ENDOCRINOLOGY AND METABOLISM

GASTROENTEROLOGY AND HEPATOLOGY

HEMATOLOGY AND ONCOLOGY

INFECTIOUS DISEASES

NEPHROLOGY

NEUROLOGY AND PSYCHIATRY

PULMONOLOGY

SYSTEMIC CONDITIONS

21st Edition

HARRISON'S®

PRINCIPLES OF

INTERNAL MEDICINE

Editors of Previous Editions

T. R. Harrison
Editor-in-Chief, Editions 1, 2, 3, 4, 5

W. R. Resnick
Editor, Editions 1, 2, 3, 4, 5

M. M. Wintrobe
Editor, Editions 1, 2, 3, 4, 5
Editor-in-Chief, Editions 6, 7

G. W. Thorn
Editor, Editions 1, 2, 3, 4, 5, 6, 7
Editor-in-Chief, Edition 8

R. D. Adams
Editor, Editions 2, 3, 4, 5, 6, 7, 8, 9, 10

P. B. Beeson
Editor, Editions 1, 2

I. L. Bennett, Jr.
Editor, Editions 3, 4, 5, 6

E. Braunwald
Editor, Editions 6, 7, 8, 9, 10, 12, 13, 14, 16, 17
Editor-in-Chief, Editions 11, 15

K. J. Isselbacher
Editor, Editions 6, 7, 8, 10, 11, 12, 14
Editor-in-Chief, Editions 9, 13

R. G. Petersdorf
Editor, Editions 6, 7, 8, 9, 11, 12
Editor-in-Chief, Edition 10

J. D. Wilson
Editor, Editions 9, 10, 11, 13, 14
Editor-in-Chief, Edition 12

J. B. Martin
Editor, Editions 10, 11, 12, 13, 14

A. S. Fauci
Editor, Editions 11, 12, 13, 15, 16, 18, 19, 20, 21
Editor-in-Chief, Editions 14, 17

R. Root
Editor, Edition 12

D. L. Kasper
Editor, Editions 13, 14, 15, 17, 18, 20, 21
Editor-in-Chief, Editions 16, 19

S. L. Hauser
Editor, Editions 14, 15, 16, 17, 18, 19, 20, 21

D. L. Longo
Editor, Editions 14, 15, 16, 17, 19, 20, 21
Editor-in-Chief, Edition 18

J. L. Jameson
Editor, Editions 15, 16, 17, 18, 19, 21
Editor-in-Chief, Edition 20

J. Loscalzo
Editor, Editions 17, 18, 19, 20
Editor-in-Chief, Edition 21

21st Edition

HARRISON'S®

PRINCIPLES OF INTERNAL MEDICINE

Editors

Joseph Loscalzo, MD, PhD
Hersey Professor of the Theory and Practice of Medicine, Harvard Medical School; Chairman, Department of Medicine; Soma Weiss MD Distinguished Chair in Medicine; Physician-in-Chief, Brigham and Women's Hospital, Boston, Massachusetts

Dennis L. Kasper, MD
William Ellery Channing Professor of Medicine and Professor of Immunology, Department of Immunology, Harvard Medical School; Division of Infectious Diseases, Brigham and Women's Hospital, Boston, Massachusetts

Dan L. Longo, MD
Professor of Medicine, Harvard Medical School; Senior Physician, Brigham and Women's Hospital; Deputy Editor, *New England Journal of Medicine,* Boston, Massachusetts

Anthony S. Fauci, MD
Chief, Laboratory of Immunoregulation; Director, National Institute of Allergy and Infectious Diseases, National Institutes of Health, Bethesda, Maryland

Stephen L. Hauser, MD
Robert A. Fishman Distinguished Professor, Department of Neurology; Director, UCSF Weill Institute for Neurosciences, University of California, San Francisco, San Francisco, California

J. Larry Jameson, MD, PhD
Robert G. Dunlop Professor of Medicine; Dean, Raymond and Ruth Perelman School of Medicine; Executive Vice President, University of Pennsylvania for the Health System, Philadelphia, Pennsylvania

VOLUME I

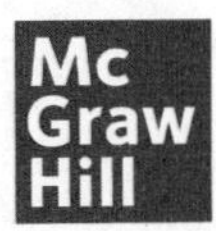

New York Chicago San Francisco Athens London Madrid Mexico City
New Delhi Milan Singapore Sydney Toronto

Note: Dr. Fauci's work as editor and author was performed outside the scope of his employment as a U.S. government employee. This work represents his personal and professional views and not necessarily those of the U.S. government.

Harrison's®
Principles of Internal Medicine
Twenty-First Edition

1 2 3 4 5 6 7 8 9 LWI 27 26 25 24 23 22

Two Volume Set ISBN 9781264268504; MHID 1264268505
Volume 1 ISBN 9781264268467; MHID 1264268467
Volume 2 ISBN 9781264268481; MHID 1264268483
eBook Two Volume Set ISBN 9781264268511; MHID 1264268513
Volume 1 eBook ISBN 9781264268474; MHID 1264268475
Volume 2 eBook ISBN 9781264268498; MHID 1264268491

FOREIGN LANGUAGE EDITIONS
Arabic: (13e): McGraw-Hill Libri Italia srl (1996)
Albanian: (20e): Life Shpk, Tirane; (17e): Tabernakul Publishing, Skopje, Macedonia
Chinese Long Form: (15e): McGraw-Hill International, Enterprises, Inc., Taiwan
Chinese Short Form: (15e, 19e): McGraw-Hill Education (Asia), Singapore
Croatian: (16e): Placebo, Split, Croatia
French: (16e, 18e): Medecine-Sciences Flammarion, Paris, France
Georgian: (19e): Tbilisi State Medical University, Tbilisi, Georgia
German: (17e, 18e, 19e, 20e): ABW Wissenschaftsverlagsgesellschaft GmbH, Berlin, Germany
Greek: (17e): Parissianos, S.A., Athens, Greece; (19e): Parisianou, S.A., Athens, Greece
Italian: (17e, 18e): The McGraw-Hill Companies, Srl, Milan, Italy; (19e, 20e): Casa Editrice Ambrosiana, Milan, Italy
Japanese: (17e, 18e, 19e): MEDSI-Medical Sciences International Ltd, Tokyo, Japan
Korean: (17e, 18e): McGraw-Hill Korea, Inc., Seoul, Korea
Macedonian: (17e): Tabernakul Publishing, Skopje, Macedonia
Polish: (17e): Czelej Publishing Company, Lubin, Poland
Portuguese: (17e, 18e): McGraw-Hill Interamericana Editores, SA de C.V., Mexico City, Mexico; (19e, 20e): AMGH Editora Ltda., Porto Alegre, Brazil
Romanian: (17e): Editura All, Bucharest, Romania; (19e): ALL Publishing House, Bucharest, Romania
Serbian: (15e): Publishing House Romanov, Bosnia & Herzegovina, Republic of Serbska; (19e): Data Status, Novi Beograd, Serbia
Spanish: (17e, 18e): McGraw-Hill Interamericana Editores, SA de C.V., Mexico City, Mexico; (19e, 20e): McGraw-Hill Mexico, Mexico City, Mexico
Turkish: (17e, 19e, 20e): Nobel Tip Kitabevleri, Ltd., Istanbul, Turkey
Vietnamese: (15e): McGraw-Hill Education (Asia), Singapore

This book was set in Palatino by KnowledgeWorks Global Ltd. The editors were James F. Shanahan and Kim J. Davis. The production manager was Jeffrey Herzich. Project management was provided by Revathi Viswanathan, KnowledgeWorks Global Ltd. The index was prepared by Susan Hunter. The text designer was Janice Bielawa; the cover design was by Anthony Landi. Figure 82-8 printed with permission from © Mount Sinai Health System.

Library of Congress Cataloging-in-Publication Data

Names: Loscalzo, Joseph, editor. | Fauci, Anthony S., 1940- editor. | Kasper, Dennis L., editor. | Hauser, Stephen L., editor. | Longo, Dan L. (Dan Louis), 1949- editor. | Jameson, J. Larry, editor.
Title: Harrison's principles of internal medicine / Joseph Loscalzo, Anthony S. Fauci, Dennis L. Kasper, Stephen L. Hauser, Dan L. Longo, J. Larry Jameson.
Other titles: Principles of internal medicine
Description: 21st edition. | New York : McGraw Hill, [2022] | Includes bibliographical references and index. | Summary: "This book presents a sharp focus on the clinical presentation of disease, expert in-depth summaries of pathophysiology and treatment, and includes highlights of emerging frontiers of science and medicine"—Provided by publisher.
Identifiers: LCCN 2021049842 (print) | LCCN 2021049843 (ebook) | ISBN 9781264268504 (hardcover ; 2 v. set) | ISBN 1264268505 (hardcover ; 2 v. set) | ISBN 9781264268467 (hardcover ; v. 1) | ISBN 1264268467 (hardcover ; v. 1) | ISBN 9781264268481 (hardcover ; v. 2) | ISBN 1264268483 (hardcover ; v. 2) | ISBN 9781264268511 (ebook ; 2 v. set) | ISBN 1264268513 (ebook ; 2 v. set) | ISBN 9781264268474 (ebook ; v. 1) | ISBN 1264268475 (ebook ; v. 1) | ISBN 9781264268498 (ebook ; v. 2) | ISBN 1264268491 (ebook ; v. 2)
Subjects: MESH: Internal Medicine
Classification: LCC RC46 (print) | LCC RC46 (ebook) | NLM WB 115 | DDC 616—dc23/eng/20211101
LC record available at https://lccn.loc.gov/2021049842
LC ebook record available at https://lccn.loc.gov/2021049843

Cover Illustration

Beginning with the 6th edition, the cover of *Harrison's* has included an image of a bright light—a patient's perception of being examined with an ophthalmoscope. This allegorical symbol of *Harrison's* is a reminder of how the light of knowledge empowers physicians to better diagnose and treat diseases that ultimately afflict all of humankind.

Author Disclosure Policy: McGraw Hill and the *Harrison's* Editorial Board require all contributors to disclose to the Editors and the Publisher any potential financial or professional conflicts that would raise the possibility of distorting the preparation of a *Harrison's* chapter.

Contents

SECTION 6 Alterations in Gastrointestinal Function

SECTION 7 Alterations in Renal and Urinary Tract Function

SECTION 8 Alterations in the Skin

SECTION 9 Hematologic Alterations

PART 3 Pharmacology

PART 4 Oncology and Hematology

SECTION 1 Neoplastic Disorders

SECTION 2 Hematopoietic Disorders

SECTION 3 Disorders of Hemostasis

PART 5 Infectious Diseases

SECTION 1 Basic Considerations in Infectious Diseases

SECTION 2 Clinical Syndromes: Community-Acquired Infections

CONTENTS

SECTION 10 Diseases Caused by Rickettsiae, Mycoplasmas, and Chlamydiae

SECTION 11 Viral Diseases: General Considerations

SECTION 12 Infections Due to DNA Viruses

SECTION 13 Infections Due to DNA and RNA Respiratory Viruses

SECTION 14 Infections Due to Human Immunodeficiency Virus and Other Human Retroviruses

SECTION 15 Infections Due to RNA Viruses

SECTION 16 Fungal Infections

SECTION 17 Protozoal and Helminthic Infections: General Considerations

SECTION 18 Protozoal Infections

PART 7 Disorders of the Respiratory System

SECTION 1 Diagnosis of Respiratory Disorders

SECTION 2 Diseases of the Respiratory System

PART 8 Critical Care Medicine

SECTION 1 Respiratory Critical Care

SECTION 2 Shock and Cardiac Arrest

SECTION 3 Neurologic Critical Care

PART 9 Disorders of the Kidney and Urinary Tract

PART 10 Disorders of the Gastrointestinal System

SECTION 1 Disorders of the Alimentary Tract

SECTION 2 Nutrition

SECTION 3 Liver and Biliary Tract Disease

SECTION 4 Disorders of the Pancreas

PART 11 Immune-Mediated, Inflammatory, and Rheumatologic Disorders

SECTION 1 The Immune System in Health and Disease

SECTION 2 Disorders of Immune-Mediated Injury

SECTION 3 Disorders of the Joints and Adjacent Tissues

PART 12 Endocrinology and Metabolism

SECTION 1 Endocrinology

SECTION 2 Sex- and Gender-Based Medicine

SECTION 3 Obesity, Diabetes Mellitus, and Metabolic Syndrome

SECTION 4 Disorders of Bone and Mineral Metabolism

PART 14 Poisoning, Drug Overdose, and Envenomation

PART 15 Disorders Associated with Environmental Exposures

PART 16 Genes, the Environment, and Disease

PART 17 Global Medicine

PART 18 Aging

PART 19 Consultative Medicine

PART 20 Frontiers

The following chapters are available online. They can be viewed by opening the table of contents of *Harrison's* 21st edition at *www.accessmedicine.com/harrisons.*

Video Collection

Supplementary Topics

Atlases

Contributors

James L. Abbruzzese, MD, FACP, FASCO, DSc (hon)
Professor, Division of Medical Oncology, Duke Cancer Institute, Durham, North Carolina [92]

Manal F. Abdelmalek, MD, MPH
Professor of Medicine, Division of Gastroenterology and Hepatology, Duke University, Durham, North Carolina [343]

John C. Achermann, MD, PhD
Wellcome Trust Senior Research Fellow in Clinical Science, Genetics & Genomic Medicine, UCL GOS Institute of Child Health, University College London, London, United Kingdom [390]

David Adams, MD, PhD
Deputy Director of Clinical Genomics, Office of the Clinical Director/NHGRI and Undiagnosed Diseases Program, National Institutes of Health, Bethesda, Maryland [492]

John W. Adamson, MD
Clinical Professor, Division of Hematology/Oncology, Department of Medicine, University of California at San Diego, San Diego, California [63, 97]

Praveen Akuthota, MD
Associate Clinical Professor, Division of Pulmonary, Critical Care & Sleep Medicine, University of California, San Diego, San Diego, California [288]

Christine Albert, MD, MPH
Chair, Department of Cardiology; Lee and Harold Kapelovitz Endowed Chair in Research Cardiology, Smidt Heart Institute, Cedars-Sinai Medical Center, Los Angeles, California [306]

Ash A. Alizadeh, MD, PhD
Professor of Medicine (Oncology), Stanford University School of Medicine, Stanford, California [490]

Anthony A. Amato, MD
Professor of Neurology, Harvard Medical School; Distinguished Chair of Neurology and Chief, Neuromuscular Division, Brigham and Women's Hospital, Boston, Massachusetts [365, 446–449]

Rachel L. Amdur, MD
Assistant Professor of Medicine, Division of General Internal Medicine and Geriatrics, Northwestern University Feinberg School of Medicine, Chicago, Illinois [35]

Neil M. Ampel, MD
Professor Emeritus of Medicine and Immunobiology, University of Arizona, Tucson, Arizona [213]

Kenneth C. Anderson, MD
Kraft Family Professor of Medicine, Harvard Medical School; Chief, Jerome Lipper Multiple Myeloma Center, Dana-Farber Cancer Institute, Boston, Massachusetts [111]

Rosa M. Andrade, MD
Assistant Professor of Medicine, University of California, Irvine School of Medicine, Irvine, California [223]

Derek C. Angus, MD, MPH
Distinguished Professor and Mitchell P. Fink Endowed Chair, Department of Critical Care Medicine; University of Pittsburgh School of Medicine, Pittsburgh, Pennsylvania [304]

Elliott M. Antman, MD
Professor of Medicine; Harvard Medical School; Senior Physician; Senior Investigator, TIMI Study Trial, Brigham and Women's Hospital, Boston, Massachusetts [273, 275]

Frederick R. Appelbaum, MD
Deputy Director, Fred Hutchinson Cancer Research Center, Seattle, Washington [114]

Cesar A. Arias, MD, PhD, MSc, FIDSA
Chief, Division of Infectious Diseases, Houston Methodist Hospital; Professor and John F. III and Ann H. Bookout Distinguished Chair; Co-Director Center for Infectious Diseases Research, Houston Methodist Research Institute and Weill Cornell Medical College, Houston, Texas [149]

Wiebke Arlt, MD, DSc, FRCP, FMedSci
William Withering Chair of Medicine, Institute of Metabolism and Systems Research, University of Birmingham; Consultant Endocrinologist, Queen Elizabeth Hospital Birmingham, Birmingham, United Kingdom [386]

Katrina A. Armstrong, MD
Physician in Chief, Massachusetts General Hospital, Boston, Massachusetts [6]

Andrew W. Artenstein, MD
Chief Physician Executive and Chief Academic Officer, Baystate Health; Regional Executive Dean and Professor of Medicine, University of Massachusetts Chan Medical School-Baystate, Springfield, Massachusetts [S6]

David A. Asch, MD, MBA
Executive Director, Penn Medicine Center for Health Care Innovation; John Morgan Professor, Perelman School of Medicine and the Wharton School, University of Pennsylvania, Philadelphia, Pennsylvania [481]

Samuel Y. Ash, MD, MPH
Assistant Professor of Medicine, Harvard Medical School; Division of Pulmonary and Critical Care Medicine, Department of Medicine, Brigham and Women's Hospital, Boston, Massachusetts [A12]

Elizabeth A. Ashley, MB, BS, MRCP, FRCPath
Professor of Tropical Medicine, Oxford University; Director, Lao-Oxford-Mahosot Hospital-Wellcome Trust Research Unit, Vientiane, Lao PDR [224, A2]

John C. Atherton, MD, FRCP
Professor of Gastroenterology and Dean of the Faculty of Medicine and Health Sciences, University of Nottingham, Nottingham, United Kingdom [163]

Eric H. Awtry, MD
Associate Professor of Medicine, Boston University School of Medicine; Associate Chair for Clinical Affairs, Section of Cardiology, Boston Medical Center, Boston, Massachusetts [271, 272]

Jamil Azzi, MD
Associate Physician, Renal Division, Brigham and Women's Hospital; Director, Renal Transplant Fellowship; Assistant Professor of Medicine, Harvard Medical School, Boston, Massachusetts [313]

Bruce R. Bacon, MD
Emeritus Professor of Internal Medicine, Saint Louis University School of Medicine, St. Louis, Missouri [344]

Jessica M. Baker, MD
Assistant Professor, Department of Neurology, University of Wisconsin School of Medicine and Public Health, Madison, Wisconsin [26]

Zoica Bakirtzief, PhD
Guest Professor of Psychology, Vocational Teacher Certification Program, Federal University of Santa Maria, Santa Maria, Rio Grande do Sul, Brazil [179]

Ruben Baler, PhD
Health Scientist, Office of Science Policy and Communications, National Institute on Drug Abuse, National Institutes of Health, Bethesda, Maryland [455]

John R. Balmes, MD
Professor of Medicine, University of California San Francisco School of Medicine, San Francisco, California [289]

Manisha Balwani, MD, MS
Professor, Department of Genetics and Genomic Sciences and Medicine, Icahn School of Medicine at Mount Sinai, New York, New York [416]

Robert L. Barbieri, MD
Kate Macy Ladd Distinguished Professor of Obstetrics, Gynecology and Reproductive Biology, Harvard Medical School; Chief of Obstetrics, Department of Obstetrics and Gynecology, Brigham and Women's Hospital, Boston, Massachusetts [479]

Alan G. Barbour, MD
Distinguished Professor of Medicine and Microbiology and Molecular Genetics, University of California, Irvine, Irvine, California [185]

Joanne M. Bargman, MD, FRCPC
Professor of Medicine, University of Toronto; Staff Nephrologist, University Health Network; Clinician Investigator, Toronto General Hospital Research Institute; Director, Peritoneal Dialysis Program, Co-Director, Renal-Rheumatology Lupus Clinic, University Health Network [311]

Tamar F. Barlam, MD, MSc
Professor of Medicine, Boston University School of Medicine; Chief, Section of Infectious Diseases, Boston Medical Center, Boston, Massachusetts [122, 158]

Richard J. Barohn, MD
Executive Vice Chancellor for Health Affairs; Executive Director, NextGen Precision Health, University of Missouri, Columbia, Missouri [440, 446]

Beverly W. Baron, MD
Professor of Pathology, Retired, University of Chicago, Chicago, Illinois [127, 290]

Rebecca M. Baron, MD
Associate Professor of Medicine, Harvard Medical School; Associate Physician, Brigham and Women's Hospital, Pulmonary Division and Critical Care, Boston, Massachusetts [37, 127, 290, 300, 301]

Miriam Baron Barshak, MD
Assistant Professor of Medicine, Harvard Medical School; Physician, Massachusetts General Hospital, Boston, Massachusetts [127, 132, 290]

Buddha Basnyat, MSc, MD, FACP, FRCP(Edinburgh)
Director, Oxford University Clinical Research Unit—Nepal, Patan Hospital, Kathmandu, Nepal [462]

Joseph Bass, MD, PhD
Division of Endocrinology, Metabolism and Molecular Medicine, Department of Medicine, Feinberg School of Medicine, Department of Neurobiology, Northwestern University, Chicago, Illinois [485]

Shari S. Bassuk, ScD
Epidemiologist, Division of Preventive Medicine, Brigham and Women's Hospital, Boston, Massachusetts [395]

David W. Bates, MD, MSc
Professor of Medicine, Harvard Medical School; Chief, Division of General Internal Medicine and Primary Care, Brigham and Women's Hospital, Phyllis Jen Center for Primary Care, Boston, Massachusetts [8]

Robert P. Baughman, MD
Department of Internal Medicine, University of Cincinnati Medical Center, Cincinnati, Ohio [367]

Laurence H. Beck, Jr., MD, PhD
Associate Professor of Medicine, Boston University School of Medicine, Boston, Massachusetts [316]

Nicholas J. Beeching, FRCP, FRACP, FFTM RCPS(Glasg), FESCMID, FISTM, DTM&H, DCH
Consultant in Tropical and Infectious Diseases, Tropical and Infectious Disease Unit, Royal Liverpool University Hospitals Foundation NHS Trust; Emeritus Professor of Tropical and Infectious Diseases, Clinical Sciences, Liverpool School of Tropical Medicine, Liverpool, United Kingdom [169]

Alex S. Befeler, MD
Medical Director Liver Transplant, Professor of Internal Medicine, Division of Gastroenterology and Hepatology, Saint Louis University, St. Louis, Missouri [344]

Michael H. Bennett, MD, MBBS, MM (Clin Epi)
Conjoint Professor in Anesthesia and Hyperbaric Medicine; Faculty of Medicine, University of New South Wales; Academic Head of Department, Wales Anaesthesia, Prince of Wales Hospital, Sydney, Australia [463]

Shelley L. Berger, PhD
Daniel S. Och University Professor, Departments of Cell and Developmental Biology; Biology; Genetics; Director, Penn Epigenetics Institute, University of Pennsylvania Perelman School of Medicine, Philadelphia, Pennsylvania [483]

Jean Bergounioux, MD, PhD
Professor of Medicine, Versailles Saint Quentin University - Paris Saclay, UFR Simone Veil - Motigney le Bretonneux, France; Director, Department of Pediatric Neurology and Intensive Care Medicine, Assistance Publique des Hôpitaux de Paris, Garches, France [166]

John L. Berk, MD
Professor of Medicine, Boston University School of Medicine, Assistant Director, Amyloidosis Center, Boston Medical Center, Boston, Massachusetts [112]

Jeffrey Berns, MD
Professor of Medicine and Pediatrics; Associate Chief, Renal Electrolyte and Hypertension Division; Vice-President and Associate Dean for Graduate Medical Education, Perelman School of Medicine of the University of Pennsylvania, Philadelphia, Pennsylvania [478]

Aaron S. Bernstein, MD, MPH
Assistant Professor of Pediatrics, Harvard Medical School; Hospitalist, Division of General Pediatrics, Boston Children's Hospital; Interim Director, Center for Climate, Health and the Global Environment, Harvard T.H. Chan School of Public Health, Boston, Massachusetts [125]

Jeanne Bertolli, PhD
Division of High-Consequence Pathogens and Pathology, National Center for Zoonotic and Emerging Infectious Diseases, Centers for Disease Control and Prevention, Atlanta, Georgia [450]

Joseph R. Betancourt, MD, MPH
Associate Professor of Medicine, Massachusetts General Hospital; Harvard Medical School, Boston, Massachusetts [10]

Emily D. Bethea, MD
Instructor in Medicine, Harvard Medical School; Associate Clinical Director of Liver Transplantation, Gastroenterology and Hepatology Division, Massachusetts General Hospital, Boston, Massachusetts [337]

Julie A. Bettinger, MPH, PhD
Professor, Department of Pediatrics, Vaccine Evaluation Center, BC Children's Hospital, University of British Columbia, Vancouver, British Columbia, Canada [3]

Atul K. Bhan, MBBS, MD
Professor of Pathology, Harvard Medical School, Associate Director, Center for the Study of Inflammatory Bowel Disease, Massachusetts General Hospital, Boston, Massachusetts [A13]

Shalender Bhasin, MB, BS
Professor of Medicine, Harvard Medical School; Director, Research Program in Men's Health: Aging and Metabolism; Director, Boston Claude D. Pepper Older Americans Independence Center; Brigham and Women's Hospital, Boston, Massachusetts [391, 399]

Deepak L. Bhatt, MD, MPH, FACC, FAHA, FSCAI, FESC
Professor of Medicine, Harvard Medical School; Executive Director of Interventional Cardiovascular Programs, Brigham and Women's Hospital Heart & Vascular Center, Boston, Massachusetts [276, A11]

Roby P. Bhattacharyya, MD, PhD
Assistant Professor of Medicine, Harvard Medical School and Massachusetts General Hospital; Associate Member, Broad Institute of MIT and Harvard, Boston, Massachusetts [121]

Daniel G. Bichet, MD
Professor of Medicine, Pharmacology and Physiology, University of Montreal; Staff Nephrologist, Hôpital du Sacré-Cœur de Montréal, Montréal, Quebec, Canada [381]

David R. Bickers, MD
Carl Truman Nelson Professor and Chair, Department of Dermatology, Columbia University Irving Medical Center, New York, New York [61]

William R. Bishai, MD, PhD
Professor of Medicine, Division of Infectious Diseases, Johns Hopkins School of Medicine, Baltimore, Maryland [150]

Bruce R. Bistrian, MD, PhD, MPH
Professor of Medicine, Harvard Medical School; Chief, Clinical Nutrition, Beth Israel Deaconess Medical Center, Boston, Massachusetts [335]

Lucas S. Blanton, MD
Assistant Professor, Division of Infectious Diseases, Department of Internal Medicine University of Texas Medical Branch, Galveston, Texas [187]

Martin J. Blaser, MD
Henry Rutgers Chair of the Human Microbiome; Director, Center for Advanced Biotechnology and Medicine, Rutgers University, Piscataway, New Jersey [163, 167]

Chantal P. Bleeker-Rovers, MD, PhD
Department of Internal Medicine, Radboud University Medical Center, Nijmegen, The Netherlands [20, 187]

William Blum, MD
Director, Acute Leukemia Program; Professor, Department of Hematology and Oncology, Winship Cancer Institute and Emory University, Atlanta, Georgia [104]

Richard S. Blumberg, MD
Vice-Chair for Research in Department of Medicine, Brigham and Women's Hospital, Professor of Medicine, Harvard Medical School, Boston, Massachusetts [326]

Yair J. Blumenfeld, MD
Associate Professor of Obstetrics and Gynecology (Maternal Fetal Medicine), Stanford University School of Medicine, Stanford, California [490]

Jean L. Bolognia, MD
Professor, Department of Dermatology, Yale University School of Medicine, New Haven, Connecticut [58]

Joseph V. Bonventre, MD, PhD
Chief, Renal Division and Engineering in Department of Medicine, Brigham and Women's Hospital, Boston, Massachusetts [310]

Joshua A. Boyce, MD
Professor of Medicine and Pediatrics; Albert L. Sheffer Professor of Medicine, Harvard Medical School; Director, Inflammation and Allergic Disease Research Section, Brigham and Women's Hospital, Boston, Massachusetts [352–354]

Emily B. Brant, MD, MS
Assistant Professor, Department of Critical Care Medicine, University of Pittsburgh School of Medicine, Pittsburgh, Pennsylvania [304]

Eugene Braunwald, MD
Distinguished Hersey Professor of the Theory and Practice of Medicine, Harvard Medical School; Brigham and Women's Hospital, BWH/Founding Chair, TIMI Group, Boston, Massachusetts [274]

Irwin M. Braverman, MD
Professor Emeritus; Senior Research Scientist, Department of Dermatology, Yale University School of Medicine, New Haven, Connecticut [58]

Otis W. Brawley, MD, MACP, FRCP(L), FASCO, FACE
Bloomberg Distinguished Professor, Johns Hopkins School of Medicine and Johns Hopkins Bloomberg School of Public Health, Baltimore, Maryland [70]

Benjamin L. Brett, PhD
Medical College of Wisconsin, Assistant Professor, Departments of Neurosurgery and Neurology (Division Neuropsychology), Milwaukee, Wisconsin [443]

Manfred Brigl, MD
Assistant Professor of Pathology, Harvard Medical School, Boston, Massachusetts [S11]

F. Richard Bringhurst, MD
Associate Professor of Medicine, Massachusetts General Hospital and Harvard Medical School, Boston, Massachusetts [409]

Steven M. Bromley, MD
Director, South Jersey MS Center, Bromley Neurology PC, Audubon, New Jersey [33]

Darron R. Brown, MD
Professor of Medicine, Microbiology, and Immunology, Division of Infectious Diseases, Indiana University School of Medicine, Indianapolis, Indiana [198]

Kevin E. Brown, MD, MRCP, FRCPath
Consultant Medical Virologist, Immunisation and Vaccine Preventable Diseases Division, UK Health Security Agency, London, United Kingdom [197]

Robert H. Brown, Jr., MD, PhD
Chairman, Department of Neurology, University of Massachusetts Medical School, Worcester, Massachusetts [437, 449]

Amy E. Bryant, PhD
Research Professor, Department of Biomedical and Pharmaceutical Sciences College of Pharmacy, Idaho State University, Meridian, Idaho [129, 154]

G. Scott Budinger, MD
Ernest S. Bazley Professor of Airway Diseases; Chief, Pulmonary and Critical Care Medicine, Department of Medicine, Northwestern University Feinberg School of Medicine, Chicago, Illinois [491]

Fred Bunz, MD, PhD
Associate Professor, Johns Hopkins University School of Medicine, Baltimore, Maryland [71]

Lucile Burgo-Black, MD, FACP
National Co-Director, VA Post-Deployment Integrated Care Initiative, Assistant Clinical Professor of Medicine, Department of General Internal Medicine, Yale University School of Medicine, New Haven, Connecticut [S7]

Maxine A. Burkett, JD
Professor of Law, William S. Richardson School of Law, University of Hawaii at Mānoa, Honolulu, Hawaii [475]

Christopher M. Burns, MD
Associate Professor of Medicine, Geisel School of Medicine at Dartmouth, Dartmouth-Hitchcock Medical Center, Lebanon, New Hampshire [417]

David M. Burns, MD
Professor Emeritus, University of California, San Diego School of Medicine Del Mar, California [454]

John C. Byrd, MD
D. Warren Brown Chair of Leukemia Research; Distinguished University Professor of Medicine, Medicinal Chemistry, and Veterinary Biosciences; Director, Division of Hematology, Department of Medicine, The Ohio State University, Columbus, Ohio [107]

Rodrigo T. Calado, MD, PhD
Associate Professor of Medicine, Ribeirão Preto Medical School, University of São Paulo, Ribeirão Preto, Brazil [469]

Michael Camilleri, MD
Atherton and Winifred W. Bean Professor; Professor of Medicine, Pharmacology, and Physiology, Mayo Clinic School of Medicine, Rochester, Minnesota [46]

Christopher P. Cannon, MD
Professor of Medicine, Harvard Medical School; Education Director, Cardiovascular Innovation, Preventive Cardiology Section, Brigham and Women's Hospital, Boston, Massachusetts [274]

Brian C. Capell, MD, PhD
Assistant Professor of Dermatology and Genetics, Departments of Dermatology and Genetics, Penn Epigenetics Institute, Abramson Cancer Center, University of Pennsylvania Perelman School of Medicine, Philadelphia, Pennsylvania [483]

Jonathan Carapetis, MBBS, FRACP, FAFPHM, PhD
Executive Director, Telethon Kids Institute, Perth Children's Hospital, Nedlands, Western Australia [359]

Arturo Casadevall, MD, PhD
Professor and Chair, Bloomberg School of Public Health, Johns Hopkins University, Baltimore, Maryland [215]

Jonathan Cedernaes, MD, PhD
Visiting Postdoctoral Fellow, Division of Endocrinology, Metabolism and Molecular Medicine, Department of Medicine, Feinberg School of Medicine, Northwestern University, Chicago, Illinois [485]

Anil K. Chandraker, MB, ChB
Associate Professor of Medicine, Harvard Medical School; Medical Director, Kidney and Pancreas Transplantation, Brigham and Women's Hospital; Boston, Massachusetts [313]

François Chappuis, MD, MCTM, PhD
Head of Division, Division of Tropical and Humanitarian Medicine, Geneva University Hospitals, Geneva, Switzerland [227]

Richelle C. Charles, MD, FIDSA
Associate Professor of Medicine, Harvard Medical School, Massachusetts General Hospital; Associate Professor of Immunology and Infectious Diseases, Harvard T.H. Chan School of Public Health, Boston, Massachusetts [133]

Justin T. Cheeley, MD, FAAD
Assistant Professor, Divisions of Dermatology and Internal Medicine and Geriatrics, Emory University School of Medicine, Atlanta, Georgia [57]

Alex Chen, MD
Associate Physician, Department of Emergency Medicine, Kaiser Permanente, South Sacramento Campus, Sacramento, California [460]

Glenn M. Chertow, MD, MPH
Professor of Medicine, Division of Nephrology, Stanford University School of Medicine, Palo Alto, California [312]

Jacques Chiaroni, MD, PhD
Professor, Aix Marseille Univ, CNRS, EFS, ADES, UMR 7268; Etablissement Francais du Sang Provence Alpes Côté d'Azur et Corse, Marseille, France [113]

Hyon K. Choi, MD, DrPH
Professor of Medicine, Harvard Medical School; Director, Gout and Crystal Arthropathy Center; Director, Clinical Epidemiology and Health Outcomes, Division of Rheumatology, Allergy, and Immunology, Department of Medicine, Massachusetts General Hospital, Boston, Massachusetts [372]

Benjamin F. Chong, MD, MSCS
Associate Professor, Department of Dermatology, University of Texas Southwestern Medical Center, Dallas, Texas [59]

Raymond T. Chung, MD
Professor of Medicine, Harvard Medical School; Director of Hepatology and Liver Center; Vice Chief, Gastroenterology Division; Kevin and Polly Maroni MGH Research Scholar, Massachusetts General Hospital, Boston, Massachusetts [345]

Jeffrey W. Clark, MD
Associate Professor of Medicine, Harvard Medical School; Medical Director, Clinical Trials Core, Dana-Farber Harvard Cancer Center; Massachusetts General Hospital, Boston, Massachusetts [72]

Bruce H. Cohen, MD, FAAN
Professor of Pediatrics, Northeast Ohio Medical University; Professor of Integrative Medical Sciences, Northeast Ohio Medical University; Considine Family Endowed Chair in Research – Akron Children's Hospital; Director; NeuroDevelopmental Science Center, Akron Children's Hospital; Divisions of Neurology, Neurosurgery, NeuroBehavioral Health, Physiatry and Developmental Pediatrics; Interim Vice President and Medical Director, Rebecca D. Considine Research Institute, Akron Children's Hospital, Akron, Ohio [468]

Jeffrey I. Cohen, MD
Chief, Laboratory of Infectious Diseases, National Institute of Allergy and Infectious Diseases, National Institutes of Health, Bethesda, Maryland [191, 194, 204]

Amanda Cohn, MD
Chief Medical Officer, National Center for Immunization and Respiratory Diseases (NCIRD), Atlanta, Georgia [123]

Jennifer P. Collins, MD, MSc
Enteric Diseases Epidemiology Branch, Division of Foodborne, Waterborne, and Environmental Diseases, National Center for Emerging and Zoonotic Infectious Diseases, Centers for Disease Control and Prevention, Atlanta, Georgia [151]

Wilson M. Compton, MD, MPE
Deputy Director, National Institute on Drug Abuse, National Institutes of Health, U.S. Department of Health and Human Services, Bethesda, Maryland [457]

Jean M. Connors, MD
Hematology Division, Brigham and Women's Hospital; Harvard Medical School, Boston, Massachusetts [116]

Darwin L. Conwell, MD, MS
Professor of Medicine, The Ohio State University College of Medicine; Director, Division of Gastroenterology, Hepatology and Nutrition; The Ohio State University Wexner Medical Center, Columbus, Ohio [347, 348]

Lawrence Corey, MD
Professor of Medicine and Laboratory Medicine and Pathology, University of Washington; Past President & Director, Fred Hutchinson Cancer Research Center; Professor, Vaccine and Infectious Disease Division, Fred Hutchinson Cancer Research Center, Seattle, Washington [192]

Jorge Cortes, MD
Jane and John Justin Distinguished Chair in Leukemia Research; Deputy Chairman; Section Chief of AML and CML, The University of Texas MD Anderson Cancer Center, Houston, Texas [105]

Sara E. Cosgrove, MD, MS
Professor of Medicine, Division of Infectious Diseases, Johns Hopkins University School of Medicine, Baltimore, Maryland [128]

James D. Crapo, MD
Professor of Medicine, Department of Medicine; Division of Pulmonary and Critical Care & Sleep Medicine, National Jewish Health, Denver, Colorado [292]

Mark A. Creager, MD
Professor of Medicine, Professor of Surgery, Geisel School of Medicine at Dartmouth; Director, Heart and Vascular Center, Dartmouth-Hitchcock Medical Center, Lebanon, New Hampshire [280–282]

Bruce A. C. Cree, MD, PhD, MAS
George A. Zimmermann Endowed Professor in Multiple Sclerosis; Professor of Clinical Neurology; Clinical Research Director, UCSF Weill Institute for Neurosciences, Department of Neurology, University of California San Francisco, San Francisco, California [444, 445]

Leslie J. Crofford, MD
Professor, Departments of Medicine and Pathology, Microbiology and Immunology, Vanderbilt University; Chief, Division of Rheumatology and Immunology, Vanderbilt University Medical Center, Nashville, Tennessee [373]

Jennifer M. Croswell, MD, MPH
Senior Program Officer, Office of the Chief Science Officer, Patient-Centered Outcomes Research Institute (PCORI), Washington, DC [70]

James E. Crowe, Jr., MD
Director, Vanderbilt Vaccine Center; Ann Scott Carell Chair and Professor, Departments of Pediatrics, Pathology, Microbiology and Immunology, Vanderbilt University Medical Center, Nashville, Tennessee [199]

Ian Crozier, MD
NIH/NIAID/DCR Integrated Research Facility at Fort Detrick, Clinical Monitoring Research Program Directorate, Frederick National Laboratory for Cancer Research, Frederick, Maryland [209, 210]

Philip E. Cryer, MD
Professor Emeritus of Medicine, Division of Endocrinology, Metabolism & Lipid Research, Washington University School of Medicine in St. Louis, St. Louis, Missouri [406]

Gary C. Curhan, MD
Professor of Medicine, Harvard Medical School; Professor of Epidemiology, Harvard School of Public Health; Channing Division of Network Medicine/Renal Division, Brigham and Women's Hospital, Boston, Massachusetts [318]

Brendan D. Curti, MD
Director, Cytokine and Adoptive Immunotherapy; Director, Genitourinary Oncology Research and Director, Melanoma Program; Robert W. Franz Endowed Chair for Clinical Research, Earle A. Chiles Research Institute, a Division of the Providence Cancer Institute, Portland, Oregon [76]

John J. Cush, MD
Executive Editor, RheumNow.com; Professor of Internal Medicine, University of Texas Southwestern Medical School, Dallas, Texas [370]

Charles A. Czeisler, MD, PhD
Frank Baldino, Jr., PhD Professor of Sleep Medicine, Professor of Medicine and Director, Division of Sleep Medicine, Harvard Medical School; Chief, Division of Sleep and Circadian Disorders, Departments of Medicine and Neurology, Brigham and Women's Hospital, Boston, Massachusetts [31]

Carolyn M. D'Ambrosio, MS, MD
Associate Professor of Medicine, Harvard Medical School; Brigham and Women's Hospital, Boston, Massachusetts [39]

Josep Dalmau, MD, PhD
ICREA Professor, Institut d'Investigacions Biomèdiques August Pi i Sunyer, Hospital Clínic, University of Barcelona, Barcelona, Spain; Adjunct Professor, University of Pennsylvania, Philadelphia, Pennsylvania [94]

Inger K. Damon, MD, PhD
Director, Division of High-Consequence Pathogens and Pathology (DHCPP), Centers for Disease Control and Prevention, Atlanta, Georgia [196]

Daniel F. Danzl, MD
Professor and Emeritus Chair, Department of Emergency Medicine, University of Louisville, Louisville, Kentucky [464, 465]

Robert B. Daroff, MD
Professor and Chair Emeritus, Department of Neurology, Case Western Reserve University School of Medicine; University Hospitals–Cleveland Medical Center, Cleveland, Ohio [22]

Jaideep Das Gupta, MD
Vascular Surgery Fellow, Vascular Surgery Division, University of California, San Diego, La Jolla, California [329]

Stephen N. Davis, MBBS, FRCP, FACE, MACP
Theodore E. Woodward Professor of Medicine; Professor of Physiology; Chairman, Department of Medicine, University of Maryland School of Medicine; Director, Institute for Clinical and Translational Research; Vice President of Clinical Translational Science
University of Maryland, Baltimore; Physician-in-Chief, University of Maryland Medical Center, Baltimore, Maryland [406]

Lisa M. DeAngelis, MD
Professor of Neurology, Weill Cornell Medical College; Physician-in-Chief and Chief Medical Officer, Memorial Sloan Kettering Cancer Center, New York, New York [90]

Rafael de Cabo, PhD
Chief, Translational Gerontology Branch, National Institute on Aging, National Institutes of Health, Baltimore, Maryland [476]

Lucia De Franceschi, MD
Department of Medicine, University of Verona and AOUI Verona, Verona, Italy [100]

John Del Valle, MD
Professor and Vice Chair of Medicine, Department of Internal Medicine, University of Michigan School of Medicine, Ann Arbor, Michigan [324]

David W. Denning, MBBS, FRCP, FRCPath, FMedSci
Professor of Infectious Diseases in Global Health, The University of Manchester, Manchester, United Kingdom [217]

Akshay S. Desai, MD, MPH
Associated Professor of Medicine, Harvard Medical School; Director, Cardiomyopathy and Heart Failure, Advanced Heart Disease Section, Cardiovascular Division, Brigham and Women's Hospital, Boston, Massachusetts [258]

Robert J. Desnick, PhD, MD
Dean for Genetic and Genomic Medicine Emeritus; Professor and Chairman Emeritus, Department of Genetics and Genomic Sciences, Icahn School of Medicine at Mount Sinai, Mount Sinai Health System, New York, New York [416]

Betty Diamond, MD
The Feinstein Institutes for Medical Research, Northwell Health System; Center for Autoimmunity and Musculoskeletal Diseases, Manhasset, New York [355]

Marcelo F. Di Carli, MD
Professor, Department of Radiology and Medicine, Harvard Medical School; Chief, Division of Nuclear Medicine and Molecular Imaging; Executive Director, Noninvasive Cardiovascular Imaging Program, Brigham and Women's Hospital, Boston, Massachusetts [241, A9]

Anna Mae Diehl, MD
Florence McAlister Professor of Medicine; Director, Duke Liver Center, Duke University, Durham, North Carolina [343]

Jules L. Dienstag, MD
Carl W. Walter Professor of Medicine, Harvard Medical School; Physician, Gastrointestinal Unit, Department of Medicine, Massachusetts General Hospital, Boston, Massachusetts [339–341, 345, A13]

William P. Dillon, MD
Professor and Executive Vice-Chair, Department of Radiology and Biomedical Imaging, University of California, San Francisco, San Francisco, California [423, A16]

Charles A. Dinarello, MD
Distinguished Professor of Medicine, University of Colorado School of Medicine, Aurora, Colorado [18]

R. Christopher Doiron, MD, FRCS(C)
Assistant Professor, Queens University at Kingston Canada; Staff Urologist, Department of Urology, Kingston Health Sciences Centre, Kingston, Ontario, Canada [51]

Anuja Dokras, MD, PhD
Professor of Obstetrics and Gynecology, Perelman School of Medicine, University of Pennsylvania, Philadelphia, Pennsylvania [392, 393, 396]

Susan M. Domchek, MD
Basser Professor of Oncology, Abramson Cancer Center, Perelman School of Medicine, University of Pennsylvania, Philadelphia, Pennsylvania [467]

Richard L. Doty, PhD
Professor, Department of Otorhinolaryngology: Head and Neck Surgery; Director, Smell and Taste Center, Perelman School of Medicine, University of Pennsylvania, Philadelphia, Pennsylvania [33]

Vanja C. Douglas, MD
Professor of Neurology and Sara and Evan Williams Foundation Endowed Neurohospitalist Chair, University of California, San Francisco, San Francisco, California [23, 441]

David F. Driscoll, PhD
Associate Professor of Medicine, University of Massachusetts Medical School, Worcester, Massachusetts [335]

Thomas D. DuBose, Jr., MD, MACP
Emeritus Professor of Medicine, Wake Forest School of Medicine, Winston Salem, North Carolina [55, S1]

J. Stephen Dumler, MD
Professor and Chairman, Department of Pathology, Uniformed Services University of the Health Sciences, Walter Reed National Military Medical Center, Joint Pathology Center, Bethesda, Maryland [187]

Andrea Dunaif, MD
Lillian and Henry M. Stratton Professor of Molecular Medicine, System Chief, Hilda and J. Lester Gabrilove Division of Endocrinology, Diabetes and Bone Disease, Icahn School of Medicine and Mount Sinai Health System, New York, New York [398]

Samuel C. Durso, MD, MBA
Mason F. Lord Professor of Medicine; Executive Vice Chair, Johns Hopkins University Department of Medicine; Director, Department of Medicine, Johns Hopkins Bayview Medical Center, Baltimore, Maryland [36, A3]

Janice P. Dutcher, MD
Associate Director, Cancer Research Foundation of New York, Chappaqua, New York; Former Professor of Medicine, New York Medical College, Valhalla, New York [75]

Johanna T. Dwyer, DSc, RD
Professor of Medicine and Community Health, Tufts Medical School; Senior Nutrition Scientist (Contractor), Office of Dietary Supplements, National Institutes of Health, Boston, Massachusetts [332]

Kim A. Eagle, MD
Albion Walter Hewett Professor of Internal Medicine; Professor of Health Management Policy, School of Public Health; Director, Samuel and Jean Frankel Cardiovascular Center, University of Michigan, Ann Arbor, Michigan [480]

Sarah Rae Easter, MD
Assistant Professor of Obstetrics, Gynecology and Reproductive Biology, Harvard Medical School; Director of Obstetric Critical Care, Brigham and Women's Hospital, Boston, Massachusetts [479]

James A. Eastham, MD
Chief, Urology Service; Peter T. Scardino Chair in Oncology, Department of Surgery, Sidney Kimmel Center for Prostate and Urologic Cancers, Memorial Sloan Kettering Cancer Center, New York, New York [87]

Robert H. Eckel, MD
Professor of Medicine, Emeritus; University of Colorado School of Medicine, Aurora, Colorado [408]

John E. Edwards, Jr., MD
Distinguished Professor of Medicine Emeritus, David Geffen School of Medicine, University of California, Los Angeles; Senior Investigator, The Lundquist Institute and Emeritus Chief, Division of Infectious Disease at Harbor-UCLA Medical Center, Torrance, California [211, 216]

David A. Ehrmann, MD
Professor of Medicine, Section of Endocrinology; Director, University of Chicago Center for PCOS, University of Chicago, Chicago, Illinois [394]

Ramy H. Elshaboury, PharmD
Clinical Pharmacy Manager; Director, PGY2 Infectious Diseases Pharmacy Residency, Massachusetts General Hospital, Boston, Massachusetts [144]

Ezekiel J. Emanuel, MD, PhD
Chair, Department of Medical Ethics and Health Policy, Levy University Professor, Perelman School of Medicine and Wharton School, University of Pennsylvania, Philadelphia, Pennsylvania [12]

Jack Ende, MD
The Schaeffer Professor of Medicine; Assistant Vice President, University of Pennsylvania Health System; Assistant Dean for Advanced Medical Practice, Perelman School of Medicine of the University of Pennsylvania, Philadelphia, Pennsylvania [478]

John W. Engstrom, MD
Betty Anker Fife Distinguished Professor and Vice-Chairman; Neurology Residency Program Director, University of California, San Francisco, San Francisco, California [17, 440]

Moshe Ephros, MD
Clinical Associate Professor of Pediatrics, Faculty of Medicine, Technion–Israel Institute of Technology, Haifa, Israel [172]

Aaron C. Ermel, MD
Assistant Professor of Clinical Medicine, Department of Internal Medicine, Division of Infectious Diseases, Indiana University School of Medicine, Indianapolis, Indiana [198]

Tim Evans, DPhil, MD
Associate Dean and Director, School of Population and Global Health, McGill University, Montreal, Quebec, Canada [474]

Carmella Evans-Molina, MD, PhD
Eli Lilly Professor of Pediatric Diabetes; Professor, Departments of Pediatrics and Medicine; Director of the Center for Diabetes and Metabolic Diseases; Director of Diabetes Research, Herman B. Wells Center for Pediatric Research; Indiana University School of Medicine; Staff Physician, Richard L. Roudebush VA Medical Center, Indianapolis, Indiana [403]

Christopher H. Fanta, MD
Professor of Medicine, Harvard Medical School; Member, Pulmonary and Critical Care Medicine Division, Brigham and Women's Hospital; Director, Partners Asthma Center, Boston, Massachusetts [38]

Paul E. Farmer, MD, PhD
Kolokotrones University Professor, Harvard University; Chair, Department of Global Health and Social Medicine, Harvard Medical School; Chief, Division of Global Health Equity, Brigham and Women's Hospital; Chief Strategist, Co-Founder, Partners In Health, Boston, Massachusetts [472, 475]

I. Sadaf Farooqi, PhD, FRCP, FMedSci, FRS
Professor of Metabolism and Medicine, Wellcome-MRC Institute of Metabolic Science, University of Cambridge, Cambridge, United Kingdom [401]

Anthony S. Fauci, MD
Chief, Laboratory of Immunoregulation; Director, National Institute of Allergy and Infectious Diseases, National Institutes of Health, Bethesda, Maryland [1, 5, 201, 202, 349, 350, 363, A14, S3]

David P. Faxon, MD
Senior Lecturer, Harvard Medical School; Associate Chief, Cardiovascular Medicine, Department of Medicine; Brigham and Women's Hospital, Boston, Massachusetts [242, 276, A11]

David Feller-Kopman, MD
Professor of Medicine, Dartmouth Geisel School of Medicine; Section Chief, Pulmonary and Critical Care Medicine, Dartmouth Hitchcock Medical Center, Lebanon, New Hampshire [299]

David T. Felson, MD, MPH
Professor of Medicine and Epidemiology, Boston University School of Medicine, Boston, Massachusetts [371]

Howard L. Fields, MD, PhD
Professor, Department of Neurology, University of California, San Francisco, San Francisco, California [13]

Gregory A. Filice, MD
Staff Physician, Veterans Affairs Medical Center, Professor of Medicine and Adjunct Professor of Public Health, University of Minnesota, Minneapolis, Minnesota [174]

Robert W. Finberg, MD‡
Richard M. Haidack Distinguished Professor of Medicine; Professor, Microbiology and Physiological Systems; Chair, Department of Medicine, University of Massachusetts Chan Medical School, Worcester, Massachusetts [74, 143]

Courtney Finlayson, MD
Associate Professor, Division of Endocrinology, Department of Pediatrics, Ann & Robert H. Lurie Children's Hospital of Chicago, Northwestern University Feinberg School of Medicine, Chicago, Illinois [390]

Alain Fischer, MD, PhD
Imagine Institute; Professor at College de France, Paris, France [351, S8]

Erik Fisher, MD
Clinical Assistant Professor of Emergency Medicine, University of South Carolina School of Medicine Greenville; Director, Medical Toxicology, Department of Emergency Medicine, Prisma Health-Update, Greenville, South Carolina [460]

Agnes B. Fogo, MD
John L. Shapiro Endowed Chair in Pathology; Professor of Pathology, Medicine and Pediatrics; Director, Renal Pathology/Electron Microscopy Laboratory, Vanderbilt University Medical Center, Nashville, Tennessee [A4]

---

‡Deceased

Gregory K. Folkers, MS, MPH
Chief of Staff, Office of the Director, National Institute of Allergy and Infectious Diseases, National Institutes of Health, Bethesda, Maryland [202]

Michael J. Fowler, MD
Associate Professor of Medicine, Division of Diabetes, Endocrinology and Metabolism, Department of Medicine; Course Director, Physical Diagnosis; Medical Director, Glucose Management Service; Director of Clinical Skills Development in Undergraduate Medical Education, Vanderbilt University School of Medicine, Nashville, Tennessee [404]

David M. Frazer, PhD
Associate Professor, Molecular Nutrition Laboratory, QIMR Berghofer Medical Research Institute, Brisbane, Queensland, Australia [414]

Jane E. Freedman, MD
Director, Division of Cardiology, Physician-in-Chief, Vanderbilt Medical Center, Nashville, Tennessee [117]

Roy Freeman, MD
Professor of Neurology, Harvard Medical School; Director, Center for Autonomic and Peripheral Nerve Disorders, Beth Israel Deaconess Medical Center, Boston, Massachusetts [21]

Lawrence S. Friedman, MD
Professor of Medicine, Harvard Medical School; Professor of Medicine, Tufts University School of Medicine; The Anton R. Fried, MD Chair, Department of Medicine, Newton-Wellesley Hospital, Newton, Massachusetts; Assistant Chief of Medicine, Massachusetts General Hospital, Boston, Massachusetts [50]

Sonia Friedman, MD
Associate Professor of Medicine, Harvard Medical School; Associate Physician, Brigham and Women's Hospital, Boston, Massachusetts [326]

Andre D. Furtado, MD
Assistant Professor, Department of Radiology, School of Medicine, University of Pittsburgh, Pittsburgh, Pennsylvania [A16]

Nicholas B. Galifianakis, MD, MPH
Associate Professor of Neurology, Movement Disorder and Neuromodulation Center Weill Institute for Neurosciences, Department of Neurology, University of California, San Francisco, San Francisco, California [V1]

John I. Gallin, MD
Associate Director for Clinical Research; Chief Scientific Officer, Clinical Center, National Institutes of Health, Bethesda, Maryland [64]

Karunesh Ganguly, MD, PhD
Department of Neurology, University of California, San Francisco; Neurology & Rehabilitation Service, San Francisco VA Medical Center, San Francisco, California [487]

Olivier Garraud, MD, PhD
Professor, INSERM 1059, University of Lyon, Faculty of Medicine of Saint-Etienne, Saint-Etienne, France [113]

Gregory M. Gauthier, MD
Associate Professor, Department of Medicine, Division of Infectious Disease, School of Medicine and Public Health, University of Wisconsin, Madison, Madison, Wisconsin [214]

Charlotte A. Gaydos, MS, MPH, DrPH
Professor of Medicine, Division of Infectious Diseases, Johns Hopkins University, Baltimore, Maryland [189]

J. Michael Gaziano, MD, MPH
Professor of Medicine, Harvard Medical School; Physician, Brigham and Women's Hospital and the VA Boston Healthcare System, Boston, Massachusetts [238]

Thomas A. Gaziano, MD, MSc
Associate Professor of Medicine, Harvard Medical School; Associate Professor, Health Policy and Management, Center for Health Decision Sciences, Harvard School of Public Health; Director, Global Cardiovascular Health Policy and Prevention Unit, Cardiovascular Medicine, Department of Medicine, Brigham and Women's Hospital, Boston, Massachusetts [238]

Susan L. Gearhart, MD
Associate Professor, Surgery, Johns Hopkins Medical Institutions, Baltimore, Maryland [328]

Jeffrey A. Gelfand, MD
Professor of Medicine (Part-Time), Harvard Medical School; Attending Physician, Infectious Diseases Division, Massachusetts General Hospital, Boston, Massachusetts [225]

Jeffrey M. Gelfand, MD, MAS, FAAN
Associate Professor of Neurology, Department of Neurology, University of California, San Francisco, San Francisco, California [23]

Lianne S. Gensler, MD
Professor of Medicine; Rheumatology Fellowship Program Director; Director, Spondyloarthritis Research Program and Clinic, University of California, San Francisco, San Francisco, California [362]

Alfred L. George, Jr., MD
Magerstadt Professor and Chair, Department of Pharmacology, Northwestern University Feinberg School of Medicine, Chicago, Illinois [309]

Dale N. Gerding, MD
Research Physician, Edward Hines Jr. VA Hospital, Hines, Illinois; Professor of Medicine (Retired), Loyola University Chicago Stritch School of Medicine, Maywood, Illinois [134]

Michael D. Geschwind, MD, PhD
Professor of Neurology; Michael J. Homer Chair in Neurology, Memory and Aging Center, University of California, San Francisco, San Francisco, California [438, V1]

Marc G. Ghany, MD, MHSc
Tenure-Track Investigator, Liver Diseases Branch, National Institute of Diabetes and Digestive and Kidney Diseases, National Institutes of Health, Bethesda, Maryland [336]

Lorenzo Giacani, PhD
Associate Professor of Medicine, Department of Medicine, Division of Allergy & Infectious Diseases, University of Washington, Seattle, Washington [183]

Matthew P. Giannetti, MD
Division of Allergy and Clinical Immunology, Brigham and Women's Hospital; Harvard Medical School, Boston, Massachusetts [354]

Michael Giladi, MD, MSc
Associate Professor of Medicine, Sackler Faculty of Medicine, Tel Aviv University; Senior Physician, The Infectious Disease Unit; Director, The Bernard Pridan Laboratory for Molecular Biology of Infectious Diseases, Tel Aviv Sourasky Medical Center, Tel Aviv, Israel [172]

Robert P. Giugliano, MD, SM, FACC, FAHA
Professor of Medicine, Harvard Medical School; Senior Investigator, TIMI Study Group, Cardiovascular Medicine, Brigham and Women's Hospital, Boston, Massachusetts [274]

Michael M. Givertz, MD
Professor of Medicine, Harvard Medical School; Medical Director, Heart Transplant and Mechanical Circulatory Support, Brigham and Women's Hospital, Boston, Massachusetts [257]

Roger I. Glass, MD, PhD
Director, Fogarty International Center; Associate Director for International Research National Institutes of Health, Bethesda, Maryland [203]

Seth R. Glassman, MD
Assistant Clinical Professor of Medicine, Division of Infectious Diseases, University at Buffalo Jacobs School of Medicine and the Biomedical Sciences, Buffalo, New York [176]

Eli Glatstein, MD‡
Professor Emeritus, Department of Radiation Oncology, Hospital of the University of Pennsylvania, Philadelphia, Pennsylvania [S5]

Ronald S. Go, MD
Chair, Core/Consultative Hematology, Division of Hematology, Mayo Clinic Rochester, Rochester, Minnesota [317]

‡Deceased

Peter J. Goadsby, MD, PhD, DSc, FRACP, FRCP, FMedSci
Professor, NIHR-Wellcome Trust King's Clinical Research Facility, King's College London, United Kingdom; Professor, Department of Neurology, University of California, Los Angeles, Los Angeles, California [16, 430]

Hilary J. Goldberg, MD, MPH
Assistant Professor of Medicine, Harvard Medical School; Medical Director, Lung Transplant Program; Clinical Director, Division of Pulmonary and Critical Care Medicine, Brigham and Women's Hospital, Boston, Massachusetts [286, 298]

Marcia B. Goldberg, MD
Professor of Medicine and Microbiology, Harvard Medical School, Massachusetts General Hospital, Boston, Massachusetts [120]

Ary L. Goldberger, MD
Professor of Medicine, Harvard Medical School & Wyss Institute for Biotechnology Inspired Engineering at Harvard University; Director, Margret and H.A. Rey Institute for Nonlinear Dynamics in Medicine; Associate Chief, Division of Interdisciplinary Medicine and Biotechnology, Beth Israel Deaconess Medical Center, Boston, Massachusetts [240, A7, A8]

David Goldblatt, MB, ChB, PhD
Professor of Vaccinology and Immunology, University College London Institute of Child Health, London, United Kingdom [146]

Samuel Z. Goldhaber, MD
Professor of Medicine, Harvard Medical School; Associate Chief and Clinical Director, Division of Cardiovascular Medicine; Director, Thrombosis Research Group, Brigham and Women's Hospital, Boston, Massachusetts [279]

Andrea Gori, MD
Full Professor of Infectious Diseases, School of Medicine and Surgery, Department of Pathophysiology and Transplantation; Co-Director, Centre for Multidisciplinary Research in Health Science (MACH), University of Milan; Director, Infectious Diseases Unit, Department of Internal Medicine, Fondazione IRCCS Ca' Granda, Ospedale Maggiore Policlinico, Milan, Italy [178]

Marga G.A. Goris, PhD, MSC
Head OIE and National Collaborating Centre for Reference and Research on Leptospirosis, Department of Medical Microbiology, Amsterdam University Medical Centers, Amsterdam, The Netherlands [184]

Maria Luisa Gorno-Tempini, MD, PhD
Professor, Department of Neurology; Language Neurobiology Lab, Memory and Aging Center; Dyslexia Center, University of California, San Francisco, San Francisco, California [V2]

Daniel J. Gottlieb, MD, MPH
Associate Professor of Medicine, Harvard Medical School; Director, Sleep Disorders Center, VA Boston Healthcare System, Sleep Medicine Division, Brigham and Women's Hospital, Boston, Massachusetts [297]

Peter A. Gottlieb, MD
Professor of Pediatrics and Medicine, Barbara Davis Center for Childhood Diabetes, University of Colorado School of Medicine, Aurora, Colorado [389]

Gregory A. Grabowski, MD
Professor Emeritus, University of Cincinnati College of Medicine; Departments of Pediatrics, and Molecular Genetics, Biochemistry and Microbiology, Division of Human Genetics, Cincinnati Children's Hospital Medical Center, Cincinnati, Ohio [418]

Yonatan H. Grad, MD, PhD
Associate Professor of Immunology and Infectious Diseases, Harvard T.H. Chan School of Public Health, Boston, Massachusetts [121]

Christine Grady, RN, PhD
Chief, Department of Bioethics, National Institutes of Health Clinical Center, Bethesda, Maryland [11]

Francesc Graus, MD, PhD
Neuroimmunology Program, Institut d'Investigacions Biomèdiques August Pi i Sunyer (IDIBAPS), Hospital Clínic, Barcelona, Spain [94]

Steven A. Greenberg, MD
Professor of Neurology, Harvard Medical School; Associate Neurologist, Brigham and Women's Hospital, Boston, Massachusetts [365]

Steven M. Greenberg, MD, PhD
Professor of Neurology, Harvard Medical School; Vice Chair of Neurology, Massachusetts General Hospital, MGH Stroke Research Center, Boston, Massachusetts [433]

Norton J. Greenberger, MD‡
Clinical Professor of Medicine, Harvard Medical School; Senior Physician, Division of Gastroenterology, Brigham and Women's Hospital, Boston, Massachusetts [346]

Daryl R. Gress, MD
Professor of Neurological Sciences; Director of Neurocritical Care, University of Nebraska Medical Center, Omaha, Nebraska [307, 429]

Patricia M. Griffin, MD
Chief, Enteric Diseases Epidemiology Branch, Division of Foodborne, Waterborne, and Environmental Diseases, National Center for Emerging and Zoonotic Infectious Diseases, Centers for Disease Control and Prevention, Atlanta, Georgia [151]

Rasim Gucalp, MD, FACP
Professor of Medicine, Albert Einstein College of Medicine; Associate Chairman for Educational Programs, Department of Oncology; Director, Hematology/Oncology Fellowship, Montefiore Medical Center, Bronx, New York [75]

Kalpana Gupta, MD, MPH
Associate Chief of Staff and Chief, Infectious Diseases, Veterans Affairs Boston Healthcare System, West Roxbury, Massachusetts; Professor of Medicine, Boston University School of Medicine, Boston, Massachusetts [135]

Chadi A. Hage, MD
Associate Professor of Clinical Medicine, Indiana University School of Medicine, Pulmonary Critical Care Medicine, Indianapolis, Indiana [212]

Bevra Hannahs Hahn, MD
Distinguished Professor of Medicine (Emeritus), University of California, Los Angeles, Los Angeles, California [356]

Noah M. Hahn, MD
Associate Professor of Oncology and Urology, Johns Hopkins University School of Medicine; Johns Hopkins University Greenberg Bladder Cancer Institute, Baltimore, Maryland [86]

Colin N. Haile, MD, PhD
Assistant Professor, Menninger Department of Psychiatry and Behavioral Sciences, Baylor College of Medicine; Michael E. DeBakey VA Medical Center, Houston, Texas [456]

Janet E. Hall, MD
Clinical Director and Senior Investigator, Division of Intramural Research, NIH/NIEHS, Research Triangle Park, North Carolina [392, 393, 396]

Scott A. Halperin, MD
Professor of Pediatrics and Microbiology & Immunology, Dalhousie University, Halifax, Nova Scotia, Canada [160]

Aidan Hampson, PhD
Program and Scientific Officer, Special Content Expert on Cannabis, Clinical Research Grants Branch, Division of Therapeutics & Medical Consequences, National Institute on Drug Abuse, National Institutes of Health, Rockville, Maryland [455]

R. Doug Hardy, MD
ID Specialists, Dallas, Texas [188]

Nigil Haroon, MD, PhD, DM, FRCPC
Associate Professor of Medicine and Rheumatology, University of Toronto; Clinician Scientist and Attending Physician, University Health Network and Mount Sinai Hospital; Scientist, Krembil Research Institute, Toronto, Ontario, Canada [362]

‡Deceased

Phil A. Hart, MD
Associate Professor of Medicine; Director, Section of Pancreatic Disorders, Division of Gastroenterology, Hepatology, and Nutrition, The Ohio State University Wexner Medical Center, Columbus, Ohio [347, 348]

William L. Hasler, MD
Professor, Division of Gastroenterology and Hepatology, University of Michigan Health System, Ann Arbor, Michigan [45, 321]

Stephen L. Hauser, MD
Robert A. Fishman Distinguished Professor, Department of Neurology, University of California, San Francisco; Director, UCSF Weill Institute for Neurosciences, San Francisco, California [1, 5, 24, 25, 28, 422, 424, 441, 442, 444, 445, 447, S9]

Thomas R. Hawn, MD, PhD
Professor, Department of Medicine, Division of Allergy & Infectious Diseases, University of Washington, Seattle, Washington [159]

Daniel F. Hayes, MD, FASCO, FACP
Stuart B. Padnos Professor of Breast Cancer Research, University of Michigan Rogel Cancer Center, Ann Arbor, Michigan [79]

Barton F. Haynes, MD
Director, Duke Human Vaccine Institute; Frederic M. Hanes Professor of Medicine; Professor of Immunology, Departments of Medicine and Immunology, Duke University Medical Center, Durham, North Carolina [349, 350]

J. Claude Hemphill, III, MD, MAS
Professor of Neurology and Neurological Surgery, University of California, San Francisco; Chief, Neurology Service, Zuckerberg San Francisco General Hospital, San Francisco, California [307, 426–429]

Dirk M. Hentschel, MD
Assistant Professor of Medicine, Harvard Medical School; Director of Interventional Nephrology, Brigham Health; Associate Physician, Brigham and Women's Hospital, Boston, Massachusetts [320]

Katherine A. High, MD
Professor Emerita, Perelman School of Medicine of the University of Pennsylvania; President, Therapeutics, Asklepios BioPharmaceuticals, Philadelphia, Pennsylvania [470]

Christine E. Hill-Kayser, MD
Assistant Professor of Radiation Oncology, Perelman School of Medicine, University of Pennsylvania, Philadelphia, Pennsylvania [S5]

Ikuo Hirano, MD
Professor of Medicine, Division of Gastroenterology, Northwestern University Feinberg School of Medicine, Chicago, Illinois [44, 323]

Martin S. Hirsch, MD
Professor of Medicine, Harvard Medical School; Senior Physician, Massachusetts General Hospital, Boston, Massachusetts [195]

Dieter Hoelzer, PhD, MD
Emeritus Director of Internal Medicine, University of Frankfurt, Frankfurt, Germany [106]

A. Victor Hoffbrand, DM
Emeritus Professor of Haematology, University College, London, United Kingdom [99]

L. John Hoffer, MD, PhD
Professor, Faculty of Medicine, McGill University; Senior Physician, Divisions of Internal Medicine and Endocrinology, Lady Davis Institute for Medical Research, Jewish General Hospital, Montreal, Quebec, Canada [335]

Charles W. Hoge, MD
Senior Scientist, Center for Psychiatry and Neuroscience, Walter Reed Army Institute of Research, Silver Spring, Maryland [S7]

Steven M. Holland, MD
Scientific Director, National Institute of Allergy and Infectious Diseases; Distinguished NIH Investigator, National Institutes of Health, Bethesda, Maryland [64, 180]

King K. Holmes, MD, PhD
Professor Emeritus, Global Health; Professor Emeritus, Medicine – Allergy and Infectious Diseases; Director, Research and Faculty Development, Department of Global Health; Co-Director, Center for AIDS Research, University of Washington – Fred Hutchinson Cancer Research Center; PI, International Training and Education Center for Health (I-TECH), University of Washington – University of California San Francisco; Director, Center for AIDS and STD, University of Washington; Infectious Disease Section Head, Harborview Medical Center; Member, National Institutes of Health (NIH) Fogarty International Center Council; Member, National Institutes of Health (NIH) Council or Councils, Seattle, Washington [136]

David Hong, MD
Assistant Professor of Medicine, Harvard Medical School; Division of Allergy & Immunology, Brigham and Women's Hospital, Boston, Massachusetts [353]

Jay H. Hoofnagle, MD
Director, Liver Diseases Research Branch, Division of Digestive Diseases and Nutrition, National Institute of Diabetes and Digestive and Kidney Diseases, National Institutes of Health, Bethesda, Maryland [336]

David C. Hooper, MD
Professor of Medicine, Harvard Medical School; Chief, Infection Control Unit, and Associate Chief, Division of Infectious Diseases, Massachusetts General Hospital, Boston, Massachusetts [144, 145]

Robert J. Hopkin, MD
Associate Professor of Clinical Pediatrics,
Cincinnati Children's Hospital Medical Center
Division of Human Genetics, Cincinnati, Ohio [418]

Leora Horn, MD, MSc
Associate Professor, Division of Hematology and Medical Oncology, Vanderbilt University School of Medicine, Nashville, Tennessee [78]

Jonathan C. Horton, MD, PhD
William F. Hoyt Professor of Neuro-ophthalmology, Professor of Ophthalmology, Neurology and Physiology, University of California, San Francisco School of Medicine, San Francisco, California [32, V3]

Howard Hu, MD, MPH, ScD
Professor & Flora L. Thornton Chair, Department of Population and Public Health Sciences, Keck School of Medicine, University of Southern California, Los Angeles, California [458]

Deborah T. Hung, MD, PhD
Professor of Genetics, Harvard Medical School, Brigham and Women's Hospital and Massachusetts General Hospital, Boston, Massachusetts; Co-Director, Infectious Disease and Microbiome Program, Broad Institute of MIT and Harvard, Cambridge, Massachusetts [121]

Gary M. Hunninghake, MD, MPH
Associate Professor of Medicine, Harvard Medical School; Division of Pulmonary & Critical Care Medicine, Brigham and Women's Hospital, Boston, Massachusetts [293]

Stephen C. Hunt, MD, MPH
National Director, VA Post-Deployment Integrated Care Initiative; Clinical Professor of Medicine, Department of Medicine, Division of General Internal Medicine, Occupational and Environmental Medicine Program, University of Washington, Seattle, Washington [S7]

Wade T. Iams, MD, MSCI
Department of Medicine, Division of Hematology/Oncology, Vanderbilt University Medical Center, Nashville, Tennessee [78]

Ashraf S. Ibrahim, PhD
Professor of Medicine, Division of Infectious Diseases, David Geffen School of Medicine at the University of California, Los Angeles; Senior Investigator and Vice Chair, Board of Directors, Director of the Graduate Studies Program, The Lindquist Institute at Harbor–UCLA Medical Center, Torrance, California [216, 218]

David H. Ingbar, MD
Professor, Medicine, Pediatrics and Integrative Biology and Physiology; Director, Pulmonary, Allergy, Critical Care and Sleep Division; CTSI Associate Director, Education, Career Development and Training; Executive Director, Center for Lung Science and Health, University of Minnesota, Minneapolis, Minnesota [305]

Elliot Israel, MD
Professor of Medicine, Harvard Medical School; Gloria M. and Anthony C. Simboli Distinguished Chair in Asthma Research; Director of Clinical Research, Pulmonary and Critical Care Division, Allergy and Immunology Division, Brigham and Women's Hospital, Boston, Massachusetts [287]

Elias Jabbour, MD
Professor, Section Chief, Acute Lymphocytic Leukemia, Department of Leukemia, Division of Cancer Medicine, MD Anderson Cancer Center, Houston, Texas [105]

Alan C. Jackson, MD
Professor of Medicine (Neurology), University of Manitoba, Winnipeg, Manitoba, Canada [208]

Yves Jackson, MD, PhD
Assistant Professor, Division of Primary Care Medicine, Geneva University Hospitals, Geneva, Switzerland [227]

Danny O. Jacobs, MD, MPH, FACS
President, Oregon Health and Science University, Portland, Oregon [15, 330, 331]

Caron A. Jacobson, MD
Assistant Professor of Medicine, Harvard Medical School; Dana-Farber Cancer Institute, Boston, Massachusetts [108, 109]

Rajesh K. Jain, MD
Assistant Professor, Department of Medicine, Section of Endocrinology, University of Chicago, Chicago, Illinois [412]

J. Larry Jameson, MD, PhD
Robert G. Dunlop Professor of Medicine; Dean, Raymond and Ruth Perelman School of Medicine; Executive Vice President, University of Pennsylvania for the Health System, Philadelphia, Pennsylvania [1, 5, 47, 93, 376–380, 382–385, 390, 391, 466, 467, A15]

Gordon L. Jensen, MD, PhD
Senior Associate Dean for Research; Professor of Medicine and Nutrition, University of Vermont Larner College of Medicine, Burlington, Vermont [334]

Savio John, MD
Chief of Gastroenterology, State University of New York Upstate Medical University, Syracuse, New York [49]

James R. Johnson, MD
Professor of Medicine, Division of Infectious Diseases and International Medicine, University of Minnesota, Minneapolis, Minnesota [161]

Stuart Johnson, MD
Professor of Medicine, Loyola University Chicago Stritch School of Medicine, Maywood, Illinois; Staff Physician, Edward Hines Jr. VA Hospital, Hines, Illinois [134]

S. Claiborne Johnston, MD, PhD
Professor of Neurology, Dell Medical School, University of Texas at Austin, Austin, Texas [426–428]

S. Andrew Josephson, MD
Professor and Chairman, Department of Neurology, University of California, San Francisco, San Francisco, California [27, 28, 307, 422, V4]

Sandeep S. Jubbal, MD
Assistant Professor of Medicine, Division of Infectious Diseases and Immunology, University of Massachusetts Chan Medical School, Worcester, Massachusetts [141]

Harald Jüppner, MD
Professor of Pediatrics, Endocrine Unit and Pediatric Nephrology Unit, Harvard Medical School; Massachusetts General Hospital, Boston, Massachusetts [410]

Joseph Kado, MBBS, DCH, MMed
University of Western Australia, Crawley, Western Australia; Clinical Research Officer, Telethon Kids Institute, Nedlands, Western Australia [359]

Peter J. Kahrilas, MD
Gilbert H. Marquardt Professor of Medicine, Feinberg School of Medicine, Northwestern University, Chicago, Illinois [44, 323]

Stephen G. Kaler, MD
CAPT, US Public Health Service (Ret); Professor of Pediatrics and Genetics, The Ohio State University College of Medicine; Principal Investigator, Center for Gene Therapy, Abigail Wexner Research Institute, Nationwide Children's Hospital, Columbus, Ohio [415]

Gail Kang, MD
Private Practice, Berkeley, California [V1]

Hagop Kantarjian, MD
Chairman, Leukemia Department; Professor of Leukemia, The University of Texas MD Anderson Cancer Center, Houston, Texas [105]

Hemanta K. Kar, MBBS, MD, MAMS
Professor and Head, Department of Dermatology, STD and Leprosy, Kalinga Institute of Medical Sciences, Bhubaneswar, Odisha, India [179]

Adolf W. Karchmer, MD
Professor of Medicine, Harvard Medical School; Emeritus Chief, Division of Infectious Diseases, Beth Israel Deaconess Medical Center, Boston, Massachusetts [128]

Dennis L. Kasper, MD
William Ellery Channing Professor of Medicine and Professor of Immunology, Department of Immunology, Harvard Medical School; Division of Infectious Diseases, Brigham and Women's Hospital, Boston, Massachusetts [1, 5, 119, 132, 177, 471]

Daniel L. Kastner, MD, PhD
Scientific Director, National Human Genome Research Institute, National Institutes of Health, Bethesda, Maryland [369]

Carol A. Kauffman, MD
Chief, Infectious Diseases Section, VA Ann Arbor Healthcare System; Professor of Internal Medicine, University of Michigan Medical School, Ann Arbor, Michigan [219]

Elaine T. Kaye, MD
Assistant Professor of Dermatology, Harvard Medical School, Boston Children's Hospital, Boston, Massachusetts [19, A1]

Kenneth M. Kaye, MD
Professor of Medicine, Harvard Medical School; Senior Physician, Division of Infectious Diseases, Brigham and Women's Hospital, Boston, Massachusetts [19, A1]

John F. Keaney, Jr., MD
Professor of Medicine, Harvard Medical School; Chief, Division of Cardiovascular Medicine; Co-Executive Director, Heart and Vascular Center, Brigham and Women's Hospital, Boston, Massachusetts [237]

David Kelsen, MD
Professor of Medicine, Weill Cornell Medical College; Edward S. Gordon Chair in Medical Oncology, Memorial Sloan Kettering Cancer Center, New York, New York [80]

John A. Kessler, MD
Davee Professor of Stem Cell Biology, Davee Department of Neurology; Director, Northwestern University Stem Cell Institute, Feinberg School of Medicine, Northwestern University, Chicago, Illinois [484]

Maryam Ali Khan, MD
Research Scholar, Division of Vascular and Endovascular Surgery, University of California, San Diego, San Diego, California [329]

Sundeep Khosla, MD
Dr. Francis Chucker and Nathan Landow Research Professor; Mayo Foundation Distinguished Investigator, Mayo Clinic College of Medicine, Rochester, Minnesota [54]

Kiran K. Khush, MD, MAS
Professor of Medicine (Cardiovascular Medicine), Stanford University School of Medicine, Stanford, California [490]

Anthony A. Killeen, MD, PhD
Professor, Department of Laboratory Medicine and Pathology, University of Minnesota, Minneapolis, Minnesota [S10]

Kami Kim, MD
Andor Szentivanyi Professor of Medicine; Director, Division of Infectious Diseases and International Medicine, Morsani College of Medicine, University of South Florida, Tampa, Florida [228]

Priya S. Kishnani, MD
C.L. and Su Chen Professor of Pediatrics; Medical Director, YT and Alice Chen Pediatrics Genetics and Genomics Center; Division Chief, Medical Genetics; Professor of Molecular Genetics and Microbiology, Duke University Medical Center, Durham, North Carolina [419]

Bruce S. Klein, MD
Gerard B. Odell Professor and Shirley S. Matchette Professor; Chief, Division of Pediatric Infectious Disease, Departments of Pediatrics, Medicine and Medical Microbiology and Immunology, University of Wisconsin, Madison, Madison, Wisconsin [214]

Christine Klein, MD
Professor of Neurology and Neurogenetics, Institute of Neurogenetics and Department of Neurology, University of Lübeck and University Hospital Schleswig-Holstein, Lübeck, Germany [436]

David M. Knipe, PhD
Higgins Professor of Microbiology and Molecular Genetics; Head, Program in Virology, Department of Microbiology, Blavatnik Institute, Harvard Medical School, Boston, Massachusetts [190]

Isaac S. Kohane, MD, PhD
Marion V. Nelson Professor and Chair, Biomedical Informatics; Harvard Medical School; Faculty Member, Informatics Program, Boston Children's Hospital, Boston, Massachusetts [488]

Barbara A. Konkle, MD
Professor of Medicine/Hematology, University of Washington; Scientific Director, Washington Center for Bleeding Disorders, Seattle, Washington [65, 115]

Bruce A. Koplan, MD, MPH
Assistant Professor of Medicine, Harvard Medical School; Director, Electrophysiology Laboratory, Brigham and Women's Hospital, Boston, Massachusetts [243–245]

Peter Kopp, MD
Professor of Medicine/Médecin Chef, Division of Endocrinology, Diabetology and Metabolism, University of Lausanne, Lausanne, Switzerland; Adjunct Professor, Division of Endocrinology, Metabolism and Molecular Medicine, Feinberg School of Medicine, Northwestern University, Chicago, Illinois [466]

Walter J. Koroshetz, MD
National Institute of Neurological Disorders and Stroke, National Institutes of Health, Bethesda, Maryland [139]

Thomas R. Kosten, MD
J. H. Waggoner Professor of Psychiatry, Pharmacology, Immunology, Neuroscience, Baylor College of Medicine, Houston, Texas [456]

Theodore A. Kotchen, MD[‡]
Professor Emeritus, Associate Dean for Clinical Research, Medical College of Wisconsin, Milwaukee, Wisconsin [277]

Camille Nelson Kotton, MD, FIDSA, FAST
Clinical Director, Transplant and Immunocompromised Host Infectious Diseases, Infectious Diseases Division, Massachusetts General Hospital, Boston, Massachusetts [195]

Barnett S. Kramer, MD, MPH, FACP
Director, Division of Cancer Prevention, National Cancer Institute, Bethesda, Maryland [70]

‡Deceased

Joel Kramer, PsyD
John Douglas French Alzheimer's Foundation Endowed Professor of Neuropsychology in Neurology; Director of Neuropsychology, Memory and Aging Center, University of California, San Francisco, San Francisco, California [V2]

Arnold R. Kriegstein, MD, PhD
Professor of Neurology, University of California, San Francisco, San Francisco, California [424]

Somashekar G. Krishna, MD, MPH
Professor of Medicine, Division of Gastroenterology, Hepatology, & Nutrition, The Ohio State University Wexner Medical Center, Columbus, Ohio [347, 348]

Henry M. Kronenberg, MD
Professor of Medicine, Massachusetts General Hospital and Harvard Medical School, Boston, Massachusetts [409]

Jens H. Kuhn, MD, PhD, MS
Principal Scientist and Director of Virology, NIH/NIAID/DCR/Integrated Research Facility at Fort Detrick, Frederick, Maryland [209, 210]

Matthew H. Kulke, MD
Zoltan Kohn Professor of Medicine, Boston University School of Medicine; Chief, Section of Hematology and Medical Oncology, Boston Medical Center; Co-Director, Boston University–Boston Medical Cancer Center, Boston, Massachusetts [84]

Sebastian G. Kurz, MD
Associate Professor of Medicine, Division of Pulmonary, Critical Care and Sleep Medicine, The Mount Sinai Hospital, New York, New York [181]

Robert F. Kushner, MD
Professor of Medicine and Medical Education, Northwestern University Feinberg School of Medicine, Chicago, Illinois [402]

Raymond Y. Kwong, MD, MPH, FACC
Professor of Medicine, Harvard Medical School; Director of Cardiac Magnetic Resonance Imaging, Cardiovascular Division, Department of Medicine, Brigham and Women's Hospital, Boston, Massachusetts [241, A9]

Loren Laine, MD
Professor of Medicine; Chief, Section of Digestive Diseases, Yale School of Medicine, New Haven, Connecticut; VA Connecticut Healthcare System, West Haven, Connecticut [48]

Neal K. Lakdawala, MD, MSc
Assistant Professor of Medicine, Harvard Medical School; Associate Physician, Brigham and Women's Hospital, Boston, Massachusetts [259]

Anil K. Lalwani, MD
Associate Dean for Student Research, Columbia University Vagelos College of Physicians and Surgeons; Professor and Vice Chair for Research; Co-Director, Columbia Cochlear Implant Center, Columbia University Vagelos College of Physicians and Surgeons; Medical Director of Perioperative Services, New York Presbyterian–Columbia University Irving Medical Center, New York, New York [34]

Michael J. Landzberg, MD
Associate Professor of Medicine, Harvard Medical School; Boston Adult Congenital Heart Disease and Pulmonary Hypertension Program, Boston Children's Hospital, Brigham and Women's Hospital, Boston, Massachusetts [269]

H. Clifford Lane, MD
Clinical Director, National Institute of Allergy and Infectious Diseases, National Institutes of Health, Bethesda, Maryland [202, S3]

Helene M. Langevin, MD
Director, National Center for Complementary and Integrative Health, National Institutes of Health, Bethesda, Maryland [482]

Carol A. Langford, MD, MHS
Harold C. Schott Endowed Chair; Director, Center for Vasculitis Care and Research, Department of Rheumatic and Immunologic Diseases, Cleveland Clinic, Cleveland, Ohio [363, 366, 374, 375, A14]

Regina C. LaRocque, MD, MPH
Associate Professor of Medicine, Harvard Medical School, Massachusetts General Hospital, Boston, Massachusetts [133]

Leslie P. Lawley, MD
Associate Professor, Department of Dermatology, School of Medicine, Emory University, Atlanta, Georgia [57]

Thomas J. Lawley, MD
William Patterson Timmie Professor of Dermatology, Former Dean, Emory University School of Medicine, Atlanta, Georgia [56, 59, A5]

David G. Le Couteur, MD, PhD
Professor of Geriatric Medicine, University of Sydney; Senior Staff Geriatrician, Concord Hospital, Sydney, Australia [476]

Sancy A. Leachman, MD, PhD
John D. Gray Endowed Chair in Melanoma Research; Professor & Chair, Department of Dermatology, Oregon Health & Science University, Center for Health & Healing, Portland, Oregon [76]

William M. Lee, MD
Professor of Internal Medicine; Meredith Mosle Chair in Liver Diseases, University of Texas Southwestern Medical Center at Dallas, Dallas, Texas [340]

Charles Lei, MD
Assistant Professor, Department of Emergency Medicine, Vanderbilt University Medical Center, Nashville, Tennessee [460]

Jane A. Leopold, MD
Associate Professor of Medicine, Harvard Medical School; Director, Women's Interventional Cardiology Health Initiative, Brigham and Women's Hospital, Boston, Massachusetts [242, A11]

Jessica Leung, MPH
Epidemiologist, Viral Vaccine Preventable Diseases Branch, Division of Viral Diseases, National Center for Immunization and Respiratory Diseases, Centers for Disease Control and Prevention, Atlanta, Georgia [207]

Nelson Leung, MD
Professor of Medicine, Division of Nephrology and Hypertension, Division of Hematology, Mayo Clinic Rochester, Rochester, Minnesota [317]

Jonathan S. Leventhal, MD
Assistant Professor of Dermatology, Yale University School of Medicine, New Haven, Connecticut [58]

Bruce D. Levy, MD
Professor of Medicine, Harvard Medical School; Pulmonary and Critical Care Medicine, Brigham and Women's Hospital, Boston, Massachusetts [284, 301]

Julia B. Lewis, MD
Professor of Medicine, Division of Nephrology and Hypertension, Vanderbilt University Medical Center, Nashville, Tennessee [314]

Peter Libby, MD
Mallinckrodt Professor of Medicine, Harvard Medical School; Brigham and Women's Hospital, Boston, Massachusetts [A10]

Richard W. Light, MD, FCCP[‡]
Professor of Medicine, Division of Allergy, Pulmonary, and Critical Care Medicine, Vanderbilt University Medical Center, Nashville, Tennessee [294, 295]

Jin-Mann S. Lin, PhD
Division of High-Consequence Pathogens and Pathology, National Center for Zoonotic and Emerging Infectious Diseases, Centers for Disease Control and Prevention, Atlanta, Georgia [450]

Jeffrey A. Linder, MD, MPH, FACP
Michael A. Gertz Professor of Medicine and Chief, Division of General Internal Medicine and Geriatrics, Department of Medicine, Northwestern University Feinberg School of Medicine, Chicago, Illinois [35]

Robert Lindsay, MD, PhD
Professor of Medicine, College of Physicians and Surgeons, Columbia University, New York, New York; Chief, Internal Medicine; Attending Physician, Helen Hayes Hospital, West Haverstraw, New York [411]

Michail S. Lionakis, MD, ScD
Chief, Fungal Pathogenesis Section, Laboratory of Clinical Immunology & Microbiology, National Institute of Allergy and Infectious Diseases, National Institutes of Health, Bethesda, Maryland [211, 216]

Marc E. Lippman, MD, MACP, FRCP
Professor of Oncology and Internal Medicine, Georgetown University, Washington, DC [79]

Peter E. Lipsky, MD
Charlottesville, Virginia [355]

Irene Litvan, MD, MSc, FAAN, FANA
Tasch Endowed Professor in Parkinson Disease Research; Director of the Parkinson and Other Movement Disorders Center, University of California, San Diego, La Jolla, California [434]

Eva S. Liu, MD
Assistant Professor of Medicine, Brigham and Women's Hospital, Harvard Medical School, Boston, Massachusetts [409]

Kathleen D. Liu, MD, PhD, MAS
Professor, Division of Nephrology, Department of Medicine, Division of Critical Care Medicine, Department of Anesthesiology, University of California, San Francisco, San Francisco, California [312]

Josep M. Llovet, MD, PhD
Liver Cancer Program, Division of Liver Diseases, Tisch Cancer Institute, Department of Medicine, Icahn School of Medicine at Mount Sinai, New York; Liver Cancer Translational Research Laboratory, Barcelona Clínic Liver Cancer Group (BCLC), Liver Unit, IDIBAPS-Hospital Clínic, CIBERehd, University of Barcelona, Catalonia, Spain; Institució Catalana de Recerca i Estudis Avançats (ICREA), Barcelona, Catalonia, Spain [82]

Donald M. Lloyd-Jones, MD, ScM, FACC, FAHA
Eileen M. Foell Professor of Heart Research; Professor of Preventive Medicine, Medicine, and Pediatrics; Chair, Department of Preventive Medicine, Northwestern University Feinberg School of Medicine; President, American Heart Association 2021–22, Chicago, Illinois [2]

Bernard Lo, MD
Professor of Medicine Emeritus and Director Emeritus of the Program in Medical Ethics, University of California, San Francisco, San Francisco, California; President Emeritus, The Greenwall Foundation, New York, New York [11]

George Loewenstein, PhD
Herbert A. Simon Professor of Economics and Psychology, Carnegie Mellon University, Pittsburgh, Pennsylvania [481]

Dan L. Longo, MD
Professor of Medicine, Harvard Medical School; Senior Physician, Brigham and Women's Hospital; Deputy Editor, *New England Journal of Medicine,* Boston, Massachusetts [1, 5, 62, 63, 66, 69, 72, 73, 93, 95, 96, 101, 108–111, 201, A6]

Nicola Longo, MD, PhD
Professor and Chief, Division of Medical Genetics, Departments of Pediatrics, Pathology, Nutrition, and Integrated Physiology; Medical Co-Director, Biochemical Genetics Laboratory, ARUP Laboratories, University of Utah, Salt Lake City, Utah [420, 421]

Lenny López, MD, MPH, MDiv
Professor of Medicine, University of California San Francisco; San Francisco VA Medical Center, San Francisco, California [10]

Joseph Loscalzo, MD, PhD
Hersey Professor of the Theory and Practice of Medicine, Harvard Medical School; Chairman, Department of Medicine, Soma Weiss MD Distinguished Chair in Medicine, Physician-in-Chief, Brigham and Women's Hospital, Boston, Massachusetts [1, 5, 40–43, 117, 236, 237, 239, 259, 261–268, 270, 273, 275, 280–283, 486, 492]

[‡]Deceased

Daniel H. Lowenstein, MD
Dr. Robert B. and Mrs. Ellinor Aird Professor of Neurology; Executive Vice Chancellor and Provost, University of California, San Francisco, San Francisco, California [422, 425, V6]

Elyse E. Lower, MD
Department of Internal Medicine, Division of Hematology-Oncology, University of Cincinnati, Cincinnati, Ohio [367]

Franklin D. Lowy, MD
Clyde '56 and Helen Wu Professor Emeritus of Medicine and Professor Emeritus of Pathology and Cell Biology (in Epidemiology), Columbia University College of Physicians and Surgeons, New York, New York [147]

Sheila A. Lukehart, PhD
Professor of Medicine, Division of Allergy & Infectious Diseases and Global Health, University of Washington, Seattle, Washington [182, 183]

Carolina Lúquez, PhD
Team Lead, National Botulism and Enteric Toxins Team, Enteric Diseases Laboratory Branch, Division of Foodborne, Waterborne, and Environmental Diseases, National Center for Emerging and Zoonotic Infectious Diseases, Centers for Disease Control and Prevention, Atlanta, Georgia [153]

Lucio Luzzatto, MD, FRCP, FRCPath
Professor of Haematology, Muhimbili University of Health and Allied Sciences, Dar-es-Salaam, Tanzania; Honorary Professor of Hematology, University of Florence, Firenze, Italy [100]

Calum A. MacRae, MD, PhD
Professor of Medicine, Harvard Medical School; Vice Chair for Scientific Innovation, Department of Medicine, Brigham and Women's Hospital, Boston, Massachusetts [237]

Lawrence C. Madoff, MD
Professor of Medicine, University of Massachusetts Chan Medical School, Worcester, Massachusetts; Medical Director, Bureau of Infectious Disease and Laboratory Sciences, Massachusetts Department of Public Health, Hinton State Laboratory Institute, Jamaica Plain, Massachusetts [130, 141]

Barry J. Make, MD
Co-Director, COPD Program; Professor, Department of Medicine, Division of Pulmonary, Critical Care and Sleep Medicine, National Jewish Health, University of Colorado Denver School of Medicine, Denver, Colorado [292]

Mahmoud Malas, MD, MHS, RPVI, FACS
Professor in Residence; Vice Chair of Surgery for Clinical Research; Chief Division Vascular and Endovascular Surgery, University of California, San Diego, Health System, La Jolla, California [329]

Fransiska Malfait, MD, PhD
Associate Professor, Center for Medical Genetics, Ghent University Hospital and Department for Biomolecular Medicine, Ghent University, Ghent, Belgium [413]

Hari R. Mallidi, MD
Associate Professor of Surgery, Harvard Medical School; Brigham and Women's Hospital, Boston, Massachusetts [298]

Susan J. Mandel, MD, MPH
Professor of Medicine; Chief, Division of Endocrinology, Diabetes and Metabolism, Perelman School of Medicine, University of Pennsylvania, Philadelphia, Pennsylvania [382–385]

Brian F. Mandell, MD, PhD
Professor and Chairman of Medicine, Cleveland Clinic Lerner College of Medicine, Department of Rheumatic and Immunologic Disease, Cleveland Clinic, Cleveland, Ohio [374]

Lionel A. Mandell, MD, FRCPC
Professor Emeritus of Medicine, McMaster University, Hamilton, Ontario, Canada [126]

Geoffrey T. Manley, MD, PhD
Professor and Vice Chairman of Neurological Surgery, University of California, San Francisco; Chief of Neurosurgery, Zuckerberg San Francisco General Hospital and Trauma Center; Co-Director, Brain and Spinal Injury Center, University of California, San Francisco, San Francisco, California [443]

Arjun K. Manrai, PhD
Assistant Professor, Harvard Medical School; Computational Health Informatics Program, Boston Children's Hospital, Boston, Massachusetts [488]

JoAnn E. Manson, MD, DrPH
Professor of Medicine and the Michael and Lee Bell Professor of Women's Health, Harvard Medical School; Chief, Division of Preventive Medicine, Brigham and Women's Hospital, Boston, Massachusetts [395]

Joan C. Marini, MD, PhD
Senior Investigator; Head, Section on Heritable Disorders of Bone and Extracellular Matrix, National Institute of Child Health and Human Development (NICHD), National Institutes of Health, Bethesda, Maryland [413]

Daniel B. Mark, MD, MPH
Professor of Medicine, Duke University Medical Center; Director, Outcomes Research, Duke Clinical Research Institute, Durham, North Carolina [4]

Mariel Marlow, PhD, MPH
Mumps Program Lead, Viral Vaccine Preventable Diseases Branch, Division of Viral Diseases, National Center for Immunization and Respiratory Diseases, Centers for Disease Control and Prevention, Atlanta, Georgia [207]

Alexander G. Marneros, MD, PhD
Associate Professor, Department of Dermatology, Harvard Medical School; Cutaneous Biology Research Center, Massachusetts General Hospital, Boston, Massachusetts [61]

Bradley A. Maron, MD
Associate Professor of Medicine, Harvard Medical School; Associate Physician, Brigham and Women's Hospital, Boston, Massachusetts [283]

Jeanne M. Marrazzo, MD, MPH
Professor of Medicine; Director, Division of Infectious Diseases, University of Alabama at Birmingham, Birmingham, Alabama [136]

Gary J. Martin, MD
Raymond J. Langenbach, MD Professor of Medicine; Senior Vice Chairman, Department of Medicine, Northwestern University Medical School, Chicago, Illinois [6]

Anthony F. Massaro, MD
Instructor, Harvard Medical School; Director, Medical Intensive Care Unit, Division of Pulmonary and Critical Care, Brigham and Women's Hospital, Boston, Massachusetts [300, 303]

Henry Masur, MD
Chief, Critical Care Medicine Department, National Institutes of Health Clinical Center, Bethesda, Maryland [220]

Max Maurin, MD, PhD
Professor of Bacteriology, Université Grenoble Alpes; Centre Hospitalier Universitaire, Institut de Biologie et Pathologie, Grenoble, France [170]

Marcela V. Maus, MD, PhD
Director, Cell Therapy Program; Paula O'Keefe Endowed Chair, Massachusetts General Hospital Cancer Center; Associate Professor of Medicine, Harvard Medical School; Attending Physician, Hematopoietic Cell Transplant & Cell Therapy Program, Massachusetts General Hospital; Associate Member, Broad Institute of MIT and Harvard; Associate Member, Ragon Institute of MGH, MIT, and Harvard, Charlestown, Massachusetts [470]

Clio P. Mavragani, MD
Rheumatologist, Associate Professor, Department of Physiology, National and Kapodistrian University of Athens, Athens, Greece [357, 361]

Robert J. Mayer, MD
Faculty Vice President for Academic Affairs, Dana-Farber Cancer Institute; Stephen B. Kay Family Professor of Medicine, Harvard Medical School, Boston, Massachusetts [81]

Jared R. Mayers, MD, PhD
Research Fellow in Medicine, Harvard Medical School; Brigham and Women's Hospital, Boston, Massachusetts [489]

Sarah Mbaeyi, MD, MPH
Medical Officer, National Center for Immunization and Respiratory Diseases, Centers for Disease Control and Prevention, Atlanta, Georgia [123]

Alexander J. McAdam, MD, PhD
Associate Professor of Pathology, Harvard Medical School; Medical Director, Infectious Diseases Diagnostic Laboratory, Boston Children's Hospital, Boston, Massachusetts [S11]

Calvin O. McCall, MD
Dermatology Section, Hunter Holmes McGuire Veterans Affairs Medical Center, Richmond, Virginia [A5]

Zachary B. R. McClain, MD
Attending Physician, Gender and Sexuality Development Clinic; Medical Director, Young Men's Clinic, Children's Hospital of Philadelphia, Philadelphia, Pennsylvania [400]

John F. McConville, MD
Associate Professor of Medicine; Director, Internal Medicine Residency Program, Vice Chair for Education, University of Chicago, Chicago, Illinois [296]

Michael McCrea, PhD, ABPP
Professor and Eminent Scholar; Vice Chair of Research; Co-Director, Center for Neurotrauma Research (CNTR), Department of Neurosurgery, Medical College of Wisconsin, Milwaukee, Wisconsin [443]

Kathleen M. McKibbin, MD
Staff Physician, Northwestern University Health Services, Evanston, Illinois [2]

Maureen McMahon, MD, MCR
Associate Chief; Associate Professor, Division of Rheumatology, David Geffen School of Medicine, University of California, Los Angeles, Los Angeles, California [356]

Kevin T. McVary, MD, FACS
Director of the Center for Male Health; Professor of Urology, Department of Urology, Stritch School of Medicine, Loyola University Medical Center, Maywood, Illinois [397]

John N. Mecchella, DO, MPH
Assistant Professor of Medicine, Geisel School of Medicine at Dartmouth, Dartmouth-Hitchcock Medical Center, Lebanon, New Hampshire [417]

Mandeep R. Mehra, MD, MSc, FRCP (London)
Professor of Medicine, Harvard Medical School; The William Harvey Distinguished Chair in Advanced Cardiovascular Medicine; Executive Director, Center for Advanced Heart Disease, Brigham and Women's Hospital, Boston, Massachusetts [257, 258, 260]

Sanjay R. Mehta, MD, DTM&H, D(ABMM)
Associate Professor of Medicine and Pathology, University of California, San Diego School of Medicine, San Diego, California [S12]

Shlomo Melmed, MBChB, MACP, FRCP
Executive Vice President and Dean of the Medical Faculty; Professor of Medicine, Cedars-Sinai Medical Center, Los Angeles, California [378–380]

Robert O. Messing, MD
Professor and Chair of Neuroscience; Professor of Neurology; Director, Waggoner Center for Alcohol and Addiction Research, University of Texas at Austin, Austin, Texas [451]

Nancy Messonnier, MD
Executive Director for Pandemic Prevention and Health Systems, Skoll Foundation, Palo Alto, California [123]

M.-Marsel Mesulam, MD
Ruth Dunbar Davee Professor of Neuroscience and Neurology, Mesulam Center for Cognitive Neurology and Alzheimer's Disease, Northwestern University Feinberg School of Medicine, Chicago, Illinois [30]

Robert G. Micheletti, MD
Associate Professor of Dermatology and Medicine, Perelman School of Medicine, University of Pennsylvania, Philadelphia, Pennsylvania [60]

Aaron W. Michels, MD
Associate Professor of Pediatrics, Medicine, and Immunology, Barbara Davis Center for Childhood Diabetes, University of Colorado School of Medicine, Aurora, Colorado [389]

Susan Miesfeldt, MD
Associate Professor of Medicine, Tufts University School of Medicine; Medical Oncology, Medical Director, Cancer Risk and Prevention Program, Maine Medical Center Cancer Institute, Scarborough, Maine [467]

Bruce L. Miller, MD
A. W. and Mary Margaret Clausen Distinguished Professor of Neurology, Memory and Aging Center, Global Brain Health Institute, University of California, San Francisco School of Medicine, San Francisco, California [27, 29, 431, 432, 434, V2]

Samuel I. Miller, MD
Professor of Medicine, Microbiology and Genome Sciences, University of Washington, Seattle, Washington [165]

William R. Miller, MD
Assistant Professor of Medicine, Division of Infectious Diseases, Houston Methodist Hospital, Center for Infectious Diseases Research, Houston Methodist Research Institute, Houston, Texas [149]

Jyoti Mishra, PhD
Department of Psychiatry, University of California, San Diego, La Jolla, California [487]

Hana Mitchell, MD, MSC
Clinical Assistant Professor, Division of Pediatric Infectious Diseases, Department of Pediatrics, The University of British Columbia, BC Children's Hospital, Vancouver, British Columbia, Canada [3]

Simon J. Mitchell, MBChB, PhD, FUHM, FANZCA
Professor, Department of Anaesthesiology, University of Auckland and Auckland City Hospital, Auckland, New Zealand [463]

Babak Mokhlesi, MD, MSc
The J. Bailey Carter, MD Professor of Medicine; Chief, Division of Pulmonary, Critical Care, and Sleep Medicine; Co-Director, Rush Lung Center, Rush University Medical Center, Chicago, Illinois [296]

Thomas A. Moore, MD, FACP, FIDSA
Clinical Professor of Medicine, University of Kansas School of Medicine-Wichita Campus, Wichita, Kansas [222]

Richard I. Morimoto, PhD
Bill and Gayle Cook Professor of Biology, Department of Molecular Biosciences, Rice Institute for Biomedical Research, Northwestern University, Evanston, Illinois [491]

Alison Morris, MD, MS
Chief, Pulmonary, Allergy and Critical Care Medicine; Professor of Medicine; UPMC Chair of Translational Pulmonary and Critical Care Medicine; Director, University of Pittsburgh Center for Medicine and the Microbiome, University of Pittsburgh School of Medicine, Pittsburgh, Pennsylvania [220]

David A. Morrow, MD, MPH
Professor of Medicine, Harvard Medical School; Director, Samuel A. Levine Cardiac Intensive Care Unit, Cardiovascular Division, Brigham and Women's Hospital, Boston, Massachusetts [14]

William J. Moss, MD, MPH
Professor, Departments of Epidemiology, International Health, and Molecular Microbiology and Immunology, Bloomberg School of Public Health, Johns Hopkins University, Baltimore, Maryland [205]

Robert J. Motzer, MD
Jack and Dorothy Byrne Chair in Clinical Oncology, Kidney Cancer Section Head; Attending Physician, Department of Medicine, Memorial Sloan Kettering Cancer Center, New York, New York [85]

David B. Mount, MD, FRCPC
Assistant Professor of Medicine, Harvard Medical School; Clinical Chief and Director, Dialysis Services Renal Divisions, Brigham and Women's Hospital and VA Boston Healthcare System; Boston, Massachusetts [52, 53, S1]

Haralampos M. Moutsopoulos, MD, FACP, FRCP(hc), Master ACR
Professor, Chair Medical Sciences-Immunology, Academy of Athens, Athens, Greece [357, 361]

Catharina M. Mulders-Manders, MD, PhD
Department of Internal Medicine, Radboud University Medical Center, Nijmegen, The Netherlands [20]

L. Silvia Munoz-Price, MD, PhD
Chief Quality and Safety Officer, Virginia Commonwealth University Health System, Richmond, Virginia [162]

Nikhil C. Munshi, MD
Professor of Medicine, Harvard Medical School; Boston VA Healthcare System; Director of Basic and Correlative Sciences; Associate Director, Jerome Lipper Myeloma Center, Dana-Farber Cancer Institute, Boston, Massachusetts [111]

Naoka Murakami, MD, PhD
Instructor in Medicine, Harvard Medical School; Associate Physician, Brigham and Women's Hospital, Boston, Massachusetts [313]

John R. Murphy, PhD
Professor of Medicine, Division of Infectious Diseases, Johns Hopkins School of Medicine, Baltimore, Maryland [150]

Timothy F. Murphy, MD
SUNY Distinguished Professor; Director, UB Clinical and Translational Science Institute; Senior Associate Dean for Clinical and Translational Research, Jacobs School of Medicine and Biomedical Sciences, University at Buffalo, The State University of New York, Buffalo, New York [157]

Barbara E. Murray, MD
J. Ralph Meadows Professor of Medicine, Division of Infectious Diseases; Professor, Microbiology and Molecular Genetics, University of Texas Medical School, Houston, Texas [149]

Joseph A. Murray, MD
Professor of Medicine, Departments of Internal Medicine and Immunology, Mayo Clinic School of Medicine, Rochester, Minnesota [46]

Mark B. Mycyk, MD
Associate Professor, Department of Emergency Medicine, Northwestern University Feinberg School of Medicine; Chair of Research, Department of Emergency Medicine, Cook County Health, Chicago, Illinois [459]

Avindra Nath, MD
Chief, Section of Infections of the Nervous System; Clinical Director, National Institute of Neurological Disorders and Stroke (NINDS), National Institutes of Health, Bethesda, Maryland [139]

Edward T. Naureckas, MD
Professor of Medicine, Section of Pulmonary and Critical Care Medicine, University of Chicago, Chicago, Illinois [285]

Eric G. Neilson, MD
Vice President for Medical Affairs; Lewis Landsberg Dean Professor of Medicine and Cell and Molecular Biology, Feinberg School of Medicine, Northwestern University, Chicago, Illinois [309, 314, A4]

Tuhina Neogi, MD, PhD
Professor of Medicine and Chief of Rheumatology, Section of Rheumatology, Department of Medicine; Professor of Epidemiology, Department of Epidemiology, Boston University School of Public Health, Boston, Massachusetts [371]

Eric J. Nestler, MD, PhD
Nash Family Professor, Department of Neuroscience; Director, Friedman Brain Institute; Dean for Academic and Scientific Affairs, Ichan School of Medicine at Mount Sinai, New York, New York [451]

Hartmut P. H. Neumann, MD
Unit for Preventive Medicine, Department of Nephrology and General Medicine, Albert-Ludwigs University of Freiburg, Freiburg, Germany [387]

Kathleen M. Neuzil, MD, MPH
Director, Center for Vaccine Development & Global Health, University of Maryland School of Medicine, Baltimore, Maryland [200]

Jonathan Newmark, MD, MM
Colonel (Retired), Medical Corps, US Army; Adjunct Professor, Neurology, F. Edward Hebert School of Medicine, Uniformed Services University of the Health Sciences, Bethesda, Maryland; Clinical Assistant Professor, Neurology, School of Medicine and Health Sciences, George Washington University, Washington, DC; Department of Neurology, Washington DC Veterans' Affairs Medical Center, Washington, DC; Senior Medical Advisor, Office of Biodefense Research and Surety, National Institute of Allergy and Infectious Diseases, National Institutes of Health, Rockville, Maryland [S4]

J. Curtis Nickel, MD, FRCS(C)
Professor, Department of Urology, Queen's University at Kingston; Staff Urologist, Kingston Health Sciences Centre, Kingston, Ontario, Canada [51]

Michael S. Niederman, MD
Professor of Clinical Medicine, Weill Cornell Medical College; Division of Pulmonary and Critical Care Medicine, New York Presbyterian/Weill Cornell Medical Center, New York, New York [126]

Kevin D. Niswender, MD, PhD
Associate Professor of Medicine, Vanderbilt University Medical Center, Nashville, Tennessee [403]

Scott A. Norton, MD, MPH, MSc
Professor of Dermatology and Pediatrics, George Washington University School of Medicine and Health Sciences; Chief of Dermatology, Division of Dermatology, Children's National Health System, Washington, DC [461]

Emily Nosova, MD
Assistant Professor of Medicine, Division of Endocrinology, Diabetes and Bone Disease, Icahn School of Medicine and Mount Sinai Health System, New York, New York [398]

Thomas B. Nutman, MD
Head, Helminth Immunology Section; Head, Clinical Parasitology Section; Chief, Laboratory of Parasitic Diseases, National Institute of Allergy and Infectious Diseases, National Institutes of Health, Bethesda, Maryland [232, 233]

Katherine L. O'Brien, MD, MPH
Director, IVB, World Health Organization, Geneva, Switzerland [146]

Max R. O'Donnell, MD, MPH
Associate Professor of Medicine & Epidemiology, Division of Pulmonary, Allergy, and Critical Care Medicine & Department of Epidemiology, Columbia University Irving Medical Center, New York, New York [181]

Nigel O'Farrell, MD, FRCP
Pasteur Suite Ealing Hospital, London, United Kingdom [173]

Jennifer Ogar, MS, CCC-SLP
Speech-Language Pathologist, Memory and Aging Center, University of California, San Francisco, San Francisco, California [V2]

Patrick T. O'Gara, MD
Professor of Medicine, Harvard Medical School; Watkins Family Distinguished Chair in Cardiology, Brigham and Women's Hospital, Boston, Massachusetts [42, 239, 261–268]

C. Warren Olanow, MD, FRCPC, FRCP(hon)
Professor and Chairman Emeritus, Department of Neurology; Professor Emeritus, Department of Neuroscience, Mount Sinai School of Medicine, New York, New York; CEO, Clintrex, LLC [435, 436]

Stephen O'Rahilly, MD, FRS, FMedSci
Professor of Clinical Biochemistry and Medicine and Director of the MRC Metabolic Disease Unit, University of Cambridge, Addenbrookes Hospital, Cambridge, United Kingdom [401]

Joseph G. Ouslander, MD
Charles E. Schmidt College of Medicine, Florida Atlantic University, Boca Raton, Florida [477]

Chung Owyang, MD
H. Marvin Pollard Professor of Internal Medicine; Professor of Molecular and Integrative Physiology; Chief, Division of Gastroenterology and Hepatology; Director, Pollard Institute for Medical Research; University of Michigan Health System, Ann Arbor, Michigan [321, 327]

Umesh D. Parashar, MBBS, MPH
Chief, Viral Gastroenteritis Branch, Division of Viral Diseases, National Center for Immunization and Respiratory Diseases, Centers for Disease Control and Prevention, Atlanta, Georgia [203]

Shreyaskumar R. Patel, MD
Robert R. Herring Distinguished Professor of Medicine; Center Medical Director, Sarcoma Center, The University of Texas MD Anderson Cancer Center, Houston, Texas [91]

Gustav Paumgartner, MD
Professor Emeritus of Medicine, University of Munich, Munich, Germany [346]

David A. Pegues, MD
Professor of Medicine, Division of Infectious Diseases, Perelman School of Medicine, University of Pennsylvania, Philadelphia, Pennsylvania [165]

Steven A. Pergam, MD, MPH
Associate Professor, Vaccine and Infectious Disease Division, Fred Hutchinson Cancer Research Center; Associate Professor, Department of Medicine, Division of Allery & Infectious Diseases, University of Washington; Medical Director, Infection Prevention, Seattle Cancer Care Alliance, Seattle, Washington [159]

Karran A. Phillips, MD, MSc
Clinical Director, National Institute on Drug Abuse, National Institutes of Health, Baltimore, Maryland [457]

Richard J. Pollack, PhD
Senior Environmental Public Health Officer, Department of Environmental Health and Safety, Harvard University, Cambridge, Massachusetts [461]

Martin R. Pollak, MD
George C. Reisman Professor of Medicine, Harvard Medical School; Beth Israel Deaconess Medical Center, Boston, Massachusetts [315]

Sir Andrew J. Pollard, BSc, MA, MBBS, MRCP(UK), FRCPCH, PhD, DIC, FHEA, FIDSA, FMedSci
Professor of Paediatric Infection and Immunity, Department of Paediatrics, University of Oxford; Children's Hospital, Oxford, United Kingdom [155]

Nongnooch Poowanawittayakom, MD, MPH
Assistant Professor, Division of Infectious Diseases, Allergy, and Immunology, St. Louis University, St. Louis, Missouri [130]

Reuven Porat, MD
Professor of Medicine, Department of Internal Medicine, Tel Aviv Souarsky Medical Center; Sackler Faculty of Medicine, Tel Aviv University, Tel Aviv, Israel [18]

John T. Potts, Jr., MD
Jackson Distinguished Professor of Clinical Medicine, Harvard Medical School; Director of Research and Physician-in-Chief Emeritus, Massachusetts General Hospital, Boston, Massachusetts [410]

Lawrie W. Powell, AC, MD, PhD
Professor Emeritus, The University of Queensland and the Royal Brisbane and Women's Hospital, Queensland, Australia [414]

Alvin C. Powers, MD
Joe C. Davis Chair in Biomedical Science; Professor of Medicine, Molecular Physiology and Biophysics; Director, Vanderbilt Diabetes Center; Chief, Division of Diabetes, Endocrinology, and Metabolism, Vanderbilt University Medical Center, Nashville, Tennessee [403–405]

Daniel S. Pratt, MD
Assistant Professor of Medicine, Harvard Medical School; Clinical Director, Liver Transplantation; Director, Autoimmune and Cholestatic Liver Center, Massachusetts General Hospital, Boston, Massachusetts [49, 337, 346]

Michael B. Prentice, MBChB, PhD, FRCP(UK), FRCPath, FFPRCPI
Professor of Medical Microbiology, School of Microbiology, University College Cork, Cork, Ireland [171]

Stanley B. Prusiner, MD
Director, Institute for Neurodegenerative Diseases; Professor, Department of Neurology, UCSF Weill Institute for Neurosciences, University of California, San Francisco; Professor, Department of Biochemistry and Biophysics, University of California, San Francisco, San Francisco, California [424, 438]

Thomas C. Quinn, MD, MSc
Professor of Medicine and Pathology, Johns Hopkins University School of Medicine; Director, Johns Hopkins Center for Global Health, Baltimore, Maryland [189]

Gil D. Rabinovici, MD
Ed Fein and Pearl Landrith Distinguished Professor, Memory and Aging Center, Department of Neurology, Department of Radiology and Biomedical Imaging, Weill Institute for Neurosciences, University of California, San Francisco, San Francisco, California [29, 431, V2]

Daniel J. Rader, MD
Seymour Gray Professor of Molecular Medicine; Chair, Department of Genetics; Chief, Division of Translational Medicine and Human Genetics, Department of Medicine, Perelman School of Medicine at the University of Pennsylvania, Philadelphia, Pennsylvania [407]

Kanwal Raghav, MBBS, MD
Associate Professor, GI Medical Oncology, The University of Texas MD Anderson Cancer Center, Houston, Texas [92]

Kaitlin Rainwater-Lovett, PhD, MPH
Senior Staff Scientist, Asymmetric Operations Sector, Johns Hopkins Applied Physics Laboratory, Laurel, Maryland [205]

Sanjay Ram, MBBS
Professor of Medicine, Division of Infectious Diseases & Immunology, University of Massachusetts Chan Medical School, Worcester, Massachusetts [156]

Prashanth S. Ramachandran, MBBS
Weill Institute for Neurosciences, Department of Neurology, University of California, San Francisco, San Francisco, California [S2]

Reuben Ramphal, MD
Courtesy Professor, Department of Medicine, University of Florida College of Medicine, Gainesville, Florida [164]

Kathryn Moynihan Ramsey, PhD
Research Assistant Professor, Division of Endocrinology, Metabolism and Molecular Medicine, Department of Medicine, Feinberg School of Medicine, Northwestern University, Chicago, Illinois [485]

Vikram R. Rao, MD, PhD
Distinguished Professor in Neurology; Associate Professor of Clinical Neurology; Chief, Epilepsy Division, Department of Neurology, University of California, San Francisco, San Francisco, California [425]

Didier Raoult, MD, PhD
Emeritus Professor, IHU Méditerranée Infection, Marseille, France. Aix-Marseille Université, Marseille, France [170]

Kumanan Rasanathan, MBChB, MPH, FAFPHM
Unit Head, Equity and Health (EQH), Department of Social Determinants of Health (SDH), World Health Organization, Phnom Penh, Cambodia [474]

James P. Rathmell, MD
Leroy D. Vandam Professor of Anaesthesia, Harvard Medical School; Chair, Department of Anesthesiology, Perioperative and Pain Medicine, Brigham and Women's Hospital, Boston, Massachusetts [13]

Mario C. Raviglione, MD, FRCP (UK), FERS, Hon RSP (RF)
Full Professor of Global Health; Co-Director, Centre for Multidisciplinary Research in Health Science (MACH), University of Milan, Milan, Italy [178]

Divya Reddy, MBBS, MPH
Associate Professor of Medicine; Program Director, Pulmonary and Critical Care Fellowship; Medical Director, Bronchiectasis and Nontuberculous Mycobacterial (NTM) Disease Program, Montefiore Medical Center, Albert Einstein College of Medicine, Bronx, New York [181]

Susan Redline, MD, MPH
Peter C. Farrell Professor of Sleep Medicine, Harvard Medical School; Brigham and Women's Hospital; Boston, Massachusetts [297]

Sharon L. Reed, MD, MScCTM
Professor of Pathology and Medicine, University of California, San Diego School of Medicine, La Jolla, California [221, 223, S12]

Susan E. Reef, MD
Medical Epidemiologist, Centers for Disease Control and Prevention, Atlanta, Georgia [206]

Michael Regner, MD
Neuroradiology Clinical Instructor, Department of Radiology & Biomedical Imaging, University of California, San Francisco, San Francisco, California [A16]

Victor I. Reus, MD
Distinguished Professor Emeritus, Department of Psychiatry and Behavioral Sciences, University of California, San Francisco School of Medicine; UCSF Weill Institute for Neurosciences, San Francisco, California [452]

Bernardo Reyes, MD
Charles E. Schmidt College of Medicine, Florida Atlantic University, Boca Raton, Florida [477]

Joseph J. Rhatigan, MD
Associate Chief, Division of Global Health Equity, Brigham and Women's Hospital; Associate Professor, Harvard Medical School and Harvard T.H. Chan School of Public Health, Boston, Massachusetts [472]

Peter A. Rice, MD
Professor of Medicine, Division of Infectious Diseases & Immunology, University of Massachusetts Chan Medical School, Worcester, Massachusetts [156]

Eugene T. Richardson, MD, PhD
Assistant Professor of Global Health and Social Medicine, Harvard Medical School, Boston, Massachusetts [475]

Jan H. Richardus, MD, PhD
Professor of Infectious Diseases and Public Health, Department of Public Health, Erasmus MC, University Medical Center Rotterdam, Rotterdam, The Netherlands [179]

Michael R. Rickels, MD, MS
Willard and Rhoda Ware Professor in Diabetes and Metabolic Diseases, Department of Medicine, Division of Endocrinology, Diabetes and Metabolism, University of Pennsylvania Perelman School of Medicine, Philadelphia, Pennsylvania [404, 405]

Elizabeth Robbins, MD
Clinical Professor, Pediatrics, Emeritus, University of California, San Francisco, San Francisco, California [S9]

Gary L. Robertson, MD
Emeritus Professor of Medicine, Northwestern University School of Medicine, Chicago, Illinois [381]

Dan M. Roden, MD
Professor of Medicine, Pharmacology, and Biomedical Informatics, Vanderbilt University School of Medicine, Nashville, Tennessee [67, 68]

James A. Romano, Jr., PhD, DABT, ATS
Principal Senior Life Scientist Advisor, Tunnell Government Services, Inc., Rockville, Maryland [S4]

Karen L. Roos, MD
John and Nancy Nelson Professor of Neurology; Professor of Neurological Surgery, Indiana University School of Medicine, Indianapolis, Indiana [137, 138, 140]

Allan H. Ropper, MD, FRCP, FACP
Professor of Neurology, Harvard Medical School; Deputy Editor, *New England Journal of Medicine*, Boston, Massachusetts [28]

Rossana Rosa, MD
Infectious Diseases Consultant, UnityPoint Clinic, Des Moines, Iowa [162]

Ivan O. Rosas, MD
Professor and Section Chief, Pulmonary, Critical Care, and Sleep Medicine, Baylor College of Medicine, Houston, Texas [293]

Mark Roschewski, MD
Clinical Director, Lymphoid Malignancies Branch, Center for Cancer Research, National Cancer Institute, National Institutes of Health, Bethesda, Maryland [95]

Misha Rosenbach, MD
Associate Professor, Perelman School of Medicine at the University of Pennsylvania, Departments of Dermatology and Internal Medicine, Hospital of the University of Pennsylvania, Philadelphia, Pennsylvania [60]

Roger N. Rosenberg, MD
Zale Distinguished Chair and Professor of Neurology, Department of Neurology, University of Texas Southwestern Medical Center, Dallas, Texas [439]

Myrna R. Rosenfeld, MD, PhD
Institut d'Investigacions Biomèdiques August Pi i Sunyer, Fundació Clínic per a la Recerca Biomèdica, Spain; Adjunct Professor, University of Pennsylvania, Philadelphia, Pennsylvania [94]

Deborah C. Rubin, MD
Professor of Medicine and of Developmental Biology; Associate Chair for Faculty Affairs and Director, Womens' GI Committee, Washington University School of Medicine, St. Louis, Missouri [325]

Thomas A. Russo, MD, CM
SUNY Distinguished Professor of Medicine and Microbiology & Immunology, Chief, Division of Infectious Diseases, Jacobs School of Medicine and the Biomedical Sciences, University at Buffalo, State University of New York, Buffalo, New York
[161, 175, 176]

George W. Rutherford, MD
Professor of Epidemiology, Preventive Medicine, Pediatrics and History, and Head, Division of Infectious Disease and Global Epidemiology, Department of Epidemiology and Biostatistics, University of California, San Francisco, San Francisco, California [473]

Edward T. Ryan, MD
Professor of Medicine, Harvard Medical School; Professor of Immunology and Infectious Diseases, Harvard T.H. Chan School of Public Health; Director, Global Infectious Diseases, Massachusetts General Hospital, Boston, Massachusetts [168]

Manish Sadarangani, MA, BM, BCh, DPhil
Associate Professor, Department of Pediatrics, University of British Columbia; Director, Vaccine Evaluation Center, BC Children's Hospital Research Institute, Vancouver, British Columbia, Canada [155]

David J. Salant, MD
Professor of Medicine, Boston University School of Medicine; Chief, Renal Section, Boston University Medical Center, Boston, Massachusetts [316]

Richard B. Saltman, PhD
Professor of Health Policy and Management, Rollins School of Public Health, Emory University, Atlanta, Georgia [7]

Blossom Samuels, MD
Attending, Westchester Medical Center; Clinical Assistant Professor, New York Medical College, Valhalla, New York [411]

Martin A. Samuels, MD, DSc (hon), FACP, FAAN, FRCP, FANA
Miriam Sydney Joseph Distinguished Professor of Neurology, Harvard Medical School; Founding Chair Emeritus, Department of Neurology, Brigham and Women's Hospital, Boston, Massachusetts [V7]

Vaishali Sanchorawala, MD
Professor of Medicine; Director, Amyloidosis Center; Director, Autologous Stem Cell Transplantation Program, Boston University School of Medicine and Boston Medical Center, Boston, Massachusetts [112]

Philippe J. Sansonetti, MD
Professor, Collège de France; Emeritus Professor, Institut Pasteur, Paris, France [166]

Clifford B. Saper, MD, PhD
James Jackson Putnam Professor of Neurology and Neuroscience, Harvard Medical School; Department of Neurology, Beth Israel Deaconess Medical Center, Boston, Massachusetts [31]

William H. Sauer, MD
Associate Professor of Medicine, Harvard Medical School; Section Chief, Cardiac Arrhythmia Service, Brigham and Women's Hospital, Boston, Massachusetts [243–256, 306]

Edward A. Sausville, MD, PhD
National Cancer Institute, Bethesda, Maryland (Retired); Marlene & Stewart Greenebaum Comprehensive Cancer Center, University of Maryland, Baltimore, Maryland [73]

David T. Scadden, MD
Gerald and Darlene Jordan Professor of Medicine; Chair Emeritus and Professor, Department of Stem Cell and Regenerative Biology, Harvard University; Director, Center for Regenerative Medicine; Massachusetts General Hospital, Co-director, Harvard Stem Cell Institute, Cambridge, Massachusetts [96]

Thomas E. Scammell, MD
Professor, Harvard Medical School; Beth Israel Deaconess Medical Center; Boston Children's Hospital, Boston, Massachusetts [31]

Anthony H. V. Schapira, MD, DSc, FRCP, FMedSci
Head and Professor, Department of Clinical and Movement Neurosciences, UCL Queen Square Institute of Neurology; Director of UCL Royal Free Campus; Vice-Dean UCL, London, United Kingdom [435]

Howard I. Scher, MD, FASCO
Professor of Medicine, Weill Cornell Medicine College; D. Wayne Calloway Chair in Urologic Oncology; Head, Biomarker Development Program, Office of the Physician in Chief; Member and Attending Physician, Genitourinary Oncology Service, Department of Medicine, Memorial Sloan Kettering Cancer Center, New York, New York [87]

Gordon Schiff, MD
Associate Professor of Medicine, Harvard Medical School; Associate Director, Brigham and Women's Hospital Center Patient Safety Research; Quality and Safety Director, HMS Center for Primary Care, Boston, Massachusetts [9]

Scott Schissel, MD, PhD
Chief of Medicine, Department of Medicine, Brigham and Women's Faulkner Hospital, Jamaica Plain, Massachusetts [302]

Bernd Schnabl, MD
Professor of Medicine, Department of Medicine, Division of Gastroenterology, University of California San Diego, La Jolla, California [342]

Marc A. Schuckit, MD
Distinguished Professor of Psychiatry, University of California, San Diego Medical School, La Jolla, California [453]

William W. Seeley, MD
Professor of Neurology and Pathology, UCSF Weill Institute for Neurosciences, University of California, San Francisco, San Francisco, California [29, 431–434]

Florencia Pereyra Segal, MD
Assistant Professor of Medicine, Brigham and Women's Hospital, Boston, Massachusetts [141]

Julian L. Seifter, MD
Associate Professor of Medicine, Harvard Medical School; Distinguished Nephrologist, Brigham and Women's Hospital, Boston, Massachusetts [308, 319]

Jaime Sepúlveda, MD, MPH, MSc, DrSc
Haile T. Debas Distinguished Professor of Global Health; Executive Director, Institute for Global Health Sciences, University of California, San Francisco, San Francisco, California [473]

Christopher W. Seymour, MD, MSc
Associate Professor of Critical Care and Emergency Medicine, Department of Critical Care and Emergency Medicine, The CRISMA Center, University of Pittsburgh School of Medicine, Pittsburgh, Pennsylvania [304]

Majid Shafiq, MD, MPH
Medical Director, Interventional Pulmonology, Division of Pulmonary and Critical Care Medicine, Brigham and Women's Hospital, Boston, Massachusetts [286]

Ankoor Shah, MD
Associate Professor, Department of Medicine, Division of Rheumatology and Immunology, Duke University Medical Center, Durham, North Carolina [358]

Erica S. Shenoy, MD, PhD
Associate Professor of Medicine, Harvard Medical School; Associate Chief, Infection Control Unit, Massachusetts General Hospital, Boston, Massachusetts [144]

Kanade Shinkai, MD, PhD
Professor, Department of Dermatology, University of California, San Francisco, San Francisco, California [60]

Edwin K. Silverman, MD, PhD
Professor of Medicine, Harvard Medical School; Chief, Channing Division of Network Medicine, Department of Medicine, Brigham and Women's Hospital, Boston, Massachusetts [292]

Shakti Singh, MSc, PhD
Research Scientist, The Lundquist Institute at Harbor-UCLA Medical Center, Torrance, California [216]

Karl Skorecki, MD, FCRPC, FASN
Dean, Azrieli Faculty of Medicine, Bar-Ilan University, Safed, Israel [311, 468]

Wade S. Smith, MD, PhD
Professor of Neurology, Department of Neurology, University of California, San Francisco, San Francisco, California [307, 426–429]

Jeremy Sobel, MD, MPH
Associate Director for Epidemiologic Science, Division of Foodborne, Waterborne, and Environmental Diseases, National Center for Emerging and Zoonotic Infectious Diseases, Centers for Disease Control and Prevention, Atlanta, Georgia [153]

Kelly A. Soderberg, PhD
Chief of Staff, Duke Human Vaccine Institute, Department of Medicine, Duke University School of Medicine; Duke University Medical Center, Durham, North Carolina [349, 350]

Scott D. Solomon, MD
The Edward D. Frohlich Distinguished Chair; Professor of Medicine, Harvard Medical School; Senior Physician, Brigham and Women's Hospital, Boston, Massachusetts [241, A9]

Julian Solway, MD
Walter L. Palmer Distinguished Service Professor of Medicine and Pediatrics; Dean for Translational Medicine, Biological Sciences Division; Vice Chair for Research, Department of Medicine; Chair, Committee on Molecular Medicine, University of Chicago, Chicago, Illinois [285, 296]

Eric J. Sorscher, MD
Hertz Endowed Professorship, Emory University School of Medicine, Children's Healthcare of Atlanta, Atlanta, Georgia [291]

Brad Spellberg, MD
Professor of Clinical Medicine, Division of Infectious Diseases, Keck School of Medicine at the University of Southern California; Chief Medical Officer, Los Angeles County + University of Southern California (LAC + USC) Medical Center, Los Angeles, California [218]

Jerry L. Spivak, MD
Professor of Medicine and Oncology, Hematology Division, Johns Hopkins University School of Medicine, Baltimore, Maryland [103]

David Spriggs, MD, FACP, FASCO
Faculty Member, Harvard Medical School; Program Director of Gynecologic Oncology, Massachusetts General Hospital Cancer Center, Boston, Massachusetts [89]

E. William St. Clair, MD
W. Lester Brooks, Jr. Professor of Medicine; Professor of Immunology, Department of Medicine, Duke University Medical Center, Durham, North Carolina [358]

John M. Stafford, MD, PhD
Associate Professor of Medicine, Diabetes and Endocrinology, Vanderbilt University School of Medicine; Tennessee Valley Health System, Veterans Affairs, Nashville, Tennessee [405]

Matthew W. State, MD, PhD
Oberndorf Family Distinguished Professor; Chair, Department of Psychiatry and Behavioral Sciences; President, Langley Porter Psychiatric Hospital and Clinics, Weill Institute for Neurosciences, University of California, San Francisco, San Francisco, California [451]

Allen C. Steere, MD
Professor of Medicine, Harvard Medical School and Massachusetts General Hospital, Boston, Massachusetts [186]

Martin H. Steinberg, MD
Professor of Medicine, Pediatrics, Pathology and Laboratory Medicine, Boston University School of Medicine, Boston, Massachusetts [98]

Dennis L. Stevens, MD, PhD
Professor of Medicine, University of Washington School of Medicine, Seattle, Washington; Director, Center of Biomedical Research Excellence in Emerging/Reemerging Infectious Diseases, Boise Veterans Affairs Medical Center, Boise, Idaho [129, 154]

Lynne Warner Stevenson, MD
Professor of Medicine; Program Director, Advanced Heart Failure Fellowship Program, Vanderbilt University Medical Center, Nashville, Tennessee [259]

Benjamin K. Stoff, MD, MAB
Associate Professor of Dermatology, Emory University School of Medicine; Senior Faculty Fellow, Emory Center for Ethics, Atlanta, Georgia [A5]

John H. Stone, MD, MPH
Professor of Medicine, Harvard Medical School; The Edward Fox Chair in Medicine, Massachusetts General Hospital, Boston, Massachusetts [368]

Shyam Sundar, MD
Distinguished Professor, Department of Medicine, Institute of Medical Sciences, Banaras Hindu University, Varanasi, India [226]

Neeraj K. Surana, MD, PhD
Assistant Professor of Pediatrics, Molecular Genetics and Microbiology, and Immunology, Duke University, Durham, North Carolina [18, 119, 177, 471]

Paolo M. Suter, MD, MS
Department of Endocrinology, Diabetology, and Clinical Nutrition, University Hospital, Zurich, Switzerland [333]

Robert A. Swerlick, MD
Department of Dermatology, Emory University School of Medicine, Atlanta, Georgia [57]

Geoffrey Tabin, MD
Director, Department of Ophthalmology, Stanford University, Stanford, California [462]

Maria Carmela Tartaglia, MD
Associate Professor, Tanz Centre for Research in Neurodegenerative Diseases, University of Toronto, Toronto, Ontario, Canada [V2]

Joel D. Taurog, MD
Professor of Internal Medicine (Retired), Rheumatic Diseases Division, University of Texas Southwestern Medical Center, Dallas, Texas [362]

Usha B. Tedrow, MD, MSc
Associate Professor of Medicine, Harvard Medical School; Director, Clinical Cardiac Electrophysiology Fellowship; Clinical Director, Ventricular Arrhythmia Program, Brigham and Women's Hospital, Boston, Massachusetts [252–256]

Ayalew Tefferi, MD
Barbara Woodward Lips Professor of Medicine and Hematology, Mayo Clinic, Rochester, Minnesota [110]

Stephen C. Textor, MD
Professor of Medicine, Division of Nephrology and Hypertension, Mayo Clinic School of Medicine, Rochester, Minnesota [278]

R. V. Thakker, MD, ScD, FRCP, FRCPath, FRS, FMedSci
May Professor of Medicine, Academic Endocrine Unit, University of Oxford; O.C.D.E.M., Churchill Hospital, Headington, Oxford, United Kingdom [388]

Holger Thiele, MD
Full Professor of Internal Medicine/Cardiology; Director, Heart Center, Department of Internal Medicine/Cardiology, University of Leipzig, Leipzig, Germany [305]

C. Louise Thwaites, MBBS, BSc, MD
Clinical Research Fellow, Oxford University Clinical Research Unit, Ho Chi Minh City, Vietnam; Clinical Lecturer, Centre for Tropical Medicine and Global Health, University of Oxford, Oxford, United Kingdom [152]

Pierre Tiberghien, MD, PhD
Professor of Medicine, Bourgogne Franche-Comté University, Besançon; Senior Advisor, Etablissement Français du Sang, Paris, France [113]

Zelig A. Tochner, MD
Professor Emeritus of Radiation Oncology, University of Pennsylvania School of Medicine, Philadelphia, Pennsylvania [S5]

Karina A. Top, MD, MSc
Associate Professor of Pediatrics and Community Health & Epidemiology, Dalhousie University, Halifax, Nova Scotia, Canada [160]

Mark Topazian, MD
Professor of Medicine, Mayo Clinic, Rochester, Minnesota [322, V5]

Camilo Toro, MD
Director, Adult NIH Undiagnosed Diseases Program, National Institutes of Health, Bethesda, Maryland [492]

Barbara W. Trautner, MD, PhD
Professor, Section of Infectious Diseases, Department of Medicine, Baylor College of Medicine; Investigator, Houston VA Center for Innovations in Quality, Effectiveness and Safety (IQuESt), Houston, Texas [135]

Katherine L. Tuttle, MD
Assistant Professor, Department of Pediatrics, Pediatric Allergy/ Immunology; Assistant Professor, Department of Medicine, Allergy/ Immunology and Rheumatology (SMD), University of Rochester Medical Center, Rochester, New York [352]

Kenneth L. Tyler, MD
Louise Baum Endowed Chair and Chairman of Neurology; Professor of Medicine and Immunology-Microbiology, University of Colorado School of Medicine, Aurora, Colorado; Neurologist, Rocky Mountain VA Medical Center, Aurora, Colorado [137, 138, 140]

Elizabeth R. Unger, PhD, MD
Division of High-Consequence Pathogens and Pathology, National Center for Zoonotic and Emerging Infectious Diseases, Centers for Disease Control and Prevention, Atlanta, Georgia [450]

Prashant Vaishnava, MD
Assistant Professor of Medicine; Director of Quality Assurance and Inpatient Services, Mount Sinai Heart, Mount Sinai Hospital, Icahn School of Medicine at Mount Sinai, New York, New York [480]

Anne Marie Valente, MD
Associate Professor of Medicine and Pediatrics, Harvard Medical School; Director, Boston Adult Congenital Heart Disease and Pulmonary Hypertension Program, Boston Children's Hospital, Brigham and Women's Hospital, Boston, Massachusetts [269]

Wim H. van Brakel, MD, MSc, PhD
Medical Director, NLR, Amsterdam, The Netherlands [179]

Jos W. M. van der Meer, MD, PhD
Emeritus Professor of Medicine, Department of Internal Medicine, Radboud University Medical Center, Nijmegen, The Netherlands [20]

Mathew G. Vander Heiden, MD, PhD
Professor and Director, Koch Institute for Integrative Cancer Research, Massachusetts Institute of Technology, Cambridge, Massachusetts [489]

Edouard Vannier, PharmD, PhD
Assistant Professor of Medicine, Division of Geographic Medicine and Infectious Diseases, Department of Medicine, Tufts Medical Center and Tufts University School of Medicine, Boston, Massachusetts [225]

Gauri R. Varadhachary, MD
Professor, GI Medical Oncology, The University of Texas MD Anderson Cancer Center, Houston, Texas [92]

John Varga, MD
Frederick Huetwell Professor; Chief, Division of Rheumatology, University of Michigan, Ann Arbor, Michigan [360]

David J. Vaughn, MD
Genitourinary Medical Oncology Professor, Perelman School of Medicine at the University of Pennsylvania, Perelman Center for Advanced Medicine, Philadelphia, Pennsylvania [88]

Birgitte Jyding Vennervald, MD, MSA
Professor, Section for Parasitology and Aquatic Pathobiology, Faculty of Health and Medical Sciences, University of Copenhagen, Frederiksberg, Denmark [234]

John T. Vetto, MD, FACS
Professor of Surgery, Division of Surgical Oncology; Director, Cutaneous Oncology Program, Department of Surgery, Oregon Health & Science University; Program Leader, Melanoma Disease Site Team, OHSU Knight Cancer Institute, Portland, Oregon [76]

Luciano Villarinho, MD
Neuroradiologist, South County Hospital, Wakefield, Rhode Island [A16]

Bert Vogelstein, MD
Professor, Ludwig Center for Cancer Genetics and Therapeutics, Johns Hopkins University School of Medicine; Investigator, Howard Hughes Medical Institute, Baltimore, Maryland [71]

Everett E. Vokes, MD
John E. Ultmann Professor; Chairman, Department of Medicine; Physician-in-Chief, University of Chicago Medicine and Biological Sciences, Chicago, Illinois [77]

Tamara J. Vokes, MD
Professor, Department of Medicine, Section of Endocrinology, University of Chicago, Chicago, Illinois [412]

Nora D. Volkow, MD
Director, National Institute on Drug Abuse (NIDA), National Institutes of Health, Rockville, Maryland [455]

Kevin G. Volpp, MD, PhD
Director, Penn Center for Health Incentives and Behavioral Economics; Founders Presidential Distinguished Professor, Perelman School of Medicine and the Wharton School, University of Pennsylvania, Philadelphia, Pennsylvania [481]

Daniel D. Von Hoff, MD, FACP, FASCO, FAACR
Distinguished Professor, Translational Genomics Research Institute (TGEN), Phoenix, Arizona; Virginia G. Piper Distinguished Chair for Innovative Cancer Research and Chief Scientific Officer, Honor Health Research Institute; Senior Consultant-Clinical Investigations, City of Hope; Professor of Medicine, Mayo Clinic, Scottsdale, Arizona [83]

Martin H. Voss, MD
Clinical Director, Genitourinary Oncology Service, Memorial Sloan Kettering Cancer Center, New York, New York [85]

Jiři F. P. Wagenaar, MD, PhD
Internist and Infectious Disease Specialist, Northwest Clinics, Alkmaar, The Netherlands [184]

Jesse Waggoner, MD
Assistant Professor, Department of Medicine, Division of Infectious Diseases, Emory University, Atlanta, Georgia [124]

Sushrut S. Waikar, MD, MPH
Chief, Section of Nephrology; Norman G. Lewinsky Professor of Medicine, Boston University School of Medicine, Boston, Massachusetts [310]

Matthew K. Waldor, MD, PhD
Edward H. Kass Professor of Medicine, Harvard Medical School, Division of Infectious Diseases, Brigham and Women's Hospital, Boston, Massachusetts [168]

David H. Walker, MD
The Carmage and Martha Walls Distinguished University Chair in Tropical Diseases; Professor, Department of Pathology; Executive Director, Center for Biodefense and Emerging Infectious Diseases, University of Texas Medical Branch, Galveston, Texas [187]

Mark F. Walker, MD
Associate Professor, Neurology, Case Western Reserve University; Director, Daroff-Dell'Osso Ocular Motility Laboratory, VA Northeast Ohio Healthcare System, Cleveland, Ohio [22]

George R. Washko, MD, MMSc
Associate Professor of Medicine, Harvard Medical School; Associate Physician, Division of Pulmonary and Critical Care Medicine, Department of Medicine, Brigham and Women's Hospital, Boston, Massachusetts [286, A12]

Michael E. Wechsler, MD, MMSc
Professor of Medicine; Director, Asthma Program, Department of Medicine, National Jewish Health, Denver, Colorado [288]

Anthony P. Weetman, MD, DSc
University of Sheffield, School of Medicine, Sheffield, United Kingdom [382–385]

Robert A. Weinstein, MD
The C. Anderson Hedberg MD Professor of Internal Medicine, Rush University Medical Center; Chairman of Medicine, Emeritus, Cook County Health, Chicago, Illinois [142]

Jeffrey I. Weitz, MD, FRCP(C), FRSC, FACP
Professor of Medicine and Biochemistry and Biomedical Sciences, McMaster University; Executive Director, Thrombosis and Atherosclerosis Research Institute, Hamilton, Ontario, Canada [118]

Peter F. Weller, MD
William Bosworth Castle Professor of Medicine, Harvard Medical School; Professor of Immunology and Infectious Diseases, Harvard T.H. Chan School of Public Health; Chief Emeritus, Infectious Diseases Division and Vice Chair of Research, Department of Medicine, Beth Israel Deaconess Medical Center, Boston, Massachusetts [229–233, 235]

Andrew Wellman, MD, PhD
Associate Professor of Medicine, Harvard Medical School; Director, Sleep Disordered Breathing Lab, Brigham and Women's Hospital, Boston, Massachusetts [297]

Patrick Y. Wen, MD
Professor of Neurology, Harvard Medical School; Director, Center for Neuro-Oncology, Dana-Farber Cancer Institute; Director, Division of Neuro-Oncology, Department of Neurology, Brigham and Women's Hospital, Boston, Massachusetts [90]

Michael R. Wessels, MD
John F. Enders Professor of Pediatrics and Professor of Medicine, Harvard Medical School; Senior Physician, Division of Infectious Diseases, Boston Children's Hospital, Boston, Massachusetts [148]

L. Joseph Wheat, MD
Medical Director, MiraVista Diagnostics, Indianapolis, Indiana [212]

A. Clinton White, Jr., MD, FACP, FIDSA, FASTMH
Professor, Infectious Disease Division, Department of Internal Medicine, University of Texas Medical Branch, Galveston, Texas [235]

Nicholas J. White, DSc, MD, FRCP, F Med Sci, FRS
Professor of Tropical Medicine, Mahidol and Oxford Universities, Bangkok, Thailand [224, A2]

Richard J. Whitley, MD
Loeb Eminent Scholar in Pediatrics; Professor of Pediatrics, Microbiology and Neurosurgery, The University of Alabama at Birmingham, Birmingham, Alabama [193]

Eleanor Wilson, MD, MHS
Associate Professor of Medicine, Associate Director of Clinical Research, Division of Clinical Care and Research, Institute of Human Virology, University of Maryland School of Medicine, Baltimore, Maryland [191]

Michael R. Wilson, MD, MAS
Rachleff Family Distinguished Associate Professor in Neurology, University of California San Francisco Weill Institute for Neurosciences; Staff Physician, University of California San Francisco Medical Center and Zuckerberg San Francisco General Hospital, San Francisco, California [137, 139, S2]

Bruce U. Wintroub, MD
Professor and Chair, Department of Dermatology, University of California, San Francisco, San Francisco, California [60]

Allan W. Wolkoff, MD
The Herman Lopata Chair in Liver Disease Research; Professor of Medicine and Anatomy and Structural Biology; Associate Chair of Medicine for Research; Chief, Division of Hepatology; Director, Marion Bessin Liver Research Center, Albert Einstein College of Medicine and Montefiore Medical Center, Bronx, New York [338]

Louis Michel Wong Kee Song, MD
Professor of Medicine, Division of Gastroenterology and Hepatology, Mayo Clinic College of Medicine, Rochester, Minnesota [322, V5]

John B. Wong, MD
Professor of Medicine, Tufts University School of Medicine; Interim Chief Scientific Officer, Tufts Medical Center, Boston, Massachusetts [4]

Thomas E. Wood, PhD
Research Fellow, Department of Medicine, Division of Infectious Diseases, Massachusetts General Hospital; Department of Microbiology, Harvard Medical School, Boston, Massachusetts [120]

Jennifer A. Woyach, MD
Professor of Medicine, Division of Hematology, The Ohio State University, Columbus, Ohio [107]

Peter F. Wright, MD
Professor of Pediatrics, Geisel School of Medicine, Dartmouth College, Hanover, New Hampshire [200]

Henry M. Wu, MD, DTM&H, FIDSA
Associate Professor of Medicine, Division of Infectious Diseases, Emory University; Director, Emory TravelWell Center, Atlanta, Georgia [124]

Kim B. Yancey, MD
Professor and Chair, Department of Dermatology, University of Texas Southwestern Medical Center in Dallas, Dallas, Texas [56, 59]

Lonny Yarmus, DO, MBA
Professor of Medicine, Division of Pulmonary and Critical Care Medicine, Johns Hopkins University School of Medicine, Baltimore, Maryland [299]

Yusuf Yazici, MD
Clinical Associate Professor of Medicine, New York University Grossman School of Medicine, New York, New York [364]

Baligh R. Yehia, MD, MPP, MSc
Ascension Health, St. Louis, Missouri [400]

Janet A. Yellowitz, DMD, MPH
Associate Professor; Director, Special Care and Geriatric Dentistry, University of Maryland School of Dentistry, Baltimore, Maryland [A3]

Lam Minh Yen, MD
Senior Clinical Researcher, Oxford University Clinical Research Unit, Ho Chi Minh City, Vietnam [152]

Neal S. Young, MD
Chief, Hematology Branch, National Heart, Lung, and Blood Institute, National Institutes of Health, Bethesda, Maryland [102, 469]

Paul C. Zei, MD, PhD
Associate Professor of Medicine, Harvard Medical School; Director, Clinical Atrial Fibrillation Program, Brigham and Women's Hospital, Boston, Massachusetts [243, 246–251]

Jing Zhou, MD, PhD, FASN
Professor of Medicine, Harvard Medical School; Director, Laboratory of Molecular Genetics and Developmental Biology of Disease, Renal Division; Director, Center for Polycystic Kidney Disease Research, Brigham and Women's Hospital; Boston, Massachusetts [315]

Werner Zimmerli, MD
Professor of Medicine, Basel University, Interdisciplinary Unit of Orthopaedic Infections, Kantonsspital Baselland, Liestal, Switzerland [131]

Laura A. Zimmerman, MPH
Epidemiologist, Centers for Disease Control and Prevention, Atlanta, Georgia [206]

The Editors are pleased to present the 21st edition of *Harrison's Principles of Internal Medicine*. This 21st edition is a true landmark in medicine, spanning 71 years and multiple generations of trainees and practicing clinicians. While medicine and medical education have evolved, readers will appreciate how this classic textbook has retained enduring features that have distinguished it among medical texts—a sharp focus on the clinical presentation of disease, expert in-depth summaries of pathophysiology and treatment, and highlights of emerging frontiers of science and medicine. Indeed, *Harrison's* retains its conviction that, in the profession of medicine, we are all perpetual students with lifelong learning as our common goal.

Harrison's is intended for learners throughout their careers. For *students*, Part 1, Chapter 1 begins with an overview of "The Practice of Medicine." In this introductory chapter, the editors continue the tradition of orienting clinicians to the *science* and the *art* of medicine, emphasizing the values of our profession while incorporating new advances in technology, science, and clinical care. Part 2, "Cardinal Manifestations and Presentation of Diseases," is a signature feature of *Harrison's*. These chapters eloquently describe how patients present with common clinical conditions, such as headache, fever, cough, palpitations, or anemia, and provide an overview of typical symptoms, physical findings, and differential diagnosis. Mastery of these topics prepares students for subsequent chapters on specific diseases they will encounter in courses on pathophysiology and in clinical clerkships. For *residents* and *fellows* caring for patients and preparing for board examinations, *Harrison's* remains a definitive source of trusted content written by internationally renowned experts. Trainees will be reassured by the depth of content, comprehensive tables, and illuminating figures and clinical algorithms. Many examination questions are based on key testing points derived from *Harrison's* chapters. A useful companion book, *Harrison's Self-Assessment and Board Review*, includes over 1000 questions, offers comprehensive explanations of the correct answer, and provides links to the relevant chapters in the textbook. *Practicing clinicians* must keep up with an ever-changing knowledge base and clinical guidelines as part of lifelong learning. Clinicians can trust that chapters are updated extensively with each edition of *Harrison's*. The text is an excellent point-of-care reference for clinical questions, differential diagnosis, and patient management. In addition to the expanded and detailed Treatment sections, *Harrison's* continues its tradition of including "Approach to the Patient" sections, which provide an expert's overview of the practical management of common but often complex clinical conditions.

This edition has been modified extensively in its structure as well as its content and offers a more consistently standardized format for each disease chapter. The authors and editors have curated rigorously and synthesized the vast amount of information that comprises general internal medicine—and each of the major specialties—into a highly readable and informative two-volume book. Readers will appreciate the concise writing style and substantive quality that have always characterized *Harrison's*. This book has a sharp focus on essential information with a goal of providing clear and definitive answers to clinical questions.

In the 21st edition, examples of new chapters include "Precision Medicine and Clinical Care," focusing on the ever-growing pool of "big data" used to provide individualized genotype-phenotype correlations; "Mechanisms of Regulation and Dysregulation of the Immune System," focusing on the extraordinary advances made over the past 5 years in understanding the complex and subtle mechanisms whereby the immune system is regulated and how perturbations in this regulation lead to disease states as well as targets for therapeutic intervention; new chapters on Alzheimer's disease and related conditions, with a special focus on vascular dementia, a common and treatable cause of cognitive loss; and a new chapter on marijuana and marijuana use disorders, as well as updated management guidelines for multiple sclerosis and the expanding array of other autoimmune nervous system diseases that can now be identified and treated.

Other new chapters include "Vaccine Opposition and Hesitancy," "Precision Medicine and Clinical Care," "Diagnosis: Reducing Errors and Improving Quality," "Approach to the Patient with Renal or Urinary Tract Disease," "Interventional Nephrology," "Health Effects of Climate Change," and "Circulating Nucleic Acids as Liquid Biopsies and Noninvasive Disease Biomarkers." In addition, many chapters have new authors.

The chapter, "Vaccine Opposition and Hesitancy," provides an overview of the current antivaccination crisis, the issues involved, and specific strategies to utilize within the clinical setting to address the lack of confidence that many patients feel toward the health care system. The chapter, "Metabolomics," outlines an emerging and important new and sensitive approach to measuring perturbations within a system or patient that will likely become a routine part of the clinical armamentarium for diagnosing, monitoring, and treating disease.

In addition to these and other new topics, the 21st edition presents important updates in the established chapters, such as the microbiology and clinical management of SARS-CoV-2 infection, the use of gene editing for sickle cell anemia and thalassemia, gene therapy for hemophilia, new immunotherapies for autoimmune diseases and cancers, and novel approaches to vaccine development, among many others. Our focus on forwarding-looking issues of emerging clinical importance continues with the series of chapters entitled "Frontiers," which foreshadows cutting-edge science that will change medical practice in the near term. Examples of new Frontier chapters include "Machine Learning and Augmented Intelligence," "Metabolomics," "Protein Folding Disorders," and "Novel Approaches to Disease of Unknown Etiology."

Harrison's content is available in a variety of print and digital formats, including eBooks, apps, and a popular, widely used online platform available at *www.accessmedicine.com*.

We have many people to thank for their efforts in producing this book. First, the authors have done a superb job of producing authoritative chapters that synthesize vast amounts of scientific and clinical data to create informative and practical approaches to managing patients. In today's information-rich, rapidly evolving environment, they have ensured that this information is current. We are most grateful to our colleagues who work closely with each editor to facilitate communication with the authors and help us keep *Harrison's* content current. In particular, we wish to acknowledge the expert support of Lauren Bauer, Patricia Conrad, Patricia L. Duffey, Gregory K. Folkers, Julie B. McCoy, Elizabeth Robbins, Marie Scurti, and Stephanie C. Tribuna. Scott Grillo and James Shanahan, our long-standing partners at McGraw Hill's Professional Publishing group, have inspired the creative and dynamic evolution of *Harrison's*, guiding the development of the book and its related products in new formats. Kim Davis, as Managing Editor, has adeptly ensured that the complex production of this multi-authored textbook proceeded smoothly and efficiently. Priscilla Beer oversaw the production of our videos and animations; Jeffrey Herzich, Elleanore Waka, and Rachel Norton, along with other members of the McGraw Hill staff; and Revathi Viswanathan of KnowledgeWorks Global Ltd., shepherded the production of this new edition.

We are privileged to have compiled this 21st edition and are enthusiastic about all that it offers our readers. We learned much in the process of editing *Harrison's* and hope that you will find this edition uniquely valuable as a clinical and educational resource.

The Editors

A complete collection to meet your educational, clinical, and board prep needs.

Harrison's Online

The online edition of *Harrison's* is available at *www.accessmedicine.com.* It requires an institutional or individual subscription separate from the purchase of the print book. The online edition of *Harrison's* features all the chapters from the print edition, plus more than two dozen supplementary chapters in print, atlas, and video formats. *Harrison's Online* includes numerous monthly updates, from the editors of *Harrison's*, on important new developments in medical research and practice. Easily search across the entire *Harrison's* content set, download images and tables for presentations and lectures, view step-by-step videos on common clinical procedures, access the text of the *Harrison's Manual of Medicine*, set up a personalized test exam for board prep, get access to chapters from new editions of *Harrison's* months before book publication, and more.

The Harrison's Manual of Medicine

The *Harrison's Manual of Medicine* provides high-yield, rapid-access clinical summaries of *Harrison's* content, suitable for use at the bedside. Chapters in the *Manual* reflect those likely to be encountered in both the inpatient and outpatient setting. The format is built for ease of use. The *Manual* is available in print, eBook, and app. In addition, the full text of the *Manual* is available to subscribers at *accessmedicine.com*. This format provides flexibility of format to customers, who can move back and forth between the full scope of *Harrison's Principles of Internal Medicine* and the high-yield clinical essentials of the *Manual.*

The *Manual* includes more than 200 chapters in 17 sections and covers presenting signs and symptoms and major conditions seen in both inpatient and outpatient settings. The full table of contents is available at *www.accessmedicine.com.*

The Harrison's Self-Assessment and Board Review

This practical resource provides more than 1000 self-assessment questions, most in board-style clinical vignette format with multiple choice answers. The explanations for the questions are comprehensive and provide detailed guidance on correct and incorrect answers. Question-and-answer sets include references to related chapters in *Harrison's Principles of Internal Medicine* for more comprehensive understanding. Use this very handy resource for primary and recertification exam prep, for rotational shelf exams, and for general assessment of understanding of the principles of clinical medicine. This resource is available as a print book, an eBook, an app, and on *accessmedicine.com*, where users can create personalized testing experiences and receive instant scores on practice tests.

Harrison's Podclass

Our podcast presents bi-weekly episodes covering clinical vignettes across internal medicine, with two expert discussants reviewing common and challenging patient presentations and a series of self-assessment Q&A choices tied to each case. The hosts work through correct and incorrect answer choices and summarize cases with practical pearls that all students and clinicians will find helpful and interesting. *Harrison's Podclass* is available in most of the common podcast outlets and on *www.accessmedicine.com.*

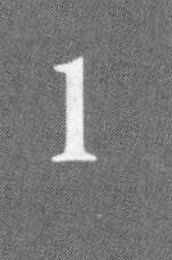

1 The Practice of Medicine

The Editors

ENDURING VALUES OF THE MEDICAL PROFESSION

No greater opportunity, responsibility, or obligation can fall to the lot of a human being than to become a physician. In the care of the suffering, [the physician] needs technical skill, scientific knowledge, and human understanding. Tact, sympathy, and understanding are expected of the physician, for the patient is no mere collection of symptoms, signs, disordered functions, damaged organs, and disturbed emotions. [The patient] is human, fearful, and hopeful, seeking relief, help, and reassurance.

—*Harrison's Principles of Internal Medicine,* 1950

The practice of medicine has changed in significant ways since the first edition of this book was published in 1950. The advent of molecular genetics, sophisticated new imaging techniques, robotics, and advances in bioinformatics and information technology have contributed to an explosion of scientific information that has changed fundamentally the way physicians define, diagnose, treat, and attempt to prevent disease. This growth of scientific knowledge continues to evolve at an accelerated pace.

The widespread use of electronic medical records and the Internet have altered the way physicians and other health care providers access and exchange information as a routine part of medical education and practice (**Fig. 1-1**). As today's physicians strive to integrate an ever-expanding body of scientific knowledge into everyday practice, it is critically important to remember two key principles: first, the ultimate goal of medicine is to prevent disease and, when it occurs, to diagnose it early and provide effective treatment; and second, despite 70 years of scientific advances since the first edition of this text, a trusting relationship between physician and patient still lies at the heart of effective patient care.

THE SCIENCE AND ART OF MEDICINE

Deductive reasoning and applied technology form the foundation for the approach and solution to many clinical problems. Extraordinary advances in biochemistry, cell biology, immunology, and genomics, coupled with newly developed imaging techniques, provide a window into the most remote recesses of the body and allow access to the innermost parts of the cell. Revelations about the nature of genes and single cells have opened a portal for formulating a new molecular basis for the physiology of systems. Researchers are deciphering the complex mechanisms by which genes are regulated, and increasingly, physicians are learning how subtle changes in many different genes, acting in an integrative contextual way, can affect the function of cells and organisms. Clinicians have developed a new appreciation of the role of stem cells in normal tissue function, in the development of cancer and other disorders, and in the treatment of certain diseases. Entirely new areas of research, including studies of the human microbiome, epigenetics, and noncoding RNAs as regulatory features of the genome, have become important for understanding both health and disease. Information technology enables the interrogation of medical records from millions of individuals, yielding new insights into the etiology, characteristics, prognosis, and stratification of many diseases. With the increasing availability of very large data sets ("big data") from omic analyses and the electronic medical record, there is now a growing need for machine learning and artificial intelligence for unbiased analyses that enhance clinical predictive accuracy. The knowledge gleaned from the ***science of medicine*** continues to enhance the understanding by physicians of complex pathologic processes and to provide new approaches to disease prevention, diagnosis, and treatment. With continued refinement of unique omic signatures coupled with nuanced clinical pathophenotypes, the profession moves ever closer to practical precision medicine. Yet, skill in the most sophisticated applications of laboratory technology and in the use of the latest therapeutic modality alone does not make a good physician. Extraordinary advances in vaccine platform technology and the use of cryo-electron microscopy for the structure-based design of vaccine immunogens have transformed the field of vaccinology, resulting in the unprecedented speed and success with which COVID-19 vaccines were developed.

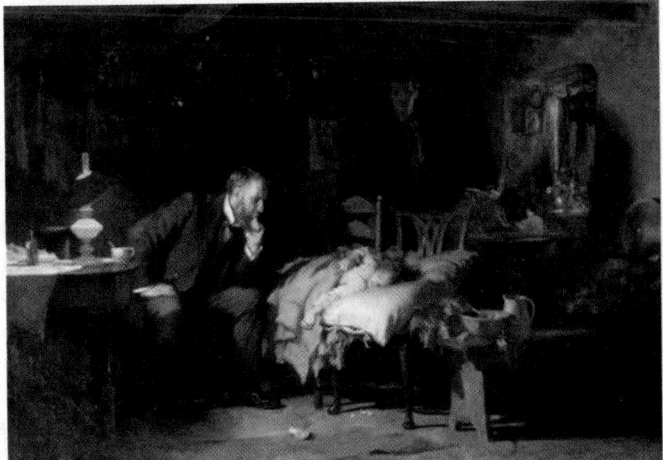

FIGURE 1-1 ***The Doctor*** **by Luke Fildes depicts the caring relationship** between this Victorian physician and a very ill child. Painted in 1891, the painting reflects the death of the painter's young son from typhoid fever and was intended to reflect the compassionate care provided by the physician even when his tools were not able to influence the course of disease. *(Source: History and Art Collection/Alamy Stock Photo.)*

When a patient poses challenging clinical problems, an effective physician must be able to identify the crucial elements in a complex history and physical examination; order the appropriate laboratory, imaging, and diagnostic tests; and extract the key results from densely populated computer screens to determine whether to treat or to "watch." As the number of tests increases, so does the likelihood that some incidental finding, completely unrelated to the clinical problem at hand, will be uncovered. Deciding whether a clinical clue is worth pursuing or should be dismissed as a "red herring" and weighing whether a proposed test, preventive measure, or treatment entails a greater risk than the disease itself are essential judgments that a skilled clinician must make many times each day. This combination of medical knowledge, intuition, experience, and judgment defines the ***art of medicine***, which is as necessary to the practice of medicine and the precision medicine of the future as is a sound scientific base, and as important for contemporary medical practice as it has been in earlier eras.

CLINICAL SKILLS

History-Taking The recorded history of an illness should include all the facts of medical significance in the life of the patient. Recent events should be given the most attention. Patients should, at some early point, have the opportunity to tell their own story of the illness without frequent interruption and, when appropriate, should receive expressions of interest, encouragement, and empathy from the physician. Any event related by a patient, however trivial or seemingly irrelevant, may provide the key to solving the medical problem. A methodical review of systems is important to elicit features of an underlying disease that might not be mentioned in the patient's narrative. In general, patients who feel comfortable with the physician will offer more complete information; thus, putting the patient at ease contributes substantially to obtaining an adequate history.

An informative history is more than eliciting an orderly listing of symptoms. By listening to patients and noting the ways in which they describe their symptoms, physicians can gain valuable insight. Inflections of voice, facial expression, gestures, and attitude (i.e., "body language") may offer important clues to patients' perception of and reaction to their symptoms. Because patients vary considerably in their medical sophistication and ability to recall facts, the reported medical history should be corroborated whenever possible. The social history also can provide important insights into the types of diseases that should be considered and can identify practical considerations for subsequent management. The family history not only identifies rare genetic disorders or common exposures, but often reveals risk factors for common disorders, such as coronary heart disease, hypertension, autoimmunity, and asthma. A thorough family history may require input from multiple relatives to ensure completeness and accuracy. An experienced clinician can usually formulate a relevant differential diagnosis from the history alone, using the physical examination and diagnostic tests to narrow the list or reveal unexpected findings that lead to more focused inquiry.

The very act of eliciting the history provides the physician with an opportunity to establish or enhance a unique bond that can form the basis for a good patient–physician relationship. This process helps the physician develop an appreciation of the patient's view of the illness, the patient's expectations of the physician and the health care system, and the financial and social implications of the illness for the patient. Although current health care settings may impose time constraints on patient visits, it is important not to rush the encounter. A hurried approach may lead patients to believe that what they are relating is not of importance to the physician, and, as a result, they may withhold relevant information. The confidentiality of the patient–physician relationship cannot be overemphasized.

Physical Examination The purpose of the physical examination is to identify physical signs of disease. The significance of these objective indications of disease is enhanced when they confirm a functional or structural change already suggested by the patient's history. At times, however, physical signs may be the only evidence of disease and may not have been suggested by the history.

The physical examination should be methodical and thorough, with consideration given to the patient's comfort and modesty. Although attention is often directed by the history to the diseased organ or part of the body, the examination of a new patient must extend from head to toe in an objective search for abnormalities. The results of the examination, like the details of the history, should be recorded at the time they are elicited—not hours later, when they are subject to the distortions of memory. Physical examination skills should be learned under direct observation of experienced clinicians. Even highly experienced clinicians can benefit from ongoing coaching and feedback. Simulation laboratories and standardized patients play an increasingly important role in the development of clinical skills. Although the skills of physical diagnosis are acquired with experience, it is not merely technique that determines success in identifying signs of disease. The detection of a few scattered petechiae, a faint diastolic murmur, or a small mass in the abdomen is not a question of keener eyes and ears or more sensitive fingers, but of a mind alert to those findings. Because physical findings can change with time, the physical examination should be repeated as frequently as the clinical situation warrants.

Given the many highly sensitive diagnostic tests now available (particularly imaging techniques), it may be tempting to place less emphasis on the physical examination. Some are critical of physical diagnosis based on perceived low levels of specificity and sensitivity. Indeed, many patients are seen by consultants only after a series of diagnostic tests have been performed and the results are known. This fact should not deter the physician from performing a thorough physical examination since important clinical findings may have escaped detection by diagnostic tests. Especially important, a thorough and thoughtful physical examination may render a laboratory finding unimportant (i.e., certain echocardiographic regurgitant lesions). The act of a hands-on examination of the patient also offers an opportunity for communication and may have reassuring effects that foster the patient–physician relationship.

Diagnostic Studies Physicians rely increasingly on a wide array of laboratory and imaging tests to make diagnoses and ultimately to solve clinical problems; however, such information does not relieve the physician from the responsibility of carefully observing and examining the patient. It is also essential to appreciate the limitations of diagnostic tests. By virtue of their apparent precision, these tests often gain an aura of certainty regardless of the fallibility of the tests themselves, the instruments used in the tests, and the individuals performing or interpreting the tests. Physicians must weigh the expense involved in laboratory procedures against the value of the information these procedures are likely to provide.

Single laboratory tests are rarely ordered. Instead, physicians generally request "batteries" of multiple tests, which often prove useful and can be performed with a single specimen at relatively low cost. For example, abnormalities of hepatic function may provide the clue to nonspecific symptoms such as generalized weakness and increased fatigability, suggesting a diagnosis of chronic liver disease. Sometimes a single abnormality, such as an elevated serum calcium level, points to a particular disease, such as hyperparathyroidism.

The thoughtful use of screening tests (e.g., measurement of low-density lipoprotein cholesterol) may allow early intervention to prevent disease (**Chap. 6**). Screening tests are most informative when they are directed toward common diseases and when their results indicate whether other potentially useful—but often costly—tests or interventions are needed. On the one hand, biochemical measurements, together with simple laboratory determinations such as routine serum chemistries, blood counts, and urinalysis, often provide a major clue to the presence of a pathologic process. On the other hand, the physician must learn to evaluate occasional screening-test abnormalities that do not necessarily connote significant disease. An in-depth workup after the report of an isolated laboratory abnormality in a person who is otherwise well is often wasteful and unproductive. Because so many tests are performed routinely for screening purposes, it is not unusual for one or two values to be slightly abnormal. Nevertheless, even if there is no reason to suspect an underlying illness, tests yielding abnormal results ordinarily are repeated to rule out laboratory error. If an abnormality is confirmed, it is important to consider its potential significance in the context of the patient's condition and other test results.

There is almost continual development of technically improved imaging studies with greater sensitivity and specificity. These tests provide remarkably detailed anatomic information that can be pivotal in informing medical decision-making. MRI, CT, ultrasonography, a variety of isotopic scans, and positron emission tomography (PET) have supplanted older, more invasive approaches and opened new diagnostic vistas. In light of their capabilities and the rapidity with which they can lead to a diagnosis, it is tempting to order a battery of imaging studies. All physicians have had experiences in which imaging studies revealed findings that led to an unexpected diagnosis. Nonetheless, patients must endure each of these tests, and the added cost of unnecessary testing is substantial. Furthermore, investigation of an unexpected abnormal finding may lead to an iatrogenic complication or to the diagnosis of an irrelevant or incidental problem. A skilled physician must learn to use these powerful diagnostic tools judiciously, always considering whether the results will alter management and benefit the patient.

MANAGEMENT OF PATIENT CARE

Team-Based Care Medical practice has long involved teams, particularly physicians working with nurses and, more recently, with physician assistants and nurse practitioners. Advances in medicine have increased our ability to manage very complex clinical situations (e.g., intensive care units [ICUs], bone marrow transplantation) and have shifted the burden of disease toward chronic illnesses. Because an individual patient may have multiple chronic diseases, he or she may be cared for by several specialists as well as a primary care physician. In the inpatient setting, care may involve multiple consultants along with the primary admitting physician. Communication through the medical record is necessary but not sufficient, particularly when patients have complex medical problems or when difficult decisions need to be made about the optimal management plan. Physicians should optimally meet face-to-face or by phone to ensure clear communication and thoughtful planning. It is important to note that patients often receive or perceive different messages from various care providers; thus, attempts should be made to provide consistency among these messages to the patient. Management plans and treatment options should be outlined succinctly and clearly for the patient.

Another dimension of team-based care involves allied health professions. It is not unusual for a hospitalized patient to encounter physical therapists, pharmacists, respiratory therapists, radiology technicians, social workers, dieticians, and transport personnel (among others) in addition to physicians and nurses. Each of these individuals contributes to clinical care as well as to the patient's experience with the health care system. In the outpatient setting, disease screening and chronic disease management are often carried out by nurses, physician assistants, or other allied health professionals.

The growth of team-based care has important implications for medical culture, student and resident training, and the organization of health care systems. Despite diversity in training, skills, and responsibilities among health care professionals, common values need to be espoused and reinforced. Many medical schools have incorporated interprofessional teamwork into their curricula. Effective communication is inevitably the most challenging aspect of implementing team-based care. While communication can be aided by electronic devices, including medical records, apps, or text messages, it is vitally important to balance efficiency with taking the necessary time to speak directly with colleagues.

The Dichotomy of Inpatient and Outpatient Internal Medicine The hospital environment has undergone sweeping changes over the past few decades. Emergency departments and critical care units have evolved to manage critically ill patients, allowing them to survive formerly fatal conditions. In parallel, there is increasing pressure to reduce the length of stay in the hospital and to manage complex disorders in the outpatient setting. This transition has been driven not only by efforts to reduce costs but also by the availability of new outpatient technologies, such as imaging and percutaneous infusion catheters for long-term antibiotics or nutrition, minimally invasive surgical procedures, and evidence that outcomes often are improved by reducing inpatient hospitalization.

In addition to traditional medical beds, hospitals now encompass multiple distinct levels of care, such as the emergency department, procedure rooms, overnight observation units, critical care units, and palliative care units. A consequence of this differentiation has been the emergence of new specialties (e.g., emergency medicine and end-of-life care) and the provision of in-hospital care by hospitalists and intensivists. Most *hospitalists* are board-certified internists who bear primary responsibility for the care of hospitalized patients and whose work is limited entirely to the hospital setting. The shortened length of hospital stay means that most patients receive only acute care while hospitalized; the increased complexities of inpatient medicine make the presence of an internist with specific training, skills, and experience in the hospital environment extremely beneficial. *Intensivists* are board-certified physicians who are further certified in critical care medicine and who direct and provide care for very ill patients in critical care units. Clearly, an important challenge in internal medicine today is to ensure the continuity of communication and information flow between a patient's primary care physician and those who are in charge of the patient's hospital care. Maintaining these channels of communication is frequently complicated by patient "handoffs"—i.e., transitions from the outpatient to the inpatient environment, from the critical care unit to a general medicine floor, from a medical to a surgical service and vice versa, from the hospital environment to the recently developed "home hospital" setting (for select patients with adequate home support), and from the hospital or home hospital to the outpatient environment.

The involvement of many care providers in conjunction with these transitions can threaten the traditional one-to-one relationship between patient and primary care physician. Of course, patients can benefit greatly from effective collaboration among a number of health care professionals; however, *it is the duty of the patient's principal or primary physician to provide cohesive guidance through an illness.* To meet this challenge, primary care physicians must be familiar with the techniques, skills, and objectives of specialist physicians and allied health professionals who care for their patients in the hospital. In addition, primary care physicians must ensure that their patients benefit from scientific advances and the expertise of specialists, both in and out of the hospital. Primary care physicians should explain the role of these specialists to reassure patients that they are in the hands of physicians best trained to manage their current illness. However, the primary care physician should assure patients and their families that decisions are being made in consultation with these specialists. The evolving concept of the "medical home" incorporates team-based primary care with subspecialty care in a cohesive environment that ensures smooth transitions of care.

Mitigating the Stress of Acute Illness Few people are prepared for a new diagnosis of cancer or anticipate the occurrence of a myocardial infarction, stroke, or major accident. The care of a frightened or distraught patient is confounded by these understandable responses to life-threatening events. The physician and other health providers can reduce the shock of life-changing events by providing information in a clear, calm, consistent, and reassuring manner. Often, information and reassurance need to be repeated. Caregivers should also recognize that, for the typical patient, hospital emergency rooms, operating rooms, ICUs, and general medical floors represent an intimidating environment. Hospitalized patients find themselves surrounded by air jets, buttons, and glaring lights; invaded by tubes and wires; and beset by the numerous members of the health care team—hospitalists, specialists, nurses, nurses' aides, physician assistants, social workers, technologists, physical therapists, medical students, house officers, attending and consulting physicians, and many others. They may be transported to special laboratories and imaging facilities replete with blinking lights, strange sounds, and unfamiliar personnel; they may be left unattended at times; and they may be obligated to share a room with other patients who have their own health problems. It is little wonder that patients may find this environment bewildering and stressful. The additive effects of an acute illness, unfamiliar environment, multiple medications, and sleep deprivation can lead to confusion or delirium, especially in older hospitalized patients. Physicians who appreciate the hospital experience from the patient's perspective and who make an effort to guide the patient through this experience may make a stressful situation more tolerable and enhance the patient's chances for an optimal recovery.

Medical Decision-Making Medical decision-making is a fundamental responsibility of the physician and occurs at each stage of the diagnostic and therapeutic process. The decision-making process involves the ordering of additional tests, requests for consultations, decisions about treatment, and predictions concerning prognosis. This process requires an in-depth understanding of the pathophysiology and natural history of disease. Formulating a differential diagnosis requires not only a broad knowledge base but also the ability to assess the relative probabilities of various diseases for a given patient. Application of the scientific method, including hypothesis formulation and data collection, is essential to the process of accepting or rejecting a particular diagnosis. Analysis of the differential diagnosis is an iterative process. As new information or test results are acquired, the group of disease processes being considered can be contracted or expanded appropriately. Whenever possible, decisions should be evidence-based, taking advantage of rigorously designed clinical trials or objective comparisons of different diagnostic tests. *Evidence-based medicine* stands in sharp contrast to anecdotal experience, which is often biased. Unless attuned to the importance of using larger, objective studies for making decisions, even the most experienced physicians can be influenced to an undue extent by recent encounters with selected patients. Evidence-based medicine has become an increasingly important part of routine medical practice and has led to the publication of many useful practice guidelines. It is important to remember, however, that only a small fraction of the many decisions made in clinical practice are based on rigorous clinical trial evidence; other guideline recommendations are, therefore, predicated on expert consensus and weaker evidentiary support.

Thus, the importance of evidence-based medicine notwithstanding, much medical decision-making still relies on good clinical judgment, an attribute that is difficult to quantify or even to assess qualitatively. Physicians must use their knowledge and experience as a basis for weighing known factors, along with the inevitable uncertainties, and then making a sound judgment; this synthesis of information is particularly important when a relevant evidence base is not available. Several quantitative tools may be invaluable in synthesizing the available information, including diagnostic tests, Bayes' theorem (the probability of an event predicated on prior knowledge of conditions possibly related to the event), and multivariate statistical models (**Chap. 4**). Diagnostic tests serve to reduce uncertainty about an individual's diagnosis or prognosis and help the physician decide how best to manage that individual's condition. The battery of diagnostic tests complements the history and physical examination. The accuracy of a particular test is ascertained by determining its sensitivity (true-positive rate) and specificity (true-negative rate), as well as the predictive value of a positive and a negative result. **See Chap. 4 for a more thorough discussion of decision-making in clinical medicine.**

Practice Guidelines Many professional organizations and government agencies have developed formal clinical-practice guidelines to aid physicians and other caregivers in making diagnostic and therapeutic decisions that are evidence-based, cost-effective, and most appropriate to a particular patient and clinical situation. As the evidence base of medicine increases, guidelines can provide a useful framework for managing patients with particular diagnoses or symptoms. Clinical guidelines can protect patients—particularly those with inadequate health care benefits—from receiving substandard care. These guidelines also can protect conscientious caregivers from inappropriate charges of malpractice and society from the excessive costs associated with the overuse of medical resources. There are, however, caveats associated with clinical-practice guidelines since they tend to oversimplify the complexities of medicine. Furthermore, groups with different perspectives may develop divergent recommendations regarding issues as basic as the need for screening of women by mammography or of men with serum prostate-specific antigen (PSA) measurements. Finally, guidelines, as the term implies, do not—and cannot be expected to—account for the uniqueness of each individual and his or her illness. The physician's challenge is to integrate into clinical practice the useful recommendations offered by experts without accepting them blindly or being inappropriately constrained by them.

Precision Medicine The concept of *precision* or *personalized medicine* reflects the growing recognition that diseases once lumped together can be further stratified on the basis of genetic, biomarker, phenotypic, and/or psychosocial characteristics that distinguish a given patient from other patients with similar clinical presentations. Inherent in this concept is the goal of targeting therapies in a more specific way to improve clinical outcomes for the individual patient and minimize unnecessary side effects for those less likely to respond to a particular treatment. In some respects, precision medicine represents the evolution of clinical practice guidelines, which are usually developed for populations of patients or a particular diagnosis (e.g., hypertension, thyroid nodule). As the pathobiology, prognosis, and treatment responses of subgroups within these diagnoses become better understood (i.e., through refined genomic analysis or enhanced deep phenotyping), the relevant clinical guidelines incorporate progressively more refined recommendations for individuals within these subgroups. The role of precision medicine is best illustrated for cancers in which genetic testing is able to predict responses (or the lack thereof) to targeted therapies (**Chap. 73**). One can anticipate similar applications of precision medicine in pharmacogenomics, immunologic disorders, and diseases in which biomarkers can predict treatment responses. **See Chap. 5 for a more thorough discussion of precision medicine.**

Evaluation of Outcomes Clinicians generally use *objective* and readily measurable parameters to judge the outcome of a therapeutic intervention. These measures may oversimplify the complexity of a clinical condition as patients often present with a major clinical problem in the context of multiple complicating background illnesses. For example, a patient may present with chest pain and cardiac ischemia, but with a background of chronic obstructive pulmonary disease and renal insufficiency. For this reason, outcome measures, such as mortality, length of hospital stay, or readmission rates, are typically risk-adjusted. An important point to remember is that patients usually seek medical attention for *subjective* reasons; they wish to obtain relief from pain, to preserve or regain function, and to enjoy life. The components of a patient's health status or quality of life can include bodily comfort, capacity for physical activity, personal and professional function, sexual function, cognitive function, and overall perception of health. Each of these important domains can be assessed through structured interviews or specially designed questionnaires. Such assessments provide useful parameters by which a physician can judge patients' subjective views of their disabilities and responses to treatment, particularly in chronic illness. The practice of medicine requires consideration and integration of both objective and subjective outcomes.

Many health systems use survey and patient feedback data to assess qualitative features such as patient satisfaction, access to care, and communication with nurses and physicians. In the United States, HCAHPS (Hospital Consumer Assessment of Healthcare Providers and Systems) surveys are used by many systems and are publicly reported. Social media is also being used to assess feedback in real time as well as to share patient experiences with health care systems, potentially enriching the information available for use in medical decisions.

Errors in the Delivery of Health Care A series of reports from the Institute of Medicine (now the National Academy of Medicine [NAM]) called for an ambitious agenda to reduce medical error rates and improve patient safety by designing and implementing fundamental changes in health care systems (**Chap. 8**). It is the responsibility of hospitals and health care organizations to develop systems to reduce risk and ensure patient safety. Medication errors can be reduced through the use of ordering systems that rely on electronic processes or, when electronic options are not available, that eliminate misreading of handwriting. Whatever the clinical situation, it is the physician's responsibility to use powerful therapeutic measures wisely, with due regard for their beneficial actions, potential dangers, and cost. Implementation of infection control systems, enforcement of hand-washing protocols, and careful oversight of antibiotic use can minimize the complications of nosocomial infections. Central-line infection rates and catheter-associated urinary tract infections have been dramatically reduced at many centers by careful adherence of trained personnel to standardized protocols for introducing and maintaining central lines and urinary catheters, respectively. Rates of surgical infection and wrong-site surgery can likewise be reduced by the use of standardized protocols and checklists. Falls by patients can be minimized by judicious use of sedatives and appropriate assistance with bed-to-chair and bed-to-bathroom transitions. Taken together, these and other measures are saving thousands of lives each year.

Electronic Medical Records Both the growing reliance on computers and the strength of information technology now play central roles in medicine, including efforts to reduce medical errors. Laboratory data are accessed almost universally through computers. Many medical centers now have electronic medical records (EMRs), computerized order entry, and bar-coded tracking of medications. Some of these systems are interactive, sending reminders or warning of potential medical errors.

EMRs offer rapid access to information that is invaluable in enhancing health care quality and patient safety, including relevant data, historical and clinical information, imaging studies, laboratory results, and medication records. These data can be used to monitor and reduce unnecessary variations in care and to provide real-time information about processes of care and clinical outcomes. Ideally, patient records are easily transferred across the health care system; however, technological limitations and concerns about privacy and cost continue to limit broad-based use of EMRs in many clinical settings.

For all of the advantages of EMRs, they can create distance between the physician and patient if care is not taken to preserve face-to-face contact. EMRs also require training and time for data entry. Many providers spend significant time entering information to generate structured data and to meet billing requirements. They may feel pressured to take short cuts, such as "cutting and pasting" parts of earlier notes into the daily record, thereby increasing the risk of errors. EMRs also structure information in a manner that disrupts the traditional narrative flow across time and among providers. These features, which may be frustrating for some providers, must be weighed against the advantages of ready access to past medical history, imaging, laboratory data, and consultant notes. Furthermore, the effort, time, and attention needed to maintain and utilize the EMR have led to a growing sense of dissatisfaction among physicians, lessening professional and personal well-being as a result. Clearly, this is an area of daily practice that requires improvement both for the delivery of safe and optimal care and physician wellness.

It is important to emphasize that information technology is merely a tool and can never replace the clinical decisions that are best made by the physician. Clinical knowledge and an understanding of a patient's needs, supplemented by quantitative tools, still represent the best approach to decision-making in the practice of medicine.

THE PATIENT–PHYSICIAN RELATIONSHIP

The significance of the intimate personal relationship between physician and patient cannot be too strongly emphasized, for in an extraordinarily large number of cases both the diagnosis and treatment are directly dependent on it. One of the essential qualities of the clinician is interest in humanity, ***for the secret of the care of the patient is in caring for the patient.***

—Francis W. Peabody, October 21, 1925, Lecture at Harvard Medical School

Physicians must never forget that patients are individuals with problems that all too often transcend their physical complaints. They are not "cases" or "admissions" or "diseases." Patients do not fail treatments; treatments fail to benefit patients. This point is particularly important in this era of high technology in clinical medicine. Most patients are anxious and fearful. Physicians should instill confidence and offer reassurance, but they must never come across as arrogant, patronizing, impatient, or hurried. A professional attitude, coupled with warmth and openness, can do much to alleviate anxiety and to encourage patients to share all aspects of their medical history. Empathy and compassion are the essential features of a caring physician. The physician needs to consider the setting in which an illness occurs—in terms not only of patients themselves but also of their familial, social, and cultural backgrounds. The ideal patient–physician relationship is based on thorough knowledge of the patient, mutual trust, and the ability to communicate.

Informed Consent The fundamental principles of medical ethics require physicians to act in the patient's best interest and to respect the patient's autonomy. Both principles are reflected in the process of informed consent. Patients are required to sign consent forms for most diagnostic or therapeutic procedures. Many patients possess limited medical knowledge and must rely on their physicians for advice. Communicating in a clear and understandable manner, physicians must fully discuss the alternatives for care and explain the risks, benefits, and likely consequences of each alternative. The physician is responsible for ensuring that the patient thoroughly understands these risks and benefits; encouraging questions is an important part of this process. It may be necessary to go over certain issues with the patient more than once. This is the very definition of *informed consent*. Complete, clear explanation and discussion of the proposed procedures and treatment can greatly mitigate the fear of the unknown that commonly accompanies hospitalization. Often the patient's understanding is enhanced by repeatedly discussing the issues in an unthreatening and supportive way, answering new questions that occur to the patient as they arise. Continuing efforts to educate the patient are essential. Patients are frequently inhibited from understanding by the fear of an uncertain future and potential impact of the illness on themselves and their families. Clear communication can also help alleviate misunderstandings in situations where complications of intervention occur. Special care should also be taken to ensure that a physician seeking a patient's informed consent has no real or apparent conflict of interest.

Approach to Grave Prognoses and Death No circumstance is more distressing than the diagnosis of an incurable disease, particularly when premature death is inevitable. What should the patient and family be told? What measures should be taken to maintain life? What can be done to optimize quality of life?

Transparency of information, delivered in an appropriate manner, is essential in the face of a terminal illness. Even patients who seem unaware of their medical circumstances, or whose family members have protected them from diagnoses or prognoses, often have keen insights into their condition. They may also have misunderstandings that can lead to additional anxiety. The patient must be given an opportunity to speak with the physician and ask questions. A wise and insightful physician uses such open communication as the basis for assessing what the patient wants to know and when he or she wants to know it. On the basis of the patient's responses, the physician can assess the most appropriate time and pace for sharing information. Ultimately, the patient must understand the expected course of the disease so that appropriate plans and preparations can be made. The patient should participate in decision-making with an understanding of the goal of treatment (palliation) and its likely effects. The patient's religious beliefs should be taken into consideration. Some patients may find it easier to share their feelings about death with their physician, nurses, or members of the clergy than with family members or friends.

The physician should provide or arrange for emotional, physical, and spiritual support, and must be compassionate, unhurried, and open. In many instances, there is much to be gained by the laying on of hands. Pain should be controlled adequately, human dignity maintained, and isolation from family and close friends avoided. These aspects of care tend to be overlooked in hospitals, where the intrusion of life-sustaining equipment can detract from attention to the individual person and encourage concentration instead on the life-threatening disease, against which the battle ultimately will be lost in any case. In the face of terminal illness, the goal of medicine must shift from *cure* to *care* in the broadest sense of the term. *Primum succurrere*, first to help, is a guiding principle. In offering care to a dying patient, a physician should be prepared to provide information to family members and deal with their grief and sometimes their feelings of guilt or even anger. It is important for the physician to assure the family that everything reasonable is being done. A substantial challenge in these discussions is that the physician often does not know exactly how to gauge the prognosis. In addition, various members of the health care team may offer different opinions. Good communication among providers is essential so that consistent information is provided to patients. This is especially important when the best path forward is uncertain. Advice from experts in palliative and terminal care should be sought whenever appropriate to ensure that clinicians are not providing patients with unrealistic expectations. **For a more complete discussion of end-of-life care, see Chap. 12.**

Maintaining Humanism and Professionalism Many trends in the delivery of health care tend to make medical care impersonal. These trends, some of which have been mentioned already, include (1) vigorous efforts to reduce the escalating costs of health care; (2) the growing number of managed-care programs, which are intended to reduce costs but where the patient may have little choice in selecting a physician; (3) increasing reliance on technological advances and computerization; and (4) the need for numerous physicians and other health professionals to be involved in the care of most patients who are seriously ill.

In light of these changes in the medical care system, it is a major challenge for physicians to maintain the *humane* aspects of medical care. The American Board of Internal Medicine, working together with the American College of Physicians–American Society of Internal Medicine and the European Federation of Internal Medicine, has published a *Charter on Medical Professionalism* that underscores three main principles in physicians' contract with society: (1) the primacy of patient welfare, (2) patient autonomy, and (3) social justice. While medical schools appropriately place substantial emphasis on professionalism, a physician's personal attributes, including integrity, respect, and compassion, also are extremely important. In the United States, the Gold Humanism Society recognizes individuals who are exemplars of humanistic patient care and serve as role models for medical education and training.

Availability to the patient, expression of sincere concern, willingness to take the time to explain all aspects of the illness, and a nonjudgmental attitude when dealing with patients whose cultures, lifestyles, attitudes, and values differ from those of the physician are just a few of the characteristics of a humane physician. Every physician will, at times, be challenged by patients who evoke strongly negative or positive emotional responses. Physicians should be alert to their own reactions to such situations and should consciously monitor and control their behavior so that the patient's best interest remains the principal motivation for their actions at all times.

Another important aspect of patient care involves an appreciation of the patient's "quality of life," a subjective assessment of what each patient values most. This assessment requires detailed, sometimes intimate knowledge of the patient, which usually can be obtained only through deliberate, unhurried, and often repeated conversations. Time pressures will always threaten these interactions, but they should not diminish the importance of understanding and seeking to fulfill the priorities of the patient.

EXPANDING FRONTIERS IN MEDICAL PRACTICE

The Era of "Omics" In the spring of 2003, announcement of the complete sequencing of the human genome officially ushered in the genomic era. However, even before that landmark accomplishment, the practice of medicine had been evolving as a result of insights into both the human genome and the genomes of a wide variety of microbes. The clinical implications of these insights are illustrated by the complete genome sequencing of H1N1 influenza virus in 2009 and even faster sequencing of COVID-19 in early 2020, leading to the swift development and dissemination of effective vaccines. Today, gene expression profiles are being used to guide therapy and inform prognosis for a number of diseases, and genotyping is providing a new means to assess the risk of certain diseases as well as variations in response to a number of drugs. Despite these advances, the use of complex genomics in the diagnosis, prevention, and treatment of disease is still in its early stages. The task of physicians is complicated by the fact that phenotypes generally are determined not by genes alone but by the complex interactions among genes and gene products, and by the interplay of genetic and environmental factors.

Rapid progress is also being made in other areas of molecular medicine. *Epigenetics* is the study of alterations in chromatin and histone proteins and methylation of DNA sequences that influence gene expression (**Chap. 483**). Every cell of the body has identical DNA sequences; the diverse phenotypes a person's cells manifest are, in part, the result of epigenetic regulation of gene expression. Epigenetic alterations are associated with a number of cancers and other diseases. *Proteomics*, the study of the entire library of proteins made in a cell or organ and the complex relationship of these proteins to disease, is enhancing the repertoire of the 23,000 genes in the human genome through alternate splicing, posttranslational processing, and posttranslational modifications that often have unique functional consequences. The presence or absence of particular proteins in the circulation or in cells is being explored for many diagnostic and disease-screening applications. *Microbiomics* is the study of the resident microbes in humans and other mammals, which together compose the microbiome. The human haploid genome has ~23,000 genes, whereas the microbes residing on and in the human body encompass more than 3–4 million genes; these resident microbes are likely to be of great significance with regard to health status. Ongoing research is demonstrating that the microbes inhabiting human mucosal and skin surfaces play a critical role in maturation of the immune system, in metabolic balance, in brain function, and in disease susceptibility. A variety of environmental factors, including the use and overuse of antibiotics, have been tied experimentally to substantial increases in disorders such as obesity, metabolic syndrome, atherosclerosis, and immune-mediated diseases in both adults and children. *Metagenomics*, of which microbiomics is a part, is the genomic study of environmental species that have the potential to influence human biology directly or indirectly. An example is the study of exposures to microorganisms in farm environments that may be responsible for the lower incidence of asthma among children raised on farms. *Metabolomics* is the study of the range of metabolites in cells or organs and the ways they are altered in disease states. The aging process itself may leave telltale metabolic footprints that allow the prediction (and possibly the prevention) of organ dysfunction and disease. It seems likely that disease-associated patterns will be found in lipids, carbohydrates, membranes, mitochondria and mitochondrial function, and other vital components of cells and tissues. *Exposomics* is the study of the exposome—i.e., the environmental exposures such as smoking, sunlight, diet, exercise, education, and violence that together have an enormous impact on health. All of this new information represents a challenge to the traditional reductionist approach to medical thinking. The variability of results in different patients, together with the large number of variables that can be assessed, creates challenges in identifying preclinical disease and defining disease states unequivocally. Accordingly, the tools of *systems biology* and *network medicine* are being applied to the enormous body of information ("big data") now obtainable for every patient and may eventually provide new approaches to classifying disease. **For a more complete discussion of a complex systems and network science approach to human disease, see Chap. 486.**

The rapidity of these advances may seem overwhelming to practicing physicians; however, physicians have an important role to play in ensuring that these powerful technologies and sources of new information are applied judiciously to patient care. Since omics are evolving so rapidly, physicians and other health care professionals must engage in continuous learning so that they can apply this new knowledge to the benefit of their patients' health and well-being. Genetic testing requires wise counsel based on an understanding of the value and limitations of the tests as well as the implications of their results for specific individuals. **For a more complete discussion of genetic testing, see Chap. 467.**

The Globalization of Medicine Physicians should be cognizant of diseases and health care services beyond local boundaries. Global travel has critical implications for disease spread, and it is not uncommon for diseases endemic to certain regions to be seen in other regions after a patient has traveled to and returned from those regions. The outbreak of Zika virus infections in the Americas is a cogent example of this phenomenon. In addition, factors such as wars, the migration of refugees, and increasing climate extremes are contributing to changing disease profiles worldwide. Patients have broader access to unique expertise or clinical trials at distant medical centers, even those in other countries, and the cost of travel may be offset by the quality of care at those distant locations. As much as any other factor influencing global aspects of medicine, the Internet has transformed the transfer of medical information throughout the world. This change has been accompanied by the transfer of technological skills through telemedicine and international consultation—for example, interpretation of radiologic images and pathologic specimens. **For a complete discussion of global issues, see Chap. 472.**

Medicine on the Internet On the whole, the Internet has had a positive effect on the practice of medicine; through personal computers, a wide range of information is available to physicians and patients almost instantaneously at any time and from anywhere in the world. This medium holds enormous potential for the delivery of current information, practice guidelines, state-of-the-art conferences, journal content, textbooks (including this text), and direct communications with other physicians and specialists, expanding the depth and breadth of information available to the physician regarding the diagnosis and care of patients. Medical journals are now accessible online, providing rapid sources of new information. By bringing them into direct and timely contact with the latest developments in medical care, this medium also serves to lessen the information gap that has hampered physicians and health care providers in remote areas.

Patients, too, are turning to the Internet in increasing numbers to acquire information about their illnesses and therapies and to join Internet-based support groups. Patients often arrive at a clinic visit with sophisticated information about their illnesses. In this regard, physicians are challenged in a positive way to keep abreast of the latest relevant information while serving as an "editor" as patients navigate this seemingly endless source of information, the accuracy and validity of which are not uniform.

A critically important caveat is that virtually anything can be published on the Internet, with easy circumvention of the peer-review process that is an essential feature of academic publications. Both physicians and patients who search the Internet for medical information must be aware of this danger. Notwithstanding this limitation, appropriate use of the Internet is revolutionizing information access for physicians and patients, and in this regard represents a remarkable resource that was not available to practitioners a generation ago.

Public Expectations and Accountability The general public's level of knowledge and sophistication regarding health issues has grown rapidly over the past few decades. As a result, expectations of the health care system in general and of physicians in particular have risen. Physicians are expected to master rapidly advancing fields (the *science* of medicine) while considering their patients' unique needs (the *art* of medicine). Thus, physicians are held accountable not only for the technical aspects of the care they provide but also for their patients' satisfaction with the delivery and costs of care.

In many parts of the world, physicians increasingly are expected to account for the way in which they practice medicine by meeting certain standards prescribed by federal and local governments. The hospitalization of patients whose health care costs are reimbursed by the government and other third parties is subjected to utilization review. Thus, a physician must defend the cause for and duration of a patient's hospitalization if it falls outside certain "average" standards. Authorization for reimbursement increasingly is based on documentation of the nature and complexity of an illness, as reflected by recorded elements of the history and physical examination. A growing "pay-for-performance" movement seeks to link reimbursement to quality of care. The goal of this movement is to improve standards of health care and contain spiraling health care costs. In many parts of the United States, managed (capitated) care contracts with insurers have replaced traditional fee-for-service care, placing the onus of managing the cost of all care directly on the providers and increasing the emphasis on preventive strategies. In addition, physicians are expected to give evidence of their current competence through mandatory continuing education, patient record audits, maintenance of certification, and relicensing.

Medical Ethics and New Technologies The rapid pace of technological advances has profound implications for medical applications that go far beyond the traditional goals of disease prevention, treatment, and cure. Cloning, genetic engineering, gene therapy, human–computer interfaces, nanotechnology, and use of targeted therapies have the potential to modify inherited predispositions to disease, select desired characteristics in embryos, augment "normal" human performance, replace failing tissues, and substantially prolong life span. Given their unique training, physicians have a responsibility to help shape the debate on the appropriate uses of and limits placed on these new technologies and to consider carefully the ethical issues associated with the implementation of such interventions. As medicine becomes more complex, shared decision-making is increasingly important, not only in areas such as genetic counseling and end-of-life care, but also in diagnostic and treatment options.

Learning Medicine More than a century has passed since the publication of the Flexner Report, a seminal study that transformed medical education and emphasized the scientific foundations of medicine as well as the acquisition of clinical skills. In an era of burgeoning information and access to medical simulation and informatics, many schools are implementing new curricula that emphasize lifelong learning and the acquisition of competencies in teamwork, communication skills, system-based practice, and professionalism. The tools of medicine also change continuously, necessitating formal training in the use of EMRs, large datasets, ultrasound, robotics, and new imaging techniques. These and other features of the medical school curriculum provide the foundation for many of the themes highlighted in this chapter and are expected to allow physicians to progress, with experience and learning over time, from competency to proficiency to mastery.

At a time when the amount of information that must be mastered to practice medicine continues to expand, increasing pressures both within and outside of medicine have led to the implementation of restrictions on the amount of time a physician-in-training can spend in the hospital and in clinics. Because the benefits associated with continuity of medical care and observation of a patient's progress over time were thought to be outstripped by the stresses imposed on trainees by long hours and by fatigue-related errors, strict limits were set on the number of patients that trainees could be responsible for at one time, the number of new patients they could evaluate in a day on call, and the number of hours they could spend in the hospital. In 1980, residents in medicine worked in the hospital more than 90 hours per week on average. In 1989, their hours were restricted to no more than 80 per week. Resident physicians' hours further decreased by ~10% between 1996 and 2008, and in 2010, the Accreditation Council for Graduate Medical Education further restricted (i.e., to 16 hours per shift) consecutive in-hospital duty hours for first-year residents. The impact of these changes is still being assessed, but the evidence that medical errors have decreased as a consequence is sparse. An unavoidable by-product of fewer hours at the bedside is an increase in the number of "handoffs" of patient responsibility from one physician to another. These transfers often involve a transition from a physician who knows the patient well, having evaluated that individual on admission, to a physician who knows the patient less well. It is imperative that these transitions of responsibility be handled with care and thoroughness, with all relevant information exchanged and acknowledged. These issues highlight the challenge our profession has in establishing a reliable measure of physician effectiveness.

The Physician as Perpetual Student From the time physicians graduate from medical school, it becomes all too apparent that this milestone is symbolic and that they must embrace the role of a "perpetual student." This realization is at the same time exhilarating and anxiety-provoking. It is exhilarating because physicians can apply constantly expanding knowledge to the treatment of their patients; it is anxiety-provoking because physicians realize that they will never know as much as they want or need to know. Ideally, physicians will translate the latter feeling into energy through which they can continue to improve and reach their potential. It is the physician's responsibility to pursue new knowledge continually by reading, attending conferences and courses, and consulting colleagues and the Internet. This is often a difficult task for a busy practitioner; however, a commitment to continued learning is an integral part of being a physician and must be given the highest priority.

The Physician as Citizen Being a physician is a privilege. The capacity to apply one's skills for the benefit of fellow human beings is a noble calling. The physician–patient relationship is inherently unbalanced in the distribution of power. In light of their influence, physicians must always be aware of the potential impact of what they do and say, and must always strive to strip away individual biases and preferences to find what is best for their patients. To the extent possible, physicians should also act within their communities to promote health and alleviate suffering. Meeting these goals begins by setting a healthy example and continues in taking action to deliver needed care even when personal financial compensation may not be available.

Research, Teaching, and the Practice of Medicine The word *doctor* is derived from the Latin *docere*, "to teach." As teachers, physicians should share information and medical knowledge with colleagues, students of medicine and related professions, and their patients. The practice of medicine is dependent on the sum total of medical knowledge, which in turn is based on an unending chain of scientific discovery, clinical observation, analysis, and interpretation. Advances in medicine depend on the acquisition of new information through research, and improved medical care requires the transmission of that information. As part of their broader societal responsibilities, physicians should encourage patients to participate in ethical and properly approved clinical investigations if these studies do not impose undue hazard, discomfort, or inconvenience. Physicians engaged in clinical research must be alert to potential conflicts of interest between their research goals and their obligations to individual patients. The best interests of the patient must always take priority.

> *To wrest from nature the secrets which have perplexed philosophers in all ages, to track to their sources the causes of disease, to correlate the vast stores of knowledge, that they may be quickly available for the prevention and cure of disease—these are our ambitions.*
>
> —William Osler, 1849–1919

FURTHER READING

Cheston CC et al: Social media use in medical education: A systematic review. Acad Med 88:893, 2013.

Cooke M et al: American medical education 100 years after the Flexner report. N Engl J Med 355:1339, 2006.

Excel JL et al: Vaccine development for emerging infectious diseases. Nat Med 27:591, 2021

Institute of Medicine: *Dying in America: Improving Quality and Honoring Individual Preferences Near the End of Life*. Washington, DC, National Academies Press, 2015.

Institute of Medicine: *Improving Diagnosis in Health Care*. Washington, DC, National Academies of Sciences, Engineering, and Medicine, 2015.

Levine DM et al: Hospital-level care at home for acutely ill adults: A qualitative evaluation of a randomized controlled trial. J Gen Intern Med 36:1965, 2021.

Stern DT, Papadakis M: The developing physician—becoming a professional. N Engl J Med 355:1794, 2006.

Vickrey BG et al: How neurologists think: A cognitive psychology perspective on missed diagnoses. Ann Neurol 67:425, 2010.

West P et al: Intervention to promote physician well-being, job satisfaction, and professionalism. A randomized clinical trial. JAMA Intern Med 174:527, 2014.

2 Promoting Good Health

Donald M. Lloyd-Jones,
Kathleen M. McKibbin

GOALS AND APPROACHES TO PREVENTION

Prevention of acute and chronic diseases before their onset has been recognized as one of the hallmarks of excellent medical practice for centuries and is now used as a metric for highly functioning health care systems. The ultimate goal of preventive strategies is to avoid premature death. However, as longevity has increased dramatically worldwide over the last century (largely as a result of public health practices), increasing emphasis is placed on prevention for the purpose of preserving quality of life and extending the health span, not just the life span. Given that all patients will eventually die, the goal of prevention ultimately becomes compression of morbidity toward the end of the life span; that is, reduction of the amount of burden and time spent with disease prior to dying. As shown in **Fig. 2-1**, normative aging tends to involve a steady decline in the stock of health, with accelerating decline over time. Successful prevention offers the opportunity both to extend life and to extend healthy life, thus "squaring the curve" of health loss during aging.

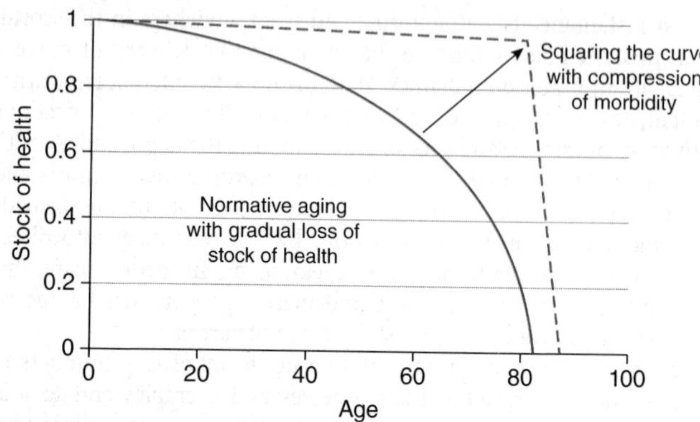

FIGURE 2-1 Loss of health with aging. Representation of normative aging with loss of the full stock of health with which individuals are born (indicating gain of morbidity), contrasted with a squared curve with greater longevity and fuller stock of health (less morbidity) until shortly before death. The "squared curve" represents the likely ideal situation for most patients.

Prevention strategies have been characterized as tertiary, secondary, primary, and primordial. *Tertiary prevention* requires rapid action to prevent imminent death in the setting of acute illness, such as through percutaneous coronary intervention in the setting of ST-segment elevation myocardial infarction. *Secondary prevention* strategies focus on avoiding the recurrence of disease and death in an individual who is already affected. For example, tamoxifen is recommended for women with surgically treated early-stage, estrogen receptor–positive breast cancer, because it reduces the risk of recurrent breast cancer (including in the contralateral breast) and death. *Primary prevention* attempts to reduce the risk of incident disease among individuals with one or more risk factors. Treatment of elevated blood pressure in individuals who have not yet experienced cardiovascular disease represents one example of primary prevention that has proven effective in reducing the incidence of stroke, heart failure, and coronary heart disease.

Primordial prevention is a more recent concept (first introduced in 1979) that focuses on prevention of the development of *risk factors* for disease, not just prevention of disease. Primordial prevention strategies emphasize upstream determinants of risk for chronic diseases, such as eating patterns, physical activity, and environmental and social determinants of health. It therefore encompasses medical treatment strategies for some individuals as well as a strong reliance on public health and social policy. It is increasingly clear that primordial prevention represents the ultimate means for reducing the burden of chronic diseases of aging. Once risk factors develop, it is difficult to restore risk to the low level of someone who never developed the risk factor. The time spent with adverse levels of the risk factor often causes irreversible damage that precludes complete restoration of low risk. For example, individuals with hypertension who are treated back to optimal levels (<120/<80 mmHg) do have a lower risk compared with untreated patients with hypertension, but they still have twice the risk of cardiovascular events as those who maintained optimal blood pressure without medications. Patients with elevated blood pressure that is subsequently treated have greater left ventricular mass index, worse renal function, and more evidence of atherosclerosis and other target organ damage as a result of the time spent with elevated blood pressure; such damage cannot be fully reversed despite efficacious therapy with antihypertensive medications. Conversely, as described below in greater detail, individuals who maintain optimal levels of all major cardiovascular risk factors into middle age through primordial prevention essentially abolish their lifetime risk of developing cardiovascular disease while also living substantially longer and having a lower burden and later onset of other comorbid illnesses (compression of morbidity).

Prevention strategies should be distinguished from disease screening strategies. Screening attempts to detect evidence of disease at its earliest stages, when treatment is likely to be more efficacious than for advanced disease (**Chap. 6**). Screening can be performed in service of prevention, especially if it aids in identifying preclinical markers, such as dyslipidemia or hyperglycemia, associated with elevated disease risk.

■ HEALTH PROMOTION

In recent decades, medical practice has increasingly focused on clinical and public health approaches to promote health, and not just prevent disease. Prevention of disease is a worthy individual and societal goal in and of itself, but it does not necessarily guarantee health. Health is a broader construct encompassing more than just absence of disease. It includes biologic, physiologic, and psychological domains (among others) in a continuum, rather than occurring as a dichotomous trait. Health is therefore somewhat subjective, but attempts have been made to use more objective criteria to define health in order to raise awareness, prevent disease, and promote healthy longevity.

For example, in 2010, the American Heart Association (AHA) defined a new construct of "cardiovascular health" based on evidence of associations with longevity, disease avoidance, healthy longevity, and quality of life. The definition of cardiovascular health is based on seven health behaviors and health factors (eating pattern, physical activity, smoking status, body mass index [BMI], and levels of blood pressure, blood cholesterol, and blood glucose) and includes a spectrum from poor to ideal. Individuals with optimal levels of all seven metrics simultaneously are considered to have ideal cardiovascular health. The state of cardiovascular health for an individual or a population can be assessed with simple scoring by counting the number of ideal metrics (out of seven) or applying 0 points for each poor metric, 1 point for each intermediate metric, and 2 points for each ideal metric, thus creating a composite cardiovascular health score ranging from 0 to 14 points. Higher cardiovascular health scores in younger and middle ages have been associated with greater longevity, lower incidence of cardiovascular disease, lower incidence of other chronic diseases of aging (including dementia, cancer, and more), compression of morbidity, greater quality of life, and lower health care costs, achieving both individual and societal goals for healthy aging and further establishing the critical importance of primordial prevention and cardiovascular health promotion.

Focusing on health promotion, rather than just disease prevention, may also provide greater motivation for patients to pursue lifestyle changes or adhere to clinician recommendations. Extensive literature suggests that providing patients solely with information regarding disease risk, or risk reduction with treatment, is unlikely to motivate desired behavior change. Empowering patients with strategies to achieve positive health goals after discussing risks can provide more effective adherence and better long-term outcomes. In the case of smoking cessation, enumerating only the risks of smoking can lead to patient inertia and therapeutic nihilism and has proven to be an ineffective approach, whereas strategies that incorporate positive health messaging, support, and feedback, with appropriate use of evidence-based therapies, have proven far more effective.

■ PRIORITIZING PREVENTION STRATEGIES

In secondary prevention, the patient already has manifest clinical disease and is therefore at high risk for progression. The approach should be to work with the patient to implement all evidence-based strategies that will help to prevent recurrence or progression. This will typically include drug therapy as well as therapeutic lifestyle changes to control ongoing risk factors that may have caused disease in the first place. Juggling priorities can be difficult, and barriers to implementation are many, including costs, time, patient health literacy, and patient and caregiver capacity to organize the regimen. Addressing these potential barriers with the patient can help to forge a therapeutic bond and may improve adherence; ignoring them will likely lead to therapeutic failure. Numerous studies demonstrate that, even in high-functioning health systems, only ~50% of patients are taking recommended, evidence-based secondary prevention medications, such as statins, by 1 year after a myocardial infarction.

In patients who are eligible for primary prevention strategies, it is important to frame the discussion around the overall evidence base as well as an individual patient's likelihood of benefit from a given preventive intervention. A first step is to understand the patient's estimated absolute risk for disease in the foreseeable future or during their remaining life span. However, absolute risk estimation and presentation of those risks are generally insufficient to motivate behavior change. It is critical to assess the patient's understanding and tolerance of the risk, their readiness to implement lifestyle changes or adhere to drug therapy, and their overall preferences regarding use of drug therapy to prevent an event (e.g., cancer, myocardial infarction, stroke). The clinician can help the patient by informing them of the risks for disease and potential for absolute benefits (and harms) from the available evidence-based choices. This may take more than one conversation, but given that diseases, such as cancer and cardiovascular disease, are the leading causes of premature death and disability, the time is well spent.

Partnering with the patient through motivational interviewing may assist in the process of selecting initial approaches to prevention. Selecting an area that the patient feels they are ready to change can lead to better adherence and greater achievement of success in the short and longer term. If the patient is uncertain what course to choose, prudence would dictate focusing on control of risk factors that may lead to the most rapid reduction in risk for acute events. For example, blood pressure is both a chronic risk factor and an acute trigger for cardiovascular events. Thus, if a patient has both significant elevations in blood pressure and dyslipidemia, it would be appropriate to focus initial efforts on blood pressure control. Likewise, a focus on smoking cessation can lead to more rapid reductions in risk for acute events than some other lifestyle interventions.

■ PREVENTION AND HEALTH PROMOTION ACROSS THE LIFE COURSE

Periodic Health Evaluations The "routine annual physical" has in many ways become an expected part of the patient-physician relationship in primary care practice. However, evidence for the efficacy of the periodic health evaluation in asymptomatic adults unselected for risk factors or disease is mixed and depends on the outcome. Systematic reviews and meta-analyses of published trials have consistently observed lack of benefit (and also lack of harm) in terms of total mortality in association with periodic health evaluations. Data are more heterogeneous but overall suggest no benefit for cancer- or cardiovascular-specific mortality, with the potential for either benefit or harm depending on number of evaluations and patient-level factors. Well-designed studies on nonfatal clinical events and morbidity have been sparsely reported, but there appear to be no large effects.

Periodic health evaluations do appear to lead to greater diagnosis of certain conditions such as hypertension and dyslipidemia, as expected. Likewise, periodic health examinations also improve the delivery of recommended preventive services, such as gynecologic examinations and Papanicolaou smears, fecal occult blood testing, and cholesterol screening. The benefits and risks associated with screening tests are discussed in detail in **Chap. 6**. Risks of routine evaluations include inappropriate testing or overtesting or false-positive findings that require follow-up and induce patients to worry. Periodic health examinations appear to be associated with less patient worry. On balance, given the lack of convincing evidence of harm and the potential for better delivery of appropriate screening, counseling, and preventive services, periodic health evaluations appear reasonable for general populations at average risk for chronic conditions.

It is important to note that routine annual comprehensive physical examinations of asymptomatic adult patients have very low yield and may take an inordinate amount of time in a wellness visit. Such time

TABLE 2-1 Guidelines and Key Recommendations from the *Dietary Guidelines for Americans, 2020–2025*

GUIDELINES	KEY RECOMMENDATIONS
1. **Follow a healthy dietary pattern at every life stage.** For the first 6 months of life, infants should exclusively be fed human milk, or iron-fortified formula if human milk is unavailable. From 6 to 12 months, infants should be introduced to a variety of complementary nutrient-dense foods. From 12 months to older adulthood, the dietary pattern should meet nutrient needs, help achieve a healthy body weight, and reduce the risk of chronic disease.	**The Dietary Guidelines' Key Recommendations for healthy eating patterns should be applied in their entirety, given the interconnected relationship that each dietary component can have with others. They are also intended as a framework to accommodate personal preferences, cultural traditions, and budgetary considerations.** **Focus on meeting food group needs with nutrient-dense foods and beverages, and stay within calorie limits to achieve a healthy weight and reduce the risk of chronic disease.** **The core elements that make up a healthy dietary pattern include:** • Vegetables of all types—dark green; red and orange; beans, peas, and lentils; starchy; and other vegetables • Fruits, especially whole fruit
2. **Customize and enjoy nutrient-dense food and beverage choices to reflect personal preferences, cultural traditions, and budgetary considerations.** The Dietary Guidelines provide a framework of several dietary patterns intended to be customized to individual needs and preferences, as well as the foodways of the diverse cultures in the United States.	• Grains, at least half of which are whole grain • Dairy, including fat-free or low-fat milk, yogurt, and cheese, and/or lactose-free versions and fortified soy beverages and yogurt as alternatives • Protein foods, including lean meats, poultry, and eggs; seafood; beans, peas, and lentils; and nuts, seeds, and soy products • Oils, including vegetable oils and oils in food, such as seafood and nuts
3. **Focus on meeting food group needs with nutrient-dense foods and beverages, and stay within calorie limits.** Nutrient-dense foods provide vitamins, minerals, and other health-promoting components and have no or little added sugars, saturated fat, and sodium. A healthy dietary pattern consists of nutrient-dense forms of foods and beverages across all food groups, in recommended amounts, and within calorie limits.	**A healthy eating pattern limits:** • Added sugars—Less than 10% of calories per day starting at age 2. Avoid foods and beverages with added sugars for those younger than age 2. • Saturated fat—Less than 10% of calories per day starting at age 2. • Sodium—Less than 2300 mg per day—and even less for children younger than age 14. • Alcoholic beverages—Adults of legal drinking age can choose not to drink or to drink in moderation by limiting intake to 2 drinks or less in a day for men and 1 drink or less in a day for women, when alcohol is consumed. Drinking less is better for health than drinking more. There are some adults who should not drink alcohol, such as women who are pregnant.
4. **Limit foods and beverages higher in added sugars, saturated fat, and sodium, and limit alcoholic beverages.** At every life stage, meeting food group recommendations, even with nutrient-dense choices, fulfills most of a person's daily calorie needs and sodium limits, with little room for extra added sugars, saturated fat, or sodium, or for alcoholic beverages.	**Meet the U.S. Department of Health and Human Services' *Physical Activity Guidelines for Americans*** In tandem with the recommendations above, Americans of all ages—children, adolescents, adults, and older adults—should meet the *Physical Activity Guidelines for Americans* to help promote health and reduce the risk of chronic disease. Americans should aim to achieve and maintain a healthy body weight. The relationship between diet and physical activity contributes to calorie balance and managing body weight.

Source: Adapted from the *Dietary Guidelines for Americans, 2020-2025.* Washington, DC: U.S. Department of Agriculture and U.S. Department of Health and Human Services; 2020. Available at *https://www.dietaryguidelines.gov/sites/default/files/2020-12/Dietary_Guidelines_for_Americans_2020-2025.pdf.*

may be better spent on assessing and counseling the patient on other aspects of their health, as discussed below. Evidence-based components that should be included in periodic evaluations focused on health and prevention include a number of age-appropriate screening tests for chronic disease and risk factors, preventive interventions including immunizations and chemoprevention for at-risk individuals, and preventive counseling. The U.S. Preventive Services Task Force publishes its *Guide to Clinical Preventive Services,* which contains evidence-based recommendations from the Task Force on preventive services for which there is a high degree of certainty that the service provides at least moderate net clinical benefit (i.e., benefits outweigh harms significantly and to a reasonable magnitude).

Healthy Behaviors and Lifestyles Owing to the paucity of evidence, the heterogeneity of study designs, and the diverse nature of interventions studied, many clinicians are uncertain as to how to deliver advice regarding healthy behaviors and lifestyles. Nevertheless, adverse behaviors and lifestyles contribute to >75% of premature, preventable deaths and disability. Estimates from the U.S. National Health and Nutrition Examination Survey indicate that fewer than 1% of Americans achieve an optimal heart-healthy eating pattern. Thus, whereas there are many demands on time during a typical patient-clinician encounter, few things may have more impact on longevity, health, and quality of life for asymptomatic patients than an efficient approach to assessing, documenting, and improving patients' health behaviors. Indeed, the mere act of assessing health behaviors has been shown to affect patients' health behaviors. Facility with tools for assessment of lifestyle and with strategies for counseling are therefore of paramount importance.

Healthy Eating Patterns (see Chap. 332) Despite the existence of numerous "fad" diets and seemingly inconsistent recommendations on dietary composition, there is remarkable agreement about what should constitute a healthy eating pattern for the broad population to avoid nutritional deficits (i.e., vitamin deficiency) and excesses (i.e., excessive caloric intake) and to maximize potential health (**Table 2-1**). Optimal eating patterns consist of whole fruits and vegetables, whole grains, lean proteins, and healthy oils, and allow for nonfat or low-fat dairy intake. They tend to exclude frequent ingestion of foods high in refined sugars and starches, saturated fat, and sodium. Since sodium and refined sugars and starches are the hallmark of much of the processed/packaged food supply, a simple rule of thumb is to provide or cook the majority of one's own meals starting from whole foods and emphasizing fruits and vegetables. Likewise, foods prepared outside of the home tend to have higher fat and sodium content, so special attention to menu choices focused on fruits, vegetables, lean proteins, and whole grains, while minimizing sauces and dressings, can help most individuals follow healthier eating patterns when eating food prepared outside the home. In all cases, sugar-sweetened beverages and nonnutritious snack foods should be minimized. If snacks are included, small amounts of healthy nuts and seeds or more fruits and vegetables should be encouraged.

Specific conditions and diseases, such as diabetes, other metabolic disorders, allergies, and gastrointestinal disorders, may require tailored approaches to diet. In counseling most patients, the general approach should focus on whole foods, eating patterns, and appropriate calorie balance, rather than on specific micronutrients such as electrolytes or selected vitamins. It should be remembered that most patients have difficulty understanding nutritional labels on packaged foods, with the attendant demands on numeracy and health literacy.

Dietary guidelines are published by the U.S. Department of Agriculture (USDA) and U.S. Department of Health and Human Services every 5 years, and these guidelines have undergone substantial evolution over time. The current U.S. Dietary Guidelines and Key Recommendations for 2020–2025 are summarized in Table 2-1 and emphasize the importance of healthy eating patterns for every stage of life, to avoid chronic diseases including obesity, diabetes, cancer, and cardiovascular disease. The core elements include eating patterns with nutrient-dense (rather than calorie-dense) whole foods and appropriate caloric intake to achieve and maintain healthy weight. The USDA guidelines focus on the concept of a healthy plate (rather than the prior food pyramid) for ease of counseling and adoption. Fifty percent of the plate should consist of vegetables and whole fruits, with remaining portions for whole grains and lean protein foods. When using fat for cooking, it should be done by sauteing in healthier oils (e.g., canola oil), and addition of judicious amounts of healthy raw oils (e.g., olive oil, nuts) to dishes is appropriate. Recommendations also focus on limitation of foods and beverages higher in added sugars, saturated fat, and sodium, and moderation or avoidance of alcohol intake.

The USDA guidelines focus on specific healthy eating patterns that adhere to these broad recommendations and are appropriate for ~97% of the general population. They identify a "Healthy U.S.-Style Dietary Pattern" that adheres closely to the evidence-based Dietary Approaches to Stop Hypertension (DASH) eating pattern but is customizable for different cultural or personal preferences. Alternative patterns, which vary more in emphasis than in content, include a "Healthy Mediterranean-Style Dietary Pattern" and a "Healthy Vegetarian Dietary Pattern."

AGE- AND SEX-SPECIFIC RECOMMENDATIONS Current dietary framework recommendations are generally similar for all life stages from ages ≥12 months, but recommended levels of caloric intake (and hence amounts of foods) differ by age, sex, and physical activity level. For example, recommended caloric intake ranges from 1000 calories/d for sedentary 2-year-old children to as high as 3200 calories/d for active 16- to 18-year-old young men. Recommended caloric intakes peak in late adolescence or early adulthood for men and women and gradually decrease over ensuing decades.

As with all lifestyle counseling aimed at behavior change, dietary approaches that partner with the patient and utilize motivational interviewing strategies and shared goals and commitments tend to work best, as described below (see "Approach to the Patient").

Physical Activity Similar to the approach to counseling regarding healthy eating patterns, recommendations on participation in physical activity emphasize the point that any physical activity is better than none. A simple rule of thumb for patients is: "If you are doing nothing, do something; and if you are doing something, do more, every day." The evidence base for physical activity indicates that the marginal benefits from physical activity are greatest in advancing from no activity to low levels of moderate activity. With increasing duration and intensity of activity, there is a continued curvilinear increase in health benefits, but the marginal gains for each additional minute of moderate-to-vigorous activity slowly diminish. Thus, for adults, the recommended amount of physical activity is 150 min of moderate-intensity or 75 min of vigorous-intensity aerobic activity per week, performed in episodes of at least 5 min, and preferably spread throughout the week, plus participation in muscle-strengthening activity at least 2 days per week. Additional health benefits can be realized by engaging in physical activity beyond this amount.

In counseling patients regarding physical activity, it is important to note that sedentary time (e.g., seated at work or at home in front of electronic screens) has adverse health consequences independent of the lack of physical activity during these episodes. Therefore, even modest efforts like standing at the desk and doing gentle stretching for periods during the day may be beneficial. It is also important to emphasize that participating in a variety of aerobic activities (biking, swimming, walking, jogging, rowing, elliptical training, stair-climbing, etc.) can be beneficial and may help to avoid overuse injuries and boredom with the exercise regimen. If patients choose to participate in muscle-strengthening activities for health improvement, emphasis should be placed on weights that allow more repetitions (e.g., 3 sets of 15–20 repetitions that can be performed comfortably, with a rest period in between) and on avoiding breath-holding and straining against a closed glottis.

SUDDEN CARDIAC DEATH RISK Patients may express concerns regarding the risk of sudden cardiac death during exercise. Whereas the risk of sudden death during exercise does increase directly with the amount of time spent exercising, this association is substantially mitigated by training effects. Thus, patients embarking on an exercise program should be encouraged to increase the duration of aerobic exercise gradually as tolerated, aiming for episodes of at least 30 min 5 times a week as an ideal. Once a comfortable duration is reached, incorporating interval training periods of more intensive activity interspersed during the exercise can provide greater fitness gains.

EXTREME ENDURANCE ACTIVITIES As with other forms of exercise, extreme endurance activities such as triathlons and marathons should be undertaken only with appropriate and graded training. Such activities tend to take a greater toll on the musculoskeletal system over time than less extreme activities, and they are also associated with measurable damage to the myocardium and greater risks for other organ damage. Athletes participating in endurance activities routinely have elevations in cardiac troponin (a specific circulating marker of myocardial cell damage and death) at the end of the race, although elevations are lower in those who are well trained. Patients and clinicians should consider the patient's overall health, specific limitations, potential for injury, and ability to train in decision-making regarding participation in endurance events.

AGE-SPECIFIC RECOMMENDATIONS The U.S. Department of Health and Human Services' *Physical Activity Guidelines for Americans*, second edition (2018) (**Table 2-2**), recommend that preschool-aged children (aged 3–5 years) should be physically active throughout the day in a variety of activity types to enhance growth and development. Children and adolescents aged 6–17 years should participate in ≥60 min of physical activity daily, most of which should be moderate- or vigorous-intensity aerobic activity, including vigorous, muscle-strengthening, and bone-strengthening activities at least 3 days a week each. As noted above, adults aged 18–64 years are recommended to pursue at least 150 min of moderate-intensity or 75 min of vigorous-intensity aerobic activity per week (or equivalent combinations), with at least 2 days of muscle-strengthening activities. Adults aged ≥65 years should follow the adult guidelines or be as active as possible as abilities and conditions allow. For older adults, special emphasis is also placed on multicomponent physical activity that includes balance training as well as aerobic and muscle-strengthening activities.

Sleep Hygiene Sleeping between 7 and 9 h per night appears to be optimal for health in adults aged ≥18 years. Sleeping <7 h is associated with adverse outcomes, including obesity, diabetes, elevated blood pressure, cardiovascular disease, depression, and all-cause mortality, as well as physiologic disturbances such as impaired immune function, increased pain sensitivity, and impaired cognitive performance. Conversely, achieving appropriate levels of sleep is associated with more success in weight loss, better blood pressure control among patients with hypertension, and improved mental health and performance. Regular sleep more than 9 h per night is appropriate for children and adolescents or individuals recovering from sleep deprivation or illness, but for most individuals, the effects on health are uncertain.

Patients often express concerns about the quantity and quality of their sleep. With aging, both aspects of sleep tend to decline, even without overt sleep disorders. Documentation of sleep using a sleep log may assist in understanding different types of insomnia and sleep disorders. Encouraging daily activity to promote fatigue, avoidance of eating and drinking alcohol too close to bedtime, and regular daily sleep habits may help patients achieve better sleep. Regular use of sedative medications should generally be discouraged given the high potential for dependence, addiction, and altered sleep quality.

DISORDERS OF SLEEP The prevalence of sleep-related breathing disorders, including obstructive sleep apnea (OSA), is poorly documented. A recent systematic review suggested that that the prevalence of clinically important OSA in the general adult population may be between 9% and 38%, with higher rates in men versus women, older versus younger adults, and those with higher versus lower BMI.

TABLE 2-2 Recommendations from *Physical Activity Guidelines for Americans*

AGE	RECOMMENDATIONS
3–5 years	• Preschool-aged children (ages 3 through 5 years) should be physically active throughout the day to enhance growth and development. • Adult caregivers of preschool-aged children should encourage active play that includes a variety of activity types.

6–17 years	• It is important to provide young people opportunities and encouragement to participate in physical activities that are appropriate for their age, that are enjoyable, and that offer variety.
	• Children and adolescents ages 6 through 17 years should do 60 min (1 h) or more of moderate-to-vigorous physical activity daily:
	  • Aerobic: Most of the 60 min or more per day should be either moderate- or vigorous-intensity aerobic physical activity and should include vigorous-intensity physical activity on at least 3 days a week.
	  • Muscle-strengthening: As part of their 60 min or more of daily physical activity, children and adolescents should include muscle-strengthening physical activity on at least 3 days a week.
	  • Bone-strengthening: As part of their 60 min or more of daily physical activity, children and adolescents should include bone-strengthening physical activity on at least 3 days a week.

18–64 years	• Adults should move more and sit less throughout the day. Some physical activity is better than none. Adults who sit less and do any amount of moderate-to-vigorous physical activity gain some health benefits. • For substantial health benefits, adults should do at least 150 min (2 h and 30 min) to 300 min (5 hours) a week of moderate-intensity or 75 min (1 h and 15 min) to 150 min (2 h and 30 min) a week of vigorous-intensity aerobic physical activity, or an equivalent combination of moderate- and vigorous-intensity aerobic activity. Preferably, aerobic activity should be spread throughout the week. • Additional health benefits are gained by engaging in physical activity beyond the equivalent of 300 min (5 h) of moderate-intensity physical activity a week. • Adults should also do muscle-strengthening activities of moderate or greater intensity and that involve all major muscle groups on 2 or more days a week, as these activities provide additional health benefits.

≥65 years	• The key guidelines for adults also apply to older adults. In addition, the following key guidelines are just for older adults:
	  • As part of their weekly physical activity, older adults should do multicomponent physical activity that includes balance training as well as aerobic and muscle-strengthening activities.
	  • Older adults should determine their level of effort for physical activity relative to their level of fitness.
	  • Older adults with chronic conditions should understand whether and how their conditions affect their ability to do regular physical activity safely.
	  • When older adults cannot do 150 min of moderate-intensity aerobic activity a week because of chronic conditions, they should be as physically active as their abilities and conditions allow.

Moderate-intensity physical activity: Aerobic activity that increases a person's heart rate and breathing to some extent. On a scale relative to a person's capacity, moderate-intensity activity is usually a 5 or 6 on a 0 to 10 scale. Brisk walking, dancing, swimming, or bicycling on a level terrain are examples. Vigorous-intensity physical activity: Aerobic activity that greatly increases a person's heart rate and breathing. On a scale relative to a person's capacity, vigorous-intensity activity is usually a 7 or 8 on a 0 to 10 scale. Jogging, singles tennis, swimming continuous laps, or bicycling uphill are examples. Muscle-strengthening activity: Physical activity, including exercise that increases skeletal muscle strength, power, endurance, and mass. It includes strength training, resistance training, and muscular strength and endurance exercises. Bone-strengthening activity: Physical activity that produces an impact or tension force on bones, which promotes bone growth and strength. Running, jumping rope, and lifting weights are examples.

Source: Adapted from U.S. Department of Health and Human Services. *Physical Activity Guidelines for Americans, 2nd edition.* Washington, DC: U.S. Department of Health and Human Services; 2018. Available at *https://health.gov/sites/default/files/2019-09/Physical_Activity_Guidelines_2nd_edition.pdf.*

Patients with persistent complaints of poor sleep quality or excessive daytime somnolence or with witnessed apneic spells may benefit from screening for sleep disorders, prior to consideration of a formal sleep study. A number of clinical tools have been developed to screen for sleep apnea, including the Epworth Sleepiness Scale, the STOP (*s*noring, *t*iredness, *o*bserved apnea, high blood *p*ressure) Questionnaire, and the STOP-Bang Questionnaire (STOP plus assessment of BMI, age, neck circumference, and gender), among others. The U.S. Preventive Services Task Force found that current evidence is insufficient to assess the balance of benefits and harms of screening for OSA in asymptomatic adults owing to a lack of validation data in primary care settings. Nonetheless, the high prevalence and significant health consequences of sleep apnea suggest that clinicians should be alert for its potential presence, particularly in patients who are obese with symptoms of excessive daytime somnolence or witnessed apnea episodes. Other sleep disorders, such as restless leg syndrome, may be identified with simple history.

Weight Management Overweight and obesity are prevalent in epidemic proportions in the United States and other industrialized nations (**Chaps. 401 and 402**). Since 1985, the prevalence of obesity in the United States has increased from ~10 to ~35%, and the prevalence of overweight is now ~40%. Overweight and obesity disproportionately affect individuals in lower socioeconomic strata and in many underserved minority populations, including black Americans, Latino Americans, and American Indians. In all race/ethnic groups, both overweight and obesity are associated with adverse health consequences, including diabetes, certain cancers, cardiovascular diseases, and degenerative joint disease. Eating disorders such as anorexia and bulimia are much less common but pose major health consequences for affected patients and should be suspected particularly in younger women with history of rapid weight shifts or underweight status.

Weight loss is one of the most difficult preventive interventions to achieve and sustain over time. However, several key factors can assist the patient and clinician, and early referral to a dietician can be very helpful. The first therapeutic goal is to aim for weight stabilization. Many of the risks of overweight and obesity are driven more strongly by continued weight gain, rather than overweight/obese status per se. Working with the patient to find initial strategies for weight maintenance can be a successful initial step with success for many patients. For those who can progress to considering weight loss, it is critical to help the patient understand that there is no standard solution. Experimentation and documentation are key. Tools to assist patients can include food and weight logs, activity logs, and smart phone apps. Some patients respond best to structured approaches such as intermittent fasting regimens or commercial dietary programs where meals are provided. Any of these approaches can be tried with or without social group supports.

The key construct for weight loss is, of course, negative calorie balance. This is achieved through a combination of reduced caloric intake and increased physical activity. Patients may already understand, from prior weight loss attempts, what combination works best for them to achieve this. Some patients find that they cannot lose weight without increasing their exercise. For many, reduction of caloric intake is most efficient. Encouraging the patient to find what works for them is most important. The same principle holds for dietary content. Well-done feeding studies indicate that weight loss is dependent far more on the reduction of caloric intake than on the relative composition of fat, protein, and carbohydrate in the diet. There may be other medical reasons to choose one approach over another, but if not, encouraging the patient to pick one approach and document the results is an important start. Once weight loss is achieved, increase in activity is often required for its successful maintenance.

Tobacco Cessation (see Chap. 454) Escaping nicotine dependence is another major, but critical, challenge to prevention and wellness efforts. The addictive effects of nicotine have been well documented, with effects that can last for years after successful cessation. Assessing a patient's past history of cessation attempts and current readiness for change are key first steps in forging a successful approach. Frequent follow-up and reinforcement, as well as use of nicotine replacement therapy and other cessation-promoting medications, are additional critical elements. Recidivism is the rule, and patients should expect to resume smoking and attempt again as they journey to tobacco cessation. Electronic cigarettes have some evidence for benefit in adult smoking cessation, but their potential for use by adolescents and young adults who are not smokers represents a major public health threat for a new generation of nicotine addiction, with unknown health consequences as a result of the high doses of nicotine delivered to developing organs, including the brain. Vaping of other substances, often in association with flavoring compounds, has also been associated with pulmonary and cardiovascular damage and should be actively discouraged.

VACCINATION (CHAP. 123)

One of the major advances in public health that has contributed to increases in health and longevity worldwide is the development of safe and effective vaccinations against endemic and epidemic infectious diseases. Patients should be counseled regarding age-appropriate vaccinations for their children and for themselves. Some individuals may be reluctant to receive a vaccination; in these cases, listening to the patient's concerns is important, followed by explanation of the benefits to the individual, their family, and their community and review of the low risk for potential harms. It is true to say that no current vaccines are ever worse than the disease they prevent, although side effects may occur rarely. Thorough knowledge of the data on side effect rates and of efficacy will aid the clinician in helping the patient make a fully informed decision.

MENTAL HEALTH AND ADDICTION

Assessment for depression and cognitive impairment is important to address when patients exhibit symptoms or they or their family members express concerns. Both of these common conditions play a major role in reducing quality of life and are high on patients' lists of concerns, even if not clearly expressed. Screening tools for depression are reviewed in **Chap. 452**. Cognitive function decline with aging or comorbid illness, including depression, should be anticipated. Assessment tools such as the General Practitioner Assessment of Cognition or the Mini-Cog™ test are widely available and effective rapid assessment tools.

Alcohol and Opioids (see Chaps. 453 and 456) Alcohol dependence and abuse are common and underdiagnosed. Rapid screening tools have proven efficacy for identifying patients with alcohol problems. In a systematic review, the CAGE (*c*ut down, *a*nnoyed, *g*uilty, *e*ye opener) questionnaire was most effective at identifying alcohol abuse and dependence, with reasonable sensitivity and high specificity. The present opioid epidemic in the United States presents a new and substantial public health challenge given the high potential for dependency and abuse of these drugs. Rapid screening tools are available to assist clinicians in screening for opioid dependence.

ACCIDENTS AND SUICIDE

Regular assessment of patient safety through simple questions about seat belt use, domestic violence, and gun safety in the home continues to be an important part of health promotion and wellness. Longstanding recommendations for assessment of suicidal ideation among patients with depression or a history of suicide attempts also continue to be relevant.

APPROACH TO THE PATIENT

In the context of a clinical visit focused on health assessment, health promotion, and prevention, the basic skills of history-taking are of paramount importance. Much of the evaluation, counseling, and management that focus on health promotion and prevention also require engagement and buy-in from the patient in order to assist with recognition of contributing behaviors and to promote adherence to therapeutic plans. Therefore, in addition to standard history-taking, additional skills such as motivational interviewing and eliciting patient commitments and contracting may prove of significant value. The availability of additional tools to assist with screening, monitoring, and chronic management, both online and through wearable devices and mobile health technologies, is rapidly expanding, with uncertain implications for the future. Major research gaps exist in our understanding of how best to employ these newer technologies to improve health outcomes. Concepts of behavioral economics are being explored to better understand the psychology of decision-making and incentives as a means to improve lifestyle choices and adherence to treatment plans (**Chap. 481**).

The limited time available to clinicians and patients during a wellness visit or periodic health examination (not driven by specific patient issues) makes it important to prioritize assessment and counseling for factors that affect longevity, health span, and quality of life over approaches that may have low yield, such as the annual comprehensive physical examination in an asymptomatic patient. Setting clear expectations for the content of a wellness visit may be a first step, and scheduling follow-up visits for findings or to continue indicated counseling are important steps to achieving better health outcomes.

FURTHER READING

Boulware LE et al: Systematic review: The value of the periodic health evaluation. Ann Intern Med 146:289, 2007.

Dietary Guidelines for Americans, 2020–2025. Washington, DC: U.S. Department of Agriculture and U.S. Department of Health and Human Services; 2020. Available at *https://www.dietaryguidelines.gov/sites/default/files/2020-12/Dietary_Guidelines_for_Americans_2020-2025.pdf.*

Irish LA et al: The role of sleep hygiene in promoting public health: A review of empirical evidence. Sleep Med Rev 22:23, 2015.

Krogsboll LT et al: General health checks in adults for reducing morbidity and mortality from disease: Cochrane systematic review and meta-analysis. BMJ 345:e7191, 2012.

U.S. Department of Health and Human Services: *Physical Activity Guidelines for Americans,* 2nd ed. Washington, DC: U.S. Department of Health and Human Services; 2018. Available at *https://health.gov/sites/default/files/2019-09/Physical_Activity_Guidelines_2nd_edition.pdf.*

U.S. Preventive Services Task Force webpage. Available at *https://www.uspreventiveservicestaskforce.org/uspstf/.*

3 Vaccine Opposition and Hesitancy

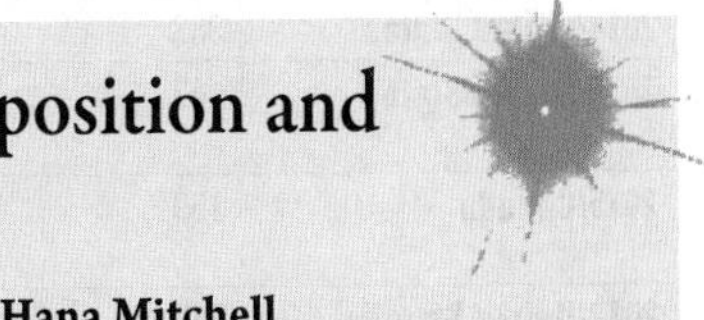

Julie A. Bettinger, Hana Mitchell

Vaccines have been recognized as one of the top public health achievements of the twentieth century. Dramatic declines in the morbidity and mortality of vaccine-preventable diseases have been observed, and the contribution of vaccines to the elimination, control, and prevention of infectious disease cannot be overstated. However, opposition and hesitancy to vaccines exist and are not new. Vaccine hesitancy has existed since Edward Jenner introduced the first vaccine against smallpox in the eighteenth century. So why did the World Health Organization rank these attitudes as one of the ten greatest threats to public health in 2019? Are current opposition and hesitancy any different from what has been seen before? Many sociologists, public health experts, and health care providers (HCPs) argue yes. Recent social and cultural trends, combined with new communication formats, have converged to create a particularly potent form of hesitancy and what some have labeled a crisis of confidence. This crisis manifests as a lack of trust in specific vaccines, vaccine programs, researchers, HCPs, the health care system, pharmaceutical companies, academics, policymakers, governments, and authority in general. (**See "Focus: COVID-19 Vaccine Hesitancy," below.**)

The roots of modern vaccine hesitancy and opposition—defined as delay or rejection of vaccines in spite of availability—vary depending on the place and the population. For some individuals and communities, pseudoscience and false claims about the safety of existing vaccines (e.g., an unsupported link between measles vaccine and autism) have driven fears, increased hesitancy, and decreased acceptance. For others, real safety events, such as the association of narcolepsy with a specific pandemic influenza vaccine (Pandemrix), have justified concerns. In a few locations (e.g., Ukraine, Pakistan), vaccine hesitancy is the result of failed health systems or even state failures. Finally, for some groups, including some fundamentalist religious groups and alternative-culture communities, vaccine hesitancy and opposition reflect exclusion from and rejection of mainstream society and allopathic health care and manifest as a deep distrust of these institutions and their HCPs. Although the genesis of modern vaccine hesitancy is multifactorial, its outcomes are uniform: a decrease in vaccine demand and uptake, a decrease in coverage by childhood and adult vaccines, and an increase in vaccine-preventable diseases, outbreaks, and epidemics of disease. Addressing this crisis and moving people from vaccine hesitancy and refusal to acceptance and active demand require intervention at multiple levels: the individual, the health system (including public health), and the state.

This chapter will define vaccine hesitancy and briefly describe its determinants and effects in North America (the United States and Canada). Physicians and other HCPs are well positioned to address the crisis of confidence many patients feel toward HCPs and the health care system. Studies demonstrate that an unambiguous, strong recommendation by trusted HCPs is most often the reason that patients, including those who are vaccine hesitant, choose to vaccinate. Strategies for counseling vaccine-hesitant and vaccine-resistant patients will be presented and examples of strong vaccine recommendations provided. Presenting strategies to increase vaccine demand at a system and policy level is beyond the scope of this chapter. While some physicians may have roles that allow them to act at this level, all physicians can act and influence their individual patients. Strategies to create active vaccine demand at the individual level alone will not solve vaccine hesitancy, but vaccine hesitancy cannot be addressed without these efforts. **For further discussion of immunization principles and vaccine use, see Chap. 123.**

■ VACCINE COVERAGE AND OUTBREAKS

The epidemiologic data from measles outbreaks over the past 10 years provide an interesting illustration of the effects of vaccine opposition and hesitancy. **For further discussion of measles, see Chap. 205.**

North America *Herd immunity* occurs when enough individuals in a population become immune to an infectious disease, usually through vaccination, that transmission of the infection stops. The level of immunity (or level of vaccine coverage) required to confer herd immunity varies with the specific infectious disease. Because measles is a highly contagious virus, a coverage rate of 93–95% must be achieved for vaccination to confer herd immunity and interrupt measles transmission. National coverage estimates place one-dose measles vaccine coverage rates in 2-year-old children at 92% in the United States and 88% in Canada. In spite of these relatively high levels of coverage in young children, numerous measles outbreaks have occurred in both countries since 2010 (**Table 3-1**).

The vast majority (>80%) of measles cases described in Table 3-1 occurred in under- or completely unvaccinated individuals. Of note, many of these outbreaks highlight pockets of significantly under- or unvaccinated individuals that are not apparent in national vaccine coverage statistics. Moreover, many of the outbreaks listed in Table 3-1 were ignited by unvaccinated returned travelers from areas with existing

TABLE 3-1 Measles Outbreaks in North America

YEAR/PLACE	NO. OF CASES	REASON
2010/Canada	70	An infected traveler to the 2010 Winter Olympics transmitted infection to an under- and unvaccinated local population in British Columbia.
2011/Canada	776	Disease was imported from France by an unvaccinated returned traveler to Quebec. The outbreak spread in a nonvaccinating religious community and outside that community. A majority of cases occurred in under- and unvaccinated persons.
2011/United States	118	Of 118 cases, 46 were in returned travelers from Europe and Asia/Pacific regions; 105 cases (89%) occurred in unvaccinated persons.
2013/United States	58	Disease was imported by a returned unvaccinated traveler from Europe. The outbreak spread in a nonvaccinating religious community in New York.
2014/Canada	433	Disease was imported from the Netherlands. The outbreak spread in a nonvaccinating religious community in British Columbia.
2014/United States	383	The outbreak occurred in nonvaccinating religious communities in Ohio.
2015/United States	147	A multistate/multicountry outbreak was linked to Disneyland amusement park. More than 80% of cases occurred in unvaccinated persons.
2015/Canada	159	Disease was imported from the United States (part of the Disneyland outbreak) by an unvaccinated traveler. The outbreak spread in a nonvaccinating religious community in Quebec.
2017/United States	75	The outbreak occurred in an under-vaccinated community in Minnesota; 95% of patients were unvaccinated.
2018/United States	375	Disease was imported by returned unvaccinated travelers from Israel. The outbreak spread in nonvaccinating religious communities in New York and New Jersey.
2019/Canada	31	Disease was imported from Vietnam by a returned traveler to British Columbia. The outbreak spread throughout local area schools in under- and unvaccinated persons and resulted in a province-wide measles mass immunization campaign for schoolchildren.
2019/United States	1282	Outbreaks occurred in 10 states; 73% of cases (~935) were linked to outbreaks in nonvaccinating religious communities in New York.

Source: Centers for Disease Control and Prevention and Public Health Agency of Canada.

outbreaks or epidemics, who spread disease into an unvaccinated or under-vaccinated community. Many of the outbreaks were contained within the nonvaccinating community, but several spread to other under-vaccinated communities geographically contiguous with the outbreak community. More concerning still are the cases and outbreaks originating in communities that had not previously been identified as nonvaccinating. These cases likely highlight pockets of unvaccinated individuals who object for cultural rather than religious reasons. In the past, these nonvaccinating individuals did not exist in large enough clusters to sustain the spread of measles. Of further concern is the number of individuals included in outbreak statistics who have had one or sometimes even two doses of vaccine and who were thought to be protected but who still end up with the disease. The assumption is that one or two doses provide full disease immunity, but this is not always true. Often, individual level characteristics (age, immune compromise, etc.) affect the individual's response to the vaccine and their level of protection. In other instances, vaccine protection can wane over time, thus leaving fully immunized individuals susceptible to infection. In fact, when herd immunity breaks (i.e., the level of immunity in a community becomes too low to prevent transmission of disease), the occurrence of cases even in fully immunized persons is seen, as reflected in outbreak statistics. As a result of decreased vaccination rates and the resulting disruption of herd immunity, these individuals may become more identifiable as non-immune.

Outside North America Although overall coverage rates may still be high in North America, they are lower in other parts of the world. In Samoa, for example, measles–mumps–rubella (MMR) vaccine coverage before a recent outbreak was 31%; in the Philippines, it was 67%. Twenty years ago, vaccine coverage was sufficiently high in some parts of the world, including Europe, that an unvaccinated traveler from a nonvaccinating community to most regions would have been protected by herd immunity at their destinations. Today that is not the case: such travelers are likely to become infected in a country with active measles transmission and return home to spread the infection into their communities and possibly beyond. Thus active measles transmission, whether at home or abroad, places individuals who rely on herd immunity (e.g., immunocompromised persons and young infants) at increased risk.

FACTORS IN VACCINE HESITANCY

Vaccination coverage rates provide an estimate of the proportion of children or adults in the population who have been vaccinated, but they do not indicate the proportion of individuals who are vaccine hesitant. An individual may be fully vaccinated but still be hesitant about the safety and effectiveness of vaccines, or an individual may be unvaccinated as a result of access issues but may not be hesitant. Therefore, in attempts to understand a patient's lack of vaccination, it is important to distinguish persons who are hesitant and refuse vaccines from those who need assistance to access the health care system and successfully complete vaccination. To this end, an understanding of vaccine hesitancy and its determinants is needed.

Vaccine hesitancy and opposition are defined by the World Health Organization's SAGE Working Group on Vaccine Hesitancy as a "delay in acceptance or refusal of vaccines despite availability of vaccination services." The SAGE group describes vaccine hesitancy as "complex and context specific, varying across time, place, and vaccines."

It is useful to frame vaccine acceptance as a continuum pyramid, with active demand for all vaccines representing the largest group at the bottom of the pyramid and outright refusal of all vaccines depicted in the smallest group at the top. In the middle lies vaccine hesitancy, in which the degree of vaccine demand and acceptance varies. Fortunately, for disease control efforts, most individuals fall within the active-demand category or, if they are hesitant, still accept all vaccines. Hesitancy can be influenced by complacency, convenience, and confidence (**Fig. 3-1**).

Complacency is self-satisfaction when accompanied by a lack of awareness for real dangers or deficiencies. Complacency exists in communities and individuals when the perceived risks of vaccine-preventable diseases are low and vaccination is not deemed a necessary preventive action. This attitude can apply to vaccination in general or to specific vaccines, such as influenza vaccines. Actual or perceived vaccine efficacy and effectiveness contribute to complacency. Patients who are complacent about vaccine-preventable diseases prioritize other lifestyle or health factors over vaccination. These individuals can be influenced toward vaccination by a strong recommendation from a trusted HCP or a local influenza outbreak. They can be influenced away from vaccination by a vaccine scare or misinformation on social

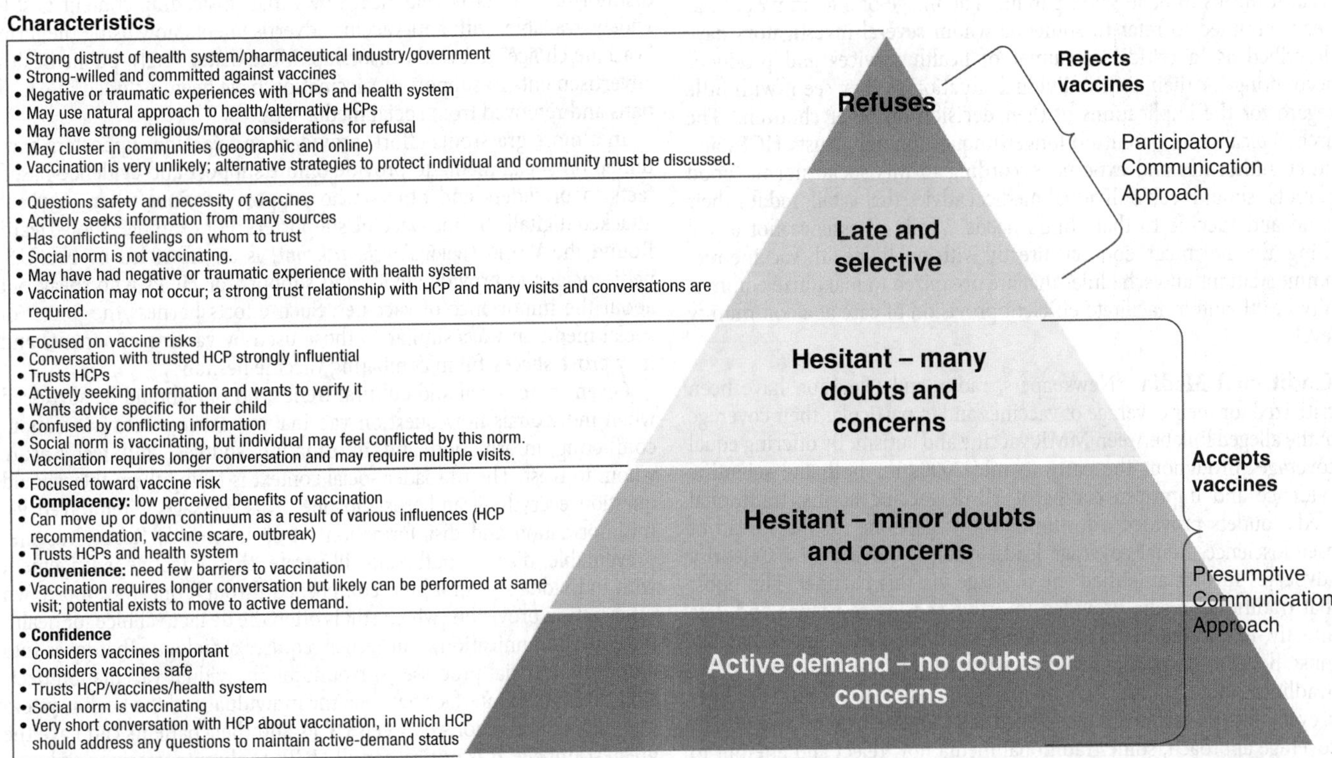

Characteristics
• Strong distrust of health system/pharmaceutical industry/government
• Strong-willed and committed against vaccines
• Negative or traumatic experiences with HCPs and health system
• May use natural approach to health/alternative HCPs
• May have strong religious/moral considerations for refusal
• May cluster in communities (geographic and online)
• Vaccination is very unlikely; alternative strategies to protect individual and community must be discussed.
• Questions safety and necessity of vaccines
• Actively seeks information from many sources
• Has conflicting feelings on whom to trust
• Social norm is not vaccinating.
• May have had negative or traumatic experience with health system
• Vaccination may not occur; a strong trust relationship with HCP and many visits and conversations are required.
• Focused on vaccine risks
• Conversation with trusted HCP strongly influential
• Trusts HCPs
• Actively seeking information and wants to verify it
• Wants advice specific for their child
• Confused by conflicting information
• Social norm is vaccinating, but individual may feel conflicted by this norm.
• Vaccination requires longer conversation and may require multiple visits.
• Focused toward vaccine risk
• Complacency: low perceived benefits of vaccination
• Can move up or down continuum as a result of various influences (HCP recommendation, vaccine scare, outbreak)
• Trusts HCPs and health system
• Convenience: need few barriers to vaccination
• Vaccination requires longer conversation but likely can be performed at same visit; potential exists to move to active demand.
• Confidence
• Considers vaccines important
• Considers vaccines safe
• Trusts HCP/vaccines/health system
• Social norm is vaccinating
• Very short conversation with HCP about vaccination, in which HCP should address any questions to maintain active-demand status
Refuses
Late and selective
Hesitant – many doubts and concerns
Hesitant – minor doubts and concerns
Active demand – no doubts or concerns
Rejects vaccines
Participatory Communication Approach
Accepts vaccines
Presumptive Communication Approach

FIGURE 3-1 Vaccine acceptance continuum. HCPs, health care providers. *(Adapted from J Leask et al: BMC Pediatrics 12:154, 2012; AL Benin et al: Pediatrics 117:1532, 2006; and E Dubé, NE MacDonald: The Vaccine Book, 2016, pp. 507-528.)*

media. Finally, the real or perceived ability of patients to take the action required for vaccination (i.e., self-efficacy) influences the role complacency plays in hesitancy and willingness to seek vaccination.

Convenience is determined by the degree to which conversations about vaccination and other services can be provided in culturally safe contexts that are convenient and comfortable for the individual. Clearly, convenience varies by community, health clinic, and even patient. Persons who are criticized or scolded for not vaccinating themselves or their children may not feel comfortable or safe accessing health services. Factors such as affordability, geographic accessibility, language, and health literacy are important considerations when evaluating the convenience of existing clinical care. Any of these factors can affect vaccine acceptance and can push a patient who has some hesitancy toward vaccinating or not vaccinating.

Confidence is based on trust in the safety and efficacy of vaccines, in the health care system that delivers vaccines (including HCPs), and in the policymakers or governments who decide which vaccines are needed and used. A continual erosion of confidence around vaccination, health systems, and governments drives today's hesitancy and has been amplified by larger social and cultural trends in medicine, parenting, and information availability.

SOCIAL AND CULTURAL TRENDS

Individualized Health Care Over the past 30 years, the focus of medicine and health care has shifted to patient-oriented, individualized care, with an increasing emphasis on treatment and prevention options tailored to the individual patient. In vaccination programs, this shift has manifested as requests for individualized vaccine recommendations and customized immunization schedules. The increasing personalization of medicine, while positive overall, has forced public health away from a focus on the community and its common good and has created tension between individual rights and community health.

Parenting Trends The desire for an individualized approach to medicine and vaccination reflects broader cultural trends concerning individual risk management: accordingly, the individual is to blame for bad outcomes, and public institutions cannot be trusted to manage technological (i.e., vaccine-related) risks. This viewpoint is directly linked with cultural shifts in parenting and social norms defining what it means to be a "good parent." The image of a good parent has been reframed to refer to someone whom several investigators have described as "a critical consumer of health services and products, accounting for their own individual situation as they see it with little regard for the implications of their decision on other children." The archetypical good parent no longer unquestioningly trusts HCPs and other authorities and experts. According to this social norm, "good parents" should seek individual medical advice that is tailored for their child and specific to that child's needs. While in essence not a bad thing, this norm can conflict directly with public health vaccine recommendations and schedules that are organized to maximize community health and to facilitate efficient provision of care at a community level.

Traditional Media Newspapers, radio, and television have been criticized for their coverage of vaccines and in particular their coverage of the alleged link between MMR vaccine and autism. By offering equal coverage throughout the early to mid-2000s for both the scientific evidence and unproven claims of MMR vaccine harms, traditional media outlets provided a forum and a megaphone for the spread of pseudoscience. Equal coverage leads to false equivalencies. Celebrity advocates further amplified the message via this channel. The boost that traditional media provided to active vaccine resistance and, less directly, to vaccine hesitancy has not been adequately measured but must be considered in any discussion of vaccine hesitancy. After headlines about multiple outbreaks of measles and other vaccine-preventable diseases and continued direct criticism of the equal-coverage approach, some traditional media now reject and attempt to discredit pseudoscience. The effect this stance will have on increasing vaccine confidence is unknown.

The Internet and Social Media Approximately 90% of Americans and 91% of Canadians use the Internet, and 80% of Americans and 60% of Canadians have a social network profile. Widespread access to social media can be empowering, but it is also problematic. The Internet and social media require users to select their information sources, creating an environment described as an "echo chamber" in which individuals choose information sources harboring beliefs or opinions similar to their own and thereby reinforcing their existing views. This situation has created a new platform for further spread of vaccine *misinformation* (inaccuracies due to error) and *disinformation* (deliberate lies) and has provided a forum for vaccine-resistant individuals, including celebrities, to organize and raise funds to support their efforts. The harmful effects of Internet and social media use on vaccine hesitancy have been well documented. Vaccine hesitancy increases for parents who seek their information from the Internet. Unfortunately, public health and health care institutions have been slow to adapt to this new communication medium and to recognize its influence and impact. In this medium, personal stories and anecdotes are now viewed as data and disproportionately influence vaccine decision-making, while traditional, more authoritative, fact-based information sources are deemphasized. Centralized monitoring by jurisdiction of vaccine misinformation and disinformation, with summaries of the relevant discourses and rebuttals provided to HCPs, has been proposed as a potential way to counter the influence of social media on vaccine hesitancy. While such strategies have been applied in single jurisdictions and appear to have had some success, their applicability to a broader context is unknown. Moreover, the resources for such a coordinated response have not been made available, and individual HCPs have been left to counter popular, shifting, viral communications on their own, patient by patient.

As with traditional media, the social media landscape appears to be shifting. In 2019, the proliferation of anti-vaccination information combined with measles outbreaks in North America and increasing pressure from health leaders led large social media companies (Facebook, Instagram, Pinterest) to deemphasize anti-vaccination information by removing relevant advertisements and recommendations and decreasing their prominence in search results. While it is too soon to determine the effects of these measures, critics are skeptical that they will have the intended result of reducing vaccine misinformation and disinformation. Early evidence shows that misleading content is still widely available, with anti-vaccine advertisements now using the term "vaccine choice" to avoid censorship. More disturbingly, public health advertisements in support of vaccination have been included in social bans and removed from social media sites.

In a more grassroots effort, providers and vaccine supporters have united on social media to provide online support and evidence-based facts to providers and others who support vaccines when they are attacked digitally by anti-vaccine supporters. For example, Shots Heard Round the World (*www.shotsheard.com*) is an effort led by two U.S. pediatricians to provide advice and support for HCPs who speak out about the importance of vaccines. Such efforts harness the power of social media in ways similar to those used by vaccine opponents and may prove successful in combating vaccine hesitancy.

Given these social and cultural trends, no one should be surprised when individuals now question vaccination, express confusion about conflicting information and information sources, and feel unsure whom to trust. Their broader social context is telling them they should question everything and trust no one. This message is reinforced via misinformation and disinformation on social media. Recent vaccine-preventable disease outbreaks illustrate that effective engagement with individuals cannot be accomplished through one-way, top-down information provision (which still is often the de facto choice for health system communication), but rather requires a dialogue that takes into account the social processes surrounding individual vaccination decisions. It is at the interface between the individual and the health system in which conversations between HCPs and their patients can have the greatest impact. It is critical for all HCPs to discuss vaccines and provide strong vaccine recommendations—including HCPs who do not administer vaccines but who have established trust with their patients.

APPROACH TO THE PATIENT

An ideal vaccine-hesitancy intervention would result in full compliance with vaccination, the patient's satisfaction with the health care encounter, and sustained trust in the HCP's recommendations. On a programmatic level, vaccine-hesitancy interventions should be multicomponent, dialogue based, and tailored to specific under-vaccinated populations.

Communicating with vaccine-hesitant individuals can be challenging and time-consuming. HCPs may feel that vaccine-hesitant patients cast doubt on their personal and professional integrity, their authority as medical experts, and their competence as communicators. Some HCPs may be reluctant to initiate conversations about vaccination because of concerns that discussing a sensitive topic may compromise their clinical rapport with their patients. Other HCPs may believe that they have not received sufficient training to confidently recommend vaccines and answer questions. Discussing vaccines with hesitant patients, while not always easy, provides an opportunity to honor the principles of patient-centered care by demonstrating an interest in patients' opinions, engaging in dialogue, and ideally increasing patients' confidence in vaccine recommendations.

FACTORS IN EFFECTIVE VACCINE RECOMMENDATIONS

Vaccine recommendations ideally should be made within an established, trusting patient–provider relationship in which patients are comfortable asking questions and voicing concerns, even if their views on vaccines contradict the HCP's recommendations. Recommending vaccines requires both provision of information and effective communication. There is no single "best practice" for how providers should approach recommending vaccines to vaccine-hesitant individuals. In general, all vaccine recommendations should be (1) strong, making it clear that the provider supports and recommends vaccination; (2) tailored, acknowledging the vaccine attitudes and potential concerns of individual patients; (3) transparent and accurate, highlighting the benefits of vaccines while also communicating the risks; (4) supported by trustworthy information resources that patients can access and review after the clinical encounter; and (5) revisited, with repetition and reinforcement during follow-up health care encounters.

Strength of the Recommendation HCPs should make it explicit (in the absence of medical contraindications) that vaccination based on the recommended schedule is the best option. While HCPs should take time to elicit patients' questions and address concerns, the recommendation for vaccination should be made in clear and unambiguous terms.

Tailored Communication Vaccine hesitancy occurs on a continuum (Fig. 3-1). Therefore, it is helpful for HCPs to have some understanding of their patients' attitudes toward vaccination at the start of the health care appointment. Unfortunately, vaccine-hesitancy surveys for use as part of vaccine consultation visits have not been validated on a large scale. However, the following are some examples of questions that can be asked, depending on the setting. (1) Did you have a chance to review the vaccine leaflet we provided? Did you have any questions about it? (2) Have you ever been reluctant or hesitant about getting a vaccination for yourself or your child? If so, what were the reasons? (3) Are there other pressures in your life that prevent you from getting yourself or your child immunized on time? (4) Whom/what resources do you trust the most for information about vaccines? Whom/what resources do you trust the least?

Communication style and content for patients in the active-demand category for vaccination will be different from those for individuals who are hesitant, late and selective, or strongly inclined to refuse vaccines. Two communication styles have been proposed for vaccine recommendations. Evidence shows that a *presumptive/directive* approach ("Your child is due for MMR vaccination.") results in higher rates of vaccine uptake than a *participatory/guiding* approach ("What are your thoughts about the MMR vaccine?"). However, adopting a strictly presumptive/directive approach may alienate some patients, especially those who are higher up on the hesitancy pyramid and who may feel that they are being pressured into vaccination before their concerns have been heard and addressed. Adopting a participatory/guiding approach and clarifying receptivity to vaccines may be more suitable for hesitant individuals with many doubts and concerns, persons with a late or selective attitude, and those who are strongly inclined to refuse vaccines. In addition, a participatory/guiding approach provides an opportunity for ongoing clinical rapport and dialogue between unvaccinated or under-vaccinated patients and their HCPs, even when it does not result in immediate vaccine uptake. Regardless of which approach is used, a strong vaccine recommendation should be made at each encounter.

Transparency and Accuracy Vaccine recommendations should be transparent, should include accurate information about both the benefits and the risks of the vaccine, and should emphasize why the benefits outweigh the risks. For example, when evidence supports an association between a vaccine and an adverse event, the occurrence of the adverse event is often very rare and the event quickly resolves (**Chap. 123**). U.S. Federal law (under the National Childhood Vaccine Injury Act) requires HCPs to provide a copy of the current Vaccine Information Statement from the Centers for Disease Control and Prevention (CDC), which describes both benefits and risks of vaccines to an adult patient or to a child's parent/legal representative before vaccination.

CDC Vaccine Information Statements should not replace a discussion with the HCP. Depending on the provider and the patient, a description of benefits and risks may include words and numbers, graphics, and personal anecdotes (e.g., why the provider vaccinates his or her own children). Personal anecdotes are powerful, and many hesitant patients seek and are influenced by them.

A discussion of benefits and risks provides an opportunity to address specific misconceptions about a particular vaccine or about vaccines overall. For example, patients may be concerned about adverse events following vaccination that are not supported by evidence, such as autism following MMR vaccination or myocardial infarction following influenza vaccination in the elderly.

Most adults—even those whose children are fully immunized—still have questions, misconceptions, or concerns about vaccines that should be addressed. A risk/benefit discussion allows HCPs to describe the vaccine safety monitoring systems in place. Providers should emphasize that vaccines are developed and approved through a highly regulated process that includes prelicensure clinical trials, review and approval by designated regulatory authorities (e.g., the U.S. Food and Drug Administration, Health Canada), strict manufacturing regulations, and ongoing postmarketing safety surveillance.

Support from Accessible Information Sources All vaccine recommendations should be supported by additional information sources patients can assess after the health care encounter. HCPs play an important role as information intermediaries for their patients. They can navigate information (and misinformation) about vaccines and direct patients toward reliable, appropriate resources. HCPs should consider what resources will be suitable for a patient or patient population. Vaccine information resources are available in different media formats and use a combination of images and text to communicate the information to various audiences. See "Further Reading," below, for suggestions or refer to resources provided by local health authorities.

Revisiting and Reinforcement of Vaccine Recommendations All health care encounters offer an opportunity to revisit and reinforce vaccine recommendations. Vaccine-hesitant individuals who do not accept vaccines but are willing to review information should be offered a follow-up appointment to reinforce previously made recommendations and address further questions. Vaccine-hesitant patients who accept vaccines should be seen at a follow-up appointment to confirm and document vaccine receipt (if vaccine is not given at the point of care), ascertain whether the vaccine was well tolerated, and reinforce the message about vaccine safety and effectiveness. Patients who actively demand vaccines usually do not require much follow-up other than to confirm and document the receipt of vaccine (if it is not given at the point of care) and to address additional questions or concerns arising subsequent to vaccination. Often this follow-up can be covered without an office visit.

WHAT TO SAY TO VACCINE-HESITANT PATIENTS

Engaging vaccine-hesitant individuals requires confidence, knowledge, skills, time, and creativity to tailor the approach to each individual patient. Examples for each part of the vaccine recommendation are listed in **Table 3-2**.

■ OTHER CONSIDERATIONS DURING CLINICAL ENCOUNTERS

Missed Opportunities The World Health Organization defines a missed opportunity for vaccination as "any contact with health services by an individual (child or person of any age) who is eligible for vaccination (e.g., unvaccinated or partially vaccinated and free of contraindications to vaccination), which does not result in the person receiving one or more of the vaccine doses for which he or she is eligible." HCPs who do not offer point-of-care vaccination frequently miss the opportunity to recommend vaccines to their patients. Missed opportunities for recommending and providing vaccines during routine health care encounters contribute to under-vaccination. Studies show that up to 45% of under-vaccinated children could be up to date with all age-appropriate vaccines and up to 90% of female adolescents could be up to date with human papillomavirus (HPV) vaccination if all opportunities to vaccinate were taken.

Vaccine counseling and vaccination should be incorporated into clinical care for individuals of all ages, not just young children. Because many adolescents and adults do not have regular health care follow-up, providers need to take advantage of every health care encounter to recommend and provide vaccines. For example, a visit to an emergency department, a routine follow-up visit at a diabetes clinic, or a visit planning for elective orthopedic surgery offer opportunities to inquire about the patient's vaccination status and to recommend vaccines.

HCPs should make preemptive vaccine recommendations (e.g., initiating discussions about infant vaccines during pregnancy, informing parents about HPV vaccine before their child becomes eligible). Such advance discussions may be especially helpful in identifying

TABLE 3-2 Sample Vaccine Conversations

STRONG VACCINE RECOMMENDATION
"We are headed into the flu season. Getting flu vaccine not only protects you, but it helps protect other people around you who can get very sick from flu. I strongly recommend you get your flu shot. Do you know where to get it?"
"You will be turning 50 next year. This means you will be eligible for a vaccine that prevents shingles, and I strongly recommend you receive it. Have you heard about this vaccine before? Can I answer your questions about it?"
"I know you are not comfortable getting vaccinated today. I do want to make it clear that I recommend vaccines because I am convinced they are the best way to protect you from some serious diseases. Is there something that would lead you to think about getting vaccinated in the future?"
TAILORED COMMUNICATION
"I recommend that children and adults stay up to date on recommended vaccines. I see from your vaccine record that you've had your childhood vaccines, but you haven't gotten any adult vaccines. I wanted to clarify whether this is because you decided not to get vaccines or something else prevented you from getting vaccinated."
"I understand that you are here for your pneumococcal vaccine. This is the best way to protect yourself and those around you from pneumonia. Do you have any questions before I give you the vaccine?"
"I understand you have some concerns about vaccines. What are you most concerned about? Would you like me to explain why I recommend giving your child these vaccines?"
TRANSPARENCY AND ACCURACY
"Serious side effects can develop after MMR vaccination but are very rare. On average, 3 out of 10,000 children who get MMR vaccine will have a febrile seizure/convulsion in the days after vaccination. Febrile seizures can be frightening, but nearly all children who have a febrile seizure recover very quickly and without any long-term consequences. On the other hand, 1 out of 1000 children who get measles will develop encephalitis (brain inflammation) that not only causes seizures but can also lead to permanent damage."
"About 10 out of every 10,000 Americans who do not get vaccinated against flu die because of influenza every year, and many more are hospitalized. While flu vaccine does not prevent all cases of influenza, it is the most effective vaccine we have. By getting the vaccine, you also help protect people around you from getting sick."
"You are correct, aluminum is used in some vaccines to help the body's immune system respond. However, aluminum is also present in food and drinking water. In fact, the amount of aluminum present in vaccines is similar to or less than what is present in breast milk or infant formulas."
SUPPORT FROM ACCESSIBLE INFORMATION SOURCES
"Your child and other boys and girls his age will be eligible for the human papillomavirus vaccine this coming school year. Have you heard about this vaccine before? What questions do you have about it? Here's a list of websites for parents and teenagers that explain what it is about."
"There's a lot of information about vaccines on the internet, and a lot of that information is not based on facts. Here is a list of websites that have been reviewed by health care professionals and accurately describe benefits and risks of each vaccine. The information is written in lay language and includes helpful illustrations."
REVISITING AND REINFORCEMENT OF THE RECOMMENDATION
"During our last visit, we talked about MMR vaccine for your son and some of the concerns you had about potential side effects. Have you had a chance to look at the take-home information I gave you? Was there anything else you would like to ask about? I recommend that we vaccinate your child today."
"During our last visit, we talked about receiving a pertussis booster during pregnancy and where you can get vaccinated. Have you had a chance to get your pertussis vaccine?"
"I see that you got your vaccines at the public health clinic last week. How did it go? Did you have any questions?"
"It's possible that the symptoms you experienced after receiving the vaccine were an adverse reaction to the vaccine. I will report this to the health authority. Let's discuss what we can do next time to prevent symptoms from occurring again."

Note: Specific vaccine recommendations, vaccine eligibility guidelines, and statistics used to communicate benefits and risks will vary with the health jurisdiction and the country. Several sample statements here are adapted from the Australian National Centre for Immunisation Research and Surveillance website (*www.talkingaboutimmunisation.org.au*). For patient vaccine information resources, see also the Immunization Action Coalition website for the public developed in partnership with the CDC (*vaccineinformation.org*).

vaccine-hesitant patients and ensuring that they have enough time to ask questions and make decisions before vaccines are due.

HCPs should ensure that a vaccine recommendation is followed by vaccination. Providers who recommend vaccines but do not vaccinate at the point of care should inform patients where they can be vaccinated. This discussion may include information about public health clinics, travel clinics, and pharmacies or a referral to another provider. HCPs should follow up with their patients at subsequent appointments to confirm that they were vaccinated.

Adverse Events Following Vaccination Although rare, adverse events (**Chap. 123**) may influence vaccine acceptance and willingness to be vaccinated in the future. It is important for providers to identify and follow up with all patients who experience an adverse event, regardless of the patients' vaccine attitudes prior to the event. Adverse events following vaccination should be reported to the relevant vaccine monitoring system: the U.S. Vaccine Adverse Event Reporting System or the Canadian Adverse Event Following Immunization Surveillance System.

Addressing Inequities In Vaccine Access Discrepancies in access to health care services create inequitable access to vaccines for children and adults and contribute to under-vaccination. A U.S. study found that socially disadvantaged individuals were more likely than other persons to be under-vaccinated, in part because of a lack of access to health care services. HCPs must recognize that socially disadvantaged individuals and populations are often at greater risk of vaccine-preventable diseases (e.g., as a result of crowded living conditions, limited access to sanitation, poor nutrition, or substance abuse) and also at greater risk of being under-vaccinated because they have limited access to health care services. In addition, specific vaccines may be recommended for some socially disadvantaged populations or communities. For example, in the wake of several outbreaks of hepatitis A among the U.S. homeless population, the CDC now recommends that everyone >1 year of age experiencing homelessness receive hepatitis A vaccine.

Depending on the setting and the patient, some recommended vaccines may not be covered through public funding or private insurance coverage. HCPs should be aware of alternative funding models, such as the Vaccines for Children Program, which provides free vaccines for U.S. children (<19 years of age) with financial barriers to vaccine access. When vaccines are not publicly funded or covered by private insurance and patients perceive that they cannot afford a vaccine, HCPs should not withhold a vaccine recommendation. The risks and benefits of vaccination still need to be communicated, with a strong recommendation, and the patient should be provided the opportunity to decide whether they can afford the vaccine.

Further Communication With Patients Who Refuse Vaccines Fortunately, the proportion of people who completely refuse all vaccines and are not willing to talk to their HCP is small. Nevertheless, in some cases, attempts to initiate discussion and address vaccine refusal may be futile. When possible, HCPs should focus on the common goals of care and preserve the therapeutic relationship. Vaccine refusal should be well documented in the patient's chart. The HCP should continue with tailored communication and be open to future discussions. Vaccine demand and vaccine refusal are rarely static over time. (**See "Focus: COVID-19 Vaccine Hesitancy," below.**)

■ CONCLUSION

In summary, vaccine hesitancy is complex and context specific. It varies with time, place, patient, and vaccine. HCPs are well positioned to address vaccine hesitancy and should develop the skills, knowledge, and confidence to make strong vaccine recommendations to their patients.

■ FOCUS: COVID-19 VACCINE HESITANCY

As COVID-19 vaccines are used to control SARS-CoV-2, some individuals will have concerns about these vaccines and a proportion of the population will reject them. While worrisome, hesitancy about COVID-19 vaccines is not unexpected; it mirrors public concerns expressed about past pandemic influenza vaccines and other newly introduced vaccines. It has been established that the newness of any vaccine, be it a pandemic influenza vaccine or a COVID-19 vaccine, raises concern in a large percentage of the population. Politicization of COVID-19 vaccines raises additional issues for some patients.

Past Experience with New Vaccines Past experience with new vaccines, including the H1N1 pandemic influenza vaccine in 2009 and the human papillomavirus vaccine in the early 2000s, provides a guide to topics that need to be addressed with regard to COVID-19 vaccines. While resistance is often framed as uncertainty about a vaccine's "newness," further discussion translates this uncertainty into concern about the new vaccine's safety. This concern encompasses both short- and long-term side effects. Frequent, acute adverse effects can be captured in clinical trial data, whereas worries about rare and long-term side effects can be addressed only by direct evidence after the initiation of a new vaccination program. In addition to queries about the overall safety of the vaccine, HCPs can expect specific questions regarding the safety of individual ingredients included in the vaccine, whether or not these ingredients are new and whether or not relevant safety data are available. Information on the incidence of common or expected health events in an unvaccinated population (i.e., background rates) over a 4-week period is helpful in distinguishing what is normal and expected from a point of concern. Studies that have examined this issue with regard to other vaccines can be used as a basis for presenting background rates of expected events in the context of COVID-19 vaccines for some groups; however, it is important to ensure that more specific background-rate information is available to HCPs with regard to the individual groups being vaccinated. HCPs, public health programs, and vaccine manufacturers can anticipate these questions and should develop answers and information to respond to them.

Specific Concerns about COVID-19 Vaccines While some concerns can be anticipated on the basis of past experience with new vaccines, several characteristics of COVID-19 vaccines require new approaches to adequately address individual concerns, and HCPs need to educate themselves in several specific areas. First, an overwhelming amount of attention has been paid to the speed of development of COVID-19 vaccines, with some jurisdictions even skipping the usual clinical-trial steps in an effort to provide vaccine more rapidly to their populations. This situation directly increases concerns about the "newness" of the vaccine and its safety and, unfortunately, raises questions about the entire vaccine development process. Education is required to explain how a process that normally requires 5–10 years was condensed to this degree. (See Lurie et al [2020] for an excellent explanation of the COVID-19 vaccine development process.) In addition, transparency with regard to clinical trial data is required to enable scientists, HCPs, and consumers to read and understand the development and evaluation processes. The usually shrouded, proprietary development process is unsuitable if the final vaccine product is to garner public trust. Education on existing vaccine-safety monitoring systems also needs to be provided. HCPs must familiarize themselves with the vaccine development process and safety monitoring systems if they are to present this information to their patients.

Second, several newer vaccine platforms that are being used for COVID-19 vaccines (e.g., nucleic acid–based vaccines, viral vector) have not been used in the past. This novelty exacerbates public concern about the unfamiliarity of new vaccines and further heightens misgivings about vaccine safety and the potential for long-term adverse effects. Again, HCPs need to familiarize themselves with the new technology and develop effective messaging for their patients. Public health officials have developed resources to address this issue (see *www.cdc.gov/vaccines/covid-19/vaccinate-with-confidence.html*), but, even in the absence of such resources, HCPs can anticipate questions about the new technology involved and become comfortable explaining it.

Third, clinical trial safety and efficacy data were lacking for all groups initially prioritized to receive the vaccine. For example, long-term-care residents were prioritized for vaccine receipt, but clinical trial data were not available for the range of chronic health conditions that exist in older adults. While observational studies have filled some of these gaps, HCPs need to extrapolate on the basis of available evidence in considering individual patients and must make a recommendation without knowing all the answers.

Fourth, some minority and marginalized communities who have been disproportionately affected by COVID-19 express hesitancy or reject COVID-19 vaccines. For some Black, Indigenous, Latinx, and other communities, COVID-19 hesitancy stems directly from systematic discrimination, racism, and mistreatment in the health care system. Black and Indigenous communities also share a horrific legacy of unethical medical experimentation,[1] which, when combined with current discrimination and overt racism, creates a powerful climate of mistrust in HCPs, the medical system, and science.

Social and Cultural Trends The social and cultural trends already discussed in this chapter—in particular, traditional media, the Internet, and social media—are exerting influence and pressure that did not affect the introduction of older vaccines, even the H1N1 pandemic vaccines. The media attention given to the development of transverse myelitis in one clinical-trial participant following receipt of COVID-19 vaccine is but one example of the intense media scrutiny of the vaccine development process. Unfortunately, in the United States, efforts to control COVID-19, including vaccine development, have become highly politicized. This degree of politicization has not occurred with past vaccines, so HCPs are in uncharted territory in terms of how to address it or even to understand its potential influence on vaccine acceptance. Again, individual HCPs need to navigate complex conversations with their patients and possibly their communities. Below are some suggestions that may prove helpful in formulating these conversations.

Tips for Discussion of COVID-19 Vaccines • **ADDRESS CONCERNS ABOUT "NEWNESS"** HCPs need to understand and be able to explain the newer vaccine platforms (mRNA, DNA, and viral vector vaccines) and to provide examples of other, older vaccines that have been developed by similar techniques. This information makes COVID-19 vaccines more familiar.

ADDRESS CONCERNS ABOUT VACCINE SAFETY HCPs need to understand and explain how vaccines are evaluated before being approved for use and how vaccine safety is monitored after vaccines are used in the population. It is important to be honest and state that potential rare and long-term effects are not yet known, but then to speak to what is from the animal and clinical trial data and to comment on background rates for rare events. Placing potential vaccine risks in the context of known COVID-19 disease risks is helpful for some patients.

Depending on the context, explain why specific high-risk groups may have been prioritized to receive the vaccine. Patients who have been prioritized may still need a strong recommendation from an HCP to accept the vaccine. An HCP recommendation is as important here as it is for acceptance of routine vaccines. As with other vaccines, many patients' decision to accept a COVID-19 vaccine rests upon whether their HCP recommends it.

[1]The Tuskegee Syphilis Study is the most infamous example of medical experimentation in Black communities in the United States. (See Brandt [1978] for details.) Numerous examples of medical experimentation on Indigenous peoples are available. For example, a 12-year trial of an experimental bacille Calmette-Guérin vaccine for tuberculosis was conducted on Cree and Nakoda Oyadebi infants in Saskatchewan during the 1930s. (See Lux [2016] for details.)

Address implicit or overt racism and systemic discrimination in the medical system and create culturally safe health care spaces. HCPs need to be aware of the legacy of discrimination, racism, and medical experimentation and the distrust it fosters in some communities. While SARS-CoV-2 has critically highlighted fractures in our health care system for minority and marginalized communities, addressing these underlying issues goes beyond addressing vaccine hesitancy and is clearly needed for all types of medical care in these communities.

EMPHASIZE THE IMPORTANCE OF KEEPING UP TO DATE WITH OTHER ROUTINE VACCINES DURING THE COVID-19 PANDEMIC These vaccines include but are not limited to seasonal influenza vaccine and the childhood primary vaccination series.

FURTHER READING

Vaccine Hesitancy

American Academy of Pediatrics: Vaccine hesitant parents. Available at *www.aap.org/en-us/advocacy-and-policy/aap-health-initiatives/immunizations/Pages/vaccine-hesitant-parents.aspx*. Accessed October 23, 2020.

DeStefano F et al: Principal controversies in vaccine safety in the United States. Clin Infect Dis 69:726, 2019.

Dudley MZ et al: The state of vaccine safety science: Systematic reviews of the evidence. Lancet Infect Dis 20:e80, 2020.

Immunization Action Coalition: For healthcare professionals. Available at *www.immunize.org*. Accessed October 23, 2020.

Immunization Action Coalition: For the public: Vaccine information you need. Available at *vaccineinformation.org*. Accessed October 23, 2020.

Jamison AM et al: Vaccine-related advertising in the Facebook Ad Archive. Vaccine 38:512, 2020.

Leask J et al: Communicating with parents about vaccination: A framework for health professionals. BMC Pediatr 12:154, 2012.

MacDonald N et al: Vaccine hesitancy: Definition, scope and determinants. Vaccine 33:4161, 2015.

World Health Organization: Vaccine hesitancy survey questions related to SAGE vaccine hesitancy. Available at *www.who.int/immunization/programmes_systems/Survey_Questions_Hesitancy.pdf*. Accessed October 23, 2020.

World Health Organization: Improving vaccination demand and addressing hesitancy. Available at *www.who.int/immunization/programmes_systems/vaccine_hesitancy/en/*. Accessed October 23, 2020.

World Health Organization: Missed opportunities for vaccination (MOV) strategy. Available at *www.who.int/immunization/programmes_systems/policies_strategies/MOV/en/*. Accessed October 23, 2020.

COVID-19 Vaccine Hesitancy

Brandt AM: Racism and research: The case of the Tuskegee Syphilis Study. Hastings Cent Rep 8:21, 1978.

Centers for Disease Control and Prevention: Vaccinate with confidence: Strategy to reinforce confidence in Covid-19 vaccines. Available at *www.cdc.gov/vaccines/covid-19/vaccinate-with-confidence.html*. Accessed April 5, 2021.

Lurie N et al: Developing Covid-19 vaccines at pandemic speed. N Engl J Med 382:21, 2020.

Lux MK: Separate beds: A history of Indian hospitals in Canada, 1920s–1980s. Toronto, University of Toronto Press, 2016.

Mosby I et al: Medical experimentation and the roots of COVID-19 vaccine hesitancy among Indigenous Peoples in Canada. CMAJ 193:E381, 2021.

4 Decision-Making in Clinical Medicine

Daniel B. Mark, John B. Wong

Practicing medicine at its core requires making decisions. What makes medical practice so difficult is not only the specialized technical knowledge required but also the intrinsic uncertainty that surrounds each decision. Mastering the technical aspects of medicine alone, unfortunately, does not ensure a mastery of the practice of medicine. Sir William Osler's familiar quote "Medicine is a science of uncertainty and an art of probability" captures well this complex duality. Although the science of medicine is often taught as if the mechanisms of the human body operate with Newtonian predictability, every aspect of medical practice is infused with an element of irreducible uncertainty that the clinician ignores at her peril. Although deeply rooted in science, more than 100 years after the practice of medicine took its modern form, it remains at its core a craft, to which individual doctors bring varying levels of skill and understanding. With the exponential growth in medical literature and other technical information and an ever-increasing number of testing and treatment options, twenty-first century physicians who seek excellence in their craft must master a more diverse and complex set of skills than any of the generations that preceded them. This chapter provides an introduction to three of the pillars upon which the craft of modern medicine rests: (1) expertise in clinical reasoning (what it is and how it can be developed); (2) rational diagnostic test use and interpretation; and (3) integration of the best available research evidence with clinical judgment in the care of individual patients (evidence-based medicine [EBM]).

■ BRIEF INTRODUCTION TO CLINICAL REASONING

Clinical Expertise Defining "clinical expertise" remains surprisingly difficult. Chess has an objective ranking system based on skill and performance criteria. Athletics, similarly, have ranking systems to distinguish novices from Olympians. But in medicine, after physicians complete training and pass the boards (or get recertified), no tests or benchmarks are used to identify those who have attained the highest levels of clinical performance. At each institution, there are often a few "elite" clinicians who are known for their "special problem-solving prowess" when particularly difficult or obscure cases have baffled everyone else. Yet despite their skill, even such master clinicians typically cannot explain their exact processes and methods, thereby limiting the acquisition and dissemination of the expertise used to achieve their impressive results. Furthermore, clinical virtuosity appears not to be generalizable, e.g., an expert on hypertrophic cardiomyopathy may be no better (and possibly worse) than a first-year medical resident at diagnosing and managing a patient with neutropenia, fever, and hypotension.

Broadly construed, clinical expertise encompasses not only cognitive dimensions involving the integration of disease knowledge with verbal and visual cues and test interpretation but also potentially the complex fine-motor skills necessary for invasive procedures and tests. In addition, "the complete package" of expertise in medicine requires effective communication and care coordination with patients and members of the medical team. Research on medical expertise remains sparse overall and mostly centered on diagnostic reasoning, so in this chapter, we focus primarily on the cognitive elements of clinical reasoning.

Because clinical reasoning occurs in the heads of clinicians, objective study of the process is difficult. One research method used for this area asks clinicians to "think out loud" as they receive increments of clinical information in a manner meant to simulate a clinical encounter. Another research approach focuses on how doctors should reason diagnostically, to identify remediable "errors," rather than on how they actually do reason. Much of what is known about clinical reasoning comes from empirical studies of nonmedical problem-solving behavior. Because of the diverse perspectives contributing to this area, with important contributions from cognitive psychology, medical education, behavioral economics, sociology, informatics, and decision sciences, no single integrated model of clinical reasoning exists, and not infrequently, different terms and reasoning models describe similar phenomena.

Intuitive Versus Analytic Reasoning A useful contemporary model of reasoning, the dual-process theory distinguishes two general conceptual modes of thinking as fast or slow. *Intuition* (System 1) provides rapid effortless judgments from memorized associations using pattern recognition and other simplifying "rules of thumb" (i.e., heuristics). For example, a very simple pattern that could be useful in certain situations is "black woman plus hilar adenopathy equals sarcoid." Because no effort is involved in recalling the pattern, the clinician is often unable to say how those judgments were formulated. In contrast, *Analysis* (System 2), the other form of reasoning in the dual-process model, is slow, methodical, deliberative, and effortful. A student might read about causes of hilar adenopathy and from that list (e.g., **Chap. 66**), identify diseases more common in black women or examine the patient for skin or eye findings that occur with sarcoid. These dual processes, of course, represent two exemplars taken from the cognitive continuum. They provide helpful descriptive insights but very little guidance in how to develop expertise in clinical reasoning. How these idealized systems interact in different decision problems, how experts use them differently from novices, and when their use can lead to errors in judgment remain the subject of study and considerable debate.

Pattern recognition, an important part of System 1 reasoning, is a complex cognitive process that appears largely effortless. One can recognize people's faces, the breed of a dog, an automobile model, or a piece of music from just a few notes within milliseconds without necessarily being able to articulate the specific features that prompted the recognition. Analogously, experienced clinicians often recognize familiar diagnostic patterns very quickly. The key here is having a large library of stored patterns that can be rapidly accessed. In the absence of an extensive stored repertoire of diagnostic patterns, students (as well as experienced clinicians operating outside their area of expertise and familiarity) often must use the more laborious System 2 analytic approach along with more intensive and comprehensive data collection to reach the diagnosis.

The following brief patient scenarios illustrate three distinct patterns associated with hemoptysis that experienced clinicians recognize without effort:

- A 46-year-old man presents to his internist with a chief complaint of hemoptysis. An otherwise healthy, nonsmoker, he is recovering from an apparent viral bronchitis. This presentation pattern suggests that the small amount of blood-streaked sputum is due to acute bronchitis, so that a chest x-ray provides sufficient reassurance that a more serious disorder is absent.
- In the second scenario, a 46-year-old patient who has the same chief complaint but with a 100-pack-year smoking history, a productive morning cough with blood-streaked sputum, and weight loss fits the pattern of carcinoma of the lung. Consequently, along with the chest x-ray, the clinician obtains a sputum cytology examination and refers this patient for a chest CT scan.
- In the third scenario, the clinician hears a soft diastolic rumbling murmur at the apex on cardiac auscultation in a 46-year-old patient with hemoptysis who immigrated from a developing country and orders an echocardiogram as well, because of possible pulmonary hypertension from suspected rheumatic mitral stenosis.

Pattern recognition by itself is not, however, sufficient for secure diagnosis. Without deliberative systematic reflection, undisciplined pattern recognition can result in premature closure: mistakenly jumping to the conclusion that one has the correct diagnosis before all the relevant data are in. A critical second step, therefore, even when the diagnosis seems obvious, is *diagnostic verification*: considering whether the diagnosis adequately accounts for the presenting symptoms and signs and can explain all the ancillary findings. The following case based on a real clinical encounter provides an example of premature closure. A 45-year-old man presents with a 3-week history of a "flulike" upper respiratory infection (URI) including dyspnea and a productive cough. The emergency department (ED) clinician pulled out a "URI assessment form," which defines and standardizes the information gathered. After quickly acquiring the requisite structured examination components and noting in particular the absence of fever and a clear chest examination, the physician prescribed a cough suppressant for acute bronchitis and reassured the patient that his illness was not serious. Following a sleepless night at home with significant dyspnea, the patient developed nausea and vomiting and collapsed. He was brought back to the ED in cardiac arrest and was unable to be resuscitated. His autopsy showed a posterior wall myocardial infarction (MI) and a fresh thrombus in an atherosclerotic right coronary artery. What went wrong? Presumably, the ED clinician felt that the patient was basically healthy (one can be misled by the way the patient appears on examination—a patient that does not appear "sick" may be incorrectly assumed to have an innocuous illness). So, in this case, the physician, upon hearing the overview of the patient from the triage nurse, elected to use the URI assessment protocol even before starting the history, closing consideration of the broader range of possibilities and associated tests required to confirm or refute these possibilities. In particular, by concentrating on the abbreviated and focused URI protocol, the clinician failed to elicit the full dyspnea history, which was precipitated by exertion and accompanied by chest heaviness and relieved by rest, suggesting a far more serious disorder.

Heuristics or rules of thumb are a part of the intuitive system. These cognitive shortcuts provide a quick and easy path to reaching conclusions and making choices, but when used improperly, they can lead to errors. Two major research programs have studied heuristics in a mostly nonmedical context and have reached very different conclusions about the value of these cognitive tools. The "heuristics and biases" program focuses on how these mental shortcuts can lead to incorrect judgments. So far, however, little evidence exists that educating physicians and other decision makers to watch for the >100 cognitive biases identified to date has had any effect on the rate of diagnostic errors. In contrast, the "fast and frugal heuristics" research program explores how and when relying on simple heuristics can produce good decisions. Although many heuristics have relevance to clinical reasoning, only four will be mentioned here.

When diagnosing patients, clinicians usually develop diagnostic hypotheses based on the similarity of that patient's symptoms, signs, and other data to their mental representations (memorized patterns) of the disease possibilities. In other words, clinicians pattern match to identify the diagnoses that share the most similar findings to the patient at hand. This cognitive shortcut is called the representativeness heuristic. Consider a patient with hypertension who has headache, palpitations, and diaphoresis. Based on the representativeness heuristic, clinicians might judge pheochromocytoma to be quite likely given this classic presenting symptom triad suggesting pheochromocytoma. Doing so, however, would be incorrect given that other causes of hypertension are much more common than pheochromocytoma and this triad of symptoms can occur in patients who do not have it. Thus, clinicians using the representativeness heuristic may overestimate the likelihood of a particular disease based on the presence of representative symptoms and signs, failing to account for its low underlying prevalence (i.e., the prior, or pretest, probabilities). Conversely, atypical presentations of common diseases may lead to underestimating the likelihood of a particular disease. Thus, inexperience with a specific disease and with the breadth of its presentations may also lead to diagnostic delays or errors, e.g., diseases that affect multiple organ systems, such as sarcoid or tuberculosis, may be particularly challenging to diagnose because of the many different patterns they may manifest.

A second commonly used cognitive shortcut, the availability heuristic, involves judgments based on how easily prior similar cases or outcomes can be brought to mind. For example, a clinician may recall a case from a morbidity and mortality conference in which an elderly patient presented with painless dyspnea of acute onset and was evaluated for a pulmonary cause but was eventually found to have acute MI, with the diagnostic delay likely contributing to the development of ischemic cardiomyopathy. If the case was associated with a malpractice accusation, such examples may be even more memorable. Errors with the availability heuristic arise from several sources of recall bias. Rare catastrophic outcomes become memorable cases with a clarity and force disproportionate to their likelihood for future diagnosis—for example, a patient with a sore throat eventually found to have leukemia or a young athlete with leg pain subsequently found to have an osteosarcoma—and those publicized in the media or recently experienced are, of course, easier to recall and therefore more influential on clinical judgments.

The third commonly used cognitive shortcut, the anchoring heuristic (also called conservatism or stickiness), involves insufficiently adjusting the initial probability of disease up (or down) following a positive (or negative test) when compared with Bayes' theorem, i.e., sticking to the initial diagnosis. For example, a clinician may still judge the probability of coronary artery disease (CAD) to be high despite a negative exercise perfusion test and go on to cardiac catheterization (see "Measures of Disease Probability and Bayes' Rule," below).

The fourth heuristic states that clinicians should use the simplest explanation possible that will adequately account for the patient's symptoms and findings (Occam's razor or, alternatively, the simplicity heuristic). Although this is an attractive and often used principle, it is important to remember that no biologic basis for it exists. Errors from the simplicity heuristic include premature closure leading to the neglect of unexplained significant symptoms or findings.

For complex or unfamiliar diagnostic problems, clinicians typically resort to analytic reasoning processes (System 2) and proceed methodically using the *hypothetico-deductive model of reasoning*. Based on the patient's stated reasons for seeking medical attention, clinicians develop an initial list of diagnostic possibilities in *hypothesis generation*. During the history of the present illness, the initial hypotheses evolve in *diagnostic refinement* as emerging information is tested against the mental models of the diseases being considered with diagnoses increasing and decreasing in likelihood or even being dropped from consideration as the working hypotheses of the moment. These mental models often generate additional questions that distinguish the diagnostic possibilities from one another. The focused physical examination contributes to further distinguishing the working hypotheses. Is the spleen enlarged? How big is the liver? Is it tender? Are there any palpable masses or nodules? *Diagnostic verification* involves testing the adequacy (whether the diagnosis accounts for all symptoms and signs) and coherency (whether the signs and symptoms are consistent with the underlying pathophysiologic causal mechanism) of the working diagnosis. For example, if the enlarged and quite tender liver felt on physical examination is due to acute hepatitis (the hypothesis), then certain specific liver function tests will be markedly elevated (the prediction). Should the tests come back normal, the hypothesis may have to be discarded and others reconsidered.

Although often neglected, negative findings are as important as positive ones because they reduce the likelihood of the diagnostic hypotheses under consideration. Chest discomfort that is not provoked or worsened by exertion and not relieved by rest in an active patient lowers the likelihood that chronic ischemic heart disease is the underlying cause. The absence of a resting tachycardia and thyroid gland enlargement reduces the likelihood of hyperthyroidism in a patient with paroxysmal atrial fibrillation.

The acuity of a patient's illness may override considerations of prevalence and the other issues described above. "Diagnostic imperatives" recognize the significance of relatively rare but potentially catastrophic conditions if undiagnosed and untreated. For example, clinicians should consider aortic dissection routinely as a possible cause of acute severe chest discomfort. Although the typical presenting symptoms of dissection differ from those of MI, dissection may mimic MI, and because it is far less prevalent and potentially fatal if mistreated, diagnosing dissection remains a challenging diagnostic imperative (**Chap. 280**).

Clinicians taking care of acute, severe chest pain patients should explicitly and routinely inquire about symptoms suggestive of dissection, measure blood pressures in both arms for discrepancies, and examine for pulse deficits. When these are all negative, clinicians may feel sufficiently reassured to discard the aortic dissection hypothesis. If, however, the chest x-ray shows a possible widened mediastinum, the hypothesis should be reinstated and an appropriate imaging test ordered (e.g., thoracic computed tomography [CT] scan or transesophageal echocardiogram). In nonacute situations, the prevalence of potential alternative diagnoses should play a much more prominent role in diagnostic hypothesis generation.

Cognitive scientists studying the thought processes of expert clinicians have observed that clinicians group data into packets, or "chunks," that are stored in short-term or "working memory" and manipulated to generate diagnostic hypotheses. Because short-term memory is limited (classically humans can accurately repeat a list of 7 ± 2 numbers read to them), the number of diagnoses that can be actively considered in hypothesis-generating activities is similarly limited. For this reason, the cognitive shortcuts discussed above play a key role in the generation of diagnostic hypotheses, many of which are discarded as rapidly as they are formed, thereby demonstrating that the distinction between analytic and intuitive reasoning is an arbitrary and simplistic, but nonetheless useful, representation of cognition.

Research into the hypothetico-deductive model of reasoning has had difficulty identifying the elements of the reasoning process that distinguish experts from novices. This has led to a shift from examining the problem-solving process of experts to analyzing the organization of their knowledge for pattern matching as exemplars, prototypes, and illness scripts. For example, diagnosis may be based on the resemblance of a new case to patients seen previously (exemplars). As abstract mental models of disease, prototypes incorporate the likelihood of various disease features. Illness scripts include risk factors, pathophysiology, and symptoms and signs. Experts have a much larger store of exemplar and prototype cases, an example of which is the visual long-term memory of experienced radiologists. However, clinicians do not simply rely on literal recall of specific cases but have constructed elaborate conceptual networks of memorized information or models of disease to aid in arriving at their conclusions (illness scripts). That is, expertise involves an enhanced ability to connect symptoms, signs, and risk factors to one another in meaningful ways; relate those findings to possible diagnoses; and identify the additional information necessary to confirm the diagnosis.

No single theory accounts for all the key features of expertise in medical diagnosis. Experts have more knowledge about presenting symptoms of diseases and a larger repertoire of cognitive tools to employ in problem solving than nonexperts. One definition of expertise highlights the ability to make powerful distinctions. In this sense, expertise involves a working knowledge of the diagnostic possibilities and those features that distinguish one disease from another. Memorization alone is insufficient, e.g., photographic memory of a medical textbook would not make one an expert. But having access to detailed case-specific relevant information is critically important. In the past, clinicians primarily acquired clinical knowledge through their patient experiences, but now clinicians have access to a plethora of information sources. Clinicians of the future will be able to leverage the experiences of large numbers of other clinicians using electronic tools, but, as with the memorized textbook, the data alone will be insufficient for becoming an expert. Nonetheless, availability of these data removes one barrier for acquiring experience with connecting symptoms, signs, and risk factors to the possible diagnoses and identifying the additional distinguishing information necessary to confirm the diagnosis, thereby potentially facilitating the development of the working knowledge necessary for becoming an expert.

Despite all of the research seeking to understand expertise in medicine and other disciplines, it remains uncertain whether any didactic program can actually accelerate the progression from novice to expert or from experienced clinician to master clinician. Deliberate effortful practice (over an extended period of time, sometimes said to be 10 years or 10,000 practice hours) and personal coaching are two strategies often used outside medicine (e.g., music, athletics, chess) to cultivate expertise. Their use in developing medical expertise and maintaining or enhancing it has not yet been adequately explored. Some studies in medicine suggest that the most beneficial approach to education exposes students to both the signs and symptoms of specific diseases (disease pattern recognition) and, in addition, the lists of diseases that can present with specific symptoms and signs (differential diagnosis). Active learning opportunities useful for those in training include developing a personal learning system, e.g., systematically reflecting on diagnostic processes used (metacognition) and following-up to identify diagnoses and treatments for patients in their care.

DIAGNOSTIC VERSUS THERAPEUTIC DECISION-MAKING

The modern ideal of medical therapeutic decision-making is to "personalize" treatment recommendations. In the abstract, personalizing treatment involves combining the best available evidence about what works with an individual patient's unique features (e.g., risk factors, genomics, and comorbidities) and his or her preferences and health goals to craft an optimal treatment recommendation with the patient. Operationally, two different and complementary levels of personalization are possible: individualizing the risk of harm and benefit for the options being considered based on the specific patient characteristics (precision medicine), and personalizing the therapeutic decision process by incorporating the patient's preferences and values for the possible health outcomes. This latter process is sometimes referred to as shared decision-making and typically involves clinicians sharing their knowledge about the options and the associated consequences and trade-offs and patients sharing their health goals (e.g., avoiding a short-term risk of dying from coronary artery bypass grafting to see their grandchild get married in a few months).

Individualizing the evidence about therapy **does not** mean relying on physician impressions of benefit and harm from their personal experience. Because of small sample sizes and rare events, the chance of drawing erroneous causal inferences from one's own clinical experience is very high. For most chronic diseases, therapeutic effectiveness is only demonstrable statistically in large patient populations. It would be incorrect to infer with any certainty, for example, that treating a hypertensive patient with angiotensin-converting enzyme (ACE) inhibitors necessarily prevented a stroke from occurring during treatment, or that an untreated patient would definitely have avoided their stroke had they been treated. For many chronic diseases, a majority of patients will remain event free regardless of treatment choices; some will have events regardless of which treatment is selected; and those who avoided having an event through treatment cannot be individually identified. Blood pressure lowering, a readily observable surrogate endpoint, does not have a tightly coupled relationship with strokes prevented. Consequently, in most situations, demonstrating therapeutic effectiveness cannot rely simply on observing the outcome of an individual patient but should instead be based on large groups of patients carefully studied and properly analyzed.

Therapeutic decision-making, therefore, should be based on the best available evidence from clinical trials and well-done outcome studies. Trustworthy clinical practice guidelines that synthesize such evidence offer normative guidance for many testing and treatment decisions. However, all guidelines recognize that "one size fits all" recommendations may not apply to individual patients. Increased research into the heterogeneity of treatment effects seeks to understand how best to adjust group-level clinical evidence of treatment harms and benefits to account for the absolute level of risks faced by subgroups and even by individual patients, using, for example, validated clinical risk scores.

NONCLINICAL INFLUENCES ON CLINICAL DECISION-MAKING

More than three decades of research on variations in clinician practice patterns has identified important nonclinical forces that shape clinical decisions. These factors can be grouped conceptually into three overlapping categories: (1) factors related to an individual physician's practice, (2) factors related to practice setting, and (3) factors related to payment systems.

Factors Related to Practice Style To ensure that necessary care is provided at a high level of quality, physicians fulfill a key role in medical care by serving as the patient's advocate. Factors that influence performance in this role include the physician's knowledge, training, and experience. Clearly, physicians cannot practice EBM if they are unfamiliar with the evidence. As would be expected, specialists generally know the evidence in their field better than do generalists. Beyond published evidence and practice guidelines, a major set of influences on physician practice can be subsumed under the general concept of "practice style." The practice style serves to define norms of clinical behavior. Differing practice styles may be based on training, personal experience, and medical evidence. Beliefs about effectiveness of different therapies and preferred patterns of diagnostic test use are examples of different facets of a practice style. For example, cardiologists evaluating patients with lower risk chest pain symptoms often conceptualize their primary diagnostic objective as maximizing the detection of ischemia. For this reason, they may strongly favor stress imaging. Internists caring for the same patients may be more comfortable with initial use of exercise ECG testing without imaging. This latter practice style focuses less on ischemia detection and more on following guideline recommendations that indicate no outcome advantage for stress imaging in this context. Cardiologist may also favor a more liberal use of coronary angiography and revascularization in patients with stable ischemic symptoms relative to general internists.

Beyond the patient's welfare, physician perceptions about the risk of a malpractice suit resulting from either an erroneous decision or a bad outcome may drive clinical decisions and create a practice referred to as defensive medicine. This practice involves ordering tests and therapies with very small marginal benefits, ostensibly to preclude future criticism should an adverse outcome occur. With conscious or unconscious awareness of a connection to the risk of litigation or to payment, however, over time, such patterns of care may become accepted as part of the practice norm, thereby perpetuating their overuse, e.g., annual cardiac exercise testing in asymptomatic patients.

Practice Setting Factors Factors in this category relate to work systems including tasks and workflow (interruptions, inefficiencies, workload), technology (poor design or implementation, errors in use, failure, misuse), organizational characteristics (e.g., culture, leadership, staffing, scheduling), and the physical environment (e.g., noise, lighting, layout). *Physician-induced demand* is a term that refers to the repeated observation that once medical facilities and technologies become available to physicians, they will find ways to use them. Other environmental factors that can influence decision-making include the local availability of specialists for consultations and procedures; "high-tech" advanced imaging or procedure facilities such as MRI machines and proton beam therapy centers; and fragmentation of care.

Payment Systems Economic incentives are closely related to the other two categories of practice-modifying factors. Financial issues can exert both stimulatory and inhibitory influences on clinical practice. Historically, physicians are paid on a fee-for-service, capitation, or salary basis. In fee-for-service, physicians who do more get paid more, thereby encouraging overuse, consciously or unconsciously. When fees are reduced (discounted reimbursement), clinicians tend to increase the number of services provided to maintain revenue. Capitation, in contrast, provides a fixed payment per patient per year to encourage physicians to consider a global population budget in managing individual patients and ideally reducing the use of interventions with small marginal benefit. To discourage volume-based excessive utilization, fixed salary compensation plans pay physicians the same regardless of the clinical effort expended but may provide an (unintended) incentive to see fewer patients. In recognition of the nonsustainability of continued growth in medical expenditures and the opportunity costs associated with that (funds that might be more beneficially applied to education, energy, social welfare, or defense), current efforts seek to transition to a value-based payment system to reduce overuse and to reflect benefit. Work to define how to actually tie payment to value has mostly focused so far on "pay for performance" models. High-quality clinical trial evidence for the effectiveness of these models is still mostly lacking.

INTERPRETATION OF DIAGNOSTIC TESTS

Despite impressive technological advances in medicine over the past century, uncertainty still abounds and challenges all aspects of medical decision-making. Compounding this challenge, massive information overload characterizes modern medicine. Clinicians on average subscribe to seven journals, presenting them with >2500 new articles each year, and need access to 2 million pieces of information to practice medicine. Of course, to be useful, this information must be sifted for quality and examined for applicability for integration into patient-specific care. Although computers appear to offer an obvious solution both for information management and for quantification of medical care uncertainties, many practical problems remain to be solved before computerized decision support can be routinely incorporated into the clinical reasoning process in a way that demonstrably improves the quality of care. For the present, understanding the nature of diagnostic test information can help clinicians become more efficient users of such data. The next section reviews select concepts related to diagnostic testing.

DIAGNOSTIC TESTING: MEASURES OF TEST ACCURACY

The purpose of performing a test on a patient is to reduce uncertainty about the patient's diagnosis or prognosis in order to facilitate appropriate management. Although diagnostic tests commonly refer to laboratory (e.g., blood count) or imaging tests or procedures (e.g., colonoscopy or bronchoscopy), any information that changes a provider's understanding of the patient's problem qualifies as a diagnostic test. Thus, even the history and physical examination can be considered as diagnostic tests. In clinical medicine, it is common to reduce the results of a test to a dichotomous outcome, such as positive or negative, normal or abnormal. Although this simplification often suppresses useful information (such as the degree of abnormality), it facilitates illustrating some important principles of test interpretation that are described below.

The accuracy of any diagnostic test is assessed relative to a "gold standard," where a positive gold standard test defines the patients who have disease and a negative test securely rules out disease (**Table 4-1**). Characterizing the diagnostic performance of a new test requires identifying an appropriate population (ideally, patients representative of those in whom the new test would be used) and applying both the new and the gold standard tests to all subjects. Biased estimates of test performance occur when diagnostic accuracy is defined using an inappropriate population or one in which gold standard determination of disease status is incomplete. The accuracy of the new test in distinguishing disease from health is determined relative to the gold standard results and summarized in four estimates. The sensitivity or true-positive rate reflects how well the new test identifies patients with disease. It is the proportion of patients with disease (defined by the gold standard) who have a positive test. The proportion of patients with disease who have a negative test is the false-negative rate, calculated as 1 – sensitivity. The specificity, or true-negative rate, reflects how well

TABLE 4-1 Measures of Diagnostic Test Accuracy

	DISEASE STATUS	
TEST RESULT	**PRESENT**	**ABSENT**
Positive	True positives (TP)	False positives (FP)
Negative	False negatives (FN)	True negatives (TN)
Test Characteristics in Patients with Disease		
True-positive rate (sensitivity) = TP/(TP + FN)		
False-negative rate = FN/(TP + FN) = 1 – true-positive rate		
Test Characteristics in Patients without Disease		
True-negative rate (specificity) = TN/(TN + FP)		
False-positive rate = FP/(TN + FP) = 1 – true-negative rate		

the new test correctly identifies patients without disease. It is the proportion of patients without disease (defined by the gold standard) who have a negative test. The proportion of patients without disease who have positive test is the false-positive rate, calculated as 1 – specificity. In theory, a perfect test would be one with a sensitivity of 100% and a specificity of 100% and would completely distinguish patients with disease from those without it. A useful mnemonic to help remember the somewhat paradoxical relationship between what the test is best at technically versus what it is most useful for clinically is: a test with a very high sensitivity (Sn) when *negative* (N) helps *rule out* (out) disease (SnNout), and a test with a very high specificity (Sp) when *positive* (P) helps *rule in* (in) disease (SpPin).

Calculating sensitivity and specificity requires selection of a threshold value or cut point above which the test is considered "positive." Making the cut point "stricter" (e.g., raising it) lowers sensitivity but improves specificity, while making it "laxer" (e.g., lowering it) raises sensitivity but lowers specificity. This dynamic trade-off between more accurate identification of subjects with disease versus those without disease is often displayed graphically as a receiver operating characteristic (ROC) curve (**Fig. 4-1**) by plotting sensitivity (*y* axis) versus 1 – specificity (*x* axis). Each point on the curve represents a potential cut point with an associated sensitivity and specificity value. The area under the ROC curve often is used as a quantitative measure of the information content of a test. Values range from 0.5 (no diagnostic information from testing at all; the test is equivalent to flipping a coin) to 1.0 (perfect test). The choice of cut point should in theory reflect the relative harms and benefits of treatment for those without versus those with disease. For example, if treatment was safe with substantial benefit, then choosing a high-sensitivity cut point (upper right of the ROC curve) for a low-risk test may be appropriate (e.g., phenylketonuria in newborns), but if treatment had substantial risk for harm, then choosing a high-specificity cut point (lower left of the ROC curve) may be appropriate (e.g., chemotherapy for cancer). The choice of cut point may also depend on the prevalence of disease, with low prevalence placing a greater emphasis on the harms of false-positive tests (e.g., HIV testing in marriage applicants) or the harms of false-negative tests (e.g., HIV testing in blood donors).

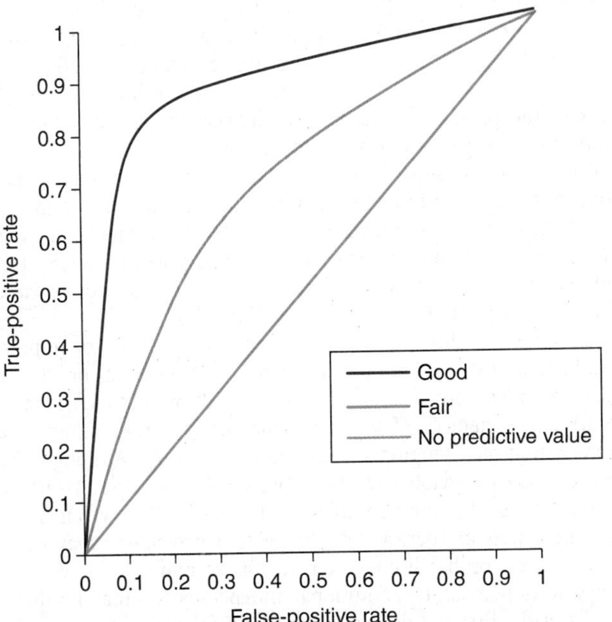

FIGURE 4-1 Each receiver operating characteristic (ROC curve) illustrates a trade-off that occurs between improved test sensitivity (accurate detection of patients with disease) and improved test specificity (accurate detection of patients without disease), as the test value defining when the test turns from "negative" to "positive" is varied. A 45° line would indicate a test with no predictive value (sensitivity = specificity at every test value). The area under each ROC curve is a measure of the information content of the test. Thus, a larger ROC area signifies increased diagnostic accuracy.

MEASURES OF DISEASE PROBABILITY AND BAYES' RULE

In the absence of perfect tests, the true disease state of the patient remains uncertain after every test. Bayes' rule provides a way to quantify the revised uncertainty using simple probability mathematics (and thereby avoid anchoring bias). It calculates the *posttest probability*, or likelihood of disease after a test result, from three parameters: the pretest probability of disease, the test sensitivity, and the test specificity. The *pretest probability* is a quantitative estimate of the likelihood of the diagnosis before the test is performed and is usually estimated from the prevalence of the disease in the underlying population (if known) or clinical context (e.g., age, sex, and type of chest pain). For some common conditions, such as CAD, existing nomograms and statistical models generate estimates of pretest probability that account for history, physical examination, and test findings. The posttest probability (also called the predictive value of the test, see below) is a recalibrated statement of the probability of the diagnosis, accounting for both pretest probability and test results. For the probability of disease following a positive test (i.e., positive predictive value), Bayes' rule is calculated as:

$$\text{Posttest probability} = \frac{\text{Pretest probability} \times \text{test sensitivity}}{\text{Pretest probability} \times \text{test sensitivity} + (1 - \text{Pretest probability}) \times (\text{false-positive test rate})}$$

For example, consider a 64-year-old woman with atypical chest pain who has a pretest probability of 0.50 and a "positive" diagnostic test result (assuming test sensitivity = 0.90 and specificity = 0.90).

$$\text{Posttest probability} = \frac{(0.50)(0.90)}{(0.50)(0.90) + (0.50)(0.10)} = 0.90$$

The term *predictive value* has often been used as a synonym for the posttest probability. Unfortunately, clinicians commonly misinterpret reported predictive values as intrinsic measures of test accuracy rather than calculated probabilities. Studies of diagnostic test performance compound the confusion by calculating predictive values from the same sample used to measure sensitivity and specificity. Such calculations are misleading unless the test is applied subsequently to populations with exactly the same disease prevalence. For these reasons, the term *predictive value* is best avoided in favor of the more descriptive posttest probability following a positive or a negative test result.

The nomogram version of Bayes' rule (**Fig. 4-2**) helps us to understand at a conceptual level how it estimates the posttest probability of disease. In this nomogram, the impact of the diagnostic test result is summarized by the likelihood ratio, which is defined as the ratio of the probability of a given test result (e.g., "positive" or "negative") in a patient with disease to the probability of that result in a patient without disease, thereby providing a measure of how well the test distinguishes those with from those without disease.

The *likelihood ratio for a positive test* is calculated as the ratio of the true-positive rate to the false-positive rate (or sensitivity/[1 – specificity]). For example, a test with a sensitivity of 0.90 and a specificity of 0.90 has a likelihood ratio of 0.90/(1 – 0.90), or 9. Thus, for this hypothetical test, a "positive" result is 9 times more likely in a patient with the disease than in a patient without it. Most tests in medicine have likelihood ratios for a positive result between 1.5 and 20. Higher values are associated with tests that more substantially increase the posttest likelihood of disease. A very high likelihood ratio positive (>10) usually implies high specificity, so a positive high specificity test helps "rule in" disease (the "SpPin" mnemonic introduced earlier). If sensitivity is excellent but specificity is less so, the likelihood ratio positive will be reduced substantially (e.g., with a 90% sensitivity but a 55% specificity, the likelihood ratio positive is 2.0).

The corresponding *likelihood ratio for a negative test* is the ratio of the false-negative rate to the true-negative rate (or [1 – sensitivity]/specificity).

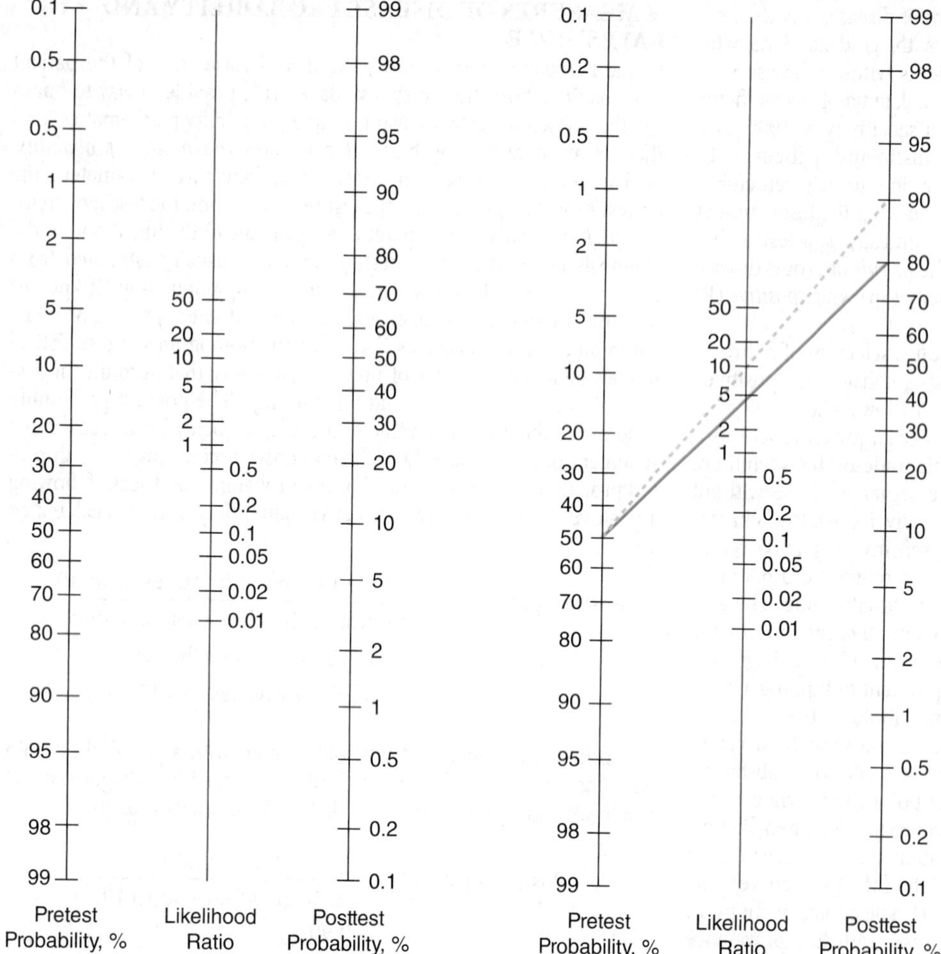

FIGURE 4-2 Nomogram version of Bayes' theorem used to predict the posttest probability of disease (right-hand scale) using the pretest probability of disease (left-hand scale) and the likelihood ratio for a positive or a negative test (middle scale). See text for information on calculation of likelihood ratios. To use, place a straightedge connecting the pretest probability and the likelihood ratio and read off the posttest probability. The right-hand part of the figure illustrates the value of a positive exercise treadmill test (likelihood ratio 4, *green line*) and a positive exercise thallium single-photon emission CT perfusion study (likelihood ratio 9, broken *yellow line*) in a patient with a pretest probability of coronary artery disease of 50%. *(Adapted from Centre for Evidence-Based Medicine: Likelihood ratios. Available at http://www.cebm.net/likelihood-ratios/.)*

Lower likelihood ratio negative values more substantially lower the posttest likelihood of disease. A very low likelihood ratio negative (falling below 0.10) usually implies high sensitivity, so a negative high sensitivity test helps "rule out" disease (the SnNout mnemonic). The hypothetical test considered above with a sensitivity of 0.9 and a specificity of 0.9 would have a likelihood ratio for a negative test result of (1 – 0.9)/0.9, or 0.11, meaning that a negative result is about one-tenth as likely in patients with disease than in those without disease (or about 10 times more likely in those without disease than in those with disease).

APPLICATIONS TO DIAGNOSTIC TESTING IN CAD

Consider two tests commonly used in the diagnosis of CAD: an exercise treadmill and an exercise single-photon emission CT (SPECT) myocardial perfusion imaging test (**Chap. 241**). A positive treadmill ST-segment response has an average sensitivity of ~60% and an average specificity of ~75%, yielding a likelihood ratio positive of 2.4 (0.60/[1 – 0.75]) (consistent with modest discriminatory ability because it falls between 2 and 5). For a 41-year-old man with nonanginal pain and a 10% pretest probability of CAD, the posttest probability of disease after a positive result rises to only ~30%. For a 60-year-old woman with typical angina and a pretest probability of CAD of 80%, a positive test result raises the posttest probability of disease to ~95%.

In contrast, exercise SPECT myocardial perfusion test is more accurate for diagnosis of CAD. For simplicity, assume that the finding of a reversible exercise-induced perfusion defect has both a sensitivity and a specificity of 90% (a bit higher than reported), yielding a likelihood ratio for a positive test of 9.0 (0.90/[1 – 0.90]) (consistent with intermediate discriminatory ability because it falls between 5 and 10). For the same 10% pretest probability patient, a positive test raises the probability of CAD to 50% (Fig. 4-2). However, despite the differences in posttest probabilities between these two tests (30 vs 50%), the more accurate test may not improve diagnostic likelihood enough to change patient management (e.g., decision to refer to cardiac catheterization) because the more accurate test has only moved the physician from being fairly certain that the patient did not have CAD to a 50:50 chance of disease. In a patient with a pretest probability of 80%, exercise SPECT test raises the posttest probability to 97% (compared with 95% for the exercise treadmill). Again, the more accurate test does not provide enough improvement in posttest confidence to alter management, and neither test has improved much on what was known from clinical data alone.

In general, positive results with an accurate test (e.g., likelihood ratio for a positive test of 10) when the pretest probability is low (e.g., 20%) do not move the posttest probability to a range high enough to rule in disease (e.g., 80%). In screening situations, pretest probabilities are often particularly low because patients are asymptomatic. In such cases, specificity becomes especially important. For example, in screening first-time female blood donors without risk factors for HIV, a positive test raised the likelihood of HIV to only 67% despite a specificity of 99.995% because the prevalence was 0.01%. Conversely, with a high pretest probability, a negative test may not rule out disease adequately if it is not sufficiently sensitive. Thus, the largest change in diagnostic likelihood following a test result occurs when the clinician is most uncertain (i.e., pretest probability between 30 and 70%). For example, in patients with a pretest probability for CAD of 50%, a positive exercise treadmill test moves the posttest probability to 80% and a positive exercise SPECT perfusion test moves it to 90% (Fig. 4-2).

As presented above, Bayes' rule employs a number of important simplifications that should be considered. First, few tests provide only "positive" or "negative" results. Many tests have multidimensional outcomes (e.g., extent of ST-segment depression, exercise duration, and exercise-induced symptoms with exercise testing). Although Bayes' theorem can be adapted to this more detailed test result format, it is computationally more complex to do so. Similarly, when multiple sequential tests are performed, the posttest probability may be used as the pretest probability to interpret the second test. However, this simplification assumes conditional independence—that is, that the results of the first test do not affect the likelihood of the second test result—and this is often not true.

Finally, many texts assert that sensitivity and specificity are prevalence-independent parameters of test accuracy. This statistically useful assumption, however, is often incorrect. A treadmill exercise test, for example, has a sensitivity of ~30% in a population of patients with one-vessel CAD, whereas its sensitivity in patients with severe three-vessel CAD approaches 80%. Thus, the best estimate of sensitivity to use in a particular decision may vary, depending on the severity of disease in the local population. A hospitalized, symptomatic, or referral population typically has a higher prevalence of disease and, in particular, a higher prevalence of more advanced disease than does an outpatient population. Consequently, test sensitivity will likely be higher in hospitalized patients and test specificity higher in outpatients.

STATISTICAL PREDICTION MODELS

Bayes' rule, when used as presented above, is useful in studying diagnostic testing concepts, but predictions based on multivariable statistical models can more accurately address these more complex problems by simultaneously accounting for additional relevant patient characteristics. In particular, these models explicitly account for multiple, even possibly overlapping, pieces of patient-specific information and assign a relative weight to each on the basis of its unique independent contribution to the prediction in question. For example, a logistic regression model to predict the probability of CAD ideally considers all the relevant independent factors from the clinical examination and diagnostic testing and their relative importance instead of the limited data that clinicians can manage in their heads or with Bayes' rule. However, despite this strength, prediction models are usually too complex computationally to use without a calculator or computer. Guideline-driven treatment recommendations based on statistical prediction models available online, e.g., the American College of Cardiology/American Heart Association risk calculator for primary prevention with statins and the CHA_2DS_2-VASC calculator for anticoagulation for atrial fibrillation, have generated more widespread usage. When electronic health records (EHRs) will provide sufficient platform support to allow for routine use of predictive models in clinical practice and increase their impact on clinical encounters and outcomes remains uncertain.

One reason for limited clinical use is that, to date, only a handful of prediction models have been validated sufficiently (for example, Wells criteria for pulmonary embolism; **Table 4-2**). The importance of independent validation in a population separate from the one used to develop the model cannot be overstated. An unvalidated prediction model should be viewed with the skepticism appropriate for any new drug or medical device that has not had rigorous clinical trial testing.

When statistical survival models in cancer and heart disease have been compared directly with clinicians' predictions, the survival models have been found to be more consistent, as would be expected, but not always more accurate. On the other hand, comparison of clinicians with websites and apps that generate lists of possible diagnoses to help patients with self-diagnosis found that physicians outperformed the currently available programs. For students and less-experienced clinicians, the biggest value of diagnostic decision support may be in extending diagnostic possibilities and triggering "rational override," but their impact on knowledge, information-seeking, and problem-solving needs additional research.

TABLE 4-2 Wells Clinical Prediction Rule for Pulmonary Embolism (PE)

CLINICAL FEATURE	POINTS
Clinical signs of deep-vein thrombosis	3
Alternative diagnosis is less likely than PE	3
Heart rate >100 beats/min	1.5
Immobilization ≥3 days or surgery in previous 4 weeks	1.5
History of deep-vein thrombosis or pulmonary embolism	1.5
Hemoptysis	1
Malignancy (with treatment within 6 months) or palliative	1
INTERPRETATION	
Score >6.0	High
Score 2.0–6.0	Intermediate
Score <2.0	Low

FORMAL DECISION SUPPORT TOOLS

DECISION SUPPORT SYSTEMS

Over the past 50 years, many attempts have been made to develop computer systems to aid clinical decision-making and patient management. Conceptually, computers offer several levels of potentially useful support for clinicians. At the most basic level, they provide ready access to vast reservoirs of information, which may, however, be quite difficult to sort through to find what is needed. At higher levels, computers can support care management decisions by making accurate predictions of outcome, or can simulate the whole decision process, and provide algorithmic guidance. Computer-based predictions using Bayesian or statistical regression models inform a clinical decision but do not actually reach a "conclusion" or "recommendation." Machine learning methods are being applied to pattern recognition tasks such as the examination of skin lesions and the interpretation of x-rays. Artificial intelligence (AI) systems attempt to simulate or replace human reasoning with a computer-based analogue. Natural language processing allows the system to access and process large amounts of data, both from the EHR and from the medical literature. To date, such approaches have achieved only limited success. The most prominent example, IBM's Watson program, introduced publicly in 2011, has yet to produce persuasive evidence of clinical decision support utility. Reminder or protocol-directed systems do not make predictions but use existing algorithms, such as guidelines or appropriate utilization criteria, to direct clinical practice. In general, however, decision support systems have so far had little impact on practice. Reminder systems built into EHRs have shown the most promise, particularly in correcting drug dosing and promoting adherence to guidelines. Checklists may also help avoid or reduce errors.

DECISION ANALYSIS

Compared with the decision support methods discussed earlier, decision analysis represents a normative prescriptive approach to decision-making in the face of uncertainty. Its principal application is in complex decisions. For example, public health policy decisions often involve *trade-offs* in length versus quality of life, benefits versus resource use, population versus individual health, and *uncertainty* regarding efficacy, effectiveness, and adverse events as well as *values* or preferences regarding mortality and morbidity outcomes.

One recent analysis using this approach involved the optimal screening strategy for breast cancer, which has remained controversial, in part because a randomized controlled trial to determine when to begin screening and how often to repeat screening mammography is impractical. In 2016, the National Cancer Institute–sponsored Cancer Intervention and Surveillance Network (CISNET) examined eight strategies differing by whether to initiate mammography screening at age 40, 45, or 50 years and whether to screen annually, biennially, or annually for women in their forties and biennially thereafter (hybrid). The six simulation models found biennial strategies to be the most efficient for average-risk women. Biennial screening for 1000 women from age 50–74 years versus no screening avoided seven breast cancer deaths. Screening annually from age 40–74 years avoided three additional deaths but required 20,000 additional mammograms and yielded 1988 more false-positive results. Factors that influenced the results included patients with a 2–4-fold higher risk for developing breast cancer in whom annual screening from age 40–74 years yielded similar benefits as biennial screening from age 50–74. For average-risk patients with moderate or severe comorbidities, screening could be stopped earlier, at age 66–68 years.

This analysis involved six models that reproduced epidemiologic trends and a screening trial result, accounted for digital technology and treatments advances, and considered quality of life, risk factors, breast density, and comorbidity. It provided novel insights into a public health problem in the absence of a randomized clinical trial and helped weigh the pros and cons of such a health policy recommendation. Although such models have been developed for selected clinical problems, their benefit and application to individual real-time clinical management has yet to be demonstrated.

DIAGNOSIS AS AN ELEMENT OF QUALITY OF CARE

High-quality medical care begins with accurate diagnosis. The incidence of diagnostic errors has been estimated by a variety of methods including postmortem examinations, medical record reviews, and medical malpractice claims, with each yielding complementary but different estimates of this quality of care patient-safety problem. In the past, diagnostic errors tended to be viewed as a failure of individual clinicians. The modern view is that they are mostly a system of care deficiencies. Current estimates suggest that nearly everyone will experience at least one diagnostic error in their lifetime, leading to mortality, morbidity, unnecessary tests and procedures, costs, and anxiety.

Solutions to the "diagnostic errors as a system of care" problem have focused on system-level approaches, such as decision support and other tools integrated into EHRs. The use of checklists has been proposed as a means of reducing some of the cognitive errors discussed earlier in the chapter, such as premature closure. While checklists have been shown to be useful in certain medical contexts, such as operating rooms and intensive care units, their value in preventing diagnostic errors that lead to patient adverse events remains to be shown.

EVIDENCE-BASED MEDICINE

Clinical medicine is defined traditionally as a practice combining medical knowledge (including scientific evidence), intuition, and judgment in the care of patients (**Chap. 1**). Evidence-based medicine (EBM) updates this construct by placing much greater emphasis on the processes by which clinicians gain knowledge of the most up-to-date and relevant clinical research to determine for themselves whether medical interventions alter the disease course and improve the length or quality of life. The phrase "evidence-based medicine" is now used so often and in so many different contexts that many practitioners are unaware of its original meaning. The intention of the EBM program, as described in the early 1990s by its founding proponents at McMaster University, becomes clearer through an examination of its four key steps:

1. Formulating the management question to be answered
2. Searching the literature and online databases for applicable research data
3. Appraising the evidence gathered with regard to its validity and relevance
4. Integrating this appraisal with knowledge about the unique aspects of the patient (including the patient's preferences about the possible outcomes)

The process of searching the world's research literature and appraising the quality and relevance of studies can be time-consuming and requires skills and training that most clinicians do not possess. In a busy clinical practice, the work required is also logistically not feasible. This has led to a focus on finding recent systematic overviews of the problem in question as a useful shortcut in the EBM process. Systematic reviews are regarded by some as the highest level of evidence in the EBM hierarchy because they are intended to comprehensively summarize the available evidence on a particular topic. To avoid the potential biases found in narrative review articles, predefined reproducible explicit search strategies and inclusion and exclusion criteria seek to find all of the relevant scientific research and grade its quality. The prototype for this kind of resource is the Cochrane Database of Systematic Reviews. When appropriate, a meta-analysis is used to quantitatively summarize the systematic review findings (discussed further below).

Unfortunately, systematic reviews are not uniformly the acme of the EBM process they were initially envisioned to be. In select circumstances, they can provide a much clearer picture of the state of the evidence than is available from any individual clinical report, but their value is less clear when only a few trials are available, when trials and observational studies are mixed, or when the evidence base is only observational. They cannot compensate for deficiencies in the underlying research available, and many are created without the requisite clinical insights. The medical literature is now flooded with systematic reviews of varying quality and clinical utility. The peer review system has, unfortunately, not proved to be an effective arbiter of quality of these papers. Therefore, systematic reviews should be used with circumspection in conjunction with selective reading of some of the best empirical studies.

■ SOURCES OF EVIDENCE: CLINICAL TRIALS AND REGISTRIES

The notion of learning from observation of patients is as old as medicine itself. Over the past 50 years, physicians' understanding of how best to turn raw observation into useful evidence has evolved considerably. Medicine has received a hard refresher lesson in this process from COVID-19 pandemic. Starting in the spring of 2020, case reports, personal and institutional anecdotal experience, and small single-center case series started appearing in the peer-reviewed literature and within months turned into a flood of confusing and often contradictory evidence. Observational reports of treatments for COVID-19 fueled the confusion. Despite >40,000 publications appearing in the first 7 months of the pandemic, an enormous amount of uncertainty around prevention, diagnosis, treatment, and prognosis of the disease remained. Many of the early 2020 publications were either small observational series or reviews of published series, neither of which can resolve the key uncertainties clinicians need to address in caring for these patients. These small observational studies often have substantial limitations in validity and generalizability, and although they may generate important hypotheses or be the first reports of adverse events or therapeutic benefit, they have no role in formulating modern standards of practice. The major tools used to develop reliable evidence consist of randomized clinical trials supplemented strategically by large (high-quality) observational registries. A registry or database typically is focused on a disease or syndrome (e.g., different types of cancer, acute or chronic CAD, pacemaker capture, or chronic heart failure), a clinical procedure (e.g., bone marrow transplantation, coronary revascularization), or an administrative process (e.g., claims data used for billing and reimbursement).

By definition, in observational data, the investigator does not control patient care. Carefully collected prospective observational data, however, can at times achieve a level of evidence quality approaching that of major clinical trial data. At the other end of the spectrum, data collected retrospectively (e.g., chart review) are limited in form and content to what previous observers recorded and may not include the specific research data being sought (e.g., claims data). Advantages of observational data include the inclusion of a broader population as encountered in practice than is typically represented in clinical trials because of their restrictive inclusion and exclusion criteria. In addition, observational data provide primary evidence for research questions when a randomized trial cannot be performed. For example, it would be difficult to randomize patients to test diagnostic or therapeutic strategies that are unproven but widely accepted in practice, and it would be unethical to randomize based on sex, racial/ethnic group, socioeconomic status, or country of residence or to randomize patients to a potentially harmful intervention, such as smoking or deliberately overeating to develop obesity.

A well-done prospective observational study of a particular management strategy differs from a well-done randomized clinical trial most importantly by its lack of protection from treatment selection bias. The use of observational data to compare diagnostic or therapeutic strategies assumes that sufficient uncertainty and heterogeneity exists in clinical practice to ensure that similar patients will be managed differently by diverse physicians. In short, the analysis assumes that a sufficient element of randomness (in the sense of disorder rather than in the formal statistical sense) exists in clinical management. In such cases, statistical models attempt to adjust for important imbalances to "level the playing field" so that a fair comparison among treatment options can be made. When management is clearly not random (e.g., all eligible left main CAD patients are referred for coronary bypass surgery), the problem may be too confounded (biased) for statistical correction, and observational data may not provide reliable evidence.

In general, the use of concurrent controls is vastly preferable to that of historical controls. For example, comparison of current surgical management of left main CAD with medically treated patients with left main CAD during the 1970s (the last time these patients were routinely treated with medicine alone) would be extremely misleading because "medical therapy" has substantially improved in the interim.

Randomized controlled clinical trials include the careful prospective design features of the best observational data studies but also include the use of random allocation of treatment. This design provides the best protection against measured and unmeasured confounding due to treatment selection bias (a major aspect of internal validity). However, the randomized trial may not have good external validity (generalizability) if the process of recruitment into the trial resulted in the exclusion of many potentially eligible subjects or if the nominal eligibility for the trial describes a very heterogeneous population.

Consumers of medical evidence need to be aware that randomized trials vary widely in their quality and applicability to practice. The process of designing such a trial often involves many compromises. For example, trials designed to gain U.S. Food and Drug Administration (FDA) approval for an investigational drug or device must fulfill regulatory requirements (such as the use of a placebo control) that may result in a trial population and design that differ substantially from what practicing clinicians would find most useful.

META-ANALYSIS

The Greek prefix *meta* signifies something at a later or higher stage of development. Meta-analysis is research that combines and summarizes the available evidence quantitatively. Although it is used to examine nonrandomized studies, meta-analysis is most useful for summarizing all available randomized trials examining a particular therapy used in a specific clinical context. Ideally, unpublished trials should be identified and included to avoid publication bias (i.e., missing "negative" trials that may not be published). Furthermore, the best meta-analyses obtain and analyze individual patient-level data from all trials rather than using only the summary data from published reports. Nonetheless, not all published meta-analyses yield reliable evidence for a particular problem, so their methodology should be scrutinized carefully to ensure proper study design and analysis. The results of a well-done meta-analysis are likely to be most persuasive if they include at least several large-scale, properly performed randomized trials. Meta-analysis can especially help detect benefits when individual trials are inadequately powered (e.g., the benefits of streptokinase thrombolytic therapy in acute MI demonstrated by ISIS-2 in 1988 were evident by the early 1970s through meta-analysis). However, in cases in which the available trials are small or poorly done, meta-analysis should not be viewed as a remedy for deficiencies in primary trial data or trial design.

Meta-analyses typically focus on summary measures of relative treatment benefit, such as odds ratios or relative risks. Clinicians should also examine what absolute risk reduction (ARR) can be expected from the therapy. A metric of absolute treatment benefit that is frequently reported is the number needed to treat (NNT) to prevent one adverse outcome event (e.g., death, stroke). NNT should not be interpreted literally as a causal statement. NNT is simply 1/ARR. For example, if a hypothetical therapy reduced mortality rates over a 5-year follow-up by 33% (the relative treatment benefit) from 12% (control arm) to 8% (treatment arm), the ARR would be 12% – 8% = 4% and the NNT would be 1/.04, or 25. This does not mean literally that 1 patient benefits and 24 do not. However, it can be conceptualized as an informal measure of treatment efficiency. If the hypothetical treatment was applied to a lower-risk population, say, with a 6% 5-year mortality, the 33% relative treatment benefit would reduce absolute mortality by 2% (from 6% to 4%), and the NNT for the same therapy in this lower-risk group of patients would be 50. Although not always made explicit, comparisons of NNT estimates from different studies should account for the duration of follow-up used to create each estimate. In addition, the NNT concept assumes a homogeneity in response to treatment that may not be accurate. The NNT is simply another way of summarizing the absolute treatment difference and does not provide any unique information.

CLINICAL PRACTICE GUIDELINES

Per the 1990 Institute of Medicine definition, clinical practice guidelines are "systematically developed statements to assist practitioner and patient decisions about appropriate health care for specific clinical circumstances." This definition emphasizes several crucial features of modern guideline development. First, guidelines are created by using the tools of EBM. In particular, the core of the development process is a systematic literature search followed by a review of the relevant peer-reviewed literature. Second, guidelines usually are focused on a clinical disorder (e.g., diabetes mellitus, stable angina pectoris) or a health care intervention (e.g., cancer screening). Third, the primary objective of guidelines is to improve the quality of medical care by identifying care practices that should be routinely implemented, based on high-quality evidence and high benefit-to-harm ratios for the interventions. Guidelines are intended to "assist" decision-making, not to define explicitly what decisions should be made in a particular situation, in part because guideline-level evidence alone is never sufficient for clinical decision-making (e.g., deciding whether to intubate and administer antibiotics for pneumonia in a terminally ill individual, in an individual with dementia, or in an otherwise healthy 30-year-old mother).

Guidelines are narrative documents constructed by expert panels whose composition often is determined by interested professional organizations. These panels vary in expertise and in the degree to which they represent all relevant stakeholders. The guideline documents consist of a series of specific management recommendations, a summary indication of the quantity and quality of evidence supporting each recommendation, an assessment of the benefit-to-harm ratio for the recommendation, and a narrative discussion of the recommendations. Many recommendations simply reflect the expert consensus of the guideline panel because literature-based evidence is insufficient or absent. A recent examination of this issue in cardiovascular guidelines showed that <15% of guideline recommendations were based on the highest level of clinical trial evidence, and this proportion had not improved in 10 years despite a substantial number of trials being conducted and published. The final step in guideline construction is peer review, followed by a final revision in response to the critiques provided.

Guidelines are closely tied to the process of quality improvement in medicine through their identification of evidence-based best practices. Such practices can be used as quality indicators. Examples include the proportion of acute MI patients who receive aspirin upon admission to a hospital and the proportion of heart failure patients with a depressed ejection fraction treated with an ACE inhibitor.

CONCLUSIONS

Thirty years after the introduction of the EBM movement, it is tempting to think that all the difficult decisions practitioners face have been or soon will be solved and digested into practice guidelines and computerized reminders. However, EBM provides practitioners with an ideal rather than a finished set of tools with which to manage patients. Moreover, even with such evidence, it is always worth remembering that the response to therapy of the "average" patient represented by the summary clinical trial outcomes may not be what can be expected for the specific patient sitting in front of a provider in the clinic or hospital. In addition, meta-analyses cannot generate evidence when there are no adequate randomized trials, and most of what clinicians confront in practice will never be thoroughly tested in a randomized trial. For the foreseeable future, excellent clinical reasoning skills and experience supplemented by well-designed quantitative tools and a keen appreciation for the role of individual patient preferences in their health care will continue to be of paramount importance in the practice of clinical medicine.

FURTHER READING

Croskerry P: A universal model of diagnostic reasoning. Acad Med 84:1022, 2009.

Dhaliwal G, Detsky AS: The evolution of the master diagnostician. JAMA 310:579, 2013.

Fanaroff AC et al: Levels of evidence supporting American College of Cardiology/American Heart Association and European Society of Cardiology Guidelines, 2008-2018. JAMA 321:1069, 2019.

Hunink MGM et al: *Decision Making in Health and Medicine: Integrating Evidence and Values*, 2nd ed. Cambridge, Cambridge University Press, 2014.

Kahneman D: *Thinking Fast and Slow*. New York, Farrar, Straus and Giroux, 2013.

Kassirer JP et al: *Learning Clinical Reasoning*, 2nd ed. Baltimore, Lippincott Williams & Wilkins, 2009.

Mandelblatt JS et al: Collaborative modeling of the benefits and harms of associated with different U.S. breast cancer screening strategies. Ann Intern Med 164:215, 2016.

Monteior S et al: The 3 faces of clinical reasoning: Epistemological explorations of disparate error reduction strategies. J Eval Clin Pract 24:666, 2018.

Murthy VK et al: An inquiry into the early careers of master clinicians. J Grad Med Educ 10:500, 2018.

Richards JB et al: Teaching clinical reasoning and critical thinking: From cognitive theory to practical application. Chest 158:1617, 2020.

Royce CS et al: Teaching critical thinking: A case for instruction in cognitive biases to reduce diagnostic errors and improve patient safety. Acad Med 94:187, 2019.

Saposnik G et al: Cognitive biases associated with medical decisions: A systematic review. BMC Med Inform Decis Mak 16:138, 2016.

Schuwirth LWT et al: Assessment of clinical reasoning: three evolutions of thought. Diagnosis (Berl) 7:191, 2020.

5 Precision Medicine and Clinical Care

The Editors

DISEASE NOSOLOGY AND PRECISION MEDICINE

Modern disease nosology arose in the late nineteenth century and represented a clear departure from the holistic, limited descriptions of disease dating to Galen. In this rubric, the definition of any disease is largely based on clinicopathologic observation. As the correlation between clinical signs and symptoms with pathoanatomy required autopsy material, diseases tended to be characterized by the end organ in which the primary syndrome was manifest and by late-stage presentations. Morgagni institutionalized this framework with the publication of *De Sedibus et Causis Morborum per Anatomen Indagatis* in 1761, in which he correlated the clinical features of patients with more than 600 autopsies at the University of Padua, demonstrating an anatomic basis for disease pathophysiology. Clinicopathologic observation served as the basis for inductive generalization coupled with the application of Occam's razor in which disease complexity was reduced to its simplest possible form. While this approach to defining human disease has held sway for over a century and facilitated the conquest of many diseases previously considered incurable, overly inclusive and simplified Oslerian diagnostics suffer from significant shortcomings. These include, but are not limited to, failure to distinguish the underlying etiology of different diseases with common pathophenotypes. For example, many different diseases can cause end-stage kidney disease or heart failure. Over time, the classification of neurodegenerative disorders or lymphomas, as well as many other diseases, is becoming more refined and precise as the underlying etiologies are identified. These distinctions are important for providing predictable prognostic information for individual patients with even highly prevalent diseases. Additionally, therapies may be ineffective owing to a lack of understanding of the often subtle molecular complexities of specific disease drivers.

Beginning in the mid-twentieth century, the era of molecular medicine offered the idealized possibility of identifying the underlying molecular basis of every disease. Using a conventional reductionist paradigm, physician-scientists explored disease mechanism at ever-increasing molecular depth, seeking the single (or limited number of) molecular cause(s) of many human diseases. Yet, as effective as this now conventional scientific approach was at uncovering many disease mechanisms, the clinical manifestations of very few diseases could be explained on the basis of a single molecular mechanism. Even knowledge of the globin β chain mutation that causes sickle cell disease does not predict the many different manifestations of the disease (stroke syndrome, painful crises, and hemolytic crisis, among others). Clearly, the profession had expected too much from oversimplified reductionism and failed to take into consideration the extraordinary biologic variety and its accompanying molecular and genetic complexity that underpin both normal and pathologic diversity. The promise of the Human Genome Project provided new tools and approaches and unleashed efforts to identify a monogenic, oligogenic, or polygenic cause for every disease (allowing for environmental modulation). Yet, once again, disappointment reigned as the pool of genomes expanded without the expected revelations (aside from rare variants). The arc of progressive reductionism (as illustrated for tuberculosis in **Fig. 5-1**) in refining and explaining disease reached a humbling plateau, revealing the need for new approaches to understand better the etiology, manifestations, and progression of most diseases. The stage was set for a return to holism. However, in contrast to the holism of ancient physicians, we adopted one that is integrative, taking genomic context into account in all dimensions. In the course of elaborating this complex pathobiologic landscape, disease definition must become more precise and progressively more individualized, setting the stage for what we term *precision medicine*.

Oversimplification of phenotype is a natural outgrowth of the observational scientific method. Categorizing individuals as falling into groups or clusters that are reasonably similar simplifies the task of the diagnostician and also facilitates the application of "specific" therapies more broadly. Biomedicine has been viewed as less quantitative and precise than other scientific disciplines, with biologic and pathobiologic diversity (biologic "noise") viewed as the norm. Thus, distilling such observational complexity to a fundamental group of symptoms or signs that are reasonably invariant across a group of sick individuals has served as the basis for the approach to disease and its treatment since the earliest days of medicine. This approach to diagnosis and therapy has remained in place into the twenty-first century, serving as the basis for the development of standard diagnostic tests and of broadly applied drug therapies. Targeting larger groups of patients is efficient when applied to large populations. As successful as this approach has been in advancing medical care, it is important to point out its limitations, which include significant predictive inaccuracies and sizeable segments of the disease population who do not respond to the most "effective" drugs (upward of 60% by some estimates). Clearly, a more nuanced approach to diagnosis and therapy is required to achieve better prognostic and therapeutic outcomes.

Turning first to phenotype, astute clinicians know full well the subtle and vivid differences in presentation that are often manifest among individuals with the same disease. In some cases, these differences in pathophenotype lead to new subclassifications of the disease, such as heart failure with preserved ejection fraction versus heart failure with reduced ejection fraction. Often, these relatively crude efforts at making diagnoses more precise are driven by new technologies or new ways of applying established technologies. In other cases, differences in pathophenotype are more subtle, not necessarily clinically apparent, and often driven by measures of endophenotype, such as distinctions among vasculitides facilitated by refinements in serologies or immunophenotyping. The impetus to create these subclasses of disease is largely determined by the need to improve prognosis and apply more precise and effective therapies. Based on these guiding principles, many experienced clinicians will argue—and rightly so—that they have been practicing personalized, precision medicine throughout their careers: they characterize each patient's illness in great detail, and choose therapies that respect and are guided by those individualized clinical and laboratory features, limited though they may be.

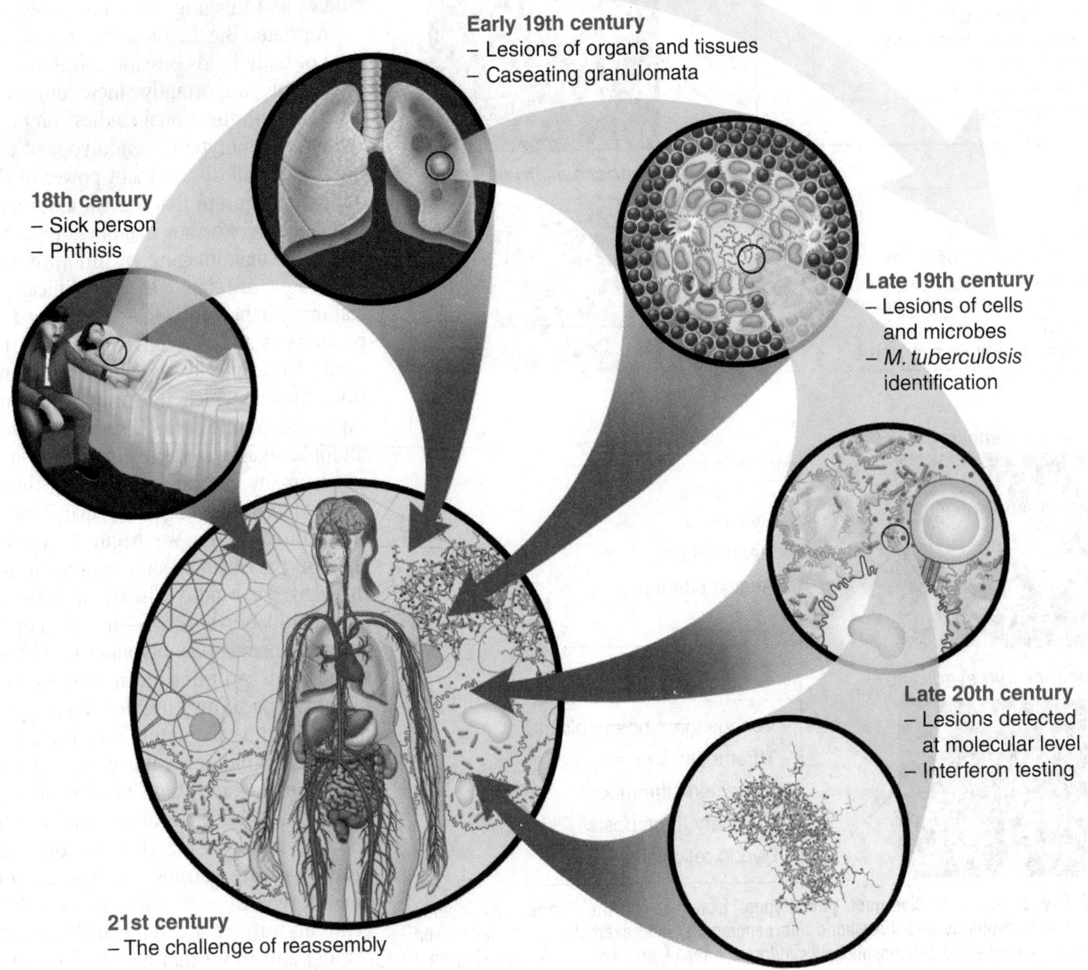

FIGURE 5-1 Arc of reductionism in medicine. *(From JA Greene, J Loscalzo. Putting the patient back together–social medicine, network medicine, and the limits of reductionism. N Engl J Med 377:2493, 2017. Copyright © 2017 Massachusetts Medical Society. Reprinted with permission from Massachusetts Medical Society.)*

For many diseases, genomic variation, whether inherited or acquired, provides opportunities to refine diagnostic precision with even greater fidelity and predictive accuracy. For this reason, the field of precision medicine has now entered a new era that couples the molecular reductionism of the last century with an integrative, systems-level understanding of the basis for pathophenotype. Equally important, modern genomics has established that genomic context, sometimes referred to as modifier genes, is distinctive for each individual person; hence, understanding that context provides the insight necessary to predict how a primary disease driver or drivers may manifest a clinical pathophenotype—e.g., why some individuals with sickle cell anemia will develop stroke, while others will develop acute chest syndrome. *This concept that primary genetic and/or environmental drivers of a disease differentially affect disease expression based on an individual's unique genomic context serves as the ultimate basis for much of what we denote as precision medicine.*

To develop a precision medicine strategy for any disease, the clinician needs to be aware of two important, confounding principles. First, patients with different diseases can manifest similar pathophenotypes, i.e., *convergent phenotypes.* Examples of this principle include the hypertrophied myocardium found in hypertrophic cardiomyopathy, infiltrative cardiomyopathies, critical aortic stenosis, and untreated, long-standing hypertension; and the thrombotic microangiopathy found in malignant hypertension, scleroderma renal crisis, thrombotic thrombocytopenic purpura, eclampsia, and antiphospholipid syndrome. Second, patients with the same basic disease can manifest very different pathophenotypes, i.e., *divergent phenotypes* **(Chap. 466)**. Examples of this principle include the different clinical manifestations of cystic fibrosis or sickle cell disease and the incomplete penetrance of many common genetic diseases. These common presentations of different diseases and different presentations of the same disease are both a consequence of genomic context coupled with unique exposures over an individual's lifetime **(Fig. 5-2)**. Understanding the interplay among these many complex molecular determinants of disease expression is essential for the success of precision medicine.

Given the complexity of the genomic and environmental context of an individual, one must ask the question: How precise do we need to be in order to practice effective precision medicine? Complete knowledge of a person's comprehensive genome (DNA, gene expression, mitochondrial function, proteome, metabolome, posttranslational modification of the proteome, and metagenome, among others) and quantitative assessments of environmental and social history are not possible to acquire; yet, this shortcoming does not render the general problem intractable. Owing to the fact that the molecular networks that govern phenotype are overdetermined (i.e., redundant) and that there are primary drivers of disease expression that are modified in a weighted way by other genomic features of an individual, the practice of precision medicine can be realized without complete knowledge of all dimensions of the genome. Examples of how best to realize this strategy are discussed later in this chapter.

REQUIREMENTS FOR PRECISION MEDICINE

The essential elements of any precision medicine effort include phenotyping, endophenotyping (defining the characteristics of a disorder that are not readily observable), and genomic profiling **(Fig. 5-3)**. While subtle distinctions among individuals with the same disease are well known to clinicians, formalizing these nuanced differences is critical for achieving more precise phenotypes. Deep phenotyping requires a

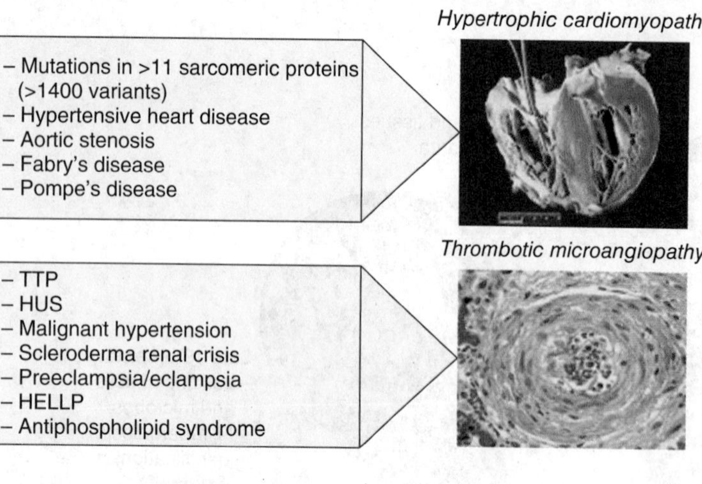

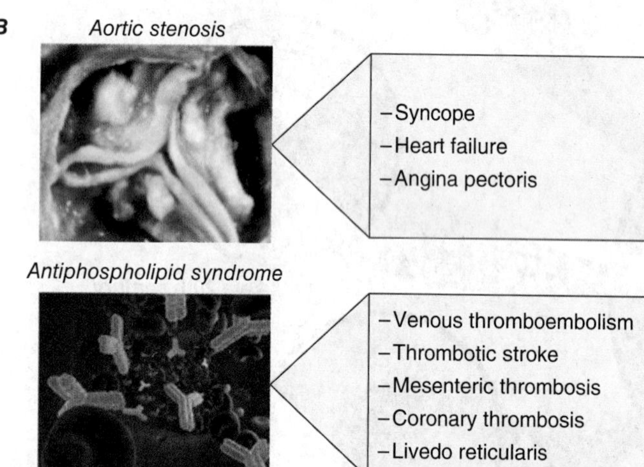

FIGURE 5-2 Convergent and divergent phenotypes. Examples of the former (***A***) include hypertrophic cardiomyopathy and thrombotic microangiopathy, and examples of the latter, and (***B***) include aortic stenosis and antiphospholipid syndrome, each of which can have several distinct clinical presentations. HELLP, hemolysis, elevated liver enzymes, and a low platelet count; HUS, hemolytic-uremic syndrome; TTP, thrombotic thrombocytopenic purpura.

detailed history, including family history and environmental exposures, as well as relevant (physiologic) functional studies and imaging, including molecular imaging where appropriate. Biochemical, immunologic, and molecular tests of body fluids provide additional detail to the overall phenotype. Importantly, these objective laboratory tests together with functional studies compose an assessment of the endophenotype (or endotype) of an individual, refining the overall discriminant power of the evaluation. One additional concept that has gained traction in recent years is the notion of orthogonal phenotyping, i.e., assessing clinical, molecular, imaging, or functional (endo)phenotypes seemingly unrelated to the clinical presentation. These features further enhance the ability to distinguish (sub) phenotypes and derive from the fact that diseases can be subtly (subclinically) manifest in organ systems different from that in which the primary symptoms or signs are expressed. While some diseases are well known to affect multiple organ systems (e.g., systemic lupus erythematosus) and in many cases involvement of those many systems is assessed at initial diagnosis, such is not the case for most other diseases. As we begin to understand the differences in the organ-specific expression of genomic variants that drive or modify disease, it is becoming increasingly apparent that orthogonal—or more appropriately, unbiased comprehensive—phenotyping should become the norm.

Genomic profiling must next be coupled to detailed phenotyping. The complex levels of genomic assessment continue to mature and include DNA sequencing (exomic, whole genome), gene expression (mRNA and protein expression), and metabolomics. In addition, the epigenome, the posttranslationally modified proteome, and the metagenome (the personal microbiome of an individual) are gaining traction as additional elements of comprehensive genomics (**Chap. 483**). Not all of these genomic features are yet available for clinical laboratory testing, and those that are available are largely confined to blood testing. While DNA sequencing using whole blood would generally apply to any organ-based disease,

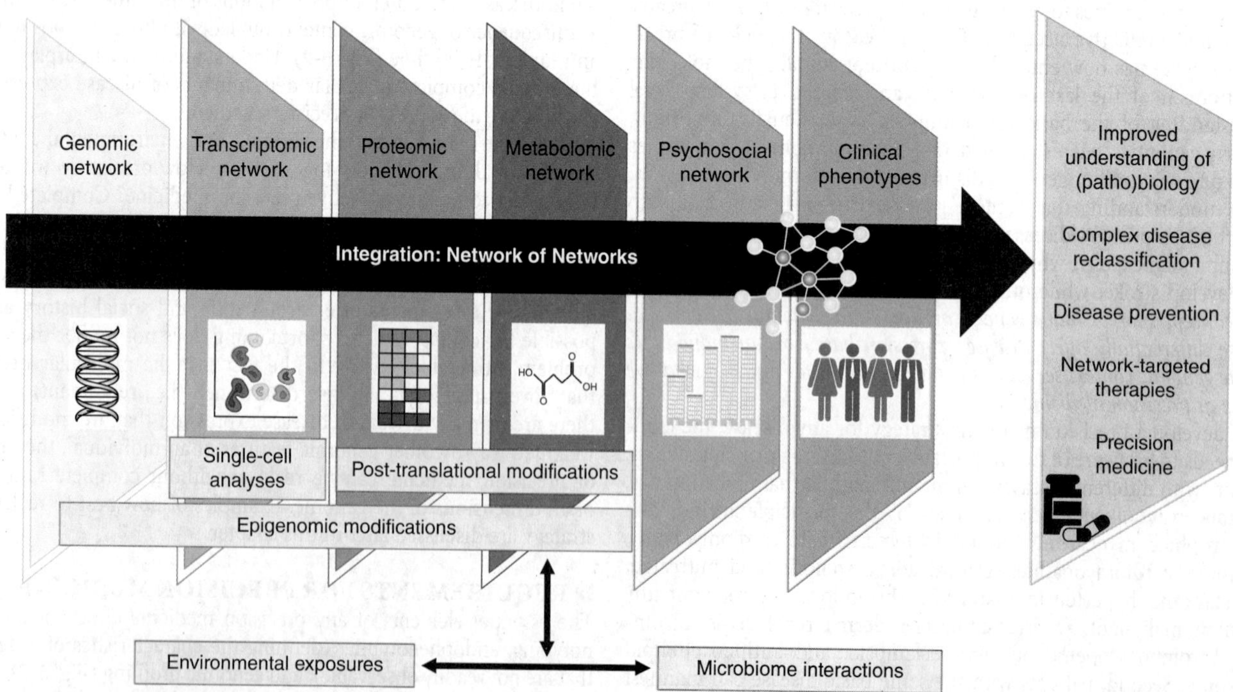

FIGURE 5-3 Universe of precision medicine. The totality of precision medicine incorporates multidimensional biologic networks, the integration of which leads to a network of networks whose components interact with each other and with environmental exposures to yield a distinctive phenotype or pathophenotype. *(Reproduced with permission from LY-H Lee, J Loscalzo: Network medicine in pathobiology. Am J Pathol 189:1311, 2019.)*

gene expression, metabolomics, and epigenetics are often tissue specific. As tissue specimens cannot always or easily be obtained from the organ of interest, attempts at correlating whole-blood mRNA, protein, or metabolite profiles with those of the involved organ are critical for precise prognostics and therapeutic choices. In many cases, systemic consequences to an organ-specific disease (e.g., systemic inflammatory responses in individuals with atherosclerosis) can be ascertained and may provide useful prognostic information or therapeutic strategies. These biomarker signatures are the subject of ongoing discovery and have provided useful guidance toward improved diagnostic precision in many diseases. However, in many diseases, the correlations between these plasma or blood markers and organ-based diseases are weak, indicating a need to analyze each condition and each resulting signature before applying it to clinical decision-making. It is important to note that one of the key determinants of the functional consequences of a genetic variant believed to drive a disease phenotype is not simply its expression in a tissue of interest but, more importantly, the coexpression of protein binding partners in that same tissue comprising specific (dys)functional pathways that govern phenotype (Fig. 5-4). An alternative strategy currently under investigation is the conversion of induced pluripotent stem cells from a patient into a cell type of interest for gene expression or metabolomics study. As rational as this approach seems from first principles, it is important to note that gene expression patterns in these induced, differentiated cell types are not completely consonant with their native counterparts, offering often limited additional information at potentially great additional expense.

While phenotype features of many chronic diseases are assessed over time, genomic features tend to be limited to single time point sampling. Time trajectories are extremely informative in precision genotyping and phenotyping, with gene expression patterns and phenotypes changing over time in different ways among different patients with the same overarching phenotype. Cost, feasible sampling frequency, predictive power, and therapeutic choices will all drive the optimal strategy for the acquisition of timed samples in any given patient; however, with continued cost reduction in genomics technologies, this limitation may be progressively mitigated and clinical application may become a reality.

One important class of diseases that does not have most of these limitations in genomic profiling is cancer. Cancers can be (and are) sampled (biopsied) frequently to monitor temporal changes in the somatically mutating oncogenome and its consequences for the limited number of well-defined oncogenic driver pathways (Chap. 68). A unique limitation of cancer in this regard, however, is that the frequency of somatic mutations over time (and, especially, with treatment) is great and the functional consequences of many of these mutations unknown. Equally important, assessment of single-cell mRNA sequencing patterns demonstrates great variability between apparently similar cells, challenging functional interpretation. Lastly, in solid tumors, stromal cells interact in a variety of ways (e.g., metabolically) with the associated malignant cells, and their gene expression signatures are also modified by the changing somatic mutational landscape of the primary malignancy. Thus, while much more information can be obtained over time in most cancer patients, the interpretation of these rich data sets continues to remain largely semi-empirical.

The possibility of identifying specific therapeutic targets remains a major goal of precision medicine. Doing so requires more than simple DNA sequencing and must include analysis of some level of gene expression, ideally in the involved organ(s). In addition to demonstrating the expression of a variant protein in the organ, one must ideally also demonstrate its functional consequences, which requires ascertaining the expression of binding partner proteins and the functional pathways they comprise. To achieve this goal, a variety of approaches have been tried, one of the most successful of which is the construction of the protein-protein interactome (the interactome), which is a comprehensive network map of the protein-protein interactions in a cell or organ of interest (Chap. 486). This template provides information on the subnetworks that govern a disease phenotype (disease modules), which can be further individualized by incorporating individual variants and differentially expressed proteins that are patient specific. This type of analysis leads to the creation of an individual "reticulome" or reticulotype, which links the genotype to the phenotype of an individual (Fig. 5-5). Using this approach, one can identify potential drug targets in a rational way or can even repurpose existing drugs by demonstrating the proximity of a known drug target to a disease module of interest (Fig. 5-6). For example, in multicentric Castleman's disease, a disorder of unclear etiology, recognition that the PI3K/Akt/mTOR pathway is highly activated led to trials with an existing, approved drug, sirolimus. Precision medicine offers additional opportunities for optimizing the utilization of a drug by assessing the individualized pharmacogenomics of its disposition and metabolism, as demonstrated for the adverse consequences of variants in *TPMT* on azathioprine metabolism and in *CYP2C19* on clopidogrel metabolism (Chap. 68).

EXAMPLES OF PRECISION MEDICINE APPLICATIONS

The field of precision medicine did not appear abruptly in medical history but, rather, evolved gradually as clinicians became more aware of differences among patients with the same disease. With the advent of modern genomics, in the ideal situation, these phenotype differences can now be mapped to genotype differences. Thus, we can consider precision medicine from the perspective of the pregenomic era and the postgenomic era. Pregenomic precision medicine was applied to many diseases as therapeutic classes expanded for those disorders. A prime example of this approach is in the field of heart failure, where diuretics, digoxin, beta blockers, afterload-reducing agents, venodilators, renin-angiotensin-aldosterone inhibitors, and brain natriuretic peptide (nesiritide) are commonly used in some combination for most patients. The choice of agents is governed by the evidence basis for their use, but tailored to the primary pathophysiologic phenotypes manifest in a patient, such as congestion, hypertension, and impaired contractility. These treatments were developed in the latter half of the last century based on empiric observation, reductionist experiments of specific pathways believed to be involved in the pathophysiology, and clinical response in prospective trials. As phenotyping became more refined (e.g., echocardiographic assessments of ventricular function and tissue Doppler characterization of ventricular relaxation), the syndrome was subclassified into heart failure with reduced ejection fraction and heart failure with preserved ejection fraction, the latter of which does not respond well to any of the classes of therapeutic agents currently available. In the postgenomic era, ever more refined and detailed methods are under investigation to characterize pathophenotypes as well as genotypes, which may then be matched to the idealized combination of therapeutic classes of agents.

Pulmonary arterial hypertension is another disease for which definitive therapies straddle the pre- and postgenomic eras of precision medicine. Prior to the 1990s, there were no effective therapies for this highly morbid and lethal condition. With the advent of molecular and biochemical characterization of vascular abnormalities in individuals with established disease, however, therapies with agents that restored normal vascular function improved morbidity and mortality. These included calcium channel blockers, prostacyclin congeners, and endothelin receptor antagonists. As genomic characterization of the disease has progressed over the past two decades, there is increasing recognition of distinct genotypes that yield unique phenotypes (Chap. 283), such as the demonstration of a primarily fibrotic endophenotype governed by the (oxidized) scaffold protein NEDD-9 and its aldosterone-dependent, TGF-β-independent enhancement of collagen III expression. This approach will continue to evolve as therapies become more effective (e.g., for perivascular fibrosis) and therapeutic choices better targeted to individual patients.

Precision genomics has also led to a new classification of the dementias, conditions previously thought to have a single cause with varied clinical expression. These disorders can now be categorized based on the genes and pathways involved and the site where aggregated proteins first form and then spread in the nervous system. For example, the varied clinical presentations of frontotemporal dementia, including progressive aphasia, behavioral disturbances, and dementia with amyotrophic lateral sclerosis, can now be linked to specific genotypes and susceptible cells (Chap. 432). In prion diseases, the clinical phenotype

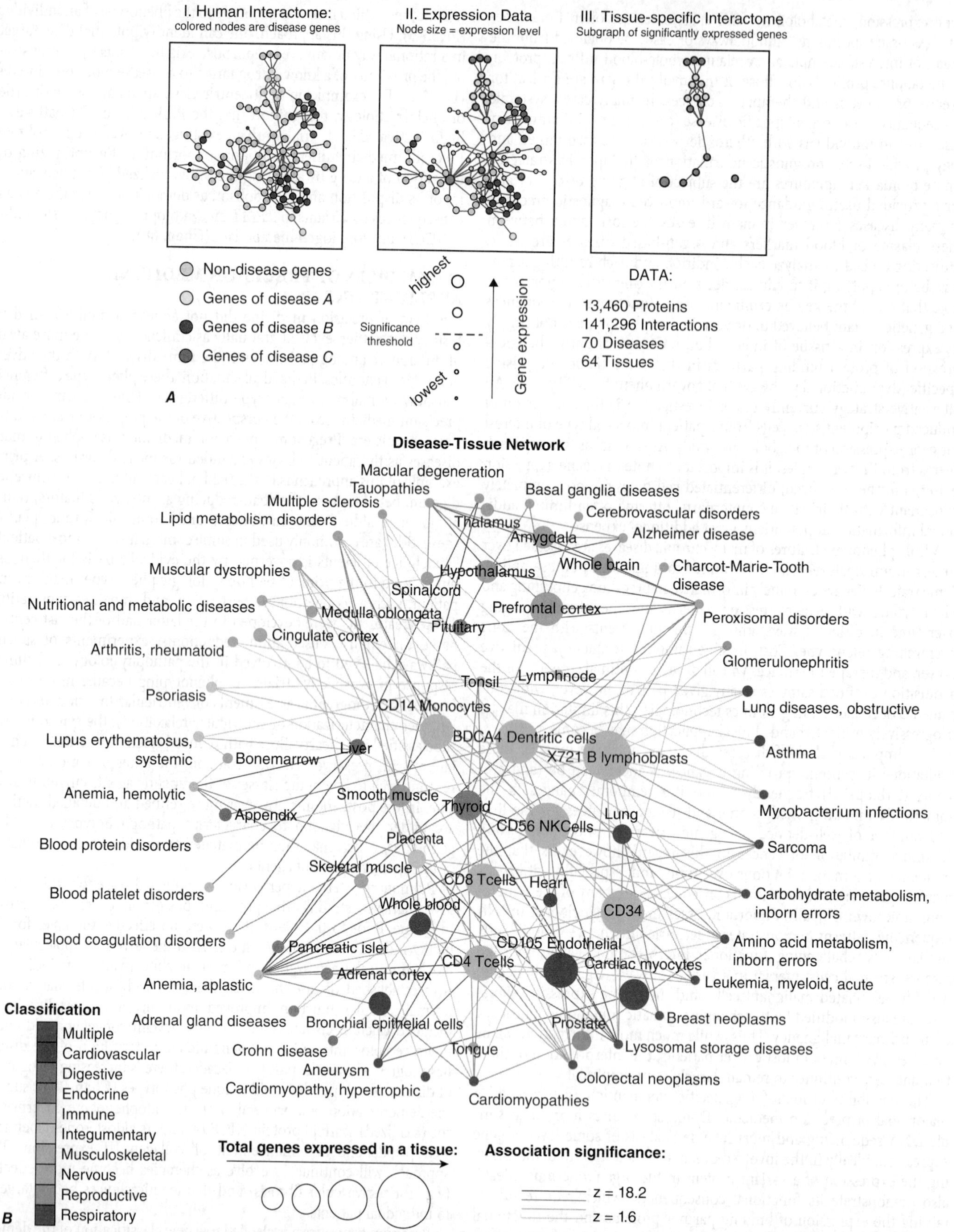

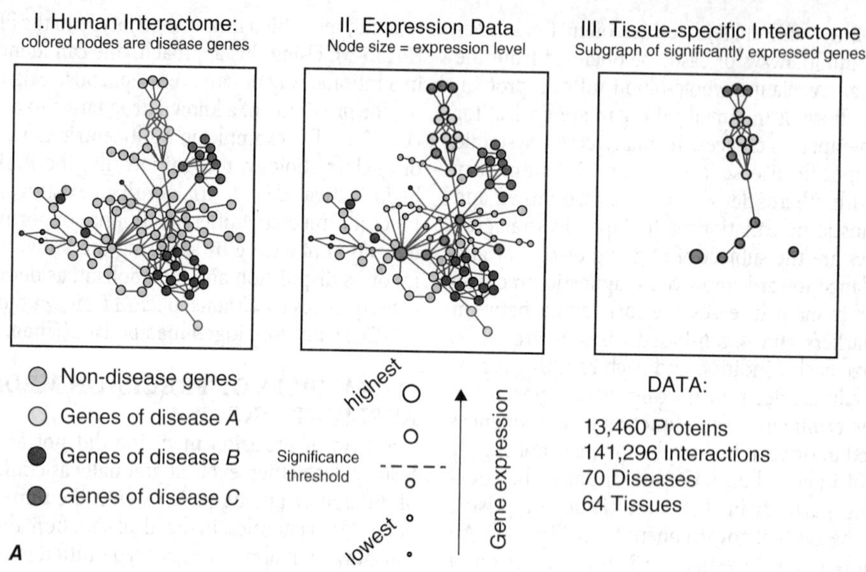

FIGURE 5-4 Gene expression and phenotype. ***A.*** The human protein-protein interactome is constructed, and a specific disease module is identified (I); gene expression within this module is ascertained (II); and the tissue specificity of gene expression is determined (III). This analysis leads to a reduction of the total number of disease module genes that govern phenotype in a specific organ, which is a reflection of the specific pathway (or pathways) that is (or are) expressed in their functional entirety in that tissue. ***B.*** A disease-tissue bipartite network is constructed wherein specific tissues are placed within the circle and linked to diseases shown on the circumference. Nodes are colored according to tissue classification, the sizes of nodes are proportional to the total number of genes expressed in them, and the widths (shades) of the lines or edges correspond to the significance of the associations with specific diseases. *(From M Kitsak et al: Tissue Specificity of Human Disease Module. Sci Rep 6: 35241, 2016, Figure 4.)*

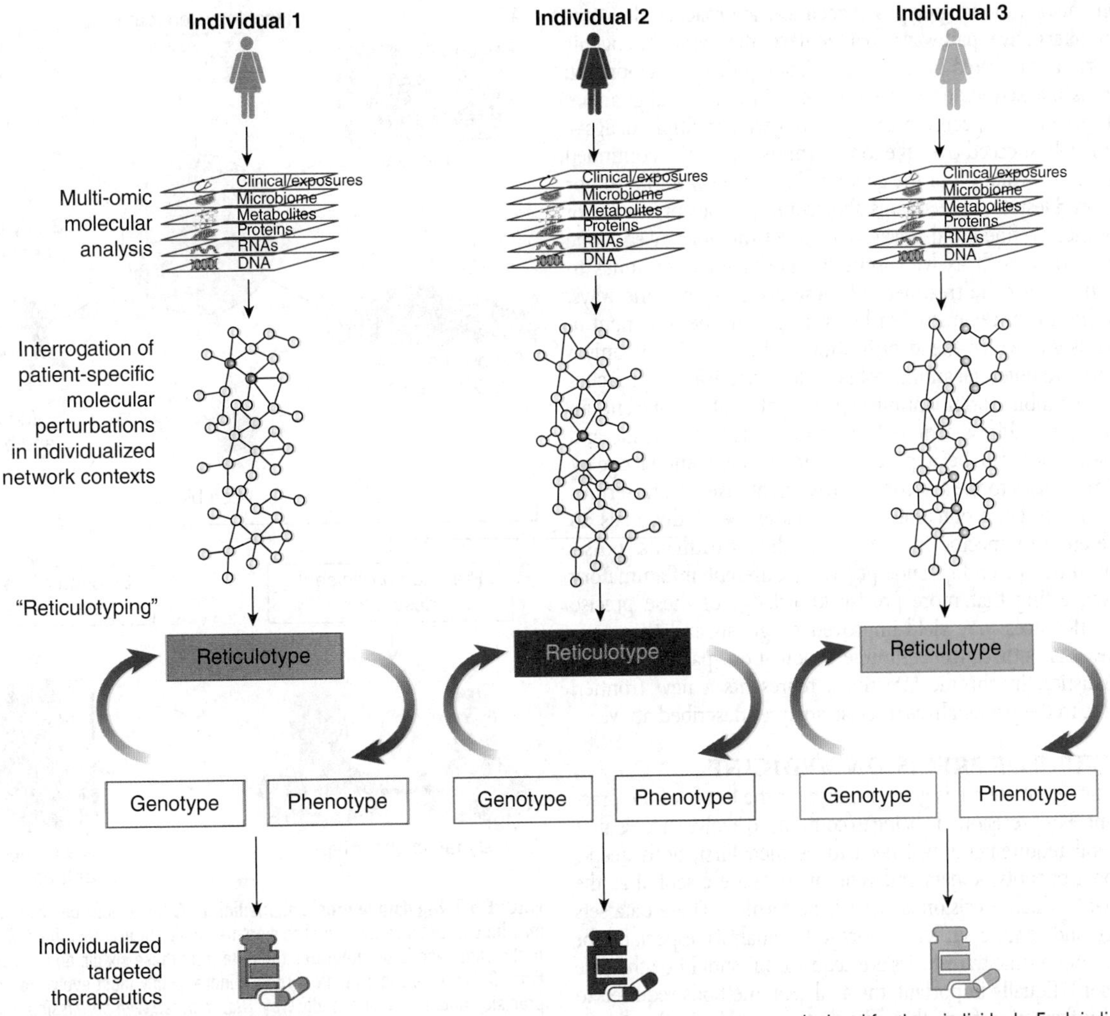

FIGURE 5-5 Reticulotype. Patient-specific genotype-phenotype relationships by multiomic network structures are depicted for three individuals. Each individual's unique molecular perturbations (genetic variants, differentially expressed genes) are examined within the context of the subject's unique integrative biologic network or reticulome derived from these multiomic analyses. These unique reticulotypes then serve as the basis for patient-specific, precision therapies. *(Reproduced with permission from LYH Lee, J Loscalzo: Network Medicine in Pathobiology. Am J Pathol 189:1311, 2019.)*

is determined by specific germline mutations present in the prion protein (**Chap. 438**). Discovery of autoantibodies against aquaporin-4 (AQP-4) and myelin oligodendrocyte glycoprotein (MOG) has allowed neuromyelitis optica, previously considered a multiple sclerosis–like disorder, to be classified as a separate entity requiring different treatment (**Chap. 445**). Similarly, in myasthenia gravis, the identification of novel autoantibodies now permits stratification and a more finely tuned precision approach to therapy (**Chap. 448**).

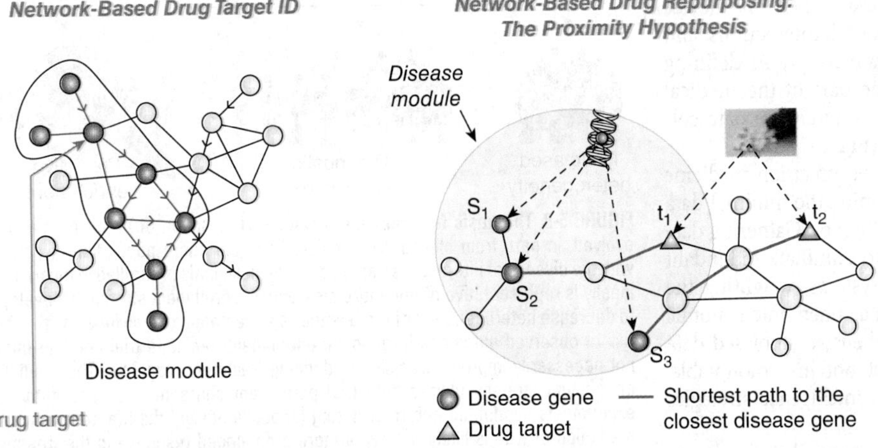

FIGURE 5-6 Network-based precision drug repurposing. *(Adapted from F Cheng et al: A genome-wide positioning systems network algorithm for in silico drug repurposing. Nat Commun 10:3476, 2019.)*

Precision medicine approaches to cancers have, of course, become the prime example of the opportunity that this strategy offers. In the pregenomic era, chemotherapy was widely used with variable success despite continued efforts to characterize the molecular features of the specific tumors and their semi-empiric responses to specific chemotherapeutic agents. As cancer genome sequencing evolved, however, it became apparent that there are a limited number of oncogenic pathways (<20) that are represented in the great majority of malignancies, without regard for the organ in which the disease was primarily manifest. These genomic signatures served as a template for precisely targeted therapies that have led to dramatic changes in response to treatment, including, for example, imatinib (and congeners) for Bcr-Abl tyrosine kinase activity in chronic myelogenous leukemia, erlotinib for *EGFR*-mutant non-small cell lung cancers, and ibrutinib for Bruton tyrosine kinase in chronic lymphocytic leukemia, among many others.

As exciting as these approaches have been, there are at least three primary challenges associated with precision therapeutics that are unique to cancer: (1) the mutational landscape continues to evolve as the disease progresses, and therapy often (if not invariably) leads to selection for resistant clones; (2) the likelihood that any cancer can be definitively cured by any single agent, no matter its exquisite precision, is quite limited, necessitating the development of rational polypharmaceutical approaches that take into account alternative pathways that achieve the same oncogenic goals as the primary targeted pathway, complicating drug development; and (3) there is marked genomic heterogeneity in many malignancies arguing that targeting a specific pathway—even with multiple drugs—may not ultimately succeed over the long term owing to the continued and heterogeneous evolution of the genomic landscape within a tumor within a patient. Despite these serious shortcomings, the application of progressively more refined and precisely targeted therapies used alone and in combination, such as with immune modulators, continues to offer great promise for the treatment of these diseases. In some ways, these approaches in cancer mirror earlier strategies in the treatment of infectious diseases in which the identification of the causative organism and its sensitivity to potential antimicrobials allows precision approaches to treatment. Combinatorial antimicrobial treatments represent an effective strategy to address acquired resistance. These diagnostic and therapeutic strategies can be applied without detailed knowledge of personalized responses to the infection or treatment (aside from serious adverse effects) with good outcomes in most cases. Yet, individuals do respond differently to specific infections and their treatments, possibly driven by different endophenotypes (e.g., different inflammatory responses), suggesting that more precise knowledge of these precise mechanistic differences may yield improved prognosis and therapeutic approaches. As with cancer, immune modulation, particularly for immune exhaustion in chronic infections, represents a new frontier, again amenable to the personalized, precise analyses described above.

THE FUTURE OF PRECISION MEDICINE

Precision medicine clearly holds great promise for the future of the practice of medicine. For precision medicine to continue to evolve successfully, however, several requirements will need to be met. First, both deeply refined personal phenotypic data and genomic data are essential as the information with which precision analysis is performed. These data sets are quite large and require sufficient storage for analysis, especially for individuals in whom time trajectories are acquired (as should be the case for every person). Equally important, the analytical methods required to extract useful information from these data sets are evolving and themselves quite complex. While great progress has been made in genomics and biochemical testing, our ability to capture meaningful immunologic endophenotypes and environmental exposures is limited by comparison. Machine learning and artificial (auxiliary) intelligence methods will be essential for extracting optimal information from these data sets, which include not only pathways that can be uniquely targeted therapeutically but also individualized genomic or phenotypic signatures that are highly predictive of outcome, with or without therapy. Gathering sufficient information on the "normal" segments of the population is also required to ensure appropriate comparison data sets for optimal prediction.

Second, phenotyping must continue to expand and become dimensionally richer. The phenotypic features included in this data gathering must incorporate not only data relevant to the clinical presentation but also orthogonal phenotypic data that may yield useful information on disease trajectory or preclinical disease markers. Personal device data, environmental exposure history, social network interactions, and health system data will all be incorporated increasingly in defining phenotype and will require great efforts on the part of the medical informatics community to harmonize data sets, standardize data collection, and optimize/standardize data analysis (Fig. 5-7).

Third, perhaps the greatest challenge to making precision medicine the standard approach to illness will be to determine the minimal data set required to predict outcome and response to therapy. Gathering data is comparatively simple; however, analyzing it to eliminate redundant information in these overdetermined biologic systems, weighting the determinants of an outcome, and using the data as phenomic/genomic signatures that are easier to collect than comprehensive, unbiased data sets are the ideal goals—a major challenge, but not insurmountable. Rapidly evolving machine learning and artificial intelligence strategies will also be essential for maximal success.

To return to the question of how precise precision medicine needs to be in order to be useful, please refer to Fig. 5-8 where the approaches

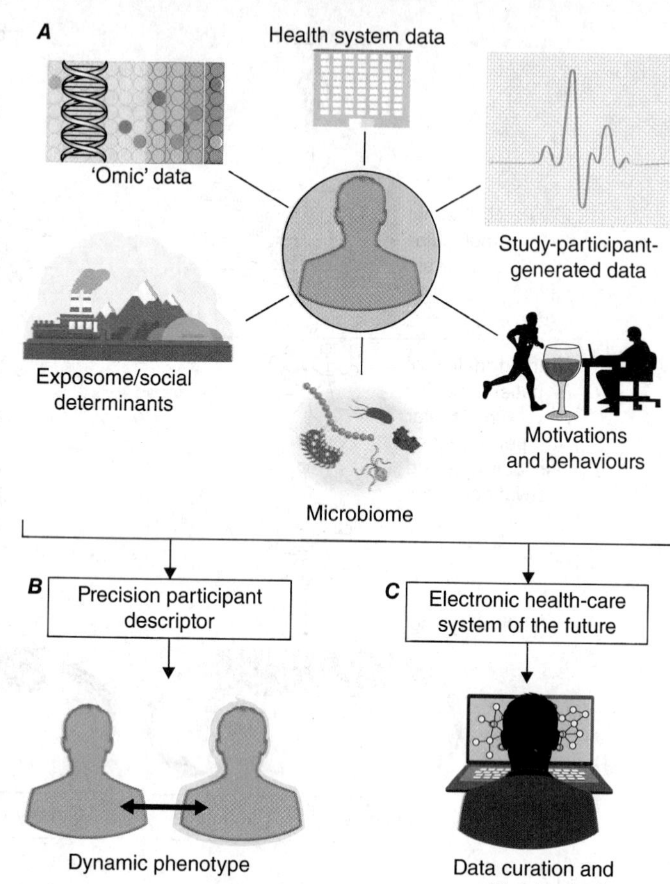

FIGURE 5-7 Big data in precision medicine. ***A.*** Six dimensions by which individuals may be characterized in the precision medicine era are described. ***B.*** The precision participant descriptor integrates the data from these six dimensions and varies over time. ***C.*** The electronic medical record increasingly must evolve to provide curated precision data in a user-friendly way. *(Reproduced with permission from EM Antman, J Loscalzo: Precision medicine in cardiology. Nat Rev Cardiol 13:591, 2016.)*

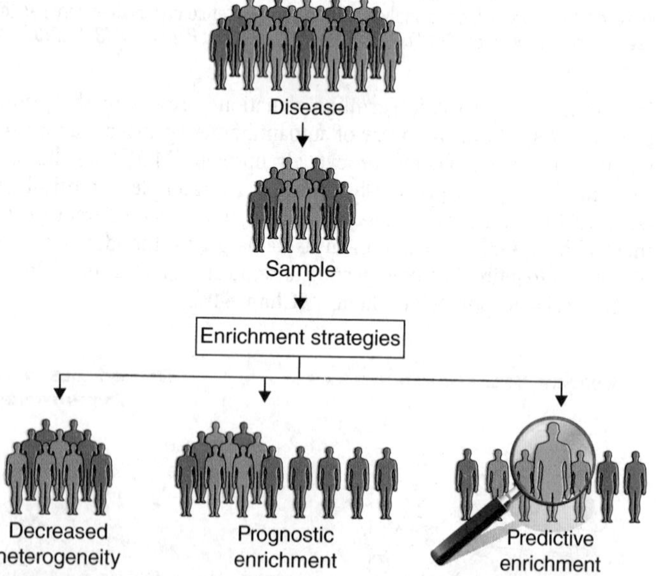

FIGURE 5-8 The basis for precision medicine. The notion of precision medicine evolved, in part, from clinical trial design. From the entire population of patients with the disease of interest, a sample cohort of individuals is enrolled in the trial that ideally is representative of the entire distribution. Enrichment strategies developed to decrease heterogeneity or increase the representation of individuals with a high risk of observed outcomes (prognostic enrichment) facilitate trial conduct but do not necessarily improve precision in defining treatment response. The predictive enrichment strategy utilizes both trial participant characteristics and data from experiments conducted before or during (adaptive design) the trial to improve the prediction of who is likely to have a more pronounced response to the treatment under study. *(Reproduced with permission from EM Antman, J Loscalzo: Precision medicine in cardiology. Nat Rev Cardiol 13:591, 2016.)*

to clinical trial design meant to improve therapeutic signal are illustrated. Decreasing heterogeneity and enriching the study population will enhance the effect size, but these strategies are based on analyses of prior data sets that define those individuals who are more likely than not to respond to a therapy. By contrast, the notion of predictive enrichment follows from the information provided by a detailed, big data–driven analysis of individuals that explores phenotypic and genomic features used to predict response. These features need not be precisely met by each patient; however, they can be collated or clustered to define a reasonably sized cohort predicted to respond in a particular way within certain confidence bounds. In this way, the boundaries to the practice of precision medicine are imprecise strictly speaking, but sufficiently predictive to be practical from the perspectives of clinical care and cost-effectiveness.

FURTHER READING

Antman EM, Loscalzo J: Precision medicine in cardiology. Nat Rev Cardiol 13:591, 2016.

Cheng F et al: Comprehensive characterization of protein-protein interactions perturbed by disease mutations. Nat Genet 53:342, 2021.

Cheng F et al: A genome-wide positioning systems network algorithm for in silico drug repurposing. Nat Commun 10:3476, 2019.

Greene JA, Loscalzo J: Putting the patient back together—Social medicine, network medicine, and the limits of reductionism. N Engl J Med 377:2493, 2017.

Kitsak M et al: Tissue specificity of human disease module. Sci Rep 6:35241, 2016.

Lee LY, Loscalzo J: Network medicine in pathobiology. Am J Pathol 189:1311, 2019.

Leopold JA et al: The application of big data to cardiovascular disease: Paths to precision medicine. J Clin Invest 130:29, 2020.

Loscalzo J et al: Human disease classification in the postgenomic era: A complex systems approach to human pathobiology. Mol Syst Biol 3:124, 2007.

Maron BA et al: Individualized interactomes for network-based precision medicine in hypertrophic cardiomyopathy with implications for other clinical pathophenotypes. Nat Commun 12:873, 2021.

Menche J et al: Disease networks. Uncovering disease-disease relationships through the incomplete interactome. Science 347:1257601, 2015.

Samokhin AO et al: NEDD9 targets *COL3A1* to promote endothelial fibrosis and pulmonary arterial hypertension. Sci Transl Med 10:eaap7294, 2018.

6 Screening and Prevention of Disease

Katrina A. Armstrong, Gary J. Martin

A primary goal of health care is to prevent disease or detect it early enough that intervention will be more effective. Tremendous progress has been made toward this goal over the past 50 years. Screening tests are available for many common diseases and encompass biochemical (e.g., cholesterol, glucose), physiologic (e.g., blood pressure, growth curves), radiologic (e.g., mammogram, bone densitometry), and cytologic (e.g., Pap smear) approaches. Effective preventive interventions have resulted in dramatic declines in mortality from many diseases, particularly infections. Preventive interventions include counseling about risk behaviors, vaccinations, medications, and, in some relatively uncommon settings, surgery. Preventive services (including screening tests, preventive interventions, and counseling) are different than other medical interventions because they are proactively administered to healthy individuals instead of in response to a symptom, sign, or diagnosis. Thus, the decision to recommend a screening test or preventive intervention requires a particularly high bar of evidence that testing and intervention are both practical and effective.

Because population-based screening and prevention strategies must be extremely low risk to have an acceptable benefit-to-harm ratio, the ability to target individuals who are more likely to develop disease could enable the application of a wider set of potential approaches and increase efficiency. Currently, there are many types of data that can predict disease incidence in an asymptomatic individual. Germline genomic data have received the most attention to date, at least in part because mutations in high-penetrance genes have clear implications for preventive care (**Chap. 467**). Women with mutations in either *BRCA1* or *BRCA2*, the two major breast cancer susceptibility genes identified to date, have a markedly increased risk (five- to twentyfold) of breast and ovarian cancer. Screening and prevention recommendations include prophylactic oophorectomy and breast magnetic resonance imaging (MRI), both of which are considered to incur too much harm for women at average cancer risk. Some women with *BRCA* mutations opt for prophylactic mastectomy to dramatically reduce their breast cancer risk. Although the proportion of common disease explained by high-penetrance genes appears to be relatively small (5–10% of most diseases), mutations in rare, moderate-penetrance genes, and variants in low-penetrance genes, also contribute to the prediction of disease risk. Most recently, polygenic risk scores combining information about variants across hundreds of genes are being evaluated for identifying individuals at high risk of coronary heart disease and other conditions. The advent of affordable whole exome/whole genome sequencing is likely to speed the dissemination of these tests into clinical practice and may transform the delivery of preventive care.

Other forms of "omic" data also have the potential to provide important predictive information. Proteomics and metabolomics can provide insight into gene function, but it has proven challenging to develop reliable, predictive measures using these platforms. More recently, it has become possible to measure the presence of mutations in DNA circulating in the bloodstream and in stool, with early promising evidence that these assays can be used to detect cancer before existing screening tests.

In addition to "omic" data, imaging data are increasingly being integrated into risk-stratified prevention approaches as evidence grows about the predictive ability of these data. For example, coronary computed tomography (CT) scans are used in many preventive cardiology programs to inform decisions about beginning statin therapy when there is conflicting or uncertain information from other risk assessment approaches. Of course, these data may also be helpful in predicting the risk of harms from screening or prevention, such as the risk of a false-positive mammogram.

In addition to advances in risk prediction, there are several other reasons that screening and prevention are likely to gain importance in medical care in the near term. New imaging modalities are being developed that promise to detect changes at the cellular and subcellular levels, greatly increasing the probability that early detection improves outcomes. The rapidly growing understanding of the biologic pathways underlying initiation and progression of many common diseases has the potential to transform the development of preventive interventions, including chemoprevention. Furthermore, screening and prevention offer the promise of both improving health and sparing the costs of disease treatment, an issue that will continue to gain importance as long as health care costs in the United States remain a concern to patients, government agencies, and insurers.

This chapter will review the basic principles of screening and prevention in the primary care setting. Recommendations for specific disorders such as cardiovascular disease, diabetes, and cancer are provided in the chapters dedicated to those topics.

BASIC PRINCIPLES OF SCREENING

The basic principles of screening populations for disease were published by the World Health Organization in 1968 (**Table 6-1**).

In general, screening is most effective when applied to relatively common disorders that carry a large disease burden (**Table 6-2**). The five leading causes of mortality in the United States are heart diseases, malignant neoplasms, chronic obstructive pulmonary disease,

TABLE 6-1 Principles of Screening

The condition should be an important health problem.
There should be a treatment for the condition.
Facilities for diagnosis and treatment should be available.
There should be a latent stage of the disease.
There should be a test or examination for the condition.
The test should be acceptable to the population.
The natural history of the disease should be adequately understood.
There should be an agreed policy on whom to treat.
The cost of finding a case should be balanced in relation to overall medical expenditure.

accidents, and cerebrovascular diseases. Thus, many screening strategies are targeted at these conditions. From a global health perspective, these conditions are priorities, but malaria, malnutrition, AIDS, tuberculosis, and violence also carry a heavy disease burden (**Chap. 472**).

Having an effective treatment for early disease has proven challenging for some common diseases. For example, although Alzheimer's disease is the sixth leading cause of death in the United States, there are no curative treatments and no evidence that early treatment improves outcomes. Lack of facilities for diagnosis and treatment is a particular challenge for developing countries and may change screening strategies, including the development of "see and treat" approaches such as those currently used for cervical cancer screening in some countries. A long latent or preclinical phase where early treatment increases the chance of cure is a hallmark of many cancers; for example, polypectomy prevents progression to colon cancer. Similarly, early identification of hypertension or hyperlipidemia allows therapeutic interventions that reduce the long-term risk of cardiovascular or cerebrovascular events. In contrast, lung cancer screening has historically proven more challenging because most tumors are not curable by the time they can be detected on a chest x-ray. However, the length of the preclinical phase also depends on the level of resolution of the screening test, and this situation changed with the development of chest CT. Low-dose chest CT scanning can detect tumors earlier and has been demonstrated to reduce lung cancer mortality by 20% in individuals who had at least a 30-pack-year history of smoking. The short interval between the ability to detect disease on a screening test and the development of incurable disease also contributes to the limited effectiveness of mammography screening in reducing deaths from some forms of breast cancer. At the other end of the spectrum, the early detection of prostate cancer may not lead to a difference in the mortality rate because the disease is often indolent and competing morbidities, such as coronary artery disease, may ultimately cause mortality (**Chap. 70**). This uncertainty about the natural history is also reflected in the controversy about treatment of prostate cancer, further contributing to the challenge of screening in this disease. Finally, screening programs can incur significant economic costs that must be considered in the context of the available resources and alternative strategies for improving health outcomes.

METHODS OF MEASURING HEALTH BENEFITS

Because screening and preventive interventions are recommended to asymptomatic individuals, they are held to a high standard for demonstrating a favorable risk-benefit ratio before implementation. In general, the principles of evidence-based medicine apply to demonstrating the efficacy of screening tests and preventive interventions, where randomized controlled trials (RCTs) with mortality outcomes are the gold standard. However, because RCTs are often not feasible, observational studies, such as case-control designs, have been used to assess the effectiveness of some interventions such as colonoscopy for colorectal cancer screening. For some strategies, such as Pap smear screening for cervical cancer, the only data available are ecologic data demonstrating dramatic declines in mortality.

Irrespective of the study design used to assess the effectiveness of screening, it is critical that disease incidence or mortality is the primary endpoint rather than length of disease survival. This is important because lead time bias and length time bias can create the appearance of an improvement in disease survival from a screening test when there is no actual effect. Lead time bias occurs because screening identifies a case before it would have presented clinically, thereby creating the perception that a patient lived longer after diagnosis simply by moving the date of diagnosis earlier rather than the date of death later. Length time bias occurs because screening is more likely to identify slowly progressive disease than rapidly progressive disease. Thus, within a fixed period of time, a screened population will have a greater proportion of these slowly progressive cases and will appear to have better disease survival than an unscreened population.

A variety of endpoints are used to assess the potential gain from screening and preventive interventions.

1. *The absolute and relative impact of screening on disease incidence or mortality*. The absolute difference in disease incidence or mortality between a screened and nonscreened group allows the comparison of size of the benefit across preventive services. A meta-analysis of Swedish mammography trials (ages 40–70) found that ~1.2 fewer women per 1000 would die from breast cancer if they were screened over a 12-year period. By comparison, at least ~3 lives per 1000 would be saved from colon cancer in a population (aged 50–75) screened with annual fecal occult blood testing (FOBT) over a 13-year period, and an estimated 20–24 lives per 1000 would be saved over the entire 25-year period. Based on this analysis, colon cancer screening may actually save more women's lives than does mammography. However, the relative impact of FOBT (30% reduction in colon cancer death) is similar to the relative impact of mammography (14–32% reduction in breast cancer death), emphasizing the importance of both relative and absolute comparisons.
2. *The number of subjects screened to prevent disease or death in one individual*. The inverse of the absolute difference in mortality is the number of subjects who would need to be screened or receive a preventive intervention to prevent one death. For example, 731 women aged 65–69 would need to be screened by dual-energy x-ray absorptiometry (DEXA) (and treated appropriately) to prevent one hip fracture from osteoporosis.
3. *Increase in average life expectancy for a population*. Predicted increases in life expectancy for various screening and preventive interventions are listed in **Table 6-3**. It should be noted, however, that the increase in life expectancy is an average that applies to a population, not to an individual. In reality, the vast majority of the population does not derive any benefit from a screening test. A small subset of patients, however, will benefit greatly. For example, Pap smears do not benefit the 98% of women who never develop cancer of the cervix. However, for the 2% who would have developed cervical cancer, Pap smears may add as much as 25 years to their lives. Some studies suggest that a 1-month gain of life expectancy is a reasonable goal for a population-based screening or prevention strategy.

TABLE 6-2 Lifetime Cumulative Risk

Breast cancer for women	10%
Colon cancer	6%
Cervical cancer for women[a]	2%
Domestic violence for women	Up to 15%
Hip fracture for white women	16%

[a]Assuming an unscreened population.

TABLE 6-3 Estimated Average Increase in Life Expectancy for a Population

SCREENING OR PREVENTIVE INTERVENTION	AVERAGE INCREASE
Mammography:	
Women, 40–50 years	0–5 days
Women, 50–70 years	1 month
Pap smears, age 18–65	2–3 months
Getting a 35-year-old smoker to quit	3–5 years
Beginning regular exercise for a 40-year-old man (30 min, 3 times a week)	9 months–2 years

■ ASSESSING THE HARMS OF SCREENING AND PREVENTION

Just as with most aspects of medical care, screening and preventive interventions also incur the possibility of adverse outcomes. These adverse outcomes include side effects from preventive medications and vaccinations, false-positive screening tests, overdiagnosis of disease from screening tests, anxiety, radiation exposure from some screening tests, and discomfort from some interventions and screening tests. The risk of side effects from preventive medications is analogous to the use of medications in therapeutic settings and is considered in the U.S. Food and Drug Administration (FDA) approval process. Side effects from currently recommended vaccinations are primarily limited to discomfort and minor immune reactions. However, the concern about associations between vaccinations and serious adverse outcomes continues to limit the acceptance of many vaccinations despite the lack of data supporting the causal nature of these associations.

The possibility of a false-positive test occurs with nearly all screening tests, although the definition of what constitutes a false-positive result often varies across settings. For some tests such as screening mammography and screening chest CT, a false-positive result occurs when an abnormality is identified that is not malignant, requiring either a biopsy diagnosis or short-term follow-up. For other tests such as Pap smears, a false-positive result occurs because the test identifies a wide range of potentially premalignant states, only a small percentage of which would ever progress to an invasive cancer. This risk is closely tied to the risk of overdiagnosis in which the screening test identifies disease that would not have presented clinically in the patient's lifetime. Assessing the degree of overdiagnosis from a screening test is very difficult given the need for long-term follow-up of an unscreened population to determine the true incidence of disease over time. Recent estimates suggest that as much as 15–40% of breast cancers identified by mammography screening and 15–37% of prostate cancers identified by prostate-specific antigen testing may never have presented clinically. Screening tests also have the potential to create unwarranted anxiety, particularly in conjunction with false-positive findings. Although multiple studies have documented increased anxiety through the screening process, there are few data suggesting this anxiety has long-term adverse consequences, including subsequent screening behavior. Screening tests that involve radiation (e.g., mammography, chest CT) add to the cumulative radiation exposure for the screened individual. The absolute amount of radiation is very small from any of these tests, but the overall impact of repeated exposure from multiple sources is still being determined. Some preventive interventions (e.g., vaccinations) and screening tests (e.g., mammography) may lead to discomfort at the time of administration, but again, there is little evidence of long-term adverse consequences.

■ WEIGHING THE BENEFITS AND HARMS

The decision to implement a population-based screening and prevention strategy requires weighing the benefits and harms, including the economic impact of the strategy. The costs include not only the expense of the intervention but also time away from work, downstream costs from false-positive results, "incidentalomas" or adverse events, and other potential harms. Cost-effectiveness is typically assessed by calculating the cost per year of life saved, with adjustment for the quality of life impact of different interventions and disease states (i.e., quality-adjusted life-year). Typically, strategies that cost $50,000–100,000 per quality-adjusted year of life saved are considered "cost-effective" (**Chap. 4**).

The U.S. Preventive Services Task Force (USPSTF) is an independent panel of experts in preventive care that provides evidence-based recommendations for screening and preventive strategies based on an assessment of the benefit-to-harm ratio (**Tables 6-4 and 6-5**). Because

TABLE 6-4 Screening Tests Recommended by the U.S. Preventive Services Task Force for Average-Risk Adults

DISEASE	TEST	POPULATION	FREQUENCY	CHAPTER
Abdominal aortic aneurysm	Ultrasound	Men 65–75 who have ever smoked	Once	
Alcohol misuse	Alcohol Use Disorders Identification Test	All adults	Unknown	453
Breast cancer	Mammography with or without clinical breast examination	Women 50–75	Every 2 years	
Cervical cancer	Pap smear	Women 21–65	Every 3 years	70
	Pap smear and/or HPV testing	Women 30–65	Every 5 years if HPV negative	
Chlamydia/gonorrhea	Nucleic acid amplification test on urine or cervical swab	Sexually active women <25	Unknown	189
Colorectal cancer	Fecal occult blood testing	45–75	Every year	70, 81
	Fecal immunochemical-DNA	45–75	Every 1–3 years	
	Sigmoidoscopy	45–75	Every 5 years	
	Colonoscopy (or occult blood testing combined with sigmoidoscopy)	45–75	Every 10 years	
Depression	Screening questions	All adults	Periodically	
Diabetes	Fasting blood glucose or HgbA1c	Adults overweight, obese, or with hypertension	Every 3 years	403
Hepatitis C	Anti-HCV antibody followed by confirmatory PCR	18–79	Once	
HIV	Reactive immunoassay or rapid HIV followed by confirmatory test	15–65	At least once	
Hyperlipidemia	Cholesterol	40–75	Unknown	407
Hypertension	Blood pressure	All adults	Periodically	277
Intimate partner violence	Screening questions	Women of childbearing age	Unknown	
Lung cancer	Low-dose computed tomography	Adults 50 to 80 years who have a 20 pack-year smoking history and currently smoke or have quit within the past 15 years	Yearly	
Obesity	Body mass index	All adults	Unknown	
Osteoporosis	DEXA	Women >65 or >60 with risk factors	Unknown	411

Abbreviations: DEXA, dual-energy x-ray absorptiometry; HCV, hepatitis C virus; HPV, human papillomavirus; PCR, polymerase chain reaction.

Source: Adapted from the U.S. Preventive Services Task Force 2017. *www.uspreventiveservicestaskforce.org/Page/Name/uspstf-a-and-b-recommendations/.*

TABLE 6-5 Preventive Interventions Recommended for Average-Risk Adults

INTERVENTION	DISEASE	POPULATION	FREQUENCY	CHAPTER
Adult immunization				123, 124
Tetanus-diphtheria		>18	Every 10 years	
Varicella		Susceptibles only, >18	Two doses	
Measles-mumps-rubella		Women, childbearing age	One dose	
Pneumococcal		>64	13 followed by 23 valent	
Influenza		>18	Yearly	
Human papillomavirus		Up to age 27	If not done prior	
Zoster		>60	Once	
Chemoprevention				
Aspirin	Cardiovascular disease	Aged 50–59 years with a ≥10% 10-year cardiovascular disease risk (bleeding risk may = benefit for some groups)		
Folic acid	Neural tube defects in baby	Women planning or capable of pregnancy		
Tamoxifen/raloxifene	Breast cancer	Women at high risk for breast cancer		
Vitamin D	Fracture/falls	>64 at increased risk for falls		

there are multiple advisory organizations providing recommendations for preventive services, the agreement among the organizations varies across the different services. For example, all advisory groups support screening for hyperlipidemia and colorectal cancer, whereas consensus is lower for breast cancer screening among women in their forties and for prostate cancer screening. Because the guidelines are only updated periodically, differences across advisory organizations may also reflect the data that were available when the guideline was issued.

For many screening tests and preventive interventions, the balance of benefits and harms may be uncertain for the average-risk population but more favorable for individuals at higher risk for disease. Although age is the most commonly used risk factor for determining screening and prevention recommendations, the USPSTF also recommends some screening tests in populations based upon the presence of other risk factors for the disease. In addition, being at increased risk for the disease often supports initiating screening at an earlier age than that recommended for the average-risk population. For example, when there is a significant family history of colon cancer, it is prudent to initiate screening 10 years before the age at which the youngest family member was diagnosed with cancer.

Although informed consent is important for all aspects of medical care, shared decision-making may be a particularly important approach to decisions about preventive services when the benefit-to-harm ratio is uncertain for a specific population. For example, many expert groups, including the American Cancer Society, recommend an individualized discussion about prostate cancer screening, because the decision-making process is complex and relies heavily on personal issues. Some men may decline screening, whereas others may be more willing to accept the risks of an early detection strategy. Recent analysis suggests that many men may be better off not screening for prostate cancer because watchful waiting was the preferred strategy when quality-adjusted life-years were considered. Another example of shared decision-making involves the choice of techniques for colon cancer screening (**Chap. 70**). In controlled studies, the use of annual FOBT reduces colon cancer deaths by 15–30%. Flexible sigmoidoscopy reduces colon cancer deaths by ~40–60%. Colonoscopy appears to offer a greater benefit than flexible sigmoidoscopy with a reduction in risk of ~70%, but its use incurs additional costs and risks. These screening procedures have not been compared directly in the same population, but models suggest that appropriate frequencies of each technique may be associated with similar numbers of lives saved and cost to society per life saved ($10,000–25,000). Thus, although one patient may prefer the ease of preparation, less time disruption, and the lower risk of flexible sigmoidoscopy, others may prefer the sedation, thoroughness, and time interval of colonoscopy.

COUNSELING ON HEALTHY BEHAVIORS

In considering the impact of preventive services, it is important to recognize that tobacco and alcohol use, diet, and exercise constitute the vast majority of factors that influence preventable deaths in developed countries. Perhaps the single greatest preventive health care measure is to help patients quit smoking (**Chap. 454**). However, efforts in these areas frequently require behavior changes (e.g., weight loss, exercise) or the management of addictive conditions (e.g., tobacco and alcohol use) that are often recalcitrant to intervention. Although these are challenging problems, evidence strongly supports the role of counseling by health care providers (**Table 6-6**) in effecting health behavior change. Educational campaigns, public policy changes, and community-based interventions have also proven to be important parts of a strategy for addressing these factors in some settings. Although the USPSTF found that the evidence was conclusive to recommend a relatively small set of counseling activities, counseling in areas such as physical activity and injury prevention (including seat belts and bicycle and motorcycle helmets) has become a routine part of primary care practice.

IMPLEMENTING DISEASE PREVENTION AND SCREENING

The implementation of disease prevention and screening strategies in practice is challenging. A number of techniques can assist physicians with the delivery of these services. An appropriately configured electronic health record can provide reminder systems that make it easier for physicians to track and meet guidelines. Some systems give patients secure access to their medical records, providing an additional means to enhance adherence to routine screening. Systems that provide nurses and other staff with standing orders are effective for immunizations. The USPSTF has developed flow sheets and electronic tools to assist clinicians (*https://www.uspreventiveservicestaskforce.org/uspstf/information-health-professionals*). Many of these tools use age categories to help guide implementation. Age-specific recommendations for screening and counseling are summarized in **Table 6-7**.

Many patients see a physician for ongoing care of chronic illnesses, and this visit provides an opportunity to include a "measure of prevention" for other health problems. For example, a patient seen for management of hypertension or diabetes can have breast cancer

TABLE 6-6 Preventive Counseling Recommended by the U.S. Preventive Services Task Force (USPSTF)

TOPIC	CHAPTER REFERENCE
Alcohol and drug use	453, 456, 457
Genetic counseling for *BRCA1/2* testing among women at increased risk for deleterious mutations	79, 467
Nutrition and diet	332, 333
Sexually transmitted infections	136, 202
Sun exposure	61
Tobacco use	454

TABLE 6-7 Age-Specific Causes of Mortality and Corresponding Preventive Options

AGE GROUP	LEADING CAUSES OF AGE-SPECIFIC MORTALITY	SCREENING PREVENTION INTERVENTIONS TO CONSIDER FOR EACH SPECIFIC POPULATION
15–24	1. Accident 2. Homicide 3. Suicide 4. Malignancy 5. Heart disease	• Counseling on routine seat belt use, bicycle/motorcycle/ATV helmets (1) • Counseling on diet and exercise (5) • Discuss dangers of alcohol use while driving, swimming, boating (1) • Assess and update vaccination status (tetanus, diphtheria, hepatitis B, MMR, rubella, varicella, meningitis, HPV) • Ask about gun use and/or gun possession (2,3) • Assess for substance abuse history including alcohol (2,3) • Screen for domestic violence (2,3) • Screen for depression and/or suicidal/homicidal ideation (2,3) • Pap smear for cervical cancer screening after age 21 (4) • Discuss skin, breast awareness, and testicular self-examinations (4) • Recommend UV light avoidance and regular sunscreen use (4) • Measurement of blood pressure, height, weight, and body mass index (5) • Discuss health risks of tobacco use, consider emphasis on cosmetic and economic issues to improve quit rates for younger smokers (4,5) • Chlamydia and gonorrhea screening and contraceptive counseling for sexually active females, discuss STD prevention • Hepatitis B, and syphilis testing if there is high-risk sexual behavior(s) or any prior history of sexually transmitted disease • Hepatitis C screening starting at age 18 to 79 • HIV testing • Continue annual influenza vaccination
25–44	1. Accident 2. Malignancy 3. Heart disease 4. Suicide 5. Homicide 6. HIV	*As above plus consider the following:* • Readdress smoking status, encourage cessation at every visit (2,3) • Obtain detailed family history of malignancies and begin early screening/prevention program if patient is at significant increased risk (2) • Assess all cardiac risk factors (including screening for diabetes and hyperlipidemia) and consider primary prevention with aspirin for patients at >3% 5-year risk of a vascular event (3) and statin therapy for higher risk patients • Assess for chronic alcohol abuse, risk factors for viral hepatitis, or other risks for development of chronic liver disease • Consider individualized breast cancer screening with mammography at age 40 (2)
45–64	1. Malignancy 2. Heart disease 3. Accident 4. Diabetes mellitus 5. Cerebrovascular disease 6. Chronic lower respiratory disease 7. Chronic liver disease and cirrhosis 8. Suicide	• Consider prostate cancer screen with annual PSA and digital rectal examination at age 50 (or possibly earlier in African Americans or patients with family history) (1) • Begin colorectal cancer screening at age 45 or 50 with fecal occult blood testing, flexible sigmoidoscopy, or colonoscopy (1) • Reassess and update vaccination status at age 50 and vaccinate all smokers against *Streptococcus pneumoniae* at age 50 (6) • Consider screening for coronary disease in higher-risk patients (2,5) • Zoster vaccination at age 60 • Begin mammography screening by age 50 • Lung cancer screening at age 50 to 80 years if a 20 pack-year smoking history and currently smoke or have quit within the past 15 years, yearly.
≥65	1. Heart disease 2. Malignancy 3. Cerebrovascular disease 4. Chronic lower respiratory disease 5. Alzheimer's disease 6. Influenza and pneumonia 7. Diabetes mellitus 8. Kidney disease 9. Accidents 10. Septicemia	*As above plus consider the following:* • Readdress smoking status, encourage cessation at every visit (1,2,3,4) • One-time ultrasound for AAA in men 65–75 who have ever smoked • Consider pulmonary function testing for all long-term smokers to assess for development of chronic obstructive pulmonary disease (4,6) • Screen all postmenopausal women (and all men with risk factors) for osteoporosis • Continue annual influenza vaccination and vaccinate against *S. pneumoniae* at age 65 (4,6) • Screen for visual and hearing problems, home safety issues, and elder abuse (9) • Consider fall prevention exercise intervention if at higher risk (9)

Note: The numbers in parentheses refer to areas of risk in the mortality column affected by the specified intervention.

Abbreviations: AAA, abdominal aortic aneurysm; ATV, all-terrain vehicle; HPV, human papillomavirus; MMR, measles-mumps-rubella; PSA, prostate-specific antigen; STD, sexually transmitted disease; UV, ultraviolet.

screening incorporated into one visit and a discussion about colon cancer screening at the next visit. Other patients may respond more favorably to a clearly defined visit that addresses all relevant screening and prevention interventions. Because of age or comorbidities, it may be appropriate with some patients to abandon certain screening and prevention activities, although there are fewer data about when to "sunset" these services. For many screening tests, the benefit of screening does not accrue until 5–10 years of follow-up, and there are generally few data to support continuing screening for most diseases past age 75. In addition, for patients with advanced diseases and limited life expectancy, there is considerable benefit from shifting the focus from screening procedures to the conditions and interventions more likely to affect quality and length of life.

FURTHER READING

BRETTHAUER M et al: America, we are confused: The updated U.S. Preventive Services Task Force recommendation on colorectal cancer screening. Ann Intern Med 166:139, 2017.

HAYES JH et al: Observation versus initial treatment for men with localized, low-risk prostate cancer: A cost-effectiveness analysis. Ann Intern Med 158:853, 2013.

HUGOSSON J et al: Mortality results from the Goteborg randomized population-based prostate-cancer screening trial. Lancet Oncol 11:725, 2010.

OEFFINGER KC et al: Breast cancer screening for women at average risk 2015. Guideline update from the American Cancer Society. JAMA 314:1599, 2015.

US PREVENTIVE SERVICES TASK FORCE: Screening for colorectal cancer. US Preventive Services Task Force recommendation statement. JAMA 315:2564, 2016.

7 Global Diversity of Health System Financing and Delivery

Richard B. Saltman

Health care systems are highly complex organizations, with many interdependent components. In developed countries, health systems have traditionally been classified by their type of financing—i.e., either predominantly tax-funded (such as the National Health Service in England and publicly operated regional care systems in the four European Nordic countries) or predominantly statutory social health insurance (SHI)-funded (such as in Germany, the Netherlands, and France). Over the past several decades, however, there has been structural convergence in the technical characteristics of both funding arrangements and in the associated delivery systems, making analytic observations about differences across national systems more difficult.

A second confounding factor has been that former Soviet Bloc countries in Central and Eastern Europe, including the Russian Federation, have, since 1991, replaced their former Soviet-style Semashko models (a top-down, national government–controlled funding and delivery structure with a parallel Communist Party administrative apparatus) with various hybrid arrangements built on national government–run SHI financing. Distinctions across developed country health systems, especially in Europe, have been further compressed by inadequate resources in many publicly funded systems in an era of rapid clinical and technological change, triggering increased private sector funding and provision.

In middle-income developing countries, institutional structures in the health sector typically reflect the country's preindependence administrative framework. Mexico, for example, has a Spanish-derived configuration with health insurance as part of social insurance for formally employed workers (via Instituto Mexicano del Seguro Social), supplemented by tax-funded health services (Seguro Popular) provided for those with informal employment and all other citizens, as well as a separate program (Instituto de Seguridad y Servicios Sociales de los Trabajadores del Estado) for public employees. Countries such as India and Egypt, reflecting British influence, have predominantly tax-funded and publicly operated health systems. China is an exception, with an internally generated system that is publicly funded and operated, although recent Communist Party policy has been to introduce SHI-based insurance with individual medical savings accounts (patterned after Singapore), promote private insurance, and expand private hospitals.

In lower-income developing countries, health services are typically provided by tax-funded public institutions, often with considerable inadequacies and sometimes with substantial copayments. It is important to note that governmentally organized systems in nearly all developing countries, as well as in former Soviet bloc countries and, to a lesser degree, in tax-funded developed countries, are supplemented to varying extents by a mix of private and/or employer-paid insurers and providers.

This chapter focuses on the individual patient care system: on the financing and delivery of individual clinical and preventive services. The individual patient care system is composed of the financing and delivery of necessary services to prevent death or serious harm ("rule of rescue"); to maintain quality of life; and to manage, reduce, and/or prevent the burden of illness on individual patients. While the technical dimensions of most clinical services are similar across countries, their organizational, social, and economic characteristics range widely. Health systems in both developed and developing countries exhibit substantial differences, for example, in access to care; in the design and reliance on quality assurance and provider payment mechanisms; in the relationship of primary care to hospital services; in the coordination of health care with home care and nursing home services; in the design and use of provider management strategies; in the way physicians work and are paid; in the decision-making roles of politically elected officials and of national, regional, and municipal governments; and in participation of both citizens and patients. These wide-ranging institutional and organizational characteristics reflect differing country contexts (geographical, social, economic, and political), differences in national culture (consisting of prioritized norms and values), and substantial variation in how health sector institutions are structured.

FINANCING INDIVIDUAL PATIENT CARE SERVICES IN DEVELOPED COUNTRIES

Funding for individual care services in developed countries comes from the particular national mix among four possible sources of revenue: national, regional, and/or municipal taxes; mandatory SHI; private health insurance (including employer-paid insurances); and out-of-pocket payments. Most countries have one preponderant payer, which then defines its funding arrangements and serves to frame the structure of its delivery system as well.

Total Health Expenditures The Organization for Economic Co-operation and Development (OECD) data from 2017 (adjusted for purchasing power parities) show that total health care expenditures in developed countries vary across a considerable range, tied to health system structure as well as national history and culture (**Table 7-1**).

Per capita health expenditure figures provide a different, specific measurement of available funds in a country's health sector (**Table 7-2**).

Tax-Funded Systems In the United Kingdom, 79% of all health care funding was furnished through general tax revenues allocated by the national government in its annual budget process (all figures from OECD for 2017). In Sweden, all public taxes combined raised 83.7% of total health care spending. Sweden's 21 regional-level elected governments provide approximately 70% of that 83.7%, with the remaining 13.7% of total health spending raised by national and municipal taxes. In Canada, 71% of total health spending was raised by tax revenues, with 66% of that 71% coming from provincial or territorial taxes, while 5% came from national and local government taxes.

In most tax-funded countries, a segment of the population also has individual-, company-, or union-purchased private complementary and/or supplemental insurance coverage. In Sweden, 2019 estimates are that about 600,000 individuals have private complementary policies in a total population of 9 million. In Denmark, 50% of the population purchase supplemental insurance, while 30% have complementary insurance (often purchased by employers) that pays for private sector services enabling them to bypass public sector queues. In Finland, many middle-class families purchase separate private health insurance for their children to enable them to bypass long waiting times

TABLE 7-1 Developed Country Total Health Expenditure (% GDP)

TAX FUNDED IN WESTERN EUROPE		SHI FUNDED IN WESTERN EUROPE		CENTRAL EUROPEAN		DEVELOPED ASIAN		DEVELOPED NORTH AMERICAN	
Ireland	7.2%	Belgium	10.3%	Latvia	6.0%	Singapore	4.5%	Canada	10.7%
Spain	8.9%	Netherlands	10.1%	Poland	6.5%	South Korea	7.6%	United States	17.1%
UK	9.6%	Germany	11.2%	Czech Republic	7.2%	Japan	10.9%		
Finland	9.6%	Switzerland	12.3%	Slovenia	8.2%				
Denmark	10.1%								
Sweden	11.0%								

Abbreviations: GDP, gross domestic product; SHI, social health insurance; UK, United Kingdom.
Source: The Organization for Economic Co-operation and Development (OECD) data.

for primary and secondary pediatric health care services. More than 400,000 Finnish children (in a total population of 5 million) have privately purchased policies. In England in 2015, individual-, employer-, and union-purchased private complementary insurance covered an estimated 10.5% of the population, or about 6 million people. In Canada, individuals are not allowed by law to purchase private complementary insurance (except for Supreme Court–ordered insurance for three backlogged surgical procedures in Quebec Province—2005 Chaoulli decision); however, approximately 65% of the population have employer-, union-, or private group–purchased supplemental insurance for non–publicly covered services such as outpatient pharmaceutical prescriptions and home care.

Social Insurance–Funded Systems In Western Europe, SHI funds have traditionally been organized on a private not-for-profit basis, but with statutory responsibilities under national law. When former Soviet Bloc countries in Eastern Europe regained their independence in 1991, they returned to pre–World War II SHI models, but because there was no remaining organizational infrastructure, these post-1991 arrangements typically became a single SHI fund, run as an arm of the national government. In the United States, the Medicare social insurance system for citizens over age 65, enacted in 1965, is organized as a single fund tied to the national Social Security (public pension) Administration, an independent agency within the national government, with reimbursement arrangements supervised by the Centers for Medicare and Medicaid Services (CMS) inside the Department of Health and Human Services. Medicare covers inpatient hospital care plus limited post-hospital nursing home services (Medicare Part A). Supplemental private insurance policies are bought by covered individuals to help pay for outpatient physician visits (Medicare Part B) and for outpatient pharmaceuticals (Medicare Part D).

In Germany, 85% of the population is enrolled in one of 120 not-for-profit, monthly premium–based private SHI funds. This figure includes all individuals with annual incomes below 54,500 euros, who are required by law to join an SHI fund, as well as those with higher incomes who choose to enroll or remain. Eleven percent of the population—all having annual incomes above the mandatory SHI enrollment ceiling of 54,500 euros—have opted out of the SHI system to voluntarily enroll in claims-based private health insurance, whereas 4% of the citizenry is enrolled in sector-specific public programs such as the military. Since 2009, all SHI members pay a flat tax on gross monthly income as a contribution (8.2% in 2018, up to an upper income limit of 49,500 euros), which is transferred by their SHI fund to a national pool, and then redistributed back to their chosen fund on an individual risk-adjusted basis. Employers send 7.3% of each employee's salary to the same national pool. Special arrangements exist for payments from self-employed, retired, and unemployed workers. Since 1995, there has been a separate mandatory social insurance fund for long-term care (LTC), with an annual premium of 1.95% of each adult's gross monthly income, split 50%–50% with their employer. Pensioners since 2004 are required to pay the full 1.95% from their pensions. Childless SHI enrollees pay a surcharge of 0.25% of monthly gross income. Overall, 78% of all health care expenditures in Germany were paid from public and/or mandatory private SHI sources.

In the Netherlands since 2006, all adult citizens pay a fixed premium (about 1453 euros in 2019) to their choice among 35 private health insurers (not-for-profit and for-profit), with four large insurance groups having over 1 million members each. In addition, employers pay 6.95% of salary below 51,400 euros for each employee into a national health insurance fund. Self-employed individuals pay 4.85% into the national fund for taxable income up to the same limit. Retired and unemployed individuals also make payments. In addition to the individual premiums paid to their choice of private insurance fund, payments from the national health insurance fund, adjusted by individual age, sex, and health characteristics, also are made to the individual's chosen insurer. The Netherlands has a separate mandatory social insurance fund for LTC (the ABWZ, since 2015 the WLZ, and now only for residential nursing home care) to which each employee pays 9.5% of taxable income beneath 33,600 euros every year. Self-employed, unemployed, and retired individuals also are required to pay premiums to the WLZ. Overall, including SHI revenues, public spending provided 87% of total health expenditures in 2014.

In Estonia, a former Soviet Republic that re-established an SHI system in 1991 upon regaining its independence, there is one national SHI fund that is an arm of the national government. This fund collects mandatory payments of 13% from salaried workers and 20% from self-employed individuals, covering both health care and retirement pensions. Overall, including SHI revenues, public spending accounted for 74.5% of total health expenditures in 2017.

Singapore, Japan, South Korea, and Taiwan have predominantly SHI systems of funding for individual care services. In these Asian countries (except Japan), there is one SHI fund that typically is operated as an arm of the national government.

In Singapore, starting in 1983, all employees up to age 50 have been required to place 20% of their income (employers add 16% more) into a personal health savings account to pay for direct health care costs,

TABLE 7-2 Developed Country Per Capita Health Expenditures

TAX FUNDED IN WESTERN EUROPE		SHI FUNDED IN WESTERN EUROPE		CENTRAL EUROPEAN		DEVELOPED ASIAN		DEVELOPED NORTH AMERICAN	
Spain	$2738	Belgium	$4149	Latvia	$874	South Korea	$2043	Canada	$4458
Italy	$2738	Germany	$4714	Poland	$809	Singapore	$4083	United States	$9869
UK	$3958	Netherlands	$4742	Czech Republic	$1321	Japan	$4233		
Denmark	$5565	Switzerland	$9835	Slovenia	$1834				
Sweden	$5710								

Abbreviations: SHI, social health insurance; UK, United Kingdom.

managed in their name by the Singapore government, called a Medisave account. Medisave accounts have a maximum amount, are tax-exempt, and receive interest payments (currently set at 4%). Consistent with a Confucian emphasis on family, the funds that accumulate in the Medisave account can be spent on health care for family members as well. If the accumulated funds are not spent on health care during the insured's life, they become part of the individual's personal estate and are distributed as a tax-free inheritance to his or her designated heirs. In addition, Singaporean citizens are also automatically enrolled into a second government-run health insurance plan called MediShield that pays for supplemental catastrophic, chronic, and long-term care. While citizens can opt out, 90% of citizens remain in the program. The Singapore government also operates a third, wholly tax-funded payer called Medifund that, with approval of a local neighborhood committee, will pay hospital costs for 3–4% of the population who are recognized as indigent. In part reflecting the high level of mandatory individual saving, public funding provided only 54.5% of total health expenditures in 2016.

In South Korea, a state-run SHI system was established in 1977, which in 1990 covered 30.9% of total health care costs. This percentage paid by the SHI system rose to 40.5% of total costs in 2017, with national tax revenue covering 16.9%, leaving out-of-pocket expenses at a relatively high 34.4% of total costs. Although there are legal ceilings on total out-of-pocket copayments for each 6-month period, over 70% of Korean adults purchase an additional private Voluntary Health Insurance policy to cover these additional direct expenditures. In 2000, three types of public SHI funds were merged into a single national state-run fund. As of 2018, 6% of an employee's salary must be paid as a social insurance contribution into this fund, with employees and employers each paying 50% of that amount. In 2008, an additional SHI fund was introduced to pay for LTC, operated by the main state-run SHI fund to reduce administrative costs. Contributions to the LTC fund are set at 6.55% of the individual's regular SHI contribution, coupled with 20% copayments for institutional care and 15% copayments for home care services.

The United States There is no single preponderant source of health care spending in the United States. The federal government's CMS reported that, for 2017, private health insurance covered 34% of total health expenditures, Medicare (mandatory SHI program for all citizens over 65) covered 20%, Medicaid (a joint federal-state welfare program for low-income citizens) covered 17%, and out-of-pocket paid 10%. Sources of funds for these programs were 28% from the federal government, 17% from state and local governments, 28% from private households, and 20% from private business (e.g., employers). The World Bank set public funding in the United States at 50.2% of total health expenditures in 2017.

In 2010, the passage of the Affordable Care Act (ACA) extended privately provided but heavily regulated and federally subsidized health insurance to many low- and middle-income uninsured individuals and families. Since the same act reduced the availability of existing individually purchased private health insurance, the total increase in the number of newly covered individuals was less than expected. Insurance premium increases for 2017 rose from 20% to over 100%, depending on the particular state, with additional increases in up-front deductible requirements, raising questions about the long-term sustainability of the ACA initiative. The recent Republican administration sought to repeal major financial and tax elements of the ACA and to replace existing subsidy arrangements with a system of refundable tax credits toward the establishment of individual health savings accounts and/or purchase of private health insurance on open cross-state markets (currently, private health insurance in the United States remains controlled at the separate 50-state level of government).

DELIVERING INDIVIDUAL PATIENT CARE SERVICES IN DEVELOPED COUNTRIES

Hospital Services In Europe, hospitals in both tax-funded and SHI-funded health systems are mostly publicly owned and operated by regional or municipal governments. In tax-funded health systems, most hospital-based physicians are civil servants, employed on a negotiated salary basis (often by a physician labor union), and subject to most of the usual advantages and disadvantages of being a public sector employee. There are somewhat more private hospitals in SHI-funded health systems. However, most larger hospitals are public institutions operated by local governments, and most hospital physicians (with the notable exception of the Netherlands, where they are private contractors organized in private group practices) are, like those in tax-funded systems, public sector employees. In most tax-funded European countries (but not continental SHI-funded countries), few specialist physicians have office-based practices, and in both tax- and SHI-funded systems, office-based specialists do not have admitting privileges to publicly operated hospitals.

Most public hospitals in both tax-funded and SHI-funded health systems are single free-standing institutions that can be classified into three broad categories by complexity of patients admitted and number of specialties available: (1) district hospitals (four specialties: internal medicine, general surgery, obstetrics, and psychiatry); (2) regional hospitals (20 specialties); and (3) university hospitals (>40 specialties). In addition, many countries have a number of small, 15- to 20-bed, freestanding, private (typically for-profit) clinics. Recently, some tax-funded countries have begun to merge district and regional hospitals in an effort to improve the quality of care and create financial efficiencies (for example, Norway; planned for Denmark, also for Ireland; however, failed Parliamentary passage and brought down the coalition government, in Finland in 2019). Institutional mergers can be difficult to negotiate among publicly operated hospitals, due to the role that these large institutions play as important care providers and as large employers in smaller cities and towns, especially given political and union concerns about maintaining current employment levels. In the United States, financial and reimbursement pressures triggered by the implementation of the 2010 ACA have generated a number of private sector hospital mergers into larger hospital groups.

In tax-funded health systems, publicly funded patients who are admitted for an elective procedure cannot choose their specialist physician (except private-pay patients in "pay beds" in National Health Service [NHS] hospitals in England). Specialists are assigned by the clinic to a patient based on availability, with both junior and senior doctors placed in rotation.

Capital costs (buildings, large medical equipment) are publicly funded in all tax-funded systems and in most traditional SHI systems. For example, in Germany, capital costs for public hospitals are paid for by the regional governments. As a result, new capital investment is often allocated politically, according to location and political priorities. In Finland, local politicians in the 1980s would say that it "takes 10 years to build a hospital," meaning that it took that long to become a political priority for the regional government that controlled capital expenditures. Local politicians would therefore regularly overbuild when they got their one opportunity to obtain new capital.

Recently, efforts have been made to make public hospitals more responsible for their use of capital. In the Netherlands, public hospitals were shifted into private not-for-profit entities that are expected either to fund new capital from operating surplus or to borrow the funds from a bank based on a viable business plan. In England, more than 100 hospitals have been built using the Public Finance Initiative (PFI) program, in which private developers build turn-key facilities (thus taking capital costs off the public borrowing limit), and then rent these facilities back to the NHS and/or the relevant NHS Foundation Trust. In Sweden and Finland, while capital equipment is now a cost on hospital operating budgets, large new capital equipment and major building renovations remain politically driven processes often with extensive delays. In Stockholm County, the New Karolinska University Hospital opened in 2018 was built and is managed by a separate nonprofit public-private company.

In Singapore and South Korea, both of which are SHI funded, larger hospitals are publicly operated. However, there are a substantial number of smaller private clinics typically owned by specialist physicians. In the United States, the passage of the 2010 ACA has triggered the selling of many private specialist group practices to hospital groups, transforming previously independent practicing physicians into hospital employees.

Primary Care Services Most primary health care in SHI-funded health systems, and also in an increasing number of tax-funded health systems (except in low-income areas of some large cities), is delivered by independent private general practitioners (GPs), working either individually or in small privately owned group practices. Recent changes in tax-funded health systems include Norway, where most primary care moved from municipally employed physicians to private-practice GPs in 2003, and Sweden, where, following a 2010 change in national reimbursement requirements, new privately owned not-for-profit and for-profit GP practices were established and now deliver 50% of all primary care visits.

In England, most primary care physicians are private GPs who are contractors to the NHS, working either independently or in small group practices. These private GPs own their own practices, which they can sell when they retire. However, as part of the original agreement to convince physicians to support the establishment of the NHS in 1948 (which most physicians strongly opposed), private GPs also receive a national government pension upon retirement. In the inner cities in England, there are some larger primary health clinics.

In 2001, England's private primary care doctors were organized into geographically based Primary Care Trusts (PCTs). These PCTs were allocated 80% of the total NHS budget to contract for elective hospital services required by their patients with both NHS hospital trusts as well as private hospitals. In 2013, PCTs were restructured into Clinical Commissioning Groups with similar contracting responsibilities.

In 2004, the Quality Outcomes Framework (QOF) was introduced as a quality of care–tied approach to providing additional income for NHS GPs. This regulatory mechanism in 2010 set 134 different standards for best practice primary care in four main domains: 86 clinical, 36 organizational, 4 preventive service, and 3 patient experience. GP income grew on average by 25% through the introduction of the QOF, with general practices averaging 96% of possible QOF points. Total spending on QOF in 2014 in England consumed 15% of all primary care expenditures.

In April 2019, a slightly revised QOF contract was implemented, which retired 28 low-value indicators, introduced 15 new more clinically appropriate indicators, added two Quality Improvement modules, and added a new personalized care adjustment option. Funding was only changed marginally.

Access for individuals to primary care services is considered good in SHI-funded systems such as those in Germany and the Netherlands. One often-cited reason is that private office-based physicians (both GPs and specialists) in these countries are paid on a modified fee-for-service basis. In Germany, office-based physicians are paid on a quarterly basis by the Sickness funds, acting jointly at the Länder (regional) level through a point-based system. A national agreement between the physician association and the association of sick funds establishes points for each clinical act. Similarly, the association of sick funds (led in each of Germany's 16 Länder by the fund with the most subscribers in that region) establishes a fixed budget for all office-based physician services for all sick fund patients each 3-month period. Retrospectively at the end of each period, the total number of points is divided into the sick funds' fixed allocation for office-based physicians for that Länder for that quarter, establishing the value of a point for that quarter. Subsequently, each office-based physician's point total is multiplied by that quarterly point value, resulting in that physician's total payment from the statutory sick funds.

In contrast to SHI systems, seeing a primary care doctor in a number of tax-funded health systems has become increasingly difficult over the past decade. In Sweden, in 2005, a "care guarantee" was introduced that required its predominantly publicly operated health centers to see a patient within 7 days after calling for an appointment. In Finland, where public primary health care centers used to provide most primary care visits, delays in getting public health center appointments have pushed up to 40% of all visits into a parallel occupational health system, as well as to publicly employed primary care physicians working privately in the afternoons.

In England in 2019, access to GP services has been labeled a "crisis," aggravated by a 6% fall in the number of practicing GPs, leading to delays of up to 30 days for an appointment in urban areas like London. A 2019 report by the King's Fund found that only 1 in 20 trainee GPs planned to work full time. Also in 2019, the Nuffield Trust published a report suggesting that future planning for primary care services in England should assume a permanent shortage of GPs, requiring large numbers of new nurse practitioners and other auxiliary personnel. In Central European countries that were formerly within the Soviet Bloc, primary care provision had to be newly established after independence was regained in 1991, since first-line care in the former Semashko model was provided in specialist polyclinics. Primary care doctors rapidly emerged as almost entirely private for-profit GPs, working on contract from the national SHI fund (Estonia, Hungary, North Macedonia), from state-regulated private insurance companies (Czech Republic), or from regional/municipal public payers (Poland). Private GPs in most Central European countries now are paid on a per-visit-tied basis. This arrangement was heavily influenced by the structure of primary care in Germany, where private office-based GPs are paid according to a point-system-tied framework.

In Asian countries such as Singapore, South Korea, and Japan, most primary care is provided by private for-profit GPs working independently or in small group practices. Private GPs are reimbursed at a set per-service fee by the national SHI fund(s). Access to primary care physicians is considered good.

Developed countries have varying policies regarding access to individual preventive services. Health systems in most countries provide vaccinations and mammography as part of funded health care services. In the United States, most insured individuals—and in Canada, most covered residents—automatically receive an annual physical exam including full blood profiles. In Norway and Denmark, adult physical exams are provided only upon special request by the individual, and in Sweden, adult physical exams are provided only to pregnant women. In Sweden, adults who wish to know their cholesterol or prostate-specific antigen (PSA) levels have begun to purchase blood tests out-of-pocket from private laboratories. In England in 2019, the NHS announced it would stop providing PSA screening tests for prostate cancer, even to men who requested one, similarly forcing concerned patients to purchase private laboratory testing.

Patients must make copayments to see a primary care doctor in some tax-funded health systems and in most SHI countries. In tax-funded systems, for example, Swedish patients are required to make a county-council-set copayment for each primary care visit up to a national-government-set annual ceiling, after which ambulatory visits (both primary and outpatient specialist) are not charged. Finland has a fixed copay for public health center visits, while Denmark's private GP visits do not have a copayment. In England, there is no copayment for GP visits.

In SHI health care systems in Europe and in Asia, patients usually are responsible for a copayment for both primary and office-based specialist care. To defray these charges (and to pay for other nonfunded services), a high percentage of citizens typically purchase additional supplemental health insurance. In France, where 95% of patients in 2015 purchased private supplemental insurance, patients paid directly the full fee for 65% of outpatient primary and specialist services, reimbursed subsequently by both their SHI fund and their supplemental insurance carrier for all payments (after deductibles), while for 35% of services (for low-income individuals and certain high-cost procedures), full agreed prices were paid directly to providers by SHI.

Access to Elective Specialist Care Approximately half of all European health care systems have a gatekeeping system that requires referrals from primary care physicians in order to book hospital specialist visits (for publicly paid visits). In most tax-funded health systems (although not in most SHI systems), there are substantial waiting times, typically several months or more, for elective specialist appointments as well as for high-tech diagnostic and treatment procedures. Waiting times can be particularly long for cancer and other elective surgical or high-demand services. In Sweden, government figures from the summer of 2017 showed that, nationally, only 5–10% of prostate cancer operations were performed within 60 days after diagnosis.

In the English NHS, waiting lists for elective surgery in 2019 were often 6 months or longer. In August 2017, there were over 4,000,000 patients on NHS waiting lists. In January 2018, what administrators termed "a severe flu season," during which hospital emergency rooms were overwhelmed with elderly patients requiring admission, led to a national-level NHS decision to cancel all elective operating room procedures in all hospitals in England (>50,000 procedures in 1200 hospitals) for the entire month of January, further lengthening waiting lists. Regarding quality of care, again in England, a March 2018 report from the national Office of Health Economics found that, in 2016 and 2017, up to three-quarters of patients who could have undergone keyhole procedures were forced to undergo open surgery, resulting in an estimated 1 million procedures each year that were more invasive than clinically necessary.

Delays in some tax-funded systems also are procedural. In England, for example, a patient who requires a further consultation with a second specialist typically has to return to their primary care physician for a second referral and then has to wait in the regular patient queue for that second appointment.

There is also substantial waiting time for radiologic imaging services in most tax-funded systems. In Malta, the tax-funded health system's recent efforts to prioritize elective MRI investigations have succeeded in reducing waiting times from 18 months to 4 months. In both the Alberta and British Columbia Provinces in Canada, waiting times for a publicly funded nonemergency MRI can extend up to several months, whereas privately paid MRIs were available in both provinces within 1 week.

This issue of waiting times for specialist services in tax-funded health systems reflects a combination of growing demand (increasing/aging populations and changing clinical indications), financial constraints, and insufficient capacity, including inadequate physician working hours. For example, in the 1980s, when several surgical procedures for the elderly became more routine practice (e.g., hip replacement, coronary artery bypass graft, corneal lens implantation), the waiting list problem worsened. It had been mitigated somewhat through increased service capacity by the early 2000s, only to return as a growing policy challenge once public sector financial resources became constrained again after the 2008 global financial crisis. Timely cancer diagnosis and care continue to be a particularly sensitive issue, with tax-funded systems often taking several months for a patient to see an oncologist and then months more to begin treatment. In 2013 in Sweden, a newspaper journalist set off a political storm when he described women patients in one large county council (Malmo) who had to wait more than 40 days to receive the results from their breast cancer biopsy. In September 2019 in England, only 76.9% of patients with suspected cancer began treatment within 2 months of an urgent referral from a GP.

In response to pressure from national patient associations, a number of tax-funded health care systems introduced maximum waiting times for elective hospital procedures in the early 2000s. (Most Western European SHI systems do not have long waiting times or treatment guarantees for hospital care.) These maximum waiting times typically include initial primary care visits as well as specialist evaluations and treatment. In Denmark, a patient has the right to go to a different Danish public hospital for care after waiting 30 days without treatment. In Sweden, under the 2005 "waiting time guarantee," an untreated patient's local county council is required to pay for care in another county's hospital after 180 days. In a parallel process at the European Union (EU) level, beginning in 1997, the EU Court of Justice steadily expanded the right of all EU citizens to travel to another EU country in order to receive "timely" care, with their home country health system required to pay for that care.

In private not-for-profit SHI-funded health systems such as in Germany and Switzerland, waiting times for specialist visits and hospital procedures are typically a few weeks to 1 month. In the SHI system in France, which is more centrally organized and funded (part of the Napoleonic tradition of public administration), ongoing disputes about insufficient central government funding for public hospitals and staff salaries led in March 2019 to 9 months of hospital staff strikes, particularly in accident and emergency departments. In November 2019, the national government announced that it would take over 10 billion euros in public hospital debt as part of an effort to reverse staff cutbacks, bed and operating theater closures, and personnel flight to the private sector.

Long-Term Care Services LTC (consisting of residential and home-based services) consumes a relatively small but increasing proportion of gross domestic product (GDP) in developed countries. In 2016, Norway (2.95% GDP), Sweden (2.87% GDP), and the Netherlands (2.64% GDP) all spent more than one-fourth of their total health expenditures on LTC (Eurostat and OECD figures). More than one-fifth of all health care expenditures went to LTC in Belgium (2.16% GDP), Ireland (1.55% GDP), and Denmark (2.5% GDP). Lower-spending countries included the United Kingdom (18% of health expenditures; 1.75% GDP), Germany (12% of expenditures; 1.33% GDP), and Spain (9% of expenditures; 0.81% GDP). In the United States, official figures put total LTC expenditures in 2016 at 4.9% of total health expenditures, or 0.9% of total GDP. (Note that these figures do not include emergency, inpatient, or outpatient hospital costs generated by elderly patients.)

Since nursing home care is more expensive than home care (nursing home care requires the provision of housing, food, and around-the-clock care providers), government policymakers seek to keep the elderly and the chronically ill out of nursing homes for as long as feasible. Moreover, in developed countries like Sweden, Norway, and the United States, some 70% of all home care services come from informal caregivers: spouses, children (typically daughters), neighbors, and nonprofit community groups. While some SHI systems (e.g., Germany) have separate public LTC insurance (funded by mandatory premiums paid by all adults) that make available cash payments for LTC that can be used to compensate informal caregivers, most policymakers work hard to not monetize what is a large amount of essentially free care. Indeed, policymakers actively seek to encourage those providing these services to continue to do so as long as possible, trying to postpone caregiver burnout by providing support services such as free respite care, special call-in lines for caregiving advice, pension points toward retirement for the informal caregiver (Nordic countries), and free day-care center services.

In most tax-funded and SHI-funded European countries, home care services are organized at the municipal government level. In tax-funded systems, these services are also delivered mostly by municipal employees, working according to union-negotiated protocols. In some European SHI systems, and recently in tax-funded Sweden and Finland, private companies also provide home care services on contract to municipal governments. In combination with national legislation, these municipal systems also provide important support for informal caregivers, since the financial costs of caring for adults in their own home are substantially less than providing housing, food, and caregiver support in publicly funded homes for the aged or in nursing homes.

A high proportion of nursing homes in European tax-funded and SHI-funded health systems are publicly owned facilities operated by municipal governments; in some instances, in SHI-funded systems (Israel, the Netherlands), they are operated by private not-for-profit organizations. Recently, in some tax-funded systems (e.g., Sweden), private for-profit chains have begun to open nursing homes that are funded on a contract basis with local municipal governments. Costs for nursing home care can be expensive: in Norway, the cost per patient is often over $100,000 per year in a publicly funded home, with the patient responsible for paying up to 80% depending on the family's economic status. In Sweden, patients living in publicly funded nursing homes in Stockholm County pay a relatively small official fee, but they also pay room rent and up to 2706 Swedish krona (SEK) per month (about $270 U.S. dollars [USD]) for food out of their monthly public pension payments.

In 2012, in an effort to reduce demand for expensive hospital and nursing home services, Norway and Denmark began elderly care reforms that shifted service delivery as well as funding responsibilities to municipal governments. Among innovations in Norway, municipalities are required to establish a municipal acute bed unit (MAU) to treat stable elderly patients and provide observation beds for evaluation. Partial funding for these units is provided by the four public regional health care administrations. Some municipalities have also embedded primary care units inside their regional hospital to arrange discharge and to coordinate care for the chronically ill elderly. Norwegian municipalities are also responsible through their contracted (mostly private) primary care physicians to implement the National Pathways Program, which established treatment protocols for cross-sector conditions such as diabetes and cardiovascular conditions.

A differently configured structural innovation to better integrate LTC for the chronically ill elderly with clinical individual health services has been to consolidate both social and health care services within the same public administrative organization. In 2019, as part of health reforms in Ireland and Denmark and a proposed (unenacted) reform in Finland, as well as a pilot decentralization program in England for 2.8 million people in Greater Manchester, social and health care programs are to be administered by a single responsible agency.

In the SHI-funded system in the Netherlands, almost 7% of the population live in a residential home. National government legislation revised the structure of nursing home funding and care in 2015. Three acts restructured the separate public LTC SHI fund, which requires mandatory payments by 100% of Dutch adults, and introduced delivery-related reforms that reduced the number and overall cost of nursing home patients paid for by the fund. Determination of eligibility for public payment for nursing home care is now made by an independent national assessment body (the Centre for Needs Assessment). Moreover, municipal governments now play a stronger role in funding and delivering home care services. The reforms created social care teams that hold "kitchen table talks" to steer the elderly first toward seeking care from family, neighbors, churches, and other local community organizations before they qualify for publicly paid in-home care. In 2012, some 1.5 million people (12% of total population) provided informal care to ill or disabled persons, averaging 22 hours per week of care per person.

Home care recipients in the Netherlands can choose to set up a "personal budget," using their public funding allocation to select their preferred individual care personnel (either publicly employed or publicly approved private providers). This arrangement also enables these home care recipients to determine the particular mix of services they want, as well as to augment the allocated public funds with personal funds. A number of innovative not-for-profit nursing homes have been created to provide additional services to elderly living in their neighborhood (primary care home visits), as well as terminal hospice care (e.g., the Saffier De Residentie Groep residences in The Haag).

In the United States, nursing home and home care are funded and delivered in a variety of different ways. For individuals who have minimal financial assets, nursing home costs are paid by a joint federal-regional (state) welfare program called Medicaid. Most state government Medicaid programs pay out more than 40% of their total budget for nursing home care. In the past, Medicaid did not pay for home care services. However, some states have programs with private for-profit and not-for-profit providers that provide home care as a way to forestall the need for the more expensive nursing home care.

Many private individuals take out private LTC insurance, typically from commercial insurance companies. These policies require individuals to make premium payments for years in advance (often 20 or more) before the individual learns whether they will, in fact, require home or nursing home care. Some private insurers have also raised premiums after individuals have paid in for many years and canceled policies if the new higher rate is not affordable. The 2010 ACA contained a new public LTC insurance program. However, the program was designed to be voluntary, and U.S. Department of Health and Human Services administrators decided in 2013 not to implement that portion of the law.

In addition to the tax-funded Medicaid program and privately purchased LTC insurance, many middle-class families pay for care from savings, by selling the elderly person's home, or by direct contribution from children and other family members. Expenses can reach between $60,000 and $100,000 per year depending on the location of a facility and who operates it.

Nursing home care in the United States is provided by a wide mix of private not-for-profit and for-profit providers, ranging from church-owned single-site homes to large stock market–listed companies. Many of these homes are purpose-built as assisted-living or memory-care facilities. Home care services are delivered by a mix of private not-for-profit and for-profit providers.

In Japan, a national LTC insurance fund was introduced in 2000. Although the new fund applies uniformly across the country, the program is administered by municipal governments and the premium level differs across municipalities, with an average monthly premium of 3000 yen (about $30 USD). In South Korea, an SHI fund for LTC is funded by mandatory contributions of 4.78% of a person's regular national health insurance contribution, with an additional 20% of total LTC expenditures provided by national government funds. The client copayment for home care is set at 15% of expenses and at 20% for residential care.

PHARMACEUTICALS

Pharmaceutical expenditures in developed countries (inpatient and outpatient combined) vary widely across different health system types, as well as between different countries within each institutional type. OECD figures for 2018 show drug expenditures in tax-funded countries in Western Europe ranging from 6.3% of total health expenditures (THE) in Denmark to 11.9% of THE in the United Kingdom and 18.6% of THE in Spain. In SHI-funded Western European systems, pharmaceuticals absorbed 7.5% of THE in the Netherlands, while in Germany, that figure was 14.1%. In the hybrid tax-funded SHI systems of Central Europe, the pharmaceutical percentage of THE is higher: 18.2% of THE in Estonia to 27.9% of THE in Hungary. Similarly, in Asian SHI systems, pharmaceuticals consumed 20.7% of THE in South Korea and 18.6% of THE in Japan. The OECD's 2018 figures for pharmaceutical spending in North America are 12.0% of THE in the United States and 16.7% in Canada.

Contributing factors to this wide-ranging variation are (1) differences in national practice and prescription patterns reflecting differing cultural expectations; (2) the ratio problem (relatively fixed level of pharmaceutical costs due to international prices—the numerator—divided by a greatly varying per capita health expenditure cost in different developed country health systems); (3) the range and type of pharmaceutical price controls in each country; and (4) the degree of limitation placed on pharmaceutical supply, tied to formularies and/or explicit forms of drug rationing.

Most European health systems have tight national controls on the cost and, in some tax-based countries, on the availability of pharmaceuticals. Most European countries also use a number of different regulatory measures to limit prices and/or availability of both inpatient and outpatient drugs, including mandatory generic prescribing, reference pricing, patient copays (sometimes with an annual ceiling, after which copayments are no longer required), and (particularly in tax-funded systems) national formularies tied to clinical effectiveness. Norway, for example, allows only about 2300 different preparations—including dosage, delivery method, and box size—to be stocked by pharmacies. Prices for drugs can vary considerably across different European countries, tied to economic development and domestic pricing patterns. One consequence of these differential national pricing controls has been the development of a parallel import market, in which drug wholesalers and pharmacists in the more expensive countries purchase supplies from a cheaper market elsewhere in Europe.

Access to expensive drugs has also been intentionally limited in some tax-funded health systems in Europe. One basis for rationing has been rationing tied to quality-adjusted life-years (QALYs). Rationing also reflects a clash between strained public drug budgets and public pressure. For example, in the case of cancer drugs in England, the recommendation of the National Institute for Health and Care Excellence (NICE) against funding the breast cancer drug trastuzumab (Herceptin) was subsequently overturned by the Minister of Health.

Expensive cancer drugs continue to be rationed in England where the NHS Cancer Drug Fund, established in 2011 to provide access to non-NHS-provided drugs on a case-by-case basis, ran out of funds in 2015, forcing it to drop 25 of 83 covered drugs and close down for 3 months to restructure its operations.

As part of earlier medical patterns in Asian countries, office-based physicians traditionally filled prescriptions as well as prescribing drugs to patients. These sales also served to supplement their income in a setting of relatively low per-visit payments from state-run SHI funds. Concerned about cost and overuse, both Taiwan (in 1997, except for emergency cases or rural regions) and South Korea (for the whole country in 2003) implemented "separation reforms," which ended these physician sales. In Japan, a series of fee and reimbursement reforms have trimmed the percentage of all prescriptions dispensed in 2016 by physicians to 26% of prescriptions filled.

GOVERNANCE AND REGULATION

Health care services in developed countries are steered, constrained, monitored, and (to varying degrees) assessed by governments and governmentally established and/or empowered bodies. Although these measures apply particularly to the financial efficiency of government-funded services, they also seek to promote patient and community safety, equity of access, and high-quality clinical outcomes. This oversight is often strongly focused on privately operated and contracted providers and insurers, although in principle, it applies to publicly operated organizations as well.

Governance consists of macro national-level policy, meso institutional-level management, and micro clinic-level care decisions. This complex mix of governance decisions is often shared among different national, regional, and local governments, depending on the degree of centralization, decentralization, or, recently, recentralization (e.g., Norway and Denmark). While most systems officially prioritize "good governance," governance activities frequently comingle with political objectives as core policy concepts are developed and transformed into concrete organizational targets.

In Sweden, health system governance is shared among national, regional (county), and local municipal governments. The national government has responsibility to pass "frame" legislation, which establishes the basic structure of the system. To cite one example, until recently, the national government had limited an adult patient's total copayments for outpatient physician care (specialist and primary care) and pharmaceuticals to 2800 SEK (about $280 USD) for a 12-month period. The 20 regional governments, in turn, made policy decisions within that legislation, deciding how to apportion the specific copayments for each primary care and specialist outpatient visit. Since Swedes can self-refer to specialists, some counties double the copayment to hospital-based doctors to discourage unnecessary appointments. Similarly, fiscal policy normally is shared between the regional government, which raises about 70% of total health expenditures through its own county-set flat income tax, and the national government, which provides additional purpose-tied funds for national objectives such as consolidating open-heart surgery across county lines as well as supplementing lower tax receipts in rural counties with smaller working populations. However, this normal funding relationship across governments can change. In the early 1990s, the national government placed a "stop" on raising county taxes prior to Sweden's admission in 1995 to the EU. In 2016, each of the 20 counties could set their own ceilings, which were almost all at 3300 SEK (about $330 USD).

In Spain's tax-funded health system (71.1% publicly funded in 2015), 17 regional "autonomous communities" were given full managerial responsibility for the provision of health services in a 1990s decentralization process, along with ownership of all publicly operated hospitals. The national government generates a substantial proportion of health care resources, which are included in the broad block grants it allocates to the regional governments, which then add regional tax revenue to make up the full public sector budget. In a mechanism to steer regional government operating policies in this decentralized environment, the national Spanish government established a joint federal-regional council to review quality and performance data (through the 2003 Health System Cohesion and Quality Act). Italy's tax-funded health system (75.8% publicly funded in 2014) similarly shares governance responsibilities between national and regional governments. Health services are provided by local health authorities (Azienda Sanitaria Locale) supervised by 20 regional governments within a nationally established governance framework, financed through a complicated mix of national and nationally stipulated but regionally collected taxes. Again, like Spain, the national government established a federal-regional government council, seeking to better coordinate care standards and information among the regions and with national government agencies. In 2006, the national government imposed strict financial plans on 10 regions that were systematically in deficit.

In Germany, where funding for its SHI-based health system is predominantly the responsibility of 120 private not-for-profit sickness funds, governance decisions are shared among these private sector sickness funds and public sector national, regional, and municipal governments. The sickness funds receive a risk-adjusted premium payment for each enrolled individual, according to a national government–determined formula, and from a national government–run health insurance pool. Most hospitals are owned and operated by municipal governments, while investment capital for structural renovations and new building comes from the 16 regional Länder taken from their tax revenues. Payment frameworks and amounts for public hospitals are negotiated between associations of these municipally owned hospitals and associations of the private sickness funds, without formal government participation.

Regulation is an essential element of an effective health care system and a key component of overall health system governance. Regulation incorporates both broad standard requirements that affect all organizations that operate in a country (e.g., hiring, firing, and wage decisions) as well as specific health sector–related regulations (e.g., proper handling, use, and disposal of low-grade nuclear waste from radiation treatments). Recent examples of health sector regulation in England, for example, include the following:

1. Requiring all cancer drugs adopted for use in the NHS to cost no more than $41,268/QALY;
2. Requiring in their employment contract that junior doctors in hospitals work a specific number of Sundays; and
3. Requiring that all emergency department patients receive care within 4 h of their arrival.

A powerful tool that has the force of law, regulation can have substantial negative as well as positive effects. A well-known political science corollary of regulatory power is that "the right to regulate is also the right to destroy." For example, in the United States, the federal Environmental Protection Agency, as part of its pursuit of cleaner air, issued wide-ranging regulatory orders setting performance standards that resulted in the closing of many West Virginia coal mines, with the loss of tens of millions of dollars of productive capacity and thousands of high-paying jobs, and likely contributing to social conditions that helped spawn that state's high rates of opioid abuse among unemployed males. Similarly, in some tax-funded European systems, such as those in Sweden and England, there is growing pressure from public health advocates for national regulations to prohibit the making of a profit from publicly paid funds. In Sweden, the national government's Reepalu report in 2016 honored a pledge made by the Social Democratic government to its Left (socialist) Party ally by calling for a legislated ban on profit-making in the provision of publicly funded health care services. The report's publication triggered substantial divestment of existing investor-owned primary care, nursing home, and home care companies.

FUTURE CHALLENGES

Health systems in developed countries face continued challenges in the coming years. These include financial, organizational, and policy dilemmas for which institutionally viable, financially sustainable, and politically supportable solutions will be complicated to develop and difficult to implement. On the delivery side, a key question is whether privately structured GP-based primary care is more efficient and effective than various clinic-based forms of primary care services. Recent movement in Northern and Central Europe toward more private GPs, along with continued private office–based primary care in much of Canada, the United States, and economically developed countries in Asia, raises complex policy issues for international organizations like the World Health Organization (WHO), as well as national policymakers. In the hospital sector, existing levels of clinical quality and patient responsiveness in publicly operated command-and-control institutions will increasingly have to compete with those of semi-autonomous public hospitals, as well as various types of private, sometimes very innovative providers. In the financing arena, continued pressure on publicly raised health system revenues is likely to erode longtime commitments in some tax-funded health systems to minimal patient copayments and low out-of-pocket funding.

An additional set of challenges will arise from recent commitments by international organizations like WHO to restructure health systems in developed countries to better address the social determinants of health. This new, incomplete strategy calls for a dramatic expansion of health sector responsibility to include a wide range of existing institutional arrangements in housing, education, work-life, and social and political decision-making. The influential 2010 Strategic Review of Health Inequalities in England entitled "Fair Society, Healthy Lives," led by Sir Michael Marmot, a British epidemiologist, called for the elimination of all "inequities in power, money, and resources." Separate from the political dimensions of this proposed new paradigm, how such fundamental societal change will be funded and implemented has yet to be addressed.

Looking forward, among the most essential challenges to national decision-makers in the coming period will be four specific health system imperatives:

1. **Finding a more sustainable balance between ethics and funding.** Policymakers in publicly funded health systems face a growing gap between patient expectations of high-quality clinical care, staff expectations of better compensation, and the economic imperative of no new taxes. Recent research has suggested that SHI-funded health systems, faced with increasing aging and thus proportionally fewer employed, face a similar gap. While the present solidaristic foundation for raising collective revenues is insufficient, available nonsolidaristic tools (copayments, supplemental insurance, private pay) inevitably contribute to overall inequality. But what then are the realistic policy alternatives? The minimalist new policy goal necessarily will have to become one of raising new revenues while doing the least economic and social harm.
2. **Developing better strategies to steer provider diversity.** Health systems in developed countries are becoming more diverse with more and different types of public owners: hospital trusts, state enterprises, and mixed public-private hospital owners/managers. There also are more and different types of private providers: not-for-profit community groups, foundations, and cooperatives, as well as for-profit small local entrepreneurs, large international companies, and risk capital funds (venture capital). Furthermore, new innovative delivery models are reorganizing traditional service boundaries: not-for-profit private nursing homes in the Netherlands also provide outpatient primary care to neighborhood elderly patients, as well as hospice care; Israeli technology companies combine high-tech home-based patient monitoring with standard medical and custodial home care services. Public pressure from citizens for more choice and better outcomes will pressure policymakers toward new, more accommodative health system arrangements. A 2019 national government report in Sweden on the hospital sector recommended a new emphasis on better access to out-of-office hours and out-of-hospital acute care by private as well as public providers.
3. **Ensuring better coordination between social and health services.** Tax-funded and SHI-funded systems alike are under intense policy pressure to develop better strategies to integrate services for the chronically ill elderly, as a way to improve the quality of services that these patients receive and to keep them at home healthier and longer, reducing expensive acute visits to hospitals and emergency departments. The clear delivery system goal will increasingly be to keep the elderly out of nursing homes and acute care facilities for as long as possible.
4. **Building labor unions into provider innovation.** In many developed countries, health sector staff, including hospital physicians, are members of labor unions. Effective policymaking will require finding mechanisms to build these personnel unions into accelerated health system restructuring processes. This process will necessarily involve integrating unions into more innovative, flexible, fiscally sustainable organizational arrangements with contracts that reward active participation in organizational change, contracts that pay incentives to more productive employees, quicker reassignment and redundancy procedures (firing health sector workers can take a year or longer in some European health systems), and establishing profit-sharing payments to teams/unions, also in public sector organizations.

While the structure and complexity of resolving these specific organizational challenges will vary depending on a country's cultural and institutional context, the commonality of these problems suggests that health systems in the developed world require a new, broader range of targeted policy strategies and solutions.

FINANCING AND PROVIDING HEALTH SERVICES IN DEVELOPING COUNTRIES (See also Chap. 474)

Health systems in developing countries reflect a complex combination of the same core elements found in developed country systems (hospitals, primary care facilities, medical staff, pharmaceuticals) adapted to different, widely varying organizational, social, political, and economic contexts and conditions. System structure and provider institutions typically vary by differing national characteristics including historical relationships (Anglophone/Francophone/Hispanic/Soviet Semashko/American institutional and educational links); GDP and per capita annual national income (low- or middle-income developing countries); political norms and values; and ethnic and/or cultural mix. Predominantly public sector funding, particularly in lower-income countries, typically generates substantially lower levels of resources per capita than in developed countries and tends to be less reliable, particularly in countries where the economy is dependent on commodity exports.

Service delivery arrangements in developing countries, in turn, typically have higher provider-to-population ratios as well as, in public sector institutions, more mixed quality of care. In a number of middle-income developing countries, migration of trained medical staff to practice in higher-paying developed country health systems (often going to countries with historical relationships and/or where they received advanced training) further depletes available medical resources. In nearly all developing countries, private sector providers play an important supplemental role, with some middle-income developing countries like China currently encouraging their further development.

Most middle- and lower-income developing countries struggle to fund high-quality individual health services. Recent emphasis on universal health coverage has intensified that struggle. In middle-income developing countries (**Table 7-3**), World Bank data from 2016 show

TABLE 7-3 Middle-Income Developing Countries: Total Health Expenditure (% of gross domestic product)

Middle-Income Developing Countries	
Kazakhstan	3.53%
Thailand	3.71%
Malaysia	3.80%
Turkey	4.31%
China	4.98%
Botswana	5.46%
Mexico	5.47%
Colombia	5.91%

TABLE 7-4 Low-Income Developing Countries: Total Health Expenditure (% of gross domestic product)

Low-Income Developing Countries	
Nigeria	3.65%
India	3.66%
Ethiopia	3.97%
Nepal	6.29%
Honduras	8.40%

a range of health expenditure rates as a percentage of GDP, including Kazakhstan at 3.53% of GDP, Thailand at 3.71%, Malaysia at 3.80%, Turkey at 4.31%, China at 4.98%, Botswana at 5.46%, Mexico at 5.47%, and Colombia at 5.91%. Total health spending in low-income developing countries (**Table 7-4**) ranges from 3.65% of GDP for Nigeria, 3.66% for India, 3.97% for Ethiopia, 6.29% for Nepal, to 8.40% for Honduras.

Given lower aggregate GDP levels, per capita annual expenditures are considerably less than those found in developed countries. In middle-income developing countries (**Table 7-5**), Thailand spent (2016 data in adjusted USD) $221 annually per person, Kazakhstan spent $262, Colombia spent $340, Malaysia spent $361, Botswana spent $379, China spent $398, Mexico spent $461, and Turkey spent $468. Among low-income developing countries (**Table 7-6**), Ethiopia spent $27 per person annually, Nepal spent $45, India spent $62, and Nigeria spent $79, whereas Honduras spent $199.

China provides an interesting example of financing and service delivery development in middle-income developing countries. Financing reforms replaced fully publicly funded services with three new arrangements tied to work status and residence: (1) Urban Employee Basic Medical Insurance in 1998 (incorporating privately funded medical savings accounts—a concept pioneered in Singapore); (2) Urban Resident Basic Medical Insurance in 2007; and (3) New Rural Cooperative Medical Scheme in 2007. The urban employee program is an SHI model reflecting the rapid rate of economic growth and increasing incomes for urban workers. Starting in 2013, the Chinese government increasingly emphasized the development of new private hospitals and promotion of private insurance in urban areas. These and other health sector reforms became possible as continued strong economic growth over 30 years raised an estimated 300 million Chinese into the middle class, generating the requisite private as well as public revenues to underpin major structural health sector change.

Service delivery in developing countries varies widely in access, quality, and outcomes across and also within many developing countries. Medical services and tertiary institutions in urban areas of China, for example, operate at a substantially higher standard of service than those typically available in poorer rural regions. Similar disparities exist in wealthier parts of India such as Rajasthan, whereas in poorer states such as Bihar, primary care is mostly delivered by community "volunteers" with basic medical training, supervised by a GP.

Two critical challenges for all developing country health systems are contingent on generating adequate future funding flows. First, the current push from United Nations agencies to achieve universal health coverage will require additional public and private sector funding to

TABLE 7-5 Middle-Income Developing Countries: Per Capita Health Expenditures

Middle-Income Developing Countries	
Thailand	$221
Kazakhstan	$262
Colombia	$340
Malaysia	$361
Botswana	$379
China	$398
Mexico	$461
Turkey	$468

TABLE 7-6 Low-Income Developing Countries: Per Capital Health Expenditures

Low-Income Developing Countries	
Ethiopia	$27
Nepal	$45
India	$62
Nigeria	$79
Honduras	$199

pay for the necessary new providers and services. Second, available funding will need to be more effectively targeted on needed and appropriate services, with minimized managerial inefficiencies and substantially less political corruption.

Both forms of expanded funding will be dependent on strong national and global economic growth, which in turn will require continued country-level economic and political reforms. Achieving both funding-related objectives will require considerable international as well as national effort.

FURTHER READING

Barber SL et al: *Price Setting and Price Regulation in Health Care: Lessons for Advancing Universal Health Coverage.* Geneva, World Health Organization, Organization for Economic Co-operation and Development, 2019. *https://apps.who.int/iris/bitstream/handle/10665/325547/9789241515924-eng.pdf.*

Figueras J, McKee M (eds): *Health Systems, Health, Wealth, and Societal Well-Being: Assessing the Case for Investing in Health Systems.* Maidenhead, Open University Press/McGraw-Hill Education, 2011. *www.euro.who.int/__data/assets/pdf_file/0007/164383/e96159.pdf.*

Haseltine W: *Affordable Excellence: The Singapore Health Story.* Washington, Brookings Institution Press, 2013. *www.brookings.edu/wp-www.brookings.edu/wp-content/uploads/2016/07/AffordableExcellencePDF.pdf.*

Kuhlmann E et al (eds): *The Palgrave International Handbook on Healthcare Policy and Governance.* London, Palgrave MacMillan, 2015.

Rice T et al: *United States of America: Health System Review.* Health in Transition (HiT) Series 15 (3). Brussels, European Observatory on Health Systems and Policies, 2013. *www.euro.who.int/__data/assets/pdf_file/0019/215155/HiT-United-States-of-America.pdf.*

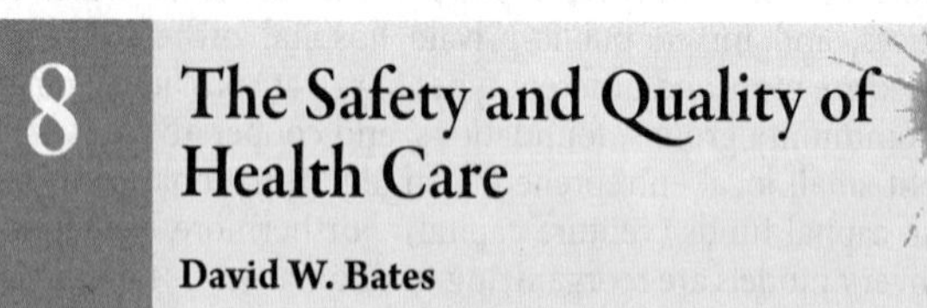

8 The Safety and Quality of Health Care

David W. Bates

Safety and quality are two of the central dimensions of health care. In recent years, it has become easier to measure safety and quality, and it is increasingly clear that performance in both dimensions could be much better. The public is—with good justification—demanding measurement and accountability, and payment for services will increasingly be based on performance in these areas. Thus, physicians must learn about these two domains, how they can be improved, and the relative strengths and limitations of the current ability to measure them.

Safety and quality are closely related but do not completely overlap. The Institute of Medicine has suggested in a seminal series of reports that safety is the first part of quality and that the health care system must first and foremost guarantee that it will deliver safe care, although quality is also pivotal. In the end, it is likely that more net clinical benefit will be derived from improving quality than from improving safety, though both are important and safety is in many ways more tangible to the public. The first section of this chapter will address issues relating to the safety of care and the second will cover quality of care.

SAFETY IN HEALTH CARE

Safety Theory and Systems Theory *Safety theory* clearly points out that individuals make errors all the time. Think of driving home from the hospital: you intend to stop and pick up a quart of milk on the way home but find yourself entering your driveway without realizing how you got there. Everybody uses low-level, semiautomatic behavior for many activities in daily life; this kind of error is called a *slip*. Slips occur often during care delivery—e.g., when people intend to write an order but forget because they must complete another action first. *Mistakes*, by contrast, are errors of a higher level; they occur in new or nonstereotypic situations in which conscious decisions are being made. An example would be dosing of a medication with which a physician is not familiar. The strategies used to prevent slips and mistakes are often different.

Systems theory suggests that most accidents occur as the result of a series of small failures that happen to line up in an individual instance so that an accident can occur (**Fig. 8-1**). It also suggests that most individuals in an industry such as health care are trying to do the right thing (e.g., deliver safe care) and that most accidents thus result from defects in systems. Systems should be designed both to make errors less likely and to identify those that do inevitably occur.

Factors That Increase the Likelihood of Errors Many factors ubiquitous in health care systems can increase the likelihood of errors, including fatigue, stress, interruptions, complexity, and transitions. The effects of fatigue in other industries are clear, but its effects in health care have been more controversial until recently. For example, the accident rate among truck drivers increases dramatically if they work over a certain number of hours in a week, especially with prolonged shifts. A recent study of house officers in the intensive care unit demonstrated that they were about one-third more likely to make errors when they were on a 24-h shift than when they were on a schedule that allowed them to sleep 8 h the previous night. The American College of Graduate Medical Education has moved to address this issue by putting in place the 80-h workweek. Although this stipulation is a step forward, it does not address the most important cause of fatigue-related errors: extended-duty shifts. High levels of stress and heavy workloads also can increase error rates. Thus, in extremely high-pressure situations, such as cardiac arrests, errors are more likely to occur. Strategies such as using protocols in these settings can be helpful, as can simple recognition that the situation is stressful.

Interruptions also increase the likelihood of error and occur frequently in health care delivery. It is common to forget to complete an action when one is interrupted partway through it by a page, for example. Approaches that may be helpful in this area include minimizing interruptions and setting up tools that help define the urgency of an interruption.

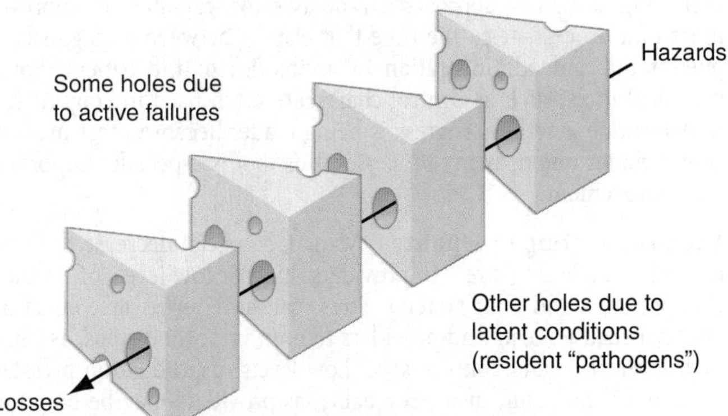

FIGURE 8-1 "Swiss cheese" diagram. Reason argues that most accidents occur when a series of "latent failures" are present in a system and happen to line up in a given instance, resulting in an accident. Examples of latent failures in the case of a fall might be that the unit is unusually busy and the floor happens to be wet. *(Adapted from J Reason: BMJ 320:768, 2000.)*

Complexity represents a key issue that contributes to errors. Providers are confronted by streams of data (e.g., laboratory tests and vital signs), many of which provide little useful information but some of which are important and require action or suggest a specific diagnosis. Tools that emphasize specific abnormalities or combinations of abnormalities may be helpful in this area.

Transitions between providers and settings are also common in health care, especially with the advent of the 80-h workweek, and generally represent points of vulnerability. Tools that provide structure in exchanging information—for example, when transferring care between providers—may be helpful.

The Frequency of Adverse Events in Health Care Most large studies focusing on the frequency and consequences of adverse events have been performed in the inpatient setting; some data are available for nursing homes, but much less information is available about the outpatient setting. The Harvard Medical Practice Study, one of the largest studies to address this issue, was performed with hospitalized patients in New York. The primary outcome was the adverse event: an injury caused by medical management rather than by the patient's underlying disease. In this study, an event either resulted in death or disability at discharge or prolonged the length of hospital stay by at least 2 days. Key findings were that the adverse event rate was 3.7% and that 58% of the adverse events were considered preventable. Although New York is not representative of the United States as a whole, the study was replicated later in Colorado and Utah, where the rates were essentially similar. Since then, other studies using analogous methodologies have been performed in various developed nations, and the rates of adverse events in these countries appear to be ~10%. Rates of safety issues appear to be even higher in developing and transitional countries; thus, this is clearly an issue of global proportions.

In the Harvard Medical Practice Study, adverse drug events (ADEs) were most common, accounting for 19% of all adverse events, and were followed in frequency by wound infections (14%) and technical complications (13%). Almost half of adverse events were associated with a surgical procedure. Among nonoperative events, 37% were ADEs, 15% were diagnostic mishaps, 14% were therapeutic mishaps, 13% were procedure-related mishaps, and 5% were falls.

ADEs have been studied more than any other error category. Studies focusing specifically on ADEs have found that they appear to be much more common than was suggested by the Harvard Medical Practice Study, although most other studies use more inclusive criteria. Detection approaches in the research setting include chart review and the use of a computerized ADE monitor, a tool that explores the database and identifies signals that suggest an ADE may have occurred. Studies that use multiple approaches find more ADEs than does any individual approach, and this discrepancy suggests that the true underlying rate in the population is higher than would be identified by a single approach. About 6–10% of patients admitted to U.S. hospitals experience an ADE.

Injuries caused by drugs are also common in the outpatient setting. One study found a rate of 21 ADEs per every 100 patients per year when patients were called to assess whether they had had a problem with one of their medications. The severity level was lower than in the inpatient setting, but approximately one-third of these ADEs were preventable.

The period immediately after a patient is discharged from the hospital appears to be very risky. A recent study of patients hospitalized on a medical service found an adverse event rate of 19%; about one-third of those events were preventable, and another one-third were ameliorable (i.e., they could have been made less severe). ADEs were the single leading error category.

Prevention Strategies Most work on strategies to prevent adverse events has targeted specific types of events in the inpatient setting, with nosocomial infections and ADEs having received the most attention. Nosocomial infection rates have been reduced greatly in intensive care settings, especially by using checklists. For ADEs, several strategies have been found to reduce the medication error rate, although it has been harder to demonstrate that they reduce the ADE rate overall, and no studies with adequate power to show a clinically meaningful reduction have been published.

Implementation of checklists to ensure that specific actions are carried out has had a major impact on rates of catheter-associated bloodstream infection and ventilator-associated pneumonia, two of the most serious complications occurring in intensive care units. The checklist concept is based on the premise that several specific actions can reduce the frequency of these issues; when these actions are all taken for every patient, the result has been an extreme reduction in the frequency of the associated complication. These practices have been disseminated across wide areas in the state of Michigan.

Computerized physician order entry (CPOE) linked with clinical decision support reduces the rate of serious medication errors, defined as those that harm someone or have the potential to do so. In one study, CPOE, even with limited decision support, decreased the serious medication error rate by 55%. CPOE can prevent medication errors by suggesting a default dose, ensuring that all orders are complete (e.g., that they include dose, route, and frequency), and checking orders for allergies, drug–drug interactions, and drug–laboratory issues. In addition, clinical decision support can suggest the right dose for a patient, tailoring it to the level of renal function and age. In one study, patients with renal insufficiency received the appropriate dose only one-third of the time without decision support, whereas that fraction increased to approximately two-thirds with decision support; moreover, with such support, patients with renal insufficiency were discharged from the hospital half a day earlier. As of 2019, over 95% of U.S. hospitals had implemented CPOE, although the decision support often is still limited.

Another technology that can improve medication safety is bar coding linked with an electronic medication administration record. Bar coding can help ensure that the right patient gets the right medication at the right time. Electronic medication administration records can make it much easier to determine what medications a patient has received. Studies to assess the impact of bar coding on medication safety are under way, and the early results are promising. Another technology to improve medication safety is "smart pumps." These pumps can be set according to which medication is being given and at what dose; the health care professional will receive a warning if too high a dose is about to be administered.

The National Safety Picture Several organizations, including the National Quality Forum and The Joint Commission, have made recommendations for improving safety. The National Quality Forum has released recommendations to U.S. hospitals about what practices will most improve the safety of care, and all hospitals are expected to implement these recommendations. Many of these practices arise frequently in routine care. One example is "readback," the practice of recording all verbal orders and immediately reading them back to the physician to verify the accuracy of what was heard. Another is the consistent use of standard abbreviations and dose designations; some abbreviations and dose designations are particularly prone to error (e.g., 7U may be read as 70).

Measurement of Safety Measuring the safety of care is difficult and expensive, since adverse events are, fortunately, rare. Most hospitals rely on spontaneous reporting to identify errors and adverse events, but the sensitivity of this approach is very low, with only ~1 in 20 ADEs reported. Promising research techniques involve searching the electronic record for signals suggesting that an adverse event has occurred. These methods are not yet in wide use but will probably be used routinely in the future. Claims data have been used to identify the frequency of adverse events; this approach works much better for surgical care than for medical care and requires additional validation. The net result is that, except for a few specific types of events (e.g., falls and nosocomial infections), hospitals have little idea about the true frequency of safety issues.

Nonetheless, all providers have the responsibility to report problems with safety as they are identified. All hospitals have spontaneous reporting systems, and if providers report events as they occur, those events can serve as lessons for subsequent improvement.

Conclusions about Safety It is abundantly clear that the safety of health care can be improved substantially. As more areas are studied closely, more problems are identified. Much more is known about the epidemiology of safety in the inpatient setting than in outpatient settings. A number of effective strategies for improving inpatient safety have been identified and are increasingly being applied. Some effective strategies are also available for the outpatient setting. Transitions appear to be especially risky. The solutions to improving care often entail the consistent use of systematic techniques such as checklists and often involve leveraging of information technology. Nevertheless, solutions will also include many other domains, such human factors techniques, team training, and a culture of safety.

QUALITY IN HEALTH CARE

Assessment of quality of care has remained somewhat elusive, although the tools for this purpose have increasingly improved. Selection of health care and measurement of its quality are components of a complex process.

Quality Theory Donabedian has suggested that quality of care can be categorized by type of measurement into structure, process, and outcome. *Structure* refers to whether a particular characteristic is applicable in a particular setting—e.g., whether a hospital has a catheterization laboratory or whether a clinic uses an electronic health record. *Process* refers to the way care is delivered; examples of process measures are whether a Pap smear was performed at the recommended interval or whether an aspirin was given to a patient with a suspected myocardial infarction. *Outcome* refers to what happens—e.g., the mortality rate in myocardial infarction. It is important to note that good structure and process do not always result in a good outcome. For instance, a patient may present with a suspected myocardial infarction to an institution with a catheterization laboratory and receive recommended care, including aspirin, but still die because of the infarction.

Quality theory also suggests that overall quality will be improved more in the aggregate if the performance level of all providers is raised rather than if a few poor performers are identified and punished. This view suggests that systems changes are especially likely to be helpful in improving quality, since large numbers of providers may be affected simultaneously.

The theory of *continuous quality improvement* suggests that organizations should be evaluating the care they deliver on an ongoing basis and continually making small changes to improve their individual processes. This approach can be very powerful if embraced over time.

Several specific tools have been developed to help improve process performance. One of the most important is the Plan-Do-Check-Act cycle (Fig. 8-2). This approach can be used for "rapid cycle" improvement of a process—e.g., the time that elapses between a diagnosis of pneumonia and administration of antibiotics to the patient. Some statistical tools, such as control charts, are often used in conjunction to determine whether progress is being made. Because most medical care includes one or many processes, this tool is especially important for improvement.

Factors Relating to Quality Many factors can decrease the level of quality, including stress to providers, high or low levels of production pressure, and poor systems. Stress can have an adverse effect on quality because it can lead providers to omit important steps, as can a high level of production pressure. Low levels of production pressure sometimes can result in worse quality, as providers may be bored or have little experience with a specific problem. Poor systems can have a tremendous impact on quality, and even extremely dedicated providers typically cannot achieve high levels of performance if they are operating within a poor system.

Data about the Current State of Quality A study published by the RAND Corporation in 2006 provided the most complete picture of

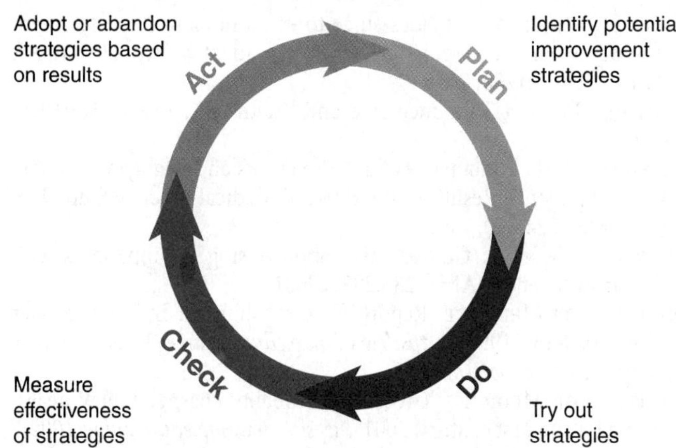

FIGURE 8-2 Plan-Do-Check-Act cycle. This approach can be used to improve a specific process rapidly. First, planning is undertaken, and several potential improvement strategies are identified. Next, these strategies are evaluated in small "tests of change." "Checking" entails measuring whether the strategies have appeared to make a difference, and "acting" refers to acting on the results.

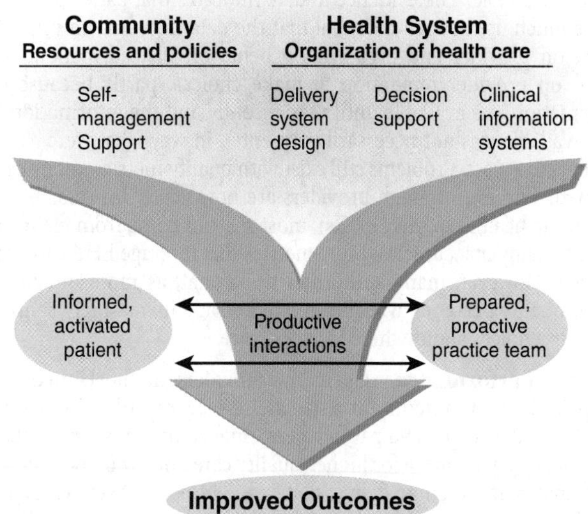

FIGURE 8-3 The Chronic Care Model, which focuses on improving care for chronic diseases, suggests that (1) delivery of high-quality care requires a range of strategies that must closely involve and engage the patient and (2) team care is essential. *(From EH Wagner et al: Eff Clin Pract 1:2, 1998.)*

quality of care delivered in the United States to date. The results were sobering. The authors found that, across a wide range of quality parameters, patients in the United States received only 55% of recommended care overall; there was little variation by subtype, with scores of 54% for preventive care, 54% for acute care, and 56% for care of chronic conditions. The authors concluded that, in broad terms, the chances of getting high-quality care in the United States were little better than those of winning a coin flip.

Work from the Dartmouth Atlas of Health Care evaluating geographic variation in use and quality of care demonstrates that, despite large variations in utilization, there is no positive correlation between the two variables at the regional level. An array of data demonstrate, however, that providers with larger volumes for specific conditions, especially for surgical conditions, do have better outcomes.

Strategies for Improving Quality and Performance Many specific strategies can be used to improve quality at the individual level, including rationing, education, feedback, incentives, and penalties. *Rationing* has been effective in some specific areas, such as persuading physicians to prescribe within a formulary, but it generally has been resisted. *Education* is effective in the short run and is necessary for changing opinions, but its effect decays fairly rapidly with time. *Feedback* on performance can be given at either the group or the individual level. Feedback is most effective if it is individualized and is given in close temporal proximity to the original events. *Incentives* can be effective, and many believe that they will prove to be a key to improving quality, especially if pay-for-performance with sufficient incentives is broadly implemented (see below). *Penalties* produce provider resentment and are rarely used in health care.

Another set of strategies for improving quality involves changing the systems of care. An example would be introducing reminders about which specific actions need to be taken at a visit for a specific patient—a strategy that has been demonstrated to improve performance in certain situations, such as the delivery of preventive services. Another approach that has been effective is the development of "bundles" or groups of quality measures that can be implemented together with a high degree of fidelity. Many hospitals have implemented a bundle for ventilator-associated pneumonia in the intensive care unit that includes five measures (e.g., ensuring that the head of the bed is elevated). These hospitals have been able to improve performance substantially. Another technique is SCAMPs, or Standardized Clinical Assessment and Management Plans. These are care guidelines developed by clinicians who identify key steps in workflow and decisions to help improve the process outcomes.

Perhaps the most pressing need is to improve the quality of care for chronic diseases. The Chronic Care Model has been developed by Wagner and colleagues (**Fig. 8-3**); it suggests that a combination of strategies is necessary (including self-management support, changes in delivery system design, decision support, and information systems) and that these strategies must be delivered by a practice team composed of several providers, not just a physician.

Available evidence about the relative efficacy of strategies in reducing hemoglobin A_{1c} (HbA_{1c}) in outpatient diabetes care supports this general premise. It is especially notable that the outcome was the HbA_{1c} level, as it has generally been much more difficult to improve outcome measures than process measures (such as whether HbA_{1c} was measured). In this meta-analysis, a variety of strategies were effective, but the most effective ones were the use of team changes and the use of a case manager. When cost-effectiveness is considered in addition, it appears likely that an amalgam of strategies will be needed. However, the more expensive strategies, such as the use of case managers, probably will be implemented widely only if pay-for-performance takes hold.

The evidence linking better performance on quality metrics assessing process and outcomes varies greatly by condition. For example, there is strong evidence that performing Pap smears results in better outcomes in patients who develop cervical cancer, but the evidence for many other conditions is far more tenuous.

National State of Quality Measurement In the inpatient setting, quality measurement is now being performed by a very large proportion of hospitals for several conditions, including myocardial infarction, congestive heart failure, pneumonia, and surgical infection prevention; 20 measures are included in all. This is the result of the Hospital Quality Initiative, which represents a collaboration among many entities, including the Hospital Quality Alliance, The Joint Commission, the National Quality Forum, and the Agency for Healthcare Research and Quality. The data are housed at the Centers for Medicare and Medicaid Services, which publicly releases performance data on the measures on a website called *Hospital Compare* (*www.cms.gov/Medicare/Quality-Initiatives-Patient-Assessment-Instruments/Hospital-QualityInits/HospitalCompare.html*). These data are reported voluntarily and are available for a very high proportion of the nation's hospitals. Analyses demonstrate substantial regional variation in quality and important differences among hospitals. Analyses by The Joint Commission for similar indicators reveal that performance on measures by hospitals has improved over time and that, as might be hoped, lower performers have improved more than higher performers.

Public Reporting Overall, public reporting of quality data is becoming increasingly common. There are now commercial websites that have quality-related data for most regions of the United States, and these data can be accessed for a fee. Similarly, national data for hospitals are available. The evidence to date indicates that patients have not made much use of such data, but that the data have had an important effect on provider and organization behavior. Instead, patients have relied on provider reputation to make choices, partly because little information was available until very recently and the information that was available was not necessarily presented in ways that were easy for patients to access. Problems still exist with quality metrics; many can be "gamed," and even though providers are now nearly universally using electronic health records (EHRs), most metrics come from claims that include many inaccuracies. More metrics that leverage EHRs are sorely needed. However, many authorities think that, as more information about quality becomes available, it will become increasingly central to patients' choices about where to access care.

Pay-for-Performance Currently, providers in the United States get paid the same amount for a specific service, regardless of the quality of care delivered. The pay-for-performance theory suggests that, if providers are paid more for higher-quality care, they will invest in strategies that enable them to deliver that care. The current key issues in the pay-for-performance debate relate to (1) how effective it is, (2) what levels of incentives are needed, and (3) what perverse consequences are produced. The evidence on effectiveness is limited, although a number of studies are ongoing. With respect to incentive levels, most quality-based performance incentives have accounted for merely 1–2% of total payment in the United States to date. In the United Kingdom, however, 40% of general practitioners' salaries have been placed at risk according to performance across a wide array of parameters; this approach has been associated with substantial improvements in reported quality performance, although it is still unclear to what extent this change represents better performance versus better reporting. The potential for perverse consequences exists with any incentive scheme. One problem is that, if incentives are tied to outcomes, there may be a tendency to transfer the sickest patients to other providers and systems. Another concern is that providers will pay too much attention to quality measures with incentives and ignore the rest of the quality picture. The validity of these concerns remains to be determined. Nonetheless, it appears likely that, under health care reform, the use of various pay-for-performance schemes is likely to increase.

CONCLUSIONS

The safety and quality of care in the United States could be improved substantially. A number of available interventions have been shown to improve the safety of care and should be used more widely; others are undergoing evaluation or soon will be. Quality also could be dramatically better, and the science of quality improvement continues to mature. Implementation of value-based approaches such as accountable care that include pay-for-performance related to safety and quality should make it much easier for organizations to justify investments in improving safety and quality parameters, including health information technology. However, many improvements will also require changing the structure of care—e.g., moving to a more team-oriented approach and ensuring that patients are more involved in their own care. Payment reform focusing on value seems very likely to progress and will likely include both positive incentives and penalties related to safety and quality performance. Measures of safety are still relatively immature and could be made much more robust; it would be particularly useful if organizations had measures they could use in routine operations to assess safety at a reasonable cost, and substantial research is addressing this. Although the quality measures available are more robust than those for safety, they still cover a relatively small proportion of the entire domain of quality, and more measures need to be developed. The public and payers are demanding better information about safety and quality as well as better performance in these areas. The clear implication is that these domains will have to be addressed directly by providers.

FURTHER READING

Bates DW et al: Effect of computerized physician order entry and a team intervention on prevention of serious medication errors. JAMA 280:1311, 1998.

Bates DW et al: Two decades since to err is human: An assessment of progress and emerging priorities in patient safety. Health Aff (Millwood) 37:1736, 2018.

Berwick DM: Era 3 for medicine and health care. JAMA 315:1329, 2016.

Brennan TA et al: Incidence of adverse events and negligence in hospitalized patients. Results of the Harvard Medical Practice Study I. N Engl J Med 324:370, 1991.

Chertow GM et al: Guided medication dosing for inpatients with renal insufficiency. JAMA 286:2839, 2001.

Institute of Medicine. Report: To err is human: Building a safer health system. 1999. *https://www.nap.edu/resource/9728/To-Err-is-Human-1999--report-brief.pdf.*

Institute of Medicine. Crossing the quality chasm: A new health system for the 21st century. 2001. *https://www.nap.edu/catalog/10027/crossing-the-quality-chasm-a-new-health-system-for-the.*

Landrigan C et al: Effect of reducing interns' work hours on serious medical errors in intensive care units. N Engl J Med 351:1838, 2004.

McGlynn EA et al: The quality of health care delivered to adults in the United States. N Engl J Med 348:2635, 2003.

Pronovost P et al: An intervention to decrease catheter-related bloodstream infections in the ICU. N Engl J Med 355:2725, 2006. Erratum in: N Engl J Med 356:2660, 2007.

Starmer AJ et al: Rates of medical errors and preventable adverse events among hospitalized children following implementation of a resident handoff bundle. JAMA 310:2262, 2013.

9 Diagnosis: Reducing Errors and Improving Quality

Gordon Schiff

Diagnosing patients' illnesses is the essence of medicine. Patients present to doctors seeking an answer to the question, "What is wrong with me?" Ideally, no clinician would want to treat a patient without knowing the diagnosis or, worse yet, erroneously treat a misdiagnosed illness. From the earliest moments of medical school, the defining quest toward becoming a knowledgeable and proficient physician is learning how to put a diagnostic label on patients' symptoms and physical findings, and clinicians pride themselves on being "good diagnosticians." Yet the centuries-old paradigm of mastering a long list of diseases, understanding their pathophysiology, and knowing the cardinal ways they manifest themselves in signs and symptoms, while still of fundamental importance, is being challenged by new insights illuminated by the glaring spotlight of diagnostic errors. Basic internal medicine diseases, such as asthma, pulmonary embolism, congestive heart failure, seizures, strokes, ruptured aneurysms, depression, and cancer, are misdiagnosed at shockingly high rates, often with 20–50% of patients either being mislabeled as having these conditions (false-positive diagnoses) or having their diagnosis missed or delayed (false negatives). How and why do physicians so often get it wrong, and what can we do to both diagnose and treat the problem of delayed diagnosis or misdiagnosis?

Diagnosis is both an ancient art and a modern science. The current science of diagnosis, however, goes far beyond what typically comes to clinicians' and patients' minds when they conjure up images of state-of-the-art molecular, genetic, or imaging technologies. Improvements in diagnosis are just as likely to come from other areas, many with origins outside of medicine, as they are from advanced diagnostic testing modalities. These diverse sciences that the field of diagnostic safety has, and must, draw from include systems and human factors engineering, reliability science, cognitive psychology, decision sciences, forensic science, clinical epidemiology, health services research, decision analysis, network medicine, learning health systems theory, medical sociology, team dynamics and communication, risk assessment and communication, information and knowledge management, and health information technology, especially artificial intelligence and clinical decision support. A clinician reading this chapter is likely to find this list of overlapping and intersecting domains quite daunting. However, rather than feeling overwhelmed, we urge readers to view them as the basic science supports that will ultimately make their lives easier and diagnosis more accurate and timely. Rather than feeling intimidated, clinicians should feel a sense of relief and assurance in understanding that good diagnosis does not rest entirely on their shoulders. Instead, it is a systems property, where an infrastructure and a team, one that especially includes the patient, can in a coordinated way work together to achieve more reliable and optimal diagnosis.

EMERGENCE OF DIAGNOSIS ERROR AS AN IMPORTANT PATIENT SAFETY ISSUE

Over the past decade, a series of studies culminating in a landmark report from the U.S. National Academy of Medicine (NAM), *Improving Diagnosis in Health Care,* have shone a spotlight on diagnostic errors. Reports from patient surveys, malpractice claims, and safety organizations, such as the ECRI and the National Patient Safety Foundation (now part of Institute for Healthcare Improvement), have found that diagnostic errors are the leading type of medical error. Although errors in diagnosis are defined in various ways, the NAM Committee defined diagnostic error as "the failure to (a) establish an accurate and timely explanation of the patient's health problem(s) or (b) communicate that explanation to the patient." One way to visualize diagnostic errors is through a Venn diagram (**Fig. 9-1**), which illustrates the fact that many things can go wrong in the diagnostic process (e.g., failure to ask an important history question, physical examination sign overlooked, laboratory specimen erroneously switched between two patients, x-ray not followed up), but this usually does not result in a wrong diagnosis or patient harm. Similarly, a patient can be misdiagnosed but unharmed, without any identifiable error in the care received. Our greatest concern is where these three circles intersect, with conservative estimates suggesting that 40,000–80,000 patients die each year in U.S. hospitals alone from diagnostic errors. The NAM report outlined eight recommendations that are the foundation for this chapter (**Table 9-1**).

NEW WAYS TO THINK ABOUT DIAGNOSIS AND DIAGNOSTIC ERRORS

Medical textbooks have historically given attention to "clinician reasoning" and associated cognitive heuristics and biases. Errors in clinical reasoning can be summarized in three broad groups: (1) hasty judgments, (2) biased judgments, and (3) inaccurate probability estimates. Research from cognitive psychology has identified scores of common mental shortcuts or "heuristics" humans are prone to use in everyday life, many of which are useful for efficient diagnosis but can also lead to biases and errors. **Table 9-2** lists some of the common cognitive biases that can lead diagnosis astray (this topic is discussed further in **Chap. 4**).

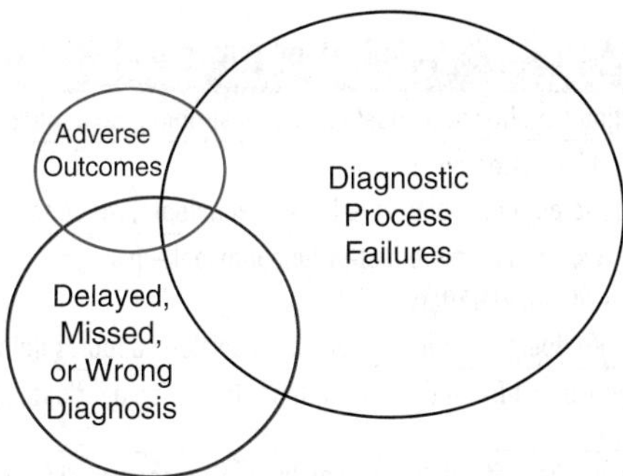

FIGURE 9-1 What is a diagnosis error? *(Adapted from GD Schiff et al: Diagnosing diagnosis errors: Lessons from a multi-institutional collaborative project, in Advances in Patient Safety: from Research to Implementation. Vol. 2 Concepts and Methodology, Rockville, MD, 2005, pp. 255-278, and GD Schiff, L Leape: Acad Med 87:135, 2012.)*

TABLE 9-1 National Academy of Medicine Recommendations for Improving Diagnosis in Health Care

1. Facilitate more effective teamwork in the diagnostic process among health care professionals, patients, and their families.
2. Enhance professional education and training in the diagnostic process in areas such as clinical reasoning; teamwork; communication with patients, families, and other health care professionals; and appropriate use of diagnostic tests.
3. Ensure that health information technologies support patients and health care professionals in the diagnostic process.
4. Develop and deploy approaches to identify, learn from, and reduce diagnostic errors and near misses in clinical practice including providing systematic feedback on diagnostic performance.
5. Establish a work system and culture that supports the diagnostic process and improvements in diagnostic performance.
6. Develop a reporting environment and medical liability system that facilitates improved diagnosis by learning from diagnostic errors and near misses.
7. Design a payment and care delivery environment that supports the diagnostic process.
8. Provide dedicated funding for research on the diagnostic process and diagnostic errors.

However, clinicians will also benefit from having a better understanding of diagnosis as a "system" rather than just what takes place in clinicians' minds. Classic teaching exhorting trainees and practicing physicians to have a broad differential and "high index of suspicion" for various diseases is challenged not only by these unconscious biases but also by limitations of human memory, information shortfalls, constrained encounter time, system process failures, and the myriad nonspecific symptoms that patients bring to clinicians. Many symptoms are self-limited, defy a precise diagnosis or etiology, and do not portend harmful outcomes. Insights from safety and cognitive sciences call for rethinking traditional approaches to diagnosis and suggest new approaches to overcome current limitations (**Table 9-3**).

UNCERTAINTY IN DIAGNOSIS

Given variations and overlap in ways patients present, illnesses evolve, and tests perform, it is often not possible or practical to "make" a definitive diagnosis, particularly in the primary care setting early in the course of a patient's illness. Clinicians need to harness these uncertainties to both engineer situational awareness of where things

TABLE 9-2 Selected Cognitive Biases Contributing to Diagnostic Errors

1. Premature closure: accepting a diagnosis before it has been fully verified
2. Anchoring: tendency to fixate on a specific symptom or piece of information early in the diagnostic process with subsequent failure to appropriately adjust
3. Confirmation bias: tendency to look for confirming evidence to support one's diagnostic hypothesis, rather than disconfirming evidence to refute it
4. Search satisficing: tendency to call off a search, satisfied once a piece of data or presumed explanation is found, and not considering/searching for additional findings or diagnoses
5. Availability bias: tendency to give too much weight to diagnoses that come more readily to mind (e.g., recent dramatic case)
6. Base-rate neglect: failing to adequately take into account prevalence of a particular disease (e.g., erroneously interpreting a positive test as indicating disease in a low-prevalence population using a test with 5% false-positive rate)
7. Knowledge deficit (on part of provider, with accompanying lack of awareness)
8. Framing bias: Judgement overly influenced by the way the problem was presented (how it was framed in words, settings, situations)
9. Social/demographic/stereotype bias: biases from personal or cultural beliefs about women, minorities, or other patient groups for whom prejudices may distort diagnostic assessment

TABLE 9-3 New Models for Conceptualizing Diagnosis and Diagnosis Improvement

TRADITIONAL WAYS OF THINKING ABOUT DIAGNOSIS AND DIAGNOSTIC ERROR	NEW PARADIGMS/BETTER WAYS TO THINK ABOUT DIAGNOSIS AND IMPROVING DIAGNOSIS
General	
A good diagnostician gets it right the first time, almost all of the time	Diagnosis is an inexact science with inherent uncertainties Goal is to minimize errors and delays via more reliable systems and follow-up
Lore of masterful/skillful academic expert diagnostician who knows/recalls everything; need to look to them if seeking diagnostic excellence	Less reliance on (fallible) human memory Quality diagnosis is based on well-coordinated distributed network/team of people and reliable processes All patients entitled to receive quality diagnosis, regardless of where and from whom they receive care
Diagnosis is the doctor's job	Co-production of diagnosis among clinicians (including lab, radiology, specialists, nurses, social workers) and, especially, the patient and family
Patients often viewed as overly anxious, exaggerating, time-consuming, questioning, with sometimes unreasonable demands and expectations	Patients are key allies in diagnosis; hold key information Need to address understandable/legitimate fears, desires for explanations Leveraging patient questions and questioning of diagnosis to stimulate rethinking the diagnosis where needed
Diagnosis and treatment as separate stages in patient care (i.e., make a diagnosis, then treat)	Prioritizing diagnostic efforts to target treatable conditions More integrated strategies and timing for testing and treatment depending on urgency for treatment
Clinical practices	
Order lots of tests to avoid missing diagnoses	Judicious ordering: targeted, well-organized data and testing Appreciation of test limitations (false positive or negative, incidental findings, overdiagnosis, test risks) and resulting harms
More referrals to avoid missing rarer/specialized diagnoses; concomitant utilization barriers (copays, prior authorization) to minimize overuse	"Pull systems" to lower barriers and make it easier to pose questions, obtain real-time virtual consults Co-management approaches to enable collaborative watch-and-wait conservative strategies where appropriate
Frequent empirical drug trials when uncertain of diagnosis	Conservative use of drugs to avoid confusing clinical picture or labeling patients with diseases they may not have
Physician attention/efforts to ensure disease screening	Automating, delegating clerical functions; teamwork to free up physician cognitive time
Diagnosis errors and challenges	
Diagnostic error viewed as a personal failing Errors classified as either "system" or "cognitive"	Many errors/delays rooted in processes and system design/failures Errors multifactorial with interwoven, interacting, and inseparable cognitive and system factors
Errors are infrequent; hit-and-miss ways to learn about errors	Errors are common; systematic proactive follow-up is needed to recognize potential for errors Surveilling of high-risk situations and one's own diagnostic performance and outcomes
Clinicians' reactions: denial, defensive, others to blame, pointing to others also making similar errors	Culture of actively and nondefensively seeking to uncover, dig deep to learn from, and share errors and lessons
Dreading complex, frustrating diagnostic dilemmas	Welcoming/enjoying intellectual/professional challenges Adequate support (time, help, consultations) for more complex patients
Diagnoses as distinct labels, events	Diagnoses can be indistinct, interacting comorbidities, socially constructed, multifactorial, evolving over time, or have overlapping genotype-phenotype expressions
Documentation/communication	
Viewed as time-consuming, mindless, primarily to document for billing code and/or bulwark against malpractice claims	Documentation as useful tool for reflecting, crafting, sharing assessments, differential diagnosis, reflecting about unanswered questions Opportunities for decision support interacting with computer Notes open for patients to read to help understand and critique diagnosis
Say and write as little as possible about uncertainties, lest it be used against you in malpractice allegation	Share uncertainties to maximize communication and engagement with other caregivers, patients
Don't let patient know about errors so they don't become angry, mistrustful, or sue	Patients have right to honest disclosure; often find out about errors anyway (e.g., cancer evolves); anticipate, engage their concerns
Patients advised to call if not better; no news is good news (test results: "We'll call if anything is abnormal.")	Systematic proactive follow-up to close loop on tests and symptoms, to check how patient is doing, monitor outcomes
Global remedies	
Knowing/memorizing more medical knowledge	Knowing more about the patient (including psychosocial, past history, environmental contexts)
Attention to the "objective" data (physical exam, tests) to reliably make diagnoses	Renewed emphasis on history, history-taking, listening Acknowledgement of ubiquitous subjective cognitive biases; efforts to anticipate, recognize, counteract
Exhortations to have "high index of suspicion" of various diagnoses	Less reliance on memory recall of lectures/reading; more just-in-time info look-up Affordances, alerts to red flags engineered into workflow Delineation of "don't miss" diagnoses with design of context-relevant decision support reminders
Ensuring physician is copied on everything, thorough/voluminous notes, widespread reminders/alerts	Biggest problem is no longer lack of access to information, but rather information overload; strategies to organize, minimize
Continuing medical education (CME) courses to expand medical knowledge	Real-time, context-aware reminders of pitfalls, critical differential diagnoses, and key differentiating features. Ready access to medical references, second opinions

(*Continued*)

TABLE 9-3 New Models for Conceptualizing Diagnosis and Diagnosis Improvement (Continued)

TRADITIONAL WAYS OF THINKING ABOUT DIAGNOSIS AND DIAGNOSTIC ERROR	NEW PARADIGMS/BETTER WAYS TO THINK ABOUT DIAGNOSIS AND IMPROVING DIAGNOSIS
Redundancies, double-checks	Recognition that single, highly reliable systems are often better than multiple halfway solutions. Clear delineation of responsibilities for follow-up tasks
Fear of malpractice suits to motivate physicians to be more careful and practice defensive medicine	Drive out fear, making it safe to learn from and share errors Shared situational awareness of where pitfalls lurk
More accountability, financial incentives, and penalties tied to performance metrics	Clinician engagement in improvement based on trust, collaboration, professionalism, financial neutrality Metric modesty, recognizing many best practices yet to be defined/proven
More rules, requirements; target outliers for better compliance	Standardization with flexibility; learning from deviations
More time with patients	Better time spent with patients: offloading distractions, more efficient history collection/organization, longitudinal continuity, and, where needed, additional time to talk/think/explain during, before, or after visits Easier access for patients to reach or be seen by clinicians when experiencing symptoms
Reflex changes in response to errors	Avoiding "tampering," which entails understanding/diagnosing difference between "special cause" versus "common cause" (random) variation

Source: Modified from GD Schiff: Quality and Safety in Health Care 2013.

can go wrong and create safety nets to protect patients against harms from delayed diagnosis and misdiagnosis. Terms such as *preliminary diagnosis, working diagnosis, differential diagnosis, deferred diagnosis, undiagnosed illness, diagnoses with uncertain or multifactorial etiologies, intermittent diagnoses, multiple/dual diagnoses, self-diagnosis*, or at times *contested diagnosis* need to be part of our vocabulary, thinking, and communications with patients to convey that diagnosis is often imprecise. Anxious patients worried about a condition, for example, cancer, COVID-19 infection, or a diagnosis to which a relative or a friend has recently succumbed, come seeking reassurance and may not welcome an uncertain answer. Thus, we have to work with patients, listen to and respect their concerns, and take their symptoms seriously yet modestly acknowledge our limitations. We need to tailor this approach to patients' differing levels of health literacy, trust in our clinical advice, and experiences with the health system.

DON'T MISS DIAGNOSES AND RED FLAGS

Uncertainty should not be a license for complacency. Particularly for diseases that (1) progress rapidly, (2) require specific treatments that depend on making the correct diagnosis, or (3) have public health or contagion implications, clinicians need to be poised, and systems designed, to consider and, where appropriate, pursue critical "don't miss" diagnoses. While clinicians are generally aware of more common "don't miss" diagnoses (e.g., acute myocardial infarction, sepsis), **Table 9-4** illustrates examples of less common diagnoses that warrant similar consideration. Throughout this textbook, readers should orient themselves to recognize such critical diagnoses and think about presentations and syndromes where they may be lurking.

An important related concept is so-called "red flags" or "alarm symptoms." This construct has its origins in guidelines for back pain but has increasingly been applied to many other problems, such as headache, red eye, swollen joint, or even abdominal pain and chest pain. Examples of widely cited red flags for back pain that should trigger consideration of more serious etiologies include fever, weight loss, history of malignancy or intravenous drug use, or neurologic signs and symptoms. In theory, many presenting syndromes could benefit from identification of such clues to more serious diagnoses. Evidence-based medicine calls for better data on the sensitivity, specificity, yield, and discriminatory ability of various clinical "red flag" clues; yet, few have been rigorously evaluated. Nonetheless, clinicians find them useful as simple ways to reassure themselves and their patients that a common symptom such as back pain or headache is, or is not, likely an indicator of more urgent or serious pathology.

Interwoven with the challenges of not missing critical diagnoses is the problem of overtesting and overdiagnosis—performing unnecessary and even potentially harmful tests whose benefit does not justify the risks or costs or that may lead to diagnoses that would have never caused any symptoms or problems. Thoughtful diagnosticians need to weigh carefully this "other side of the coin" of missed diagnosis to avoid such harms and expenses.

DIAGNOSTIC PITFALLS

One of the important ways of learning in medicine is learning from the missteps of those who have walked the path ahead of us. By learning about commonly missed diagnoses and the ways accurate, timely diagnosis went astray, we can avoid making similar mistakes. Anticipating the potential for similar types of errors can both create situational awareness of traps to avoid and contribute to learning from our own personal and collective patterns of mistakes. Several studies have examined common or recurring pitfalls in diagnosis. An example of a common disease-specific diagnostic pitfall in breast cancer diagnosis is ordering a mammogram for a woman with a palpable breast lump and, when the mammogram returns as normal, reassuring her that cancer has been "ruled out" by the negative test. Any mass or lesion palpable

TABLE 9-4 Examples of "Don't Miss" Diagnoses

INFECTIONS/ INFLAMMATION	CARDIAC/ISCHEMIC/ BLEEDING	METABOLIC/ HEMATOLOGIC/ ENVIRONMENTAL
Spinal epidural abscess	Aortic dissection Leaking/ruptured abdominal aortic aneurysm	Diabetes ketoacidosis Hyperosmolar hyperglycemia
Necrotizing fasciitis	Pericardial tamponade	Myxedema/ thyrotoxicosis
Meningitis	Wolff-Parkinson-White Prolonged QT	Addison's disease
Endocarditis	Pulmonary embolism	B_{12} deficiency anemia
Peritonsillar abscess	Tension pneumothorax	von Willebrand's disease
Tuberculosis-active pulmonary, other	Acute mesenteric ischemia Sigmoid volvulus	Hemochromatosis
COVID-19 infection	Esophageal, bowel perforation	Celiac sprue
Guillain-Barré syndrome	Cerebellar hemorrhage	Carbon monoxide poisoning
Ebola infection	Spinal cord compression	Food poisoning
Temporal arteritis	Testicular, ovarian torsion	Malignant hyperthermia
Rhabdomyolysis	Ectopic pregnancy	Alcohol, benzodiazepine, barbiturate withdrawal
Angioedema	Retroperitoneal hemorrhage	Tumor lysis syndrome Hypo-/hypercalcemia

TABLE 9-5 Generic Types of Diagnostic Pitfalls

PITFALL	EXAMPLES
Disease A mistaken for disease B Diseases often mistaken/misdiagnosed with each other	• Aortic dissection misdiagnosed as acute myocardial infarction • Bipolar disorder misdiagnosed as depression
Misinterpretation of test result(s) False-positive or false-negative results with failure to recognize test limitations	• Breast lump dismissed after negative mammogram • Negative COVID-19 test early or late in course
Failure to recognize atypical presentation, signs, and symptoms	• Apathetic hyperthyroidism • Sepsis in elderly patient who is afebrile or hypothermic
Failure to assess appropriately the urgency of diagnosis Urgency of the clinical situation was not appreciated and/or delays critical diagnoses	• Compartment syndrome • Pericardial tamponade • Tension pneumothorax
Perils of intermittent symptoms or misleading evolution Intermittent symptoms dismissed due to normal findings (exam, lab, electrocardiogram) when initially seen	• "Lucid interval" in traumatic epidural hematoma • Paroxysmal arrhythmias • Intermittent hydrocephalus (Bruns' syndrome)
Confusion arising from response/masking by empiric treatment	• Empiric treatment with steroids, proton pump inhibitors, antibiotics, pain medication erroneously masking serious diagnosis
Chronic disease or comorbidity presumed to account for new symptoms Especially in medically complex patients	• Septic joint signs misattributed to chronic rheumatoid arthritis • Mental status change due to infection or medication misattributed to underlying dementia
Rare diagnosis: failure to consider or know	• Many; fortunately, by definition, rare, but still warrant consideration especially if urgent or treatable
Drug or environmental factor not considered/overlooked Underlying etiology causing/contributing to symptoms, or disease progression not sought, uncovered	• Ventricular arrhythmia related to QT-prolonging drug • Achilles tendon rupture related to quinolone drugs
Failure to appreciate risk factors for particular disease	• Family history of breast, colorectal cancer not solicited and/or weighed in diagnostic evaluation or screening
Failure to appreciate limitations of physical exam Now with ↑ telemedicine, missing physical exam entirely	• Overweighing absence of tenderness, swelling in deep vein thrombosis • Missing pill-rolling tremor during telemedicine visit

on physical examination probably needs more careful assessment proceeding all the way to invasive biopsy, if necessary. Diagnostic pitfalls can be classified into a number of generic scenarios (**Table 9-5**). We now have large databases that have the potential to track "diagnoses outcomes"—i.e., whether a new diagnosis emerges that suggests an initial diagnosis was incorrect or a diagnosis of a patient's symptoms was suboptimally delayed. This should, in the future, allow us to more rigorously focus on these cases, to identify contributing factors and recurring patterns, and to help point the way for systemwide improvement strategies.

■ DIAGNOSIS SAFETY CULTURE

Just as diagnosing bacterial infections relies on a proper culture medium to grow and identify etiologic organisms, good diagnosis also requires a healthy safety culture that will allow it to grow and flourish. While clinicians may be inclined to view "safety culture" as something too subjective to be important in their quest to make a definitive diagnosis, this view is misguided. Multiple studies have demonstrated adverse consequences resulting from organizational cultures that inhibit openness, learning, and sharing and create a climate where staff and patients are afraid to speak up when they observe problems or have questions. Most importantly, patients need to be encouraged to question diagnoses and be heard, particularly when they are not responding to treatment as expected or developing symptoms that are either not consistent with the diagnosis or represent possible red flags for other diagnoses or complications.

Studies examining "high-reliability organizations" outside of medicine and "learning health care organizations" have distilled a series of fundamental properties that are correlated with more reliable and safer outcomes. Just as a thermometer or recording of a pulse can suggest how ill a patient is, we now have instruments that can measure safety culture. These safety measurement tools typically are validated staff surveys that assess (1) communication about errors with staff willingness to report mistakes because they do not feel these mistakes are held against them; (2) openness and encouragement to talk about hospital/office problems; (3) existence of a learning culture that seeks to learn from errors and improve based on lessons learned; (4) leadership commitment to safety, prioritizing safety over production speed and the "bottom line" by providing adequate staffing and resources to operate safely; and (5) accountability and transparency for following up safety events and concerns. Each of these generic culture attributes translates into specific implications for diagnostic safety. These include the following:

- Making it "safe" for clinicians to admit and share diagnostic errors
- Proactive identification, ownership, and accountability regarding error-prone diagnostic workflow processes (particularly around test results, referrals, and patient follow-up)
- Leadership making diagnosis improvement a top priority based on recognition that patients and malpractice insurers report that diagnostic errors are the leading patient safety problem
- Mutual trust and respect for challenges that clinicians often face in making diagnoses and caution in applying the lens of hindsight bias in judging what in retrospect might seem like an "obvious" diagnosis that a clinician initially missed

■ HEALTH INFORMATION TECHNOLOGY AND THE FUTURE OF DIAGNOSIS

Clinicians now spend more time interacting with computers than they do interacting with patients. This is especially true for diagnosis and will likely be even more so in the future. Interactions with patients, consultants, and other staff are increasingly mediated through the computer. Key activities, such as collecting patients' history (past and current), interpreting data to make a diagnosis, conveying diagnostic assessments (to others on the team and, increasingly, to the patient via open notes), and tracking diagnostic trajectories as they evolve over time, are now computer based. With the rise of telemedicine, even elements of the physical examination have been rerouted to electronic encounters.

While many complain the computer has "gotten in the way" of good diagnosis, distracting clinicians from quality time listening to patients and miring doctors in reading and writing notes filled with copied/pasted/templated information of questionable currency and accuracy, medicine needs to harness the computer's capabilities to improve diagnosis (**Table 9-6**). Although these basic diagnosis-supporting capabilities should be the foundation of the design of health information technology and everyday workflow, electronic medical records have historically been largely designed around other needs, such as ordering medications and billing and malpractice documentation. They need to be radically redesigned to better support diagnostic processes, as well as save, rather than squander, clinicians' time.

■ DIAGNOSIS OF DIAGNOSIS ERRORS AND SAFETY: PRACTICAL CONCLUSIONS

In practice, there are frequent and meaningful opportunities for improving diagnosis in each of the three NAM-defined areas to make it a) more reliable, b) timely, and c) to improve diagnosis-related communication with patients. Clinicians in training, practicing physicians, nurses, and others should develop the habit of regularly asking

TABLE 9-6 Areas Where Health Information Technology Has Potential to Help Improve Diagnosis and Reduce Errors

FUNCTION	EXAMPLES
Facilitate collection/gathering of information	• Quickly access past history from prior care at same and outside institutions • Electronic collection of history of present illness, review of systems, and social determinant risks in advance of visits
Enhanced information entry, organization, and display	• Visually enhanced flowsheets showing trends, relationships to treatment • Reorganized notes to facilitate summarization and simplification and prevent items from getting lost
Generating differential diagnosis	• Automated creation of lists of diagnoses to consider based on patient's symptoms, demographics, risks
Weighing diagnoses likelihoods	• Tools to assist in calculation of posttest (Bayesian) probabilities
Aids for formulating diagnostic plan, intelligent test ordering	• Entering a diagnostic consideration (e.g., celiac disease, pheochromocytoma) and computer suggests most appropriate diagnostic test(s) and how to order
Access to diagnostic reference information	• Info-buttons instantly linking symptom or diagnosis relevant questions to Harrison's, Up-to-Date chapters, references
Ensuring more reliable follow-up	• Hardwiring "closed loops" to ensure abnormal labs, missed referrals, worrisome symptoms are tracked and followed up
Support screening for early detection	• Collaborative tools that patients, clinicians, and offices can use to know when due, order and track screening based on individualized demographics, risk factors, prior tests
Collaborative diagnosis; access to specialist	• Real-time posing/answering of questions • Electronic consults; virtual co-management
Facilitating feedback on diagnoses	• Feeding back new diagnoses (from downstream providers, patients) that emerge suggesting potential misdiagnosis/errors to clinicians, ERs who saw patient previously

Abbreviation: ERs, emergency rooms.

Source: Modified from G Schiff, DW Bates: N Engl J Med 362:1066, 2010, and R El-Karah et al: BMJ Qual Saf Suppl 2:ii40, 2013.

themselves three questions about individual patients in their care, and another three questions regarding the systems in which they work. For each patient being assessed, clinicians should ask:

1. What else might this be? (forcing a differential diagnosis to be made)
2. What doesn't fit? (making sure unexplained abnormal findings are not dismissed)
3. What critical diagnoses are important not to miss? (injecting consideration of "don't miss" diagnoses, red flags, and known pitfalls)

and to diagnose safely, each practitioner must recognize that he or she is working within a larger system. Questions to be asking continually, ensuring we are maximizing reliability and timeliness and minimizing potential for errors, include:

1. Do we have reliable "closed loop" systems to provide reliable, ideally automated tracking and following up of patients' symptoms, abnormal laboratory or imaging findings, and critical referrals that we order?
2. What is the culture-of-safety climate in our organization, office, or clinic?
3. How does the electronic (or even paper) medical record as currently implemented help versus impair efficient, timely, accurate, and fail-safe diagnosis, and how can it be improved?

To take these questions to the next stage, an international movement dedicated to studying and improving diagnosis has emerged. These efforts include annual conferences of clinicians, researchers, and patients; the formation of the Society for Improving Diagnosis in Medicine (SIDM); and convening of a broad coalition of organizations, including the American Board of Internal Medicine (ABIM), the American College of Physicians (ACP), and the Society of Hospital Medicine (SHM), committed to increasing awareness and action. Ultimately, collectively tackling the challenges of improving the quality of diagnosis will transform the way clinicians and patients work together to co-produce better diagnoses.

FURTHER READING

Gandhi TK, Singh H: Reducing the risk of diagnostic error in the COVID-19 era. J Hosp Med 15:363, 2020.

Graber ML et al: The impact of electronic health records on diagnosis. Diagnosis (Berl) 4:211, 2017.

National Academies of Sciences, Engineering, and Medicine. 2015. *Improving Diagnosis in Health Care. https://doi.org/10.17226/21794.* Adapted and reproduced with permission from the National Academy of Sciences, Courtesy of the National Academies Press, Washington, DC.

Newman-Toker DE et al: Serious misdiagnosis-related harms in malpractice claims: The "big three"—Vascular events, infections, and cancers. Diagnosis (Berl) 6:227, 2019.

Schiff GD et al: Diagnosing diagnosis errors: Lessons from a multi-institutional collaborative project, in *Advances in Patient Safety: From Research to Implementation. Vol 2: Concepts and Methodology.* Rockville, MD, Agency for Healthcare Research and Quality, 2005.

Schiff GD et al: Ten principles for more conservative, care-full diagnosis. Ann Intern Med 169:643, 2018.

10 Racial and Ethnic Disparities in Health Care

Lenny López, Joseph R. Betancourt

Over the course of its history, the United States has experienced dramatic improvements in overall health and life expectancy, largely as a result of initiatives in public health, health promotion, disease prevention, and chronic care management. Our ability to prevent, detect, and treat diseases in their early stages has allowed us to target and reduce rates of morbidity and mortality. Despite interventions that have improved the overall health of the majority of Americans, racial and ethnic minorities (blacks, Hispanics/Latinos, Native Americans/Alaskan Natives, Asian/Pacific Islanders) have benefited less from these advances than whites and have suffered poorer health outcomes from many major diseases, including cardiovascular disease, cancer, and diabetes. These disparities highlight the importance of recognizing and addressing the multiple factors that impact health outcomes, including structural racism, *social determinants of health* (SDOH), access to care, and health care quality. On this last point, research has revealed that minorities may receive less care and lower-quality care than whites, even when confounders such as stage of presentation, comorbidities, and health insurance are controlled. These differences in quality are called *racial and ethnic disparities in health care.* These health care disparities have taken on greater importance with the significant transformation of the U.S. health care system and value-based purchasing. The shift toward creating financial incentives and disincentives to achieve quality goals makes focusing on those who receive lower-quality care more important than ever before. This chapter will provide an overview of racial and ethnic disparities in health and health care, identify root causes, and provide key recommendations to address these disparities at both the clinical and health system levels.

NATURE AND EXTENT OF DISPARITIES

Life expectancy at birth is an important measure of the health of a nation's population. Although the overall life expectancy in the United States has been increasing since 1900, differences due to

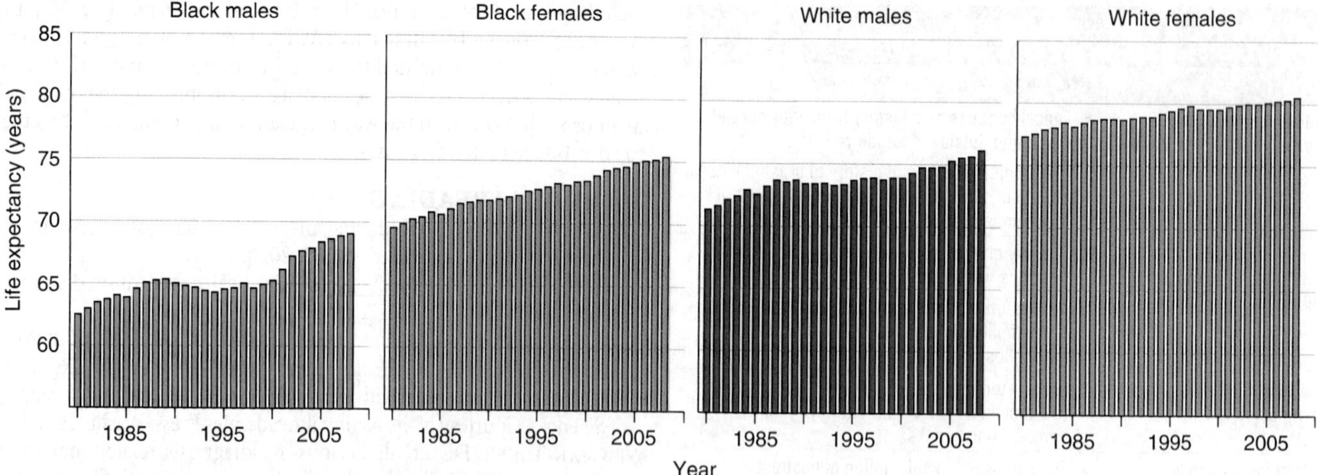

FIGURE 10-1 Life expectancy at birth among black and white males and females in the United States, 1975–2003. *(Adapted from S Harper, J Lynch, S Burris, GD Smith: Trends in the black-white life expectancy gap in the United States, 1983-2003. JAMA 297:1224, 2007.)*

race/ethnicity, education, and socioeconomic status have persisted. For example, at every level of education and income, African Americans have lower life expectancy at age 25 than whites and Hispanics/Latinos. Blacks with a college degree or more education have lower life expectancy than whites and Hispanics who graduated from high school. Blacks have had lower life expectancy compared to whites for as long as data have been collected. From 1975 to 2003, the largest difference in life expectancy between blacks and whites was substantial (6.3 years for males and 4.5 years for females) (**Fig. 10-1**). The gap in life expectancy between the black and white populations decreased by 2.3 years between 1999 and 2013 from 5.9 to 3.6 years (4.4 years for males and 3.0 years for women) (**Fig. 10-2**).

The life expectancy gap is augmented by worse health and higher disease burden. Cardiovascular-related diseases remain the leading cause of black-white differences in life expectancy. If all cardiovascular causes and diabetes are considered together, they account for 35% and 52% of the gap for males and females, respectively. Finally, place matters for health. Analysis of data from 2010 to 2015 demonstrate large geographic life expectancy gap variation at the census tract level (**Fig. 10-3**). Socioeconomic and race/ethnicity factors, behavioral and metabolic risk factors (prevalence of obesity, leisure-time physical inactivity, cigarette smoking, hypertension, diabetes), and health care factors (percentage of the population younger than 65 years who are insured, primary care access and quality, number of physicians per capita) explained 60%, 74%, and 27% of county-level variation in life expectancy, respectively. Combined, these factors explained 74% of this variation. Most of the association between socioeconomic and race/ethnicity factors and life expectancy was mediated through behavioral and metabolic risk factors.

In addition to racial and ethnic disparities in *health*, there are racial and ethnic disparities in the *quality of care* for persons with access to the health care system. Seminal studies over several decades have consistently documented disparities in health care. For instance, studies have documented disparities in the treatment of pneumonia and congestive heart failure, with blacks receiving less optimal care than whites when hospitalized for these conditions. Moreover, blacks with end-stage renal disease are referred less often to the transplant list than are their white counterparts (**Fig. 10-4**). Disparities have been found, for example, in the use of cardiac diagnostic and therapeutic procedures (with blacks being referred less often than whites for cardiac catheterization and bypass grafting), prescription of analgesia for pain control (with blacks and Hispanics/Latinos receiving less pain medication than whites for long-bone fractures and cancer), and surgical treatment of lung cancer (with blacks receiving less curative surgery than whites for non-small-cell lung cancer). Again, many of these disparities have occurred even when variations in factors such as insurance status, income, age, comorbid conditions, and symptom expression are taken into account. Finally, disparities in the quality of care provided at the sites where minorities tend to receive care have been shown to be an important additional contributor to overall disparities.

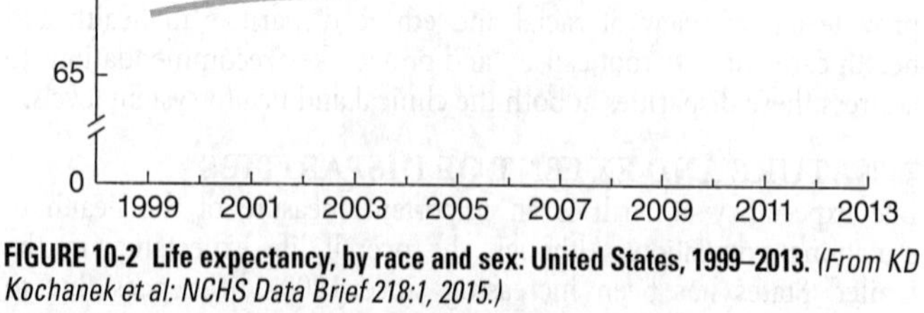

The 2019 National Healthcare Quality and Disparities Report, released by the Agency for Healthcare Research and Quality, tracks about 250 health care process, outcome, and access measures, across many diseases and settings. This annual report is particularly important because most studies of disparities have not been longitudinally repeated with the same methodology to document trends and changes in disparities over time. This report found that some disparities were getting smaller from 2000 through 2016–2018, but disparities persisted and some even worsened, especially for poor and uninsured populations. For about 40% of quality measures, blacks (82 of 202 measures) and American Indians and Alaska Natives (47 of 116 measures) received worse care than whites. For more than one-third of quality measures, Hispanics (61 of 177 measures) received worse care than whites. Asians and Native Hawaiians/Pacific Islanders received worse care than whites for about 30% of quality measures, but Asians also received better care for about 30% of quality measures (**Fig. 10-5**). Of note, for those quality measures that demonstrated disparities at baseline, >90% of these measures showed no improvement since 2000 (**Fig. 10-6**).

FIGURE 10-2 Life expectancy, by race and sex: United States, 1999–2013. *(From KD Kochanek et al: NCHS Data Brief 218:1, 2015.)*

ROOT CAUSES OF DISPARITIES

Race, Racism, and Health Race and racism are core elements of any explanatory model on racial and ethnic disparities in health and health care. Our nation's history of slavery, segregation, separate but "equal" health care, and medical experimentation, among a myriad of other ways in which racism has manifested in the United States, has played a key role in the existence and persistence of these disparities. It is now well accepted that race is a social category without biologic foundation and a product of historical racism. Nevertheless, it is clear that racism has a biologic impact as a form of psychosocial stress. It is now well established

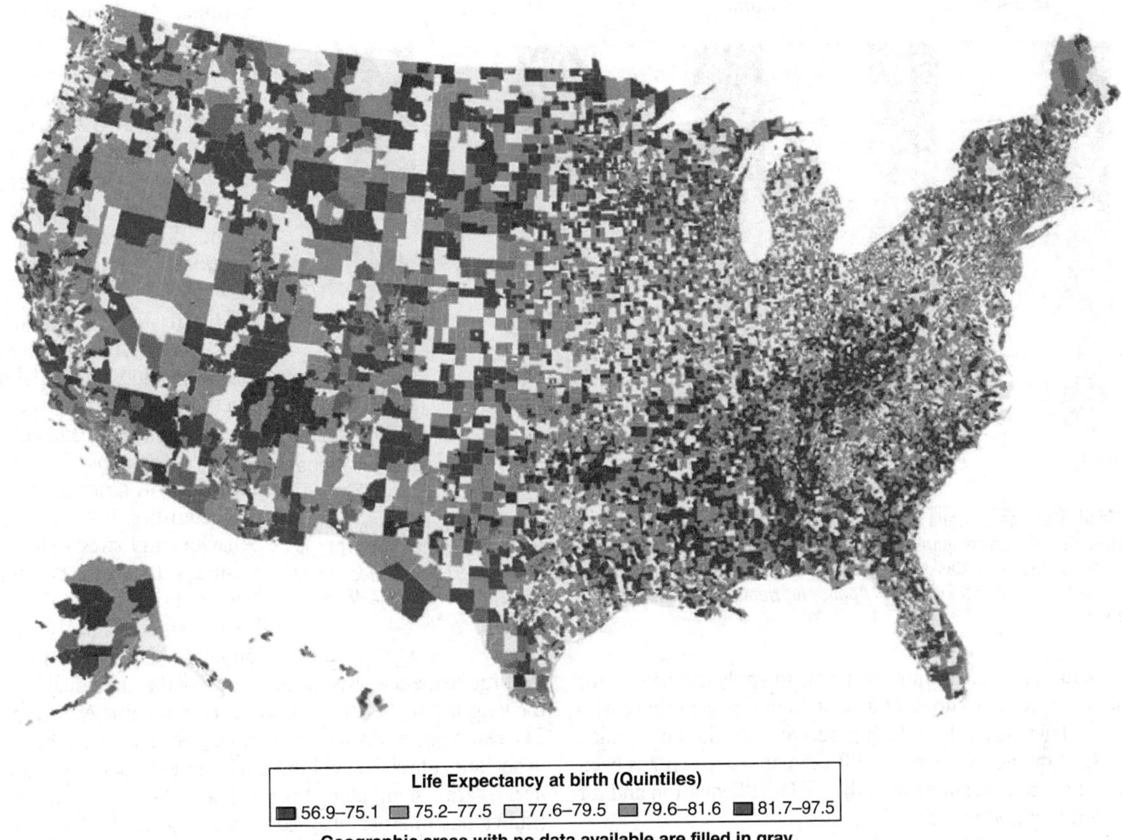

FIGURE 10-3 Life expectancy at birth for U.S. census tracts, 2010-2015. *(A New View of Life Expectancy, Surveillance and Data - Blogs and Stories, Centers for Disease Control and Prevention. Retrieved from https://www.cdc.gov/surveillance/blogs-stories/life-expectancy.html.)*

that psychosocial stress negatively impacts health through psychophysiologic reactivity causing hyperstimulation of the sympathetic-adrenal-medullary system and the hypothalamic-pituitary-adrenal axis, leading to vascular inflammation, endothelial dysfunction, and neurohormonal dysregulation causing an acceleration of cardiovascular disease. Behavioral changes occurring as adaptations or coping responses to stressors such as increased smoking, decreased exercise and sleep, and poorer adherence to medical regimens provide an additional important pathway through which stressors influence disease risk. This accelerated disease risk, aging, and premature death has been termed the *weathering effect*.

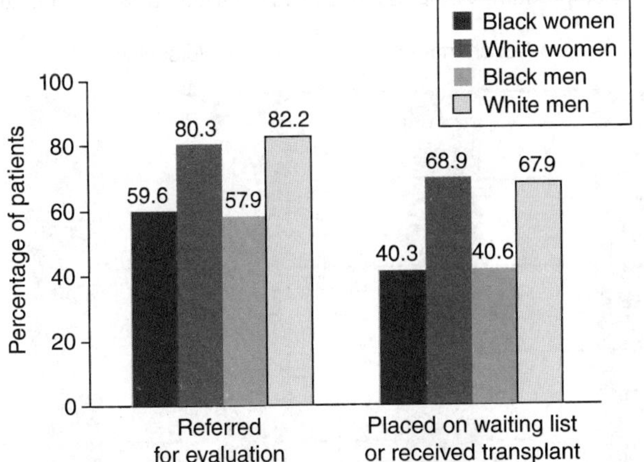

FIGURE 10-4 Referral for evaluation at a transplantation center or placement on a waiting list/receipt of a renal transplant within 18 months after the start of dialysis among patients who wanted a transplant, according to race and sex. The reference population consisted of 239 black women, 280 white women, 271 black men, and 271 white men. Racial differences were statistically significant among both the women and the men ($p < .0001$ for each comparison). *(From JZ Ayanian, PD Cleary, JS Weissman, AM Epstein: The effect of patients' preferences on racial differences in access to renal transplantation. N Engl J Med 341:1661,1999. Copyright © 1999 Massachusetts Medical Society. Reprinted with permission from Massachusetts Medical Society.)*

While most empiric research focuses on interpersonal racial/ethnic discrimination, structural racism (sometimes called institutional racism) provides a more holistic framework. Structural racism refers to the totality of ways that a society fosters, sustains, and reinforces discrimination through sociopolitical, legal, economic, and health structures that determine differential access to risks, opportunities, and resources that drive health and health care disparities. Structural racism explains how racism's structure and ideology can persist in governmental and institutional policies in the absence of individual actors who are explicitly racially prejudiced. For example, the history of residential segregation has had lasting negative effects generationally on equal access for racial/ethnic minorities to employment, banking, earnings, high-quality education, and health care. Policies that do not address root structural causes will not address health and health care inequities.

With the promise of individualizing clinical decisions, the use of race in clinical and risk assessment algorithms has long been a part of modern medicine. The evidence is now clear that race is not a reliable proxy for genetic difference and that race adjustment has the potential to create inadvertent disparities in health care. One clinical example is from nephrology. Blacks have higher rates of end-stage kidney disease and death due to kidney failure than the overall population. The most widely used cohort-derived equation to estimate glomerular filtration rate (GFR), the Chronic Kidney Disease Epidemiology Collaboration (CKD-EPI) equation, has the limitation that it produces 80–90% estimated GFR (eGFR) values that are within ±30% of a patient's measured GFR. In addition, this equation uses a black race-related factor, which increases eGFR for any given serum creatinine by 15.9% compared to a nonblack patient with the same age, sex, and serum creatinine. The increase in eGFR is likely to disadvantage blacks for early referral to a nephrologist, early treatment of advanced chronic kidney disease, and

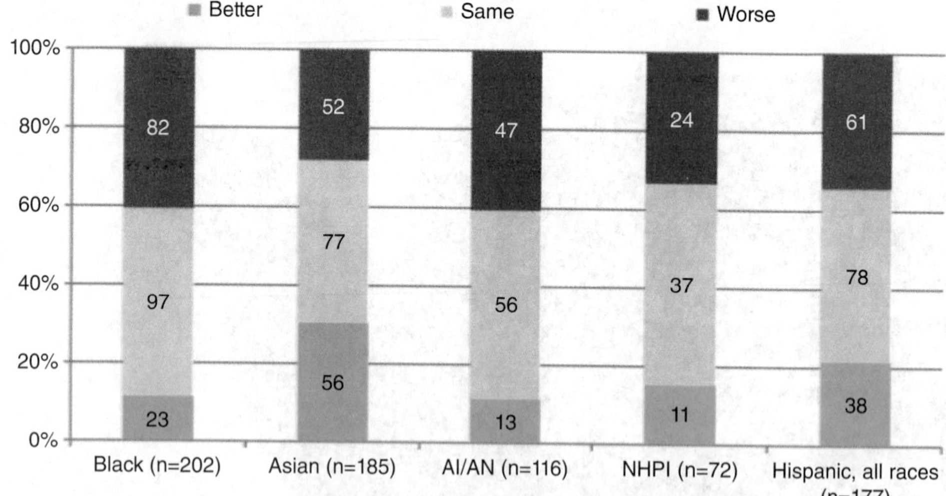

FIGURE 10-5 Number and percentage of quality measures for which members of selected groups experienced better, same, or worse quality of care compared with reference group (white) for the most recent data year, 2014, 2016, 2017, or 2018. AI/AN, American Indian or Alaska Native; NHPI, Native Hawaiian/Pacific Islander *(From 2019 National Healthcare Quality and Disparities Report. Rockville, MD: Agency for Healthcare Research and Quality; December 2020. AHRQ Pub. No. 20(21)-0045-EF.)*

kidney transplantation. It is also not clear how to apply the race factor when the patient's race is unknown and/or ambiguous, as in those who are multiracial. This disparity-inducing scenario could be avoided through the use of cystatin C–based eGFR estimation, which has been demonstrated to be more accurate than the CKD-EPI equation and for which race is not required in estimation.

The application of artificial intelligence (AI) analytics to large amounts of clinical electronic data—big data—holds the promise to better understand health care costs, utilization, resource allocation, and population health monitoring. Machine learning models can identify the statistical patterns in large amounts of historically collected data. These data naturally contain the patterning of preexisting health care disparities created by socially and historically structured inequities. This biased patterning can lead to incorrect predictions, withholding of resources, and worse outcomes for vulnerable populations. Recently, analysis of a commercial, national, proprietary prediction algorithm, affecting millions of patients, exhibited racial bias. Historical cost data were used to predict clinical risk and allocate additional clinical services for high-cost patients. Algorithmic bias arose because black patients historically have less access to health care and thus less money is spent on their care compared to white patients. Thus, blacks, who tended to be sicker than white patients, received lower clinical risk scores and thus were less likely to receive additional clinical services. The observed allocation bias was remedied using direct measures of illness and illness severity. Thus, machine learning algorithms are not inherently free of bias and should be assessed for accuracy and fairness.

In summary, there are many ways in which racism has contributed and does and will continue to contribute to racial and ethnic disparities in health and health care.

SOCIAL DETERMINANTS OF HEALTH

Minority Americans have poorer health outcomes than whites from preventable and treatable conditions such as cardiovascular disease, diabetes, asthma, cancer, and HIV/AIDS. Multiple factors contribute to these racial and ethnic disparities in health. The landmark National Academy of Medicine (formerly, the Institute of Medicine [IOM]) report, *Unequal Treatment: Confronting Racial and Ethnic Disparities in Health Care*, published in 2002, summarized the scientific evidence on health disparities and provided an important framework for conceptualizing and defining racial/ethnic disparities. Since the *Unequal Treatment* report, there has been a growing empiric evidence base on how racism and the SDOH, often working in synergy, create and sustain disparities. Mechanistically, the biopsychosocial model brings together the social and physical characteristics of the environment with individual physical and psychological attributes. These environmental and individual characteristics, in turn, influence health behaviors and stress-related physiologic pathways that directly impact health. The National Institute on Minority Health and Health Disparities SDOH model builds on prior models and adds the time element across the life course of the individual in recognition of the long-lasting health effects of socioeconomic exposures (**Fig. 10-7**). The resulting matrix has the domains of influence of health (biological, behavioral, physical and built environment, sociocultural environment, health care system) along the y-axis and the levels of influence on health (individual, interpersonal, community, societal) along the x-axis. Cells are not mutually exclusive, and examples of factors within each cell are illustrative and not comprehensive. This framework emphasizes the complex multidomain etiologies of disparities across the factors in the conceptual matrix thus highlighting the limitation of individual-level focused research and policy.

In addition to race and racism, *Unequal Treatment* identified a set of root causes that included health system, provider-level, and patient-level factors.

Health System Factors • HEALTH SYSTEM COMPLEXITY Even among persons who are insured and educated and who have a high degree of health literacy, navigating the U.S. health care system can be complicated and confusing. Some individuals may be at higher risk for receiving substandard care because of their difficulty navigating the system's complexities. These individuals may include those from cultures

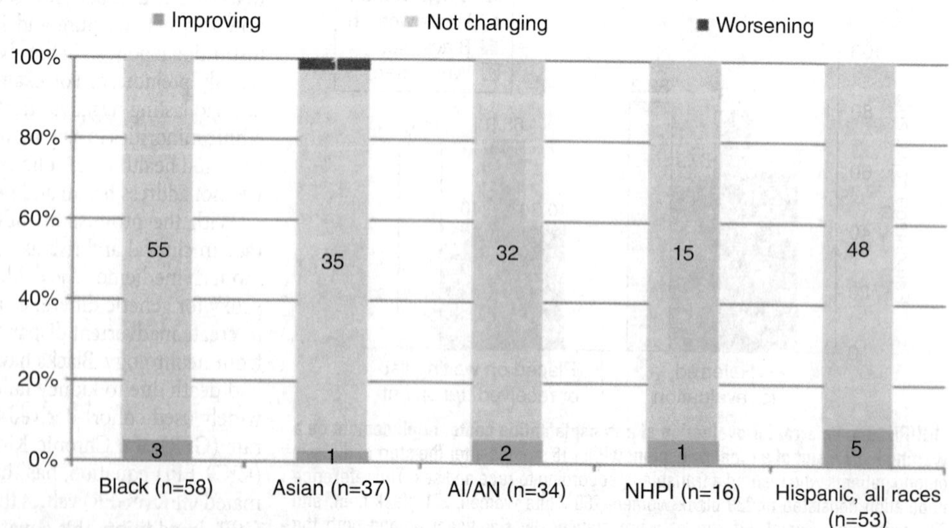

FIGURE 10-6 Number and percentage of quality measures with disparity at baseline for which disparities related to race and ethnicity were improving, not changing, or worsening over time, 2000 through 2014, 2015, 2016, 2017, or 2018. AI/AN, American Indian or Alaska Native; NHPI, Native Hawaiian/Pacific Islander. *(From 2019 National Healthcare Quality and Disparities Report. Rockville, MD: Agency for Healthcare Research and Quality; December 2020. AHRQ Pub. No. 20(21)-0045-EF.)*

Domains of Influence (Over the Lifecourse)	Levels of Influence*			
	Individual	Interpersonal	Community	Societal
Biological	Biological Vulnerability and Mechanisms	Caregiver–Child Interaction Family Microbiome	Community Illness Exposure Herd Immunity	Sanitation Immunization Pathogen Exposure
Behavioral	Health Behaviors Coping Strategies	Family Functioning School/Work Functioning	Community Functioning	Policies and Laws
Physical/Built Environment	Personal Environment	Household Environment School/Work Environment	Community Environment Community Resources	Societal Structure
Sociocultural Environment	Sociodemographics Limited English Cultural Identity Response to Discrimination	Social Networks Family/Peer Norms Interpersonal Discrimination	Community Norms Local Structural Discrimination	Social Norms Societal Structural Discrimination
Health Care System	Insurance Coverage Health Literacy Treatment Preferences	Patient–Clinician Relationship Medical Decision-Making	Availability of Services Safety Net Services	Quality of Care Health Care Policies
Health Outcomes	Individual Health	Family/ Organizational Health	Community Health	Population Health

FIGURE 10-7 National Institute on Minority Health and Health Disparities social determinants research framework. *Health disparity populations: race/ethnicity, low socioeconomic status, rural, sexual and gender minority. Other fundamental characteristics: sex and gender, disability, geographic region. *(From National Institute on Minority Health and Health Disparities. NIMHD Research Framework. 2017. Retrieved from https://www.nimhd.nih.gov/about/overview/research-framework.html.)*

unfamiliar with the Western model of health care delivery, those with limited English proficiency, those with low health literacy, and those who are mistrustful of the health care system. These individuals may have difficulty knowing how and where to go for a referral to a specialist; how to prepare for a procedure such as a colonoscopy; or how to follow up on an abnormal test result such as a mammogram. Since people of color in the United States tend to be overrepresented among the groups listed above, the inherent complexity of navigating the health care system has been seen as a root cause for racial/ethnic disparities in health care.

OTHER HEALTH SYSTEM FACTORS Racial/ethnic disparities are due not only to differences in care provided within hospitals but also to where and from whom minorities receive their care; i.e., certain specific providers, geographic regions, or hospitals are lower-performing on certain aspects of quality. For example, one study showed that 25% of hospitals cared for 90% of black Medicare patients in the United States and that these hospitals tended to have lower performance scores on certain quality measures than other hospitals. That said, health systems generally are not well prepared to measure, report, and intervene to reduce disparities in care. Few hospitals or health plans stratify their quality data by race/ethnicity or language to measure disparities, and even fewer use data of this type to develop disparity-targeted interventions. Similarly, despite regulations concerning the need for professional interpreters, research demonstrates that many health care organizations and providers fail to routinely provide this service for patients with limited English proficiency. Despite the link between limited English proficiency and health care quality and safety, few providers or institutions monitor performance for patients in these areas.

Provider-Level Factors • PROVIDER-PATIENT COMMUNICATION Significant evidence highlights the impact of sociocultural factors, race, ethnicity, and limited English proficiency on health and clinical care. Health care professionals frequently care for diverse populations with varied perspectives, values, beliefs, and behaviors regarding health and well-being. The differences include variations in the recognition of symptoms, thresholds for seeking care, comprehension of management strategies, expectations of care (including preferences for or against diagnostic and therapeutic procedures), and adherence to preventive measures and medications. In addition, sociocultural differences between patient and provider influence communication and clinical decision-making and are especially pertinent: evidence clearly links provider–patient communication to improved patient satisfaction, regimen adherence, and better health outcomes (**Fig. 10-8**). Thus, when sociocultural differences between patient and provider are not appreciated, explored, understood, or communicated effectively during the medical encounter, patient dissatisfaction, poor adherence, poorer health outcomes, and racial/ethnic disparities in care may result.

A survey of 6722 Americans ≥18 years of age is particularly relevant to this important link between provider–patient communication and health outcomes. Whites, African Americans, Hispanics/Latinos, and Asian Americans who had made a medical visit in the past 2 years were asked whether they had trouble understanding their doctors; whether they felt the doctors did not listen; and whether they had medical questions they were afraid to ask. The survey found that 19% of all patients experienced one or more of these problems, yet whites experienced them 16% of the time as opposed to 23% of the time for African Americans, 33% for Hispanics/Latinos, and 27% for Asian Americans (**Fig. 10-9**).

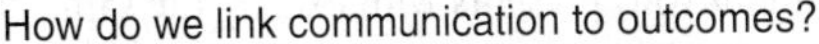

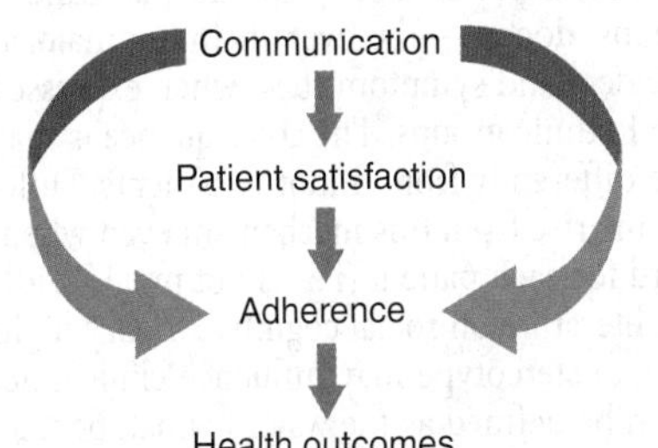

FIGURE 10-8 The link between effective communication and patient satisfaction, adherence, and health outcomes. *(Institute of Medicine. 2003. Unequal Treatment: Confronting Racial and Ethnic Disparities in Health Care. https://doi.org/10.17226/12875. Adapted and reproduced with permission from the National Academy of Sciences, Courtesy of the National Academies Press, Washington, D.C.)*

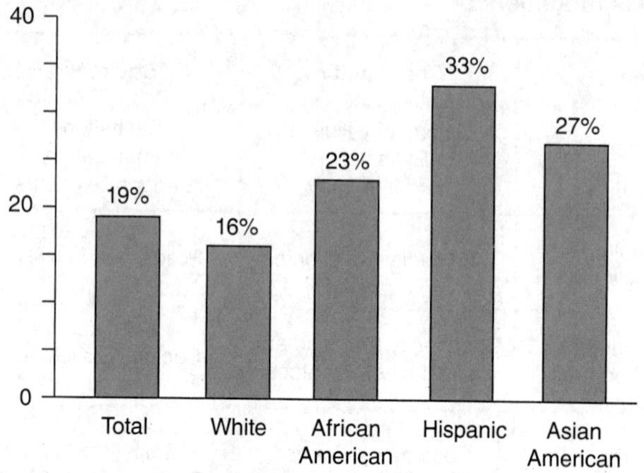

FIGURE 10-9 Communication difficulties with physicians, by race/ethnicity. The reference population consisted of 6722 Americans ≥18 years of age who had made a medical visit in the previous 2 years and were asked whether they had had trouble understanding their doctors, whether they felt that the doctors had not listened, and whether they had had medical questions they were afraid to ask. *(Reproduced with permission from the Commonwealth Fund Health Care Quality Survey, 2001.)*

In addition, in the setting of even a minimal language barrier, provider–patient communication without an interpreter is recognized as a major challenge to effective health care delivery. These communication barriers for patients with limited English proficiency lead to frequent misunderstanding of diagnosis, treatment, and follow-up plans; inappropriate use of medications; lack of informed consent for surgical procedures; high rates of adverse events with more serious clinical consequences; and a lower-quality health care experience than is provided to patients who speak fluent English. Physicians who have access to trained interpreters report a significantly higher quality of patient–physician communication than physicians who use other methods. Communication issues related to discordant language disproportionately affect minorities and likely contribute to racial/ethnic disparities in health care.

CLINICAL DECISION-MAKING Theory and research suggest that variations in clinical decision-making may contribute to racial and ethnic disparities in health care. Two factors are central to this process: clinical uncertainty and stereotyping.

First, a doctor's decision-making process is nested in *clinical uncertainty*. Doctors depend on inferences about severity based on what they understand about illness and the information obtained from the patient. A doctor caring for a patient whose symptoms he or she has difficulty understanding and whose "signals"—the set of clues and indications that physicians rely on to make clinical decisions—are hard to read may make a decision different from the one that would be made for another patient who presents with exactly the same clinical condition. Given that the expression of symptoms may differ among cultural and racial groups, doctors—the overwhelming majority of whom are white—may understand symptoms best when expressed by patients of their own racial/ethnic groups. The consequence is that white patients may be treated differently from minority patients. Differences in clinical decisions can arise from this mechanism even when the doctor has the same regard for each patient (i.e., is not prejudiced).

Second, the literature on social cognitive theory highlights how natural tendencies to stereotype may influence clinical decision-making. *Stereotyping* can be defined as the way in which people use social categories (e.g., race, gender, age) in acquiring, processing, and recalling information about others. Faced with enormous information loads and the need to make many decisions, people often subconsciously simplify the decision-making process and lessen cognitive effort by using "categories" or "stereotypes" that bundle information into groups or types that can be processed more quickly. Although functional, stereotyping can be systematically biased, as people are automatically classified into social categories based on dimensions such as *race*, *gender*, and *age*. Many people may not be aware of their attitudes, may not consciously endorse specific stereotypes, and paradoxically may consider themselves egalitarian and not prejudiced.

Stereotypes may be strongly influenced by the messages presented consciously and unconsciously in society. For instance, if the media and our social/professional contacts tend to present images of minorities as being less educated, more violent, and nonadherent to health care recommendations, these impressions may generate stereotypes that unnaturally and unjustly impact clinical decision-making. As signs of racism, classism, gender bias, and ageism are experienced (consciously or unconsciously) in our society, stereotypes may be created that impact the way doctors manage patients from these groups. On the basis of training or practice location, doctors may develop certain perceptions about race/ethnicity, culture, and class that may evolve into stereotypes. For example, many medical students and residents are trained—and minorities cared for—in academic health centers or public hospitals located in socioeconomically disadvantaged areas. As a result, doctors may begin to equate certain races and ethnicities with specific health beliefs and behaviors (e.g., "these patients" engage in risky behaviors, "those patients" tend to be noncompliant) that are more associated with the social environment (e.g., poverty) than with a patient's racial/ethnic background or cultural traditions. This "conditioning" phenomenon may also be operative if doctors are faced with certain racial/ethnic patient groups who frequently do not choose aggressive forms of diagnostic or therapeutic intervention. The result over time may be that doctors begin to believe that "these patients" do not like invasive procedures; thus, they may not offer these procedures as options. A wide range of studies have documented the potential for provider biases to contribute to racial/ethnic disparities in health care. For example, one study measured physicians' unconscious (or implicit) biases and showed that these were related to differences in decisions to provide thrombolysis for a hypothetical black or white patient with a myocardial infarction.

It is important to differentiate stereotyping from prejudice and discrimination. *Prejudice* is a conscious prejudgment of individuals that may lead to disparate treatment, and *discrimination* is conscious and intentional disparate treatment. All individuals *stereotype* subconsciously, yet, if left unquestioned, these subconscious assumptions may lead to lower-quality care for certain groups because of differences in clinical decision-making or differences in communication and patient-centeredness. For example, one study tested physicians' unconscious racial/ethnic biases and showed that patients perceived more biased physicians as being less patient-centered in their communication. What is particularly salient is that stereotypes tend to be activated most in environments where the individual is stressed, multitasking, and under time pressure—the hallmarks of the clinical encounter. In fact, in a survey of close to 16,000 physicians, 42% admitted that bias—including by race and ethnicity—impacted their clinical decision-making. Interestingly, emergency medicine physicians, who work in environments of stress, time pressure, risk, and where they are multitasking, topped the list by discipline at 62%.

Patient-Level Factors Lack of trust has become a major concern for many health care institutions today. For example, an IOM report, *To Err Is Human: Building a Safer Health System*, documented alarming rates of medical errors that made patients feel vulnerable and less trustful of the U.S. health care system. The increased media and academic attention to problems related to quality of care (and of disparities themselves) has clearly diminished trust in doctors and nurses.

Trust is a crucial element in the therapeutic alliance between patient and health care provider. It facilitates open communication and is directly correlated with adherence to the physician's recommendations and the patient's satisfaction. In other words, patients who mistrust their health care providers are less satisfied with the care they receive, and mistrust of the health care system greatly affects patients' use of services. Mistrust can also result in inconsistent care, "doctor-shopping,"

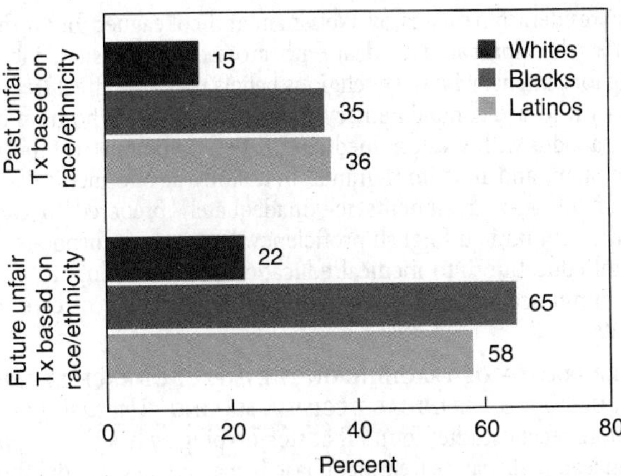

FIGURE 10-10 Patient perspectives regarding unfair treatment (Tx) based on race/ethnicity. The reference population consisted of 3884 individuals surveyed about how fairly they had been treated in the health care system in the past and how fairly they felt they would be treated in the future on the basis of their race/ethnicity. *(From Race, Ethnicity & Medical Care: A Survey of Public Perceptions and Experiences. Kaiser Family Foundation, 2005.)*

self-medication, and an increased demand by patients for referrals and diagnostic tests.

On the basis of historic factors such as discrimination, segregation, and medical experimentation, blacks may be especially mistrustful of providers. The exploitation of blacks by the U.S. Public Health Service during the Tuskegee syphilis study from 1932 to 1972 left a legacy of mistrust that persists even today among this population. Other populations, including Native Americans/Alaskan Natives, Hispanics/Latinos, and Asian Americans, also harbor significant mistrust of the health care system. A national survey conducted by the Kaiser Family Foundation found that there is significant mistrust for the health care system among minority populations. Of the 3884 individuals surveyed, 36% of Hispanics and 35% of blacks (compared to 15% of whites) felt they were treated unfairly in the health care system in the past based on their race and ethnicity. Perhaps even more alarming—65% of blacks and 58% of Hispanics (compared to 22% of whites) were afraid of being treated unfairly in the future based on their race/ethnicity (Fig. 10-10).

This mistrust may contribute to wariness in accepting or following recommendations, undergoing invasive procedures, or participating in clinical research, and these choices, in turn, may lead to misunderstanding and the perpetuation of stereotypes among health professionals.

■ KEY RECOMMENDATIONS TO ADDRESS RACIAL/ETHNIC DISPARITIES IN HEALTH CARE

Unequal Treatment provides recommendations to address the root causes of racial/ethnic disparities organized as *health system interventions, provider interventions, patient interventions,* and *general recommendations.*

Health System Interventions • COLLECTING, REPORTING, AND TRACKING OF DATA ON HEALTH CARE ACCESS AND USE, BY PATIENTS' RACE/ETHNICITY *Unequal Treatment* found that the appropriate systems to track and monitor racial and ethnic disparities in health care are lacking and that less is known about the disparities affecting minority groups other than African Americans (Hispanics, Asian Americans, Pacific Islanders, Native Americans, and Alaskan Natives). For instance, only in the mid-1980s did the Medicare database begin to collect data on patient groups outside the standard categories of "white," "black," and "other." Federal, private, and state-supported data-collection efforts are scattered and unsystematic, and many health care systems and hospitals still do not collect data on the race, ethnicity, or primary language of enrollees or patients. A survey by the Institute for Diversity in Health Management and the Health Research and Educational Trust in 2015 found that 98% of 1083 U.S. hospitals collected information on race, 95% collected data on ethnicity, and 94% collected data on primary language. However, only 45% collected data on race, 40% collected data on ethnicity, and 38% collected data on primary language to benchmark gaps in care. A survey by America's Health Insurance Plans Foundation in 2008 and 2010 showed that the proportion of enrollees in plans that collected race/ethnicity data of some type increased from 75 to 79%; however, the total percentage of plan enrollees whose race/ethnicity and language are recorded is still much lower than these figures.

COLLECTING, REPORTING, AND TRACKING OF SDOH DATA In 2014, the IOM Committee on Recommended Social and Behavioral Domains and Measures for Electronic Health Records recommended the routine collection, in the electronic health record, of a parsimonious panel of clinically significant SDOH measures that may be obtained by self-report in advance of or during the health care encounter and, when used together, provide a psychosocial vital sign. The IOM-recommended questionnaire includes 25 items addressing the following domains: race and ethnicity, education, financial resource strain, stress, depression, physical activity, tobacco use, alcohol use, social connection or isolation, intimate partner violence, residential address, and geocoded census tract median income. Implementation studies have demonstrated that collection of these data takes about 5 minutes, and both patients and providers saw this data collection as appropriate and important. Given that data access and monitoring is an essential component to disparities elimination, we highlight several important sources of up-to-date racial/ethnic disparities monitoring initiatives that are available to the general public and are updated regularly. We highlight only three examples of national data sources.

- Since 2003, the Agency for Healthcare Research and Quality has led the yearly compilation of *The National Healthcare Quality and Disparities Report*, which reports trends for measures related to access to health care, affordable care, care coordination, healthy living, patient safety, and the quality of care across acute and chronic disease management by race/ethnicity, income, and other SDOH (*https://www.ahrq.gov/research/findings/nhqrdr/index.html*).
- Since 2011, the Geospatial Research, Analysis, and Services Program (GRASP) created and maintains the Centers for Disease Control and Prevention Social Vulnerability Index. This database maps, for all U.S. Census tracts, 15 social factors (grouped in four SDOH categories: socioeconomic status, housing composition and disability, minority status and language, and housing and transportation) and is updated every 2 years (*https://www.atsdr.cdc.gov/placeandhealth/svi/index.html*).
- Launched in 2018, the Health Opportunity and Equity (HOPE) Initiative benchmarks and tracks 27 indicators by race, ethnicity, and socioeconomic status. The indicators measure social and economic factors, community and safety, physical environment, access to health care, and health outcomes for the United States (*https://www.nationalcollaborative.org/our-programs/hope-initiative-project/*).

INCREASE INSURANCE COVERAGE AND ACCESS Lack of access to high-quality health care is an important driver of racial/ethnic disparities. Signed into law in 2010, the Affordable Care Act (ACA) fundamentally transformed health insurance by decreasing the uninsured population from 16.3% in 2010 (~49.9 million) to 8.8.% in 2016 (~28.1 million). This represents the largest expansion of health insurance since the creation of Medicare and Medicaid in 1965. Prior to the ACA, non-Hispanic blacks were 70% and Hispanics nearly three times more likely to be uninsured than non-Hispanic whites. Of note, Medicaid expansion accounted for an estimated 60% of the ACA's effect through a combination of expanded eligibility and increased enrollment of previously eligible but unenrolled people. This is important given the higher number of racial/ethnic minorities who obtain insurance through Medicaid. Many studies have demonstrated that increased insurance coverage has also translated to greater improvement for blacks and Hispanics in access to care, more access to a usual source of care, and improved health outcomes.

ENCOURAGEMENT OF THE USE OF EVIDENCE-BASED GUIDELINES AND QUALITY IMPROVEMENT *Unequal Treatment* highlights the subjectivity of clinical decision-making as a potential cause of racial and ethnic disparities in health care by describing how clinicians—despite the existence of well-delineated practice guidelines—may offer (consciously or unconsciously) different diagnostic and therapeutic options to different patients on the basis of their race or ethnicity. Therefore, the widespread adoption and implementation of evidence-based guidelines is a key recommendation in eliminating disparities. For instance, evidence-based guidelines are now available for the management of diabetes, HIV/AIDS, cardiovascular diseases, cancer screening and management, and asthma—all areas where significant disparities exist. As part of ongoing quality-improvement efforts, particular attention should be paid to the implementation of evidence-based guidelines for all patients, regardless of their race and ethnicity.

SUPPORT FOR THE USE OF LANGUAGE INTERPRETATION SERVICES IN THE CLINICAL SETTING As described previously, a lack of efficient and effective interpreter services in a health care system can lead to patient dissatisfaction, to poor comprehension and adherence, and thus to ineffective/lower-quality care for patients with limited English proficiency. *Unequal Treatment*'s recommendation to support the use of interpretation services has clear implications for delivery of quality health care by improving doctors' ability to communicate effectively with these patients.

INCREASES IN THE PROPORTION OF UNDERREPRESENTED MINORITIES IN THE HEALTH CARE WORKFORCE Data for 2018 from the Association of American Medical Colleges indicate that of active physicians, 56.2% identified as white, 5.8% identified as Hispanic, 5.0% identified as black or African American, and 0.3% identified as Native American or Alaskan Natives. Furthermore, U.S. national data show that only 3.6% of full-time faculty are black or African American, and 5.5% are Hispanic, Latino, or of Spanish origin (alone or in combination with another race/ethnicity), compared to 63.9% who identified as white. Longitudinal data demonstrate that minority faculty are more likely to be at or below the rank of assistant professor, while whites composed the highest proportion of full professors. Similarly, several studies have found that both Hispanic and black faculty were promoted at lower rates than their white counterparts. Despite representing ~30% of the U.S. population (a number projected to almost double by 2050), minority students are still underrepresented in medical schools. In 2018, matriculates to U.S. medical schools were 6.2% Latino, 7.1% African American, 0.1% Native Hawaiian or Other Pacific Islander, and 0.2% Native American or Alaskan Native. These percentages have decreased or remained nearly the same since 2007. It will be difficult to develop a diverse physician workforce that can meet the needs of an increasingly diverse population without dramatic changes in the racial and ethnic composition of medical student bodies. Long-term investment in pipeline programs and the nearly universal adoption of holistic admissions (a process by which schools consider each applicant individually to determine how they might contribute to the learning environment and the workforce instead of relying just on test scores and grades) have produced modest results. Institutional change in medical schools, focused on creating nurturing, inclusive, and equity-focused environments that dismantle the structural racism that has created the opportunity gap faced by many minority students, is needed to address this important workforce challenge.

Provider Interventions • INTEGRATION OF CROSS-CULTURAL EDUCATION INTO THE TRAINING OF ALL HEALTH CARE PROFESSIONALS The goal of cross-cultural education is to improve providers' ability to understand, communicate with, and care for patients from diverse backgrounds. Such education focuses on enhancing awareness of sociocultural influences on health beliefs and behaviors and on building skills to facilitate understanding and management of these factors in the medical encounter. Cross-cultural education includes curricula on health care disparities, use of interpreters, and effective communication and negotiation across cultures. These curricula can be incorporated into health professions training in medical schools, residency programs, nursing schools, and other health professions programs, and can be offered as a component of continuing education. Despite the importance of this area of education and the attention it has attracted from medical education accreditation bodies, a national survey of senior resident physicians by Weissman and colleagues found that up to 28% felt unprepared to deal with cross-cultural issues, including caring for patients who have religious beliefs that may affect treatment, patients who use complementary medicine, patients who have health beliefs at odds with Western medicine, patients who mistrust the health care system, and new immigrants. In a study at one medical school, 70% of fourth-year students felt inadequately prepared to care for patients with limited English proficiency. Efforts to incorporate cross-cultural education into medical education will contribute to improving communication and to providing a better quality of care for all patients.

INCORPORATION OF TEACHING ON THE IMPACT OF RACE, ETHNICITY, AND CULTURE ON CLINICAL DECISION-MAKING *Unequal Treatment* and more recent studies found that stereotyping by health care providers can lead to disparate treatment based on a patient's race or ethnicity. The Liaison Committee on Medical Education, which accredits medical schools, issued a directive that medical education should include instruction on how a patient's race, ethnicity, and culture might unconsciously impact communication and clinical decision-making.

Patient Interventions Difficulty navigating the health care system and obtaining access to care can be a hindrance to all populations, particularly to minorities. Similarly, lack of empowerment or involvement in the medical encounter by minorities can be a barrier to care. Patients need to be educated on how to navigate the health care system and how best to access care. Interventions should be used to increase patients' participation in treatment decisions.

General Recommendations • INCREASE AWARENESS OF RACIAL/ETHNIC DISPARITIES IN HEALTH CARE Efforts to raise awareness of racial/ethnic health care disparities have done little for the general public but have been fairly successful among physicians, according to a Kaiser Family Foundation report. In 2006, nearly 6 in 10 people surveyed believed that blacks received the same quality of care as whites, and 5 in 10 believed that Latinos received the same quality of care as whites. These estimates are similar to findings in a 1999 survey. Despite this lack of awareness, most people believed that all Americans deserve quality care, regardless of their background. In contrast, the level of awareness among physicians has risen sharply. In 2002, the majority (69%) of physicians said that the health care system "rarely or never" treated people unfairly on the basis of their racial/ethnic background. In 2005, less than one-quarter (24%) of physicians disagreed with the statement that "minority patients generally receive lower-quality care than white patients." More recently, a survey by WebMD showed that 42% of 16,000 physicians admitted that their own personal biases impact their clinical decision-making, including on characteristics such as race and ethnicity. Increasing awareness of racial and ethnic health disparities, and their root causes, among health care professionals and the public is an important first step in addressing these disparities. The ultimate goals are to generate discourse and to mobilize action to address disparities at multiple levels, including health policymakers, health systems, and the community.

CONDUCT FURTHER RESEARCH TO IDENTIFY SOURCES OF DISPARITIES AND PROMISING INTERVENTIONS While the literature that formed the basis for the findings reported and recommendations made in *Unequal Treatment* provided significant evidence for racial and ethnic disparities, additional research is needed in several areas. First, most of the literature on disparities focuses on black-versus-white differences; much less is known about the experiences of other minority groups. Improving the ability to collect racial and ethnic patient data should facilitate this process. However, in instances where the necessary systems are not yet in place, racial and ethnic patient data may be collected prospectively in the setting of clinical or health services research to more fully elucidate disparities for other populations. Second, much of the literature on disparities to date has focused on defining areas in which these disparities exist, but less has been done to identify the multiple factors that contribute to the disparities or to test interventions to address these factors. There is clearly a need for research that identifies promising practices and solutions to disparities.

IMPLICATIONS FOR CLINICAL PRACTICE

Individual health care providers can do several things in the clinical encounter to address racial and ethnic disparities in health care.

Be Aware That Disparities Exist Increasing awareness of racial and ethnic disparities among health care professionals is an important first step in addressing disparities in health care. Only with greater awareness can care providers be attuned to their behavior in clinical practice and thus monitor that behavior and ensure that all patients receive the highest quality of care, regardless of race, ethnicity, or culture.

Practice Culturally Competent Care Previous efforts have been made to teach clinicians about the attitudes, values, beliefs, and behaviors of certain cultural groups—the key practice "dos and don'ts" in caring for "the Hispanic patient" or the "Asian patient," for example. In certain situations, learning about a particular local community or cultural group, with a goal of following the principles of community-oriented primary care, can be helpful; when broadly and uncritically applied, however, this approach can actually lead to stereotyping and oversimplification of culture, without respect for its complexity.

Cultural competence has thus evolved from merely learning information and making assumptions about patients on the basis of their backgrounds to focusing on the development of skills that follow the principles of patient-centered care. *Patient-centeredness* encompasses the qualities of compassion, empathy, and responsiveness to the needs, values, and expressed preferences of the individual patient. *Cultural competence* aims to take things a step further by expanding the repertoire of knowledge and skills classically defined as "patient-centered" to include those that are especially useful in cross-cultural interactions (and that, in fact, are vital in all clinical encounters). This repertoire includes effectively using interpreter services, eliciting the patient's understanding of his or her condition, assessing decision-making preferences and the role of family, determining the patient's views about biomedicine versus complementary and alternative medicine, recognizing sexual and gender issues, and building trust. For example, while it is important to understand all patients' beliefs about health, it may be particularly crucial to understand the health beliefs of patients who come from a different culture or have a different health care experience. With the individual patient as teacher, the physician can adjust his or her practice style to meet the patient's specific needs.

Avoid Stereotyping Several strategies can allow health care providers to counteract, both systemically and individually, the normal tendency to stereotype. For example, when racially/ethnically/culturally/socially diverse teams in which each member is given equal power are assembled and are tasked to achieve a common goal, a sense of camaraderie develops and prevents the development of stereotypes based on race/ethnicity, gender, culture, or class. Thus, health care providers should aim to gain experiences working with and learning from a diverse set of colleagues. In addition, simply being aware of the operation of social cognitive factors allows providers to actively check up on or monitor their behavior. Physicians can constantly reevaluate to ensure that they are offering the same things, in the same ways, to all patients. Understanding one's own susceptibility to stereotyping—and how disparities may result—is essential in providing equitable, high-quality care to all patients.

Work to Build Trust Patients' mistrust of the health care system and of health care providers impacts multiple facets of the medical encounter, with effects ranging from decreased patient satisfaction to delayed care. Although the historic legacy of discrimination can never be erased, several steps can be taken to build trust with patients and to address disparities. First, providers must be aware that mistrust exists and is more prevalent among minority populations, given the history of discrimination in the United States and other countries. Second, providers must reassure patients that they come first, that everything possible will be done to ensure that they always get the best care available, and that their caregivers will serve as their advocates. Third, interpersonal skills and communication techniques that demonstrate honesty, openness, compassion, and respect on the part of the health care provider are essential tools in dismantling mistrust. Finally, patients indicate that trust is built when there is shared, participatory decision-making and the provider makes a concerted effort to understand the patient's background. When the doctor–patient relationship is reframed as one of solidarity, the patient's sense of vulnerability can be transformed into one of trust. The successful elimination of disparities requires trust-building interventions and strengthening of this relationship.

CONCLUSION

The issue of racial and ethnic disparities in health care has gained national prominence, both with the release of the IOM report *Unequal Treatment* and with more recent articles that have confirmed their persistence and explored their root causes. Furthermore, another influential IOM report, *Crossing the Quality Chasm*, has highlighted the importance of equity—i.e., no variations in quality of care due to personal characteristics, including race and ethnicity—as a central principle of quality. Current efforts in health care reform and transformation, including a greater focus on value (high-quality care and cost-control), will sharpen the nation's focus on the care of populations who experience low-quality, costly care. Addressing disparities will become a major focus, and there will be many obvious opportunities for interventions to eliminate them. Greater attention to addressing the root causes of disparities will improve the care provided to all patients, not just those who belong to racial and ethnic minorities.

FURTHER READING

Buchmueller TC et al: The ACA's impact on racial and ethnic disparities in health insurance coverage and access to care. Health Aff (Millwood) 39:395, 2020.

Carnethon MR et al: Cardiovascular health in African Americans: A scientific statement from the American Heart Association. Circulation 136:e393, 2017.

Dwyer-Lindgren L et al: Inequalities in life expectancy among us counties, 1980 to 2014: Temporal trends and key drivers. JAMA Intern Med 177:1003, 2017.

Kreuter MW et al: Addressing social needs in health care settings: Evidence, challenges and opportunities for public health. Annu Rev Public Health 42:11, 2021.

Krieger N: Measures of racism, sexism, heterosexism, and gender binarism for health equity research: from structural injustice to embodied harm: An ecosocial analysis. Annu Rev Public Health 41:37, 2020.

Medscape: Medscape Lifestyle Report 2016: Bias and burnout. *http://www.medscape.com/features/slideshow/lifestyle/2016/public/overview.*

Vyas DA et al: Hidden in plain sight: Reconsidering the use of race correction in clinical algorithms. N Engl J Med 383:874, 2020.

Williams DR et al: Racism and health: Evidence and needed research. Annu Rev Public Health 40:105, 2019.

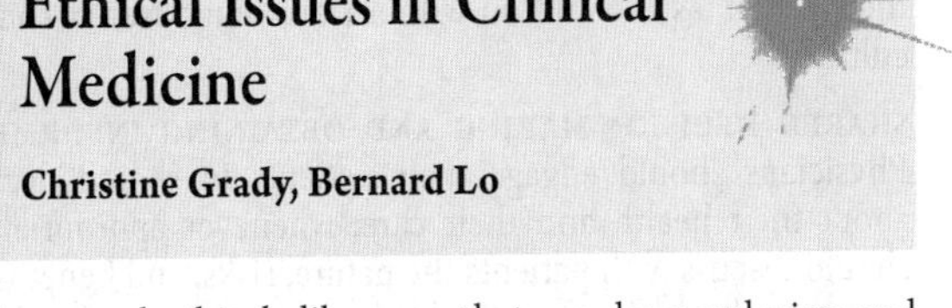

11 Ethical Issues in Clinical Medicine

Christine Grady, Bernard Lo

Physicians face novel ethical dilemmas that can be perplexing and emotionally draining. For example, telemedicine, artificial intelligence, handheld personal devices, and learning health care systems all hold the promise of more coordinated and comprehensive care, but also raise concerns about confidentiality, the doctor–patient relationship, and responsibility. This chapter presents approaches and principles that physicians can use to address important vexing ethical issues they encounter in their work. Physicians make ethical judgments about clinical situations every day. They should prepare for lifelong learning about ethical issues so they can respond appropriately. Traditional professional codes and ethical principles provide instructive guidance for physicians but need to be interpreted and applied to each situation. When facing or struggling with a challenging ethical issue, physicians may need to reevaluate their basic convictions, tolerate uncertainty, and maintain their integrity while respecting the opinions of others. Physicians should articulate their concerns and reasoning, discuss and listen to the views of others involved in the case, and utilize available resources, including other health care team members, palliative care, social work, and spiritual care. Moreover, ethics consultation services or a hospital ethics committee can help to clarify issues and identify strategies for resolution, including improving communication and dealing with strong or conflicting emotions. Through these efforts, physicians can gain deeper insight into the ethical issues they face and usually reach mutually acceptable resolutions to complex problems.

APPROACHES TO ETHICAL PROBLEMS

Several approaches are useful for resolving ethical issues, including approaches based on ethical principles, virtue ethics, professional oaths, and personal values. These various sources of guidance may seem to conflict in a particular case, leaving the physician in a quandary. In a diverse society, different individuals may turn to different sources of moral guidance. In addition, general moral precepts often need to be interpreted and applied to a particular clinical situation.

■ ETHICAL PRINCIPLES

Ethical principles can serve as general guidelines to help physicians determine the right thing to do.

Respecting Patients Physicians should always treat patients with respect, which entails understanding patients' goals, providing information, communicating effectively, obtaining informed and voluntary consent, respecting informed refusals, and protecting confidentiality. Different clinical goals and approaches are often feasible, and interventions can result in both benefit and harm. Individuals differ in how they value health and medical care and how they weigh the benefits and risks of medical interventions. Generally, physicians should respect patients' values and informed choices. Treating patients with respect is especially important when patients are responding to experiences of, or fears about, disrespect and discrimination.

GOALS AND TREATMENT DECISIONS Physicians should provide relevant and accurate information for patients about diagnoses, current clinical circumstances, expected future course, prognosis, treatment options, and uncertainties, and discuss patients' goals of care. Physicians may be tempted to withhold a serious diagnosis, misrepresent it by using ambiguous terms, or limit discussions of prognosis or risks for fear that patients will become anxious or depressed. Providing honest information about clinical situations promotes patients' autonomy and trust as well as sound communication with patients and colleagues. When physicians have to share bad news with patients, they should adjust the pace of disclosure, offer empathy and hope, provide emotional support, and call on other resources such as spiritual care or social work to help patients cope. Some patients may choose not to receive such information or may ask surrogates to make decisions on their behalf, as is common with serious diagnoses in some traditional cultures.

SHARED DECISION-MAKING AND OBTAINING INFORMED CONSENT Physicians should engage their patients in shared decision-making about their health and their care, whenever appropriate. Physicians should discuss with patients the nature, risks, and benefits of proposed care; any alternative; and the likely consequences of each option. Physicians promote shared decision-making by informing and educating patients, answering their questions, checking that they understand key issues, making recommendations, and helping them to deliberate. Medical jargon, needlessly complicated explanations, or the provision of too much information at once may overwhelm patients. Increasingly, decision aids can assist patients in playing a more active role in decision-making, improving the accuracy of their perception of risk and benefit, and helping them feel better informed and clearer about their values. Informed consent is more than obtaining signatures on consent forms and involves disclosure of honest and understandable information to promote understanding and choice. Competent, informed patients may refuse recommended interventions and choose among reasonable alternatives. In an emergency, treatment can be given without informed consent if patients cannot give their own consent and delaying treatment while surrogates are contacted would jeopardize patients' lives or health. People are presumed to want such emergency care unless they have previously indicated otherwise.

Respect for patients does not entitle patients to insist on any care or treatment that they want. Physicians are not obligated to provide interventions that have no physiologic rationale, that have already failed, or that are contrary to evidence-based practice recommendations or good clinical judgment. Public policies and laws also dictate certain decisions—e.g., allocation of scarce medical resources during a public health crisis such as the COVID-19 pandemic, use of cadaveric organs for transplantation, and requests for physician aid in dying.

CARING FOR PATIENTS WHO LACK DECISION-MAKING CAPACITY Some patients are unable to make informed decisions because of unconsciousness, advanced dementia, delirium, or other medical conditions. Courts have the legal authority to determine that a patient is legally incompetent, but in practice, physicians usually determine when patients lack the capacity to make particular health care decisions and arrange for authorized surrogates to make decisions, without involving the courts. Patients with decision-making capacity can express a choice and appreciate their medical situation; the nature, risks, and benefits of proposed care; and the consequences of each alternative. Patient choices should be consistent with their values and not the result of delusions, hallucinations, or misinformation. Physicians should use available and validated assessment tools, resources such as psychiatry or ethics consultation, and clinical judgment to ascertain whether individuals have the capacity to make decisions for themselves. Patients should not be assumed to lack capacity if they disagree with recommendations or refuse treatment. Such decisions should be probed, however, to ensure the patient is not deciding based on misunderstandings and has the capacity to make an informed decision. When impairments are fluctuating or reversible, decisions should be postponed if possible until the patient recovers decision-making capacity.

When a patient lacks decision-making capacity, physicians seek an appropriate surrogate. Patients may designate a health care proxy through an advance directive or on a Physician Orders for Life-Sustaining Treatment form; such choices should be respected (see **Chap. 12**). For patients who lack decision-making capacity and have not previously designated a health care proxy, family members usually serve as surrogates. Statutes in most U.S. states delineate a prioritized list of relatives to make medical decisions. Patients' values, goals, and previously expressed preferences guide surrogate decisions. However, the patient's current best interests may sometimes justify overriding earlier preferences if an intervention is likely to provide significant benefit, previous statements do not fit the situation well, or the patient gave the surrogate leeway in decisions.

MAINTAINING CONFIDENTIALITY Maintaining confidentiality is essential to respecting patients' autonomy and privacy; it encourages patients to seek treatment and to discuss problems candidly. However, confidentiality may be overridden to prevent serious harm to third parties or the patient. Exceptions to confidentiality are justified when the risk to others is serious and probable, no less restrictive measures can avert risk, and the adverse effects of overriding confidentiality are minimized and deemed acceptable by society. For example, laws require physicians to report cases of tuberculosis, sexually transmitted infection, elder or child abuse, and domestic violence.

Beneficence or Acting in Patients' Best Interests The principle of *beneficence* requires physicians to act for the patient's benefit. Patients typically lack medical expertise, and illness may make them vulnerable. Patients rely on and trust physicians to treat them with compassion and provide sound recommendations and treatments aimed to promote their well-being. Physicians encourage such trust and have a fiduciary duty to act in the best interests of patients, which should prevail over physicians' self-interest or the interests of third parties such as hospitals or insurers. A principle related to beneficence, "first do no harm," obliges physicians to prevent unnecessary harm by recommending interventions that maximize benefit and minimize harm and forbids physicians from providing known ineffective interventions or acting without due care. Although often cited, this precept alone provides limited guidance because many beneficial interventions also pose serious risks.

Physicians increasingly provide care within interdisciplinary teams and rely on consultation with or referral to specialists. Team members and consultants contribute different types of expertise to the provision of comprehensive, high-quality care for patients. Physicians should collaborate with and respect the contributions of the various interdisciplinary team members and should initiate and participate in regular communication and planning to avoid diffusion of responsibility and ensure accountability for quality patient care.

INFLUENCES ON PATIENTS' BEST INTERESTS Conflicts arise when patients' refusal or request of interventions thwarts their own goals for care, causes serious harm, or conflicts with their best medical interests. For example, simply accepting a young asthmatic adult's refusal of mechanical ventilation for reversible respiratory failure, in the name of respecting autonomy, is morally constricted. Physicians should elicit patients' expectations and concerns, correct their misunderstandings, and try to persuade them to accept beneficial therapies. If disagreements persist after such efforts, physicians should call on institutional resources for assistance, but patients' informed choices and views of their own best interests should prevail.

Drug prices and out-of-pocket expenses for patients have been escalating in many parts of the world and may compromise care that is in the patients' best interests. Physicians should recognize that patients, especially those with high copayments or inadequate insurance, may not be able to afford prescribed tests and interventions. Physicians should strive to prescribe medications that are affordable and acceptable to the patient. Knowing what kind of insurance, if any, the patient has and whether certain medications are likely to be covered may help in determining appropriate prescriptions. Available alternatives should be considered and discussed. Physicians should follow up with patients who don't fill prescriptions, don't take their medications, or skip doses to explore whether cost and affordability are obstacles. It may be reasonable for physicians to advocate for coverage of nonformulary products for sound reasons, such as when the formulary drugs are less effective or not tolerated or are too costly for the patient to pay for out of pocket. These should be shared decisions with the patient to the extent possible.

Organizational policies and workplace conditions may sometimes conflict with patients' best interests. Physicians' focus and dedication to the well-being and interests of patients may be negatively influenced by perceived or actual staffing inadequacies, unfair wages, infrastructural deficiencies or lack of equipment, work-hour limitations, corporate culture, and threats to personal security in the workplace. Physicians should work with institutional leaders to ensure that policies and practices support their ability to provide quality care focused on patients' best interests.

Patients' interests are served by improvements in overall quality of care and the increasing use of evidence-based practice guidelines and performance benchmarking. However, practice guideline recommendations may not serve the interests of each individual patient, especially when another plan of care may provide substantially greater benefits. In prioritizing their duty to act in the patient's best interests, physicians should be familiar with relevant practice guidelines, be able to recognize situations that might justify exceptions, and advocate for reasonable exceptions.

Acting Justly The principle of *justice* provides guidance to physicians about how to ethically treat patients and make decisions about allocating important resources, including their own time. *Justice* in a general sense means fairness: people should receive what they deserve. In addition, it is important to act consistently in cases that are similar in ethically relevant ways, in order to avoid arbitrary, biased, and unfair decisions. Justice forbids discrimination in health care based on race, religion, gender, sexual orientation, disability, age, or other personal characteristics (**Chap. 10**).

ALLOCATION OF RESOURCES Justice also requires fair allocation of limited health care resources. Universal access to medically needed health care remains an unrealized moral aspiration in the United States and many countries around the world. Patients with no or inadequate health insurance often cannot afford health care and lack access to safety-net services. Even among insured patients, insurers may deny coverage for interventions recommended by their physician. In this situation, physicians should advocate for patients' affordable access to indicated care, try to help patients obtain needed care, and work with institutions and policies to promote wider access. Doctors might consider—or patients might request—the use of lies or deception to obtain such benefits, for example, signing a disability form for a patient who does not meet disability criteria. Although motivated by a desire to help the patient, such deception breaches basic ethical guidelines and undermines physicians' credibility and trustworthiness.

Allocation of health care resources is unavoidable when resources are limited. Allocation policies should be fair, transparent, accountable, responsive to the concerns of those affected, and proportionate to the situation, including the supply relative to the need. In the 2019–2020 SARS-CoV-2/COVID-19 pandemic, some epicenters anticipated or faced shortages of staff, protective equipment, hospital and critical care beds, and ventilators, even after increasing supplies and modifying usual clinical procedures. Many jurisdictions developed guidelines for implementing crisis standards of care to allocate limited interventions and services. Under crisis standards of care, some aspects of conventional care are not possible and interventions may not be provided to all who might benefit or wish to receive them. Crisis standards of care aim to promote the good of the community by saving the most lives in the short term, using evidence-based criteria.

When demand for medications or other interventions exceeds the supply, allocation should be fair, strive to avoid discrimination, and mitigate health disparities. First-come, first-served allocation is not fair, because it disadvantages patients who experience barriers to accessing care. To avoid discrimination, allocation decisions should not consider personal social characteristics such as race, gender, or disability, nor consider insurance status or wealth. Allocation policies also should aspire to reduce health care disparities. U.S. African-American, Latino-American, and Native-American patients suffered a disproportionate number of COVID-19 cases and deaths, likely due in part to being employed in jobs that cannot be done remotely or with physical distancing, crowded housing, lack of health benefits, and poor access to health care.

Fair and well-considered guidelines help mitigate any emotional and moral distress that clinicians may experience making difficult allocation decisions. Authorizing triage officers or committees to make allocation decisions according to policies determined with public input allows treating physicians and nurses to dedicate their efforts to their patients. Ad hoc resource allocation by physicians at the bedside may be inconsistent, unfair, and ineffective. At the bedside, physicians should act as patient advocates within constraints set by society, reasonable insurance policies, and evidence-based practice. Many allocation decisions are made at the level of public policy, with physician and public input. For example, the United Network for Organ Sharing (*www.unos.org*) provides criteria for allocating scarce organs.

VIRTUE ETHICS

Virtue ethics focuses on physicians' character and qualities, with the expectation that doctors will cultivate virtues such as compassion, trustworthiness, intellectual honesty, humility, and integrity. Proponents argue that, if such characteristics become ingrained, they help guide physicians in unforeseen situations. Moreover, following ethical precepts or principles without any of these virtues could lead to uncaring doctor–patient relationships.

■ PROFESSIONAL OATHS AND CODES

Professional oaths and codes are useful guides for physicians. Most physicians take oaths during their medical training, and many are members of professional societies that have professional codes. Physicians pledge to the public and to their patients that they will be guided by the principles and values in these oaths or codes and commit to the spirit of the ethical ideals and precepts represented in oaths and professional codes of ethics.

■ PERSONAL VALUES

Personal values, cultural traditions, and religious beliefs are important sources of personal morality that help physicians address ethical issues and cope with any moral distress they may experience in practice. While essential, personal morality alone is a limited ethical guide in clinical practice. Physicians have role-specific ethical obligations that go beyond their obligations as good people, including the duties to obtain informed consent and maintain confidentiality discussed earlier. Furthermore, in a culturally and religiously diverse world, physicians should expect that some patients and colleagues will have personal moral beliefs that differ from their own.

ETHICALLY COMPLEX PROFESSIONAL ISSUES FOR PHYSICIANS

■ CLAIMS OF CONSCIENCE

Some physicians, based on their personal values, have conscientious objections to providing, or referring patients for, certain treatments such as contraception or physician aid in dying. Although physicians should not be asked to violate deeply held moral beliefs or religious convictions, patients need medically appropriate, timely care and should always be treated with respect. Institutions such as clinics and hospitals have a collective ethical duty to provide care that patients need while making reasonable attempts to accommodate health care workers' conscientious objections—for example, when possible by arranging for another professional to provide the service in question. Patients seeking a relationship with a doctor or health care institution should be notified in advance of any conscientious objections to the provision of specific interventions. Since insurance often constrains patients' selection of physicians or health care facilities, switching providers can be burdensome. There are also important limits on claims of conscience. Health care workers may not insist that patients receive unwanted medical interventions. They also may not refuse to treat or discriminate against patients because of their race, ethnicity, disability, genetic information, or diagnosis. Such discrimination is illegal and violates physicians' duties to respect patients. Refusal to treat patients for other reasons such as sexual orientation, gender identity, or other personal characteristics is legally more controversial, yet ethically inappropriate because it falls short of helping patients in need and respecting them as persons.

■ PHYSICIAN AS GATEKEEPER

In some cases, patients may ask their physicians to facilitate access to services that the physician has ethical qualms about providing. For example, a patient might request a prescription for a cognitively enhancing medication to temporarily augment his cognitive abilities in order to take an exam or apply for employment. Patients may request more pain medication than the physician believes is warranted for the given situation or marijuana to facilitate sleep. Patients may ask their physician to sign a waiver to avoid vaccines for reasons that are not included in state exceptions (see **Chap. 3**). A physician may feel uncomfortable prescribing attention-deficit/hyperactivity disorder medications to a young child because she is not convinced that the possible benefit justifies the risks to the child despite the parent's request. In these circumstances, the physician should work with the patient or parent to understand the reasons for their requests, some of which might be legitimate. In addition to considering possible risks and benefits to the patient, the physician should consider how meeting the request might affect other patients, societal values, and public trust in the medical profession. If the physician determines that fulfilling the request requires deception, is unfair, jeopardizes her professional responsibilities, or is inconsistent with the patient's best medical interests, the physician should decline and explain the reasons to the patient.

■ MORAL DISTRESS

Health care providers, including residents, medical students, and experienced physicians, may experience moral distress when they feel that ethically appropriate action is hindered by institutional policies or culture, decision-making hierarchies, limited resources, or other reasons. Moral distress can lead to anger, anxiety, depression, frustration, fatigue, work dissatisfaction, and burnout. A physician's health and well-being can affect how he or she cares for patients. Discussing complex or unfamiliar clinical situations with colleagues and seeking assistance with difficult decisions can help alleviate moral distress, as can a healthy work environment characterized by open communication, mutual respect, and emphasis on the common goal of good patient care. In addition, physicians should take good care of their own well-being and be aware of the personal and system factors associated with stress, burnout, and depression. Health care organizations should provide a supportive work environment, counseling, and other support services when needed.

■ OCCUPATIONAL RISKS AND BURDENS

Physicians accept some physical risk in fulfilling their professional responsibilities, including exposure to infectious agents or toxic substances, violence in the workplace, and musculoskeletal injury. Nonetheless, most physicians, nurses, and other hospital staff willingly care for patients, despite personal risk and fear, grueling hours, and sometimes inadequate personal protective equipment or information. During the COVID-19 pandemic, many communities honored clinicians' dedication to professional ideals, and some medical students who were relieved from in-person patient care responsibilities volunteered to support front-line workers in other ways. The burdens of navigating professional and personal responsibilities fall more heavily on women health care providers. Health care institutions are responsible for reducing occupational risk and burden by providing proper information, training and supervision, protective equipment, infrastructure and workflow modifications, and emotional and psychological support to physicians. Clinical leaders need to acknowledge fears about personal safety and take steps to mitigate the impact of work on family responsibilities, moral distress, and burnout.

■ USE OF SOCIAL MEDIA AND PATIENT PORTALS

Increasingly, physicians use social and electronic media to share information and advice with patients and other providers. Social networking may be especially useful in reaching young or otherwise hard-to-access patients. Patients increasingly access their physicians' notes through patient portals, which aim to transparently share information, promote patient engagement, and increase adherence. Physicians should be professional and respectful and consider patient confidentiality, professional boundaries, and therapeutic relationships when posting to social media or writing notes for the portal. Overall, appropriate use of these platforms can enhance communication and transparency while avoiding misunderstandings or harmful consequences for patients, physicians, or their colleagues. Unprofessional or careless posts that express frustration or anger over work incidents, disparage patients or colleagues, use offensive or discriminatory language, or reveal inappropriate personal information about the physician can have negative consequences. Physicians should separate professional from personal websites and accounts and follow institutional and professional society guidelines when communicating with patients.

CONFLICTS OF INTEREST

Acting in patients' best interests may sometimes conflict with a physician's self-interest or the interests of third parties such as insurers or hospitals. From an ethical viewpoint, patients' interests are paramount. Transparency, appropriate disclosure, and management of conflicts of interest are essential to maintain the trust of colleagues and the public. Disclosure requirements vary for different purposes, and software has been developed to assist physicians in complying with specific requirements. Importantly, not all conflicts are financial. Physicians sometimes face conflicts of commitment between their patient's interests and their own personal interests, professional goals, responsibilities, and aspirations. As mentioned earlier, physicians should prioritize patients' interests while recognizing possible conflicts and using disclosure, discussion with the chief of service, and management of the conflict or recusal when appropriate.

In addition to individual physicians, medical institutions may have conflicts of interest arising from patent rights, industry-funded research programs, and donations from individuals and companies. Institutions need to be transparent about the presence and amount of such relationships and make clear the steps taken to prevent such relationships from having an impact on clinical or financial decisions. If there is good evidence that a donor acted in ways that breached ethical or legal standards, the institution should take steps not to benefit from the donation or honor the donor.

■ FINANCIAL INCENTIVES

Physicians have financial incentives to improve the quality or efficiency of care that might lead some to avoid patients who are older, are chronically ill, or have more complicated problems, or to focus on benchmarked outcomes even when not in the best interests of individual patients. In contrast, fee-for-service payments might encourage physicians to order more interventions than necessary or to refer patients to laboratory, imaging, or surgical facilities in which they have a financial stake. Regardless of financial incentives, physicians should recommend available care that is in the patient's best interests—no more and no less.

■ RELATIONSHIPS WITH PHARMACEUTICAL COMPANIES

Financial relationships between physicians and industry are increasingly scrutinized. Many academic medical centers have banned drug-company gifts, including branded pens and notepads and meals to physicians, to reduce inappropriate risk of undue influence or subconscious feelings of reciprocity and to decrease possible influences on public trust or the costs of health care.

The federal Open Payments website provides public information on the payments and amounts that drug and device companies give to individual physicians by name. The challenge is to distinguish payments for scientific consulting and research contracts—which should be encouraged as consistent with professional and academic missions—from those for promotional speaking and consulting whose goal is to increase sales of company products.

■ LEARNING CLINICAL SKILLS

Medical students', residents', and physicians' interests in learning, which fosters the long-term goal of benefiting future patients, may sometimes conflict with the short-term goal of providing optimal care to current patients. When trainees are learning procedures on patients, they lack the proficiency of experienced physicians, and patients may experience inconvenience, discomfort, longer procedures, or increased risk. Increasingly, institutions are developing clinical skills laboratories for simulation-based medical education and requiring students to demonstrate proficiency before carrying out procedures such as venipuncture and intravenous lines in patients. Furthermore, teaching hospitals are establishing proceduralist services in which procedure-specialist faculty members directly supervise interns for procedures such as lumbar puncture and thoracentesis and certify their proficiency. Medical students may need to defer learning such invasive procedures until internship. Seeking patients' consent for trainee participation in their care is always important and is particularly important for intimate examinations, such as pelvic, rectal, breast, and testicular examinations, and for invasive procedures. Patients should be told who is providing care and how trainees are supervised. Failing to introduce students or not telling patients that trainees will be performing procedures undermines trust, may lead to more elaborate deception, and makes it difficult for patients to make informed choices about their care. Most patients, when informed, allow trainees to play an active role in their care.

■ RESPONSE TO MEDICAL ERRORS

Errors are inevitable in clinical medicine, and some errors cause harm to patients. Most errors are caused by lapses of attention or flaws in the system of delivering health care; only a small number result from blameworthy individual behavior. Many health care institutions have adopted a just culture system, which encourages open and honest reporting of errors as essential to quality learning and shifts the focus from individual blame to system design for improvement in quality and safety (**Chap. 8**). This approach is more likely than a punitive approach to improve patient safety. However, professional discipline is appropriate for cases of gross incompetence, reckless behavior, physician impairment, and boundary violations. Physicians and students may fear that disclosing errors will damage their careers. Physicians and health care institutions show respect for patients by disclosing and explaining errors, offering an apology, offering appropriate compensation for harm done, and using errors as opportunities to improve the quality of care.

■ PHYSICIAN IMPAIRMENT

Physicians may hesitate to intervene when colleagues impaired by alcohol, drugs, or psychiatric or medical illness place patients at risk. However, society relies on physicians to regulate themselves. Colleagues of an impaired physician should take steps to protect patients and help their impaired colleague, starting with reporting their concerns to their clinical supervisor or director.

ETHICAL ISSUES IN CLINICAL RESEARCH

Clinical research is essential to translate scientific discoveries into beneficial interventions for patients. However, clinical research raises ethical concerns because participants face inconvenience and risks in research designed to advance scientific knowledge and not specifically to benefit them. Ethical guidelines require researchers to rigorously design and conduct research, minimize risk to participants, and obtain informed and voluntary consent from participants and approval from an institutional review board (IRB). IRBs determine that risks to participants are acceptable and have been minimized and recommend appropriate additional protections when research includes vulnerable participants.

Physicians may be clinical research investigators themselves or may be in a position to refer or recommend clinical trial participation to their patients. Physician-investigators are likely to feel some inherent tension between conducting research and providing health care. Awareness of this tension, familiarity with research ethics, collaboration with research and clinical team members, and utilizing research ethics consultation can help to mitigate tensions. Before starting clinical research, investigators should complete training in the ethics of clinical research, which is widely available.

Physicians also should be critical consumers of clinical research results and keep up with research advances that change standards of practice. Precision medicine initiatives aim to individualize clinical care by combining clinical information from electronic health records, genomic sequencing, and data from personal mobile devices. Furthermore, physicians and health care institutions are analyzing data routinely collected and available in electronic health records, leftover clinical specimens, and administrative data. Such studies encompass traditional discovery research as well as quality improvement, comparative effectiveness research, and learning health care systems. Efforts to improve the quality of care in real-world clinical settings are important but also raise new issues about informed consent, privacy, and risk.

EMERGING TECHNOLOGIES

Scientific advances in genome sequencing, gene editing (e.g., with CRISPR-Cas9), machine learning, artificial intelligence, computer-brain interfaces, and other technologies offer great promise for research and clinical care with the ultimate goal of improving the prediction, prevention, and treatment of disease. Groundbreaking innovations that have strong scientific plausibility need to be evaluated in rigorous clinical studies for efficacy and safety.

Physicians should keep up to date on the status of novel and often complex technologies as research evolves, data emerge, and technologies are incorporated into clinical practice. They can help their patients understand research findings and the evidence for clinical use, correct any misunderstandings, facilitate shared decision-making, and advocate for fair access to such therapies. Further, physicians should engage in professional and public discussion related to allocation of resources and fair access to expensive new therapies and emerging technologies and their impact on overall health care affordability.

Certain cell-based therapies, such as peripheral blood stem cell transplantation (**Chap. 114**) and chimeric antigen receptor (CAR)-T cell therapy (**Chap. 69**), are approved for use in several serious hematologic cancers, and gene therapies have been approved as safe and effective for clinical use in certain serious inherited diseases and cancers. Patients may request these and other complex, highly technical, and expensive therapies for unproven indications. Yet, claims of cures through unproven stem cell or gene-based "therapies" pose significant health and financial risks to patients without evidence of benefit. Physicians should help patients distinguish approved therapies from unproven claims and refer interested patients to well-designed clinical trials.

Medical applications of CRISPR-Cas9 are promising, and their safety and efficacy for particular clinical conditions are being carefully evaluated in clinical trials. Applications of CRISPR genome editing in somatic cells to modify or correct problematic genes could lay the foundation for treating a variety of serious diseases, including blood disorders, HIV, cancer, and hereditary blindness. Germline gene editing in blastocysts or embryos raises many ethical questions and is currently not permitted in the United States in clinical trials or clinical practice.

In artificial intelligence (AI), computers carry out tasks typically done by humans. Machine learning (ML) is a type of AI that automatically learns and improves its performance without explicit programming. Clinical algorithms using AI and ML can make diagnoses from radiology images, retinal scans, or skin photographs and identify patients at increased risk for surgical complications, critical care, or hospital readmission. However, such algorithms can also pose risks. Bias may occur if an algorithm was derived or validated from a data set in which groups who suffer from health disparities or poor health outcomes are underrepresented or if the algorithm predicts outcomes that are not clinically meaningful. To address these ethical concerns, researchers should assess AI algorithms in well-designed randomized clinical trials with clinical endpoints. Institutions should integrate validated and unbiased algorithms into clinical workflow without unduly burdening physicians and nurses and should check effectiveness and safety in their particular settings and patient populations.

Physicians should stay informed of emerging evidence about such technologies and the ethical challenges that accompany their use and always keep their patients' best interests and preferences at the forefront.

GLOBAL CONSIDERATIONS

■ INTERNATIONAL RESEARCH

Clinical research is often conducted across multiple sites and across national borders. Societal, legal, and cultural norms and perspectives about research may vary, and there are many ethical challenges. Physician-investigators involved in international research should be familiar with international guidelines, such as the Declaration of Helsinki, the Council for International Organizations of Medical Sciences (CIOMS) guidelines, and the International Council on Harmonisation Good Clinical Practice guidelines, as well as national and local laws where research is taking place. Partnering with local researchers and communities is essential not only to demonstrate respect but also to facilitate successful clinical research.

■ INTERNATIONAL CLINICAL EXPERIENCES

Many physicians and trainees gain valuable experience providing patient care in international settings through international training opportunities or volunteering for humanitarian or other international clinical work. Such arrangements, however, raise ethical challenges—for example, as a result of differences in beliefs about health and illness, expectations regarding health care and physicians' roles, standards of clinical practice, resource limitations, and norms for disclosure of serious diagnoses. Additional dilemmas arise if visiting physicians and trainees take on responsibilities beyond their expertise or if donated drugs and equipment are not appropriate to local needs. Visiting physicians and trainees should prepare well for these experiences, receive training and mentoring, learn about cultural and clinical practices in the host community, respect local customs and values, collaborate closely with local professionals and staff, and be explicit and humble about their own skills, knowledge, and limits. Leaders of global health field experiences should ensure that participating physicians receive training on ethical and cultural issues, as well as mentoring, backup, and debriefing upon return home.

■ CONCLUSION

Ethical issues are common in clinical medicine and occur in circumstances that may be foreseeable, novel, or unexpected. Physicians address these ethical issues by being prepared, informed, and thoughtful and using appropriate available resources.

■ FURTHER READING

Beauchamp T, Childress J: *Principles of Biomedical Ethics*, 8th ed. New York, Oxford University Press, 2019.

DeJong C et al: An ethical framework for allocating scarce medications for COVID-19 in the US. JAMA 323:2367, 2020.

Matheny M et al (eds): *Artificial Intelligence in Health Care: The Hope, the Hype, the Promise, the Peril.* NAM Special Publication. Washington, DC, National Academy of Medicine, 2019.

Ulrich C, Grady C: *Moral Distress in the Health Professions*. Cham, Switzerland, Springer-Nature International, 2018.

Wasserman J et al: Responding to unprofessional behavior by trainees: a "just culture" framework. N Engl J Med 382:773, 2020.

Wicclair MR: Conscientious objection, moral integrity, and professional obligations. Perspect Biol Med 62:543, 2019.

12 Palliative and End-of-Life Care

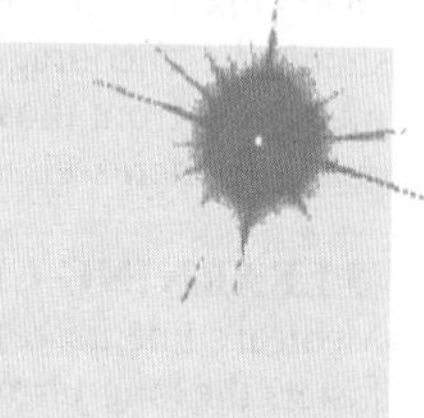

Ezekiel J. Emanuel

EPIDEMIOLOGY

■ CAUSES OF DEATH

In 2019, 2,854,838 individuals died in the United States (**Table 12-1**). Approximately 74% of these deaths occurred in those aged ≥65 years. The epidemiology of death has changed significantly since 1900 and even since 1980. In 1900, heart disease caused ~8% of all deaths, and cancer accounted for <4% of all deaths. In 1980, heart disease accounted for 38.2% of all deaths, cancer 20.9%, and cerebrovascular disease 8.6% of all deaths. By 2019, there had been a dramatic drop in deaths from cardiovascular and cerebrovascular diseases. In 2019, 23.1% of all deaths were from cardiovascular disease and just 5.3% from cerebrovascular disease. Deaths attributable to cancer, however, had increased slightly to 21.0%. The proportions of deaths due to chronic lower respiratory disease, diabetes, Alzheimer's, and suicide have increased. Interestingly, in 2019, HIV/AIDS accounted for <0.18% of all U.S. deaths. While unlikely to continue being a leading cause of death in the future, COVID-19 was also the cause for >600,000 deaths in 2020–2021, and the official figure is almost certainly an undercount of the actual death toll.

TABLE 12-1 Ten Leading Causes of Death in the United States and Britain

CAUSE OF DEATH	UNITED STATES (2019)		ENGLAND AND WALES (2019)	
	NUMBER OF DEATHS, ALL AGES (%)	NUMBER OF DEATHS, PEOPLE ≥65 YEARS OF AGE	NUMBER OF DEATHS, ALL AGES (%)	NUMBER OF DEATHS, PEOPLE ≥65 YEARS OF AGE
All deaths	2,854,838	2,117,332	530,841	449,047
Heart disease[a]	659,041 (23.1)	531,583 (25.1)	87,095 (16.4)	74,967 (16.7)
Malignant neoplasms	599,601 (21.0)	435,462 (20.6)	147,419 (27.8)	118,982 (26.5)
Chronic lower respiratory diseases	156,979 (5.5)	133,246 (6.3)	31,221 (5.9)	28,235 (6.3)
Accidents	173,040 (6.1)	60,527 (2.9)	15,141 (2.9)	8999 (2.0)
Cerebrovascular diseases	150,005 (5.3)	129,193 (6.1)	29,816 (5.6)	27,210 (6.0)
Alzheimer's disease	121,499 (4.3)	120,090 (5.7)	20,400 (3.8)	20,279 (4.5)
Diabetes mellitus	87,647 (3.1)	62,397 (2.9)	6528 (1.2)	5552 (1.2)
Influenza and pneumonia	49,783 (1.7)	40,399 (1.9)	26,398 (5.0)	24,269 (5.4)
Nephritis, nephritic syndrome, nephrosis	51,565 (1.8)	42,230 (2.0)	3575 (0.7)	3323 (0.7)
Intentional self-harm	47,511 (1.7)	—	4832 (0.9)	751 (0.2)

[a]Calculated using International Classification of Diseases codes I00–I09, I11, I13, I20–I51.
Source: National Center for Health Statistics (United States, 2019), *http://www.cdc.gov/nchs;* National Statistics (Great Britain, 2019), *http://www.statistics.gov.uk.*

This change in the epidemiology of death is also reflected in the costs of illness. In the United States, ~84% of all health care spending goes to patients with chronic illnesses, and 12% of total personal health care spending—slightly less than $400 billion in 2015—goes to the 0.83% of the population in the last year of their lives.

In upper-middle- and upper-income countries, an estimated 70% of all deaths are preceded by a disease or condition, making it reasonable to plan for dying in the foreseeable future. Cancer has served as the paradigm for terminal care, but it is not the only type of illness with a recognizable and predictable terminal phase. Since heart failure, chronic obstructive pulmonary disease (COPD), chronic liver failure, dementia, and many other conditions have recognizable terminal phases, a systematic approach to end-of-life care should be part of all medical specialties. Many patients with chronic illness–related symptoms and suffering also can benefit from palliative care regardless of prognosis. Ideally, palliative care should be considered part of comprehensive care for all chronically ill patients. Strong evidence demonstrates that palliative care can be improved by coordination between caregivers, doctors, and patients for advance care planning, as well as dedicated teams of physicians, nurses, and other providers.

SITE OF DEATH

Where patients die varies by country. In Belgium and Canada, for instance, over half of all cancer patients still die in the hospital. The past few decades have seen a steady shift, both in the United States and other countries like the Netherlands, out of the hospital, as patients and their families list their own homes as the preferred site of death. In the early 1980s, ~70% of American cancer patients died in the hospital. Today, that percentage is ~25% (**Fig. 12-1**). A recent report shows that since 2000, there has been a shift in the United States from inpatient to home deaths, especially for patients with cancer, COPD, and dementia. For instance, among Medicare beneficiaries, 30.1% of deaths due to cancer in 2000 occurred in acute care hospitals; by 2009, this figure had dropped to 22.1%; by 2015, it was 19.8%.

Paradoxically, while deaths in acute care hospitals have declined in the United States since 2000, both hospitalizations in the last 90 days of life and—even more troublingly—admission to the intensive care unit (ICU) in the last 30 days have actually increased. Over 40% of cancer patients in the United States are admitted to the ICU in their last 6 months of life, and >25% of cancer patients are admitted to the hospital in the last 30 days.

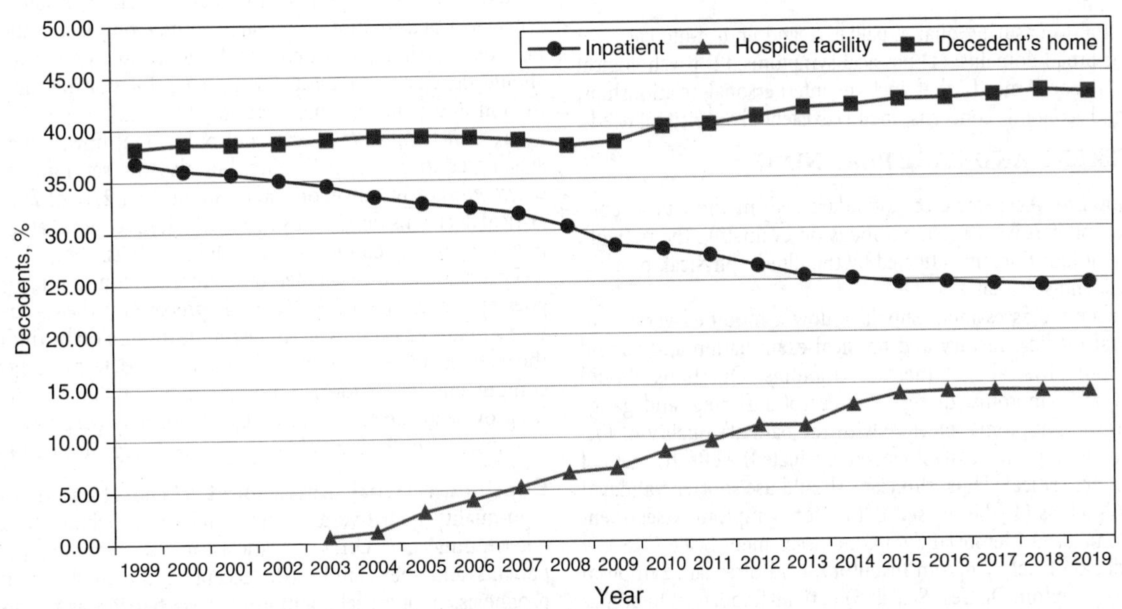

FIGURE 12-1 Graph showing trends in cancer decedents' site of death 1999–2019. *(Source: Centers for Disease Control and Prevention, National Center for Health Statistics. Underlying Cause of Death 1999-2019 on CDC WONDER Online Database. http://wonder.cdc.gov.)*

The shift in deaths out of the hospital has been accompanied by an increase in the use of hospice in the United States. In 2000, 21.6% of Medicare decedents used hospice at the time of death; by 2009, 42.2% were using hospice; and by 2018, 50.7% of Medicare decedents were enrolled in hospice at the time of death. Among cancer patients, ~60% were using hospice at the time of death. Hospice is also increasingly being used by noncancer patients. Today, cancer patients constitute ~20% of hospice users. But since 2014, the proportion of patients with other diagnoses using hospice has grown substantially, including those with circulatory/heart disease (17.4% in 2018 vs 13.8% in 2014), stroke (9.5% vs 6.2%), and respiratory disease (11.0% vs 9.4%). Of 2018 Medicare hospice decedents, 51.5% died at home, 17.4% in a nursing facility, 12.8% in a hospice inpatient facility, and 12.3% in assisted living.

Unfortunately, significant racial disparities exist in end-of-life care and the use of hospice, especially for noncancer deaths. Racial and ethnic minorities are less likely to receive hospice services than white decedents and are more likely to receive invasive or aggressive care in end-of-life treatment. Of people who died of head and neck cancers between 1999 and 2017, African Americans and Asians/Pacific Islanders were less likely to die at home or in hospice. Among Medicare beneficiaries who had a pancreatectomy for pancreatic cancer and lived at least 30 days, racial and ethnic minority patients remained 22% less likely than white patients to initiate hospice before death.

In 2008, for the first time, the American Board of Medical Specialties (ABMS) offered certification in hospice and palliative medicine. With the shortening of hospital stays, many serious conditions are now being treated at home or on an outpatient basis. Consequently, providing optimal palliative and end-of-life care requires ensuring that appropriate services are available in a variety of settings, including noninstitutional settings.

HOSPICE AND THE PALLIATIVE CARE FRAMEWORK

Central to this type of care is an interdisciplinary team approach that typically encompasses pain and symptom management, spiritual and psychological care for the patient, and support for family caregivers during the patient's illness and the bereavement period.

One of the more important changes in this field is beginning palliative care many months before death in order to focus on symptom relief and then switching to hospice in the patient's last few months. This approach avoids leaving hospice until the very end by introducing palliative care earlier, thereby allowing patients and families time to accommodate and transition. Phasing palliative care into end-of-life care means that patients will often receive palliative interventions long before they are formally diagnosed as terminally ill, or likely to die within 6 months.

Fundamental to ensuring quality palliative and end-of-life care is a focus on four broad domains: (1) physical symptoms; (2) psychological symptoms; (3) social needs that include interpersonal relationships, caregiving, and economic concerns; and (4) existential or spiritual needs.

ASSESSMENT AND CARE PLANNING

Comprehensive Assessment Standardized methods for conducting a comprehensive assessment focus on evaluating the patient's condition in all four domains affected by the illness: physical, psychological, social, and spiritual.

A comprehensive assessment should follow a modified version of the traditional medical history and physical examination and should emphasize both physical and mental symptoms. Questions should aim to elucidate symptoms, discern sources of suffering, and gauge how much those symptoms interfere with the patient's quality of life. Standardized and repeated assessments to evaluate the effectiveness of interventions are critical. Thus, clinicians should use shorter, validated instruments, such as (1) the revised Edmonton Symptom Assessment Scale; (2) Condensed Memorial Symptom Assessment Scale (MSAS); (3) MD Anderson Brief Symptom Inventory; (4) Rotterdam Symptom Checklist; (5) Symptom Distress Scale; (6) Patient-Reported Outcomes Measurement Information System; and (7) Interactive Symptom Assessment and Collection (ISAAC) tool.

MENTAL HEALTH With respect to mental health, many practices use the Patient Health Questionnaire-9 (PHQ-9) to screen for depression and the Generalized Anxiety Disorder-7 (GAD-7) to screen for anxiety. Using such tools ensures that the assessment is comprehensive and does not focus excessively on only pain.

INVASIVE TESTS Invasive tests are best avoided in end-of-life care, and even minimally invasive tests should be evaluated carefully for their benefit-to-burden ratio for the patient. Aspects of the physical examination that are uncomfortable and unlikely to yield useful information that change patient management should be omitted.

SOCIAL NEEDS Health care providers should also assess the status of important relationships, financial burdens, caregiving needs, and access to medical care. Relevant questions include the following: *How often is there someone to feel close to? How has this illness been for your family? How has it affected your relationships? How much help do you need with things like getting meals and getting around? How much trouble do you have getting the medical care you need?*

EXISTENTIAL NEEDS To determine a patient's existential needs, providers should assess distress, the patient's sense of emotional and existential well-being, and whether the patient believes he or she has found purpose or meaning. Helpful assessment questions can include the following: *How much are you able to find meaning since your illness began? What things are most important to you at this stage?*

PERCEPTION OF CARE In addition, it can be helpful to ask how the patient perceives his or her care: *How much do you feel your doctors and nurses respect you? How clear is the information from us about what to expect regarding your illness? How much do you feel that the medical care you are getting fits with your goals?* If concern is detected in any of these areas, deeper evaluative questions are warranted.

Communication Particularly when an illness is life-threatening, there exists the potential for many emotionally charged and potentially conflict-creating moments—collectively called "bad news" situations—in which empathic and effective communication skills are essential. Those moments include the sharing of a terminal diagnosis with the patient and/or family, the discussion of the patient's prognosis and any treatment failures, the consideration of deemphasizing efforts to cure and prolong life while focusing more on symptom management and palliation, advance care planning, and the patient's actual death. Although these conversations can be difficult, research indicates that end-of-life discussions can lead to earlier hospice referrals, rather than overly aggressive treatment, ultimately benefiting quality of life for patients and improving the bereavement process for families.

Just as surgeons prepare for major operations and investigators rehearse a presentation of research results, physicians and health care providers caring for patients with significant or advanced illnesses should develop a standardized approach for sharing important information and planning interventions. In addition, physicians must be aware that families often care not only about how prepared the physician was to deliver bad news, but also the setting in which it was delivered. For instance, one study found that 27% of families making critical decisions for patients in an ICU desired better and more private physical space to communicate with physicians.

One structured seven-step procedure for communicating bad news goes by the acronym P-SPIKES: (1) ***p***repare for the discussion, (2) ***s***et up a suitable environment, (3) begin the discussion by finding out what the ***p***atient and/or family understand, (4) determine how they will comprehend new ***i***nformation best and how much they want to know, (5) provide needed new ***k***nowledge accordingly, (6) allow for ***e***motional responses, and (7) ***s***hare plans for the next steps in care (**Table 12-2**).

Continuous Goal Assessment Major barriers to providing high-quality palliative and end-of-life care include the difficulty in determining an accurate prognosis and the emotional resistance of patients and their families to accepting the implications of a poor prognosis. A practical solution to these barriers is to integrate palliative care interventions or home visits from a palliative care visiting nurse months before the estimated final 6 months of life. Under this

TABLE 12-2 Elements of Communicating Bad News—The P-SPIKES Approach

ACRONYM	STEPS	AIM OF THE INTERACTION	PREPARATIONS, QUESTIONS, OR PHRASES
P	Preparation	Mentally prepare for the interaction with the patient and/or family.	Review what information needs to be communicated. Plan how you will provide emotional support. Rehearse key steps and phrases in the interaction.
S	Setting of the interaction	Ensure the appropriate setting for a serious and potentially emotionally charged discussion.	Ensure that patient, family, and appropriate social supports are present. Devote sufficient time. Ensure privacy and prevent interruptions by people or beeper. Bring a box of tissues.
P	Patient's perception and preparation	Begin the discussion by establishing the baseline and whether the patient and family can grasp the information. Ease tension by having the patient and family contribute.	Start with open-ended questions to encourage participation. Possible questions to use: *What do you understand about your illness?* *When you first had symptom X, what did you think it might be?* *What did Dr. X tell you when he or she sent you here?* *What do you think is going to happen?*
I	Invitation and information needs	Discover what information needs the patient and/or family have and what limits they want regarding the bad information.	Possible questions to use: *If this condition turns out to be something serious, do you want to know?* *Would you like me to tell you all the details of your condition? If not, who would you like me to talk to?*
K	Knowledge of the condition	Provide the bad news or other information to the patient and/or family sensitively.	Do not just dump the information on the patient and family. Check for patient and family understanding. Possible phrases to use: *I feel badly to have to tell you this, but...* *Unfortunately, the tests showed...* *I'm afraid the news is not good...*
E	Empathy and exploration	Identify the cause of the emotions—e.g., poor prognosis. Empathize with the patient's and/or family's feelings. Explore by asking open-ended questions.	Strong feelings in reaction to bad news are normal. Acknowledge what the patient and family are feeling. Remind them such feelings are normal, even if frightening. Give them time to respond. Remind the patient and family you won't abandon them. Possible phrases to use: *I imagine this is very hard for you to hear.* *You look very upset. Tell me how you are feeling.* *I wish the news were different.* *We'll do whatever we can to help you.*
S	Summary and planning	Delineate for the patient and the family the next steps, including additional tests or interventions.	It is the unknown and uncertain that can increase anxiety. Recommend a schedule with goals and landmarks. Provide your rationale for the patient and/or family to accept (or reject). If the patient and/or family are not ready to discuss the next steps, schedule a follow-up visit.

Source: Adapted from R Buckman: *How to Break Bad News: A Guide for Health Care Professionals.* Baltimore, Johns Hopkins University Press, 1992.

approach, palliative care no longer conveys the message of failure, having no more treatments, or "giving up hope." The transition from palliative to end-of-life care or hospice also feels less hasty and unexpected to the family. Fundamental to integrating palliative care with curative therapy is the inclusion of a continuous goal assessment as part of the routine patient reassessments that occur at most patient-physician encounters.

Goals for care are numerous, ranging from curing a specific disease, to prolonging life, to relieving a particular symptom, to adapting to a progressive disability without disrupting the family, to finding peace of mind or personal meaning, to dying in a manner that leaves loved ones with positive memories. Discerning a patient's goals for care can be approached through a seven-step protocol: (1) ensure that medical and other information is as complete as reasonably possible and is understood by all relevant parties (see above); (2) explore what the patient and/or family is hoping for, while also identifying relevant and realistic goals; (3) share all the options with the patient and family; (4) respond with empathy as they adjust to changing expectations; (5) make a plan that emphasizes what can be done to achieve the realistic goals; (6) follow through with the plan; and (7) periodically review the plan and consider at every encounter whether the goals of care should be revised with the patient and/or family. Each of these steps need not be followed in rote order, but together they provide a helpful framework for interactions with patients and their families regarding their goals for care. Such interactions can be especially challenging if a patient or family member has difficulty letting go of an unrealistic goal. In such cases, the provider should help them refocus on more realistic goals and should also suggest that while it is fine to hope for the best, it is still prudent to plan for other outcomes as well.

Advance Care Planning • PRACTICES Advance care planning is the process of planning for future medical care in case the patient becomes incapable of making medical decisions. A 2010 study of adults aged ≥60 who died between 2000 and 2006 found that while 42% of adults were required to make treatment decisions in their final days of life, 70% lacked decision-making capacity. Among those lacking decision-making capacity, approximately one-third did not have advance planning directives. Ideally, such planning would occur before a health care crisis or the terminal phase of an illness. Unfortunately, diverse barriers prevent this. Approximately 80% of Americans endorse advance care planning and living wills. However, according to a 2013 Pew survey, only 35% of adults have written down their end-of-life wishes. Other studies report that even fewer Americans—with some estimates as low as 26% of adults—have filled out advance care directives. A review of studies suggests that the percentage of Americans who had written advance directives did not change between 2011 and 2016 and remains slightly over one-third of Americans. Larger numbers of adults, between 50 and 70%, claim to have talked with someone about their treatment wishes. Americans aged 65 and older are more likely to complete an advance directive compared to younger adults (46% vs 32%).

Effective advance care planning should follow six key steps: (1) introducing the topic, (2) structuring a discussion, (3) reviewing plans that have been discussed by the patient and family, (4) documenting the plans, (5) updating them periodically, and (6) implementing the advance care directives (**Table 12-3**). Two of the main barriers to advance care planning are problems in raising the topic and difficulty in structuring a succinct discussion. Raising the topic can be done efficiently as a routine matter, noting that it is recommended for all patients, analogous to purchasing insurance or estate planning. Many of the most difficult cases have involved unexpected, acute episodes of brain damage in young individuals.

Structuring a focused discussion is an important communication skill. To do so, a provider must first identify the health care proxy and recommend his or her involvement in the advance care planning process. Next, a worksheet must be selected that has been demonstrated to produce reliable and valid expressions of patient preferences, and the patient and proxy must be oriented to it. Such worksheets exist for both general and disease-specific situations. The provider should then discuss with the patient and proxy one example scenario to demonstrate how to think about the issues. It is often helpful to begin with a scenario in which the patient is likely to have settled preferences for care, such as being in a persistent vegetative state. Once the patient's preferences for interventions in this scenario are determined, the provider should suggest that the patient and proxy discuss and complete the worksheet for each other. If appropriate, the patient and proxy should consider involving other family members in the discussion. During a subsequent return visit, the provider should go over the patient's preferences, checking and resolving any inconsistencies. After having the patient and proxy sign the document, the provider should place the document in the patient's medical chart and make sure that copies are provided to relevant family members and care sites. Since patients' preferences can change, these documents must be reviewed periodically.

TYPES OF DOCUMENTS Advance care planning documents are of two broad types. The first includes living wills, also known as instructional directives; these are advisory documents that describe the types of decisions that should direct a patient's care. Some are more specific, delineating different scenarios and interventions for the patient to choose from. Among these, some are for general use and others are designed for use by patients with a specific type of disease, such as cancer, renal failure, or HIV. Less specific directives can be general statements, such as not wanting life-sustaining interventions, or forms that describe the values that should guide specific discussions about terminal care. The second type of advance directive allows the designation of a health care proxy (sometimes also referred to as a durable attorney for health care), an individual selected by the patient to make decisions. The choice is not either/or; a combined directive that includes a living

TABLE 12-3 Steps in Advance Care Planning

STEP	GOALS TO BE ACHIEVED AND MEASURES TO COVER	USEFUL PHRASES OR POINTS TO MAKE
Introduce advance care planning	Ask the patient what he or she knows about advance care planning and if he or she has already completed an advance care directive.	*I'd like to talk with you about something I try to discuss with all my patients. It's called advance care planning. In fact, I feel that this is such an important topic that I have done this myself. Are you familiar with advance care planning or living wills?*
	Indicate that you as a physician have completed advance care planning.	*Have you thought about the type of care you would want if you ever became too sick to speak for yourself? That is the purpose of advance care planning.*
	Indicate that you try to perform advance care planning with all patients regardless of prognosis.	*There is no change in health that we have not discussed. I am bringing this up now because it is sensible for everyone, no matter how well or ill, old or young.*
	Explain the goals of the process as empowering the patient and ensuring that you and the proxy understand the patient's preferences.	*Have many copies of advance care directives available, including in the waiting room, for patients and families.*
	Provide the patient relevant literature, including the advance care directive that you prefer to use.	*Know resources for state-specific forms (available at www.nhpco.org).*
	Recommend the patient identify a proxy decision-maker who should attend the next meeting.	
Have a structured discussion of scenarios with the patient	Affirm that the goal of the process is to follow the patient's wishes if the patient loses decision-making capacity.	*Use a structured worksheet with typical scenarios.*
	Elicit the patient's overall goals related to health care. Elicit the patient's preferences for specific interventions in a few salient and common scenarios. Help the patient define the threshold for withdrawing and withholding interventions. Define the patient's preference for the role of the proxy.	*Begin the discussion with persistent vegetative state and consider other scenarios, such as recovery from an acute event with serious disability; then ask the patient about his or her preferences regarding specific interventions, such as ventilators, artificial nutrition, and CPR; finally, proceeding to less invasive interventions, such as blood transfusions and antibiotics.*
Review the patient's preferences	After the patient has made choices of interventions, review them to ensure they are consistent and the proxy is aware of them.	
Document the patient's preferences	Formally complete the advance care directive and have a witness sign it.	
	Provide a copy for the patient and the proxy.	
	Insert a copy into the patient's medical record and summarize it in a progress note.	
Update the directive	Periodically, and with major changes in health status, review the directive with the patient and make any modifications.	
Apply the directive	The directive goes into effect only when the patient becomes unable to make medical decisions for himself or herself.	
	Reread the directive to be sure about its content.	
	Discuss your proposed actions based on the directive with the proxy.	

Abbreviation: CPR, cardiopulmonary resuscitation.

will and designates a proxy is often used, and the directive should indicate clearly whether the specified patient preferences or the proxy's choice takes precedence if they conflict. Some states have begun to put into practice a "Physician Orders for Life-Sustaining Treatment (POLST)" directive, which builds on communication between providers and patients by including guidance for end-of-life care in a color-coordinated form that follows the patient across treatment settings. The procedures for completing advance care planning documents vary according to state law.

A potentially misleading distinction relates to statutory, as opposed to advisory, documents. Statutory documents are drafted to fulfill relevant state laws. Advisory documents are drafted to reflect the patient's wishes. Both are legal, the former under state law and the latter under common or constitutional law.

LEGAL ASPECTS As of 2021, 48 states and the District of Columbia had enacted living will legislation. Massachusetts and Michigan are the two states without living will legislation. Indiana has a life-prolonging procedures declaration. States differ in the requirements for advanced directives, including whether they need to be witnessed and, if so, by how many witnesses and whether they need to be notarized. Importantly, in 25 states, the laws state that the living will is not valid if a woman is pregnant. All states except Alaska have enacted durable power of attorney for health care laws that permit patients to designate a proxy decision-maker with authority to terminate life-sustaining treatments. Only in Alaska does the law prohibit proxies from terminating life-sustaining treatments for pregnant women.

The U.S. Supreme Court has ruled that patients have a constitutional right to decide any issues related to refusing or terminating medical interventions, including life-sustaining interventions, and that mentally incompetent patients can exercise this right by providing "clear and convincing evidence" of their preferences. Since advance care directives permit patients to provide such evidence, commentators agree that they are constitutionally protected. Most commentators believe that a state is required to honor any clear advance care directive, regardless of whether it is written on an "official" form. Many states have enacted laws for the explicit purpose of honoring out-of-state directives. If a patient is not using a statutory form, it may be advisable to attach a statutory form to the advance care directive being used. State-specific forms are readily available free of charge for health care providers, patients, and families through the website of the National Hospice and Palliative Care Organization (*http://www.nhpco.org*).

REIMBURSEMENT As of January 1, 2016, the Centers for Medicare and Medicaid Services amended the physician fee schedule to reimburse discussions of advance care planning under Current Procedural Terminology codes 99497 and 99498. The session must be voluntary and include an explanation of advance care planning but need not include a completed advance care document. There can be multiple bills for the discussion if it extends over several encounters. A study found that patients who engaged in a billed advance care planning encounter were more likely to be enrolled in hospice and less likely to receive intensive therapies, despite being more likely to be hospitalized in the ICU. However, a billing incentive in and of itself may not increase advance care planning discussions by clinicians. In 2016, just 1.6% of Medicare Advantage patients had a discussion of advance care planning that was billed. Factors beyond reimbursement, such as clinicians' lack of comfort and skill in carrying out advance care planning discussions and lack of time, appear to impede discussions of advance care planning.

INTERVENTIONS

PHYSICAL SYMPTOMS AND THEIR MANAGEMENT

Great emphasis has been placed on addressing dying patients' pain. In order to emphasize its importance, pain assessment has frequently been included as the fifth vital sign. Heightened consideration of pain has been advocated by large health care systems such as the Veterans' Administration and accrediting bodies such as The Joint Commission. Although this embrace of pain has been symbolically important, available data suggest that making pain the fifth vital sign does not lead to improved pain management practices. In light of the opioid crisis in the United States, the emphasis on pain management has begun to be reexamined. For instance, in 2017 draft standards, The Joint Commission recommends nonpharmacologic pain treatment as well as identification of psychosocial risk factors for addiction. Importantly, good palliative care requires much more than good pain management. The frequency of symptoms varies by disease and other factors. The most common physical and psychological symptoms among all terminally ill patients include pain, fatigue, insomnia, anorexia, dyspnea, depression, anxiety, nausea, and vomiting. In the last days of life, terminal delirium is also common. Assessments of patients with advanced cancer have shown that patients experienced an average of 11.5 different physical and psychological symptoms (**Table 12-4**).

TABLE 12-4 Common Physical and Psychological Symptoms of Terminally Ill Patients

PHYSICAL SYMPTOMS	PSYCHOLOGICAL SYMPTOMS
Pain	Anxiety
Fatigue and weakness	Depression
Dyspnea	Hopelessness
Insomnia	Meaninglessness
Dry mouth	Irritability
Anorexia	Impaired concentration
Nausea and vomiting	Confusion
Constipation	Delirium
Cough	Loss of libido
Swelling of arms or legs	
Itching	
Diarrhea	
Dysphagia	
Dizziness	
Fecal and urinary incontinence	
Numbness/tingling in hands/feet	

In the vast majority of cases, evaluations to determine the etiology of these symptoms should be limited to the history and physical examination. In some cases, radiologic or other diagnostic examinations will provide sufficient benefit in directing optimal palliative care to warrant the risks, potential discomfort, and inconvenience, especially to a seriously ill patient. Only a few of the common symptoms that present difficult management issues will be addressed in this chapter. **Additional information on the management of other symptoms, such as nausea and vomiting, insomnia, and diarrhea, can be found in Chaps. 45, 31, and 46, respectively. Information on the management of patients with cancer is provided in Chap. 69.**

Pain • **FREQUENCY** The frequency of pain among terminally ill patients varies significantly. Cancer (~85%), congestive heart failure (CHF; ~75%), and AIDS have been associated with a higher prevalence of pain compared to other advanced illnesses, such as COPD (~45%), chronic kidney disease (~40%), and dementia (~40%). One meta-analysis of adults with advanced or terminal illness found pain prevalence of 30–94% in patients with cancer, compared to 21–77% for COPD, 14–78% for CHF, 11–83% for end-stage renal disease, 14–63% for dementia, and 30–98% for AIDS.

ETIOLOGY There are two types of pain: nociceptive and neuropathic. Nociceptive pain is further divided into somatic or visceral pain. *Somatic pain* is the result of direct mechanical or chemical stimulation of nociceptors and normal neural signaling to the brain. It tends to be localized, aching, throbbing, and cramping. The classic example is bone metastases. *Visceral pain* is caused by nociceptors in gastrointestinal (GI), respiratory, and other organ systems. It is a deep or colicky type of pain classically associated with pancreatitis, myocardial infarction, or tumor invasion of viscera. *Neuropathic pain* arises from disordered nerve signals. It is described by patients as burning, electrical, or shock-like pain. Classic examples are post-stroke pain, tumor invasion of the brachial plexus, and herpetic neuralgia.

ASSESSMENT Pain is a subjective experience. Depending on the patient's circumstances, perspective, and physiologic condition, the same physical lesion or disease state can produce different levels of reported pain and need for pain relief. Systematic assessment includes eliciting the following: (1) type: throbbing, cramping, burning, etc.; (2) periodicity: continuous, with or without exacerbations, or incident; (3) location; (4) intensity; (5) modifying factors; (6) effects of treatments; (7) functional impact; and (8) impact on patient. Several validated pain assessment measures may be used, including the Visual Analogue Scale (VAS), the Brief Pain Inventory (BPI), or the Numerical Pain Rating Scale (NRS-11). Other scales have been developed for neuropathic pain, such as the Neuropathic Pain Scale and the DN4 Questionnaire. Frequent reassessments on a consistent scale are essential to assess the impact of and need to readjust interventions.

INTERVENTIONS Interventions for pain must be tailored to each individual, with the goal of preempting chronic pain and relieving breakthrough pain. At the end of life, there is rarely reason to doubt a patient's report of pain. With the opioid crisis in the United States, there is more emphasis on making opioids one component of multimodal analgesia. Nevertheless, at the end of life, pain medications, especially opioids, remain the cornerstone of management (**Fig. 12-2**). If they are failing and nonpharmacologic interventions—including radiotherapy and anesthetic or neurosurgical procedures such as peripheral nerve blocks or epidural medications—are required, a pain consultation is appropriate.

Pharmacologic interventions still largely follow the World Health Organization three-step, "analgesic ladder" approach, which involves nonopioid analgesics, "mild" opioids, and "strong" opioids, with or without adjuvants (**Chap. 13**). Nonopioid analgesics, especially nonsteroidal anti-inflammatory drugs (NSAIDs), are the initial treatments for mild pain. They work primarily by inhibiting peripheral prostaglandins and reducing inflammation but may also have central nervous system (CNS) effects. Additionally, NSAIDs have a ceiling effect. Ibuprofen, up to 2400 mg/d qid, has a minimal risk of causing bleeding and renal impairment and is a good initial choice. In patients with a history of severe GI or other bleeding, however, ibuprofen should be avoided. In patients with a history of mild gastritis or gastroesophageal reflux disease (GERD), acid-lowering therapy, such as a proton pump inhibitor, should be used. Acetaminophen is an alternative in patients with a history of GI bleeding and can be used safely at up to 4 g/d qid. In patients with liver dysfunction due to metastases or other causes and in patients with heavy alcohol use, doses should be reduced.

If nonopioid analgesics are insufficient, opioids should be introduced. Opioids primarily work by interacting with μ opioid receptors to activate pain-inhibitory neurons in the CNS, although they also interact variably with δ and κ receptors. Receptor agonists, such as morphine, codeine, and fentanyl, produce analgesia by activating pain-inhibitory neurons in the CNS. Partial agonists, such as buprenorphine, have a ceiling effect for analgesia and a lower potential for abuse. They are useful for postacute pain but should not be used for chronic pain in end-of-life care. Pure antagonists, such as naloxone and methylnaltrexone, are used for reversal of opioid effects.

Traditionally, "weak" opioids such as codeine were used first. If they failed to relieve pain after dose escalation, "strong" opioids like morphine were used in doses of 5–10 mg every 4 h. However, this breakdown between "weak" and "strong" opioids is no longer commonly accepted, with smaller doses of "stronger" opioids frequently being preferred over similar or larger doses of "weaker" opioids, and different pain syndromes having different preferred therapies. Regardless, nonopioid analgesics should be combined with opioids, as they potentiate the effect of opioids.

Importantly, the goal is to prevent patients from experiencing pain. Consequently, for continuous pain, opioids should be administered on a regular, around-the-clock basis consistent with their duration of analgesia, and the next dose should occur before the effect of the previous dose wears off. They should not be provided only when the patient

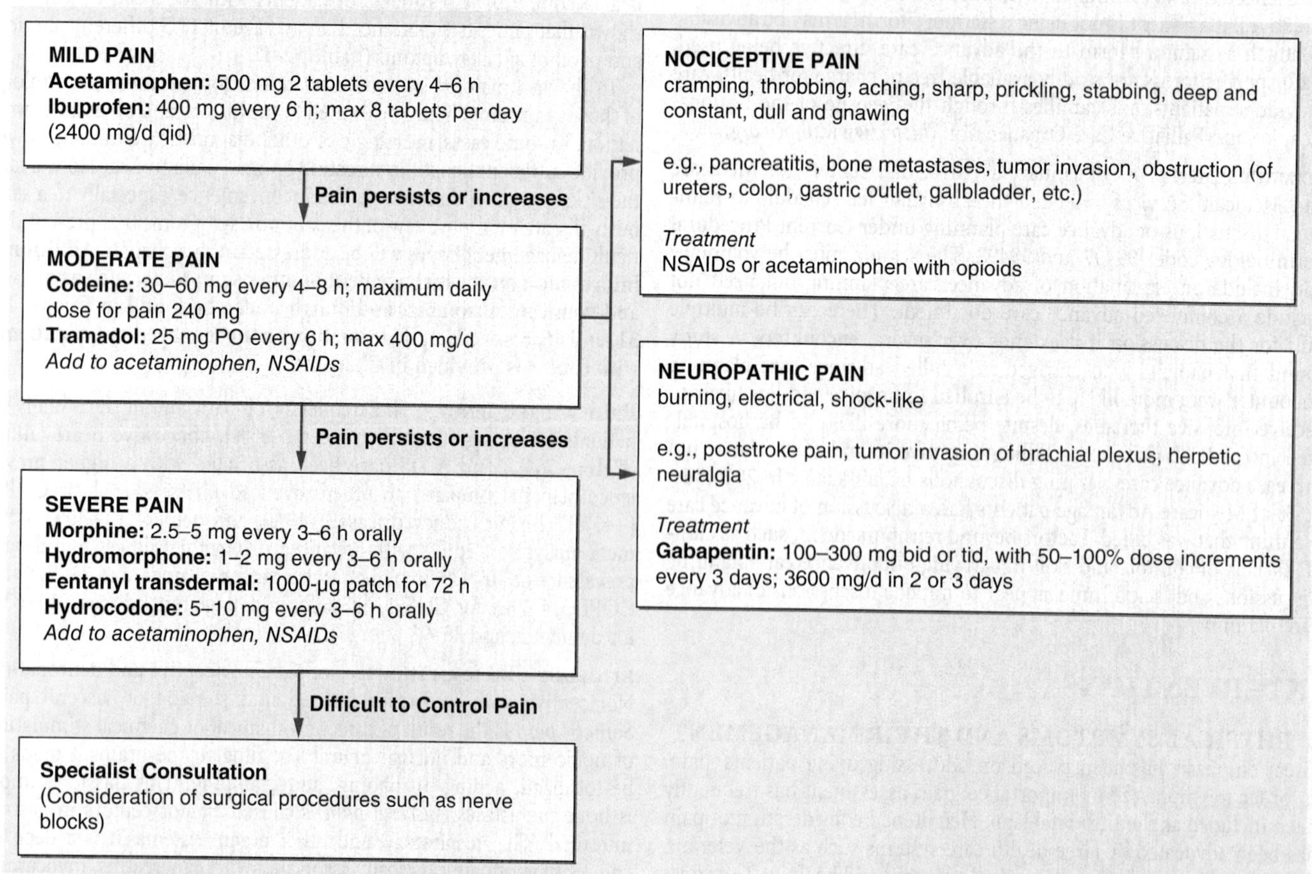

MILD PAIN
Acetaminophen: 500 mg 2 tablets every 4–6 h
Ibuprofen: 400 mg every 6 h; max 8 tablets per day (2400 mg/d qid)
Pain persists or increases
MODERATE PAIN
Codeine: 30–60 mg every 4–8 h; maximum daily dose for pain 240 mg
Tramadol: 25 mg PO every 6 h; max 400 mg/d
Add to acetaminophen, NSAIDs
Pain persists or increases
SEVERE PAIN
Morphine: 2.5–5 mg every 3–6 h orally
Hydromorphone: 1–2 mg every 3–6 h orally
Fentanyl transdermal: 1000-μg patch for 72 h
Hydrocodone: 5–10 mg every 3–6 h orally
Add to acetaminophen, NSAIDs
Difficult to Control Pain
Specialist Consultation
(Consideration of surgical procedures such as nerve blocks)
NOCICEPTIVE PAIN
cramping, throbbing, aching, sharp, prickling, stabbing, deep and constant, dull and gnawing
e.g., pancreatitis, bone metastases, tumor invasion, obstruction (of ureters, colon, gastric outlet, gallbladder, etc.)
Treatment
NSAIDs or acetaminophen with opioids
NEUROPATHIC PAIN
burning, electrical, shock-like
e.g., poststroke pain, tumor invasion of brachial plexus, herpetic neuralgia
Treatment
Gabapentin: 100–300 mg bid or tid, with 50–100% dose increments every 3 days; 3600 mg/d in 2 or 3 days

FIGURE 12-2 Terminal pain management flow chart. NSAIDs, nonsteroidal anti-inflammatory drugs.

experiences pain. Patients should also be provided rescue medication, such as liquid morphine, for breakthrough pain, generally at 20% of the baseline dose. Patients should be informed that using the rescue medication does not obviate the need to take the next standard dose of pain medication. If the patient's pain remains uncontrolled after 24 h and recurs before the next dose, requiring the patient to utilize the rescue medication, the daily opioid dose can be increased by the total dose of rescue medications used by the patient, or by 50% of the standing opioid daily dose for moderate pain and 100% for severe pain.

It is inappropriate to start with extended-release preparations. Instead, an initial focus on using short-acting preparations to determine how much is required in the first 24–48 h will allow clinicians to determine opioid needs. Once pain relief is obtained using short-acting preparations, the switch should be made to extended-release preparations. Even with a stable extended-release preparation regimen, the patient may experience incident pain, such as during movement or dressing changes. Short-acting preparations should be taken before such predictable episodes. Although less common, patients may have "end-of-dose failure" with long-acting opioids, meaning that they develop pain after 8 h in the case of an every-12-h medication. In these cases, a trial of giving an every-12-h medication every 8 h is appropriate.

Due to differences in opioid receptors, cross-tolerance among opioids is incomplete, and patients may experience different side effects with different opioids. Therefore, if a patient is not experiencing pain relief or is experiencing too many side effects, a change to another opioid preparation is appropriate. When switching, one should begin with 50–75% of the published equianalgesic dose of the new opioid.

Unlike NSAIDs, opioids have no ceiling effect; therefore, there is no maximum dose, no matter how many milligrams the patient is receiving. The appropriate dose is the dose needed to achieve pain relief. This is an important point for clinicians to explain to patients and families. Addiction or excessive respiratory depression is extremely unlikely in the terminally ill; fear of these side effects should neither prevent escalating opioid medications when the patient is experiencing insufficient pain relief nor justify using opioid antagonists.

Opioid side effects should be anticipated and treated preemptively. Nearly all patients experience constipation that can be debilitating (see below). Failure to prevent constipation often results in noncompliance with opioid therapy. The preferred treatment is prevention. Cathartics (senna 2 tbsp qHS), stool softeners (docusate 100 mg PO qd), and/or laxatives (laxtulose 30 mL qd) are considered first-line treatment. For refractory cases, opioid antagonists or other therapies, such as lubiprostone, should be considered.

Methylnaltrexone is the best-studied opioid antagonist for use in refractory opioid-induced constipation. It reverses opioid-induced constipation by blocking peripheral opioid receptors, but not central receptors, for analgesia. In placebo-controlled trials, it has been shown to cause laxation within 24 h of administration. As with the use of opioids, about a third of patients using methylnaltrexone experience nausea and vomiting, but unlike with opioid usage, tolerance usually develops within a week. Therefore, when one is beginning opioids, an antiemetic such as metoclopramide or a serotonin antagonist is often prescribed prophylactically and stopped after 1 week. Olanzapine has also been shown to have antinausea properties and can be effective in countering delirium or anxiety, with the advantage of some weight gain.

Drowsiness, a common side effect of opioids, also usually abates within a week. For refractory or severe cases, pharmacologic therapy should be considered. The best-studied agents are the psychostimulants dextroamphetamine, methylphenidate, and modafinil, although evidence regarding their efficacy is weak. Modafinil has the advantage of once-a-day dosing compared to methyphenidate's twice daily dosing.

Seriously ill patients who require chronic pain relief rarely become addicted. Suspicion of addiction should not be a reason to withhold pain medications from terminally ill patients. Nonetheless, patients and families may withhold prescribed opioids for fear of addiction or dependence. Physicians and health care providers should reassure patients and families that the patient will not become addicted to opioids if they are used as prescribed for pain relief; this fear should not prevent the patient from taking the medications around the clock. However, diversion of drugs for use by other family members or illicit sale may occur. It may be necessary to advise the patient and caregiver about secure storage of opioids. Contract writing with the patient and family can help. If that fails, transfer to a safe facility may be necessary.

Tolerance describes the need to increase medication dosage for the same pain relief without a concurrent change in disease. In the case of patients with advanced disease, the need for increasing opioid dosage for pain relief usually is caused by disease progression rather than tolerance. Physical dependence is indicated by symptoms resulting from the abrupt withdrawal of opioids and should not be confused with addiction.

In recent years, the potential dangers of opioid drugs have become increasingly apparent. To help mitigate the risk of these powerful drugs, several strategies should be used to reduce the risk of aberrant drug use. To start, all patients should be assessed for their individual levels of risk. While there are multiple surveys available, including the Opioid Risk Tool, none have gained widespread use or validation. In general, however, it is important to screen for prior substance abuse and major psychiatric disorders.

For patients deemed to be high risk, a multidisciplinary effort should be pursued to reduce the risk of adverse consequences, such as addiction and diversion. Prescribing strategies include selecting opioids with longer durations of action and lower street values, such as methadone, and prescribing smaller quantities with more frequent follow-up. Monitoring options include periodic urine screening and referral to pain specialists. In some cases, it may also be reasonable to consider not offering short-acting opioids for breakthrough pain. In no situation, however, should adequate pain relief be withheld due to risk.

Adjuvant analgesic medications are nonopioids that potentiate the analgesic effects of opioids. They are especially important in the management of neuropathic pain. Gabapentin, an anticonvulsant initially studied in the setting of herpetic neuralgia, is now the first-line treatment for neuropathic pain resulting from a variety of causes. It is begun at 100–300 mg bid or tid, with 50–100% dose increments every 3 days. Usually 900–3600 mg/d in two or three doses is effective. The combination of gabapentin and nortriptyline may be more effective than gabapentin alone. Two potential side effects of gabapentin to be aware of are confusion and drowsiness, especially in the elderly. Other effective adjuvant medications include pregabalin, which has the same mechanism of action as gabapentin but is absorbed more efficiently from the GI tract. Lamotrigine is a novel agent whose mechanism of action is unknown but has been shown to be effective. It is recommended to begin at 25–50 mg/d, increasing to 100 mg/d. Carbamazepine, a first-generation agent, has been proven effective in randomized trials for neuropathic pain. Other potentially effective anticonvulsant adjuvants include topiramate (25–50 mg qd or bid, rising to 100–300 mg/d) and oxcarbazepine (75–300 mg bid, rising to 1200 mg bid).

Glucocorticoids, preferably dexamethasone given once a day, can be useful in reducing inflammation that causes pain, while also elevating mood, energy, and appetite. Its main side effects include confusion, sleep difficulties, and fluid retention. Glucocorticoids are especially effective for bone pain and abdominal pain from distention of the GI tract or liver. Other drugs, including clonidine and baclofen, can be effective in providing pain relief. These drugs are adjuvants and generally should be used in conjunction with—not instead of—opioids. Methadone, carefully dosed because of its unpredictable half-life in many patients, has activity at the *N*-methyl-D-aspartamate (NMDA) receptor and is useful for complex pain syndromes and neuropathic pain. It is generally reserved for cases in which first-line opioids (morphine, oxycodone, hydromorphone) are either ineffective or unavailable.

Radiation therapy can treat bone pain from single metastatic lesions. Bone pain from multiple metastases can be amenable to radiopharmaceuticals such as strontium-89 and samarium-153. Bisphosphonates, such as pamidronate (90 mg every 4 weeks) and calcitonin (200 IU intranasally once or twice a day), also provide relief from bone pain but have multiday onsets of action.

Constipation • **FREQUENCY** Constipation is reported in up to 70–100% of patients requiring palliative care.

ETIOLOGY Although hypercalcemia and other factors can cause constipation, it is most frequently a predictable consequence of the use of opioids for pain and dyspnea relief and of the anticholinergic effects of tricyclic antidepressants, as well as due to the inactivity and poor diets common among seriously ill patients. If left untreated, constipation can cause substantial pain and vomiting and also is associated with confusion and delirium. Whenever opioids and other medications known to cause constipation are used, preemptive treatment for constipation should be instituted.

ASSESSMENT Assessing constipation can be difficult because people describe it differently. Four commonly used assessment scales are the Bristol Stool Form Scale, the Constipation Assessment Scale, the Constipation Visual Analogue Scale, and the Eton Scale Risk Assessment for Constipation. The Bowel Function Index can be used to quantify opioid-induced constipation. The physician should establish the patient's previous bowel habits, as well as any changes in subjective and objective qualities such as bloating or decreased frequency. Abdominal and rectal examinations should be performed to exclude impaction or an acute abdomen. Radiographic assessments beyond a simple flat plate of the abdomen in cases in which obstruction is suspected are rarely necessary.

INTERVENTION Any measure to address constipation during end-of-life care should include interventions to reestablish comfortable bowel habits and to relieve pain or discomfort. Although physical activity, adequate hydration, and dietary treatments with fiber can be helpful, each is limited in its effectiveness for most seriously ill patients, and fiber may exacerbate problems in the setting of dehydration or if impaired motility is the etiology. Fiber is contraindicated in the presence of opioid use. Stimulant and osmotic laxatives, stool softeners, fluids, and enemas are the mainstays of therapy (**Table 12-5**). To prevent constipation from opioids and other medications, a combination of a laxative and a stool softener (such as senna and docusate) should be used. If after several days of treatment a bowel movement has not occurred, a rectal examination to remove impacted stool and place a suppository is necessary. For patients with impending bowel obstruction or gastric stasis, octreotide to reduce secretions can be helpful. For patients in whom the suspected mechanism is dysmotility, metoclopramide can be helpful.

TABLE 12-5 Medications for the Management of Constipation

INTERVENTION	DOSE	COMMENT
Stimulant laxatives		These agents directly stimulate peristalsis and may reduce colonic absorption of water.
Prune juice	120–240 mL/d	Work in 6–12 h.
Senna (Senokot)	2–8 tablets PO bid	
Bisacodyl	5–15 mg/d PO, PR	
Osmotic laxatives		These agents are not absorbed. They attract and retain water in the gastrointestinal tract.
Lactulose	15–30 mL PO q4–8h	Lactulose may cause flatulence and bloating.
Magnesium hydroxide (Milk of Magnesia)	15–30 mL/d PO	Lactulose works in 1 day, magnesium products in 6 h.
Magnesium citrate	125–250 mL/d PO	
Stool softeners		These agents work by increasing water secretion and as detergents, increasing water penetration into the stool.
Sodium docusate (Colace)	300–600 mg/d PO	Work in 1–3 days.
Calcium docusate	300–600 mg/d PO	
Suppositories and enemas		
Bisacodyl	10–15 PR qd	
Sodium phosphate enema	PR qd	Fixed dose, 4.5 oz, Fleet's.

Nausea • **FREQUENCY** Up to 70% of patients with advanced cancer have nausea, defined as the subjective sensation of wanting to vomit.

ETIOLOGY Nausea and vomiting are both caused by stimulation at one of four sites: the GI tract, the vestibular system, the chemoreceptor trigger zone (CTZ), and the cerebral cortex. Medical treatments for nausea are aimed at receptors at each of these sites: the GI tract contains mechanoreceptors, chemoreceptors, and 5-hydroxytryptamine type 3 (5-HT_3) receptors; the vestibular system probably contains histamine and acetylcholine receptors; and the CTZ contains chemoreceptors, dopamine type 2 receptors, and 5-HT3 receptors. An example of nausea that most likely is mediated by the cortex is anticipatory nausea before a dose of chemotherapy or other noxious stimuli.

Specific causes of nausea include metabolic changes (liver failure, uremia from renal failure, hypercalcemia), bowel obstruction, constipation, infection, GERD, vestibular disease, brain metastases, medications (including antibiotics, NSAIDs, proton pump inhibitors, opioids, and chemotherapy), and radiation therapy. Anxiety can also contribute to nausea.

INTERVENTION Medical treatment of nausea is directed at the anatomic and receptor-mediated cause revealed by a careful history and physical examination. When no specific cause of nausea is identified, many advocate beginning treatment with metoclopramide; a serotonin type 3 (5-HT_3) receptor antagonist such as ondansetron, granisetron, palonosetron, dolasetron, tropisetron, or ramosetron; or a dopamine antagonist such as chlorpromazine, haloperidol, or prochlorperazine. When decreased motility is suspected, metoclopramide can be an effective treatment. When inflammation of the GI tract is suspected, glucocorticoids, such as dexamethasone, are an appropriate treatment. For nausea that follows chemotherapy and radiation therapy, one of the 5-HT_3 receptor antagonists or neurokinin-1 antagonists, such as aprepitant or fosaprepitant, is recommended. Clinicians should attempt prevention of postchemotherapy nausea, rather than simply providing treatment after the fact. Current clinical guidelines recommend tailoring the strength of treatments to the specific emetic risk posed by a specific chemotherapy drug. When a vestibular cause (such as "motion sickness" or labyrinthitis) is suspected, antihistamines, such as meclizine (whose primary side effect is drowsiness), or anticholinergics, such as scopolamine, can be effective. In anticipatory nausea, patients can benefit from nonpharmacologic interventions, such as biofeedback and hypnosis. The most common pharmacologic intervention for anticipatory nausea is a benzodiazepine, such as lorazepam. As with antihistamines, drowsiness and confusion are the main side effects.

The use of medical marijuana or oral cannabinoids for palliative treatment of nausea is controversial, as there are no controlled trials showing its effectiveness for patients at the end of life. A 2015 meta-analysis showed "low-quality evidence suggesting that cannabinoids were associated with improvements in nausea and vomiting due to chemotherapy," and such treatments are not as good as 5-HT_3 receptor antagonists and can sometimes even cause cannabis hyperemesis syndrome. Older patients, who compose the vast majority of dying patients, seem to tolerate cannabinoids poorly.

Dyspnea • **FREQUENCY** Dyspnea is the subjective experience of being short of breath. Over 50%, and as many as 75%, of dying patients, especially those with lung cancer, metastases to the lung, CHF, and COPD, experience dyspnea at some point near the end of life. Dyspnea is among the most distressing of physical symptoms and can be even more distressing than pain.

ASSESSMENT As with pain, dyspnea is a subjective experience that may not correlate with objective measures of PO_2, PCO_2, or respiratory rate. Consequently, measurements of oxygen saturation through pulse oximetry or blood gases are rarely helpful in guiding therapy. Despite the limitations of existing assessment methods, physicians should regularly assess and document patients' experience of dyspnea and its intensity. Guidelines recommend visual analogue dyspnea scales to assess the severity of symptoms and the effects of treatment. Potentially reversible or treatable causes of dyspnea include infection, pleural effusions, pulmonary emboli, pulmonary edema, asthma, and tumor encroachment on the airway. However, the risk-versus-benefit ratio of the diagnostic and therapeutic interventions for patients with little time left to live must be considered carefully before undertaking diagnostic steps. Frequently, the specific etiology cannot be identified, and dyspnea is the consequence of progression of the underlying disease that cannot be treated. The anxiety caused by dyspnea and the choking sensation can significantly exacerbate the underlying dyspnea in a negatively reinforcing cycle.

INTERVENTIONS When reversible or treatable etiologies are diagnosed, they should be treated as long as the side effects of treatment, such as repeated drainage of effusions or anticoagulants, are less burdensome than the dyspnea itself. More aggressive treatments such as stenting a bronchial lesion may be warranted if it is clear that the dyspnea is due to tumor invasion at that site and if the patient and family understand the risks of such a procedure.

Usually, treatment will be symptomatic (**Table 12-6**). Supplemental oxygen does not appear to be effective. "A systematic review of the literature failed to demonstrate a consistent beneficial effect of oxygen inhalation over air inhalation for study participants with dyspnea due to end-stage cancer or cardiac failure." Therefore, oxygen may be no more than an expensive placebo. Low-dose opioids reduce the sensitivity of the central respiratory center and relieve the sensation of dyspnea. If patients are not receiving opioids, weak opioids can be initiated; if patients are already receiving opioids, morphine or other stronger opioids should be used. Controlled trials do not support the use of nebulized opioids for dyspnea at the end of life. Phenothiazines and chlorpromazine may be helpful when combined with opioids. Benzodiazepines can be helpful in treating dyspnea, but only if anxiety is present. Benzodiazepines should not be used as first-line therapy or if there is no anxiety. If the patient has a history of COPD or asthma, inhaled bronchodilators and glucocorticoids may be helpful. If the patient has pulmonary edema due to heart failure, diuresis with a medication such as furosemide is indicated. Excess secretions can be transdermally or intravenously dried with scopolamine. More general interventions that medical staff can perform include sitting the patient upright, removing smoke or other irritants like perfume, ensuring a supply of fresh air with sufficient humidity, and minimizing other factors that can increase anxiety.

TABLE 12-6 Medications for the Management of Dyspnea

INTERVENTION	DOSE	COMMENTS
Weak opioids		For patients with mild dyspnea
Codeine (or codeine with 325 mg acetaminophen)	30 mg PO q4h	For opioid-naïve patients
Hydrocodone	5 mg PO q4h	
Strong opioids		For opioid-naïve patients with moderate to severe dyspnea
Morphine	5–10 mg PO q4h	For patients already taking opioids for pain or other symptoms
	30–50% of baseline opioid dose q4h	
Oxycodone	5–10 mg PO q4h	
Hydromorphone	1–2 mg PO q4h	
Anxiolytics		Give a dose every hour until the patient is relaxed; then provide a dose for maintenance
Lorazepam	0.5–2.0 mg PO/SL/IV qh then q4–6h	
Clonazepam	0.25–2.0 mg PO q12h	
Midazolam	0.5 mg IV q15min	

Fatigue • **FREQUENCY** Fatigue is one of the most commonly reported symptoms not only of cancer treatment but also of the palliative care of multiple sclerosis, COPD, heart failure, and HIV. More than 90% of terminally ill patients experience fatigue and/or weakness. Fatigue is frequently cited as one of the most distressing symptoms in these patients.

ETIOLOGY The multiple causes of fatigue in the terminally ill can be categorized as resulting from the underlying disease; from disease-induced factors such as tumor necrosis factor and other cytokines; and from secondary factors such as dehydration, anemia, infection, hypothyroidism, and drug side effects. In addition to low caloric intake, loss of muscle mass and changes in muscle enzymes may play an important role in fatigue during terminal illness. The importance of changes in the CNS, especially the reticular activating system, have been hypothesized based on reports of fatigue in patients receiving cranial radiation, experiencing depression, or having chronic pain in the absence of cachexia or other physiologic changes. Finally, depression and other causes of psychological distress can contribute to fatigue.

ASSESSMENT Like pain and dyspnea, fatigue is subjective, as it represents a patient's sense of tiredness and decreased capacity for physical work. Objective changes, even in body mass, may be absent. Consequently, assessment must rely on patient self-reporting. Scales used to measure fatigue, such as the Edmonton Functional Assessment Tool, the Fatigue Self-Report Scales, and the Rhoten Fatigue Scale, are usually appropriate for research but not clinical purposes. In clinical practice, a simple performance assessment such as the Karnofsky performance status or the Eastern Cooperative Oncology Group (ECOG)'s question "How much of the day does the patient spend in bed?" may be the best measure. In the ECOG 0–4 performance status assessment, 0 = normal activity; 1 = symptomatic without being bedridden; 2 = requiring some, but <50%, bed time; 3 = bedbound more than half the day; and 4 = bedbound all the time. Such a scale allows for assessment over time and correlates with overall disease severity and prognosis. A 2008 review by the European Association of Palliative Care also described several longer assessment tools that contained 9–20 items, including the Piper Fatigue Inventory, the Multidimensional Fatigue Inventory, and the Brief Fatigue Inventory (BFI).

INTERVENTIONS Reversible causes of fatigue, such as anemia and infection, should be treated. However, at the end of life, it must be realistically acknowledged that fatigue will not be "cured." The goal is to ameliorate fatigue and help patients and families adjust expectations. Behavioral interventions should be utilized to avoid blaming the patient for inactivity and to educate both the family and the patient that the underlying disease causes physiologic changes that produce low energy levels. Understanding that the problem is physiologic and not psychological can help alter expectations regarding the patient's level of physical activity. Practically, this may mean reducing routine activities such as housework, cooking, and social events outside the house and making it acceptable to receive guests while lying on a couch. At the same time, the implementation of exercise regimens and physical therapy can raise endorphins, reduce muscle wasting, and decrease the risk of depression. In addition, ensuring good hydration without worsening edema may help reduce fatigue. Discontinuing medications that worsen fatigue may help, including cardiac medications, benzodiazepines, certain antidepressants, or opioids if the patient's pain is well-controlled. As end-of-life care proceeds into its final stages, fatigue may protect patients from further suffering, and continued treatment could be detrimental.

Only a few pharmacologic interventions target fatigue and weakness. Randomized controlled trials suggest glucocorticoids can increase energy and enhance mood. Dexamethasone (8 mg/d) is preferred for its once-a-day dosing and minimal mineralocorticoid activity. Benefit, if any, is usually seen within the first month. For fatigue related to anorexia, megestrol (480–800 mg) can be helpful. Psychostimulants such as dextroamphetamine (5–10 mg PO) and methylphenidate (2.5–5 mg PO) may enhance energy levels, although controlled trials have not shown these drugs to be effective for fatigue induced by mild to moderate cancer. Doses should be given in the morning and at noon to minimize the risk of counterproductive insomnia. Modafinil and armodafinil, developed for narcolepsy, have shown promise in the treatment of fatigue and have the advantage of once-daily dosing. Their precise role in fatigue at the end of life has not been documented but may be worth trying if other interventions are not beneficial. Anecdotal evidence suggests that L-carnitine may improve fatigue, depression, and sleep disruption.

■ PALLIATIVE SEDATION

Palliative sedation is used in distressing situations that cannot be addressed in other ways. When patients experience severe symptoms, such as pain or dyspnea, that cannot be relieved by conventional interventions or experience acute catastrophic symptoms, such as uncontrolled seizures, then palliative sedation should be considered as an intervention of last resort. It can be abused if done to hasten death (which it usually does not), when done at the request of the family rather than according to the patient's wishes, or when there are other interventions that could still be tried. The use of palliative sedation in cases of extreme existential or spiritual distress remains controversial. Typically, palliative sedation should be introduced only after the patient and family have been assured that all other interventions have been tried and after the patient and their loved ones have been able to "say goodbye."

Palliative sedation can be achieved by significantly increasing opioid doses until patients become unconscious and then putting them on a continuous infusion. Another commonly used medication for palliative sedation is midazolam at 1–5 mg IV every 5–15 min to calm the patient, followed by a continuous IV or subcutaneous infusion of 1 mg/h. In hospital settings, a continuous propofol infusion of 5 μg/kg per min can be used. There are also other, less commonly used medications for palliative sedation that include levomepromazine, chlorpromazine, and phenobarbital.

PSYCHOLOGICAL SYMPTOMS AND THEIR MANAGEMENT

Depression • **FREQUENCY AND IMPACT** Depression at the end of life presents an apparently paradoxical situation. Many people believe that depression is normal among seriously ill patients because they are dying. People frequently say, "Wouldn't you be depressed?" Although sadness, anxiety, anger, and irritability are normal responses to a serious condition, they are typically of modest intensity and transient. Persistent sadness and anxiety and the physically disabling symptoms that they can lead to are abnormal and suggestive of major depression. The precise number of terminally ill patients who are depressed is uncertain, primarily due to a lack of consistent diagnostic criteria and screening. Careful follow-up of patients suggests that while as many as 75% of terminally ill patients experience depressive symptoms, ~25% of terminally ill patients have major depression. Depression at the end of life is concerning because it can decrease the quality of life, interfere with closure in relationships and other separation work, obstruct adherence to medical interventions, and amplify the suffering associated with pain and other symptoms.

ETIOLOGY Previous history of depression, family history of depression or bipolar disorder, and prior suicide attempts are associated with increased risk for depression among terminally ill patients. Other symptoms, such as pain and fatigue, are associated with higher rates of depression; uncontrolled pain can exacerbate depression, and depression can cause patients to be more distressed by pain. Many medications used in the terminal stages, including glucocorticoids, and some anticancer agents, such as tamoxifen, interleukin 2, interferon α, and vincristine, also are associated with depression. Some terminal conditions, such as pancreatic cancer, certain strokes, and heart failure, have been reported to be associated with higher rates of depression, although this is controversial. Finally, depression may be attributable to grief over the loss of a role or function, social isolation, or loneliness.

ASSESSMENT Unfortunately, many studies suggest that most depressed patients at the end of life are not diagnosed, or if they are diagnosed, they are not properly treated. Diagnosing depression among seriously ill patients is complicated, as many of the vegetative symptoms in the *DSM-V* (*Diagnostic and Statistical Manual of Mental Disorders, Fifth Edition*) criteria for clinical depression—insomnia, anorexia and weight loss, fatigue, decreased libido, and difficulty concentrating—are associated with the process of dying itself. The assessment of depression in seriously ill patients therefore should focus on the dysphoric mood, helplessness, hopelessness, and lack of interest, enjoyment, and concentration in normal activities. It is now recommended that patients near the end of life should be screened with either the PHQ-9 or the PHQ-2, which asks "Over the past 2 weeks, how often have you been bothered by any of the following problems? (1) Little interest or pleasure in doing things and (2) feeling down, depressed or hopeless." The answer categories are as follows: not at all, several days, more than half the days, nearly every day. Other possible diagnostic tools include the short form of the Beck Depression Index or a visual analogue scale.

Certain conditions may be confused with depression. Endocrinopathies, such as hypothyroidism and Cushing's syndrome, electrolyte abnormalities, such as hypercalcemia, and akathisia, especially from dopamine-blocking antiemetics such as metoclopramide and prochlorperazine, can mimic depression and should be excluded.

INTERVENTIONS Undertreatment of depressed, terminally ill patients is common. Physicians must treat any physical symptom, such as pain, that may be causing or exacerbating depression. Fostering adaptation to the many losses that the patient is experiencing can also be helpful. Unfortunately, there are few randomized trials to guide such interventions. Thus, treatment typically follows the treatment used for non–terminally ill depressed patients.

In the absence of randomized controlled trials, nonpharmacologic interventions, including group or individual psychological counseling, and behavioral therapies such as relaxation and imagery can be helpful, especially in combination with drug therapy.

Pharmacologic interventions remain at the core of therapy. The same medications are used to treat depression in terminally ill as in non–terminally ill patients. Psychostimulants may be preferred for patients with a poor prognosis or for those with fatigue or opioid-induced somnolence. Psychostimulants are comparatively fast-acting, working within a few days instead of the weeks required for selective serotonin reuptake inhibitors (SSRIs). Dextroamphetamine or methylphenidate should be started at 2.5–5.0 mg in the morning and at noon, the same starting doses used for treating fatigue. The doses can eventually be escalated up to 15 mg bid. Modafinil is started at 100 mg qd and can be increased to 200 mg if there is no effect at the lower dose. Pemoline is a nonamphetamine psychostimulant with minimal abuse potential. It is also effective as an antidepressant beginning at 18.75 mg in the morning and at noon. Because it can be absorbed through the buccal mucosa, it is preferred for patients with intestinal obstruction or dysphagia. If it is used for prolonged periods, liver function must be monitored. The psychostimulants can also be combined with more traditional antidepressants while waiting for the antidepressants to become effective, then tapered down after a few weeks if necessary. Psychostimulants have side effects, particularly initial anxiety, insomnia, and very rarely paranoia, which may necessitate lowering the dose or discontinuing treatment.

Mirtazapine, an antagonist at the postsynaptic serotonin receptors, is a promising psychostimulant. It should be started at 7.5 mg before bed and titrated up no more than once every 1–2 weeks to a maximal dose of 45 mg/d. It has sedating, antiemetic, and anxiolytic properties, with few drug interactions. Its side effect of weight gain may be beneficial for seriously ill patients; it is available in orally disintegrating tablets.

For patients with a prognosis of several months or longer, SSRIs, including fluoxetine, sertraline, paroxetine, escitalopram, and citalopram, and serotonin-noradrenaline reuptake inhibitors, such as venlafaxine and duloxetine, are the preferred treatments, due to their efficacy and comparatively few side effects. Because low doses of these medications may be effective for seriously ill patients, one should use half the usual starting dose as for healthy adults. The starting dose for fluoxetine is 10 mg once a day. In most cases, once-a-day dosing is possible. The choice of which SSRI to use should be driven by (1) the patient's past success or failure with the specific medication and (2) the most favorable side effect profile for that specific agent. For instance, for a patient in whom fatigue is a major symptom, a more activating SSRI (fluoxetine) would be appropriate. For a patient in whom anxiety and sleeplessness are major symptoms, a more sedating SSRI (paroxetine) would be appropriate. Importantly, it can take up to 4 weeks for these drugs to have an effect.

Atypical antidepressants are recommended only in select circumstances, usually with the assistance of a specialty consultation. Trazodone can be an effective antidepressant but is sedating and can cause orthostatic hypotension and, occasionally, priapism. Therefore, it should be used before bed and only when a sedating effect is desired and is often used for patients with insomnia at a dose starting at 25 mg. Bupropion can also be used. In addition to its antidepressant effects, bupropion is energizing, making it useful for depressed patients who experience fatigue. However, it can cause seizures, preventing its use for patients with a risk of CNS neoplasms or terminal delirium. Finally, alprazolam, a benzodiazepine, starting at 0.25–1.0 mg tid, can be effective in seriously ill patients who have a combination of anxiety and depression. Although it is potent and works quickly, it has many drug interactions and may cause delirium, especially among very ill patients, because of its strong binding to the benzodiazepine–γ-aminobutyric acid (GABA) receptor complex.

Unless used as adjuvants for the treatment of pain, tricyclic antidepressants are not recommended. While they can be effective, their therapeutic window and serious side effects typically limit their utility. Similarly, monoamine oxidase (MAO) inhibitors are not recommended because of their side effects and dangerous drug interactions.

Delirium (See Chap. 27) • **FREQUENCY** In the weeks or months before death, delirium is uncommon, although it may be significantly underdiagnosed. However, delirium becomes relatively common in the days and hours immediately before death. Up to 85% of patients dying from cancer may experience terminal delirium.

ETIOLOGY Delirium is a global cerebral dysfunction characterized by alterations in cognition and consciousness. It is frequently preceded by anxiety, changes in sleep patterns (especially reversal of day and night), and decreased attention. In contrast to dementia, delirium has an acute onset, is characterized by fluctuating consciousness and inattention, and is reversible, although reversibility may be more theoretical than real for patients near death. Delirium may occur in a patient with dementia; indeed, patients with dementia are more vulnerable to delirium.

Causes of delirium include metabolic encephalopathy arising from liver or renal failure, hypoxemia, or infection; electrolyte imbalances such as hypercalcemia; paraneoplastic syndromes; dehydration; and primary brain tumors, brain metastases, or leptomeningeal spread of tumor. Among dying patients, delirium is commonly caused by side effects of treatments, including radiation for brain metastases and medications, such as opioids, glucocorticoids, anticholinergic drugs, antihistamines, antiemetics, benzodiazepines, and chemotherapeutic agents. The etiology may be multifactorial; e.g., dehydration may exacerbate opioid-induced delirium.

ASSESSMENT Delirium should be recognized in any terminally ill patient exhibiting new onset of disorientation, impaired cognition, somnolence, fluctuating levels of consciousness, or delusions with or without agitation. Delirium must be distinguished from acute anxiety, depression, and dementia. The central distinguishing feature is altered consciousness, which usually is not noted in anxiety, depression, or dementia. Although "hyperactive" delirium, characterized by overt confusion and agitation, is probably more common, patients should also be assessed for "hypoactive" delirium, which is characterized by sleep-wake reversal and decreased alertness.

In some cases, use of formal assessment tools such as the Mini-Mental Status Examination (which does not distinguish delirium from dementia) and the Delirium Rating Scale (which does distinguish delirium from dementia) may be helpful in distinguishing delirium from other processes. The patient's list of medications must be evaluated carefully. Nonetheless, a reversible etiologic factor for delirium is found in fewer than half of all terminally ill patients. Given that most terminally ill patients experiencing delirium are very close to death and often at home, extensive diagnostic evaluations such as lumbar punctures and neuroradiologic examinations are inappropriate.

INTERVENTIONS One of the most important objectives of terminal care is to provide terminally ill patients the lucidity to say goodbye to the people they love. Delirium, especially when in combination with agitation during the final days, is distressing to family and caregivers. A strong determinant of bereavement difficulties is witnessing a difficult death. Thus, terminal delirium should be treated aggressively.

At the first sign of delirium, such as day-night reversal with slight changes in mentation, the physician should let the family members know that it is time to be sure that everything they want to say has been said. The family should be informed that delirium is common just before death.

If medications are suspected of being a cause of the delirium, unnecessary agents should be discontinued. Other potentially reversible causes, such as constipation, urinary retention, and metabolic abnormalities, should be treated. Supportive measures aimed at providing a familiar environment should be instituted, including restricting visits only to individuals with whom the patient is familiar and eliminating new experiences; orienting the patient, if possible, by providing a clock and calendar; and gently correcting the patient's hallucinations or cognitive mistakes.

Pharmacologic management focuses on the use of neuroleptics and, in extreme cases, anesthetics (**Table 12-7**). Haloperidol remains the first-line therapy. Usually, patients can be controlled with a low dose (1–3 mg/d), given every 6 h, although some may require as much as 20 mg/d. Haloperidol can be administered PO, SC, or IV. IM injections should not be used, except when this is the only way to address a patient's delirium. Olanzapine, an atypical neuroleptic, has shown significant effectiveness in completely resolving delirium in cancer patients. It also has other beneficial effects for terminally ill patients, including antinausea, antianxiety, and weight gain. Olanzapine is useful for patients with longer anticipated life expectancies because it is less likely to cause dysphoria and has a lower risk of dystonic reactions. Additionally, because olanzapine is metabolized through multiple pathways, it can be used in patients with hepatic and renal dysfunction. Olanzapine has the disadvantage that it is only available orally and takes a week to reach steady state. The usual dose is 2.5–5 mg PO bid. Chlorpromazine (10–25 mg every 4–6 h) can be useful if sedation is desired and can be administered IV or PR in addition to PO. Dystonic reactions resulting from dopamine blockade are a side effect of neuroleptics, although they are reported to be rare when these drugs are used to treat terminal delirium. If patients develop dystonic reactions, benztropine should be administered. Neuroleptics may be

TABLE 12-7 Medications for the Management of Delirium

INTERVENTIONS	DOSE
Neuroleptics	
Haloperidol	0.5–5 mg q2–12h, PO/IV/SC/IM
Thioridazine	10–75 mg q4–8h, PO
Chlorpromazine	12.5–50 mg q4–12h, PO/IV/IM
Atypical neuroleptics	
Olanzapine	2.5–5 mg qd or bid, PO
Risperidone	1–3 mg q12h, PO
Anxiolytics	
Lorazepam	0.5–2 mg q1–4h, PO/IV/IM
Midazolam	1–5 mg/h continuous infusion, IV/SC
Anesthetics	
Propofol	0.3–2.0 mg/h continuous infusion, IV

combined with lorazepam to reduce agitation when the delirium is the result of alcohol or sedative withdrawal.

If no response to first-line therapy is observed, a specialty consultation should be obtained with a goal to change to a different medication. If the patient fails to improve after a second neuroleptic, sedation with either an anesthetic such as propofol or continuous-infusion midazolam may be necessary. By some estimates, as many as 25% of patients at the very end of life who experience delirium, especially restless delirium with myoclonus or convulsions, may require sedation.

Physical restraints should be used with great reluctance and only when patients' violence is threatening to themselves or others. If restraints are used, their appropriateness should be frequently reevaluated.

Insomnia • FREQUENCY Sleep disorders, defined as difficulty initiating sleep or maintaining sleep, sleep difficulty at least 3 nights a week, or sleep difficulty that causes impairment of daytime functioning, occurs in 19–63% of patients with advanced cancer. Some 30–74% of patients with other end-stage conditions, including AIDS, heart disease, COPD, and renal disease, experience insomnia.

ETIOLOGY Patients with cancer may experience changes in sleep efficiency, such as an increase in stage I sleep. Insomnia may also coexist with both physical illnesses, like thyroid disease, and psychological illnesses, like depression and anxiety. Medications, including antidepressants, psychostimulants, glucocorticoids, and β agonists, are significant contributors to sleep disorders, as are caffeine and alcohol. Multiple over-the-counter medications contain caffeine and antihistamines, which can contribute to sleep disorders.

ASSESSMENT Assessments should include specific questions concerning sleep onset, sleep maintenance, and early-morning wakening, as these will provide clues to both the causative agents and management of insomnia. Patients should be asked about previous sleep problems, screened for depression and anxiety, and asked about symptoms of thyroid disease. Caffeine and alcohol are prominent causes of sleep problems, and a careful history of the use of these substances should be obtained. Both excessive use and withdrawal from alcohol can be causes of sleep problems.

INTERVENTIONS The mainstays of any intervention include improvement of sleep hygiene (encouragement of regular time for sleep, decreased nighttime distractions, elimination of caffeine and other stimulants and alcohol), interventions to treat anxiety and depression, and treatment for the insomnia itself. For patients with depression who have insomnia and anxiety, a sedating antidepressant such as mirtazapine can be helpful. In the elderly, trazodone, beginning at 25 mg at nighttime, is an effective sleep aid at doses lower than those that cause its antidepressant effect. Zolpidem may have a decreased incidence of delirium in patients compared with traditional benzodiazepines, but this has not been clearly established. When benzodiazepines are prescribed, short-acting ones (such as lorazepam) are favored over longer-acting ones (such as diazepam). Patients who receive these medications should be observed for signs of increased confusion and delirium.

SOCIAL NEEDS AND THEIR MANAGEMENT

Financial Burdens • FREQUENCY Dying can impose substantial economic strains on patients and families, potentially causing distress. This is known as financial toxicity. In the United States, which has the least comprehensive health insurance systems among wealthy countries, a quarter of families coping with end-stage cancer report that care was a major financial burden and a third used up most of their savings. Among Medicare beneficiaries, average out-of-pocket costs were >$8000. Between 10% and 30% of families are forced to sell assets, use savings, or take out a mortgage to pay for the patient's health care costs.

The patient is likely to reduce hours worked and eventually stop working altogether. In 20% of cases, a family member of the terminally ill patient also must stop working to provide care. The major underlying causes of economic burden are related to poor physical functioning and care needs, such as the need for housekeeping, nursing, and personal care. More debilitated patients and poor patients experience greater economic burdens.

INTERVENTION The economic burden of end-of-life care should not be ignored as a private matter. It has been associated with a number of adverse health outcomes, including preferring comfort care over life-prolonging care, as well as consideration of euthanasia or physician-assisted suicide (PAS). Economic burdens increase the psychological distress of the families and caregivers of terminally ill patients, and poverty is associated with many adverse health outcomes. Importantly, studies have found that "patients with advanced cancer who reported having end-of-life conversations with physicians had significantly lower health care costs in their final week of life. Higher costs were associated with worse quality of death." Assistance from a social worker, early on if possible, to ensure access to all available benefits may be helpful. Many patients, families, and health care providers are unaware of options for long-term care insurance, respite care, the Family Medical Leave Act (FMLA), and other sources of assistance. Some of these options (such as respite care) may be part of a formal hospice program, but others (such as the FMLA) do not require enrollment in a hospice program.

Relationships • FREQUENCY Settling personal issues and closing the narrative of lived relationships are universal needs. When asked if sudden death or death after an illness is preferable, respondents often initially select the former, but soon change to the latter as they reflect on the importance of saying goodbye. Bereaved family members who have not had the chance to say goodbye often have a more difficult grief process.

INTERVENTIONS Care of seriously ill patients requires efforts to facilitate the types of encounters and time spent with family and friends that are necessary to meet those needs. Family and close friends may need to be accommodated in hospitals and other facilities with unrestricted visiting hours, which may include sleeping near the patient, even in otherwise regimented institutional settings. Physicians and other health care providers may be able to facilitate and resolve strained interactions between the patient and other family members. Assistance for patients and family members who are unsure about how to create or help preserve memories, whether by providing materials such as a scrapbook or memory box or by offering them suggestions and informational resources, can be deeply appreciated. Taking photographs and creating videos can be especially helpful to terminally ill patients who have younger children or grandchildren.

Family Caregivers • FREQUENCY Caring for seriously ill patients places a heavy burden on families. Families are frequently required to provide transportation and homemaking, as well as other services. Typically, paid professionals, such as home health nurses and hospice workers, supplement family care; only about a quarter of all caregiving consists of exclusively paid professional assistance. Over the past 40 years, there has been a significant decline in the United States of deaths occurring in hospitals, with a simultaneous increase in deaths in other facilities and at home. Over a third of deaths occur in patients' homes. This increase in out-of-hospital deaths increases reliance on families for end-of-life care. Increasingly, family members are being called upon to provide physical care (such as moving and bathing patients) and medical care (such as assessing symptoms and giving medications) in addition to emotional care and support.

Three-quarters of family caregivers of terminally ill patients are women—wives, daughters, sisters, and even daughters-in-law. Since many are widowed, women tend to be able to rely less on family for caregiving assistance and may need more paid assistance. About 20% of terminally ill patients report substantial unmet needs for nursing and personal care. The impact of caregiving on family caregivers is substantial: both bereaved and current caregivers have a higher mortality rate than that of non-caregiving controls.

INTERVENTIONS It is imperative to inquire about unmet needs and to try to ensure that those needs are met either through the family or by paid professional services when possible. Community assistance through houses of worship or other community groups often can be mobilized by telephone calls from the medical team to someone the patient or family identifies. Sources of support specifically for family caregivers should be identified through local sources or nationally through groups such as the National Family Caregivers Association (*www.nfcacares.org*), the American Cancer Society (*www.cancer.org*), and the Alzheimer's Association (*www.alz.org*).

EXISTENTIAL NEEDS AND THEIR MANAGEMENT

Frequency Religion and spirituality are often important to dying patients. Nearly 70% of patients report becoming more religious or spiritual when they became terminally ill, and many find comfort in religious or spiritual practices such as prayer. However, ~20% of terminally ill patients become less religious, frequently feeling cheated or betrayed by becoming terminally ill. For other patients, the need is for existential meaning and purpose that is distinct from, and may even be antithetical to, religion or spirituality. When asked, patients and family caregivers frequently report wanting their professional caregivers to be more attentive to religion and spirituality.

Assessment Health care providers are often hesitant about involving themselves in the religious, spiritual, and existential experiences of their patients because it may seem private or not relevant to the current illness. But physicians and other members of the care team should be able at least to detect spiritual and existential needs. Screening questions have been developed for a physician's spiritual history taking. Spiritual distress can amplify other types of suffering and even masquerade as intractable physical pain, anxiety, or depression. The screening questions in the comprehensive assessment are usually sufficient. Deeper evaluation and intervention are rarely appropriate for the physician unless no other member of a care team is available or suitable. Pastoral care providers may be helpful, whether from the medical institution or from the patient's own community.

Interventions Precisely how religious practices, spirituality, and existential explorations can be facilitated and improve end-of-life care is not well established. What is clear is that for physicians, one main intervention is to inquire about the role and importance of spirituality and religion in a patient's life. This will help a patient feel heard and help physicians identify specific needs. In one study, only 36% of respondents indicated that a clergy member would be comforting. Nevertheless, the increase in religious and spiritual interest among a substantial fraction of dying patients suggests inquiring of individual patients how this need can be addressed. Some evidence supports specific methods of addressing existential needs in patients, ranging from establishing a supportive group environment for terminal patients to individual treatments emphasizing a patient's dignity and sources of meaning.

MANAGING THE LAST STAGES

PALLIATIVE CARE SERVICES: HOW AND WHERE

Determining the best approach to providing palliative care to patients will depend on patient preferences, the availability of caregivers and specialized services in close proximity, institutional resources, and reimbursement. Hospice is a leading, but not the only, model of palliative care services. In the United States, slightly more than a third—35.7%—of hospice care is provided in private residential homes with 14.5% of hospice care in nursing homes. In the United States, Medicare pays for hospice services under Part A, the hospital insurance part of reimbursement. Two physicians must certify that the patient has a prognosis of ≤6 months if the disease runs its usual course. Prognoses are probabilistic by their nature; patients are not required to die within 6 months but rather to have a condition from which half the individuals with it would not be alive within 6 months. Patients sign a hospice enrollment form that states their intent to forgo curative services related to their terminal illness but can still receive medical services for other comorbid conditions. Patients also can withdraw enrollment and reenroll later; the hospice Medicare benefit can be revoked later to secure traditional Medicare benefits. Payments to the hospice are per diem (or capitated), not fee-for-service. Payments are intended to cover physician services for the medical direction of the care team; regular home care visits by registered nurses and licensed practical nurses; home health aide and homemaker services; chaplain services; social work services; bereavement counseling; and medical equipment, supplies, and medications. No specific therapy is excluded, and the goal is for each therapy to be considered for its symptomatic (as opposed to disease-modifying) effect. Additional clinical care, including services of the primary physician, is covered by Medicare Part B even while the hospice Medicare benefit is in place.

The Affordable Care Act directs the secretary of Health and Human Services to gather data on Medicare hospice reimbursement with the goal of reforming payment rates to account for resource use over an entire episode of care. The legislation also requires additional evaluations and reviews of eligibility for hospice care by hospice physicians or nurses. The Center for Medicare and Medicaid Innovation (CMMI) sponsors and carries out demonstration projects to test models and evaluate the potential of new methods. In 2016, CMMI started a 5-year test of concurrent hospice and palliative care services with curative treatment for terminally ill patients who have a life expectancy of ≤6 months. A 4-year test initiated in 2021 will examine the inclusion of hospice in Medicare Advantage covering 8% of the market and include important health plans.

By 2018, the average length of enrollment in a hospice for Medicare beneficiaries was 90 days. However, the median length of stay was just 18 days, suggesting most patients are in hospice for a short time. Such short stays create barriers to establishing high-quality palliative services in patients' homes and also place financial strains on hospice providers since the initial assessments are resource intensive. Physicians should initiate early referrals to the hospice to allow more time for patients to receive palliative care.

In the United States, hospice care has been the main method for securing palliative services for terminally ill patients. However, leading physicians have increasingly emphasized the need to introduce palliative care much earlier in patients' illness, and efforts are being made to develop palliative care services that can be provided before the last 6 months of life and across a variety of settings. Studies of terminally ill patients indicate that those who received in-home palliative care delivered by an interdisciplinary team compared to usual care were more satisfied, more likely to die at home, and had fewer visits to the emergency room and lower per-day costs. More companies and home health agencies are now offering nonhospice palliative care services in patients' homes in an effort to increase quality of life and forestall emergency room visits and hospitalizations. Similarly, palliative care services are increasingly available via consultation, rather than being available only in hospital, day care, outpatient, and nursing home settings. Palliative care consultations for nonhospice patients can be billed as for other consultations under Medicare Part B. It is argued that using palliative care earlier in patients' illness allows patients and family members to become more acculturated to avoiding life-sustaining treatments, facilitating a smoother transition to hospice care closer to death.

WITHDRAWING AND WITHHOLDING LIFE-SUSTAINING TREATMENT

Legal Aspects For centuries, it has been deemed ethical to withhold or withdraw life-sustaining interventions. The current legal consensus in the United States and most wealthy countries is that patients have a moral as well as legal right to refuse medical interventions. American courts also have held that incompetent patients have a right to refuse medical interventions. For patients who are incompetent and terminally ill and who have not completed an advance care directive, next of kin can exercise that right, although this may be restricted in some states, depending on how clear and convincing the evidence is of the patient's preferences. Courts have limited families' ability to terminate life-sustaining treatments in patients who are conscious and incompetent but not terminally ill. In theory, patients' right to refuse medical therapy can be limited by four countervailing interests: (1) preservation of life, (2) prevention of suicide, (3) protection of third parties such as children, and (4) preservation of the integrity of the medical profession. In practice, these interests almost never override the right of competent patients and incompetent patients who have left explicit wishes or advance care directives.

For incompetent patients who either appointed a proxy without specific indications of their wishes or never completed an advance care directive, three criteria have been suggested to guide the decision to terminate medical interventions. First, some commentators suggest that ordinary care should be administered but extraordinary care could be terminated. Because the ordinary/extraordinary distinction is too vague, courts and commentators widely agree that it should not be used to justify decisions about stopping treatment. Second, many courts have advocated the use of the substituted-judgment criterion, which holds that the proxy decision-makers should try to imagine what the incompetent patient would do if he or she were competent. However, multiple studies indicate that many proxies, even close family members, cannot accurately predict what the patient would have wanted. Therefore, substituted judgment becomes more of a guessing game than a way of fulfilling the patient's wishes. Finally, the best-interests criterion holds that proxies should evaluate treatments by balancing their benefits and risks and select those treatments where the benefits maximally outweigh the burdens of treatment. Clinicians have a clear and crucial role in this by carefully and dispassionately explaining the known benefits and burdens of specific treatments. Yet even when that information is as clear as possible, different individuals can have very different views of what is in the patient's best interests, and families may have disagreements or even overt conflicts. This criterion has been criticized because there is no single way to determine the balance between benefits and burdens; it depends on a patient's personal values. For instance, for some people, being alive even if mentally incapacitated is a benefit, whereas for others, it may be the worst possible existence. As a matter of practice, physicians rely on family members to make decisions that they feel are best and object only if those decisions seem to demand treatments that the physicians consider not beneficial.

Practices Withholding and withdrawing acutely life-sustaining medical interventions from terminally ill patients are now standard practice. More than 90% of American patients die without cardiopulmonary resuscitation (CPR), and just as many forgo other potentially life-sustaining interventions. For instance, in ICUs in the period of 1987–1988, CPR was performed 49% of the time, but it was performed only 10% of the time in 1992–1993 and on just 1.8% of admissions from 2001 to 2008. On average, 3.8 interventions, such as vasopressors and transfusions, were stopped for each dying ICU patient. However, up to 19% of decedents in hospitals received interventions such as extubation, ventilation, and surgery in the 48 h preceding death. There is wide variation in practices among hospitals and ICUs, suggesting an important element of physician preferences rather than consistent adherence to professional society recommendations.

Mechanical ventilation may be the most challenging intervention to withdraw. The two approaches are *terminal extubation*, which is the removal of the endotracheal tube, and *terminal weaning*, which is the gradual reduction of the fraction of inspired oxygen (FIO_2) or ventilator rate. One-third of ICU physicians prefer to use the terminal weaning technique, and 13% extubate; the majority of physicians utilize both techniques. The American Thoracic Society's 2008 clinical policy guidelines note that there is no single correct process of ventilator withdrawal and that physicians use and should be proficient in both methods but that the chosen approach should carefully balance benefits and burdens as well as patient and caregiver preferences. Some recommend terminal weaning because patients do not develop upper airway obstruction and the distress caused by secretions or stridor; however, terminal weaning can prolong the dying process and not allow a patient's family to be with the patient unencumbered by an endotracheal tube. To ensure comfort for conscious or semiconscious patients before withdrawal of the ventilator, neuromuscular blocking agents should be terminated and sedatives and analgesics administered. Removing the neuromuscular blocking agents permits patients to show discomfort, facilitating the titration of sedatives and analgesics; it also permits interactions between patients and their families. A common practice is to inject a bolus of midazolam (2–4 mg) or lorazepam (2–4 mg) before withdrawal, followed by a bolus of 5–10 mg of morphine and continuous infusion of morphine (50% of the bolus dose per hour) during weaning. In patients who have significant upper airway secretions, IV scopolamine at a rate of 100 μg/h can be administered. Additional boluses of morphine or increases in the infusion rate should be administered for respiratory distress or signs of pain. Higher doses will be needed for patients already receiving sedatives and opioids.

The median time to death after stopping of the ventilator is 1 h. However, up to 10% of patients unexpectedly survive for 1 day or more after mechanical ventilation is stopped. Women and older patients tend to survive longer after extubation. Families need to be reassured about both the continuations of treatments for common symptoms, such as dyspnea and agitation, after withdrawal of ventilatory support and the uncertainty of length of survival after withdrawal of ventilatory support.

FUTILE CARE

Beginning in the late 1980s, some commentators argued that physicians could terminate futile treatments demanded by the families of terminally ill patients. Although no objective definition or standard of futility exists, several categories have been proposed. Physiologic futility means that an intervention will have no physiologic effect. Some have defined qualitative futility as applying to procedures that "fail to end a patient's total dependence on intensive medical care." Quantitative futility occurs "when physicians conclude (through personal experience, experiences shared with colleagues, or consideration of reported empiric data) that in the last 100 cases, a medical treatment has been useless." The term conceals subjective value judgments about when a treatment is "not beneficial." Deciding whether a treatment that obtains an additional 6 weeks of life or a 1% survival advantage confers benefit depends on patients' preferences and goals. Furthermore, physicians' predictions of when treatments are futile deviate markedly from the quantitative definition. When residents thought CPR was quantitatively futile, more than one in five patients had a >10% chance of survival to hospital discharge. Most studies that purport to guide determinations of futility are based on insufficient data and therefore cannot provide statistical confidence for clinical decision-making. Quantitative futility rarely applies in ICU settings.

Many commentators reject using futility as a criterion for withdrawing care, preferring instead to consider futility situations as ones that represent conflict that calls for careful negotiation between families and health care providers. The American Medical Association and other professional societies have developed process-based approaches to resolving cases clinicians feel are futile. These process-based measures mainly suggest involving consultants and/or ethics committees when there are seemingly irresolvable differences. Some hospitals have enacted "unilateral do-not-resuscitate" policies to allow clinicians to provide a do-not-resuscitate order in cases in which consensus cannot be reached with families and medical opinion is that resuscitation would be futile if attempted. This type of a policy is not a replacement for careful and patient communication and negotiation but recognizes that agreement cannot always be reached.

In 1999, Texas enacted the so-called Futile Care Act. Other states, such as Virginia, Maryland, and California, have also enacted such laws that provide physicians a "safe harbor" from liability if they refuse a patient's or family's request for life-sustaining interventions. For instance, in Texas, when a disagreement about terminating interventions between the medical team and the family has not been resolved by an ethics consultation, the physician is tasked with trying to facilitate transfer of the patient to an institution willing to provide treatment. If this fails after 10 days, the hospital and physician may unilaterally withdraw treatments determined to be futile. The family may appeal to a state court. Early data suggest that the law increases futility consultations for the ethics committee and that, although most families concur with withdrawal, ~10–15% of families refuse to withdraw treatment. As of 2007, there had been 974 ethics committee consultations on medical futility cases and 65 in which committees ruled against families and gave notice that treatment would be terminated. In 2007, a survey of Texas hospitals showed that 30% of hospitals had used the futility law in 213 adult cases and 42 pediatric cases. Treatment was withdrawn for 27 of those patients, and the remainder were transferred to other facilities or died while awaiting transfer.

EUTHANASIA AND PHYSICIAN-ASSISTED SUICIDE

Euthanasia and PAS are defined in **Table 12-8**. Terminating life-sustaining care and providing opioid medications to manage symptoms such as pain or dyspnea have long been considered ethical by the medical profession and legal by courts and should not be conflated with euthanasia or PAS.

Legal Aspects Euthanasia and PAS are legal in the Netherlands, Belgium, Luxembourg, Colombia, Canada, Spain, Western Australia, and New Zealand. Euthanasia was legalized in the Northern Territory of Australia in 1996, but that legislation was repealed 9 months later in 1997. Under certain conditions, a layperson in Switzerland or Germany can legally elect assisted suicide. In the United States, PAS is legal in Washington, D.C., and 10 states: Oregon, Washington State, Montana, Vermont, California, Colorado, Hawaii, Maine, New Jersey, and New Mexico. No state in the United States has legalized euthanasia. In the United States, multiple criteria must be met for PAS: the patient must have a terminal condition of <6 months and must be determined eligible through a process that includes a 15-day waiting period. In 2009, the state supreme court of Montana ruled that state law permits PAS for terminally ill patients. Many other countries, such as Portugal, are actively debating the legalization of euthanasia and/or PAS.

Practices Fewer than 10–20% of terminally ill patients actually consider euthanasia and/or PAS for themselves. Use of euthanasia and PAS is increasing but remains relatively rare. In all countries, even the Netherlands and Belgium where these practices have been tolerated and legal for many years, <5% of death occur by euthanasia or PAS. As of the most recent data, 4.7% of all deaths were by euthanasia or PAS in the Netherlands (2015) and 4.6% in Belgium (2013). Just 0.50% of all deaths in Oregon in 2019 (188 of 37,397 deaths) and 0.36% of all deaths in Washington State in 2018 (203 of 56,913 deaths) were reported to be by PAS, although these may be underestimates since the cause of some deaths of patients who received medications could not be verified.

In Belgium, the Netherlands, Oregon, and Washington, >70% of patients utilizing these interventions are dying of cancer; <10% of deaths by euthanasia or PAS involve patients with AIDS or amyotrophic lateral sclerosis. While the numbers are small, in the Netherlands, the numbers of euthanasia or PAS cases in patients with psychiatric disorders, dementia, and the accumulation of health issues are increasing.

TABLE 12-8 Definitions of Physician-Assisted Suicide and Euthanasia

TERM	DEFINITION	LEGAL STATUS
Voluntary active euthanasia	Intentionally administering medications or other interventions to cause the patient's death with the patient's informed consent	Netherlands, Belgium, Luxembourg, Canada, Colombia, Spain, Western Australia, New Zealand
Involuntary active euthanasia	Intentionally administering medications or other interventions to cause the patient's death when the patient was competent to consent but did not—e.g., the patient may not have been asked	Nowhere
Passive euthanasia	Withholding or withdrawing life-sustaining medical treatments from a patient to let him or her die (terminating life-sustaining treatments)	Everywhere
Physician-assisted suicide	A physician provides medications or other interventions to a patient with the understanding that the patient can use them to commit suicide	Netherlands, Belgium, Luxembourg, Canada, Colombia, Germany, Switzerland, Oregon, Washington, Montana, Vermont, California, Colorado, District of Columbia, Hawaii, Maine, New Jersey, New Mexico

Pain is not the primary motivator for patients' requests for or interest in euthanasia and/or PAS. Among the first patients to receive PAS in Oregon, only 1 of the 15 patients had inadequate pain control, compared with 15 of the 43 patients in a control group who experienced inadequate pain relief. About 33% of patients in Oregon seeking PAS currently cite pain or fear of pain as their main reason for doing so. Conversely, depression and hopelessness are strongly associated with patient interest in euthanasia and PAS. Concerns about loss of dignity or autonomy or being a burden on family members appear to be more important factors motivating a desire for euthanasia or PAS. Losing autonomy (87% Oregon [OR], 85% Washington [WA]), not being able to enjoy activities (90% OR, 84% WA), and fear of losing dignity (72% OR, 69% WA) are the most-cited end-of-life concerns in both states. A high percentage of patients seeking PAS note being a burden on family (59% OR, 51% WA). A study from the Netherlands showed that depressed terminally ill cancer patients were four times more likely to request euthanasia and confirmed that uncontrolled pain was not associated with greater interest in euthanasia.

Euthanasia and PAS are no guarantee of a painless, quick death. Data from the Netherlands indicate that in as many as 20% of euthanasia and PAS cases technical and other problems arose, including patients waking from coma, not becoming comatose, regurgitating medications, and experiencing a prolonged time to death. Data from Oregon between 1998 and 2017 and Washington between 2009 and 2017 indicate that of patients who received PAS prescriptions, 81% died at home and prescribers were present in 9.7% of cases. The time between drug intake and coma ranged from 1 min to 11 h, and the time from drug intake to death ranged from 1 min to 104 h. The median time from ingestion to coma was 5 min and from ingestion to death was 25 min. In Oregon between 1998 and 2015, 53% of patients had no complications, 44% of patients had no data on complications, and 2.4% of patients had regurgitation after taking the prescribed medicine as the only complication. In addition, six patients awakened. In Washington State between 2014 and 2015, 1.4% of patients had regurgitation, one patient had a seizure, and the reported range of time to death extended to 30 h. In the Netherlands, problems were significantly more common in PAS, sometimes requiring the physician to intervene and provide euthanasia.

Regardless of whether they practice in a setting where euthanasia is legal or not, many physicians over the course of their careers will receive a patient request for euthanasia or PAS. In the United States, 18% of physicians have received a request for PAS and 11% have received a request for euthanasia. Three percent complied with a request for PAS, while 5% complied with a request for euthanasia. In the Netherlands, where the practices are legal, 77% of physicians have received a request for PAS or euthanasia and 60% have performed these interventions.

Competency in dealing with such a request is crucial. Although challenging, the request can also provide a chance to address intense suffering. After receiving a request for euthanasia and/or PAS, health care providers should carefully clarify the request with empathic, open-ended questions to help elucidate the underlying cause for the request, such as, "What makes you want to consider this option?" Endorsing either moral opposition or moral support for the act tends to be counterproductive, giving an impression of being judgmental or of endorsing the idea that the patient's life is worthless. Health care providers must reassure the patient of continued care and commitment. The patient should be educated about alternative, less laden options, such as symptom management and withdrawing any unwanted treatments, and the reality of euthanasia and/or PAS, since the patient may have misconceptions about their effectiveness as well as the legal implications of the choice. Depression, hopelessness, and other symptoms of psychological distress, as well as physical suffering and economic burdens, are likely factors motivating the request, and such factors should be assessed and treated aggressively. After these interventions and clarification of options, most patients proceed with another approach, declining life-sustaining interventions, possibly including refusal of nutrition and hydration.

CARE DURING THE LAST HOURS

Most laypersons have limited experiences with the actual dying process and death. They frequently do not know what to expect of the final hours and afterward. The family and other caregivers must be prepared, especially if the plan is for the patient to die at home.

Patients in the last days of life typically experience extreme weakness and fatigue and become bedbound; this can lead to pressure sores. The issue of turning patients who are near the end of life, however, must be balanced against the potential discomfort that movement may cause. Patients stop eating and drinking with drying of mucosal membranes and dysphagia. Careful attention to oral swabbing, lubricants for lips, and use of artificial tears can provide a form of care to substitute for attempts at feeding the patient. With loss of the gag reflex and dysphagia, patients may also experience accumulation of oral secretions, producing noises during respiration sometimes called "the death rattle." Scopolamine can reduce the secretions. Patients also experience changes in respiration with periods of apnea or Cheyne-Stokes breathing. Decreased intravascular volume and cardiac output cause tachycardia, hypotension, peripheral coolness, and livedo reticularis (skin mottling). Patients can have urinary and, less frequently, fecal incontinence. Changes in consciousness and neurologic function generally lead to two different paths to death.

Each of these terminal changes can cause patients and families distress, requiring reassurance and targeted interventions (**Table 12-9**). Informing families that these changes might occur and providing them with an information sheet can help preempt problems and minimize distress. Understanding that patients stop eating because they are dying, not dying because they have stopped eating, can reduce family and caregiver anxiety. Similarly, informing the family and caregivers that the "death rattle" may occur and that it is not indicative of suffocation, choking, or pain can reduce their worry from the breathing sounds.

Families and caregivers may also feel guilty about stopping treatments, fearing that they are "killing" the patient. This may lead to demands for interventions, such as feeding tubes, that may be ineffective. In such cases, the physician should remind the family and caregivers about the inevitability of events and the palliative goals.

TABLE 12-9 Managing Changes in the Patient's Condition during the Final Days and Hours

CHANGES IN THE PATIENT'S CONDITION	POTENTIAL COMPLICATION	FAMILY'S POSSIBLE REACTION AND CONCERN	ADVICE AND INTERVENTION
Profound fatigue	Bedbound with development of pressure ulcers that are prone to infection, malodor, and pain, and joint pain	Patient is lazy and giving up.	Reassure family and caregivers that terminal fatigue will not respond to interventions and should not be resisted. Use an air mattress if necessary.
Anorexia	None	Patient is giving up; patient will suffer from hunger and will starve to death.	Reassure family and caregivers that the patient is not eating because he or she is dying; not eating at the end of life does not cause suffering or death. Forced feeding, whether oral, parenteral, or enteral, does not reduce symptoms or prolong life.
Dehydration	Dry mucosal membranes (see below)	Patient will suffer from thirst and die of dehydration.	Reassure family and caregivers that dehydration at the end of life does not cause suffering because patients lose consciousness before any symptom distress. Intravenous hydration can worsen symptoms of dyspnea by pulmonary edema and peripheral edema as well as prolong the dying process.
Dysphagia	Inability to swallow oral medications needed for palliative care		Do not force oral intake. Discontinue unnecessary medications that may have been continued, including antibiotics, diuretics, antidepressants, and laxatives. If swallowing pills is difficult, convert essential medications (analgesics, antiemetics, anxiolytics, and psychotropics) to oral solutions, buccal, sublingual, or rectal administration.
"Death rattle"—noisy breathing		Patient is choking and suffocating.	Reassure the family and caregivers that this is caused by secretions in the oropharynx and the patient is not choking. Reduce secretions with scopolamine (0.2–0.4 mg SC q4h or 1–3 patches q3d). Reposition patient to permit drainage of secretions. Do not suction. Suction can cause patient and family discomfort and is usually ineffective.
Apnea, Cheyne-Stokes respirations, dyspnea		Patient is suffocating.	Reassure family and caregivers that unconscious patients do not experience suffocation or air hunger. Apneic episodes are frequently a premorbid change. Opioids or anxiolytics may be used for dyspnea. Oxygen is unlikely to relieve dyspneic symptoms and may prolong the dying process.
Urinary or fecal incontinence	Skin breakdown if days until death Potential transmission of infectious agents to caregivers	Patient is dirty, malodorous, and physically repellent.	Remind family and caregivers to use universal precautions. Frequent changes of bedclothes and bedding. Use diapers, urinary catheter, or rectal tube if diarrhea or high urine output.
Agitation or delirium	Day/night reversal Hurt self or caregivers	Patient is in horrible pain and going to have a horrible death.	Reassure family and caregivers that agitation and delirium do not necessarily connote physical pain. Depending on the prognosis and goals of treatment, consider evaluating for causes of delirium and modifying medications. Manage symptoms with haloperidol, chlorpromazine, diazepam, or midazolam.
Dry mucosal membranes	Cracked lips, mouth sores, and candidiasis can also cause pain. Odor	Patient may be malodorous, physically repellent.	Use baking soda mouthwash or saliva preparation q15–30 min. Use topical nystatin for candidiasis. Coat lips and nasal mucosa with petroleum jelly q60–90 min. Use ophthalmic lubricants q4h or artificial tears q30 min.

Interventions may prolong the dying process and cause discomfort. Physicians also should emphasize that withholding treatments is both legal and ethical and that the family members are not the cause of the patient's death. This reassurance may have to be provided multiple times.

Hearing and touch are said to be the last senses to stop functioning. Whether this is the case or not, families and caregivers can be encouraged to communicate with the dying patient. Encouraging them to talk directly to the patient, even if he or she is unconscious, and hold the patient's hand or demonstrate affection in other ways can be an effective way to channel their urge "to do something" for the patient.

When the plan is for the patient to die at home, the physician must inform the family and caregivers how to determine that the patient has died. The cardinal signs are cessation of cardiac function and respiration; the pupils become fixed; the body becomes cool; muscles relax; and incontinence may occur. Remind the family and caregivers that the eyes may remain open even after the patient has died.

The physician should establish a plan for who the family or caregivers will contact when the patient is dying or has died. Without a plan, family members may panic and call 911, unleashing a cascade of unwanted events, from arrival of emergency personnel and resuscitation to hospital admission. The family and caregivers should be instructed to contact the hospice (if one is involved), the covering physician, or the on-call member of the palliative care team. They should also be told that the medical examiner need not be called unless the state requires it for all deaths. Unless foul play is suspected, the health care team need not contact the medical examiner either.

Just after the patient dies, even the best-prepared family may experience shock and loss and be emotionally distraught. They need time to assimilate the event and be comforted. Health care providers are likely to find it meaningful to write a bereavement card or letter to the family. The purpose is to communicate about the patient, perhaps emphasizing the patient's virtues and the honor it was to care for the patient, and to express concern for the family's hardship. Some physicians attend the funerals of their patients. Although this is beyond any medical obligation, the presence of the physician can be a source of support to the grieving family and provides an opportunity for closure for the physician.

Death of a spouse is a strong predictor of poor health, and even mortality, for the surviving spouse. It may be important to alert the spouse's physician about the death so that he or she is aware of symptoms that might require professional attention.

FURTHER READING

Emanuel E et al: Attitudes and practices of euthanasia and physician-assisted suicide in the United States, Canada, and Europe. JAMA 316:79, 2016.

Kelley AS, Meier DE: Palliative care—A shifting paradigm. N Engl J Med 363:781, 2010.

Kelley AS et al: Hospice enrollment saves money for Medicare and improves care quality across a number of different lengths-of-stay. Health Aff 32:552, 2012.

Kelley AS et al: Palliative care for the seriously ill. N Engl J Med 373:747, 2015.

Mack JW et al: Associations between end-of-life discussion characteristics and care received near death: A prospective cohort study. J Clin Oncol 30:4387, 2012.

Murray SA et al: Illness trajectories and palliative care. BMJ 330:1007, 2005.

Neuman P et al: Medicare per capita spending by age and service: New data highlights oldest beneficiaries. Health Aff (Millwood) 34:335, 2015.

Nicholas LH et al: Regional variation in the association between advance directives and end-of-life Medicare expenditures. JAMA 306:1447, 2011.

Ornstein KA et al: Evaluation of racial disparities in hospice use and end-of-life treatment intensity in the REGARDS cohort. JAMA Netw Open 3(8):e2014639, 2020.

Quinn KL et al: Association of receipt of palliative care interventions with health care use, quality of life, and symptom burden among adults with chronic noncancer illness: A systematic review and meta-analysis. JAMA 324:1439, 2020.

Teno JM et al: Change in end-of-life care for medicare beneficiaries: Site of death, place of care, and health transitions in 2000, 2005, and 2009. JAMA 309:470, 2013.

Teno JM et al: Site of death, place of care, and health care transitions among US Medicare beneficiaries, 2000-2015. JAMA 320:264, 2018.

Van Den Beuken-VanEverdingen MH et al: Update on prevalence of pain in patients with cancer: Systematic review and meta-analysis. J Pain Symptom Manage 51:1070, 2016.

WEBSITES

American Academy of Hospice and Palliative Medicine: *www.aahpm.org*

Center to Advance Palliative Care: *http://www.capc.org*

Education in Palliative and End of Life Care (EPEC): *http://www.epec.net*

Family Caregiver Alliance: *http://www.caregiver.org*

National Hospice and Palliative Care Organization (including state-specific advance directives): *http://www.nhpco.org*

Nccn: The National Comprehensive Cancer Network palliative care guidelines: *http://www.nccn.org*

Our Care Wishes Advance Care Planning Tool: *https://www.ourcarewishes.org*

Section 1 Pain

13 Pain: Pathophysiology and Management

James P. Rathmell, Howard L. Fields

The province of medicine is to preserve and restore health and to relieve suffering. Understanding pain is essential to both of these goals. Because pain is universally understood as a signal of disease, it is the most common symptom that brings a patient to a physician's attention. The function of the pain sensory system is to protect the body and maintain homeostasis. It does this by detecting, localizing, and identifying potential or actual tissue-damaging processes. Because different diseases produce characteristic patterns of tissue damage, the quality, time course, and location of a patient's pain lend important diagnostic clues. It is the physician's responsibility to assess each patient promptly for any remediable cause underlying the pain and to provide rapid and effective pain relief whenever possible.

THE PAIN SENSORY SYSTEM

Pain is an unpleasant sensation localized to a part of the body. It is often described in terms of a penetrating or tissue-destructive process (e.g., stabbing, burning, twisting, tearing, squeezing) and/or of a bodily or emotional reaction (e.g., terrifying, nauseating, sickening). Furthermore, any pain of moderate or higher intensity is accompanied by anxiety and the urge to escape or terminate the feeling. These properties illustrate the duality of pain: it is both sensation and emotion. When it is acute, pain is characteristically associated with behavioral arousal and a stress response consisting of increased blood pressure, heart rate, pupil diameter, and plasma cortisol levels. In addition, local muscle contraction (e.g., limb flexion, abdominal wall rigidity) is often present.

PERIPHERAL MECHANISMS

The Primary Afferent Nociceptor A peripheral nerve consists of the axons of three different types of neurons: primary sensory afferents, motor neurons, and sympathetic postganglionic neurons (Fig. 13-1). The cell bodies of primary sensory afferents are located in the dorsal root ganglia within the vertebral foramina. The primary afferent axon has two branches: one projects centrally into the spinal cord and the other projects peripherally to innervate tissues. Primary afferents are classified by their diameter, degree of myelination, and conduction velocity. The largest diameter afferent fibers, A-beta (Aβ), respond maximally to light touch and/or moving stimuli; they are present primarily in nerves that innervate the skin. In normal individuals, the activity of these fibers does not produce pain. There are two other classes of primary afferent nerve fibers: the small diameter myelinated A-delta (Aδ) and the unmyelinated (C) axons (Fig. 13-1). These fibers are present in nerves to the skin and to deep somatic and visceral structures. Some tissues, such as the cornea, are innervated only by Aδ and C fiber afferents. Most Aδ and C fiber afferents respond maximally to intense (painful) stimuli and produce the subjective experience of pain when they are activated; this defines them as *primary afferent nociceptors* (*pain receptors*). The ability to detect painful stimuli is completely abolished when conduction in Aδ and C fiber axons is blocked.

Individual primary afferent nociceptors can respond to several different types of noxious stimuli. For example, most nociceptors respond to heat; intense cold; intense mechanical distortion, such as a pinch; changes in pH, particularly an acidic environment; and application of chemical irritants including adenosine triphosphate (ATP), serotonin, bradykinin (BK), and histamine. The transient receptor potential cation channel subfamily V member 1 (TrpV1), also known as the vanilloid receptor, mediates perception of some noxious stimuli, especially heat sensations, by nociceptive neurons; it is activated by heat, acidic pH, endogenous mediators, and capsaicin, a component of hot chili peppers.

Sensitization When intense, repeated, or prolonged stimuli are applied to damaged or inflamed tissues, the threshold for activating primary afferent nociceptors is lowered, and the frequency of firing is higher for all stimulus intensities. Inflammatory mediators such as BK, nerve-growth factor, some prostaglandins (PGs), and leukotrienes contribute to this process, which is called *sensitization*. Sensitization occurs at the level of the peripheral nerve terminal (*peripheral sensitization*) as well as at the level of the dorsal horn of the spinal cord (*central sensitization*). Peripheral sensitization occurs in damaged or inflamed tissues, when inflammatory mediators activate intracellular signal transduction in nociceptors, prompting an increase in the production, transport, and membrane insertion of chemically gated and voltage-gated ion channels. These changes increase the excitability of nociceptor terminals and lower their threshold for activation by mechanical, thermal, and chemical stimuli. Central sensitization occurs when activity, generated by nociceptors during inflammation, enhances the excitability of nerve cells in the dorsal horn of the spinal cord. Following injury and resultant sensitization, normally innocuous stimuli can produce pain (termed *allodynia*). Sensitization is a clinically important process that contributes to tenderness, soreness, and *hyperalgesia* (increased pain intensity in response to the same noxious stimulus; e.g., pinprick causes severe pain). A striking example of sensitization is sunburned skin, in which severe pain can be produced by a gentle slap or a warm shower.

Sensitization is of particular importance for pain and tenderness in deep tissues. Viscera are normally relatively insensitive to noxious mechanical and thermal stimuli, although hollow viscera do generate

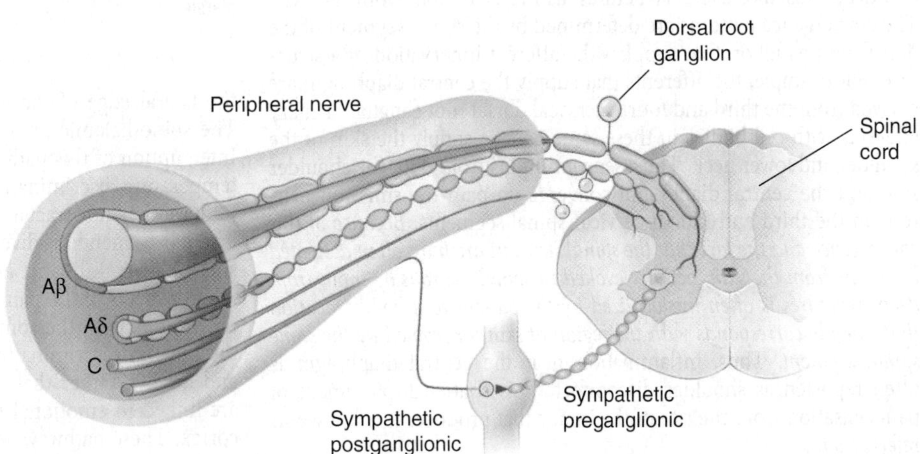

FIGURE 13-1 Components of a typical cutaneous nerve. There are two distinct functional categories of axons: primary afferents with cell bodies in the dorsal root ganglion and sympathetic postganglionic fibers with cell bodies in the sympathetic ganglion. Primary afferents include those with large-diameter myelinated (Aβ), small-diameter myelinated (Aδ), and unmyelinated (C) axons. All sympathetic postganglionic fibers are unmyelinated.

significant discomfort when distended. In contrast, when affected by a disease process with an inflammatory component, deep structures such as joints or hollow viscera characteristically become exquisitely sensitive to mechanical stimulation.

A large proportion of Aδ and C fiber afferents innervating viscera are completely insensitive in normal noninjured, noninflamed tissue. That is, they cannot be activated by known mechanical or thermal stimuli and are not spontaneously active. However, in the presence of inflammatory mediators, these afferents become sensitive to mechanical stimuli. Such afferents have been termed *silent nociceptors*, and their characteristic properties may explain how, under pathologic conditions, the relatively insensitive deep structures can become the source of severe and debilitating pain and tenderness. Low pH, PGs, leukotrienes, and other inflammatory mediators such as BK play a significant role in sensitization.

Nociceptor-Induced Inflammation Primary afferent nociceptors are not simply passive messengers of threats to tissue injury but also play an active role in tissue protection through a neuroeffector function. Most nociceptors contain polypeptide mediators, including substance P, calcitonin gene related peptide (CGRP), and cholecystokinin, that are released from their peripheral terminals when they are activated (**Fig. 13-2**). Substance P is an 11-amino-acid peptide that is released in peripheral tissues from primary afferent nociceptors and has multiple biologic activities. It is a potent vasodilator, causes mast cell degranulation, is a chemoattractant for leukocytes, and increases the production and release of inflammatory mediators. Interestingly, depletion of substance P from joints reduces the severity of experimental arthritis.

■ CENTRAL MECHANISMS

The Spinal Cord and Referred Pain The axons of primary afferent nociceptors enter the spinal cord via the dorsal root. They terminate in the dorsal horn of the spinal gray matter (**Fig. 13-3**). The terminals of primary afferent axons contact spinal neurons that transmit the pain signal to brain sites involved in pain perception. When primary afferents are activated by noxious stimuli, they release neurotransmitters from their terminals that excite the spinal cord neurons. The major neurotransmitter released is glutamate, which rapidly excites the second-order dorsal horn neurons. Primary afferent nociceptor terminals also release substance P and CGRP, which produce a slower and longer-lasting excitation of the dorsal horn neurons. The axon of each primary afferent contacts many spinal neurons, and each spinal neuron receives convergent inputs from many primary afferents.

The convergence of sensory inputs to a single spinal pain-transmission neuron is of great importance because it underlies the phenomenon of referred pain. All spinal neurons that receive input from the viscera and deep musculoskeletal structures also receive input from the skin. The convergence patterns are determined by the spinal segment of the dorsal root ganglion that supplies the afferent innervation of a structure. For example, the afferents that supply the central diaphragm are derived from the third and fourth cervical dorsal root ganglia. Primary afferents with cell bodies in these same ganglia supply the skin of the shoulder and lower neck. Thus, sensory inputs from both the shoulder skin and the central diaphragm converge on pain-transmission neurons in the third and fourth cervical spinal segments. *Because of this convergence and the fact that the spinal neurons are most often activated by inputs from the skin, activity evoked in spinal neurons by input from deep structures is often mislocalized by the patient to a bodily location that roughly corresponds with the region of skin innervated by the same spinal segment.* Thus, inflammation near the central diaphragm is often reported as shoulder discomfort. This spatial displacement of pain sensation from the site of the injury that produces it is known as *referred pain*.

Ascending Pathways for Pain A majority of spinal neurons contacted by primary afferent nociceptors send their axons to the contralateral thalamus. These axons form the contralateral spinothalamic tract, which lies in the anterolateral white matter of the spinal cord,

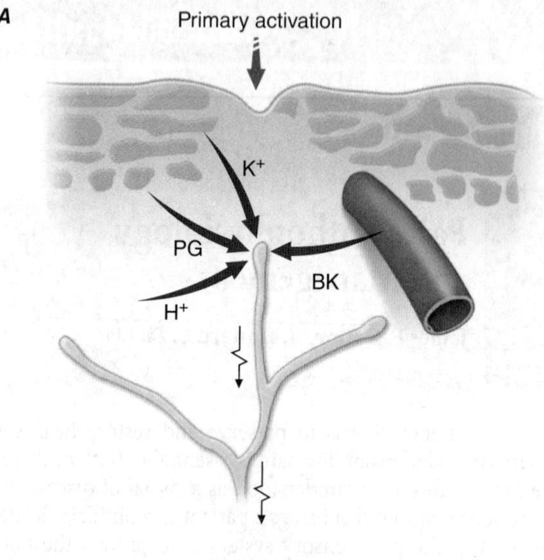

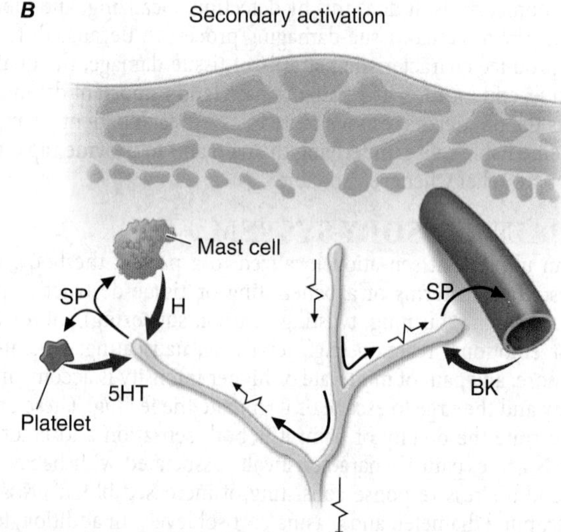

FIGURE 13-2 Events leading to activation, sensitization, and spread of sensitization of primary afferent nociceptor terminals. *A*. Direct activation by intense pressure and consequent cell damage. Cell damage induces lower pH (H^+) and leads to release of potassium (K^+) and to synthesis of prostaglandins (PGs) and bradykinin (BK). PGs increase the sensitivity of the terminal to BK and other pain-producing substances. ***B*.** Secondary activation. Impulses generated in the stimulated terminal propagate not only to the spinal cord but also into other terminal branches where they induce the release of peptides, including substance P (SP). Substance P causes vasodilation and neurogenic edema with further accumulation of BK. Substance P also causes the release of histamine (H) from mast cells and serotonin (5HT) from platelets.

the lateral edge of the medulla, and the lateral pons and midbrain. The spinothalamic pathway is crucial for pain sensation in humans. Interruption of this pathway produces permanent deficits in pain and temperature discrimination.

Spinothalamic tract axons ascend to several regions of the thalamus. There is tremendous divergence of the pain signal from these thalamic sites to several distinct areas of the cerebral cortex that subserve different aspects of the pain experience (**Fig. 13-4**). One of the thalamic projections is to the somatosensory cortex. This projection mediates the sensory discriminative aspects of pain, i.e., its location, intensity, and quality. Other thalamic neurons project to cortical regions that are linked to emotional responses, such as the cingulate and insular cortex. These pathways to the frontal cortex subserve the affective or unpleasant emotional dimension of pain. This affective dimension of pain produces suffering and exerts potent control of behavior. Because of this dimension, fear is a constant companion of pain. As a consequence, injury or surgical lesions to areas of the frontal cortex activated by painful stimuli can diminish the emotional impact of pain while

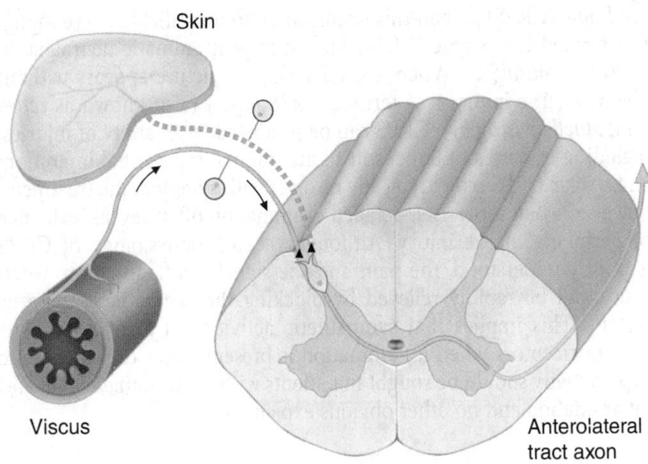

FIGURE 13-3 The convergence-projection hypothesis of referred pain. According to this hypothesis, visceral afferent nociceptors converge on the same pain-projection neurons as the afferents from the somatic structures in which the pain is perceived. The brain has no way of knowing the actual source of input and mistakenly "projects" the sensation to the somatic structure.

largely preserving the individual's ability to recognize noxious stimuli as painful.

PAIN MODULATION

The pain produced by injuries of similar magnitude is remarkably variable in different situations and in different individuals. For example, athletes have been known to sustain serious fractures with only minor pain, and Beecher's classic World War II survey revealed that many soldiers in battle were unbothered by injuries that would have produced agonizing pain in civilian patients. Furthermore, even the suggestion that a treatment will relieve pain can have a significant analgesic effect (the *placebo effect*). On the other hand, many patients find even minor injuries such as venipuncture frightening and unbearable, and the expectation of pain can induce pain even without a noxious stimulus. The suggestion that pain will worsen following administration of an inert substance can increase its perceived intensity (the *nocebo effect*).

The powerful effect of expectation and other psychological variables on the perceived intensity of pain is explained by brain circuits that modulate the activity of the pain-transmission pathways. One of these circuits has links to the hypothalamus, midbrain, and medulla, and it selectively controls spinal pain-transmission neurons through a descending pathway (Fig. 13-4).

Human brain-imaging studies have implicated this pain-modulating circuit in the pain-relieving effect of attention, suggestion, and opioid analgesic medications (**Fig. 13-5**). Furthermore, each of the component structures of the pathway contains opioid receptors and is sensitive to the direct application of opioid drugs. In animals, lesions of this descending modulatory system reduce the analgesic effect of

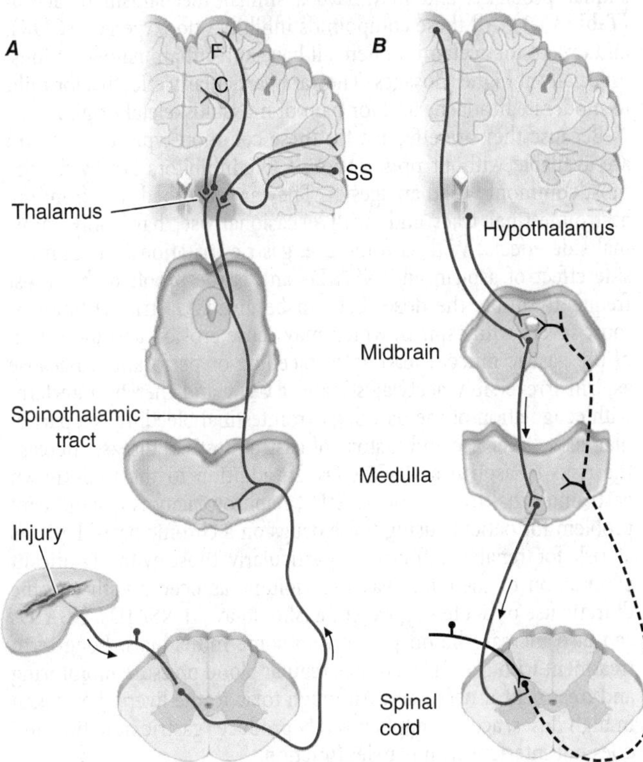

FIGURE 13-4 Pain-transmission and modulatory pathways. *A*. Transmission system for nociceptive messages. Noxious stimuli activate the sensitive peripheral ending of the primary afferent nociceptor by the process of transduction. The message is then transmitted over the peripheral nerve to the spinal cord, where it synapses with cells of origin of the major ascending pain pathway, the spinothalamic tract. The message is relayed in the thalamus to the anterior cingulate (C), frontal insular (F), and somatosensory cortex (SS). ***B*.** Pain-modulation network. Inputs from frontal cortex and hypothalamus activate cells in the midbrain that control spinal pain-transmission cells via cells in the medulla.

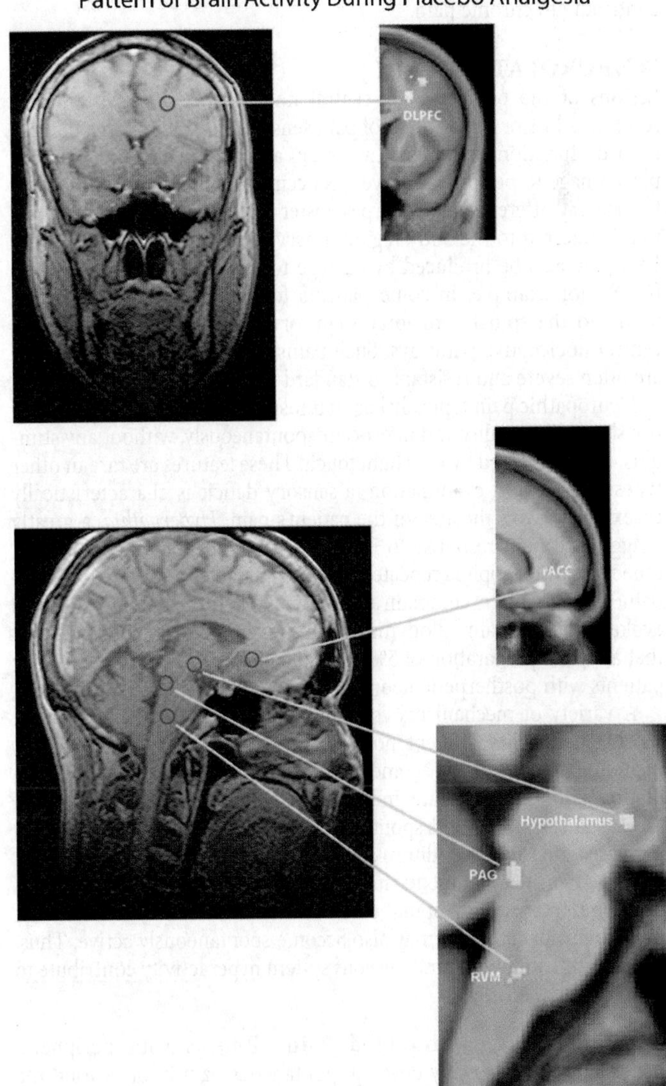

FIGURE 13-5 Functional magnetic resonance imaging (fMRI) demonstrates placebo-enhanced brain activity in anatomic regions correlating with the opioidergic descending pain control system. *Top panel:* Frontal fMRI image shows placebo-enhanced brain activity in the dorsal lateral prefrontal cortex (DLPFC). *Bottom panel:* Sagittal fMRI images show placebo-enhanced responses in the rostral anterior cingulate cortex (rACC), the rostral ventral medullae (RVM), the periaqueductal gray (PAG) area, and the hypothalamus. The placebo-enhanced activity in all areas was reduced by naloxone, demonstrating the link between the descending opioidergic system and the placebo analgesic response. *(F Eippert et al: Activation of the opioidergic descending pain control system underlies placebo analgesia. Neuron 63(4):533-543, 2009.)*

systemically administered opioids such as morphine. Along with the opioid receptor, the component nuclei of this pain-modulating circuit contain endogenous opioid peptides such as the enkephalins and β-endorphin.

The most reliable way to activate this endogenous opioid-mediated modulating system is by suggestion of pain relief or by intense emotion directed away from the pain-causing injury (e.g., during severe threat or an athletic competition). In fact, pain-relieving endogenous opioids are released following surgical procedures and in patients given a placebo for pain relief.

Pain-modulating circuits can enhance as well as suppress pain. Both pain-inhibiting and pain-facilitating neurons in the medulla project to and control spinal pain-transmission neurons. Because pain-transmission neurons can be activated by modulatory neurons, it is theoretically possible to generate a pain signal with no peripheral noxious stimulus. In fact, human functional imaging studies have demonstrated increased activity in this circuit during migraine headaches. A central circuit that facilitates pain could account for the finding that pain can be induced by suggestion or enhanced by expectation and provides a framework for understanding how psychological factors can contribute to chronic pain.

■ NEUROPATHIC PAIN

Lesions of the peripheral or central nociceptive pathways typically result in a loss or impairment of pain sensation. Paradoxically, damage to or dysfunction of these pathways can also produce pain. For example, damage to peripheral nerves, as occurs in diabetic neuropathy, or to primary afferents, as in herpes zoster infection, can result in pain that is referred to the body region innervated by the damaged nerves. Pain may also be produced by damage to the central nervous system (CNS), for example, in some patients following trauma or vascular injury to the spinal cord, brainstem, or thalamic areas that contain central nociceptive pathways. Such pains are termed *neuropathic* and are often severe and resistant to standard treatments for pain.

Neuropathic pain typically has an unusual burning, tingling, or electric shock-like quality and may occur spontaneously, without any stimulus, or be triggered by very light touch. These features are rare in other types of pain. On examination, a sensory deficit is characteristically co-extensive with the area of the patient's pain. *Hyperpathia*, a greatly exaggerated pain response to innocuous or mild nociceptive stimuli, especially when applied repeatedly, is also characteristic of neuropathic pain; patients often complain that the very lightest moving stimulus evokes exquisite pain (allodynia). In this regard, it is of clinical interest that a topical preparation of 5% lidocaine in patch form is effective for patients with postherpetic neuralgia who have prominent allodynia.

A variety of mechanisms contribute to neuropathic pain. As with sensitized primary afferent nociceptors, damaged primary afferents, including nociceptors, become highly sensitive to mechanical stimulation and may generate impulses in the absence of stimulation. Increased sensitivity and spontaneous activity are due, in part, to an increased density of sodium channels in the damaged nerve fiber. Damaged primary afferents may also develop sensitivity to norepinephrine. Interestingly, spinal cord pain-transmission neurons cut off from their normal input may also become spontaneously active. Thus, both central and peripheral nervous system hyperactivity contribute to neuropathic pain.

Sympathetically Maintained Pain Patients with peripheral nerve injury occasionally develop spontaneous pain in or beyond the region innervated by the nerve. This pain is often described as having a burning quality. The pain typically begins after a delay of hours to days or even weeks and is accompanied by swelling of the extremity, periarticular bone loss, and arthritic changes in the distal joints. Early in the course of the condition, the pain may be relieved by a local anesthetic block of the sympathetic innervation to the affected extremity. Damaged primary afferent nociceptors acquire adrenergic sensitivity and can be activated by stimulation of the sympathetic outflow. This constellation of spontaneous pain and signs of sympathetic dysfunction following injury has been termed *complex regional pain syndrome* (CRPS). When this occurs after an identifiable nerve injury, it is termed CRPS type II (also known as posttraumatic neuralgia or, if severe, *causalgia*). When a similar clinical picture appears without obvious nerve injury, it is termed CRPS type I (also known as *reflex sympathetic dystrophy*). CRPS can be produced by a variety of injuries, including fractures of bone, soft tissue trauma, myocardial infarction, and stroke. CRPS type I typically resolves with symptomatic treatment; however, when it persists, detailed examination often reveals evidence of peripheral nerve injury. Although the pathophysiology of CRPS is poorly understood, the pain and the signs of inflammation, when acute, can be rapidly relieved by blocking the sympathetic nervous system. This implies that sympathetic activity can activate undamaged nociceptors when inflammation is present. Signs of sympathetic hyperactivity should be sought in patients with posttraumatic pain and inflammation and no other obvious explanation.

TREATMENT

Acute Pain

The ideal treatment for any pain is to remove the cause; thus, while treatment can be initiated immediately, efforts to establish the underlying etiology should always proceed as treatment begins. Sometimes, treating the underlying condition does not immediately relieve pain. Furthermore, some conditions are so painful that rapid and effective analgesia is essential (e.g., the postoperative state, burns, trauma, cancer, or sickle cell crisis). Analgesic medications are a first line of treatment in these cases, and all practitioners should be familiar with their use.

ASPIRIN, ACETAMINOPHEN, AND NONSTEROIDAL ANTI-INFLAMMATORY AGENTS (NSAIDS)

These drugs are considered together because they are used for similar problems and may have a similar mechanism of action (**Table 13-1**). All these compounds inhibit cyclooxygenase (COX), and except for acetaminophen, all have anti-inflammatory actions, especially at higher dosages. They are particularly effective for mild to moderate headache and for pain of musculoskeletal origin.

Because they are effective for these common types of pain and are available without prescription, COX inhibitors are by far the most commonly used analgesics. They are absorbed well from the gastrointestinal tract and, with occasional use, have only minimal side effects. With chronic use, gastric irritation is a common side effect of aspirin and NSAIDs and is the problem that most frequently limits the dose that can be given. Gastric irritation is most severe with aspirin, which may cause erosion and ulceration of the gastric mucosa leading to bleeding or perforation. Because aspirin irreversibly acetylates platelet COX and thereby interferes with coagulation of the blood, gastrointestinal bleeding is a particular risk. Older age and history of gastrointestinal disease increase the risks of aspirin and NSAIDs. In addition to the well-known gastrointestinal toxicity of NSAIDs, nephrotoxicity is a significant problem for patients using these drugs on a chronic basis. Patients at risk for renal insufficiency, particularly those with significant contraction of their intravascular volume as occurs with chronic diuretic use or acute hypovolemia, should avoid NSAIDs. NSAIDs can also increase blood pressure in some individuals. Long-term treatment with NSAIDs requires regular blood pressure monitoring and treatment if necessary. Although toxic to the liver when taken in high doses, acetaminophen rarely produces gastric irritation and does not interfere with platelet function.

The introduction of parenteral forms of NSAIDs, ketorolac and diclofenac, extends the usefulness of this class of compounds in the management of acute severe pain. Both agents are sufficiently potent and rapid in onset to supplant opioids as first-line treatment for many patients with acute severe headache and musculoskeletal pain.

There are two major classes of COX: COX-1 is constitutively expressed, and COX-2 is induced in the inflammatory state.

TABLE 13-1 Drugs for Relief of Pain

GENERIC NAME	DOSE, mg	INTERVAL	COMMENTS
Nonnarcotic Analgesics: Usual Doses and Intervals			
Acetylsalicylic acid	650 PO	q4h	Enteric-coated preparations available
Acetaminophen	650 PO	q4h	Side effects uncommon
Ibuprofen	400 PO	q4–6h	Available without prescription
Naproxen	250–500 PO	q12h	Naproxen is the common NSAID that poses the least cardiovascular risk, but it has a somewhat higher incidence of gastrointestinal bleeding
Fenoprofen	200 PO	q4–6h	Contraindicated in renal disease
Indomethacin	25–50 PO	q8h	Gastrointestinal side effects common
Ketorolac	15–60 IM/IV	q4–6h	Available for parenteral use
Celecoxib	100–200 PO	q12–24h	Useful for arthritis
Valdecoxib	10–20 PO	q12–24h	Removed from U.S. market in 2005

GENERIC NAME	PARENTERAL DOSE, mg	PO DOSE, mg	COMMENTS
Narcotic Analgesics: Usual Doses and Intervals			
Codeine	30–60 q4h	30–60 q4h	Nausea common
Oxycodone	—	5–10 q4–6h	Usually available with acetaminophen or aspirin
Oxycodone extended-release	—	10-40 q12h	Oral extended-release tablet; high potential for misuse
Morphine	5 q4h	30 q4h	
Morphine sustained release	—	15–60 bid to tid	Oral slow-release preparation
Hydromorphone	1–2 q4h	2–4 q4h	Shorter acting than morphine sulfate
Levorphanol	2 q6–8h	4 q6–8h	Longer acting than morphine sulfate; absorbed well PO
Methadone	5–10 q6–8h	5–20 q6–8h	Due to long half-life, respiratory depression and sedation may persist after analgesic effect subsides; therapy should not be initiated with >40 mg/d, and dose escalation should be made no more frequently than every 3 days
Meperidine	50–100 q3–4h	300 q4h	Poorly absorbed PO; normeperidine is a toxic metabolite; routine use of this agent is not recommended
Butorphanol	—	1–2 q4h	Intranasal spray
Fentanyl	25–100 μg/h	—	72-h transdermal patch
Buprenorphine	5–20 μg/h		7-day transdermal patch
Buprenorphine	0.3 q6–8h		Parenteral administration
Tramadol	—	50–100 q4–6h	Mixed opioid/adrenergic action

GENERIC NAME	UPTAKE BLOCKADE 5-HT	UPTAKE BLOCKADE NE	SEDATIVE POTENCY	ANTICHOLINERGIC POTENCY	ORTHOSTATIC HYPOTENSION	CARDIAC ARRHYTHMIA	AVERAGE DOSE, mg/d	RANGE, mg/d
Antidepressants[a]								
Doxepin	++	+	High	Moderate	Moderate	Less	200	75–400
Amitriptyline	++++	++	High	Highest	Moderate	Yes	150	25–300
Imipramine	++++	++	Moderate	Moderate	High	Yes	200	75–400
Nortriptyline	+++	++	Moderate	Moderate	Low	Yes	100	40–150
Desipramine	+++	++++	Low	Low	Low	Yes	150	50–300
Venlafaxine	+++	++	Low	None	None	No	150	75–400
Duloxetine	+++	+++	Low	None	None	No	40	30–60

GENERIC NAME	PO DOSE, mg	INTERVAL	COMMENTS
Anticonvulsants and Antiarrythmics[a]			
Carbamazepine	200–300	q6h	Rare aplastic anemia, GI irritation, hepatoitoxicity
Oxcarbamazepine	300	bid	Similar to carbamazepine
Gabapentin[b]	600–1200	q8h	Dizziness, GI irritation; useful in trigeminal neuralgia
Pregabalin	150–600	bid	Similar to gabapentin; dry mouth, edema

[a]Antidepressants, anticonvulsants, and antiarrhythmics have not been approved by the U.S. Food and Drug Administration (FDA) for the treatment of pain. [b]Gabapentin in doses up to 1800 mg/d is FDA approved for postherpetic neuralgia.

Abbreviations: 5-HT, serotonin; NE, norepinephrine; NSAID, nonsteroidal anti-inflammatory agent.

COX-2-selective drugs have similar analgesic potency and produce less gastric irritation than the nonselective COX inhibitors. The use of COX-2-selective drugs does not appear to lower the risk of nephrotoxicity compared to nonselective NSAIDs. On the other hand, COX-2-selective drugs offer a significant benefit in the management of acute postoperative pain because they do not affect blood coagulation. Nonselective COX inhibitors (especially aspirin) are usually contraindicated postoperatively because they impair platelet-mediated blood clotting and are thus associated with increased bleeding at the operative site. COX-2 inhibitors, including celecoxib (Celebrex), are associated with increased cardiovascular risk, including cardiovascular death, myocardial infarction, stroke, heart failure, or a thromboembolic event. It appears that this is a class effect of NSAIDs, excluding aspirin. These drugs are contraindicated in patients in the immediate period after coronary artery bypass surgery and should be used with caution in elderly patients and those with a history of or significant risk factors for cardiovascular disease.

OPIOID ANALGESICS

Opioids are the most potent pain-relieving drugs currently available. Of all analgesics, they have the broadest range of efficacy and provide the most reliable and effective treatment for rapid pain relief. Although side effects are common, most are reversible: nausea, vomiting, pruritus, sedation, and constipation are the most frequent and bothersome side effects. Respiratory depression is uncommon at standard analgesic doses but can be life-threatening. Opioid-related side effects can be reversed rapidly with the narcotic antagonist naloxone. Many physicians, nurses, and patients have a certain trepidation about using opioids that is based on a fear of initiating addiction in their patients. In fact, there is a very small chance of patients becoming addicted to narcotics as a result of their appropriate medical use. For chronic pain, particularly chronic noncancer pain, the risk of addiction in patients taking opioids on a chronic basis remains small, but the risk does appear to increase with dose escalation. The physician should not hesitate to use opioid analgesics in patients with acute severe pain. Table 13-1 lists the most commonly used opioid analgesics.

Opioids produce analgesia by actions in the CNS. They activate pain-inhibitory neurons and directly inhibit pain-transmission neurons. Most of the commercially available opioid analgesics act at the same opioid receptor (μ-receptor), differing mainly in potency, speed of onset, duration of action, and optimal route of administration. Some side effects are due to accumulation of nonopioid metabolites that are unique to individual drugs. One striking example of this is normeperidine, a metabolite of meperidine. At higher doses of meperidine, typically >1 g/d, accumulation of normeperidine can produce hyperexcitability and seizures that are not reversible with naloxone. Normeperidine accumulation is increased in patients with renal failure.

The most rapid pain relief is obtained by intravenous administration of opioids; relief with oral administration is significantly slower. Because of the potential for respiratory depression, patients with any form of respiratory compromise must be kept under close observation following opioid administration; an oxygen-saturation monitor may be useful, but only in a setting where the monitor is under constant surveillance. Opioid-induced respiratory depression is primarily manifest as a reduction in respiratory rate and is typically accompanied by sedation. A fall in oxygen saturation represents a critical level of respiratory depression and the need for immediate intervention to prevent life-threatening hypoxemia. Newer monitoring devices that incorporate capnography or pharyngeal air flow can detect apnea at the point of onset and should be used in hospitalized patients. Ventilatory assistance should be maintained until the opioid-induced respiratory depression has resolved. The opioid antagonist naloxone should be readily available whenever opioids are used at high doses or in patients with compromised pulmonary function. Opioid effects are dose-related, and there is great variability among patients in the doses that relieve pain and produce side effects. Synergistic respiratory depression is common when opioids are administered with other CNS depressants. Co-administration of benzodiazepines is particularly likely to produce respiratory depression and should be avoided, especially in outpatient pain management. Because of this variability in patient response, initiation of therapy requires titration to optimal dose and interval. The most important principle is to provide adequate pain relief. This requires determining whether the drug has adequately relieved the pain and timely reassessment to determine the optimal interval for dosing. *The most common error made by physicians in managing severe pain with opioids is to prescribe an inadequate dose. Because many patients are reluctant to complain, this practice leads to needless suffering.* In the absence of sedation at the expected time of peak effect, a physician should not hesitate to repeat the initial dose to achieve satisfactory pain relief.

A now standard approach to the problem of achieving adequate pain relief is the use of patient-controlled analgesia (PCA). PCA uses a microprocessor-controlled infusion device that can deliver a baseline continuous dose of an opioid drug as well as preprogrammed additional doses whenever the patient pushes a button. The patient can then titrate the dose to the optimal level. This approach is used most extensively for the management of postoperative pain, but there is no reason why it should not be used for any hospitalized patient with persistent severe pain. PCA is also used for short-term home care of patients with intractable pain, such as that caused by metastatic cancer.

It is important to understand that the PCA device delivers small, repeated doses to maintain pain relief; in patients with severe pain, the pain must first be brought under control with a loading dose before transitioning to the PCA device. The bolus dose of the drug (typically 1 mg of morphine, 0.2 mg of hydromorphone, or 10 μg of fentanyl) can then be delivered repeatedly as needed. To prevent overdosing, PCA devices are programmed with a lockout period after each demand dose is delivered (typically starting at 10 min) and a limit on the total dose delivered per hour. Although some have advocated the use of a simultaneous continuous or basal infusion of the PCA drug, this may increase the risk of respiratory depression and has not been shown to increase the overall efficacy of the technique.

The availability of new routes of administration has extended the usefulness of opioid analgesics. Most important is the availability of spinal administration. Opioids can be infused through a spinal catheter placed either intrathecally or epidurally. By applying opioids directly to the spinal or epidural space adjacent to the spinal cord, regional analgesia can be obtained using relatively low total doses. Indeed, the dose required to produce effective analgesia when using morphine intrathecally (0.1–0.3 mg) is a fraction of that required to produce similar analgesia when administered intravenously (5–10 mg). In this way, side effects such as sedation, nausea, and respiratory depression can be minimized. This approach has been used extensively during labor and delivery and for postoperative pain relief following surgical procedures. Continuous intrathecal delivery via implanted spinal drug-delivery systems is now commonly used, particularly for the treatment of cancer-related pain that would require sedating doses for adequate pain control if given systemically. Opioids can also be given intranasally (butorphanol), rectally, and transdermally (fentanyl and buprenorphine), or through the oral mucosa (fentanyl), thus avoiding the discomfort of frequent injections in patients who cannot be given oral medication. The fentanyl and buprenorphine transdermal patches have the advantage of providing fairly steady plasma levels, which may improve patient comfort.

Recent additions to the armamentarium for treating opioid-induced side effects are the peripherally acting opioid antagonists alvimopan (Entereg) and methylnaltrexone (Rellistor). Alvimopan is available as an orally administered agent that is restricted to the intestinal lumen by limited absorption; methylnaltrexone is available in a subcutaneously administered form that has virtually no penetration into the CNS. Both agents act by binding to peripheral μ-receptors, thereby inhibiting or reversing the effects of opioids at these peripheral sites. The action of both agents is restricted to receptor sites outside of the CNS; thus, these drugs can reverse the adverse effects of opioid analgesics that are mediated through their peripheral receptors without reversing their CNS-mediated analgesic effects. Alvimopan has proven effective in lowering the duration of persistent ileus following abdominal surgery in patients receiving opioid analgesics for postoperative pain control. Methylnaltrexone has proven effective for relief of opioid-induced constipation in patients taking opioid analgesics on a chronic basis.

Opioid and COX Inhibitor Combinations When used in combination, opioids and COX inhibitors have additive effects. Because a lower dose of each can be used to achieve the same degree of pain relief and their side effects are nonadditive, such combinations are used to lower the severity of dose-related side effects. However, fixed-ratio combinations of an opioid with acetaminophen carry an important risk. Dose escalation as a result of increased severity of pain or decreased opioid effect as a result of tolerance may lead to ingestion of levels of acetaminophen that are toxic to the liver. Although acetaminophen-related hepatotoxicity is uncommon, it remains a significant cause for liver failure. Thus, many practitioners have moved away from the use of opioid-acetaminophen combination analgesics to avoid the risk of excessive acetaminophen exposure as the dose of the analgesic is escalated.

CHRONIC PAIN

Managing patients with chronic pain is intellectually and emotionally challenging. Sensitization of the nervous system can occur without an obvious precipitating cause, e.g., fibromyalgia, or chronic headache. In many patients, chronic pain becomes a distinct disease unto itself. The pain-generating mechanism is often difficult or impossible to determine with certainty; such patients are demanding of the physician's time and often appear emotionally distraught. The traditional medical approach of seeking an obscure organic pathology is often unhelpful. On the other hand, psychological evaluation and behaviorally based treatment paradigms are frequently helpful, particularly in the setting of a multidisciplinary pain-management center. Unfortunately, this approach, while effective, remains largely underused in current medical practice.

There are several factors that can cause, perpetuate, or exacerbate chronic pain. First, of course, the patient may simply have a disease that is characteristically painful for which there is presently no cure. Arthritis, cancer, chronic daily headaches, fibromyalgia, and diabetic neuropathy are examples of this. Second, there may be secondary perpetuating factors that are initiated by disease and persist after that disease has resolved. Examples include damaged sensory nerves, sympathetic efferent activity, and painful reflex muscle contraction (spasm). Finally, a variety of psychological conditions can exacerbate or even cause pain.

There are certain areas to which special attention should be paid in a patient's medical history. Because depression is the most common emotional disturbance in patients with chronic pain, patients should be questioned about their mood, appetite, sleep patterns, and daily activity. A simple standardized questionnaire, such as the Beck Depression Inventory, can be a useful screening device. It is important to remember that major depression is a common, treatable, and potentially fatal illness.

Other clues that a significant emotional disturbance is contributing to a patient's chronic pain complaint include pain that occurs in multiple, unrelated sites; a pattern of recurrent, but separate, pain problems beginning in childhood or adolescence; pain beginning at a time of emotional trauma, such as the loss of a parent or spouse; a history of physical or sexual abuse; and past or present substance abuse.

On examination, special attention should be paid to whether the patient guards the painful area and whether certain movements or postures are avoided because of pain. Discovering a mechanical component to the pain can be useful both diagnostically and therapeutically. Painful areas should be examined for deep tenderness, noting whether this is localized to muscle, ligamentous structures, or joints. Chronic myofascial pain is very common, and in these patients, deep palpation may reveal highly localized trigger points that are firm bands or knots in muscle. Relief of the pain following injection of local anesthetic into these trigger points supports the diagnosis. A neuropathic component to the pain is indicated by evidence of nerve damage, such as sensory impairment, exquisitely sensitive skin (allodynia), weakness, and muscle atrophy, or loss of deep tendon reflexes. Evidence suggesting sympathetic nervous system involvement includes the presence of diffuse swelling, changes in skin color and temperature, and hypersensitive skin and joint tenderness compared with the normal side. Relief of the pain with a sympathetic block supports the diagnosis, but once the condition becomes chronic, the response to sympathetic blockade is of variable magnitude and duration; the role for repeated sympathetic blocks in the overall management of CRPS is unclear.

A guiding principle in evaluating patients with chronic pain is to assess both emotional and somatic causal and perpetuating factors before initiating therapy. Addressing these issues together, rather than waiting to address emotional issues after somatic causes of pain have been ruled out, improves compliance in part because it assures patients that a psychological evaluation does not mean that the physician is questioning the validity of their complaint. Even when a somatic cause for a patient's pain can be found, it is still wise to look for other factors. For example, a cancer patient with painful bony metastases may have additional pain due to nerve damage and may also be depressed. Optimal therapy requires that each of these factors be assessed and treated.

TREATMENT
Chronic Pain

Once the evaluation process has been completed and the likely causative and exacerbating factors identified, an explicit treatment plan should be developed. An important part of this process is to identify specific and realistic functional goals for therapy, such as getting a good night's sleep, being able to go shopping, or returning to work. A multidisciplinary approach that uses medications, counseling, physical therapy, nerve blocks, and even surgery may be required to improve the patient's quality of life. There are also some newer, minimally invasive procedures that can be helpful for some patients with intractable pain. These include image-guided interventions such as epidural injection of glucocorticoids for acute radicular pain and radiofrequency treatment of the facet joints for chronic facet-related back and neck pain. For patients with severe and persistent pain that is unresponsive to more conservative treatment, placement of electrodes on peripheral nerves or within the spinal canal on nerve roots or in the space overlying the dorsal columns of the spinal cord (spinal cord stimulation) or implantation of intrathecal drug-delivery systems has shown significant benefit. The criteria for predicting which patients will respond to these procedures continue to evolve. They are generally reserved for patients who have not responded to conventional pharmacologic approaches. Referral to a multidisciplinary pain clinic for a full evaluation should precede any invasive procedure. Such referrals are clearly not necessary for all chronic pain patients. For some, pharmacologic management alone can provide adequate relief.

ANTIDEPRESSANT MEDICATIONS

The tricyclic antidepressants (TCAs), particularly nortriptyline and desipramine (Table 13-1), are useful for the management of chronic pain. Although developed for the treatment of depression, the TCAs have a spectrum of dose-related biologic activities that include analgesia in a variety of chronic clinical conditions. Although the mechanism is unknown, the analgesic effect of TCAs has a more rapid onset and occurs at a lower dose than is typically required for the treatment of depression. Furthermore, patients with chronic pain who are not depressed obtain pain relief with antidepressants. There is evidence that TCAs potentiate opioid analgesia, so they may be useful adjuncts for the treatment of severe persistent pain such as occurs with malignant tumors. **Table 13-2** lists some of the painful conditions that respond to TCAs. TCAs are of particular value in the management of neuropathic pain such as occurs in diabetic neuropathy and postherpetic neuralgia, for which there are few other therapeutic options.

The TCAs that have been shown to relieve pain have significant side effects (Table 13-1; **Chap. 452**). Some of these side effects,

TABLE 13-2 Painful Conditions That Respond to Tricyclic Antidepressants

Postherpetic neuralgia[a]
Diabetic neuropathy[a]
Fibromyalgia[a]
Tension headache[a]
Migraine headache[a]
Rheumatoid arthritis[a,b]
Chronic low back pain[b]
Cancer
Central poststroke pain

[a]Controlled trials demonstrate analgesia. [b]Controlled studies indicate benefit but not analgesia.

such as orthostatic hypotension, drowsiness, cardiac conduction delay, memory impairment, constipation, and urinary retention, are particularly problematic in elderly patients, and several are additive to the side effects of opioid analgesics. The selective serotonin reuptake inhibitors such as fluoxetine (Prozac) have fewer and less serious side effects than TCAs, but they are much less effective for relieving pain. It is of interest that venlafaxine (Effexor) and duloxetine (Cymbalta), which are nontricyclic antidepressants that block both serotonin and norepinephrine reuptake, appear to retain most of the pain-relieving effect of TCAs with a side effect profile more like that of the selective serotonin reuptake inhibitors. These drugs may be particularly useful in patients who cannot tolerate the side effects of TCAs.

ANTICONVULSANTS AND ANTIARRHYTHMICS

These drugs are useful primarily for patients with neuropathic pain. Phenytoin (Dilantin) and carbamazepine (Tegretol) were first shown to relieve the pain of trigeminal neuralgia (**Chap. 441**). This pain has a characteristic brief, shooting, electric shock-like quality. In fact, anticonvulsants seem to be particularly helpful for pains that have such a lancinating quality. Newer anticonvulsants, the calcium channel alpha-2-delta subunit ligands gabapentin (Neurontin) and pregabalin (Lyrica), are effective for a broad range of neuropathic pains. Furthermore, because of their favorable side effect profile, these newer anticonvulsants are often used as first-line agents.

CANNABINOIDS

These agents are widely used for their analgesic properties, although published evidence suggests that any effects are likely to be modest, with small increases in pain threshold reported and variable reductions in clinical pain intensity. Cannabis more consistently reduces the unpleasantness of the pain experience and, in cancer-related pain, can lessen the nausea and vomiting associated with chemotherapy use. *Marijuana and related compounds are discussed in* ***Chap. 455***.

CHRONIC OPIOID MEDICATION

The long-term use of opioids is accepted for patients with pain due to malignant disease. Although opioid use for chronic pain of nonmalignant origin is controversial, it is clear that, for many patients, opioids are the only option that produces meaningful pain relief. This is understandable because opioids are the most potent and have the broadest range of efficacy of any analgesic medications. Although addiction is rare in patients who first use opioids for pain relief, some degree of tolerance and physical dependence is likely with long-term use. Furthermore, studies suggest that long-term opioid therapy may worsen pain in some individuals, termed *opioid-induced hyperalgesia*. Therefore, before embarking on opioid therapy, other options should be explored, and the limitations and risks of opioids should be explained to the patient. It is also important to point out that some opioid analgesic medications have mixed agonist-antagonist properties (e.g., butorphanol and buprenorphine). From a practical standpoint, this means that they may worsen pain by inducing an abstinence syndrome in patients who are actively being treated with other opioids and are physically dependent.

With long-term outpatient use of orally administered opioids, it may be desirable to use long-acting compounds such as levorphanol, methadone, extended-release morphine or oxycodone, or transdermal fentanyl (Table 13-1). The pharmacokinetic profiles of these drug preparations enable the maintenance of sustained analgesic blood levels, potentially minimizing side effects such as sedation that are associated with high peak plasma levels, and reducing the likelihood of rebound pain associated with a rapid fall in plasma opioid concentration. Extended-release opioid formulations are approved primarily for patients who are already taking other opioids and should not be used as first-line opioids for pain. Although long-acting opioid preparations may provide superior pain relief in patients with a continuous pattern of ongoing pain, others suffer from intermittent severe episodic pain and experience superior pain control and fewer side effects with the periodic use of short-acting opioid analgesics. Constipation is a virtually universal side effect of opioid use and should be treated expectantly. As noted earlier in the discussion of acute pain treatment, a recent advance for patients is the development of peripherally acting opioid antagonists that can reverse the constipation associated with opioid use without interfering with analgesia.

Soon after the introduction of an extended-release oxycodone formulation (OxyContin) in the late 1990s, a dramatic rise in emergency department visits and deaths associated with oxycodone ingestion appeared. This appears to be due primarily to individuals using a prescription opioid nonmedically. Drug-induced deaths have rapidly risen and are now the second leading cause of death in Americans, just behind motor vehicle fatalities. In 2011, the Office of National Drug Control Policy established a multifaceted approach to address prescription drug abuse, including prescription drug monitoring programs (PDMPs) that allow practitioners to determine if patients are receiving prescriptions from multiple providers and use of law enforcement to eliminate improper prescribing practices. In 2016, the Centers for Disease Control and Prevention (CDC) released the *CDC Guideline for Prescribing Opioids for Chronic Pain*, with recommendations for primary care clinicians who are prescribing opioids for chronic noncancer pain. A modified approach to opioid prescribing was published in 2019 by the Health and Human Services Task Force on chronic pain best medical practices. These guidelines address (1) when to initiate or continue opioids for chronic pain; (2) opioid selection, dosage, duration, follow-up, and discontinuation; and (3) assessing risk and addressing harms of opioid use. The recent increase in scrutiny leaves many practitioners hesitant to prescribe opioid analgesics, other than for brief periods to control pain associated with illness or injury. For now, the choice to begin chronic opioid therapy for a given patient is left to the individual practitioner. Pragmatic guidelines for properly selecting and monitoring patients receiving chronic opioid therapy are shown in **Table 13-3**; a checklist for primary care clinicians prescribing opioids for noncancer pain is shown in **Table 13-4**.

TREATMENT OF NEUROPATHIC PAIN

It is important to individualize treatment for patients with neuropathic pain. Several general principles should guide therapy: the first is to move quickly to provide relief, and the second is to minimize drug side effects. For example, in patients with postherpetic neuralgia and significant cutaneous hypersensitivity, topical lidocaine (Lidoderm patches) can provide immediate relief without side effects. The anticonvulsants gabapentin or pregabalin (see above) or antidepressants (nortriptyline, desipramine, duloxetine, or venlafaxine) can be used as first-line drugs for patients with neuropathic pain. Systemically administered antiarrhythmic drugs such as lidocaine and mexiletine are less likely to be effective. Although intravenous infusion of lidocaine can provide analgesia for patients with different types of neuropathic pain, the relief is usually transient,

TABLE 13-3 Guidelines for Selecting and Monitoring Patients Receiving Chronic Opioid Therapy (COT) for the Treatment of Chronic, Noncancer Pain

Patient Selection
• Conduct a history, physical examination, and appropriate testing, including an assessment of risk of substance abuse, misuse, or addiction. • Consider a trial of COT if pain is moderate or severe, pain is having an adverse impact on function or quality of life, and potential therapeutic benefits outweigh potential harms. • A benefit-to-harm evaluation, including a history, physical examination, and appropriate diagnostic testing, should be performed and documented before and on an ongoing basis during COT.
Informed Consent and Use of Management Plans
• Informed consent should be obtained. A continuing discussion with the patient regarding COT should include goals, expectations, potential risks, and alternatives to COT. • Consider using a written COT management plan to document patient and clinician responsibilities and expectations and assist in patient education.
Initiation and Titration
• Initial treatment with opioids should be considered as a therapeutic trial to determine whether COT is appropriate. • Opioid selection, initial dosing, and titration should be individualized according to the patient's health status, previous exposure to opioids, attainment of therapeutic goals, and predicted or observed harms.
Monitoring
• Reassess patients on COT periodically and as warranted by changing circumstances. Monitoring should include documentation of pain intensity and level of functioning, assessments of progress toward achieving therapeutic goals, presence of adverse events, and adherence to prescribed therapies. • In patients on COT who are at high risk or who have engaged in aberrant drug-related behaviors, clinicians should periodically obtain urine drug screens or other information to confirm adherence to the COT plan of care. • In patients on COT not at high risk and not known to have engaged in aberrant drug-related behaviors, clinicians should consider periodically obtaining urine drug screens or other information to confirm adherence to the COT plan of care.

Source: Adapted with permission from R Chou et al: Clinical guidelines for the use of chronic opioid therapy in chronic noncancer pain. J Pain 10:113, 2009.

typically lasting just hours after the cessation of the infusion. The oral lidocaine congener mexiletine is poorly tolerated, producing frequent gastrointestinal adverse effects. There is no consensus on which class of drug should be used as a first-line treatment for any chronically painful condition. However, because relatively high doses of anticonvulsants are required for pain relief, sedation is not uncommon. Sedation is also a problem with TCAs but is much less of a problem with serotonin/norepinephrine reuptake inhibitors (SNRIs; e.g., venlafaxine and duloxetine). Thus, in the elderly or in patients whose daily activities require high-level mental activity, these drugs should be considered the first line. In contrast, opioid medications should be used as a second- or third-line drug class. Although highly effective for many painful conditions, opioids are sedating, and their effect tends to lessen over time, leading to dose escalation and, occasionally, a worsening of pain. A couple of interesting alternatives to pure opioids are two drugs with mixed opioid and norepinephrine reuptake action: tramadol and tapentadol. Tramadol is a relatively weak opioid but is sometimes effective for pain unresponsive to nonopioid analgesics. Tapentadol is a stronger opioid, but its analgesic action is apparently enhanced by the norepinephrine reuptake blockade. Similarly, drugs of different classes can be used in combination to optimize pain control. Repeated injection of botulinum toxin is an emerging approach that is showing some promise in treating focal neuropathic pain, particularly post-herpetic, trigeminal, and post-traumatic neuralgias.

It is worth emphasizing that many patients, especially those with chronic pain, seek medical attention primarily because they are

TABLE 13-4 Centers for Disease Control and Prevention Checklist for Prescribing Opioids for Chronic Pain

For Primary Care Providers Treating Adults (18+) with Chronic Pain ≥3 months, Excluding Cancer, Palliative, and End-of-Life Care
CHECKLIST
WHEN CONSIDERING LONG-TERM OPIOID THERAPY

• Set realistic goals for pain and function based on diagnosis (e.g., walk around the block).
• Check that nonopioid therapies tried and optimized.
• Discuss benefits and risks (e.g., addiction, overdose) with patient.
• Evaluate risk of harm or misuse.
  • Discuss risk factors with patient.
  • Check prescription drug monitoring program (PDMP) data.
  • Check urine drug screen.
• Set criteria for stopping or continuing opioids.
• Assess baseline pain and function (e.g., Pain, Enjoyment, General Activity [PEG] scale).
• Schedule initial reassessment within 1–4 weeks.
• Prescribe short-acting opioids using lowest dosage on product labeling; match duration to scheduled reassessment.

IF RENEWING WITHOUT A PATIENT VISIT
• Check that return visit is scheduled ≤3 months from last visit.
WHEN REASSESSING AT A PATIENT VISIT

• Continue opioids only after confirming clinically meaningful improvements in pain and function without significant risks or harm.
• Assess pain and function (e.g., PEG); compare results to baseline.
• Evaluate risk of harm or misuse:
  • Observe patient for signs of oversedation or overdose risk. If yes: Taper dose.
  • Check PDMP.
  • Check for opioid use disorder if indicated (e.g., difficulty controlling use). If yes: Refer for treatment.
• Check that nonopioid therapies optimized. Determine whether to continue, adjust, taper, or stop opioids.
• Calculate opioid dosage morphine milligram equivalent (MME).
  • If ≥50 MME/day total (≥50 mg hydrocodone; ≥33 mg oxycodone), increase frequency of follow-up; consider offering naloxone.
  • Avoid ≥90 MME/day total (≥90 mg hydrocodone; ≥60 mg oxycodone), or carefully justify; consider specialist referral.
• Schedule reassessment at regular intervals (≤3 months).

Source: Centers for Disease Control and Prevention, available at: *https://stacks.cdc.gov/view/cdc/38025*. Accessed May 25, 2017 (Public Domain).

suffering and because only physicians can provide the medications required for pain relief. A primary responsibility of all physicians is to minimize the physical and emotional discomfort of their patients. Familiarity with pain mechanisms and analgesic medications is an important step toward accomplishing this aim.

FURTHER READING

De Vita MJ et al: Association of cannabinoid administration with experimental pain in healthy adults a systematic review and meta-analysis. JAMA Psychiatry 75:1118, 2018.

Dowell D et al: CDC guideline for prescribing opioids for chronic pain—United States, 2016. JAMA 315:1624, 2016.

Finnerup NB et al: Pharmacotherapy for neuropathic pain in adults: A systematic review and meta-analysis. Lancet Neurol 14:162, 2015.

Sun EC et al: Incidence of and risk factors for chronic opioid use among opioid-naive patients in the postoperative period. JAMA Intern Med 176:1286, 2016.

U.S. Department of Health and Human Services: Pain management best practices inter-agency task force report: Updates, gaps, inconsistencies, and recommendations. May 2019. *https://www.hhs.gov/ash/advisory-committees/pain/reports/index.html.*

14 Chest Discomfort

David A. Morrow

Chest discomfort is among the most common reasons for which patients present for medical attention at either an emergency department (ED) or an outpatient clinic. The evaluation of nontraumatic chest discomfort is inherently challenging owing to the broad variety of possible causes, a minority of which are life-threatening conditions that should not be missed. It is helpful to frame the initial diagnostic assessment and triage of patients with acute chest discomfort around three categories: (1) myocardial ischemia; (2) other cardiopulmonary causes (myopericardial disease, aortic emergencies, and pulmonary conditions); and (3) noncardiopulmonary causes. Although rapid identification of high-risk conditions is a priority of the initial assessment, strategies that incorporate routine liberal use of testing carry the potential for adverse effects of unnecessary investigations.

EPIDEMIOLOGY AND NATURAL HISTORY

Chest discomfort is one of the three most common reason for visits to the ED in the United States, resulting in 6 to 7 million emergency visits each year. More than 60% of patients with this presentation are hospitalized for further testing, and most of the remainder undergo additional investigation in the ED. Fewer than 15% of evaluated patients are eventually diagnosed with acute coronary syndrome (ACS), with rates of 10–20% in most series of unselected populations, and a rate as low as 5% in some studies. The most common diagnoses are gastrointestinal causes (**Fig. 14-1**), and as few as 5% are other life-threatening cardiopulmonary conditions. In a large proportion of patients with transient acute chest discomfort, ACS or another acute cardiopulmonary cause is excluded but the cause is not determined. Therefore, the resources and time devoted to the evaluation of chest discomfort *in the absence of a severe cause* are substantial. Nevertheless, historically, a disconcerting 2–6% of patients with chest discomfort of presumed nonischemic etiology who are discharged from the ED were later deemed to have had a missed myocardial infarction (MI). Patients with a missed diagnosis of MI have a 30-day risk of death that is double that of their counterparts who are hospitalized.

The natural histories of ACS, myocarditis, acute pericardial diseases, pulmonary embolism, and aortic emergencies are discussed in **Chaps. 270, 273, 274, 275, 279, and 280**, respectively. In a study of more than 350,000 patients with unspecified presumed noncardiopulmonary chest discomfort, the mortality rate 1 year after discharge was <2% and did not differ significantly from age-adjusted mortality in the general population. The estimated rate of major cardiovascular events through 30 days in patients with acute chest pain who had been stratified as low risk was 2.5% in a large population-based study that excluded patients with ST-segment elevation or definite noncardiac chest pain.

CAUSES OF CHEST DISCOMFORT

The major etiologies of chest discomfort are discussed in this section and summarized in **Table 14-1**. Additional elements of the history, physical examination, and diagnostic testing that aid in distinguishing these causes are discussed in a later section (see "Approach to the Patient").

■ MYOCARDIAL ISCHEMIA/INJURY

Myocardial ischemia causing chest discomfort, termed *angina pectoris*, is a primary clinical concern in patients presenting with chest symptoms. Myocardial ischemia is precipitated by an imbalance between myocardial oxygen requirements and myocardial oxygen supply, resulting in insufficient delivery of oxygen to meet the heart's metabolic demands. Myocardial oxygen consumption may be elevated by increases in heart rate, ventricular wall stress, and myocardial contractility, whereas myocardial oxygen supply is determined by coronary blood flow and coronary arterial oxygen content. When myocardial ischemia is sufficiently severe and prolonged in duration (as little as 20 min), irreversible cellular injury occurs, resulting in MI.

Ischemic heart disease is most commonly caused by atheromatous plaque that obstructs one or more of the epicardial coronary arteries. Stable ischemic heart disease (**Chap. 273**) usually results from the gradual atherosclerotic narrowing of the coronary arteries. *Stable angina* is characterized by ischemic episodes that are typically precipitated by a superimposed increase in oxygen demand during physical exertion and relieved upon resting. Ischemic heart disease becomes unstable, manifest by ischemia at rest or with an escalating pattern, most commonly when rupture or erosion of one or more atherosclerotic lesions triggers coronary thrombosis. Unstable ischemic heart disease is further classified clinically by the presence or absence of detectable acute myocardial injury and the presence or absence of ST-segment elevation on the patient's electrocardiogram (ECG). When acute coronary atherothrombosis occurs, the intracoronary thrombus may be partially obstructive, generally leading to myocardial ischemia in the absence of ST-segment elevation. Unstable ischemic heart disease is classified as *unstable angina* when there is no detectable acute myocardial injury and as *non–ST elevation MI* (NSTEMI) when there is evidence of acute myocardial necrosis (**Chap. 274**). When the coronary thrombus is acutely and completely occlusive, transmural myocardial ischemia usually ensues, with ST-segment elevation on the ECG and myocardial necrosis leading to a diagnosis of *ST elevation MI* (STEMI; see **Chap. 275**).

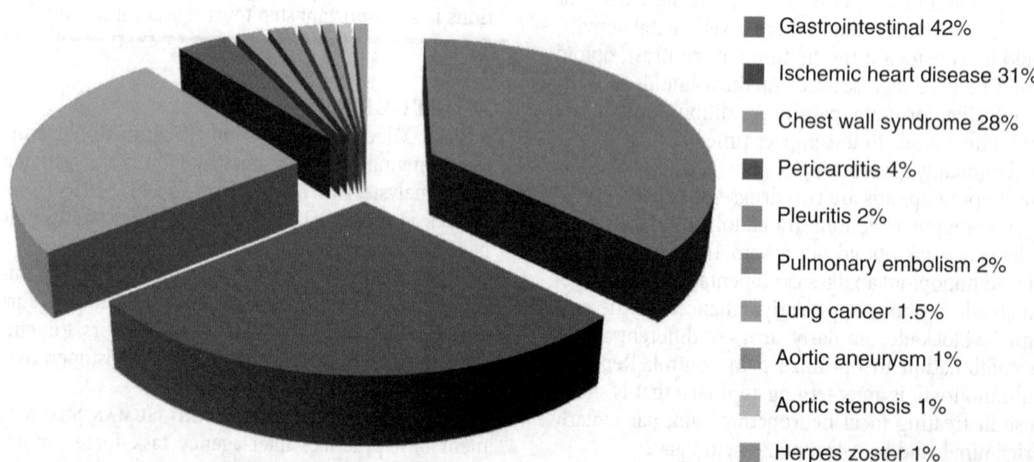

FIGURE 14-1 Distribution of final discharge diagnoses in patients with nontraumatic acute chest pain. *(Figure prepared from data in P Fruergaard et al: Eur Heart J 17:1028, 1996.)*

PART 2 Cardinal Manifestations and Presentation of Diseases

TABLE 14-1 Typical Clinical Features of Major Causes of Acute Chest Discomfort

SYSTEM	CONDITION	ONSET/DURATION	QUALITY	LOCATION	ASSOCIATED FEATURES
Cardiopulmonary					
Cardiac	Myocardial ischemia	*Stable angina:* Precipitated by exertion, cold, or stress; 2–10 min *Unstable angina:* Increasing pattern or at rest *Myocardial infarction:* Usually >30 min	Pressure, tightness, squeezing, heaviness, burning	Retrosternal; often radiation to neck, jaw, shoulders, or arms; sometimes epigastric	S_4 gallop or mitral regurgitation murmur (rare) during pain; S_3 or rales if severe ischemia or complication of myocardial infarction
	Pericarditis	Variable; hours to days; may be episodic	Pleuritic, sharp	Retrosternal or toward cardiac apex; may radiate to left shoulder	May be relieved by sitting up and leaning forward; pericardial friction rub
Vascular	Acute aortic syndrome	Sudden onset of unrelenting pain	Tearing or ripping; knifelike	Anterior chest, often radiating to back, between shoulder blades	Associated with hypertension and/or underlying connective tissue disorder; murmur of aortic insufficiency; loss of peripheral pulses
	Pulmonary embolism	Sudden onset	Pleuritic; may manifest as heaviness with massive pulmonary embolism	Often lateral, on the side of the embolism	Dyspnea, tachypnea, tachycardia, and hypotension
	Pulmonary hypertension	Variable; often exertional	Pressure	Substernal	Dyspnea, signs of increased venous pressure
Pulmonary	Pneumonia or pleuritis	Variable	Pleuritic	Unilateral, often localized	Dyspnea, cough, fever, rales, occasional rub
	Spontaneous pneumothorax	Sudden onset	Pleuritic	Lateral to side of pneumothorax	Dyspnea, decreased breath sounds on side of pneumothorax
Noncardiopulmonary					
Gastrointestinal	Esophageal reflux	10–60 min	Burning	Substernal, epigastric	Worsened by postprandial recumbency; relieved by antacids
	Esophageal spasm	2–30 min	Pressure, tightness, burning	Retrosternal	Can closely mimic angina
	Peptic ulcer	Prolonged; 60–90 min after meals	Burning	Epigastric, substernal	Relieved with food or antacids
	Gallbladder disease	Prolonged	Aching or colicky	Epigastric, right upper quadrant; sometimes to the back	May follow meal
Neuromuscular	Costochondritis	Variable	Aching	Sternal	Sometimes swollen, tender, warm over joint; may be reproduced by localized pressure on examination
	Cervical disk disease	Variable; may be sudden	Aching; may include numbness	Arms and shoulders	May be exacerbated by movement of neck
	Trauma or strain	Usually constant	Aching	Localized to area of strain	Reproduced by movement or palpation
	Herpes zoster	Usually prolonged	Sharp or burning	Dermatomal distribution	Vesicular rash in area of discomfort
Psychological	Emotional and psychiatric conditions	Variable; may be fleeting or prolonged	Variable; often manifests as tightness and dyspnea with feeling of panic or doom	Variable; may be retrosternal	Situational factors may precipitate symptoms; history of panic attacks, depression

Clinicians should be aware that unstable ischemic symptoms may also occur predominantly because of increased myocardial oxygen demand (e.g., during intense psychological stress or fever) or because of decreased oxygen delivery due to anemia, hypoxia, or hypotension. However, the term *acute coronary syndrome*, which encompasses unstable angina, NSTEMI, and STEMI, is in general reserved for ischemia precipitated by acute coronary atherothrombosis. In order to guide therapeutic strategies, a standardized system for classification of MI has been expanded to discriminate MI resulting from acute coronary thrombosis (type 1 MI) from MI occurring secondary to other imbalances of myocardial oxygen supply and demand (type 2 MI; see **Chap. 274**). These conditions are additionally distinguished from nonischemic causes of acute myocardial injury, such as myocarditis.

Other contributors to stable and unstable ischemic heart disease, such as endothelial dysfunction, microvascular disease, and vasospasm, may exist alone or in combination with coronary atherosclerosis and may be the dominant cause of myocardial ischemia in some patients. Moreover, nonatherosclerotic processes, including congenital abnormalities of the coronary vessels, myocardial bridging, coronary arteritis, and radiation-induced coronary disease, can lead to coronary obstruction. In addition, conditions associated with extreme myocardial oxygen demand and impaired endocardial blood flow, such as aortic valve disease (**Chap. 280**), hypertrophic cardiomyopathy, or idiopathic dilated cardiomyopathy (**Chap. 259**), can precipitate myocardial ischemia in patients with or without underlying obstructive atherosclerosis.

Characteristics of Ischemic Chest Discomfort The clinical characteristics of angina pectoris, often referred to simply as "angina," are highly similar whether the ischemic discomfort is a manifestation of stable ischemic heart disease, unstable angina, or MI; the exceptions are differences in the pattern and duration of symptoms associated with these syndromes (Table 14-1). Heberden initially described angina as a sense of "strangling and anxiety." Chest discomfort characteristic of myocardial ischemia is typically described as aching, heavy, squeezing, crushing, or constricting. However, in a substantial minority of patients, the quality of discomfort is extremely vague and may be described as a mild tightness, or merely an uncomfortable feeling, that sometimes is experienced as numbness or a burning sensation. The site of the discomfort is usually retrosternal, but radiation is common and generally occurs down the ulnar surface of the left arm; the right arm, both arms, neck, jaw, or shoulders may also be involved. These and other characteristics of ischemic chest discomfort pertinent to discrimination from other causes of chest pain are discussed later in this chapter (see "Approach to the Patient").

Stable angina usually begins gradually and reaches its maximal intensity over a period of minutes before dissipating within several minutes with rest or with nitroglycerin. The discomfort typically occurs predictably at a characteristic level of exertion or psychological stress. By definition, unstable angina is manifest by anginal chest discomfort that occurs with progressively lower intensity of physical activity or even at rest. Chest discomfort associated with MI is commonly more severe, is prolonged (usually lasting ≥30 min), and is not relieved by rest.

Mechanisms of Cardiac Pain The neural pathways involved in ischemic cardiac pain are poorly understood. Ischemic episodes are thought to excite local chemosensitive and mechanoreceptive receptors that, in turn, stimulate release of adenosine, bradykinin, and other substances that activate the sensory ends of sympathetic and vagal afferent fibers. The afferent fibers traverse the nerves that connect to the upper five thoracic sympathetic ganglia and upper five distal thoracic roots of the spinal cord. From there, impulses are transmitted to the thalamus. Within the spinal cord, cardiac sympathetic afferent impulses may converge with impulses from somatic thoracic structures, and this convergence may be the basis for referred cardiac pain. In addition, cardiac vagal afferent fibers synapse in the nucleus tractus solitarius of the medulla and then descend to the upper cervical spinothalamic tract, and this route may contribute to anginal pain experienced in the neck and jaw.

OTHER CARDIOPULMONARY CAUSES

Pericardial and Other Myocardial Diseases (See also Chap. 270) Inflammation of the pericardium due to infectious or noninfectious causes can be responsible for acute or chronic chest discomfort. The visceral surface and most of the parietal surface of the pericardium are insensitive to pain. Therefore, the pain of pericarditis is thought to arise principally from associated pleural inflammation. Because of this pleural association, the discomfort of pericarditis is usually pleuritic pain that is exacerbated by breathing, coughing, or changes in position. Moreover, owing to the overlapping sensory supply of the central diaphragm via the phrenic nerve with somatic sensory fibers originating in the third to fifth cervical segments, the pain of pleural and pericardial inflammation is often referred to the shoulder and neck. Involvement of the pleural surface of the lateral diaphragm can lead to pain in the upper abdomen.

Acute inflammatory and other nonischemic myocardial diseases can also produce chest discomfort. The symptoms of acute myocarditis are highly varied. Chest discomfort may either originate with inflammatory injury of the myocardium or be due to severe increases in wall stress related to poor ventricular performance. The symptoms of *Takotsubo (stress-related) cardiomyopathy* often start abruptly with chest pain and shortness of breath. This form of cardiomyopathy, in its most recognizable form, is triggered by an emotionally or physically stressful event and may mimic acute MI because of its commonly associated ECG abnormalities, including ST-segment elevation, and elevated biomarkers of myocardial injury. Observational studies support a predilection for women >50 years of age.

Diseases of the Aorta (See also Chap. 280) Acute aortic dissection (Fig. 14-1) is a less common cause of chest discomfort but is important because of the catastrophic natural history of certain subsets of cases when recognized late or left untreated. Acute aortic syndromes encompass a spectrum of acute aortic diseases related to disruption of the media of the aortic wall. *Aortic dissection* involves a tear in the aortic intima, resulting in separation of the media and creation of a separate "false" lumen. A *penetrating ulcer* has been described as ulceration of an aortic atheromatous plaque that extends through the intima and into the aortic media, with the potential to initiate an intramedial dissection or rupture into the adventitia. *Intramural hematoma* is an aortic wall hematoma with no demonstrable intimal flap, no radiologically apparent intimal tear, and no false lumen. Intramural hematoma can occur due to either rupture of the vasa vasorum or, less commonly, a penetrating ulcer.

Each of these subtypes of acute aortic syndrome typically presents with chest discomfort that is often severe, sudden in onset, and sometimes described as "tearing" in quality. Acute aortic syndromes involving the *ascending* aorta tend to cause pain in the midline of the anterior chest, whereas *descending* aortic syndromes most often present with pain in the back. Therefore, dissections that begin in the ascending aorta and extend to the descending aorta tend to cause pain in the front of the chest that extends toward the back, between the shoulder blades. Proximal aortic dissections that involve the ascending aorta (type A in the Stanford nomenclature) are at high risk for major complications that may influence the clinical presentation, including (1) compromise of the aortic ostia of the coronary arteries, resulting in MI; (2) disruption of the aortic valve, causing acute aortic insufficiency; and (3) rupture of the hematoma into the pericardial space, leading to pericardial tamponade.

Knowledge of the epidemiology of acute aortic syndromes can be helpful in maintaining awareness of this relatively uncommon group of disorders (estimated annual incidence, 3 cases per 100,000 population). Nontraumatic aortic dissections are very rare in the absence of hypertension or conditions associated with deterioration of the elastic or muscular components of the aortic media, including pregnancy, bicuspid aortic disease, or inherited connective tissue diseases, such as Marfan and Ehlers-Danlos syndromes.

Although aortic aneurysms are most often asymptomatic, thoracic aortic aneurysms can cause chest pain and other symptoms by compressing adjacent structures. This pain tends to be steady, deep, and occasionally severe. Aortitis, whether of noninfectious or infectious etiology, in the absence of aortic dissection is a rare cause of chest or back discomfort.

Pulmonary Conditions Pulmonary and pulmonary-vascular conditions that cause chest discomfort usually do so in conjunction with dyspnea and often produce symptoms that have a pleuritic nature.

PULMONARY EMBOLISM (SEE ALSO CHAP. 279) Pulmonary emboli (annual incidence, ~1 per 1000) can produce dyspnea and chest discomfort that is sudden in onset. Typically pleuritic in pattern, the chest discomfort associated with pulmonary embolism may result from (1) involvement of the pleural surface of the lung adjacent to a resultant pulmonary infarction; (2) distention of the pulmonary artery; or (3) possibly, right ventricular wall stress and/or subendocardial ischemia related to acute pulmonary hypertension. The pain associated with small pulmonary emboli is often lateral and pleuritic and is believed to be related to the first of these three possible mechanisms. In contrast, massive pulmonary emboli may cause severe substernal pain that may mimic an MI and that is plausibly attributed to the second and third of these potential mechanisms. Massive or submassive pulmonary embolism may also be associated with syncope, hypotension, and signs of right heart failure. Other typical characteristics that aid in the recognition of pulmonary embolism are discussed later in this chapter (see "Approach to the Patient").

PNEUMOTHORAX (SEE ALSO CHAP. 294) *Primary spontaneous pneumothorax* is a rare cause of chest discomfort, with an estimated annual incidence in the United States of 7 per 100,000 among men and <2 per 100,000 among women. Risk factors include male sex, smoking, family history, and Marfan syndrome. The symptoms are usually sudden in onset, and dyspnea may be mild; thus, presentation to medical attention is sometimes delayed. *Secondary spontaneous pneumothorax* may occur in patients with underlying lung disorders, such as chronic obstructive pulmonary disease, asthma, or cystic fibrosis, and usually produces symptoms that are more severe. Tension pneumothorax is a medical emergency caused by trapped intrathoracic air that precipitates hemodynamic collapse.

Other Pulmonary Parenchymal, Pleural, or Vascular Disease (See also Chaps. 283, 284, and 294) Most pulmonary diseases that produce chest pain, including pneumonia and malignancy, do so because of involvement of the pleura or surrounding structures. Pleurisy is typically described as a knifelike pain that is worsened by inspiration or coughing. In contrast, chronic pulmonary hypertension can manifest as chest pain that may be very similar to angina in its characteristics, suggesting right ventricular myocardial ischemia in some cases. Reactive airways diseases similarly can cause chest tightness associated with breathlessness rather than pleurisy.

NONCARDIOPULMONARY CAUSES

Gastrointestinal Conditions (See also Chap. 321) Gastrointestinal disorders are the most common cause of nontraumatic chest discomfort and often produce symptoms that are difficult to discern from more serious causes of chest pain, including myocardial ischemia. Esophageal disorders, in particular, may simulate angina in the character and location of the pain. Gastroesophageal reflux and disorders of esophageal motility are common and should be considered in the differential diagnosis of chest pain (Fig. 14-1 and Table 14-1). The pain of esophageal spasm is commonly an intense, squeezing discomfort that is retrosternal in location and, like angina, may be relieved by nitroglycerin or dihydropyridine calcium channel antagonists. Chest pain can also result from injury to the esophagus, such as a Mallory-Weiss tear or even an esophageal rupture (Boerhaave's syndrome) caused by severe vomiting. Peptic ulcer disease is most commonly epigastric in location but can radiate into the chest (Table 14-1).

Hepatobiliary disorders, including cholecystitis and biliary colic, may mimic acute cardiopulmonary diseases. Although the pain arising from these disorders usually localizes to the right upper quadrant of the abdomen, it is variable and may be felt in the epigastrium and radiate to the back and lower chest. This discomfort is sometimes referred to the scapula or may in rare cases be felt in the shoulder, suggesting diaphragmatic irritation. The pain is steady, usually lasts several hours, and subsides spontaneously, without symptoms between attacks. Pain resulting from pancreatitis is typically aching epigastric pain that radiates to the back.

Musculoskeletal and Other Causes (See also Chap. 360) Chest discomfort can be produced by any musculoskeletal disorder involving the chest wall or the nerves of the chest wall, neck, or upper limbs. Costochondritis causing tenderness of the costochondral junctions (*Tietze's syndrome*) is relatively common. Cervical radiculitis may manifest as a prolonged or constant aching discomfort in the upper chest and limbs. The pain may be exacerbated by motion of the neck. Occasionally, chest pain can be caused by compression of the brachial plexus by the cervical ribs, and tendinitis or bursitis involving the left shoulder may mimic the radiation of angina. Pain in a dermatomal distribution can also be caused by cramping of intercostal muscles or by herpes zoster (**Chap. 193**).

Emotional and Psychiatric Conditions As many as 10% of patients who present to EDs with acute chest discomfort have a panic disorder or related condition (Table 14-1). The symptoms may include chest tightness or aching that is associated with a sense of anxiety and difficulty breathing. The symptoms may be prolonged or fleeting.

APPROACH TO THE PATIENT

Chest Discomfort

Given the broad set of potential causes and the heterogeneous risk of serious complications in patients who present with acute nontraumatic chest discomfort, the priorities of the initial clinical encounter include assessment of (1) the patient's clinical stability and (2) the probability that the patient has an underlying cause of the discomfort that may be life-threatening. The high-risk conditions of principal concern are acute cardiopulmonary processes, including ACS, acute aortic syndrome, pulmonary embolism, tension pneumothorax, and pericarditis with tamponade. Fulminant myocarditis also carries a poor prognosis but is usually also manifest by heart failure symptoms. Among noncardiopulmonary causes of chest pain, esophageal rupture likely holds the greatest urgency for diagnosis. Patients with these conditions may deteriorate rapidly despite initially appearing well. The remaining population with noncardiopulmonary conditions has a more favorable prognosis during completion of the diagnostic workup. A rapid targeted assessment for a serious cardiopulmonary cause is of particular relevance for patients with acute ongoing pain who have presented for emergency evaluation. Among patients presenting in the outpatient setting with chronic pain or pain that has resolved, a general diagnostic assessment is reasonably undertaken (see "Outpatient Evaluation of Chest Discomfort," below). A series of questions that can be used to structure the clinical evaluation of patients with chest discomfort is shown in **Table 14-2**.

HISTORY

The evaluation of nontraumatic chest discomfort relies heavily on the clinical history and physical examination to direct subsequent diagnostic testing. The evaluating clinician should assess the quality, location (including radiation), and pattern (including onset and duration) of the pain as well as any provoking or alleviating factors. The presence of associated symptoms may also be useful in establishing a diagnosis.

Quality of Pain The quality of chest discomfort alone is never sufficient to establish a diagnosis. However, the characteristics of the pain are pivotal in formulating an initial clinical impression and assessing the likelihood of a serious cardiopulmonary process

TABLE 14-2 Considerations in the Assessment of the Patient with Chest Discomfort

1. Could the chest discomfort be due to an acute, potentially life-threatening condition that warrants urgent evaluation and management?			
Unstable ischemic heart disease	Aortic dissection	Pneumothorax	Pulmonary embolism
2. If not, could the discomfort be due to a chronic condition likely to lead to serious complications?			
Stable angina	Aortic stenosis	Pulmonary hypertension	
3. If not, could the discomfort be due to an acute condition that warrants specific treatment?			
Pericarditis	Pneumonia/pleuritis	Herpes zoster	
4. If not, could the discomfort be due to another treatable chronic condition?			
Esophageal reflux		Cervical disk disease	
Esophageal spasm		Arthritis of the shoulder or spine	
Peptic ulcer disease		Costochondritis	
Gallbladder disease		Other musculoskeletal disorders	
Other gastrointestinal conditions		Anxiety state	

Source: Developed by Dr. Thomas H. Lee for the 18th edition of *Harrison's Principles of Internal Medicine*.

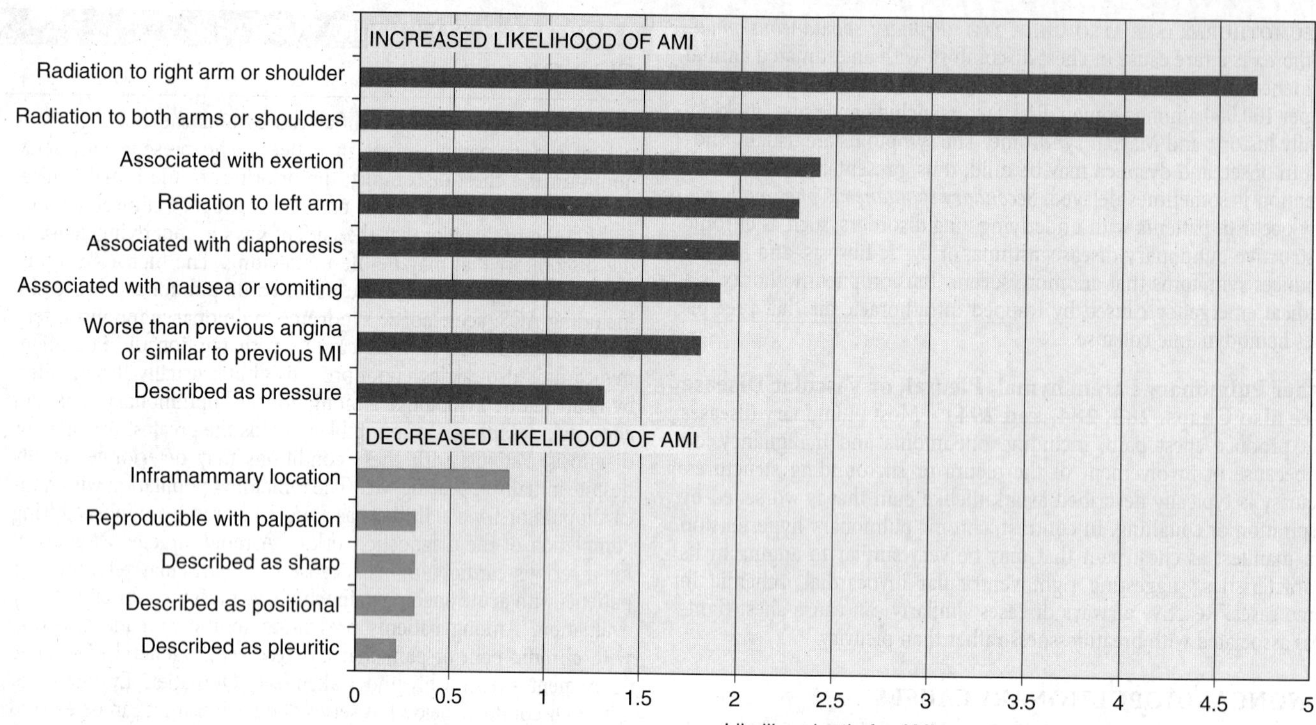

FIGURE 14-2 Association of chest pain characteristics with the probability of acute myocardial infarction (AMI). Note that a subsequent larger study showed a nonsignificant association with radiation to the right arm. *(Figure prepared from data in CJ Swap, JT Nagurney: JAMA 294:2623, 2005.)*

(Table 14-1), including ACS in particular (Fig. 14-2). Pressure or tightness is consistent with a typical presentation of myocardial ischemic pain. Nevertheless, the clinician must remember that some patients with ischemic chest symptoms deny any "pain" but rather complain of dyspnea or a vague sense of anxiety. The severity of the discomfort has poor diagnostic accuracy. It is often helpful to ask about the similarity of the discomfort to previous definite ischemic symptoms. It is unusual for angina to be sharp, as in knifelike, stabbing, or pleuritic; however, patients sometimes use the word "sharp" to convey the intensity of discomfort rather than the quality. Pleuritic discomfort is suggestive of a process involving the pleura, including pericarditis, pulmonary embolism, or pulmonary parenchymal processes. Less frequently, the pain of pericarditis or massive pulmonary embolism is a steady severe pressure or aching that can be difficult to discriminate from myocardial ischemia. "Tearing" or "ripping" pain is often described by patients with acute aortic dissection. However, acute aortic emergencies also present commonly with knifelike pain. A burning quality can suggest acid reflux or peptic ulcer disease but may also occur with myocardial ischemia. Esophageal pain, particularly with spasm, can be a severe squeezing discomfort identical to angina.

Location of Discomfort A substernal location with radiation to the neck, jaw, shoulder, or arms is typical of myocardial ischemic discomfort. Radiation to both arms has a particularly high association with MI as the etiology. Some patients present with aching in sites of radiated pain as their only symptoms of ischemia. However, pain that is highly localized—e.g., that which can be demarcated by the tip of one finger—is highly unusual for angina. A retrosternal location should prompt consideration of esophageal pain; however, other gastrointestinal conditions usually present with pain that is most intense in the abdomen or epigastrium, with possible radiation into the chest. Angina may also occur in an epigastric location. Pain that occurs solely above the mandible or below the epigastrium is rarely angina. Severe pain radiating to the back, particularly between the shoulder blades, should prompt consideration of an acute aortic syndrome. Radiation to the trapezius ridge is characteristic of pericardial pain and does not usually occur with angina.

Pattern Myocardial ischemic discomfort usually builds over minutes and is exacerbated by activity and mitigated by rest. In contrast, pain that reaches its peak intensity immediately is more suggestive of aortic dissection, pulmonary embolism, or spontaneous pneumothorax. Pain that is fleeting (lasting only a few seconds) is rarely ischemic in origin. Similarly, pain that is constant in intensity for a prolonged period (many hours to days) is unlikely to represent myocardial ischemia if it occurs in the absence of other clinical consequences, such as abnormalities of the ECG, elevation of cardiac biomarkers, or clinical sequelae (e.g., heart failure or hypotension). Both myocardial ischemia and acid reflux may have their onset in the morning.

Provoking and Alleviating Factors Patients with myocardial ischemic pain usually prefer to rest, sit, or stop walking. However, clinicians should be aware of the phenomenon of "warm-up angina" in which some patients experience relief of angina as they continue at the same or even a greater level of exertion (Chap. 273). Alterations in the intensity of pain with changes in position or movement of the upper extremities and neck are less likely with myocardial ischemia and suggest a musculoskeletal etiology. The pain of pericarditis, however, often is worse in the supine position and relieved by sitting upright and leaning forward. Gastroesophageal reflux may be exacerbated by alcohol, some foods, or a reclined position. Relief can occur with sitting.

Exacerbation by eating suggests a gastrointestinal etiology such as peptic ulcer disease, cholecystitis, or pancreatitis. Peptic ulcer disease tends to become symptomatic 60–90 min after meals. However, in the setting of severe coronary atherosclerosis, redistribution of blood flow to the splanchnic vasculature after eating can trigger postprandial angina. The discomfort of acid reflux and peptic ulcer disease is usually diminished promptly by acid-reducing therapies. In contrast with its impact in some patients with angina, physical exertion is very unlikely to alter symptoms from gastrointestinal causes of chest pain. Relief of chest discomfort within minutes after administration of nitroglycerin is suggestive of but not sufficiently sensitive or specific for a definitive diagnosis of myocardial ischemia. Esophageal spasm may also be relieved promptly with nitroglycerin. A delay of >10 min before relief is obtained after nitroglycerin suggests that the symptoms either are not caused by ischemia or are caused by severe ischemia, such as during acute MI.

Associated Symptoms Symptoms that accompany myocardial ischemia may include diaphoresis, dyspnea, nausea, fatigue, faintness, and eructations. In addition, these symptoms may exist in isolation as anginal equivalents (i.e., symptoms of myocardial ischemia other than typical angina), particularly in women and the elderly. Dyspnea may occur with multiple conditions considered in the differential diagnosis of chest pain and thus is not discriminative, but the presence of dyspnea is important because it suggests a cardiopulmonary etiology. Sudden onset of significant respiratory distress should lead to consideration of pulmonary embolism and spontaneous pneumothorax. Hemoptysis may occur with pulmonary embolism or as blood-tinged frothy sputum in severe heart failure but usually points toward a pulmonary parenchymal etiology of chest symptoms. Presentation with syncope or presyncope should prompt consideration of hemodynamically significant pulmonary embolism or aortic dissection as well as ischemic arrhythmias. Although nausea and vomiting suggest a gastrointestinal disorder, these symptoms may occur in the setting of MI (more commonly inferior MI), presumably because of activation of the vagal reflex or stimulation of left ventricular receptors as part of the Bezold-Jarisch reflex.

Past Medical History The past medical history is useful in assessing the patient for risk factors for coronary atherosclerosis and venous thromboembolism (**Chap. 279**) as well as for conditions that may predispose the patient to specific disorders. For example, a history of connective tissue diseases such as Marfan syndrome should heighten the clinician's suspicion of an acute aortic syndrome or spontaneous pneumothorax. A careful history may elicit clues about depression or prior panic attacks.

PHYSICAL EXAMINATION

In addition to providing an initial assessment of the patient's clinical stability, the physical examination of patients with chest discomfort can provide direct evidence of specific etiologies of chest pain (e.g., unilateral absence of lung sounds) and can identify potential precipitants of acute cardiopulmonary causes of chest pain (e.g., uncontrolled hypertension), relevant comorbid conditions (e.g., obstructive pulmonary disease), and complications of the presenting syndrome (e.g., heart failure). However, because the findings on physical examination may be normal in patients with unstable ischemic heart disease, an unremarkable physical exam is not definitively reassuring.

General The patient's general appearance is helpful in establishing an initial impression of the severity of illness. Patients with acute MI or other acute cardiopulmonary disorders often appear anxious, uncomfortable, pale, cyanotic, or diaphoretic. Patients who are massaging or clutching their chests may describe their pain with a clenched fist held against the sternum (*Levine's sign*). Occasionally, body habitus is helpful—e.g., in patients with Marfan syndrome or the prototypical young, tall, thin man with spontaneous pneumothorax.

Vital Signs Significant tachycardia and hypotension are indicative of important hemodynamic consequences of the underlying cause of chest discomfort and should prompt a rapid survey for the most severe conditions, such as acute MI with cardiogenic shock, massive pulmonary embolism, pericarditis with tamponade, or tension pneumothorax. Acute aortic emergencies usually present with severe hypertension but may be associated with profound hypotension when there is coronary arterial compromise or dissection into the pericardium. Sinus tachycardia is an important manifestation of submassive pulmonary embolism. Tachypnea and hypoxemia point toward a pulmonary cause. The presence of low-grade fever is nonspecific because it may occur with MI and with thromboembolism in addition to infection.

Pulmonary Examination of the lungs may localize a primary pulmonary cause of chest discomfort, as in cases of pneumonia, asthma, or pneumothorax. Left ventricular dysfunction from severe ischemia/infarction as well as acute valvular complications of MI or aortic dissection can lead to pulmonary edema, which is an indicator of high risk.

Cardiac The jugular venous pulse is often normal in patients with acute myocardial ischemia but may reveal characteristic patterns with pericardial tamponade or acute right ventricular dysfunction (**Chaps. 239 and 270**). Cardiac auscultation may reveal a third or, more commonly, a fourth heart sound, reflecting myocardial systolic or diastolic dysfunction. Murmurs of mitral regurgitation or a ventricular-septal defect may indicate mechanical complications of STEMI. A murmur of aortic insufficiency may be a complication of ascending aortic dissection. Other murmurs may reveal underlying cardiac disorders contributory to ischemia (e.g., aortic stenosis or hypertrophic cardiomyopathy). Pericardial friction rubs reflect pericardial inflammation.

Abdominal Localizing tenderness on the abdominal exam is useful in identifying a gastrointestinal cause of the presenting syndrome. Abdominal findings are infrequent with purely acute cardiopulmonary problems, except in the case of right-sided heart failure leading to hepatic congestion.

Extremities Vascular pulse deficits may reflect underlying chronic atherosclerosis, which increases the likelihood of coronary artery disease. However, evidence of acute limb ischemia with loss of the pulse and pallor, particularly in the upper extremities, can indicate catastrophic consequences of aortic dissection. Unilateral lower-extremity swelling should raise suspicion about venous thromboembolism.

Musculoskeletal Pain arising from the costochondral and chondrosternal articulations may be associated with localized swelling, redness, or marked localized tenderness. Pain on palpation of these joints is usually well localized and is a useful clinical sign, although deep palpation may elicit pain in the absence of costochondritis. Although palpation of the chest wall often elicits pain in patients with various musculoskeletal conditions, it should be appreciated that chest wall tenderness does not exclude myocardial ischemia. Sensory deficits in the upper extremities may be indicative of cervical disk disease.

ELECTROCARDIOGRAPHY

Electrocardiography is crucial in the evaluation of nontraumatic chest discomfort. The ECG is pivotal for identifying patients with ongoing ischemia as the principal reason for their presentation as well as secondary cardiac complications of other disorders. Professional society guidelines recommend that an ECG be obtained within 10 min of presentation, with the primary goal of identifying patients with ST-segment elevation diagnostic of MI who are candidates for immediate interventions to restore flow in the occluded coronary artery. ST-segment depression and symmetric T-wave inversions at least 0.2 mV in depth are useful for detecting myocardial ischemia in the absence of STEMI and are also indicative of higher risk of death or recurrent ischemia. Serial performance of ECGs (every 30–60 min) is recommended in the ED evaluation of suspected ACS. In addition, an ECG with right-sided lead placement should be considered in patients with clinically suspected ischemia and a nondiagnostic standard 12-lead ECG. Despite the value of the resting ECG, its sensitivity for ischemia is poor—as low as 20% in some studies.

Abnormalities of the ST segment and T wave may occur in a variety of conditions, including pulmonary embolism, ventricular hypertrophy, acute and chronic pericarditis, myocarditis, electrolyte imbalance, and metabolic disorders. Notably, hyperventilation associated with panic disorder can also lead to nonspecific ST and T-wave abnormalities. Pulmonary embolism is most often associated with sinus tachycardia but can also lead to rightward shift of the ECG axis, manifesting as an S-wave in lead I, with a Q-wave and T-wave in lead III (**Chaps. 240 and 279**). In patients with ST-segment elevation, the presence of diffuse lead involvement not corresponding to a specific coronary anatomic distribution and PR-segment depression can aid in distinguishing pericarditis from acute MI.

CHEST RADIOGRAPHY

(See **Chap. A12**) Plain radiography of the chest is performed routinely when patients present with acute chest discomfort and selectively when individuals who are being evaluated as outpatients have subacute or chronic pain. The chest radiograph is most useful for identifying pulmonary processes, such as pneumonia or pneumothorax. Findings are often unremarkable in patients with ACS, but pulmonary edema may be evident. Other specific findings include widening of the mediastinum in some patients with aortic dissection, Hampton's hump or Westermark's sign in patients with pulmonary embolism (**Chaps. 279 and A12**), or pericardial calcification in chronic pericarditis.

CARDIAC BIOMARKERS

Laboratory testing in patients with acute chest pain is focused on the detection of myocardial injury. Such injury can be detected by the presence of circulating proteins released from damaged cardiomyocytes. Owing to the time necessary for this release, initial biomarkers of injury may be in the normal range, even in patients with STEMI. Cardiac troponin is the preferred biomarker for the diagnosis of MI and should be measured in all patients with suspected ACS. It is not necessary or advisable to measure troponin in patients without suspicion of ACS unless this test is being used specifically for risk stratification (e.g., in pulmonary embolism or heart failure).

The development of cardiac troponin assays with progressively greater analytical sensitivity has facilitated detection of substantially lower blood concentrations of troponin than was previously possible. This evolution permits earlier detection of myocardial injury and more reliable discrimination of changing values, enhances the overall accuracy of a diagnosis of MI, and improves risk stratification in suspected ACS. For these reasons, high-sensitivity assays are generally preferred over prior generation troponin assays. The greater negative predictive value of a negative troponin result with high-sensitivity assays is an advantage in the evaluation of chest pain in the ED. Rapid rule-out protocols that use serial testing and changes in troponin concentration over as short a period as 1–2 h appear to perform well for diagnosis of ACS when using a high-sensitivity troponin assay. Troponin should be measured at presentation and repeated at 1–3 h using high-sensitivity troponin and 3–6 h using conventional troponin assays. Additional troponin measurements may be warranted beyond 3–6 h when the clinical condition still suggests possible ACS or if there is diagnostic uncertainty. In patients presenting more than 2–3 h after symptom onset, a concentration of cardiac troponin, at the time of hospital presentation, below the limit of detection using a high-sensitivity assay may be sufficient to exclude MI with a negative predictive value >99%.

With the use of high-sensitivity assays for troponin, myocardial injury is detected in a larger proportion of patients who have non-ACS cardiopulmonary conditions than with previous, less sensitive assays. Therefore, other aspects of the clinical evaluation are critical to the practitioner's determination of the probability that the symptoms represent ACS. In addition, observation of a change in cardiac troponin concentration between serial samples is necessary for discriminating acute causes of myocardial injury from chronic elevation due to underlying structural heart disease, end-stage renal disease, or the rare presence of interfering antibodies. The diagnosis of MI is reserved for acute myocardial injury that is marked by a rising and/or falling pattern—with at least one value exceeding the 99th percentile reference limit—*and that is caused by ischemia*. Other nonischemic insults, such as myocarditis, may result in acute myocardial injury but should not be labeled MI (**Fig. 14-3**).

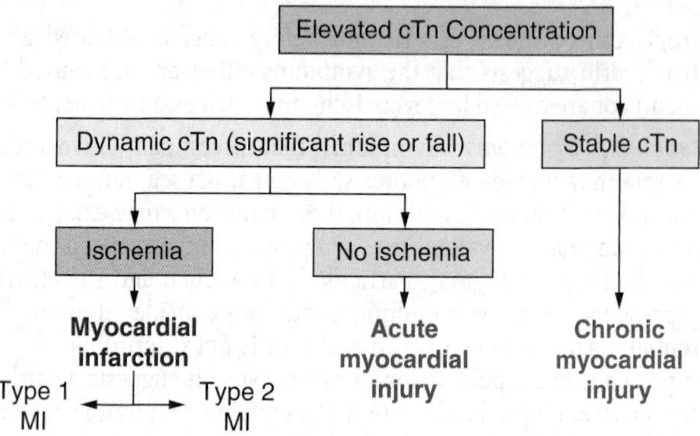

FIGURE 14-3 Clinical classification of patients with elevated cardiac troponin (cTn). MI, myocardial infarction.

Other laboratory assessments may include the D-dimer test to aid in exclusion of pulmonary embolism (**Chap. 279**). Measurement of a B-type natriuretic peptide is useful when considered in conjunction with the clinical history and exam for the diagnosis of heart failure. B-type natriuretic peptides also provide prognostic information among patients with ACS and those with pulmonary embolism.

INTEGRATIVE DECISION-AIDS

Multiple clinical algorithms have been developed to aid in decision-making during the evaluation and disposition of patients with acute nontraumatic chest pain. Such decision-aids estimate either of two closely related but not identical probabilities: (1) the probability of a final diagnosis of ACS and (2) the probability of major cardiac events during short-term follow-up. Such decision-aids are used most commonly to identify patients with a low clinical probability of ACS who are candidates for discharge from the ED, with or without additional noninvasive testing. Goldman and Lee developed one of the first such decision-aids, using only the ECG and risk indicators—hypotension, pulmonary rales, and known ischemic heart disease—to categorize patients into four risk categories ranging from a <1% to a >16% probability of a major cardiovascular complication. Decision-aids used more commonly in current practice are shown in **Fig. 14-4**. Elements common across multiple risk stratification tools are (1) symptoms typical for ACS; (2) older age; (3) risk factors for or known atherosclerosis; (4) ischemic ECG abnormalities; and (5) elevated cardiac troponin level. Although, because of very low specificity, the overall diagnostic performance of such decision-aids is poor (area under the receiver operating curve, 0.55–0.65), in conjunction with the ECG and serial high-sensitivity cardiac troponin, they can help identify patients with a very low probability of ACS (e.g., <1%) or adverse cardiovascular events (<2% at 30 days). Clinical application of such integrated decision-aids or "accelerated diagnostic protocols" has been reported to achieve overall "miss rates" for ACS of <0.5% and may be useful for identifying patients who may be discharged without the need for additional cardiac testing.

Clinicians should differentiate between the algorithms discussed above and risk scores derived for stratification of prognosis (e.g., the TIMI and GRACE risk scores, **Chap. 275**) in patients *who already have an established diagnosis of ACS*. The latter risk scores were not designed to be used for *diagnostic* assessment.

CORONARY AND MYOCARDIAL STRESS IMAGING

Among patients for whom other life-threatening causes of chest pain have been reasonably excluded and serial biomarker and clinical assessment have determined the patient to remain eligible for further testing because of intermediate or undetermined risk, diagnostic coronary imaging with coronary computed tomographic (CT) angiography or functional testing, preferably with nuclear or echocardiographic imaging, is recommended. Patient characteristics (e.g., body habitus and renal function), prior cardiac testing,

HEART Score (without cTn)		
History	Highly suspicious Moderately suspicious Slightly suspicious	2 1 0
ECG	Significant ST depression Nonspecific abnormality Normal	2 1 0
Age	≥65 y 45–<65 y <45 y	2 1 0
Risk factors	≥3 risk factors 1–2 risk factors None	2 1 0
	TOTAL	
	Low risk: 0–3 **Not low risk:** ≥4	

EDACS Score		
Age	86+ y 81–85 y 76–80 y Step down by 5-y increments 46–50 y 18–45 y	20 18 16 (–2) 4 2
Known CAD or risk factors	Known CAD (prior MI, PCI, or CABG) or ≥3 cardiac risk factors in patient aged ≤50 y	4
Sex	Male Female	6 0
Symptoms	Radiation to arm, shoulder, neck, or jaw Diaphoresis Pain with inspiration Reproduced by palpation	5 3 –4 –6
	TOTAL	
	Low risk: 0–15 **Not low risk:** ≥16	

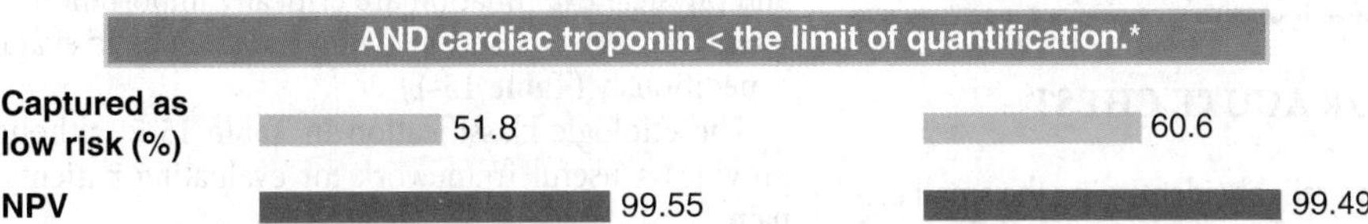

FIGURE 14-4 Examples of decision-aids used in conjunction with serial measurement of cardiac troponin (cTn) for evaluation of acute chest pain. The HEART score was modified by the authors in the presented study and omitting the assignment of 0, 1, or 2 points based on troponin. The negative predictive value (NPV) reported is for the composite endpoint of myocardial infarction (MI), cardiogenic shock, cardiac arrest, and all-cause mortality by 60 days. *Limit of quantification is the lowest analyte concentration that can be quantitatively detected with a total imprecision of ≤20%. CABG, coronary artery bypass graft; CAD, coronary artery disease; ECG, electrocardiogram; PCI, percutaneous coronary intervention. *(Figure prepared from data in DG Mark et al: J Am Coll Cardiol 13:606, 2018.)*

history of known coronary artery disease, existing contraindications for a given test modality, and patient preferences are considerations when choosing among these diagnostic tests (**Chaps. 241 and A9**).

CT Angiography (See Chap. 241) CT angiography has emerged as a preferred modality for the evaluation of patients with acute chest discomfort who are candidates for further testing after biomarker and clinical risk assessment. Coronary CT angiography is a sensitive technique for detection of obstructive coronary disease. CT appears to enhance the speed to disposition of patients with a low-intermediate probability for ACS, with its major strength being the negative predictive value of a finding of no significant stenosis or coronary plaque. In addition, contrast-enhanced CT can detect focal areas of myocardial injury in the acute setting. At the same time, CT angiography can exclude aortic dissection, pericardial effusion, and pulmonary embolism.

Stress Nuclear Perfusion Imaging or Stress Echocardiography (See Chaps. 241 and A9) Functional testing with stress nuclear perfusion imaging and stress echocardiography are alternatives for the evaluation of patients with acute chest pain who are candidates for further testing and are preferred over coronary CT angiography in patients with known obstructive epicardial disease. The selection of stress test modality may depend on institutional availability and expertise. Stress testing with myocardial imaging, either with nuclear perfusion imaging or echocardiography, offers superior diagnostic performance over exercise ECG. In patients selected for stress myocardial imaging who are able to exercise, exercise stress is preferred over pharmacologic testing. When available, positron emission tomography offers advantages of improved diagnostic performance and fewer nondiagnostic studies than single-photon emission CT.

Although functional testing is generally contraindicated in patients with ongoing chest pain, in selected patients with persistent pain and nondiagnostic ECG and biomarker data, resting myocardial perfusion images can be obtained; the absence of any perfusion abnormality substantially reduces the likelihood of coronary artery disease. In such a strategy, used in some centers, those with abnormal rest perfusion imaging, which cannot discriminate between old or new myocardial defects, usually must undergo additional evaluation.

EXERCISE ELECTROCARDIOGRAPHY

Exercise electrocardiography has historically been commonly employed for completion of risk stratification of patients who have undergone an initial evaluation that has not revealed a specific cause of chest discomfort and has identified a low risk of ACS. Early exercise testing is safe in patients without ongoing chest pain or high-risk findings and may assist in refining their prognostic assessment. However, for patients with chest pain for whom both cardiac troponin and clinical risk stratification have determined the patient to have *low* probability of ACS, there is insufficient evidence that stress testing or cardiac imaging improves their outcomes. This evolution in evidence supports a change from past practice in which outpatient stress testing within 72 hours was broadly used for patients with acute chest pain.

OTHER NONINVASIVE STUDIES

Other noninvasive imaging studies of the chest can be used selectively to provide additional diagnostic and prognostic information on patients with chest discomfort.

Echocardiography Echocardiography (nonstress) is not necessarily routine in patients with chest discomfort. However, in patients with an uncertain diagnosis, particularly those with nondiagnostic ST elevation, ongoing symptoms, or hemodynamic instability, detection of abnormal regional wall motion provides evidence of possible ischemic dysfunction. Echocardiography is diagnostic in patients with mechanical complications of MI or in patients with pericardial tamponade. Transthoracic echocardiography is poorly sensitive for aortic dissection, although an intimal flap may sometimes be detected in the ascending aorta.

MRI (See Chap. 241) Cardiac magnetic resonance (CMR) imaging is an evolving, versatile technique for structural and functional evaluation of the heart and the vasculature of the chest. CMR can be performed as a modality for pharmacologic stress perfusion imaging. Gadolinium-enhanced CMR can provide early detection of MI, defining areas of myocardial necrosis accurately, and can delineate patterns of myocardial disease that are often useful in discriminating ischemic from nonischemic myocardial injury. Although usually not practical for the urgent evaluation of acute chest discomfort, CMR can be a useful modality for cardiac structural evaluation of patients with elevated cardiac troponin levels in the absence of definite coronary artery disease. CMR coronary angiography is in its early stages. MRI also permits highly accurate assessment for aortic dissection but is infrequently used as the first test because CT and transesophageal echocardiography are usually more practical.

CRITICAL PATHWAYS FOR ACUTE CHEST DISCOMFORT

Because of the challenges inherent in reliably identifying the small proportion of patients with serious causes of acute chest discomfort while not exposing the larger number of low-risk patients to unnecessary testing and extended ED or hospital evaluations, many medical centers have adopted critical pathways to expedite the assessment and management of patients with nontraumatic chest pain, often in dedicated chest pain units. Such pathways are generally aimed at (1) rapid identification, triage, and treatment of high-risk cardiopulmonary conditions (e.g., STEMI); (2) accurate identification of low-risk patients who can be safely observed in units with less intensive monitoring, undergo early noninvasive testing, or be discharged home; and (3) through more efficient and systematic accelerated diagnostic protocols, safe reduction in costs associated with overuse of testing and unnecessary hospitalizations. In some studies, provision of protocol-driven care in chest pain units has decreased costs and overall duration of hospital evaluation with no detectable excess of adverse clinical outcomes.

OUTPATIENT EVALUATION OF CHEST DISCOMFORT

Chest pain is common in outpatient practice, with a lifetime prevalence of 20–40% in the general population. More than 25% of patients with MI have had a related visit with a primary care physician in the previous month. The diagnostic principles are the same as in the ED. However, the pretest probability of an acute cardiopulmonary cause is significantly lower. Therefore, testing paradigms are less intense, with an emphasis on the history, physical examination, and ECG. Moreover, decision-aids developed for settings with a high prevalence of significant cardiopulmonary disease have lower positive predictive value when applied in the practitioner's office. However, in general, if the level of clinical suspicion of ACS is sufficiently high to consider troponin testing, the patient should be referred to the ED for evaluation.

FURTHER READING

Amsterdam EA et al: Testing of low-risk patients presenting to the emergency department with chest pain: A scientific statement from the American Heart Association. Circulation 122:1756, 2010.

Chapman AR et al: Association of high-sensitivity cardiac troponin I concentration with cardiac outcomes in patients with suspected acute coronary syndrome. JAMA 318:1913, 2017.

Fanaroff AC et al: Does this patient with chest pain have acute coronary syndrome? JAMA 314:1955, 2015.

Hsia RY et al: A national study of the prevalence of life-threatening diagnoses in patients with chest pain. JAMA Intern Med 176:1029, 2016.

Mahler SA et al: Safely identifying emergency department patients with acute chest pain for early discharge: HEART pathway accelerated diagnostic protocol. Circulation 138:2456, 2018.

15 Abdominal Pain

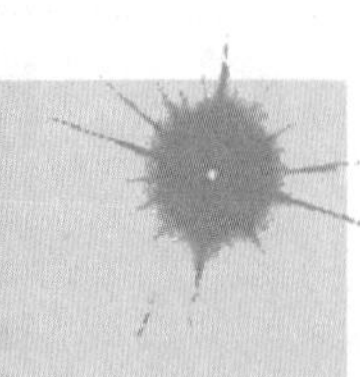

Danny O. Jacobs

Correctly diagnosing acute abdominal pain can be quite challenging. Few clinical situations require greater judgment, because the most catastrophic of events may be forecast by the subtlest of symptoms and signs. In every instance, the clinician must distinguish those conditions that require urgent intervention from those that do not and can best be managed nonoperatively. A meticulously executed, detailed history and physical examination are critically important for focusing the differential diagnosis and allowing the diagnostic evaluation to proceed expeditiously (**Table 15-1**).

The etiologic classification in **Table 15-2**, although not complete, provides a useful framework for evaluating patients with abdominal pain.

Any patient with abdominal pain of recent onset requires an early and thorough evaluation. The most common causes of abdominal pain on admission are nonspecific abdominal pain, acute appendicitis, pain of urologic origin, and intestinal obstruction. A diagnosis of "acute or surgical abdomen" is not acceptable because of its often misleading and erroneous connotations. Most patients who present with acute abdominal pain will have self-limited disease processes. However, it is important to remember that pain severity does not necessarily correlate with the severity of the underlying condition. And, the presence or absence of various degrees of "hunger" is unreliable as a sole indicator of the severity of intraabdominal disease. The most obvious of "acute abdomens" may not require operative intervention, and the mildest of abdominal pains may herald an urgently correctable disease.

SOME MECHANISMS OF PAIN ORIGINATING IN THE ABDOMEN

Inflammation of the Parietal Peritoneum The pain of parietal peritoneal inflammation is steady and aching in character and is located directly over the inflamed area, its exact reference being possible because it is transmitted by somatic nerves supplying the parietal peritoneum. The intensity of the pain is dependent on the type and amount of material to which the peritoneal surfaces are exposed in a given time period. For example, the sudden release of a small quantity

TABLE 15-1 Some Key Components of the Patient's History
Age
Time and mode of onset of the pain
Pain characteristics
Duration of symptoms
Location of pain and sites of radiation
Associated symptoms and their relationship to the pain
Nausea, emesis, and anorexia
Diarrhea, constipation, or other changes in bowel habits
Menstrual history

TABLE 15-2 Some Important Causes of Abdominal Pain

Pain Originating in the Abdomen	
Parietal peritoneal inflammation	Vascular disturbances
Bacterial contamination	Embolism or thrombosis
Perforated appendix or other perforated viscus	Vascular rupture
Pelvic inflammatory disease	Pressure or torsional occlusion
Chemical irritation	Sickle cell anemia
Perforated ulcer	Abdominal wall
Pancreatitis	Distortion or traction of mesentery
Mittelschmerz	Trauma or infection of muscles
Mechanical obstruction of hollow viscera	Distension of visceral surfaces, e.g., by hemorrhage
Obstruction of the small or large intestine	Hepatic or renal capsules
Obstruction of the biliary tree	Inflammation
Obstruction of the ureter	Appendicitis
	Typhoid fever
	Neutropenic enterocolitis or "typhlitis"
Pain Referred from Extraabdominal Source	
Cardiothoracic	Pleurodynia
Acute myocardial infarction	Pneumothorax
Myocarditis, endocarditis, pericarditis	Empyema
Congestive heart failure	Esophageal disease, including spasm, rupture, or inflammation
Pneumonia (especially lower lobes)	Genitalia
Pulmonary embolus	Torsion of the testis
Metabolic Causes	
Diabetes	Acute adrenal insufficiency
Uremia	Familial Mediterranean fever
Hyperlipidemia	Porphyria
Hyperparathyroidism	C1 esterase inhibitor deficiency (angioneurotic edema)
Neurologic/Psychiatric Causes	
Herpes zoster	Spinal cord or nerve root compression
Tabes dorsalis	Functional disorders
Causalgia	Psychiatric disorders
Radiculitis from infection or arthritis	
Toxic Causes	
Lead poisoning	
Insect or animal envenomation	
Black widow spider bites	
Snake bites	
Uncertain Mechanisms	
Narcotic withdrawal	
Heat stroke	

of *sterile* acidic gastric juice into the peritoneal cavity causes much more pain than the same amount of grossly contaminated neutral feces. Enzymatically active pancreatic juice incites more pain and inflammation than does the same amount of sterile bile containing no potent enzymes. Blood is normally only a mild irritant, and the response to urine is also typically bland, so exposure of blood and urine to the peritoneal cavity may go unnoticed unless it is sudden and massive. Bacterial contamination, such as may occur with pelvic inflammatory disease or perforated distal intestine, causes low-intensity pain until multiplication causes significant amounts of inflammatory mediators to be released. Patients with perforated upper gastrointestinal ulcers may present entirely differently depending on how quickly gastric juices enter the peritoneal cavity and their pH. Thus, the rate at which any inflammatory material irritates the peritoneum is important.

The pain of peritoneal inflammation is invariably accentuated by pressure or changes in tension of the peritoneum, whether produced by palpation or by movement such as with coughing or sneezing. The patient with peritonitis characteristically lies quietly in bed, preferring to avoid motion, in contrast to the patient with colic, who may be thrashing in discomfort.

Another characteristic feature of peritoneal irritation is tonic reflex spasm of the abdominal musculature, localized to the involved body segment. Its intensity depends on the integrity of the nervous system, the location of the inflammatory process, and the rate at which it develops. Spasm over a perforated retrocecal appendix or perforation into the lesser peritoneal sac may be minimal or absent because of the protective effect of overlying viscera. Catastrophic abdominal emergencies may be associated with minimal or no detectable pain or muscle spasm in obtunded, seriously ill, debilitated, immunosuppressed, or psychotic patients. A slowly developing process also often greatly attenuates the degree of muscle spasm.

Obstruction of Hollow Viscera Intraluminal obstruction classically elicits intermittent or colicky abdominal pain that is not as well localized as the pain of parietal peritoneal irritation. However, the absence of cramping discomfort can be misleading because distention of a hollow viscus may also produce steady pain with only rare paroxysms.

Small-bowel obstruction often presents as poorly localized, intermittent periumbilical or supraumbilical pain. As the intestine progressively dilates and loses muscular tone, the colicky nature of the pain may diminish. With superimposed strangulating obstruction, pain may spread to the lower lumbar region if there is traction on the root of the mesentery. The colicky pain of colonic obstruction is of lesser intensity, is commonly located in the infraumbilical area, and may often radiate to the lumbar region.

Sudden distention of the biliary tree produces a steady rather than colicky type of pain; hence, the term *biliary colic* is misleading. Acute distention of the gallbladder typically causes pain in the right upper quadrant with radiation to the right posterior region of the thorax or to the tip of the right scapula, but discomfort is also not uncommonly found near the midline. Distention of the common bile duct often causes epigastric pain that may radiate to the upper lumbar region. Considerable variation is common, however, so that differentiation between gallbladder or common ductal disease may be impossible.

Gradual dilatation of the biliary tree, as can occur with carcinoma of the head of the pancreas, may cause no pain or only a mild aching sensation in the epigastrium or right upper quadrant. The pain of distention of the pancreatic ducts is similar to that described for distention of the common bile duct but, in addition, is very frequently accentuated by recumbency and relieved by the upright position.

Obstruction of the urinary bladder usually causes dull, low-intensity pain in the suprapubic region. Restlessness, without specific complaint of pain, may be the only sign of a distended bladder in an obtunded patient. In contrast, acute obstruction of the intravesicular portion of the ureter is characterized by severe suprapubic and flank pain that radiates to the penis, scrotum, or inner aspect of the upper thigh. Obstruction of the ureteropelvic junction manifests as pain near the costovertebral angle, whereas obstruction of the remainder of the ureter is associated with flank pain that often extends into the same side of the abdomen.

Vascular Disturbances A frequent misconception is that pain due to intraabdominal vascular disturbances is sudden and catastrophic in nature. Certain disease processes, such as embolism or thrombosis of the superior mesenteric artery or impending rupture of an abdominal aortic aneurysm, can certainly be associated with diffuse, severe pain. Yet, just as frequently, the patient with occlusion of the superior mesenteric artery only has mild continuous or cramping diffuse pain for 2 or 3 days before vascular collapse or findings of peritoneal inflammation appear. The early, seemingly insignificant discomfort is caused by hyperperistalsis rather than peritoneal inflammation. Indeed, absence of tenderness and rigidity in the presence of continuous, diffuse pain (e.g., "pain out of proportion to physical findings") in a patient likely to have vascular disease is quite characteristic of occlusion of the superior mesenteric artery. Abdominal pain with radiation to the sacral region, flank, or genitalia should always signal the possible presence of a rupturing abdominal aortic aneurysm. This pain may persist over a period of several days before rupture and collapse occur.

Abdominal Wall Pain arising from the abdominal wall is usually constant and aching. Movement, prolonged standing, and pressure accentuate the discomfort and associated muscle spasm. In the relatively rare case of hematoma of the rectus sheath, now most frequently encountered in association with anticoagulant therapy, a mass may be present in the lower quadrants of the abdomen. Simultaneous involvement of muscles in other parts of the body usually serves to differentiate myositis of the abdominal wall from other processes that might cause pain in the same region.

REFERRED PAIN IN ABDOMINAL DISEASE

Pain referred to the abdomen from the thorax, spine, or genitalia may present a diagnostic challenge because diseases of the upper part of the abdominal cavity such as acute cholecystitis or perforated ulcer may be associated with intrathoracic complications. A most important, yet often forgotten, dictum is that the possibility of intrathoracic disease must be considered in every patient with abdominal pain, especially if the pain is in the upper abdomen.

Systematic questioning and examination directed toward detecting myocardial or pulmonary infarction, pneumonia, pericarditis, or esophageal disease (the intrathoracic diseases that most often masquerade as abdominal emergencies) will often provide sufficient clues to establish the proper diagnosis. Diaphragmatic pleuritis resulting from pneumonia or pulmonary infarction may cause pain in the right upper quadrant and pain in the supraclavicular area, the latter radiation to be distinguished from the referred subscapular pain caused by acute distention of the extrahepatic biliary tree. The ultimate decision as to the origin of abdominal pain may require deliberate and planned observation over a period of several hours, during which repeated questioning and examination will provide the diagnosis or suggest the appropriate studies.

Referred pain of thoracic origin is often accompanied by splinting of the involved hemithorax with respiratory lag and a decrease in excursion more marked than that seen in the presence of intraabdominal disease. In addition, apparent abdominal muscle spasm caused by referred pain will diminish during the inspiratory phase of respiration, whereas it persists throughout both respiratory phases if it is of abdominal origin. Palpation over the area of referred pain in the abdomen also does not usually accentuate the pain and, in many instances, actually seems to relieve it.

Thoracic disease and abdominal disease frequently coexist and may be difficult or impossible to differentiate. For example, the patient with known biliary tract disease often has epigastric pain during myocardial infarction, or biliary colic may be referred to the precordium or left shoulder in a patient who has suffered previously from angina pectoris. **For an explanation of the radiation of pain to a previously diseased area, see Chap. 13.**

Referred pain from the spine, which usually involves compression or irritation of nerve roots, is characteristically intensified by certain motions such as cough, sneeze, or strain and is associated with hyperesthesia over the involved dermatomes. Pain referred to the abdomen from the testes or seminal vesicles is generally accentuated by the slightest pressure on either of these organs. The abdominal discomfort experienced is of dull, aching character and is poorly localized.

METABOLIC ABDOMINAL CRISES

Pain of metabolic origin may simulate almost any other type of intraabdominal disease. Several mechanisms may be at work. In certain instances, such as hyperlipidemia, the metabolic disease itself may be accompanied by an intraabdominal process such as pancreatitis, which can lead to unnecessary laparotomy unless recognized. C1 esterase deficiency associated with angioneurotic edema is often associated with episodes of severe abdominal pain. Whenever the cause of abdominal pain is obscure, a metabolic origin always must be considered. Abdominal pain is also the hallmark of familial Mediterranean fever **(Chap. 369)**.

The pain of porphyria and of lead colic is usually difficult to distinguish from that of intestinal obstruction, because severe hyperperistalsis is a prominent feature of both. The pain of uremia or diabetes is nonspecific, and the pain and tenderness frequently shift in location and intensity. Diabetic acidosis may be precipitated by acute appendicitis or intestinal obstruction, so if prompt resolution of the abdominal pain does not result from correction of the metabolic abnormalities, an underlying organic problem should be suspected. Black widow spider bites produce intense pain and rigidity of the abdominal muscles and back, an area infrequently involved in intraabdominal disease.

IMMUNOCOMPROMISE

Evaluating and diagnosing causes of abdominal pain in immunosuppressed or otherwise immunocompromised patients is very difficult. This includes those who have undergone organ transplantation; who are receiving immunosuppressive treatments for autoimmune diseases, chemotherapy, or glucocorticoids; who have AIDS; and who are very old. In these circumstances, normal physiologic responses may be absent or masked. In addition, unusual infections may cause abdominal pain where the etiologic agents include cytomegalovirus, mycobacteria, protozoa, and fungi. These pathogens may affect all gastrointestinal organs, including the gallbladder, liver, and pancreas, as well as the gastrointestinal tract, causing occult or overtly symptomatic perforations of the latter. Splenic abscesses due to *Candida* or *Salmonella* infection should also be considered, especially when evaluating patients with left upper quadrant or left flank pain. Acalculous cholecystitis may be observed in immunocompromised patients or those with AIDS, where it is often associated with cryptosporidiosis or cytomegalovirus infection.

Neutropenic enterocolitis (typhlitis) is often identified as a cause of abdominal pain and fever in some patients with bone marrow suppression due to chemotherapy. Acute graft-versus-host disease should be considered in this circumstance. Optimal management of these patients requires meticulous follow-up including serial examinations to assess the need for more surgical intervention, for example, to address perforation.

NEUROGENIC CAUSES

Diseases that injure sensory nerves may cause causalgic pain. This pain has a burning character and is usually limited to the distribution of a given peripheral nerve. Stimuli that are normally not painful such as touch or a change in temperature may be causalgic and are often present even at rest. The demonstration of irregularly spaced cutaneous "pain spots" may be the only indication that an old nerve injury exists. Even though the pain may be precipitated by gentle palpation, rigidity of the abdominal muscles is absent, and the respirations are not usually disturbed. Distention of the abdomen is uncommon, and the pain has no relationship to food intake.

Pain arising from spinal nerves or roots comes and goes suddenly and is of a lancinating type **(Chap. 17)**. It may be caused by herpes zoster, impingement by arthritis, tumors, a herniated nucleus pulposus, diabetes, or syphilis. It is not associated with food intake, abdominal distention, or changes in respiration. Severe muscle spasms, when present, may be relieved by, but are certainly not accentuated by, abdominal palpation. The pain is made worse by movement of the spine and is usually confined to a few dermatomes. Hyperesthesia is very common.

Pain due to functional causes conforms to none of the aforementioned patterns. Mechanisms of disease are not clearly established. Irritable bowel syndrome (IBS) is a functional gastrointestinal disorder characterized by abdominal pain and altered bowel habits. The diagnosis is made on the basis of clinical criteria **(Chap. 327)** and after exclusion of demonstrable structural abnormalities. The episodes of abdominal pain may be brought on by stress, and the pain varies considerably in type and location. Nausea and vomiting are rare. Localized tenderness and muscle spasm are inconsistent or absent. The causes of IBS or related functional disorders are not yet fully understood.

APPROACH TO THE PATIENT

Abdominal Pain

Few abdominal conditions require such urgent operative intervention that an orderly approach needs to be abandoned, no matter how ill the patient is. Only patients with exsanguinating intraabdominal hemorrhage (e.g., ruptured aneurysm) must be rushed to the operating room immediately, but in such instances, only a few minutes are required to assess the critical nature of the problem. Under these circumstances, all obstacles must be swept aside, adequate venous access for fluid replacement obtained, and the operation begun. Unfortunately, many of these patients may die in the radiology department or the emergency room while awaiting unnecessary examinations. *There are no absolute contraindications to operation when massive intraabdominal hemorrhage is present.* Fortunately, this situation is relatively rare. This statement does not necessarily apply to patients with intraluminal gastrointestinal hemorrhage, who can often be managed by other means (**Chap. 48**). In these patients, obtaining a *detailed history when possible* can be extremely helpful even though it can be laborious and time-consuming. Decision-making regarding next steps is facilitated and a reasonably accurate diagnosis can be made before any further diagnostic testing is undertaken.

In cases of *acute* abdominal pain, a diagnosis can be readily established in most instances, whereas success is not so frequent in patients with *chronic* pain. IBS is one of the most common causes of abdominal pain and must always be kept in mind (**Chap. 327**). The location of the pain can assist in narrowing the differential diagnosis (**Table 15-3**); however, the *chronological sequence of events* in the patient's history is often more important than the pain's location. Careful attention should be paid to the extraabdominal regions. Narcotics or analgesics should *not* be withheld until a definitive diagnosis or a definitive plan has been formulated; obfuscation of the diagnosis by adequate analgesia is unlikely.

An accurate menstrual history in a female patient is essential. It is important to remember that normal anatomic relationships can be significantly altered by the gravid uterus. Abdominal and pelvic pain may occur during pregnancy due to conditions that do not require operation. Lastly, some otherwise noteworthy laboratory values (e.g., leukocytosis) may represent the normal physiologic changes of pregnancy.

In the examination, simple critical inspection of the patient, for example, of facies, position in bed, and respiratory activity, provides valuable clues. The amount of information to be gleaned is directly proportional to the *gentleness* and thoroughness of the examiner. Once a patient with peritoneal inflammation has been examined brusquely, accurate assessment by the next examiner becomes almost impossible. Eliciting rebound tenderness by sudden release of a deeply palpating hand in a patient with suspected peritonitis is cruel and unnecessary. The same information can be obtained by gentle percussion of the abdomen (rebound tenderness on a miniature scale), a maneuver that can be far more precise and localizing. Asking the patient to cough will elicit true rebound tenderness without the need for placing a hand on the abdomen. Furthermore, the forceful demonstration of rebound tenderness will startle and induce protective spasm in a nervous or worried patient in whom true rebound tenderness is not present. A palpable gallbladder will be missed if palpation is so aggressive that voluntary muscle spasm becomes superimposed on involuntary muscular rigidity.

As with history taking, sufficient time should be spent in the examination. Abdominal signs may be minimal but, nevertheless, if accompanied by consistent symptoms, may be exceptionally meaningful. Abdominal signs may be virtually or totally absent in cases of pelvic peritonitis, so careful *pelvic and rectal examinations are mandatory in every patient with abdominal pain.* Tenderness on pelvic or rectal examination in the absence of other abdominal signs can be caused by operative indications such as perforated appendicitis, diverticulitis, twisted ovarian cyst, and many others. Much attention has been paid to the presence or absence of peristaltic sounds, their quality, and their frequency. Auscultation of the abdomen is one of the least revealing aspects of the physical examination of a patient with abdominal pain. Catastrophes such as a strangulating small-intestinal obstruction or perforated appendicitis may occur in the presence of normal peristaltic sounds. Conversely, when the proximal part of the intestine above obstruction becomes markedly distended and edematous, peristaltic sounds may lose the characteristics of borborygmi and become weak or absent, even when peritonitis is not present. It is usually the severe chemical peritonitis of sudden onset that is associated with the truly silent abdomen.

Laboratory examinations may be valuable in assessing the patient with abdominal pain, yet, with few exceptions, they rarely establish a diagnosis. Leukocytosis should never be the single deciding factor as to whether or not operation is indicated. A white blood cell count >20,000/μL may be observed with perforation of a viscus, but pancreatitis, acute cholecystitis, pelvic inflammatory disease, and intestinal infarction may also be associated with marked leukocytosis. A normal white blood cell count is not rare in cases of perforation of abdominal viscera. A diagnosis of anemia may be more helpful than the white blood cell count, especially when combined with the history.

The urinalysis may reveal the state of hydration or rule out severe renal disease, diabetes, or urinary infection. Blood urea nitrogen, glucose, and serum bilirubin levels and liver function tests may be

TABLE 15-3 Differential Diagnoses of Abdominal Pain by Location

Right Upper Quadrant	Epigastric	Left Upper Quadrant
Cholecystitis Cholangitis Pancreatitis Pneumonia/empyema Pleurisy/pleurodynia Subdiaphragmatic abscess Hepatitis Budd-Chiari syndrome	Peptic ulcer disease Gastritis GERD Pancreatitis Myocardial infarction Pericarditis Ruptured aortic aneurysm Esophagitis	Splenic infarct Splenic rupture Splenic abscess Gastritis Gastric ulcer Pancreatitis Subdiaphragmatic abscess
Right Lower Quadrant	**Periumbilical**	**Left Lower Quadrant**
Appendicitis Salpingitis Inguinal hernia Ectopic pregnancy Nephrolithiasis Inflammatory bowel disease Mesenteric lymphadenitis Typhlitis	Early appendicitis Gastroenteritis Bowel obstruction Ruptured aortic aneurysm	Diverticulitis Salpingitis Inguinal hernia Ectopic pregnancy Nephrolithiasis Irritable bowel syndrome Inflammatory bowel disease
Diffuse Nonlocalized Pain		
Gastroenteritis Mesenteric ischemia Bowel obstruction Irritable bowel syndrome Peritonitis Diabetes	Malaria Familial Mediterranean fever Metabolic diseases Psychiatric disease	

Abbreviation: GERD, gastroesophageal reflux disease.

helpful. Serum amylase levels may be increased by many diseases other than pancreatitis, for example, perforated ulcer, strangulating intestinal obstruction, and acute cholecystitis; thus, elevations of serum amylase do not rule in or rule out the need for an operation.

Plain and upright or lateral decubitus radiographs of the abdomen have limited utility and may be unnecessary in some patients who have substantial evidence of some diseases such as acute appendicitis or strangulated external hernia. Where the indications for surgical or medical intervention are not clear, low-dose computed tomography is preferred to abdominal radiography when evaluating nontraumatic acute abdominal pain.

Very rarely, barium or water-soluble contrast study of the upper part of the gastrointestinal tract is an appropriate radiographic investigation and may demonstrate partial intestinal obstruction that may elude diagnosis by other means. If there is any question of obstruction of the colon, oral administration of barium sulfate should be avoided. On the other hand, in cases of suspected colonic obstruction (without perforation), a contrast enema may be diagnostic.

In the absence of trauma, peritoneal lavage has been replaced as a diagnostic tool by CT scanning and laparoscopy. Ultrasonography has proved to be useful in detecting an enlarged gallbladder or pancreas, the presence of gallstones, an enlarged ovary, or a tubal pregnancy. Laparoscopy is especially helpful in diagnosing pelvic conditions, such as ovarian cysts, tubal pregnancies, salpingitis, acute appendicitis, and other disease processes. Laparoscopy has a particular advantage over imaging in that the underlying etiologic condition can often be definitively addressed.

Radioisotopic hepatobiliary iminodiacetic acid scans (HIDAs) may help differentiate acute cholecystitis or biliary colic from acute pancreatitis. A CT scan may demonstrate an enlarged pancreas, ruptured spleen, or thickened colonic or appendiceal wall and streaking of the mesocolon or mesoappendix characteristic of diverticulitis or appendicitis.

Sometimes, even under the best circumstances with all available aids and with the greatest of clinical skill, a definitive diagnosis cannot be established at the time of the initial examination. And, in some cases, operation may be indicated based on clinical grounds alone. Should that decision be questionable, watchful waiting with repeated questioning and examination will often elucidate the true nature of the illness and indicate the proper course of action.

Acknowledgment

The author gratefully acknowledges the enormous contribution to this chapter and the approach it espouses of William Silen, who wrote this chapter for many editions.

FURTHER READING

Bhangu A et al: Acute appendicitis: Modern understanding of pathogenesis, diagnosis and management. Lancet 386:1278, 2015.

Cartwright SL, Knudson MP: Diagnostic imaging of acute abdominal pain in adults. Am Fam Phys 91:452, 2015.

Huckins DS et al: Diagnostic performance of a biomarker panel as a negative predictor for acute appendicitis in acute emergency department patients with abdominal pain. Am J Emerg Med 35:418, 2017.

Nayor J et al: Tracing the cause of abdominal pain. N Engl J Med 375:e8, 2016.

Phillips MT: Clinical yield of computed tomography scans in the emergency department for abdominal pain. J Invest Med 64:542, 2016.

Silen W, Cope Z: *Cope's Early Diagnosis of the Acute Abdomen*, 22nd ed. New York, Oxford University Press, 2010.

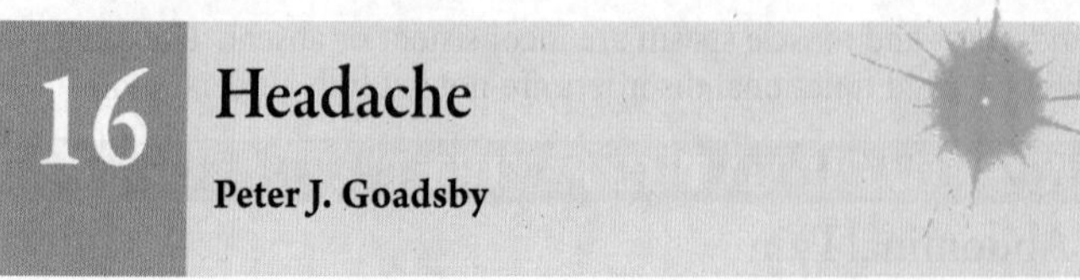

16 Headache

Peter J. Goadsby

Headache is among the most common reasons patients seek medical attention and is responsible, on a global basis, for more disability than any other neurologic problem. Diagnosis and management are based on a careful clinical approach augmented by an understanding of the anatomy, physiology, and pharmacology of the nervous system pathways mediating the various headache syndromes. This chapter will focus on the general approach to a patient with headache; migraine and other primary headache disorders are discussed in **Chap. 430**.

GENERAL PRINCIPLES

A classification system developed by the International Headache Society (*www.ihs-headache.org/en/resources/guidelines/*) characterizes headache as primary or secondary (**Table 16-1**). *Primary headaches* are those in which headache and its associated features are the disorder itself, whereas *secondary headaches* are those caused by exogenous disorders (Headache Classification Committee of the International Headache Society, 2018). Primary headache often results in considerable disability and a decrease in the patient's quality of life. Mild secondary headache, such as that seen in association with upper respiratory tract infections, is common but rarely worrisome. Life-threatening headache is relatively uncommon, but vigilance is required in order to recognize and appropriately treat such patients.

ANATOMY AND PHYSIOLOGY OF HEADACHE

Pain usually occurs when peripheral nociceptors are stimulated in response to tissue injury, visceral distension, or other factors (**Chap. 13**). In such situations, pain perception is a normal physiologic response mediated by a healthy nervous system. Pain can also result when pain-producing pathways of the peripheral or central nervous system (CNS) are damaged or activated inappropriately. Headache may originate from either or both mechanisms. Relatively few cranial structures are pain producing; these include the scalp, meningeal arteries, dural sinuses, falx cerebri, and proximal segments of the large pial arteries. The ventricular ependyma, choroid plexus, pial veins, and much of the brain parenchyma are not pain producing.

The key structures involved in primary headache are the following:

- The large intracranial vessels and dura mater, and the peripheral terminals of the trigeminal nerve that innervate these structures
- The caudal portion of the trigeminal nucleus, which extends into the dorsal horns of the upper cervical spinal cord and receives input from the first and second cervical nerve roots (the trigeminocervical complex)
- Rostral pain-processing regions, such as the ventroposteromedial thalamus and the cortex
- The pain-modulatory systems in the brain that modulate input from the trigeminal nociceptors at all levels of the pain-processing pathways and influence vegetative functions, such as the hypothalamus and brainstem

TABLE 16-1 Common Causes of Headache

PRIMARY HEADACHE		SECONDARY HEADACHE	
TYPE	%	TYPE	%
Tension-type	69	Systemic infection	63
Migraine	16	Head injury	4
Idiopathic stabbing	2	Vascular disorders	1
Exertional	1	Subarachnoid hemorrhage	<1
Cluster	0.1	Brain tumor	0.1

Source: After J Olesen et al: *The Headaches*. Philadelphia, Lippincott Williams & Wilkins, 2005.

The *trigeminovascular system* innervates the large intracranial vessels and dura mater via the trigeminal nerve. Cranial autonomic symptoms, such as lacrimation, conjunctival injection, nasal congestion, rhinorrhea, periorbital swelling, aural fullness, and ptosis, are prominent in the trigeminal autonomic cephalalgias (TACs), including cluster headache and paroxysmal hemicrania, and may also be seen in migraine, even in children. These autonomic symptoms reflect activation of cranial parasympathetic pathways, and functional imaging studies indicate that vascular changes in migraine and cluster headache, when present, are similarly driven by these cranial autonomic systems. Thus, they are secondary, and not causative, events in the headache cascade. Moreover, they can often be mistaken for symptoms or signs of cranial sinus inflammation, which is then overdiagnosed and inappropriately managed. Migraine and other primary headache types are not "vascular headaches"; these disorders do not reliably manifest vascular changes, and treatment outcomes cannot be predicted by vascular effects. Migraine is a brain disorder and is best understood and managed as such.

CLINICAL EVALUATION OF ACUTE, NEW-ONSET HEADACHE

The patient who presents with a new, severe headache has a differential diagnosis that is quite different from the patient with recurrent headaches over many years. In new-onset and severe headache, the probability of finding a potentially serious cause is considerably greater than in recurrent headache. Patients with recent onset of pain require prompt evaluation and appropriate treatment. Serious causes to be considered include meningitis, subarachnoid hemorrhage, epidural or subdural hematoma, glaucoma, tumor, and purulent sinusitis. When worrisome symptoms and signs are present (Table 16-2), rapid diagnosis and management are critical.

A careful neurologic examination is an essential first step in the evaluation. In most cases, patients with an abnormal examination or a history of recent-onset headache should be evaluated by a computed tomography (CT) or magnetic resonance imaging (MRI) study of the brain. As an initial screening procedure for intracranial pathology in this setting, CT and MRI methods appear to be equally sensitive. In some circumstances, a lumbar puncture (LP) is also required, unless a benign etiology can be otherwise established. A general evaluation of acute headache might include cranial arteries by palpation; cervical spine by the effect of passive movement of the head and by imaging; the investigation of cardiovascular and renal status by blood pressure monitoring and urine examination; and eyes by funduscopy, intraocular pressure measurement, and refraction.

The patient's psychological state should also be evaluated because a relationship exists between head pain, depression, and anxiety. This is intended to identify comorbidity rather than provide an explanation for the headache, because troublesome headache is seldom simply caused by mood change. Although it is notable that medicines with antidepressant actions are also effective in the preventive treatment of both tension-type headache and migraine, each symptom must be treated optimally.

TABLE 16-2 Headache Symptoms That Suggest a Serious Underlying Disorder

Sudden-onset headache
First severe headache
"Worst" headache ever
Vomiting that precedes headache
Subacute worsening over days or weeks
Pain induced by bending, lifting, coughing
Pain that disturbs sleep or presents immediately upon awakening
Known systemic illness
Onset after age 55
Fever or unexplained systemic signs
Abnormal neurologic examination
Pain associated with local tenderness, e.g., region of temporal artery

Underlying recurrent headache disorders may be activated by pain that follows otologic or endodontic surgical procedures. Thus, pain about the head as the result of diseased tissue or trauma may reawaken an otherwise quiescent migraine syndrome. Treatment of the headache is largely ineffective until the cause of the primary problem is addressed.

Serious underlying conditions that are associated with headache are described below. Brain tumor is a rare cause of headache and even less commonly a cause of severe pain. The vast majority of patients presenting with severe headache have a benign cause.

SECONDARY HEADACHE

The management of secondary headache focuses on diagnosis and treatment of the underlying condition.

MENINGITIS

Acute, severe headache with stiff neck and fever suggests meningitis. LP is mandatory. Often there is striking accentuation of pain with eye movement. Meningitis can be easily mistaken for migraine in that the cardinal symptoms of pounding headache, photophobia, nausea, and vomiting are frequently present, perhaps reflecting the underlying biology of some of the patients.

Meningitis is discussed in Chaps. 138 and 139.

INTRACRANIAL HEMORRHAGE

Acute, maximal in <5 min, severe headache lasting >5 min with stiff neck but without fever suggests subarachnoid hemorrhage. A ruptured aneurysm, arteriovenous malformation, or intraparenchymal hemorrhage may also present with headache alone. Rarely, if the hemorrhage is small or below the foramen magnum, the head CT scan can be normal. Therefore, LP may be required to diagnose definitively subarachnoid hemorrhage.

Subarachnoid hemorrhage is discussed in Chap. 429, and intracranial hemorrhage in Chap. 428.

BRAIN TUMOR

Approximately 30% of patients with brain tumors consider headache to be their chief complaint. The head pain is usually nondescript—an intermittent deep, dull aching of moderate intensity, which may worsen with exertion or change in position and may be associated with nausea and vomiting. This pattern of symptoms results from migraine far more often than from brain tumor. The headache of brain tumor disturbs sleep in about 10% of patients. Vomiting that precedes the appearance of headache by weeks is highly characteristic of posterior fossa brain tumors. A history of amenorrhea or galactorrhea should lead one to question whether a prolactin-secreting pituitary adenoma (or polycystic ovary syndrome) is the source of headache. Headache arising de novo in a patient with known malignancy suggests either cerebral metastases or carcinomatous meningitis. Head pain appearing abruptly after bending, lifting, or coughing can be due to a posterior fossa mass, a Chiari malformation, or low cerebrospinal fluid (CSF) volume.

Brain tumors are discussed in Chap. 90.

TEMPORAL ARTERITIS (SEE ALSO CHAPS. 32 AND 363)

Temporal (giant cell) arteritis is an inflammatory disorder of arteries that frequently involves the extracranial carotid circulation. It is a common disorder of the elderly; its annual incidence is 77 per 100,000 individuals aged ≥50. The average age of onset is 70 years, and women account for 65% of cases. About half of patients with untreated temporal arteritis develop blindness due to involvement of the ophthalmic artery and its branches; indeed, the ischemic optic neuropathy induced by giant cell arteritis is the major cause of rapidly developing bilateral blindness in patients >60 years. Because treatment with glucocorticoids is effective in preventing this complication, prompt recognition of the disorder is important.

Typical presenting symptoms include headache, polymyalgia rheumatica (Chap. 363), jaw claudication, fever, and weight loss. Headache is the dominant symptom and often appears in association with malaise and muscle aches. Head pain may be unilateral or bilateral and is located temporally in 50% of patients but may involve any and all aspects of the cranium. Pain usually appears gradually over a few hours before peak intensity is reached; occasionally, it is explosive in onset. The quality of pain is infrequently throbbing; it is almost invariably described as dull and boring, with superimposed episodic stabbing pains similar to the sharp pains that appear in migraine. Most patients can recognize that the origin of their head pain is superficial, external to the skull, rather than originating deep within the cranium (the pain site usually identified by migraineurs). Scalp tenderness is present, often to a marked degree; brushing the hair or resting the head on a pillow may be impossible because of pain. Headache is usually worse at night and often aggravated by exposure to cold. Additional findings may include reddened, tender nodules or red streaking of the skin overlying the temporal arteries, and tenderness of the temporal or, less commonly, the occipital arteries.

The erythrocyte sedimentation rate (ESR) is often, although not always, elevated; a normal ESR does not exclude giant cell arteritis. A temporal artery biopsy followed by immediate treatment with prednisone 80 mg daily for the first 4–6 weeks should be initiated when clinical suspicion is high; treatment should not be unreasonably delayed to obtain a biopsy. The prevalence of migraine among the elderly is substantial, considerably higher than that of giant cell arteritis. Migraineurs often report amelioration of their headache with prednisone; thus, caution must be used when interpreting the therapeutic response.

GLAUCOMA

Glaucoma may present with a prostrating headache associated with nausea and vomiting. The headache often starts with severe eye pain. On physical examination, the eye is often red with a fixed, moderately dilated pupil.

Glaucoma is discussed in Chap. 32.

PRIMARY HEADACHE DISORDERS

Primary headaches are disorders in which headache and associated features occur in the absence of any exogenous cause. The most common are migraine, tension-type headache, and the TACs, notably cluster headache. These entities are discussed in detail in **Chap. 430**.

CHRONIC DAILY OR NEAR-DAILY HEADACHE

The broad description of chronic daily headache (CDH) can be applied when a patient experiences headache on 15 days or more per month. CDH is neither a single entity nor a diagnosis; it encompasses a number of different headache syndromes, both primary and secondary (**Table 16-3**). In aggregate, this group presents considerable disability and is thus specially mentioned here. Population-based estimates suggest that about 4% of adults have daily or near-daily headache.

TABLE 16-3 Classification of Daily or Near-Daily Headache

Primary		
>4 H DAILY	**<4 H DAILY**	**SECONDARY**
Chronic migraine[a]	Chronic cluster headache[b]	Posttraumatic Head injury Iatrogenic Postinfectious
Chronic tension-type headache[a]	Chronic paroxysmal hemicrania	Inflammatory, such as Giant cell arteritis Sarcoidosis Behçet's syndrome
Hemicrania continua[a]	SUNCT/SUNA	Chronic CNS infection
New daily persistent headache[a]	Hypnic headache	Medication-overuse headache[a]

[a]May be complicated by medication overuse. [b]Some patients may have headache >4 h/d.

Abbreviations: CNS, central nervous system; SUNA, short-lasting unilateral neuralgiform headache attacks with cranial autonomic symptoms; SUNCT, short-lasting unilateral neuralgiform headache attacks with conjunctival injection and tearing.

APPROACH TO THE PATIENT

Chronic Daily Headache

The first step in the management of patients with CDH is to diagnose any secondary headache and treat that problem (Table 16-3). This can sometimes be a challenge when the underlying cause triggers worsening of a primary headache. For patients with primary headaches, diagnosis of the headache type will guide therapy. Preventive treatments such as tricyclics, either amitriptyline or nortriptyline, at doses up to 1 mg/kg, are very useful in patients with CDH arising from migraine or tension-type headache or where the secondary cause has activated the underlying primary headache. Tricyclics are started in low doses (10–25 mg daily) and may be given 12 h before the expected time of awakening in order to avoid excessive morning sleepiness. Medicines including topiramate, valproate, propranolol, flunarizine (not available in the United States), candesartan, and the newer calcitonin gene-related peptide (CGRP) pathway monoclonal antibodies, or gepants-CGRP receptor antagonists (see **Chap. 430**) are also useful when the underlying issue is migraine.

MANAGEMENT OF MEDICALLY INTRACTABLE DISABLING PRIMARY HEADACHE

The management of medically intractable headache is difficult, although recent developments in therapy are at hand. Monoclonal antibodies to CGRP or its receptor have been reported to be effective and well tolerated in chronic migraine and are now licensed for use in clinical practice. Noninvasive neuromodulatory approaches, such as single-pulse transcranial magnetic stimulation and noninvasive vagal nerve stimulation, which appear to modulate thalamic processing or brainstem mechanisms, respectively, in migraine have been used in clinical practice with success. Noninvasive vagal nerve stimulation has also shown promise particularly in chronic cluster headache, chronic paroxysmal hemicrania, and hemicrania continua, and possibly in short-lasting unilateral neuralgiform headache attacks with cranial autonomic symptoms (SUNA) and short-lasting unilateral neuralgiform headache attacks with conjunctival injection and tearing (SUNCT) (**Chap. 430**). Other modalities are discussed in **Chap. 430**.

MEDICATION-RELATED AND MEDICATION-OVERUSE HEADACHE

Overuse of analgesic medication for headache can aggravate headache frequency, markedly impair the effect of preventive medicines, and induce a state of refractory daily or near-daily headache called *medication-overuse headache*. A proportion of patients who stop taking analgesics will experience substantial improvement in the severity and frequency of their headache. However, even after cessation of analgesic use, many patients continue to have headache, although they may feel clinically improved in some way, especially if they have been using opioids or barbiturates regularly. The residual symptoms probably represent the underlying primary headache disorder, and most commonly this issue occurs in patients prone to migraine.

Management of Medication Overuse: Outpatients For patients who overuse analgesic medications, it is often helpful to reduce and eliminate the medications, although this approach is far from universally effective. One approach is to reduce the medication dose by 10% every 1–2 weeks. Immediate cessation of analgesic use is possible for some patients, provided there is no contraindication. Both approaches are facilitated by use of a medication diary maintained during the month or two before cessation; this helps to identify the scope of the problem. A small dose of a nonsteroidal anti-inflammatory drug (NSAID) such as naproxen, 500 mg bid, if tolerated, will help relieve residual pain as analgesic use is reduced.

NSAID overuse is not usually a problem for patients with daily headache when an NSAID with a longer half-life is taken once or twice daily; however, overuse problems may develop with shorter-acting NSAIDS. Once the patient has substantially reduced analgesic use, a preventive medication should be introduced. Another widely used approach is to commence the preventive at the same time the analgesic reduction is started. It must be emphasized that *preventives may not work in the presence of analgesic overuse, particularly with opioids.* The most common cause of unresponsiveness to treatment is the use of a preventive when analgesics continue to be used regularly. For some patients, discontinuing analgesics is very difficult; often the best approach is to inform the patient that some degree of headache is inevitable during this initial period.

Management of Medication Overuse: Inpatients Some patients will require hospitalization for detoxification. Such patients have typically failed efforts at outpatient withdrawal or have a significant medical condition, such as diabetes mellitus or epilepsy, which would complicate withdrawal as an outpatient. Following admission to the hospital, medications are withdrawn completely on the first day, in the absence of a contraindication. Antiemetics and fluids are administered as required; clonidine is used for opioid withdrawal symptoms. For acute intolerable pain during the waking hours, aspirin, 1 g IV (not approved in the United States), is useful. IM chlorpromazine can be helpful at night; patients must be adequately hydrated. Three to five days into the admission, as the effect of the withdrawn substance wears off, a course of IV dihydroergotamine (DHE) can be used. DHE, administered every 8 h for 5 consecutive days, a treatment that is not stopped short if headache settles, can induce a significant remission that allows a preventive treatment to be established. Serotonin 5-HT$_3$ receptor antagonists, such as ondansetron or granisetron, or the neurokinin receptor antagonist, aprepitant, may be required with DHE to prevent significant nausea, and domperidone (not approved in the United States) orally or by suppository can be very helpful. Avoiding sedating or otherwise side effect–prone antiemetics is helpful.

NEW DAILY PERSISTENT HEADACHE

New daily persistent headache (NDPH) is a clinically distinct syndrome with important secondary causes; these are listed in **Table 16-4**.

Clinical Presentation NDPH presents with headache on most if not all days, and the patient can clearly, and often vividly, recall the moment of onset. The headache usually begins abruptly, but onset may be more gradual; evolution over 3 days has been proposed as the upper limit for this syndrome. Patients typically recall the exact day and circumstances of the onset of headache; the new, persistent head pain does not remit. The first priority is to distinguish between a primary and a secondary cause of this syndrome. Subarachnoid hemorrhage is the most serious of the secondary causes and must be excluded either by history or appropriate investigation **(Chap. 429)**.

Secondary NDPH • **Low CSF Volume Headache** In these syndromes, head pain is positional: it begins when the patient sits or stands upright and resolves upon reclining. The pain, which is occipitofrontal, is usually a dull ache but may be throbbing. Patients with chronic low CSF volume headache typically present with a history of headache from one day to the next that is generally not present on waking but worsens during the day. Recumbency usually improves the headache within minutes, and it can take only minutes to an hour for the pain to return when the patient resumes an upright position.

The most common cause of headache due to persistent low CSF volume is CSF leak following LP **(Chap. S9)**. Post-LP headache usually begins within 48 h but may be delayed for up to 12 days. Its incidence is between 10% and 30%. Beverages with caffeine may provide temporary relief. Besides LP, index events may include epidural injection or a vigorous Valsalva maneuver, such as from lifting, straining, coughing, clearing the eustachian tubes in an airplane, or multiple orgasms. Spontaneous CSF leaks are well recognized, and the diagnosis should be considered whenever the headache history is typical, even when there is no obvious index event. As time passes from the index event, the postural nature may become less apparent; cases in which the index event occurred several years before the eventual diagnosis have been recognized. Symptoms appear to result from low volume rather than low pressure: although low CSF pressures, typically 0–50 mm CSF, are usually identified, a pressure as high as 140 mm CSF has been noted with a documented leak.

Postural orthostatic tachycardia syndrome (POTS; **Chap. 440**) can present with orthostatic headache similar to low CSF volume headache and is a diagnosis that needs consideration in this setting.

When imaging is indicated to identify the source of a presumed leak, an MRI with gadolinium is the initial study of choice **(Fig. 16-1)**. A striking pattern of diffuse meningeal enhancement is so typical that in the appropriate clinical context the diagnosis is established. Chiari malformations may sometimes be noted on MRI; in such cases, surgery to decompress the posterior fossa is *not* indicated and usually worsens the headache. Spinal MRI with T2 weighting may reveal a leak, and spinal MRI may demonstrate spinal meningeal cysts whose role in these syndromes is yet to be elucidated. The source of CSF leakage may be identified by spinal MRI with appropriate sequences, or by CT, preferably digital subtraction, myelography. In the absence of a directly identified site of leakage, 111In-DTPA CSF studies may demonstrate early emptying of the tracer into the bladder or slow progress of tracer across the brain suggesting a CSF leak; this procedure is now only rarely employed.

TABLE 16-4 Differential Diagnosis of New Daily Persistent Headache

PRIMARY	SECONDARY
Migrainous-type	Subarachnoid hemorrhage
Featureless (tension-type)	Low cerebrospinal fluid (CSF) volume headache
	Raised CSF pressure headache
	Posttraumatic headache[a]
	Chronic meningitis

[a]Includes postinfectious forms.

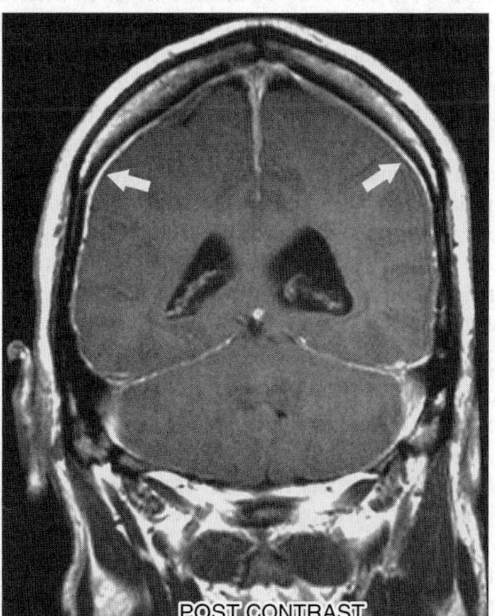

FIGURE 16-1 Magnetic resonance image showing diffuse meningeal enhancement after gadolinium administration in a patient with low cerebrospinal fluid (CSF) volume headache.

Initial treatment for low CSF volume headache is bed rest. For patients with persistent pain, IV caffeine (500 mg in 500 mL of saline administered over 2 h) can be very effective. An electrocardiogram (ECG) to screen for arrhythmia should be performed before administration. It is reasonable to administer at least two infusions of caffeine before embarking on additional tests to identify the source of the CSF leak. Because IV caffeine is safe and can be curative, it spares many patients the need for further investigations. If unsuccessful, an abdominal binder may be helpful. If a leak can be identified, an autologous blood patch is usually curative. A blood patch is also effective for post-LP headache; in this setting, the location is empirically determined to be the site of the LP. In patients with intractable headache, oral theophylline is a useful alternative that can take some months to be effective.

Raised CSF Pressure Headache Raised CSF pressure is well recognized as a cause of headache. Brain imaging can often reveal the cause, such as a space-occupying lesion.

Idiopathic intracranial hypertension (pseudotumor cerebri) NDPH due to raised CSF pressure can be the presenting symptom for patients with idiopathic intracranial hypertension, a disorder associated with obesity, female gender, and, on occasion, pregnancy. The syndrome can also occur without visual problems, particularly when the fundi are normal. These patients typically present with a history of generalized headache that is present on waking and improves as the day goes on. It is generally present on awakening in the morning and is worse with recumbency. Transient visual obscurations are frequent and may occur when the headaches are most severe. The diagnosis is relatively straightforward when papilledema is present, but the possibility must be considered even in patients without funduscopic changes. Formal visual field testing should be performed even in the absence of overt ophthalmic involvement. Partial obstructions of the cerebral venous sinuses are found in a small number of cases. In addition, persistently raised intracranial pressure can trigger a syndrome of chronic migraine. Other conditions that characteristically produce headache on rising in the morning or nocturnal headache are obstructive sleep apnea or poorly controlled hypertension.

Evaluation of patients suspected to have raised CSF pressure requires brain imaging. It is most efficient to obtain an MRI, including an MR venogram, as the initial study. If there are no contraindications, the CSF pressure should be measured by LP; this should be done when the patient is symptomatic so that both the pressure and the response to removal of 20–30 mL of CSF can be determined. An elevated opening pressure and improvement in headache following removal of CSF are diagnostic in the absence of fundal changes.

Initial treatment is with acetazolamide (250–500 mg bid); the headache may improve within weeks. If ineffective, topiramate is the next treatment of choice; it has many actions that may be useful in this setting, including carbonic anhydrase inhibition, weight loss, and neuronal membrane stabilization, likely mediated via effects on phosphorylation pathways. Severely disabled patients who do not respond to medical treatment require intracranial pressure monitoring and may require shunting. If appropriate, weight loss should be encouraged.

Posttraumatic Headache A traumatic event can trigger a headache process that lasts for many months or years after the event. The term *trauma* is used here in a very broad sense: headache can develop following an injury to the head, but it can also develop after an infectious episode, typically viral meningitis; a flulike illness; or a parasitic infection. Complaints of dizziness, vertigo, and impaired memory can accompany the headache. Symptoms may remit after several weeks or persist for months and even years after the injury. Typically, the neurologic examination is normal and CT or MRI studies are unrevealing. Chronic subdural hematoma may on occasion mimic this disorder. Posttraumatic headache may also be seen after carotid dissection and subarachnoid hemorrhage and after intracranial surgery. The underlying theme appears to be that a traumatic event involving the pain-producing meninges can trigger a headache process that lasts for many years.

Other Causes In one series, one-third of patients with NDPH reported headache beginning after a transient flulike illness characterized by fever, neck stiffness, photophobia, and marked malaise. Evaluation typically reveals no apparent cause for the headache. There is no convincing evidence that persistent Epstein-Barr virus infection plays a role in NDPH. A complicating factor is that many patients undergo LP during the acute illness; iatrogenic low CSF volume headache must be considered in these cases.

Treatment Treatment is largely empirical and directed at the headache phenotype. Tricyclic antidepressants, notably amitriptyline, and anticonvulsants, such as topiramate, valproate, candesartan, and gabapentin, have been used with reported benefit. The monoamine oxidase inhibitor phenelzine may also be useful in carefully selected patients. The headache usually resolves within 3–5 years, but it can be quite disabling.

PRIMARY CARE AND HEADACHE MANAGEMENT

Most patients with headache will be seen first in a primary care setting. The challenging task of the primary care physician is to identify the very few worrisome secondary headaches from the very great majority of primary and less dangerous secondary headaches (Table 16-2).

Absent any warning signs, a reasonable approach is to treat when a diagnosis is established. As a general rule, the investigation should focus on identifying worrisome causes of headache or on helping the patient to gain confidence if no primary headache diagnosis can be made.

After treatment has been initiated, follow-up care is essential to identify whether progress has been made against the headache complaint. Not all headaches will respond to treatment, but, in general, worrisome headaches will progress and will be easier to identify.

When a primary care physician feels the diagnosis is a primary headache disorder, it is worth noting that >90% of patients who present to primary care with a complaint of headache will have migraine (Chap. 430).

In general, patients who do not have a clear diagnosis, have a primary headache disorder other than migraine or tension-type headache, or are unresponsive to two or more standard therapies for the considered headache type, should be considered for referral to a specialist. In a practical sense, the threshold for referral is also determined by the experience of the primary care physician in headache medicine and the availability of secondary care options.

Acknowledgment

The editors acknowledge the contributions of Neil H. Raskin to earlier editions of this chapter.

FURTHER READING

Headache Classification Committee of the International Headache Society: The International Classification of Headache Disorders, 3rd ed. Cephalalgia 33:629, 2018.

Kernick D, Goadsby PJ: *Headache: A Practical Manual.* Oxford: Oxford University Press, 2008.

Lance JW, Goadsby PJ: *Mechanism and Management of Headache*, 7th ed. New York, Elsevier, 2005.

Olesen J et al: *The Headaches.* Philadelphia, Lippincott, Williams & Wilkins, 2005.

Silberstein SD, Lipton RB, Dodick DW: *Wolff's Headache and Other Head Pain*, 9th ed. New York, Oxford University Press, 2021.

17 Back and Neck Pain

John W. Engstrom

The importance of back and neck pain in our society is underscored by the following: (1) the cost of chronic back pain in the United States is estimated at more than $200 billion annually; approximately one-third of this cost is due to direct health care expenses and two-thirds are indirect costs resulting from loss of wages and productivity; (2) back symptoms are the most common cause of disability in individuals <45 years of age; (3) low back pain (LBP) is the second most common reason for visiting a physician in the United States; and (4) more than four out of five people will experience significant back pain at some point in their lives.

ANATOMY OF THE SPINE

The anterior spine consists of cylindrical vertebral bodies separated by intervertebral disks and stabilized by the anterior and posterior longitudinal ligaments. The intervertebral disks are composed of a central gelatinous nucleus pulposus surrounded by a tough cartilaginous ring, the annulus fibrosis. Disks are responsible for 25% of spinal column length and allow the bony vertebrae to move easily upon each other (**Figs. 17-1 and 17-2**). Desiccation of the nucleus pulposus and degeneration of the annulus fibrosus worsen with age, resulting in loss of disk height. The disks are largest in the cervical and lumbar regions where movements of the spine are greatest. The anterior spine absorbs the shock of bodily movements such as walking and running, and with the posterior spine protects the spinal cord and nerve roots in the spinal canal.

The posterior spine consists of the vertebral arches and processes. Each arch consists of paired cylindrical pedicles anteriorly and paired lamina posteriorly. The vertebral arch also gives rise to two transverse processes laterally, one spinous process posteriorly, plus two superior and two inferior articular facets. The apposition of a superior and inferior facet constitutes a *facet joint*. The posterior spine provides an anchor for the attachment of muscles and ligaments. The contraction of muscles attached to the spinous and transverse processes and lamina works like a system of pulleys and levers producing flexion, extension, rotation, and lateral bending movements of the spine.

Nerve root injury (*radiculopathy*) is a common cause of pain in the neck and arm, or low back and buttock, or leg (**see dermatomes in Figs. 25-2 and 25-3**). Each nerve root exits just above its corresponding vertebral body in the cervical region (e.g., the C7 nerve root exits at the C6-C7 level), and just below the vertebral body in the thoracic and lumbar spine (e.g., the T1 nerve root exits at the T1-T2 level). The cervical nerve roots follow a short intraspinal course before exiting. In contrast, because the spinal cord ends at the L1 or L2 vertebral level, the lumbar nerve roots follow a long intraspinal course and can be injured anywhere along its path. For example, disk herniation at the L4-L5 level can produce L4 root compression laterally, but more often compression of the traversing L5 nerve root occurs (**Fig. 17-3**). The lumbar nerve roots are mobile in the spinal canal, but eventually pass through the narrow *lateral recess* of the spinal canal and *intervertebral*

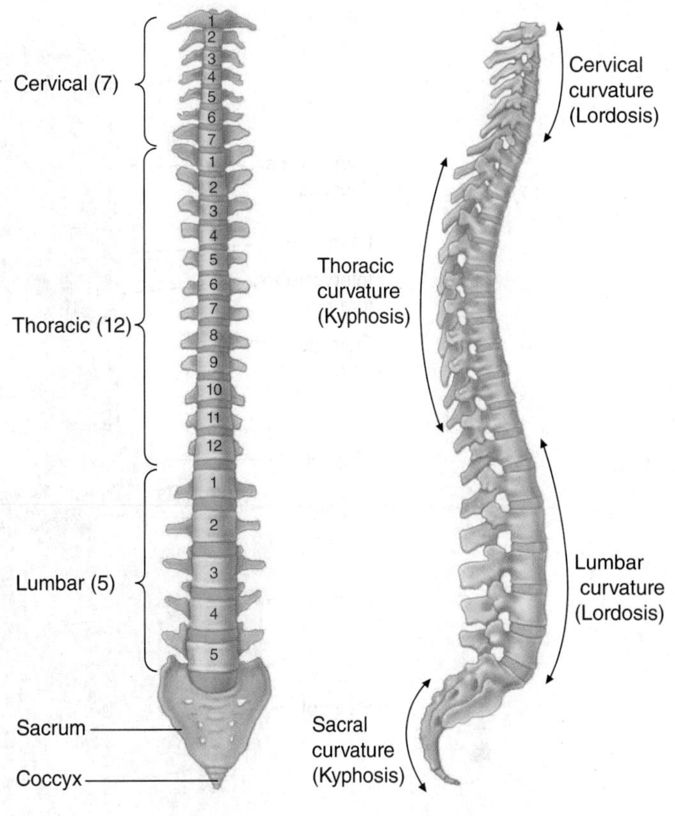

FIGURE 17-2 Spinal column. *(Reproduced with permission from AG Cornuelle, DH Gronefeld: Radiographic Anatomy Positioning. New York, McGraw-Hill, 1998.)*

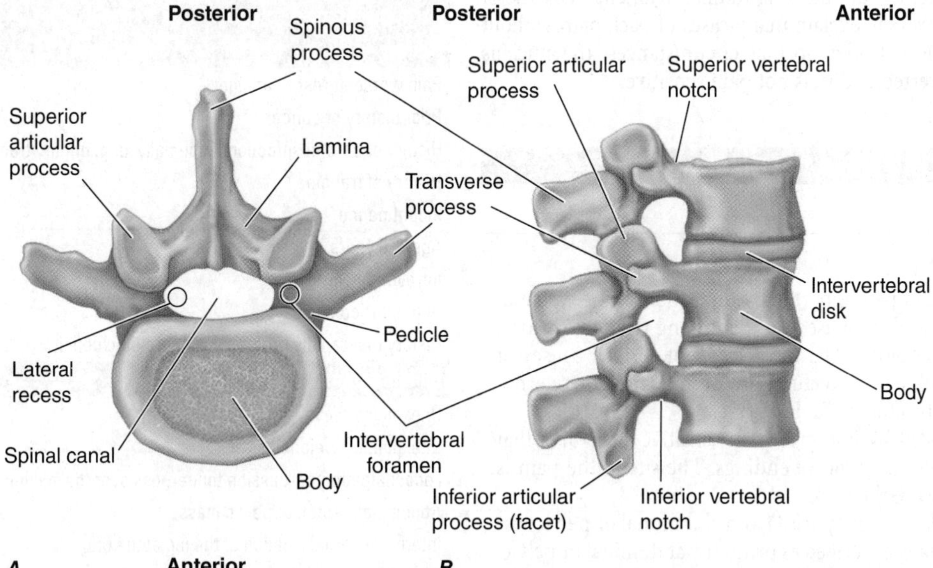

FIGURE 17-1 Vertebral anatomy. ***A.*** Vertebral body—axial view; ***B.*** vertebral column—sagittal view. *(Reproduced with permission from AG Cornuelle, DH Gronefeld: Radiographic Anatomy Positioning. New York, McGraw-Hill, 1998.)*

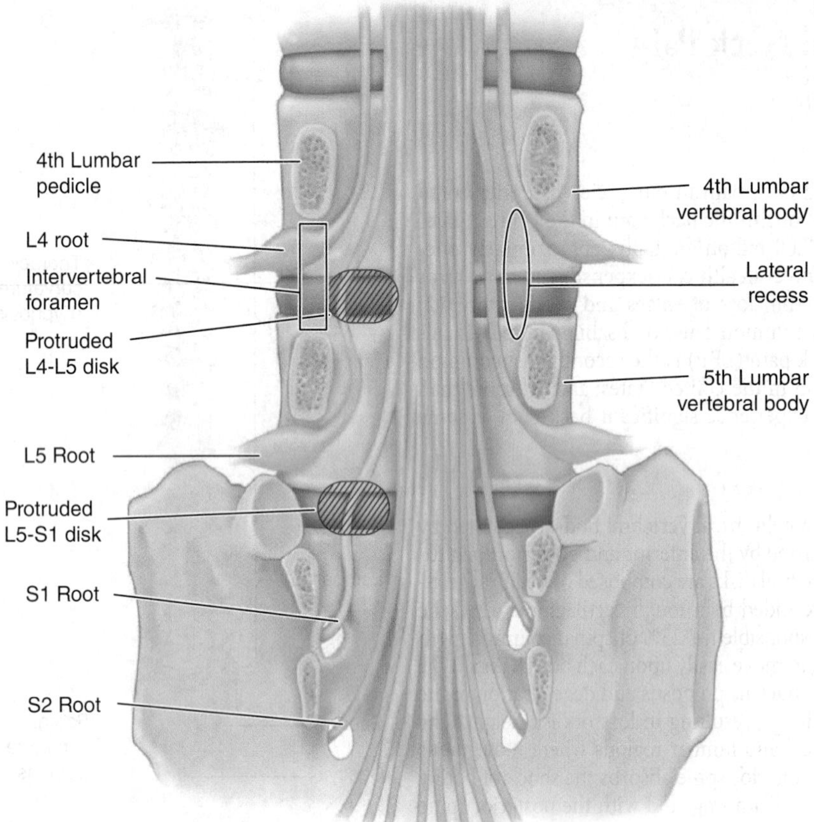

FIGURE 17-3 Compression of L5 and S1 roots by herniated disks. *(Reproduced with permission from AH Ropper, MA Samuels: Adams and Victor's Principles of Neurology, 9th ed. New York, McGraw-Hill, 2009.)*

foramen (Figs. 17-2 and 17-3). When imaging the spine, both sagittal and axial views are needed to assess possible compression at these sites.

Beginning at the C3 level, each cervical (and the first thoracic) vertebral body projects a lateral bony process upward—the uncinate process. The uncinate process articulates with the cervical vertebral body above via the uncovertebral joint. The uncovertebral joint can hypertrophy with age and contribute to neural foraminal narrowing and cervical radiculopathy.

Pain-sensitive structures of the spine include the periosteum of the vertebrae, dura, facet joints, annulus fibrosus of the intervertebral disk, epidural veins and arteries, and the longitudinal ligaments. Disease of these diverse structures may explain many cases of back pain without nerve root compression. Under normal circumstances, the nucleus pulposus of the intervertebral disk is not pain sensitive.

APPROACH TO THE PATIENT

Back Pain

TYPES OF BACK PAIN

Delineating the type of pain reported by the patient is the essential first step. Attention is also focused on identifying risk factors for a serious underlying etiology. The most frequent serious causes of back pain are radiculopathy, fracture, tumor, infection, or referred pain from visceral structures (Table 17-1).

Local pain is caused by injury to pain-sensitive structures that compress or irritate sensory nerve endings. The site of the pain is near the affected part of the back.

Pain referred to the back may arise from abdominal or pelvic viscera. The pain is usually described as primarily abdominal or pelvic, accompanied by back pain, and usually unaffected by posture. The patient may occasionally complain of back pain only.

Pain of spine origin may be located in the back or referred to the buttocks or legs. Diseases affecting the upper lumbar spine tend to refer pain to the lumbar region, groin, or anterior thighs. Diseases affecting the lower lumbar spine tend to produce pain referred to the buttocks, posterior thighs, calves, or feet. Referred pain often explains pain syndromes that cross multiple dermatomes without evidence of nerve or nerve root injury.

TABLE 17-1 Acute Low Back Pain: Risk Factors for an Important Structural Cause

History
Pain worse at rest or at night
Prior history of cancer
History of chronic infection (especially lung, urinary tract, skin, poor dentition)
History of trauma
Incontinence
Age >70 years
Intravenous drug use
Glucocorticoid use
History of a rapidly progressive neurologic deficit
Examination
Unexplained fever
Unexplained weight loss
Focal palpation/percussion tenderness over the midline spine
Abdominal, rectal, or pelvic mass
Internal/external rotation of the leg at the hip
Straight-leg or reverse straight-leg raising signs
Progressive focal neurologic deficit

Radicular pain is typically sharp and radiates from the low back to a leg within the territory of a nerve root (see "Lumbar Disk Disease," below). Coughing, sneezing, or voluntary contraction of abdominal muscles (lifting heavy objects or straining at stool) may elicit or worsen the radiating pain. The pain may also increase in postures that stretch the nerves and nerve roots. Sitting with the leg outstretched places traction on the sciatic nerve and L5 and S1 roots because the sciatic nerve passes posterior to the hip. The femoral nerve (L2, L3, and L4 roots) passes anterior to the hip and is not stretched by sitting. The description of the pain alone often fails to distinguish between referred pain and radiculopathy, although a burning or electric quality favors radiculopathy.

Pain associated with muscle spasm is commonly associated with many spine disorders. The spasms may be accompanied by an abnormal posture, tense paraspinal muscles, and dull or achy pain in the paraspinal region.

Knowledge of the circumstances associated with the onset of back pain is important when weighing possible serious underlying causes for the pain. Some patients involved in accidents or work-related injuries may exaggerate their pain for the purpose of compensation or for psychological reasons.

EXAMINATION

A complete physical examination including vital signs, heart and lungs, abdomen and rectum, and limbs is advisable. Back pain referred from visceral organs may be reproduced during palpation of the abdomen (pancreatitis, abdominal aortic aneurysm [AAA]) or percussion over the costovertebral angles (pyelonephritis).

The normal spine has a cervical and lumbar lordosis and a thoracic kyphosis. Exaggeration of these normal alignments may result in hyperkyphosis of the thoracic spine or hyperlordosis of the lumbar spine. Inspection of the back may reveal a lateral curvature of the spine (scoliosis). A midline hair tuft, skin dimpling or pigmentation, or a sinus tract may indicate a congenital spine anomaly. Asymmetry in the prominence of the paraspinal muscles suggests muscle spasm. Palpation over the spinous process transmits force to the entire vertebrae and suggests vertebral pathology.

Flexion at the hips is normal in patients with lumbar spine disease, but flexion of the lumbar spine is limited and sometimes painful. Lateral bending to the side opposite the injured spinal element may stretch the damaged tissues, worsen pain, and limit motion. Hyperextension of the spine (with the patient prone or standing) is limited when nerve root compression, facet joint pathology, or other bony spine disease is present.

Pain from hip disease may mimic the pain of lumbar spine disease. Hip pain can be reproduced by passive internal and external rotation at the hip with the knee and hip in flexion or by percussing the heel with the examiner's palm with the leg extended (heel percussion sign).

The *straight-leg raising (SLR)* maneuver is a simple bedside test for nerve root disease. With the patient supine, passive straight-leg flexion at the hip stretches the L5 and S1 nerve roots and the sciatic nerve; dorsiflexion of the foot during the maneuver adds to the stretch. In healthy individuals, flexion to at least 80° is normally possible without causing pain, although a tight, stretching sensation in the hamstring muscles is common. The SLR test is positive if the maneuver reproduces the patient's usual back or limb pain. Eliciting the SLR sign in both the supine and sitting positions can help determine if the finding is reproducible. The patient may describe pain in the low back, buttocks, posterior thigh, or lower leg, but the *key feature is reproduction of the patient's usual pain*. The *crossed SLR sign* is present when flexion of one leg reproduces the usual pain in the opposite leg or buttocks. In disk herniation, the crossed SLR sign is less sensitive but more specific than the SLR sign. The *reverse SLR sign* is elicited by standing the patient next to the examination table and passively extending each leg with the knee fully extended. This maneuver, which stretches the L2-L4 nerve roots, lumbosacral plexus, and femoral nerve, is considered positive if the patient's usual back or limb pain is reproduced. For all of these tests, the nerve or nerve root lesion is always on the side of the pain. Examination of the unaffected leg first provides a control test, ensures mutual understanding of test parameters, and enhances test utility.

The neurologic examination includes a search for focal weakness or muscle atrophy, localized reflex changes, diminished sensation in the legs, or signs of spinal cord injury. The examiner should be alert to the possibility of breakaway weakness, defined as fluctuations in the maximum power generated during muscle testing. Breakaway weakness may be due to pain, inattention, or a combination of pain and underlying true weakness. Breakaway weakness without pain is usually due to a lack of effort. In uncertain cases, electromyography (EMG) can determine if true weakness due to nerve tissue injury is present. Findings with specific lumbosacral nerve root lesions are shown in **Table 17-2** and are discussed below.

LABORATORY, IMAGING, AND EMG STUDIES

Laboratory studies are rarely needed for the initial evaluation of nonspecific acute (<3 months duration) low back pain (ALBP).

TABLE 17-2 Lumbosacral Radiculopathy: Neurologic Features

LUMBOSACRAL NERVE ROOT	EXAMINATION FINDINGS			PAIN DISTRIBUTION
	REFLEX	SENSORY	MOTOR	
L2[a]	—	Upper anterior thigh	Psoas (hip flexors)	Anterior thigh
L3[a]	—	Lower anterior thigh Anterior knee	Psoas (hip flexors) Quadriceps (knee extensors) Thigh adductors	Anterior thigh, knee
L4[a]	Quadriceps (knee)	Medial calf	Quadriceps (knee extensors)[b] Thigh adductors	Knee, medial calf Anterolateral thigh
L5[c]	—	Dorsal surface—foot Lateral calf	Peronei (foot evertors)[b] Tibialis anterior (foot dorsiflexors) Gluteus medius (leg abductors) Toe dorsiflexors	Lateral calf, dorsal foot, posterolateral thigh, buttocks
S1[c]	Gastrocnemius/soleus (ankle)	Plantar surface—foot Lateral aspect—foot	Gastrocnemius/soleus (foot plantar flexors)[b] Abductor hallucis (toe flexors)[b] Gluteus maximus (leg extensors)	Bottom foot, posterior calf, posterior thigh, buttocks

[a]Reverse straight-leg raising sign may be present—see "Examination of the Back." [b]These muscles receive the majority of innervation from this root. [c]Straight-leg raising sign may be present—see "Examination of the Back."

Risk factors for a serious underlying cause and for infection, tumor, or fracture in particular should be sought by history and examination. If risk factors are present (Table 17-1), then laboratory studies (complete blood count [CBC], erythrocyte sedimentation rate [ESR], urinalysis) are indicated. If risk factors are absent, then management is conservative (see "Treatment," below).

CT scanning is used as a primary screening modality for acute trauma that is moderate to severe. CT is superior to x-rays for detection of fractures involving posterior spine structures, craniocervical and cervicothoracic junctions, C1 and C2 vertebrae, bone fragments in the spinal canal, or misalignment. MRI or CT myelography is the radiologic test of choice for evaluation of most serious diseases involving the spine. MRI is superior for the definition of soft tissue structures, whereas CT myelography provides optimal imaging of the lateral recess of the spinal canal, defines bony abnormalities, and is tolerated by claustrophobic patients.

Population surveys in the United States suggest that patients with back pain report greater functional limitations in recent years, despite rapid increases in spine imaging, opioid prescribing, injections, and spine surgery. This suggests that more selective use of diagnostic and treatment modalities may be reasonable for many patients. One prospective case-control study found that older adults with back pain of less than 6 weeks duration who received spine imaging as part of a primary care visit had no better outcomes than the control group.

Spine imaging often reveals abnormalities of dubious clinical relevance that may alarm clinicians and patients alike and prompt further testing and unnecessary therapy. When imaging tests are reviewed, it is important to remember that degenerative findings are common in normal, pain-free individuals. Randomized trials and observational studies have suggested that imaging can have a "cascade effect," creating a gateway to other unnecessary care. Interventions have included physician education and computerized decision support within the electronic medical record to require specific indications for approval of imaging tests. Other strategies have included audit and feedback of individual practitioners' rates of ordering, more rapid access to physical therapy, or consultation with spine experts for patients without imaging indications.

Educational tools created by the America College of Physicians for patients and the public have included "Five Things Physicians and Patients Should Question": (1) Do not recommend advanced imaging (e.g., MRI) of the spine within the first 6 weeks in patients with nonspecific ALBP in the absence of red flags. (2) Do not perform elective spinal injections without imaging guidance, unless contraindicated. (3) Do not use bone morphogenetic protein (BMP) for routine anterior cervical spine fusion surgery. (4) Do not use EMG and nerve conduction studies (NCSs) to determine the cause of purely midline lumbar, thoracic, or cervical spine pain. (5) Do not recommend bed rest for >48 h when treating LBP. In an observational study, application of this strategy was associated with lower rates of repeat imaging, opioid use, and referrals for physical therapy.

Electrodiagnostic studies can be used to assess the functional integrity of the peripheral nervous system (**Chap. 446**). Sensory NCSs are normal when focal sensory loss confirmed by examination is due to nerve root damage because the nerve roots are proximal to the nerve cell bodies in the dorsal root ganglia. Injury to nerve tissue distal to the dorsal root ganglion (e.g., plexus or peripheral nerve) results in reduced sensory nerve signals. Needle EMG complements NCSs by detecting denervation or reinnervation changes in a myotomal (segmental) distribution. Multiple muscles supplied by different nerve roots and nerves are sampled; the pattern of muscle involvement indicates the nerve root(s) responsible for the injury. Needle EMG provides objective information about motor nerve fiber injury when clinical evaluation of weakness is limited by pain or poor effort. EMG and NCSs will be normal when sensory nerve root injury or irritation is the pain source.

The COVID-19 pandemic has disrupted and complicated the care of patients with LBP. Paraspinal myalgias may result in LBP. The sedentary lifestyle resulting from quarantine is associated with an increased frequency or severity of LBP. Fear of infection risk has also prevented many patients from seeking needed care. Video-telemedicine visits can help identify patients with underlying risks for a serious cause and inform appropriate next steps in management.

CAUSES OF BACK PAIN (TABLE 17-3)

LUMBAR DISK DISEASE

Lumbar disk disease is a common cause of acute, chronic, or recurrent low back and leg pain (**Figs. 17-3 and 17-4**). Disk disease is most likely to occur at the L4-L5 or L5-S1 levels, but upper lumbar levels can also be involved. The cause is often unknown, but the risk is increased in overweight individuals. Disk herniation is unusual prior to age 20 years and is rare in the fibrotic disks of the elderly. Complex genetic factors may play a role in predisposition. The pain may be located in the low back only or referred to a leg, buttock, or hip. A sneeze, cough, or trivial movement may cause the nucleus pulposus to prolapse, pushing the frayed and weakened annulus posteriorly. With severe disk disease, the nucleus can protrude through the annulus (herniation) or become extruded to lie as a free fragment in the spinal canal.

TABLE 17-3 Causes of Back or Neck Pain
Lumbar or Cervical Disk Disease
Degenerative Spine Disease
Lumbar spinal stenosis without or with neurogenic claudication
Intervertebral foraminal or lateral recess narrowing
Disk-osteophyte complex
Facet or uncovertebral joint hypertrophy
Lateral disk protrusion
Spondylosis (osteoarthritis), spondylolisthesis, or spondylolysis
Spine Infection
Vertebral osteomyelitis
Spinal epidural abscess
Septic disk (diskitis)
Meningitis
Lumbar arachnoiditis
Neoplasms
Metastatic with/without pathologic fracture
Primary Nervous System: Meningioma, neurofibroma, schwannoma
Primary Bone: chordoma, osteoma
Trauma
Strain or sprain
Whiplash injury
Trauma/falls, motor vehicle accidents
Metabolic Spine Disease
Osteoporosis with/without pathologic fracture—hyperparathyroidism, immobility
Osteosclerosis (e.g., Paget's disease)
Congenital/Developmental
Spondylolysis
Kyphoscoliosis
Spina bifida occulta
Tethered spinal cord
Autoimmune Inflammatory Arthritis
Other Causes of Back Pain
Referred pain from visceral disease (e.g., abdominal aortic aneurysm)
Postural
Psychiatric, malingering, chronic pain syndromes

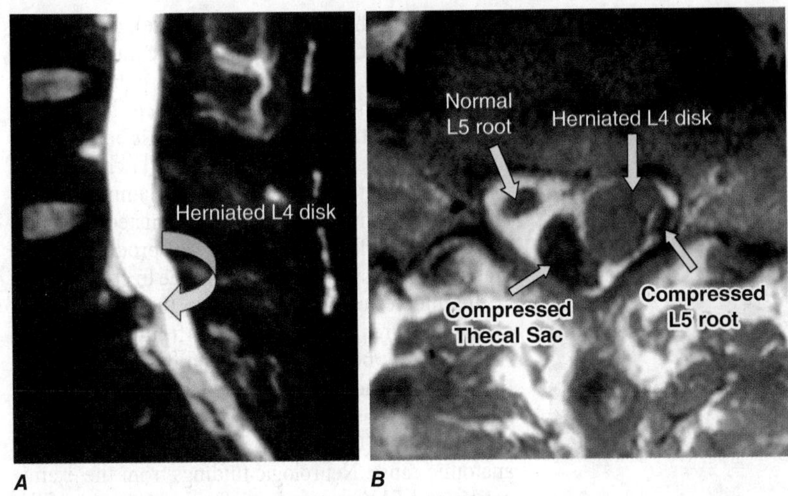

FIGURE 17-4 Disk herniation. ***A.*** Sagittal T2-weighted image on the left side of the spinal canal reveals disk herniation at the L4-L5 level. ***B.*** Axial T1-weighted image shows paracentral disk herniation with displacement of the thecal sac medially and the left L5 nerve root posteriorly in the left lateral recess.

The mechanism by which intervertebral disk injury causes back pain is uncertain. The inner annulus fibrosus and nucleus pulposus are normally devoid of innervation. Inflammation and production of proinflammatory cytokines within a ruptured nucleus pulposus may trigger or perpetuate back pain. Ingrowth of nociceptive (pain) nerve fibers into the nucleus pulposus of a diseased disk may be responsible for some cases of chronic "diskogenic" pain. Nerve root injury (radiculopathy) from disk herniation is usually due to inflammation, but lateral herniation may produce compression in the lateral recess or intervertebral foramen.

A ruptured disk may be asymptomatic or cause back pain, limited spine motion (particularly flexion), a focal neurologic deficit, or radicular pain. A dermatomal pattern of sensory loss or a reduced or absent deep tendon reflex is more suggestive of a specific root lesion than is the pattern of pain. Motor findings (focal weakness, muscle atrophy, or fasciculations) occur less frequently than focal sensory or reflex changes. Symptoms and signs are usually unilateral, but bilateral involvement does occur with large central disk herniations that involve roots bilaterally or cause inflammation of nerve roots within the spinal canal. Clinical manifestations of specific nerve root lesions are summarized in Table 17-2.

The differential diagnosis covers a variety of serious and treatable conditions, including epidural abscess, hematoma, fracture, or tumor. Fever, constant pain uninfluenced by position, sphincter abnormalities, or signs of myelopathy suggest an etiology other than lumbar disk disease. Absent ankle reflexes can be a normal finding in persons >60 years or a sign of bilateral S1 radiculopathies. An absent deep tendon reflex or focal sensory loss may indicate injury to a nerve root, but other sites of injury along the nerve must also be considered. As examples, an absent knee reflex may be due to a femoral neuropathy or an L4 nerve root injury; loss of sensation over the foot and lateral lower calf may result from a peroneal or lateral sciatic neuropathy, or an L5 nerve root injury. Focal muscle atrophy may reflect injury to the anterior horn cells of the spinal cord, a nerve root, peripheral nerve, or disuse.

A lumbar spine MRI scan or CT myelogram can often confirm the location and type of pathology. Spine MRIs yield exquisite views of intraspinal and adjacent soft tissue anatomy, whereas bony lesions of the lateral recess or intervertebral foramen are optimally visualized by CT myelography. The correlation of neuroradiologic findings to clinical symptoms, particularly pain, is not simple. Contrast-enhancing tears in the annulus fibrosus or disk protrusions are widely accepted as common sources of back pain; however, studies have found that many asymptomatic adults have similar radiologic findings. Entirely asymptomatic disk protrusions are also common, occurring in up to one-third of adults, and these may also enhance with contrast. Furthermore, in patients with known disk herniation treated either medically or surgically, persistence of the herniation 10 years later had no relationship to the clinical outcome. In summary, MRI findings of disk protrusion, tears in the annulus fibrosus, or hypertrophic facet joints are common incidental findings that, by themselves, should not dictate management decisions for patients with back pain.

The diagnosis of nerve root injury is most secure when the history, examination, results of imaging studies, and the EMG are concordant. There is often good correlation between CT and EMG findings for localization of nerve root injury.

Management of lumbar disk disease is discussed below.

Cauda equina syndrome (CES) signifies an injury of multiple lumbosacral nerve roots within the spinal canal distal to the termination of the spinal cord at L1-L2. LBP, weakness and areflexia in the legs, saddle anesthesia, or loss of bladder function may occur. The problem must be distinguished from disorders of the lower spinal cord (conus medullaris syndrome), acute transverse myelitis (**Chap. 442**), and Guillain-Barré syndrome (**Chap. 447**). Combined involvement of the conus medullaris and cauda equina can occur. CES is most commonly due to a large ruptured lumbosacral intervertebral disk, but other causes include lumbosacral spine fracture, hematoma within the spinal canal (sometimes following lumbar puncture in patients with coagulopathy), and tumor or other compressive mass lesions. Treatment is usually surgical decompression, sometimes on an urgent basis in an attempt to restore or preserve motor or sphincter function, or radiotherapy for metastatic tumors (**Chap. 90**).

DEGENERATIVE CONDITIONS

Lumbar spinal stenosis (LSS) describes a narrowed lumbar spinal canal. *Neurogenic claudication* consists of pain, typically in the back and buttocks or legs, that is brought on by walking or standing and relieved by sitting. Unlike vascular claudication, symptoms are often provoked by standing without walking. Unlike lumbar disk disease, symptoms are usually relieved by sitting. Patients with neurogenic claudication can often walk much farther when leaning over a shopping cart and can pedal a stationary bike with ease while sitting. These flexed positions increase the anteroposterior spinal canal diameter and reduce intraspinal venous hypertension, producing pain relief. Focal weakness, sensory loss, or reflex changes may occur when spinal stenosis is associated with neural foraminal narrowing and radiculopathy. Severe neurologic deficits, including paralysis and urinary incontinence, occur only rarely.

LSS by itself is common (6–7% of adults) and is usually asymptomatic. Symptoms are correlated with severe spinal canal stenosis. LSS is most often acquired (75%) but can also be congenital or due to a mixture of both etiologies. Congenital forms (achondroplasia and idiopathic) are characterized by short, thick pedicles that produce both spinal canal and lateral recess stenosis. Acquired factors that contribute to spinal stenosis include degenerative diseases (spondylosis, spondylolisthesis, and scoliosis), trauma, spine surgery, metabolic or endocrine disorders (epidural lipomatosis, osteoporosis, acromegaly, renal osteodystrophy, and hypoparathyroidism), and Paget's disease. MRI provides the best definition of the abnormal anatomy (**Fig. 17-5**).

LSS accompanied by neurogenic claudication responds to surgical decompression of the stenotic segments. The same processes leading to LSS may cause lumbar foraminal or lateral recess narrowing resulting in coincident lumbar radiculopathy that may require treatment as well.

Conservative treatment of symptomatic LSS can include nonsteroidal anti-inflammatory drugs (NSAIDs), acetaminophen, exercise programs, and symptomatic treatment of acute pain episodes. There is insufficient evidence to support the routine use of epidural glucocorticoid injections. Surgery is considered when medical therapy does not relieve symptoms sufficiently to allow for resumption of activities of

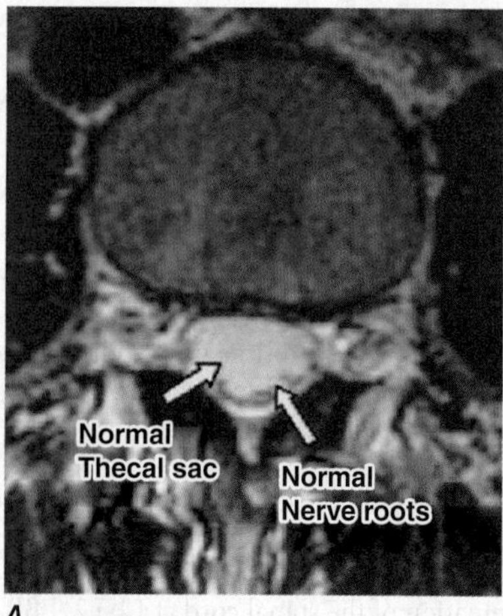

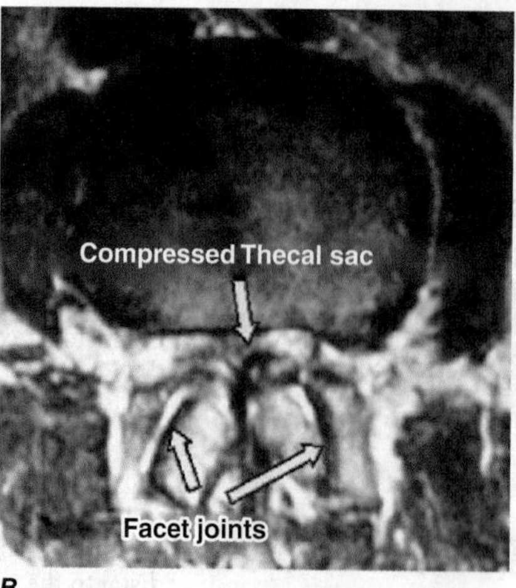

A B

FIGURE 17-5 Spinal stenosis. ***A.*** An axial T2-weighted image of the normal lumbar spine shows a normal thecal sac within the lumbar spinal canal. The thecal sac is bright. The lumbar roots are seen as dark punctate dots located posteriorly in the thecal sac. ***B.*** The thecal sac is not well visualized due to severe lumbar spinal canal stenosis, partially the result of hypertrophic facet joints.

daily living or when focal neurologic signs are present. Most patients with neurogenic claudication who are treated medically do not improve over time. Surgical management with laminectomy, which increases the spinal canal diameter and reduces venous hypertension, can produce significant relief of exertional back and leg pain, leading to less disability and improved functional outcomes. Laminectomy and fusion is usually reserved for patients with LSS and spondylolisthesis. Predictors of a poor surgical outcome include impaired walking preoperatively, depression, cardiovascular disease, and scoliosis. Up to one-quarter of surgically treated patients develop recurrent stenosis at the same or an adjacent spinal level within 7–10 years; recurrent symptoms usually respond to a second surgical decompression.

Neural foraminal narrowing or lateral recess stenosis with radiculopathy is a common consequence of osteoarthritic processes that cause LSS (**Figs.** 17-1 and 17-6), including osteophytes, lateral disk protrusion, calcified disk-osteophytes, facet joint hypertrophy, uncovertebral joint hypertrophy (in the cervical spine), congenitally shortened pedicles, or, frequently, a combination of these processes. Neoplasms (primary or metastatic), fractures, infections (epidural abscess), or hematomas are less frequent causes. Most common is bony foraminal narrowing leading to nerve root ischemia and persistent symptoms, in contrast to inflammation that is associated with a paracentral herniated disk and radiculopathy. These conditions can produce unilateral nerve root symptoms or signs due to compression at the intervertebral foramen or in the lateral recess; symptoms are indistinguishable from disk-related radiculopathy, but treatment may differ depending on the etiology. The history and neurologic examination alone cannot distinguish between these possibilities. Neuroimaging (CT or MRI) is required to identify the anatomic cause. Neurologic findings from the examination and EMG can help direct the attention of the radiologist to specific nerve roots, especially on axial images. For *facet joint hypertrophy with foraminal stenosis,* surgical foraminotomy produces long-term relief of leg and back pain in 80–90% of patients. Facet joint or medial branch blocks for back or neck pain are sometimes used to help determine the anatomic origin of back pain or for treatment, but there is a lack of clinical data to support their utility. Medical causes of lumbar or cervical radiculopathy unrelated to primary spine disease include infections (e.g., herpes zoster and Lyme disease), carcinomatous meningitis, diabetes, and root avulsion or traction (trauma).

SPONDYLOSIS AND SPONDYLOLISTHESIS

Spondylosis, or osteoarthritic spine disease, typically occurs in later life and primarily involves the cervical and lumbosacral spine. Patients often complain of back pain that increases with movement, is associated with stiffness, and is better with inactivity. The relationship between clinical symptoms and radiologic findings is usually not straightforward. Pain may be prominent when MRI, CT, or x-ray findings are minimal, and prominent degenerative spine disease can be seen in asymptomatic patients. Osteophytes, combined

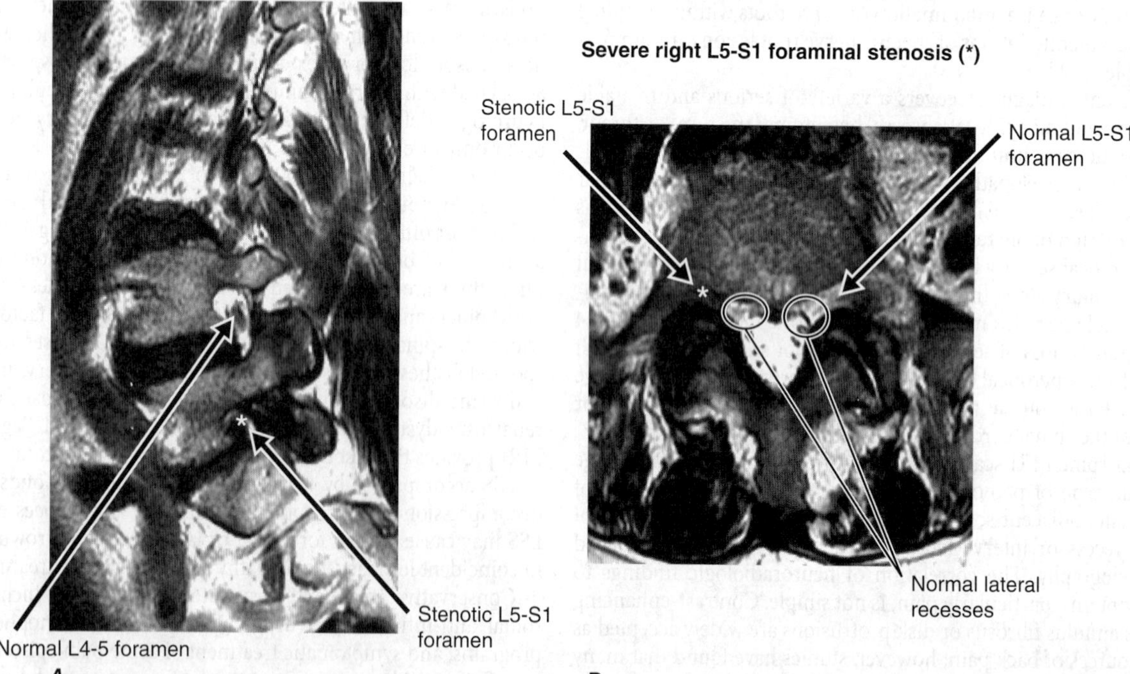

FIGURE 17-6 Foraminal stenosis. ***A.*** Sagittal T2-weighted image reveals normal high signal around the exiting right L4 nerve root in the right neural foramen at L4-L5; effacement of the high signal is noted one level below at L5-S1, due to severe foraminal stenosis. ***B.*** Axial T2-weighted image at the L5-S1 level demonstrates normal lateral recesses bilaterally, a normal intervertebral foramen on the left, but a severely stenotic foramen (*) on the right.

disk-osteophytes, or a thickened ligamentum flavum may cause or contribute to central spinal canal stenosis, lateral recess stenosis, or neural foraminal narrowing.

Spondylolisthesis is the anterior slippage of the vertebral body, pedicles, and superior articular facets, leaving the posterior elements behind. Spondylolisthesis can be associated with spondylolysis, congenital anomalies, degenerative spine disease, or other causes of mechanical weakness of the pars interarticularis (e.g., infection, osteoporosis, tumor, trauma, earlier surgery). The slippage may be asymptomatic or may cause LBP, nerve root injury (the L5 root most frequently), symptomatic spinal stenosis, or CES in rare severe cases. A "step-off" on palpation or tenderness may be elicited near the segment that has "slipped" (most often L4 on L5 or occasionally L5 on S1). Focal anterolisthesis or retrolisthesis can occur at any cervical or lumbar level and be the source of neck or LBP. Plain x-rays of the low back or neck in flexion and extension will reveal movement at the abnormal spinal segment. Surgery is performed for spinal instability (slippage 5–8 mm) and considered for pain symptoms that do not respond to conservative measures (e.g., rest, physical therapy), cases with a progressive neurologic deficit, or scoliosis.

■ NEOPLASMS

Back pain is the most common neurologic symptom in patients with systemic cancer and is the presenting symptom in 20%. The cause is usually vertebral body metastasis (85–90%) but can also result from spread of cancer through the intervertebral foramen (especially with lymphoma), carcinomatous meningitis, or metastasis to the spinal cord. The thoracic spine is most often affected. Cancer-related back pain tends to be constant, dull, unrelieved by rest, and worse at night. By contrast, mechanical causes of LBP usually improve with rest. MRI, CT, and CT myelography are the studies of choice when spinal metastasis is suspected. Once a metastasis is found, imaging of the entire spine is essential, as it reveals additional tumor deposits in one-third of patients. MRI is preferred for soft tissue definition, but the most rapidly available imaging modality is best because the patient's condition may worsen quickly without intervention. Early diagnosis is crucial. A strong predictor of outcome is baseline neurologic function prior to diagnosis. Half to three-quarters of patients are nonambulatory at the time of diagnosis and few regain the ability to walk. **The management of spinal metastasis is discussed in detail in Chap. 90.**

■ INFECTIONS/INFLAMMATION

Vertebral osteomyelitis is most often caused by hematogenous seeding of staphylococci, but other bacteria or tuberculosis (Pott's disease) may be responsible. The primary source of infection is usually the skin or urinary tract. Other common sources of bacteremia are IV drug use, poor dentition, endocarditis, lung abscess, IV catheters, or postoperative wound sites. Back pain at rest, tenderness over the involved vertebra, and an elevated erythrocyte sedimentation rate (ESR) or C-reactive protein (CRP) are the most common findings in vertebral osteomyelitis. Fever or an elevated white blood cell count is found in a minority of patients. MRI and CT are sensitive and specific for early detection of osteomyelitis. The intervertebral disk can also be affected by infection (diskitis) and almost never by tumor. Extension of the infection posteriorly from the vertebral body can produce a spinal epidural abscess.

Spinal epidural abscess **(Chap. 442)** presents with back pain (aggravated by movement or palpation of the spinous process), fever, radiculopathy, or signs of spinal cord compression. The subacute development of two or more of these findings should increase suspicion for spinal epidural abscess. The abscess is best delineated by spine MRI and may track over multiple spinal levels.

Lumbar adhesive arachnoiditis with radiculopathy is due to fibrosis following inflammation within the subarachnoid space. The fibrosis results in nerve root adhesions and presents as back and leg pain associated with multifocal motor, sensory, or reflex changes. Causes of arachnoiditis include multiple lumbar operations (most common in the United States), chronic spinal infections (especially tuberculosis in the developing world), spinal cord injury, intrathecal hemorrhage, myelography (rare), intrathecal injections (glucocorticoids, anesthetics, or other agents), and foreign bodies. The MRI shows clumped nerve roots on axial views or loculations of cerebrospinal fluid within the thecal sac. Clumped nerve roots should be distinguished from enlarged nerve roots seen with demyelinating polyneuropathy or neoplastic infiltration. Treatment is usually unsatisfactory. Microsurgical lysis of adhesions, dorsal rhizotomy, dorsal root ganglionectomy, and epidural glucocorticoids have been tried, but outcomes have been poor. Dorsal column stimulation for pain relief has produced varying results.

■ TRAUMA

A patient complaining of back pain and an inability to move the legs may have a spine fracture or dislocation; fractures above L1 place the spinal cord at risk for compression. Care must be taken to avoid further damage to the spinal cord or nerve roots by immobilizing the back or neck pending the results of radiologic studies. Vertebral fractures frequently occur in the absence of trauma in association with osteoporosis, glucocorticoid use, osteomyelitis, or neoplastic infiltration.

Sprains and Strains The terms *low back sprain, strain,* and *mechanically induced muscle spasm* refer to minor, self-limited injuries associated with lifting a heavy object, a fall, or a sudden deceleration such as in an automobile accident. These terms are used loosely and do not correlate with specific underlying pathologies. The pain is usually confined to the lower back. Patients with paraspinal muscle spasm often assume unusual postures.

Traumatic Vertebral Fractures Most traumatic fractures of the lumbar vertebral bodies result from injuries producing anterior wedging or compression. With severe trauma, the patient may sustain a fracture-dislocation or a "burst" fracture involving the vertebral body and posterior elements. Traumatic vertebral fractures are caused by falls from a height, sudden deceleration in an automobile accident, or direct injury. Neurologic impairment is common, and early surgical treatment is indicated. In victims of blunt trauma, CT scans of the chest, abdomen, or pelvis can be reformatted to detect associated vertebral fractures. Rules have been developed to avoid unnecessary spine imaging associated with low-risk trauma, but these studies typically exclude patients aged >65 years—a group that can sustain fractures with minor trauma.

■ METABOLIC CAUSES

Osteoporosis and Osteosclerosis Immobilization, osteomalacia, the postmenopausal state, renal disease, multiple myeloma, hyperparathyroidism, hyperthyroidism, metastatic carcinoma, or glucocorticoid use may accelerate osteoporosis and weaken the vertebral body, leading to compression fractures and pain. Up to two-thirds of compression fractures seen on radiologic imaging are asymptomatic. The most common nontraumatic vertebral body fractures are due to a postmenopausal cause, or to osteoporosis in adults >75 years old **(Chap. 411)**. The risk of an additional vertebral fracture 1 year following a first vertebral fracture is 20%. The presence of fever, weight loss, fracture at a level above T4, any fracture in a young adult, or the predisposing conditions described above should increase suspicion for a cause other than typical osteoporosis. The sole manifestations of a compression fracture may be localized back or radicular pain exacerbated by movement and often reproduced by palpation over the spinous process of the affected vertebra.

Relief of acute pain can often be achieved with acetaminophen, NSAIDs, opioids, or a combination of these medications. Both pain and disability are improved with bracing. Antiresorptive drugs are not recommended in the setting of acute pain but are the preferred treatment to prevent additional fractures. Less than one-third of patients with prior compression fractures are adequately treated for osteoporosis despite the increased risk for future fractures; even fewer at-risk patients without a history of fracture are adequately treated. The literature for percutaneous vertebroplasty (PVP) or kyphoplasty for osteoporotic compression fractures associated with debilitating pain does not support their use.

Osteosclerosis, an abnormally increased bone density often due to Paget's disease, is readily identifiable on routine x-ray studies and can sometimes be a source of back pain. It may be associated with an isolated increase in alkaline phosphatase in an otherwise healthy older person. Spinal cord or nerve root compression can result from bony encroachment. The diagnosis of Paget's disease as the cause of a patient's back pain is a diagnosis of exclusion.

For further discussion of these bone disorders, see Chaps. 410, 411, and 412.

■ AUTOIMMUNE INFLAMMATORY ARTHRITIS

Autoimmune inflammatory disease of the spine can present with the insidious onset of low back, buttock, or neck pain. Examples include rheumatoid arthritis (RA) **(Chap. 358)**, ankylosing spondylitis, reactive arthritis and psoriatic arthritis **(Chap. 355)**, or inflammatory bowel disease **(Chap. 326)**.

■ CONGENITAL ANOMALIES OF THE LUMBAR SPINE

Spondylolysis is a bony defect in the vertebral pars interarticularis (a segment near the junction of the pedicle with the lamina), a finding present in up to 6% of adolescents. The cause is usually a stress microfracture in a congenitally abnormal segment. Multislice CT with multiplanar reformation is the most accurate modality for detecting spondylolysis in adults. Symptoms may occur in the setting of a single injury, repeated minor injuries, or during a growth spurt. Spondylolysis is the most common cause of persistent LBP in adolescents and is often associated with sports-related activities.

Scoliosis refers to an abnormal curvature in the coronal (lateral) plane of the spine. With *kyphoscoliosis,* there is, in addition, a forward curvature of the spine. The abnormal curvature may be congenital, due to abnormal spine development, acquired in adulthood due to degenerative spine disease, or progressive due to paraspinal neuromuscular disease. The deformity can progress until ambulation or pulmonary function is compromised.

Spina bifida occulta (closed spinal dysraphism) is a failure of closure of one or several vertebral arches posteriorly; the meninges and spinal cord are normal. A dimple or small lipoma may overlie the defect, but the skin is intact. Most cases are asymptomatic and discovered incidentally during a physical examination for back pain.

Tethered cord syndrome usually presents as a progressive cauda equina disorder (see below), although myelopathy may also be the initial manifestation. The patient is often a child or young adult who complains of perineal or perianal pain, sometimes following minor trauma. MRI studies typically reveal a low-lying conus (below L1 and L2) and a short and thickened filum terminale. The MRI findings also occur as incidental findings, sometimes during evaluation of unrelated LBP in adults.

■ REFERRED PAIN FROM VISCERAL DISEASE

Diseases of the thorax, abdomen, or pelvis may refer pain to the spinal segment that innervates the diseased organ. Occasionally, back pain may be the first and only manifestation. Upper abdominal diseases generally refer pain to the lower thoracic or upper lumbar region (eighth thoracic to the first and second lumbar vertebrae), lower abdominal diseases to the midlumbar region (second to fourth lumbar vertebrae), and pelvic diseases to the sacral region. Local signs (pain with spine palpation, paraspinal muscle spasm) are absent, and little or no pain accompanies routine movements.

Low Thoracic or Lumbar Pain with Abdominal Disease Tumors of the posterior wall of the stomach or duodenum typically produce epigastric pain **(Chaps. 80 and 324)**, but back pain may occur if retroperitoneal extension is present. Fatty foods occasionally induce back pain associated with biliary or pancreatic disease. Pathology in retroperitoneal structures (hemorrhage, tumors, and pyelonephritis) can produce paraspinal pain that radiates to the lower abdomen, groin, or anterior thighs. A mass in the iliopsoas region can produce unilateral lumbar pain with radiation toward the groin, labia, or testicle. The sudden appearance of lumbar pain in a patient receiving anticoagulants should prompt consideration of retroperitoneal hemorrhage.

Isolated LBP occurs in some patients with a contained rupture of an AAA. The classic clinical triad of abdominal pain, shock, and back pain occurs in <20% of patients. The diagnosis may be missed because the symptoms and signs can be nonspecific. Misdiagnoses include nonspecific back pain, diverticulitis, renal colic, sepsis, and myocardial infarction. A careful abdominal examination revealing a pulsatile mass (present in 50–75% of patients) is an important physical finding. Patients with suspected AAA should be evaluated with abdominal ultrasound, CT, or MRI **(Chap. 280)**.

Sacral Pain with Gynecologic and Urologic Disease Pelvic organs rarely cause isolated LBP. Uterine malposition (retroversion, descensus, and prolapse) may cause traction on the uterosacral ligament. The pain is referred to the sacral region, sometimes appearing after prolonged standing. Endometriosis or uterine cancers can invade the uterosacral ligaments. Pain associated with endometriosis is typically premenstrual and often continues until it merges with menstrual pain.

Menstrual pain with poorly localized, cramping pain can radiate down the legs. LBP that radiates into one or both thighs is common in the last weeks of pregnancy. Continuous and worsening pain unrelieved by rest or at night may be due to neoplastic infiltration of nerves or nerve roots.

Urologic sources of lumbosacral back pain include chronic prostatitis, prostate cancer with spinal metastasis **(Chap. 87)**, and diseases of the kidney or ureter. Infectious, inflammatory, or neoplastic renal diseases may produce ipsilateral lumbosacral pain, as can renal artery or vein thrombosis. Paraspinal lumbar pain may be a symptom of ureteral obstruction due to nephrolithiasis.

■ OTHER CAUSES OF BACK PAIN

Postural Back Pain There is a group of patients with nonspecific chronic low back pain (CLBP) in whom no specific anatomic lesion can be found despite exhaustive investigation. Exercises to strengthen the paraspinal and abdominal muscles are sometimes helpful. CLBP may be encountered in patients who seek financial compensation; in malingerers; or in those with concurrent substance abuse. Many patients with CLBP have a history of psychiatric illness (depression, anxiety states) or childhood trauma (physical or sexual abuse) that antedates the onset of back pain. Preoperative psychological assessment has been used to exclude patients with marked psychological impairments that predict a poor surgical outcome from spine surgery.

Idiopathic The cause of LBP occasionally remains unclear. Some patients have had multiple operations for disk disease. The original indications for surgery may have been questionable, with back pain only, no definite neurologic signs, or a minor disk bulge noted on CT or MRI. Scoring systems based on neurologic signs, psychological factors, physiologic studies, and imaging studies have been devised to minimize the likelihood of unsuccessful surgery.

■ GLOBAL CONSIDERATIONS

While many of the history and examination features described in this chapter apply to all patients, information regarding the global epidemiology and prevalence of LBP is limited. The Global Burden of Diseases Study 2019 reported that LBP represented the #1 cause overall for total years lived with disability (YLD), and #9 overall as a cause of disability-related life years (DALYs). These numbers increased substantially from 1990 estimates, and with the aging of the population worldwide, the numbers of individuals suffering from LBP are expected to increase further in the future. Although rankings for LBP generally were higher in developed regions, a high burden exists in every part of the world. An area of uncertainty is the degree to which regional differences exist in terms of the specific etiologies of LBP and how these are managed. For example, the most common cause of arachnoiditis in developing countries is a prior spinal infection, but in developed countries the most frequent cause is multiple lumbar spine surgeries.

TREATMENT

Back Pain

Management is considered separately for acute and chronic low back pain syndromes without radiculopathy, and for back pain with radiculopathy.

ACUTE LOW BACK PAIN WITHOUT RADICULOPATHY

This is defined as pain of <12 weeks duration. Full recovery can be expected in >85% of adults with ALBP without leg pain. Most have purely "mechanical" symptoms (i.e., pain that is aggravated by motion and relieved by rest).

The initial assessment is focused on excluding serious causes of spine pathology that require urgent intervention, including infection, cancer, or trauma. Risk factors for a serious cause of ALBP are shown in Table 17-1. Laboratory and imaging studies are unnecessary if risk factors are absent. CT, MRI, or plain spine films are rarely indicated in the first month of symptoms unless a spine fracture, tumor, or infection is suspected.

The prognosis of ALBP is generally excellent; however, episodes tend to recur, and as many as two-thirds of patients will experience a second episode within 1 year. Most patients do not seek medical care and improve on their own. Even among those seen in primary care, two-thirds report substantial improvement after 7 weeks. This high likelihood of spontaneous improvement can mislead clinicians and patients about the efficacy of treatment interventions, highlighting the importance of rigorous prospective trials. Many treatments commonly used in the past are now known to be ineffective, including bed rest and lumbar traction.

Clinicians should reassure and educate patients that improvement is very likely and instruct them in self-care. Satisfaction and the likelihood of follow-up increase when patients are educated about prognosis, evidence-based treatments, appropriate activity modifications, and strategies to prevent future exacerbations. Counseling patients about the risks of overtreatment is another important part of the discussion. Patients who report that they did not receive an adequate explanation for their symptoms are likely to request further diagnostic tests.

In general, bed rest should be avoided for relief of severe symptoms or limited to a day or two at most. Several randomized trials suggest that bed rest does not hasten the pace of recovery. In general, early resumption of normal daily physical activity should be encouraged, avoiding only strenuous manual labor. Advantages of early ambulation for ALBP also include maintenance of cardiovascular conditioning; improved bone, cartilage, and muscle strength; and increased endorphin levels. Specific back exercises or early vigorous exercise have not shown benefits for acute back pain. Empiric use of heating pads or blankets is sometimes helpful.

NSAIDs and Acetaminophen Evidence-based guidelines recommend over-the-counter medicines such as NSAIDs and acetaminophen as first-line options for treatment of ALBP. In otherwise healthy patients, a trial of NSAIDs can be followed by acetaminophen for time-limited periods. In theory, the anti-inflammatory effects of NSAIDs might provide an advantage over acetaminophen to suppress inflammation that accompanies many causes of ALBP, but in practice there is no clinical evidence to support the superiority of NSAIDs. The risk of renal and gastrointestinal toxicity with NSAIDs is increased in patients with preexisting medical comorbidities (e.g., renal insufficiency, cirrhosis, prior gastrointestinal hemorrhage, use of anticoagulants or glucocorticoids, heart failure). Some patients elect to take acetaminophen and an NSAID together in hopes of a more rapid benefit.

Muscle Relaxants Skeletal muscle relaxants, such as cyclobenzaprine or methocarbamol, may be useful, but sedation is a common side effect. Limiting the use of muscle relaxants to nighttime only may be an option for patients with back pain that interferes with sleep.

Opioids There is no good evidence to support the use of opioid analgesics or tramadol as first-line therapy for ALBP. Their use is best reserved for patients who cannot tolerate acetaminophen or NSAIDs and for those with severe refractory pain. Also, the duration of opioid treatment for ALBP should be strictly limited to 3–7 days. As with muscle relaxants, these drugs are often sedating, so it may be useful to prescribe them at nighttime only. Side effects of short-term opioid use include nausea, constipation, and pruritus; risks of long-term opioid use include hypersensitivity to pain, hypogonadism, and dependency. Falls, fractures, driving accidents, and fecal impaction are other risks. The clinical efficacy of opioids for chronic pain beyond 16 weeks of use is unproven.

Mounting evidence of morbidity from long-term opioid therapy (including overdose, dependency, addiction, falls, fractures, accident risk, and sexual dysfunction) has prompted efforts to reduce its use for chronic pain, including back pain (**Chap. 13**). When used, safety may be improved with automated notices for high doses, early refills, prescriptions from multiple pharmacies, overlapping opioid and benzodiazepine prescriptions, and in the United States by state-based prescription drug monitoring programs (PDMPs). A recent study indicated that most patients with opioid use disorder presenting to emergency departments had no prescriptions recorded in the PDMP, reflecting other methods used to obtain opioids. Greater access to alternative treatments for chronic pain, such as tailored exercise programs and cognitive behavioral therapy (CBT), may also reduce opioid prescribing.

Other Approaches There is no evidence to support use of oral or injected glucocorticoids, antiepileptics, antidepressants, or therapies for neuropathic pain such as gabapentin or herbal therapies. Commonly used nonpharmacologic treatments for ALBP are also of unproven benefit, including spinal manipulation, physical therapy, massage, acupuncture, laser therapy, therapeutic ultrasound, corsets, transcutaneous electrical nerve stimulation (TENS), special mattresses, or lumbar traction. Although important for chronic pain, use of back exercises for ALBP are generally not supported by clinical evidence. There is no convincing evidence regarding the value of ice or heat applications for ABLP; however, many patients report temporary symptomatic relief from ice or frozen gel packs just before sleep, and heat may produce a short-term reduction in pain after the first week. Patients often report improved satisfaction with the care that they receive when they actively participate in the selection of symptomatic approaches.

CHRONIC LOW BACK PAIN WITHOUT RADICULOPATHY

Back pain is considered chronic when the symptoms last >12 weeks; it accounts for 50% of total back pain costs. Risk factors include obesity, female gender, older age, prior history of back pain, restricted spinal mobility, pain radiating into a leg, high levels of psychological distress, poor self-rated health, minimal physical activity, smoking, job dissatisfaction, and widespread pain. In general, the same treatments that are recommended for ALBP can be useful for patients with CLBP. In this setting, however, the benefit of opioid therapy or muscle relaxants is less clear. In general, improved activity tolerance is the primary goal, while pain relief is secondary.

Some observers have raised concerns that CLBP may often be overtreated. For CLBP without radiculopathy, multiple guidelines explicitly recommend against use of SSRIs, any type of injection, TENS, lumbar supports, traction, radiofrequency facet joint denervation, intradiskal electrothermal therapy, or intradiskal radiofrequency thermocoagulation. On the other hand, exercise therapy and treatment of depression appear to be useful and underused.

Exercise Programs Evidence supports the use of exercise therapy to alleviate pain symptoms and improve function. Exercise can be one of the mainstays of treatment for CLBP. Effective regimens have generally included a combination of core-strengthening exercises, stretching, and gradually increasing aerobic exercise. A program of supervised exercise can improve compliance. Supervised intensive physical exercise or "work hardening" regimens have been effective in returning some patients to work, improving walking distance, and reducing pain. In addition, some forms of yoga have been evaluated in randomized trials and may be helpful for patients who are interested.

Intensive multidisciplinary rehabilitation programs can include daily or frequent physical therapy, exercise, CBT, a workplace evaluation, and other interventions. For patients who have not responded to other approaches, such programs appear to offer some benefit. Systematic reviews, however, suggest that the evidence and benefits are limited.

Nonopioid Medications Medications for CLBP may include short courses of NSAIDs or acetaminophen. Duloxetine is approved for the treatment of CLBP (60 mg daily) and may also treat coincident depression. Tricyclic antidepressants can provide modest pain relief for some patients without evidence of depression. Depression is common among patients with chronic pain and should be appropriately treated.

Cognitive Behavioral Therapy CBT is based on evidence that psychological and social factors, as well as somatic pathology, are important in the genesis of chronic pain and disability; CBT focuses on efforts to identify and modify patients' thinking about their condition. In one randomized trial, CBT reduced disability and pain in patients with CLBP. Such behavioral treatments appear to provide benefits similar in magnitude to exercise therapy.

Complementary Medicine Back pain is the most frequent reason for seeking complementary and alternative treatments. Spinal manipulation or massage therapy may provide short-term relief, but long-term benefit is unproven. Biofeedback has not been studied rigorously. There is no convincing evidence that either TENS, laser therapy, or ultrasound are effective in treating CLBP. Rigorous trials of acupuncture suggest that true acupuncture is not superior to sham acupuncture, but that both may offer an advantage over routine care. Whether this is due entirely to placebo effects provided even by sham acupuncture is uncertain.

Injections and Other Interventions Various injections, including epidural glucocorticoid injections, facet joint injections, and trigger point injections, have been used for treating CLBP. However, in the absence of radiculopathy, there is no clear evidence that these approaches are sustainably effective.

Injection studies are sometimes used diagnostically to help determine the anatomic source of back pain. Pain relief following a glucocorticoid and anesthetic injection into a facet or medial branch block are used as evidence that the facet joint is the pain source; however, the possibility that the response was a placebo effect or due to systemic absorption of the glucocorticoids is difficult to exclude.

Another category of intervention for CLBP is electrothermal and radiofrequency therapy. Intradiskal therapy has been proposed using energy to thermocoagulate and destroy nerves in the intervertebral disk, using specially designed catheters or electrodes. Current evidence does not support the use of discography to identify a specific disk as the pain source, or the use of intradiskal electrothermal or radiofrequency therapy for CLBP.

Radiofrequency denervation is sometimes used to destroy nerves that are thought to mediate pain, and this technique has been used for facet joint pain (with the target nerve being the medial branch of the primary dorsal ramus), for back pain thought to arise from the intervertebral disk (ramus communicans), and radicular back pain (dorsal root ganglia). These interventional therapies have not been studied in sufficient detail to draw firm conclusions regarding their value for CLBP.

Surgery Surgical intervention for CLBP without radiculopathy has been evaluated in a number of randomized trials. The case for fusion surgery for CLBP without radiculopathy is weak. While some studies have shown modest benefit, there has been no benefit when compared to an active medical treatment arm, often including highly structured, rigorous rehabilitation combined with CBT. The use of bone matrix protein (BMP) instead of iliac crest graft for the fusion was shown to increase hospital costs and length of stay but not improve clinical outcomes.

Guidelines suggest that referral for an opinion on spinal fusion can be considered for patients who have completed an optimal nonsurgical treatment program (including combined physical and psychological treatment) and who have persistent severe back pain for which they would consider surgery. The high cost, wide geographic variations, and rapidly increasing rates of spinal fusion surgery have prompted scrutiny regarding the lack of standardization of appropriate indications. Some insurance carriers have begun to limit coverage for the most controversial indications, such as LBP without radiculopathy.

Lumbar disk replacement with prosthetic disks is US Food and Drug Administration–approved for uncomplicated patients needing single-level surgery at the L3-S1 levels. The disks are generally designed as metal plates with a polyethylene cushion sandwiched in between. The trials that led to approval of these devices were not blinded. When compared to spinal fusion, the artificial disks were "not inferior." Long-term follow-up is needed to determine device failure rates over time. Serious complications are somewhat more likely with the artificial disk. This treatment remains controversial for CLBP.

LOW BACK PAIN WITH RADICULOPATHY

A common cause of back pain with radiculopathy is a herniated disk affecting the nerve root and producing back pain with radiation down the leg. The term *sciatica* is used when the leg pain radiates posteriorly in a sciatic or L5/S1 distribution. The prognosis for acute low back and leg pain with radiculopathy due to disk herniation is generally favorable, with most patients showing substantial improvement over months. Serial imaging studies suggest spontaneous regression of the herniated portion of the disk in two-thirds of patients over 6 months. Nonetheless, several important treatment options provide symptomatic relief while the healing process unfolds.

Resumption of normal activity is recommended. Randomized trial evidence suggests that bed rest is ineffective for treating sciatica as well as back pain alone. Acetaminophen and NSAIDs are useful for pain relief, although severe pain may require short courses (3–7 days) of opioid analgesics. Opioids are superior for acute pain relief in the emergency department.

Epidural glucocorticoid injections have a role in providing symptom relief for acute lumbar radiculopathy due to a herniated disk, but do not reduce the use of subsequent surgical intervention. A brief course of high-dose oral glucocorticoids (methylprednisolone dose pack) for 3 days followed by a rapid taper over 4 more days can be helpful for some patients with acute disk-related radiculopathy, although this specific regimen has not been studied rigorously.

Diagnostic nerve root blocks have been advocated to determine if pain originates from a specific nerve root. However, improvement may result even when the nerve root is not responsible for the pain; this may occur as a placebo effect, from a pain-generating lesion located distally along the peripheral nerve, or from effects of systemic absorption.

Urgent surgery is recommended for patients who have evidence of CES or spinal cord compression, generally manifesting as combinations of bowel or bladder dysfunction, diminished sensation in a saddle distribution, a sensory level on the trunk, and bilateral leg weakness or spasticity. Surgical intervention is also indicated for patients with progressive motor weakness due to nerve root injury demonstrated on clinical examination or EMG.

Surgery is also an important option for patients who have disabling radicular pain despite optimal conservative treatment. Because patients with a herniated disk and sciatica generally experience rapid improvement over weeks, most experts do not recommend considering surgery unless the patient has failed to respond to a minimum of 6–8 weeks of nonsurgical management. For patients who have not improved, randomized trials show that surgery results in more rapid pain relief than nonsurgical treatment. However, after

2 years of follow-up, patients appear to have similar pain relief and functional improvement with or without surgery. Thus, both treatment approaches are reasonable, and patient preferences and needs (e.g., rapid return to employment) strongly influence decision-making. Some patients will want the fastest possible relief and find surgical risks acceptable. Others will be more risk-averse and more tolerant of symptoms and will choose watchful waiting, especially if they understand that improvement is likely in the end.

The usual surgical procedure is a partial hemilaminectomy with excision of the prolapsed disk (diskectomy). Minimally invasive techniques have gained in popularity in recent years, but some evidence suggests they may be less effective than standard surgical techniques, with more residual back pain, leg pain, and higher rates of rehospitalization. Fusion of the involved lumbar segments should be considered only if significant spinal instability is present (i.e., degenerative spondylolisthesis). The costs associated with lumbar interbody fusion have increased dramatically in recent years. There are no large prospective, randomized trials comparing fusion to other types of surgical intervention. In one study, patients with persistent LBP despite an initial diskectomy fared no better with spine fusion than with a conservative regimen of cognitive intervention and exercise. Artificial disks, as discussed above, are used in Europe; their utility remains controversial in the United States.

PAIN IN THE NECK AND SHOULDER

Neck pain, which usually arises from diseases of the cervical spine and soft tissues of the neck, is common, typically precipitated by movement, and may be accompanied by focal tenderness and limitation of motion. Many of the earlier comments made regarding causes of LBP also apply to disorders of the cervical spine. The text below will emphasize differences. Pain arising from the brachial plexus, shoulder, or peripheral nerves can be confused with cervical spine disease (**Table 17-4**), but the history and examination usually identify a more distal origin for the pain. When the site of nerve tissue injury is unclear, EMG studies can localize the lesion. Cervical spine trauma, disk disease, or spondylosis with intervertebral foraminal narrowing may be asymptomatic or painful and can produce a myelopathy, radiculopathy, or both. The same risk factors for serious causes of LBP also apply to neck pain with the additional feature that neurologic signs of myelopathy (incontinence, sensory level, spastic legs) may also occur. Lhermitte's sign, an electrical shock down the spine with neck flexion, suggests involvement of the cervical spinal cord.

TRAUMA TO THE CERVICAL SPINE

Trauma (fractures, subluxation) places the spinal cord at risk for compression. Motor vehicle accidents, violent crimes, or falls account for 87% of cervical spinal cord injuries (**Chap. 442**). Immediate immobilization of the neck is essential to minimize further spinal cord injury from movement of unstable cervical spine segments. A CT scan is the diagnostic procedure of choice for detection of acute fractures following severe trauma; plain x-rays are used for lesser degrees of trauma or in settings where CT is unavailable. When traumatic injury to the vertebral arteries or cervical spinal cord is suspected, visualization by MRI with magnetic resonance angiography is preferred.

The decision to obtain imaging should be based on the clinical context of the injury. The National Emergency X-Radiography Utilization Study (NEXUS) low-risk criteria established that normally alert patients without palpation tenderness in the midline; intoxication; neurologic deficits; or painful distracting injuries were very unlikely to have sustained a clinically significant traumatic injury to the cervical spine. The Canadian C-spine rule recommends that imaging should be obtained following neck region trauma if the patient is >65 years old or has limb paresthesias or if there was a dangerous mechanism for the injury (e.g., bicycle collision with tree or parked car, fall from height >3 ft or five stairs, diving accident). These guidelines are helpful but must be tailored to individual circumstances; for example, patients with advanced osteoporosis, glucocorticoid use, or cancer may warrant imaging after even mild trauma.

Whiplash injury is due to rapid flexion and extension of the neck, usually from automobile accidents. The likely mechanism involves injury to the facet joints. This diagnosis should not be applied to patients with fractures, disk herniation, head injury, focal neurologic findings, or altered consciousness. Up to 50% of persons reporting whiplash injury acutely have persistent neck pain 1 year later. When personal compensation for pain and suffering was removed from the Australian health care system, the prognosis for recovery at 1 year improved. Imaging of the cervical spine is not cost-effective acutely but is useful to detect disk herniations when symptoms persist for >6 weeks following the injury. Severe initial symptoms have been associated with a poor long-term outcome.

CERVICAL DISK DISEASE

Degenerative cervical disk disease is very common and usually asymptomatic. Herniation of a lower cervical disk is a common cause of pain or tingling in the neck, shoulder, arm, or hand. Neck pain, stiffness, and a range of motion limited by pain are the usual manifestations.

TABLE 17-4 Cervical Radiculopathy: Neurologic Features

CERVICAL NERVE ROOT	EXAMINATION FINDINGS			PAIN DISTRIBUTION
	REFLEX	SENSORY	MOTOR	
C5	Biceps	Lateral deltoid	Rhomboids[a] (elbow extends backward with hand on hip)	Lateral arm, medial scapula
			Infraspinatus[a] (arm rotates externally with elbow flexed at the side)	
			Deltoid[a] (arm raised laterally 30°–45° from the side)	
C6	Biceps	Palmar thumb/index finger	Biceps[a] (arm flexed at the elbow in supination)	Lateral forearm, thumb/index fingers
		Dorsal hand/lateral forearm	Pronator teres (forearm pronated)	
C7	Triceps	Middle finger	Triceps[a] (forearm extension, flexed at elbow)	Posterior arm, dorsal forearm, dorsal hand
		Dorsal forearm	Wrist/finger extensors[a]	
C8	Finger flexors	Palmar surface of little finger	Abductor pollicis brevis (abduction of thumb)	Fourth and fifth fingers, medial hand and forearm
		Medial hand and forearm	First dorsal interosseous (abduction of index finger)	
			Abductor digiti minimi (abduction of little finger)	
T1	Finger flexors	Axilla, medial arm, anteromedial forearm	Abductor pollicis brevis (abduction of thumb)	Medial arm, axilla
			First dorsal interosseous (abduction of index finger)	
			Abductor digiti minimi (abduction of little finger)	

[a]These muscles receive the majority of innervation from this root.

Herniated cervical disks are responsible for ~25% of cervical radiculopathies. Extension and lateral rotation of the neck narrow the ipsilateral intervertebral foramen and may reproduce radicular symptoms (Spurling's sign). In young adults, acute nerve root compression from a ruptured cervical disk is often due to trauma. Cervical disk herniations are usually posterolateral near the lateral recess. Typical patterns of reflex, sensory, and motor changes that accompany cervical nerve root lesions are summarized in Table 17-4. Although the classic patterns are clinically helpful, there are numerous exceptions because (1) there is overlap in sensory function between adjacent nerve roots, (2) symptoms and signs may be evident in only part of the injured nerve root territory, and (3) the location of pain is the most variable of the clinical features.

CERVICAL SPONDYLOSIS

Osteoarthritis of the cervical spine may produce neck pain that radiates into the back of the head, shoulders, or arms, or may be the source of headaches in the posterior occipital region (supplied by the C2-C4 nerve roots). Osteophytes, disk protrusions, or hypertrophic facet or uncovertebral joints may alone or in combination compress one or several nerve roots at the intervertebral foramina; these causes together account for 75% of cervical radiculopathies. The roots most commonly affected are C7 and C6. Narrowing of the spinal canal by osteophytes, ossification of the posterior longitudinal ligament (OPLL), or a large central disk may compress the cervical spinal cord and produce signs of myelopathy alone or radiculopathy with myelopathy (myeloradiculopathy). When little or no neck pain accompanies cervical cord involvement, other diagnoses to be considered include amyotrophic lateral sclerosis (**Chap. 437**), multiple sclerosis (**Chap. 444**), spinal cord tumors, or syringomyelia (**Chap. 442**). Cervical spondylotic myelopathy should be considered even when the patient presents with symptoms or spinal cord signs in the legs only. MRI is the study of choice to define soft tissues in the cervical region including the spinal cord, whereas plain CT is optimal to identify bone pathology including foraminal, lateral recess, OPLL, or spinal canal stenosis. In spondylotic myelopathy, focal enhancement by MRI, sometimes in a characteristic "pancake pattern," may be present at the site of maximal cord compression.

There is no evidence to support prophylactic surgery for asymptomatic cervical spinal stenosis unaccompanied by myelopathic signs or abnormal spinal cord findings on MRI, except in the setting of *dynamic instability* (see spondylolisthesis above). If the patient has postural neck pain, a prior history of whiplash or other spine/head injury, a Lhermitte sign, or preexisting listhesis at the stenotic segment on cervical MRI or CT, then cervical spine flexion-extension x-rays or MRI are indicated to look for dynamic instability. Surgical intervention is not recommended for patients with listhesis alone, unaccompanied by dynamic instability.

OTHER CAUSES OF NECK PAIN

Rheumatoid arthritis (RA) (**Chap. 358**) of the cervical facet joints produces neck pain, stiffness, and limitation of motion. Synovitis of the atlantoaxial joint (C1-C2; Fig. 17-2) may damage the transverse ligament of the atlas, producing forward displacement of the atlas on the axis (atlantoaxial subluxation). Radiologic evidence of atlantoaxial subluxation occurs in up to 30% of patients with RA and plain x-ray films of the neck should be routinely performed preoperatively to assess the risk of neck hyperextension in patients requiring intubation. The degree of subluxation correlates with the severity of erosive disease. When subluxation is present, careful assessment is important to identify early signs of myelopathy that could be a harbinger of life-threatening spinal cord compression. Surgery should be considered when myelopathy or spinal instability is present. *Ankylosing spondylitis* is another cause of neck pain and less commonly atlantoaxial subluxation.

Acute *herpes zoster* can present as acute posterior occipital or neck pain prior to the outbreak of vesicles. *Neoplasms* metastatic to the cervical spine, *infections* (osteomyelitis and epidural abscess), and *metabolic bone diseases* may be the cause of neck pain, as discussed above. Neck pain may also be referred from the heart with coronary artery ischemia (cervical angina syndrome). Rheumatologic disease should be considered if the neck pain is accompanied by shoulder or hip girdle pain.

THORACIC OUTLET SYNDROMES

The thoracic outlet contains the first rib, the subclavian artery and vein, the brachial plexus, the clavicle, and the lung apex. Injury to these structures may result in postural or movement-induced pain around the shoulder and supraclavicular region, classified as follows.

True neurogenic thoracic outlet syndrome (*TOS*) is an uncommon disorder resulting from compression of the lower trunk of the brachial plexus or ventral rami of the C8 or T1 nerve roots, caused most often by an anomalous band of cartilaginous tissue connecting an elongate transverse process at C7 with the first rib. Pain is mild or may be absent. Signs include weakness and wasting of intrinsic muscles of the hand and diminished sensation on the palmar aspect of the fifth digit. An anteroposterior cervical spine x-ray will show an elongate C7 transverse process (an anatomic marker for the anomalous cartilaginous band), and EMG and NCSs confirm the diagnosis. Treatment consists of surgical resection of the anomalous band. The weakness and wasting of intrinsic hand muscles typically do not improve, but surgery halts the insidious progression of weakness.

Arterial TOS results from compression of the subclavian artery by a cervical rib, resulting in poststenotic dilatation of the artery and in some cases secondary thrombus formation. Blood pressure is reduced in the affected limb, and signs of emboli may be present in the hand. Neurologic signs are absent. Ultrasound can confirm the diagnosis noninvasively. Treatment is with thrombolysis or anticoagulation (with or without embolectomy) and surgical excision of the cervical rib compressing the subclavian artery.

Venous TOS is due to subclavian vein thrombosis resulting in swelling of the arm and pain. The vein may be compressed by a cervical rib or anomalous scalene muscle. Venography is the diagnostic test of choice.

Disputed TOS accounts for 95% of patients diagnosed with TOS; chronic arm and shoulder pain are prominent and of unclear cause. The lack of sensitive and specific findings on physical examination or specific markers for this condition results in diagnostic uncertainty. The role of surgery in disputed TOS is controversial. Major depression, chronic symptoms, work-related injury, and diffuse arm symptoms predict poor surgical outcomes. Multidisciplinary pain management is a conservative approach, although treatment is often unsuccessful.

BRACHIAL PLEXUS AND NERVES

Pain from injury to the brachial plexus or peripheral nerves of the arm can occasionally mimic referred pain of cervical spine origin, including cervical radiculopathy, but the pain typically begins distal to the posterior neck region in the shoulder girdle or upper arm. Neoplastic infiltration of the lower trunk of the brachial plexus may produce shoulder or supraclavicular pain radiating down the arm, numbness of the fourth and fifth fingers or medial forearm, and weakness of intrinsic hand muscles innervated by the lower trunk and medial cord of the brachial plexus. Delayed radiation injury may produce weakness in the upper arm or numbness of the lateral forearm or arm due to involvement of the upper trunk and lateral cord of the plexus. Pain is less common and less severe than with neoplastic infiltration. A Pancoast tumor of the lung (**Chap. 78**) is another cause and should be considered, especially when a concurrent Horner's syndrome is present. *Acute brachial neuritis* is often confused with radiculopathy; the acute onset of severe shoulder or scapular pain is followed typically over days by weakness of the proximal arm and shoulder girdle muscles innervated by the upper brachial plexus. The onset may be preceded by an infection, vaccination, or minor surgical procedure. The long thoracic nerve may be affected, resulting in a winged scapula. Brachial neuritis may also present as an isolated paralysis of the diaphragm with or without involvement of other nerves of the upper limb. Recovery may take up to 3 years, and full functional recovery can be expected in the majority of patients.

Occasional cases of carpal tunnel syndrome produce pain and paresthesias extending into the forearm, arm, and shoulder resembling a C5 or C6 root lesion. Lesions of the radial or ulnar nerve can also mimic radiculopathy, at C7 or C8, respectively. EMG and NCSs can accurately localize lesions to the nerve roots, brachial plexus, or peripheral nerves.

For further discussion of peripheral nerve disorders, see Chap. 446.

SHOULDER

Pain arising from the shoulder can on occasion mimic pain from the spine. If symptoms and signs of radiculopathy are absent, then the differential diagnosis includes mechanical shoulder pain (bicipital tendonitis, frozen shoulder, bursitis, rotator cuff tear, dislocation, adhesive capsulitis, or rotator cuff impingement under the acromion) and referred pain (subdiaphragmatic irritation, angina, Pancoast tumor). Mechanical pain is often worse at night, associated with local shoulder tenderness and aggravated by passive abduction, internal rotation, or extension of the arm. Demonstrating normal passive full range of motion of the arm at the shoulder without worsening the usual pain can help exclude mechanical shoulder pathology as a cause of neck region pain. Pain from shoulder disease may radiate into the arm or hand, but focal neurologic signs (sensory, motor, or reflex changes) are absent.

GLOBAL CONSIDERATIONS

Many of the considerations described above for LBP also apply to neck pain. The Global Burden of Diseases Study 2019 reported that neck pain ranked second only to back pain as a cause of total years lived with disability (YLD). In general, neck pain rankings were also higher in developed regions of the world.

TREATMENT

Neck Pain Without Radiculopathy

The evidence regarding treatment for neck pain is less comprehensive than that for LBP, but the approach is remarkably similar in many respects. As with LBP, spontaneous improvement is the norm for acute neck pain. The usual goals of therapy are to promote a rapid return to normal function and provide pain relief while healing proceeds.

Acute neck pain is often treated with NSAIDs, acetaminophen, cold packs, or heat, alone or in combination while awaiting recovery. Patients should be specifically educated regarding the favorable natural history of acute neck pain to avoid unrealistic fear and inappropriate requests for imaging and other tests. For patients kept awake by symptoms, cyclobenzaprine (5–10 mg) at night can help relieve muscle spasm and promote drowsiness. For patients with neck pain unassociated with trauma, supervised exercise with or without mobilization appears to be effective. Exercises often include shoulder rolls and neck stretches. The evidence in support of nonsurgical treatments for whiplash-associated disorders is generally of limited quality and neither supports nor refutes the common treatments used for symptom relief. Gentle mobilization of the cervical spine combined with exercise programs may be beneficial. Evidence is insufficient to recommend the use of cervical traction, TENS, ultrasound, trigger point injections, botulinum toxin injections, tricyclic antidepressants, and SSRIs for acute or chronic neck pain. Some patients obtain modest pain relief using a soft neck collar; there is little risk or cost. Massage can produce temporary pain relief.

For patients with chronic neck pain, supervised exercise programs can provide symptom relief and improve function. Acupuncture provided short-term benefit for some patients when compared to a sham procedure and is an option. Spinal manipulation alone has not been shown to be effective and carries a risk for injury. Surgical treatment for chronic neck pain without radiculopathy or spine instability is not recommended.

Neck Pain With Radiculopathy

The natural history of acute neck pain with radiculopathy due to disk disease is favorable, and many patients will improve without specific therapy. Although there are no randomized trials of NSAIDs for neck pain, a course of NSAIDs, acetaminophen, or both, with or without muscle relaxants, and avoidance of activities that trigger symptoms are reasonable as initial therapy. Gentle supervised exercise and avoidance of inactivity are reasonable as well. A short course of high-dose oral glucocorticoids with a rapid taper, or epidural steroids administered under imaging guidance can be effective for acute or subacute disk-related cervical radicular pain, but have not been subjected to rigorous trials. The risk of injection-related complications is higher in the neck than the low back; vertebral artery dissection, dural puncture, spinal cord injury, and embolism in the vertebral arteries have all been reported. Opioid analgesics can be used in the emergency department and for short courses as an outpatient. Soft cervical collars can be modestly helpful by limiting spontaneous and reflex neck movements that exacerbate pain; hard collars are in general poorly tolerated.

If cervical radiculopathy is due to bony compression from cervical spondylosis with foraminal narrowing, periodic follow-up to assess for progression is indicated and consideration of surgical decompression is reasonable. Surgical treatment can produce rapid pain relief, although it is unclear if long-term functional outcomes are improved over nonsurgical therapy. Indications for cervical disk surgery include a progressive motor deficit due to nerve root compression, functionally limiting pain that fails to respond to conservative management, or spinal cord compression. In other circumstances, clinical improvement over time regardless of therapeutic intervention is common.

Surgical treatments include anterior cervical diskectomy alone, laminectomy with diskectomy, or diskectomy with fusion. The risk of subsequent radiculopathy or myelopathy at cervical segments adjacent to a fusion is ~3% per year and 26% per decade. Although this risk is sometimes portrayed as a late complication of surgery, it may also reflect the natural history of degenerative cervical disk disease.

FURTHER READING

Agency for Healthcare Research and Quality (AHRQ): Noninvasive treatments for low back pain. AHRQ Publication No. 16-EHC004-EF. February 2016, *https://effectivehealthcare.ahrq.gov/ehc/products/553/2178/back-pain-treatment-report-160229.pdf*

Austevoll IM et al: Decompression with or without fusion in degenerative lumbar spondylolisthesis. N Engl J Med 385:526, 2021.

Bailey CS et al: Surgery versus conservative care for persistent sciatica lasting 4 to 12 months. N Engl J Med 19;382:1093, 2020.

Cieza A et al: Global estimates of the need for rehabilitation based on the Global Burden of Disease study 2019: A systematic analysis for the Global Burden of Disease Study 2019. Lancet 396:2006, 2021.

Engstrom JW: Physical and Neurologic Examination. In Steinmetz et al (eds). *Benzel's Spine Surgery*, 5th ed. Philadelphia, Elsevier, 2021.

Goldberg H et al: Oral steroids for acute radiculopathy due to a herniated lumbar disk. JAMA 313:1915, 2015.

Hawk K et al: Past-year prescription drug monitoring program opioid prescriptions and self-reported opioid use in an emergency department population with opioid use disorder. Acad Emerg Med 25:508, 2018.

Jarvik JG et al: Association of early imaging for back pain with clinical outcomes in older adults. JAMA 313:1143, 2015.

Katz JN, Harris MB: Clinical practice. Lumbar spinal stenosis. N Engl J Med 358:818, 2008.

Theodore N: Degenerative cervical spondylosis. N Engl J Med 383:159, 2020.

Zygourakis CC et al: Geographic and hospital variation in cost of lumbar laminectomy and lumbar fusion for degenerative conditions. Neurosurgery 81:331, 2017.

Section 2 Alterations in Body Temperature

18 Fever

Neeraj K. Surana, Charles A. Dinarello, Reuven Porat

Body temperature is controlled by the hypothalamus. Neurons in both the preoptic anterior hypothalamus and the posterior hypothalamus receive two kinds of signals: one from peripheral nerves that transmit information from warmth/cold receptors in the skin and the other from the temperature of the blood bathing the region. These two types of signals are integrated by the thermoregulatory center of the hypothalamus to maintain normal temperature. In a neutral temperature environment, the human metabolic rate produces more heat than is necessary to maintain the core body temperature in the range of 36.5–37.5°C (97.7–99.5°F).

A normal body temperature is ordinarily maintained despite environmental variations because the hypothalamic thermoregulatory center balances the excess heat production derived from metabolic activity in muscle and the liver with heat dissipation from the skin and lungs. According to a study of >35,000 individuals ≥18 years of age seen in routine medical visits, the mean oral temperature is 36.6°C (95% confidence interval, 35.7–37.3°C). In light of this study, *a temperature of >37.7°C (>99.9°F), which represents the 99th percentile for healthy individuals, defines a fever.* Importantly, higher ambient temperatures are linked to higher baseline body temperatures. Additionally, body temperatures have diurnal and seasonal variation, with low levels at 8 A.M. and during summer and higher levels at 4 P.M. and during winter. Baseline temperatures are also affected by age (lower by 0.02°C for every 10-year increase in age), demographics (African-American women have temperatures 0.052°C higher than white men), and comorbid conditions (cancer is associated with 0.02°C higher temperatures; hypothyroidism is linked to temperatures lower by 0.01°C). After controlling for age, sex, race, vital signs, and comorbidities, an increase in baseline temperature of 0.15°C (or 1 standard deviation) intriguingly translates into a 0.52% absolute increase in 1-year mortality.

Rectal temperatures are generally 0.4°C (0.7°F) higher than oral readings. The lower oral readings are probably attributable to mouth breathing, which is a factor in patients with respiratory infections and rapid breathing. Lower-esophageal temperatures closely reflect core temperature. Tympanic membrane thermometers measure radiant heat from the tympanic membrane and nearby ear canal and display that absolute value (*unadjusted mode*) or a value automatically calculated from the absolute reading on the basis of nomograms relating the radiant temperature measured to actual core temperatures obtained in clinical studies (*adjusted mode*). These measurements, although convenient, may be more variable than directly determined oral or rectal values. Studies in adults show that readings are lower with unadjusted-mode than with adjusted-mode tympanic membrane thermometers and that unadjusted-mode tympanic membrane values are 0.8°C (1.6°F) lower than rectal temperatures.

In women who menstruate, the A.M. temperature is generally lower during the 2 weeks before ovulation; it then rises by ~0.6°C (1°F) with ovulation and stays at that level until menses occur. During the luteal phase, the amplitude of the circadian rhythm remains the same.

FEVER VERSUS HYPERTHERMIA

Fever is an elevation of body temperature that exceeds the normal daily variation and occurs *in conjunction with an increase in the hypothalamic set point* (e.g., from 37°C to 39°C). This shift of the set point from "normothermic" to febrile levels very much resembles the resetting of the home thermostat to a higher level in order to raise the ambient temperature in a room. Once the hypothalamic set point is raised, neurons in the vasomotor center are activated and vasoconstriction commences. The individual first notices vasoconstriction in the hands and feet. Shunting of blood away from the periphery to the internal organs essentially decreases heat loss from the skin, and the person feels cold. For most fevers, body temperature increases by 1–2°C. Shivering, which increases heat production from the muscles, may begin at this time; however, shivering is not required if mechanisms of heat conservation raise blood temperature sufficiently. Nonshivering heat production from the liver also contributes to increasing core temperature. Behavioral adjustments (e.g., putting on more clothing or bedding) help raise body temperature by decreasing heat loss.

The processes of heat conservation (vasoconstriction) and heat production (shivering and increased nonshivering thermogenesis) continue until the temperature of the blood bathing the hypothalamic neurons matches the new "thermostat setting." Once that point is reached, the hypothalamus maintains the temperature at the febrile level by the same mechanisms of heat balance that function in the afebrile state. When the hypothalamic set point is again reset downward (in response to either a reduction in the concentration of pyrogens or the use of antipyretics), the processes of heat loss through vasodilation and sweating are initiated. Loss of heat by sweating and vasodilation continues until the blood temperature at the hypothalamic level matches the lower setting. Behavioral changes (e.g., removal of clothing) facilitate heat loss.

A fever of >41.5°C (>106.7°F) is called *hyperpyrexia*. This extraordinarily high fever can develop in patients with severe infections but most commonly occurs in patients with central nervous system (CNS) hemorrhages. In the preantibiotic era, fever due to a variety of infectious diseases rarely exceeded 106°F, and there has been speculation that this natural "thermal ceiling" is mediated by neuropeptides functioning as central antipyretics.

In rare cases, the hypothalamic set point is elevated as a result of local trauma, hemorrhage, tumor, or intrinsic hypothalamic malfunction. The term *hypothalamic fever* is sometimes used to describe elevated temperature caused by abnormal hypothalamic function. However, most patients with hypothalamic damage have *sub*normal, not *supra*normal, body temperatures.

Although most patients with elevated body temperature have fever, there are circumstances in which elevated temperature represents not fever but *hyperthermia* (*heat stroke*). Hyperthermia is characterized by an uncontrolled increase in body temperature that exceeds the body's ability to lose heat. The setting of the hypothalamic thermoregulatory center is unchanged. In contrast to fever in infections, hyperthermia does not involve pyrogenic molecules. Exogenous heat exposure and endogenous heat production are two mechanisms by which hyperthermia can result in dangerously high internal temperatures. Excessive heat production can easily cause hyperthermia despite physiologic and behavioral control of body temperature. For example, work or exercise in hot environments can produce heat faster than peripheral mechanisms can lose it. **For a detailed discussion of hyperthermia, see Chap. 465.**

It is important to distinguish between fever and hyperthermia since hyperthermia can be rapidly fatal and characteristically does not respond to antipyretics. In an emergency situation, however, making this distinction can be difficult. For example, in systemic sepsis, fever (hyperpyrexia) can be rapid in onset, and temperatures can exceed 40.5°C (104.9°F). Hyperthermia is often diagnosed on the basis of the events immediately preceding the elevation of core temperature—e.g., heat exposure or treatment with drugs that interfere with thermoregulation. In patients with heat stroke syndromes and in those taking drugs that block sweating, the skin is hot but dry, whereas in fever, the skin can be cold as a consequence of vasoconstriction. Antipyretics do not reduce the elevated temperature in hyperthermia, whereas in fever—and even in hyperpyrexia—adequate doses of either aspirin or acetaminophen usually result in some decrease in body temperature.

PATHOGENESIS OF FEVER

PYROGENS

The term *pyrogen* (Greek *pyro*, "fire") is used to describe any substance that causes fever. *Exogenous* pyrogens are derived from outside the patient; most are microbial products, microbial toxins, or whole microorganisms (including viruses). The classic example of an exogenous pyrogen is the lipopolysaccharide (endotoxin) produced by all gram-negative bacteria. Pyrogenic products of gram-positive organisms include the enterotoxins of *Staphylococcus aureus* and the groups A and B streptococcal toxins, also called *superantigens*. One staphylococcal toxin of clinical importance is that associated with isolates of *S. aureus* from patients with toxic shock syndrome. These products of staphylococci and streptococci cause fever in experimental animals when injected intravenously at concentrations of 1–10 μg/kg. Endotoxin is a highly pyrogenic molecule in humans: when injected intravenously into volunteers, a dose of 2–3 ng/kg produces fever, leukocytosis, acute-phase proteins, and generalized symptoms of malaise.

PYROGENIC CYTOKINES

Cytokines are small proteins (molecular mass, 10,000–20,000 Da) that regulate immune, inflammatory, and hematopoietic processes. For example, the elevated leukocytosis seen in several infections with an absolute neutrophilia is attributable to the cytokines interleukin (IL) 1 and IL-6. Some cytokines also cause fever; formerly referred to as *endogenous pyrogens*, they are now called *pyrogenic cytokines*. The pyrogenic cytokines include IL-1, IL-6, tumor necrosis factor (TNF), and ciliary neurotropic factor, a member of the IL-6 family. Fever is a prominent side effect of interferon α therapy. Each pyrogenic cytokine is encoded by a separate gene, and each has been shown to cause fever in laboratory animals and in humans. When injected into humans at low doses (10–100 ng/kg), IL-1 and TNF produce fever; in contrast, for IL-6, a dose of 1–10 μg/kg is required for fever production.

A wide spectrum of bacterial and fungal products induce the synthesis and release of pyrogenic cytokines. However, fever can be a manifestation of disease in the absence of microbial infection. For example, inflammatory processes such as pericarditis, trauma, stroke, and routine immunizations induce the production of IL-1, TNF, and/or IL-6; individually or in combination, these cytokines trigger the hypothalamus to raise the set point to febrile levels.

ELEVATION OF THE HYPOTHALAMIC SET POINT BY CYTOKINES

During fever, levels of prostaglandin E_2 (PGE_2) are elevated in hypothalamic tissue and the third cerebral ventricle. The concentrations of PGE_2 are highest near the circumventricular vascular organs (organum vasculosum of lamina terminalis)—networks of enlarged capillaries surrounding the hypothalamic regulatory centers. Destruction of these organs reduces the ability of pyrogens to produce fever. Most studies in animals have failed to show, however, that pyrogenic cytokines pass from the circulation into the brain itself. Thus, it appears that both exogenous pyrogens and pyrogenic cytokines interact with the endothelium of these capillaries and that this interaction is the first step in initiating fever—i.e., in raising the set point to febrile levels.

The key events in the production of fever are illustrated in **Fig. 18-1**. Myeloid and endothelial cells are the primary cell types that produce pyrogenic cytokines. Pyrogenic cytokines such as IL-1, IL-6, and TNF are released from these cells and enter the systemic circulation. Although these circulating cytokines lead to fever by inducing the synthesis of PGE_2, they also induce PGE_2 in peripheral tissues. The increase in PGE_2 in the periphery accounts for the nonspecific myalgias and arthralgias that often accompany fever. It is thought that some systemic PGE_2 escapes destruction by the lung and gains access to the hypothalamus via the internal carotid. However, it is the elevation of PGE_2 in the brain that starts the process of raising the hypothalamic set point for core temperature.

There are four receptors for PGE_2, and each signals the cell in different ways. Of the four receptors, the third (EP-3) is essential for fever: when the gene for this receptor is deleted in mice, no fever follows the

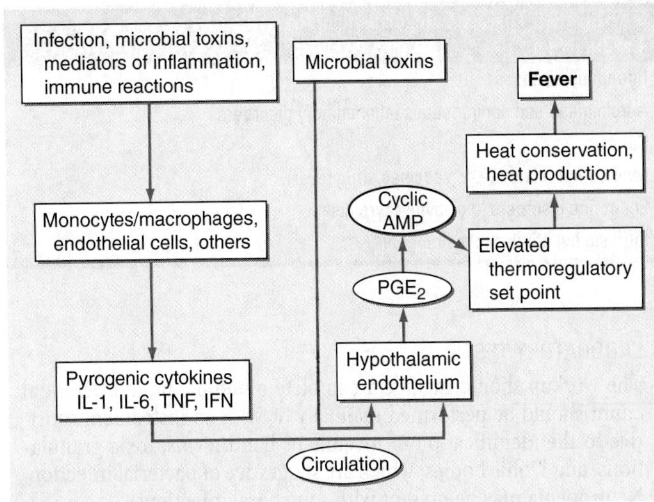

FIGURE 18-1 Chronology of events required for the induction of fever. AMP, adenosine 5′-monophosphate; IFN, interferon; IL, interleukin; PGE_2, prostaglandin E_2; TNF, tumor necrosis factor.

injection of IL-1 or endotoxin. Deletion of the other PGE_2 receptor genes leaves the fever mechanism intact. Although PGE_2 is essential for fever, it is not a neurotransmitter. Rather, the release of PGE_2 from the brain side of the hypothalamic endothelium triggers the PGE_2 receptor on glial cells, and this stimulation results in the rapid release of cyclic adenosine 5′-monophosphate (cAMP), which is a neurotransmitter. As shown in Fig. 18-1, the release of cAMP from glial cells activates neuronal endings from the thermoregulatory center that extend into the area. The elevation of cAMP is thought to account for changes in the hypothalamic set point either directly or indirectly (by inducing the release of neurotransmitters). Distinct receptors for microbial products are located on the hypothalamic endothelium. These receptors are called *Toll-like receptors* and are similar in many ways to IL-1 receptors. IL-1 receptors and Toll-like receptors share the same signal-transducing mechanism. Thus, the direct activation of Toll-like receptors or IL-1 receptors results in PGE_2 production and fever.

PRODUCTION OF CYTOKINES IN THE CNS

Cytokines produced in the brain may account for the hyperpyrexia of CNS hemorrhage, trauma, or infection. Viral infections of the CNS induce microglial and possibly neuronal production of IL-1, TNF, and IL-6. In experimental animals, the concentration of a cytokine required to cause fever is several orders of magnitude lower with direct injection into the brain substance or brain ventricles than with systemic injection. Therefore, cytokines produced in the CNS can raise the hypothalamic set point, bypassing the circumventricular organs. CNS cytokines likely account for the hyperpyrexia of CNS hemorrhage, trauma, or infection.

APPROACH TO THE PATIENT

Fever

HISTORY AND PHYSICAL EXAMINATION

There are a range of disease processes that present with fever as a cardinal manifestation, and a thorough history can help distinguish between these broad categories (**Table 18-1**). The chronology of events preceding fever, including exposure to other symptomatic individuals or to vectors of disease, should be ascertained. Electronic devices for measuring oral, tympanic membrane, or rectal temperatures are reliable, but the same site should be used consistently to monitor a febrile disease. Moreover, physicians should be aware that newborns, elderly patients, patients with chronic hepatic or renal failure, and patients taking glucocorticoids or being treated with an anticytokine may have active disease in the absence of fever because of a blunted febrile response.

TABLE 18-1 Disease Categories That Present with Fever as a Cardinal Sign

Infectious diseases
Autoimmune and noninfectious inflammatory disorders
Cancer
Medication related (e.g., vaccines, drug fever)
Endocrine disorders (e.g., hyperthyroidism)
Intrinsic hypothalamic malfunction

LABORATORY TESTS

The workup should include a complete blood count; a differential count should be performed manually or with an instrument sensitive to the identification of juvenile or band forms, toxic granulations, and Döhle bodies, which are suggestive of bacterial infection. Neutropenia may be present with some viral infections.

Measurement of circulating cytokines in patients with fever is not helpful since levels of cytokines such as IL-1 and TNF in the circulation often are below the detection limit of the assay or do not coincide with fever. However, in patients with low-grade fevers or with suspected occult disease, the most valuable measurements are the C-reactive protein (CRP) level and the erythrocyte sedimentation rate. These markers of inflammatory processes are particularly helpful in detecting occult disease. Measurement of circulating IL-6, which induces CRP, can be useful. However, whereas IL-6 levels may vary during a febrile disease, CRP levels remain elevated. Acute-phase reactants are discussed in **Chap. 304**.

FEVER IN PATIENTS RECEIVING ANTICYTOKINE THERAPY

Patients receiving long-term treatment with anticytokine-based regimens are at increased risk of infection because of lowered host defenses. For example, latent *Mycobacterium tuberculosis* infection can disseminate in patients receiving anti-TNF therapy. With the increasing use of anticytokines to reduce the activity of IL-1, IL-6, IL-12, IL-17, or TNF in patients with Crohn's disease, rheumatoid arthritis, or psoriasis, the possibility that these therapies blunt the febrile response should be kept in mind.

The blocking of cytokine activity has the distinct clinical drawback of lowering the level of host defenses against both routine bacterial and opportunistic infections such as *M. tuberculosis* and fungal infections. The use of monoclonal antibodies to reduce IL-17 in psoriasis increases the risk of systemic candidiasis.

In nearly all reported cases of infection associated with anticytokine therapy, fever is among the presenting signs. However, the extent to which the febrile response is blunted in these patients remains unknown. Therefore, low-grade fever in patients receiving anticytokine therapies is of considerable concern. The physician should conduct an early and rigorous diagnostic evaluation in these cases. The febrile response is also blunted in patients receiving chronic glucocorticoid therapy or anti-inflammatory agents such as nonsteroidal anti-inflammatory drugs (NSAIDs).

TREATMENT

Fever

THE DECISION TO TREAT FEVER

In deciding whether to treat fever, it is important to remember that fever itself is not an illness: it is an ordinary response to a perturbation of normal host physiology. Most fevers are associated with self-limited infections, such as common viral diseases. The use of antipyretics is not contraindicated in these infections: no significant clinical evidence indicates either that antipyretics delay the resolution of viral or bacterial infections or that fever facilitates recovery from infection or acts as an adjuvant to the immune system. In short, treatment of fever and its symptoms with routine antipyretics does no harm and does not slow the resolution of common viral and bacterial infections.

However, in bacterial infections, the withholding of antipyretic therapy can be helpful in evaluating the effectiveness of a particular antibiotic, especially in the absence of positive cultures of the infecting organism, and the routine use of antipyretics can mask an inadequately treated bacterial infection. Withholding antipyretics in some cases may facilitate the diagnosis of an unusual febrile disease. Temperature–pulse dissociation (*relative bradycardia*) occurs in typhoid fever, brucellosis, leptospirosis, some drug-induced fevers, and factitious fever. As stated earlier, in newborns, elderly patients, patients with chronic liver or kidney failure, and patients taking glucocorticoids, fever may not be present despite infection. Hypothermia can develop in patients with septic shock.

Some infections have characteristic patterns in which febrile episodes are separated by intervals of normal temperature. For example, *Plasmodium vivax* causes fever every third day, whereas fever occurs every fourth day with *Plasmodium malariae*. Another relapsing fever is related to *Borrelia* infection, with days of fever followed by a several-day afebrile period and then a relapse into additional days of fever. In the Pel-Ebstein pattern, fever lasting 3–10 days is followed by afebrile periods of 3–10 days; this pattern can be classic for Hodgkin's disease and other lymphomas. In cyclic neutropenia, fevers occur every 21 days and accompany the neutropenia. There are also a number of periodic fever syndromes (e.g., familial Mediterranean fever, TNF receptor–associated periodic syndrome [TRAPS]) that differ in their periodicity, duration of attack, constellation of clinical features, genetic causes, and therapies **(Chap. 369)**. Understanding these clinical differences can help tailor diagnostic testing to confirm the diagnosis and guide therapy.

ANTICYTOKINE THERAPY TO REDUCE FEVER IN AUTOIMMUNE AND AUTOINFLAMMATORY DISEASES

Recurrent fever is documented at some point in most autoimmune diseases and many autoinflammatory diseases, which include the periodic fever syndromes as well as disorders of inflammasomes (e.g., NLRP3, pyrin) and other components of the innate immune system **(Chap. 349)**. Although fever can be a manifestation of autoimmune diseases, recurrent fevers are characteristic of autoinflammatory diseases, including uncommon diseases such as adult and juvenile Still's disease, familial Mediterranean fever, and hyper-IgD syndrome but also common diseases such as idiopathic pericarditis and gout. In addition to recurrent fevers, neutrophilia and serosal inflammation characterize autoinflammatory diseases. The fevers associated with many of these illnesses are dramatically reduced by blocking of IL-1 activity with anakinra or canakinumab. Anticytokines therefore reduce fever in autoimmune and autoinflammatory diseases. Although fevers in autoinflammatory diseases are mediated by IL-1β, patients also respond to antipyretics.

MECHANISMS OF ANTIPYRETIC AGENTS

The reduction of fever by lowering of the elevated hypothalamic set point is a direct function of reduction of the PGE_2 level in the thermoregulatory center. The synthesis of PGE_2 depends on the constitutively expressed enzyme cyclooxygenase. The substrate for cyclooxygenase is arachidonic acid released from the cell membrane, and this release is the rate-limiting step in the synthesis of PGE_2. Therefore, inhibitors of cyclooxygenase are potent antipyretics. The antipyretic potency of various drugs is directly correlated with the inhibition of brain cyclooxygenase. Acetaminophen is a poor cyclooxygenase inhibitor in peripheral tissue and lacks noteworthy anti-inflammatory activity; in the brain, however, acetaminophen is oxidized by the P450 cytochrome system, and the oxidized form inhibits cyclooxygenase activity. Moreover, in the brain, the inhibition of another enzyme, COX-3, by acetaminophen may account for the antipyretic effect of this agent. However, COX-3 is not found outside the CNS.

Oral aspirin and acetaminophen are equally effective in reducing fever in humans. NSAIDs such as ibuprofen and specific inhibitors of COX-2 also are excellent antipyretics. Chronic, high-dose therapy with antipyretics such as aspirin or any NSAID does not reduce normal core body temperature. Thus, PGE_2 appears to play no role in normal thermoregulation.

As effective antipyretics, glucocorticoids act at two levels. First, similar to the cyclooxygenase inhibitors, glucocorticoids reduce PGE_2 synthesis by inhibiting the activity of phospholipase A_2, which is needed to release arachidonic acid from the cell membrane. Second, glucocorticoids block the transcription of the mRNA for the pyrogenic cytokines. Limited experimental evidence indicates that ibuprofen and COX-2 inhibitors reduce IL-1-induced IL-6 production and may contribute to the antipyretic activity of NSAIDs.

REGIMENS FOR THE TREATMENT OF FEVER

The objectives in treating fever are first to reduce the elevated hypothalamic set point and second to facilitate heat loss. Reducing fever with antipyretics also reduces systemic symptoms of headache, myalgias, and arthralgias.

Oral aspirin and NSAIDs effectively reduce fever but can adversely affect platelets and the gastrointestinal tract. Therefore, acetaminophen is preferred as an antipyretic. In children, acetaminophen or oral ibuprofen must be used because aspirin increases the risk of Reye's syndrome. If the patient cannot take oral antipyretics, parenteral preparations of NSAIDs and rectal suppositories of various antipyretics can be used.

Treatment of fever in some patients is highly recommended. Fever increases the demand for oxygen (i.e., for every increase of 1°C over 37°C, there is a 13% increase in oxygen consumption) and can aggravate the condition of patients with preexisting impairment of cardiac, pulmonary, or CNS function. Children with a history of febrile or nonfebrile seizure should be aggressively treated to reduce fever. However, it is unclear what triggers the febrile seizure, and there is no correlation between absolute temperature elevation and onset of a febrile seizure in susceptible children.

In hyperpyrexia, the use of cooling blankets facilitates the reduction of temperature; however, cooling blankets should not be used without oral antipyretics. In hyperpyretic patients with CNS disease or trauma (CNS bleeding), reducing core temperature mitigates the detrimental effects of high temperature on the brain.

For a discussion of treatment for hyperthermia, see Chap. 465.

FURTHER READING

DINARELLO CA et al: Treating inflammation by blocking interleukin-1 in a broad spectrum of diseases. Nature Rev 11:633, 2012.

GATTORNO M et al: Classification criteria for autoinflammatory recurrent fevers. Ann Rheum Dis 78:1025, 2019.

KULLENBERG T et al: Long-term safety profile of anakinra in patients with severe cryopyrin-associated periodic syndromes. Rheumatology 55:1499, 2016.

SAKKAT A et al: Temperature control in critically ill patients with fever: A meta-analysis of randomized controlled trials. J Crit Care 61:89, 2021.

19 Fever and Rash

Elaine T. Kaye, Kenneth M. Kaye

The acutely ill patient with fever and rash often presents a diagnostic challenge for physicians, yet the distinctive appearance of an eruption in concert with a clinical syndrome can facilitate a prompt diagnosis and the institution of life-saving therapy or critical infection-control interventions. **Representative images of many of the rashes discussed in this chapter are included in Chap. A1.**

APPROACH TO THE PATIENT

Fever and Rash

A thorough history of patients with fever and rash includes the following relevant information: immune status, medications taken within the previous month, specific travel history, immunization status, exposure to domestic pets and other animals, history of animal (including arthropod) bites, recent dietary exposures, existence of cardiac abnormalities, presence of prosthetic material, recent exposure to ill individuals, and sexual exposures. The history should also include the site of onset of the rash and its direction and rate of spread.

PHYSICAL EXAMINATION

A thorough physical examination entails close attention to the rash, with an assessment and precise definition of its salient features. First, it is critical to determine what *type* of lesions make up the eruption. *Macules* are flat lesions defined by an area of changed color (i.e., a blanchable erythema). *Papules* are raised, solid lesions <5 mm in diameter; *plaques* are lesions >5 mm in diameter with a flat, plateau-like surface; and *nodules* are lesions >5 mm in diameter with a more rounded configuration. *Wheals* (urticaria, hives) are papules or plaques that are pale pink and may appear annular (ringlike) as they enlarge; classic (nonvasculitic) wheals are transient, lasting only 24 h in any defined area. *Vesicles* (<5 mm) and *bullae* (>5 mm) are circumscribed, elevated lesions containing fluid. *Pustules* are raised lesions containing purulent exudate; vesicular processes such as varicella or herpes simplex may evolve to pustules. *Nonpalpable purpura* is a flat lesion that is due to bleeding into the skin. If <3 mm in diameter, the purpuric lesions are termed *petechiae*; if >3 mm, they are termed *ecchymoses*. *Palpable purpura* is a raised lesion that is due to inflammation of the vessel wall (vasculitis) with subsequent hemorrhage. An *ulcer* is a defect in the skin extending at least into the upper layer of the dermis, and an *eschar* (tâche noire) is a necrotic lesion covered with a black crust.

Other pertinent features of rashes include their *configuration* (i.e., annular or target), the *arrangement* of their lesions, and their *distribution* (i.e., central or peripheral).

For further discussion, see Chaps. 56, 58, 122, and 129.

CLASSIFICATION OF RASH

This chapter reviews rashes that reflect systemic disease, but it does not include localized skin eruptions (i.e., cellulitis, impetigo) that may also be associated with fever (**Chap. 129**). The chapter is not intended to be all-inclusive, but it covers the most important and most common diseases associated with fever and rash. Rashes are classified herein on the basis of lesion morphology and distribution. For practical purposes, this classification system is based on the most typical disease presentations. However, morphology may vary as rashes evolve, and the presentation of diseases with rashes is subject to many variations (**Chap. 58**). For instance, the classic petechial rash of Rocky Mountain spotted fever (**Chap. 187**) may initially consist of blanchable erythematous macules distributed peripherally; at times, however, the rash associated with this disease may not be predominantly acral, or no rash may develop at all.

Diseases with fever and rash may be classified by type of eruption: centrally distributed maculopapular, peripheral, confluent desquamative erythematous, vesiculobullous, urticaria-like, nodular, purpuric, ulcerated, or with eschars. Diseases are listed by these categories in **Table 19-1**, and many are highlighted in the text. However, for a more detailed discussion of each disease associated with a rash, the reader is referred to the chapter dealing with that specific disease. **(Reference chapters are cited in the text and listed in Table 19-1.)**

CENTRALLY DISTRIBUTED MACULOPAPULAR ERUPTIONS

Centrally distributed rashes, in which lesions are primarily truncal, are the most common type of eruption. The rash of *rubeola* (measles) starts

TABLE 19-1 Diseases Associated with Fever and Rash

DISEASE	ETIOLOGY	DESCRIPTION	GROUP AFFECTED/ EPIDEMIOLOGIC FACTORS	CLINICAL SYNDROME	CHAPTER
Centrally Distributed Maculopapular Eruptions					
Acute meningococcemia[a]	—	—	—	—	155
Drug reaction with eosinophilia and systemic symptoms (DRESS); also termed drug-induced hypersensitivity syndrome (DIHS)[b]; Chikungunya[c]; COVID-19[c]	—	—	—	—	60
Rubeola (measles, first disease) (**Fig. 19-1, Fig. A1-2, Fig. A1-3**)	Paramyxovirus	Discrete lesions that become confluent as rash spreads from hairline downward, usually sparing palms and soles; lasts ≥3 days; Koplik's spots	Nonimmune individuals	Cough, conjunctivitis, coryza, severe prostration	205
Rubella (German measles, third disease) (**Fig. A1-4**)	Togavirus	Spreads from hairline downward, clearing as it spreads; Forchheimer spots	Nonimmune individuals	Adenopathy, arthritis	206
Erythema infectiosum (fifth disease) (**Fig. A1-1**)	Human parvovirus B19	Bright-red "slapped-cheeks" appearance followed by lacy reticular rash that waxes and wanes over 3 weeks; rarely, papular-purpuric "gloves-and-socks" syndrome on hands and feet	Most common among children 3–12 years old; occurs in winter and spring	Mild fever; arthritis in adults; rash following resolution of fever	197
Exanthem subitum (roseola, sixth disease) (**Fig. A1-5**)	Human herpesvirus 6 or, less commonly, the closely related human herpesvirus 7	Diffuse maculopapular eruption over trunk and neck; resolves within 2 days	Usually affects children <3 years old	Rash following resolution of fever; similar to Boston exanthem (echovirus 16); febrile seizures may occur	195
Primary HIV infection (**Fig. A1-6**)	HIV	Nonspecific diffuse macules and papules most commonly on upper thorax, face, collar region; less commonly, urticarial or vesicular lesions; oral or genital ulcers	Individuals recently infected with HIV	Pharyngitis, adenopathy, arthralgias	202
Infectious mononucleosis	Epstein-Barr virus	Diffuse maculopapular eruption (5% of cases; 30–90% if ampicillin is given); urticaria, petechiae in some cases; periorbital edema (50%); palatal petechiae (25%)	Adolescents, young adults	Hepatosplenomegaly, pharyngitis, cervical lymphadenopathy, atypical lymphocytosis, heterophile antibody	194
Other viral exanthems	Echoviruses 2, 4, 9, 11, 16, 19, 25; coxsackieviruses A9, B1, B5; etc.	Wide range of skin findings that may mimic rubella or measles	Affect children more commonly than adults	Nonspecific viral syndromes	204
Exanthematous drug-induced eruption (**Fig. A1-7**)	Drugs (antibiotics, anticonvulsants, diuretics, etc.)	Intensely pruritic, bright-red macules and papules, symmetric on trunk and extremities; may become confluent	Occurs 2–3 days after exposure in previously sensitized individuals; otherwise, after 2–3 weeks (but can occur anytime, even shortly after drug is discontinued)	Variable findings: fever and eosinophilia	60
Epidemic typhus	*Rickettsia prowazekii*	Maculopapular eruption appearing in axillae, spreading to trunk and later to extremities; usually spares face, palms, soles; evolves from blanchable macules to confluent eruption with petechiae; rash evanescent in recrudescent typhus (Brill-Zinsser disease)	Exposure to body lice; occurrence of recrudescent typhus as relapse after 30–50 years	Headache, myalgias; mortality rates 10–40% if untreated; milder clinical presentation in recrudescent form	187
Endemic (murine) typhus	*Rickettsia typhi*	Maculopapular eruption, usually sparing palms, soles	Exposure to rat or cat fleas	Headache, myalgias	187
Scrub typhus	*Orientia tsutsugamushi*	Diffuse macular rash starting on trunk; eschar at site of mite bite	Endemic in South Pacific, Australia, Asia; transmitted by mites	Headache, myalgias, regional adenopathy; mortality rates up to 30% if untreated	187
Rickettsial spotted fevers (**Fig. 19-8**)	*Rickettsia conorii* (boutonneuse fever), *Rickettsia australis* (North Queensland tick typhus), *Rickettsia sibirica* (Siberian tick typhus), *Rickettsia africae* (African tick-bite fever), and others	Eschar common at bite site; maculopapular (rarely, vesicular and petechial) eruption on proximal extremities, spreading to trunk and face	Exposure to ticks; *R. conorii* in Mediterranean region, India, Africa; *R. australis* in Australia; *R. sibirica* in Siberia, Mongolia; *R. africae* in Africa, Caribbean	Headache, myalgias, regional adenopathy	187

(Continued)

TABLE 19-1 Diseases Associated with Fever and Rash (Continued)

DISEASE	ETIOLOGY	DESCRIPTION	GROUP AFFECTED/ EPIDEMIOLOGIC FACTORS	CLINICAL SYNDROME	CHAPTER
Human monocytotropic ehrlichiosis[d]	*Ehrlichia chaffeensis*	Maculopapular eruption (40% of cases), involves trunk and extremities; may be petechial	Tick-borne; most common in U.S. Southeast, southern Midwest, and mid-Atlantic regions	Headache, myalgias, leukopenia	187
Leptospirosis	*Leptospira interrogans* and other *Leptospira* species	Maculopapular eruption; conjunctivitis; scleral hemorrhage in some cases	Exposure to water contaminated with animal urine	Myalgias; aseptic meningitis; *fulminant form*: icterohemorrhagic fever (Weil's disease)	184
Lyme disease **(Fig. A1-8)**	*Borrelia burgdorferi* (sole cause in U.S.), *Borrelia afzelii, Borrelia garinii*	Papule expanding to erythematous annular lesion with central clearing (erythema migrans; average diameter, 15 cm), sometimes with concentric rings, sometimes with indurated or vesicular center; multiple secondary erythema migrans lesions in some cases	Bite of *Ixodes* tick vector	Headache, myalgias, chills, photophobia occurring acutely; CNS disease, myocardial disease, arthritis weeks to months later in some cases	186
Southern tick-associated rash illness (STARI, Master's disease)	Unknown (possibly *Borrelia lonestari* or other *Borrelia* spirochetes)	Similar to erythema migrans of Lyme disease with several differences, including: multiple secondary lesions less likely; lesions tending to be smaller (average diameter, ~8 cm); central clearing more likely	Bite of tick vector *Amblyomma americanum* (Lone Star tick); often found in regions where Lyme disease is uncommon, including southern United States	Compared with Lyme disease: fewer constitutional symptoms, tick bite more likely to be recalled; other Lyme disease sequelae lacking	186
Typhoid fever **(Fig. A1-9)**	*Salmonella typhi*	Transient, blanchable erythematous macules and papules, 2–4 mm, usually on trunk (rose spots)	Ingestion of contaminated food or water (rare in U.S.)	Variable abdominal pain and diarrhea; headache, myalgias, hepatosplenomegaly	165
Dengue fever[e] **(Fig. A1-53)**	Dengue virus (4 serotypes; flaviviruses)	Rash in 50% of cases; initially diffuse flushing; midway through illness, onset of maculopapular rash, which begins on trunk and spreads centrifugally to extremities and face; pruritus, hyperesthesia in some cases; after defervescence, petechiae on extremities may occur	Occurs in tropics and subtropics; transmitted by mosquito	Headache; musculoskeletal pain ("breakbone fever"); leukopenia; occasionally biphasic ("saddleback") fever	209
Rat-bite fever (sodoku)	*Spirillum minus*	Eschar at bite site; then blotchy violaceous or red-brown rash involving trunk and extremities	Rat bite; primarily found in Asia; rare in U.S.	Regional adenopathy; recurrent fevers if untreated	141
Relapsing fever	*Borrelia* species	Central rash at end of febrile episode; petechiae in some cases	Exposure to ticks or body lice	Recurrent fever, headache, myalgias, hepatosplenomegaly	185
Erythema marginatum (rheumatic fever)	Group A *Streptococcus*	Erythematous annular papules and plaques occurring as polycyclic lesions in waves over trunk, proximal extremities; evolving and resolving within hours	Patients with rheumatic fever	Pharyngitis preceding polyarthritis, carditis, subcutaneous nodules, chorea	388
Systemic lupus erythematosus (SLE) **(Fig. A1-10, Fig. A1-11, Fig. A1-12)**	Autoimmune disease	Macular and papular erythema, often in sun-exposed areas; discoid lupus lesions (local atrophy, scale, pigmentary changes); periungual telangiectasis; malar rash; vasculitis sometimes causing urticaria, palpable purpura; oral erosions in some cases	Most common in young to middle-aged women; flares precipitated by sun exposure	Arthritis; cardiac, pulmonary, renal, hematologic, and vasculitic disease	359
Still's disease **(Fig. A1-13)**	Autoimmune disease	Transient 2- to 5-mm erythematous papules appearing at height of fever on trunk, proximal extremities; lesions evanescent	Children and young adults	High spiking fever, polyarthritis, splenomegaly; erythrocyte sedimentation rate >100 mm/h	—
African trypanosomiasis **(Fig. A1-47)**	*Trypanosoma brucei rhodesiense/gambiense*	Blotchy or annular erythematous macular and papular rash (trypanid), primarily on trunk; pruritus; chancre at site of tsetse fly bite may precede rash by several weeks	Tsetse fly bite in eastern (*T. brucei rhodesiense*) or western (*T. brucei gambiense*) Africa	Hemolymphatic disease followed by meningoencephalitis; Winterbottom's sign (posterior cervical lymphadenopathy) (*T. brucei gambiense*)	227
Arcanobacterial pharyngitis	*Arcanobacterium (Corynebacterium) haemolyticum*	Diffuse, erythematous, maculopapular eruption involving trunk and proximal extremities; may desquamate	Children and young adults	Exudative pharyngitis, lymphadenopathy	150

(*Continued*)

TABLE 19-1 Diseases Associated with Fever and Rash (Continued)

DISEASE	ETIOLOGY	DESCRIPTION	GROUP AFFECTED/ EPIDEMIOLOGIC FACTORS	CLINICAL SYNDROME	CHAPTER
West Nile virus infection	West Nile virus	Maculopapular eruption involving the trunk, extremities, and head or neck; rash in 20–50% of cases	Mosquito bite; rarely, blood transfusion or transplanted organ	Headache, weakness, malaise, myalgia, neuroinvasive disease (encephalitis, meningitis, flaccid paralysis)	209
Zika virus infection (Fig. A1-51)	Zika virus	Pruritic macular and papular erythema; rash may begin on trunk and descend to lower body; conjunctival injection; palatal petechiae may occur	Mosquito bite; sexual transmission or blood transfusion less common	Arthralgia (especially of small joints), myalgia, lymphadenopathy, headache, low-grade fever; illness in pregnancy may cause severe birth defects, including microcephaly; neurologic complications, including Guillain-Barré, may occur	209
Peripheral Eruptions					
Chronic meningococcemia, disseminated gonococcal infection,[e] human parvovirus B19 infection,[f] MIRM[g]	—	—	—	—	155, 156, 197
Rocky Mountain spotted fever (Fig. 19-2, Fig. A1-16)	*Rickettsia rickettsii*	Rash beginning on wrists and ankles and spreading centripetally; appears on palms and soles later in disease; lesion evolution from blanchable macules to petechiae	Tick vector; widespread but more common in southeastern and southwest-central U.S.	Headache, myalgias, abdominal pain; mortality rates up to 40% if untreated	187
Secondary syphilis (Figs. A1-18, Fig. A1-19, Fig. A1-20, Fig. A1-21)	*Treponema pallidum*	Coincident primary chancre in 10% of cases; copper-colored, scaly papular eruption, diffuse but prominent on palms and soles; rash never vesicular in adults; condyloma latum, mucous patches, and alopecia in some cases	Sexually transmitted	Fever, constitutional symptoms	182
Chikungunya fever (Fig. A1-54)	Chikungunya virus	Maculopapular eruption; typically occurs on trunk, but also occurs on extremities and face	*Aedes aegypti* and *A. albopictus* mosquito bites; tropical and subtropical regions	Severe polyarticular, migratory arthralgias, especially involving small joints (e.g., hands, wrists, ankles)	209
Hand-foot-and-mouth disease (Fig. A1-22)	Coxsackievirus A16 and enterovirus 71 most common causes; coxsackievirus A6 associated with atypical syndrome	Tender vesicles, erosions in mouth; 0.25-cm papules on hands and feet with rim of erythema evolving into tender vesicles; shedding of nails (onychomadesis) can occur 1–2 months after acute illness; coxsackievirus A6 lesions may also be maculopapular, petechial, purpuric, or erosive; atypical form often extends to perioral area, extremities, trunk, buttocks, genitals, and areas affected by eczema (eczema coxsackium)	Summer and fall; primarily children <10 years old; multiple family members; coxsackievirus A6 infection also occurs in young adults	Transient fever; enterovirus 71 can be associated with brain stem encephalitis, flaccid paralysis resembling polio, or aseptic meningitis	204
Erythema multiforme (EM) (Fig. A1-24)	Infection, drugs, idiopathic causes	Target lesions (central erythema surrounded by area of clearing and another rim of erythema) up to 2 cm; symmetric on knees, elbows, palms, soles; spreads centripetally; papular, sometimes vesicular; when extensive and involving mucous membranes, termed *EM major*	Herpes simplex virus or *Mycoplasma pneumoniae* infection; drug intake (i.e., sulfa, phenytoin, penicillin)	50% of patients <20 years old; fever more common in most severe form, EM major, which can be confused with Stevens-Johnson syndrome (but EM major lacks prominent skin sloughing)	—[h]
Rat-bite fever (Haverhill fever)	*Streptobacillus moniliformis*	Maculopapular eruption over palms, soles, and extremities; tends to be more severe at joints; eruption sometimes becoming generalized; may be purpuric; may desquamate	Rat bite, ingestion of contaminated food	Myalgias; arthritis (50%); fever recurrence in some cases	141

(Continued)

TABLE 19-1 Diseases Associated with Fever and Rash (Continued)

DISEASE	ETIOLOGY	DESCRIPTION	GROUP AFFECTED/ EPIDEMIOLOGIC FACTORS	CLINICAL SYNDROME	CHAPTER
Bacterial endocarditis (**Fig. A1-23**)	*Streptococcus, Staphylococcus,* etc.	*Subacute course* (e.g., viridans streptococci): Osler's nodes (tender pink nodules on finger or toe pads); petechiae on skin and mucosa; splinter hemorrhages. *Acute course* (e.g., *Staphylococcus aureus*): Janeway lesions (painless erythematous or hemorrhagic macules, usually on palms and soles)	Abnormal heart valve (e.g., viridans streptococci), intravenous drug use	New or changing heart murmur	128
COVID-19 (**Fig. A1-57**)	SARS-CoV-2	*Mild or asymptomatic COVID-19:* Pernio (macules, papules, or plaques that are tender, erythematous/violaceous; acral, feet more common than hands); *Moderate/severe COVID-19:* vesicles, urticaria, maculopapular erythema; often pruritic; occur on trunk, extremities; *Severe COVID-19:* Retiform purpura (net-like, purple patches/ plaques often with necrosis); lesions often asymptomatic; occur on extremities, buttocks; *Multisystem inflammatory syndrome in children (MIS-C):* findings similar to Kawasaki disease	Infection with SARS-CoV-2; MIS-C in older children/adolescents	Ranging from asymptomatic to mild/ moderate with loss of taste/smell, pharyngitis, cough, fever, to severe with dyspnea, ARDS; complications include thrombosis, especially with retiform purpura; lesions may be delayed compared to other COVID-19 symptoms; MIS-C occurs ~2-6 weeks following acute (often asymptomatic) infection	
Confluent Desquamative Erythemas					
Scarlet fever (second disease) (**Fig. A1-25**)	Group A *Streptococcus* (pyrogenic exotoxins A, B, C)	Diffuse blanchable erythema beginning on face and spreading to trunk and extremities; circumoral pallor; "sandpaper" texture to skin; accentuation of linear erythema in skin folds (Pastia's lines); enanthem of white evolving into red "strawberry" tongue; desquamation in second week	Most common among children 2–10 years old; usually follows group A streptococcal pharyngitis	Fever, pharyngitis, headache	148
Kawasaki disease (**Fig. A1-29**)	Idiopathic	Rash similar to scarlet fever (scarlatiniform) or EM; fissuring of lips, strawberry tongue; conjunctivitis; edema of hands, feet; desquamation later in disease	Children <8 years old	Cervical adenopathy, pharyngitis, coronary artery vasculitis	58, 363
Streptococcal toxic shock syndrome	Group A *Streptococcus* (associated with pyrogenic exotoxin A and/ or B or certain M types)	When present, rash often scarlatiniform	May occur in setting of severe group A streptococcal infections (e.g., necrotizing fasciitis, bacteremia, pneumonia)	Multiorgan failure, hypotension; mortality rate 30%	148
Staphylococcal toxic shock syndrome	*S. aureus* (toxic shock syndrome toxin 1, enterotoxins B and others)	Diffuse erythema involving palms; pronounced erythema of mucosal surfaces; conjunctivitis; desquamation 7–10 days into illness	Colonization with toxin-producing *S. aureus*	Fever >39°C (>102°F), hypotension, multiorgan dysfunction	147
Staphylococcal scalded-skin syndrome (**Fig. 19-3, Fig. A1-28**)	*S. aureus,* phage group II	Diffuse tender erythema, often with bullae and desquamation; Nikolsky's sign	Colonization with toxin-producing *S. aureus*; occurs in children <10 years old (termed *Ritter's disease* in neonates) or adults with renal dysfunction	Irritability; nasal or conjunctival secretions	147
Exfoliative erythroderma syndrome (**Fig. A1-27**)	Underlying psoriasis, eczema, drug eruption, mycosis fungoides	Diffuse erythema (often scaling) interspersed with lesions of underlying condition	Usually occurs in adults over age 50; more common among men	Fever, chills (i.e., difficulty with thermoregulation); lymphadenopathy	58, 60
DRESS (drug-induced hypersensitivity syndrome [DIHS]) (**Fig. A1-48**)	Aromatic anticonvulsants; other drugs, including sulfonamides, minocycline	Maculopapular eruption (mimicking exanthematous drug rash), sometimes progressing to exfoliative erythroderma; profound edema, especially facial; pustules may occur	Individuals genetically unable to detoxify arene oxides (anticonvulsant metabolites), patients with slow *N*-acetylating capacity (sulfonamides)	Lymphadenopathy, multiorgan failure (especially hepatic), eosinophilia, atypical lymphocytes; mimics sepsis	60
Stevens-Johnson syndrome (SJS), toxic epidermal necrolysis (TEN) (**Fig. A1-26**)	Drugs (80% of cases; often allopurinol, anticonvulsants, antibiotics), infection, idiopathic factors	Erythematous and purpuric macules, sometimes targetoid, or diffuse erythema progressing to bullae, with sloughing and necrosis of entire epidermis; Nikolsky's sign; involves mucosal surfaces; TEN (>30% epidermal necrosis) is maximal form; SJS involves <10% of epidermis; SJS/TEN overlap involves 10–30% of epidermis	Uncommon among children; more common among patients with HIV infection, systemic lupus erythematosus, certain HLA types, or slow acetylators	Dehydration, sepsis sometimes resulting from lack of normal skin integrity; mortality rates up to 30%	60

(Continued)

TABLE 19-1 Diseases Associated with Fever and Rash (Continued)

DISEASE	ETIOLOGY	DESCRIPTION	GROUP AFFECTED/ EPIDEMIOLOGIC FACTORS	CLINICAL SYNDROME	CHAPTER
Vesiculobullous or Pustular Eruptions					
Hand-foot-and-mouth syndrome[c]; staphylococcal scalded-skin syndrome[b]; TEN[b]; DRESS[b]; COVID-19[c]	—	—	—	—	—[h]
Varicella (chickenpox) (**Fig. 19-4, Fig. A1-30**)	Varicella-zoster virus (VZV)	Macules (2–3 mm) evolving into papules, then vesicles (sometimes umbilicated), on an erythematous base ("dewdrops on a rose petal"); pustules then forming and crusting; lesions appearing in crops; may involve scalp, mouth; intensely pruritic	Usually affects children; 10% of adults susceptible; most common in late winter and spring; incidence down by 90% in U.S. as a result of varicella vaccination	Malaise; generally mild disease in healthy children; more severe disease with complications in adults and immunocompromised children	193
Pseudomonas "hot-tub" folliculitis (**Fig. A1-55**)	*Pseudomonas aeruginosa*	Pruritic erythematous follicular, papular, vesicular, or pustular lesions that may involve axillae, buttocks, abdomen, and especially areas occluded by bathing suits; can manifest as tender isolated nodules on palmar or plantar surfaces (the latter designated "*Pseudomonas* hot-foot syndrome")	Bathers in hot tubs or swimming pools; occurs in outbreaks	Earache, sore eyes and/or throat; fever may be absent; generally self-limited	164
Variola (smallpox) (**Fig. A1-50**)	Variola major virus	Red macules on tongue and palate evolving to papules and vesicles; skin macules evolving to papules, then vesicles, then pustules over 1 week, with subsequent lesion crusting; lesions initially appearing on face and spreading centrifugally from trunk to extremities; differs from varicella in that (1) skin lesions in any given area are at same stage of development and (2) there is a prominent distribution of lesions on face and extremities (including palms, soles)	Nonimmune individuals exposed to smallpox	Prodrome of fever, headache, backache, myalgias; vomiting in 50% of cases	S3
Primary herpes simplex virus (HSV) infection	HSV	Erythema rapidly followed by hallmark painful *grouped vesicles* that may evolve into pustules that ulcerate, especially on mucosal surfaces; lesions at site of inoculation: commonly gingivostomatitis for HSV-1 and genital lesions for HSV-2; recurrent disease milder (e.g., herpes labialis does not involve oral mucosa)	Primary infection most common among children and young adults for HSV-1 and among sexually active young adults for HSV-2; no fever in recurrent infection	Regional lymphadenopathy	192
Disseminated herpesvirus infection (**Fig. A1-31**)	VZV or HSV	Generalized vesicles that can evolve to pustules and ulcerations; individual lesions similar for VZV and HSV. *Zoster cutaneous dissemination*: >25 lesions extending outside involved dermatome. *HSV*: extensive, progressive mucocutaneous lesions that may occur in absence of dissemination, sometimes disseminate in eczematous skin (eczema herpeticum); HSV visceral dissemination may occur with only localized mucocutaneous disease; in disseminated neonatal disease, skin lesions diagnostically helpful when present, but rash absent in a substantial minority of cases	Patients with immunosuppression, eczema; neonates	Visceral organ involvement (e.g., liver, lungs) in some cases; neonatal disease particularly severe	138, 192, 193
Rickettsialpox (**Fig. A1-33**)	*Rickettsia akari*	Eschar found at site of mite bite; generalized rash involving face, trunk, extremities; may involve palms and soles; <100 papules and plaques (2–10 mm); centers of papules develop vesicles or pustules	Seen in urban settings; transmitted by mouse mites	Headache, myalgias, regional adenopathy; mild disease	187
Acute generalized exanthematous pustulosis (**Fig. A1-49**)	Drugs (mostly anticonvulsants or antimicrobials); also viral	Tiny, sterile, nonfollicular pustules on erythematous, edematous skin; begins on face and in body folds, then becomes generalized	Appears 2–21 days after start of drug therapy, depending on whether patient has been sensitized	Acute fever, pruritus, leukocytosis	60

(Continued)

TABLE 19-1 Diseases Associated with Fever and Rash (Continued)

DISEASE	ETIOLOGY	DESCRIPTION	GROUP AFFECTED/ EPIDEMIOLOGIC FACTORS	CLINICAL SYNDROME	CHAPTER
Disseminated *Vibrio vulnificus* infection	*V. vulnificus*	Erythematous lesions evolving into hemorrhagic bullae and then into necrotic ulcers	Patients with cirrhosis, diabetes, renal failure; exposure by ingestion of contaminated saltwater, seafood	Hypotension; mortality rate 50%	168
Ecthyma gangrenosum (Fig. A1-34)	*P. aeruginosa*, other gram-negative rods, fungi	Indurated plaque evolving into hemorrhagic bulla or pustule that sloughs, resulting in eschar formation; erythematous halo; most common in axillary, groin, perianal regions	Usually affects neutropenic patients; occurs in up to 28% of individuals with *Pseudomonas* bacteremia	Clinical signs of sepsis	164
Mycoplasma-induced rash and mucositis (MIRM)	*Mycoplasma pneumoniae*	Severe mucositis of at least two sites (e.g., oropharynx, ocular, genital) with nearly universal hemorrhagic crusting of lips; sparse, vesiculobullous, or atypical targetoid rash over <10% of body; lesions typically on extremities but can be truncal; rash sometimes absent (MIRM sine rash)	More common in males; usually children (mean age 11–12 years old)	Evidence of *M. pneumoniae* infection (typically pneumonia); good prognosis; distinct from SJS/TEN; rarely *Chlamydophila pneumoniae* can cause similar syndrome	
Urticaria-Like Eruptions					
COVID-19[c]					
Urticarial vasculitis (Fig. 19-5, Fig. A1-35)	Serum sickness, often due to infection (including acute hepatitis B, enteroviral, parasitic), drugs; connective tissue disease	Erythematous, edematous "urticaria-like" plaques, pruritic or burning; unlike urticaria: typical lesion duration >24 h (up to 5 days) and lack of complete lesion blanching with compression due to hemorrhage	Patients with serum sickness (including acute hepatitis B), connective tissue disease	Fever variable; arthralgias/arthritis	363[h]
Nodular Eruptions					
Disseminated infection (Fig. 19-6, Fig. A1-36, Fig. A1-37, Fig. A1-38)	Fungal infections (e.g., candidiasis, histoplasmosis, cryptococcosis, sporotrichosis, coccidioidomycosis); mycobacteria	Subcutaneous nodules (up to 3 cm); fluctuance, draining common with mycobacteria; necrotic nodules (extremities, periorbital or nasal regions) common with *Aspergillus, Mucor*	Immunocompromised hosts (e.g., bone marrow transplant recipients, patients undergoing chemotherapy, HIV-infected patients)	Features vary with organism	—[h]
Erythema nodosum (septal panniculitis) (Fig. A1-39)	Infections (e.g., streptococcal, fungal, mycobacterial, yersinial); drugs (e.g., sulfas, penicillins, oral contraceptives); sarcoidosis; idiopathic causes	Large, violaceous, nonulcerative, subcutaneous nodules; exquisitely tender; usually on lower legs but also on upper extremities	More common among females 15–30 years old	Arthralgias (50%); features vary with associated condition	—[h]
Sweet syndrome (acute febrile neutrophilic dermatosis) (Fig. A1-40)	*Yersinia* infection; upper respiratory infection; inflammatory bowel disease; pregnancy; malignancy (usually hematologic); drugs (G-CSF)	Tender red or blue edematous nodules giving impression of vesiculation; usually on face, neck, upper extremities; when on lower extremities, may mimic erythema nodosum	More common among women and among persons 30–60 years old; 20% of cases associated with malignancy (men and women equally affected in this group)	Headache, arthralgias, leukocytosis	58
Bacillary angiomatosis	*Bartonella henselae, B. quintana*	Many forms, including erythematous, smooth vascular nodules; friable, exophytic lesions; erythematous plaques (may be dry, scaly); subcutaneous nodules (may be erythematous)	Immunosuppressed individuals, especially those with advanced HIV infection	Peliosis of liver and spleen in some cases; lesions sometimes involving multiple organs; bacteremia	172
Purpuric Eruptions					
Rocky Mountain spotted fever, rat-bite fever, endocarditis[c]; epidemic typhus[f]; dengue fever[e,f]; human parvovirus B19 infection[f]; COVID-19[c]	—	—	—	—	—[h]
Acute meningococcemia	*Neisseria meningitidis*	Initially pink maculopapular lesions evolving into petechiae; petechiae rapidly becoming numerous, sometimes enlarging and becoming vesicular; trunk, extremities most commonly involved; may appear on face, hands, feet; may include purpura fulminans (see below) reflecting DIC	Most common among children, individuals with asplenia or terminal complement component deficiency (C5–C8)	Hypotension, meningitis (sometimes preceded by upper respiratory infection)	155

(Continued)

TABLE 19-1 Diseases Associated with Fever and Rash (Continued)

DISEASE	ETIOLOGY	DESCRIPTION	GROUP AFFECTED/ EPIDEMIOLOGIC FACTORS	CLINICAL SYNDROME	CHAPTER
Purpura fulminans **(Fig. 19-7, Fig. A1-41)**	Severe DIC	Large ecchymoses with sharply irregular shapes evolving into hemorrhagic bullae and then into black necrotic lesions	Individuals with sepsis (e.g., involving *N. meningitidis*), malignancy, or massive trauma; asplenic patients at high risk for sepsis	Hypotension	**155, 304**
Chronic meningococcemia **(Fig. A1-42)**	*N. meningitidis*	Variety of recurrent eruptions, including pink maculopapular; nodular (usually on lower extremities); petechial (sometimes developing vesicular centers); purpuric areas with pale blue-gray centers	Individuals with complement deficiencies	Fevers, sometimes intermittent; arthritis, myalgias, headache	**155**
Disseminated gonococcal infection **(Fig. A1-43)**	*Neisseria gonorrhoeae*	Papules (1–5 mm) evolving over 1–2 days into hemorrhagic pustules with gray necrotic centers; hemorrhagic bullae occurring rarely; lesions (usually <40) distributed peripherally near joints (more commonly on upper extremities)	Sexually active individuals (more often females), some with complement deficiency	Low-grade fever, tenosynovitis, arthritis	**156**
Enteroviral petechial rash	Usually echovirus 9 or coxsackievirus A9	Disseminated petechial lesions (may also be maculopapular, vesicular, or urticarial)	Often occurs in outbreaks	Pharyngitis, headache; aseptic meningitis with echovirus 9	**204**
Viral hemorrhagic fever	Arenaviruses, bunyaviruses, filoviruses (including Ebola), flaviviruses (including dengue)	Petechial rash	Residence in or travel to endemic areas, other virus exposure	Triad of fever, shock, hemorrhage from mucosa or gastrointestinal tract	**209, 210**
Thrombotic thrombocytopenic purpura/hemolytic-uremic syndrome	Idiopathic, bloody diarrhea caused by Shiga toxin–generating bacteria (e.g., *Escherichia coli* O157:H7), deficiency in ADAMTS13 (cleaves von Willebrand factor), drugs (e.g., quinine, chemotherapy, immunosuppression)	Petechiae	Individuals with *E. coli* O157:H7 gastroenteritis (especially children), cancer chemotherapy, HIV infection, autoimmune diseases, pregnant/postpartum women, those with ADAMTS13 deficiency	Fever (not always present), microangiopathic hemolytic anemia, thrombocytopenia, renal dysfunction, neurologic dysfunction; coagulation studies normal	**58, 100, 115, 161, 166**
Cutaneous small-vessel vasculitis (leukocytoclastic vasculitis) **(Fig. A1-44)**	Infections (including group A streptococcal infection, hepatitis B or C), drugs, idiopathic factors	Palpable purpuric lesions appearing in crops on legs or other dependent areas; may become vesicular or ulcerative	Occurs in a wide spectrum of diseases, including connective tissue disease, cryoglobulinemia, malignancy, Henoch-Schönlein purpura (HSP); more common among children	Fever (not always present), malaise, arthralgias, myalgias; systemic vasculitis in some cases; renal, joint, and gastrointestinal involvement common in HSP	**58**
Eruptions with Ulcers and/or Eschars					
Scrub typhus, rickettsial spotted fevers, rat-bite fever, African trypanosomiasis[f]; rickettsialpox, ecthyma gangrenosum[g]	—	—	—	—	—[h]
Tularemia **(Fig. A1-45, Fig. A1-46)**	*Francisella tularensis*	Ulceroglandular form: erythematous, tender papule evolves into necrotic, tender ulcer with raised borders; in 35% of cases, eruptions (maculopapular, vesiculopapular, acneiform, or urticarial; erythema nodosum; or EM) may occur	Exposure to ticks, biting flies, infected animals	Fever, headache, lymphadenopathy	**170**
Anthrax **(Fig. A1-52)**	*Bacillus anthracis*	Pruritic papule enlarging and evolving into a 1- by 3-cm painless ulcer surrounded by vesicles and then developing a central eschar with edema; residual scar	Exposure to infected animals or animal products, other exposure to anthrax spores	Lymphadenopathy, headache	**S3**

[a]See "Purpuric Eruptions." [b]See "Confluent Desquamative Erythemas." [c]See "Peripheral Eruptions." [d]Rash is rare in human granulocytotropic ehrlichiosis or anaplasmosis (caused by *Anaplasma phagocytophilum*; most common in the upper midwestern and northeastern United States). [e]See "Viral hemorrhagic fever" under "Purpuric Eruptions" for dengue hemorrhagic fever/dengue shock syndrome. [f]See "Centrally Distributed Maculopapular Eruptions." [g]See "Vesiculobullous or Pustular Eruptions." [h]See etiology-specific chapters.

Abbreviations: CNS, central nervous system; DIC, disseminated intravascular coagulation; G-CSF, granulocyte colony-stimulating factor; HLA, human leukocyte antigen.

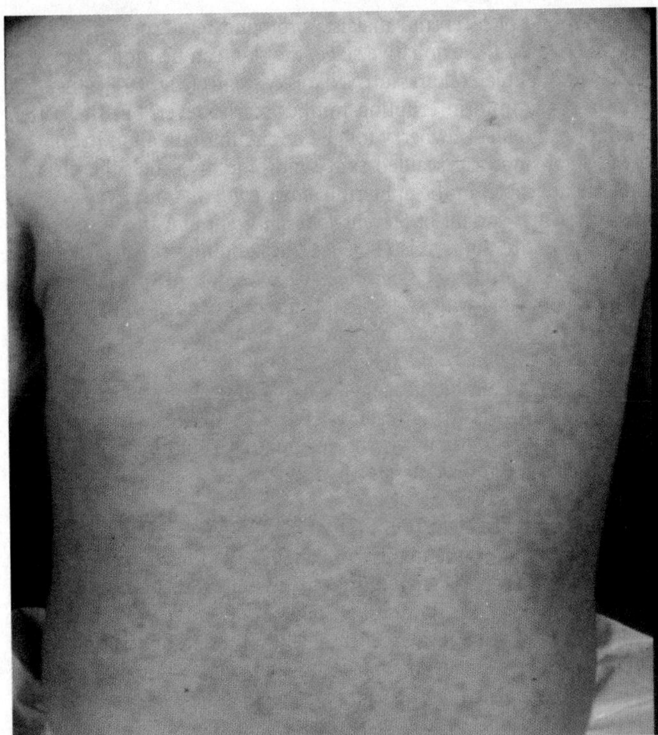

FIGURE 19-1 Centrally distributed, maculopapular eruption on the trunk in a patient with measles. *(From EJ Mayeaux Jr et al: Measles, in Usatine RP et al [eds]: Color Atlas and Synopsis of Family Medicine, 3rd ed. New York, McGraw-Hill, 2019, p. 797, Figure 132-2. Reproduced with permission from Richard P. Usatine, MD.)*

at the hairline 2–3 days into the illness and moves down the body, typically sparing the palms and soles (Fig. 19-1; see also Fig. A1-3) (Chap. 205). It begins as discrete erythematous lesions, which become confluent as the rash spreads. Koplik's spots (1- to 2-mm white or bluish lesions with an erythematous halo on the buccal mucosa) (Fig. A1-2) are pathognomonic for measles and are generally seen during the first 2 days of symptoms. They should not be confused with Fordyce's spots (ectopic sebaceous glands), which have no erythematous halos and are found in the mouth of healthy individuals. Koplik's spots may briefly overlap with the measles exanthem.

Rubella (German measles) (Fig. A1-4) also spreads from the hairline downward; unlike that of measles, however, the rash of rubella tends to clear from originally affected areas as it migrates, and it may be pruritic (Chap. 206). Forchheimer spots (palatal petechiae) may develop but are nonspecific because they also develop in *infectious mononucleosis* (Chap. 194), *scarlet fever* (Chap. 148), and *Zika virus infection* (Chap. 209) (Fig. A1-51D). Postauricular and suboccipital adenopathy and arthritis are common among adults with rubella. Exposure of pregnant women to ill individuals should be avoided, as rubella causes severe congenital abnormalities. Numerous strains of *enteroviruses* (Chap. 204), primarily echoviruses and coxsackieviruses, cause nonspecific syndromes of fever and eruptions that may mimic rubella or measles. Patients with *infectious mononucleosis* caused by Epstein-Barr virus (Chap. 194) or with *primary HIV infection* (Fig. A1-6; see also Chapter 202) may exhibit pharyngitis, lymphadenopathy, and a nonspecific maculopapular exanthem.

The rash of *erythema infectiosum* (fifth disease), which is caused by human parvovirus B19, primarily affects children 3–12 years old; it develops after fever has resolved as a bright blanchable erythema on the cheeks ("slapped cheeks") (Fig. A1-1A) with perioral pallor (Chap. 197). A more diffuse rash (often pruritic) appears the next day on the trunk and extremities and then rapidly develops into a lacy reticular eruption (Fig. A1-1B) that may wax and wane (especially with temperature change) over 3 weeks. Adults with fifth disease often have arthritis, and fetal hydrops can develop in association with this condition in pregnant women.

Exanthem subitum (roseola) is caused by human herpesvirus 6, or less commonly by the closely related human herpesvirus 7, and is most common among children <3 years of age (Chap. 195). As in erythema infectiosum, the rash usually appears after fever has subsided. It consists of 2- to 3-mm rose-pink macules and papules that coalesce only rarely, occur initially on the trunk (Fig. A1-5) and sometimes on the extremities (sparing the face), and fade within 2 days.

Although drug reactions have many manifestations, including urticaria, exanthematous *drug-induced eruptions* (Chap. 60) (Fig. A1-7) are most common and are often difficult to distinguish from viral exanthems. Eruptions elicited by drugs are usually more intensely erythematous and pruritic than viral exanthems, but this distinction is not reliable. A history of new medications and an absence of prostration may help to distinguish a drug-related rash from an eruption of another etiology. Rashes may persist for up to 2 weeks after administration of the offending agent is discontinued. Certain populations are more prone than others to drug rashes. Of HIV-infected patients, 50–60% develop a rash in response to sulfa drugs; 30–90% of patients with mononucleosis due to Epstein-Barr virus develop a rash when given ampicillin.

Rickettsial illnesses (Chap. 187) should be considered in the evaluation of individuals with centrally distributed maculopapular eruptions. The usual setting for *epidemic typhus* is a site of war or natural disaster in which people are exposed to body lice. Endemic typhus or *leptospirosis* (the latter caused by a spirochete) (Chap. 184) may be seen in urban environments where rodents proliferate. Outside the United States, other rickettsial diseases cause a spotted-fever syndrome and should be considered in residents of or travelers to endemic areas. Similarly, *typhoid fever*, a nonrickettsial disease caused by *Salmonella typhi* (Chap. 165) (Fig. A1-9), is usually acquired during travel outside the United States. *Dengue fever* (Fig. A1-53), caused by a mosquito-transmitted flavivirus, occurs in tropical and subtropical regions of the world (Chap. 209).

Some centrally distributed maculopapular eruptions have distinctive features. Erythema migrans (Fig. A1-8), the rash of *Lyme disease* (Chap. 186), typically manifests as single or multiple annular lesions. Untreated erythema migrans lesions usually fade within a month but may persist for more than a year. *Southern tick-associated rash illness* (STARI) (Chap. 186) has an erythema migrans–like rash, but is less severe than Lyme disease and often occurs in regions where Lyme is not endemic. Erythema marginatum, the rash of *acute rheumatic fever* (Chap. 359), has a distinctive pattern of enlarging and shifting transient annular lesions.

Collagen vascular diseases may cause fever and rash. Patients with *systemic lupus erythematosus* (Chap. 356) typically develop a sharply defined, erythematous eruption in a butterfly distribution on the cheeks (malar rash) (Fig. A1-10) as well as many other skin manifestations (Figs. A1-11, A1-12). *Still's disease* presents as an evanescent, salmon-colored rash on the trunk and proximal extremities that coincides with fever spikes (Fig. A1-13).

Hemophagocytic lymphohistiocytosis may be familial or triggered by infection, autoimmunity, or neoplasia. Cutaneous manifestations are protean and can present as an erythematous maculopapular eruption, pyoderma gangrenosum, purpura, panniculitis, or Stevens Johnson syndrome.

Zika virus is a mosquito-transmitted flavivirus that is associated with severe birth defects (Chap. 209). Zika is widespread among tropical and subtropical regions of the world. The eruption of Zika virus infection (Fig. A1-51A, A1-51B) is typically pruritic and often accompanied by conjunctival injection (Fig. A1-51C).

PERIPHERAL ERUPTIONS

These rashes are alike in that they are most prominent peripherally or begin in peripheral (acral) areas before spreading centripetally. Early diagnosis and therapy are critical in *Rocky Mountain spotted fever* (Chap. 187) because of its grave prognosis if untreated. Lesions (Fig. 19-2; see also Fig. A1-16) evolve from macular to petechial, start on the wrists and ankles, spread centripetally, and appear on the palms and soles only later in the disease. The rash of *secondary syphilis* (Chap. 182), which may be generalized (Fig. A1-18) but is prominent on the palms and soles (Fig. A1-19), should be considered in the differential diagnosis of pityriasis rosea, especially in sexually active patients. *Chikungunya fever* (Chap. 209), which is transmitted by mosquito bite

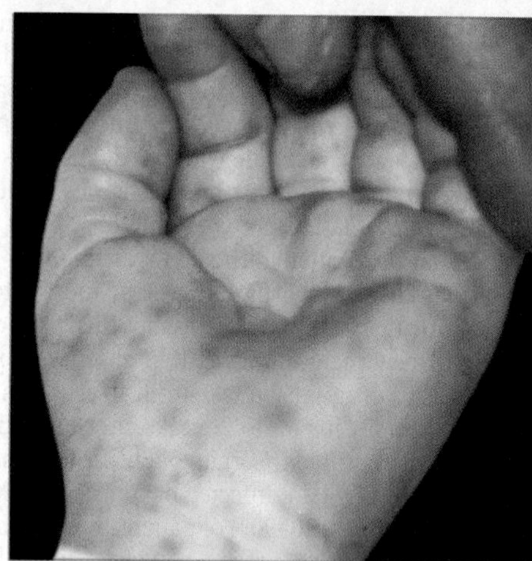

FIGURE 19-2 Peripheral eruption on the wrist and palm exhibiting erythematous macules in the process of evolving into petechial lesions in a patient with Rocky Mountain spotted fever. *(From K Wolff et al [eds]: Fitzpatrick's Color Atlas and Synopsis of Clinical Dermatology, 8th ed. New York, McGraw-Hill, 2017, p. 562, Figure 25-50; with permission.)*

in tropical and subtropical regions, is associated with a maculopapular eruption **(Fig. A1-54)** and severe polyarticular small-joint arthralgias. *Hand-foot-and-mouth disease* **(Chap. 204)**, most commonly caused by coxsackievirus A16 or enterovirus 71, is distinguished by tender vesicles distributed on the hands and feet and in the mouth **(Fig. A1-22)**; coxsackievirus A6 causes an atypical syndrome with more extensive lesions. The classic target lesions of *erythema multiforme* **(Fig. A1-24)** appear symmetrically on the elbows, knees, palms, soles, and face. In severe cases, these lesions spread diffusely and involve mucosal surfaces. Lesions may develop on the hands and feet in *endocarditis* **(Fig. A1-23) (Chap. 128)**. Pernio, tender violaceous lesions that are acral **(Fig. A1-57)**, occur most commonly on the feet, in asymptomatic or mild COVID-19. Vesicles, urticaria, or maculopapular eruptions, often pruritic, may occur on the trunk and extremities in moderate or severe disease, while retiform purpura occurs on the extremities and buttocks in severe COVID-19.

■ CONFLUENT DESQUAMATIVE ERYTHEMAS

These eruptions consist of diffuse erythema frequently followed by desquamation. The eruptions caused by group A *Streptococcus* or *Staphylococcus aureus* are toxin-mediated. *Scarlet fever* **(Chap. 148) (Fig. A1-25)** usually follows pharyngitis; patients have a facial flush, a "strawberry" tongue, and accentuated petechiae in body folds (Pastia's lines). *Kawasaki disease* **(Fig. A1-29) (Chaps. 58 and 363)** presents in the pediatric population as fissuring of the lips, a strawberry tongue, conjunctivitis, adenopathy, and sometimes cardiac abnormalities. *Streptococcal toxic shock syndrome* **(Chap. 148)** manifests with hypotension, multiorgan failure, and, often, a severe group A streptococcal infection (e.g., necrotizing fasciitis). *Staphylococcal toxic shock syndrome* **(Chap. 147)** also presents with hypotension and multiorgan failure, but usually only *S. aureus* colonization—not a severe *S. aureus* infection—is documented. *Staphylococcal scalded-skin syndrome* **(Fig. A1-28) (Chap. 147)** is seen primarily in children and in immunocompromised adults. Generalized erythema is often evident during the prodrome of fever and malaise; profound tenderness of the skin is distinctive. In the exfoliative stage, the skin can be induced to form bullae with light lateral pressure (Nikolsky's sign) **(Fig. 19-3)**. In a mild form, a scarlatiniform eruption mimics scarlet fever, but the patient does not exhibit a strawberry tongue or circumoral pallor. In contrast to the staphylococcal scalded-skin syndrome, in which the cleavage plane is superficial in the epidermis, *toxic epidermal necrolysis* **(Chap. 60)**, a maximal variant of *Stevens-Johnson syndrome*, involves sloughing of the entire epidermis **(Fig. A1-26)**, resulting in severe disease. *Exfoliative erythroderma syndrome* **(Chaps. 58 and 60)** is a serious reaction associated with systemic toxicity that is often due to eczema, psoriasis **(Fig. A1-27)**, a drug reaction, or mycosis fungoides. *Drug rash with eosinophilia and systemic symptoms (DRESS)*, often due to antiepileptic and antibiotic agents **(Chap. 60)**, initially appears similar to an exanthematous drug reaction **(Fig. A1-48)** but may progress to exfoliative erythroderma; it is accompanied by multiorgan failure and has an associated mortality rate of ~10%.

■ VESICULOBULLOUS OR PUSTULAR ERUPTIONS

Varicella **(Chap. 193)** is highly contagious, often occurring in winter or spring, and is characterized by pruritic lesions that, within a given region of the body, are in different stages of development at any point in time **(Fig. 19-4; see also Fig. A1-30)**. In immunocompromised hosts, varicella vesicles may lack the characteristic erythematous base or may appear hemorrhagic. Lesions of *Pseudomonas "hot-tub" folliculitis* **(Chap. 164)** are also pruritic and may appear similar to those of varicella **(Fig. A1-55)**. However, hot-tub folliculitis generally occurs in outbreaks after bathing in hot tubs or swimming pools, and lesions occur in regions occluded by bathing suits. Lesions of *variola (smallpox)* **(Chap. S3)** also appear similar to those of varicella but are

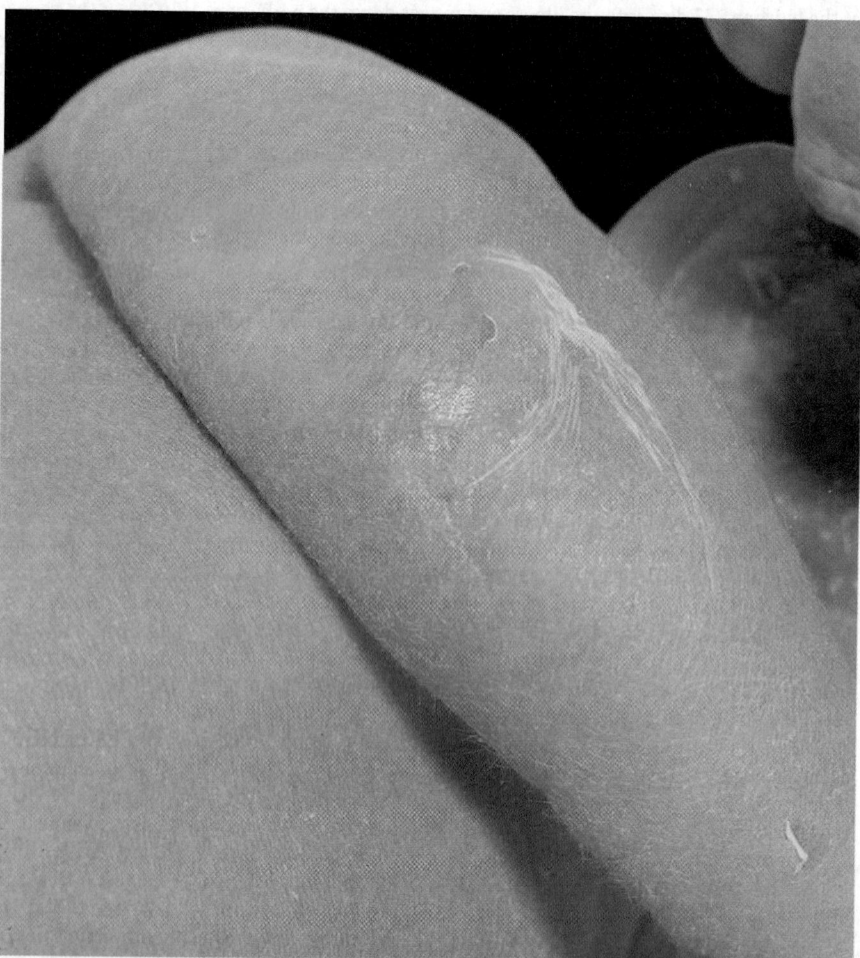

FIGURE 19-3 Confluent desquamative erythema in a patient with Staphylococcal scalded-skin syndrome. Nikolsky sign evident as shearing of epidermis due to gentle, lateral pressure. *(From K Wolff et al [eds]: Fitzpatrick's Color Atlas and Synopsis of Clinical Dermatology, 8th ed. New York, McGraw-Hill, 2017, p. 554, Figure 25-42; with permission.)*

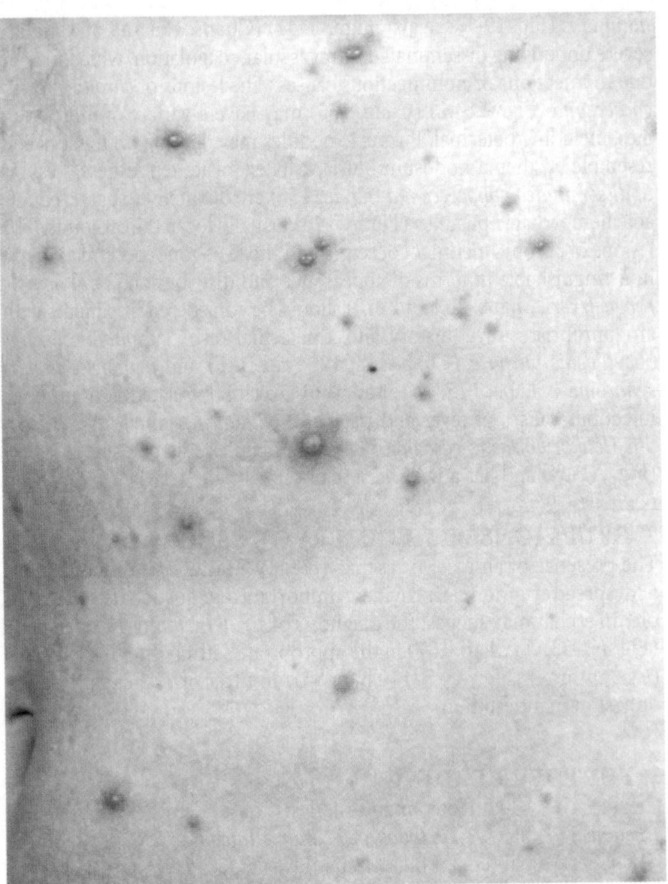

FIGURE 19-4 Vesicular and pustular lesions on the chest in a patient with varicella. *(From K Wolff et al [eds]: Fitzpatrick's Color Atlas and Synopsis of Clinical Dermatology, 8th ed. New York, McGraw-Hill, 2017, p. 695, Figure 27-48; with permission.)*

all at the same stage of development in a given region of the body (**Figs. A1-50B, A1-50C**). Variola lesions are most prominent on the face (**Fig. A1-50A**) and extremities, while varicella lesions are most prominent on the trunk. *Herpes simplex virus infection* (**Chap. 192**) is characterized by hallmark grouped vesicles on an erythematous base. Primary herpes infection is accompanied by fever and toxicity, while recurrent disease is milder. *Rickettsialpox* (**Chap. 187**) is often documented in urban settings and is characterized by vesicles followed by pustules (**Figs. A1-33B, A1-33C**). It can be distinguished from varicella by an eschar at the site of the mouse-mite bite (**Fig. A1-33A**) and the papule/plaque base of each vesicle. *Acute generalized exanthematous pustulosis* (**Fig. A1-49**) should be considered in individuals who are acutely febrile and are taking new medications, especially anticonvulsant or antimicrobial agents (**Chap. 60**). Disseminated *Vibrio vulnificus* infection (**Chap. 168**) or *ecthyma gangrenosum* due to *Pseudomonas aeruginosa* (**Fig. A1-34**) (**Chap. 164**) should be considered in immunosuppressed individuals with sepsis and hemorrhagic bullae. In children, *Mycoplasma pneumoniae*–induced rash and mucositis (MIRM) (**Fig. A1-56**) is characterized by a sparse, often vesiculobullous eruption with prominent oral, ocular, or urogenital mucositis.

URTICARIA-LIKE ERUPTIONS

Individuals with classic urticaria ("hives") (**Fig. 19-5; see also Fig. A1-35**) usually have a hypersensitivity reaction without associated fever. In the presence of fever, urticaria-like eruptions are most often due to *urticarial vasculitis* (**Chap. 363**). Unlike individual lesions of classic urticaria, which last up to 24 h, these lesions may last 3–5 days. Etiologies include serum sickness (often induced by drugs such as penicillins, sulfas, salicylates, or barbiturates), connective-tissue disease (e.g., systemic lupus erythematosus or Sjögren's syndrome), and infection (e.g., with hepatitis B virus, enteroviruses, or parasites). Malignancy, especially lymphoma, may be associated with fever and chronic urticaria (**Chap. 58**).

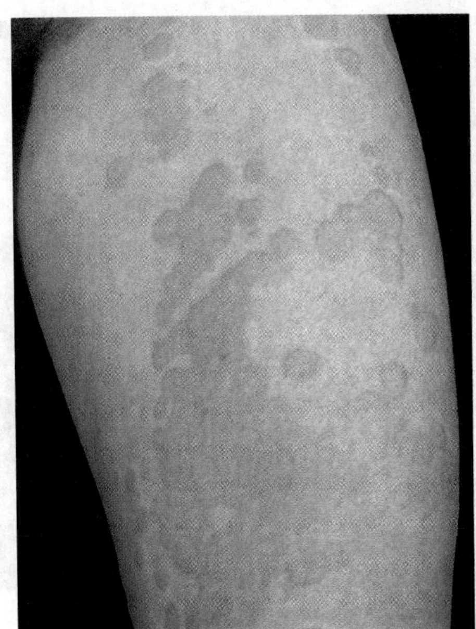

FIGURE 19-5 Urticarial eruption. *(From K Wolff et al [eds]: Fitzpatrick's Color Atlas and Synopsis of Clinical Dermatology, 8th ed. New York, McGraw-Hill, 2017, p. 299, Figure 14-2; with permission.)*

NODULAR ERUPTIONS

In immunocompromised hosts, nodular lesions often represent disseminated infection. Patients with disseminated *candidiasis* (**Fig. A1-37**) (often due to *Candida tropicalis*) may have a triad of fever, myalgias, and eruptive nodules (**Chap. 216**). Disseminated *cryptococcosis* lesions (**Fig. 19-6; see also Fig. A1-36**) (**Chap. 215**) may resemble molluscum contagiosum (**Chap. 196**). Necrosis of nodules should raise the suspicion of *aspergillosis* (**Fig. A1-38**) (**Chap. 217**) or *mucormycosis*

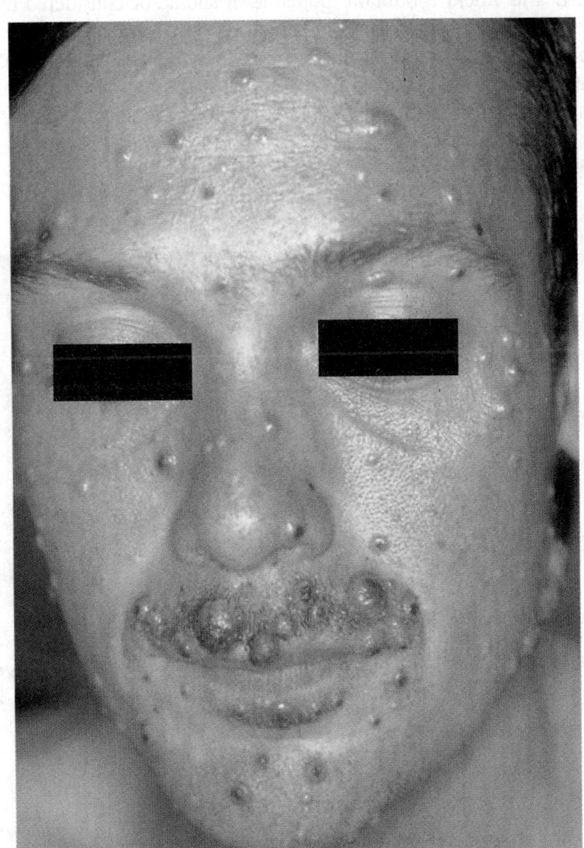

FIGURE 19-6 Nodular eruption on the face due to disseminated Cryptococcus in a patient with HIV infection. *(From K Wolff et al [eds]: Fitzpatrick's Color Atlas and Synopsis of Clinical Dermatology, 8th ed. New York, McGraw-Hill, 2017, p. 641, Figure 26-57. Used with permission from Loïc Vallant, MD.)*

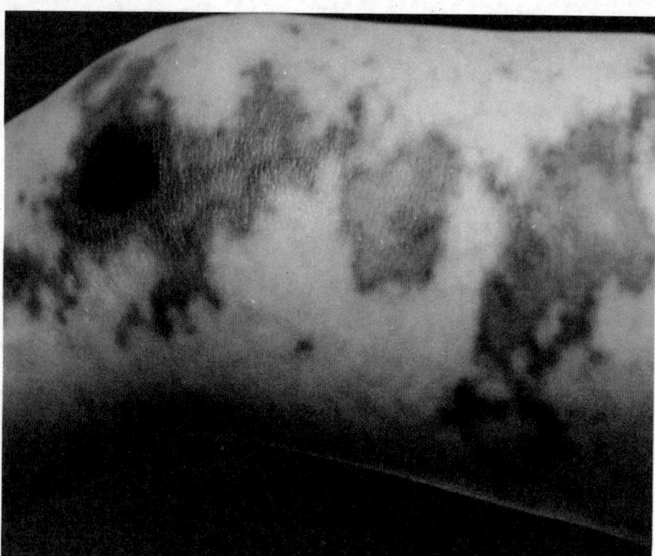

FIGURE 19-7 Purpura fulminans in a patient with acute meningococcemia. *(From K Wolff et al [eds]: Fitzpatrick's Color Atlas and Synopsis of Clinical Dermatology, 8th ed. New York, McGraw-Hill, 2017, p. 568, Figure 25-59; with permission.)*

(Chap. 218). *Erythema nodosum* presents with exquisitely tender nodules on the lower extremities (Fig. A1-39). *Sweet syndrome* (Chap. 58) should be considered in individuals with multiple nodules and plaques, often so edematous (Fig. A1-40) that they give the appearance of vesicles or bullae. Sweet syndrome may occur in individuals with infection, inflammatory bowel disease, or malignancy and can also be induced by drugs.

■ PURPURIC ERUPTIONS

Acute meningococcemia (Chap. 155) classically presents in children as a petechial eruption, but initial lesions may appear as blanchable macules or urticaria. Rocky Mountain spotted fever should be considered in the differential diagnosis of acute meningococcemia. *Echovirus 9 infection* (Chap. 204) may mimic acute meningococcemia; patients should be treated as if they have bacterial sepsis because prompt differentiation of these conditions may be impossible. Large ecchymotic areas of *purpura fulminans* (Fig. 19-7; see also Fig. A1-41) (Chaps. 155 and 304) reflect severe underlying disseminated intravascular coagulation, which may be due to infectious or noninfectious causes. The lesions of *chronic meningococcemia* (Fig. A1-42) (Chap. 155) may have a variety of morphologies, including petechial. Purpuric nodules may develop on the legs and resemble erythema nodosum but lack its exquisite tenderness. Lesions of *disseminated gonococcemia* (Chap. 156) are distinctive, sparse, countable hemorrhagic pustules (Fig. A1-43), usually located near joints. The lesions of chronic meningococcemia and those of gonococcemia may be indistinguishable in terms of appearance and distribution. *Viral hemorrhagic fever* (Chaps. 209 and 210) should be considered in patients with an appropriate travel history and a petechial rash. *Thrombotic thrombocytopenic purpura* (Chaps. 58, 100, and 115) and *hemolytic-uremic syndrome* (Chaps. 115, 161, and 166) are closely related and are noninfectious causes of fever and petechiae. *Cutaneous small-vessel vasculitis (leukocytoclastic vasculitis)* typically manifests as palpable purpura (Fig. A1-44) and has a wide variety of causes (Chap. 58).

■ ERUPTIONS WITH ULCERS OR ESCHARS

The presence of an ulcer or eschar (Fig. 19-8) in the setting of a more widespread eruption can provide an important diagnostic clue. For example, an eschar may suggest the diagnosis of *scrub typhus* or *rickettsialpox* (Fig. A1-33A) (Chap. 187) in the appropriate setting. In other illnesses (e.g., anthrax) (Fig. A1-52) (Chap. S3), an ulcer or eschar may be the only skin manifestation.

■ FURTHER READING

Cherry JD: Cutaneous manifestations of systemic infections, in *Feigin and Cherry's Textbook of Pediatric Infectious Diseases*, 8th ed. JD Cherry et al (eds). Philadelphia, Elsevier, 2019, pp 539–559.

Juliano JJ et al: The acutely ill patient with fever and rash, in *Mandell, Douglas, and Bennett's Principles and Practice of Infectious Diseases*, vol 1, 9th ed. JI Bennett et al (eds). Philadelphia, Elsevier, 2020, pp 801–818.

Kang S et al (eds): *Fitzpatrick's Dermatology*, 9th ed. New York, McGraw-Hill, 2019.

Wolff K et al: *Fitzpatrick's Color Atlas and Synopsis of Clinical Dermatology*, 8th ed. New York, McGraw-Hill, 2017.

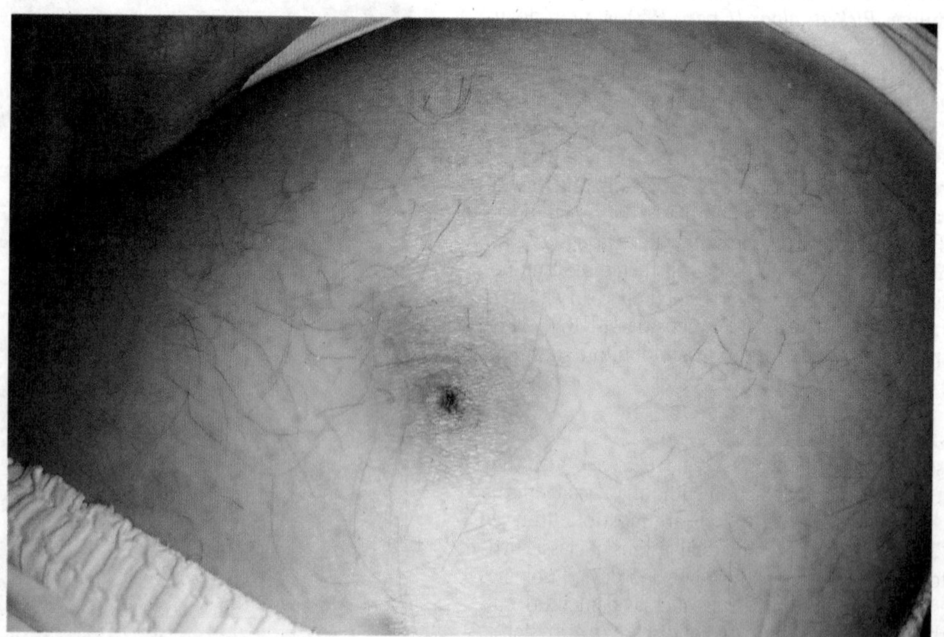

FIGURE 19-8 Eschar with surrounding erythema at the site of a tick bite in a patient with African tick-bite fever. *(From K Wolff et al [eds]: Fitzpatrick's Color Atlas and Synopsis of Clinical Dermatology, 8th ed. New York, McGraw-Hill, 2017, p. 561, Figure 25-49; with permission.)*

20 Fever of Unknown Origin

Chantal P. Bleeker-Rovers,
Catharina M. Mulders-Manders,
Jos W. M. van der Meer

DEFINITION

Clinicians commonly refer to any febrile illness without an initially obvious etiology as *fever of unknown origin* (FUO). Most febrile illnesses either resolve before a diagnosis can be made or develop distinguishing characteristics that lead to a diagnosis. The term *FUO* should be reserved for prolonged febrile illnesses without an established etiology despite intensive evaluation and diagnostic testing. This chapter focuses on FUO in the adult patient.

FUO was originally defined by Petersdorf and Beeson in 1961 as an illness of >3 weeks' duration with fever of ≥38.3°C (≥101°F) on two occasions and an uncertain diagnosis despite 1 week of inpatient evaluation. Nowadays, most patients with FUO are hospitalized only if their clinical condition requires it, and not for diagnostic purposes alone; thus the in-hospital evaluation requirement has been eliminated from the definition. The definition of FUO has been further modified by the exclusion of immunocompromised patients, whose workup requires an entirely different diagnostic and therapeutic approach. For optimal comparison of patients with FUO in different geographic areas, it has been proposed that the quantitative criterion (diagnosis uncertain after 1 week of evaluation) be changed to a qualitative criterion that requires the performance of a specific list of investigations. Accordingly, FUO is now defined as follows:

1. Fever ≥38.3°C (≥101°F) on at least two occasions
2. Illness duration of ≥3 weeks
3. No known immunocompromised state
4. Diagnosis that remains uncertain after a thorough history-taking, physical examination, and the following obligatory investigations: determination of erythrocyte sedimentation rate (ESR) and C-reactive protein (CRP) level; platelet count; leukocyte count and differential; measurement of levels of hemoglobin, electrolytes, creatinine, total protein, alkaline phosphatase, alanine aminotransferase, aspartate aminotransferase, lactate dehydrogenase, creatine kinase, ferritin, antinuclear antibodies, and rheumatoid factor; protein electrophoresis; urinalysis; blood cultures (n = 3); urine culture; chest x-ray; abdominal ultrasonography; and tuberculin skin test (TST) or interferon γ release assay (IGRA).

Closely related to FUO is *inflammation of unknown origin (IUO)*, which has the same definition as FUO, except for the body temperature criterion: IUO is defined as the presence of elevated inflammatory parameters (CRP or ESR) on multiple occasions for a period of at least 3 weeks in an immunocompetent patient with normal body temperature, for which a final explanation is lacking despite history-taking, physical examination, and the obligatory tests listed above. It has been shown that the causes and workup for IUO are the same as for FUO. Therefore, for convenience, the term FUO will refer to both FUO and IUO within the remainder of this chapter.

ETIOLOGY AND EPIDEMIOLOGY

Table 20-1 summarizes the findings of large studies on FUO conducted over the past 20 years.

The range of FUO etiologies has evolved since its first definition as a result of changes in the spectrum of diseases causing FUO, the widespread use of antibiotics, and especially the availability of new diagnostic techniques. The proportion of cases caused by intraabdominal abscesses and tumors, for example, has decreased because of earlier detection by CT and ultrasound. In addition, infective endocarditis is a less frequent cause because blood culture and echocardiographic techniques have improved. Conversely, some diagnoses such as acute HIV infection were unknown six decades ago.

Roughly comparable to 60 years ago, in non-Western cohorts infections remain the most common cause of FUO. Up to half of all infections in patients with FUO outside Western nations are caused by *Mycobacterium tuberculosis*, which is a less common cause in Western Europe and probably also in the United States. Recent data from the latter, however, have not been reported. In Western cohorts, noninfectious inflammatory diseases (NIIDs), including autoimmune, autoinflammatory, and granulomatous diseases, as well as vasculitides, form the most common cause of FUO. More than one-third of Western patients with FUO have a diagnosis that falls within the category of NIIDs. The number of FUO patients diagnosed with NIIDs probably will not decrease in the near future, as fever may precede more typical manifestations or laboratory evidence of these diseases by months. Moreover, many NIIDs can be diagnosed only after prolonged observation and exclusion of other diseases.

In Western cohorts, FUO remains unexplained in more than one-third of patients. This is much higher than 60 years ago. This difference can be explained by the fact that in patients with fever a diagnosis is often established before 3 weeks have elapsed because these patients tend to seek medical advice earlier, and because better diagnostic techniques, such as CT, MRI, and positron emission tomography (PET)/CT, are now available. Therefore, only the cases that are most difficult to diagnose continue to meet the criteria for FUO. Furthermore, most patients who have FUO without a diagnosis currently do well. A less aggressive diagnostic approach may be used in clinically stable patients once diseases with immediate therapeutic or prognostic consequences have been ruled out. In patients with recurrent fever (defined as repeated episodes of fever

TABLE 20-1 Etiology of FUO: Pooled Results of Large Studies Published in the Past 20 Years (1999–2019)

GEOGRAPHIC AREA	NO. OF COHORTS (INCLUSION PERIOD)	NO. OF PATIENTS	INFECTIONS, MEDIAN % (RANGE)	NONINFECTIOUS INFLAMMATORY DISEASES, MEDIAN % (RANGE)	MALIGNANCY, MEDIAN % (RANGE)	MISCELLANEOUS, MEDIAN % (RANGE)	NO DIAGNOSIS, MEDIAN % (RANGE)
Western Europe	10 (1990–2014)	1820	17 (11–32)	25 (12–32)	10 (3–20)	10 (0–15)	37 (26–51)
Other European and Turkey	13 (1984–2015)	1316	38 (26–59)	25 (15–38)	14 (5–19)	6 (2–18)	16 (4–35)
Middle East	3 2009–2010 and ?[a]	1235	66 (42–79)	15 (7–17)	7 (1–30)	1 (0–12)	8 (2–12)
Asia	20 (1994–2017)	3802	42 (11–58)	20 (7–57)	13 (6–22)	9 (0–15)	18 (0–36)

[a]One study (published in 2015) did not report the inclusion period.

Abbreviation: NIID, non-infectious inflammatory disease.

For references, see supplementary material at *www.accessmedicine.com/harrisons.*

interspersed with fever-free intervals of at least 2 weeks and apparent remission of the underlying disease), the chance of attaining an etiologic diagnosis is <50%.

DIFFERENTIAL DIAGNOSIS

The differential diagnosis for FUO is extensive. It is important to remember that FUO is far more often caused by an atypical presentation of a rather common disease than by a very rare disease. **Table 20-2** presents an overview of possible causes of FUO. Atypical presentations of endocarditis, diverticulitis, vertebral osteomyelitis, and extrapulmonary tuberculosis are the more common infectious disease diagnoses. Q fever and Whipple's disease (*Tropheryma whipplei* infection) are quite rare but should always be kept in mind as a cause of FUO since the presenting symptoms can be nonspecific. Serologic testing for Q fever, which results from exposure to animals or animal products, should be performed by immunofluorescence assay (IFA) when the patient lives in a rural area or has a history of heart valve disease, an aortic aneurysm, or a vascular prosthesis. In patients with unexplained symptoms localized to the central nervous system, gastrointestinal tract, or joints, polymerase chain reaction testing for *Tropheryma whipplei* should be performed. Travel to or (former) residence in tropical countries or the American Southwest should lead to consideration

TABLE 20-2 All Reported Causes of Fever of Unknown Origin (FUO)[a]

Infections	
Bacterial, nonspecific	Abdominal abscess, adnexitis, apical granuloma, appendicitis, cholangitis, cholecystitis, diverticulitis, endocarditis, endometritis, epidural abscess, infected joint prosthesis, infected vascular catheter, infected vascular prosthesis, infectious arthritis, infective myonecrosis, intracranial abscess, liver abscess, lung abscess, malakoplakia, mastoiditis, mediastinitis, mycotic aneurysm, osteomyelitis, pelvic inflammatory disease, prostatitis, pyelonephritis, pylephlebitis, renal abscess, septic phlebitis, sinusitis, spondylodiscitis, xanthogranulomatous urinary tract infection
Bacterial, specific	Actinomycosis, atypical mycobacterial infection, bartonellosis, brucellosis, *Campylobacter* infection, *Chlamydia pneumoniae* infection, chronic meningococcemia, ehrlichiosis, gonococcemia, legionellosis, leptospirosis, listeriosis, louse-borne relapsing fever (*Borrelia recurrentis*), Lyme disease, melioidosis (*Pseudomonas pseudomallei*), *Mycoplasma* infection, nocardiosis, psittacosis, Q fever (*Coxiella burnetii*), rickettsiosis, *Spirillum minor* infection, *Streptobacillus moniliformis* infection, syphilis, tick-borne relapsing fever (*Borrelia duttonii*), tuberculosis, tularemia, typhoid fever and other salmonelloses, Whipple's disease (*Tropheryma whipplei*), yersiniosis
Fungal	Aspergillosis, blastomycosis, candidiasis, coccidioidomycosis, cryptococcosis, histoplasmosis, *Malassezia furfur* infection, paracoccidioidomycosis, *Pneumocystis jirovecii* pneumonia, sporotrichosis, zygomycosis
Parasitic	Amebiasis, babesiosis, echinococcosis, fascioliasis, malaria, schistosomiasis, strongyloidiasis, toxocariasis, toxoplasmosis, trichinellosis, trypanosomiasis, visceral leishmaniasis
Viral	Colorado tick fever, coxsackievirus infection, cytomegalovirus infection, dengue, Epstein-Barr virus infection, hantavirus infection, hepatitis (A, B, C, D, E), herpes simplex, HIV infection, human herpesvirus 6 infection, parvovirus infection, West Nile virus infection
Noninfectious Inflammatory Diseases	
Systemic rheumatic and autoimmune diseases	Ankylosing spondylitis, antiphospholipid syndrome, autoimmune hemolytic anemia, autoimmune hepatitis, Behçet's disease, cryoglobulinemia, dermatomyositis, Felty syndrome, gout, mixed connective-tissue disease, polymyositis, pseudogout, reactive arthritis, relapsing polychondritis, rheumatic fever, rheumatoid arthritis, Sjögren's syndrome, systemic lupus erythematosus, Vogt-Koyanagi-Harada syndrome
Vasculitis	Allergic vasculitis, eosinophilic granulomatosis with polyangiitis, giant cell vasculitis/polymyalgia rheumatica, granulomatosis with polyangiitis, hypersensitivity vasculitis, Kawasaki disease, polyarteritis nodosa, Takayasu arteritis, urticarial vasculitis
Granulomatous diseases	Idiopathic granulomatous hepatitis, sarcoidosis
Autoinflammatory syndromes	Adult-onset Still's disease, Blau syndrome, CAPS[b] (cryopyrin-associated periodic syndromes), Crohn's disease, DIRA (deficiency of the interleukin 1 receptor antagonist), familial Mediterranean fever, hemophagocytic syndrome, hyper-IgD syndrome (HIDS, also known as mevalonate kinase deficiency), juvenile idiopathic arthritis, PAPA syndrome (pyogenic sterile arthritis, pyoderma gangrenosum, and acne), PFAPA syndrome (periodic fever, aphthous stomatitis, pharyngitis, adenitis), recurrent idiopathic pericarditis, SAPHO (synovitis, acne, pustulosis, hyperostosis, osteomyelitis), Schnitzler syndrome, TRAPS (tumor necrosis factor receptor–associated periodic syndrome)
Neoplasms	
Hematologic malignancies	Amyloidosis, angioimmunoblastic lymphoma, Castleman's disease, Hodgkin's disease, hypereosinophilic syndrome, leukemia, lymphomatoid granulomatosis, malignant histiocytosis, multiple myeloma, myelodysplastic syndrome, myelofibrosis, non-Hodgkin's lymphoma, plasmacytoma, systemic mastocytosis, vaso-occlusive crisis in sickle cell disease
Solid tumors	Most solid tumors and metastases can cause fever. Those most commonly causing FUO are breast, colon, hepatocellular, lung, pancreatic, and renal cell carcinomas.
Benign tumors	Angiomyolipoma, cavernous hemangioma of the liver, craniopharyngioma, necrosis of dermoid tumor in Gardner's syndrome
Miscellaneous Causes	
	ADEM (acute disseminated encephalomyelitis), adrenal insufficiency, aneurysms, anomalous thoracic duct, aortic dissection, aortic-enteral fistula, aseptic meningitis (Mollaret's syndrome), atrial myxoma, brewer's yeast ingestion, Caroli disease, cholesterol emboli, cirrhosis, complex partial status epilepticus, cyclic neutropenia, drug fever, Erdheim-Chester disease, extrinsic allergic alveolitis, Fabry's disease, factitious disease, fire-eater's lung, fraudulent fever, Gaucher disease, Hamman-Rich syndrome (acute interstitial pneumonia), Hashimoto's encephalopathy, hematoma, hypersensitivity pneumonitis, hypertriglyceridemia, hypothalamic hypopituitarism, idiopathic normal-pressure hydrocephalus, inflammatory pseudotumor, Kikuchi's disease, linear IgA dermatosis, mesenteric fibromatosis, metal fume fever, milk protein allergy, myotonic dystrophy, nonbacterial osteitis, organic dust toxic syndrome, panniculitis, POEMS (polyneuropathy, organomegaly, endocrinopathy, monoclonal protein, skin changes), polymer fume fever, post–cardiac injury syndrome, primary biliary cirrhosis, primary hyperparathyroidism, pulmonary embolism, pyoderma gangrenosum, retroperitoneal fibrosis, Rosai-Dorfman disease, sclerosing mesenteritis, silicone embolization, subacute thyroiditis (de Quervain's), Sweet syndrome (acute febrile neutrophilic dermatosis), thrombosis, tubulointerstitial nephritis and uveitis syndrome (TINU), ulcerative colitis
Thermoregulatory Disorders	
Central	Brain tumor, cerebrovascular accident, encephalitis, hypothalamic dysfunction
Peripheral	Anhidrotic ectodermal dysplasia, exercise-induced hyperthermia, hyperthyroidism, pheochromocytoma

[a]This table includes all causes of FUO that have been described in the literature. [b]CAPS includes chronic infantile neurologic cutaneous and articular syndrome (CINCA, also known as neonatal-onset multisystem inflammatory disease, or NOMID), familial cold autoinflammatory syndrome (FCAS), and Muckle-Wells syndrome.

of infectious diseases such as malaria, leishmaniasis, histoplasmosis, or coccidioidomycosis. Fever with signs of endocarditis and negative blood culture results poses a special problem. Culture-negative endocarditis (**Chap. 128**) may be due to difficult-to-culture bacteria such as nutritionally variant bacteria, HACEK organisms (including *Haemophilus parainfluenzae*, *H. paraphrophilus*, *Aggregatibacter actinomycetemcomitans*, *A. aphrophilus*, *A. paraphrophilus*, *Cardiobacterium hominis*, *C. valvarum*, *Eikenella corrodens*, and *Kingella kingae*; discussed below), *Coxiella burnetii*, *T. whipplei*, and *Bartonella* species. Marantic endocarditis is a sterile thrombotic disease that occurs as a paraneoplastic phenomenon, especially with adenocarcinomas. Sterile endocarditis is also seen in the context of systemic lupus erythematosus and antiphospholipid syndrome.

Of the NIIDs, adult-onset Still's disease, large-vessel vasculitis, polymyalgia rheumatica, systemic lupus erythematodus (SLE), and sarcoidosis are rather common diagnoses in patients with FUO. The hereditary autoinflammatory syndromes are very rare (with the exception of familial Mediterranean fever in specific geographic regions) and usually present in young patients. Schnitzler syndrome, which can present at any age, is uncommon but can often be diagnosed easily in a patient with FUO who presents with urticaria, bone pain, and monoclonal gammopathy.

Although most tumors can present with fever, malignant lymphoma is by far the most common diagnosis of FUO among the neoplasms. Sometimes the fever even precedes lymphadenopathy detectable by physical examination.

Apart from drug-induced fever and exercise-induced hyperthermia, none of the miscellaneous causes of fever is found very frequently in patients with FUO. Virtually all drugs can cause fever, even after long-term use. *Drug-induced fever*, including DRESS (drug reaction with eosinophilia and systemic symptoms; **Fig. A1-48**), is often accompanied by eosinophilia and also by lymphadenopathy, which can be extensive. More common causes of drug-induced fever are allopurinol, carbamazepine, lamotrigine, phenytoin, sulfasalazine, furosemide, antimicrobial drugs (especially sulfonamides, minocycline, vancomycin, β-lactam antibiotics, and isoniazid), some cardiovascular drugs (e.g., quinidine), and some antiretroviral drugs (e.g., nevirapine). *Exercise-induced hyperthermia* (**Chaps. 18 and 465**) is characterized by an elevated body temperature that is associated with moderate to strenuous exercise lasting from half an hour up to several hours without an increase in CRP level or ESR. Unlike patients with fever, these patients typically sweat during the temperature elevation. *Factitious fever* (fever artificially induced by the patient—for example, by IV injection of contaminated water) should be considered in all patients but is more common among young women in health-care professions. In *fraudulent fever*, the patient is normothermic but manipulates the thermometer. Simultaneous measurements at different body sites (rectum, ear, mouth) should rapidly identify this diagnosis. Another clue to fraudulent fever is dissociation between pulse rate and temperature.

Previous studies of FUO have shown that a cause is more likely to be found in elderly patients than in younger age groups. In many cases, FUO in the elderly results from an atypical manifestation of a common disease, among which giant cell arteritis and polymyalgia rheumatica are most frequently involved. Tuberculosis is the most common infectious disease associated with FUO in elderly patients, occurring much more often than in younger patients. As many of these diseases are treatable, it is well worth pursuing the cause of fever in elderly patients.

APPROACH TO THE PATIENT

Fever of Unknown Origin

FIRST-STAGE DIAGNOSTIC TESTS

Figure 20-1 shows a structured approach to patients presenting with FUO. The most important step in the diagnostic workup is the search for potentially diagnostic clues (PDCs) through complete and repeated history-taking and physical examination and the obligatory investigations listed above and in the figure. *PDCs* are defined as all localizing signs, symptoms, and abnormalities potentially pointing toward a diagnosis. Although PDCs are often misleading, only with their help can a concise list of probable diagnoses be made. The history should include information about the fever pattern (continuous or recurrent) and duration, previous medical history, present and recent drug use, family history, sexual history, country of origin, recent and remote travel, unusual environmental exposures associated with travel or hobbies, and animal contacts. A complete physical examination should be performed, with special attention to the eyes, lymph nodes, temporal arteries, liver, spleen, sites of previous surgery, entire skin surface, and mucous membranes. Before further diagnostic tests are initiated, antibiotic and glucocorticoid treatment, which can mask many diseases, should be stopped. For example, blood and other cultures are not reliable when samples are obtained during antibiotic treatment, and the size of enlarged lymph nodes usually decreases during glucocorticoid treatment, regardless of the cause of lymphadenopathy. Despite the high percentage of false-positive ultrasounds and the relatively low sensitivity of chest x-rays, the performance of these simple, low-cost diagnostic tests remains obligatory in all patients with FUO in order to separate cases that are caused by easily diagnosed diseases from those that are not. Abdominal ultrasound is preferred to abdominal CT as an obligatory test because of relatively low cost, lack of radiation burden, and absence of side effects.

Only rarely do biochemical tests (beyond the obligatory tests needed to classify a patient's fever as FUO) lead directly to a definitive diagnosis in the absence of PDCs. The diagnostic yield of immunologic serology other than that included in the obligatory tests is relatively low. These tests more often yield false-positive rather than true-positive results and are of little use without PDCs pointing to specific immunologic disorders. Given the absence of specific symptoms in many patients and the relatively low cost of the test, investigation of cryoglobulins appears to be a valuable screening test in patients with FUO.

Multiple blood samples should be cultured in the laboratory long enough to ensure ample growth time for any fastidious organisms, such as HACEK organisms. It is critical to inform the laboratory of the intent to test for unusual organisms. Specialized media should be used when the history suggests uncommon microorganisms, such as *Histoplasma* or *Legionella*. Performing more than three blood cultures or more than one urine culture is useless in patients with FUO in the absence of PDCs (e.g., a high level of clinical suspicion of endocarditis). Repeating blood or urine cultures is useful only when previously cultured samples were collected during antibiotic treatment or within 1 week after its discontinuation. FUO with headache should prompt microbiologic examination of cerebrospinal fluid (CSF) for organisms including herpes simplex virus (especially type 2), *Cryptococcus neoformans*, and *Mycobacterium tuberculosis*. In central nervous system tuberculosis, the CSF typically has elevated protein and lowered glucose concentrations, with a mononuclear pleocytosis. CSF protein levels range from 100 to 500 mg/dL in most patients, the CSF glucose concentration is <45 mg/dL in 80% of cases, and the usual CSF cell count is between 100 and 500 cells/μL.

Microbiologic serology should not be included in the diagnostic workup of patients without PDCs for specific infections. A tuberculin skin test (TST) or interferon γ release assay (IGRA, QuantiFERON test) is included in the obligatory investigations, but it may yield false-negative results in patients with miliary tuberculosis, malnutrition, or immunosuppression. Although the IGRA is less influenced by prior vaccination with bacille Calmette-Guérin (BCG) or by infection with nontuberculous mycobacteria, its sensitivity is similar to that of the TST; a negative TST or IGRA therefore does not exclude a diagnosis of tuberculosis. Miliary tuberculosis is especially difficult to diagnose. Granulomatous disease in liver or bone marrow biopsy samples, for example, should always lead to a (re)consideration of this diagnosis. If miliary tuberculosis is suspected, liver biopsy for acid-fast smear, culture, and polymerase chain reaction probably still has the highest diagnostic yield;

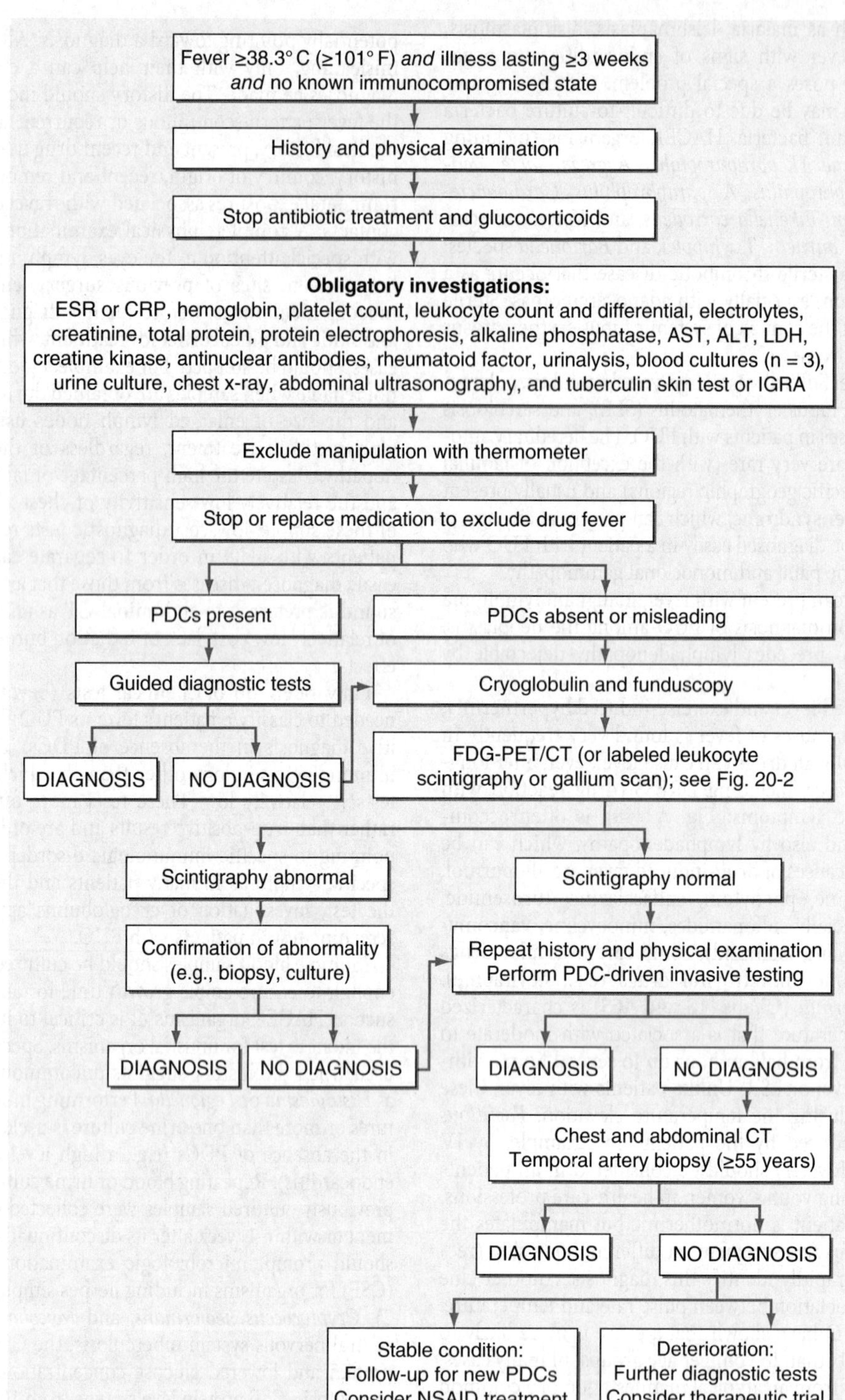

FIGURE 20-1 Structured approach to patients with FUO. ALT, alanine aminotransferase; AST, aspartate aminotransferase; CRP, C-reactive protein; ESR, erythrocyte sedimentation rate; FDG-PET/CT, ^{18}F-fluorodeoxyglucose positron emission tomography combined with low-dose CT; IGRA, interferon γ release assay; LDH, lactate dehydrogenase; NSAID, nonsteroidal anti-inflammatory drug; PDCs, potentially diagnostic clues (all localizing signs, symptoms, and abnormalities potentially pointing toward a diagnosis).

however, biopsies of bone marrow, lymph nodes, or other involved organs also can be considered.

The diagnostic yield of echocardiography, sinus radiography, radiologic or endoscopic evaluation of the gastrointestinal tract, and bronchoscopy is very low in the absence of PDCs. Therefore, these tests should not be used as screening procedures.

After identification of all PDCs retrieved from the history, physical examination, and obligatory tests, a limited list of the most probable diagnoses should be made. Since most investigations are helpful only for patients who have PDCs for the diagnoses sought, further diagnostic procedures should be limited to specific investigations aimed at confirming or excluding diseases on this list. In FUO, the diagnostic pointers are numerous and diverse but may be missed on initial examination, often being detected only by a very careful examination performed subsequently. In the absence of PDCs, the history and physical examination should therefore be repeated regularly. One of the first steps should be to rule out factitious or fraudulent fever, particularly in patients without signs of inflammation in laboratory tests. All medications, including nonprescription drugs and nutritional supplements, should be discontinued early in the evaluation to exclude drug fever. If fever persists beyond 72 h after discontinuation of the suspected drug, it is unlikely that this drug is the cause. In patients without PDCs or with only misleading PDCs, fundoscopy by an ophthalmologist may be useful in the early stage of the diagnostic workup to exclude retinal vasculitis. When the first-stage diagnostic tests do not lead to a diagnosis, ^{18}F-fluorodeoxyglucose (^{18}F-FDG) positron emission tomography combined with computed tomography (PET/CT) or, if the former is not available, radiolabeled leukocyte scintigraphy should be performed, especially when the ESR or the CRP level is elevated.

Recurrent Fever In patients with recurrent fever, the diagnostic workup should consist of thorough history-taking, physical examination, and obligatory tests. The search for PDCs should be directed toward clues matching known recurrent syndromes (**Table 20-3**). Patients should be asked to return during a febrile episode so that the history, physical examination, and laboratory tests can be repeated during a symptomatic phase. Further diagnostic tests, such as PET/CT or scintigraphic imaging (see below), should be performed only during a febrile episode or when inflammatory parameters are abnormal because abnormalities may be absent between episodes. In patients with recurrent fever lasting >2 years, it is very unlikely that the fever is caused by infection or malignancy. Further diagnostic tests in that direction should be considered only when PDCs for infections, vasculitis syndromes, or malignancy are present or when the patient's clinical condition is deteriorating.

Fluorodeoxyglucose Positron Emission Tomography ^{18}F-FDG PET/CT has become an established imaging procedure in FUO. FDG accumulates in tissues with a high rate of glycolysis, which occurs not only in malignant cells but also in activated leukocytes and thus permits the imaging of acute and chronic inflammatory processes. Compared with conventional scintigraphy (see below), FDG-PET/CT offers the advantages of higher resolution, greater sensitivity in chronic low-grade infections, and a high degree of accuracy in the central skeleton. Furthermore, vascular uptake of FDG is increased in patients with vasculitis (**Fig. 20-2**). The mechanisms responsible for FDG uptake do not allow differentiation among infection, sterile inflammation, and malignancy. However, since all of these disorders are causes of FUO, FDG-PET/CT can be used to guide additional diagnostic tests (e.g., targeted biopsies) that may yield the final diagnosis. It is important to realize that physiologic uptake of FDG may obscure pathologic foci in the brain, heart, bowel, kidneys, and bladder. FDG uptake in the heart, which obscures endocarditis, may be prevented by consumption of a low-carbohydrate diet before the PET investigation. In patients with fever, bone marrow uptake is frequently increased in a nonspecific way due to cytokine activation, which upregulates glucose transporters in bone marrow cells.

TABLE 20-3 All Reported Causes of Recurrent Fever[a]

Infections	
Bacterial, nonspecific	Apical granuloma, diverticulitis, prostatitis, recurrent bacteremia caused by colonic neoplasia or persistent focal infection, recurrent cellulitis, recurrent cholangitis or cholecystitis, recurrent pneumonia, recurrent sinusitis, recurrent urinary tract infection
Bacterial, specific	Bartonellosis, brucellosis, chronic gonococcemia, chronic meningococcemia, louse-borne relapsing fever (*Borrelia recurrentis*), melioidosis (*Pseudomonas pseudomallei*), Q fever (*Coxiella burnetii*), salmonellosis, *Spirillum minor* infection, *Streptobacillus moniliformis* infection, syphilis, tick-borne relapsing fever (*Borrelia duttonii*), tularemia, Whipple's disease (*Tropheryma whipplei*), yersiniosis
Fungal	Coccidioidomycosis, histoplasmosis, paracoccidioidomycosis
Parasitic	Babesiosis, malaria, toxoplasmosis, trypanosomiasis, visceral leishmaniasis
Viral	Cytomegalovirus infection, Epstein-Barr virus infection, herpes simplex
Noninfectious Inflammatory Diseases	
Systemic rheumatic and autoimmune diseases	Ankylosing spondylitis, antiphospholipid syndrome, autoimmune hemolytic anemia, autoimmune hepatitis, Behçet's disease, cryoglobulinemia, gout, polymyositis, pseudogout, reactive arthritis, relapsing polychondritis, systemic lupus erythematosus
Vasculitis	Churg-Strauss syndrome, giant cell vasculitis/polymyalgia rheumatica, hypersensitivity vasculitis, polyarteritis nodosa, urticarial vasculitis
Granulomatous diseases	Idiopathic granulomatous hepatitis, sarcoidosis
Autoinflammatory syndromes	Adult-onset Still's disease, Blau syndrome, CANDLE (chronic atypical neutrophilic dermatitis with lipodystrophy and elevated temperature syndrome), CAPS[b] (cryopyrin-associated periodic syndrome), CRMO (chronic recurrent multifocal osteomyelitis), Crohn's disease, DIRA (deficiency of the interleukin 1 receptor antagonist), familial Mediterranean fever, hemophagocytic syndrome, hyper-IgD syndrome (HIDS, also known as mevalonate kinase deficiency), juvenile idiopathic arthritis, NLRC4-activating mutations, PAPA syndrome (pyogenic sterile arthritis, pyoderma gangrenosum, and acne), PFAPA syndrome (periodic fever, aphthous stomatitis, pharyngitis, adenitis), recurrent idiopathic pericarditis, SAPHO (synovitis, acne, pustulosis, hyperostosis, osteomyelitis), SAVI (stimulator of interferon genes [STING]–associated vasculopathy with onset in infancy), Schnitzler syndrome, TRAPS (tumor necrosis factor receptor–associated periodic syndrome)
Neoplasms	
	Angioimmunoblastic lymphoma, Castleman's disease, colon carcinoma, craniopharyngioma, Hodgkin's disease, malignant histiocytosis, mesothelioma, non-Hodgkin's lymphoma
Miscellaneous Causes	
	Adrenal insufficiency, aortic-enteral fistula, aseptic meningitis (Mollaret's syndrome), atrial myxoma, brewer's yeast ingestion, cholesterol emboli, cyclic neutropenia, drug fever, extrinsic allergic alveolitis, Fabry's disease, factitious disease, fraudulent fever, Gaucher disease, hypersensitivity pneumonitis, hypertriglyceridemia, hypothalamic hypopituitarism, inflammatory pseudotumor, metal fume fever, milk protein allergy, polymer fume fever, pulmonary embolism, sclerosing mesenteritis
Thermoregulatory Disorders	
Central	Hypothalamic dysfunction
Peripheral	Anhidrotic ectodermal dysplasia, exercise-induced hyperthermia, pheochromocytoma

[a]This table includes all causes of recurrent fever that have been described in the literature. [b]CAPS includes chronic infantile neurologic cutaneous and articular syndrome (CINCA, also known as neonatal-onset multisystem inflammatory disease, or NOMID), familial cold autoinflammatory syndrome (FCAS), and Muckle-Wells syndrome.

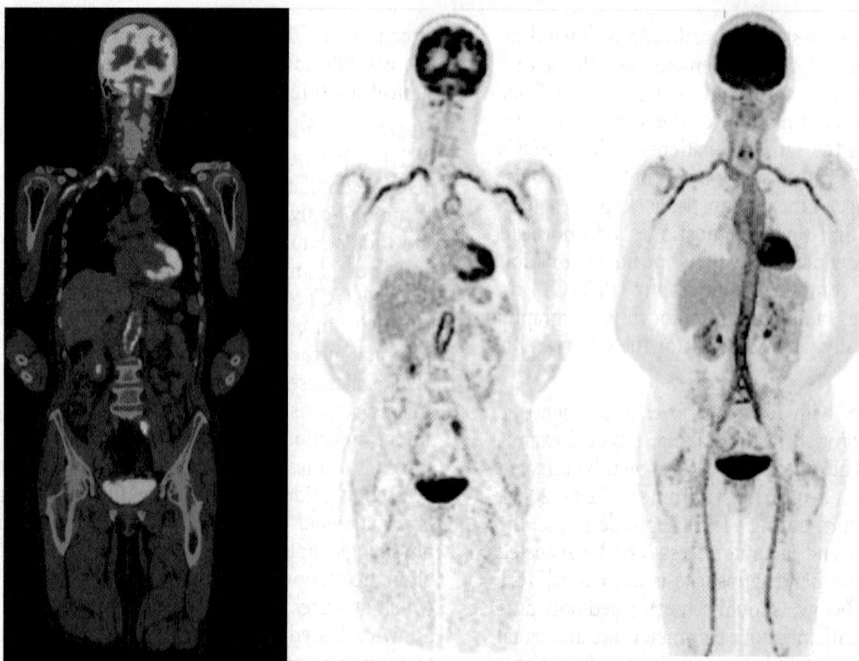

FIGURE 20-2 FDG-PET/CT in a patient with FUO. This 72-year-old woman presented with a low-grade fever and severe fatigue of almost 3 months' duration. An extensive history was taken, but the patient had no specific complaints and had not traveled recently. Her previous history was unremarkable, and she did not use any drugs. Physical examination, including palpation of the temporal arteries, yielded completely normal results. Laboratory examination showed normocytic anemia, a C-reactive protein level of 43 mg/L, an erythrocyte sedimentation rate of 87 mm/h, and mild hypoalbuminemia. Results of the other obligatory tests were all normal. Since there were no potentially diagnostic clues, FDG-PET/CT was performed. This test showed increased FDG uptake in all major arteries (carotid, jugular, and subclavian arteries; thoracic and abdominal aorta; iliac, femoral, and popliteal arteries) and in the soft tissue around the shoulders, hips, and knees—findings compatible with large-vessel vasculitis and polymyalgia rheumatica. Within 1 week after the initiation of treatment with prednisone (60 mg once daily), the patient completely recovered. After 1 month, the prednisone dose was slowly tapered.

In recent years, many cohort studies and several meta-analyses have focused on the diagnostic yield of PET and PET/CT in FUO. These studies are highly variable in terms of the selection of patients, the follow-up, and the selection of a gold-standard reference. Indirect comparisons of test performance suggested that FDG-PET/CT outperformed stand-alone FDG-PET, gallium scintigraphy, and leukocyte scintigraphy. Similarly, indirect comparisons of diagnostic yield suggested that FDG-PET/CT was more likely than alternative tests to correctly identify the cause of FUO. Meta-analyses report a high diagnostic yield for PET and PET/CT in the workup of FUO patients, with pooled sensitivity and specificity figures of ~85% and ~50%, respectively, and a total diagnostic yield of ~50% for PET/CT and ~40% for PET.

As many patients with FUO present with periodic fever, correct timing of PET/CT increases its diagnostic value. Few studies on the use of biomarkers such as elevated CRP or ESR for a contributory outcome of PET/CT have been performed. When both CRP and ESR are normal at the time of FDG-PET/CT, outcome may only be contributory when a patient does have fever at the time of the scan.

Although PET/CT and other scintigraphic techniques do not directly provide a definitive diagnosis (with the exception of some patients with, for instance, large vessel vasculitis), they often identify the anatomic location of a particular ongoing metabolic process. With the help of other techniques such as biopsy and culture, a timely diagnosis and treatment can be facilitated. Pathologic FDG uptake is quickly eradicated by treatment with glucocorticoids in many diseases, including vasculitis and lymphoma; therefore, glucocorticoid use should be stopped or postponed until after FDG-PET/CT is performed.

FDG-PET/CT is a relatively expensive procedure whose availability is still limited compared with that of CT and conventional scintigraphy. Nevertheless, FDG-PET/CT can be cost-effective in the FUO diagnostic workup if used at an early stage, helping to establish an early diagnosis, reducing days of hospitalization for diagnostic purposes, and obviating unnecessary and unhelpful tests. When FDG-PET/CT has been made under the right conditions (i.e., when elevated CRP or ESR or fever were present during the scan) but has not contributed to the final diagnosis, repeating PET/CT is probably of little value, unless new signs or symptoms appear.

Conventional scintigraphic imaging other than PET/CT Conventional scintigraphic methods used in clinical practice are ^{67}Ga-citrate scintigraphy and ^{111}In- or ^{99m}Tc-labeled leukocyte scintigraphy. Sensitivity and specificity of conventional scintigraphic studies are lower than for PET/CT: the diagnostic yield of gallium scintigraphy ranges from 21% to 54%, and on average the location of a source of fever can correctly be localized in approximately one-third of patients. The diagnostic value of leukocyte scintigraphy ranges from 8% to 31%, and overall the cause of FUO can correctly be identified in one-fifth of patients. When PET/CT is not available, these techniques are the only alternative.

LATER-STAGE DIAGNOSTIC TESTS

In some cases, more invasive tests are appropriate. Abnormalities found with imaging often need to be confirmed by pathology and/or culture of biopsy specimens. If lymphadenopathy is found, lymph node biopsy is necessary, even when the affected lymph nodes are hard to reach or when previous biopsies were inconclusive. In the case of skin lesions, skin biopsy should be undertaken.

If no diagnosis is reached despite PET/CT and PDC-driven histologic investigations or culture, second-stage screening diagnostic tests should be considered (Fig. 20-1). In three studies, the diagnostic yield of screening chest and abdominal CT in patients with FUO was ~20%. The specificity of chest CT was ~80%, but that of abdominal CT varied between 63% and 80%. Despite the relatively limited specificity of abdominal CT and the probably limited additional value of chest CT after normal FDG-PET/CT, chest and abdominal CT may be used as screening procedures at a later stage of the diagnostic protocol because of their noninvasive nature and high sensitivity. Bone marrow aspiration is seldom useful in the absence of PDCs for bone marrow disorders. With addition of FDG-PET/CT, which is highly sensitive in detecting lymphoma, carcinoma, and osteomyelitis, the value of bone marrow biopsy as a screening procedure is probably further reduced. Several studies have shown a high prevalence of giant cell arteritis among patients with FUO, with rates up to 17% among elderly patients. Giant cell arteritis often involves large arteries and in most cases can be diagnosed by FDG-PET/CT. However, temporal artery biopsy is still recommended for patients ≥55 years of age in a later stage of the diagnostic protocol: FDG-PET/CT will not be useful in vasculitis limited to the temporal arteries because of the small diameter of these vessels and the high levels of FDG uptake in the brain. In the past, liver biopsies were often performed as a screening procedure in patients with FUO. In each of two studies, liver biopsy as part of the later stage of a screening diagnostic protocol was helpful in only one patient. Moreover, abnormal liver tests are not predictive of a diagnostic liver biopsy in FUO. Liver biopsy is an invasive procedure that carries the possibility of complications and even death. Therefore, it should not be used for screening purposes in patients with FUO except in those with PDCs for liver disease or miliary tuberculosis.

In patients with unexplained fever after all of the above procedures, the last steps in the diagnostic workup—with only a marginal diagnostic yield—come at an extraordinarily high cost in terms of both expense and discomfort for the patient. Repetition of a thorough history-taking and physical examination and review of laboratory results and imaging studies (including those from other hospitals) are recommended. Diagnostic delay often results from a failure to recognize PDCs in the available information. In these patients with persisting FUO, waiting for new PDCs to appear probably is better than ordering more screening investigations. Only when a patient's condition deteriorates without providing new PDCs should a further diagnostic workup be performed.

SECOND OPINION IN AN EXPERT CENTER

When despite the workup described above no explanation for FUO is found, second opinion in an expert center on FUO should be considered. The single study on the value of second opinion in FUO reported that in 57.3% of patients with unexplained FUO, a diagnosis could be found in an expert center. Additionally, of all patients who remained without a diagnosis even after second opinion, 10.9% became fever-free upon empirical treatment, adding up to a beneficial outcome in 68.2% of patients.

TREATMENT

Fever of Unknown Origin

Empirical therapeutic trials with antibiotics, glucocorticoids, or antituberculous agents should be avoided in FUO except when a patient's condition is rapidly deteriorating after the aforementioned diagnostic tests have failed to provide a definite diagnosis.

ANTIBIOTICS AND ANTITUBERCULOUS THERAPY

Antibiotic or antituberculous therapy may irrevocably diminish the ability to culture fastidious bacteria or mycobacteria. However, hemodynamic instability or neutropenia is a good indication for empirical antibiotic therapy. If the TST or IGRA is positive or if granulomatous disease is present with anergy and sarcoidosis seems unlikely, a trial of therapy for tuberculosis should be started. Especially in miliary tuberculosis, it may be very difficult to obtain a rapid diagnosis. If the fever does not respond after 6 weeks of empirical antituberculous treatment, another diagnosis should be considered.

COLCHICINE, NONSTEROIDAL ANTI-INFLAMMATORY DRUGS, AND GLUCOCORTICOIDS

Colchicine is highly effective in preventing attacks of familial Mediterranean fever (FMF) but is not always effective once an attack is well under way. When FMF is suspected, the response to colchicine is not a completely reliable diagnostic tool in the acute phase, but with colchicine treatment most patients show remarkable improvements in the frequency and severity of subsequent febrile episodes within weeks to months. Therefore, colchicine may be tried in patients with features compatible with FMF, especially when these patients originate from a high-prevalence region.

If the fever persists and the source remains elusive after completion of the later-stage investigations, supportive treatment with nonsteroidal anti-inflammatory drugs (NSAIDs) can be helpful. The response of adult-onset Still's disease to NSAIDs is dramatic in some cases.

The effects of glucocorticoids on giant cell arteritis and polymyalgia rheumatica are equally impressive. Early empirical trials with glucocorticoids, however, decrease the chances of reaching a diagnosis for which more specific and sometimes life-saving treatment might be more appropriate, such as malignant lymphoma. The ability of NSAIDs and glucocorticoids to mask fever while permitting the spread of infection or lymphoma dictates that their use should be avoided unless infectious diseases and malignant lymphoma have been largely ruled out and inflammatory disease is probable and is likely to be debilitating or threatening.

INTERLEUKIN 1 INHIBITION

Interleukin (IL) 1 is a key cytokine in local and systemic inflammation and the febrile response. The availability of specific IL-1-targeting agents has revealed a pathologic role of IL-1-mediated inflammation in a growing list of diseases. Anakinra, a recombinant form of the naturally occurring IL-1 receptor antagonist (IL-1Ra), blocks the activity of both IL-1α and IL-1β. Anakinra is extremely effective in the treatment of many autoinflammatory syndromes, such as FMF, cryopyrin-associated periodic syndrome, tumor necrosis factor receptor–associated periodic syndrome, mevalonate kinase deficiency (hyper IgD syndrome), Schnitzler syndrome, and adult onset Still's disease. There are many other chronic inflammatory disorders in which anti-IL-1 therapy is highly effective. A therapeutic trial with anakinra can be considered in patients whose FUO has not been diagnosed after later-stage diagnostic tests. Although most chronic inflammatory conditions without a known basis can be controlled with glucocorticoids, monotherapy with IL-1 blockade can provide improved control without the metabolic, immunologic, and gastrointestinal side effects of glucocorticoid administration.

PROGNOSIS

In patients in whom FUO remains unexplained, prognosis is favorable. Two large studies on mortality in these patients have been performed. The first study included 436 patients of whom 168 remained without a diagnosis. Of these, 4 (2.4%) died during follow-up. All 4 patients died during the index admission, and in 2 of them a diagnosis was made upon autopsy (1 had intravascular lymphoma and 1 had bilateral pneumonia). The second study included 131 patients with unexplained FUO. Of these patients, 9 (6.9%) died during a median follow-up of 5 years. In 6 of these patients the cause of death was known, and in 5 of them death was considered unrelated to the febrile disease. Overall, FUO-related mortality rates have continuously declined over recent decades. The majority of fevers are caused by treatable diseases, and the risk of death related to FUO is, of course, dependent on the underlying disease.

FURTHER READING

Bleeker-Rovers CP et al: A prospective multicenter study on fever of unknown origin: The yield of a structured diagnostic protocol. Medicine (Baltimore) 86:26, 2007.

Kouijzer IJE et al: Fever of unknown origin: The value of FDG-PET/CT. Semin Nucl Med 48:100, 2018.

Mulders-Manders C et al: Fever of unknown origin. Clin Med 15:280, 2015.

Mulders-Manders C et al: Long-term prognosis, treatment, and outcome of patients with fever of unknown origin in whom no diagnosis was made despite extensive investigation: A questionnaire based study. Medicine (Baltimore) 97:e11241, 2018.

Vanderschueren S et al: Inflammation of unknown origin versus fever of unknown origin: Two of a kind. Eur J Intern Med 20:4, 2009.

Vanderschueren S et al: Mortality in patients presenting with fever of unknown origin. Acta Clin Belg 69:12, 2014.

Section 3 Nervous System Dysfunction

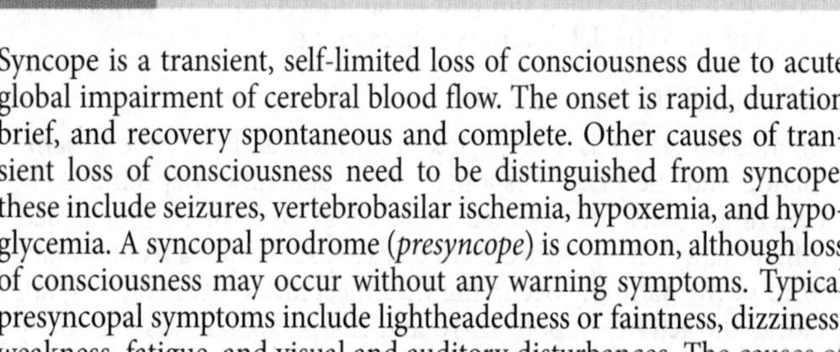

21 Syncope

Roy Freeman

Syncope is a transient, self-limited loss of consciousness due to acute global impairment of cerebral blood flow. The onset is rapid, duration brief, and recovery spontaneous and complete. Other causes of transient loss of consciousness need to be distinguished from syncope; these include seizures, vertebrobasilar ischemia, hypoxemia, and hypoglycemia. A syncopal prodrome (*presyncope*) is common, although loss of consciousness may occur without any warning symptoms. Typical presyncopal symptoms include lightheadedness or faintness, dizziness, weakness, fatigue, and visual and auditory disturbances. The causes of syncope can be divided into three general categories: (1) neurally mediated syncope (also called *reflex or vasovagal syncope*), (2) orthostatic hypotension, and (3) cardiac syncope.

Neurally mediated syncope comprises a heterogeneous group of functional disorders that are characterized by a transient change in the reflexes responsible for maintaining cardiovascular homeostasis. Episodic vasodilation (or loss of vasoconstrictor tone), decreased cardiac output, and bradycardia occur in varying combinations, resulting in temporary failure of blood pressure control. In contrast, in patients with orthostatic hypotension due to autonomic failure, these cardiovascular homeostatic reflexes are chronically impaired. Cardiac syncope may be due to arrhythmias or structural cardiac diseases that cause a decrease in cardiac output. The clinical features, underlying pathophysiologic mechanisms, therapeutic interventions, and prognoses differ markedly among these three causes.

EPIDEMIOLOGY AND NATURAL HISTORY

Syncope is a common presenting problem, accounting for ~3% of all emergency department (ED) visits and 1% of all hospital admissions. The annual cost for syncope-related hospitalization in the United States is ~$2.4 billion. Syncope has a lifetime cumulative incidence of up to 35% in the general population. The peak incidence in the young occurs between ages 10 and 30 years, with a median peak around 15 years. Neurally mediated syncope is the etiology in the vast majority of these cases. In older adults, there is a sharp rise in the incidence of syncope after 70 years of age.

In population-based studies, neurally mediated syncope is the most common cause of syncope. The incidence is higher in women than men. In young subjects, there is often a family history in first-degree relatives. Cardiovascular disease due to structural disease or arrhythmias is the next most common cause in most series, particularly in ED settings and in older patients. Orthostatic hypotension also increases in prevalence with age because of the reduced baroreflex responsiveness, decreased cardiac compliance, and attenuation of the vestibulosympathetic reflex associated with aging. Other contributors are reduced fluid intake and vasoactive medications, also more likely in this age group. In the elderly, orthostatic hypotension is more common in institutionalized than community-dwelling individuals, most likely explained by a greater prevalence of predisposing neurologic disorders, physiologic impairment, and vasoactive medication use among institutionalized patients.

TABLE 21-1 High-Risk Features Indicating Hospitalization or Intensive Evaluation of Syncope
Chest pain suggesting coronary ischemia
Features of congestive heart failure
Moderate or severe valvular disease
Moderate or severe structural cardiac disease
Electrocardiographic features of ischemia
History of ventricular arrhythmias
Prolonged QT interval (>500 ms)
Repetitive sinoatrial block or sinus pauses
Persistent sinus bradycardia
Bi- or trifascicular block or intraventricular conduction delay with QRS duration ≥120 ms
Atrial fibrillation
Nonsustained ventricular tachycardia
Family history of sudden death
Preexcitation syndromes
Brugada pattern on ECG
Palpitations at time of syncope
Syncope at rest or during exercise

Syncope of noncardiac and unexplained origin in younger individuals has an excellent prognosis; life expectancy is unaffected. By contrast, syncope due to a cardiac cause, either structural heart disease or a primary arrhythmic disorder, is associated with an increased risk of sudden cardiac death and mortality from other causes. Similarly, the mortality rate is increased in individuals with syncope due to orthostatic hypotension related to age and the associated comorbid conditions (**Table 21-1**). The likelihood of hospitalization and mortality risk are higher in older adults.

PATHOPHYSIOLOGY

The upright posture imposes a unique physiologic stress upon humans; most, although not all, syncopal episodes occur from a standing position. Standing results in pooling of 500–1000 mL of blood in the lower extremities, buttocks, and splanchnic circulation. The dependent pooling leads to a decrease in venous return to the heart and reduced ventricular filling that result in diminished cardiac output and blood pressure. These hemodynamic changes provoke a compensatory reflex response, initiated by the baroreceptors in the carotid sinus and aortic arch, resulting in increased sympathetic outflow and decreased vagal nerve activity (**Fig. 21-1**). The reflex increases peripheral resistance, venous return to the heart, and cardiac output and thus limits the fall in blood pressure. If this response fails, as is the case chronically in orthostatic hypotension and transiently in neurally mediated syncope, hypotension and cerebral hypoperfusion occur.

Syncope is a consequence of global cerebral hypoperfusion and thus represents a failure of cerebral blood flow autoregulatory mechanisms. Myogenic factors, local metabolites, and to a lesser extent autonomic neurovascular control are responsible for the autoregulation of cerebral blood flow (**Chap. 307**). The latency of the autoregulatory response is 5–10 s. Typically, cerebral blood flow ranges from 50–60 mL/min per 100 g brain tissue and remains relatively constant over perfusion pressures ranging from 50–150 mmHg. Cessation of blood flow for 6–8 s

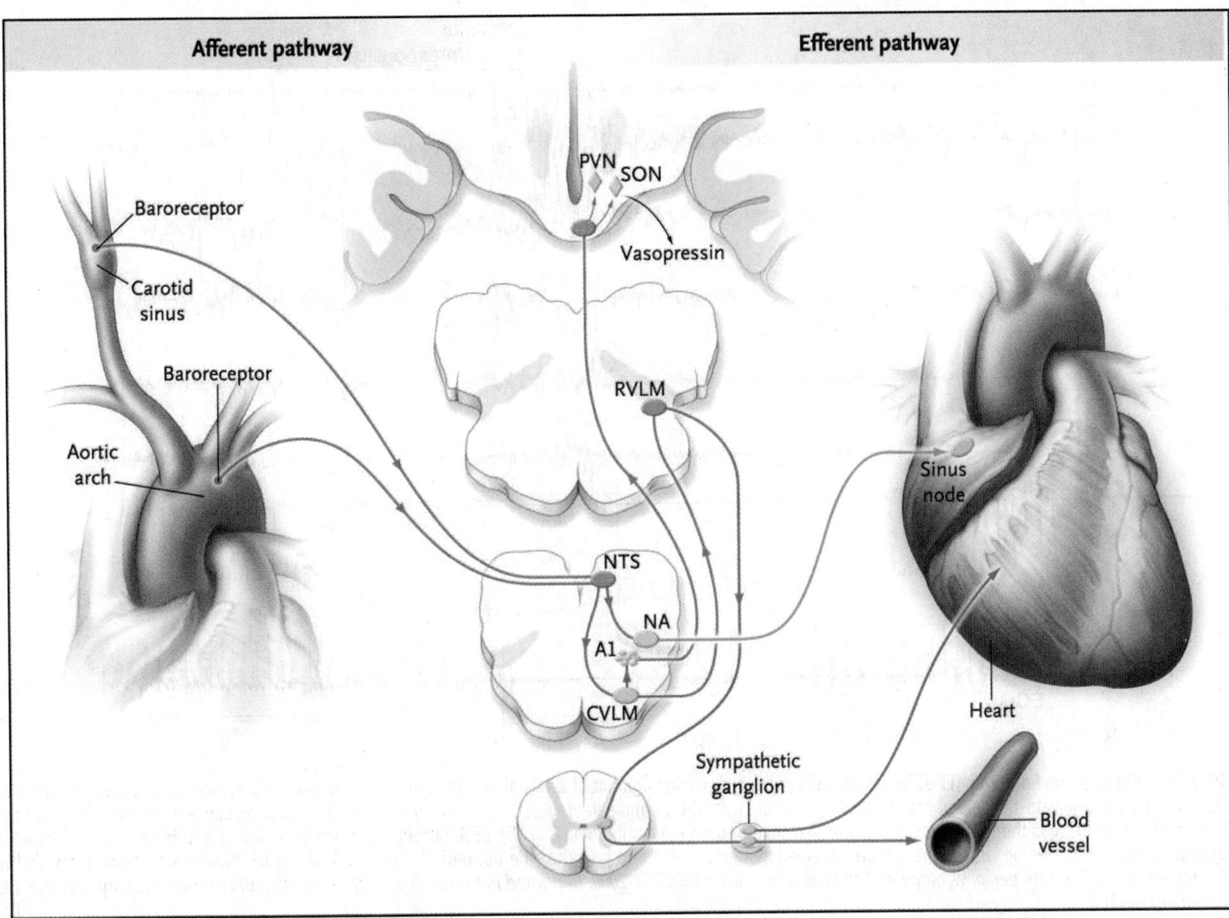

FIGURE 21-1 The baroreflex. A decrease in arterial pressure unloads the baroreceptors—the terminals of afferent fibers of the glossopharyngeal and vagus nerves—that are situated in the carotid sinus and aortic arch. This leads to a reduction in the afferent impulses that are relayed from these mechanoreceptors through the glossopharyngeal and vagus nerves to the nucleus of the tractus solitarius (NTS) in the dorsomedial medulla. The reduced baroreceptor afferent activity produces a decrease in vagal nerve input to the sinus node that is mediated via connections of the NTS to the nucleus ambiguus (NA). There is an increase in sympathetic efferent activity that is mediated by the NTS projections to the caudal ventrolateral medulla (CVLM) (an excitatory pathway) and from there to the rostral ventrolateral medulla (RVLM) (an inhibitory pathway). The activation of RVLM presympathetic neurons in response to hypotension is thus predominantly due to disinhibition. In response to a sustained fall in blood pressure, vasopressin release is mediated by projections from the A1 noradrenergic cell group in the ventrolateral medulla. This projection activates vasopressin-synthesizing neurons in the magnocellular portion of the paraventricular nucleus (PVN) and the supraoptic nucleus (SON) of the hypothalamus. *Blue* denotes sympathetic neurons, and *green* denotes parasympathetic neurons. *(From R Freeman: Neurogenic orthostatic hypotension. N Engl J Med 358:615, 2008. Copyright © 2008 Massachusetts Medical Society. Reprinted with permission.)*

will result in loss of consciousness, while impairment of consciousness ensues when blood flow decreases to 25 mL/min per 100 g brain tissue.

From the clinical standpoint, a fall in systemic systolic blood pressure to ~50 mmHg or lower will result in syncope. A decrease in cardiac output and/or systemic vascular resistance—the determinants of blood pressure—thus underlies the pathophysiology of syncope. Common causes of impaired cardiac output include decreased effective circulating blood volume, increased thoracic pressure, massive pulmonary embolus, cardiac brady- and tachyarrhythmias, valvular heart disease, and myocardial dysfunction. Systemic vascular resistance may be decreased by central and peripheral autonomic nervous system diseases, sympatholytic medications, and transiently during neurally mediated syncope. Increased cerebral vascular resistance, most frequently due to hypocarbia induced by hyperventilation, may also contribute to the pathophysiology of syncope.

Two patterns of electroencephalographic (EEG) changes occur in syncopal subjects. The first is a "slow-flat-slow" pattern (**Fig. 21-2**) in which normal background activity is replaced with high-amplitude slow delta waves. This is followed by sudden flattening of the EEG—a cessation or attenuation of cortical activity—followed by the return of slow waves, and then normal activity. A second pattern, the "slow pattern," is characterized by increasing and decreasing slow wave activity only. The EEG flattening that occurs in the slow-flat-slow pattern is a marker of more severe cerebral hypoperfusion. Despite the presence of myoclonic movements and other motor activity during some syncopal events, EEG seizure discharges are not detected.

CLASSIFICATION

NEURALLY MEDIATED SYNCOPE

Neurally mediated (reflex; vasovagal) syncope is the final pathway of a complex central and peripheral nervous system reflex arc. There is a transient change in autonomic efferent activity with increased parasympathetic outflow, plus sympathoinhibition, resulting in bradycardia, vasodilation, and/or reduced vasoconstrictor tone (the vasodepressor response) and reduced cardiac output. The resulting fall in systemic blood pressure can then reduce cerebral blood flow to below the compensatory limits of autoregulation (**Fig. 21-3**). In order to develop neurally mediated syncope, a functioning autonomic nervous system is necessary, in contrast to syncope resulting from autonomic failure (discussed below).

Multiple triggers of the afferent limb of the reflex arc can result in neurally mediated syncope. In some situations, these can be clearly defined, e.g., orthostatic stress and stimulus of the carotid sinus, the gastrointestinal tract, or the bladder. Often, however, the trigger is less easily recognized and the cause is multifactorial. Under these circumstances, it is likely that different afferent pathways converge on the central autonomic network within the medulla that integrates the neural impulses and mediates the vasodepressor-bradycardic response.

Classification of Neurally Mediated Syncope Neurally mediated syncope may be subdivided based on the afferent pathway and provocative trigger. Vasovagal syncope (the common faint) is provoked

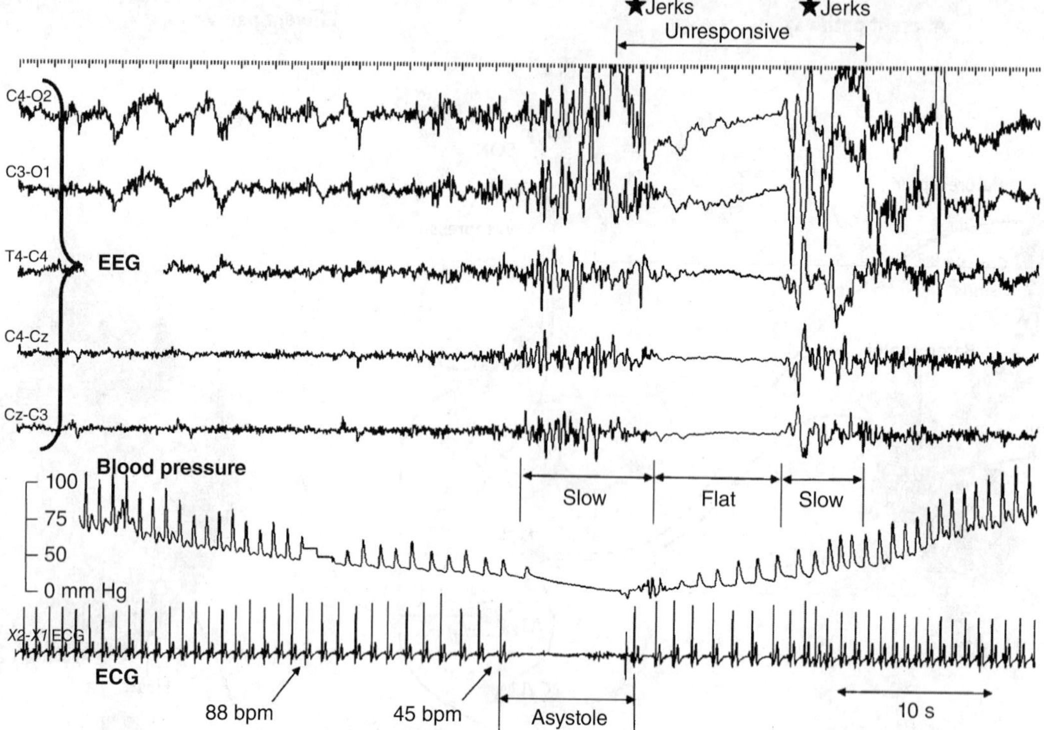

FIGURE 21-2 The electroencephalogram (EEG) in vasovagal syncope. A 1-min segment of a tilt-table test with typical vasovagal syncope demonstrating the "slow-flat-slow" EEG pattern. Finger beat-to-beat blood pressure, electrocardiogram (ECG), and selected EEG channels are shown. EEG slowing starts when systolic blood pressure drops to ~50 mmHg; heart rate is then ~45 beats/min (bpm). Asystole occurred, lasting about 8 s. The EEG flattens for a similar period, but with a delay. A transient loss of consciousness, lasting 14 s, was observed. There were muscle jerks just before and just after the flat period of the EEG. *(From W Wieling et al: Symptoms and signs of syncope: a review of the link between physiology and clinical clues. Brain 132:2630, 2009. Reprinted (and translated) by permission of Oxford University Press on behalf of the Guarantors of Brain.)*

by intense emotion, pain, and/or orthostatic stress, whereas the situational reflex syncopes have specific localized stimuli that provoke the reflex vasodilation and bradycardia that leads to syncope. The underlying mechanisms have been identified and pathophysiology delineated for most of these situational reflex syncopes. The afferent trigger may originate in the pulmonary system, gastrointestinal system, urogenital system, heart, and carotid sinus in the carotid artery (**Table 21-2**). Hyperventilation leading to hypocarbia and cerebral vasoconstriction, and raised intrathoracic pressure that impairs venous return to the heart, play a central role in many of the situational reflex syncopes. The afferent pathway of the reflex arc differs among these disorders, but the efferent response via the vagus and sympathetic pathways is similar.

Alternately, neurally mediated syncope may be subdivided based on the predominant efferent pathway. Vasodepressor syncope describes syncope predominantly due to efferent, sympathetic, vasoconstrictor failure; cardioinhibitory syncope describes syncope predominantly associated with bradycardia or asystole due to increased vagal outflow;

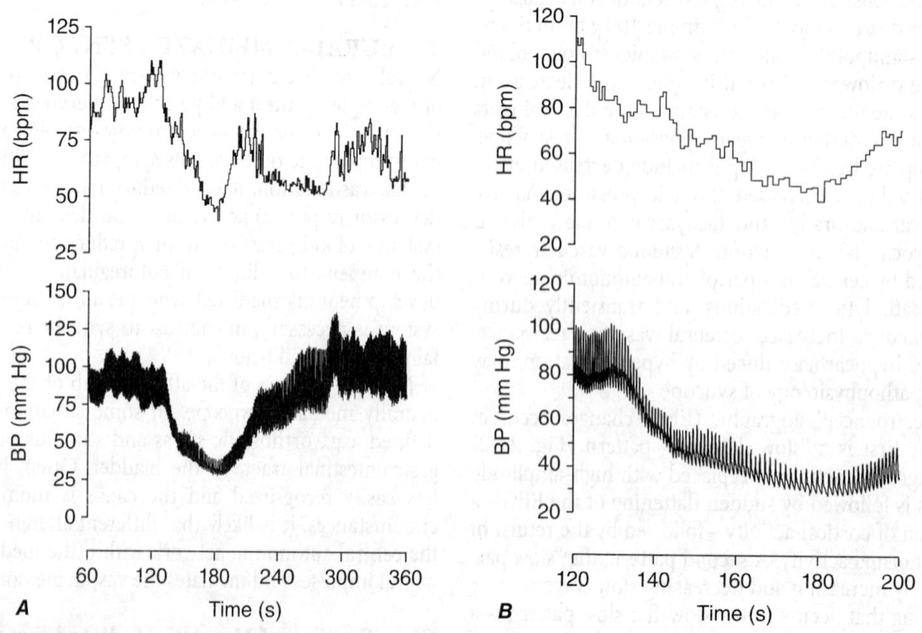

FIGURE 21-3 ***A.*** The paroxysmal hypotensive-bradycardic response that is characteristic of neurally mediated syncope. Noninvasive beat-to-beat blood pressure and heart rate are shown >5 min (from 60 to 360 s) of an upright tilt on a tilt table. ***B.*** The same tracing expanded to show 80 s of the episode (from 80 to 200 s). BP, blood pressure; bpm, beats per minute; HR, heart rate.

TABLE 21-2 Causes of Syncope

A. Neurally Mediated Syncope
Vasovagal syncope
Provoked fear, pain, anxiety, intense emotion, sight of blood, unpleasant sights and odors, orthostatic stress
Situational reflex syncope
Pulmonary
Cough syncope, wind instrument player's syncope, weightlifter's syncope, "mess trick"[a] and "fainting lark,"[b] sneeze syncope, airway instrumentation
Urogenital
Postmicturition syncope, urogenital tract instrumentation, prostatic massage
Gastrointestinal
Swallow syncope, glossopharyngeal neuralgia, esophageal stimulation, gastrointestinal tract instrumentation, rectal examination, defecation syncope
Cardiac
Bezold-Jarisch reflex, cardiac outflow obstruction
Carotid sinus
Carotid sinus sensitivity, carotid sinus massage
Ocular
Ocular pressure, ocular examination, ocular surgery
B. Orthostatic Hypotension
Primary autonomic failure due to idiopathic central and peripheral neurodegenerative diseases—the "synucleinopathies"
Lewy body diseases
Parkinson's disease
Lewy body dementia
Pure autonomic failure
Multiple system atrophy (Shy-Drager syndrome)
Secondary autonomic failure due to autonomic peripheral neuropathies
Diabetes
Hereditary amyloidosis (familial amyloid polyneuropathy)
Primary amyloidosis (AL amyloidosis; immunoglobulin light chain associated)
Hereditary sensory and autonomic neuropathies (HSAN) (especially type III—familial dysautonomia)
Idiopathic immune-mediated autonomic neuropathy
Autoimmune autonomic ganglionopathy
Sjögren's syndrome
Paraneoplastic autonomic neuropathy
HIV neuropathy
Postprandial hypotension
Iatrogenic (drug-induced)
Volume depletion
C. Cardiac Syncope
Arrhythmias
Sinus node dysfunction
Atrioventricular dysfunction
Supraventricular tachycardias
Ventricular tachycardias
Inherited channelopathies
Cardiac structural disease
Valvular disease
Myocardial ischemia
Obstructive and other cardiomyopathies
Atrial myxoma
Pericardial effusions and tamponade

[a]Hyperventilation for ~1 min, followed by sudden chest compression. [b]Hyperventilation (~20 breaths) in a squatting position, rapid rise to standing, then Valsalva maneuver.

and mixed syncope describes syncope in which there are both vagal and sympathetic reflex changes.

Features of Neurally Mediated Syncope In addition to symptoms of orthostatic intolerance such as dizziness, lightheadedness, and fatigue, premonitory features of autonomic activation may be present in patients with neurally mediated syncope. These include diaphoresis, pallor, palpitations, nausea, hyperventilation, and yawning. During the syncopal event, proximal and distal myoclonus (typically arrhythmic and multifocal) may occur, raising the possibility of a seizure. The eyes typically remain open and usually deviate upward. Pupils are usually dilated. Roving eye movements may occur. Grunting, moaning, snorting, and stertorous breathing may be present. Urinary incontinence may occur. Fecal incontinence is very rare, however. Postictal confusion is also rare, although visual and auditory hallucinations and near-death and out-of-body experiences are sometimes reported.

Although some predisposing factors and provocative stimuli are well established (for example, motionless upright posture, warm ambient temperature, intravascular volume depletion, alcohol ingestion, hypoxemia, anemia, pain, the sight of blood, venipuncture, and intense emotion), the underlying basis for the widely different thresholds for syncope among individuals exposed to the same provocative stimulus is not known. A genetic basis for neurally mediated syncope may exist; several studies have reported an increased incidence of syncope in first-degree relatives of fainters, but no gene or genetic marker has been identified, and environmental, social, and cultural factors have not been excluded by these studies.

TREATMENT

Neurally Mediated Syncope

Reassurance, education, avoidance of provocative stimuli, and plasma volume expansion with fluid and salt are the cornerstones of the management of neurally mediated syncope. Isometric counterpressure maneuvers of the limbs (tensing of the abdominal and leg muscles, handgrip and arm tensing, and leg crossing) may raise blood pressure by increasing central blood volume and cardiac output. Of these, abdominal muscle tensing is the most effective. By maintaining pressure in the autoregulatory zone, these maneuvers, which may be particularly helpful in patients with a long prodrome, avoid or delay the onset of syncope. Randomized controlled trials support this intervention.

Fludrocortisone, vasoconstricting agents, and β-adrenoreceptor antagonists are widely used by experts to treat refractory patients, although there is no consistent evidence from randomized controlled trials for any pharmacotherapy to treat neurally mediated syncope. Because vasodilation, decreased central blood volume, decreased stroke volume and cardiac output are the dominant pathophysiologic syncopal mechanisms in most patients, use of a cardiac pacemaker is rarely beneficial. A systematic review of the literature examining whether cardiac pacing reduces risk of recurrent syncope and relevant clinical outcomes in adults with neurally mediated syncope, concluded that the existing evidence does not support the use of routine cardiac pacing. Possible exceptions are (1) older patients (>40 years), with at least three prior episodes associated with asystole (of at least 3 s associated with syncope or at least 6 s associated with presyncope) documented by an implantable loop recorder; and (2) patients with prominent cardioinhibition due to carotid sinus syndrome. In these patients, dual-chamber pacing may be helpful, although this continues to be an area of uncertainty.

■ ORTHOSTATIC HYPOTENSION

Orthostatic hypotension, defined as a reduction in systolic blood pressure of at least 20 mmHg or diastolic blood pressure of at least 10 mmHg after 3 min of standing or head-up tilt on a tilt table, is a manifestation of sympathetic vasoconstrictor (autonomic) failure (Fig. 21-4). In many (but not all) cases, there is no compensatory

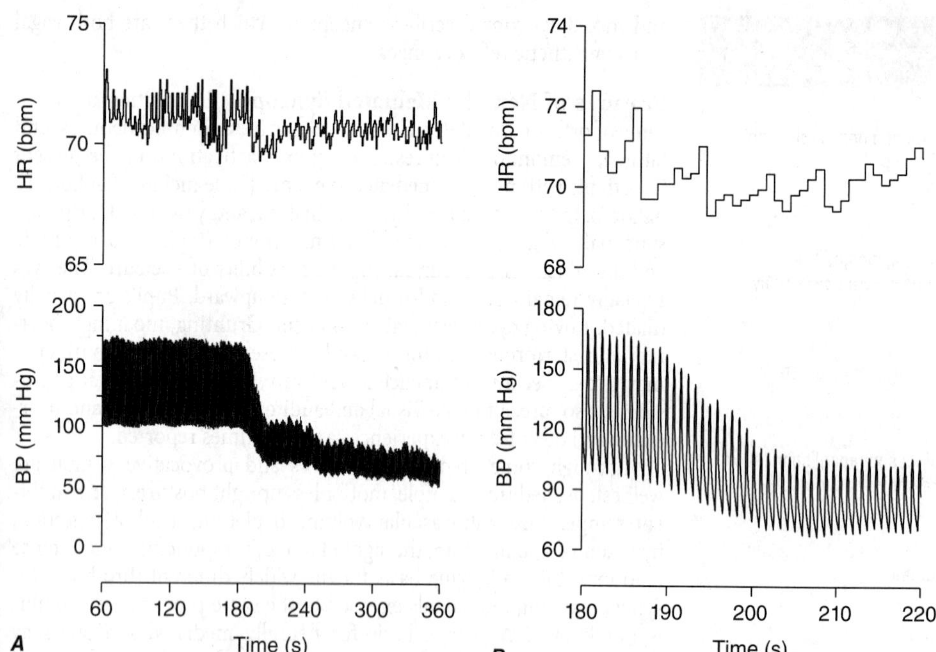

FIGURE 21-4 ***A.*** The gradual fall in blood pressure without a compensatory heart rate increase that is characteristic of orthostatic hypotension due to autonomic failure. Blood pressure and heart rate are shown >5 min (from 60 to 360 s) of an upright tilt on a tilt table. ***B.*** The same tracing expanded to show 40 s of the episode (from 180 to 220 s). BP, blood pressure; bpm, beats per minute; HR, heart rate.

increase in heart rate despite hypotension; with partial autonomic failure, heart rate may increase to some degree but is insufficient to maintain cardiac output. A variant of orthostatic hypotension is "delayed" orthostatic hypotension, which occurs beyond 3 min of standing; this may reflect a mild or early form of sympathetic adrenergic dysfunction. In some cases, orthostatic hypotension occurs within 15 s of standing (so-called initial orthostatic hypotension), a finding that may reflect a transient mismatch between cardiac output and peripheral vascular resistance and does not represent autonomic failure.

Characteristic symptoms of orthostatic hypotension include light-headedness, dizziness, and presyncope (near-faintness) occurring in response to sudden postural change. However, symptoms may be absent or nonspecific, such as generalized weakness, fatigue, cognitive slowing, leg buckling, or headache. Visual blurring may occur, likely due to retinal or occipital lobe ischemia. Neck pain, typically in the suboccipital, posterior cervical, and shoulder region (the "coat-hanger headache"), most likely due to neck muscle ischemia, may be the only symptom. Patients may report orthostatic dyspnea (thought to reflect ventilation-perfusion mismatch due to inadequate perfusion of ventilated lung apices) or angina (attributed to impaired myocardial perfusion even with normal coronary arteries). Symptoms may be exacerbated by exertion, prolonged standing, increased ambient temperature, or meals. Syncope is usually preceded by warning symptoms, but may occur suddenly, suggesting the possibility of a seizure or cardiac cause. Some patients have profound decreases in blood pressure, sometimes without symptoms but placing them at risk for falls and injuries if the autoregulatory threshold is crossed with ensuing cerebral hypoperfusion.

Supine hypertension is common in patients with orthostatic hypotension due to autonomic failure, affecting >50% of patients in some series. Orthostatic hypotension may present after initiation of therapy for hypertension, and supine hypertension may follow treatment of orthostatic hypotension. However, in other cases, the association of the two conditions is unrelated to therapy; it may in part be explained by baroreflex dysfunction in the presence of residual sympathetic outflow, particularly in patients with central autonomic degeneration.

Causes of Neurogenic Orthostatic Hypotension Causes of neurogenic orthostatic hypotension include central and peripheral autonomic nervous system dysfunction (**Chap. 440**). Autonomic dysfunction of other organ systems (including the bladder, bowels, sexual organs, and sudomotor system) of varying severity frequently accompanies orthostatic hypotension in these disorders (Table 21-2).

The primary autonomic degenerative disorders are multiple system atrophy (Shy-Drager syndrome; **Chap. 440**), Parkinson's disease (**Chap. 435**), dementia with Lewy bodies (**Chap. 434**), and pure autonomic failure (**Chap. 440**). These are often grouped together as "synucleinopathies" due to the presence of α-synuclein, a protein that aggregates predominantly in the cytoplasm of neurons in the Lewy body disorders (Parkinson's disease, dementia with Lewy bodies, and pure autonomic failure) and in the glia in multiple system atrophy.

Peripheral autonomic dysfunction may also accompany small-fiber peripheral neuropathies such as those associated with diabetes mellitus, acquired and hereditary amyloidosis, immune-mediated neuropathies, and hereditary sensory and autonomic neuropathies (HSAN; particularly HSAN type III, familial dysautonomia) (**Chaps. 446 and 447**). Less frequently, orthostatic hypotension is associated with the peripheral neuropathies that accompany vitamin B_{12} deficiency, neurotoxin exposure, HIV and other infections, and porphyria.

Patients with autonomic failure and the elderly are susceptible to falls in blood pressure associated with meals. The magnitude of the blood pressure fall is exacerbated by large meals, meals high in carbohydrate, and alcohol intake. The mechanism of postprandial syncope is not fully elucidated.

Orthostatic hypotension is often iatrogenic. Drugs from several classes may lower peripheral resistance (e.g., α-adrenoreceptor antagonists used to treat hypertension and prostatic hypertrophy; antihypertensive agents of several classes; nitrates and other vasodilators; tricyclic agents and phenothiazines). Iatrogenic volume depletion due to diuresis and volume depletion due to medical causes (hemorrhage, vomiting, diarrhea, or decreased fluid intake) may also result in decreased effective circulatory volume, orthostatic hypotension, and syncope.

TREATMENT

Orthostatic Hypotension

The first step is to remove reversible causes—usually vasoactive medications (**see Table 440-6**). Next, nonpharmacologic interventions should be introduced. These include patient education regarding staged moves from supine to upright; warnings about the hypotensive effects of large meals; instructions about the isometric counterpressure maneuvers that increase intravascular pressure (see above); and raising the head of the bed to reduce supine hypertension and nocturnal diuresis. Intravascular volume should be expanded by increasing dietary fluid and salt. If these nonpharmacologic measures fail, pharmacologic intervention with fludrocortisone acetate and vasoconstricting agents such as midodrine and L-dihydroxyphenylserine should be introduced. Some patients with intractable symptoms require additional therapy with supplementary agents that include pyridostigmine, atomoxetine, yohimbine, octreotide, desmopressin acetate (DDAVP), and erythropoietin (**Chap. 440**).

■ CARDIAC SYNCOPE

Cardiac (or cardiovascular) syncope is caused by arrhythmias and structural heart disease. These may occur in combination because structural disease renders the heart more vulnerable to abnormal electrical activity.

Arrhythmias Bradyarrhythmias that cause syncope include those due to severe sinus node dysfunction (e.g., sinus arrest or sinoatrial block) and atrioventricular (AV) block (e.g., Mobitz type II, high-grade, and complete AV block). The bradyarrhythmias due to sinus node dysfunction are often associated with an atrial tachyarrhythmia, a disorder known as the tachycardia-bradycardia syndrome. A prolonged pause following the termination of a tachycardic episode is a frequent cause of syncope in patients with the tachycardia-bradycardia syndrome. Medications of several classes may also cause bradyarrhythmias of sufficient severity to cause syncope. Syncope due to bradycardia or asystole has been referred to as a Stokes-Adams attack.

Ventricular tachyarrhythmias frequently cause syncope. The likelihood of syncope with ventricular tachycardia is in part dependent on the ventricular rate; rates <200 beats/min are less likely to cause syncope. The compromised hemodynamic function during ventricular tachycardia is caused by ineffective ventricular contraction, reduced diastolic filling due to abbreviated filling periods, loss of AV synchrony, and concurrent myocardial ischemia.

Several disorders associated with cardiac electrophysiologic instability and arrhythmogenesis are due to mutations in ion channel subunit genes. These include the long QT syndrome, Brugada syndrome, and catecholaminergic polymorphic ventricular tachycardia. The long QT syndrome is a genetically heterogeneous disorder associated with prolonged cardiac repolarization and a predisposition to ventricular arrhythmias. Syncope and sudden death in patients with long QT syndrome result from a unique polymorphic ventricular tachycardia called *torsades des pointes* that degenerates into ventricular fibrillation. The long QT syndrome has been linked to genes encoding K^+ channel α-subunits, K^+ channel β-subunits, voltage-gated Na^+ channel, and a scaffolding protein, ankyrin B (ANK2). Brugada syndrome is characterized by idiopathic ventricular fibrillation in association with right ventricular electrocardiogram (ECG) abnormalities without structural heart disease. This disorder is also genetically heterogeneous, although it is most frequently linked to mutations in the Na^+ channel α-subunit, SCN5A. Catecholaminergic polymorphic tachycardia is an inherited, genetically heterogeneous disorder associated with exercise- or stress-induced ventricular arrhythmias, syncope, or sudden death. Acquired QT interval prolongation, most commonly due to drugs, may also result in ventricular arrhythmias and syncope. **These disorders are discussed in detail in Chap. 255.**

Structural Disease Structural heart disease (e.g., valvular disease, myocardial ischemia, hypertrophic and other cardiomyopathies, cardiac masses such as atrial myxoma, and pericardial effusions) may lead to syncope by compromising cardiac output. Structural disease may also contribute to other pathophysiologic mechanisms of syncope. For example, cardiac structural disease may predispose to arrhythmogenesis; aggressive treatment of cardiac failure with diuretics and/or vasodilators may lead to orthostatic hypotension; and inappropriate reflex vasodilation may occur with structural disorders such as aortic stenosis and hypertrophic cardiomyopathy, possibly provoked by increased ventricular contractility.

TREATMENT

Cardiac Syncope

Treatment of cardiac disease depends on the underlying disorder. Therapies for arrhythmias include cardiac pacing for sinus node disease and AV block, and ablation, antiarrhythmic drugs, and cardioverter-defibrillators for atrial and ventricular tachyarrhythmias. These disorders are best managed by physicians with specialized skills in this area.

APPROACH TO THE PATIENT

Syncope

DIFFERENTIAL DIAGNOSIS

Syncope is easily diagnosed when the characteristic features are present; however, several disorders with transient real or apparent loss of consciousness may create diagnostic confusion.

Generalized and partial seizures may be confused with syncope; however, there are a number of differentiating features. Whereas tonic-clonic movements are the hallmark of a generalized seizure, myoclonic and other movements also may occur in up to 90% of syncopal episodes. Myoclonic jerks associated with syncope may be multifocal or generalized. They are typically arrhythmic and of short duration (<30 s). Mild flexor and extensor posturing also may occur. Partial or partial-complex seizures with secondary generalization are usually preceded by an aura, commonly an unpleasant smell; fear; anxiety; abdominal discomfort; or other visceral sensations. These phenomena should be differentiated from the premonitory features of syncope.

Autonomic manifestations of seizures (autonomic epilepsy) may provide a more difficult diagnostic challenge. Autonomic seizures have cardiovascular, gastrointestinal, pulmonary, urogenital, pupillary, and cutaneous manifestations that are similar to the premonitory features of syncope. Furthermore, the cardiovascular manifestations of autonomic epilepsy include clinically significant tachycardias and bradycardias that may be of sufficient magnitude to cause loss of consciousness. The presence of accompanying non-autonomic auras may help differentiate these episodes from syncope.

Loss of consciousness associated with a seizure usually lasts >5 min and is associated with prolonged postictal drowsiness and disorientation, whereas reorientation occurs almost immediately after a syncopal event. Muscle aches may occur after both syncope and seizures, although they tend to last longer and be more severe following a seizure. Seizures, unlike syncope, are rarely provoked by emotions or pain. Incontinence of urine may occur with both seizures and syncope; however, fecal incontinence occurs very rarely with syncope.

Hypoglycemia may cause transient loss of consciousness, typically in individuals with type 1 or type 2 diabetes **(Chap. 403)** treated with insulin. The clinical features associated with impending or actual hypoglycemia include tremor, palpitations, anxiety, diaphoresis, hunger, and paresthesias. These symptoms are due to autonomic activation to counter the falling blood glucose. Hunger, in particular, is not a typical premonitory feature of syncope. Hypoglycemia also impairs neuronal function, leading to fatigue, weakness, dizziness, and cognitive and behavioral symptoms. Diagnostic difficulties may occur in individuals in strict glycemic control; repeated hypoglycemia impairs the counterregulatory response and leads to a loss of the characteristic warning symptoms that are the hallmark of hypoglycemia.

Patients with cataplexy **(Chap. 31)** experience an abrupt partial or complete loss of muscular tone triggered by strong emotions, typically anger or laughter. Unlike syncope, consciousness is maintained throughout the attacks, which typically last between 30 s and 2 min. There are no premonitory symptoms. Cataplexy occurs in 60%–75% of patients with narcolepsy.

The clinical interview and interrogation of eyewitnesses usually allow differentiation of syncope from falls due to vestibular dysfunction, cerebellar disease, extrapyramidal system dysfunction, and other gait disorders. A diagnosis of syncope can be particularly challenging in patients with dementia who experience repeated falls and are unable to provide a clear history of the episodes. If the fall is accompanied by head trauma, a postconcussive syndrome, amnesia for the precipitating events, and/or a loss or alteration of consciousness, this may also contribute to diagnostic difficulty.

Apparent loss of consciousness can be a manifestation of psychiatric disorders such as generalized anxiety, panic disorders, major depression, and somatization disorder. These possibilities should be considered in individuals who faint frequently without prodromal symptoms. Such patients are rarely injured despite numerous falls. There are no clinically significant hemodynamic changes concurrent with these episodes. In contrast, transient loss of consciousness due to vasovagal syncope precipitated by fear, stress, anxiety, and emotional distress is accompanied by hypotension, bradycardia, or both.

INITIAL EVALUATION

The goals of the initial evaluation are to determine whether the transient loss of consciousness was due to syncope; to identify the cause; and to assess risk for future episodes and serious harm (Table 21-1). The initial evaluation should include a detailed history, thorough questioning of eyewitnesses, and a complete physical and neurologic examination. Blood pressure and heart rate should be measured in the supine position and after 3 min of standing to determine whether orthostatic hypotension is present. High-risk features on history include: the new onset of chest discomfort, abdominal pain, shortness of breath or headache; syncope during exertion or while supine; sudden onset of palpitations followed by syncope; severe coronary artery or structural heart disease.

High-risk features on examination include an unexplained systolic BP of <90 mmHg; suggestion of gastrointestinal hemorrhage; persistent bradycardia (<40 beats/min); and an undiagnosed systolic murmur.

An ECG should be performed if there is suspicion of syncope due to an arrhythmia or underlying cardiac disease. Relevant electrocardiographic abnormalities include bradyarrhythmias or tachyarrhythmias, AV block, acute myocardial ischemia, old myocardial infarction, long QT_c, and bundle branch block. This initial assessment will lead to the identification of a cause of syncope in ~50% of patients and also allows stratification of patients at risk for cardiac mortality.

Laboratory Tests Baseline laboratory blood tests are rarely helpful in identifying the cause of syncope. Blood tests should be performed when specific disorders, e.g., myocardial infarction, anemia, and secondary autonomic failure, are suspected (Table 21-2).

Autonomic Nervous System Testing (Chap. 440) Autonomic testing, including tilt-table testing, can be performed in specialized centers. Autonomic testing is helpful to uncover objective evidence of autonomic failure and also to demonstrate a predisposition to neurally mediated syncope. Autonomic testing includes assessments of parasympathetic autonomic nervous system function (e.g., heart rate variability to deep respiration and a Valsalva maneuver), sympathetic cholinergic function (e.g., thermoregulatory sweat response and quantitative sudomotor axon reflex test), and sympathetic adrenergic function (e.g., blood pressure response to a Valsalva maneuver and a tilt-table test with beat-to-beat blood pressure measurement). The hemodynamic abnormalities demonstrated on the tilt-table test (Figs. 21-3 and 21-4) may be useful in distinguishing orthostatic hypotension due to autonomic failure from the hypotensive bradycardic response of neurally mediated syncope. Similarly, the tilt-table test may help identify patients with syncope due to immediate or delayed orthostatic hypotension.

Carotid sinus massage should be considered in patients with symptoms suggestive of carotid sinus syncope and in patients >40 years with recurrent syncope of unknown etiology. This test should only be carried out under continuous ECG and blood pressure monitoring and should be avoided in patients with carotid bruits, possible or known plaques, or stenosis.

Cardiac Evaluation ECG monitoring is indicated for patients with a high pretest probability of arrhythmia causing syncope. Patients should be monitored in the hospital if the likelihood of a life-threatening arrhythmia is high, e.g., patients with severe coronary artery or structural heart disease, nonsustained ventricular tachycardia, supraventricular tachycardia, paroxysmal atrial fibrillation, trifascicular heart block, prolonged QT interval, Brugada syndrome ECG pattern, syncope during exertion, syncope while seated or supine, and family history of sudden cardiac death (Table 21-1). Outpatient Holter monitoring is recommended for patients who experience frequent syncopal episodes (e.g., one or more per week), whereas loop recorders, which continually record and erase cardiac rhythm, are indicated for patients with suspected arrhythmias with low risk of sudden cardiac death. Loop recorders may be external (e.g., for evaluation of episodes that occur at a frequency of >1 per month) or implantable (e.g., if syncope occurs less frequently).

Echocardiography should be performed in patients with a history of cardiac disease or if abnormalities are found on physical examination or the ECG. Echocardiographic diagnoses that may be responsible for syncope include aortic stenosis, hypertrophic cardiomyopathy, cardiac tumors, aortic dissection, and pericardial tamponade. Echocardiography also has a role in risk stratification based on the left ventricular ejection fraction.

Treadmill exercise testing with ECG and blood pressure monitoring should be performed in patients who have experienced syncope during or shortly after exercise. Treadmill testing may help identify exercise-induced arrhythmias (e.g., tachycardia-related AV block) and exercise-induced exaggerated vasodilation.

Electrophysiologic studies are indicated in patients with structural heart disease and ECG abnormalities in whom noninvasive investigations have failed to yield a diagnosis. Electrophysiologic studies have low sensitivity and specificity and should only be performed when a high pretest probability exists. Currently, these tests are rarely performed to evaluate patients with syncope.

Psychiatric Evaluation Screening for psychiatric disorders may be appropriate in patients with recurrent unexplained syncope episodes. Tilt-table testing, with demonstration of symptoms in the absence of hemodynamic change, may be useful in reproducing syncope in patients with suspected psychogenic syncope.

FURTHER READING

Brignole M et al: 2018 ESC Guidelines for the diagnosis and management of syncope. Eur Heart J 39:1883, 2018.

Cheshire WP et al: Electrodiagnostic assessment of the autonomic nervous system: a consensus statement endorsed by the American Autonomic Society, American Academy of Neurology, and the International Federation of Clinical Neurophysiology. Clin Neurophysiol 132:666, 2021.

Freeman R et al: Consensus statement on the definition of orthostatic hypotension, neurally mediated syncope and the postural tachycardia syndrome. Auton Neurosci 161:46, 2011.

Freeman R et al: Orthostatic Hypotension: JACC State-of-the-Art Review. J Am Coll Cardiol 72:1294, 2018.

Gibbons CH et al: The recommendations of a consensus panel for the screening, diagnosis, and treatment of neurogenic orthostatic hypotension and associated supine hypertension. J Neurol 264:1567, 2017.

Sheldon RS, Raj SR: Pacing and vasovagal syncope: back to our physiologic roots. Clin Auton Res 27:213, 2017.

Shen WK et al: 2017 ACC/AHA/HRS Guideline for the Evaluation and Management of Patients With Syncope: A Report of the American College of Cardiology/American Heart Association Task Force on Clinical Practice Guidelines and the Heart Rhythm Society. Circulation 136:e60, 2017.

Varosy PD et al: Pacing as a treatment for reflex-mediated (vasovagal, situational, or carotid sinus hypersensitivity) syncope: a systematic review for the 2017 ACC/AHA/HRS guideline for the evaluation and management of patients with syncope: A report of the American College of Cardiology/American Heart Association Task Force on Clinical Practice Guidelines and the Heart Rhythm Society. J Am Coll Cardiol 70:664, 2017.

22 Dizziness and Vertigo

Mark F. Walker, Robert B. Daroff

Dizziness is an imprecise symptom used to describe a variety of common sensations that include vertigo, light-headedness, faintness, and imbalance. *Vertigo* refers to a sense of spinning or other motion that may be physiological, occurring during or after a sustained head rotation, or pathological, due to vestibular dysfunction. The term *light-headedness* is classically applied to presyncopal sensations resulting from brain hypoperfusion but as used by patients has little specificity, as it may also refer to other symptoms such as disequilibrium and imbalance. A challenge to diagnosis is that patients often have difficulty distinguishing among these various symptoms, and the words they choose do not reliably indicate the underlying etiology.

There are many causes of dizziness. Vestibular dizziness (vertigo or imbalance) may be due to peripheral disorders that affect the labyrinths or vestibular nerves, or it may result from disruption of central vestibular pathways. It may be paroxysmal or due to a fixed unilateral or bilateral vestibular deficit. Acute unilateral lesions cause vertigo due to a sudden imbalance in vestibular inputs from the two labyrinths. Bilateral lesions cause imbalance and instability of vision when the head moves (*oscillopsia*) due to loss of normal vestibular reflexes.

Presyncopal dizziness occurs when cardiac dysrhythmia, orthostatic hypotension, medication effects, or another cause leads to brain hypoperfusion. Such presyncopal sensations vary in duration; they may increase in severity until loss of consciousness occurs, or they may resolve before loss of consciousness if the cerebral ischemia is corrected. Faintness and syncope, which are discussed in detail in **Chap. 21**, should always be considered when one is evaluating patients with brief episodes of dizziness or dizziness that occurs with upright posture. Other causes of dizziness include nonvestibular imbalance, gait disorders (e.g., loss of proprioception from sensory neuropathy, parkinsonism), and anxiety.

When evaluating patients with dizziness, questions to consider include the following: (1) Is it dangerous (e.g., arrhythmia, transient ischemic attack/stroke)? (2) Is it vestibular? (3) If vestibular, is it peripheral or central? A careful history and examination often provide sufficient information to answer these questions and determine whether additional studies or referral to a specialist is necessary.

APPROACH TO THE PATIENT

Dizziness

HISTORY

When a patient presents with dizziness, the first step is to delineate more precisely the nature of the symptom. In the case of vestibular disorders, the physical symptoms depend on whether the lesion is unilateral or bilateral, and whether it is acute or chronic. Vertigo, an illusion of self or environmental motion, implies an acute asymmetry of vestibular inputs from the two labyrinths or in their central pathways. Symmetric bilateral vestibular hypofunction causes imbalance but no vertigo. Because of the ambiguity in patients' descriptions of their symptoms, diagnosis based simply on symptom characteristics is typically unreliable. Thus the history should focus closely on other features, including whether this is the first attack, the duration of this and any prior episodes, provoking factors, and accompanying symptoms.

Dizziness can be divided into episodes that last for seconds, minutes, hours, or days. Common causes of brief dizziness (seconds) include benign paroxysmal positional vertigo (BPPV) and orthostatic hypotension, both of which typically are provoked by changes in head and/or body position relative to gravity. Attacks of vestibular migraine and Ménière's disease often last hours. When episodes are of intermediate duration (minutes), transient ischemic attacks of the posterior circulation should be considered, although migraine and other causes are also possible.

Symptoms that accompany vertigo may be helpful in distinguishing peripheral vestibular lesions from central causes. Unilateral hearing loss and other acute aural symptoms (ear pain, pressure, fullness, new tinnitus) typically point to a peripheral cause. Because the auditory pathways quickly become bilateral upon entering the brainstem, central lesions are unlikely to cause unilateral hearing loss unless the lesion lies near the root entry zone of the auditory nerve. Symptoms such as double vision, numbness, and limb ataxia suggest a brainstem or cerebellar lesion.

EXAMINATION

Because dizziness and imbalance can be a manifestation of a variety of neurologic disorders, the neurologic examination is important in the evaluation of these patients. Focus should be given to assessment of eye movements, vestibular function, and hearing. The range of eye movements and whether they are equal in each eye should be observed. Peripheral eye movement disorders (e.g., cranial neuropathies, eye muscle weakness) are usually disconjugate (different in the two eyes). One should check pursuit (the ability to follow a smoothly moving target) and saccades (the ability to look back and forth accurately between two targets). Poor pursuit or inaccurate (dysmetric) saccades usually indicate central pathology, often involving the cerebellum. Alignment of the two eyes can be checked with a cover test: while the patient is looking at a target, alternately cover the eyes and observe for corrective saccades. A vertical misalignment may indicate a brainstem or cerebellar lesion. Finally, one should look for spontaneous nystagmus, an involuntary back-and-forth movement of the eyes. Nystagmus is most often of the jerk type, in which a slow drift (slow phase) in one direction alternates with a rapid saccadic movement (quick phase or fast phase) in the opposite direction that resets the position of the eyes in the orbits. Except in the case of acute vestibulopathy (e.g., vestibular neuritis), if primary position nystagmus is easily seen in the light, it is probably due to a central cause. Two forms of nystagmus that are characteristic of lesions of the cerebellar pathways are vertical nystagmus with downward fast phases (downbeat nystagmus) and horizontal nystagmus that changes direction with gaze (gaze-evoked nystagmus). By contrast, peripheral lesions typically cause unidirectional horizontal nystagmus. Use of Frenzel eyeglasses (self-illuminated goggles with convex lenses that blur the patient's vision but allow the examiner to see the eyes greatly magnified) or infrared video goggles can aid in the detection of peripheral vestibular nystagmus, because they reduce the patient's ability to use visual fixation to suppress nystagmus. **Table 22-1** outlines key findings that help distinguish peripheral from central causes of vertigo.

The most useful bedside test of peripheral vestibular function is the head impulse test, in which the vestibulo-ocular reflex (VOR) is assessed with small-amplitude (~20 degrees) rapid head rotations. While the patient fixates on a target, the head is rotated quickly to the left or right. If the VOR is deficient, the rotation is followed by a catch-up saccade in the opposite direction (e.g., a leftward saccade

TABLE 22-1 Features of Peripheral and Central Vertigo

- Nystagmus from an acute peripheral lesion is unidirectional, with fast phases beating away from the ear with the lesion. Nystagmus that changes direction with gaze is due to a central lesion.
- Transient mixed vertical-torsional nystagmus occurs in benign paroxysmal positional vertigo (BPPV), but pure vertical or pure torsional nystagmus is a central sign.
- Nystagmus from a peripheral lesion may be inhibited by visual fixation, whereas central nystagmus is not suppressed.
- Absence of a head impulse sign in a patient with acute prolonged vertigo should suggest a central cause.
- Unilateral hearing loss suggests peripheral vertigo. Findings such as diplopia, dysarthria, and limb ataxia suggest a central disorder.

after a rightward rotation). The head impulse test can identify both unilateral (catch-up saccades after rotations toward the weak side) and bilateral (catch-up saccades after rotations in both directions) vestibular hypofunction.

All patients with episodic dizziness, especially if provoked by positional change, should be tested with the Dix-Hallpike maneuver. The patient begins in a sitting position with the head turned 45 degrees; holding the back of the head, the examiner then lowers the patient into a supine position with the head extended backward by about 20 degrees while watching the eyes. Posterior canal BPPV can be diagnosed confidently if transient upbeating-torsional nystagmus is seen. If no nystagmus is observed after 15–20 s, the patient is raised to the sitting position, and the procedure is repeated with the head turned to the other side. Again, Frenzel goggles may improve the sensitivity of the test.

Dynamic visual acuity is a functional test that can be useful in assessing vestibular function. Visual acuity is measured with the head still and when the head is rotated back and forth by the examiner (about 1–2 Hz). A drop in visual acuity during head motion of more than one line on a near card or Snellen chart is abnormal and indicates vestibular dysfunction.

ANCILLARY TESTING

The choice of ancillary tests should be guided by the history and examination findings. Audiometry should be performed whenever a vestibular disorder is suspected. Unilateral sensorineural hearing loss supports a peripheral disorder (e.g., vestibular schwannoma). Predominantly low-frequency hearing loss is characteristic of Ménière's disease. Videonystagmography includes recordings of spontaneous nystagmus (if present) and measurement of positional nystagmus. Caloric testing compares the responses of the two horizontal semicircular canals, while video head-impulse testing measures the integrity of each of the six semicircular canals. Vestibular evoked potentials assess otolith reflexes. The test battery often includes recording of saccades and pursuit to evaluate central ocular motor function. Neuroimaging is important if a central vestibular disorder is suspected. In addition, patients with unexplained unilateral hearing loss or vestibular hypofunction should undergo MRI of the internal auditory canals, including administration of gadolinium, to rule out a schwannoma.

DIFFERENTIAL DIAGNOSIS AND TREATMENT

Treatment of vestibular symptoms should be driven by the underlying diagnosis. Simply treating dizziness with vestibular suppressant medications is often not helpful and may make the symptoms worse and prolong recovery. The diagnostic and specific treatment approaches for the most commonly encountered vestibular disorders are discussed below.

ACUTE PROLONGED VERTIGO (VESTIBULAR NEURITIS)

An acute unilateral vestibular lesion causes constant vertigo, nausea, vomiting, oscillopsia (motion of the visual scene), and imbalance. These symptoms are due to a sudden asymmetry of inputs from the two labyrinths or in their central connections, simulating a continuous rotation of the head. Unlike BPPV, continuous vertigo persists even when the head remains still.

When a patient presents with an acute vestibular syndrome, the most important question is whether the lesion is central (e.g., a cerebellar or brainstem infarct or hemorrhage), which may be life-threatening, or peripheral, affecting the vestibular nerve or labyrinth (vestibular neuritis). Attention should be given to any symptoms or signs that point to central dysfunction (diplopia, weakness or numbness, dysarthria). The pattern of spontaneous nystagmus, if present, may be helpful (Table 22-1). If the head impulse test is normal, an acute peripheral vestibular lesion is unlikely. A central lesion cannot always be excluded with certainty based on symptoms and examination alone; thus older patients with vascular risk factors who present with an acute vestibular syndrome should be evaluated for the possibility of stroke even when there are no specific findings that indicate a central lesion.

Most patients with vestibular neuritis recover spontaneously, although chronic dizziness, motion sensitivity, and disequilibrium may persist. The role of early glucocorticoid therapy is uncertain, as studies have yielded disparate results. Antiviral medications are of no proven benefit and are not typically given unless there is evidence to suggest herpes zoster oticus (Ramsay Hunt syndrome). Vestibular suppressant medications may reduce acute symptoms but should be avoided after the first several days because they may impede central compensation and recovery. Patients should be encouraged to resume a normal level of activity as soon as possible, and directed vestibular rehabilitation therapy may accelerate improvement.

BENIGN PAROXYSMAL POSITIONAL VERTIGO

BPPV is a common cause of recurrent vertigo. Episodes are brief (<1 min and typically 15–20 s) and are always provoked by changes in head position relative to gravity, such as lying down, rising from a supine position, and extending the head to look upward. Rolling over in bed is a common trigger that may help to distinguish BPPV from orthostatic hypotension. The attacks are caused by free-floating otoconia (calcium carbonate crystals) that have been dislodged from the utricular macula and have moved into one of the semicircular canals, usually the posterior canal. When head position changes, gravity causes the otoconia to move within the canal, producing vertigo and nystagmus. With posterior canal BPPV, the nystagmus beats upward and torsionally (the upper poles of the eyes beat toward the affected lower ear). Less commonly, the otoconia enter the horizontal canal, resulting in a horizontal nystagmus when the patient is lying with either ear down. Superior (also called anterior) canal involvement is rare. BPPV is treated with repositioning maneuvers that use gravity to remove the otoconia from the semicircular canal. For posterior canal BPPV, the Epley maneuver (**Fig. 22-1**) is the most commonly used procedure. For more refractory cases of BPPV, patients can be taught a variant of this maneuver that they can perform alone at home. A demonstration of the Epley maneuver is available online (*http://www.dizziness-and-balance.com/disorders/bppv/bppv.html*).

VESTIBULAR MIGRAINE

Vestibular migraine is a common yet underdiagnosed cause of episodic vertigo. Vertigo sometimes precedes a typical migraine headache but more often occurs without headache or with only a mild headache. Some patients who have had frequent migraine headaches in the past present later in life with vestibular migraine as the predominant problem. In vestibular migraine, the duration of vertigo may be from minutes to hours, and some migraineurs also experience more prolonged periods of disequilibrium (lasting days to weeks). Motion sensitivity and sensitivity to visual motion (e.g., movies) are common. Even in the absence of headache, other migraine features may be present, such as photophobia, phonophobia, or a visual aura. Although data from controlled studies are generally lacking, vestibular migraine typically is treated with medications that are used for prophylaxis of migraine headaches (**Chap. 430**). Antiemetics may be helpful to relieve symptoms at the time of an attack.

MÉNIÈRE'S DISEASE

Attacks of Ménière's disease consist of vertigo and hearing loss, as well as pain, pressure, and/or fullness in the affected ear. Low-frequency hearing loss and aural symptoms are key features that distinguish Ménière's disease from other peripheral vestibulopathies and from vestibular migraine. Audiometry at the time of an attack shows a characteristic asymmetric low-frequency hearing loss; hearing commonly improves between attacks, although permanent hearing loss may eventually occur. Ménière's disease is associated with excess endolymph fluid in the inner ear; hence the term *endolymphatic hydrops*. The exact pathophysiological mechanism, however, remains unclear. Patients suspected of having Ménière's disease should be referred to an otolaryngologist for further evaluation. Diuretics and sodium restriction are typically the initial treatments. If attacks persist, injections of

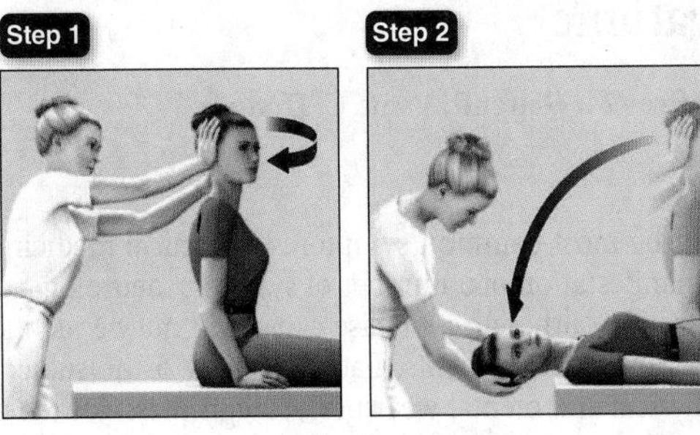

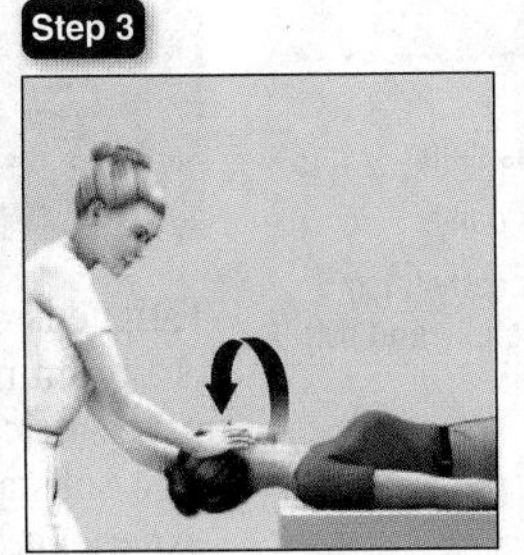

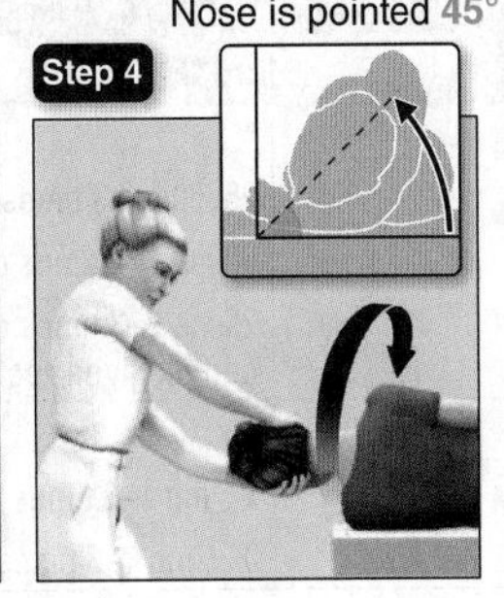

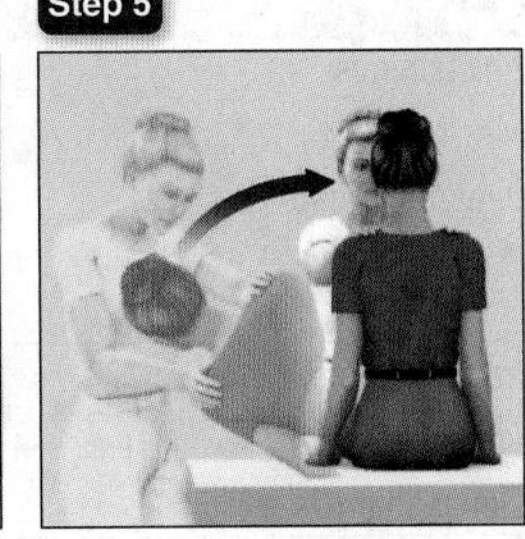

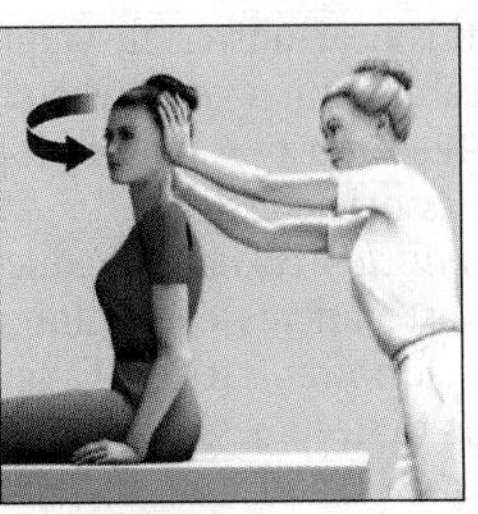
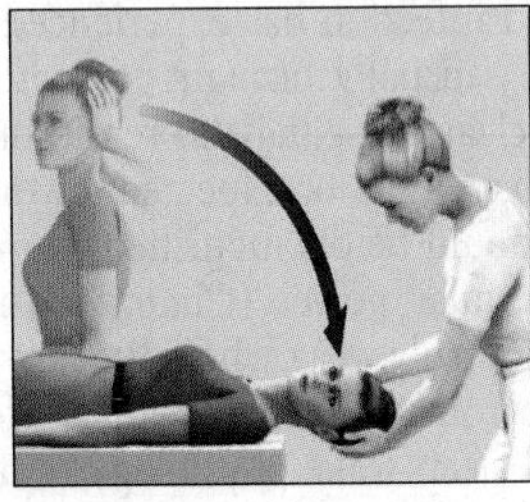
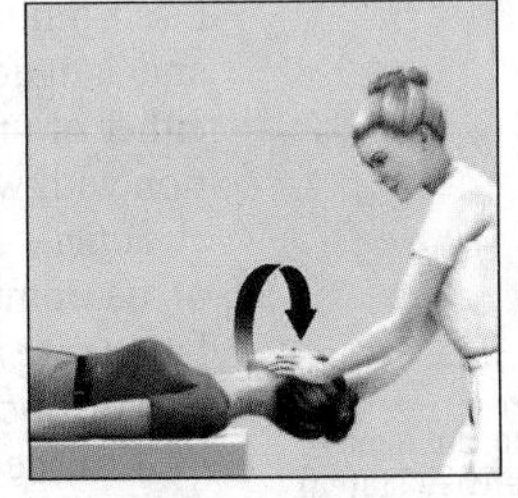
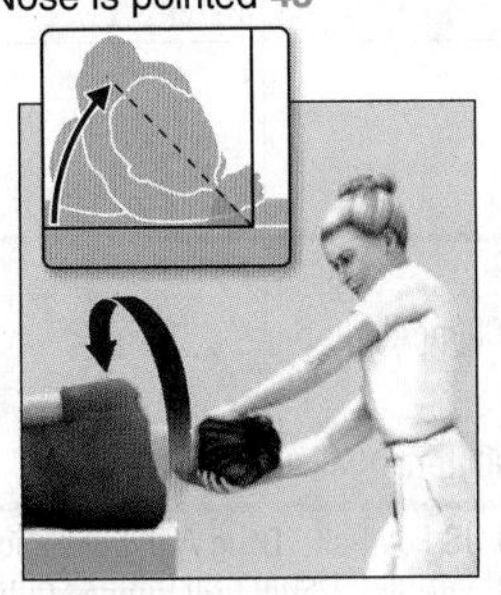

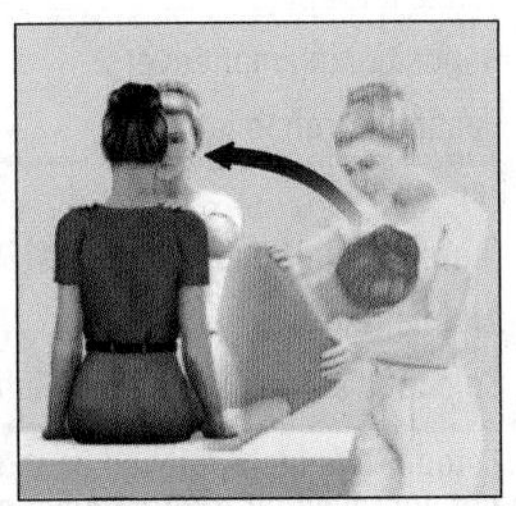

FIGURE 22-1 Modified Epley maneuver for treatment of benign paroxysmal positional vertigo of the right (*top panels*) and left (*bottom panels*) posterior semicircular canals. **Step 1.** With the patient seated, turn the head 45 degrees toward the affected ear. **Step 2.** Keeping the head turned, lower the patient to the head-hanging position and hold for at least 30 s and until nystagmus disappears. **Step 3.** Without lifting the head, turn it 90 degrees toward the other side. Hold for another 30 s. **Step 4.** Rotate the patient onto her side while turning the head another 90 degrees, so that the nose is pointed down 45 degrees. Hold again for 30 s. **Step 5.** Have the patient sit up on the side of the table. After a brief rest, the maneuver should be repeated to confirm successful treatment. *(Reproduced with permission from Chicago dizziness and Hearing (CDH). Figure adapted from http://www.dizziness-and-balance.com/disorders/bppv/movies/Epley-480x640.avi)*

glucocorticoids or gentamicin into the middle ear may be considered. Nonablative surgical options include decompression and shunting of the endolymphatic sac. Full ablative procedures (vestibular nerve section, labyrinthectomy) are seldom required.

VESTIBULAR SCHWANNOMA

Vestibular schwannomas (sometimes termed *acoustic neuromas*) and other tumors at the cerebellopontine angle cause slowly progressive unilateral sensorineural hearing loss and vestibular hypofunction. These patients typically do not have vertigo, because the gradual vestibular deficit is compensated centrally as it develops. The diagnosis often is not made until there is sufficient hearing loss to be noticed. The vestibular examination will show a deficient response to the head impulse test when the head is rotated toward the affected side, but nystagmus will not be prominent. As noted above, patients with unexplained unilateral sensorineural hearing loss or vestibular hypofunction require MRI of the internal auditory canals to look for a schwannoma.

BILATERAL VESTIBULAR HYPOFUNCTION

Patients with bilateral loss of vestibular function also typically do not have vertigo, because vestibular function is lost on both sides simultaneously, and there is no asymmetry of vestibular input. Symptoms include loss of balance, particularly in the dark, where vestibular input is most critical, and oscillopsia during head movement, such as while walking or riding in a car. Bilateral vestibular hypofunction may be (1) idiopathic and progressive, (2) part of a neurodegenerative disorder, or (3) iatrogenic due to medication ototoxicity (most commonly gentamicin or other aminoglycoside antibiotics). Other causes include bilateral vestibular schwannomas (neurofibromatosis type 2), autoimmune disease, superficial siderosis, and meningeal-based infection or tumor. It also may occur in patients with peripheral polyneuropathy; in these patients, both vestibular loss and impaired proprioception may contribute to poor balance. Finally, unilateral processes such as vestibular neuritis and Ménière's disease may involve both ears sequentially, resulting in bilateral vestibulopathy.

Examination findings include diminished *dynamic visual acuity* (see above) due to loss of stable vision when the head is moving, abnormal head impulse responses in both directions, and a Romberg sign. Responses to caloric testing are reduced. Patients with bilateral vestibular hypofunction should be referred for vestibular rehabilitation therapy. Vestibular suppressant medications should not be used, as they will increase the imbalance. Evaluation by a neurologist is important not only to confirm the diagnosis but also to consider any other associated neurologic abnormalities that may clarify the etiology.

CENTRAL VESTIBULAR DISORDERS

Central lesions causing vertigo typically involve vestibular pathways in the brainstem and/or cerebellum. They may be due to discrete lesions, such as from ischemic or hemorrhagic stroke (**Chaps. 426–428**), demyelination (**Chap. 444**), or tumors (**Chap. 90**), or they may be due to neurodegenerative conditions that include the vestibulocerebellum (**Chaps. 431–434**). Subacute cerebellar degeneration may be due to immune, including paraneoplastic, processes (**Chaps. 94 and 439**). Table 22-1 outlines important features of the history and examination that help to identify central vestibular disorders. Acute central vertigo is a medical emergency, due to the possibility of life-threatening stroke or hemorrhage. All patients with suspected central vestibular disorders should undergo brain MRI, and the patient should be referred for full neurologic evaluation.

PSYCHOSOMATIC AND FUNCTIONAL DIZZINESS

Psychological factors play an important role in chronic dizziness. First, dizziness may be a somatic manifestation of a psychiatric condition such as major depression, anxiety, or panic disorder (**Chap. 452**). Second, patients may develop anxiety and autonomic symptoms as a consequence or comorbidity of an independent vestibular disorder. One particular form of this has been termed variously *phobic postural vertigo*, *psychophysiologic vertigo*, or *chronic subjective dizziness*, but is now referred to as *persistent postural-perceptual dizziness (PPPD)*. These patients have a chronic feeling (3 months or longer) of fluctuating dizziness and disequilibrium that is present at rest but worse while standing. There is an increased sensitivity to self-motion and visual motion (e.g., watching movies), and a particular intensification of symptoms when moving through complex visual environments such as supermarkets. Although there may be a past history of an acute vestibular disorder (e.g., vestibular neuritis), the neuro-otologic examination

TABLE 22-2 Treatment of Vertigo

AGENT[a]	DOSE[b]
Antihistamines	
Meclizine	25–50 mg 3 times daily
Dimenhydrinate	50 mg 1–2 times daily
Promethazine	25 mg 2–3 times daily (also can be given rectally and IM)
Benzodiazepines	
Diazepam	2.5 mg 1–3 times daily
Clonazepam	0.25 mg 1–3 times daily
Anticholinergic	
Scopolamine transdermal[c]	Patch
Physical therapy	
Repositioning maneuvers[d]	
Vestibular rehabilitation	
Other	
Diuretics and/or low-sodium (1000 mg/d) diet[e]	
Antimigrainous drugs[f]	
Selective serotonin reuptake inhibitors[g]	

[a]All listed drugs are approved by the US Food and Drug Administration, but most are not approved for the treatment of vertigo. [b]Usual oral (unless otherwise stated) starting dose in adults; a higher maintenance dose can be reached by a gradual increase. [c]For motion sickness only. [d]For benign paroxysmal positional vertigo. [e]For Ménière's disease. [f]For vestibular migraine. [g]For persistent postural-perceptual vertigo and anxiety.

and vestibular testing are normal or indicative of a compensated vestibular deficit, indicating that the ongoing subjective dizziness cannot be explained by a primary vestibular pathology. Anxiety disorders are particularly common in patients with chronic dizziness; when present, they contribute substantially to the morbidity. Treatment approaches for PPPD include pharmacological therapy with selective serotonin reuptake inhibitors (SSRIs), cognitive-behavioral psychotherapy, and vestibular rehabilitation. Vestibular suppressant medications generally should be avoided.

TREATMENT

Vertigo

Table 22-2 provides a list of commonly used medications for suppression of vertigo. As noted, these medications should be reserved for short-term control of active vertigo, such as during the first few days of acute vestibular neuritis, or for acute attacks of Ménière's disease. They are less helpful for chronic dizziness and, as previously stated, may hinder central compensation. An exception is that benzodiazepines may attenuate psychosomatic dizziness and the associated anxiety, although SSRIs are generally preferable in such patients.

Vestibular rehabilitation therapy promotes central adaptation processes that compensate for vestibular loss and also may help habituate motion sensitivity and other symptoms of psychosomatic dizziness. The general approach is to use a graded series of exercises that progressively challenge gaze stabilization and balance.

■ FURTHER READING

Altissimi G et al: Drugs inducing hearing loss, tinnitus, dizziness and vertigo: An updated guide. Eur Rev Med Pharmacol Sci 24:7946, 2020.

Huang TC et al: Vestibular migraine: An update on current understanding and future directions. Cephalalgia 40:107, 2020.

Kim JS, Zee DS: Benign paroxysmal positional vertigo. N Engl J Med 370:1138, 2014.

Popkirov S et al: Persistent postural-perceptual dizziness (PPPD): a common, characteristic and treatable cause of chronic dizziness. Pract Neurol 18:5, 2018.

23 Fatigue

Jeffrey M. Gelfand, Vanja C. Douglas

Fatigue is one of the most common symptoms in clinical medicine. It is a prominent manifestation of a number of systemic, neurologic, and psychiatric syndromes, although a precise cause will not be identified in a substantial minority of patients. Fatigue refers to the subjective experience of physical and mental weariness, sluggishness, low energy, and exhaustion. In the context of clinical medicine, fatigue is most practically defined as difficulty initiating or maintaining voluntary mental or physical activity. Nearly everyone who has ever been ill with a self-limited infection has experienced this near-universal symptom, and fatigue is usually brought to medical attention only when it is either of unclear cause, fails to remit, or the severity is out of proportion with what would be expected for the associated trigger.

Fatigue should be distinguished from *muscle weakness*, a reduction of neuromuscular power (**Chap. 24**); most patients complaining of fatigue are not truly weak when direct muscle power is tested. Fatigue is also distinct from *somnolence*, which refers to sleepiness in the context of disturbed sleep-wake physiology (**Chap. 31**), and from *dyspnea on exertion*, although patients may use the word fatigue to describe any of these symptoms. The task facing clinicians when a patient presents with fatigue is to identify the underlying cause and develop a therapeutic alliance, the goal of which is to spare patients expensive and fruitless diagnostic workups and steer them toward effective therapy.

■ EPIDEMIOLOGY AND GLOBAL CONSIDERATIONS

Variability in the definitions of fatigue and the survey instruments used in different studies makes it difficult to arrive at precise figures about the global burden of fatigue. The point prevalence of fatigue was 6.7% and the lifetime prevalence was 25% in a large National Institute of Mental Health survey of the U.S. general population. In primary care clinics in Europe and the United States, between 10 and 25% of patients surveyed endorsed symptoms of prolonged (present for >1 month) or chronic (present for >6 months) fatigue, but in only a minority was fatigue the primary reason for seeking medical attention. In a community survey of women in India, 12% reported chronic fatigue. By contrast, the prevalence of chronic fatigue syndrome (**Chap. 450**), as defined by the U.S. Centers for Disease Control and Prevention, is low.

■ DIFFERENTIAL DIAGNOSIS

Psychiatric Disease Fatigue is a common somatic manifestation of many major psychiatric syndromes, including depression, anxiety, and somatoform disorders (**Chap. 452**). Psychiatric symptoms are reported in more than three-quarters of patients with unexplained chronic fatigue. Even in patients with systemic or neurologic disorders in which fatigue is independently recognized as a symptom, comorbid psychiatric disease may still be an important contributor.

Neurologic Disease Patients complaining of fatigue often say they feel weak, but upon careful examination, objective muscle weakness is rarely discernible. If found, muscle weakness must then be localized to the central nervous system, peripheral nervous system, neuromuscular junction, or muscle, and appropriate follow-up studies obtained (**Chap. 24**). *Fatigability* of muscle power is a cardinal manifestation of some neuromuscular disorders such as myasthenia gravis and is distinguished from *fatigue* by finding clinically evident diminution of the amount of force that a muscle generates upon repeated contraction (**Chap. 448**). Fatigue is one of the most common and bothersome symptoms reported in multiple sclerosis (MS) (**Chap. 444**), affecting nearly 90% of patients; fatigue in MS can persist between MS attacks and does not necessarily correlate with magnetic resonance imaging (MRI) disease activity. Fatigue is also increasingly identified as a troublesome feature of many neurodegenerative diseases, including Parkinson's disease (**Chap. 435**), amyotrophic lateral sclerosis

(Chap. 437), and central nervous system dysautonomias (Chap. 440). Fatigue after stroke (Chap. 426) is a well-described but poorly understood entity with a widely varying prevalence. Episodic fatigue can be a premonitory symptom of migraine (Chap. 430). Fatigue is also a frequent consequence of traumatic brain injury (Chap. 443), often occurring in association with depression and sleep disorders.

Sleep Disorders Obstructive sleep apnea is an important cause of excessive daytime sleepiness in association with fatigue and should be investigated using overnight polysomnography, particularly in those with prominent snoring, obesity, or other predictors of obstructive sleep apnea (Chap. 297). Whether the cumulative sleep deprivation that is common in modern society contributes to clinically apparent fatigue is not known (Chap. 31).

Endocrine Disorders Fatigue, sometimes in association with true muscle weakness, can be a heralding symptom of hypothyroidism (Chap. 383), particularly in the context of hair loss, dry skin, cold intolerance, constipation, and weight gain. Fatigue associated with heat intolerance, sweating, and palpitations is typical of hyperthyroidism (Chap. 384). Adrenal insufficiency (Chap. 386) can also manifest with unexplained fatigue as a primary or prominent symptom, often with anorexia, weight loss, nausea, myalgias, and arthralgias; hyponatremia, hyperkalemia, and hyperpigmentation may be present at time of diagnosis. Mild hypercalcemia can cause fatigue, which may be relatively vague, whereas severe hypercalcemia can lead to lethargy, stupor, and coma (Chap. 410). Both hypoglycemia and hyperglycemia can cause lethargy, often in association with confusion; diabetes mellitus, and in particular type 1 diabetes, is also associated with fatigue independent of glucose levels (Chap. 403). Fatigue may also accompany Cushing's disease, hypoaldosteronism, and hypogonadism. Low vitamin D status has also been associated with fatigue.

Liver and Kidney Disease Both chronic liver failure and chronic kidney disease can cause fatigue. Over 80% of hemodialysis patients complain of fatigue, which makes it one of the most common symptoms reported by patients in chronic kidney disease (Chap. 311).

Obesity Obesity (Chap. 401) is associated with fatigue and sleepiness independent of the presence of obstructive sleep apnea. Obese patients undergoing bariatric surgery experience improvement in daytime sleepiness sooner than would be expected if the improvement were solely the result of weight loss and resolution of sleep apnea. A number of other factors common in obese patients are likely contributors as well, including physical inactivity, diabetes, and depression.

Physical Inactivity Physical inactivity is associated with fatigue, and increasing physical activity can improve fatigue in some patients.

Malnutrition Although fatigue can be a presenting feature of malnutrition (Chap. 334), nutritional status may also be an important comorbidity and contributor to fatigue in other chronic illnesses, including cancer-associated fatigue.

Infection Both acute and chronic infections commonly lead to fatigue as part of the broader infectious syndrome. Evaluation for undiagnosed infection as the cause of unexplained fatigue, and particularly prolonged or chronic fatigue, should be guided by the history, physical examination, and infectious risk factors, with particular attention to risk for tuberculosis, HIV, chronic hepatitis, and endocarditis. Infectious mononucleosis may cause prolonged fatigue that persists for weeks to months following the acute illness, but infection with the Epstein-Barr virus is only very rarely the cause of unexplained chronic fatigue. Postinfectious fatigue may also occur following a variety of acute infections. For example, a substantial minority of patients who have recovered from SARS-CoV-1, SARS-CoV-2, and Ebola virus complain of persistent fatigue.

Drugs Many medications, drugs, drug withdrawal, and chronic alcohol use can all lead to fatigue. Medications that are more likely to be causative include antidepressants, antipsychotics, anxiolytics, opiates, antispasticity agents, antiseizure agents, and beta blockers.

Cardiovascular and Pulmonary Disorders Fatigue is one of the most taxing symptoms reported by patients with congestive heart failure and chronic obstructive pulmonary disease and negatively affects quality of life. In a population-based cohort study in Norfolk, United Kingdom, fatigue was associated with an increased hazard of all-cause mortality in the general population, but particularly for deaths related to cardiovascular disease.

Malignancy Fatigue, particularly in association with unexplained weight loss, can be a sign of occult malignancy, but cancer is rarely identified in patients with unexplained chronic fatigue in the absence of other telltale signs or symptoms. Cancer-related fatigue is experienced by 40% of patients at the time of diagnosis and by >80% at some time in the disease course.

Hematologic Disorders Chronic or progressive anemia may present with fatigue, sometimes in association with exertional tachycardia and breathlessness. Anemia may also contribute to fatigue in chronic illness. Low serum ferritin in the absence of anemia may also cause fatigue that is reversible with iron replacement.

Immune-Mediated Disorders Fatigue is a prominent complaint in many chronic inflammatory disorders, including systemic lupus erythematosus, polymyalgia rheumatica, rheumatoid arthritis, inflammatory bowel disease, antineutrophil cytoplasmic antibody (ANCA)–associated vasculitis, sarcoidosis, and Sjögren's syndrome, but is not usually an isolated symptom. Fatigue is also associated with primary immunodeficiency diseases.

Pregnancy Fatigue is very commonly reported by women during all stages of pregnancy and postpartum.

Disorders of Unclear Cause Myalgic encephalomyelitis (ME)/chronic fatigue syndrome (CFS) (Chap. 450) and fibromyalgia (Chap. 373) incorporate chronic fatigue as part of the syndromic definition when fatigue is present in association with other criteria, as discussed in the respective chapters. Chronic multisymptom illness, also known as Gulf-War syndrome, is another symptom complex with prominent fatigue; it is most commonly, although not exclusively, observed in veterans of the 1991 Gulf War conflict (Chap. S7). Idiopathic chronic fatigue is used to describe the syndrome of unexplained chronic fatigue in the absence of enough additional clinical features to meet the diagnostic criteria for ME/CFS.

APPROACH TO THE PATIENT
Fatigue

A detailed history focusing on the quality, pattern, time course, associated symptoms, and alleviating factors of fatigue is necessary to define the syndrome and help direct further evaluation and treatment. It is important to determine if fatigue is the appropriate designation, whether symptoms are acute or chronic, and if the impairment is primarily mental, physical, or a combination of the two. The review of systems should attempt to distinguish fatigue from excessive sleepiness, dyspnea on exertion, exercise intolerance, and muscle weakness. The presence of fever, chills, night sweats, or weight loss should raise suspicion for an occult infection or malignancy. A careful review of prescription, over-the-counter, herbal, and recreational drug and alcohol use is required. Circumstances surrounding the onset of symptoms and potential triggers should be investigated. The social history is important, with attention paid to life stressors and adverse experiences, workhours, the social support network, and domestic affairs including a screen for intimate partner violence. Sleep habits and sleep hygiene should be questioned. The impact of fatigue on daily functioning is important to understand the patient's experience and gauge recovery and the success of treatment.

The physical examination of patients with fatigue is guided by the history and differential diagnosis. A detailed mental status examination should be performed with particular attention to symptoms of depression and anxiety. A formal neurologic examination is required to determine whether objective muscle weakness is present. This is usually a straightforward exercise, although occasionally patients with fatigue have difficulty sustaining effort against resistance and sometimes report that generating full power requires substantial mental effort. On confrontational testing, full power may be generated for only a brief period before the patient suddenly gives way to the examiner. This type of weakness is often referred to as *breakaway weakness* and may or may not be associated with pain. This is contrasted with weakness due to lesions in the motor tracts or lower motor unit, in which the patient's resistance can be overcome in a smooth and steady fashion and full power can never be generated. Occasionally, a patient may demonstrate fatigable weakness, in which power is full when first tested but becomes weak upon repeat evaluation without interval rest. Fatigable weakness, which usually indicates a problem of neuromuscular transmission, never has the sudden breakaway quality that one occasionally observes in patients with fatigue. If the presence or absence of muscle weakness cannot be determined with the physical examination, electromyography with nerve conductions studies can be a helpful ancillary test.

The general physical examination should screen for signs of cardiopulmonary disease, malignancy, lymphadenopathy, organomegaly, infection, liver failure, kidney disease, malnutrition, endocrine abnormalities, and connective tissue disease. In patients with associated widespread musculoskeletal pain, assessment of tender points may help to reveal fibromyalgia. Although the diagnostic yield of the general physical examination may be relatively low in the context of evaluation of unexplained chronic fatigue, elucidating the cause of only 2% of cases in one prospective analysis, the yield of a detailed neuropsychiatric and mental status evaluation is likely to be much higher, revealing a potential explanation for fatigue in up to 75–80% of patients in some series. Furthermore, a complete physical examination demonstrates a serious and systematic approach to the patient's complaint and helps build trust and a therapeutic alliance.

Laboratory testing is likely to identify the cause of chronic fatigue in only about 5% of cases. Beyond a few standard screening tests, laboratory evaluation should be guided by the history and physical examination; extensive testing is likely to lead to incidental findings that require explanation and unnecessary follow-up investigation, and should be avoided in lieu of frequent clinical follow-up. A reasonable approach to screening includes a complete blood count with differential (to screen for anemia, infection, and malignancy), electrolytes (including sodium, potassium, and calcium), glucose, renal function, liver function, and thyroid function. Testing for HIV and adrenal function can also be considered. Published guidelines for chronic fatigue syndrome also recommend an erythrocyte sedimentation rate (ESR) as part of the evaluation for mimics, but unless the value is very high, such nonspecific testing in the absence of other features is unlikely to clarify the situation. Routine screening with an antinuclear antibody (ANA) test is also unlikely to be informative in isolation and is frequently positive at low titers in otherwise healthy adults. Additional unfocused studies, such as whole-body imaging scans, are usually not indicated; in addition to their inconvenience, potential risk, and cost, they often reveal unrelated incidental findings that can prolong the workup unnecessarily.

TREATMENT

Fatigue

The first priority is to address the underlying disorder or disorders that account for fatigue, because this can be curative in select contexts and palliative in others. Unfortunately, in many chronic illnesses, fatigue may be refractory to traditional disease-modifying therapies, but it is nevertheless important in such cases to evaluate for other potential contributors because the cause may be multifactorial. Antidepressants **(Chap. 452)** may be helpful for treatment of chronic fatigue when symptoms of depression are present and are generally most effective as part of a multimodal approach. However, antidepressants can also cause fatigue and should be discontinued if they are not clearly effective. Cognitive-behavioral therapy has also been demonstrated to be helpful in ME/CFS as well as cancer-associated fatigue. Both cognitive-behavioral therapy and graded exercise therapy, in which physical exercise, most typically walking, is gradually increased with attention to target heart rates to avoid overexertion, were shown to modestly improve walking times and self-reported fatigue measures when compared to standard medical care in patients in the United Kingdom with chronic fatigue. These benefits were maintained after a median follow-up of 2.5 years. Psychostimulants such as amphetamines, modafinil, and armodafinil can help increase alertness and concentration and reduce excessive daytime sleepiness in certain clinical contexts, which may in turn help with symptoms of fatigue in a minority of patients, but they have generally proven to be unhelpful in randomized trials for treating fatigue in posttraumatic brain injury, Parkinson's disease, cancer, and MS. In patients with low vitamin D status, vitamin D replacement may lead to improvement in fatigue.

Development of more effective therapy for fatigue is hampered by limited knowledge of the biologic basis of this symptom, including how fatigue is detected and registered in the nervous system. Proinflammatory cytokines, such as interleukin 1α and 1β and tumor necrosis factor α, might mediate fatigue in some patients. While preliminary studies of biologic therapies that inhibit cytokines have suggested a benefit against fatigue in some patients with inflammatory conditions, this approach has largely not led to improvement in clinical trials that focused on fatigue as the primary endpoint. Nonetheless, specific targeting with cytokine antagonists could represent a possible future approach for some patients.

PROGNOSIS

Acute fatigue significant enough to require medical evaluation is more likely to lead to an identifiable medical, neurologic, or psychiatric cause than is unexplained chronic fatigue. Evaluation of unexplained chronic fatigue most commonly leads to diagnosis of a psychiatric condition or remains unexplained. Identification of a previously undiagnosed serious or life-threatening culprit etiology is rare, even with longitudinal follow-up of patients with unexplained chronic fatigue. Complete resolution is uncommon, at least over the short term, but multidisciplinary treatment approaches can lead to symptomatic improvements that substantially improve quality of life.

FURTHER READING

Basu N et al: Fatigue is associated with excess mortality in the general population: Results from the EPIC-Norfolk study. BMC Med 14:122, 2016.

Dukes JC et al: Approach to fatigue: Best practice. Med Clin North Am 105:137, 2021.

Roerink ME et al: Interleukin-1 as a mediator of fatigue in disease: A narrative review. J Neuroinflammation 14:16, 2017.

Sharpe M et al: Rehabilitative treatments for chronic fatigue syndrome: Long-term follow-up from the PACE trial. Lancet Psychiatry 2:1067, 2015.

White PD et al: Comparison of adaptive pacing therapy, cognitive behaviour therapy, graded exercise therapy, and specialist medical care for chronic fatigue syndrome (PACE): A randomised trial. Lancet 377:823, 2011.

24 Neurologic Causes of Weakness and Paralysis

Stephen L. Hauser

Normal motor function involves integrated muscle activity that is modulated by the activity of the cerebral cortex, basal ganglia, cerebellum, red nucleus, brainstem reticular formation, lateral vestibular nucleus, and spinal cord. Motor system dysfunction leads to weakness or paralysis, discussed in this chapter, or to ataxia (**Chap. 439**) or abnormal movements (**Chap. 436**). *Weakness* is a reduction in the power that can be exerted by one or more muscles. It must be distinguished from increased *fatigability* (i.e., the inability to sustain the performance of an activity that should be normal for a person of the same age, sex, and size), limitation in function due to pain or articular stiffness, or impaired motor activity because severe *proprioceptive sensory loss* prevents adequate feedback information about the direction and power of movements. It is also distinct from *bradykinesia* (in which increased time is required for full power to be exerted) and *apraxia*, a disorder of planning and initiating a skilled or learned movement unrelated to a significant motor or sensory deficit (**Chap. 30**).

Paralysis or the suffix "-plegia" indicates weakness so severe that a muscle cannot be contracted at all, whereas *paresis* refers to less severe weakness. The prefix "hemi-" refers to one-half of the body, "para-" to both legs, and "quadri-" to all four limbs.

The *distribution* of weakness helps to localize the underlying lesion. Weakness from involvement of upper motor neurons occurs particularly in the extensors and abductors of the upper limb and the flexors of the lower limb. Lower motor neuron weakness depends on whether involvement is at the level of the anterior horn cells, nerve root, limb plexus, or peripheral nerve—only muscles supplied by the affected structure are weak. Myopathic weakness is generally most marked in proximal muscles. Weakness from impaired neuromuscular transmission has no specific pattern of involvement.

Weakness often is accompanied by other neurologic abnormalities that help indicate the site of the responsible lesion (**Table 24-1**).

Tone is the resistance of a muscle to passive stretch. Increased tone may be of several types. *Spasticity* is the increase in tone associated with disease of upper motor neurons. It is velocity dependent, has a sudden release after reaching a maximum (the "clasp-knife" phenomenon), and predominantly affects the antigravity muscles (i.e., upper-limb flexors and lower-limb extensors). *Rigidity* is hypertonia that is present throughout the range of motion (a "lead pipe" or "plastic" stiffness) and affects flexors and extensors equally; it sometimes has a cogwheel quality that is enhanced by voluntary movement of the contralateral limb (reinforcement). Rigidity occurs with certain extrapyramidal disorders, such as Parkinson's disease. *Paratonia* (or *gegenhalten*) is increased tone that varies irregularly in a manner seemingly related to the degree of relaxation, is present throughout the range of motion, and affects flexors and extensors equally; it usually results from disease of the frontal lobes. Weakness with *decreased tone (flaccidity)* or normal tone occurs with disorders of *motor units*. A motor unit consists of a single lower motor neuron and all the muscle fibers that it innervates.

Muscle bulk generally is not affected by upper motor neuron lesions, although mild disuse atrophy eventually may occur. By contrast, atrophy is often conspicuous when a lower motor neuron lesion is responsible for weakness and also may occur with advanced muscle disease.

Muscle stretch (tendon) reflexes are usually increased with upper motor neuron lesions but may be decreased or absent for a variable period immediately after onset of an acute lesion. Hyperreflexia is usually—but not invariably—accompanied by loss of *cutaneous reflexes* (such as superficial abdominals; **Chap. 422**) and, in particular, by an extensor plantar (Babinski) response. The muscle stretch reflexes are depressed with lower motor neuron lesions directly involving specific reflex arcs. They generally are preserved in patients with myopathic weakness except in advanced stages, when they sometimes are attenuated. In disorders of the neuromuscular junction, reflex responses may be affected by preceding voluntary activity of affected muscles; such activity may lead to enhancement of initially depressed reflexes in Lambert-Eaton myasthenic syndrome and, conversely, to depression of initially normal reflexes in myasthenia gravis (**Chap. 448**).

The distinction of *neuropathic* (lower motor neuron) from *myopathic* weakness is sometimes difficult clinically, although distal weakness is likely to be neuropathic, and symmetric proximal weakness myopathic. *Fasciculations* (visible or palpable twitches within a muscle due to the spontaneous discharge of a motor unit) and early atrophy indicate that weakness is neuropathic.

PATHOGENESIS

Upper Motor Neuron Weakness Lesions of the upper motor neurons or their descending axons to the spinal cord (**Fig. 24-1**) produce weakness through decreased activation of lower motor neurons. In general, distal muscle groups are affected more severely than proximal ones, and axial movements are spared unless the lesion is severe and bilateral. Spasticity is typical but may not be present acutely. Rapid repetitive movements are slowed and coarse, but normal rhythmicity is maintained. With corticobulbar involvement, weakness occurs in the lower face and tongue; extraocular, upper facial, pharyngeal, and jaw muscles are typically spared. Bilateral corticobulbar lesions produce a *pseudobulbar palsy*: dysarthria, dysphagia, dysphonia, and emotional lability accompany bilateral facial weakness and a brisk jaw jerk. Electromyogram (EMG) (**Chap. 446**) shows that with weakness of the upper motor neuron type, motor units have a diminished maximal discharge frequency.

Lower Motor Neuron Weakness This pattern results from disorders of lower motor neurons in the brainstem motor nuclei and the anterior horn of the spinal cord or from dysfunction of the axons of these neurons as they pass to skeletal muscle (**Fig. 24-2**). Weakness is due to a decrease in the number of muscle fibers that can be activated through a loss of α motor neurons or disruption of their connections to muscle. Loss of γ motor neurons does not cause weakness but decreases tension on the muscle spindles, which decreases muscle tone and attenuates the stretch reflexes. An absent stretch reflex suggests involvement of spindle afferent fibers.

When a motor unit becomes diseased, especially in anterior horn cell diseases, it may discharge spontaneously, producing *fasciculations*. When α motor neurons or their axons degenerate, the denervated muscle fibers also may discharge spontaneously. These single muscle

TABLE 24-1 Signs That Distinguish the Origin of Weakness

SIGN	UPPER MOTOR NEURON	LOWER MOTOR NEURON	MYOPATHIC	PSYCHOGENIC
Atrophy	None	Severe	Mild	None
Fasciculations	None	Common	None	None
Tone	Spastic	Decreased	Normal/decreased	Variable/paratonia
Distribution of weakness	Pyramidal/regional	Distal/segmental	Proximal	Variable/inconsistent with daily activities
Muscle stretch reflexes	Hyperactive	Hypoactive/absent	Normal/hypoactive	Normal
Babinski sign	Present	Absent	Absent	Absent

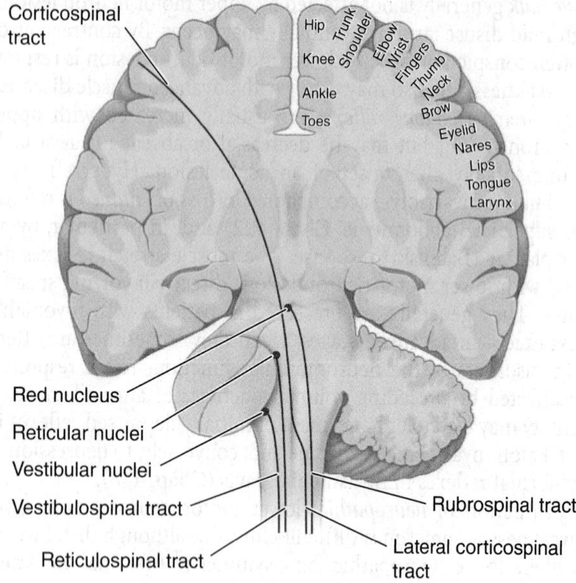

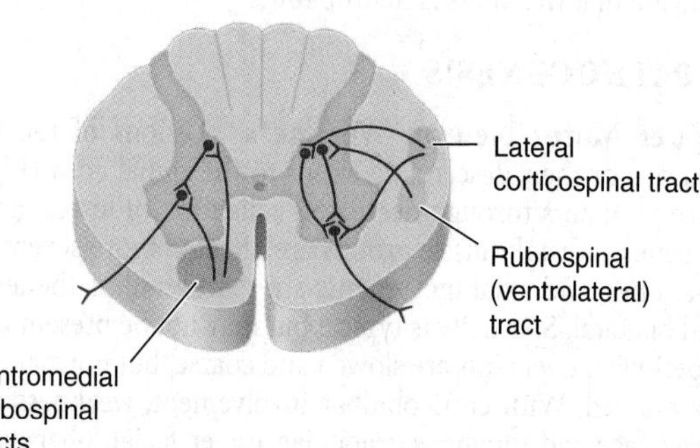

FIGURE 24-1 The corticospinal and bulbospinal upper motor neuron pathways. Upper motor neurons have their cell bodies in layer V of the primary motor cortex (the precentral gyrus, or Brodmann area 4) and in the premotor and supplemental motor cortex (area 6). The upper motor neurons in the primary motor cortex are somatotopically organized (*right side of figure*). Axons of the upper motor neurons descend through the subcortical white matter and the posterior limb of the internal capsule. Axons of the pyramidal or corticospinal system descend through the brainstem in the cerebral peduncle of the midbrain, the basis pontis, and the medullary pyramids. At the cervicomedullary junction, most corticospinal axons decussate into the contralateral corticospinal tract of the lateral spinal cord, but 10–30% remain ipsilateral in the anterior spinal cord. Corticospinal neurons synapse on premotor interneurons, but some—especially in the cervical enlargement and those connecting with motor neurons to distal limb muscles—make direct monosynaptic connections with lower motor neurons. They innervate most densely the lower motor neurons of hand muscles and are involved in the execution of learned, fine movements. Corticobulbar neurons are similar to corticospinal neurons but innervate brainstem motor nuclei. Bulbospinal upper motor neurons influence strength and tone but are not part of the pyramidal system. The descending ventromedial bulbospinal pathways originate in the tectum of the midbrain (tectospinal pathway), the vestibular nuclei (vestibulospinal pathway), and the reticular formation (reticulospinal pathway). These pathways influence axial and proximal muscles and are involved in the maintenance of posture and integrated movements of the limbs and trunk. The descending ventrolateral bulbospinal pathways, which originate predominantly in the red nucleus (rubrospinal pathway), facilitate distal limb muscles. The bulbospinal system sometimes is referred to as the extrapyramidal upper motor neuron system. In all figures, nerve cell bodies and axon terminals are shown, respectively, as *closed circles* and *forks*.

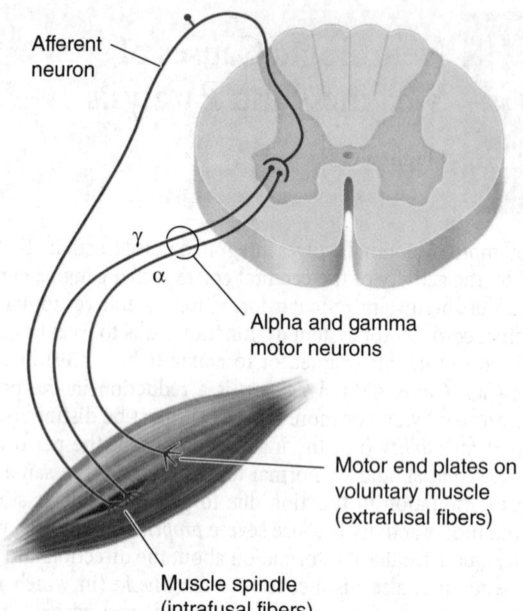

FIGURE 24-2 Lower motor neurons are divided into α and γ types. The larger α motor neurons are more numerous and innervate the extrafusal muscle fibers of the motor unit. Loss of α motor neurons or disruption of their axons produces lower motor neuron weakness. The smaller, less numerous γ motor neurons innervate the intrafusal muscle fibers of the muscle spindle and contribute to normal tone and stretch reflexes. The α motor neuron receives direct excitatory input from corticomotoneurons and primary muscle spindle afferents. The α and γ motor neurons also receive excitatory input from other descending upper motor neuron pathways, segmental sensory inputs, and interneurons. The α motor neurons receive direct inhibition from Renshaw cell interneurons, and other interneurons indirectly inhibit the α and γ motor neurons. A muscle stretch (tendon) reflex requires the function of all the illustrated structures. A tap on a tendon stretches muscle spindles (which are tonically activated by γ motor neurons) and activates the primary spindle afferent neurons. These neurons stimulate the α motor neurons in the spinal cord, producing a brief muscle contraction, which is the familiar tendon reflex.

fiber discharges, or *fibrillation potentials*, cannot be seen but can be recorded with EMG. Weakness leads to delayed or reduced recruitment of motor units, with fewer than normal activated at a particular discharge frequency.

Neuromuscular Junction Weakness Disorders of the neuromuscular junction produce weakness of variable degree and distribution. The number of muscle fibers that are activated varies over time, depending on the state of rest of the neuromuscular junctions. Strength is influenced by preceding activity of the affected muscle. In myasthenia gravis, for example, sustained or repeated contractions of affected muscle decline in strength despite continuing effort (**Chap. 440**). Thus, fatigable weakness is suggestive of disorders of the neuromuscular junction, which cause functional loss of muscle fibers due to failure of their activation.

Myopathic Weakness Myopathic weakness is produced by a decrease in the number or contractile force of muscle fibers activated within motor units. With muscular dystrophies, inflammatory myopathies, or myopathies with muscle fiber necrosis, the number of muscle fibers is reduced within many motor units. On EMG, the size of each motor unit action potential is decreased, and motor units must be recruited more rapidly than normal to produce the desired power. Some myopathies produce weakness through loss of contractile force of muscle fibers or through relatively selective involvement of type II (fast) fibers. These myopathies may not affect the size of individual motor unit action potentials and are detected by a discrepancy between the electrical activity and force of a muscle.

Psychogenic Weakness Weakness may occur without a recognizable organic basis. It tends to be variable, inconsistent, and with a pattern of distribution that cannot be explained on a neuroanatomic basis. On formal testing, antagonists may contract when the patient is supposedly activating the agonist muscle. The severity of weakness is out of keeping with the patient's daily activities.

DISTRIBUTION OF WEAKNESS

Hemiparesis Hemiparesis results from an upper motor neuron lesion above the midcervical spinal cord; most such lesions are above the foramen magnum. The presence of other neurologic deficits helps localize the lesion. Thus language disorders, for example, point to a cortical lesion. Homonymous visual field defects reflect either a cortical or a subcortical hemispheric lesion. A "pure motor" hemiparesis of the face, arm, and leg often is due to a small, discrete lesion in the posterior limb of the internal capsule, cerebral peduncle in the midbrain, or upper pons. Some brainstem lesions produce "crossed paralyses," consisting of ipsilateral cranial nerve signs and contralateral hemiparesis (**Chap. 426**). The absence of cranial nerve signs or facial weakness suggests that a hemiparesis is due to a lesion in the high cervical spinal cord, especially if associated with Brown-Séquard syndrome, consisting of loss of joint position and vibration sense on the side of the weakness, and loss of pain and temperature sense on the opposite side (**Chap. 442**).

Acute or episodic hemiparesis usually results from focal structural lesions, particularly vascular etiologies, rapidly expanding lesions, or an inflammatory process. *Subacute hemiparesis* that evolves over days or weeks may relate to subdural hematoma, infectious or inflammatory disorders (e.g., cerebral abscess, fungal granuloma or meningitis, parasitic infection, multiple sclerosis, sarcoidosis), or primary or metastatic neoplasms. AIDS may present with subacute hemiparesis due to toxoplasmosis or primary central nervous system (CNS) lymphoma. *Chronic hemiparesis* that evolves over months usually is due to a neoplasm or vascular malformation, a chronic subdural hematoma, or a degenerative disease.

Investigation of hemiparesis (**Fig. 24-3**) of acute origin usually starts with a CT scan of the brain and laboratory studies. If the CT is normal, or in subacute or chronic cases of hemiparesis, MRI of the brain and/or cervical spine (including the foramen magnum) is performed, depending on the clinical accompaniments.

Paraparesis ***Acute paraparesis*** is caused most commonly by an intraspinal lesion, but its spinal origin may not be recognized initially if the legs are flaccid and areflexic. Usually, however, there is sensory loss in the legs with an upper level on the trunk; a dissociated sensory loss (loss of pain and temperature but not touch, position, and vibration sense) suggestive of a central cord syndrome; or hyperreflexia in the legs with normal reflexes in the arms (**Chap. 442**). Imaging the spinal cord (Fig. 24-3) may reveal compressive lesions, infarction (proprioception usually is spared), arteriovenous fistulas or other vascular anomalies, or transverse myelitis (**Chap. 442**).

Diseases of the cerebral hemispheres that produce acute paraparesis include anterior cerebral artery ischemia (shoulder shrug also is affected), superior sagittal sinus or cortical venous thrombosis, and acute hydrocephalus.

Paraparesis may also result from a cauda equina syndrome, for example, after trauma to the low back, a midline disk herniation, or an intraspinal tumor. The sphincters are commonly affected, whereas hip flexion often is spared, as is sensation over the anterolateral thighs. Rarely, paraparesis is caused by a rapidly evolving anterior horn cell disease (such as poliovirus or West Nile virus infection), peripheral neuropathy (such as Guillain-Barré syndrome; **Chap. 447**), or myopathy (**Chap. 449**).

Subacute or chronic spastic paraparesis is caused by upper motor neuron disease. When associated with lower-limb sensory loss and sphincter involvement, a chronic spinal cord disorder should be considered (**Chap. 442**). If hemispheric signs are present, a parasagittal meningioma or chronic hydrocephalus is likely. The absence of spasticity in a long-standing paraparesis suggests a lower motor neuron or myopathic etiology.

Investigations typically begin with spinal MRI, but when upper motor neuron signs are associated with drowsiness, confusion, seizures, or other hemispheric signs, brain MRI should also be performed, sometimes as the initial investigation. Electrophysiologic studies are diagnostically helpful when clinical findings suggest an underlying neuromuscular disorder.

Quadriparesis or Generalized Weakness Generalized weakness may be due to disorders of the CNS or the motor unit. Although the terms often are used interchangeably, *quadriparesis* is commonly used when an upper motor neuron cause is suspected, and *generalized weakness* is used when a disease of the motor units is likely. Weakness from CNS disorders usually is associated with changes in consciousness or cognition and accompanied by spasticity, hyperreflexia, and sensory disturbances. Most neuromuscular causes of generalized weakness are associated with normal mental function, hypotonia, and hypoactive muscle stretch reflexes. The major causes of intermittent weakness are listed in **Table 24-2**. A patient with generalized fatigability without objective weakness may have chronic fatigue syndrome (**Chap. 450**).

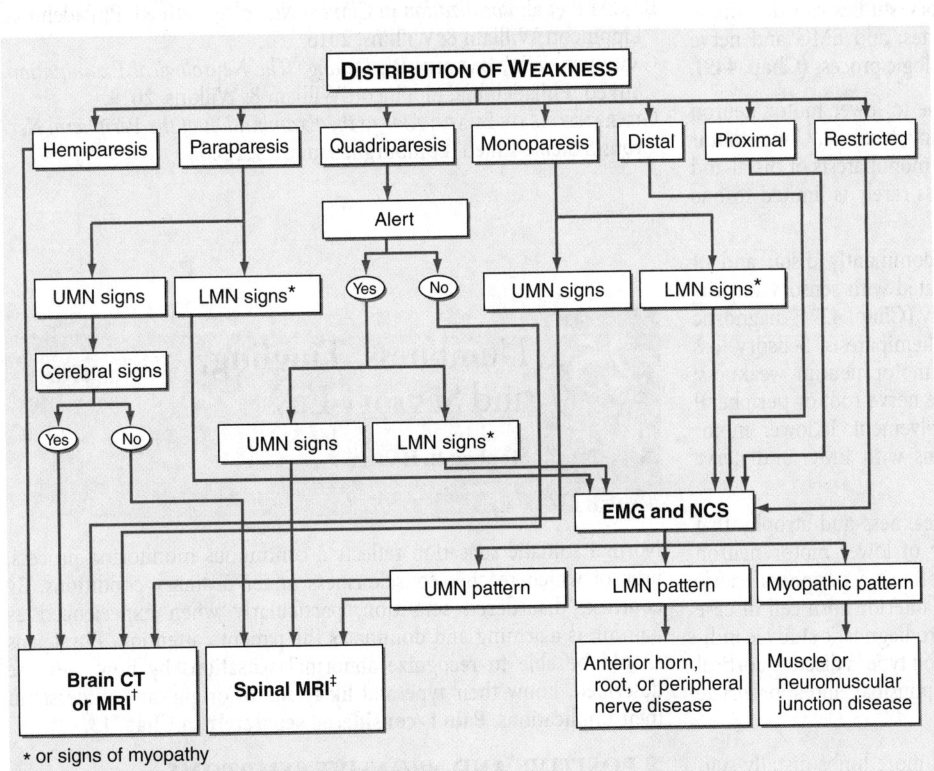

FIGURE 24-3 An algorithm for the initial workup of a patient with weakness. CT, computed tomography; EMG, electromyography; LMN, lower motor neuron; MRI, magnetic resonance imaging; NCS, nerve conduction studies; UMN, upper motor neuron.

ACUTE QUADRIPARESIS Quadriparesis with onset over minutes may result from disorders of upper motor neurons (such as from anoxia, hypotension, brainstem or cervical cord ischemia, trauma, and systemic metabolic abnormalities) or muscle (electrolyte disturbances, certain inborn errors of muscle energy metabolism, toxins, and periodic paralyses). Onset over hours to weeks may, in addition to these disorders, be due to lower motor neuron disorders such as Guillain-Barré syndrome (**Chap. 447**).

In obtunded patients, evaluation begins with a CT or MRI scan of the brain. If upper motor neuron signs are present but the patient is alert, the initial test is usually an MRI of the cervical cord. If weakness is lower motor neuron, myopathic, or uncertain in origin, the clinical approach begins with blood studies to determine the level of muscle enzymes and electrolytes and with EMG and nerve conduction studies.

TABLE 24-2 Causes of Episodic Generalized Weakness

1. Electrolyte disturbances, e.g., hypokalemia, hyperkalemia, hypercalcemia, hypernatremia, hyponatremia, hypophosphatemia, hypermagnesemia
2. Muscle disorders
   a. Channelopathies (periodic paralyses)
   b. Metabolic defects of muscle (impaired carbohydrate or fatty acid utilization; abnormal mitochondrial function)
3. Neuromuscular junction disorders
   a. Myasthenia gravis
   b. Lambert-Eaton myasthenic syndrome
4. Central nervous system disorders
   a. Transient ischemic attacks of the brainstem
   b. Transient global cerebral ischemia
   c. Multiple sclerosis
5. Lack of voluntary effort
   a. Anxiety
   b. Pain or discomfort
   c. Somatization disorder

SUBACUTE OR CHRONIC QUADRIPARESIS Quadriparesis due to upper motor neuron disease may develop over weeks to years from chronic myelopathies, multiple sclerosis, brain or spinal tumors, chronic subdural hematomas, and various metabolic, toxic, and infectious disorders. It may also result from lower motor neuron disease, a chronic neuropathy (in which weakness is often most profound distally), or myopathic weakness (typically proximal).

When quadriparesis develops acutely in obtunded patients, evaluation begins with a CT scan of the brain. If upper motor neuron signs have developed acutely but the patient is alert, the initial test is usually an MRI of the cervical cord. When onset has been gradual, disorders of the cerebral hemispheres, brainstem, and cervical spinal cord can usually be distinguished clinically, and imaging is directed first at the clinically suspected site of pathology. If weakness is lower motor neuron, myopathic, or uncertain in origin, laboratory studies can determine the levels of muscle enzymes and electrolytes, and EMG and nerve conduction studies help to localize the pathologic process (**Chap. 449**).

Monoparesis Monoparesis usually is due to lower motor neuron disease, with or without associated sensory involvement. Upper motor neuron weakness occasionally presents as a monoparesis of distal and nonantigravity muscles. Myopathic weakness rarely is limited to one limb.

ACUTE MONOPARESIS If weakness is predominantly distal and of upper motor neuron type and is not associated with sensory impairment or pain, focal cortical ischemia is likely (**Chap. 427**); diagnostic possibilities are similar to those for acute hemiparesis. Sensory loss and pain usually accompany acute lower motor neuron weakness; the weakness commonly localizes to a single nerve root or peripheral nerve, but occasionally reflects plexus involvement. If lower motor neuron weakness is likely, evaluation begins with EMG and nerve conduction studies.

SUBACUTE OR CHRONIC MONOPARESIS Weakness and atrophy that develop over weeks or months are usually of lower motor neuron origin. When associated with sensory symptoms, a peripheral cause (nerve, root, or plexus) is likely; otherwise, anterior horn cell disease should be considered. In either case, an electrodiagnostic study is indicated. If weakness is of the upper motor neuron type, a discrete cortical (precentral gyrus) or cord lesion may be responsible, and appropriate imaging is performed.

Distal Weakness Involvement of two or more limbs distally suggests lower motor neuron or peripheral nerve disease. Acute distal lower-limb weakness results occasionally from an acute toxic polyneuropathy or cauda equina syndrome. Distal symmetric weakness usually develops over weeks, months, or years and, when associated with numbness, is due to peripheral neuropathy (**Chap. 446**). Anterior horn cell disease may begin distally but is typically asymmetric and without accompanying numbness (**Chap. 437**). Rarely, myopathies present with distal weakness (**Chap. 449**). Electrodiagnostic studies help localize the disorder (Fig. 24-3).

Proximal Weakness Myopathy often produces symmetric weakness of the pelvic or shoulder girdle muscles (**Chap. 449**). Diseases of the neuromuscular junction, such as myasthenia gravis (**Chap. 448**), may present with symmetric proximal weakness often associated with ptosis, diplopia, or bulbar weakness and fluctuate in severity during the day. In anterior horn cell disease, proximal weakness is usually asymmetric, but it may be symmetric especially in genetic forms. Numbness does not occur with any of these diseases. The evaluation usually begins with determination of the serum creatine kinase level and electrophysiologic studies.

Weakness in a Restricted Distribution Weakness may not fit any of these patterns, being limited, for example, to the extraocular, hemifacial, bulbar, or respiratory muscles. If it is unilateral, restricted weakness usually is due to lower motor neuron or peripheral nerve disease, such as in a facial palsy. Weakness of part of a limb is commonly due to a peripheral nerve lesion such as an entrapment neuropathy. Relatively symmetric weakness of extraocular or bulbar muscles frequently is due to a myopathy (**Chap. 449**) or neuromuscular junction disorder (**Chap. 448**). Bilateral facial palsy with areflexia suggests Guillain-Barré syndrome (**Chap. 447**). Worsening of relatively symmetric weakness with fatigue is characteristic of neuromuscular junction disorders. Asymmetric bulbar weakness usually is due to motor neuron disease. Weakness limited to respiratory muscles is uncommon and usually is due to motor neuron disease, myasthenia gravis, or polymyositis/dermatomyositis (**Chap. 365**).

ACKNOWLEDGMENT
The editors acknowledge the contributions of Michael J. Aminoff to earlier editions of this chapter.

■ FURTHER READING

Brazis P et al: *Localization in Clinical Neurology*, 7th ed. Philadelphia, Lippincott William & Wilkins, 2016.

Campbell WW, Barohn RJ: *DeJong's The Neurological Examination*, 8th ed. Philadelphia, Lippincott William & Wilkins, 2019.

Guarantors of Brain: *Aids to the Examination of the Peripheral Nervous System*, 4th ed. Edinburgh, Saunders, 2000.

25 Numbness, Tingling, and Sensory Loss

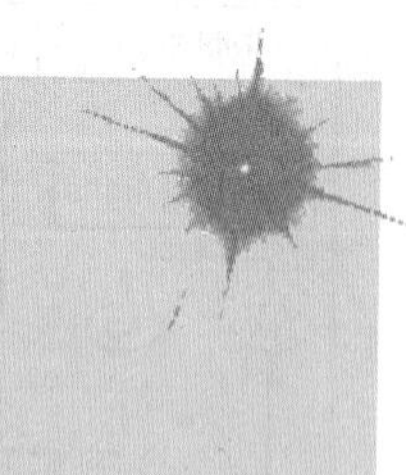

Stephen L. Hauser

Normal somatic sensation reflects a continuous monitoring process, little of which reaches consciousness under ordinary conditions. By contrast, disordered sensation, particularly when experienced as painful, is alarming and dominates the patient's attention. Physicians should be able to recognize abnormal sensations by how they are described, know their type and likely site of origin, and understand their implications. **Pain is considered separately in Chap. 13.**

■ POSITIVE AND NEGATIVE SYMPTOMS

Abnormal sensory symptoms can be divided into two categories: positive and negative. The prototypical positive symptom is tingling (pins and needles); other positive sensory phenomena include itch and altered sensations that are described as pricking, bandlike, lightning-like shooting feelings (lancinations), aching, knifelike, twisting, drawing, pulling, tightening, burning, searing, electrical, or raw feelings. Such symptoms are often painful.

Positive phenomena usually result from trains of impulses generated at sites of lowered threshold or heightened excitability along a peripheral or central sensory pathway. The nature and severity of the abnormal sensation depend on the number, rate, timing, and distribution of ectopic impulses and the type and function of nervous tissue in which they arise. Because positive phenomena represent excessive activity in sensory pathways, they are not necessarily associated with a sensory deficit (loss) on examination.

Negative phenomena represent loss of sensory function and are characterized by diminished or absent feeling that often is experienced as numbness and by abnormal findings on sensory examination. In disorders affecting peripheral sensation, at least one-half of the afferent axons innervating a particular site are probably lost or functionless before a sensory deficit can be demonstrated by clinical examination. If the rate of loss is slow, however, lack of cutaneous feeling may be unnoticed by the patient and difficult to demonstrate on examination, even though few sensory fibers are functioning; if it is rapid, both positive and negative phenomena are usually conspicuous. Subclinical degrees of sensory dysfunction may be revealed by sensory nerve conduction studies or somatosensory-evoked potentials.

Whereas sensory symptoms may be either positive or negative, sensory signs on examination are always a measure of negative phenomena.

■ TERMINOLOGY

Paresthesias and dysesthesias are general terms used to denote positive sensory symptoms. The term *paresthesias* typically refers to tingling or pins-and-needles sensations but may include a wide variety of other abnormal sensations, except pain; it sometimes implies that the abnormal sensations are perceived spontaneously. The more general term *dysesthesias* denotes all types of abnormal sensations, including painful ones, regardless of whether a stimulus is evident.

Another set of terms refers to sensory abnormalities found on examination. *Hypesthesia* or *hypoesthesia* refers to a reduction of cutaneous sensation to a specific type of testing such as pressure, light touch, and warm or cold stimuli; *anesthesia,* to a complete absence of skin sensation to the same stimuli plus pinprick; and *hypalgesia* or *analgesia*, to reduced or absent pain perception (nociception). *Hyperesthesia* means pain or increased sensitivity in response to touch. Similarly, *allodynia* describes the situation in which a nonpainful stimulus, once perceived, is experienced as painful, even excruciating. An example is elicitation of a painful sensation by application of a vibrating tuning fork. *Hyperalgesia* denotes severe pain in response to a mildly noxious stimulus, and *hyperpathia*, a broad term, encompasses all the phenomena described by hyperesthesia, allodynia, and hyperalgesia. With hyperpathia, the threshold for a sensory stimulus is increased and perception is delayed, but once felt, it is unduly painful.

Disorders of deep sensation arising from muscle spindles, tendons, and joints affect proprioception (position sense). Manifestations include imbalance (particularly with eyes closed or in the dark), clumsiness of precision movements, and unsteadiness of gait, which are referred to collectively as *sensory ataxia*. Other findings on examination usually, but not invariably, include reduced or absent joint position and vibratory sensibility and absent deep tendon reflexes in the affected limbs. The Romberg sign is positive, which means that the patient sways markedly or topples when asked to stand with feet close together and eyes closed. In severe states of deafferentation involving deep sensation, the patient cannot walk or stand unaided or even sit unsupported. Continuous involuntary movements (*pseudoathetosis*) of the outstretched hands and fingers occur, particularly with eyes closed.

■ ANATOMY OF SENSATION

Cutaneous receptors are classified by the type of stimulus that optimally excites them. They consist of naked nerve endings (nociceptors, which respond to tissue-damaging stimuli, and thermoreceptors, which respond to noninjurious thermal stimuli) and encapsulated terminals (several types of mechanoreceptor, activated by physical deformation of the skin or stretch of muscles). Each type of receptor has its own set of sensitivities to specific stimuli, size and distinctness of receptive fields, and adaptational qualities.

Afferent peripheral nerve fibers conveying somatosensory information from the limbs and trunk traverse the dorsal roots and enter the dorsal horn of the spinal cord (**Fig. 25-1**); the cell bodies of first-order neurons are located in the dorsal root ganglia (DRG). In an analogous fashion, sensations from the face and head are conveyed through the trigeminal system (**Fig. 441-2**). Once fiber tracts enter the spinal cord, the polysynaptic projections of the smaller fibers (unmyelinated and small myelinated), which subserve mainly nociception, itch, temperature sensibility, and touch, cross and ascend in the opposite anterior and lateral columns of the spinal cord, through the brainstem, to the ventral posterolateral (VPL) nucleus of the thalamus and ultimately project to the postcentral gyrus of the parietal cortex and other cortical areas (**Chap. 13**). This is the *spinothalamic pathway* or *anterolateral system*. The larger fibers, which subserve tactile and position sense and kinesthesia, project rostrally in the posterior and posterolateral columns on the same side of the spinal cord and make their first synapse in the gracile or cuneate nucleus of the lower medulla. Axons of second-order neurons decussate and ascend in the medial lemniscus located medially in the medulla and in the tegmentum of the pons and midbrain and synapse in the VPL nucleus; third-order neurons project to parietal cortex as well as to other cortical areas. This large-fiber system is referred to as the *posterior column–medial lemniscal pathway* (lemniscal, for short). Although the fiber types and functions that make up the spinothalamic and lemniscal systems are relatively well known, many other fibers, particularly those associated with touch, pressure, and position sense, ascend in a diffusely distributed pattern both ipsilaterally and contralaterally in the anterolateral quadrants of the spinal cord. This explains why a complete lesion of the posterior columns of the spinal cord may be associated with little sensory deficit on examination.

APPROACH TO THE PATIENT

Clinical Examination of Sensation

The main components of the sensory examination are tests of primary sensation (pain, touch, vibration, joint position, and thermal sensation) (**Table 25-1**). The examiner must depend on patient responses, and this complicates interpretation. Further, examination may be limited in some patients. In a stuporous patient, for example, sensory examination is reduced to observing the briskness of withdrawal in response to a pinch or another noxious stimulus. Comparison of responses on the two sides of the body is essential. In an alert but uncooperative patient, it may not be possible to examine cutaneous sensation, but some idea of proprioceptive function may be gained by noting the patient's best performance of movements requiring balance and precision.

In patients with sensory complaints, testing should begin in the center of the affected region and proceed radially until sensation is perceived as normal. The distribution of any abnormality is defined and compared to root and peripheral nerve territories (**Figs. 25-2 and 25-3**). Some patients present with sensory symptoms that do not fit an anatomic localization and are accompanied by either no abnormalities or gross inconsistencies on examination. The examiner should consider in such cases the possibility of a psychologic cause (see "Psychogenic Symptoms," below). Sensory examination of a patient who has no neurologic complaints can be brief and consist of pinprick, touch, and vibration testing in the hands and feet plus evaluation of stance and gait, including the Romberg maneuver (**Chap. V6**). Evaluation of stance and gait also tests the integrity of motor and cerebellar systems.

PRIMARY SENSATION

The sense of pain usually is tested with a clean pin, which is then discarded. The patient is asked to close the eyes and focus on the pricking or unpleasant quality of the stimulus, not just the pressure

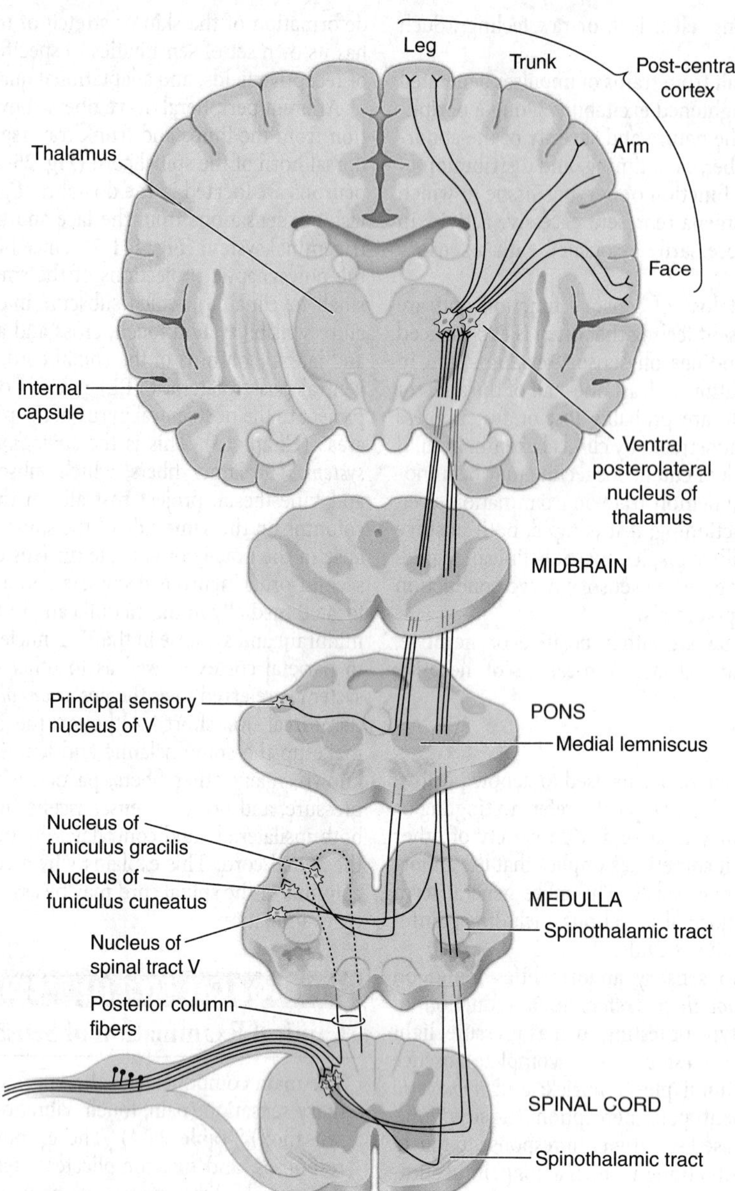

FIGURE 25-1 The main somatosensory pathways. The spinothalamic tract (pain, thermal sense) and the posterior column–lemniscal system (touch, pressure, joint position) are shown. Offshoots from the ascending anterolateral fasciculus (spinothalamic tract) to nuclei in the medulla, pons, and mesencephalon and nuclear terminations of the tract are indicated. *(Reproduced with permission from AH Ropper, MA Samuels: Adams and Victor's Principles of Neurology, 9th ed. New York, McGraw-Hill, 2009.)*

or touch sensation elicited. Areas of hypalgesia should be mapped by proceeding radially from the most hypalgesic site. Temperature sensation to both hot and cold is best tested with small containers filled with water of the desired temperature. An alternative way to test cold sensation is to touch a metal object, such as a tuning fork at room temperature, to the skin. For testing warm temperatures, the tuning fork or another metal object may be held under warm water of the desired temperature and then used. The appreciation of both cold and warmth should be tested because different receptors respond to each. Touch usually is tested with a wisp of cotton,

TABLE 25-1 Testing Primary Sensation

SENSE	TEST DEVICE	ENDINGS ACTIVATED	FIBER SIZE MEDIATING	CENTRAL PATHWAY
Pain	Pinprick	Cutaneous nociceptors	Small	SpTh, also D
Temperature, heat	Warm metal object	Cutaneous thermoreceptors for hot	Small	SpTh
Temperature, cold	Cold metal object	Cutaneous thermoreceptors for cold	Small	SpTh
Touch	Cotton wisp, fine brush	Cutaneous mechanoreceptors, also naked endings	Large and small	Lem, also D and SpTh
Vibration	Tuning fork, 128 Hz	Mechanoreceptors, especially pacinian corpuscles	Large	Lem, also D
Joint position	Passive movement of specific joints	Joint capsule and tendon endings, muscle spindles	Large	Lem, also D

Abbreviations: D, diffuse ascending projections in ipsilateral and contralateral anterolateral columns; Lem, posterior column and lemniscal projection, ipsilateral; SpTh, spinothalamic projection, contralateral.

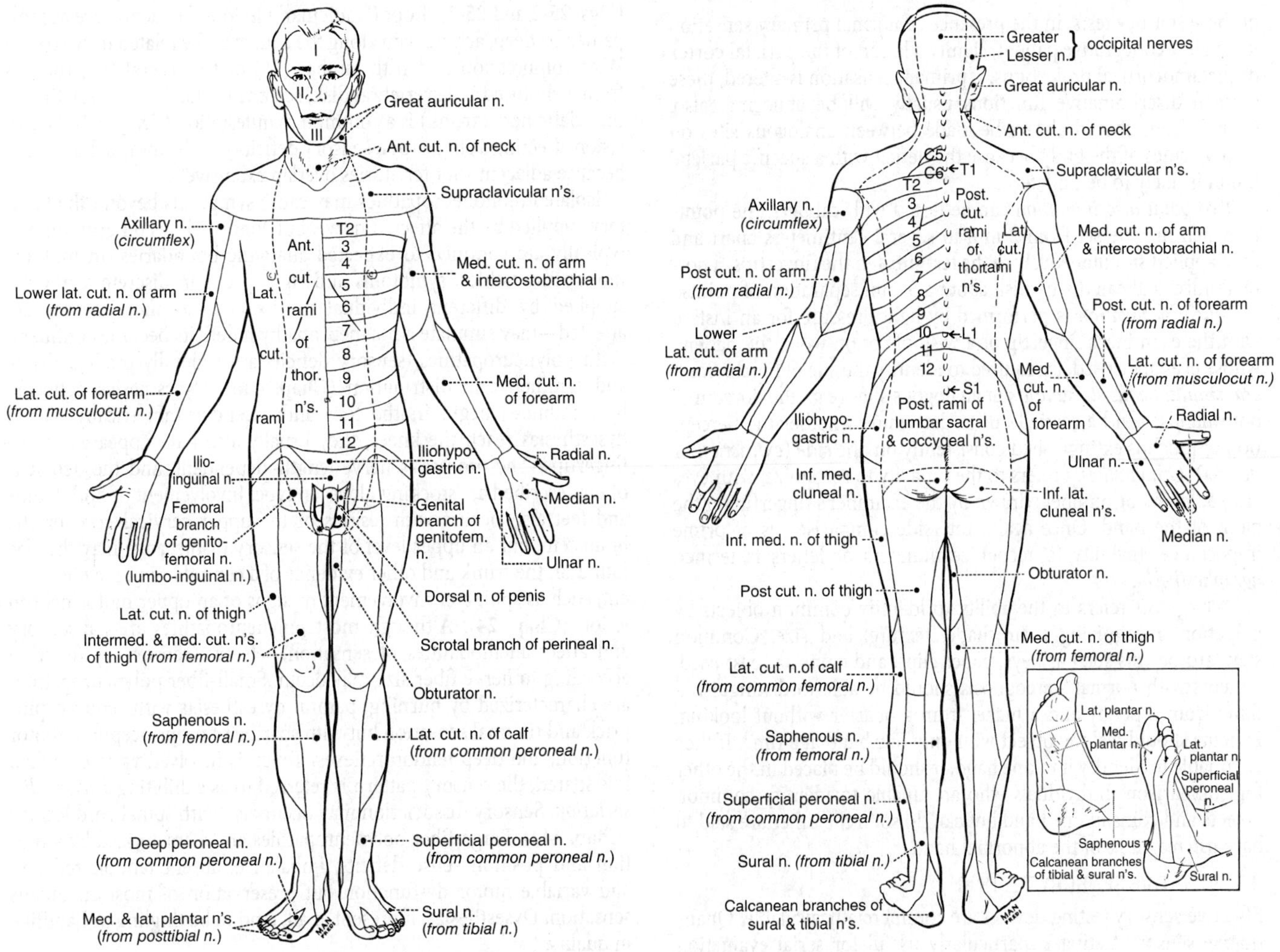

FIGURE 25-2 The cutaneous fields of peripheral nerves. *(Reproduced with permission from W Haymaker, B Woodhall: Peripheral Nerve Injuries, 2nd ed. Philadelphia, Saunders, 1953.)*

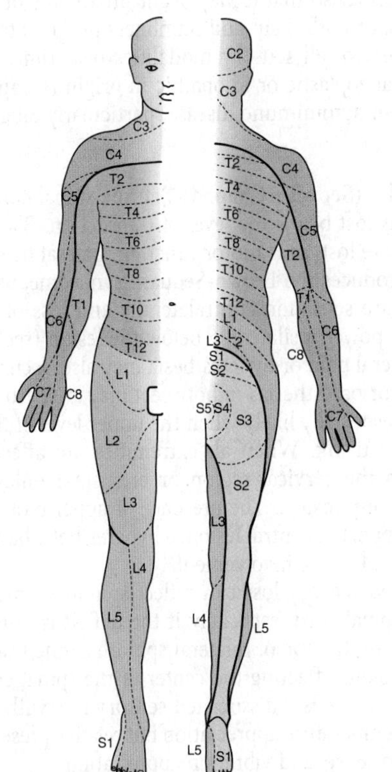

FIGURE 25-3 Distribution of the sensory spinal roots on the surface of the body (dermatomes). *(Reproduced with permission from D Sinclair: Mechanisms of Cutaneous Sensation. Oxford, UK, Oxford University Press, 1981 through PLS Clear.)*

minimizing pressure on the skin. In general, it is better to avoid testing touch on hairy skin because of the profusion of the sensory endings that surround each hair follicle. The patient is tested with the eyes closed and should respond as soon as the stimulus is perceived, indicating its location.

Joint position testing is a measure of proprioception. With the patient's eyes closed, joint position is tested in the distal interphalangeal joint of the great toe and fingers. The digit is held by its sides, distal to the joint being tested, and moved passively while more proximal joints are stabilized—the patient indicates the change in position or direction of movement. If errors are made, more proximal joints are tested. A test of proximal joint position sense, primarily at the shoulder, is performed by asking the patient to bring the two index fingers together with arms extended and eyes closed. Normal individuals can do this accurately, with errors of 1 cm or less.

The sense of vibration is tested with an oscillating tuning fork that vibrates at 128 Hz. Vibration is tested over bony points, beginning distally; in the feet, it is tested over the dorsal surface of the distal phalanx of the big toes and at the malleoli of the ankles, and in the hands, it is tested dorsally at the distal phalanx of the fingers. If abnormalities are found, more proximal sites should be examined. Vibratory thresholds at the same site in the patient and the examiner may be compared for control purposes.

CORTICAL SENSATION

The most commonly used tests of cortical function are two-point discrimination, touch localization, and bilateral simultaneous stimulation, and tests for graphesthesia and stereognosis. Abnormalities of these sensory tests, in the presence of normal primary sensation in an alert cooperative patient, signify a lesion of the parietal cortex or thalamocortical projections. If primary sensation is altered, these cortical discriminative functions usually will be abnormal also. Comparisons should always be made between analogous sites on the two sides of the body because the deficit with a specific parietal lesion is likely to be unilateral.

Two-point discrimination can be tested with calipers, the points of which may be set from 2 mm to several centimeters apart and then applied simultaneously to the test site. On the fingertips, a normal individual can distinguish about a 3-mm separation of points.

Touch localization is performed by light pressure for an instant with the examiner's fingertip or a wisp of cotton wool; the patient, whose eyes are closed, is required to identify the site of touch. *Bilateral simultaneous stimulation* at analogous sites (e.g., the dorsum of both hands) can be carried out to determine whether the perception of touch is extinguished consistently on one side (*extinction* or *neglect*). *Graphesthesia* refers to the capacity to recognize, with eyes closed, letters or numbers drawn by the examiner's fingertip on the palm of the hand. Once again, interside comparison is of prime importance. Inability to recognize numbers or letters is termed *agraphesthesia*.

Stereognosis refers to the ability to identify common objects by palpation, recognizing their shape, texture, and size. Common standard objects such as keys, paper clips, and coins are best used. Patients with normal stereognosis should be able to distinguish a dime from a penny and a nickel from a quarter without looking. Patients should feel the object with only one hand at a time. If they are unable to identify it in one hand, it should be placed in the other for comparison. Individuals who are unable to identify common objects and coins in one hand but can do so in the other are said to have *astereognosis* of the abnormal hand.

QUANTITATIVE SENSORY TESTING

Effective sensory testing devices are commercially available. Quantitative sensory testing is particularly useful for serial evaluation of cutaneous sensation in clinical trials. Threshold testing for touch and vibratory and thermal sensation is the most widely used application.

ELECTRODIAGNOSTIC STUDIES AND NERVE BIOPSY

Nerve conduction studies and nerve biopsy are important means of investigating the peripheral nervous system, but they do not evaluate the function or structure of cutaneous receptors and free nerve endings or of unmyelinated or thinly myelinated nerve fibers in the nerve trunks. Skin biopsy can be used to evaluate these structures in the dermis and epidermis.

■ LOCALIZATION OF SENSORY ABNORMALITIES

Sensory symptoms and signs can result from lesions at many different levels of the nervous system from the parietal cortex to the peripheral sensory receptor. Noting their distribution and nature is the most important way to localize their source. Their extent, configuration, symmetry, quality, and severity are the key observations.

Dysesthesias without sensory findings by examination may be difficult to interpret. To illustrate, tingling dysesthesias in an acral distribution (hands and feet) can be systemic in origin, for example, secondary to hyperventilation, or induced by a medication such as acetazolamide. Distal dysesthesias can also be an early event in an evolving polyneuropathy or may herald a myelopathy, such as from vitamin B_{12} deficiency. Sometimes, distal dysesthesias have no definable basis. In contrast, dysesthesias that correspond in distribution to that of a particular peripheral nerve structure denote a lesion at that site. For instance, dysesthesias restricted to the fifth digit and the adjacent one-half of the fourth finger on one hand reliably point to disorder of the ulnar nerve, most commonly at the elbow.

Nerve and Root In focal nerve trunk lesions, sensory abnormalities are readily mapped and generally have discrete boundaries (**Figs. 25-2 and 25-3**). Root ("radicular") lesions frequently are accompanied by deep, aching pain along the course of the related nerve trunk. With compression of a fifth lumbar (L5) or first sacral (S1) root, as from a ruptured intervertebral disk, sciatica (radicular pain relating to the sciatic nerve trunk) is a common manifestation (**Chap. 17**). With a lesion affecting a single root, sensory deficits may be minimal or absent because adjacent root territories overlap extensively.

Isolated mononeuropathies may cause symptoms beyond the territory supplied by the affected nerve, but abnormalities on examination typically are confined to expected anatomic boundaries. In multiple mononeuropathies, symptoms and signs occur in discrete territories supplied by different individual nerves and—as more nerves are affected—may simulate a polyneuropathy if deficits become confluent. With polyneuropathies, sensory deficits are generally graded, distal, and symmetric in distribution (**Chap. 446**). Dysesthesias, followed by numbness, begin in the toes and ascend symmetrically. When dysesthesias reach the knees, they usually also have appeared in the fingertips. The process is nerve length–dependent, and the deficit is often described as "stocking glove" in type. Involvement of both hands and feet also occurs with lesions of the upper cervical cord or the brainstem, but an upper level of the sensory disturbance may then be found on the trunk and other evidence of a central lesion may be present, such as sphincter involvement or signs of an upper motor neuron lesion (**Chap. 24**). Although most polyneuropathies are pansensory and affect all modalities of sensation, selective sensory dysfunction according to nerve fiber size may occur. Small-fiber polyneuropathies are characterized by burning, painful dysesthesias with reduced pinprick and thermal sensation but with sparing of proprioception, motor function, and deep tendon reflexes. Touch is involved variably; when it is spared, the sensory pattern is referred to as exhibiting *sensory dissociation*. Sensory dissociation may occur also with spinal cord lesions (**Chap. 442**). Large-fiber polyneuropathies are characterized by vibration and position sense deficits, imbalance, absent tendon reflexes, and variable motor dysfunction but preservation of most cutaneous sensation. Dysesthesias, if present at all, tend to be tingling or bandlike in quality.

Sensory neuronopathy (or ganglionopathy) is characterized by widespread but asymmetric sensory loss occurring in a non-length-dependent manner so that it may occur proximally or distally, and in the arms, legs, or both. Pain and numbness progress to sensory ataxia and impairment of all sensory modalities over time. This condition is usually paraneoplastic or idiopathic in origin (**Chaps. 94 and 445**) or related to an autoimmune disease, particularly Sjögren's syndrome (**Chap. 361**).

Spinal Cord (See also **Chap. 442**) If the spinal cord is transected, all sensation is lost below the level of transection. Bladder and bowel function also are lost, as is motor function. Lateral hemisection of the spinal cord produces the Brown-Séquard syndrome, with absent pain and temperature sensation contralaterally and loss of proprioceptive sensation and power ipsilaterally below the lesion (see **Figs. 25-1 and 442-1**); ipsilateral pain or hyperesthesia may also occur.

Numbness or paresthesias in both feet may arise from a spinal cord lesion; this is especially likely when the upper level of the sensory loss extends to the trunk. When all extremities are affected, the lesion is probably in the cervical region or brainstem unless a peripheral neuropathy is responsible. The presence of upper motor neuron signs (**Chap. 24**) supports a central lesion; a hyperesthetic band on the trunk may suggest the level of involvement.

A dissociated sensory loss can reflect spinothalamic tract involvement in the spinal cord, especially if the deficit is unilateral and has an upper level on the torso. Bilateral spinothalamic tract involvement occurs with lesions affecting the center of the spinal cord, such as in syringomyelia. There is a dissociated sensory loss with impairment of pinprick and temperature appreciation but relative preservation of light touch, position sense, and vibration appreciation.

Dysfunction of the posterior columns in the spinal cord or of the posterior root entry zone may lead to a bandlike sensation around the trunk or a feeling of tight pressure in one or more limbs. Flexion of the neck sometimes leads to an electric shock–like sensation that radiates down the back and into the legs (Lhermitte's sign) in patients with a cervical lesion affecting the posterior columns, such as from multiple sclerosis, cervical spondylosis, or following irradiation to the cervical region.

Brainstem Crossed patterns of sensory disturbance, in which one side of the face and the opposite side of the body are affected, localize to the lateral medulla. Here a small lesion may damage both the ipsilateral descending trigeminal tract and the ascending spinothalamic fibers subserving the opposite arm, leg, and hemitorso (see "Lateral medullary syndrome" in **Fig. 426-7**). A lesion in the tegmentum of the pons and midbrain, where the lemniscal and spinothalamic tracts merge, causes pansensory loss contralaterally.

Thalamus Hemisensory disturbance with tingling numbness from head to foot is often thalamic in origin but also can arise from the anterior parietal region. If abrupt in onset, the lesion is likely to be due to a small stroke (lacunar infarction), particularly if localized to the thalamus. Occasionally, with lesions affecting the VPL nucleus or adjacent white matter, a syndrome of thalamic pain, also called *Déjerine-Roussy syndrome*, may ensue. The persistent, unrelenting unilateral pain often is described in dramatic terms.

Cortex With lesions of the parietal lobe involving either the cortex or subjacent white matter, the most prominent symptoms are contralateral hemineglect, hemi-inattention, and a tendency not to use the affected hand and arm. On cortical sensory testing (e.g., two-point discrimination, graphesthesia), abnormalities are often found but primary sensation is usually intact. Anterior parietal infarction may present as a pseudothalamic syndrome with contralateral loss of primary sensation from head to toe. Dysesthesias or a sense of numbness and, rarely, a painful state may also occur.

Focal Sensory Seizures These seizures generally are due to lesions in the area of the postcentral or precentral gyrus. The principal symptom of focal sensory seizures is tingling, but additional, more complex sensations may occur, such as a rushing feeling, a sense of warmth, or a sense of movement without detectable motion. Symptoms typically are unilateral; commonly begin in the arm or hand, face, or foot; and often spread in a manner that reflects the cortical representation of different bodily parts, as in a Jacksonian march. Their duration is variable; seizures may be transient, lasting only for seconds, or persist for an hour or more. Focal motor features may supervene, often becoming generalized with loss of consciousness and tonic-clonic jerking.

Psychogenic Symptoms Sensory symptoms may have a psychogenic basis. Such symptoms may be generalized or have an anatomic boundary that is difficult to explain neurologically, for example, circumferentially at the groin or shoulder or around a specific joint. Pain is common, but the nature and intensity of any sensory disturbances are variable. The diagnosis should not be one of exclusion but based on suggestive findings that are otherwise difficult to explain, such as midline splitting of impaired vibration, pinprick, or light touch appreciation; variability or poor reproducibility of sensory deficits; or normal performance of tasks requiring sensory input that is seemingly abnormal on formal testing, such as good performance with eyes closed of the finger-to-nose test despite an apparent loss of position sense in the upper limb. The side with abnormal sensation may be confused when the limbs are placed in an unusual position, such as crossed behind the back. Sensory complaints should not be regarded as psychogenic simply because they are unusual.

TREATMENT

Management is based on treatment of the underlying condition. Symptomatic treatment of acute and chronic pain is discussed in **Chap. 13**. Dysesthesias, when severe and persistent, may respond to anticonvulsants (carbamazepine, 100–1000 mg/d; gabapentin, 300–3600 mg/d; or pregabalin, 50–300 mg/d), antidepressants (amitriptyline, 25–150 mg/d; nortriptyline, 25–150 mg/d; desipramine, 100–300 mg/d; or venlafaxine, 75–225 mg/d).

ACKNOWLEDGMENTS

The editors acknowledge the contributions of Michael J. Aminoff to earlier editions of this chapter.

FURTHER READING

Brazis P et al: *Localization in Clinical Neurology*, 7th ed. Philadelphia, Lippincott William & Wilkins, 2016.

Campbell WW, Barohn RJ: *DeJong's the Neurologic Examination*, 8th ed. Philadelphia, Wolters Kluwer, 2020.

Waxman S: *Clinical Neuroanatomy*, 29th ed. New York, McGraw Hill Education, 2020.

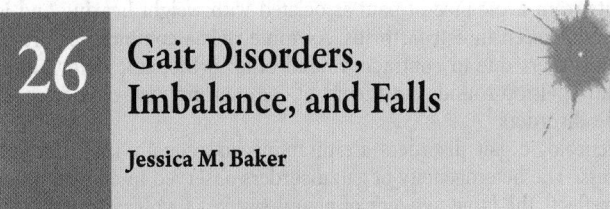

26 Gait Disorders, Imbalance, and Falls

Jessica M. Baker

PREVALENCE, MORBIDITY, AND MORTALITY

Gait and balance problems are common in the elderly and contribute to the risk of falls and injury. Gait disorders have been described in 15% of individuals aged >65. By age 80, one person in four will use a mechanical aid to assist with ambulation. Among those aged ≥85, the prevalence of gait abnormality approaches 40%. In epidemiologic studies, gait disorders are consistently identified as a major risk factor for falls and injury.

ANATOMY AND PHYSIOLOGY

An upright bipedal gait depends on the successful integration of postural control and locomotion. These functions are widely distributed in the central nervous system. The biomechanics of bipedal walking are complex, and the performance is easily compromised by a neurologic deficit at any level. Command and control centers in the brainstem, cerebellum, and forebrain modify the action of spinal pattern generators to promote stepping. While a form of "fictive locomotion" can be elicited from quadrupedal animals after spinal transection, this capacity is limited in primates. Step generation in primates is dependent on locomotor centers in the pontine tegmentum, midbrain, and subthalamic region. Locomotor synergies are executed through the reticular formation and descending pathways in the ventromedial spinal cord. Cerebral control provides a goal and purpose for walking and is involved in avoidance of obstacles and adaptation of locomotor programs to context and terrain.

Postural control requires the maintenance of the center of mass over the base of support through the gait cycle. Unconscious postural adjustments maintain standing balance: long latency responses are measurable in the leg muscles, beginning 110 milliseconds after a perturbation. Forward motion of the center of mass provides propulsive force for stepping, but failure to maintain the center of mass within stability limits results in falls. The anatomic substrate for dynamic balance has not been well defined, but the vestibular nucleus and midline cerebellum contribute to balance control in animals. Patients with damage to these structures have impaired balance while standing and walking.

Standing balance depends on good-quality sensory information about the position of the body center with respect to the environment, support surface, and gravitational forces. Sensory information for postural control is primarily generated by the visual system, the vestibular system, and proprioceptive receptors in the muscle spindles and joints. A healthy redundancy of sensory afferent information is generally available, but loss of two of the three pathways is sufficient to compromise standing balance. Balance disorders in older individuals sometimes result from multiple insults in the peripheral sensory systems (e.g., visual loss, vestibular deficit, peripheral neuropathy) that critically degrade the quality of afferent information needed for balance stability.

Older patients with cognitive impairment appear to be particularly prone to falls and injury. There is a growing body of literature on the use of attentional resources to manage gait and balance. Walking is generally considered to be unconscious and automatic, but the ability to walk while attending to a cognitive task (*dual-task walking*) may be compromised in the elderly. Older patients with deficits in executive function may have particular difficulty in managing the attentional resources needed for dynamic balance when distracted.

DISORDERS OF GAIT

Disorders of gait may be attributed to neurologic and nonneurologic causes, although significant overlap often exists. The *antalgic gait* results from avoidance of pain associated with weight bearing and is commonly seen in osteoarthritis. Asymmetry is a common feature of gait disorders due to contractures and other orthopedic deformities. Impaired vision rounds out the list of common nonneurologic causes of gait disorders.

Neurologic gait disorders are disabling and equally important to address. The heterogeneity of gait disorders observed in clinical practice reflects the large network of neural systems involved in the task. Walking is vulnerable to neurologic disease at every level. Gait disorders have been classified descriptively on the basis of abnormal physiology and biomechanics. One problem with this approach is that many failing gaits look fundamentally similar. This overlap reflects common patterns of adaptation to threatened balance stability and declining performance. *The gait disorder observed clinically must be viewed as the product of a neurologic deficit and a functional adaptation.* Unique features of the failing gait are often overwhelmed by the adaptive response. Some common patterns of abnormal gait are summarized next. Gait disorders can also be classified by etiology **(Table 26-1)**.

■ CAUTIOUS GAIT

The term *cautious gait* is used to describe the patient who walks with an abbreviated stride, widened base, and lowered center of mass, as if walking on a slippery surface. Arms are often held abducted. This disorder is both common and nonspecific. It is, in essence, an adaptation to a perceived postural threat. There may be an associated fear of falling. This disorder can be observed in more than one-third of older patients with gait impairment. Physical therapy often improves walking to the degree that follow-up observation may reveal a more specific underlying disorder.

■ STIFF-LEGGED GAIT

Spastic gait is characterized by stiffness in the legs, an imbalance of muscle tone, and a tendency to circumduct and scuff the feet. The disorder reflects compromise of corticospinal command and overactivity of spinal reflexes. The patient may walk on the toes. In extreme instances, the legs cross due to increased tone in the adductors ("scissoring" gait). Upper motor neuron signs are present on physical examination. The disorder may be cerebral or spinal in origin.

Myelopathy from cervical spondylosis is a common cause of spastic or spastic-ataxic gait in the elderly. Demyelinating disease and trauma are the leading causes of myelopathy in younger patients. In chronic progressive myelopathy of unknown cause, a workup with laboratory and imaging tests may establish a diagnosis. A structural lesion, such as a tumor or a spinal vascular malformation, should be excluded with appropriate testing. **Spinal cord disorders are discussed in detail in Chap. 442.**

With cerebral spasticity, asymmetry is common, the upper extremities are usually involved, and dysarthria is often an associated feature. Common causes include vascular disease (stroke), multiple sclerosis, motor neuron disease, and perinatal nervous system injury (cerebral palsy).

Other stiff-legged gaits include dystonia **(Chap. 436)** and stiff-person syndrome **(Chap. 94)**. Dystonia is a disorder characterized by sustained muscle contractions resulting in repetitive twisting movements and abnormal posture. It often has a genetic basis. Dystonic spasms can produce plantar flexion and inversion of the feet, sometimes with torsion of the trunk. In autoimmune stiff-person syndrome, exaggerated lordosis of the lumbar spine and overactivation of antagonist muscles restrict trunk and lower-limb movement and result in a wooden or fixed posture.

■ PARKINSONISM, FREEZING GAIT, AND OTHER MOVEMENT DISORDERSS

Parkinson's disease **(Chap. 435)** is common, affecting 1% of the population >65 years of age. The stooped posture, shuffling gait, and decreased arm swing are characteristic and distinctive features. Patients sometimes accelerate (festinate) with walking, display retropulsion, or exhibit a tendency to turn en bloc. The step-to-step variability

TABLE 26-1 Prevalence of Neurologic Gait Disorders

NEUROLOGIC GAIT DISORDER	NO. (%)[a]	TOTAL NUMBER[b]	CAUSES (NO.)
Single neurologic gait disorder	81 (69%)		
Sensory ataxic	22 (18%)	46	Peripheral sensory neuropathy (46)
Parkinsonian	19 (16%)	34	Parkinson's disease (18), drug-induced parkinsonism (8), dementia with parkinsonism (4), parkinsonism (4)
Higher level	9 (8%)	31	Vascular encephalopathy (20), normal pressure hydrocephalus (1), severe dementia (7), hypoxic ischemic encephalopathy (1), unknown (1)
Cerebellar ataxic	7 (6%)	10	Cerebellar stroke (3), cerebellar lesion due to multiple sclerosis (1), severe essential tremor (3), postvaccinal cerebellitis (1), chronic alcohol abuse (1), multiple system atrophy (1)
Cautious	7 (6%)	7	Idiopathic, associated fear of falling (7)
Paretic/hypotonic	6 (5%)	14	Neurogenic claudication (7), diabetic neuropathy (1), nerve lesion due to trauma or surgery (4), distal paraparesis after Guillain-Barré syndrome (1), unknown (2)
Spastic	6 (5%)	7	Ischemic stroke (3), intracerebral hemorrhage (3), congenital (1)
Vestibular ataxic	4 (3%)	6	Bilateral vestibulopathy (3), recent vestribular neuronitis (1), recent Ménière's attack (1), acoustic neuroma with surgery (1)
Dyskinetic	1 (1%)	4	Levodopa-induced dyskinesia (3), chorea (1)
Multiple neurologic gait disorders	36 (30%)		
Total	117		

[a]Percentage of individuals with a single gait disorder. [b]Includes individuals with multiple gait disorders.

Note: Of 117 patients with a neurologic gait disorder, 81 had a single neurologic gait disorder; the remainder (36) had multiple neurologic gait disorders.

Source: Reproduced with modifications from P Mahlknecht et al: PLoS One 8:e69627, 2013.

of the parkinsonian gait also contributes to falls, which are a major source of morbidity, particularly later in the disease course. Dopamine replacement improves step length, arm swing, turning speed, and gait initiation. There is increasing evidence that deficits in cholinergic circuits in the pedunculopontine nucleus and cortex contribute to the gait disorder of Parkinson's disease. Cholinesterase inhibitors such as donepezil and rivastigmine have been shown in early studies to significantly decrease gait variability, instability, and fall frequency, even in the absence of cognitive impairment, perhaps through improvement in attention.

Freezing is defined as a brief, episodic absence of forward progression of the feet, despite the intention to walk. Freezing may be triggered by approaching a narrow doorway or crowd, may be overcome by visual cueing, and contributes to fall risk. Gait freezing is present in approximately one-quarter of Parkinson's patients within 5 years of onset, and its frequency increases further over time. In treated patients, end-of-dose gait freezing is a common problem that may improve with more frequent administration of dopaminergic drugs or with use of monoamine oxidase type B inhibitors such as rasagiline or selegiline (**Chap. 435**).

Freezing of gait is also common in other neurodegenerative disorders associated with parkinsonism, including progressive supranuclear palsy (PSP), multiple-system atrophy, and corticobasal degeneration. Patients with these disorders frequently present with axial stiffness, postural instability, and a shuffling, freezing gait while lacking the characteristic pill-rolling tremor of Parkinson's disease. The gait of PSP is typically more erect compared with the stooped posture of typical Parkinson's disease, and falls within the first year also suggest the possibility of PSP. The gait of vascular parkinsonism tends to be broad-based and shuffling with reduced arm swing bilaterally; disproportionate involvement of gait early in the disease course differentiates this entity from Parkinson's disease.

Hyperkinetic movement disorders also produce characteristic and recognizable disturbances in gait. In Huntington's disease (**Chap. 436**), the unpredictable occurrence of choreic movements gives the gait a dancing quality. Tardive dyskinesia is the cause of many odd, stereotypic gait disorders seen in patients chronically exposed to antipsychotics and other drugs that block the D_2 dopamine receptor. *Orthostatic tremor* is a high-frequency, low-amplitude tremor predominantly involving the lower extremities. Patients often report shakiness or unsteadiness on standing and improvement with sitting or walking. Falls are common. The tremor is often only appreciable by palpating the legs while standing.

FRONTAL GAIT DISORDER

Frontal gait disorder, also known as higher-level gait disorder, is common in the elderly and has a variety of causes. The term is used to describe a shuffling, freezing gait with imbalance, and other signs of higher cerebral dysfunction. Typical features include a wide base of support, a short stride, shuffling along the floor, and difficulty with starts and turns. Many patients exhibit a difficulty with gait initiation that is descriptively characterized as the "slipping clutch" syndrome or gait ignition failure. The term *lower-body parkinsonism* is also used to describe such patients. Strength is generally preserved, and patients are able to make stepping movements when not standing and maintaining their balance at the same time. This disorder is best considered a higher-level motor control disorder, as opposed to an apraxia (**Chap. 30**), though the term *gait apraxia* persists in the literature.

The most common cause of frontal gait disorder is vascular disease, particularly subcortical small-vessel disease in the deep frontal white matter and centrum ovale. Over three-quarters of patients with subcortical vascular dementia demonstrate gait abnormalities; decreased arm swing and a stooped posture are particularly prevalent features. The clinical syndrome also includes dysarthria, pseudobulbar affect (emotional disinhibition), increased tone, and hyperreflexia in the lower limbs.

Normal pressure (communicating) hydrocephalus (NPH) in adults also presents with a similar gait disorder (**Chap. 431**). Other features of the diagnostic triad (mental changes, incontinence) may be absent in a substantial number of patients. MRI demonstrates ventricular enlargement, an enlarged flow void about the aqueduct, periventricular white matter change, and high-convexity tightness (disproportionate widening of the sylvian fissures versus the cortical sulci). A lumbar puncture or dynamic test is necessary to confirm a diagnosis of NPH. Neurodegenerative dementias and mass lesions of the frontal lobes cause a similar clinical picture and can be differentiated from vascular disease and hydrocephalus by neuroimaging.

CEREBELLAR GAIT ATAXIA

Disorders of the cerebellum (**Chap. 439**) have a dramatic impact on gait and balance. Cerebellar gait ataxia is characterized by a wide base of support, lateral instability of the trunk, erratic foot placement, and decompensation of balance when attempting to walk on a narrow base. Difficulty maintaining balance when turning is often an early feature. Patients are unable to walk tandem heel to toe and display truncal sway in narrow-based or tandem stance. They show considerable variation in their tendency to fall in daily life.

Causes of cerebellar ataxia in older patients include stroke, trauma, tumor, and neurodegenerative disease such as multiple-system atrophy (**Chap. 440**) and various forms of hereditary cerebellar degeneration (**Chap. 439**). A short expansion at the site of the fragile X mutation (*fragile X premutation*) has been associated with gait ataxia in older men. Alcohol causes an acute and chronic cerebellar ataxia. In patients with ataxia due to cerebellar degeneration, MRI demonstrates the extent and topography of cerebellar atrophy.

SENSORY ATAXIA

As reviewed earlier in this chapter, balance depends on high-quality afferent information from the visual and the vestibular systems and proprioception. When this information is lost or degraded, balance during locomotion is impaired and instability results. The sensory ataxia of tabetic neurosyphilis is a classic example. The contemporary equivalent is the patient with neuropathy affecting large fibers. Vitamin B_{12} deficiency is a treatable cause of large-fiber sensory loss in the spinal cord and peripheral nervous system. Joint position and vibration sense are diminished in the lower limbs. The stance in such patients is destabilized by eye closure; they often look down at their feet when walking and do poorly in the dark. **Table 26-2** compares sensory ataxia with cerebellar ataxia and frontal gait disorder.

TABLE 26-2 Features of Cerebellar Ataxia, Sensory Ataxia, and Frontal Gait Disorders

FEATURE	CEREBELLAR ATAXIA	SENSORY ATAXIA	FRONTAL GAIT
Base of support	Wide-based	Narrow base, looks down	Wide-based
Velocity	Variable	Slow	Very slow
Stride	Irregular, lurching	Regular with path deviation	Short, shuffling
Romberg test	+/–	Unsteady, falls	+/–
Heel → shin	Abnormal	+/–	Normal
Initiation	Normal	Normal	Hesitant
Turns	Unsteady	+/–	Hesitant, multistep
Postural instability	+	+++	++++ Poor postural synergies rising from a chair
Falls	Late event	Frequent	Frequent

NEUROMUSCULAR DISEASE

Patients with neuromuscular disease often have an abnormal gait, occasionally as a presenting feature. With distal weakness (peripheral neuropathy), the step height is increased to compensate for foot drop, and the sole of the foot may slap on the floor during weight acceptance, termed the *steppage gait*. Patients with myopathy or muscular dystrophy more typically exhibit proximal weakness. Weakness of the hip girdle may result in some degree of excess pelvic sway during locomotion. The stooped posture of lumbar spinal stenosis ameliorates pain from the compression of the cauda equina occurring with a more upright posture while walking and may mimic early parkinsonism.

TOXIC AND METABOLIC DISORDERS

Chronic toxicity from medications and metabolic disturbances can impair motor function and gait. Examination may reveal mental status changes, asterixis, or myoclonus. Static equilibrium is disturbed, and such patients are easily thrown off balance. Disequilibrium is particularly evident in patients with chronic renal disease and those with hepatic failure, in whom asterixis may impair postural support. Sedative drugs, especially neuroleptics and long-acting benzodiazepines, affect postural control and increase the risk for falls. These disorders are especially important to recognize because they are often treatable.

FUNCTIONAL GAIT DISORDER

Functional neurologic disorders (formerly "psychogenic") are common in practice, and the presentation often involves gait. Sudden onset, inconsistent deficits, waxing and waning course, incongruence of symptoms with an organic lesion, and improvement with distraction are key features. Phenomenology is variable; extreme slow motion, an inappropriately overcautious gait, odd gyrations of posture with wastage of muscular energy, astasia-abasia (inability to stand and walk), bouncing, and foot stiffness (dystonia) have been described. Falls are rare, and there are often discrepancies between examination findings and the patient's functional status. Preceding stress or trauma is variably present, and its absence does not preclude the diagnosis of a functional gait disorder. Functional gait disorders may be challenging to diagnose and should be differentiated from the slowness and psychomotor retardation seen in certain patients with major depression.

APPROACH TO THE PATIENT

Slowly Progressive Disorder of Gait

When reviewing the history, it is helpful to inquire about the onset and progression of disability. Initial awareness of an unsteady gait often follows a fall. Stepwise evolution or sudden progression suggests vascular disease. Gait disorder may be associated with urinary urgency and incontinence, particularly in patients with cervical spine disease or hydrocephalus. It is always important to review the use of alcohol and medications that affect gait and balance. Information on localization derived from the neurologic examination can be helpful in narrowing the list of possible diagnoses.

Gait observation provides an immediate sense of the patient's degree of disability. Arthritic and antalgic gaits are recognized by observation, although neurologic and orthopedic problems may coexist. Characteristic patterns of abnormality are sometimes seen, although, as stated previously, failing gaits often look fundamentally similar. Cadence (steps per minute), velocity, and stride length can be recorded by timing a patient over a fixed distance. Watching the patient rise from a chair provides a good functional assessment of balance.

Brain imaging studies may be informative in patients with an undiagnosed disorder of gait. MRI is sensitive for cerebral lesions of vascular or demyelinating disease and is a good screening test for occult hydrocephalus. Patients with recurrent falls are at risk for subdural hematoma. As mentioned earlier, many elderly patients with gait and balance difficulty have white matter abnormalities in the periventricular region and centrum semiovale. While these lesions may be an incidental finding, a substantial burden of white matter disease will ultimately impact cerebral control of locomotion.

DISORDERS OF BALANCE

DEFINITION, ETIOLOGY, AND MANIFESTATIONS

Balance is the ability to maintain equilibrium—a dynamic state in which one's center of mass is controlled with respect to the lower extremities, gravity, and the support surface despite external perturbations. The reflexes required to maintain upright posture require input from cerebellar, vestibular, and somatosensory systems; the premotor cortex and corticospinal and reticulospinal tracts mediate output to axial and proximal limb muscles. These responses are physiologically complex, and the anatomic representation they entail is not well understood. Failure can occur at any level and presents as difficulty maintaining posture while standing and walking.

The history and physical examination may differentiate underlying causes of imbalance. Patients with *cerebellar* ataxia do not generally complain of dizziness, although balance is visibly impaired. Neurologic examination reveals a variety of cerebellar signs. Postural compensation may prevent falls early on, but falls are inevitable with disease progression. The progression of neurodegenerative ataxia is often measured by the number of years to loss of stable ambulation.

Vestibular disorders (**Chap. 22**) have symptoms and signs that fall into three categories: (1) vertigo (the subjective inappropriate perception or illusion of movement); (2) nystagmus (involuntary eye movements); and (3) impaired standing balance. Not every patient has all manifestations. Patients with vestibular deficits related to ototoxic drugs may lack vertigo or obvious nystagmus, but their balance is impaired on standing and walking, and they cannot navigate in the dark. Laboratory testing is available to investigate vestibular deficits.

Somatosensory deficits also produce imbalance and falls. There is often a subjective sense of insecure balance and fear of falling. Postural control is compromised by eye closure (*Romberg's sign*); these patients also have difficulty navigating in the dark. A dramatic example is provided by the patient with autoimmune subacute sensory neuropathy, which is sometimes a paraneoplastic disorder (**Chap. 94**). Compensatory strategies enable such patients to walk in the virtual absence of proprioception, but the task requires active visual monitoring.

Patients with *higher-level disorders of equilibrium* have difficulty maintaining balance in daily life and may present with falls. Their awareness of balance impairment may be reduced. Patients taking sedating medications are in this category.

FALLS

Falls are common in the elderly; over one-third of people aged >65 who are living in the community fall each year. This number is even higher in nursing homes and hospitals. Elderly people are not only at higher risk for falls but are also more likely to suffer serious complications due to medical comorbidities such as osteoporosis. Hip fractures result in hospitalization, can lead to nursing home admission, and are associated with an increased mortality risk in the subsequent year. Falls may result in brain or spinal injury, the history of which may be difficult for the patient to provide. The proportion of spinal cord injuries due to falls in individuals aged >65 years has doubled in the past decade, perhaps due to increasing activity in this age group. Some falls result in a prolonged time lying on the ground; fractures and CNS injury are a particular concern in this context.

For each person who is physically disabled, there are others whose functional independence is limited by anxiety and fear of falling. Nearly one in five elderly individuals voluntarily restricts his or her activity because of fear of falling. With loss of ambulation, the quality of life diminishes, and rates of morbidity and mortality increase.

RISK FACTORS FOR FALLS

Risk factors for falls may be *intrinsic* (e.g., gait and balance disorders) or *extrinsic* (e.g., polypharmacy, environmental factors); some risk factors are modifiable. The presence of multiple risk factors is associated with a substantially increased risk of falls. **Table 26-3** summarizes a meta-analysis of studies establishing the principal risk factors for falls. Polypharmacy (use of four or more prescription medications) has also been identified as an important risk factor.

TABLE 26-3 Meta-Analysis of Risk Factors for Falls in Older Persons

RISK FACTOR	MEAN RR (OR)	RANGE
Muscle weakness	4.4	1.5–10.3
History of falls	3.0	1.7–7.0
Gait deficit	2.9	1.3–5.6
Balance deficit	2.9	1.6–5.4
Use assistive device	2.6	1.2–4.6
Visual deficit	2.5	1.6–3.5
Arthritis	2.4	1.9–2.9
Impaired ADL	2.3	1.5–3.1
Depression	2.2	1.7–2.5
Cognitive impairment	1.8	1.0–2.3
Age >80 years	1.7	1.1–2.5

Abbreviations: ADL, activity of daily living; OR, odds ratio from retrospective studies; RR, relative risk from prospective studies.

Source: Reproduced with permission from Guideline for the Prevention of Falls in Older Persons. J Am Geriatr Soc 49:664, 2001.

ASSESSMENT OF THE PATIENT WITH FALLS

The most productive approach is to identify the high-risk patient prospectively, before there is a serious injury. All community-dwelling adults should be asked annually about falls and whether or not fear of falling limits daily activities. The Timed Up and Go ("TUG") test involves timing a patient as they stand up from a chair, walk 10 feet, turn, and then sit down. Patients with a history of falls or those requiring >12 s to complete the TUG test are at high risk for falls and should undergo further assessment.

History The history surrounding a fall is often problematic or incomplete, and the underlying mechanism or cause may be difficult to establish in retrospect. Patients should be queried about any provoking factors (including head turn, standing) or prodromal symptoms, such as dizziness, vertigo, presyncopal symptoms, or focal weakness. A history of baseline mobility and medical comorbidities should be elicited. Patients at particular risk include those with mental status changes or dementia. Medications should be reviewed, with particular attention to benzodiazepines, opioids, antipsychotics, antiepileptics, antidepressants, antiarrhythmics, and diuretics, all of which are associated with an increased risk of falls. It is equally important to distinguish *mechanical falls* (those caused by tripping or slipping) due to purely extrinsic or environmental factors from those in which a modifiable intrinsic factor contributes. *Recurrent falls* may indicate an underlying gait or balance disorder. Falls associated with loss of consciousness (syncope, seizure) may require appropriate cardiac or neurologic evaluation and intervention **(Chaps. 21 and 425)**, although a patient's report of change in consciousness may be unreliable.

Physical Examination Examination of the patient with falls should include a basic cardiac examination, including orthostatic blood pressure if indicated by history, and observation of any orthopedic abnormalities. Mental status is easily assessed while obtaining a history from the patient; the remainder of the neurologic examination should include visual acuity, strength and sensation in the lower extremities, muscle tone, and cerebellar function, with particular attention to gait and balance as described earlier in this chapter.

Fall Patterns The description of a fall event may provide further clues to the underlying etiology. While there is no standard nosology of falls, some common clinical patterns may emerge and provide a clue.

DROP ATTACKS AND COLLAPSING FALLS Drop attacks and collapsing falls are associated with a sudden loss of postural tone. Patients may report that their legs just "gave out" underneath them or that they "collapsed in a heap." Syncope or orthostatic hypotension may be a factor in some such falls. Neurologic causes are relatively rare but include atonic seizures, myoclonus, and intermittent obstruction of the foramen of Monro by a colloid cyst of the third ventricle causing acute obstructive hydrocephalus. An emotional trigger suggests cataplexy. While collapsing falls are more common among older patients with vascular risk factors, drop attacks should not be confused with vertebrobasilar ischemic attacks.

TOPPLING FALLS Some patients maintain tone in antigravity muscles but fall over like a tree trunk, as if postural defenses had disengaged. Causes include cerebellar pathology and lesions of the vestibular system. There may be a consistent direction to such falls. Toppling falls are an early feature of progressive supranuclear palsy, and a late feature of Parkinson's disease, once postural instability has developed. Thalamic lesions causing truncal instability (*thalamic astasia*) may also contribute to this type of fall.

FALLS DUE TO GAIT FREEZING Freezing of gait is seen in Parkinson's disease and related disorders. The feet stick to the floor and the center of mass keeps moving, resulting in a disequilibrium from which the patient has difficulty recovering, resulting in a forward fall. Similarly, patients with Parkinson's disease and festinating gait may find their feet unable to keep up and may thus fall forward.

FALLS RELATED TO SENSORY LOSS Patients with somatosensory, visual, or vestibular deficits are prone to falls. These patients have particular difficulty dealing with poor illumination or walking on uneven ground. They often report subjective imbalance, apprehension, and fear of falling. These patients may be especially responsive to a rehabilitation-based intervention.

FALLS RELATED TO WEAKNESS Patients who lack strength in antigravity muscles have difficulty rising from a chair or maintaining their balance after a perturbation. These patients are often unable to get up after a fall and may have to remain on the floor for a prolonged period until help arrives. If due to deconditioning, this is often treatable. Resistance strength training can increase muscle mass and leg strength, even for people in their eighties and nineties.

TREATMENT

Interventions to Reduce the Risk of Falls and Injury

Efforts should be made to define the mechanism underlying falls in a given patient, as specific treatment may be possible once a diagnosis is established. Orthostatic changes in blood pressure and pulse should be recorded. Medications (including over-the-counter) should be reviewed, reevaluating benefits and burdens of medications that might increase fall risk. Treatment of cataracts and avoidance of multifocal lenses could be considered for patients whose falls result from vision impairment. A home visit to look for environmental hazards can be helpful. A variety of modifications may be recommended to improve safety, including improved lighting, installation of grab bars and nonslip surfaces, and use of adaptive equipment.

Home- and group-based exercise programs focusing on leg strength and balance, physical therapy, and use of assistive devices reduce fall risk in individuals with a history of falls or disorders of gait and balance. Rehabilitative interventions aim to improve muscle strength and balance stability and to make the patient more resistant to injury. High-intensity resistance strength training with weights and machines is useful to improve muscle mass, even in frail older patients. Improvements realized in posture and gait should translate to reduced risk of falls and injury. Sensory balance training is another approach to improving balance stability. Measurable gains can be made in a few weeks of training, and benefits can be maintained over 6 months by a 10- to 20-min home exercise program. This strategy is particularly successful in patients with vestibular and somatosensory balance disorders. The National Institute on Aging provides online examples of balance exercises for older adults. A Tai Chi exercise program has been demonstrated to reduce the risk of falls and injury in patients with Parkinson's disease. Cognitive training, including dual-task training, may improve mobility in older adults with cognitive impairment.

Acknowledgements

I am grateful to Dr. Lewis R. Sudarsky for his substantial contributions to earlier versions of this chapter.

FURTHER READING

American Geriatrics Society, British Geriatrics Society, American Academy of Orthopedic Surgeons Panel on Falls Prevention: Guideline for the prevention of falls in older persons. J Am Geriatr Soc 49:664, 2001.

Ganz D, Latham N: Prevention of falls in community-dwelling older adults. N Engl J Med 382:734, 2020.

National Institute on Aging: Exercise and Physical Activity. Available from *https://www.nia.nih.gov/health/exercise-physical-activity*. Accessed April 25, 2021.

Nutt JG: Classification of gait and balance disorders. Adv Neurol 87:135, 2001.

Pirker W, Katzenschlager R: Gait disorders in adults and the elderly. Wien Klin Wochenschr 129:81, 2017.

27 Confusion and Delirium

S. Andrew Josephson, Bruce L. Miller

Confusion, a mental and behavioral state of reduced comprehension, coherence, and capacity to reason, is one of the most common problems encountered in medicine, accounting for a large number of emergency department visits, hospital admissions, and inpatient consultations. *Delirium*, a term used to describe an acute confusional state, remains a major cause of morbidity and mortality, costing billions of dollars yearly in health care costs in the United States alone. Despite increased efforts targeting awareness of this condition, delirium often goes unrecognized in the face of evidence that it is usually the cognitive manifestation of serious underlying medical or neurologic illness.

CLINICAL FEATURES OF DELIRIUM

A multitude of terms are used to describe patients with delirium, including *encephalopathy, acute brain failure, acute confusional state*, and *postoperative* or *intensive care unit (ICU) psychosis*. Delirium has many clinical manifestations, but it is defined as a relatively acute decline in cognition that fluctuates over hours or days. The hallmark of delirium is a deficit of attention, although all cognitive domains—including memory, executive function, visuospatial tasks, and language—are variably involved. Associated symptoms that may be present in some cases include altered sleep-wake cycles, perceptual disturbances such as hallucinations or delusions, affect changes, and autonomic findings that include heart rate and blood pressure instability.

Delirium is a clinical diagnosis that is made only at the bedside. Two subtypes have been described—hyperactive and hypoactive—based on differential psychomotor features. The cognitive syndrome associated with severe alcohol withdrawal (i.e., "delirium tremens") remains the classic example of the hyperactive subtype, featuring prominent hallucinations, agitation, and hyperarousal, often accompanied by life-threatening autonomic instability. In striking contrast is the hypoactive subtype, exemplified by benzodiazepine intoxication, in which patients are withdrawn and quiet, with prominent apathy and psychomotor slowing.

This dichotomy between subtypes of delirium is a useful construct, but patients often fall somewhere along a spectrum between the hyperactive and hypoactive extremes, sometimes fluctuating from one to the other. Therefore, clinicians must recognize this broad range of presentations of delirium to identify all patients with this potentially reversible cognitive disturbance. Hyperactive patients are often easily recognized by their characteristic severe agitation, tremor, hallucinations, and autonomic instability. Patients who are quietly hypoactive are more often overlooked on the medical wards and in the ICU.

The reversibility of delirium is emphasized because many etiologies, such as infection and medication effects, can be treated easily. The long-term cognitive consequences of delirium remain an area of active research. Some episodes of delirium continue for weeks, months, or even years. The persistence of delirium in some patients and its high recurrence rate may be due to inadequate initial treatment of the underlying etiology. In other instances, delirium appears to cause permanent neuronal damage and long-term cognitive decline. Therefore, prevention strategies are important to implement. Even if an episode of delirium completely resolves, there may be lingering effects of the disorder; a patient's recall of events after delirium varies widely, ranging from complete amnesia to repeated reexperiencing of the frightening period of confusion, similar to what is seen in patients with posttraumatic stress disorder.

RISK FACTORS

An effective primary prevention strategy for delirium begins with identification of high-risk patients. Some hospital systems have initiated comprehensive delirium programs that screen most or all patients upon admission or before elective surgery; positive screens trigger a host of focused prevention measures. Multiple validated scoring systems have been developed as a screen for asymptomatic patients, many of which emphasize well-established risk factors for delirium.

The two most consistently identified risk factors are older age and baseline cognitive dysfunction. Individuals who are aged >65 or exhibit low scores on standardized tests of cognition develop delirium upon hospitalization at a rate approaching 50%. Whether age and baseline cognitive dysfunction are truly independent risk factors is uncertain. Other predisposing factors include sensory deprivation, such as preexisting hearing and visual impairment, as well as indices for poor overall health, including baseline immobility, malnutrition, and underlying medical or neurologic illness.

In-hospital risks for delirium include the use of bladder catheterization, physical restraints, sleep and sensory deprivation, and the addition of three or more new medications. Avoiding such risks remains a key component of delirium prevention as well as treatment. Surgical and anesthetic risk factors for the development of postoperative delirium include procedures such as those involving cardiopulmonary bypass, inadequate or excessive treatment of pain in the immediate postoperative period, and perhaps specific agents such as inhalational anesthetics.

The relationship between delirium and dementia (**Chap. 29**) is complicated by significant overlap between the two conditions, and it is not always simple to distinguish between them. Dementia and preexisting cognitive dysfunction serve as major risk factors for delirium, and at least two-thirds of cases of delirium occur in patients with coexisting underlying dementia. A form of dementia with parkinsonism, *dementia with Lewy bodies* (**Chap. 434**), is characterized by a fluctuating course, prominent visual hallucinations, parkinsonism, and an attentional deficit that clinically resembles hyperactive delirium; patients with this condition are particularly vulnerable to delirium. Delirium in the elderly often reflects an insult to a brain that is vulnerable due to an underlying neurodegenerative condition. Therefore, the development of delirium sometimes heralds the onset of a previously unrecognized brain disorder, and after the acute delirious episode has cleared, careful screening for an underlying condition should occur in the outpatient setting.

EPIDEMIOLOGY

Delirium is common, but its reported incidence has varied widely with the criteria used to define this disorder. Estimates of delirium in hospitalized patients range from 10% to >50%, with higher rates reported for elderly patients and patients undergoing hip surgery. Older patients in the ICU have especially high rates of delirium that approach 75%. The condition is not recognized in up to one-third of delirious inpatients, and the diagnosis is especially problematic in the ICU environment, where cognitive dysfunction is often difficult to appreciate in the setting of serious systemic illness and sedation. Delirium in the ICU should be viewed as an important manifestation of organ dysfunction not unlike liver, kidney, or heart failure. Outside the acute hospital setting, delirium occurs in nearly one-quarter of patients in nursing homes and in 50–80% of those at the end of life. These estimates emphasize the remarkably high frequency of this cognitive syndrome in older patients, a population that continues to grow.

An episode of delirium was previously viewed as a transient condition that carried a benign prognosis. It is now recognized as a disorder with substantial morbidity and mortality, and that often represents the first manifestation of a serious underlying illness. Estimates of in-hospital mortality rates among delirious patients range from 25% to 33%, similar to mortality rates due to sepsis. Patients with an in-hospital episode of delirium have a fivefold higher mortality rate in the months after their illness compared with age matched nondelirious hospitalized patients. Delirious hospitalized patients also have a longer length of stay, are more likely to be discharged to a nursing home, have a higher frequency of readmission, and are more likely to experience subsequent episodes of delirium and cognitive decline; as a result, this condition has an enormous economic cost.

PATHOGENESIS

The pathogenesis and anatomy of delirium are incompletely understood. The attentional deficit that serves as the neuropsychological hallmark of delirium has a diffuse localization within the brainstem, thalamus, prefrontal cortex, and parietal lobes. Rarely, focal lesions such as ischemic strokes have led to delirium in otherwise healthy persons; right parietal and medial dorsal thalamic lesions have been reported most commonly, pointing to the importance of these areas in delirium pathogenesis. In most cases, however, delirium results from widespread disturbances in cortical and subcortical regions of the brain. Electroencephalogram (EEG) usually reveals symmetric slowing, a nonspecific finding that supports diffuse cerebral dysfunction.

Multiple neurotransmitter abnormalities, proinflammatory factors, and specific genes likely play a role in the pathogenesis of delirium. Deficiency of acetylcholine may play a key role, and medications with anticholinergic properties can commonly precipitate delirium. As noted earlier, patients with preexisting dementia are particularly susceptible to episodes of delirium. Alzheimer's disease **(Chap. 431)**, dementia with Lewy bodies **(Chap. 434)**, and Parkinson's disease dementia **(Chap. 435)** are all associated with cholinergic deficiency due to degeneration of acetylcholine-producing neurons in the basal forebrain. In addition, other neurotransmitters are also likely to be involved in this diffuse cerebral disorder. For example, increases in dopamine can lead to delirium, and patients with Parkinson's disease treated with dopaminergic medications can develop a delirium-like state that features visual hallucinations, fluctuations, and confusion.

Not all individuals exposed to the same insult will develop signs of delirium. A low dose of an anticholinergic medication may have no cognitive effects on a healthy young adult but produce a florid delirium in an elderly person with known underlying dementia, although even healthy young persons develop delirium with very high doses of anticholinergic medications. This concept of delirium developing as the result of an insult in predisposed individuals is currently the most widely accepted pathogenic construct. Therefore, if a previously healthy individual with no known history of cognitive illness develops delirium in the setting of a relatively minor insult such as elective surgery or hospitalization, an unrecognized underlying neurologic illness such as a neurodegenerative disease, multiple previous strokes, or another diffuse cerebral cause should be considered. In this context, delirium can be viewed as a "stress test for the brain" whereby exposure to known inciting factors such as systemic infection and offending drugs can unmask a decreased cerebral reserve and herald a serious underlying and potentially treatable illness. New blood-based biomarkers for specific dementias may soon be available to help predict people at risk for delirium before surgical procedures or hospitalization.

APPROACH TO THE PATIENT

Delirium

Because the diagnosis of delirium is clinical and is made at the bedside, a careful history and physical examination are necessary in evaluating patients with possible confusional states. Screening tools can aid physicians and nurses in identifying patients with delirium, including the Confusion Assessment Method (CAM); the Nursing Delirium Screening Scale (NuDESC); the Organic Brain Syndrome Scale; the Delirium Rating Scale; and, in the ICU, the ICU version of the CAM and the Delirium Detection Score. Using the well-validated CAM, a diagnosis of delirium is made if there is (1) an acute onset and fluctuating course and (2) inattention accompanied by either (3) disorganized thinking or (4) an altered level of consciousness **(Table 27-1)**. These scales may not identify the full spectrum of patients with delirium, and all patients who are acutely confused should be presumed delirious regardless of their presentation due to the wide variety of possible clinical features. A course that fluctuates over hours or days and may worsen at night (termed *sundowning*) is typical but not essential for the diagnosis. Observation will usually reveal an altered level of consciousness or a deficit of attention. Other features that are sometimes present include alteration of sleep-wake cycles, thought disturbances such as hallucinations or delusions, autonomic instability, and changes in affect.

HISTORY

It may be difficult to elicit an accurate history in delirious patients who have altered levels of consciousness or impaired attention. Information from a collateral source such as a spouse or another family member is therefore invaluable. The three most important pieces of history are the patient's baseline cognitive function, the time course of the present illness, and current medications.

Premorbid cognitive function can be assessed through the collateral source or, if needed, via a review of outpatient records. Delirium by definition represents a change that is relatively acute and usually developing over hours to days, from a cognitive baseline. An acute confusional state is nearly impossible to diagnose without some knowledge of baseline cognitive function. Without

TABLE 27-1 The Confusion Assessment Method (CAM) Diagnostic Algorithm[a]

The diagnosis of delirium requires the presence of features 1 and 2 **and** *either* feature 3 or 4.
Feature 1. Acute Onset and Fluctuating Course
This feature is satisfied by positive responses to the following questions: Is there evidence of an acute change in mental status from the patient's baseline? Did the (abnormal) behavior fluctuate during the day, that is, tend to come and go, or did it increase and decrease in severity?
Feature 2. Inattention
This feature is satisfied by a positive response to the following question: Did the patient have difficulty focusing attention, for example, being easily distractible, or have difficulty keeping track of what was being said?
Feature 3. Disorganized Thinking
This feature is satisfied by a positive response to the following question: Was the patient's thinking disorganized or incoherent, such as rambling or irrelevant conversation, unclear or illogical flow of ideas, or unpredictable switching from subject to subject?
Feature 4. Altered Level of Consciousness
This feature is satisfied by any answer other than "alert" to the following question: Overall, how would you rate the patient's level of consciousness: alert (normal), vigilant (hyperalert), lethargic (drowsy, easily aroused), stupor (difficult to arouse), or coma (unarousable)?

[a]Information is usually obtained from a reliable reporter, such as a family member, caregiver, or nurse.

Source: From Annals of Internal Medicine, SK Inouye et al: Clarifying confusion: The Confusion Assessment Method. A new method for detection of delirium. 113(12):941, 1990.

this information, many patients with dementia or longstanding depression may be mistaken as delirious during a single initial evaluation. Patients with a more hypoactive, apathetic presentation with psychomotor slowing may be identified as being different from baseline only through conversations with family members. A number of validated instruments have been shown to diagnose cognitive dysfunction accurately using a collateral source, including the modified Blessed Dementia Rating Scale and the Clinical Dementia Rating (CDR). Baseline cognitive impairment is common in patients with delirium. Even when no such history of cognitive impairment is elicited, there should still be a high suspicion for a previously unrecognized underlying neurologic disorder.

Establishing the time course of cognitive change is important not only to make a diagnosis of delirium but also to correlate the onset of the illness with potentially treatable etiologies such as recent medication changes or symptoms of systemic infection.

Medications remain a common cause of delirium, especially compounds with anticholinergic or sedative properties. It is estimated that nearly one-third of all cases of delirium are secondary to medications, especially in the elderly. Medication histories should include all prescription as well as over-the-counter and herbal substances taken by the patient and any recent changes in dosing or formulation, including substitution of generics for brand-name medications.

Other important elements of the history include screening for symptoms of organ failure or systemic infection, which often contributes to delirium in the elderly. A history of illicit drug use, alcoholism, or toxin exposure is common in younger delirious patients. Finally, asking the patient and collateral source about other symptoms that may accompany delirium, such as depression, may help identify potential therapeutic targets.

PHYSICAL EXAMINATION

The general physical examination in a delirious patient should include careful screening for signs of infection such as fever, tachypnea, pulmonary consolidation, heart murmur, and meningismus. The patient's fluid status should be assessed; both dehydration and fluid overload with resultant hypoxemia have been associated with delirium, and each is usually easily rectified. The appearance of the skin can be helpful, showing jaundice in hepatic encephalopathy, cyanosis in hypoxemia, or needle tracks in patients using intravenous drugs.

The neurologic examination requires a careful assessment of mental status. Patients with delirium often present with a fluctuating course; therefore, the diagnosis can be missed when one relies on a single time point of evaluation. For patients who worsen in the evening (sundowning), assessment only during morning rounds may be falsely reassuring.

An altered level of consciousness ranging from hyperarousal to lethargy to coma is present in most patients with delirium and can be assessed easily at the bedside. In a patient with a relatively normal level of consciousness, a screen for an attentional deficit is in order, because this deficit is the classic neuropsychological hallmark of delirium. Attention can be assessed while taking a history from the patient. Tangential speech, a fragmentary flow of ideas, or inability to follow complex commands often signifies an attentional problem. There are formal neuropsychological tests to assess attention, but a simple bedside test of digit span forward is quick and fairly sensitive. In this task, patients are asked to repeat successively longer random strings of digits beginning with two digits in a row, said to the patient at one per second intervals. Healthy adults can repeat a string of five to seven digits before faltering; a digit span of four or less usually indicates an attentional deficit unless hearing or language barriers are present, and many patients with delirium have digit spans of three or fewer digits.

More formal neuropsychological testing can be helpful in assessing a delirious patient, but it is usually too cumbersome and time-consuming in the inpatient setting. A Mini-Mental State Examination (MMSE) provides information regarding orientation, language, and visuospatial skills **(Chap. 29)**; however, performance of many tasks on the MMSE, including the spelling of "world" backward and serial subtraction of digits, will be impaired by delirious patients' attentional deficits, rendering the test unreliable.

The remainder of the screening neurologic examination should focus on identifying new focal neurologic deficits. Focal strokes or mass lesions in isolation are rarely the cause of delirium, but patients with underlying extensive cerebrovascular disease or neurodegenerative conditions may not be able to cognitively tolerate even relatively small new insults. Patients should be screened for other signs of neurodegenerative conditions such as parkinsonism, which is seen not only in idiopathic Parkinson's disease but also in other dementing conditions including Alzheimer's disease, dementia with Lewy bodies, and progressive supranuclear palsy. The presence of multifocal myoclonus or asterixis on the motor examination is nonspecific but usually indicates a metabolic or toxic etiology of the delirium.

ETIOLOGY

Some etiologies can be easily discerned through a careful history and physical examination, whereas others require confirmation with laboratory studies, imaging, or other ancillary tests. A large, diverse group of insults can lead to delirium, and the cause in many patients is multifactorial. Common etiologies are listed in **Table 27-2**.

Prescribed, over-the-counter, and herbal medications all can precipitate delirium. Drugs with anticholinergic properties, narcotics, and benzodiazepines are particularly common offenders, but nearly any compound can lead to cognitive dysfunction in a predisposed patient. Whereas an elderly patient with baseline dementia may become delirious upon exposure to a relatively low dose of a medication, in less susceptible individuals, delirium occurs only with very high doses of the same medication. This observation emphasizes the importance of correlating the timing of recent medication changes, including dose and formulation, with the onset of cognitive dysfunction.

In younger patients, illicit drugs and toxins are common causes of delirium. In addition to more classic drugs of abuse, the availability of "bath salts," synthetic cannabis **(Chap. 455)**, methylenedioxymethamphetamine (MDMA, ecstasy), γ-hydroxybutyrate (GHB), and the phencyclidine (PCP)-like agent ketamine has led to an increase in delirious young persons presenting to acute care settings **(Chap. 457)**. Many common prescription drugs such as oral narcotics and benzodiazepines are often abused and readily available on the street. Alcohol abuse leading to high serum levels causes confusion, but more commonly, it is withdrawal from alcohol that leads to a hyperactive delirium **(Chap. 453)**. Alcohol and benzodiazepine withdrawal should be considered in all cases of delirium, including in the elderly, because even patients who drink only a few servings of alcohol every day can experience relatively severe withdrawal symptoms upon hospitalization.

Metabolic abnormalities such as electrolyte disturbances of sodium, calcium, magnesium, or glucose can cause delirium, and mild derangements can lead to substantial cognitive disturbances in susceptible individuals. Other common metabolic etiologies include liver and renal failure, hypercarbia and hypoxemia, vitamin deficiencies of thiamine and B_{12}, autoimmune disorders including central nervous system (CNS) vasculitis, and endocrinopathies such as thyroid and adrenal disorders.

Systemic infections often cause delirium, especially in the elderly. A common scenario involves the development of an acute cognitive decline in the setting of a urinary tract infection in a patient with baseline dementia. Pneumonia, skin infections such as cellulitis, and frank sepsis also lead to delirium. This so-called septic encephalopathy, often seen in the ICU, is probably due to the release of proinflammatory cytokines and their diffuse cerebral effects. CNS infections such as meningitis, encephalitis, and abscess are less common etiologies of delirium, as are cases of autoimmune or

TABLE 27-2 Differential Diagnosis of Delirium

Toxins
Prescription medications: especially those with anticholinergic properties, narcotics, and benzodiazepines
Drugs of abuse: alcohol intoxication and alcohol withdrawal, opiates, ecstasy, LSD, GHB, PCP, ketamine, cocaine, "bath salts," marijuana and its synthetic forms
Poisons: inhalants, carbon monoxide, ethylene glycol, pesticides
Metabolic Conditions
Electrolyte disturbances: hypoglycemia, hyperglycemia, hyponatremia, hypernatremia, hypercalcemia, hypocalcemia, hypomagnesemia
Hypothermia and hyperthermia
Pulmonary failure: hypoxemia and hypercarbia
Liver failure/hepatic encephalopathy
Renal failure/uremia
Cardiac failure
Vitamin deficiencies: B_{12}, thiamine, folate, niacin
Dehydration and malnutrition
Anemia
Infections
Systemic infections: urinary tract infections, pneumonia, skin and soft tissue infections, sepsis
CNS infections: meningitis, encephalitis, brain abscess
Endocrine Conditions
Hyperthyroidism, hypothyroidism
Hyperparathyroidism
Adrenal insufficiency
Cerebrovascular Disorders
Global hypoperfusion states
Hypertensive encephalopathy
Focal ischemic strokes and hemorrhages (rare): especially nondominant parietal and thalamic lesions
Autoimmune Disorders
CNS vasculitis
Cerebral lupus
Neurologic paraneoplastic and autoimmune encephalitis
Seizure-Related Disorders
Nonconvulsive status epilepticus
Intermittent seizures with prolonged postictal states
Neoplastic Disorders
Diffuse metastases to the brain
Gliomatosis cerebri
Carcinomatous meningitis
CNS lymphoma
Hospitalization
Terminal end-of-life delirium

Abbreviations: CNS, central nervous system; GHB, γ-hydroxybutyrate; LSD, lysergic acid diethylamide; PCP, phencyclidine.

paraneoplastic encephalitis; however, in light of the high morbidity and mortality rates associated with these conditions when they are not treated, clinicians must always maintain a high index of suspicion.

In some susceptible individuals, exposure to the unfamiliar environment of a hospital itself can contribute to delirium. This etiology usually occurs as part of a multifactorial delirium and should be considered a diagnosis of exclusion after all other causes have been thoroughly investigated. Many primary prevention and treatment strategies for delirium involve relatively simple methods to address the aspects of the inpatient setting that are most confusing.

Cerebrovascular etiologies of delirium are usually due to global hypoperfusion in the setting of systemic hypotension from heart failure, septic shock, dehydration, or anemia. Focal strokes in the right parietal lobe and medial dorsal thalamus rarely can lead to a delirious state. A more common scenario involves a new focal stroke or hemorrhage causing confusion in a patient who has decreased cerebral reserve. In these individuals, it is sometimes difficult to distinguish between cognitive dysfunction resulting from the new neurovascular insult itself and delirium due to the infectious, metabolic, and pharmacologic complications that can accompany hospitalization after stroke.

Because a fluctuating course often is seen in delirium, intermittent seizures may be overlooked when one is considering potential etiologies. Both nonconvulsive status epilepticus and recurrent focal or generalized seizures followed by postictal confusion can cause delirium; EEG remains essential for this diagnosis and should be considered whenever the etiology of delirium remains unclear following initial workup. Seizure activity spreading from an electrical focus in a mass or infarct can explain global cognitive dysfunction caused by relatively small lesions.

It is extremely common for patients to experience delirium at the end of life in palliative care settings. This condition must be identified and treated aggressively because it is an important cause of patient and family discomfort at the end of life. It should be remembered that these patients also may be suffering from more common etiologies of delirium such as systemic infection.

LABORATORY AND DIAGNOSTIC EVALUATION

A cost-effective approach allows the history and physical examination to guide further tests. No single algorithm will fit all delirious patients due to the staggering number of potential etiologies, but one stepwise approach is detailed in **Table 27-3**. If a clear precipitant such as an offending medication is identified, further testing may not be required. If, however, no likely etiology is uncovered with initial evaluation, an aggressive search for an underlying cause should be initiated.

Basic screening labs, including a complete blood count, electrolyte panel, and tests of liver and renal function, should be obtained in all patients with delirium. In elderly patients, screening for systemic infection, including chest radiography, urinalysis and culture, and possibly blood cultures, is important. In younger individuals, serum and urine drug and toxicology screening may be appropriate earlier in the workup. Additional laboratory tests addressing other autoimmune, endocrinologic, metabolic, and infectious etiologies should be reserved for patients in whom the diagnosis remains unclear after initial testing.

Multiple studies have demonstrated that brain imaging in patients with delirium is often unhelpful. If, however, the initial workup is unrevealing, most clinicians quickly move toward imaging of the brain to exclude structural causes. A noncontrast computed tomography (CT) scan can identify large masses and hemorrhages but is otherwise unlikely to help determine an etiology of delirium. The ability of magnetic resonance imaging (MRI) to identify most acute ischemic strokes as well as to provide neuroanatomic detail that gives clues to possible infectious, inflammatory, neurodegenerative, and neoplastic conditions makes it the test of choice. Because MRI techniques are limited by availability, speed of imaging, patient's cooperation, and contraindications, many clinicians begin with CT scanning and proceed to MRI if the etiology of delirium remains elusive.

Lumbar puncture (LP) must be obtained immediately after neuroimaging for all patients in whom CNS infection is suspected. Spinal fluid examination can also be useful in identifying autoimmune, other inflammatory, and neoplastic conditions. As a result, LP should be considered in any delirious patient with a negative workup. EEG remains invaluable if seizures are considered or if there is no cause readily identified.

TABLE 27-3 Stepwise Evaluation of a Patient with Delirium
Initial Evaluation
History with special attention to medications (including over-the-counter and herbals)
General physical examination and neurologic examination
Complete blood count
Electrolyte panel including calcium, magnesium, phosphorus
Liver function tests, including albumin
Renal function tests
First-Tier Further Evaluation Guided by Initial Evaluation
Systemic infection screen
Urinalysis and culture
Chest radiograph
Blood cultures
Electrocardiogram
Arterial blood gas
Serum and/or urine toxicology screen (perform earlier in young persons)
Brain imaging with MRI with diffusion and gadolinium (preferred) or CT
Suspected CNS infection or other inflammatory disorder: lumbar puncture after brain imaging
Suspected seizure-related etiology: electroencephalogram (EEG) (if high suspicion, should be performed immediately)
Second-Tier Further Evaluation
Vitamin levels: B_{12}, folate, thiamine
Endocrinologic laboratories: thyroid-stimulating hormone (TSH) and free T_4; cortisol
Serum ammonia
Sedimentation rate
Autoimmune serologies: antinuclear antibodies (ANA), complement levels; p-ANCA, c-ANCA, consider paraneoplastic/autoimmune encephalitis serologies
Infectious serologies: rapid plasmin reagin (RPR); fungal and viral serologies if high suspicion; HIV antibody
Lumbar puncture (if not already performed)
Brain MRI with and without gadolinium (if not already performed)

Abbreviations: c-ANCA, cytoplasmic antineutrophil cytoplasmic antibody; CNS, central nervous system; CT, computed tomography; MRI, magnetic resonance imaging; p-ANCA, perinuclear antineutrophil cytoplasmic antibody.

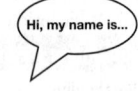

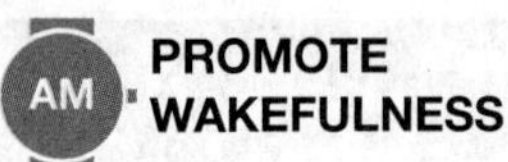
AM
PROMOTE WAKEFULNESS
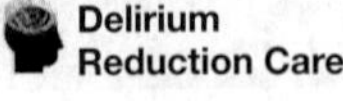
Delirium Reduction Care
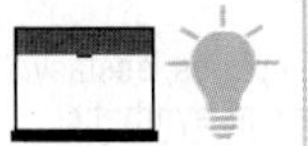
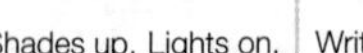
Shades up. Lights on.

Write date and staff names on board to orient patient.
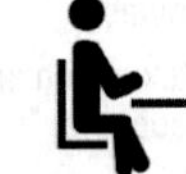
Patient out of bed to chair for all 3 meals. Ask for assistance if you need help.
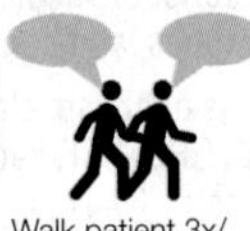
Walk patient 3x/ day. Engage patient in conversation.
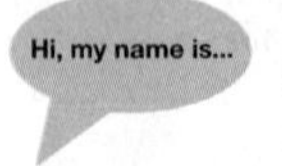
Hi, my name is...
Each visit, introduce yourself; remind patient where they are, what day and time it is.
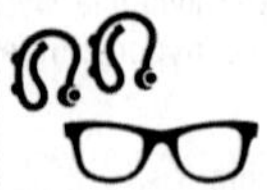
Patient is wearing hearing aids/glasses (if needed) to hear and see appropriately.

Provide activities like games and reading materials to keep patient's mind active while awake.
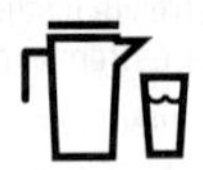
Make sure your patient has water within reach at all times. Dehydration is the #1 complaint in the hospital!

Make sure family members have been provided the pamphlet about delirium and discuss any questions they have. It is ok to refer to the nurse or doctor if you are unsure.
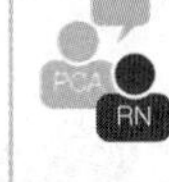
PCA
RN
Discuss with the nurse at each shift if the patient truly needs the following: nasal cannula on their nose, Foley catheter, telemetry, and CPO. These "tethers" make it difficult for the patient to move and can contribute to confusion.
A

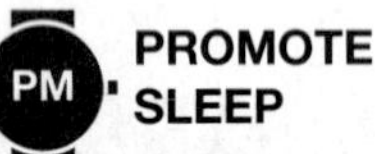
PM
PROMOTE SLEEP

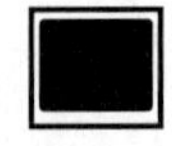
Shades closed. Lights off. TV off. Make room as dark and quiet as possible.
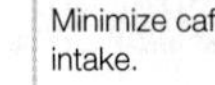
Minimize caffeine intake.

Offer eye mask, ear plugs to help with sleep.
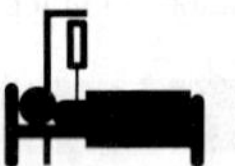
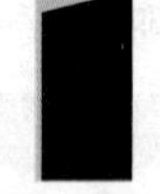
Group your nighttime tasks so that you are entering the room and waking the patient as few times as possible.
Discuss with the nurse each shift if they need vital signs done overnight.
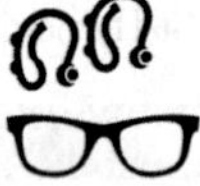
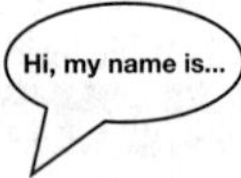
Hi, my name is...
If you communicate with the patient during the night, make sure glasses and hearing aids are on. Remember to introduce yourself, remind the patient where they are.
B

FIGURE 27-1 Delirium management and prevention: a checklist for hospitalized patients. Effective management of delirium relies on broad efforts to promote wakefulness (***A***) and sleep (***B***). CPO, continuous pulse oximetry.

TREATMENT

Delirium

Management of delirium begins with treatment of the underlying inciting factor (e.g., patients with systemic infections should be given appropriate antibiotics, and underlying electrolyte disturbances should be judiciously corrected). These treatments often lead to prompt resolution of delirium. Blindly targeting the symptoms of delirium pharmacologically only serves to prolong the time patients remain in the confused state and may mask important diagnostic information.

Relatively simple methods of supportive care can be highly effective (**Fig. 27-1**). Reorientation by the nursing staff and family combined with visible clocks, calendars, and outside-facing windows can reduce confusion. Sensory isolation should be prevented by providing glasses and hearing aids to patients who need them. Sundowning can be addressed to a large extent through vigilance to appropriate sleep-wake cycles. During the day, a well-lit room should be accompanied by activities or exercises to prevent napping. At night, a quiet, dark environment with limited interruptions by staff can assure proper rest; melatonin can be considered before bed to promote sleep. These sleep-wake cycle interventions are especially important in the ICU setting as the usual constant 24-h activity commonly provokes delirium. Attempting to mimic the home environment as much as possible also has been shown to help treat and even prevent delirium. Visits from friends and family throughout the day minimize the anxiety associated with the constant flow of new faces of staff and physicians. Allowing hospitalized patients to have access to home bedding, clothing, and nightstand objects makes the hospital environment less foreign and therefore less confusing. Simple standard nursing practices such as maintaining proper nutrition and volume status as well as managing pain, incontinence, and skin breakdown also help alleviate discomfort and resulting confusion.

In some instances, patients pose a threat to their own safety or to the safety of staff members, and acute management is required. Bed alarms and personal sitters are more effective and much less disorienting than physical restraints. Chemical restraints should be avoided, but when necessary, very-low-dose typical or atypical antipsychotic medications administered on an as-needed basis can be used, recognizing that clinical trials have consistently shown that these medications are ineffective in treating delirium. Therefore, they should be reserved for patients who display severe agitation and significant potential to harm themselves or staff. The association of antipsychotic use in the elderly with increased mortality rates underscores the importance of using these medications judiciously and only as a last resort. Benzodiazepines often worsen confusion through their sedative properties. Although many clinicians use benzodiazepines to treat acute confusion, their use should be limited to cases in which delirium is caused by alcohol or benzodiazepine withdrawal.

PREVENTION

In light of the high morbidity associated with delirium and the tremendously increased health care costs that accompany it, development of an effective strategy to prevent delirium in hospitalized patients is extremely important. Successful identification of high-risk patients is the first step, followed by initiation of appropriate interventions. Increasingly, hospitals are using nursing or physician-administered tools to screen for high-risk individuals, triggering simple standardized protocols used to manage risk factors for delirium, including sleep-wake cycle reversal, immobility, visual impairment, hearing impairment, sleep deprivation, and dehydration. No specific medications have been definitively shown to be effective for delirium prevention, including trials of cholinesterase inhibitors and antipsychotic agents. Melatonin and its agonist ramelteon have shown some promising results in small preliminary trials. Recent studies in the ICU have focused both on identifying sedatives, such as dexmedetomidine, that are less likely to lead to delirium in critically ill patients and on developing protocols for daily awakenings in which infusions of sedative medications are interrupted and the patient is reorientated by the staff. All hospitals and health care systems should work toward decreasing the incidence of delirium and promptly recognizing and treating the disorder when it occurs.

FURTHER READING

Brown EG et al: Evaluation of a multicomponent pathway to address inpatient delirium on a neurosciences ward. BMC Health Serv Res 18:106, 2018.

Constantin JM et al: Efficacy and safety of sedation with dexmedetomidine in critical care patients: A meta-analysis of randomized controlled trials. Anaesth Crit Care Pain Med 35:7, 2016.

Girard TD et al: Haloperidol and ziprasidone for treatment of delirium in critical illness. N Engl J Med 379:2506, 2018.

Goldberg TE et al: Association of delirium with long-term cognitive decline: A meta-analysis. JAMA Neurol 77:1, 2020.

Hatta K et al: Preventive effects of ramelteon on delirium: A randomized placebo-controlled trial. JAMA Psychiatry 71:397, 2014.

28 Coma

S. Andrew Josephson, Allan H. Ropper, Stephen L. Hauser

Coma is among the most common neurologic emergencies encountered general medicine and requires an organized approach. It accounts for a substantial portion of admissions to emergency wards and occurs on all hospital services.

There exists a continuum of states of reduced alertness, the most severe form being coma, defined as a deep sleeplike state with eyes closed, from which the patient cannot be aroused. Stupor refers to a lower threshold for arousability, in which the patient can be transiently awakened by vigorous stimuli, accompanied by motor behavior that leads to avoidance or withdrawal from noxious stimuli. Drowsiness simulates light sleep and is characterized by easy arousal that may persist for brief periods. Stupor and drowsiness are usually accompanied by some degree of confusion when the patient is alerted (**Chap. 27**). A precise narrative description of the level of arousal and of the type of responses evoked by various stimuli as observed at the bedside is preferable to use of ambiguous terms such as lethargy, semicoma, or obtundation.

Several conditions that render patients unresponsive and simulate coma are considered separately because of their special significance. The *vegetative state* signifies an awake-appearing but nonresponsive state, usually encountered in a patient who has emerged from coma. In the vegetative state, the eyelids may open periodically, giving the appearance of wakefulness. Respiratory and autonomic functions are retained. Yawning, coughing, swallowing, and limb and head movements persist, but there are few, if any, meaningful responses to the external and internal environment. There are typically accompanying signs that indicate extensive damage in both cerebral hemispheres, e.g., decerebrate or decorticate limb posturing and absent responses to visual stimuli (see below). In the closely related but less severe *minimally conscious state*, the patient displays rudimentary vocal or motor behaviors, often spontaneous, but sometimes in response to touch, visual stimuli, or command. Cardiac arrest with cerebral hypoperfusion and head trauma are the most common causes of the vegetative and minimally conscious states (**Chap. 307**).

The prognosis for regaining meaningful mental faculties once the vegetative state has supervened for several months is poor, and after a year, almost nil; hence the term *persistent vegetative state*. Most reports of dramatic recovery, when investigated carefully, are found to yield to the usual rules for prognosis, but there have been rare instances in which recovery has occurred to a severely disabled condition and, in rare childhood cases, to an even better state. Patients in the minimally conscious state carry a better prognosis for some recovery compared to those in a persistent vegetative state, but even in these patients, dramatic recovery after 12 months is unusual.

The possibility of incorrectly attributing meaningful behavior to patients in the vegetative and minimally conscious states creates problems and anguish for families and physicians. The question of whether some of these patients have the capability for cognition has been investigated by functional MRI and electroencephalogram (EEG) studies that have demonstrated cerebral activation that is temporally consistent in response to verbal and other stimuli, as discussed in more detail below. This finding suggests at a minimum that some of these patients could in the future be able to communicate their needs using technological advances and that further research could shed light on treatment approaches targeting areas of the brain and their connections that seem to be preserved in individual patients.

Several syndromes that affect alertness are prone to be misinterpreted as stupor or coma, and clinicians should be aware of these pitfalls when diagnosing coma at the bedside. Akinetic mutism refers to a partially or fully awake state in which the patient remains virtually immobile and mute but can form impressions and think, as demonstrated by later recounting of events. This condition results from damage in the regions of the medial thalamic nuclei or the frontal lobes (particularly lesions situated deeply or on the orbitofrontal surfaces) or from extreme hydrocephalus. The term *abulia* describes a milder form of akinetic mutism characterized by mental and physical slowness and diminished ability to initiate activity. It is also usually the result of damage to the medial frontal lobes and their connections (**Chap. 30**).

Catatonia is a hypomobile and mute syndrome that occurs usually as part of a major psychosis, typically schizophrenia or major depression. Catatonic patients make few voluntary or responsive movements, although they blink, swallow, and may not appear distressed. There are nevertheless signs that the patient is responsive, although it takes a careful examination to demonstrate these features. For example, eyelid elevation is actively resisted, blinking occurs in response to a visual threat, and the eyes move concomitantly with head rotation, all of which are inconsistent with the presence of a brain lesion causing unresponsiveness. The limbs may retain postures in which they have been placed by the examiner ("waxy flexibility," or catalepsy). With recovery from catatonia, patients often have some memory of events that occurred during their stupor. Catatonia is superficially similar to akinetic mutism, but clinical evidence of cerebral damage such as hyperreflexia and hypertonicity of the limbs is lacking in the former. The special problem of coma in brain death is discussed below.

The locked-in state describes a type of pseudocoma in which an awake but paralyzed patient has no means of producing speech or volitional limb movement but retains voluntary vertical eye movements and lid elevation, thus allowing the patient to communicate. The pupils are normally reactive. The usual cause is an infarction (e.g., basilar artery thrombosis) or hemorrhage of the bilateral ventral pons that transects all descending motor (corticospinal and corticobulbar) pathways. Another awake but de-efferented state occurs as a result of total paralysis of the musculature in severe cases of neuromuscular weakness such as in Guillain-Barré syndrome (**Chap. 447**), critical illness neuropathy (**Chap. 307**), or pharmacologic neuromuscular blockade.

THE ANATOMY AND PHYSIOLOGY OF COMA

Almost all instances of coma can be traced to either (1) widespread abnormalities of the cerebral hemispheres or (2) reduced activity of the thalamocortical alerting system, the reticular activating system (RAS), which is an assemblage of neurons located diffusely in the upper brainstem and thalamus. The proper functioning of this system, its ascending projections to the cortex, and the cortex itself are required to maintain alertness and coherence of thought. In addition to structural damage to either or both of these systems, suppression of reticulocerebral function commonly occurs by drugs, toxins, or metabolic derangements such as hypoglycemia, anoxia, uremia, and hepatic failure, or by seizures; these types of metabolic causes of coma are far more common than structural injuries.

Coma Due to Cerebral Mass Lesions and Herniation Syndromes The skull prevents outward expansion of the brain, and infoldings of the dura create compartments that restrict displacement of brain tissue within the cranium. The two cerebral hemispheres are separated by the falx and the anterior and posterior fossae by the tentorium. Herniation refers to displacement of brain tissue by an intracerebral or overlying mass into a contiguous compartment that it normally does not occupy. Coma from mass lesions, and many of its associated signs, are attributable to these tissue shifts, and certain clinical features are characteristic of specific configurations of herniation (**Fig. 28-1**).

In the most common form of herniation, brain tissue is displaced from the supratentorial to the infratentorial compartment through the tentorial opening, referred to as transtentorial herniation. The cause is often a mass hemispheral lesion, with accompanying contralateral hemiparesis. Uncal transtentorial herniation refers to impaction of the anterior medial temporal gyrus (the uncus) into the tentorial opening just anterior to and adjacent to the midbrain (**Fig. 28-1*A***). The uncus can compress the third nerve as the nerve traverses the subarachnoid space, causing enlargement of the ipsilateral pupil as the first sign (the fibers subserving parasympathetic pupillary function are located peripherally in the nerve). The coma that typically follows is due to lateral displacement of the midbrain (and therefore the RAS) against the opposite tentorial edge by the displaced parahippocampal gyrus (**Fig. 28-2**), compressing the opposite cerebral peduncle and producing a Babinski sign and ipsilateral hemiparesis (the Kernohan-Woltman sign). Herniation may also compress the anterior and posterior cerebral arteries as they pass over the tentorial reflections, with resultant brain infarction. These distortions may also entrap portions of the ventricular system, causing hydrocephalus.

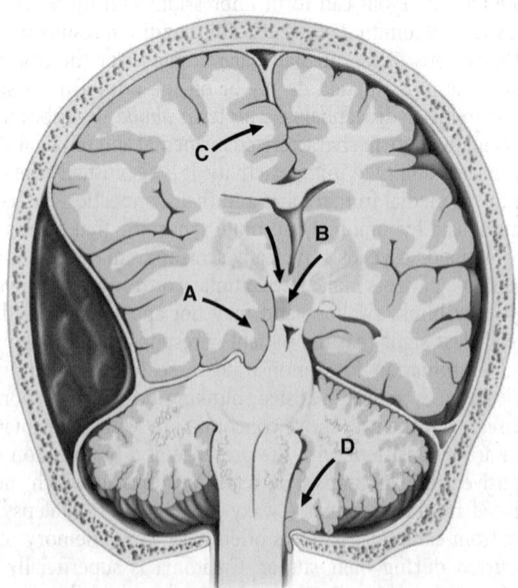

FIGURE 28-1 Types of cerebral herniation: (*A*) uncal; (*B*) central; (*C*) transfalcial; and (*D*) foraminal.

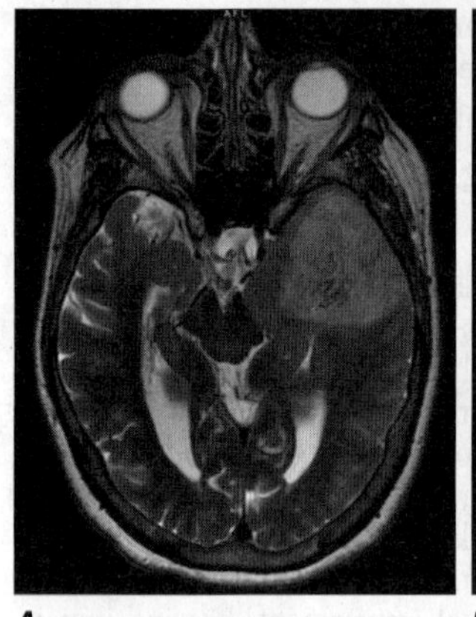

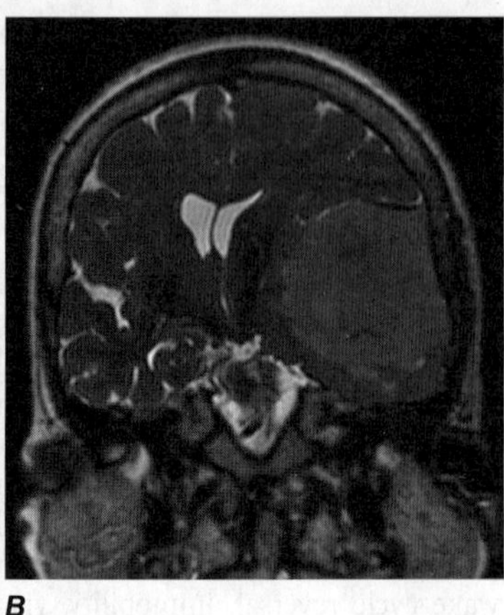

A ***B***

FIGURE 28-2 Axial (A) and coronal (B) T2-weighted magnetic resonance images from a stuporous patient with a left third nerve palsy from a large left-sided meningioma. A. The upper midbrain is compressed and displaced horizontally away from the mass, and there is transtentorial herniation of the medial temporal lobe structures, including the uncus. **B.** The lateral ventricle opposite to the mass has become enlarged as a result of compression of the third ventricle.

Central transtentorial herniation denotes a symmetric downward movement of the thalamic structures through the tentorial opening with compression of the upper midbrain (**Fig. 28-1*B***). Miotic pupils and drowsiness are the heralding signs, in contrast to a unilaterally enlarged pupil of the uncal syndrome. Both uncal and central transtentorial herniations cause progressive compression of the brainstem and RAS, with initial damage to the midbrain, then the pons, and finally the medulla. The result is an approximate sequence of neurologic signs that corresponds to each affected level, with respiratory centers in the brainstem often spared until late in the herniation syndrome. Other forms of herniation include transfalcial herniation (displacement of the cingulate gyrus under the falx and across the midline, **Fig. 28-1*C***) and foraminal herniation (downward forcing of the cerebellar tonsils into the foramen magnum, **Fig. 28-1*D***), which causes early compression of the medulla, respiratory arrest, and death.

Coma Due to Metabolic, Drug, and Toxic Disorders Many systemic metabolic abnormalities cause coma by interrupting the delivery of energy substrates (e.g., oxygen, glucose) or by altering neuronal excitability (drugs and alcohol, anesthesia, and epilepsy). These are the most common causes of coma in large case series. The metabolic abnormalities that produce coma may, in milder forms, induce a confusional state (metabolic encephalopathy) in which clouded consciousness and coma are in a continuum.

Cerebral neurons are dependent on cerebral blood flow (CBF) and the delivery of oxygen and glucose. Brain stores of glucose are able to provide energy for ~2 min after blood flow is interrupted, and oxygen stores last 8–10 s after the cessation of blood flow. Simultaneous hypoxia and ischemia exhaust glucose more rapidly. The EEG rhythm in these circumstances becomes diffusely slowed, typical of metabolic encephalopathies, and as substrate delivery worsens, eventually brain electrical activity ceases.

Unlike hypoxia-ischemia, which first causes a metabolic encephalopathy due to reduced energy substrate but ultimately causes neuronal destruction, most metabolic disorders such as hypoglycemia, hyponatremia, hyperosmolarity, hypercapnia, hypercalcemia, and hepatic and renal failure cause no or only minor neuropathologic changes in the brain. The reversible effects of these conditions are not fully understood but may result from impaired energy supplies, changes in ion fluxes across neuronal membranes, and neurotransmitter abnormalities. In hepatic encephalopathy (HE), high ammonia concentrations lead to increased synthesis of glutamine in astrocytes and osmotic swelling of the cells, mitochondrial energy failure, production of reactive nitrogen and oxygen species, increases in the inhibitory neurotransmitter GABA, and synthesis of putative "false" neurotransmitters. Over time, development of a diffuse astrocytosis is typical of chronic HE. Which, if any, of these is responsible for coma is not known.

The mechanism of the encephalopathy of renal failure is also uncertain and likely to be multifactorial; unlike ammonia, urea does not produce central nervous system (CNS) depression. Contributors to uremic encephalopathy may include accumulation of neurotoxic substances such as creatinine, guanidine, and related compounds; depletion of catecholamines; altered glutamate and GABA tone; increases in brain calcium; inflammation with disruption of the blood-brain barrier; and frequent coexisting vascular disease.

Coma and seizures are common accompaniments of large shifts in sodium and water balance in the brain. These changes in osmolarity arise from systemic medical disorders, including diabetic ketoacidosis, the nonketotic hyperosmolar state, and hyponatremia from any cause (e.g., water intoxication, excessive secretion of antidiuretic hormone, or atrial natriuretic peptides). Sodium levels <125 mmol/L, especially if achieved quickly, induce confusion, and levels <119 mmol/L are typically associated with coma and convulsions. In hyperosmolar coma, the serum osmolarity is generally >350 mosmol/L. Hypercapnia depresses the level of consciousness in proportion to the rise in carbon dioxide (CO_2) in the blood. In all of these metabolic encephalopathies, the degree of neurologic change depends on the rapidity with which the serum changes occur. The pathophysiology of other metabolic encephalopathies such as those due to hypercalcemia, hypothyroidism, vitamin B_{12} deficiency, and hypothermia are incompletely understood but must reflect derangements of CNS biochemistry, membrane function, or neurotransmitters.

Comas due to drugs and toxins are typically reversible and leave no residual damage provided there has not been hypoxia or severe hypotension. Many drugs and toxins are capable of depressing nervous system function. Some produce coma by affecting both the RAS and the cerebral cortex. The combination of cortical and brainstem signs, which occurs occasionally in certain drug overdoses, may lead to an incorrect diagnosis of structural brainstem disease. Overdose of medications that have atropinic actions produces signs such as dilated pupils, tachycardia, and dry skin; opiate overdose produces pinpoint pupils <1 mm in diameter. Some drug intoxications, typified by barbiturates, can mimic all of the signs of brain death; thus, toxic etiologies should be excluded prior to making a diagnosis of brain death.

Epileptic Coma Generalized electrical seizures are associated with coma, even in the absence of motor convulsions (nonconvulsive status epilepticus). As a result, EEG monitoring is often used in the evaluation of unexplained coma to exclude this treatable etiology. The self-limited coma that follows a seizure, the postictal state, may be due to exhaustion of energy reserves or effects of locally toxic molecules that are the by-product of seizures. The postictal state produces continuous, generalized slowing of the background EEG activity similar to that of metabolic encephalopathies. It typically lasts for a few minutes but in some cases can be prolonged for hours or even rarely for days.

Coma Due to Widespread Structural Damage to the Cerebral Hemispheres This category, comprising several unrelated disorders, results from extensive bilateral structural cerebral damage. The clinical appearance simulates a metabolic encephalopathy. Hypoxia-ischemia is perhaps the best characterized form of this type of injury, in which it is not possible initially to distinguish the acute reversible effects of oxygen deprivation of the brain from the subsequent effects of anoxic neuronal damage. Similar cerebral damage may be produced by disorders that occlude widespread small blood vessels throughout the brain; examples include thrombotic thrombocytopenic purpura, hyperviscosity, and cerebral malaria. Diffuse white matter damage from cranial trauma or inflammatory demyelinating diseases can cause a similar coma syndrome.

APPROACH TO THE PATIENT

Coma

A video examination of the comatose patient is shown in Chap. V4. Acute respiratory and cardiovascular problems should be attended to prior to neurologic assessment. In most instances, a complete medical evaluation, except for vital signs, funduscopy, and examination for nuchal rigidity, may be deferred until the neurologic evaluation has established the severity and nature of coma. **The approach to the patient with coma from cranial trauma is discussed in Chap. 443.**

HISTORY

The cause of coma may be immediately evident as in cases of trauma, cardiac arrest, or observed drug ingestion. In the remainder, certain points are useful: (1) the circumstances and rapidity with which neurologic symptoms developed; (2) antecedent symptoms (confusion, weakness, headache, fever, seizures, dizziness, double vision, or vomiting); (3) the use of medications, drugs, or alcohol; and (4) chronic liver, kidney, lung, heart, or other medical disease. Direct interrogation of family, observers, and emergency medical technicians on the scene, in person or by telephone, is an important part of the evaluation when possible.

GENERAL PHYSICAL EXAMINATION

Signs of head trauma raise the possibility of coexisting spinal cord injury, and in such cases, immobilization of the cervical spine is essential to prevent further injury. Fever suggests a systemic infection, bacterial meningitis, encephalitis, heat stroke, neuroleptic malignant syndrome, malignant hyperthermia due to anesthetics, or anticholinergic drug intoxication. Only rarely is fever attributable to a lesion that has disturbed hypothalamic temperature-regulating centers ("central fever"), and this diagnosis should only be considered after an exhaustive search for other causes fails to reveal an explanation for fever. A slight elevation in temperature may follow vigorous convulsions. Hypothermia is observed with alcohol, barbiturate, sedative, or phenothiazine intoxication; hypoglycemia; peripheral circulatory failure; or extreme hypothyroidism. Hypothermia itself causes coma when the temperature is <31°C (87.8°F) regardless of the underlying etiology; less dramatically low body temperatures can also cause coma in some instances. Tachypnea may indicate systemic acidosis or pneumonia. Aberrant respiratory patterns that reflect brainstem disorders are discussed below. Marked hypertension suggests hypertensive encephalopathy, cerebral hemorrhage, large cerebral infarction, or head injury. Hypotension is characteristic of coma from alcohol or barbiturate intoxication, internal hemorrhage or myocardial infarction causing poor delivery of blood to the brain, sepsis, profound hypothyroidism, or Addisonian crisis. The funduscopic examination can detect increased intracranial pressure (ICP) (papilledema), subarachnoid hemorrhage (subhyaloid hemorrhages), and hypertensive encephalopathy (exudates, hemorrhages, vessel-crossing changes, papilledema). Cutaneous petechiae suggest thrombotic thrombocytopenic purpura, meningococcemia, or a bleeding diathesis associated with an intracerebral hemorrhage. Cyanosis and reddish or anemic skin coloration are other indications of an underlying systemic disease or carbon monoxide as responsible for the coma.

NEUROLOGIC EXAMINATION

The patient should first be observed without intervention by the examiner. Spontaneously moving about the bed, reaching up toward the face, crossing legs, yawning, swallowing, coughing, and moaning reflect a drowsy state that is close to normal awakeness. Lack of restless movements on one side or an outturned leg suggests hemiplegia. Subtle, intermittent twitching movements of a foot, finger, or facial muscle may be the only sign of seizures. Multifocal myoclonus usually indicates a metabolic disorder, particularly uremia, anoxia, drug intoxication, or rarely a prion disease (**Chap. 438**). In a drowsy and confused patient, bilateral asterixis is a sign of metabolic encephalopathy or drug intoxication.

Decorticate rigidity and decerebrate rigidity, or "posturing," describe stereotyped arm and leg movements occurring spontaneously or elicited by sensory stimulation. Flexion of the elbows and wrists and supination of the arm (decorticate posturing) classically suggest bilateral damage rostral to the midbrain, whereas extension of the elbows and wrists with pronation (decerebrate posturing) indicates damage to motor tracts caudal to the midbrain. However, these localizations have been adapted from animal work and cannot be applied with precision to coma in humans. In fact, acute and widespread disorders of any type, regardless of location, frequently cause limb extension.

LEVEL OF AROUSAL

A sequence of increasingly intense stimuli is first used to determine the threshold for arousal and the motor response of each side of the body. The results of testing may vary from minute to minute, and serial examinations are useful. Tickling the nostrils with a cotton wisp is a moderate stimulus to arousal—all but deeply stuporous and comatose patients will move the head away and arouse to some degree. An even greater degree of responsiveness is present if the patient uses his hand to remove an offending stimulus. Pressure on bony prominences and pinprick stimulation, when necessary, are humane forms of noxious stimuli; pinching the skin causes ecchymoses and is generally not performed but may be useful in eliciting abduction withdrawal movements of the limbs. Posturing in response to noxious stimuli indicates severe damage to the corticospinal system, whereas abduction-avoidance movement of a limb is usually purposeful and denotes an intact corticospinal system. Posturing may also be unilateral and coexist with purposeful limb movements, reflecting incomplete damage to the motor system.

BRAINSTEM REFLEXES

Assessment of brainstem function is essential to localization of the lesion in coma (**Fig. 28-3**). Patients with preserved brainstem reflexes typically have a bihemispheric localization to coma, including toxic or drug intoxication, whereas patients with abnormal brainstem reflexes either have a lesion in the brainstem or a herniation syndrome from a cerebral mass lesion impacting the brainstem secondarily. The most important brainstem reflexes are pupillary size and reaction to light, spontaneous and elicited eye movements, corneal responses, and the respiratory pattern.

Pupillary Signs Pupillary reactions are examined with a bright, diffuse light. Reactive and round pupils of midsize (2.5–5 mm) essentially exclude upper midbrain damage, either primary or secondary to compression from herniation. A response to light may be difficult to appreciate in pupils <2 mm in diameter, and bright room lighting may mute pupillary reactivity. One enlarged (>6 mm) and poorly reactive pupil signifies compression of the third nerve from the effects of a cerebral mass above. Enlargement of the pupil contralateral to a hemispheral mass may occur but is infrequent. An oval and slightly eccentric pupil is a transitional sign that accompanies early midbrain–third nerve compression. The most extreme pupillary sign, bilaterally dilated and unreactive pupils, indicates severe midbrain damage, usually from compression by a supratentorial mass. Ingestion of drugs with anticholinergic activity, the use of mydriatic eye drops, nebulizer treatments, and direct ocular trauma are other causes of pupillary enlargement.

Reactive and bilaterally small (1–2.5 mm) but not pinpoint pupils are seen in metabolic encephalopathies or in deep bilateral hemispheral lesions such as hydrocephalus or thalamic hemorrhage. Even smaller reactive pupils (<1 mm) characterize opioid overdoses but also occur with extensive pontine hemorrhage. The response to naloxone and the presence of reflex eye movements (see below) assist in distinguishing between these. Unilateral miosis in coma has been attributed to dysfunction of sympathetic efferents originating in the posterior hypothalamus and descending in the tegmentum of the brainstem to the cervical cord. It is an occasional finding in patients with a large cerebral hemorrhage that affects the thalamus.

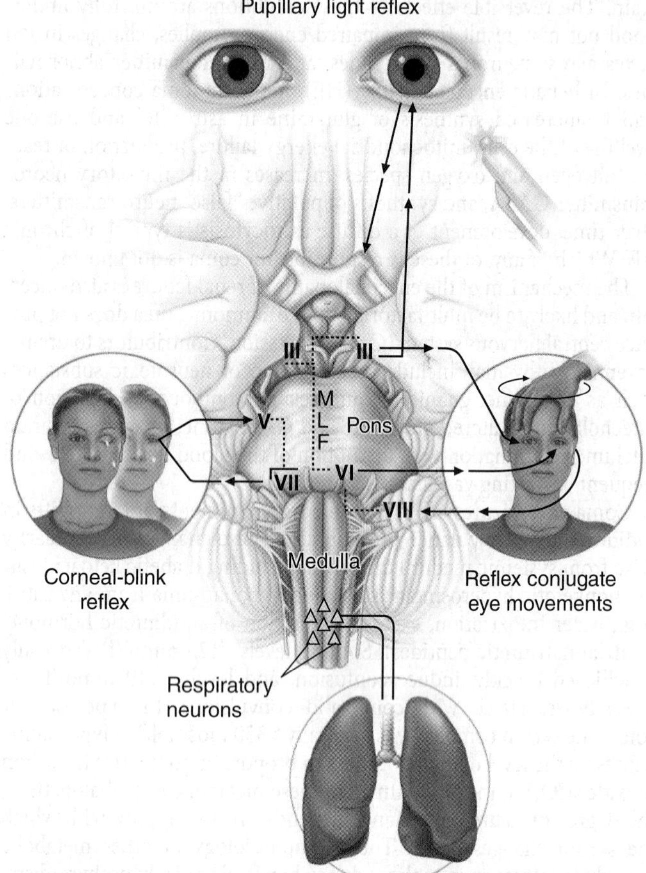

FIGURE 28-3 Examination of brainstem reflexes in coma. Midbrain and third nerve function are tested by pupillary reaction to light, pontine function by spontaneous and reflex eye movements and corneal responses, and medullary function by respiratory and pharyngeal responses. Reflex conjugate, horizontal eye movements are dependent on the medial longitudinal fasciculus (MLF) interconnecting the sixth and contralateral third nerve nuclei. Head rotation (oculocephalic reflex) or caloric stimulation of the labyrinths (oculovestibular reflex) elicits contraversive eye movements (for details, see text).

Ocular Movements The eyes are first observed by elevating the lids and observing the resting position and spontaneous movements of the globes. Horizontal divergence of the eyes at rest is normal in drowsiness. As coma deepens, the ocular axes may become parallel again.

Spontaneous eye movements in coma often take the form of conjugate horizontal roving. This finding alone exonerates extensive damage in the midbrain and pons and has the same significance as normal reflex eye movements (see below). Conjugate horizontal ocular deviation to one side indicates damage to the frontal lobe on the same side or less commonly the pons on the opposite side. This phenomenon is summarized by the following maxim: *The eyes look toward a hemispheral lesion and away from a brainstem lesion*. Seizures involving the frontal lobe drive the eyes to the opposite side, simulating a pontine destructive lesion. The eyes may occasionally turn paradoxically away from the side of a deep hemispheral lesion ("wrong-way eyes"). The eyes turn down and inward with thalamic and upper midbrain lesions, typically thalamic hemorrhage. "Ocular bobbing" describes brisk downward and slow upward movements of the eyes associated with loss of horizontal eye movements and is diagnostic of bilateral pontine damage, usually from thrombosis of the basilar artery. "Ocular dipping" is a slower, arrhythmic downward movement followed by a faster upward movement in patients with normal reflex horizontal gaze; it usually indicates diffuse cortical anoxic damage.

The oculocephalic reflexes, elicited by moving the head from side to side or vertically and observing eye movements in the direction opposite to the head movement, depend on the integrity of the ocular motor nuclei and their interconnecting tracts that extend from the midbrain to the pons and medulla (Fig. 28-3). The movements, called somewhat inaccurately "doll's eyes," are normally suppressed in the awake patient with intact frontal lobes. The ability to elicit them therefore reflects both reduced cortical influence on the brainstem and intact brainstem pathways. The opposite, an absence of reflex eye movements, usually signifies damage within the brainstem but can result from overdoses of certain drugs. In this circumstance, normal pupillary size and light reaction distinguishes most drug-induced comas from structural brainstem damage. Oculocephalic maneuvers should not be attempted in patients with neck trauma, as vigorous head movements can precipitate or worsen a spinal cord injury.

Thermal, or "caloric," stimulation of the vestibular apparatus (oculovestibular response) provides a more intense stimulus for the oculocephalic reflex but provides essentially the same information. The test is performed by irrigating the external auditory canal with cold water in order to induce convection currents in the labyrinths. After a brief latency, the result is tonic deviation of both eyes to the side of cold-water irrigation. In comatose patients, nystagmus in the opposite direction may not occur. The acronym "COWS" has been used to remind generations of medical students of the direction of nystagmus—cold water opposite, warm water same—but since nystagmus is often absent in the opposite direction due to frontal lobe dysfunction in coma, this mnemonic does not often hold true.

The corneal reflex, elicited by touching the cornea with a wisp of cotton and observing bilateral lid closure, depends on the integrity of pontine pathways between the fifth (afferent) and both seventh (efferent) cranial nerves; it is a useful test of pontine function. CNS-depressant drugs diminish or eliminate the corneal responses soon after reflex eye movements are paralyzed but before the pupils become unreactive to light. The corneal response may be lost for a time on the side of an acute hemiplegia.

Respiratory Patterns These are of less localizing value in comparison to other brainstem signs. Shallow, slow, but regular breathing suggests metabolic or drug-induced depression of the medullary respiratory centers. Cheyne-Stokes respiration in its typical cyclic form, ending with a brief apneic period, signifies bihemispheral damage or metabolic suppression and commonly accompanies light coma. Rapid, deep (Kussmaul) breathing usually implies metabolic acidosis but may also occur with pontomesencephalic lesions. Agonal gasps are the result of lower brainstem (medullary) damage and are recognized as the terminal respiratory pattern of severe brain damage. Other cyclic breathing patterns have been described but are of lesser significance.

■ LABORATORY STUDIES AND IMAGING

The studies that are most useful in the diagnosis of coma are chemical-toxicologic analysis of blood and urine, cranial CT or MRI, EEG, and cerebrospinal fluid (CSF) examination. Arterial blood gas analysis is helpful in patients with lung disease and acid-base disorders. The metabolic aberrations commonly encountered in clinical practice are usually revealed by measurement of electrolytes, glucose, calcium, magnesium, osmolarity, and renal (blood urea nitrogen) and hepatic (NH_3) function. Toxicologic analysis may be necessary in cases of acute coma, when the diagnosis is not immediately clear. However, the presence of exogenous drugs or toxins, especially alcohol, does not exclude the possibility that other factors, particularly head trauma, are contributing to the clinical state. An ethanol level of 43 mmol/L (0.2 g/dL) in nonhabituated patients generally causes impaired mental activity; a level of >65 mmol/L (0.3 g/dL) is associated with stupor. The development of tolerance may allow some chronic alcoholics to remain awake at levels >87 mmol/L (0.4 g/dL).

The availability of cranial CT and MRI has focused attention on causes of coma that are detectable by imaging (e.g., hemorrhage, tumor, or hydrocephalus). Resorting primarily to this approach, although at times expedient, is imprudent because most cases of coma (and confusion) are metabolic or toxic in origin. Furthermore, a normal CT scan does not exclude an anatomic lesion as the cause of coma; for example, early bilateral hemisphere infarction, acute brainstem infarction, encephalitis, meningitis, mechanical shearing of axons as a result of closed head trauma, sagittal sinus thrombosis, hypoxic injury, and subdural hematoma isodense to adjacent brain are some of the disorders that may not be detected. Sometimes imaging results can be misleading such as when small subdural hematomas or old strokes are found, but the patient's coma is due to intoxication. Additional imaging with CT angiography or MRI can be obtained if acute posterior circulation stroke is considered.

The EEG (**Chap. 425**) provides clues in metabolic or drug-induced states but is rarely diagnostic in these disorders. However, it is the essential test to reveal coma due to nonconvulsive seizures and shows fairly characteristic patterns in herpesvirus encephalitis and prion disease. The EEG may be further helpful in disclosing generalized slowing of the background activity, a reflection of the severity of an encephalopathy. Predominant high-voltage slowing (δ or triphasic waves) in the frontal regions is typical of metabolic coma, as from hepatic failure, and widespread fast (β) activity implicates overdose with sedative drugs (e.g., benzodiazepines). A special pattern of "alpha coma," defined by widespread, variable 8- to 12-Hz activity, superficially resembles the normal α rhythm of waking but, unlike normal α activity, is not altered by environmental stimuli. Alpha coma results from pontine or diffuse cortical damage and is associated with a poor prognosis. A unique EEG pattern in adults of "extreme delta brush" is characteristic of a specific (anti–*N*-methyl-D-aspartate [NMDA] receptor) form of autoimmune encephalitis. Normal α activity on the EEG, which is suppressed by stimulating the patient, also alerts the clinician to the locked-in syndrome, hysteria, or catatonia.

Lumbar puncture should be performed if no cause is readily apparent, as examination of the CSF remains indispensable in the diagnosis of various forms of meningitis and encephalitis. An imaging study should be performed prior to lumbar puncture to exclude a large intracranial mass lesion, which could lead to herniation with lumbar puncture. Blood cultures and administration of antibiotics should precede the imaging study if infectious meningitis is suspected (**Chap. 138**).

■ DIFFERENTIAL DIAGNOSIS OF COMA

(**Table 28-1**) The causes of coma can be divided into three broad categories: those without focal neurologic signs (e.g., metabolic and toxic encephalopathies); those with prominent focal signs (e.g., stroke, cerebral hemorrhage); and meningitis syndromes, characterized by fever or stiff neck and an excess of cells in the spinal fluid (e.g., bacterial meningitis, subarachnoid hemorrhage, encephalitis). Causes of sudden coma include drug ingestion, cerebral hemorrhage, trauma, cardiac arrest, epilepsy, and basilar artery occlusion. Coma that appears subacutely is usually related to a preexisting medical or neurologic problem or, less often, to secondary brain swelling surrounding a mass such as tumor or cerebral infarction.

The diagnosis of coma due to cerebrovascular disease can be difficult (**Chap. 426**). The most common diseases in this category are (1) basal ganglia and thalamic hemorrhage (acute but not instantaneous onset, vomiting, headache, hemiplegia, and characteristic eye signs); (2) pontine hemorrhage (sudden onset, pinpoint pupils, loss of reflex eye movements and corneal responses, ocular bobbing, posturing, and hyperventilation); (3) cerebellar hemorrhage (occipital headache, vomiting, gaze paresis, and inability to stand and walk); (4) basilar artery thrombosis (neurologic prodrome or transient ischemic attack warning spells, diplopia, dysarthria, vomiting, eye movement and corneal response abnormalities, and asymmetric limb paresis); and

TABLE 28-1 Differential Diagnosis of Coma

1. Diseases that cause no focal brainstem or lateralizing neurologic signs (CT scan is often normal)
   a. Intoxications: alcohol, sedative drugs, opiates, etc.
   b. Metabolic disturbances: anoxia, hyponatremia, hypernatremia, hypercalcemia, diabetic acidosis, nonketotic hyperosmolar hyperglycemia, hypoglycemia, uremia, hepatic coma, hypercarbia, Addisonian crisis, hypo- and hyperthyroid states, profound nutritional deficiency
   c. Severe systemic infections: pneumonia, septicemia, typhoid fever, malaria, Waterhouse-Friderichsen syndrome
   d. Shock from any cause
   e. Status epilepticus, nonconvulsive status epilepticus, postictal states
   f. Hyperperfusion syndromes including hypertensive encephalopathy, eclampsia, posterior reversible encephalopathy syndrome (PRES)
   g. Severe hyperthermia, hypothermia
   h. Concussion
   i. Acute hydrocephalus
2. Diseases that cause focal brainstem or lateralizing cerebral signs (CT scan is typically abnormal)
   a. Hemispheral hemorrhage (basal ganglionic, thalamic) or infarction (large middle cerebral artery territory) with secondary brainstem compression
   b. Brainstem infarction due to basilar artery thrombosis or embolism
   c. Brain abscess, subdural empyema
   d. Epidural and subdural hemorrhage, brain contusion
   e. Brain tumor with surrounding edema
   f. Cerebellar and pontine hemorrhage and infarction
   g. Widespread traumatic brain injury
   h. Metabolic coma (see above) in the setting of preexisting focal damage
3. Diseases that cause meningeal irritation with or without fever, and with an excess of white blood cells or red blood cells in the CSF
   a. Subarachnoid hemorrhage from ruptured aneurysm, arteriovenous malformation, trauma
   b. Infectious meningitis and meningoencephalitis
   c. Paraneoplastic and autoimmune encephalitis
   d. Carcinomatous and lymphomatous meningitis

(5) subarachnoid hemorrhage (precipitous coma after sudden severe headache and vomiting). The most common stroke, infarction in the territory of the middle cerebral artery, does not cause coma, but edema surrounding large infarctions may expand over several days and cause coma from mass effect.

The syndrome of acute hydrocephalus accompanies many intracranial diseases, particularly subarachnoid hemorrhage. It is characterized by headache and sometimes vomiting that may progress quickly to coma with extensor posturing of the limbs, bilateral Babinski signs, small unreactive pupils, and impaired oculocephalic movements in the vertical direction. At times, the coma may be featureless without lateralizing signs, although papilledema is often present.

BRAIN DEATH

Brain death is a state of irreversible cessation of all cerebral and brainstem function with preservation of cardiac activity and maintenance of respiratory and somatic function by artificial means. It is the only type of brain damage recognized as morally, ethically, and legally equivalent to death. Criteria have been advanced for the diagnosis of brain death, and it is essential to adhere to consensus standards as multiple studies have shown variability in local practice. Given the implications of the diagnosis, clinicians must be thorough and precise in determining brain death. It is advisable to delay clinical testing for at least 24 h if a cardiac arrest has caused brain death or if the inciting disease is not known. Some centers advocate a brief period of observation between two examiners' tests during which the clinical signs of brain death are sustained.

Established criteria contain two essential elements, after assuring that no confounding factors (e.g., hypothermia, drug intoxication) are present: (1) widespread cortical destruction that is reflected by deep coma and unresponsiveness to all forms of stimulation; and (2) global brainstem damage as demonstrated by absent pupillary light reaction, absent corneal reflexes, loss of oculovestibular reflexes, and destruction of the medulla, manifested by complete and irreversible apnea. Diabetes insipidus is often present but may only develop hours or days after the other clinical signs of brain death appear. The pupils are usually midsized but may be enlarged. Loss of deep tendon reflexes is not required because the spinal cord remains functional. Occasionally, other reflexes that originate from the spine may be present and should not preclude a diagnosis of brain death.

Demonstration that apnea is due to medullary damage requires that the P_{CO_2} be high enough to stimulate respiration during a test of spontaneous breathing. Apnea testing can be done by the use of preoxygenation with 100% oxygen prior to and following removal of the ventilator. CO_2 tension increases ~0.3–0.4 kPa/min (2–3 mmHg/min) during apnea. Apnea is confirmed if no respiratory effort has been observed in the presence of a sufficiently elevated P_{CO_2}. The apnea test is usually stopped if there is cardiovascular instability and alternative means of testing can be employed.

An isoelectric EEG may be used as an optional confirmatory test for total cerebral damage. Radionuclide brain scanning, cerebral angiography, or transcranial Doppler measurements may be used to demonstrate the absence of blood flow when a confirmatory study is desired.

It is largely accepted in Western society that the ventilator can be disconnected from a brain-dead patient and that organ donation is subsequently possible. Good communication between the physician and the family is important with appropriate preparation of the family for brain death testing and diagnosis.

TREATMENT

Coma

The immediate goal in a comatose patient is prevention of further nervous system damage. Hypotension, hypoglycemia, hypercalcemia, hypoxia, hypercapnia, and hyperthermia should be corrected rapidly. Hyponatremia should be corrected slowly to avoid injury from osmotic demyelination (**Chap. 307**). An oropharyngeal airway is adequate to keep the pharynx open in a drowsy patient who is breathing normally. Tracheal intubation is indicated if there is apnea, upper airway obstruction, hypoventilation, or emesis, or if the patient is at risk for aspiration. Mechanical ventilation is required if there is hypoventilation or a need to induce hypocapnia in order to lower ICP. **The management of raised ICP is discussed in Chap. 307.** IV access is established and naloxone and dextrose are administered if opioid overdose or hypoglycemia are possibilities; thiamine is given along with glucose to avoid provoking Wernicke's encephalopathy in malnourished patients. In cases of suspected ischemic stroke including basilar thrombosis with brainstem ischemia, IV tissue plasminogen activator or mechanical embolectomy is often used after cerebral hemorrhage has been excluded and when the patient presents within established time windows for these interventions (**Chap. 427**). Physostigmine may awaken patients with anticholinergic-type drug overdose but should be used only with careful monitoring; many physicians believe that it should only be used to treat anticholinergic overdose–associated cardiac arrhythmias. The use of benzodiazepine antagonists offers some prospect of improvement after overdose; however, these drugs are not commonly used empirically in part due to their tendency to provoke seizures. Certain other toxic and drug-induced comas have specific treatments such as fomepizole for ethylene glycol ingestion.

Administration of hypotonic IV solutions should be monitored carefully in any serious acute brain illness because of the potential for exacerbating brain swelling. Cervical spine injuries must not be overlooked, particularly before attempting intubation or evaluation of oculocephalic responses. Fever and meningismus indicate an urgent need for examination of the CSF to diagnose meningitis. Whenever acute bacterial meningitis is suspected, antibiotics including at least vancomycin and a third-generation cephalosporin are typically administered rapidly along with dexamethasone (**see Chap. 138**).

■ PROGNOSIS

Some patients, especially children and young adults, may have ominous early clinical findings such as abnormal brainstem reflexes and yet recover; early prognostication outside of brain death therefore is unwise. Metabolic comas have a far better prognosis than traumatic ones. Systems for estimating prognosis in adults should be taken as approximations, and medical judgments must be tempered by factors such as age, underlying systemic disease, and general medical condition. In an attempt to collect prognostic information from large numbers of patients with head injury, the Glasgow Coma Scale was devised; it has predictive value in cases of brain trauma **(see Chap. 443)**. For anoxic coma, clinical signs such as the pupillary and motor responses after 1 day, 3 days, and 1 week have predictive value; however, some prediction rules are less reliable in the setting of therapeutic hypothermia, and therefore, serial examinations and multimodal prognostication approaches are advised in this setting. For example, the absence of the cortical responses of the somatosensory evoked potentials has been shown to be a strong indicator of poor outcome following hypoxic injury.

The poor outcome of persistent vegetative and minimally conscious states has already been mentioned, but reports of a small number of patients displaying cortical activation on functional MRI in response to salient stimuli have begun to alter the perception of such individuals. In one series, about 10% of vegetative patients (mainly following traumatic brain injury) could activate their frontal or temporal lobes in response to requests by an examiner to imagine certain visuospatial tasks. Another series demonstrated that up to 15% of patients with various forms of acute brain injury and absence of behavioral responses to motor commands showed EEG activation in response to these commands. It is prudent to avoid generalizations from these findings, but the need for future studies of novel techniques to help communication and possibly recovery is needed.

■ FURTHER READING

Claasen J et al: Detection of brain activation in unresponsive patients with acute brain injury. N Engl J Med 380:2497, 2019.

Edlow JA et al: Diagnosis of reversible causes of coma. Lancet 384:2064, 2014.

Greer DM et al: Determination of brain death/death by neurologic criteria: The World Brain Death Project. JAMA 324:1078, 2020.

Monti MM et al: Willful modulation of brain activity in disorders of consciousness. N Engl J Med 362:579, 2010.

Posner JB et al: *Plum and Posner's Diagnosis of Stupor and Coma*, 5th ed. New York, Oxford University Press, 2019.

Wijdicks EFM: Predicting the outcome of a comatose patient at the bedside. Pract Neurol 20:26, 2020.

29 Dementia

William W. Seeley, Gil D. Rabinovici, Bruce L. Miller

Dementia, a syndrome with many causes, affects nearly 6 million people in the United States and results in a total annual health care cost in excess of $300 billion. Dementia is defined as an acquired deterioration in cognitive abilities that impairs the successful performance of activities of daily living. Episodic memory, the ability to recall events specific in time and place, is the cognitive function most commonly lost; 10% of persons age >70 years and 20–40% of individuals age >85 years have clinically identifiable memory loss. In addition to memory, dementia may erode other mental faculties, including language, visuospatial, praxis, calculation, judgment, and problem-solving abilities. Neuropsychiatric and social deficits also arise in many dementia syndromes, manifesting as depression, apathy, anxiety, hallucinations, delusions, agitation, insomnia, sleep disturbances, compulsions, or disinhibition. The clinical course may be slowly progressive, as in Alzheimer's disease (AD); static, as in anoxic encephalopathy; or may fluctuate from day to day or minute to minute, as in dementia with Lewy bodies (DLB). Most patients with AD, the most prevalent form of dementia, begin with episodic memory impairment, but in other dementias, such as frontotemporal dementia (FTD), memory loss is not typically a presenting feature. **Focal cerebral disorders are discussed in Chap. 30 and illustrated in a video library in Chap. V2; detailed discussions of AD can be found in Chap. 431; FTD and related disorders in Chap. 432; vascular dementia in Chap. 433; DLB in Chap. 434; Huntington's disease (HD) in Chap. 436; and prion diseases in Chap. 438.**

FUNCTIONAL ANATOMY OF THE DEMENTIAS

Dementia syndromes result from the disruption of specific large-scale neuronal networks; the location and severity of synaptic and neuronal loss combine to produce the clinical features **(Chap. 30)**. Behavior, mood, and attention are modulated by ascending noradrenergic, serotonergic, and dopaminergic pathways, whereas cholinergic signaling is critical for attention and memory functions. The dementias differ in the relative neurotransmitter deficit profiles; accordingly, accurate diagnosis guides effective pharmacologic therapy.

AD typically begins in the entorhinal region of the medial temporal lobe, spreads to the hippocampus and other limbic structures, and moves through the basal temporal areas and then into the lateral and posterior temporal and parietal neocortex, eventually causing a more widespread degeneration. Vascular dementia is associated with focal damage in a variable patchwork of cortical and subcortical regions or white matter tracts that disconnects nodes within distributed networks. In keeping with its anatomy, AD typically presents with episodic memory loss accompanied later by aphasia, executive dysfunction, or navigational problems. In contrast, dementias that begin in frontal or subcortical regions, such as FTD or HD, are less likely to begin with memory problems and more likely to present with difficulties with judgment, mood, executive control, movement, and behavior.

Lesions of frontal-striatal[1] pathways produce specific and predictable effects on behavior. The dorsolateral prefrontal cortex has connections with a central band of the caudate nucleus. Lesions of either the caudate or dorsolateral prefrontal cortex, or their connecting white matter pathways, may result in executive dysfunction, manifesting as poor organization and planning, decreased cognitive flexibility, and impaired working memory. The lateral orbital frontal cortex connects with the ventromedial caudate, and lesions of this system cause impulsiveness, distractibility, and disinhibition. The anterior cingulate cortex and adjacent medial prefrontal cortex project to the nucleus accumbens, and interruption of this system produces apathy, poverty of speech, emotional blunting, or even akinetic mutism. All corticostriatal systems also include topographically organized projections through the globus pallidus and thalamus, and damage to these nodes can likewise reproduce the clinical syndrome associated with the corresponding cortical or striatal injuries. Involvement of brainstem nuclei and cerebellar structures can further contribute to cognitive, behavioral, and motor manifestations.

■ THE CAUSES OF DEMENTIA

The single strongest risk factor for dementia is increasing age. The prevalence of disabling memory loss increases with each decade over age 50 and is usually associated with the microscopic changes of AD at autopsy. Yet some centenarians have intact memory function and no evidence of clinically significant dementia. Whether dementia is an inevitable consequence of normal human aging remains controversial although the prevalence increases with every decade of life.

[1]The striatum comprises the caudate/putamen/nucleus accumbens.

TABLE 29-1 Differential Diagnosis of Dementia

Most Common Causes of Dementia	
Alzheimer's disease Vascular dementia Multi-infarct Diffuse white matter disease (Binswanger's)	Alcoholism[a] PDD/LBD spectrum Drug/medication intoxication[a] Limbic-predominant age-related TDP-43 encephalopathy
Less Common Causes of Dementia	
Vitamin deficiencies Thiamine (B_1): Wernicke's encephalopathy[a] B_{12} (subacute combined degeneration)[a] Nicotinic acid (pellagra)[a] Endocrine and other organ failure Hypothyroidism[a] Adrenal insufficiency and Cushing's syndrome[a] Hypo- and hyperparathyroidism[a] Renal failure[a] Liver failure[a] Pulmonary failure[a] Chronic infections HIV Neurosyphilis[a] Papovavirus (JC virus) (progressive multifocal leukoencephalopathy) Tuberculosis, fungal, and protozoal[a] Whipple's disease[a] Head trauma and diffuse brain damage Chronic traumatic encephalopathy Chronic subdural hematoma[a] Postanoxia Postencephalitis Normal-pressure hydrocephalus[a] Intracranial hypotension Neoplastic Primary brain tumor[a] Metastatic brain tumor[a] Autoimmune (paraneoplastic) encephalitis[a]	Toxic disorders Drug, medication, and narcotic poisoning[a] Heavy metal intoxication[a] Organic toxins Psychiatric Depression (pseudodementia)[a] Schizophrenia[a] Conversion disorder[a] Degenerative disorders Huntington's disease Multisystem atrophy Hereditary ataxias (some forms) Frontotemporal lobar degeneration spectrum Multiple sclerosis Adult Down's syndrome with Alzheimer's disease ALS-parkinsonism-dementia complex of Guam Prion (Creutzfeldt-Jakob and Gerstmann-Sträussler-Scheinker diseases) Miscellaneous Sarcoidosis[a] Vasculitis[a] CADASIL, etc. Acute intermittent porphyria[a] Recurrent nonconvulsive seizures[a] Additional conditions in children or adolescents Pantothenate kinase–associated neurodegeneration Subacute sclerosing panencephalitis Metabolic disorders (e.g., Wilson's and Leigh's diseases, leukodystrophies, lipid storage diseases, mitochondrial mutations)

[a]Potentially reversible dementia.

Abbreviations: ALS, amyotrophic lateral sclerosis; CADASIL, cerebral autosomal dominant arteriopathy with subcortical infarcts and leukoencephalopathy; LBD, Lewy body disease; PDD, Parkinson's disease dementia.

The many causes of dementia are listed in **Table 29-1**. The frequency of each condition depends on the age group under study, access of the group to medical care, country of origin, and perhaps racial or ethnic background. AD is the most common cause of dementia in Western countries, accounting for more than half of all patients. Vascular disease is the second most frequent cause for dementia and is particularly common in elderly patients or populations with limited access to medical care, where vascular risk factors are undertreated. Often, vascular brain injury is mixed with neurodegenerative disorders, particularly AD, making it difficult, even for the neuropathologist, to estimate the contribution of cerebrovascular disease to the cognitive disorder in an individual patient. Dementias associated with Parkinson's disease (PD) are common and may develop years after onset of a parkinsonian disorder, as seen with PD-related dementia (PDD), or they can occur concurrently with or preceding the motor syndrome, as in DLB. Limbic-predominant aging-related TDP-43 encephalopathy (LATE) is common after age 70 and has been linked to declining episodic memory function. Chronic traumatic encephalopathy (CTE), a unique disease found in individuals with a history of repetitive head impacts (e.g., professional athletes in collision or fighting sports, military veterans exposed to multiple blasts), presents with changes in cognition, mood, behavior, or motor function. Mixed pathology is common, especially in older individuals. In patients under the age of 65, FTD rivals AD as the most common cause of dementia. Chronic intoxications, including those resulting from alcohol and prescription drugs, are an important and often treatable cause of dementia. Other disorders listed in Table 29-1 are uncommon but important because many are reversible. The classification of dementing illnesses into reversible and irreversible disorders is a useful approach to differential diagnosis. When effective treatments for the neurodegenerative conditions emerge, this dichotomy will become obsolete.

In a study of 1000 persons attending a memory disorders clinic, 19% had a potentially reversible cause of the cognitive impairment and 23% had a potentially reversible concomitant condition that may have contributed to the patient's impairment. The three most common potentially reversible diagnoses were depression, normal pressure hydrocephalus (NPH), and alcohol dependence; medication side effects are also common and should be considered in every patient (Table 29-1).

The term *rapidly progressive dementia (RPD)* is applied to illnesses that progress from initial symptom onset to dementia within a year or less; confusional states related to toxic/metabolic conditions are excluded. Although the prion proteinopathy Creutzfeldt-Jakob disease (CJD) (**Chap. 438**) is the classic cause of a rapidly progressive dementia, especially when associated with myoclonus, more often cases of RPD are due to AD or another neurodegenerative disorder, or to an autoimmune encephalitis.

Subtle cumulative decline in episodic memory is a common part of aging. This frustrating experience, often the source of jokes and humor, has historically been referred to as *benign forgetfulness of the elderly. Benign* means that it is not so progressive or serious that it impairs successful and productive daily functioning, although the distinction between benign and significant memory loss can be subtle. At age 85, the average person is able to learn and recall approximately one-half of the items (e.g., words on a list) that he or she could at age 18. The term *subjective cognitive decline* describes individuals who experience a subjective decline from their cognitive baseline but perform within normal limits for their age and educational attainment on formal neuropsychological testing. *Mild cognitive impairment (MCI)* is defined as a decline in cognition that is confirmed on objective cognitive testing but does not disrupt normal daily activities. MCI can be further subcategorized based on the presenting complaints and deficits (e.g., amnestic MCI, executive MCI). Factors that predict progression from MCI to an AD dementia include a prominent memory deficit, family history of dementia, presence of an apolipoprotein ε4 (Apo ε4) allele, small hippocampal volumes, an AD-like signature of cortical atrophy, low cerebrospinal fluid Aβ and elevated tau, or evidence of brain amyloid and tau deposition on positron emission tomography (PET) imaging.

The major degenerative dementias include AD, DLB, FTD and related disorders, HD, and prion diseases, including CJD. All are associated with the abnormal aggregation of a specific protein: $Aβ_{42}$ and tau in AD; α-synuclein in DLB; tau, TAR DNA-binding protein of 43 kDa (TDP-43), or the FET family of proteins (*fu*sed in sarcoma [FUS], Ewing sarcoma [EWS], and TBP-associated factor 15 [TAF15]) in FTD; huntingtin in HD; and misfolded prion protein (PrP^{sc}) in CJD (**Table 29-2**).

The risk of developing dementia in late-life is associated with exposures and lifestyle factors that can operate across the life span. Modifiable risk factors include low education, hearing loss, traumatic brain injury, hypertension, diabetes mellitus, obesity, heavy alcohol use, smoking, depression, physical inactivity, and air pollution. Improved management of midlife vascular risk factors has been credited with a decreasing incidence of dementia observed in North America and Western Europe.

TABLE 29-2 The Molecular Basis for Degenerative Dementia

DEMENTIA	MOLECULAR BASIS	CAUSAL GENES (CHROMOSOME)	SUSCEPTIBILITY GENES	PATHOLOGIC FINDINGS
AD	Aβ/tau	*APP* (21), *PS-1* (14), *PS-2* (1) (<2% carry these mutations, most often in *PS-1*)	*Apo* ε*4* (19)	Amyloid plaques, neurofibrillary tangles, and neuropil threads
FTD	Tau	*MAPT* exon and intron mutations (17) (about 10% of familial cases)	H1 *MAPT* haplotype	Tau neuronal and glial inclusions varying in morphology and distribution
	TDP-43	*GRN* (10% of familial cases), *C9ORF72* (20%–30% of familial cases), rare *VCP*, very rare *TARDBP, TBK1, TIA1*		TDP-43 neuronal and glial inclusions varying in morphology and distribution
	FET	Very rare *FUS*		FET neuronal and glial inclusions varying in morphology and distribution
DLB	α-Synuclein	Very rare *SNCA* (4)	Unknown	α-Synuclein neuronal inclusions (Lewy bodies)
CJD	PrP^{SC}	*PRNP* (20) (up to 15% of patients carry these dominant mutations)	Codon 129 homozygosity for methionine or valine	PrP^{SC} deposition, panlaminar spongiosis

Abbreviations: AD, Alzheimer's disease; CJD, Creutzfeldt-Jakob disease; DLB, dementia with Lewy bodies; FET, FUS/EWS/TAF-15; FTD, frontotemporal dementia.

APPROACH TO THE PATIENT

Dementias

Three major issues should be kept at the forefront: (1) What is the clinical diagnosis? (2) What component of the dementia syndrome is treatable or reversible? (3) Can the physician help to alleviate the burden on caregivers? A broad overview of the approach to dementia is shown in **Table 29-3**. The major degenerative dementias can usually be distinguished by the initial symptoms; neuropsychological, neuropsychiatric, and neurologic findings; and neuroimaging features **(Table 29-4)**.

HISTORY

The history should concentrate on the onset, duration, and tempo of progression. An acute or subacute onset of confusion may be due to delirium **(Chap. 27)** and should trigger a search for intoxication, infection, or metabolic derangement. An elderly person with slowly progressive memory loss over several years is likely to suffer from AD. Nearly 75% of patients with AD begin with memory symptoms, but other early symptoms include anxiety or depression as well as difficulty managing money, driving, shopping, following instructions, finding words, or navigating. Personality change, disinhibition, and weight gain or compulsive eating suggest FTD, not AD. FTD is also suggested by prominent apathy, compulsivity, loss of empathy for others, or progressive loss of speech fluency or single-word comprehension with relative sparing of memory and visuospatial abilities. The diagnosis of DLB is suggested by early visual hallucinations; parkinsonism; proneness to delirium or sensitivity to psychoactive medications; rapid eye movement (REM) behavior disorder (RBD; dramatic, sometimes violent, limb movements during dreaming **[Chap. 31]**); or Capgras syndrome, the delusion that a familiar person has been replaced by an impostor.

A history of stroke with irregular stepwise progression suggests vascular dementia. Vascular dementia is also commonly seen in the setting of hypertension, atrial fibrillation, peripheral vascular disease, smoking, and diabetes. In patients suffering from cerebrovascular disease, it can be difficult to determine whether the dementia is due to AD, vascular disease, or a mixture of the two because many of the risk factors for vascular dementia, including diabetes, high cholesterol, elevated homocysteine, and low exercise, are also risk factors for AD. Moreover, many patients with a major vascular contribution to their dementia lack a history of stepwise decline. Rapid progression with motor rigidity and myoclonus suggests CJD **(Chap. 438)**. Seizures may indicate strokes or neoplasm but also occur in AD, particularly early-age-of-onset AD. Gait disturbance is common in vascular dementia, PD/DLB, or NPH. A history of high-risk sexual behaviors or intravenous drug use should trigger a search for central nervous system (CNS) infection, especially HIV or syphilis. A history of recurrent head trauma could indicate chronic subdural hematoma, CTE, intracranial hypotension, or NPH. Subacute onset of severe amnesia and psychosis with mesial temporal T2/fluid-attenuated inversion recovery (FLAIR) hyperintensities on MRI should raise concern for autoimmune (paraneoplastic) encephalitis, sometimes in long-term smokers or other patients at risk for cancer. The spectrum of autoimmune etiologies producing

TABLE 29-3 Evaluation of the Patient with Dementia

ROUTINE EVALUATION	OPTIONAL FOCUSED TESTS	OCCASIONALLY HELPFUL TESTS
History	Psychometric testing	EEG
Physical examination	Chest x-ray	Parathyroid function
Laboratory tests	Lumbar puncture	Adrenal function
Thyroid function (TSH)	Liver function	Urine heavy metals
Vitamin B_{12}	Renal function	RBC sedimentation rate
Complete blood count	Urine toxin screen	Angiogram
Electrolytes	HIV	Brain biopsy
CT/MRI	Apolipoprotein E	SPECT
	RPR or VDRL	PET
		Autoantibodies
Diagnostic Categories		
REVERSIBLE CAUSES	**IRREVERSIBLE/ DEGENERATIVE DEMENTIAS**	**PSYCHIATRIC DISORDERS**
Examples	Examples	Depression
Hypothyroidism	Alzheimer's	Schizophrenia
Thiamine deficiency	Frontotemporal dementia	Conversion reaction
Vitamin B_{12} deficiency	Huntington's	
Normal pressure hydrocephalus	Dementia with Lewy bodies	
Subdural hematoma	Vascular	
Chronic infection	Leukoencephalopathies	
Brain tumor	Parkinson's	
Drug intoxication		
Autoimmune encephalopathy		
Associated Treatable Conditions		
	Depression	Agitation
	Seizures	Caregiver "burnout"
	Insomnia	Drug side effects

Abbreviations: CT, computed tomography; EEG, electroencephalogram; MRI, magnetic resonance imaging; PET, positron emission tomography; RBC, red blood cell; RPR, rapid plasma reagin (test); SPECT, single-photon emission computed tomography; TSH, thyroid-stimulating hormone; VDRL, venereal disease research laboratory (test for syphilis).

TABLE 29-4 Clinical Differentiation of the Major Dementias

DISEASE	FIRST SYMPTOM	MENTAL STATUS	NEUROPSYCHIATRY	NEUROLOGY	IMAGING
AD	Memory loss	Episodic memory loss	Irritability, anxiety, depression	Initially normal	Entorhinal cortex and hippocampal atrophy
FTD	Apathy, poor judgment/ insight, speech/language, hyperorality	Frontal/executive and/or language; spares drawing	Apathy, disinhibition, overeating, compulsivity	May have vertical gaze palsy, axial rigidity, dystonia, alien hand, or MND	Frontal, insular, and/or temporal atrophy; usually spares posterior parietal lobe
DLB	Visual hallucinations, REM sleep behavior disorder, delirium, Capgras syndrome, parkinsonism	Drawing and frontal/ executive, spares memory, delirium-prone	Visual hallucinations, depression, sleep disorder, delusions	Parkinsonism	Posterior parietal atrophy, hippocampi larger than in AD
CJD	Dementia, mood, anxiety, movement disorders	Variable, frontal/ executive, focal cortical, memory	Depression, anxiety, psychosis in some	Myoclonus, rigidity, parkinsonism	Cortical ribboning and basal ganglia or thalamus hyperintensity on diffusion/ FLAIR MRI
Vascular	Often but not always sudden, variable, apathy, falls, focal weakness	Frontal/executive, cognitive slowing, can spare memory	Apathy, delusions, anxiety	Usually motor slowing, spasticity, can be normal	Cortical and/or subcortical infarctions, confluent white matter disease

Abbreviations: AD, Alzheimer's disease; CBD, cortical basal degeneration; CJD, Creutzfeldt-Jakob disease; DLB, dementia with Lewy bodies; FLAIR, fluid-attenuated inversion recovery; FTD, frontotemporal dementia; MND, motor neuron disease; MRI, magnetic resonance imaging; REM, rapid eye movement.

RPD has rapidly expanded, and includes antibodies targeting leucine-rich glioma-inactivated 1 (LGI1; faciobrachial dystonic seizures); contactin-associated protein-like 2 (Caspr2; insomnia, ataxia, myotonia); *N-methyl-*D*-aspartate* (NMDA)-receptor (psychosis, insomnia, dyskinesias); and α-amino-3-hydroxy-5-methylisoxazole-4-propionic acid (AMPA)-receptor (limbic encephalitis with relapses), among others (**Chap. 94**). Alcohol abuse creates risk for malnutrition and thiamine deficiency. Veganism, bowel irradiation, an autoimmune diathesis, a remote history of gastric surgery, and chronic therapy with histamine H2-receptor antagonists for dyspepsia or gastroesophageal reflux predispose to B_{12} deficiency. Certain occupations, such as working in a battery or chemical factory, might indicate heavy metal intoxication. Careful review of medication intake, especially for sedatives and analgesics, may raise the issue of chronic drug intoxication. An autosomal dominant family history is found in HD and in familial forms of AD, FTD, DLB, or prion disorders. A history of mood disorder, the recent death of a loved one, or depressive signs such as insomnia or weight loss, raise the possibility of depression-related cognitive impairment.

PHYSICAL AND NEUROLOGIC EXAMINATION

A thorough general and neurologic examination is essential to identify signs of nervous system involvement and search for clues suggesting a systemic disease that might be responsible for the cognitive disorder. Typical AD spares motor systems until late in the course. In contrast, patients with FTD often develop axial rigidity, supranuclear gaze palsy, or a motor neuron disease reminiscent of amyotrophic lateral sclerosis (ALS). In DLB, the initial symptoms may include a parkinsonian syndrome (resting tremor, cogwheel rigidity, bradykinesia, festinating gait), but DLB often starts with visual hallucinations or cognitive impairment, and symptoms referable to the lower brainstem (RBD, gastrointestinal, or autonomic problems) may arise years or even decades before parkinsonism or dementia. Corticobasal syndrome (CBS) features asymmetric akinesia and rigidity, dystonia, myoclonus, alien limb phenomena, pyramidal signs, and prefrontal deficits such as nonfluent aphasia with or without motor speech impairment, executive dysfunction, apraxia, or a behavioral disorder. Progressive supranuclear palsy (PSP) is associated with unexplained falls, axial rigidity, dysphagia, and vertical gaze deficits. CJD is suggested by the presence of diffuse rigidity, an akinetic mute state, and prominent, often startle-sensitive, myoclonus.

Hemiparesis or other focal neurologic deficits suggest vascular dementia or brain tumor. Dementia with a myelopathy and peripheral neuropathy suggests vitamin B_{12} deficiency. Peripheral neuropathy could also indicate another vitamin deficiency, heavy metal intoxication, thyroid dysfunction, Lyme disease, or vasculitis. Dry cool skin, hair loss, and bradycardia suggest hypothyroidism. Fluctuating confusion associated with repetitive stereotyped movements may indicate ongoing limbic, temporal, or frontal seizures. In the elderly, hearing impairment or visual loss may produce confusion and disorientation misinterpreted as dementia. Profound bilateral sensorineural hearing loss in a younger patient with short stature or myopathy, however, should raise concern for a mitochondrial disorder.

COGNITIVE AND NEUROPSYCHIATRIC EXAMINATION

Brief screening tools such as the Mini-Mental State Examination (MMSE), the Montreal Cognitive Assessment (MOCA), the Tablet Based Cognitive Assessment Tool, and Cognistat can be used to capture dementia and follow progression. None of these tests is highly sensitive to early-stage dementia or reliably discriminates between dementia syndromes. The MMSE is a 30-point test of cognitive function, with each correct answer being scored as 1 point. It includes tests of: orientation (e.g., identify season/date/month/year/floor/hospital/town/state/country); registration (e.g., name and restate 3 objects); recall (e.g., remember the same three objects 5 minutes later); and language (e.g., name pencil and watch; repeat "no ifs ands or buts"; follow a 3-step command; obey a written command; and write a sentence and copy a design). In most patients with MCI and some with clinically apparent AD, bedside screening tests may be normal, and a more challenging and comprehensive set of neuropsychological tests will be required. When the etiology for the dementia syndrome remains in doubt, a specially tailored evaluation should be performed that includes tasks of working and episodic memory, executive function, language, and visuospatial and perceptual abilities. In AD, the early deficits involve episodic memory, category generation ("name as many animals as you can in 1 minute"), and visuoconstructive ability. Usually deficits in verbal or visual episodic memory are the first neuropsychological abnormalities detected, and tasks that require the patient to recall a long list of words or a series of pictures after a predetermined delay will demonstrate deficits in most patients. In FTD, the earliest deficits on cognitive testing involve executive control or language (speech or naming) functions, but some patients lack either finding despite profound social-emotional deficits. PDD or DLB patients have more severe deficits in executive and visuospatial function but do better on episodic memory tasks than patients with AD. Patients with vascular dementia often demonstrate a mixture of executive and visuospatial deficits, with prominent psychomotor slowing. In delirium, the most prominent deficits involve attention, working

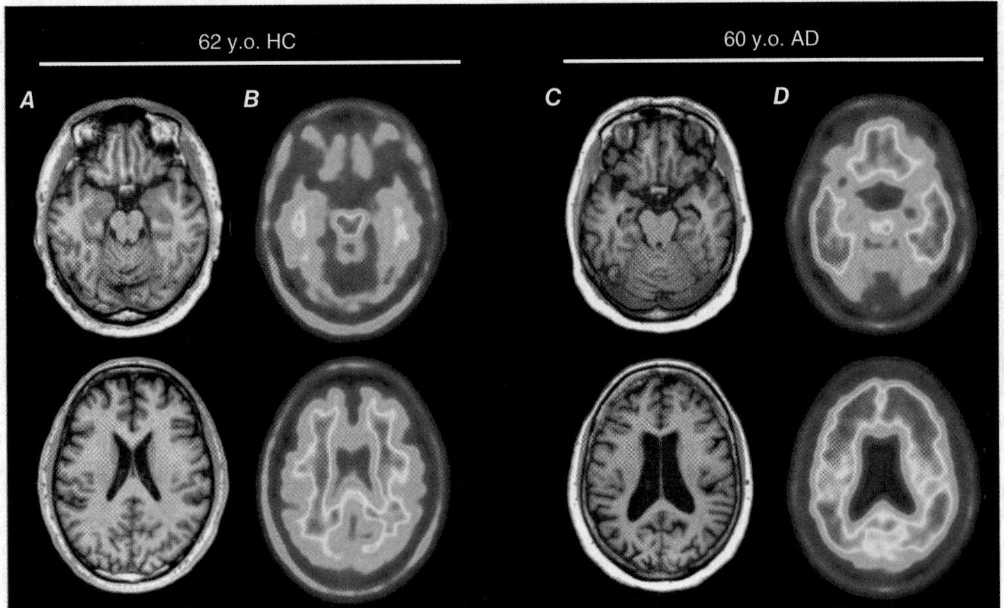

FIGURE 29-1 Alzheimer's disease (AD). Axial T1-weighted magnetic resonance images of a healthy 62-year-old (***A, B***) and a 60-year-old with AD (***C, D***). Note the diffuse atrophy, plus temporal lobe volume loss, in the patient with AD. Aβ positron emission tomography (PET) with [^{11}C]PIB (***B*** and ***D***) reveals extensive radiotracer retention in neocortex bilaterally in AD, consistent with the known distribution of amyloid plaques. HC, healthy control. *(Source: Gil Rabinovici, University of California, San Francisco and William Jagust, University of California, Berkeley.)*

memory, and executive function, making the assessment of other cognitive domains challenging and often uninformative.

A functional assessment should also be performed to help the physician determine the day-to-day impact of the disorder on the patient's memory, community affairs, hobbies, judgment, dressing, and eating. Knowledge of the patient's functional abilities will help the clinician and the family to organize a therapeutic approach.

Neuropsychiatric assessment is important for diagnosis, prognosis, and treatment. In the early stages of AD, mild depressive features, social withdrawal, and irritability or anxiety are the most prominent psychiatric changes, but patients often maintain core social graces into the middle or late stages, when delusions, agitation, and sleep disturbance may emerge. In FTD, dramatic personality change with apathy, overeating, compulsions, disinhibition, and loss of empathy are early and common. DLB is associated with visual hallucinations, delusions related to person or place identity, RBD, and excessive daytime sleepiness. Dramatic fluctuations occur not only in cognition but also in arousal. Vascular dementia can present with psychiatric symptoms such as depression, anxiety, delusions, disinhibition, or apathy.

LABORATORY TESTS

The choice of laboratory tests in the evaluation of dementia is complex and should be tailored to the individual patient. The physician must take measures to avoid missing a reversible or treatable cause, yet no single treatable etiology is common; thus a screen must use multiple tests, each of which has a low yield. Cost/benefit ratios are difficult to assess, and many laboratory screening algorithms for dementia discourage multiple tests. Nevertheless, even a test with only a 1–2% positive rate is worth undertaking if the alternative is missing a treatable cause of dementia. Table 29-3 lists most screening tests for dementia. The American Academy of Neurology recommends the routine measurement of a complete blood count; electrolytes; glucose; renal, liver, and thyroid functions; a vitamin B_{12} level; and a structural neuroimaging study (MRI or CT).

Neuroimaging studies, especially MRI, help to rule out primary and metastatic neoplasms, locate areas of infarction or inflammation, detect subdural hematomas, and suggest NPH or diffuse white matter disease. They also help to establish a regional pattern of atrophy. Support for the diagnosis of AD includes hippocampal atrophy in addition to posterior-predominant cortical atrophy (**Fig. 29-1**). Focal frontal, insular, and/or anterior temporal atrophy suggests FTD (**Chap. 432**). DLB often features less prominent atrophy, with greater involvement of the amygdala than the hippocampus. In CJD, magnetic resonance (MR) diffusion-weighted imaging reveals restricted diffusion within the cortical ribbon and/or basal ganglia in most patients. Extensive multifocal white matter abnormalities suggest a vascular etiology (**Fig. 29-2**). Communicating hydrocephalus with vertex effacement (crowding of dorsal convexity gyri/sulci), gaping Sylvian fissures despite minimal cortical atrophy, and additional features shown in **Fig. 29-3** suggest NPH. Single-photon emission computed tomography (SPECT) and fluoro-deoxyglucose PET scanning show temporal-parietal hypoperfusion or hypometabolism in AD and frontotemporal deficits in FTD, but abnormalities in these patterns can be detected with MRI alone in many patients. Recently, amyloid- and tau-PET imaging have shown promise for the diagnosis of AD. There are currently

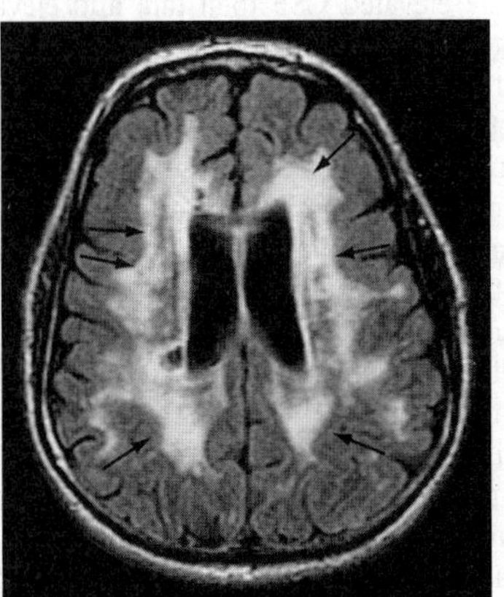

FIGURE 29-2 Diffuse white matter disease. Axial fluid-attenuated inversion recovery (FLAIR) magnetic resonance image through the lateral ventricles reveals multiple areas of hyperintensity (*arrows*) involving the periventricular white matter as well as the corona radiata and striatum. Although seen in some individuals with normal cognition, this appearance is more pronounced in patients with dementia of a vascular etiology.

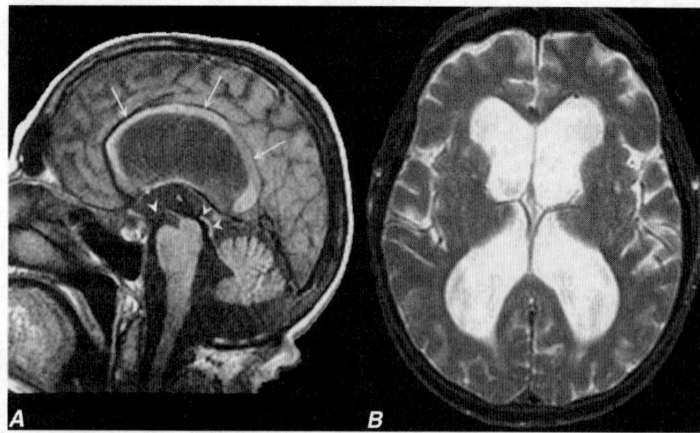

FIGURE 29-3 Normal pressure hydrocephalus. ***A.*** Sagittal T1-weighted MRI demonstrates dilation of the lateral ventricle and stretching of the corpus callosum (*arrows*), depression of the floor of the third ventricle (*single arrowhead*), and enlargement of the aqueduct (*double arrowheads*). Note the diffuse dilation of the lateral, third, and fourth ventricles with a patent aqueduct, typical of communicating hydrocephalus. ***B.*** Axial T2-weighted MRIs demonstrate dilation of the lateral ventricles. This patient underwent successful ventriculoperitoneal shunting.

three amyloid PET ligands (F18-florbetapir, F18-florbetaben, F18-flutametamol) and one tau PET ligand (F18-flortaucipir) approved by the US Food and Drug Administration for clinical use. Amyloid PET ligands bind to diffuse and neuritic amyloid plaques, as well as to vascular amyloid deposits (prominent in cerebral amyloid angiopathy), while tau PET ligands bind to the paired helical filaments of tau characteristic of neurofibrillary tangles in AD (**Chap. 431**). Because amyloid plaques are also commonly found in cognitively normal older persons (~25% of individuals at age 65), the main clinical value of amyloid imaging is to exclude AD as the likely cause of dementia in patients who have negative scans. The spread of tau is more tightly linked to cognitive state (**Chap. 431**), and thus may be more useful than amyloid imaging for "ruling in" AD, as well as for disease staging. Once disease-modifying therapies become available, CSF or molecular PET biomarkers will likely be used to identify treatment candidates. In the meantime, the prognostic value of detecting brain amyloid in an asymptomatic elder to assess preclinical disease and risk of future cognitive decline remains a topic of vigorous investigation.

Lumbar puncture need not be done routinely in the evaluation of dementia, but it is indicated when CNS infection or inflammation are credible diagnostic possibilities. Cerebrospinal fluid (CSF) levels of $A\beta_{42}$ and tau proteins show differing patterns with the various dementias, and the presence of low $A\beta_{42}$ (or a low $A\beta_{42}/A\beta_{40}$ ratio), mild-moderately elevated CSF total tau, and elevated CSF phosphorylated tau (at residues 181 or 217) is highly suggestive of AD. Novel fully automated CSF Aβ and tau assays perform comparably to amyloid and tau PET respectively, though, as with PET, their routine use in the diagnosis of dementia is debated. Blood-based biomarkers for AD show promise as a less invasive screening tool but remain under development (**Chap. 431**). Formal psychometric testing helps to document the severity of cognitive disturbance, suggests psychogenic causes, and provides a more formal method for following the disease course. Electroencephalogram (EEG) is not routinely used but can help to suggest CJD (repetitive bursts of diffuse high-amplitude sharp waves, or "periodic complexes") or an underlying nonconvulsive seizure disorder (epileptiform discharges). Brain biopsy (including meninges) is not advised except to diagnose vasculitis, neoplasms, or unusual infections when the diagnosis is uncertain. Systemic disorders with CNS manifestations, such as sarcoidosis, can often be confirmed through biopsy of lymph node or solid organ rather than brain. MR angiography should be considered when cerebral vasculitis or cerebral venous thrombosis is a possible cause of the dementia.

GLOBAL CONSIDERATIONS

Vascular dementia (**Chap. 433**) is more common in Asia due to the higher prevalence of intracranial atherosclerosis. Rates of vascular dementia are also on the rise in developing countries as vascular risk factors such as hypertension, hypercholesterolemia, and diabetes mellitus become more widespread. CNS infections, HIV (and associated opportunistic infections), syphilis, cysticercosis, and tuberculosis, likewise represent major contributors to dementia in the developing world. Systemic infection with SARS-CoV-2 may, in some individuals, have lasting effects on cognition due to involvement of brain microvasculature or to immunologically mediated white matter injury (acute disseminated encephalomyelitis [ADEM]) (**Chap. 444**). Some individuals complain of lasting fatigue, changes in mood, and cognitive difficulties, but the long-term prognosis for SARS-CoV-2-related cognitive impairment remains unknown. Isolated populations have also contributed to our understanding of neurodegenerative dementia. Kuru, the cannibalism-associated rapidly progressive dementia seen in tribal New Guinea, played a role in the discovery of human prion disease. Amyotrophic lateral sclerosis-parkinsonism-dementia complex of Guam (or, Lytico-bodig disease) is a poly-proteinopathy, often with tau, TDP-43, and alpha-synuclein aggregation. The root cause of the disease remains uncertain, but its incidence has declined sharply over the past 60 years.

TREATMENT

Dementia

The major goals of dementia management are to treat reversible causes and provide comfort and support to the patient and caregivers. Treatment of underlying causes includes thyroid replacement for hypothyroidism; vitamin therapy for thiamine or B_{12} deficiency or for elevated serum homocysteine; antimicrobials for opportunistic infections or antiretrovirals for HIV; ventricular shunting for NPH; or surgical, radiation, and/or chemotherapeutic treatment for CNS neoplasms. Removal of cognition-impairing drugs or medications is essential when appropriate. If the patient's cognitive complaints stem from a psychiatric disorder, vigorous treatment of the condition should be tried to eliminate the cognitive complaint or to confirm that it persists despite adequate resolution of the mood or anxiety symptoms. Patients with degenerative diseases may also be depressed or anxious, and those aspects of their condition often respond to therapy while not necessarily improving cognition. Antidepressants, such as selective serotonin reuptake inhibitors (SSRIs) or serotonin-norepinephrine reuptake inhibitors (SNRIs) (**Chap. 452**), which feature anxiolytic properties but few cognitive side effects, provide the mainstay of treatment when necessary. Anticonvulsants are used to control AD-associated seizures.

Agitation, hallucinations, delusions, and confusion are difficult to treat. These behavioral problems represent major causes for nursing home placement and institutionalization. Before treating these behaviors with medications, the clinician should aggressively seek out modifiable environmental or metabolic factors. Hunger, lack of exercise, toothache, constipation, urinary tract or respiratory infection, electrolyte imbalance, and drug toxicity all represent easily correctable causes that can be remedied without psychoactive drugs. Drugs such as phenothiazines and benzodiazepines may ameliorate the behavior problems but have untoward side effects such as sedation, rigidity, or dyskinesia; benzodiazepines can occasionally produce paradoxical disinhibition. Despite their unfavorable side effect profile, second-generation antipsychotics such as quetiapine (starting dose, 12.5–25 mg daily) can be used for patients with agitation, aggression, and psychosis, although the risk profile for these compounds is significant, including increased mortality in patients with dementia. When patients do not respond to treatment, it is usually a mistake to advance to higher doses or to use anticholinergic drugs (like diphenhydramine) or sedatives (such as barbiturates or benzodiazepines). It is important to recognize and treat depression; treatment can begin with a low dose of an

SSRI (e.g., escitalopram, starting dose 5 mg daily, target dose 5–10 mg daily) while monitoring for efficacy and toxicity. Sometimes apathy, visual hallucinations, depression, and other psychiatric symptoms respond to cholinesterase inhibitors, especially in DLB, obviating the need for other more toxic therapies.

Cholinesterase inhibitors are being used to treat AD (donepezil, rivastigmine, galantamine) and PDD (rivastigmine). Memantine is useful for some patients with moderate to severe AD; its major benefit relates to decreasing caregiver burden, most likely by decreasing resistance to dressing and grooming support. In moderate to severe AD, the combination of memantine and a cholinesterase inhibitor delayed nursing home placement in several studies, although other studies have not supported the efficacy of adding memantine to the regimen. Memantine should be used with great caution, or not at all, in patients with DLB, due to risk of worsening agitation and confusion. Therapies targeting the production, aggregation, and spread of misfolded proteins associated with dementia are under development. Recently the first drug in this class, the amyloid-beta targeting monoclonal antibody aducanumab, was approved by the United States Food & Drug Administration for treatment of Alzheimer's disease (Chap. 431). Other drugs under development target disease-associated neuroinflammation metabolic changes, synaptic loss, and neurotransmitter changes.

Proactive approaches reduce the occurrence of delirium in hospitalized patients. Frequent orientation, cognitive activities, sleep-enhancement measures, vision and hearing aids, and correction of dehydration are all valuable in decreasing the likelihood of delirium.

Nondrug behavior therapy has an important place in dementia management. The primary goals are to make the patient's life comfortable, uncomplicated, and safe. Preparing lists, schedules, calendars, and labels can be helpful in the early stages. It is also useful to stress familiar routines, walks, and simple physical exercises. For many demented patients, memory for events is worse than their ability to carry out routine activities, and they may still be able to take part in their favorite hobbies, sports, and social activities. Demented patients often object to losing control over familiar tasks such as driving, cooking, and handling finances. Attempts to help may be greeted with complaints, depression, or anger. Hostile responses on the part of the caregiver are counterproductive and sometimes even harmful. Reassurance, distraction, and calm positive statements are more productive when resistance is present. Eventually, tasks such as finances and driving must be assumed by others, and the patient will conform and adjust. Safety is an important issue that includes not only driving but controlling the kitchen, bathroom, and sleeping area environments, as well as stairways. These areas need to be monitored, supervised, and made as safe as possible. A move to a retirement complex, assisted-living center, or nursing home can initially increase confusion and agitation. Repeated reassurance, reorientation, and careful introduction to the new personnel will help to smooth the process. Providing activities that are known to be enjoyable to the patient can also help.

The clinician must pay special attention to frustration and depression among family members and caregivers. Caregiver guilt and burnout are common. Family members often feel overwhelmed and helpless and may vent their frustrations on the patient, each other, and health care providers. Caregivers should be encouraged to take advantage of day-care facilities and respite services. Education and counseling about dementia are important. Local and national support groups, such as the Alzheimer's Association (*www.alz.org*), can provide considerable help.

■ FURTHER READING

Barton C et al: Non-pharmacological management of behavioral symptoms in frontotemporal and other dementias. Curr Neurol Neurosci Rep 16:14, 2016.

Griem J et al: Psychologic/functional forms of memory disorder. Handb Clin Neurol 139:407, 2017.

Wesley SF, Ferguson D: Autoimmune encephalitides and rapidly progressive dementias. Semin Neurol 39:283, 2019.

30 Aphasia, Memory Loss, and Other Cognitive Disorders

M.-Marsel Mesulam

The cerebral cortex of the human brain contains ~20 billion neurons spread over an area of 2.5 m². The primary sensory and motor areas constitute 10% of the cerebral cortex. The rest is subsumed by modality-selective, heteromodal, paralimbic, and limbic areas collectively known as the *association cortex* (**Fig. 30-1**). The association cortex mediates the integrative processes that subserve cognition, emotion, and comportment. A systematic testing of these mental functions is necessary for the effective clinical assessment of the association cortex and its diseases. According to current thinking, there are no centers for "hearing words," "perceiving space," or "storing memories." Cognitive

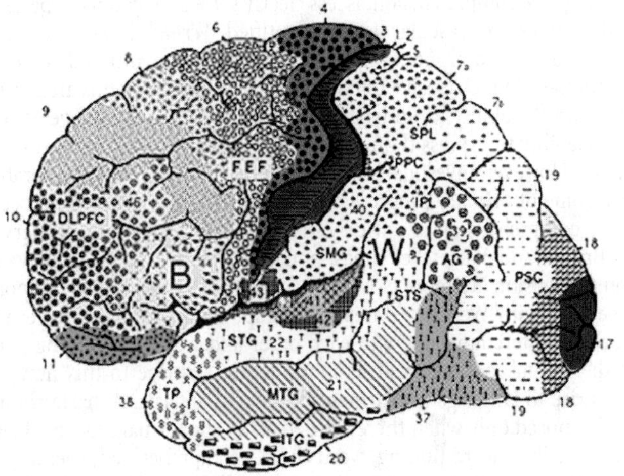

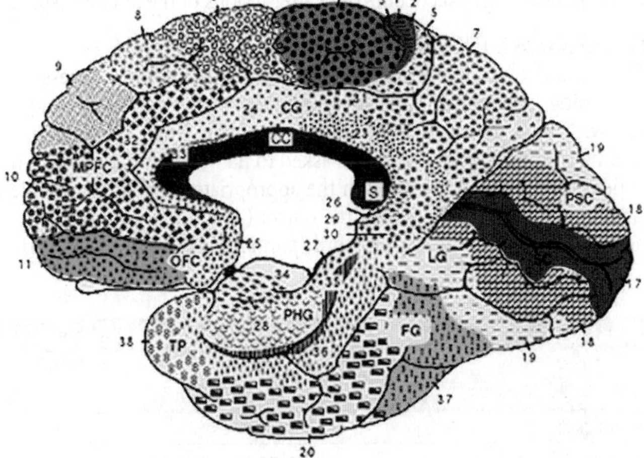

FIGURE 30-1 Lateral (*top*) and medial (*bottom*) views of the cerebral hemispheres. The numbers refer to the Brodmann cytoarchitectonic designations. Area 17 corresponds to the primary visual cortex, 41–42 to the primary auditory cortex, 1–3 to the primary somatosensory cortex, and 4 to the primary motor cortex. The rest of the cerebral cortex contains association areas. AG, angular gyrus; B, Broca's area; CC, corpus callosum; CG, cingulate gyrus; DLPFC, dorsolateral prefrontal cortex; FEF, frontal eye fields (premotor cortex); FG, fusiform gyrus; IPL, inferior parietal lobule; ITG, inferior temporal gyrus; LG, lingual gyrus; MPFC, medial prefrontal cortex; MTG, middle temporal gyrus; OFC, orbitofrontal cortex; PHG, parahippocampal gyrus; PPC, posterior parietal cortex; PSC, peristriate cortex; SC, striate cortex; SMG, supramarginal gyrus; SPL, superior parietal lobule; STG, superior temporal gyrus; STS, superior temporal sulcus; TP, temporopolar cortex; W, Wernicke's area.

and behavioral functions (domains) are coordinated by intersecting *large-scale neural networks* that contain interconnected cortical and subcortical components. Five anatomically defined *large-scale networks* are most relevant to clinical practice: (1) a left-dominant perisylvian network for language, (2) a right-dominant parietofrontal network for spatial orientation, (3) an occipitotemporal network for face and object recognition, (4) a limbic network for episodic memory and emotional modulation, and (5) a prefrontal network for the executive control of cognition and comportment. Investigations based on functional imaging have also identified a *default mode network*, which becomes activated when the person is not engaged in a specific task requiring attention to external events. The clinical consequences of damage to this network are not yet fully defined.

THE LEFT PERISYLVIAN NETWORK FOR LANGUAGE AND APHASIAS

The production and comprehension of words and sentences is dependent on the integrity of a distributed network located along the perisylvian region of the language-dominant (usually left) hemisphere. One hub, situated in the inferior frontal gyrus, is known as *Broca's area.* Damage to this region impairs fluency of verbal output and the grammatical structure of sentences. The location of a second hub, critical for language comprehension, is less clearly settled. Accounts of patients with focal cerebrovascular lesions identified *Wernicke's area*, located at the parietotemporal junction, as a critical hub for word and sentence comprehension. Occlusive or embolic strokes involving this area interfere with the ability to understand spoken or written language as well as the ability to express thoughts through meaningful words and statements. However, investigations of patients with the neurodegenerative syndrome of primary progressive aphasia (PPA) have shown that sentence comprehension is a widely distributed faculty jointly subserved by Broca's and Wernicke's areas, and that the areas critical for word comprehension are more closely associated with the anterior temporal lobe than with Wernicke's area. All components of the language network are interconnected with each other and with surrounding parts of the frontal, parietal, and temporal lobes. Damage to this network gives rise to language impairments known as aphasia. Aphasia should be diagnosed only when there are deficits in the formal aspects of language, such as word finding, word choice, comprehension, spelling, or grammar. Dysarthria, apraxia of speech, and mutism do not by themselves lead to a diagnosis of aphasia. In ~90% of right-handers and 60% of left-handers, aphasia occurs only after lesions of the left hemisphere.

■ CLINICAL EXAMINATION

The clinical examination of language should include the assessment of naming, spontaneous speech, comprehension, repetition, reading, and writing. A deficit of naming (*anomia*) is the single most common finding in aphasic patients. When asked to name a common object, the patient may fail to come up with the appropriate word, may provide a circumlocutious description of the object ("the thing for writing"), or may come up with the wrong word (*paraphasia*). If the patient offers an incorrect but related word ("pen" for "pencil"), the naming error is known as a *semantic paraphasia*; if the word approximates the correct answer but is phonetically inaccurate ("plentil" for "pencil"), it is known as a *phonemic paraphasia*. In most anomias, the patient cannot retrieve the appropriate name when shown an object but can point to the appropriate object when the name is provided by the examiner. This is known as a one-way (or retrieval-based) naming deficit. A two-way (comprehension-based or semantic) naming deficit exists if the patient can neither provide nor recognize the correct name. *Spontaneous speech* is described as "fluent" if it maintains appropriate output volume, phrase length, and melody or as "nonfluent" if it is sparse and halting and average utterance length is below four words. The examiner also should note the integrity of *grammar* as manifested by word order (syntax), tenses, suffixes, prefixes, plurals, and possessives. *Comprehension* can be tested by assessing the patient's ability to follow conversation, asking yes-no questions ("Can a dog fly?" "Does it snow in summer?"), asking the patient to point to appropriate objects ("Where is the source of illumination in this room?"), or asking for verbal definitions of single words. *Repetition* is assessed by asking the patient to repeat single words, short sentences, or strings of words such as "No ifs, ands, or buts." The testing of repetition with tongue twisters such as "hippopotamus" and "Irish constabulary" provides a better assessment of dysarthria and apraxia of speech than of aphasia. It is important to make sure that the number of words does not exceed the patient's attention span. Otherwise, the failure of repetition becomes a reflection of the narrowed attention span (auditory working memory) rather than an indication of an aphasic deficit caused by dysfunction of a hypothetical *phonological loop* in the language network. *Reading* should be assessed for deficits in reading aloud as well as comprehension. *Alexia* describes an inability to either read aloud or comprehend written words and sentences; *agraphia* (or dysgraphia) is used to describe an acquired deficit in spelling.

Aphasias can arise acutely in cerebrovascular accidents (CVAs) or gradually in neurodegenerative diseases. In CVAs, damage encompasses cerebral cortex as well as deep white matter pathways interconnecting otherwise unaffected cortical areas. The syndromes listed in **Table 30-1** are most applicable to this group, where gray matter and white matter at the lesion site are abruptly and jointly destroyed. Progressive neurodegenerative diseases can have cellular, laminar, and regional specificity for the cerebral cortex, giving rise to a different set of aphasias that will be described separately.

Wernicke's Aphasia Comprehension is impaired for spoken and written words and sentences. Language output is fluent but is highly paraphasic and circumlocutious. Paraphasic errors may lead to strings of neologisms, which lead to "jargon aphasia." Speech contains few substantive nouns. The output is therefore voluminous but uninformative. For example, a patient attempts to describe how his wife accidentally threw away something important, perhaps his dentures: "We don't need it anymore, she says. And with it when that was downstairs was my teeth-tick ... a ... den ... dentith ... my dentist. And they happened

TABLE 30-1 Clinical Features of Aphasias and Related Conditions Commonly Seen in Cerebrovascular Accidents

	COMPREHENSION	REPETITION OF SPOKEN LANGUAGE	NAMING	FLUENCY
Wernicke's	Impaired	Impaired	Impaired	Preserved or increased
Broca's	Preserved (except grammar)	Impaired	Impaired	Decreased
Global	Impaired	Impaired	Impaired	Decreased
Conduction	Preserved	Impaired	Impaired	Preserved
Nonfluent (anterior) transcortical	Preserved	Preserved	Impaired	Impaired
Fluent (posterior) transcortical	Impaired	Preserved	Impaired	Preserved
Isolation	Impaired	Echolalia	Impaired	No purposeful speech
Anomic	Preserved	Preserved	Impaired	Preserved except for word-finding pauses
Pure word deafness	Impaired only for spoken language	Impaired	Preserved	Preserved
Pure alexia	Impaired only for reading	Preserved	Preserved	Preserved

to be in that bag ... see? ...Where my two ... two little pieces of dentist that I use ... that I ... all gone. If she throws the whole thing away ... visit some friends of hers and she can't throw them away."

Gestures and pantomime do not improve communication. The patient may not realize that his or her language is incomprehensible and may appear angry and impatient when the examiner fails to decipher the meaning of a severely paraphasic statement. In some patients, this type of aphasia can be associated with severe agitation and paranoia. The ability to follow commands aimed at axial musculature may be preserved. The dissociation between the failure to understand simple questions ("What is your name?") in a patient who rapidly closes his or her eyes, sits up, or rolls over when asked to do so is characteristic of Wernicke's aphasia and helps differentiate it from deafness, psychiatric disease, or malingering. Patients with Wernicke's aphasia cannot express their thoughts in meaning-appropriate words and cannot decode the meaning of words in any modality of input. This aphasia therefore has expressive as well as receptive components. Repetition, naming, reading, and writing also are impaired.

The lesion site most commonly associated with Wernicke's aphasia caused by CVAs is the posterior portion of the language network. An embolus to the inferior division of the middle cerebral artery (MCA), to the posterior temporal or angular branches in particular, is the most common etiology **(Chap. 426)**. Intracerebral hemorrhage, head trauma, and neoplasm are other causes of Wernicke's aphasia. A coexisting right hemianopia or superior quadrantanopia is common, and mild right nasolabial flattening may be found, but otherwise, the examination is often unrevealing. The paraphasic, neologistic speech in an agitated patient with an otherwise unremarkable neurologic examination may lead to the suspicion of a primary psychiatric disorder such as schizophrenia or mania, but the other components characteristic of acquired aphasia and the absence of prior psychiatric disease usually settle the issue. Prognosis for recovery of language function is guarded.

Broca's Aphasia Speech is nonfluent, labored, interrupted by many word-finding pauses, and usually dysarthric. It is impoverished in function words but enriched in meaning-appropriate nouns. Abnormal word order and the inappropriate deployment of *bound morphemes* (word endings used to denote tenses, possessives, or plurals) lead to a characteristic agrammatism. Speech is telegraphic and pithy but quite informative. In the following passage, a patient with Broca's aphasia describes his medical history: "I see ... the dotor, dotor sent me ... Bosson. Go to hospital. Dotor ... kept me beside. Two, tee days, doctor send me home."

Output may be reduced to a grunt or single word ("yes" or "no"), which is emitted with different intonations in an attempt to express approval or disapproval. In addition to fluency, naming and repetition are impaired. Comprehension of spoken language is intact except for syntactically difficult sentences with a passive voice structure or embedded clauses, indicating that Broca's aphasia is not just an "expressive" or "motor" disorder and that it also may involve a comprehension deficit in decoding syntax. Patients with Broca's aphasia can be tearful, easily frustrated, and profoundly depressed. Insight into their condition is preserved, in contrast to Wernicke's aphasia. Even when spontaneous speech is severely dysarthric, the patient may be able to display a relatively normal articulation of words when singing. This dissociation has been used to develop specific therapeutic approaches (melodic intonation therapy) for Broca's aphasia. Additional neurologic deficits include right facial weakness, hemiparesis or hemiplegia, and a buccofacial apraxia characterized by an inability to carry out motor commands involving oropharyngeal and facial musculature (e.g., patients are unable to demonstrate how to blow out a match or suck through a straw). The cause is most often infarction of Broca's area (the inferior frontal convolution; "B" in Fig. 30-1) and surrounding anterior perisylvian and insular cortex due to occlusion of the superior division of the MCA **(Chap. 426)**. Mass lesions, including tumor, intracerebral hemorrhage, and abscess, also may be responsible. When the cause of Broca's aphasia is stroke, recovery of language function generally peaks within 2–6 months, after which time further progress is limited. Speech therapy is more successful than in Wernicke's aphasia.

Conduction Aphasia Speech output is fluent but contains many phonemic paraphasias, comprehension of spoken language is intact, and repetition is severely impaired. Naming elicits phonemic paraphasias, and spelling is impaired. Reading aloud is impaired, but reading comprehension is preserved. The responsible lesion, usually a CVA in the temporoparietal or dorsal perisylvian region, interferes with the function of the phonological loop interconnecting Broca's area with Wernicke's area. Occasionally, a transient Wernicke's aphasia may rapidly resolve into a conduction aphasia. The paraphasic and circumlocutious output in conduction aphasia interferes with the ability to express meaning, but this deficit is not nearly as severe as the one displayed by patients with Wernicke's aphasia. Associated neurologic signs in conduction aphasia vary according to the primary lesion site.

Transcortical Aphasias: Fluent and Nonfluent Clinical features of *fluent (posterior) transcortical aphasia* are similar to those of Wernicke's aphasia, but repetition is intact. The lesion site disconnects the intact core of the language network from other temporoparietal association areas. Associated neurologic findings may include hemianopia. Cerebrovascular lesions (e.g., infarctions in the posterior watershed zone) and neoplasms that involve the temporoparietal cortex posterior to Wernicke's area are common causes. The features of *nonfluent (anterior) transcortical aphasia* are similar to those of Broca's aphasia, but repetition is intact and agrammatism is less pronounced. The neurologic examination may be otherwise intact, but a right hemiparesis also can exist. The lesion site disconnects the intact language network from prefrontal areas of the brain and usually involves the anterior watershed zone between anterior and MCA territories or the supplementary motor cortex in the territory of the anterior cerebral artery.

Global and Isolation Aphasias *Global aphasia* represents the combined dysfunction of Broca's and Wernicke's areas and usually results from strokes that involve the entire MCA distribution in the left hemisphere. Speech output is nonfluent, and comprehension of language is severely impaired. Related signs include right hemiplegia, hemisensory loss, and homonymous hemianopia. *Isolation aphasia* represents a combination of the two transcortical aphasias. Comprehension is severely impaired, and there is no purposeful speech output. The patient may parrot fragments of heard conversations (*echolalia*), indicating that the neural mechanisms for repetition are at least partially intact. This condition represents the pathologic function of the language network when it is isolated from other regions of the brain. Broca's and Wernicke's areas tend to be spared, but there is damage to the surrounding frontal, parietal, and temporal cortex. Lesions are patchy and can be associated with anoxia, carbon monoxide poisoning, or complete watershed zone infarctions.

Anomic Aphasia This form of aphasia may be considered the "minimal dysfunction" syndrome of the language network. Articulation, comprehension, and repetition are intact, but confrontation naming, word finding, and spelling are impaired. Word-finding pauses are uncommon, so language output is fluent but paraphasic, circumlocutious, and uninformative. The lesion sites can be anywhere within the left hemisphere language network, including the middle and inferior temporal gyri. *Anomic aphasia is the single most common language disturbance seen in head trauma, metabolic encephalopathy, and Alzheimer's disease.*

Pure Word Deafness The most common causes are either bilateral or left-sided MCA strokes affecting the superior temporal gyrus. The net effect of the underlying lesion is to interrupt the flow of information from the auditory association cortex to the language network. Patients have no difficulty understanding written language and can express themselves well in spoken or written language. They have no difficulty interpreting and reacting to environmental sounds if the primary auditory cortex and auditory association areas of the right hemisphere are spared. Because auditory information cannot be conveyed to the language network, however, it cannot be decoded into neural word representations, and the patient reacts to speech as if it were in an alien tongue that cannot be deciphered. Patients cannot repeat spoken language but have no difficulty naming objects. In time, patients with pure word deafness teach themselves lipreading and may appear to have improved. There may be no additional neurologic findings, but agitated paranoid reactions are common in the acute stages. Cerebrovascular lesions are the most common cause.

Pure Alexia Without Agraphia This is the visual equivalent of pure word deafness. The lesions (usually a combination of damage to the left occipital cortex and to a posterior sector of the corpus callosum—the splenium) interrupt the flow of visual input into the language network. There is usually a right hemianopia, but the core language network remains unaffected. The patient can understand and produce spoken language, name objects in the left visual hemifield, repeat, and write. However, the patient acts as if illiterate when asked to read even the simplest sentence because the visual information from the written words (presented to the intact left visual hemifield) cannot reach the language network. Objects in the left hemifield may be named accurately because they activate nonvisual associations in the right hemisphere, which in turn can access the language network through transcallosal pathways anterior to the splenium. Patients with this syndrome also may lose the ability to name colors, although they can match colors. This is known as a *color anomia*. The most common etiology of pure alexia is a vascular lesion in the territory of the posterior cerebral artery or an infiltrating neoplasm in the left occipital cortex that involves the optic radiations as well as the crossing fibers of the splenium. Because the posterior cerebral artery also supplies medial temporal components of the limbic system, a patient with pure alexia also may experience an amnesia, but this is usually transient because the limbic lesion is unilateral.

Apraxia and Aphemia *Apraxia* designates a complex motor deficit that cannot be attributed to pyramidal, extrapyramidal, cerebellar, or sensory dysfunction and that does not arise from the patient's failure to understand the nature of the task. *Apraxia of speech* is used to designate articulatory abnormalities in the duration, fluidity, and stress of syllables that make up words. It can arise with CVAs in the posterior part of Broca's area or in the course of frontotemporal lobar degeneration (FTLD) with tauopathy. *Aphemia* is a severe form of acute speech apraxia that presents with severely impaired fluency (often mutism). Recovery is the rule and involves an intermediate stage of hoarse whispering. Writing, reading, and comprehension are intact, and so this is not a true aphasic syndrome. CVAs in parts of Broca's area or subcortical lesions that undercut its connections with other parts of the brain may be present. Occasionally, the lesion site is on the medial aspects of the frontal lobes and may involve the supplementary motor cortex of the left hemisphere. *Ideomotor apraxia* is diagnosed when commands to perform a specific motor act ("cough," "blow out a match") or pantomime the use of a common tool (a comb, hammer, straw, or toothbrush) in the absence of the real object cannot be followed. The patient's ability to comprehend the command is ascertained by demonstrating multiple movements and establishing that the correct one can be recognized. Some patients with this type of apraxia can imitate the appropriate movement when it is demonstrated by the examiner and show no impairment when handed the real object, indicating that the sensorimotor mechanisms necessary for the movement are intact. Some forms of ideomotor apraxia represent a disconnection of the language network from pyramidal motor systems so that commands to execute complex movements are understood but cannot be conveyed to the appropriate motor areas. *Buccofacial apraxia* involves apraxic deficits in movements of the face and mouth. Ideomotor *limb apraxia* encompasses apraxic deficits in movements of the arms and legs. Ideomotor apraxia almost always is caused by lesions in the left hemisphere and is commonly associated with aphasic syndromes, especially Broca's aphasia and conduction aphasia. Because the handling of real objects is not impaired, ideomotor apraxia by itself causes no major limitation of daily living activities. Patients with lesions of the anterior corpus callosum can display ideomotor apraxia confined to the left side of the body, a sign known as *sympathetic dyspraxia*. A severe form of sympathetic dyspraxia, known as the *alien hand* syndrome, is characterized by additional features of motor disinhibition on the left hand. *Ideational apraxia* refers to a deficit in the sequencing of goal-directed movements in patients who have no difficulty executing the individual components of the sequence. For example, when the patient is asked to pick up a pen and write, the sequence of uncapping the pen, placing the cap at the opposite end, turning the point toward the writing surface, and writing may be disrupted, and the patient may be seen trying to write with the wrong end of the pen or even with the removed cap. These motor sequencing problems usually are seen in the context of confusional states and dementias rather than focal lesions associated with aphasic conditions. *Limb-kinetic apraxia* involves clumsiness in the use of tools or objects that cannot be attributed to sensory, pyramidal, extrapyramidal, or cerebellar dysfunction. This condition can emerge in the context of focal premotor cortex lesions or *corticobasal degeneration* and can interfere with the use of tools and utensils.

Gerstmann's Syndrome The combination of *acalculia* (impairment of simple arithmetic), *dysgraphia* (impaired writing), *finger anomia* (an inability to name individual fingers such as the index and thumb), and *right-left confusion* (an inability to tell whether a hand, foot, or arm of the patient or examiner is on the right or left side of the body) is known as Gerstmann's syndrome. In making this diagnosis, it is important to establish that the finger and left-right naming deficits are not part of a more generalized anomia and that the patient is not otherwise aphasic. When Gerstmann's syndrome arises acutely and in isolation, it is commonly associated with damage to the inferior parietal lobule (especially the angular gyrus) in the left hemisphere.

Pragmatics and Prosody *Pragmatics* refers to aspects of language that communicate attitude, affect, and the figurative rather than literal aspects of a message (e.g., "green thumb" does not refer to the actual color of the finger). One component of pragmatics, *prosody*, refers to variations of melodic stress and intonation that influence attitude and the inferential aspect of verbal messages. For example, the two statements "He *is* clever." and "He is *clever*?" contain an identical word choice and syntax but convey vastly different messages because of differences in the intonation with which the statements are uttered. Damage to right hemisphere regions corresponding to Broca's area impairs the ability to introduce meaning-appropriate prosody into spoken language. The patient produces grammatically correct language with accurate word choice, but the statements are uttered in a monotone that interferes with the ability to convey the intended stress and effect. Patients with this type of *aprosodia* give the mistaken impression of being depressed or indifferent. Other aspects of pragmatics, especially the ability to infer the figurative aspect of a message, become impaired by damage to the right hemisphere or frontal lobes.

Subcortical Aphasia Damage to subcortical components of the language network (e.g., the striatum and thalamus of the left hemisphere) also can lead to aphasia. The resulting syndromes contain combinations of deficits in the various aspects of language but rarely fit the specific patterns described in Table 30-1. In a patient with a CVA, an anomic aphasia accompanied by dysarthria or a fluent aphasia with hemiparesis should raise the suspicion of a subcortical lesion site.

CLINICAL PRESENTATION AND DIAGNOSIS OF PPA Aphasias caused by CVAs start suddenly and display maximal deficits at the onset. These are the "classic" aphasias described above. Aphasias caused by neurodegenerative diseases have an insidious onset and relentless progression. The neuropathology can be selective not only for gray matter but also for specific layers and cell types. The clinico-anatomic patterns are therefore different from those described in Table 30-1.

Several neurodegenerative syndromes, such as typical Alzheimer-type (amnestic; **Chap. 431**) and frontotemporal (behavioral; **Chap. 432**) dementias, can also include language impairments as the disease progresses. In these cases, the aphasia is an ancillary component of the overall syndrome. A diagnosis of primary progressive aphasia (PPA) is justified only if the language disorder (i.e., aphasia) arises in relative isolation, becomes the primary concern that brings the patient to medical attention, and remains the most salient deficit for 1–2 years. PPA can be caused by either FTLD or Alzheimer's disease (AD) pathology. Rarely, an identical syndrome can be caused by Creutzfeldt-Jacob disease (CJD) but with a more rapid progression (**Chap. 438**).

LANGUAGE IN PPA The impairments of language in PPA have slightly different patterns from those seen in CVA-caused aphasias. For example, the full syndrome of Wernicke's aphasia is almost never seen in PPA, confirming the view that sentence comprehension and word comprehension are controlled by different regions of the language network. Three major subtypes of PPA can be recognized.

Agrammatic PPA The *agrammatic variant* is characterized by consistently low fluency and impaired grammar but intact word comprehension. It most closely resembles Broca's aphasia or anterior transcortical aphasia but usually lacks the right hemiparesis or dysarthria and may have more profound impairments of grammar. Peak sites of neuronal loss (gray matter atrophy) include the left inferior frontal gyrus where Broca's area is located. The neuropathology is usually a FTLD with tauopathy but can also be an atypical form of AD pathology.

Semantic PPA The *semantic variant* is characterized by preserved fluency and syntax but poor single-word comprehension and profound two-way naming impairments. This kind of aphasia is not seen with CVAs. It differs from Wernicke's aphasia or posterior transcortical aphasia because speech is usually informative and repetition is intact. Comprehension of sentences is relatively preserved if the meaning is not too dependent on words that fail to be understood allowing the patient to surmise the gist of the conversation through contextual cues. Such patients may appear unimpaired in the course of casual small talk but become puzzled upon encountering an undecipherable word such as "pumpkin" or "umbrella." Peak atrophy sites are located in the left anterior temporal lobe, indicating that this part of the brain plays a critical role in the comprehension of words, especially words that denote concrete objects. This is a part of the brain that was not included within the classic language network, probably because it is not a common site for focal CVAs. The neuropathology is frequently an FTLD with abnormal precipitates of the 43-kDa transactive response DNA-binding protein TDP-43 of type C.

Logopenic PPA The *logopenic variant* is characterized by preserved syntax and comprehension but frequent and severe word-finding pauses, anomia, circumlocutions, and simplifications during spontaneous speech. Repetition is usually impaired. Peak atrophy sites are located in the temporoparietal junction and posterior temporal lobe, partially overlapping with traditional location of Wernicke's area. However, the comprehension impairment of *Wernicke's aphasia* is absent probably because the underlying deep white matter, frequently damaged by CVAs, remains relatively intact in PPA. The repetition impairment suggests that parts of Wernicke's area are critical for phonological loop functionality. In contrast to Broca's aphasia or agrammatic PPA, the interruption of fluency is variable so that speech may appear entirely normal if the patient is allowed to engage in small talk. Logopenic PPA resembles the anomic aphasia of Table 30-1 but usually has longer and more frequent word-finding pauses. When repetition is impaired, the aphasia resembles the *conduction aphasia* in Table 30-1. Of all PPA subtypes, this is the one most commonly associated with the pathology of AD, but FTLD can also be the cause. In addition to these three major subtypes, there is also a *mixed* type of PPA where grammar, fluency, and word comprehension are jointly impaired. This is most like the global aphasia of Table 30-1. Rarely, PPA can present with patterns reminiscent of *pure word deafness* or *Gerstmann's syndrome*.

THE PARIETOFRONTAL NETWORK FOR SPATIAL ORIENTATION

Adaptive spatial orientation is subserved by a large-scale network containing three major cortical components. The *cingulate cortex* provides access to a motivational mapping of the extrapersonal space, the *posterior parietal cortex* to a sensorimotor representation of salient extrapersonal events, and the *frontal eye fields* to motor strategies for attentional behaviors (**Fig. 30-2**). Subcortical components of this network include the striatum and the thalamus. Damage to this network can undermine the distribution of attention within the extrapersonal space, giving rise to hemispatial neglect, simultanagnosia, and object finding failures. The integration of egocentric (self-centered) with allocentric (object-centered) coordinates can also be disrupted, giving rise to impairments in route finding, the ability to avoid obstacles, and the ability to dress.

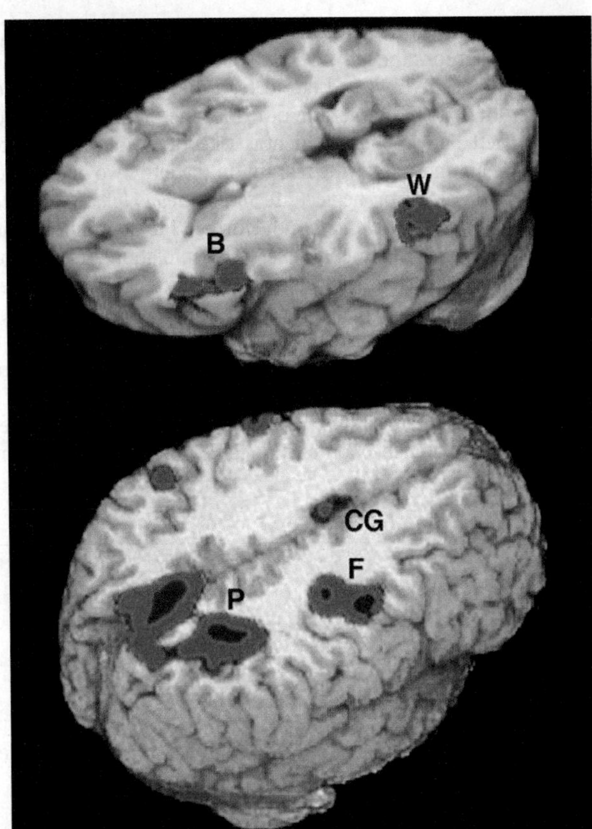

FIGURE 30-2 Functional magnetic resonance imaging of language and spatial attention in neurologically intact subjects. The red and black areas show regions of task-related significant activation. (*Top*) The subjects were asked to determine if two words were synonymous. This language task led to the simultaneous activation of the two components of the language network, Broca's area (B) and Wernicke's area (W). The activations are exclusively in the left hemisphere. (*Bottom*) The subjects were asked to shift spatial attention to a peripheral target. This task led to the simultaneous activation of the three epicenters of the attentional network: the posterior parietal cortex (P), the frontal eye fields (F), and the cingulate gyrus (CG). The activations are predominantly in the right hemisphere. *(Courtesy of Darren Gitelman, MD.)*

HEMISPATIAL NEGLECT

Contralesional hemispatial neglect represents one outcome of damage to the cortical or subcortical components of this network. *The traditional view that hemispatial neglect always denotes a parietal lobe lesion is inaccurate.* According to one model of spatial cognition, the right hemisphere directs attention within the *entire* extrapersonal space, whereas the left hemisphere directs attention mostly within the contralateral right hemispace. Consequently, left hemisphere lesions do not give rise to much contralesional neglect because the global attentional mechanisms of the right hemisphere can compensate for the loss of the *contralaterally* directed attentional functions of the left hemisphere. Right hemisphere lesions, however, give rise to severe contralesional left hemispatial neglect because the unaffected left hemisphere does not contain ipsilateral attentional mechanisms. This model is consistent with clinical experience, which shows that contralesional neglect is more common, more severe, and longer lasting after damage to the right hemisphere than after damage to the left hemisphere. Severe neglect for the right hemispace is rare, even in left-handers with left hemisphere lesions.

Clinical Examination Patients with severe neglect may fail to dress, shave, or groom the left side of the body; fail to eat food placed on the left side of the tray; and fail to read the left half of sentences. When asked to copy a simple line drawing, the patient fails to copy detail on the left, and when the patient is asked to write, there is a tendency to leave an unusually wide margin on the left. Two bedside tests that are useful in assessing neglect are *simultaneous bilateral stimulation* and *visual target cancellation*. In the former, the examiner provides either unilateral or simultaneous bilateral stimulation in the visual, auditory, and tactile modalities. After right hemisphere injury, patients who have no difficulty detecting unilateral stimuli on either side experience the bilaterally presented stimulus as coming only from the right. This phenomenon is known as *extinction* and is a manifestation of the sensory-representational aspect of hemispatial neglect. In the target detection task, targets (e.g., A's) are interspersed with foils (e.g., other letters of the alphabet) on a 21.5- to 28.0-cm (8.5–11 in.) sheet of paper, and the patient is asked to circle all the targets. A failure to detect targets on the left is a manifestation of the exploratory (motor) deficit in hemispatial neglect (**Fig. 30-3*A***). Hemianopia is not by itself sufficient to cause the target detection failure because the patient is free to turn the head and eyes to the left. Target detection failures therefore reflect a distortion of spatial attention, not just of sensory input. Some patients with neglect also may deny the existence of hemiparesis and may even deny ownership of the paralyzed limb, a condition known as *anosognosia*.

BÁLINT'S SYNDROME, SIMULTANAGNOSIA, DRESSING APRAXIA, CONSTRUCTION APRAXIA, AND ROUTE-FINDING IMPAIRMENTS

Bilateral involvement of the network for spatial attention, especially its parietal components, leads to a state of severe spatial disorientation known as *Bálint's syndrome*. Bálint's syndrome involves deficits in the

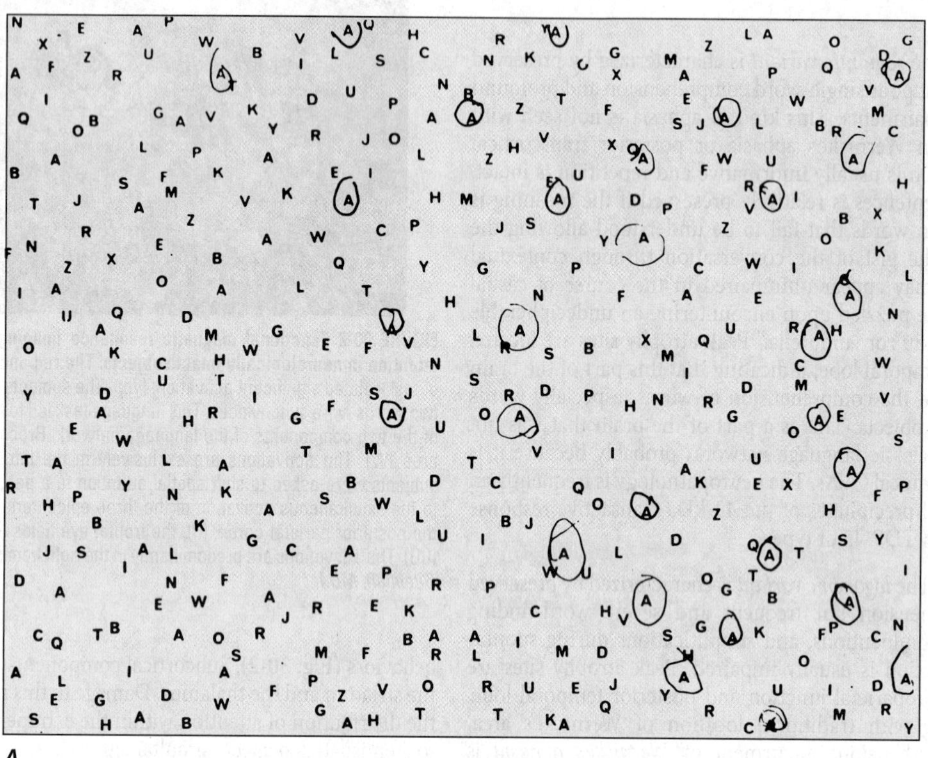

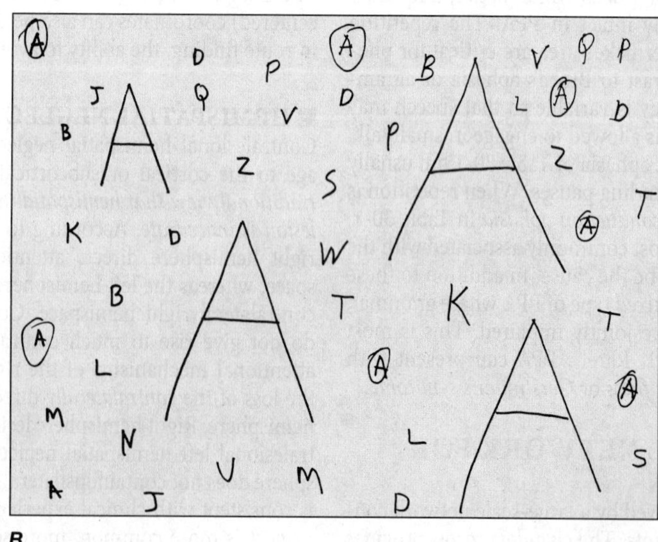

FIGURE 30-3 ***A.*** A 47-year-old man with a large frontoparietal lesion in the right hemisphere was asked to circle all the A's. Only targets on the right are circled. This is a manifestation of left hemispatial neglect. ***B.*** A 70-year-old woman with a 2-year history of degenerative dementia was able to circle most of the small targets but ignored the larger ones. This is a manifestation of simultanagnosia.

orderly visuomotor scanning of the environment (*oculomotor apraxia*), accurate manual reaching toward visual targets (*optic ataxia*), and the ability to integrate visual information in the center of gaze with more peripheral information (*simultanagnosia*). A patient with simultanagnosia "misses the forest for the trees." For example, a patient who is shown a table lamp and asked to name the object may look at its circular base and call it an ashtray. Some patients with simultanagnosia report that objects they look at may vanish suddenly, probably indicating an inability to compute the oculomotor return to the original point of gaze after brief saccadic displacements. Movement and distracting stimuli greatly exacerbate the difficulties of visual perception. Simultanagnosia can occur without the other two components of Bálint's syndrome, especially in association with AD.

A modification of the letter cancellation task described above can be used for the bedside diagnosis of simultanagnosia. In this modification, some of the targets (e.g., A's) are made to be much larger than the others (7.5–10 cm vs 2.5 cm [3–4 in. vs 1 in.] in height), and all targets are embedded among foils. Patients with simultanagnosia display a counterintuitive but characteristic tendency to miss the larger targets (**Fig. 30-3*B***). This occurs because the information needed for the identification of the larger targets cannot be confined to the immediate line of gaze and requires the integration of visual information across multiple fixation points. The greater difficulty in the detection of the larger targets also indicates that poor acuity is not responsible for the impairment of visual function and that the problem is central rather than peripheral. The test shown in Fig. 30-3*B* is not by itself sufficient to diagnose simultanagnosia as some patients with a frontal network syndrome may omit the letters that appear incongruous for the size of the paper. This may happen because they lack the mental flexibility to realize that the two types of targets are symbolically identical despite being superficially different.

Bilateral parietal lesions can impair the integration of egocentric with allocentric spatial coordinates. One manifestation is *dressing apraxia*. A patient with this condition is unable to align the body axis with the axis of the garment and can be seen struggling as he or she holds a coat from its bottom or extends his or her arm into a fold of the garment rather than into its sleeve. Lesions that involve the posterior parietal cortex also lead to severe difficulties in copying simple line drawings. This is known as a *construction apraxia* and is much more severe if the lesion is in the right hemisphere. In some patients with right hemisphere lesions, the drawing difficulties are confined to the left side of the figure and represent a manifestation of hemispatial neglect; in others, there is a more universal deficit in reproducing contours and three-dimensional perspective. Impairments of route finding can be included in this group of disorders, which reflect an inability to orient the self with respect to external objects and landmarks.

Causes of Spatial Disorientation and the Posterior Cortical Atrophy Syndrome Cerebrovascular lesions and neoplasms in the right hemisphere are common causes of hemispatial neglect. Depending on the site of the lesion, a patient with neglect also may have hemiparesis, hemihypesthesia, and hemianopia on the left, but these are not invariant findings. The majority of these patients display considerable improvement of hemispatial neglect, usually within the first several weeks. Bálint's syndrome, dressing apraxia, and route-finding impairments are more likely to result from bilateral dorsal parietal lesions; common settings for acute onset include watershed infarction between the middle and posterior cerebral artery territories, hypoglycemia, and sagittal sinus thrombosis.

A progressive form of spatial disorientation, known as the *posterior cortical atrophy* (PCA) syndrome, most commonly represents a variant of AD with unusual concentrations of neurofibrillary degeneration in the parieto-occipital cortex and the superior colliculus (**Fig. 30-4**). Lewy body disease (LBD), CJD, and FTLD (corticobasal degeneration type) are other possible causes. The patient displays progressive hemispatial neglect, Bálint's syndrome, and route-finding impairments, usually accompanied by dressing and construction apraxia.

THE OCCIPITOTEMPORAL NETWORK FOR FACE AND OBJECT RECOGNITION

A patient with *prosopagnosia* cannot recognize familiar faces, including, sometimes, the reflection of their own face in the mirror. This is not a perceptual deficit because prosopagnosic patients easily can tell whether two faces are identical. Furthermore, a prosopagnosic patient who cannot recognize a familiar face by visual inspection alone can use auditory cues to reach appropriate recognition if allowed to listen to the person's voice. The deficit in prosopagnosia is therefore modality-specific and reflects the existence of a lesion that prevents the activation of otherwise intact multimodal associative templates by relevant visual input. Prosopagnosic patients characteristically have no difficulty with the generic identification of a face as a face or a car as a car, but may not recognize the identity of an individual face or the make of an individual car. This reflects a visual recognition deficit for proprietary features that characterize individual members of an object class. When recognition problems become more generalized and extend to the generic identification of common objects, the condition is known as *visual object agnosia*. A patient with anomia cannot name the object but can describe its use. In contrast, a patient with visual agnosia is unable either to name a visually presented object or to describe its use. Face and object recognition disorders also can result from the simultanagnosia of Bálint's syndrome, in which case they are known as *apperceptive* agnosias as opposed to the *associative* agnosias that result from inferior temporal lobe lesions.

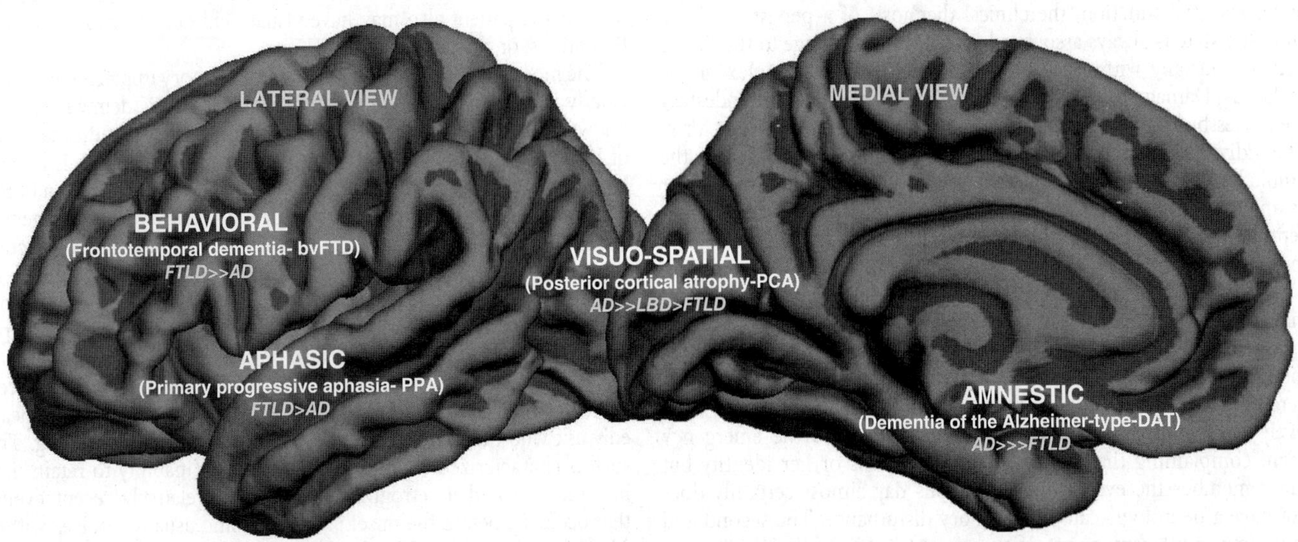

FIGURE 30-4 Four focal dementia syndromes and their most likely neuropathologic correlates. AD, Alzheimer's disease; bvFTD, behavioral variant frontotemporal dementia; DAT, amnestic dementia of the Alzheimer type; FTLD, frontotemporal lobar degeneration (tau or TDP-43 type); LBD, Lewy body disease; PCA, posterior cortical atrophy syndrome; PPA, primary progressive aphasia.

CAUSES AND RELATION TO SEMANTIC DEMENTIA

The characteristic lesions in prosopagnosia and visual object agnosia of acute onset consist of bilateral infarctions in the territory of the posterior cerebral arteries that involve the fusiform gyrus. Associated deficits can include visual field defects (especially superior quadrantanopias) and a centrally based color blindness known as achromatopsia. Rarely, the responsible lesion is unilateral. In such cases, prosopagnosia is associated with lesions in the right hemisphere, and object agnosia with lesions in the left. Degenerative diseases of anterior and inferior temporal cortex can cause progressive associative prosopagnosia and object agnosia. The combination of progressive associative agnosia and a fluent aphasia with word comprehension impairment is known as *semantic dementia*. Patients with semantic dementia fail to recognize faces and objects and cannot understand the meaning of words denoting objects. This needs to be differentiated from the semantic type of PPA where there is severe impairment in understanding words that denote objects and in naming faces and objects but a relative preservation of face and object recognition. The anterior temporal lobe atrophy is usually bilateral in semantic dementia whereas it tends to affect mostly the left hemisphere in semantic PPA. Acute onset of the semantic dementia syndrome can be associated with herpes simplex encephalitis.

LIMBIC NETWORK FOR EXPLICIT MEMORY AND AMNESIA

Limbic areas (e.g., the hippocampus, amygdala, and entorhinal cortex), paralimbic areas (e.g., the cingulate gyrus, insula, temporopolar cortex, and parts of orbitofrontal regions), the anterior and medial nuclei of the thalamus, the medial and basal parts of the striatum, and the hypothalamus collectively constitute a distributed network known as the *limbic system*. The behavioral affiliations of this network can be classified into two groups. One includes the coordination of emotion, motivation, affiliative behaviors, autonomic tone, and endocrine function. These functions are under the influence of the amygdala and anterior paralimbic areas. They make up the salience network. The two neurologic conditions that most frequently interfere with this group of limbic functions are temporal lobe epilepsy and behavioral variant frontotemporal dementia (bvFTD). An additional area of specialization for the limbic network and the one that is of most relevance to clinical practice is that of declarative (explicit) memory for recent episodes and experiences. This function is under the influence of the hippocampus, entorhinal cortex, posterior paralimbic areas, and limbic nuclei of the thalamus. This part of the limbic system is also known as the Papez circuit. A disturbance of explicit memory is known as an *amnestic state*. In the absence of deficits in motivation, attention, language, or visuospatial function, the clinical diagnosis of a persistent global amnestic state is always associated with bilateral damage to the limbic network, usually within the hippocampo-entorhinal complex or the thalamus. Damage to the limbic network does not necessarily destroy memories but interferes with their conscious recall in coherent form. The individual fragments of information remain preserved despite the limbic lesions and can sustain what is known as *implicit memory*. For example, patients with amnestic states can acquire new motor or perceptual skills even though they may have no conscious knowledge of the experiences that led to the acquisition of these skills.

The memory disturbance in the amnestic state is multimodal and includes retrograde and anterograde components. The *retrograde amnesia* involves an inability to recall experiences that occurred before the onset of the amnestic state. Relatively recent events are more vulnerable to retrograde amnesia than are more remote and more extensively consolidated events. A patient who comes to the emergency room complaining that he cannot remember his or her identity but can remember the events of the previous day almost certainly does not have a neurologic cause of memory disturbance. The second and most important component of the amnestic state is the *anterograde amnesia*, which indicates an inability to store, retain, and recall new knowledge. Patients with amnestic states cannot remember what they ate a few hours ago or the details of an important event they may have experienced in the recent past. In the acute stages, there also may be a tendency to fill in memory gaps with inaccurate, fabricated, and often implausible information. This is known as *confabulation*. Patients with the amnestic syndrome forget that they forget and tend to deny the existence of a memory problem when questioned. Confabulation is more common in cases where the underlying lesion also interferes with parts of the frontal network, as in the case of the Wernicke-Korsakoff syndrome or traumatic head injury.

CLINICAL EXAMINATION

A patient with an amnestic state is almost always disoriented, especially to time, and has little knowledge of current news. The anterograde component of an amnestic state can be tested with a list of four to five words read aloud by the examiner up to five times or until the patient can immediately repeat the entire list without an intervening delay. The next phase of the recall occurs after a period of 5–10 min during which the patient is engaged in other tasks. Amnestic patients fail this phase of the task and may even forget that they were given a list of words to remember. Accurate recognition of the words by multiple choice in a patient who cannot recall them indicates a less severe memory disturbance that affects mostly the retrieval stage of memory. The retrograde component of an amnesia can be assessed with questions related to autobiographical or historic events. The anterograde component of amnestic states is usually much more prominent than the retrograde component. In rare instances, occasionally associated with temporal lobe epilepsy or herpes simplex encephalitis, the retrograde component may dominate. Confusional states caused by toxic-metabolic encephalopathies and some types of frontal lobe damage lead to secondary memory impairments, especially at the stages of encoding and retrieval, even in the absence of limbic lesions. This sort of memory impairment can be differentiated from the amnestic state by the presence of additional impairments in the attention-related tasks described below in the section on the frontal lobes.

CAUSES, INCLUDING ALZHEIMER'S DISEASE

Neurologic diseases that give rise to an amnestic state include tumors (of the sphenoid wing, posterior corpus callosum, thalamus, or medial temporal lobe), infarctions (in the territories of the anterior or posterior cerebral arteries), head trauma, herpes simplex encephalitis, Wernicke-Korsakoff encephalopathy, autoimmune limbic encephalitis, and degenerative dementias such as AD and Pick's disease. The one common denominator of all these diseases is the presence of bilateral lesions within one or more components in the limbic network. Occasionally, unilateral left-sided hippocampal lesions can give rise to an amnestic state, but the memory disorder tends to be transient. Depending on the nature and distribution of the underlying neurologic disease, the patient also may have visual field deficits, eye movement limitations, or cerebellar findings.

The most common cause of progressive memory impairments in the elderly is AD. This is why a predominantly amnestic dementia is also known as a dementia of the Alzheimer type (DAT). A prodromal stage of DAT, when daily living activities are generally preserved, is known as amnestic mild cognitive impairment (MCI). The predilection of the entorhinal cortex and hippocampus for early neurofibrillary degeneration by typical AD pathology is responsible for the initially selective impairment of episodic memory. In time, additional impairments in language, attention, and visuospatial skills emerge as the neurofibrillary degeneration spreads to additional neocortical areas. Less frequently, amnestic dementias can also be caused by FTLD.

Transient global amnesia is a distinctive syndrome usually seen in late middle age. Patients become acutely disoriented and repeatedly ask who they are, where they are, and what they are doing. The spell is characterized by anterograde amnesia (inability to retain new information) and a retrograde amnesia for relatively recent events that occurred before the onset. The syndrome usually resolves within 24–48 h and is followed by the filling in of the period affected by the retrograde amnesia, although there is persistent loss of memory for the events that occurred during the ictus. Recurrences are noted in

~20% of patients. Migraine, temporal lobe seizures, and perfusion abnormalities in the posterior cerebral territory have been postulated as causes of transient global amnesia. The absence of associated neurologic findings occasionally may lead to the incorrect diagnosis of a psychiatric disorder.

THE PREFRONTAL NETWORK FOR EXECUTIVE FUNCTION AND BEHAVIOR

The frontal lobes can be subdivided into motor-premotor, dorsolateral prefrontal, medial prefrontal, and orbitofrontal components. The terms *frontal lobe syndrome* and *prefrontal cortex* refer only to the last three of these four components. These are the parts of the cerebral cortex that show the greatest phylogenetic expansion in primates, especially in humans. The dorsolateral prefrontal, medial prefrontal, and orbitofrontal areas, along with the subcortical structures with which they are interconnected (i.e., the head of the caudate and the dorsomedial nucleus of the thalamus), collectively make up a large-scale network that coordinates exceedingly complex aspects of human cognition and behavior. The prefrontal network overlaps with the salience network through the anterior cingulate gyrus and parts of the orbitofrontal region. Impairments of social conduct and empathy seen in neurodegenerative frontal dementias (such as bvFTD) are attributed to pathology of the prefrontal and salience networks.

The prefrontal network plays an important role in behaviors that require multitasking and the integration of thought with emotion. Cognitive operations impaired by prefrontal cortex lesions often are referred to as "executive functions." The most common clinical manifestations of damage to the prefrontal network take the form of two relatively distinct syndromes. In the *frontal abulic syndrome*, the patient shows a loss of initiative, creativity, and curiosity and displays a pervasive emotional blandness, apathy, and lack of empathy. In the *frontal disinhibition syndrome*, the patient becomes socially disinhibited and shows severe impairments of judgment, insight, foresight, and the ability to mind rules of conduct. The dissociation between intact intellectual function and a total lack of even rudimentary common sense is striking. Despite the preservation of all essential memory functions, the patient cannot learn from experience and continues to display inappropriate behaviors without appearing to feel emotional pain, guilt, or regret when those behaviors repeatedly lead to disastrous consequences. The impairments may emerge only in real-life situations when behavior is under minimal external control and may not be apparent within the structured environment of the medical office. Testing judgment by asking patients what they would do if they detected a fire in a theater or found a stamped and addressed envelope on the road is not very informative because patients who answer these questions wisely in the office may still act very foolishly in real-life settings. The physician must therefore be prepared to make a diagnosis of frontal lobe disease based on historic information alone even when the mental state is quite intact in the office examination.

■ CLINICAL EXAMINATION

The emergence of developmentally primitive reflexes, also known as frontal release signs, such as grasping (elicited by stroking the palm) and sucking (elicited by stroking the lips) are seen primarily in patients with large structural lesions that extend into the premotor components of the frontal lobes or in the context of metabolic encephalopathies. The vast majority of patients with prefrontal lesions and frontal lobe behavioral syndromes do not display these reflexes. Damage to the frontal lobe disrupts a variety of attention-related functions, including working memory (the transient online holding and manipulation of information), concentration span, the effortful scanning and retrieval of stored information, the inhibition of immediate but inappropriate responses, and mental flexibility. Digit span (which should be seven forward and five reverse) is decreased, reflecting poor working memory; the recitation of the months of the year in reverse order (which should take <15 s) is slowed as another indication of poor working memory; and the fluency in producing words starting with the letter a, f, or s that can be generated in 1 min (normally ≥12 per letter) is diminished even in nonaphasic patients, indicating an impairment in the ability to search and retrieve information from long-term stores. In "go–no go" tasks (where the instruction is to raise the finger upon hearing one tap but keep it still upon hearing two taps), the patient shows a characteristic inability to inhibit the response to the "no go" stimulus. Mental flexibility (tested by the ability to shift from one criterion to another in sorting or matching tasks) is impoverished; distractibility by irrelevant stimuli is increased; and there is a pronounced tendency for impersistence and perseveration. The ability for abstracting similarities and interpreting proverbs is also undermined.

The attentional deficits disrupt the orderly registration and retrieval of new information and lead to *secondary* deficits of explicit memory. The distinction of the underlying neural mechanisms is illustrated by the observation that severely amnestic patients who cannot remember events that occurred a few minutes ago may have intact if not superior working memory capacity as shown in tests of digit span. The use of the term *memory* to designate two completely different mental faculties is confusing. Working memory depends on the on-line holding of information for brief periods of time, whereas explicit memory depends on the off-line storage and subsequent retrieval of the information.

■ CAUSES: TRAUMA, NEOPLASM, AND FRONTOTEMPORAL DEMENTIA

The abulic syndrome tends to be associated with damage in dorsolateral or dorsomedial prefrontal cortex, and the disinhibition syndrome with damage in orbitofrontal or ventromedial cortex. These syndromes tend to arise almost exclusively after bilateral lesions. Unilateral lesions confined to the prefrontal cortex may remain silent until the pathology spreads to the other side; this explains why thromboembolic CVA is an unusual cause of the frontal lobe syndrome. When behavioral syndromes of the frontal network arise in conjunction with asymmetric disease, the lesion tends to be predominantly on the right side of the brain. Common settings for frontal lobe syndromes include head trauma, ruptured aneurysms, hydrocephalus, tumors (including metastases, glioblastoma, and falx or olfactory groove meningiomas), and focal degenerative diseases, especially FTLD. The most prominent neurodegenerative frontal syndrome is bvFTD. In many patients with bvFTD, the atrophy includes orbitofrontal cortex and also extends into the anterior temporal lobes, insula, and anterior cingulate cortex. Occasionally, atrophy predominantly in the right anterior temporal lobe presents with the bvFTD syndrome. The behavioral changes in these patients can range from apathy to shoplifting, compulsive gambling, sexual indiscretions, remarkable lack of common sense, new ritualistic behaviors, and alterations in dietary preferences, usually leading to increased taste for sweets or rigid attachment to specific food items. In many patients with AD, neurofibrillary degeneration eventually spreads to prefrontal cortex and gives rise to components of the frontal lobe syndrome, but almost always on a background of severe memory impairment. Rarely, the bvFTD syndrome can arise in isolation in the context of an atypical form of AD pathology.

Lesions in the caudate nucleus or in the dorsomedial nucleus of the thalamus (subcortical components of the prefrontal network) also can produce a frontal lobe syndrome affecting mostly executive functions. This is one reason why the changes in mental state associated with degenerative basal ganglia diseases such as Parkinson's disease and Huntington's disease display components of the frontal lobe syndrome. Bilateral multifocal lesions of the cerebral hemispheres, none of which are individually large enough to cause specific cognitive deficits such as aphasia and neglect, can collectively interfere with the connectivity and therefore integrating (executive) function of the prefrontal cortex. A frontal lobe syndrome, usually of the abulic form, is therefore the single most common behavioral profile associated with a variety of bilateral multifocal brain diseases, including metabolic encephalopathy, multiple sclerosis, and vitamin B_{12} deficiency, among others. Many patients with the clinical diagnosis of a frontal lobe syndrome tend to have lesions that do not involve prefrontal cortex but involve either the subcortical components of the prefrontal network or its connections with other parts of the brain. To avoid making a diagnosis of "frontal lobe syndrome" in a patient with no evidence of frontal cortex disease, it is advisable to use the diagnostic term *frontal network syndrome*, with the understanding that the responsible lesions can lie anywhere within this distributed network. A patient with frontal lobe disease raises potential dilemmas in differential diagnosis: the abulia and blandness may be misinterpreted as depression, and the disinhibition as idiopathic mania or acting out. Appropriate intervention may be delayed while a treatable tumor keeps expanding.

CARING FOR PATIENTS WITH DEFICITS OF HIGHER CEREBRAL FUNCTION

Spontaneous improvement of cognitive deficits following stroke or trauma is common. It is most rapid in the first few weeks but may continue for up to 2 years, especially in young individuals with single brain lesions. Some of the initial deficits in such cases appear to arise from remote dysfunction (diaschisis) in brain regions that are interconnected with the site of initial injury. Improvement in these patients may reflect, at least in part, a normalization of the remote dysfunction. Other mechanisms may involve functional reorganization in surviving neurons adjacent to the injury or the compensatory use of homologous structures, e.g., the right superior temporal gyrus with recovery from Wernicke's aphasia. In contrast, neurodegenerative diseases show a progression of impairment but at rates that vary greatly from patient to patient.

Pharmacologic and Nonpharmacologic Interventions Some of the deficits described in this chapter are so complex that they may bewilder not only the patient and family but also the physician. The care of patients with such deficits requires a careful evaluation of the history, cognitive test results, and diagnostic procedures. Each piece of information needs to be interpreted cautiously and placed in context. A complaint of "poor memory," for example, may reflect an anomia; poor scores on a learning task may reflect a weakness of attention rather than explicit memory; a report of depression or indifference may reflect impaired prosody rather than a change in mood or empathy; jocularity may arise from poor insight rather than good mood. Although there are few well-controlled studies, several nonpharmacologic interventions have been used to treat higher cortical deficits. These include speech therapy for aphasias, behavioral modification for compartmental disorders, and cognitive training for visuospatial disorientation and amnestic syndromes. More practical interventions, usually delivered through occupational therapy, aim to improve daily living activities through assistive devices and modifications of the home environment. Determining driving competence is challenging, especially in the early stages of dementing diseases. An on-the-road driving test and reports from family members may help time decisions related to this very important activity. In neurodegenerative conditions such as PPA, transcranial magnetic (or direct current) stimulation has had mixed success in eliciting symptomatic improvement. The goal is to activate remaining neurons at sites of atrophy or in unaffected regions of the contralateral hemisphere. Depression and sleep disorders can intensify the cognitive disorders and should be treated with appropriate modalities. If neuroleptics become absolutely necessary for the control of agitation, atypical neuroleptics are preferable because of their lower extrapyramidal side effects. Treatment with neuroleptics in elderly patients with dementia requires weighing the potential benefits against the potentially serious side effects. This is especially relevant to the case of patients with Lewy body dementia, who can be unusually sensitive to side effects.

As in all other branches of medicine, a crucial step in patient care is to identify the underlying cause of the impairment. This is easily done in cases of CVA, head trauma, or encephalitis but becomes particularly challenging in the dementias because the same progressive clinical syndrome can be caused by one of several neuropathologic entities. The advent of imaging, blood, and cerebrospinal fluid biomarkers now makes it possible to address this question with reasonable success and to make specific diagnoses of AD, LBD, CJD, and FTLD. A specific etiologic diagnosis allows the physician to recommend medications or clinical trials that are the most appropriate for the underlying disease process. A clinical assessment that identifies the principal domain of behavioral and cognitive impairment followed by the judicious use of biomarker information to surmise the nature of the underlying disease allows a personalized approach to patients with higher cognitive impairment.

FURTHER READING

Ghetti B et al: *Frontotemporal Dementias: Emerging Milestones of the 21st Century*. New York, Springer, 2021.

Henry ML et al: Retraining speech production and fluency in non-fluent/agrammatic primary progressive aphasia. Brain 141:1799, 2018.

Mesulam M-M: Behavioral neuroanatomy: Large-scale networks, association cortex, frontal syndromes, the limbic system and hemispheric specialization, in *Principles of Behavioral and Cognitive Neurology*, M-M Mesulam (ed). New York, Oxford University Press, 2000, pp 1–120.

Mesulam M-M et al: Word comprehension in temporal cortex and Wernicke area: A PPA perspective. Neurology 92:e224, 2019.

Miller BL, Boeve BF (eds): *The Behavioral Neurology of Dementia*, 2nd ed. Cambridge, Cambridge University Press, 2017.

31 Sleep Disorders

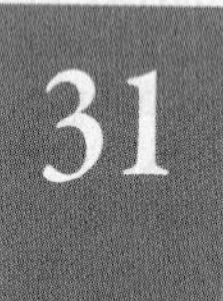

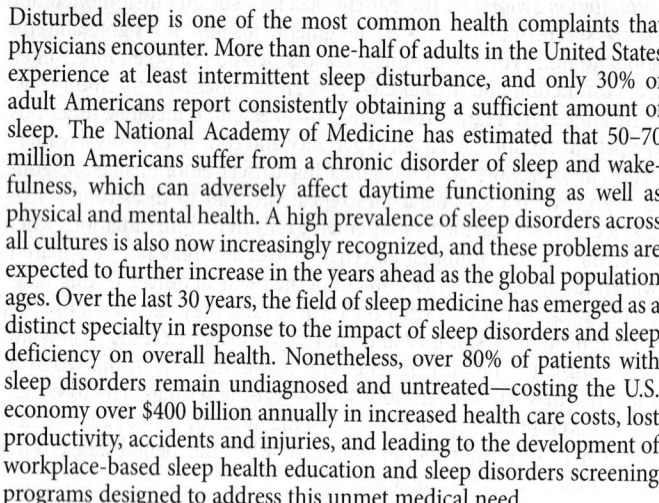

Thomas E. Scammell, Clifford B. Saper, Charles A. Czeisler

Disturbed sleep is one of the most common health complaints that physicians encounter. More than one-half of adults in the United States experience at least intermittent sleep disturbance, and only 30% of adult Americans report consistently obtaining a sufficient amount of sleep. The National Academy of Medicine has estimated that 50–70 million Americans suffer from a chronic disorder of sleep and wakefulness, which can adversely affect daytime functioning as well as physical and mental health. A high prevalence of sleep disorders across all cultures is also now increasingly recognized, and these problems are expected to further increase in the years ahead as the global population ages. Over the last 30 years, the field of sleep medicine has emerged as a distinct specialty in response to the impact of sleep disorders and sleep deficiency on overall health. Nonetheless, over 80% of patients with sleep disorders remain undiagnosed and untreated—costing the U.S. economy over $400 billion annually in increased health care costs, lost productivity, accidents and injuries, and leading to the development of workplace-based sleep health education and sleep disorders screening programs designed to address this unmet medical need.

PHYSIOLOGY OF SLEEP AND WAKEFULNESS

Most adults need 7–9 h of sleep per night to promote optimal health, although the timing, duration, and internal structure of sleep vary among individuals. In the United States, adults tend to have one consolidated sleep episode each night, although in some cultures sleep may be divided into a mid-afternoon nap and a shortened night sleep. This pattern changes considerably over the life span, as infants and young children sleep considerably more than older people, while individuals >70 years of age sleep on average about an hour less than young adults.

The stages of human sleep are defined on the basis of characteristic patterns in the electroencephalogram (EEG), the electrooculogram (EOG—a measure of eye-movement activity), and the surface electromyogram (EMG) measured on the chin, neck, and legs. The continuous recording of these electrophysiologic parameters to define sleep and wakefulness is termed *polysomnography*.

Polysomnographic profiles define two basic states of sleep: (1) rapid eye movement (REM) sleep and (2) non–rapid eye movement (NREM)

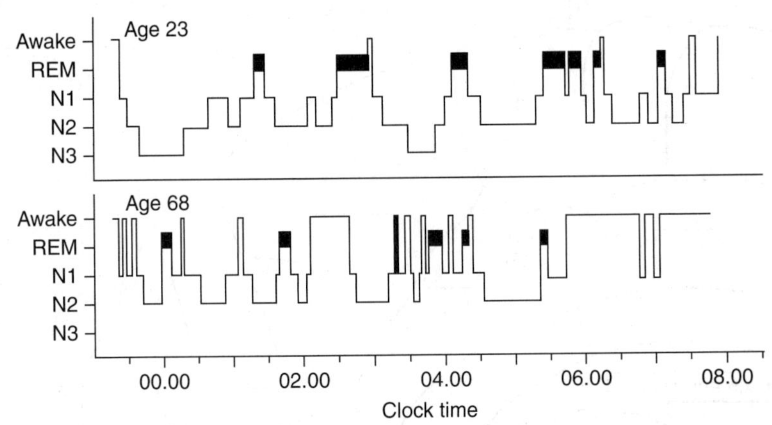

FIGURE 31-1 Wake-sleep architecture. Alternating stages of wakefulness, the three stages of non–rapid eye movement sleep (N1–N3), and rapid eye movement (REM) sleep (*solid bars*) occur over the course of the night for representative young and older adult men. Characteristic features of sleep in older people include reduction of N3 slow-wave sleep, frequent spontaneous awakenings, early sleep onset, and early morning awakening.

sleep. NREM sleep is further subdivided into three stages: N1, N2, and N3, characterized by an increasing threshold for arousal and slowing of the cortical EEG. REM sleep is characterized by a low-amplitude, mixed-frequency EEG, similar to NREM stage N1 sleep, and an EOG pattern of REMs that tend to occur in flurries or bursts. EMG activity is absent in nearly all skeletal muscles except those involved in respiration, reflecting the brainstem-mediated muscle paralysis that is characteristic of REM sleep.

ORGANIZATION OF HUMAN SLEEP

Normal nocturnal sleep in adults displays a consistent organization from night to night (**Fig. 31-1**). After sleep onset, sleep usually progresses through NREM stages N1–N3 sleep within 45–60 min. NREM stage N3 sleep (also known as slow-wave sleep) predominates in the first third of the night and comprises 15–25% of total nocturnal sleep time in young adults. Sleep deprivation increases the rapidity of sleep onset and both the intensity and amount of slow-wave sleep.

The first REM sleep episode usually occurs in the second hour of sleep. NREM and REM sleep alternate through the night with an average period of 90–110 min (the "ultradian" sleep cycle). Overall, in a healthy young adult, REM sleep constitutes 20–25% of total sleep, and NREM stages N1 and N2 constitute 50–60%.

Age has a profound impact on sleep state organization (Fig. 31-1). N3 sleep is most intense and prominent during childhood, decreasing with puberty and across the second and third decades of life. In older adults, N3 sleep may be completely absent, and the remaining NREM sleep typically becomes more fragmented, with frequent awakenings from NREM sleep. It is the increased frequency of awakenings, rather than a decreased ability to fall back asleep, that accounts for the increased wakefulness during the sleep episode in older people. While REM sleep may account for 50% of total sleep time in infancy, the percentage falls off sharply over the first postnatal year as a mature REM-NREM cycle develops; thereafter, REM sleep occupies about 25% of total sleep time.

Sleep deprivation degrades cognitive performance, particularly on tests that require continual vigilance. Paradoxically, older people are less vulnerable than young adults to the neurobehavioral performance impairment induced by acute sleep deprivation, maintaining their reaction time and sustaining vigilance with fewer lapses of attention. However, it is more difficult for older adults to obtain recovery sleep after staying awake all night, as the ability to sleep during the daytime declines with age.

After sleep deprivation, NREM sleep generally recovers first, followed by REM sleep. However, because REM sleep tends to be most prominent in the second half of the night, sleep truncation (e.g., by an alarm clock) results in selective REM sleep deprivation. This may increase REM sleep pressure to the point where the first REM sleep may occur much earlier in the nightly sleep episode. Because several disorders (see below) also cause sleep fragmentation, it is important that the patient have sufficient sleep opportunity (at least 8 h per night) for several nights prior to a diagnostic polysomnogram.

There is growing evidence that inadequate sleep in humans is associated with glucose intolerance that may contribute to the development of diabetes, obesity, and the metabolic syndrome, as well as impaired immune responses, accelerated atherosclerosis, and increased risk of cardiac disease, cognitive impairment, Alzheimer's disease, and stroke. For these reasons, the National Academy of Medicine declared sleep deficiency and sleep disorders "an unmet public health problem."

WAKE AND SLEEP ARE REGULATED BY BRAIN CIRCUITS

Two principal neural systems govern the expression of sleep and wakefulness. The ascending arousal system, illustrated in *green* in **Fig. 31-2**, consists of clusters of nerve cells extending from the upper pons to the hypothalamus and basal forebrain that activate the cerebral cortex, thalamus (which is necessary to relay sensory information to the cortex), and other forebrain regions. The ascending arousal neurons use monoamines (norepinephrine, dopamine, serotonin, and histamine), glutamate, or acetylcholine as neurotransmitters to activate their target neurons. Some basal forebrain neurons use γ-aminobutyric acid (GABA) to inhibit cortical inhibitory interneurons, thus promoting arousal. Additional wake-promoting neurons in the hypothalamus use the peptide neurotransmitter orexin (also known as hypocretin, shown in Fig. 31-2 in *blue*) to reinforce activity in the other arousal cell groups.

Damage to the arousal system at the level of the rostral pons and lower midbrain causes coma, indicating that the ascending arousal influence from this level is critical in maintaining wakefulness. Injury to the hypothalamic branch of the arousal system causes profound sleepiness but usually not coma. Specific loss of the orexin neurons produces the sleep disorder narcolepsy (see below). Isolated damage to the thalamus causes loss of the content of wakefulness, known as a persistent vegetative state, but wake-sleep cycles are largely preserved.

The arousal system is turned off during sleep by inhibitory inputs from cell groups in the sleep-promoting system, shown in Fig. 31-2 in *red*. These neurons in the preoptic area and pons use GABA to inhibit the arousal system. Additional neurons in the lateral hypothalamus containing the peptide melanin-concentrating hormone promote REM sleep. Many sleep-promoting neurons are themselves inhibited by inputs from the arousal system. This mutual inhibition between the arousal- and sleep-promoting systems forms a neural circuit akin to what electrical engineers call a "flip-flop switch." A switch of this type tends to promote rapid transitions between the on (wake) and off (sleep) states, while avoiding intermediate states. The relatively rapid transitions between waking and sleeping states, as seen in the EEG of humans and animals, is consistent with this model.

Neurons in the ventrolateral preoptic nucleus, one of the key sleep-promoting sites, are lost during normal human aging, correlating with reduced ability to maintain sleep (sleep fragmentation). The ventrolateral preoptic neurons are also injured in Alzheimer's disease, which may in part account for the poor sleep quality in those patients.

Transitions between NREM and REM sleep appear to be governed by a similar switch in the brainstem. GABAergic REM-Off neurons have been identified in the lower midbrain that inhibit REM-On neurons in the upper pons. The REM-On group contains both GABAergic neurons that inhibit the REM-Off group (thus satisfying the conditions for a REM sleep flip-flop switch) as well as glutamatergic neurons that project widely in the central nervous system (CNS) to cause the key phenomena associated with REM sleep. REM-On neurons that project to the medulla and spinal cord activate inhibitory (GABA and glycine-containing) interneurons, which in turn hyperpolarize the motor neurons, producing the paralysis of REM sleep. REM-On neurons that project to the forebrain may be important in producing dreams.

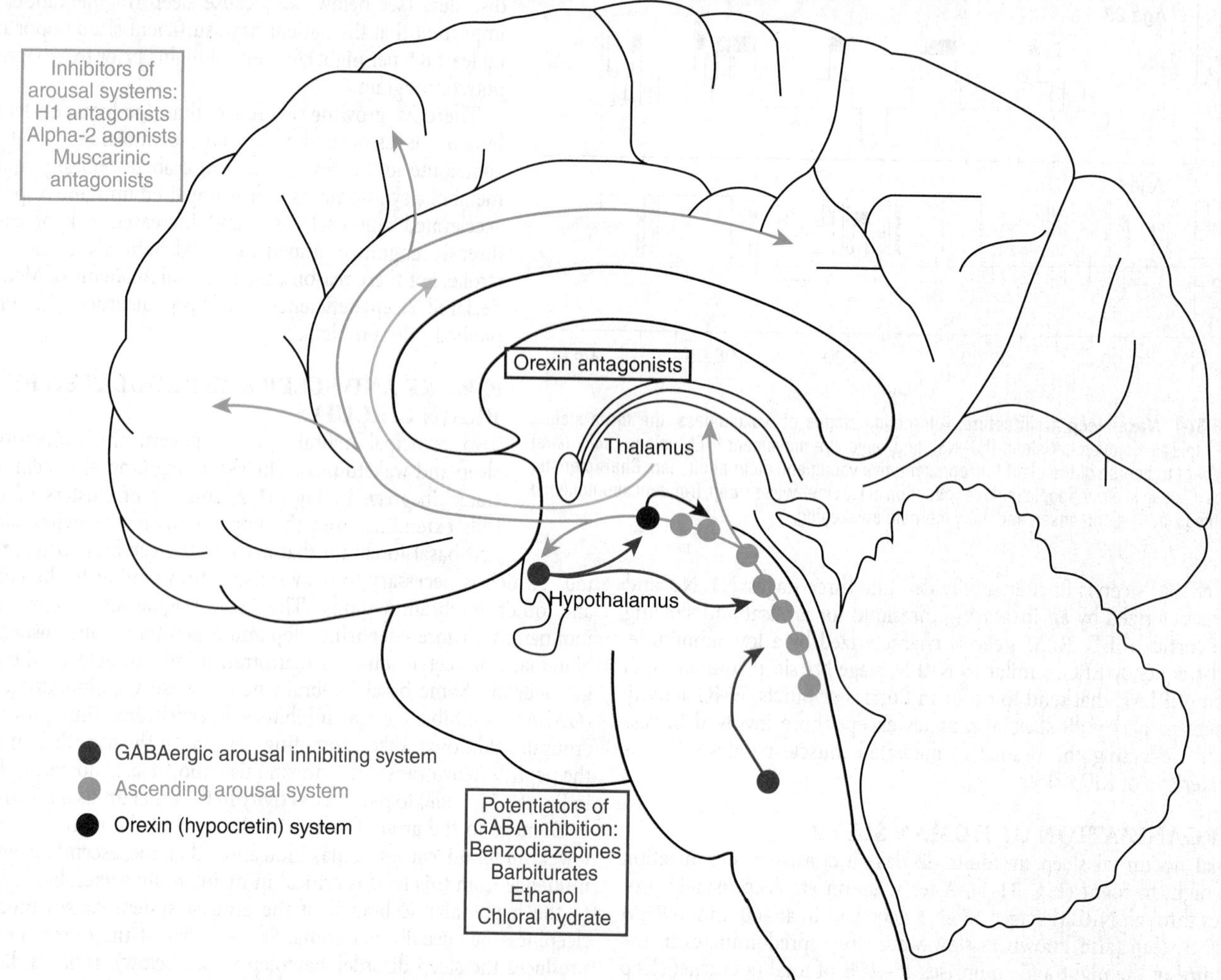

FIGURE 31-2 Relationship of drugs for insomnia with wake-sleep systems. The arousal system in the brain (*green*) includes monoaminergic, glutamatergic, and cholinergic neurons in the brainstem that activate neurons in the hypothalamus, thalamus, basal forebrain, and cerebral cortex. Orexin neurons (*blue*) in the hypothalamus, which are lost in narcolepsy, reinforce and stabilize arousal by activating other components of the arousal system. The sleep-promoting system (*red*) consists of GABAergic neurons in the preoptic area and brainstem that inhibit the components of the arousal system, thus allowing sleep to occur. Drugs used to treat insomnia include those that block the effects of arousal system neurotransmitters (*green* and *blue*) and those that enhance the effects of γ-aminobutyric acid (GABA) produced by the sleep system (*red*).

The REM sleep switch receives cholinergic input, which favors transitions to REM sleep, and monoaminergic (norepinephrine and serotonin) input that prevents REM sleep. As a result, drugs that increase monoamine tone (e.g., serotonin or norepinephrine reuptake inhibitors) tend to reduce the amount of REM sleep. Damage to the neurons that promote REM sleep paralysis can produce REM sleep behavior disorder, a condition in which patients act out their dreams (see below).

■ SLEEP-WAKE CYCLES ARE DRIVEN BY HOMEOSTATIC, ALLOSTATIC, AND CIRCADIAN INPUTS

The gradual increase in sleep drive with prolonged wakefulness, followed by deeper slow-wave sleep and prolonged sleep episodes, demonstrates that there is a *homeostatic* mechanism that regulates sleep. The neurochemistry of sleep homeostasis is only partially understood, but with prolonged wakefulness, adenosine levels rise in parts of the brain. Adenosine may act through A1 receptors to directly inhibit many arousal-promoting brain regions. In addition, adenosine promotes sleep through A2a receptors; blockade of these receptors by caffeine is one of the chief ways in which people fight sleepiness. Other humoral factors, such as prostaglandin D_2, have also been implicated in this process. Both adenosine and prostaglandin D_2 activate the sleep-promoting neurons in the ventrolateral preoptic nucleus.

Allostasis is the physiologic response to a challenge such as physical danger or psychological threat that cannot be managed by homeostatic mechanisms. These stress responses can severely impact the need for and ability to sleep. For example, insomnia is very common in patients with anxiety and other psychiatric disorders. Stress-induced insomnia is even more common, affecting most people at some time in their lives. Positron emission tomography (PET) studies in patients with chronic insomnia show hyperactivation of components of the ascending arousal system, as well as their limbic system targets in the forebrain (e.g., cingulate cortex and amygdala). The limbic areas are not only targets for the arousal system, but they also send excitatory outputs back to the arousal system, which contributes to a vicious cycle of anxiety about insomnia that makes it more difficult to sleep. Approaches to treating insomnia may employ drugs that either inhibit the output of the ascending arousal system (*green* and *blue* in Fig. 31-2) or potentiate the output of the sleep-promoting system (*red* in Fig. 31-2). However, behavioral approaches (cognitive behavioral therapy [CBT] and sleep hygiene) that may reduce forebrain limbic activity at bedtime are often the best long-term treatment.

Sleep is also regulated by a strong *circadian* timing signal, driven by the suprachiasmatic nuclei (SCN) of the hypothalamus, as described below. The SCN sends outputs to key sites in the hypothalamus, which impose 24-h rhythms on a wide range of behaviors and body systems, including the wake-sleep cycle.

■ PHYSIOLOGY OF CIRCADIAN RHYTHMICITY

The wake-sleep cycle is the most evident of many 24-h rhythms in humans. Prominent daily variations also occur in endocrine, thermoregulatory, cardiac, pulmonary, renal, immune, gastrointestinal, and neurobehavioral functions. In evaluating daily rhythms in humans, it is important to distinguish between diurnal components passively evoked by periodic environmental or behavioral changes (e.g., the increase in blood pressure and heart rate that occurs upon assumption of the upright posture) and circadian rhythms actively driven by an endogenous oscillatory process (e.g., the circadian variations in adrenal cortisol and pineal melatonin secretion that persist across a variety of environmental and behavioral conditions).

At the cellular level, endogenous circadian rhythmicity is driven by self-sustaining feedback loops. While it is now recognized that most cells in the body have circadian clocks that regulate diverse physiologic processes, these clocks in different tissues, or even in different cells in the same tissue, when placed in isolation in a tissue explant are unable to maintain the long-term synchronization with each other that is required to produce useful 24-h rhythms aligned with the external light-dark cycle. The only tissue that maintains this rhythm in vitro is the SCN, whose neurons are interconnected with one another in such a way as to produce a near-24-h synchronous rhythm of neural activity even in prolonged slice culture. SCN neurons are located just above the optic chiasm in the hypothalamus, from which they receive visual input to synchronize them with the external world, and they have outputs to transmit that signal to the rest of the body. Bilateral destruction of the SCN results in a loss of most endogenous circadian rhythms including wake-sleep behavior and rhythms in endocrine and metabolic systems. The genetically determined period of this endogenous neural oscillator, which averages ~24.15 h in humans, is normally synchronized to the 24-h period of the environmental light-dark cycle through direct input from intrinsically photosensitive ganglion cells in the retina to the SCN. Humans are exquisitely sensitive to the resetting effects of light, particularly the shorter wavelengths (~460–500 nm) in the blue part of the visible spectrum. Small differences in circadian period contribute to variations in diurnal preference. Changes in homeostatic sleep regulation may underlie age-related changes in sleep-wake timing.

The timing and internal architecture of sleep are directly coupled to the output of the endogenous circadian pacemaker. Paradoxically, the endogenous circadian rhythm for wake propensity peaks just before the habitual bedtime, whereas that of sleep propensity peaks near the habitual wake time. These rhythms are thus timed to oppose the rise of sleep tendency throughout the usual waking day and the decline of sleep propensity during the habitual sleep episode, respectively, thus promoting consolidated sleep and wakefulness. Misalignment of the endogenous circadian pacemaker with the desired wake-sleep cycle can, therefore, induce insomnia, decrease alertness, and impair performance, posing health problems for night-shift workers and airline travelers.

BEHAVIORAL AND PHYSIOLOGIC CORRELATES OF SLEEP STATES AND STAGES

Polysomnographic staging of sleep correlates with behavioral changes during specific states and stages. During the transitional state (stage N1) between wakefulness and deeper sleep, individuals may respond to faint auditory or visual signals. Formation of short-term memories is inhibited at the onset of NREM stage N1 sleep, which may explain why individuals aroused from that transitional sleep stage frequently lack situational awareness. After sleep deprivation, such transitions may intrude upon behavioral wakefulness notwithstanding attempts to remain continuously awake (for example, see "Shift-Work Disorder," below).

Subjects awakened from REM sleep recall vivid dream imagery >80% of the time, especially later in the night. Less vivid imagery may also be reported after NREM sleep interruptions. Certain disorders may occur during specific sleep stages and are described below under "Parasomnias." These include sleepwalking, night terrors, and enuresis (bed wetting), which occur most commonly in children during deep (N3) NREM sleep, and REM sleep behavior disorder, which occurs mainly among older men who fail to maintain full paralysis during REM sleep, and often call out, thrash around, or even act out fragments of dreams.

All major physiologic systems are influenced by sleep. Blood pressure and heart rate decrease during NREM sleep, particularly during N3 sleep. During REM sleep, bursts of eye movements are associated with large variations in both blood pressure and heart rate mediated by the autonomic nervous system. Cardiac dysrhythmias may occur selectively during REM sleep. Respiratory function also changes. In comparison to relaxed wakefulness, respiratory rate becomes slower but more regular during NREM sleep (especially N3 sleep) and becomes irregular during bursts of eye movements in REM sleep. Decreases in minute ventilation during NREM sleep are out of proportion to the decrease in metabolic rate, resulting in a slightly higher P_{CO_2}.

Within the brain itself, neurotransmission is supported by ion gradients across the cell membranes of neurons and astrocytes. These ion flows are accompanied by increases in intracellular volume, so that during wake, there is very little extracellular space in the brain. During sleep, intracellular volume is reduced, resulting in increased extracellular space, which has higher calcium and lower potassium concentrations, supporting hyperpolarization and reduced firing of neurons. This expansion of the extracellular space during sleep increases diffusion of substances that accumulate extracellularly, like β-amyloid peptide, enhancing their clearance from the brain via cerebrospinal fluid (CSF) flow. Recent evidence suggests that lack of adequate sleep may contribute to extracellular accumulation of β-amyloid peptide, a key step in the pathogenesis of Alzheimer's disease.

Endocrine function also varies with sleep. N3 sleep is associated with secretion of growth hormone in men, while sleep in general is associated with augmented secretion of prolactin in both men and women. Sleep has a complex effect on the secretion of luteinizing hormone (LH): during puberty, sleep is associated with increased LH secretion, whereas sleep in postpubertal women inhibits LH secretion in the early follicular phase of the menstrual cycle. Sleep onset (and probably N3 sleep) is associated with inhibition of thyroid-stimulating hormone and of the adrenocorticotropic hormone–cortisol axis, an effect that is superimposed on the prominent circadian rhythms in the two systems.

The pineal hormone melatonin is secreted predominantly at night in both day- and night-active species, reflecting the direct modulation of pineal activity by the SCN via the sympathetic nervous system, which innervates the pineal gland. Melatonin secretion does not require sleep, but melatonin secretion is inhibited by ambient light, an effect mediated by the neural connection from the retina to the pineal gland via the SCN. In humans, sleep efficiency is highest when sleep coincides with endogenous melatonin secretion. When endogenous melatonin levels are low, such as during the biological day or at the desired bedtime in people with delayed sleep-wake phase disorder (DSWPD), administration of exogenous melatonin can hasten sleep onset and increase sleep efficiency, but it does not increase sleep efficiency if administered when endogenous melatonin levels are elevated. This may explain why melatonin is often ineffective in the treatment of patients with primary insomnia. On the other hand, patients with sympathetic denervation of the pineal gland, such as occurs in cervical spinal cord injury or in patients with Parkinson's disease, often have low melatonin levels, and administration of melatonin (3 mg 30 min before bedtime) may help them sleep.

Sleep is accompanied by alterations of thermoregulatory function. NREM sleep is associated with an increase in the firing of warm-responsive neurons in the preoptic area and a fall in body temperature; conversely, skin warming without increasing core body temperature has been found to increase NREM sleep. REM sleep is associated with reduced thermoregulatory responsiveness.

DISORDERS OF SLEEP AND WAKEFULNESS

APPROACH TO THE PATIENT

Sleep Disorders

Patients may seek help from a physician because of: (1) sleepiness or tiredness during the day; (2) difficulty initiating or maintaining sleep at night (insomnia); or (3) unusual behaviors during sleep itself (parasomnias).

Obtaining a careful history is essential. In particular, the duration, severity, and consistency of the symptoms are important, along with the patient's estimate of the consequences of the sleep disorder on waking function. Information from a bed partner or family member is often helpful because some patients may be unaware of symptoms such as heavy snoring or may underreport symptoms such as falling asleep at work or while driving. Physicians should inquire about when the patient typically goes to bed, when they fall asleep and wake up, whether they awaken during sleep, whether they feel rested in the morning, and whether they nap during the day. Depending on the primary complaint, it may be useful to ask about snoring, witnessed apneas, restless sensations in the legs, movements during sleep, depression, anxiety, and behaviors around the sleep episode. The physical examination may provide evidence of a small airway, large tonsils, or a neurologic or medical disorder that contributes to the main complaint.

It is important to remember that, rarely, seizures may occur exclusively during sleep, mimicking a primary sleep disorder; such sleep-related seizures typically occur during episodes of NREM sleep and may take the form of generalized tonic-clonic movements (sometimes with urinary incontinence or tongue biting) or stereotyped movements in partial complex epilepsy (**Chap. 418**).

It is often helpful for the patient to complete a daily sleep log for 1–2 weeks to define the timing and amounts of sleep. When relevant, the log can also include information on levels of alertness, work times, and drug and alcohol use, including caffeine and hypnotics.

Polysomnography is necessary for the diagnosis of several disorders such as sleep apnea, narcolepsy, and periodic limb movement disorder (PLMD). A conventional polysomnogram performed in a clinical sleep laboratory allows measurement of sleep stages, respiratory effort and airflow, oxygen saturation, limb movements, heart rhythm, and additional parameters. A home sleep test usually focuses on just respiratory measures and is helpful in patients with a moderate to high likelihood of having obstructive sleep apnea. The multiple sleep latency test (MSLT) is used to measure a patient's propensity to sleep during the day and can provide crucial evidence for diagnosing narcolepsy and some other causes of sleepiness. The maintenance of wakefulness test is used to measure a patient's ability to sustain wakefulness during the daytime and can provide important evidence for evaluating the efficacy of therapies for improving sleepiness in conditions such as narcolepsy and obstructive sleep apnea.

EVALUATION OF DAYTIME SLEEPINESS

Up to 25% of the adult population has persistent daytime sleepiness that impairs an individual's ability to perform optimally in school, at work, while driving, and in other conditions that require alertness. Sleepy students often have trouble staying alert and performing well in school, and sleepy adults struggle to stay awake and focused on their work. More than half of Americans have fallen asleep while driving. An estimated 1.2 million motor vehicle crashes per year are due to drowsy drivers, causing about 20% of all serious crash injuries and deaths. One need not fall asleep to have a motor vehicle crash, as the inattention and slowed responses of drowsy drivers are major contributors. Twenty-four hours of continuous wakefulness impairs reaction time as much as a blood alcohol concentration of 0.10 g/dL (which is legally drunk in all 50 states).

Identifying and quantifying sleepiness can be challenging. First, patients may describe themselves as "sleepy," "fatigued," or "tired," and the meanings of these words may differ between patients. For clinical purposes, it is best to use the term "sleepiness" to describe a propensity to fall asleep, whereas "fatigue" is best used to describe a feeling of low physical or mental energy but without a tendency to actually sleep. Sleepiness is usually most evident when the patient is sedentary, whereas fatigue may interfere with more active pursuits. Sleepiness generally occurs with disorders that reduce the quality or quantity of sleep or that interfere with the neural mechanisms of arousal, whereas fatigue is more common in inflammatory disorders such as cancer, multiple sclerosis (**Chap. 444**), fibromyalgia (**Chap. 373**), chronic fatigue syndrome (**Chap. 450**), or endocrine deficiencies such as hypothyroidism (**Chap. 383**) or Addison's disease (**Chap. 386**). Second, sleepiness can affect judgment in a manner analogous to ethanol, such that patients may have limited insight into the condition and the extent of their functional impairment. Finally, patients may be reluctant to admit that sleepiness is a problem because they may have become unfamiliar with feeling fully alert, and because sleepiness is sometimes viewed pejoratively as reflecting poor motivation or bad sleep habits.

Table 31-1 outlines the diagnostic and therapeutic approach to the patient with a complaint of excessive daytime sleepiness.

To determine the extent and impact of sleepiness on daytime function, it is helpful to ask patients about the occurrence of sleep episodes during normal waking hours, both intentional and unintentional. Specific areas to be addressed include the occurrence of inadvertent sleep episodes while driving or in other safety-related settings, sleepiness while at work or school (and its impact on performance), and the effect of sleepiness on social and family life. Standardized questionnaires such as the Epworth Sleepiness Scale are often used clinically to measure sleepiness.

TABLE 31-1 Evaluation of the Patient with Excessive Daytime Sleepiness

FINDINGS ON HISTORY AND PHYSICAL EXAMINATION	DIAGNOSTIC EVALUATION	DIAGNOSIS	THERAPY
Difficulty waking in the morning, rebound sleep on weekends and vacations with improvement in sleepiness	Sleep log	Insufficient sleep	Sleep education and behavioral modification to increase amount of sleep
Obesity, snoring, hypertension	Polysomnogram or home sleep test	Obstructive sleep apnea (**Chap. 297**)	Continuous positive airway pressure; upper airway surgery (e.g., uvulopalatopharyngoplasty); dental appliance; weight loss
Cataplexy, hypnagogic hallucinations, sleep paralysis	Polysomnogram and multiple sleep latency test	Narcolepsy	Stimulants (e.g., modafinil, methylphenidate); REM sleep-suppressing antidepressants (e.g., venlafaxine); pitolisant; solriamfetol; sodium oxybate
Restless legs, kicking movements during sleep	Assessment for predisposing medical conditions (e.g., iron deficiency or renal failure)	Restless legs syndrome with or without periodic limb movements	Treatment of predisposing condition; dopamine agonists (e.g., pramipexole, ropinirole); gabapentin; pregabalin; opiates
Sedating medications, stimulant withdrawal, head trauma, systemic inflammation, Parkinson's disease and other neurodegenerative disorders, hypothyroidism, encephalopathy	Thorough medical history and examination including detailed neurologic examination	Sleepiness due to a drug or medical condition	Change medications, treat underlying condition, consider stimulants

Eliciting a history of daytime sleepiness is usually adequate, but objective quantification is sometimes necessary. The MSLT measures a patient's propensity to sleep under quiet conditions. An overnight polysomnogram should precede the MSLT to establish that the patient has had an adequate amount of good-quality nighttime sleep. The MSLT consists of five 20-min nap opportunities every 2 h across the day. The patient is instructed to try to fall asleep, and the major endpoints are the average latency to sleep and the occurrence of REM sleep during the naps. An average sleep latency across the naps of <8 min is considered objective evidence of excessive daytime sleepiness. REM sleep normally occurs only during nighttime sleep, and the occurrence of REM sleep in two or more of the MSLT daytime naps provides support for the diagnosis of narcolepsy.

For the safety of the individual and the general public, physicians have a responsibility to help manage issues around driving in patients with sleepiness. Legal reporting requirements vary between states and countries, but at a minimum, physicians should inform sleepy patients about their increased risk of having an accident and advise such patients not to drive a motor vehicle until the sleepiness has been treated effectively. This discussion is especially important for commercial drivers, and it should be documented in the patient's medical record.

INSUFFICIENT SLEEP

Insufficient sleep is probably the most common cause of excessive daytime sleepiness. The average adult needs 7.5–8 h of sleep, but on weeknights the average U.S. adult gets only 6.75 h of sleep. Only 30% of the U.S. adult population reports consistently obtaining sufficient sleep. Insufficient sleep is especially common among shift workers, individuals working multiple jobs, and people in lower socioeconomic groups. Most teenagers need ≥9 h of sleep, but many fail to get enough sleep because of circadian phase delay, plus social pressures to stay up late coupled with early school start times. Late evening light exposure, television viewing, video-gaming, social media, texting, and smartphone use often delay bedtimes, despite the fixed early wake times required for work or school. As is typical with any disorder that causes sleepiness, individuals with chronically insufficient sleep may feel inattentive, irritable, unmotivated, and depressed, and have difficulty with school, work, and driving. Individuals differ in their optimal amount of sleep, and it can be helpful to ask how much sleep the patient obtains on a quiet vacation when he or she can sleep without restrictions. Some patients may think that a short amount of sleep is normal or advantageous, and they may not appreciate their biological need for more sleep, especially if coffee and other stimulants mask the sleepiness. A 2-week sleep log documenting the timing of sleep and daily level of alertness is diagnostically useful and provides helpful feedback for the patient. Extending sleep to the optimal amount on a regular basis can resolve the sleepiness and other symptoms. As with any lifestyle change, extending sleep requires commitment and adjustments, but the improvements in daytime alertness make this change worthwhile.

SLEEP APNEA SYNDROMES

Respiratory dysfunction during sleep is a common, serious cause of excessive daytime sleepiness as well as of disturbed nocturnal sleep. At least 24% of middle-aged men and 9% of middle-aged women in the United States have a reduction or cessation of breathing dozens or more times each night during sleep, with 9% of men and 4% of women doing so more than a hundred times per night. These episodes may be due to an occlusion of the airway (*obstructive sleep apnea*), absence of respiratory effort (*central sleep apnea*), or a combination of these factors. Failure to recognize and treat these conditions appropriately may reduce daytime alertness and increase the risk of sleep-related motor vehicle crashes, depression, hypertension, myocardial infarction, diabetes, stroke, and mortality. Sleep apnea is particularly prevalent in overweight men and in the elderly, yet it is estimated to go undiagnosed in most affected individuals. This is unfortunate because several effective treatments are available. **Readers are referred to Chap. 297 for a comprehensive review of the diagnosis and treatment of patients with sleep apnea.**

NARCOLEPSY

Narcolepsy is characterized by difficulty sustaining wakefulness, poor regulation of REM sleep, and disturbed nocturnal sleep. All patients with narcolepsy have excessive daytime sleepiness. This sleepiness is usually moderate to severe, and in contrast to patients with disrupted sleep (e.g., sleep apnea), people with narcolepsy usually feel well rested upon awakening and then feel tired throughout much of the day. They may fall asleep at inappropriate times, but then feel refreshed again after a nap. In addition, they often experience symptoms related to an intrusion of REM sleep characteristics into wakefulness. REM sleep is characterized by dreaming and muscle paralysis, and people with narcolepsy can have: (1) sudden muscle weakness without a loss of consciousness, which is usually triggered by strong emotions (cataplexy; **Video 31-1**); (2) dream-like hallucinations at sleep onset (hypnagogic hallucinations) or upon awakening (hypnopompic hallucinations); and (3) muscle paralysis upon awakening (sleep paralysis). With severe cataplexy, an individual may be laughing at a joke and then suddenly collapse to the ground, immobile but awake for 1–2 min. With milder episodes, patients may have partial weakness of the face or neck. Narcolepsy is one of the more common causes of chronic sleepiness and affects about 1 in 2000 people in the United States. Narcolepsy typically begins between age 10 and 20; once established, the disease persists for life.

Narcolepsy is caused by loss of the hypothalamic neurons that produce the orexin neuropeptides (also known as hypocretins). Research in mice and dogs first demonstrated that a loss of orexin signaling due to null mutations of either the orexin neuropeptides or one of the orexin receptors causes sleepiness and cataplexy nearly identical to that seen in people with narcolepsy. Although genetic mutations rarely cause human narcolepsy, researchers soon discovered that patients with narcolepsy with cataplexy (now called type 1 narcolepsy) have very low or undetectable levels of orexins in their CSF, and autopsy studies showed a nearly complete loss of the orexin-producing neurons in the hypothalamus. The orexins normally promote long episodes of wakefulness and suppress REM sleep, and thus loss of orexin signaling results in frequent intrusions of sleep during the usual waking episode, with REM sleep and fragments of REM sleep at any time of day (**Fig. 31-3**). Patients with narcolepsy but no cataplexy (type 2 narcolepsy) usually have normal orexin levels and may have other yet uncharacterized causes of their excessive daytime sleepiness.

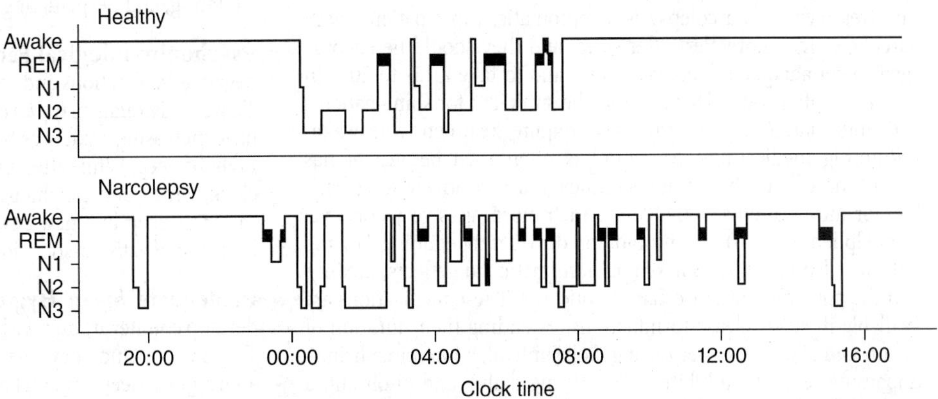

FIGURE 31-3 Polysomnographic recordings of a healthy individual and a patient with narcolepsy. The healthy individual has a long period or NREM sleep before entering REM sleep, but the individual with narcolepsy enters rapid eye movement (REM) sleep quickly at night and has moderately fragmented sleep. During the day, the healthy subject stays awake from 8:00 A.M. until midnight, but the patient with narcolepsy dozes off frequently, with many daytime naps that include REM sleep.

Extensive evidence suggests that an autoimmune process likely causes this selective loss of the orexin-producing neurons. Certain human leukocyte antigens (HLAs) can increase the risk of autoimmune disorders **(Chap. 350)**, and narcolepsy has the strongest known HLA association. HLA DQB1*06:02 is found in >90% of people with type 1 narcolepsy, whereas it occurs in only 12–25% of the general population. Researchers now hypothesize that in people with DQB1*06:02, an immune response against influenza, *Streptococcus*, or other infections may also damage the orexin-producing neurons through a process of molecular mimicry. This mechanism may account for the eight- to twelvefold increase in new cases of narcolepsy among children in Europe who received a particular brand of H1N1 influenza A vaccine (Pandemrix). In support of this hypothesis, people with type 1 narcolepsy have heightened T cell responses against orexin peptides.

On rare occasions, narcolepsy can occur with neurologic disorders such as tumors or strokes that directly damage the orexin-producing neurons in the hypothalamus or their projections.

Diagnosis Narcolepsy is most commonly diagnosed by the history of chronic sleepiness plus cataplexy or other symptoms. Many disorders can cause feelings of weakness, but with true cataplexy patients will describe definite functional weakness (e.g., slurred speech, dropping a cup, slumping into a chair) that has consistent emotional triggers such as laughing at a joke, happy surprise at unexpectedly seeing a friend, or intense anger. Cataplexy occurs in about half of all narcolepsy patients and is diagnostically very helpful because it occurs in almost no other disorder. In contrast, occasional hypnagogic hallucinations and sleep paralysis occur in about 20% of the general population, and these symptoms are not as diagnostically specific.

When narcolepsy is suspected, the diagnosis should be firmly established with a polysomnogram followed the next day by an MSLT. The polysomnogram helps rule out other possible causes of sleepiness such as sleep apnea and establishes that the patient had adequate sleep the night before, and the MSLT provides essential, objective evidence of sleepiness plus REM sleep dysregulation. Across the five naps of the MSLT, most patients with narcolepsy will fall asleep in <8 min on average, and they will have episodes of REM sleep in at least two of the naps. Abnormal regulation of REM sleep is also manifested by the appearance of REM sleep within 15 min of sleep onset at night, which is rare in healthy individuals sleeping at their habitual bedtime. Stimulants should be stopped 1 week before the MSLT and antidepressants should be stopped 3 weeks prior, because these medications can affect the MSLT. In addition, patients should be encouraged to obtain a fully adequate amount of sleep each night for the week prior to the test to eliminate any effects of insufficient sleep.

TREATMENT

Narcolepsy

The treatment of narcolepsy is symptomatic. Most patients with narcolepsy feel more alert after sleep, and they should be encouraged to get adequate sleep each night and to take a 15- to 20-min nap in the afternoon. This nap may be sufficient for some patients with mild narcolepsy, but most also require treatment with wake-promoting medications. Modafinil is often used because it has fewer side effects than amphetamines and a relatively long half-life; for most patients, 200–400 mg each morning is very effective. Methylphenidate (10–20 mg bid) or dextroamphetamine (10 mg bid) are also effective, but sympathomimetic side effects, anxiety, and the potential for abuse can be concerns. These medications are available in slow-release formulations, extending their duration of action and allowing easier dosing. Solriamfetol, a norepinephrine-dopamine reuptake inhibitor (75–150 mg daily), and pitolisant, a selective histamine 3 (H_3) receptor antagonist (8.9–35.6 mg daily), also improve sleepiness and have relatively few side effects. Sodium oxybate (gamma hydroxybutyrate), given at bedtime and 3–4 h later, is often very valuable in improving alertness, but it can produce excessive sedation, nausea, and confusion.

Cataplexy is usually much improved with antidepressants that increase noradrenergic or serotonergic tone because these neurotransmitters strongly suppress REM sleep and cataplexy. Venlafaxine (37.5–150 mg each morning) and fluoxetine (10–40 mg each morning) are often quite effective. The tricyclic antidepressants, such as protriptyline (10–40 mg/d) or clomipramine (25–50 mg/d) are potent suppressors of cataplexy, but their anticholinergic effects, including sedation and dry mouth, make them less attractive.[1] Sodium oxybate, twice each night, is also very helpful in reducing cataplexy.

[1]No antidepressant has been approved by the US Food and Drug Administration (FDA) for treating narcolepsy.

EVALUATION OF INSOMNIA

Insomnia is the complaint of poor sleep and usually presents as difficulty initiating or maintaining sleep. People with insomnia are dissatisfied with their sleep and feel that it impairs their ability to function well in work, school, and social situations. Affected individuals often experience fatigue, decreased mood, irritability, malaise, and cognitive impairment.

Chronic insomnia, lasting >3 months, occurs in about 10% of adults and is more common in women, older adults, people of lower socioeconomic status, and individuals with medical, psychiatric, and substance abuse disorders. Acute or short-term insomnia affects over 30% of adults and is often precipitated by stressful life events such as a major illness or loss, change of occupation, medications, and substance abuse. If the acute insomnia triggers maladaptive behaviors such as increased nocturnal light exposure, frequently checking the clock, or attempting to sleep more by napping, it can lead to chronic insomnia.

Most insomnia begins in adulthood, but many patients may be predisposed and report easily disturbed sleep predating the insomnia, suggesting that their sleep is lighter than usual. Clinical studies and animal models indicate that insomnia is associated with activation during sleep of brain areas normally active only during wakefulness. The polysomnogram is rarely used in the evaluation of insomnia, as it typically confirms the patient's subjective report of long latency to sleep and numerous awakenings but usually adds little new information. Many patients with insomnia have increased fast (beta) activity in the EEG during sleep; this fast activity is normally present only during wakefulness, which may explain why some patients report feeling awake for much of the night. The MSLT is rarely used in the evaluation of insomnia because, despite their feelings of low energy, most people with insomnia do not easily fall asleep during the day, and on the MSLT, their average sleep latencies are usually longer than normal.

Many factors can contribute to insomnia, and obtaining a careful history is essential so one can select therapies targeting the underlying factors. The assessment should focus on identifying predisposing, precipitating, and perpetuating factors.

Psychophysiological Factors Many patients with insomnia have negative expectations and conditioned arousal that interfere with sleep. These individuals may worry about their insomnia during the day and have increasing anxiety as bedtime approaches if they anticipate a poor night of sleep. While attempting to sleep, they may frequently check the clock, which only heightens anxiety and frustration. They may find it easier to sleep in a new environment rather than their bedroom, as it lacks the negative associations.

Inadequate Sleep Hygiene Patients with insomnia sometimes develop counterproductive behaviors that contribute to their insomnia. These can include daytime napping that reduces sleep drive at night; an irregular sleep-wake schedule that disrupts their circadian rhythms; use of wake-promoting substances (e.g., caffeine, tobacco) too close to bedtime; engaging in alerting or stressful activities close to bedtime (e.g., arguing with a partner, work-related emailing and texting while in bed, sleeping with a smartphone or tablet at the bedside); and routinely using the bedroom for activities other than sleep or sex (e.g., email, television, work), so the bedroom becomes associated with arousing or stressful feelings.

Psychiatric Conditions About 80% of patients with psychiatric disorders have sleep complaints, and about half of all chronic insomnia occurs in association with a psychiatric disorder. Depression is classically associated with early morning awakening, but it can also interfere with the onset and maintenance of sleep. Mania and hypomania can disrupt sleep and often are associated with substantial reductions in the total amount of sleep. Anxiety disorders can lead to racing thoughts and rumination that interfere with sleep and can be very problematic if the patient's mind becomes active midway through the night. Panic attacks can arise from sleep and need to be distinguished from other parasomnias. Insomnia is common in schizophrenia and other psychoses, often resulting in fragmented sleep, less deep NREM sleep, and sometimes reversal of the day-night sleep pattern.

Medications and Drugs of Abuse A wide variety of psychoactive drugs can interfere with sleep. Caffeine, which has a half-life of 6–9 h, can disrupt sleep for up to 8–14 h, depending on the dose, variations in metabolism, and an individual's caffeine sensitivity. Insomnia can also result from use of prescription medications too close to bedtime (e.g., antidepressants, stimulants, glucocorticoids, theophylline). Conversely, withdrawal of sedating medications such as alcohol, narcotics, or benzodiazepines can cause insomnia. Alcohol taken just before bed can shorten sleep latency, but it often produces rebound insomnia 2–3 h later as it wears off. This same problem with sleep maintenance can occur with short-acting medications such as alprazolam or zolpidem.

Medical Conditions A large number of medical conditions disrupt sleep. Pain from rheumatologic disorders or a painful neuropathy commonly disrupts sleep. Some patients may sleep poorly because of respiratory conditions such as asthma, chronic obstructive pulmonary disease, cystic fibrosis, congestive heart failure, or restrictive lung disease, and some of these disorders are worse at night due to circadian variations in airway resistance and postural changes in bed that can result in nocturnal dyspnea. Many women experience poor sleep with the hormonal changes of menopause. Gastroesophageal reflux is also a common cause of difficulty sleeping.

Neurologic Disorders Dementia (**Chap. 29**) is often associated with poor sleep, probably due to a variety of factors, including napping during the day, altered circadian rhythms, and perhaps a weakened output of the brain's sleep-promoting mechanisms. In fact, insomnia and nighttime wandering are some of the most common causes for institutionalization of patients with dementia, because they place a larger burden on caregivers. Conversely, in cognitively intact elderly men, fragmented sleep and poor sleep quality are associated with subsequent cognitive decline. Patients with Parkinson's disease may sleep poorly due to rigidity, dementia, and other factors. Fatal familial insomnia is a very rare neurodegenerative condition caused by mutations in the prion protein gene (**Chap. 438**), and although insomnia is a common early symptom, most patients present with other obvious neurologic signs such as dementia, myoclonus, dysarthria, or autonomic dysfunction.

TREATMENT

Insomnia

Treatment of insomnia improves quality of life and can promote long-term health. With improved sleep, patients often report less daytime fatigue, improved cognition, and more energy. Treating the insomnia can also improve comorbid disease. For example, management of insomnia at the time of diagnosis of major depression often improves the response to antidepressants and reduces the risk of relapse. Sleep loss can heighten the perception of pain, so a similar approach is warranted in acute and chronic pain management.

The treatment plan should target all putative contributing factors: establish good sleep hygiene, treat medical disorders, use behavioral therapies for anxiety and negative conditioning, and use pharmacotherapy and/or psychotherapy for psychiatric disorders. Behavioral therapies should be the first-line treatment, followed by judicious use of sleep-promoting medications if needed.

TREATMENT OF MEDICAL AND PSYCHIATRIC DISEASE

If the history suggests that a medical or psychiatric disease contributes to the insomnia, then it should be addressed by, for example, treating the pain or depression, improving breathing, and switching or adjusting the timing of medications.

IMPROVE SLEEP HYGIENE

Attention should be paid to improving sleep hygiene and avoiding counterproductive, arousing behaviors before bedtime. Patients should establish a regular bedtime and wake time, even on weekends, to help synchronize their circadian rhythms and sleep patterns. The amount of time allocated for sleep should not be more than their actual total amount of sleep. In the 30 min before bedtime, patients should establish a relaxing "wind-down" routine that can include a warm bath, listening to music, meditation, or other relaxation techniques. The bedroom should be off-limits to computers, televisions, radios, smartphones, videogames, and tablets. If an e-reader is used, the light should be adjusted for evening use (dimmer and reduced blue light) if possible, because light itself, especially in the blue spectrum, suppresses melatonin secretion and is arousing. Once in bed, patients should try to avoid thinking about anything stressful or arousing such as problems with relationships or work. If they cannot fall asleep within 20 min, it often helps to get out of bed and read or listen to relaxing music in dim light as a form of distraction from any anxiety, but artificial light, including light from a television, cell phone, or computer, should be avoided.

Table 31-2 outlines some of the key aspects of good sleep hygiene to improve insomnia.

COGNITIVE BEHAVIORAL THERAPY

Cognitive behavioral therapy (CBT) uses a combination of the techniques above plus additional methods to improve insomnia. A trained therapist may use cognitive psychology techniques to reduce excessive worrying about sleep and to reframe faulty beliefs about the insomnia and its daytime consequences. The therapist may also teach the patient relaxation techniques, such as progressive muscle relaxation or meditation, to reduce autonomic arousal, intrusive thoughts, and anxiety.

MEDICATIONS FOR INSOMNIA

If insomnia persists after treatment of these contributing factors, pharmacotherapy is often used on a nightly or intermittent basis. A variety of sedatives can improve sleep.

Antihistamines, such as diphenhydramine, are the primary active ingredient in most over-the-counter sleep aids. These may be of

TABLE 31-2 Methods to Improve Sleep Hygiene in Insomnia Patients

HELPFUL BEHAVIORS	BEHAVIORS TO AVOID
Use the bed only for sleep and sex • If you cannot sleep within 20 min, get out of bed and read or do other relaxing activities in dim light before returning to bed	Avoid behaviors that interfere with sleep physiology, including: • Napping, especially after 3:00 PM • Attempting to sleep too early • Caffeine after lunchtime
Make quality sleep a priority • Go to bed and get up at the same time each day • Ensure a restful environment (comfortable bed, bedroom quiet and dark)	In the 2–3 h before bedtime, avoid: • Heavy eating • Smoking or alcohol • Vigorous exercise
Develop a consistent bedtime routine. For example: • Prepare for sleep with 20–30 min of relaxation (e.g., soft music, meditation, yoga, pleasant reading) • Take a warm bath	When trying to fall asleep, avoid: • Solving problems • Thinking about life issues • Reviewing events of the day

benefit when used intermittently but can produce tolerance and anticholinergic side effects such as dry mouth and constipation, which limit their use, particularly in the elderly.

Benzodiazepine receptor agonists (BzRAs) are an effective and well-tolerated class of medications for insomnia. BzRAs bind to the $GABA_A$ receptor and potentiate the postsynaptic response to GABA. $GABA_A$ receptors are found throughout the brain, and BzRAs may globally reduce neural activity and enhance the activity of specific sleep-promoting GABAergic pathways. Classic BzRAs include lorazepam, triazolam, and clonazepam, whereas newer agents such as zolpidem and zaleplon have more selective affinity for the α_1 subunit of the $GABA_A$ receptor.

Specific BzRAs are often chosen based on the desired duration of action. The most commonly prescribed agents in this family are zaleplon (5–20 mg), with a half-life of 1–2 h; zolpidem (5–10 mg) and triazolam (0.125–0.25 mg), with half-lives of 2–4 h; eszopiclone (1–3 mg), with a half-life of 5–8 h; and temazepam (15–30 mg), with a half-life of 8–20 h. Generally, side effects are minimal when the dose is kept low and the serum concentration is minimized during the waking hours (by using the shortest-acting effective agent). For chronic insomnia, intermittent use is recommended, unless the consequences of untreated insomnia outweigh concerns regarding chronic use.

The heterocyclic antidepressants (trazodone, amitriptyline,[2] and doxepin) are the most commonly prescribed alternatives to BzRAs due to their lack of abuse potential and low cost. Trazodone (25–100 mg) is used more commonly than the tricyclic antidepressants, because it has a much shorter half-life (5–9 h) and less anticholinergic activity.

The orexin receptor antagonists suvorexant (10–20 mg) and lemborexant (5–10 mg) can also improve insomnia by blocking the wake-promoting effects of the orexin neuropeptides. These have long half-lives and can produce morning sedation, and as they reduce orexin signaling, they can rarely produce hypnagogic hallucinations and sleep paralysis (see narcolepsy section above).

Medications for insomnia are now among the most commonly prescribed medications, but they should be used cautiously. All sedatives increase the risk of injurious falls and confusion in the elderly, and therefore if needed these medications should be used at the lowest effective dose. Morning sedation can interfere with driving and judgment, and when selecting a medication, one should consider the duration of action. Benzodiazepines carry a risk of addiction and abuse, especially in patients with a history of alcohol or sedative abuse. In patients with depression, all sedatives can worsen the depression. Like alcohol, some sleep-promoting medications can worsen sleep apnea. Sedatives can also produce complex behaviors during sleep, such as sleepwalking and sleep eating, especially at higher doses.

[2]Trazodone and amitriptyline have not been approved by the FDA for treating insomnia.

RESTLESS LEGS SYNDROME

Patients with restless legs syndrome (RLS) report an irresistible urge to move the legs. Many patients report a creepy-crawly or unpleasant deep ache within the thighs or calves, and those with more severe RLS may have discomfort in the arms as well. For most patients with RLS, these dysesthesias and restlessness are much worse in the evening and first half of the night. The symptoms appear with inactivity and can make sitting still in an airplane or when watching a movie a miserable experience. The sensations are temporarily relieved by movement, stretching, or massage. This nocturnal discomfort usually interferes with sleep, and patients may report daytime sleepiness as a consequence. RLS is very common, affecting 5–10% of adults, and is more common in women and older adults.

A variety of factors can cause RLS. Iron deficiency is the most common treatable cause, and iron replacement should be considered if the ferritin level is <75 ng/mL. RLS can also occur with peripheral neuropathies and uremia and can be worsened by pregnancy, caffeine, alcohol, antidepressants, lithium, neuroleptics, and antihistamines. Genetic factors contribute to RLS, and polymorphisms in a variety of genes (*BTBD9, MEIS1, MAP2K5/LBXCOR*, and *PTPRD*) have been linked to RLS, although as yet, the mechanism through which they cause RLS remains unknown. Roughly one-third of patients (particularly those with an early age of onset) have multiple affected family members.

RLS is treated by addressing the underlying cause such as iron deficiency if present. Otherwise, treatment is symptomatic, and dopamine agonists or alpha-2-delta calcium channel ligands are used most frequently. Agonists of dopamine $D_{2/3}$ receptors such as pramipexole (0.25–0.5 mg q7PM) or ropinirole (0.5–4 mg q7PM) are usually quite effective, but about 25% of patients taking dopamine agonists develop augmentation, a worsening of RLS such that symptoms begin earlier in the day and can spread to other body regions. Other possible side effects of dopamine agonists include nausea, morning sedation, and increases in rewarding behaviors such as sex and gambling. Alpha-2-delta calcium channel ligands such as gabapentin (300–600 mg q7PM) and pregabalin (150–450 mg q7PM) can also be quite effective; these are less likely to cause augmentation, and they can be especially helpful in patients with concomitant pain, neuropathy, or anxiety. Opioids and benzodiazepines may also be of therapeutic value. Most patients with restless legs also experience PLMD, although the reverse is not the case.

PERIODIC LIMB MOVEMENT DISORDER

PLMD involves rhythmic twitches of the legs that disrupt sleep. The movements resemble a triple flexion reflex with extensions of the great toe and dorsiflexion of the foot for 0.5–5.0 s, which recur every 20–40 s during NREM sleep, in episodes lasting from minutes to hours. PLMD is diagnosed by a polysomnogram that includes recordings of the anterior tibialis and sometimes other muscles. The EEG shows that the movements of PLMD frequently cause brief arousals that disrupt sleep and can cause insomnia and daytime sleepiness. PLMD can be caused by the same factors that cause RLS (see above), and the frequency of leg movements improves with the same medications used for RLS, including dopamine agonists. Genetic studies identified polymorphisms associated with both RLS and PLMD, suggesting that they may have a common pathophysiology.

PARASOMNIAS

Parasomnias are abnormal behaviors or experiences that arise from or occur during sleep. A variety of parasomnias can occur during NREM sleep, from brief confusional arousals to sleepwalking and night terrors. The presenting complaint is usually related to the behavior itself, but the parasomnias can disturb sleep continuity or lead to mild impairments in daytime alertness. Two main parasomnias occur in REM sleep: REM sleep behavior disorder (RBD) and nightmares.

Sleepwalking (Somnambulism) Patients affected by this disorder carry out automatic motor activities that range from simple to complex. Individuals may walk, urinate inappropriately, eat, exit the house, or drive a car with minimal awareness. It may be difficult to arouse the patient to wakefulness, and some individuals may respond to attempted awakening with agitation or violence. In general, it is safest to lead the patient back to bed, at which point he or she will often fall back asleep. Sleepwalking arises from NREM stage N3 sleep, usually in the first few hours of the night, and the EEG initially shows the slow cortical activity of deep NREM sleep even when the patient is moving about. Sleepwalking is most common in children and adolescents, when deep NREM sleep is most abundant. About 15% of children have occasional sleepwalking, and it persists in about 1% of adults. Episodes are usually isolated but may be recurrent in 1–6% of patients. The cause is unknown, although it has a familial basis in roughly one-third of cases. Sleepwalking can be worsened by stress, alcohol, and insufficient sleep, which subsequently causes an increase in deep NREM sleep. These should be addressed if present. Small studies have shown some efficacy of antidepressants and benzodiazepines;

relaxation techniques and hypnosis can also be helpful. Patients and their families should improve home safety (e.g., replace glass doors, remove low tables to avoid tripping) to minimize the chance of injury if sleepwalking occurs.

Sleep Terrors This disorder occurs primarily in young children during the first few hours of sleep during NREM stage N3 sleep. The child often sits up during sleep and screams, exhibiting autonomic arousal with sweating, tachycardia, large pupils, and hyperventilation. The individual may be difficult to arouse and rarely recalls the episode on awakening in the morning. Treatment usually consists of reassuring parents that the condition is self-limited and benign, and like sleepwalking, it may improve by avoiding insufficient sleep.

Sleep Enuresis Bedwetting, like sleepwalking and night terrors, is another parasomnia that occurs during sleep in the young. Before age 5 or 6 years, nocturnal enuresis should be considered a normal feature of development. The condition usually improves spontaneously by puberty, persists in 1–3% of adolescents, and is rare in adulthood. Treatment consists of bladder training exercises and behavioral therapy. Symptomatic pharmacotherapy is usually accomplished in adults with desmopressin (0.2 mg qhs), oxybutynin chloride (5 mg qhs), or imipramine (10–25 mg qhs). Important causes of nocturnal enuresis in patients who were previously continent for 6–12 months include urinary tract infections or malformations, cauda equina lesions, emotional disturbances, epilepsy, sleep apnea, and certain medications.

Sleep Bruxism Bruxism is an involuntary, forceful grinding of teeth during sleep that affects 10–20% of the population. The patient is usually unaware of the problem. The typical age of onset is 17–20 years, and spontaneous remission usually occurs by age 40. In many cases, the diagnosis is made during dental examination, damage is minor, and no treatment is indicated. In more severe cases, treatment with a mouth guard is necessary to prevent tooth injury. Stress management, benzodiazepines, and biofeedback can be useful when bruxism is a manifestation of psychological stress.

REM Sleep Behavior Disorder (RBD) RBD (**Video 31-2**) is distinct from other parasomnias in that it occurs during REM sleep. The patient or the bed partner usually reports agitated or violent behavior during sleep, and upon awakening, the patient can often report a dream that matches the accompanying movements. During normal REM sleep, nearly all nonrespiratory skeletal muscles are paralyzed, but in patients with RBD, dramatic limb movements such as punching or kicking lasting seconds to minutes occur during REM sleep, and it is not uncommon for the patient or the bed partner to be injured.

The prevalence of RBD increases with age, afflicting about 2% of adults aged >70, and is about twice as common in men. Within 12 years of disease onset, half of RBD patients develop a synucleinopathy such as Parkinson's disease (**Chap. 435**) or dementia with Lewy bodies (**Chap. 434**), or occasionally multiple system atrophy (**Chap. 440**), and over 90% develop a synucleinopathy by 25 years. RBD can occur in patients taking antidepressants, and in some, these medications may unmask this early indicator of neurodegeneration. Synucleinopathies probably cause neuronal loss in brainstem regions that regulate muscle paralysis during REM sleep, and loss of these neurons permits movements to break through during REM sleep. RBD also occurs in about 30% of patients with narcolepsy, but the underlying cause is probably different, as they seem to be at no increased risk of a neurodegenerative disorder.

Many patients with RBD have sustained improvement with clonazepam (0.5–2.0 mg qhs).[3] Melatonin at doses up to 9 mg nightly may also prevent attacks.

■ CIRCADIAN RHYTHM SLEEP DISORDERS

A subset of patients presenting with either insomnia or hypersomnia may have a disorder of sleep *timing* rather than sleep *generation*. Disorders of sleep timing can be either organic (i.e., due to an abnormality of circadian pacemaker[s]) or environmental/behavioral (i.e., due to a disruption of environmental synchronizers). Effective therapies aim to entrain the circadian rhythm of sleep propensity to the appropriate behavioral phase.

Delayed Sleep-Wake Phase Disorder DSWPD is characterized by: (1) sleep onset and wake times persistently later than desired; (2) actual sleep times at nearly the same clock hours daily; and (3) if conducted at the habitual delayed sleep time, essentially normal sleep on polysomnography (except for delayed sleep onset). About half of patients with DSWPD exhibit an abnormally delayed endogenous circadian phase, which can be assessed by measuring the onset of secretion of melatonin in either the blood or saliva; this is best done in a dimly lit environment as light suppresses melatonin secretion. Dim-light melatonin onset (DLMO) in DSWPD patients occurs later in the evening than normal, which is about 8:00–9:00 P.M. (i.e., about 1–2 h before habitual bedtime). Patients tend to be young adults. The delayed circadian phase could be due to: (1) an abnormally long, genetically determined intrinsic period of the endogenous circadian pacemaker; (2) reduced phase-advancing capacity of the pacemaker; (3) slower buildup of homeostatic sleep drive during wakefulness; or (4) an irregular prior sleep-wake schedule, characterized by frequent nights when the patient chooses to remain awake while exposed to artificial light well past midnight (for personal, social, school, or work reasons). In most cases, it is difficult to distinguish among these factors, as patients with either a behaviorally induced or biologically driven circadian phase delay may both exhibit a similar circadian phase delay in DLMO, and both factors make it difficult to fall asleep at the desired hour. Late onset of dim-light melatonin secretion can help distinguish DSWPD from other forms of sleep-onset insomnia. DSWPD is a chronic condition that can persist for years and may not respond to attempts to reestablish normal bedtime hours. Treatment methods involving phototherapy with blue-enriched light during the morning hours and/or melatonin administration in the evening hours show promise in these patients, although the relapse rate is high.

Advanced Sleep-Wake Phase Disorder Advanced sleep-wake phase disorder (ASWPD) is the converse of DSWPD. Most commonly, this syndrome occurs in older people, 15% of whom report that they cannot sleep past 5:00 A.M., with twice that number complaining that they wake up too early at least several times per week. Patients with ASWPD are sleepy during the evening hours, even in social settings. Sleep-wake timing in ASWPD patients can interfere with a normal social life. Patients with this circadian rhythm sleep disorder can be distinguished from those who have early wakening due to insomnia because ASWPD patients show early onset of dim-light melatonin secretion.

In addition to age-related ASWPD, an early-onset familial variant of this condition has also been reported. In two families in which ASWPD was inherited in an autosomal dominant pattern, the syndrome was due to missense mutations in a circadian clock component (in the casein kinase binding domain of *PER2* in one family, and in casein kinase I delta in the other) that shortens the circadian period. Patients with ASWPD may benefit from bright light and/or blue enriched phototherapy during the evening hours to reset the circadian pacemaker to a later hour.

Non-24-h Sleep-Wake Rhythm Disorder Non-24-h sleep-wake rhythm disorder (N24SWD) most commonly occurs when the primary synchronizing input (i.e., the light-dark cycle) from the environment to the circadian pacemaker is lost (as occurs in many blind people with no light perception), and the maximal phase-advancing capacity of the circadian pacemaker in response to nonphotic cues cannot accommodate the difference between the 24-h geophysical day and the intrinsic period of the patient's circadian pacemaker, resulting in loss of entrainment to the 24-h day. The sleep of most blind patients with N24SWD is restricted to the nighttime hours due to social or occupational demands. Despite this regular sleep-wake schedule, affected patients with N24SWD are nonetheless unable to maintain

[3]No medications have been approved by the FDA for the treatment of RBD.

a stable phase relationship between the output of the non-entrained circadian pacemaker and the 24-h day. Therefore, most blind patients present with intermittent bouts of insomnia. When the blind patient's endogenous circadian rhythms are out of phase with the local environment, nighttime insomnia coexists with excessive daytime sleepiness. Conversely, when the endogenous circadian rhythms of those same patients are in phase with the local environment, symptoms remit. The interval between symptomatic phases may last several weeks to several months in blind patients with N24SWD, depending on the period of the underlying nonentrained rhythm and the 24-h day. Nightly low-dose (0.5 mg) melatonin administration may improve sleep and, in some cases, induce synchronization of the circadian pacemaker. In sighted patients, N24SWD can be caused by self-selected exposure to artificial light that inadvertently entrains the circadian pacemaker to a >24-h schedule, and these individuals present with an incremental pattern of successive delays in sleep timing, progressing in and out of phase with local time—a clinical presentation that is seldom seen in blind patients with N24SWD.

Shift-Work Disorder More than 7 million workers in the United States regularly work at night, either on a permanent or rotating schedule. Many more begin the commute to work or school between 4:00 A.M. and 7:00 A.M., requiring them to commute and then work during a time of day that they would otherwise be asleep. In addition, each week, millions of "day" workers and students elect to remain awake at night or awaken very early in the morning to work or study to meet work or school deadlines, drive long distances, compete in sporting events, or participate in recreational activities. Such schedules can result in both sleep loss and misalignment of circadian rhythms with respect to the sleep-wake cycle.

The circadian timing system usually fails to adapt successfully to the inverted schedules required by overnight work or the phase advance required by early morning (4:00 A.M. to 7:00 A.M.) start times. This leads to a misalignment between the desired work-rest schedule and the output of the pacemaker, resulting in disturbed daytime sleep in most such individuals. Excessive work hours (per day or per week), insufficient time off between consecutive days of work or school, and frequent travel across time zones may be contributing factors. Sleep deficiency, increased length of time awake prior to work, and misalignment of circadian phase impair alertness and performance, increase reaction time, and increase risk of performance lapses, thereby resulting in greater safety hazards among night workers and other sleep-deprived individuals. Sleep disturbance nearly doubles the risk of a fatal work accident. In addition, long-term night-shift workers have higher rates of breast, colorectal, and prostate cancer and of cardiac, gastrointestinal, metabolic, and reproductive disorders. The World Health Organization has added night-shift work to its list of probable carcinogens.

Sleep onset begins in local brain regions before gradually sweeping over the entire brain as sensory thresholds rise and consciousness is lost. A sleepy individual struggling to remain awake may attempt to continue performing routine and familiar motor tasks during the transition state between wakefulness and stage N1 sleep, while unable to adequately process sensory input from the environment. Such sleep-related attentional failures typically last only seconds but are known on occasion to persist for longer durations. Motor vehicle operators who fail to heed the warning signs of sleepiness are especially vulnerable to sleep-related accidents, as sleep processes can slow reaction times, induce automatic behavior, and intrude involuntarily upon the waking brain, causing catastrophic consequences—including 6400 fatalities and 50,000 debilitating injuries in the United States annually. For this reason, an expert consensus panel has concluded that individuals who have slept <2 h in the prior 24 h are unfit to drive a motor vehicle. There is a significant increase in the risk of sleep-related, fatal-to-the-driver highway crashes in the early morning and late afternoon hours, coincident with bimodal peaks in the daily rhythm of sleep tendency.

Physicians who work prolonged shifts, especially intermittent overnight shifts, constitute another group of workers at greater risk for accidents and other adverse consequences of lack of sleep and misalignment of the circadian rhythm. Recurrent scheduling of resident physicians to work shifts of ≥24 consecutive hours impairs psychomotor performance to a degree that is comparable to alcohol intoxication, doubles the risk of attentional failures among intensive care unit resident physicians working at night, and significantly increases the risk of serious medical errors in intensive care units, including a fivefold increase in the risk of serious diagnostic mistakes. Some 20% of hospital resident physicians report making a fatigue-related mistake that injured a patient, and 5% admit making a fatigue-related mistake that resulted in the death of a patient. Moreover, working for >24 consecutive hours increases the risk of percutaneous injuries and more than doubles the risk of motor vehicle crashes during the commute home. For these reasons, in 2008, the National Academy of Medicine concluded that the practice of scheduling resident physicians to work for >16 consecutive hours without sleep is hazardous for both resident physicians and their patients.

Of individuals scheduled to work at night or in the early morning hours, 5–15% have much greater-than-average difficulties remaining awake during night work and sleeping during the day; these individuals are diagnosed with chronic and severe shift-work disorder (SWD). Patients with this disorder have a level of excessive sleepiness during work at night or in the early morning and insomnia during day sleep that the physician judges to be clinically significant; the condition is associated with an increased risk of sleep-related accidents and with some of the illnesses associated with night-shift work. Patients with chronic and severe SWD are profoundly sleepy at work. In fact, their sleep latencies during night work average just 2 min, comparable to mean daytime sleep latency durations of patients with narcolepsy or severe sleep apnea.

TREATMENT

Shift-Work Disorder

Caffeine is frequently used by night workers to promote wakefulness. However, it cannot forestall sleep indefinitely, and it does not shield users from sleep-related performance lapses. Postural changes, exercise, and strategic placement of nap opportunities can sometimes temporarily reduce the risk of fatigue-related performance lapses. Properly timed exposure to blue-enriched light or bright white light can directly enhance alertness and facilitate more rapid adaptation to night-shift work.

Modafinil (200 mg) or armodafinil (150 mg) 30–60 min before the start of an 8-h overnight shift is an effective treatment for the excessive sleepiness during night work in patients with SWD. Although treatment with modafinil or armodafinil significantly improves performance and reduces sleep propensity and the risk of lapses of attention during night work, affected patients remain excessively sleepy.

Fatigue risk management programs for night-shift workers should promote education about sleep, increase awareness of the hazards associated with sleep deficiency and night work, and screen for common sleep disorders. Work schedules should be designed to minimize: (1) exposure to night work; (2) the frequency of shift rotations; (3) the number of consecutive night shifts; and (4) the duration of night shifts.

Jet Lag Disorder Each year, >60 million people fly from one time zone to another, often resulting in excessive daytime sleepiness, sleep-onset insomnia, and frequent arousals from sleep, particularly in the latter half of the night. The syndrome is transient, typically lasting 2–14 d depending on the number of time zones crossed, the direction of travel, and the traveler's age and phase-shifting capacity. Travelers who spend more time outdoors at their destination reportedly adapt more quickly than those who remain in hotel or seminar rooms, presumably due to brighter (outdoor) light exposure. Avoidance of antecedent sleep loss or napping on the afternoon prior to overnight travel can reduce the difficulties associated with extended wakefulness. Laboratory studies suggest that low doses of melatonin can enhance sleep efficiency, but only if taken when endogenous melatonin concentrations are low (i.e., during the biologic daytime).

In addition to jet lag associated with travel across time zones, many patients report a behavioral pattern that has been termed *social jet lag*, in which bedtimes and wake times on weekends or days off occur 4–8 h later than during the week. Such recurrent displacement of the timing of the sleep-wake cycle is common in adolescents and young adults and is associated with delayed circadian phase, sleep-onset insomnia, excessive daytime sleepiness, poorer academic performance, and increased risk of both obesity and depressive symptoms.

MEDICAL IMPLICATIONS OF CIRCADIAN RHYTHMICITY

Prominent circadian variations have been reported in the incidence of acute myocardial infarction, sudden cardiac death, and stroke, the leading causes of death in the United States. Platelet aggregability is increased in the early morning hours, coincident with the peak incidence of these cardiovascular events. Recurrent circadian disruption combined with chronic sleep deficiency, such as occurs during night-shift work, is associated with increased plasma glucose concentrations after a meal due to inadequate pancreatic insulin secretion. Night-shift workers with elevated fasting glucose have an increased risk of progressing to diabetes. Blood pressure of night workers with sleep apnea is higher than that of day workers. A better understanding of the possible role of circadian rhythmicity in the acute destabilization of a chronic condition such as atherosclerotic disease could improve the understanding of its pathophysiology.

Diagnostic and therapeutic procedures may also be affected by the time of day at which data are collected. Examples include blood pressure, body temperature, the dexamethasone suppression test, and plasma cortisol levels. The timing of chemotherapy administration has been reported to have an effect on the outcome of treatment. In addition, both the toxicity and effectiveness of drugs can vary with time of day. For example, more than a fivefold difference has been observed in mortality rates after administration of toxic agents to experimental animals at different times of day. Anesthetic agents are particularly sensitive to time-of-day effects. Finally, the physician must be aware of the public health risks associated with the ever-increasing demands made by the 24/7 schedules in our round-the-clock society.

Acknowledgment

John W. Winkelman, MD, PhD, and Gary S. Richardson, MD, contributed to this chapter in prior editions, and some material from their work has been retained here.

FURTHER READING

Cash RE et al: Association between sleep duration and ideal cardiovascular health among US adults, National Health and Nutrition Examination Survey. Prev Chronic Dis 17:E43, 2020.

Chinoy ED et al: Unrestricted evening use of light-emitting tablet computers delays self-selected bedtime and disrupts circadian timing and alertness. Physiol Rep 6:e13692, 2018.

Fultz NE et al: Coupled electrophysiological, hemodynamic, and cerebrospinal fluid oscillations in human sleep. Science 366:628, 2019.

Holth JK et al: The sleep-wake cycle regulates brain interstitial fluid tau in mice and CSF tau in humans. Science 363:880, 2019.

Landrigan CP et al: Effect on patient safety of a resident physician schedule without 24-hour shifts. N Engl J Med 382:2514, 2020.

Lee ML et al: High risk of near-crash driving events following night-shift work. Proc Natl Acad Sci USA 113:176, 2016.

Lim AS et al: Sleep is related to neuron numbers in the ventrolateral preoptic/intermediate nucleus in older adults with and without Alzheimer's disease. Brain 137:2847, 2014.

McAlpine CS et al: Sleep modulates haematopoiesis and protects against atherosclerosis. Nature 566:383, 2019.

Riemann D et al: The neurobiology, investigation, and treatment of chronic insomnia. Lancet Neurol 14:547, 2015.

Scammell TE: Narcolepsy. N Engl J Med 373:2654, 2015.

Scammell TE et al: Neural circuitry of wakefulness and sleep. Neuron 93:747, 2017.

Sletten TL et al: Efficacy of melatonin with behavioural sleep-wake scheduling for delayed sleep-wake phase disorder: a double-blind, randomised clinical trial. PLoS Med 15:e1002587, 2018.

VIDEO 31-1 A typical episode of severe cataplexy. The patient is joking and then falls to the ground with an abrupt loss of muscle tone. The electromyogram recordings (*four lower traces on the right*) show reductions in muscle activity during the period of paralysis. The electroencephalogram (*top two traces*) shows wakefulness throughout the episode. *(Video courtesy of Giuseppe Plazzi, University of Bologna.)*

VIDEO 31-2 Typical aggressive movements in rapid eye movement (REM) sleep behavior disorder. *(Video courtesy of Dr. Carlos Schenck, University of Minnesota Medical School.)*

Section 4 Disorders of Eyes, Ears, Nose, and Throat

32 Disorders of the Eye

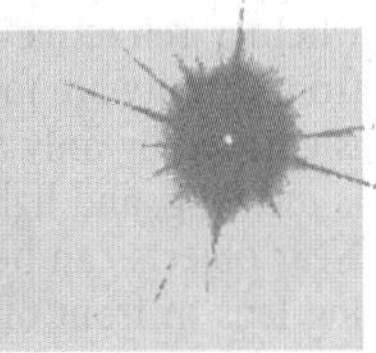

Jonathan C. Horton

THE HUMAN VISUAL SYSTEM

The visual system provides a supremely efficient means for the rapid assimilation of information from the environment to aid in the guidance of behavior. The act of seeing begins with the capture of images focused by the cornea and lens on a light-sensitive membrane in the back of the eye called the *retina*. The retina is actually part of the brain, banished to the periphery to serve as a transducer for the conversion of patterns of light energy into neuronal signals. Light is absorbed by pigment in two types of photoreceptors: rods and cones. In the human retina, there are 100 million rods and 5 million cones. The rods operate in dim (scotopic) illumination. The cones function under daylight (photopic) conditions. The cone system is specialized for color perception and high spatial resolution. The majority of cones are within the macula, the portion of the retina that serves the central 10° of vision. In the middle of the macula, a small pit termed the *fovea*, packed exclusively with cones, provides the best visual acuity.

Photoreceptors hyperpolarize in response to light, activating bipolar, amacrine, and horizontal cells in the inner nuclear layer. After processing of photoreceptor responses by this complex retinal circuit, the flow of sensory information ultimately converges on a final common pathway: the ganglion cells. These cells translate the visual image impinging on the retina into a continuously varying barrage of action potentials that propagates along the primary optic pathway to visual centers within the brain. There are a million ganglion cells in each retina and hence a million fibers in each optic nerve.

Ganglion cell axons sweep along the inner surface of the retina in the nerve fiber layer, exit the eye at the optic disc, and travel through the optic nerve, optic chiasm, and optic tract to reach targets in the brain. The majority of fibers synapse on cells in the lateral geniculate body, a thalamic relay station. Cells in the lateral geniculate body project in turn to the primary visual cortex. This afferent retinogeniculocortical sensory pathway provides the neural substrate for visual perception. Although the lateral geniculate body is the main target of the retina, separate classes of ganglion cells project to other subcortical visual nuclei involved in different functions. Ganglion cells that mediate pupillary constriction and circadian rhythms are light sensitive owing to a novel visual pigment, melanopsin. Pupil responses are mediated by input to the pretectal olivary nuclei in the midbrain. The pretectal nuclei send their output to the Edinger-Westphal nuclei, which in turn provide parasympathetic innervation to the iris sphincter via an interneuron in the ciliary ganglion. Circadian rhythms are timed by a retinal projection to the suprachiasmatic nucleus. Visual orientation and eye movements are served by retinal input to the superior colliculus. Gaze stabilization and optokinetic reflexes are governed by a group of small retinal targets known collectively as the *brainstem accessory optic system*.

The eyes must be rotated constantly within their orbits to place and maintain targets of visual interest on the fovea. This activity, called *foveation*, or looking, is governed by an elaborate efferent motor system. Each eye is moved by six extraocular muscles that are supplied by cranial nerves from the oculomotor (III), trochlear (IV), and abducens (VI) nuclei. Activity in these ocular motor nuclei is coordinated by pontine and midbrain mechanisms for smooth pursuit, saccades, and gaze stabilization during head and body movements. Large regions of the frontal and parietooccipital cortex control these brainstem eye movement centers by providing descending supranuclear input.

CLINICAL ASSESSMENT OF VISUAL FUNCTION

■ REFRACTIVE STATE

In approaching a patient with reduced vision, the first step is to decide whether refractive error is responsible. In *emmetropia*, parallel rays from infinity are focused perfectly on the retina. Sadly, this condition is enjoyed by only a minority of the population. In *myopia*, the globe is too long, and light rays come to a focal point in front of the retina. Near objects can be seen clearly, but distant objects require a diverging lens in front of the eye. In *hyperopia*, the globe is too short, and hence, a converging lens is used to supplement the refractive power of the eye. In *astigmatism*, the corneal surface is not perfectly spherical, necessitating a cylindrical corrective lens. Most patients elect to wear eyeglasses or contact lenses to neutralize refractive error. An alternative is to permanently alter the refractive properties of the cornea by performing laser in situ keratomileusis (LASIK) or photorefractive keratectomy (PRK).

With the onset of middle age, *presbyopia* develops as the lens within the eye becomes unable to increase its refractive power to accommodate on near objects. To compensate for presbyopia, an emmetropic patient must use reading glasses. A patient already wearing glasses for distance correction usually switches to bifocals. The only exception is a myopic patient, who may achieve clear vision at near simply by removing glasses containing the distance prescription.

Refractive errors usually develop slowly and remain stable after adolescence, except in unusual circumstances. For example, the acute onset of diabetes mellitus can produce sudden myopia because of lens edema induced by hyperglycemia. Testing vision through a pinhole aperture is a useful way to screen quickly for refractive error. If visual acuity is better through a pinhole than it is with the unaided eye, the patient needs refraction to obtain best corrected visual acuity.

■ VISUAL ACUITY

The Snellen chart is used to test acuity at a distance of 6 m (20 ft). For convenience, a scale version of the Snellen chart called the Rosenbaum card is held at 36 cm (14 in.) from the patient (**Fig. 32-1**). All subjects should be able to read the 6/6 m (20/20 ft) line with each eye using their refractive correction, if any. Patients who need reading glasses because of presbyopia must wear them for accurate testing with the Rosenbaum card. If 6/6 (20/20) acuity is not present in each eye, the deficiency in vision must be explained. If it is worse than 6/240 (20/800), acuity should be recorded in terms of counting fingers, hand motions, light perception, or no light perception. Legal blindness is defined by the Internal Revenue Service as a best corrected acuity of 6/60 (20/200) or less in the better eye or a binocular visual field subtending 20° or less. Loss of vision in one eye only does not constitute legal blindness. For driving, the laws vary by state, but most require a corrected acuity of 6/12 (20/40) in at least one eye for unrestricted privileges. Patients who develop a homonymous hemianopia should not drive.

■ PUPILS

The pupils should be tested individually in dim light with the patient fixating on a distant target. There is no need to check the near response

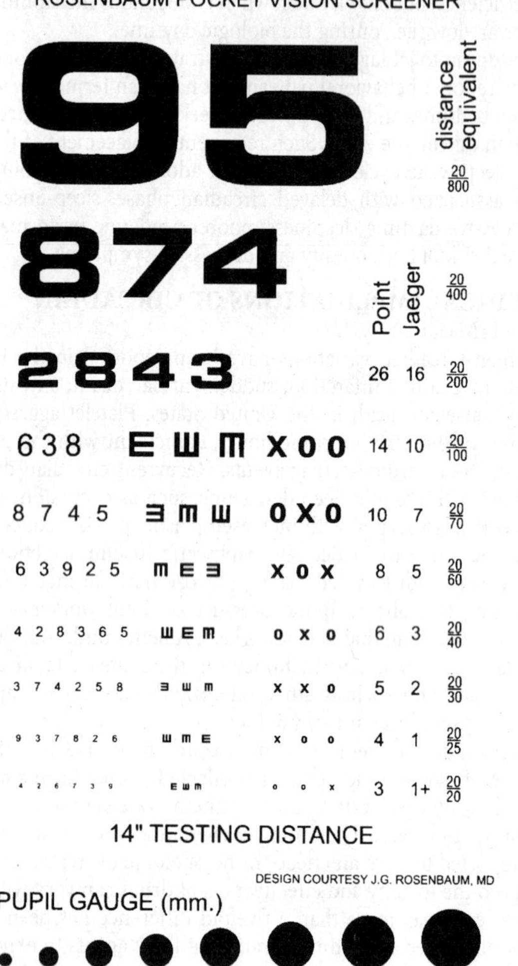

FIGURE 32-1 The Rosenbaum card is a miniature, scale version of the Snellen chart for testing visual acuity at near. When the visual acuity is recorded, the Snellen distance equivalent should bear a notation indicating that vision was tested at near, not at 6 m (20 ft), or else the Jaeger number system should be used to report the acuity. *(Design Courtesy J.G. Rosenbaum MD.)*

if the pupils respond briskly to light, because isolated loss of constriction (miosis) to accommodation does not occur. For this reason, the ubiquitous abbreviation PERRLA (pupils equal, round, and reactive to light and accommodation) implies a wasted effort with the last step. However, it is important to test the near response if the light response is poor or absent. Light-near dissociation occurs with neurosyphilis (Argyll Robertson pupil), with lesions of the dorsal midbrain (*Parinaud's syndrome*), and after aberrant regeneration (oculomotor nerve palsy, Adie's tonic pupil).

An eye with no light perception has no pupillary response to direct light stimulation. If the retina or optic nerve is only partially injured, the direct pupillary response will be weaker than the consensual pupillary response evoked by shining a light into the healthy fellow eye. A *relative afferent pupillary defect* (Marcus Gunn pupil) is elicited with the swinging flashlight test (**Fig. 32-2**). It is an extremely useful sign in retrobulbar optic neuritis and other optic nerve diseases, in which it may be the sole objective evidence for disease. In bilateral optic neuropathy, no afferent pupil defect is present if the optic nerves are affected equally.

Subtle inequality in pupil size, up to 0.5 mm, is a fairly common finding in normal persons. The diagnosis of essential or physiologic anisocoria is secure as long as the relative pupil asymmetry remains constant as ambient lighting varies. Anisocoria that increases in dim light indicates a sympathetic paresis of the iris dilator muscle. The triad of miosis with ipsilateral ptosis and anhidrosis constitutes *Horner's*

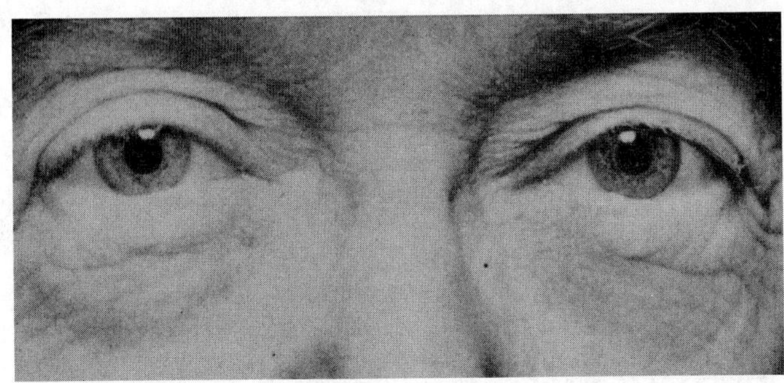

A

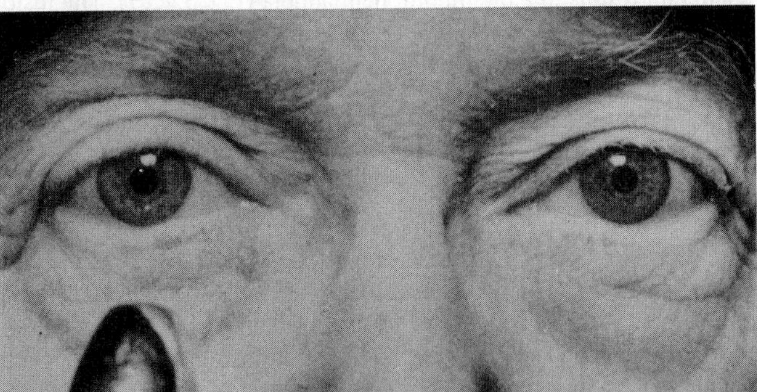

B

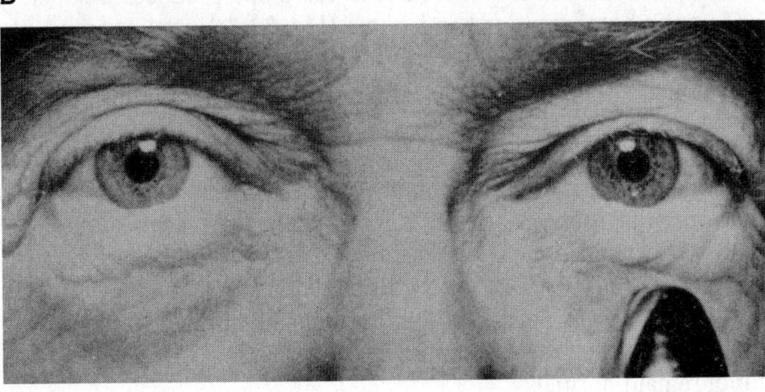

C

FIGURE 32-2 Demonstration of a relative afferent pupil defect (Marcus Gunn pupil) in the left eye, done with the patient fixating on a distant target. *A.* With dim background lighting, the pupils are equal and relatively large. ***B.*** Shining a flashlight into the right eye evokes equal, strong constriction of both pupils. ***C.*** Swinging the flashlight over to the damaged left eye causes dilation of both pupils, although they remain smaller than in ***A.*** Swinging the flashlight back over to the healthy right eye would result in symmetric constriction back to the appearance shown in ***B.*** Note that the pupils always remain equal; the damage to the left retina/optic nerve is revealed by weaker bilateral pupil constriction to a flashlight in the left eye compared with the right eye. *(From P Levatin: Arch Ophthalmol 62:768, 1959. Copyright © 1959 American Medical Association. All rights reserved.)*

syndrome, although anhidrosis is an inconstant feature. A drop of 1% apraclonidine produces no effect on the normal pupil, but the miotic pupil dilates because of denervation hypersensitivity. Brainstem stroke, carotid dissection, and neoplasm impinging on the sympathetic chain occasionally are identified as the cause of Horner's syndrome, but most cases are idiopathic.

Anisocoria that increases in bright light suggests a parasympathetic palsy. The first concern is an oculomotor nerve paresis. This possibility is excluded if the eye movements are full and the patient has no ptosis or diplopia. Acute pupillary dilation (mydriasis) can result from damage to the ciliary ganglion in the orbit. Common mechanisms are infection (herpes zoster, influenza), trauma (blunt, penetrating, surgical), and ischemia (diabetes, temporal arteritis). After denervation of the iris sphincter, the pupil does not respond well to light, but the response to near is often relatively intact. When the near stimulus is removed, the pupil redilates very slowly compared with the normal pupil, hence the term *tonic pupil.* In *Adie's syndrome*, a tonic pupil is present, sometimes in conjunction with weak or absent tendon reflexes in the lower extremities. This benign disorder, which occurs predominantly in healthy young women, is assumed to represent a mild dysautonomia. Tonic pupils are also associated with multiple system atrophy, segmental hypohidrosis, diabetes, and amyloidosis. Occasionally, a tonic pupil is discovered incidentally in an otherwise completely normal, asymptomatic individual. The diagnosis is confirmed by placing a drop of dilute (0.125%) pilocarpine into each eye. Denervation hypersensitivity produces pupillary constriction in a tonic pupil, whereas the normal pupil shows no response. Pharmacologic dilatation from accidental or deliberate instillation of anticholinergic (atropine, scopolamine) drops can produce pupillary mydriasis. Gardener's pupil refers to mydriasis induced by exposure to tropane alkaloids, contained in plants such as deadly nightshade, jimsonweed, or angel's trumpet. When an anticholinergic agent is responsible for pupil dilation, 1% pilocarpine causes no constriction.

Both pupils are affected equally by systemic medications. They are small with narcotic use (morphine, oxycodone) and large with anticholinergics (scopolamine). Parasympathetic agents (pilocarpine) used to treat glaucoma produce miosis. In any patient with an unexplained pupillary abnormality, a slit-lamp examination is helpful to exclude surgical trauma to the iris, an occult foreign body, perforating injury, intraocular inflammation, adhesions (synechia), angle-closure glaucoma, and iris sphincter rupture from blunt trauma.

EYE MOVEMENTS AND ALIGNMENT

Eye movements are tested by asking the patient, with both eyes open, to pursue a small target such as a pen tip into the cardinal fields of gaze. Normal ocular versions are smooth, symmetric, full, and maintained in all directions without nystagmus. Saccades, or quick refixation eye movements, are assessed by having the patient look back and forth between two stationary targets. The eyes should move rapidly and accurately in a single jump to their target. Ocular alignment can be judged by holding a penlight directly in front of the patient at about 1 m. If the eyes are straight, the corneal light reflex will be centered in the middle of each pupil. To test eye alignment more precisely, the cover test is useful. The patient is instructed to look at a small fixation target in the distance. One eye is occluded with a paddle or hand, while the other eye is observed. If the viewing eye shifts position to take up fixation on the target, it was misaligned. If it remains motionless, the first eye is uncovered and the test is repeated on the second eye. If neither eye moves, the eyes are aligned orthotropically. If the eyes are orthotropic in primary gaze but the patient complains of diplopia, the cover test should be performed with the head tilted or turned in whatever direction elicits diplopia. With practice, the examiner can detect an ocular deviation (heterotropia) as small as 1–2° with the cover test. In a patient with vertical diplopia, a small deviation can be difficult to detect and easy to dismiss. The magnitude of the deviation can be measured by placing a prism in front of the misaligned eye to determine the power required to neutralize the fixation shift evoked by covering the other eye. Temporary press-on plastic Fresnel prisms, prism eyeglasses, or eye muscle surgery can be used to restore binocular alignment.

STEREOPSIS

Stereoacuity is determined by presenting targets with retinal disparity separately to each eye by using polarized images. The most popular office tests measure a range of thresholds from 800 to 40 s of arc. Normal stereoacuity is 40 s of arc. If a patient achieves this level of stereoacuity, one is assured that the eyes are aligned orthotropically and that vision is intact in each eye. Random dot stereograms have no monocular depth cues and provide an excellent screening test for strabismus.

COLOR VISION

The retina contains three classes of cones, with visual pigments of differing peak spectral sensitivity: red (560 nm), green (530 nm), and blue (430 nm). The red and green cone pigments are encoded on the X chromosome, and the blue cone pigment on chromosome 7. Mutations of the blue cone pigment are exceedingly rare. Mutations of the red and green pigments cause congenital X-linked color blindness in 8% of males. Affected individuals are not truly color blind; rather, they differ from normal subjects in the way they perceive color and how they combine primary monochromatic lights to match a particular color. Anomalous trichromats have three cone types, but a mutation in one cone pigment (usually red or green) causes a shift in peak spectral sensitivity, altering the proportion of primary colors required to achieve a color match. Dichromats have only two cone types and therefore will accept a color match based on only two primary colors. Anomalous trichromats and dichromats have 6/6 (20/20) visual acuity, but their hue discrimination is impaired. Ishihara color plates can be used to detect red-green color blindness. The test plates contain a hidden number that is visible only to subjects with color confusion from red-green color blindness. Because color blindness is almost exclusively X-linked, it is worthwhile screening only male children.

The Ishihara plates often are used to detect acquired defects in color vision, although they are intended as a screening test for congenital color blindness. Acquired defects in color vision frequently result from disease of the macula or optic nerve. For example, patients with a history of optic neuritis often complain of color desaturation long after their visual acuity has returned to normal. Color blindness also can result from bilateral strokes involving the ventral portion of the occipital lobe (cerebral achromatopsia). Such patients can perceive only shades of gray and also may have difficulty recognizing faces (prosopagnosia) (**Chap. 30**). Infarcts of the dominant occipital lobe sometimes give rise to color anomia. Affected patients can discriminate colors but cannot name them.

VISUAL FIELDS

Vision can be impaired by damage to the visual system anywhere from the eyes to the occipital lobes. One can localize the site of the lesion with considerable accuracy by mapping the visual field deficit by finger confrontation and then correlating it with the topographic anatomy of the visual pathway (**Fig. 32-3**). Quantitative visual field mapping is performed by computer-driven perimeters that present a target of variable intensity at fixed positions in the visual field (**Fig. 32-3*A***). By generating an automated printout of light thresholds, these static perimeters provide a sensitive means of detecting scotomas in the visual field. They are exceedingly useful for serial assessment of visual function in chronic diseases such as glaucoma and pseudotumor cerebri.

The crux of visual field analysis is to decide whether a lesion is before, at, or behind the optic chiasm. If a scotoma is confined to one eye, it must be due to a lesion anterior to the chiasm, involving either the optic nerve or the retina. Retinal lesions produce scotomas that correspond optically to their location in the fundus. For example, a superior-nasal retinal detachment results in an inferior-temporal field cut. Damage to the macula causes a central scotoma (**Fig. 32-3*B***).

Optic nerve disease produces characteristic patterns of visual field loss. Glaucoma selectively destroys axons that enter the superotemporal or inferotemporal poles of the optic disc, resulting in arcuate scotomas shaped like a Turkish scimitar, which emanate from the blind spot and curve around fixation to end flat against the horizontal meridian (**Fig. 32-3*C***). This type of field defect mirrors the arrangement of the nerve fiber layer in the temporal retina. Arcuate or nerve fiber layer scotomas also result from optic neuritis, ischemic optic neuropathy, optic disc drusen, and branch retinal artery or vein occlusion.

Damage to the entire upper or lower pole of the optic disc causes an altitudinal field cut that follows the horizontal meridian (**Fig. 32-3*D***). This pattern of visual field loss is typical of ischemic optic neuropathy but also results from retinal vascular occlusion, advanced glaucoma, and optic neuritis.

About half the fibers in the optic nerve originate from ganglion cells serving the macula. Damage to papillomacular fibers causes a cecocentral scotoma that encompasses the blind spot and macula (**Fig. 32-3*E***). If the damage is irreversible, pallor eventually appears in the temporal portion of the optic disc. Temporal pallor from a cecocentral scotoma may develop in optic neuritis, nutritional optic neuropathy, toxic optic neuropathy, Leber's hereditary optic neuropathy, Kjer's dominant optic atrophy, and compressive optic neuropathy. It is worth mentioning that the temporal side of the optic disc is slightly paler than the nasal side in most normal individuals. Therefore, it sometimes can be difficult to decide whether the temporal pallor visible on fundus examination represents a pathologic change. Pallor of the nasal rim of the optic disc is a less equivocal sign of optic atrophy.

At the optic chiasm, fibers from nasal ganglion cells decussate into the contralateral optic tract. Crossed fibers are damaged more by compression than are uncrossed fibers. As a result, mass lesions of the sellar region cause a temporal hemianopia in each eye. Tumors anterior to the optic chiasm, such as meningiomas of the tuberculum sella, produce a junctional scotoma characterized by an optic neuropathy in one eye and a superior-temporal field cut in the other eye (**Fig. 32-3*G***). More symmetric compression of the optic chiasm by a pituitary adenoma (**see Fig. 380-1**), meningioma, craniopharyngioma, glioma, or aneurysm results in a bitemporal hemianopia (**Fig. 32-3*H***). The insidious development of a bitemporal hemianopia often goes unnoticed by the patient and will escape detection by the physician unless each eye is tested separately.

It is difficult to localize a postchiasmal lesion accurately, because injury anywhere in the optic tract, lateral geniculate body, optic radiations, or visual cortex can produce a homonymous hemianopia (i.e., a temporal hemifield defect in the contralateral eye and a matching nasal hemifield defect in the ipsilateral eye) (**Fig. 32-3*I***). A unilateral postchiasmal lesion leaves the visual acuity in each eye unaffected, although the patient may read the letters on only the left or right half of the eye chart. Lesions of the optic radiations tend to cause poorly matched or incongruous field defects in each eye. Damage to the optic radiations in the temporal lobe (Meyer's loop) produces a superior quadrantic homonymous hemianopia (**Fig. 32-3*J***), whereas injury to the optic radiations in the parietal lobe results in an inferior quadrantic homonymous hemianopia (**Fig. 32-3*K***). Lesions of the primary visual cortex give rise to dense, congruous hemianopic field defects. Occlusion of the posterior cerebral artery supplying the occipital lobe is a common cause of total homonymous hemianopia. Some patients have macular sparing, because the central field representation at the tip of the occipital lobe is supplied by collaterals from the middle cerebral artery (**Fig. 32-3*L***). Destruction of both occipital lobes produces cortical blindness. This condition can be distinguished from bilateral prechiasmal visual loss by noting that the pupil responses and optic fundi remain normal.

Partial recovery of homonymous hemianopia has been reported through computer-based rehabilitation therapy. During daily training sessions, patients fixate a central target while visual stimuli are presented within the blind region. The premise of vision restoration programs is that extra stimulation can promote recovery of partially damaged tissue located at the fringe of a cortical lesion. When fixation is controlled rigorously, however, no improvement of the visual fields can be demonstrated. No effective treatment exists for homonymous hemianopia caused by permanent brain damage.

DISORDERS

RED OR PAINFUL EYE

Corneal Abrasions Corneal abrasions are seen best by placing a drop of fluorescein in the eye and looking with the slit lamp, using a cobalt-blue light. A penlight with a blue filter will suffice if a slit lamp is not available. Damage to the corneal epithelium is revealed by yellow fluorescence of the basement membrane exposed by loss of the overlying epithelium. It is important to check for foreign bodies. To search the conjunctival fornices, the lower lid should be pulled down and the upper lid everted. A foreign body can be removed with a moistened cotton-tipped applicator after a drop of a topical anesthetic such as proparacaine has been placed in the eye. Alternatively, it may be possible to flush the foreign body from the eye by irrigating copiously with saline or artificial tears. If the corneal epithelium has been abraded, antibiotic ointment and a patch may be applied to the eye. A drop of an intermediate-acting cycloplegic such as cyclopentolate hydrochloride 1% helps reduce pain by relaxing the ciliary body. The eye should be reexamined the next day. Minor abrasions may not require patching, antibiotics, or cycloplegia.

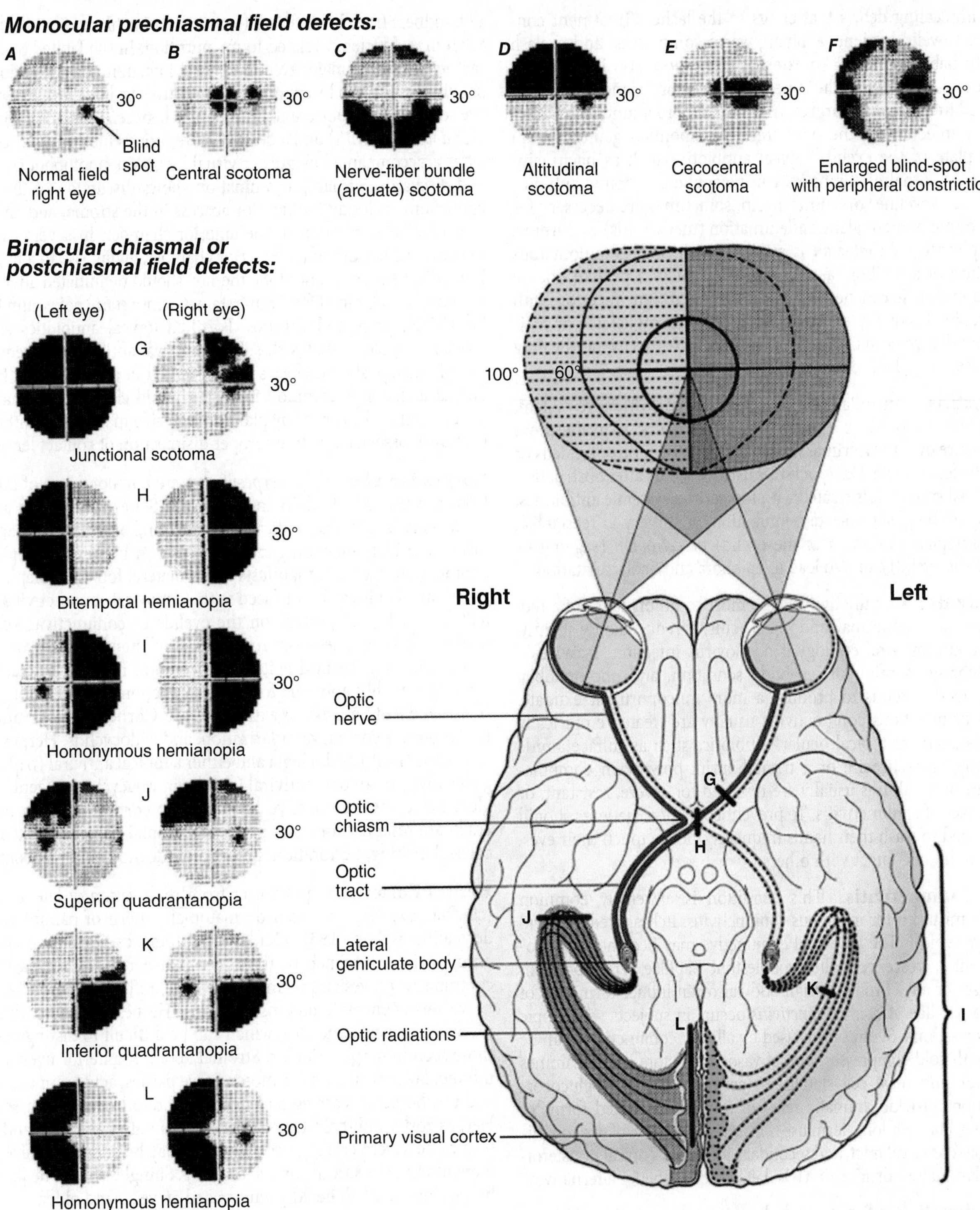

FIGURE 32-3 Ventral view of the brain, correlating patterns of visual field loss with the sites of lesions in the visual pathway. The visual fields overlap partially, creating 120° of central binocular field flanked by a 40° monocular crescent on either side. The visual field maps in this figure were done with a computer-driven perimeter (Humphrey Instruments, Carl Zeiss, Inc.). It plots the retinal sensitivity to light in the central 30° by using a gray scale format. Areas of visual field loss are shown in black. The examples of common monocular, prechiasmal field defects are all shown for the right eye. By convention, the visual fields are always recorded with the left eye's field on the left and the right eye's field on the right, just as the patient sees the world.

Subconjunctival Hemorrhage This results from rupture of small vessels bridging the potential space between the episclera and the conjunctiva. Blood dissecting into this space can produce a spectacular red eye, but vision is not affected and the hemorrhage resolves without treatment. Subconjunctival hemorrhage is usually spontaneous but can result from blunt trauma, eye rubbing, or vigorous coughing. Occasionally, it is a clue to an underlying bleeding disorder.

Pinguecula Pinguecula is a small, raised conjunctival nodule, usually at the nasal limbus. In adults, such lesions are extremely common and have little significance unless they become inflamed (pingueculitis). They are more apt to occur in workers with outdoor exposure. A *pterygium* resembles a pinguecula but has crossed the limbus to encroach on the corneal surface. Removal is justified when symptoms of irritation or blurring develop, but recurrence is common.

Blepharitis This refers to inflammation of the eyelids. The most common form occurs in association with acne rosacea or seborrheic dermatitis. The eyelid margins usually are colonized heavily by staphylococci. Upon close inspection, they appear greasy, ulcerated, and crusted with scaling debris that clings to the lashes. Treatment consists of strict eyelid hygiene, applying warm compresses, and eyelash scrubs with baby shampoo. An external *hordeolum* (sty) is caused by staphylococcal infection of the superficial accessory glands of Zeis or Moll located in the eyelid margins. An internal hordeolum occurs after suppurative infection of the oil-secreting meibomian glands within the tarsal plate of the eyelid. Topical antibiotics such as bacitracin/polymyxin B ophthalmic ointment can be applied. Systemic antibiotics, usually tetracyclines or azithromycin, sometimes are necessary for treatment of meibomian gland inflammation (meibomitis) or chronic, severe blepharitis. A *chalazion* is a painless, chronic granulomatous inflammation of a meibomian gland that produces a pealike nodule within the eyelid. It can be incised and drained, but injection with glucocorticoids is equally effective. Basal cell, squamous cell, or meibomian gland carcinoma should be suspected with any nonhealing ulcerative lesion of the eyelids.

Dacryocystitis An inflammation of the lacrimal drainage system, dacryocystitis can produce epiphora (tearing) and ocular injection. Gentle pressure over the lacrimal sac evokes pain and reflux of mucus or pus from the tear puncta. Dacryocystitis usually occurs after obstruction of the lacrimal system. It is treated with topical and systemic antibiotics, followed by probing, silicone stent intubation, or surgery to reestablish patency. *Entropion* (inversion of the eyelid) or *ectropion* (sagging or eversion of the eyelid) can also lead to epiphora and ocular irritation.

Conjunctivitis Conjunctivitis is the most common cause of a red, irritated eye. Pain is minimal, and visual acuity is reduced only slightly. The most common viral etiology is adenovirus infection. It causes a watery discharge, a mild foreign-body sensation, and photophobia. Bacterial infection tends to produce a more mucopurulent exudate. Mild cases of infectious conjunctivitis usually are treated empirically with broad-spectrum topical ocular antibiotics such as sulfacetamide 10%, polymyxin-bacitracin, or a trimethoprim-polymyxin combination. Smears and cultures usually are reserved for severe, resistant, or recurrent cases of conjunctivitis. To prevent contagion, patients should be admonished to wash their hands frequently, not to touch their eyes, and to avoid direct contact with others.

Allergic Conjunctivitis This condition is extremely common and often is mistaken for infectious conjunctivitis. Itching, redness, and epiphora are typical. The palpebral conjunctiva may become hypertropic with giant excrescences called cobblestone papillae. Irritation from contact lenses or any chronic foreign body also can induce formation of cobblestone papillae. *Atopic conjunctivitis* occurs in subjects with atopic dermatitis or asthma. Symptoms caused by allergic conjunctivitis can be alleviated with cold compresses, topical vasoconstrictors, antihistamines (olopatadine), and mast cell stabilizers (cromolyn). Topical glucocorticoid solutions provide dramatic relief of immune-mediated forms of conjunctivitis, but their long-term use is ill advised because of the complications of glaucoma, cataract, and secondary infection. Topical nonsteroidal anti-inflammatory drugs (NSAIDs; ketorolac) are better alternatives.

Keratoconjunctivitis Sicca Also known as dry eye, this produces a burning foreign-body sensation, injection, and photophobia. In mild cases, the eye appears surprisingly normal, but tear production measured by wetting of a filter paper (Schirmer strip) is deficient. A variety of systemic drugs, including antihistaminic, anticholinergic, and psychotropic medications, result in dry eye by reducing lacrimal secretion. Disorders that involve the lacrimal gland directly, such as sarcoidosis and Sjögren's syndrome, also cause dry eye. Patients may develop dry eye after radiation therapy if the treatment field includes the orbits. Problems with ocular drying are also common after lesions affecting cranial nerve V or VII. Corneal anesthesia is particularly dangerous, because the absence of a normal blink reflex exposes the cornea to injury without pain to warn the patient. Dry eye is managed by frequent and liberal application of artificial tears and ocular lubricants. In severe cases, the tear puncta can be plugged or cauterized to reduce lacrimal outflow.

Keratitis Keratitis is a threat to vision because of the risk of corneal clouding, scarring, and perforation. Worldwide, the two leading causes of blindness from keratitis are trachoma from chlamydial infection and vitamin A deficiency related to malnutrition. In the United States, contact lenses play a major role in corneal infection and ulceration. They should not be worn by anyone with an active eye infection. In evaluating the cornea, it is important to differentiate between a superficial infection (*keratoconjunctivitis*) and a deeper, more serious ulcerative process. The latter is accompanied by greater visual loss, pain, photophobia, redness, and discharge. Slit-lamp examination shows disruption of the corneal epithelium, a cloudy infiltrate or abscess in the stroma, and an inflammatory cellular reaction in the anterior chamber. In severe cases, pus settles at the bottom of the anterior chamber, giving rise to a hypopyon. Immediate empirical antibiotic therapy should be initiated after corneal scrapings are obtained for Gram's stain, Giemsa stain, potassium hydroxide (KOH) prep, and cultures. Fortified topical antibiotics are most effective, supplemented with subconjunctival antibiotics as required. A fungal etiology should always be considered in a patient with keratitis. Fungal infection is common in warm humid climates, especially after penetration of the cornea by plant or vegetable material. Acanthamoeba keratitis is associated with improper disinfection of contact lenses.

Herpes Simplex The *herpesviruses* are a major cause of blindness from keratitis. Most adults in the United States have serum antibodies to herpes simplex, indicating prior viral infection (**Chap. 192**). Primary ocular infection generally is caused by herpes simplex type 1 rather than type 2. It manifests as a unilateral follicular blepharoconjunctivitis that is easily confused with adenoviral conjunctivitis, unless telltale vesicles are present on the eyelids or conjunctiva. Recurrent ocular infection arises from reactivation of latent herpesvirus. A dendritic pattern of corneal epithelial ulceration revealed by fluorescein staining is pathognomonic for herpes infection but often not present. Involvement of both eyes is extremely rare. Corneal stromal inflammation produces edema, vascularization, and iridocyclitis. Herpes keratitis is treated with cycloplegia and either a topical antiviral (trifluridine, ganciclovir) or an oral antiviral (acyclovir, valacyclovir) agent. Topical glucocorticoids are effective in mitigating corneal scarring but generally are reserved for cases involving stromal damage. Risks include corneal melting, perforation, prolonged infection, and glaucoma.

Herpes Zoster Herpes zoster from reactivation of latent varicella (chickenpox) virus causes a dermatomal pattern of painful vesicular dermatitis (**Chap. 193**). Ocular symptoms can occur after zoster eruption in any branch of the trigeminal nerve but are particularly common when vesicles form on the nose, reflecting nasociliary (V1) nerve involvement (Hutchinson's sign). Herpes zoster ophthalmicus produces corneal dendrites, which can be difficult to distinguish from those seen in herpes simplex. Stromal keratitis, anterior uveitis, raised intraocular pressure, ocular motor nerve palsies, acute retinal necrosis, and postherpetic scarring and neuralgia are other common sequelae. Herpes zoster ophthalmicus is treated with antiviral agents and cycloplegics. In severe cases, glucocorticoids may be added to prevent permanent visual loss from corneal scarring. Shingles should be prevented by vaccination of all healthy adults aged 50 years and older.

Episcleritis This is an inflammation of the episclera, a thin layer of connective tissue between the conjunctiva and the sclera. Episcleritis resembles conjunctivitis, but it is a more localized process and discharge is absent. Most cases of episcleritis are idiopathic, but some occur in the setting of an autoimmune disease. *Scleritis* refers to a deeper, more severe inflammatory process that frequently is associated with a connective tissue disease such as rheumatoid arthritis, lupus erythematosus, polyarteritis nodosa, granulomatosis with polyangiitis, or relapsing polychondritis. The inflammation and thickening of the sclera can be diffuse or nodular. In anterior forms of scleritis, the globe assumes a violet hue and the patient complains of severe ocular tenderness and pain. With posterior scleritis, the pain and redness may be less marked, but there is often proptosis, choroidal effusion, reduced motility, and visual loss. Episcleritis and scleritis should be treated with NSAIDs. If these agents fail, topical or even systemic glucocorticoid therapy may be necessary, especially if an underlying autoimmune process is active.

Anterior Uveitis Involving the anterior structures of the eye, uveitis was previously called *iritis* or *iridocyclitis*. The diagnosis requires slit-lamp examination to identify inflammatory cells floating in the aqueous humor or deposited on the corneal endothelium (keratic precipitates). Anterior uveitis develops in sarcoidosis, ankylosing spondylitis, juvenile idiopathic arthritis, inflammatory bowel disease, psoriasis, reactive arthritis, and Behçet's disease. It also is associated with herpes infections, syphilis, Lyme disease, onchocerciasis, tuberculosis, and leprosy. Although anterior uveitis can occur in conjunction with many diseases, no cause is found to explain the majority of cases. For this reason, laboratory evaluation usually is reserved for patients with recurrent or severe anterior uveitis. Treatment is aimed at reducing inflammation and scarring by judicious use of topical glucocorticoids. Dilatation of the pupil reduces pain and prevents the formation of synechiae.

Posterior Uveitis This diagnosis is made by observing inflammation of the vitreous, retina, or choroid on fundus examination. It is more likely than anterior uveitis to be associated with an identifiable systemic disease. Some patients have panuveitis, or inflammation of both the anterior and posterior segments of the eye. Posterior uveitis is a manifestation of autoimmune diseases such as sarcoidosis, Behçet's disease, Vogt-Koyanagi-Harada syndrome, and inflammatory bowel disease. It also accompanies diseases such as toxoplasmosis, onchocerciasis, cysticercosis, coccidioidomycosis, toxocariasis, and histoplasmosis; infections caused by organisms such as *Candida*, *Pneumocystis carinii*, *Cryptococcus*, *Aspergillus*, herpes, and cytomegalovirus (see Fig. 195-1); and other diseases, such as syphilis, Lyme disease, tuberculosis, cat-scratch disease, Whipple's disease, and brucellosis. In multiple sclerosis, chronic inflammatory changes can develop in the extreme periphery of the retina (pars planitis or intermediate uveitis). Glucocorticoids have been the mainstay of treatment for noninfectious uveitis. Biologic agents that target proinflammatory cytokines, such as the tumor necrosis factor alpha (TNF-α) inhibitor adalimumab, are effective at preventing vision loss in chronic uveitis.

Acute Angle-Closure Glaucoma This is an unusual but frequently misdiagnosed cause of a red, painful eye. Asian populations have a particularly high risk of angle-closure glaucoma. Susceptible eyes have a shallow anterior chamber because the eye has either a short axial length (hyperopia) or a lens enlarged by the gradual development of cataract. When the pupil becomes mid-dilated, the peripheral iris blocks aqueous outflow via the anterior chamber angle and the intraocular pressure rises abruptly, producing pain, injection, corneal edema, obscurations, and blurred vision. In some patients, ocular symptoms are overshadowed by nausea, vomiting, or headache, prompting a fruitless workup for abdominal or neurologic disease. The diagnosis is made by measuring the intraocular pressure during an acute attack or by performing gonioscopy, a procedure that allows one to observe a narrow chamber angle with a mirrored contact lens. Acute angle closure is treated with acetazolamide (PO or IV), topical beta blockers, prostaglandin analogues, α_2-adrenergic agonists, and pilocarpine to induce miosis. If these measures fail, a laser can be used to create a hole in the peripheral iris to relieve pupillary block. Many physicians are reluctant to dilate patients routinely for fundus examination because they fear precipitating an angle-closure glaucoma. The risk is actually remote and more than outweighed by the potential benefit to patients of discovering a hidden fundus lesion visible only through a fully dilated pupil. Moreover, a single attack of angle closure after pharmacologic dilatation rarely causes any permanent damage to the eye and serves as an inadvertent provocative test to identify patients with narrow angles who would benefit from prophylactic laser iridectomy.

Endophthalmitis This results from bacterial, viral, fungal, or parasitic infection of the internal structures of the eye. It usually is acquired by hematogenous seeding from a remote site. Chronically ill, diabetic, or immunosuppressed patients, especially those with a history of indwelling IV catheters or positive blood cultures, are at greatest risk for endogenous endophthalmitis. Although most patients have ocular pain and injection, visual loss is sometimes the only symptom. Septic emboli from a diseased heart valve or a dental abscess that lodge in the retinal circulation can give rise to endophthalmitis. White-centered retinal hemorrhages known as Roth's spots (Fig. 32-4) are considered pathognomonic for subacute bacterial endocarditis, but they also appear in leukemia, diabetes, and many other conditions. Endophthalmitis occurs as a complication of ocular surgery, especially glaucoma filtering, occasionally months or even years after the operation. An occult penetrating foreign body or unrecognized trauma to the globe should be considered in any patient with unexplained intraocular infection or inflammation.

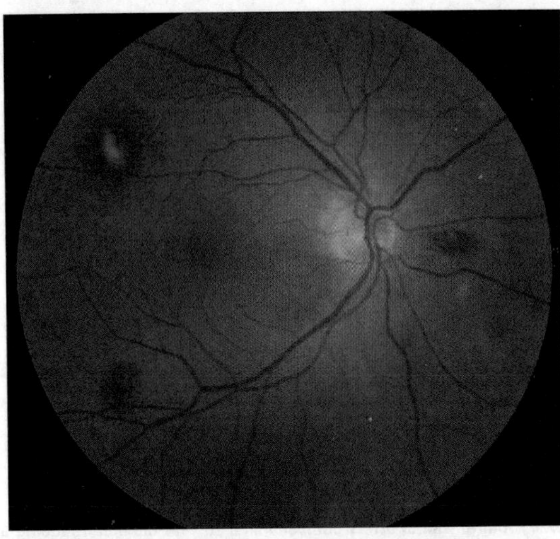

FIGURE 32-4 Roth's spot, cotton-wool spot, and retinal hemorrhages in a 48-year-old liver transplant patient with candidemia from immunosuppression.

TRANSIENT OR SUDDEN VISUAL LOSS

Amaurosis Fugax This term refers to a transient ischemic attack of the retina (Chap. 427). Because neural tissue has a high rate of metabolism, interruption of blood flow to the retina for more than a few seconds results in *transient monocular blindness*, a term used interchangeably with amaurosis fugax. Patients describe a rapid fading of vision like a curtain descending, sometimes affecting only a portion of the visual field. Amaurosis fugax usually results from an embolus that becomes stuck within a retinal arteriole (Fig. 32-5). If the embolus breaks up or passes, flow is restored and vision returns quickly to normal without permanent damage. With prolonged interruption of blood flow, the inner retina suffers infarction. Ophthalmoscopy reveals zones of whitened, edematous retina following the distribution of branch retinal arterioles. Complete occlusion of the central retinal artery

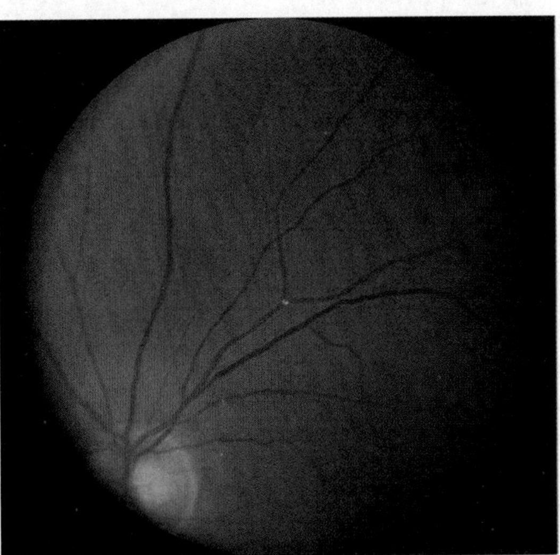

FIGURE 32-5 Hollenhorst plaque lodged at the bifurcation of a retinal arteriole proves that a patient is shedding emboli from the carotid artery, great vessels, or heart.

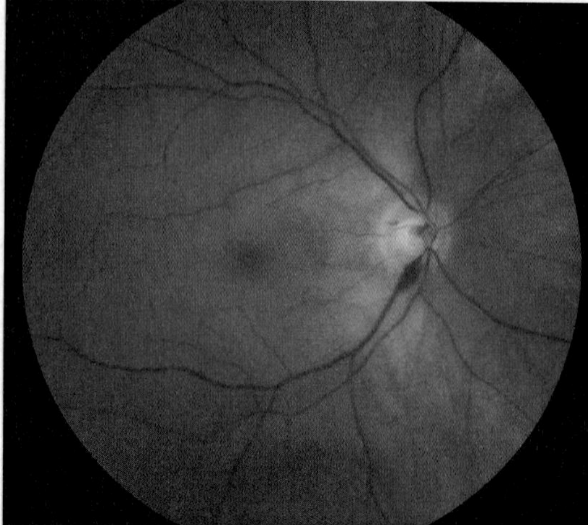

FIGURE 32-6 Central retinal artery occlusion in a 78-year-old man reducing acuity to counting fingers in the right eye. Note the splinter hemorrhage on the optic disc and the slightly milky appearance to the macula with a cherry-red fovea.

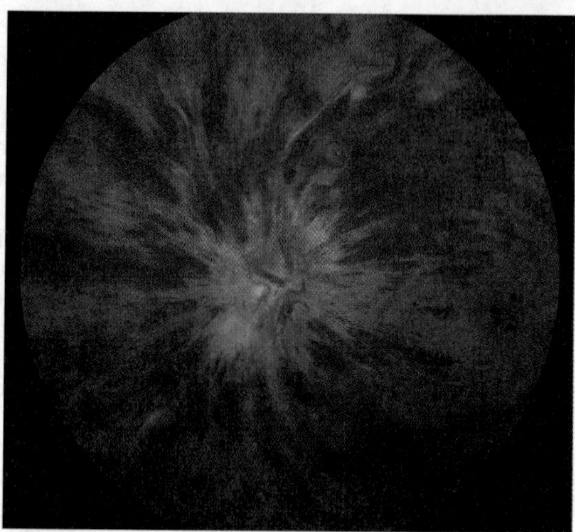

FIGURE 32-8 Central retinal vein occlusion can produce massive retinal hemorrhage ("blood and thunder"), ischemia, and vision loss.

produces arrest of blood flow and a milky retina with a cherry-red fovea (**Fig. 32-6**). Emboli are composed of cholesterol (Hollenhorst plaque), calcium, or platelet-fibrin debris. The most common source is an atherosclerotic plaque in the carotid artery or aorta, although emboli also can arise from the heart, especially in patients with diseased valves, atrial fibrillation, or wall motion abnormalities.

In rare instances, amaurosis fugax results from low central retinal artery perfusion pressure in a patient with a critical stenosis of the ipsilateral carotid artery and poor collateral flow via the circle of Willis. In this situation, amaurosis fugax develops when there is a dip in systemic blood pressure or a slight worsening of the carotid stenosis. Sometimes there is contralateral motor or sensory loss, indicating concomitant hemispheric cerebral ischemia.

Retinal arterial occlusion also occurs rarely in association with retinal migraine, lupus erythematosus, anticardiolipin antibodies, anticoagulant deficiency states (protein S, protein C, and antithrombin deficiency), Susac's syndrome, pregnancy, IV drug abuse, blood dyscrasias, dysproteinemias, and temporal arteritis.

Marked *systemic hypertension* causes sclerosis of retinal arterioles, splinter hemorrhages, focal infarcts of the nerve fiber layer (cotton-wool spots), and leakage of lipid and fluid (hard exudate) into the macula (**Fig. 32-7**). In hypertensive crisis, sudden visual loss can result from ischemia induced by vasospasm of retinal arterioles. In addition, visual loss can occur from ischemic optic disc swelling. Patients with acute hypertensive retinopathy should be treated by lowering the blood pressure. However, the blood pressure should not be reduced precipitously, because there is a danger of optic disc infarction from sudden hypoperfusion.

Impending *branch* or *central retinal vein occlusion* can produce prolonged visual obscurations that resemble those described by patients with amaurosis fugax. The veins appear engorged and phlebitic, with numerous retinal hemorrhages (**Fig. 32-8**). In some patients, venous blood flow recovers spontaneously, whereas others evolve a frank obstruction with extensive retinal bleeding ("blood and thunder" appearance), infarction, and visual loss. Venous occlusion of the retina is often idiopathic, but hypertension, diabetes, and glaucoma are prominent risk factors. Polycythemia, thrombocythemia, or other factors leading to an underlying hypercoagulable state should be corrected; aspirin treatment may be beneficial.

Anterior Ischemic Optic Neuropathy (AION) This is caused by insufficient blood flow through the posterior ciliary arteries that supply the optic disc. It produces painless monocular visual loss that is sudden in onset, followed sometimes by stuttering progression. The optic disc is edematous and usually bordered by nerve fiber layer splinter hemorrhages (**Fig. 32-9**). AION is divided into two forms: arteritic and nonarteritic. The nonarteritic form is most common. No specific cause is known, although diabetes, renal failure, and hypertension are common risk factors. Case reports have linked erectile dysfunction

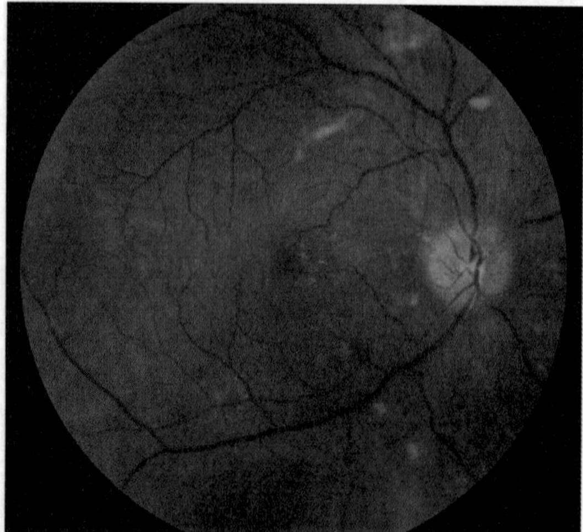

FIGURE 32-7 Hypertensive retinopathy with blurred optic disc, scattered hemorrhages, cotton-wool spots (nerve fiber layer infarcts), and foveal exudate in a 62-year-old man with chronic renal failure and a systolic blood pressure of 220.

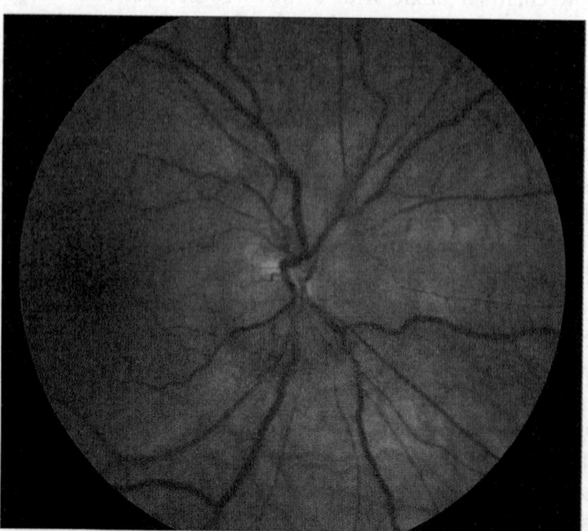

FIGURE 32-9 Anterior ischemic optic neuropathy from temporal arteritis in a 64-year-old woman with acute disc swelling, splinter hemorrhages, visual loss, and an erythrocyte sedimentation rate of 60 mm/h.

drugs to AION, but a causal association is doubtful. Evidence is strong that a crowded disc architecture and small optic cup predispose to the development of nonarteritic AION. In patients with such a "disc-at-risk," the advent of AION in one eye increases the likelihood of the same event occurring in the other eye. No treatment is available for nonarteritic AION; glucocorticoids should not be prescribed.

About 5% of patients, especially Caucasian females aged >60, have the arteritic form of AION in conjunction with giant cell (temporal) arteritis **(Chap. 363)**. It is urgent to recognize arteritic AION so that high doses of glucocorticoids can be instituted immediately to prevent blindness in the second eye. Tocilizumab, a monoclonal antibody against interleukin 6 receptor, is an effective alternative to glucocorticoids for sustained suppression of symptoms of giant cell arteritis. Symptoms of polymyalgia rheumatica may be present; the sedimentation rate and C-reactive protein level are usually elevated. In a patient with visual loss from suspected arteritic AION, temporal artery biopsy is mandatory to confirm the diagnosis. Administer glucocorticoids immediately, without waiting for the biopsy to be completed. The biopsy should be obtained as soon as practical, because prolonged glucocorticoid treatment can hide inflammatory changes. It is important to harvest an arterial segment at least 3 cm long and to examine a sufficient number of tissue sections. The histologic features of granulomatous inflammation are often quite subtle in temporal artery specimens. If the biopsy is declared negative by an experienced pathologist, the diagnosis of arteritic AION is highly unlikely and glucocorticoids should usually be discontinued.

Posterior Ischemic Optic Neuropathy This is an uncommon cause of acute visual loss, induced by the combination of severe anemia and hypotension. Cases have been reported after major blood loss during surgery (especially in patients undergoing cardiac or lumbar spine operations), shock, gastrointestinal bleeding, and renal dialysis. The fundus usually appears normal, although optic disc swelling develops if the process extends anteriorly far enough to reach the globe. Vision can be salvaged in some patients by immediate blood transfusion and reversal of hypotension.

Optic Neuritis This is a common inflammatory disease of the optic nerve. In the Optic Neuritis Treatment Trial (ONTT), the mean age of patients was 32 years, 77% were female, 92% had ocular pain (especially with eye movements), and 35% had optic disc swelling. In most patients, the demyelinating event was retrobulbar and the ocular fundus appeared normal on initial examination **(Fig. 32-10)**, although optic disc pallor slowly developed over subsequent months.

Virtually all patients experience a gradual recovery of vision after a single episode of optic neuritis, even without treatment. This rule is so reliable that failure of vision to improve after a first attack of optic neuritis casts doubt on the original diagnosis. Treatment with high-dose IV methylprednisolone (250 mg every 6 h for 3 days) followed by oral prednisone (1 mg/kg per day for 11 days) makes no difference in ultimate acuity 6 months after the attack, but the recovery of visual function occurs more rapidly. Therefore, when visual loss is severe (worse than 20/100), IV followed by PO glucocorticoids are often recommended.

For some patients, optic neuritis remains an isolated event. However, the ONTT showed that the 15-year cumulative probability of developing clinically definite multiple sclerosis after optic neuritis is 50%. A brain magnetic resonance (MR) scan is advisable in every patient with a first attack of optic neuritis. If two or more plaques are present on initial imaging, treatment should be considered to prevent the development of additional demyelinating lesions **(Chap. 444)**.

A particularly severe optic neuritis, often involving a long segment of nerve, occurs in neuromyelitis optica (NMO); it may be bilateral and associated with myelitis. NMO can occur as a primary disorder, in the setting of systemic autoimmune disease, or rarely, as a paraneoplastic condition. Detection of circulating antibodies directed against aquaporin-4 or myelin oligodendrocyte glycoprotein (MOG) is diagnostic. Treatment for acute episodes consists of glucocorticoids followed by satralizumab, eculizumab, or inebilizumab to prevent relapse. **Neuromyelitis optica is discussed in detail in Chap. 445.**

LEBER'S HEREDITARY OPTIC NEUROPATHY

This disease usually affects young men, causing progressive, painless, severe central visual loss in one eye, followed weeks to years later by the same process in the other eye. Acutely, the optic disc appears mildly plethoric with surface capillary telangiectasias but no vascular leakage on fluorescein angiography. Eventually, optic atrophy ensues. Leber's optic neuropathy is caused by a point mutation at codon 11778 in the mitochondrial gene encoding nicotinamide adenine dinucleotide dehydrogenase (NADH) subunit 4. Additional mutations responsible for the disease have been identified, most in mitochondrial genes that encode proteins involved in electron transport. Mitochondrial mutations that cause Leber's neuropathy are maternally inherited by all children, but for unknown reasons, only 10% of cases occur in females. Clinical trials of gene therapy for this condition have been unsuccessful.

Toxic Optic Neuropathy This can result in acute visual loss with bilateral optic disc swelling and cecocentral scotomas. Cases have been reported from exposure to ethambutol, methyl alcohol (moonshine), ethylene glycol (antifreeze), or carbon monoxide. In toxic optic neuropathy, visual loss also can develop gradually and produce optic atrophy **(Fig. 32-11)** without a phase of acute optic disc edema. Many agents have been implicated in toxic optic neuropathy, but evidence supporting the association is often weak. The following is a partial list of potential offending drugs or toxins: disulfiram, ethchlorvynol, chloramphenicol,

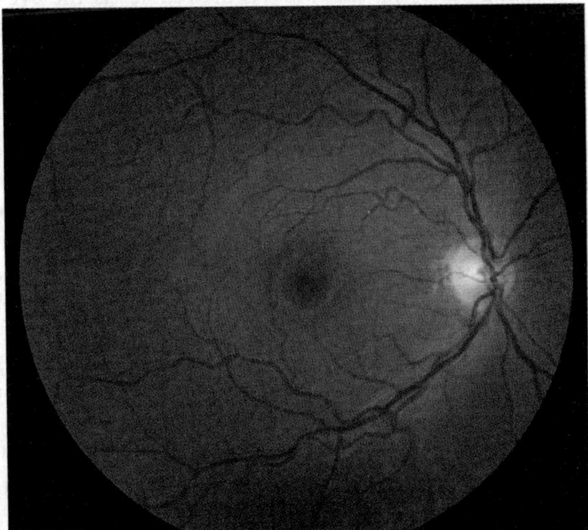

FIGURE 32-10 Retrobulbar optic neuritis is characterized by a normal fundus examination initially, hence the rubric "the doctor sees nothing, and the patient sees nothing." Optic atrophy develops after severe or repeated attacks.

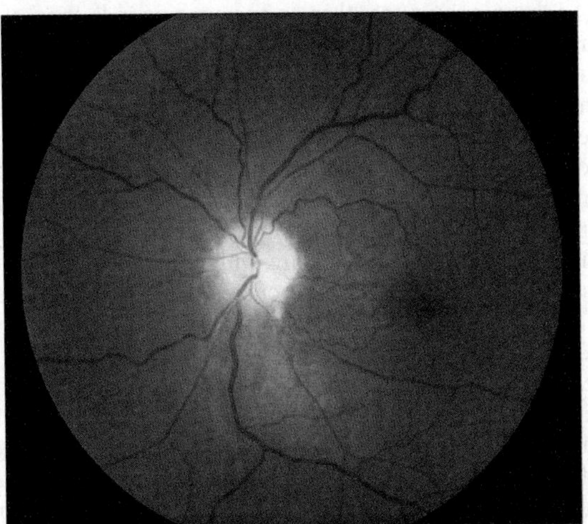

FIGURE 32-11 Optic atrophy is not a specific diagnosis but refers to the combination of optic disc pallor, arteriolar narrowing, and nerve fiber layer destruction produced by a host of eye diseases, especially optic neuropathies.

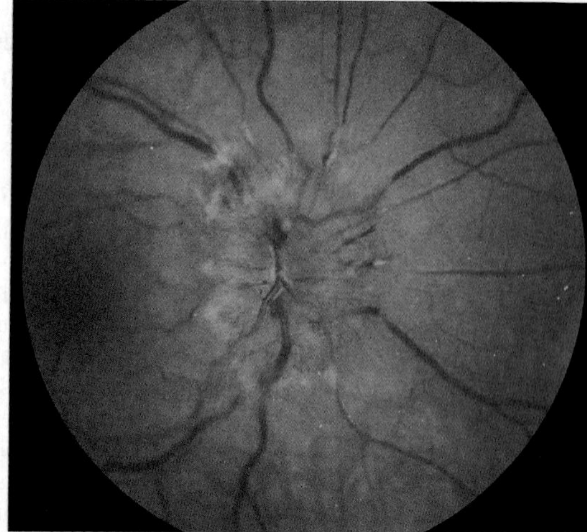

FIGURE 32-12 Papilledema means optic disc edema from raised intracranial pressure. This young woman developed acute papilledema, with hemorrhages and cotton-wool spots, as a rare side effect of treatment with tetracycline for acne.

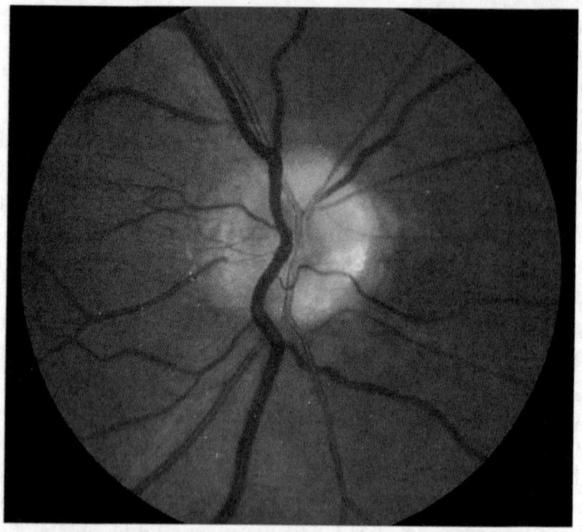

FIGURE 32-13 Optic disc drusen are calcified, mulberry-like deposits of unknown etiology within the optic disc, giving rise to "pseudopapilledema."

amiodarone, monoclonal anti-CD3 antibody, ciprofloxacin, digitalis, streptomycin, lead, arsenic, thallium, D-penicillamine, isoniazid, emetine, and sulfonamides. Metallosis (chromium, cobalt, nickel) from hip implant failure is a rare cause of toxic optic neuropathy. Deficiency states induced by starvation, malabsorption, alcoholism, or gastric bypass can lead to insidious visual loss. Thiamine, vitamin B_{12}, and folate levels should be checked in any patient with unexplained bilateral central scotomas and optic pallor.

Papilledema This connotes bilateral optic disc swelling from raised intracranial pressure (**Fig. 32-12**). Headache is a common but not invariable accompaniment. All other forms of optic disc swelling (e.g., from optic neuritis or ischemic optic neuropathy) should be called "optic disc edema." This convention is arbitrary but serves to avoid confusion. Often it is difficult to differentiate papilledema from other forms of optic disc edema by fundus examination alone. Transient visual obscurations are a classic symptom of papilledema. They occur in only one eye or simultaneously in both eyes. They usually last seconds but can persist longer. Obscurations follow abrupt shifts in posture or happen spontaneously. When obscurations are prolonged or spontaneous, the papilledema is more threatening. Visual acuity is not affected by papilledema unless the papilledema is severe, longstanding, or accompanied by macular edema and hemorrhage. Visual field testing shows enlarged blind spots and peripheral constriction (Fig. 32-3*F*). With unremitting papilledema, peripheral visual field loss progresses in an insidious fashion while the optic nerve develops atrophy. In this setting, reduction of optic disc swelling is an ominous sign of a dying nerve rather than an encouraging indication of resolving papilledema.

Evaluation of papilledema requires neuroimaging to exclude an intracranial lesion. Noninvasive MR vascular imaging may be useful in selected cases to search for a dural venous sinus thrombosis or an arteriovenous shunt. If neuroradiologic studies are negative, the subarachnoid opening pressure should be measured in the lateral decubitus position by lumbar puncture. Inaccurate pressure readings are a common pitfall. An elevated pressure, with normal cerebrospinal fluid, points by exclusion to the diagnosis of *pseudotumor cerebri* (idiopathic intracranial hypertension). Almost all patients are female, and most are obese. Treatment with a carbonic anhydrase inhibitor such as acetazolamide lowers intracranial pressure by reducing the production of cerebrospinal fluid and improves the visual fields. Weight reduction is vital: bariatric surgery should be considered in patients who cannot lose weight by diet control. If vision loss is severe or progressive, a shunt should be performed without delay to prevent blindness. Placement of a stent across the junction of the transverse and sigmoid dural sinuses, where stenosis is usually present, has emerged as a new treatment option. Optic nerve sheath fenestration is a less effective approach and does not address other neurologic symptoms. Occasionally, fulminant papilledema produces rapid onset of blindness. In such patients, emergency surgery should be performed to install a shunt.

Optic Disc Drusen These are refractile, glittering particles within the substance of the optic nerve head (**Fig. 32-13**). They are unrelated to drusen of the retina, which occur in age-related macular degeneration. Optic disc drusen are most common in people of northern European descent. Their diagnosis is obvious when they are visible on the surface of the optic disc. However, in many patients, they are hidden beneath the surface, producing pseudopapilledema. It is important to recognize optic disc drusen to avoid an unnecessary evaluation for papilledema. When optic disc drusen are buried, B-ultrasound is the most sensitive way to detect them. They appear hyperechoic because they contain calcium. They are also visible on computed tomography (CT) or optical coherence tomography (OCT), a technique for acquiring cross-section images of the retina. In most patients, optic disc drusen are an incidental, innocuous finding, but they can produce visual obscurations. On perimetry, they give rise to enlarged blind spots and arcuate scotomas from damage to the optic disc. With increasing age, drusen tend to become more exposed on the disc surface as optic atrophy develops. Hemorrhage, choroidal neovascular membrane, and AION are more likely to occur in patients with optic disc drusen. No treatment is available.

Vitreous Degeneration This occurs in all individuals with advancing age, leading to visual symptoms. Opacities develop in the vitreous, casting annoying shadows on the retina. As the eye moves, these distracting "floaters" move synchronously, with a slight lag caused by inertia of the vitreous gel. Vitreous traction on the retina causes mechanical stimulation, resulting in perception of flashing lights. This photopsia is brief and is confined to one eye, in contrast to the bilateral, prolonged scintillations of cortical migraine. Contraction of the vitreous can result in sudden separation from the retina, heralded by an alarming shower of floaters and photopsia. This process, known as *vitreous detachment*, is a common involutional event in the elderly. It is not harmful unless it damages the retina. A careful examination of the dilated fundus is important in any patient complaining of floaters or photopsia to search for peripheral tears or holes. If such a lesion is found, laser application can forestall a retinal detachment. Occasionally a tear ruptures a retinal blood vessel, causing vitreous hemorrhage and sudden loss of vision. On attempted ophthalmoscopy the fundus is hidden by a dark haze of blood. Ultrasound is required to examine the interior of the eye for a retinal tear or detachment. If the hemorrhage does not resolve spontaneously, the vitreous can be removed surgically. Vitreous hemorrhage also results from the fragile neovascular vessels that proliferate on the surface of the retina in diabetes, sickle cell anemia, and other ischemic ocular diseases.

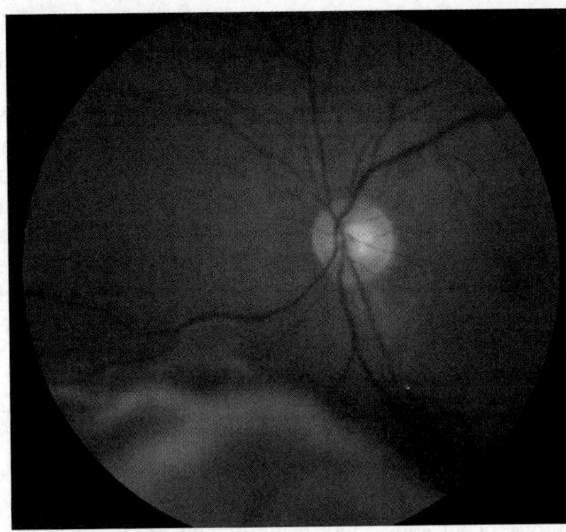

FIGURE 32-14 Retinal detachment appears as an elevated sheet of retinal tissue with folds. In this patient, the fovea was spared, so acuity was normal, but an inferior detachment produced a superior scotoma.

Retinal Detachment This produces symptoms of floaters, flashing lights, and a scotoma in the peripheral visual field corresponding to the detachment (Fig. 32-14). If the detachment includes the fovea, there is an afferent pupil defect and the visual acuity is reduced. In most eyes, retinal detachment starts with a hole, flap, or tear in the peripheral retina (rhegmatogenous retinal detachment). Patients with peripheral retinal thinning (lattice degeneration) are particularly vulnerable to this process. Once a break has developed in the retina, liquefied vitreous is free to enter the subretinal space, separating the retina from the pigment epithelium. The combination of vitreous traction on the retinal surface and passage of fluid behind the retina leads inexorably to detachment. Patients with a history of myopia, trauma, or prior cataract extraction are at greatest risk for retinal detachment. The diagnosis is confirmed by ophthalmoscopic examination of the dilated eye.

Classic Migraine (See also Chap. 430) This usually occurs with a visual aura lasting about 20 min. In a typical attack, a small central disturbance in the field of vision marches toward the periphery, leaving a transient scotoma in its wake. The expanding border of migraine scotoma has a scintillating, dancing, or zigzag edge, resembling the bastions of a fortified city, hence the term *fortification spectra*. Patients' descriptions of fortification spectra vary widely and can be confused with amaurosis fugax. Migraine patterns usually last longer and are perceived in both eyes, whereas amaurosis fugax is briefer and occurs in only one eye. Migraine phenomena also remain visible in the dark or with the eyes closed. Generally, they are confined to either the right or the left visual hemifield, but sometimes, both fields are involved simultaneously. Patients often have a long history of stereotypic attacks. After the visual symptoms recede, headache develops in most patients.

Transient Ischemic Attacks Vertebrobasilar insufficiency may result in acute homonymous visual symptoms. Many patients mistakenly describe symptoms in the left or right eye when in fact the symptoms are occurring in the left or right hemifield of both eyes. Interruption of blood supply to the visual cortex causes a sudden fogging or graying of vision, occasionally with flashing lights or other positive phenomena that mimic migraine. Cortical ischemic attacks are briefer in duration than migraine, occur in older patients, and are not followed by headache. There may be associated signs of brainstem ischemia, such as diplopia, vertigo, numbness, weakness, and dysarthria.

Stroke Stroke occurs when interruption of blood supply from the posterior cerebral artery to the visual cortex is prolonged. The only finding on examination is a homonymous visual field defect that stops abruptly at the vertical meridian. Occipital lobe stroke usually is due to thrombotic occlusion of the vertebrobasilar system, embolus, or dissection. Lobar hemorrhage, tumor, abscess, and arteriovenous malformation are other common causes of hemianopic cortical visual loss.

Factitious (Functional, Nonorganic) Visual Loss This is claimed by hysterics or malingerers. The latter account for the vast majority, seeking sympathy, special treatment, or financial gain by feigning loss of sight. The diagnosis is suspected when the history is atypical, physical findings are lacking or contradictory, inconsistencies emerge on testing, and a secondary motive can be identified. In our litigious society, the fraudulent pursuit of recompense has spawned an epidemic of factitious visual loss.

CHRONIC VISUAL LOSS

Cataract Cataract is a clouding of the lens sufficient to reduce vision. Most cataracts develop slowly as a result of aging, leading to gradual impairment of vision. The formation of cataract occurs more rapidly in patients with a history of uveitis, diabetes mellitus, ocular trauma, or vitrectomy. Cataracts are acquired in a variety of genetic diseases, such as myotonic dystrophy, neurofibromatosis type 2, and galactosemia. Radiation therapy and glucocorticoid treatment can induce cataract as a side effect. The cataracts associated with radiation or glucocorticoids have a typical posterior subcapsular location. Cataract can be detected by noting an impaired red reflex when viewing light reflected from the fundus with an ophthalmoscope or by examining the dilated eye with the slit lamp.

The only treatment for cataract is surgical extraction of the opacified lens. Millions of cataract operations are performed each year around the globe. The operation generally is done under local anesthesia on an outpatient basis. A plastic or silicone intraocular lens is placed within the empty lens capsule in the posterior chamber, substituting for the natural lens and leading to rapid recovery of sight. More than 95% of patients who undergo cataract extraction can expect an improvement in vision. In some patients, the lens capsule remaining in the eye after cataract extraction eventually turns cloudy, causing secondary loss of vision. A small opening, called a posterior capsulotomy, is made in the lens capsule with a laser to restore clarity.

Glaucoma Glaucoma is a slowly progressive, insidious optic neuropathy that usually is associated with chronic elevation of intraocular pressure. After cataract, it is the most common cause of blindness in the world. It is especially prevalent in people of African descent. The mechanism by which raised intraocular pressure injures the optic nerve is not understood. Axons entering the inferotemporal and superotemporal aspects of the optic disc are damaged first, producing typical nerve fiber bundle defects called arcuate scotomas. As fibers are destroyed, the neural rim of the optic disc shrinks and the physiologic cup within the optic disc enlarges (Fig. 32-15). This process is referred to as pathologic "cupping." The cup-to-disc diameter is expressed as a fraction (e.g., 0.2). The cup-to-disc ratio ranges widely in normal individuals, making it difficult to diagnose glaucoma reliably simply by

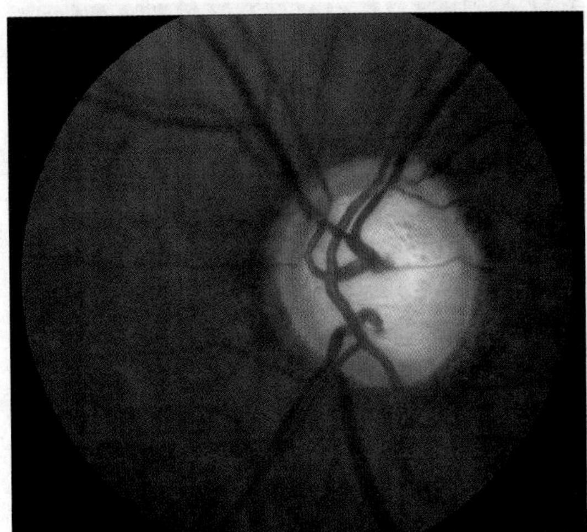

FIGURE 32-15 Glaucoma results in "cupping" as the neural rim is destroyed and the central cup becomes enlarged and excavated. The cup-to-disc ratio is about 0.8 in this patient.

observing an unusually large or deep optic cup. Careful documentation of serial examinations is helpful. In a patient with physiologic cupping, the large cup remains stable, whereas in a patient with glaucoma, it expands relentlessly over the years. Observation of progressive cupping and detection of an arcuate scotoma or a nasal step on computerized visual field testing is sufficient to establish the diagnosis of glaucoma. OCT reveals corresponding loss of fibers along the arcuate pathways in the nerve fiber layer.

The preponderance of patients with glaucoma have open anterior chamber angles. In most affected individuals, the intraocular pressure is elevated. The cause of elevated intraocular pressure is unknown, but it is associated with gene mutations in the heritable forms. Surprisingly, a third of patients with open-angle glaucoma have an intraocular pressure within the normal range of 10–20 mmHg. For this so-called normal or low-tension form of glaucoma, high myopia is a risk factor.

Chronic angle-closure glaucoma and chronic open-angle glaucoma are usually asymptomatic. Only acute angle-closure glaucoma causes a red or painful eye, from abrupt elevation of intraocular pressure. In all forms of glaucoma, foveal acuity is spared until end-stage disease is reached. For these reasons, severe and irreversible damage can occur before either the patient or the physician recognizes the diagnosis. Screening of patients for glaucoma by noting the cup-to-disc ratio on ophthalmoscopy and by measuring intraocular pressure is vital. Glaucoma is treated with topical adrenergic agonists, cholinergic agonists, beta blockers, prostaglandin analogues, and carbonic anhydrase inhibitors. Occasionally, systemic absorption of beta blocker from eyedrops can be sufficient to cause side effects of bradycardia, hypotension, heart block, bronchospasm, or depression. Laser treatment of the trabecular meshwork in the anterior chamber angle improves aqueous outflow from the eye. If medical or laser treatments fail to halt optic nerve damage from glaucoma, a filter must be constructed surgically (trabeculectomy) or a drainage device placed to release aqueous from the eye in a controlled fashion.

Macular Degeneration This is a major cause of gradual, painless, bilateral central visual loss in the elderly. It occurs in a nonexudative (dry) form and an exudative (wet) form. Inflammation may be important in both forms of macular degeneration; susceptibility is associated with variants in the gene for complement factor H, an inhibitor of the alternative complement pathway. The nonexudative process begins with the accumulation of extracellular deposits called drusen underneath the retinal pigment epithelium. On ophthalmoscopy, they are pleomorphic but generally appear as small discrete yellow lesions clustered in the macula (**Fig. 32-16**). With time, they become larger, more numerous, and confluent. The retinal pigment epithelium becomes focally detached and atrophic, causing visual loss by interfering with photoreceptor function. Treatment with vitamins C and E, beta-carotene, and zinc may retard dry macular degeneration.

Exudative macular degeneration, which develops in only a minority of patients, occurs when neovascular vessels from the choroid grow through defects in Bruch's membrane and proliferate underneath the retinal pigment epithelium or the retina. Leakage from these vessels produces elevation of the retina, with distortion (metamorphopsia) and blurring of vision. Although the onset of these symptoms is usually gradual, bleeding from a subretinal choroidal neovascular membrane sometimes causes acute visual loss. Neovascular membranes can be difficult to see on fundus examination because they are located beneath the retina. Fluorescein angiography and OCT are extremely useful for their detection. Major or repeated hemorrhage under the retina from neovascular membranes results in fibrosis, development of a round (disciform) macular scar, and permanent loss of central vision.

A major therapeutic advance has occurred with the discovery that exudative macular degeneration can be treated with intraocular injection of antagonists to vascular endothelial growth factor. Bevacizumab, ranibizumab, aflibercept, or brolucizumab is administered by direct injection into the vitreous cavity, beginning on a monthly basis. These antibodies cause the regression of neovascular membranes by blocking the action of vascular endothelial growth factor, thereby improving visual acuity.

Central Serous Chorioretinopathy This primarily affects males between the ages of 20 and 50 years. Leakage of serous fluid from the choroid causes small, localized detachment of the retinal pigment epithelium and the neurosensory retina. These detachments produce acute or chronic symptoms of metamorphopsia and blurred vision when the macula is involved. They are difficult to visualize with a direct ophthalmoscope because the detached retina is transparent and only slightly elevated. OCT shows fluid beneath the retina, and fluorescein angiography shows dye streaming into the subretinal space. The cause of central serous chorioretinopathy is unknown. Symptoms may resolve spontaneously if the retina reattaches, but recurrent detachment is common. Laser photocoagulation has benefited some patients with this condition.

Diabetic Retinopathy A rare disease until 1921, when the discovery of insulin resulted in a dramatic improvement in life expectancy for patients with diabetes mellitus, diabetic retinopathy is now a leading cause of blindness in the United States. The retinopathy takes years to develop but eventually appears in nearly all cases. Regular surveillance of the dilated fundus is crucial for any patient with diabetes. In advanced diabetic retinopathy, the proliferation of neovascular vessels leads to blindness from vitreous hemorrhage, retinal detachment, and glaucoma (**Fig. 32-17**). These complications can be avoided in most patients by administration of panretinal laser photocoagulation at the appropriate point in the evolution of the disease. Anti-vascular

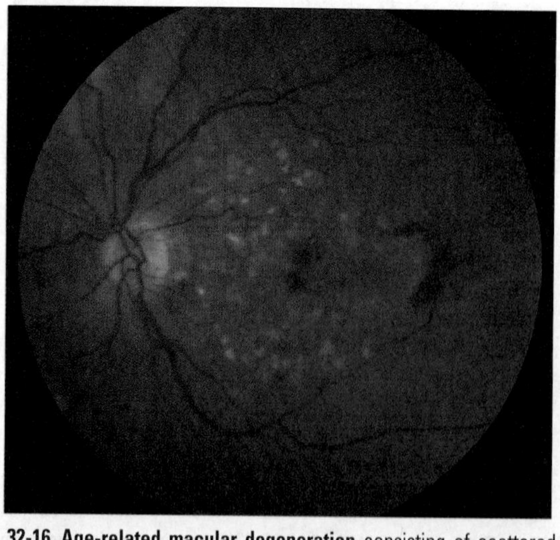

FIGURE 32-16 Age-related macular degeneration consisting of scattered yellow drusen in the macula (dry form) and a crescent of fresh hemorrhage temporal to the fovea from a subretinal neovascular membrane (wet form).

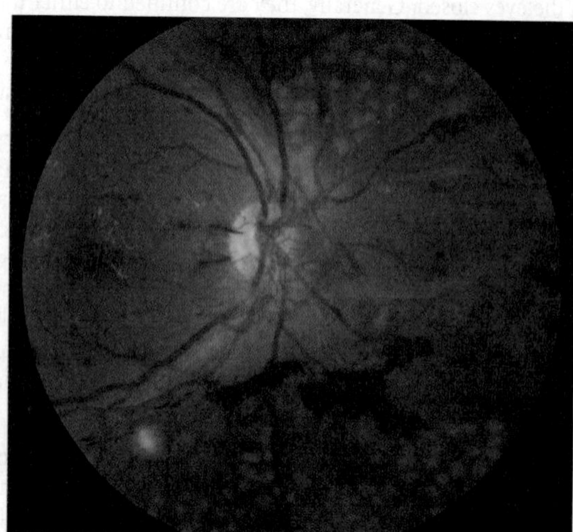

FIGURE 32-17 Proliferative diabetic retinopathy in a 25-year-old man with an 18-year history of diabetes, showing neovascular vessels emanating from the optic disc, retinal and vitreous hemorrhage, cotton-wool spots, and macular exudate. Round spots in the periphery represent recently applied panretinal photocoagulation.

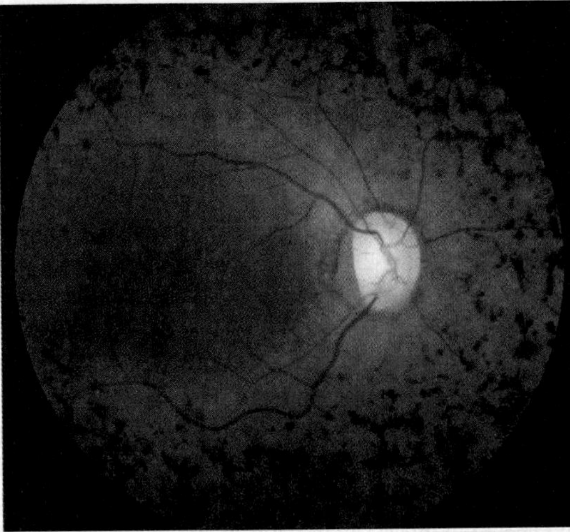

FIGURE 32-18 Retinitis pigmentosa with black clumps of pigment known as "bone spicules." The patient had peripheral visual field loss with sparing of central (macular) vision.

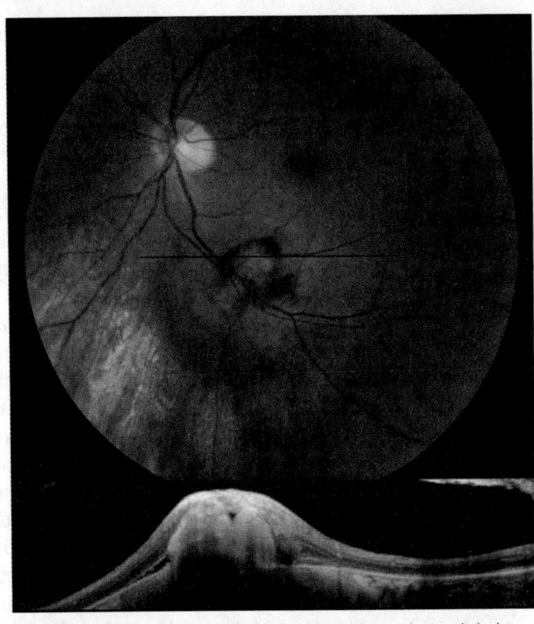

FIGURE 32-19 Melanoma of the choroid, appearing as an elevated dark mass in the inferior fundus, with overlying hemorrhage. The black line denotes the plane of the optical coherence tomography scan (*below*) showing the subretinal tumor.

endothelial growth factor antibody treatment is equally effective, but intraocular injections must be given repeatedly. **For further discussion of the manifestations and management of diabetic retinopathy, see Chaps. 403–405.**

Retinitis Pigmentosa This is a general term for a disparate group of rod-cone dystrophies characterized by progressive night blindness, visual field constriction with a ring scotoma, loss of acuity, and an abnormal electroretinogram (ERG). It occurs sporadically or in an autosomal recessive, dominant, or X-linked pattern. Irregular black deposits of clumped pigment in the peripheral retina, called *bone spicules* because of their vague resemblance to the spicules of cancellous bone, give the disease its name **(Fig. 32-18)**. The name is actually a misnomer because retinitis pigmentosa is not an inflammatory process. Genetic testing usually identifies a mutation in the gene for rhodopsin, the rod photopigment, or in the gene for peripherin, a glycoprotein located in photoreceptor outer segments. Vitamin A (15,000 IU/d) slightly retards the deterioration of the ERG in patients with retinitis pigmentosa but has no beneficial effect on visual acuity or fields.

Leber's congenital amaurosis, a rare cone dystrophy, has been treated by replacement of the missing RPE65 protein through gene therapy, resulting in slight improvement in visual function. Some forms of retinitis pigmentosa occur in association with rare, hereditary systemic diseases (olivopontocerebellar degeneration, Bassen-Kornzweig disease, Kearns-Sayre syndrome, Refsum's disease). Chronic treatment with chloroquine, hydroxychloroquine, and phenothiazines (especially thioridazine) can produce visual loss from a toxic retinopathy that resembles retinitis pigmentosa. Patients receiving long-term treatment with hydroxychloroquine require regular eye examinations to monitor for potential development of a bull's eye maculopathy.

Epiretinal Membrane This is a fibrocellular tissue that grows across the inner surface of the retina, causing metamorphopsia and reduced visual acuity from distortion of the macula. A crinkled, cellophane-like membrane is visible on the retinal examination. Epiretinal membrane is most common in patients aged >50 years and is usually unilateral. Most cases are idiopathic, but some occur as a result of hypertensive retinopathy, diabetes, retinal detachment, or trauma. When visual acuity is reduced to the level of about 6/24 (20/80), vitrectomy and surgical peeling of the membrane to relieve macular puckering are recommended. Contraction of an epiretinal membrane sometimes gives rise to a *macular hole*. Most macular holes, however, are caused by local vitreous traction within the fovea. Vitrectomy can improve acuity in selected cases.

Melanoma and Other Tumors Melanoma is the most common primary tumor of the eye **(Fig. 32-19)**. Approximately 2000 cases occur annually in the United States. It causes photopsia, an enlarging scotoma, and loss of vision. A small melanoma is often difficult to differentiate from a benign choroidal nevus. Serial examinations are required to document a malignant pattern of growth. Risk factors include light skin, hair, and eyes. Uveal origin accounts for 85% of cases. *GNAQ* and *GNA11* mutations are common. About half metastasize, mainly to the liver. Small and medium-sized tumors may be treated with radiation therapy; enucleation is the best treatment for large tumors. *Metastatic tumors* to the eye outnumber primary tumors. Breast and lung carcinomas have a special propensity to spread to the choroid or iris. Leukemia and lymphoma also commonly invade ocular tissues. Sometimes their only sign on eye examination is cellular debris in the vitreous, which can masquerade as a chronic posterior uveitis.

In a patient with vision loss, CT or MR scanning should be considered if the cause remains unknown after careful review of the history, visual fields, and thorough examination of the eye. Optic nerve sheath meningioma is a common retrobulbar tumor. It produces the classic triad of optociliary shunt vessels, optic atrophy, and progressive visual loss. Optic disc swelling and proptosis are also frequent signs. Optic nerve glioma in young patients is usually a pilocytic astrocytoma and has a good prognosis for preservation of vision, especially in neurofibromatosis type 1 **(Chap. 90)**. In adults, optic nerve glioma is rare and highly malignant. Chiasmal tumors (pituitary adenoma, meningioma, craniopharyngioma) produce visual loss with few objective findings except for optic disc pallor. Loss of the temporal visual field in each eye is typically described, but in fact, patients complain of vision loss in just one eye. A high degree of vigilance is necessary to avoid missing chiasmal tumors. Although symptoms progress gradually, in rare instances, the sudden expansion of a pituitary adenoma from infarction and bleeding (*pituitary apoplexy*) causes acute retrobulbar visual loss, with headache, nausea, and ocular motor nerve palsies.

PROPTOSIS

When the globes appear asymmetric, the clinician must first decide which eye is abnormal. Is one eye recessed within the orbit (*enophthalmos*), or is the other eye protuberant (*exophthalmos*, or *proptosis*)? A small globe or Horner's syndrome can give the appearance of enophthalmos. True enophthalmos occurs commonly after trauma, from atrophy of retrobulbar fat, or from fracture of the orbital floor. The position of the eyes within the orbits is measured by using a Hertel exophthalmometer, a handheld instrument that records the position of the anterior corneal surface relative to the lateral orbital rim. If this instrument is not available, relative eye position can be judged by bending the patient's head forward and looking down upon the orbits.

A proptosis of only 2 mm in one eye is detectable from this perspective. The development of proptosis implies a space-occupying lesion in the orbit and usually warrants CT or MR imaging.

Graves' Ophthalmopathy This is the leading cause of proptosis in adults (**Chap. 382**). The proptosis is often asymmetric and can even appear to be unilateral. Orbital inflammation and engorgement of the extraocular muscles, particularly the medial rectus and the inferior rectus, account for the protrusion of the globe. Corneal exposure, lid retraction, lid lag on downgaze, conjunctival injection, restriction of gaze, diplopia, and visual loss from optic nerve compression are cardinal symptoms. Graves' eye disease is a clinical diagnosis, but laboratory testing can be useful. The serum level of thyroid-stimulating immunoglobulins is often elevated. Orbital imaging usually reveals enlarged extraocular eye muscles, but not always. Topical lubricants, taping the eyelids closed at night, and moisture chambers are helpful to limit exposure of ocular tissues. Graves' ophthalmopathy can be treated with oral prednisone (60 mg/d) for 1 month, followed by a taper over several months, but worsening of symptoms upon glucocorticoid withdrawal is common. Infusions of teprotumumab, an inhibitor of the insulin-like growth factor I receptor, reduce proptosis and diplopia. Radiation therapy is not effective. Orbital decompression should be performed for severe, symptomatic exophthalmos or if visual function is reduced by optic nerve compression. In patients with diplopia, prisms or eye muscle surgery can be used to restore ocular alignment in primary gaze.

Orbital Pseudotumor This is an idiopathic, inflammatory orbital syndrome that is distinguished from Graves' ophthalmopathy by the prominent complaint of pain. Other symptoms include diplopia, ptosis, proptosis, and orbital congestion. Evaluation for sarcoidosis, granulomatosis with polyangiitis, and other types of orbital vasculitis or collagen-vascular disease is negative. Imaging often shows swollen eye muscles (orbital myositis) with enlarged tendons. By contrast, in Graves' ophthalmopathy, the tendons of the eye muscles usually are spared. The Tolosa-Hunt syndrome (**Chap. 441**) may be regarded as an extension of orbital pseudotumor through the superior orbital fissure into the cavernous sinus. The diagnosis of orbital pseudotumor is difficult. Biopsy of the orbit frequently yields nonspecific evidence of fat infiltration by lymphocytes, plasma cells, and eosinophils. A dramatic response to a therapeutic trial of systemic glucocorticoids indirectly provides the best confirmation of the diagnosis.

Orbital Cellulitis This causes pain, lid erythema, proptosis, conjunctival chemosis, restricted motility, decreased acuity, afferent pupillary defect, fever, and leukocytosis. It often arises from the paranasal sinuses, especially by contiguous spread of infection from the ethmoid sinus through the lamina papyracea of the medial orbit. A history of recent upper respiratory tract infection, chronic sinusitis, thick mucus secretions, or dental disease is significant in any patient with suspected orbital cellulitis. Blood cultures should be obtained, but they are usually negative. Most patients respond to empirical therapy with broad-spectrum IV antibiotics. Occasionally, orbital cellulitis follows an overwhelming course, with massive proptosis, blindness, septic cavernous sinus thrombosis, and meningitis. To avert this disaster, orbital cellulitis should be managed aggressively in the early stages, with immediate imaging of the orbits and antibiotic therapy that includes coverage of methicillin-resistant *Staphylococcus aureus* (MRSA). Prompt surgical drainage of an orbital abscess or paranasal sinusitis is indicated if optic nerve function deteriorates despite antibiotics.

Tumors Tumors of the orbit cause painless, progressive proptosis. The most common primary tumors are cavernous hemangioma, lymphangioma, neurofibroma, schwannoma, dermoid cyst, adenoid cystic carcinoma, optic nerve glioma, optic nerve meningioma, and benign mixed tumor of the lacrimal gland. Metastatic tumor to the orbit occurs frequently in breast carcinoma, lung carcinoma, and lymphoma. Diagnosis by fine-needle aspiration followed by urgent radiation therapy sometimes can preserve vision.

Carotid Cavernous Fistulas With anterior drainage through the orbit, these fistulas produce proptosis, diplopia, glaucoma, and corkscrew, arterialized conjunctival vessels. Direct fistulas usually result from trauma. They are easily diagnosed because of the prominent signs produced by high-flow, high-pressure shunting. Indirect fistulas, or dural arteriovenous malformations, are more likely to occur spontaneously, especially in older women. The signs are more subtle, and the diagnosis frequently is missed. The combination of slight proptosis, diplopia, enlarged muscles, and an injected eye often is mistaken for thyroid ophthalmopathy. A bruit heard upon auscultation of the head or reported by the patient is a valuable diagnostic clue. Imaging shows an enlarged superior ophthalmic vein in the orbits. Carotid cavernous shunts can be eliminated by intravascular embolization.

PTOSIS

Blepharoptosis This is an abnormal drooping of the eyelid. Unilateral or bilateral ptosis can be congenital, from dysgenesis of the levator palpebrae superioris, or from abnormal insertion of its aponeurosis into the eyelid. Acquired ptosis can develop so gradually that the patient is unaware of the problem. Inspection of old photographs is helpful in dating the onset. A history of prior trauma, eye surgery, contact lens use, diplopia, systemic symptoms (e.g., dysphagia or peripheral muscle weakness), or a family history of ptosis should be sought. Fluctuating ptosis that worsens late in the day is typical of myasthenia gravis. Ptosis evaluation should focus on evidence for proptosis, eyelid masses or deformities, inflammation, pupil inequality, or limitation of motility. The width of the palpebral fissures is measured in primary gaze to determine the degree of ptosis. The ptosis will be underestimated if the patient compensates by lifting the brow with the frontalis muscle.

Mechanical Ptosis This occurs in many elderly patients from stretching and redundancy of eyelid skin and subcutaneous fat (dermatochalasis). The extra weight of these sagging tissues causes the lid to droop. Enlargement or deformation of the eyelid from infection, tumor, trauma, or inflammation also results in ptosis on a purely mechanical basis.

Aponeurotic Ptosis This is an acquired dehiscence or stretching of the aponeurotic tendon, which connects the levator muscle to the tarsal plate of the eyelid. It occurs commonly in older patients, presumably from loss of connective tissue elasticity. Aponeurotic ptosis is also a common sequela of eyelid swelling from infection or blunt trauma to the orbit, cataract surgery, or contact lens use.

Myogenic Ptosis The causes of *myogenic ptosis* include myasthenia gravis (**Chap. 448**) and a number of rare myopathies that manifest with ptosis. The term *chronic progressive external ophthalmoplegia* refers to a spectrum of systemic diseases caused by mutations of mitochondrial DNA. As the name implies, the most prominent findings are symmetric, slowly progressive ptosis and limitation of eye movements. In general, diplopia is a late symptom because all eye movements are reduced equally. In the *Kearns-Sayre* variant, retinal pigmentary changes and abnormalities of cardiac conduction develop. Peripheral muscle biopsy shows characteristic "ragged-red fibers." *Oculopharyngeal dystrophy* is a distinct autosomal dominant disease with onset in middle age, characterized by ptosis, limited eye movements, and trouble swallowing. *Myotonic dystrophy*, another autosomal dominant disorder, causes ptosis, ophthalmoparesis, cataract, and pigmentary retinopathy. Patients have muscle wasting, myotonia, frontal balding, and cardiac abnormalities.

Neurogenic Ptosis This results from a lesion affecting the innervation to either of the two muscles that open the eyelid: Müller's muscle or the levator palpebrae superioris. Examination of the pupil helps distinguish between these two possibilities. In Horner's syndrome, the eye with ptosis has a smaller pupil and the eye movements are full. In an oculomotor nerve palsy, the eye with the ptosis has a larger or a normal pupil. If the pupil is normal but there is limitation of adduction, elevation, and depression, a pupil-sparing oculomotor nerve palsy is likely (see next section). Rarely, a lesion affecting the small, central subnucleus of the oculomotor complex will cause bilateral ptosis with normal eye movements and pupils.

DOUBLE VISION (DIPLOPIA)

The first point to clarify is whether diplopia persists in either eye after the opposite eye is covered. If it does, the diagnosis is monocular diplopia. The cause is usually intrinsic to the eye and therefore has no dire implications for the patient. Corneal aberrations (e.g., keratoconus, pterygium), uncorrected refractive error, cataract, or foveal traction may give rise to monocular diplopia. Occasionally, it is a symptom of malingering or psychiatric disease. Diplopia alleviated by covering one eye is binocular diplopia and is caused by disruption of ocular alignment. Inquiry should be made into the nature of the double vision (purely side-by-side versus partial vertical displacement of images), mode of onset, duration, intermittency, diurnal variation, and associated neurologic or systemic symptoms. If the patient has diplopia while being examined, motility testing should reveal a deficiency corresponding to the patient's symptoms. However, subtle limitation of ocular excursions is often difficult to detect. For example, a patient with a slight left abducens nerve paresis may appear to have full eye movements despite a complaint of horizontal diplopia upon looking to the left. In this situation, the cover test provides a more sensitive method for demonstrating the ocular misalignment. It should be conducted in primary gaze and then with the head turned and tilted in each direction while the patient fixates a central, distant target. In the above example, a cover test with the head turned to the right bringing the eyes into left gaze will maximize the fixation shift evoked by the cover test.

Occasionally, a cover test performed in an asymptomatic patient during a routine examination will reveal an ocular deviation. If the eye movements are full and the ocular misalignment is equal in all directions of gaze (comitant deviation), the diagnosis is strabismus. In this condition, which affects about 1% of the population, fusion is disrupted in infancy or early childhood. To avoid diplopia, retinal input from the nonfixating eye may be partially suppressed. In some children, this leads to impaired vision (amblyopia, or "lazy" eye) in the deviated eye.

Binocular diplopia results from a wide range of processes: infectious, neoplastic, metabolic, degenerative, inflammatory, and vascular. One must decide whether the diplopia is neurogenic in origin or is due to restriction of globe rotation by local disease in the orbit. Orbital pseudotumor, myositis, infection, tumor, thyroid disease, and muscle entrapment (e.g., from a blowout fracture) cause restrictive diplopia. The diagnosis of restriction is usually made by recognizing other associated signs and symptoms of local orbital disease. Dedicated, high-resolution orbital imaging is helpful when the cause of diplopia is not evident.

Myasthenia Gravis **(See also Chap. 448)** This is a major cause of painless diplopia. The diplopia is often intermittent, variable, and not confined to any single ocular motor nerve distribution. The pupils are always normal. Serial observation of a fatigable ptosis, often accompanied by diplopia from fluctuating ocular misalignment, establishes the diagnosis. Many patients have a purely ocular form of the disease, with no evidence of systemic muscular weakness. Classically, the diagnosis was confirmed by an IV edrophonium injection, which produces a transient reversal of eyelid or eye muscle weakness, but this drug is discontinued in the United States. Blood tests for antibodies against the acetylcholine receptor or the MuSK protein are frequently negative in the purely ocular form of myasthenia gravis. *Botulism* from food or wound poisoning can mimic ocular myasthenia.

If restrictive orbital disease and myasthenia gravis are excluded, a lesion of a cranial nerve supplying innervation to the extraocular muscles is the most likely cause of binocular diplopia.

Oculomotor Nerve The third cranial nerve innervates the medial, inferior, and superior recti; inferior oblique; levator palpebrae superioris; and the iris sphincter. Total palsy of the oculomotor nerve causes ptosis, a dilated pupil, and leaves the eye "down and out" because of the unopposed action of the lateral rectus and superior oblique. This combination of findings is obvious. More challenging is the diagnosis of early or partial oculomotor nerve palsy. In this setting, any combination of ptosis, pupil dilation, and weakness of the eye muscles supplied by the oculomotor nerve may be encountered. Frequent serial examinations during the rapidly evolving phase of the palsy help ensure that the diagnosis is not missed. The advent of an oculomotor nerve palsy with a pupil involvement, especially when accompanied by pain, suggests a compressive lesion, such as a tumor or circle of Willis aneurysm. Urgent neuroimaging should be obtained, along with a CT or MR angiogram. The resolution of these noninvasive techniques has advanced to the point that catheter angiography is rarely necessary to exclude an aneurysm.

A lesion of the oculomotor nucleus in the rostral midbrain produces signs that differ from those caused by a lesion of the nerve itself. There is bilateral ptosis because the levator muscle is innervated by a single central subnucleus. There is also weakness of the contralateral superior rectus, because it is supplied by the oculomotor nucleus on the other side. Occasionally both superior recti are weak. Isolated nuclear oculomotor palsy is rare. Usually, neurologic examination reveals additional signs that suggest brainstem damage from infarction, hemorrhage, tumor, or infection.

Injury to structures surrounding fascicles of the oculomotor nerve descending through the midbrain has given rise to a number of classic eponymic designations. In *Nothnagel's syndrome*, injury to the superior cerebellar peduncle causes ipsilateral oculomotor palsy and contralateral cerebellar ataxia. In *Benedikt's syndrome*, injury to the red nucleus results in ipsilateral oculomotor palsy and contralateral tremor, chorea, and athetosis. *Claude's syndrome* incorporates features of both of these syndromes, by injury to both the red nucleus and the superior cerebellar peduncle. Finally, in *Weber's syndrome*, injury to the cerebral peduncle causes ipsilateral oculomotor palsy with contralateral hemiparesis.

In the subarachnoid space, the oculomotor nerve is vulnerable to aneurysm, meningitis, tumor, infarction, and compression. In cerebral herniation, the nerve becomes trapped between the edge of the tentorium and the uncus of the temporal lobe. Oculomotor palsy also can result from midbrain torsion and hemorrhage during herniation. In the cavernous sinus, oculomotor palsy arises from carotid aneurysm, carotid cavernous fistula, cavernous sinus thrombosis, tumor (pituitary adenoma, meningioma, metastasis), herpes zoster infection, and the Tolosa-Hunt syndrome.

The etiology of an isolated, pupil-sparing oculomotor palsy often remains an enigma even after neuroimaging and extensive laboratory testing. Most cases are thought to result from microvascular infarction of the nerve somewhere along its course from the brainstem to the orbit. Usually, the patient complains of pain. Diabetes, hypertension, and vascular disease are major risk factors. Spontaneous recovery over a period of months is the rule. If this fails to occur or if new findings develop, the diagnosis of microvascular oculomotor nerve palsy should be reconsidered. Aberrant regeneration is common when the oculomotor nerve is injured by trauma or compression (tumor, aneurysm). Miswiring of sprouting fibers to the levator muscle and the rectus muscles results in elevation of the eyelid upon downgaze or adduction. The pupil also constricts upon attempted adduction, elevation, or depression of the globe. Aberrant regeneration is not seen after oculomotor palsy from microvascular infarct and hence vitiates that diagnosis.

Trochlear Nerve The fourth cranial nerve originates in the midbrain, just caudal to the oculomotor nerve complex. Fibers exit the brainstem dorsally and cross to innervate the contralateral superior oblique. The principal actions of this muscle are to depress and intort the globe. A palsy therefore results in hypertropia and excyclotorsion. The cyclotorsion seldom is noticed by patients. Instead, they complain of vertical diplopia, especially upon reading or looking down. Vertical diplopia is exacerbated by tilting the head toward the side with the muscle palsy and alleviated by tilting it away. This "head tilt test" is a cardinal diagnostic feature. Review of old photographs will sometimes reveal a habitual head tilt, signifying a patient with a decompensated, congenital trochlear nerve palsy.

New, isolated trochlear nerve palsy results from all the causes listed above for the oculomotor nerve except aneurysm. The trochlear nerve is particularly apt to suffer injury after closed head trauma. The free edge of the tentorium impinges on the nerve during a concussive blow.

Most isolated trochlear nerve palsies are idiopathic and hence are diagnosed by exclusion as "microvascular." Spontaneous improvement occurs over a period of months in most patients. A base-down prism (conveniently applied to the patient's glasses as a stick-on Fresnel lens) may serve as a temporary measure to alleviate diplopia. If the palsy does not resolve, the eyes can be realigned by weakening the inferior oblique muscle.

Abducens Nerve The sixth cranial nerve innervates the lateral rectus muscle. A palsy produces horizontal diplopia, worse on gaze to the side of the lesion. A nuclear lesion has different consequences, because the abducens nucleus contains interneurons that project via the medial longitudinal fasciculus to the medial rectus subnucleus of the contralateral oculomotor complex. Therefore, an abducens nuclear lesion produces a complete lateral gaze palsy from weakness of both the ipsilateral lateral rectus and the contralateral medial rectus. *Foville's syndrome* after dorsal pontine injury includes lateral gaze palsy, ipsilateral facial palsy, and contralateral hemiparesis incurred by damage to descending corticospinal fibers. *Millard-Gubler syndrome* from ventral pontine injury is similar except for the eye findings. There is lateral rectus weakness only, instead of gaze palsy, because the abducens fascicle is injured rather than the nucleus. Infarct, tumor, hemorrhage, vascular malformation, and multiple sclerosis are the most common etiologies of brainstem abducens palsy.

After leaving the ventral pons, the abducens nerve runs forward along the clivus to pierce the dura at the petrous apex, where it enters the cavernous sinus. Along its subarachnoid course, it is susceptible to meningitis, tumor (meningioma, chordoma, carcinomatous meningitis), subarachnoid hemorrhage, trauma, and compression by aneurysm or dolichoectatic vessels. At the petrous apex, mastoiditis can produce deafness, pain, and ipsilateral abducens palsy (*Gradenigo's syndrome*). In the cavernous sinus, the nerve can be affected by carotid aneurysm, carotid cavernous fistula, tumor (pituitary adenoma, meningioma, nasopharyngeal carcinoma), herpes infection, and Tolosa-Hunt syndrome.

Unilateral or bilateral abducens palsy is a classic sign of raised intracranial pressure. The diagnosis can be confirmed if papilledema is observed on fundus examination. The mechanism is still debated but probably is related to rostral-caudal displacement of the brainstem. The same phenomenon accounts for abducens palsy from Chiari malformation or low intracranial pressure (e.g., after lumbar puncture, spinal anesthesia, or spontaneous dural cerebrospinal fluid leak).

Treatment of abducens palsy is aimed at prompt correction of the underlying cause. However, the cause remains obscure in many instances despite diligent evaluation. As was mentioned above for isolated trochlear or oculomotor palsy, most cases are assumed to represent microvascular infarcts because they often occur in the setting of diabetes or other vascular risk factors. Some cases may develop as a postinfectious mononeuritis (e.g., after a viral flu). Patching one eye, occluding one eyeglass lens with tape, or applying a temporary prism will provide relief of diplopia until the palsy resolves. If recovery is incomplete, eye muscle surgery nearly always can realign the eyes, at least in primary position. A patient with an abducens palsy that fails to improve should be reevaluated for an occult etiology (e.g., chordoma, carcinomatous meningitis, carotid cavernous fistula, myasthenia gravis). Skull base tumors are easily missed even on contrast-enhanced neuroimaging studies.

Multiple Ocular Motor Nerve Palsies These should not be attributed to spontaneous microvascular events affecting more than one cranial nerve at a time. This remarkable coincidence does occur, especially in diabetic patients, but the diagnosis is made only in retrospect after all other diagnostic alternatives have been exhausted. Neuroimaging should focus on the cavernous sinus, superior orbital fissure, and orbital apex, where all three ocular motor nerves are in close proximity. In a diabetic or immunocompromised host, fungal infection (*Aspergillus*, Mucorales, *Cryptococcus*) is a common cause of multiple nerve palsies. In a patient with systemic malignancy, carcinomatous meningitis is a likely diagnosis. Cytologic examination may be negative despite repeated sampling of the cerebrospinal fluid. The cancer-associated Lambert-Eaton myasthenic syndrome also can produce ophthalmoplegia. Giant cell (temporal) arteritis occasionally manifests as diplopia from ischemic palsies of extraocular muscles. Fisher's syndrome, an ocular variant of Guillain-Barré, produces ophthalmoplegia with areflexia and ataxia. Often the ataxia is mild, and the reflexes are normal. Antiganglioside antibodies (GQ1b) can be detected in about 50% of cases.

Supranuclear Disorders of Gaze These are often mistaken for multiple ocular motor nerve palsies. For example, Wernicke's encephalopathy can produce nystagmus and a partial deficit of horizontal and vertical gaze that mimics a combined abducens and oculomotor nerve palsy. The disorder occurs in patients who are malnourished, alcoholic, or following bariatric surgery, and can be reversed by thiamine. Infarct, hemorrhage, tumor, multiple sclerosis, encephalitis, vasculitis, and Whipple's disease are other important causes of supranuclear gaze palsy. Disorders of vertical gaze, especially downward saccades, are an early feature of progressive supranuclear palsy. Smooth pursuit is affected later in the course of the disease. Parkinson's disease, Huntington's disease, and olivopontocerebellar degeneration also can affect vertical gaze.

The *frontal eye field* of the cerebral cortex is involved in generation of saccades to the contralateral side. After hemispheric stroke, the eyes usually deviate toward the lesioned side because of the unopposed action of the frontal eye field in the normal hemisphere. With time, this deficit resolves. Seizures generally have the opposite effect: the eyes deviate conjugately away from the irritative focus. *Parietal lesions* disrupt smooth pursuit of targets moving toward the side of the lesion. Bilateral parietal lesions produce *Bálint's syndrome*, which is characterized by impaired eye-hand coordination (optic ataxia), difficulty initiating voluntary eye movements (ocular apraxia), and visuospatial disorientation (simultanagnosia).

Horizontal Gaze Descending cortical inputs mediating horizontal gaze ultimately converge at the level of the pons. Neurons in the paramedian pontine reticular formation are responsible for controlling conjugate gaze toward the same side. They project directly to the ipsilateral abducens nucleus. A lesion of either the paramedian pontine reticular formation or the abducens nucleus causes an ipsilateral conjugate gaze palsy. Lesions at either locus produce nearly identical clinical syndromes, with the following exception: vestibular stimulation (oculocephalic maneuver or caloric irrigation) will succeed in driving the eyes conjugately to the side in a patient with a lesion of the paramedian pontine reticular formation but not in a patient with a lesion of the abducens nucleus.

INTERNUCLEAR OPHTHALMOPLEGIA This results from damage to the medial longitudinal fasciculus ascending from the abducens nucleus in the pons to the oculomotor nucleus in the midbrain (hence, "internuclear"). Damage to fibers carrying the conjugate signal from abducens interneurons to the contralateral medial rectus motoneurons results in a failure of adduction on attempted lateral gaze. For example, a patient with a left internuclear ophthalmoplegia (INO) will have slowed or absent adducting movements of the left eye (**Fig. 32-20**). A patient with bilateral injury to the medial longitudinal fasciculus will have bilateral INO. Multiple sclerosis is the most common cause, although tumor, stroke, trauma, or any brainstem process may be responsible. *One-and-a-half syndrome* is due to a lesion of the medial longitudinal fasciculus combined with a lesion of either the abducens nucleus or the paramedian pontine reticular formation on the same side. The patient's only horizontal eye movement is abduction of the eye on the other side.

Vertical Gaze This is controlled at the level of the midbrain. The neuronal circuits affected in disorders of vertical gaze are not fully elucidated, but lesions of the rostral interstitial nucleus of the medial longitudinal fasciculus and the interstitial nucleus of Cajal cause supranuclear paresis of upgaze, downgaze, or all vertical eye movements. Distal basilar artery ischemia is the most common etiology.

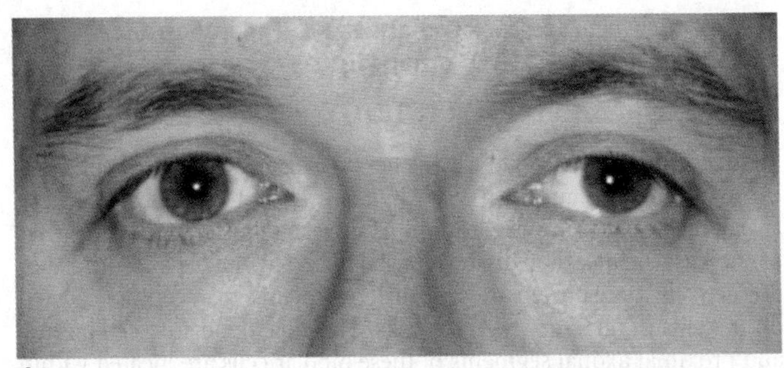

A

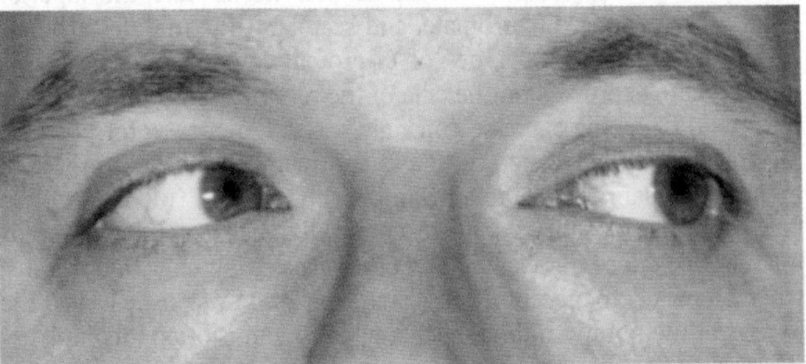

B

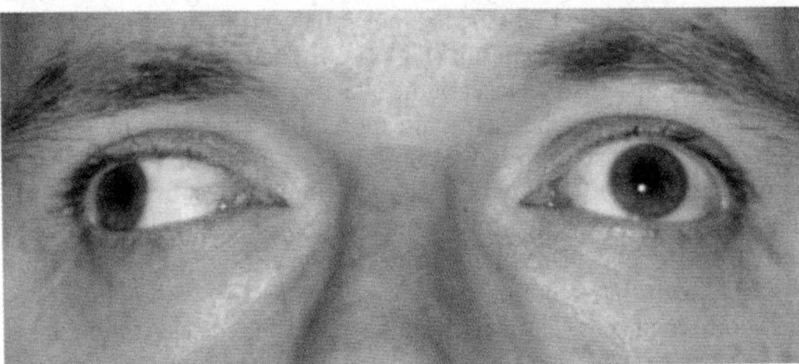

C

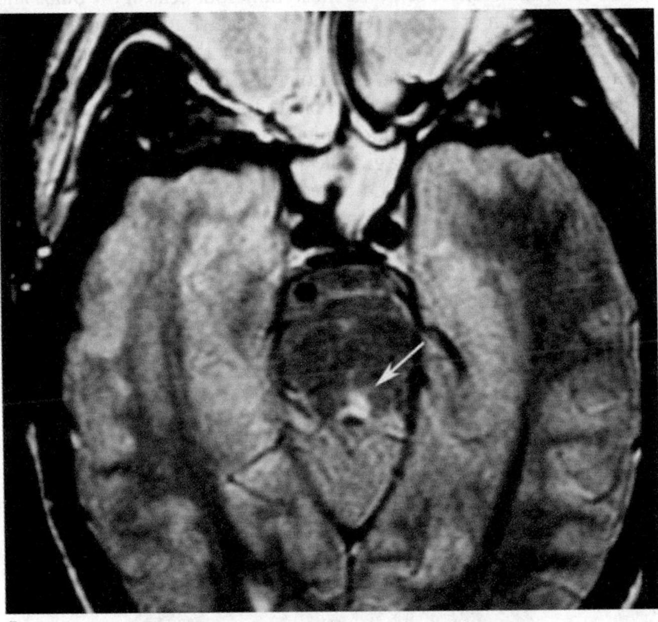

D

FIGURE 32-20 Left internuclear ophthalmoplegia (INO). ***A.*** In primary position of gaze, the eyes appear normal. ***B.*** Horizontal gaze to the left is intact. ***C.*** On attempted horizontal gaze to the right, the left eye fails to adduct. In mildly affected patients, the eye may adduct partially or more slowly than normal. Nystagmus is usually present in the abducted eye. ***D.*** T2-weighted axial magnetic resonance image through the pons showing a demyelinating plaque in the left medial longitudinal fasciculus (*arrow*).

Skew deviation refers to a vertical misalignment of the eyes, usually constant in all positions of gaze. The finding has poor localizing value because skew deviation has been reported after lesions in widespread regions of the brainstem and cerebellum.

PARINAUD'S SYNDROME Also known as dorsal midbrain syndrome, this is a distinct supranuclear vertical gaze disorder caused by damage to the posterior commissure. It is a classic sign of hydrocephalus from aqueductal stenosis. Pineal region or midbrain tumors, cysticercosis, and stroke also cause Parinaud's syndrome. Features include loss of upgaze (and sometimes downgaze), convergence-retraction nystagmus on attempted upgaze, downward ocular deviation ("setting sun" sign), lid retraction (Collier's sign), skew deviation, pseudoabducens palsy, and light-near dissociation of the pupils.

Nystagmus This is a rhythmic oscillation of the eyes, occurring physiologically from vestibular and optokinetic stimulation or pathologically in a wide variety of diseases (**Chap. 22**). Abnormalities of the eyes or optic nerves, present at birth or acquired in childhood, can produce a complex, searching nystagmus with irregular pendular (sinusoidal) and jerk features. Examples are albinism, Leber's congenital amaurosis, and bilateral cataract. This nystagmus is commonly referred to as *congenital sensory nystagmus*. This is a poor term because even in children with congenital lesions, the nystagmus does not appear until weeks after birth. *Congenital motor nystagmus*, which looks similar to congenital sensory nystagmus, develops in the absence of any abnormality of the sensory visual system. Visual acuity also is reduced in congenital motor nystagmus, probably by the nystagmus itself, but seldom below a level of 20/200.

JERK NYSTAGMUS This is characterized by a slow drift off the target, followed by a fast corrective saccade. By convention, the nystagmus is named after the quick phase. Jerk nystagmus can be downbeat, upbeat, horizontal (left or right), and torsional. The pattern of nystagmus may vary with gaze position. Some patients will be oblivious to their nystagmus. Others will complain of blurred vision or a subjective to-and-fro movement of the environment (oscillopsia) corresponding to the nystagmus. Fine nystagmus may be difficult to see on gross examination of the eyes. Observation of nystagmoid movements of the optic disc on ophthalmoscopy is a sensitive way to detect subtle nystagmus.

GAZE-EVOKED NYSTAGMUS This is the most common form of jerk nystagmus. When the eyes are held eccentrically in the orbits, they have a natural tendency to drift back to primary position. The subject compensates by making a corrective saccade to maintain the deviated eye position. Many normal patients have mild gaze-evoked nystagmus. Exaggerated gaze-evoked nystagmus can be induced by drugs (sedatives, anticonvulsants, alcohol); muscle paresis; myasthenia gravis; demyelinating disease; and cerebellopontine angle, brainstem, and cerebellar lesions.

VESTIBULAR NYSTAGMUS *Vestibular nystagmus* results from dysfunction of the labyrinth (Ménière's disease), vestibular nerve, or vestibular nucleus in the brainstem. Peripheral vestibular nystagmus often occurs in discrete attacks, with symptoms of nausea and vertigo. There may be associated tinnitus and hearing loss. Sudden shifts in head position may provoke or exacerbate symptoms.

DOWNBEAT NYSTAGMUS *Downbeat nystagmus* results from lesions near the craniocervical junction (Chiari malformation, basilar invagination). It also has been reported in brainstem or cerebellar stroke, lithium or anticonvulsant intoxication, alcoholism, and multiple sclerosis. *Upbeat nystagmus* is associated with damage to the pontine tegmentum from stroke, demyelination, or tumor.

Opsoclonus This rare, dramatic disorder of eye movements consists of bursts of consecutive saccades (saccadomania). When the saccades are confined to the horizontal plane, the term *ocular flutter* is preferred. It can result from viral encephalitis, trauma, or a paraneoplastic effect of neuroblastoma, breast carcinoma, and other malignancies. It has also been reported as a benign, transient phenomenon in otherwise healthy patients.

FURTHER READING

Adamis AP et al: Building on the success of anti-vascular endothelial growth factor therapy: A vision for the next decade. Eye 34:1966, 2020.

Douglas RS: Teprotumumab for the treatment of active thyroid eye disease. N Engl J Med 382:341, 2020.

Dowling JE: Restoring vision to the blind. Science 368:827, 2020.

Gross JG et al: Panretinal photocoagulation vs intravitreous ranibizumab for proliferative diabetic retinopathy. JAMA 314:2137, 2015.

Jaffe GJ et al: Adalimumbab in patients with active noninfectious uveitis. N Engl J Med 375:932, 2016.

Maeder ML: Development of a gene-editing approach to restore vision loss in Leber congenital amaurosis type 10. Nat Med 25:229, 2019.

Pioro MH: Primary care vasculitis: Polymyalgia rheumatica and giant cell arteritis. Prim Care 45:305, 2018.

Stone JH et al: Trial of tocilizumab in giant-cell arteritis. N Engl J Med 377:317, 2017.

Yanoff M, Duker J: *Ophthalmology*, 5th ed. Atlanta, Saunders, 2019.

33 Disorders of Smell and Taste

Richard L. Doty, Steven M. Bromley

All environmental chemicals necessary for life enter the body by the nose and mouth. The senses of smell (olfaction) and taste (gustation) monitor such chemicals, determine the flavor and palatability of foods and beverages, and warn of dangerous environmental conditions, including fire, air pollution, leaking natural gas, and bacteria-laden foodstuffs. These senses contribute significantly to quality of life and, when dysfunctional, can have untoward physical and psychological consequences. A longitudinal study of 1162 nondemented elderly persons found, even after controlling for confounders, that those with the lowest baseline olfactory test scores had a 45% mortality rate over a 4-year period, compared to an 18% mortality rate for those with the highest olfactory test scores. A basic understanding of these senses in health and disease is critical for the physician, because thousands of patients present to doctors' offices each year with complaints of chemosensory dysfunction. Among the more important recent developments in neurology is the discovery that decreased smell function is among the first signs of such neurodegenerative diseases as Parkinson's disease (PD) and Alzheimer's disease (AD), signifying their "presymptomatic" phase.

ANATOMY AND PHYSIOLOGY

Olfactory System Odorous chemicals enter the front of nose during inhalation and active sniffing, as well as the back of the nose (nasopharynx) during deglutition. After reaching the highest recesses of the nasal cavity, they dissolve in the olfactory mucus and diffuse or are actively transported by specialized proteins to receptors located on the cilia of olfactory receptor cells. The cilia, dendrites, cell bodies, and proximal axonal segments of these bipolar cells are located within a unique neuroepithelium covering the cribriform plate, the superior nasal septum, superior turbinate, and sectors of the middle turbinate (**Fig. 33-1**). Nearly 400 types of G-protein-coupled odor receptors (GPCRs) are expressed on the cilia of the receptor cells, with only one type of GPCR being expressed on a given cell. Other receptors, including trace amine-associated receptors and members of the non-GPCR membrane-spanning 4-domain family, subfamily A (MS4A) protein family, are also present on some receptor cells. Such a plethora of receptor cell types does not exist in any other sensory system. Importantly, when damaged, the receptor cells can be replaced by stem cells near the basement membrane, although such replacement is often incomplete.

After coalescing into bundles surrounded by glia-like ensheathing cells (termed fila), the receptor cell axons pass through the cribriform plate to the olfactory bulbs, where they synapse with dendrites of other cell types within the glomeruli (**Fig. 33-2**). These spherical structures, which make up a distinct layer of the olfactory bulb, are a site of convergence of information, because many more fibers enter than leave them. Receptor cells that express the same type of receptor project to the same glomeruli, effectively making each glomerulus a functional unit. The major projection neurons of the olfactory system—the mitral and tufted cells—send primary dendrites into the glomeruli, connecting not only with the incoming receptor cell axons, but with dendrites of periglomerular cells. The activity of the mitral/tufted cells is modulated by the periglomerular cells, secondary dendrites from other mitral/tufted cells, and granule cells, the most numerous cells of the bulb. The latter cells, which are largely GABAergic, receive inputs from central brain structures and modulate the output of the mitral/tufted cells. Interestingly, like the olfactory receptor cells, some cells within the bulb undergo replacement. Thus, neuroblasts formed within the anterior subventricular zone of the brain migrate along the rostral migratory stream, ultimately becoming granule and periglomerular cells.

The axons of the mitral and tufted cells synapse within secondary olfactory structures, which largely compose the primary olfactory cortex (POC) (**Fig. 33-3**). The POC is defined as those cortical structures that receive direct projections from the olfactory bulb, most notably the piriform and entorhinal cortices. Although olfaction is unique

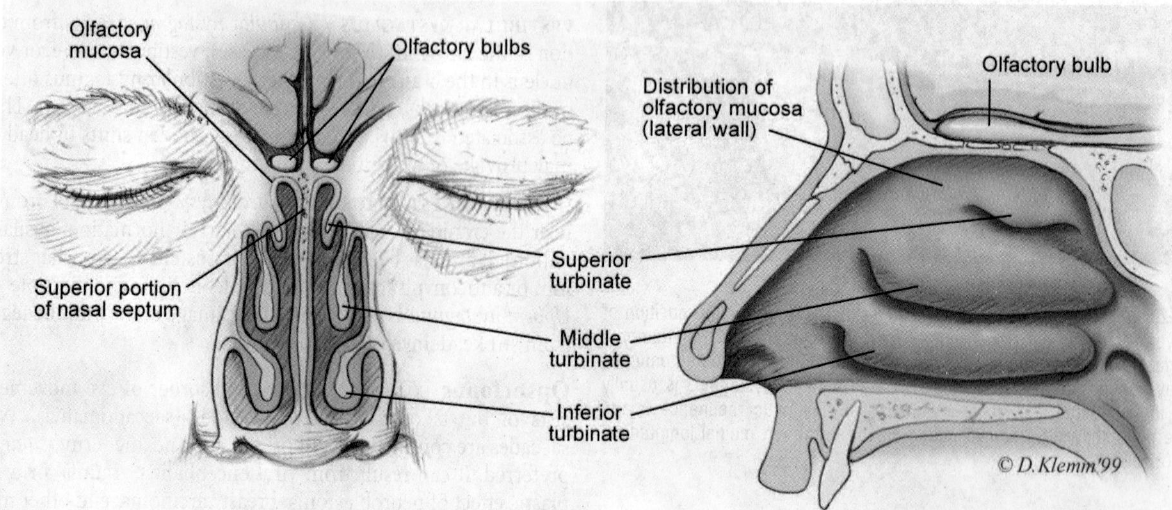

FIGURE 33-1 Anatomy of the nose, showing the distribution of olfactory receptors in the roof of the nasal cavity. *(Copyright David Klemm, Faculty and Curriculum Support [FACS], Georgetown University Medical Center.)*

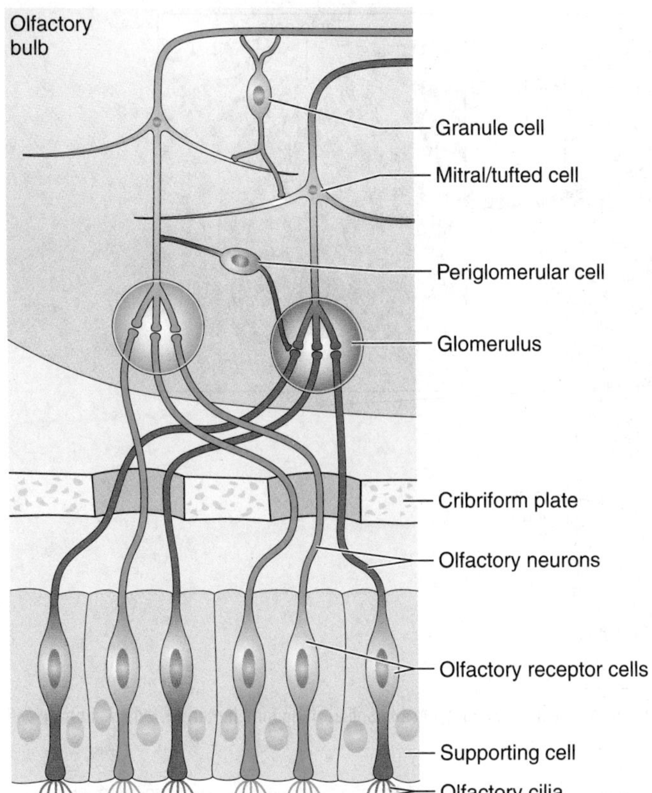

FIGURE 33-2 Schematic of the layers and wiring of the olfactory bulb. Each receptor type (red, green, blue) projects to a common glomerulus. The neural activity within each glomerulus is modulated by periglomerular cells. The activity of the primary projection cells, the mitral and tufted cells, is modulated by granule cells, periglomerular cells, and secondary dendrites from adjacent mitral and tufted cells. *(Adapted from www.med.yale.edu/neurosurg/treloar/index.html)*

in that its initial afferent projections bypass the thalamus, persons with damage to the thalamus can exhibit olfactory deficits, particularly ones of odor identification. Such deficits likely reflect the involvement of thalamic connections between the POC and the orbitofrontal cortex (OFC), where odor identification largely occurs. The close anatomic ties between the olfactory system and the amygdala, hippocampus, and hypothalamus help to explain the intimate associations between odor perception and cognitive functions such as memory, motivation, arousal, autonomic activity, digestion, and sex.

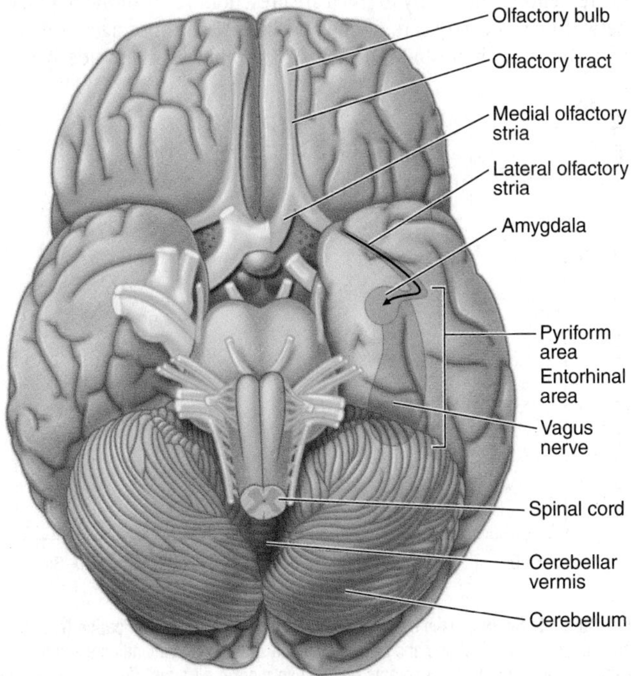

FIGURE 33-3 Anatomy of the base of the brain showing the primary olfactory cortex.

Taste System Tastants are sensed by specialized receptor cells present within taste buds—small grapefruit-like segmented structures located on the lateral margins and dorsum of the tongue, roof of the mouth, pharynx, larynx, and superior esophagus **(Fig. 33-4)**. Lingual taste buds are embedded in well-defined protuberances, termed fungiform, foliate, and circumvallate papillae. After dissolving in a liquid, tastants enter the opening of the taste bud—the taste pore—and bind to receptors on microvilli, small extensions of receptor cells within each taste bud. Such binding changes the electrical potential across the taste cell, resulting in neurotransmitter release onto the first-order taste neurons. Although humans have ~7500 taste buds, not all harbor taste-sensitive cells; some contain only one class of receptor (e.g., cells responsive only to sugars), whereas others contain cells sensitive to more than one class. The number of taste receptor cells per taste bud ranges from zero to well over 100. A small family of three GPCRs, namely T1R1, T1R2, and T1R3, mediate sweet and umami taste sensations. Bitter sensations, on the other hand, depend on T2R receptors, a family of ~30 GPCRs expressed on cells different from those that express the sweet and umami receptors. T2Rs sense a wide range of bitter substances but do not distinguish among them. Sour tastants are sensed by the PKD2L1 receptor, a member of the transient receptor potential protein (TRP) family. Perception of salty sensations, such as induced by sodium chloride, arises from the entry of Na^+ ions into the cells via specialized membrane channels, such as the amiloride-sensitive Na^+ channel.

It is now well established that both bitter and sweet taste-related receptors are also present elsewhere in the body, most notably in the alimentary and respiratory tracts. This important discovery generalizes the concept of taste-related chemoreception to areas of the body beyond the mouth and throat, with α-gustducin, the taste-specific G-protein α-subunit, expressed in so-called brush cells found specifically within the human trachea, lung, pancreas, and gallbladder. These brush cells are rich in nitric oxide (NO) synthase, known to defend against xenobiotic organisms, protect the mucosa from acid-induced lesions, and, in the case of the gastrointestinal tract, stimulate vagal and splanchnic afferent neurons. NO further acts on nearby cells, including enteroendocrine cells, absorptive or secretory epithelial cells, mucosal blood vessels, and cells of the immune system. Members of the T2R family of bitter receptors and the sweet receptors of the T1R family have been identified within the gastrointestinal tract and in enteroendocrine cell lines. In some cases, these receptors are important for metabolism, with the T1R3 receptors and gustducin playing decisive roles in the sensing and transport of dietary sugars from the intestinal lumen into absorptive enterocytes via a sodium-dependent glucose transporter and in regulation of hormone release from gut enteroendocrine cells. In other cases, these receptors may be important for airway protection, with a number of T2R bitter receptors in the motile cilia of the human airway that respond to bitter compounds by increasing their beat frequency. One specific T2R38 taste receptor is expressed in human upper respiratory epithelia and responds to acyl-monoserine lactone quorum-sensing molecules secreted by *Pseudomonas aeruginosa* and other gram-negative bacteria. Differences in T2R38 functionality, as related to TAS2R38 genotype, correlate with susceptibility to upper respiratory infections in humans.

Taste information is sent to the brain via three cranial nerves (CNs): CN VII (the *facial nerve*, which involves the intermediate nerve with its branches, the greater petrosal and chorda tympani nerves), CN IX (the *glossopharyngeal nerve*), and CN X (the *vagus nerve*) **(Fig. 33-5)**. CN VII innervates the anterior tongue and all of the soft palate, CN IX innervates the posterior tongue, and CN X innervates the laryngeal surface of the epiglottis, larynx, and proximal portion of the esophagus. The mandibular branch of CN V (V_3) conveys somatosensory information (e.g., touch, burning, cooling, irritation) to the brain. Although not technically a gustatory nerve, CN V shares primary nerve routes with many of the gustatory nerve fibers and adds temperature, texture, pungency, and spiciness to the taste experience. The chorda tympani

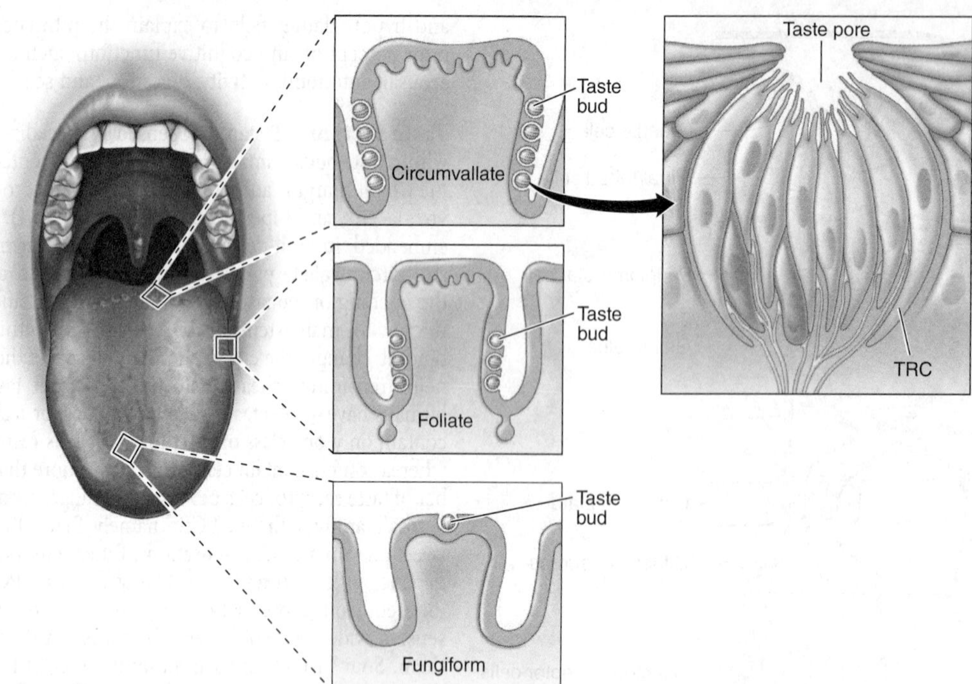

FIGURE 33-4 Schematic of the taste bud and its opening (pore), as well as the location of buds on the three major types of papillae: fungiform (anterior), foliate (lateral), and circumvallate (posterior). TRC, taste receptor cell.

nerve is famous for taking a recurrent course through the facial canal in the petrosal portion of the temporal bone, passing through the middle ear, and then exiting the skull via the petrotympanic fissure, where it joins the lingual nerve (a division of CN V) near the tongue. This nerve also carries parasympathetic fibers to the submandibular and sublingual glands, whereas the greater petrosal nerve supplies the palatine glands, thereby influencing saliva production.

The axons of the projection cells, which synapse with taste buds, enter the rostral portion of the nucleus of the solitary tract (NTS) within the medulla of the brainstem (Fig. 33-5). From the NTS, neurons then project to a division of the ventroposteromedial thalamic nucleus (VPM) via the medial lemniscus. From here, projections are made to the rostral part of the frontal operculum and adjoining insula, a brain region considered the *primary taste cortex* (PTC). Projections from the PTC then go to the *secondary taste cortex*, namely the caudolateral OFC. This brain region is involved in the conscious recognition of taste qualities. Moreover, because it contains cells that are activated by several sensory modalities, it is likely a center for establishing "flavor."

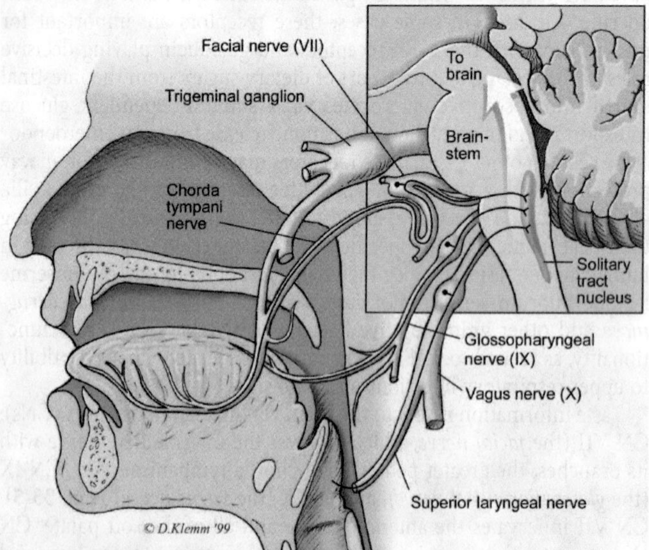

FIGURE 33-5 Schematic of the cranial nerves (CNs) that mediate taste function, including the chorda tympani nerve (CN VII), the glossopharyngeal nerve (CN IX), and the vagus nerve (CN X). *(Copyright David Klemm, Faculty and Curriculum Support [FACS], Georgetown University Medical Center.)*

DISORDERS OF OLFACTION

The ability to smell is influenced, in everyday life, by such factors as age, gender, general health, nutrition, smoking, and reproductive state. Women typically outperform men on tests of olfactory function and retain normal smell function to a later age than do men.

Estimates of the prevalence of olfactory dysfunction in the general population vary; a cross-sectional analysis from the National Health and Nutrition Examination Survey (NHANES 2013–2014) found an overall prevalence of 13.5%. However, it is apparent that significant decrements in the ability to smell are present in >50% of the population between 65 and 80 years of age and in 75% of those aged ≥80 years (**Fig. 33-6**). Such presbyosmia helps to explain why many elderly report

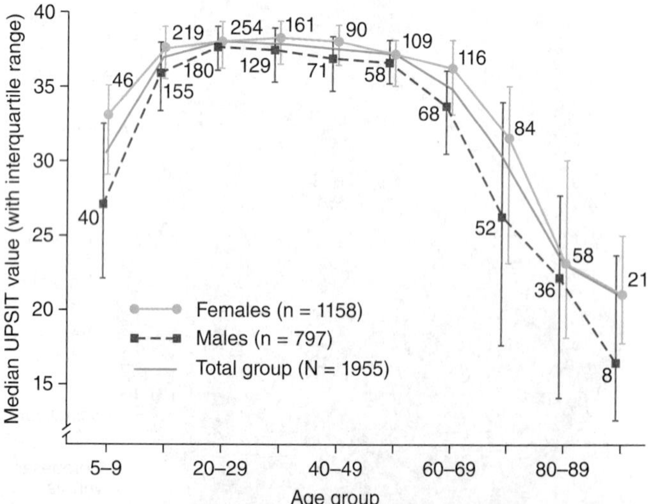

FIGURE 33-6 Scores on the University of Pennsylvania Smell Identification Test (UPSIT) as a function of subject age and sex. Numbers by each data point indicate sample sizes. Note that women identify odorants better than men at all ages. *(RL Doty et al: Smell identification ability: Changes with age. Science 226:4681, 1984. Copyright © 1984 American Association for the Advancement of Science. Reprinted with permission from AAAS.)*

TABLE 33-1 Disorders and Conditions Associated with Compromised Olfactory Function, as Measured by Olfactory Testing

Endocrine and Metabolic Conditions	Nasosinus Disorders	Viral, Bacterial, and Fungal Infections
Adrenal cortical insufficiency (Addison's disease)	Adenoid hypertrophy	Candidiasis
Chromatin-negative gonadal dysgenesis (Turner's syndrome)	Bacterial and viral upper respiratory infections	COVID-19
Cushing's syndrome	Laryngopharyngeal reflux disease	Hepatitis C
Diabetes	Rhinosinusitis/polyposis	Herpetic meningoencephalitis
Hypertension	**Neurologic Diseases/Disorders**	Human immunodeficiency virus
Hypothyroidism	Alzheimer's disease	Legionnaires' disease
Idiopathic hypogonadotropic hypogonadism	Amyotrophic lateral sclerosis (ALS)	Leprosy (Hansen's disease)
Kallmann's syndrome	Bell's palsy	Lyme disease
Liver disease	Degenerative ataxias	Poliomyelitis
Renal disease/kidney failure	Down's syndrome	Rhinosinusitis
Pregnancy	Epilepsy	Upper respiratory infections
Pseudohypoparathyroidism	Facial paralysis	**Other Disorders or Factors**
Wilson's disease	Fibromyalgia	Alcoholism
Immune-Related Diseases	Frontotemporal lobe degeneration	Bardet-Biedl syndrome
Acute disseminated encephalomyelitis	Guamanian ALS/Parkinson's disease/dementia syndrome	Chemical exposure
Allergic rhinitis	Head trauma	Congenital
Asthma	Huntington's disease	Iatrogenesis, including chemotherapy and radiation
Autoimmune pancreatitis	Idiopathic inflammatory myopathies	Nutritional deficiencies
Behçet's disease	Korsakoff psychosis	Obesity
Churg-Strauss syndrome	Lubag disease	Tobacco smoking
Cystic fibrosis	Migraine	Toxic chemical exposures
Fibromyalgia	Multi-infarct dementia	Vitamin B_{12} deficiency
Giant cell arteritis	Narcolepsy with cataplexy	
Hereditary angioedema	Neoplasms, cranial/nasal	
Idiopathic inflammatory myopathies	Orthostatic tremor	
Inflammatory bowel diseases	Parkinson's disease	
Lupus	Pick's disease	
Mikulicz's disease	Rapid eye movement behavioral sleep disorder	
Multiple sclerosis	Stroke	
Myasthenia gravis	**Psychiatric-Related Diseases/Disorders**	
Neuromyelitis optica	Anorexia nervosa	
Pemphigus vulgaris	Asperger's syndrome	
Psoriasis vulgaris	Attention deficit/hyperactivity disorder	
Rheumatoid arthritis	Depression	
Sjögren's syndrome	Obsessive compulsive disorder	
Systemic sclerosis (scleroderma)	Panic disorder	
Wegener's granulomatosis	Posttraumatic stress disorder	
	Psychopathy	
	Schizophrenia	
	Seasonal affective disorder	
	22q11 deletion syndrome	

Note: These disease/disorder classifications are not necessarily mutually exclusive.

that food has little flavor, a problem that can result in nutritional disturbances. This also helps to explain why a disproportionate number of elderly die in accidental gas poisonings. A relatively complete listing of conditions and disorders that have been associated with olfactory dysfunction is presented in **Table 33-1**.

Aside from aging, the three most common identifiable causes of long-lasting or permanent smell loss seen in the clinic are, in order of frequency, severe upper respiratory infections, head trauma, and chronic rhinosinusitis. The physiologic basis for most head trauma–related losses is the shearing and subsequent scarring of the olfactory fila as they pass from the nasal cavity into the brain cavity. The cribriform plate does not have to be fractured or show pathology for smell loss to be present. Severity of trauma, as indexed by a poor Glasgow Coma Scale score on presentation and the length of posttraumatic amnesia, is associated with higher risk of olfactory impairment. Less than 10% of posttraumatic anosmic patients will recover age-related normal function over time. This increases to nearly 25% of those with less-than-total loss. Respiratory infections, such as those associated with the common cold, influenza, pneumonia, HIV, and COVID-19 can directly and permanently damage the olfactory epithelium, decreasing receptor cell number, damaging cilia on remaining receptor cells, and inducing the replacement of sensory epithelium with respiratory epithelium. The smell loss associated with chronic rhinosinusitis is related to disease severity, with most loss occurring in cases where rhinosinusitis and polyposis are both present. Smell loss is among the first signs of the SARS-CoV-2 infection responsible for COVID-19, a loss that is seemingly independent of nasal inflammation. Although in rhinosinusitis cases systemic glucocorticoid therapy can usually induce short-term functional improvement, it does not, on average, return smell test scores to normal, implying that chronic permanent neural loss is present and/or that short-term administration of systemic glucocorticoids does not completely mitigate the inflammation. It is well established that microinflammation in an otherwise seemingly normal epithelium can influence smell function.

A number of neurodegenerative diseases are accompanied by olfactory impairment, including PD, AD, Huntington's disease, parkinsonism-dementia complex of Guam, dementia with Lewy bodies (DLB), multiple system atrophy, corticobasal degeneration, frontotemporal dementia, and Down's syndrome; smell loss can also occur in idiopathic rapid eye movement (REM) behavioral sleep disorder (iRBD), as well as in multiple sclerosis (MS) related to lesions within olfaction-related structures. Olfactory impairment in PD often predates the clinical diagnosis by a number of years. In staged cases, studies of the sequence of formation of abnormal α-synuclein aggregates and Lewy bodies suggest that the olfactory bulbs may be, along with the dorsomotor nucleus of the vagus, the first site of neural damage in PD. In postmortem studies of patients with very mild "presymptomatic" signs of AD, poorer smell function has been associated with higher levels of AD-related pathology. Smell loss is more marked in patients with early clinical manifestations of DLB than in those with mild AD. Interestingly, smell loss is minimal or nonexistent in progressive supranuclear palsy and 1-methyl-4-phenyl-1,2,3,6-tetrahydropyridine (MPTP)-induced parkinsonism. The relative contributions of disease-specific pathology or differential damage to forebrain neuromodulator/neurotransmitter systems in explaining different degrees of olfactory dysfunction among the various neurodegenerative diseases are presently unknown.

The smell loss seen in iRBD is of the same magnitude as that found in PD. This is of particular interest because patients with iRBD frequently develop PD and hyposmia. REM behavior disorder is not only seen in its idiopathic form, but can also be associated with narcolepsy (**Chap. 31**). A study of narcoleptic patients with and without REM behavior disorder demonstrated that narcolepsy, independent of REM behavior disorder, was associated with impairments in olfactory function. Loss of hypothalamic neurons expressing orexin (also known as hypocretin) neuropeptides is believed to be responsible for narcolepsy and cataplexy. Orexin-containing neurons project throughout the entire olfactory system (from the olfactory epithelium to the olfactory cortex), and damage to these projections may be one underlying mechanism for impaired olfactory performance in narcoleptic patients. Administration of intranasal orexin A (hypocretin-1) improved olfactory function, supporting the notion that mild olfactory impairment is not only a primary feature of narcolepsy with cataplexy, but that orexin deficiency may be directly responsible for the loss of smell in this condition.

DISORDERS OF TASTE

The majority of patients who present with taste dysfunction exhibit olfactory, not taste, loss. This is because most flavors attributed to taste actually depend on retronasal stimulation of the olfactory receptors during deglutition. As noted earlier, taste buds only mediate basic tastes such as sweet, sour, bitter, salty, and umami. Significant impairment of whole-mouth gustatory function is rare outside of generalized metabolic disturbances or systemic use of some medications, because taste bud regeneration occurs and peripheral damage alone would require the involvement of multiple CN pathways. Taste function can be influenced by age, diet, smoking behavior, use of medications, and other subject-related factors including (1) the release of foul-tasting materials from the oral cavity from oral medical conditions (e.g., gingivitis, purulent sialadenitis) or appliances; (2) transport problems of tastants to the taste buds (e.g., drying, infections, or inflammatory conditions of the orolingual mucosa), (3) damage to the taste buds themselves (e.g., local trauma, invasive carcinomas), (4) damage to the neural pathways innervating the taste buds (e.g., middle ear infections), (5) damage to central structures (e.g., multiple sclerosis, tumor, epilepsy, stroke), and (6) systemic disturbances of metabolism (e.g., diabetes, thyroid disease, medications).

Unlike CN VII, CN IX is relatively protected along its path, although iatrogenic interventions such as tonsillectomy, bronchoscopy, laryngoscopy, endotracheal intubation, and radiation therapy can result in selective injury. CN VII damage commonly results from mastoidectomy, tympanoplasty, and stapedectomy, in some cases inducing persistent metallic sensations. Bell's palsy (**Chap. 441**) is one of the most common causes of CN VII injury that results in taste disturbance. On rare occasions, migraine (**Chap. 430**) is associated with a gustatory prodrome or aura, and in some cases, tastants can trigger a migraine attack. Interestingly, dysgeusia occurs in some cases of *burning mouth syndrome* (also termed *glossodynia* or *glossalgia*), as does dry mouth and thirst. Burning mouth syndrome is likely associated with dysfunction of the trigeminal nerve (CN V). Some of the etiologies suggested for this poorly understood syndrome are amenable to treatment, including (1) nutritional deficiencies (e.g., iron, folic acid, B vitamins, zinc), (2) diabetes mellitus (possibly predisposing to oral candidiasis), (3) denture allergy, (4) mechanical irritation from dentures or oral devices, (5) repetitive movements of the mouth (e.g., tongue thrusting, teeth grinding, jaw clenching), (6) tongue ischemia as a result of temporal arteritis, (7) periodontal disease, (8) reflux esophagitis, and (9) geographic tongue.

Although both taste and smell can be adversely influenced by drugs, taste alterations are more common. Indeed, >250 medications have been reported to alter the ability to taste. Major offenders include antineoplastic agents, antirheumatic drugs, antibiotics, and blood pressure medications. Terbinafine, a commonly used antifungal, has been linked to taste disturbance lasting up to 3 years. In a recent controlled trial, nearly two-thirds of individuals taking eszopiclone (Lunesta) for insomnia experienced a bitter dysgeusia that was stronger in women, systematically related to the time since drug administration, and positively correlated with both blood and saliva levels of the drug. Intranasal use of nasal gels and sprays containing zinc, which are common over-the-counter prophylactics for upper respiratory viral infections, has been implicated in loss of smell function. Whether their efficacy in preventing such infections, which are the most common cause of anosmia and hyposmia, outweighs their potential detriment to smell function requires study. Dysgeusia occurs commonly in the context of drugs used to treat or minimize symptoms of cancer, with a weighted prevalence from 56% to 76% depending on the type of cancer treatment. Attempts to prevent taste problems from such drugs using prophylactic zinc sulfate or amifostine have proven to be minimally beneficial. Although antiepileptic medications are occasionally used to treat smell or taste disturbances, the use of topiramate has been reported to result in a reversible loss of an ability to detect and recognize tastes and odors during treatment.

As with olfaction, a number of systemic disorders can affect taste. These include, but are not limited to, chronic renal failure, end-stage liver disease, vitamin and mineral deficiencies, diabetes mellitus, and hypothyroidism. In diabetes, there appears to be a progressive loss of taste beginning with glucose and then extending to other sweeteners, salty stimuli, and then all stimuli. Psychiatric conditions can be associated with chemosensory alterations (e.g., depression, schizophrenia, bulimia). A recent review of tactile, gustatory, and olfactory hallucinations demonstrated that no one type of hallucinatory experience is pathognomonic to any given diagnosis.

Pregnancy is a unique condition with regard to taste function. There appears to be an increase in dislike and intensity of bitter tastes during the first trimester that may help to ensure that pregnant women avoid poisons during a critical phase of fetal development. Similarly, a relative increase in the preference for salt and bitter in the second and third trimesters may support the ingestion of much needed electrolytes to expand fluid volume and support a varied diet.

CLINICAL EVALUATION

In most cases, a careful clinical history will establish the probable etiology of a chemosensory problem, including questions about its nature, onset, duration, and pattern of fluctuations. *Sudden loss* suggests the possibility of head trauma, ischemia, infection, or a psychiatric condition. *Gradual loss* can reflect the development of a progressive obstructive lesion, although gradual loss can also follow head trauma. *Intermittent loss* suggests the likelihood of an inflammatory process. The patient should be asked about potential precipitating events, such as cold or flu infections, prior to symptom onset, because these often go underappreciated. Information regarding head trauma, smoking habits, drug and alcohol abuse (e.g., intranasal cocaine, chronic alcoholism), exposures to pesticides and other toxic agents, and medical interventions is also informative. A determination of all the medications that the patient was taking before and at the time of symptom onset is important, because many can cause chemosensory disturbances. Comorbid medical conditions associated with smell impairment, such as renal failure, liver disease, hypothyroidism, diabetes, or dementia, should be assessed. Delayed puberty in association with anosmia (with or without midline craniofacial abnormalities, deafness, and renal anomalies) suggests the possibility of Kallmann's syndrome. Recollection of epistaxis, discharge (clear, purulent, or bloody), nasal obstruction, allergies, and somatic symptoms, including headache or irritation, may have localizing value. Questions related to memory, parkinsonian symptoms, and seizure activity (e.g., automatisms, blackouts, auras, déjà vu) should be posed. Pending litigation and the possibility of malingering should be considered. Modern forced-choice olfactory tests can detect malingering from improbable responses.

Neurologic and otorhinolaryngologic (ORL) examinations, along with appropriate brain and nasosinus imaging, aid in the evaluation of patients with olfactory or gustatory complaints. The neural evaluation should focus on CN function, with particular attention to possible skull base and intracranial lesions. Visual acuity, field, and optic disc examinations aid in detection of intracranial mass lesions that produce raised intracranial pressure (papilledema) and optic atrophy. Foster Kennedy syndrome refers to raised intracranial pressure plus a compressive optic neuropathy; typical causes are olfactory groove meningiomas or other frontal lobe tumors. The ORL examination should thoroughly assess the intranasal architecture and mucosal surfaces. Polyps, masses, and adhesions of the turbinates to the septum may compromise the flow of air to the olfactory receptors, because less than a fifth of the inspired air traverses the olfactory cleft in the unobstructed state. Blood tests may be helpful to identify such conditions as diabetes, infection, heavy metal exposure, nutritional deficiency (e.g., vitamin B_6 or B_{12}), allergy, and thyroid, liver, and kidney disease.

As with other sensory disorders, quantitative sensory testing is advised. Self-reports of patients can be misleading, and a number of patients who complain of chemosensory dysfunction have normal function for their age and gender. Quantitative smell and taste testing provides objective information for worker's compensation and other legal claims, as well as a way to accurately assess the effects of treatment interventions. A number of standardized olfactory and taste tests are commercially available. The most widely used olfactory test, the 40-item University of Pennsylvania Smell Identification Test (UPSIT), uses norms based on nearly 4000 normal subjects. A determination is made of both absolute dysfunction (i.e., mild loss, moderate loss, severe loss, total loss, probable malingering) and relative dysfunction (percentile rank for age and gender). Although electrophysiologic testing is available at some smell and taste centers (e.g., odor event-related potentials), they require complex stimulus presentation and recording equipment and rarely provide additional diagnostic information. With the exception of electrogustometers, commercially available taste tests have only recently become available. Most use filter paper strips or similar materials impregnated with tastants, so no stimulus preparation is required.

■ TREATMENT AND MANAGEMENT

Given the various mechanisms by which olfactory and gustatory disturbance can occur, management of patients tends to be condition-specific. For example, patients with hypothyroidism, diabetes, or infections often benefit from specific treatments to correct the underlying disease process that is adversely influencing chemoreception. For most patients who present primarily with obstructive/transport loss affecting the nasal and paranasal regions (e.g., allergic rhinitis, polyposis, intranasal neoplasms, nasal deviations), medical and/or surgical intervention is often beneficial. Antifungal and antibiotic treatments may reverse taste problems secondary to candidiasis or other oral infections. Chlorhexidine mouthwash mitigates some salty or bitter dysgeusias, conceivably as a result of its strong positive charge. Excessive dryness of the oral mucosa is a problem with many medications and conditions, and artificial saliva (e.g., Xerolube) or oral pilocarpine treatments may prove beneficial. Other methods to improve salivary flow include the use of mints, lozenges, or sugarless gum. Flavor enhancers may make food more palatable (e.g., monosodium glutamate), but caution is advised to avoid overusing ingredients containing sodium or sugar, particularly in circumstances when a patient also has underlying hypertension or diabetes. Medications that induce distortions of taste can often be discontinued and replaced with other types of medications or modes of therapy. As mentioned earlier, pharmacologic agents result in taste disturbances much more frequently than smell disturbances. It is important to note, however, that many drug-related effects are long lasting and not reversed by short-term drug discontinuance.

A study of endoscopic sinus surgery in patients with chronic rhinosinusitis and hyposmia revealed that patients with severe olfactory dysfunction prior to the surgery had a more dramatic and sustained improvement over time compared to patients with more mild olfactory dysfunction prior to intervention. In the case of intranasal and sinus-related inflammatory conditions, such as seen with allergy, viruses, and traumas, the use of intranasal or systemic glucocorticoids may also be helpful. One common approach is to use a tapering course of oral prednisone. Topical intranasal administration of glucocorticoids was found to be less effective in general than systemic administration; however, the effects of different nasal administration techniques were not analyzed. For example, intranasal glucocorticoids are more effective if administered in the Moffett's position (head in the inverted position such as over the edge of the bed with the bridge of the nose perpendicular to the floor). After head trauma, an initial trial of glucocorticoids may help to reduce local edema and the potential deleterious deposition of scar tissue around olfactory fila at the level of the cribriform plate.

Treatments are limited for patients with chemosensory loss or primary injury to neural pathways. Nonetheless, spontaneous recovery can occur. In a follow-up study of 542 patients presenting to our center with smell loss from a variety of causes, modest improvement occurred over an average time period of 4 years in about half of the participants. However, only 11% of the anosmic and 23% of the hyposmic patients regained normal age-related function. Interestingly, the amount of dysfunction at the time of presentation, not etiology, was the best predictor of prognosis. Other predictors were age and the duration of dysfunction prior to initial testing.

Several studies have reported that patients with hyposmia may benefit from repeated smelling of odors over the course of weeks or months, although it remains to be determined how much improvement, if any, occurs over that known to occur spontaneously. The usual paradigm is to smell odors such as eucalyptol, citronella, eugenol, and phenyl ethyl alcohol before going to bed and immediately upon awakening each day. The rationale for such an approach comes from animal studies demonstrating that prolonged exposure to odorants can induce increased neural activity within the olfactory bulb. There is also limited evidence that α-lipoic acid (400 mg/d), an essential cofactor for many enzyme complexes with possible antioxidant effects, may be beneficial in mitigating smell loss following viral infection of the upper respiratory tract. However, double-blind studies are needed to confirm this observation. α-Lipoic acid has also been suggested to be useful in some cases of hypogeusia and burning mouth syndrome.

The use of zinc and vitamin A in treating olfactory disturbances is controversial, and there does not appear to be much benefit beyond replenishing established deficiencies. However, zinc has been shown to improve taste function secondary to hepatic deficiencies, and retinoids (bioactive vitamin A derivatives) are known to play an essential role in the survival of olfactory neurons. One protocol in which zinc was infused with chemotherapy treatments suggested a possible protective effect against developing taste impairment. Diseases of the alimentary tract can not only influence chemoreceptive function but also occasionally influence vitamin B_{12} absorption. This can result in a relative deficiency of vitamin B_{12}, theoretically contributing to olfactory nerve disturbance. Vitamin B_2 (riboflavin) and magnesium supplements are reported in the alternative literature to aid in the management of migraine that, in turn, may be associated with smell dysfunction. Because vitamin D deficiency is a cofactor of chemotherapy-induced mucocutaneous toxicity and dysgeusia, adding vitamin D_3, 1000–2000 units per day, may benefit some patients with smell and taste complaints during or following chemotherapy.

A number of medications have reportedly been used with success in ameliorating olfactory symptoms, although strong scientific evidence for efficacy is generally lacking. A report that theophylline improved smell function was uncontrolled and failed to account for the fact that some meaningful improvement occurs without treatment; indeed, the percentage of responders was about the same (~50%) as that noted by others to show spontaneous improvement over a similar time period. Antiepileptics and some antidepressants (e.g., amitriptyline) have been used to treat dysosmias and smell distortions, particularly following head trauma. Ironically, amitriptyline is also frequently on the list of medications that can ultimately distort smell and taste function, possibly from its anticholinergic effects. One study suggested that the centrally acting acetylcholinesterase inhibitor donepezil in AD resulted in improvements on smell identification measures that correlated with overall clinician-based impressions of change in dementia severity scores.

Alternative therapies, such as acupuncture, meditation, cognitive-behavioral therapy, and yoga, can help patients manage uncomfortable experiences associated with chemosensory disturbance and oral pain syndromes and to cope with the psychosocial stressors surrounding the impairment. Additionally, modification of diet and eating habits is also important. By accentuating the other sensory experiences of a meal, such as food texture, aroma, temperature, and color, one can optimize the overall eating experience for a patient. In some cases, a flavor enhancer like monosodium glutamate (MSG) can be added to foods to increase palatability and encourage intake.

Proper oral and nasal hygiene and routine dental care are extremely important ways for patients to protect themselves from disorders of the mouth and nose that can ultimately result in chemosensory disturbance. Patients should be warned not to overcompensate for their taste loss by adding excessive amounts of sugar or salt. Smoking cessation and the discontinuance of oral tobacco use are essential in the management of any patient with smell and/or taste disturbance and should be repeatedly emphasized.

A major and often overlooked element of therapy comes from chemosensory testing itself. Confirmation or lack of conformation of loss is beneficial to patients who come to believe, in light of unsupportive family members and medical providers, that they may be "crazy." In cases where the loss is minor, patients can be informed of the likelihood of a more positive prognosis. Importantly, quantitative testing places the patient's problem into overall perspective. Thus, it is often therapeutic for an older person to know that, while his or her smell function is not what it used to be, it still falls above the average of his or her peer group. Without testing, many such patients are simply told that they are getting old and nothing can be done for them, leading in some cases to depression and decreased self-esteem.

FURTHER READING

Devanand DP et al: Olfactory identification deficits are associated with increased mortality in a multiethnic urban community. Ann Neurol 78:401, 2015.

Doty RL: Olfaction in Parkinson's disease and related disorders. Neurobiol Dis 46:527, 2012.

Doty RL et al: Taste function in early stage treated and untreated Parkinson's disease. J Neurol 262:547, 2015.

Doty RL et al: Systemic diseases and disorders. Handbook Clin Neurol 164:361, 2019.

Doty RL et al: Treatments for smell and taste disorders: A critical review. Handbook Clin Neurol 164:455, 2019.

Fornazieri MA et al: Adherence and efficacy of olfactory training as a treatment for persistent olfactory loss. Am J Rhinol Allergy 34:238, 2020.

Hawkes CH, Doty RL: *Smell and Taste Disorders.* Cambridge, Cambridge University Press, 2018.

Liu G et al: Prevalence and risk factors of taste and smell impairment in a nationwide sample of the US population: A cross-sectional study. BMJ Open 6:e013246, 2016.

London B et al: Predictors of prognosis in patients with olfactory disturbance. Ann Neurol 63:159, 2008.

Moein ST et al: Smell dysfunction: A biomarker for COVID-19. Int Forum Allergy Rhinol 10:944, 2020.

Perricone C et al: Smell and autoimmunity: A comprehensive review. Clin Rev Allergy Immunol 45:87, 2013.

34 Disorders of Hearing

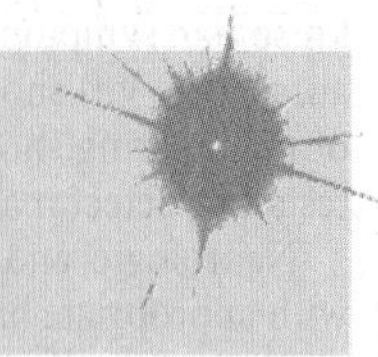

Anil K. Lalwani

Hearing loss can present at any age and is one of the most common sensory disorders in humans. Nearly 10% of the adult population has some hearing loss, and one-third of individuals age >65 years have a hearing loss of sufficient magnitude to require a hearing aid.

PHYSIOLOGY OF HEARING

The function of the external and middle ear is to amplify sound to facilitate conversion of the mechanical energy of the sound wave into an electrical signal by the inner-ear hair cells, a process called mechanotransduction (**Fig. 34-1**). Sound waves enter the external auditory canal and set the tympanic membrane (eardrum) in motion, which in turn moves the malleus, incus, and stapes of the middle ear. Movement of the footplate of the stapes causes pressure changes in the fluid-filled inner ear, eliciting a traveling wave in the basilar membrane of the cochlea. The tympanic membrane and the ossicular chain in the middle ear serve as an impedance-matching mechanism, improving the efficiency of energy transfer from air to the fluid-filled inner ear. In its absence, nearly 99.9% of the acoustical energy would be reflected and thus not heard. Instead, the eardrum and the ossicles boost the sound energy nearly 200-fold by the time it reaches the inner ear.

Within the cochlea of the inner ear, there are two types of hair cells that aid in hearing: inner and outer. The inner and outer hair cells of the organ of Corti have different innervation patterns, but both are mechanoreceptors; they detect the mechanical energy of the acoustic signal and aid its conversion to an electrical signal that travels by the auditory nerve. The afferent innervation relates principally to the inner hair cells while the efferent innervation relates principally to the outer hair cells. The outer hair cells outnumber the inner hair cells by nearly 6:1 (20,000 vs 3500). The motility of the outer hair cells alters the micromechanics of the inner hair cells, creating a cochlear amplifier, which explains the exquisite sensitivity and frequency selectivity of the cochlea.

Stereocilia of the hair cells of the organ of Corti, which rests on the basilar membrane, are in contact with the tectorial membrane and are deformed by the traveling wave. The deformation stretches tiny filamentous connections (tip links) between stereocilia, leading to opening of ion channels, influx of potassium, and hair cell depolarization and subsequent neurotransmission. A point of maximal displacement of the basilar membrane is determined by the frequency of the stimulating tone. High-frequency tones cause maximal displacement of the basilar membrane near the base of the cochlea, whereas for low-frequency sounds, the point of maximal displacement is toward the apex of the cochlea.

Beginning in the cochlea, the frequency specificity is maintained at each point of the central auditory pathway: dorsal and ventral cochlear nuclei, trapezoid body, superior olivary complex, lateral lemniscus, inferior colliculus, medial geniculate body, and auditory cortex. At low frequencies, individual auditory nerve fibers can respond more or less synchronously with the stimulating tone. At higher frequencies, phase-locking occurs so that neurons alternate in response to particular phases of the cycle of the sound wave. Intensity is encoded by the

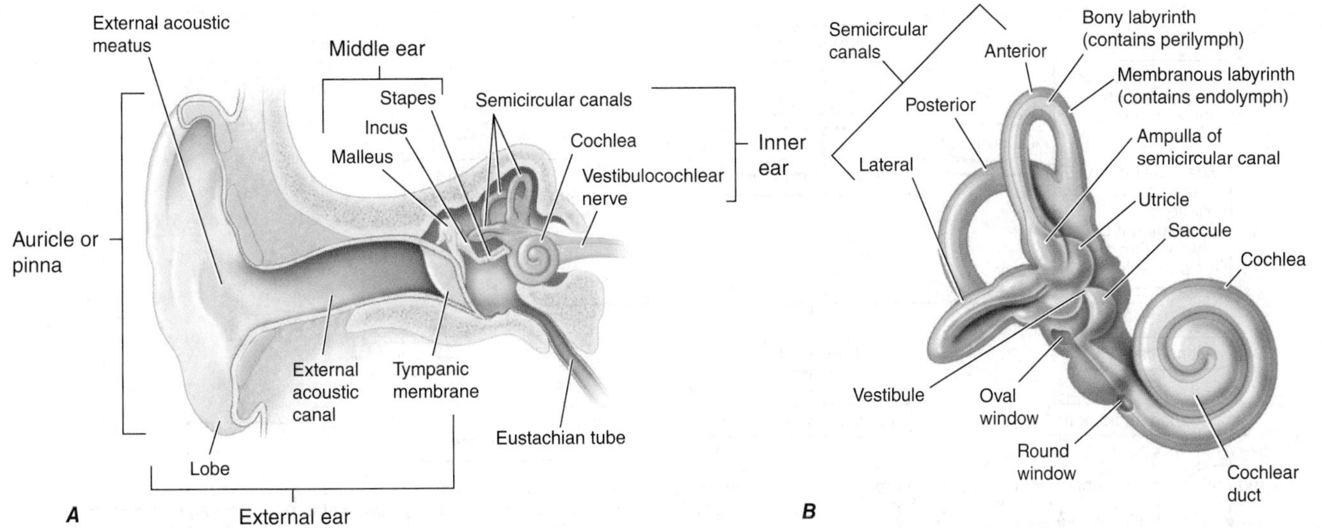

FIGURE 34-1 Ear anatomy. ***A.*** Drawing of modified coronal section through external ear and temporal bone, with structures of the middle and inner ear demonstrated. ***B.*** High-resolution view of inner ear.

amount of neural activity in individual neurons, the number of neurons that are active, and the specific neurons that are activated.

There is evidence that the right and left ears as well as the central nervous system may process speech asymmetrically. Generally, a sound is processed symmetrically from the peripheral to the central auditory system. However, a "right ear advantage" exists for dichotic listening tasks, in which subjects are asked to report on competing sounds presented to each ear. In most individuals, a perceptual right ear advantage for consonant-vowel syllables, stop consonants, and words also exists. Similarly, whereas central auditory processing for sounds is symmetric with minimal lateral specialization for the most part, speech processing is lateralized. There is specialization of the left auditory cortex for speech recognition and production, and of the right hemisphere for emotional and tonal aspects of speech. Left hemisphere dominance for speech is found in 95–98% of right-handed persons and 70–80% of left-handed persons.

DISORDERS OF THE SENSE OF HEARING

Hearing loss can result from disorders of the auricle, external auditory canal, middle ear, inner ear, or central auditory pathways (**Fig. 34-2**). In general, lesions in the auricle, external auditory canal, or middle ear that impede the transmission of sound from the external environment to the inner ear cause conductive hearing loss, whereas lesions that impair mechanotransduction in the inner ear or transmission of the electrical signal along the eighth nerve to the brain cause sensorineural hearing loss.

Conductive Hearing Loss The external ear, the external auditory canal, and the middle-ear apparatus are designed to collect and amplify sound and efficiently transfer the mechanical energy of the sound wave to the fluid-filled cochlea. Factors that obstruct the transmission of sound or dampen the acoustic energy result in conductive hearing loss. Conductive hearing loss can occur from obstruction of the external auditory canal by cerumen, debris, and foreign bodies; swelling of the lining of the canal; atresia or neoplasms of the canal; perforations of the tympanic membrane; disruption of the ossicular chain, as occurs with necrosis of the long process of the incus in trauma or infection; otosclerosis; or fluid, scarring, or neoplasms in the middle ear. Rarely, inner-ear malformations or pathologies that create a "third window" in the inner ear such as superior semicircular canal dehiscence, lateral semicircular canal dysplasia, incomplete partition of the inner ear, and large vestibular aqueduct, are also associated with conductive hearing loss. This pathologic third window is associated with loss of mechanical energy associated with the sound wave leading to conductive hearing loss (see below).

Eustachian tube dysfunction is extremely common in adults and may predispose to acute otitis media (AOM) or serous otitis media (SOM). Recently, Eustachian tube balloon dilation has been shown to relieve acquired inflammatory obstruction of the Eustachian tube orifice and improve symptoms due to Eustachian tube dysfunction. Trauma, AOM, and chronic otitis media are the usual factors responsible for tympanic membrane perforation. While small perforations often heal spontaneously, larger defects usually require surgical intervention. Tympanoplasty is highly effective (>90%) in the repair of tympanic membrane perforations. Otoscopy is usually sufficient to diagnose AOM, SOM, chronic otitis media, cerumen impaction, tympanic membrane perforation, and Eustachian tube dysfunction; tympanometry and Eustachian tube function testing can be useful to confirm the clinical suspicion of these conditions.

Cholesteatoma, a benign tumor composed of stratified squamous epithelium in the middle ear or mastoid, occurs frequently in adults, often in the setting of severe Eustachian tube dysfunction. This is a slowly growing lesion that destroys bone and normal ear tissue. Theories of pathogenesis include traumatic immigration and invasion of squamous epithelium through a retraction pocket of the tympanic membrane, implantation of squamous epithelia in the middle ear through a perforation or surgery, and metaplasia following chronic infection and irritation. A chronically draining ear that fails to respond to appropriate antibiotic therapy should raise suspicion of a cholesteatoma. On examination, there is often a perforation of the tympanic membrane filled with cheesy white squamous debris. The presence of an aural polyp obscuring the tympanic membrane is highly suggestive of an underlying cholesteatoma. Conductive hearing loss secondary to ossicular erosion is common. Bony destruction visualized on CT of the temporal bone is also highly suggestive of cholesteatoma. Surgery is required to remove this destructive process and reconstruct the ossicles.

Conductive hearing loss with a normal ear canal and intact tympanic membrane suggests either ossicular pathology or the presence of a "third window" in the inner ear (see below). Fixation of the stapes from *otosclerosis* is a common cause of low-frequency conductive hearing loss. It occurs equally in men and women and is inherited as an autosomal dominant trait with incomplete penetrance; in some cases, it may be a manifestation of osteogenesis imperfecta. Hearing impairment usually presents between the late teens and the forties. In women, the otosclerotic process is accelerated during pregnancy, and the hearing loss is often first noticeable at this time. A hearing aid or a simple outpatient surgical procedure (stapedectomy) can provide excellent auditory rehabilitation. Extension of otosclerosis beyond the stapes footplate to involve the cochlea (cochlear otosclerosis) can lead to mixed or sensorineural hearing loss. Fluoride therapy to prevent hearing loss from cochlear otosclerosis is of uncertain value.

Disorders that lead to the formation of a pathologic "third window" in the inner ear can be associated with conductive hearing loss. There

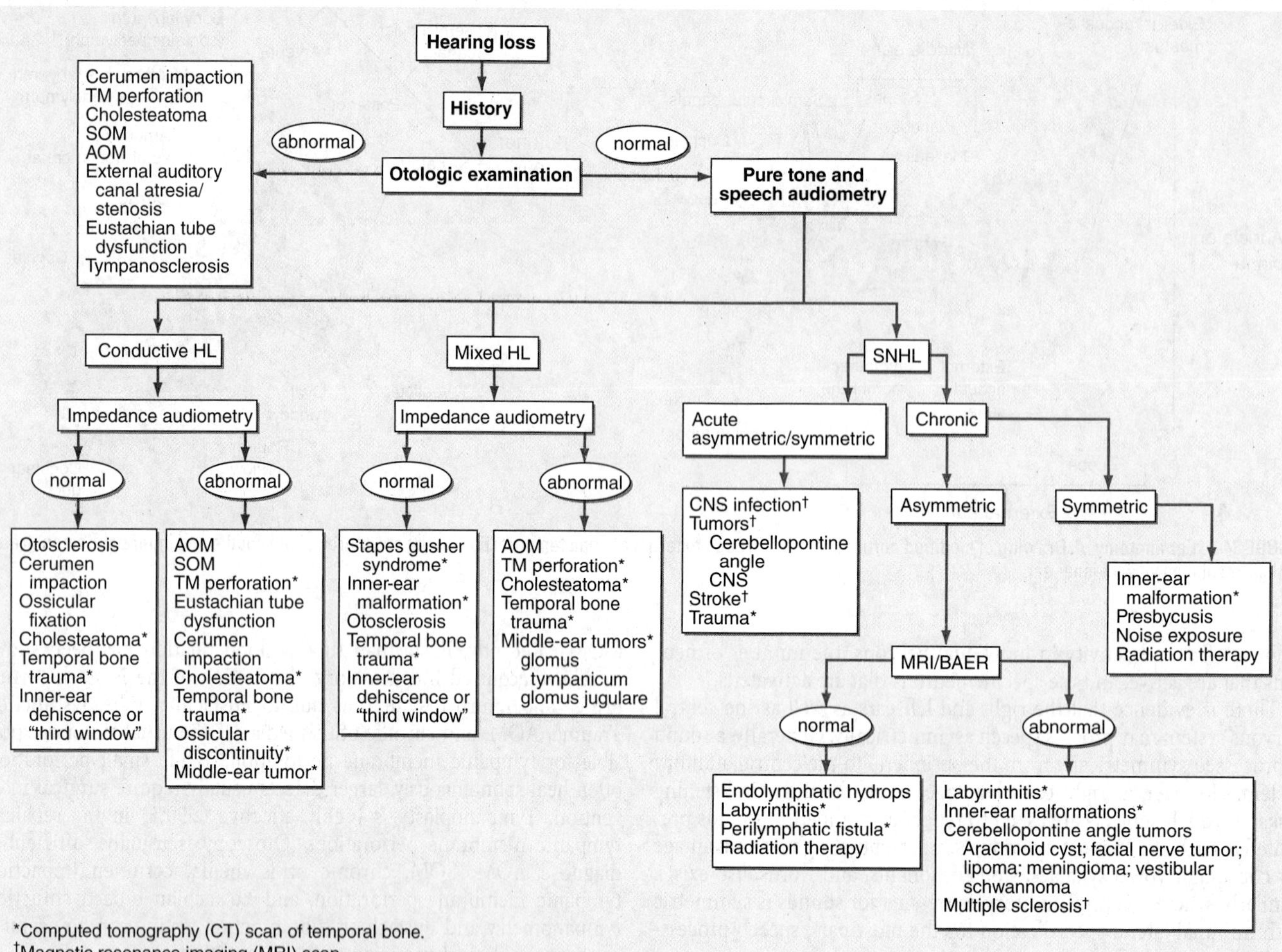

FIGURE 34-2 An algorithm for the approach to hearing loss. AOM, acute otitis media; BAER, brainstem auditory-evoked response; CNS, central nervous system; HL, hearing loss; SNHL, sensorineural hearing loss; SOM, serous otitis media; TM, tympanic membrane.

are normally two major openings, or windows, that connect the inner ear with the middle ear and serve as conduits for transmission of sound; these are, respectively, the oval and round windows. A third window is formed where the normally hard otic bone surrounding the inner ear is eroded; dissipation of the acoustic energy at the third window is responsible for the "inner-ear conductive hearing loss." The superior semicircular canal dehiscence syndrome resulting from erosion of the otic bone over the superior circular canal can present with conductive hearing loss that mimics otosclerosis. A common symptom is vertigo evoked by loud sounds (Tullio phenomenon), by Valsalva maneuvers that change middle-ear pressure, or by applying positive pressure on the tragus (the cartilage anterior to the external opening of the ear canal). Patients with this syndrome also complain of fullness of the ear, pulsatile tinnitus, and being able to hear the movement of their eyes and neck. A large jugular bulb or jugular bulb diverticulum can create a "third window" by eroding into the vestibular aqueduct or posterior semicircular canal; the symptoms are similar to those of the superior semicircular canal dehiscence syndrome. Other inner-ear malformations such as lateral semicircular canal dysplasia, large vestibular aqueduct, or incomplete partition seen in stapes gusher syndrome can also be associated with inner-ear conductive hearing loss as a result of the third window. Low activation threshold on the vestibular-evoked myogenic potential test (VEMP test, see below) and inner-ear erosion on CT are diagnostic. Recalcitrant vertigo and dizziness may respond to surgical repair of the dehiscence.

Sensorineural Hearing Loss Sensorineural hearing loss results from either damage to the mechanotransduction apparatus of the cochlea or disruption of the electrical conduction pathway from the inner ear to the brain. Thus, injury to hair cells, supporting cells, auditory neurons, or the central auditory pathway can cause sensorineural hearing loss. Damage to the hair cells of the organ of Corti may be caused by intense noise, viral infections, ototoxic drugs (e.g., salicylates, quinine and its synthetic analogues, aminoglycoside antibiotics, loop diuretics such as furosemide and ethacrynic acid, and cancer chemotherapeutic agents such as cisplatin), fractures of the temporal bone, meningitis, cochlear otosclerosis (see above), Ménière's disease, and aging. Congenital malformations of the inner ear may be the cause of hearing loss in some adults. Genetic predisposition alone or in concert with environmental exposures may also be responsible (see below).

Noise-Induced Hearing Loss Exposure to loud noise, either a short burst or over a more prolonged period of time, can lead to noise-induced hearing loss. Acute exposure to noise can lead to either temporary or permanent threshold shifts, depending on the intensity and duration of sound, due to hair cell injury and/or death. Typically, with permanent hearing loss there is a "noise notch" with elevated hearing thresholds at 3000–4000 Hz. More recently, loud noise exposure has also been associated with "hidden hearing loss"—hidden, because routine audiometry shows the pure tone hearing to be normal. Patients usually complain of not being able to hear clearly and are more bothered by the presence of background noise. In contrast to hair cell loss, hidden hearing loss is thought to be due to loss of auditory synapses on hair cells following noise exposure. In an increasingly noisy world, avoiding acoustic trauma with earplugs or earmuffs is highly recommended to prevent noise-induced or hidden hearing loss.

Presbycusis (age-associated hearing loss) is the most common cause of sensorineural hearing loss in adults. It is estimated to affect over half of adults aged >75 years in the United States, a population that is expected to double in size over the next 40 years. In the early stages, it is

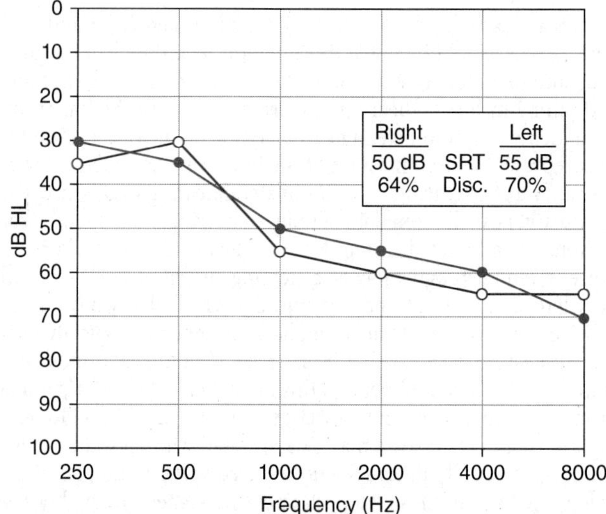

FIGURE 34-3 Presbycusis or age-related hearing loss. The audiogram shows a moderate to severe downsloping sensorineural hearing loss typical of presbycusis. The loss of high-frequency hearing is associated with a decreased speech discrimination score; consequently, patients complain of lack of clarity of hearing, especially in a noisy background. HL, hearing threshold level; SRT, speech reception threshold.

characterized by symmetric, gentle to sharply sloping, high-frequency hearing loss (**Fig. 34-3**). With progression, the hearing loss involves all frequencies. More importantly, the hearing impairment is associated with significant loss in clarity. There is a loss of discrimination for phonemes, recruitment (abnormal growth of loudness), and particular difficulty in understanding speech in noisy environments such as at restaurants and social events. Poor hearing is also associated with an increased incidence of cognitive impairment, rate of cognitive decline, and falls. In the elderly, left untreated, hearing loss leads to diminished quality of life, and has been shown to increase overall morbidity and mortality through falls and accidents. Hearing aids are helpful in enhancing the signal-to-noise ratio by amplifying sounds that are close to the listener. Hearing aid use has been shown to reduce cognitive decline and risk of falls. Although hearing aids are able to amplify sounds, they cannot restore the clarity of hearing. Thus, amplification with hearing aids may provide only limited rehabilitation once the word recognition score deteriorates below 50%. Cochlear implants are the treatment of choice when hearing aids prove inadequate, even when hearing loss is incomplete (see below).

Ménière's disease is characterized by episodic vertigo, fluctuating sensorineural hearing loss, tinnitus, and aural fullness. An absence of vertigo is inconsistent with the diagnosis of Ménière's disease, and the presence of fluctuating sensorineural hearing loss, tinnitus, and fullness without vertigo is more suggestive of cochlear hydrops. Tinnitus and/or deafness may be absent during the initial attacks of vertigo, but invariably appear as the disease progresses and increases in severity during acute attacks. The annual incidence of Ménière's disease is 0.5–7.5 per 1000; onset is most frequently in the fifth decade of life but may also occur in young adults or the elderly. Histologically, there is distention of the endolymphatic system (endolymphatic hydrops) leading to degeneration of vestibular and cochlear hair cells. This may result from endolymphatic sac dysfunction secondary to infection, trauma, autoimmune disease, inflammatory causes, or tumor; an idiopathic etiology constitutes the largest category and is most accurately referred to as Ménière's disease. Endolymphatic sac tumors, often associated with von Hippel Lindau disease, may clinically mimic Ménière's disease. Although any pattern of hearing loss can be observed, typically, low-frequency, unilateral sensorineural hearing impairment is present. An abnormal VEMP test (see below) may be helpful in detecting Ménière's disease in a clinically unaffected contralateral ear. MRI should be obtained to exclude retrocochlear pathology such as a cerebellopontine angle tumor, endolymphatic sac tumor, or demyelinating disorder. Therapy is directed toward the control of vertigo. A 2-g/d low-salt diet is the mainstay of treatment for control of rotatory vertigo. Diuretics, a short course of oral glucocorticoids, intratympanic glucocorticoids, or intratympanic gentamicin may also be useful adjuncts in recalcitrant cases. Surgical therapy of vertigo is reserved for unresponsive cases and includes endolymphatic sac decompression, labyrinthectomy, and vestibular nerve section. Both labyrinthectomy and vestibular nerve section abolish rotatory vertigo in >90% of cases. Unfortunately, there is no effective therapy for hearing loss, tinnitus, or aural fullness from Ménière's disease.

Sensorineural hearing loss may also result from any neoplastic, vascular, demyelinating, infectious, degenerative disease, or trauma affecting the central auditory pathways. Characteristically, in hearing loss due to central nervous system pathology, a reduction in clarity of hearing and speech comprehension is much greater than the loss of the ability to hear pure tone. Auditory testing is consistent with an auditory neuropathy; normal otoacoustic emissions (OAEs) and an abnormal auditory brainstem response (ABR) are typical (see below). Hearing loss can accompany hereditary sensorimotor neuropathies and inherited disorders of myelin. Tumors of the cerebellopontine angle such as vestibular schwannoma and meningioma (**Chap. 90**) usually present with asymmetric sensorineural hearing loss with greater deterioration of speech understanding than pure tone hearing. Multiple sclerosis (**Chap. 444**) may present with acute unilateral or bilateral hearing loss; typically, pure tone testing remains relatively stable while speech understanding fluctuates. Isolated labyrinthine infarction can present with acute hearing loss and vertigo due to a cerebrovascular accident involving the posterior circulation, usually the anterior inferior cerebellar artery; it may also be the heralding sign of impending catastrophic basilar artery infarction (**Chap. 426**). HIV (**Chap. 202**), which can produce both peripheral and central auditory system pathology, is another consideration in the evaluation of sensorineural hearing impairment.

A finding of conductive and sensorineural hearing loss in combination is termed *mixed hearing loss*. Mixed hearing losses can result from pathology of both the middle and inner ear, as can occur in otosclerosis involving the ossicles and the cochlea, head trauma, chronic otitis media, cholesteatoma, middle-ear tumors, and some inner-ear malformations.

Trauma resulting in temporal bone fractures may be associated with conductive, sensorineural, or mixed hearing loss. If the fracture spares the inner ear, there may simply be conductive hearing loss due to rupture of the tympanic membrane or disruption of the ossicular chain. These abnormalities can be surgically corrected. Profound hearing loss and severe vertigo are associated with temporal bone fractures involving the inner ear. A perilymphatic fistula associated with leakage of inner-ear fluid into the middle ear can occur and may require surgical repair. An associated facial nerve injury is not uncommon. CT is best suited to assess fracture of the traumatized temporal bone, evaluate the ear canal, and determine the integrity of the ossicular chain and involvement of the inner ear. Cerebrospinal fluid leaks that accompany temporal bone fractures are usually self-limited; the value of prophylactic antibiotics is uncertain.

Tinnitus Tinnitus is defined as the perception of a sound when there is no sound in the environment. It can have a buzzing, roaring, or ringing quality and may be pulsatile (synchronous with the heartbeat). Tinnitus is often associated with either a conductive or sensorineural hearing loss. The pathophysiology of tinnitus is not well understood. The cause of the tinnitus can usually be determined by finding the cause of the associated hearing loss. Tinnitus may be the first symptom of a serious condition such as a vestibular schwannoma. Pulsatile tinnitus requires evaluation of the vascular system of the head to exclude vascular tumors such as glomus jugulare tumors, aneurysms, dural arteriovenous fistulas, and stenotic arterial lesions; it may also occur with SOM, superior semicircular dehiscence, and inner-ear dehiscence. It is most commonly associated with some abnormality of the jugular bulb such as a large jugular bulb or jugular bulb diverticulum. In absence of demonstrated pathology on MRA/MRV or CT angiography, pulsatile tinnitus is usually attributed to turbulent venous blood flow through the transverse sinus, sigmoid sinus, and the jugular bulb.

GENETIC CAUSES OF HEARING LOSS

More than half of childhood hearing impairment is thought to be hereditary; hereditary hearing impairment (HHI) can also manifest later in life. HHI may be classified as either nonsyndromic, when hearing loss is the only clinical abnormality, or syndromic, when hearing loss is associated with anomalies in other organ systems. Nearly two-thirds of HHIs are nonsyndromic. Between 70% and 80% of nonsyndromic HHI is inherited in an autosomal recessive manner and designated DFNB; another 15–20% is autosomal dominant (DFNA). Less than 5% is X-linked (DFNX) or maternally inherited via the mitochondria.

More than 150 loci harboring genes for nonsyndromic HHI have been mapped, with recessive loci outnumbering dominant ones; numerous genes have now been identified (**Table 34-1**). The hearing genes fall into the categories of structural proteins (*MYH9, MYO7A, MYO15, TECTA, DIAPH1*), transcription factors (*POU3F4, POU4F3*), ion channels (*KCNQ4, SLC26A4*), and gap junction proteins (*GJB2, GJB3, GJB6*). Several of these genes, including *GJB2, TECTA*, and *TMC1*, cause both autosomal dominant and recessive forms of nonsyndromic HHI. In general, the hearing loss associated with dominant genes has its onset in adolescence or adulthood, varies in severity, and progresses with age, whereas the hearing loss associated with recessive inheritance is congenital and profound. Connexin 26, a product of the *GJB2* gene, is particularly important because it is responsible for nearly 20% of all cases of childhood deafness; half of genetic deafness in children is *GJB2* related. Two frameshift mutations, 35delG and 167delT, account for >50% of the cases; however, screening for these two mutations alone is insufficient, and sequencing of the entire gene is required to fully capture *GJB2*-related recessive deafness. The 167delT mutation is highly prevalent in Ashkenazi Jews; ~1 in 1765 individuals in this population is homozygous and affected. *GJB2* hearing loss can also vary among the members of the same family, suggesting that other genes or factors influence the auditory phenotype. A single mutation in *GJB2* in combination with a single mutation in *GJB6* (connexin 30) can also lead to hearing loss and is an example of digenic inheritance of hearing loss.

In addition to *GJB2*, several other nonsyndromic genes are associated with hearing loss that progresses with age. The contribution of genetics to presbycusis is also becoming better understood and likely reflects a combination of genetic susceptibility impacted by environmental exposure to sound. Sensitivity to aminoglycoside ototoxicity can be maternally transmitted through a mitochondrial mutation. Susceptibility to noise-induced hearing loss may also be genetically determined.

There are >400 syndromic forms of hearing loss. These include Usher's syndrome (retinitis pigmentosa and hearing loss), Waardenburg's syndrome (pigmentary abnormality and hearing loss), Pendred's syndrome (thyroid organification defect and hearing loss), Alport's syndrome (renal disease and hearing loss), Jervell and Lange-Nielsen syndrome (prolonged QT interval and hearing loss), neurofibromatosis type 2 (bilateral acoustic schwannoma), and mitochondrial disorders (mitochondrial encephalopathy, lactic acidosis, and stroke-like episodes [MELAS]; myoclonic epilepsy and ragged red fibers [MERRF]; and progressive external ophthalmoplegia [PEO]) (**Table 34-2**).

APPROACH TO THE PATIENT

Disorders of the Sense of Hearing

The goal in the evaluation of a patient with auditory complaints is to determine (1) the nature of the hearing impairment (conductive vs sensorineural vs mixed), (2) the severity of the impairment (mild, moderate, severe, or profound), (3) the anatomy of the impairment (external ear, middle ear, inner ear, or central auditory pathway), and (4) the etiology. The presence of signs and symptoms associated with hearing loss should be ascertained (**Table 34-3**). The history should elicit characteristics of the hearing loss, including the duration of deafness, unilateral versus bilateral involvement, nature of onset (sudden vs insidious), and rate of progression (rapid vs slow). Symptoms of tinnitus, vertigo, imbalance, aural fullness, otorrhea, headache, facial nerve dysfunction, and head and neck paresthesias should be noted. Information regarding head trauma, exposure to ototoxins, occupational or recreational noise exposure, and family history of hearing impairment may also be important. A sudden onset of unilateral hearing loss, with or without tinnitus, may represent a viral infection of the inner ear, vestibular schwannoma, or a stroke. Patients with unilateral hearing loss (sensory or conductive) usually complain of reduced hearing, poor sound localization, and difficulty hearing clearly in the presence of background noise. Gradual progression of a hearing deficit is common with otosclerosis, noise-induced hearing loss, vestibular schwannoma, or Ménière's disease. Small vestibular schwannomas typically present with asymmetric hearing impairment, tinnitus, and imbalance (rarely vertigo); cranial neuropathy, in particular of the trigeminal or facial nerve, may accompany larger tumors. In addition to hearing loss, Ménière's disease may be associated with episodic vertigo, tinnitus, and aural fullness. Sound-induced vertigo, autophony, and being able to hear one's own neck or eye movement are highly suggestive of superior semicircular canal dehiscence. Hearing loss with otorrhea is most likely due to chronic otitis media or cholesteatoma.

Examination should include the auricle, external ear canal, and tympanic membrane. In the elderly, the external ear canal is often dry and fragile; it is preferable to clean cerumen with wall-mounted suction or cerumen loops and to avoid irrigation. Irrigation should also be avoided when a tympanic membrane perforation is present or the integrity of the eardrum cannot be established. In examining the eardrum, the topography of the tympanic membrane is more important than the presence or absence of the light reflex. In addition to the pars tensa (the lower two-thirds of the tympanic membrane), the pars flaccida (upper one-third of the tympanic membrane) above the short process of the malleus should also be examined for retraction pockets that may be evidence of chronic Eustachian tube dysfunction or cholesteatoma. Insufflation of the ear canal is necessary to assess tympanic membrane mobility and compliance. Careful inspection of the nose, nasopharynx, and upper respiratory tract is important. Unilateral serous effusion or unexplained otalgia should prompt a fiberoptic examination of the nasopharynx and larynx to exclude neoplasms. Cranial nerves should be evaluated with special attention to facial and trigeminal nerves, which are commonly affected with tumors involving the cerebellopontine angle.

The Rinne and Weber tuning fork tests, with a 512-Hz tuning fork, are used to screen for hearing loss, differentiate conductive from sensorineural hearing losses, and confirm the findings of audiologic evaluation. The Rinne test compares the ability to hear by air conduction with the ability to hear by bone conduction. The tines of a vibrating tuning fork are held near the opening of the external auditory canal, and then the stem is placed on the mastoid process; for direct contact, it may be placed on teeth or dentures. The patient is asked to indicate whether the tone is louder by air conduction or bone conduction. Normally, and in the presence of sensorineural hearing loss, a tone is heard louder by air conduction than by bone conduction; however, with conductive hearing loss of ≥30 dB (see "Audiologic Assessment," below), the bone-conduction stimulus is perceived as louder than the air-conduction stimulus. For the Weber test, the stem of a vibrating tuning fork is placed on the head in the midline and the patient is asked whether the tone is heard in both ears or better in one ear than in the other. With a unilateral conductive hearing loss, the tone is perceived in the affected ear. With a unilateral sensorineural hearing loss, the tone is perceived in the unaffected ear. A 5-dB difference in hearing between the two ears is required for lateralization.

LABORATORY ASSESSMENT OF HEARING

Audiologic Assessment The minimum audiologic assessment for hearing loss should include the measurement of pure tone air-conduction and bone-conduction thresholds, speech reception threshold, word recognition score, tympanometry, acoustic reflexes, and

TABLE 34-1 Hereditary Hearing Impairment Genes

DESIGNATION	GENE	FUNCTION
Autosomal Dominant		
DFNA1	*DIAPH1*	Cytoskeletal protein
DFNA2A	*KCNQ4*	Potassium channel
DFNA2B	*GJB3*	Gap junction
DFNA2C	*IFNLR1*	Class II cytokine receptor
DFNA3A	*GJB2*	Gap junction
DFNA3B	*GJB6*	Gap junction
DFNA4A	*MYH14*	Class II nonmuscle myosin
DFNA4B	*CEACAM16*	Cell adhesion molecule
DFNA5	*GSDME/DFNA5*	Executioner of pyroptosis
DFNA6/14/38	*WFS1*	Transmembrane protein
DFNA7	*LMX1A*	Transcription factor
DFNA8/12	*TECTA*	Tectorial membrane protein
DFNA9	*COCH*	Unknown
DFNA10	*EYA4*	Developmental gene
DFNA11	*MYO7A*	Cytoskeletal protein
DFNA13	*COL11A2*	Cytoskeletal protein
DFNA15	*POU4F3*	Transcription factor
DFNA17	*MYH9*	Cytoskeletal protein
DFNA20/26	*ACTG1*	Cytoskeletal protein
DFNA22	*MYO6*	Unconventional myosin
DFNA23	*SIX1*	Developmental gene
DFNA25	*SLC17A8*	Vesicular glutamate transporter
DFNA27	*REST*	Transcriptional repressor
DFNA28	*GRHL2*	Transcription factor
DFNA34	*NLRP3*	Pyrin-like protein involved in inflammation
DFNA36	*TMC1*	Transmembrane protein
DNA37	*COL11A1*	Cytoskeletal protein
DFNA40	*CRYM*	Thyroid hormone–binding protein
DFNA41	*P2RX2*	Purinergic receptor
DFNA44	*CCDC50*	Effector of epidermal growth factor–mediated signaling
DFNA50	*MIRN96*	MicroRNA
DFNA51	*TJP2*	Tight junction protein
DFNA56	*TNC*	Extracellular matrix protein
DFNA64	*SMAC/DIABLO*	Mitochondrial proapoptotic protein
DFNA65	*TBC1D24*	ARF6-interacting protein
DFNA66	*CD164*	Sialomucin
DFNA67	*OSBPL2*	Intracellular lipid receptor
DFNA68	*HOMER2*	Stereociliary scaffolding protein
DFNA69	*KITLG*	Ligand for KIT receptor
DFNA70	*MCM2*	Initiation and elongation during DNA replication
DFNA73	*PTPRQ*	Member of type III receptor-like protein-tyrosine phosphatase (PTPase) family
	DMXL2	Regulator of Notch signaling
	MYO3A	Member of myosin superfamily
	PDE1C	Catalyze hydrolysis of cAMP and cGMP
	TRRAP	Transformation/transcription domain associated protein
	PLS1	Actin-bundling protein
	SCD5	Catalyzes formation of monounsaturated fatty acids from saturated fatty acids
	SLC12A2	Sodium-potassium-chloride transporter
	MAP1B	Microtubule binding protein
	RIPOR2/FAM65B	Membrane-associated protein in stereocilia

DESIGNATION	GENE	FUNCTION
Autosomal Recessive		
DFNB1A	*GJB2*	Gap junction
DFNB1B	*GJB6*	Gap junction
DFNB2	*MYO7A*	Cytoskeletal protein
DFNB3	*MYO15A*	Cytoskeletal protein
DFNB4	*SLC26A4*	Chloride/iodide transporter
DFNB6	*TMIE*	Transmembrane protein
DFNB7/B11	*TMC1*	Transmembrane protein
DFNB8/10	*TMPRSS3*	Transmembrane serine protease
DFNB9	*OTOF*	Trafficking of membrane vesicles
DFNB12	*CDH23*	Intercellular adherence protein
DFNB15/72/95	*GIPC3*	PDZ domain–containing protein
DFNB16	*STRC*	Stereocilia protein
DFNB18	*USH1C*	Unknown
DFNB18B	*OTOG*	Tectorial membrane protein
DFNB21	*TECTA*	Tectorial membrane protein
DFNB22	*OTOA*	Gel attachment to nonsensory cell
DFNB23	*PCDH15*	Morphogenesis and cohesion
DFNB24	*RDX*	Cytoskeletal protein
DFNB25	*GRXCR1*	Reversible S-glutathionylation of proteins
DFNB26	*GAB1*	Member of insulin receptor substrate 1–like multisubstrate docking adapter protein family
DFNB28	*TRIOBP*	Cytoskeletal-organizing protein
DFNB29	*CLDN14*	Tight junctions
DFNB30	*MYO3A*	Hybrid motor-signaling myosin
DFNB31	*WHRN*	PDZ domain–containing protein
DFNB32/105	*CDC14A*	Protein phosphatase involved in hair cell ciliogenesis
DFNB35	*ESRRB*	Estrogen-related receptor beta protein
DFNB36	*ESPN*	Ca-insensitive actin-bundling protein
DFNB37	*MYO6*	Unconventional myosin
DFNB39	*HFG*	Hepatocyte growth factor
DFNB42	*ILDR1*	Ig-like domain–containing receptor
DFNB44	*ADCY1*	Adenylate cyclase
DFNB48	*CIB2*	Calcium and integrin binding protein
DFNB49	*BDP1*	Subunit of RNA polymerase
DFNB49	*MARVELD2*	Tight junction protein
DFNB53	*COL11A2*	Collagen protein
DFNB59	*PJVK*	Zn-binding protein
DFNB60	*SLC22A4*	Prestin, motor protein of cochlear outer hair cell
DFNB61	*SLC26A5*	Motor protein
DFNB63	*LRTOMT/COMT2*	Putative methyltransferase
DFNB66	*DCDC2*	Ciliary protein
DFNB66/67	*LHFPL5*	Tetraspan protein
DFNB68	*S1PR2*	Tetraspan membrane protein of hair cell stereocilia
DFNB70	*PNPT1*	Mitochondrial–RNA–import protein
DFNB73	*BSND*	Beta subunit of chloride channel
DFNB74	*MSRB3*	Methionine sulfoxide reductase
DFNB76	*SYNE4*	Part of *LINC* tethering complex
DFNB77	*LOXHD1*	Stereociliary protein
DFNB79	*TPRN*	Unknown
DFNB82	*GPSM2*	G protein signaling modulator
DFNB84	*PTPRQ*	Type III receptor-like protein-tyrosine phosphatase family

(Continued)

TABLE 34-1 Hereditary Hearing Impairment Genes (Continued)

DESIGNATION	GENE	FUNCTION
DFNB84	*OTOGL*	Otogelin-like protein
DFNB86	*TBC1D24*	GTPase-activating protein
DFNB88	*ELMOD3*	GTPase-activating protein
DFNB89	*KARS*	Lysyl-tRNA synthetase
DFNB91	*SERPINB6*	Protease inhibitor
DFNB93	*CABP2*	Calcium-binding protein
DFN94	*NARS2*	Mitochondrial asparaginyl-tRNA synthetase
DFNA97	*MET*	Oncogene/hepatocyte growth factor receptor
DFNB98	*TSPEAR*	Epilepsy-associated repeats containing protein
DFNB99	*TMEM132E*	Transmembrane protein
DFNB100	*PPIP5K2*	Diphosphoinositol-pentakisphosphate kinase
DFNB101	*GRXCR2*	Maintaining stereocilia bundles
DFNB102	*EPS8*	Epidermal growth factor receptor
DFNB103	*CLIC5*	Chloride ion transport
DFNB104	*FAM65B/RIPOR2*	Membrane-associated protein in stereocilia
DFNB106	*EPS8L2*	Actin remodeling in response to EGF stimulation
DFNB108	*ROR1*	Receptor tyrosine kinase-like orphan receptor
	WBP2	Transcriptional coactivator for estrogen receptor-alpha and progesterone receptor
	ESRP1	Modulates activation of G proteins
	MPZL2	Mediates epithelial cell-cell interactions in developing tissues
	CEACAM16	Cell adhesion molecule
	GRAP	Cytoplasmic signaling protein
	SPNS2	Sphingosine-1-phosphate (S1P) transporter
	CLDN9	Tight junctions
	CLRN2	Maintenance of transducing stereocilia in auditory hair cells
X-linked		
DFNX1	PRPS1	Catalyzes phosphoribosylation of ribose 5-phosphate to 5-phosphoribosyl-1-pyrophosphate
DFNX2	POU3F4	Transcription factor
DFNX4	SMPX	Small muscle protein
DFNX5	AIFM1	Mitochondrial flavin adenine dinucleotide (FAD)-dependent oxidoreductase
DFNX6	COL4A6	Collagen protein

TABLE 34-2 Syndromic Hereditary Hearing Impairment Genes

SYNDROME	GENE	FUNCTION
Alport's syndrome	*COL4A3-5*	Cytoskeletal protein
BOR syndrome	*EYA1*	Developmental gene
	SIX5	Developmental gene
	SIX1	Developmental gene
Jervell and Lange-Nielsen syndrome	*KCNQ1*	Delayed rectifier K^+ channel
	KCNE1	Delayed rectifier K^+ channel
Norrie's disease	*NDP*	Cell–cell interactions
Pendred's syndrome	*SLC26A4*	Chloride/iodide transporter
	FOXI1	Transcriptional activator of *SLC26A4*
	KCNJ10	Inwardly rectifying K^+ channel
Treacher Collins syndrome	*TCOF1*	Nucleolar-cytoplasmic transport
	POLR1D	Subunit of RNA polymerases I and III
	POLR1C	Subunit of RNA polymerases I and III
Usher's syndrome	*MYO7A*	Cytoskeletal protein
	USH1C	Unknown
	CDH23	Intercellular adherence protein
	PCDH15	Cell adhesion molecule
	SANS	Harmonin-associated protein
	CIB2	Calcium- and integrin-binding protein
	USH2A	Cell adhesion molecule
	VLGR1	G protein–coupled receptor
	WHRN	PDZ domain–containing protein
	CLRN1	Cellular synapse protein
	HARS	Histidyl-tRNA synthetase
	PDZD7	PDZ domain–containing protein
WS type I, III	*PAX3*	Transcription factor
WS type II	*MITF*	Transcription factor
	SNAI2	Transcription factor
WS type IV	*EDNRB*	Endothelin B receptor
	EDN3	Endothelin B receptor ligand
	SOX10	Transcription factor

Abbreviations: BOR, branchio-oto-renal syndrome; WS, Waardenburg's syndrome.

acoustic-reflex decay. This test battery provides a screening evaluation of the entire auditory system and allows one to determine whether further differentiation of a sensory (cochlear) from a neural (retrocochlear) hearing loss is indicated.

Pure tone audiometry assesses hearing acuity for pure tones. The test is administered by an audiologist and is performed in a sound-attenuated chamber. The pure tone stimulus is delivered with an audiometer, an electronic device that allows the presentation of specific frequencies (generally between 250–8000 Hz) at specific intensities. Air- and bone-conduction thresholds are established for each ear. Air-conduction thresholds are determined by presenting the stimulus in air with the use of headphones. Bone-conduction thresholds are determined by placing the stem of a vibrating tuning fork or an oscillator of an audiometer in contact with the head. In the presence of a hearing loss, broad-spectrum noise is presented to the nontest ear for masking purposes so that responses are based on perception from the ear under test.

The responses are measured in decibels (dBs). An *audiogram* is a plot of intensity in dBs of hearing threshold versus frequency. A dB is equal to 20 times the logarithm of the ratio of the sound pressure required to achieve threshold in the patient to the sound pressure required to achieve threshold in a normal-hearing person. Therefore, a change of 6 dB represents doubling of sound pressure, and a change of 20 dB represents a tenfold change in sound pressure. Loudness, which depends on the frequency, intensity, and duration of a sound, doubles with approximately each 10-dB increase in sound pressure level. Pitch, on the other hand, does not directly correlate with frequency. The

TABLE 34-3 Signs and Symptoms Suggestive of Hearing Loss

Saying "huh" a great deal
Reduced clarity of hearing
Difficulty understanding conversations in background noise
Family complaining of hearing loss
Tinnitus
Turning the volume up on radio or television
Sensitivity to noises
Fullness in the ear
Avoiding social settings

perception of pitch changes slowly in the low and high frequencies. In the middle tones, which are important for human speech, pitch varies more rapidly with changes in frequency.

Pure tone audiometry establishes the presence and severity of hearing impairment, unilateral versus bilateral involvement, and the type of hearing loss. Conductive hearing losses with a large mass component, as is often seen in middle-ear effusions, produce elevation of thresholds that predominate in the higher frequencies. Conductive hearing losses with a large stiffness component, as in fixation of the footplate of the stapes in early otosclerosis, produce threshold elevations in the lower frequencies. Often, the conductive hearing loss involves all frequencies, suggesting involvement of both stiffness and mass. In general, sensorineural hearing losses such as presbycusis affect higher frequencies more than lower frequencies (Fig. 34-3). An exception is Ménière's disease, which is characteristically associated with low-frequency sensorineural hearing loss (though any frequency can be affected). Noise-induced hearing loss has an unusual pattern of hearing impairment in which the loss at 3000–4000 Hz is greater than at higher frequencies. Vestibular schwannomas characteristically affect the higher frequencies, but any pattern of hearing loss can be observed.

Speech recognition requires greater synchronous neural firing than is necessary for appreciation of pure tones. *Speech audiometry* tests the clarity with which one hears. The *speech reception threshold* (*SRT*) is defined as the intensity at which speech is recognized as a meaningful symbol and is obtained by presenting two-syllable words with an equal accent on each syllable. The intensity at which the patient can repeat 50% of the words correctly is the SRT. Once the SRT is determined, discrimination or word recognition ability is tested by presenting one-syllable words at 25–40 dB above the SRT. The words are phonetically balanced in that the phonemes (speech sounds) occur in the list of words at the same frequency that they occur in ordinary conversational English. An individual with normal hearing or conductive hearing loss can repeat 88–100% of the phonetically balanced words correctly. Patients with a sensorineural hearing loss have variable loss of discrimination. As a general rule, neural lesions produce greater deficits in discrimination than do cochlear lesions. For example, in a patient with mild asymmetric sensorineural hearing loss, a clue to the diagnosis of vestibular schwannoma is the presence of greater than expected deterioration in discrimination ability. Deterioration in discrimination ability at higher intensities above the SRT also suggests a lesion in the eighth nerve or central auditory pathways.

Tympanometry measures the impedance of the middle ear to sound and is useful in diagnosis of middle-ear effusions. A *tympanogram* is the graphic representation of change in impedance or compliance as the pressure in the ear canal is changed. Normally, the middle ear is most compliant at atmospheric pressure, and the compliance decreases as the pressure is increased or decreased (type A); this pattern is seen with normal hearing or in the presence of sensorineural hearing loss. Compliance that does not change with change in pressure suggests middle-ear effusion (type B). With a negative pressure in the middle ear, as with Eustachian tube obstruction, the point of maximal compliance occurs with negative pressure in the ear canal (type C). A tympanogram in which no point of maximal compliance can be obtained is most commonly seen with discontinuity of the ossicular chain (type A_d). A reduction in the maximal compliance peak can be seen in otosclerosis (type A_s).

During tympanometry, an intense tone elicits contraction of the stapedius muscle. The change in compliance of the middle ear with contraction of the stapedius muscle can be detected. The presence or absence of this *acoustic reflex* is important in determining the etiology of hearing loss as well as in the anatomic localization of facial nerve paralysis. The acoustic reflex can help differentiate between conductive hearing loss due to otosclerosis and that caused by an inner-ear "third window": it is absent in otosclerosis and present in inner-ear conductive hearing loss. Normal or elevated acoustic reflex thresholds in an individual with sensorineural hearing impairment suggest a cochlear hearing loss. An absent acoustic reflex in the setting of sensorineural hearing loss is not helpful in localizing the site of lesion. Assessment of *acoustic reflex decay* helps differentiate sensory from neural hearing losses. In neural hearing loss, such as with vestibular schwannoma, the reflex adapts or decays with time.

OAEs generated by outer hair cells only can be measured with microphones inserted into the external auditory canal. The emissions may be spontaneous or evoked with sound stimulation. The presence of OAEs indicates that the outer hair cells of the organ of Corti are intact and can be used to assess auditory thresholds and to distinguish sensory from neural hearing losses.

Evoked Responses *Electrocochleography* measures the earliest evoked potentials generated in the cochlea and the auditory nerve. Receptor potentials recorded include the cochlear microphonic, generated by the outer hair cells of the organ of Corti, and the summating potential, generated by the inner hair cells in response to sound. The whole nerve action potential representing the composite firing of the first-order neurons can also be recorded during electrocochleography. Clinically, the test is useful in the diagnosis of Ménière's disease, in which an elevation of the ratio of summating potential to action potential is seen.

Brainstem auditory-evoked responses (*BAERs*), also known as ABRs, are useful in differentiating the site of sensorineural hearing loss. In response to sound, five distinct electrical potentials arising from different stations along the peripheral and central auditory pathway (eighth nerve, cochlear nucleus, superior olivary complex, lateral lemniscus, and inferior colliculus) can be identified using computer averaging from scalp surface electrodes. BAERs are valuable in situations in which patients cannot or will not give reliable voluntary thresholds. They are also used to assess the integrity of the auditory nerve and brainstem in various clinical situations, including intraoperative monitoring, and in determination of brain death.

The *VEMP test* investigates otolith and vestibular nerve function by presenting a high-level acoustic stimulus and evoking a short-latency electromyographic potential; cVEMP (or cervical VEMP) and oVEMP (or ocular VEMP) have been described. The cVEMP elicits a vestibulocollic reflex whose afferent limb arises from acoustically sensitive cells in the saccule, with signals conducted via the inferior vestibular nerve. cVEMP is a biphasic, short-latency response recorded from the tonically contracted sternocleidomastoid muscle in response to loud auditory clicks or tones. cVEMPs may be diminished or absent in patients with early and late Ménière's disease, vestibular neuritis, benign paroxysmal positional vertigo, and vestibular schwannoma. On the other hand, the threshold for VEMPs may be lower in cases of superior canal dehiscence, other inner-ear dehiscence ("third window"), and perilymphatic fistula. The oVEMP, in contrast, is a response involving the utricle primarily and superior vestibular nerve. The oVEMP excitatory response is recorded from the extraocular muscle. The oVEMP is abnormal in superior vestibular neuritis.

Imaging Studies The choice of radiologic tests is largely determined by whether the goal is to evaluate the bony anatomy of the external, middle, and inner ear or to image the auditory nerve and brain. Axial and coronal CT of the temporal bone with fine 0.3-mm cuts is ideal for determining the caliber of the external auditory canal, integrity of the ossicular chain, and presence of middle-ear or mastoid disease; it can also detect inner-ear malformations. CT is also ideal for the detection of bone erosion with chronic otitis media and cholesteatoma. Pöschl reformatting in the plane of the superior semicircular canal is required for the identification of dehiscence or absence of bone over the superior semicircular canal. MRI is superior to CT for imaging of retrocochlear pathology such as vestibular schwannoma, meningioma, other lesions of the cerebellopontine angle, demyelinating lesions of the brainstem, and brain tumors. Both CT and MRI are equally capable of identifying inner-ear malformations and assessing cochlear patency for preoperative evaluation of patients for cochlear implantation.

TREATMENT

Disorders of the Sense of Hearing

In general, conductive hearing losses are amenable to surgical correction, whereas sensorineural hearing losses are usually managed medically. Atresia of the ear canal can be surgically repaired, often with significant improvement in hearing. Alternatively, the conductive hearing loss associated with atresia can be addressed with a bone-anchored hearing aid (BAHA). Tympanic membrane perforations due to chronic otitis media or trauma can be repaired with an outpatient tympanoplasty. Likewise, conductive hearing loss associated with otosclerosis can be treated by stapedectomy, which is successful in >95% of cases. Tympanostomy tubes allow the prompt return of normal hearing in individuals with middle-ear effusions. Hearing aids are effective and well tolerated in patients with conductive hearing losses.

Patients with mild, moderate, and severe sensorineural hearing losses are regularly rehabilitated with hearing aids of varying configuration and strength. Hearing aids have been improved to provide greater fidelity and have been miniaturized. The current generation of hearing aids is nearly invisible, thus reducing stigma associated with their use. In general, the more severe the hearing impairment, the larger the hearing aid required for auditory rehabilitation. Digital hearing aids lend themselves to individual programming, and multiple and directional microphones at the ear level may be helpful in noisy surroundings. Because all hearing aids amplify noise as well as speech, the only absolute solution to the problem of noise is to place the microphone closer to the speaker than the noise source. This arrangement is not possible with a self-contained, cosmetically acceptable device. A significant limitation of rehabilitation with a hearing aid is that although it is able to enhance detection of sound with amplification, it cannot restore clarity of hearing that is lost with presbycusis.

The cost of a single hearing aid (~$2300 US) is a significant obstacle for many hearing-impaired individuals and usually bilateral amplification is recommended. To reduce cost and spur innovation, a new category of over-the-counter amplification devices that can be purchased similar to reading eyeglasses by simply walking into a store has recently been approved by the US Food and Drug Administration. By reducing the cost of amplification devices to consumers, promoting innovation, and increasing competition, this new class of devices could fundamentally change the way hearing rehabilitation is delivered.

Patients with unilateral deafness have difficulty with sound localization and reduced clarity of hearing in background noise. They may benefit from a contralateral routing of signal (CROS) hearing aid in which a microphone is placed on the hearing-impaired side, and the sound is transmitted to the receiver placed on the contralateral ear. The same result may be obtained with a BAHA, in which a hearing aid clamps to a screw integrated into the skull on the hearing-impaired side. Like the CROS hearing aid, the BAHA transfers the acoustic signal to the contralateral hearing ear, but it does so by vibrating the skull. Patients with profound deafness on one side and some hearing loss in the better ear are candidates for a BICROS hearing aid; it differs from the CROS hearing aid in that the patient wears a hearing aid, and not simply a receiver, in the better ear. Unfortunately, while CROS and BAHA devices provide benefit, they do not restore hearing in the deaf ear. Only cochlear implants can restore hearing (see below). Increasingly, cochlear implants are being used for the treatment of patients with single-sided deafness; they show great promise in not only restoring hearing and reducing tinnitus, but also improving sound localization and performance in background noise.

In many situations, including lectures and the theater, hearing-impaired persons benefit from assistive devices that are based on the principle of having the speaker closer to the microphone than any source of noise. Assistive devices include infrared and frequency-modulated (FM) transmission as well as an electromagnetic loop around the room for transmission to the individual's hearing aid. Hearing aids with telecoils can also be used with properly equipped telephones in the same way. Bluetooth technology has revolutionized connectivity between hearing aids and other devices such as smart phones.

In the event that the hearing aid provides inadequate rehabilitation, cochlear implants may be appropriate (**Fig. 34-4**). Criteria for implantation include severe to profound hearing loss with open-set sentence cognition of ≤40% under best-aided conditions.

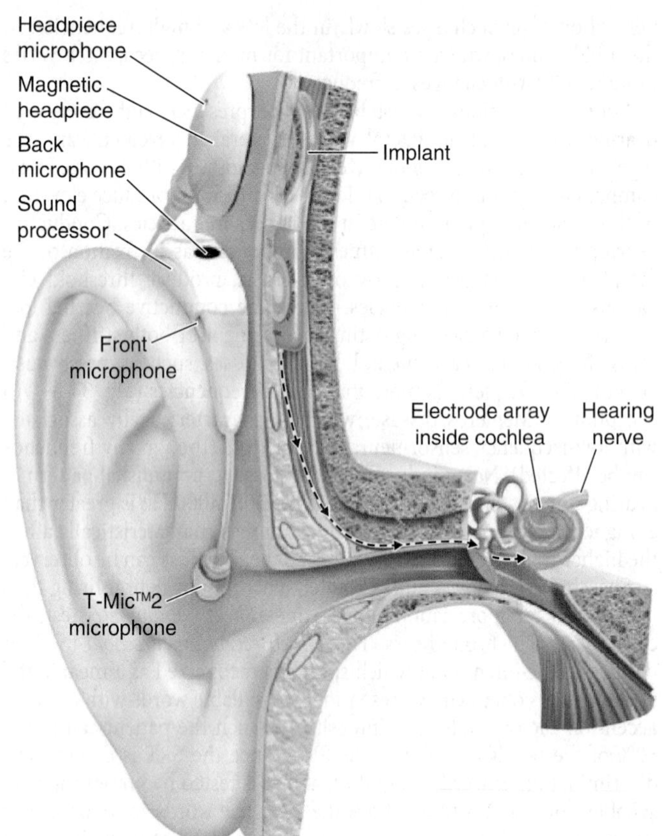

FIGURE 34-4 A cochlear implant is composed of an external microphone and speech processor worn on the ear and a receiver implanted underneath the temporalis muscle. The internal receiver is attached to an electrode that is placed surgically in the cochlea.

Worldwide, >600,000 hearing-impaired individuals have received cochlear implants. Cochlear implants are neural prostheses that convert sound energy to electrical energy and can be used to stimulate the auditory division of the eighth nerve directly. In most cases of profound hearing impairment, the auditory hair cells are lost but the ganglionic cells of the auditory division of the eighth nerve are preserved. Cochlear implants consist of electrodes that are inserted into the cochlea through the round window, speech processors that extract acoustic elements of speech for conversion to electrical currents, and a means of transmitting the electrical energy through the skin. Patients with implants experience sound that helps with speech reading, allows open-set word recognition, and helps in modulating the person's own voice. Usually, within the first 3–6 months after implantation, adult patients can understand speech without visual cues. With the current generation of multichannel cochlear implants, nearly 75% of patients are able to converse on the telephone. Bilateral cochlear implantations are commonly performed, especially in children; these patients perform better in background noise, have better sound localization, and are less fatigued by the "work" compared to monaural hearing.

Hybrid cochlear implants are indicated for the treatment of high-frequency hearing loss in patients who do not have profound hearing loss and yet do not benefit from hearing aids. Patients with presbycusis typically have normal low-frequency hearing while suffering from high-frequency hearing loss associated with loss of clarity that cannot always be adequately rehabilitated with a hearing aid. However, these patients are not candidates for conventional cochlear implants because they have too much residual hearing. The hybrid implant has been specifically designed for this patient population; it has a shorter electrode than a conventional cochlear implant and can be introduced into the cochlea atraumatically, thus preserving low-frequency hearing. Individuals with a hybrid implant use their own natural low-frequency "acoustic" hearing and rely on the implant for providing "electrical" high-frequency hearing. Patients who have received the hybrid implant perform better on speech discrimination tests in both quiet and noisy backgrounds.

For individuals who were born without cochlea or have had both eighth nerves destroyed by trauma or bilateral vestibular schwannomas (e.g., neurofibromatosis type 2), brainstem auditory implants placed near the cochlear nucleus may provide auditory rehabilitation. Currently, brainstem implants provide sound awareness but unfortunately speech understanding remains elusive.

Tinnitus often accompanies hearing loss. Similar to background noise, tinnitus can degrade speech comprehension in individuals with hearing impairment. Patients with tinnitus should be advised to minimize caffeine ingestion, avoid high dosage of nonsteroidal anti-inflammatory drugs (NSAIDs), and reduce stress. Therapy for tinnitus is usually directed toward minimizing the appreciation of tinnitus. Relief of the tinnitus may be obtained by masking it with background music or white noise. Hearing aids are also helpful in tinnitus suppression, as are tinnitus maskers, devices that present a sound to the affected ear that is more pleasant to listen to than the tinnitus. The use of a tinnitus masker is often followed by several hours of inhibition of the tinnitus. Antidepressants have also been shown to be beneficial in helping patients cope with tinnitus.

Hard-of-hearing individuals often benefit from a reduction in unnecessary noise in the environment (e.g., radio or television) to enhance the signal-to-noise ratio. Speech comprehension is aided by lip reading; therefore, the impaired listener should be seated so that the face of the speaker is well illuminated and easily seen. Although speech should be in a loud, clear voice, one should be aware that in sensorineural hearing losses in general and in hard-of-hearing elderly in particular, recruitment (abnormal perception of loud sounds) may be troublesome. Above all, optimal communication cannot take place without both parties giving it their full and undivided attention.

PREVENTION

Conductive hearing losses may be prevented by prompt antibiotic therapy of adequate duration for AOM and by ventilation of the middle ear with tympanostomy tubes in middle-ear effusions lasting ≥12 weeks. Loss of vestibular function and deafness due to aminoglycoside antibiotics can largely be prevented by careful monitoring of serum peak and trough levels.

Some 10 million Americans have noise-induced hearing loss, and 20 million are exposed to hazardous noise in their employment. Noise-induced hearing loss can be prevented by avoidance of exposure to loud noise or by regular use of earplugs or fluid-filled ear muffs to attenuate intense sound. **Table 34-4** lists loudness levels for a variety of environmental sounds. High-risk activities for noise-induced hearing loss include use of electrical equipment for wood- and metalworking, and target practice or hunting with small firearms. All internal-combustion and electric engines, including snow and leaf blowers, snowmobiles, outboard motors, and chainsaws, require protection of the user with hearing protectors. Virtually all noise-induced hearing loss is preventable through education, which should begin before the teenage years. Programs for conservation of hearing in the workplace are required by the Occupational Safety and Health Administration (OSHA) whenever the exposure over an 8-h period averages 85 dB. OSHA mandates that workers in such noisy environments have hearing monitoring and protection programs that include a preemployment screen, an annual audiologic assessment, and the mandatory use of hearing protectors. Exposure to loud sounds above 85 dB in the work environment is restricted by OSHA, with halving of allowed exposure time for each increment of 5 dB above this threshold; for example, exposure to 90 dB is permitted for 8 h; 95 dB for 4 h, and 100 dB for 2 h (**Table 34-5**).

TABLE 34-4 Decibel (Loudness) Level of Common Environmental Noise

SOURCE	DECIBEL (dB)
Weakest sound heard	0
Whisper	30
Normal conversation	55–65
City traffic inside car	85
OSHA Monitoring Requirement Begins	**90**
Jackhammer	95
Subway train at 200 ft	95
Power mower	107
Power saw	110
Painful Sound	**125**
Jet engine at 100 ft	140
12-gauge shotgun blast	165
Loudest sound that can occur	194

Abbreviation: OSHA, Occupational Safety and Health Administration.

TABLE 34-5 OSHA Daily Permissible Noise Level Exposure

SOUND LEVEL (dB)	DURATION PER DAY (h)
90	8
92	6
95	4
97	3
100	2
102	1.5
105	1
110	0.5
115	≤0.25

Note: Exposure to impulsive or impact noise should not exceed 140-dB peak sound pressure level.

Source: From *https://www.osha.gov/pls/oshaweb/owadisp.show_document?p_table=standards&p_id=9735.*

FURTHER READING

Carlson ML: Cochlear implantation in adults. N Engl J Med 382:1531, 2020.

Espinosa-Sanchez JM, Lopez-Escamez JA: Menière's disease. Handb Clin Neurol 137:257, 2016.

Moser T, Starr A: Auditory neuropathy—neural and synaptic mechanisms. Nat Rev Neurol 12:135, 2016.

Patel M et al: Intratympanic methylprednisolone versus gentamicin in patients with unilateral Ménière's disease: a randomised, double-blind, comparative effectiveness trial. Lancet 388:2753, 2016.

Tikka C et al: Interventions to prevent occupational noise-induced hearing loss. Cochrane Database Syst Rev 7:CD006396, 2017.

Wilson BS et al: Global hearing health care: new findings and perspectives. Lancet 390:2503, 2017.

35 Upper Respiratory Symptoms, Including Earache, Sinus Symptoms, and Sore Throat

Rachel L. Amdur, Jeffrey A. Linder

Upper respiratory symptoms are most commonly caused by viral infection but also can be caused by other infectious, inflammatory, allergic, autoimmune, and neoplastic conditions. This chapter will discuss ambulatory antibiotic prescribing and review the most common causes of upper respiratory symptoms, including nonspecific upper respiratory infections.

Ear pain is most commonly caused by otitis externa, acute otitis media (AOM), otitis media with effusion (OME), and acute mastoiditis. Sinus symptoms can be caused by acute sinusitis, invasive fungal sinusitis, nosocomial sinusitis, and chronic sinusitis. Sore throat and neck pain can be caused by streptococcal pharyngitis, nonstreptococcal pharyngitis, acute infectious mononucleosis, other types of bacterial pharyngitis, Lemierre's syndrome, gonococcal pharyngitis, diphtheria, acute HIV infection, head and neck abscesses, epiglottitis, and laryngitis. At the time of presentation, upper respiratory symptoms of most common viral and bacterial etiologies have generally lasted from hours up to a few days.

UPPER RESPIRATORY INFECTIONS

Upper respiratory infections (URIs) are acute respiratory infections that occur above the vocal cords. URIs, including nonspecific upper respiratory tract infection, otitis media, sinusitis, and pharyngitis, are collectively the most common symptomatic reason for seeking care in the United States. In terms of etiology, symptoms, and signs, URIs overlap with lower acute respiratory infections that occur below the vocal cords, such as influenza **(Chap. 200)**, acute bronchitis, and pneumonia **(Chap. 126)**, as well as with noninfectious cough **(Chap. 38)**. The average adult has 2–4 URIs per year; children can have 6–10 URIs annually. URIs can be prevented by hand washing or sanitization, physical distancing, use of facial masks, isolation of persons who are ill, and environmental cleaning **(Chap. 199)**.

SARS-CoV-2, the pathogen that causes COVID-19, can cause virtually any upper respiratory symptom **(Chap. 199)**. COVID-19 symptoms appear 2–14 days after exposure and may include fever, chills, cough, shortness of breath, fatigue, myalgias, headaches, rhinorrhea, sore throat, nausea, vomiting, or diarrhea. New loss of taste or smell appears to be specific for COVID-19. Until there is widespread natural or vaccine-induced immunity, any respiratory symptom occurring in areas where SARS-CoV-2 is circulating should be considered a potential manifestation of COVID-19.

■ IMPROVING AMBULATORY ANTIBIOTIC PRESCRIBING

The only common acute respiratory infections that should be treated with antibiotics are AOM, sinusitis, streptococcal pharyngitis, and pneumonia. Even for AOM, sinusitis, and pharyngitis, only a minority of cases meet the criteria for antibiotic prescribing. Common respiratory viruses **(Chap. 199)** cause the overwhelming majority of acute respiratory infections, and these infections are generally self-limited; antibiotics neither speed resolution nor prevent complications for the majority of acute respiratory infections. Unfortunately, for this reason, at least half of ambulatory antibiotic prescriptions for acute respiratory infections in the United States are inappropriate. Internationally, population rates of antibiotic prescribing vary nearly threefold, with no differences in infectious complications. Antibiotics cause adverse drug effects, alter the microbiome, cause *Clostridioides difficile* infection **(Chap. 134)**, increase health care costs, and increase the prevalence of antibiotic-resistant bacteria **(Chap. 145)**.

Clinicians prescribe inappropriate antibiotics because of time pressure; fear of missing a rare bacterial diagnosis; concern about preventing a rare bacterial complication; a lack of salience of adverse antibiotic effects; or a mistaken belief that most patients expect, demand, or will not be satisfied without an antibiotic prescription.

■ AMBULATORY ANTIBIOTIC STEWARDSHIP

Antibiotic stewardship has traditionally been an inpatient concern **(Chap. 144)**, but ambulatory antibiotic use accounts for ~85% of antibiotic use by patients in most developed countries. In 2016, the Centers for Disease Control and Prevention published the "Core Elements of Outpatient Antibiotic Stewardship." The core elements include (1) committing to improving antibiotic prescribing; (2) implementing at least one policy or practice to improve antibiotic prescribing and assessing its effectiveness; (3) monitoring antibiotic prescribing and providing feedback; and (4) providing educational resources to clinicians and patients on antibiotic prescribing. Effective interventions to decrease inappropriate ambulatory antibiotic prescribing include peer comparison, accountable justification, precommitment, clinical decision support, patient education, and multifaceted interventions. Communication training has been particularly effective when it includes making a clear diagnosis, focusing on positive actions patients can take to feel better, reviewing the expected course of illness, and informing patients about concerning symptoms (red flags) for which they should seek or reconnect with care. Telemedicine—synchronous telephone or video or asynchronous electronic messaging—has the potential to improve patient convenience and reduce inappropriate antibiotic prescribing.

Several techniques that seemed promising for the reduction of ambulatory antibiotic prescribing remain unproven, have been ineffective (e.g., procalcitonin testing), or are not durable (e.g., C-reactive protein testing). The practice of delayed antibiotic prescription—i.e., a prescription given to a patient who is asked not to fill it unless symptoms do not improve in a few days—is conceptually flawed and should be avoided. Delayed antibiotic prescriptions are usually given for antibiotic-inappropriate diagnoses (e.g., viral infections); they ignore the natural history of acute respiratory infections, which are self-limited and generally last from 5 to 14 days; they put the burden of clinical decision-making on patients; and they send a confusing, mixed message to patients about the appropriateness of antibiotics for respiratory infections.

NONSPECIFIC UPPER RESPIRATORY INFECTION ("THE COMMON COLD")

■ DEFINITION AND ETIOLOGY

Nonspecific URI, or the common cold, is a respiratory tract infection in which no single symptom predominates. Nonspecific URI is most commonly caused by respiratory viruses that are acquired through direct contact with infected individuals, contaminated surfaces, and large and small respiratory droplets. The most common viral causes of nonspecific URIs are rhinoviruses (well over 100 serotypes; **Chap. 199**), coronaviruses, parainfluenza virus, respiratory syncytial virus, influenza virus **(Chap. 199)**, adenovirus (57 serotypes; **Chap. 199**), metapneumovirus, and bocavirus **(Chap. 199)**. Making a specific viral diagnosis is not practical, cost-effective, or necessary. Multiplex panels of reverse transcription polymerase chain reaction are available but may be overly sensitive, as prior recent infection can cause false-positive results. Although the diagnosis is usually obvious, clinicians diagnosing a nonspecific URI should also consider influenza **(Chap. 200)**, measles (cough, coryza, and conjunctivitis; **Chap. 205**), acute HIV infection (in which sore throat and rash often predominate; see below and **Chap. 202**), and COVID-19 **(Chap. 199)**.

Individual susceptibility to nonspecific URIs depends on prior exposure, immunity, general health, genetics, microbiome-related factors, and mental health and social factors, including stress. Prior exposure leads to immunity to specific rhinoviruses and adenoviruses, but the number of serotypes makes reinfection likely. Immunity to non-COVID-19 coronaviruses, parainfluenza virus, respiratory syncytial virus, and metapneumoviruses is generally weak or of short duration.

■ SYMPTOMS AND SIGNS

Common respiratory viruses have incubation periods of 2–8 days after exposure. Symptoms generally begin gradually and include nasal fullness or obstruction, rhinorrhea, sore throat, laryngitis, lymphadenopathy, cough, and low-grade fever. Patients may have myalgias, but this feature usually is not as prominent as it is in influenza. Epistaxis is common with frequent nose blowing.

On physical examination, findings vary, but patients may have conjunctivitis, pharyngeal erythema, pharyngeal exudates, or pharyngeal cobblestoning. Depending on the phase of illness, the nasal mucosa may be pale, boggy, or red and swollen. Nasal mucus can range from watery to purulent. On auscultation, the lungs may be clear, or the patient may have diffuse wheezing or bronchial breath sounds consistent with a viral infection. Symptoms usually last 5–10 days but often last up to 14 days.

TREATMENT

Nonspecific Upper Respiratory Infection

For adults and older children, treatment of nonspecific URI is symptom-based. Fever, myalgias, and sore throat can be treated with acetaminophen or a nonsteroidal anti-inflammatory drug (NSAID) such as ibuprofen. Rhinorrhea can be treated with ipratropium bromide. Nasal congestion can be managed with nasal decongestants such as oxymetazoline (two sprays into each nostril twice a day for up to 5 days) or systemic decongestants such as pseudoephedrine. Products that combine a decongestant with analgesics, antihistamines, or both help relieve symptoms. Although supporting data are weak, cough may be relieved with dextromethorphan or benzonatate (Tessalon Perles). Opioids, while effective at relieving cough, are associated with somnolence, dysphoria, constipation, and addiction.

For children <6 years old, cough and cold medicines should not be prescribed, recommended, or used because of the risks of adverse effects. Honey can help soothe a sore throat for children >1 year old. Cool-mist humidifiers may help with breathing, and saline nasal drops and bulb suctioning can help with nasal congestion.

Patients need to be informed that symptoms generally peak early but can last for up to 14 days; that they are infectious as long as they have symptoms; and that they should rest and drink plenty of fluids to avoid dehydration. Red flags for which patients should seek care include a fever of >102°F, chest pain (other than from a pulled muscle), shortness of breath, dizziness, confusion, new ear or sinus pain, and symptoms lasting >14 days. Although nonspecific URI can be complicated by otitis media and bacterial sinusitis, for an individual patient, an antibiotic is more likely to cause an adverse reaction than to prevent complications.

Other remedies that are ineffective, of questionable benefit, or associated with significant adverse effects include echinacea, zinc, inhaled steam, vitamin C, vitamin D, garlic, antihistamines, Chinese medicinal herbs, intranasal glucocorticoids, *Pelargonium sidoides* herbal extract, saline nasal irrigation, and antiviral drugs.

EAR PAIN

Ear pain is most commonly caused by otitis externa and otitis media. In adults, otologic disease is almost always associated with hearing changes. At >50 years of age, temporal arteritis should be considered in patients who have headache, malaise, weight loss, fever, anorexia, and a normal ear exam. Head and neck cancers should be considered in persons with a history of smoking and alcohol use. In children, the presence of a foreign body should be considered.

Ear pain can also result from other causes of local infection, inflammation, trauma, or tumors or can be referred. Innervation of the ear and surrounding areas includes cranial nerves V, VII, IX, and X and cervical nerves C2 and C3. Neuropathic and myopathic pain syndromes (e.g., trigeminal neuralgia) can cause ear pain. Ramsay Hunt syndrome (herpes zoster oticus) (**Chap. 441**) and Bell's palsy (**Chap. 441**) are both associated with ear pain.

Dental pathology can cause pain that radiates to the ear; caries and abscesses are most common. Bruxism, malocclusion, and temporomandibular disorder may be associated with tenderness in muscular attachments and the temporomandibular joint. Salivary gland pathology and cervical adenopathy can cause pain that radiates to the ear.

Sinusitis, tonsillitis, and pharyngitis cause pain that can radiate to the ear via cranial nerve IX. Gastroesophageal reflux disease (**Chap. 321**) is often associated with ear symptoms. Myocardial infarction can cause ear pain via cranial nerve X.

Relapsing polychondritis (**Chap. 366**) is a rare condition associated with recurrent, sometimes bilateral, erythematous, or violaceous swelling of the auricle (sparing the earlobe). Inflammation from relapsing polychondritis can involve nasal septal, laryngeal, or respiratory cartilage and can cause ocular inflammation, audiovestibular damage, and nonerosive seronegative inflammatory arthritis.

■ OTITIS EXTERNA

Etiology and Clinical Manifestations Otitis externa is an inflammation or infection of the external auditory canal manifesting as pain, redness, swelling, aural discharge, and hearing impairment. It is often associated with bacterial infection (frequently by *Pseudomonas aeruginosa* or *Staphylococcus aureus*), but fungi like *Aspergillus* or *Candida* can be implicated.

Otitis externa is most common among preteen and teenage children. Risk factors for otitis externa include swimming (with the resulting condition referred to as "swimmer's ear," which is more common in the summer), mechanical trauma (from cotton swabs or hearing aids), narrow ear canals, cerumen obstruction, eczema, and psoriasis. Classic swimmer's ear is associated with bacterial infection. Physical exam is notable for pain on movement of the auricle or tragus and an external auditory canal that is erythematous, edematous, inflamed, and sometimes coated with exudate on otoscopy. In contrast, fungal otitis externa often manifests with pruritus and ear discharge but without much pain.

Otitis externa can co-occur with otitis media. Preauricular, mastoid, parotid, or cervical lymphadenopathy may be present. AOM with tympanic membrane rupture (see below) can be associated with ear discharge and debris in the ear canal but (unlike otitis externa) without sensitivity to movement of the auricle.

Malignant Otitis Externa Malignant otitis externa is a potentially life-threatening form of otitis externa that involves the temporal bone and occurs in patients with diabetes or other types of immunosuppression, often in older adults. Patients may have fever. Progression of malignant otitis externa can affect cranial nerve VII, IX, XI, or XII.

TREATMENT

Otitis Externa

Analgesia should be provided with acetaminophen or an NSAID. The mainstay of treatment is one or more topical antibacterial drugs with a glucocorticoid for 7–10 days. Polymyxin B–neomycin–hydrocortisone is often used but should be avoided in patients with tympanic membrane perforation because of ototoxicity. Ciprofloxacin–hydrocortisone is an alternative.

Topical aluminum acetate may be as effective as a topical antibacterial–glucocorticoid regimen. For patients whose condition does not improve within 2–4 days with topical treatment, ear wicks or gauze impregnated with or soaked in anti-infective agents can be placed. Ineffective treatments include oral antibiotics and topical antifungals. Otitis externa frequently recurs; its recurrence may be prevented with periodic acetic acid or aluminum acetate drops.

For malignant otitis externa, oral antipseudomonal antibiotics are often prescribed. Patients sometimes require IV pain medication, fluids, or other antimicrobials.

■ ACUTE OTITIS MEDIA

Epidemiology and Etiology AOM—for which patients almost always present within days—is predominantly a disease of children, with incidence peaking at 6–24 months of age. By age 6, ~60% of children will have had an episode of AOM. Younger children appear to be susceptible because of a shorter, more horizontal eustachian tube that more easily accumulates fluid than it does in older children and adults and because their immune system is still developing.

AOM is caused by a viral URI leading to edema and inflammation of the nasopharynx and eustachian tube, collection of fluid, and infection by bacteria that colonize the nasopharynx. Viruses isolated include respiratory syncytial virus, rhinoviruses, enteroviruses, coronaviruses, influenza virus, adenoviruses, and human metapneumovirus. The bacteria most commonly isolated are *Streptococcus pneumoniae*, nontypeable *Haemophilus influenzae*, and *Moraxella catarrhalis*.

Symptoms and Signs Symptoms of AOM include ear pain, fever, irritability, otorrhea, and anorexia. Physical examination may be notable for a bulging, inflamed, cloudy tympanic membrane, with obscured landmarks, and immobility of the membrane on pneumatoscopy, the Valsalva maneuver, or swallowing while holding the nose shut. (An immobile tympanic membrane is also indicative of perforation, old middle-ear adhesions, a blocked auditory tube, or the presence of middle-ear fluid.) Patients have conductive hearing loss. Severe signs and symptoms include moderate to severe otalgia, otalgia lasting at least 2 days, and a temperature of >102.2°F.

AOM should be diagnosed in children with moderate to severe bulging of the tympanic membrane or new-onset otorrhea (not due to otitis externa). With mild bulging of the tympanic membrane, AOM can also be diagnosed if the patient has had symptoms for <48 h or if there is intense erythema of the tympanic membrane. AOM should *not* be diagnosed in children who do not have middle-ear effusion.

TREATMENT

Acute Otitis Media

Pain from AOM should be treated with NSAIDs or acetaminophen, which are effective for mild to moderate pain. Topical agents like benzocaine, procaine, or lidocaine may provide some additional, brief benefit beyond that offered by NSAIDs or acetaminophen.

In up to 80% of children, AOM resolves without antibiotics. Indications for antibiotic treatment in children include an age of <6 months, bilateral ear findings in children 6 months to 2 years old, otorrhea in children >6 months old, and—in children of all ages—ear findings with severe otalgia, ear pain for >48 h, or a fever of >102.2°F (**Table 35-1**).

The benefits of antibiotics are modest and are offset by adverse effects. Antibiotics do not result in early resolution of pain but do decrease pain by day 2 or 3 (number needed to treat, 20 patients treated with antibiotics for 1 patient to have decreased pain by day 2 or 3). More children who receive antibiotics have vomiting, diarrhea, and rash (number needed to harm, 14 patients treated with antibiotics for 1 to have vomiting, diarrhea, or rash). Severe complications like mastoiditis are rare, and the number needed to treat to prevent a case of mastoiditis is ~5000 (i.e., 5000 otitis media patients treated with antibiotics to prevent 1 case of mastoiditis). The American Academy of Family Physicians recommends not routinely prescribing antibiotics for otitis media in children 2–12 years old who have nonsevere symptoms and for whom the observation option is reasonable.

The antibiotic of choice for AOM is high-dose amoxicillin (90 mg/kg per d, up to 3 g). Alternatives include cefdinir, cefuroxime, cefpodoxime, or IM ceftriaxone. If the patient has received amoxicillin in the prior 30 days, clinicians should prescribe amoxicillin/clavulanate (90/6.4 mg/kg per d) in two divided doses. The duration of antibiotic treatment is 10 days for children <2 years old or children with severe symptoms; 5–7 days for children 2–5 years old with mild to moderate AOM; and 5 days for children ≥6 years old with mild or moderate symptoms.

If a patient's condition is not better after 48–72 h of treatment, the antibiotic regimen should be changed to amoxicillin/clavulanate, a second- or third-generation oral cephalosporin, or IM ceftriaxone for 3 days. If, despite a change in antibiotics, the patient's condition still does not improve, that patient should be referred to a specialist. Middle-ear effusions are present in 60–70% of children with AOM; these should resolve over 3 months. Tympanostomy tubes should be considered for recurrent AOM (i.e., three episodes in 6 months or four episodes in 1 year). Mastoiditis is a rare complication of AOM that is suggested by postauricular tenderness, a postauricular mass, or protrusion of the ear lobe.

In adults, AOM is rare and there is little high-quality evidence to guide treatment. For adults, it remains important to differentiate AOM from OME, but AOM is generally treated with antibiotics, regardless of bilaterality or otorrhea. Amoxicillin is the drug of choice. Adults should also be treated with decongestants and analgesics. Adults with more than two episodes in a year or persistent effusion should be referred to an otolaryngologist.

TABLE 35-1 Indications for Antibiotic Treatment of Acute Otitis Media

AGE	INDICATION
<6 months	Antibiotic treatment reasonable for all
6 months to 2 years	Bilateral ear findings
≥6 months	Otorrhea
>2 years	Symptoms worsening or not improving within 48–72 h
All ages	Ear findings with severe otalgia, otalgia lasting at least 2 days, or temperature of >102.2°F

OTITIS MEDIA WITH EFFUSION

Definition and Etiology OME, also called serous otitis media, occurs when there is fluid in the middle ear but no acute infection. Most patients with OME are young children; >60% of cases occur in children <2 years old. Many children have recurrent episodes.

OME is most often a sequela of a viral infection causing AOM, but it can also be caused by allergies. In addition to allergies, predisposing factors include craniofacial abnormalities, gastroesophageal reflux, and enlarged adenoids.

Symptoms and Signs The most common symptoms are decreases in sound conduction and hearing. Children with OME may exhibit impaired language development or communication difficulties. More rarely, patients complain of intermittent ear fullness or earache, tinnitus, or balance problems. On examination, the tympanic membrane may be translucent or gray with fluid (often colorless or amber), air-fluid levels, or bubbles behind the membrane. There is a loss of the light reflex. The tympanic membrane has decreased mobility on pneumatic otoscopy. The evaluation may include audiometry, tympanometry, and, in infants, measurement of auditory brainstem responses.

OME usually resolves spontaneously within 4–6 weeks. If it persists for >3 months, the condition is referred to as chronic OME or chronic serous otitis media.

Cholesteatomas are accumulations of epithelium or keratin in the middle ear that can enlarge, perforate the tympanic membrane, envelop the ossicles, or destroy surrounding tissue. Cholesteatomas can cause labyrinthitis, hearing loss, cranial nerve palsies, vertigo, meningitis, extradural or brain abscess, and lateral sinus thrombophlebitis.

TREATMENT

Otitis Media with Effusion

OME is treated with myringotomy with tympanostomy tube insertion. For young children with nasal obstruction or recurrent infection, adenoidectomy may be considered. Medications, including antihistamines, glucocorticoids, or antibiotics, do not reliably help. Children at risk for speech or language delay may need earlier referral for more aggressive treatment.

ACUTE MASTOIDITIS

Etiology Acute mastoiditis is a serious infection with significant morbidity despite antibiotic and surgical treatment. This condition is most common among children <2 years old but can occur at any age. Acute mastoiditis is often a complication of AOM but may develop without clinically apparent, prior AOM. In older children with acute mastoiditis, clinicians should suspect cholesteatoma.

The pathogenesis of mastoiditis involves spread of organisms from the middle-ear spaces through the aditus ad antrum to the mastoid air cells. *Incipient* mastoiditis consists of fluid within the mastoid air cells, without bony destruction of the bony septa, and can progress to *coalescent* mastoiditis, with destruction of the bony septa. Acute mastoiditis often causes subperiosteal abscess laterally. The organisms most commonly involved in mastoiditis are *S. pneumoniae*, *Streptococcus pyogenes*, *H. influenzae*, *S. aureus* (including methicillin-resistant *S. aureus* [MRSA] strains), and *P. aeruginosa*.

Symptoms and Signs Symptoms of acute mastoiditis include ear pain, fever, lethargy, or fussiness despite adequate treatment of AOM. Patients—especially those with subperiosteal abscess—may have postauricular erythema, tenderness, warmth, fluctuance, and protrusion of the auricle. Otoscopic examination most often yields findings of AOM and may show superoposterior protrusion of the external auditory canal. Complications of mastoiditis include facial nerve palsy, labyrinthitis, skull osteomyelitis, temporal lobe abscess, cerebellar abscess, meningitis, epidural abscess, subdural abscess, venous sinus thrombosis, or Bezold's abscess (an abscess medial to the sternocleidomastoid that tracks into the deep cervical fascia).

Evaluation Laboratory evaluation reveals elevation of inflammatory markers and white blood cells with neutrophilia. Imaging is not necessary in children with a classic history and presentation but may be required if there is concern about complications or severity. CT may show disruption of bony septations, fluid, mucosal thickening, periosteal thickening, disruption of the periosteum, or subperiosteal abscess. MRI with gadolinium permits better visualization of abscesses and vascular problems.

Differential Diagnosis The differential diagnosis of acute mastoiditis includes cellulitis, otitis externa, postauricular lymphadenopathy, perichondritis, and tumors, including rhabdomyosarcoma, Ewing sarcoma, and myofibroblastic tumor.

TREATMENT

Mastoiditis

Patients with mastoiditis should be admitted to the hospital and treated with IV antibiotics and myringotomy, with or without tympanostomy tubes; if there is no improvement within 48 h, mastoidectomy should be undertaken. Tympanostomy or myringotomy samples or subperiosteal abscess drainage should be sent for culture and sensitivity testing. Depending on complications, additional drainage and surgical procedures may be necessary.

Empirical IV antibiotic therapy for children without recurrent AOM or recent antibiotic treatment consists of vancomycin (if there is concern about antibiotic-resistant *S. pneumoniae* or MRSA) or a cephalosporin (e.g., cefepime or ceftazidime). Patients with recurrent AOM or recent antibiotic treatment should be given vancomycin plus an antipseudomonal penicillin. Culture and sensitivity results will guide antibiotic changes. IV antibiotic therapy should be continued for 7–10 days, and patients should complete a 4-week course of oral antibiotics.

SINUS SYMPTOMS

Sinus symptoms are commonly due to respiratory viruses. These symptoms are considered acute if they last <4 weeks, subacute if they last 4–12 weeks, and chronic if they last ≥12 weeks. Beyond sinus infection, the differential diagnosis of rhinitis includes the common cold, allergic rhinitis (**Chap. 352**), vasomotor rhinitis, rhinitis medicamentosa due to topical decongestants, drug-induced rhinitis (e.g., due to aspirin, ibuprofen, or beta blockers), autoimmune disease (e.g., granulomatosis with polyangiitis), and cerebrospinal fluid leak. Pain over the sinuses can be caused by headaches (**Chap. 430**), facial pain syndromes, temporomandibular disorder (**Chap. 36**), and dental pathology. Gastroesophageal reflux can cause referral of symptoms to the sinuses. Patients who have uncontrolled diabetes or are otherwise immunocompromised can have rapidly progressing invasive fungal infections (**Chap. 211**). More indolent fungal infections should be considered in the event of recurrent or nonresolving sinusitis. In children, it is important to consider the presence of a foreign body as a cause of sinus symptoms.

ACUTE SINUSITIS

Definition and Etiology *Sinusitis* is an inflammation of the paranasal sinuses; *rhinosinusitis* also involves the nasal passages. The majority of acute sinusitis cases are caused by respiratory viruses. A diagnosis of sinusitis is a major reason for unnecessary antibiotic prescribing in adults: although <2% of sinusitis episodes are due to bacteria (most often *S. pneumoniae, H. influenzae*, or *M. catarrhalis*), antibiotics are prescribed at >70% of office visits for sinusitis. According to guideline criteria, no more than 50% of adults—and probably closer to 20%—meet the criteria for antibiotic prescribing.

Symptoms and Signs Sinusitis symptoms commonly include purulent nasal discharge, facial congestion or fullness, and facial pain or pressure. Other symptoms include fever; hyposmia or anosmia; ear pain, pressure, or fullness; postnasal drip; halitosis; maxillary toothache; cough; and fatigue. Risk factors for developing sinusitis include an age of 45–65 years, smoking, asthma, air travel, and allergies.

On physical examination, direct rhinoscopy reveals excess mucus or purulence. Patients may have tenderness over the maxillary sinuses and, in severe cases, erythema and swelling of the maxilla. Sinus transillumination is not accurate in diagnosing sinusitis.

Complications Complications from sinusitis can be dramatic but are extremely rare. These complications may include orbital cellulitis, osteomyelitis, meningitis, intracranial abscesses, and cavernous sinus thrombosis. New symptoms that might indicate a sinusitis complication include confusion, unilateral weakness, proptosis, limited ocular movements, and acute vision changes.

RECURRENT ACUTE SINUSITIS Patients who have four or more episodes of acute sinusitis in a year, without signs or symptoms between episodes, are said to have recurrent acute sinusitis.

INVASIVE FUNGAL SINUSITIS Invasive fungal sinusitis may develop in immunocompromised patients, such as those with uncontrolled diabetes or transplant recipients, and should be considered an emergency. Invasive fungal sinusitis is caused by Mucorales fungi or *Aspergillus* (**Chap. 217**). Patients may appear to have a rapidly progressive case of rhinosinusitis, with facial pain and pressure, headaches, and fever followed within days by cranial nerve involvement, orbital swelling, cellulitis, proptosis, chemosis, and ophthalmoplegia. Patients may be critically ill. Evaluation should include nasal endoscopy with biopsy and imaging with gadolinium-enhanced MRI as the preferred modality.

NOSOCOMIAL SINUSITIS Nosocomial sinusitis occurs in critically ill patients, often those who are nasotracheally intubated. Nosocomial sinusitis should be suspected in hospitalized patients who have fever without another identifiable cause.

TREATMENT

Acute Sinusitis

All patients with acute sinusitis should be counseled about symptom-based treatments, which may include decongestants, analgesic/antipyretics, nasal saline, or intranasal glucocorticoids. Intranasal decongestants (e.g., oxymetazoline, two sprays in each nostril twice a day for no more than 5 days) and oral decongestants (e.g., 12-h pseudoephedrine [120 mg] during the day) relieve pain, pressure, and rhinorrhea. Analgesics and antipyretics like acetaminophen or NSAIDs (e.g., ibuprofen), nasal saline spray, and nasal washes provide relief. Intranasal glucocorticoids may help, particularly for

TABLE 35-2 Indications for Antibiotic Treatment of Acute Sinusitis

INDICATION	DEFINITION
Persistent	Symptoms lasting ≥10 days
Severe	Fever of >102°F and either purulent nasal discharge or nasal pain for at least 3–4 consecutive days
Worsening	New fever, headache, or increase in nasal discharge following an upper respiratory tract infection that lasted for 5–6 days and was initially improving

Note: In typical populations, roughly 20% and no more than 50% of adults with sinusitis will meet the criteria for antibiotic prescribing.

patients with an allergic cause of sinusitis. Because patients may be accustomed to receiving antibiotics, provision of a clear explanation, symptom-based treatments, and reasons for reconsultation are important. Red flags for which patients should reconsult include recurrent fever of >102°F, sinus symptoms that worsen after initial improvement, and rapid worsening of facial pain that becomes persistent, as well as any other concerning symptoms.

Antibiotic prescribing criteria for sinusitis are based on symptoms (**Table 35-2**). Only patients with persistent, severe, or worsening symptoms, especially those who have already used decongestants and analgesics for 2–4 days, meet the criteria for antibiotic prescribing. The antibiotic of choice is amoxicillin/clavulanate (875 mg/125 mg bid for 7 days). Amoxicillin (875 mg PO bid for 7 days) is an alternative. For patients with mild penicillin allergies, cefuroxime is a reasonable choice. For those with severe penicillin allergies, doxycycline is a reasonable alternative. Macrolides are specifically not recommended for sinusitis because of high rates of macrolide-resistant *S. pneumoniae*.

Patients who meet the criteria for antibiotic prescribing should show signs of improvement after 3–5 days of therapy. If not, second-line regimens include amoxicillin/clavulanate (2000 mg/125 mg bid for 7 days) or levofloxacin, although fluoroquinolones are associated with dysglycemia, neuropathy, and tendon and aortic rupture. For patients whose condition still is not improving after 3–5 days of treatment with a second-line antibiotic or in whom a complication or an alternative diagnosis is suspected, clinicians should consider referral to an otorhinolaryngologist and/or the performance of imaging tests. The imaging modality of choice is noncontrast CT. Patients with recurrent acute sinusitis may benefit from nasal culture during episodes; imaging between episodes to identify predisposing anatomic abnormalities; and allergic or immunologic evaluation.

Patients with acute fungal sinusitis should be treated with IV antifungal agents and often require surgical debridement. Patients with nosocomial sinusitis should have precipitating factors (e.g., nasotracheal intubation) addressed and should be empirically treated with broad-spectrum antibiotics until culture and susceptibility results are available.

CHRONIC SINUSITIS

Definition and Etiology Chronic sinusitis is defined as inflammation of the paranasal sinuses that lasts >12 weeks. Chronic sinusitis is primarily an inflammatory disease and can also be associated with acute or chronic infection or allergic, structural (e.g., deviated nasal septum or polyps), and immunologic etiologies. Repeated viral infections may lead to chronic sinusitis. Bacterial colonization or chronic infection plays a role in some cases of chronic sinusitis. *S. aureus* and gram-negative bacteria are commonly identified. Commonly involved allergens and irritants are dust mites, mold, tobacco smoke, occupational factors, and other airborne toxins. Functional or immunologic problems can include impaired mucociliary clearance (e.g., due to cystic fibrosis) or immunodeficiency due to acquired conditions or medications. Chronic sinusitis often coexists with allergic rhinitis and asthma.

Symptoms and Signs Cardinal symptoms of chronic sinusitis are facial pain or pressure, nasal discharge or postnasal drip, congestion, and hyposmia or anosmia. Associated symptoms may include fatigue, malaise, ear pressure, hoarseness, and cough. The diagnosis of sinus inflammation must be confirmed with anterior rhinoscopy, nasal endoscopy, or imaging because up to 40% of patients with chronic sinus symptoms do not have mucosal changes evidencing disease.

In practical terms, chronic sinusitis can be divided into three main types (in decreasing order of frequency): (1) chronic sinusitis without polyps, (2) chronic sinusitis with polyps, and (3) allergic fungal sinusitis. In general, chronic sinusitis without polyps is more common among women, develops in childhood and young adulthood, is characterized by presentations with facial pain, and is often due to T_H1 lymphocyte predominance associated with bacterial infection or colonization. Chronic sinusitis with polyps is more common among men; develops in adulthood; is characterized by presentations with decrease or loss of smell, asthma, or aspirin sensitivity (**Chap. 287**); and is often due to T_H2 lymphocyte predominance associated with eosinophilic inflammation, asthma, or aspirin sensitivity. Allergic fungal rhinosinusitis is also associated with polyp formation; typically occurs in patients in their 20s and 30s who are from warm, humid regions and who have other atopic diseases; and is associated with IgE-mediated allergy and eosinophils (**Chap. 217**). The mucus in allergic fungal rhinosinusitis is classically greenish-brown, has a peanut butter–like consistency, and includes viable hyphae from *Aspergillus* or other fungal species. Allergic fungal rhinosinusitis is resistant to medical treatments.

Evaluation On anterior rhinoscopy, polyps are seen as white, gray, tan, or yellow translucent growths in the middle meatus. The imaging modality of choice is noncontrast CT. Allergic fungal rhinosinusitis may be unilateral; however, unilateral symptoms or polyps on exam or imaging, especially if associated with bloody discharge, should raise concern about tumors.

TREATMENT
Chronic Sinusitis

Treatment includes avoidance of identifiable triggers such as allergens, smoke, and irritants. Saline sprays and washes provide symptom relief, and higher-volume saline washes are probably more effective. Intranasal glucocorticoids, including mometasone and fluticasone sprays or higher-potency and higher-volume budesonide rinses, are mainstays of treatment, especially for chronic sinusitis with polyps. Intranasal glucocorticoids reduce polyp size. Oral administration of glucocorticoids for 2–3 weeks is sometimes effective against chronic sinusitis that is unresponsive to intranasal steroids—again, especially for patients with polyps. Intranasal or systemic antihistamines may help patients whose illness has an allergic component. Likewise, leukotriene antagonists like montelukast may help.

Although antibiotics are frequently prescribed for 2–4 weeks to patients with chronic sinusitis, there is little evidence that these drugs are effective. Evidence of modest quality supports the use of 3 months of macrolide treatment for patients who have chronic sinusitis without polyps. Antifungal agents have not shown benefit against any subtype of chronic sinusitis. Decongestants should be used only sparingly and briefly.

Endoscopic sinus surgery improves quality of life in patients who have had inadequate responses to medical therapy. Patients with more limited, focal disease may more reliably have better results. The goals of surgery are to remove polyps from the nasal cavity and paranasal sinuses. For patients with allergic fungal rhinosinusitis, medical therapy is classically ineffective, surgery produces good results, and patients should be treated with perioperative glucocorticoids. In children, adenoidectomy may be effective in some cases. In the future, immune endotyping may allow selection of more individualized biological treatments.

TABLE 35-3 Clinical Findings That Suggest Various Forms of Nonstreptococcal Pharyngitis

CLINICAL FINDING(S) OR BEHAVIORAL FACTOR	SUSPECTED DIAGNOSIS
Scarlatiniform rash	Group A β-hemolytic streptococci or *Arcanobacterium haemolyticum*
Cough and otitis media	*Haemophilus influenzae*
Sex between men with associated urogenital symptoms, fellatio between a woman and a man who has current urogenital symptoms, persistent sore throat unresponsive to penicillin	*Neisseria gonorrhoeae*
Travel to endemic areas, pseudomembrane on examination	*Corynebacterium diphtheriae*
Persistent sore throat with bronchopulmonary symptoms	*Mycoplasma pneumoniae*
Marked adenopathy (especially that involving posterior cervical or auricular nodes), splenomegaly, palatine petechiae, gelatinous uvula	Acute infectious mononucleosis
New sexual partner in the previous month; fever, rash, myalgias, headache	Acute HIV infection

SORE THROAT AND NECK PAIN

Sore throat is not synonymous with pharyngitis and can also be caused by submandibular space, retropharyngeal and peritonsillar abscesses, thyroiditis, gastroesophageal reflux, tumors, and postnasal drainage.

Acute pharyngitis, in which symptoms are generally present for days, is most often caused by respiratory viruses; is often caused by group A β-hemolytic streptococci (GAS); and can be caused by other bacteria (including *Neisseria gonorrhoeae*), Epstein-Barr virus (EBV), and HIV. On physical examination, pharyngeal erythema is associated most commonly with viral infections, including the common cold and influenza. Pharyngeal exudate should not be confused with *Candida* infection, which looks like cottage-cheese, can be scraped off, and leaves a bleeding surface, or leukoplakia, which cannot be scraped off. History and exam findings may help differentiate sore throat and pharyngitis of various etiologies (**Table 35-3**).

STREPTOCOCCAL PHARYNGITIS

GAS is the only common cause of sore throat that should be treated with antibiotics. The principal goal in the evaluation of adults with sore throat is to identify patients likely to have GAS pharyngitis, or "strep throat." Prompt antibiotic treatment of adults likely to have strep throat has the potential to reduce symptoms, prevent the spread of disease, and reduce suppurative complications (e.g., peritonsillar abscess). Nonsuppurative complications are rare. In developed countries, the prevalence of rheumatic fever (**Chap. 148**) is extremely low, and antibiotic treatment does not prevent poststreptococcal glomerulonephritis (**Chap. 148**).

Most patients with non-GAS pharyngitis have various forms of viral pharyngitis and do not require antibiotics. Nevertheless, clinicians prescribe antibiotics to a majority of adults with sore throats. By using a simple clinical scoring algorithm, clinicians can predict the presence or absence of GAS with sufficient accuracy and avoid prescribing antibiotics to patients who are unlikely to have strep throat. Although there is a role for testing (see "Evaluation," below), most adults with sore throat do not need to have a GAS test.

About 10% of adults with sore throat are infected with GAS. Among children with sore throat, the prevalence of GAS can be as high as 35%, with rates peaking from 5 to 15 years of age. The prevalence of GAS is higher in winter and early spring. The risk of streptococcal pharyngitis is elevated among health care and child care workers, teachers, parents of young children, and patients exposed to individuals with strep throat. Clinicians need to be aware of local outbreaks of GAS infection, particularly in military and institutional settings, where the prevalence of GAS and the risk of acute rheumatic fever may be elevated.

TABLE 35-4 The Centor Criteria and the Probability of Streptococcal Pharyngitis for Adults[a]

NO. OF CRITERIA MET[b]	POSTEVALUATION PROBABILITY (%)	RECOMMENDATION
0	2	No test, no antibiotic
1	3	No test, no antibiotic
2	8	Rapid test
3	19	Rapid test
4	41	Empirical antibiotic treatment or rapid test

[a]Assuming a pretest probability of strep throat for adults of 10%. [b]The criteria are (1) a history of fever, (2) an absence of cough, (3) tender anterior cervical lymphadenopathy, and (4) tonsillar swelling or exudate. Each criterion gets 1 point. Roughly 40–60% of adults will meet no criteria or one criterion; ~20% will meet the criteria for antibiotic prescribing.

Evaluation The Centor criteria consist of four findings, each of which is assigned 1 point: (1) history of fever, (2) absence of cough, (3) tender anterior cervical lymphadenopathy, and (4) tonsillar exudate or swelling. The Centor criteria are easy to assess and accurately stratify adult patients with suspected streptococcal pharyngitis. Patients with no points have a 2% probability of being infected with GAS, whereas those with 4 points have a probability of 41% (**Table 35-4**). The Centor criteria have an area under the curve of 0.79. Other clinical decision algorithms similar to the Centor criteria may not perform as well, are not as simple, or have not been as rigorously evaluated.

If the test/no treatment threshold is set at 5%, for a GAS prevalence of ~10%, adults meeting no criteria or only one Centor criterion have a probability of GAS pharyngitis so low that they should neither be tested nor be treated with an antibiotic. Adults meeting two or three Centor criteria have an intermediate probability of GAS pharyngitis; they should have a rapid antigen test performed, and the results should guide antibiotic treatment. For adults meeting four Centor criteria, it is reasonable either to perform a rapid test or to institute empirical antibiotic treatment. However, some guidelines recommend—and some ambulatory quality measures require—a GAS test to be associated with antibiotic prescribing in adults, regardless of the number of Centor criteria met.

In children, the Centor criteria are less specific, and streptococcal pharyngitis should be confirmed with testing. Children who have signs of pharyngitis without signs of viral infection (conjunctivitis, runny nose, cough, hoarseness, nonexudative oral lesions) should have testing performed.

Outside of the United States, because complications are rare and even streptococcal pharyngitis is self-limited in the vast majority of cases, some guidelines do not recommend use of rapid GAS testing or routine antibiotic treatment of sore throat.

Clinicians should have a lower threshold for diagnosing and treating GAS pharyngitis in patients with a history of acute rheumatic fever, patients with documented streptococcal exposure in the past week, patients who live in a community with a current strep throat epidemic, and patients who are diabetic or otherwise immunocompromised.

RAPID STREP TESTS Rapid GAS-specific antigen tests have a sensitivity of ~80% and a specificity of ~95%. Results are available within minutes and can be used to make therapeutic decisions before the patient leaves the office. Improper collection technique can adversely affect the sensitivity of rapid strep tests: clinicians should rub the tonsils and pharynx, touching any areas where exudate or ulceration are present.

THROAT CULTURES A single-swab throat culture has a sensitivity of ~85–90%, as defined by isolation of GAS on a second swab. A throat culture can also be falsely positive for true infection: some patients with a culture positive for GAS may be only uninfected carriers, as defined by their failure to exhibit a fourfold increase in antibodies to GAS—the gold standard test. Among adults and children seeking medical care for a sore throat, test specificity may be as low as 50–70% because of patients who do not exhibit serologic evidence of infection. Throat cultures are not recommended for the routine evaluation of adults with sore throat. The modest gain in sensitivity over rapid testing is outweighed by the 24- to 48-h delay in test results, with a consequent delay in the symptomatic relief associated with antibiotic treatment.

Indiscriminate strep testing in adults with sore throat or respiratory symptoms should be discouraged. Rapid strep tests and culture do not differentiate between patients who have true infection and those who are carriers of GAS (with carriage rates as high as 20% among schoolchildren and ~5% among adolescents and young adults). In adults who meet no Centor criteria or only one criterion—40–60% of adults with pharyngitis—a positive test is highly likely to be falsely positive and/or to represent GAS carriage.

Complications Complications of streptococcal pharyngitis are rare but include acute rheumatic fever (**Chap. 148**), poststreptococcal glomerulonephritis (**Chap. 148**), scarlet fever (**Chap. 148**), sinusitis, peritonsillar abscess, and other invasive GAS infections.

TREATMENT

Streptococcal Pharyngitis

All patients with pharyngitis—nonstreptococcal and streptococcal—should receive analgesics (acetaminophen or NSAIDs). Saline gargles, humidification, soft foods, and tea with honey soothe a painful throat.

Penicillin is the antibiotic of choice for streptococcal pharyngitis (**Table 35-5**). Penicillin is a narrow-spectrum, low-cost, and well-tolerated drug to which no GAS isolate has been resistant. Amoxicillin is an acceptable alternative in children as it comes in a palatable liquid form. For patients with mild penicillin allergy, cephalexin and cefadroxil are good alternatives. For patients with severe penicillin allergies, clinicians should prescribe erythromycin, clarithromycin, or clindamycin. Unlike other infections for which emerging evidence supports progressively shorter antibiotic courses, streptococcal pharyngitis requires longer courses (7–10 days), which are more effective.

Glucocorticoids (e.g., dexamethasone, 10 mg as a single oral dose) have so far been poorly studied as an adjunctive treatment for sore throat and strep throat and are not recommended. These drugs may result in decreased pain within 24 h but do not decrease school or work absenteeism or relapse rates. Even short courses of steroids are associated with increased rates of sepsis, gastrointestinal bleeding, congestive heart failure, venous thromboembolism, and fracture within 30 days.

Streptococcal and nonstreptococcal pharyngitis should resolve in 3–5 days. Symptoms that should lead patients to seek further care include shaking chills (rigors), neck swelling (beyond lymphadenopathy), trouble swallowing, drooling, or symptoms that persist for >5 days without improvement.

TABLE 35-5 Antibiotic Treatment of Group A Streptococcal Pharyngitis

ANTIBIOTIC	DOSING
Antibiotic of Choice	
Penicillin	500 mg PO qid or 1000 mg PO bid × 10 days
Alternative for Non-Penicillin-Allergic Patients	
Amoxicillin	500 mg PO bid or 1000 mg qd × 10 days
Alternatives for Non-Anaphylactic Penicillin-Allergic Patients	
Cephalexin	500 mg PO bid × 10 days
Cefadroxil	1 g PO qd × 10 days
Alternatives for Patients with Severe Penicillin Allergy	
Erythromycin	250–500 mg PO qid or 500–1000 mg PO bid × 5 days
Clarithromycin	500 mg PO bid × 5 days
Clindamycin	300 mg PO tid × 10 days

NONSTREPTOCOCCAL PHARYNGITIS

Acute Infectious Mononucleosis New EBV infection may be the cause of pharyngitis in 1–6% of young adults (**Chap. 194**). EBV is rarely the cause of pharyngitis in adults >40 years of age. The full-blown acute syndrome, which is present in only about one-fourth of patients with infectious mononucleosis ("mono"), is characterized by a triad of clinical, hematologic, and serologic findings. The clinical presentation is typified by the development over several days of malaise, fever, sore throat, and marked adenopathy that is particularly evident in the cervical lymph nodes. On physical examination, marked adenopathy is virtually always documented and is most specific for mononucleosis when the posterior cervical or posterior auricular nodes are involved. Splenomegaly and exudative pharyngitis with prominent tonsillar swelling, palatine petechiae, and a gelatinous uvula are often noted. The classic hematologic findings are an absolute lymphocyte count of >4000/μL or a relative lymphocyte count of >50% with "atypical" morphologic features in >10% of the lymphocytes. The characteristic serologic finding is the heterophil antibody, which is detectable in only 40% of patients during the first week of illness but in 80–90% of patients by the third week.

Other Bacterial Pharyngitis Non–group A streptococci (especially group C and group G streptococci), *Mycoplasma pneumoniae, Chlamydia pneumoniae, N. gonorrhoeae*, and *H. influenzae* have all been associated with sore throat in some studies. Although antibacterial treatment has not been proven to speed the resolution of symptoms and signs of any of these types of nonstreptococcal pharyngitis, antibiotic treatment is indicated if throat cultures from a patient with persistent sore throat yield group C or group G streptococci.

LEMIERRE'S SYNDROME Lemierre's syndrome consists of septic thrombophlebitis of the internal jugular vein accompanied by metastatic infections, most commonly of the lung but with possible involvement of the joints, bones, liver, meninges, and brain. Lemierre's syndrome is most commonly caused by *Fusobacterium necrophorum*, although it can also be caused by species of *Bacteroides, Eikenella, Streptococcus, Peptostreptococcus*, or other bacterial genera. This syndrome probably occurs predominantly in male patients. Clinicians should consider Lemierre's syndrome in a teenage or young adult patient who has non-GAS pharyngitis that is not resolving, particularly if it is accompanied by rigors, neck pain or swelling, or other extrapharyngeal symptoms.

GONOCOCCAL PHARYNGITIS *N. gonorrhoeae* may be the cause of pharyngitis in 1% of adult patients seeking primary care for a sore throat, although gonococcal infection of the pharynx is more often asymptomatic. When symptomatic, pharyngeal gonorrhea may range from mild to severe, with protracted pharyngitis characterized by pain, fever, and pharyngeal exudate. Gonococcal pharyngitis should be suspected in men who have sex with men with associated symptoms of urogenital infection, women who have practiced fellatio with a man with genital gonorrhea, and anyone who has persistent sore throat that has been unresponsive to treatment for presumptive streptococcal pharyngitis.

DIPHTHERIA Diphtheria, caused by *Corynebacterium diphtheriae*, is endemic in developing countries (**Chap. 150**). Diphtheria produces only mild pharyngitis beneath its characteristic grayish pseudomembrane.

ACUTE HIV INFECTION Clinicians should consider acute HIV infection in patients with sore throat, particularly when it is associated with headache, fever, myalgias, lymphadenopathy, anorexia, and rash (**Chap. 202**). Of patients with acute HIV infection, roughly half have a sore throat. However, in most settings in the United States, only ~1% of patients with viral or mononucleosis-like symptoms have acute HIV infection.

HEAD AND NECK ABSCESSES

Head and neck abscesses are more common among patients with diabetes, who are immunocompromised, and among older adults. Such abscesses are often a complication of infections of the teeth and gums, throat, or salivary ducts; lymphadenitis; ear infections; sinus infections; congenital cysts; and IV drug use. Prompt recognition is important, as head and neck abscesses can cause airway compromise due to edema or mass effect. Head and neck abscesses can follow fascial planes and spread to the mediastinum (where they can cause mediastinitis, pleural effusions, empyema, or pericarditis), the carotid sheath, the skull base, and the meninges. Head and neck abscesses have also been associated with aspiration pneumonia, necrotizing fasciitis, Lemierre's syndrome, and toxic shock syndrome.

Submandibular abscesses generally result from an infected or extracted tooth and can cause Ludwig angina, a swelling of the floor of the mouth that can enlarge and displace the tongue posteriorly.

Peritonsillar abscesses, which may occur predominantly in male patients, generally result from complicated bacterial pharyngitis and present with fever, dysphagia, profound throat pain (necessitating drooling to avoid swallowing saliva), trismus, and "hot potato voice" (inability to articulate, as if patients have hot food in their mouths). Patients are likely to have unilateral palate bulging, often with uvular deviation. Peritonsillar abscesses are caused by viridans group streptococci, β-hemolytic streptococci, *F. necrophorum, S. aureus, Prevotella,* and *Bacteroides.*

Retropharyngeal abscesses often present after an antecedent URI in children with sore throat, dysphagia, deep neck pain, neck stiffness, trismus, and drooling. The pharyngeal wall may be displaced, but swelling or abscess may not be apparent on examination. In severe cases, patients may have dyspnea and stridor.

Patients with suspected head and neck abscesses, with the possible exception of patients who have obvious peritonsillar abscesses, should undergo imaging by CT.

TREATMENT

Head and Neck Abscesses

The mainstays of treatment for head and neck abscesses are securing the airway, surgical drainage, and IV antibiotic administration. To secure the airway, mask ventilation or oral intubation may not be effective, and oral fiberoptic intubation or tracheotomy may be necessary. Peritonsillar abscess may be managed with needle aspiration and/or tonsillectomy. Other head and neck abscesses require incision and drainage. The selected IV antibiotics should cover streptococci, anaerobes, and possibly *S. aureus*. Frequently used antibiotics include ampicillin/sulbactam, clindamycin plus ceftriaxone, or meropenem. For some abscesses with adequate source control with incision and drainage, penicillin may be as effective as broader-spectrum agents.

■ EPIGLOTTITIS

Along with associated dysphagia, odynophagia, hoarseness, and stridor or tachypnea, supraglottitis or epiglottitis must be considered in adults presenting with sore throat. The inflamed and enlarged epiglottis protrudes up into the oropharynx. Patients may extend their neck or lean forward and drool oral secretions to avoid swallowing. Epiglottitis can cause "hot potato voice." Attempts to examine or swab the posterior pharynx or obtain a culture can provoke laryngospasm and should only be done carefully in a controlled setting. Because obstruction of the airway may become acutely life-threatening, the patient with epiglottitis must be observed in a hospital setting, and examination in an operating room, where an airway can be established immediately by an experienced operator, should be strongly considered. Although not necessary for the diagnosis, a lateral neck radiograph can demonstrate epiglottal swelling referred to as the "thumb sign."

In adults, conservative therapy under observation is sufficient in most cases, but intubation by an experienced clinician or tracheostomy may become necessary. Treatments also include humidification with nebulized normal saline or humidified oxygen and administration of glucocorticoids, IV antibiotics, and nebulized epinephrine.

H. influenzae, the most common cause of supraglottitis in children, is less common in adults. Other responsible organisms in adults are *S. pneumoniae*, *S. pyogenes*, and *S. aureus*. The *H. influenzae* type b vaccine has led to a dramatic decrease in epiglottitis overall, with large reductions in young children; however, the incidence of supraglottitis and epiglottitis in adults may be increasing.

■ LARYNGITIS

Laryngitis—inflammation of the larynx and surrounding structures—is most commonly caused by viral URIs. In children, parainfluenza virus can cause croup, or laryngotracheobronchitis, which is characterized by a "barking" cough but can also include laryngitis.

Beyond viruses, laryngitis can be caused in rare cases by bacteria and fungi. Bacterial laryngitis can be a complication of viral laryngitis, occurring about 7 days into the illness. The most common bacteria involved are *S. pneumoniae, H. influenzae,* and *M. catarrhalis.* Fungal laryngitis is probably rarer but should be considered in patients who are immunosuppressed or who have recently been treated with antibacterial drugs.

Noninfectious causes of laryngitis include vocal trauma (e.g., due to yelling, screaming, or loud singing), inhalation injuries, allergies, gastroesophageal reflux disease (laryngopharyngeal reflux), asthma, and pollution. Immunosuppressed patients are at risk for infections with herpesvirus, HIV, and coxsackievirus. Smokers are at elevated risk for malignancy and other infections.

Laryngitis is characterized by a raspy, hoarse, or breathy voice, sometimes progressing to a complete loss of voice. Laryngitis can have associated dry cough and anterior throat pain; patients often feel a need to clear their throats. The physical examination in patients who may have laryngitis should focus on the head, neck, and lungs, but the diagnosis of laryngitis is generally based on history. If visualization of the vocal cords is necessary, indirect examination with a mirror or flexible laryngoscopy usually shows erythema and edema of the vocal cords and surrounding structures.

TREATMENT

Laryngitis

Laryngitis is generally self-limited, usually lasting 3–7 days, but may last up to 14 days. Vocal rest is crucial. Airway humidification and hydration should help. Patients likely to have laryngopharyngeal reflux should avoid gastroesophageal reflux–inducing foods and behaviors and should take antireflux medications. In randomized controlled trials, antibiotics were not effective in decreasing objective symptoms of laryngitis.

Red flags for emergency evaluation and monitoring include shortness of breath, stridor, dysphagia, odynophagia, drooling, and posturing that could indicate epiglottitis. Referral to an otolaryngologist should be considered for patients who rely on their voice for work, such as singers and teachers. A history of smoking or weight loss should raise suspicion of malignancy. Symptoms lasting >3 weeks should prompt referral to an otolaryngologist or speech specialist.

■ FURTHER READING

Centor RM, Linder JA: Web exclusive. Annals on call—*Fusobacterium* pharyngitis debate. Ann Intern Med 171:OC1, 2019.

Chua KP et al: Appropriateness of outpatient antibiotic prescribing among privately insured US patients: ICD-10-CM based cross sectional study. BMJ 364:k5092, 2019.

Lieberthal AS et al: Clinical practice guideline: The diagnosis and management of acute otitis media. Pediatrics 131:e964, 2013.

Rowe TA, Linder JA: Novel approaches to decrease inappropriate ambulatory antibiotic use. Expert Rev Anti Infect Ther 17:511, 2019.

Sanchez GV et al: Core elements of outpatient antibiotic stewardship. MMWR Recomm Rep 65:1, 2016.

36 Oral Manifestations of Disease

Samuel C. Durso

As primary care physicians and consultants, internists are often asked to evaluate patients with disease of the oral soft tissues, teeth, and pharynx. Knowledge of the oral milieu and its unique structures is necessary to guide preventive services and recognize oral manifestations of local or systemic disease (**Chap. A3**). Furthermore, internists frequently collaborate with dentists in the care of patients who have a variety of medical conditions that affect oral health or who undergo dental procedures that increase their risk of medical complications.

DISEASES OF THE TEETH AND PERIODONTAL STRUCTURES

Tooth formation begins during the sixth week of embryonic life and continues through 17 years of age. Teeth start to develop in utero and continue to develop until after the tooth erupts. Normally, all 20 deciduous teeth have erupted by age 3 and have been shed by age 13. Permanent teeth, eventually totaling 32, begin to erupt by age 6 and have completely erupted by age 14, though third molars ("wisdom teeth") may erupt later.

The erupted tooth consists of the visible *crown* covered with enamel and the root submerged below the gum line and covered with bonelike *cementum. Dentin*, a material that is denser than bone and exquisitely sensitive to pain, forms the majority of the tooth substance, surrounding a core of myxomatous *pulp* containing the vascular and nerve supply. The tooth is held firmly in the alveolar socket by the *periodontium*, supporting structures that consist of the gingivae, alveolar bone, cementum, and periodontal ligament. The periodontal ligament tenaciously binds the tooth's cementum to the alveolar bone. Above this ligament is a collar of attached gingiva just below the crown. A few millimeters of unattached or free gingiva (1–3 mm) overlap the base of the crown, forming a shallow sulcus along the gum-tooth margin.

Dental Caries, Pulpal and Periapical Disease, and Complications Dental caries usually begin asymptomatically as a destructive infectious process of the enamel. Bacteria—principally *Streptococcus mutans*—colonize the organic buffering biofilm (*plaque*) on the tooth surface. If not removed by brushing or by the natural cleansing and antibacterial action of saliva, bacterial acids can demineralize the enamel. Fissures and pits on the occlusal surfaces are the most frequent sites of early decay. Surfaces between the teeth, adjacent to tooth restorations and exposed roots, are also vulnerable, particularly as individuals age. Over time, dental caries extend to the underlying dentin, leading to cavitation of the enamel. Without management, the caries will penetrate to the tooth pulp, producing *acute pulpitis*. At this stage, when the pulp infection is limited, the tooth may become sensitive to percussion and to hot or cold, and pain resolves immediately when the irritating stimulus is removed. Should the infection spread throughout the pulp, *irreversible pulpitis* occurs, leading to *pulp necrosis*. At this later stage, pain can be severe and has a sharp or throbbing visceral quality that may be worse when the patient lies down. Once pulp necrosis is complete, pain may be constant or intermittent, but cold sensitivity is lost.

Treatment of caries involves removal of the softened and infected hard tissue and restoration of the tooth structure with silver amalgam, glass ionomer, composite resin, or gold. Once irreversible pulpitis occurs, root canal therapy becomes necessary; removal of the contents of the pulp chamber and root canal is followed by thorough cleaning and filling with an inert material. Alternatively, the tooth may be extracted.

Pulpal infection leads to *periapical abscess* formation, which can produce pain on chewing. If the infection is mild and chronic, a *periapical granuloma* or eventually a *periapical cyst* forms, either of which produces radiolucency at the root apex. When unchecked, a periapical abscess can erode into the alveolar bone, producing osteomyelitis; penetrate and drain through the gingivae, producing a parulis (gumboil); or track along deep fascial planes, producing virulent cellulitis (Ludwig's angina) involving the submandibular space and floor of the mouth (**Chap. 177**). Elderly patients, patients with diabetes mellitus, and patients taking glucocorticoids may experience little or no pain or fever as these complications develop.

Periodontal Disease Periodontal disease and dental caries are the primary causes of tooth loss. Like dental caries, chronic infection of the gingiva and anchoring structures of the tooth begins with formation of bacterial plaque. The process begins at the gum line. Plaque and *calculus* (calcified plaque) are preventable by appropriate daily oral hygiene, including periodic professional cleaning. Left undisturbed, chronic inflammation can ensue and produce hyperemia of the free and attached gingivae (*gingivitis*), which then typically bleed with brushing. If this issue is ignored, severe *periodontitis* can develop, leading to deepening of the physiologic sulcus and destruction of the periodontal ligament. Gingival pockets develop around the teeth. As the periodontium (including the supporting bone) is destroyed, the teeth loosen. A role for chronic inflammation due to chronic periodontal disease in promoting coronary heart disease and stroke has been proposed. Epidemiologic studies have demonstrated a moderate but significant association between chronic periodontal inflammation and atherogenesis, though a causal role remains unproven.

Acute and aggressive forms of periodontal disease are less common than the chronic forms described above. However, if the host is stressed or exposed to a new pathogen, rapidly progressive and destructive disease of the periodontal tissue can occur. A virulent example is *acute necrotizing ulcerative gingivitis*. The presentation includes sudden gingival inflammation, ulceration, bleeding, interdental gingival necrosis, and fetid halitosis. *Localized juvenile periodontitis*, which is seen in adolescents, is particularly destructive and appears to be associated with impaired neutrophil chemotaxis. *AIDS-related periodontitis* resembles acute necrotizing ulcerative gingivitis in some patients and a more destructive form of adult chronic periodontitis in others. It may also produce a gangrene-like destructive process of the oral soft tissues and bone that resembles *noma*, an infectious condition seen in severely malnourished children in developing nations.

Prevention of Tooth Decay and Periodontal Infection Despite the reduced prevalences of dental caries and periodontal disease in the United States (due in large part to water fluoridation and improved dental care, respectively), both diseases constitute a major public health problem worldwide, particularly in certain groups. The internist should promote preventive dental care and hygiene as part of health maintenance. Populations at high risk for dental caries and periodontal disease include those with hyposalivation and/or xerostomia, diabetics, alcoholics, tobacco users, persons with Down syndrome, and those with gingival hyperplasia. Furthermore, patients lacking access to dental care (e.g., as a result of low socioeconomic status) and patients with a reduced ability to provide self-care (e.g., individuals with disabilities, nursing home residents, and persons with dementia or upper-extremity disability) suffer at a disproportionate rate. It is important to provide counseling regarding regular dental hygiene and professional cleaning, use of fluoride-containing toothpaste, professional fluoride treatments, and (for patients with limited dexterity) use of electric toothbrushes and also to instruct persons caring for those who are not capable of self-care. Cost, fear of dental care, and differences in language and culture create barriers that prevent some people from seeking preventive dental services.

Developmental and Systemic Disease Affecting the Teeth and Periodontium In addition to posing cosmetic issues, *malocclusion*, the most common developmental oral problem, can interfere with mastication unless corrected through orthodontic and surgical techniques. Impacted third molars are common and can become infected or erupt into an insufficient space. Acquired prognathism due to *acromegaly* may also lead to malocclusion, as may deformity of the maxilla and mandible due to *Paget's disease* of the bone. Delayed tooth eruption, a receding chin, and a protruding tongue are occasional features of *cretinism* and *hypopituitarism*. Congenital syphilis produces tapering, notched (*Hutchinson's*) incisors and finely nodular (*mulberry*) molar crowns. *Enamel hypoplasia* results in crown defects ranging from pits to deep fissures of primary or permanent teeth. Intrauterine infection (syphilis, rubella), vitamin deficiency (A, C, or D), disorders of calcium metabolism (malabsorption, vitamin D–resistant rickets, hypoparathyroidism), prematurity, high fever, and rare inherited defects (*amelogenesis imperfecta*) are all causes. Tetracycline, given in sufficiently high doses during the first 8 years of life, may produce enamel hypoplasia and discoloration. Doxycycline does not cause permanent tooth staining in children despite warnings included for all tetracycline-class antibiotics. Exposure to endogenous pigments can discolor developing teeth; etiologies include *erythroblastosis fetalis* (green or bluish-black), congenital liver disease (green or yellow-brown), and porphyria (red or brown that fluoresces with ultraviolet light). *Mottled enamel* occurs if excessive fluoride is ingested during development. Worn enamel is seen with age, bruxism, or excessive acid exposure (e.g., chronic gastric reflux or bulimia). Celiac disease is associated with nonspecific enamel defects in children but not in adults.

Total or partial tooth loss resulting from periodontitis is seen with cyclic neutropenia, Papillon-Lefévre syndrome, Chédiak-Higashi syndrome, and leukemia. Rapid focal tooth loosening is most often due to infection, but rarer causes include Langerhans cell histiocytosis, Ewing's sarcoma, osteosarcoma, and Burkitt's lymphoma. Early loss of primary teeth is a feature of *hypophosphatasia*, a rare congenital error of metabolism.

Pregnancy may produce gingivitis and localized *pyogenic granulomas*. Severe periodontal disease occurs in uncontrolled diabetes mellitus. *Drug-induced gingival overgrowth* may be caused by anticonvulsants, calcium channel blockers, and immunosuppressants, although excellent daily oral care can prevent or reduce its occurrence. *Idiopathic familial gingival fibromatosis* and several syndrome-related disorders cause similar conditions. Discontinuation of the medication may reverse the drug-induced form, although surgery may be needed to control both of the latter entities. *Linear gingival erythema* is variably seen in patients with advanced HIV infection and probably represents immune deficiency and decreased neutrophil activity. Diffuse or focal gingival swelling may be a feature of early or late acute myelomonocytic leukemia as well as of other lymphoproliferative disorders. A rare but pathognomonic sign of granulomatosis with polyangiitis is a red-purplish, granular gingivitis (*strawberry gums*).

DISEASES OF THE ORAL MUCOSA

Infections Most oral mucosal diseases involve microorganisms (**Table 36-1**).

Pigmented Lesions See **Table 36-2**.

Dermatologic Diseases See Tables 36-1, 36-2, and **36-3** and **Chaps. 56–61**.

Diseases of the Tongue See **Table 36-4**.

HIV Disease and AIDS See Tables 36-1, 36-2, 36-3, and **36-5**; **Chap. 202**.

Ulcers Ulceration is the most common oral mucosal lesion. Although there are many causes, the host and the pattern of lesions, including the presence of organ system features, narrow the differential diagnosis (Table 36-1). Most acute ulcers are painful and self-limited. Recurrent aphthous ulcers and herpes simplex account for the majority. Persistent and deep aphthous ulcers can be idiopathic or can accompany HIV/AIDS. Aphthous lesions are often the presenting symptom in *Behçet's syndrome* (**Chap. 364**). Similar-appearing, though less painful, lesions may occur in reactive arthritis, and aphthous ulcers are occasionally present during phases of *discoid* or *systemic lupus erythematosus* (**Chap. 360**). Aphthous-like ulcers are seen in *Crohn's disease* (**Chap. 326**), but, unlike the common aphthous variety, they may exhibit granulomatous inflammation on histologic examination. Recurrent aphthae are more prevalent in patients with *celiac disease* and have been reported to remit with elimination of gluten.

Of major concern are chronic, relatively painless ulcers and mixed red/white patches (erythroplakia and leukoplakia) of >2 weeks' duration. Squamous cell carcinoma and premalignant dysplasia should be considered early and a diagnostic biopsy performed. This awareness and this procedure are critically important because early-stage malignancy is vastly more treatable than late-stage disease. High-risk sites include the lower lip, floor of the mouth, ventral and lateral tongue, and soft palate–tonsillar pillar complex. Significant risk factors for oral cancer in Western countries include sun exposure (lower lip), tobacco and alcohol use, and human papillomavirus infection. In India and some other Asian countries, smokeless tobacco mixed with betel nut, slaked lime, and spices is a common cause of oral cancer. Rarer causes of chronic oral ulcer, such as tuberculosis, fungal infection, granulomatosis with polyangiitis, and midline granuloma, may look identical to carcinoma. Making the correct diagnosis depends on recognizing other clinical features and performing a biopsy of the lesion. The syphilitic chancre is typically painless and therefore easily missed. Regional lymphadenopathy is invariably present. The syphilitic etiology is confirmed with appropriate bacterial and serologic tests.

Disorders of mucosal fragility often produce painful oral ulcers that fail to heal within 2 weeks. *Mucous membrane pemphigoid* and *pemphigus vulgaris* are the major acquired disorders. While their clinical features are often distinctive, a biopsy or immunohistochemical examination should be performed to diagnose these entities and to distinguish them from *lichen planus* and drug reactions.

Hematologic and Nutritional Disease Internists are more likely to encounter patients with acquired, rather than congenital, bleeding disorders. Bleeding should stop 15 min after minor trauma and within an hour after tooth extraction if local pressure is applied. More prolonged bleeding, if not due to continued injury or rupture of a large vessel, should lead to investigation for a clotting abnormality. In addition to bleeding, petechiae and ecchymoses are prone to occur at the vibrating line between the soft and hard palates in patients with platelet dysfunction or thrombocytopenia.

All forms of leukemia, but particularly *acute myelomonocytic leukemia*, can produce gingival bleeding, ulcers, and gingival enlargement. Oral ulcers are a feature of agranulocytosis, and ulcers and mucositis are often severe complications of chemotherapy and radiation therapy for hematologic and other malignancies. *Plummer-Vinson syndrome* (iron deficiency, angular stomatitis, glossitis, and dysphagia) raises the risk of oral squamous cell cancer and esophageal cancer at the postcricoidal tissue web. Atrophic papillae and a red, burning tongue may occur with pernicious anemia. Deficiencies in B-group vitamins produce many of these same symptoms as well as oral ulceration and cheilosis. Consequences of *scurvy* include swollen, bleeding gums; ulcers; and loosening of the teeth.

NONDENTAL CAUSES OF ORAL PAIN

Most, but not all, oral pain emanates from inflamed or injured tooth pulp or periodontal tissues. Nonodontogenic causes are often overlooked. In most instances, toothache is predictable and proportional to the stimulus applied, and an identifiable condition (e.g., caries, abscess) is found. Local anesthesia eliminates pain originating from dental or periodontal structures, but not referred pains. The most common nondental source of pain is myofascial pain referred from muscles of mastication, which become tender and ache with increased use. Many sufferers exhibit *bruxism* (grinding of the teeth) secondary to stress and anxiety. *Temporomandibular joint disorder* is closely related. It affects both sexes, with a higher prevalence among women. Features include pain, limited mandibular movement, and temporomandibular joint sounds. The etiologies are complex; malocclusion does not play the primary role once attributed to it. *Osteoarthritis* is a common cause of masticatory pain. Anti-inflammatory medication, jaw rest, soft foods, and heat provide relief. The temporomandibular joint is involved in 50% of patients with *rheumatoid arthritis*, and its involvement is

TABLE 36-1 Vesicular, Bullous, or Ulcerative Lesions of the Oral Mucosa

CONDITION	USUAL LOCATION	CLINICAL FEATURES	COURSE
Viral Diseases			
Primary acute herpetic gingivostomatitis (HSV type 1; rarely type 2)	Lip and oral mucosa (buccal, gingival, lingual mucosa)	Labial vesicles that rupture and crust, and intraoral vesicles that quickly ulcerate; extremely painful; acute gingivitis, fever, malaise, foul odor, and cervical lymphadenopathy; occurs primarily in infants, children, and young adults	Heals spontaneously in 10–14 days; unless secondarily infected, lesions lasting >3 weeks are not due to primary HSV infection
Recurrent herpes labialis	Mucocutaneous junction of lip, perioral skin	Eruption of groups of vesicles that may coalesce, then rupture and crust; painful to pressure or spicy foods	Lasts ~1 week, but condition may be prolonged if secondarily infected; if severe, topical or oral antiviral treatment may reduce healing time
Recurrent intraoral herpes simplex	Palate and gingiva	Small vesicles on keratinized epithelium that rupture and coalesce; painful	Heals spontaneously in ~1 week; if severe, topical or oral antiviral treatment may reduce healing time
Chickenpox (VZV)	Gingiva and oral mucosa	Skin lesions may be accompanied by small vesicles on oral mucosa that rupture to form shallow ulcers; may coalesce to form large bullous lesions that ulcerate; mucosa may have generalized erythema	Lesions heal spontaneously within 2 weeks
Herpes zoster (VZV reactivation)	Cheek, tongue, gingiva, or palate	Unilateral vesicular eruptions and ulceration in linear pattern following sensory distribution of trigeminal nerve or one of its branches	Gradual healing without scarring unless secondarily infected; postherpetic neuralgia is common; oral acyclovir, famciclovir, or valacyclovir reduces healing time and postherpetic neuralgia
Infectious mononucleosis (Epstein-Barr virus)	Oral mucosa	Fatigue, sore throat, malaise, fever, and cervical lymphadenopathy; numerous small ulcers usually appear several days before lymphadenopathy; gingival bleeding and multiple petechiae at junction of hard and soft palates	Oral lesions disappear during convalescence; no treatment is given, though glucocorticoids are indicated if tonsillar swelling compromises the airway
Herpangina (coxsackievirus A; also possibly coxsackievirus B and echovirus)	Oral mucosa, pharynx, tongue	Sudden onset of fever, sore throat, and oropharyngeal vesicles, usually in children <4 years old, during summer months; diffuse pharyngeal congestion and vesicles (1–2 mm), grayish-white surrounded by red areola; vesicles enlarge and ulcerate	Incubation period of 2–9 days; fever for 1–4 days; recovery uneventful
Hand-foot-and-mouth disease (most commonly coxsackievirus A16)	Oral mucosa, pharynx, palms, and soles	Fever, malaise, headache with oropharyngeal vesicles that become painful, shallow ulcers; highly infectious; usually affects children under age 10	Incubation period 2–18 days; lesions heal spontaneously in 2–4 weeks
Primary HIV infection	Gingiva, palate, and pharynx	Acute gingivitis and oropharyngeal ulceration, associated with febrile illness resembling mononucleosis and including lymphadenopathy	Followed by HIV seroconversion, asymptomatic HIV infection, and usually ultimately by HIV disease
Bacterial or Fungal Diseases			
Acute necrotizing ulcerative gingivitis ("trench mouth")	Gingiva	Painful, bleeding gingiva characterized by necrosis and ulceration of gingival papillae and margins plus lymphadenopathy and foul breath	Debridement and diluted (1:3) peroxide lavage provide relief within 24 h; antibiotics in acutely ill patients; relapse may occur
Prenatal (congenital) syphilis	Palate, jaws, tongue, and teeth	Gummatous involvement of palate, jaws, and facial bones; Hutchinson's incisors, mulberry molars, glossitis, mucous patches, and fissures at corner of mouth	Tooth deformities in permanent dentition irreversible
Primary syphilis (chancre)	Lesion appearing where organism enters body; may occur on lips, tongue, or tonsillar area	Small papule developing rapidly into a large, painless ulcer with indurated border; unilateral lymphadenopathy; chancre and lymph nodes containing spirochetes; serologic tests positive by third to fourth weeks	Healing of chancre in 1–2 months, followed by secondary syphilis in 6–8 weeks
Secondary syphilis	Oral mucosa frequently involved with mucous patches, which occur primarily on palate and also at commissures of mouth	Maculopapular lesions of oral mucosa, 5–10 mm in diameter with central ulceration covered by grayish membrane; eruptions occurring on various mucosal surfaces and skin, accompanied by fever, malaise, and sore throat	Lesions may persist from several weeks to a year
Tertiary syphilis	Palate and tongue	Gummatous infiltration of palate or tongue followed by ulceration and fibrosis; atrophy of tongue papillae produces characteristic bald tongue and glossitis	Gumma may destroy palate, causing complete perforation
Gonorrhea	Lesions may occur in mouth at site of inoculation or secondarily by hematogenous spread from a primary focus	Most pharyngeal infection is asymptomatic; may produce burning or itching sensation; oropharynx and tonsils may be ulcerated and erythematous; saliva viscous and fetid	More difficult to eradicate than urogenital infection, though pharyngitis usually resolves with appropriate antimicrobial treatment
Tuberculosis	Tongue, tonsillar area, soft palate	Painless, solitary, 1- to 5-cm, irregular ulcer covered with persistent exudate; ulcer has firm undermined border	Autoinoculation from pulmonary infection is usual; lesions resolve with appropriate antimicrobial therapy
Cervicofacial actinomycosis	Swellings in region of face, neck, and floor of mouth	Infection may be associated with extraction, jaw fracture, or eruption of molar tooth; in acute form, resembles acute pyogenic abscess, but contains yellow "sulfur granules" (gram-positive mycelia and their hyphae)	Typically, swelling is hard and grows painlessly; multiple abscesses with draining tracts develop; penicillin first choice; surgery usually necessary

(*Continued*)

TABLE 36-1 Vesicular, Bullous, or Ulcerative Lesions of the Oral Mucosa (Continued)

CONDITION	USUAL LOCATION	CLINICAL FEATURES	COURSE
Bacterial or Fungal Diseases (Continued)			
Histoplasmosis	Any area of the mouth, particularly tongue, gingiva, or palate	Nodular, verrucous, or granulomatous lesions; ulcers are indurated and painful; usual source hematogenous or pulmonary, but may be primary	Systemic antifungal therapy necessary
Candidiasis[a]			
Dermatologic Diseases			
Mucous membrane pemphigoid	Typically produces marked gingival erythema and ulceration; other areas of oral cavity, esophagus, and vagina may be affected	Painful, grayish-white collapsed vesicles or bullae of full-thickness epithelium with peripheral erythematous zone; gingival lesions desquamate, leaving ulcerated area	Protracted course with remissions and exacerbations; involvement of different sites develops slowly; glucocorticoids may temporarily reduce symptoms but do not control disease
EM minor and EM major (Stevens-Johnson syndrome)	Primarily oral mucosa and skin of hands and feet	Intraoral ruptured bullae surrounded by inflammatory area; lips may show hemorrhagic crusts; "iris" or "target" lesion on skin is pathognomonic; patient may have severe signs of toxicity	Onset very rapid; usually idiopathic, but may be associated with trigger such as drug reaction; condition may last 3–6 weeks; mortality rate for untreated EM major is 5–15%
Pemphigus vulgaris	Oral mucosa and skin; sites of mechanical trauma (soft/hard palate, frenulum, lips, buccal mucosa)	Usually (>70%) presents with oral lesions; fragile, ruptured bullae and ulcerated oral areas; mostly in older adults	With repeated occurrence of bullae, toxicity may lead to cachexia, infection, and death within 2 years; often controllable with oral glucocorticoids
Lichen planus	Oral mucosa and skin	White striae in mouth; purplish nodules on skin at sites of friction; occasionally causes oral mucosal ulcers and erosive gingivitis	White striae alone usually asymptomatic; erosive lesions often difficult to treat, but may respond to glucocorticoids
Other Conditions			
Recurrent aphthous ulcers	Usually on nonkeratinized oral mucosa (buccal and labial mucosa, floor of mouth, soft palate, lateral and ventral tongue)	Single or clustered painful ulcers with surrounding erythematous border; lesions may be 1–2 mm in diameter in crops (herpetiform), 1–5 mm (minor), or 5–15 mm (major)	Lesions heal in 1–2 weeks but may recur monthly or several times a year; protective barrier with benzocaine and topical glucocorticoids relieve symptoms; systemic glucocorticoids may be needed in severe cases
Behçet's syndrome	Oral mucosa, eyes, genitalia, gut, and CNS	Multiple aphthous ulcers in mouth; inflammatory ocular changes, ulcerative lesions on genitalia; inflammatory bowel disease and CNS disease	Oral lesions often first manifestation; persist several weeks and heal without scarring
Traumatic ulcers	Anywhere on oral mucosa; dentures frequently responsible for ulcers in vestibule	Localized, discrete ulcerated lesions with red border; produced by accidental biting of mucosa, penetration by foreign object, or chronic irritation by dentures	Lesions usually heal in 7–10 days when irritant is removed, unless secondarily infected
Squamous cell carcinoma	Any area of mouth, most commonly on lower lip, lateral borders of tongue, and floor of mouth	Red, white, or red and white ulcer with elevated or indurated border; failure to heal; pain not prominent in early lesions	Invades and destroys underlying tissues; frequently metastasizes to regional lymph nodes
Acute myeloid leukemia (usually monocytic)	Gingiva	Gingival swelling and superficial ulceration followed by hyperplasia of gingiva with extensive necrosis and hemorrhage; deep ulcers may occur elsewhere on mucosa, complicated by secondary infection	Usually responds to systemic treatment of leukemia; occasionally requires local irradiation
Lymphoma	Gingiva, tongue, palate, and tonsillar area	Elevated, ulcerated area that may proliferate rapidly, giving appearance of traumatic inflammation	Fatal if untreated; may indicate underlying HIV infection
Chemical or thermal burns	Any area in mouth	White slough due to contact with corrosive agents (e.g., aspirin, hot cheese) applied locally; removal of slough leaves raw, painful surface	Lesion heals in several weeks if not secondarily infected

[a]See Table 36-3.

Abbreviations: CNS, central nervous system; EM, erythema multiforme; HSV, herpes simplex virus; VZV, varicella-zoster virus.

usually a late feature of severe disease. Bilateral preauricular pain, particularly in the morning, limits range of motion.

Migrainous neuralgia may be localized to the mouth. Episodes of pain and remission without an identifiable cause and a lack of relief with local anesthesia are important clues. *Trigeminal neuralgia* (*tic douloureux*) can involve the entire branch or part of the mandibular or maxillary branch of the fifth cranial nerve and can produce pain in one or a few teeth. Pain may occur spontaneously or may be triggered by touching the lip or gingiva, brushing the teeth, or chewing. *Glossopharyngeal neuralgia* produces similar acute neuropathic symptoms in the distribution of the ninth cranial nerve. Swallowing, sneezing, coughing, or pressure on the tragus of the ear triggers pain that is felt in the base of the tongue, pharynx, and soft palate and may be referred to the temporomandibular joint. *Neuritis* involving the maxillary and mandibular divisions of the trigeminal nerve (e.g., maxillary sinusitis, neuroma, and leukemic infiltrate) is distinguished from ordinary toothache by the neuropathic quality of the pain. Occasionally, *phantom pain* follows tooth extraction. Pain and hyperalgesia behind the ear and on the side of the face in the day or so before facial weakness develops often constitute the earliest symptom of *Bell's palsy*. Likewise,

TABLE 36-2 Pigmented Lesions of the Oral Mucosa

CONDITION	USUAL LOCATION	CLINICAL FEATURES	COURSE
Oral melanotic macule	Any area of mouth	Discrete or diffuse, localized, brown to black macule	Remains indefinitely; no growth
Diffuse melanin pigmentation	Any area of mouth	Diffuse pale to dark-brown pigmentation; may be physiologic ("racial") or due to smoking	Remains indefinitely
Nevi	Any area of mouth	Discrete, localized, brown to black pigmentation	Remains indefinitely
Malignant melanoma	Any area of mouth	Can be flat and diffuse, painless, brown to black; or can be raised and nodular	Expands and invades early; metastasis leads to death
Addison's disease	Any area of mouth, but mostly buccal mucosa	Blotches or spots of bluish-black to dark-brown pigmentation occurring early in disease, accompanied by diffuse pigmentation of skin; other symptoms of adrenal insufficiency	Condition controlled by adrenal steroid replacement
Peutz-Jeghers syndrome	Any area of mouth	Dark-brown spots on lips, buccal mucosa, with characteristic distribution of pigment around lips, nose, and eyes and on hands; concomitant intestinal polyposis	Oral pigmented lesions remain indefinitely; gastrointestinal polyps may become malignant
Drug ingestion (neuroleptics, oral contraceptives, minocycline, zidovudine, quinine derivatives)	Any area of mouth	Brown, black, or gray areas of pigmentation	Gradually disappears following cessation of drug intake
Amalgam tattoo	Gingiva and alveolar mucosa	Small blue-black pigmented areas associated with embedded amalgam particles in soft tissues; may show up on radiographs as radiopaque particles in some cases	Remains indefinitely
Heavy metal pigmentation (bismuth, mercury, lead)	Gingival margin	Thin blue-black pigmented line along gingival margin; rarely seen except in children exposed to lead-based paint	Indicative of systemic absorption; no significance for oral health
Black hairy tongue	Dorsum of tongue	Elongation of filiform papillae of tongue, which become stained by coffee, tea, tobacco, or pigmented bacteria	Improves within 1–2 weeks with gentle brushing of tongue or (if due to bacterial overgrowth) discontinuation of antibiotic
Fordyce spots	Buccal and labial mucosa	Numerous small yellowish spots just beneath mucosal surface; no symptoms; due to hyperplasia of sebaceous glands	Benign; remains without apparent change
Kaposi's sarcoma	Palate most common, but may occur at any other site	Red or blue plaques of variable size and shape; often enlarge, become nodular, and may ulcerate	Usually indicative of HIV infection or non-Hodgkin's lymphoma; rarely fatal, but may require treatment for comfort or cosmesis
Mucous retention cysts	Buccal and labial mucosa	Bluish, clear fluid–filled cyst due to extravasated mucus from injured minor salivary gland	Benign; painless unless traumatized; may be removed surgically

TABLE 36-3 White Lesions of Oral Mucosa

CONDITION	USUAL LOCATION	CLINICAL FEATURES	COURSE
Lichen planus	Buccal mucosa, tongue, gingiva, and lips; skin	Striae, white plaques, red areas, ulcers in mouth; purplish papules on skin; may be asymptomatic, sore, or painful; lichenoid drug reactions may look similar	Protracted; responds to topical glucocorticoids
White sponge nevus	Oral mucosa, vagina, anal mucosa	Painless white thickening of epithelium; adolescence/early adulthood onset; familial	Benign and permanent
Smoker's leukoplakia and smokeless tobacco lesions	Any area of oral mucosa, sometimes related to location of habit	White patch that may become firm, rough, or red-fissured and ulcerated; may become sore and painful but is usually painless	May or may not resolve with cessation of habit; 2% of patients develop squamous cell carcinoma; early biopsy essential
Erythroplakia with or without white patches	Floor of mouth commonly affected in men; tongue and buccal mucosa in women	Velvety, reddish plaque; occasionally mixed with white patches or smooth red areas	High risk of squamous cell cancer; early biopsy essential
Candidiasis	Any area in mouth	*Pseudomembranous type* ("thrush"): creamy white curdlike patches that reveal a raw, bleeding surface when scraped; found in sick infants, debilitated elderly patients receiving high-dose glucocorticoids or broad-spectrum antibiotics, and patients with AIDS	Responds favorably to antifungal therapy and correction of predisposing causes where possible
		Erythematous type: flat, red, sometimes sore areas in same groups of patients	Course same as for pseudomembranous type
		Candidal leukoplakia: nonremovable white thickening of epithelium due to *Candida*	Responds to prolonged antifungal therapy
		Angular cheilitis: sore fissures at corner of mouth	Responds to topical antifungal therapy
Hairy leukoplakia	Usually on lateral tongue, rarely elsewhere on oral mucosa	White areas ranging from small and flat to extensive accentuation of vertical folds; found in HIV carriers (all risk groups for AIDS)	Due to Epstein-Barr virus; responds to high-dose acyclovir but recurs; rarely causes discomfort unless secondarily infected with *Candida*
Warts (human papillomavirus)	Anywhere on skin and oral mucosa	Single or multiple papillary lesions with thick, white, keratinized surfaces containing many pointed projections; cauliflower lesions covered with normal-colored mucosa or multiple pink or pale bumps (focal epithelial hyperplasia)	Lesions grow rapidly and spread; squamous cell carcinoma must be ruled out with biopsy; excision or laser therapy; may regress in HIV-infected patients receiving antiretroviral therapy

TABLE 36-4 Alterations of the Tongue

TYPE OF CHANGE	CLINICAL FEATURES
Size or Morphology	
Macroglossia	Enlarged tongue that may be part of a syndrome found in developmental conditions such as Down syndrome, Simpson-Golabi-Behmel syndrome, or Beckwith-Wiedemann syndrome; may be due to tumor (hemangioma or lymphangioma), metabolic disease (e.g., primary amyloidosis), or endocrine disturbance (e.g., acromegaly or cretinism); may occur when all teeth are removed
Fissured ("scrotal") tongue	Dorsal surface and sides of tongue covered by painless shallow or deep fissures that may collect debris and become irritated
Median rhomboid glossitis	Congenital abnormality with ovoid, denuded area in median posterior portion of tongue; may be associated with candidiasis and may respond to antifungal treatment
Color	
"Geographic" tongue (benign migratory glossitis)	Asymptomatic inflammatory condition of tongue, with rapid loss and regrowth of filiform papillae leading to appearance of denuded red patches "wandering" across surface
Hairy tongue	Elongation of filiform papillae of medial dorsal surface area due to failure of keratin layer of papillae to desquamate normally; brownish-black coloration may be due to staining by tobacco, food, or chromogenic organisms
"Strawberry" and "raspberry" tongue	Appearance of tongue during scarlet fever due to hypertrophy of fungiform papillae as well as changes in filiform papillae
"Bald" tongue	Atrophy may be associated with xerostomia, pernicious anemia, iron-deficiency anemia, pellagra, or syphilis; may be accompanied by painful burning sensation; may be an expression of erythematous candidiasis and respond to antifungal treatment

TABLE 36-5 Oral Lesions Associated with HIV Infection

LESION MORPHOLOGY	ETIOLOGIES
Papules, nodules, plaques	Candidiasis (hyperplastic and pseudomembranous)[a]
	Condyloma acuminatum (human papillomavirus infection)
	Squamous cell carcinoma (preinvasive and invasive)
	Non-Hodgkin's lymphoma[a]
	Hairy leukoplakia[a]
Ulcers	Recurrent aphthous ulcers[a]
	Angular cheilitis
	Squamous cell carcinoma
	Acute necrotizing ulcerative gingivitis[a]
	Necrotizing ulcerative periodontitis[a]
	Necrotizing ulcerative stomatitis
	Non-Hodgkin's lymphoma[a]
	Viral infection (herpes simplex, herpes zoster, cytomegalovirus infection)
	Infection caused by *Mycobacterium tuberculosis* or *Mycobacterium avium-intracellulare*
	Fungal infection (histoplasmosis, cryptococcosis, candidiasis, geotrichosis, aspergillosis)
	Bacterial infection (*Escherichia coli, Enterobacter cloacae, Klebsiella pneumoniae, Pseudomonas aeruginosa*)
	Drug reactions (single or multiple ulcers)
Pigmented lesions	Kaposi's sarcoma[a]
	Bacillary angiomatosis (skin and visceral lesions more common than oral)
	Zidovudine pigmentation (skin, nails, and occasionally oral mucosa)
	Addison's disease
Miscellaneous	Linear gingival erythema[a]

[a]Strongly associated with HIV infection.

similar symptoms may precede visible lesions of herpes zoster infecting the seventh nerve (*Ramsey-Hunt syndrome*) or trigeminal nerve. *Postherpetic neuralgia* may follow either condition. *Coronary ischemia* may produce pain exclusively in the face and jaw; as in typical angina pectoris, this pain is usually reproducible with increased myocardial demand. Aching in several upper molar or premolar teeth that is unrelieved by anesthetizing the teeth may point to *maxillary sinusitis*.

Giant cell arteritis is notorious for producing headache, but it may also produce facial pain or sore throat without headache. Jaw and tongue claudication with chewing or talking is relatively common. Tongue infarction is rare. Patients with subacute thyroiditis often experience pain referred to the face or jaw before the tenderness of the thyroid gland and transient hyperthyroidism are appreciated.

"Burning mouth syndrome" (*glossodynia*) occurs in the absence of an identifiable cause (e.g., vitamin B_{12} deficiency, iron deficiency, diabetes mellitus, low-grade *Candida* infection, food sensitivity, or subtle xerostomia) and predominantly affects postmenopausal women. The etiology may be neuropathic. Clonazepam, α-lipoic acid, and cognitive-behavioral therapy have benefited some patients. Some cases associated with an angiotensin-converting enzyme inhibitor have remitted when treatment with the drug was discontinued.

■ DISEASES OF THE SALIVARY GLANDS

Saliva is essential to oral health. Its absence leads to dental caries, periodontal disease, and difficulties in wearing dental prostheses, masticating, and speaking. Its major components, water and mucin, serve as a cleansing solvent and lubricating fluid. In addition, saliva contains antimicrobial factors (e.g., lysozyme, lactoperoxidase, secretory IgA), epidermal growth factor, minerals, and buffering systems. The major salivary glands secrete intermittently in response to autonomic stimulation, which is high during a meal but low otherwise. Hundreds of minor glands in the lips and cheeks secrete mucus continuously throughout the day and night. Consequently, oral function becomes impaired when salivary function is reduced. The sensation of a dry mouth (*xerostomia*) is perceived when salivary flow is reduced by 50%. The most common etiology is medication, especially drugs with anticholinergic properties but also alpha and beta blockers, calcium channel blockers, and diuretics. Other causes include Sjögren's syndrome, chronic parotitis, salivary duct obstruction, diabetes mellitus, HIV/AIDS, and radiation therapy that includes the salivary glands in the field (e.g., for Hodgkin's lymphoma and for head and neck cancer). Management involves the elimination or limitation of drying medications, preventive dental care, and supplementation with oral liquid or salivary substitutes. Sugarless mints or chewing gum may stimulate salivary secretion if dysfunction is mild. When sufficient exocrine tissue remains, pilocarpine or cevimeline has been shown to increase secretions. Commercial saliva substitutes or gels relieve dryness. Fluoride supplementation is critical to prevent caries.

Sialolithiasis presents most often as painful swelling but in some instances as only swelling or only pain. Conservative therapy consists of local heat, massage, and hydration. Promotion of salivary secretion with mints or lemon drops may flush out small stones. Antibiotic treatment is necessary when bacterial infection in suspected. In adults, *acute bacterial parotitis* is typically unilateral and most commonly affects postoperative, dehydrated, and debilitated patients. *Staphylococcus aureus* (including methicillin-resistant strains) and anaerobic bacteria are the most common pathogens. Chronic bacterial *sialadenitis* results from lowered salivary secretion and recurrent bacterial infection. When suspected bacterial infection is not responsive to therapy, the differential diagnosis should be expanded to include benign and malignant neoplasms, lymphoproliferative disorders, Sjögren's syndrome, sarcoidosis, tuberculosis, lymphadenitis, actinomycosis, and granulomatosis with polyangiitis. Bilateral nontender parotid enlargement occurs with diabetes mellitus, cirrhosis, bulimia, HIV/AIDS, and drugs (e.g., iodide, propylthiouracil).

Pleomorphic adenoma composes two-thirds of all salivary neoplasms. The parotid is the principal salivary gland affected, and the tumor presents as a firm, slow-growing mass. Although this tumor is benign, its recurrence is common if resection is incomplete. Malignant tumors such as mucoepidermoid carcinoma, adenoid cystic carcinoma, and adenocarcinoma tend to grow relatively fast, depending upon grade. They may ulcerate and invade nerves, producing numbness and facial paralysis. Surgical resection is the primary treatment. Radiation therapy (particularly neutron-beam therapy) is used when surgery is not feasible and after resection for certain histologic types with a high risk of recurrence. Malignant salivary gland tumors have a 5-year survival rate of 94% when the stage is local and 35% when distant.

Dental Care for Medically Complex Patients Routine dental care (e.g., uncomplicated extraction, scaling and cleaning, tooth restoration, and root canal) is remarkably safe. The most common concerns regarding care of dental patients with medical disease are excessive bleeding for patients taking anticoagulants, infection of the heart valves and prosthetic devices from hematogenous seeding by the oral flora, and cardiovascular complications resulting from vasopressors used with local anesthetics during dental treatment. Experience confirms that the risk of any of these complications is very low.

Patients undergoing tooth extraction or alveolar and gingival surgery rarely experience uncontrolled bleeding when warfarin anticoagulation is maintained within the therapeutic range currently recommended for prevention of venous thrombosis, atrial fibrillation, or mechanical heart valve. Embolic complications and death, however, have been reported during subtherapeutic anticoagulation. Therapeutic anticoagulation should be confirmed before and continued through the procedure. Likewise, low-dose aspirin (e.g., 81–325 mg) can safely be continued. For patients taking aspirin and another antiplatelet medication (e.g., clopidogrel), the decision to continue the second antiplatelet medication should be based on individual consideration of the risks of thrombosis and bleeding. The newer target-specific oral anticoagulants (dabigatran, apixaban, rivaroxaban, and edoxaban) are in increasingly common use. Simple extractions of one to three teeth, periodontal surgery, abscess drainage, and implant positioning do not typically require interruption of therapy. More extensive surgery may necessitate delaying or holding a dose of the anticoagulant or more elaborate measures to manage the risk of thrombosis and bleeding.

Patients at risk for bacterial endocarditis (**Chap. 128**) should maintain optimal oral hygiene, including flossing, and have regular professional cleanings. Currently, guidelines recommend that prophylactic antibiotics be restricted to those patients at high risk for bacterial endocarditis who undergo dental and oral procedures involving significant manipulation of gingival or periapical tissue or penetration of the oral mucosa. If unexpected bleeding occurs, antibiotics given within 2 h after the procedure provide effective prophylaxis.

Hematogenous bacterial seeding from oral infection can undoubtedly produce late prosthetic-joint infection and therefore requires removal of the infected tissue (e.g., drainage, extraction, root canal) and appropriate antibiotic therapy. However, evidence that late prosthetic-joint infection follows routine dental procedures is lacking. For this reason, antibiotic prophylaxis is generally not recommended before oral surgery or oral mucosal manipulation for patients who have undergone joint replacement surgery. Exceptions to this may be considered for patients who have experienced joint replacement complications.

Concern often arises regarding the use of vasoconstrictors to treat patients with hypertension and heart disease. Vasoconstrictors enhance the depth and duration of local anesthesia, thus reducing the anesthetic dose and potential toxicity. If intravascular injection is avoided, 2% lidocaine with 1:100,000 epinephrine (limited to a total of 0.036 mg of epinephrine) can be used safely in patients with controlled hypertension and stable coronary heart disease, arrhythmia, or congestive heart failure. Precautions should be taken with patients taking tricyclic antidepressants and nonselective beta blockers because these drugs may potentiate the effect of epinephrine.

Elective dental treatments should be postponed for at least 1 month and preferably for 6 months after myocardial infarction, after which the risk of reinfarction is low provided the patient is medically stable (e.g., stable rhythm, stable angina, and no heart failure). Patients who have suffered a stroke should have elective dental care deferred for 9 months. In both situations, effective stress reduction requires good pain control, including the use of the minimal amount of vasoconstrictor necessary to provide good hemostasis and local anesthesia.

Bisphosphonate therapy is associated with *osteonecrosis* of the jaw. However, the risk with oral bisphosphonate therapy is very low. Most patients affected have received high-dose aminobisphosphonate therapy for multiple myeloma or metastatic breast cancer and have undergone tooth extraction or dental surgery. Intraoral lesions, of which two-thirds are painful, appear as exposed yellow-white hard bone involving the mandible or maxilla. Screening tests for determining risk of osteonecrosis are unreliable. Patients slated for aminobisphosphonate therapy should receive preventive dental care that reduces the risk of infection and the need for future dentoalveolar surgery.

Halitosis Halitosis typically emanates from the oral cavity or nasal passages. Volatile sulfur compounds resulting from bacterial decay of food and cellular debris account for the malodor. Periodontal disease, caries, acute forms of gingivitis, poorly fitting dentures, oral abscess, and tongue coating are common causes. Treatment includes correcting poor hygiene, treating infection, and tongue brushing. Hyposalivation can produce and exacerbate halitosis. Pockets of decay in the tonsillar crypts, esophageal diverticulum, esophageal stasis (e.g., achalasia, stricture), sinusitis, and lung abscess account for some instances. A few systemic diseases produce distinctive odors: renal failure (ammoniacal), hepatic (fishy), and ketoacidosis (fruity). *Helicobacter pylori* gastritis can also produce ammoniacal breath. If a patient presents because of concern about halitosis but no odor is detectable, then pseudohalitosis or halitophobia must be considered.

Aging and Oral Health While tooth loss and dental disease are not normal consequences of aging, a complex array of structural and functional changes that occur with age can affect oral health. Subtle changes in tooth structure (e.g., diminished pulp space and volume, sclerosis of dentinal tubules, and altered proportions of nerve and vascular pulp content) result in the elimination or diminution of pain sensitivity and a reduction in the reparative capacity of the teeth. In addition, age-associated fatty replacement of salivary acini may reduce physiologic reserve, thus increasing the risk of hyposalivation. In healthy older adults, there is minimal, if any, reduction in salivary flow.

Poor oral hygiene often results when general health fails or when patients lose manual dexterity and upper-extremity flexibility. This situation is particularly common among frail older adults and nursing home residents and must be emphasized because regular oral cleaning and dental care reduce the incidence of pneumonia and oral disease as well as the mortality risk in this population. Other risks for dental decay include limited lifetime fluoride exposure. Without assiduous care, decay can become quite advanced yet remain asymptomatic. Consequently, much of a tooth—or the entire tooth—can be destroyed before the patient is aware of the process.

Periodontal disease, a leading cause of tooth loss, is indicated by loss of alveolar bone height. More than 90% of the U.S. population has some degree of periodontal disease by age 50. Healthy adults who have not had significant alveolar bone loss by the sixth decade of life do not typically experience significant worsening with advancing age.

With the passing of those born in the first half of the twentieth century, complete edentulousness in the United States is becoming increasingly restricted to impoverished populations. When it is present, speech, mastication, and facial contours are dramatically affected. Edentulousness may also exacerbate obstructive sleep apnea, particularly in asymptomatic individuals who wear dentures. Dentures can improve verbal articulation and restore diminished facial contours. Mastication can also be restored; however, patients expecting dentures to facilitate oral intake are often disappointed. Accommodation to dentures requires a period of adjustment. Pain can result from friction or traumatic lesions produced by loose dentures. Poor fit and poor oral hygiene may permit the development of candidiasis. This fungal infection may be either asymptomatic or painful and is suggested by erythematous smooth or granular tissue conforming to an area covered by the appliance. Individuals with dentures and no natural teeth need regular (annual) professional oral examinations.

FURTHER READING

Durso SC: Interaction with other health team members in caring for elderly patients. Dent Clin North Am 49:377, 2005.

Kaplovitch E, Dounaevskaia V: Treatment in the dental practice of the patient receiving anticoagulant therapy. J Am Dent Assoc 150:602, 2019.

Weintraub JA et al: Improving nursing home residents' oral hygiene: Results of a cluster randomized intervention trial. J Am Med Dir Assoc 19:1086, 2018.

Section 5 Alterations in Circulatory and Respiratory Functions

37 Dyspnea

Rebecca M. Baron

DYSPNEA

DEFINITION

The American Thoracic Society consensus statement defines *dyspnea* as a "subjective experience of breathing discomfort that consists of qualitatively distinct sensations that vary in intensity. The experience derives from interactions among multiple physiological, psychological, social, and environmental factors and may induce secondary physiological and behavioral responses." Dyspnea, a symptom, can be perceived only by the person experiencing it and, therefore, must be self-reported. In contrast, signs of increased work of breathing, such as tachypnea, accessory muscle use, and intercostal retraction, can be measured and reported by clinicians.

EPIDEMIOLOGY

Dyspnea is common. It has been reported that up to one-half of inpatients and one-quarter of ambulatory patients experience dyspnea, with a prevalence of 9–13% in the community that increases to as high as 37% for adults aged ≥70 years. Dyspnea is a frequent cause for emergency room visits, accounting for as many as 3–4 million visits per year. Furthermore, it is increasingly appreciated that the degree of dyspnea may better predict outcomes in chronic obstructive pulmonary disease (COPD) than does the forced expiratory volume in 1 s (FEV_1), and formal measures of dyspnea have been incorporated into the Global Initiative for Chronic Obstructive Lung Disease (GOLD) COPD severity assessment guidelines. Dyspnea may also predict outcomes in other chronic heart and lung diseases as well. Dyspnea can arise from a diverse array of pulmonary, cardiac, and neurologic underlying causes, and elucidation of particular symptoms may point toward a specific etiology and/or mechanism driving dyspnea (although additional diagnostic testing is often required, as will be further discussed below).

MECHANISMS UNDERLYING DYSPNEA

The mechanisms underlying dyspnea are complex, as it can arise from different contributory respiratory sensations. Although a large body of research has increased our understanding of mechanisms underlying particular respiratory sensations such as "chest tightness" or "air hunger," it is likely that a given disease state might produce the sensation of dyspnea via more than one underlying mechanism. Dyspnea can arise from a variety of pathways, including generation of *afferent* signals from the respiratory system to the central nervous system (CNS), *efferent* signals from the CNS to the respiratory muscles, and particularly when there is a mismatch in the integrative signaling between these two pathways, termed *efferent-reafferent mismatch* (Fig. 37-1).

Afferent signals trigger the CNS (brainstem and/or cortex) and include primarily: (1) peripheral chemoreceptors in the carotid body and aortic arch and central chemoreceptors in the medulla that are activated by hypoxemia, hypercapnia, or acidemia, and might produce a sense of "air hunger"; and (2) mechanoreceptors in the upper airways, lungs (including stretch receptors, irritant receptors, and J receptors), and chest wall (including muscle spindles as stretch receptors and tendon organs that monitor force generation) that are activated in the setting of an increased work load from a disease state producing an increase in airway resistance that may be associated with symptoms of chest tightness (e.g., asthma or COPD) or decreased lung or chest wall compliance (e.g., pulmonary fibrosis). Other afferent signals that trigger dyspnea within the respiratory system can arise from pulmonary vascular receptor responses to changes in pulmonary artery pressure and skeletal muscle (termed metaboreceptors) that are believed to sense changes in the biochemical environment.

Efferent signals are sent from the CNS (motor cortex and brainstem) to the respiratory muscles and are also transmitted by corollary discharge to the sensory cortex; they are believed to underlie sensations of respiratory effort (or "work of breathing") and perhaps contribute to sensations of "air hunger," especially in response to an increased ventilatory load in a disease state such as COPD. In addition, fear or anxiety may heighten the sense of dyspnea by exacerbating the underlying physiologic disturbance in response to an increased respiratory rate or disordered breathing pattern.

ASSESSING DYSPNEA

While it is well appreciated that dyspnea is a difficult quality to reliably measure due to multiple relevant possible domains that can be measured (e.g., sensory-perceptual experience, affective distress, and symptom impact or burden), and there exist no uniformly agreed upon tools for dyspnea assessment, consensus opinion is that dyspnea should be formally assessed in a context most relevant and beneficial for patient management and, furthermore, that the specific domains being measured are adequately described. There are a number of emerging tools that have been developed for formal dyspnea assessment. As an example, the GOLD criteria advocate use of a dyspnea assessment tool such as the Modified Medical Research Council Dyspnea Scale (**Table 37-1**) to assess symptom/impact burden in COPD.

DIFFERENTIAL DIAGNOSIS

This chapter focuses largely on chronic dyspnea, which is defined as symptoms lasting longer than 1 month and can arise from a broad array of different underlying conditions, most commonly attributable to pulmonary or cardiac conditions that account for as many as 85% of the underlying causes of dyspnea. However, as many as one-third of patients may have multifactorial reasons underlying dyspnea. Examples of a wide array of conditions that underlie dyspnea with possible mechanisms underlying the presenting symptoms are described in **Table 37-2**.

Respiratory system causes include diseases of the airways (e.g., asthma and COPD), diseases of the parenchyma (more commonly, interstitial lung diseases are seen in the setting of chronic dyspnea, but alveolar filling processes, such as hypersensitivity pneumonitis or bronchiolitis obliterans organizing pneumonia [BOOP], can also

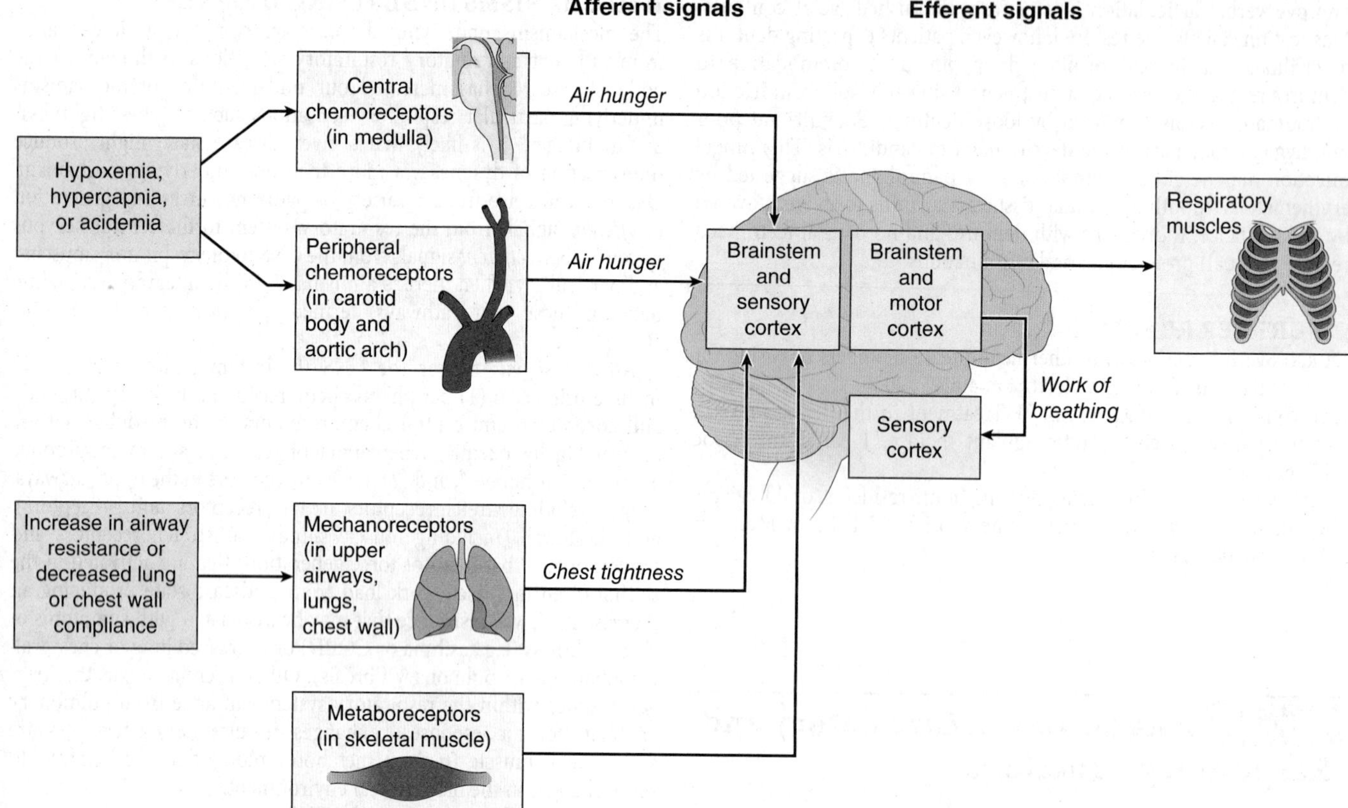

FIGURE 37-1 Signaling pathways underlying dyspnea. Dyspnea arises from a range of sensory inputs, many of which lead to distinct descriptive phrases used by patients (shown in italics in the figure). The sensation of respiratory effort (or work of breathing) likely arises from signals transmitted from the motor cortex to the sensory cortex when outgoing motor commands are sent to the respiratory muscles. Motor output from the brain stem may also be accompanied by signals transmitted to the sensory cortex and contribute to the sensation of work of breathing. The sensation of air hunger likely derives from stimuli that increase the drive to breathe (e.g., hypoxemia, hypercapnia, acidemia; mediated by signals from central and peripheral chemoreceptors), as well as airway and interstitial inflammation (mediated by pulmonary afferent signals) and pulmonary vascular receptors. Dyspnea arises, in part, from a perceived mismatch between the outgoing efferent messages to the respiratory muscles and incoming afferent signals from the lungs and chest wall. Chest tightness, often associated with bronchospasm, is largely mediated by simulation of vagal-irritant receptors. Afferent signals from airway, lung, and chest wall mechanoreceptors most likely pass through the brain stem before being transmitted to the sensory cortex, although it is possible that some afferent information bypasses the brain stem and goes directly to the sensory cortex. *(Adapted from RM Schwartzstein: Approach to the patient with dyspnea. In: UpToDate, TW Post (Ed), UpToDate, Waltham, MA. (Accessed on 7 December 2021) 2018 UpToDate, Inc. For more information visit www.uptodate.com.)*

present with similar symptoms), diseases affecting the chest wall (e.g., bony abnormalities such as kyphoscoliosis, or neuromuscular weakness conditions such as amyotrophic lateral sclerosis), and diseases affecting the pulmonary vasculature (e.g., pulmonary hypertension that can arise from a variety of underlying causes, or chronic thromboemolic disease). Diseases affecting the cardiovascular system that can present with dyspnea include processes affecting left heart function, such as coronary artery disease and cardiomyopathy, as well as disease processes affecting the pericardium, including constrictive pericarditis and cardiac tamponade. Other conditions underyling dyspnea that might not directly emanate from the pulmonary or cardiovascular systems include anemia (thereby potentially affecting oxygen-carrying capacity), deconditioning, and psychological processes such as anxiety. Distinguishing between the myriad of underlying processes that might present with dyspnea can be challenging. A graded approach that begins with a history and physical examination, followed by selected laboratory testing that might then advance to additional diagnostics and potentially subspecialty referral, may help elucidate the underlying cause of dyspnea. However, a substantial proportion of patients may have persistent dyspnea despite treatment for an underlying process or may not have a specific underlying process identified that is driving the dyspnea.

TABLE 37-1 An Example of a Clinical Method for Rating Dyspnea: The Modified Medical Research Council Dyspnea Scale[a]

GRADE OF DYSPNEA	DESCRIPTION
0	Not troubled by breathlessness, except with strenuous exercise
1	Shortness of breath walking on level ground or with walking up a slight hill
2	Walks slower than people of similar age on level ground due to breathlessness, or has to stop to rest when walking at own pace on level ground
3	Stops to rest after walking 100 m or after walking a few minutes on level ground
4	Too breathless to leave the house, or breathless with activities of daily living (e.g., dressing/undressing)

[a]Which has been incorporated into the Global Initiative for Chronic Obstructive Lung Disease (GOLD) guidelines as a possible tool for rating dyspnea in chronic obstructive pulmonary disease.

Source: Reproduced with permission from DA Mahler, CK Wells: Evaluation of clinical methods for rating dyspnea. Chest 93:580, 1988.

APPROACH TO THE PATIENT

Dyspnea (See Fig. 37-2)

OVERALL

For patients with a known prior pulmonary, cardiac, or neuromuscular condition and worsening dyspnea, the initial focus of the

TABLE 37-2 Differential Diagnosis of Disease Processes Underlying Dyspnea

SYSTEM	TYPE OF PROCESS	EXAMPLE OF DISEASE PROCESS	POSSIBLE PRESENTING DYSPNEA SYMPTOMS	POSSIBLE PHYSICAL FINDINGS	POSSIBLE MECHANISMS UNDERLYING DYSPNEA	INITIAL DIAGNOSTIC STUDIES (AND POSSIBLE FINDINGS)
Pulmonary	Airways disease	Asthma, COPD, upper airway obstruction	Chest tightness, tachypnea, increased WOB, air hunger, inability to get a deep breath	Wheezing, accessory muscle use, exertional hypoxemia (especially with COPD)	Increased WOB, hypoxemia, hypercapnia, stimulation of pulmonary receptors	Peak flow (reduced); spirometry (OVD); CXR (hyperinflation; loss of lung parenchyma in COPD), chest CT and airway examination for upper airway obstruction
	Parenchymal disease	Interstitial lung disease[a]	Air hunger, inability to get a deep breath	Dry end-inspiratory crackles, clubbing, exertional hypoxemia	Increased WOB, increased respiratory drive, hypoxemia, hypercapnia, stimulation of pulmonary receptors	Spirometry and lung volumes (RVD); CXR and chest CT (interstitial lung disease)
	Chest wall disease	Kyphoscoliosis, neuromuscular (NM) weakness	Increased WOB, inability to get a deep breath	Decreased diaphragm excursion; atelectasis	Increased WOB; stimulation of pulmonary receptors (if atelectasis is present)	Spirometry and lung volumes (RVD); MIP and MEPs (reduced in NM weakness)
Pulmonary and cardiac	Pulmonary vasculature	Pulmonary hypertension	Tachypnea	Elevated right heart pressures, exertional hypoxemia	Increased respiratory drive, hypoxemia, stimulation of vascular receptors	Diffusion capacity (reduced); ECG; ECHO (to evaluate pulmonary artery pressures)[b]
Cardiac	Left heart failure	Coronary artery disease, cardiomyopathy[c]	Chest tightness, air hunger	Elevated left heart pressures; wet crackles on lung examination; pulsus paradoxus (pericardial disease)	Increased WOB and drive, hypoxemia, stimulation of vascular and pulmonary receptors[d]	Consider BNP testing, especially in the acute setting; ECG, ECHO, may need stress testing and/or LHC
	Pericardial disease	Constrictive pericarditis; cardiac tamponade				
Other	Variable	Anemia Deconditioning Psychological Metabolic disturbances Gastrointestinal (e.g., gastroesophageal reflux disease [GERD], aspiration pneumonitis)	Exertional breathlessness Poor fitness Anxiety	Variable	Metaboreceptors (anemia, poor fitness); chemoreceptors (anaerobic metabolism from poor fitness); some subjects may have increased sensitivity to hypercapnia	Hematocrit for anemia; laboratory studies (e.g., metabolic panel, thyroid hormone testing for metabolic disturbances); consider upper gastrointestinal endoscopy and/or esophageal pH probe testing for GERD and concerns for aspiration; exclude other causes

[a]Differential diagnosis of interstitial lung disease includes idiopathic pulmonary fibrosis, collagen vascular disease, drug- or occupation-induced pneumonitis, lymphangitic spread of malignancy; processes that are more alveolar rather than interstitial in nature can also less commonly contribute to parenchymal lung disease underlying chronic dyspnea and include entities such as hypersensitivity pneumonitis, bronchiolitis obliterans organizing pneumonia, etc. [b]Would additionally consider these patients for CT angiography to evaluate for presence of thromboemboli, ventilation/perfusion scanning to evaluate for the presence of chronic thromboembolic disease, and right heart catheterization to further evaluate for pulmonary hypertension. [c]Diastolic dysfunction in the setting of a stiff left ventricle is often seen and contributes significantly to insidious dyspnea that can be difficult to treat. [d]May stimulate metaboreceptors if cardiac output is sufficiently reduced to result in a lactic acidosis.

Abbreviations: BNP, brain natriuretic peptide; COPD, chronic obstructive pulmonary disease; CT, computed tomography; CXR, chest x-ray; ECG, electrocardiogram; ECHO, echocardiogram; GERD, gastroesophageal reflux disease; LHC, left heart catheterization; MIP/MEP, maximal inspiratory and maximal expiratory pressures (obtained in the pulmonary function testing laboratory); OVD, obstructive ventilatory defect; RVD, restrictive ventilatory defect; WOB, work of breathing.

evaluation will usually address determining whether the known condition has progressed or whether a new process has developed that is causing dyspnea. For patients without a prior known potential cause of dyspnea, the initial evaluation will focus on determining an underlying etiology. Determining the underlying cause, if possible, is extremely important, as the treatment may vary dramatically based on the predisposing condition. An initial history and physical examination remain fundamental to the evaluation followed by initial diagnostic testing as indicated that might prompt subspecialty referral (e.g., pulmonary, cardiology, neurology, sleep, and/or specialized dyspnea clinic) if the cause of dyspnea remains elusive (Fig. 37-2). As many as two-thirds of patients will require diagnostic testing beyond the initial clinical presentation.

HISTORY

The patient should be asked to describe in his or her own words what the discomfort feels like as well as the effect of position, infections, and environmental stimuli on the dyspnea, as descriptors may be helpful in pointing toward an etiology. For example, symptoms of chest tightness might suggest the possibility of bronchoconstriction, and the sensation of inability to take a deep breath may correlate with dynamic hyperinflation from COPD. Orthopnea is a common indicator of congestive heart failure (CHF), mechanical impairment of the diaphragm associated with obesity, or asthma triggered by esophageal reflux. Nocturnal dyspnea suggests CHF or asthma. Acute, intermittent episodes of dyspnea are more likely to reflect episodes of myocardial ischemia, bronchospasm, or pulmonary embolism, while chronic persistent dyspnea is more typical of COPD, interstitial lung disease, and chronic thromboembolic disease. Information on risk factors for drug-induced or occupational lung disease and for coronary artery disease should be elicited. Left atrial myxoma or hepatopulmonary syndrome should be considered when the patient complains of *platypnea*—i.e., dyspnea in the upright position with relief in the supine position.

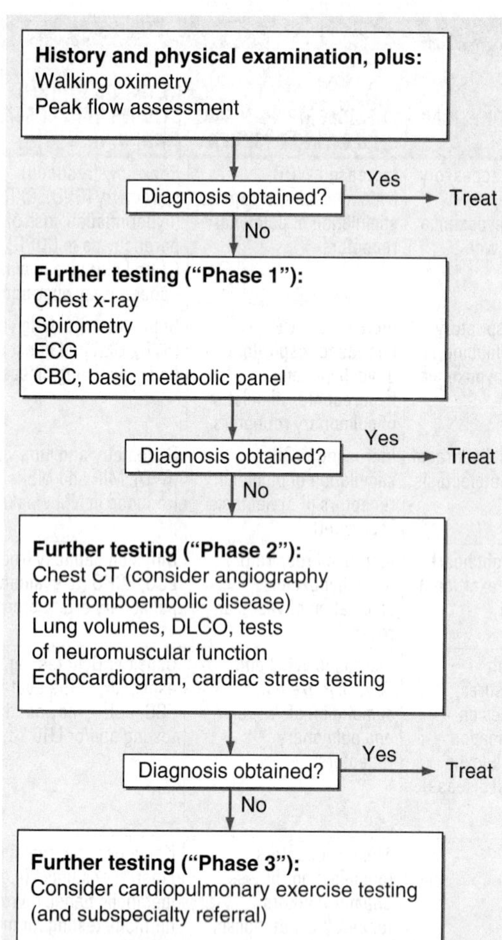

FIGURE 37-2 Possible algorithm for the evaluation of the patient with dyspnea. As described in the text, the approach should begin with a detailed history and physical examination, followed by progressive testing and ultimately more invasive testing and subspecialty referral as is indicated to determine the underlying cause of dyspnea. CBC, complete blood count; DLCO, diffusing capacity of the lungs for carbon monoxide; ECG, electrocardiogram. *(Adapted from NG Karnani et al: Am Fam Physician 71:1529, 2005.)*

PHYSICAL EXAMINATION

Initial vital signs might be helpful in pointing toward an underlying etiology in the context of the remainder of the evaluation. For example, the presence of fever might point toward an underlying infectious or inflammatory process; the presence of hypertension in the setting of a heart failure might point toward diastolic dysfunction; the presence of tachycardia might be associated with many different underlying processes including fever, cardiac dysfunction, and deconditioning; and the presence of resting hypoxemia suggests processes involving hypercapnia, ventilation-perfusion mismatch, shunt, or impairment in diffusion capacity might be involved. An exertional oxygen saturation should also be obtained as described below. The physical examination should begin during the interview of the patient. Inability of the patient to speak in full sentences before stopping to get a deep breath suggests a condition that leads to stimulation of the controller or impairment of the ventilatory pump with reduced vital capacity. Evidence of increased work of breathing (supraclavicular retractions; use of accessory muscles of ventilation; and the tripod position, characterized by sitting with the hands braced on the knees) is indicative of increased airway resistance or stiffness of the lungs and the chest wall. When measuring the vital signs, the physician should accurately assess the respiratory rate and measure the pulsus paradoxus (**Chap. 270**); if the systolic pressure decreases by >10 mmHg on inspiration, the presence of COPD, acute asthma, or pericardial disease should be considered. During the general examination, signs of anemia (pale conjunctivae), cyanosis, and cirrhosis (spider angiomata, gynecomastia) should be sought. Examination of the chest should focus on symmetry of movement; percussion (dullness is indicative of pleural effusion; hyperresonance is a sign of pneumothorax and emphysema); and auscultation (wheezes, rhonchi, prolonged expiratory phase, and diminished breath sounds are clues to disorders of the airways; rales suggest interstitial edema or fibrosis). The cardiac examination should focus on signs of elevated right heart pressures (jugular venous distention, edema, accentuated pulmonic component to the second heart sound); left ventricular dysfunction (S3 and S4 gallops); and valvular disease (murmurs). When examining the abdomen with the patient in the supine position, the physician should note whether there is paradoxical movement of the abdomen as well as the presence of increased respiratory distress in the supine position: inward motion during inspiration is a sign of diaphragmatic weakness, and rounding of the abdomen during exhalation is suggestive of pulmonary edema. Clubbing of the digits may be an indication of interstitial pulmonary fibrosis or bronchiectasis, and joint swelling or deformation as well as changes consistent with Raynaud's disease may be indicative of a collagen-vascular process that can be associated with pulmonary disease.

Patients should be asked to walk under observation with oximetry in order to reproduce the symptoms. The patient should be examined during and at the end of exercise for new findings that were not present at rest (e.g., presence of wheezing) and for changes in oxygen saturation.

CHEST IMAGING

After the history elicitation and the physical examination, a chest radiograph should be obtained if the diagnosis remains elusive. The lung volumes should be assessed: hyperinflation is consistent with obstructive lung disease, whereas low lung volumes suggest interstitial edema or fibrosis, diaphragmatic dysfunction, or impaired chest wall motion. The pulmonary parenchyma should be examined for evidence of interstitial disease, infiltrates, and emphysema. Prominent pulmonary vasculature in the upper zones indicates pulmonary venous hypertension, while enlarged central pulmonary arteries may suggest pulmonary arterial hypertension. An enlarged cardiac silhouette can point toward dilated cardiomyopathy or valvular disease. Bilateral pleural effusions are typical of CHF and some forms of collagen-vascular disease. Unilateral effusions raise the specter of carcinoma and pulmonary embolism but may also occur in heart failure or in the case of a parapneumonic effusion. CT of the chest is generally reserved for further evaluation of the lung parenchyma (interstitial lung disease) and possible pulmonary embolism if there remains diagnostic uncertainty.

LABORATORY STUDIES

Initial laboratory testing should include a hematocrit to exclude occult anemia as an underlying cause of reduced oxygen-carrying capacity contributing to dyspnea, and a basic metabolic panel may be helpful to exclude a significant underlying metabolic acidosis (and conversely, an elevated bicarbonate might point toward the possibility of carbon dioxide retention that might be seen in chronic respiratory failure—in such a setting, an arterial blood gas may provide useful additional information). Additional laboratory studies should include electrocardiography to seek evidence of ventricular hypertrophy and prior myocardial infarction and spirometry, which can be diagnostic of the presence of an obstructive ventilatory defect and suggest the possibility of a restrictive ventilatory defect (that then might prompt additional pulmonary function laboratory testing, including lung volumes, diffusion capacity, and possible tests of neuromuscular function). Echocardiography is indicated when systolic dysfunction, pulmonary hypertension, or valvular heart disease is suspected. Bronchoprovocation testing and/or home peak-flow monitoring may be useful in patients with intermittent symptoms suggestive of asthma who have a normal physical examination and spirometry; up to one-third of patients with the clinical diagnosis of asthma do not have reactive airways disease when formally tested. Measurement of brain natriuretic peptide levels in serum is increasingly used to assess for CHF in patients presenting with acute dyspnea but may be elevated in the presence of right ventricular strain as well.

DISTINGUISHING CARDIOVASCULAR FROM RESPIRATORY SYSTEM DYSPNEA

If a patient has evidence of both pulmonary and cardiac disease that is not responsive to treatment or it remains unclear what factors are primarily driving the dyspnea, a cardiopulmonary exercise test (CPET) can be carried out to determine which system is responsible for the exercise limitation. CPET includes incremental symptom-limited exercise (cycling or treadmill) with measurements of ventilation and pulmonary gas exchange and, in some cases, includes noninvasive and invasive measures of pulmonary vascular pressures and cardiac output. If, at peak exercise, the patient achieves predicted maximal ventilation, demonstrates an increase in dead space or hypoxemia, or develops bronchospasm, the respiratory system may be the cause of the problem. Alternatively, if the heart rate is >85% of the predicted maximum, if the anaerobic threshold occurs early, if the blood pressure becomes excessively high or decreases during exercise, if the O_2 pulse (O_2 consumption/heart rate, an indicator of stroke volume) falls, or if there are ischemic changes on the electrocardiogram, an abnormality of the cardiovascular system is likely the explanation for the breathing discomfort. Additionally, a CPET may also help point toward a peripheral extraction deficit or metabolic/neuromuscular disease as potential underlying processes driving dyspnea.

TREATMENT

Dyspnea

The first goal is to correct the underlying condition(s) driving dyspnea and address potentially reversible causes with appropriate treatment for the particular condition. Multiple different interventions may be necessary, given that dyspnea often arises from multifactorial causes. If relief of dyspnea with treatment of the underlying condition(s) is not fully possible, an effort is made to lessen the intensity of the symptom and its effect on the patient's quality of life. More recent work at the consensus conference level has sought to define an identifiable entity of persistent dyspnea in order to develop an approach to improving efforts to address symptom management for this condition. In 2017, an international group of experts defined "chronic breathlessness syndrome" as "the experience of breathlessness that persists despite optimal treatment of the underlying pathophysiology and results in disability for the patient." Despite an increased understanding of the mechanisms underlying dyspnea, there has been limited progress in treatment strategies for dyspnea. Supplemental O_2 should be administered if the resting O_2 saturation is ≤88% or if the patient's saturation drops to these levels with activity or sleep. In particular, for patients with COPD, supplemental oxygen for those with hypoxemia has been shown to improve mortality, and pulmonary rehabilitation programs (including some community-based exercise programs such as yoga and Tai Chi) have demonstrated positive effects on dyspnea, exercise capacity, and rates of hospitalization. Opioids have been shown to reduce symptoms of dyspnea, largely through reducing air hunger, thus likely suppressing respiratory drive and influencing cortical activity. However, opioids should be considered for each patient individually based on the risk-benefit profile in regard to the effects of respiratory depression. Studies of anxiolytics for dyspnea have not demonstrated consistent benefit. Additional approaches are under study for dyspnea, including inhaled furosemide that might alter afferent sensory information.

FURTHER READING

Banzett RB et al: Multidimensional dyspnea profile: An instrument for clinical and laboratory research. Eur Respir J 45:1681, 2015.

Ferry OR et al: Diagnostic approach to chronic dyspnea in adults. J Thorac Dis 11(Suppl 17):S2117, 2019.

Johnson M et al: Toward an expert consensus to delineate a clinical syndrome of chronic breathlessness: Chronic breathlessness syndrome. Eur Respir J 49:1602277, 2017.

Laviolette L, Laveneziana P on behalf of the ERS Research Seminar Faculty: Dyspnoea: A multidimensional and multidisciplinary approach. Eur Respir J 43:1750, 2014.

O'Donnell DE et al: Unraveling the causes of unexplained dyspnea. Clin Chest Med 40:471, 2019.

Parshall MB et al: An Official American Thoracic Society Statement: Update on the mechanisms, assessment, and management of dyspnea. Am J Respir Crit Care Med 185:435, 2012.

Ratarasarn K et al: Yoga and Tai Chi: A mind-body approach in managing respiratory symptoms in obstructive lung diseases. Curr Opin Pulm Med 26:186, 2020.

38 Cough

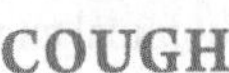

Christopher H. Fanta

COUGH

Cough performs an essential protective function for human airways and lungs. Without an effective cough reflex, we are at risk for retained airway secretions and aspirated material predisposing to infection, atelectasis, and respiratory compromise. At the other extreme, excessive coughing can be exhausting; can be complicated by emesis, syncope, muscular pain, or rib fractures; can aggravate low back pain, abdominal or inguinal hernias, and urinary incontinence; and can be a major impediment to social interactions. Cough is often a clue to the presence of respiratory disease. In many instances, cough is an expected and accepted manifestation of disease, as in acute respiratory tract infection. However, persistent cough in the absence of other respiratory symptoms commonly causes patients to seek medical attention.

COUGH MECHANISM

Both chemical (e.g., capsaicin) and mechanical (e.g., mucus, particulates in air pollution) stimuli can initiate the cough reflex. Cationic channels (e.g., transient receptor potential channels) and adenosine triphosphate–activated ion channels (P2X3) function as sensory neuronal receptors, with signals transmitted centrally via Aδ (mechanosensory) and C fibers (chemosensory). Afferent nerve endings richly innervate the pharynx, larynx, and airways to the level of the terminal bronchioles and extend into the lung parenchyma. They are also located in the external auditory canal (the auricular branch of the vagus nerve, or Arnold's nerve) and in the esophagus. Sensory signals travel via the vagus and superior laryngeal nerves to a region of the brainstem in the nucleus tractus solitarius. Integrated neural networks process this input into a conscious sensation referred to as the "urge to cough." The efferent limb of the cough reflex involves a highly orchestrated series of involuntary muscular actions, with the potential for input from cortical pathways as well, making possible voluntary cough. The vocal

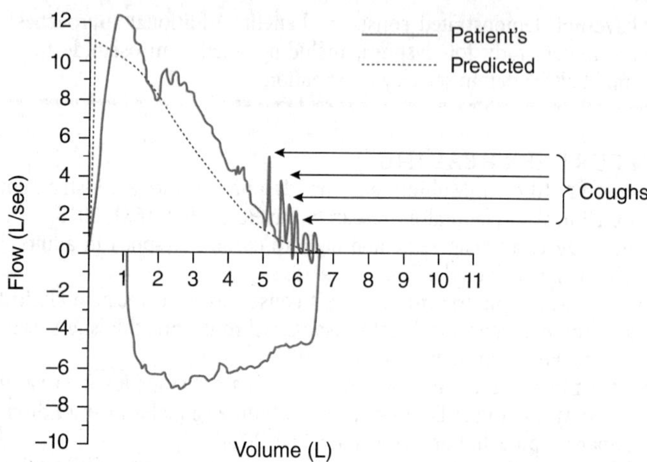

FIGURE 38-1 Flow-volume curve shows spikes of high expiratory flow achieved with cough.

cords adduct, leading to transient upper-airway occlusion. Expiratory muscles contract, generating positive intrathoracic pressures as high as 300 mmHg. With sudden release of the laryngeal contraction, rapid expiratory flows are generated, exceeding the normal "envelope" of maximal expiratory flow seen on the flow-volume curve (**Fig. 38-1**). Bronchial smooth-muscle contraction together with dynamic compression of airways narrows airway lumens and maximizes the velocity of exhalation. The kinetic energy available to dislodge mucus from the inside of airway walls is directly proportional to the square of the velocity of expiratory airflow. A deep breath preceding a cough optimizes the function of the expiratory muscles; a series of repetitive coughs at successively lower lung volumes sweeps the point of maximal expiratory velocity progressively further into the lung periphery.

IMPAIRED COUGH

Weak or ineffective cough compromises the ability to clear lower respiratory tract secretions, predisposing to more serious infections and their sequelae. Weakness or paralysis of the expiratory (abdominal and intercostal) muscles and pain in the chest wall or abdomen are foremost on the list of causes of impaired cough (**Table 38-1**). Cough strength is generally assessed qualitatively; peak expiratory flow or maximal expiratory pressure at the mouth can be used as a surrogate marker for cough strength. A variety of assistive devices and techniques have been developed to improve cough efficacy, running the gamut from simple (splinting of the abdominal muscles with a tightly held pillow to reduce postoperative pain while coughing) to complex (a mechanical cough-assist device supplied via face mask or tracheal tube that applies a cycle of positive pressure followed rapidly by negative pressure). Cough may fail to clear secretions completely despite a preserved ability to generate normal expiratory velocities; such failure may be due to abnormal airway secretions (e.g., abnormally viscous secretions of cystic fibrosis), ciliary dysfunction (e.g., primary ciliary dyskinesia), or structural abnormalities of the airways (e.g., tracheomalacia with excessive expiratory collapse of the trachea during cough).

TABLE 38-1 Causes of Impaired Cough and Airway Clearance
Respiratory muscle weakness
Chest wall or abdominal pain
Chest wall deformity (e.g., severe kyphoscoliosis)
Impaired glottic closure or tracheostomy
Central respiratory depression (e.g., anesthesia, sedation, or neurologic disease)
Abnormal airway secretions
Ciliary dysfunction
Tracheobronchomalacia
Bronchiectasis
Tracheal or bronchial stenoses

SYMPTOMATIC COUGH

Cough may occur in the context of other respiratory symptoms that together point to a diagnosis; for example, cough accompanied by wheezing, shortness of breath, and chest tightness after exposure to a cat or other sources of allergens suggests asthma. At times, however, cough is the dominant or sole symptom of disease, and it may be of sufficient duration and severity that relief is sought. The duration of cough is a clue to its etiology, at least retrospectively. Acute cough (<3 weeks) is most commonly due to a respiratory tract infection, aspiration, or inhalation of noxious chemicals or smoke. Subacute cough (3–8 weeks in duration) is a common residuum of tracheobronchitis, as in pertussis or "postviral tussive syndrome." Chronic cough (>8 weeks) may be caused by a wide variety of cardiopulmonary diseases, including those of inflammatory, infectious, neoplastic, and cardiovascular etiologies. When initial assessment with chest examination and radiography is normal, cough-variant asthma, gastroesophageal reflux, rhinosinusitis with excessive nasopharyngeal drainage, and medications (angiotensin-converting enzyme [ACE] inhibitors) are the most common identifiable causes of chronic cough. In a long-time cigarette smoker, an early-morning, productive cough suggests chronic bronchitis. A dry, irritative cough that lingers for >2 months following one or more respiratory tract infections ("postbronchitic cough") is a very common cause of chronic cough, especially in the winter months. Chronic cough in the absence of identifiable etiology has been recognized with increasing frequency, is thought to be due to exaggerated neurologic signaling via sensory cough-reflex pathways, and is referred to as "chronic cough hypersensitivity syndrome."

ASSESSMENT OF CHRONIC COUGH

Except for our ability to detect the sound of excess airway secretions, details as to the resonance of the cough, its time of occurrence during the day, and the pattern of coughing (e.g., occurring in paroxysms) infrequently provide useful etiologic clues. Regardless of cause, cough often worsens upon first lying down at night, with talking, or with the hyperpnea of exercise; it frequently improves with sleep. An exception may involve the cough that occurs only with certain allergic exposures or exercise in cold air, as in asthma. Useful historical questions include what circumstances surrounded the onset of cough, what makes the cough better or worse, and whether the cough produces sputum.

The physical examination seeks clues suggesting the presence of cardiopulmonary disease, including findings such as wheezing or crackles on chest examination. Examination of the auditory canals and tympanic membranes (for irritation of the latter resulting in stimulation of Arnold's nerve), the nasal passageways (for rhinitis or polyps), and the nails (for clubbing) may also provide etiologic clues. Because cough can be a manifestation of a systemic disease such as sarcoidosis or vasculitis, a thorough general examination is likewise important.

In virtually all instances, evaluation of chronic cough merits a chest radiograph. The list of diseases that can cause persistent cough without other symptoms and without detectable abnormalities on physical examination is long. It includes serious illnesses such as sarcoidosis or Hodgkin's disease in young adults, lung cancer in older patients, and (worldwide) pulmonary tuberculosis. An abnormal chest film prompts an evaluation aimed at explaining the radiographic abnormality. In a patient with chronic productive cough, examination of expectorated sputum is warranted, because determining the cause of mucus hypersecretion is a crucial clue to etiology. Purulent-appearing sputum should be sent for routine bacterial culture and, in certain circumstances, mycobacterial culture as well. Cytologic examination of mucoid sputum may be useful to assess for malignancy and oropharyngeal aspiration and to distinguish neutrophilic from eosinophilic bronchitis. Expectoration of blood—whether streaks of blood, blood mixed with airway secretions, or pure blood—deserves a special approach to assessment and management (**Chap. 39**).

CHRONIC COUGH WITH A NORMAL CHEST RADIOGRAPH

It is commonly held that (alone or in combination) the use of an ACE inhibitor; postnasal drainage; gastroesophageal reflux; and asthma account for >90% of cases of chronic cough with a normal or noncontributory chest radiograph. However, clinical experience does not support this contention, and strict adherence to this concept discourages the search for alternative explanations by both clinicians and researchers. In recent years, the concept of a distinct "cough hypersensitivity syndrome" has emerged, emphasizing the putative role of sensitized sensory nerve endings and afferent neural pathways in causing chronic refractory cough, akin to chronic neuropathic pain. It presents with a dry or minimally productive cough and a tickle or sensitivity in the throat, made worse with talking, laughing, or exertion. It is more common in women than men and can last for years. Specific diagnostic criteria are lacking; the diagnosis is suspected when alternative etiologies are excluded by diagnostic testing or failed therapeutic trials. It is uncertain whether persistent daily coughing elicits an inflammatory response and is thereby self-perpetuating.

ACE inhibitor–induced cough occurs in 5–30% of patients taking these agents and is not dose-dependent. ACE metabolizes bradykinin and other tachykinins, such as substance P. The mechanism of ACE inhibitor–associated cough may involve sensitization of sensory nerve endings due to accumulation of bradykinin. Any patient with chronic unexplained cough who is taking an ACE inhibitor should have a trial period off the medication, regardless of the timing of the onset of cough relative to the initiation of ACE inhibitor therapy. In most instances, a safe alternative is available; angiotensin receptor blockers do not cause cough. Failure to observe a decrease in cough after 1 month off medication argues strongly against this etiology.

Postnasal drainage of any etiology can cause cough as a response to stimulation of sensory receptors of the cough-reflex pathway in the hypopharynx or aspiration of draining secretions into the trachea. The term *upper airway cough syndrome* has been coined to encompass the concept that chronic inflammation in the nose and sinuses can cause cough even in the absence of physical drainage into the pharynx. Historical clues suggesting this etiology include a sensation of postnasal drip, frequent throat clearing, and sneezing and rhinorrhea. On speculum examination of the nose, excess mucoid or purulent secretions, inflamed and edematous nasal mucosa, and/or polyps may be seen; in addition, secretions or a cobblestoned appearance of the mucosa along the posterior pharyngeal wall may be noted. Unfortunately, there is no means by which to quantitate postnasal drainage. In many instances, this diagnosis must rely on subjective information provided by the patient. Furthermore, this assessment must also be counterbalanced by the fact that many people who have chronic postnasal drainage do not experience cough.

Linking gastroesophageal reflux to chronic cough poses similar challenges. It is thought that reflux of gastric contents into the lower esophagus may trigger cough via reflex pathways initiated in the esophageal mucosa. Reflux to the level of the pharynx (laryngopharyngeal reflux), with consequent aspiration of gastric contents, causes a chemical bronchitis and possibly pneumonitis that can elicit cough for days afterward, but it is a rare finding among persons with chronic cough. Retrosternal burning after meals or on recumbency, frequent eructation, hoarseness, and throat pain may be indicative of gastroesophageal reflux. Nevertheless, reflux may also elicit minimal or no symptoms. Glottic inflammation detected on laryngoscopy may be a manifestation of recurrent reflux to the level of the throat, but it is a nonspecific finding. Quantification of the frequency and level of reflux requires a somewhat invasive procedure to measure esophageal pH (either nasopharyngeal placement of a catheter with a pH probe into the esophagus for 24 h or endoscopic placement of a radiotransmitter capsule into the esophagus) and, with newer techniques, esophageal pressures (manometry) and nonacid reflux. The precise interpretation of test results that permits an etiologic linking of reflux events and cough remains debated. Again, assigning the cause of cough to gastroesophageal reflux must be weighed against the observation that many people with symptomatic reflux do not experience chronic cough.

Cough alone as a manifestation of asthma is common among children but not among adults. Cough due to asthma in the absence of wheezing, shortness of breath, and chest tightness is referred to as "cough-variant asthma." A history suggestive of cough-variant asthma ties the onset of cough to exposure to typical triggers for asthma and the resolution of cough to discontinuation of exposure. Objective testing can establish the diagnosis of asthma (airflow obstruction on spirometry that varies over time or reverses in response to a bronchodilator) or exclude it with certainty (a negative response to a bronchoprovocation challenge—e.g., with methacholine). In a patient capable of taking reliable measurements, home expiratory peak flow monitoring can be a cost-effective method to support or discount a diagnosis of asthma.

Eosinophilic bronchitis causes chronic cough with a normal chest radiograph. This uncommon condition is characterized by sputum eosinophilia in excess of 3% without airflow obstruction or bronchial hyperresponsiveness and is successfully treated with inhaled glucocorticoids. Measurement of an elevated concentration of nitric oxide in exhaled breath has the potential to detect eosinophilic airway inflammation (in asthma or eosinophilic bronchitis) and predict a favorable response to inhaled steroids in persons with chronic cough.

Treatment of chronic cough in a patient with a normal chest radiograph is often empirical and is targeted at the most likely cause(s) of cough as determined by history, physical examination, and possibly pulmonary function testing. Therapy for postnasal drainage depends on the presumed etiology (infection, allergy, or vasomotor rhinitis) and may include systemic antihistamines; decongestants; antibiotics; nasal saline irrigation; and nasal pump sprays with glucocorticoids, antihistamines, or anticholinergics. Antacids histamine type 2 (H_2) receptor antagonists, and proton pump inhibitors are used to neutralize or decrease the production of gastric acid in gastroesophageal reflux disease; dietary changes, elevation of the head and torso during sleep, and medications to improve gastric emptying or impede the flow of refluxate (e.g., alginates) are additional therapeutic measures. Cough-variant asthma typically responds well to inhaled glucocorticoids and intermittent use of inhaled β-agonist bronchodilators.

Patients who fail to respond to treatment targeting the common causes of chronic cough or who have had these causes excluded by appropriate diagnostic testing should, in the opinion of the author, undergo chest CT. Diseases causing cough that may be missed on chest x-ray include tumors, early interstitial lung disease, bronchiectasis, and atypical mycobacterial pulmonary infection. On the other hand, patients with chronic cough who have normal findings on chest examination, lung function testing, oxygenation assessment, and chest CT can be reassured as to the absence of serious pulmonary pathology.

GLOBAL CONSIDERATIONS

Regular exposure to air pollution can cause chronic cough and throat clearing, as well as lower respiratory tract disease. Smoke from cooking and heating fuels in poorly ventilated homes; toxic exposures in work settings lacking implementation of occupational safety standards; and ambient chemicals and particulates in highly polluted outdoor air are all forms of air pollution causing cough. Limited therapeutic options are available; treatment focuses on improving environmental air quality (e.g., use of a stove chimney in the home), removal from the exposure, and use of an appropriate face mask.

In areas of the world where tuberculosis is endemic, chronic cough conjures the possibility of active pulmonary tuberculosis and mandates appropriate evaluation, including chest imaging and sputum analysis.

SYMPTOM-BASED TREATMENT OF COUGH

Empiric treatment of chronic idiopathic cough with inhaled corticosteroids, inhaled anticholinergic bronchodilators, and macrolide antibiotics has been tried without consistent success. Currently available cough suppressants are only modestly effective. Most potent are narcotic cough suppressants, such as codeine, hydrocodone, or morphine, which are thought to act in the "cough center" in the brainstem. The tendency of narcotic cough suppressants to cause drowsiness and constipation and their potential for addictive dependence limit their appeal for long-term use. Dextromethorphan is an over-the-counter, centrally acting cough suppressant with fewer side effects and less efficacy than the narcotic cough suppressants. Dextromethorphan is thought to have a different site of action than narcotic cough suppressants and can be used in combination with them if necessary. Benzonatate is thought to inhibit neural activity of sensory nerves in the cough-reflex pathway. It is generally free of side effects; however, its effectiveness in suppressing cough is variable and unpredictable. Inhaled lidocaine, an inhibitor of voltage-gated sodium channels, provides transient cough suppression, but because of associated oropharyngeal anesthesia, it poses the risk of aspiration.

Attempts to treat cough hypersensitivity syndrome have focused on inhibition of neural pathways. Small case series and randomized clinical trials have indicated benefit from off-label use of gabapentin, pregabalin, or amitriptyline. Recent studies suggest a role for behavioral modification using specialized speech therapy techniques, but widespread application of this modality is currently not practical. Novel cough suppressants without the limitations of currently available agents are greatly needed. Approaches that are being explored include the development of neurokinin-1 receptor antagonists, transient receptor protein vanilloid-1 (TRPV1) channel antagonists, a promising P2X3 channel antagonist (gefapixant), and novel opioid and opioid-like receptor agonists.

■ FURTHER READING

Brightling CE et al: Eosinophilic bronchitis as an important cause of chronic cough. Am J Respir Crit Care Med 160:406, 1999.

Carroll TL (ed): *Chronic Cough*. San Diego, Plural Publishing, Inc., 2019.

Gibson P et al: Treatment of unexplained chronic cough: CHEST guideline and expert panel report. Chest 149:27, 2016.

Kahrilas PJ et al: Chronic cough due to gastroesophageal reflux in adults: CHEST Guideline and Expert Panel Report. Chest 150:1381, 2016.

Morice AH et al: ERS guidelines on the diagnosis and treatment of chronic cough in adults and children. Eur Respir J 55: 1901136, 2020.

Ramsay LE et al: Double-blind comparison of losartan, lisinopril and hydrochlorothiazide in hypertensive patients with previous angiotensin converting enzyme inhibitor-associated cough. J Hypertens Suppl 13:S73, 1995.

Ryan NM et al: Gabapentin for refractory chronic cough: A randomized, double-blind, placebo-controlled trial. Lancet 380:1583, 2012.

Smith JA, Woodcock A: Chronic cough. N Engl J Med 375:1544, 2016.

39 Hemoptysis

Carolyn M. D'Ambrosio

Hemoptysis is the expectoration of blood from the respiratory tract. Bleeding from the gastrointestinal tract (hematemesis) or nasal cavities (epistaxis) can mimic hemoptysis. Once established as hemoptysis, the degree of blood that is being expectorated (volume and frequency) is the next step as massive or life-threatening hemoptysis (>400 mL of blood in 24 h or >150 mL at one time) requires emergent intervention. This chapter will focus predominantly on non–life-threatening hemoptysis. The source of the bleeding as well as the cause are the next steps when approaching a patient with hemoptysis.

ANATOMY AND PHYSIOLOGY OF HEMOPTYSIS

Hemoptysis can arise from anywhere in the respiratory tract, from the glottis to the alveolus. Most commonly, bleeding arises from the bronchi or medium-sized airways, but a thorough evaluation of the entire respiratory tree is important.

The dual blood supply of the lungs makes it unique. The lungs have both the pulmonary and bronchial circulations. The pulmonary circulation is a low-pressure system that is essential for gas exchange at the alveolar level; in contrast, the bronchial circulation originates from the aorta and, therefore, is a higher-pressure system. The bronchial arteries supply the airways and can neovascularize tumors, dilated airways of bronchiectasis, and cavitary lesions. Most hemoptysis originates from the bronchial circulation, and bleeding from the higher-pressure system makes it more difficult to stop.

ETIOLOGY

Hemoptysis commonly results from infection, malignancy, or vascular disease; however, the differential for bleeding from the respiratory tree is varied and broad. In the United States, the most common causes are viral bronchitis, bronchiectasis, or malignancy. In other parts of the world, infections such as tuberculosis are the most common causes.

Infections Most blood-tinged sputum and small-volume hemoptysis are due to viral bronchitis. Patients with chronic bronchitis are at risk for bacterial superinfection with organisms such as *Streptococcus pneumoniae, Haemophilus influenzae,* or *Moraxella catarrhalis,* increasing airway inflammation and potential for bleeding. Similarly, patients with bronchiectasis are prone to hemoptysis during exacerbations. Due to recurrent bacterial infection, bronchiectatic airways are dilated, inflamed, and highly vascular, supplied by the bronchial circulation. In several case series, bronchiectasis is the leading cause of massive hemoptysis and subsequent death.

Tuberculosis had long been the most common cause of hemoptysis worldwide, but it is now surpassed in industrialized countries by bronchitis and bronchiectasis. In patients with tuberculosis, development of cavitary disease is frequently the source of bleeding, but rarer complications such as the erosion of a pulmonary artery aneurysm into a preexisting cavity (i.e., Rasmussen's aneurysm) can also be the source.

Other infectious agents such as endemic fungi, *Nocardia*, and nontuberculous mycobacteria can present as cavitary lung disease complicated by hemoptysis. In addition, *Aspergillus* species can develop into mycetomas within preexisting cavities, with neovascularization to these inflamed spaces leading to bleeding. Pulmonary abscesses and necrotizing pneumonia can cause bleeding by devitalizing lung parenchyma. Common responsible organisms include *Staphylococcus aureus, Klebsiella pneumoniae*, and oral anaerobes.

Paragonimiasis can mimic tuberculosis and is another significant cause of hemoptysis seen globally; it is common in Southeast Asia and China, although cases have been reported in North America from raw crayfish ingestion. It should be considered as a cause of hemoptysis in recent immigrants from endemic areas.

Vascular Hemoptysis from a vascular cause can be associated with cardiac disease, pulmonary embolism, arteriovenous malformation, or diffuse alveolar hemorrhage (DAH). While the classic description of the sputum expectorated in pulmonary edema (from elevated left end-diastolic pressure) is "pink and frothy," a spectrum of hemoptysis including frank blood can be seen. This observation is particularly true now with the more widespread use of anticoagulants and antiplatelet medications.

Pulmonary embolism with parenchymal infarction can present with hemoptysis, but pulmonary emboli do not commonly cause hemoptysis. An ectatic vessel in an airway or a pulmonary arteriovenous malformation can be a source of bleeding. A rare vascular cause of hemoptysis is the rupture of an aortobronchial fistula; these fistulae arise in the setting of aortic pathology such as aneurysm or pseudoaneurysm and can cause small bleeding episodes that herald massive hemoptysis.

DAH causes significant bleeding into the lung parenchyma but, interestingly, is not often associated with hemoptysis. DAH typically presents with diffuse ground glass opacities on chest imaging. A range of insults cause DAH, including immune-mediated capillaritis from diseases such as systemic lupus erythematosus, toxicity from cocaine and other inhalants, and stem cell transplantation. The so-called "pulmonary-renal" syndromes, including granulomatosis with polyangiitis and anti-glomerular basement membrane disease, may lead to both hemoptysis and hematuria (though one manifestation may be present without the other). A recently identified cause of hemoptysis and DAH is vaping-induced lung injury.

Malignancy Bronchogenic carcinoma of any histology is a common cause of hemoptysis (both massive and nonmassive). Hemoptysis can indicate airway involvement of the tumor and can be a presenting symptom of carcinoid tumors, vascular lesions that frequently arise in the proximal airways. Small cell and squamous cell carcinomas are frequently central in nature and more likely to erode into major pulmonary vessels, resulting in massive hemoptysis. Pulmonary metastases from distant tumors (e.g., melanoma, sarcoma, adenocarcinomas of the breast and colon) can also cause bleeding. Kaposi's sarcoma, seen in advanced acquired immunodeficiency syndrome, is very vascular and can develop anywhere along the respiratory tract, from the bronchi to the oral cavity.

Mechanical and Other Causes In addition to infection, vascular disease, and malignancy, other insults to the pulmonary system can cause hemoptysis. Pulmonary endometriosis causes cyclical bleeding known as catamenial hemoptysis. Foreign body aspiration can lead to airway irritation and bleeding. Diagnostic and therapeutic procedures are also potential offenders: pulmonary vein stenosis can result from left atrial procedures, such as pulmonary vein isolation, and pulmonary artery catheters can lead to rupture of the pulmonary artery if the distal balloon is kept inflated. Finally, in the setting of thrombocytopenia, coagulopathy, anticoagulation, or antiplatelet therapy, even minor insults can cause hemoptysis.

EVALUATION AND MANAGEMENT

History The amount or severity of bleeding is the first step in assessing a patient with hemoptysis. A patient's description of the sputum (e.g., flecks of blood, pink-tinged, or frank blood or clot) is helpful if you cannot examine it. An approach to management of hemoptysis is outlined in **Fig. 39-1**.

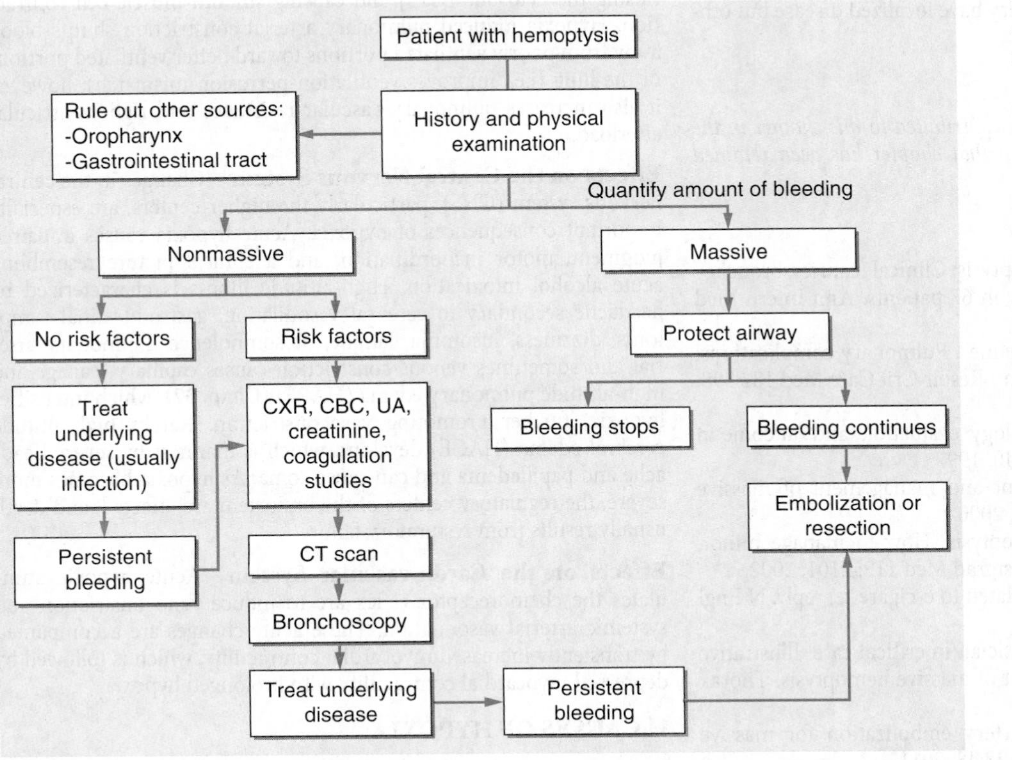

While there is no agreed-upon volume, blood loss of 400 mL in 24 h or 100–150 mL expectorated at one time should be considered *life-threatening hemoptysis*. These numbers derive from the blood volume of the tracheobronchial tree (generally 100–200 mL). Patients rarely die of exsanguination but, rather, are at risk of death due to asphyxiation from blood filling the airways and airspaces. Most patients cannot describe the volume of their hemoptysis in milliliters, so using referents like cups (one U.S. cup is 236 mL) can be helpful. Fortunately, life-threatening hemoptysis only accounts for 5–15% of cases of hemoptysis.

The history may point to the cause of hemoptysis. Fever, chills, or antecedent cough may suggest infection. A history of smoking or unintentional weight loss makes malignancy more likely. Patients should be asked about inhalational exposures, including vaping. A thorough medical history with careful attention to chronic pulmonary disease should be obtained, with evaluation of risk factors for malignancy and bronchiectatic lung disease (e.g., cystic fibrosis, sarcoidosis).

Physical Examination Reviewing the vital signs is an important first step. Patients who have life-threatening hemoptysis can have hypoxemia, tachycardia, and hemodynamic instability. As the site of bleeding is important, evaluation of the nasal and oral cavities is imperative. In addition, auscultation of the lungs and seeking other relevant physical findings such as clubbing can point to a cause of the hemoptysis. A focal area of wheezing could suggest a foreign body aspiration. Other signs of a bleeding diathesis (e.g., skin or mucosal ecchymoses and petechiae) or telangiectasias may suggest other etiologies of the hemoptysis.

Diagnostic Studies Initial studies should include measurement of a complete blood count to assess for infection, anemia, or thrombocytopenia; coagulation parameters; measurement of electrolytes and renal function; and urinalysis to exclude pulmonary-renal disease. Chest imaging is necessary for every patient.

A chest radiograph is usually obtained first, although it frequently does not localize bleeding and can appear normal. In patients without risk factors for malignancy or other abnormalities in the initial evaluation and with a normal chest radiograph, treating for bronchitis and ensuring close follow-up is a reasonable strategy, with further diagnostic workup.

In contrast, patients with risk factors for malignancy (i.e., age >40 or a smoking history) should undergo additional testing. First, chest computed tomography (CT) with contrast should be obtained to better identify masses, bronchiectasis, and parenchymal lesions. A CT looking for pulmonary embolism should be considered if the history and physical examination are consistent with that diagnosis. Following a CT, a flexible bronchoscopy should be performed to exclude bronchogenic carcinoma unless imaging reveals a lesion that can be sampled without bronchoscopy. Small case series show that patients with hemoptysis and unrevealing bronchoscopies have good outcomes.

Interventions When the amount of hemoptysis is massive or life-threatening, there are three simultaneous goals: first, protect the nonbleeding lung; second, locate the site of bleeding; and third, control the bleeding.

FIGURE 39-1 Approach to the management of hemoptysis. CBC, complete blood count; CT, computed tomography; CXR, chest x-ray; UA, urinalysis.

Protecting the airway and nonbleeding lung is paramount in the management of massive hemoptysis because asphyxiation can happen quickly. If the side of bleeding is known, the patient should be positioned with the bleeding side down to use gravitational advantage to keep blood out of the nonbleeding lung. Endotracheal intubation should be avoided unless truly necessary, since suctioning through an endotracheal tube is a less effective means of removing blood and clot than the cough reflex. If intubation is required, take steps to protect the nonbleeding lung either by selective intubation of one lung (i.e., the nonbleeding lung) or insertion of a double-lumen endotracheal tube.

Locating the bleeding site is sometimes obvious, but frequently, it can be difficult to determine. A chest radiograph, if it shows new opacities, can be helpful in localizing the side or site of bleeding, although this test is not adequate by itself. CT angiography helps by localizing active extravasation. Flexible bronchoscopy may be useful to identify the side of bleeding (although it has only a 50% chance of locating the site). Experts do not agree on the timing of bronchoscopy, although in some cases—cystic fibrosis, for instance—bronchoscopy is *not* recommended because it may delay definitive management. Finally, proceeding directly to angiography is also a reasonable strategy given that it has both diagnostic and therapeutic capabilities.

Controlling the bleeding during an episode of life-threatening hemoptysis can be accomplished in one of three ways: from the airway lumen, from the involved blood vessel, or by surgical resection of both airway and vessel involved. Bronchoscopic measures are generally only temporizing: a flexible bronchoscope can be used to suction clot and insert a balloon catheter or bronchial blocker that occludes the involved airway. Rigid bronchoscopy, done by an interventional pulmonologist or thoracic surgeon, may allow therapeutic interventions of bleeding airway lesions such as photocoagulation and cautery. Because most life-threatening cases of hemoptysis arise from the bronchial circulation, bronchial artery embolization is the procedure of choice for control of the bleeding. However, bronchial artery embolization can have significant complications such as embolization of the anterior spinal artery. However, it is generally successful in the short term, with >80% success rate at controlling bleeding immediately, although bleeding can recur if the underlying disease (e.g., a mycetoma) is not treated. Surgical resection has a high mortality rate (up to 15–40%) and should not be pursued unless initial measures have failed and bleeding is ongoing. Ideal candidates for surgery have localized disease but otherwise normal lung parenchyma.

Acknowledgment

Anna K. Brady and Patricia A. Kritek contributed to this chapter in the 20th edition, and some material from that chapter has been retained here.

■ FURTHER READING

Adelman M et al: Cryptogenic hemoptysis: Clinical features, bronchoscopic findings, and natural history in 67 patients. Ann Intern Med 102:829, 1985.

Flume PA et al: CF pulmonary guidelines. Pulmonary complications: Hemoptysis and pneumothorax. Am J Respir Crit Care Med 182:298, 2010.

Hirshberg B et al: Hemoptysis: Etiology, evaluation, and outcome in a tertiary care hospital. Chest 112:440, 1997.

Jean-Baptiste E: Clinical assessment and management of massive hemoptysis. Crit Care Med 28:1642, 2000.

Johnson JL: Manifestations of hemoptysis: How to manage minor, moderate, and massive bleeding. Postgrad Med 112:4:101, 2002.

Layden JE et al: Pulmonary illness related to e-cigarette, reply. N Engl J Med 382:903, 2020.

Lordan JL et al: The pulmonary physician in critical care: Illustrative case 7. Assessment and management of massive hemoptysis. Thorax 58:814, 2003.

Sopko DR, Smith TP: Bronchial artery embolization for massive hemoptysis. Semin Intervent Radiol 28:48, 2011.

40 Hypoxia and Cyanosis

Joseph Loscalzo

HYPOXIA

The fundamental purpose of the cardiorespiratory system is to deliver O_2 and nutrients to cells and to remove CO_2 and other metabolic products from them. Proper maintenance of this function depends not only on intact cardiovascular and respiratory systems, but also on an adequate number of red blood cells and hemoglobin and a supply of inspired gas containing adequate O_2.

■ RESPONSES TO HYPOXIA

Decreased O_2 availability to cells typically results in an inhibition of oxidative phosphorylation and increased anaerobic glycolysis. This switch from aerobic to anaerobic metabolism, the Pasteur effect, reduces the rate of adenosine 5′-triphosphate (ATP) production. In severe hypoxia, when ATP production is inadequate to meet the energy requirements of ionic and osmotic equilibrium, cell membrane depolarization leads to uncontrolled Ca^{2+} influx and activation of Ca^{2+}-dependent phospholipases and proteases. These events, in turn, cause cell swelling, activation of apoptotic pathways, and, ultimately, cell death.

The adaptations to hypoxia are mediated, in part, by the upregulation of genes encoding a variety of proteins, including glycolytic enzymes, such as phosphoglycerate kinase and phosphofructokinase, as well as the glucose transporters Glut-1 and Glut-2; and by growth factors, such as vascular endothelial growth factor (VEGF) and erythropoietin, which enhance erythrocyte production. The hypoxia-induced increase in expression of these and other key proteins is governed by the hypoxia-sensitive transcription factor, hypoxia-inducible factor-1 (HIF-1).

During hypoxia, systemic arterioles dilate, at least in part, by opening of K_{ATP} channels in vascular smooth-muscle cells due to the hypoxia-induced reduction in ATP concentration. By contrast, in pulmonary vascular smooth-muscle cells, inhibition of K^+ channels causes depolarization, which, in turn, activates voltage-gated Ca^{2+} channels, raising the cytosolic $[Ca^{2+}]$ and causing smooth-muscle cell contraction. Hypoxia-induced pulmonary arterial constriction shunts blood away from poorly ventilated portions toward better ventilated portions of the lung (i.e., improves ventilation-perfusion mismatch); however, it also increases pulmonary vascular resistance and right ventricular afterload.

Effects on the Central Nervous System Changes in the central nervous system (CNS), particularly the higher centers, are especially important consequences of hypoxia. Acute hypoxia causes impaired judgment, motor incoordination, and a clinical picture resembling acute alcohol intoxication. High-altitude illness is characterized by headache secondary to cerebral vasodilation, gastrointestinal symptoms, dizziness, insomnia, fatigue, or somnolence. Pulmonary arterial and sometimes venous constriction causes capillary leakage and high-altitude pulmonary edema (HAPE) (**Chap. 37**), which intensifies hypoxia, further promoting vasoconstriction. Rarely, high-altitude cerebral edema (HACE) develops, which is manifest by severe headache and papilledema and can cause coma. As hypoxia becomes more severe, the regulatory centers of the brainstem are affected, and death usually results from respiratory failure.

Effects on the Cardiovascular System Acute hypoxia stimulates the chemoreceptor reflex arc to induce venoconstriction and systemic arterial vasodilation. These acute changes are accompanied by transiently increased myocardial contractility, which is followed by depressed myocardial contractility with prolonged hypoxia.

■ CAUSES OF HYPOXIA

Respiratory Hypoxia When hypoxia occurs from respiratory failure, $Pa{O_2}$ declines, and when respiratory failure is persistent, the hemoglobin-oxygen (Hb-O_2) dissociation curve (**see Fig. 98-2**) is displaced to the right, with greater quantities of O_2 released at any level of tissue Po_2. Arterial hypoxemia, that is, a reduction of O_2 saturation of arterial blood (Sao_2), and consequent cyanosis are likely to be more marked when such depression of Pao_2 results from pulmonary disease than when the depression occurs as the result of a decline in the fraction of oxygen in inspired air (Fio_2). In this latter situation, $Paco_2$ falls secondary to anoxia-induced hyperventilation and the Hb-O_2 dissociation curve is displaced to the left, limiting the decline in Sao_2 at any level of Pao_2.

The most common cause of respiratory hypoxia is *ventilation-perfusion mismatch* resulting from perfusion of poorly ventilated alveoli. Respiratory hypoxemia may also be caused by *hypoventilation*, in which case it is associated with an elevation of $Paco_2$ (**Chap. 285**). These two forms of respiratory hypoxia are usually correctable by inspiring 100% O_2 for several minutes. A third cause of respiratory hypoxia is shunting of blood across the lung from the pulmonary arterial to the venous bed (*intrapulmonary right-to-left shunting*) by perfusion of nonventilated portions of the lung, as in pulmonary atelectasis or through pulmonary arteriovenous connections. The low Pao_2 in this situation is only partially corrected by an Fio_2 of 100%.

Hypoxia Secondary to High Altitude As one ascends rapidly to 3000 m (~10,000 ft), the reduction of the O_2 content of inspired air (Fio_2) leads to a decrease in alveolar Po_2 to ~60 mmHg, and a condition termed *high-altitude illness* develops (see above). At higher altitudes, arterial saturation declines rapidly and symptoms become more serious; and at 5000 m, unacclimated individuals usually cease to be able to function normally owing to the changes in CNS function described above.

Hypoxia Secondary to Right-to-Left Extrapulmonary Shunting From a physiologic viewpoint, this cause of hypoxia resembles intrapulmonary right-to-left shunting but is caused by congenital cardiac malformations, such as tetralogy of Fallot, transposition of the great arteries, atrial or ventricular septal defect, patent ductus arteriosus, and Eisenmenger's syndrome (**Chap. 269**). As in pulmonary right-to-left shunting, the Pao_2 cannot be restored to normal with inspiration of 100% O_2.

Anemic Hypoxia A reduction in hemoglobin concentration of the blood is accompanied by a corresponding decline in the O_2-carrying capacity of the blood. Although the Pao_2 is normal in anemic hypoxia, the absolute quantity of O_2 transported per unit volume of blood is diminished. As the anemic blood passes through the capillaries and the usual quantity of O_2 is removed from it, the Po_2 and saturation in the venous blood decline to a greater extent than normal.

Carbon Monoxide (CO) Intoxication (**See also Chap. 463**) Hemoglobin that binds with CO (carboxy-hemoglobin [COHb]) is unavailable for O_2 transport. In addition, the presence of COHb shifts the Hb-O_2 dissociation curve to the left (**see Fig. 98-2**) so that O_2 is unloaded only at lower tensions, further contributing to tissue hypoxia.

Circulatory Hypoxia As in anemic hypoxia, the Pao_2 is usually normal, but venous and tissue Po_2 values are reduced as a consequence of reduced tissue perfusion and greater tissue O_2 extraction. This pathophysiology leads to an increased arterial-mixed venous O_2 difference (a-v-O_2 difference), or gradient. Generalized circulatory hypoxia occurs in heart failure (**Chap. 257**) and in most forms of shock (**Chap. 303**).

Specific Organ Hypoxia Localized circulatory hypoxia may occur as a result of decreased perfusion secondary to arterial obstruction, as in localized atherosclerosis in any vascular bed, or as a consequence of vasoconstriction, as observed in Raynaud's phenomenon (**Chap. 281**). Localized hypoxia may also result from venous obstruction and the resultant expansion of interstitial fluid causing arteriolar compression and, thereby, reduction of arterial inflow. Edema, which increases the distance through which O_2 must diffuse before it reaches cells, can also cause localized hypoxia. In an attempt to maintain adequate perfusion to more vital organs in patients with reduced cardiac output secondary to heart failure or hypovolemic shock, vasoconstriction may reduce perfusion in the limbs and skin, causing hypoxia of these regions.

Increased O_2 Requirements If the O_2 consumption of tissues is elevated without a corresponding increase in perfusion, tissue hypoxia ensues and the Po_2 in venous blood declines. Ordinarily, the clinical picture of patients with hypoxia due to an elevated metabolic rate, as in fever or thyrotoxicosis, is quite different from that in other types of hypoxia: the skin is warm and flushed owing to increased cutaneous blood flow that dissipates the excessive heat produced, and cyanosis is usually absent.

Exercise is a classic example of increased tissue O_2 requirements. These increased demands are normally met by several mechanisms operating simultaneously: (1) increase in the cardiac output and ventilation and, thus, O_2 delivery to the tissues; (2) a preferential shift in blood flow to the exercising muscles by changing vascular resistances in the circulatory beds of exercising tissues, directly and/or reflexly; (3) an increase in O_2 extraction from the delivered blood and a widening of the arteriovenous O_2 difference; and (4) a reduction in the pH of the tissues and capillary blood, shifting the Hb-O_2 curve to the right (**see Fig. 98-2**), and unloading more O_2 from hemoglobin. If the capacity of these mechanisms is exceeded, then hypoxia, especially of the exercising muscles, will result.

Improper Oxygen Utilization Cyanide (**Chap. 459**) and several other similarly acting poisons cause cellular hypoxia by impairing electron transport in mitochondria, thereby limiting oxidative phosphorylation and ATP production. The tissues are unable to use O_2, and as a consequence, the venous blood tends to have a high O_2 tension. This condition has been termed *histotoxic hypoxia*.

ADAPTATION TO HYPOXIA

An important component of the respiratory response to hypoxia originates in special chemosensitive cells in the carotid and aortic bodies and in the respiratory center in the brainstem. The stimulation of these cells by hypoxia increases ventilation, with a loss of CO_2, and can lead to respiratory alkalosis. When combined with the metabolic acidosis resulting from the production of lactic acid, the serum bicarbonate level declines (**Chap. 55**).

With the reduction of Pao_2, cerebrovascular resistance decreases and cerebral blood flow increases in an attempt to maintain O_2 delivery to the brain. However, when the reduction of Pao_2 is accompanied by hyperventilation and a reduction of $Paco_2$, cerebrovascular resistance rises, cerebral blood flow falls, and tissue hypoxia intensifies.

The diffuse, systemic vasodilation that occurs in generalized hypoxia increases the cardiac output. In patients with underlying heart disease, the requirements of peripheral tissues for an increase of cardiac output with hypoxia may precipitate congestive heart failure. In patients with ischemic heart disease, a reduced Pao_2 may intensify myocardial ischemia and further impair left ventricular function.

One of the important compensatory mechanisms for chronic hypoxia is an increase in the hemoglobin concentration and in the number of red blood cells in the circulating blood, that is, the development of polycythemia induced by erythropoietin production (**Chap. 103**). In persons with chronic hypoxemia secondary to prolonged residence at a high altitude (>13,000 ft, 4200 m), a condition termed *chronic mountain sickness* develops. This disorder is characterized by a blunted respiratory drive, reduced ventilation, erythrocytosis, cyanosis, weakness, right ventricular enlargement secondary to pulmonary hypertension, and even stupor.

CYANOSIS

Cyanosis refers to a bluish color of the skin and mucous membranes resulting from an increased quantity of reduced hemoglobin (i.e., deoxygenated hemoglobin) or of hemoglobin derivatives (e.g., methemoglobin or sulfhemoglobin) in the small blood vessels of those tissues. It is usually most marked in the lips, nail beds, ears, and malar eminences. Cyanosis, especially if developed recently, is more commonly detected by a family member than the patient. The florid skin characteristic of polycythemia vera (**Chap. 103**) must be distinguished from the true cyanosis discussed here. A cherry-colored flush, rather than cyanosis, is caused by COHb (**Chap. 459**).

The degree of cyanosis is modified by the color of the cutaneous pigment and the thickness of the skin, as well as by the state of the cutaneous capillaries. The accurate clinical detection of the presence and degree of cyanosis is difficult, as proved by oximetric studies. In some instances, central cyanosis can be detected reliably when the Sa_{O_2} has fallen to 85%; in others, particularly in dark-skinned persons, it may not be detected until it has declined to 75%. In the latter case, examination of the mucous membranes in the oral cavity and the conjunctivae rather than examination of the skin is more helpful in the detection of cyanosis.

The increase in the quantity of reduced hemoglobin in the mucocutaneous vessels that produces cyanosis may be brought about either by an increase in the quantity of venous blood as a result of dilation of the venules (including precapillary venules) or by a reduction in the Sa_{O_2} in the capillary blood. In general, cyanosis becomes apparent when the concentration of reduced hemoglobin in capillary blood exceeds 40 g/L (4 g/dL).

It is the *absolute*, rather than the *relative*, quantity of reduced hemoglobin that is important in producing cyanosis. Thus, in a patient with severe anemia, the *relative* quantity of reduced hemoglobin in the venous blood may be very large when considered in relation to the total quantity of hemoglobin in the blood. However, since the concentration of the latter is markedly reduced, the *absolute* quantity of reduced hemoglobin may still be low, and, therefore, patients with severe anemia and even *marked* arterial desaturation may not display cyanosis. Conversely, the higher the total hemoglobin content, the greater is the tendency toward cyanosis; thus, patients with marked polycythemia tend to be cyanotic at higher levels of Sa_{O_2} than patients with normal hematocrit values. Likewise, local passive congestion, which causes an increase in the total quantity of reduced hemoglobin in the vessels in a given area, may cause cyanosis. Cyanosis is also observed when nonfunctional hemoglobin, such as methemoglobin (consequential or acquired) or sulfhemoglobin (**Chap. 98**), is present in blood.

Cyanosis may be subdivided into central and peripheral types. In *central* cyanosis, the Sa_{O_2} is reduced or an abnormal hemoglobin derivative is present, and the mucous membranes and skin are both affected. *Peripheral* cyanosis is due to a slowing of blood flow and abnormally great extraction of O_2 from normally saturated arterial blood; it results from vasoconstriction and diminished peripheral blood flow, such as occurs in cold exposure, shock, congestive failure, and peripheral vascular disease. Often in these conditions, the mucous membranes of the oral cavity, including the sublingual mucosa, may be spared. Clinical differentiation between central and peripheral cyanosis may not always be straightforward, and in conditions such as cardiogenic shock with pulmonary edema, there may be a mixture of both types.

DIFFERENTIAL DIAGNOSIS

Central Cyanosis (Table 40-1) Decreased Sa_{O_2} results from a marked reduction in the Pa_{O_2}. This reduction may be brought about by a decline in the F_{IO_2} without sufficient compensatory alveolar hyperventilation to maintain alveolar P_{O_2}. Cyanosis usually becomes manifest in an ascent to an altitude of 4000 m (13,000 ft).

Seriously *impaired pulmonary function*, through perfusion of unventilated or poorly ventilated areas of the lung or alveolar hypoventilation, is a common cause of central cyanosis (**Chap. 285**). This condition may occur acutely, as in extensive pneumonia or pulmonary edema, or chronically, with chronic pulmonary diseases (e.g., emphysema). In the latter situation, secondary polycythemia is generally present and clubbing of the fingers (see below) may occur. Another cause of reduced Sa_{O_2} is *shunting of systemic venous blood into the arterial circuit*. Certain forms of congenital heart disease are associated with cyanosis on this basis (see above and **Chap. 269**).

Pulmonary arteriovenous fistulae may be congenital or acquired, solitary or multiple, and microscopic or massive. The severity of cyanosis produced by these fistulae depends on their size and number. They occur with some frequency in hereditary hemorrhagic telangiectasia. Sa_{O_2} reduction and cyanosis may also occur in some patients with cirrhosis, presumably as a consequence of pulmonary arteriovenous fistulae or portal vein–pulmonary vein anastomoses.

TABLE 40-1 Causes of Cyanosis

Central Cyanosis
Decreased arterial oxygen saturation
Decreased atmospheric pressure—high altitude
Impaired pulmonary function
Alveolar hypoventilation
Inhomogeneity in pulmonary ventilation and perfusion (perfusion of hypoventilated alveoli)
Impaired oxygen diffusion
Anatomic shunts
Certain types of congenital heart disease
Pulmonary arteriovenous fistulas
Multiple small intrapulmonary shunts
Hemoglobin with low affinity for oxygen
Hemoglobin abnormalities
Methemoglobinemia—hereditary, acquired
Sulfhemoglobinemia—acquired
Carboxyhemoglobinemia (not true cyanosis)
Peripheral Cyanosis
Reduced cardiac output
Cold exposure
Redistribution of blood flow from extremities
Arterial obstruction
Venous obstruction

In patients with cardiac or pulmonary right-to-left shunts, the presence and severity of cyanosis depend on the size of the shunt relative to the systemic flow and on the Hb-O_2 saturation of the venous blood. With increased extraction of O_2 from the blood by the exercising muscles, the venous blood returning to the right side of the heart is more unsaturated than at rest, and shunting of this blood intensifies the cyanosis. Secondary polycythemia occurs frequently in patients in this setting and contributes to the cyanosis.

Cyanosis can be caused by small quantities of circulating methemoglobin (Hb Fe^{3+}) and by even smaller quantities of sulfhemoglobin (**Chap. 98**); both of these hemoglobin derivatives impair oxygen delivery to the tissues. Although they are uncommon causes of cyanosis, these abnormal hemoglobin species should be sought by spectroscopy when cyanosis is not readily explained by malfunction of the circulatory or respiratory systems. Generally, digital clubbing does not occur with them.

Peripheral Cyanosis Probably the most common cause of peripheral cyanosis is the normal vasoconstriction resulting from exposure to cold air or water. When cardiac output is reduced, cutaneous vasoconstriction occurs as a compensatory mechanism so that blood is diverted from the skin to more vital areas such as the CNS and heart, and cyanosis of the extremities may result even though the arterial blood is normally saturated.

Arterial obstruction to an extremity, as with an embolus, or arteriolar constriction, as in cold-induced vasospasm (Raynaud's phenomenon) (**Chap. 281**), generally results in pallor and coldness, and there may be associated cyanosis. Venous obstruction, as in thrombophlebitis or deep venous thrombosis, dilates the subpapillary venous plexuses and thereby intensifies cyanosis.

APPROACH TO THE PATIENT

Cyanosis

Certain features are important in arriving at the cause of cyanosis:

1. It is important to ascertain the time of onset of cyanosis. Cyanosis present since birth or infancy is usually due to congenital heart disease.

2. Central and peripheral cyanosis must be differentiated. Evidence of disorders of the respiratory or cardiovascular systems is helpful. Massage or gentle warming of a cyanotic extremity will increase peripheral blood flow and abolish peripheral, but not central, cyanosis.
3. The presence or absence of clubbing of the digits (see below) should be ascertained. The combination of cyanosis and clubbing is frequent in patients with congenital heart disease and right-to-left shunting and is seen occasionally in patients with pulmonary disease, such as lung abscess or pulmonary arteriovenous fistulae. In contrast, peripheral cyanosis or acutely developing central cyanosis is *not* associated with clubbed digits.
4. Pao_2 and Sao_2 should be determined, and in patients with cyanosis in whom the mechanism is obscure, spectroscopic examination of the blood should be performed to look for abnormal types of hemoglobin (critical in the differential diagnosis of cyanosis).

CLUBBING

The selective bulbous enlargement of the distal segments of the fingers and toes due to proliferation of connective tissue, particularly on the dorsal surface, is termed *clubbing*; there is also increased sponginess of the soft tissue at the base of the clubbed nail. Clubbing may be hereditary, idiopathic, or acquired and associated with a variety of disorders, including cyanotic congenital heart disease (see above), infective endocarditis, and a variety of pulmonary conditions (among them primary and metastatic lung cancer, bronchiectasis, asbestosis, sarcoidosis, lung abscess, cystic fibrosis, tuberculosis, and mesothelioma), as well as with some gastrointestinal diseases (including inflammatory bowel disease and hepatic cirrhosis). In some instances, it is occupational, for example, in jackhammer operators.

Clubbing in patients with primary and metastatic lung cancer, mesothelioma, bronchiectasis, or hepatic cirrhosis may be associated with *hypertrophic osteoarthropathy*. In this condition, the subperiosteal formation of new bone in the distal diaphyses of the long bones of the extremities causes pain and symmetric arthritis-like changes in the shoulders, knees, ankles, wrists, and elbows. The diagnosis of hypertrophic osteoarthropathy may be confirmed by bone radiograph or magnetic resonance imaging (MRI). Although the mechanism of clubbing is unclear, it appears to be secondary to humoral substances that cause dilation of the vessels of the distal digits as well as growth factors released from platelet precursors in the digital circulation. In certain circumstances, clubbing is reversible, such as following lung transplantation for cystic fibrosis.

FURTHER READING

Callemeyn J et al: Clubbing and hypertrophic osteoarthropathy: Insights into diagnosis, pathophysiology, and clinical significance. Acta Clin Belg 22:1, 2016.

MacIntyre NR: Tissue hypoxia: Implications for the respiratory clinician. Respir Care 59:1590, 2014.

41 Edema

Joseph Loscalzo

PLASMA AND INTERSTITIAL FLUID EXCHANGE

Approximately two-thirds of total body water is intracellular and one-third is extracellular. One-fourth of the latter is in the plasma, and the remainder comprises the interstitial fluid. Edema represents an excess of interstitial fluid that has become evident clinically.

There is constant interchange of fluid between the two compartments of the extracellular fluid. The hydrostatic pressure within the capillaries and the colloid oncotic pressure in the interstitial fluid promote the movement of water and diffusible solutes from plasma to the interstitium. This movement is most prominent at the arterial origin of the capillary and falls progressively with the decline in intracapillary pressure and the rise in oncotic pressure toward the venular end. Fluid is returned from the interstitial space into the vascular system largely through the lymphatic system. These interchanges of fluids are normally balanced so that the volumes of the intravascular and interstitial compartments remain constant. However, a net movement of fluid from the intravascular to the interstitial spaces takes place and may be responsible for the development of edema under the following conditions: (1) an increase in intracapillary hydrostatic pressure; (2) inadequate lymphatic drainage; (3) reductions in the oncotic pressure in the plasma; (4) damage to the capillary endothelial barrier; and (5) increases in the oncotic pressure in the interstitial space.

REDUCTION OF EFFECTIVE ARTERIAL VOLUME

In many forms of edema, the effective arterial blood volume, a parameter that represents the filling of the arterial tree and that effectively perfuses the tissues, is reduced. Underfilling of the arterial tree may be caused by a reduction of cardiac output and/or systemic vascular resistance, by the pooling of blood in the splanchnic veins (as in cirrhosis), and by hypoalbuminemia (**Fig. 41-1A**). As a consequence of this underfilling, a series of physiologic responses designed to restore the effective arterial volume to normal are set into motion. A key element of these responses is the renal retention of sodium and, therefore, water, thereby restoring effective arterial volume, but sometimes also leading to the development or intensification of edema.

RENAL FACTORS AND THE RENIN-ANGIOTENSIN-ALDOSTERONE SYSTEM

The diminished renal blood flow characteristic of states in which the effective arterial blood volume is reduced is translated by the renal juxtaglomerular cells (specialized myoepithelial cells surrounding the afferent arteriole) into a signal for increased renin release. Renin is an enzyme with a molecular mass of about 40,000 Da that acts on its substrate, angiotensinogen, an α_2-globulin synthesized by the liver, to release angiotensin I, a decapeptide, which in turn is converted to angiotensin II (AII), an octapeptide. AII has generalized vasoconstrictor properties, particularly on the renal efferent arterioles. This action reduces the hydrostatic pressure in the peritubular capillaries, whereas the increased filtration fraction raises the colloid osmotic pressure in these vessels, thereby enhancing salt and water reabsorption in the proximal tubule as well as in the ascending limb of the loop of Henle.

The renin-angiotensin-aldosterone system (RAAS) operates as both a hormonal and paracrine system. Its activation causes sodium and water retention and thereby contributes to edema formation. Blockade of the conversion of angiotensin I to AII and blockade of the AII receptors enhance sodium and water excretion and reduce many forms of edema. AII that enters the systemic circulation stimulates the production of aldosterone by the zona glomerulosa of the adrenal cortex. Aldosterone in turn enhances sodium reabsorption (and potassium excretion) by the collecting tubule, further favoring edema formation. Blockade of the action of aldosterone by spironolactone or eplerenone (aldosterone antagonists) or by amiloride (a blocker of epithelial sodium channels) often induces a moderate diuresis in edematous states.

ARGININE VASOPRESSIN

(See also Chap. 381) The secretion of arginine vasopressin (AVP) by the posterior pituitary gland occurs in response to increased intracellular osmolar concentration; by stimulating V_2 receptors, AVP increases the reabsorption of free water in the distal tubules and collecting ducts of the kidneys, thereby increasing total-body water. Circulating AVP is elevated in many patients with heart failure secondary to a nonosmotic stimulus associated with decreased effective arterial volume and reduced compliance of the left atrium. Such patients fail to show the normal reduction of AVP with a reduction of osmolality, contributing to edema formation and hyponatremia.

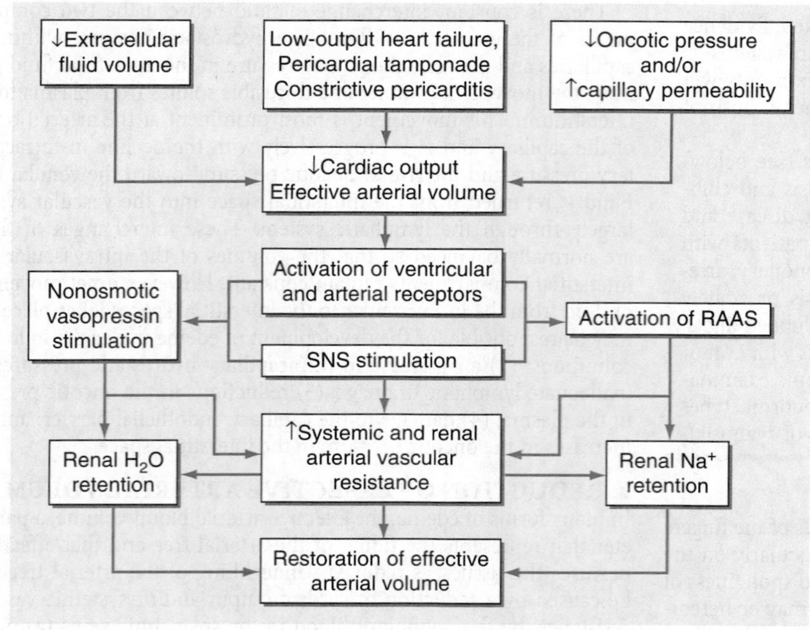

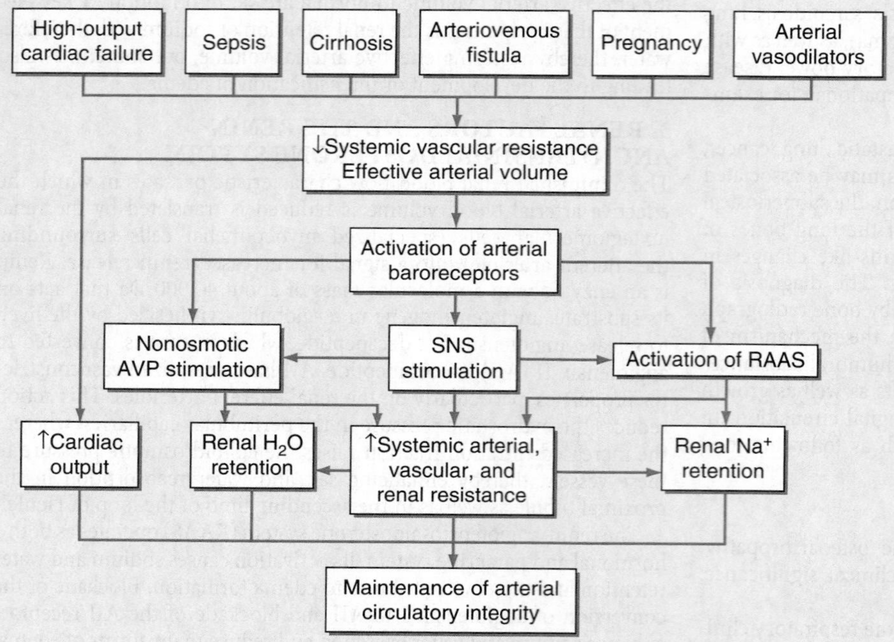

FIGURE 41-1 Clinical conditions in which a decrease in cardiac output (*A*) and systemic vascular resistance (*B*) cause arterial underfilling with resulting neurohumoral activation and renal sodium and water retention. In addition to activating the neurohumoral axis, adrenergic stimulation causes renal vasoconstriction and enhances sodium and fluid transport by the proximal tubule epithelium. AVP, arginine vasopressin; RAAS, renin-angiotensin aldosterone system; SNS, sympathetic nervous system. *(From Annals of Internal Medicine, RW Schrier: Body fluid volume regulation in health and disease: A unifying hypothesis. 113(2):155-159, 1990. Copyright © 1990, American College of Physicians. All Rights Reserved. Reprinted with the permission of American College of Physicians, Inc.)*

ENDOTHELIN-1

This potent peptide vasoconstrictor is released by endothelial cells. Its concentration in the plasma is elevated in patients with severe heart failure and contributes to renal vasoconstriction, sodium retention, and edema.

NATRIURETIC PEPTIDES

Atrial distention causes release into the circulation of atrial natriuretic peptide (ANP), a polypeptide. A high-molecular-weight precursor of ANP is stored in secretory granules within atrial myocytes. A closely related natriuretic peptide (pre-prohormone brain natriuretic peptide [BNP]) is stored primarily in ventricular myocytes and is released when ventricular diastolic pressure rises. Released ANP and BNP (which is derived from its precursor) bind to the natriuretic receptor-A, which causes (1) excretion of sodium and water by augmenting glomerular filtration rate, inhibiting sodium reabsorption in the proximal tubule, and inhibiting release of renin and aldosterone; and (2) dilation of arterioles and venules by antagonizing the vasoconstrictor actions of AII, AVP, and sympathetic stimulation. Thus, elevated levels of natriuretic peptides have the capacity to oppose sodium retention in hypervolemic and edematous states.

Although circulating levels of ANP and BNP are elevated in heart failure and in cirrhosis with ascites, these natriuretic peptides are not sufficiently potent to prevent edema formation. Indeed, in edematous states, resistance to the actions of natriuretic peptides may be increased, further reducing their effectiveness.

Further discussion of the control of sodium and water balance is found in **Chap. S1**.

CLINICAL CAUSES OF EDEMA

A weight gain of several kilograms usually precedes overt manifestations of generalized edema. *Anasarca* refers to gross, generalized edema. *Ascites* **(Chap. 50)** and *hydrothorax* refer to accumulation of excess fluid in the peritoneal and pleural cavities, respectively, and are considered special forms of edema.

Edema is recognized by the persistence of an indentation of the skin after pressure known as "pitting" edema. In its more subtle form, edema may be detected by noting that after the stethoscope is removed from the chest wall, the rim of the bell leaves an indentation on the skin of the chest for a few minutes. Edema may be present when the ring on a finger fits more snugly than in the past or when a patient complains of difficulty putting on shoes, particularly in the evening. Edema may also be recognized by puffiness of the face, which is most readily apparent in the periorbital areas owing to relative tissue laxity.

GENERALIZED EDEMA

The differences among the major causes of generalized edema are shown in **Table 41-1**. Cardiac, renal, hepatic, or nutritional disorders are responsible for a large majority of patients with generalized edema. Consequently, the differential diagnosis of generalized edema should be directed toward identifying or excluding these several conditions.

Heart Failure **(See also Chap. 257)** In heart failure, the impaired systolic emptying of the ventricle(s) and/or the impairment of ventricular relaxation promotes an accumulation of blood in the venous circulation at the expense of the effective arterial volume. In addition, the activation of the sympathetic nervous system and the RAAS (see above) acts in concert to cause renal vasoconstriction and reduction of glomerular filtration and salt and water retention. Sodium and water retention continue, and the increment in blood volume accumulates in

TABLE 41-1 Principal Causes of Generalized Edema: History, Physical Examination, and Laboratory Findings

ORGAN SYSTEM	HISTORY	PHYSICAL EXAMINATION	LABORATORY FINDINGS
Cardiac	Dyspnea with exertion prominent—often associated with orthopnea—or paroxysmal nocturnal dyspnea	Elevated jugular venous pressure, ventricular (S_3) gallop; occasionally with displaced or dyskinetic apical pulse; peripheral cyanosis, cool extremities, small pulse pressure when severe	Elevated urea nitrogen-to-creatinine ratio common; serum sodium often diminished; elevated natriuretic peptides
Hepatic	Dyspnea uncommon, except if associated with significant degree of ascites; most often a history of ethanol abuse	Frequently associated with ascites; jugular venous pressure normal or low; blood pressure lower than in renal or cardiac disease; one or more additional signs of chronic liver disease (jaundice, palmar erythema, Dupuytren's contracture, spider angiomata, male gynecomastia; asterixis and other signs of encephalopathy) may be present	If severe, reductions in serum albumin, cholesterol, other hepatic proteins (transferrin, fibrinogen); liver enzymes elevated, depending on the cause and acuity of liver injury; tendency toward hypokalemia, respiratory alkalosis; macrocytosis from folate deficiency
Renal (CRF)	Usually chronic: may be associated with uremic signs and symptoms, including decreased appetite, altered (metallic or fishy) taste, altered sleep pattern, difficulty concentrating, restless legs, or myoclonus; dyspnea can be present, but generally less prominent than in heart failure	Elevated blood pressure; hypertensive retinopathy; nitrogenous fetor; pericardial friction rub in advanced cases with uremia	Elevation of serum creatinine and cystatin C; albuminuria; hyperkalemia, metabolic acidosis, hyperphosphatemia, hypocalcemia, anemia (usually normocytic)
Renal (NS)	Childhood diabetes mellitus; plasma cell dyscrasias	Periorbital edema; hypertension	Proteinuria (≥3.5 g/d); hypoalbuminemia; hypercholesterolemia; microscopic hematuria

Abbreviations: CRF, chronic renal failure; NS, nephrotic syndrome.
Source: Reproduced with permission from GM Chertow, in E Braunwald, L Goldman (eds): Approach to the patient with edema, in Primary Cardiology, 2nd ed. Philadelphia, Saunders, 2003.

the venous circulation, raising venous and intracapillary pressure and resulting in edema (Fig. 41-1).

The presence of overt cardiac disease, as manifested by cardiac enlargement and/or ventricular hypertrophy, together with clinical evidence of cardiac failure, such as dyspnea, basilar rales, venous distention, and hepatomegaly, usually indicates that edema results from heart failure. Noninvasive tests such as electrocardiography, echocardiography, and measurements of BNP (or N-terminal proBNP [NT-proBNP]) are helpful in establishing the diagnosis of heart disease. The edema of heart failure typically occurs in the dependent portions of the body.

Edema of Renal Disease **(See also Chap. 314)** The edema that occurs during the acute phase of glomerulonephritis is characteristically associated with hematuria, proteinuria, and hypertension. In most instances, the edema results from primary retention of sodium and water by the kidneys owing to renal dysfunction. This state differs from most forms of heart failure in that it is characterized by a normal (or sometimes even increased) cardiac output. Patients with *chronic* renal failure may also develop edema due to primary renal retention of sodium and water.

Nephrotic Syndrome and Other Hypoalbuminemic States The primary alteration in the nephrotic syndrome is a diminished colloid oncotic pressure due to losses of large quantities (≥3.5 g/d) of protein into the urine and hypoalbuminemia (<3.0 g/dL). As a result of the reduced colloid osmotic pressure, the sodium and water that are retained cannot be confined within the vascular compartment, and total and effective arterial blood volumes decline. This process initiates the edema-forming sequence of events described above, including activation of the RAAS. The nephrotic syndrome may occur during the course of a variety of kidney diseases, including glomerulonephritis, diabetic glomerulosclerosis, and hypersensitivity reactions. The edema is diffuse, symmetric, and most prominent in the dependent areas; periorbital edema is most prominent in the morning.

Hepatic Cirrhosis **(See also Chap. 344)** This condition is characterized, in part, by hepatic venous outflow obstruction, which in turn expands the splanchnic blood volume, and hepatic lymph formation. Intrahepatic hypertension acts as a stimulus for renal sodium retention and causes a reduction of effective arterial blood volume. These alterations are frequently complicated by hypoalbuminemia secondary to reduced hepatic synthesis, as well as peripheral arterial vasodilation. These effects reduce the effective arterial blood volume, leading to activation of the sodium- and water-retaining mechanisms described above (**Fig. 41-1*B***). The concentration of circulating aldosterone often is elevated by the failure of the liver to metabolize this hormone. Initially, the excess interstitial fluid is localized preferentially proximal (upstream) to the congested portal venous system, causing ascites (**Chap. 50**). In later stages, particularly when there is severe hypoalbuminemia, peripheral edema may develop. A sizable accumulation of ascitic fluid may increase intraabdominal pressure and impede venous return from the lower extremities and contribute to the accumulation of the edema.

Drug-Induced Edema A large number of widely used drugs can cause edema (**Table 41-2**). Mechanisms include renal vasoconstriction

TABLE 41-2 Drugs Associated with Edema Formation

Nonsteroidal anti-inflammatory drugs
Antihypertensive agents
Direct arterial/arteriolar vasodilators
Hydralazine
Clonidine
Methyldopa
Guanethidine
Minoxidil
Calcium channel antagonists
α-Adrenergic antagonists
Thiazolidinediones
Steroid hormones
Glucocorticoids
Anabolic steroids
Estrogens
Progestins
Cyclosporine
Growth hormone
Immunotherapies
Interleukin 2
OKT3 monoclonal antibody

Source: Reproduced with permission from GM Chertow, in E Braunwald, L Goldman (eds): Approach to the patient with edema, in Primary Cardiology, 2nd ed. Philadelphia, Saunders, 2003.

(nonsteroidal anti-inflammatory drugs and cyclosporine), arteriolar dilation (vasodilators), augmented renal sodium reabsorption (steroid hormones), and capillary damage.

Edema of Nutritional Origin A diet grossly deficient in calories and particularly in protein over a prolonged period may produce hypoproteinemia and edema. The latter may be intensified by the development of beriberi heart disease, which also is of nutritional origin, in which multiple peripheral arteriovenous fistulae result in reduced effective systemic perfusion and effective arterial blood volume, thereby enhancing edema formation **(Chap. 333)** (Fig. 41-1*B*). Edema develops or becomes intensified when famished subjects are first provided with an adequate diet. The ingestion of more food may increase the quantity of sodium ingested, which is then retained along with water. So-called refeeding edema also may be linked to increased release of insulin, which directly increases tubular sodium reabsorption. In addition to hypoalbuminemia, hypokalemia and caloric deficits may be involved in the edema of starvation.

LOCALIZED EDEMA

In thrombophlebitis, varicose veins, and primary venous valve failure, the hydrostatic pressure in the capillary bed upstream (proximal) of the obstruction increases so that an abnormal quantity of fluid is transferred from the vascular to the interstitial space, which may give rise to localized edema. The latter may also occur in lymphatic obstruction caused by chronic lymphangitis, resection of regional lymph nodes, filariasis, and genetic (frequently called primary) lymphedema. The latter is particularly intractable because restriction of lymphatic flow results in both an increase in intracapillary pressure and increased protein concentration in the interstitial fluid, which act in concert to aggravate fluid retention.

Other Causes of Edema These causes include hypothyroidism (myxedema) due to deposition of hyaluronic acid; hyperthyroidism (pretibial myxedema secondary to Graves' disease), in which edema is typically nonpitting and, in Graves' disease, exogenous hypercortisolism; pregnancy; and administration of estrogens and vasodilators, particularly dihydropyridines such as nifedipine.

DISTRIBUTION OF EDEMA

The distribution of edema is an important guide to its cause. Edema associated with heart failure tends to be more extensive in the legs and to be accentuated in the evening, a feature also determined largely by posture. When patients with heart failure are confined to bed, edema may be most prominent in the presacral region.

Edema resulting from hypoproteinemia, as occurs in the nephrotic syndrome, characteristically is generalized, but it is especially evident in the very soft tissues of the eyelids and face and tends to be most pronounced in the morning owing to the recumbent posture assumed during the night. Less common causes of facial edema include trichinosis, allergic reactions, and myxedema. Edema limited to one leg or to one or both arms is usually the result of venous and/or lymphatic obstruction. Unilateral paralysis reduces lymphatic and venous drainage on the affected side and may also be responsible for unilateral edema. In patients with obstruction of the superior vena cava, edema is confined to the face, neck, and upper extremities in which the venous pressure is elevated compared with that in the lower extremities.

APPROACH TO THE PATIENT

Edema

An important first question is whether the edema is localized or generalized. If it is localized, the local phenomena that may be responsible should be identified. If the edema is generalized, one should determine if there is serious hypoalbuminemia, e.g., serum albumin <3.0 g/dL. If so, the history, physical examination, urinalysis, and other laboratory data will help evaluate the question of cirrhosis, severe malnutrition, or the nephrotic syndrome as the underlying disorder. If hypoalbuminemia is not present, it should be determined if there is evidence of heart failure severe enough to promote generalized edema. Finally, it should be ascertained as to whether or not the patient has an adequate urine output or if there is significant oliguria or anuria. **These abnormalities are discussed in Chaps. 52, 310, and 311.**

FURTHER READING

Clark AL, Cleland JG: Causes and treatment of oedema in patients with heart failure. Nature Rev Cardiol 10:156, 2013.

Damman K et al: Congestion in chronic systolic heart failure is related to renal dysfunction and increased mortality. Eur J Heart Fail 12:974, 2010.

Ferrell RE et al: *GJC2* missense mutations cause human lymphedema. Am J Hum Genet 86:943, 2010.

Frison S et al: Omitting edema measurement: How much acute malnutrition are we missing? Am J Clin Nutr 102:1176, 2015.

Levick JR, Michel CC: Microvascular fluid exchange and the revised Starling principle. Cardiovascular Res 87:198, 2010.

Telinius N, Hjortdal VE: Role of the lymphatic vasculature in cardiovascular medicine. Heart 105:1777, 2019.

42 Approach to the Patient with a Heart Murmur

Patrick T. O'Gara, Joseph Loscalzo

The differential diagnosis of a heart murmur begins with a careful assessment of its major attributes and response to bedside maneuvers. The history, clinical context, and associated physical examination findings provide additional clues to help establish the significance of a heart murmur. Accurate bedside identification of a heart murmur can inform decisions regarding the indications for noninvasive testing and the need for referral to a cardiovascular specialist. Preliminary discussions can be held with the patient regarding antibiotic or rheumatic fever prophylaxis, the need to restrict various forms of physical activity, and the potential role for family screening.

Heart murmurs are caused by audible vibrations that are due to increased turbulence from accelerated blood flow through normal or abnormal orifices; flow through a narrowed or irregular orifice into a dilated vessel or chamber; or backward flow through an incompetent valve, ventricular septal defect, or patent ductus arteriosus. They traditionally are defined by their timing within the cardiac cycle **(Fig. 42-1)**. *Systolic murmurs* begin with or after the first heart sound (S_1) and terminate at or before the component (A_2 or P_2) of the second heart sound (S_2) that corresponds to their site of origin (left or right, respectively). *Diastolic murmurs* begin with or after the associated component of S_2 and end at or before the subsequent S_1. *Continuous murmurs* are not confined to either phase of the cardiac cycle but instead begin in early systole and proceed through S_2 into all or part of diastole. The accurate timing of heart murmurs is the first step in their identification. The distinction between S_1 and S_2, and therefore systole and diastole, is usually a straightforward process but can be difficult in the setting of a tachyarrhythmia, in which case the heart sounds can be distinguished by simultaneous palpation of the carotid upstroke, which should closely follow S_1.

Duration and Character The duration of a heart murmur depends on the length of time over which a pressure difference exists between two cardiac chambers, the left ventricle and the aorta, the right ventricle and the pulmonary artery, or the great vessels. The magnitude and

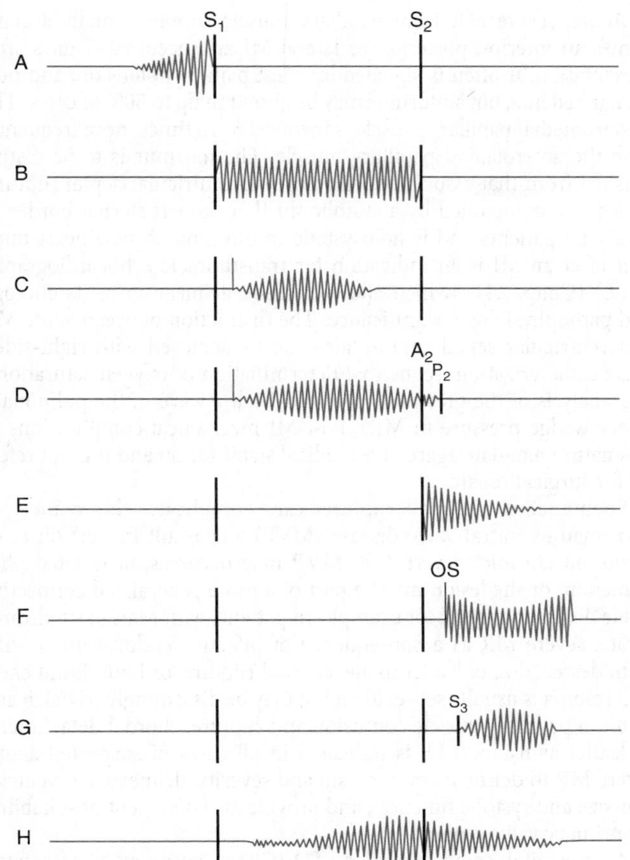

FIGURE 42-1 **Diagram depicting principal heart murmurs.** ***A.*** Presystolic murmur of mitral or tricuspid stenosis. ***B.*** Holosystolic (pansystolic) murmur of mitral or tricuspid regurgitation or of ventricular septal defect. ***C.*** Aortic ejection murmur beginning with an ejection click and fading before the second heart sound. ***D.*** Systolic murmur in pulmonic stenosis spilling through the aortic second sound, pulmonic valve closure being delayed. ***E.*** Aortic or pulmonary diastolic murmur. ***F.*** Long diastolic murmur of mitral stenosis after the opening snap (OS). ***G.*** Short mid-diastolic inflow murmur after a third heart sound. ***H.*** Continuous murmur of patent ductus arteriosus. *(Courtesy of Antony and Julie Wood.)*

variability of this pressure difference, coupled with the geometry and compliance of the involved chambers or vessels, dictate the velocity of flow; the degree of turbulence; and the resulting frequency, configuration, and intensity of the murmur. The diastolic murmur of chronic aortic regurgitation (AR) is a blowing, high-frequency event, whereas the murmur of mitral stenosis (MS), indicative of the left atrial–left ventricular diastolic pressure gradient, is a low-frequency event, heard as a rumbling sound with the bell of the stethoscope. The frequency components of a heart murmur may vary at different sites of auscultation. The coarse systolic murmur of aortic stenosis (AS) may sound higher pitched and more acoustically pure at the apex, a phenomenon eponymously referred to as the *Gallavardin effect*. Some murmurs may have a distinct or unusual quality, such as the "honking" sound appreciated in some patients with mitral regurgitation (MR) due to mitral valve prolapse (MVP).

The configuration of a heart murmur may be described as crescendo, decrescendo, crescendo-decrescendo, or plateau. The decrescendo configuration of the murmur of chronic AR (**Fig. 42-1*E***) can be understood in terms of the progressive decline in the diastolic pressure gradient between the aorta and the left ventricle. The crescendo-decrescendo configuration of the murmur of AS reflects the changes in the systolic pressure gradient between the left ventricle and the aorta as ejection occurs, whereas the plateau configuration of the murmur of chronic MR (**Fig. 42-1*B***) is consistent with the large and nearly constant pressure difference between the left ventricle and the left atrium.

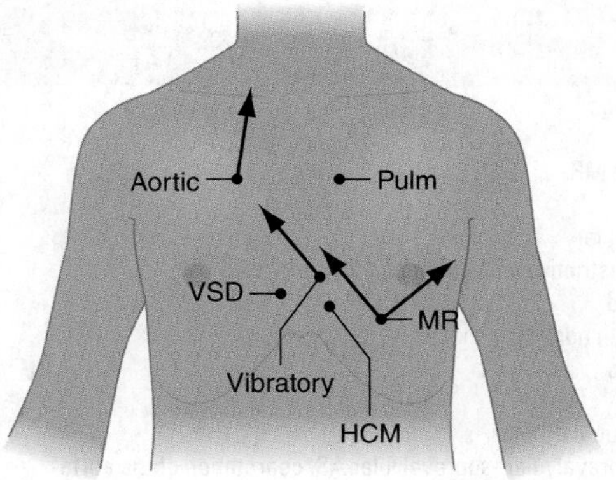

FIGURE 42-2 **Maximal intensity and radiation of six isolated systolic murmurs.** Aortic, aortic stenosis; HCM, hypertrophic obstructive cardiomyopathy; MR, mitral regurgitation; Pulm, pulmonary stenosis; VSD, ventricular septal defect. *(From JB Barlow: Perspectives on the Mitral Valve. Philadelphia, FA Davis, 1987, p 140.)*

Intensity The intensity of a heart murmur is graded on a scale of 1–6 (or I–VI). A grade 1 murmur is very soft and is heard only with great effort. A grade 2 murmur is easily heard but not particularly loud. A grade 3 murmur is loud but is not accompanied by a palpable thrill over the site of maximal intensity. A grade 4 murmur is very loud and accompanied by a thrill. A grade 5 murmur is loud enough to be heard with only the edge of the stethoscope touching the chest, whereas a grade 6 murmur is loud enough to be heard with the stethoscope slightly off the chest. Murmurs of grade 3 or greater intensity usually signify important structural heart disease and indicate high blood flow velocity at the site of murmur production. Small, restrictive ventricular septal defects (VSDs), for example, are accompanied by loud, usually grade 4 or greater, systolic murmurs as blood is ejected at high velocity from the left ventricle to the right ventricle. Low-velocity events, such as left-to-right shunting across an atrial septal defect (ASD), are usually silent. The intensity of a heart murmur may be diminished by any process that increases the distance between the intracardiac source and the stethoscope on the chest wall, such as obesity, obstructive lung disease, or a large pericardial effusion. The intensity of a murmur also may be misleadingly soft when cardiac output is reduced significantly or when the pressure gradient between the involved cardiac structures is low.

Location and Radiation Recognition of the location and radiation of the murmur helps facilitate its accurate identification (**Fig. 42-2**). Adventitious sounds, such as a systolic click or diastolic snap, or abnormalities of S_1 or S_2 may provide additional clues. Careful attention to the characteristics of the murmur and other heart sounds during the respiratory cycle and the performance of simple bedside maneuvers complete the auscultatory examination. These features, along with recommendations for further testing, are discussed below in the context of specific systolic, diastolic, and continuous heart murmurs (**Table 42-1**).

SYSTOLIC HEART MURMURS

Early Systolic Murmurs Early systolic murmurs begin with S_1 and extend for a variable period, ending well before S_2. Their causes are relatively few. *Acute, severe MR* into a normal-sized, relatively noncompliant left atrium results in an early, decrescendo systolic murmur best heard at or just medial to the apical impulse. These characteristics reflect the progressive attenuation of the pressure gradient between the left ventricle and the left atrium during systole owing to the rapid rise in left atrial pressure caused by the sudden volume load into an unprepared, noncompliant chamber, and contrast sharply with the auscultatory features of chronic MR. Clinical settings in which acute, severe MR occur include (1) papillary muscle rupture complicating acute myocardial infarction (MI) (**Chap. 275**), (2) rupture of chordae tendineae in the setting of myxomatous mitral valve disease (MVP, **Chap. 265**), (3) infective endocarditis (**Chap. 128**), and (4) blunt chest wall trauma.

TABLE 42-1 Principal Causes of Heart Murmurs

Systolic Murmurs

Early systolic
- Mitral
  - Acute MR
- VSD
  - Muscular
  - Nonrestrictive with pulmonary hypertension
- Tricuspid
  - TR with normal pulmonary artery pressure

Midsystolic
- Aortic
  - Obstructive
    - Supravalvular–supravalvular AS, coarctation of the aorta
    - Valvular–AS and aortic sclerosis
    - Subvalvular–discrete, tunnel or HOCM
  - Increased flow, hyperkinetic states, AR, complete heart block
  - Dilation of ascending aorta, atheroma, aortitis
- Pulmonary
  - Obstructive
    - Supravalvular–pulmonary artery stenosis
    - Valvular–pulmonic valve stenosis
    - Subvalvular–infundibular stenosis (dynamic)
  - Increased flow, hyperkinetic states, left-to-right shunt (e.g., ASD)
  - Dilation of pulmonary artery

Late systolic
- Mitral
  - MVP, acute myocardial ischemia
- Tricuspid
  - TVP

Holosystolic
- Atrioventricular valve regurgitation (MR, TR)
- Left-to-right shunt at ventricular level (VSD)

Early Diastolic Murmurs

AR
- Valvular: congenital (bicuspid valve), rheumatic deformity, endocarditis, prolapse, trauma, post-valvotomy
- Dilation of valve ring: aorta dissection, annuloaortic ectasia, medial degeneration, hypertension, ankylosing spondylitis
- Widening of commissures: syphilis

Pulmonic regurgitation
- Valvular: post-valvotomy, endocarditis, rheumatic fever, carcinoid
- Dilation of valve ring: pulmonary hypertension; Marfan syndrome
- Congenital: isolated or associated with tetralogy of Fallot, VSD, pulmonic stenosis

Mid-Diastolic Murmurs

Mitral
- MS
- Carey-Coombs murmur (mid-diastolic apical murmur in acute rheumatic fever)
- Increased flow across nonstenotic mitral valve (e.g., MR, VSD, PDA, high-output states, and complete heart block)

Tricuspid
- Tricuspid stenosis
- Increased flow across nonstenotic tricuspid valve (e.g., TR, ASD, and anomalous pulmonary venous return)

Left and right atrial tumors (myxoma)

Severe AR (Austin Flint murmur)

Continuous Murmurs

Patent ductus arteriosus	Proximal coronary artery stenosis
Coronary AV fistula	Mammary souffle of pregnancy
Ruptured sinus of Valsalva aneurysm	Pulmonary artery branch stenosis
Aortic septal defect	Bronchial collateral circulation
Cervical venous hum	Small (restrictive) ASD with MS
Anomalous left coronary artery	Intercostal AV fistula

Abbreviations: AR, aortic regurgitation; AS, aortic stenosis; ASD, atrial septal defect; AV, arteriovenous; HOCM, hypertrophic obstructive cardiomyopathy; MR, mitral regurgitation; MS, mitral stenosis; MVP, mitral valve prolapse; PDA, patent ductus arteriosus; TR, tricuspid regurgitation; TVP, tricuspid valve prolapse; VSD, ventricular septal defect.

Source: E Braunwald, JK Perloff, in D Zipes et al (eds): *Braunwald's Heart Disease*, 7th ed. Philadelphia, Elsevier, 2005; PJ Norton, RA O'Rourke, in E Braunwald, L Goldman (eds): *Primary Cardiology*, 2nd ed. Philadelphia, Elsevier, 2003.

Acute, severe MR from papillary muscle rupture usually accompanies an inferior, posterior, or lateral MI and occurs 2–7 days after presentation. It often is signaled by chest pain, hypotension, and pulmonary edema, but a murmur may be absent in up to 50% of cases. The posteromedial papillary muscle is involved 6–10 times more frequently than the anterolateral papillary muscle. The murmur is to be distinguished from that associated with post-MI ventricular septal rupture, which is accompanied by a systolic thrill at the left sternal border in nearly all patients and is holosystolic in duration. A new heart murmur after an MI is an indication for transthoracic echocardiography (TTE) (**Chap. 241**), which allows bedside delineation of its etiology and pathophysiologic significance. The distinction between acute MR and ventricular septal rupture also can be achieved with right-sided heart catheterization, sequential determination of oxygen saturations, and analysis of the pressure waveforms (tall *v* wave in the pulmonary artery wedge pressure in MR). Post-MI mechanical complications of this nature mandate aggressive medical stabilization and prompt referral for surgical repair.

Spontaneous chordal rupture can complicate the course of myxomatous mitral valve disease (MVP) and result in new-onset or "acute on chronic" severe MR. MVP may occur as an isolated phenomenon, or the lesion may be part of a more generalized connective tissue disorder as seen, for example, in patients with Marfan syndrome. Acute, severe MR as a consequence of infective endocarditis results from destruction of leaflet tissue, chordal rupture, or both. Blunt chest wall trauma is usually self-evident but may be disarmingly trivial; it can result in papillary muscle contusion and rupture, chordal detachment, or leaflet avulsion. TTE is indicated in all cases of suspected acute, severe MR to define its mechanism and severity, delineate left ventricular size and systolic function, and provide an assessment of suitability for primary valve repair.

A congenital, small muscular VSD (**Chap. 269**) may be associated with an early systolic murmur. The defect closes progressively during septal contraction, and thus the murmur is confined to early systole. It is localized to the left sternal border (Fig. 42-2) and is usually of grade 4 or 5 intensity. Signs of pulmonary hypertension or left ventricular volume overload are absent. Anatomically large and uncorrected VSDs, which usually involve the membranous portion of the septum, may lead to pulmonary hypertension. The murmur associated with the left-to-right shunt, which earlier may have been holosystolic, becomes limited to the first portion of systole as the elevated pulmonary vascular resistance leads to an abrupt rise in right ventricular pressure and an attenuation of the interventricular pressure gradient during the remainder of the cardiac cycle. In such instances, signs of pulmonary hypertension (right ventricular lift, loud and single or closely split S_2) may predominate. The murmur is best heard along the left sternal border but is softer. Suspicion of a VSD is an indication for TTE.

Tricuspid regurgitation (TR) with normal pulmonary artery pressures, as may occur with infective endocarditis, may produce an early systolic murmur. The murmur is soft (grade 1 or 2), is best heard at the lower left sternal border, and may increase in intensity with inspiration (Carvallo's sign). Regurgitant *c-v* waves may be visible in the jugular venous pulse. TR in this setting is not associated with signs of right heart failure, such as ascites or lower extremity edema.

Midsystolic Murmurs Midsystolic murmurs begin at a short interval after S_1, end before S_2 (**Fig. 42-1C**) and are usually crescendo-decrescendo in configuration. AS is the most common cause of a midsystolic murmur in an adult. The murmur of AS is usually loudest to the right of the sternum in the second intercostal space (aortic area, Fig. 42-2) and radiates into the carotids. Transmission of the midsystolic murmur to the apex, where it becomes higher-pitched, is common (Gallavardin effect; see above).

Differentiation of this apical systolic murmur from MR can be difficult. The murmur of AS will increase in intensity or become louder, in the beat after a premature beat, whereas the murmur of MR will have constant intensity from beat to beat. The intensity of the AS murmur also varies directly with the cardiac output. With a normal cardiac output, a systolic thrill at the second right intercostal space and a grade 4 or higher murmur suggest severe AS. The murmur is softer in the setting of heart failure and low cardiac output. Other auscultatory findings of severe AS include a soft or absent A_2, paradoxical splitting of S_2, an apical S_4, and a late-peaking systolic murmur. In children, adolescents, and young adults with congenital valvular AS, an early ejection sound (click) is usually audible, more often along the left sternal border than at the base. Its presence signifies a flexible, noncalcified bicuspid valve (or one of its variants) and localizes the left ventricular outflow obstruction to the valvular (rather than sub- or supravalvular) level.

Assessment of the volume and rate of rise of the carotid pulse can provide additional information. A small and delayed upstroke (*parvus et tardus*) is consistent with severe AS. The carotid pulse examination is less discriminatory, however, in older patients with stiffened arteries. The electrocardiogram (ECG) shows signs of left ventricular hypertrophy (LVH) as the severity of the stenosis increases. TTE is indicated to assess the anatomic features of the aortic valve, the severity of the stenosis, left ventricular size, wall thickness and function, and the size and contour of the aortic root and proximal ascending aorta.

The obstructive form of hypertrophic cardiomyopathy (HOCM) is associated with a midsystolic murmur that is usually loudest along the left sternal border or between the left lower sternal border and the apex **(Chap. 259**, Fig. 42-2). The murmur is produced by both dynamic left ventricular outflow tract obstruction and MR, and thus, its configuration is a hybrid between ejection and regurgitant phenomena. The intensity of the murmur may vary from beat to beat and after provocative maneuvers but usually does not exceed grade 3. The murmur classically will increase in intensity with maneuvers that result in increasing degrees of outflow tract obstruction, such as a reduction in preload or afterload (Valsalva, standing, vasodilators), or with an augmentation of contractility (inotropic stimulation). Maneuvers or medications that increase preload (squatting, passive leg raising, volume administration) or afterload (squatting, vasopressors) or that reduce contractility (β-adrenoreceptor blockers) decrease the intensity of the murmur. In rare patients, there may be reversed splitting of S_2. A sustained left ventricular apical impulse and an S_4 may be appreciated. In contrast to AS, the carotid upstroke is rapid and of normal volume. Rarely, it is bisferiens or bifid in contour **(see Fig. 239-2*D*)** due to midsystolic closure of the aortic valve. LVH is present on the ECG, and the diagnosis is confirmed by TTE. Although the systolic murmur associated with MVP behaves similarly to that due to HOCM in response to the Valsalva maneuver and to standing/squatting **(Fig. 42-3)**, these two lesions can be distinguished on the basis of their associated findings, such as the presence of LVH in HOCM or a nonejection click in MVP.

The midsystolic, crescendo-decrescendo murmur of congenital pulmonic stenosis (PS; **Chap. 269**) is best appreciated in the second and third left intercostal spaces (pulmonic area) **(Figs. 42-2 and 42-4)**. The duration of the murmur lengthens and the intensity of P_2 diminishes with increasing degrees of valvular stenosis **(Fig. 42-1*D*)**. An early ejection sound, the intensity of which *decreases* with inspiration, is heard in younger patients. A parasternal lift and ECG evidence of right ventricular hypertrophy indicate severe pressure overload. If obtained, the chest x-ray may show poststenotic dilation of the main pulmonary artery. TTE is recommended for complete characterization.

Significant left-to-right intracardiac shunting due to an ASD **(Chap. 269)** leads to an increase in pulmonary blood flow and a grade 2–3 midsystolic murmur at the middle to upper left sternal border attributed to increased flow rates across the pulmonic valve with fixed splitting of S_2. Ostium secundum ASDs are the most common cause of these shunts in adults. Features suggestive of a primum ASD include the coexistence of MR due to a cleft anterior mitral valve leaflet and left axis deviation of the QRS complex on the ECG. With sinus venosus ASDs, the left-to-right shunt is usually not large enough to result in a systolic murmur, although the ECG may show abnormalities of sinus node function. A grade 2 or 3 midsystolic murmur may also be heard best at the upper left sternal border in patients with idiopathic dilation of the pulmonary artery; a pulmonary ejection sound is also present in these patients. TTE is indicated to evaluate a grade 2 or 3 midsystolic murmur when there are other signs of cardiac disease.

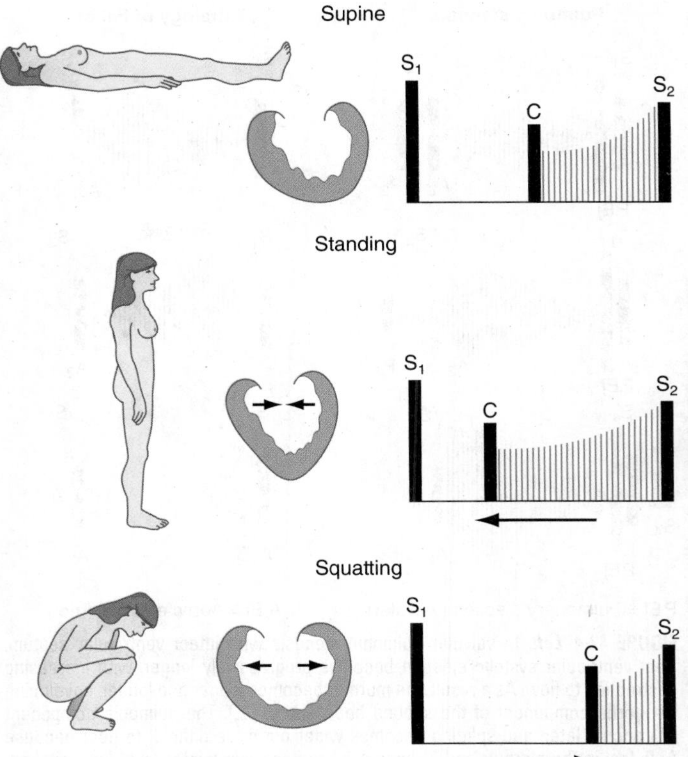

FIGURE 42-3 A midsystolic nonejection sound (C) occurs in mitral valve prolapse and is followed by a late systolic murmur that crescendos to the second heart sound (S_2). Standing decreases venous return; the heart becomes smaller; C moves closer to the first heart sound (S_1), and the mitral regurgitant murmur has an earlier onset. With prompt squatting, venous return and afterload increase; the heart becomes larger; C moves toward S_2; and the duration of the murmur shortens. The systolic murmur of hypertrophic obstructive cardiomyopathy behaves similarly. *(Reprinted with permission Examination of the Heart, Part IV: Auscultation of the Heart ©American Heart Association, Inc.)*

An isolated grade 1 or 2 midsystolic murmur, heard in the absence of symptoms or signs of heart disease, is most often a benign finding for which no further evaluation, including TTE, is necessary. The most common example of a murmur of this type in an older adult patient is the crescendo-decrescendo murmur of aortic valve sclerosis, heard at the second right interspace (Fig. 42-2). Aortic sclerosis is defined as focal thickening and calcification of the aortic valve to a degree that does not interfere with leaflet opening. The carotid upstrokes are normal, and electrocardiographic LVH is not present. A grade 1 or 2 midsystolic murmur often can be heard at the left sternal border with pregnancy, hyperthyroidism, or anemia, physiologic states that are associated with accelerated blood flow. *Still's murmur* refers to a benign grade 2, vibratory or musical midsystolic murmur at the mid or lower left sternal border in normal children and adolescents, best heard in the supine position (Fig. 42-2).

Late Systolic Murmurs A late systolic murmur that is best heard at the left ventricular apex is usually due to MVP **(Chap. 265)**. Often, this murmur is introduced by one or more nonejection clicks. The radiation of the murmur can help identify the specific mitral leaflet involved in the process of prolapse or flail. The term *flail* refers to the movement made by an unsupported portion of the leaflet (usually the tip) after loss of its chordal attachment(s). With posterior leaflet prolapse or flail, the resultant jet of MR is directed anteriorly and medially, as a result of which the murmur radiates to the base of the heart and masquerades as AS. Anterior leaflet prolapse or flail results in a posteriorly directed MR jet that radiates to the axilla or left infrascapular region. Leaflet flail is associated with a murmur of grade 3 or 4 intensity that can be heard throughout the precordium in thin-chested patients. The presence of an S_3 or a short, rumbling mid-diastolic murmur due to enhanced flow signifies severe MR.

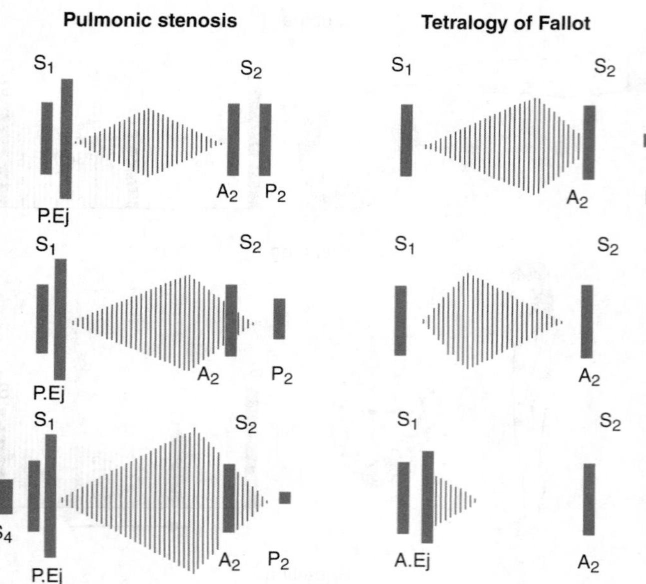

FIGURE 42-4 ***Left.*** In valvular pulmonic stenosis with intact ventricular septum, right ventricular systolic ejection becomes progressively longer, with increasing obstruction to flow. As a result, the murmur becomes longer and louder, enveloping the aortic component of the second heart sound (A_2). The pulmonic component (P_2) occurs later, and splitting becomes wider but more difficult to hear because A_2 is lost in the murmur and P_2 becomes progressively fainter and lower pitched. As the pulmonic gradient increases, the isometric contraction phase shortens until the pulmonic valve ejection sound fuses with the first heart sound (S_1). In severe pulmonic stenosis with concentric hypertrophy and decreasing right ventricular compliance, a fourth heart sound appears. ***Right.*** In tetralogy of Fallot with increasing obstruction at the pulmonic infundibular area, an increasing amount of right ventricular blood is shunted across the silent ventricular septal defect and flow across the obstructed outflow tract decreases. Therefore, with increasing obstruction, the murmur becomes shorter, earlier, and fainter. P_2 is absent in severe tetralogy of Fallot. A large aortic root receives almost all cardiac output from both ventricular chambers, and the aorta dilates and is accompanied by a root ejection sound that does not vary with respiration. *(Reprinted with permission Examination of the Heart, Part IV: Auscultation of the Heart ©American Heart Association, Inc.)*

Bedside maneuvers that decrease left ventricular preload, such as standing, will cause the click and murmur of MVP to move closer to the first heart sound, as leaflet prolapse occurs earlier in systole. Standing also causes the murmur to become louder and longer. With squatting, left ventricular preload and afterload are increased abruptly, leading to an increase in left ventricular volume, and the click and murmur move away from the first heart sound as leaflet prolapse is delayed; the murmur becomes softer and shorter in duration (Fig. 42-3). As noted above, these responses to standing and squatting are directionally similar to those observed in patients with HOCM.

A late, apical systolic murmur indicative of MR may be heard transiently in the setting of acute myocardial ischemia; it is due to apical tethering and malcoaptation of the leaflets in response to structural and functional changes of the ventricle and mitral annulus. The intensity of the murmur varies as a function of left ventricular afterload and will increase in the setting of hypertension. TTE is recommended for assessment of late systolic murmurs.

Holosystolic Murmurs (Figs. 42-1*B* and 42-5) Holosystolic murmurs begin with S_1 and continue through systole to S_2. They are usually indicative of chronic mitral or tricuspid valve regurgitation or a VSD and warrant TTE for further characterization. The holosystolic murmur of chronic MR is best heard at the left ventricular apex and radiates to the axilla (Fig. 42-2); it is usually high-pitched and plateau in configuration because of the wide difference between left ventricular and left atrial pressure throughout systole. In contrast to acute MR, left atrial compliance is normal or even increased in chronic MR. As a result, there is only a small increase in left atrial pressure for any increase in regurgitant volume.

Several conditions are associated with chronic MR and an apical holosystolic murmur, including rheumatic scarring of the leaflets, mitral annular calcification, postinfarction left ventricular remodeling, and severe left ventricular chamber enlargement in the setting of a dilated cardiomyopathy **(Chap. 259)**. The severity of the MR is worsened by any contribution from apical displacement of the papillary muscles and leaflet tethering (remodeling). Because the mitral annulus is contiguous with the left atrial endocardium, gradual enlargement of the left atrium from chronic MR will result in further stretching of the annulus and more MR; thus, "MR begets MR." Chronic severe MR results in enlargement and leftward displacement of the left ventricular

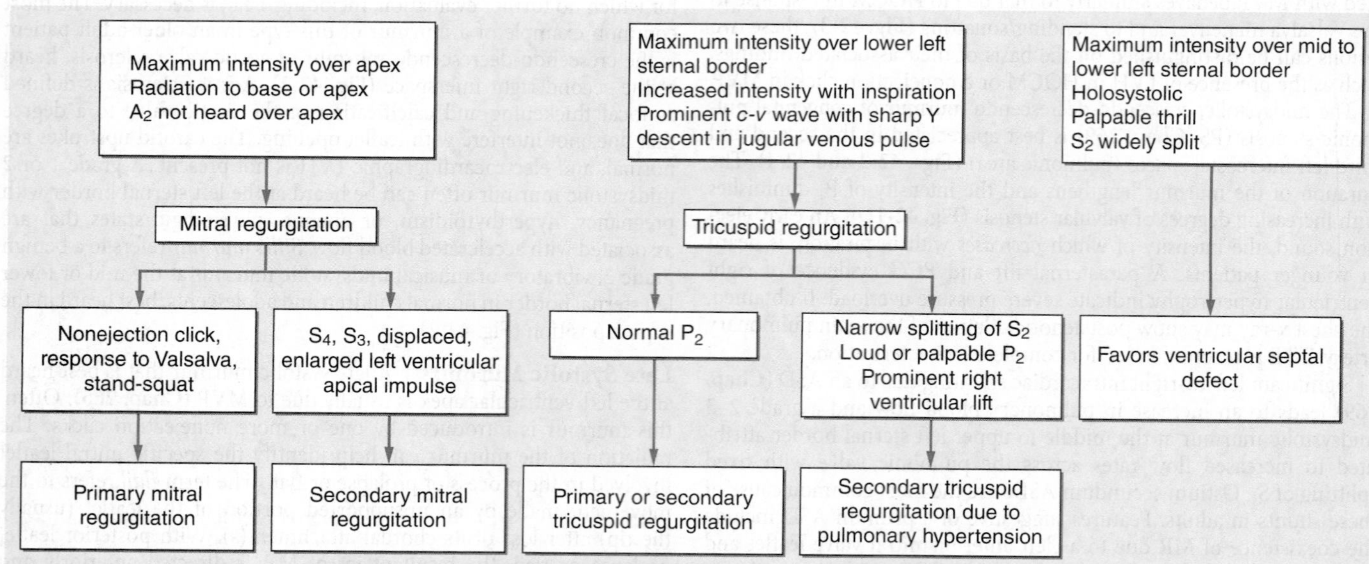

FIGURE 42-5 Differential diagnosis of a holosystolic murmur. The murmur of mitral regurgitation is best heard over the left ventricular apex. The radiation of the murmur depends on the direction in which the jet of mitral regurgitation enters into the left atrium. Differentiation of primary and secondary causes of mitral regurgitation is usually accomplished with transthoracic echocardiography, although the presence of a nonejection click and a mid-late apical systolic murmur, for example, can establish a bedside diagnosis of mitral valve prolapse (primary mitral regurgitation). Secondary mitral regurgitation can occur as a result of left ventricular remodeling. The murmur may be soft and difficult to hear. Other signs of left ventricular dysfunction may be present. Greater than 80% of the tricuspid regurgitation encountered clinically is due to a secondary cause. Severe pulmonary hypertension can be appreciated by a loud, single P_2. Primary tricuspid regurgitation may be present in the setting of pacemaker leads or in patients with carcinoid syndrome who usually have signs of liver involvement. A ventricular septal defect is usually manifested by a holosystolic murmur with a palpable thrill along the mid- to lower left sternal edge.

apex beat and, in some patients, a diastolic filling complex, as described previously (Fig. 42-1G).

The holosystolic murmur of chronic TR is generally softer than that of MR, is loudest at the left lower sternal border, and usually increases in intensity with inspiration (Carvallo's sign). Associated signs include *c-v* waves in the jugular venous pulse, an enlarged and pulsatile liver, ascites, and peripheral edema. The abnormal jugular venous waveforms are the predominant finding and seen very often in the absence of an audible murmur despite Doppler echocardiographic verification of TR. Causes of *primary* TR include myxomatous disease (prolapse), endocarditis, rheumatic disease, radiation, carcinoid, Ebstein's anomaly, leaflet trauma due to intracardiac device leads, or chordal detachment as a complication of right ventricular endomyocardial biopsy. TR is much more commonly a passive process that results secondarily from annular enlargement due to right ventricular dilation in the face of volume or pressure overload or adverse right ventricular remodeling.

The holosystolic murmur of a VSD is loudest at the mid- to lower-left sternal border (Fig. 42-2) and radiates widely. A thrill is present at the site of maximal intensity in the majority of patients. There is no change in the intensity of the murmur with inspiration. The intensity of the murmur varies as a function of the anatomic size of the defect. Small, restrictive VSDs, as exemplified by the *maladie de Roger*, create a very loud murmur due to the significant and sustained systolic pressure gradient between the left and right ventricles. With large defects, the ventricular pressures tend to equalize, shunt flow is balanced, and a murmur is not appreciated. The distinction between post-MI ventricular septal rupture and MR has been reviewed previously.

DIASTOLIC HEART MURMURS

Early Diastolic Murmurs (Fig. 42-1*E*) Chronic AR results in a high-pitched, blowing, decrescendo, early- to mid-diastolic murmur that begins after the aortic component of S_2 (A_2) and is best heard at the second right interspace and along the left sternal border. The murmur may be soft and difficult to hear unless auscultation is performed with the patient leaning forward at end expiration. This maneuver brings the aortic root closer to the anterior chest wall. Radiation of the murmur may provide a clue to the cause of the AR. With primary valve disease, such as that due to congenital bicuspid disease, prolapse, or endocarditis, the diastolic murmur tends to radiate along the left sternal border, where it is often louder than appreciated in the second right interspace. When AR is caused by aortic root disease, the diastolic murmur may radiate along the right sternal border. Diseases of the aortic root cause dilation or distortion of the aortic annulus and failure of leaflet coaptation. Causes include Marfan syndrome with aneurysm formation, annuloaortic ectasia, ankylosing spondylitis, and aortic dissection.

Chronic, severe AR also may produce a lower-pitched mid to late, grade 1 or 2 diastolic murmur at the apex (Austin Flint murmur), which is thought to reflect turbulence at the mitral inflow area from the admixture of regurgitant (aortic) and forward (mitral) blood flow. This lower-pitched, apical diastolic murmur can be distinguished from that due to MS by the absence of an opening snap and the response of the murmur to a vasodilator challenge. Lowering afterload with an agent such as amyl nitrite will decrease the duration and magnitude of the aortic–left ventricular diastolic pressure gradient, and thus, the Austin Flint murmur of severe AR will become shorter and softer. The intensity of the diastolic murmur of MS (Fig. 42-6) may either remain constant or increase with afterload reduction because of the reflex increase in cardiac output and mitral valve flow.

Although AS and AR may coexist, a grade 2 or 3 crescendo-decrescendo midsystolic murmur frequently is heard at the base of the heart in patients with isolated, severe AR and is due to an increased volume and rate of systolic flow. Accurate bedside identification of coexistent AS can be difficult unless the carotid pulse examination is abnormal or the midsystolic murmur is of grade 4 or greater intensity. In the absence of heart failure, chronic severe AR is accompanied by several peripheral signs of significant diastolic runoff, including a wide pulse pressure, a "water-hammer" carotid upstroke (Corrigan's pulse), and Quincke's pulsations of the nail beds. The diastolic murmur of

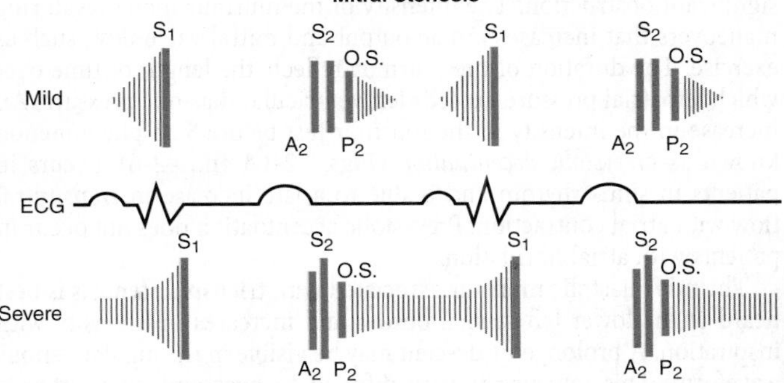

FIGURE 42-6 Diastolic filling murmur (rumble) in mitral stenosis. In mild mitral stenosis, the diastolic gradient across the valve is limited to the phases of rapid ventricular filling in early diastole and presystole. The rumble may occur during either or both periods. As the stenotic process becomes severe, a large pressure gradient exists across the valve during the entire diastolic filling period, and the rumble persists throughout diastole. As the left atrial pressure becomes greater, the interval between A_2 (or P_2) and the opening snap (O.S.) shortens. In severe mitral stenosis, secondary pulmonary hypertension develops and results in a loud P_2 and the splitting interval usually narrows. ECG, electrocardiogram. *(Reprinted with permission Examination of the Heart, Part IV: Auscultation of the Heart ©American Heart Association, Inc.)*

acute, severe AR is notably shorter in duration and lower pitched than the murmur of chronic AR. It can be very difficult to appreciate in the presence of a rapid heart rate. These attributes reflect the abrupt rate of rise of diastolic pressure within the unprepared and noncompliant left ventricle and the correspondingly rapid decline in the aortic–left ventricular diastolic pressure gradient. Left ventricular diastolic pressure may increase sufficiently to result in premature closure of the mitral valve and a soft first heart sound. Peripheral signs of significant diastolic runoff are generally not present.

Pulmonic regurgitation (PR) results in a decrescendo, early to mid-diastolic murmur (*Graham Steell murmur*) that begins after the pulmonic component of S_2 (P_2), is best heard at the second left interspace, and radiates along the left sternal border. The intensity of the murmur may increase with inspiration. PR is most commonly due to dilation of the valve annulus from chronic elevation of the pulmonary artery pressure. Signs of pulmonary hypertension, including a right ventricular lift and a loud, single or narrowly split S_2, are present. These features also help distinguish PR from AR as the cause of a decrescendo diastolic murmur heard along the left sternal border. PR in the absence of pulmonary hypertension can occur with endocarditis or a congenitally deformed valve. It is usually present after repair of tetralogy of Fallot in childhood. When pulmonary hypertension is not present, the diastolic murmur is softer and lower pitched than the classic Graham Steell murmur, and the severity of the PR can be difficult to appreciate.

TTE is indicated for the further evaluation of a patient with an early to mid-diastolic murmur. Longitudinal assessment of lesion severity, ventricular size, and systolic function helps guide a potential decision for surgical management. TTE also can provide anatomic information regarding the root and proximal ascending aorta, although computed tomographic or magnetic resonance angiography may be indicated for more precise characterization (Chap. 241).

Mid-Diastolic Murmurs (Figs. 42-1*F* and 42-1*G*) Mid-diastolic murmurs result from obstruction and/or augmented flow at the level of the mitral or tricuspid valve. Rheumatic fever is the most common cause of MS (Fig. 42-6). In younger patients with pliable valves, S_1 is loud and the murmur begins after an opening snap, which is a high-pitched sound that occurs shortly after S_2. The interval between the pulmonic component of the second heart sound (P_2) and the opening snap is inversely related to the magnitude of the left atrial–left ventricular pressure gradient. The murmur of MS is low-pitched and thus is best heard with the bell of the stethoscope. It is loudest at the left ventricular apex and often is appreciated only when the patient is turned in the left lateral decubitus position. It is usually of grade 1 or 2 intensity but may be absent when the cardiac output is severely reduced despite significant obstruction. The intensity of the murmur increases during maneuvers that increase cardiac output and mitral valve flow, such as exercise. The duration of the murmur reflects the length of time over which left atrial pressure exceeds left ventricular diastolic pressure. An increase in the intensity of the murmur just before S_1, a phenomenon known as *presystolic accentuation* (**Figs. 42-1*A* and 42-6**), occurs in patients in sinus rhythm and is due to a late increase in transmitral flow with atrial contraction. Presystolic accentuation does not occur in patients with atrial fibrillation.

The mid-diastolic murmur associated with tricuspid stenosis is best heard at the lower left sternal border and increases in intensity with inspiration. A prolonged *y* descent may be visible in the jugular venous waveform. This murmur is very difficult to hear and most often is obscured by left-sided acoustical events.

There are several other causes of mid-diastolic murmurs. Large left atrial myxomas may prolapse across the mitral valve and cause variable degrees of obstruction to left ventricular inflow (**Chap. 271**). The murmur associated with an atrial myxoma may change in duration and intensity with changes in body position. An opening snap is not present, and there is no presystolic accentuation. Augmented mitral diastolic flow can occur with isolated severe MR or with a large left-to-right shunt at the ventricular or great vessel level and produce a soft, rapid filling sound (S_3) followed by a short, low-pitched mid-diastolic apical murmur (Fig. 42-1*G*). The Austin Flint murmur of severe, chronic AR has already been described.

A short, mid-diastolic murmur is rarely heard during an episode of acute rheumatic fever (Carey-Coombs murmur) and probably is due to flow through an edematous mitral valve. An opening snap is not present in the acute phase, and the murmur dissipates with resolution of the acute attack. Complete heart block with dyssynchronous atrial and ventricular activation may be associated with intermittent mid- to late diastolic murmurs if atrial contraction occurs when the mitral valve is partially closed. Mid-diastolic murmurs indicative of increased tricuspid valve flow can occur with severe, isolated TR and with large ASDs and significant left-to-right shunting. Other signs of an ASD are present (**Chap. 269**), including fixed splitting of S_2 and a midsystolic murmur at the mid- to upper left sternal border. TTE is indicated for evaluation of a patient with a mid- to late diastolic murmur. Findings specific to the diseases discussed above will help guide management.

CONTINUOUS MURMURS

(**Figs. 42-1*H* and 42-7**) Continuous murmurs begin in systole, peak near the second heart sound, and continue into all or part of diastole. Their presence throughout the cardiac cycle implies a pressure gradient between two chambers or vessels during both systole and diastole. The continuous murmur associated with a patent ductus arteriosus is best heard lateral to the upper left sternal border. Large, uncorrected shunts may lead to pulmonary hypertension, attenuation or obliteration of the diastolic component of the murmur, reversal of shunt flow, and differential cyanosis of the lower extremities. A ruptured sinus of Valsalva aneurysm creates a continuous murmur of abrupt onset at the upper right sternal border. Rupture typically occurs into a right heart chamber, and the murmur is indicative of a continuous pressure difference between the aorta and either the right atrium or the right ventricle. A continuous murmur also may be audible along the left sternal border with a coronary arteriovenous fistula and at the site of an arteriovenous fistula used for hemodialysis access. Enhanced flow through enlarged intercostal collateral arteries in patients with aortic coarctation may produce a continuous murmur along the course of one or more ribs. A cervical bruit with both systolic and diastolic components (a to-fro murmur, Fig. 42-7) usually indicates a high-grade carotid artery stenosis.

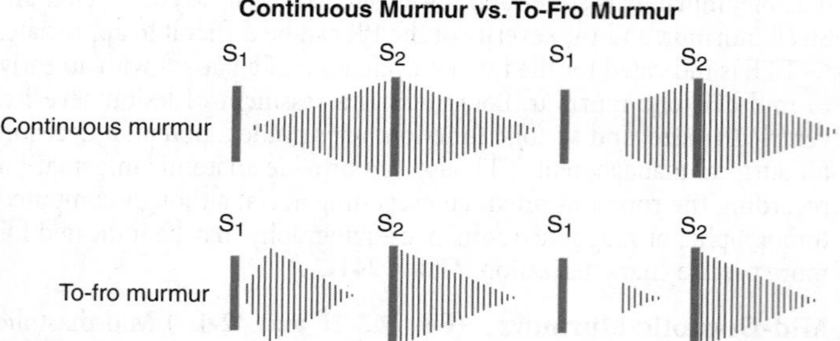

FIGURE 42-7 Comparison of the continuous murmur and the to-fro murmur. During abnormal communication between high-pressure and low-pressure systems, a large pressure gradient exists throughout the cardiac cycle, producing a continuous murmur. A classic example is patent ductus arteriosus. At times, this type of murmur can be confused with a to-fro murmur, which is a combination of systolic ejection murmur and a murmur of semilunar valve incompetence. A classic example of a to-fro murmur is aortic stenosis and regurgitation. A continuous murmur crescendos to near the second heart sound (S_2), whereas a to-fro murmur has two components. The midsystolic ejection component decrescendos and disappears as it approaches S_2. *(Reprinted with permission Examination of the Heart, Part IV: Auscultation of the Heart ©American Heart Association, Inc.)*

Not all continuous murmurs are pathologic. A continuous venous hum can be heard in healthy children and young adults, especially during pregnancy; it is best appreciated in the right supraclavicular fossa and can be obliterated by pressure over the right internal jugular vein or by having the patient turn his or her head toward the examiner. The continuous mammary souffle of pregnancy is created by enhanced arterial flow through engorged breasts and usually appears during the late third trimester or early puerperium. The murmur is louder in systole. Firm pressure with the diaphragm of the stethoscope can eliminate the diastolic portion of the murmur.

DYNAMIC AUSCULTATION

(**Table 42-2; see Table 239-1**) Careful attention to the behavior of heart murmurs during simple maneuvers that alter cardiac hemodynamics can provide important clues to their cause and significance.

Respiration Auscultation should be performed during quiet respiration or with a modest increase in inspiratory effort, as more forceful movement of the chest tends to obscure the heart sounds. Left-sided murmurs may be best heard at end expiration, when lung volumes are minimized, and the heart and great vessels are brought closer to the chest wall. This phenomenon is characteristic of the murmur of AR. Murmurs of right-sided origin, such as tricuspid or pulmonic regurgitation, increase in intensity during inspiration. The intensity of left-sided murmurs either remains constant or decreases with inspiration.

Bedside assessment also should evaluate the behavior of S_2 with respiration and the dynamic relationship between the aortic and pulmonic components (**Fig. 42-8**). Reversed splitting can be a feature of severe AS, HOCM, left bundle branch block, right ventricular pacing, or acute myocardial ischemia. Fixed splitting of S_2 in the presence of a grade 2 or 3 midsystolic murmur at the mid- or upper left sternal border indicates an ASD. Physiologic but wide splitting during the respiratory cycle implies either premature aortic valve closure, as can occur with severe MR, or delayed pulmonic valve closure due to PS or right bundle branch block.

Alterations of Systemic Vascular Resistance Murmurs can change characteristics after maneuvers that alter systemic vascular

TABLE 42-2 Dynamic Auscultation: Bedside Maneuvers That can be Used to Change the Intensity of Cardiac Murmurs (See Text)
1. Respiration
2. Isometric exercise (handgrip)
3. Transient arterial occlusion
4. Pharmacologic manipulation of preload and/or afterload
5. Valsalva maneuver
6. Rapid standing/squatting
7. Passive leg raising
8. Post-premature beat

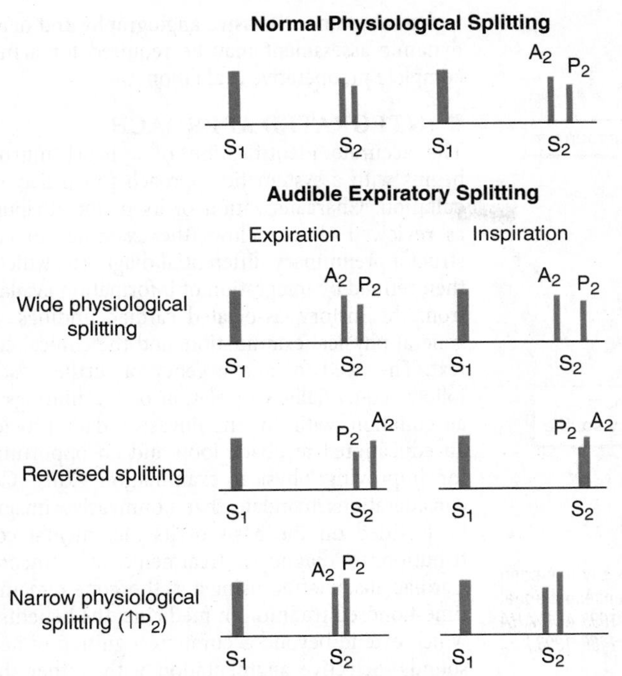

FIGURE 42-8 ***Top.*** Normal physiologic splitting of the second heart sound. During expiration, the aortic (A_2) and pulmonic (P_2) components of the second heart sound are separated by <30 ms and are appreciated as a single sound. During inspiration, the splitting interval widens, and A_2 and P_2 are clearly separated into two distinct sounds. ***Bottom.*** Audible expiratory splitting. Wide physiologic splitting is caused by a delay in P_2 (as, for example, with right bundle branch block) or by early closure of the aortic valve (A_2, as for example with severe mitral regurgitation). Reversed splitting is caused by a delay in A_2, resulting in paradoxical movement; i.e., with inspiration P_2 moves toward A_2, and the splitting interval narrows. Narrow physiologic splitting occurs in pulmonary hypertension, and both A_2 and P_2 are heard during expiration at a narrow splitting interval because of the increased intensity and high-frequency composition of P_2. *(Reprinted with permission Examination of the Heart, Part IV: Auscultation of the Heart ©American Heart Association, Inc.)*

resistance and left ventricular afterload. The systolic murmurs of MR and VSD become louder during sustained handgrip, simultaneous inflation of blood pressure cuffs on both upper extremities to pressures 20–40 mmHg above systolic pressure for 20 s, or infusion of a vasopressor agent. The murmurs associated with AS or HOCM will become softer or remain unchanged with these maneuvers. The diastolic murmur of AR becomes louder in response to interventions that raise systemic vascular resistance.

Opposite changes in systolic and diastolic murmurs may occur with the use of pharmacologic agents that lower systemic vascular resistance. Inhaled amyl nitrite is now rarely used for this purpose but can help distinguish the murmur of AS or HOCM from that of either MR or VSD, if necessary. The former two murmurs increase in intensity, whereas the latter two become softer after exposure to amyl nitrite. As noted previously, the Austin Flint murmur of severe AR becomes softer, but the mid-diastolic rumble of MS becomes louder, in response to the abrupt lowering of systemic vascular resistance with amyl nitrite and enhanced transmitral valve flow.

Changes in Venous Return The Valsalva maneuver results in an increase in intrathoracic pressure, followed by a decrease in venous return, ventricular filling, and cardiac output. The majority of murmurs decrease in intensity during the strain phase of the maneuver. Two notable exceptions are the murmurs associated with MVP and HOCM, both of which become louder during the Valsalva maneuver. The murmur of MVP may also become longer as leaflet prolapse occurs earlier in systole at smaller ventricular volumes. These murmurs behave in a similar and parallel fashion with standing. Both the click and the murmur of MVP move closer in timing to S_1 on rapid standing from a squatting position (Fig. 42-3). The increase in the intensity of the murmur of HOCM is predicated on the augmentation of the dynamic left ventricular outflow tract gradient that occurs with reduced ventricular filling. Squatting results in abrupt increases in both venous return (preload) and left ventricular afterload that increase ventricular volume, changes that predictably cause a decrease in the intensity and duration of the murmurs associated with MVP and HOCM; the click and murmur of MVP move away from S_1 with squatting. Passive leg raising can be used to increase venous return in patients who are unable to squat and stand. This maneuver may lead to a decrease in the intensity of the murmur associated with HOCM but has less effect in patients with MVP.

Post-Premature Ventricular Contraction A change in the intensity of a systolic murmur in the first beat after a premature beat, or in the beat after a long cycle length in patients with atrial fibrillation, can help distinguish AS from MR, particularly in an older patient in whom the murmur of AS is well transmitted to the apex. Systolic murmurs due to left ventricular outflow obstruction, including that due to AS, increase in intensity in the beat after a premature beat because of the combined effects of enhanced left ventricular filling and post-extrasystolic potentiation of contractile function. Forward flow accelerates, causing an increase in the gradient and a louder murmur. The intensity of the murmur of MR does not change in the post-premature beat as there is relatively little further increase in mitral valve flow or change in the left ventricular–left atrial gradient.

THE CLINICAL CONTEXT

Additional clues to the etiology and importance of a heart murmur can be gleaned from the history and other physical examination findings. Symptoms suggestive of cardiovascular, neurologic, or pulmonary disease help focus the differential diagnosis, as do findings relevant to the jugular venous pressure and waveforms, the arterial pulses, other heart sounds, the lungs, the abdomen, the skin, and the extremities. In many instances, laboratory studies, an ECG, and/or a chest x-ray may have been obtained earlier and may contain valuable information. A patient with suspected infective endocarditis, for example, may have a murmur in the setting of fever, chills, anorexia, fatigue, dyspnea, splenomegaly, petechiae, and positive blood cultures. A new systolic murmur in a patient with a marked fall in blood pressure after a recent MI suggests myocardial rupture. By contrast, an isolated grade 1 or 2 midsystolic murmur at the left sternal border in a healthy, active, and asymptomatic young adult is most likely a benign finding for which no further evaluation is indicated. The context in which the murmur is appreciated often dictates the need for further testing and the pace of the evaluation.

ECHOCARDIOGRAPHY

(Fig. 42-9; Chaps. 239 and 241) Echocardiography with color flow and spectral Doppler is a valuable tool for the assessment of cardiac murmurs. Information regarding valve structure and function, chamber size, wall thickness, ventricular function, estimated pulmonary artery pressures, intracardiac shunt flow, pulmonary and hepatic vein flow, and aortic flow can be ascertained readily. It is important to note that Doppler signals of trace or mild valvular regurgitation of no clinical consequence can be detected with structurally normal tricuspid, pulmonic, and mitral valves. Such signals are not likely to generate enough turbulence to create an audible murmur.

Echocardiography is indicated for the evaluation of patients with early, late, or holosystolic murmurs and patients with grade 3 or louder midsystolic murmurs. Patients with grade 1 or 2 midsystolic murmurs but other symptoms or signs of cardiovascular disease, including those from ECG or chest x-ray, should also undergo echocardiography. Echocardiography is also indicated for the evaluation of any patient with a diastolic murmur and for patients with continuous murmurs not due to a venous hum or mammary souffle. Echocardiography should be considered when there is a clinical need to verify normal cardiac structure and function in a patient whose symptoms and signs are probably noncardiac in origin. The performance of serial

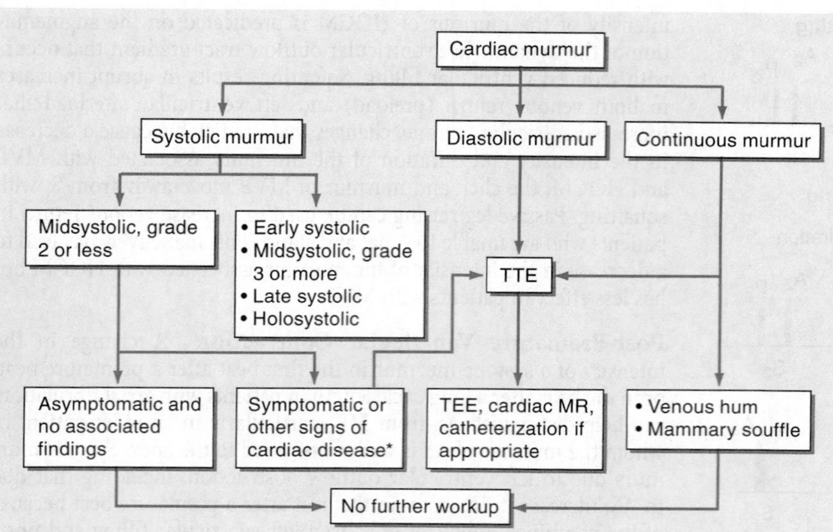

FIGURE 42-9 Strategy for evaluating heart murmurs. *If an electrocardiogram or chest x-ray has been obtained and is abnormal, echocardiography is indicated. MR, magnetic resonance; TEE, transesophageal echocardiography; TTE, transthoracic echocardiography. *(Adapted from RO Bonow et al: 1998 ACC/AHA Guideline for the management of patients with valvular heart disease. J Am Coll Cardiol 32:1486, 1998.)*

echocardiography to follow the course of asymptomatic individuals with valvular heart disease is a central feature of their longitudinal assessment, and it provides valuable information that may have an impact on decisions regarding the timing of surgery. Routine echocardiography is *not* recommended for asymptomatic patients with a grade 1 or 2 midsystolic murmur without other signs of heart disease. For this category of patients, referral to a cardiovascular specialist could be considered if there is doubt about the significance of the murmur after the initial examination.

The selective use of echocardiography outlined above has not been subjected to rigorous analysis of its cost-effectiveness. For some clinicians, handheld or miniaturized cardiac ultrasound devices have replaced the stethoscope. Although several reports attest to the improved sensitivity of such devices for the detection of valvular heart disease (e.g., rheumatic heart disease in susceptible populations), accuracy is highly operator-dependent, and incremental cost considerations and outcomes have not been addressed adequately for most patient scenarios. The use of electronic or digital stethoscopes with spectral display capabilities has also been proposed as a method to improve the characterization of heart murmurs and the mentored teaching of cardiac auscultation.

OTHER CARDIAC TESTING

(Chap. 241, Fig. 42-9) In relatively few patients, clinical assessment and TTE do not adequately characterize the origin and significance of a heart murmur. Transesophageal echocardiography (TEE) can be considered for further evaluation, especially when the TTE windows are limited by body size, chest configuration, or intrathoracic pathology. TEE offers enhanced sensitivity for the detection of a wide range of structural cardiac disorders. Electrocardiographically gated cardiac magnetic resonance (CMR) imaging can provide quantitative information regarding valvular function, regurgitant fraction, regurgitant volume, shunt flow, chamber and great vessel size, ventricular function, and myocardial perfusion. CMR imaging has largely supplanted the need for cardiac catheterization and invasive hemodynamic assessment when there is a discrepancy between the clinical and echocardiographic findings in patients with regurgitant heart valve disease, such as MR or AR. Both CMR and cardiac CT can provide assessment of aortic valve leaflet number when there is uncertainty by TTE regarding whether the valve is bi- or tricuspid, as well as provide information on aortic root and ascending aortic anatomy. The use of coronary CT angiography to exclude coronary artery disease in selected patients with a low pretest probability of disease before valve surgery has gained wider acceptance. Invasive angiography and hemodynamic assessment may be required for a more complete preoperative evaluation.

INTEGRATED APPROACH

The accurate identification of a heart murmur begins with a systematic approach to cardiac auscultation. Characterization of its major attributes, as reviewed above, allows the examiner to construct a preliminary differential diagnosis, which is then refined by integration of information available from the history, associated cardiac findings, the general physical examination, and the clinical context. The need for and urgency of further testing follow sequentially. Correlation of the findings on auscultation with the noninvasive data provides an educational feedback loop and an opportunity for improving physical examination skills. Cost considerations mandate that noninvasive imaging be justified on the basis of its incremental contribution to diagnosis, treatment, and outcome. Cardiac auscultation using a stethoscope remains a time-honored tradition in medicine, the benefits of which extend beyond accurate recognition of heart sounds. Selective augmentation with, rather than wholesale replacement by, handheld ultrasound and newer technologies may improve diagnostic accuracy and better guide therapeutic decisions.

FURTHER READING

Edelman ER, Weber BN: Tenuous tether. N Engl J Med 373:2199, 2015.

Evangelista A et al: Hand-held cardiac ultrasound screening performed by family doctors with remote expert support interpretation. Heart 102:376, 2016.

Fang LC, O'Gara PT: The history and physical examination. An evidence-based approach, in *Braunwald's Heart Disease. A Textbook of Cardiovascular Medicine*, 11th ed, DP Zipes et al (eds). Philadelphia, Elsevier/Saunders, 2019, pp 83-101.

Fuster V: The stethoscope's prognosis. Very much alive and very necessary. J Am Coll Cardiol 67:1118, 2016.

Otto CM et al: 2020 AHA/ACC guideline for the management of patients with valvular heart disease. J Am Coll Cardiol 143:e72, 2021.

Stokke TM et al: Brief group training of medical students in focused cardiac ultrasound may improve diagnostic accuracy of physical examination. J Am Soc Echocardiogr 27:1238, 2014.

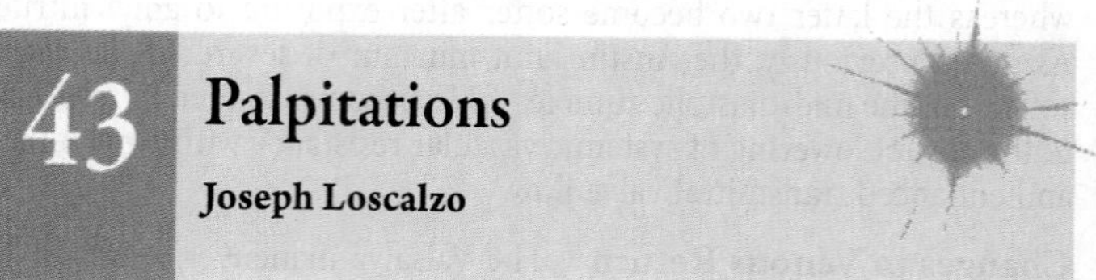

43 Palpitations

Joseph Loscalzo

Palpitations are extremely common among patients who present to their internists and can best be defined as a "thumping," "pounding," or "fluttering" sensation in the chest. This sensation can be either intermittent or sustained and either regular or irregular. Most patients interpret palpitations as an unusual awareness of the heartbeat and become especially concerned when they sense that they have had "skipped" or "missing" heartbeats. Palpitations are often noted when the patient is quietly resting, during which time other stimuli are minimal. Palpitations that are positional generally reflect a structural process within (e.g., atrial myxoma) or adjacent to (e.g., mediastinal mass) the heart.

Palpitations are brought about by cardiac (43%), psychiatric (31%), miscellaneous (10%), and unknown (16%) causes, according to one large series. Among the cardiovascular causes are premature atrial and ventricular contractions, supraventricular and ventricular arrhythmias, mitral valve prolapse (with or without associated arrhythmias), aortic insufficiency, atrial myxoma, myocarditis, and pulmonary embolism. Intermittent palpitations are commonly caused by premature atrial or ventricular contractions: the post-extrasystolic beat is sensed by the patient owing to the increase in ventricular end-diastolic dimension following the pause in the cardiac cycle and the increased strength of contraction (post-extrasystolic potentiation) of that beat. Regular, sustained palpitations can be caused by regular supraventricular and ventricular tachycardias. Irregular, sustained palpitations can be caused by atrial fibrillation. It is important to note that most arrhythmias are not associated with palpitations. In those that are, it is often useful either to ask the patient to "tap out" the rhythm of the palpitations or to take his or her pulse during palpitations. In general, hyperdynamic cardiovascular states caused by catecholaminergic stimulation from exercise, stress, or pheochromocytoma can lead to palpitations. Palpitations are common among athletes, especially older endurance athletes. In addition, the enlarged ventricle of aortic regurgitation and accompanying hyperdynamic precordium frequently lead to the sensation of palpitations. Other factors that enhance the strength of myocardial contraction, including tobacco, caffeine, aminophylline, atropine, thyroxine, cocaine, and amphetamines, can cause palpitations.

Psychiatric causes of palpitations include panic attacks or disorders, anxiety states, and somatization, alone or in combination. Patients with psychiatric causes for palpitations more commonly report a longer duration of the sensation (>15 min) and other accompanying symptoms than do patients with other causes. Among the miscellaneous causes of palpitations are thyrotoxicosis, drugs (see above) and ethanol, spontaneous skeletal muscle contractions of the chest wall, pheochromocytoma, and systemic mastocytosis.

APPROACH TO THE PATIENT

Palpitations

The principal goal in assessing patients with palpitations is to determine whether the symptom is caused by a life-threatening arrhythmia. Patients with preexisting coronary artery disease (CAD) or risk factors for CAD are at greatest risk for ventricular arrhythmias (**Chap. 246**) as a cause for palpitations. In addition, the association of palpitations with other symptoms suggesting hemodynamic compromise, including syncope or lightheadedness, supports this diagnosis. Palpitations caused by sustained tachyarrhythmias in patients with CAD can be accompanied by angina pectoris or dyspnea, and, in patients with ventricular dysfunction (systolic or diastolic), aortic stenosis, hypertrophic cardiomyopathy, or mitral stenosis (with or without CAD), can be accompanied by dyspnea from increased left atrial and pulmonary venous pressure.

Key features of the physical examination that will help confirm or refute the presence of an arrhythmia as a cause for palpitations (as well as its adverse hemodynamic consequences) include measurement of the vital signs, assessment of the jugular venous pressure and pulse, and auscultation of the chest and precordium. A resting electrocardiogram can be used to document the arrhythmia. If exertion is known to induce the arrhythmia and accompanying palpitations, exercise electrocardiography can be used to make the diagnosis. If the arrhythmia is sufficiently infrequent, other methods must be used, including continuous electrocardiographic (Holter) monitoring; telephonic monitoring, through which the patient can transmit an electrocardiographic tracing during a sensed episode; loop recordings (external or implantable), which can capture the electrocardiographic event for later review; and mobile (self-monitoring) cardiac outpatient telemetry. Data suggest that Holter monitoring is of limited clinical utility, while the implantable loop recorder and mobile cardiac outpatient telemetry are safe and possibly more cost-effective in the assessment of patients with (infrequent) recurrent, unexplained palpitations. The use of a diary or an electronic marker to indicate the timing of palpitations sensed by the patient is essential for appropriate interpretation of these studies.

Most patients with palpitations do not have serious arrhythmias or underlying structural heart disease. If sufficiently troubling to the patient, occasional benign atrial or ventricular premature contractions can often be managed with beta-blocker therapy. Palpitations incited by alcohol, tobacco, or illicit drugs need to be managed by abstention, while those caused by pharmacologic agents should be addressed by considering alternative therapies when appropriate or possible. Psychiatric causes of palpitations may benefit from cognitive therapy or pharmacotherapy. The physician should note that palpitations are at the very least bothersome and, on occasion, frightening to the patient. Once serious causes for the symptom have been excluded, the patient should be reassured that the palpitations will not adversely affect prognosis.

FURTHER READING

Crossland S, Berkin L: Problem based review: The patient with palpitations. Acute Med 11:169, 2012.

Jamshed N et al: Emergency management of palpitations in the elderly: Epidemiology, diagnostic approaches, and therapeutic options. Clin Geriatr Med 29:205, 2013.

Martson HR et al: Mobile self-monitoring ECG devices to diagnose arrhythmias that coincide with palpitations: A scoping review. Healthcare (Basel) 7:pii: E96, 2019.

Sakh R et al: Insertable cardiac monitors: current indications and devices. Expert Rev Med Devices 16:45, 2019.

Weber BE, Kapoor WN: Evaluation and outcomes of patients with palpitations. Am J Med 100:138, 1996.

Section 6 Alterations in Gastrointestinal Function

44 Dysphagia

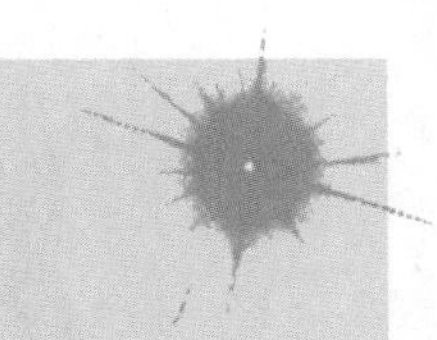

Ikuo Hirano, Peter J. Kahrilas

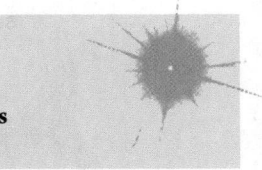

Dysphagia—difficulty with swallowing—refers to problems with the transit of food or liquid from the mouth to the hypopharynx or through the esophagus. Severe dysphagia can compromise nutrition, cause aspiration, and reduce quality of life. Additional terminology pertaining to swallowing dysfunction is as follows. *Aphagia* (inability to swallow) typically denotes complete esophageal obstruction, most commonly encountered in the acute setting of a food bolus or foreign body impaction. *Odynophagia* refers to painful swallowing, typically resulting from mucosal ulceration within the oropharynx or esophagus. It commonly is accompanied by dysphagia, but the converse is not true. *Globus pharyngeus* is a foreign body sensation localized in the neck that does not interfere with swallowing and sometimes is relieved by swallowing. *Transfer dysphagia* frequently results in nasal regurgitation or pulmonary aspiration during swallowing and is characteristic of oropharyngeal dysphagia. *Phagophobia* (fear of swallowing) and *refusal to swallow* may be psychogenic or related to anticipatory anxiety about food bolus obstruction, odynophagia, or aspiration.

PHYSIOLOGY OF SWALLOWING

Swallowing begins with a voluntary (oral) phase that includes preparation during which food is masticated and mixed with saliva. This is followed by a transfer phase during which the bolus is pushed into the pharynx by the tongue. Bolus entry into the hypopharynx initiates the pharyngeal swallow response, which is centrally mediated and involves a complex series of actions, the net result of which is to propel food through the pharynx into the esophagus while preventing its entry into the airway. To accomplish this, the larynx is elevated and pulled forward, actions that also facilitate upper esophageal sphincter (UES) opening. Tongue pulsion then propels the bolus through the UES, followed by a peristaltic contraction that clears residue from the pharynx and through the esophagus. The lower esophageal sphincter (LES) relaxes as the food enters the esophagus and remains relaxed until the peristaltic contraction has delivered the bolus into the stomach. Peristaltic contractions elicited in response to a swallow are called *primary peristalsis* and involve sequenced inhibition followed by contraction of the musculature along the entire length of the esophagus. The inhibition that precedes the peristaltic contraction is called *deglutitive inhibition*. Local distention of the esophagus anywhere along its length, as may occur with gastroesophageal reflux, activates *secondary peristalsis* that begins at the point of distention and proceeds distally. Tertiary esophageal contractions are nonperistaltic, disordered esophageal contractions that may be observed to occur spontaneously during fluoroscopic observation.

The musculature of the oral cavity, pharynx, UES, and cervical esophagus is striated and directly innervated by lower motor neurons carried in cranial nerves (**Fig. 44-1**). Oral cavity muscles are innervated by the fifth (trigeminal) and seventh (facial) cranial nerves; the tongue, by the twelfth (hypoglossal) cranial nerve. Pharyngeal muscles are innervated by the ninth (glossopharyngeal) and tenth (vagus) cranial nerves.

Physiologically, the UES consists of the cricopharyngeus muscle, the adjacent inferior pharyngeal constrictor, and the proximal portion of the cervical esophagus. UES innervation is derived from the vagus nerve, whereas the innervation to the musculature acting on the UES to facilitate its opening during swallowing comes from the fifth, seventh, and twelfth cranial nerves. The UES remains closed at rest owing to both its inherent elastic properties and neurogenically mediated contraction of the cricopharyngeus muscle. UES opening during swallowing involves both cessation of vagal excitation to the cricopharyngeus and simultaneous contraction of the suprahyoid and geniohyoid muscles that pull open the UES in conjunction with the upward and forward displacement of the larynx.

The neuromuscular apparatus for peristalsis is distinct in proximal and distal parts of the esophagus. The cervical esophagus, like the pharyngeal musculature, consists of striated muscle and is directly innervated by lower motor neurons of the vagus nerve. Peristalsis in the proximal esophagus is governed by the sequential activation of the vagal motor neurons in the nucleus ambiguus. In contrast, the distal esophagus and LES are composed of smooth muscle and are controlled by excitatory and inhibitory neurons within the esophageal myenteric plexus. Medullary preganglionic neurons from the dorsal motor nucleus of the vagus trigger peristalsis via these ganglionic neurons during primary peristalsis. Neurotransmitters of the excitatory ganglionic neurons are acetylcholine and substance P; those of the inhibitory neurons are vasoactive intestinal peptide and nitric oxide. Peristalsis results from the patterned activation of inhibitory followed by excitatory ganglionic neurons, with progressive dominance of the inhibitory neurons distally. Similarly, LES relaxation occurs with the onset of deglutitive inhibition and persists until the peristaltic sequence is complete. At rest, the LES is contracted because of excitatory ganglionic stimulation and its intrinsic myogenic tone, a property that distinguishes it from the adjacent esophagus. The function of the LES is supplemented by the surrounding muscle of the right diaphragmatic crus, which acts as an external sphincter during inspiration, cough, or abdominal straining.

PATHOPHYSIOLOGY OF DYSPHAGIA

Dysphagia can be subclassified both by location and by the circumstances in which it occurs. With respect to location, distinct considerations apply to oral, pharyngeal, or esophageal dysphagia. Normal transport of an ingested bolus depends on the consistency and size of the bolus, the caliber of the lumen, the integrity of peristaltic contraction, and deglutitive inhibition of both the UES and the LES. Dysphagia caused by an oversized bolus or a narrow lumen is called *structural dysphagia*, whereas dysphagia due to abnormalities of peristalsis or impaired sphincter relaxation after swallowing is called *propulsive* or

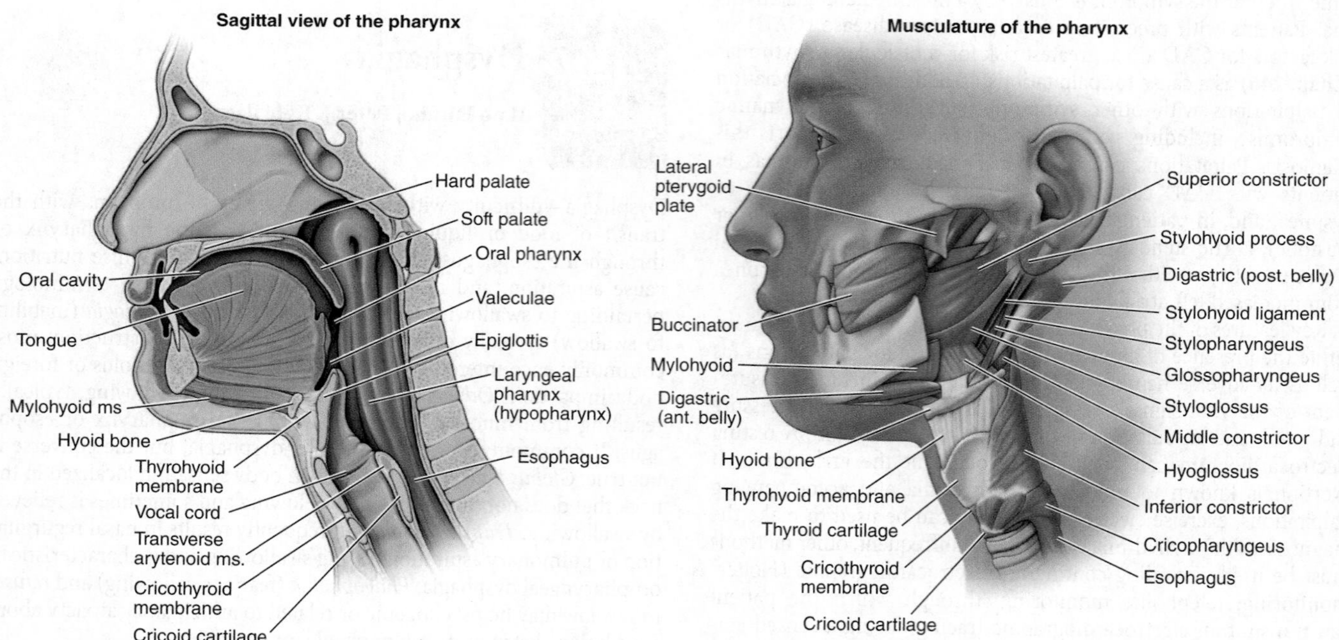

FIGURE 44-1 Sagittal and diagrammatic views of the musculature involved in enacting oropharyngeal swallowing. Note the dominance of the tongue in the sagittal view and the intimate relationship between the entrance to the larynx (airway) and the esophagus. In the resting configuration illustrated, the esophageal inlet is closed. This is transiently reconfigured such that the esophageal inlet is open and the laryngeal inlet closed during swallowing. *(Adapted from PJ Kahrilas, in DW Gelfand and JE Richter [eds]: Dysphagia: Diagnosis and Treatment. New York, Igaku-Shoin Medical Publishers, 1989, pp. 11–28.)*

motor dysphagia. More than one mechanism may be operative in a patient with dysphagia. Scleroderma commonly presents with absent peristalsis as well as a weakened LES that predisposes patients to peptic stricture formation. Likewise, radiation therapy for head and neck cancer may compound the functional deficits in the oropharyngeal swallow attributable to the tumor and cause cervical esophageal stenosis. It is worth noting that in addition to bolus transit, symptom reporting of dysphagia is dependent upon intact sensory innervation and central nervous system perception.

Oral and Pharyngeal (Oropharyngeal) Dysphagia Oral-phase dysphagia is associated with poor bolus formation and control so that food has prolonged retention within the oral cavity and may seep out of the mouth. Drooling and difficulty in initiating swallowing are other characteristic signs. Poor bolus control also may lead to premature spillage of food into the hypopharynx with resultant aspiration into the trachea or regurgitation into the nasal cavity. Pharyngeal-phase dysphagia is associated with retention of food in the pharynx due to poor tongue or pharyngeal propulsion or obstruction at the UES. Signs and symptoms of concomitant hoarseness or cranial nerve dysfunction may be associated with oropharyngeal dysphagia.

Oropharyngeal dysphagia may be due to neurologic, muscular, structural, iatrogenic, infectious, and metabolic causes. Iatrogenic, neurologic, and structural pathologies are most common. Iatrogenic causes include surgery and radiation, often in the setting of head and neck cancer. Neurogenic dysphagia resulting from cerebrovascular accidents, Parkinson's disease, and amyotrophic lateral sclerosis is a major source of morbidity related to aspiration and malnutrition. Medullary nuclei directly innervate the oropharynx. Lateralization of pharyngeal dysphagia implies either a structural pharyngeal lesion or a neurologic process that selectively targeted the ipsilateral brainstem nuclei or cranial nerve. Advances in functional brain imaging have elucidated an important role of the cerebral cortex in swallow function and dysphagia. Asymmetry in the cortical representation of the pharynx provides an explanation for the dysphagia that occurs as a consequence of unilateral cortical cerebrovascular accidents.

Oropharyngeal structural lesions causing dysphagia include Zenker's diverticulum, cricopharyngeal bar, and neoplasia. Zenker's diverticulum typically is encountered in elderly patients. In addition to dysphagia, patients may present with regurgitation of particulate food debris, aspiration, and halitosis. The pathogenesis is related to stenosis of the cricopharyngeus that causes diminished opening of the UES and results in increased hypopharyngeal pressure during swallowing with development of a pulsion diverticulum immediately above the cricopharyngeus in a region of potential weakness known as Killian's dehiscence. A cricopharyngeal bar, appearing as a prominent indentation behind the lower third of the cricoid cartilage, is related to Zenker's diverticulum in that it involves limited distensibility of the cricopharyngeus and can lead to the formation of a Zenker's diverticulum. However, a cricopharyngeal bar is a common radiographic finding, and most patients with transient cricopharyngeal bars are asymptomatic, making it important to rule out alternative etiologies of dysphagia before treatment. Furthermore, cricopharyngeal bars may be secondary to other neuromuscular disorders that impair opening of the UES.

Since the pharyngeal phase of swallowing occurs in less than a second, rapid-sequence fluoroscopy is necessary to evaluate for functional abnormalities. Adequate fluoroscopic examination requires that the patient be conscious and cooperative. The study incorporates recordings of swallow sequences during ingestion of food and liquids of varying consistencies. The pharynx is examined to detect bolus retention, regurgitation into the nose, or aspiration into the trachea. Timing and integrity of pharyngeal contraction and opening of the UES with a swallow are analyzed to assess both aspiration risk and the potential for swallow therapy. Structural abnormalities of the oropharynx, especially those that may require biopsies, also should be assessed by direct laryngoscopic examination.

Esophageal Dysphagia The adult esophagus measures 18–26 cm in length and is anatomically divided into the cervical esophagus, extending from the pharyngoesophageal junction to the suprasternal notch, and the thoracic esophagus, which continues to the diaphragmatic hiatus. When distended, the esophageal lumen has internal dimensions of about 2 cm in the anteroposterior plane and 3 cm in the lateral plane. Solid food dysphagia becomes common when the lumen is narrowed to <13 mm, but also can occur with larger diameters in the setting of poorly masticated food or motor dysfunction. Circumferential lesions are more likely to cause dysphagia than are lesions that involve only a partial circumference of the esophageal wall. The most common structural causes of dysphagia are Schatzki's rings, eosinophilic esophagitis, and peptic strictures. Dysphagia also occurs in the setting of gastroesophageal reflux disease without a stricture, perhaps on the basis of altered esophageal sensation, reduced esophageal mural distensibility, or motor dysfunction.

Propulsive disorders leading to esophageal dysphagia result from abnormalities of peristalsis and/or deglutitive inhibition, potentially affecting the cervical or thoracic esophagus. Since striated muscle pathology usually involves both the oropharynx and the cervical esophagus, the clinical manifestations usually are dominated by oropharyngeal dysphagia. Diseases affecting smooth muscle involve both the thoracic esophagus and the LES. A dominant manifestation of this, absent peristalsis, refers to either the complete absence of swallow-induced contraction (absent contractility) or the presence of nonperistaltic, disordered contractions. Absent peristalsis and failure of deglutitive LES relaxation are the defining features of achalasia. In diffuse esophageal spasm (DES), LES function is normal, with the disordered motility restricted to the esophageal body. Absent contractility combined with severe weakness of the LES is a pattern commonly found in patients with scleroderma.

APPROACH TO THE PATIENT

Dysphagia

Figure 44-2 shows an algorithm for the approach to a patient with dysphagia.

HISTORY

The patient history is extremely valuable in making a presumptive diagnosis or at least substantially limiting the differential diagnoses in most patients. Key elements of the history are the localization of dysphagia, the circumstances in which dysphagia is experienced, other symptoms associated with dysphagia, and progression. Dysphagia that localizes to the suprasternal notch may indicate either an oropharyngeal or an esophageal etiology as distal dysphagia is referred proximally about 30% of the time. Dysphagia that localizes to the chest is esophageal in origin. Nasal regurgitation and tracheobronchial aspiration manifest by coughing with swallowing are hallmarks of oropharyngeal dysphagia. Severe cough with swallowing may also be a sign of a tracheoesophageal fistula. The presence of hoarseness may be another important diagnostic clue. When hoarseness precedes dysphagia, the primary lesion is usually laryngeal; hoarseness that occurs after the development of dysphagia may result from compromise of the recurrent laryngeal nerve by a malignancy. The type of food causing dysphagia is an important consideration. Intermittent dysphagia that occurs only with solid food implies structural dysphagia, whereas constant dysphagia with both liquids and solids strongly suggests an esophageal motor abnormality. Two caveats to this pattern are that despite having a motor abnormality, patients with scleroderma generally develop mild dysphagia for solids only and that patients with oropharyngeal dysphagia often have greater difficulty managing liquids than solids. Dysphagia that is progressive over the course of weeks to months raises concern for neoplasia. Episodic dysphagia to solids that is unchanged or slowly progressive over years indicates a benign disease process such as a Schatzki ring or eosinophilic

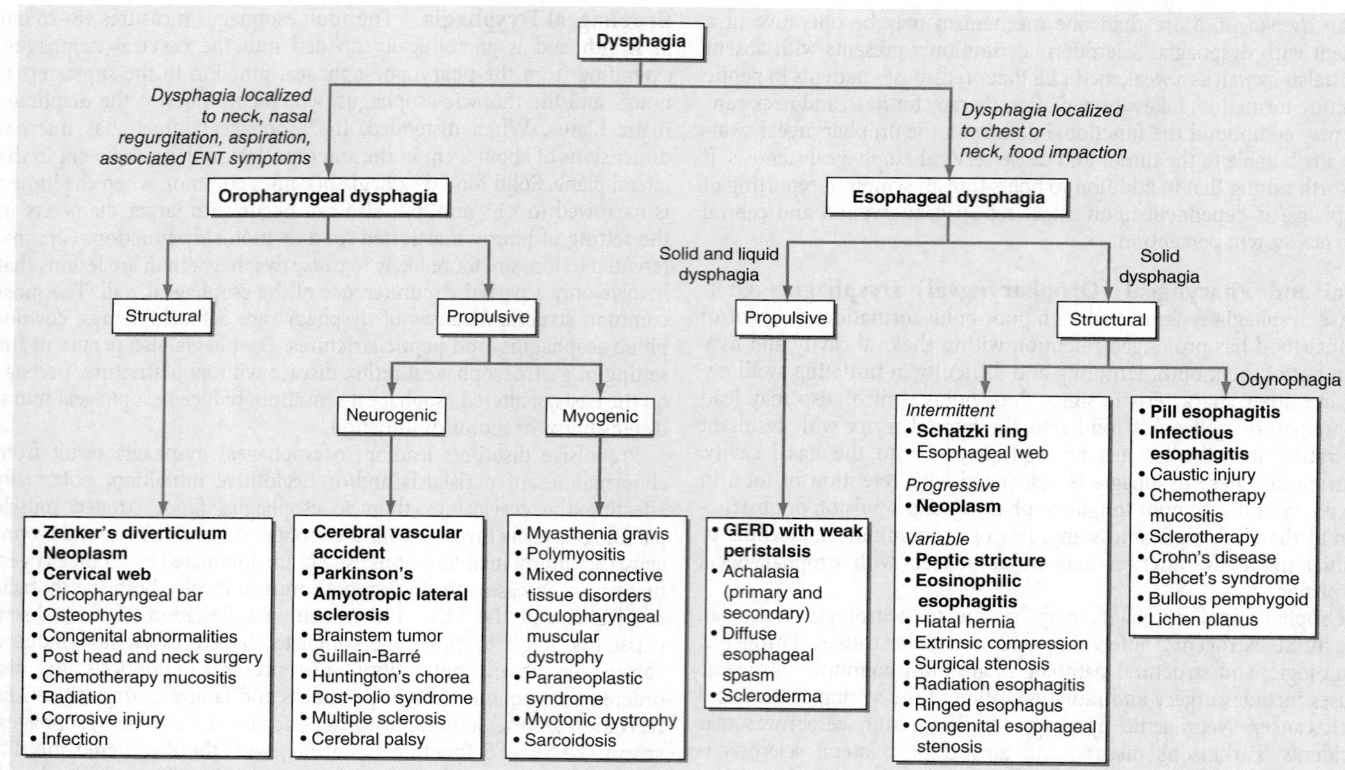

FIGURE 44-2 Approach to the patient with dysphagia. Etiologies in bold print are the most common. ENT, ear, nose, and throat; GERD, gastroesophageal reflux disease.

esophagitis. Food impaction with a prolonged inability to pass an ingested bolus even with ingestion of liquid is typical of a structural dysphagia. Chest pain may accompany dysphagia whether it is related to motor disorders, structural disorders, or reflux disease. A prolonged history of heartburn preceding the onset of dysphagia is suggestive of peptic stricture and, infrequently, esophageal adenocarcinoma. A history of prolonged nasogastric intubation, esophageal or head and neck surgery, ingestion of caustic agents or pills, previous radiation or chemotherapy, or associated mucocutaneous diseases may help isolate the cause of dysphagia. With accompanying odynophagia, which usually is indicative of ulceration, infectious or pill-induced esophagitis should be suspected. In patients with AIDS or other immunocompromised states, esophagitis due to opportunistic infections such as *Candida*, herpes simplex virus, or cytomegalovirus and to tumors such as Kaposi's sarcoma and lymphoma should be considered. A history of atopy increases concerns for eosinophilic esophagitis, which is most prevalent in Caucasian male patients between the ages of 20 and 40 years. Medication use should identify agents associated with pill esophagitis and narcotics that are associated with opioid-induced esophageal dysmotility.

PHYSICAL EXAMINATION

Physical examination is important in the evaluation of oral and pharyngeal dysphagia because dysphagia is usually only one of many manifestations of a more global disease process. Signs of bulbar or pseudobulbar palsy, including dysarthria, dysphonia, ptosis, and tongue atrophy, in addition to evidence of generalized neuromuscular disease, should be elicited. The neck should be examined for thyromegaly or lymphadenopathy. A careful inspection of the mouth and pharynx should disclose inflammatory or infectious lesions. Missing dentition can interfere with mastication and exacerbate an existing cause of dysphagia. Physical examination is less helpful in the evaluation of esophageal dysphagia as most relevant pathology is restricted to the esophagus. The notable exception is skin disease. Changes in the skin and oral mucosa may suggest a diagnosis of scleroderma or mucocutaneous diseases such as pemphigoid, lichen planus, and epidermolysis bullosa, all of which can involve the esophagus.

DIAGNOSTIC PROCEDURES

Although most instances of dysphagia are attributable to benign disease processes, dysphagia is also a cardinal symptom of several malignancies, making it an important symptom to evaluate. Cancer may result in dysphagia most commonly as the result of intraluminal obstruction (esophageal or proximal gastric cancer, metastatic deposits) and less commonly due to extrinsic compression (lymphoma, lung cancer) or paraneoplastic syndromes. Even when not attributable to malignancy, dysphagia is usually a manifestation of an identifiable and treatable disease entity, making its evaluation beneficial to the patient and gratifying to the practitioner. The specific diagnostic algorithm to pursue is guided by the details of the history (Fig. 44-2). If oral or pharyngeal dysphagia is suspected, a fluoroscopic swallow study, usually done by a swallow therapist, is the procedure of choice. Otolaryngoscopic and neurologic evaluation also can be important, depending on the circumstances. For suspected esophageal dysphagia, upper endoscopy is the single most useful test. Endoscopy allows better visualization of mucosal lesions than does barium radiography and also allows for procurement of mucosal biopsies. Endoscopic or histologic abnormalities are evident in the leading causes of esophageal dysphagia: Schatzki's ring, gastroesophageal reflux disease, and eosinophilic esophagitis. Furthermore, therapeutic intervention with esophageal dilation can be done as part of the procedure if it is deemed necessary. The emergence of eosinophilic esophagitis as a leading cause of dysphagia in both children and adults has led to the recommendation that esophageal mucosal biopsies be obtained routinely in the evaluation of unexplained dysphagia even if characteristic, endoscopically identified esophageal mucosal features are absent. For cases of suspected esophageal motility disorders, endoscopy is still the appropriate initial evaluation as neoplastic and inflammatory conditions can secondarily produce patterns of either achalasia or esophageal spasm. Esophageal manometry is done if dysphagia is not adequately explained by endoscopy or to confirm the diagnosis of a suspected esophageal motor disorder. Barium radiography can provide useful adjunctive information in cases of subtle or complex esophageal strictures, prior esophageal surgery, esophageal diverticula, or paraesophageal herniation. Use of a barium tablet in conjunction with fluoroscopy can identify strictures and esophageal motility disorders that may be overlooked with liquid barium. In specific cases, computed tomography (CT) examination, esophageal manometry with solid meal challenge, and endoscopic ultrasonography may be useful.

TREATMENT

Treatment of dysphagia depends on both the locus and the specific etiology. Oropharyngeal dysphagia most commonly results from functional deficits caused by neurologic disorders. In such circumstances, the treatment focuses on utilizing postures or maneuvers devised to reduce pharyngeal residue and enhance airway protection learned under the direction of a swallow therapist. Aspiration risk may be reduced by altering the consistency of ingested food and liquid. Dysphagia resulting from a cerebrovascular accident usually, but not always, spontaneously improves within the first few weeks after the event. More severe and persistent cases may require consideration of gastrostomy and enteral feeding. Patients with myasthenia gravis (**Chap. 448**) and polymyositis (**Chap. 365**) may respond to medical treatment of the primary neuromuscular disease. Surgical intervention with cricopharyngeal myotomy is usually not helpful, with the exception of specific disorders such as symptomatic cricopharyngeal bar, Zenker's diverticulum, and oculopharyngeal muscular dystrophy. Chronic neurologic disorders such as Parkinson's disease and amyotrophic lateral sclerosis may manifest with severe oropharyngeal dysphagia. Feeding by a nasogastric tube or an endoscopically placed gastrostomy tube may be considered for nutritional support; however, these maneuvers do not provide protection against aspiration of salivary secretions or refluxed gastric contents.

Treatment of esophageal dysphagia is covered in detail in **Chap. 323**. The majority of causes of structural, esophageal dysphagia are effectively managed by means of esophageal dilation using bougie or balloon dilators. Cancer and achalasia are often managed surgically, although endoscopic techniques are available for both palliation and primary therapy, respectively. Infectious etiologies respond to antimicrobial medications or treatment of the underlying immunosuppressive state. Finally, eosinophilic esophagitis is an important and increasingly recognized cause of dysphagia that is amenable to treatment by elimination of dietary allergens, proton pump inhibition or swallowed, topically acting glucocorticoids in combination with esophageal dilation for persistent strictures.

FURTHER READING

Hirano I: Esophagus: Anatomy and structural anomalies, in *Yamada Atlas of Gastroenterology*, 6th ed. New York, Wiley-Blackwell Publishing Co., 2016, pp 42–59.

Kahrilas PJ et al: The Chicago Classification of esophageal motility disorders, v3.0. Neurogastroenterol Motil 27:160, 2015.

Kim JP, Kahrilas PJ: How I approach dysphagia. Curr Gastroenterol Rep 21:49, 2019.

Pandolfino JP, Kahrilas PJ: Esophageal neuromuscular function and motility disorders, in *Sleisenger and Fordtran's Gastrointestinal and Liver Disease*, 10th ed, Feldman M, Friedman LS, Brandt LJ (eds). Philadelphia, Elsevier, 2016, pp 701–732.

Shaker R et al (eds): *Principles of Deglutition: A Multidisciplinary Text for Swallowing and Its Disorders*. New York, Springer, 2013.

45 Nausea, Vomiting, and Indigestion

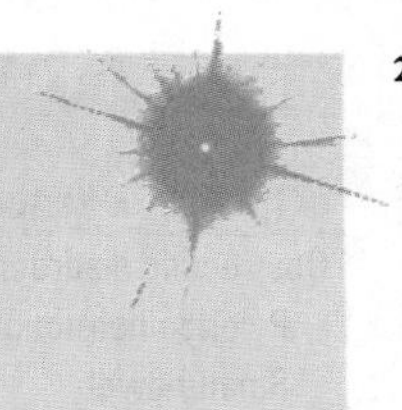

William L. Hasler

Nausea is the feeling of a need to vomit. *Vomiting* (emesis) is the oral expulsion of gastrointestinal contents resulting from gut and thoracoabdominal wall contractions. Vomiting is contrasted with *regurgitation*, the effortless passage of gastric contents into the mouth. *Rumination* is the repeated regurgitation of food residue, which may be rechewed and reswallowed. In contrast to emesis, these phenomena exhibit volitional control. *Indigestion* encompasses a range of complaints including nausea, vomiting, heartburn, regurgitation, and dyspepsia (symptoms thought to originate in the gastroduodenal region). Some individuals with dyspepsia experience postprandial fullness, early satiety (inability to complete a meal due to premature fullness), bloating, eructation (belching), and anorexia. Others report predominantly epigastric burning or pain. Nausea, vomiting, and dyspepsia have been correlated with a condition now called avoidant/restrictive food intake disorder.

NAUSEA AND VOMITING

MECHANISMS

Vomiting is coordinated by the brainstem and is effected by responses in the gut, pharynx, and somatic musculature. Mechanisms underlying nausea are poorly understood but likely involve the cerebral cortex, as nausea requires cognitive and emotional input and is associated with autonomic responses including diaphoresis, pallor, and altered heart rate. Functional brain imaging studies support this idea showing activation of cerebral regions including the insula, anterior cingulate cortex, and amygdala during nausea.

Coordination of Emesis Brainstem nuclei—including the nucleus tractus solitarius; dorsal vagal and phrenic nuclei; medullary nuclei regulating respiration; and nuclei that control pharyngeal, facial, and tongue movements—coordinate initiation of emesis involving neurokinin NK_1, serotonin 5-HT_3, endocannabinoid, and vasopressin pathways.

Somatic and visceral muscles respond stereotypically during emesis. Inspiratory thoracic and abdominal wall muscles contract, increasing intrathoracic and intraabdominal pressures to evacuate the stomach. Under normal conditions, distally migrating gut contractions are coordinated by an electrical phenomenon, the slow wave, which cycles at 3 cycles/min in the stomach and 11 cycles/min in the duodenum. During emesis, slow waves are abolished and replaced by orally propagating spikes that evoke retrograde contractions to facilitate expulsion of gut contents.

Activators of Emesis Emetic stimuli act at several sites. Emesis evoked by unpleasant thoughts or smells originates in the brain. Motion sickness and inner ear disorders act on labyrinthine pathways. Gastric irritants and cytotoxic agents like cisplatin stimulate gastroduodenal vagal afferent nerves. Nongastric afferents are activated by bowel obstruction and mesenteric ischemia. The area postrema, in the medulla, responds to bloodborne stimuli (emetogenic drugs, bacterial toxins, uremia, hypoxia, ketoacidosis) and is termed the *chemoreceptor trigger zone*.

Neurotransmitters mediating vomiting are selective for different sites. Labyrinthine disorders stimulate vestibular muscarinic M_1 and histaminergic H_1 receptors. Vagal afferent stimuli activate 5-HT_3 receptors. The area postrema is served by nerves acting on 5-HT_3, M_1, H_1, and dopamine D_2 subtypes. NK_1 receptors in the central nervous system (CNS) mediate both nausea and vomiting. Cannabinoid CB_1 pathways may participate in the cerebral cortex and brainstem. Therapies for vomiting act on these receptor-mediated pathways.

TABLE 45-1 Causes of Nausea and Vomiting

INTRAPERITONEAL	EXTRAPERITONEAL	MEDICATIONS/ METABOLIC DISORDERS
Obstructing disorders	Cardiopulmonary disease	Drugs
Pyloric obstruction	Cardiomyopathy	Cancer chemotherapy
Small-bowel obstruction	Myocardial infarction	Analgesics
Colonic obstruction	Labyrinthine disease	Opioids
Superior mesenteric artery syndrome	Motion sickness	Antibiotics
Enteric infections	Labyrinthitis	Cardiac antiarrhythmics
Viral	Malignancy	Digoxin
Bacterial	Intracerebral disorders	Oral hypoglycemics
Inflammatory diseases	Malignancy	Oral contraceptives
Cholecystitis	Hemorrhage	Antidepressants
Pancreatitis	Abscess	Restless legs/ Parkinson's therapies
Appendicitis	Hydrocephalus	Smoking cessation agents
Hepatitis	Psychiatric illness	Endocrine/metabolic disease
Altered sensorimotor function	Anorexia and bulimia nervosa	Pregnancy
Gastroparesis	Depression	Uremia
Intestinal pseudoobstruction	Postoperative vomiting	Ketoacidosis
Gastroesophageal reflux		Thyroid and parathyroid disease
Chronic nausea vomiting syndrome		Adrenal insufficiency
Cyclic vomiting syndrome		Toxins
Cannabinoid hyperemesis syndrome		Liver failure
Rumination syndrome		Ethanol
Mesenteric insufficiency		
Celiac artery stenosis		
Median arcuate ligament syndrome		
Biliary colic		
Abdominal irradiation		

DIFFERENTIAL DIAGNOSIS

Nausea and vomiting are caused by conditions within and outside the gut, drugs, and circulating toxins (**Table 45-1**). Unexplained chronic nausea and vomiting is reported by 2–3% of the population.

Intraperitoneal Disorders Obstruction and inflammation of hollow and solid viscera may elicit vomiting. Ulcers and malignancy cause gastric obstruction, while adhesions, benign or malignant tumors, volvulus, intussusception, or inflammatory diseases like Crohn's disease cause small intestinal and colonic obstruction. The superior mesenteric artery syndrome, occurring after weight loss or prolonged bed rest, results when the duodenum is compressed by the overlying superior mesenteric artery. Median arcuate ligament syndrome, with compression of the celiac artery, is a rare cause of vomiting. Abdominal irradiation impairs intestinal motility and induces strictures. Biliary colic causes nausea by acting on afferent nerves. Vomiting with pancreatitis, cholecystitis, and appendicitis results from visceral irritation and induction of ileus. Enteric infectious causes of vomiting include viruses (norovirus, rotavirus), bacteria (*Staphylococcus aureus*, *Bacillus cereus*), and opportunistic organisms like cytomegalovirus or herpes simplex in immunocompromised individuals.

Gut sensorimotor dysfunction often causes nausea and vomiting. *Gastroparesis* presents with these symptoms with evidence of delayed gastric emptying and occurs after vagotomy or with pancreatic carcinoma, mesenteric vascular insufficiency, or organic diseases like diabetes, scleroderma, and amyloidosis. Idiopathic gastroparesis is the most prevalent etiology; it occurs in the absence of systemic illness and follow a viral illness in ~15–20% of cases. Rapid gastric emptying is associated with nausea and vomiting in some conditions. *Intestinal pseudoobstruction* is characterized by disrupted intestinal motility with retention of food residue and secretions; bacterial overgrowth; nutrient malabsorption; and symptoms of nausea, vomiting, bloating, pain, and altered defecation. Intestinal pseudoobstruction may be idiopathic, inherited, result from systemic disease like scleroderma or an infiltrative process like amyloidosis, or occur as a paraneoplastic consequence of malignancy (e.g., small-cell lung carcinoma). Patients with gastroesophageal reflux, irritable bowel syndrome (IBS), or chronic constipation often report nausea and vomiting.

Other functional gastroduodenal disorders without organic abnormalities have been characterized. *Chronic nausea vomiting syndrome* is defined as bothersome nausea at least 1 day and/or one or more vomiting episodes weekly in the absence of an eating disorder or psychiatric disease. *Cyclic vomiting syndrome (CVS)* causes 3–14% of cases of unexplained nausea and vomiting and presents with discrete episodes of relentless vomiting and is associated with migraines. Some adult cases have been associated with rapid gastric emptying. A related condition, *cannabinoid hyperemesis syndrome (CHS)*, presents with cyclical vomiting in individuals (mostly men) with long-standing use of large quantities of cannabis and resolves with its discontinuation. *Rumination syndrome* is often misdiagnosed as refractory vomiting.

Extraperitoneal Disorders Myocardial infarction and congestive heart failure may cause nausea and vomiting. Postoperative emesis occurs after 25% of surgeries, especially abdominal and orthopedic surgery. Increased intracranial pressure from tumors, bleeding, abscess, or blockage of cerebrospinal fluid outflow produces vomiting with or without nausea. Patients with anorexia nervosa, bulimia nervosa, anxiety, and depression often report significant nausea associated with delayed gastric emptying.

Medications and Metabolic Disorders Drugs evoke vomiting by action on the stomach (analgesics, erythromycin) or area postrema (opioids, anti-parkinsonian drugs). Other emetogenic agents include antibiotics, cardiac antiarrhythmics, antihypertensives, oral hypoglycemics, antidepressants (selective serotonin and serotonin norepinephrine reuptake inhibitors), smoking cessation drugs (varenicline, nicotine), and contraceptives. Cancer chemotherapy causes acute (within hours of administration), delayed (after 1 or more days), or anticipatory vomiting. Acute emesis from highly emetogenic agents (e.g., cisplatin) is mediated by 5-HT_3 pathways. Delayed emesis is more dependent on NK_1 mechanisms. Anticipatory nausea may respond to anxiolytic therapy rather than antiemetics.

Metabolic disorders elicit nausea and vomiting. Nausea affects 70% of women in the first trimester of pregnancy. Hyperemesis gravidarum is a severe form of nausea of pregnancy that produces dehydration and electrolyte disturbances and has been proposed to result from excessive amounts of a blood protein—growth differentiation factor 15. Uremia, ketoacidosis, adrenal insufficiency, and parathyroid and thyroid disease are other metabolic etiologies.

Circulating toxins evoke emesis via effects on the area postrema. Endogenous toxins are generated in fulminant liver failure, whereas exogenous enterotoxins may be produced by enteric bacterial infection. Ethanol intoxication is a common toxic etiology of nausea and vomiting.

APPROACH TO THE PATIENT

Nausea and Vomiting

HISTORY AND PHYSICAL EXAMINATION

The history helps define the etiology of nausea and vomiting. Drugs, toxins, and infections often cause acute symptoms, whereas established illnesses evoke chronic complaints. Gastroparesis and pyloric obstruction elicit vomiting within an hour of eating. Emesis from intestinal blockage occurs later. Vomiting occurring minutes after meal consumption prompts consideration of rumination syndrome. With severe gastric emptying delays, vomitus may contain food residue ingested days before. Hematemesis raises suspicion of ulcer, malignancy, or Mallory-Weiss tear. Feculent emesis is noted with distal intestinal or colonic obstruction. Bilious vomiting excludes gastric obstruction, whereas emesis of undigested food is consistent with a Zenker's diverticulum or achalasia. Vomiting can relieve abdominal pain from a bowel obstruction but has no effect in pancreatitis or cholecystitis. Weight loss raises concern about malignancy. Taking prolonged hot baths or showers is associated with CHS and CVS. Intracranial sources are considered if there are headaches or visual changes. Vertigo or tinnitus indicates labyrinthine disease.

The physical examination complements the history. Orthostatic hypotension and reduced skin turgor indicate intravascular fluid loss. Pulmonary abnormalities raise concern for aspiration of vomitus. Bowel sounds are absent with ileus. High-pitched rushes suggest bowel obstruction, whereas a succussion splash is found with gastroparesis or pyloric obstruction. Involuntary guarding raises suspicion of inflammation. Fecal blood suggests ulcer, ischemia, or tumor. Neurologic disease presents with papilledema, visual loss, or focal neural abnormalities. Neoplasm is suggested by palpable masses or adenopathy.

DIAGNOSTIC TESTING

For intractable symptoms or an elusive diagnosis, screening testing can direct care. Electrolyte replacement is indicated for hypokalemia or metabolic alkalosis. Iron-deficiency anemia mandates exclusion of mucosal causes. Abnormal pancreatic or liver biochemistries are found with pancreaticobiliary disease. Endocrinologic, rheumatologic, or paraneoplastic etiologies are suggested by hormone or serologic abnormalities. Supine and upright abdominal radiographs may show intestinal air-fluid levels and reduced colonic air with small-bowel obstruction. Ileus is characterized by diffusely dilated air-filled bowel loops.

Anatomic studies are indicated if initial testing is nondiagnostic. Upper endoscopy detects ulcers, malignancy, and retained food in gastroparesis. Small-bowel barium radiography or computed tomography (CT) diagnoses partial bowel obstruction. Colonoscopy or contrast enema radiography detects colonic obstruction. Ultrasound or CT defines intraperitoneal inflammation; CT and magnetic resonance imaging (MRI) enterography define inflammation in Crohn's disease. Brain CT or MRI delineates intracranial disease. Mesenteric angiography, CT, or MRI is useful for suspected ischemia.

Gastrointestinal motility testing can detect an underlying motor disorder. Gastroparesis commonly is diagnosed by gastric scintigraphy, which measures emptying of a radiolabeled meal. A nonradioactive ^{13}C-labeled gastric emptying breath test is an alternative to scintigraphy. Intestinal pseudoobstruction is suggested by luminal dilation on imaging or abnormal transit on contrast radiography or intestinal scintigraphy. Wireless motility capsules diagnose gastroparesis or small-bowel dysmotility by detecting local or generalized transit delays in the stomach or small bowel from characteristic pH changes between regions. Small-intestinal manometry confirms a diagnosis of pseudoobstruction and discriminates between neuropathic or myopathic disease based on contractile patterns. Manometry can obviate the need for surgical intestinal biopsy to detect smooth muscle or neuronal degeneration. Combined ambulatory esophageal pH/impedance testing and high-resolution manometry facilitates diagnosis of rumination syndrome. Impedance planimetry detects reduced pyloric distensibility in some cases of gastroparesis.

TREATMENT
Nausea and Vomiting

GENERAL PRINCIPLES

Therapy of vomiting is tailored to correct remediable abnormalities if possible. Patients with severe dehydration should be hospitalized if oral fluid replenishment is unsustainable. Once oral intake is tolerated, low-fat liquid nutrients are restarted because lipids delay gastric emptying. Low-residue, small-particle diets have shown efficacy in gastroparesis. Glycemic control should be optimized to reduce diabetic gastroparesis symptoms.

ANTIEMETIC MEDICATIONS

Most antiemetic agents act on CNS sites (**Table 45-2**). Antihistamines like dimenhydrinate and meclizine and anticholinergics like scopolamine act on vestibular pathways to treat motion sickness and labyrinthine disorders. D_2 antagonists treat emesis evoked by area postrema stimuli including medications, toxins, and metabolic disturbances. Dopamine antagonists cross the blood-brain barrier and cause anxiety, movement disorders, and hyperprolactinemic effects (galactorrhea, sexual dysfunction).

Other classes exhibit antiemetic properties. 5-HT_3 antagonists like ondansetron and granisetron prevent postoperative vomiting, radiation therapy–induced symptoms, and cancer chemotherapy–induced emesis, but also are used for other conditions. NK_1 antagonists like aprepitant are approved for chemotherapy-induced vomiting. Aprepitant reduces gastroparesis symptoms. Tricyclic antidepressants reduce symptoms in some patients with functional causes of vomiting, but did not show benefits in a controlled trial in gastroparesis. Other antidepressants such as mirtazapine and olanzapine and the pain-modulating agent gabapentin also exhibit antiemetic effects in some clinical settings.

GASTROINTESTINAL MOTOR STIMULANTS

Drugs that stimulate gastric emptying are used for gastroparesis (Table 45-2). Metoclopramide, a combined 5-HT_4 agonist and D_2 antagonist, is effective in gastroparesis, but antidopaminergic side effects, including dystonias and mood disturbances, limit use in ~25% of cases. Erythromycin increases gastroduodenal motility by action on receptors for motilin, an endogenous transmitter that regulates fasting motility. Intravenous erythromycin is useful for inpatients with refractory gastroparesis. Benefits of long-term oral erythromycin are limited by development of tolerance. Domperidone, a D_2 antagonist not available in the United States, exhibits prokinetic and antiemetic effects but does not cross into most brain regions. The drug rarely causes dystonic reactions but can induce hyperprolactinemic side effects via penetration of pituitary regions served by a porous blood-brain barrier. Prucalopride, a 5-HT_4 agonist, has shown efficacy in accelerating gastric emptying and improving symptoms in idiopathic gastroparesis.

Refractory motility disorders pose challenges. Intestinal pseudoobstruction may respond to the somatostatin analogue octreotide, which induces propagative small-intestinal motor complexes. Acetylcholinesterase inhibitors like pyridostigmine benefit some patients with small-bowel dysmotility. Pyloric botulinum toxin injections reduced gastroparesis symptoms in uncontrolled studies, but small controlled trials observed benefits no greater than sham treatments. Surgical pyloroplasty and gastric peroral endoscopic myotomy (G-POEM) of the pylorus improved symptoms in case series. Enteral feedings through a jejunostomy reduce hospitalizations and improve overall health in some patients with refractory gastroparesis. Subtotal gastric resection may improve some cases of postvagotomy gastroparesis, but its utility for other gastroparesis etiologies is unproven. Implanted gastric electrical stimulators may reduce symptoms, enhance nutrition, improve quality of life, and decrease health care expenditures in medication-refractory gastroparesis; a controlled trial has confirmed modest improvement in vomiting.

SAFETY CONSIDERATIONS

Safety concerns have been raised about selected antiemetics. Metoclopramide can cause irreversible movement disorders like tardive dyskinesia, particularly in older patients. This complication should be explained and documented in the medical record. Domperidone, erythromycin, tricyclic antidepressants, and 5-HT_3 antagonists increase risk of cardiac arrhythmias and sudden cardiac death in

TABLE 45-2 Treatment of Nausea and Vomiting

TREATMENT	MECHANISM	EXAMPLES	CLINICAL INDICATIONS
Antiemetic agents	Antihistaminergic	Dimenhydrinate, meclizine	Motion sickness, inner ear disease
	Anticholinergic	Scopolamine	Motion sickness, inner ear disease
	Antidopaminergic	Prochlorperazine, thiethylperazine, haloperidol	Medication-, toxin-, or metabolic-induced emesis, chemotherapy-induced nausea and vomiting, ?cannabinoid hyperemesis syndrome
	5-HT_3 antagonist	Ondansetron, granisetron	Chemotherapy- and radiation-induced emesis, postoperative emesis, opioid-induced nausea and vomiting
	Cannabinoids	Tetrahydrocannabinol	Chemotherapy-induced emesis
	Tricyclic antidepressant	Amitriptyline, nortriptyline	Functional vomiting, chronic idiopathic nausea, cyclic vomiting syndrome, ?gastroparesis
	Other antidepressant	Mirtazapine, olanzapine	Functional dyspepsia, ?gastroparesis
	Neuropathic modulator	Gabapentin	Chemotherapy-induced nausea and vomiting
	Neurokinin (NK1) receptor antagonists	Aprepitant, fosaprepitant, netupitant, rolapitant	Chemotherapy-induced emesis
Prokinetic agents	5-HT_4 agonist and antidopaminergic	Metoclopramide	Gastroparesis
	Motilin agonist	Erythromycin	Gastroparesis, ?intestinal pseudoobstruction
	Peripheral antidopaminergic	Domperidone	Gastroparesis
	Pure 5-HT_4 agonist	Prucalopride	?Idiopathic gastroparesis
	Somatostatin analogue	Octreotide	Intestinal pseudoobstruction
	Acetylcholinesterase inhibitor	Pyridostigmine	?Small-intestinal dysmotility/pseudoobstruction
Special settings	Benzodiazepines	Lorazepam	Anticipatory nausea and vomiting with chemotherapy, cyclic vomiting syndrome
	5-HT_{1A} agonist	Buspirone	Functional dyspepsia
	Glucocorticoids	Methylprednisolone, dexamethasone	Chemotherapy-induced emesis
	Anticonvulsants	Topiramate, zonisamide, levetiracetam	Cyclic vomiting syndrome
	Antimigraine agents	Sumatriptan	Cyclic vomiting syndrome
	Topical analgesic	Capsaicin cream	?Cannabinoid hyperemesis syndrome
	Atypical antipsychotic agent	Olanzapine	Chemotherapy-induced and breakthrough emesis

Note: ?, indication is uncertain.

those with QTc interval prolongation on electrocardiography (ECG). Surveillance ECG testing is advocated for some of these agents.

OTHER CLINICAL SETTINGS

Some cancer chemotherapies are intensely emetogenic **(Chap. 73)**. Combining a 5-HT_3 antagonist, an NK_1 antagonist, and a glucocorticoid can control both acute and delayed vomiting after highly emetogenic chemotherapy. Benzodiazepines like lorazepam reduce anticipatory nausea and vomiting. Other therapies with benefit in chemotherapy-induced emesis include cannabinoids, olanzapine, gabapentin, and alternative therapies like ginger. Most antiemetic regimens produce greater reductions in chemotherapy-induced vomiting than nausea.

Clinicians should exercise caution in managing nausea of pregnancy. Studies of the teratogenic effects of antiemetic agents provide conflicting results. Antihistamines like meclizine and doxylamine, antidopaminergics like prochlorperazine, and antiserotonergics like ondansetron demonstrate limited efficacy. Some obstetricians recommend alternative therapies including pyridoxine, acupressure, or ginger.

Managing CVS and CHS is challenging. Prophylaxis with tricyclic antidepressants or anticonvulsants (topiramate, zonisamide, levetiracetam) reduces the severity and frequency of CVS attacks in uncontrolled reports. Combining intravenous 5-HT_3 antagonists with the sedating effects of a benzodiazepine like lorazepam are mainstays for aborting acute flares. Small studies report benefits with aprepitant and injectable or intranasal forms of the 5-HT_1 agonist sumatriptan to manage acute CVS episodes. These treatments are reportedly less effective for CHS, but haloperidol and topical capsaicin cream may reduce acute CHS attacks.

INDIGESTION

■ MECHANISMS

Several mechanisms may contribute to indigestion, including acid reflux, altered gut motility or sensation, inflammation, and microbial processes.

Gastroesophageal Reflux Gastroesophageal reflux results from many defects. Reduced lower esophageal sphincter (LES) tone causes reflux in scleroderma and pregnancy and may be a factor in some patients without systemic illness. Other cases exhibit frequent transient LES relaxations (TLESRs). Reductions in esophageal body motility or saliva production prolong esophageal fluid clearance. Increased intragastric pressure promotes gastroesophageal reflux with obesity. Many reflux patients have hiatal hernias, and large hernias can increase symptomatic reflux.

Gastric Motor Dysfunction Disturbed gastric motility may contribute to gastroesophageal reflux in up to one-third of cases. Delayed gastric emptying is found in ~30% of functional dyspeptics, while rapid gastric emptying affects 5%. Impaired gastric fundus relaxation after eating (i.e., accommodation) may underlie selected dyspeptic symptoms like bloating, nausea, and early satiety in ~40% of patients and may predispose to TLESRs and acid reflux.

Visceral Afferent Hypersensitivity Disturbed gastric sensation is another pathogenic factor in functional dyspepsia. Approximately 35% of dyspeptic patients note discomfort with fundic distention to lower pressures than in healthy controls. Other individuals with dyspepsia exhibit hypersensitivity to chemical stimulation of the stomach with capsaicin or with duodenal acid or lipid perfusion. Some cases of functional heartburn without increased acid or nonacid reflux exhibit heightened perception of normal esophageal acidity.

Immune Activation Increases in duodenal epithelial permeability in functional dyspepsia may relate to increases in eosinophils and mast cells adjacent to submucosal neurons. Increased activation of these cells is proposed to contribute to gastric emptying delays and altered sensory function in functional dyspepsia and may selectively elicit early satiety and epigastric pain. Proliferations in duodenal bacteria were shown to correlate with meal-induced symptoms in functional dyspepsia, suggesting a role for microbiome alterations. Intestinal bile salt release also is proposed to worsen dyspeptic symptoms after eating. Both dysbiosis and bile may contribute to mucosal permeability defects.

Other Factors *Helicobacter pylori* has a proven etiologic role in peptic ulcer disease but is a minor factor in the genesis of functional dyspepsia. Anxiety and depression may play contributing roles in some functional dyspepsia cases. Functional MRI studies show increased activation of several brain regions, emphasizing CNS contributions. Up to 20% of functional dyspepsia patients report symptom onset after a viral illness, suggesting an infectious trigger. Analgesics cause dyspepsia, whereas nitrates, calcium channel blockers, theophylline, and progesterone promote gastroesophageal reflux. Ethanol, tobacco, and caffeine induce LES relaxation and reflux. Genetic factors predispose to development of reflux and dyspepsia in some cases.

DIFFERENTIAL DIAGNOSIS

Gastroesophageal Reflux Disease Heartburn or regurgitation is reported weekly by 18–28% of the population, highlighting the prevalence of gastroesophageal reflux disease (GERD). Most cases of heartburn result from excess acid reflux, but reflux of weakly acidic or nonacidic fluid can produce similar symptoms. Alkaline reflux esophagitis elicits GERD symptoms in patients who have had surgery for peptic ulcer disease. Ten percent of patients with heartburn exhibit no acidic or nonacidic esophageal reflux and are considered to have functional heartburn.

Functional Dyspepsia Approximately 20% of the populace has dyspepsia at least six times yearly, but only 10–20% present to clinicians. Functional dyspepsia, the cause of symptoms in 70–80% of dyspeptic patients, is defined as bothersome postprandial fullness, early satiety, or epigastric pain or burning with symptom onset ≥6 months before diagnosis in the absence of organic cause. Functional dyspepsia is subdivided into postprandial distress syndrome (61% of cases), characterized by meal-induced fullness and early satiety, and epigastric pain syndrome (18% of cases), with epigastric pain or burning that may or may not be meal related. Twenty-one percent of individuals present with overlapping postprandial distress and epigastric pain syndromes. Functional dyspepsia is associated with other functional gut disorders including irritable bowel syndrome and nongastrointestinal disorders like fibromyalgia, chronic fatigue, and anxiety. Most cases follow a benign course, but some with *H. pylori* infection or on nonsteroidal anti-inflammatory drugs (NSAIDs) develop ulcers.

Ulcer Disease Most GERD patients do not exhibit esophageal injury, but 5% develop esophageal ulcers. Symptoms cannot distinguish nonerosive from erosive or ulcerative esophagitis. A minority of cases of dyspepsia stem from gastric or duodenal ulcers. The most common causes of ulcers are *H. pylori* infection and NSAID use. Other rare causes of gastroduodenal ulcers include Crohn's disease **(Chap. 326)** and Zollinger-Ellison syndrome **(Chap. 324)**, resulting from gastrin overproduction by an endocrine tumor.

Malignancy Dyspeptic patients may seek care because of fear of cancer, but few cases result from malignancy. Esophageal squamous cell carcinoma occurs most often with long-standing tobacco or ethanol intake. Other risks include prior caustic ingestion, achalasia, and the hereditary disorder tylosis. Esophageal adenocarcinoma usually complicates prolonged acid reflux. Eight to 20% of GERD patients exhibit esophageal intestinal metaplasia, termed *Barrett's metaplasia,* which predisposes to esophageal adenocarcinoma **(Chap. 80)**. Gastric malignancies include adenocarcinoma, which is prevalent in certain Asian societies, and lymphoma.

Other Causes Opportunistic fungal or viral esophageal infections may produce heartburn but more often cause odynophagia. Other causes of esophageal inflammation include eosinophilic esophagitis and pill esophagitis. Biliary colic is a potential cause unexplained upper abdominal pain, but most patients report discrete acute episodes of right upper quadrant or epigastric pain rather than chronic burning or fullness. Twenty percent of gastroparesis patients note a predominance of pain rather than nausea and vomiting. Intestinal lactase deficiency may cause gas, bloating, and discomfort and occurs more commonly in blacks and Asians. Intolerance of other carbohydrates (e.g., fructose, sorbitol) produces similar symptoms. Small-intestinal bacterial overgrowth may cause dyspepsia, as well as bowel dysfunction, distention, and malabsorption. Celiac disease, nonceliac gluten sensitivity, pancreatic disease (chronic pancreatitis, malignancy), hepatocellular carcinoma, Ménétrier's disease, infiltrative diseases (sarcoidosis, mastocytosis, eosinophilic gastroenteritis), mesenteric ischemia, thyroid and parathyroid disease, and abdominal wall strain cause dyspepsia. Extraperitoneal etiologies of indigestion include congestive heart failure and tuberculosis.

APPROACH TO THE PATIENT

Indigestion

HISTORY AND PHYSICAL EXAMINATION

Managing indigestion requires a thorough interview. GERD classically produces heartburn, a substernal warmth that moves toward the neck. Heartburn often is exacerbated by meals and may awaken the patient. Associated symptoms include regurgitation of acid or nonacidic fluid and water brash, the reflex release of salty saliva into the mouth. Atypical symptoms include pharyngitis, asthma, cough, bronchitis, hoarseness, and chest pain that mimics angina. Some patients with acid reflux on esophageal pH testing note abdominal pain instead of heartburn.

Dyspeptic patients report symptoms referable to the upper abdomen that may be meal-related (postprandial distress syndrome) or independent of food ingestion (epigastric pain syndrome). The history in functional dyspepsia may also report symptoms of GERD, IBS, or idiopathic gastroparesis.

The physical exam with GERD and functional dyspepsia usually is normal. In atypical GERD, pharyngeal erythema and wheezing may be noted. Recurrent regurgitation may cause poor dentition. Dyspeptics may exhibit epigastric tenderness or distention.

Discriminating functional from organic causes of indigestion mandates excluding certain historic and exam features. Odynophagia suggests esophageal infection. Dysphagia is concerning for a benign or malignant esophageal blockage. Other alarm features include unexplained weight loss, recurrent vomiting, dysphagia, occult or gross bleeding, nocturnal symptoms, jaundice, palpable mass or adenopathy, and a family history of gastrointestinal neoplasm. Patients with an abdominal wall source of upper abdominal pain may exhibit a positive Carnett's sign of increased tenderness with tensing of abdominal muscles upon lifting the head from the exam table.

DIAGNOSTIC TESTING

Because indigestion is prevalent and most cases result from GERD or functional dyspepsia, it is generally recommended to perform no more than limited and directed diagnostic testing in most individuals.

After excluding alarm factors **(Table 45-3)**, patients with typical GERD do not need further evaluation and are treated empirically. Upper endoscopy is indicated only in cases with atypical symptoms or these alarm factors. For heartburn >5 years in duration,

TABLE 45-3 Alarm Symptoms in Gastroesophageal Reflux Disease

Odynophagia or dysphagia
Unexplained weight loss
Recurrent vomiting
Occult or gross gastrointestinal bleeding
Jaundice
Palpable mass or adenopathy
Family history of gastroesophageal malignancy

especially in patients >50 years old, endoscopy is advocated to screen for Barrett's metaplasia. Endoscopy is not needed in low-risk patients who respond to acid suppressants. Ambulatory esophageal pH testing using a catheter method or a wireless capsule endoscopically attached to the esophageal wall is considered for drug-refractory symptoms and atypical symptoms like unexplained chest pain. High-resolution esophageal manometry is ordered when surgical treatment of GERD is considered. A low LES pressure predicts failure of drug therapy and provides a rationale to proceed to surgery. Poor esophageal body peristalsis raises concern about postoperative dysphagia and directs the choice of surgical technique. Nonacidic reflux may be detected by combined esophageal impedance-pH testing in medication-unresponsive patients.

Upper endoscopy is recommended as the initial test in patients with unexplained dyspepsia who are >60 years old to exclude malignancy—a finding in only 0.3% of endoscopies performed for uninvestigated dyspepsia. Management of patients <60 years old depends on the local *H. pylori* prevalence. In regions with low prevalence (<10%), a 4-week trial of an acid-suppressing medication such as a proton pump inhibitor (PPI) is recommended. If empiric acid suppression fails, a "test and treat" approach for *H. pylori* status is initiated with urea breath testing or stool antigen measurement. Those who are *H. pylori* positive are given therapy to eradicate infection. For patients in areas with high *H. pylori* prevalence (>10%), an initial "test and treat" approach is advocated, and empiric PPI therapy is reserved for those who are negative for infection or who fail to respond to *H. pylori* treatment. Patients who are treated for *H. pylori* should undergo confirmation of eradication with repeat urea breath testing or fecal antigen testing 4–6 weeks after completing therapy. Those under age 60 only warrant upper endoscopy if their symptoms fail to respond to these therapies. Some advocate initial endoscopy for patients <60 years old who report alarm symptoms, but some guidelines have not endorsed this practice unless symptoms persist despite treatment.

Further testing is indicated in some settings. For suspected bleeding, a blood count can exclude anemia. Thyroid chemistries or calcium levels screen for metabolic disease. Specific serologies may suggest celiac disease. Pancreatic and liver chemistries are obtained for suspected pancreaticobiliary causes, which are further investigated with ultrasound, CT, or MRI. Gastric emptying testing is considered to exclude gastroparesis for dyspeptic symptoms resembling postprandial distress when therapy fails. Breath testing after carbohydrate ingestion detects lactase deficiency, intolerance to other carbohydrates, or small-intestinal bacterial overgrowth.

TREATMENT

Indigestion

LIFESTYLE, DIET, AND NONMEDICATION RECOMMENDATIONS

Patients with mild indigestion can be reassured that a careful evaluation revealed no serious disease and are offered no other intervention. If possible, drugs that cause gastroesophageal reflux or dyspepsia should be stopped. GERD patients should limit ethanol, caffeine, chocolate, and tobacco use and can ingest a low-fat diet, avoid snacks before bedtime, and elevate the head of the bed. Functional dyspepsia patients can be advised to reduce intake of fat, spicy foods, caffeine, and alcohol. Dietary lactose restriction is appropriate for lactase deficiency, while gluten exclusion is indicated for celiac disease. Low FODMAP (fermentable oligosaccharide, disaccharide, monosaccharide, and polyol) diets are effective for gaseous symptoms in IBS. In a systematic review, FODMAP intake correlated with functional dyspepsia symptoms, suggesting potential utility in this disorder as well.

ACID-SUPPRESSING OR -NEUTRALIZING MEDICATIONS

Drugs that reduce or neutralize gastric acid are often prescribed for GERD. Histamine H_2 antagonists like cimetidine, ranitidine, famotidine, and nizatidine are useful in mild to moderate GERD. For severe symptoms or for many cases of erosive or ulcerative esophagitis, PPIs like omeprazole, lansoprazole, rabeprazole, pantoprazole, esomeprazole, or dexlansoprazole are needed. These drugs inhibit gastric H^+, K^+-ATPase and are more potent than H_2 antagonists. Up to one-third of GERD patients do not respond to standard PPI doses; one-third of these patients have nonacidic reflux, whereas 10% have persistent acid-related disease. Heartburn responds better to PPI therapy than regurgitation or atypical GERD symptoms. Some individuals respond to doubling of the PPI dose or adding an H_2 antagonist. Complications of long-term PPI therapy include diarrhea (*Clostridium difficile* infection, microscopic colitis), small-intestinal bacterial overgrowth, nutrient deficiency (vitamin B_{12}, iron, calcium), hypomagnesemia, bone demineralization, interstitial nephritis, and impaired medication absorption (clopidogrel). Many patients started on a PPI can be stepped down to an H_2 antagonist or switched to on-demand use.

Acid suppressants also are effective for both the postprandial distress and epigastric pain subtypes of functional dyspepsia. A meta-analysis of 18 controlled trials calculated a risk ratio of 0.88, with a 95% confidence interval of 0.82–0.94, favoring PPI therapy over placebo in functional dyspepsia. H_2 antagonists also improve symptoms in functional dyspepsia, but a guideline has advocated PPIs over H_2 antagonists as first-line therapies for functional dyspepsia. In addition to acid suppression, PPIs may have the additional action of reducing duodenal eosinophil counts in dyspepsia.

Antacids are useful for short-term control of mild GERD but have less benefit in severe cases unless given at high doses that cause side effects (diarrhea and constipation with magnesium- and aluminum-containing agents, respectively). Alginic acid combined with antacids forms a floating barrier to reflux in patients with upright symptoms. Sucralfate, a salt of aluminum hydroxide and sucrose octasulfate that buffers acid and binds pepsin and bile salts, shows efficacy in GERD similar to H_2 antagonists.

HELICOBACTER PYLORI ERADICATION

H. pylori eradication is indicated for peptic ulcer and mucosa-associated lymphoid tissue gastric lymphoma. The benefits of eradication therapy in functional dyspepsia are limited but are statistically significant. A systematic review of 25 controlled trials calculated a pooled risk ratio of 1.24, with a 95% confidence interval of 1.12–1.37, favoring *H. pylori* eradication over placebo. Most drug combinations **(Chaps. 163 and 324)** include 7–14 days of a PPI with two or three antibiotics with or without bismuth products. *H. pylori* infection is associated with reduced prevalence of GERD. However, eradication of infection does not worsen GERD symptoms. No consensus recommendations regarding *H. pylori* eradication in GERD patients have been offered.

AGENTS THAT MODIFY GASTROINTESTINAL MOTOR ACTIVITY

The γ-aminobutyric acid B (GABA-B) agonist baclofen reduces esophageal exposure to acid and nonacidic fluids by reducing TLESRs by 40%. This drug can be used in patients with refractory acid or nonacid reflux. Several studies have promoted the efficacy of agents that stimulate gastric emptying in functional dyspepsia with 33% relative risk reductions, but publication bias and small sample sizes raise questions about reported benefits of these agents. Some clinicians suggest that patients with the postprandial distress subtype may respond preferentially to such prokinetic drugs. The newer 5-HT_4 agonist prucalopride was reported to reduce symptoms in patients with idiopathic gastroparesis, but no similar studies have been conducted in functional dyspepsia. The 5-HT_{1A} agonists buspirone and tandospirone may improve some functional dyspepsia symptoms by enhancing meal-induced gastric accommodation. Acotiamide stimulates gastric emptying and augments accommodation by enhancing acetylcholine release via muscarinic receptor antagonism and acetylcholinesterase inhibition. This agent is approved for functional dyspepsia in Japan and India.

ANTIDEPRESSANTS

Some patients with refractory functional heartburn may respond to antidepressants in the tricyclic and selective serotonin reuptake inhibitor (SSRI) classes, although studies are limited. Their mechanism of action may involve blunting of visceral pain processing in the brain. In a controlled trial in functional dyspepsia, the tricyclic drug amitriptyline produced symptom reductions, whereas the SSRI escitalopram had no benefit in a three-way comparison with placebo. In another controlled trial in functional dyspepsia, the antidepressant mirtazapine produced superior symptom reductions versus placebo. However, in a meta-analysis of 13 trials, SSRIs and serotonin-norepinephrine reuptake inhibitors showed no benefits in functional dyspepsia.

OTHER OPTIONS

Antireflux surgery (fundoplication) to enhance the barrier function of the LES may be offered to GERD patients who are young and require lifelong therapy, have typical heartburn, are responsive to PPIs, and show acid reflux on pH monitoring. Surgery also is effective for some cases of nonacidic reflux. Individuals who respond less well to fundoplication include those with atypical symptoms, those who have functional heartburn without reflux on testing, or those who have esophageal body motor disturbances. Dysphagia, gas-bloat syndrome, and gastroparesis are long-term complications of fundoplication; ~60% develop recurrent GERD symptoms over time. Magnetic sphincter augmentation may be appropriate for GERD treatment, while endoscopic radiofrequency therapies can be considered for some patients. Other endoscopic options including transoral incisionless fundoplication, endoscopic stapling, and antireflux mucosectomy are not yet advocated.

Gas and bloating are bothersome in some patients with indigestion and are difficult to treat. Simethicone, activated charcoal, and alpha-galactosidase provide benefits in some cases. One trial suggested possible benefits of the nonabsorbable antibiotic rifaximin in functional dyspepsia, while another reported improvement with the probiotic *Lactobacillus gasseri*. Herbal remedies like STW 5 (Iberogast, a mixture of nine herbal agents) and formulations of caraway oil and menthol are useful in some dyspeptic patients. Psychological treatments (e.g., behavioral therapy, psychotherapy, hypnotherapy) may be offered for refractory functional dyspepsia; a meta-analysis of four trials reported benefits in patients with persistent dyspepsia.

FURTHER READING

Gyawali CP et al: ACG Clinical Guidelines: clinical use of esophageal physiologic testing. Am J Gastroenterol 115:1412, 2020.

Maret-Ouda J et al: Gastroesophageal reflux disease: a review. JAMA 324:2536, 2020.

Sharaf RN et al: Management of cyclic vomiting syndrome in adults: evidence review. Neurogastroenterol Motil 31(Suppl 2):e13605, 2019.

Venkatesan T et al: Role of chronic cannabis use: cyclic vomiting syndrome vs. cannabinoid hyperemesis syndrome. Neurogastroenterol Motil 31(Suppl 2):e13606, 2019.

Wauters L et al: Novel concepts in the pathophysiology and treatment of functional dyspepsia. Gut 69:591, 2020.

46 Diarrhea and Constipation

Michael Camilleri, Joseph A. Murray

Diarrhea and constipation are exceedingly common and, together, exact an enormous toll in terms of mortality, morbidity, social inconvenience, loss of work productivity, and consumption of medical resources. Worldwide, >1 billion individuals suffer one or more episodes of acute diarrhea each year. Among the 100 million persons affected annually by acute diarrhea in the United States, nearly half must restrict activities, 10% consult physicians, ~250,000 require hospitalization, and ~5000 die (primarily the elderly). Updated 2014–2015 annual disease burden data from the United States show 3.4 million annual clinic or emergency department visits, about 130,000 hospital admissions, and annual economic burden to society (excluding all costs for inflammatory bowel disease) exceeding $8 billion. Acute infectious diarrhea remains one of the most common causes of mortality in developing countries, particularly among impoverished infants, accounting for 1.8 million deaths per year. Recurrent, acute diarrhea in children in tropical countries results in environmental enteropathy with long-term impacts on physical and intellectual development.

Constipation, by contrast, is rarely associated with mortality and is exceedingly common in developed countries, leading to frequent self-medication and, in a third of those, to medical consultation. Annual disease burden data for 2014–2015 show about 5 million clinic or emergency department visits for constipation or hemorrhoids, 50,000 admissions to hospital, and average cost of $3500 per patient, about double that of controls in a nested controlled study.

Population statistics on chronic diarrhea and constipation are more uncertain, perhaps due to variable definitions and reporting, but the frequency of these conditions is also high. U.S. population surveys put prevalence rates for chronic diarrhea at 2–7% and for chronic constipation at 12–19%, with women being affected twice as often as men, reaching parity at 70 years of age. Diarrhea and constipation are among the most common patient complaints presenting in primary care and account for nearly 50% of referrals to gastroenterologists.

Although diarrhea and constipation may present as mere nuisance symptoms at one extreme, they can be severe or life threatening at the other. Even mild symptoms may signal a serious underlying gastrointestinal (GI) lesion, such as colorectal cancer, or systemic disorder, such as thyroid disease. Given the heterogeneous causes and potential severity of these common complaints, it is imperative for clinicians to appreciate the pathophysiology, etiologic classification, diagnostic strategies, and principles of management of diarrhea and constipation so that rational and cost-effective care can be delivered.

NORMAL PHYSIOLOGY

While the primary function of the small intestine is the digestion and assimilation of nutrients from food, the small intestine and colon together perform important functions that regulate the secretion and absorption of water and electrolytes, the storage and subsequent transport of intraluminal contents aborally, and the salvage of some nutrients that are not absorbed in the small intestine after bacterial metabolism of carbohydrate allows salvage of short-chain fatty acids. The main motor functions are summarized in **Table 46-1**. Alterations in fluid and electrolyte handling contribute significantly to diarrhea. Alterations in motor and sensory functions of the colon result in highly prevalent syndromes such as irritable bowel syndrome (IBS), chronic diarrhea, and chronic constipation.

NEURAL CONTROL

The small intestine and colon have intrinsic and extrinsic innervation. The *intrinsic innervation*, also called the enteric nervous system, comprises myenteric, submucosal, and mucosal neuronal layers. The function of these layers is modulated by interneurons through the actions

TABLE 46-1 Normal Gastrointestinal Motility: Functions at Different Anatomic Levels

Stomach and Small Bowel
Synchronized MMC in fasting
Accommodation, trituration, mixing, transit
Stomach ~3 h
Small bowel ~3 h
Ileal reservoir empties boluses
Colon: Irregular Mixing, Fermentation, Absorption, Transit
Ascending, transverse: reservoirs
Descending: conduit
Sigmoid/rectum: volitional reservoir

Abbreviation: MMC, migrating motor complex.

of neurotransmitter amines or peptides, including acetylcholine, vasoactive intestinal peptide (VIP), opioids, norepinephrine, serotonin, adenosine triphosphate (ATP), and nitric oxide (NO). The myenteric plexus regulates smooth-muscle function through intermediary pacemaker-like cells called the interstitial cells of Cajal, and the submucosal plexus affects secretion, absorption, and mucosal blood flow. The enteric nervous system receives input from the extrinsic nerves, but it is capable of independent control of these functions.

The *extrinsic innervations* of the small intestine and colon are part of the autonomic nervous system and also modulate motor and secretory functions. The parasympathetic nerves convey visceral sensory pathways from and excitatory pathways to the small intestine and colon. Parasympathetic fibers via the vagus nerve reach the small intestine and proximal colon along the branches of the superior mesenteric artery. The distal colon is supplied by sacral parasympathetic nerves (S_{2-4}) via the pelvic plexus; these fibers course through the wall of the colon as ascending intracolonic fibers as far as, and in some instances including, the proximal colon. The chief excitatory neurotransmitters controlling motor function are acetylcholine and the tachykinins, such as substance P. The sympathetic nerve supply modulates motor functions and reaches the small intestine and colon alongside their arterial vessels. Sympathetic input to the gut is generally excitatory to sphincters and inhibitory to nonsphincteric muscle. Visceral afferents convey sensation from the gut to the central nervous system (CNS). Some afferent fibers synapse in the prevertebral ganglia and reflexly modulate intestinal motility, blood flow, and secretion.

INTESTINAL FLUID ABSORPTION AND SECRETION

On an average day, 9 L of fluid enter the GI tract, ~1 L of residual fluid reaches the colon, and the stool excretion of fluid constitutes about 0.2 L/d. The colon has a large capacitance and functional reserve and may recover up to four times its usual volume of 0.8 L/d, provided the rate of flow permits reabsorption to occur. Thus, the colon can partially compensate for excess fluid delivery to the colon that may result from intestinal absorptive or secretory disorders.

In the small intestine and colon, sodium absorption is predominantly electrogenic (i.e., it can be measured as an ionic current across the membrane because there is not an equivalent loss of a cation from the cell), and uptake takes place at the apical membrane; it is compensated for by the export functions of the basolateral sodium pump. There are several active transport proteins at the apical membrane, especially in the small intestine, whereby sodium ion entry is coupled to monosaccharides (e.g., glucose through the transporter SGLT1, or fructose through GLUT-5). Glucose then exits the basal membrane through a specific transport protein, GLUT-2, creating a glucose concentration and osmotic gradient between the lumen and the intercellular space, drawing water and electrolytes passively from the lumen. Several channels mediate the secretion of chloride ions in diarrheal diseases or in response to medications administered for the treatment of constipation. The diverse ion channels (chloride channels and cystic fibrosis transmembrane regulator), transporters (SGLT1, GLUT-2), and receptors (e.g., guanylate cyclase C receptor) are summarized in **Figure 46-1**.

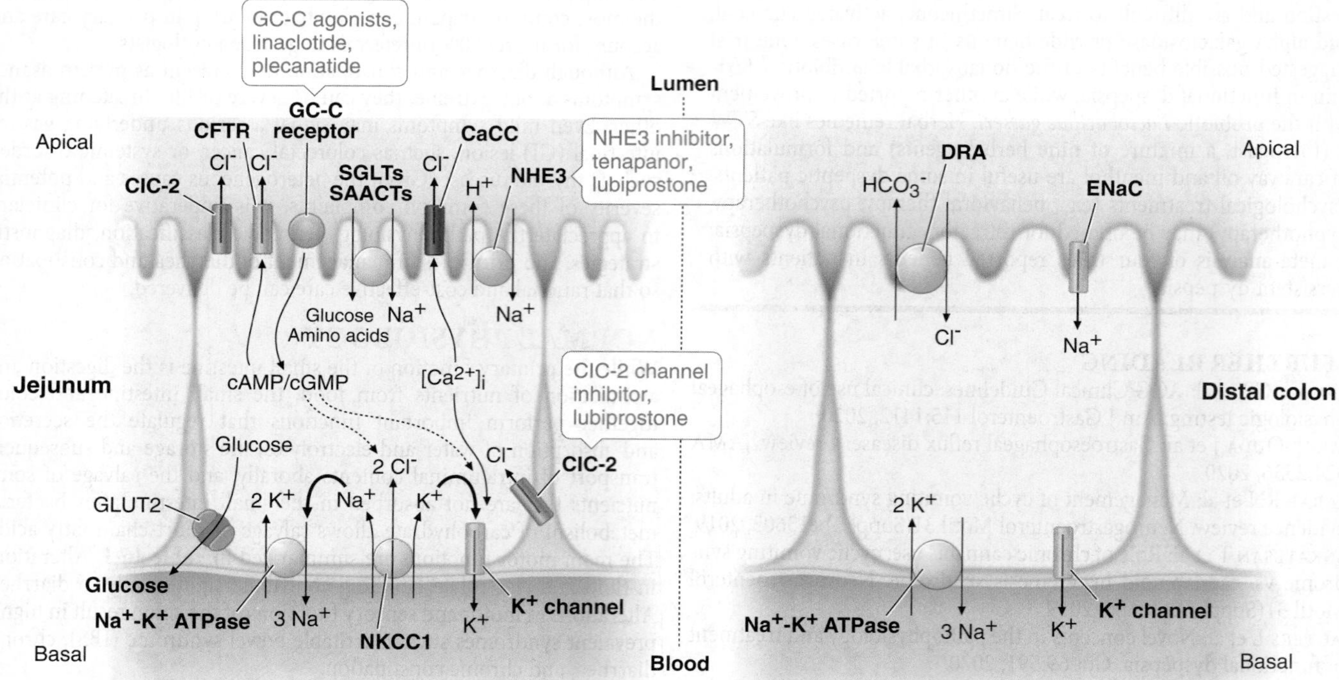

FIGURE 46-1 Important ion transport mechanisms in the jejunum and colon, and the site of action of medications used as secretagogues in the treatment of chronic constipation. CFTR, cystic fibrosis transmembrane regulator; ClC2, type 2 chloride channel, DRA, downregulated in adenoma (also called SLC26A3); ENaC, epithelial sodium channel; GC-C, guanylate cyclase C; Na^+-K^+ ATPase, sodium potassium adenosine triphosphatase; NHE3, sodium-hydrogen exchanger; NKCC1, Na-K-Cl cotransporter; SAACT, sodium amino acid co- transporters; SGLT, sodium glucose transporters.

A variety of neural and nonneural mediators regulate colonic fluid and electrolyte balance, including cholinergic, adrenergic, and serotonergic mediators. Angiotensin and aldosterone also influence colonic absorption, reflecting the common embryologic development of the distal colonic epithelium and the renal tubules.

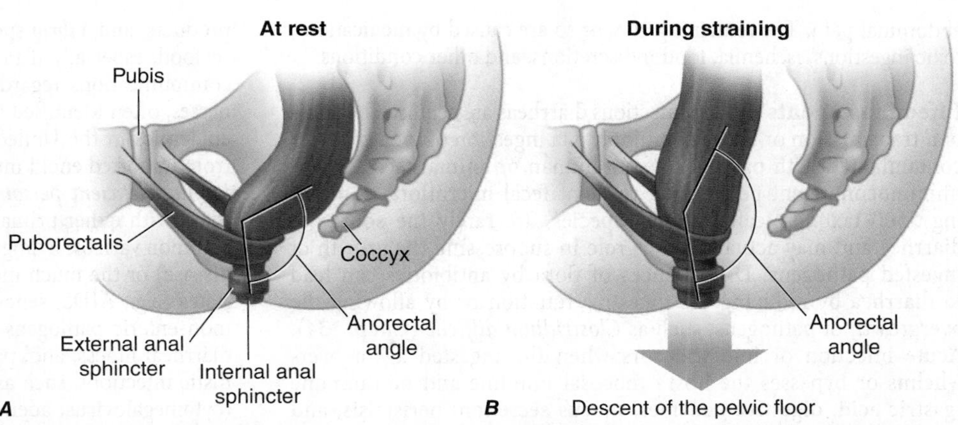

FIGURE 46-2 Sagittal view of the anorectum (*A*) at rest and (*B*) during straining to defecate. Continence is maintained by normal rectal sensation and tonic contraction of the internal anal sphincter and the puborectalis muscle, which wraps around the anorectum, maintaining an anorectal angle between 80° and 110°. During defecation, the pelvic floor muscles (including the puborectalis) relax, allowing the anorectal angle to straighten by at least 15°, and the perineum descends by 1–3.5 cm. The external anal sphincter also relaxes and reduces pressure on the anal canal. *(From A Lembo, M Camilleri: Chronic constipation. N Engl J Med 349:1360, 2003 Massachusetts Medical Society. Reprinted with permission.)*

SMALL-INTESTINAL MOTILITY

During the fasting period, the motility of the small intestine is characterized by a cyclical event called the migrating motor complex (MMC), which serves to clear nondigestible residue from the small intestine (the intestinal "housekeeper"). This organized, propagated series of contractions lasts, on average, 4 min, occurs every 60–90 min, and usually involves the entire small intestine. After food ingestion, the small intestine produces irregular, mixing contractions of relatively low amplitude, except in the distal ileum where more powerful contractions occur intermittently and empty the ileum by bolus transfers.

ILEOCOLONIC STORAGE AND SALVAGE

The distal ileum acts as a reservoir, emptying intermittently by bolus movements. This action allows time for salvage of fluids, electrolytes, and nutrients. Segmentation by haustra compartmentalizes the colon and facilitates mixing, retention of residue, and formation of solid stools. There is increased appreciation of the intimate interaction between the colonic function and the luminal ecology. The resident microorganisms, predominantly anaerobic bacteria, in the colon are necessary for the digestion of unabsorbed carbohydrates that reach the colon even in health, thereby providing a vital source of nutrients to the mucosa. Normal intestinal flora also keeps pathogens at bay by a variety of mechanisms including a crucial role in the development and maintenance of a potent but well-regulated immune response capacity to pathogens and tolerance to normal ingesta. In health, the ascending and transverse regions of colon function as reservoirs (average transit time, 15 h), and the descending colon acts as a conduit (average transit time, 3 h). The colon is efficient at conserving sodium and water, a function that is particularly important in sodium-depleted patients in whom the small intestine alone is unable to maintain sodium balance. Diarrhea or constipation may result from alteration in the reservoir function of the proximal colon or the propulsive function of the left colon. Constipation may also result from disturbances of the rectal or sigmoid reservoir, typically as a result of dysfunction of the pelvic floor, the anal sphincters, the coordination of defecation, or dehydration.

COLONIC MOTILITY AND TONE

The small-intestinal MMC only rarely continues into the colon. However, short duration or phasic contractions mix colonic contents, and high-amplitude (>75 mmHg) propagated contractions (HAPCs) are sometimes associated with mass movements through the colon and normally occur approximately five times per day, usually on awakening in the morning and postprandially. Increased frequency of HAPCs may result in diarrhea or urgency. The predominant phasic contractions in the colon are irregular and nonpropagated and serve a "mixing" function.

Colonic tone refers to the background contractility upon which phasic contractile activity (typically contractions lasting <15 s) is superimposed. It is an important cofactor in the colon's capacitance (volume accommodation) and sensation.

COLONIC MOTILITY AFTER MEAL INGESTION

After meal ingestion, colonic phasic and tonic contractility increase for a period of ~2 h. The initial phase (~10 min) is mediated by the vagus nerve in response to mechanical distention of the stomach. The subsequent response of the colon requires caloric stimulation (e.g., intake of at least 500 kcal) and is mediated, at least in part, by hormones (e.g., gastrin and serotonin).

DEFECATION

Tonic contraction of the puborectalis muscle, which forms a sling around the rectoanal junction, is important to maintain continence; during defecation, sacral parasympathetic nerves relax this muscle, facilitating the straightening of the rectoanal angle (**Fig. 46-2**). Distention of the rectum results in transient relaxation of the internal anal sphincter via intrinsic and reflex sympathetic innervation. As sigmoid and rectal contractions, as well as straining (Valsalva maneuver), which increases intraabdominal pressure, increase the pressure within the rectum, the rectosigmoid angle opens by >15°. Voluntary relaxation of the external anal sphincter (striated muscle innervated by the pudendal nerve) in response to the sensation produced by distention permits the evacuation of feces. Defecation can also be delayed voluntarily by contraction of the external anal sphincter.

DIARRHEA

DEFINITION

Diarrhea is loosely defined as passage of abnormally liquid or unformed stools at an increased frequency. For adults on a typical Western diet, stool weight >200 g/d can generally be considered diarrheal. Diarrhea may be further defined as *acute* if <2 weeks, *persistent* if 2–4 weeks, and *chronic* if >4 weeks in duration.

Two common conditions, usually associated with the passage of stool totaling <200 g/d, must be distinguished from diarrhea, because diagnostic and therapeutic algorithms differ. *Pseudodiarrhea*, or the frequent passage of small volumes of stool, is often associated with rectal urgency, tenesmus, or a feeling of incomplete evacuation and accompanies IBS or proctitis. *Fecal incontinence* is the involuntary discharge of rectal contents and is most often caused by neuromuscular disorders or structural anorectal problems. Diarrhea and urgency, especially if severe, may aggravate or cause incontinence. Pseudodiarrhea and fecal incontinence occur at prevalence rates comparable to or higher than that of chronic diarrhea and should always be considered in patients complaining of "diarrhea." Overflow diarrhea may occur in nursing home patients due to fecal impaction that is readily detectable by rectal examination. A careful history and physical examination generally allow these conditions to be discriminated from true diarrhea.

ACUTE DIARRHEA

More than 90% of cases of acute diarrhea are caused by infectious agents; these cases are often accompanied by vomiting, fever, and abdominal pain. The remaining 10% or so are caused by medications, toxic ingestions, ischemia, food indiscretions, and other conditions.

Infectious Agents Most infectious diarrheas are acquired by fecal-oral transmission or, more commonly, via ingestion of food or water contaminated with pathogens from human or animal feces. In the immunocompetent person, the resident fecal microflora, containing >500 taxonomically distinct species, are rarely the source of diarrhea and may actually play a role in suppressing the growth of ingested pathogens. Disturbances of flora by antibiotics can lead to diarrhea by reducing the digestive function or by allowing the overgrowth of pathogens, such as *Clostridium difficile* **(Chap. 134)**. Acute infection or injury occurs when the ingested agent overwhelms or bypasses the host's mucosal immune and nonimmune (gastric acid, digestive enzymes, mucus secretion, peristalsis, and suppressive resident flora) defenses. Established clinical associations with specific enteropathogens may offer diagnostic clues. Diarrhea occasionally is an early symptom of infection such as SARS-CoV-2 and *Legionella*.

In the United States, five high-risk groups are recognized:

1. *Travelers.* Nearly 40% of tourists to endemic regions of Latin America, Africa, and Asia develop so-called traveler's diarrhea, most commonly due to enterotoxigenic or enteroaggregative *Escherichia coli* as well as to *Campylobacter, Shigella, Aeromonas,* norovirus, *Coronavirus,* and *Salmonella.* Visitors to Russia (especially St. Petersburg) may have increased risk of *Giardia*-associated diarrhea; visitors to Nepal may acquire *Cyclospora.* Campers, backpackers, and swimmers in wilderness areas may become infected with *Giardia.* Cruise ships may be affected by outbreaks of gastroenteritis caused by agents such as norovirus.
2. *Consumers of certain foods.* Diarrhea closely following food consumption at a picnic, banquet, or restaurant may suggest infection with *Salmonella, Campylobacter,* or *Shigella* from chicken; enterohemorrhagic *E. coli* (O157:H7) from undercooked hamburger; *Bacillus cereus* from fried rice or other reheated food; *Staphylococcus aureus* or *Salmonella* from mayonnaise or creams; *Salmonella* from eggs; *Listeria* from fresh or frozen uncooked foods, mushrooms, or dairy products; and *Vibrio* species, *Salmonella,* or acute hepatitis A from seafood, especially if raw. State departments of public health issue communications regarding domestic and foreign food-related illnesses, often identified by rapid DNA typing (PulseNet), that cause epidemics in the United States (e.g., the *Listeria* epidemic of 2020 from imported enoki mushrooms).
3. *Immunodeficient persons.* Individuals at risk for diarrhea include those with either primary immunodeficiency (e.g., IgA deficiency, common variable hypogammaglobulinemia, chronic granulomatous disease) or the much more common secondary immunodeficiency states (e.g., AIDS, senescence, pharmacologic suppression). Common enteric pathogens often cause a more severe and protracted diarrheal illness, and, particularly in persons with AIDS, opportunistic infections, such as by *Mycobacterium* species, certain viruses (cytomegalovirus, adenovirus, and herpes simplex), and protozoa (*Cryptosporidium, Isospora belli,* Microsporidia, and *Blastocystis hominis*) may also play a role **(Chap. 202)**. In patients with AIDS, agents transmitted venereally per rectum or by extension from vaginal infection (e.g., *Neisseria gonorrhoeae, Treponema pallidum, Chlamydia*) may contribute to proctocolitis. Symptoms suggesting anorectal disease, particularly pain, may result from constipation occurring coincidentally in a person with immunodeficiency. Persons with hemochromatosis are especially prone to invasive, even fatal, enteric infections with *Vibrio* species and *Yersinia* infections and should avoid raw fish and exposing open wounds to seawater.
4. *Daycare attendees and their family members.* Infections with *Shigella, Giardia, Cryptosporidium,* rotavirus, and other agents are very common and should be considered.
5. *Institutionalized persons.* Infectious diarrhea is one of the most frequent categories of nosocomial infections in many hospitals and long-term care facilities; the causes are a variety of microorganisms but most commonly *C. difficile. C. difficile* can affect those with no history of antibiotic use and is often community acquired.

The pathophysiology underlying acute diarrhea by infectious agents produces specific clinical features that may also be helpful in diagnosis **(Table 46-2)**. Profuse, watery diarrhea secondary to small-bowel hypersecretion occurs with ingestion of preformed bacterial toxins,

TABLE 46-2 Association Between Pathobiology of Causative Agents and Clinical Features in Acute Infectious Diarrhea

PATHOBIOLOGY/AGENTS	INCUBATION PERIOD	VOMITING	ABDOMINAL PAIN	FEVER	DIARRHEA
Toxin producers					
Preformed toxin					
Bacillus cereus, Staphylococcus aureus, Clostridium perfringens	1–8 h 8–24 h	3–4+	1–2+	0–1+	3–4+, watery
Enterotoxin					
Vibrio cholerae, enterotoxigenic *Escherichia coli, Klebsiella pneumoniae, Aeromonas* species	8–72 h	2–4+	1–2+	0–1+	3–4+, watery
Enteroadherent					
Enteropathogenic and enteroadherent *E. coli, Giardia* organisms, cryptosporidiosis, helminths	1–8 d	0–1+	1–3+	0–2+	1–2+, watery, mushy
Cytotoxin producers					
Clostridium difficile	1–3 d	0–1+	3–4+	1–2+	1–3+, usually watery, occasionally bloody
Hemorrhagic *E. coli*	12–72 h	0–1+	3–4+	1–2+	1–3+, initially watery, quickly bloody
Invasive organisms					
Minimal inflammation					
Rotavirus and norovirus	1–3 d	1–3+	2–3+	3–4+	1–3+, watery
Variable inflammation					
Salmonella, Campylobacter, and *Aeromonas* species, *Vibrio parahaemolyticus, Yersinia*	12 h–11 d	0–3+	2–4+	3–4+	1–4+, watery or bloody
Severe inflammation					
Shigella species, enteroinvasive *E. coli, Entamoeba histolytica*	12 h–8 d	0–1+	3–4+	3–4+	1–2+, bloody

Source: Adapted from DW Powell, in T Yamada (ed): *Textbook of Gastroenterology and Hepatology,* 4th ed. Philadelphia, Lippincott Williams & Wilkins, 2003.

enterotoxin-producing bacteria, and enteroadherent pathogens. Diarrhea associated with marked vomiting and minimal or no fever may occur abruptly within a few hours after ingestion of the former two types; vomiting is usually less, abdominal cramping or bloating is greater, and fever is higher with the latter. Cytotoxin-producing and invasive microorganisms all cause high fever and abdominal pain. Invasive bacteria and *Entamoeba histolytica* often cause bloody diarrhea (referred to as *dysentery*). *Yersinia* invades the terminal ileal and proximal colon mucosa and may cause especially severe abdominal pain with tenderness mimicking acute appendicitis.

Finally, infectious diarrhea may be associated with systemic manifestations. Reactive arthritis (formerly known as Reiter's syndrome), arthritis, urethritis, and conjunctivitis may accompany or follow infections by *Salmonella*, *Campylobacter*, *Shigella*, and *Yersinia*. Yersiniosis may also lead to an autoimmune-type thyroiditis, pericarditis, and glomerulonephritis. Both enterohemorrhagic *E. coli* (O157:H7) and *Shigella* can lead to the *hemolytic-uremic syndrome* with an attendant high mortality rate. The syndrome of postinfectious IBS has now been recognized as a complication of infectious diarrhea. Similarly, acute gastroenteritis may precede the diagnosis of celiac disease or Crohn's disease. Acute diarrhea can also be a major symptom of several systemic infections including *viral hepatitis*, *listeriosis*, *legionellosis*, and *toxic shock syndrome*.

Other Causes Side effects from medications are probably the most common noninfectious causes of acute diarrhea, and etiology may be suggested by a temporal association between use and symptom onset. Although innumerable medications may produce diarrhea, some of the more frequently incriminated include antibiotics, cardiac antidysrhythmics, antihypertensives, nonsteroidal anti-inflammatory drugs (NSAIDs), certain antidepressants, chemotherapeutic agents, bronchodilators, antacids, and laxatives. Occlusive or nonocclusive ischemic colitis typically occurs in persons aged >50 years; often presents as acute lower abdominal pain preceding watery, then bloody diarrhea; and generally results in acute inflammatory changes in the sigmoid or left colon while sparing the rectum. Acute diarrhea may accompany colonic diverticulitis and graft-versus-host disease. Acute diarrhea, often associated with systemic compromise, can follow ingestion of toxins including organophosphate insecticides, amanita and other mushrooms, arsenic, and preformed toxins in seafood such as ciguatera (from algae that the fish eat) and scombroid (an excess of histamine due to inadequate refrigeration). Acute anaphylaxis to food ingestion can have a similar presentation. Conditions causing chronic diarrhea can also be confused with acute diarrhea early in their course. This confusion may occur with inflammatory bowel disease (IBD) and some of the other inflammatory chronic diarrheas that may have an abrupt rather than insidious onset and exhibit features that mimic infection.

APPROACH TO THE PATIENT

Acute Diarrhea

The decision to evaluate acute diarrhea depends on its severity and duration and on various host factors (Fig. 46-3). Most episodes of acute diarrhea are mild and self-limited and do not justify the cost and potential morbidity rate of diagnostic or pharmacologic interventions. Indications for evaluation include profuse diarrhea with dehydration, grossly bloody stools, fever ≥38.5°C (≥101°F), duration >48 h without improvement, recent antibiotic use, new community outbreaks, associated severe abdominal pain in patients aged >50 years, and elderly (≥70 years) or immunocompromised patients. In some cases of moderately severe febrile diarrhea associated with fecal leukocytes (or increased fecal levels of the leukocyte proteins, such as calprotectin) or with gross blood, a diagnostic evaluation might be avoided in favor of an empirical antibiotic trial (see below).

The cornerstone of diagnosis in those suspected of severe acute infectious diarrhea is microbiologic analysis of the stool. Workup

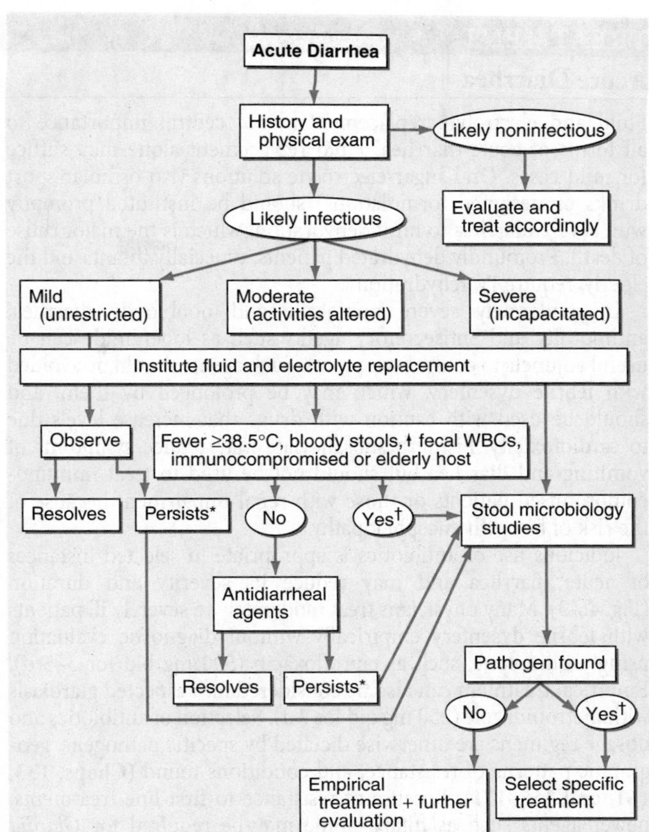

FIGURE 46-3 Algorithm for the management of acute diarrhea. Consider empirical treatment before evaluation with (*) metronidazole and with (†) quinolone. WBCs, white blood cells.

includes cultures for bacterial and viral pathogens; direct inspection for ova and parasites; and immunoassays for certain bacterial toxins (*C. difficile*), viral antigens (rotavirus), and protozoal antigens (*Giardia*, *E. histolytica*). The aforementioned clinical and epidemiologic associations may assist in focusing the evaluation. If a particular pathogen or set of possible pathogens is so implicated, either the whole panel of routine studies may not be necessary or, in some instances, special cultures may be appropriate, as for enterohemorrhagic and other types of *E. coli*, *Vibrio* species, and *Yersinia*. Molecular diagnosis of pathogens in stool can be made by identification of unique DNA sequences, and evolving microarray technologies have led to more rapid, sensitive, specific, and cost-effective diagnosis.

Persistent diarrhea is commonly due to *Giardia* (Chap. 223), but additional causative organisms that should be considered include *C. difficile* (especially if antibiotics had been administered), *E. histolytica*, *Cryptosporidium*, *Campylobacter*, and others. If stool studies are unrevealing, flexible sigmoidoscopy with biopsies and upper endoscopy with duodenal aspirates and biopsies may be indicated. Brainerd diarrhea is an increasingly recognized entity characterized by an abrupt-onset diarrhea that persists for at least 4 weeks, but may last 1–3 years, and is thought to be of infectious origin. It may be associated with subtle inflammation of the distal small intestine or proximal colon.

Structural examination by sigmoidoscopy, colonoscopy, or abdominal computed tomography (CT) scanning (or other imaging approaches) may be appropriate in patients with uncharacterized persistent diarrhea to exclude IBD or as an initial approach in patients with suspected noninfectious acute diarrhea such as might be caused by ischemic colitis, diverticulitis, or partial bowel obstruction.

TREATMENT
Acute Diarrhea

Fluid and electrolyte replacement are of central importance to all forms of acute diarrhea. Fluid replacement alone may suffice for mild cases. Oral sugar-electrolyte solutions (iso-osmolar sport drinks or designed formulations) should be instituted promptly with severe diarrhea to limit dehydration, which is the major cause of death. Profoundly dehydrated patients, especially infants and the elderly, require IV rehydration.

In moderately severe nonfebrile and nonbloody diarrhea, antimotility and antisecretory agents such as loperamide can be useful adjuncts to control symptoms. Such agents should be avoided with febrile dysentery, which may be prolonged by them, and should be used with caution with drugs that increase levels due to cardiotoxicity. Bismuth subsalicylate may reduce symptoms of vomiting and diarrhea but should not be used to treat immunocompromised patients or those with renal impairment because of the risk of bismuth encephalopathy.

Judicious use of antibiotics is appropriate in selected instances of acute diarrhea and may reduce its severity and duration (Fig. 46-3). Many physicians treat moderately to severely ill patients with febrile dysentery empirically without diagnostic evaluation using a quinolone, such as ciprofloxacin (500 mg bid for 3–5 d). Empirical treatment can also be considered for suspected giardiasis with metronidazole (250 mg qid for 7 d). Selection of antibiotics and dosage regimens are otherwise dictated by specific pathogens, geographic patterns of resistance, and conditions found **(Chaps. 133, 161, and 165–171)**. Because of resistance to first-line treatments, newer agents such as nitazoxanide may be required for *Giardia* and *Cryptosporidium* infections. Antibiotic coverage is indicated, whether or not a causative organism is discovered, in patients who are immunocompromised, have mechanical heart valves or recent vascular grafts, or are elderly. Bismuth subsalicylate may reduce the frequency of traveler's diarrhea. Antibiotic prophylaxis is only indicated for certain patients traveling to high-risk countries in whom the likelihood or seriousness of acquired diarrhea would be especially high, including those with immunocompromise, IBD, hemochromatosis, or gastric achlorhydria. Use of ciprofloxacin, azithromycin, or rifaximin may reduce bacterial diarrhea in such travelers by 90%, though rifaximin is not suitable for invasive disease but rather as treatment for uncomplicated traveler's diarrhea. There is little role for endoscopic evaluation in most circumstances except in immunocompromised patients. Finally, physicians should be vigilant to identify if an outbreak of diarrheal illness is occurring and to alert the public health authorities promptly. This may reduce the ultimate size of the affected population.

■ CHRONIC DIARRHEA

Diarrhea lasting >4 weeks warrants evaluation to exclude serious underlying pathology. In contrast to acute diarrhea, most of the causes of chronic diarrhea are noninfectious. The classification of chronic diarrhea by pathophysiologic mechanism facilitates a rational approach to management, although many diseases cause diarrhea by more than one mechanism **(Table 46-3)**.

TABLE 46-3 Major Causes of Chronic Diarrhea According to Predominant Pathophysiologic Mechanism

Secretory Causes
Exogenous stimulant laxatives
Chronic ethanol ingestion
Other drugs and toxins
Endogenous laxatives (dihydroxy bile acids)
Idiopathic secretory diarrhea or bile acid diarrhea
Certain bacterial infections
Bowel resection, disease, or fistula (↓ absorption)
Partial bowel obstruction or fecal impaction
Hormone-producing tumors (carcinoid, VIPoma, medullary cancer of thyroid, mastocytosis, gastrinoma, colorectal villous adenoma)
Addison's disease
Congenital electrolyte absorption defects
Osmotic Causes
Osmotic laxatives (Mg^{2+}, PO_4^{-3}, SO_4^{-2})
Lactase and other disaccharide deficiencies
Nonabsorbable carbohydrates (sorbitol, lactulose, polyethylene glycol)
Gluten and FODMAP intolerance
Steatorrheal Causes
Intraluminal maldigestion (pancreatic exocrine insufficiency, bacterial overgrowth, bariatric surgery, liver disease)
Mucosal malabsorption (celiac sprue, Whipple's disease, infections, abetalipoproteinemia, ischemia, drug-induced enteropathy)
Postmucosal obstruction (1° or 2° lymphatic obstruction)
Inflammatory Causes
Idiopathic inflammatory bowel disease (Crohn's, chronic ulcerative colitis)
Lymphocytic and collagenous colitis
Immune-related mucosal disease (1° or 2° immunodeficiencies, food allergy, eosinophilic gastroenteritis, graft-versus-host disease)
Infections (invasive bacteria, viruses, and parasites, Brainerd diarrhea)
Radiation injury
Gastrointestinal malignancies
Dysmotile Causes
Irritable bowel syndrome (including postinfectious IBS)
Visceral neuromyopathies
Hyperthyroidism
Drugs (prokinetic agents)
Postvagotomy
Factitial Causes
Munchausen
Eating disorders
Iatrogenic Causes
Cholecystectomy
Ileal resection
Bariatric surgery
Vagotomy, fundoplication

Abbreviations: FODMAP, fermentable oligosaccharides, disaccharides, monosaccharides, and polyols; IBS, irritable bowel syndrome.

Secretory Causes Secretory diarrheas are due to derangements in fluid and electrolyte transport across the enterocolonic mucosa. They are characterized clinically by watery, large-volume fecal outputs that are typically painless and persist with fasting. Because there is no malabsorbed solute, stool osmolality is accounted for by normal endogenous electrolytes with no fecal osmotic gap.

MEDICATIONS Side effects from regular ingestion of drugs and toxins are the most common secretory causes of chronic diarrhea. Hundreds of prescription and over-the-counter medications (see earlier section, "Acute Diarrhea, Other Causes") may produce diarrhea. Surreptitious or habitual use of stimulant laxatives (e.g., senna, cascara, bisacodyl, ricinoleic acid [castor oil]) must also be considered. Chronic ethanol consumption may cause a secretory-type diarrhea due to enterocyte injury with impaired sodium and water absorption as well as rapid transit and other alterations. Inadvertent ingestion of certain environmental toxins (e.g., arsenic) may lead to chronic rather than acute forms of diarrhea. Certain bacterial infections may occasionally persist and be associated with a secretory-type diarrhea. The oral angiotensin receptor blocker olmesartan is associated with diarrhea due to sprue-like enteropathy.

BOWEL RESECTION, MUCOSAL DISEASE, OR ENTEROCOLIC FISTULA These conditions may result in a secretory-type diarrhea because of inadequate surface for reabsorption of secreted fluids and electrolytes. Unlike other secretory diarrheas, this subset of conditions tends to worsen with eating. With disease (e.g., Crohn's ileitis) or resection of <100 cm of terminal ileum, dihydroxy bile acids may escape absorption and stimulate colonic secretion (cholerheic diarrhea). This mechanism may contribute to so-called *idiopathic secretory diarrhea or bile acid diarrhea (BAD)*, in which bile acids are functionally malabsorbed from a normal-appearing terminal ileum. This *idiopathic bile acid malabsorption (BAM)* may account for an average of 40% of unexplained chronic diarrhea. Reduced negative feedback regulation of bile acid synthesis in hepatocytes by fibroblast growth factor 19 (FGF-19) produced by ileal enterocytes results in a degree of bile-acid synthesis that exceeds the normal capacity for ileal reabsorption, producing BAD. An alternative cause of BAD is a genetic variation in the receptor proteins (β-klotho and fibroblast growth factor 4) on the hepatocyte that normally mediate the effect of FGF-19. Dysfunction of these proteins prevents FGF-19 inhibition of hepatocyte bile acid synthesis. Another mechanism is based on genetic variation in the bile acid receptor (TGR5) in the colon, resulting in accelerated colonic transit.

Partial bowel obstruction, ostomy stricture, or fecal impaction may paradoxically lead to increased fecal output due to fluid hypersecretion.

HORMONES Although uncommon, the classic examples of secretory diarrhea are those mediated by hormones. *Metastatic gastrointestinal carcinoid tumors* or, rarely, *primary bronchial carcinoids* may produce watery diarrhea alone or as part of the carcinoid syndrome that comprises episodic flushing, wheezing, dyspnea, and right-sided valvular heart disease. Diarrhea is due to the release into the circulation of potent intestinal secretagogues including serotonin, histamine, prostaglandins, and various kinins. Pellagra-like skin lesions may rarely occur as the result of serotonin overproduction with niacin depletion. *Gastrinoma*, one of the most common neuroendocrine tumors, most typically presents with refractory peptic ulcers, but diarrhea occurs in up to one-third of cases and may be the only clinical manifestation in 10%. While other secretagogues released with gastrin may play a role, the diarrhea most often results from fat maldigestion owing to pancreatic enzyme inactivation by low intraduodenal pH. The watery diarrhea hypokalemia achlorhydria syndrome, also called *pancreatic cholera*, is due to a non-β cell pancreatic adenoma, referred to as a *VIPoma*, that secretes VIP and a host of other peptide hormones including pancreatic polypeptide, secretin, gastrin, gastrin-inhibitory polypeptide (also called glucose-dependent insulinotropic peptide), neurotensin, calcitonin, and prostaglandins. The secretory diarrhea is often massive with stool volumes >3 L/d; daily volumes as high as 20 L have been reported. Life-threatening dehydration; neuromuscular dysfunction from associated hypokalemia, hypomagnesemia, or hypercalcemia; flushing; and hyperglycemia may accompany a VIPoma. *Medullary carcinoma of the thyroid* may present with watery diarrhea caused by calcitonin, other secretory peptides, or prostaglandins. Prominent diarrhea is often associated with metastatic disease and poor prognosis. *Systemic mastocytosis*, which may be associated with the skin lesion urticaria pigmentosa, may cause diarrhea that is either secretory and mediated by histamine or inflammatory due to intestinal infiltration by mast cells. Large *colorectal villous adenomas* may rarely be associated with a secretory diarrhea that may cause hypokalemia, can be inhibited by NSAIDs, and are apparently mediated by prostaglandins.

CONGENITAL DEFECTS IN ION ABSORPTION Rarely, defects in specific carriers associated with ion absorption cause watery diarrhea from birth. These disorders include defective Cl^-/HCO_3^- exchange (*congenital chloridorrhea*) with alkalosis (which results from a mutated *DRA* [down-regulated in adenoma] gene) and defective Na^+/H^+ exchange (*congenital sodium diarrhea*), which results from a mutation in the *NHE3* (sodium-hydrogen exchanger) gene and results in acidosis.

Some hormone deficiencies may be associated with watery diarrhea, such as occurs with adrenocortical insufficiency (Addison's disease) that may be accompanied by skin hyperpigmentation.

Osmotic Causes Osmotic diarrhea occurs when ingested, poorly absorbable, osmotically active solutes draw enough fluid into the lumen to exceed the reabsorptive capacity of the colon. Fecal water output increases in proportion to such a solute load. Osmotic diarrhea characteristically ceases with fasting or with discontinuation of the causative agent.

OSMOTIC LAXATIVES Ingestion of magnesium-containing antacids, health supplements, or laxatives may induce osmotic diarrhea typified by a stool osmotic gap (>50 mosmol/L): serum osmolarity (typically 290 mosmol/kg) − (2 × [fecal sodium + potassium concentration]). Measurement of fecal osmolarity is no longer recommended because, even when measured immediately after evacuation, it may be erroneous because carbohydrates are metabolized by colonic bacteria, causing an increase in osmolarity.

CARBOHYDRATE MALABSORPTION Carbohydrate malabsorption due to acquired or congenital defects in brush-border disaccharidases and other enzymes leads to osmotic diarrhea with a low pH. One of the most common causes of chronic diarrhea in adults is *lactase deficiency*, which affects three-fourths of nonwhites worldwide and 5–30% of persons in the United States; the total lactose load at any one time influences the symptoms experienced. Most patients learn to avoid milk products without requiring treatment with enzyme supplements. Some sugars, such as sorbitol, lactulose, or fructose, are frequently malabsorbed, and diarrhea ensues with ingestion of medications, gum, or candies sweetened with these poorly or incompletely absorbed sugars.

WHEAT AND FODMAP INTOLERANCE Chronic diarrhea, bloating, and abdominal pain are recognized as symptoms of nonceliac gluten intolerance (which is associated with impaired intestinal or colonic barrier function) and intolerance of fermentable oligosaccharides, disaccharides, monosaccharides, and polyols (FODMAPs). The latter's effects represent the interaction between the GI microbiome and the nutrients.

Steatorrheal Causes Fat malabsorption may lead to greasy, foul-smelling, difficult-to-flush diarrhea often associated with weight loss and nutritional deficiencies due to concomitant malabsorption of amino acids and vitamins. Increased fecal output is caused by the osmotic effects of fatty acids, especially after bacterial hydroxylation, and, to a lesser extent, by the neutral fat. Quantitatively, steatorrhea is defined as stool fat exceeding the normal 7 g/d; rapid-transit diarrhea may result in fecal fat up to 14 g/d; daily fecal fat averages 15–25 g with small-intestinal diseases and is often >32 g with pancreatic exocrine insufficiency. Intraluminal maldigestion, mucosal malabsorption, or lymphatic obstruction may produce steatorrhea.

INTRALUMINAL MALDIGESTION This condition most commonly results from pancreatic exocrine insufficiency, which occurs when >90% of pancreatic secretory function is lost. *Chronic pancreatitis*, usually a sequel of ethanol abuse, most frequently causes pancreatic insufficiency. Other causes include *cystic fibrosis*, *pancreatic duct obstruction*, and, rarely, *somatostatinoma*. Bacterial overgrowth in the small intestine may deconjugate bile acids and alter micelle formation, impairing fat digestion; it occurs with stasis from a blind-loop, small-bowel diverticulum or dysmotility and is especially likely in the elderly. Finally, cirrhosis or biliary obstruction may lead to mild steatorrhea due to deficient intraluminal bile acid concentration.

MUCOSAL MALABSORPTION Mucosal malabsorption occurs from a variety of enteropathies, but it most commonly occurs from *celiac disease*. This gluten-sensitive enteropathy affects all ages and is characterized by villous atrophy and crypt hyperplasia in the proximal small bowel and can present with fatty diarrhea associated with multiple nutritional deficiencies of varying severity. Celiac disease is much more frequent than previously thought; it affects ~1% of the population, frequently presents without steatorrhea, can mimic IBS, and has many other GI and extraintestinal manifestations. *Tropical sprue* may produce a similar histologic and clinical syndrome but occurs in residents of or travelers to tropical climates; abrupt onset and response to antibiotics suggest an infectious etiology. *Whipple's disease*, due to the bacillus *Tropheryma whipplei* and histiocytic infiltration of the small-bowel mucosa, is a less common cause of steatorrhea that most typically occurs in young or middle-aged men; it is frequently associated with arthralgias, fever, lymphadenopathy, and extreme fatigue, and it may affect the CNS and endocardium. A similar clinical and histologic picture results from *Mycobacterium avium-intracellulare* infection in patients with AIDS. *Abetalipoproteinemia* is a rare defect of chylomicron formation and fat malabsorption in children, associated with acanthocytic erythrocytes, ataxia, and retinitis pigmentosa. Several other conditions may cause mucosal malabsorption including infections, especially with protozoa such as *Giardia*, numerous medications (e.g., olmesartan, mycophenolate mofetil, colchicine, cholestyramine, neomycin), idiopathic enteropathies, amyloidosis, and chronic ischemia.

POSTMUCOSAL LYMPHATIC OBSTRUCTION The pathophysiology of this condition, which is due to the rare *congenital intestinal lymphangiectasia* or to *acquired lymphatic obstruction* secondary to trauma, tumor, cardiac disease, or infection, leads to the unique constellation of fat malabsorption with enteric losses of protein (often causing edema) and lymphocytopenia. Carbohydrate and amino acid absorption are preserved.

Inflammatory Causes Inflammatory diarrheas are generally accompanied by pain, fever, bleeding, or other manifestations of inflammation. The mechanism of diarrhea may not only be exudation but, depending on lesion site, may include fat malabsorption, disrupted fluid/electrolyte absorption, and hypersecretion or hypermotility from release of cytokines and other inflammatory mediators. The unifying feature on stool analysis is the presence of leukocytes or leukocyte-derived proteins such as calprotectin. With severe inflammation, exudative protein loss can lead to anasarca (generalized edema). Any middle-aged or older person with chronic inflammatory-type diarrhea, especially with blood, should be carefully evaluated to exclude a colorectal tumor.

IDIOPATHIC INFLAMMATORY BOWEL DISEASE The illnesses in this category, which include *Crohn's disease* and *chronic ulcerative colitis*, are among the most common organic causes of chronic diarrhea in adults and range in severity from mild to fulminant and life-threatening. They may be associated with uveitis, polyarthralgias, cholestatic liver disease (primary sclerosing cholangitis), and skin lesions (erythema nodosum, pyoderma gangrenosum). *Microscopic colitis*, including both lymphocytic and *collagenous colitis*, is an increasingly recognized cause of chronic watery diarrhea, especially in middle-aged women and those on NSAIDs, statins, proton pump inhibitors (PPIs), and selective serotonin reuptake inhibitors (SSRIs); biopsy of a normal-appearing colon is required for histologic diagnosis. It may coexist with symptoms suggesting IBS or with celiac sprue or drug-induced enteropathy. It typically responds well to anti-inflammatory drugs (e.g., bismuth), the opioid agonist loperamide, or budesonide.

PRIMARY OR SECONDARY FORMS OF IMMUNODEFICIENCY Immunodeficiency may lead to prolonged infectious diarrhea. With selective IgA deficiency or common variable *hypogammaglobulinemia*, diarrhea is particularly prevalent and often the result of giardiasis, bacterial overgrowth, or sprue.

EOSINOPHILIC GASTROENTERITIS Eosinophil infiltration of the mucosa, muscularis, or serosa at any level of the GI tract may cause diarrhea, pain, vomiting, or ascites. Affected patients often have an atopic history, Charcot-Leyden crystals due to extruded eosinophil contents may be seen on microscopic inspection of stool, and peripheral eosinophilia is present in 50–75% of patients. While hypersensitivity to certain foods occurs in adults, true food allergy causing chronic diarrhea is rare.

OTHER CAUSES Chronic inflammatory diarrhea may be caused by *radiation enterocolitis*, *chronic graft-versus-host disease*, autoimmune or idiopathic enteropathies, *Behçet's syndrome*, and *Cronkhite-Canada syndrome*, among others.

Dysmotility Causes Rapid transit may accompany many diarrheas as a secondary or contributing phenomenon, but primary dysmotility is an unusual etiology of true diarrhea. Stool features often suggest a secretory diarrhea, but mild steatorrhea of up to 14 g of fat per day can be produced by maldigestion from rapid transit alone. *Hyperthyroidism*, *carcinoid syndrome*, and certain drugs (e.g., prostaglandins, prokinetic agents) may produce hypermotility with resultant diarrhea. Primary visceral neuromyopathies or idiopathic acquired intestinal pseudoobstruction may lead to stasis with secondary bacterial overgrowth causing diarrhea. *Diabetic diarrhea*, often accompanied by peripheral and generalized autonomic neuropathies, may occur in part because of intestinal dysmotility.

The exceedingly common IBS (10% point prevalence, 1–2% per year incidence) is characterized by disturbed intestinal and colonic motor and sensory responses to various stimuli. Symptoms of stool frequency typically cease at night, alternate with periods of constipation, are accompanied by abdominal pain relieved with defecation, and rarely result in weight loss.

Factitial Causes Factitial diarrhea accounts for up to 15% of unexplained diarrheas referred to tertiary care centers. Either as a form of *Munchausen syndrome* (deception or self-injury for secondary gain) or *eating disorders*, some patients covertly self-administer laxatives alone or in combination with other medications (e.g., diuretics) or surreptitiously add water or urine to stool sent for analysis. Such patients are typically women, often with histories of psychiatric illness, and disproportionately from careers in health care. Hypotension and hypokalemia are common co-presenting features. The evaluation of such patients may be difficult: contamination of the stool with water or urine is suggested by very low or high stool osmolarity, respectively. Such patients often deny this possibility when confronted, but they do benefit from psychiatric counseling when they acknowledge their behavior.

APPROACH TO THE PATIENT

CHRONIC DIARRHEA

The laboratory tools available to evaluate the very common problem of chronic diarrhea are extensive, and many are costly and invasive. As such, the diagnostic evaluation must be rationally directed by a careful history, including medications, and physical examination (**Fig. 46-4**). When this strategy is unrevealing, simple triage tests are often warranted to direct the choice of more complex investigations (Fig. 46-4). The history, physical examination (**Table 46-4**), and routine blood studies should attempt to characterize the mechanism of diarrhea, identify diagnostically helpful associations, and assess the patient's fluid/electrolyte and nutritional status. Patients should be questioned about the onset, duration, pattern, aggravating (especially diet) and relieving factors, and stool characteristics of their diarrhea. The presence or absence of fecal incontinence, fever, weight loss, pain, certain exposures (travel, medications, contacts with diarrhea), and common extraintestinal manifestations (skin changes, arthralgias, oral aphthous ulcers) should be noted. A family history of IBD or celiac disease may indicate those possibilities. Physical findings may offer clues such as a thyroid mass, wheezing, heart murmurs, edema, hepatomegaly, abdominal masses, lymphadenopathy, mucocutaneous abnormalities, perianal fistulas, or anal sphincter laxity. Peripheral blood leukocytosis, elevated sedimentation rate, or C-reactive protein suggests inflammation; anemia reflects blood loss or nutritional deficiencies; or eosinophilia may occur with parasitoses, neoplasia, collagen-vascular disease, allergy, or eosinophilic gastroenteritis. Blood chemistries may demonstrate electrolyte, hepatic, or other metabolic disturbances. Measuring IgA tissue transglutaminase antibodies

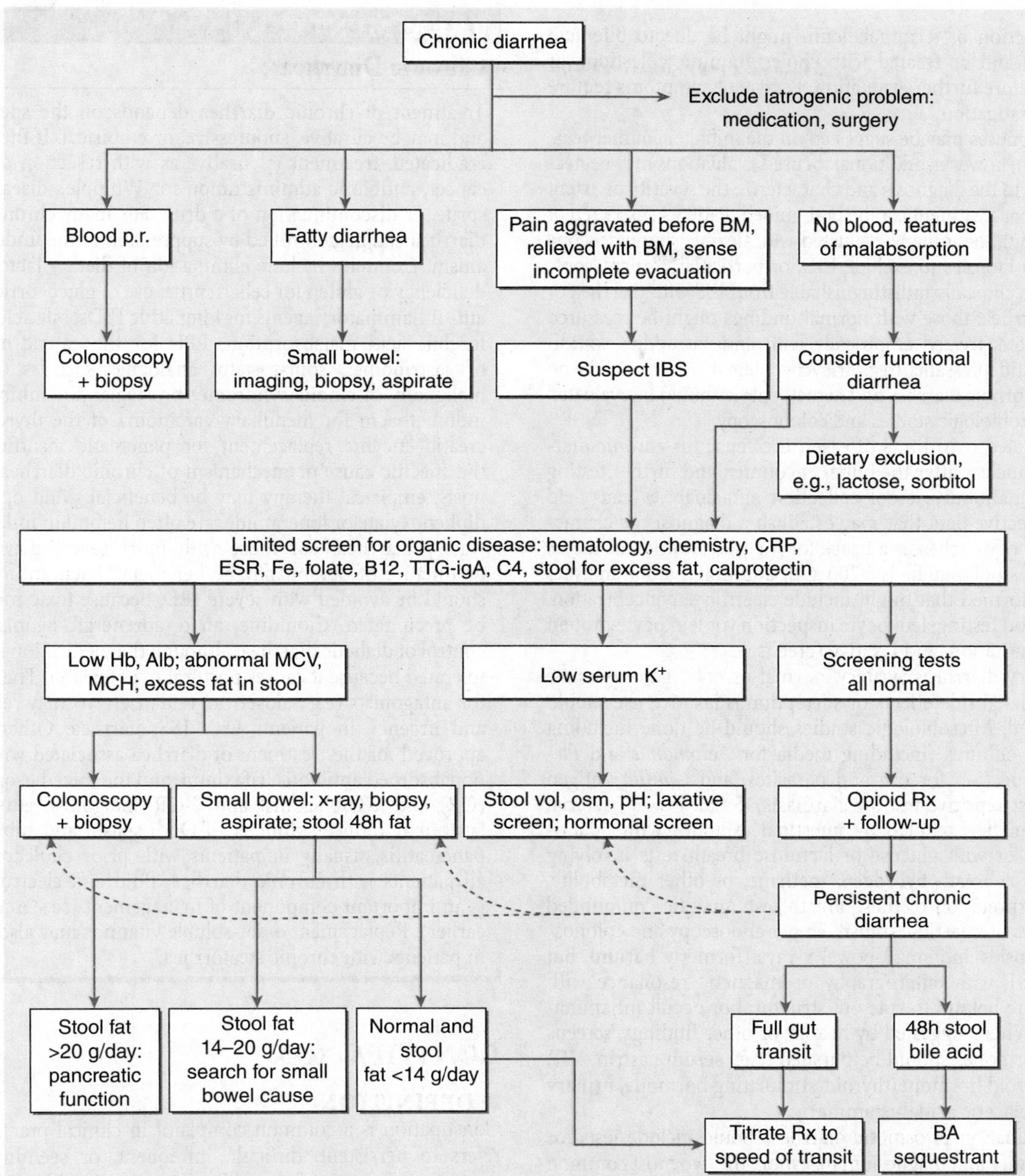

FIGURE 46-4 Algorithm for management of chronic diarrhea. Patients undergo an initial evaluation based on different symptom presentations, leading to selection of patients for imaging, biopsy analysis, and limited screens for organic diseases. Alb, albumin; BA, bile acid; BM, bowel movement; C4, 7 α-hydroxy-4-cholesten-3-one; CRP, C-reactive protein; ESR, erythrocyte sedimentation rate; Hb, hemoglobin; Hx, history; IBS, irritable bowel syndrome; MCH, mean corpuscular hemoglobin; MCV, mean corpuscular volume; osm, osmolality; p.r., per rectum; Rx, treatment; TTG, tissue transglutaminase. *(Reproduced with permission from M Camilleri, JH Sellin, KE Barrett: Pathophysiology, evaluation, and management of chronic watery diarrhea. Gastroenterology 152:515, 2017.)*

TABLE 46-4 Physical Examination in Patients with Chronic Diarrhea

1. Are there general features to suggest malabsorption or inflammatory bowel disease (IBD) such as anemia, dermatitis herpetiformis, edema, or clubbing?
2. Are there features to suggest underlying autonomic neuropathy or collagen-vascular disease in the pupils, orthostasis, skin, hands, or joints?
3. Is there an abdominal mass or tenderness?
4. Are there any abnormalities of rectal mucosa, rectal defects, or altered anal sphincter functions?
5. Are there any mucocutaneous manifestations of systemic disease such as dermatitis herpetiformis (celiac disease), erythema nodosum (ulcerative colitis), flushing (carcinoid), or oral ulcers for IBD or celiac disease?

may help detect celiac disease. Bile acid diarrhea is confirmed by a scintigraphic radiolabeled bile acid retention test; however, this is not available in many countries. Alternative approaches are a screening blood test (serum C4 or FGF-19), measurement of fecal bile acids, or a therapeutic trial with a bile acid sequestrant (e.g., cholestyramine, colestipol or colesevelam).

A therapeutic trial is often appropriate, definitive, and highly cost-effective when a specific diagnosis is suggested on the initial physician encounter. For example, chronic watery diarrhea, which ceases with fasting in an otherwise healthy young adult, may justify a trial of a lactose-restricted diet; bloating and diarrhea persisting since a mountain backpacking trip may warrant a trial of metronidazole for likely giardiasis; and postprandial diarrhea persisting following resection of terminal ileum might be due to bile acid malabsorption and be treated with cholestyramine, colestipol, or colesevelam before further evaluation. Persistent symptoms require additional investigation.

Certain diagnoses may be suggested on the initial encounter (e.g., idiopathic IBD); however, additional focused evaluations may be necessary to confirm the diagnosis and characterize the severity or extent of disease so that treatment can be best guided. Patients suspected of having IBS should be initially evaluated with flexible sigmoidoscopy with colorectal biopsies to exclude IBD, or particularly microscopic colitis, which is clinically indistinguishable from IBS with diarrhea or functional diarrhea; those with normal findings might be reassured and, as indicated, treated empirically with antispasmodics, antidiarrheals, or antidepressants (e.g., tricyclic agents). Any patient who presents with chronic diarrhea and hematochezia should be evaluated with stool microbiologic studies and colonoscopy.

In an estimated two-thirds of cases, the cause for chronic diarrhea remains unclear after the initial encounter, and further testing is required. Quantitative stool collection and analyses can yield important objective data that may establish a diagnosis or characterize the type of diarrhea as a triage for focused additional studies (Fig. 46-4). If stool weight is >200 g/d, additional stool analyses should be performed that might include electrolyte concentration, pH, occult blood testing, leukocyte inspection (or leukocyte protein assay), fat quantitation, and laxative screens.

For secretory diarrheas (watery, normal osmotic gap), possible medication-related side effects or surreptitious laxative use should be reconsidered. Microbiologic studies should be done including fecal bacterial cultures (including media for *Aeromonas* and *Plesiomonas*), inspection for ova and parasites, and *Giardia* antigen assay (the most sensitive test for giardiasis). Small-bowel bacterial overgrowth can be excluded by intestinal aspirates with quantitative cultures or with glucose or lactulose breath tests involving measurement of breath hydrogen, methane, or other metabolite. However, interpretation of these breath tests may be confounded by disturbances of intestinal transit. Upper endoscopy and colonoscopy with biopsies and small-bowel x-rays (formerly barium, but increasingly CT with enterography or magnetic resonance with enteroclysis) are helpful to rule out structural or occult inflammatory disease. When suggested by history or other findings, screens for peptide hormones should be pursued (e.g., serum gastrin, VIP, calcitonin, thyroid hormone/thyroid-stimulating hormone, urinary 5-hydroxyindolacetic acid, histamine).

Further evaluation of osmotic diarrhea should include tests for lactose intolerance and magnesium ingestion, the two most common causes. Low fecal pH suggests carbohydrate malabsorption; lactose malabsorption can be confirmed by lactose breath testing or by a therapeutic trial with lactose exclusion and observation of the effect of lactose challenge (e.g., a liter of milk). Lactase determination on small-bowel biopsy is not generally available. If fecal magnesium or laxative levels are elevated, inadvertent or surreptitious ingestion should be considered and psychiatric help should be sought.

For those with proven fatty diarrhea, endoscopy with small-bowel biopsy (including aspiration for quantitative cultures, if available) should be performed; if this procedure is unrevealing, a small-bowel radiograph is often an appropriate next step. If small-bowel studies are negative or if pancreatic disease is suspected, pancreatic exocrine insufficiency should be excluded with direct tests, such as the secretin-cholecystokinin stimulation test or a variation that could be performed endoscopically. In general, indirect tests such as assay of fecal elastase or chymotrypsin activity or a bentiromide test have fallen out of favor because of low sensitivity and specificity.

Chronic inflammatory-type diarrheas should be suspected by the presence of blood or leukocytes in the stool. Such findings warrant stool cultures; inspection for ova and parasites; *C. difficile* toxin assay; colonoscopy with biopsies; and, if indicated, small-bowel imaging studies.

TREATMENT

Chronic Diarrhea

Treatment of chronic diarrhea depends on the specific etiology and may be curative, suppressive, or empirical. If the cause can be eradicated, treatment is curative as with resection of a colorectal cancer, antibiotic administration for Whipple's disease or tropical sprue, or discontinuation of a drug. For many chronic conditions, diarrhea can be controlled by suppression of the underlying mechanism. Examples include elimination of dietary lactose for lactase deficiency or gluten for celiac sprue, use of glucocorticoids or other anti-inflammatory agents for idiopathic IBDs, bile acid sequestrants for bile acid malabsorption, PPIs for the gastric hypersecretion of gastrinomas, somatostatin analogues such as octreotide for malignant carcinoid syndrome, prostaglandin inhibitors such as indomethacin for medullary carcinoma of the thyroid, and pancreatic enzyme replacement for pancreatic insufficiency. When the specific cause or mechanism of chronic diarrhea evades diagnosis, empirical therapy may be beneficial. Mild opiates, such as diphenoxylate or loperamide, are often helpful in mild or moderate watery diarrhea. For those with more severe diarrhea, codeine or tincture of opium may be beneficial. Such antimotility agents should be avoided with severe IBD, because toxic megacolon may be precipitated. Clonidine, an α_2-adrenergic agonist, may allow control of diabetic diarrhea, although the medication may be poorly tolerated because it causes postural hypotension. The 5-HT_3 receptor antagonists (e.g., alosetron, ondansetron) may relieve diarrhea and urgency in patients with IBS diarrhea. Other medications approved for the treatment of diarrhea associated with IBS are the nonabsorbed antibiotic, rifaximin, and the mixed μ-opioid receptor (OR) and κ-OR agonist and δ-OR antagonist, eluxadoline. The latter may induce sphincter of Oddi spasm and subsequent acute pancreatitis, usually in patients with prior cholecystectomy. For all patients with chronic diarrhea, fluid and electrolyte repletion is an important component of management (see "Acute Diarrhea," earlier). Replacement of fat-soluble vitamins may also be necessary in patients with chronic steatorrhea.

CONSTIPATION

DEFINITION

Constipation is a common complaint in clinical practice and usually refers to persistent, difficult, infrequent, or seemingly incomplete defecation. Because of the wide range of normal bowel habits, constipation is difficult to define precisely. Most persons have at least three bowel movements per week; however, low stool frequency alone is not the sole criterion for the diagnosis of constipation. Many constipated patients have a normal frequency of defecation but complain of excessive straining, hard stools, lower abdominal fullness, or a sense of incomplete evacuation. The individual patient's symptoms must be analyzed in detail to ascertain what is meant by "constipation" or "difficulty" with defecation.

Stool form and consistency are well correlated with the time elapsed from the preceding defecation. Hard, pellety stools occur with slow transit, whereas loose, watery stools are associated with rapid transit. Both small pellety or very large stools are more difficult to expel than normal stools.

The perception of hard stools or excessive straining is more difficult to assess objectively, and the need for enemas or digital disimpaction is a clinically useful way to corroborate the patient's perceptions of difficult defecation.

Psychosocial or cultural factors may also be important. A person whose parents attached great importance to daily defecation will become greatly concerned when he or she misses a daily bowel movement; some children withhold stool to gain attention or because of fear of pain from anal irritation; and some adults habitually ignore or delay the call to have a bowel movement.

CAUSES

Pathophysiologically, chronic constipation generally results from inadequate fiber or fluid intake or from disordered colonic transit or anorectal function. These result from neurogastroenterologic disturbance, certain drugs, advancing age, or in association with a large number of systemic diseases that affect the GI tract (**Table 46-5**). Constipation of recent onset may be a symptom of significant organic disease such as tumor, anorectal irritation, or stricture. In *idiopathic constipation*, a subset of patients exhibits delayed emptying of the ascending and transverse colon with prolongation of transit (often in the proximal colon) and a reduced frequency of propulsive HAPCs. *Outlet obstruction to defecation* (also called *evacuation disorders*) accounts for about a quarter of cases presenting with constipation in tertiary care and may cause delayed colonic transit, which is usually corrected by biofeedback retraining of the disordered defecation. Constipation of any cause may be exacerbated by hospitalization or chronic illnesses that lead to physical or mental impairment and result in inactivity or physical immobility.

APPROACH TO THE PATIENT

Constipation

A careful history should explore the patient's symptoms and confirm whether she or he is indeed constipated based on frequency (e.g., fewer than three bowel movements per week), consistency (lumpy/hard), excessive straining, prolonged defecation time, or need to support the perineum or digitate the anorectum to facilitate stool evacuation. These latter items identified in the history suggest the presence of a rectal evacuation disorder. In the vast majority of cases (probably >90%), there is no underlying cause (e.g., cancer, depression, or hypothyroidism), and constipation responds to ample hydration, exercise, and supplementation of dietary fiber (15–25 g/d). A good diet and medication history and attention to psychosocial issues are key. Physical examination and, particularly, rectal examination are mandatory and should exclude fecal impaction and most of the important diseases that present with constipation and possibly indicate features suggesting an evacuation disorder (e.g., high anal sphincter tone, failure of perineal descent, or paradoxical puborectalis contraction or puborectalis tenderness during straining to simulate stool evacuation).

The presence of weight loss, rectal bleeding, or anemia with constipation mandates either flexible sigmoidoscopy plus barium enema or colonoscopy alone, particularly in patients aged >40 years, to exclude structural diseases such as cancer or strictures. Colonoscopy alone is most cost-effective in this setting because it provides an opportunity to biopsy mucosal lesions, perform polypectomy, or dilate strictures. Barium enema has advantages over colonoscopy in the patient with isolated constipation because it is less costly and identifies colonic dilation and all significant mucosal lesions or strictures that are likely to present with constipation. Melanosis coli, or pigmentation of the colon mucosa, indicates the use of anthraquinone laxatives such as cascara or senna; however, this is usually apparent from a careful history. An unexpected disorder such as megacolon or cathartic colon may also be detected by colonic radiographs. Measurement of serum calcium, potassium, and thyroid-stimulating hormone levels will identify rare patients with metabolic disorders.

Patients with more troublesome constipation may not respond to fiber alone and may be helped by a bowel-training regimen, which involves taking an osmotic laxative (e.g., magnesium salts, lactulose, sorbitol, polyethylene glycol) and evacuating with enema or suppository (e.g., glycerin or bisacodyl) as needed. After breakfast, a distraction-free 15–20 min on the toilet without straining is encouraged. Excessive straining may lead to development of hemorrhoids and, if there is weakness of the pelvic floor or injury to the pudendal nerve, may result in obstructed defecation from descending perineum syndrome several years later. Those few who do not benefit from the simple measures delineated above or require long-term treatment or fail to respond to potent laxatives should undergo further investigation (**Fig. 46-5**). Novel agents that induce secretion (e.g., lubiprostone, a chloride channel activator, or linaclotide, a guanylate cyclase C agonist that activates chloride secretion) are also available.

TABLE 46-5 Causes of Constipation in Adults

TYPES OF CONSTIPATION AND CAUSES	EXAMPLES
Recent Onset	
Colonic obstruction	Neoplasm; stricture: ischemic, diverticular, inflammatory
Anal sphincter spasm	Anal fissure, painful hemorrhoids
Medications	
Chronic	
Irritable bowel syndrome	Constipation-predominant, alternating
Medications	Ca^{2+} blockers, antidepressants
Colonic pseudoobstruction	Slow-transit constipation, megacolon (rare Hirschsprung's, Chagas' diseases)
Disorders of rectal evacuation	Pelvic floor dysfunction; anismus; descending perineum syndrome; rectal mucosal prolapse; rectocele
Endocrinopathies	Hypothyroidism, hypercalcemia, pregnancy
Psychiatric disorders	Depression, eating disorders, drugs
Neurologic disease	Parkinsonism, multiple sclerosis, spinal cord injury
Generalized muscle disease	Progressive systemic sclerosis

INVESTIGATION OF SEVERE CONSTIPATION

A small minority (probably <5%) of patients have severe or "intractable" constipation; about 25% have evacuation disorders. These are the patients most likely to require evaluation by gastroenterologists or in referral centers. Further observation of the patient may occasionally

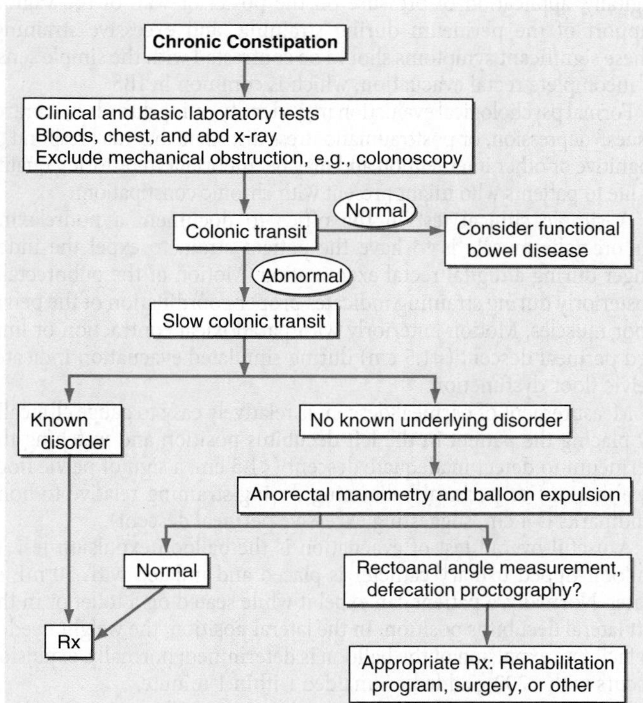

FIGURE 46-5 Algorithm for the management of constipation. abd, abdominal; Rx, treatment.

reveal a previously unrecognized cause, such as an evacuation disorder, laxative abuse, malingering, or psychological disorder. In these patients, evaluations of the physiologic function of the colon and pelvic floor and of psychological status aid in the rational choice of treatment. Even among these highly selected patients with severe constipation, a cause can be identified in only about one-third of tertiary referral patients, with the others being diagnosed with normal transit constipation. Since evacuation disorders also retard colonic transit through the left colon or the entire colon, anorectal and pelvic floor testing should precede transit measurements if there is clinical suspicion of an evacuation disorder. If an evacuation disorder is identified on testing, colonic transit may be unnecessary.

Measurement of Colonic Transit Radiopaque marker transit tests are easy, repeatable, generally safe, inexpensive, reliable, and highly applicable in evaluating constipated patients in clinical practice. Several validated methods are very simple. For example, radiopaque markers are ingested; an abdominal flat film taken 5 days later should indicate passage of 80% of the markers out of the colon without the use of laxatives or enemas. This test does not provide useful information about the transit profile of the stomach and small bowel. An alternative approach involves ingestion of 24 radiopaque markers on 3 successive days and an abdominal radiograph on the fourth day. The number of markers counted in the radiograph is an estimate of the colonic transit in hours. The collection of gas in the rectum between the level of the ischial spines and the lower border of the sacroiliac joints may suggest the presence of a rectal evacuation disorder as the cause of constipation.

Radioscintigraphy with a delayed-release capsule containing radiolabeled particles has been used to noninvasively characterize normal, accelerated, or delayed colonic function over 24–48 h with low radiation exposure. This approach simultaneously assesses gastric, small bowel (which may be important in ~20% of patients with delayed colonic transit because they reflect a more generalized GI motility disorder), and colonic transit. The disadvantages are the greater cost and the need for specific materials prepared in a nuclear medicine laboratory.

Anorectal and Pelvic Floor Tests Pelvic floor dysfunction is suggested by the inability to evacuate the rectum, a feeling of persistent rectal fullness, rectal pain, the need to extract stool from the rectum digitally, application of pressure on the posterior wall of the vagina, support of the perineum during straining, and excessive straining. These significant symptoms should be contrasted with the simple sense of incomplete rectal evacuation, which is common in IBS.

Formal psychological evaluation may identify eating disorders, "control issues," depression, or posttraumatic stress disorders that may respond to cognitive or other intervention and may be important in restoring quality of life to patients who might present with chronic constipation.

A simple clinical test in the office to document a nonrelaxing puborectalis muscle is to have the patient strain to expel the index finger during a digital rectal examination. Motion of the puborectalis posteriorly during straining indicates proper coordination of the pelvic floor muscles. Motion anteriorly with paradoxical contraction or limited perineal descent (<1.5 cm) during simulated evacuation indicates pelvic floor dysfunction.

Measurement of perineal descent is relatively easy to gauge clinically by placing the patient in the left decubitus position and watching the perineum to detect inadequate descent (<1.5 cm, a sign of pelvic floor dysfunction) or perineal ballooning during straining relative to bony landmarks (>4 cm, suggesting excessive perineal descent).

A useful overall test of evacuation is the balloon expulsion test. A balloon-tipped urinary catheter is placed and inflated with 50 mL of water. Normally, a patient can expel it while seated on a toilet or in the left lateral decubitus position. In the lateral position, the weight needed to facilitate expulsion of the balloon is determined; normally, expulsion occurs with <200 g added or unaided within 1 minute.

Anorectal manometry, when used in the evaluation of patients with severe constipation, may find an excessively high resting (>80 mmHg) or squeeze anal sphincter tone, suggesting anismus (anal sphincter spasm). This test also identifies rare syndromes, such as adult Hirschsprung's disease, by the absence of the rectoanal inhibitory reflex.

Defecography (a dynamic barium enema including lateral views obtained during barium expulsion or a magnetic resonance defecogram) reveals "soft abnormalities" in many patients; the most relevant findings are the measured changes in rectoanal angle, anatomic defects of the rectum such as internal mucosal prolapse, and enteroceles or rectoceles. Surgically remediable conditions are identified in only a few patients. These include severe, whole-thickness intussusception with complete outlet obstruction due to funnel-shaped plugging at the anal canal or an extremely large rectocele that fills preferentially during attempts at defecation instead of expulsion of the barium through the anus. In summary, defecography requires an interested and experienced radiologist, and abnormalities are not pathognomonic for pelvic floor dysfunction. The most common cause of outlet obstruction is failure of the puborectalis muscle to relax; this is not identified by barium defecography but can be demonstrated by magnetic resonance defecography, which provides more information about the structure and function of the pelvic floor, distal colorectum, and anal sphincters.

Neurologic testing (electromyography) is more helpful in the evaluation of patients with incontinence than of those with symptoms suggesting obstructed defecation. The absence of neurologic signs in the lower extremities suggests that any documented denervation of the puborectalis results from pelvic (e.g., obstetric) injury or from stretching of the pudendal nerve by chronic, long-standing straining. Constipation is common among patients with spinal cord injuries, neurologic diseases such as Parkinson's disease, multiple sclerosis, and diabetic neuropathy.

Spinal-evoked responses during electrical rectal stimulation or stimulation of external anal sphincter contraction by applying magnetic stimulation over the lumbosacral cord identify patients with limited sacral neuropathies with sufficient residual nerve conduction to attempt biofeedback training.

In summary, a balloon expulsion test is an important screening test for anorectal dysfunction. Rarely, an anatomic evaluation of the rectum or anal sphincters and an assessment of pelvic floor relaxation are the tools for evaluating patients in whom obstructed defecation is suspected and is associated with symptoms of rectal mucosal prolapse, pressure of the posterior wall of the vagina to facilitate defecation (suggestive of anterior rectocele), or prior pelvic surgery that may be complicated by enterocele.

TREATMENT

Constipation

After the cause of constipation is characterized, a treatment decision can be made. Slow-transit constipation requires aggressive medical or surgical treatment; anismus or pelvic floor dysfunction usually responds to biofeedback management (Fig. 46-5). The remaining ~60% of patients with constipation have normal colonic transit and can be treated symptomatically. Patients with spinal cord injuries or other neurologic disorders require a dedicated bowel regimen that often includes rectal stimulation, enema therapy, and carefully timed laxative therapy.

Patients with constipation are treated with bulk (fiber, psyllium), osmotic (milk of magnesia, lactulose, polyethylene glycol), secretory (lubiprostone, linaclotide, plecanatide, tenapanor), and prokinetic or stimulant laxatives (including diphenyl methanes such as bisacodyl and sodium picosulfate and 5-HT$_4$ agonists prucalopride and tegaserod). If a 3- to 6-month trial of medical therapies fails, unassociated with obstructed defecation, the patient should be considered for laparoscopic colectomy with ileorectostomy; however, this should not be undertaken for pain or if there is continued evidence of an evacuation disorder or a generalized GI dysmotility. Referral to a specialized center for further tests of colonic motor function is warranted. The decision to resort to surgery is facilitated by the presence of megacolon and megarectum. The complications after surgery include small-bowel obstruction (11%) and fecal soiling, particularly at night during the first postoperative year. Frequency of defecation is 3–8 per day during the first year, dropping to 1–3 per day from the second year after surgery.

Patients who have a combined (evacuation and transit/motility) disorder should first pursue pelvic floor retraining (biofeedback and muscle relaxation), psychological counseling, and dietetic advice. If symptoms are intractable despite biofeedback and optimized medical therapy, colectomy and ileorectostomy could be considered as long as the evacuation disorder is resolved and optimized medical therapy is unsuccessful. In patients with pelvic floor dysfunction alone, biofeedback training has a 70–80% success rate, measured by the acquisition of comfortable stool habits. Attempts to manage pelvic floor dysfunction with operations (internal anal sphincter or puborectalis muscle division) or injections with botulinum toxin have achieved only mediocre success and have been largely abandoned.

FURTHER READING

Assi R et al: Sexually transmitted infections of the anus and rectum. World J Gastroenterol 20:15262, 2014.

Bharucha AE, Rao SS: An update on anorectal disorders for gastroenterologists. Gastroenterology 146:37, 2014.

Bharucha AE et al: American Gastroenterological Association technical review on constipation. Gastroenterology 144:218, 2013.

Boeckxstaens G et al: Fundamentals of neurogastroenterology: Physiology/motility—sensation. Gastroenterology 150:1292, 2016.

Camilleri M et al: Chronic constipation. Nat Rev Dis Primers 3:17095, 2017.

Camilleri M et al: Pathophysiology, evaluation, and management of chronic watery diarrhea. Gastroenterology 152:515, 2017.

Peery AF et al: Burden and cost of gastrointestinal, liver, and pancreatic diseases in the United States: Update 2018. Gastroenterology 156:254, 2019.

Riddle MS et al: ACG Clinical Guideline: Diagnosis, treatment, and prevention of acute diarrheal infections in adults. Am J Gastroenterol 111:602, 2016.

Rubio-Tapia A et al: American College of Gastroenterology. ACG clinical guidelines: Diagnosis and management of celiac disease. Am J Gastroenterol 108:656, 2013.

Smalley W et al: AGA Clinical Practice Guidelines on the laboratory evaluation of functional diarrhea and diarrhea-predominant irritable bowel syndrome in adults (IBS-D). Gastroenterology 157:851, 2019.

Uzzan M et al: Gastrointestinal disorders associated with common variable immune deficiency (CVID) and chronic granulomatous disease (CGD). Curr Gastroenterol Rep 18:17, 2016.

47 Unintentional Weight Loss

J. Larry Jameson

Involuntary or unintentional weight loss (UWL) is frequently insidious and can have important implications, often serving as a harbinger of serious underlying disease. Clinically important weight loss is defined as the loss of 10 pounds (4.5 kg) or >5% of one's body weight over a period of 6–12 months. UWL is encountered in up to 8% of all adult outpatients and 27% of frail persons aged ≥65 years. There is no identifiable cause in up to one-quarter of patients despite extensive investigation. Conversely, up to half of people who claim to have lost weight have no documented evidence of weight loss. People with no known cause of weight loss generally have a better prognosis than do those with known causes, particularly when the source is neoplastic. Weight loss in older persons is associated with a variety of deleterious effects, including falls and fractures, pressure ulcers, impaired immune function, and decreased functional status. Not surprisingly, significant weight loss is associated with increased mortality, which can range from 9% to as high as 38% within 1–2.5 years in the absence of clinical awareness and attention.

PHYSIOLOGY OF WEIGHT REGULATION WITH AGING

(See also Chaps. 401 and 476) Among healthy aging people, total body weight peaks in the sixth decade of life and generally remains stable until the ninth decade, after which it gradually falls. In contrast, lean body mass (fat-free mass) begins to decline at a rate of 0.3 kg per year in the third decade, and the rate of decline increases further beginning at age 60 in men and age 65 in women. These changes in lean body mass largely reflect the age-dependent decline in growth hormone secretion and, consequently, circulating levels of insulin-like growth factor type I (IGF-I) that occur with normal aging. Loss of sex steroids, at menopause in women and more gradually in men, also contributes to these changes in body composition. In the healthy elderly, an increase in fat tissue balances the loss in lean body mass until very old age, when loss of both fat and skeletal muscle occurs. Age-dependent changes also occur at the cellular level. Telomeres shorten, and body cell mass—the fat-free portion of cells—declines steadily with aging.

Between ages 20 and 80, mean energy intake is reduced by up to 1200 kcal/d in men and 800 kcal/d in women. Decreased hunger is a reflection of reduced physical activity and loss of lean body mass, producing lower demand for calories and food intake. Several important age-associated physiologic changes also predispose elderly persons to weight loss, such as declining chemosensory function (smell and taste), reduced efficiency of chewing, slowed gastric emptying, and alterations in the neuroendocrine axis, including changes in levels of leptin, cholecystokinin, neuropeptide Y, and other hormones and peptides. These changes are associated with early satiety and a decline in both appetite and the hedonistic appreciation of food. Collectively, they contribute to the "anorexia of aging." As noted below, these physiologic changes with aging may be accompanied by social isolation, poverty, and immobility, further contributing to undernutrition.

CAUSES OF UNINTENTIONAL WEIGHT LOSS

Most causes of UWL belong to one of four categories: (1) malignant neoplasms, (2) chronic inflammatory or infectious diseases, (3) metabolic disorders (e.g., hyperthyroidism and diabetes), or (4) psychiatric disorders **(Table 47-1)**. Not infrequently, more than one of these causes can be responsible for UWL. Depending upon patient populations, UWL is caused by malignant disease in a quarter of patients and by organic disease in one-third, with the remainder due to psychiatric disease, medications, or uncertain causes. Risk factors for undiagnosed cancer include a history of smoking, particularly for men, localizing symptoms, and abnormal laboratory tests.

The most common malignant causes of UWL are gastrointestinal, hepatobiliary, hematologic, lung, breast, genitourinary, ovarian, and prostate. Half of all patients with cancer lose some body weight; one-third lose more than 5% of their original body weight, and up to 20% of all cancer deaths are caused directly by cachexia (through immobility and/or cardiac/respiratory failure). The greatest incidence of weight loss is seen among patients with solid tumors. Malignancy that reveals itself through significant weight loss usually has a very poor prognosis.

In addition to malignancies, gastrointestinal diseases are among the most prominent causes of UWL. Peptic ulcer disease, inflammatory bowel disease, dysmotility syndromes, chronic pancreatitis, celiac disease, constipation, and atrophic gastritis are some of the more common entities. Oral and dental problems are easily overlooked and may manifest with halitosis, poor oral hygiene, xerostomia, inability to chew, reduced masticatory force, nonocclusion, temporomandibular joint syndrome, edentulousness, and pain due to caries or abscesses.

Tuberculosis, fungal diseases, parasites, subacute bacterial endocarditis, and HIV are well-documented causes of UWL. Cardiovascular

TABLE 47-1 Causes of Involuntary Weight Loss

Cancer	**Medications**
Colon	Sedatives
Hepatobiliary	Antibiotics
Hematologic	Nonsteroidal anti-inflammatory drugs
Lung	Serotonin reuptake inhibitors
Breast	Metformin
Genitourinary	Levodopa
Ovarian	Angiotensin-converting enzyme inhibitors
Prostate	Other drugs
Gastrointestinal disorders	**Disorders of the mouth and teeth**
Difficulty swallowing	Caries
Malabsorption	Dysgeusia
Peptic ulcer	**Age-related factors**
Inflammatory bowel disease	Physiologic changes
Pancreatitis	Visual impairment
Obstruction/constipation	Decreased taste and smell
Pernicious anemia	Functional disabilities
Endocrine and metabolic	**Neurologic**
Hyperthyroidism	Stroke
Diabetes mellitus	Parkinson's disease
Pheochromocytoma	Neuromuscular disorders
Adrenal insufficiency	Dementia
Cardiac disorders	**Social**
Chronic ischemia	Isolation
Chronic congestive heart failure	Poverty
Respiratory disorders	**Psychiatric and behavioral**
Emphysema	Depression
Chronic obstructive pulmonary disease	Anxiety
Renal insufficiency	Paranoia
Rheumatologic disease	Bereavement
Infections	Alcoholism
HIV	Eating disorders
Tuberculosis	Increased activity or exercise
Parasitic infection	**Idiopathic**
Subacute bacterial endocarditis	

and pulmonary diseases cause UWL through increased metabolic demand and decreased appetite and caloric intake. Repeated surgeries may lead to weight loss because of reduced caloric intake and increased metabolic demands resulting from a systemic inflammatory response. Uremia produces nausea, anorexia, and vomiting. Connective tissue diseases may increase metabolic demand and disrupt nutritional balance. As the incidence of diabetes mellitus increases with aging, the associated glucosuria can contribute to weight loss. Hyperthyroidism in the elderly may have less prominent sympathomimetic features and may present as "apathetic hyperthyroidism" or T_3 toxicosis **(Chap. 382)**.

Neurologic injuries such as stroke, quadriplegia, and multiple sclerosis may lead to visceral and autonomic dysfunction that can impair caloric intake. Dysphagia from these neurologic insults is a common mechanism. Functional disability that compromises activities of daily living (ADLs) is a common cause of undernutrition in the elderly. Visual impairment from ophthalmic or central nervous system disorders such as a tremor can limit the ability of people to prepare and eat meals. UWL may be one of the earliest manifestations of Alzheimer's dementia.

Isolation and depression are significant causes of UWL that may manifest as an inability to care for oneself, including nutritional needs. A cytokine-mediated inflammatory metabolic cascade can be both a cause of and a manifestation of depression. Bereavement can be a cause of UWL and, when present, is often more pronounced in men. More intense forms of mental illness such as paranoid disorders may lead to delusions about food and cause weight loss. Alcoholism can be a significant source of weight loss and malnutrition.

Elderly persons living in poverty may have to choose whether to purchase food or use the money for other expenses, including medications. Screening questions can probe whether patients have run out of food or whether they routinely purchase less than they need. Institutionalization is an independent risk factor, as up to 30–50% of nursing home patients have inadequate food intake.

Medications can cause anorexia, nausea, vomiting, gastrointestinal distress, diarrhea, dry mouth, and changes in taste. This is particularly an issue in the elderly, many of whom take five or more medications.

ASSESSMENT

The four major manifestations of UWL are (1) anorexia (loss of appetite), (2) sarcopenia (loss of muscle mass), (3) cachexia (a syndrome that combines weight loss, loss of muscle and adipose tissue, anorexia, and weakness), and (4) dehydration. The current obesity epidemic adds complexity, as excess adipose tissue can mask the development of sarcopenia and delay awareness of the development of cachexia. If it is not possible to measure weight directly, a change in clothing size, corroboration of weight loss by a relative or friend, and a numeric estimate of weight loss provided by the patient are suggestive of true weight loss.

Initial assessment includes a comprehensive history and physical, a complete blood count, tests of liver enzyme levels, C-reactive protein, erythrocyte sedimentation rate, renal function studies, thyroid function tests, chest radiography, and an abdominal ultrasound **(Table 47-2)**. Age-, sex-, and risk factor–specific cancer screening tests, such as mammography and colonoscopy, should be performed **(Chap. 70)**. Patients at risk should have HIV testing. All elderly patients with weight loss should undergo screening for dementia and depression by using instruments such as the Mini-Mental State Examination and the Geriatric Depression Scale, respectively **(Chap. 477)**. The Mini Nutritional Assessment (*www.mna-elderly.com*) and the Nutrition Screening Initiative (*http://www.ncbi.nlm.nih.gov/pmc/articles/PMC1694757/*) are also available for the nutritional assessment of elderly patients. Almost all patients with a malignancy and >90% of those with other organic diseases have at least one laboratory abnormality. In patients presenting with substantial UWL, major organic and malignant diseases are unlikely when

TABLE 47-2 Assessment and Testing for Involuntary Weight Loss

Indications	Laboratory
5% weight loss in 30 d	Complete blood count
10% weight loss in 180 d	Comprehensive electrolyte and metabolic panel, including liver and renal function tests
Body mass index <21	Thyroid function tests
25% of food left uneaten after 7 d	Erythrocyte sedimentation rate
Change in fit of clothing	C-reactive protein
Change in appetite, smell, or taste	Ferritin
Abdominal pain, nausea, vomiting, diarrhea, constipation, dysphagia	HIV testing, if indicated
Assessment	**Radiology**
Complete physical examination, including dental evaluation	Chest x-ray Abdominal ultrasound
Medication review	
Recommended cancer screening	
Mini-Mental State Examination[a]	
Mini-Nutritional Assessment[a]	
Nutrition Screening Initiative[a]	
Simplified Nutritional Assessment Questionnaire[a]	
Observation of eating[a]	
Activities of daily living[a]	
Instrumental activities of daily living[a]	

[a]May be more specific to assess weight loss in the elderly.

a baseline evaluation is completely normal. Careful follow-up rather than undirected testing is advised because the prognosis of weight loss of undetermined cause is generally favorable.

TREATMENT
Unintentional Weight Loss

The first priority in managing weight loss is to identify and treat the underlying causes. Treatment of underlying metabolic, psychiatric, infectious, or other systemic disorders may be sufficient to restore weight and functional status gradually. Medications that cause nausea or anorexia should be withdrawn or changed, if possible. For those with unexplained UWL, oral nutritional supplements such as high-energy drinks sometimes reverse weight loss. Advising patients to consume supplements between meals rather than with a meal may help minimize appetite suppression and facilitate increased overall intake. Orexigenic, anabolic, and anticytokine agents are under investigation. In selected patients, the antidepressant mirtazapine results in a significant increase in body weight, body fat mass, and leptin concentration. Patients with wasting conditions who can comply with an appropriate exercise program gain muscle protein mass, strength, and endurance and may be more capable of performing ADLs.

Acknowledgment
The author is grateful to Russell G. Robertson, MD, for contributions to this chapter in prior editions.

FURTHER READING

Alibhai SM et al: An approach to the management of unintentional weight loss in elderly people. CMAJ 172:773, 2005.

Gaddey HL, Holder K: Unintentional weight loss in older adults. Am Fam Physician 89:718, 2014.

McMinn J et al: Investigation and management of unintentional weight loss in older adults. BMJ 342:d1732, 2011.

Nicholson BD et al: Prioritising primary care patients with unexpected weight loss for cancer investigation. BMJ 370:m2651, 2020.

Vanderschueren S et al: The diagnostic spectrum of unintentional weight loss. Eur J Intern Med 16:160, 2005.

Wong CJ: Involuntary weight loss. Med Clin North Am 98:625, 2014.

48 Gastrointestinal Bleeding

Loren Laine

Gastrointestinal bleeding (GIB) presents as either overt or occult bleeding. *Overt GIB* is manifested by *hematemesis*, vomitus of red blood or "coffee-grounds" material; *melena*, black, tarry stool; and/or *hematochezia*, passage of red or maroon blood from the rectum. In the absence of overt bleeding, *occult GIB* may present with *symptoms of blood loss or anemia* such as lightheadedness, syncope, angina, or dyspnea; with iron-deficiency anemia; or a positive fecal occult blood test on colorectal cancer screening. GIB is also categorized by the site of bleeding as upper, from the esophagus, stomach, or duodenum; lower, from the colon; small intestinal; or obscure GIB if the source is unclear.

GIB is the most common gastrointestinal condition leading to hospitalization in the United States, accounting for ~513,000 admissions and $5 billion in direct costs annually. The case fatality of patients hospitalized with GIB is ~2% in the United States. Patients generally die from decompensation of other underlying illnesses rather than exsanguination.

SOURCES OF GASTROINTESTINAL BLEEDING

Upper Gastrointestinal Sources of Bleeding • PEPTIC ULCERS Peptic ulcers are the most common cause of upper GIB (UGIB), accounting for ~50% of UGIB hospitalizations. Features of an ulcer at endoscopy provide important prognostic information that guides subsequent management decisions (**Fig. 48-1**). Approximately 20% of patients with bleeding ulcers have the highest-risk findings of active bleeding or a nonbleeding visible vessel; one-third of such patients have further bleeding that requires urgent surgery if they are treated conservatively. These patients benefit from endoscopic therapy such as bipolar electrocoagulation, heater probe, injection therapy (e.g., absolute alcohol, 1:10,000 epinephrine), and/or clips with reductions in bleeding, hospital stay, mortality, and costs. In contrast, patients with clean-based ulcers have rates of serious recurrent bleeding approaching zero. If stable with no other reason for hospitalization, such patients may be discharged home after endoscopy.

Randomized controlled trials document that high-dose, constant-infusion IV proton pump inhibitor (PPI) (80-mg bolus and 8-mg/h infusion), designed to sustain intragastric pH >6 and enhance clot stability, decreases further bleeding and mortality in patients with high-risk ulcers (active bleeding, nonbleeding visible vessel, adherent clot) when given after endoscopic therapy. Meta-analysis of randomized trials indicates that high-dose intermittent PPIs are noninferior to constant-infusion PPI therapy and thus may be substituted. Patients with lower-risk findings (flat pigmented spot or clean base) do not require endoscopic therapy and receive standard doses of oral PPI.

Approximately 10–50% of patients with bleeding ulcers rebleed within the next year if no preventive strategies are employed. Prevention of recurrent bleeding focuses on the three main factors in ulcer pathogenesis, *Helicobacter pylori*, nonsteroidal anti-inflammatory drugs (NSAIDs), and acid. Eradication of *H. pylori* in patients with bleeding ulcers decreases rebleeding rates to <5%. If a bleeding ulcer develops in a patient taking NSAIDs, the NSAIDs should be discontinued. If NSAIDs must be given, a cyclooxygenase (COX)-2 selective NSAID plus a PPI is recommended, based on results of a randomized trial. Patients with established cardiovascular disease who develop bleeding ulcers while taking low-dose aspirin for secondary prevention should restart aspirin as soon as possible after their bleeding episode (1–7 days). A randomized trial showed that immediate reinstitution of aspirin was associated with a lower 8-week mortality compared to not restarting aspirin (1% vs 13%; hazard ratio, 0.2; 95% CI, 0.1–0.6). In contrast, aspirin probably should be discontinued in most patients taking aspirin for primary prevention of cardiovascular events who develop UGIB. Patients with bleeding ulcers unrelated to *H. pylori* or NSAIDs should remain on PPI therapy indefinitely given a 42% incidence of rebleeding at 7 years without protective therapy. **Peptic ulcers are discussed in Chap. 324.**

MALLORY-WEISS TEARS Mallory-Weiss tears account for ~2–10% of UGIB hospitalizations. The classic history is vomiting, retching, or coughing preceding hematemesis, especially in an alcoholic patient. Bleeding from these tears, which are usually on the gastric side of the gastroesophageal junction, stops spontaneously in ~80–90% of patients and recurs in only 0–10%. Endoscopic therapy is indicated for actively bleeding Mallory-Weiss tears. **Mallory-Weiss tears are discussed in Chap. 323.**

ESOPHAGEAL VARICES The proportion of UGIB hospitalizations due to varices varies widely, from ~2–40%, depending on the population. Patients with variceal hemorrhage have poorer outcomes than patients with other sources of UGIB. Esophageal varices are treated with endoscopic ligation and an IV vasoactive medication (octreotide, somatostatin, vapreotide, terlipressin) for 2–5 days. Combination of endoscopic and medical therapy is superior to either therapy alone in decreasing rebleeding. Over the long term, treatment with nonselective beta blockers plus endoscopic ligation is recommended because the combination is more effective than either alone in reduction of recurrent esophageal variceal bleeding. Transjugular intrahepatic portosystemic shunt (TIPS) is recommended in patients who have persistent or

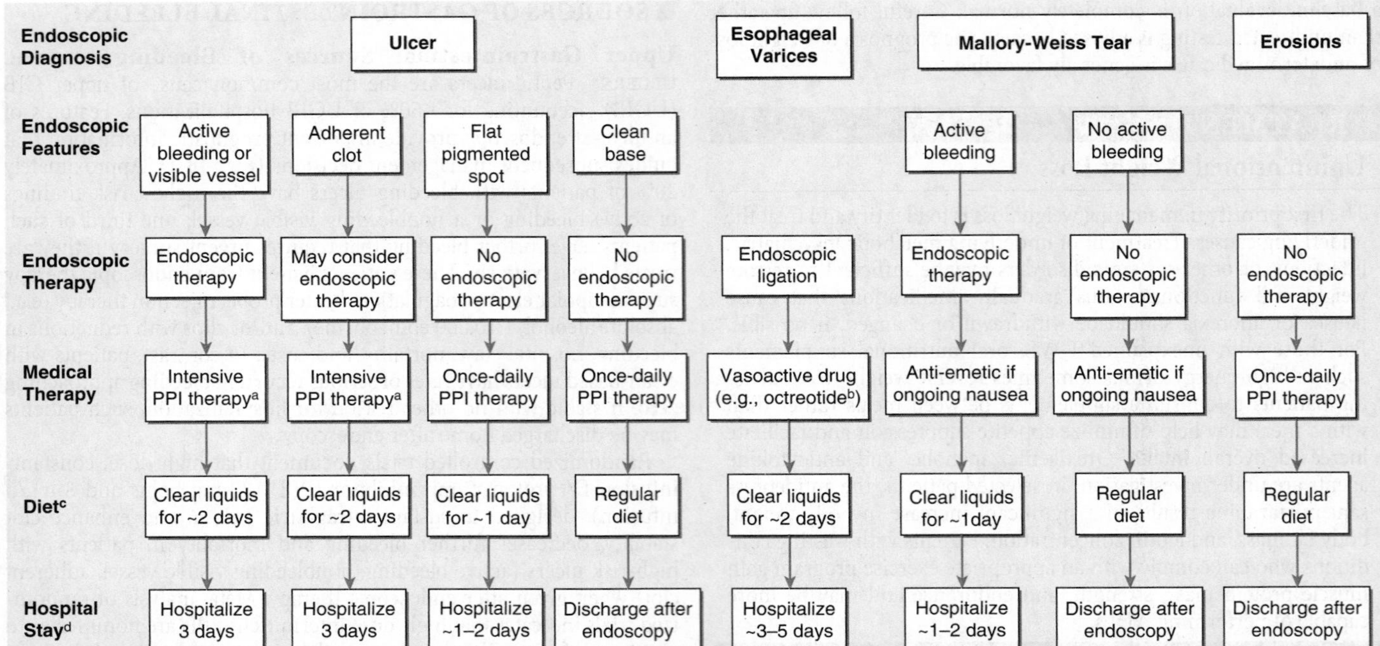

[a]Intravenous bolus (80 mg) followed by infusion (8 mg/h) for 3 days; or oral or intravenous bolus (e.g., 80 mg) followed by intermittent high doses (e.g., 40–80 mg bid or 40 mg tid) for 3 days.Then twice-daily PPI on days 4–14 followed by once-daily PPI.
[b]Intravenous 50 μg bolus followed by 50 μg/h infusion for 2–5 days.
[c]Diet after endoscopy, assuming no nausea or vomiting.
[d]Duration after endoscopy assuming patient stable without further bleeding or concurrent medical conditions requiring hospitalization; PPI, proton pump inhibitor.

FIGURE 48-1 Suggested algorithm for patients with acute upper gastrointestinal bleeding based on endoscopic findings.

recurrent bleeding despite endoscopic and medical therapy. TIPS also should be considered in the first 1–2 days of hospitalization for acute variceal bleeding in patients with advanced liver disease (Child-Pugh class B, Child-Pugh class C with score 10–13), because randomized trials show significant decreases in rebleeding and mortality compared with standard endoscopic and medical therapy.

Portal hypertension is also responsible for bleeding from gastric varices, varices in the small and large intestine, and portal hypertensive gastropathy and enterocolopathy. Bleeding gastric varices are treated with endoscopic injection of tissue adhesive (e.g., *n*-butyl cyanoacrylate), if available; if not, TIPS is performed.

EROSIVE DISEASE Erosions are endoscopically visualized breaks that are confined to the mucosa and do not cause major bleeding because arteries and veins are not present in the mucosa. Erosions in the esophagus, stomach, or duodenum commonly cause mild UGIB, with erosive gastritis and duodenitis accounting for perhaps ~10–15% and erosive esophagitis (primarily due to gastroesophageal reflux disease) accounting for ~1–10% of UGIB hospitalizations. The most important cause of gastric and duodenal erosions is NSAID use: ~50% of patients who chronically ingest NSAIDs may have gastric erosions. Other potential causes of gastric erosions include alcohol intake, *H. pylori* infection, and stress-related mucosal injury.

Stress-related gastric mucosal injury occurs only in extremely sick patients, such as those with serious trauma, major surgery, burns covering more than one-third of the body surface area, major intracranial disease, or severe medical illness (e.g., ventilator dependence, coagulopathy). Severe bleeding should not develop unless ulceration occurs. The mortality rate in these patients is high because of their serious underlying illnesses.

The incidence of bleeding from stress-related gastric mucosal injury has decreased dramatically in recent years, most likely due to better care of critically ill patients. A recent double-blind placebo-controlled randomized trial in 3282 intensive care patients with risk factors for GIB showed a small benefit of PPI in clinically important bleeding (2.5% vs 4.2%) without a difference in mortality or infections (e.g., *Clostridium difficile*, pneumonia). Thus, pharmacologic prophylaxis for bleeding has limited benefit but may be considered in the high-risk patients mentioned above. Meta-analyses of randomized trials suggest PPIs are more effective than H_2-receptor antagonists in reduction of overt and clinically important UGIB without differences in mortality or nosocomial pneumonia.

OTHER CAUSES Less common causes of UGIB include neoplasms, vascular ectasias (including hereditary hemorrhagic telangiectasias [Osler-Weber-Rendu] and gastric antral vascular ectasia ["watermelon stomach"]), Dieulafoy's lesion (in which an aberrant vessel in the mucosa bleeds from a pinpoint mucosal defect), prolapse gastropathy (prolapse of proximal stomach into esophagus with retching, especially in alcoholics), aortoenteric fistulas, and hemobilia or hemosuccus pancreaticus (bleeding from the bile duct or pancreatic duct).

Small-Intestinal Sources of Bleeding Patients without a source of GIB identified on upper endoscopy and colonoscopy were previously labeled as having obscure GIB. With the advent of improved diagnostic modalities, ~75% of GIB previously labeled obscure is now estimated to originate in the small intestine beyond the extent of a standard upper endoscopic exam. Small-intestinal GIB may account for ~5% of GIB cases. The most common causes in adults include vascular ectasias, neoplasm (e.g., gastrointestinal stromal tumor, carcinoid, adenocarcinoma, lymphoma, metastases), and NSAID-induced erosions and ulcers. Meckel's diverticulum is the most common cause of significant small-intestinal GIB in children, decreasing in frequency as a cause of bleeding with age. Other less common causes of small-intestinal GIB include Crohn's disease, infection, ischemia, vasculitis, small-bowel varices, diverticula, intussusception, Dieulafoy's lesions, aortoenteric fistulas, and duplication cysts.

Small-intestinal vascular ectasias are treated with endoscopic therapy, if possible, based on observational studies suggesting initial efficacy. However, rebleeding is common: 45% over a mean follow-up of 26 months in a systematic review. Estrogen/progesterone compounds are not recommended because a multicenter double-blind trial found no benefit in prevention of recurrent bleeding. Octreotide is used, based on positive results from case series but no randomized trials. A randomized trial reported significant benefit of thalidomide and awaits further confirmation. Other isolated lesions, such as tumors, generally require surgical resection.

Colonic Sources of Bleeding Hemorrhoids are probably the most common cause of lower GIB (LGIB); anal fissures also cause minor bleeding and pain. If these local anal processes, which rarely require hospitalization, are excluded, the most common cause of LGIB in adults is diverticulosis. Other causes include vascular ectasias (especially in the proximal colon of patients >70 years), neoplasms (primarily adenocarcinoma), colitis (ischemic, infectious, Crohn's or ulcerative colitis, NSAID-induced colitis or ulcers), postpolypectomy bleeding, and radiation proctopathy. Rarer causes include solitary rectal ulcer syndrome, varices (most commonly rectal), lymphoid nodular hyperplasia, vasculitis, trauma, and aortocolic fistulas. In children and adolescents, the most common colonic causes of significant GIB are inflammatory bowel disease and juvenile polyps.

Diverticular bleeding is abrupt in onset, usually painless, sometimes massive, and often from the right colon; chronic or occult bleeding is not characteristic. Case series from the United States and Europe suggest colonic diverticula stop bleeding spontaneously in ≥90% of patients, with rebleeding on long-term follow-up as low as ~15% over 4-5 years. Rebleeding is substantially higher in reports from Asia. Case series suggest endoscopic therapy may decrease recurrent bleeding in the uncommon case when colonoscopy identifies the specific bleeding diverticulum. When diverticular bleeding is found at angiography, transcatheter arterial embolization by superselective technique stops bleeding in a majority of patients. Segmental surgical resection is recommended for persistent or refractory diverticular bleeding.

Bleeding from colonic vascular ectasias may be overt or occult; it tends to be chronic and only occasionally hemodynamically significant. Endoscopic hemostatic therapy may be used in the treatment of vascular ectasias, as well as discrete bleeding ulcers and postpolypectomy bleeding. Transcatheter arterial embolization also may be attempted for persistent bleeding from vascular ectasias and other discrete lesions. Surgical therapy is generally required for major persistent or recurrent bleeding from colonic sources that cannot be treated medically, endoscopically, or angiographically. Patients with Heyde's syndrome (bleeding vascular ectasias and aortic stenosis) appear to benefit from aortic valve replacement.

APPROACH TO THE PATIENT

Gastrointestinal Bleeding

INITIAL ASSESSMENT

Measurement of the heart rate and blood pressure is the best way to initially assess a patient with GIB. Clinically significant bleeding leads to postural changes in heart rate or blood pressure, tachycardia, and, finally, recumbent hypotension. In contrast, hemoglobin does not fall immediately with acute GIB, due to proportionate reductions in plasma and red cell volumes ("people bleed whole blood"). Thus, hemoglobin may be normal or only minimally decreased at initial presentation of a severe bleeding episode. As extravascular fluid enters the vascular space to restore volume, the hemoglobin falls, but this process may take up to 72 h. Transfusion is recommended when the hemoglobin drops below 7 g/dL, based on a large randomized trial showing this restrictive transfusion strategy decreases rebleeding and death in acute UGIB compared with a transfusion threshold of 9 g/dL. Patients with slow, chronic GIB may have very low hemoglobin values despite normal blood pressure and heart rate. With the development of iron-deficiency anemia, the mean corpuscular volume is low and red blood cell distribution width is increased.

DIFFERENTIATION OF UGIB FROM LGIB

Hematemesis indicates an UGIB source. Melena indicates blood has been present in the gastrointestinal (GI) tract for ≥14 h and as long as 3–5 days. The more proximal the bleeding site, the more likely melena will occur. Hematochezia usually represents a lower GI source of bleeding, although an upper GI lesion may bleed so briskly that blood transits the bowel before melena develops. When hematochezia is the presenting symptom of UGIB, it is associated with hemodynamic instability and dropping hemoglobin. Bleeding lesions of the small bowel may present as melena or hematochezia. Other clues to UGIB include hyperactive bowel sounds and an elevated blood urea nitrogen (due to volume depletion and blood proteins absorbed in the small intestine).

A nonbloody nasogastric aspirate may be seen in ~15% of patients with UGIB who present with clinically serious hematochezia. A bile-stained appearance does not exclude UGIB because reports of bile in the aspirate are incorrect in ~50% of cases. Testing of aspirates that are not grossly bloody for occult blood is not useful.

EVALUATION AND MANAGEMENT OF UGIB (FIG. 48-1)

Initial Risk Assessment Baseline characteristics predictive of rebleeding and death include hemodynamic compromise (tachycardia or hypotension), increasing age, and comorbidities. Risk assessment tools may be used to identify patients with very low risk. Discharge from the emergency room with outpatient management has been suggested for patients with a Glasgow-Blatchford score (possible range 0–23, **Table 48-1**) of 0–1 because only ~1% of patients who require transfusion, require hemostatic intervention, or die have a score of 0–1.

Pre-Endoscopic Medications PPI infusion may be considered at presentation; it decreases high-risk ulcer stigmata (e.g., active bleeding) and need for endoscopic therapy but does not improve clinical outcomes such as further bleeding, surgery, or death. The promotility agent erythromycin, 250 mg intravenously ~30–90 min before endoscopy, is suggested to improve visualization at endoscopy, thereby reducing the need for repeat endoscopy and hospital stay. Cirrhotic patients presenting with UGIB should be given an antibiotic (e.g., ceftriaxone) and IV vasoactive medication (e.g., octreotide) upon presentation. Antibiotics decrease bacterial infections, rebleeding, and mortality, and vasoactive medications may improve control of bleeding in the 12 h after presentation.

Endoscopy Upper endoscopy should be performed within 24 h in most patients hospitalized with UGIB whether they have clinical features predicting low risk or high risk of further bleeding

TABLE 48-1 Glasgow-Blatchford Score

RISK FACTORS AT ADMISSION	SCORE
Blood urea nitrogen (mg/dL)	
18.2 to <22.4	2
22.4 to <28.0	3
28.0 to <70.0	4
≥70.0	6
Hemoglobin (g/dL)	
12.0 to <13.0 (men); 10.0 to <12.0 (women)	1
10.0 to <12.0 (men)	3
<10.0	6
Systolic blood pressure (mmHg)	
100–109	1
90–99	2
<90	3
Heart rate (beats per minute)	
≥100	1
Melena	1
Syncope	2
Hepatic disease	2
Cardiac failure	2

and death. Even in high-risk patients, more urgent endoscopy (performed within 6 h of gastroenterology consultation) does not improve clinical outcomes. Early endoscopy in low-risk patients (e.g., hemodynamically stable without severe comorbidities) identifies low-risk findings (e.g., clean-based ulcers, erosions, nonbleeding Mallory-Weiss tears) that allow discharge in ≥40% of patients, thereby reducing hospital stay and costs. Patients with high-risk endoscopic findings (e.g., varices, ulcers with active bleeding or a visible vessel) benefit from hemostatic therapy at endoscopy.

EVALUATION AND MANAGEMENT OF LGIB (FIG. 48-2)

Patients with hematochezia and hemodynamic instability should have upper endoscopy to rule out an upper GI source before evaluation of the lower GI tract.

Colonoscopy after an oral lavage solution is the procedure of choice in most patients admitted with LGIB unless bleeding is too massive, in which case angiography is recommended. Computed tomography (CT) angiography is often suggested prior to angiography to document evidence and location of active bleeding. Sigmoidoscopy is used primarily in patients <40 years old with minor bleeding. In patients with no source identified on colonoscopy, imaging studies may be employed. ^{99m}Tc-labeled red cell scan allows repeated imaging for up to 24 h and may identify the general location of bleeding. However, CT angiography is increasingly used instead because it is likely superior and more readily available. In active LGIB, angiography can detect the site of bleeding (extravasation of contrast into the gut) and permits treatment with transcatheter arterial embolization.

EVALUATION AND MANAGEMENT OF SMALL-INTESTINAL OR OBSCURE GIB

In patients with massive bleeding suspected to be from the small intestine, current guidelines suggest angiography as the initial test, with CT angiography or ^{99m}Tc-labeled red cell scan prior to angiography if the patient's clinical status permits. For others, repeat upper and lower endoscopy may be considered as the initial evaluation because second-look procedures identify a source in up to ~25% of upper endoscopies and colonoscopies; a push enteroscopy, usually performed with a pediatric colonoscope to inspect the entire duodenum and proximal jejunum, may be substituted for a repeat standard upper endoscopy. If second-look procedures are negative, evaluation of the entire small intestine is performed, usually with video capsule endoscopy. A systematic review of comparative studies showed the yield of "clinically significant findings" to be greater with capsule than push enteroscopy (56% vs 26%) or small bowel barium radiography (42% vs 6%). However, capsule endoscopy does not allow full visualization of the small intestine, tissue sampling, or application of therapy.

CT enterography may be used initially instead of video capsule in patients with possible small bowel narrowing (e.g., stricture, prior surgery or radiation, Crohn's disease) and may follow a negative video capsule for suspected small-intestinal GIB, given its higher sensitivity for small-intestinal masses.

If capsule endoscopy is positive, management is dictated by the finding. If capsule endoscopy is negative, clinically stable patients may be observed and treated with iron if iron deficiency is present, while those with ongoing bleeding (e.g., need for transfusions) undergo further testing. A second capsule endoscopy may be considered because it is reported to identify a source in up to ~50% of cases. "Deep" enteroscopy (double-balloon, single-balloon, or spiral enteroscopy) is commonly the next test after capsule endoscopy for clinically important GIB documented or suspected to be from the small intestine because it allows the endoscopist to examine, obtain specimens from, and provide therapy to much or all of the small intestine. Other imaging techniques sometimes used in evaluation of obscure GIB include ^{99m}Tc-labeled red blood cell scintigraphy, CT angiography, angiography, and ^{99m}Tc-pertechnetate scintigraphy for Meckel's

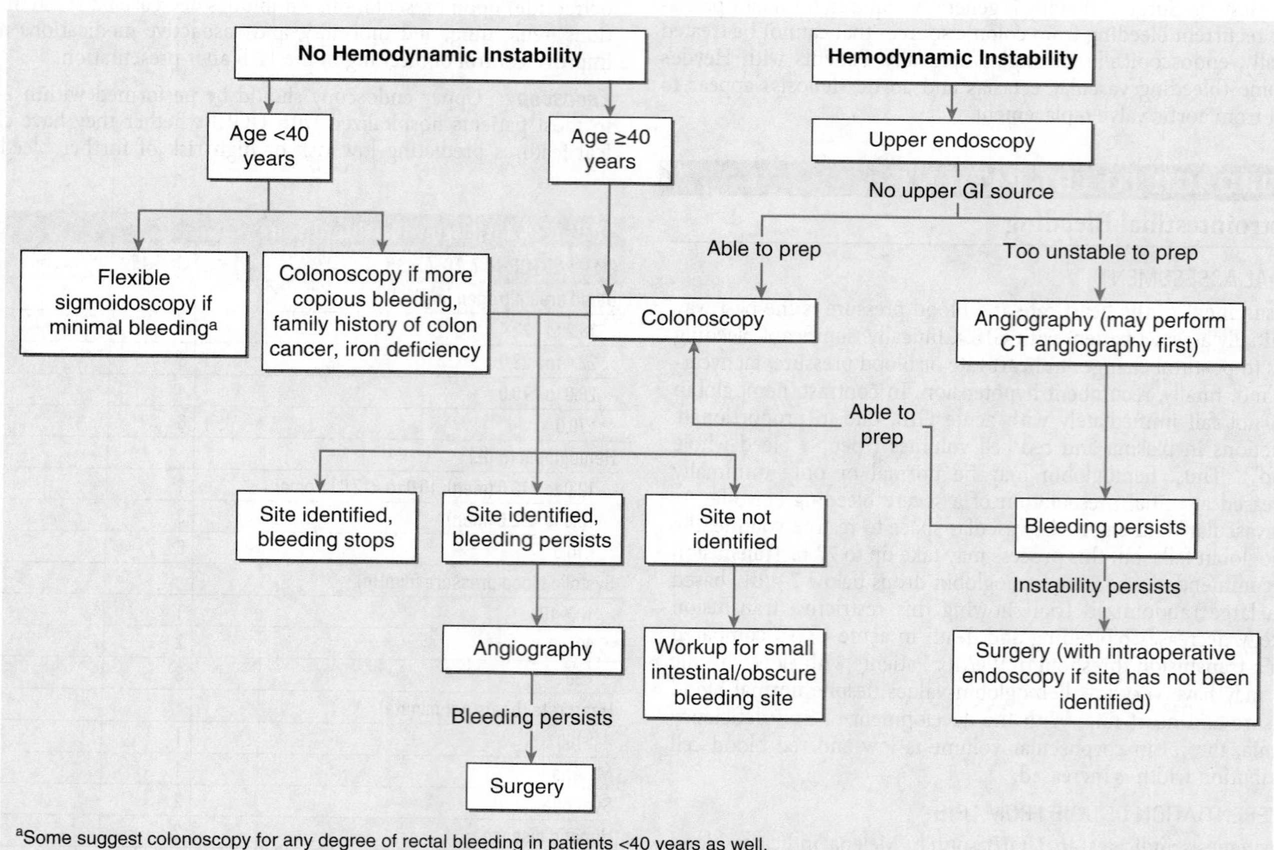

FIGURE 48-2 Suggested algorithm for patients with acute lower gastrointestinal bleeding.

diverticulum (especially in young patients). If all tests are unrevealing, intraoperative endoscopy is indicated in patients with severe recurrent or persistent bleeding requiring repeated transfusions.

POSITIVE FECAL OCCULT BLOOD TEST

Fecal occult blood testing is recommended only for colorectal cancer screening, beginning at age 45–50 years in average-risk adults. A positive test necessitates colonoscopy. If evaluation of the colon is negative, further workup is not recommended unless iron-deficiency anemia or GI symptoms are present.

FURTHER READING

GARCIA-TSAO G et al: Portal hypertensive bleeding in cirrhosis: Risk stratification, diagnosis, and management: 2016 practice guidance by the American Association for the Study of Liver Diseases. Hepatology 65:310, 2017.

GURUDU SR et al: The role of endoscopy in the management of suspected small-bowel bleeding. Gastrointest Endosc 85:22, 2017.

KRAG M et al: Pantoprazole in patients at risk for gastrointestinal bleeding in the ICU. N Engl J Med 379:2199, 2018.

LAINE L et al: ACG clinical guideline: Upper gastrointestinal and ulcer bleeding. Am J Gastroenterol 116:899, 2021.

LAU JYW et al: Timing of endoscopy for acute upper gastrointestinal bleeding. N Engl J Med 382:1299, 2020.

PEERY AF et al: Burden and cost of gastrointestinal, liver, and pancreatic diseases in the United States: Update 2018. Gastroenterology 156:254, 2019.

STANLEY AJ, LAINE L: Management of acute upper gastrointestinal bleeding. BMJ 364:l536, 2019.

STRATE LL, GRALNEK KM: ACG clinical guideline: Management of patients with acute lower gastrointestinal bleeding. Am J Gastroenterol 111:459, 2016.

VILLANEUVA C et al: Transfusion strategies for acute upper gastrointestinal bleeding. N Engl J Med 368:11, 2013.

49 Jaundice

Savio John, Daniel S. Pratt

Jaundice is a yellowish discoloration of body tissues resulting from the deposition of bilirubin. Tissue deposition of bilirubin occurs only in the presence of serum hyperbilirubinemia and is a sign of either liver disease or, less often, a hemolytic disorder or disorder of bilirubin metabolism. The degree of serum bilirubin elevation can be estimated by physical examination. Slight increases in serum bilirubin level are best detected by examining the sclerae for icterus. Sclerae have a particular affinity for bilirubin due to their high elastin content, and the presence of scleral icterus indicates a serum bilirubin level of at least 51 μmol/L (3 mg/dL). The ability to detect scleral icterus is made more difficult if the examining room has fluorescent lighting. If the examiner suspects scleral icterus, a second site to examine is underneath the tongue. As serum bilirubin levels rise, the skin will eventually become yellow in light-skinned patients and even green if the process is long-standing; the green color is produced by oxidation of bilirubin to biliverdin.

The differential diagnosis for yellowing of the skin is limited. In addition to jaundice, it includes carotenoderma; the use of drugs including quinacrine, sunitinib, and sorafenib; and excessive exposure to phenols. Carotenoderma, a yellow coloring of the skin, is associated with diabetes, hypothyroidism, and anorexia nervosa, but most commonly, it is caused by the ingestion of an excessive amounts of vegetables and fruits such as carrots, leafy vegetables, squash, peaches, and oranges that contain carotene. In jaundice, the yellow coloration of the skin is uniformly distributed over the body, whereas in carotenoderma, the pigment is concentrated on the palms, soles, forehead, and nasolabial folds. Carotenoderma can be distinguished from jaundice by the sparing of the sclerae. Quinacrine causes a yellow discoloration of the skin in 4–37% of patients treated with it. It has also been reported with the use of the tyrosine kinase inhibitors sunitinib and sorafenib.

Another sensitive indicator of increased serum bilirubin is darkening of the urine, which is due to the renal excretion of conjugated bilirubin. Patients often describe their urine as tea- or cola-colored. Bilirubinuria indicates an elevation of the direct serum bilirubin fraction and, therefore, the presence of liver or biliary disease.

Serum bilirubin levels increase when an imbalance exists between bilirubin production and clearance. A logical evaluation of the patient who is jaundiced requires an understanding of bilirubin production and metabolism.

PRODUCTION AND METABOLISM OF BILIRUBIN

(See Chap. 338) Bilirubin, a tetrapyrrole pigment, is a breakdown product of heme (ferroprotoporphyrin IX). About 80–85% of the 4 mg/kg body weight of bilirubin produced each day is derived from the breakdown of hemoglobin in senescent red blood cells. The remainder comes from prematurely destroyed erythroid cells in bone marrow and from the turnover of hemoproteins such as myoglobin and cytochromes found in tissues throughout the body.

The formation of bilirubin occurs in reticuloendothelial cells, primarily in the spleen and liver. The first reaction, catalyzed by the microsomal enzyme heme oxygenase, oxidatively cleaves the α bridge of the porphyrin group and opens the heme ring. The end products of this reaction are biliverdin, carbon monoxide, and iron. The second reaction, catalyzed by the cytosolic enzyme biliverdin reductase, reduces the central methylene bridge of biliverdin and converts it to bilirubin. Bilirubin formed in the reticuloendothelial cells is virtually insoluble in water due to tight internal hydrogen bonding between the water-soluble moieties of bilirubin—that is, the bonding of the propionic acid carboxyl groups of one dipyrrolic half of the molecule with the imino and lactam groups of the opposite half. This configuration blocks solvent access to the polar residues of bilirubin and places the hydrophobic residues on the outside. To be transported in blood, bilirubin must be solubilized. Solubilization is accomplished by the reversible, noncovalent binding of bilirubin to albumin. Unconjugated bilirubin bound to albumin is transported to the liver. There, the bilirubin—but not the albumin—is taken up by hepatocytes via a process that at least partly involves carrier-mediated membrane transport. No specific bilirubin transporter has yet been identified **(Chap. 338, Fig. 338-1)**.

After entering the hepatocyte, unconjugated bilirubin is bound in the cytosol to several proteins including proteins in the glutathione-S-transferase superfamily. These proteins serve both to reduce efflux of bilirubin back into the serum and to present the bilirubin for conjugation. In the endoplasmic reticulum, bilirubin is made aqueous soluble by conjugation to glucuronic acid, a process that disrupts the hydrophobic internal hydrogen bonds and yields bilirubin monoglucuronide and diglucuronide. The conjugation of glucuronic acid to bilirubin is catalyzed by bilirubin uridine diphosphate-glucuronosyl transferase (UDPGT). The now-hydrophilic bilirubin conjugates diffuse from the endoplasmic reticulum to the canalicular membrane, where bilirubin monoglucuronide and diglucuronide are actively transported into canalicular bile by an energy-dependent mechanism involving the multidrug resistance–associated protein 2 (MRP2). A portion of bilirubin glucuronides is transported into the sinusoids and portal circulation by MRP3 and is subjected to reuptake into the hepatocyte by the sinusoidal organic anion transport protein 1B1 (OATP1B1) and OATP1B3. The conjugated bilirubin excreted into bile drains into the duodenum and passes unchanged through the proximal small bowel. Conjugated bilirubin is not reabsorbed by the intestinal mucosa due to its hydrophilicity and increased molecular size. When the conjugated bilirubin reaches the distal ileum and colon, it is hydrolyzed to unconjugated bilirubin by bacterial β-glucuronidases.

The unconjugated bilirubin is reduced by normal gut bacteria to form a group of colorless tetrapyrroles called *urobilinogens* and other products, the nature and relative amounts of which depend on the bacterial flora. About 80–90% of these products are excreted in feces, either unchanged or oxidized to orange derivatives called *urobilins.* The remaining 10–20% of the urobilinogens undergo enterohepatic cycling. A small fraction (usually <3 mg/dL) escapes hepatic uptake, filters across the renal glomerulus, and is excreted in urine. Increased urinary excretion of urobilinogen can be due to increased bilirubin production, increased hepatic reabsorption of urobilinogen from the colon, or decreased hepatic clearance of urobilinogen.

MEASUREMENT OF SERUM BILIRUBIN

The terms *direct* and *indirect* bilirubin—that is, conjugated and unconjugated bilirubin, respectively—are based on the original van den Bergh reaction. This assay, or a variation of it, is still used in most clinical chemistry laboratories to determine the serum bilirubin level. In this assay, bilirubin is exposed to diazotized sulfanilic acid and splits into two relatively stable dipyrrylmethene azopigments that absorb maximally at 540 nm, allowing photometric analysis. The direct fraction is that which reacts with diazotized sulfanilic acid in the absence of an accelerator substance such as alcohol. The direct fraction provides an approximation of the conjugated bilirubin level in serum. The *total* serum bilirubin is the amount that reacts after the addition of alcohol. The indirect fraction is the difference between the total and the direct bilirubin levels and provides an estimate of the unconjugated bilirubin in serum. Unconjugated bilirubin also reacts with diazo reagents, albeit slowly, even when the accelerator is absent. Thus, the calculated indirect bilirubin may underestimate the true amount of unconjugated bilirubin in circulation.

With the van den Bergh method, the normal serum bilirubin concentration usually is between 17 and 26 μmol/L (1 and 1.5 mg/dL). Total serum bilirubin concentrations are between 3.4 and 15.4 μmol/L (0.2 and 0.9 mg/dL) in 95% of a normal population. Unconjugated hyperbilirubinemia is present when the direct fraction is <15% of the total serum bilirubin. The presence of even limited amounts of true conjugated bilirubin in serum suggests significant hepatobiliary pathology. As conjugated hyperbilirubinemia is always associated with bilirubinuria (except in the presence of delta bilirubin in prolonged cholestasis when jaundice is overt), detection of bilirubin in urine via dipstick test is extremely helpful to confirm the presence of conjugated hyperbilirubinemia in a patient with mildly elevated direct fraction.

Several new techniques, although less convenient to perform, have added considerably to our understanding of bilirubin metabolism. First, studies using these methods demonstrate that, in normal persons or those with Gilbert's syndrome, almost 100% of the serum bilirubin is unconjugated; <3% is monoconjugated bilirubin. Second, in jaundiced patients with hepatobiliary disease, the total serum bilirubin concentration measured by these new, more accurate methods is lower than the values found with diazo methods. This finding suggests that there are diazo-positive compounds distinct from bilirubin in the serum of patients with hepatobiliary disease. Third, these studies indicate that, in jaundiced patients with hepatobiliary disease, monoglucuronides of bilirubin predominate over diglucuronides. Fourth, part of the direct-reacting bilirubin fraction includes conjugated bilirubin that is covalently linked to albumin. This albumin-linked fraction of conjugated bilirubin (*delta fraction, delta bilirubin,* or *biliprotein*) represents an important fraction of total serum bilirubin in patients with cholestasis and hepatobiliary disorders. The delta bilirubin is formed in serum when hepatic excretion of bilirubin glucuronides is impaired and the glucuronides accumulate in serum. By virtue of its tight binding to albumin, the clearance rate of delta bilirubin from serum approximates the half-life of albumin (12–14 days) rather than the short half-life of bilirubin (about 4 h).

The prolonged half-life of albumin-bound conjugated bilirubin accounts for two previously unexplained enigmas in jaundiced patients with liver disease: (1) that some patients with conjugated hyperbilirubinemia do not exhibit bilirubinuria during the recovery phase of their disease because the delta bilirubin, although conjugated, is covalently bound to albumin and therefore not filtered by the renal glomeruli, and (2) that the elevated serum bilirubin level declines more slowly than expected in some patients who otherwise appear to be recovering satisfactorily. Late in the recovery phase of hepatobiliary disorders, all the conjugated bilirubin may be in the albumin-linked form.

MEASUREMENT OF URINE BILIRUBIN

Unconjugated bilirubin is always bound to albumin in the serum, is not filtered by the kidney, and is not found in the urine. Conjugated bilirubin is filtered at the glomerulus, and the majority is reabsorbed by the proximal tubules; a small fraction is excreted in the urine. Any bilirubin found in the urine is conjugated bilirubin. The presence of bilirubinuria on urine dipstick test (Ictotest) indicates an elevation of the conjugated bilirubin fraction that cannot be excreted from the liver and implies the presence of hepatobiliary disease. A false-negative result is possible in patients with prolonged cholestasis due to the predominance of delta bilirubin, which is covalently bound to albumin and therefore not filtered by the renal glomeruli.

APPROACH TO THE PATIENT

Jaundice

The goal of this chapter is not to provide an encyclopedic review of every condition that causes jaundice. Rather, the chapter is intended to offer a framework that helps a physician to evaluate the patient with jaundice in a logical way (**Fig. 49-1**).

The initial step is to perform appropriate blood tests in order to determine whether the patient has an isolated elevation of serum bilirubin. If so, is the bilirubin elevation due to an increased unconjugated or conjugated fraction? If the hyperbilirubinemia is accompanied by other liver test abnormalities, is the disorder hepatocellular or cholestatic? If cholestatic, is it intra- or extrahepatic? These questions can all be answered with a thoughtful history, physical examination, and interpretation of laboratory and radiologic tests and procedures.

The bilirubin present in serum represents a balance between input from the production of bilirubin and hepatic/biliary removal of the pigment. Hyperbilirubinemia may result from (1) overproduction of bilirubin; (2) impaired uptake, conjugation, or excretion of bilirubin; or (3) regurgitation of unconjugated or conjugated bilirubin from damaged hepatocytes or bile ducts. An increase in unconjugated bilirubin in serum results from overproduction, impaired uptake, or conjugation of bilirubin. An increase in conjugated bilirubin is due to decreased excretion into the bile ductules or backward leakage of the pigment. The initial steps in evaluating the patient with jaundice are to determine (1) whether the hyperbilirubinemia is predominantly conjugated or unconjugated in nature and (2) whether other biochemical liver tests are abnormal. The thoughtful interpretation of limited data permits a rational evaluation of the patient (Fig. 49-1). The following discussion will focus solely on the evaluation of the adult patient with jaundice.

ISOLATED ELEVATION OF SERUM BILIRUBIN

Unconjugated Hyperbilirubinemia The differential diagnosis of isolated unconjugated hyperbilirubinemia is limited (**Table 49-1**). The critical determination is whether the patient is suffering from a hemolytic process resulting in an overproduction of bilirubin (hemolytic disorders and ineffective erythropoiesis) or from impaired hepatic uptake/conjugation of bilirubin (drug effect or genetic disorders).

Hemolytic disorders that cause excessive heme production may be either inherited or acquired. Inherited disorders include spherocytosis, sickle cell anemia, thalassemia, and deficiency of red cell enzymes such as pyruvate kinase and glucose-6-phosphate dehydrogenase. In these conditions, the serum bilirubin level rarely exceeds 86 μmol/L (5 mg/dL). Higher levels may occur when there

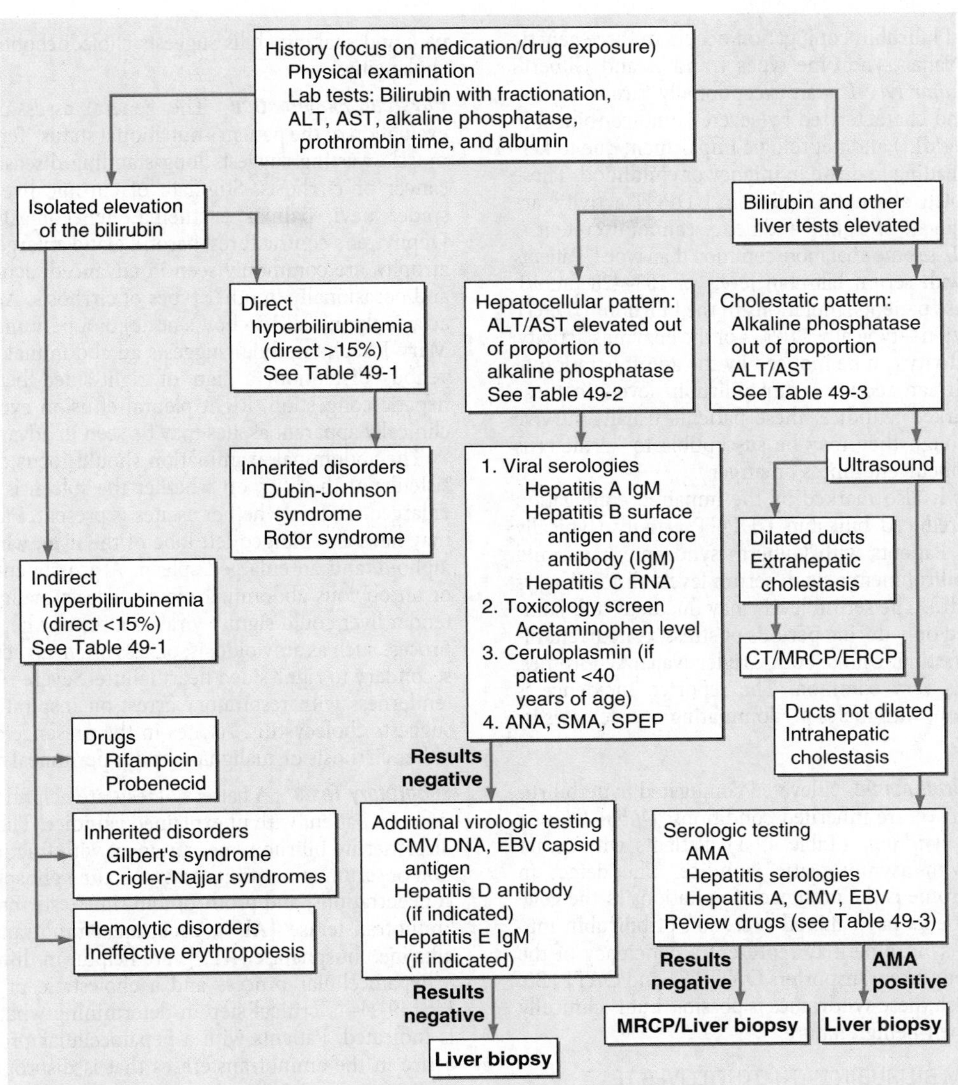

FIGURE 49-1 Evaluation of the patient with jaundice. ALT, alanine aminotransferase; AMA, antimitochondrial antibody; ANA, antinuclear antibody; AST, aspartate aminotransferase; CMV, cytomegalovirus; EBV, Epstein-Barr virus; ERCP, endoscopic retrograde cholangiopancreatography; LKM, liver-kidney microsomal antibody; MRCP, magnetic resonance cholangiopancreatography; SMA, smooth-muscle antibody; SPEP, serum protein electrophoresis.

TABLE 49-1 Causes of Isolated Hyperbilirubinemia

- I. Indirect hyperbilirubinemia
  - A. Hemolytic disorders
  - B. Ineffective erythropoiesis
  - C. Increased bilirubin production
    1. Massive blood transfusion
    2. Resorption of hematoma
  - D. Drugs
    1. Rifampin
    2. Probenecid
    3. Antibiotics—cephalosporins and penicillins
  - E. Inherited conditions
    1. Crigler-Najjar types I and II
    2. Gilbert's syndrome
- II. Direct hyperbilirubinemia (inherited conditions)
  - A. Dubin-Johnson syndrome
  - B. Rotor syndrome

is coexistent renal or hepatocellular dysfunction or in acute hemolysis, such as a sickle cell crisis. In evaluating jaundice in patients with chronic hemolysis, it is important to remember the high incidence of pigmented (calcium bilirubinate) gallstones found in these patients, which increases the likelihood of choledocholithiasis as an alternative explanation for hyperbilirubinemia.

Acquired hemolytic disorders include microangiopathic hemolytic anemia (e.g., hemolytic-uremic syndrome), paroxysmal nocturnal hemoglobinuria, spur cell anemia, immune hemolysis, and parasitic infections (e.g., malaria and babesiosis). Ineffective erythropoiesis occurs in cobalamin, folate, and iron deficiencies. Resorption of hematomas and massive blood transfusions both can result in increased hemoglobin release and overproduction of bilirubin.

In the absence of hemolysis, the physician should consider a problem with the hepatic uptake or conjugation of bilirubin. Certain drugs, including rifampin and probenecid, may cause unconjugated hyperbilirubinemia by diminishing hepatic uptake of bilirubin. Impaired bilirubin conjugation occurs in three genetic conditions: Crigler-Najjar syndrome types I and II and Gilbert's syndrome. *Crigler-Najjar type I* is an exceptionally rare condition found in neonates and characterized by severe jaundice (bilirubin >342 μmol/L [>20 mg/dL]) and neurologic impairment due to kernicterus, frequently leading to death in infancy or childhood. These patients have a complete absence of bilirubin UDPGT activity; are totally unable to conjugate bilirubin; and hence cannot excrete it.

Crigler-Najjar type II is somewhat more common than type I. Patients live into adulthood with serum bilirubin levels of 103–428 μmol/L (6–25 mg/dL). In these patients, mutations in the bilirubin *UDPGT* gene cause the reduction—typically ≤10%—of the enzyme's activity. Bilirubin UDPGT activity can be induced by the administration of phenobarbital, which can reduce serum bilirubin levels in these patients. Despite marked jaundice, these patients usually survive into adulthood, although they may be susceptible to kernicterus under the stress of concurrent illness or surgery.

Gilbert's syndrome is also marked by the impaired conjugation of bilirubin due to reduced bilirubin UDPGT activity (typically 10–35% of normal). Patients with Gilbert's syndrome have mild unconjugated hyperbilirubinemia, with serum levels almost always <103 μmol/L (6 mg/dL). The serum levels may fluctuate, and jaundice is often identified only during periods of stress, concurrent illness, alcohol use, or fasting. Unlike both Crigler-Najjar syndromes, Gilbert's syndrome is very common. The reported incidence is 3–7% of the population, with males predominating over females by a ratio of 1.5–7:1.

Conjugated Hyperbilirubinemia Elevated conjugated hyperbilirubinemia is found in two rare inherited conditions: *Dubin-Johnson syndrome* and *Rotor syndrome* (Table 49-1). Patients with either condition present with asymptomatic jaundice. The defect in Dubin-Johnson syndrome is the presence of mutations in the gene for MRP2. These patients have altered excretion of bilirubin into the bile ducts. Rotor syndrome may represent a deficiency of the major hepatic drug reuptake transporters OATP1B1 and OATP1B3. Differentiating between these syndromes is possible but is clinically unnecessary due to their benign nature.

ELEVATION OF SERUM BILIRUBIN WITH OTHER LIVER TEST ABNORMALITIES

The remainder of this chapter will focus on the evaluation of patients with conjugated hyperbilirubinemia in the setting of other liver test abnormalities. This group of patients can be divided into those with a primary hepatocellular process and those with intra- or extrahepatic cholestasis. This distinction, which is based on the history and physical examination as well as the pattern of liver test abnormalities, guides the clinician's evaluation (Fig. 49-1).

History A complete medical history is perhaps the single most important part of the evaluation of the patient with unexplained jaundice. Important considerations include the use of or exposure to any chemical or medication, whether physician-prescribed, over-the-counter, complementary, or alternative medicines (e.g., herbal and vitamin preparations) or other drugs such as anabolic steroids. The patient should be carefully questioned about possible parenteral exposures, including transfusions, intravenous and intranasal drug use, tattooing, and sexual activity. Other important points include recent travel history; exposure to people with jaundice; exposure to possibly contaminated foods; occupational exposure to hepatotoxins; alcohol consumption; the duration of jaundice; and the presence of any accompanying signs and symptoms, such as arthralgias, myalgias, rash, anorexia, weight loss, abdominal pain, fever, pruritus, and changes in the urine and stool. While none of the latter manifestations is specific for any one condition, any of them can suggest a diagnosis. A history of arthralgias and myalgias predating jaundice suggests hepatitis, either viral or drug related. Jaundice associated with the sudden onset of severe right-upper-quadrant pain and shaking chills suggests choledocholithiasis and ascending cholangitis.

Physical Examination The general assessment should include evaluation of the patient's nutritional status. Temporal and proximal muscle wasting suggests long-standing disease such as pancreatic cancer or cirrhosis. Stigmata of chronic liver disease, including spider nevi, palmar erythema, gynecomastia, caput medusae, Dupuytren's contractures, parotid gland enlargement, and testicular atrophy, are commonly seen in advanced alcohol-related cirrhosis and occasionally in other types of cirrhosis. An enlarged left supraclavicular node (Virchow's node) or a periumbilical nodule (Sister Mary Joseph's nodule) suggests an abdominal malignancy. Jugular venous distention, a sign of right-sided heart failure, suggests hepatic congestion. Right pleural effusion even in the absence of clinically apparent ascites may be seen in advanced cirrhosis.

The abdominal examination should focus on the size and consistency of the liver, on whether the spleen is palpable and hence enlarged, and on whether ascites is present. Patients with cirrhosis may have an enlarged left lobe of the liver, which is felt below the xiphoid, and an enlarged spleen. A grossly enlarged nodular liver or an obvious abdominal mass suggests malignancy. An enlarged tender liver could signify viral or alcoholic hepatitis; an infiltrative process such as amyloidosis; or, less often, an acutely congested liver secondary to right-sided heart failure. Severe right-upper-quadrant tenderness with respiratory arrest on inspiration (Murphy's sign) suggests cholecystitis. Ascites in the presence of jaundice suggests either cirrhosis or malignancy with peritoneal spread.

Laboratory Tests A battery of tests are helpful in the initial evaluation of a patient with unexplained jaundice. These include total and direct serum bilirubin measurement with fractionation; determination of serum aminotransferase, alkaline phosphatase, and albumin concentrations; and prothrombin time tests. Enzyme tests (alanine aminotransferase [ALT], aspartate aminotransferase [AST], and alkaline phosphatase [ALP]) are helpful in differentiating between a hepatocellular process and a cholestatic process (**Table 337-1**; Fig. 49-1)—a critical step in determining what additional workup is indicated. Patients with a hepatocellular process generally have a rise in the aminotransferases that is disproportionate to that in ALP, whereas patients with a cholestatic process have a rise in ALP that is disproportionate to that of the aminotransferases. The serum bilirubin can be prominently elevated in both hepatocellular and cholestatic conditions and therefore is not necessarily helpful in differentiating between the two.

In addition to enzyme tests, all jaundiced patients should have additional blood tests—specifically, an albumin level and a prothrombin time—to assess liver function. A low albumin level suggests a chronic process such as cirrhosis or cancer. A normal albumin level is suggestive of a more acute process such as viral hepatitis or choledocholithiasis. An elevated prothrombin time indicates either vitamin K deficiency due to prolonged jaundice and malabsorption of vitamin K or significant hepatocellular dysfunction. The failure of the prothrombin time to correct with parenteral administration of vitamin K indicates severe hepatocellular injury.

The results of the bilirubin, enzyme, albumin, and prothrombin time tests will usually indicate whether a jaundiced patient has a hepatocellular or a cholestatic disease and offer some indication of the duration and severity of the disease. The causes and evaluations of hepatocellular and cholestatic diseases are quite different.

Hepatocellular Conditions Hepatocellular diseases that can cause jaundice include viral hepatitis, drug or environmental toxicity, alcohol, and end-stage cirrhosis from any cause (**Table 49-2**). Wilson's disease occurs primarily in young adults. Autoimmune hepatitis is typically seen in young to middle-aged women but may affect men and women of any age. Alcoholic hepatitis can be differentiated from viral and toxin-related hepatitis by the pattern of the aminotransferases: patients with alcoholic hepatitis typically have

TABLE 49-2 Hepatocellular Conditions That May Produce Jaundice

Viral hepatitis
Hepatitis A, B, C, D, and E
Epstein-Barr virus
Cytomegalovirus
Herpes simplex virus
Alcoholic hepatitis
Chronic liver disease and cirrhosis
Drug toxicity
Predictable, dose-dependent (e.g., acetaminophen)
Unpredictable, idiosyncratic (e.g., isoniazid)
Environmental toxins
Vinyl chloride
Jamaica bush tea—pyrrolizidine alkaloids
Kava kava
Wild mushrooms—*Amanita phalloides, A. verna*
Wilson's disease
Autoimmune hepatitis

an AST-to-ALT ratio of at least 2:1, and the AST level rarely exceeds 300 U/L. Patients with acute viral hepatitis and toxin-related injury severe enough to produce jaundice typically have aminotransferase levels >500 U/L, with the ALT greater than or equal to the AST. While ALT and AST values <8 times normal may be seen in either hepatocellular or cholestatic liver disease, values 25 times normal or higher are seen primarily in acute hepatocellular diseases. Patients with jaundice from cirrhosis can have normal or only slightly elevated aminotransferase levels.

When the clinician determines that a patient has a hepatocellular disease, appropriate testing for acute viral hepatitis includes a hepatitis A IgM antibody assay, a hepatitis B surface antigen and core IgM antibody assay, a hepatitis C viral RNA test, and, depending on the circumstances, a hepatitis E IgM antibody assay. The hepatitis C antibody can take up to 6 weeks to become detectable, making it an unreliable test if acute hepatitis C is suspected. Studies for hepatitis D, Epstein-Barr virus (EBV), and cytomegalovirus (CMV) may also be indicated. Ceruloplasmin is the initial screening test for Wilson's disease. Testing for autoimmune hepatitis usually includes antinuclear antibody and anti-smooth muscle antibody assays and measurement of specific immunoglobulins.

Drug-induced hepatocellular injury can be classified as either predictable or unpredictable. Predictable drug reactions are dose-dependent and affect all patients who ingest a toxic dose of the drug in question. The classic example is acetaminophen hepatotoxicity. Unpredictable or idiosyncratic drug reactions are not dose-dependent and occur in a minority of patients. A great number of drugs can cause idiosyncratic hepatic injury. Environmental toxins are also an important cause of hepatocellular injury. Examples include industrial chemicals such as vinyl chloride, herbal preparations containing pyrrolizidine alkaloids (Jamaica bush tea) or kava, and the mushrooms *Amanita phalloides* and *A. verna*, which contain highly hepatotoxic amatoxins.

Cholestatic Conditions When the pattern of the liver tests suggests a cholestatic disorder, the first step is to determine whether it is intra- or extrahepatic cholestasis (Fig. 49-1). Distinguishing intrahepatic from extrahepatic cholestasis may be difficult. History, physical examination, and laboratory tests often are not helpful. The next appropriate test is an ultrasound. The ultrasound is inexpensive, does not expose the patient to ionizing radiation, and can detect dilation of the intra- and extrahepatic biliary tree with a high degree of sensitivity and specificity. The absence of biliary dilation suggests intrahepatic cholestasis, while its presence indicates extrahepatic cholestasis. False-negative results occur in patients with partial obstruction of the common bile duct or in patients with cirrhosis or primary sclerosing cholangitis (PSC), in which scarring prevents the intrahepatic ducts from dilating.

Although ultrasonography may indicate extrahepatic cholestasis, it rarely identifies the site or cause of obstruction. The distal common bile duct is a particularly difficult area to visualize by ultrasound because of overlying bowel gas. Appropriate next tests include computed tomography (CT), magnetic resonance cholangiopancreatography (MRCP), endoscopic retrograde cholangiopancreatography (ERCP), percutaneous transhepatic cholangiography (PTC), and endoscopic ultrasound (EUS). CT and MRCP are better than ultrasonography for assessing the head of the pancreas and for identifying choledocholithiasis in the distal common bile duct, particularly when the ducts are not dilated. ERCP is the "gold standard" for identifying choledocholithiasis. Beyond its diagnostic capabilities, ERCP allows therapeutic interventions, including the removal of common bile duct stones and the placement of stents. PTC can provide the same information as ERCP and it also allows for intervention in patients in whom ERCP is unsuccessful due to proximal biliary obstruction or altered gastrointestinal anatomy. MRCP has replaced ERCP as the initial diagnostic test in most cases. EUS displays sensitivity and specificity comparable to that of MRCP in the detection of bile duct obstruction and allows biopsy of suspected malignant lesions.

In patients with apparent *intrahepatic cholestasis*, the diagnosis is often made by serologic testing in combination with a liver biopsy. The list of possible causes of intrahepatic cholestasis is long and varied (**Table 49-3**). A number of conditions that typically cause a hepatocellular pattern of injury can also present as a cholestatic variant. Both hepatitis B and C viruses can cause cholestatic hepatitis (fibrosing cholestatic hepatitis). This disease variant has been reported in patients who have undergone solid organ transplantation. Hepatitis A and E, alcoholic hepatitis, and EBV or CMV infections may also present as cholestatic liver disease.

Drugs may cause intrahepatic cholestasis that is usually reversible after discontinuation of the offending agent, although it may take many months for cholestasis to resolve. Drugs most commonly associated with cholestasis are the anabolic and contraceptive steroids. Cholestatic hepatitis has been reported with chlorpromazine, imipramine, tolbutamide, sulindac, cimetidine, and erythromycin estolate. It also occurs in patients taking trimethoprim; sulfamethoxazole; and penicillin-based antibiotics such as ampicillin, dicloxacillin, and clavulanic acid. Rarely, cholestasis may be chronic and associated with progressive fibrosis despite early discontinuation of the offending drug. Chronic cholestasis has been associated with chlorpromazine and prochlorperazine.

Primary biliary cholangitis is an autoimmune disease predominantly affecting women and characterized by progressive destruction of interlobular bile ducts. The diagnosis is made by the detection of antimitochondrial antibody, which is found in 95% of patients. *Primary sclerosing cholangitis* is characterized by the destruction and fibrosis of larger bile ducts. The diagnosis of PSC is made with cholangiography (either MRCP or ERCP), which demonstrates the pathognomonic segmental strictures. Approximately 75% of patients with PSC also have inflammatory bowel disease.

The *vanishing bile duct syndrome* and *adult bile ductopenia* are rare conditions in which a decreased number of bile ducts are seen in liver biopsy specimens. This histologic picture is also seen in patients who develop chronic rejection after liver transplantation and in those who develop graft-versus-host disease after bone marrow transplantation. Vanishing bile duct syndrome also occurs in rare cases of sarcoidosis, in patients taking certain drugs (including chlorpromazine), and idiopathically.

There are also familial forms of intrahepatic cholestasis. The familial intrahepatic cholestatic syndromes include *progressive familial intrahepatic cholestasis* (PFIC) *types 1–3* and *benign recurrent intrahepatic cholestasis* (BRIC) *types 1 and 2*. BRIC is characterized

TABLE 49-3 Cholestatic Conditions That May Produce Jaundice

I. Intrahepatic
- A. Viral hepatitis
  1. Fibrosing cholestatic hepatitis—hepatitis B and C
  2. Hepatitis A, Epstein-Barr virus infection, cytomegalovirus infection
- B. Alcoholic hepatitis
- C. Drug toxicity
  1. Pure cholestasis—anabolic and contraceptive steroids
  2. Cholestatic hepatitis—chlorpromazine, erythromycin estolate
  3. Chronic cholestasis—chlorpromazine and prochlorperazine
- D. Primary biliary cholangitis
- E. Primary sclerosing cholangitis
- F. Vanishing bile duct syndrome
  1. Chronic rejection of liver transplants
  2. Sarcoidosis
  3. Drugs
- G. Congestive hepatopathy and ischemic hepatitis
- H. Inherited conditions
  1. Progressive familial intrahepatic cholestasis
  2. Benign recurrent intrahepatic cholestasis
- I. Cholestasis of pregnancy
- J. Total parenteral nutrition
- K. Nonhepatobiliary sepsis
- L. Benign postoperative cholestasis
- M. Paraneoplastic syndrome
- N. Veno-occlusive disease
- O. Graft-versus-host disease
- P. Infiltrative disease
  1. Tuberculosis
  2. Lymphoma
  3. Amyloidosis
- Q. Infections
  1. Malaria
  2. Leptospirosis

II. Extrahepatic
- A. Malignant
  1. Cholangiocarcinoma
  2. Pancreatic cancer
  3. Gallbladder cancer
  4. Ampullary cancer
  5. Malignant involvement of the porta hepatis lymph nodes
- B. Benign
  1. Choledocholithiasis
  2. Postoperative biliary strictures
  3. Primary sclerosing cholangitis
  4. Chronic pancreatitis
  5. AIDS cholangiopathy
  6. Mirizzi's syndrome
  7. Parasitic disease (ascariasis)

by episodic attacks of pruritus, cholestasis, and jaundice beginning at any age, which can be debilitating but does not lead to chronic liver disease. Serum bile acids are elevated during episodes, but serum γ-glutamyltransferase (γ-GT) activity is normal. PFIC disorders begin at childhood and are progressive in nature. All three types of PFIC are associated with progressive cholestasis, elevated levels of serum bile acids, and similar phenotypes but different genetic mutations. Only type 3 PFIC is associated with high levels of γ-GT. *Cholestasis of pregnancy* occurs in the second and third trimesters and resolves after delivery. Its cause is unknown, but the condition is probably inherited, and cholestasis can be triggered by estrogen administration.

Other causes of intrahepatic cholestasis include total parenteral nutrition (TPN); nonhepatobiliary sepsis; benign postoperative cholestasis; and a paraneoplastic syndrome associated with a number of different malignancies, including Hodgkin's disease, medullary thyroid cancer, renal cell cancer, renal sarcoma, T-cell lymphoma, prostate cancer, and several gastrointestinal malignancies. The term *Stauffer's syndrome* has been used for intrahepatic cholestasis specifically associated with renal cell cancer. In patients developing cholestasis in the intensive care unit, the major considerations should be sepsis, ischemic hepatitis ("shock liver"), and TPN-related jaundice. Jaundice occurring after bone marrow transplantation is most likely due to veno-occlusive disease or graft-versus-host disease. In addition to hemolysis, sickle cell disease may cause intrahepatic and extrahepatic cholestasis. Jaundice is a late finding in heart failure caused by hepatic congestion and hepatocellular hypoxia. Ischemic hepatitis is a distinct entity of acute hypoperfusion characterized by an acute and dramatic elevation in the serum aminotransferases followed by a gradual peak in serum bilirubin.

Jaundice with associated liver dysfunction can be seen in severe cases of *Plasmodium falciparum* malaria. The jaundice in these cases is due to a combination of indirect hyperbilirubinemia from hemolysis and both cholestatic and hepatocellular jaundice. Weil's disease, a severe presentation of leptospirosis, is marked by jaundice with renal failure, fever, headache, and muscle pain.

Causes of *extrahepatic cholestasis* can be split into malignant and benign (Table 49-3). Malignant causes include pancreatic, gallbladder, and ampullary cancers as well as cholangiocarcinoma. This last malignancy is most commonly associated with PSC and is exceptionally difficult to diagnose because its appearance is often identical to that of PSC. Pancreatic and gallbladder tumors as well as cholangiocarcinoma are rarely resectable and have poor prognoses. Ampullary carcinoma has the highest surgical cure rate of all the tumors that present as painless jaundice. Hilar lymphadenopathy due to metastases from other cancers may cause obstruction of the extrahepatic biliary tree.

Choledocholithiasis is the most common cause of extrahepatic cholestasis. The clinical presentation can range from mild right-upper-quadrant discomfort with only minimal elevations of enzyme test values to ascending cholangitis with jaundice, sepsis, and circulatory collapse. PSC may occur with clinically important strictures limited to the extrahepatic biliary tree. IgG4-associated cholangitis is marked by stricturing of the biliary tree. It is critical that the clinician differentiate this condition from PSC as it is responsive to glucocorticoid therapy. In rare instances, chronic pancreatitis causes strictures of the distal common bile duct, where it passes through the head of the pancreas. AIDS cholangiopathy is a condition that is usually due to infection of the bile duct epithelium with CMV or cryptosporidia and has a cholangiographic appearance similar to that of PSC. The affected patients usually present with greatly elevated serum alkaline phosphatase levels (mean, 800 IU/L), but the bilirubin level is often near normal. These patients do not typically present with jaundice.

GLOBAL CONSIDERATIONS

While extrahepatic biliary obstruction and drugs are common causes of new-onset jaundice in developed countries, infections remain the leading cause in developing countries. Liver involvement and jaundice are observed with numerous infections, particularly malaria, babesiosis, severe leptospirosis, infections due to *Mycobacterium tuberculosis* and the *Mycobacterium avium* complex, typhoid fever, infection with hepatitis viruses A–E, EBV, CMV, viral hemorrhagic fevers including Ebola virus, late phases of yellow fever, dengue fever, schistosomiasis, fascioliasis, clonorchiasis, opisthorchiasis, ascariasis, echinococcosis, hepatosplenic candidiasis, disseminated histoplasmosis, cryptococcosis, coccidioimycosis, ehrlichiosis, chronic Q fever, yersiniosis, brucellosis, syphilis, and leprosy. Bacterial infections that do not necessarily involve the liver and bile ducts may also lead to jaundice, as in cholestasis of sepsis. The presence of fever or abdominal pain suggests concurrent infection, sepsis, or complications from gallstones. The development of encephalopathy and coagulopathy in a jaundiced patient with no preexisting liver disease signifies acute liver failure, which warrants urgent liver transplant evaluation.

ACKNOWLEDGMENT

This chapter is a revised version of chapters that have appeared in prior editions of Harrison's in which Marshall M. Kaplan was a co-author with Daniel Pratt.

FURTHER READING

ERLINGER S et al: Inherited disorders of bilirubin transport and conjugation: New insights into molecular mechanisms and consequences. Gastroenterology 146:1625, 2014.

WOLKOFF AW et al: Bilirubin metabolism and jaundice, in *Schiff's Diseases of the Liver*, 11th ed, Schiff ER et al (eds). Oxford, UK, John Wiley & Sons, Ltd, 2012, pp 120–150.

50 Abdominal Swelling and Ascites

Lawrence S. Friedman

ABDOMINAL SWELLING

Abdominal swelling is a manifestation of numerous diseases. Patients may complain of bloating or abdominal fullness and may note increasing abdominal girth on the basis of increased clothing or belt size. Abdominal discomfort is often reported, but pain is less frequent. When abdominal pain does accompany swelling, it is frequently the result of an intraabdominal infection, peritonitis, or pancreatitis. Patients with abdominal distention from *ascites* (fluid in the abdomen) may report the new onset of an inguinal or umbilical hernia. Dyspnea may result from pressure against the diaphragm and the inability to expand the lungs fully.

CAUSES

The causes of abdominal swelling can be remembered conveniently as the *six Fs*: flatus, fat, fluid, fetus, feces, or a "fatal growth" (often a neoplasm).

Flatus Abdominal swelling may be the result of increased intestinal gas. The normal small intestine contains ~200 mL of gas made up of nitrogen, oxygen, carbon dioxide, hydrogen, and methane. Nitrogen and oxygen are consumed (swallowed), whereas carbon dioxide, hydrogen, and methane are produced intraluminally by bacterial fermentation. Increased intestinal gas can occur in a number of conditions. *Aerophagia*, the swallowing of air, can result in increased amounts of oxygen and nitrogen in the small intestine and lead to abdominal swelling. Aerophagia typically results from gulping food; chewing gum; smoking; or as a response to anxiety, which can lead to repetitive belching. In some cases, increased intestinal gas is the consequence of bacterial metabolism of excess fermentable substances such as lactose and other oligosaccharides, which can lead to production of hydrogen, carbon dioxide, or methane. In many cases, the precise cause of abdominal distention cannot be determined. In some persons, particularly those with irritable bowel syndrome and bloating, the subjective sense of abdominal pressure is attributable to impaired intestinal transit of gas rather than increased gas volume. Abdominal distention—an objective increase in girth—is the result of a lack of coordination between diaphragmatic contraction and anterior abdominal wall relaxation, a response in some cases to intraluminal bowel stimuli; dietary alterations, manipulation of the intestinal microbiota, or biofeedback may be effective therapy. Occasionally, increased lumbar lordosis accounts for apparent abdominal distention.

Fat Weight gain with an increase in abdominal fat can result in an increase in abdominal girth and can be perceived as abdominal swelling. Abdominal fat may be caused by an imbalance between caloric intake and energy expenditure associated with a poor diet and sedentary lifestyle; it also can be a manifestation of certain diseases, such as Cushing's syndrome. Excess abdominal fat has been associated with an increased risk of insulin resistance and cardiovascular disease.

Fluid The accumulation of fluid within the abdominal cavity (ascites) often results in abdominal distention and is discussed in detail below. Grade 1 ascites is detectable only by ultrasonography; grade 2 ascites is detectable by physical examination; and grade 3 ascites results in marked abdominal distention.

Fetus Pregnancy results in increased abdominal girth. Typically, an increase in abdominal size is first noted at 12–14 weeks of gestation, when the uterus moves from the pelvis into the abdomen. Abdominal distention may be seen before this point as a result of fluid retention and relaxation of the abdominal muscles.

Feces In the setting of severe constipation or intestinal obstruction, increased stool in the colon leads to increased abdominal girth. These conditions are often accompanied by abdominal discomfort or pain, nausea, and vomiting and can be diagnosed by imaging studies.

Fatal Growth An abdominal mass can result in abdominal swelling. Neoplasms, abscesses, or cysts can grow to sizes that lead to increased abdominal girth. Enlargement of the intraabdominal organs, specifically the liver (hepatomegaly) or spleen (splenomegaly), or an abdominal aortic aneurysm can result in abdominal distention. Bladder distention also may result in abdominal swelling.

APPROACH TO THE PATIENT

Abdominal Swelling

HISTORY

Determining the etiology of abdominal swelling begins with history-taking and a physical examination. Patients should be questioned regarding symptoms suggestive of malignancy, including weight loss, night sweats, and anorexia. Inability to pass stool or flatus together with nausea or vomiting suggests bowel obstruction, severe constipation, or an ileus (lack of peristalsis). Increased eructation and flatus may point toward aerophagia or increased intestinal production of gas. Patients should be questioned about risk factors for or symptoms of chronic liver disease, including excessive alcohol use and jaundice, which suggest ascites. Patients should also be asked about symptoms of other medical conditions, including heart failure and tuberculosis, which may cause ascites.

PHYSICAL EXAMINATION

Physical examination should include an assessment for signs of systemic disease. The presence of lymphadenopathy, especially supraclavicular lymphadenopathy (*Virchow's node*), suggests metastatic abdominal malignancy. Care should be taken during the cardiac examination to evaluate for elevation of jugular venous pressure (JVP); *Kussmaul's sign* (elevation of the JVP during inspiration); a pericardial knock, which may be seen in heart failure or constrictive pericarditis; or a murmur of tricuspid regurgitation. Spider angiomas, palmar erythema, dilated superficial veins around the umbilicus (*caput medusae*), and gynecomastia suggest liver disease.

The abdominal examination should begin with inspection for the presence of uneven distention or an obvious mass. Auscultation should follow. The absence of bowel sounds or the presence of high-pitched localized bowel sounds points toward an ileus or intestinal obstruction. An umbilical venous hum may suggest the presence of portal hypertension, and a harsh bruit over the liver is heard rarely in patients with hepatocellular carcinoma or alcohol-associated hepatitis. Abdominal swelling caused by intestinal gas can be differentiated from swelling caused by fluid or a solid mass by percussion; an abdomen filled with gas is tympanic, whereas an abdomen containing a mass or fluid is dull to percussion. The absence of abdominal dullness, however, does not exclude ascites, because a minimum of 1500 mL of ascitic fluid is required for detection on physical examination. Finally, the abdomen should be palpated to assess for tenderness, a mass, enlargement of the spleen or liver, or presence of a nodular liver suggesting cirrhosis or tumor. Light palpation of the liver may detect pulsations suggesting retrograde vascular flow from the heart in patients with right-sided heart failure, particularly tricuspid regurgitation.

IMAGING AND LABORATORY EVALUATION

Abdominal x-rays can be used to detect dilated loops of bowel suggesting intestinal obstruction or ileus. Abdominal ultrasonography can detect as little as 100 mL of ascitic fluid, hepatosplenomegaly, a nodular liver, or a mass. Ultrasonography is often inadequate to detect retroperitoneal lymphadenopathy or a pancreatic lesion because of overlying bowel gas. If malignancy or pancreatic disease is suspected, CT can be performed. CT may also detect changes associated with advanced cirrhosis and portal hypertension (**Fig. 50-1**).

Laboratory evaluation should include liver biochemical testing, serum albumin level measurement, and prothrombin time determination (international normalized ratio) to assess hepatic function as well as a complete blood count to evaluate for the presence of cytopenias that may result from portal hypertension or of leukocytosis, anemia, and thrombocytosis that may result from systemic infection. Serum amylase and lipase levels should be checked to evaluate the patient for acute pancreatitis. Urinary protein quantitation is indicated when nephrotic syndrome, which may cause ascites, is suspected. Hydrogen and methane absorbed from the intestine are not metabolized by the host and are excreted in expired air, and detection of increased amounts of these gases in expired breath is the basis for tests used to diagnose carbohydrate (e.g., lactose) malabsorption and small intestinal bacterial overgrowth.

In selected cases, the hepatic venous pressure gradient (pressure across the liver between the portal and hepatic veins) can be measured via cannulation of the hepatic vein to confirm that ascites is caused by cirrhosis (**Chap. 344**). In some cases, a liver biopsy may be necessary to confirm cirrhosis.

ASCITES

PATHOGENESIS IN THE PRESENCE OF CIRRHOSIS

Ascites in patients with cirrhosis is the result of portal hypertension and renal salt and water retention. Similar mechanisms contribute to ascites formation in heart failure. Portal hypertension signifies elevation of the pressure within the portal vein. According to Ohm's law, pressure is the product of resistance and flow. Increased hepatic resistance occurs by several mechanisms. First, the development of hepatic fibrosis, which defines cirrhosis, disrupts the normal architecture of the hepatic sinusoids and impedes normal blood flow through the liver. Second, activation of hepatic stellate cells, which mediate fibrogenesis, leads to smooth-muscle contraction and fibrosis. Finally, cirrhosis is associated with a decrease in endothelial nitric oxide synthetase (eNOS) production, which results in decreased nitric oxide production and increased intrahepatic vasoconstriction.

The development of cirrhosis is also associated with increased systemic circulating levels of nitric oxide (in contrast to the decrease seen intrahepatically), as well as increased levels of vascular endothelial growth factor and tumor necrosis factor, that result in splanchnic arterial vasodilation. Vasodilation of the splanchnic circulation results in pooling of blood and a decrease in the effective circulating volume, which is perceived by the kidneys as hypovolemia. Compensatory vasoconstriction via release of antidiuretic hormone ensues; the consequences are free water retention and activation of the sympathetic nervous system and the renin-angiotensin-aldosterone system, which lead in turn to renal sodium and water retention.

PATHOGENESIS IN THE ABSENCE OF CIRRHOSIS

Ascites in the absence of cirrhosis generally results from peritoneal carcinomatosis, peritoneal infection, or pancreatic disease. Peritoneal carcinomatosis can result from primary peritoneal malignancies such as mesothelioma or sarcoma, abdominal malignancies such as gastric or colonic adenocarcinoma, or metastatic disease from breast or lung carcinoma or melanoma (**Fig. 50-2**). The tumor cells lining the

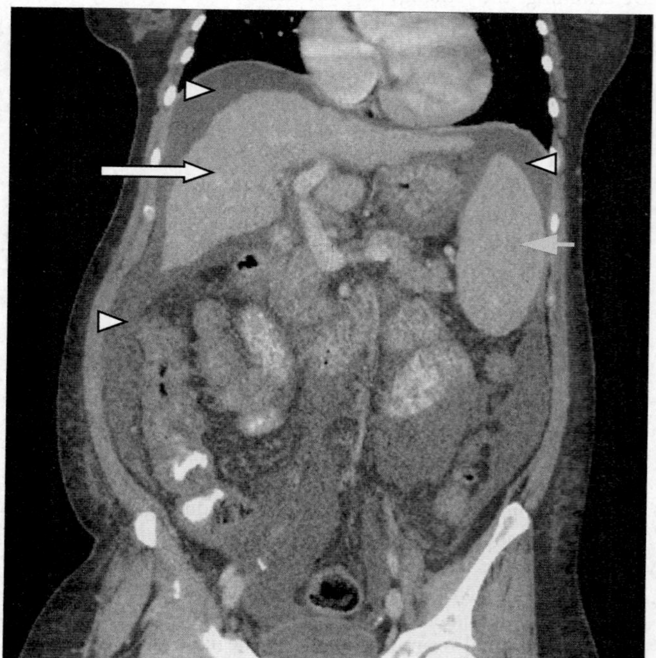

FIGURE 50-1 CT of a patient with a cirrhotic, nodular liver (*white arrow*), splenomegaly (*yellow arrow*), and ascites (*arrowheads*).

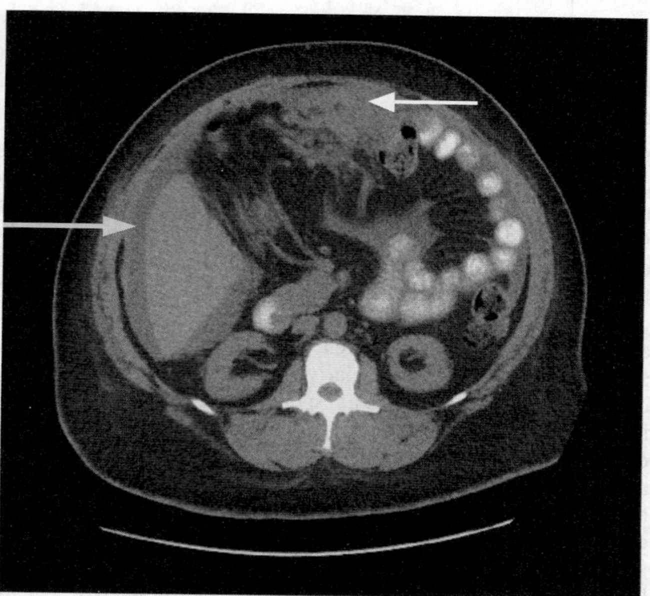

FIGURE 50-2 CT of a patient with peritoneal carcinomatosis (*white arrow*) and ascites (*yellow arrow*).

peritoneum produce a protein-rich fluid that contributes to the development of ascites. Fluid from the extracellular space is drawn into the peritoneum, further contributing to the development of ascites. Tuberculous peritonitis causes ascites via a similar mechanism; tubercles deposited on the peritoneum exude a proteinaceous fluid. Pancreatic ascites results from leakage of pancreatic enzymes into the peritoneum.

■ CAUSES

Cirrhosis accounts for 84% of cases of ascites. Cardiac ascites, peritoneal carcinomatosis, and "mixed" ascites resulting from cirrhosis and a second disease account for 10–15% of cases. Less common causes of ascites include massive hepatic metastasis, infection (tuberculosis, *Chlamydia* infection), pancreatitis, and renal disease (nephrotic syndrome). Rare causes of ascites include hypothyroidism and familial Mediterranean fever.

■ EVALUATION

Once the presence of ascites has been confirmed, the etiology of the ascites is best determined by *paracentesis*, a bedside procedure in which a needle or small catheter is passed transcutaneously to extract ascitic fluid from the peritoneum. The lower quadrants are the most frequent sites for paracentesis. The left lower quadrant is preferred because of the greater depth of ascites and the thinner abdominal wall. Paracentesis is a safe procedure even in patients with coagulopathy; complications, including abdominal wall hematomas, hypotension, hepatorenal syndrome, and infection, are infrequent.

Once ascitic fluid has been extracted, its gross appearance should be examined. Turbid fluid can result from the presence of infection or tumor cells. White, milky fluid indicates a triglyceride level >200 mg/dL (and often >1000 mg/dL), which is the hallmark of *chylous ascites*. Chylous ascites results from lymphatic disruption that may occur with trauma, cirrhosis, tumor, tuberculosis, or certain congenital abnormalities. Dark brown fluid can reflect a high bilirubin concentration and indicates biliary tract perforation. Black fluid may indicate the presence of pancreatic necrosis or metastatic melanoma.

The ascitic fluid should be sent for measurement of albumin and total protein levels, cell and differential counts, and, if infection is suspected, Gram's stain and culture, with inoculation into blood culture bottles at the patient's bedside to maximize the yield. A serum albumin level should be measured simultaneously to permit calculation of the *serum-ascites albumin gradient* (SAAG).

The SAAG is useful for distinguishing ascites caused by portal hypertension from nonportal hypertensive ascites (**Fig. 50-3**). The SAAG reflects the pressure within the hepatic sinusoids and correlates with the hepatic venous pressure gradient. The SAAG is calculated by subtracting the ascitic albumin concentration from the serum albumin level and does not change with diuresis. A SAAG ≥1.1 g/dL reflects the presence of portal hypertension and indicates that the ascites is due to increased pressure in the hepatic sinusoids. According to Starling's law, a high SAAG reflects the oncotic pressure that counterbalances the portal pressure. Possible causes include cirrhosis, cardiac ascites, hepatic vein thrombosis (Budd-Chiari syndrome), sinusoidal obstruction syndrome (veno-occlusive disease), or massive liver metastases. A SAAG <1.1 g/dL indicates that the ascites is not related to portal hypertension, as in tuberculous peritonitis, peritoneal carcinomatosis, or pancreatic ascites.

For high-SAAG (≥1.1) ascites, the ascitic protein level can provide further clues to the etiology (Fig. 50-3). An ascitic protein level of ≥2.5 g/dL indicates that the hepatic sinusoids are normal and are allowing passage of protein into the ascites, as occurs in cardiac ascites, early Budd-Chiari syndrome, or sinusoidal obstruction syndrome. An ascitic protein level <2.5 g/dL indicates that the hepatic sinusoids have been damaged and scarred and no longer allow passage of protein, as occurs with cirrhosis, late Budd-Chiari syndrome, or massive liver metastases. Pro-brain-type natriuretic peptide (BNP) is a natriuretic hormone released by the heart as a result of increased volume and ventricular wall stretch. High levels of BNP in serum occur in heart failure and may be useful in identifying heart failure as the cause of high-SAAG ascites.

Further tests are indicated only in specific clinical circumstances. When secondary peritonitis resulting from a perforated hollow viscus is suspected, ascitic glucose and lactate dehydrogenase (LDH) levels can be measured. In contrast to "spontaneous" bacterial peritonitis, which may complicate cirrhotic ascites (see "Complications," below), secondary peritonitis is suggested by an ascitic glucose level <50 mg/dL, an ascitic LDH level higher than the serum LDH level, and the detection of multiple pathogens on ascitic fluid culture. When pancreatic ascites is suspected, the ascitic amylase level should be measured and is typically >1000 mg/dL. Cytology can be useful in the diagnosis of peritoneal carcinomatosis. At least 50 mL of fluid should be obtained and sent for immediate processing. Tuberculous peritonitis is typically associated with ascitic fluid lymphocytosis but can be difficult to diagnose by paracentesis. A smear for acid-fast bacilli has a diagnostic sensitivity of only 0–3%; a culture increases the sensitivity to 35–50%. In patients without cirrhosis, an elevated ascitic adenosine deaminase level has a sensitivity of >90% for tuberculous ascites when a cut-off value of 30–45 U/L is used. When the cause of ascites remains uncertain, laparotomy or laparoscopy with peritoneal biopsies for histology and culture remains the gold standard.

TREATMENT

Ascites

The initial treatment for cirrhotic ascites is restriction of sodium intake to 2 g/d. When sodium restriction alone is inadequate to control ascites, oral diuretics—typically the combination of spironolactone and furosemide—are used to increase urinary sodium excretion. Spironolactone is an aldosterone antagonist that inhibits sodium resorption in the distal convoluted tubule of the kidney. Use of spironolactone may be limited by hyponatremia, hyperkalemia, and painful gynecomastia. If the gynecomastia is

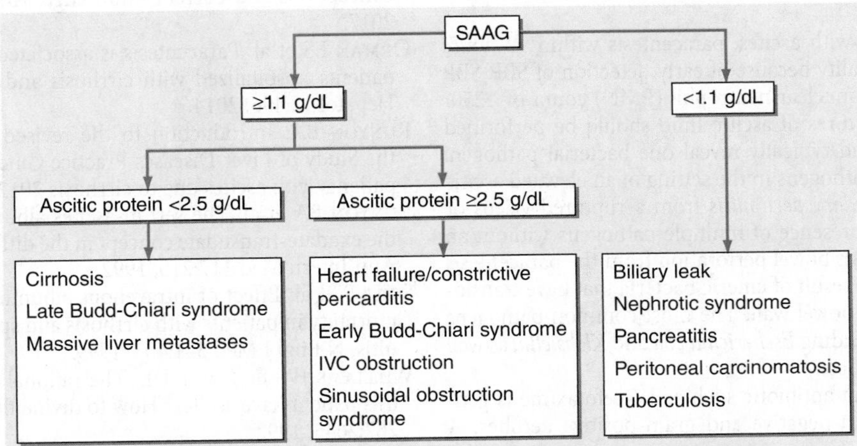

FIGURE 50-3 Algorithm for the diagnosis of ascites according to the serum-ascites albumin gradient (SAAG). IVC, inferior vena cava.

distressing, amiloride (5–40 mg/d) may be substituted for spironolactone. Furosemide is a loop diuretic that is generally combined with spironolactone in a ratio of 40:100; maximal daily doses of spironolactone and furosemide are 400 mg and 160 mg, respectively. Fluid intake may be restricted in patients with hyponatremia.

Refractory cirrhotic ascites is defined by the persistence of ascites despite sodium restriction and maximal (or maximally tolerated) diuretic use. Pharmacologic therapy for refractory ascites includes the addition of midodrine, an α_1-adrenergic agonist, or clonidine, an α_2-adrenergic agonist, to diuretic therapy. These agents act as vasoconstrictors, counteracting splanchnic vasodilation. Midodrine alone or in combination with clonidine improves systemic hemodynamics and control of ascites over that obtained with diuretics alone. Although β-adrenergic blocking agents (beta blockers) are often prescribed to prevent variceal hemorrhage in patients with cirrhosis, the use of beta blockers in patients with refractory ascites may be associated with decreased survival rates.

When medical therapy alone is insufficient, refractory cirrhotic ascites can be managed by repeated large-volume paracentesis (LVP) or a transjugular intrahepatic peritoneal shunt (TIPS)—a radiologically placed portosystemic shunt that decompresses the hepatic sinusoids. Intravenous (IV) infusion of albumin accompanying LVP decreases the risk of "postparacentesis circulatory dysfunction" and death. Patients undergoing LVP should receive IV albumin infusions of 6–8 g/L of ascitic fluid removed. TIPS placement is superior to LVP in reducing the reaccumulation of ascites but is associated with an increased frequency of hepatic encephalopathy, with no difference in mortality rates. The Alfapump system, which consists of an automated pump and tunneled peritoneal catheter that transports ascites from the peritoneal cavity to the urinary bladder, has shown promise in the management of refractory ascites but is associated with a higher frequency of technical difficulties and renal dysfunction.

Malignant ascites does not respond to sodium restriction or diuretics. Patients must undergo serial LVPs, transcutaneous drainage catheter placement, or, rarely, creation of a peritoneovenous shunt (a shunt from the abdominal cavity to the vena cava) or placement of the Alfapump system, if available.

Ascites caused by tuberculous peritonitis is treated with standard antituberculosis therapy. Noncirrhotic ascites of other causes is treated by correction of the precipitating condition.

COMPLICATIONS

Spontaneous bacterial peritonitis (SBP; **Chap. 132**) is a common and potentially lethal complication of cirrhotic ascites. Occasionally, SBP also complicates ascites caused by nephrotic syndrome, heart failure, acute hepatitis, and acute liver failure but is rare in malignant ascites. Patients with SBP generally note an increase in abdominal girth; however, abdominal tenderness is found in only 40% of patients, and rebound tenderness is uncommon. Patients may present with fever, nausea, vomiting, or the new onset or an exacerbation of preexisting hepatic encephalopathy.

In hospitalized patients with ascites, paracentesis within 12 hours of admission reduces mortality because of early detection of SBP. SBP is defined by a polymorphonuclear neutrophil (PMN) count of ≥250/μL in the ascitic fluid. Cultures of ascitic fluid should be performed in blood culture bottles and typically reveal one bacterial pathogen. The presence of multiple pathogens in the setting of an elevated ascitic PMN count suggests *secondary peritonitis* from a ruptured viscus or abscess (**Chap. 132**). The presence of multiple pathogens without an elevated PMN count suggests bowel perforation from the paracentesis needle. SBP is generally the result of enteric bacteria that have translocated across an edematous bowel wall. The most common pathogens are gram-negative rods, including *Escherichia coli* and *Klebsiella*, as well as streptococci and enterococci.

Treatment of SBP with an antibiotic such as IV cefotaxime is generally effective against gram-negative and gram-positive aerobes. A 5-day course of treatment is sufficient if the patient improves clinically. Nosocomial or health care–acquired SBP is frequently caused by multidrug-resistant bacteria, and initial antibiotic therapy should be guided by the local bacterial epidemiology.

Cirrhotic patients with a history of SBP, an ascitic fluid total protein concentration <1 g/dL, or active gastrointestinal bleeding should receive prophylactic antibiotics to prevent SBP; oral daily ciprofloxacin or, where available, norfloxacin is commonly used. IV ceftriaxone may be used in hospitalized patients. Diuresis increases the activity of ascitic fluid protein opsonins and may decrease the risk of SBP.

Hepatic hydrothorax occurs when ascites, often caused by cirrhosis, migrates via fenestrae in the diaphragm into the pleural space. This condition can result in shortness of breath, hypoxia, and infection. Treatment is similar to that for cirrhotic ascites and includes sodium restriction, diuretics, and, if needed, thoracentesis or TIPS placement. Chest tube placement should be avoided.

ACKNOWLEDGMENT

The author thanks Dr. Kathleen E. Corey for contributions to this chapter in prior editions of the textbook.

FURTHER READING

ADEBAYO D et al: Refractory ascites in liver cirrhosis. Am J Gastroenterol 114:40, 2019.

BARBA E et al: Correction of abdominal distention by biofeedback-guided control of abdominothoracic muscular activity in a randomized, placebo-controlled trial. Clin Gastroenterol Hepatol 15:1922, 2017.

BERNARDI M et al: Albumin infusion in patients undergoing large-volume paracentesis: A meta-analysis of randomized trials. Hepatology 55:1172, 2012.

EUROPEAN ASSOCIATION FOR THE STUDY OF THE LIVER: EASL Clinical Practice Guidelines for the management of patients with decompensated cirrhosis. J Hepatol 69:406, 2018.

FARIAS AQ et al: Serum B-type natriuretic peptide in the initial workup of patients with new onset ascites: A diagnostic accuracy study. Hepatology 59:1043, 2014.

FERNANDEZ J et al: Prevalence and risk factors of infections by multiresistant bacteria in cirrhosis: A prospective study. Hepatology 55:1551, 2012.

GE PS, RUNYON BA: Role of plasma BNP in patients with ascites: Advantages and pitfalls. Hepatology 59:751, 2014.

JOHN S, FRIEDMAN LS: Portal hypertensive ascites: Current status. Curr Hepatol Rep 19:226, 2020.

JOHN S, THULUVATH PJ: Hyponatremia in cirrhosis: Pathophysiology and management. World J Gastroenterol 21:3197, 2015.

LIZAOLA B et al: Review article: the diagnostic approach and current management of chylous ascites. Aliment Pharmacol Ther 46:816, 2017.

MALAGELADA JR et al: Bloating and abdominal distension: Old misconceptions and current knowledge. Am J Gastroenterol 112:1221, 2017.

ORMAN ES et al: Paracentesis is associated with reduced mortality in patients hospitalized with cirrhosis and ascites. Clin Gastroenterol Hepatol 12:496, 2014.

RUNYON BA: Introduction to the revised American Association for the Study of Liver Diseases Practice Guideline management of adult patients with ascites due to cirrhosis 2012. Hepatology 57:165, 2013.

RUNYON BA et al: The serum-ascites albumin gradient is superior to the exudate-transudate concept in the differential diagnosis of ascites. Ann Intern Med 117:215, 1992.

SORT P et al: Effect of intravenous albumin on renal impairment and mortality in patients with cirrhosis and spontaneous bacterial peritonitis. N Engl J Med 341:403, 1999.

WILLIAMS JW JR, SIMEL DL: The rational clinical examination. Does this patient have ascites? How to divine fluid in the abdomen. JAMA 267:2645, 1992.

51 Interstitial Cystitis/Bladder Pain Syndrome

R. Christopher Doiron, J. Curtis Nickel

DEFINITION

A condition associated with bladder inflammation and pain, with what were thought to be discrete bladder ulcerations, was first described in 1887. The description of the classic bladder-wall ulcer—now referred to as a *Hunner lesion*—became known as *interstitial cystitis* (IC). The first generally accepted definition of IC was derived from a National Institute for Diabetes and Digestive and Kidney Diseases (NIDDK) consensus of experts in the field in 1998. The NIDDK criteria used to define IC included typical cystoscopic findings such as glomerulations (submucosal petechial hemorrhages of the urothelium) or Hunner lesions. However, over time, the syndrome experienced by patients, including bladder and/or pelvic pain with associated urinary storage symptoms of urinary frequency and urgency, negative urine cultures, and no specific identifiable causes, became known as *interstitial cystitis/bladder pain syndrome* (IC/BPS).

The nomenclature and definitions have evolved, but the contemporary definitions accepted by the American Urological Association, the Canadian Urological Association, the International Continence Society, the Society for Urodynamics and Female Urology, and the European Society for the Study of IC/BPS, although they all differ somewhat in language and specifics, generally reflect several fundamental concepts common in the disease: (1) it is chronic in nature; (2) it causes pain perceived to be attributable to the bladder; (3) this pain occurs in the presence of lower urinary tract symptoms (LUTS); and (4) pain outside the bladder—in the pelvis, perineum, genitals, abdomen, and beyond—is common.

The following definition incorporates the major descriptions by all international groups interested in the diagnosis and management of IC/BPS: an unpleasant sensation (pain, pressure, discomfort) perceived to be related to the urinary bladder, associated with LUTS of >6 weeks' duration, in the absence of infection or other identifiable causes.

A generalized urologic chronic pelvic pain syndrome (UCPPS) is referenced in the literature and is thought to encompass two distinct urologic chronic pain disorders: IC/BPS, which may be present in men and women, and chronic prostatitis/chronic pelvic pain syndrome (CP/CPPS), which is present only in men. The latter refers to a urologic pain disorder with pain localized to the perineum and/or male genitals, with or without LUTS. IC/BPS can exist independent of CP/CPPS in men. In reality, the urologic chronic pain disorders often have overlapping symptom presentations and may share common etiologic and pathophysiologic origins, but the focus of the current chapter will be on IC/BPS.

ETIOLOGY AND PATHOGENESIS

Pinning a single etiology to a diagnosis of IC/BPS has been an endeavor fraught with uncertainty that ultimately has failed thus far. Instead, it is much more likely and widely accepted that IC/BPS represents a syndrome or constellation of interrelated disease processes that manifest in a spectrum of disease that reaches beyond the bladder. While the search for a single etiology soldiers on, we will review here a collection of proposed theories.

INFECTION AND THE URINARY MICROBIOTA

Bacterial infection of the urothelium has long been regarded as a major suspect in the etiology of IC/BPS but has never been definitively shown to cause the disease. It is not uncommon for patients presenting with IC/BPS to describe a long history of "urinary tract infections" (UTIs); these patients often have undergone multiple courses of treatment with one or multiple antibiotics prescribed by their physicians. Often, however, in patients with IC/BPS, the benefit of antibiotic treatment is short-lived, urine culture results are negative, and the return of symptoms is inevitable.

Although studies examining the role of microbiologic organisms in this patient population are numerous and the results conflicting, far more studies have yielded negative results rather than positive findings. Furthermore, our understanding of the urinary microbiota continues to expand, rendering older studies using outdated and insensitive cultivation techniques less relevant.

Using state-of-the-art, culture-independent techniques for microorganism identification, investigators observe subtle differences between the urinary microbiota of IC/BPS patients and that of healthy controls and between IC/BPS patients experiencing symptom flares and IC/BPS patients not in flare. The clinical relevance of these findings is still not fully understood. As the study of the urinary microbiota continues to unfold, researchers and clinicians believe that although a single causative microbe is unlikely, dysbiosis or disturbance in the microbial ecology of the lower urinary tract may be responsible for flares or symptom patterns experienced by IC/BPS patients.

AUTOIMMUNITY

The consideration of IC/BPS as a disorder of the immune system stems from the observation of a significant prevalence of autoimmune disorders in IC/BPS patients; several historical studies have identified anti-urothelial antibodies within the bladder mucosa of IC/BPS patients. Furthermore, although IC/BPS is not a pathologic diagnosis, there are widely accepted, recognizable patterns of inflammatory infiltration in the bladder mucosa of this patient population, including lymphoplasmacytic infiltrates, stromal edema and fibrosis, urothelial denudation, and detrusor mastocytosis. Thus, although it is likely that immune disturbances cause the condition in a subset of patients (for example, in those with associated Sjögren's syndrome), researchers and clinicians have been unable to leverage this knowledge into a clear description, and its clinical relevance is not fully understood.

INFLAMMATION

It is well established that a subset of patients suffering from IC/BPS clearly have associated bladder inflammation of unknown etiology. The best described of these patients are those with Hunner lesions—discrete inflammatory lesions, previously believed to be ulcers, that have a well-characterized inflammatory profile on histologic and pathologic analysis. While Hunner lesions are easily identified under direct vision by cystoscopy, a spectrum of other, less obvious inflammatory patterns in the bladder is associated with infiltration of acute and chronic inflammatory cells and mast cells. This inflammation observed on histologic analysis can be so subtle that it cannot be recognized under direct visual examination of the bladder with cystoscopy.

Investigators in the Multidisciplinary Approach to the Study of Chronic Pelvic Pain (MAPP) Research Network have found that, among patients with UCPPS, women exhibit more robust inflammatory responses to stimulation of Toll-like receptor 2 (TLR2) and TLR4. Furthermore, an increased response to stimulation of TLR4 predicts more severe symptoms, widespread pain (vs pelvic/bladder pain only), and a higher number of chronic overlapping pain conditions (COPCs). Further studies aimed at a better understanding of these findings are under way.

UROTHELIAL DYSFUNCTION

Urothelial Permeability and the Glycosaminoglycan Layer The stratified epithelium of the bladder—the urothelium—is composed of basal precursor cells, intermediate cells, and a layer of specialized, superficial epithelial cells called *umbrella cells*. Collectively, these layers are responsible for the various functions of the bladder lining. One important function of the urothelium is to provide a robust barrier layer. This function is fulfilled by the dense layering of glycosaminoglycans (GAGs) on the luminal surface of the urothelium along with a complex arrangement of numerous intercellular tight junctions among urothelial cells that protects the underlying bladder interstitium from the constituents of the urine resting in the bladder.

Defects in this barrier function—either disruptions in the GAG layer or disruptions in the epithelial layer itself or its cellular junctions—have been proposed as a possible mechanism for bladder pain in IC/BPS patients. This theory, while still popular, lacks definitive evidence supporting it as the etiology of this disease.

Antiproliferative Factor The discovery that urothelial cells from IC/BPS patients appear to grow far more slowly than urothelial cells from a healthy control population led to the identification of antiproliferative factor (APF). Although APF initially showed promise as a sensitive and specific urine biomarker for IC/BPS, this idea has not been widely adopted, and the etiologic role of APF is not yet fully understood.

■ PELVIC ORGAN CROSSTALK

The observation of dysfunction and symptoms in multiple organ systems, including gastrointestinal, gynecologic, and genital organs, in patients with IC/BPS is so common that it might be considered the norm. Mechanisms of neural sensitization in patients with chronic pain have been reported, and abnormalities in the autonomic nervous system have been observed among IC/BPS patients. Again, although these observations apply in a subset of patients, their broader application to the heterogeneous IC/BPS patient population as a clear cause of disease is not warranted.

■ NEUROBIOLOGIC CONTRIBUTIONS AND CENTRAL SENSITIZATION

One breakthrough by the MAPP Research Network is an investigation of the role of structural and functional alterations in the brains of patients with UCPPS. The network's innovative methods of correlating clinical and deep phenotyping data with functional MRI data identified such structural and functional differences. These differences were later shown to successfully predict the progression of symptoms in a cohort of 52 patients with UCPPS. Although the relevant study did not differentiate between IC/BPS and CP/CPPS patients, the findings are nevertheless informative, and further longitudinal studies are ongoing.

In addition to the novel MAPP-led findings using neuroimaging, quantitative sensory testing (QST) methods have been used to investigate the sensory processing mechanisms in UCPPS patients. The findings—generalized pain hypersensitivity and altered endogenous inhibitory pain control systems among UCPPS patients—further support a hypothesis of a central sensitization phenotype in urologic chronic pelvic pain. The clinical implications of observed neural alterations and multisensory hypersensitivity remain under investigation.

Although a single etiology for this clinically heterogeneous pain syndrome may never be identified, efforts to do so have revealed much about its pathogenesis in subsets of patients and have provided valuable insight into specific patient phenotypes. The challenge for researchers and clinicians moving forward will be to unify clinical phenotypes with these proposed underlying mechanisms of disease and to integrate this knowledge into clinically actionable interventions that may provide meaningful outcomes.

EPIDEMIOLOGY

The prevalence of IC/BPS has been difficult to determine because definitions and diagnostic criteria (in the absence of a definitive diagnostic test or biomarker) are constantly evolving. In addition, the various methods used in attempting to describe the syndrome's epidemiology (patient self-reports, symptom-based surveys, physician visits, population-based databases) have been problematic and have made comparisons of results challenging. Many studies have historically been performed only in female populations. Currently, it is estimated that 2.7–6.5% of North American women experience symptoms consistent with a diagnosis of IC/BPS. Fewer than 10% of women who experience these symptoms actually have a diagnosis of IC/BPS. The syndrome does occur in men, with a reported 10:1 female-to-male ratio, but it is thought that the condition is dramatically underreported in men.

Some predictors of the development of IC/BPS have been suggested through an analysis of retrospective observational studies of childhood disorders and adverse childhood experiences (ACEs), including childhood UTI, childhood bowel and bladder dysfunction, and childhood sexual trauma. Furthermore, it has been well established that IC/BPS patients exhibit a remarkable prevalence of COPCs such as fibromyalgia, irritable bowel syndrome (IBS), chronic back pain, and chronic fatigue syndrome (CFS). Recent MAPP-led studies have shown that more than one-third of IC/BPS patients have one COPC (IBS, fibromyalgia, or CFS), while up to 10% have multiple COPCs. Thus, these conditions might be considered risk factors for the development of IC/BPS.

CLINICAL MANIFESTATIONS

Patients with IC/BPS, both female and male, present with varying degrees of discomfort and/or pain perceived to be related to the bladder and associated with urinary storage symptoms, including daytime and nighttime urinary frequency and urinary urgency. For some patients, urinary symptoms (the most common complaint after bladder pain) are the most bothersome, while for most patients, bladder pain causes the most distress and most significantly affects quality of life. Unfortunately, the majority of patients with IC/BPS present with both types of symptoms, as patients void frequently to relieve pain (or because of fear of bladder pain). Typically, this combination of bladder pain and urinary frequency severely impacts patients' quality of life, social interactions, and physical activities.

Pain-mapping studies have been used to identify different pain phenotypes within the disease. Nickel and colleagues first described a bladder-only phenotype present in 20% of a cohort of female IC/BPS patients, whereas up to 80% of patients described pain in the pelvis and at least one site beyond. Common associated conditions include IBS (40%), pelvic floor dysfunctional pain syndrome (40–60%), vulvodynia (17%), fibromyalgia (36%), CFS (10%), and chronic back pain (47%). As described above, these multiorgan symptoms may be due to central nervous system sensitization and associated spinal crosstalk, which may promote phenotypic progression as patients with one pain syndrome slowly progress to another. Subsequent MAPP-led studies among a more heterogeneous UCPPS cohort of men and women have supported this concept of specific pain phenotypes, reporting a pelvic-pain-only phenotype in 25% of participants and pain in the pelvis and beyond in up to 75%.

Another important finding from the MAPP investigations is their identification of not just a pelvic-pain-only phenotype but also of a bladder-focused phenotype. The latter phenotype was identified by patients' responses to two RAND Interstitial Cystitis Epidemiology (RICE) survey questions: whether they had "painful bladder filling" and/or "painful urinary urgency." Most female UCPPS patients (88%) responded "yes" to at least one of these questions. The bladder-focused phenotype was associated with more severe urologic symptoms and worse quality of life.

Patients present with unique pain trajectories. Some initially have mild discomfort that progresses over many years to pain with bladder filling and finally to chronic unremitting pelvic pain with only short periods of relief with urination. Other patients begin with UTI-like symptoms and acute bladder and urethral pain with urinary frequency and urgency; these manifestations persist as a chronic cystitis–like syndrome despite negative cultures and no benefit from antimicrobial therapy. Still other patients report a waxing and waning of pain over time, with flares exacerbated by diet, anxiety/stress, infection, or hormone cycle (typically with increased pain prior to menses). In a longitudinal study of UCPPS patients followed over a 12-month period during routine care for their disease, MAPP investigators described 60% of patients' symptoms as stable, 20% as improved, and 20% as worsened.

TABLE 51-1 Workup of Patients by a Primary Care Practitioner or General Internist

STEPS IN WORKUP	SPECIFICS
History/physical examination	Conduct a pelvic exam (recommended). Categorize symptoms as bladder/pelvis focused and/or extending beyond the pelvis.
Urinalysis	Perform a urine culture. If the culture is positive, conduct sensitivity testing.
Consideration of patient-centered treatment options if satisfied with diagnosis[a]	Begin with conservative measures. Introduce further symptom-specific treatments as needed.
Referral to an appropriate specialist under certain conditions	Referral should follow if: • the diagnosis is unclear • microscopic or gross hematuria is present • the condition is refractory to treatment • symptoms are severe • the presentation is complex

[a]See text.

APPROACH TO THE PATIENT

Interstitial Cystitis/Bladder Pain Syndrome

Patients with IC/BPS present to their family physician or internist with pelvic pain that typically increases in severity with bladder filling, other associated pain, and various degrees of urinary symptomatology. The course that should be followed by primary care practitioners or general internists during the patient's workup and before referral to a specialist is outlined in **Table 51-1**. Most of these physicians will not move beyond a suspected diagnosis and conservative advice; that is acceptable. Patients with IC/BPS can often represent diagnostic challenges, and referral to an appropriate subspecialist is warranted if any diagnostic uncertainty remains.

A diagnosis of IC/BPS is often missed and delayed for many years because physicians tend to silo patients into various medical-specialty streams on the basis of the predominant or most bothersome symptom. For example, patients presenting with pelvic pain in which flares are associated with monthly menstrual cycles may be referred to gynecologists. Patients with abdominal/pelvic pain associated with diarrhea and/or constipation tend to be referred to gastroenterologists, while those with generalized muscle and joint pain, perhaps associated with fatigue, are referred to rheumatologists. Patients with urinary symptoms and bladder pain are treated for UTIs (even with negative urine cultures) or overactive bladder—a common bladder condition associated with urinary frequency and urgency, but not pain.

It would be simple if the approach to patients presenting with pelvic pain was only to determine the actual pelvic organ and/or disease causing the symptoms. However, spinal crosstalk, phenotype progression over time, central sensitization, and COPCs complicate the picture. Since only ~20–25% of patients eventually diagnosed with IC/BPS have bladder-only disease, one must not be bladder-centric in approach but rather must consider the entire patient. The provider must determine the patient's "clinical picture"—that is, the patient's unique presenting clinical phenotype.

Urologists have adapted a system of clinical symptom categorization for patients with UCPPS. UPOINT, which includes documenting the contribution of six distinct domains—*U*rinary, *P*sychosocial, *O*rgan-specific, *I*nfection, *N*eurologic, and *T*enderness (as in pelvic floor muscle tenderness)—has helped categorize patient symptoms and allows the practitioner to focus their management on the most bothersome domain, while helping to avoid neglecting domains that are often forgotten. While used by many urologists managing this condition, UPOINT is not as effective in IC/BPS as it is in male CP/CPPS, probably because all IC/BPS patients would be categorized, by definition, in the U and O domains.

A further simplified clinical approach to the assessment of patients with symptoms of IC/BPS is to classify patients with perceived bladder pain (a mandatory criterion for diagnosis) into one of two categories: (1) a "pelvic-pain-only" category, which would include the "bladder-pain-only," pelvic floor dysfunctional pain, and associated gynecologic pain groups; or (2) a "pelvic pain and beyond" category, which would include patients with associated COPCs (such as IBS and fibromyalgia). This approach has been supported by recent observations from the MAPP investigators.

The contribution of psychosocial parameters, such as depression, catastrophizing, anxiety, and stress, and their impact on pain and disability cannot be overlooked and are important to ascertain in all cases. This approach to clinical phenotyping will let the physician tailor a unique treatment plan for each individual patient, using combinations of local bladder, pelvic floor, or more general systemic therapies.

DIAGNOSIS

IC/BPS is a clinically heterogeneous condition whose lack of a clear etiopathogenesis presents difficulties in diagnosis. In making a diagnosis of exclusion, clinicians must rule out other confusable diseases and identify to the best of their ability the phenotypic presentation of the presenting patient. Although attempts have been made to establish a set of diagnostic criteria in the past, the specified criteria have proven overly stringent and too exclusive to be clinically useful. Furthermore, although several guidelines exist to aide in decision making in diagnostic investigations, most investigations serve merely to rule out other pathology. In contrast, history and physical examination, along with some simple laboratory testing, are the most reliable tools with which to establish a diagnosis of IC/BPS. Details of relevant investigations, some of which may be beyond the scope of the general practitioner or internist, are presented here. Table 51-1 offers an approach for the general practitioner, and **Table 51-2** provides a more complete summary of diagnostic recommendations.

HISTORY AND PHYSICAL (INCLUDING FREQUENCY/VOLUME CHARTS)

A thorough history and physical examination are of utmost importance in diagnosing IC/BPS. A history of the patient's pain symptoms is a logical place to start. The nature, intensity, and timing of the pain are all significant factors. Some patients will be less explicit than others in describing their pain and may instead describe a sense of pressure, burning, or vague fullness in the pelvis or bladder area.

All aspects of the patient's pain should be explored, as many patients' pain will not be limited to the pelvis or bladder but will be associated with the genitals, anus or rectum, perineum, abdomen, and beyond. Furthermore, although pain is commonly experienced with bladder filling, patients may also have suprapubic tenderness or pressure with voiding or burning or pain in the bladder, urethra, or perineum, with radiation into the vagina for women or the prostate, penis, and testicles

TABLE 51-2 Recommendations for Investigations in Patients with Suspected Interstitial Cystitis/Bladder Pain Syndrome

MANDATORY	RECOMMENDED	OPTIONAL	NOT RECOMMENDED
History	Frequency/volume chart	Ultrasound/pelvic imaging	Potassium sensitivity test
Physical examination	Urinalysis	Postvoid residual	Urodynamics
	Urine culture	Urine cytology	Bladder biopsy
	Symptom scores	Intravesical anesthetic bladder challenge	
	Cystoscopy	Hydrodistension	

Source: Adapted from A Cox et al: CUA guideline: Diagnosis and treatment of interstitial cystitis/bladder pain syndrome. Can Urol Assoc J 10:E136, 2016.

for men. In male patients, distinguishing IC/BPS from CP/CPPS can be challenging. Physicians must assess for more widespread pain locations outside the pelvis; screening for COPCs, particularly IBS, fibromyalgia, CFS, back pain, and headache, is important in adequately addressing the clinical impact of IC/BPS.

Eliciting and understanding associated LUTS—specifically urinary frequency, urgency, and nocturia—should be another focus of the history. While several confusable diseases can present with LUTS, the manifestation of IC/BPS as voiding dysfunction can help guide treatment decisions and is often a significant focus of bother for the patient. Having patients complete frequency/volume charts, noting the time and volume of each urination over a 24-hour period, can help provide objective evidence of a LUTS history and facilitate follow-up during and after treatment.

Physical examination should focus on the abdomen, pelvis, genitals, and pelvic floor. The degree of pelvic floor relaxation (i.e., degree of muscle tension and/or spasm) during examination is important to note. Trigger points in the pelvic floor musculature and any areas of localized spasticity should be identified. In women, an examination of the vulva, vaginal mucosa, and urethral meatus is essential to identify the presence of vulvodynia (vulvar mucosal pain with no identifiable cause) or any signs of genitourinary syndrome of menopause. In men, an examination of the external genitalia and a digital rectal (prostate) examination as well as a similar pelvic floor examination should be included to rule out related pathology.

■ SYMPTOM SCORES

The quality of a history can be elevated by an accompanying validated, objective measurement of the patient's symptoms. Although several relevant tools exist, the Interstitial Cystitis Symptom Index (ICSI) and the Interstitial Cystitis Problem Index (ICPI) are the most widely used, are commonly employed in research trials as outcome measures, and are straightforward enough for the practitioner to perform in an outpatient setting. These short questionnaires document pain severity, urinary frequency, urgency, and nocturia as well as the bother experienced from each of these symptoms.

More recently, MAPP investigators have suggested that pain and urinary symptoms should be assessed independently using two separate questionnaires: the Genitourinary Pain Index (GUPI) to assess pain and the ICSI to separately assess urinary symptoms. This suggestion is based on their finding of variable effects of urologic pain versus urinary symptoms on quality of life and mental health. Although symptom scores should not be relied on as diagnostic tools, their utility in establishing objective baseline measures to monitor response to treatment and symptoms over time can be valuable to the patient and the practitioner.

■ URINE STUDIES

Urine studies (urinalysis, culture, sensitivity, and cytology) should be included in the workup of a patient in whom IC/BPS is suspected. However, their role is mostly in ruling out other confusable disease rather than in aiding in the diagnosis of IC/BPS. A microscopic examination of the urine can reveal abnormalities attributable to the kidney that may warrant referral to a nephrologist; microscopic hematuria may trigger cystoscopic examination and referral to a urologist. The presenting symptoms of IC/BPS often mimic those of UTI, which must be ruled out by urine cultures. It is important to recognize that IC/BPS patients are subject to at least as great a risk of UTIs as the general population and that UTI should be considered when a flare in symptoms is reported. Finally, urine cytology should be considered if a diagnosis of bladder cancer is suspected or if there is a history of hematuria.

■ IMAGING, CYSTOSCOPY, AND URODYNAMICS

More intensive investigations and imaging studies should be considered in specific scenarios but need not be routinely performed. Abdominal and pelvic imaging studies in selected patients can help identify anatomic abnormalities of the upper or lower urinary tracts, diagnose urolithiasis or masses in the upper urinary tract, and rule out hydronephrosis, which may suggest obstructive uropathy. Furthermore, brain imaging with functional MRI and quantitative sensory testing may prove beneficial in establishing a central sensitization phenotype; however, this is an emerging field of investigation, and routine brain imaging and sensory testing are currently not recommended.

Cystoscopy is used to rule out bladder pathology—most importantly, bladder cancer. Moreover, cystoscopy plays an important role in phenotyping IC/BPS and is required for identification of Hunner lesions. Although a broad consensus is lacking, the authors and others advocate for routine cystoscopic evaluation when IC/BPS is suspected, given the potential therapeutic implications and the ability of this measure to make phenotype-directed therapies possible. Finally, urodynamics testing should be reserved for specific scenarios—for example, cases in which complex voiding dysfunction may be contributing to the presentation.

■ INTRAVESICAL ANESTHETIC BLADDER CHALLENGE AND HYDRODISTENSION

An intravesical anesthetic bladder challenge (using intravesical lidocaine) can be done in the outpatient setting and can help distinguish bladder-focused pain from pelvic pain of other causes. It can further be harnessed as a therapeutic strategy if the patient experiences an improvement in symptoms. Similarly, hydrodistension, which requires a general or regional anesthetic, can play a diagnostic or therapeutic role. Bladder capacities of <400 mL under general anesthesia have correlated with worse pain and poor prognosis. The diagnostic role of post-hydrodistension inspection for bladder glomerulations has been suggested as a possible important clinical differentiation, although the utility of identifying and grading glomerulations is debated.

TREATMENT

Clinical Phenotyping

The UPOINT phenotyping tool introduced in 2009 was the first clinical tool to recognize that patients presenting with pelvic pain syndromes are a heterogeneous population with disease of unclear etiology that makes it difficult to predict outcomes in individuals with standard therapies. UPOINT is based on a patient-centered approach: individualized treatments are matched to patient evaluations by phenotyping of patients using six distinct clinical domains—*u*rinary, *p*sychosocial, *o*rgan-specific, *i*nfectious, *n*eurologic, and *t*enderness. Since its initial publication, follow-up phenotyping studies have indicated that UPOINT is likely better than other methods in establishing phenotypic pain patterns in the clinic setting as local (bladder specific or pelvic pain only) or widespread (pelvic pain and beyond). Similarly, identifying inflammatory subtypes (e.g., Hunner lesion patients) and psychological parameters can help organize a patient's management plan and make it more likely that interventions will be successful. Applying an individualized multimodal treatment approach has proven beneficial in clinical practice. A collection of treatment options that might be directed at different domains of disease is presented in **Fig. 51-1**.

Although many of these treatments would be considered outside the scope of a general practitioner or general internist, it is important for the practitioner to be aware of them. In general, treatment should begin with more conservative measures, moving on to oral regimens or more invasive procedures if the patient's condition does not improve. A patient-centered approach is paramount in considering treatment escalation. The American Urological Association's IC/BPS guidelines provide a measure of overall efficacy of each individual therapy and a suggested order of implementation (tiered approach), but, because of the inability to predict the response to specific therapies, it is more clinically pragmatic to choose a multimodal approach based on the individual patient's presenting clinical phenotype or "clinical picture." Physicians are better positioned to implement this approach than are surgeons (urologists and gynecologists), who tend to be more organ- and surgery-focused when treating IC/BPS patients.

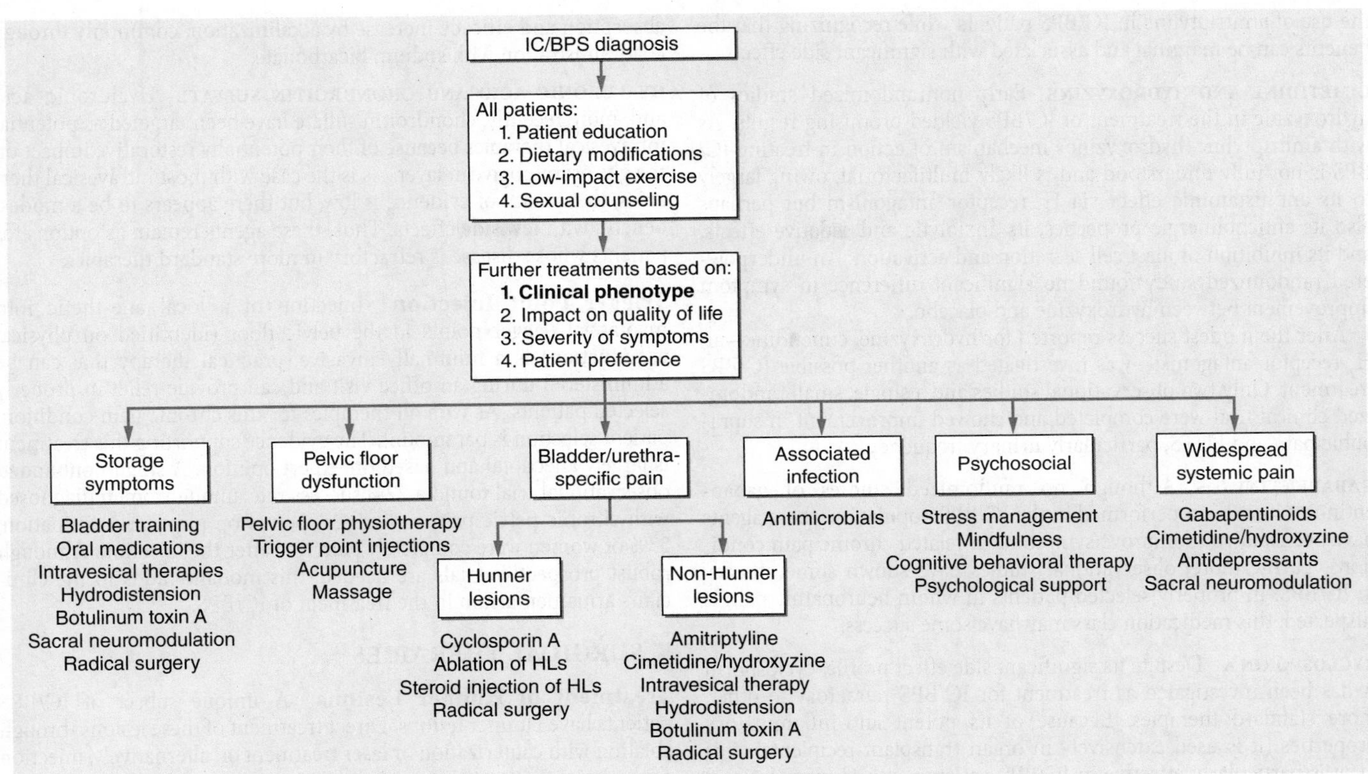

FIGURE 51-1 Proposed management paradigm for the treatment of interstitial cystitis (IC)/bladder pain syndrome (BPS). HLs, Hunner lesions.

CONSERVATIVE MEASURES

Conservative measures should be implemented for all patients with a diagnosis of IC/BPS. These therapies tend to be simple and inexpensive to introduce, pose little risk of significant side effects, and can be intensified or abandoned on the basis of the patient's response.

Patient Education Patient education and empowerment are paramount in this chronic pain disorder. Patients have often seen multiple practitioners prior to their diagnosis of IC/BPS. Acknowledging their suffering while educating them about their disease can go a long way in terms of relieving stress and anxiety related to an unknown and poorly understood problem. This acknowledgement also helps to develop a therapeutic patient–provider relationship. Setting realistic expectations and understanding that cure is not the goal constitute an important first step. Several resources are available for patients to explore at their own leisure.

Dietary Modifications Although limited evidence supports the role of dietary modifications, it has long been recognized that certain foods can trigger flares in IC/BPS patients and that simple dietary modifications can result in meaningful improvements in symptoms. Common dietary triggers include acidic and spicy foods and/or drinks, caffeinated or alcoholic beverages, artificial sweeteners, and/or gluten products; this list is by no means exhaustive, and dietary modifications should be made on an individual basis.

Pelvic Floor Physiotherapy Involvement of the pelvic floor in the pain syndrome can be ascertained on physical examination. Randomized studies have shown that, for patients who are found to have dysfunctional pelvic floors—muscle spasm, trigger points, or tenderness—contributing to their pain syndrome, pelvic floor physiotherapy may be beneficial. The musculoskeletal anatomy of the pelvic floor is complex; finding a provider with training specifically on the pelvic floor can be difficult but is crucial. Because accessing this resource may be financially burdensome for the patient, working together to find a way to obtain this helpful adjunctive therapy is important.

Psychological Interventions Mental health and psychosocial factors have long been identified as significantly prevalent in the IC/BPS population and can impact disease and quality-of-life outcomes. There is some indication that, in IC/BPS and other related chronic pain conditions, mindfulness and cognitive behavioral therapy may improve outcomes. Challenges in accessing these therapies are a major barrier, and there is a general lack of consensus on which specific interventions are best suited to individual patients.

MEDICAL THERAPIES

Only two medications are currently approved by the U.S. Food and Drug Administration (FDA) for the treatment of IC/BPS: pentosan polysulfate sodium (PPS) given orally and dimethyl sulfoxide (DMSO) given intravesically. However, a collection of medications, administered orally or intravesically, are commonly used (albeit off-label) for this purpose.

Oral Therapies • PPS The only FDA-approved oral medication for IC/BPS has recently come under scrutiny because of reports regarding its association with vision-threatening maculopathy. Although causation has yet to be established, given its marginal benefit in the treatment of IC/BPS, the authors recommend against the long-term use of this medication. For patients currently taking PPS, the risks and benefits of treatment must be weighed. Consideration of a trial of weaning off the medication may be in the best interest of the patient. Any patients experiencing vision-related complaints while taking PPS should undergo immediate ophthalmologic assessment.

ANTIBIOTICS IC/BPS is not an infectious condition, and thus, antibiotics should have no role in treatment. Furthermore, the overwhelming majority of IC/BPS patients will have received at least one course, if not several courses, of antibiotics at some point in the course of their disease. Nevertheless, it is not unreasonable to administer a single course of antibiotics (after obtaining a sample for urine culture and sensitivity testing) if the patient has never previously received such therapy.

AMITRIPTYLINE Amitriptyline's pharmacologic activity is attributable primarily to its anticholinergic properties, its serotonin and norepinephrine uptake–inhibiting activity, and its sedative effects, which may include an antihistaminic pathway. Amitriptyline has been used to treat IC/BPS and other chronic pain syndromes. Studies support the use of amitriptyline in IC/BPS patients while recognizing that the benefits can be marginal and associated with significant side effects.

CIMETIDINE AND HYDROXYZINE Early nonrandomized studies of hydroxyzine in the treatment of IC/BPS yielded promising results. As with amitriptyline, hydroxyzine's mechanism of action in treating IC/BPS is not fully understood and is likely multifactorial, owing largely to its antihistaminic effect via H_1-receptor antagonism but perhaps also its anticholinergic properties, its anxiolytic and sedative effects, and its inhibition of mast cell secretion and activation. An underpowered randomized study found no significant difference in symptom improvement between hydroxyzine and placebo.

After the modest success reported for hydroxyzine, cimetidine—an H_2-receptor antagonist—was investigated as another possible IC/BPS treatment. Only two observational studies and a single, small randomized clinical trial were completed and showed improvement in suprapubic pain and LUTS, particularly urinary frequency.

GABAPENTINOIDS Although no randomized studies of gabapentinoids have been performed in the IC/BPS population, these agents have been shown to improve symptoms in related chronic pain conditions. Furthermore, observational studies have shown some efficacy in IC/BPS. In properly selected patients in whom neuropathic pain is suspected, this medication class may have some success.

CYCLOSPORIN A Despite its significant side effect profile, cyclosporin A has been investigated as treatment for IC/BPS refractory to other, more standard therapies. Because of its potent anti-inflammatory properties (it is used extensively in organ transplant recipients), this drug is particularly effective in IC/BPS patients with Hunner lesions, although the improvement in symptoms is modest. Side effects, including hypertension and nephrotoxicity, must be carefully monitored for, and the medication is typically reserved for patients in whom standard therapies have failed.

Intravesical Therapies Intravesical instillations remain a mainstay in the management of bladder-specific pain. Although this treatment modality typically requires an office visit, able and motivated patients can be trained to administer the medication at home. Patients' responses are variable, and the treatment is not curative, but it can significantly change the trajectory of disease in some patients and can rescue those experiencing symptom flares. Intravesical instillations can be administered as induction therapy; maintenance strategies have been proposed and can be effective for properly selected patients. A plethora of agents—most of them used off-label for this indication—have been investigated. The best-studied options are reviewed here.

DMSO DMSO, a solvent with anti-inflammatory properties, has been used in intravesical treatment for IC/BPS for several years. Despite a lack of high-quality evidence (with efficacy documented in only one placebo-controlled randomized clinical trial), DMSO remains the only FDA-approved intravesical medication for IC/BPS treatment. Its use has fallen out of favor, however, largely because of its unpleasant side effect of halitosis (its elimination via the lungs is associated with a garlic-like odor). Although the degree of improvement in symptoms is highly variable (60–95%), DMSO remains in the armamentarium of intravesical therapies.

HEPARIN Heparin, a glycosaminoglycan, was first investigated as a treatment for IC/BPS in light of the glycosaminoglycan layer deficiency theory of IC/BPS etiology; in animal models, heparin was shown to restore areas of damaged urothelium. Although there are no randomized clinical trials showing its efficacy, several observational studies have suggested benefit. Furthermore, in current practice, heparin is commonly administered with other medications as part of an intravesical "cocktail." Systemic absorption is minimal and appears not to affect coagulation parameters.

LIDOCAINE Lidocaine is commonly used as a local anesthetic and has been investigated as an option for intravesical treatment for IC/BPS. This agent works by blocking sensory nerves in the urothelium. Its absorption and efficacy increase by alkalinization, commonly through coadministration with sodium bicarbonate.

HYALURONIC ACID AND CHONDROITIN SULFATE Hyaluronic acid and, more recently, chondroitin sulfate have been targeted as potential intravesical therapies because of their potentially restorative impact on the glycosaminoglycan layer. As is the case with most intravesical therapies, the quality of evidence is low, but there appears to be a modest benefit, with few side effects. Thus, these agents remain as options for patients whose disease is refractory to more standard therapies.

Trigger Point Injection Injection of a local anesthetic into myofascial trigger points in the pelvic floor (identified on physical examination) is a minimally invasive, practical therapy that can be administered during an office visit and can provide relief in properly selected patients. As with all therapies for this chronic pain condition, patient selection is paramount. The evidence supporting this treatment is largely anecdotal and based on expert opinion. A small nonblinded observational trial found a 72% success rate among women diagnosed with chronic pelvic pain and trigger points on physical examination; 33% of women were completely pain free after the injection. Although robust prospective trials are needed, this modality adds to the clinician's armamentarium in the treatment of IC/BPS.

SURGICAL THERAPIES

Treatment of Hunner Lesions A unique subset of IC/BPS patients have Hunner lesions. Direct treatment of these lesions through ablation with cauterization or laser treatment or, alternatively, injection of the lesion with a glucocorticoid improves symptoms in 70–90% of these patients. Hunner lesions tend to be recurrent, however; thus, treated patients still require follow-up, with consideration of a multimodal approach to their disease.

Hydrodistension Recent reports confirm that one of the oldest therapies for IC/BPS, hydrodistension under general anesthesia, provides some benefit in up to 54% of patients. Short- and long-term adverse effects (including bladder perforation and long-term bladder wall fibrosis) and the temporary nature of the benefit (with symptoms typically recurring within 3–12 months) mean that repeated bladder distension may not be an ideal long-term management strategy.

Onabotulinum Toxin A Onabotulinum toxin A (i.e., Botox) has been used to treat IC/BPS. There has, however, never been a randomized, placebo-controlled study evaluating onabotulinum toxin A injection into the detrusor muscle as monotherapy in this disease. Several randomized studies have evaluated this agent's efficacy and have shown improvements in symptoms; unfortunately, these trials often use onabotulinum toxin A in combination with hydrodistension, lack a placebo arm, and do not control for LUTS. Attributing benefit to this treatment is thus challenging. Furthermore, the side effect of acute urinary retention can be catastrophic in IC/BPS patients, whose pain is often secondary to bladder filling.

Sacral Neuromodulation In properly selected patients, sacral neuromodulation (SNM) can provide symptom relief in IC/BPS. Its use for this purpose is off-label, and it is not FDA approved for pain therapy. Nevertheless, SNM is FDA approved for treatment of bladder overactivity—a common symptom in IC/BPS patients—that is refractory to standard therapies. Although studies evaluating improvements in pain have shown variable results, a recent meta-analysis examining 17 observational trials (but no randomized clinical trials) of the use of SNM for IC/BPS does support its efficacy, with a statistically significant pooled treatment success rate of up to 84%. Side effects related to SNM must be considered, and the procedure carries with it a high rate of revision surgery, which is needed in up to half of patients undergoing this treatment.

Radical Surgery Radical surgery for the treatment of IC/BPS is reserved as a modality of desperation for the most refractory patients.

Options range from substitution cystoplasty to cystectomy with urinary diversion. Although improved symptoms and quality of life may result, such surgery is a potentially morbid operation and patient selection must be very specific.

COMPLICATIONS AND PROGNOSIS

IC/BPS is not unlike other chronic pain conditions in that, although a clear link has not been established with higher mortality, this condition is certainly associated with significant disability, decreased quality of life, and significant mental health morbidity. The economic impact of the disability associated with IC/BPS is similar to that of fibromyalgia, low back pain, rheumatoid arthritis, and peripheral neuropathy. Suicidal ideation is a reality in this patient population, with a reported prevalence as high as 11–23%.

For most patients, IC/BPS onset is subacute, with continuous development of the classic symptom complex over a short time and rapid (within 5 years) progression to its final stage. Symptoms then continue to wax and wane without significant overall change in symptomatology for the majority of patients. However, spontaneous improvement and/or resolution occurs in some patients, while a small subset experience subsequent deterioration to a small-capacity, fibrotic, noncompliant bladder ("end-stage bladder"). A multimodal approach to therapy, interdisciplinary involvement in patient care, particular attention to psychosocial parameters, and check-ins on mental health are important aspects of ongoing care.

GLOBAL CONSIDERATIONS

Significant challenges have been encountered in confirming the prevalence of IC/BPS, particularly globally. Prevalence estimates have ranged widely from as low as 3.5 per 100,000 women in a study of a Japanese population to as high as 20,000 per 100,000 in a self-report questionnaire study of a U.S. population. Despite these challenges, it has been recognized that IC/BPS is not simply a disease of the global West. Although robust epidemiologic studies outside North America, Europe, and some regions of Asia are lacking, it is presumed that this disease occurs at similar rates globally. This presumption may be extrapolated from epidemiologic studies of a related population and its male counterpart: CP/CPPS. These studies have shown rates of CP/CPPS in African and Asian populations that are similar to rates in North American populations.

There is no evidence to suggest that IC/BPS is phenotypically distinct in various geographic regions. Thus, this condition should be diagnosed and treated in the same ways globally. Given that its diagnosis of exclusion is based largely on history and physical examination and its treatment is based on a minimally invasive algorithm, with the focus on the patient's clinical phenotype and the initial implementation of conservative therapeutic measures, IC/BPS can be well managed even in resource-poor settings. As with many poorly understood and difficult-to-treat conditions, the greatest barrier to its diagnosis and treatment may perhaps be its recognition.

■ FURTHER READING

Clemens JQ et al: Urologic chronic pelvic pain syndrome: Insights from the MAPP Research Network. Nat Rev Urol 16:187, 2019.

Cox A et al: CUA guideline: Diagnosis and treatment of interstitial cystitis/bladder pain syndrome. Can Urol Assoc J 10:E136, 2016.

Hanno PM et al: AUA guideline for the diagnosis and treatment of interstitial cystitis/bladder pain syndrome. J Urol 185:2162, 2011.

Hanno P et al: Incontinence, in *International Consultation on Incontinence, September 2016*, vol 2, 6th ed, P Abrams et al (eds). Tokyo, ICUD ICS, 2017, pp 2203–2301.

van de Merwe JP et al: Diagnostic criteria, classification, and nomenclature for painful bladder syndrome/interstitial cystitis: An ESSIC proposal. Eur Urol 53:60, 2008.

52 Azotemia and Urinary Abnormalities

David B. Mount

Normal kidney functions occur through numerous cellular processes to maintain body homeostasis. Disturbances in any of these functions can lead to abnormalities that may be detrimental to survival. Clinical manifestations of these disorders depend on the pathophysiology of renal injury and often are identified as a complex of symptoms, abnormal physical findings, and laboratory changes that constitute specific syndromes. These renal syndromes **(Table 52-1)** may arise from systemic illness or as primary renal disease. Nephrologic syndromes usually consist of several elements that reflect the underlying pathologic processes, typically including one or more of the following: (1) reduction in glomerular filtration rate (GFR), (2) abnormalities of urine sediment (red blood cells [RBCs], white blood cells [WBCs], casts, and crystals), (3) abnormal urinary excretion of serum proteins (proteinuria), (4) disturbances in urine volume (oliguria, anuria, polyuria), (5) presence of hypertension and/or expanded total body fluid volume (edema), (6) electrolyte abnormalities, and (7) in some syndromes, fever/pain. The specific combination of these findings should permit identification of one of the major nephrologic syndromes (Table 52-1) and allow differential diagnoses to be narrowed so that the appropriate diagnostic and therapeutic course can be determined. All these syndromes and their associated diseases are discussed in more detail in subsequent chapters. This chapter focuses on several aspects of renal abnormalities that are critically important for distinguishing among those processes: (1) reduction in GFR, (2) alterations of the urinary sediment and/or protein excretion, and (3) abnormalities of urinary volume.

AZOTEMIA

■ ASSESSMENT OF GFR

Monitoring the GFR is important in both hospital and outpatient settings, and several different methodologies are available. GFR is the primary metric for kidney "function," and its direct measurement involves administration of a radioactive isotope (such as inulin or iothalamate) that is filtered at the glomerulus into the urinary space but is neither reabsorbed nor secreted throughout the tubule. GFR—i.e., the clearance of inulin or iothalamate in milliliters per minute—is calculated from the rate of appearance of the isotope in the urine over several hours. In most clinical circumstances, direct GFR measurement is not feasible, and the plasma creatinine level is used as a surrogate to estimate GFR. Plasma creatinine (P_{Cr}) is the most widely used marker for GFR, which is related directly to urine creatinine (U_{Cr}) excretion and inversely to P_{Cr}. On the basis of this relationship (with some important caveats, as discussed below), GFR will fall in roughly inverse proportion to the rise in P_{Cr}. Failure to account for GFR reductions in drug dosing can lead to significant morbidity and death from drug toxicities (e.g., digoxin, imipenem). In the outpatient setting, P_{Cr} serves as an estimate for GFR (although much less accurate; see below). In patients with chronic progressive renal disease, there is an approximately linear relationship between $1/P_{Cr}$ (*y* axis) and time (*x* axis). The slope of that line will remain constant for an individual; when values deviate, an investigation for a superimposed acute process (e.g., volume depletion, drug reaction) should be initiated. Signs and symptoms of uremia, the clinical symptom complex associated with renal failure, develop at significantly different levels of P_{Cr}, depending on the patient (size, age, and sex), underlying renal disease, existence of concurrent diseases, and true GFR. Generally, patients do not develop symptomatic uremia until renal insufficiency is severe (GFR <15 mL/min).

A significantly reduced GFR (either acute or chronic) is usually reflected in a rise in P_{Cr}, leading to retention of nitrogenous waste products (defined as azotemia) such as urea. Azotemia may result from

TABLE 52-1 Initial Clinical and Laboratory Database for Defining Major Syndromes in Nephrology

SYNDROME	IMPORTANT CLUES TO DIAGNOSIS	COMMON FINDINGS	CHAP(S). DISCUSSING DISEASE-CAUSING SYNDROME
Acute or rapidly progressive renal failure	Anuria	Hypertension, hematuria	310, 314, 316, 319
	Oliguria	Proteinuria, pyuria	
	Documented recent decline in GFR	Casts, edema	
Acute nephritis	Hematuria, RBC casts	Proteinuria	314
	Azotemia, reduced GFR, oliguria	Pyuria	
	Edema, hypertension	Circulatory congestion	
Chronic renal failure	Azotemia for >3 months	Proteinuria, casts	311
	Symptoms or signs of uremia, (late manifestation), casts	Hypocalcemia, hyperphosphatemia, hyperparathyroidism	
	Symptoms or signs of renal osteodystrophy	Polyuria, nocturia	
	Kidneys reduced in size bilaterally	Edema, hypertension	
	Broad casts in urinary sediment	Hyperkalemia, metabolic acidosis	
Nephrotic syndrome	Proteinuria, with >3.5 g/24 h per 1.73 m^2	Casts	314
	Hypoalbuminemia	Lipiduria	
	Edema	Hypercoagulable state	
	Hyperlipidemia		
Asymptomatic urinary abnormalities	Hematuria		314
	Proteinuria (below nephrotic range)		
	Sterile pyuria, casts		
Urinary tract infection/ pyelonephritis	Bacteriuria, with >10^5 cfu/mL	Hematuria	135
	Other infectious agent documented in urine	Mild azotemia and reduced GFR	
	Pyuria, leukocyte casts	Mild proteinuria	
	Frequency, urgency	Fever	
	Bladder tenderness, flank tenderness		
Renal tubular defects	Electrolyte disorders	Hematuria	315, 316
	Polyuria, nocturia	"Tubular" proteinuria (<1 g/24 h)	
	Renal calcification	Enuresis	
	Large kidneys	Electrolyte and/or acid-base abnormalities	
	Renal transport defects	Other electrolyte issues, e.g., hypomagnesemia	
Hypertension	Systolic/diastolic hypertension	Proteinuria	277, 317
		Casts	
		Azotemia	
Nephrolithiasis	Previous history of stone passage or removal	Hematuria	318
	Previous history of stone seen by x-ray	Pyuria	
	Renal colic	Frequency, urgency	
Urinary tract obstruction	Azotemia, oliguria, anuria	Hematuria	319
	Polyuria, nocturia, urinary retention	Pyuria	
	Slowing of urinary stream	Enuresis, dysuria	
	Large prostate, large kidneys		
	Flank tenderness, full bladder after voiding		

Abbreviations: cfu, colony-forming units; GFR; glomerular filtration rate; RBC, red blood cell.

reduced renal perfusion, intrinsic renal disease, or postrenal processes (ureteral obstruction; see below and **Fig. 52-1**). Precise determination of GFR is problematic, as both commonly measured indices (urea and creatinine) have characteristics that affect their accuracy as markers of clearance. Urea clearance may underestimate GFR significantly because of urea reabsorption by the tubule. In contrast, creatinine is derived from muscle metabolism of creatine, and its generation varies little from day to day.

Creatinine clearance (CrCl), an approximation of GFR, is measured from plasma and urinary creatinine excretion rates for a defined period (usually 24 h) and is expressed in milliliters per minute: $CrCl = (U_{vol} \times U_{Cr})/(P_{Cr} \times T_{min})$. The "adequacy" or "completeness" of the urinary collection is estimated by the urinary volume and creatinine content; creatinine is produced from muscle and excreted at a relatively constant rate. For a 20- to 50-year-old man, creatinine excretion should be 18.5–25.0 mg/kg body weight; for a woman of the same age, it should be 16.5–22.4 mg/kg body weight. For example, an 80-kg man should excrete between ~1500 and 2000 mg of creatinine in an "adequate" collection. Creatinine is useful for estimating GFR because it is a small, freely filtered solute that is not reabsorbed by the tubules. P_{Cr} levels can increase acutely from dietary ingestion of cooked meat, however, and creatinine can be secreted into the proximal tubule through an organic cation pathway (especially in advanced progressive chronic kidney disease [CKD]), leading to overestimation of GFR. When a timed collection for CrCl is not available, decisions about drug dosing must be based on P_{Cr} alone. Two formulas are used widely to estimate kidney function from P_{Cr}: (1) Cockcroft-Gault and (2) four-variable MDRD (Modification of Diet in Renal Disease).

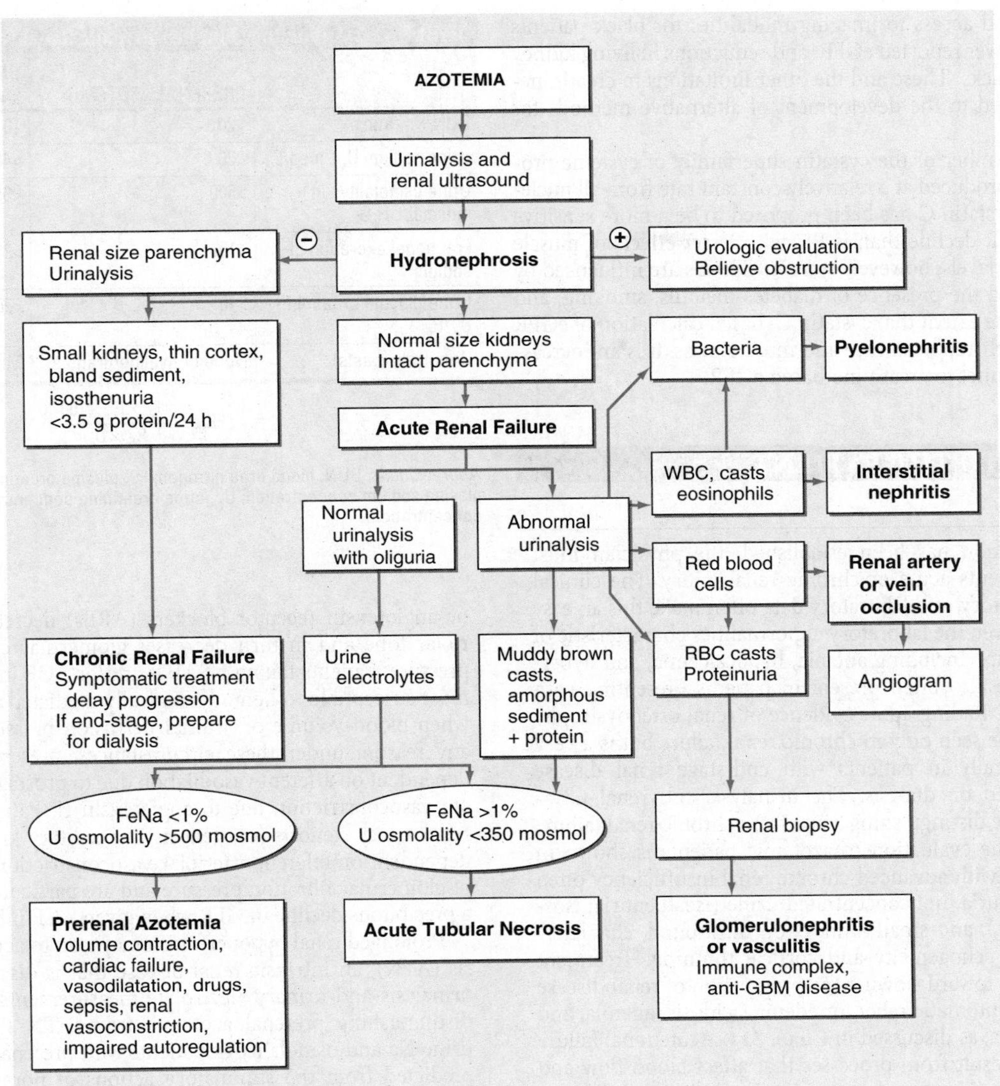

FIGURE 52-1 Approach to the patient with azotemia. FeNa, fractional excretion of sodium; GBM, glomerular basement membrane; RBC, red blood cell; U, urine; WBC, white blood cell.

Cockcroft-Gault:

$$\textbf{CrCl(mL/min)} = \frac{(140-\text{age})\times\text{Lean Body Weight (kg)}}{\text{Serum Creatinine (mg/dL)}\times 72}(\times 0.85 \text{ if female})$$

$$\text{MDRD: eGFR (mL/min per 1.73 m}^2) = 186.3 \times P_{Cr}\,(e^{-1.154}) \times \text{age}\,(e^{-0.203}) \times (0.742 \text{ if female}) \times (1.21 \text{ if black}).$$

Numerous websites are available to assist with these calculations (*www.kidney.org/professionals/kdoqi/gfr_calculator.cfm*). A newer Chronic Kidney Disease Epidemiology Collaboration (CKD-EPI) estimated GFR (eGFR), which was developed by pooling several cohorts with and without kidney disease who had data on directly measured GFR, appears to be more accurate:

$$\text{CKD-EPI: eGFR} = 141 \times \min(P_{Cr}/k, 1)^a \times \max(P_{Cr}/k, 1)^{-1.209} \times 0.993^{Age} \times 1.018\ [\text{if female}] \times 1.159\ [\text{if black}],$$

where P_{Cr} is plasma creatinine, *k* is 0.7 for females and 0.9 for males, *a* is –0.329 for females and –0.411 for males, *min* indicates the minimum of P_{Cr}/k or 1, and *max* indicates the maximum of P_{Cr}/k or 1 (*https://www.mdcalc.com/ckd-epi-equations-glomerular-filtration-rate-gfr*).

There are limitations to all creatinine-based estimates of GFR. Each equation, along with 24-h urine collection for measurement of creatinine clearance, is based on the assumption that the patient is in *steady state*, without daily increases or decreases in P_{Cr} as a result of rapidly changing GFR. The MDRD equation is better correlated with true GFR when the GFR is <60 mL/min per 1.73 m^2. The gradual loss of muscle from chronic illness, chronic use of glucocorticoids, or malnutrition can mask significant changes in GFR with small or imperceptible changes in P_{Cr}.

The coefficient of 1.159 in the CKD-EPI equation to adjust for self-reported black race reflects that measured GFR was 16% higher in blacks than nonblacks with similar age, sex, and creatinine in the data set used to develop the equation. Race is a social rather than a biological construct, for which reason the use of the "race modifier" in calculating eGFR using CKD-EPI and other equations has come under scrutiny. In particular, given the implications of utilizing self-reported race to modify clinical laboratory results, many medical centers have recently stopped reporting eGFRs that have been calculated using a race modifier. This change is projected to have positive consequences, in particular, improved access to waitlisting for renal transplantation in black patients at an earlier stage of CKD. Potential negative consequences include "overdiagnosis" of CKD, inadequate or inaccurate dosing of drugs that are eliminated through the kidney (e.g., metformin), reduced access to imaging modalities for black patients with CKD with a lower reported eGFR, and reductions in living kidney donation among blacks. These and the other limitations in creatinine-based eGFR have led to the development of alternative methods for estimating GFR.

Cystatin C, a member of the cystatin superfamily of cysteine protease inhibitors, is produced at a relatively constant rate from all nucleated cells. Serum cystatin C has been proposed to be a more sensitive marker of early GFR decline than is P_{Cr}, with lesser effects of muscle mass on circulating levels; however, cystatin C levels are influenced by the patient's sex and the presence of diabetes mellitus, smoking, and inflammation. To the extent that cystatin C–based calculation of eGFR is less affected by self-reported race and muscle mass, it is an increasingly important adjunct to creatinine-based eGFR.

TABLE 52-2 Laboratory Findings in Acute Renal Failure

INDEX	PRERENAL AZOTEMIA	OLIGURIC ACUTE RENAL FAILURE
BUN/P_{Cr} ratio	>20:1	10–15:1
Urine sodium U_{Na}, meq/L	<20	>40
Urine osmolality, mosmol/L H_2O	>500	<350
Fractional excretion of sodium[a]	<1%	>2%
Urine/plasma creatinine U_{Cr}/P_{Cr}	>40	<20
Urinalysis (casts)	None or hyaline/granular	Muddy brown

$$^{a}FE_{Na} = \frac{U_{Na} \times P_{Cr} \times 100}{P_{Na} \times U_{Cr}}$$

Abbreviations: BUN, blood urea nitrogen; P_{Cr}, plasma creatinine concentration; P_{Na}, plasma sodium concentration; U_{Cr}, urine creatinine concentration; U_{Na}, urine sodium concentration.

APPROACH TO THE PATIENT

Azotemia

Once GFR reduction has been established, the physician must decide if it represents acute or chronic renal injury. The clinical circumstances, history, and laboratory data often make this an easy distinction. However, the laboratory abnormalities characteristic of chronic renal failure, including anemia, hypocalcemia, and hyperphosphatemia, are also often present in patients presenting with acute renal failure. Radiographic evidence of renal osteodystrophy (**Chap. 311**) can be seen only in chronic renal failure but is a very late finding, typically in patients with end-stage renal disease (ESRD) maintained on dialysis. The urinalysis and renal ultrasound can facilitate distinguishing acute from chronic renal failure. An approach to the evaluation of azotemic patients is shown in Fig. 52-1. Patients with advanced chronic renal insufficiency often have some proteinuria, nonconcentrated urine (isosthenuria; isosmotic with plasma), and small kidneys on ultrasound, characterized by increased echogenicity and cortical thinning. Treatment should be directed toward slowing the progression of renal disease and providing symptomatic relief for edema, acidosis, anemia, and hyperphosphatemia, as discussed in **Chap. 311**. Acute renal failure (**Chap. 310**) can result from processes that affect blood flow and glomerular perfusion (prerenal azotemia), intrinsic renal diseases (affecting small vessels, glomeruli, or tubules), or postrenal processes (obstruction of urine flow in ureters, bladder, or urethra) (**Chap. 319**).

PRERENAL FAILURE

Decreased renal perfusion accounts for 40–80% of cases of acute renal failure and, if appropriately treated, is readily reversible. The etiologies of prerenal azotemia include any cause of decreased circulating blood volume (gastrointestinal hemorrhage, burns, diarrhea, diuretics), volume sequestration (pancreatitis, peritonitis, rhabdomyolysis), or decreased effective arterial volume (cardiogenic shock, sepsis). Renal and glomerular perfusion also can be affected by reductions in cardiac output from peripheral vasodilation (sepsis, drugs) or profound renal vasoconstriction (severe heart failure, hepatorenal syndrome, agents such as nonsteroidal anti-inflammatory drugs [NSAIDs]). True or "effective" arterial hypovolemia leads to a fall in mean arterial pressure, which in turn triggers a series of neural and humoral responses, including activation of the sympathetic nervous and renin-angiotensin-aldosterone systems and vasopressin (AVP) release. GFR is maintained by prostaglandin-mediated dilatation of afferent arterioles and angiotensin II–mediated constriction of efferent arterioles. Once the mean arterial pressure falls below 80 mmHg, GFR declines steeply.

Blockade of prostaglandin production by NSAIDs can result in severe vasoconstriction and acute renal failure. Blocking angiotensin action with angiotensin-converting enzyme (ACE) inhibitors or angiotensin receptor blockers (ARBs) decreases efferent arteriolar tone and in turn decreases glomerular capillary perfusion pressure. Patients taking NSAIDs and/or ACE inhibitors/ARBs are most susceptible to hemodynamically mediated acute renal failure when blood volume or arterial perfusion pressure is reduced for any reason; under these circumstances, preservation of GFR is dependent on afferent vasodilation due to prostaglandins and efferent vasoconstriction due to angiotensin II. Patients with bilateral renal artery stenosis (or stenosis in a solitary kidney) can also be dependent on efferent arteriolar vasoconstriction for maintenance of glomerular filtration pressure and are particularly susceptible to a precipitous decline in GFR when given ACE inhibitors or ARBs.

Prolonged renal hypoperfusion may lead to acute tubular necrosis (ATN), an intrinsic renal disease that is discussed below. The urinalysis and urinary electrolyte measurements can be useful in distinguishing prerenal azotemia from ATN (**Table 52-2**). The urine Na and osmolality of patients with prerenal azotemia can be predicted from the stimulatory actions of norepinephrine, angiotensin II, AVP, aldosterone, and low tubule fluid flow rate. In prerenal conditions, the tubules are intact, leading to a concentrated urine (>500 mosmol), avid Na retention (urine Na concentration, <20 mmol/L; fractional excretion of Na [FE_{Na}], <1%), and U_{Cr}/P_{Cr} >40 (Table 52-2). The FE_{Na} is typically >1% in ATN, but may be <1% in patients with milder, nonoliguric ATN (e.g., from rhabdomyolysis) and in patients with underlying "prerenal" disorders, such as congestive heart failure (CHF) or cirrhosis or hepatorenal syndrome. The prerenal urine sediment is usually normal or has hyaline and granular casts, whereas the sediment of ATN usually is filled with cellular debris, tubular epithelial casts, and dark (muddy brown) granular casts. The measurement of urinary biomarkers associated with tubular injury is a promising technique to detect subclinical ATN and/or help further diagnose the exact cause of acute renal failure.

POSTRENAL AZOTEMIA

Urinary tract obstruction accounts for <5% of cases of acute renal failure but is usually reversible and must be ruled out early in the evaluation (Fig. 52-1). Since a single kidney is capable of adequate clearance, complete obstructive acute renal failure requires obstruction at the urethra or bladder outlet, bilateral ureteral obstruction, or unilateral obstruction in a patient with a single functioning kidney. Obstruction is usually diagnosed by the presence of ureteral and renal pelvic dilation on renal ultrasound. However, early in the course of obstruction or if the ureters are unable to dilate (e.g., encasement by pelvic or periureteral tumors or by retroperitoneal fibrosis), the ultrasound examination may be negative. Other imaging, such as a furosemide renogram (MAG3 nuclear medicine study), may be required to better define the presence or absence of obstructive uropathy. The specific urologic conditions that cause obstruction are discussed in **Chap. 319**.

INTRINSIC RENAL DISEASE

When prerenal and postrenal azotemia have been excluded as etiologies of renal failure, an intrinsic parenchymal renal disease is present. Intrinsic renal disease can arise from processes involving large renal vessels, intrarenal microvasculature and glomeruli, or the tubulointerstitium. Ischemic and toxic ATN account for ~90% of cases of acute intrinsic renal failure. As outlined in Fig. 52-1, the clinical setting and urinalysis are helpful in separating the possible etiologies. Prerenal azotemia and ATN are part of a spectrum of renal hypoperfusion; evidence of structural tubule injury is present in ATN, whereas prompt reversibility occurs with prerenal azotemia upon restoration of adequate renal perfusion. Thus, ATN often can be distinguished from prerenal azotemia by urinalysis and urine electrolyte composition (Table 52-2 and Fig. 52-1). Ischemic ATN is observed most frequently in patients who have undergone major surgery, trauma, severe hypovolemia, overwhelming sepsis, or extensive burns. Nephrotoxic ATN complicates the administration of many common medications, usually by inducing a combination of intrarenal vasoconstriction, direct tubule toxicity, and/or tubular obstruction. The kidney is vulnerable to toxic injury by virtue of its rich blood supply (25% of cardiac output) and its ability to concentrate and metabolize toxins. A diligent search for hypotension and nephrotoxins usually uncovers the specific etiology of ATN. Discontinuation of nephrotoxins and stabilization of blood pressure often suffice without the need for dialysis, with ongoing regeneration of tubular cells. **An extensive list of potential drugs and toxins implicated in ATN is found in Chap. 310.**

Processes involving the tubules and interstitium can lead to acute kidney injury (AKI), a subtype of acute renal failure. These processes include drug-induced interstitial nephritis (especially by antibiotics, NSAIDs, and diuretics), severe infections (both bacterial and viral), systemic diseases (e.g., systemic lupus erythematosus), and systemic disorders (e.g., sarcoidosis, Sjögren's syndrome, lymphoma, or leukemia). A list of drugs associated with allergic interstitial nephritis is found in **Chap. 316**. Urinalysis usually shows mild to moderate proteinuria, hematuria, and pyuria (~75% of cases) and occasionally WBC casts. The finding of RBC casts in interstitial nephritis has been reported but should prompt a search for glomerular diseases (Fig. 52-1). Occasionally, renal biopsy will be needed to distinguish among these possibilities. The classic sediment finding in allergic interstitial nephritis is a predominance (>10%) of urinary eosinophils with Wright's or Hansel's stain; however, urinary eosinophils can be increased in several other causes of AKI, such that measurement of urine eosinophils has no diagnostic utility in renal disease.

Occlusion of large renal vessels, including arteries and veins, is an uncommon cause of acute renal failure. A significant reduction in GFR by this mechanism suggests bilateral processes or, in a patient with a single functioning kidney, a unilateral process. In patients with preexisting renal artery stenosis, a substantial renal collateral circulation can develop over time and sustain renal perfusion—typically not enough to sustain glomerular filtration—in the event of total renal artery occlusion. Renal arteries can be occluded with atheroemboli, thromboemboli, in situ thrombosis, aortic dissection, or vasculitis. Atheroembolic renal failure can occur spontaneously but most often is associated with recent aortic instrumentation. The emboli are cholesterol-rich and lodge in medium and small renal arteries, with a consequent eosinophil-rich inflammatory reaction. Patients with atheroembolic acute renal failure often have a normal urinalysis, but the urine may contain eosinophils and casts. The diagnosis can be confirmed by renal biopsy, but this procedure is often unnecessary when other stigmata of atheroemboli are present (livedo reticularis, distal peripheral infarcts, eosinophilia). Renal artery thrombosis may lead to mild proteinuria and hematuria, whereas renal vein thrombosis typically occurs in the context of heavy proteinuria and hematuria. These vascular complications often require angiography for confirmation and are discussed in **Chap. 317**.

Diseases of the glomeruli (glomerulonephritis and vasculitis) and the renal microvasculature (hemolytic-uremic syndromes, thrombotic thrombocytopenic purpura, and malignant hypertension) usually present with various combinations of glomerular injury: proteinuria, hematuria, reduced GFR, and alterations of sodium excretion that lead to hypertension, edema, and circulatory congestion (acute nephritic syndrome). These findings may occur as primary renal diseases or as renal manifestations of systemic diseases. The clinical setting and other laboratory data help distinguish primary renal diseases from systemic diseases. The finding of RBC casts in the urine is an indication for early renal biopsy (Fig. 52-1), as the pathologic pattern has important implications for diagnosis, prognosis, and treatment. Hematuria without RBC casts can also be an indication of glomerular disease, since RBC casts are highly specific but very insensitive for glomerulonephritis. The specificity of urine microscopy can be enhanced by examining urine with a phase contrast microscope capable of detecting dysmorphic red cells ("acanthocytes") that are associated with glomerular disease. This evaluation is summarized in **Fig. 52-2**. A detailed discussion of glomerulonephritis and diseases of the microvasculature is found in **Chap. 316**.

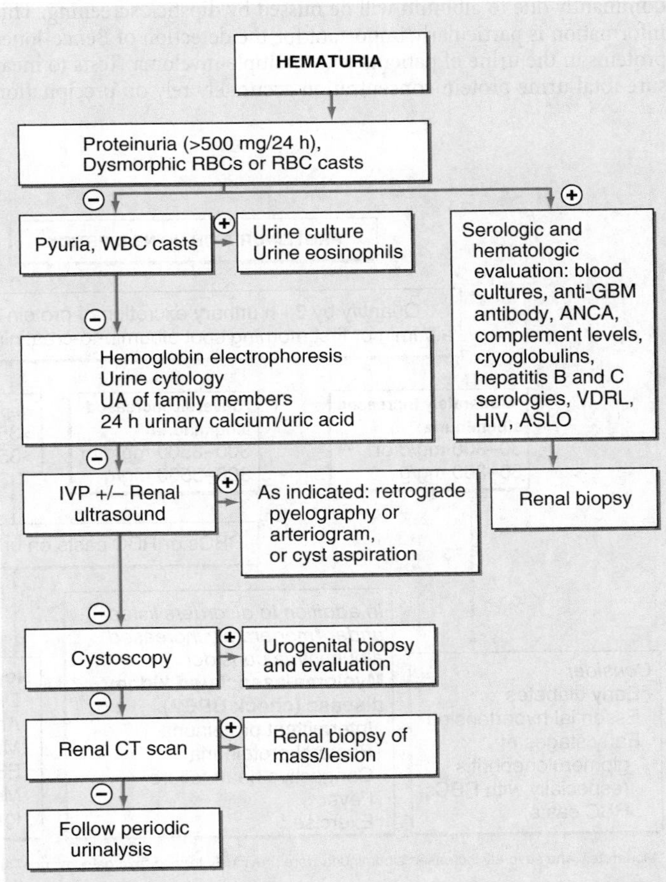

FIGURE 52-2 Approach to the patient with hematuria. ANCA, antineutrophil cytoplasmic antibody; ASLO, antistreptolysin O; CT, computed tomography; GBM, glomerular basement membrane; IVP, intravenous pyelography; RBC, red blood cell; UA, urinalysis; VDRL, Venereal Disease Research Laboratory; WBC, white blood cell.

OLIGURIA AND ANURIA

Oliguria refers to a 24-h urine output <400 mL, and *anuria* is the complete absence of urine formation (<100 mL). Anuria can be caused by complete bilateral urinary tract obstruction; a vascular catastrophe (dissection or arterial occlusion); renal vein thrombosis; acute cast nephropathy in myeloma; renal cortical necrosis; severe ATN; combined therapy with NSAIDs, ACE inhibitors, and/or ARBs; and hypovolemic, cardiogenic, or septic shock. Oliguria is never normal, since at least 400 mL of maximally concentrated urine must be produced to excrete the obligate daily osmolar load. *Nonoliguria* refers to urine output >400 mL/d in patients with acute or chronic azotemia. With nonoliguric ATN, disturbances of potassium and hydrogen balance are less severe than in oliguric patients, and recovery to normal renal function is usually more rapid.

ABNORMALITIES OF THE URINE

PROTEINURIA

The evaluation of proteinuria is shown schematically in **Fig. 52-3** and typically is initiated after detection of proteinuria by dipstick examination. The dipstick measurement detects only albumin and gives false-positive results at pH >7.0 or when the urine is very concentrated or contaminated with blood. Because the dipstick relies on urinary albumin concentration, a very dilute urine may obscure significant proteinuria on dipstick examination. Quantification of urinary albumin on a spot urine sample (ideally from a first morning void) by measurement of an albumin-to-creatinine ratio (ACR) is helpful in approximating a 24-h albumin excretion rate (AER), where ACR (mg/g) ≈ AER (mg/24 h). Furthermore, proteinuria that is not predominantly due to albumin will be missed by dipstick screening. This information is particularly important for the detection of Bence-Jones proteins in the urine of patients with multiple myeloma. Tests to measure total urine protein concentration accurately rely on precipitation with sulfosalicylic or trichloroacetic acid (Fig. 52-3). As with albuminuria, the ratio of protein to creatinine in a random, "spot" urine can also provide a rough estimate of protein excretion; for example, a protein/creatinine ratio of 3.0 correlates to ~3.0 g of proteinuria per day. Formal assessment of urinary protein excretion requires a 24-h urine protein collection (see "Measurement of GFR," above).

The magnitude of proteinuria and its composition in the urine depend on the mechanism of renal injury that leads to protein losses. Both charge and size selectivity normally prevent virtually all plasma albumin, globulins, and other high-molecular-weight proteins from crossing the glomerular wall; however, if this barrier is disrupted, plasma proteins may leak into the urine (glomerular proteinuria; Fig. 52-3). Smaller proteins (<20 kDa) are freely filtered but are readily reabsorbed by the proximal tubule. Typically, healthy individuals excrete <150 mg/d of total protein and <30 mg/d of albumin. However, even at albuminuria levels <30 mg/d, risk for progression to overt nephropathy or subsequent cardiovascular disease is increased. The remainder of the protein in the urine is secreted by the tubules (Tamm-Horsfall, IgA, and urokinase) or represents small amounts of filtered β_2-microglobulin, apoproteins, enzymes, and peptide hormones. Another mechanism of proteinuria entails excessive production of an abnormal protein that exceeds the capacity of the tubule for reabsorption. This situation most commonly occurs with plasma cell dyscrasias, such as multiple myeloma, amyloidosis, and lymphomas, that are associated with monoclonal production of immunoglobulin light chains.

The normal glomerular endothelial cell forms a barrier composed of pores of ~100 nm that retain blood cells but offer little impediment to passage of most proteins. The glomerular basement membrane traps most large proteins (>100 kDa), and the foot processes of epithelial cells (podocytes) cover the urinary side of the glomerular basement membrane and produce a series of narrow channels (slit diaphragms) to allow molecular passage of small solutes and water but not proteins. Some glomerular diseases, such as minimal change disease, cause fusion of glomerular epithelial cell foot processes, resulting in predominantly "selective" (Fig. 52-3) loss of albumin. Other glomerular diseases can present with disruption of the basement membrane and slit diaphragms (e.g., by immune complex deposition), resulting in losses of albumin and other plasma proteins. The fusion of foot processes causes increased pressure across the capillary basement membrane, resulting in areas with larger pore sizes (and more severe "nonselective" proteinuria) (Fig. 52-3).

When the total daily urinary excretion of protein is >3.5 g, hypoalbuminemia, hyperlipidemia, and edema (nephrotic syndrome; Fig. 52-3) are often present as well. However, total daily urinary protein excretion >3.5 g can occur without the other features of the nephrotic syndrome in a variety of other renal diseases, including diabetes (Fig. 52-3). Plasma cell dyscrasias (multiple myeloma) can be associated with large amounts of excreted light chains in the urine, which may not be detected by dipstick. The light chains are filtered by the glomerulus and overwhelm the reabsorptive capacity of the proximal tubule. Renal failure from these disorders occurs through a variety of mechanisms, including but not limited to proximal tubule injury, tubule obstruction (cast nephropathy), amyloid deposition, and light chain deposition (**Chap. 316**). The specific renal lesion is dictated by the sequence and structural

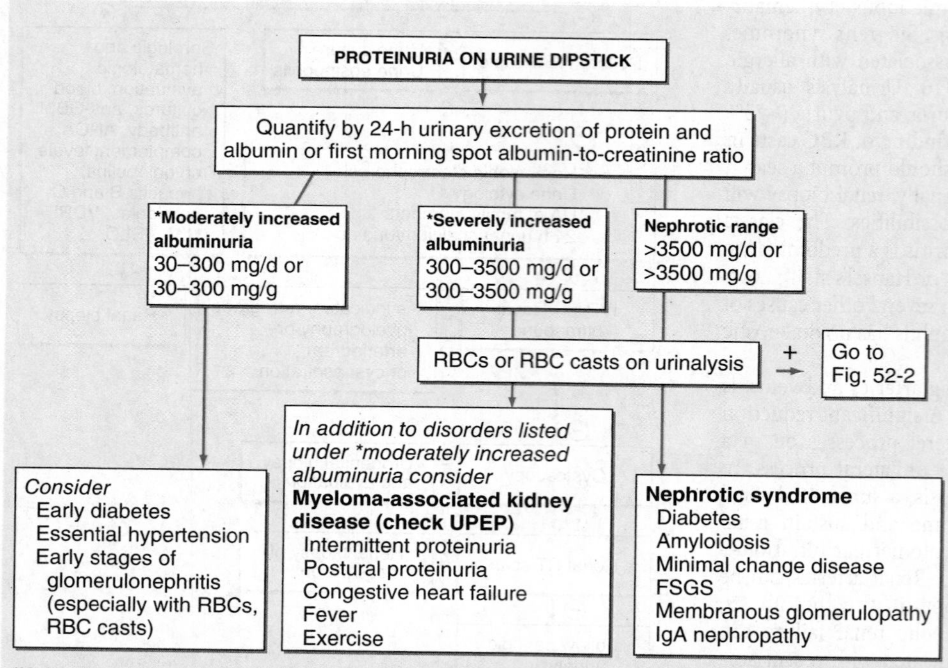

FIGURE 52-3 Approach to the patient with proteinuria. Investigation of proteinuria is often initiated by a positive dipstick on routine urinalysis. Conventional dipsticks detect predominantly albumin and provide a semiquantitative assessment (trace, 1+, 2+, or 3+), which is influenced by urinary concentration as reflected by urine specific gravity (minimum, <1.005; maximum, 1.030). However, more exact determination of proteinuria should employ a spot morning protein/creatinine ratio (mg/g) or a 24-h urine collection (mg/24 h). FSGS, focal segmental glomerulosclerosis; RBC, red blood cell; UPEP, urine protein electrophoresis.

characteristics of the monoclonal light chain; however, not all excreted light chains are nephrotoxic.

Hypoalbuminemia in nephrotic syndrome occurs through excessive urinary losses and increased proximal tubule catabolism of filtered albumin. Edema results from renal sodium retention and reduced plasma oncotic pressure, which favors fluid movement from capillaries to interstitium. To compensate for the perceived decrease in effective intravascular volume, activation of the renin-angiotensin system, stimulation of AVP, and activation of the sympathetic nervous system take place, promoting continued renal salt and water reabsorption and progressive edema. Filtered proteases, normally retained by the glomerular filtration barrier, can also directly activate sodium reabsorption by the epithelial Na channels in principal cells (ENaC) in nephrotic syndrome. Despite these changes, hypertension is uncommon in primary kidney diseases resulting in the nephrotic syndrome (Fig. 52-3 and **Chap. 314**). The urinary loss of regulatory proteins and changes in hepatic synthesis contribute to the other manifestations of the nephrotic syndrome. A hypercoagulable state may arise from urinary losses of antithrombin III, reduced serum levels of proteins S and C, hyperfibrinogenemia, and enhanced platelet aggregation. Hypercholesterolemia may be severe and results from increased hepatic lipoprotein synthesis. Loss of immunoglobulins contributes to an increased risk of infection. Many diseases (some listed in Fig. 52-3) and drugs can cause the nephrotic syndrome; a complete list is found in **Chap. 314**.

HEMATURIA, PYURIA, AND CASTS

Isolated hematuria without proteinuria, other cells, or casts is often indicative of bleeding from the urinary tract. Hematuria is defined as two to five RBCs per high-power field (HPF) and can be detected by dipstick. A false-positive dipstick for hematuria (where no RBCs are seen on urine microscopy) may occur when myoglobinuria is present, often in the setting of rhabdomyolysis. Common causes of isolated hematuria include stones, neoplasms, tuberculosis, trauma, and prostatitis. Gross hematuria with blood clots usually is not an intrinsic renal process; rather, it suggests a postrenal source in the urinary collecting system. Evaluation of patients presenting with microscopic hematuria is outlined in Fig. 52-2. A single urinalysis with hematuria is common and can result from menstruation, viral illness, allergy, exercise, or mild trauma. Persistent or significant hematuria (>3 RBCs/HPF on three urinalyses, a single urinalysis with >100 RBCs, or gross hematuria) is associated with significant renal or urologic lesions in 9.1% of cases. The level of suspicion for urogenital neoplasms in patients with isolated painless hematuria and nondysmorphic RBCs increases with age. Neoplasms are rare in the pediatric population, and isolated hematuria is more likely to be "idiopathic" or associated with a congenital anomaly. Hematuria with pyuria and bacteriuria is typical of infection and should be treated with antibiotics after appropriate cultures. Acute cystitis or urethritis in women can cause gross hematuria. Hypercalciuria and hyperuricosuria are also risk factors for unexplained isolated hematuria in both children and adults. In some of these patients (50–60%), reducing calcium and uric acid excretion through dietary interventions can eliminate the microscopic hematuria.

Isolated microscopic hematuria can be a manifestation of glomerular diseases. The RBCs of glomerular origin are often dysmorphic when examined by phase-contrast microscopy. Irregular shapes of RBCs may also result from pH and osmolarity changes produced along the distal nephron. Observer variability in detecting dysmorphic RBCs is common. The most common etiologies of isolated glomerular hematuria are IgA nephropathy, hereditary nephritis, and thin basement membrane disease. IgA nephropathy and hereditary nephritis can lead to episodic gross hematuria. A family history of renal failure is often present in hereditary nephritis, and patients with thin basement membrane disease often have family members with microscopic hematuria. A renal biopsy is needed for the definitive diagnosis of these disorders, which are discussed in more detail in **Chap. 314**. Hematuria with dysmorphic RBCs, RBC casts, and protein excretion >500 mg/d is virtually diagnostic of glomerulonephritis. RBC casts form as RBCs that enter the tubule fluid and become trapped in a cylindrical mold of gelled Tamm-Horsfall protein. Even in the absence of azotemia, these patients should undergo serologic evaluation and renal biopsy as outlined in Fig. 52-2.

Isolated pyuria is unusual since inflammatory reactions in the kidney or collecting system also are associated with hematuria. The presence of bacteria suggests infection, and WBC casts with bacteria are indicative of pyelonephritis; "sterile pyuria" with negative urinary bacterial cultures can be seen in urogenital tuberculosis. WBCs and/or WBC casts also may be seen in acute glomerulonephritis as well as in tubulointerstitial processes such as interstitial nephritis and transplant rejection.

Casts can be seen in chronic renal diseases. Degenerated cellular casts called *waxy casts* or *broad casts* (arising in the dilated tubules that have undergone compensatory hypertrophy in response to reduced renal mass) may be seen in the urine.

ABNORMALITIES OF URINE VOLUME

POLYURIA

By history, it is often difficult for patients to distinguish urinary frequency (often of small volumes) from true polyuria (>3 L/d), and a quantification of volume by 24-h urine collection may be needed (**Fig. 52-4**). Polyuria results from two potential mechanisms: (1) excretion of nonabsorbable solutes (such as glucose) or (2) excretion of water (usually from a defect in AVP production or renal responsiveness). To distinguish a solute diuresis from a water diuresis and to determine whether the diuresis is appropriate for the clinical circumstances, urine osmolality is measured. The average person excretes between 600 and 800 mosmol of solutes per day, primarily as urea and electrolytes. If the urine output is >3 L/d and the urine is dilute (<250 mosmol/L), total osmolar excretion is normal and a water diuresis is present. This circumstance could arise from polydipsia, inadequate secretion of AVP (*central diabetes*

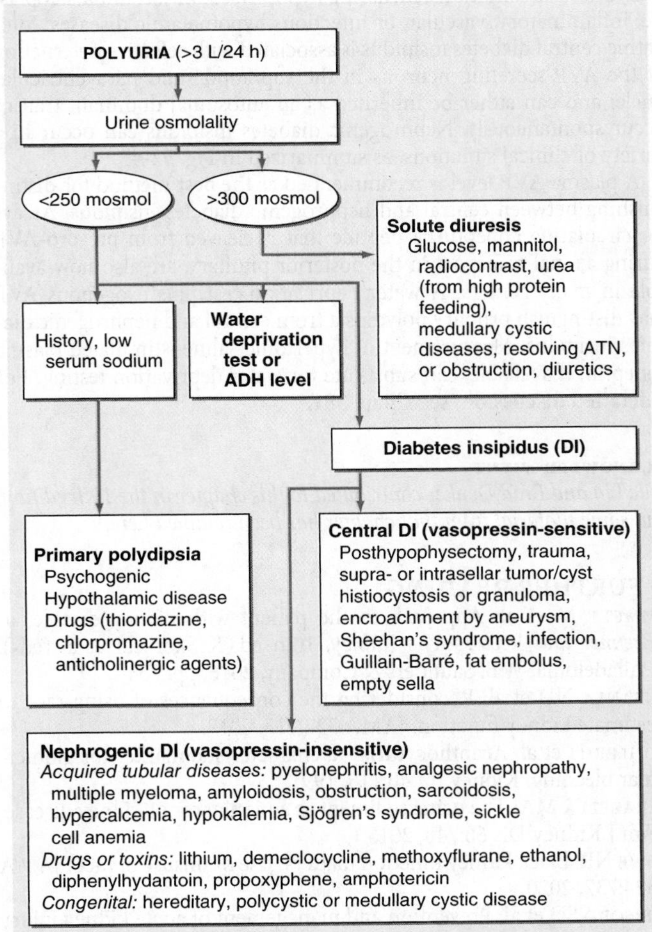

FIGURE 52-4 Approach to the patient with polyuria. ADH, antidiuretic hormone; ATN, acute tubular necrosis.

insipidus), or failure of renal tubules to respond to AVP (*nephrogenic diabetes insipidus*). If the urine volume is >3 L/d and urine osmolality is >300 mosmol/L, a solute diuresis is clearly present and a search for the responsible solute(s) is mandatory.

Excessive filtration of a poorly reabsorbed solute such as glucose or mannitol can depress reabsorption of NaCl and water in the proximal tubule and lead to enhanced excretion in the urine. Poorly controlled diabetes mellitus with glucosuria is the most common cause of a solute diuresis, leading to volume depletion and serum hypertonicity. Since the urine sodium concentration is less than that of blood, more water than sodium is lost, causing hypernatremia and hypertonicity. Common iatrogenic solute diuresis occurs in association with mannitol administration, radiocontrast media, and high-protein feedings (enteral or parenteral), leading to increased urea production and excretion. Less commonly, excessive sodium loss may result from cystic renal diseases or Bartter's syndrome or may develop during a tubulointerstitial process (such as resolving ATN). In these so-called salt-wasting disorders, the tubule damage results in direct impairment of sodium reabsorption and indirectly reduces the responsiveness of the tubule to aldosterone. Usually, the sodium losses are mild, and the obligatory urine output is <2 L/d; resolving ATN and postobstructive diuresis are exceptions and may be associated with significant natriuresis and polyuria.

Formation of large volumes of dilute urine is usually due to polydipsic states or diabetes insipidus. Primary polydipsia can result from habit, psychiatric disorders, neurologic lesions, or medications. During deliberate polydipsia, extracellular fluid volume is normal or expanded and plasma AVP levels are reduced because serum osmolality tends to be near the lower limits of normal. Urine osmolality is also maximally dilute at 50 mosmol/L.

Central diabetes insipidus may be idiopathic in origin or secondary to a variety of conditions, including hypophysectomy, trauma, neoplastic, inflammatory, vascular, or infectious hypothalamic diseases. Idiopathic central diabetes insipidus is associated with selective destruction of the AVP-secreting neurons in the supraoptic and paraventricular nuclei and can either be inherited as an autosomal dominant trait or occur spontaneously. Nephrogenic diabetes insipidus can occur in a variety of clinical situations, as summarized in Fig. 52-4.

A plasma AVP level is recommended as the best method for distinguishing between central and nephrogenic diabetes insipidus. Assays for circulating copeptin, a peptide that is cleaved from pre-pro-AVP during axonal transport in the posterior pituitary, are also now available in many centers. A water deprivation test plus exogenous AVP may distinguish primary polydipsia from central and nephrogenic diabetes insipidus. Measurement of hypertonic saline–stimulated plasma copeptin, if available, can substitute for water deprivation testing. **For a detailed discussion, see Chap. 381.**

ACKNOWLEDGMENT

Julie Lin and Brad Denker contributed to this chapter in the 19th edition, and some material from that chapter has been retained here.

FURTHER READING

EMMETT M et al: Approach to the patient with kidney disease, in *Brenner and Rector's The Kidney*, 10th ed, K Skorecki et al (eds). Philadelphia, W.B. Saunders & Company, 2016, pp. 754–779.

ENEANYA ND et al: Reconsidering the consequences of using race to estimate kidney function. JAMA 322:113, 2019.

KÖHLER H et al: Acanthocyturia—a characteristic marker for glomerular bleeding. Kidney Int 40:115, 1991.

PERAZELLA MA: The urine sediment as a biomarker of kidney disease. Am J Kidney Dis 66:748, 2015.

POWE NR: Black kidney function matters: Use or misuse of race? JAMA 324:737, 2020.

WEISORD SD et al: Prevention and management of acute kidney injury in *Brenner and Rector's The Kidney*, 11th ed, ASL Yu et al: (eds). Philadelphia, W.B. Saunders & Company, 2020, pp. 940–977.

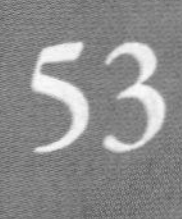

53 Fluid and Electrolyte Disturbances

David B. Mount

SODIUM AND WATER

COMPOSITION OF BODY FLUIDS

Water is the most abundant constituent in the body, comprising ~50% of body weight in women and 60% in men. Total-body water is distributed in two major compartments: 55–75% is intracellular (intracellular fluid [ICF]), and 25–45% is extracellular (extracellular fluid [ECF]). The ECF is further subdivided into intravascular (plasma water) and extravascular (interstitial) spaces in a ratio of 1:3. Fluid movement between the intravascular and interstitial spaces occurs across the capillary wall and is determined by Starling forces, i.e., capillary hydraulic pressure and colloid osmotic pressure. The transcapillary hydraulic pressure gradient exceeds the corresponding oncotic pressure gradient, thereby favoring the movement of plasma ultrafiltrate into the extravascular space. The return of fluid into the intravascular compartment occurs via lymphatic flow.

The solute or particle concentration of a fluid is known as its osmolality, expressed as milliosmoles per kilogram of water (mOsm/kg). Water easily diffuses across most cell membranes to achieve osmotic equilibrium (ECF osmolality = ICF osmolality). Notably, the extracellular and intracellular solute compositions differ considerably owing to the activity of various transporters, channels, and ATP-driven membrane pumps. The major ECF particles are Na^+ and its accompanying anions Cl^- and HCO_3^-, whereas K^+ and organic phosphate esters (ATP, creatine phosphate, and phospholipids) are the predominant ICF osmoles. Solutes that are restricted to the ECF or the ICF determine the "tonicity" or effective osmolality of that compartment. Certain solutes, particularly urea, do not contribute to water shifts across most membranes and are thus known as *ineffective osmoles*.

Water Balance Vasopressin secretion, water ingestion, and renal water transport collaborate to maintain human body fluid osmolality between 280 and 295 mOsm/kg. Vasopressin (AVP) is synthesized in magnocellular neurons within the hypothalamus; the distal axons of these neurons project to the posterior pituitary or neurohypophysis, from which AVP is released into the circulation. A network of central "osmoreceptor" neurons, which includes the AVP-expressing magnocellular neurons themselves, sense circulating osmolality via nonselective, stretch-activated cation channels. These osmoreceptor neurons are activated or inhibited by modest increases and decreases in circulating osmolality, respectively; activation leads to AVP release and thirst.

AVP secretion is stimulated as systemic osmolality increases above a threshold level of ~285 mOsm/kg, above which there is a linear relationship between osmolality and circulating AVP (**Fig. 53-1**). Thirst and thus water ingestion are also activated at ~285 mOsm/kg, beyond which there is an equivalent linear increase in the perceived intensity of thirst as a function of circulating osmolality. Changes in blood volume and blood pressure are also direct stimuli for AVP release and thirst, albeit with a less sensitive response profile. Of perhaps greater clinical relevance to the pathophysiology of water homeostasis, ECF volume strongly modulates the relationship between circulating osmolality and AVP release, such that hypovolemia reduces the osmotic threshold and increases the slope of the response curve to osmolality; *hypervolemia* has an opposite effect, increasing the osmotic threshold and reducing the slope of the response curve (Fig. 53-1). Notably, AVP has a half-life in the circulation of only 10–20 min; thus, changes in ECF volume and/or circulating osmolality can rapidly affect water homeostasis. In addition to volume status, a number of other "nonosmotic" stimuli have potent activating effects on osmosensitive neurons and AVP

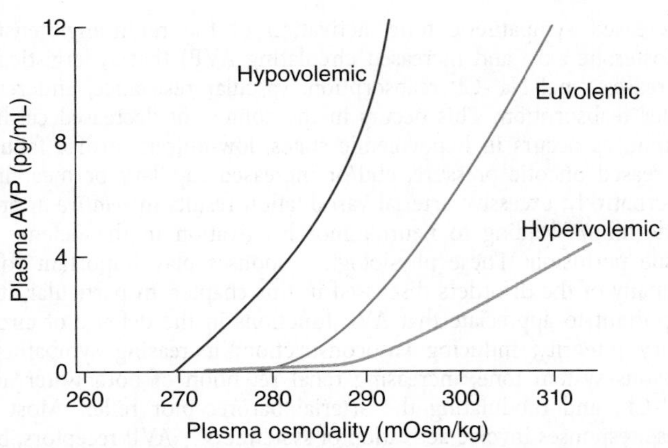

FIGURE 53-1 Circulating levels of vasopressin (AVP) in response to changes in osmolality. Plasma AVP becomes detectable in euvolemic, healthy individuals at a threshold of ~285 mOsm/kg, above which there is a linear relationship between osmolality and circulating AVP. The AVP response to osmolality is modulated strongly by volume status. The osmotic threshold is thus slightly lower in hypovolemia, with a steeper response curve; hypervolemia reduces the sensitivity of circulating AVP levels to osmolality.

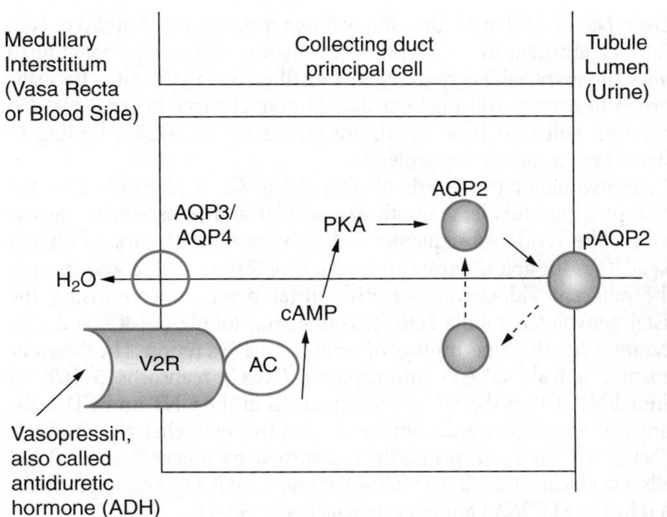

FIGURE 53-3 Vasopressin and the regulation of water permeability in the renal collecting duct. Vasopressin binds to the type 2 vasopressin receptor (V2R) on the basolateral membrane of principal cells, activates adenylyl cyclase (AC), increases intracellular cyclic adenosine monophosphatase (cAMP), and stimulates protein kinase A (PKA) activity. Cytoplasmic vesicles carrying aquaporin-2 (AQP) water channel proteins are inserted into the luminal membrane in response to vasopressin, thereby increasing the water permeability of this membrane. When vasopressin stimulation ends, water channels are retrieved by an endocytic process and water permeability returns to its low basal rate. The AQP3 and AQP4 water channels are expressed on the basolateral membrane and complete the transcellular pathway for water reabsorption. pAQP2, phosphorylated aquaporin-2. *(From Annals of Internal Medicine JM Sands, DG Bichet: Nephrogenic diabetes insipidus. 144(3):186, 2006. Copyright © 2006 American College of Physicians. All Rights Reserved. Reprinted with the permission of American College of Physicians, Inc.)*

release, including nausea, intracerebral angiotensin II, serotonin, and multiple drugs.

The excretion or retention of electrolyte-free water by the kidney is modulated by circulating AVP. AVP acts on renal, V_2-type receptors in the thick ascending limb of Henle and principal cells of the collecting duct (CD), increasing intracellular levels of cyclic AMP and activating protein kinase A (PKA)–dependent phosphorylation of multiple transport proteins. The AVP- and PKA-dependent activation of Na^+-Cl^- and K^+ transport by the thick ascending limb of the loop of Henle (TALH) is a key participant in the countercurrent mechanism (**Fig. 53-2**). The countercurrent mechanism ultimately increases the interstitial osmolality in the inner medulla of the kidney, driving water absorption across the renal CD. However, water, salt, and solute transport by both proximal and distal nephron segments participates in the renal concentrating mechanism (Fig. 53-2). Water transport across apical and basolateral aquaporin-1 water channels in the descending thin limb of the loop of Henle is thus involved, as is passive absorption of Na^+-Cl^- by the thin ascending limb, via apical and basolateral CLC-K1 chloride channels and paracellular Na^+ transport. Renal urea transport in turn plays important roles in the generation of the medullary osmotic gradient and the ability to excrete solute-free water under conditions of both high and low protein intake (Fig. 53-2).

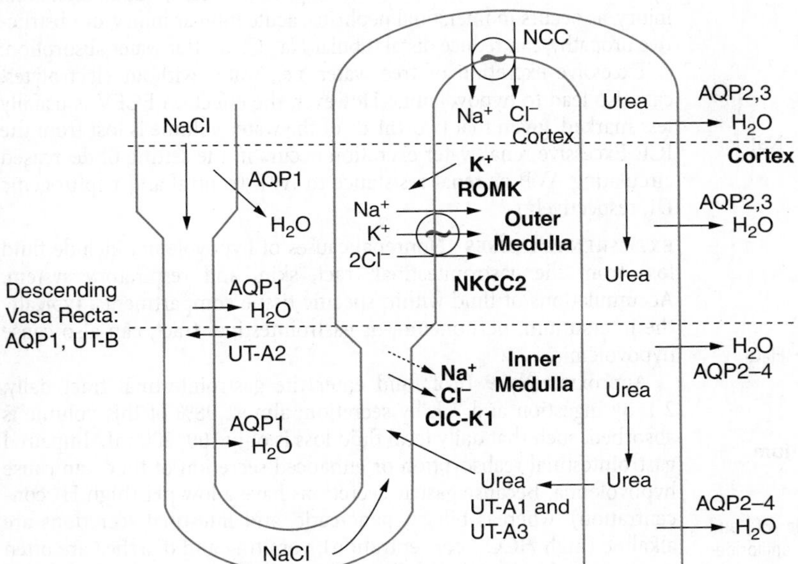

FIGURE 53-2 The renal concentrating mechanism. Water, salt, and solute transport by both proximal and distal nephron segments participates in the renal concentrating mechanism (see text for details). Diagram showing the location of the major transport proteins involved; a loop of Henle is depicted on the *left,* collecting duct on the *right.* AQP, aquaporin; CLC-K1, chloride channel; NKCC2, Na-K-2Cl cotransporter; ROMK, renal outer medullary K^+ channel; UT, urea transporter. *(Republished with permission of American Society of Nephrology, from Molecular approaches to urea transporters, JM Sands, 13(11), 2002; permission conveyed through Copyright Clearance Center, Inc.)*

AVP-induced, PKA-dependent phosphorylation of the aquaporin-2 water channel in principal cells stimulates the insertion of active water channels into the lumen of the CD, resulting in transepithelial water absorption down the medullary osmotic gradient (**Fig. 53-3**). Under "antidiuretic" conditions, with increased circulating AVP, the kidney reabsorbs water filtered by the glomerulus, equilibrating the osmolality across the CD epithelium to excrete a hypertonic, "concentrated" urine (osmolality of up to 1200 mOsm/kg). In the absence of circulating AVP, insertion of aquaporin-2 channels and water absorption across the CD is essentially abolished, resulting in secretion of a hypotonic, dilute urine (osmolality as low as 30–50 mOsm/kg). Abnormalities in this "final common pathway" are involved in most disorders of water homeostasis, e.g., a reduced or absent insertion of active aquaporin-2 water channels into the membrane of principal cells in diabetes insipidus (DI).

Maintenance of Arterial Circulatory Integrity

Sodium is actively pumped out of cells by the Na^+/K^+-ATPase membrane pump. In consequence, 85–90% of body Na^+ is extracellular, and the ECF volume (ECFV) is a function of total-body Na^+ content. Arterial perfusion and circulatory integrity are, in turn, determined by renal Na^+ retention or excretion, in addition to the modulation of systemic arterial resistance. Within the kidney, Na^+ is filtered by the glomeruli and then sequentially reabsorbed by the renal tubules. The Na^+ cation is typically reabsorbed with the chloride anion (Cl^-), and thus, chloride homeostasis also affects the ECFV. On a quantitative level, at a glomerular filtration rate (GFR) of 180 L/d and serum Na^+ of ~140 m*M*, the kidney filters some 25,200 mmol/d of Na^+. This is equivalent to ~1.5 kg of salt, which would occupy roughly 10 times the extracellular space; 99.6% of filtered Na^+-Cl^- must be reabsorbed to excrete 100 m*M* per day. Minute changes in renal Na^+-Cl^- excretion will thus have significant effects on the ECFV, leading to edema syndromes or hypovolemia.

Approximately two-thirds of filtered Na^+-Cl^- is reabsorbed by the renal proximal tubule, via both paracellular and transcellular mechanisms. The TALH subsequently reabsorbs another 25–30% of filtered Na^+-Cl^- via the apical, furosemide-sensitive Na^+-K^+-$2Cl^-$ cotransporter. The adjacent aldosterone-sensitive distal nephron, comprising the distal convoluted tubule (DCT), connecting tubule (CNT), and CD, accomplishes the "fine-tuning" of renal Na^+-Cl^- excretion. The thiazide-sensitive apical Na^+-Cl^- cotransporter (NCC) reabsorbs 5–10% of filtered Na^+-Cl^- in the DCT. Principal cells in the CNT and CD reabsorb Na^+ via electrogenic, amiloride-sensitive epithelial Na^+ channels (ENaC); Cl^- ions are primarily reabsorbed by adjacent intercalated cells, via apical Cl^- exchange (Cl^--OH^- and Cl^--HCO_3^- exchange, mediated by the SLC26A4 anion exchanger) (**Fig. 53-4**).

Renal tubular reabsorption of filtered Na^+-Cl^- is regulated by multiple circulating and paracrine hormones, in addition to the activity of renal nerves. Angiotensin II activates proximal Na^+-Cl^- reabsorption, as do adrenergic receptors under the influence of renal sympathetic innervation; locally generated dopamine, in contrast, has a *natriuretic* effect. Aldosterone primarily activates Na^+-Cl^- reabsorption within the aldosterone-sensitive distal nephron. In particular, aldosterone activates the ENaC channel in principal cells, inducing Na^+ absorption and promoting K^+ excretion (Fig. 53-4).

Circulatory integrity is critical for the perfusion and function of vital organs. "Underfilling" of the arterial circulation is sensed by ventricular and vascular pressure receptors, resulting in a neurohumoral activation (increased sympathetic tone, activation of the renin-angiotensin-aldosterone axis, and increased circulating AVP) that synergistically increases renal Na^+-Cl^- reabsorption, vascular resistance, and renal water reabsorption. This occurs in the context of decreased cardiac output, as occurs in hypovolemic states, low-output cardiac failure, decreased oncotic pressure, and/or increased capillary permeability. Alternatively, excessive arterial vasodilation results in *relative* arterial underfilling, leading to neurohumoral activation in the defense of tissue perfusion. These physiologic responses play important roles in many of the disorders discussed in this chapter. In particular, it is important to appreciate that AVP functions in the defense of circulatory integrity, inducing vasoconstriction, increasing sympathetic nervous system tone, increasing renal retention of both water and Na^+-Cl^-, and modulating the arterial baroreceptor reflex. Most of these responses involve activation of systemic V_{1A} AVP receptors, but concomitant activation of V_2 receptors in the kidney can result in renal water retention and hyponatremia.

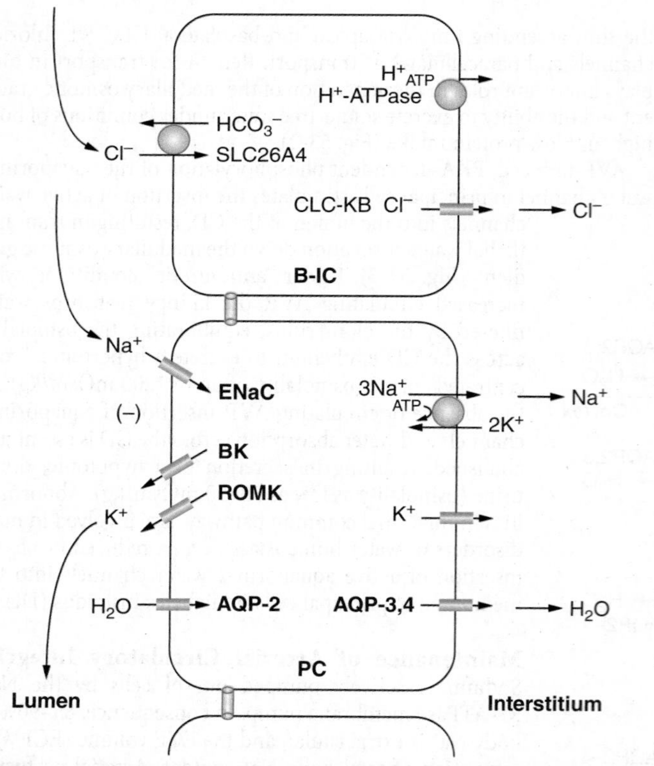

FIGURE 53-4 Sodium, water, and potassium transport in principal cells (PC) and adjacent β-intercalated cells (B-IC). The absorption of Na^+ via the amiloride-sensitive epithelial sodium channel (ENaC) generates a lumen-negative potential difference, which drives K^+ excretion through the apical secretory K^+ channel ROMK (renal outer medullary K^+ channel) and/or the flow-dependent BK channel. Transepithelial Cl^- transport occurs in adjacent β-intercalated cells, via apical Cl^--HCO_3^- and Cl^--OH^- exchange (SLC26A4 anion exchanger, also known as pendrin) basolateral CLC chloride channels. Water is absorbed down the osmotic gradient by principal cells, through the apical aquaporin-2 (AQP-2) and basolateral aquaporin-3 and aquaporin-4 (Fig. 53-3).

HYPOVOLEMIA

Etiology True volume depletion, or hypovolemia, generally refers to a state of combined salt and water loss, leading to contraction of the ECFV. The loss of salt and water may be renal or nonrenal in origin.

RENAL CAUSES Excessive urinary Na^+-Cl^- and water loss is a feature of several conditions. A high filtered load of endogenous solutes, such as glucose and urea, can impair tubular reabsorption of Na^+-Cl^- and water, leading to an osmotic diuresis. Exogenous mannitol, often used to decrease intracerebral pressure, is filtered by glomeruli but not reabsorbed by the proximal tubule, thus causing an osmotic diuresis. Pharmacologic diuretics selectively impair Na^+-Cl^- reabsorption at specific sites along the nephron, leading to increased urinary Na^+-Cl^- excretion. Other drugs can induce natriuresis as a side effect. For example, acetazolamide can inhibit proximal tubular Na^+-Cl^- absorption via its inhibition of carbonic anhydrase; other drugs, such as the antibiotics trimethoprim (TMP) and pentamidine, inhibit distal tubular Na^+ reabsorption through the amiloride-sensitive ENaC channel, leading to urinary Na^+-Cl^- loss. Hereditary defects in renal transport proteins are also associated with reduced reabsorption of filtered Na^+-Cl^- and/or water. Alternatively, mineralocorticoid deficiency, mineralocorticoid resistance, or inhibition of the mineralocorticoid receptor (MLR) can reduce Na^+-Cl^- reabsorption by the aldosterone-sensitive distal nephron. Finally, tubulointerstitial injury, as occurs in interstitial nephritis, acute tubular injury, or obstructive uropathy, can reduce distal tubular Na^+-Cl^- and/or water absorption.

Excessive excretion of free water, i.e., water without electrolytes, can also lead to hypovolemia. However, the effect on ECFV is usually less marked, given that two-thirds of the water volume is lost from the ICF. Excessive renal water excretion occurs in the setting of decreased circulating AVP or renal resistance to AVP (central and nephrogenic DI, respectively).

EXTRARENAL CAUSES Nonrenal causes of hypovolemia include fluid loss from the gastrointestinal tract, skin, and respiratory system. Accumulations of fluid within specific tissue compartments, typically the interstitium, peritoneum, or gastrointestinal tract, can also cause hypovolemia.

Approximately 9 L of fluid enter the gastrointestinal tract daily, 2 L by ingestion and 7 L by secretion; almost 98% of this volume is absorbed, such that daily fecal fluid loss is only 100–200 mL. Impaired gastrointestinal reabsorption or enhanced secretion of fluid can cause hypovolemia. Because gastric secretions have a low pH (high H^+ concentration), whereas biliary, pancreatic, and intestinal secretions are alkaline (high HCO_3^- concentration), vomiting and diarrhea are often accompanied by metabolic alkalosis and acidosis, respectively.

Evaporation of water from the skin and respiratory tract (so-called "insensible losses") constitutes the major route for loss of solute-free water, which is typically 500–650 mL/d in healthy adults. This evaporative loss can increase during febrile illness or prolonged heat exposure. Hyperventilation can also increase insensible losses via the respiratory tract, particularly in ventilated patients; the humidity of inspired air is another determining factor. In addition, increased exertion and/or ambient temperature will increase insensible losses via sweat, which is hypotonic to plasma. Profuse sweating without adequate repletion of water and Na^+-Cl^- can thus lead to both hypovolemia and hypertonicity. Alternatively, replacement of these insensible losses with a surfeit of free water, without adequate replacement of electrolytes, may lead to hypovolemic hyponatremia.

Excessive fluid accumulation in interstitial and/or peritoneal spaces can also cause intravascular hypovolemia. Increases in vascular permeability and/or a reduction in oncotic pressure (hypoalbuminemia) alter Starling forces, resulting in excessive "third spacing" of the ECFV. This occurs in sepsis syndrome, burns, pancreatitis, nutritional hypoalbuminemia, and peritonitis. Alternatively, distributive hypovolemia can occur due to accumulation of fluid within specific compartments, for example, within the bowel lumen in gastrointestinal obstruction or ileus. Hypovolemia can also occur after extracorporeal hemorrhage or after significant hemorrhage into an expandable space, for example, the retroperitoneum.

Diagnostic Evaluation A careful history will usually determine the etiologic cause of hypovolemia. Symptoms of hypovolemia are nonspecific and include fatigue, weakness, thirst, and postural dizziness; more severe symptoms and signs include oliguria, cyanosis, abdominal and chest pain, and confusion or obtundation. Associated electrolyte disorders may cause additional symptoms, for example, muscle weakness in patients with hypokalemia. On examination, diminished skin turgor and dry oral mucous membranes are less than ideal markers of a decreased ECFV in adult patients; more reliable signs of hypovolemia include a decreased jugular venous pressure (JVP), orthostatic tachycardia (an increase of >15–20 beats/min upon standing), and orthostatic hypotension (a >10–20 mmHg drop in blood pressure on standing). More severe fluid loss leads to hypovolemic shock, with hypotension, tachycardia, peripheral vasoconstriction, and peripheral hypoperfusion; these patients may exhibit peripheral cyanosis, cold extremities, oliguria, and altered mental status.

Routine chemistries may reveal an increase in blood urea nitrogen (BUN) and creatinine, reflective of a decrease in GFR. Creatinine is the more dependable measure of GFR, because BUN levels may be influenced by an increase in tubular reabsorption ("prerenal azotemia"), an increase in urea generation in catabolic states, hyperalimentation, or gastrointestinal bleeding, and/or a decreased urea generation in decreased protein intake. In hypovolemic shock, liver function tests and cardiac biomarkers may show evidence of hepatic and cardiac ischemia, respectively. Routine chemistries and/or blood gases may reveal evidence of acid-base disorders. For example, bicarbonate loss due to diarrheal illness is a very common cause of metabolic acidosis; alternatively, patients with severe hypovolemic shock may develop lactic acidosis with an elevated anion gap.

The neurohumoral response to hypovolemia stimulates an increase in renal tubular Na^+ and water reabsorption. Therefore, the urine Na^+ concentration is typically <20 m*M* in nonrenal causes of hypovolemia, with a urine osmolality of >450 mOsm/kg. The reduction in both GFR and distal tubular Na^+ delivery may cause a defect in renal potassium excretion, with an increase in plasma K^+ concentration. Of note, patients with hypovolemia and a hypochloremic alkalosis due to vomiting, diarrhea, or diuretics will typically have a urine Na^+ concentration >20 m*M* and urine pH of >7.0, due to the increase in filtered HCO_3^-; the urine Cl^- concentration in this setting is a more accurate indicator of volume status, with a level <25 m*M* suggestive of hypovolemia. The urine Na^+ concentration is often >20 m*M* in patients with *renal* causes of hypovolemia, such as acute tubular necrosis; similarly, patients with DI will have an inappropriately dilute urine.

TREATMENT

Hypovolemia

The therapeutic goals in hypovolemia are to restore normovolemia and replace ongoing fluid losses. Mild hypovolemia can usually be treated with oral hydration and resumption of a normal maintenance diet. More severe hypovolemia requires intravenous hydration, tailoring the choice of solution to the underlying pathophysiology. Isotonic, "normal" saline (0.9% NaCl, 154 m*M* Na^+) is the most appropriate resuscitation fluid for normonatremic or hyponatremic patients with severe hypovolemia; colloid solutions such as intravenous albumin are not demonstrably superior for this purpose. Hypernatremic patients should receive a hypotonic solution, 5% dextrose if there has only been water loss (as in DI), or hypotonic saline (1/2 or 1/4 normal saline) if there has been water and Na^+-Cl^- loss; changes in free water administration should be made if necessary, based on frequent measuring of serum chemistries. Patients with bicarbonate loss and metabolic acidosis, as occur frequently in diarrhea, should receive intravenous bicarbonate, either an isotonic solution (150 meq of Na^+-HCO_3^- in 5% dextrose) or a more hypotonic bicarbonate solution in dextrose or dilute saline. Patients with severe hemorrhage or anemia should receive red cell transfusions, without increasing the hematocrit beyond 35%.

SODIUM DISORDERS

Disorders of serum Na^+ concentration are caused by abnormalities in water homeostasis, leading to changes in the relative ratio of Na^+ to body water. Water intake and circulating AVP constitute the two key effectors in the defense of serum osmolality; defects in one or both of these two defense mechanisms cause most cases of hyponatremia and hypernatremia. In contrast, abnormalities in sodium homeostasis per se lead to a deficit or surplus of whole-body Na^+-Cl^- content, a key determinant of the ECFV and circulatory integrity. Notably, volume status also modulates the release of AVP by the posterior pituitary, such that hypovolemia is associated with higher circulating levels of the hormone at each level of serum osmolality. Similarly, in "hypervolemic" causes of arterial underfilling, e.g., heart failure and cirrhosis, the associated neurohumoral activation encompasses an increase in circulating AVP, leading to water retention and hyponatremia. Therefore, a key concept in sodium disorders is that the absolute plasma Na^+ concentration tells one nothing about the volume status of a given patient, which furthermore must be taken into account in the diagnostic and therapeutic approach.

HYPONATREMIA

Hyponatremia, which is defined as a plasma Na^+ concentration <135 m*M*, is a very common disorder, occurring in up to 22% of hospitalized patients. This disorder is almost always the result of an increase in circulating AVP and/or increased renal sensitivity to AVP, combined with an intake of free water; a notable exception is hyponatremia due to low solute intake (see below). The underlying pathophysiology for the exaggerated or "inappropriate" AVP response differs in patients with hyponatremia as a function of their ECFV. Hyponatremia is thus subdivided diagnostically into three groups, depending on clinical history and volume status, i.e., "hypovolemic," "euvolemic," and "hypervolemic" (**Fig. 53-5**).

Hypovolemic Hyponatremia Hypovolemia causes a marked neurohumoral activation, increasing circulating levels of AVP. The increase in circulating AVP helps preserve blood pressure via vascular and baroreceptor V_{1A} receptors and increases water reabsorption via renal V_2 receptors; activation of V_2 receptors can lead to hyponatremia in the setting of increased free water intake. Nonrenal causes of hypovolemic hyponatremia include gastrointestinal loss (e.g., vomiting, diarrhea, tube drainage) and insensible loss (sweating, burns) of Na^+-Cl^- and water, in the absence of adequate oral replacement; urine Na^+ concentration is typically <20 m*M*. Notably, these patients may be clinically classified as euvolemic, with only the reduced urinary Na^+ concentration to indicate the cause of their hyponatremia. Indeed, a urine Na^+ concentration <20 m*M*, in the absence of a cause of hypervolemic hyponatremia, predicts a rapid increase in plasma Na^+ concentration in response to intravenous normal saline; saline therapy thus induces a water diuresis in this setting, as circulating AVP levels plummet.

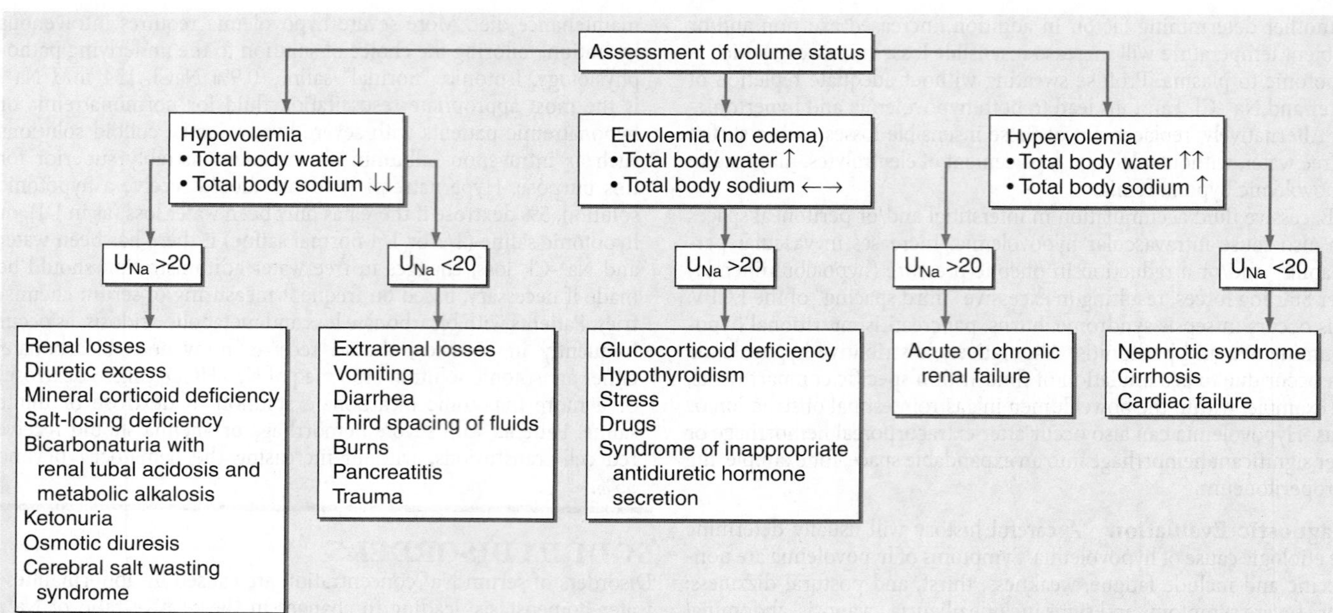

FIGURE 53-5 The diagnostic approach to hyponatremia. *(Reproduced with permission from S Kumar, T Berl: Diseases of water metabolism, in RW Schrier [ed], Atlas of Diseases of the Kidney, Philadelphia, Current Medicine, Inc, 1999.)*

The *renal* causes of hypovolemic hyponatremia share an inappropriate loss of Na^+-Cl^- in the urine, leading to volume depletion and an increase in circulating AVP; urine Na^+ concentration is typically >20 m*M* (Fig. 53-5). A deficiency in circulating aldosterone and/or its renal effects can lead to hyponatremia in primary adrenal insufficiency and other causes of hypoaldosteronism; hyperkalemia and hyponatremia in a hypotensive and/or hypovolemic patient with high urine Na^+ concentration (much greater than 20 m*M*) should strongly suggest this diagnosis. Salt-losing nephropathies may lead to hyponatremia when sodium intake is reduced, due to impaired renal tubular function; typical causes include reflux nephropathy, interstitial nephropathies, postobstructive uropathy, medullary cystic disease, and the recovery phase of acute tubular necrosis. Thiazide diuretics cause hyponatremia via a number of mechanisms, including polydipsia and diuretic-induced volume depletion. Notably, thiazides do not inhibit the renal concentrating mechanism, such that circulating AVP retains a full effect on renal water retention. In contrast, loop diuretics, which are less frequently associated with hyponatremia, inhibit Na^+-Cl^- and K^+ absorption by the TALH, blunting the countercurrent mechanism and reducing the ability to concentrate the urine. Increased excretion of an osmotically active nonreabsorbable or poorly reabsorbable solute can also lead to volume depletion and hyponatremia; important causes include glycosuria, ketonuria (e.g., in starvation or in diabetic or alcoholic ketoacidosis), and bicarbonaturia (e.g., in renal tubular acidosis or metabolic alkalosis, where the associated bicarbonaturia leads to loss of Na^+).

Finally, the syndrome of "cerebral salt wasting" is a rare cause of hypovolemic hyponatremia, encompassing hyponatremia with clinical hypovolemia and inappropriate natriuresis in association with intracranial disease; associated disorders include subarachnoid hemorrhage, traumatic brain injury, craniotomy, encephalitis, and meningitis. Distinction from the more common syndrome of inappropriate antidiuresis (SIAD) is critical because cerebral salt wasting will typically respond to aggressive Na^+-Cl^- repletion.

Hypervolemic Hyponatremia Patients with hypervolemic hyponatremia develop an increase in total-body Na^+-Cl^- that is accompanied by a proportionately *greater* increase in total-body water, leading to a reduced plasma Na^+ concentration. As in hypovolemic hyponatremia, the causative disorders can be separated by the effect on urine Na^+ concentration, with acute or chronic renal failure uniquely associated with an increase in urine Na^+ concentration (Fig. 53-5). The pathophysiology of hyponatremia in the sodium-avid edematous disorders (congestive heart failure [CHF], cirrhosis, and nephrotic syndrome) is similar to that in hypovolemic hyponatremia, except that arterial filling and circulatory integrity is decreased due to the specific etiologic factors (e.g., cardiac dysfunction in CHF, peripheral vasodilation in cirrhosis). Urine Na^+ concentration is typically very low, i.e., <10 m*M*, even after hydration with normal saline; this Na^+-avid state may be obscured by diuretic therapy. The degree of hyponatremia provides an indirect index of the associated neurohumoral activation and is an important prognostic indicator in hypervolemic hyponatremia.

Euvolemic Hyponatremia Euvolemic hyponatremia can occur in moderate to severe hypothyroidism, with correction after achieving a euthyroid state. Severe hyponatremia can also be a consequence of secondary adrenal insufficiency due to pituitary disease; whereas the deficit in circulating aldosterone in primary adrenal insufficiency causes *hypovolemic* hyponatremia, the predominant glucocorticoid deficiency in secondary adrenal failure is associated with *euvolemic* hyponatremia. Glucocorticoids exert a negative feedback on AVP release by the posterior pituitary such that hydrocortisone replacement in these patients can rapidly normalize the AVP response to osmolality, reducing circulating AVP.

The SIAD is the most frequent cause of euvolemic hyponatremia (**Table 53-1**). The generation of hyponatremia in SIAD requires an intake of free water, with persistent intake at serum osmolalities that are lower than the usual threshold for thirst; as one would expect, the osmotic threshold and osmotic response curves for the sensation of thirst are shifted downward in patients with SIAD. Four distinct patterns of AVP secretion have been recognized in patients with SIAD, independent for the most part of the underlying cause. Unregulated, erratic AVP secretion is seen in about a third of patients, with no obvious correlation between serum osmolality and circulating AVP levels. Other patients fail to suppress AVP secretion at lower serum osmolalities, with a normal response curve to hyperosmolar conditions; others have a "reset osmostat," with a lower threshold osmolality and a left-shifted osmotic response curve. Finally, the fourth subset of patients have essentially no detectable circulating AVP, suggesting either a gain in function in renal water reabsorption or a circulating antidiuretic substance that is distinct from AVP. Gain-in-function mutations of a single specific residue in the V_2 AVP receptor have been described in some of these patients, leading to constitutive activation of the receptor in the absence of AVP and "nephrogenic" SIAD.

TABLE 53-1 Causes of the Syndrome of Inappropriate Antidiuresis (SIAD)

MALIGNANT DISEASES	PULMONARY DISORDERS	DISORDERS OF THE CENTRAL NERVOUS SYSTEM	DRUGS	OTHER CAUSES
Carcinoma	Infections	Infection	Drugs that stimulate release of AVP or enhance its action	Hereditary (gain-of-function mutations in the vasopressin V_2 receptor)
Lung	Bacterial pneumonia	Encephalitis	Chlorpropamide	Idiopathic
Small cell	Viral pneumonia	Meningitis	SSRIs	Transient
Mesothelioma	Pulmonary abscess	Brain abscess	Tricyclic antidepressants	Endurance exercise
Oropharynx	Tuberculosis	Rocky Mountain spotted fever	Clofibrate	General anesthesia
Gastrointestinal tract	Aspergillosis	AIDS	Carbamazepine	Nausea
Stomach	Asthma	Bleeding and masses	Vincristine	Pain
Duodenum	Cystic fibrosis	Subdural hematoma	Nicotine	Stress
Pancreas	Respiratory failure associated with positive-pressure breathing	Subarachnoid hemorrhage	Narcotics	
Genitourinary tract		Cerebrovascular accident	Antipsychotic drugs	
Ureter		Brain tumors	Ifosfamide	
Bladder		Head trauma	Cyclophosphamide	
Prostate		Hydrocephalus	Nonsteroidal anti-inflammatory drugs	
Endometrium		Cavernous sinus thrombosis	MDMA ("Ecstasy", "Molly")	
Endocrine thymoma		Other	AVP analogues	
Lymphomas		Multiple sclerosis	Desmopressin	
Sarcomas		Guillain-Barré syndrome	Oxytocin	
Ewing's sarcoma		Shy-Drager syndrome	Vasopressin	
		Delirium tremens		
		Acute intermittent porphyria		

Abbreviations: AVP, vasopressin; MDMA, 3,4-methylenedioxymethamphetamine; SSRI, selective serotonin reuptake inhibitor.
Source: From DH Ellison, T Berl: The syndrome of inappropriate antidiuresis. N Engl J Med 356:2064, 2007. Copyright © 2007 Massachusetts Medical Society. Reprinted with permission from Massachusetts Medical Society.

Strictly speaking, patients with SIAD are not euvolemic but are subclinically volume-expanded, due to AVP-induced water and Na^+-Cl^- retention; "AVP escape" mechanisms invoked by sustained increases in AVP serve to limit distal renal tubular transport, preserving a modestly hypervolemic steady state. Serum uric acid is often low (<4 mg/dL) in patients with SIAD, consistent with suppressed proximal tubular transport in the setting of increased distal tubular Na^+-Cl^- and water transport; in contrast, patients with hypovolemic hyponatremia will often be hyperuricemic due to a shared activation of proximal tubular Na^+-Cl^- and urate transport.

Common causes of SIAD include pulmonary disease (e.g., pneumonia, tuberculosis, pleural effusion) and central nervous system (CNS) diseases (e.g., tumor, subarachnoid hemorrhage, meningitis). SIAD also occurs with malignancies, most commonly with small-cell lung carcinoma (75% of malignancy-associated SIAD); ~10% of patients with this tumor will have a plasma Na^+ concentration of <130 m*M* at presentation. SIAD is also a frequent complication of certain drugs, most commonly the selective serotonin reuptake inhibitors (SSRIs). Other drugs can potentiate the renal effect of AVP, without exerting direct effects on circulating AVP levels (Table 53-1).

Low Solute Intake and Hyponatremia Hyponatremia can occasionally occur in patients with a very low intake of dietary solutes. Classically, this occurs in alcoholics whose sole nutrient is beer, hence the diagnostic label of *beer potomania*; beer is very low in protein and salt content, containing only 1–2 m*M* of Na^+. The syndrome has also been described in nonalcoholic patients with highly restricted solute intake due to nutrient-restricted diets, e.g., extreme vegetarian diets. Patients with hyponatremia due to low solute intake typically present with a very low urine osmolality (<100–200 mOsm/kg) with a urine Na^+ concentration that is <10–20 m*M*. The fundamental abnormality is the inadequate dietary intake of solutes; the reduced urinary solute excretion limits water excretion such that hyponatremia ensues after relatively modest polydipsia. AVP levels have not been reported in patients with beer potomania but are expected to be suppressed or rapidly suppressible with saline hydration; this fits with the overly rapid correction in plasma Na^+ concentration that can be seen with saline hydration. Resumption of a normal diet and/or saline hydration will also correct the causative deficit in urinary solute excretion, such that patients with beer potomania typically correct their plasma Na^+ concentration promptly after admission to the hospital.

Clinical Features of Hyponatremia Hyponatremia induces generalized cellular swelling, a consequence of water movement down the osmotic gradient from the hypotonic ECF to the ICF. The symptoms of hyponatremia are primarily neurologic, reflecting the development of cerebral edema within a rigid skull. The initial CNS response to acute hyponatremia is an increase in interstitial pressure, leading to shunting of ECF and solutes from the interstitial space into the cerebrospinal fluid and then on into the systemic circulation. This is accompanied by an efflux of the major intracellular ions, Na^+, K^+, and Cl^-, from brain cells. Acute hyponatremic encephalopathy ensues when these volume regulatory mechanisms are overwhelmed by a rapid decrease in tonicity, resulting in acute cerebral edema. Early symptoms can include nausea, headache, and vomiting. However, severe complications can rapidly evolve, including seizure activity, brainstem herniation, coma, and death. A key complication of acute hyponatremia is normocapneic or hypercapneic respiratory failure; the associated hypoxia may amplify the neurologic injury. Normocapneic respiratory failure in this setting is typically due to noncardiogenic, "neurogenic" pulmonary edema, with a normal pulmonary capillary wedge pressure.

Acute symptomatic hyponatremia is a medical emergency, occurring in a number of specific settings **(Table 53-2)**. Women, particularly

TABLE 53-2 Causes of Acute Hyponatremia

Iatrogenic
Postoperative: premenopausal women
Hypotonic fluids with cause of ↑ vasopressin
Glycine irrigation: TURP, uterine surgery
Colonoscopy preparation
Recent institution of thiazides
Polydipsia
MDMA ("ecstasy," "Molly") ingestion
Exercise induced
Multifactorial, e.g., thiazide and polydipsia

Abbreviations: MDMA, 3,4-methylenedioxymethamphetamine; TURP, transurethral resection of the prostate.

before menopause, are much more likely than men to develop encephalopathy and severe neurologic sequelae. Acute hyponatremia often has an iatrogenic component, e.g., when hypotonic intravenous fluids are given to postoperative patients with an increase in circulating AVP. Exercise-associated hyponatremia, an important clinical issue at marathons and other endurance events, has similarly been linked to both a "nonosmotic" increase in circulating AVP and excessive free water intake. The recreational drugs Molly and Ecstasy, which share an active ingredient (MDMA, 3,4-methylenedioxymethamphetamine), cause a rapid and potent induction of both thirst and AVP, leading to severe acute hyponatremia.

Persistent, chronic hyponatremia results in an efflux of organic osmolytes (creatine, betaine, glutamate, myoinositol, and taurine) from brain cells; this response reduces intracellular osmolality and the osmotic gradient favoring water entry. This reduction in intracellular osmolytes is largely complete within 48 h, the time period that clinically defines chronic hyponatremia; this temporal definition has considerable relevance for the treatment of hyponatremia (see below). The cellular response to chronic hyponatremia does not fully protect patients from symptoms, which can include vomiting, nausea, confusion, and seizures, usually at plasma Na^+ concentration <125 m*M*. Even patients who are judged "asymptomatic" can manifest subtle gait and cognitive defects that reverse with correction of hyponatremia; notably, chronic "asymptomatic" hyponatremia increases the risk of falls. Chronic hyponatremia also increases the risk of bony fractures owing to the associated neurologic dysfunction and to a hyponatremia-associated reduction in bone density. Therefore, every attempt should be made to safely correct the plasma Na^+ concentration in patients with chronic hyponatremia, even in the absence of overt symptoms (see the section on treatment of hyponatremia below).

The management of chronic hyponatremia is complicated significantly by the asymmetry of the cellular response to correction of plasma Na^+ concentration. Specifically, the *reaccumulation* of organic osmolytes by brain cells is attenuated and delayed as osmolality increases after correction of hyponatremia, sometimes resulting in degenerative loss of oligodendrocytes and an osmotic demyelination syndrome (ODS). Overly rapid correction of hyponatremia (>8–10 m*M* in 24 h or 18 m*M* in 48 h) causes hypertonic stress in astrocytes within brain regions prone to ODS, leading to generalized protein ubiquitination and endoplasmic reticulum stress due to activation of the unfolded protein response; this is accompanied by apoptotic and autophagic cell death. Rapid correction of hyponatremia also causes a disruption in integrity of the blood-brain barrier, allowing the entry of immune mediators that may contribute to demyelination. The lesions of ODS classically affect the pons, a neuroanatomic structure wherein the delay in the reaccumulation of osmotic osmolytes is particularly pronounced; clinically, patients with central pontine myelinolysis can present 1 or more days after overcorrection of hyponatremia with paraparesis or quadriparesis, dysphagia, dysarthria, diplopia, a "locked-in syndrome," and/or loss of consciousness. Other regions of the brain can also be involved in ODS, most commonly in association with lesions of the pons but occasionally in isolation; in order of frequency, the lesions of extrapontine myelinolysis can occur in the cerebellum, lateral geniculate body, thalamus, putamen, and cerebral cortex or subcortex. Clinical presentation of ODS can, therefore, vary as a function of the extent and localization of extrapontine myelinolysis, with the reported development of ataxia, mutism, parkinsonism, dystonia, and catatonia. Relowering of plasma Na^+ concentration after overly rapid correction can prevent or attenuate ODS (see the section on treatment of hyponatremia below). However, even appropriately slow correction can be associated with ODS, particularly in patients with additional risk factors; these include alcoholism, malnutrition, hypokalemia, and liver transplantation.

Diagnostic Evaluation of Hyponatremia Clinical assessment of hyponatremic patients should focus on the underlying cause; a detailed drug history is particularly crucial (Table 53-1). A careful clinical assessment of volume status is obligatory for the classical diagnostic approach to hyponatremia (Fig. 53-5). Hyponatremia is frequently multifactorial, particularly when severe; clinical evaluation should consider *all* the possible causes for excessive circulating AVP, including volume status, drugs, and the presence of nausea and/or pain. Radiologic imaging may also be appropriate to assess whether patients have a pulmonary or CNS cause for hyponatremia. A screening chest x-ray may fail to detect a small-cell carcinoma of the lung; computed tomography (CT) scanning of the thorax should be considered in patients at high risk for this tumor (e.g., patients with a smoking history).

Laboratory investigation should include a measurement of serum osmolality to exclude pseudohyponatremia, which is defined as the coexistence of hyponatremia with a normal or increased plasma tonicity. Most clinical laboratories measure plasma Na^+ concentration by testing diluted samples with automated ion-sensitive electrodes, correcting for this dilution by assuming that plasma is 93% water. This correction factor can be inaccurate in patients with pseudohyponatremia due to extreme hyperlipidemia and/or hyperproteinemia, in whom serum lipid or protein makes up a greater percentage of plasma volume. The measured osmolality should also be converted to the effective osmolality (tonicity) by subtracting the measured concentration of urea (divided by 2.8, if in mg/dL); patients with hyponatremia have an effective osmolality of <275 mOsm/kg.

Elevated BUN and creatinine in routine chemistries can also indicate renal dysfunction as a potential cause of hyponatremia, whereas hyperkalemia may suggest adrenal insufficiency or hypoaldosteronism. Serum glucose should also be measured; plasma Na^+ concentration falls by ~1.6–2.4 m*M* for every 100-mg/dL increase in glucose, due to glucose-induced water efflux from cells; this "true" hyponatremia resolves after correction of hyperglycemia. Measurement of serum uric acid should also be performed; whereas patients with SIAD-type physiology will typically be hypouricemic (serum uric acid <4 mg/dL), volume-depleted patients will often be hyperuricemic. In the appropriate clinical setting, thyroid, adrenal, and pituitary function should also be tested; hypothyroidism and secondary adrenal failure due to pituitary insufficiency are important causes of euvolemic hyponatremia, whereas primary adrenal failure causes hypovolemic hyponatremia. A cosyntropin stimulation test is necessary to assess for primary adrenal insufficiency.

Urine electrolytes and osmolality are crucial tests in the initial evaluation of hyponatremia. A urine Na^+ concentration <20–30 m*M* is consistent with hypovolemic hyponatremia, in the clinical absence of a hypervolemic, Na^+-avid syndrome such as CHF (Fig. 53-5). In contrast, patients with SIAD will typically excrete urine with an Na^+ concentration that is >30 m*M*. However, there can be substantial overlap in urine Na^+ concentration values in patients with SIAD and hypovolemic hyponatremia, particularly in the elderly; the ultimate "gold standard" for the diagnosis of hypovolemic hyponatremia is the demonstration that plasma Na^+ concentration corrects after hydration with normal saline. Patients with thiazide-associated hyponatremia may also present with higher than expected urine Na^+ concentration and other findings suggestive of SIAD; one should defer making a diagnosis of SIAD in these patients until 1–2 weeks after discontinuing the thiazide. A urine osmolality <100 mOsm/kg is suggestive of polydipsia; urine osmolality >400 mOsm/kg indicates that AVP excess is playing a more dominant role, whereas intermediate values are more consistent with multifactorial pathophysiology (e.g., AVP excess with a significant component of polydipsia). Patients with hyponatremia due to decreased solute intake (beer potomania) typically have urine Na^+ concentration <20 m*M* and urine osmolality in the range of <100 to the low 200s. Finally, the measurement of urine K^+ concentration is required to calculate the urine-to-plasma electrolyte ratio, which is useful to predict the response to fluid restriction (see the section on treatment of hyponatremia below).

TREATMENT

Hyponatremia

Three major considerations guide the therapy of hyponatremia. First, the presence and/or severity of symptoms determine the urgency and goals of therapy. Patients with acute hyponatremia

(Table 53-2) present with symptoms that can range from headache, nausea, and/or vomiting, to seizures, obtundation, and central herniation; patients with chronic hyponatremia, present for >48 h, are less likely to have severe symptoms. Second, patients with chronic hyponatremia are at risk for ODS if plasma Na^+ concentration is corrected by >8–10 m*M* within the first 24 h and/or by >18 m*M* within the first 48 h. Third, the response to interventions such as hypertonic saline, isotonic saline, or AVP antagonists can be highly unpredictable, such that frequent monitoring of plasma Na^+ concentration during corrective therapy is imperative.

Once the urgency in correcting the plasma Na^+ concentration has been established and appropriate therapy instituted, the focus should be on treatment or withdrawal of the underlying cause. Patients with euvolemic hyponatremia due to SIAD, hypothyroidism, or secondary adrenal failure will respond to successful treatment of the underlying cause, with an increase in plasma Na^+ concentration. However, not all causes of SIAD are immediately reversible, necessitating pharmacologic therapy to increase the plasma Na^+ concentration (see below). Hypovolemic hyponatremia will respond to intravenous hydration with isotonic normal saline, with a rapid reduction in circulating AVP and a brisk water diuresis; it may be necessary to reduce the rate of correction if the history suggests that hyponatremia has been chronic, i.e., present for >48 h (see below). Hypervolemic hyponatremia due to CHF will often respond to improved therapy of the underlying cardiomyopathy, e.g., following the institution or intensification of angiotensin-converting enzyme (ACE) inhibition. Finally, patients with hyponatremia due to beer potomania and low solute intake will respond very rapidly to intravenous saline and the resumption of a normal diet. Notably, patients with beer potomania have a very high risk of developing ODS, due to the associated hypokalemia, alcoholism, malnutrition, and high risk of overcorrecting the plasma Na^+ concentration.

Water deprivation has long been a cornerstone of the therapy of chronic hyponatremia. However, patients who are excreting minimal electrolyte-free water will require aggressive fluid restriction; this can be very difficult for patients with SIAD to tolerate, given that their thirst is also inappropriately stimulated. The urine-to-plasma electrolyte ratio (urinary $[Na^+]$ + $[K^+]$/plasma $[Na^+]$) can be exploited as a quick indicator of electrolyte-free water excretion (**Table 53-3**); patients with a ratio of >1 should be more aggressively restricted (<500 mL/d) if possible, those with a ratio of ~1 should be restricted to 500–700 mL/d, and those with a ratio <1 should be restricted to <1 L/d. In hypokalemic patients, potassium replacement will serve to increase plasma Na^+ concentration, given that the plasma Na^+ concentration is a function of both exchangeable Na^+ and exchangeable K^+ divided by total-body water; a corollary is that aggressive repletion of K^+ has the potential to overcorrect the plasma Na^+ concentration even in the absence of hypertonic saline. Plasma Na^+ concentration will also tend to respond to an increase in dietary solute intake, which increases the ability to excrete free water; this can be accomplished with oral salt tablets and with newly available, palatable preparations of oral urea.

Patients in whom therapy with fluid restriction, potassium replacement, and/or increased solute intake fails may merit pharmacologic therapy to increase their plasma Na^+ concentration. Some patients with SIAD initially respond to combined therapy with oral furosemide, 20 mg twice a day (higher doses may be necessary in renal insufficiency), and oral salt tablets; furosemide serves to inhibit the renal countercurrent mechanism and blunt urinary concentrating ability, whereas the salt tablets counteract diuretic-associated natriuresis. The risk of hypokalemia and/or renal dysfunction limits enthusiasm for this approach, which requires careful titration of diuretic and salt tablets. Demeclocycline is a potent inhibitor of principal cells and can be used in patients whose Na levels do not increase in response to furosemide and salt tablets. However, this agent can be associated with a reduction in GFR, due to excessive natriuresis and/or direct renal toxicity; it should be avoided in cirrhotic patients in particular, who are at higher risk of nephrotoxicity due to drug accumulation. If available, palatable preparations of oral urea can also be used to manage SIAD, with comparable efficacy to AVP antagonists (vaptans); the increase in solute excretion with oral urea ingestion increases free water excretion, thus reducing the plasma Na^+.

AVP antagonists (vaptans) are highly effective in SIAD and in hypervolemic hyponatremia due to heart failure or cirrhosis, reliably increasing plasma Na^+ concentration due to their "aquaretic" effects (augmentation of free water clearance). Most of these agents specifically antagonize the V_2 AVP receptor; tolvaptan is currently the only oral V_2 antagonist to be approved by the U.S. Food and Drug Administration. Conivaptan, the only available intravenous vaptan, is a mixed V_{1A}/V_2 antagonist, with a modest risk of hypotension due to V_{1A} receptor inhibition. Therapy with vaptans must be initiated in a hospital setting, with a liberalization of fluid restriction (>2 L/d) and close monitoring of plasma Na^+ concentration. Although approved for the management of all but hypovolemic hyponatremia and acute hyponatremia, the clinical indications are limited. Oral tolvaptan is perhaps most appropriate for the management of significant and persistent SIAD (e.g., in small-cell lung carcinoma) that has not responded to water restriction and/or oral furosemide and salt tablets. Abnormalities in liver function tests have been reported with chronic tolvaptan therapy; hence, the use of this agent should be restricted to <1–2 months.

Treatment of acute symptomatic hyponatremia should include hypertonic 3% saline (513 m*M*) to acutely increase plasma Na^+ concentration by 1–2 m*M*/h to a total of 4–6 m*M*; this modest increase is typically sufficient to alleviate severe acute symptoms, after which corrective guidelines for chronic hyponatremia are appropriate (see below). A bolus of 100 mL of hypertonic saline is more effective than an infusion, rapidly improving both serum sodium and mental status. For ongoing infusions, a number of equations have been developed to estimate the required rate of hypertonic saline, which has an Na^+-Cl^- concentration of 513 m*M*. The traditional approach is to calculate an Na^+ deficit, where the Na^+ deficit = 0.6 × body weight × (target plasma Na^+ concentration – starting plasma Na^+ concentration), followed by a calculation of the required rate. Regardless of the method used to determine the rate of administration, the increase in plasma Na^+ concentration can be highly unpredictable during treatment with hypertonic saline, due to rapid changes in the underlying physiology; plasma Na^+ concentration should be monitored every 2–4 h during treatment, with appropriate changes in therapy based on the observed rate of change. The administration of supplemental oxygen and ventilatory support is also critical in acute hyponatremia, in the event

TABLE 53-3 Management of Hypernatremia

Water Deficit
1. Estimate total-body water (TBW): 50% of body weight in women and 60% in men
2. Calculate free-water deficit: $[(Na^+ - 140)/140] \times TBW$
3. Administer deficit over 48–72 h, without decrease in plasma Na^+ concentration by >10 m*M*/24 h
Ongoing Water Losses
4. Calculate free-water clearance, C_eH_2O: $$C_eH_2O = V \times \left(1 - \frac{U_{Na} + U_K}{P_{Na}}\right)$$ where V is urinary volume, U_{Na} is urinary $[Na^+]$, U_K is urinary $[K^+]$, and P_{Na} is plasma $[Na^+]$
Insensible Losses
5. ~10 mL/kg per day: less if ventilated, more if febrile
Total
6. Add components to determine water deficit and ongoing water loss; correct the water deficit over 48–72 h and replace daily water loss. Avoid correction of plasma $[Na^+]$ by >10 m*M*/d.

that patients develop acute pulmonary edema or hypercapneic respiratory failure. Intravenous loop diuretics will help treat acute pulmonary edema and will also increase free water excretion, by interfering with the renal countercurrent multiplication system. AVP antagonists do *not* have an approved role in the management of acute hyponatremia.

The rate of correction should be comparatively slow in *chronic* hyponatremia (<6-8 m*M* in the first 24 h and <6 m*M* each subsequent 24h), so as to avoid ODS; lower target rates are appropriate in patients at particular risk for ODS, such as alcoholics or hypokalemic patients. Overcorrection of the plasma Na^+ concentration can occur when AVP levels rapidly normalize, for example, following the treatment of patients with chronic hypovolemic hyponatremia with intravenous saline or following glucocorticoid replacement of patients with hypopituitarism and secondary adrenal failure. Approximately 10% of patients treated with vaptans will overcorrect; the risk is increased if water intake is not liberalized. In the event that the plasma Na^+ concentration overcorrects following therapy, be it with hypertonic saline, isotonic saline, or a vaptan, hyponatremia can be safely reinduced or stabilized by the administration of the AVP *agonist* desmopressin acetate (DDAVP) and/or the administration of free water, typically intravenous D_5W; the goal is to prevent or reverse the development of ODS. Alternatively, the treatment of patients with marked hyponatremia can be initiated with the twice-daily administration of DDAVP to maintain constant AVP bioactivity, combined with the administration of hypertonic saline to slowly correct the serum sodium in a more controlled fashion, thus reducing upfront the risk of overcorrection.

HYPERNATREMIA

Etiology Hypernatremia is defined as an increase in the plasma Na^+ concentration to >145 m*M*. Considerably less common than hyponatremia, hypernatremia is nonetheless associated with mortality rates of as high as 40–60%, mostly due to the severity of the associated underlying disease processes. Hypernatremia is usually the result of a combined water and electrolyte deficit, with losses of H_2O in excess of Na^+. Less frequently, the ingestion or iatrogenic administration of excess Na^+ can be causative, for example, after IV administration of excessive hypertonic Na^+-Cl^- or Na^+-HCO_3^- **(Fig. 53-6)**.

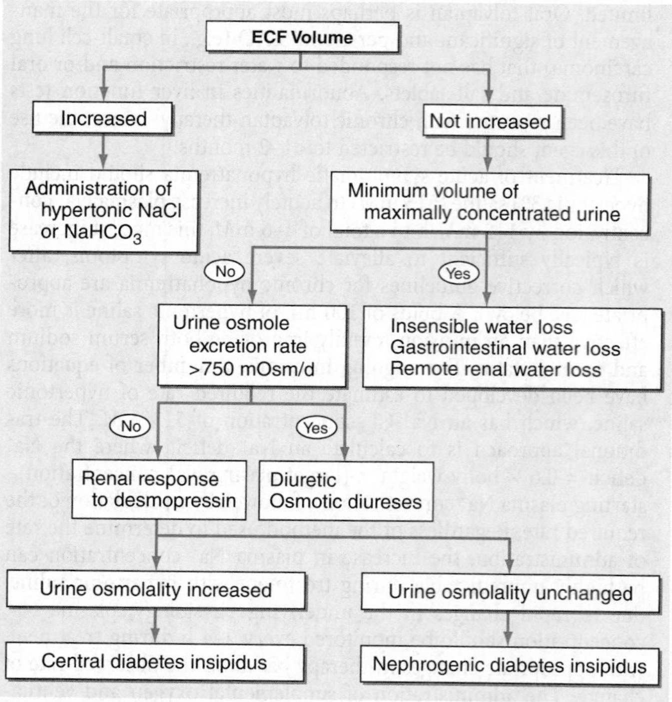

FIGURE 53-6 The diagnostic approach to hypernatremia. ECF, extracellular fluid.

Elderly individuals with reduced thirst and/or diminished access to fluids are at the highest risk of developing hypernatremia. Patients with hypernatremia may rarely have a central defect in hypothalamic osmoreceptor function, with a mixture of both decreased thirst and reduced AVP secretion. Causes of this adipsic DI include primary or metastatic tumor, occlusion or ligation of the anterior communicating artery, trauma, hydrocephalus, and inflammation.

Hypernatremia can develop following the loss of water via both renal and nonrenal routes. Insensible losses of water may increase in the setting of fever, exercise, heat exposure, severe burns, or mechanical ventilation. Diarrhea is, in turn, the most common gastrointestinal cause of hypernatremia. Notably, osmotic diarrhea and viral gastroenteritides typically generate stools with Na^+ and K^+ <100 m*M*, thus leading to water loss and hypernatremia; in contrast, secretory diarrhea typically results in isotonic stool and thus hypovolemia with or without hypovolemic hyponatremia.

Common causes of renal water loss include osmotic diuresis secondary to hyperglycemia, excess urea, postobstructive diuresis, or mannitol; these disorders share an increase in urinary solute excretion and urinary osmolality (see "Diagnostic Approach," below). Hypernatremia due to a water diuresis occurs in central or nephrogenic DI (NDI).

NDI is characterized by renal resistance to AVP, which can be partial or complete (see "Diagnostic Approach," below). Genetic causes include loss-of-function mutations in the X-linked V_2 receptor; mutations in the AVP-responsive aquaporin-2 water channel can cause autosomal recessive and autosomal dominant NDI, whereas recessive deficiency of the aquaporin-1 water channel causes a more modest concentrating defect (Fig. 53-2). Hypercalcemia can also cause polyuria and NDI; calcium signals directly through the calcium-sensing receptor to downregulate Na^+, K^+, and Cl^- transport by the TALH and water transport in principal cells, thus reducing renal concentrating ability in hypercalcemia. Another common acquired cause of NDI is hypokalemia, which inhibits the renal response to AVP and downregulates aquaporin-2 expression. Several drugs can cause acquired NDI, in particular, lithium, ifosfamide, and several antiviral agents. Lithium causes NDI by multiple mechanisms, including direct inhibition of renal glycogen synthase kinase-3 (GSK3), a kinase thought to be the pharmacologic target of lithium in bipolar disease; GSK3 is required for the response of principal cells to AVP. The entry of lithium through the amiloride-sensitive Na^+ channel ENaC (Fig. 53-4) is required for the effect of the drug on principal cells, such that combined therapy within lithium and amiloride can mitigate lithium-associated NDI. However, lithium causes chronic tubulointerstitial scarring and chronic kidney disease after prolonged therapy, such that patients may have a persistent NDI long after stopping the drug, with a reduced therapeutic benefit from amiloride.

Finally, gestational DI is a rare complication of late-term pregnancy wherein increased activity of a circulating placental protease with "vasopressinase" activity leads to reduced circulating AVP and polyuria, often accompanied by hypernatremia. DDAVP is an effective therapy for this syndrome, given its resistance to the vasopressinase enzyme.

Clinical Features Hypernatremia increases osmolality of the ECF, generating an osmotic gradient between the ECF and ICF, an efflux of intracellular water, and cellular shrinkage. As in hyponatremia, the symptoms of hypernatremia are predominantly neurologic. Altered mental status is the most frequent manifestation, ranging from mild confusion and lethargy to deep coma. The sudden shrinkage of brain cells in acute hypernatremia may lead to parenchymal or subarachnoid hemorrhages and/or subdural hematomas; however, these vascular complications are primarily encountered in pediatric and neonatal patients. Rarely, osmotic demyelination may occur in acute hypernatremia. Osmotic damage to muscle membranes can also lead to hypernatremic rhabdomyolysis. Brain cells accommodate to a chronic increase in ECF osmolality (>48 h) by activating membrane transporters that mediate influx and intracellular accumulation of organic osmolytes (creatine, betaine, glutamate, myoinositol, and taurine); this results in an increase in ICF water and normalization of brain parenchymal volume. In consequence, patients with *chronic* hypernatremia are less likely to develop severe neurologic compromise. However, the cellular response to chronic hypernatremia predisposes pediatric patients with hypernatremia, particularly infants, to the development of cerebral edema and seizures during overly rapid hydration (overcorrection of plasma Na^+ concentration by >10 m*M*/d). In critically ill adults, however, recent evidence does not indicate that rapid correction of hypernatremia is associated with a higher risk for mortality, seizure, alteration of consciousness, and/or cerebral edema. Given that restricting the rate of correction to <10 m*M*/d has no physiologic sequelae, it seems prudent to restrict correction in adults to this rate; however, should that rate be exceeded, hypernatremia does not need to be reinduced.

Diagnostic Approach The history should focus on the presence or absence of thirst, polyuria, and/or an extrarenal source for water loss, such as diarrhea. The physical examination should include a detailed neurologic exam and an assessment of the ECFV; patients with a particularly large water deficit and/or a combined deficit in electrolytes and water may be hypovolemic, with reduced JVP and orthostasis. Accurate documentation of daily fluid intake and daily urine output is also critical for the diagnosis and management of hypernatremia.

Laboratory investigation should include a measurement of serum and urine osmolality, in addition to urine electrolytes. The appropriate response to hypernatremia and a serum osmolality >295 mOsm/kg is an increase in circulating AVP and the excretion of low volumes (<500 mL/d) of maximally concentrated urine, i.e., urine with osmolality >800 mOsm/kg; should this be the case, then an extrarenal source of water loss is primarily responsible for the generation of hypernatremia. Many patients with hypernatremia are polyuric; should an osmotic diuresis be responsible, with excessive excretion of Na^+-Cl^-, glucose, and/or urea, then daily solute excretion will be >750–1000 mOsm/d (>15 mOsm/kg body water per day) (Fig. 53-6). More commonly, patients with hypernatremia and polyuria will have a predominant water diuresis, with excessive excretion of hypotonic, dilute urine.

Adequate differentiation between nephrogenic and central causes of DI requires the measurement of the response in urinary osmolality to DDAVP, combined with measurement of circulating AVP in the setting of hypertonicity. If measurement of serum copeptin is available, an "indirect water deprivation" test can be performed in patients with hypotonic polyuria without hypernatremia; if an infusion of hypertonic saline increases the level of circulating copeptin, a peptide co-secreted with AVP, then the patient suffers from polydipsia rather than central DI. By definition, patients with baseline hypernatremia are hypertonic, with an adequate stimulus for AVP by the posterior pituitary. Therefore, in contrast to polyuric patients with a normal or reduced baseline plasma Na^+ concentration and osmolality, a water deprivation test (**Chap. 52**) is unnecessary in hypernatremia; indeed, water deprivation is absolutely contraindicated in this setting, given the risk for worsening the hypernatremia. Hypernatremic patients with NDI will have high serum levels of AVP and copeptin. Their low urine osmolality will also fail to respond to DDAVP, increasing by <50% or <150 mOsm/kg from baseline; patients with central DI will respond to DDAVP, with a reduced circulating AVP and copeptin. Patients may exhibit a partial response to DDAVP, with a >50% rise in urine osmolality that nonetheless fails to reach 800 mOsm/kg; the level of circulating AVP will help differentiate the underlying cause, i.e., NDI versus central DI. In pregnant patients, AVP assays should be drawn in tubes containing the protease inhibitor 1,10-phenanthroline to prevent in vitro degradation of AVP by placental vasopressinase.

For patients with hypernatremia due to renal loss of water, it is critical to quantify *ongoing* daily losses using the calculated electrolyte-free water clearance, in addition to calculation of the baseline water deficit (the relevant formulas are discussed in Table 53-3). This requires daily measurement of urine electrolytes, combined with accurate measurement of daily urine volume.

TREATMENT

Hypernatremia

The underlying cause of hypernatremia should be withdrawn or corrected, be it drugs, hyperglycemia, hypercalcemia, hypokalemia, or diarrhea. The approach to the correction of hypernatremia is outlined in Table 53-3. It is imperative to correct hypernatremia slowly to avoid cerebral edema, typically replacing the calculated free water deficit over 48 h. Notably, the plasma Na^+ concentration should be corrected by no more than 10 m*M*/d, which may take longer than 48 h in patients with severe hypernatremia (>160 m*M*). A rare exception is patients with acute hypernatremia (<48 h) due to sodium loading, who can safely be corrected rapidly at a rate of 1 m*M*/h.

Water should ideally be administered by mouth or by nasogastric tube, as the most direct way to provide free water, i.e., water without electrolytes. Alternatively, patients can receive free water in dextrose-containing IV solutions, such as 5% dextrose (D_5W); blood glucose should be monitored in case hyperglycemia occurs. Depending on the history, blood pressure, or clinical volume status, it may be appropriate to initially treat with hypotonic saline solutions (1/4 or 1/2 normal saline); normal saline is usually inappropriate in the absence of very severe hypernatremia, where normal saline is proportionally more hypotonic relative to plasma, or frank hypotension. Calculation of urinary electrolyte-free water clearance (Table 53-3) is required to estimate daily, ongoing loss of free water in patients with NDI or central DI, which should be replenished daily.

Additional therapy may be feasible in specific cases. Patients with central DI should respond to the administration of intravenous, intranasal, or oral DDAVP. Patients with NDI due to lithium may reduce their polyuria with amiloride (2.5–10 mg/d), which decreases entry of lithium into principal cells by inhibiting ENaC (see above); in practice, however, most patients with lithium-associated DI are able to compensate for their polyuria by simply increasing their daily water intake. Thiazides may reduce polyuria due to NDI, ostensibly by inducing hypovolemia and increasing proximal tubular water reabsorption. Occasionally, nonsteroidal anti-inflammatory drugs (NSAIDs) have been used to treat polyuria associated with NDI, reducing the negative effect of intrarenal prostaglandins on urinary concentrating mechanisms; however, this assumes the risks of NSAID-associated gastric and/or renal toxicity. Furthermore, it must be emphasized that thiazides, amiloride, and NSAIDs are only appropriate for *chronic* management of polyuria from NDI and have *no* role in the acute management of associated hypernatremia, where the focus is on replacing free water deficits and ongoing free water loss.

POTASSIUM DISORDERS

Homeostatic mechanisms maintain plasma K^+ concentration between 3.5 and 5.0 m*M*, despite marked variation in dietary K^+ intake. In a healthy individual at steady state, the entire daily intake of potassium is excreted, ~90% in the urine and 10% in the stool; thus, the kidney plays a dominant role in potassium homeostasis. However, >98% of total-body potassium is intracellular, chiefly in muscle; buffering of extracellular K^+ by this large intracellular pool plays a crucial role in the regulation of plasma K^+ concentration. Changes in the exchange and distribution of intra- and extracellular K^+ can thus lead to marked hypo- or hyperkalemia. A corollary is that massive necrosis and the attendant release of tissue K^+ can cause severe hyperkalemia, particularly in the setting of acute kidney injury and reduced excretion of K^+.

Changes in whole-body K^+ content are primarily mediated by the kidney, which *reabsorbs* filtered K^+ in hypokalemic, K^+-deficient states and *secretes* K^+ in hyperkalemic, K^+-replete states. Although K^+ is transported along the entire nephron, it is the principal cells of the connecting segment (CNT) and cortical CD that play a dominant role in renal K^+ secretion, whereas alpha-intercalated cells of the outer medullary CD function in renal tubular reabsorption of filtered K^+ in K^+-deficient states. In principal cells, apical Na^+ entry via the amiloride-sensitive ENaC generates a lumen-negative potential difference, which drives passive K^+ exit through apical K^+ channels (Fig. 53-4). Two major K^+ channels mediate distal tubular K^+ secretion: the secretory K^+ channel ROMK (renal outer medullary K^+ channel; also known as Kir1.1 or KcnJ1) and the flow-sensitive "big potassium" (BK) or maxi-K

K$^+$ channel. ROMK is thought to mediate the bulk of constitutive K$^+$ secretion, whereas increases in distal flow rate and/or genetic absence of ROMK activate K$^+$ secretion via the BK channel.

An appreciation of the relationship between ENaC-dependent Na$^+$ entry and distal K$^+$ secretion (Fig. 53-4) is required for the bedside interpretation of potassium disorders. For example, decreased distal delivery of Na$^+$, as occurs in hypovolemic, prerenal states, tends to blunt the ability to excrete K$^+$, leading to hyperkalemia; on the other hand, an *increase* in distal delivery of Na$^+$ and distal flow rate, as occurs after treatment with thiazide and loop diuretics, can enhance K$^+$ secretion and lead to hypokalemia. Hyperkalemia is also a predictable consequence of drugs that directly inhibit ENaC, due to the role of this Na$^+$ channel in generating a lumen-negative potential difference. Aldosterone in turn has a major influence on potassium excretion, increasing the activity of ENaC channels and thus amplifying the driving force for K$^+$ secretion across the luminal membrane of principal cells. Abnormalities in the renin-angiotensin-aldosterone system can thus cause both hypokalemia and hyperkalemia. Notably, however, potassium excess and potassium restriction have opposing, aldosterone-independent effects on the density and activity of apical K$^+$ channels in the distal nephron, i.e., factors other than aldosterone modulate the renal capacity to secrete K$^+$. In addition, potassium restriction and hypokalemia activate aldosterone-independent distal *reabsorption* of filtered K$^+$, activating apical H$^+$/K$^+$-ATPase activity in intercalated cells within the outer medullary CD. Reflective perhaps of this physiology, changes in plasma K$^+$ concentration are not universal in disorders associated with changes in aldosterone activity.

HYPOKALEMIA

Hypokalemia, defined as a plasma K$^+$ concentration of <3.5 m*M*, occurs in up to 20% of hospitalized patients. Hypokalemia is associated with a tenfold increase in in-hospital mortality, due to adverse effects on cardiac rhythm, blood pressure, and cardiovascular morbidity. Mechanistically, hypokalemia can be caused by redistribution of K$^+$ between tissues and the ECF or by renal and nonrenal loss of K$^+$ (**Table 53-4**). Systemic hypomagnesemia can also cause treatment-resistant hypokalemia, due to a combination of reduced cellular uptake of K$^+$ and exaggerated renal secretion. Spurious hypokalemia or "pseudohypokalemia" can occasionally result from in vitro cellular uptake of K$^+$ after venipuncture, for example, due to profound leukocytosis in acute leukemia.

Redistribution and Hypokalemia Insulin, β_2-adrenergic activity, thyroid hormone, and alkalosis promote Na$^+$/K$^+$-ATPase-mediated cellular uptake of K$^+$, leading to hypokalemia. Inhibition of the passive *efflux* of K$^+$ can also cause hypokalemia, albeit rarely; this typically occurs in the setting of systemic inhibition of K$^+$ channels by toxic barium ions. Exogenous insulin can cause iatrogenic hypokalemia, particularly during the management of K$^+$-deficient states such as diabetic ketoacidosis. Alternatively, the stimulation of *endogenous* insulin can provoke hypokalemia, hypomagnesemia, and/or hypophosphatemia in malnourished patients given a carbohydrate load. Alterations in the activity of the endogenous sympathetic nervous system can cause hypokalemia in several settings, including alcohol withdrawal, hyperthyroidism, acute myocardial infarction, and severe head injury. β_2 agonists, including both bronchodilators and tocolytics (ritodrine), are powerful activators of cellular K$^+$ uptake; "hidden" sympathomimetics, such as pseudoephedrine and ephedrine in cough syrup or dieting agents, may also cause unexpected hypokalemia. Finally, xanthine-dependent activation of cAMP-dependent signaling, downstream of the β_2 receptor, can lead to hypokalemia, usually in the setting of overdose (theophylline) or marked overingestion (dietary caffeine).

Redistributive hypokalemia can also occur in the setting of hyperthyroidism, with periodic attacks of hypokalemic paralysis (thyrotoxic periodic paralysis [TPP]). Similar episodes of hypokalemic weakness in the absence of thyroid abnormalities occur in *familial* hypokalemic periodic paralysis, usually caused by missense mutations of voltage sensor domains within the α_1 subunit of L-type calcium channels or the skeletal Na$^+$ channel; these mutations generate an abnormal gating pore current activated by hyperpolarization. TPP develops more frequently in patients of Asian or Hispanic origin; this shared predisposition has been linked to genetic variation in Kir2.6, a muscle-specific, thyroid hormone–responsive K$^+$ channel. Genome-wide association studies have also implicated variation in the *KCNJ2* gene, which encodes a related muscle K$^+$ channel, Kir 2.1, in predisposition to TPP. Patients with TPP typically present with weakness of the extremities and limb girdles, with paralytic episodes that occur most frequently between 1 and 6 A.M. Signs and symptoms of hyperthyroidism are not invariably present. Hypokalemia is usually profound and almost invariably accompanied by hypophosphatemia and hypomagnesemia. The hypokalemia in TPP is also attributed to both direct and indirect activation of the Na$^+$/K$^+$-ATPase, resulting in increased uptake of K$^+$ by muscle

TABLE 53-4 Causes of Hypokalemia

I. Decreased intake
  A. Starvation
  B. Clay ingestion
II. Redistribution into cells
  A. Acid-base
    1. Metabolic alkalosis
  B. Hormonal
    1. Insulin
    2. Increased β_2-adrenergic sympathetic activity: post–myocardial infarction, head injury
    3. β_2-Adrenergic agonists—bronchodilators, tocolytics
    4. α-Adrenergic antagonists
    5. Thyrotoxic periodic paralysis
    6. Downstream stimulation of Na$^+$/K$^+$-ATPase: theophylline, caffeine
  C. Anabolic state
    1. Vitamin B_{12} or folic acid administration (red blood cell production)
    2. Granulocyte-macrophage colony-stimulating factor (white blood cell production)
    3. Total parenteral nutrition
  D. Other
    1. Pseudohypokalemia
    2. Hypothermia
    3. Familial hypokalemic periodic paralysis
    4. Barium toxicity: systemic inhibition of "leak" K$^+$ channels
III. Increased loss
  A. Nonrenal
    1. Gastrointestinal loss (diarrhea)
    2. Integumentary loss (sweat)
  B. Renal
    1. Increased distal flow and distal Na+ delivery: diuretics, osmotic diuresis, salt-wasting nephropathies
    2. Increased secretion of potassium
      a. Mineralocorticoid excess: primary hyperaldosteronism (aldosterone-producing adenomas, primary or unilateral adrenal hyperplasia, idiopathic hyperaldosteronism due to bilateral adrenal hyperplasia, and adrenal carcinoma), genetic hyperaldosteronism (familial hyperaldosteronism types I/II/III, congenital adrenal hyperplasias), secondary hyperaldosteronism (malignant hypertension, renin-secreting tumors, renal artery stenosis, hypovolemia), Cushing's syndrome, Bartter's syndrome, Gitelman's syndrome
      b. Apparent mineralocorticoid excess: genetic deficiency of 11β-dehydrogenase-2 (syndrome of apparent mineralocorticoid excess), inhibition of 11β-dehydrogenase-2 (glycyrrhetinic/glycyrrhizinic acid and/or carbenoxolone; itraconazole and posaconazole; licorice, food products, drugs), Liddle's syndrome (genetic activation of epithelial Na$^+$ channels)
      c. Distal delivery of nonreabsorbed anions: vomiting, nasogastric suction, proximal renal tubular acidosis, diabetic ketoacidosis, glue-sniffing (toluene abuse), penicillin derivatives (penicillin, nafcillin, dicloxacillin, ticarcillin, oxacillin, and carbenicillin)
    3. Magnesium deficiency

and other tissues. Increases in β-adrenergic activity play an important role in that high-dose propranolol (3 mg/kg) rapidly reverses the associated hypokalemia, hypophosphatemia, and paralysis. Outward-directed inward-rectifying K^+ current, mediated by KIR channels (primarily Kir2.1 and Kir2.2 tetramers), is also reduced in skeletal muscles of patients with TPP, providing an additional mechanism for hypokalemia. Together with increased Na^+/K^+-ATPase activity and increased circulating insulin, this reduced KIR current may trigger a "feedforward" cycle of hypokalemia leading to inactivation of muscle Na^+ channels, paradoxical depolarization, and paralysis.

Nonrenal Loss of Potassium The loss of K^+ in sweat is typically low, except under extremes of physical exertion. Direct gastric losses of K^+ due to vomiting or nasogastric suctioning are also minimal; however, the ensuing hypochloremic alkalosis results in persistent kaliuresis due to secondary hyperaldosteronism and bicarbonaturia, i.e., a *renal* loss of K^+. Diarrhea is a globally important cause of hypokalemia, given the worldwide prevalence of infectious diarrheal disease. Noninfectious gastrointestinal processes such as celiac disease, ileostomy, villous adenomas, inflammatory bowel disease, colonic pseudo-obstruction (Ogilvie's syndrome), VIPomas, and chronic laxative abuse can also cause significant hypokalemia; an exaggerated intestinal secretion of potassium by upregulated colonic BK channels has been directly implicated in the pathogenesis of hypokalemia in many of these disorders.

Renal Loss of Potassium Drugs can increase renal K^+ excretion by a variety of different mechanisms. Diuretics are a particularly common cause, due to associated increases in distal tubular Na^+ delivery and distal tubular flow rate, in addition to secondary hyperaldosteronism. Thiazides have a greater effect on plasma K^+ concentration than loop diuretics, despite their lesser natriuretic effect. The diuretic effect of thiazides is largely due to inhibition of the Na^+-Cl^- cotransporter NCC in DCT cells. This leads to a direct increase in the delivery of luminal Na^+ to the principal cells immediately downstream in the CNT and cortical CD, which augments Na^+ entry via ENaC, increases the lumen-negative potential difference, and amplifies K^+ secretion. The higher propensity of thiazides to cause hypokalemia may also be secondary to thiazide-associated hypocalciuria, versus the *hypercalciuria* seen with loop diuretics; the increases in downstream luminal calcium in response to loop diuretics inhibit ENaC in principal cells, thus reducing the lumen-negative potential difference and attenuating distal K^+ excretion. High doses of penicillin-related antibiotics (nafcillin, dicloxacillin, ticarcillin, oxacillin, and carbenicillin) can increase obligatory K^+ excretion by acting as nonreabsorbable anions in the distal nephron. Finally, several renal tubular toxins cause renal K^+ and magnesium wasting, leading to hypokalemia and hypomagnesemia; these drugs include aminoglycosides, amphotericin, foscarnet, cisplatin, and ifosfamide (see also "Magnesium Deficiency and Hypokalemia," below).

Aldosterone activates the ENaC channel in principal cells via multiple synergistic mechanisms, thus increasing the driving force for K^+ excretion. In consequence, increases in aldosterone bioactivity and/or gains in function of aldosterone-dependent signaling pathways are associated with hypokalemia. Increases in circulating aldosterone (hyperaldosteronism) may be primary or secondary. Increased levels of circulating renin in secondary forms of hyperaldosteronism lead to increased angiotensin II and thus aldosterone; renal artery stenosis is perhaps the most frequent cause (Table 53-4). Primary hyperaldosteronism may be genetic or acquired. Hypertension and hypokalemia, due to increases in circulating 11-deoxycorticosterone, occur in patients with congenital adrenal hyperplasia caused by defects in either steroid 11β-hydroxylase or steroid 17α-hydroxylase; deficient 11β-hydroxylase results in associated virilization and other signs of androgen excess, whereas reduced sex steroids in 17α-hydroxylase deficiency lead to hypogonadism.

The major forms of *isolated* primary genetic hyperaldosteronism are familial hyperaldosteronism type I (FH-I, also known as glucocorticoid-remediable hyperaldosteronism [GRA]) and familial hyperaldosteronism types II and III (FH-II and FH-III), in which aldosterone production is not repressible by exogenous glucocorticoids. FH-I is caused by a chimeric gene duplication between the homologous 11β-hydroxylase (*CYP11B1*) and aldosterone synthase (*CYP11B2*) genes, fusing the adrenocorticotropic hormone (ACTH)–responsive 11β-hydroxylase promoter to the coding region of aldosterone synthase; this chimeric gene is under the control of ACTH and thus repressible by glucocorticoids. FH-III is caused by mutations in the *KCNJ5* gene, which encodes the G protein–activated inward rectifier K^+ channel 4 (GIRK4); these mutations lead to the acquisition of sodium permeability in the mutant GIRK4 channels, causing an exaggerated membrane depolarization in adrenal glomerulosa cells and the activation of voltage-gated calcium channels. The resulting calcium influx is sufficient to produce aldosterone secretion and cell proliferation, leading to adrenal adenomas and hyperaldosteronism.

Acquired causes of primary hyperaldosteronism include aldosterone-producing adenomas (APAs), primary or unilateral adrenal hyperplasia (PAH), idiopathic hyperaldosteronism (IHA) due to bilateral adrenal hyperplasia, and adrenal carcinoma; APA and IHA account for close to 60% and 40%, respectively, of diagnosed hyperaldosteronism. Acquired somatic mutations in *KCNJ5* or less frequently in the *ATP1A1* (an Na^+/K^+ ATPase α subunit) and *ATP2B3* (a Ca^{2+} ATPase) genes can be detected in APAs; as in FH-III (see above), the exaggerated depolarization of adrenal glomerulosa cells caused by these mutations is implicated in the excessive adrenal proliferation and the exaggerated release of aldosterone.

Random testing of plasma renin activity (PRA) and aldosterone is a helpful screening tool in hypokalemic and/or hypertensive patients, with an aldosterone:PRA ratio of >50 suggestive of primary hyperaldosteronism. Hypokalemia and multiple antihypertensive drugs may alter the aldosterone:PRA ratio by suppressing aldosterone or increasing PRA, leading to a ratio of <50 in patients who do in fact have primary hyperaldosteronism; therefore, the clinical context should always be considered when interpreting these results.

The glucocorticoid cortisol has equal affinity for the MLR to that of aldosterone, with resultant "mineralocorticoid-like" activity. However, cells in the aldosterone-sensitive distal nephron are protected from this "illicit" activation by the enzyme 11β-hydroxysteroid dehydrogenase-2 (11βHSD-2), which converts cortisol to cortisone; cortisone has minimal affinity for the MLR. Recessive loss-of-function mutations in the *11βHSD-2* gene are thus associated with cortisol-dependent activation of the MLR and the syndrome of apparent mineralocorticoid excess (SAME), encompassing hypertension, hypokalemia, hypercalciuria, and metabolic alkalosis, with suppressed PRA and suppressed aldosterone. A similar syndrome is caused by biochemical inhibition of 11βHSD-2 by glycyrrhetinic/glycyrrhizinic acid and/or carbenoxolone. Glycyrrhizinic acid is a natural sweetener found in licorice root, typically encountered in licorice and its many guises or as a flavoring agent in tobacco and food products. More recently, the antifungals itraconazole and posaconazole have been shown to inhibit 11βHSD-2, leading to hypertension and hypokalemia.

Finally, hypokalemia may also occur with systemic increases in glucocorticoids. In Cushing's syndrome caused by increases in pituitary ACTH (**Chap. 386**), the incidence of hypokalemia is only 10%, whereas it is 60–100% in patients with ectopic secretion of ACTH, despite a similar incidence of hypertension. Indirect evidence suggests that the activity of renal 11βHSD-2 is reduced in patients with ectopic ACTH compared with Cushing's syndrome, resulting in SAME.

Finally, defects in multiple renal tubular transport pathways are associated with hypokalemia. For example, loss-of-function mutations in subunits of the acidifying H^+-ATPase in alpha-intercalated cells cause hypokalemic distal renal tubular acidosis, as do many acquired disorders of the distal nephron. Liddle's syndrome is caused by autosomal dominant gain-in-function mutations of ENaC subunits. Disease-associated mutations either activate the channel directly or abrogate aldosterone-inhibited retrieval of ENaC subunits from the plasma membrane; the end result is increased expression of activated ENaC channels at the plasma membrane of principal cells. Patients with Liddle's syndrome classically manifest severe hypertension with hypokalemia, unresponsive to spironolactone yet sensitive to amiloride. Hypertension and hypokalemia are, however, variable aspects of the Liddle's phenotype; more consistent features include a blunted aldosterone response to ACTH and reduced urinary aldosterone excretion.

Loss of the transport functions of the TALH and DCT nephron segments causes hereditary hypokalemic alkalosis and Bartter's syndrome (BS) and Gitelman's syndrome (GS), respectively. Patients with classic BS typically suffer from polyuria and polydipsia, due to the reduction in renal concentrating ability. They may have an increase in urinary calcium excretion, and 20% are hypomagnesemic. Other features include marked activation of the renin-angiotensin-aldosterone axis. Patients with antenatal BS suffer from a severe systemic disorder characterized by marked electrolyte wasting, polyhydramnios, and hypercalciuria with nephrocalcinosis; renal prostaglandin synthesis and excretion are significantly increased, accounting for much of the systemic symptoms. There are five disease genes for BS, all of them functioning in some aspect of regulated Na^+, K^+, and Cl^- transport by the TALH. In contrast, GS is genetically homogeneous, caused almost exclusively by loss-of-function mutations in the thiazide-sensitive Na^+-Cl^- cotransporter of the DCT. Patients with GS are uniformly hypomagnesemic and exhibit marked hypocalciuria, rather than the hypercalciuria typically seen in BS; urinary calcium excretion is thus a critical diagnostic test in GS. GS is a milder phenotype than BS; however, patients with GS may suffer from chondrocalcinosis, an abnormal deposition of calcium pyrophosphate dihydrate (CPPD) in joint cartilage (**Chap. 315**).

Magnesium Deficiency and Hypokalemia Magnesium depletion has inhibitory effects on muscle Na^+/K^+-ATPase activity, reducing influx into muscle cells and causing a secondary kaliuresis. In addition, magnesium depletion causes exaggerated K^+ secretion by the distal nephron; this effect is attributed to a reduction in the magnesium-dependent, intracellular block of K^+ efflux through the secretory K^+ channel of principal cells (ROMK; Fig. 53-4). In consequence, hypomagnesemic patients are clinically refractory to K^+ replacement in the absence of Mg^{2+} repletion. Notably, magnesium deficiency is also a common concomitant of hypokalemia because many disorders of the distal nephron may cause both potassium and magnesium wasting (**Chap. 315**).

Clinical Features Hypokalemia has prominent effects on cardiac, skeletal, and intestinal muscle cells. In particular, hypokalemia is a major risk factor for both ventricular and atrial arrhythmias. Hypokalemia predisposes to digoxin toxicity by a number of mechanisms, including reduced competition between K^+ and digoxin for shared binding sites on cardiac Na^+/K^+-ATPase subunits. Electrocardiographic changes in hypokalemia include broad flat T waves, ST depression, and QT prolongation; these are most marked when serum K^+ is <2.7 mmol/L. Hypokalemia can thus be an important precipitant of arrhythmia in patients with additional genetic or acquired causes of QT prolongation. Hypokalemia also results in hyperpolarization of skeletal muscle, thus impairing the capacity to depolarize and contract; weakness and even paralysis may ensue. It also causes a skeletal myopathy and predisposes to rhabdomyolysis. Finally, the paralytic effects of hypokalemia on intestinal smooth muscle may cause intestinal ileus.

The functional effects of hypokalemia on the kidney can include Na^+-Cl^- and HCO_3^- retention, polyuria, phosphaturia, hypocitraturia, and an activation of renal ammoniagenesis. Bicarbonate retention and other acid-base effects of hypokalemia can contribute to the generation of metabolic alkalosis. Hypokalemic polyuria is due to a combination of central polydipsia and an AVP-resistant renal concentrating defect. Structural changes in the kidney due to hypokalemia include a relatively specific vacuolizing injury to proximal tubular cells, interstitial nephritis, and renal cysts. Hypokalemia also predisposes to acute kidney injury and can lead to end-stage renal disease (ESRD) in patients with long-standing hypokalemia due to eating disorders and/or laxative abuse.

Hypokalemia and/or reduced dietary K^+ are implicated in the pathophysiology and progression of hypertension, heart failure, vascular disease, and stroke. For example, short-term K^+ restriction in healthy humans and patients with essential hypertension induces Na^+-Cl^- retention and hypertension. Correction of hypokalemia is particularly important in hypertensive patients treated with diuretics, in whom blood pressure improves with potassium supplementation and the establishment of normokalemia.

Diagnostic Approach The cause of hypokalemia is usually evident from history, physical examination, and/or basic laboratory tests. The history should focus on medications (e.g., laxatives, diuretics, antibiotics), diet and dietary habits (e.g., licorice), and/or symptoms that suggest a particular cause (e.g., periodic weakness, diarrhea). The physical examination should pay particular attention to blood pressure, volume status, and signs suggestive of specific hypokalemic disorders, e.g., hyperthyroidism and Cushing's syndrome. Initial laboratory evaluation should include electrolytes, BUN, creatinine, serum osmolality, Mg^{2+}, Ca^{2+}, a complete blood count, and urinary pH, osmolality, creatinine, and electrolytes (**Fig. 53-7**). The presence of a non–anion gap acidosis suggests a distal, hypokalemic renal tubular acidosis or diarrhea; calculation of the urinary anion gap can help differentiate these two diagnoses. Renal K^+ excretion can be assessed with a 24-h urine collection; a 24-h K^+ excretion of <15 mmol is indicative of an extrarenal cause of hypokalemia (Fig. 53-7). If only a random, spot urine sample is available, serum and urine osmolality can be used to calculate the transtubular K^+ gradient (TTKG), which should be <3 in the presence of hypokalemia (see also "Hyperkalemia"). Alternatively, a urinary K^+-to-creatinine ratio of >13 mmol/g creatinine (>1.5 mmol/mmol creatinine) is compatible with excessive renal K^+ excretion. Urine Cl^- is usually decreased in patients with hypokalemia from a nonreabsorbable anion, such as antibiotics or HCO_3^-. The most common causes of chronic hypokalemic alkalosis are surreptitious vomiting, diuretic abuse, and GS; these can be distinguished by the pattern of urinary electrolytes. Hypokalemic patients with vomiting due to bulimia will thus typically have a urinary Cl^- <10 mmol/L; urine Na^+, K^+, and Cl^- are persistently elevated in GS, due to loss of function in the thiazide-sensitive Na^+-Cl^- cotransporter, but less elevated in diuretic abuse and with greater variability. Urine diuretic screens for loop diuretics and thiazides may be necessary to further exclude diuretic abuse.

Other tests, such as urinary Ca^{2+}, thyroid function tests, and/or PRA and aldosterone levels, may also be appropriate in specific cases. A plasma aldosterone:PRA ratio of >50, due to suppression of circulating renin and an elevation of circulating aldosterone, is suggestive of hyperaldosteronism. Patients with hyperaldosteronism or apparent mineralocorticoid excess may require further testing, for example, adrenal vein sampling (**Chap. 386**) or the clinically available testing for specific genetic causes (e.g., FH-I, SAME, Liddle's syndrome). Patients with primary aldosteronism should thus be tested for the chimeric FH-I/GRA gene (see above) if they are younger than 20 years of age or have a family history of primary aldosteronism or stroke at a young age (<40 years). Preliminary differentiation of Liddle's syndrome due to mutant ENaC channels from SAME due to mutant 11βHSD-2 (see above), both of which cause hypokalemia and hypertension with aldosterone suppression, can be made on a clinical basis and then confirmed by genetic analysis; patients with Liddle's syndrome should respond to amiloride (ENaC inhibition) but not spironolactone, whereas patients with SAME will respond to spironolactone.

TREATMENT

Hypokalemia

The goals of therapy in hypokalemia are to prevent life-threatening and/or serious chronic consequences, to replace the associated K^+ deficit, and to correct the underlying cause and/or mitigate future hypokalemia. The urgency of therapy depends on the severity of hypokalemia, associated clinical factors (e.g., cardiac disease, digoxin therapy), and the rate of decline in serum K^+. Patients with a prolonged QT interval and/or other risk factors for arrhythmia should be monitored by continuous cardiac telemetry during repletion. Urgent but cautious K^+ replacement should be considered in patients with severe redistributive hypokalemia (plasma K^+ concentration <2.5 m*M*) and/or when serious complications ensue; however, this approach has a risk of rebound hyperkalemia following

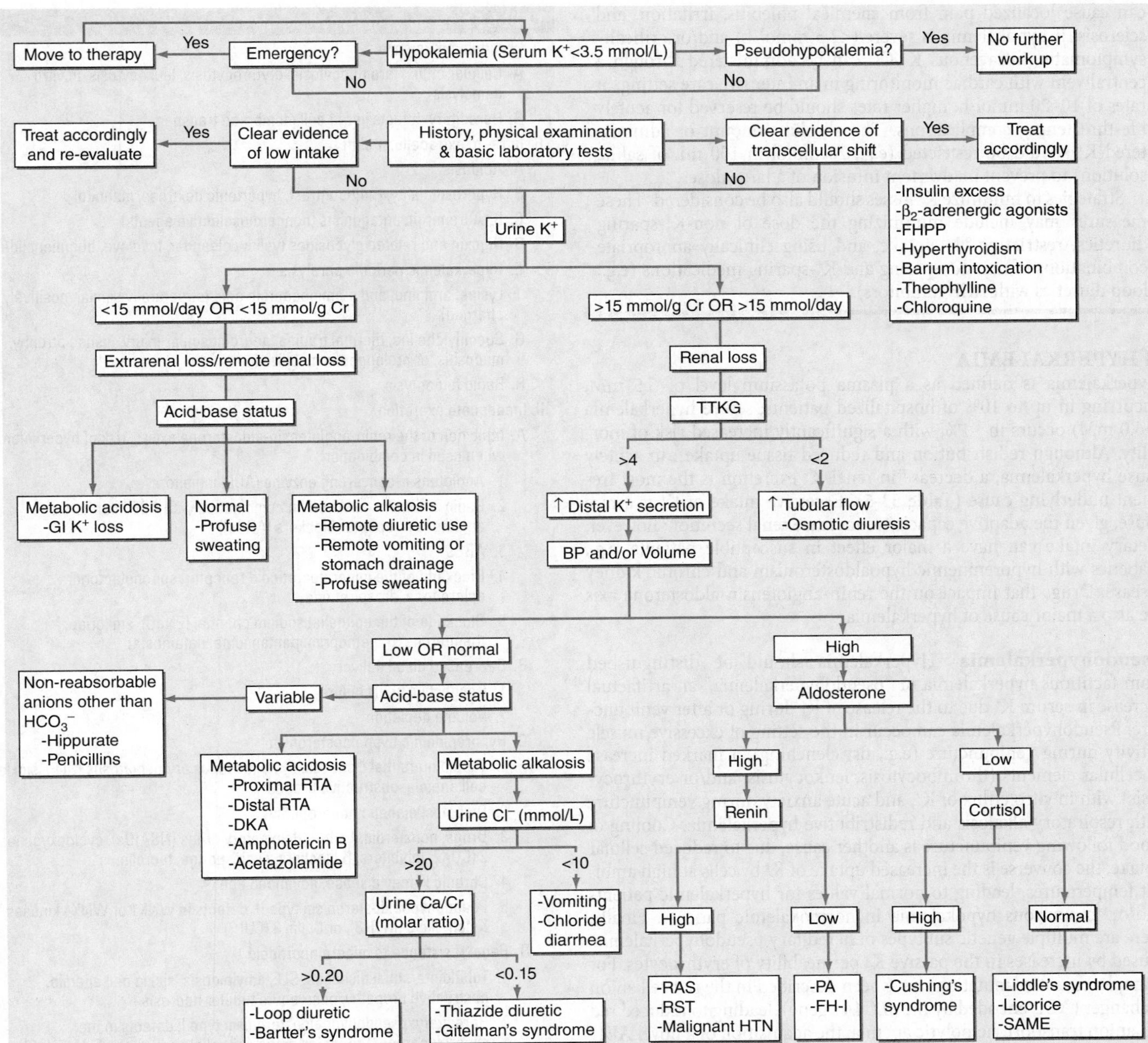

FIGURE 53-7 The diagnostic approach to hypokalemia. See text for details. AME, apparent mineralocorticoid excess; BP, blood pressure; CCD, cortical collecting duct; DKA, diabetic ketoacidosis; FH-I, familial hyperaldosteronism type I; FHPP, familial hypokalemic periodic paralysis; GI, gastrointestinal; GRA, glucocorticoid remediable aldosteronism; HTN, hypertension; PA, primary aldosteronism; RAS, renal artery stenosis; RST, renin-secreting tumor; RTA, renal tubular acidosis; SAME, syndrome of apparent mineralocorticoid excess; TTKG, transtubular potassium gradient. *(Reproduced with permission from DB Mount, K Zandi-Nejad: Disorders of potassium balance, in BM Brenner [ed], Brenner and Rector's The Kidney, 8th ed, Philadelphia, W.B. Saunders & Company, 2008.)*

acute resolution of the underlying cause. When excessive activity of the sympathetic nervous system is thought to play a dominant role in redistributive hypokalemia, as in TPP, theophylline overdose, and acute head injury, high-dose propranolol (3 mg/kg) should be considered; this nonspecific β-adrenergic blocker will correct hypokalemia without the risk of rebound hyperkalemia.

Oral replacement with K^+-Cl^- is the mainstay of therapy in hypokalemia. Potassium phosphate, oral or IV, may be appropriate in patients with combined hypokalemia and hypophosphatemia. Potassium bicarbonate or potassium citrate should be considered in patients with concomitant metabolic acidosis. Notably, hypomagnesemic patients are refractory to K^+ replacement alone, such that concomitant Mg^{2+} deficiency should *always* be corrected with oral or intravenous repletion. The deficit of K^+ and the rate of correction should be estimated as accurately as possible; renal function, medications, and comorbid conditions such as diabetes should also be considered, so as to gauge the risk of overcorrection. In the absence of abnormal K^+ redistribution, the total deficit correlates with serum K^+, such that serum K^+ drops by ~0.27 m*M* for every 100-mmol reduction in total-body stores; loss of 400–800 mmol of total-body K^+ results in a reduction in serum K^+ by ~2.0 m*M*. Notably, given the delay in redistributing potassium into intracellular compartments, this deficit must be replaced gradually over 24–48 h, with frequent monitoring of plasma K^+ concentration to avoid transient overrepletion and transient hyperkalemia.

The use of intravenous administration should be limited to patients unable to use the enteral route or in the setting of severe complications (e.g., paralysis, arrhythmia). Intravenous K^+-Cl^- should always be administered in saline solutions, rather than dextrose, because the dextrose-induced increase in insulin can acutely exacerbate hypokalemia. The peripheral intravenous dose is usually 20–40 mmol of K^+-Cl^- per liter; higher concentrations can cause localized pain from chemical phlebitis, irritation, and sclerosis. If hypokalemia is severe (<2.5 mmol/L) and/or critically symptomatic, intravenous K^+-Cl^- can be administered through a central vein with cardiac monitoring in an intensive care setting, at rates of 10–20 mmol/h; higher rates should be reserved for acutely life-threatening complications. The absolute amount of administered K^+ should be restricted (e.g., 20 mmol in 100 mL of saline solution) to prevent inadvertent infusion of a large dose.

Strategies to minimize K^+ losses should also be considered. These measures may include minimizing the dose of non-K^+-sparing diuretics, restricting Na^+ intake, and using clinically appropriate combinations of non-K^+-sparing and K^+-sparing medications (e.g., loop diuretics with ACE inhibitors).

HYPERKALEMIA

Hyperkalemia is defined as a plasma potassium level of 5.5 m*M*, occurring in up to 10% of hospitalized patients; severe hyperkalemia (>6.0 m*M*) occurs in ~1%, with a significantly increased risk of mortality. Although redistribution and reduced tissue uptake can acutely cause hyperkalemia, a decrease in renal K^+ excretion is the most frequent underlying cause (**Table 53-5**). Excessive intake of K^+ is a rare cause, given the adaptive capacity to increase renal secretion; however, dietary intake can have a major effect in susceptible patients, e.g., diabetics with hyporeninemic hypoaldosteronism and chronic kidney disease. Drugs that impact on the renin-angiotensin-aldosterone axis are also a major cause of hyperkalemia.

Pseudohyperkalemia Hyperkalemia should be distinguished from factitious hyperkalemia or "pseudohyperkalemia," an artifactual increase in serum K^+ due to the release of K^+ during or after venipuncture. Pseudohyperkalemia can occur in the setting of excessive muscle activity during venipuncture (e.g., fist clenching), a marked increase in cellular elements (thrombocytosis, leukocytosis, and/or erythrocytosis) with in vitro efflux of K^+, and acute anxiety during venipuncture with respiratory alkalosis and redistributive hyperkalemia. Cooling of blood following venipuncture is another cause, due to reduced cellular uptake; the converse is the increased uptake of K^+ by cells at high ambient temperatures, leading to normal values for hyperkalemic patients and/or to spurious hypokalemia in normokalemic patients. Finally, there are multiple genetic subtypes of hereditary pseudohyperkalemia, caused by increases in the passive K^+ permeability of erythrocytes. For example, causative mutations have been described in the red cell anion exchanger (AE1, encoded by the *SLC4A1* gene), leading to reduced red cell anion transport, hemolytic anemia, the acquisition of a novel AE1-mediated K^+ leak, and pseudohyperkalemia.

Redistribution and Hyperkalemia Several different mechanisms can induce an efflux of intracellular K^+ and hyperkalemia. Acidemia is associated with cellular uptake of H^+ and an associated efflux of K^+; it is thought that this effective K^+-H^+ exchange serves to help maintain extracellular pH. Notably, this effect of acidosis is limited to non–anion gap causes of metabolic acidosis and, to a lesser extent, respiratory causes of acidosis; hyperkalemia due to an acidosis-induced shift of potassium from the cells into the ECF does *not* occur in the anion gap acidoses lactic acidosis and ketoacidosis. Hyperkalemia due to hypertonic mannitol, hypertonic saline, and intravenous immune globulin is generally attributed to a "solvent drag" effect, as water moves out of cells along the osmotic gradient. Diabetics are also prone to osmotic hyperkalemia in response to intravenous hypertonic glucose, when given without adequate insulin. Cationic amino acids, specifically lysine, arginine, and the structurally related drug epsilon-aminocaproic acid, cause efflux of K^+ and hyperkalemia, through an effective cation-K^+ exchange of unknown identity and mechanism. Digoxin inhibits Na^+/K^+-ATPase and impairs the uptake of K^+ by skeletal muscle, such that digoxin overdose predictably results in hyperkalemia. Structurally related glycosides are found in specific plants (e.g., yellow oleander, foxglove) and in the cane toad, *Bufo marinus* (bufadienolide); ingestion of these substances and extracts thereof can also

TABLE 53-5 Causes of Hyperkalemia

I. Pseudohyperkalemia
   - A. Cellular efflux; thrombocytosis, erythrocytosis, leukocytosis, in vitro hemolysis
   - B. Hereditary defects in red cell membrane transport

II. Intra- to extracellular shift
   - A. Acidosis
   - B. Hyperosmolality; radiocontrast, hypertonic dextrose, mannitol
   - C. β_2-Adrenergic antagonists (noncardioselective agents)
   - D. Digoxin and related glycosides (yellow oleander, foxglove, bufadienolide)
   - E. Hyperkalemic periodic paralysis
   - F. Lysine, arginine, and ε-aminocaproic acid (structurally similar, positively charged)
   - G. Succinylcholine; thermal trauma, neuromuscular injury, disuse atrophy, mucositis, or prolonged immobilization
   - H. Rapid tumor lysis

III. Inadequate excretion
   - A. Inhibition of the renin-angiotensin-aldosterone axis; ↑ risk of hyperkalemia when used in combination
     1. Angiotensin-converting enzyme (ACE) inhibitors
     2. Renin inhibitors; aliskiren (in combination with ACE inhibitors or angiotensin receptor blockers [ARBs])
     3. ARBs
     4. Blockade of the mineralocorticoid receptor: spironolactone, eplerenone, drospirenone
     5. Blockade of the epithelial sodium channel (ENaC): amiloride, triamterene, trimethoprim, pentamidine, nafamostat
   - B. Decreased distal delivery
     1. Congestive heart failure
     2. Volume depletion
   - C. Hyporeninemic hypoaldosteronism
     1. Tubulointerstitial diseases: systemic lupus erythematosus (SLE), sickle cell anemia, obstructive uropathy
     2. Diabetes, diabetic nephropathy
     3. Drugs: nonsteroidal anti-inflammatory drugs (NSAIDs), cyclooxygenase 2 (COX2) inhibitors, β blockers, cyclosporine, tacrolimus
     4. Chronic kidney disease, advanced age
     5. Pseudohypoaldosteronism type II: defects in WNK1 or WNK4 kinases, Kelch-like 3 (KLHL3), or Cullin 3 (CUL3)
   - D. Renal resistance to mineralocorticoid
     1. Tubulointerstitial diseases: SLE, amyloidosis, sickle cell anemia, obstructive uropathy, post–acute tubular necrosis
     2. Hereditary: pseudohypoaldosteronism type I; defects in the mineralocorticoid receptor *or* the epithelial sodium channel (ENaC)
   - E. Advanced renal insufficiency
     1. Chronic kidney disease
     2. End-stage renal disease
     3. Acute oliguric kidney injury
   - F. Primary adrenal insufficiency
     1. Autoimmune: Addison's disease, polyglandular endocrinopathy
     2. Infectious: HIV, cytomegalovirus, tuberculosis, disseminated fungal infection
     3. Infiltrative: amyloidosis, malignancy, metastatic cancer
     4. Drug-associated: heparin, low-molecular-weight heparin
     5. Hereditary: adrenal hypoplasia congenita, congenital lipoid adrenal hyperplasia, aldosterone synthase deficiency
     6. Adrenal hemorrhage or infarction, including in antiphospholipid syndrome

cause hyperkalemia. Finally, fluoride ions also inhibit Na^+/K^+-ATPase, such that fluoride poisoning is typically associated with hyperkalemia.

Succinylcholine depolarizes muscle cells, causing an efflux of K^+ through acetylcholine receptors (AChRs). The use of this agent is contraindicated in patients who have sustained thermal trauma, neuromuscular injury, disuse atrophy, mucositis, or prolonged immobilization.

These disorders share a marked increase and redistribution of AChRs at the plasma membrane of muscle cells; depolarization of these upregulated AChRs by succinylcholine leads to an exaggerated efflux of K^+ through the receptor-associated cation channels, resulting in acute hyperkalemia.

Hyperkalemia Caused by Excess Intake or Tissue Necrosis Increased intake of even small amounts of K^+ may provoke severe hyperkalemia in patients with predisposing factors; hence, an assessment of dietary intake is crucial. Foods rich in potassium include tomatoes, bananas, and citrus fruits; occult sources of K^+, particularly K^+-containing salt substitutes, may also contribute significantly. Iatrogenic causes include simple overreplacement with K^+-Cl^- or the administration of a potassium-containing medication (e.g., K^+-penicillin) to a susceptible patient. Red cell transfusion is a well-described cause of hyperkalemia, typically in the setting of massive transfusions. Finally, severe tissue necrosis, as in acute tumor lysis syndrome and rhabdomyolysis, will predictably cause hyperkalemia from the release of intracellular K^+.

Hypoaldosteronism and Hyperkalemia Aldosterone release from the adrenal gland may be reduced by hyporeninemic hypoaldosteronism, medications, primary hypoaldosteronism, or isolated deficiency of ACTH (secondary hypoaldosteronism). Primary hypoaldosteronism may be genetic or acquired **(Chap. 386)** but is commonly caused by autoimmunity, either in Addison's disease or in the context of a polyglandular endocrinopathy. HIV has surpassed tuberculosis as the most important infectious cause of adrenal insufficiency. The adrenal involvement in HIV disease is usually subclinical; however, adrenal insufficiency may be precipitated by stress, drugs such as ketoconazole that inhibit steroidogenesis, or the acute withdrawal of steroid agents such as megestrol. Among medications associated with hyperkalemia, heparin preparations can cause selective inhibition of aldosterone synthesis by zona glomerulosa cells, leading to hyperreninemic hypoaldosteronism.

Hyporeninemic hypoaldosteronism is a very common predisposing factor in several overlapping subsets of hyperkalemic patients: diabetics, the elderly, and patients with renal insufficiency. Classically, patients should have suppressed PRA and aldosterone; ~50% have an associated acidosis, with a reduced renal excretion of NH_4^+, a positive urinary anion gap, and urine pH <5.5. Most patients are volume expanded, with secondary increases in circulating atrial natriuretic peptide (ANP) that inhibit both renal renin release and adrenal aldosterone release.

Renal Disease and Hyperkalemia Chronic kidney disease and end-stage kidney disease are very common causes of hyperkalemia, due to the associated deficit or absence of functioning nephrons. Hyperkalemia is more common in oliguric acute kidney injury; distal tubular flow rate and Na^+ delivery are less limiting factors in nonoliguric patients. Hyperkalemia out of proportion to GFR can also be seen in the context of tubulointerstitial disease that affects the distal nephron, such as amyloidosis, sickle cell anemia, interstitial nephritis, and obstructive uropathy.

Hereditary renal causes of hyperkalemia have overlapping clinical features with hypoaldosteronism, hence the diagnostic label *pseudohypoaldosteronism* (PHA). PHA type I (PHA-I) has both an autosomal recessive and an autosomal dominant form. The autosomal dominant form is due to loss-of-function mutations in the MLR; the recessive form is caused by various combinations of mutations in the three subunits of ENaC, resulting in impaired Na^+ channel activity in principal cells and other tissues. Patients with recessive PHA-I suffer from lifelong salt wasting, hypotension, and hyperkalemia, whereas the phenotype of autosomal dominant PHA-I due to MLR dysfunction improves in adulthood. PHA type II (PHA-II; also known as *hereditary hypertension with hyperkalemia*) is in every respect the mirror image of GS caused by loss of function in NCC, the thiazide-sensitive Na^+-Cl^- cotransporter (see above); the clinical phenotype includes hypertension, hyperkalemia, hyperchloremic metabolic acidosis, suppressed PRA and aldosterone, hypercalciuria, and reduced bone density. PHA-II thus behaves like a gain of function in NCC, and treatment with thiazides results in resolution of the entire clinical phenotype. However, the NCC gene is not directly involved in PHA-II, which is caused by mutations in the WNK1 and WNK4 serine-threonine kinases or the upstream Kelch-like 3 (KLHL3) and Cullin 3 (CUL3) proteins, two components of an E3 ubiquitin ligase complex that regulates these kinases; these proteins collectively regulate NCC activity, with PHA-II-associated activation of the transporter.

Medication-Associated Hyperkalemia Most medications associated with hyperkalemia cause inhibition of some component of the renin-angiotensin-aldosterone axis. ACE inhibitors, angiotensin receptor blockers, renin inhibitors, and MLRs are predictable and common causes of hyperkalemia, particularly when prescribed in combination. The oral contraceptive agent Yasmin-28 contains the progestin drospirenone, which inhibits the MLR and can cause hyperkalemia in susceptible patients. Cyclosporine, tacrolimus, NSAIDs, and cyclooxygenase 2 (COX2) inhibitors cause hyperkalemia by multiple mechanisms, but share the ability to cause hyporeninemic hypoaldosteronism. Notably, most drugs that affect the renin-angiotensin-aldosterone axis also block the local adrenal response to hyperkalemia, thus attenuating the *direct* stimulation of aldosterone release by increased plasma K^+ concentration.

Inhibition of apical ENaC activity in the distal nephron by amiloride and other K^+-sparing diuretics results in hyperkalemia, often with a voltage-dependent hyperchloremic acidosis and/or hypovolemic hyponatremia. Amiloride is structurally similar to the antibiotics TMP and pentamidine, which also block ENaC; risk factors for TMP-associated hyperkalemia include the administered dose, renal insufficiency, and hyporeninemic hypoaldosteronism. Indirect inhibition of ENaC at the plasma membrane is also a cause of drug-associated hyperkalemia; nafamostat, a protease inhibitor used in some countries for anticoagulation and for the management of pancreatitis, inhibits aldosterone-induced renal proteases that activate ENaC by proteolytic cleavage.

Clinical Features Hyperkalemia is a medical emergency due to its effects on the heart. Cardiac arrhythmias associated with hyperkalemia include sinus bradycardia, sinus arrest, slow idioventricular rhythms, ventricular tachycardia, ventricular fibrillation, and asystole. Mild increases in extracellular K^+ affect the repolarization phase of the cardiac action potential, resulting in changes in T-wave morphology; further increase in plasma K^+ concentration depresses intracardiac conduction, with progressive prolongation of the PR and QRS intervals. Severe hyperkalemia results in loss of the P wave and a progressive widening of the QRS complex; development of a sine-wave sinoventricular rhythm suggests impending ventricular fibrillation or asystole. Hyperkalemia can also cause a type I Brugada pattern in the electrocardiogram (ECG), with a pseudo–right bundle branch block and persistent coved ST-segment elevation in at least two precordial leads. This hyperkalemic Brugada's sign occurs in critically ill patients with severe hyperkalemia and can be differentiated from genetic Brugada's syndrome by an absence of P waves, marked QRS widening, and an abnormal QRS axis. Classically, the ECG manifestations in hyperkalemia progress from tall peaked T waves (5.5–6.5 m*M*), to a loss of P waves (6.5–7.5 m*M*), to a widened QRS complex (7.0–8.0 m*M*), and, ultimately, a to a sine wave pattern (>8.0 m*M*). However, these changes are notoriously insensitive, particularly in patients with chronic kidney disease or ESRD.

Hyperkalemia from a variety of causes can also present with ascending paralysis, denoted *secondary hyperkalemic paralysis* to differentiate it from familial hyperkalemic periodic paralysis (HYPP). The presentation may include diaphragmatic paralysis and respiratory failure. Patients with familial HYPP develop myopathic weakness during hyperkalemia induced by increased K^+ intake or rest after heavy exercise. Depolarization of skeletal muscle by hyperkalemia unmasks an inactivation defect in skeletal Na^+ channel; autosomal dominant mutations in the *SCN4A* gene encoding this channel are the predominant cause.

Within the kidney, hyperkalemia has negative effects on the ability to excrete an acid load, such that hyperkalemia per se can contribute to metabolic acidosis. This defect appears to be due in part to competition between K^+ and NH_4^+ for reabsorption by the TALH and subsequent countercurrent multiplication, ultimately reducing the medullary gradient for NH_3/NH_4 excretion by the distal nephron. Regardless of the underlying mechanism, restoration of normokalemia can, in many instances, correct hyperkalemic metabolic acidosis.

Diagnostic Approach The first priority in the management of hyperkalemia is to assess the need for emergency treatment, followed by a comprehensive workup to determine the cause (**Fig. 53-8**). History and physical examination should focus on medications, diet and dietary supplements, risk factors for kidney failure, reduction in urine output, blood pressure, and volume status. Initial laboratory tests should include electrolytes, BUN, creatinine, serum osmolality, Mg^{2+} and Ca^{2+}, a complete blood count, and urinary pH, osmolality, creatinine, and electrolytes. A urine Na^+ concentration of <20 m*M* indicates that distal Na^+ delivery is a limiting factor in K^+ excretion; volume repletion with 0.9% saline or treatment with furosemide may be effective in reducing plasma K^+ concentration. Serum and urine osmolality are required for calculation of the transtubular K^+ gradient (TTKG) (Fig. 53-8). The expected values of the TTKG are largely based on historical data, and are <3 in the presence of hypokalemia and >7–8 in the presence of hyperkalemia. Notably, some authors have opined that the TTKG does not consider the effects of distal tubular urea reabsorption on potassium excretion, concluding that the TTKG is, thus, an unreliable test in the assessment of hyperkalemia. These criticisms are theoretical and not supported by animal experiments; the TTKG remains a helpful bedside test of urinary potassium excretion in hyperkalemia.

$$\text{TTKG} = \frac{[K^+]_{\text{urine}} \times \text{Osm}_{\text{serum}}}{[K^+]_{\text{serum}} \times \text{Osm}_{\text{urine}}}$$

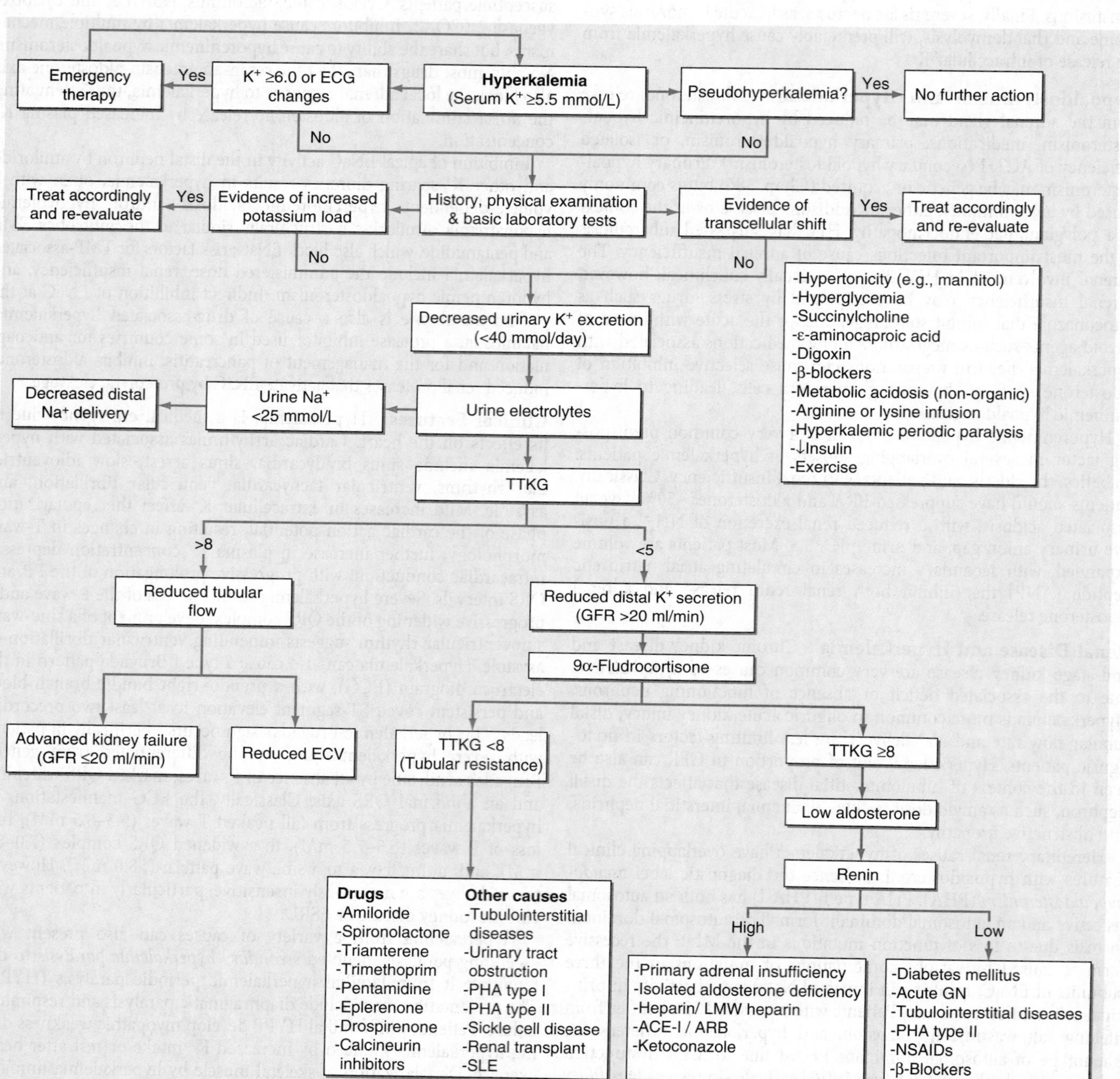

FIGURE 53-8 The diagnostic approach to hyperkalemia. See text for details. ACE-I, angiotensin-converting enzyme inhibitor; ARB, angiotensin II receptor blocker; CCD, cortical collecting duct; ECG, electrocardiogram; ECV, effective circulatory volume; GFR, glomerular filtration rate; GN, glomerulonephritis; HIV, human immunodeficiency virus; LMW heparin, low-molecular-weight heparin; NSAIDs, nonsteroidal anti-inflammatory drugs; PHA, pseudohypoaldosteronism; SLE, systemic lupus erythematosus; TTKG, transtubular potassium gradient. *(Reproduced with permission from DB Mount, K Zandi-Nejad: Disorders of potassium balance, in BM Brenner [ed], Brenner and Rector's The Kidney, 8th ed, Philadelphia, W.B. Saunders & Company, 2008.)*

TREATMENT

Hyperkalemia

ECG manifestations of hyperkalemia should be considered a medical emergency and treated urgently. However, patients with significant hyperkalemia (plasma K^+ concentration ≥6.5 m*M*) in the absence of ECG changes should also be aggressively managed, given the limitations of ECG changes as a predictor of cardiac toxicity. Urgent management of hyperkalemia includes admission to the hospital, continuous cardiac monitoring, and immediate treatment. The treatment of hyperkalemia is divided into three stages:

1. *Immediate antagonism of the cardiac effects of hyperkalemia.* Intravenous calcium serves to protect the heart, whereas other measures are taken to correct hyperkalemia. Calcium raises the action potential threshold and reduces excitability, without changing the resting membrane potential. By restoring the difference between resting and threshold potentials, calcium reverses the depolarization blockade due to hyperkalemia. The recommended dose is 10 mL of 10% calcium gluconate (3–4 mL of calcium chloride), infused intravenously over 2–3 min with cardiac monitoring. The effect of the infusion starts in 1–3 min and lasts 30–60 min; the dose should be repeated if there is no change in ECG findings or if they recur after initial improvement. Hypercalcemia potentiates the cardiac toxicity of digoxin; hence, intravenous calcium should be used with extreme caution in patients taking this medication; if judged necessary, 10 mL of 10% calcium gluconate can be added to 100 mL of 5% dextrose in water and infused over 20–30 min to avoid acute hypercalcemia.
2. *Rapid reduction in plasma K^+ concentration by redistribution into cells.* Insulin lowers plasma K^+ concentration by shifting K^+ into cells. The recommended dose is 10 units of intravenous regular insulin followed immediately by 50 mL of 50% dextrose ($D_{50}W$, 25 g of glucose total); the effect begins in 10–20 min, peaks at 30–60 min, and lasts for 4–6 h. Bolus $D_{50}W$ without insulin is *never* appropriate, given the risk of acutely worsening hyperkalemia due to the osmotic effect of hypertonic glucose. Hypoglycemia is common with insulin plus glucose; hence, this should be followed by an infusion of 10% dextrose at 50–75 mL/h, with close monitoring of plasma glucose concentration. In hyperkalemic patients with glucose concentrations of ≥200–250 mg/dL, insulin should be administered *without* glucose, again with close monitoring of glucose concentrations.

   β_2-Agonists, most commonly albuterol, are effective but underused agents for the acute management of hyperkalemia. Albuterol and insulin with glucose have an additive effect on plasma K^+ concentration; however, ~20% of patients with ESRD are resistant to the effect of β_2-agonists; hence, these drugs should not be used without insulin. The recommended dose for inhaled albuterol is 10–20 mg of nebulized albuterol in 4 mL of normal saline, inhaled over 10 min; the effect starts at about 30 min, reaches its peak at about 90 min, and lasts for 2–6 h. Hyperglycemia is a side effect, along with tachycardia. β_2-Agonists should be used with caution in hyperkalemic patients with known cardiac disease.

   Intravenous bicarbonate has no role in the acute treatment of hyperkalemia, but may slowly attenuate hyperkalemia with sustained administration over several hours. It should not be given repeatedly as a hypertonic intravenous bolus of undiluted ampules, given the risk of associated hypernatremia and hypertonicity, but should instead be infused in an isotonic or hypotonic fluid (e.g., 150 milliequivalents of sodium bicarbonate in 1 L of D_5W). In patients with metabolic acidosis, a delayed drop in plasma K^+ concentration can be seen after 4–6 h of isotonic bicarbonate infusion.
3. *Removal of potassium.* This is typically accomplished using cation exchange resins, diuretics, and/or dialysis. The cation exchange resin sodium polystyrene sulfonate (SPS) exchanges Na^+ for K^+ in the gastrointestinal tract and increases the fecal excretion of K^+. The recommended dose of SPS is 15–30 g of powder, almost always given in a premade suspension with 33% sorbitol. The effect of SPS on plasma K^+ concentration is slow; the full effect may take up to 24 h and usually requires repeated doses every 4–6 h. Intestinal necrosis, typically of the colon or ileum, is a rare but usually fatal complication of SPS. Intestinal necrosis is more common in patients with reduced intestinal motility (e.g., in the postoperative state or after treatment with opioids). The coadministration of SPS with sorbitol appears to increase the risk of intestinal necrosis; however, this complication can also occur with SPS alone, and in animal models, SPS is the causative agent. The low but real risk of intestinal necrosis with SPS, which can sometimes be the only available or appropriate therapy for the removal of potassium, must be weighed against the delayed onset of efficacy. Whenever possible, alternative therapies for the acute management of hyperkalemia (i.e., alternative potassium binders, aggressive redistributive therapy, isotonic bicarbonate infusion, diuretics, and/or hemodialysis) should be used instead of SPS.

   Novel intestinal potassium binders have recently become available for the management of hyperkalemia. These agents lack the intestinal toxicity of SPS and are preferred over SPS for the management of hyperkalemia. Patiromer is a nonabsorbed polymer provided as a powder for suspension, which binds K^+ in exchange for Ca^{2+}. In healthy adults, patiromer causes a decrease in urinary potassium, magnesium, and sodium excretion, suggesting the binding of the polymer to these cations in the intestine; notably, a major side effect of the medication is hypomagnesemia. ZS-9 (sodium zirconium cyclosilicate) is an inorganic, nonabsorbable crystalline compound that exchanges both Na^+ and H^+ ions in exchange for K^+ and NH_4^+ in the intestine. These agents have revolutionized the management of both chronic and acute hyperkalemia. In particular, the availability of safe, well-tolerated potassium binders allows for greater intensity of renin-angiotensin-aldosterone system inhibition in both renal and cardiac disease.

   Therapy with intravenous saline may be beneficial in hypovolemic patients with oliguria and decreased distal delivery of Na^+, with the associated reductions in renal K^+ excretion. Loop and thiazide diuretics can be used to reduce plasma K^+ concentration in volume-replete or hypervolemic patients with sufficient renal function for a diuretic response; this may need to be combined with intravenous saline or isotonic bicarbonate to achieve or maintain euvolemia.

   Hemodialysis is the most effective and reliable method to reduce plasma K^+ concentration; peritoneal dialysis is considerably less effective. Patients with acute kidney injury require temporary, urgent venous access for hemodialysis, with the attendant risks; in contrast, patients with ESRD or advanced chronic kidney disease may have a preexisting venous access. The amount of K^+ removed during hemodialysis depends on the relative distribution of K^+ between ICF and ECF (potentially affected by prior therapy for hyperkalemia), the type and surface area of the dialyzer used, dialysate and blood flow rates, dialysate flow rate, dialysis duration, and the plasma-to-dialysate K^+ gradient.

FURTHER READING

CHOI M et al: K^+ channel mutations in adrenal aldosterone-producing adenomas and hereditary hypertension. Science 331:768, 2011.

FENSKE W et al: A copeptin-based approach in the diagnosis of diabetes insipidus. N Engl J Med 379:428, 2018.

GANKAM-KENGNE F et al: Osmotic stress–induced defective glial proteostasis contributes to brain demyelination after hyponatremia treatment. J Am Soc Nephrol 28:1802, 2017.

MOUNT DB: Disorders of potassium balance, in *Brenner and Rector's The Kidney*, 11th ed, ASL Yu et al: (eds). Philadelphia, W.B. Saunders & Company, 2020, pp. 537–579.

PACKHAM DK et al: Sodium zirconium cyclosilicate in hyperkalemia. N Engl J Med 372:222, 2015.

Perianayagam A et al: DDAVP is effective in preventing and reversing inadvertent overcorrection of hyponatremia. Clin J Am Soc Nephrol 3:331, 2008.

Schrier RW: Decreased effective blood volume in edematous disorders: What does this mean? J Am Soc Nephrol 18:2028, 2007.

Sood L et al: Hypertonic saline and desmopressin: A simple strategy for safe correction of severe hyponatremia. Am J Kidney Dis 61:571, 2013.

Soupart A et al: Efficacy and tolerance of urea compared with vaptans for long-term treatment of patients with SIADH. Clin J Am Soc Nephrol 7:742, 2012.

54 Hypercalcemia and Hypocalcemia

Sundeep Khosla

The calcium ion plays a critical role in normal cellular function and signaling, regulating diverse physiologic processes such as neuromuscular signaling, cardiac contractility, hormone secretion, and blood coagulation. Thus, extracellular calcium concentrations are maintained within an exquisitely narrow range through a series of feedback mechanisms that involve parathyroid hormone (PTH) and the active vitamin D metabolite 1,25-dihydroxyvitamin D [1,25(OH)$_2$D]. These feedback mechanisms are orchestrated by integrating signals between the parathyroid glands, kidney, intestine, and bone **(Fig. 54-1; Chap. 409)**.

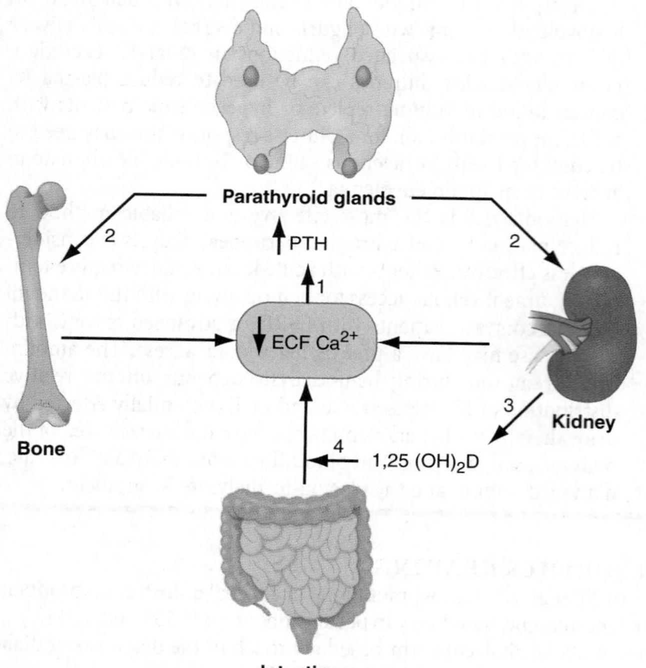

FIGURE 54-1 Feedback mechanisms maintaining extracellular calcium concentrations within a narrow, physiologic range (8.9–10.1 mg/dL [2.2–2.5 m*M*]). A decrease in extracellular (ECF) calcium (Ca^{2+}) triggers an increase in parathyroid hormone (PTH) secretion (1) via the calcium sensor receptor on parathyroid cells. PTH, in turn, results in increased tubular reabsorption of calcium by the kidney (2) and resorption of calcium from bone (2) and also stimulates renal 1,25(OH)$_2$D production (3). 1,25(OH)$_2$D, in turn, acts principally on the intestine to increase calcium absorption (4). Collectively, these homeostatic mechanisms serve to restore serum calcium levels to normal.

Disorders of serum calcium concentration are relatively common and often serve as a harbinger of underlying disease. This chapter provides a brief summary of the approach to patients with altered serum calcium levels. **See Chap. 410 for a detailed discussion of this topic.**

HYPERCALCEMIA

ETIOLOGY

The causes of hypercalcemia can be understood and classified based on derangements in the normal feedback mechanisms that regulate serum calcium **(Table 54-1)**. Excess PTH production, which is not appropriately suppressed by increased serum calcium concentrations, occurs in primary neoplastic disorders of the parathyroid glands (parathyroid adenomas; hyperplasia; or, rarely, carcinoma) that are associated with increased parathyroid cell mass and impaired feedback inhibition by calcium. Inappropriate PTH secretion for the ambient level of serum calcium also occurs in familial hypocalciuric hypercalcemia (FHH), which is an autosomal dominant syndrome most commonly involving inactivating mutations in the calcium sensor receptor (*CaSR*; FHH type 1), with rare families having mutations in the Gα_{11} protein (*GNA11*; FHH type 2) or the adaptor-related protein complex 2, σ-2 subunit (*AP2S1*; FHH type 3); all of these mutations impair extracellular calcium sensing by the parathyroid glands and the kidneys, leading to inappropriate PTH secretion and increased renal tubular calcium reabsorption. Although PTH secretion by tumors is extremely rare, many solid tumors produce PTH-related peptide (PTHrP), which shares homology with PTH in the first 13 amino acids and binds the PTH receptor, thus mimicking effects of PTH on bone and the kidney. In PTHrP-mediated hypercalcemia of malignancy, PTH levels are suppressed by the high serum calcium levels. Hypercalcemia associated with granulomatous disease (e.g., sarcoidosis) or lymphomas is caused by enhanced conversion of 25(OH)D to the potent 1,25(OH)$_2$D. In these disorders, 1,25(OH)$_2$D enhances intestinal calcium absorption, resulting in hypercalcemia and suppressed PTH. Disorders that directly increase calcium mobilization from bone, such as hyperthyroidism or osteolytic metastases, also lead to hypercalcemia

TABLE 54-1 Causes of Hypercalcemia

Excessive PTH production
Primary hyperparathyroidism (adenoma, hyperplasia, rarely carcinoma)
Tertiary hyperparathyroidism (long-term stimulation of PTH secretion in renal insufficiency)
Ectopic PTH secretion (very rare)
FHH
Alterations in CaSR function (lithium therapy)
Hypercalcemia of malignancy
Overproduction of PTHrP (many solid tumors)
Lytic skeletal metastases (breast, myeloma)
Excessive 1,25(OH)$_2$D production
Granulomatous diseases (sarcoidosis, tuberculosis, silicosis)
Lymphomas
Vitamin D intoxication
Primary increase in bone resorption
Hyperthyroidism
Immobilization
Excessive calcium intake
Milk-alkali syndrome
Total parenteral nutrition
Other causes
Endocrine disorders (adrenal insufficiency, pheochromocytoma, VIPoma)
Medications (thiazides, vitamin A, antiestrogens)

Abbreviations: CaSR, calcium sensor receptor; FHH, familial hypocalciuric hypercalcemia; PTH, parathyroid hormone; PTHrP, PTH-related peptide.

with suppressed PTH secretion as does exogenous calcium overload, as in milk-alkali syndrome, or total parenteral nutrition with excessive calcium supplementation.

CLINICAL MANIFESTATIONS

Mild hypercalcemia (up to 11–11.5 mg/dL) is usually asymptomatic and recognized only on routine calcium measurements. Some patients may complain of vague neuropsychiatric symptoms, including trouble concentrating, personality changes, or depression. Other presenting symptoms may include peptic ulcer disease or nephrolithiasis, and fracture risk may be increased. More severe hypercalcemia (>12–13 mg/dL), particularly if it develops acutely, may result in lethargy, stupor, or coma, as well as gastrointestinal symptoms (nausea, anorexia, constipation, or pancreatitis). Hypercalcemia decreases renal concentrating ability, which may cause polyuria and polydipsia. With long-standing hyperparathyroidism, patients may present with bone pain or pathologic fractures. Finally, hypercalcemia can result in significant electrocardiographic changes, including bradycardia, atrioventricular (AV) block, and short QT interval; changes in serum calcium can be monitored by following the QT interval.

DIAGNOSTIC APPROACH

The first step in the diagnostic evaluation of hyper- or hypocalcemia is to ensure that the alteration in serum calcium levels is not due to abnormal albumin concentrations. About 50% of total calcium is ionized, and the rest is bound principally to albumin. Although direct measurements of ionized calcium are possible, they are easily influenced by collection methods and other artifacts; thus, it is generally preferable to measure total calcium and albumin to "correct" the serum calcium. When serum albumin concentrations are reduced, a corrected calcium concentration is calculated by adding 0.2 m*M* (0.8 mg/dL) to the total calcium level for every decrement in serum albumin of 1.0 g/dL below the reference value of 4.1 g/dL for albumin, and, conversely, for elevations in serum albumin.

A detailed history may provide important clues regarding the etiology of the hypercalcemia (Table 54-1). Chronic hypercalcemia is most commonly caused by primary hyperparathyroidism, as opposed to the second most common etiology of hypercalcemia, an underlying malignancy. The history should include medication use, previous neck surgery, and systemic symptoms suggestive of sarcoidosis or lymphoma.

Once true hypercalcemia is established, the second most important laboratory test in the diagnostic evaluation is a PTH level using a two-site assay for the intact hormone. Increases in PTH are often accompanied by hypophosphatemia. In addition, serum creatinine should be measured to assess renal function; hypercalcemia may impair renal function, and renal clearance of PTH may be altered depending on the fragments detected by the assay. If the PTH level is increased (or "inappropriately normal") in the setting of elevated calcium and low phosphorus, the diagnosis is almost always primary hyperparathyroidism. Because individuals with FHH may also present with mildly elevated PTH levels and hypercalcemia, this diagnosis should be considered and excluded because parathyroid surgery is ineffective in this condition. A calcium/creatinine clearance ratio (calculated as urine calcium/serum calcium divided by urine creatinine/serum creatinine) of <0.01 is suggestive of FHH, particularly when there is a family history of mild, asymptomatic hypercalcemia. In addition, sequence analysis of the *CASR* gene is now commonly performed for the definitive diagnosis of FHH, although as noted above, in rare families, FHH may be caused by mutations in the *GNA11* or *AP2S1* genes, and patients may have to pay out-of-pocket for the genetic analysis. Ectopic PTH secretion is extremely rare.

A suppressed PTH level in the face of hypercalcemia is consistent with non-parathyroid-mediated hypercalcemia, most often due to underlying malignancy. Although a tumor that causes hypercalcemia is generally overt, a PTHrP level may be needed to establish the diagnosis of hypercalcemia of malignancy. Serum $1,25(OH)_2D$ levels are increased in granulomatous disorders, and clinical evaluation in combination with laboratory testing will generally provide a diagnosis for the various disorders listed in Table 54-1.

TREATMENT
Hypercalcemia

Mild, asymptomatic hypercalcemia does not require immediate therapy, and management should be dictated by the underlying diagnosis. By contrast, significant, symptomatic hypercalcemia usually requires therapeutic intervention independent of the etiology of hypercalcemia. Initial therapy of significant hypercalcemia begins with volume expansion because hypercalcemia invariably leads to dehydration; 4–6 L of intravenous saline may be required over the first 24 h, keeping in mind that underlying comorbidities (e.g., congestive heart failure) may require the use of loop diuretics to enhance sodium and calcium excretion. However, loop diuretics should not be initiated until the volume status has been restored to normal. If there is increased calcium mobilization from bone (as in malignancy or severe hyperparathyroidism), drugs that inhibit bone resorption should be considered. Although salmon calcitonin (4–8 IU/kg intramuscularly or subcutaneously every 6–12 h) is sometimes used, the mainstays of therapy are bisphosphonates, which are potent inhibitors of bone resorption. Zoledronic acid (e.g., 4 mg intravenously over ~30 min) and pamidronate (e.g., 60–90 mg intravenously over 2–4 h) are bisphosphonates that are commonly used for the treatment of hypercalcemia of malignancy in adults. Onset of action is within 1–3 days, with normalization of serum calcium levels occurring in 60–90% of patients. Bisphosphonate infusions may need to be repeated if hypercalcemia relapses. Denosumab (120 mg subcutaneously on days 1, 8, 15, and 29, and then every 4 weeks), an antibody to RANKL, is a potent inhibitor of bone resorption and has been shown to be effective in treating hypercalcemia refractory to bisphosphonates. An alternative to the bisphosphonates or denosumab is gallium nitrate (200 mg/m^2 intravenously daily for 5 days), which is also effective, but has potential nephrotoxicity. In rare instances, dialysis may be necessary. Finally, although intravenous phosphate chelates calcium and decreases serum calcium levels, this therapy can be toxic because calcium-phosphate complexes may deposit in tissues and cause extensive organ damage.

In patients with $1,25(OH)_2D$-mediated hypercalcemia, glucocorticoids are the preferred therapy, as they decrease $1,25(OH)_2D$ production. Intravenous hydrocortisone (100–300 mg daily) or oral prednisone (40–60 mg daily) for 3–7 days is used most often. Other drugs, such as ketoconazole, chloroquine, and hydroxychloroquine, may also decrease $1,25(OH)_2D$ production and are used occasionally.

HYPOCALCEMIA

ETIOLOGY

The causes of hypocalcemia can be differentiated according to whether serum PTH levels are low (hypoparathyroidism) or high (secondary hyperparathyroidism). Although there are many potential causes of hypocalcemia, impaired PTH production and impaired vitamin D production are the most common etiologies **(Table 54-2) (Chap. 410)**. Because PTH is the main defense against hypocalcemia, disorders associated with deficient PTH production or secretion may be associated with profound, life-threatening hypocalcemia. In adults, hypoparathyroidism most commonly results from inadvertent damage to all four glands during thyroid or parathyroid gland surgery. Hypoparathyroidism is a cardinal feature of autoimmune endocrinopathies **(Chap. 388)**; rarely, it may be associated with infiltrative diseases such as sarcoidosis. Impaired PTH secretion may be secondary to magnesium deficiency or to activating mutations in the CaSR or in the G proteins that mediate CaSR signaling (autosomal dominant hypocalcemia), which suppress PTH, leading to effects that are opposite to those that occur in FHH.

Vitamin D deficiency, impaired $1,25(OH)_2D$ production (primarily secondary to renal insufficiency), or vitamin D resistance also cause hypocalcemia. However, the degree of hypocalcemia in these disorders is generally not as severe as that seen with hypoparathyroidism because the parathyroids are capable of mounting a compensatory increase in

TABLE 54-2 Causes of Hypocalcemia

Low Parathyroid Hormone Levels (Hypoparathyroidism)
Parathyroid agenesis
Isolated
DiGeorge's syndrome
Parathyroid destruction
Surgical
Radiation
Infiltration by metastases or systemic diseases
Autoimmune
Reduced parathyroid function
Hypomagnesemia
Autosomal dominant hypocalcemia
High Parathyroid Hormone Levels (Secondary Hyperparathyroidism)
Vitamin D deficiency or impaired $1,25(OH)_2D$ production/action
Nutritional vitamin D deficiency (poor intake or absorption)
Renal insufficiency with impaired $1,25(OH)_2D$ production
Vitamin D resistance, including receptor defects
Parathyroid hormone resistance syndromes
PTH receptor mutations
Pseudohypoparathyroidism (G protein mutations)
Drugs
Calcium chelators
Inhibitors of bone resorption (bisphosphonates, plicamycin)
Altered vitamin D metabolism (phenytoin, ketoconazole)
Miscellaneous causes
Acute pancreatitis
Acute rhabdomyolysis
Hungry bone syndrome after parathyroidectomy
Osteoblastic metastases with marked stimulation of bone formation (prostate cancer)

Abbreviation: PTH, parathyroid hormone.

PTH secretion. Hypocalcemia may also occur in conditions associated with severe tissue injury such as burns, rhabdomyolysis, tumor lysis, or pancreatitis. The cause of hypocalcemia in these settings may include a combination of low albumin, hyperphosphatemia, tissue deposition of calcium, and impaired PTH secretion.

CLINICAL MANIFESTATIONS

Patients with hypocalcemia may be asymptomatic if the decreases in serum calcium are relatively mild and chronic, or they may present with life-threatening complications. Moderate to severe hypocalcemia is associated with paresthesias, usually of the fingers, toes, and circumoral regions, and is caused by increased neuromuscular irritability. On physical examination, a Chvostek's sign (twitching of the circumoral muscles in response to gentle tapping of the facial nerve just anterior to the ear) may be elicited, although it is also present in ~10% of normal individuals. Carpal spasm may be induced by inflation of a blood pressure cuff to 20 mmHg above the patient's systolic blood pressure for 3 min (Trousseau's sign). Severe hypocalcemia can induce seizures, carpopedal spasm, bronchospasm, laryngospasm, and prolongation of the QT interval.

DIAGNOSTIC APPROACH

In addition to measuring serum calcium, it is useful to determine albumin, phosphorus, and magnesium levels. As for the evaluation of hypercalcemia, determining the PTH level is central to the evaluation of hypocalcemia. A suppressed (or "inappropriately low") PTH level in the setting of hypocalcemia establishes absent or reduced PTH secretion (hypoparathyroidism) as the cause of the hypocalcemia. Further history will often elicit the underlying cause (i.e., parathyroid agenesis vs destruction). By contrast, an elevated PTH level (secondary hyperparathyroidism) should direct attention to the vitamin D axis as the cause of the hypocalcemia. Nutritional vitamin D deficiency is best assessed by obtaining serum 25-hydroxyvitamin D levels, which reflect vitamin D stores. In the setting of renal insufficiency or suspected vitamin D resistance, serum $1,25(OH)_2D$ levels are informative.

TREATMENT

Hypocalcemia

The approach to treatment depends on the severity of the hypocalcemia, the rapidity with which it develops, and the accompanying complications (e.g., seizures, laryngospasm). Acute, symptomatic hypocalcemia is initially managed with calcium gluconate, 10 mL 10% wt/vol (90 mg or 2.2 mmol) intravenously, diluted in 50 mL of 5% dextrose or 0.9% sodium chloride, given intravenously over 5 min. Continuing hypocalcemia often requires a constant intravenous infusion (typically 10 ampules of calcium gluconate or 900 mg of calcium in 1 L of 5% dextrose or 0.9% sodium chloride administered over 24 h). Accompanying hypomagnesemia, if present, should be treated with appropriate magnesium supplementation.

Chronic hypocalcemia due to hypoparathyroidism is treated with calcium supplements (1000–1500 mg/d elemental calcium in divided doses) and either vitamin D_2 or D_3 (25,000–100,000 U daily) or calcitriol [$1,25(OH)_2D$, 0.25–2 μg/d]. Other vitamin D metabolites (dihydrotachysterol, alfacalcidiol) are now used less frequently. Importantly, PTH (1-84) (Natpara) is now approved by the Food and Drug Administration for the treatment of refractory hypoparathyroidism, representing an important advance in treatment of these patients. Vitamin D deficiency is best treated using vitamin D supplementation, with the dose depending on the severity of the deficit and the underlying cause. Thus, nutritional vitamin D deficiency generally responds to relatively low doses of vitamin D (50,000 IU, 2–3 times per week for several months), whereas vitamin D deficiency due to malabsorption may require much higher doses (100,000 IU/d or more). The treatment goal is to bring serum calcium into the low normal range and to avoid hypercalciuria, which may lead to nephrolithiasis.

GLOBAL CONSIDERATIONS

In countries with more limited access to health care or screening laboratory testing of serum calcium levels, primary hyperparathyroidism often presents in its severe form with skeletal complications (osteitis fibrosa cystica) in contrast to the asymptomatic form that is common in developed countries. In addition, vitamin D deficiency is paradoxically common in some countries despite extensive sunlight (e.g., India) due to avoidance of sun exposure and poor dietary vitamin D intake.

FURTHER READING

Bilezikian JP et al: Hyperparathyroidism. Lancet 391:168, 2018.

Brandi ML et al: Management of hypoparathyroidism: Summary statement and guidelines. J Clin Endocrinol Metab 101:2273, 2016.

Hannan FM et al: The calcium-sensing receptor in physiology and in calcitropic and noncalcitropic diseases. Nat Rev Endocrinol 15:33, 2018.

Minisola S et al: The diagnosis and management of hypercalcemia. BMJ 350:h2723, 2015.

Acidosis and Alkalosis

Thomas D. DuBose, Jr.

NORMAL ACID-BASE HOMEOSTASIS

Systemic arterial pH is maintained between 7.35 and 7.45 by extracellular and intracellular chemical buffering together with respiratory and renal regulatory mechanisms. The control of arterial CO_2 tension ($Paco_2$) by the central nervous system (CNS) and respiratory system and the control of plasma bicarbonate by the kidneys stabilize the arterial pH by excretion or retention of acid or alkali. The metabolic and respiratory components that regulate systemic pH are described by the Henderson-Hasselbalch equation and solved for pH when the solubility of CO_2 is considered (dissolved CO_2 in mmol/L = 0.03 × $Paco_2$ in mmHg), at a pK' of 6.1:

$$\text{pH} = pK' + \log_{10}\frac{[\text{HCO}_3^-]}{\alpha_{\text{CO}_2}\text{PCO}_2}$$

Under most circumstances, CO_2 production and excretion are matched, and the usual steady-state $Paco_2$ is maintained at ~40 mmHg. Underexcretion of CO_2 produces hypercapnia, and overexcretion causes hypocapnia. Nevertheless, production and excretion are again matched at a new steady-state $Paco_2$. Therefore, the $Paco_2$ is regulated primarily by neural respiratory factors and is not subject to regulation by the rate of CO_2 production. Hypercapnia is usually the result of hypoventilation rather than of increased CO_2 production. Increases or decreases in $Paco_2$ represent derangements of neural respiratory control or are due to compensatory changes in response to a primary alteration in the plasma $[HCO_3^-]$.

DIAGNOSIS OF GENERAL TYPES OF DISTURBANCES

The most common clinical disturbances are simple acid-base disorders; i.e., metabolic acidosis or alkalosis or respiratory acidosis or alkalosis occurring individually. Recognition of simple acid-base disorders requires appreciation of the limits of physiologic compensation for a primary disturbance.

■ SIMPLE ACID-BASE DISORDERS

Primary respiratory disturbances (primary changes in $Paco_2$) invoke compensatory metabolic responses (secondary changes in $[HCO_3^-]$), and primary metabolic disturbances elicit predictable compensatory respiratory responses (secondary changes in $Paco_2$). Physiologic compensation can be predicted from the relationships displayed in **Table 55-1**. In general, with one exception, compensatory responses return the pH toward, but not to, the normal value. Chronic respiratory alkalosis when prolonged is an exception to this rule and may return the pH to a normal value. Metabolic acidosis due to an increase in endogenous acid production (e.g., ketoacidosis or lactic acid acidosis) lowers extracellular fluid $[HCO_3^-]$ and decreases extracellular pH. This stimulates the medullary chemoreceptors to increase ventilation and to return the ratio of $[HCO_3^-]$ to $Paco_2$, and thus pH, toward, but not typically to, the normal value. The degree of respiratory compensation expected in a metabolic acidosis can be predicted from the relationship: $Paco_2$ = (1.5 × $[HCO_3^-]$) + 8 ± 2 (Winter's equation). Thus, applying this equation, a patient with metabolic acidosis and $[HCO_3^-]$ of 12 mmol/L would be expected to have a $Paco_2$ of approximately 26 mmHg. In this example, if values for $Paco_2$ were <24 or >28 mmHg, values that exceed the boundaries for compensation for a simple disorder, a *mixed* disturbance should be recognized (metabolic acidosis plus respiratory alkalosis or metabolic acidosis plus respiratory acidosis, respectively). Compensatory responses for primary metabolic disorders move the $Paco_2$ in the same direction as the change in $[HCO_3^-]$, while compensation for primary respiratory disorders moves the $[HCO_3^-]$ in the same direction as the primary change in $Paco_2$ (Table 55-1). Therefore, changes in $Paco_2$ and $[HCO_3^-]$ in **opposite directions** (i.e., $Paco_2$ or $[HCO_3^-]$ is increased, whereas the other value is decreased) indicate a **mixed acid-base disturbance**. Another way to judge the appropriateness of the response in $[HCO_3^-]$ or $Paco_2$ is to use an acid-base nomogram (**Fig. 55-1**). While the shaded areas of the nomogram show the 95% confidence limits for physiologic

TABLE 55-1 Prediction of Compensatory Responses to Simple Acid-Base Disturbances and Pattern of Changes

DISORDER	PREDICTION OF COMPENSATION	RANGE OF VALUES		
		pH	HCO_3^-	$Paco_2$
Metabolic acidosis	$Paco_2$ = (1.5 × HCO_3^-) + 8 ± 2 *or* $Paco_2$ will ↓ 1.25 mmHg per mmol/L ↓ in $[HCO_3^-]$ *or* $Paco_2$ = $[HCO_3^-]$ + 15	Low	Low	Low
Metabolic alkalosis	$Paco_2$ will ↑ 0.75 mmHg per mmol/L ↑ in $[HCO_3^-]$ *or* $Paco_2$ will ↑ 6 mmHg per 10 mmol/L ↑ in $[HCO_3^-]$ *or* $Paco_2$ = $[HCO_3^-]$ + 15	High	High	High
Respiratory alkalosis		High	Low	Low
Acute	$[HCO_3^-]$ will ↓ 0.2 mmol/L per mmHg ↓ in $Paco_2$			
Chronic	$[HCO_3^-]$ will ↓ 0.4 mmol/L per mmHg ↓ in $Paco_2$			
Respiratory acidosis		Low	High	High
Acute	$[HCO_3^-]$ will ↑ 0.1 mmol/L per mmHg ↑ in $Paco_2$			
Chronic	$[HCO_3^-]$ will ↑ 0.4 mmol/L per mmHg ↑ in $Paco_2$			

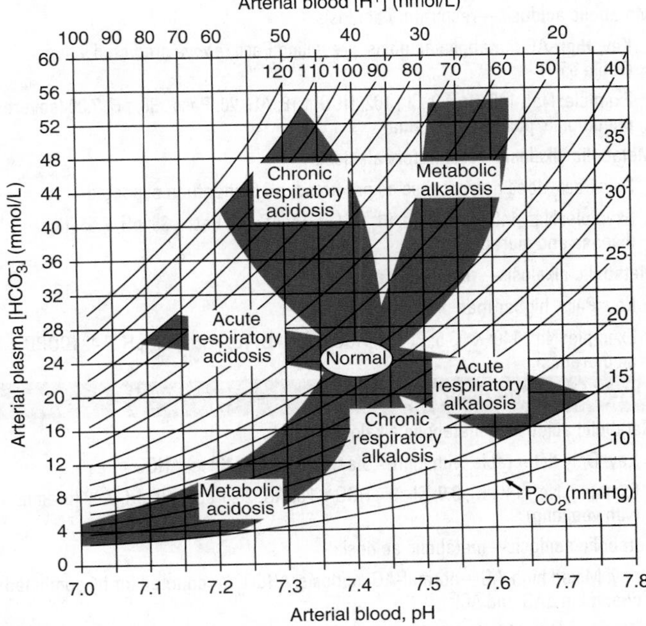

FIGURE 55-1 Acid-base nomogram. Shown are the 90% confidence limits (range of values) of the normal respiratory and metabolic compensations for primary acid-base disturbances. *(Reproduced with permission from LL Hamm and TD DuBose Jr, in Alan S.L. Yu, et al (eds): Brenner and Rector's The Kidney, 11th ed. Philadelphia, Elsevier, 2020.)*

compensation in simple disturbances, finding acid-base values within the shaded area does not necessarily rule out a mixed disturbance. Imposition of one disorder over another may result in values lying within the area of a third. Thus, the nomogram, while convenient, is not a substitute for the equations in Table 55-1.

MIXED ACID-BASE DISORDERS

Mixed acid-base disorders—defined as independently coexisting disorders, not merely compensatory responses—are often seen in patients in critical care units and can lead to dangerous extremes of pH (**Table 55-2**). The diagnosis of mixed acid-base disorders requires consideration of the anion gap (AG). To be accurate, the AG requires the presence of, or correction to, a normal serum albumin of 4.5 g/dL (see below, "Evaluate the Anion Gap"). If a patient with diabetic ketoacidosis (metabolic acidosis) and a high AG has an independent and concomitant respiratory disorder (e.g., pneumonia), the latter may lead to a superimposed respiratory acidosis or alkalosis and the $Paco_2$ will deviate from the predicted value for the response to a pure high-AG metabolic acidosis (Table 55-2). Patients with underlying chronic obstructive pulmonary disease may not respond to metabolic acidosis with an appropriate ventilatory response because of insufficient respiratory reserve (Table 55-2). Such imposition of respiratory acidosis on metabolic acidosis can lead to severe acidemia. When metabolic acidosis and metabolic alkalosis coexist in the same patient, the pH may be in the normal range. In this circumstance, it is the presence of an elevated AG (see below) that denotes the presence of a metabolic acidosis. Assuming a normal value for the AG of 10 mmol/L, incongruity in the ΔAG (existing minus normal AG) and the ΔHCO_3^- (normal value of 25 mmol/L minus abnormal HCO_3^- in the patient) indicates the presence of a mixed high-gap acidosis—metabolic alkalosis (see example below). A diabetic patient with ketoacidosis may have acute or chronic kidney failure resulting in a combination of metabolic acidoses from accumulation of both ketoacids and uremic acids. Patients who have ingested an overdose of drug combinations such as sedatives and salicylates may have mixed disturbances as a result of the acid-base response to the individual drugs (metabolic acidosis mixed with respiratory acidosis or respiratory alkalosis, respectively). Triple acid-base disturbances are more complex. For example, patients with metabolic acidosis due to alcoholic ketoacidosis may develop metabolic alkalosis due to vomiting and superimposed respiratory alkalosis due to the hyperventilation of hepatic dysfunction or alcohol withdrawal.

TABLE 55-2 Examples of Mixed Acid-Base Disorders

Mixed Metabolic and Respiratory
Metabolic acidosis—respiratory alkalosis
Key: High-AG metabolic acidosis; prevailing $Paco_2$ *below* predicted value (Table 55-1)
Example: Na^+, 140; K^+, 4.0; Cl^-, 106; HCO_3^-, 14; AG, 20; $Paco_2$, 24; pH, 7.39 (lactic acidosis, sepsis in ICU)
Metabolic acidosis—respiratory acidosis
Key: High-AG metabolic acidosis; prevailing $Paco_2$ *above* predicted value (Table 55-1)
Example: Na^+, 140; K^+, 4.0; Cl^-, 102; HCO_3^-, 18; AG, 20; $Paco_2$, 38; pH, 7.30 (severe pneumonia, pulmonary edema)
Metabolic alkalosis—respiratory alkalosis
Key: $Paco_2$ does not increase as predicted; pH higher than expected
Example: Na^+, 140; K^+, 4.0; Cl^-, 91; HCO_3^-, 33; AG, 16; $Paco_2$, 38; pH, 7.55 (liver disease and diuretics)
Metabolic alkalosis—respiratory acidosis
Key: $Paco_2$ higher than predicted; pH normal
Example: Na^+, 140; K^+, 3.5; Cl^-, 88; HCO_3^-, 42; AG, 10; $Paco_2$, 67; pH, 7.42 (COPD on diuretics)
Mixed Metabolic Disorders
Metabolic acidosis—metabolic alkalosis
Key: Only detectable with high-AG acidosis; ΔAG (10) >> ΔHCO_3^- (0)
Example: Na^+, 140; K^+, 3.0; Cl^-, 95; HCO_3^-, 25; AG, 20; $Paco_2$, 40; pH, 7.42 (uremia with vomiting)
Metabolic acidosis—metabolic acidosis
Key: Mixed high-AG—normal-AG acidosis; ΔHCO_3^- accounted for by combined change in ΔAG and ΔCl^-
Example: Na^+, 135; K^+, 3.0; Cl^-, 110; HCO_3^-, 10; AG, 15; $Paco_2$, 25; pH, 7.20 (diarrhea and lactic acidosis, toluene toxicity, treatment of diabetic ketoacidosis)

Abbreviations: AG, anion gap; COPD, chronic obstructive pulmonary disease; ICU, intensive care unit.

APPROACH TO THE PATIENT

Acid-Base Disorders

The diagnosis of acid-base disorders follows a stepwise approach (**Table 55-3**). Blood for electrolytes and arterial blood gases should be drawn simultaneously, prior to therapy. An increase in $[HCO_3^-]$ occurs with either metabolic alkalosis or respiratory acidosis. Conversely, a decrease in $[HCO_3^-]$ occurs with either metabolic acidosis or respiratory alkalosis. In the determination of arterial blood gases by the clinical laboratory, both pH and $Paco_2$ are measured, and the $[HCO_3^-]$ is calculated from the Henderson-Hasselbalch equation. This *calculated* value should be compared with the *measured* $[HCO_3^-]$ (or total CO_2) on the electrolyte panel. These two values should agree within 2 mmol/L. If they do not, the values may not have been drawn simultaneously, or a laboratory error may be present. After verifying the blood acid-base values, the precise acid-base disorder can then be classified.

EVALUATE THE ANION GAP

Evaluations of acid-base disorders should involve acknowledgement of the AG. The AG is calculated, either by the clinical laboratory or the clinician, as follows: $AG = Na^+ - (Cl^- + HCO_3^-)$. The value for plasma $[K^+]$ is typically omitted from the calculation of the AG in the United States. The "normal" value for the AG reported by clinical laboratories has declined with improved methodology for measuring plasma electrolytes and ranges from 6–12 mmol/L, with an average of approximately 10 mmol/L. The unmeasured anions normally present in plasma include anionic proteins (e.g., albumin), phosphate, sulfate, and organic anions. When acid anions, such as acetoacetate and lactate, accumulate in extracellular fluid, the AG increases, causing a **high-AG acidosis**. An increase in the AG is most often due to an increase in unmeasured anions but, less commonly, may be due to a decrease in unmeasured cations (calcium, magnesium, potassium). In addition, the AG may increase with an increase in anionic albumin (e.g., severe dehydration). A decrease in the AG can be due to (1) an increase in unmeasured cations; (2) the addition to the blood of abnormal cations, such as lithium (lithium intoxication) or cationic immunoglobulins (plasma cell dyscrasias); (3) a reduction in the plasma anion albumin concentration (nephrotic syndrome, liver disease, or malabsorption); or (4) hyperviscosity and severe hyperlipidemia, which can lead to an underestimation of sodium and chloride concentrations. Because the normal AG of 10 mmol/L assumes that the serum albumin is normal, if hypoalbuminemia is present, the value for the AG must

TABLE 55-3 Steps in Acid-Base Diagnosis

1. Obtain arterial blood gas (ABG) and electrolytes simultaneously.
2. Compare $[HCO_3^-]$ on ABG and electrolytes to verify accuracy.
3. Evaluate anion gap (AG); if not normal, correct to albumin concentration of 4.5 g/dL (see text).
4. Know four causes of high-AG acidosis (ketoacidosis, lactic acid acidosis, renal failure, and toxins).
5. Know two causes of hyperchloremic or nongap acidosis (bicarbonate loss from gastrointestinal tract, renal tubular acidosis).
6. Estimate compensatory response (Table 55-1).
7. Compare ΔAG and ΔHCO_3^-.
8. Compare change in $[Cl^-]$ with change in $[Na^+]$.

be corrected. For example, for each g/dL of serum albumin below the normal value (4.5 g/dL), 2.5 mmol/L should be added to the reported (uncorrected) AG. Thus, in a patient with a serum albumin of 2.5 g/dL (2 g/dL below the normal value) and an uncorrected AG of 15, the corrected AG is calculated by adding 5 mmol/L (2.5 × 2 = 5; 5 + 15 = corrected AG of 20 mmol/L). Clinical laboratories do not correct the AG for coexisting hypoalbuminemia and typically report the uncorrected value, requiring the attention of the clinician to the prevailing serum albumin concentration. The clinical disorders that may cause a high-AG acidosis are displayed in Table 55-3.

A high AG is usually due to accumulation of non–chloride-containing acids that contain inorganic (phosphate, sulfate), organic (ketoacids, lactate, uremic organic anions), exogenous (salicylate or ingested toxins with organic acid production), or unidentified anions. The high AG is meaningful even if the [HCO_3^-] or pH is normal. Simultaneous metabolic acidosis of the high-AG variety plus either chronic respiratory acidosis or metabolic alkalosis represents a situation in which [HCO_3^-] may be normal or even high (Table 55-3). In cases of high-AG metabolic acidosis, it is valuable to compare the decline in [HCO_3^-] (ΔHCO_3^-: 25 – patient's [HCO_3^-]) with the increase in the AG (ΔAG: patient's AG – 10).

Similarly, normal values for [HCO_3^-], $Paco_2$, and pH do not ensure the absence of an acid-base disturbance. For instance, an alcoholic who has been vomiting may develop a metabolic alkalosis with a pH of 7.55, $Paco_2$ of 47 mmHg, [HCO_3^-] of 40 mmol/L, [Na^+] of 135, [Cl^-] of 80, and [K^+] of 2.8. If such a patient were then to develop a superimposed alcoholic ketoacidosis with a β-hydroxybutyrate concentration of 15 mmol/L, arterial pH would fall to 7.40, the [HCO_3^-] to 25 mmol/L, and the $Paco_2$ to 40 mmHg. Although these blood gases are normal, the AG is elevated at 30 mmol/L, indicating a mixed metabolic alkalosis and metabolic acidosis is present. A mixture of high-gap acidosis and metabolic alkalosis is recognized easily by comparing the differences (Δ values) in the normal to prevailing patient values. In this example, the ΔHCO_3^- is 0 (25 – 25 mmol/L), but the ΔAG is 20 (30 – 10 mmol/L). Therefore, 20 mmol/L is unaccounted for in the Δ/Δ value (ΔAG to ΔHCO_3^-).

METABOLIC ACIDOSIS

Metabolic acidosis can occur because of an increase in endogenous acid production (such as lactate and ketoacids), loss of bicarbonate (as in diarrhea), or accumulation of endogenous acids because of inappropriately low excretion of net acid by the kidney (as in chronic kidney disease). Metabolic acidosis has profound effects on the respiratory, cardiac, and nervous systems. The fall in blood pH is accompanied by a characteristic increase in ventilation, especially the tidal volume (Kussmaul respiration). Intrinsic cardiac contractility may be depressed, but inotropic function can be normal because of catecholamine release. Both peripheral arterial vasodilation and central venoconstriction may be present; the decrease in central and pulmonary vascular compliance predisposes to pulmonary edema with even minimal volume overload. CNS function is depressed, with headache, lethargy, stupor, and, in some cases, even coma. Glucose intolerance may also occur.

There are two major categories of clinical metabolic acidosis: high-AG and non-AG acidosis (Table 55-3 and **Table 55-4**). The presence of metabolic acidosis, a normal AG, and hyperchloremia denotes the presence of a non-AG metabolic acidosis.

TABLE 55-4 Causes of High-Anion Gap Metabolic Acidosis

Lactic acidosis	Toxins
Ketoacidosis	Ethylene glycol
Diabetic	Methanol
Alcoholic	Salicylates
Starvation	Propylene glycol
	Pyroglutamic acid (5-oxoproline)
	Renal failure (acute and chronic)

TREATMENT
Metabolic Acidosis

Treatment of metabolic acidosis with alkali should be reserved for severe acidemia except when the patient has no "potential HCO_3^-" in plasma. The potential [HCO_3^-] can be estimated from the increment (Δ) in the AG (ΔAG = patient's AG – 10), only if the acid anion that has accumulated in plasma is metabolizable (i.e., β-hydroxybutyrate, acetoacetate, and lactate). Conversely, nonmetabolizable anions that may accumulate in advanced-stage chronic kidney disease or after toxin ingestion are not metabolizable and do not represent "potential" HCO_3^-. In patients with acute kidney failure or acute-on-chronic kidney failure, improvement in kidney function after volume resuscitation may improve the serum [HCO_3^-], but this is a slow and unpredictable process. Consequently, patients with a non-AG acidosis (hyperchloremic acidosis) or an AG acidosis attributable to a nonmetabolizable anion due to advanced kidney failure ("uremic" acidosis) should receive alkali therapy, either PO ($NaHCO_3$ tablets or Shohl's solution) or IV ($NaHCO_3$), in an amount necessary to slowly increase the plasma [HCO_3^-] to a target value of 22 mmol/L. Importantly, overcorrection should be avoided.

Bicarbonate therapy in diabetic ketoacidosis (DKA) is reserved for adult patients with severe acidemia (pH <7.00) and/or evidence of shock. In such circumstances, bicarbonate may be administered IV, as a slow infusion of 50 meq of $NaHCO_3$ diluted in 300 mL of a saline solution, over 30–45 min, during the initial 1–2 h of therapy. Bolus administration should be avoided. Administration of $NaHCO_3$ requires careful monitoring of plasma electrolytes during the course of therapy because of the risk for hypokalemia as urine output is established. A reasonable initial goal in DKA is to increase the [HCO_3^-] to 10–12 mmol/L and the pH to approximately 7.20, but clearly not to increase these values to normal.

HIGH-ANION GAP ACIDOSES

APPROACH TO THE PATIENT
High-Anion Gap Acidoses

There are four principal causes of a high-AG acidosis: (1) lactic acidosis, (2) ketoacidosis, (3) ingested toxins, and (4) acute and chronic kidney failure (Table 55-4). Initial screening to differentiate the high-AG acidoses should include (1) a probe of the history for evidence of drug and toxin ingestion and measurement of arterial blood gas to detect coexistent respiratory alkalosis (salicylates); (2) determination of whether a history of diabetes mellitus is present (DKA); (3) a search for evidence of alcoholism or increased levels of β-hydroxybutyrate (alcoholic ketoacidosis); (4) observation for clinical signs of uremia and determination of the blood urea nitrogen (BUN) and creatinine (uremic acidosis); (5) inspection of the urine for oxalate crystals (ethylene glycol ingestion); and (6) recognition of the numerous clinical settings in which lactate levels may be increased (hypotension, shock, cardiac failure, leukemia, cancer, and drug or toxin ingestion).

Lactic Acidosis An increase in plasma L-lactate may be secondary to poor tissue perfusion (type A)—circulatory insufficiency (shock, cardiac failure), severe anemia, mitochondrial enzyme defects, and inhibitors (carbon monoxide, cyanide)—or to aerobic disorders (type B)—malignancies, nucleoside analogue reverse transcriptase inhibitors in HIV, diabetes mellitus, renal or hepatic failure, thiamine deficiency, severe infections (cholera, malaria), seizures, or drugs/toxins (biguanides, ethanol, and the toxic alcohols: ethylene glycol, methanol, or propylene glycol). Unrecognized bowel ischemia or infarction in a patient with severe atherosclerosis or cardiac decompensation receiving vasopressors is a common cause of lactic acidosis in elderly patients. Pyroglutamic acidemia may occur in critically ill patients receiving acetaminophen, which causes depletion of glutathione and accumulation of 5-oxyprolene. D-Lactic acid acidosis, which may be associated with jejunoileal bypass, short bowel syndrome, or intestinal obstruction, is due to formation of D-lactate by gut bacteria.

APPROACH TO THE PATIENT

L-Lactic Acid Acidosis

The overarching goal of treatment is to correct the underlying condition that disrupts lactate metabolism; tissue perfusion should be restored when inadequate, but vasoconstrictors should be avoided, or used cautiously, because they may worsen tissue perfusion. Alkali therapy is generally advocated for acute, severe acidemia (pH <7.00) to improve cardiovascular function. However, $NaHCO_3$ therapy may paradoxically depress cardiac performance and exacerbate acidosis by enhancing lactate production (HCO_3^- stimulates phosphofructokinase). While the use of alkali in moderate lactic acidosis is controversial, it is generally agreed that attempts to return the pH or [HCO_3^-] to normal by administration of exogenous $NaHCO_3$ are deleterious. A reasonable approach with severe acidemia is to infuse sufficient $NaHCO_3$ to raise arterial pH to no more than 7.2 or the [HCO_3^-] to no more than 12 mmol/L.

$NaHCO_3$ therapy can cause fluid overload, hypercapnia, and hypertension because the amount required can be massive when accumulation of lactic acid is relentless. Fluid administration is poorly tolerated, especially in the oliguric patient, when central venoconstriction coexists. If the underlying cause of the lactic acidosis can be remedied, blood lactate will be converted to HCO_3^- and may result in an overshoot alkalosis if exogenous $NaHCO_3$ has been administered excessively.

Ketoacidosis • DIABETIC KETOACIDOSIS (DKA) This condition is caused by increased fatty acid metabolism and the accumulation of ketoacids (acetoacetate and β-hydroxybutyrate). DKA usually occurs in insulin-dependent diabetes mellitus in association with cessation of insulin or an intercurrent illness such as an infection, gastroenteritis, pancreatitis, or myocardial infarction, which increases insulin requirements temporarily and acutely, and is characterized by hyperglycemia, ketonemia, and a high-AG acidosis. Nevertheless, the plasma glucose may be normal or only slightly elevated in the setting of starvation ketoacidosis or in diabetics receiving antagonists of the proximal tubule sodium-glucose co-transporter 2 (SGLT2). These agents cause glycosuria, an osmotic diuresis, and lower the plasma glucose. Ketoacidosis can occur in patients receiving SGLT2 antagonists for the same reasons as in classical DKA, but the plasma glucose is typically normal or only slightly elevated. The accumulation of ketoacids in plasma accounts for the increment in the AG in both classical DKA and euglycemic DKA. Measurement of urine ketones (by the dipstick nitroprusside reaction) does not detect β-hydroxybutyrate and may underestimate the degree of ketosis (see below). Excretion of ketoacids obligates the excretion of cations, such as Na^+ and K^+, contributing to volume depletion and Cl^- retention. In some circumstances, a mixed non-AG–high-AG acidosis may occur simultaneously and is recognized when the ΔHCO_3^- exceeds the ΔAG. It should be noted that bicarbonate therapy is rarely necessary in DKA except with extreme acidemia (pH <7.00) or if the patient is in shock. If administered, $NaHCO_3$ should be administered in only limited amounts because of the risk for cerebral edema. Patients with DKA are typically volume depleted and require fluid resuscitation with isotonic saline. Volume overexpansion should be avoided, however, because overly aggressive saline administration may cause hyperchloremic acidosis during or following treatment of DKA. Regular insulin should be administered IV as an initial bolus of 0.1 U/kg followed by an infusion of 0.1 U/kg/h until the AG returns to normal; see **Chap. 403** for more detail.

ALCOHOLIC KETOACIDOSIS (AKA) AKA is usually associated with chronic alcoholism, binge drinking, vomiting, abdominal pain, poor nutrition, and volume depletion. The glucose concentration is variable, and acidosis may be severe because of elevated ketones, predominantly β-hydroxybutyrate. The presence of a high-AG acidosis, in the absence of hyperglycemia, in a patient with chronic alcoholism suggests the diagnosis of AKA. Mixed acid-base disorders are common in AKA. Hypoperfusion may enhance lactic acid production (mixed high-AG acidosis), chronic respiratory alkalosis may accompany liver disease (mixed high-AG acidosis and respiratory alkalosis), and metabolic alkalosis can result from vomiting (mixed high-AG acidosis and metabolic alkalosis: ΔAG exceeds ΔHCO_3^-). As the circulation is restored by administration of IV fluids, the preferential accumulation of β-hydroxybutyrate is then shifted to acetoacetate. This explains the common clinical observation of an increasingly positive nitroprusside reaction (ketones) as the circulation is restored. The nitroprusside reaction can detect acetoacetic acid but not β-hydroxybutyrate, so that the degree of ketosis and ketonuria can not only change with therapy, but can be underestimated initially. Therefore, the plasma β-hydroxybutyrate level should be measured. Patients with AKA usually present with relatively normal renal function, as opposed to DKA, where renal function is often compromised because of volume depletion (osmotic diuresis) or diabetic nephropathy. The AKA patient with normal renal function may excrete relatively large quantities of ketoacids and retain Cl^- and, therefore, may have a mixed high-AG–non-AG metabolic acidosis (ΔHCO_3^- exceeds ΔAG).

TREATMENT

Alcoholic Ketoacidosis

Extracellular fluid deficits almost always accompany AKA and should be repaired by IV administration, initially, of saline and glucose (5% dextrose in 0.9% NaCl). Hypophosphatemia, hypokalemia, and hypomagnesemia may coexist and should be monitored carefully and corrected when indicated. Hypophosphatemia may emerge 12–24 h after admission, exacerbated by glucose infusion, and, if severe, may induce marked muscle weakness, hemolysis, rhabdomyolysis, or respiratory arrest. Upper gastrointestinal hemorrhage, pancreatitis, and pneumonia may accompany this disorder.

Drug- and Toxin-Induced Acidosis • SALICYLATES **(See also Chap. 458)** Salicylate intoxication in adults usually causes respiratory alkalosis or a mixture of high-AG metabolic acidosis and respiratory alkalosis. Only a portion of the AG is due to salicylates. Lactic acid production is also often increased.

TREATMENT

Salicylate-Induced Acidosis

Vigorous gastric lavage with isotonic saline (not $NaHCO_3$) should be initiated immediately. All patients should receive at least one round of activated charcoal per nasogastric tube (1 g/kg up to 50 g). To facilitate excretion of salicylate in the acidotic patient, IV $NaHCO_3$ is administered in amounts adequate to alkalinize the urine (urine pH >7.5) and to maintain urine output. Raising urine pH from 6.5 to 7.5 increases salicylate clearance fivefold. Patients with coexisting respiratory alkalosis should also receive $NaHCO_3$ cautiously to avoid excessive alkalemia. Acetazolamide may be administered in the face of alkalemia, when an alkaline diuresis cannot be achieved, or to ameliorate volume overload associated with $NaHCO_3$ administration. Acetazolamide may cause systemic metabolic acidosis if the excreted HCO_3^- is not replaced, a circumstance that can markedly reduce salicylate clearance. **Hypokalemia should be anticipated** with vigorous bicarbonate therapy and should be treated promptly and aggressively. Glucose-containing fluids should be administered because of the danger of hypoglycemia. Excessive insensible fluid losses may cause severe volume depletion and hypernatremia. If renal failure prevents rapid clearance of salicylate, hemodialysis should be performed against a standard bicarbonate dialysate ($[HCO_3^-]$ = 30–35 meq/L).

ALCOHOLS Under most physiologic conditions, sodium, urea, and glucose generate the osmotic pressure of blood. Plasma osmolality is calculated according to the following expression: $P_{osm} = 2Na^+ + Glu + BUN$ (all in mmol/L), or, using conventional laboratory values in which glucose and BUN are expressed in mg/dL: $P_{osm} = 2Na^+ + Glu/18 + BUN/2.8$. The calculated and determined osmolality should agree within 10–15 mmol/kg H_2O. When the measured osmolality exceeds the calculated osmolality by >10–15 mmol/kg H_2O, one of two circumstances prevails. Either the serum sodium is spuriously low, as with hyperlipidemia or hyperproteinemia (pseudohyponatremia), or osmolytes other than sodium salts, glucose, or urea have accumulated in plasma. Examples of such osmolytes include mannitol, radiocontrast media, ethanol, isopropyl alcohol, ethylene glycol, propylene glycol, methanol, and acetone. In this situation, the difference between the calculated osmolality and the measured osmolality (*osmolar gap*) is proportional to the concentration of the unmeasured solute. With an appropriate clinical history and index of suspicion, identification of an osmolar gap is helpful in identifying the presence of toxic alcohol-associated AG acidosis. Three alcohols may cause fatal intoxications: ethylene glycol, methanol, and isopropyl alcohol. All cause an elevated osmolal gap, but only the first two cause a high-AG acidosis. Isopropyl alcohol ingestion does not typically elevate the AG unless extreme overdose causes hypotension and lactic acid acidosis.

ETHYLENE GLYCOL (See also Chap. 458) Ethylene glycol (EG) (commonly used in antifreeze, but also in brake fluid and windshield washer fluid deicers) is metabolized by alcohol dehydrogenase, and ingestion of EG leads to a metabolic acidosis and severe damage to the CNS, heart, lungs, and kidneys. The combination of both a high AG and osmolar gap is highly suspicious for EG or methanol intoxication. The combination of a high AG and high osmolar gap in a patient suspected of EG ingestion should be taken as evidence of EG toxicity prior to measurement of EG levels, and treatment should not be delayed. The osmolar gap may be elevated earlier than the AG, and as the osmolar gap declines, the AG increases. The increased AG and osmolar gap in EG intoxication are attributable to EG and its metabolites, glycolate, oxalate, and other organic acids. Lactic acid production increases secondary to inhibition of the tricarboxylic acid cycle and altered intracellular redox state and may contribute to the high AG. Acute tubule injury is caused initially by glycolate and later is amplified by tubule obstruction from oxalate crystals.

TREATMENT
Ethylene Glycol Intoxication

This includes the prompt institution of IV isotonic fluids, thiamine and pyridoxine supplements, fomepizole, and usually, hemodialysis. Both fomepizole and ethanol compete with EG for metabolism by alcohol dehydrogenase. Fomepizole (4-methylpyrazole; 15 mg/kg IV over 30 min as a loading dose, then 10 mg/kg for four doses every 12 h) is the agent of choice and offers the advantages of a predictable decline in EG levels without excessive obtundation, as seen during ethyl alcohol infusion. Fomepizole should be continued until blood pH is normal or the osmolar gap is <10 mOsm/kg H_2O. Hemodialysis is indicated when the arterial pH is <7.3, a high-AG acidosis is present, the osmolar gap exceeds 20 mOsm/kg H_2O, or there is evidence of end organ damage such as CNS manifestations and kidney failure.

METHANOL (See also Chap. 458) The ingestion of methanol (wood alcohol) causes metabolic acidosis, and its metabolites formaldehyde and formic acid cause severe optic nerve and CNS damage. Lactic acid, ketoacids, and other unidentified organic acids may contribute to the acidosis. Due to its low molecular mass (32 Da), an osmolar gap is present and may precede the elevation of the AG.

TREATMENT
Methanol Intoxication

Treatment of methanol intoxication is similar to that for EG intoxication, including general supportive measures, fomepizole, and hemodialysis.

PROPYLENE GLYCOL Propylene glycol is the vehicle used in IV administration of diazepam, lorazepam, phenobarbital, nitroglycerine, etomidate, enoximone, and phenytoin. Propylene glycol is generally safe for limited use in these IV preparations, but toxicity has been reported in the setting of the intensive care unit in patients receiving frequent or continuous therapy, where the propylene glycol vehicle may accumulate in the plasma. This form of high-gap acidosis should be considered in patients with unexplained high-gap acidosis, hyperosmolality, and clinical deterioration, especially in the setting of treatment for alcohol withdrawal. Propylene glycol, like EG and methanol, is metabolized by alcohol dehydrogenase. With intoxication by propylene glycol, the first response is to stop the offending infusion. Additionally, fomepizole should also be administered in acidotic patients.

ISOPROPYL ALCOHOL Ingested isopropanol is absorbed rapidly and may be fatal when as little as 150 mL of rubbing alcohol, solvent, or deicer is consumed. A plasma level >400 mg/dL is life-threatening. Isopropyl alcohol is metabolized by alcohol dehydrogenase to acetone. The characteristic features differ significantly from EG and methanol intoxication in that the parent compound, not the metabolites, causes toxicity, and a high-AG acidosis is ***not*** present because acetone is rapidly excreted. Both isopropyl alcohol and acetone increase the osmolar gap, and hypoglycemia is common. Alternative diagnoses should be considered if the patient does not improve significantly within a few hours. Patients with hemodynamic instability with plasma levels above 400 mg/dL should be considered for hemodialysis.

TREATMENT
Isopropyl Alcohol Toxicity

Isopropanol alcohol toxicity is treated by supportive therapy, IV fluids, pressors, ventilatory support if needed, and acute hemodialysis for prolonged coma, hemodynamic instability, or levels >400 mg/dL.

PYROGLUTAMIC ACID Acetaminophen-induced high-AG metabolic acidosis is uncommon but is recognized in either patients with acetaminophen overdose or malnourished or critically ill patients receiving acetaminophen in typical dosage. 5-Oxoproline accumulation after acetaminophen should be suspected in the setting of an unexplained high-AG acidosis without elevation of the osmolar gap in patients receiving acetaminophen. The first step in treatment is to immediately discontinue acetaminophen. Additionally, sodium bicarbonate IV should be given. Although *N*-acetylcysteine has been suggested, it is not proven that it hastens the metabolism of 5-oxoproline by increasing intracellular glutathione concentrations in this setting, as assumed.

Chronic Kidney Disease (See also Chap. 311) The hyperchloremic acidosis of moderate chronic kidney disease (CKD; stage 3) is eventually converted to the high-AG acidosis of advanced renal failure (stages 4 and 5 CKD). Poor filtration and reabsorption of organic anions contribute to the pathogenesis. As renal disease progresses, the number of functioning nephrons eventually becomes insufficient to keep pace with net acid production. Uremic acidosis in advanced CKD is characterized, therefore, by a reduced rate of NH_4^+ production and excretion. Alkaline salts from bone buffer the acid retained in CKD. Despite significant retention of acid (up to 20 mmol/d), the serum $[HCO_3^-]$ does not typically decrease further, indicating participation of buffers outside the extracellular compartment. Therefore, the trade-off in untreated chronic metabolic acidosis of CKD stages 3 and 4 is significant loss of bone mass due to reduction in bone calcium carbonate.

Chronic acidosis also contributes significantly to muscle wasting and disability in advancing CKD.

TREATMENT

Metabolic Acidosis of Chronic Kidney Disease

Because of the association of metabolic acidosis in advanced CKD with muscle catabolism, bone disease, and more rapid progression of CKD, both the "uremic acidosis" of end-stage renal disease and the non-AG metabolic acidosis of stages 3 and 4 CKD require oral alkali replacement to increase and maintain the $[HCO_3^-]$ to a value >22 mmol/L. This can be accomplished with relatively modest amounts of alkali (1.0–1.5 mmol/kg body weight per day) and has been shown to slow the progression of CKD. Either $NaHCO_3$ tablets (650-mg tablets contain 7.8 meq) or oral sodium citrate (Shohl's solution) is effective. Moreover, addition of fruits and vegetables (citrate) to the diet may increase the plasma $[HCO_3^-]$ and slow progression.

NON-ANION GAP METABOLIC ACIDOSES

Alkali can be lost from the gastrointestinal tract as a result of diarrhea or from the kidneys due to renal tubular abnormalities (e.g., renal tubular acidosis [RTA]). In these disorders **(Table 55-5)**, reciprocal changes in $[Cl^-]$ and $[HCO_3^-]$ result in a normal AG. In non–AG acidosis, therefore, the increase in $[Cl^-]$ above the normal value approximates the decrease in $[HCO_3^-]$. The absence of such a relationship suggests a mixed disturbance.

TABLE 55-5 Causes of Non–Anion Gap Acidosis

I. Gastrointestinal bicarbonate loss
  A. Diarrhea
  B. External pancreatic or small-bowel drainage
  C. Ureterosigmoidostomy, jejunal loop, ileal loop
  D. Drugs
    1. Calcium chloride (acidifying agent)
    2. Magnesium sulfate (diarrhea)
    3. Cholestyramine (bile acid diarrhea)

II. Renal acidosis
  A. Hypokalemia
    1. Proximal RTA (type 2)
       Drug-induced: acetazolamide, topiramate
    2. Distal (classic) RTA (type 1)
       Drug-induced: amphotericin B, ifosfamide
  B. Hyperkalemia
    1. Generalized distal nephron dysfunction (type 4 RTA)
      a. Selective aldosterone deficiency
      b. Mineralocorticoid resistance (PHA I, autosomal dominant)
      c. Voltage defect (PHA I, autosomal recessive, and PHA II)
      d. Hyporeninemic hypoaldosteronism
      e. Tubulointerstitial disease
  C. Normokalemia
    1. Chronic progressive kidney disease

III. Drug-induced hyperkalemia (with renal insufficiency)
  A. Potassium-sparing diuretics (amiloride, triamterene, spironolactone, eplerenone)
  B. Trimethoprim
  C. Pentamidine
  D. ACE-Is and ARBs
  E. Nonsteroidal anti-inflammatory drugs
  F. Calcineurin inhibitors
  G. Heparin in critically ill patients

IV. Other
  A. Acid loads (ammonium chloride, hyperalimentation)
  B. Loss of potential bicarbonate: ketosis with ketone excretion
  C. Expansion acidosis (rapid saline administration)
  D. Hippurate
  E. Cation exchange resins

Abbreviations: ACE-I, angiotensin-converting enzyme inhibitor; ARB, angiotensin receptor blocker; PHA, pseudohypoaldosteronism; RTA, renal tubular acidosis.

Stool contains a higher concentration of HCO_3^- and decomposed HCO_3^- than plasma so that metabolic acidosis develops in diarrhea. Instead of an acid urine pH (as anticipated with systemic acidosis), urine pH is usually >6 because metabolic acidosis and hypokalemia increase renal synthesis and excretion of NH_4^+, thus providing a urinary buffer that increases urine pH. Metabolic acidosis due to gastrointestinal losses with a high urine pH can be differentiated from RTA because urinary NH_4^+ excretion is typically low in RTA and high with diarrhea. Urinary NH_4^+ levels are not routinely measured by clinical laboratories but can be estimated by calculating the urine anion gap (UAG): UAG = $[Na^+ + K^+]_u - [Cl^-]_u$. When $[Cl^-]_u > [Na^+ + K^+]_u$, the UAG is negative by definition. This suggests that the urine ammonium level is appropriately increased, suggesting an extrarenal cause of the acidosis. Conversely, when the UAG is positive, the urine ammonium level is predictably low, suggesting a renal tubular origin of the acidosis. Recent studies have shown a poor correlation between the UAG and the measured urine ammonium, thus calling the estimation of urine ammonium by calculation of the UAG into question. Therefore, clinical laboratories should be encouraged to measure urine ammonium by adaptation of automated plasma ammonium assays, using the enzymatic method, if the urine sample is diluted 1:200 in normal saline.

Proximal RTA (type 2 RTA) **(Chap. 315)** is most often due to generalized proximal tubular dysfunction manifested by glycosuria, generalized aminoaciduria, and phosphaturia (Fanconi syndrome). When the plasma $[HCO_3^-]$ is low, the urine pH is acid (pH <5.5) but exceeds 5.5 with alkali therapy. The fractional excretion of $[HCO_3^-]$ may exceed 10–15% when the serum HCO_3^- is >20 mmol/L. Because of the defect in HCO_3^- reabsorption by the proximal tubule, therapy with $NaHCO_3$ will enhance delivery of HCO_3^- to the distal nephron and enhance renal potassium secretion, thereby causing hypokalemia.

The typical findings in acquired or inherited forms of **classic distal RTA** (type 1 RTA) include hypokalemia, a non-AG metabolic acidosis, low urinary NH_4^+ excretion (positive UAG, low urine $[NH_4^+]$), and inappropriately high urine pH (pH >5.5). Most patients have hypocitraturia and hypercalciuria; nephrolithiasis, nephrocalcinosis, and bone disease are common. In **generalized distal RTA** (type 4 RTA), hyperkalemia is disproportionate to the reduction in glomerular filtration rate (GFR) because of coexisting dysfunction of potassium and acid secretion. Urinary ammonium excretion is invariably depressed, and kidney function may be compromised secondary to diabetic nephropathy, obstructive uropathy, or chronic tubulointerstitial disease.

Hyporeninemic hypoaldosteronism typically presents as a non-AG metabolic acidosis in older adults with diabetes mellitus or tubulointerstitial disease and CKD (estimated GFR 20–50 mL/min) with hyperkalemia ($[K^+]$ 5.2–6.0 mmol/L), concurrent hypertension, and congestive heart failure. Both the metabolic acidosis and the hyperkalemia are out of proportion to impairment in GFR. Nonsteroidal anti-inflammatory drugs, trimethoprim, pentamidine, angiotensin-converting enzyme (ACE) inhibitors, and angiotensin receptor blockers (ARBs) can also increase the risk for hyperkalemia and a non-AG metabolic acidosis in patients with CKD, especially from diabetic nephropathy (Table 55-5).

TREATMENT

Non–Anion Gap Metabolic Acidoses

For non-AG acidosis due to gastrointestinal losses of bicarbonate, $NaHCO_3$ may be administered intravenously or orally, as determined by the severity of both the acidosis and the accompanying volume depletion. Proximal RTA is the most challenging of the RTAs to treat if the goal is to restore the serum $[HCO_3^-]$ to normal because administration of oral alkali increases urinary excretion of bicarbonate and potassium. In patients with proximal RTA (type 2), potassium administration is typically required. An oral solution of sodium and potassium citrate (citric acid 334 mg, sodium citrate 500 mg, and potassium citrate 550 mg per 5 mL) may be prescribed for this purpose (Virtrate or Cytra-3). In classical distal RTA (type 1), hypokalemia should be corrected first. When accomplished, alkali therapy with either sodium citrate (Shohl's solution) or $NaHCO_3$ tablets (650-mg tablets contain 7.8 meq) should be initiated to correct and maintain the serum $[HCO_3^-]$ in the range of 24–26 meq/L. Type 1 RTA patients typically respond to chronic alkali therapy readily, and the benefits of adequate alkali therapy include a decrease in the frequency of nephrolithiasis, improvement in bone density, resumption of normal growth patterns in children, and preservation of kidney function in both adults and children. For type 4 RTA, attention must be paid to the dual goals of correction of the metabolic acidosis, using the same approach as for classical distal renal tubular acidosis (type 1 RTA), and also correction of the plasma $[K^+]$. Restoration of normokalemia increases urinary net acid excretion and consequently can greatly improve the metabolic acidosis. Chronic administration of oral sodium polystyrene sulfonate (15 g of power prepared as an oral solution, without sorbitol, once daily 2–3 times per week) is sometimes used but is unpalatable, and patient compliance is low. The nonabsorbed, calcium-potassium cation exchange polymer, patiromer, may be considered for type 4 RTA patients with hyperkalemia because it is more palatable. It is administered as 8.4-g packets of powder for suspension PO twice daily with dose adjustment at weekly intervals, based on the plasma $[K^+]$, not to exceed 25.2 g/d. Additionally, the diet should be low in potassium-containing foods or supplements (salt substitute), all potassium-retaining medications should be discontinued, and a loop diuretic may be administered. Finally, patients with documented isolated hypoaldosteronism should receive fludrocortisone, but the dose varies with the cause of the hormone deficiency. This agent should be administered very cautiously and in combination with furosemide in patients with edema and hypertension because of possible aggravation of these conditions.

METABOLIC ALKALOSIS

Metabolic alkalosis is established by an elevated arterial pH, an increase in the serum $[HCO_3^-]$, and an increase in $Paco_2$ as a result of compensatory alveolar hypoventilation (Table 55-1). It is often accompanied by hypochloremia and hypokalemia. The elevation in arterial pH establishes the diagnosis because pH is decreased in respiratory acidosis, even though both have an elevated $Paco_2$. Metabolic alkalosis frequently occurs as a mixed acid-base disorder in association with either respiratory acidosis, respiratory alkalosis, or metabolic acidosis.

ETIOLOGY AND PATHOGENESIS

Metabolic alkalosis occurs as a result of net gain of $[HCO_3^-]$ or loss of nonvolatile acid (usually HCl by vomiting) from the extracellular fluid. When vomiting causes loss of HCl from the stomach, HCO_3^- secretion cannot be initiated in the small bowel, and thus, HCO_3^- is retained in the extracellular fluid. Thus, vomiting or nasogastric suction is an example of the *generation stage* of metabolic alkalosis, in which the loss of acid typically causes alkalosis. Upon cessation of vomiting, the *maintenance stage* ensues because secondary factors prevent the kidneys from excreting HCO_3^- appropriately.

Maintenance of metabolic alkalosis, therefore, represents a failure of the kidneys to eliminate excess HCO_3^- from the extracellular compartment. The kidneys will retain, rather than excrete, the excess alkali and maintain the alkalosis if (1) volume deficiency, chloride deficiency, and K^+ deficiency exist in combination with a reduced GFR (associated with a low urine $[Cl^-]$) or (2) hypokalemia exists because of autonomous hyperaldosteronism (normal urine $[Cl^-]$). In the first example, saline-responsive metabolic alkalosis is corrected by extracellular fluid volume (ECFV) restoration (IV administration of NaCl and KCl), whereas, in the latter, it may be necessary to repair the alkalosis by pharmacologic or surgical intervention, not with saline administration (saline-unresponsive metabolic alkalosis).

TABLE 55-6 Causes of Metabolic Alkalosis

I. Exogenous HCO_3^- loads
   A. Acute alkali administration
   B. Milk-alkali syndrome
II. Effective ECFV contraction, normotension, K^+ deficiency, and secondary hyperreninemic hyperaldosteronism
   A. Gastrointestinal origin
      1. Vomiting
      2. Gastric aspiration
      3. Congenital chloridorrhea
      4. Gastrocystoplasty
      5. Villous adenoma
   B. Renal origin
      1. Diuretic use (thiazides and loop diuretics)
      2. Posthypercapnic state
      3. Hypercalcemia/hypoparathyroidism
      4. Recovery from lactic acidosis or ketoacidosis
      5. Nonreabsorbable anions including penicillin, carbenicillin
      6. Mg^{2+} deficiency
      7. K^+ depletion
      8. Bartter's syndrome (loss-of-function mutations of transporters and ion channels in TALH)
      9. Gitelman's syndrome (loss-of-function mutation of Na^+-Cl^- cotransporter in DCT)
III. ECFV expansion, hypertension, K^+ deficiency, and mineralocorticoid excess
   A. High renin
      1. Renal artery stenosis
      2. Accelerated hypertension
      3. Renin-secreting tumor
      4. Estrogen therapy
   B. Low renin
      1. Primary aldosteronism
         a. Adenoma
         b. Hyperplasia
         c. Carcinoma
      2. Adrenal enzyme defects
         a. 11β-Hydroxylase deficiency
         b. 17α-Hydroxylase deficiency
      3. Cushing's syndrome or disease
      4. Other
         a. Licorice
         b. Carbenoxolone
         c. Chewer's tobacco
IV. Gain-of-function mutation of sodium channel in DCT with ECFV expansion, hypertension, K^+ deficiency, and hyporeninemic-hypoaldosteronism
   A. Liddle's syndrome

Abbreviations: DCT, distal convoluted tubule; ECFV, extracellular fluid volume; TALH, thick ascending limb of Henle's loop.

DIFFERENTIAL DIAGNOSIS

To establish the cause of metabolic alkalosis **(Table 55-6)**, it is necessary to assess the status of the ECFV, the recumbent and upright blood pressure (to determine if orthostasis is present), the serum $[K^+]$, the urine $[Cl^-]$, and in some circumstances, the renin-aldosterone system. For example, the presence of chronic hypertension and chronic hypokalemia in an alkalotic patient suggests either mineralocorticoid excess or that the hypertensive patient is receiving diuretics. Low plasma renin activity and values for urine $[Cl^-]$ >20 meq/L in a patient who is not taking diuretics suggest primary mineralocorticoid excess. The combination of hypokalemia and alkalosis in a normotensive, nonedematous patient can be due to Bartter's or Gitelman's syndrome, magnesium deficiency, vomiting, exogenous alkali, or diuretic ingestion. Measurement of urine electrolytes (especially the urine $[Cl^-]$) and screening of the urine for diuretics are recommended. If the urine is alkaline, with an elevated $[Na^+]_u$ and $[K^+]_u$ but low $[Cl^-]_u$, the diagnosis is usually either vomiting (overt or surreptitious) or alkali ingestion. If the urine is relatively acid with low concentrations of Na^+, K^+, and Cl^-, the most likely possibilities are prior vomiting, the posthypercapnic state, or prior diuretic ingestion. If the urine sodium, potassium, and chloride concentrations are not depressed, magnesium deficiency, Bartter's or Gitelman's syndrome, or current diuretic ingestion should be considered. Bartter's syndrome is distinguished from Gitelman's syndrome by the presence of hypocalciuria in the latter disorder.

Alkali Administration Chronic administration of alkali to individuals with normal renal function rarely causes alkalosis. However, in patients with coexistent hemodynamic disturbances associated with effective ECFV depletion (e.g., heart failure), alkalosis can develop because of diminished capacity to excrete HCO_3^- or enhanced reabsorption of HCO_3^-. Such patients include those who receive $NaHCO_3$ (PO or IV), citrate loads IV (transfusions of whole blood, or therapeutic apheresis), or antacids plus cation-exchange resins (aluminum hydroxide and sodium polystyrene sulfonate). Nursing home patients receiving enteral tube feedings have a higher incidence of metabolic alkalosis than nursing home patients receiving regular diets.

METABOLIC ALKALOSIS ASSOCIATED WITH ECFV CONTRACTION, K^+ DEPLETION, AND SECONDARY HYPERRENINEMIC HYPERALDOSTERONISM

Gastrointestinal Origin Gastrointestinal loss of H^+ from vomiting or gastric aspiration causes simultaneous addition of HCO_3^- into the extracellular fluid. During active vomiting, the filtered load of bicarbonate reaching the kidneys is acutely increased and will exceed the reabsorptive capacity of the proximal tubule for HCO_3^- absorption. Subsequently, enhanced delivery of HCO_3^- to the distal nephron, where the capacity for HCO_3^- reabsorption is lower, will result in excretion of alkaline urine that stimulates potassium secretion. When vomiting ceases, the persistence of volume, potassium, and chloride depletion triggers maintenance of the alkalosis because these conditions promote HCO_3^- reabsorption. Correction of the contracted ECFV with NaCl and repair of K^+ deficits with KCl corrects the acid-base disorder by restoring the ability of the kidney to excrete the excess bicarbonate.

Renal Origin • DIURETICS **(See also Chap. 258)** Diuretics such as thiazides and loop diuretics (furosemide, bumetanide, torsemide) increase excretion of salt and acutely diminish the ECFV without altering the total body bicarbonate content. The serum $[HCO_3^-]$ increases because the reduced ECFV "contracts" around the $[HCO_3^-]$ in plasma (contraction alkalosis). The chronic administration of diuretics tends to generate an alkalosis by increasing distal salt delivery so that both K^+ and H^+ secretion are stimulated. The alkalosis is maintained by persistence of the contraction of the ECFV, secondary hyperaldosteronism, K^+ deficiency, and the direct effect of the diuretic (as long as diuretic administration continues). Discontinuing the diuretic and providing isotonic saline to correct the ECFV deficit will repair the alkalosis.

SOLUTE LOSING DISORDERS: BARTTER'S SYNDROME AND GITELMAN'S SYNDROME See Chap. 315.

NON-REABSORBABLE ANIONS AND MAGNESIUM DEFICIENCY Administration of large quantities of the penicillin derivatives carbenicillin or ticarcillin cause their non-reabsorbable anions to appear in the distal tubule. This increases the transepithelial potential difference in the collecting tubule and thereby enhances H^+ and K^+ secretion. Mg^{2+} deficiency may occur with chronic administration of thiazide diuretics, alcoholism, and malnutrition, and in Gitelman's syndrome, it potentiates the development of hypokalemic alkalosis by enhancing distal acidification through stimulation of renin and hence aldosterone secretion.

POTASSIUM DEPLETION Chronic K^+ depletion as a result of extreme dietary potassium insufficiency, diuretics, or alcohol abuse may initiate metabolic alkalosis by increasing urinary net acid excretion. The renal generation of NH_4^+ (ammoniagenesis) is upregulated directly by hypokalemia. Chronic K^+ deficiency also upregulates the H^+, K^+-ATPases in the distal tubule and collecting duct to increase K^+ absorption while simultaneously increasing H^+ secretion. Alkalosis associated with severe K^+ depletion is resistant to salt administration, but repair of the K^+ deficiency corrects the alkalosis. Potassium depletion often occurs concurrent with magnesium deficiency in alcoholics with malnutrition.

AFTER TREATMENT OF LACTIC ACIDOSIS OR KETOACIDOSIS When an underlying stimulus for the generation of lactic acid or ketoacid is corrected, such as shock or severe volume depletion by volume restoration, or with insulin therapy, the lactate or ketones are metabolized to yield an equivalent amount of HCO_3^-. Exogenous sources of HCO_3^- will be additive to that amount generated by organic anion metabolism and may create a surfeit of HCO_3^- ("rebound alkalosis").

POSTHYPERCAPNIA Prolonged CO_2 retention with chronic respiratory acidosis enhances renal HCO_3^- absorption and the generation of new HCO_3^- (increased net acid excretion). Metabolic alkalosis results from the persistently elevated $[HCO_3^-]$ when the elevated $Paco_2$ is abruptly returned toward normal.

METABOLIC ALKALOSIS ASSOCIATED WITH ECFV EXPANSION, HYPERTENSION, AND MINERALOCORTICOID EXCESS

Increased aldosterone levels may be the result of autonomous primary adrenal overproduction or of secondary aldosterone release due to renal overproduction of renin. Mineralocorticoid excess increases net acid excretion and may result in metabolic alkalosis, which is typically exacerbated by associated K^+ deficiency. Salt retention and hypertension are due to upregulation of the epithelial Na^+ channel (ENaC) in the collecting tubule in response to aldosterone. The kaliuresis persists because of mineralocorticoid excess and stimulation of ENaC, causing an increase in transepithelial voltage, which enhances K^+ excretion. Persistent K^+ depletion may cause polydipsia and polyuria.

Liddle's syndrome **(Chap. 315)** results from an inherited gain-of-function mutation of genes that regulate the collecting duct Na^+ channel, ENaC. This rare monogenic form of hypertension is the result of volume expansion that secondarily suppresses aldosterone elaboration. Patients typically present with hypertension, hypokalemia, and metabolic alkalosis.

Symptoms With metabolic alkalosis, changes in CNS and peripheral nervous system function are similar to those of hypocalcemia **(Chap. 409)**; symptoms include mental confusion; obtundation; and a predisposition to seizures, paresthesias, muscular cramping, tetany, aggravation of arrhythmias, and hypoxemia in chronic obstructive pulmonary disease. Related electrolyte abnormalities include hypokalemia and hypophosphatemia.

TREATMENT

Metabolic Alkalosis

The first goal of therapy is to correct the underlying stimulus for HCO_3^- generation. If primary aldosteronism or Cushing's syndrome is present, correction of the underlying cause will reverse the hypokalemia and alkalosis. $[H^+]$ loss by the stomach or kidneys can be mitigated by the use of proton pump inhibitors or the discontinuation of diuretics. The second aspect of treatment is to eliminate factors that sustain the inappropriate increase in HCO_3^- reabsorption, such as ECFV contraction or K^+ deficiency. K^+ deficits should always be repaired. Isotonic saline is recommended to reverse the alkalosis when ECFV contraction is present. If associated conditions, such as congestive heart failure, preclude infusion of isotonic saline, renal HCO_3^- loss can be accelerated by administration of acetazolamide (125–250 mg IV), a carbonic anhydrase inhibitor, which is usually effective in patients with adequate renal function. However, acetazolamide triggers urinary K^+

losses and may cause hypokalemia that should be corrected. Dilute hydrochloric acid IV (0.1 *N* HCl) has been advocated in extreme cases of metabolic alkalosis but causes hemolysis and must be delivered slowly in a central vein. This preparation is not available generally and must be prepared in the pharmacy. Because serious errors or harm may occur, its use is not advised. Therapy in Liddle's syndrome should include a potassium-sparing diuretic (amiloride or triamterene) to inhibit ENaC and correct both the hypertension and the hypokalemia.

RESPIRATORY ACIDOSIS

Respiratory acidosis occurs as a result of severe pulmonary disease, respiratory muscle fatigue, or abnormalities in ventilatory control and is recognized by an increase in $Paco_2$ and decrease in pH (**Table 55-7**). In acute respiratory acidosis, there is a compensatory elevation in HCO_3^- (due to cellular buffering mechanisms) that increases 1 mmol/L for every 10-mmHg increase in $Paco_2$. In chronic respiratory acidosis (>24 h), renal adaptation increases the $[HCO_3^-]$ by 4 mmol/L for every 10-mmHg increase in $Paco_2$. The serum HCO_3^- usually does not increase above 38 mmol/L.

The clinical features vary according to the severity and duration of the respiratory acidosis, the underlying disease, and whether there is accompanying hypoxemia. A rapid increase in $Paco_2$ (acute hypercapnia) may cause anxiety, dyspnea, confusion, psychosis, and hallucinations and may progress to coma. However, chronic hypercapnia may cause sleep disorders; loss of memory; daytime somnolence; personality changes; impairment of coordination; and motor disturbances such as tremor, myoclonic jerks, and asterixis. Headaches and other signs that mimic raised intracranial pressure, such as papilledema, abnormal reflexes, and focal muscle weakness, are also seen.

Depression of the respiratory center by a variety of drugs, injury, or disease can produce respiratory acidosis. This may occur acutely with general anesthetics, sedatives, and head trauma or chronically with sedatives, alcohol, intracranial tumors, and the syndromes of sleep-disordered breathing including the primary alveolar and obesity-hypoventilation syndromes **(Chaps. 296 and 297)**. Abnormalities or disease in the motor neurons, neuromuscular junction, and skeletal muscle can cause hypoventilation via respiratory muscle fatigue. Mechanical ventilation, when not properly adjusted, may result in respiratory acidosis, particularly if CO_2 production suddenly rises (because of fever, agitation, sepsis, or overfeeding) or alveolar ventilation decreases because of worsening pulmonary function. High levels of positive end-expiratory pressure in the presence of reduced cardiac output may cause hypercapnia as a result of large increases in alveolar dead space **(Chap. 285)**. Permissive hypercapnia may be used to minimize intrinsic positive end-expiratory pressure in respiratory distress syndrome, but the consequential respiratory acidosis may require administration of $NaHCO_3$ to increase the arterial pH to approximately 7.20, but not to the normal value.

Acute hypercapnia follows sudden occlusion of the upper airway or generalized bronchospasm as in severe asthma, anaphylaxis, inhalational burn, or toxin injury. Chronic hypercapnia and respiratory acidosis occur in end-stage obstructive lung disease. Restrictive disorders involving both the chest wall and the lungs can cause respiratory acidosis because the high metabolic cost of respiration causes ventilatory muscle fatigue. Advanced stages of intrapulmonary and extrapulmonary restrictive defects present as chronic respiratory acidosis.

The diagnosis of respiratory acidosis requires the measurement of $Paco_2$ and arterial pH. A detailed history and physical examination often indicate the cause. Pulmonary function studies **(Chap. 285)**, including spirometry, diffusion capacity for carbon monoxide, lung volumes, and arterial $Paco_2$ and O_2 saturation, usually make it possible to determine if respiratory acidosis is secondary to lung disease. The workup for nonpulmonary causes should include a detailed drug history, measurement of hematocrit, and assessment of upper airway, chest wall, pleura, and neuromuscular function.

TABLE 55-7 Respiratory Acid-Base Disorders

I. Alkalosis
- A. Central nervous system stimulation
  1. Pain
  2. Anxiety, psychosis
  3. Fever
  4. Cerebrovascular accident
  5. Meningitis, encephalitis
  6. Tumor
  7. Trauma
- B. Hypoxemia or tissue hypoxia
  1. High altitude
  2. Pneumonia, pulmonary edema
  3. Aspiration
  4. Severe anemia
- C. Drugs or hormones
  1. Pregnancy, progesterone
  2. Salicylates
  3. Cardiac failure
- D. Stimulation of chest receptors
  1. Hemothorax
  2. Flail chest
  3. Cardiac failure
  4. Pulmonary embolism
- E. Miscellaneous
  1. Septicemia
  2. Hepatic failure
  3. Mechanical hyperventilation
  4. Heat exposure
  5. Recovery from metabolic acidosis

II. Acidosis
- A. Central
  1. Drugs (anesthetics, morphine, sedatives)
  2. Stroke
  3. Infection
- B. Airway
  1. Obstruction
  2. Asthma
- C. Parenchyma
  1. Emphysema
  2. Pneumoconiosis
  3. Bronchitis
  4. Adult respiratory distress syndrome
  5. Barotrauma
- D. Neuromuscular
  1. Poliomyelitis
  2. Kyphoscoliosis
  3. Myasthenia
  4. Muscular dystrophies
- E. Miscellaneous
  1. Obesity
  2. Hypoventilation
  3. Permissive hypercapnia

TREATMENT

Respiratory Acidosis

The management of respiratory acidosis depends on its severity and rate of onset. Acute respiratory acidosis can be life-threatening, and measures to reverse the underlying cause should be undertaken simultaneously with restoration of adequate alveolar ventilation. This may necessitate tracheal intubation and assisted mechanical ventilation. Oxygen administration should be titrated carefully in patients with severe obstructive pulmonary disease and chronic CO_2 retention who are breathing spontaneously **(Chap. 292)**. When oxygen is used injudiciously, these patients may experience progression of the respiratory acidosis causing severe acidemia. Aggressive and rapid correction of hypercapnia should be avoided, because the falling $Paco_2$ may provoke the same complications noted with acute respiratory alkalosis (i.e., cardiac arrhythmias, reduced cerebral perfusion, and seizures). The $Paco_2$ should be lowered gradually in chronic respiratory acidosis, aiming to restore the $Paco_2$ to baseline levels and to provide sufficient Cl^- and K^+ to enhance the renal excretion of HCO_3^-.

Chronic respiratory acidosis is frequently difficult to correct, but the primary goal is to institute measures that may improve lung function **(Chap. 292)**.

RESPIRATORY ALKALOSIS

Alveolar hyperventilation decreases $Paco_2$ and increases the $HCO_3^-/Paco_2$ ratio, thus increasing pH (Table 55-7). Nonbicarbonate cellular buffers respond by consuming HCO_3^-. Hypocapnia develops when a sufficiently strong ventilatory stimulus causes CO_2 output in the lungs to exceed its metabolic production by tissues. Plasma pH and $[HCO_3^-]$ appear to vary proportionately with $Paco_2$ over a range from 40–15 mmHg. The relationship between arterial $[H^+]$ concentration and $Paco_2$ is ~0.7 mmol/L per mmHg (or 0.01 pH unit/mmHg), and that for plasma $[HCO_3^-]$ is 0.2 mmol/L per mmHg. Hypocapnia sustained for >2–6 h is further compensated by a decrease in renal ammonium and titratable acid excretion and a reduction in filtered HCO_3^- reabsorption. Full renal adaptation to respiratory alkalosis may take several days and requires normal volume status and renal function. The kidneys appear to respond directly to the lowered $Paco_2$ rather than to alkalosis per se. In chronic respiratory alkalosis, a 1-mmHg decrease in $Paco_2$ causes a 0.4-to 0.5-mmol/L drop in $[HCO_3^-]$ and a 0.3-mmol/L decrease in $[H^+]$ (or 0.003 increase in pH).

The effects of respiratory alkalosis vary according to duration and severity but are primarily those of the underlying disease. Reduced cerebral blood flow as a consequence of a rapid decline in $Paco_2$ may cause dizziness, mental confusion, and seizures, even in the absence of hypoxemia. The cardiovascular effects of acute hypocapnia in the conscious human are generally minimal, but in the anesthetized or mechanically ventilated patient, cardiac output and blood pressure may fall because of the depressant effects of anesthesia and positive-pressure ventilation on heart rate, systemic resistance, and venous return. Cardiac arrhythmias may occur in patients with heart disease as a result of changes in oxygen unloading by blood from a left shift in the hemoglobin-oxygen dissociation curve (Bohr effect). Acute respiratory alkalosis causes intracellular shifts of Na^+, K^+, and PO_4^{2-} and reduces free $[Ca^{2+}]$ by increasing the protein-bound fraction. Hypocapnia-induced hypokalemia is usually minor.

Chronic respiratory alkalosis is the most common acid-base disturbance in critically ill patients and, when severe, portends a poor prognosis. Many cardiopulmonary disorders manifest respiratory alkalosis in their early to intermediate stages, and the finding of normocapnia and hypoxemia in a patient with hyperventilation may herald the onset of rapid respiratory failure and should prompt an assessment to determine if the patient is becoming fatigued. Respiratory alkalosis is common during mechanical ventilation.

The hyperventilation syndrome may be disabling. Paresthesia; circumoral numbness; chest wall tightness or pain; dizziness; inability to take an adequate breath; and, rarely, tetany may be sufficiently stressful to perpetuate the disorder. Arterial blood-gas analysis demonstrates an acute or chronic respiratory alkalosis, often with hypocapnia in the range of 15–30 mmHg and no hypoxemia. CNS diseases or injury can produce several patterns of hyperventilation and sustained $Paco_2$ levels of 20–30 mmHg. Hyperthyroidism, high caloric loads, and exercise raise the basal metabolic rate, but ventilation usually rises in proportion so that arterial blood gases are unchanged and respiratory alkalosis does not develop. Salicylates are the most common cause of drug-induced respiratory alkalosis because of direct stimulation of the medullary chemoreceptor **(Chap. 458)**. In addition, the methylxanthines, theophylline, and aminophylline stimulate ventilation and increase the ventilatory response to CO_2. Progesterone increases ventilation and lowers arterial $Paco_2$ by as much as 5–10 mmHg. Therefore, chronic respiratory alkalosis is a common feature of pregnancy. Respiratory alkalosis is also prominent in liver failure, and the severity correlates with the degree of hepatic insufficiency. Respiratory alkalosis is often an early finding in gram-negative septicemia, before fever, hypoxemia, or hypotension develops.

The diagnosis of respiratory alkalosis depends on measurement of arterial pH and $Paco_2$. The plasma $[K^+]$ is often reduced and the $[Cl^-]$ increased. In the acute phase, respiratory alkalosis is not associated with increased renal HCO_3^- excretion, but within hours, net acid excretion is reduced. In general, the HCO_3^- concentration falls by 2.0 mmol/L for each 10-mmHg decrease in $Paco_2$. Chronic respiratory alkalosis occurs when hypocapnia persists for greater than 3–5 days. The decline in $Paco_2$ reduces the serum $[HCO_3^-]$ by 4.0–5 mmol/L for each 10-mmHg decrease in $Paco_2$. It is unusual to observe a plasma HCO_3^- <12 mmol/L as a result of a pure respiratory alkalosis. The compensatory reduction in plasma $[HCO_3^-]$ is so effective in chronic respiratory alkalosis that the pH may not decline significantly from the normal value. Therefore, chronic respiratory alkalosis is the only acid-base disorder for which compensation can return the pH to the normal value.

When the diagnosis of respiratory alkalosis is made, its cause should be investigated. The diagnosis of hyperventilation syndrome is made by exclusion. In difficult cases, it may be important to rule out other conditions such as pulmonary embolism, coronary artery disease, and hyperthyroidism.

TREATMENT
Respiratory Alkalosis

The management of respiratory alkalosis is directed toward alleviation of the underlying disorder. If respiratory alkalosis complicates ventilator management, changes in dead space and tidal volume can minimize the hypocapnia. Patients with the hyperventilation syndrome may benefit from reassurance, rebreathing from a paper bag during symptomatic attacks, and attention to underlying psychological stress. Antidepressants and sedatives are not recommended. β-Adrenergic blockers may ameliorate peripheral manifestations of the hyperadrenergic state.

REFERENCES

Berend K et al: Physiological approach to assessment of acid-base disturbances. N Engl J Med 371:1434, 2014.

DuBose TD: Etiologic causes of metabolic acidosis II: The normal anion gap acidosis. In *Metabolic Acidosis*. Wesson DE (ed). New York, Springer, 2016, pp. 27–38.

Hamm LL, DuBose TD: Disorders of acid-base balance. In *Brenner and Rector's The Kidney*, 11th ed. Yu A et al (eds). Philadelphia, Elsevier, 2020, pp 496–536.

Kraut JA, Madias NE: Metabolic acidosis of CKD: An update. Am J Kidney Dis 67:307, 2016.

Kraut JA, Madias NE: Re-evaluation of the normal range of serum total CO_2 concentration. Clin J Am Soc Nephrol 13:343, 2018.

Palmer BF, Clegg DJ: Electrolyte and acid–base disturbances in patients with diabetes mellitus. N Engl J Med 373:548, 2015.

Wesson DE et al: Mechanisms of metabolic acidosis-induced kidney injury in chronic kidney disease. J Am Soc Nephrol 31:469, 2020.

Section 8 Alterations in the Skin

56 Approach to the Patient with a Skin Disorder

Kim B. Yancey, Thomas J. Lawley

The challenge of examining the skin lies in distinguishing normal from abnormal findings, distinguishing significant findings from trivial ones, and integrating pertinent signs and symptoms into an appropriate differential diagnosis. The fact that the largest organ in the body is visible is both an advantage and a disadvantage to those who examine it. It is advantageous because no special instrumentation is necessary and because the skin can be biopsied with little morbidity. However, the casual observer can be misled by a variety of stimuli and overlook important, subtle signs of skin or systemic disease. For instance, the sometimes minor differences in color and shape that distinguish a melanoma (Fig. 56-1) from a benign nevomelanocytic nevus (Fig. 56-2) can be difficult to recognize. A variety of descriptive terms have been developed that characterize cutaneous lesions (**Tables 56-1, 56-2, and 56-3; Fig. 56-3**), thereby aiding in their interpretation and in the formulation of a differential diagnosis (**Table 56-4**). For example, the finding of scaling papules, which are present in psoriasis or atopic dermatitis, places the patient in a different diagnostic category than would hemorrhagic papules, which may indicate vasculitis or sepsis (**Figs. 56-4 and 56-5, respectively**). It is also important to differentiate primary from secondary skin lesions. If the examiner focuses on linear erosions overlying an area of erythema and scaling, he or she may incorrectly assume that the erosion is the primary lesion and that the redness and scale are secondary, whereas the correct interpretation would be that the patient has a pruritic eczematous dermatitis with erosions caused by scratching.

APPROACH TO THE PATIENT

Skin Disorder

In examining the skin, it is usually advisable to assess the patient before taking an extensive history. This approach ensures that the entire cutaneous surface will be evaluated, and objective findings can be integrated with relevant historical data. Four basic features of a skin problem must be noted and considered during a physical examination: the *distribution* of the eruption, the *types* of primary

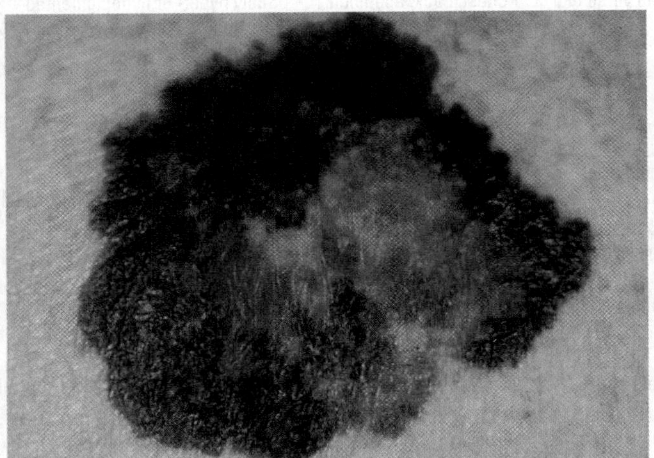

FIGURE 56-1 Superficial spreading melanoma. This is the most common type of melanoma. Such lesions usually demonstrate asymmetry, border irregularity, color variegation (black, blue, brown, pink, and white), a diameter >6 mm, and a history of change (e.g., an increase in size or development of associated symptoms such as pruritus or pain).

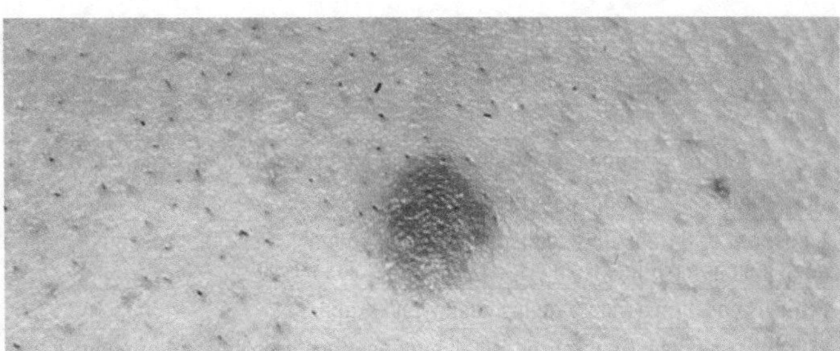

FIGURE 56-2 Nevomelanocytic nevus. Nevi are benign proliferations of nevomelanocytes characterized by regularly shaped hyperpigmented macules or papules of a uniform color.

TABLE 56-1 Description of Primary Skin Lesions
Macule: A flat, colored lesion, <2 cm in diameter, not raised above the surface of the surrounding skin. A "freckle," or ephelid, is a prototypical pigmented macule.
Patch: A large (>2 cm) flat lesion with a color different from the surrounding skin. This differs from a macule only in size.
Papule: A small, solid lesion, <0.5 cm in diameter, raised above the surface of the surrounding skin and thus palpable (e.g., a closed comedone, or whitehead, in acne).
Nodule: A larger (0.5–5.0 cm), firm lesion raised above the surface of the surrounding skin. This differs from a papule only in size (e.g., a large dermal nevomelanocytic nevus).
Tumor: A solid, raised growth >5 cm in diameter.
Plaque: A large (>1 cm), flat-topped, raised lesion; edges may either be distinct (e.g., in psoriasis) or gradually blend with surrounding skin (e.g., in eczematous dermatitis).
Vesicle: A small, fluid-filled lesion, <0.5 cm in diameter, raised above the plane of surrounding skin. Fluid is often visible, and the lesions are translucent (e.g., vesicles in allergic contact dermatitis caused by *Toxicodendron* [poison ivy]).
Pustule: A vesicle filled with leukocytes. Note: The presence of pustules does not necessarily signify the existence of an infection.
Bulla: A fluid-filled, raised, often translucent lesion >0.5 cm in diameter.
Wheal: A raised, erythematous, edematous papule or plaque, usually representing short-lived vasodilation and vasopermeability.
Telangiectasia: A dilated, superficial blood vessel.

TABLE 56-2 Description of Secondary Skin Lesions
Lichenification: A distinctive thickening of the skin that is characterized by accentuated skinfold markings.
Scale: Excessive accumulation of stratum corneum.
Crust: Dried exudate of body fluids that may be either yellow (i.e., serous crust) or red (i.e., hemorrhagic crust).
Erosion: Loss of epidermis without an associated loss of dermis.
Ulcer: Loss of epidermis and at least a portion of the underlying dermis.
Excoriation: Linear, angular erosions that may be covered by crust and are caused by scratching.
Atrophy: An acquired loss of substance. In the skin, this may appear as a depression with intact epidermis (i.e., loss of dermal or subcutaneous tissue) or as sites of shiny, delicate, wrinkled lesions (i.e., epidermal atrophy).
Scar: A change in the skin secondary to trauma or inflammation. Sites may be erythematous, hypopigmented, or hyperpigmented depending on their age or character. Sites on hair-bearing areas may be characterized by destruction of hair follicles.

TABLE 56-3 Common Dermatologic Terms

Alopecia: Hair loss, partial or complete.

Annular: Ring-shaped.

Cyst: A soft, raised, encapsulated lesion filled with semisolid or liquid contents.

Herpetiform: In a grouped configuration.

Lichenoid eruption: Violaceous to purple, polygonal lesions that resemble those seen in lichen planus.

Milia: Small, firm, white papules filled with keratin.

Morbilliform rash: Generalized, small erythematous macules and/or papules that resemble lesions seen in measles.

Nummular: Coin-shaped.

Poikiloderma: Skin that displays variegated pigmentation, atrophy, and telangiectasias.

Polycyclic lesions: A configuration of skin lesions formed from coalescing rings or incomplete rings.

Pruritus: A sensation that elicits the desire to scratch. Pruritus is often the predominant symptom of inflammatory skin diseases (e.g., atopic dermatitis, allergic contact dermatitis); it is also commonly associated with xerosis and aged skin. Systemic conditions that can be associated with pruritus include chronic renal disease, cholestasis, pregnancy, malignancy, thyroid disease, polycythemia vera, and delusions of parasitosis.

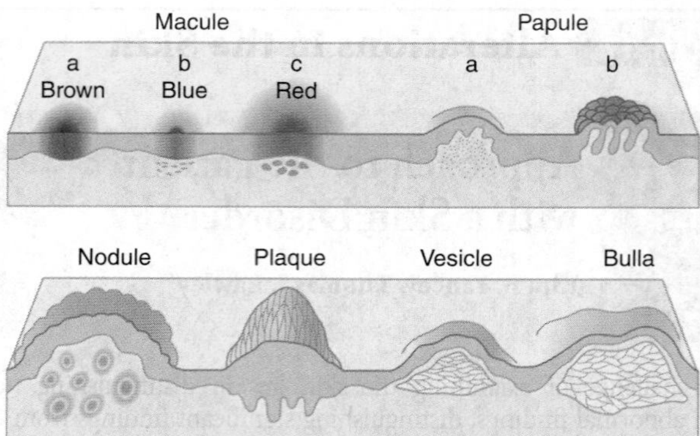

FIGURE 56-3 A schematic representation of several common primary skin lesions (see Table 56-1).

TABLE 56-4 Selected Common Dermatologic Conditions

DIAGNOSIS	COMMON DISTRIBUTION	USUAL MORPHOLOGY	DIAGNOSIS	COMMON DISTRIBUTION	USUAL MORPHOLOGY
Acne vulgaris	Face, upper back, chest	Open and closed comedones, erythematous papules, pustules, cysts	Seborrheic keratosis	Trunk, face, extremities	Brown plaques with adherent, greasy scale; "stuck on" appearance
Rosacea	Blush area of cheeks, nose, forehead, chin	Erythema, telangiectasias, papules, pustules	Folliculitis Impetigo	Any hair-bearing area Anywhere	Follicular pustules Papules, vesicles, pustules, often with honey-colored crusts
Seborrheic dermatitis	Scalp, eyebrows, perinasal areas	Erythema with greasy yellow-brown scale	Herpes simplex	Lips, genitalia	Grouped vesicles progressing to crusted erosions
Atopic dermatitis	Antecubital and popliteal fossae; may be widespread	Patches and plaques of erythema, scaling, and lichenification; pruritus	Herpes zoster	Dermatomal, usually trunk but may be anywhere	Vesicles limited to a dermatome (often painful)
Stasis dermatitis	Ankles, lower legs over medial malleoli	Patches of erythema and scaling on background of hyperpigmentation associated with signs of venous insufficiency	Varicella	Face, trunk, relative sparing of extremities	Lesions arise in crops and quickly progress from erythematous macules, to papules, to vesicles, to pustules, to crusted sites
Dyshidrotic eczema	Palms, soles, sides of fingers, and toes	Deep vesicles	Pityriasis rosea	Trunk (Christmas tree pattern); herald patch followed by multiple smaller lesions	Symmetric erythematous papules and plaques with a collarette of scale
Allergic contact dermatitis	Anywhere	Localized erythema, vesicles, scale, and pruritus (e.g., fingers, earlobes—nickel; dorsal aspect of foot—shoe; exposed surfaces—poison ivy)	Tinea versicolor	Chest, back, abdomen, proximal extremities	Scaly hyper- or hypopigmented macules
Psoriasis	Elbows, knees, scalp, lower back, fingernails (may be generalized)	Papules and plaques covered with silvery scale; nails have pits	Candidiasis	Groin, beneath breasts, vagina, oral cavity	Erythematous macerated areas with satellite pustules; white, friable patches on mucous membranes
Lichen planus	Wrists, ankles, mouth (may be widespread)	Violaceous flat-topped papules and plaques	Dermatophytosis	Feet, groin, beard, or scalp	Varies with site (e.g., tinea corporis—scaly annular plaque)
Keratosis pilaris	Extensor surfaces of arms and thighs, buttocks	Keratotic follicular papules with surrounding erythema	Scabies	Groin, axillae, between fingers and toes, beneath breasts	Excoriated papules, burrows, pruritus
Melasma	Forehead, cheeks, temples, upper lip	Tan to brown patches	Insect bites	Anywhere	Erythematous papules with central puncta
Vitiligo	Periorificial, trunk, extensor surfaces of extremities, flexor wrists, axillae	Chalk-white macules	Cherry angioma Keloid Dermatofibroma	Trunk Anywhere (site of previous injury) Anywhere	Red, blood-filled papules Firm tumor, pink, purple, or brown Firm red to brown nodule that shows dimpling of overlying skin with lateral compression

(*Continued*)

TABLE 56-4 Selected Common Dermatologic Conditions (Continued)

DIAGNOSIS	COMMON DISTRIBUTION	USUAL MORPHOLOGY	DIAGNOSIS	COMMON DISTRIBUTION	USUAL MORPHOLOGY
Actinic keratosis	Sun-exposed areas	Skin-colored or red-brown macule or papule with dry, rough, adherent scale	Acrochordons (skin tags)	Groin, axilla, neck	Fleshy papules
Basal cell carcinoma	Face	Papule with pearly, telangiectatic border on sun-damaged skin	Urticaria	Anywhere	Wheals, sometimes with surrounding flare; pruritus
Squamous cell carcinoma	Face, especially lower lip, ears	Indurated and possibly hyperkeratotic lesions often showing ulceration and/or crusting	Transient acantholytic dermatosis	Trunk, especially anterior chest	Erythematous papules
			Xerosis	Extensor extremities, especially legs	Dry, erythematous, scaling patches; pruritus

and secondary lesions, the *shape* of individual lesions, and the *arrangement* of the lesions. An ideal skin examination includes evaluation of the skin, hair, and nails as well as the mucous membranes of the mouth, eyes, nose, nasopharynx, and anogenital region. In the initial examination, it is important that the patient be disrobed as completely as possible to minimize chances of missing important individual skin lesions and permit accurate assessment of the distribution of the eruption. The patient should first be viewed from a distance of about 1.5–2 m (4–6 ft) so that the general character of the skin and the distribution of lesions can be evaluated. Indeed, the distribution of lesions often correlates highly with diagnosis (Fig. 56-6). For example, a hospitalized patient with a generalized erythematous exanthem is more likely to have a drug eruption than is a patient with a similar rash limited to the sun-exposed portions of the face. Once the distribution of the lesions has been established, the nature of the primary lesion must be determined. Thus, when lesions are distributed on elbows, knees, and scalp, the most likely possibility based solely on distribution is psoriasis or dermatitis herpetiformis (**Figs. 56-7 and 56-8, respectively**). The primary lesion in psoriasis is a scaly papule that soon forms erythematous plaques covered with a white scale, whereas that of dermatitis herpetiformis is an urticarial papule that quickly becomes a small vesicle. In this manner, identification of the primary lesion directs the examiner toward the proper diagnosis. Secondary changes in skin can also be quite helpful. For example, scale represents excessive epidermis, while crust is the result of a discontinuous epithelial cell layer. Palpation of skin lesions can yield insight into the character of an eruption. Thus, red papules on the lower extremities that blanch with pressure can be a manifestation of many different diseases, but hemorrhagic red papules that do not blanch with pressure indicate palpable purpura characteristic of necrotizing vasculitis (Fig. 56-4).

The shape of lesions is also an important feature. Flat, round, erythematous papules and plaques are common in many cutaneous diseases. However, target-shaped lesions that consist in part of erythematous plaques are specific for erythema multiforme (**Fig. 56-9**). Likewise, the arrangement of individual lesions is important. Erythematous papules and vesicles can occur in many conditions, but their arrangement in a specific linear array suggests an external etiology such as allergic contact dermatitis (**Fig. 56-10**) or primary irritant dermatitis. In contrast, lesions with a generalized arrangement are common and suggest a systemic etiology.

As in other branches of medicine, a complete history should be obtained to emphasize the following features:

1. Evolution of lesions
   a. Site of onset
   b. Manner in which the eruption progressed or spread
   c. Duration
   d. Periods of resolution or improvement in chronic eruptions
2. Symptoms associated with the eruption
   a. Itching, burning, pain, numbness
   b. What, if anything, has relieved symptoms
   c. Time of day when symptoms are most severe
3. Current or recent medications (prescribed as well as over-the-counter)
4. Associated systemic symptoms (e.g., malaise, fever, arthralgias)
5. Ongoing or previous illnesses
6. History of allergies
7. Presence of photosensitivity
8. Review of systems
9. Family history (particularly relevant for patients with melanoma, atopy, psoriasis, or acne)
10. Social, sexual, or travel history

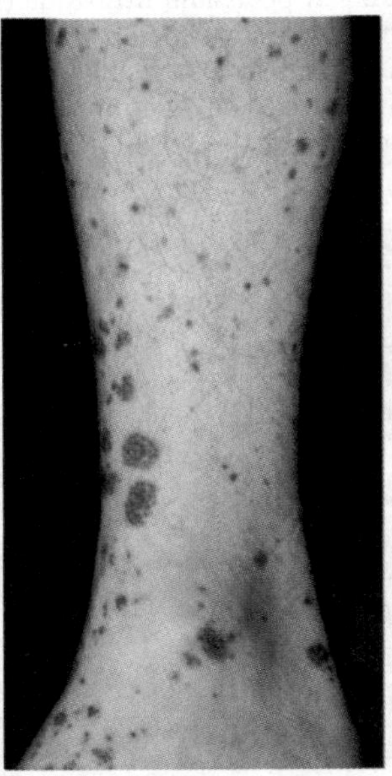

FIGURE 56-4 Necrotizing vasculitis. Palpable purpuric papules on the lower legs are seen in this patient with cutaneous small-vessel vasculitis. *(Courtesy of Robert Swerlick, MD; with permission.)*

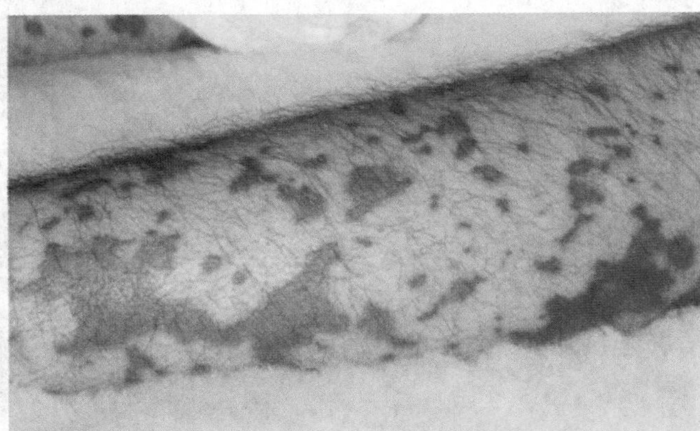

FIGURE 56-5 Meningococcemia. An example of fulminant meningococcemia with extensive angular purpuric patches. *(Courtesy of Stephen E. Gellis, MD; with permission.)*

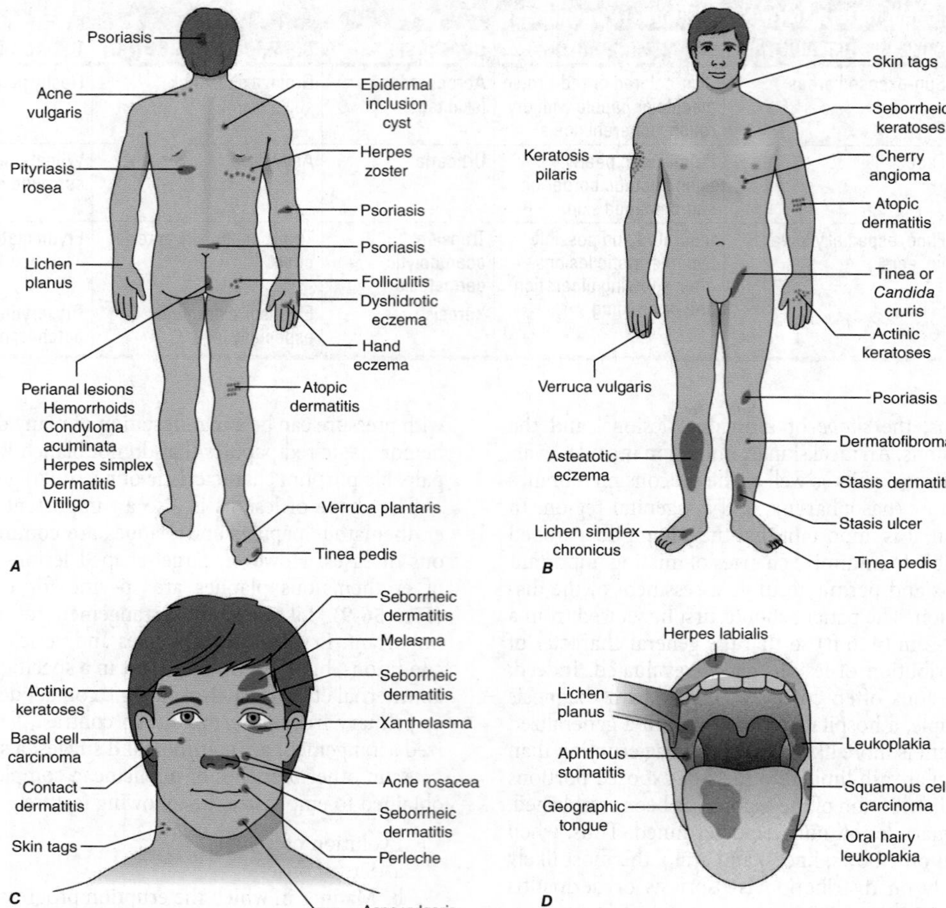

FIGURE 56-6 Distribution of some common dermatologic diseases and lesions.

■ DIAGNOSTIC TECHNIQUES

Many skin diseases can be diagnosed on the basis of gross clinical appearance, but sometimes relatively simple diagnostic procedures can yield valuable information. In most instances, they can be performed at the bedside with a minimum of equipment.

Skin Biopsy A skin biopsy is a straightforward minor surgical procedure; however, it is important to biopsy a lesion that is most likely to yield diagnostic findings. This decision may require expertise in skin diseases and knowledge of superficial anatomic structures in selected areas of the body. In this procedure, a small area of skin is anesthetized with 1% lidocaine with or without epinephrine. The skin lesion in question can be excised or saucerized with a scalpel or removed by punch biopsy. In the latter technique, a punch is pressed against the surface of the skin and rotated with downward pressure until it penetrates to the subcutaneous tissue. The circular biopsy is then lifted with forceps, and the bottom is cut with iris scissors. Biopsy sites may or may not need suture closure, depending on size and location.

KOH Preparation A potassium hydroxide (KOH) preparation is performed on scaling skin lesions where a fungal infection is suspected. The edge of such a lesion is scraped gently with a no. 15 scalpel blade. The removed scale is collected on a glass microscope slide, treated with 1 or 2 drops of a solution of 10–20% KOH, and placement of a cover

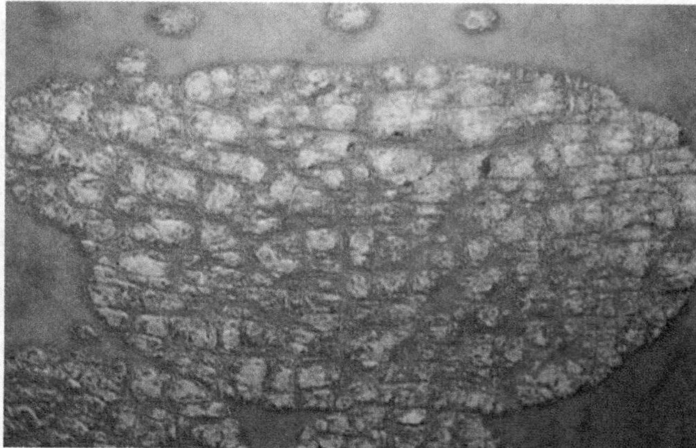

FIGURE 56-7 Psoriasis. This papulosquamous skin disease is characterized by small and large erythematous papules and plaques with overlying adherent silvery scale.

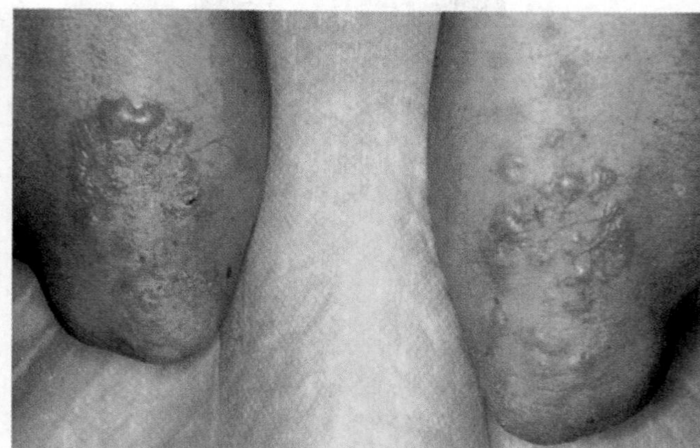

FIGURE 56-8 Dermatitis herpetiformis. This disorder typically displays pruritic, grouped papulovesicles on elbows, knees, buttocks, and posterior scalp. Vesicles are often excoriated due to associated pruritus.

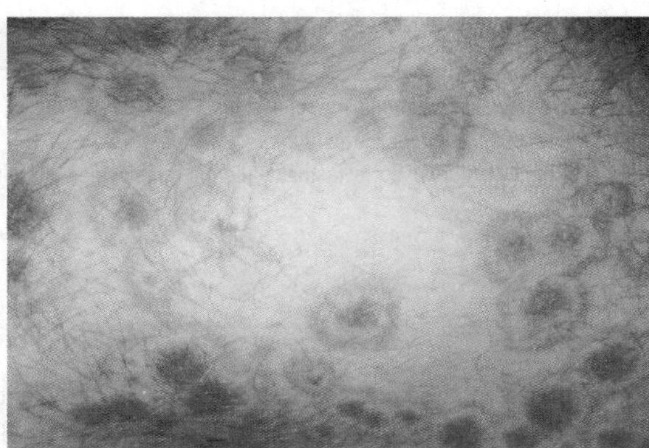

FIGURE 56-9 Erythema multiforme. This eruption is characterized by multiple erythematous plaques with a target or iris morphology. It usually represents a hypersensitivity reaction to drugs (e.g., sulfonamides) or infections (e.g., HSV). *(Courtesy of the Yale Resident's Slide Collection; with permission.)*

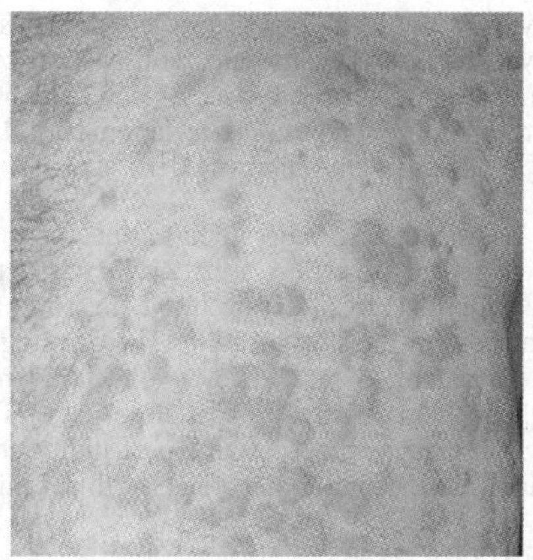

FIGURE 56-11 Urticaria. Discrete and confluent, edematous, erythematous papules and plaques are characteristic of this whealing eruption.

slip. KOH dissolves keratin and allows easier visualization of fungal elements. Brief heating of the slide accelerates dissolution of keratin. When the preparation is viewed under the microscope, the refractile hyphae are seen more easily when the light intensity is reduced and the condenser is lowered. This technique can be used to identify hyphae in dermatophyte infections, pseudohyphae and budding yeasts in *Candida* infections, and "spaghetti and meatballs" yeast forms in tinea versicolor. The same sampling technique can be used to obtain scale for culture of selected pathogenic organisms.

Tzanck Smear A Tzanck smear is a cytologic technique most often used in the diagnosis of herpesvirus infections (herpes simplex virus [HSV] or varicella-zoster virus [VZV]) **(see Figs. 193-1 and 193-3)**. An early vesicle, not a pustule or crusted lesion, is unroofed, and the base of the lesion is scraped gently with a scalpel blade. The material is placed on a glass slide, air-dried, and stained with Giemsa or Wright's stain. Multinucleated epithelial giant cells suggest the presence of HSV or VZV; culture, immunofluorescence microscopy, or genetic testing must be performed to identify the specific virus.

Diascopy Diascopy is designed to assess whether a skin lesion will blanch with pressure as, for example, in determining whether a red lesion is hemorrhagic or simply blood-filled. Urticaria **(Fig. 56-11)** will blanch with pressure, whereas a purpuric lesion caused by necrotizing vasculitis (Fig. 56-4) will not. Diascopy is performed by pressing a microscope slide or magnifying lens against a lesion and noting the amount of blanching that occurs. Granulomas often have an opaque to transparent, brown-pink "apple jelly" appearance on diascopy.

Dermoscopy Dermoscopy is a noninvasive method of examining the skin surface that uses a high-quality magnifying lens and a specialized light source (i.e., a dermatoscope). Dermoscopy identifies skin structures, colors, and patterns that are not visible to the naked eye. It is particularly useful in the evaluation of pigmented skin lesions.

Wood's Light A Wood's lamp generates 360-nm ultraviolet ("black") light that can be used to aid the evaluation of certain skin disorders. For example, a Wood's lamp will cause erythrasma (a superficial, intertriginous infection caused by *Corynebacterium minutissimum*) to show a characteristic coral pink color, and wounds colonized by *Pseudomonas* will appear pale blue. Tinea capitis caused by certain dermatophytes (e.g., *Microsporum canis* or *M. audouinii*) exhibits a yellow fluorescence. Pigmented lesions of the epidermis such as freckles are accentuated, while dermal pigment such as postinflammatory hyperpigmentation fades under a Wood's light. Vitiligo **(Fig. 56-12)**

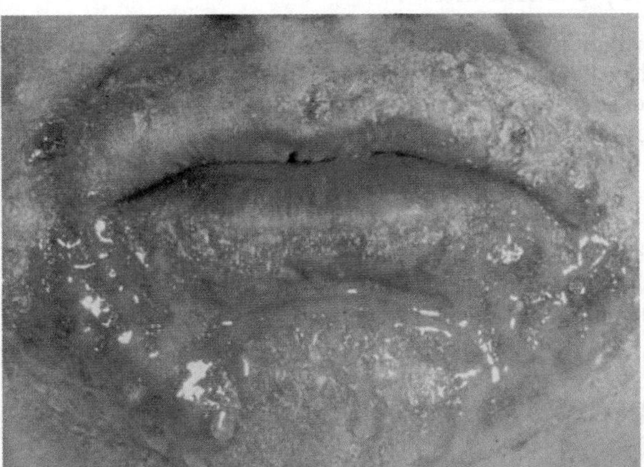

A

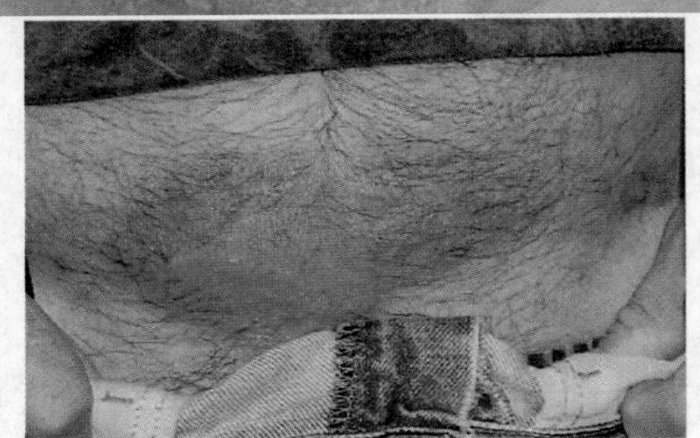

B

FIGURE 56-10 Allergic contact dermatitis (ACD). ***A.*** An example of ACD in its acute phase, with sharply demarcated, weeping, eczematous plaques in a perioral distribution. ***B.*** ACD in its chronic phase, with an erythematous, lichenified, weeping plaque on skin chronically exposed to nickel in a metal snap. *(B, Courtesy of Robert Swerlick, MD; with permission.)*

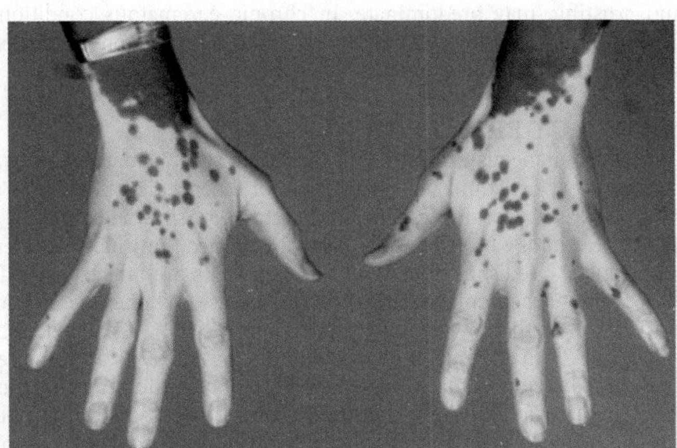

FIGURE 56-12 Vitiligo. Characteristic lesions display an acral distribution and striking depigmentation as a result of loss of melanocytes.

appears totally white under a Wood's lamp, and previously unsuspected areas of involvement often become apparent. A Wood's lamp may also aid in the demonstration of tinea versicolor, detection of sites of depigmentation within and/or surrounding melanomas, and recognition of ash leaf spots in patients with tuberous sclerosis.

Patch Tests Patch testing is designed to document sensitivity to a specific antigen. In this procedure, a battery of suspected allergens is applied to the patient's back under occlusive dressings and allowed to remain in contact with the skin for 48 h. The dressings are removed, and the area is examined for evidence of delayed hypersensitivity reactions (e.g., erythema, edema, or papulovesicles). This test is best performed by physicians with special expertise in patch testing and is often helpful in the evaluation of patients with chronic dermatitis.

FURTHER READING

Bolognia JL et al (eds): *Dermatology*, 4th ed. Philadelphia, Elsevier, 2018.

James WD: *Andrews' Diseases of the Skin: Clinical Dermatology*, 13th ed. Philadelphia, Elsevier, 2019.

Kang S et al (eds): *Fitzpatrick's Dermatology in General Medicine*, 9th ed. New York, McGraw-Hill, 2019.

57 Eczema, Psoriasis, Cutaneous Infections, Acne, and Other Common Skin Disorders

Leslie P. Lawley, Justin T. Cheeley, Robert A. Swerlick

ECZEMA AND DERMATITIS

Eczema is a type of dermatitis, and these terms are often used synonymously (e.g., atopic eczema or atopic dermatitis [AD]). Eczema is a reaction pattern that presents with variable clinical findings and the common histologic finding of *spongiosis* (intercellular edema of the epidermis). Eczema is the final common expression for a number of disorders, including those discussed in the following sections. Primary lesions may include erythematous macules, papules, and vesicles, which can coalesce to form patches and plaques. In severe eczema, secondary lesions from infection or excoriation, marked by weeping and crusting, may predominate. In chronic eczematous conditions, *lichenification* (cutaneous hypertrophy and accentuation of normal skin markings) may alter the characteristic appearance of eczema.

ATOPIC DERMATITIS

AD is the cutaneous expression of the atopic state, characterized by a family history of asthma, allergic rhinitis, or eczema. The prevalence of AD is increasing worldwide. Some of its features are shown in **Table 57-1**.

The etiology of AD is only partially defined, but there is a clear genetic predisposition. When both parents are affected by AD, >80% of their children manifest the disease. When only one parent is affected, the prevalence drops to slightly >50%. A characteristic defect in AD that contributes to the pathophysiology is an impaired epidermal barrier. In many patients, a mutation in the gene encoding filaggrin, a structural protein in the stratum corneum, is responsible. Patients with AD may display a variety of immunoregulatory abnormalities, including increased IgE synthesis; increased serum IgE levels; and impaired, delayed-type hypersensitivity reactions.

TABLE 57-1 Clinical Features of Atopic Dermatitis

1. Pruritus and scratching
2. Course marked by exacerbations and remissions
3. Lesions typical of eczematous dermatitis
4. Personal or family history of atopy (asthma, allergic rhinitis, food allergies, or eczema)
5. Clinical course lasting >6 weeks
6. Lichenification of skin
7. Presence of dry skin

The clinical presentation often varies with age. Half of patients with AD present within the first year of life, and 80% present by 5 years of age. About 80% ultimately coexpress allergic rhinitis or asthma. The infantile pattern is characterized by weeping inflammatory patches and crusted plaques on the face, neck, and extensor surfaces. The childhood and adolescent patterns are typified by dermatitis of flexural skin, particularly in the antecubital and popliteal fossae (**Fig. 57-1**). AD may resolve spontaneously, but approximately 40% of all individuals affected as children will have dermatitis in adult life. The distribution of lesions in adults may be similar to those seen in childhood; however, adults frequently have localized disease manifesting as lichen simplex chronicus or hand eczema (see below). In patients with localized disease, AD may be suspected because of a typical personal or family history or the presence of cutaneous stigmata of AD such as perioral pallor, an extra fold of skin beneath the lower eyelid (Dennie-Morgan folds), increased palmar skin markings, and an increased incidence of cutaneous infections, particularly with *Staphylococcus aureus*. Regardless of other manifestations, pruritus is a prominent characteristic of AD in all age groups and is exacerbated by dry skin. Many of the cutaneous findings in affected patients, such as lichenification, are secondary to rubbing and scratching.

TREATMENT

Atopic Dermatitis

Therapy for AD should include avoidance of cutaneous irritants, adequate moisturization through the application of emollients, judicious use of topical anti-inflammatory agents, and prompt treatment of secondary infection. Patients should be instructed to bathe no more often than daily, using warm or cool water, and to use only mild bath soap. Immediately after bathing, while the skin is still moist, a topical anti-inflammatory agent in a cream or ointment base should be applied to areas of dermatitis, and all other skin areas should be lubricated with a moisturizer. Approximately 30 g of a topical agent is required to cover the entire body surface of an average adult.

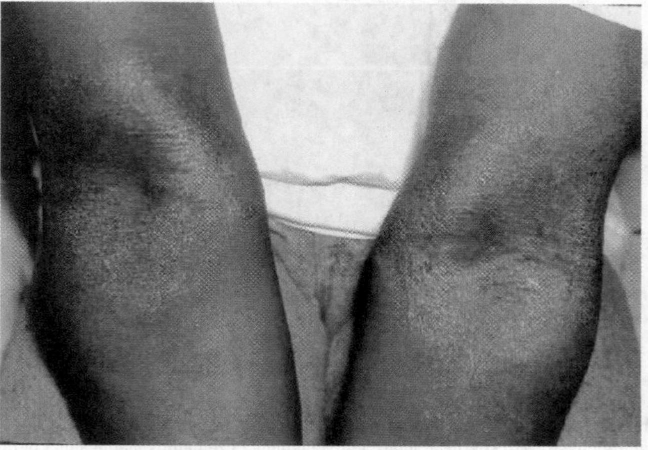

FIGURE 57-1 Atopic dermatitis. Hyperpigmentation, lichenification, and scaling in the antecubital fossae are seen in this patient with atopic dermatitis. *(Courtesy of Robert Swerlick, MD.)*

Low- to mid-potency topical glucocorticoids are employed in most treatment regimens for AD. Skin atrophy and the potential for systemic absorption are constant concerns, especially with more potent agents. Low-potency topical glucocorticoids or nonglucocorticoid anti-inflammatory agents should be selected for use on the face and in intertriginous areas to minimize the risk of skin atrophy. Three nonglucocorticoid anti-inflammatory agents approved by the U.S. Food and Drug Administration (FDA) are available for topical use in AD: tacrolimus ointment, pimecrolimus cream, and crisaborole ointment. These agents do not cause skin atrophy, nor do they suppress the hypothalamic-pituitary-adrenal axis. The first two agents are topical calcineurin inhibitors (TCIs), whereas crisaborole is a phosphodiesterase-4 inhibitor. Concerns regarding the potential for lymphomas in patients treated with TCIs have largely been unfounded. Currently, all three agents are more costly than topical glucocorticoids. Barrier-repair products that attempt to restore the impaired epidermal barrier are also nonglucocorticoid agents and are gaining popularity in the treatment of AD.

Secondary infection of eczematous skin may lead to exacerbation of AD. Crusted and weeping skin lesions may be infected with *S. aureus*. When secondary infection is suspected, eczematous lesions should be cultured and patients treated with systemic antibiotics active against *S. aureus*. The initial use of penicillinase-resistant penicillins or cephalosporins is preferable. Dicloxacillin or cephalexin (250 mg qid for 7–10 days) is generally adequate for adults; however, antibiotic selection must be directed by culture results and clinical response. More than 50% of *S. aureus* isolates are now methicillin resistant in some communities. Current recommendations for the treatment of infection with these community-acquired methicillin-resistant *S. aureus* (CA-MRSA) strains in adults include trimethoprim-sulfamethoxazole (one double-strength tablet bid), minocycline (100 mg bid), doxycycline (100 mg bid), or clindamycin (300–450 mg qid). Duration of therapy should be 7–10 days. Inducible resistance may limit clindamycin's usefulness. Such resistance can be detected by the double-disk diffusion test, which should be ordered if the isolate is erythromycin resistant and clindamycin sensitive. As an adjunct, antibacterial washes or dilute sodium hypochlorite baths (0.005% bleach) and intermittent nasal mupirocin may be useful.

Control of pruritus is essential for treatment, as AD often represents "an itch that rashes." Antihistamines are most often used to control pruritus. Diphenhydramine (25 mg every 4–6 h), hydroxyzine (10–25 mg every 6 h), and doxepin (10–25 mg at bedtime) are useful primarily due to their sedating action. Higher doses of these agents may be required, but sedation can become bothersome. Patients need to be counseled about driving or operating heavy equipment after taking these medications. When used at bedtime, sedating antihistamines may improve the patient's sleep. Although they are effective in urticaria, nonsedating antihistamines and selective H_2 blockers are of little use in controlling the pruritus of AD.

Treatment with systemic glucocorticoids should be limited to severe exacerbations unresponsive to topical therapy. In the patient with chronic AD, therapy with systemic glucocorticoids will generally clear the skin only briefly, and cessation of the systemic therapy will invariably be accompanied by a return, if not a worsening, of the dermatitis. For chronic severe AD poorly responsive to standard topical regimens, systemic agents may be considered. Cyclosporine is approved for treatment of severe recalcitrant AD in some European countries. Monitoring of renal function and secondary infections is required. Dupilumab, an interleukin 4 receptor blocker, is FDA approved for use in patients 6 years of age and older and provides more targeted immunomodulation and a better safety profile than cyclosporine. Patients who do not respond to conventional therapies should be considered for patch testing to rule out allergic contact dermatitis (ACD). The role of dietary allergens in AD is controversial, and there is little evidence that they play any role outside of infancy, during which a small percentage of patients with AD may be affected by food allergens.

LICHEN SIMPLEX CHRONICUS

Lichen simplex chronicus may represent the end stage of a variety of pruritic and eczematous disorders, including AD. It consists of a circumscribed plaque or plaques of lichenified skin due to chronic scratching or rubbing. Common areas involved include the posterior nuchal region, dorsum of the feet, and ankles. Treatment of lichen simplex chronicus centers on breaking the cycle of chronic itching and scratching. High-potency topical glucocorticoids are helpful in most cases, but, in recalcitrant cases, application of topical glucocorticoids under occlusion or intralesional injection of glucocorticoids may be required.

CONTACT DERMATITIS

Contact dermatitis is an inflammatory skin process caused by an exogenous agent or agents that directly or indirectly injure the skin. In *irritant* contact dermatitis (ICD), this injury is caused by an inherent characteristic of a compound—for example, a concentrated acid or base. Agents that cause *allergic* contact dermatitis (ACD) induce an antigen-specific immune response (e.g., poison ivy dermatitis). The clinical lesions of contact dermatitis may be acute (wet and edematous) or chronic (dry, thickened, and scaly), depending on the persistence of the insult **(see Chap. 56, Fig. 56-10)**.

Irritant Contact Dermatitis ICD is generally well demarcated and often localized to areas of thin skin (eyelids, intertriginous areas) or areas where the irritant was occluded. Lesions may range from minimal skin erythema to areas of marked edema, vesicles, and ulcers. Prior exposure to the offending agent is not necessary, and the reaction develops in minutes to a few hours. Chronic low-grade irritant dermatitis is the most common type of ICD, and the most common area of involvement is the hands (see below). The most common irritants encountered are chronic wet work, soaps, and detergents. Treatment should be directed toward the avoidance of irritants and the use of protective gloves or clothing.

Allergic Contact Dermatitis ACD is a manifestation of delayed-type hypersensitivity mediated by memory T lymphocytes in the skin. Prior exposure to the offending agent is necessary to develop the hypersensitivity reaction, which may take as little as 12 h or as long as 72 h to develop. The most common cause of ACD is exposure to plants, especially to members of the family Anacardiaceae, including the genus *Toxicodendron*. Poison ivy, poison oak, and poison sumac are members of this genus and cause an allergic reaction marked by erythema, vesiculation, and severe pruritus. The eruption is often linear or angular, corresponding to areas where plants have touched the skin. The sensitizing antigen common to these plants is urushiol, an oleoresin containing the active ingredient pentadecylcatechol. The oleoresin may adhere to skin, clothing, tools, and pets, and contaminated articles may cause dermatitis even after prolonged storage. Blister fluid does not contain urushiol and is not capable of inducing skin eruption in exposed subjects.

TREATMENT

Contact Dermatitis

If contact dermatitis is suspected and an offending agent is identified and removed, the eruption will resolve. Usually, treatment with high-potency topical glucocorticoids is enough to relieve symptoms while the dermatitis runs its course. For patients who require systemic therapy, daily oral prednisone—beginning at 1 mg/kg, but usually ≤60 mg/d—is sufficient. The dose should be tapered over 2–3 weeks, and each daily dose should be taken in the morning with food.

Identification of a contact allergen can be a difficult and time-consuming task. ACD should be suspected in patients with dermatitis unresponsive to conventional therapy or with an unusual and patterned distribution. Patients should be questioned carefully regarding occupational exposures and topical medications. Common sensitizers include preservatives in topical preparations,

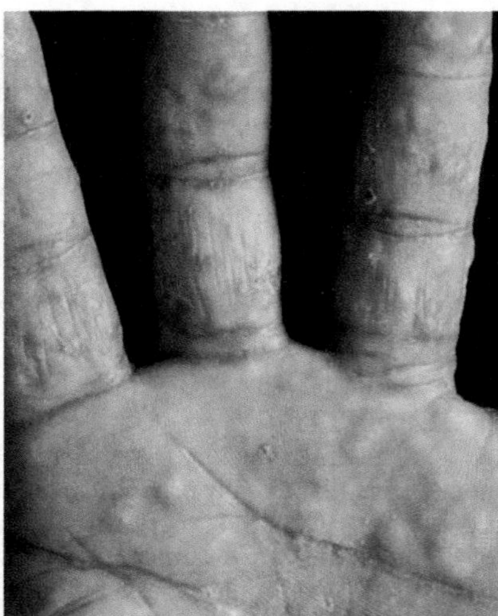

FIGURE 57-2 Dyshidrotic eczema. This example is characterized by deep-seated vesicles and scaling on palms and lateral fingers, and the disease is often associated with an atopic diathesis.

nickel sulfate, potassium dichromate, thimerosal, neomycin sulfate, fragrances, formaldehyde, and rubber-curing agents. Patch testing is helpful in identifying these agents but should not be attempted when patients have widespread active dermatitis or are taking systemic glucocorticoids.

HAND ECZEMA

Hand eczema is a very common, chronic skin disorder in which both exogenous and endogenous factors play important roles. It may be associated with other cutaneous disorders such as AD, and contact with various agents may be involved. Hand eczema represents a large proportion of cases of occupation-associated skin disease. Chronic, excessive exposure to water and detergents, harsh chemicals, or allergens may initiate or aggravate this disorder. It may present with dryness and cracking of the skin of the hands as well as with variable amounts of erythema and edema. Often, the dermatitis will begin under rings, where water and irritants are trapped. *Dyshidrotic* eczema, a variant of hand eczema, presents with multiple, intensely pruritic, small papules and vesicles on the thenar and hypothenar eminences and the sides of the fingers **(Fig. 57-2)**. Lesions tend to occur in crops that slowly form crusts and then heal.

The evaluation of a patient with hand eczema should include an assessment of potential occupation-associated exposures. The history should be directed to identifying possible irritant or allergen exposures.

TREATMENT

Hand Eczema

Therapy for hand eczema is directed toward avoidance of irritants, identification of possible contact allergens, treatment of coexistent infection, and application of topical glucocorticoids. Whenever possible, the hands should be protected by gloves, preferably vinyl. The use of rubber gloves (latex) to protect dermatitic skin is sometimes associated with the development of hypersensitivity reactions to components of the gloves, which could be either a type I hypersensitivity reaction to the latex (manifested by the development of hives, itching, angioedema, and possibly anaphylaxis within minutes to hours of exposure) or a type IV hypersensitivity reaction to rubber accelerators (with worsening of eczematous eruptions days after exposure). Patients can be treated with cool moist compresses followed by application of a mid- to high-potency topical glucocorticoid in a cream or ointment base. As in AD, treatment of secondary infection is essential for good control. In addition, patients with hand eczema should be examined for dermatophyte infection by potassium hydroxide (KOH) preparation and culture (see below).

NUMMULAR ECZEMA

Nummular eczema is characterized by circular or oval "coinlike" lesions, beginning as small edematous papules that become crusted and scaly. The etiology of nummular eczema is unknown, but dry skin is a contributing factor. Common locations are the trunk or the extensor surfaces of the extremities, particularly on the pretibial areas or dorsum of the hands. Nummular eczema occurs more frequently in men and is most common in middle age. The treatment of nummular eczema is similar to that for AD.

ASTEATOTIC ECZEMA

Asteatotic eczema, also known as *xerotic eczema* or "winter itch," is a mildly inflammatory dermatitis that develops in areas of extremely dry skin, especially during the dry winter months. Clinically, there may be considerable overlap with nummular eczema. This form of eczema accounts for many physician visits because of the associated pruritus. Fine cracks and scale, with or without erythema, characteristically develop in areas of dry skin, especially on the anterior surfaces of the lower extremities in elderly patients. Asteatotic eczema responds well to topical moisturizers and the avoidance of cutaneous irritants. Overbathing and the use of harsh soaps exacerbate asteatotic eczema.

STASIS DERMATITIS AND STASIS ULCERATION

Stasis dermatitis develops on the lower extremities secondary to venous incompetence and chronic edema. Patients may give a history of deep venous thrombosis and may have evidence of vein removal or varicose veins. Early findings in stasis dermatitis consist of mild erythema and scaling associated with pruritus. The typical initial site of involvement is the medial aspect of the ankle, often over a distended vein **(Fig. 57-3)**.

Stasis dermatitis may become acutely inflamed, with crusting and exudate. In this state, it is easily confused with cellulitis. Of note, symmetrical and bilateral involvement is more likely stasis dermatitis, whereas unilateral involvement may represent cellulitis. Chronic stasis dermatitis is often associated with dermal fibrosis that is recognized clinically as brawny edema of the skin. As the disorder progresses, the dermatitis becomes progressively pigmented due to chronic erythrocyte extravasation leading to cutaneous hemosiderin deposition. Stasis dermatitis may be complicated by secondary infection and contact dermatitis. Severe stasis dermatitis may precede the development of stasis ulcers.

TREATMENT

Stasis Dermatitis and Stasis Ulceration

Patients with stasis dermatitis and stasis ulceration benefit greatly from leg elevation and the routine use of compression stockings with a gradient of at least 30–40 mmHg. Stockings providing less

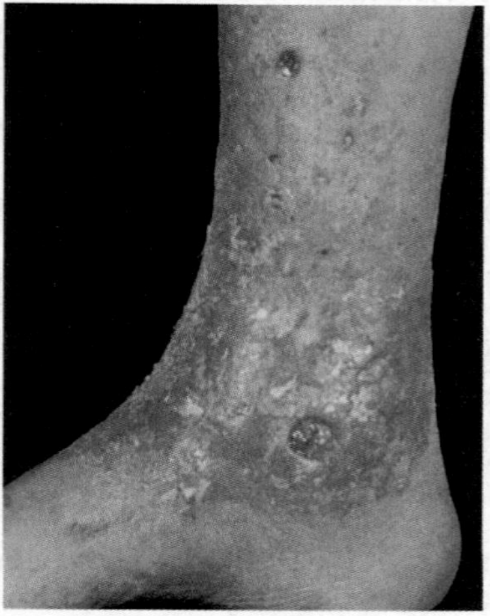

FIGURE 57-3 Stasis dermatitis. An example of stasis dermatitis showing erythematous, scaly, and oozing patches over the lower leg. Several stasis ulcers are also seen in this patient.

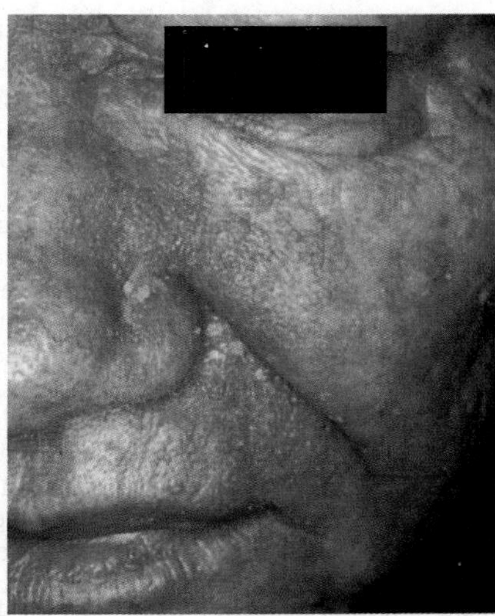

FIGURE 57-4 Seborrheic dermatitis. Central facial erythema with overlying greasy, yellowish scale is seen in this patient. *(Courtesy of Jean Bolognia, MD; with permission.)*

compression, such as antiembolism hose, are poor substitutes. Use of emollients and/or mid-potency topical glucocorticoids and avoidance of irritants are also helpful in treating stasis dermatitis. Protection of the legs from injury, including scratching, and control of chronic edema are essential to prevent ulcers. Diuretics may be required to adequately control chronic edema.

Stasis ulcers are difficult to treat, and resolution is slow. It is extremely important to elevate the affected limb as much as possible. The ulcer should be kept clear of necrotic material by gentle debridement and covered with a semipermeable dressing and a compression dressing or compression stocking. Glucocorticoids should not be applied to ulcers, because they may retard healing; however, they may be applied to the surrounding skin to control itching, scratching, and additional trauma. Superficial bacterial cultures of chronic stasis ulcers often yield polymicrobial colonizers and are of little utility in determination of secondary infection. Care must be taken to exclude treatable causes of leg ulcers (hypercoagulation, vasculitis, arterial insufficiency) before beginning the chronic management outlined above.

SEBORRHEIC DERMATITIS

Seborrheic dermatitis is a common, chronic disorder characterized by greasy scales overlying erythematous patches or plaques. Induration and scale are generally less prominent than in psoriasis, but clinical overlap exists between these diseases ("sebopsoriasis"). The most common location is in the scalp, where it may be recognized as severe dandruff. On the face, seborrheic dermatitis affects the eyebrows, eyelids, glabella, and nasolabial folds (**Fig. 57-4**). Scaling of the external auditory canal is common in seborrheic dermatitis. In addition, the postauricular areas often become macerated and tender. Seborrheic dermatitis may also develop in the central chest, axilla, groin, submammary folds, and gluteal cleft. Rarely, it may cause widespread generalized dermatitis. Pruritus is variable.

Seborrheic dermatitis may be evident within the first few weeks of life, and within this context, it typically occurs in the scalp ("cradle cap"), face, or groin. It is rarely seen in children beyond infancy but becomes evident again during adolescent and adult life. Although it is frequently seen in patients with Parkinson's disease, in those who have had cerebrovascular accidents, and in those with HIV infection, the overwhelming majority of individuals with seborrheic dermatitis have no underlying disorder.

TREATMENT
Seborrheic Dermatitis

Treatment with low-potency topical glucocorticoids in conjunction with a topical antifungal agent, such as ketoconazole cream or ciclopirox cream, is often effective. The scalp and beard areas may benefit from antidandruff shampoos, which should be left in place 3–5 min before rinsing. High-potency topical glucocorticoid solutions (betamethasone or clobetasol) are effective for control of severe scalp involvement. High-potency glucocorticoids should not be used on the face because this treatment is often associated with steroid-induced rosacea or atrophy.

PAPULOSQUAMOUS DISORDERS (TABLE 57-2)

PSORIASIS

Psoriasis is one of the most common dermatologic diseases, affecting up to 2% of the world's population. It is an immune-mediated disease clinically characterized by erythematous, sharply demarcated papules and rounded plaques covered by silvery micaceous scale. The skin lesions of psoriasis are variably pruritic. Traumatized areas often develop lesions of psoriasis (the *Koebner* or isomorphic phenomenon). In addition, other external factors may exacerbate psoriasis, including infections, stress, and medications (lithium, beta blockers, and antimalarial drugs).

The most common variety of psoriasis is called *plaque-type*. Patients with plaque-type psoriasis have stable, slowly enlarging plaques, which remain basically unchanged for long periods of time. The most commonly involved areas are the elbows, knees, gluteal cleft, and scalp. Involvement tends to be symmetric. Plaque psoriasis generally develops slowly and runs an indolent course. It rarely remits spontaneously. *Inverse psoriasis* affects the intertriginous regions, including the axilla, groin, submammary region, and navel; it also tends to affect the scalp, palms, and soles. The individual lesions are sharply demarcated plaques (**see Chap. 56, Fig. 56-7**), but they may be moist and without scale due to their locations.

TABLE 57-2 Papulosquamous Disorders

	CLINICAL FEATURES	OTHER NOTABLE FEATURES	HISTOLOGIC FEATURES
Psoriasis	Sharply demarcated, erythematous plaques with mica-like scale; predominantly on elbows, knees, and scalp; atypical forms may localize to intertriginous areas; eruptive forms may be associated with infection	May be aggravated by certain drugs, infection; severe forms seen in association with HIV	Acanthosis, vascular proliferation
Lichen planus	Purple polygonal papules marked by severe pruritus; lacy white markings, especially associated with mucous membrane lesions	Certain drugs may induce: thiazides, antimalarial drugs	Interface dermatitis
Pityriasis rosea	Rash often preceded by herald patch; oval to round plaques with trailing scale; most often affects trunk; eruption lines up in skinfolds giving a "fir tree–like" appearance; generally spares palms and soles	Variable pruritus; self-limited, resolving in 2–8 weeks; may be imitated by secondary syphilis	Pathologic features often nonspecific
Dermatophytosis	Polymorphous appearance depending on dermatophyte, body site, and host response; sharply defined to ill-demarcated scaly plaques with or without inflammation; may be associated with hair loss	KOH preparation may show branching hyphae; culture helpful	Hyphae and neutrophils in stratum corneum

Abbreviations: HIV, human immunodeficiency virus; KOH, potassium hydroxide.

Guttate psoriasis (eruptive psoriasis) is most common in children and young adults. It develops acutely in individuals without psoriasis or in those with chronic plaque psoriasis. Patients present with many small erythematous, scaling papules, frequently after upper respiratory tract infection with β-hemolytic streptococci. The differential diagnosis should include pityriasis rosea and secondary syphilis.

In *pustular psoriasis*, patients may have disease localized to the palms and soles, or the disease may be generalized. Regardless of the extent of disease, the skin is erythematous, with pustules and variable scale. Localized to the palms and soles, it is easily confused with dishydrotic eczema. When it is generalized, episodes are characterized by fever (39°–40°C [102.2°–104.0°F]) lasting several days, an accompanying generalized eruption of sterile pustules, and a background of intense erythema; patients may become erythrodermic. Episodes of fever and pustules are recurrent. Local irritants, pregnancy, medications, infections, and systemic glucocorticoid withdrawal can precipitate this form of psoriasis. Oral retinoids are the treatment of choice in nonpregnant patients.

Fingernail involvement, appearing as punctate pitting, onycholysis, nail thickening, or subungual hyperkeratosis, may be a clue to the diagnosis of psoriasis when the clinical presentation is not classic.

According to the National Psoriasis Foundation, up to 30% of patients with psoriasis have psoriatic arthritis (PsA). It develops most commonly between the ages of 30 and 50 years. There are five subtypes of PsA: symmetric PsA, asymmetric PsA, distal PsA, spondylitis, and arthritis mutilans. Approximately 50% of PsA is classified as symmetric, which may resemble rheumatoid arthritis. Asymmetric arthritis comprises about 35% of cases. It can involve any joint and may present as "sausage digits." Distal PsA is the classic form; however, it occurs in only about 5% of patients with PsA. It can involve fingers and toes; fingernails and toenails are often dystrophic, including nail pitting. Spondylitis also occurs in ~5% of patients with PsA. Arthritis mutilans is severe and deforming and affects primarily the small joints of the hands and feet. It accounts for fewer than 5% of PsA cases.

An increased risk of metabolic syndrome, including increased morbidity and mortality from cardiovascular events, has been demonstrated in psoriasis patients. Appropriate screening tests should be performed. The etiology of psoriasis is still poorly understood, but there is clearly a genetic component to the disease. In various studies, 30–50% of patients with psoriasis report a positive family history. Psoriatic lesions contain infiltrates of activated T cells that are thought to elaborate cytokines responsible for keratinocyte hyperproliferation, which results in the characteristic clinical findings. Agents inhibiting T-cell activation, clonal expansion, or release of proinflammatory cytokines are often effective for the treatment of severe psoriasis (see below).

TREATMENT
Psoriasis

Treatment of psoriasis depends on the type, location, and extent of disease. All patients should be instructed to avoid excess drying or irritation of their skin and to maintain adequate cutaneous hydration. Most cases of localized, plaque-type psoriasis can be managed with mid-potency topical glucocorticoids, although their long-term use is often accompanied by loss of effectiveness (tachyphylaxis) and atrophy of the skin. A topical vitamin D analogue (calcipotriene) and a retinoid (tazarotene) are also efficacious in the treatment of limited psoriasis and have largely replaced other topical agents such as coal tar, salicylic acid, and anthralin.

Ultraviolet (UV) light, natural or artificial, is an effective therapy for many patients with widespread psoriasis. Ultraviolet B (UVB), narrowband UVB, and ultraviolet A (UVA) light with either oral or topical psoralens (PUVA) are used clinically. UV light's immunosuppressive properties are thought to be responsible for its therapeutic activity in psoriasis. It is also mutagenic, potentially leading to an increased incidence of nonmelanoma and melanoma skin cancer. UV-light therapy is contraindicated in patients receiving cyclosporine and should be used with great care in all immunocompromised patients due to the increased risk of skin cancer.

Various systemic agents can be used for severe, widespread psoriatic disease **(Table 57-3)**. Oral glucocorticoids should not be used for the treatment of psoriasis due to the potential for development of life-threatening pustular psoriasis when therapy is discontinued. Methotrexate is an effective agent, especially in patients with PsA. The synthetic retinoid acitretin is useful, especially when immunosuppression must be avoided; however, teratogenicity limits its use. Apremilast inhibits phosphodiesterase type 4. It is approved for both psoriasis and PsA. It must be used cautiously in the presence of renal failure or depression.

The evidence implicating psoriasis as a T-cell–mediated disorder has directed therapeutic efforts to immunoregulation. Cyclosporine and other immunosuppressive agents can be very effective in the treatment of psoriasis, and much attention is currently directed toward the development of biologic agents with more selective immunosuppressive properties and better safety profiles **(Table 57-4)**. These biologic agents appear to be quite efficacious in treatment of psoriasis and are well tolerated; however, caution with certain patient comorbidities must be exercised. Use of tumor necrosis factor-α (TNF-α) inhibitors may worsen congestive heart failure (CHF), and they should be used with caution in patients at risk for or known to have CHF. Further, none of the immunosuppressive agents used in the treatment of psoriasis should be initiated if the patient has a severe infection (including tuberculosis, HIV, hepatitis B or C); patients on such therapy should be routinely screened for tuberculosis. There have been reports of progressive multifocal leukoencephalopathy and lupus erythematosus in association with treatment with the TNF-α inhibitors. Malignancies, including a risk or history of certain malignancies, may limit the use of these systemic agents. In general, immunosuppressive agents have also been linked to an increase risk of skin cancer, and patients receiving these agents should be monitored for the development of skin cancer.

LICHEN PLANUS

Lichen planus (LP) is a papulosquamous disorder that may affect the skin, scalp, nails, and mucous membranes. The primary cutaneous lesions are pruritic, polygonal, flat-topped, violaceous papules. Close

TABLE 57-3 FDA-Approved Systemic Therapy for Psoriasis

		ADMINISTRATION		
AGENT	MEDICATION CLASS	ROUTE	FREQUENCY	ADVERSE EVENTS (SELECTED)
Methotrexate	Antimetabolite	Oral	Weekly[a]	Hepatotoxicity, pulmonary toxicity, pancytopenia, potential for increased malignancies, ulcerative stomatitis, nausea, diarrhea, teratogenicity
Acitretin	Retinoid	Oral	Daily	Teratogenicity, hepatotoxicity, hyperostosis, hyperlipidemia/pancreatitis, depression, ophthalmologic effects, pseudotumor cerebri
Cyclosporine	Calcineurin inhibitor	Oral	Twice daily	Renal dysfunction, hypertension, hyperkalemia, hyperuricemia, hypomagnesemia, hyperlipidemia, increased risk of malignancies
Apremilast	Phosphodiesterase type 4 inhibitor	Oral	Twice daily[b]	Hypersensitivity reaction, depression, nausea, diarrhea, vomiting, dyspepsia, weight loss, headache, fatigue

[a]Initial test dose is required. [b]Initial dose escalation is required.

Abbreviation: FDA, Food and Drug Administration.

TABLE 57-4 FDA-Approved Biologics for Psoriasis or Psoriatic Arthritis

MECHANISM OF ACTION	AGENTS (INDICATION; ROUTE)	FREQUENCY	WARNINGS, SELECTED
Anti-TNF-α	Etanercept (Ps, PsA; SC) Adalimumab (Ps, PsA; SC) Certolizumab (Ps, PsA; SC) Infliximab (Ps, PsA; IV) Golimumab (PsA; SC)	Ranges from once or twice weekly[a] to every 8 weeks[a]	Serious infections, hepatotoxicity, CHF, hematologic events, hypersensitivity reactions, neurologic events, potential for increased malignancies
Anti-IL-12 and anti-IL-23	Ustekinumab (Ps, PsA; SC)	Every 12 weeks[a]	Serious infections, neurologic events, potential for increased malignancies
Anti-IL-23	Risankizumab (Ps; SC) Tildrakizumab (Ps; SC) Guselkumab (Ps; SC)	Ranges from every 8–12 weeks[a]	Serious infections, headaches
Anti-IL-17	Secukinumab (Ps, PsA; SC) Ixekizumab (Ps; SC) Brodalumab (Ps; SC)	Ranges from every 2–4 weeks[a]	Serious infections, hypersensitivity reaction, inflammatory bowel disease

[a]Initial dose modifications required.

Abbreviations: CHF, congestive heart failure; IL, interleukin; IV, intravenous; Ps, psoriasis; PsA, psoriatic arthritis; SC, subcutaneous; TNF-α, tumor necrosis factor-α.

examination of the surface of these papules often reveals a network of gray lines (*Wickham's striae*). The skin lesions may occur anywhere but have a predilection for the wrists, shins, lower back, and genitalia (**Fig. 57-5**). Involvement of the scalp (*lichen planopilaris*) may lead to scarring alopecia, and nail involvement may lead to permanent deformity or loss of fingernails and toenails. LP commonly involves mucous membranes, particularly the buccal mucosa, where it can present on a spectrum ranging from a mild, white, reticulate eruption of the mucosa to a severe, erosive stomatitis. Erosive stomatitis may persist for years and may be linked to an increased risk of oral squamous cell carcinoma. Cutaneous eruptions clinically resembling LP have been observed after administration of numerous drugs, including thiazide diuretics, gold, antimalarial agents, penicillamine, and phenothiazines, and in patients with skin lesions of chronic graft-versus-host disease. In addition, LP may be associated with hepatitis C infection. The course of LP is variable, but most patients have spontaneous remissions 6 months to 2 years after the onset of disease. Topical glucocorticoids are the mainstay of therapy.

■ PITYRIASIS ROSEA

Pityriasis rosea (PR) is a papulosquamous eruption of unknown etiology occurring more commonly in the spring and fall. Its first manifestation is the development of a 2- to 6-cm annular lesion (the herald patch). This is followed in a few days to a few weeks by the appearance of many smaller annular or papular lesions with a predilection to occur on the trunk (**Fig. 57-6**). The lesions are generally oval, with their long axis parallel to the skinfold lines. Individual lesions may range in color from red to brown and have a trailing scale. PR shares many clinical features with the eruption of secondary syphilis, but palm and sole lesions are extremely rare in PR and common in secondary syphilis. The eruption tends to be moderately pruritic and lasts 3–8 weeks. Treatment is directed at alleviating pruritus and consists of oral antihistamines; mid-potency topical glucocorticoids; and, in some cases, UVB phototherapy.

CUTANEOUS INFECTIONS (TABLE 57-5)

■ IMPETIGO, ECTHYMA, AND FURUNCULOSIS

Impetigo is a common superficial bacterial infection of skin caused most often by *S. aureus* (**Chap. 147**) and in some cases by group A β-hemolytic streptococci (**Chap. 148**). The primary lesion is a superficial pustule that ruptures and forms a characteristic yellow-brown honey-colored crust (**see Chap. 148, Fig. 148-3**). Lesions may occur on normal skin (primary infection) or in areas already affected by another skin disease (secondary infection). Lesions caused by staphylococci may be tense, clear bullae, and this less common form of the disease is called *bullous impetigo*. Blisters are caused by the production of exfoliative toxin by *S. aureus* phage type II. This is the same toxin responsible for staphylococcal scalded-skin syndrome, often resulting in dramatic loss of the superficial epidermis due to blistering. The latter syndrome is much more common in children than in adults; however, it should be considered along with toxic epidermal necrolysis

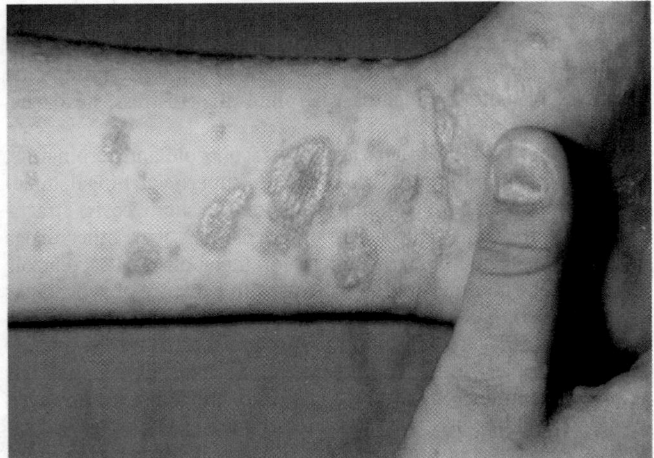

FIGURE 57-5 Lichen planus. An example of lichen planus showing multiple flat-topped, violaceous papules and plaques. Nail dystrophy, as seen in this patient's thumbnail, may also be a feature. *(Courtesy of Robert Swerlick, MD; with permission.)*

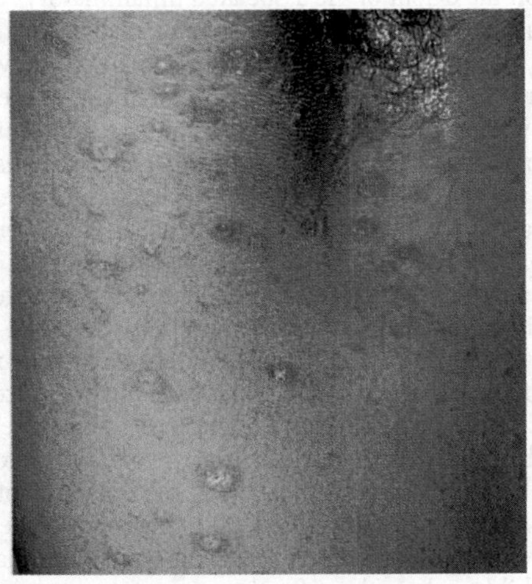

FIGURE 57-6 Pityriasis rosea. In this patient with pityriasis rosea, multiple round to oval erythematous patches with fine central scale are distributed along the skin tension lines on the trunk.

TABLE 57-5 Common Skin Infections

	CLINICAL FEATURES	ETIOLOGIC AGENT	TREATMENT
Impetigo	Honey-colored crusted papules, plaques, or bullae	Group A *Streptococcus* and *Staphylococcus aureus*	Systemic or topical antistaphylococcal and antistreptococcal antibiotics
Dermatophytosis	Inflammatory or noninflammatory annular scaly plaques; may involve hair loss; groin involvement spares scrotum; hyphae on KOH preparation	*Trichophyton, Epidermophyton,* or *Microsporum* spp.	Topical azoles, systemic griseofulvin, terbinafine, or azoles
Candidiasis	Inflammatory papules and plaques with satellite pustules, frequently in intertriginous areas; may involve scrotum; pseudohyphae on KOH preparation	*Candida albicans* and other *Candida* spp.	Topical nystatin or azoles; systemic azoles for resistant disease
Tinea versicolor	Hyper- or hypopigmented scaly patches on trunk; characteristic mixture of hyphae and spores ("spaghetti and meatballs") on KOH preparation	*Malassezia furfur*	Topical selenium sulfide lotion or azoles

Abbreviation: KOH, potassium hydroxide.

and severe drug eruptions in patients with widespread blistering of the skin. *Ecthyma* is a deep nonbullous variant of impetigo that causes punched-out ulcerative lesions. It is more often caused by a primary or secondary infection with *Streptococcus pyogenes*. Ecthyma is a deeper infection than typical impetigo and resolves with scars. Treatment of both ecthyma and impetigo involves gentle debridement of adherent crusts, facilitated by using soaks and topical antibiotics in conjunction with appropriate oral antibiotics.

Furunculosis is also caused by *S. aureus*, and this disorder has gained prominence in the past few decades because of CA-MRSA. A furuncle, or boil, is a painful, erythematous nodule that can occur on any cutaneous surface. The lesions may be solitary but are most often multiple. Patients frequently believe they have been bitten by spiders or insects. Family members or close contacts may also be affected. Furuncles can rupture and drain spontaneously or may need incision and drainage, which may be adequate therapy for small solitary furuncles without cellulitis or systemic symptoms. Whenever possible, lesional material should be sent for culture. Current recommendations for methicillin-sensitive infections are β-lactam antibiotics. Therapy for CA-MRSA is discussed previously (see "Atopic Dermatitis"). Warm compresses and nasal mupirocin are helpful therapeutic additions. Severe infections may require IV antibiotics.

ERYSIPELAS AND CELLULITIS

See Chap. 129.

DERMATOPHYTOSIS

Dermatophytes are fungi that infect skin, hair, and nails and include members of the genera *Trichophyton*, *Microsporum*, and *Epidermophyton* **(Chap. 219)**. *Tinea corporis*, or infection of the relatively hairless skin of the body (glabrous skin), may have a variable appearance depending on the extent of the associated inflammatory reaction. Typical infections consist of erythematous, scaly plaques, with an annular appearance that accounts for the common name "ringworm." Deep inflammatory nodules or granulomas occur in some infections, most often those inappropriately treated with mid- to high-potency topical glucocorticoids. Involvement of the groin (*tinea cruris*) is more common in males than in females. It presents as a scaling, erythematous eruption sparing the scrotum. Infection of the foot (*tinea pedis*) is the most common dermatophyte infection and is often chronic; it is characterized by variable erythema, edema, scaling, pruritus, and occasionally vesiculation. The infection may be widespread or localized but generally involves the web space between the fourth and fifth toes. Infection of the nails (*tinea unguium* or *onychomycosis*) occurs in many patients with tinea pedis and is characterized by opacified, thickened nails and subungual debris. The distal-lateral variant is most common. Proximal subungual onychomycosis may be a marker for HIV infection or other immunocompromised states. Dermatophyte infection of the scalp (*tinea capitis*) continues to be common, particularly affecting inner-city children but also affecting immunocompromised adults. The predominant organism is *Trichophyton tonsurans*, which can produce a relatively noninflammatory infection with mild scale and hair loss that is diffuse or localized. *T. tonsurans* and *Microsporum canis* can also cause a markedly inflammatory dermatosis with edema and nodules. This latter presentation is a *kerion*.

The diagnosis of tinea can be made from skin scrapings, nail scrapings, or hair by culture or direct microscopic examination with KOH. Nail clippings may be sent for histologic examination with periodic acid–Schiff (PAS) stain.

TREATMENT

Dermatophytosis

Both topical and systemic therapies may be used in dermatophyte infections. Treatment depends on the site involved and the type of infection. Topical therapy is generally effective for uncomplicated tinea corporis, tinea cruris, and limited tinea pedis. Topical agents are not effective as monotherapy for tinea capitis or onychomycosis (see below), and nystatin is not active against dermatophytes. Topicals are generally applied twice daily, and treatment should continue for 1 week beyond clinical resolution of the infection. Tinea pedis often requires longer treatment courses and frequently relapses. Oral antifungal agents may be required for recalcitrant tinea pedis or tinea corporis.

For dermatophyte infections involving the hair and nails and for other infections unresponsive to topical therapy, oral antifungal agents are often used. Markedly inflammatory tinea capitis may result in scarring and hair loss, and a systemic antifungal agent plus systemic or topical glucocorticoids may be helpful in preventing these sequelae. A fungal etiology should be confirmed by direct microscopic examination or by culture before oral antifungal agents are prescribed for any infection. All the oral agents may cause hepatotoxicity. They should not be used in women who are pregnant or breast-feeding.

Griseofulvin is approved in the United States for dermatophyte infections involving the skin, hair, or nails. Common side effects of griseofulvin include gastrointestinal distress, headache, and urticaria.

Two other oral antifungal agents, itraconazole and terbinafine, are sometimes prescribed "off-label" for superficial fungal infections. Oral itraconazole is approved for onychomycosis. Itraconazole has the potential for serious interactions with other drugs requiring the P450 enzyme system for metabolism. Itraconazole should not be administered to patients with evidence of ventricular dysfunction or patients with known CHF.

Terbinafine is also approved for onychomycosis, and the granule version is approved for treatment of tinea capitis. Terbinafine has fewer interactions with other drugs than itraconazole; however, caution should be used with patients who are on multiple medications. The risk/benefit ratio should be considered when an asymptomatic toenail infection is treated with systemic agents.

The FDA has limited the use of a third oral agent due to potential hepatotoxicity and published the following: "Nizoral [ketoconazole] oral tablets should not be a first-line treatment for any fungal infection." The topical form of ketoconazole is not affected by this action.

TINEA (PITYRIASIS) VERSICOLOR

Tinea versicolor is caused by a nondermatophytic, dimorphic fungus, *Malassezia furfur*, a normal inhabitant of the skin. The expression of infection is promoted by heat and humidity. The typical lesions consist of oval scaly macules, papules, and patches concentrated on the chest, shoulders, and back but only rarely on the face or distal extremities. On dark skin, the lesions often appear as hypopigmented areas, whereas on light skin, they are slightly erythematous or hyperpigmented. A KOH preparation from scaling lesions will demonstrate a confluence of short hyphae and round spores ("spaghetti and meatballs"). Lotions or shampoos containing sulfur, salicylic acid, or selenium sulfide are the treatments of choice and will clear the infection if used daily for 1–2 weeks and then weekly thereafter. These preparations are irritating if left on the skin for >10 min; thus, they should be washed off completely. Treatment with some oral antifungal agents is also effective, but they do not provide lasting results and are not FDA approved for this indication.

CANDIDIASIS

Candidiasis is a fungal infection caused by a related group of yeasts whose manifestations may be localized to the skin and mucous membranes or, rarely, may be systemic and life-threatening (**Chap. 216**). The causative organism is usually *Candida albicans*. These organisms are normal saprophytic inhabitants of the gastrointestinal tract but may overgrow due to broad-spectrum antibiotic therapy, diabetes mellitus, or immunosuppression and cause disease. Candidiasis is a very common infection in HIV-infected individuals (**Chap. 202**). The oral cavity is commonly involved. Lesions may occur on the tongue or buccal mucosa (*thrush*) and appear as white plaques. Fissured, macerated lesions at the corners of the mouth (*perlèche*) are often seen in individuals with poorly fitting dentures and may also be associated with candidal infection. In addition, candidal infections have an affinity for sites that are chronically wet and macerated, including the skin around nails (onycholysis and paronychia), and in intertriginous areas. Intertriginous lesions are characteristically edematous, erythematous, and scaly, with scattered "satellite pustules." In males, there is often involvement of the penis and scrotum as well as the inner aspect of the thighs. In contrast to dermatophyte infections, candidal infections are frequently painful and accompanied by a marked inflammatory response. Diagnosis of candidal infection is based on the clinical pattern and demonstration of yeast on KOH preparation or culture.

TREATMENT
Candidiasis

Treatment involves removal of any predisposing factors such as antibiotic therapy or chronic moisture and the use of appropriate topical or systemic antifungal agents. Effective topicals include nystatin or azoles (miconazole, clotrimazole, econazole, or ketoconazole). The associated inflammatory response accompanying candidal infection on glabrous skin can be treated with a mild glucocorticoid lotion or cream (2.5% hydrocortisone). Systemic therapy is usually reserved for immunosuppressed patients or individuals with chronic or recurrent disease who fail to respond to appropriate topical therapy. Oral fluconazole is most commonly prescribed for cutaneous candidiasis. Oral nystatin is effective only for candidiasis of the gastrointestinal tract.

WARTS

Warts are cutaneous neoplasms caused by papillomaviruses. More than 100 different human papillomaviruses (HPVs) have been described. A typical wart, *verruca vulgaris*, is sessile, dome-shaped, and usually about a centimeter in diameter. Its surface is hyperkeratotic, consisting of many small filamentous projections. HPV also causes typical plantar warts, flat warts (*verruca plana*), and filiform warts. Plantar warts are endophytic and are covered by thick keratin. Paring of the wart will generally reveal a central core of keratinized debris and punctate bleeding points. Filiform warts are commonly seen on the face, neck, and skinfolds and present as papillomatous lesions on a narrow base. Flat warts are only slightly elevated and have a velvety, nonverrucous surface. They have a propensity for the face, arms, and legs, and are often spread by shaving.

Genital warts begin as small papillomas that may grow to form large, fungating lesions. In women, they may involve the labia, perineum, or perianal skin. In addition, the mucosa of the vagina, urethra, and anus can be involved as well as the cervical epithelium. In men, the lesions often occur initially in the coronal sulcus but may be seen on the shaft of the penis, the scrotum, or the perianal skin or in the urethra.

Appreciable evidence has accumulated indicating that HPV plays a role in the development of neoplasia of the uterine cervix and anogenital skin (**Chap. 89**). HPV types 16 and 18 have been most intensely studied and are the major risk factors for intraepithelial neoplasia and squamous cell carcinoma of the cervix, anus, vulva, and penis. The risk is higher among patients immunosuppressed after solid organ transplantation and among those infected with HIV. Recent evidence also implicates other HPV types. Histologic examination of biopsied samples from affected sites may reveal changes associated with typical warts and/or features typical of intraepidermal carcinoma (Bowen's disease). Squamous cell carcinomas associated with HPV infections have also been observed in extragenital skin (**Chap. 76**), most commonly in patients immunosuppressed after organ transplantation. Patients on long-term immunosuppression should be monitored for the development of squamous cell carcinoma and other cutaneous malignancies.

TREATMENT
Warts

Treatment of warts, other than anogenital warts, should be tempered by the observation that most warts in normal individuals resolve spontaneously within 1–2 years. There are many modalities available to treat warts, but no single therapy is universally effective. Factors that influence the choice of therapy include the location of the wart, the extent of disease, the age and immunologic status of the patient, and the patient's desire for therapy. Perhaps the most useful and convenient method for treating warts in almost any location is cryotherapy with liquid nitrogen. Equally effective for nongenital warts, but requiring much more patient compliance, is the use of keratolytic agents such as salicylic acid plasters or solutions. For genital warts, in-office application of a podophyllin solution is moderately effective but may be associated with marked local reactions. Prescription preparations of dilute, purified podophyllin are available for home use. Topical imiquimod, a potent inducer of local cytokine release, has been approved for treatment of genital warts. A topical compound composed of green tea extracts (sinecatechins) is also available. Conventional and laser surgical procedures may be required for recalcitrant warts. Recurrence of warts appears to be common with all these modalities. A highly effective vaccine for selected types of HPV has been approved by the FDA, and its use is reported to reduce the incidence of anogenital and cervical carcinoma.

HERPES SIMPLEX

See Chap. 192.

HERPES ZOSTER

See Chap. 193.

ACNE

ACNE VULGARIS

Acne vulgaris is a self-limited disorder primarily of teenagers and young adults, although perhaps 10–20% of adults may continue to experience some form of the disorder. The permissive factor for the expression of the disease in adolescence is the increase in sebum production by sebaceous glands with puberty. Small cysts, called *comedones*, form in hair follicles due to blockage of the follicular orifice by retention of keratinous material and sebum. The activity of bacteria (*Cutibacterium acnes*) within the comedones releases free fatty acids from sebum, causes inflammation within the cyst, and results in rupture of the cyst wall. An inflammatory foreign-body reaction develops as result of extrusion of oily and keratinous debris from the cyst.

The clinical hallmark of acne vulgaris is the comedone, which may be closed (*whitehead*) or open (*blackhead*). Closed comedones appear as 1- to 2-mm pebbly white papules, which are accentuated when the skin is stretched. They are the precursors of inflammatory lesions of acne vulgaris. The contents of closed comedones are not easily expressed. Open comedones, which rarely result in inflammatory acne lesions, have a dilated follicular orifice and are filled with easily expressible oxidized, darkened, oily debris. Comedones are usually accompanied by inflammatory lesions: papules, pustules, or nodules.

The earliest lesions seen in adolescence are generally mildly inflamed or noninflammatory comedones on the forehead. Subsequently, more typical inflammatory lesions develop on the cheeks, nose, and chin (**Fig. 57-7**). The most common location for acne is the face, but involvement of the chest and back is common. Most disease remains mild and does not lead to scarring. A small number of patients develop large inflammatory cysts and nodules, which may drain and result in significant scarring. Regardless of the severity, acne may affect a patient's quality of life. With adequate treatment, this effect may be transient. In the case of severe, scarring acne, the effects can be permanent and profound. Early therapeutic intervention in severe acne is essential.

Exogenous and endogenous factors can alter the expression of acne vulgaris. Friction and trauma (from headbands or chin straps of athletic helmets), application of comedogenic topical agents (cosmetics or hair preparations), or chronic topical exposure to certain industrial compounds may elicit or aggravate acne. Glucocorticoids, topical or systemic, may also elicit acne. Other systemic medications such as progestin-only contraception, lithium, isoniazid, androgenic steroids, halogens, phenytoin, and phenobarbital may produce acneiform eruptions or aggravate preexisting acne. Genetic factors and polycystic ovary disease may also play a role.

TREATMENT
Acne Vulgaris

Treatment of acne vulgaris is directed toward elimination of comedones by normalizing follicular keratinization and decreasing sebaceous gland activity, the population of *C. acnes*, and inflammation. Minimal to moderate pauci-inflammatory disease may respond adequately to local therapy alone. Although areas affected with acne should be kept clean, overly vigorous scrubbing may aggravate acne due to mechanical rupture of comedones. Topical agents such as retinoic acid, benzoyl peroxide, or salicylic acid may alter the pattern of epidermal desquamation, preventing the formation of comedones and aiding in the resolution of preexisting cysts. Topical antibacterial agents (such as benzoyl peroxide, azelaic acid, erythromycin, clindamycin, or dapsone) are also useful adjuncts to therapy. Topical antibiotics (erythromycin and clindamycin) should be used in combination with benzoyl peroxide to prevent development of bacterial resistance.

Patients with moderate to severe acne with a prominent inflammatory component will benefit from the addition of systemic therapy, such as minocycline or doxycycline in doses of 100 mg bid or in lower dose, extended-release preparations. Such antibiotics appear to have anti-inflammatory effects independent of their antibacterial effects. Female patients who do not respond to oral antibiotics may benefit from hormonal therapy. Several oral contraceptives are now approved by the FDA for use in the treatment of acne vulgaris. Spironolactone is emerging as a safe, effective, and durable antiandrogen treatment in women.

Patients with severe nodulocystic acne unresponsive to the therapies discussed above may benefit from treatment with the synthetic retinoid isotretinoin. Dosing is weight-based and cumulative, with duration of therapy dictated by summative dose or acne lesion remission. Results are excellent in appropriately selected patients. Its use is highly regulated due to its potential for severe adverse events, primarily teratogenicity and depression. In addition, patients receiving this medication develop dry skin and cheilitis and must be followed for development of hypertriglyceridemia.

At present, prescribers must enroll in a program designed to prevent pregnancy and adverse events while patients are taking isotretinoin. These measures are imposed to ensure that all prescribers are familiar with the risks of isotretinoin, that all female patients have two negative pregnancy tests prior to initiation of therapy and a negative pregnancy test prior to each refill, and that all patients have been warned about the risks associated with isotretinoin.

ACNE ROSACEA

Acne rosacea, commonly referred to simply as *rosacea*, is an inflammatory disorder predominantly affecting the central face. Persons most often affected are Caucasians of northern European background, but rosacea also occurs in patients with dark skin. Rosacea is seen almost exclusively in adults, only rarely affecting patients <30 years old. Rosacea is more common in women, but those most severely affected are men. It is characterized by the presence of erythema, telangiectasias, and superficial pustules (**Fig. 57-8**) but is not associated with the presence of comedones. Rosacea rarely involves the chest or back.

There is a relationship between the tendency for facial flushing and the subsequent development of acne rosacea. Often, individuals with rosacea initially demonstrate a pronounced flushing reaction. This may be in response to heat, emotional stimuli, alcohol, hot drinks, or spicy foods. As the disease progresses, the flush persists longer and longer and may eventually become permanent. Papules, pustules, and

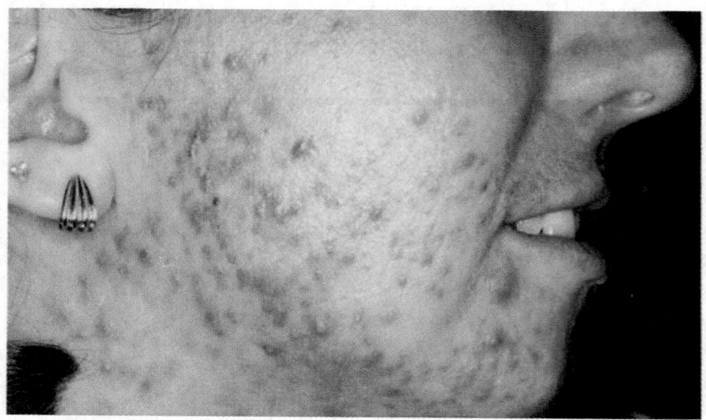

FIGURE 57-7 Acne vulgaris. An example of acne vulgaris with inflammatory papules, pustules, and comedones. *(Courtesy of Kalman Watsky, MD; with permission.)*

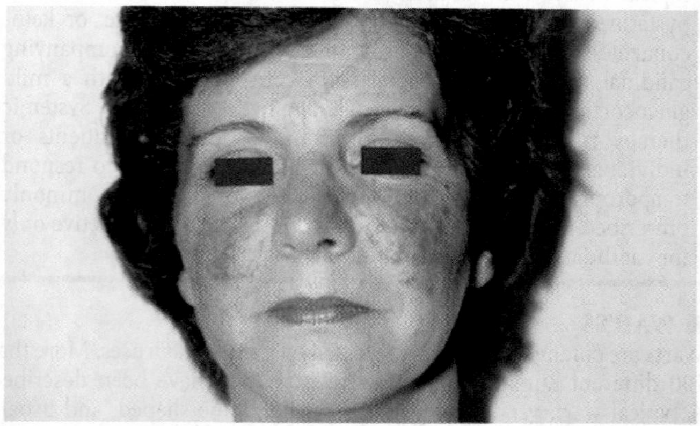

FIGURE 57-8 Acne rosacea. Prominent facial erythema, telangiectasia, scattered papules, and small pustules are seen in this patient with acne rosacea. *(Courtesy of Robert Swerlick, MD; with permission.)*

telangiectasias can become superimposed on the persistent flush. Rosacea of very long standing may lead to connective tissue overgrowth, particularly of the nose (*rhinophyma*). Rosacea may also be complicated by various inflammatory disorders of the eye, including keratitis, blepharitis, iritis, and recurrent chalazion. These ocular problems are potentially sight-threatening and warrant ophthalmologic evaluation.

TREATMENT

Acne Rosacea

Acne rosacea can be treated topically or systemically. Mild disease often responds to topical preparations of metronidazole, sodium sulfacetamide, azelaic acid, ivermectin, brimonidine, or oxymetazoline. More severe disease requires oral tetracyclines in subantimicrobial, modified-release preparations. Residual telangiectasia may respond to laser therapy. Topical glucocorticoids, especially potent agents, should be avoided because chronic use of these preparations may elicit rosacea. Application of topical agents to the skin is not effective treatment for ocular disease.

SKIN DISEASES AND SMALLPOX VACCINATION

Although smallpox vaccinations were discontinued several decades ago for the general population, they are still required for certain military personnel and first responders. In the absence of a bioterrorism attack and a real or potential exposure to smallpox, such vaccination is contraindicated in persons with a history of skin diseases, such as AD, eczema, and psoriasis, who have a higher incidence of adverse events associated with smallpox vaccination. In the case of such exposure, the risk of smallpox infection outweighs that of adverse events from the vaccine (**Chap. S3**).

FURTHER READING

BOLOGNIA JL et al (eds): *Dermatology*, 4th ed. Philadelphia, Elsevier, 2018.

JAMES WD et al (eds): *Andrew's Diseases of the Skin Clinical Dermatology*, 13th ed. Philadelphia, Elsevier, 2020.

KANG S et al (eds): *Fitzpatrick's Dermatology in General Medicine*, 9th ed. New York, McGraw-Hill, 2019.

WOLFF K et al (eds): *Fitzpatrick's Color Atlas and Synopsis of Clinical Dermatology*, 8th ed. New York, McGraw-Hill, 2017.

58 Skin Manifestations of Internal Disease

Jean L. Bolognia, Jonathan S. Leventhal, Irwin M. Braverman

It is a generally accepted concept in medicine that the skin can develop signs of internal disease. Therefore, in textbooks of medicine, one finds a chapter describing in detail the major systemic disorders that can be identified by cutaneous signs. The underlying assumption of such a chapter is that the clinician has been able to identify the specific disorder in the patient and needs only to read about it in the textbook. In reality, concise differential diagnoses and the identification of these disorders are actually difficult for the nondermatologist because he or she is not well-versed in the recognition of cutaneous lesions or their spectrum of presentations. Therefore, this chapter covers this particular topic of cutaneous medicine not by simply focusing on individual diseases, but by describing the various presenting clinical signs and symptoms that point to specific disorders. Concise differential diagnoses will be generated in which the significant diseases will be distinguished from the more common cutaneous disorders that have minimal or no significance with regard to associated internal disease. The latter disorders are reviewed in table form and always need to be excluded when considering the former. For a detailed description of individual diseases, the reader should consult a dermatologic text.

PAPULOSQUAMOUS SKIN LESIONS

(**Table 58-1**) When an eruption is characterized by elevated lesions, either papules (<1 cm) or plaques (>1 cm), in association with scale, it is referred to as *papulosquamous*. The most common papulosquamous diseases—*tinea, psoriasis, pityriasis rosea*, and *lichen planus*—are primary cutaneous disorders (**Chap. 57**). When psoriatic lesions are accompanied by arthritis, the possibility of psoriatic arthritis or reactive arthritis should be considered. A history of oral ulcers, conjunctivitis, uveitis, and/or urethritis points to the latter diagnosis. Lithium, beta blockers, anti-PD-1/PD-L1 antibodies, HIV or streptococcal infections, and a rapid taper of systemic glucocorticoids are known to exacerbate psoriasis; despite being used to treat psoriasis, tumor necrosis factor (TNF) inhibitors can also induce psoriatic lesions. Comorbidities in patients with psoriasis include cardiovascular disease and metabolic syndrome.

Whenever the clinical diagnosis of pityriasis rosea or lichen planus is made, it is important to review the patient's medications because the eruption may resolve by simply discontinuing the offending agent. Pityriasis rosea–like drug eruptions are seen most commonly with beta blockers, angiotensin-converting enzyme (ACE) inhibitors, and metronidazole, whereas the drugs that can produce a lichenoid eruption include thiazides, antimalarials, quinidine, beta blockers, TNF inhibitors, anti-PD-1/PD-L1 antibodies, and ACE inhibitors. In some populations (e.g., Europeans), there is a higher prevalence of hepatitis C viral infection in patients with oral lichen planus. Lichen planus–like lesions are also observed in chronic graft-versus-host disease.

In its early stages, the mycosis fungoides (MF) form of *cutaneous T-cell lymphoma* (CTCL) may be confused with eczema or psoriasis, but it often eventually fails to respond to appropriate therapy for those inflammatory diseases. MF can develop within lesions of large-plaque parapsoriasis and is suggested by an increase in the thickness of the lesions. The diagnosis of MF is established by skin biopsy in which

TABLE 58-1 Selected Causes of Papulosquamous Skin Lesions

1. Primary cutaneous disorders
   a. Tinea[a]—widespread disease may be sign of immunosuppression
   b. Psoriasis[a]—widespread or resistant disease may be sign of HIV infection
   c. Pityriasis rosea[a]
   d. Lichen planus[a]
   e. Parapsoriasis, small plaque and large plaque
   f. Bowen's disease (squamous cell carcinoma in situ)[b]
2. Drugs
3. Systemic diseases
   a. Lupus erythematosus, primarily subacute or chronic (discoid) lesions[c]
   b. Cutaneous T-cell lymphoma, in particular, mycosis fungoides[d]
   c. Secondary syphilis
   d. Reactive arthritis
   e. Sarcoidosis[e]—with scale less common than without scale
   f. Bazex syndrome (acrokeratosis paraneoplastica)[f]

[a]Discussed in detail in **Chap. 57**; cardiovascular disease and the metabolic syndrome are comorbidities in psoriasis; primarily in Europe, hepatitis C virus is associated with oral lichen planus. [b]Associated with chronic sun exposure more often than exposure to arsenic; usually one or a few lesions. [c]See also Red Lesions in "Papulonodular Skin Lesions." [d]Also cutaneous lesions of HTLV-1-associated adult T-cell leukemia/lymphoma. [e]See also Red-Brown Lesions in "Papulonodular Skin Lesions." [f]Psoriasiform lesions of the helices, nose, and acral sites; squamous cell carcinoma of the upper aerodigestive tract most common underlying malignancy.

Abbreviation: HIV, human immunodeficiency virus.

TABLE 58-2 Causes of Erythroderma

1. Primary cutaneous disorders
   a. Psoriasis[a]
   b. Dermatitis (atopic > contact >> stasis [with autosensitization] or seborrheic [primarily infants])[a]
   c. Pityriasis rubra pilaris
2. Drugs
3. Systemic diseases
   a. Cutaneous T-cell lymphoma (Sézary syndrome, erythrodermic mycosis fungoides)
   b. Other lymphomas
   c. Rarely, late-stage solid tumors
4. Idiopathic (usually older men)

[a]Discussed in detail in **Chap. 57**.

collections of atypical T lymphocytes are found in the epidermis and dermis. As the disease progresses, cutaneous tumors and lymph node involvement may appear.

In *secondary syphilis*, there are scattered pink to red-brown papules with thin scale. The eruption often involves the palms and soles and can resemble pityriasis rosea. Associated findings are helpful in making the diagnosis and include nonscarring alopecia, annular plaques on the face, mucous patches, condyloma lata (broad-based and moist), and lymphadenopathy, as well as malaise, fever, headache, and myalgias. The interval between the primary chancre and the secondary stage is usually 4–8 weeks, and spontaneous resolution without appropriate therapy occurs.

ERYTHRODERMA

(Table 58-2) *Erythroderma* is the term used when the majority of the skin surface is erythematous (red in color). There may be associated scale, erosions, or pustules as well as shedding of the hair and nails. Potential systemic manifestations include fever, chills, hypothermia, reactive lymphadenopathy, peripheral edema, hypoalbuminemia, and high-output cardiac failure. The major etiologies of erythroderma are (1) cutaneous diseases such as psoriasis and dermatitis **(Table 58-3)**; (2) drugs; (3) systemic diseases, most commonly CTCL; and (4) idiopathic. In the first three groups, the location and description of the initial lesions, prior to the development of the erythroderma, aid in the diagnosis. For example, a history of red scaly plaques on the elbows and knees would point to psoriasis. It is also important to examine the skin carefully for a migration of the erythema and associated secondary changes such as pustules or erosions. Migratory waves of erythema studded with superficial pustules are seen in *pustular psoriasis*.

Drug-induced erythroderma may begin as an exanthematous (morbilliform) eruption **(Chap. 60)** or may arise as diffuse erythema. A number of drugs can produce an erythroderma, including penicillins, sulfonamides, aromatic anticonvulsants (e.g., carbamazepine, phenytoin), and allopurinol. Fever and peripheral eosinophilia often accompany the eruption, and there may also be facial swelling, hepatitis, myocarditis, thyroiditis, and allergic interstitial nephritis; this constellation is frequently referred to as *drug reaction with eosinophilia and systemic symptoms* (DRESS) or *drug-induced hypersensitivity syndrome* (DIHS). In addition, these reactions, especially to aromatic anticonvulsants, can lead to a pseudolymphoma syndrome with adenopathy and circulating atypical lymphocytes, while reactions to allopurinol may be accompanied by gastrointestinal bleeding.

The most common malignancy that is associated with erythroderma is CTCL; in some series, up to 25% of the cases of erythroderma were due to CTCL. The patient may progress from isolated plaques and tumors, but more commonly, the erythroderma is present throughout the course of the disease (Sézary syndrome). In Sézary syndrome, there are circulating clonal atypical T lymphocytes, pruritus, and lymphadenopathy. In cases of erythroderma where there is no apparent cause (idiopathic), longitudinal evaluation is mandatory to monitor for the possible development of CTCL.

ALOPECIA

(Table 58-4) The two major forms of alopecia are scarring and nonscarring. *Scarring alopecia* is associated with fibrosis, inflammation, and loss of hair follicles. A smooth scalp with a decreased number of follicular openings is usually observed clinically, but in some patients, the changes are seen only in biopsy specimens from affected areas. In *nonscarring alopecia*, the hair shafts are absent or miniaturized, but the hair follicles are preserved, explaining the reversible nature of nonscarring alopecia.

The most common causes of nonscarring alopecia include *androgenetic alopecia, telogen effluvium, alopecia areata, tinea capitis*, and the early phase of *traumatic alopecia* **(Table 58-5)**. In women with androgenetic alopecia, an elevation in circulating levels of androgens may be seen as a result of ovarian or adrenal gland dysfunction or neoplasm. When there are signs of virilization, such as a deepened voice and/or enlarged clitoris, the possibility of an ovarian or adrenal gland tumor should be considered.

Exposure to various drugs can also cause diffuse hair loss, usually by inducing a telogen effluvium. An exception is the anagen effluvium observed with chemotherapeutic agents such as daunorubicin. Alopecia is a side effect of the following drugs: warfarin, heparin, propylthiouracil, carbimazole, isotretinoin, acitretin, lithium, beta blockers, interferons, colchicine, and amphetamines. Fortunately, spontaneous regrowth usually follows discontinuation of the offending agent.

Less commonly, nonscarring alopecia is associated with *lupus erythematosus* and *secondary syphilis*. In systemic lupus, there are two forms of alopecia—one is scarring secondary to discoid lesions (see below), and the other is nonscarring. The latter form coincides with flares of systemic disease and may involve the entire scalp or just the frontal scalp, with the appearance of multiple short hairs ("lupus hairs") as a sign of initial regrowth. Scattered, poorly circumscribed patches of alopecia with a "moth-eaten" appearance are a manifestation of the secondary stage of syphilis. Diffuse thinning of the hair is also associated with hypothyroidism and hyperthyroidism (Table 58-4).

Scarring alopecia is more frequently the result of a primary cutaneous disorder such as *lichen planus, chronic cutaneous (discoid) lupus, central centrifugal cicatricial alopecia, folliculitis decalvans*, or *linear scleroderma (morphea)* than it is a sign of systemic disease. Although the scarring lesions of *discoid lupus* can be seen in patients with systemic lupus, in the majority of patients, the disease process is limited to the skin. Less common causes of scarring alopecia include *sarcoidosis* (see "Papulonodular Skin Lesions," below), chemotherapeutic agents, and *cutaneous metastases*.

In the early phases of discoid lupus, lichen planus, and folliculitis decalvans, there are circumscribed areas of alopecia. Fibrosis and subsequent loss of hair follicles are observed primarily in the center of these alopecic patches, whereas the inflammatory process is most prominent at the periphery. The areas of active inflammation in discoid lupus are erythematous with scale, whereas the areas of previous inflammation are often hypopigmented with a rim of hyperpigmentation. In lichen planus, perifollicular macules at the periphery are usually violet-colored. A complete examination of the skin and oral mucosa combined with a biopsy and direct immunofluorescence microscopy of inflamed skin will aid in distinguishing these two entities. The peripheral active lesions in folliculitis decalvans are follicular pustules; these patients can develop a reactive arthritis.

FIGURATE SKIN LESIONS

(Table 58-6) In *figurate eruptions*, the lesions form rings and arcs that are usually erythematous but can be skin-colored to brown. Most commonly, they are due to primary cutaneous diseases such as *tinea, urticaria, granuloma annulare*, and *erythema annulare centrifugum* **(Chaps. 57 and 59)**. An underlying systemic illness is found in a second, less common group of migratory annular erythemas. It includes *erythema migrans, erythema gyratum repens, erythema marginatum*, and *necrolytic migratory erythema*.

In erythema gyratum repens, one sees numerous mobile concentric arcs and wavefronts that resemble the grain in wood. A search for an

TABLE 58-3 Erythroderma (Primary Cutaneous Disorders)

	INITIAL LESIONS	LOCATION OF INITIAL LESIONS	OTHER FINDINGS	DIAGNOSTIC AIDS	TREATMENT
Psoriasis[a]	Pink-red, silvery scale, sharply demarcated	Elbows, knees, scalp, presacral area, intergluteal fold	Nail dystrophy (e.g., pits, oil drop sign), arthritis, pustules, SAPHO syndrome[b]	Skin biopsy	Topical glucocorticoids, vitamin D analogs; UV-B (narrowband) > PUVA; oral retinoids; MTX; anti-TNF agents, anti-IL-12/23 Ab, anti-IL-23 Ab, anti-IL-17A or -IL-17 receptor A Ab; apremilast; cyclosporine
Dermatitis[a]					
Atopic	Acute: Erythema, fine scale, crust, indistinct borders, excoriations Chronic: Lichenification (increased skin markings), excoriations	Antecubital and popliteal fossae, neck, hands, eyelids	Pruritus Personal and/or family history of atopy, including asthma, allergic rhinitis or conjunctivitis, and atopic dermatitis Exclude secondary infection with *Staphylococcus aureus* or HSV Exclude superimposed irritant or allergic contact dermatitis	Skin biopsy	Topical glucocorticoids, tacrolimus, pimecrolimus, tar, crisaborole, and antipruritics; oral antihistamines for sedation; open wet dressings; UV-B ± UV-A > PUVA; anti-IL-4/13 Ab; oral/IM glucocorticoids (short-term); MTX; mycophenolate mofetil; azathioprine; cyclosporine Topical or oral antibiotics
Contact	Local: Erythema, crusting, vesicles, and bullae	Depends on offending agent	Irritant—onset often within hours Allergic—delayed-type hypersensitivity; lag time of 48 h with rechallenge	Patch testing; repeat open application test	Remove irritant or allergen; topical glucocorticoids; oral antihistamines; oral/IM glucocorticoids (short-term)
	Systemic: Erythema, fine scale, crust	Generalized vs major intertriginous zones (especially groin)	Patient has history of allergic contact dermatitis to topical agent and then receives systemic medication that is structurally related, e.g., formaldehyde (skin), aspartame (oral)	Patch testing	Same as local
Seborrheic (rare in adults)	Pink-red to pink-orange, greasy scale	Scalp, nasolabial folds, eyebrows, intertriginous zones	Flares with stress, HIV infection Associated with Parkinson's disease	Skin biopsy	Topical glucocorticoids and imidazoles
Stasis (with autosensitization)	Erythema, crusting, excoriations	Lower extremities	Pruritus, lower extremity edema, varicosities, hemosiderin deposits, lipodermatosclerosis History of venous ulcers, thrombophlebitis, and/or cellulitis Exclude cellulitis Exclude superimposed contact dermatitis, e.g., topical neomycin	Skin biopsy	Topical glucocorticoids; open wet dressings; leg elevation; pressure stockings; pressure wraps if associated ulcers
Pityriasis rubra pilaris	Orange-red (salmon-colored), perifollicular papules	Generalized, but characteristic "skip" areas of normal skin	Wax-like palmoplantar keratoderma Exclude cutaneous T-cell lymphoma	Skin biopsy	Isotretinoin or acitretin; MTX; anti-IL-12/23 Ab, anti-IL-23 Ab, anti-TNF agents, anti-IL-17A or -IL-17 receptor A Ab

[a]Discussed in detail in **Chap. 57**. [b]SAPHO syndrome occurs more commonly in patients with palmoplantar pustulosis than in those with erythrodermic psoriasis.

Abbreviations: Ab, antibody; HSV, herpes simplex virus; IL, interleukin; IM, intramuscular; MTX, methotrexate; PUVA, psoralens plus ultraviolet A irradiation; SAPHO, *s*ynovitis, *a*cne, *p*ustulosis, *h*yperostosis, and *o*steitis (a subtype is chronic recurrent multifocal osteomyelitis); TNF, tumor necrosis factor; UV-A, ultraviolet A irradiation; UV-B, ultraviolet B irradiation.

underlying malignancy is mandatory in a patient with this eruption. Erythema migrans is the cutaneous manifestation of Lyme disease, which is caused by the spirochete *Borrelia burgdorferi*. In the initial stage (3–30 days after tick bite), a single annular lesion is usually seen, which can expand to ≥10 cm in diameter. Within several days, up to half of the patients develop multiple smaller erythematous lesions at sites distant from the bite. Associated symptoms include fever, headache, photophobia, myalgias, arthralgias, and malar rash. Erythema marginatum is seen in patients with rheumatic fever, primarily on the trunk. Lesions are pink-red in color, flat to minimally elevated, and transient.

There are additional cutaneous diseases that present as annular eruptions but lack an obvious migratory component. Examples include *CTCL*, *subacute cutaneous lupus*, *secondary syphilis*, and *sarcoidosis* (see "Papulonodular Skin Lesions," below).

ACNE

(Table 58-7) In addition to *acne vulgaris* and *acne rosacea*, the two major forms of acne **(Chap. 57)**, there are drugs and systemic diseases that can lead to acneiform eruptions.

Patients with the *carcinoid syndrome* have episodes of flushing of the head, neck, and sometimes the trunk. Resultant skin changes of the

TABLE 58-4 Causes of Alopecia

I. Nonscarring alopecia
   A. Primary cutaneous disorders
      1. Androgenetic alopecia (female pattern, male pattern)
      2. Telogen effluvium
      3. Alopecia areata
      4. Tinea capitis
      5. Traumatic alopecia[a]
      6. Psoriasiform alopecia, including TNF inhibitor–induced
   B. Drugs
      1. Telogen effluvium—see text for most common causes
      2. Anagen effluvium—chemotherapeutic agents (e.g., anthracyclines)
   C. Systemic diseases
      1. Systemic lupus erythematosus
      2. Secondary syphilis
      3. Hypothyroidism
      4. Hyperthyroidism
      5. Hypopituitarism
      6. Deficiencies of protein, biotin, zinc, and perhaps iron
II. Scarring alopecia
   A. Primary cutaneous disorders
      1. Cutaneous lupus (chronic discoid lesions)[b]
      2. Lichen planus, including frontal fibrosing alopecia
      3. Central centrifugal cicatricial alopecia
      4. Folliculitis decalvans
      5. Dissecting cellulitis
      6. Linear morphea (linear scleroderma)[c]
   B. Drugs
      1. Chemotherapeutic agents (e.g., taxanes, busulfan)
   C. Systemic diseases
      1. Discoid lesions in the setting of systemic lupus erythematosus[b]
      2. Sarcoidosis
      3. Cutaneous metastases

[a]Most patients with trichotillomania or early stages of traction alopecia and some patients with pressure-induced alopecia. [b]While the majority of patients with discoid lesions have only cutaneous disease, these lesions do represent one of the criteria in the European League Against Rheumatism (EULAR)/American College of Rheumatology (ACR) [2019] and ACR [1982] classification schemes for systemic lupus erythematosus. [c]Can involve underlying muscles and osseous structures, and rarely in linear morphea of the frontal scalp (*en coup de sabre*), there is involvement of the meninges and brain.

face, in particular telangiectasias, may mimic the clinical appearance of erythematotelangiectatic acne rosacea.

PUSTULAR LESIONS

Acneiform eruptions (see "Acne," above) and *folliculitis* represent the most common pustular dermatoses. An important consideration in the evaluation of follicular pustules is a determination of the associated pathogen, for example, normal flora (culture-negative), *Staphylococcus aureus*, *Pseudomonas aeruginosa* ("hot tub" folliculitis), *Malassezia*, dermatophytes (Majocchi's granuloma), and *Demodex* spp. Noninfectious forms of folliculitis include HIV- or immunosuppression-associated eosinophilic folliculitis and folliculitis secondary to drugs such as glucocorticoids, lithium, and epidermal growth factor receptor (EGFR) or MEK inhibitors. Administration of high-dose systemic glucocorticoids can result in a widespread eruption of follicular pustules on the trunk, characterized by lesions in the same stage of development. With regard to underlying systemic diseases, nonfollicular-based pustules are a characteristic component of pustular psoriasis (sterile) and can be seen in septic emboli of bacterial or fungal origin (see "Purpura," below). In patients with acute generalized exanthematous pustulosis (AGEP) due primarily to medications (e.g., cephalosporins), there are large areas of erythema studded with multiple sterile pustules in addition to neutrophilia.

TELANGIECTASIAS

(Table 58-8) To distinguish the various types of telangiectasias, it is important to examine the shape and configuration of the dilated blood vessels. *Linear telangiectasias* are seen on the face of patients with *actinically damaged skin* and *acne rosacea*, and they are found on the legs of patients with *venous hypertension* and first appear on the legs in *generalized essential telangiectasia*. Patients with an unusual form of *mastocytosis* (telangiectasia macularis eruptiva perstans) and the *carcinoid syndrome* (see "Acne," above) also have linear telangiectasias. Lastly, linear telangiectasias are found in areas of cutaneous inflammation. For example, longstanding lesions of discoid lupus frequently have telangiectasias within them.

Poikiloderma is a term used to describe a patch of skin with: (1) reticulated hypo- and hyperpigmentation, (2) wrinkling secondary to epidermal atrophy, and (3) telangiectasias. Poikiloderma does not imply a single disease entity—although it is becoming less common, it is seen in skin damaged by *ionizing radiation* as well as in patients with autoimmune connective tissue diseases, primarily *dermatomyositis* (DM), and rare genodermatoses (e.g., Kindler syndrome).

In *systemic sclerosis (scleroderma)*, the dilated blood vessels have a unique configuration and are known as *mat telangiectasias*. The lesions are broad macules that usually measure 2–7 mm in diameter but occasionally are larger. Mats have a polygonal or oval shape, and their erythematous color may appear uniform, but, upon closer inspection, the erythema is the result of delicate telangiectasias. The most common locations for mat telangiectasias are the face, oral mucosa, and hands—peripheral sites that are prone to intermittent ischemia. The limited form of systemic sclerosis, also referred to as the CREST (*c*alcinosis cutis, *R*aynaud's phenomenon, *e*sophageal dysmotility, *s*clerodactyly, and *t*elangiectasia) variant **(Chap. 360)**, is associated with a chronic course and anticentromere antibodies. Mat telangiectasias are an important clue to the diagnosis of this variant as well as the diffuse form of systemic sclerosis because they may be the only cutaneous finding.

Nailfold telangiectasias are pathognomonic signs of the three major autoimmune connective tissue diseases: *lupus erythematosus*, *systemic sclerosis*, and *DM*. They are easily visualized by the naked eye and occur in at least two-thirds of these patients. In both DM and lupus, there is associated nailfold erythema, and in DM, the erythema is often accompanied by "ragged" cuticles and fingertip tenderness. Under 10× magnification or by dermoscopy, the blood vessels in the nailfolds of lupus patients are tortuous and resemble "glomeruli," whereas in systemic sclerosis and DM, there is a loss of capillary loops and those that remain are markedly dilated.

In *hereditary hemorrhagic telangiectasia* (Osler-Rendu-Weber disease), the lesions usually appear during adolescence (mucosal) and adulthood (cutaneous) and are most commonly seen on the mucous membranes (nasal, orolabial), face, and distal extremities, including under the nails. They represent arteriovenous (AV) malformations of the dermal microvasculature, are dark red in color, and are usually slightly elevated. When the skin is stretched over an individual lesion, an eccentric punctum with radiating legs is seen. Although the degree of systemic involvement varies in this autosomal dominant disease (due primarily to mutations in either the endoglin or activin receptor–like kinase gene), the major symptoms are recurrent epistaxis and gastrointestinal bleeding. The fact that these mucosal telangiectasias are actually AV communications helps to explain their tendency to bleed.

HYPOPIGMENTATION

(Table 58-9) Disorders of hypopigmentation are often classified as either diffuse or localized. The classic example of *diffuse hypopigmentation* is *oculocutaneous albinism* (OCA). The most common forms are due to mutations in the tyrosinase gene (type I) or the *P* gene (type II); patients with type IA OCA have a total lack of enzyme activity. At birth, different forms of OCA can appear similar—white hair, gray-blue eyes, and pink-white skin. However, the patients with no tyrosinase activity maintain this phenotype, whereas those with decreased activity will acquire some pigmentation of the eyes, hair, and skin as they age.

TABLE 58-5 Nonscarring Alopecia (Primary Cutaneous Disorders)

	CLINICAL CHARACTERISTICS	PATHOGENESIS	TREATMENT
Telogen effluvium	Diffuse shedding of normal hairs Follows major stress (high fever, severe infection) or change in hormone levels (postpartum) Reversible without treatment	Stress causes more of the asynchronous growth cycles of individual hairs to become synchronous; therefore, larger numbers of growing (anagen) hairs simultaneously enter the dying (telogen) phase	Observation; discontinue any drugs that have alopecia as a side effect; must exclude underlying metabolic causes, e.g., hypothyroidism, hyperthyroidism
Androgenetic alopecia (male pattern; female pattern)	Miniaturization of hairs along the midline of the scalp Recession of the anterior scalp line in men and some women	Increased sensitivity of affected hairs to the effects of androgens—most common Increased levels of circulating androgens (ovarian or adrenal source in women)—less common	If no evidence of hyperandrogenemia, then topical minoxidil; finasteride[a]; spironolactone (women); hair transplant; low-dose oral minoxidil
Alopecia areata	Well-circumscribed, circular areas of hair loss, 2–5 cm in diameter In extensive cases, coalescence of lesions and/or involvement of other hair-bearing surfaces of the body Pitting or sandpapered appearance of the nails	The germinative zones of the hair follicles are surrounded by T lymphocytes Occasional associated diseases: hyperthyroidism, hypothyroidism, vitiligo, Down syndrome	Topical anthralin or tazarotene; intralesional glucocorticoids; topical contact sensitizers; JAK inhibitors
Tinea capitis	Varies from scaling with minimal hair loss to discrete patches with "black dots" (sites of broken infected hairs) to boggy plaque with pustules (kerion)[b]	Invasion of hairs by dermatophytes, most commonly *Trichophyton tonsurans*	Oral griseofulvin or terbinafine plus 2.5% selenium sulfide or ketoconazole shampoo; examine family members
Traumatic alopecia[c]	Broken hairs, often of varying lengths Irregular outline in trichotillomania and traction alopecia Fringe sign in traction alopecia	Traction with curlers, rubber bands, tight braiding Exposure to heat or chemicals (e.g., hair straighteners) Mechanical pulling (trichotillomania)	Discontinuation of offending hair style or chemical treatments; diagnosis of trichotillomania may require observation of shaved hairs (for growth) or biopsy, possibly followed by psychotherapy

[a]To date, Food and Drug Administration–approved for men. [b]Scarring alopecia can occur at sites of kerions. [c]May also be scarring, especially late-stage traction alopecia.

The degree of pigment formation is also a function of racial background, and the pigmentary dilution is more readily apparent when patients are compared to their first-degree relatives. The ocular findings in OCA correlate with the degree of hypopigmentation and include decreased visual acuity, nystagmus, photophobia, strabismus, and a lack of normal binocular vision.

TABLE 58-6 Causes of Figurate Skin Lesions

I. Primary cutaneous disorders
  A. Tinea
  B. Urticaria (primary in ≥90% of patients)
  C. Granuloma annulare
  D. Erythema annulare centrifugum
  E. Psoriasis, annular pustular psoriasis
  F. Interstitial granulomatous drug reaction
II. Systemic diseases
  A. Migratory
    1. Erythema migrans (CDC case definition is ≥5 cm in diameter)
    2. Urticaria (≤10% of patients)
    3. Erythema gyratum repens
    4. Erythema marginatum
    5. Pustular psoriasis (generalized and annular forms)
    6. Necrolytic migratory erythema (glucagonoma syndrome)[a]
  B. Nonmigratory (may slowly expand)
    1. Subacute cutaneous LE, LE tumidus
    2. Sarcoidosis
    3. Leprosy (borderline, tuberculoid)
    4. Secondary syphilis (especially the face)
    5. Cutaneous T-cell lymphoma (especially mycosis fungoides)
    6. Interstitial granulomatous dermatitis[b]
    7. Annular erythema of Sjögren's syndrome

[a]Migratory erythema with erosions; favors lower extremities and girdle area.
[b]Underlying diseases include rheumatoid arthritis, LE, and granulomatosis with polyangiitis.

Abbreviations: CDC, Centers for Disease Control and Prevention; LE, lupus erythematosus.

The differential diagnosis of *localized hypomelanosis* includes the following primary cutaneous disorders: *postinflammatory hypopigmentation*, *idiopathic guttate hypomelanosis*, *pityriasis (tinea) versicolor*, *vitiligo*, *chemical- or drug-induced leukoderma*, *nevus depigmentosus* (see below), *progressive macular hypomelanosis*, and *piebaldism* (**Table 58-10**). In this group of diseases, the areas of involvement are macules or patches with a decrease or absence of pigmentation. Patients with vitiligo also have an increased incidence of several autoimmune disorders, including Hashimoto's thyroiditis, Graves' disease, pernicious anemia, Addison's disease, uveitis, alopecia areata, chronic mucocutaneous candidiasis, and the autoimmune polyendocrine syndromes (types I and II). Diseases of the thyroid gland are the most frequently associated disorders, occurring in up to 30% of patients with vitiligo. Circulating autoantibodies are often found, and the most common ones are antithyroglobulin, antimicrosomal, and antithyroid-stimulating hormone receptor antibodies.

There are four systemic diseases that should be considered in a patient with skin findings suggestive of vitiligo—*systemic sclerosis*, *melanoma-associated leukoderma*, *onchocerciasis*, and *Vogt-Koyanagi-Harada syndrome*. The vitiligo-like leukoderma seen in patients with

TABLE 58-7 Causes of Acneiform Eruptions

I. Primary cutaneous disorders
  A. Acne vulgaris
  B. Acne rosacea
II. Drugs, e.g., anabolic steroids, glucocorticoids, lithium, EGFR inhibitors, HER2 inhibitors, MEK inhibitors, iodides
III. Systemic diseases
  A. Increased androgen production
    1. Adrenal origin, e.g., Cushing's disease, 21-hydroxylase deficiency
    2. Ovarian origin, e.g., polycystic ovary syndrome, ovarian hyperthecosis
  B. Cryptococcosis, disseminated
  C. Dimorphic fungal infections
  D. Behçet's disease

Abbreviations: EGFR, epidermal growth factor receptor; HER2, human epidermal growth factor receptor 2; MEK, MAP (mitogen activated protein) kinase.

TABLE 58-8 Causes of Telangiectasias

- I. Primary cutaneous disorders
  - A. Linear/branching
    1. Acne rosacea (face)
    2. Actinically damaged skin (face, neck, V of chest)
    3. Venous hypertension (legs)
    4. Generalized essential telangiectasia
    5. Cutaneous collagenous vasculopathy
    6. Within basal cell carcinomas or cutaneous lymphoma
  - B. Poikiloderma
    1. Ionizing radiation[a]
  - C. Spider angioma
    1. Idiopathic
    2. Pregnancy
- II. Systemic diseases
  - A. Linear/branching
    1. Carcinoid (head, neck, upper trunk)
    2. Ataxia-telangiectasia (bulbar conjunctivae, head and neck)
    3. Mastocytosis (within lesions)
  - B. Poikiloderma
    1. Dermatomyositis, lupus erythematosus
    2. Mycosis fungoides, patch stage
    3. Genodermatoses, e.g., xeroderma pigmentosum, Kindler syndrome
  - C. Mat
    1. Systemic sclerosis (scleroderma)
  - D. Nailfold
    1. Lupus erythematosus
    2. Systemic sclerosis (scleroderma)
    3. Dermatomyositis
    4. Hereditary hemorrhagic telangiectasia
  - E. Papular
    1. Hereditary hemorrhagic telangiectasia
  - F. Spider angioma
    1. Cirrhosis[b]

[a]Becoming less common. [b]Due to hyperestrogenic state.

TABLE 58-9 Causes of Hypopigmentation

- I. Primary cutaneous disorders
  - A. Diffuse
    1. Generalized vitiligo[a]
  - B. Localized
    1. Postinflammatory
    2. Idiopathic guttate hypomelanosis
    3. Pityriasis (tinea) versicolor
    4. Vitiligo[a]
    5. Chemical- or drug-induced leukoderma, e.g., topical imiquimod, oral imatinib
    6. Nevus depigmentosus and pigmentary mosaicism
    7. Progressive macular hypomelanosis
    8. Piebaldism[a]
- II. Systemic diseases
  - A. Diffuse
    1. Oculocutaneous albinism[b]
    2. Hermansky-Pudlak syndrome[b,c]
    3. Chédiak-Higashi syndrome[b,d]
    4. Phenylketonuria
  - B. Localized
    1. Systemic sclerosis (scleroderma)[e]
    2. Melanoma-associated vitiligo-like leukoderma, immunotherapy-induced or spontaneous[e]
    3. Sarcoidosis
    4. Cutaneous T-cell lymphoma (especially mycosis fungoides)
    5. Tuberculoid and indeterminate leprosy
    6. Onchocerciasis[e]
    7. Linear nevoid hypopigmentation (pigmentary mosaicism)[b,f]
    8. Incontinentia pigmenti (stage IV)
    9. Tuberous sclerosis
    10. Waardenburg syndrome and Shah-Waardenburg syndrome
    11. Vogt-Koyanagi-Harada syndrome[e]

[a]Absence of melanocytes in areas of leukoderma; congenital in piebaldism. [b]Normal number of melanocytes. [c]Platelet storage defect and restrictive lung disease secondary to deposits of ceroid-like material or immunodeficiency; due to mutations in β or δ subunit of adaptor-related protein complex 3 as well as subunits of *b*iogenesis of *l*ysosome-related *o*rganelles *c*omplex (BLOC)-1, -2, and -3. [d]Giant lysosomal granules and recurrent infections. [e]Can resemble vitiligo due to acquired complete loss of pigment. [f]Minority of patients in a nonreferral setting have systemic abnormalities (musculoskeletal, central nervous system, ocular), previously referred to as hypomelanosis of Ito.

systemic sclerosis has a clinical resemblance to idiopathic vitiligo that has begun to repigment as a result of treatment; that is, perifollicular macules of normal pigmentation are seen within areas of depigmentation. The basis of this leukoderma is unknown; there is no evidence of inflammation in areas of involvement, but it can resolve if the underlying connective tissue disease becomes inactive. In contrast to idiopathic vitiligo, melanoma-associated vitiligo-like leukoderma often begins on the trunk, and its appearance, if spontaneous, should prompt a search for metastatic disease. It is also seen in patients undergoing immunotherapy for melanoma, including immune checkpoint-blocking antibodies, with cytotoxic T lymphocytes presumably recognizing cell surface antigens common to melanoma cells and melanocytes, and is associated with a greater likelihood of a clinical response. A history of aseptic meningitis, nontraumatic uveitis, tinnitus, hearing loss, and/or dysacousia points to the diagnosis of the Vogt-Koyanagi-Harada syndrome. In these patients, the face and scalp are the most common locations of pigment loss.

There are two systemic disorders (neurocristopathies) that may have the cutaneous findings of piebaldism (Table 58-9). They are *Shah-Waardenburg syndrome* and *Waardenburg syndrome*. A possible explanation for both disorders is an abnormal embryonic migration or survival of two neural crest–derived elements, one of them being melanocytes and the other myenteric ganglion cells (leading to Hirschsprung disease in Shah-Waardenburg syndrome) or auditory nerve cells (Waardenburg syndrome). The latter syndrome is characterized by congenital sensorineural hearing loss, dystopia canthorum (lateral displacement of the inner canthi but normal interpupillary distance), heterochromic irises, and a broad nasal root, in addition to the piebaldism. The facial dysmorphism can be explained by the neural crest origin of the connective tissues of the head and neck. Patients with Waardenburg syndrome have been shown to have mutations in four genes, including *PAX-3* and *MITF*, all of which encode transcription factors, whereas patients with Hirschsprung disease plus white spotting have mutations in one of three genes—endothelin 3, endothelin B receptor, and *SOX-10*.

In *tuberous sclerosis*, the earliest cutaneous sign is macular hypomelanosis, referred to as an ash leaf spot. These lesions are often present at birth and are usually multiple; however, detection may require Wood's lamp examination, especially in lightly pigmented individuals. The pigment within them is reduced, but not absent. The average size is 1–3 cm, and the common shapes are polygonal and lance-ovate. Examination of the patient for additional cutaneous signs such as multiple angiofibromas of the face (adenoma sebaceum), ungual and intraoral fibromas, fibrous cephalic plaques, and connective tissue nevi (shagreen patches) is recommended. It is important to remember that an ash leaf spot on the scalp will result in a circumscribed patch of lightly pigmented hair. Internal manifestations include seizures, intellectual disability, central nervous system (CNS) and retinal hamartomas, pulmonary lymphangioleiomyomatosis (women), renal angiomyolipomas, and cardiac rhabdomyomas. The latter can be detected in up to 60% of children (<18 years) with tuberous sclerosis by echocardiography.

Nevus depigmentosus is a stable, well-circumscribed hypomelanosis that is present at birth. There is usually a single oval or rectangular

TABLE 58-10 Hypopigmentation (Primary Cutaneous Disorders, Localized)

	CLINICAL CHARACTERISTICS	WOOD'S LAMP EXAMINATION (UV-A; PEAK = 365 NM)	SKIN BIOPSY SPECIMEN	PATHOGENESIS	TREATMENT
Postinflammatory hypopigmentation	Can develop within active lesions, as in subacute cutaneous lupus, or after the lesion fades, as in atopic dermatitis	Depends on particular disease Usually less enhancement than in vitiligo	Type of inflammatory infiltrate depends on specific disease	Block in transfer of melanin from melanocytes to keratinocytes could be secondary to edema or decrease in contact time Destruction of melanocytes if inflammatory cells attack basal layer of epidermis	Treat underlying inflammatory disease
Idiopathic guttate hypomelanosis	Common; acquired; usually 2–4 mm in diameter Shins and extensor forearms	Less enhancement than vitiligo	Abrupt decrease in epidermal melanin content	Possible somatic mutations as a reflection of aging or UV exposure	None
Pityriasis (tinea) versicolor[a]	Common disorder Upper trunk and neck (shawl-like distribution), groin Young adults Macules have fine white scale when scratched	Golden fluorescence	Hyphal forms and budding yeast in stratum corneum	Invasion of stratum corneum by the yeast *Malassezia* Yeast is lipophilic and produces C_9 and C_{11} dicarboxylic acids, which in vitro inhibit tyrosinase	Selenium sulfide 2.5% shampoo; topical imidazoles; oral triazoles
Vitiligo	Acquired; progressive Symmetric areas of complete pigment loss Periorificial—around mouth, nose, eyes, nipples, umbilicus, anus Other areas—flexor wrists, extensor distal extremities Segmental form is less common—unilateral, dermatomal-like	More apparent Chalk-white	Absence of melanocytes in well-developed lesions Mild inflammation	Autoimmune phenomenon that results in destruction of melanocytes—primarily cellular (circulating skin-homing autoreactive T cells)	Topical glucocorticoids; topical calcineurin inhibitors; UV-B (narrowband); PUVA; JAK inhibitors; transplants, if stable; depigmentation (topical MBEH), if widespread and treatment-resistant
Chemical- or drug-induced leukoderma	Similar appearance to vitiligo Often begins on hands when associated with chemical exposure Satellite lesions in areas not exposed to chemicals	More apparent Chalk-white	Decreased number or absence of melanocytes	Exposure to chemicals that selectively destroy melanocytes, in particular phenols and catechols (germicides; rubber products) or ingestion of drugs such as imatinib Release of cellular antigens and activation of circulating lymphocytes may explain satellite phenomenon Possible inhibition of KIT receptor	Avoid exposure to offending agent, then treat as vitiligo Drug-induced variant may undergo repigmentation when medication is discontinued
Piebaldism	Autosomal dominant Congenital, stable White forelock Areas of amelanosis contain normally pigmented and hyperpigmented macules of various sizes Symmetric involvement of central forehead, ventral trunk, and mid regions of upper and lower extremities	Enhancement of leukoderma and hyperpigmented macules	Amelanotic areas—few to no melanocytes	Defect in migration of melanoblasts from neural crest to involved skin or failure of melanoblasts to survive or differentiate in these areas Mutations within the *KIT* protooncogene that encodes the tyrosine kinase receptor for stem cell growth factor (kit ligand)	None; occasionally transplants

[a]If potassium hydroxide (KOH) examination of scale is negative, consider the possibility of progressive macular hypomelanosis.

Abbreviations: MBEH, monobenzylether of hydroquinone; PUVA, psoralens plus ultraviolet A irradiation; UV-B, ultraviolet B irradiation.

lesion, but when there are multiple lesions, the possibility of tuberous sclerosis needs to be considered. In *linear nevoid hypopigmentation*, a term that is replacing hypomelanosis of Ito and segmental or systematized nevus depigmentosus, streaks and swirls of hypopigmentation are observed. Up to one-third of patients in a tertiary care setting had associated abnormalities involving the musculoskeletal system (asymmetry), the CNS (seizures and intellectual disability), and the eyes (strabismus and hypertelorism). Chromosomal mosaicism has been detected in these patients, lending support to the hypothesis that the cutaneous pattern is the result of the migration of two clones of primordial melanocytes, each with a different pigment potential.

Localized areas of decreased pigmentation are commonly seen as a result of cutaneous inflammation (Table 58-10) and have been observed in the skin overlying active lesions of sarcoidosis (see "Papulonodular Skin Lesions," below) as well as in CTCL. Cutaneous infections also present as disorders of hypopigmentation, and in *tuberculoid leprosy*, there are a few asymmetric patches of hypomelanosis that have associated anesthesia, anhidrosis, and alopecia. Biopsy specimens of the palpable border show dermal granulomas that contain rare, if any, *Mycobacterium leprae* organisms.

HYPERPIGMENTATION

(Table 58-11) Disorders of hyperpigmentation are also divided into two major groups—localized and diffuse. The localized forms are due to an epidermal alteration, a proliferation of melanocytes, or an increase in pigment production. Both acanthosis nigricans and seborrheic keratoses belong to the first group. *Acanthosis nigricans* can be a reflection of an internal malignancy, most commonly of the gastrointestinal tract, and it appears as velvety hyperpigmentation, primarily in flexural areas. However, in the majority of patients, acanthosis nigricans is associated with obesity and insulin resistance, although it may be a reflection of an endocrinopathy such as acromegaly, Cushing's syndrome, polycystic ovary syndrome, or insulin-resistant diabetes mellitus (type A, type B, and lipodystrophic forms). *Seborrheic keratoses* are common lesions, but in one rare clinical setting, they are a sign of systemic disease, and that setting is the sudden appearance of multiple lesions, often with an inflammatory base and in association with acrochordons (skin tags) and acanthosis nigricans. This is termed the *sign of Leser-Trélat* and alerts the clinician to search for an internal malignancy.

A proliferation of melanocytes results in the following pigmented lesions: *lentigo*, *melanocytic nevus*, and *melanoma* (**Chap. 76**). In an adult, the majority of lentigines are related to sun exposure, which explains their distribution. However, in the Peutz-Jeghers and LEOPARD (*l*entigines; *E*CG abnormalities, primarily conduction defects; *o*cular hypertelorism; *p*ulmonary stenosis and subaortic valvular stenosis; *a*bnormal genitalia [cryptorchidism, hypospadias]; *r*etardation of growth; and *d*eafness [sensorineural]) syndromes, lentigines do serve as a clue to systemic disease. In *LEOPARD/Noonan with multiple lentigines syndrome*, hundreds of lentigines develop during childhood and are scattered over the entire surface of the body. The lentigines in patients with *Peutz-Jeghers syndrome* are located primarily around the nose and mouth, on the hands and feet, and within the oral cavity. While the pigmented macules on the face may fade with age, the oral lesions persist. However, similar intraoral lesions are also seen in Addison's disease, in Laugier-Hunziker syndrome (no internal manifestations), and as a normal finding in darkly pigmented individuals. Patients with this autosomal dominant syndrome (due to mutations in a novel serine threonine kinase gene) have multiple benign polyps of the gastrointestinal tract, testicular or ovarian tumors, and an increased risk of developing gastrointestinal (primarily colon) and pancreatic cancers.

In the *Carney complex*, numerous lentigines are also seen, but they are in association with cardiac myxomas. This autosomal dominant disorder is also known as the *LAMB* (*l*entigines, *a*trial myxomas, *m*ucocutaneous myxomas, and *b*lue nevi) *syndrome* or *NAME* (*n*evi, *a*trial myxoma, *m*yxoid neurofibroma, and *e*phelides [freckles]) *syndrome*. These patients can also have evidence of endocrine overactivity in the form of Cushing's syndrome (pigmented nodular adrenocortical disease) and acromegaly.

The third type of localized hyperpigmentation is due to a local increase in pigment production, and it includes *ephelides* and *café au lait macules* (CALMs). While a single CALM can be seen in up to 10% of the normal population, the presence of multiple or large-sized CALMs raises the possibility of an associated genodermatosis, for example, neurofibromatosis (NF) or McCune-Albright syndrome. *CALMs* are flat, uniformly brown in color (usually two shades darker than uninvolved skin), and can vary in size from 0.5 to 12+ cm. More than 90% of adult patients with *type I NF* will have six or more CALMs measuring ≥1.5 cm in diameter. Additional findings are discussed in the section on neurofibromas (see "Papulonodular Skin Lesions," below). In comparison with NF, the CALMs in patients with *McCune-Albright syndrome* (polyostotic fibrous dysplasia with precocious puberty in females due to mosaicism for an activating mutation

TABLE 58-11 Causes of Hyperpigmentation

- I. Primary cutaneous disorders
  - A. Localized
    - 1. Epidermal alteration
      - a. Seborrheic keratosis
      - b. Pigmented actinic keratosis
    - 2. Proliferation of melanocytes
      - a. Lentigo
      - b. Melanocytic nevus (mole)
      - c. Melanoma
    - 3. Increased pigment production
      - a. Ephelide (freckle)
      - b. Café au lait macule
      - c. Postinflammatory hyperpigmentation (also dermal)
      - d. Melasma (also dermal)
    - 4. Dermal pigmentation
      - a. Fixed drug eruption
  - B. Localized and diffuse
    - 1. Drugs (e.g., minocycline, hydroxychloroquine, bleomycin)
- II. Systemic diseases
  - A. Localized
    - 1. Epidermal alteration
      - a. Acanthosis nigricans (insulin resistance > other endocrine disorders, paraneoplastic)
      - b. Seborrheic keratoses (sign of Leser-Trélat)
    - 2. Proliferation of melanocytes
      - a. Lentigines (Peutz-Jeghers and LEOPARD/Noonan with multiple lentigines syndromes; xeroderma pigmentosum)
      - b. Melanocytic nevi (Carney complex [LAMB and NAME syndromes])[a]
    - 3. Increased pigment production
      - a. Café au lait macules (neurofibromatosis, Legius syndrome, McCune-Albright syndrome[b])
      - b. Urticaria pigmentosa[c]
    - 4. Dermal pigmentation
      - a. Incontinentia pigmenti (stage III)
      - b. Dyskeratosis congenita
    - 5. Dermal deposits
      - a. Exogenous ochronosis
      - b. Localized argyria
  - B. Diffuse
    - 1. Endocrinopathies
      - a. Addison's disease
      - b. Nelson syndrome
      - c. Ectopic ACTH syndrome
      - d. Hyperthyroidism
    - 2. Metabolic
      - a. Porphyria cutanea tarda
      - b. Hemochromatosis
      - c. Vitamin B_{12}, folate deficiency
      - d. Pellagra
      - e. Malabsorption, including Whipple's disease
    - 3. Melanosis secondary to metastatic melanoma
    - 4. Autoimmune
      - a. Primary biliary cholangitis
      - b. Systemic sclerosis (scleroderma)
      - c. POEMS syndrome
      - d. Eosinophilia-myalgia syndrome[d]
    - 5. Drugs (e.g., cyclophosphamide) and metals (e.g., silver)

[a]Also lentigines. [b]Polyostotic fibrous dysplasia. [c]See also "Papulonodular Skin Lesions." [d]Late 1980s.

Abbreviations: LAMB, *l*entigines, *a*trial *m*yxomas, *m*ucocutaneous myxomas, and *b*lue nevi; LEOPARD, *l*entigines, *E*CG abnormalities, *o*cular hypertelorism, *p*ulmonary stenosis and subaortic valvular stenosis, *a*bnormal genitalia, *r*etardation of growth, and *d*eafness (sensorineural); NAME, *n*evi, *a*trial myxoma, *m*yxoid neurofibroma, and *e*phelides (freckles); POEMS, *p*olyneuropathy, *o*rganomegaly, *e*ndocrinopathies, *M*-protein, and *s*kin changes.

in a G protein [$G_s\alpha$] gene) are usually larger, are more irregular in outline, and tend to respect the midline.

In incontinentia pigmenti, dyskeratosis congenita, and bleomycin pigmentation, the areas of localized hyperpigmentation form a pattern—swirls and streaks in the first, reticulated in the second, and flagellate in the third. In *dyskeratosis congenita*, atrophic reticulated hyperpigmentation is seen on the neck, trunk, and thighs and is accompanied by nail dystrophy, pancytopenia, and leukoplakia of the oral and anal mucosae. The latter often develops into squamous cell carcinoma. In addition to the flagellate pigmentation (linear streaks) on the trunk, patients receiving bleomycin often have hyperpigmentation overlying the elbows, knees, and small joints of the hand.

Localized hyperpigmentation is seen as a side effect of several other *systemic medications*, including those that produce fixed drug reactions (nonsteroidal anti-inflammatory drugs [NSAIDs], sulfonamides, barbiturates, and tetracyclines) and those that can complex with melanin or iron (antimalarials and minocycline). Fixed drug eruptions recur in the exact same location as circular areas of erythema that can become bullous and then resolve as brown macules. The eruption usually appears within hours of readministration of the offending agent, and common locations include the genitalia, distal extremities, and perioral region. Chloroquine and hydroxychloroquine produce gray-brown to blue-black discoloration of the shins, hard palate, and face, while blue macules (often misdiagnosed as bruises) can be seen on the lower extremities and in sites of inflammation with prolonged minocycline administration. Estrogen in oral contraceptives can induce melasma—symmetric brown patches on the face, especially the cheeks, upper lip, and forehead. Similar changes are seen in pregnancy and in patients receiving phenytoin.

In the diffuse forms of hyperpigmentation, the darkening of the skin may be of equal intensity over the entire body or may be accentuated in sun-exposed areas. The causes of diffuse hyperpigmentation can be divided into four major groups—endocrine, metabolic, autoimmune, and drugs. The endocrinopathies that frequently have associated hyperpigmentation include *Addison's disease, Nelson's syndrome,* and *ectopic adrenocorticotropic hormone (ACTH) syndrome*. In these diseases, the increased pigmentation is diffuse but is accentuated in sun-exposed areas, as well as in the palmar creases, sites of friction, and scars. An overproduction of the pituitary hormones α-MSH (melanocyte-stimulating hormone) and ACTH can lead to an increase in melanocyte activity. These peptides are products of the proopiomelanocortin gene and exhibit homology, for example, α-MSH and ACTH share 13 amino acids. A minority of patients with Cushing's disease or hyperthyroidism have generalized hyperpigmentation.

The metabolic causes of hyperpigmentation include *porphyria cutanea tarda* (PCT), *hemochromatosis, vitamin* B_{12} *deficiency, folic acid deficiency, pellagra,* and *malabsorption,* including *Whipple's disease*. In patients with PCT (see "Vesicles/Bullae," below), the skin darkening is seen in sun-exposed areas and is a reflection of the photoreactive properties of porphyrins. The increased level of iron in the skin of patients with type 1 hemochromatosis stimulates melanin pigment production and leads to the classic bronze color. Patients with pellagra have a brown discoloration of the skin, especially in sun-exposed areas, as a result of nicotinic acid (niacin) deficiency. In the areas of increased pigmentation, there is a thin, varnish-like scale. These changes are also seen in patients who are vitamin B_6 deficient, have functioning carcinoid tumors (increased consumption of niacin), or take isoniazid. Approximately 50% of the patients with Whipple's disease have an associated generalized hyperpigmentation in association with diarrhea, weight loss, arthritis, and lymphadenopathy. A diffuse, slate-blue to gray-brown color is seen in patients with *melanosis secondary to metastatic melanoma*. The color reflects widespread deposition of melanin within the dermis as a result of the high concentration of circulating melanin precursors.

Of the autoimmune diseases associated with diffuse hyperpigmentation, *primary biliary cholangitis* and *systemic sclerosis* are the most common, and occasionally, both disorders are seen in the same patient. The skin is dark brown in color, especially in sun-exposed areas. In primary biliary cholangitis, the hyperpigmentation is accompanied by pruritus, jaundice, and xanthomas, whereas in systemic sclerosis, it is accompanied by sclerosis of the extremities, face, and, less commonly, the trunk. Additional clues to the diagnosis of systemic sclerosis are mat and cuticular telangiectasias, calcinosis cutis, Raynaud's phenomenon, and distal ulcerations (see "Telangiectasias," above). The differential diagnosis of cutaneous sclerosis with hyperpigmentation includes POEMS (*p*olyneuropathy; *o*rganomegaly [liver, spleen, lymph nodes]; *e*ndocrinopathies [impotence, gynecomastia]; *M*-protein; and *s*kin changes) syndrome. The skin changes include hyperpigmentation, induration, hypertrichosis, angiomas, clubbing, and facial lipoatrophy.

Diffuse hyperpigmentation that is due to drugs or metals can result from one of several mechanisms—induction of melanin pigment formation, complexing of the drug or its metabolites to melanin, and deposits of the drug in the dermis. Busulfan, cyclophosphamide, 5-fluorouracil, and inorganic arsenic induce pigment production. Complexes containing melanin or iron plus the drug or its metabolites are seen in patients receiving minocycline, and a diffuse, brown-gray, muddy appearance within sun-exposed areas may develop, in addition to pigmentation of the mucous membranes, teeth, nails, bones, and thyroid. Administration of amiodarone can result in both a phototoxic eruption (exaggerated sunburn) and/or a slate-gray to violaceous discoloration of sun-exposed skin. Biopsy specimens of the latter show yellow-brown granules in dermal macrophages, which represent intralysosomal accumulations of lipids, amiodarone, and its metabolites. Actual deposits of a particular drug or metal in the skin are seen with silver (argyria), where the skin appears blue-gray in color; gold (chrysiasis), where the skin has a brown to blue-gray color; and clofazimine, where the skin appears reddish brown. The associated pigmentation is accentuated in sun-exposed areas, and discoloration of the eye is seen with gold (sclerae) and clofazimine (conjunctivae).

VESICLES/BULLAE

(**Table 58-12**) Depending on their size, cutaneous blisters are referred to as *vesicles* (<1 cm) or *bullae* (>1 cm). The primary autoimmune blistering disorders include *pemphigus vulgaris, pemphigus foliaceus, paraneoplastic pemphigus, bullous pemphigoid, gestational pemphigoid, cicatricial pemphigoid, epidermolysis bullosa acquisita, linear IgA bullous dermatosis* (*LABD*), and *dermatitis herpetiformis* (**Chap. 59**).

Vesicles and bullae are also seen in *contact dermatitis*, both allergic and irritant forms (**Chap. 57**). When there is a linear arrangement of vesicular lesions, an exogenous cause or herpes zoster should be suspected. Bullous disease secondary to the ingestion of drugs can take one of several forms, including phototoxic eruptions, isolated bullae, Stevens-Johnson syndrome (SJS), and toxic epidermal necrolysis (TEN) (**Chap. 60**). Clinically, phototoxic eruptions resemble an exaggerated sunburn with diffuse erythema and bullae in sun-exposed areas. The most commonly associated drugs are doxycycline, quinolones, voriconazole, thiazides, NSAIDs, vemurafenib, and psoralens. The development of a phototoxic eruption is dependent on the doses of both the drug and ultraviolet (UV)-A irradiation.

Toxic epidermal necrolysis is characterized by bullae that arise on widespread areas of tender erythema and then slough. This results in large areas of denuded skin. The associated morbidity, such as sepsis, and mortality rates are relatively high and are a function of the extent of epidermal necrosis. In addition, these patients may also have involvement of the mucous membranes and respiratory and intestinal tracts. Drugs are the primary cause of TEN, and the most common offenders are aromatic anticonvulsants (phenytoin, barbiturates, carbamazepine), sulfonamides, aminopenicillins, allopurinol, and NSAIDs. Generalized bullous fixed drug eruption, severe acute graft-versus-host disease (grade 4), vancomycin-induced LABD, and flares of cutaneous lupus can also resemble TEN.

In *erythema multiforme* (EM), the primary lesions are pink-red macules and edematous papules, the centers of which may become vesicular. In contrast to a morbilliform exanthem, the clue to the diagnosis of EM, and especially SJS, is the development of a "dusky" violet color in the center of the lesions. Target lesions are also characteristic of EM and arise as a result of active centers and borders in combination

TABLE 58-12 Causes of Vesicles/Bullae

I. Primary mucocutaneous diseases
  A. Primary blistering diseases (autoimmune)
    1. Pemphigus, foliaceus and vulgaris[a]
    2. Bullous pemphigoid[b]
    3. Gestational pemphigoid[b]
    4. Cicatricial pemphigoid[b]
    5. Dermatitis herpetiformis[b,c]
    6. Linear IgA bullous dermatosis[b]
    7. Epidermolysis bullosa acquisita[b,d]
  B. Secondary blistering diseases
    1. Contact dermatitis[a,b]
    2. Erythema multiforme[e]
    3. Stevens-Johnson syndrome[e]
    4. Toxic epidermal necrolysis[e]
    5. Bullous fixed drug eruption, including generalized variant[e]
    6. Pseudoporphyria, drug- or tanning booth–induced
  C. Infections
    1. Varicella-zoster virus[a,f]
    2. Herpes simplex virus[a,f]
    3. Enteroviruses, e.g., hand-foot-and-mouth disease[f]
    4. SARS-CoV-2
    5. Staphylococcal scalded-skin syndrome[a,g]
    6. Bullous impetigo[a]
    7. Bullous tinea
II. Systemic diseases
  A. Autoimmune
    1. Paraneoplastic pemphigus[a] (bronchiolitis obliterans)
  B. Infections
    1. Cutaneous emboli[b]
  C. Metabolic
    1. Diabetic bullae[a,b]
    2. Porphyria cutanea tarda[b]
    3. Porphyria variegata[b]
    4. Bullous dermatosis of hemodialysis[b] (less often associated with peritoneal dialysis and also referred to as pseudoporphyria)
  D. Ischemia
    1. Coma bullae
  E. Secondary blistering diseases
    1. Toxic epidermal necrolysis[e] (respiratory and gastrointestinal tracts can be involved)

[a]Intraepidermal. [b]Subepidermal. [c]Associated with gluten enteropathy. [d]Associated with inflammatory bowel disease. [e]Degeneration of cells within the basal layer of the epidermis can give impression split is subepidermal. [f]Also systemic. [g]In adults, associated with renal failure and immunocompromised state.

with centrifugal spread. However, target lesions need not be present to make the diagnosis of EM.

EM has been subdivided into two major groups: (1) EM minor due to herpes simplex virus (HSV); and (2) EM major due to HSV, *Mycoplasma pneumonia*, or, occasionally, other viruses, *Chlamydia*, or drugs. Involvement of the mucous membranes (ocular, nasal, oral, and genital) is seen more commonly in the latter form, and in patients with *Mycoplasma pneumoniae*-induced rash and mucositis (MIRM), there may be minimal cutaneous involvement. Hemorrhagic crusts of the lips are characteristic of EM major and SJS as well as herpes simplex, pemphigus vulgaris, and paraneoplastic pemphigus. Fever, malaise, myalgias, sore throat, and cough may precede or accompany the eruption. The lesions of EM usually resolve over 2–4 weeks but may be recurrent, especially when due to HSV. In addition to HSV (in which lesions usually appear 7–12 days after the viral eruption), EM can also follow vaccinations, radiation therapy, and exposure to environmental toxins, including the oleoresin in poison ivy.

Induction of SJS is most often due to drugs, especially sulfonamides, aromatic anticonvulsants, lamotrigine, aminopenicillins, and nonnucleoside reverse transcriptase inhibitors (e.g., nevirapine). Widespread dusky macules and significant mucosal involvement are characteristic of SJS, and the cutaneous lesions may or may not develop epidermal detachment. If the latter occurs, by definition, it is limited to <10% of the body surface area (BSA). Greater involvement leads to the diagnosis of SJS/TEN overlap (10–30% BSA) or TEN (>30% BSA).

In addition to primary blistering disorders and hypersensitivity reactions, bacterial and viral infections can lead to vesicles and bullae. The most common infectious agents are HSV **(Chap. 192)**, varicella-zoster virus **(Chap. 193)**, and *S. aureus* **(Chap. 147)**.

Staphylococcal scalded-skin syndrome (SSSS) and *bullous impetigo* are two blistering disorders associated with staphylococcal (phage group II) infection. In SSSS, the initial findings are redness and tenderness of the central face, neck, trunk, and intertriginous zones. This is followed by short-lived flaccid bullae and a slough or exfoliation of the superficial epidermis. Crusted areas then develop, characteristically around the mouth in a radial pattern. SSSS is distinguished from TEN by the following features: younger age group (primarily infants and toddlers), more superficial site of blister formation, no oral lesions, shorter course, lower morbidity and mortality rates, and an association with staphylococcal exfoliative toxin ("exfoliatin"), not drugs. A rapid diagnosis of SSSS versus TEN can be made by a frozen section of the blister roof or exfoliative cytology of the blister contents. In SSSS, the site of staphylococcal infection is usually extracutaneous (conjunctivitis, rhinorrhea, otitis media, pharyngitis, tonsillitis), and the cutaneous lesions are sterile, whereas in bullous impetigo, the skin lesions are the site of infection. Impetigo is more localized than SSSS and usually presents with honey-colored crusts. Occasionally, superficial purulent blisters also form. *Cutaneous emboli* from gram-negative infections may present as isolated bullae, but the base of the lesion is purpuric or necrotic, and it may develop into an ulcer (see "Purpura," below).

Several metabolic disorders are associated with blister formation, including diabetes mellitus, renal failure, and porphyria. Local hypoxemia secondary to decreased cutaneous blood flow can also produce blisters, which explains the presence of bullae over pressure points in comatose patients (coma bullae). In *diabetes mellitus*, tense bullae with clear sterile viscous fluid arise on normal skin. The lesions can be as large as 6 cm in diameter and are located on the distal extremities. There are several types of porphyria, but the most common form with cutaneous findings is *porphyria cutanea tarda* (PCT). In sun-exposed areas (primarily the hands), the skin is very fragile, with trauma leading to erosions mixed with tense vesicles. These lesions then heal with scarring and formation of milia; the latter are firm, 1- to 2-mm white or yellow papules that represent epidermoid cysts. Associated findings can include hypertrichosis of the lateral malar region (men) or face (women) and, in sun-exposed areas, hyperpigmentation and firm sclerotic plaques. An elevated level of urinary uroporphyrins confirms the diagnosis and is due to a decrease in uroporphyrinogen decarboxylase activity. PCT can be exacerbated by alcohol, hemochromatosis and other forms of iron overload, chlorinated hydrocarbons, hepatitis C virus and HIV infections, and hepatomas.

The differential diagnosis of PCT includes (1) *porphyria variegata*—the skin signs of PCT plus the systemic findings of acute intermittent porphyria; it has a diagnostic plasma porphyrin fluorescence emission at 626 nm; (2) *drug-induced pseudoporphyria*—the clinical and histologic findings are similar to PCT, but porphyrins are normal; etiologic agents include naproxen and other NSAIDs, furosemide, tetracycline, and voriconazole; (3) *bullous dermatosis of hemodialysis*—the same appearance as PCT, but porphyrins are usually normal or occasionally borderline elevated; patients have chronic renal failure and are on hemodialysis; (4) *PCT associated with hepatomas and hemodialysis;* and (5) *epidermolysis bullosa acquisita* **(Chap. 59)**.

EXANTHEMS

(Table 58-13) Exanthems are characterized by an acute generalized eruption. The most common presentation is erythematous macules and papules (morbilliform) and less often confluent blanching erythema (scarlatiniform). *Morbilliform* eruptions are usually due to either drugs or viral infections. For example, up to 5% of patients receiving penicillins,

TABLE 58-13 Causes of Exanthems

I. Morbilliform
- A. Drugs
- B. Viral
  1. Rubeola (measles)
  2. Rubella
  3. Erythema infectiosum (erythema of cheeks; reticulated on extremities)
  4. Epstein-Barr virus, echovirus, coxsackievirus, CMV, adenovirus, HHV-6/HHV-7[a], dengue, Zika, chikungunya, SARS-CoV-2, and West Nile virus infections
  5. HIV seroconversion exanthem (plus mucosal ulcerations)
- C. Bacterial
  1. Typhoid fever
  2. Early secondary syphilis
  3. Early *Rickettsia* infections
  4. Early meningococcemia
  5. Ehrlichiosis
- D. Acute graft-versus-host disease
- E. Kawasaki disease

II. Scarlatiniform
- A. Scarlet fever
- B. Toxic shock syndrome
- C. Kawasaki disease
- D. Early staphylococcal scalded-skin syndrome

[a]Primary infection in infants and reactivation in the setting of immunosuppression.
Abbreviations: CMV, cytomegalovirus; HHV, human herpesvirus; HIV, human immunodeficiency virus.

sulfonamides, phenytoin, or nevirapine will develop a maculopapular eruption. Accompanying signs may include pruritus, fever, eosinophilia, transaminitis, and transient lymphadenopathy **(Chap. 60)**. Similar maculopapular eruptions are seen in the classic childhood viral exanthems, including (1) *rubeola* (measles)—a prodrome of coryza, cough, and conjunctivitis followed by Koplik's spots on the buccal mucosa; the eruption begins behind the ears, at the hairline, and on the forehead and then spreads down the body, often becoming confluent; (2) *rubella*—the eruption begins on the forehead and face and then spreads down the body; it resolves in the same order and is associated with retroauricular and suboccipital lymphadenopathy; and (3) *erythema infectiosum* (fifth disease)—erythema of the cheeks is followed by a reticulated pattern on the extremities; it is secondary to a parvovirus B19 infection, and an associated arthritis is seen in adults.

Both measles and rubella can occur in unvaccinated adults, and an atypical form of measles is seen in adults immunized with either killed measles vaccine or killed vaccine followed in time by live vaccine. In contrast to classic measles, the eruption of atypical measles begins on the palms, soles, wrists, and ankles, and the lesions may become purpuric. The patient with atypical measles can have pulmonary involvement and be quite ill. Rubelliform and roseoliform eruptions are also associated with *Epstein-Barr virus* (5–15% of patients), *echovirus, coxsackievirus, cytomegalovirus, adenovirus*, SARS-CoV-2, and *dengue, chikungunya*, and *West Nile virus* infections. Detection of specific IgM antibodies or fourfold elevations in IgG antibodies often allows the proper diagnosis, but polymerase chain reaction (PCR) is gradually replacing serologic assays. Occasionally, a maculopapular drug eruption is a reflection of an underlying viral infection. For example, ~95% of the patients with infectious mononucleosis who are given ampicillin will develop a rash.

Of note, early in the course of infections with *Rickettsia* and meningococcus, prior to the development of petechiae and purpura, the lesions may be erythematous macules and papules. This is also the case in chickenpox prior to the development of vesicles. Maculopapular eruptions are associated with early *HIV infection*, early secondary *syphilis, typhoid fever*, and *acute graft-versus-host disease*. In the last, lesions frequently begin on the dorsal hands and forearms; the macular rose spots of typhoid fever involve primarily the anterior trunk.

The prototypic *scarlatiniform* eruption is seen in *scarlet fever* and is due to an erythrogenic toxin produced by bacteriophage-containing group A β-hemolytic streptococci, most commonly in the setting of pharyngitis. This eruption is characterized by diffuse erythema, which begins on the neck and upper trunk, and red follicular puncta. Additional findings include a white strawberry tongue (white coating with red papillae) followed by a red strawberry tongue (red tongue with red papillae); petechiae of the palate; a facial flush with circumoral pallor; linear petechiae in the antecubital fossae; and desquamation of the involved skin, palms, and soles 5–20 days after onset of the eruption. A similar desquamation of the palms and soles is seen in toxic shock syndrome (TSS), in Kawasaki disease, and after severe febrile illnesses. Certain strains of staphylococci also produce an erythrotoxin that leads to the same clinical findings as in streptococcal scarlet fever, except that the anti-streptolysin O or DNase B titers are not elevated.

In *toxic shock syndrome*, staphylococcal (phage group I) infections produce an exotoxin (TSST-1) that causes the fever and rash as well as enterotoxins. Initially, the majority of cases were reported in menstruating women who were using tampons. However, other sites of infection, including wounds and nasal packing, can lead to TSS. The diagnosis of TSS is based on clinical criteria **(Chap. 147)**, and three of these involve mucocutaneous sites (diffuse erythema of the skin, desquamation of the palms and soles 1–2 weeks after onset of illness, and involvement of the mucous membranes). The latter is characterized as hyperemia of the vagina, oropharynx, or conjunctivae. Similar systemic findings have been described in *streptococcal toxic shock syndrome* **(Chap. 148)**, and although an exanthem is seen less often than in TSS due to a staphylococcal infection, the underlying infection is often in the soft tissue (e.g., cellulitis).

The cutaneous eruption in *Kawasaki disease* **(Chap. 363)** is polymorphous, but the two most common forms are morbilliform and scarlatiniform. Additional mucocutaneous findings include bilateral conjunctival injection; erythema and edema of the hands and feet followed by desquamation; and diffuse erythema of the oropharynx, red strawberry tongue, and dry fissured lips. This clinical picture can resemble TSS and scarlet fever, but clues to the diagnosis of Kawasaki disease are cervical lymphadenopathy, cheilitis, and thrombocytosis. The most serious associated systemic finding in this disease is coronary aneurysms secondary to arteritis. Seen primarily in children, SARS-CoV-2-associated multisystem inflammatory syndrome must be distinguished from Kawasaki disease. Scarlatiniform eruptions are also seen in the early phase of SSSS (see "Vesicles/Bullae," above), in young adults with *Arcanobacterium haemolyticum* infection, and as reactions to drugs.

URTICARIA

(Table 58-14) *Urticaria* (hives) are transient lesions that are composed of a central wheal surrounded by an erythematous halo or flare. Individual lesions are round, oval, or figurate and are often pruritic. Acute and chronic urticarias have a wide variety of allergic etiologies

TABLE 58-14 Causes of Urticaria and Angioedema

I. Primary cutaneous disorders
- A. Acute and chronic urticaria[a]
- B. Physical urticaria
  1. Dermographism
  2. Solar urticaria[b]
  3. Cold urticaria[b]
  4. Cholinergic urticaria[b]
- C. Angioedema (hereditary and acquired)[b,c]

II. Systemic diseases
- A. Urticarial vasculitis
- B. Hepatitis B or C viral infection, SARS-CoV-2 infection
- C. Serum sickness
- D. Angioedema (hereditary and acquired)

[a]A small minority develop anaphylaxis. [b]Also systemic. [c]Acquired angioedema can be idiopathic, associated with a lymphoproliferative disorder, or due to a drug, e.g., angiotensin-converting enzyme (ACE) inhibitors.

and reflect edema in the dermis. Urticarial lesions can also be seen in patients with mastocytosis (urticaria pigmentosa), hypo- or hyperthyroidism, Schnitzler's syndrome, and systemic-onset juvenile idiopathic arthritis (Still's disease). In both juvenile- and adult-onset Still's disease, the lesions coincide with the fever spike, are transient, and are due to dermal infiltrates of neutrophils; the latter is also referred to as neutrophilic urticarial dermatosis.

The common *physical urticarias* include dermographism, solar urticaria, cold urticaria, and cholinergic urticaria. Patients with *dermographism* exhibit linear wheals following minor pressure or scratching of the skin and may be a contributing factor to pruritic dermatoses. It is a common disorder, affecting ~5% of the population. *Solar urticaria* characteristically occurs within minutes of sun exposure and is a skin sign of one systemic disease—erythropoietic protoporphyria. In addition to the urticaria, these patients have subtle pitted scarring of the nose and hands. *Cold urticaria* is precipitated by exposure to the cold, and therefore, exposed areas are usually affected. In occasional patients, the disease is associated with abnormal circulating proteins—more commonly cryoglobulins and less commonly cryofibrinogens. Additional systemic symptoms include wheezing and syncope, thus explaining the need for these patients to avoid swimming in cold water. Autosomal dominantly inherited cold urticaria is associated with dysfunction of cryopyrin. *Cholinergic urticaria* is precipitated by heat, exercise, or emotion and is characterized by small wheals with relatively large flares. It is occasionally associated with wheezing.

Whereas urticarias are the result of dermal edema, subcutaneous edema leads to the clinical picture of *angioedema*. Sites of involvement include the eyelids, lips, tongue, larynx, and gastrointestinal tract as well as the subcutaneous tissue. Angioedema occurs alone or in combination with urticaria, including urticarial vasculitis and the physical urticarias. Both acquired and hereditary (autosomal dominant) forms of angioedema occur **(Chap. 354)**, and in the latter, urticaria is rarely, if ever, seen.

Urticarial vasculitis is an immune complex disease that may be confused with simple urticaria. In contrast to simple urticaria, individual lesions tend to last longer than 24 h and usually develop central petechiae that can be observed even after the urticarial phase has resolved. The patient may also complain of burning rather than pruritus. On biopsy, there is a leukocytoclastic vasculitis of the small dermal blood vessels. Although urticarial vasculitis may be idiopathic in origin, it can be a reflection of an underlying systemic illness such as lupus erythematosus, Sjögren's syndrome, or hereditary complement deficiency. There is a spectrum of urticarial vasculitis that ranges from purely cutaneous to multisystem involvement. The most common systemic signs and symptoms are arthralgias and/or arthritis, nephritis, and crampy abdominal pain, with asthma and chronic obstructive lung disease seen less often. Hypocomplementemia occurs in one- to two-thirds of patients, even in the idiopathic cases. Urticarial vasculitis can also be seen in patients with *hepatitis B* and *hepatitis C* infections and *serum sickness*, but is usually not seen in *serum sickness–like illnesses* (e.g., due to cefaclor, minocycline).

PAPULONODULAR SKIN LESIONS

(Table 58-15) In the *papulonodular diseases*, the lesions are elevated above the surface of the skin and may coalesce to form larger plaques. The location, consistency, and color of the lesions are the keys to their diagnosis; this section is organized on the basis of color.

■ WHITE LESIONS

In *calcinosis cutis*, there are firm white to white-yellow papules with an irregular surface. When the contents are expressed, a chalky white material is seen. *Dystrophic calcification* is seen at sites of previous inflammation or damage to the skin. It develops in acne scars as well as on the distal extremities of patients with systemic sclerosis and in the subcutaneous tissue and intermuscular fascial planes in DM. The latter is more extensive and is more commonly seen in children. An elevated calcium phosphate product, most commonly due to secondary hyperparathyroidism in the setting of renal failure, can lead to nodules of *metastatic calcinosis cutis*, which tend to be subcutaneous and

TABLE 58-15 Papulonodular Skin Lesions According to Color Groups

I. White
  A. Calcinosis cutis
  B. Osteoma cutis (also skin-colored or blue)
II. Skin-colored
  A. Rheumatoid nodules
  B. Neurofibromas (von Recklinghausen's disease [NF1])
  C. Angiofibromas (tuberous sclerosis, MEN syndrome, type 1; also pink-red)
  D. Neuromas (MEN syndrome, type 2b)
  E. Adnexal tumors
    1. Basal cell carcinomas (basal cell nevus syndrome)
    2. Tricholemmomas (Cowden disease)
    3. Fibrofolliculomas (Birt-Hogg-Dubé syndrome)
  F. Osteomas (arise in skull and jaw in Gardner syndrome)
  G. Primary cutaneous disorders
    1. Epidermal inclusion cysts[a]
    2. Lipomas
III. Pink/translucent[b]
  A. Amyloidosis, primary systemic
  B. Papular mucinosis/scleromyxedema
  C. Multicentric reticulohistiocytosis
IV. Yellow
  A. Xanthomas
  B. Tophi
  C. Necrobiosis lipoidica
  D. Pseudoxanthoma elasticum
  E. Sebaceous adenomas (Muir-Torre syndrome)
V. Red[b]
  A. Papules
    1. Angiokeratomas (Fabry disease and related lysosomal storage diseases)[c]
    2. Bacillary angiomatosis (primarily in AIDS)
  B. Papules/plaques
    1. Cutaneous lupus erythematosus
    2. Lymphoma cutis
    3. Leukemia cutis
    4. Sweet syndrome
  C. Nodules
    1. Panniculitis
    2. Medium-sized vessel vasculitis (e.g., cutaneous polyarteritis nodosa)
  D. Primary cutaneous disorders
    1. Arthropod bites
    2. Cherry hemangiomas
    3. Infections, e.g., streptococcal cellulitis, sporotrichosis
    4. Polymorphous light eruption
    5. Cutaneous lymphoid hyperplasia (lymphocytoma cutis, pseudolymphoma)
VI. Red-brown[b]
  A. Sarcoidosis
  B. Urticaria pigmentosa
  C. Erythema elevatum diutinum (chronic leukocytoclastic vasculitis)
  D. Lupus vulgaris
VII. Blue[b]
  A. Venous malformations (e.g., blue rubber bleb syndrome)
  B. Primary cutaneous disorders
    1. Venous lake
    2. Blue nevus
VIII. Violaceous
  A. Lupus pernio (sarcoidosis)
  B. Lymphoma cutis
  C. Cutaneous lupus erythematosus
IX. Purple
  A. Kaposi's sarcoma, acral angiodermatitis (pseudo-Kaposi's sarcoma)
  B. Angiosarcoma
  C. Palpable purpura (see Table 58-16)
  D. Primary cutaneous disorders
    1. Angiokeratomas of the scrotum and vulva
X. Brown-black[d]
XI. Any color
  A. Metastases

[a]If multiple with childhood onset, consider Gardner syndrome. [b]May have darker hue in more darkly pigmented individuals. [c]More widespread, especially lower trunk and girdle region, and often red-purple in color. [d]See also "Hyperpigmentation."
Abbreviations: MEN, multiple endocrine neoplasia; NF1, neurofibromatosis type 1.

periarticular. These patients can also develop calcification of muscular arteries and subsequent ischemic necrosis (calciphylaxis). *Osteoma cutis*, in the form of small papules, most commonly occurs on the face of individuals with a history of acne vulgaris, whereas plate-like lesions occur in rare genetic syndromes.

SKIN-COLORED LESIONS

There are several types of skin-colored lesions, including epidermoid cysts, lipomas, rheumatoid nodules, neurofibromas, angiofibromas, neuromas, and adnexal tumors such as tricholemmomas. Both *epidermoid cysts* and *lipomas* are very common mobile subcutaneous nodules—the former are rubbery and drain cheeselike material (sebum and keratin) if incised. Lipomas are firm and somewhat lobulated on palpation. When extensive facial epidermoid cysts develop during childhood or there is a family history of such lesions, the patient should be examined for other signs of Gardner syndrome, including osteomas and desmoid tumors. *Rheumatoid nodules* are firm 0.5- to 4-cm nodules that favor the extensor aspect of joints, especially the elbows. They are seen in ~20% of patients with rheumatoid arthritis and 6% of patients with Still's disease. Biopsies of the nodules show palisading granulomas. Similar lesions that are smaller and shorter-lived are seen in rheumatic fever.

Neurofibromas (benign Schwann cell tumors) are soft papules or nodules that exhibit the "button-hole" sign; that is, they invaginate into the skin with pressure in a manner similar to a hernia. Single lesions are seen in normal individuals, but multiple neurofibromas, usually in combination with six or more CALMs measuring >1.5 cm (see "Hyperpigmentation," above), axillary freckling, and multiple Lisch nodules, are seen in von Recklinghausen's disease (NF type I) (**Chap. 90**). In some patients, the neurofibromas are localized and unilateral due to somatic mosaicism.

Angiofibromas are firm pink-red to skin-colored papules that measure from 3 mm to 1.5 cm in diameter. When multiple lesions are located on the central cheeks (adenoma sebaceum), the patient has tuberous sclerosis or multiple endocrine neoplasia (MEN) syndrome, type 1. The former is an autosomal disorder due to mutations in two different genes, and the associated findings are discussed in the section on ash leaf spots as well as in **Chap. 90**.

Neuromas (benign proliferations of nerve fibers) are also firm, skin-colored papules. They are more commonly found at sites of amputations and in rudimentary polydactyly. However, when there are multiple neuromas on the eyelids, lips, distal tongue, and/or oral mucosa, the patient should be investigated for other signs of MEN syndrome, type 2b. Associated findings include marfanoid habitus, protuberant lips, intestinal ganglioneuromas, and medullary thyroid carcinoma (>75% of patients; **Chap. 388**).

Adnexal tumors are derived from pluripotent cells of the epidermis that can differentiate toward hair, sebaceous, or apocrine or eccrine glands, or remain undifferentiated. *Basal cell carcinomas* (BCCs) are examples of adnexal tumors that have little or no evidence of differentiation. Clinically, they are translucent papules with rolled borders, telangiectasias, and central erosion. BCCs commonly arise in sun-damaged skin of the head and neck as well as the upper trunk. When a patient has multiple BCCs, especially prior to age 30, the possibility of the basal cell nevus syndrome should be raised. It is inherited as an autosomal dominant trait and is associated with jaw cysts, palmar and plantar pits, frontal bossing, medulloblastomas, and calcification of the falx cerebri and diaphragma sellae. *Tricholemmomas* are also skin-colored adnexal tumors but differentiate toward hair follicles and can have a wartlike appearance. The presence of multiple tricholemmomas on the face and cobblestoning of the oral mucosa points to the diagnosis of Cowden disease (multiple hamartoma syndrome) due to mutations in the phosphatase and tensin homolog (*PTEN*) gene. Internal organ involvement (in decreasing order of frequency) includes fibrocystic disease and carcinoma of the breast, adenomas and carcinomas of the thyroid, and gastrointestinal polyposis. Keratoses of the palms, soles, and dorsal aspect of the hands are also seen. *Fibrofolliculomas* are skin-colored to white, smooth papules that favor the face, ears, and neck and, when multiple, are associated with Birt-Hogg-Dubé syndrome, which is associated with renal lesions including cancer (**Chap. 85**).

PINK LESIONS

The cutaneous lesions associated with primary systemic *amyloidosis* are often pink to pink-orange in color and translucent. Common locations are the face, especially the periorbital and perioral regions, and flexural areas. On biopsy, homogeneous deposits of amyloid are seen in the dermis and in the walls of blood vessels; the latter lead to an increase in vessel wall fragility. As a result, petechiae and purpura develop in clinically normal skin as well as in lesional skin following minor trauma, hence the term *pinch purpura*. Amyloid deposits are also seen in the striated muscle of the tongue and result in macroglossia.

Even though specific mucocutaneous lesions are present in only ~30% of the patients with primary systemic (AL) amyloidosis, the diagnosis can be made via histologic examination of abdominal subcutaneous fat, in conjunction with a serum free light chain assay. By special staining, amyloid deposits are seen around blood vessels or individual fat cells in 40–50% of patients. There are also three forms of amyloidosis that are limited to the skin and that should not be construed as cutaneous lesions of systemic amyloidosis. They are macular amyloidosis (upper back), lichen amyloidosis (usually lower extremities), and nodular amyloidosis. In macular and lichen amyloidosis, the deposits are composed of altered epidermal keratin. Early-onset macular and lichen amyloidosis have been associated with MEN syndrome, type 2a.

Patients with *multicentric reticulohistiocytosis* also have pink-colored papules and nodules on the face and mucous membranes as well as on the extensor surface of the hands and forearms. They have a polyarthritis that can mimic rheumatoid arthritis clinically. On histologic examination, the papules have characteristic giant cells that are not seen in biopsies of rheumatoid nodules. Pink to skin-colored papules that are firm, 2–5 mm in diameter, and often in a linear arrangement are seen in patients with *papular mucinosis*. This disease is also referred to as *scleromyxedema*. The latter name comes from the induration of the face and extremities that may accompany the papular eruption. Biopsy specimens of the papules show localized mucin deposition, and serum protein electrophoresis plus immunofixation electrophoresis demonstrates a monoclonal spike of IgG, usually with a λ light chain.

YELLOW LESIONS

Several systemic disorders are characterized by yellow-colored cutaneous papules or plaques—hyperlipidemia (xanthomas), gout (tophi), diabetes (necrobiosis lipoidica), pseudoxanthoma elasticum, and Muir-Torre syndrome (sebaceous tumors). Eruptive xanthomas are the most common form of *xanthomas* and are associated with hypertriglyceridemia (primarily hyperlipoproteinemia types I, IV, and V). Crops of yellow papules with erythematous halos occur primarily on the extensor surfaces of the extremities and the buttocks, and they spontaneously involute with a fall in serum triglycerides. Types II and III result in one or more of the following types of xanthoma: xanthelasma, tendon xanthomas, and plane xanthomas. Xanthelasma are found on the eyelids, whereas tendon xanthomas are frequently associated with the Achilles and extensor finger tendons; plane xanthomas are flat and favor the palmar creases and flexural folds. Tuberous xanthomas are frequently associated with hypercholesterolemia; however, they are also seen in patients with hypertriglyceridemia and are found most frequently over the large joints or hand. Biopsy specimens of xanthomas show collections of lipid-containing macrophages (foam cells).

Patients with several disorders, including biliary cirrhosis, can have a secondary form of hyperlipidemia with associated tuberous and plane xanthomas. However, patients with plasma cell dyscrasias have *normolipemic plane xanthomas*. This latter form of xanthoma may be ≥12 cm in diameter and is most frequently seen on the neck, upper trunk, and flexural folds. It is important to note that the most common setting for eruptive xanthomas is uncontrolled diabetes mellitus. The least specific sign for hyperlipidemia is xanthelasma, because at least 50% of the patients with this finding have normal lipid profiles.

In *tophaceous gout*, there are deposits of monosodium urate in the skin around the joints, particularly those of the hands and feet. Additional sites of *tophi* formation include the helix of the ear and the olecranon and prepatellar bursae. The lesions are firm, yellow to yellow-white in color, and occasionally discharge a chalky material. Their size varies from 1 mm to 7 cm, and the diagnosis can be established by polarized light microscopy of the aspirated contents of a tophus. Lesions of *necrobiosis lipoidica* are found primarily on the shins (90%), and patients can have diabetes mellitus or develop it subsequently. Characteristic findings include a central yellow color, atrophy (transparency), telangiectasias, and a red to red-brown border. Ulcerations can also develop within the plaques. Biopsy specimens show necrobiosis of collagen and granulomatous inflammation.

In *pseudoxanthoma elasticum* (PXE), due to mutations in the gene *ABCC6*, there is an abnormal deposition of calcium on the elastic fibers of the skin, eye, and blood vessels. In the skin, the flexural areas such as the neck, axillae, antecubital fossae, and inguinal area are the primary sites of involvement. Yellow papules coalesce to form reticulated plaques that have an appearance similar to that of plucked chicken skin. In severely affected skin, hanging, redundant folds develop. Biopsy specimens of involved skin show swollen and irregularly clumped elastic fibers with deposits of calcium. In the eye, the calcium deposits in Bruch's membrane lead to angioid streaks and choroiditis; in the arteries of the heart, kidney, gastrointestinal tract, and extremities, the deposits lead to angina, hypertension, gastrointestinal bleeding, and claudication, respectively.

Adnexal tumors that have differentiated toward sebaceous glands include sebaceous adenoma, sebaceous carcinoma, and sebaceous hyperplasia. Except for sebaceous hyperplasia, which is commonly seen on the face, these tumors are fairly rare. Patients with Muir-Torre syndrome have one or more *sebaceous adenoma(s)*, and they can also have sebaceous carcinomas and sebaceous hyperplasia as well as keratoacanthomas. The internal manifestations of Muir-Torre syndrome include *multiple* carcinomas of the gastrointestinal tract (primarily colon) as well as cancers of the genitourinary tract.

■ RED LESIONS

Cutaneous lesions that are red in color have a wide variety of etiologies; in an attempt to simplify their identification, they will be subdivided into papules, papules/plaques, and subcutaneous nodules. Common red papules include *arthropod bites* and *cherry hemangiomas*; the latter are small, bright-red, dome-shaped papules that represent a benign proliferation of capillaries. In patients with AIDS (**Chap. 202**), the development of multiple red hemangioma-like lesions points to bacillary angiomatosis, and biopsy specimens show clusters of bacilli that stain positively with the Warthin-Starry stain; the pathogens have been identified as *Bartonella henselae* and *Bartonella quintana*. Disseminated visceral disease is seen primarily in immunocompromised hosts but can occur in immunocompetent individuals.

Multiple *angiokeratomas* are seen in Fabry disease, an X-linked recessive lysosomal storage disease that is due to a deficiency of α-galactosidase A. The lesions are red to red-purple in color and can be quite small in size (1–3 mm), with the most common location being the lower trunk. Associated findings include chronic renal disease, peripheral neuropathy, and corneal opacities (cornea verticillata). While electron photomicrographs demonstrate lamellar lipid deposits in dermal fibroblasts, pericytes, and endothelial cells, nowadays, genetic analysis is more frequently performed for diagnosis. Widespread acute eruptions of erythematous papules are discussed in the section on exanthems.

There are several infectious diseases that present as erythematous papules or nodules in a lymphocutaneous or sporotrichoid pattern, that is, in a linear arrangement along the lymphatic channels. The two most common etiologies are *Sporothrix schenckii* (sporotrichosis) and the atypical mycobacterium *Mycobacterium marinum*. The organisms are introduced as a result of trauma, and a primary inoculation site is often seen in addition to the lymphatic nodules. Additional causes include *Nocardia*, *Leishmania*, and other atypical mycobacteria and dimorphic fungi; culture or PCR of lesional tissue will aid in the diagnosis.

The diseases that are characterized by erythematous plaques with scale are reviewed in the papulosquamous section, and the various forms of dermatitis are discussed in the section on erythroderma. Additional disorders in the differential diagnosis of red papules/plaques include *cellulitis*, *polymorphous light eruption* (PMLE), *cutaneous lymphoid hyperplasia* (lymphocytoma cutis), *cutaneous lupus*, *lymphoma cutis*, and *leukemia cutis*. The first three diseases represent primary cutaneous disorders, although cellulitis may be accompanied by a bacteremia. PMLE is characterized by erythematous papules and plaques in a primarily sun-exposed distribution—dorsum of the hand, extensor forearm, and upper trunk. Lesions follow exposure to UV-B and/or UV-A, and in higher latitudes, PMLE is most severe in the late spring and early summer. A process referred to as "hardening" occurs with continued UV exposure, and the eruption fades, but in temperate climates, it recurs the next spring. PMLE must be differentiated from cutaneous lupus, and this is accomplished by observation of the natural history, histologic examination, and sometimes direct immunofluorescence of the lesions. Cutaneous lymphoid hyperplasia (pseudolymphoma) is a *benign* polyclonal proliferation of lymphocytes within the skin that presents as infiltrated pink-red to red-purple papules and plaques; it must be distinguished from lymphoma cutis.

Several types of red plaques are seen in patients with systemic *lupus*, including (1) erythematous urticarial plaques across the cheeks and nose in the classic butterfly rash; (2) erythematous discoid lesions with fine or "carpet-tack" scale, telangiectasias, central hypopigmentation, peripheral hyperpigmentation, follicular plugging, and atrophy located on the scalp, face, external ears, arms, and upper trunk; and (3) psoriasiform or annular lesions of subacute cutaneous lupus with hypopigmented centers located primarily on the extensor arms and upper trunk. Additional mucocutaneous findings include (1) a violaceous flush on the face and V of the neck; (2) photosensitivity; (3) urticarial vasculitis (see "Urticaria," above); (4) lupus panniculitis (see below); (5) diffuse alopecia; (6) alopecia secondary to discoid lesions; (7) nailfold telangiectasias and erythema; (8) EM- or TEN-like lesions that may become bullous; (9) oral or nasal ulcers; (10) livedo reticularis; and (11) distal ulcerations secondary to Raynaud's phenomenon, vasculitis, or livedoid vasculopathy. Patients with only discoid lesions usually have the form of lupus that is limited to the skin. However, up to 10–15% of these patients eventually develop systemic lupus. Direct immunofluorescence of involved skin, in particular discoid lesions, shows deposits of IgG or IgM and C3 in a granular distribution along the dermal-epidermal junction.

In *lymphoma cutis*, there is a clonal proliferation of malignant lymphocytes within the skin, and the clinical appearance resembles that of cutaneous lymphoid hyperplasia—infiltrated pink-red to red-purple papules and plaques. Lymphoma cutis can occur anywhere on the surface of the skin, whereas the sites of predilection for lymphocytomas include the malar ridge, tip of the nose, and earlobes. Patients with non-Hodgkin's lymphomas have specific cutaneous lesions more often than those with Hodgkin's lymphoma, and, occasionally, the skin nodules precede the development of extracutaneous non-Hodgkin's lymphoma or represent the only site of involvement (e.g., primary cutaneous B-cell lymphoma). Arcuate lesions are sometimes seen in lymphoma and lymphocytoma cutis as well as in CTCL. *Adult T-cell leukemia/lymphoma* that develops in association with HTLV-1 infection is characterized by cutaneous plaques, hypercalcemia, and circulating CD25+ lymphocytes. *Leukemia cutis* has the same appearance as lymphoma cutis, and specific lesions are seen more commonly in monocytic leukemias than in lymphocytic or granulocytic leukemias. Cutaneous chloromas (granulocytic sarcomas) may precede the appearance of circulating blasts in acute myelogenous leukemia and, as such, represent a form of aleukemic leukemia cutis.

Sweet syndrome is characterized by pink-red to red-brown edematous plaques that are frequently painful and occur primarily on the head, neck, and upper extremities. The patients also have fever, neutrophilia, and a dense dermal infiltrate of neutrophils in the lesions. In ~10% of the patients, there is an associated malignancy, most commonly acute myelogenous leukemia. Sweet syndrome has also been reported with inflammatory bowel disease, systemic lupus erythematosus, and solid tumors (primarily of the genitourinary tract) as well as drugs (e.g., granulocyte colony-stimulating factor [G-CSF], hypomethylating agents, all-*trans*-retinoic acid). The differential diagnosis includes neutrophilic eccrine hidradenitis; bullous forms of pyoderma gangrenosum; and, occasionally, cellulitis. Extracutaneous sites of involvement include joints, muscles, eyes, kidneys (proteinuria, occasionally glomerulonephritis), and lungs (neutrophilic infiltrates). The idiopathic form of Sweet syndrome is seen more often in women, following a respiratory tract infection.

Common causes of erythematous subcutaneous nodules include inflamed epidermoid cysts, acne cysts, and furuncles. *Panniculitis*, an inflammation of the fat, also presents as subcutaneous nodules and is frequently a sign of systemic disease. There are several forms of panniculitis, including erythema nodosum, erythema induratum/nodular vasculitis, lupus panniculitis, lipodermatosclerosis, α_1-antitrypsin deficiency, factitial, and fat necrosis secondary to pancreatic disease. Except for erythema nodosum, these lesions may break down and ulcerate or heal with a scar. The shin is the most common location for the nodules of erythema nodosum, whereas the calf is the most common location for lesions of erythema induratum. In erythema nodosum, the nodules are initially red but then develop a blue bruise-like color as they resolve. Patients with erythema nodosum but no underlying systemic illness can still have fever, malaise, leukocytosis, arthralgias, and/or arthritis. However, the possibility of an underlying illness should be excluded, and the most common associations are streptococcal infections, upper respiratory viral infections, sarcoidosis, and inflammatory bowel disease, in addition to drugs (oral contraceptives, sulfonamides, penicillins, bromides, iodides, BRAF inhibitors). Less common associations include bacterial gastroenteritis (*Yersinia*, *Salmonella*) and coccidioidomycosis followed by tuberculosis, histoplasmosis, brucellosis, and infections with *Chlamydia pneumoniae*, *Chlamydia trachomatis*, *Mycoplasma pneumoniae*, or hepatitis B virus.

Erythema induratum and nodular vasculitis have overlapping features clinically and histologically, and whether they represent two separate entities or the ends of a single disease spectrum is a point of debate; in general, the latter is usually idiopathic and the former is associated with the presence of *Mycobacterium tuberculosis* DNA by PCR within skin lesions. The lesions of lupus panniculitis are found primarily on the cheeks, upper arms, and buttocks (sites of abundant fat) and are seen in both the cutaneous and systemic forms of lupus. The overlying skin may be normal, erythematous, or have the changes of discoid lupus. The subcutaneous fat necrosis that is associated with pancreatic disease is presumably secondary to circulating lipases and is seen in patients with pancreatic carcinoma as well as in patients with acute and chronic pancreatitis. In this disorder, there may be an associated arthritis, fever, and inflammation of visceral fat. Histologic examination of deep incisional biopsy specimens will aid in the diagnosis of the particular type of panniculitis.

Subcutaneous erythematous nodules are also seen in cutaneous polyarteritis nodosa and as a manifestation of *systemic vasculitis* when there is involvement of medium-sized vessels, for example, systemic polyarteritis nodosa, eosinophilic granulomatosis with polyangiitis, or granulomatosis with polyangiitis (**Chap. 363**). Cutaneous polyarteritis nodosa presents with painful subcutaneous nodules and ulcers within a red-purple, netlike pattern of livedo reticularis. The latter is due to slowed blood flow through the superficial horizontal venous plexus. The majority of lesions are found on the lower extremities, and while arthralgias and myalgias may accompany cutaneous polyarteritis nodosa, there is no evidence of systemic involvement. In both the cutaneous and systemic forms of vasculitis, skin biopsy specimens of the associated nodules will show the changes characteristic of a necrotizing vasculitis and/or granulomatous inflammation.

RED-BROWN LESIONS

The cutaneous lesions in *sarcoidosis* (**Chap. 367**) are classically red to red-brown in color, and with diascopy (pressure with a glass slide), a yellow-brown residual color is observed that is secondary to the granulomatous infiltrate. The waxy papules and plaques may be found anywhere on the skin, but the face is the most common location. Usually there are no surface changes, but occasionally, the lesions will have scale. Biopsy specimens of the papules show "naked" granulomas in the dermis, that is, granulomas surrounded by a minimal number of lymphocytes. Other cutaneous findings in sarcoidosis include annular lesions with an atrophic or scaly center, papules within scars, hypopigmented papules and patches, subcutaneous plaques, alopecia, acquired ichthyosis, erythema nodosum, and lupus pernio (see below).

The differential diagnosis of sarcoidosis includes foreign-body granulomas produced by chemicals such as beryllium and zirconium, late secondary syphilis, and *lupus vulgaris*. Lupus vulgaris is a form of cutaneous tuberculosis that is seen in previously infected and sensitized individuals. There is often underlying active tuberculosis elsewhere, usually in the lungs or lymph nodes. Lesions occur primarily in the head and neck region and are red-brown plaques with a yellow-brown color on diascopy. Secondary scarring can develop within the central portion of the plaques. Cultures or PCR analysis of the lesions should be performed, along with an interferon γ release assay of peripheral blood, because it is rare for the acid-fast stain to show bacilli within the dermal granulomas.

A generalized distribution of red-brown macules and papules is seen in the form of mastocytosis known as *urticaria pigmentosa* (**Chap. 354**). Each lesion represents a collection of mast cells in the dermis, with hyperpigmentation of the overlying epidermis. Stimuli such as rubbing cause these mast cells to degranulate, and this leads to the formation of localized urticaria (Darier's sign). Additional symptoms can result from mast cell degranulation and include headache, flushing, diarrhea, and pruritus. Mast cells also infiltrate various organs such as the liver, spleen, and gastrointestinal tract, and accumulations of mast cells in the bones may produce either osteosclerotic or osteolytic lesions on radiographs. In the majority of these patients, however, the internal involvement remains indolent. A subtype of chronic cutaneous small-vessel vasculitis, *erythema elevatum diutinum* (EED), also presents with papules that are red-brown in color. The papules coalesce into plaques on the extensor surfaces of knees, elbows, and the small joints of the hand. Flares of EED have been associated with streptococcal infections.

BLUE LESIONS

Lesions that are blue in color are the result of vascular ectasias, hyperplasias, and tumors or melanin pigment within the dermis. *Venous lakes* (ectasias) are compressible dark-blue lesions that are found commonly in the head and neck region. *Venous malformations* are also compressible blue papulonodules and plaques that can occur anywhere on the body, including the oral mucosa. When there are multiple papulonodules rather than a single congenital lesion, the patient may have the blue rubber bleb syndrome or Maffucci's syndrome. Patients with the blue rubber bleb syndrome also have vascular anomalies of the gastrointestinal tract that may bleed, whereas patients with Maffucci's syndrome have associated osteochondromas. *Blue nevi* (moles) are seen when there are collections of pigment-producing nevus cells in the dermis. These benign papular lesions are dome-shaped and occur most commonly on the dorsum of the hand or foot or in the head and neck region.

VIOLACEOUS LESIONS

Violaceous papules and plaques are seen in *lupus pernio*, *lymphoma cutis*, and *cutaneous lupus*. Lupus pernio is a particular type of sarcoidosis that involves the tip and alar rim of the nose as well as the earlobes, with lesions that are violaceous in color rather than red-brown. This form of sarcoidosis is associated with involvement of the upper respiratory tract. The plaques of lymphoma cutis and cutaneous lupus may be red or violaceous in color and were discussed above.

PURPLE LESIONS

Purple-colored papules and plaques are seen in vascular tumors, such as *Kaposi's sarcoma* (**Chap. 202**) and *angiosarcoma*, and when there is extravasation of red blood cells into the skin in association with inflammation, as in *palpable purpura* (see "Purpura," below). Patients with congenital or acquired AV fistulas and venous hypertension can develop purple papules on the lower extremities that can resemble Kaposi's sarcoma clinically and histologically; this condition is referred to as pseudo-Kaposi's sarcoma (acral angiodermatitis). Angiosarcoma is found most commonly on the scalp and face of elderly patients or within areas of chronic lymphedema and presents as purple papules and plaques. In the head and neck region, the tumor often extends beyond the clinically defined borders and may be accompanied by facial edema.

■ BROWN AND BLACK LESIONS

Brown- and black-colored papules are reviewed in "Hyperpigmentation," above.

■ CUTANEOUS METASTASES

These are discussed last because they can have a wide range of colors. Most commonly, they present as either firm, skin-colored subcutaneous nodules or firm, red to red-brown papulonodules, whereas metastatic melanoma can be pink, blue, or black in color. Cutaneous metastases develop from hematogenous or lymphatic spread and are most often due to the following primary carcinomas: in men, melanoma, oropharynx, lung, and colon; and in women, breast, melanoma, and ovary. These metastatic lesions may be the initial presentation of the carcinoma, especially when the primary site is the lung.

TABLE 58-16 Causes of Purpura

- I. Primary cutaneous disorders
  - A. Nonpalpable
    - 1. Trauma
    - 2. Solar (actinic, senile) purpura
    - 3. Steroid purpura
    - 4. Stasis purpura due to venous hypertension
    - 5. Capillaritis
    - 6. Livedoid vasculopathy in the setting of venous hypertension[a]
- II. Drugs (e.g., antiplatelet agents, anticoagulants)
- III. Systemic diseases
  - A. Nonpalpable
    - 1. Clotting disturbances
      - a. Thrombocytopenia (including ITP)
      - b. Abnormal platelet function
      - c. Clotting factor defects
    - 2. Vascular fragility
      - a. Amyloidosis (within normal-appearing skin)
      - b. Ehlers-Danlos syndrome
      - c. Scurvy
    - 3. Thrombi
      - a. Disseminated intravascular coagulation, purpura fulminans
      - b. Warfarin (Coumadin)-induced necrosis
      - c. Heparin-induced thrombocytopenia and thrombosis
      - d. Antiphospholipid antibody syndrome
      - e. Monoclonal cryoglobulinemia
      - f. Vasculopathy induced by levamisole-adulterated cocaine[b]
      - g. SARS-CoV-2 infection
      - h. Thrombotic thrombocytopenic purpura
      - i. Thrombocytosis
      - j. Homozygous protein C or protein S deficiency
    - 4. Emboli
      - a. Cholesterol
      - b. Fat
    - 5. Possible immune complex
      - a. Gardner-Diamond syndrome (autoerythrocyte sensitivity)
      - b. Waldenström's hypergammaglobulinemic purpura
  - B. Palpable
    - 1. Vasculitis
      - a. Cutaneous small-vessel vasculitis, including in the setting of systemic vasculitides
    - 2. Emboli[c]
      - a. Acute meningococcemia
      - b. Disseminated gonococcal infection
      - c. Rocky Mountain spotted fever
      - d. Ecthyma gangrenosum

[a]Also associated with underlying disorders that lead to hypercoagulability/thrombophilia, e.g., factor V Leiden, protein C dysfunction/deficiency. [b]Combined vasculopathy/vasculitis can be seen. [c]Bacterial (including rickettsial), fungal, or parasitic.

Abbreviation: ITP, idiopathic thrombocytopenic purpura.

PURPURA

(Table 58-16) *Purpura* are seen when there is an extravasation of red blood cells into the dermis and, as a result, the lesions do not blanch with pressure. This is in contrast to those erythematous or violet-colored lesions that are due to localized vasodilatation—they do blanch with pressure. Purpura (≥3 mm) and petechiae (≤2 mm) are divided into two major groups: palpable and nonpalpable. The most frequent causes of *nonpalpable* purpura and petechiae are primary cutaneous disorders such as *trauma*, *solar* (*actinic*) *purpura*, *stasis purpura*, and *capillaritis*. Less common causes are *steroid purpura* and *livedoid vasculopathy* (see "Ulcers," below). Solar purpura are seen primarily on the extensor forearms, whereas steroid purpura secondary to potent topical glucocorticoids or endogenous or exogenous Cushing's syndrome can be more widespread. In both cases, there is alteration of the supporting connective tissue that surrounds the dermal blood vessels. In contrast, the petechiae that result from capillaritis are found primarily on the lower extremities. In capillaritis, there is an extravasation of erythrocytes as a result of perivascular lymphocytic inflammation. The petechiae are bright red, 1–2 mm in size, and scattered within yellow-brown patches. The yellow-brown color is caused by hemosiderin deposits within the dermis.

Systemic causes of nonpalpable purpura fall into several categories, and those secondary to clotting disturbances and vascular fragility will be discussed first. The former group includes *thrombocytopenia* **(Chap. 115)**, *abnormal platelet function* as is seen in uremia, and *clotting factor defects*. The initial site of presentation for thrombocytopenia-induced petechiae is the distal lower extremity. Capillary fragility leads to nonpalpable purpura in patients with systemic *amyloidosis* (see "Papulonodular Skin Lesions," above), disorders of collagen production such as *Ehlers-Danlos syndrome*, and *scurvy*. In scurvy, there are flattened corkscrew hairs with surrounding hemorrhage on the lower extremities, in addition to gingivitis. Vitamin C is a cofactor for lysyl hydroxylase, an enzyme involved in the posttranslational modification of procollagen that is necessary for cross-link formation.

In contrast to the previous group of disorders, the noninflammatory purpura seen in the following group of diseases are associated with thrombi formation within vessels and have a retiform configuration. It is important to note that these thrombi are demonstrable in skin biopsy specimens. This group of disorders includes disseminated intravascular coagulation (DIC), monoclonal cryoglobulinemia, thrombocytosis, thrombotic thrombocytopenic purpura, antiphospholipid antibody syndrome, and reactions to warfarin and heparin (heparin-induced thrombocytopenia and thrombosis). DIC is triggered by several types of infection (gram-negative, gram-positive, viral, and rickettsial) as well as by tissue injury and neoplasms. Widespread purpura and hemorrhagic infarcts of the distal extremities are seen. Similar lesions are found in purpura fulminans, which is a form of DIC associated with fever and hypotension that occurs more commonly in children following an infectious illness such as varicella, scarlet fever, or an upper respiratory tract infection. In both disorders, hemorrhagic bullae can develop in involved skin.

Monoclonal cryoglobulinemia is associated with plasma cell dyscrasias, chronic lymphocytic leukemia, and lymphoma. Purpura, primarily of the lower extremities, and hemorrhagic infarcts of the fingers, toes, nose and ears are seen in these patients. Exacerbations of disease activity can follow cold exposure or an increase in serum viscosity. Biopsy specimens show precipitates of the cryoglobulin within dermal vessels. Similar deposits have been found in the lung, brain, and renal glomeruli. Patients with *thrombotic thrombocytopenic purpura* can also have hemorrhagic infarcts as a result of intravascular thromboses.

Additional signs include microangiopathic hemolytic anemia and fluctuating neurologic abnormalities, especially headaches and confusion.

Administration of *warfarin* can result in painful areas of erythema that become purpuric and then necrotic with an adherent black eschar; the condition is also referred to as Coumadin-induced necrosis. This reaction is seen more often in women and in areas with abundant subcutaneous fat—breasts, abdomen, buttocks, thighs, and calves. The erythema and purpura develop between the third and tenth day of therapy, most likely as a result of a transient imbalance in the levels of anticoagulant and procoagulant vitamin K–dependent factors. Continued therapy does not exacerbate preexisting lesions, and patients with an inherited or acquired deficiency of protein C are at increased risk for this particular reaction as well as for purpura fulminans and calciphylaxis.

Purpura secondary to *cholesterol emboli* are usually seen on the lower extremities of patients with atherosclerotic vascular disease. They often follow anticoagulant therapy or an invasive vascular procedure such as an arteriogram but also occur spontaneously from disintegration of atheromatous plaques. Associated findings include livedo reticularis, gangrene, cyanosis, and ischemic ulcerations. Multiple step sections of the biopsy specimen may be necessary to demonstrate the cholesterol clefts within the vessels. Petechiae are also an important sign of *fat embolism* and occur primarily on the upper body 2–3 days after a major injury. By using special fixatives, the emboli can be demonstrated in biopsy specimens of the petechiae. Rarely, emboli of tumor or thrombus are seen in patients with atrial myxomas and marantic endocarditis.

In the *Gardner-Diamond syndrome* (autoerythrocyte sensitivity), female patients develop large ecchymoses within areas of painful, warm erythema. Intradermal injections of autologous erythrocytes or phosphatidyl serine derived from the red cell membrane can reproduce the lesions in some patients; however, there are instances where a reaction is seen at an injection site of the forearm but not in the midback region. The latter has led some observers to view Gardner-Diamond syndrome as a cutaneous manifestation of severe emotional stress. More recently, the possibility of platelet dysfunction (as assessed via aggregation studies) has been raised. *Waldenström's hypergammaglobulinemic purpura* is a chronic disorder characterized by recurrent crops of petechiae and larger purpuric macules on the lower extremities. There are circulating complexes of IgG–anti-IgG molecules, and exacerbations are associated with prolonged standing or walking. Patients may have an underlying autoimmune connective tissue disease, e.g., Sjögren's syndrome.

Palpable purpura are further subdivided into vasculitic and embolic. In the group of vasculitic disorders, cutaneous small-vessel vasculitis, also known as *leukocytoclastic vasculitis* (LCV), is the one most commonly associated with palpable purpura (**Chap. 363**). Underlying etiologies include drugs (e.g., antibiotics), infections (e.g., hepatitis C virus), and autoimmune connective tissue diseases (e.g., rheumatoid arthritis, Sjögren's syndrome, lupus). *Henoch-Schönlein purpura* (HSP) is a subtype of acute LCV that is seen more commonly in children and adolescents following an upper respiratory infection. The majority of lesions are found on the lower extremities and buttocks. Systemic manifestations include fever, arthralgias (primarily of the knees and ankles), abdominal pain, gastrointestinal bleeding, and nephritis. Direct immunofluorescence examination shows deposits of IgA within dermal blood vessel walls. Renal disease is of particular concern in adults with IgA vasculitis.

Several types of infectious emboli can give rise to palpable purpura. These embolic lesions are usually *irregular* in outline as opposed to the lesions of LCV, which are *circular* in outline. The irregular outline is indicative of a cutaneous infarct, and the size corresponds to the area of skin that received its blood supply from that particular arteriole or artery. The palpable purpura in LCV are circular because the erythrocytes simply diffuse out evenly from the postcapillary venules as a result of inflammation. Infectious emboli are most commonly due to gram-negative cocci (meningococcus, gonococcus), gram-negative rods (Enterobacteriaceae), and gram-positive cocci (*Staphylococcus*). Additional causes include *Rickettsia* and, in immunocompromised patients, *Aspergillus* and other opportunistic fungi.

The embolic lesions in *acute meningococcemia* are found primarily on the trunk, lower extremities, and sites of pressure, and a gunmetal-gray color often develops within them. Their size varies from a few millimeters to several centimeters, and the organisms can be cultured from the lesions. Associated findings include a preceding upper respiratory tract infection; fever; meningitis; DIC; and, in some patients, a deficiency of the terminal components of complement. In *disseminated gonococcal infection* (arthritis-dermatitis syndrome), a small number of inflammatory papules and vesicopustules, often with central purpura or hemorrhagic necrosis, are found on the distal extremities. Additional symptoms include arthralgias, tenosynovitis, and fever. To establish the diagnosis, a Gram stain of these lesions should be performed. *Rocky Mountain spotted fever* is a tick-borne disease that is caused by *Rickettsia rickettsii*. A several-day history of fever, chills, severe headache, and photophobia precedes the onset of the cutaneous eruption. The initial lesions are erythematous macules and papules on the wrists, ankles, palms, and soles. With time, the lesions spread centripetally and become purpuric.

Lesions of *ecthyma gangrenosum* begin as edematous, erythematous papules or plaques and then develop central purpura and necrosis. Bullae formation also occurs in these lesions, and they are frequently found in the girdle region. The organism that is classically associated with ecthyma gangrenosum is *Pseudomonas aeruginosa*, but other gram-negative rods such as *Klebsiella*, *Escherichia coli*, and *Serratia* can produce similar lesions. In immunocompromised hosts, the list of potential pathogens is expanded to include *Candida* and other opportunistic fungi (e.g., *Aspergillus*, *Fusarium*).

ULCERS

The approach to the patient with a cutaneous ulcer is outlined in **Table 58-17**. Peripheral vascular diseases of the extremities are reviewed in **Chap. 281**, as is Raynaud's phenomenon.

Livedoid vasculopathy (livedoid vasculitis; atrophie blanche) represents a combination of a vasculopathy plus intravascular thrombosis. Purpuric lesions and livedo reticularis are found in association with *painful* ulcerations of the lower extremities. These ulcers are often slow to heal, but when they do, irregularly shaped white scars form. The majority of cases are secondary to venous hypertension, but possible underlying illnesses include disorders of hypercoagulability, for example, antiphospholipid syndrome and factor V Leiden (**Chaps. 117 and 357**).

In *pyoderma gangrenosum*, the border of untreated active ulcers has a characteristic appearance consisting of an undermined necrotic violaceous edge and a peripheral erythematous halo. The ulcers often begin as pustules that then expand rather rapidly to a size as large as 20 cm. Although these lesions are most commonly found on the lower extremities, they can arise anywhere on the surface of the body, including at sites of trauma (pathergy). An estimated 30–50% of cases are idiopathic, and the most common associated disorders are ulcerative colitis and Crohn's disease. Less commonly, pyoderma gangrenosum is associated with seropositive rheumatoid arthritis, acute and chronic myelogenous leukemia, myelodysplasia, a monoclonal gammopathy (usually IgA), or an autoinflammatory disorder. Because the histology of pyoderma gangrenosum may be nonspecific (dermal infiltrate of neutrophils when in untreated state), the diagnosis requires clinicopathologic correlation, in particular, the exclusion of similar-appearing ulcers such as necrotizing vasculitis, Meleney's ulcer (synergistic infection at a site of trauma or surgery), dimorphic fungi, cutaneous amebiasis, spider bites, and factitial. In the myeloproliferative disorders, the ulcers may be more superficial with a pustulobullous border, and these lesions provide a connection between classic pyoderma gangrenosum and acute febrile neutrophilic dermatosis (Sweet syndrome).

FEVER AND RASH

The major considerations in a patient with a fever and a rash are inflammatory diseases versus infectious diseases. In the hospital setting, the most common scenario is a patient who has a drug rash plus a fever secondary to an underlying infection. However, it should be emphasized that a drug reaction can lead to both a cutaneous eruption and a fever ("drug fever"), especially in the setting of DRESS, AGEP, or serum

TABLE 58-17 Causes of Mucocutaneous Ulcers

I. Primary cutaneous disorders
A. Peripheral vascular disease **(Chap. 281)**
1. Venous
2. Arterial[a]
B. Livedoid vasculopathy in the setting of venous hypertension[b]
C. Squamous cell carcinoma (e.g., within scars), basal cell carcinomas
D. Infections, e.g., ecthyma caused by *Streptococcus* **(Chap. 148)**
E. Physical, e.g., trauma, pressure
F. Drugs, e.g., hydroxyurea
II. Systemic diseases
A. Lower legs
1. Small-vessel and medium-vessel vasculitis[c]
2. Hemoglobinopathies **(Chap. 98)**
3. Cryoglobulinemia,[c] cryofibrinogenemia
4. Cholesterol emboli[a,c]
5. Necrobiosis lipoidica[d]
6. Antiphospholipid syndrome **(Chap. 116)**
7. Neuropathic[e] **(Chap. 403)**
8. Panniculitis
9. Kaposi's sarcoma, acral angiodermatitis (pseudo-Kaposi's sarcoma)
10. Diffuse dermal angiomatosis
B. Hands and feet
1. Raynaud's phenomenon **(Chap. 281)**
2. Buerger disease
C. Generalized
1. Pyoderma gangrenosum, but most commonly legs
2. Calciphylaxis **(Chap. 410)**
3. Infections, e.g., dimorphic fungi, leishmaniasis
4. Lymphoma
D. Face, especially perioral, and anogenital
1. Chronic herpes simplex[f]
III. Mucosal
A. Aphthae
B. Drug-induced mucositis
C. Behçet's disease **(Chap. 364)**
D. Erythema multiforme major, Stevens-Johnson syndrome, TEN
E. Primary blistering disorders **(Chap. 59)**
F. Lupus erythematosus, lichen planus, lichenoid GVHD
G. Inflammatory bowel disease
H. Acute HIV infection
I. Reactive arthritis

[a]Underlying atherosclerosis. [b]Also associated with underlying disorders that lead to hypercoagulability/thrombophilia, e.g., factor V Leiden, protein C dysfunction/deficiency, antiphospholipid antibodies. [c]Reviewed in section on purpura. [d]Reviewed in section on papulonodular skin lesions. [e]Favors plantar surface of the foot. [f]Sign of immunosuppression.

Abbreviations: GVHD, graft versus host disease; HIV, human immunodeficiency virus; TEN, toxic epidermal necrolysis.

sickness–like reaction. Additional inflammatory diseases that are often associated with a fever include pustular psoriasis, erythroderma, and Sweet syndrome. Lyme disease, secondary syphilis, and viral and bacterial exanthems (see "Exanthems," above) are examples of infectious diseases that produce a rash and a fever. Lastly, it is important to determine whether or not the cutaneous lesions represent septic emboli (see "Purpura," above). Such lesions usually have evidence of ischemia in the form of purpura, necrosis, or impending necrosis (gunmetal-gray color). In the patient with thrombocytopenia, however, purpura can be seen in inflammatory reactions such as morbilliform drug eruptions and infectious lesions.

FURTHER READING

Bolognia JL, Schaffer JV, Cerroni L (eds): *Dermatology*, 4th ed. Philadelphia, Elsevier, 2018.

Callen JP et al (eds): *Dermatological Signs of Systemic Disease*, 5th ed. Edinburgh, Elsevier, 2017.

Fazel N (ed): *Oral Signs of Systemic Disease*. Switzerland, Springer, 2019.

Kurtzman D: Rheumatologic dermatology. Clin Dermatol 36:439, 2018.

Taylor SC et al (eds): *Taylor and Kelly's Dermatology for Skin of Color*, 2nd ed. New York, McGraw-Hill, 2016.

59 Immunologically Mediated Skin Diseases

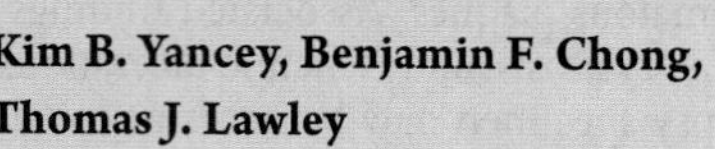

Kim B. Yancey, Benjamin F. Chong, Thomas J. Lawley

A number of immunologically mediated skin diseases and immunologically mediated systemic disorders with cutaneous manifestations are now recognized as distinct entities with consistent clinical, histologic, and immunopathologic findings. Clinically, these disorders are characterized by morbidity (pain, pruritus, disfigurement) and, in some instances, result in death (largely due to loss of epidermal barrier function and/or secondary infection). The major features of the more common immunologically mediated skin diseases are summarized in this chapter (**Table 59-1**), as are autoimmune systemic disorders with cutaneous manifestations.

AUTOIMMUNE CUTANEOUS DISEASES

PEMPHIGUS VULGARIS

Pemphigus refers to a group of autoantibody-mediated intraepidermal blistering diseases characterized by loss of cohesion between epidermal cells (a process termed *acantholysis*). Manual pressure to the skin of these patients may elicit the separation of the epidermis (*Nikolsky's sign*). This finding, while characteristic of pemphigus, is not specific to this group of disorders and is also seen in toxic epidermal necrolysis, Stevens-Johnson syndrome, and a few other skin diseases.

Pemphigus vulgaris (PV) is a mucocutaneous blistering disease that predominantly occurs in patients >40 years of age. PV typically begins on mucosal surfaces and often progresses to involve the skin. This disease is characterized by fragile, flaccid blisters that rupture to produce extensive denudation of mucous membranes and skin (**Fig. 59-1**). The mouth, scalp, face, neck, axilla, groin, and trunk are typically involved. PV may be associated with severe skin pain; some patients experience pruritus as well. Lesions usually heal without scarring except at sites complicated by secondary infection or mechanically induced dermal wounds. Postinflammatory hyperpigmentation is usually present for some time at sites of healed lesions.

Biopsies of early lesions demonstrate intraepidermal vesicle formation secondary to loss of cohesion between epidermal cells (i.e., acantholytic blisters). Blister cavities contain acantholytic epidermal cells, which appear as round homogeneous cells containing hyperchromatic nuclei. Basal keratinocytes remain attached to the epidermal basement membrane; hence, blister formation takes place within the suprabasal portion of the epidermis. Lesional skin may contain focal collections of intraepidermal eosinophils within blister cavities; dermal alterations are slight, often limited to an eosinophil-predominant leukocytic infiltrate. Direct immunofluorescence microscopy of lesional or intact patient skin shows deposits of IgG on the surface of keratinocytes; deposits of complement components are typically found in lesional but not in uninvolved skin. Deposits of IgG on keratinocytes are derived from circulating autoantibodies to cell-surface autoantigens.

TABLE 59-1 Immunologically Mediated Blistering Diseases

DISEASE	CLINICAL MANIFESTATIONS	HISTOLOGY	IMMUNOPATHOLOGY	AUTOANTIGENS[a]
Pemphigus vulgaris	Flaccid blisters, denuded skin, oromucosal lesions	Acantholytic blister formed in suprabasal layer of epidermis	Cell surface deposits of IgG on keratinocytes	Dsg3 (plus Dsg1 in patients with skin involvement)
Pemphigus foliaceus	Crusts and shallow erosions on scalp, central face, upper chest, and back	Acantholytic blister formed in superficial layer of epidermis	Cell surface deposits of IgG on keratinocytes	Dsg1
Paraneoplastic pemphigus	Painful stomatitis with papulosquamous or lichenoid eruptions that may progress to blisters	Acantholysis, keratinocyte necrosis, and vacuolar interface dermatitis	Cell surface deposits of IgG and C3 on keratinocytes and (variably) similar immunoreactants in epidermal BMZ	Plakin protein family members and desmosomal cadherins (see text for details)
Bullous pemphigoid	Large tense blisters on flexor surfaces and trunk	Subepidermal blister with eosinophil-rich infiltrate	Linear band of IgG and/or C3 in epidermal BMZ	BPAG1, BPAG2
Pemphigoid gestationis	Pruritic, urticarial plaques rimmed by vesicles and bullae on the trunk and extremities	Teardrop-shaped, subepidermal blisters in dermal papillae; eosinophil-rich infiltrate	Linear band of C3 in epidermal BMZ	BPAG2 (plus BPAG1 in some patients)
Dermatitis herpetiformis	Extremely pruritic small papules and vesicles on elbows, knees, buttocks, and posterior neck	Subepidermal blister with neutrophils in dermal papillae	Granular deposits of IgA in dermal papillae	Epidermal transglutaminase
Linear IgA disease	Pruritic small papules on extensor surfaces; occasionally larger, arciform blisters	Subepidermal blister with neutrophil-rich infiltrate	Linear band of IgA in epidermal BMZ	BPAG2 (see text for specific details)
Epidermolysis bullosa acquisita	Blisters, erosions, scars, and milia on sites exposed to trauma; widespread, inflammatory, tense blisters may be seen initially	Subepidermal blister that may or may not include a leukocytic infiltrate	Linear band of IgG and/or C3 in epidermal BMZ	Type VII collagen
Mucous membrane pemphigoid	Erosive and/or blistering lesions of mucous membranes and possibly the skin; scarring of some sites	Subepidermal blister that may or may not include a leukocytic infiltrate	Linear band of IgG, IgA, and/or C3 in epidermal BMZ	BPAG2, laminin-332, or others

[a]Autoantigens bound by these patients' autoantibodies are defined as follows: Dsg1, desmoglein 1; Dsg3, desmoglein 3; BPAG1, bullous pemphigoid antigen 1; BPAG2, bullous pemphigoid antigen 2.
Abbreviation: BMZ, basement membrane zone.

Such circulating autoantibodies can be demonstrated in 80–90% of PV patients by indirect immunofluorescence microscopy; monkey esophagus is the optimal substrate for these studies. Patients with PV have IgG autoantibodies to *desmogleins* (Dsgs), transmembrane desmosomal glycoproteins that belong to the cadherin family of calcium-dependent adhesion molecules. Such autoantibodies can be precisely quantitated by enzyme-linked immunosorbent assay (ELISA). Patients with early PV (i.e., mucosal disease) have IgG autoantibodies to Dsg3; patients with advanced PV (i.e., mucocutaneous disease) have IgG autoantibodies to both Dsg3 and Dsg1. Experimental studies have shown that autoantibodies from patients with PV are pathogenic (i.e., responsible for blister formation) and that their titer correlates with disease activity. Recent studies have shown that the anti-Dsg autoantibody profile in these patients' sera as well as the tissue distribution of Dsg3 and Dsg1 determine the site of blister formation in patients with PV. Coexpression of Dsg3 and Dsg1 by epidermal cells protects against pathogenic IgG antibodies to either of these cadherins but not against pathogenic autoantibodies to both.

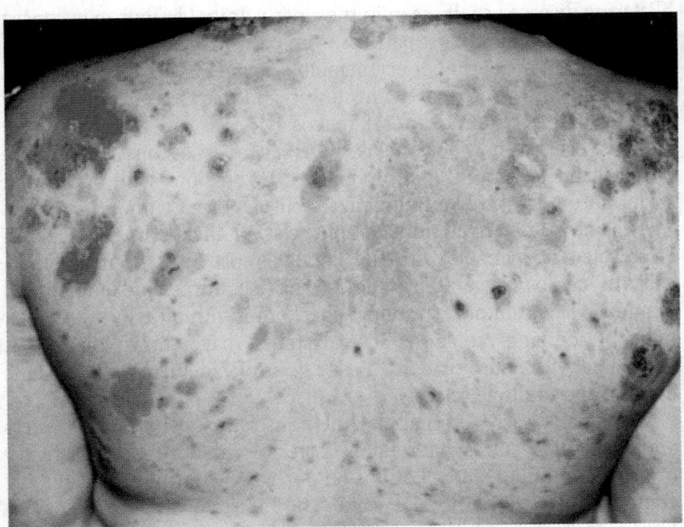
A

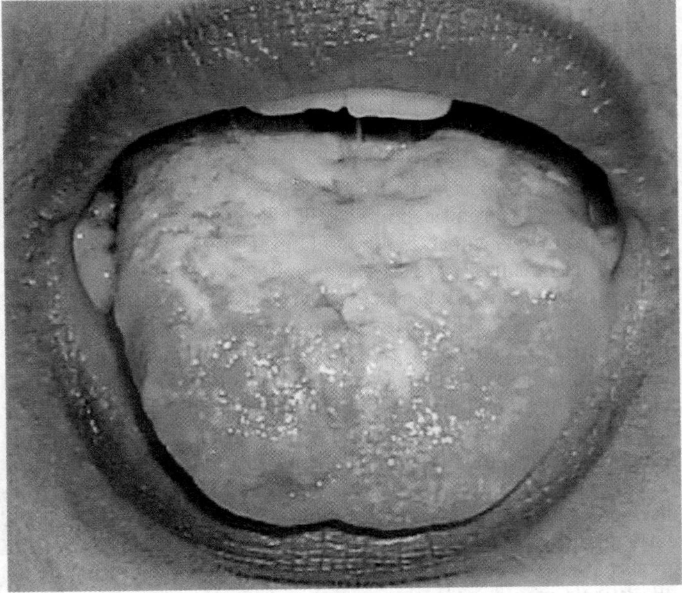
B

FIGURE 59-1 Pemphigus vulgaris. ***A.*** Flaccid bullae are easily ruptured, resulting in multiple erosions and crusted plaques. ***B.*** Involvement of the oral mucosa, which is almost invariable, may present with erosions on the gingiva, buccal mucosa, palate, posterior pharynx, or tongue. *(Figure B: Courtesy of Robert Swerlick, MD.)*

PV can be life-threatening. Prior to the availability of glucocorticoids, mortality rates ranged from 60% to 90%; the current figure is ~5%. Common causes of morbidity and death are infection and complications of treatment. Bad prognostic factors include advanced age, widespread involvement, and the requirement for high doses of glucocorticoids (with or without other immunosuppressive agents) for control of disease. The course of PV in individual patients is variable and difficult to predict. Some patients experience remission, while others may require long-term treatment or succumb to complications of their disease or its treatment. The mainstay of treatment is systemic glucocorticoids alone or in combination with other immunosuppressive agents. Patients with moderate to severe PV are usually started on prednisone at doses ≤1 mg/kg per day (single morning dose). If new lesions continue to appear after 1–2 weeks of treatment, the dose of prednisone may need to be increased and/or combined with another immunosuppressive agent. Among these, rituximab in combination with prednisone often achieves remission (though maintenance therapy may be required to prevent relapse). Other immunosuppressive agents sometimes combined with prednisone to treat PV include azathioprine, mycophenolate mofetil, or cyclophosphamide. Patients with severe, treatment-resistant disease may derive benefit from plasmapheresis (six high-volume exchanges [i.e., 2–3 L per exchange] over ~2 weeks) and/or IV immunoglobulin (IVIg). It is important to bring severe or progressive disease under control quickly in order to lessen the severity and/or duration of this disorder. Increasingly, rituximab and daily glucocorticoids are used early in PV patients to avert the development of advanced and/or treatment-resistant disease.

PEMPHIGUS FOLIACEUS

Pemphigus foliaceus (PF) is distinguished from PV by several features. In PF, acantholytic blisters are located high within the epidermis, usually just beneath the stratum corneum. Hence, PF is a more superficial blistering disease than PV. The distribution of lesions in the two disorders is much the same, except that in PF mucous membranes are almost always spared. Patients with PF rarely have intact blisters but rather exhibit shallow erosions associated with erythema, scale, and crust formation. Mild cases of PF can resemble severe seborrheic dermatitis; severe PF may cause extensive exfoliation. Sun exposure (ultraviolet irradiation) may be an aggravating factor.

PF has immunopathologic features in common with PV. Specifically, direct immunofluorescence microscopy of perilesional skin demonstrates IgG on the surface of keratinocytes. Similarly, patients with PF have circulating IgG autoantibodies directed against the surface of keratinocytes. In PF, autoantibodies are directed against Dsg1, a 160-kDa desmosomal cadherin. These autoantibodies can be quantitated by ELISA. As noted for PV, the autoantibody profile in patients with PF (i.e., anti-Dsg1 IgG) and the tissue distribution of this autoantigen (i.e., expression in oral mucosa that is compensated by coexpression of Dsg3) are thought to account for the distribution of lesions in this disease.

Endemic forms of PF are found in south-central rural Brazil, where the disease is known as *fogo salvagem* (FS), as well as in selected sites in Latin America and Tunisia. Endemic PF, like other forms of this disease, is mediated by IgG autoantibodies to Dsg1. Clusters of FS overlap with those of leishmaniasis, a disease transmitted by bites of the sand fly *Lutzomyia longipalis*. Studies have shown that sand fly salivary antigens (specifically, the LJM11 salivary protein) are recognized by IgG autoantibodies from FS patients (as well as by monoclonal antibodies to Dsg1 derived from these patients). The demonstration that mice immunized with LJM11 produce antibodies to Dsg1 suggests that insect bites may deliver salivary antigens, initiate a cross-reactive humoral immune response, and lead to FS in genetically susceptible individuals.

Although pemphigus has been associated with several autoimmune diseases, its association with thymoma and/or myasthenia gravis is particularly notable. To date, >30 cases of thymoma and/or myasthenia gravis have been reported in association with pemphigus, usually with PF. Patients may also develop pemphigus as a consequence of drug exposure; drug-induced pemphigus usually resembles PF rather than PV. Drugs containing a thiol group in their chemical structure (e.g., penicillamine, captopril, enalapril) are most commonly associated with drug-induced pemphigus. Nonthiol drugs linked to pemphigus include penicillins, cephalosporins, and piroxicam. Some cases of drug-induced pemphigus are durable and require treatment with systemic glucocorticoids and/or immunosuppressive agents.

PF is generally a less severe disease than PV and usually carries a better prognosis. Localized disease can sometimes be treated with topical or intralesional glucocorticoids; more active cases can usually be controlled with systemic glucocorticoids either alone or in combination with other immunosuppressive agents. Patients with severe, treatment-resistant disease may require more aggressive interventions, as described above for patients with PV.

PARANEOPLASTIC PEMPHIGUS

Paraneoplastic pemphigus (PNP) is an autoimmune acantholytic mucocutaneous disease associated with an occult or confirmed neoplasm. Patients with PNP typically have painful stomatitis in association with papulosquamous and/or lichenoid eruptions that often progress to blisters. Palm and sole involvement are common in these patients and raise the possibility that prior reports of neoplasia-associated erythema multiforme may have represented unrecognized cases of PNP. Biopsies of lesional skin from these patients show varying combinations of acantholysis, keratinocyte necrosis, and vacuolar-interface dermatitis. Direct immunofluorescence microscopy of a patient's skin shows deposits of IgG and complement on the surface of keratinocytes and (variably) similar immunoreactants in the epidermal basement membrane zone. Patients with PNP have IgG autoantibodies to cytoplasmic proteins that are members of the plakin family (e.g., desmoplakins I and II, bullous pemphigoid antigen [BPAG] 1, envoplakin, periplakin, and plectin) and to cell-surface proteins that are members of the cadherin family (e.g., Dsg1 and Dsg3). Passive transfer studies have shown that autoantibodies from patients with PNP are pathogenic in animal models.

The predominant neoplasms associated with PNP are non-Hodgkin's lymphoma, chronic lymphocytic leukemia, thymoma, spindle cell tumors, Waldenström's macroglobulinemia, and Castleman's disease; the last-mentioned neoplasm is particularly common among children with PNP. Rare cases of seronegative PNP have been reported in patients with B-cell malignancies previously treated with rituximab. In addition to severe skin lesions, many patients with PNP develop life-threatening bronchiolitis obliterans. PNP is generally resistant to conventional therapies (i.e., those used to treat PV); rarely, a patient's disease may ameliorate or even remit following ablation or removal of underlying neoplasms.

BULLOUS PEMPHIGOID

Bullous pemphigoid (BP) is a polymorphic autoimmune subepidermal blistering disease usually seen in the elderly. Initial lesions may consist of urticarial plaques; most patients eventually display tense blisters on either normal-appearing or erythematous skin (**Fig. 59-2**). The lesions are usually distributed over the lower abdomen, groin, and flexor surface of the extremities; oral mucosal lesions are found in some patients. Pruritus may be nonexistent or severe. As lesions evolve, tense blisters tend to rupture and be replaced by erosions with or without surmounting crust. Nontraumatized blisters heal without scarring. The major histocompatibility complex class II allele HLA-DQβ1*0301 is prevalent in patients with BP. Though most cases occur sporadically, BP can be triggered by medications (e.g., furosemide, dipeptidyl peptidase-4 inhibitors, immune checkpoint inhibitors), ultraviolet light, or ionizing radiation. Several studies have shown that BP is associated with neurologic diseases (e.g., stroke, dementia, Parkinson's disease, and multiple sclerosis).

Biopsies of early lesional skin demonstrate subepidermal blisters and histologic features that roughly correlate with the clinical character of the lesion under study. Lesions on normal-appearing skin generally contain a sparse perivascular leukocytic infiltrate with some eosinophils; conversely, biopsies of inflammatory lesions typically show an eosinophil-rich infiltrate at sites of vesicle formation and in perivascular areas. In addition to eosinophils, cell-rich lesions also contain mononuclear cells and neutrophils. It is not possible to distinguish

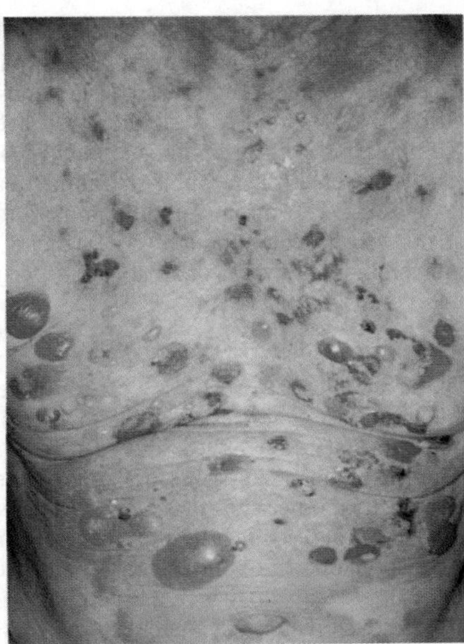

FIGURE 59-2 Bullous pemphigoid with tense vesicles and bullae on erythematous, urticarial bases. *(Courtesy of the Yale Resident's Slide Collection; with permission.)*

BP from other subepidermal blistering diseases by routine histologic studies alone.

Direct immunofluorescence microscopy of normal-appearing perilesional skin from patients with BP shows linear deposits of IgG and/or C3 in the epidermal basement membrane. The sera of ~70% of these patients contain circulating IgG autoantibodies that bind the epidermal basement membrane of normal human skin in indirect immunofluorescence microscopy. IgG from an even higher percentage of patients reacts with the epidermal side of 1 *M* NaCl split skin (an alternative immunofluorescence microscopy test substrate used to distinguish circulating IgG autoantibodies to the basement membrane in patients with BP from those in patients with similar, yet different, subepidermal blistering diseases; see below). In BP, circulating autoantibodies recognize 230- and 180-kDa hemidesmosome-associated proteins in basal keratinocytes (i.e., BPAG1 and BPAG2, respectively). Autoantibodies to BPAG2 are thought to deposit in situ, activate complement, produce dermal mast-cell degranulation, and generate granulocyte-rich infiltrates that cause tissue damage and blister formation.

BP may persist for months to years, with exacerbations or remissions. Extensive involvement may result in widespread erosions and compromise cutaneous integrity; elderly and/or debilitated patients may die. Local or minimal disease can sometimes be controlled with potent topical glucocorticoids alone; more extensive lesions generally respond to systemic glucocorticoids either alone or in combination with other agents. Adjuncts to systemic glucocorticoids include doxycycline, azathioprine, mycophenolate mofetil, and rituximab.

■ PEMPHIGOID GESTATIONIS

Pemphigoid gestationis (PG), also known as *herpes gestationis*, is a rare, nonviral, subepidermal blistering disease of pregnancy and the puerperium. PG may begin during any trimester of pregnancy or present shortly after delivery. Lesions are usually distributed over the abdomen, trunk, and extremities; mucous membrane lesions are rare. Skin lesions in these patients may be quite polymorphic and consist of erythematous urticarial papules and plaques, vesiculopapules, and/or frank bullae. Lesions are almost always extremely pruritic. Severe exacerbations of PG frequently follow delivery, typically within 24–48 h. PG tends to recur in subsequent pregnancies, often beginning earlier during such gestations. Brief flare-ups of disease may occur with resumption of menses and may develop in patients later exposed to oral contraceptives. Occasionally, infants of affected mothers have transient skin lesions.

Biopsies of early lesional skin show teardrop-shaped subepidermal vesicles forming in dermal papillae in association with an eosinophil-rich leukocytic infiltrate. Differentiation of PG from other subepidermal bullous diseases by light microscopy is difficult. However, direct immunofluorescence microscopy of perilesional skin from PG patients reveals the immunopathologic hallmark of this disorder: linear deposits of C3 in the epidermal basement membrane. These deposits develop as a consequence of complement activation produced by low-titer IgG anti–basement membrane autoantibodies directed against BPAG2, the same hemidesmosome-associated protein that is targeted by autoantibodies in patients with BP—a subepidermal bullous disease that resembles PG clinically, histologically, and immunopathologically.

The goals of therapy in patients with PG are to prevent the development of new lesions, relieve intense pruritus, and care for erosions at sites of blister formation. Many patients require treatment with moderate doses of daily glucocorticoids (i.e., 20–40 mg of prednisone) at some point in their course. Mild cases (or brief flare-ups) may be controlled by vigorous use of potent topical glucocorticoids. Infants born of mothers with PG appear to be at increased risk of being born slightly premature or "small for dates." Current evidence suggests that there is no difference in the incidence of uncomplicated live births between PG patients treated with systemic glucocorticoids and those managed more conservatively. If systemic glucocorticoids are administered, newborns are at risk for development of reversible adrenal insufficiency.

■ DERMATITIS HERPETIFORMIS

Dermatitis herpetiformis (DH) is an intensely pruritic, papulovesicular skin disease characterized by lesions symmetrically distributed over extensor surfaces (i.e., elbows, knees, buttocks, back, scalp, and posterior neck) **(see Fig. 56-8)**. Primary lesions in this disorder consist of papules, papulovesicles, or urticarial plaques. Because pruritus is prominent, patients may present with excoriations and crusted papules but no observable primary lesions. Patients sometimes report that their pruritus has a distinctive burning or stinging component; the onset of such local symptoms reliably heralds the development of distinct clinical lesions 12–24 h later. Almost all DH patients have associated, usually subclinical, gluten-sensitive enteropathy **(Chap. 325)**, and >90% express the HLA-B8/DRw3 and HLA-DQw2 haplotypes. DH may present at any age, including in childhood; onset in the second to fourth decades is most common. The disease is typically chronic.

Biopsy of early lesional skin reveals neutrophil-rich infiltrates within dermal papillae. Neutrophils, fibrin, edema, and microvesicle formation at these sites are characteristic of early disease. Older lesions may demonstrate nonspecific features of a subepidermal bulla or an excoriated papule. Because the clinical and histologic features of this disease can be variable and resemble those of other subepidermal blistering disorders, the diagnosis is confirmed by direct immunofluorescence microscopy of normal-appearing perilesional skin. Such studies demonstrate granular deposits of IgA (with or without complement components) in the papillary dermis and along the epidermal basement membrane zone. IgA deposits in the skin are unaffected by control of disease with medication; however, these immunoreactants diminish in intensity or disappear in patients maintained for long periods on a strict gluten-free diet (see below). Patients with DH have granular deposits of IgA in their epidermal basement membrane zone and should be distinguished from individuals with linear IgA deposits at this site (see below).

Although most DH patients do not report overt gastrointestinal symptoms or have laboratory evidence of malabsorption, biopsies of the small bowel usually reveal blunting of intestinal villi and a lymphocytic infiltrate in the lamina propria. As is true for patients with celiac disease, this gastrointestinal abnormality can be reversed by a gluten-free diet. Moreover, if maintained, this diet alone may control the skin disease and eventuate in clearance of IgA deposits from these patients' epidermal basement membrane zones. Subsequent gluten exposure in such patients alters the morphology of their small bowel, elicits a flare-up of their skin disease, and is associated with the reappearance of IgA in their epidermal basement membrane zones. As in patients with celiac disease, dietary gluten sensitivity in patients with DH is associated with IgA anti-endomysial autoantibodies that target tissue transglutaminase. Studies indicate that patients with DH also have high-avidity IgA autoantibodies to epidermal transglutaminase and that the latter is co-localized with granular deposits of IgA in the papillary dermis of DH patients. Patients with DH also have an increased incidence of thyroid abnormalities, achlorhydria, atrophic gastritis, and autoantibodies to gastric parietal cells. These associations likely relate to the high frequency of the HLA-B8/DRw3 haplotype in these patients, since this marker is commonly linked to autoimmune disorders. The mainstay of treatment of DH is dapsone, a sulfone. Patients respond rapidly (24–48 h) to dapsone, but require careful pre-treatment evaluation (e.g., screening for glucose-6-phosphate dehydrogenase deficiency) and close follow-up to ensure that complications are avoided or controlled. All patients taking dapsone at >100 mg/d will have some hemolysis and methemoglobinemia, which are expected pharmacologic side effects of this agent. Gluten restriction can control DH and lessen dapsone requirements; this diet must rigidly exclude gluten to be of maximal benefit. Many months of dietary restriction may be necessary before a beneficial result is achieved. Good dietary counseling by a trained dietitian is essential.

LINEAR IGA DISEASE

Linear IgA disease, once considered a variant form of DH, is actually a separate and distinct entity. Clinically, patients with linear IgA disease may resemble individuals with DH, BP, or other subepidermal blistering diseases. Lesions typically consist of papulovesicles, bullae, and/or urticarial plaques that develop predominantly on central or flexural sites. Oral mucosal involvement occurs in some patients. Severe pruritus resembles that seen in patients with DH. Patients with linear IgA disease do not have an increased frequency of the HLA-B8/DRw3 haplotype or an associated enteropathy and therefore are not candidates for treatment with a gluten-free diet.

Histologic alterations in early lesions may be virtually indistinguishable from those in DH. However, direct immunofluorescence microscopy of normal-appearing perilesional skin reveals a linear band of IgA (and often C3) in the epidermal basement membrane zone. Most patients with linear IgA disease have circulating IgA anti-basement membrane autoantibodies directed against neoepitopes in the proteolytically processed extracellular domain of BPAG2. These patients generally respond to treatment with dapsone (50–200 mg/d) alone or in combination with low daily doses of prednisone.

EPIDERMOLYSIS BULLOSA ACQUISITA

Epidermolysis bullosa acquisita (EBA) is a rare, noninherited, polymorphic, chronic, subepidermal blistering disease. **(The inherited form is discussed in Chap. 413.)** Patients with classic or noninflammatory EBA have blisters on noninflamed skin, atrophic scars, milia, nail dystrophy, hair loss, and oral lesions. Because lesions generally occur at sites exposed to minor trauma, classic EBA is considered a mechanobullous disease. Other patients with EBA have widespread inflammatory scarring and bullous lesions that resemble severe BP. Inflammatory EBA may evolve into the classic, noninflammatory form of this disease. Rarely, patients present with lesions that predominate on mucous membranes. The HLA-DR2 haplotype is found with increased frequency in EBA patients. Studies suggest that EBA is sometimes associated with inflammatory bowel disease (especially Crohn's disease).

The histology of lesional skin varies with the character of the lesion being studied. Noninflammatory bullae are subepidermal, feature a sparse leukocytic infiltrate, and resemble the lesions in patients with porphyria cutanea tarda. Inflammatory lesions consist of neutrophil-rich subepidermal blisters. EBA patients have continuous deposits of IgG (and frequently C3) in a linear pattern within the epidermal basement membrane zone. Ultrastructurally, these immunoreactants are found in the sublamina densa region in association with anchoring fibrils. Approximately 50% of EBA patients have demonstrable circulating IgG anti-basement membrane autoantibodies directed against type VII collagen—the collagen species that makes up anchoring fibrils. Such IgG autoantibodies bind the dermal side of 1 *M* NaCl split skin (in contrast to IgG autoantibodies in patients with BP). Studies have shown that passive transfer of experimental or patient IgG against type VII collagen can produce lesions in mice that clinically, histologically, and immunopathologically resemble those in patients with EBA.

Treatment of EBA is generally unsatisfactory. Some patients with inflammatory EBA may respond to systemic glucocorticoids, either alone or in combination with immunosuppressive agents. Other patients (especially those with neutrophil-rich inflammatory lesions) may respond to dapsone. The chronic, noninflammatory form of EBA is largely resistant to treatment, although some patients may respond to prednisone in combination with rituximab, cyclosporine, mycophenolate mofetil, azathioprine, or IVIg.

MUCOUS MEMBRANE PEMPHIGOID

Mucous membrane pemphigoid (MMP) is a rare, acquired, subepithelial immunobullous disease characterized by erosive lesions of mucous membranes and skin that result in scarring of at least some sites of involvement. Common sites include the oral mucosa (especially the gingiva) and conjunctiva; other sites that may be affected include the nasopharyngeal, laryngeal, esophageal, and anogenital mucosa. Skin lesions (present in about one-third of patients) tend to predominate on the scalp, face, and upper trunk and generally consist of a few scattered erosions or tense blisters on an erythematous or urticarial base. MMP is typically a chronic and progressive disorder. Serious complications may arise as a consequence of ocular, laryngeal, esophageal, or anogenital lesions. Erosive conjunctivitis may result in shortened fornices, symblepharon, ankyloblepharon, entropion, corneal opacities, and (in severe cases) blindness. Similarly, erosive lesions of the larynx may cause hoarseness, pain, and tissue loss that, if unrecognized and untreated, may eventuate in complete destruction of the airway. Esophageal lesions may result in stenosis and/or strictures that could place patients at risk for aspiration. Strictures may also complicate anogenital involvement.

Biopsies of lesional tissue generally show subepithelial vesiculobullae and a mononuclear leukocytic infiltrate. Neutrophils and eosinophils may be seen in biopsies of early lesions; older lesions may demonstrate a scant leukocytic infiltrate and fibrosis. Direct immunofluorescence microscopy of perilesional tissue typically reveals deposits of IgG, IgA, and/or C3 in the epidermal basement membrane. Because many patients with MMP exhibit no evidence of circulating anti-basement membrane autoantibodies, testing of perilesional skin is important diagnostically. Although MMP was once thought to be a single nosologic entity, it is now largely regarded as a disease phenotype that may develop as a consequence of an autoimmune reaction to a variety of molecules in the epidermal basement membrane (e.g., BPAG2, laminin-332, type VII collagen, $\alpha_6\beta_4$ integrin) and other antigens yet to be completely defined. Studies suggest that MMP patients with autoantibodies to laminin-332 have an increased relative risk for cancer. Treatment of MMP is largely dependent upon the sites of involvement. Due to potentially severe complications, patients with ocular, laryngeal, esophageal, and/or anogenital involvement require aggressive systemic treatment with dapsone, prednisone, or the latter in combination with another immunosuppressive agent (e.g., rituximab, azathioprine, mycophenolate mofetil, or cyclophosphamide), or IVIg. Less threatening forms of the disease may be managed with topical or intralesional glucocorticoids.

AUTOIMMUNE SYSTEMIC DISEASES WITH PROMINENT CUTANEOUS FEATURES

DERMATOMYOSITIS

The cutaneous manifestations of dermatomyositis **(Chap. 365)** are often distinctive but at times may resemble those of systemic lupus erythematosus (SLE) **(Chap. 356)**, scleroderma **(Chap. 360)**, or other overlapping connective tissue diseases **(Chap. 360)**. The extent and severity of cutaneous disease may or may not correlate with the extent and severity of the myositis. The cutaneous manifestations of dermatomyositis are similar, whether the disease appears in children or in the elderly, except that calcification of subcutaneous tissue is a common late sequela in childhood dermatomyositis. Dermatomyositis may be associated with interstitial lung disease or cancer.

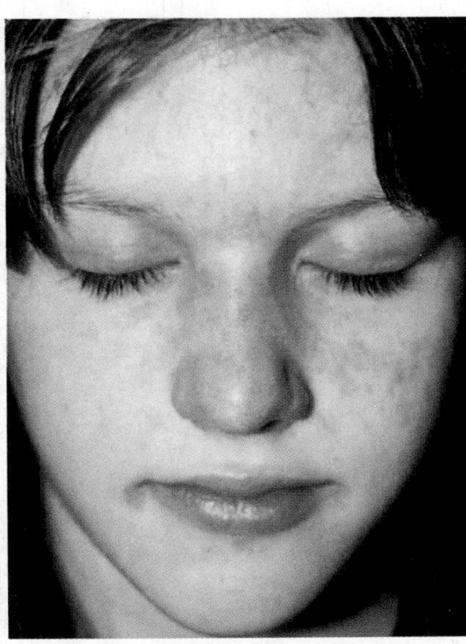

FIGURE 59-3 Dermatomyositis. Periorbital violaceous erythema characterizes the classic heliotrope rash. *(Courtesy of James Krell, MD; with permission.)*

The cutaneous signs of dermatomyositis may precede or follow the development of myositis by weeks to years. Cases lacking muscle involvement (i.e., *dermatomyositis sine myositis* or *amyopathic dermatomyositis*) have also been reported. The most common manifestation is a purple-red discoloration of the upper eyelids, sometimes associated with scaling ("heliotrope" erythema; **Fig. 59-3**) and periorbital edema. Erythema on the cheeks and nose in a "butterfly" distribution may resemble the malar eruption of SLE. Erythematous or violaceous thin, scaly plaques are common on the upper trunk and neck (shawl sign), the scalp, lateral aspects of the thighs (holster sign), and the extensor surfaces of the forearms and hands (tendon streaking). Approximately one-third of patients have violaceous, flat-topped papules over the dorsal interphalangeal joints that are pathognomonic of dermatomyositis (Gottron's papules) (**Fig. 59-4**). Thin violaceous papules and plaques on the elbows and knees of patients with dermatomyositis are referred to as *Gottron's sign*. These lesions can be contrasted with the erythema and scaling on the dorsum of the fingers that spares the skin over the interphalangeal joints of some SLE patients. Periungual telangiectasias and edema may be prominent in patients with dermatomyositis. Other patients, particularly those with long-standing disease, develop areas of hypopigmentation, hyperpigmentation, mild atrophy, and telangiectasia known as *poikiloderma*. Poikiloderma is rare in both SLE and scleroderma and thus can serve as a clinical sign that distinguishes dermatomyositis from these two diseases. Cutaneous changes may be similar in dermatomyositis and various overlap syndromes where thickening and binding down of the skin of the hands (*sclerodactyly*) as well as Raynaud's phenomenon can be seen. However, the presence of severe muscle disease, Gottron's papules, heliotrope erythema, and poikiloderma serves to distinguish patients with dermatomyositis. Skin biopsy of the erythematous, scaling lesions of dermatomyositis may reveal only mild nonspecific inflammation, but sometimes may show changes indistinguishable from those found in cutaneous lupus erythematosus (LE), including epidermal atrophy, hydropic degeneration of basal keratinocytes, and dermal changes consisting of interstitial mucin deposition and a mild mononuclear cell perivascular infiltrate. Direct immunofluorescence microscopy of lesional skin is usually negative, although granular deposits of immunoglobulin(s) and complement in the epidermal basement membrane zone have been described in some patients. Treatment should be stratified based on the relative severity of disease. Topical treatments include glucocorticoids, sunscreens, and aggressive photoprotective measures. Treatment of systemic disease includes antimalarials (though some patients may develop a drug eruption upon initiation of therapy) or systemic glucocorticoids in conjunction with methotrexate, mycophenolate mofetil, azathioprine, rituximab, or IVIg.

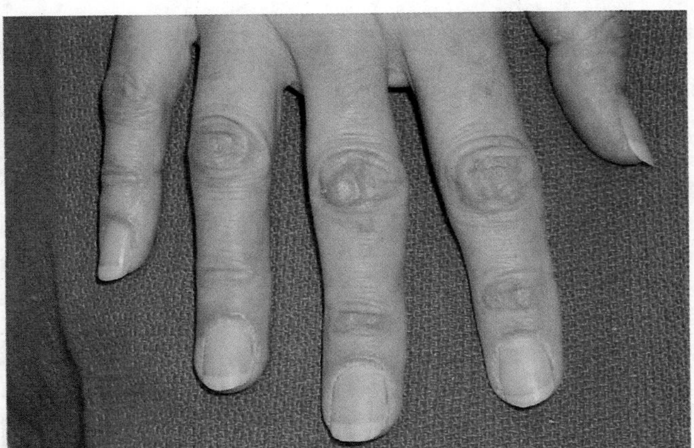

FIGURE 59-4 Gottron's papules. Dermatomyositis often involves the hands as erythematous flat-topped papules over the knuckles. Periungual telangiectasias are also evident.

LUPUS ERYTHEMATOSUS

The cutaneous manifestations of LE (**Chap. 356**) can be divided into acute, subacute, and chronic types. *Acute cutaneous LE* is characterized by erythema of the nose and malar eminences in a "butterfly" distribution (**Fig. 59-5*A***). The erythema is often sudden in onset, accompanied

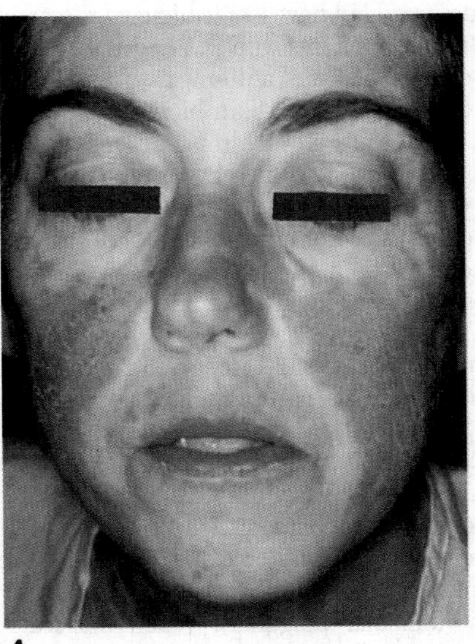

A

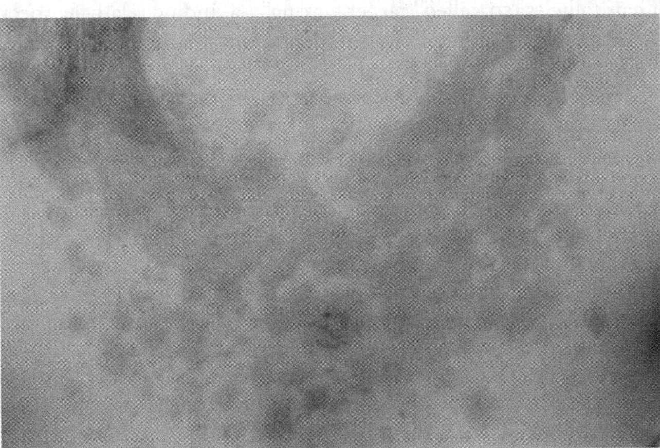

B

FIGURE 59-5 Acute cutaneous lupus erythematosus (LE). ***A.*** Acute cutaneous LE on the face, showing prominent, scaly, malar erythema. Involvement of other sun-exposed sites is also common. ***B.*** Acute cutaneous LE on the upper chest, demonstrating brightly erythematous and slightly edematous papules and plaques. *(Source: B, Courtesy of Robert Swerlick, MD; with permission.)*

by edema and fine scale, and correlated with systemic involvement. Patients may have widespread involvement of the face as well as erythema and scaling of the extensor surfaces of the extremities and upper chest (**Fig. 59-5*B***). These acute lesions, while sometimes evanescent, usually last for days and are often associated with exacerbations of systemic disease. Skin biopsy of acute lesions typically shows hydropic degeneration of basal keratinocytes, dermal edema, and (in some cases) a sparse perivascular infiltrate of mononuclear cells in the upper dermis as well as dermal mucin. Direct immunofluorescence microscopy of lesional skin frequently reveals deposits of immunoglobulin(s) and complement in the epidermal basement membrane zone. Treatment of cutaneous disease includes topical glucocorticoids, aggressive photoprotection, antimalarials, and control of systemic disease. Treatment of systemic disease associated with acute cutaneous LE includes systemic glucocorticoids in conjunction with other immunosuppressive agents.

Subacute cutaneous lupus erythematosus (SCLE) is characterized by a widespread photosensitive, nonscarring eruption. In most patients, renal and central nervous system involvement is mild or absent. SCLE may present as a papulosquamous eruption that resembles psoriasis or as annular polycyclic lesions. In the papulosquamous form, discrete erythematous papules arise on the back, chest, shoulders, extensor surfaces of the arms, and dorsum of the hands; lesions are uncommon on the central face and the flexor surfaces of the arms as well as below the waist. These slightly scaling papules tend to merge into plaques. The annular form involves the same areas and presents with erythematous papules that evolve into oval, circular, or polycyclic lesions. The lesions of SCLE are more widespread but have less tendency for scarring than lesions of discoid LE. In many patients with SCLE, drugs (e.g., hydrochlorothiazide, calcium channel blockers, antifungals, proton pump inhibitors) may induce or exacerbate disease. Skin biopsy typically reveals epidermal changes that include atrophy, hydropic degeneration of basal keratinocytes, and apoptosis accompanied by an infiltrate of mononuclear cells in the upper dermis. Direct immunofluorescence microscopy of lesional skin reveals deposits of immunoglobulin(s) in the epidermal basement membrane zone in about one-half of these cases. A particulate pattern of IgG deposition throughout the epidermis has been associated with SCLE. Most SCLE patients have anti-Ro autoantibodies. Local therapy alone is usually unsuccessful. Most patients require treatment with aminoquinoline antimalarial drugs. Low-dose therapy with oral glucocorticoids is sometimes necessary. Photoprotective measures against both ultraviolet B and ultraviolet A wavelengths are very important.

Chronic cutaneous LE has multiple subtypes; *discoid LE* (DLE) is the most common. DLE is characterized by discrete lesions, most often found on the face, scalp, and/or external ears. The lesions are erythematous papules or plaques with a thick, adherent scale that occludes hair follicles (follicular plugging). When the scale is removed, its underside shows small excrescences that correlate with the openings of hair follicles (so-called "carpet tacking"), a finding relatively specific for DLE. Long-standing lesions develop central atrophy, scarring, and hypopigmentation but frequently have erythematous, sometimes raised borders (**Fig. 59-6**). These lesions persist for years and tend to expand slowly. Up to 20% of patients with DLE eventually meet the American College of Rheumatology criteria for SLE. Typical discoid lesions are frequently seen in patients with SLE. Biopsy of DLE lesions shows hyperkeratosis, follicular plugging, atrophy of the epidermis, hydropic degeneration of basal keratinocytes, thickening of the epidermal basement membrane zone, and a mononuclear cell infiltrate adjacent to epidermal, adnexal, and microvascular basement membranes. Direct immunofluorescence microscopy demonstrates immunoglobulin(s) and complement deposits at the basement membrane zone in ~90% of cases. Treatment is focused on control of local cutaneous disease and consists mainly of photoprotection and topical or intralesional glucocorticoids. If local therapy is ineffective, use of aminoquinoline antimalarial agents may be indicated.

SCLERODERMA AND MORPHEA

The skin changes of scleroderma (**Chap. 360**) may be limited or diffuse. In both instances, disease usually begin on the fingers, hands, toes, feet, and face, with episodes of recurrent nonpitting edema. Sclerosis of the skin commences distally on the fingers (sclerodactyly) and spreads proximally, usually accompanied by resorption of bone of the fingertips, which may have punched out ulcers, stellate scars, or areas of hemorrhage (**Fig. 59-7**). The fingers may shrink and become sausage-shaped, and, because the fingernails are usually unaffected, they may curve over the end of the fingertips. Periungual telangiectasias are usually present, but periungual erythema is rare. In diffuse disease, the extremities show contractures and calcinosis cutis; facial involvement includes a smooth, unwrinkled brow, taut skin over the nose, shrinkage of tissue around the mouth, and perioral radial furrowing (**Fig. 59-8**). Matlike telangiectasias are often present, particularly on the face and hands. Involved skin feels indurated, smooth, and bound to underlying structures; hyper- and hypopigmentation are common as well. *Raynaud's phenomenon* (i.e., cold-induced blanching, cyanosis, and reactive hyperemia) is documented in almost all patients and can precede development of scleroderma by many years. The combination of calcinosis cutis, Raynaud's phenomenon, esophageal dysmotility, sclerodactyly, and telangiectasias has been termed as the *CREST syndrome*. Anti-centromere autoantibodies have been reported in a very high percentage of patients with CREST syndrome but in only a small minority of patients with scleroderma. Skin biopsy reveals thickening of the dermis, homogenization of collagen bundles, atrophic pilosebaceous and eccrine glands, and a sparse mononuclear cell infiltrate in the dermis and subcutaneous fat. Direct immunofluorescence microscopy of lesional skin is usually negative. Treatments for

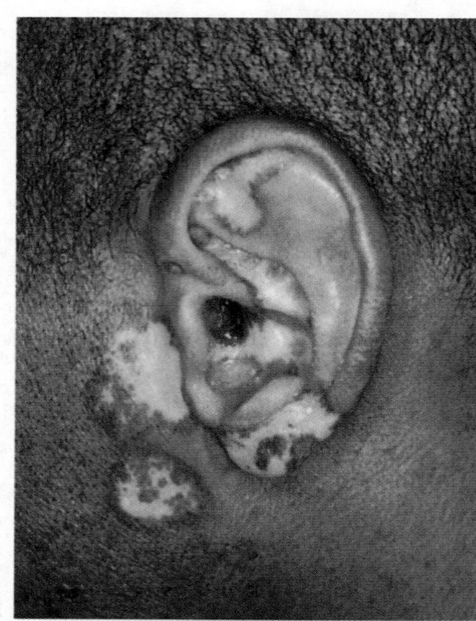

FIGURE 59-6 Discoid lupus erythematosus (DLE). Violaceous, hyperpigmented, atrophic plaques, follicular plugging, and scarring are typical features of DLE.

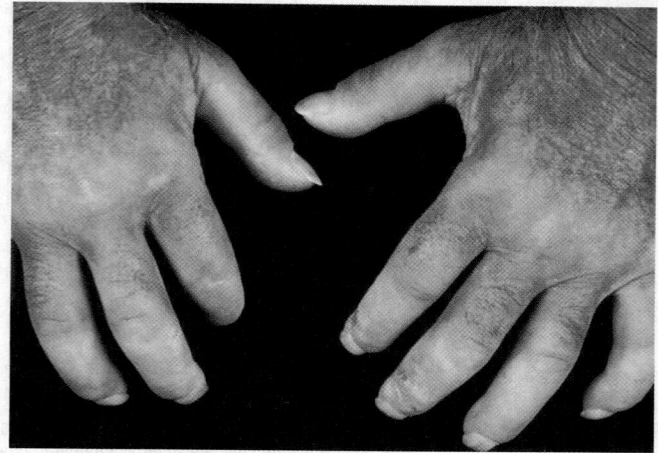

FIGURE 59-7 Scleroderma showing acral sclerosis and focal digital ulcers.

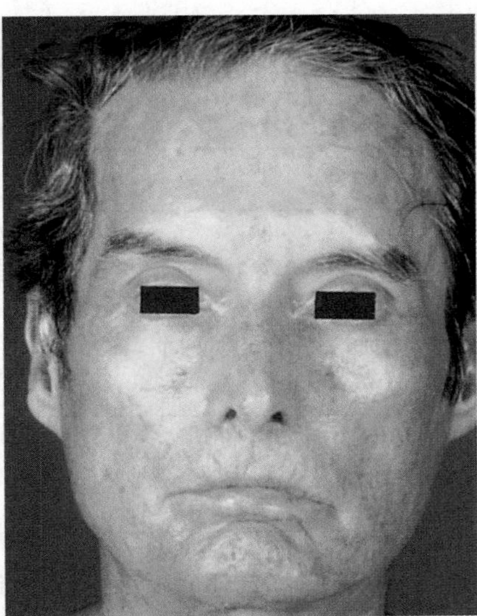

FIGURE 59-8 Scleroderma often eventuates in development of an expressionless, masklike facies.

cutaneous disease include emollients, antipruritics, and phototherapy (UVA1 [ultraviolet A1 irradiation] or PUVA [psoralens + ultraviolet A irradiation]). Treatment of systemic disease includes vascular modifying agents, immunosuppressives, and antifibrotics.

Morphea is characterized by localized thickening and sclerosis of skin; it dominates on the trunk. This disorder may affect children or adults. Morphea begins as erythematous or flesh-colored plaques that become sclerotic, develop central hypopigmentation, and have an erythematous border. In most cases, patients have one or a few lesions, and the disease is termed *circumscribed morphea*. In some patients, widespread cutaneous lesions may occur without systemic involvement (*generalized morphea*). Many adults with generalized morphea have concomitant rheumatic or other autoimmune disorders. Skin biopsy of morphea is generally indistinguishable from that of scleroderma. Scleroderma and morphea are usually quite resistant to therapy. For this reason, physical therapy to prevent joint contractures and to maintain function is employed and is often helpful. Treatment options for early, rapidly progressive disease include phototherapy (UVA1 or PUVA) or methotrexate alone or in combination with daily glucocorticoids.

Diffuse fasciitis with eosinophilia is a clinical entity that can sometimes be confused with scleroderma. There is usually a sudden onset of swelling, induration, and erythema of the extremities, frequently following significant physical exertion, initiation of hemodialysis, exposure to certain medications, or other triggers. The proximal portions of the extremities (upper arms, forearms, thighs, calves) are more often involved than are the hands and feet. While the skin is indurated, it usually displays a woody, dimpled, or "pseudocellulite" appearance rather than being bound down as in scleroderma; contractures may occur early secondary to fascial involvement. The latter may also cause muscle groups to be separated and veins to appear depressed (i.e., the "groove sign"). These skin findings are accompanied by peripheral-blood eosinophilia, increased erythrocyte sedimentation rate, and sometimes hypergammaglobulinemia. Deep biopsy of affected areas of skin reveals inflammation and thickening of the deep fascia overlying muscle. An inflammatory infiltrate composed of eosinophils and mononuclear cells is usually found. Patients with eosinophilic fasciitis appear to be at increased risk for developing bone marrow failure or other hematologic abnormalities. While the ultimate course of eosinophilic fasciitis is variable, most patients respond favorably to treatment with prednisone. Relapses may occur and require treatment with prednisone in combination with other immunosuppressive or immunomodulatory agents.

The *eosinophilia-myalgia syndrome*, a disorder with epidemic numbers of cases reported in 1989 and linked to ingestion of L-tryptophan manufactured by a single company in Japan, is a multisystem disorder characterized by debilitating myalgias and absolute eosinophilia in association with varying combinations of arthralgias, pulmonary symptoms, and peripheral edema. In a later phase (3–6 months after initial symptoms), these patients often develop localized sclerodermatous skin changes, weight loss, and/or neuropathy (**Chap. 360**).

FURTHER READING

Bolognia JL et al (eds): *Dermatology*, 4th ed. Philadelphia, Elsevier, 2018.

Hammers CM, Stanley JR: Mechanisms of disease: Pemphigus and bullous pemphigoid. Annu Rev Pathol 11:175, 2016.

Kang S et al (eds): *Fitzpatrick's Dermatology in General Medicine*, 9th ed. New York, McGraw-Hill, 2019.

Schmidt E, Zillikens D: Pemphigoid diseases. Lancet 381:320, 2013.

60 Cutaneous Drug Reactions

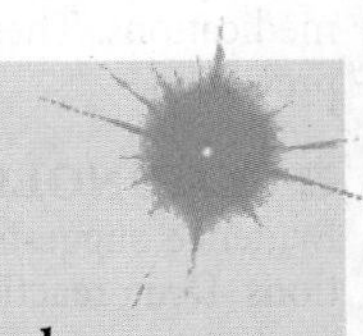

Robert G. Micheletti, Misha Rosenbach, Bruce U. Wintroub, Kanade Shinkai

Cutaneous reactions are the most frequent adverse reactions to medications, representing 10–15% of reported adverse drug reactions. Most are benign, but a few can be life threatening. Prompt recognition of severe reactions, drug withdrawal, and appropriate therapeutic interventions can minimize toxicity. This chapter focuses on adverse cutaneous reactions to systemic medications; it covers their incidence, patterns, and pathogenesis, and provides some practical guidelines on treatment, assessment of causality, and future use of drugs.

USE OF PRESCRIPTION DRUGS IN THE UNITED STATES

In the United States, more than 4 billion prescriptions for >60,000 drug products are dispensed annually. Hospital inpatients alone annually receive about 120 million courses of drug therapy, and half of adult Americans receive prescription drugs on a regular outpatient basis. Adverse effects of a prescription medication may result in 4.5 million urgent or emergency care visits and over 7000 deaths each year in the United States. Many patients use over-the-counter medicines that may cause adverse cutaneous reactions.

INCIDENCE OF CUTANEOUS REACTIONS

Several recent prospective studies reported that acute cutaneous reactions to drugs affect between 2.2 and 10 per 1000 hospitalized patients. Reactions usually occur a few days to 4 weeks after initiation of therapy.

In a series of 48,005 inpatients over a 20-year period, morbilliform rash (91%) and urticaria (6%) were the most frequent skin reactions, and antimicrobials, radiocontrast, and nonsteroidal anti-inflammatory drugs (NSAIDs) were the most common drug associations. Severe hypersensitivity reactions to medications have been reported to occur in between 1 in 1000 to 2 per million users, depending on the reaction type. Although rare, severe cutaneous reactions to drugs have an important impact on health because of significant sequelae; in addition, they may require hospitalization, increase the duration of hospital stay, or be life threatening. Some populations are at increased risk of drug reactions, including elderly patients, patients with autoimmune disease, hematopoietic stem cell transplant recipients, and those with acute Epstein-Barr virus (EBV) or human immunodeficiency virus (HIV) infection. The pathophysiology underlying this association is unknown but may be related to immune dysregulation. Individuals with advanced HIV disease (e.g., CD4 T lymphocyte count <200 cells/μL) have a 40- to 50-fold increased risk of adverse reactions to sulfamethoxazole (**Chap. 202**) and increased risk of severe hypersensitivity reactions.

In addition to acute eruptions, a variety of skin diseases can be induced or exacerbated by prolonged use of drugs (e.g., pruritus, pigmentation, nail or hair disorders, psoriasis, bullous pemphigoid, photosensitivity, and even cutaneous neoplasms). These drug reactions are not frequent; however, neither their incidence nor their impact on public health has been evaluated.

PATHOGENESIS OF DRUG REACTIONS

Adverse cutaneous responses to drugs can arise as a result of immunologic or nonimmunologic mechanisms.

■ NONIMMUNOLOGIC DRUG REACTIONS

Examples of nonimmunologic drug reactions are pigmentary changes due to dermal accumulation of medications or their metabolites, alteration of hair follicles by antimetabolites and signaling inhibitors, and lipodystrophy associated with metabolic effects of anti-HIV medications. These side effects are predictable and sometimes can be prevented.

■ IMMUNOLOGIC DRUG REACTIONS

Evidence suggests an immunologic basis for most acute drug eruptions. Drug reactions may result from immediate release of preformed mediators (e.g., urticaria, anaphylaxis), antibody-mediated reactions, immune complex deposition, and antigen-specific responses. Drug-specific CD4+ and CD8+ T-cell clones can be derived from the blood or from skin lesions of patients with a variety of drug allergies, strongly suggesting that these T cells mediate drug allergy in an antigen-specific manner. Drug presentation to T cells is major histocompatibility complex (MHC)-restricted and likely involves drug-peptide complex recognition by specific T-cell receptors (TCRs).

Once a drug has induced an immune response, the phenotype of the reaction is determined by the nature of effectors: cytotoxic (CD8+) T cells in blistering and certain hypersensitivity reactions, chemokines for reactions mediated by neutrophils or eosinophils, and B cell collaboration for production of specific antibodies for urticarial reactions. Immunologic reactions have recently been classified into further subtypes that provide a useful framework for designating adverse drug reactions based on involvement of specific immune pathways **(Table 60-1)**.

TABLE 60-1 Classification of Adverse Drug Reactions Based on Immune Pathway

TYPE	KEY PATHWAY	KEY IMMUNE MEDIATORS	ADVERSE DRUG REACTION TYPE
Type I	IgE	IgE	Urticaria, angioedema, anaphylaxis
Type II	IgG-mediated cytotoxicity	IgG	Drug-induced hemolysis, thrombocytopenia (e.g., penicillin)
Type III	Immune complex	IgG + antigen	Vasculitis, serum sickness, drug-induced lupus
Type IVa	T lymphocyte–mediated macrophage inflammation	IFN-γ, TNF-α T_H1 cells	Tuberculin skin test, contact dermatitis
Type IVb	T lymphocyte–mediated eosinophil inflammation	IL-4, IL-5, IL-13 T_H2 cells Eosinophils	DIHS Morbilliform eruption
Type IVc	T lymphocyte–mediated cytotoxic T lymphocyte inflammation	Cytotoxic T lymphocytes Granzyme Perforin Granulysin (SJS/TEN] only)	SJS/TEN Morbilliform eruption
Type IVd	T lymphocyte–mediated neutrophil inflammation	CXCL8, IL-17, GM-CSF Neutrophils	AGEP

Abbreviations: AGEP, acute generalized exanthematous pustulosis; DIHS, drug-induced hypersensitivity syndrome; GM-CSF, granulocyte-macrophage colony-stimulating factor; IFN, interferon; IL, interleukin; SJS, Stevens-Johnson syndrome; TEN, toxic epidermal necrolysis; TNF, tumor necrosis factor.

Immediate Reactions Immediate reactions depend on the release of mediators of inflammation by tissue mast cells or circulating basophils. These mediators include histamine, leukotrienes, prostaglandins, bradykinins, platelet-activating factor, enzymes, and proteoglycans. Drugs can trigger mediator release either directly ("anaphylactoid" reaction) or through IgE-specific antibodies. These reactions usually manifest in the skin and gastrointestinal, respiratory, and cardiovascular systems **(Chap. 353)**. Primary symptoms and signs include pruritus, urticaria, nausea, vomiting, abdominal cramps, bronchospasm, laryngeal edema, and, occasionally, anaphylactic shock with hypotension and death. They occur within minutes of drug exposure. NSAIDs, including aspirin, and radiocontrast media are frequent causes of direct mast cell degranulation or anaphylactoid reactions, which can occur on first exposure. Penicillins and muscle relaxants used in general anesthesia are the most frequent causes of IgE-dependent reactions to drugs, which require prior sensitization. Release of mediators is triggered when polyvalent drug protein conjugates cross-link IgE molecules fixed to sensitized cells. Certain routes of administration favor different clinical patterns (e.g., gastrointestinal effects from oral route, circulatory effects from intravenous route).

Immune Complex–Dependent Reactions Serum sickness is produced by tissue deposition of circulating immune complexes with consumption of complement. It is characterized by fever, arthritis, nephritis, neuritis, edema, and an urticarial, papular, or purpuric rash **(Chap. 363)**. First described following administration of nonhuman sera, it currently occurs in the setting of monoclonal antibodies and similar medications. In classic serum sickness, symptoms develop 6 or more days after drug exposure, the latent period representing the time needed to synthesize antibody. Vasculitis, a relatively rare complication of drugs, may also be a result of immune complex deposition **(Chap. 363)**. Penicillin, cefaclor, amoxicillin, trimethoprim/sulfamethoxazole, and monoclonal antibodies such as infliximab, rituximab, and omalizumab may be associated with clinically similar "serum sickness–like" reactions (SSLR). The mechanism of this reaction is unknown but is unrelated to immune complex formation and complement activation, and systemic involvement is rare. Whereas serum sickness most commonly occurs in adults, SSLR is more frequently observed in children.

Delayed Hypersensitivity While not completely understood, delayed hypersensitivity directed by drug-specific T cells is an important mechanism underlying the most common drug eruptions, that is, morbilliform eruptions, and also rare and severe forms such as drug-induced hypersensitivity syndrome (DIHS) (also known as drug rash with eosinophilia and systemic symptoms [DRESS]), acute generalized exanthematous pustulosis (AGEP), Stevens-Johnson syndrome (SJS), and toxic epidermal necrolysis (TEN) (Table 60-1). Drug-specific T cells have been detected in these types of drug eruptions. In TEN, skin lesions contain T lymphocytes reactive to autologous lymphocytes and keratinocytes in a drug-specific, human leukocyte antigen (HLA)-restricted, and perforin/granzyme-mediated pathway. In the case of carbamazepine, studies have identified cytotoxic T lymphocytes (CTLs) reactive to carbamazepine that use highly restricted V-alpha and V-beta TCR repertoires in patients with carbamazepine hypersensitivity that are not found in carbamazepine-tolerant individuals.

The mechanism(s) by which medications result in T-cell activation is unknown. Two hypotheses prevail: first, that the antigens driving these reactions may be the native drug itself or components of the drug covalently complexed with endogenous proteins, presented in association with HLA molecules to T cells through the classic antigen presentation pathway or, alternatively, through direct interaction of the drug/metabolite with the TCR or peptide-loaded HLA (e.g., the pharmacologic interaction of drugs with immune receptors, or p-i hypothesis). Recent x-ray crystallography data characterizing binding between specific HLA molecules to drugs known to cause hypersensitivity reactions demonstrate unique alterations to the MHC peptide-binding groove, suggesting a molecular basis for T-cell activation in the development of hypersensitivity reactions.

GENETIC FACTORS AND CUTANEOUS DRUG REACTIONS

Genetic determinants may predispose individuals to severe drug reactions by affecting either drug metabolism or immune responses to drugs. Polymorphisms in cytochrome P450 enzymes, drug acetylation, methylation (such as thiopurine methyltransferase activity and azathioprine), and other forms of metabolism (such as glucose-6-phosphate dehydrogenase and dapsone) may increase susceptibility to drug toxicity or underdosing and increase risk for medication interactions, highlighting a role for differential pharmacokinetic or pharmacodynamic effects. The value of routine screening of P450 enzymes for prediction of cutaneous reactions has not been determined, though its cost-effectiveness in certain populations (e.g., patients with seizure disorder, depression) as well as patients considering specific therapies (e.g., tamoxifen, warfarin) has been suggested.

Associations between drug hypersensitivities and HLA haplotypes suggest a key role for immune mechanisms, especially those leading to skin involvement. Hypersensitivity to the anti-HIV medication abacavir is strongly associated with HLA-B*57:01 **(Chap. 202)**. In Taiwan, within a homogeneous Han Chinese population, a strong association was observed between SJS/TEN (but not DIHS) related to carbamazepine and HLA-B*15:02. In the same population, a strong association was found between HLA-B*58:01 and SJS, TEN, or DIHS related to allopurinol. These associations are drug and phenotype specific; that is, HLA-specific T cell stimulation by medications leads to distinct reactions. However, while this genetic association is strong, it is not sufficient to cause severe drug hypersensitivity reactions.

GLOBAL CONSIDERATIONS

Recognition of HLA associations with drug hypersensitivity has resulted in recommendations to screen high-risk populations. Genetic screening for HLA-B*57:01 to prevent abacavir hypersensitivity, which carries a 100% negative predictive value when patch test confirmed and 55% positive predictive value generalizable across races, is becoming the clinical standard of care worldwide (number needed to treat = 13). The U.S. Food and Drug Administration has recommended HLA-B*15:02 screening of Asian individuals prior to a new prescription of carbamazepine. The American College of Rheumatology has recommended HLA-B*58:01 screening of Han Chinese patients prescribed allopurinol. To date, screening for a single HLA (but not multiple HLA haplotypes) in specific populations has been determined to be cost-effective (e.g., HLA-B*1301 screening in Chinese patients with leprosy treated with dapsone). Genetic testing for specific HLA haplotypes and functional screening for TCR repertoire to identify patients at risk is becoming more widely available and heralds the era of personalized medicine and pharmacogenomics.

CLINICAL PRESENTATION OF CUTANEOUS DRUG REACTIONS

NONIMMUNE CUTANEOUS REACTIONS

Exacerbation or Induction of Dermatologic Diseases A variety of drugs can exacerbate preexisting diseases or induce—or unmask—a disease that may or may not disappear after withdrawal of the inducing medication. For example, NSAIDs, lithium, beta blockers, tumor necrosis factor (TNF) antagonists, interferon (IFN) α, and angiotensin-converting enzyme (ACE) inhibitors can exacerbate plaque psoriasis, whereas antimalarials and withdrawal of systemic glucocorticoids can worsen pustular psoriasis. The situation of TNF-α inhibitors is unusual, as this class of medications is used to treat psoriasis; however, they may induce psoriasis (especially palmoplantar) in patients being treated for other conditions. Acne may be induced by glucocorticoids, androgens, lithium, and antidepressants. Follicular papular or pustular eruptions of the face and trunk resembling acne frequently occur with epidermal growth factor receptor (EGFR) antagonists, mitogen-activated protein kinase (MEK) inhibitors, and other targeted inhibitors. With EGFR antagonists, the severity of the eruption correlates with a better anticancer effect. This rash is typically responsive to and prevented by tetracycline antibiotics.

Several medications induce or exacerbate autoimmune disease. Checkpoint inhibitors induce a wide array of systemic autoimmune reactions, including in skin. Interleukin (IL) 2, IFN-α, and anti-TNF-α are associated with new-onset systemic lupus erythematosus (SLE). Drug-induced lupus is classically marked by antinuclear and antihistone antibodies and, in some cases, anti-double-stranded DNA (D-penicillamine, anti-TNF-α) or perinuclear antineutrophil cytoplasmic antibodies (p-ANCA) (minocycline). Subacute cutaneous lupus erythematosus (SCLE) can be induced by a growing list of drugs, including thiazide diuretics, proton pump inhibitors, TNF inhibitors, terbinafine, and minocycline. Drug-induced dermatomyositis may rarely occur with TNF inhibitors or capecitabine; hydroxyurea can induce skin findings of dermatomyositis. IFN and TNF inhibitors, as well as checkpoint inhibitors, can induce granulomatous disease and sarcoidosis. Autoimmune blistering diseases may be drug induced as well: pemphigus by D-penicillamine and ACE inhibitors; bullous pemphigoid by DPP4 inhibitors, furosemide, and PD-1 inhibitors; and linear IgA bullous dermatosis by vancomycin. Other medications may cause highly specific cutaneous reactions. Gadolinium contrast has been associated with nephrogenic systemic fibrosis, a condition of sclerosing skin with rare internal organ involvement; advanced renal compromise may be an important risk factor. Granulocyte colony-stimulating factor, azacitidine, all-*trans*-retinoic acid, the *FLT3* inhibitor class of drugs, and rarely levamisole-contaminated cocaine may induce neutrophilic dermatoses. In this setting, the hypothesis that a drug may be responsible should always be considered, even after the treatment is complete. In addition, reactions may develop in cases of long-term medication therapy due to changes in dosing or host metabolism. Resolution of the cutaneous reaction may be delayed upon discontinuation of the medication.

Photosensitivity Eruptions Photosensitivity eruptions are usually most marked in sun-exposed areas, but they may extend to sun-protected areas. The mechanism is almost always phototoxicity. Phototoxic reactions resemble sunburn and can occur with first exposure to a drug. Blistering may occur in drug-related pseudoporphyria, most commonly with NSAIDs. The severity of the reaction depends on the tissue level of the drug, its efficiency as a photosensitizer, and the extent of exposure to the activating wavelengths of ultraviolet (UV) light **(Chap. 61)**.

Common orally administered photosensitizing drugs include fluoroquinolones, tetracycline antibiotics, and trimethoprim/sulfamethoxazole. Other drugs less frequently implicated are chlorpromazine, thiazides, NSAIDs, and BRAF inhibitors. Voriconazole may result in severe photosensitivity, accelerated photoaging, and cutaneous carcinogenesis.

Because UV-A and visible light, which trigger these reactions, are not easily absorbed by nonopaque sunscreens and are transmitted through window glass, photosensitivity reactions may be difficult to block. Photosensitivity reactions abate with removal of either the drug or UV radiation, use of sunscreens that block UV-A light, and treatment of the reaction as one would a sunburn. Rarely, individuals develop persistent reactivity to light, necessitating long-term avoidance of sun exposure. Some chemotherapeutic agents, such as methotrexate, can induce a UV-recall reaction characterized by an erythematous, slightly scaly eruption at sites of prior severe sun exposure.

Pigmentation Changes Drugs, either systemic or topical, may cause a variety of pigmentary changes in the skin by triggering melanocyte production of melanin (as in the case of oral contraceptives causing melasma) or due to deposition of drug or drug metabolites. Long-term minocycline and amiodarone may cause blue-gray pigmentation. Phenothiazine, gold, and bismuth result in gray-brown pigmentation of sun-exposed areas. Numerous cancer chemotherapeutic agents

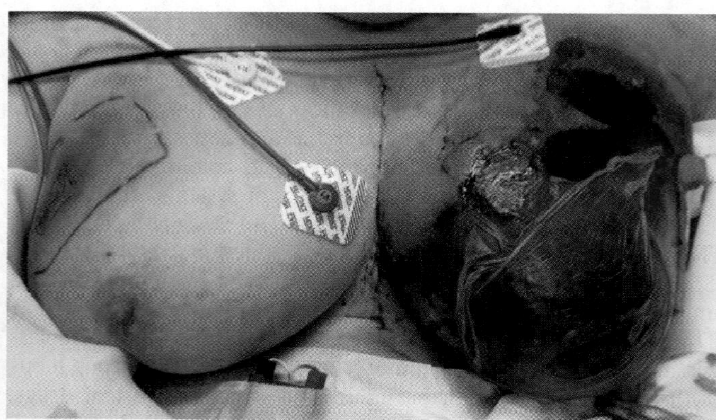

FIGURE 60-1 Warfarin necrosis involving the breasts.

may be associated with characteristic patterns of pigmentation (e.g., bleomycin, busulfan, daunorubicin, cyclophosphamide, hydroxyurea, fluorouracil, and methotrexate). Clofazimine causes a drug-induced lipofuscinosis with characteristic red-brown coloration. Hyperpigmentation of the face, mucous membranes, and pretibial and subungual areas occurs with antimalarials. Quinacrine causes generalized yellow discoloration. Pigmentation changes may also occur in mucous membranes (busulfan, bismuth), conjunctiva (chlorpromazine, thioridazine, imipramine, clomipramine), nails (zidovudine, doxorubicin, cyclophosphamide, bleomycin, fluorouracil, hydroxyurea), hair, and teeth (tetracyclines).

Warfarin Necrosis of Skin This rare reaction (0.01–0.1%) usually occurs between the third and tenth days of therapy with warfarin, usually in women. Common sites are breasts, thighs, and buttocks (**Fig. 60-1**). Lesions are sharply demarcated, erythematous, or purpuric, and may progress to form large, hemorrhagic bullae with necrosis and eschar formation.

Warfarin anticoagulation in protein C or S deficiency causes an additional reduction in already low circulating levels of endogenous anticoagulants, permitting hypercoagulability and thrombosis in the cutaneous microvasculature, with consequent areas of necrosis. Heparin-induced necrosis may have clinically similar features but is probably due to heparin-induced platelet aggregation with subsequent occlusion of blood vessels; it can affect areas adjacent to the injection site or more distant sites if infused. Levamisole-tainted cocaine (and more recently, heroin) can induce similar skin necrosis; however, the distribution tends to involve the ears and cheeks predominantly, with stellate or retiform purpura. Patients may have abnormal white blood cell counts and may be dual P- and C-ANCA positive.

Drug-Induced Hair Disorders • DRUG-INDUCED HAIR LOSS Medications may affect hair follicles at two different phases of their growth cycle: anagen (growth) or telogen (resting). *Anagen effluvium* occurs within days of drug administration, especially with antimetabolite or other chemotherapeutic drugs. In contrast, in *telogen effluvium*, the delay is 2–4 months following initiation of a new medication. Both present as diffuse, nonscarring alopecia most often reversible after discontinuation of the responsible agent.

A considerable number of drugs have been associated with hair loss. These include antineoplastic agents (alkylating agents, bleomycin, vinca alkaloids, platinum compounds), anticonvulsants (carbamazepine, valproate), beta blockers, antidepressants, antithyroid drugs, IFNs, oral contraceptives, and cholesterol-lowering agents.

DRUG-INDUCED HAIR GROWTH Medications may also cause hair growth. Hirsutism is an excessive growth of terminal hair with masculine hair growth pattern in a female, most often on the face and trunk, due to androgenic stimulation of hormone-sensitive hair follicles (anabolic steroids, oral contraceptives, testosterone, corticotropin). Hypertrichosis is a distinct pattern of hair growth, not in a masculine pattern, typically located on the forehead and temporal regions of the face. Drugs responsible for hypertrichosis include anti-inflammatory drugs, glucocorticoids, vasodilators (diazoxide, minoxidil), diuretics (acetazolamide), anticonvulsants (phenytoin), immunosuppressive agents (cyclosporine A), psoralens, and zidovudine.

Changes in hair color or structure are uncommon adverse effects from medications. Hair discoloration may occur with chloroquine, IFN-α, chemotherapeutic agents, and tyrosine kinase inhibitors. Changes in hair structure have been observed in patients given EGFR inhibitors, BRAF inhibitors, tyrosine kinase inhibitors, and acitretin.

Drug-Induced Nail Disorders Drug-related nail disorders usually involve all 20 nails and need months to resolve after withdrawal of the medication. The pathogenesis is most often toxic. Drug-induced nail changes include Beau's line (transverse depression of the nail plate), onycholysis (detachment of the distal part of the nail plate), onychomadesis (detachment of the proximal part of the nail plate), pigmentation, and paronychia (inflammation of periungual skin).

ONYCHOLYSIS Onycholysis occurs with tetracyclines, fluoroquinolones, retinoids, NSAIDs, and others, including many chemotherapeutic agents, and may be triggered by exposure to sunlight.

ONYCHOMADESIS Onychomadesis is caused by temporary arrest of nail matrix mitotic activity. Common drugs reported to induce onychomadesis include carbamazepine, lithium, retinoids, and chemotherapeutic agents such as taxanes.

PARONYCHIA Paronychia and multiple pyogenic granulomas with progressive and painful periungual abscess of fingers and toes are side effects of systemic retinoids, lamivudine, indinavir, and anti-EGFR monoclonal antibodies.

NAIL DISCOLORATION Some drugs—including anthracyclines, taxanes, fluorouracil, psoralens, and zidovudine—may induce nail bed hyperpigmentation through melanocyte stimulation. It appears to be reversible and dose dependent.

Toxic Erythema of Chemotherapy and Other Chemotherapy Reactions Because many agents used in cancer chemotherapy inhibit cell division, rapidly proliferating elements of the skin, including hair, mucous membranes, and appendages, are sensitive to their effects. A broad spectrum of chemotherapy-related skin toxicities has been reported, including neutrophilic eccrine hidradenitis, sterile cellulitis, exfoliative dermatitis, and flexural erythema; recent nomenclature classifies these under the unifying diagnosis of toxic erythema of chemotherapy (TEC) (**Fig. 60-2**). Acral erythema is marked by dysesthesia and an erythematous, edematous eruption of the palms and soles. Common causes include cytarabine, doxorubicin, methotrexate, hydroxyurea, fluorouracil, and capecitabine.

The recent introduction of many new monoclonal antibody and small molecular signaling inhibitors for the treatment of cancer has been accompanied by numerous reports of skin and hair toxicity; only the most common of these are mentioned here. EGFR antagonists induce follicular eruptions and nail toxicity after a mean interval of 10 days in a majority of patients. Xerosis, eczematous eruptions, acneiform eruptions, and pruritus are common. Erlotinib is associated with marked hair textural changes. Sorafenib, a tyrosine kinase inhibitor, may result in follicular eruptions and focal bullous eruptions at palmoplantar, flexural sites or areas of frictional pressure. BRAF inhibitors are associated with photosensitivity, palmoplantar hyperkeratosis, hair curling, dyskeratotic (Grover's-like) rash, hyperkeratotic benign cutaneous neoplasms, and keratoacanthoma-like squamous cell carcinomas. Rash, pruritus, and vitiliginous depigmentation have been reported in association with ipilimumab (anti-CTLA4) treatment. Up to 50% of patients experience immune-mediated skin eruptions, including granulomatous reactions, dermatomyositis, panniculitis, and vasculitis. The checkpoint inhibitor class of drugs (including anti-CTLA4, anti-PD-1, and anti-PD-L1 agents) can induce a wide range of cutaneous eruptions beyond vitiligo, including lichenoid, eczematous, granulomatous, papulosquamous, and panniculitis eruptions.

IMMUNE CUTANEOUS REACTIONS: COMMON

Maculopapular Eruptions Morbilliform or maculopapular eruptions (**Fig. 60-3**) are the most common of all drug-induced reactions,

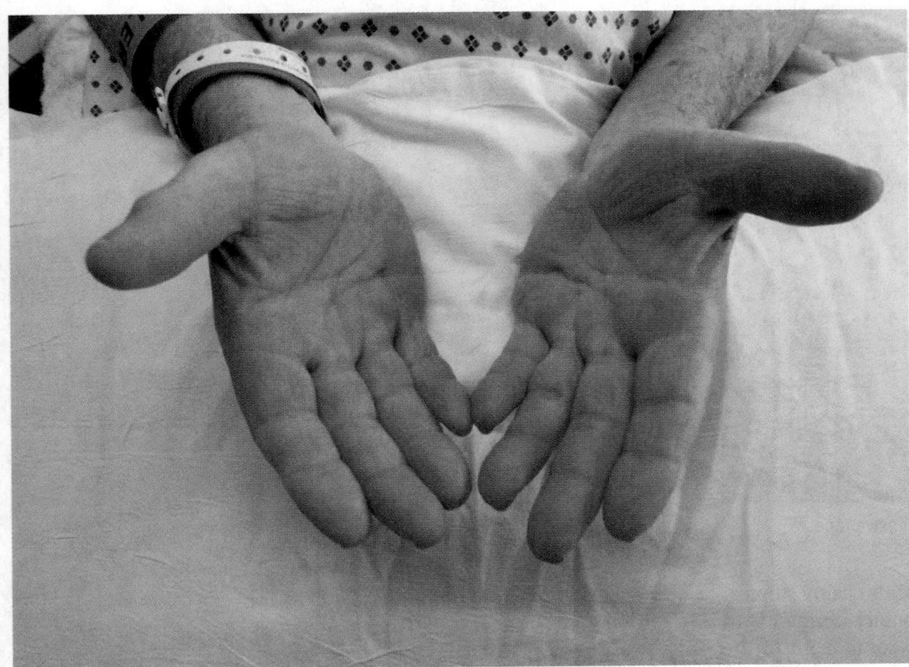

FIGURE 60-2 Toxic erythema of chemotherapy.

often start on the trunk or intertriginous areas, and consist of blanching erythematous macules and papules that are symmetric and confluent. Nonblanching, dusky, or bright-red macules as well as mucosal involvement should raise concern for a more severe reaction. Facial involvement in morbilliform eruptions is also uncommon, and the presence of extensive facial lesions with facial edema suggests DIHS. Diagnosis of morbilliform eruptions is rarely assisted by laboratory testing or skin biopsy.

Morbilliform eruptions may be associated with moderate to severe pruritus and fever. A viral exanthem is another differential diagnostic consideration, especially in children, and graft-versus-host disease is also a consideration in the proper clinical setting. Absence of enanthems; absence of ear, nose, throat, and upper respiratory tract symptoms; and polymorphism of the skin lesions support a drug rather than a viral eruption. Common offenders include aminopenicillins, cephalosporins, antibacterial sulfonamides, allopurinol, and antiepileptic drugs. Beta blockers, calcium channel blockers, and ACE inhibitors are rarely the culprit; however, any drug can cause a morbilliform exanthem. Certain medications carry very high rates of morbilliform eruption, including nevirapine and lamotrigine, even in the absence of DIHS reactions. Lamotrigine morbilliform rash is associated with higher starting doses, rapid dose escalation, concomitant use of valproate (which increases lamotrigine levels and half-life), and use in children.

Maculopapular reactions usually develop within 1 week of initiation of therapy and last less than 2 weeks. Occasionally, these eruptions resolve despite continued use of the responsible drug. Because the eruption may also worsen, the suspect drug should be discontinued unless it is essential. It is important to note that the rash may continue to progress for a few days up to 1 week following medication discontinuation. Oral antihistamines and emollients may help relieve pruritus. Short courses of potent topical glucocorticoids can reduce inflammation and symptoms. Systemic glucocorticoid treatment is rarely indicated.

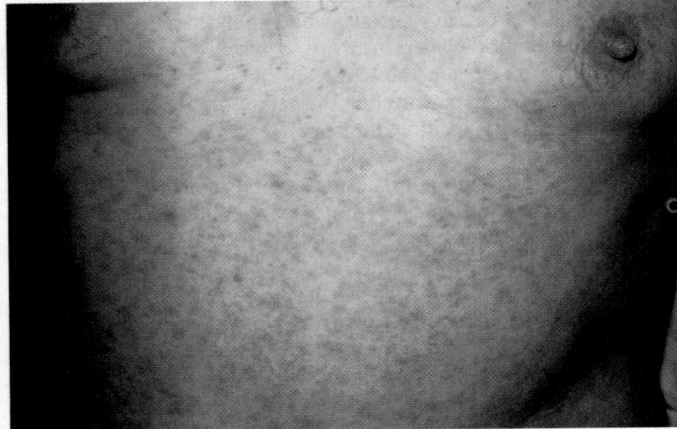

FIGURE 60-3 Morbilliform drug eruption.

Pruritus Pruritus is associated with almost all drug eruptions and, in some cases, may represent the only symptom of the adverse cutaneous reaction. It may be alleviated by antihistamines such as hydroxyzine or diphenhydramine. Pruritus stemming from specific medications may require distinct treatment, such as selective opiate antagonists for opiate-related pruritus.

Urticaria/Angioedema/Anaphylaxis Urticaria, the second most frequent type of cutaneous reaction to drugs, is characterized by pruritic, red wheals of varying size rarely lasting more than 24 hours. It has been observed in association with nearly all drugs, most frequently ACE inhibitors, aspirin, NSAIDs, penicillin, and blood products. However, medications account for no more than 10–20% of acute urticaria cases. Deep edema within dermal and subcutaneous tissues is known as angioedema and may involve respiratory and gastrointestinal mucous membranes. Urticaria and angioedema may be part of a life-threatening anaphylactic reaction.

Drug-induced urticaria may be caused by three mechanisms: an IgE-dependent mechanism, circulating immune complexes (serum sickness), and nonimmunologic activation of effector pathways. IgE-dependent urticarial reactions usually occur within 36 hours of drug exposure but can occur within minutes. Immune complex–induced urticaria associated with serum sickness reactions usually occurs 6–12 days after first exposure. In this syndrome, the urticarial eruption (typically polycyclic plaques over distal joints) may be accompanied by fever, hematuria, arthralgias, hepatic dysfunction, and neurologic symptoms. Certain drugs, such as NSAIDs, ACE inhibitors, angiotensin II antagonists, radiographic dye, and opiates, may induce urticarial reactions, angioedema, and anaphylaxis in the absence of drug-specific antibodies through direct mast-cell degranulation.

Radiocontrast agents are a common cause of urticaria and, in rare cases, can cause anaphylaxis. High-osmolality radiocontrast media are about five times more likely to induce urticaria (1%) or anaphylaxis than are newer low-osmolality media. About one-third of those with mild reactions to previous exposure react on reexposure. Pretreatment with prednisone and diphenhydramine reduces reaction rates.

The treatment of urticaria or angioedema depends on the severity of the reaction. In severe cases with respiratory or cardiovascular compromise, epinephrine and intravenous glucocorticoids are the mainstay of therapy. For patients with urticaria without symptoms of angioedema or anaphylaxis, drug withdrawal and oral antihistamines are usually sufficient. Future drug avoidance is recommended; rechallenge, especially in individuals with severe reactions, should only occur in an intensive care setting.

Anaphylactoid Reactions Vancomycin is associated with red man syndrome, a histamine-related anaphylactoid reaction characterized by flushing, diffuse maculopapular eruption, and hypotension. In rare cases, cardiac arrest may be associated with rapid intravenous (IV) infusion of the medication.

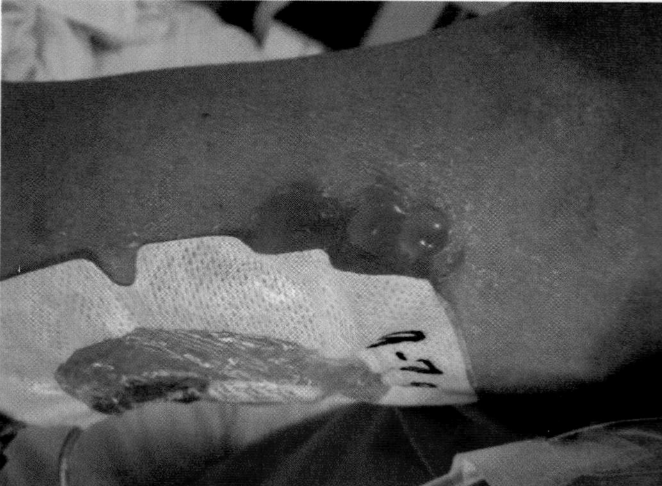

FIGURE 60-4 Allergic contact dermatitis (bullous) due to adhesive tape.

Irritant/Allergic Contact Dermatitis Patients using topical medications may develop an irritant or allergic contact dermatitis to the medication itself or to a preservative or other component of the formulation. Reactions to neomycin sulfate, bacitracin, and polymyxin B are common. Contact dermatitis may be seen to adhesive tapes, leading to irritation or blisters around ports and IV sites (Fig. 60-4). Harsh disinfectant skin cleansers may lead to localized irritant dermatitis.

Fixed Drug Eruptions These less common reactions are characterized by one or more sharply demarcated, dull red to brown lesions, sometimes with central dusky violaceous erythema and central bulla (Fig. 60-5). Hyperpigmentation often results after resolution of the acute inflammation. With rechallenge, the process recurs in the same (fixed) location but may spread to new areas as well. Lesions often involve the lips, hands, legs, face, genitalia, and oral mucosa, and cause a burning sensation. Most patients have multiple lesions. Fixed drug eruptions have been associated with pseudoephedrine (frequently a nonpigmenting reaction), phenolphthalein (in laxatives), sulfonamides, tetracyclines, NSAIDs, barbiturates, and others.

IMMUNE CUTANEOUS REACTIONS: RARE AND SEVERE

Drug-Induced Hypersensitivity Syndrome DIHS is a systemic drug reaction also known as DRESS (drug reaction with eosinophilia and systemic symptoms) syndrome; because eosinophilia is not always present, the term *DIHS* is preferred. Clinically, DIHS presents with a prodrome of fever and flu-like symptoms for several days, followed by the appearance of a diffuse morbilliform eruption, usually involving the face (Fig. 60-6). Facial swelling and hand/foot swelling are often present. Systemic manifestations include lymphadenopathy, fever, and leukocytosis (often with eosinophilia or atypical lymphocytosis), as well as hepatitis, nephritis, pneumonitis, myositis, and gastroenteritis, in descending order. Distinct patterns of timing of onset and organ involvement may exist. For example, allopurinol classically induces DIHS with renal involvement; cardiac and lung involvement are more common with minocycline; gastrointestinal involvement is almost exclusively seen with abacavir; and some medications typically do not induce eosinophilia (abacavir, dapsone, lamotrigine). The cutaneous reaction usually begins 2–8 weeks after the drug is started and persists after drug cessation. Signs and symptoms may continue for several weeks, especially those associated with hepatitis. The eruption recurs with rechallenge, and cross-reactions among aromatic anticonvulsants, including phenytoin, carbamazepine, and phenobarbital, are common. Other drugs causing DIHS include antibacterial sulfonamides and other antibiotics. Hypersensitivity to reactive drug metabolites, hydroxylamine for sulfamethoxazole and arene oxide for aromatic anticonvulsants, may be involved in the pathogenesis of DIHS. Recent research suggests that inciting drugs may reactivate quiescent human herpes viruses, including herpesviruses 6 and 7, EBV, and cytomegalovirus (CMV), resulting in expansion of viral-specific CD8+ T lymphocytes and subsequent end-organ damage. Viral reactivation may be associated with a worse clinical prognosis. Mortality rates as high as 10% have been reported, with most fatalities resulting from liver failure. Systemic glucocorticoids (1.5–2 mg/kg/d prednisone equivalent) should be started and tapered slowly over 8–12 weeks, during which time clinical symptoms and labs (including complete blood count with differential, basic metabolic panel, and liver function tests) should be followed carefully. A steroid-sparing agent such as mycophenolate mofetil, IV immunoglobulin, or cyclosporine may be indicated in cases of rapid recurrence upon steroid taper. In all cases, immediate

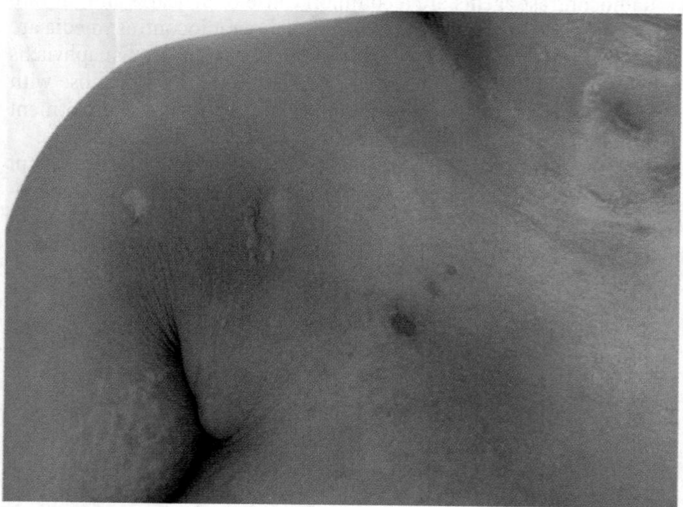

FIGURE 60-5 Fixed drug eruption.

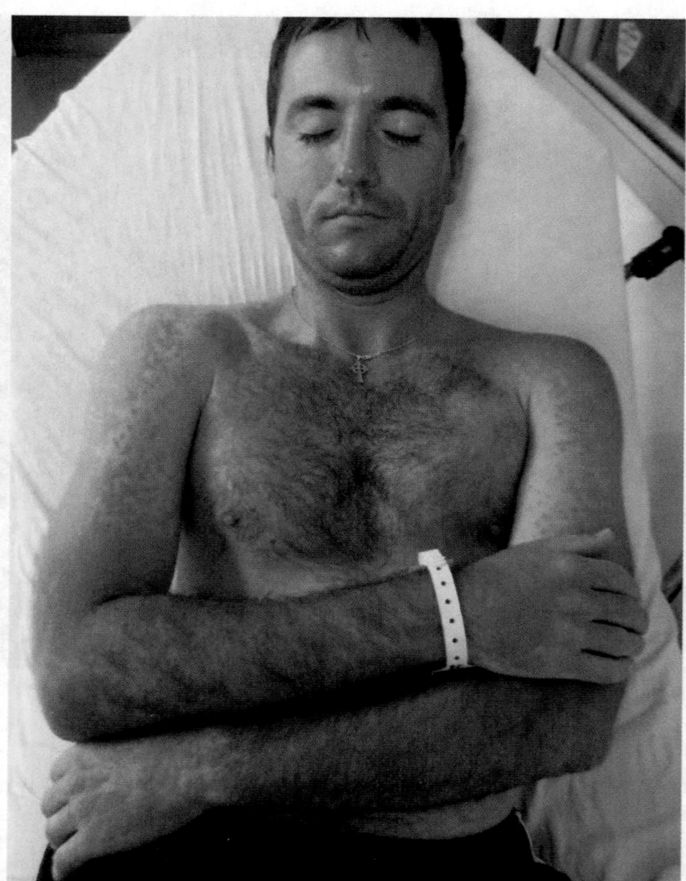

FIGURE 60-6 Drug-induced hypersensitivity syndrome/drug rash with eosinophilia and systemic symptoms (DIHS/DRESS). *(Courtesy of Gildo Micheletti, MD.)*

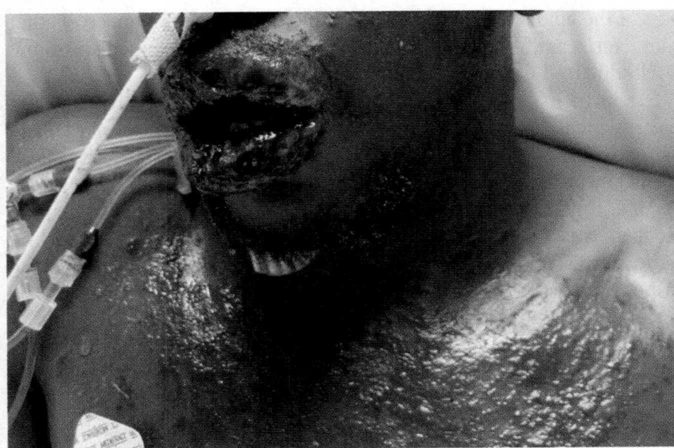

FIGURE 60-7 Stevens-Johnson syndrome (SJS).

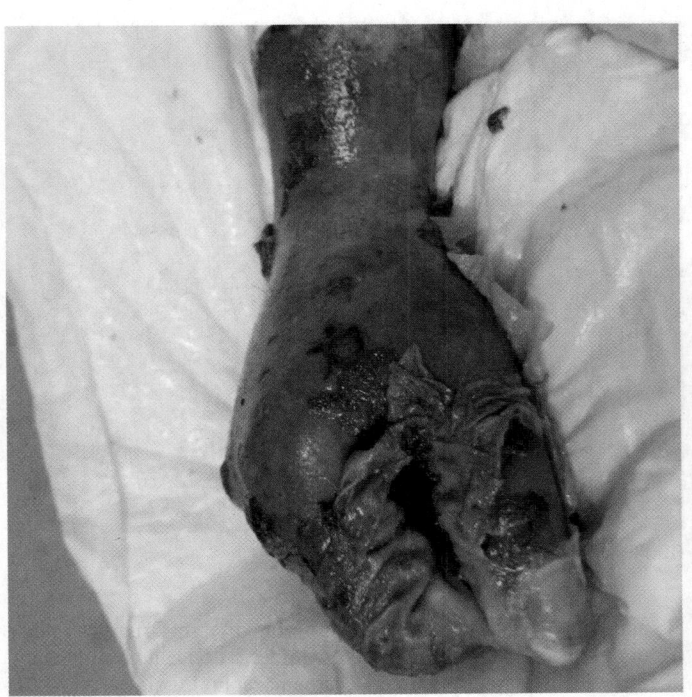

FIGURE 60-9 Toxic epidermal necrolysis, hand.

withdrawal of the suspected culprit drug is required. Given the severe long-term complications of myocarditis, patients should undergo cardiac evaluation in cases of severe DIHS or if heart involvement is suspected due to hypotension or arrhythmia. Patients should be closely monitored for resolution of organ dysfunction and for development of late-onset autoimmune thyroiditis and diabetes (up to 6 months).

Stevens-Johnson Syndrome and Toxic Epidermal Necrolysis

SJS and *TEN* are characterized by blisters and mucosal/epidermal detachment resulting from full-thickness epidermal necrosis in the absence of substantial dermal inflammation. The term *Stevens-Johnson syndrome* (SJS) describes cases in which the total body surface area of blistering and eventual detachment is <10% (Fig. 60-7). The term *Stevens-Johnson syndrome/toxic epidermal necrolysis (SJS/TEN) overlap* is used to describe cases with 10–30% epidermal detachment (Fig. 60-8), and the term *toxic epidermal necrolysis (TEN)* is used to describe cases with >30% detachment (Figs. 60-9 and 60-10).

Other blistering eruptions with concomitant mucositis may be confused with SJS/TEN. Erythema multiforme (EM) associated with herpes simplex virus is characterized by painful mucosal erosions and target lesions, typically with an acral distribution and limited skin detachment. *Mycoplasma* and other respiratory infections in children cause a clinically distinct presentation with prominent mucositis and limited cutaneous involvement. The term *reactive infectious mucocutaneous eruption (RIME)* has been proposed to help differentiate this clinical entity, which some believe may be the syndrome originally described by Stevens and Johnson.

Patients with SJS/TEN initially present with fever >39°C (102.2°F); sore throat; conjunctivitis; and acute onset of painful dusky, atypical, target-like lesions (Fig. 60-11). Intestinal and upper respiratory tract involvement are associated with a poor prognosis, as are older age and greater extent of epidermal detachment. At least 10% of those with

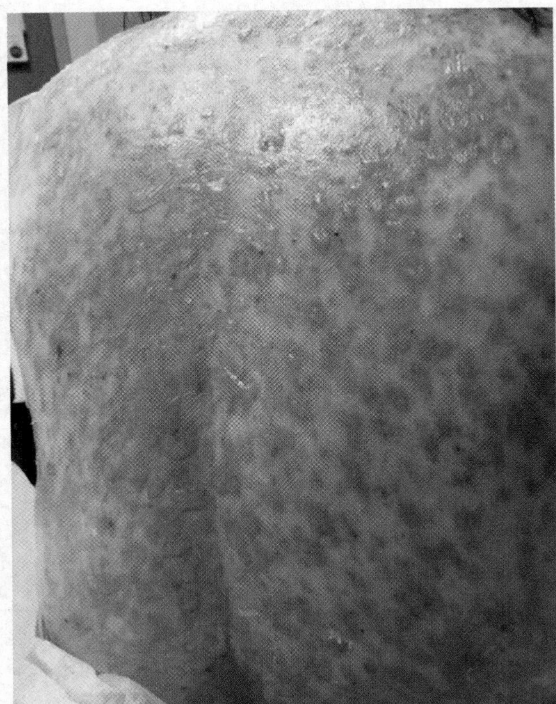

FIGURE 60-8 SJS-TEN overlap.

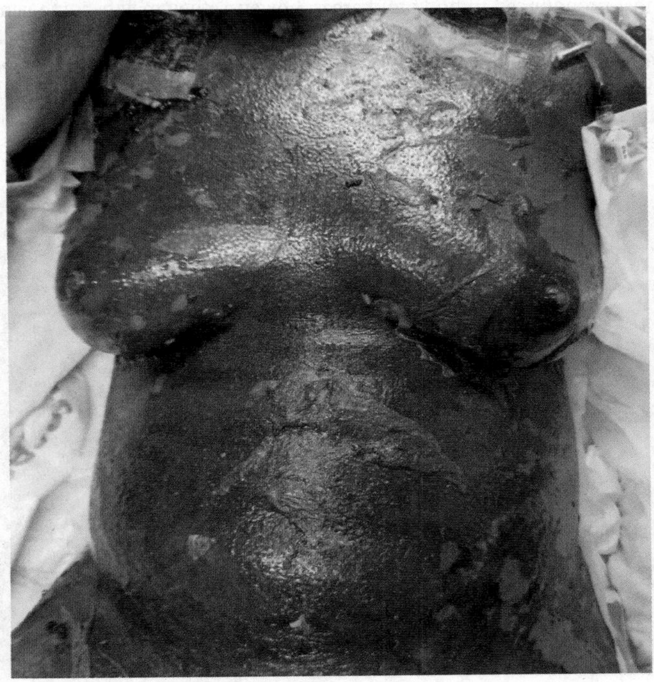

FIGURE 60-10 Toxic epidermal necrolysis.

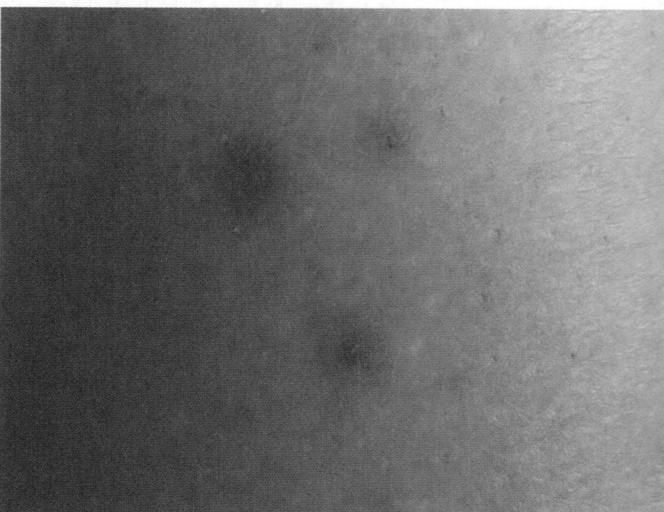

FIGURE 60-11 Target-like lesion in SJS.

SJS and 30% of those with TEN die from the disease. Drugs that most commonly cause SJS/TEN are sulfonamides, allopurinol, antiepileptics (e.g., lamotrigine, phenytoin, carbamazepine), oxicam NSAIDs, β-lactam and other antibiotics, and nevirapine. Frozen-section skin biopsy may aid in rapid diagnosis.

At this time, there is no consensus on the most effective treatment for SJS/TEN. The best outcomes stem from early diagnosis, immediate discontinuation of the suspected drug, and meticulous supportive therapy in an intensive care or burn unit. Fluid management, atraumatic wound care, infection prevention and treatment, and ophthalmologic and respiratory support are critical. Early administration of systemic glucocorticoids, intravenous immunoglobulin, cyclosporine, or etanercept may improve disease outcomes, but randomized studies to evaluate potential therapies are lacking and difficult to perform.

Pustular Eruptions AGEP is a rare reaction pattern affecting 3–5 people per million per year. It is thought to be secondary to medication exposure in >90% of cases (**Fig. 60-12**). Patients typically present with diffuse erythema or erythroderma, as well as high spiking fevers and leukocytosis with neutrophilia. One to two days later, innumerable pinpoint pustules develop overlying the erythema. The pustules are most pronounced in body fold areas; however, they may become generalized and, when coalescent, can lead to superficial erosion. In such cases, differentiating the eruption from SJS in its initial stages may be difficult, although in AGEP, any erosions tend to be more superficial, and prominent mucosal involvement is lacking. Skin biopsy shows collections of neutrophils and sparse necrotic keratinocytes in the upper part of the epidermis, unlike the full-thickness epidermal necrosis that characterizes SJS. Before the pustules appear, AGEP may also mimic DIHS due to the prominent fever and erythroderma.

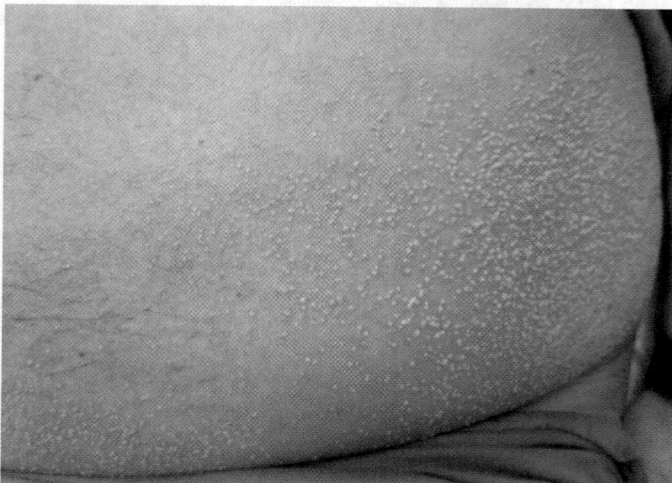

FIGURE 60-12 Acute generalized exanthematous pustulosis.

The principal differential diagnosis for AGEP is acute pustular psoriasis, which has an identical clinical and histologic appearance. Many patients with AGEP have a personal or family history of psoriasis. AGEP classically begins within 24–48 hours of drug exposure, although it may occur as much as 1–2 weeks later. β-Lactam antibiotics, calcium channel blockers, macrolide antibiotics, and other inciting agents (including radiocontrast and dialysates) have been reported. Patch testing with the responsible drug often results in a localized pustular eruption.

Overlap Hypersensitivity Syndromes An important concept in the clinical approach to severe drug eruptions is the presence of "overlap syndromes," most notably DIHS with TEN-like features, DIHS with pustular eruption (AGEP-like), and AGEP with TEN-like features. In several case series of AGEP, 50% of cases had TEN-like or DRESS-like features, and 20% of cases had mucosal involvement resembling SJS/TEN. In one study, up to 20% of all severe drug eruptions had overlap features, suggesting that AGEP, DIHS, and SJS/TEN represent a clinical spectrum with some common pathophysiologic mechanisms. Designation of a single diagnosis based on cutaneous and extracutaneous involvement may not always be possible in cases of hypersensitivity; in such instances, treatment should be geared toward addressing the dominant clinical features. The timing of rash onset with respect to drug administration, which is usually much more delayed in DIHS, and the presence of systemic manifestations such as hepatitis are helpful clues to that diagnosis.

Vasculitis Cutaneous small-vessel vasculitis (CSVV) typically presents with purpuric papules and macules involving the lower extremities and other dependent areas (**Fig. 60-13**) (**Chap. 363**). Pustular and hemorrhagic vesicles as well as rounded ulcers also occur. Importantly, vasculitis may involve other organs, including the kidneys,

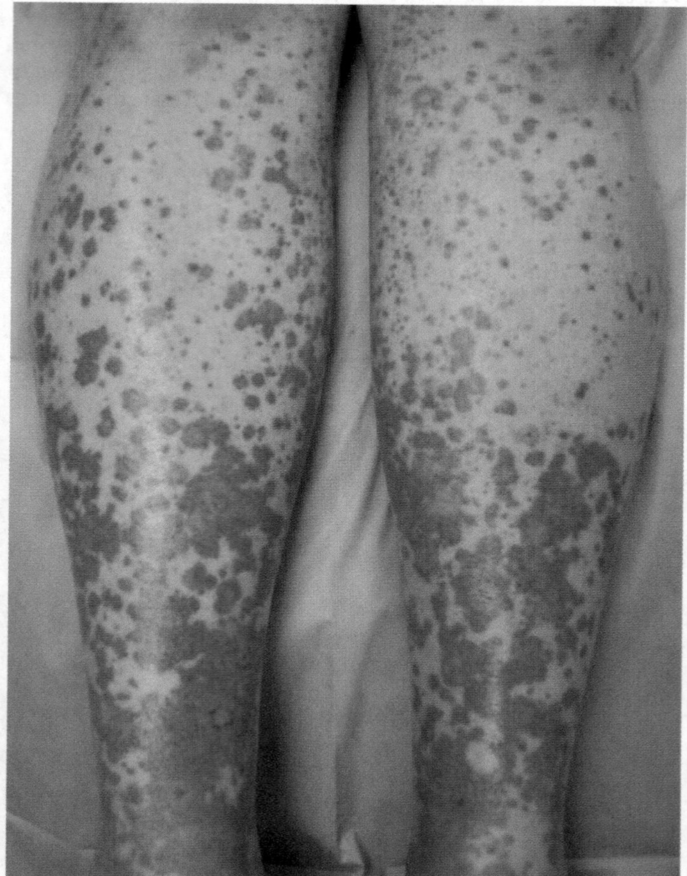

FIGURE 60-13 Cutaneous small-vessel vasculitis (CSVV, leukocytoclastic vasculitis).

joints, gastrointestinal tract, and lungs, necessitating a thorough clinical evaluation for systemic involvement. Drugs are implicated as a cause of roughly 15% of all cases of small-vessel vasculitis. Antibiotics, particularly β-lactams, are commonly implicated; however, almost any drug can cause vasculitis. Vasculitis may also be idiopathic or due to underlying infection, connective tissue disease, or (rarely) malignancy.

Rare but important types of drug-induced vasculitis include drug-induced ANCA vasculitis. Such patients commonly present with cutaneous manifestations but can develop the full range of symptoms associated with ANCA-associated vasculitis, including crescentic glomerulonephritis and alveolar hemorrhage. Propylthiouracil, methimazole, and hydralazine are common culprits. Drug-induced polyarteritis nodosa has been associated with long-term exposure to minocycline. The presence of perivascular eosinophils on skin biopsy can be a clue to possible drug etiology.

MANAGEMENT OF THE PATIENT WITH SUSPECTED DRUG ERUPTION

There are four main questions to answer regarding a suspected drug eruption:

1. Is the observed rash caused by a medication?
2. Is the reaction severe or evolving with systemic involvement?
3. Which drug or drugs are suspected, and should they be withdrawn?
4. What recommendation can be made for future medication use?

EARLY DIAGNOSIS OF SEVERE ERUPTIONS

Rapid recognition of potentially serious or life-threatening reactions is paramount. In this regard, a suspected drug eruption is best defined initially by what it is not (e.g., SJS/TEN, DIHS). **Table 60-2** lists clinical and laboratory features that, if present, suggest the presence of a severe reaction. **Table 60-3** lists the most important of these reactions, along with their key features and commonly associated medications. Any concern for a serious reaction should prompt immediate consultation with a dermatologist and/or referral of the patient to a specialized center.

CONFIRMATION OF DRUG REACTION

The probability of drug etiology varies with the pattern of the reaction. Only fixed drug eruptions are always drug-induced. Morbilliform eruptions are usually viral in children and drug-induced in adults. Among severe reactions, drugs account for 10–20% of anaphylaxis and vasculitis and between 70% and 90% of AGEP, DIHS, SJS, and TEN. Skin biopsy helps characterize the reaction but does not indicate drug causality. Blood counts and liver and renal function tests are important for evaluating organ involvement. The association of mild elevation of liver enzymes and high eosinophil count is frequent but not specific for a drug reaction. Blood tests that could identify an alternative cause, serologic tests (to rule out drug-induced lupus), and serology or polymerase chain reaction for infections may be of great importance to determine a cause.

WHAT DRUG(S) TO SUSPECT AND WITHDRAW

Most cases of drug eruptions occur during the first course of treatment with a new medication. A notable exception is IgE-mediated urticaria and anaphylaxis that need presensitization and develop a few minutes to a few hours after rechallenge. Characteristic timing of onset following drug administration is as follows: 4–14 days for morbilliform eruption, 2–4 days for AGEP, 5–28 days for SJS/TEN, and 14–48 days for DIHS. A drug chart, compiling information of all current and past medications/supplements and the timing of administration relative to the rash, is a key diagnostic tool for identifying the inciting drug. Medications introduced for the first time in the relevant time frame are prime suspects. Two other important elements to suspect causality at this stage are (1) previous experience with the drug (or related members of the same pharmacologic class) and (2) alternative etiologic candidates.

The decision to continue or discontinue any medication depends on the severity of the reaction, the severity of the primary disease undergoing treatment, the degree of suspicion of causality, and the feasibility of finding an alternative safer treatment. In any potentially fatal drug reaction, elimination of all possible suspect drugs or unnecessary medications should be immediately attempted. Some rashes may resolve when "treating through" a benign drug-related eruption. The decision to treat through an eruption should, however, remain the exception and withdrawal of every suspect drug the general rule. On the other hand, drugs that are not suspected and are important for the patient (e.g., antihypertensive agents) generally should not be quickly withdrawn. This approach may permit judicious use of these agents in the future.

RECOMMENDATION FOR FUTURE USE OF DRUGS

The aims are to (1) prevent the recurrence of the drug eruption and (2) avoid compromising future treatment by inaccurately excluding otherwise useful medications.

A thorough assessment of drug causality is based on timing of the reaction, evaluation of other possible causes, and effect of drug withdrawal or continuation. The RegiSCAR group has proposed the Algorithm of Drug Causality for Epidermal Necrolysis (ALDEN) to rank likelihood of drug causality in SJS/TEN; validation of this and other instruments, such as the Naranjo adverse drug reaction probability scale, is limited. Medication(s) with a "definite" or "probable" causality should be contraindicated, a warning card or medical alert tag (e.g., wristband) should be given to the patient, and the drugs should be listed in the patient's medical chart as allergies.

CROSS-SENSITIVITY

Because of possible cross-sensitivity among chemically related drugs, many physicians recommend avoidance of not only the medication that induced the reaction but also all drugs of the same pharmacologic class.

There are two types of cross-sensitivity. Reactions that depend on a pharmacologic interaction may occur with all drugs that target the same pathway, whether the drugs are structurally similar or not. This is the case with angioedema caused by NSAIDs and ACE inhibitors. In this situation, the risk of recurrence varies from drug to drug in a particular class; however, avoidance of all drugs in the class is usually recommended. Immune recognition of structurally related drugs is the second mechanism by which cross-sensitivity occurs. A classic example

TABLE 60-2 Clinical and Laboratory Findings Suggestive of Severe Cutaneous Adverse Drug Reaction

Cutaneous
Generalized erythema
Facial edema
Skin pain
Palpable purpura
Dusky or target-like lesions
Skin necrosis
Blisters or epidermal detachment
Positive Nikolsky sign
Mucous membrane erosions
Swelling of lips or tongue
General
High fever
Enlarged lymph nodes
Arthralgias or arthritis
Shortness of breath, hoarseness, wheezing, hypotension
Laboratory Results
Eosinophil count >1000/μL
Lymphocytosis with atypical lymphocytes
Abnormal liver or kidney function tests

Source: From JC Roujeau, RS Stern: Severe adverse cutaneous reactions to drugs. N Engl J Med 331:1272, 1994.

TABLE 60-3 Clinical Features of Severe Cutaneous Drug Reactions

DIAGNOSIS	MUCOSAL LESIONS	TYPICAL SKIN LESIONS	FREQUENT SIGNS AND SYMPTOMS	MOST COMMON CULPRIT DRUGS
Stevens-Johnson syndrome (SJS)	Erosions usually at two or more sites	Small blisters form from dusky macules or atypical targets; rare areas of confluence; detachment ≤10% body surface area	Most cases involve fever	Sulfonamides, anticonvulsants, allopurinol, nonsteroidal anti-inflammatory drugs (NSAIDs)
Toxic epidermal necrolysis (TEN)[a]	Erosions usually at two or more sites	Individual lesions like those seen in SJS; confluent dusky erythema; large sheets of necrotic epidermis; total detachment of >30% body surface area	Nearly all cases involve fever, "acute skin failure," leukopenia	Same as for SJS
Drug-induced hypersensitivity syndrome/drug rash with eosinophilia and systemic symptoms (DIHS/DRESS)	Mucositis reported in as many as 30%	Diffuse, deep red morbilliform eruption with facial involvement; facial and acral swelling	Fever, lymphadenopathy, hepatitis, nephritis, myocarditis, eosinophilia, atypical lymphocytosis	Anticonvulsants, sulfonamides, allopurinol, minocycline
Acute generalized exanthematous pustulosis (AGEP)	Oral erosions in perhaps 20%	Innumerable pinpoint pustules overlying a diffuse erythematous eruption; may develop superficial erosions	High fever, leukocytosis (neutrophilia), hypocalcemia	β-Lactam antibiotics, calcium channel blockers, macrolide antibiotics
Serum sickness or serum sickness–like reaction	Absent	Urticarial serpiginous or polycyclic rash; purpuric eruption along the sides of the feet and hands is characteristic	Fever, arthralgias	Antithymocyte globulin, cephalosporins, monoclonal antibodies
Anticoagulant-induced necrosis	Infrequent	Purpura and necrosis, especially of central, fatty areas	Pain in affected areas	Warfarin, heparin
Angioedema	Often involved	Urticaria or swelling of the central face, other areas	Respiratory distress, cardiovascular collapse	Angiotensin-converting enzyme (ACE) inhibitors, NSAIDs, contrast dye

[a]Overlap of SJS and TEN have features of both, and attachment of 10–30% of body surface area may occur.

Source: From JC Roujeau, RS Stern: Severe adverse cutaneous reactions to drugs. N Engl J Med 331:1272, 1994. Copyright © 1994 Massachusetts Medical Society. Reprinted with permission from Massachusetts Medical Society.

is hypersensitivity to aromatic antiepileptics (barbiturates, phenytoin, carbamazepine) with up to 50% reaction to a second drug in patients who reacted to one. For other drugs, in vitro and in vivo data have suggested that cross-reactivity exists only between compounds with very similar chemical structures. Sulfamethoxazole-specific lymphocytes may be activated by other antibacterial sulfonamides but not diuretics, antidiabetic drugs, or anti-COX2 NSAIDs with a sulfonamide group. Though it has been previously reported that 10% of patients with penicillin allergies will also develop allergic reactions to cephalosporin class antibiotics, the cross-reactivity is likely much lower, as is the incidence of true penicillin allergy itself, and severe reactions are very rare.

Recent data suggest that although the risk of developing a drug eruption to another drug is increased in persons with a prior reaction, "cross-sensitivity" is probably not the explanation. As an example, those with a history of an allergic-like reaction to penicillin are at greater risk of developing a reaction to antibacterial sulfonamides than to cephalosporins.

These data suggest that the list of drugs to avoid after a drug reaction should be limited to the causative one(s) and to a few very similar medications.

Because of growing evidence that some severe cutaneous reactions to drugs are associated with HLA genes, it is recommended that first-degree family members of patients with severe cutaneous reactions also should avoid causative agents. This may be most relevant for sulfonamides and antiepileptic medications.

ROLE OF TESTING FOR CAUSALITY AND DRUG RECHALLENGE

The usefulness of laboratory tests, skin-prick, or patch testing to determine causality is debated and may be of limited practical value. Many in vitro immunologic assays have been developed for research purposes; however, the predictive value of these tests has not been validated in large series of affected patients. In some cases, diagnostic rechallenge may be appropriate, even for drugs with high rates of adverse reactions.

Skin-prick testing has clinical value in specific settings. In patients with a history suggesting immediate IgE-mediated reactions to penicillin, skin-prick testing with penicillins or cephalosporins has proven useful for identifying patients at risk of anaphylactic reactions to these agents. Negative skin tests do not totally rule out IgE-mediated reactivity; however, the risk of anaphylaxis in response to penicillin administration in patients with negative skin tests is about 1%. In contrast, two-thirds of patients with a positive skin test experience an allergic response upon rechallenge. The skin tests themselves carry a small risk of anaphylaxis.

For patients with delayed-type hypersensitivity, the clinical utility of skin tests remains questionable. At least one of a combination of several tests (prick, patch, and intradermal) is positive in 50–70% of patients with a reaction "definitely" attributed to a single medication. This low sensitivity corresponds to the observation that readministration of drugs with negative skin testing results in eruptions in 17% of cases.

Desensitization can be considered in those with a history of reaction to a medication that must be used again. Efficacy of such procedures has been demonstrated in cases of immediate reaction to penicillin and positive skin tests, anaphylactic reactions to platinum chemotherapy, and delayed reactions to sulfonamides in patients with AIDS. Desensitization is often successful in HIV-infected patients with morbilliform eruptions to sulfonamides but is not recommended in HIV-infected patients who developed erythroderma or a bullous reaction in response to prior sulfonamide exposure. Various protocols are available, including oral and parenteral approaches. Oral desensitization appears to have a lower risk of serious anaphylactic reaction. Desensitization carries the risk of anaphylaxis regardless of how it is performed and should be performed in monitored clinical settings such as an intensive care unit. After desensitization, many patients experience non-life-threatening reactions during therapy with the culprit drug.

REPORTING

Any severe reaction to drugs should be reported to a regulatory agency or to pharmaceutical companies. Because severe reactions are too rare to be detected in premarketing clinical trials, spontaneous reports are of critical importance for early detection of unexpected life-threatening events. To be useful, the report should contain enough details to permit ascertainment of severity and drug causality.

Acknowledgments

We acknowledge the contribution of Drs. Jean-Claude Roujeau and Robert S. Stern to this chapter in previous editions.

FURTHER READING

Alfirevic A et al: Genetic testing for prevention of severe drug-induced skin rash. Cochrane Database Syst Rev 7:CD010891, 2019.

Cornejo-Garcia JA et al: The genetics of drug hypersensitivity reactions. J Investig Allergol Clin Immunol 26:222, 2016.

Duong TA et al: Severe cutaneous adverse reactions to drugs. Lancet 390:1996, 2017.

Ko TM et al: Use of HLA-B*5801 genotyping to prevent allopurinol induced severe cutaneous adverse reactions in Taiwan: National prospective cohort study. BMJ 351:h4848, 2015.

Lee S et al: Association of dipeptidyl peptidase 4 inhibitor use with risk of bullous pemphigoid in patients with diabetes. JAMA Dermatol 155:172, 2018.

Mayorga C et al: In vitro tests for drug hypersensitivity reactions: An ENDA/EAACI Drug Allergy Interest Group position paper. Allergy 71:1103, 2016.

Oussalah A et al: Genetic variants associated with drug-induced immediate hypersensitivity reactions: A PRISMA-compliant systematic review. Allergy 71:443, 2016.

Peter JG et al: Severe delayed cutaneous and systemic reactions to drugs: A global perspective on the science and art of current practice. J Allergy Clin Immunol Pract 5:547, 2017.

Petrelli F et al: Antibiotic prophylaxis for skin toxicity induced by antiepidermal growth factor receptor agents: A systematic review and meta-analysis. Br J Dermatol 175:1166, 2016.

Sassolas B et al: ALDEN, an algorithm for assessment of drug causality in Stevens-Johnson syndrome and toxic epidermal necrolysis: Comparison with case-control analysis. Clin Pharmacol Ther 88:60, 2010.

Seminario-Vidal L et al: Society of Dermatology Hospitalists supportive care guidelines for the management of Stevens-Johnson syndrome/toxic epidermal necrolysis in adults. J Am Acad Dermatol 82:1553, 2020.

Simonsen A et al: Cutaneous adverse reactions to anti-PD-1 treatment: A systematic review. J Am Acad Dermatol 83:1415, 2020.

Zimmermann S et al: Systemic immunomodulating therapies for Stevens-Johnson syndrome and toxic epidermal necrolysis: A systematic review and meta-analysis. JAMA Dermatol 153:514, 2017.

61 Photosensitivity and Other Reactions to Sunlight

Alexander G. Marneros, David R. Bickers

SOLAR RADIATION

Sunlight is the most visible and obvious source of comfort in the environment. The sun provides the beneficial effects of warmth and vitamin D synthesis. However, acute and chronic sun exposure also has pathologic consequences. Cutaneous exposure to sunlight is a major cause of human skin cancer and can have immunosuppressive effects as well.

The sun's energy reaching the Earth's surface is limited to components of the ultraviolet (UV) spectrum, the visible spectrum, and portions of the infrared spectrum. The cutoff at the short end of the UV spectrum at ~290 nm is due primarily to stratospheric ozone—formed by highly energetic ionizing radiation—that prevents penetration to the earth's surface of the shorter, more energetic, potentially more harmful wavelengths of solar radiation. Indeed, concern about destruction of the ozone layer by chlorofluorocarbons released into the atmosphere has led to international agreements to reduce production of those chemicals.

Measurements of solar flux showed a 20-fold regional variation in the amount of energy at 300 nm that reaches the earth's surface. This variability relates to seasonal effects, the path that sunlight traverses through ozone and air, the altitude (a 4% increase for each 300 m of elevation), the latitude (increasing intensity with decreasing latitude), and the amount of cloud cover, fog, and pollution.

The major components of the photobiologic action spectrum that can affect human skin include the UV and visible wavelengths between 290 and 700 nm. In addition, the wavelengths beyond 700 nm in the infrared spectrum primarily emit heat and in certain circumstances may exacerbate the pathologic effects of energy in the UV and visible spectra.

The UV spectrum reaching the Earth represents <10% of total incident solar energy and is arbitrarily divided into two major segments, UV-B and UV-A, which constitute the wavelengths from 290 to 400 nm. UV-B consists of wavelengths between 290 and 320 nm. This portion of the photobiologic action spectrum is the most efficient in producing redness or erythema in human skin and thus is sometimes known as the "sunburn spectrum." UV-A includes wavelengths between 320 and 400 nm and is ~1000-fold less efficient in producing skin redness than is UV-B.

The wavelengths between 400 and 700 nm are visible to the human eye. The photon energy in the visible spectrum is not capable of damaging human skin in the absence of a photosensitizing chemical. Without the absorption of energy by a molecule, there can be no photosensitivity. Thus, the *absorption spectrum* of a molecule is defined as the range of wavelengths it absorbs, whereas the *action spectrum* for an effect of incident radiation is defined as the range of wavelengths that evoke the response.

Photosensitivity occurs when a photon-absorbing chemical (*chromophore*) present in the skin absorbs incident energy, becomes excited, and transfers the absorbed energy to various structures or to molecular oxygen.

UV RADIATION (UVR) AND SKIN STRUCTURE AND FUNCTION

Human skin consists of two major compartments: the outer epidermis, which is a stratified squamous epithelium, and the underlying dermis, which is rich in matrix proteins such as collagens and elastin. Both compartments are susceptible to damage from sun exposure. The epidermis and the dermis contain several chromophores capable of absorbing incident solar energy, including nucleic acids, proteins, and lipids. The outermost epidermal layer, the stratum corneum, is a major absorber of UV-B, and <10% of incident UV-B wavelengths penetrate through the epidermis to the dermis. Approximately 3% of radiation below 300 nm, 20% of radiation below 360 nm, and 33% of short visible radiation reach the basal cell layer in untanned human skin. UV-A readily penetrates to the dermis and is capable of altering structural and matrix proteins that contribute to photoaging of chronically sun-exposed skin, particularly in individuals of light complexion. Thus, longer wavelengths can penetrate more deeply into the skin.

Molecular Targets for UVR-Induced Skin Effects Epidermal DNA—predominantly in keratinocytes and in Langerhans cells (dendritic antigen-presenting cells)—absorbs UV-B and undergoes structural changes between adjacent pyrimidine bases (thymine or cytosine), including the formation of cyclobutane dimers and 6,4-photoproducts. These structural changes are potentially mutagenic and are found in nonmelanoma skin cancers (NMSCs), including basal cell carcinoma (BCC), squamous cell carcinoma (SCC), and Merkel cell carcinoma (MCC). They can be repaired by cellular mechanisms that result in their recognition and excision and the restoration of normal base sequences. The efficient repair of these structural aberrations is crucial, since individuals with defective DNA repair are at high risk for the development of cutaneous cancer. For example, patients with xeroderma pigmentosum, an autosomal recessive disorder, have a variably deficient repair of UV-induced photoproducts. The skin of these patients often shows the dry, leathery appearance of prematurely photoaged skin, and these patients have an increased frequency of skin cancer already in the first two decades of life. Studies in transgenic mice have verified the importance of functional genes that regulate these repair pathways in preventing the development of UV-induced skin cancer. DNA damage to Langerhans cells may also contribute to the known immunosuppressive effects of UV-B (see "Photoimmunology," later).

In addition to DNA, molecular oxygen is a target for incident solar UVR, leading to the generation of reactive oxygen species (ROS). These ROS can damage skin components through oxidative damage to DNA, oxidation of polyunsaturated fatty acids in lipids (lipid peroxidation), or oxidation of amino acids in proteins, or they can lead to oxidative deactivation of specific enzymes. UVR can also promote increased cross-linking and degradation of dermal matrix proteins and accumulation of abnormal dermal elastin, leading to photoaging changes known as *solar elastosis*.

Cutaneous Optics and Chromophores *Chromophores* are endogenous or exogenous chemicals that can absorb physical energy. Endogenous chromophores are of two types: (1) normal components of skin, including nucleic acids, proteins, lipids, and 7-dehydrocholesterol (the precursor of vitamin D); and (2) components that are synthesized elsewhere in the body and that circulate in the bloodstream and diffuse into the skin, such as porphyrins. Normally, only trace amounts of porphyrins are present in the skin, but, in selected diseases known as the *porphyrias* (**Chap. 416**), porphyrins are released into the circulation in increased amounts from the bone marrow and/or the liver and are transported to the skin, where they absorb incident energy both in the Soret band (~400 nm; short visible) and, to a lesser extent, in the red portion of the visible spectrum (580–660 nm). This energy absorption results in the generation of ROS that can mediate structural damage to the skin, manifested as erythema, edema, urticaria, or blister formation. It is of interest that photoexcited porphyrins are currently used in the treatment of BCCs and SCCs and their precursor lesions, actinic keratoses. Known as *photodynamic therapy* (PDT), this modality generates ROS in the skin, leading to cell death. Topical photosensitizers used in PDT are the porphyrin precursors 5-aminolevulinic acid and methyl aminolevulinate, which are readily converted to porphyrins in the skin. It is believed that PDT targets tumor cells for destruction more selectively than it targets adjacent nonneoplastic cells. The efficacy of such therapy requires appropriate timing of the application of methyl aminolevulinate or 5-aminolevulinic acid to the affected skin followed by exposure to artificial sources of visible light. High-intensity blue light has been used successfully for PDT of thin actinic keratoses. Red light PDT penetrates more deeply into the skin and is more beneficial in the treatment of superficial BCCs.

Acute Effects of Sun Exposure The acute effects of skin exposure to sunlight include sunburn and vitamin D synthesis.

SUNBURN This painful skin condition is an acute inflammatory response of the skin, predominantly to UV-B. Generally, an individual's ability to tolerate sunlight is inversely proportional to that individual's degree of melanin pigmentation. Melanin, a complex polymer of tyrosine derivatives, is synthesized in specialized epidermal dendritic cells known as *melanocytes* and is packaged into *melanosomes* that are transferred via dendritic processes into *keratinocytes*, thereby providing photoprotection (dissipating the vast majority of absorbed UVR in the skin) and simultaneously darkening the skin. Sun-induced melanogenesis is a consequence of increased tyrosinase activity in melanocytes. Central to the suntan response is the melanocortin-1 receptor (*MC1R*), and mutations in this gene contribute to the wide variation in human skin and hair color; individuals with red hair and fair skin typically have low MC1R activity. In the skin, there are two main types of melanin: eumelanin (providing brown and black pigmentation associated with high MC1R activity) and pheomelanin (providing red pigmentation associated with low MC1R activity). Pheomelanin is a cysteine-containing red polymer of benzothiazine units and has much weaker shielding capacity against UVR compared to eumelanin. This may explain why individuals with a higher proportion of pheomelanin (red hair/fair skin appearance) have an increased risk of melanoma formation. In addition, pheomelanin may also promote melanoma formation through induction of oxidative damage by amplifying UV-A–induced ROS but also through UVR-independent mechanisms.

The human *MC1R* gene encodes a G protein–coupled receptor that binds α-melanocyte-stimulating hormone (α-MSH), which is secreted in the skin mainly by keratinocytes in response to UVR. The UV-induced expression of this hormone is controlled by the tumor suppressor p53, and absence of functional p53 attenuates the tanning response. Activation of the melanocortin receptor leads to increased intracellular cyclic adenosine 5′-monophosphate (cAMP) and protein kinase A activation, resulting in an increased transcription of the microphthalmia-associated transcription factor (MITF), which stimulates melanogenesis. Since the precursor of α-MSH, proopiomelanocortin produced by keratinocytes, is also the precursor of β-endorphins, UVR may result in not only increased pigmentation but also increased β-endorphin production in the skin, an effect that has been hypothesized to promote sun-seeking behaviors and even mediate addiction to tanning.

The Fitzpatrick classification of human skin phototypes is based on the efficiency of the epidermal-melanin unit, which usually can be ascertained by asking an individual two questions: (1) Do you burn after sun exposure? (2) Do you tan after sun exposure? The answers to these questions permit division of the population into six skin types, varying from type I (always burn, never tan) to type VI (never burn, always tan) (**Table 61-1**).

Sunburn erythema is due to vasodilation of dermal blood vessels. There is a lag time (usually 4–12 h) between skin exposure to sunlight and the development of visible redness. The action spectrum for sunburn erythema includes UV-B and UV-A, although UV-B is much more efficient than UV-A in evoking the response. However, UV-A may contribute to sunburn erythema at midday, when much more UV-A than UV-B is present in the solar spectrum. The erythema that accompanies the inflammatory response induced by UVR results from the orchestrated release of cytokines along with growth factors and the generation of ROS. Furthermore, UV-induced activation of nuclear factor κB–dependent gene transcription can augment release of several proinflammatory cytokines and vasoactive mediators. These cytokines and mediators accumulate locally in sunburned skin, providing chemotactic factors that attract neutrophils, macrophages, and T lymphocytes, which promote the inflammatory response. UVR also stimulates infiltration of inflammatory cells through induced expression of adhesion molecules such as E-selectin and intercellular adhesion molecule 1 on endothelial cells and keratinocytes. UVR has been shown to activate phospholipase A_2, resulting in increases in eicosanoids such as prostaglandin E_2, which is known to be a potent inducer of sunburn erythema. The role of eicosanoids in this reaction has been verified by studies showing that nonsteroidal anti-inflammatory drugs (NSAIDs) can reduce sunburn erythema.

Epidermal changes in sunburn include the induction of "sunburn cells," which are keratinocytes undergoing p53-dependent apoptosis as a defense, with elimination of cells that harbor UV-B–induced structural DNA damage.

VITAMIN D SYNTHESIS AND PHOTOCHEMISTRY Cutaneous exposure to UV-B causes photolysis of epidermal 7-dehydrocholesterol,

TABLE 61-1 Skin Type and Sunburn Sensitivity (Fitzpatrick Classification)

TYPE	DESCRIPTION
I	Always burn, never tan
II	Always burn, sometimes tan
III	Sometimes burn, sometimes tan
IV	Sometimes burn, always tan
V	Never burn, sometimes tan
VI	Never burn, always tan

converting it to pre–vitamin D_3, which then undergoes temperature-dependent isomerization to form the stable hormone vitamin D_3. This compound diffuses to the dermal vasculature and circulates to the liver and kidney, where it is converted to the dihydroxylated functional hormone 1,25-dihydroxyvitamin D_3. Vitamin D metabolites from the circulation and those produced in the skin itself can augment epidermal differentiation signaling and inhibit keratinocyte proliferation. These effects are exploited therapeutically in psoriasis with the topical application of synthetic vitamin D analogues. In addition, vitamin D is increasingly thought to have beneficial effects in several other inflammatory conditions, and some evidence suggests that—besides its classic physiologic effects on calcium metabolism and bone homeostasis—it is associated with a reduced risk of various internal malignancies. There is controversy regarding the risk-to-benefit ratio of sun exposure for vitamin D homeostasis. At present, it is important to emphasize that no clear-cut evidence suggests that the use of sunscreens substantially diminishes vitamin D levels. Since aging also substantially decreases the ability of human skin to photocatalytically produce vitamin D_3, the widespread use of sunscreens that filter out UV-B has led to concerns that the elderly might be unduly susceptible to vitamin D deficiency. However, the amount of sunlight needed to produce sufficient vitamin D is small and does not justify the risks of skin cancer and other types of photodamage linked to increased sun exposure or tanning behavior. Nutritional supplementation of vitamin D is a preferable strategy for patients with vitamin D deficiency.

Chronic Effects of Sun Exposure: Nonmalignant The clinical features of photoaging (*dermatoheliosis*) consist of wrinkling, blotchiness, and telangiectasia, as well as a roughened, irregular, "weather-beaten" leathery appearance.

UVR is important in the pathogenesis of photoaging in human skin, and ROS are likely involved. The dermis and its connective tissue matrix are major targets for sun-associated chronic damage that manifests as solar elastosis, a massive increase in thickened irregular masses of abnormal-appearing elastic fibers. Collagen fibers are also abnormally clumped in the deeper dermis of sun-damaged skin. The chromophores, the action spectra, and the specific biochemical events orchestrating these changes are only partially understood, although more deeply penetrating UV-A seems to be primarily involved. Chronologically aged sun-protected skin and photoaged skin share important molecular features, including connective tissue damage and elevated levels of matrix metalloproteinases (MMPs). MMPs are enzymes involved in the degradation of the extracellular matrix. UV-A induces expression of some MMPs, including MMP-1 and MMP-3, leading to increased collagen breakdown. In addition, UV-A reduces type I procollagen messenger RNA (mRNA) expression. Thus, chronic UVR alters the structure and function of dermal collagen both by inhibiting its synthesis and enhancing its breakdown. Based on these observations, it is not surprising that high-dose UV-A phototherapy may have beneficial effects in some patients with localized fibrotic diseases of the skin, such as localized scleroderma.

Chronic Effects of Sun Exposure: Malignant One of the major known consequences of chronic excessive skin exposure to sunlight is NMSC, including SCCs, BCCs and MCCs (**Chap. 76**). A model for skin cancer induction involves three major steps: initiation, promotion, and progression. Exposure of human skin to sunlight results in *initiation*, a step by which structural (mutagenic) changes in DNA evoke an irreversible alteration in the target cell (keratinocyte) that begins the tumorigenic process. Exposure to a tumor initiator such as UV-B is believed to be a necessary but not a sufficient step in the malignant process, since initiated skin cells not exposed to tumor promoters generally do not develop into tumors. The second stage in tumor development is *promotion*, a multistep process by which chronic exposure to sunlight evokes further changes that culminate in the clonal expansion of initiated cells and cause the development of premalignant growths known as *actinic keratoses*, which may progress to form SCCs. As a result of extensive studies, it seems clear that UV-B is a *complete carcinogen*, meaning that it can act as both a tumor initiator and a tumor promoter. The third and final step in the malignant process is *malignant conversion* of benign precursors into cancers, a process thought to enhance genetic instability.

On a molecular level, skin carcinogenesis results from the accumulation of gene mutations that cause inactivation of tumor suppressors, activation of oncogenes, or reactivation of cellular signaling pathways that normally are expressed only during embryologic epidermal development that drive cell proliferation. Interestingly, a large number of UV-induced oncogenic driver mutations that are present in SCCs can already be found in aged sun-exposed normal skin, leading to a growth advantage and innumerable precancerous clones carrying cancer-causing mutations. These mutations occur particularly often in genes that affect proliferation of epidermal stem cells (e.g., NOTCH receptor genes). The pattern of oncogenic gene mutations in aged sun-exposed skin shows considerable overlap with the mutations identified in SCCs, while there is little overlap with the mutations identified in BCCs or melanomas. For example, ~20% of normal aged sun-exposed skin cells and ~60% of SCCs carry driver mutations in *NOTCH1*. Additionally, the accumulation of mutations in the tumor-suppressor gene *p53* can also promote skin carcinogenesis. Indeed, the majority of both human and murine UV-induced skin cancers have characteristic UVR-induced *p53* mutations (C → T and CC → TT transitions). Studies in mice have shown that sunscreens can substantially reduce the frequency of these signature mutations in *p53* and inhibit the induction of tumors. The comparison of UVR-induced gene mutations between aged sun-exposed normal skin and SCCs supports the hypothesis of a progressive accumulation of additional oncogenic mutations that eventually lead to the transition from precancerous cell clones to SCCs. It has been estimated that SCCs harbor ~10 times more oncogenic driver mutations per cell than cells in aged sun-exposed normal skin. Furthermore, while aged sun-exposed skin and SCCs carry similar UVR-induced mutations in *p53* or NOTCH receptors, oncogenic mutations in other genes (e.g., *CDKN2A*) were mainly found in SCCs and not in aged sun-exposed skin, which are thus likely to play a critical role in malignant progression.

Compared to SCCs, BCCs carry a distinct mutational profile in specific genes. BCCs harbor inactivating mutations particularly in the tumor-suppressor gene *patched* or activating mutations in the oncogene *smoothened*, which result in the constitutive activation of the sonic hedgehog signaling pathway and increased cell proliferation. There is also evidence linking alterations in the Wnt/β-catenin signaling pathway, which is known to be critical for hair follicle development, to skin cancer as well. Thus, interactions between this pathway and the hedgehog signaling pathway appear to be involved in both skin carcinogenesis and embryologic development of the skin and hair follicles.

Clonal analysis in mouse models of BCC revealed that tumor cells arise from stem cells of the interfollicular epidermis and the upper infundibulum of the hair follicle. These BCC-initiating cells are reprogrammed to resemble embryonic hair follicle progenitors, whose tumor-initiating ability depends on activation of the Wnt/β-catenin signaling pathway.

SCC initiation occurs both in the interfollicular epidermis and in the hair follicle bulge stem cell populations. In mouse models, the combination of mutant K-Ras and p53 is sufficient to induce invasive SCCs from these cell populations.

The transcription factor Myc is important for stem cell maintenance in the skin, and oncogenic activation of Myc has been implicated in the development of BCCs and SCCs.

The third NMSC is MCC, which is named after its resemblance to Merkel cells in the skin. The incidence of MCCs has been increasing in recent years for unknown reasons. The age-adjusted global incidence is about 1 in 100,000. Just like SCC and BCC, patients with MCCs are usually fair-skinned males in the sixth to eighth decades of life who are living in geographic regions with greater solar UVR. These tumors occur predominantly on the head and neck in older individuals and on the trunk in younger people. MCCs also have a higher incidence among immunosuppressed patients. MCCs are aggressive and life-threatening, poorly differentiated neuroendocrine carcinomas. Overall survival at 5 years is around 50% for local disease, 35% for nodal disease, and 15% for metastatic disease. While the majority of MCCs present locally, nodal and metastatic disease can occur simultaneously. The pathogenesis of MCCs is closely connected to the Merkel cell polyoma virus (MCPyV). It is now recognized that MCCs can either be MCPyV positive or MCPyV negative. MCPyV-negative MCCs manifest high levels of classic UV-induced signature mutations (C to T or CC to TT) and inactivation of tumor suppressor genes, which could explain the growth of these viral-negative lesions. MCPyV-positive tumors are thought to grow secondary to viral integration into the host genome and acquisition of a truncating mutation of the large T antigen that results in the production of viral oncoproteins. The growth of MCPyV-positive tumors may be further promoted by UVR-induced local immunosuppression. Both forms of MCC are immunogenic, and metastatic MCC has been treated in some patients successfully with PD-1/PD-L1 immune checkpoint inhibitors.

In summary, NMSC involves mutations and alterations in multiple genes and pathways that occur as a result of their chronic accumulation driven by exposure to environmental factors such as solar UVR.

Epidemiologic studies have linked excessive sun exposure to an increased risk of NMSCs and melanoma of the skin; the evidence is far more direct for NMSCs (BCCs, SCCs, and MCCs) than for melanoma. Approximately 80% of NMSCs develop on sun-exposed body areas, including the face, neck, and hands. Major risk factors include male sex, childhood sun exposures, older age, fair skin, and residence at latitudes relatively close to the equator. Individuals with darker-pigmented skin have a lower risk of skin cancer than do fair-skinned individuals. More than 2 million individuals in the United States develop NMSC annually, and the lifetime risk that a fair-skinned individual will develop such a neoplasm is estimated at ~15%. The incidence of NMSC in the population is increasing at a rate of 2–3% per year, likely due to earlier detection and increased opportunities for outdoor activities.

The relationship of sun exposure to melanoma development is less direct, but strong evidence supports an association. Clear-cut risk factors include a positive family or personal history of melanoma and multiple dysplastic nevi. Melanomas can occur during adolescence; the implication is that the latent period for tumor growth is shorter than that for NMSC. For reasons that are only partially understood, melanomas are among the most rapidly increasing human malignancies (Chap. 76). One potential explanation is the widespread use of indoor tanning. It is estimated that 30 million people tan indoors in the United States annually, including >2 million adolescents. Furthermore, epidemiologic studies suggest that life in a sunny climate from birth or early childhood may increase the risk of melanoma development. In general, risk does not correlate with cumulative sun exposure but may be related to the duration and extent of exposure in childhood.

However, in contrast to NMSCs, melanoma frequently develops in non–sun-exposed skin, and oncogenic mutations in melanoma may also not be UVR-signature mutations. These observations suggest that UVR-independent factors may contribute to melanomagenesis, which is consistent with findings in mouse models showing that pheomelanin is less efficient in protecting against melanoma than is eumelanin and may promote melanoma through UVR-independent mechanisms.

Importantly, mutations in BRAF and NRAS that lead to activation of a growth-promoting signaling cascade are frequently found in melanoma (but not in SCCs or BCCs), which has led to the development of specific inhibitors of this pathway for the treatment of BRAF-mutant melanoma. However, a high mutational load in melanoma may not be equated with a more unfavorable prognosis. Tumor-specific missense mutations in melanomas can result in neoantigens that facilitate an immune response to the tumor cell. A major advance in treating melanoma, termed immune checkpoint blockade, targets inhibitors of cytotoxic T effector function. For example, the PD-1/PD-L1 interaction inhibits tumor cell apoptosis, promotes peripheral T effector cell exhaustion, and induces conversion of T effector cells to regulatory T cells. Checkpoint inhibitor treatment (e.g., with antibodies that inhibit PD-1 or PD-L1) disrupts this interaction and has resulted in a durable and potent immune destruction of melanoma cells in a subset of patients, leading to prolonged survival of patients with locally advanced or metastatic melanoma. It has recently been shown that a high mutational load in melanomas correlates with improved therapeutic outcome to immune checkpoint blockade, consistent with the hypothesis that acquired missense mutations in the tumor cells lead to neoantigens that increase the vulnerability of these melanoma cells to attack by activated T cells.

GLOBAL CONSIDERATIONS The frequency of skin cancer shows strong geographic variation, depending on the skin phototype of the majority of the population in these geographic areas, but also depending on the intensity of UVR. For example, both melanoma and NMSCs are particularly common in Australia.

Photoimmunology Exposure to solar radiation causes both local and systemic immunosuppression and involves both the innate and adaptive immune systems. Local immunosuppression is defined as inhibition of immune responses to antigens applied at the irradiated site, whereas systemic immunosuppression is defined as inhibition of immune responses to antigens applied at remote, unirradiated sites. An example of local immunosuppression is that human skin exposure to modest doses of UV-B can deplete the epidermal antigen-presenting Langerhans cells, thereby reducing the degree of allergic sensitization to topical application of the potent contact allergen dinitrochlorobenzene at the irradiated skin site. An example of the systemic immunosuppressive effects of higher doses of UVR is the diminished immunologic response to antigens introduced either epicutaneously or intracutaneously at sites remote from the irradiated site.

The major chromophores in the upper epidermis that are known to initiate UV-mediated immunosuppression include DNA, *trans*-urocanic acid, and membrane components. The action spectrum for UV-induced immunosuppression closely mimics the absorption spectrum of DNA. UVR-induced cyclobutane pyrimidine dimers in Langerhans cells may inhibit antigen presentation. The absorption spectrum of epidermal urocanic acid closely mimics the action spectrum for UV-B–induced immunosuppression. Urocanic acid is a metabolic product of the essential amino acid histidine and accumulates in the upper epidermis through breakdown of the histidine-rich protein filaggrin due to the absence of its catabolizing enzyme in keratinocytes. Urocanic acid is synthesized as a *trans*-isomer, and UV-induced *trans-cis* isomerization of urocanic acid in the stratum corneum drives immunosuppression. *Cis*-urocanic acid may exert its immunosuppressive effects through a variety of mechanisms, including inhibition of antigen presentation by Langerhans cells.

Various additional immunomodulatory factors and cytokines have been implicated in UVR-induced systemic immunosuppression, including tumor necrosis factor-α, interleukin 4 (IL-4), interleukin 10 (IL-10), and eicosanoids. Keratinocytes can release multiple immunomodulators as a response to UVR-induced cell damage that result in an immunosuppressive environment. Induction of IL-4–producing natural killer T cells and of regulatory T cells and B cells has been linked to cell-mediated and humoral immunosuppression as a consequence of UVR damage to skin. Moreover, UVR-induced formation of damage-associated molecular patterns (DAMPs) from necrotic keratinocytes can lead to a type I interferon innate immune response via activation of Toll-like receptor signaling.

One important consequence of chronic sun exposure and associated immunosuppression is an enhanced risk of skin cancer. In part, UV-B activates regulatory T cells that suppress antitumor immune responses via IL-10 expression, whereas in the absence of high UV-B exposure, epidermal Langerhans cells present tumor-associated antigens and induce protective immunity, thereby inhibiting skin tumorigenesis. UV-induced DNA damage is a major molecular trigger of this immunosuppressive effect.

Perhaps the most graphic demonstration of the role of long-term immunosuppression in enhancing the risk of NMSC comes from studies of organ transplant recipients who require lifelong immunosuppressive/antirejection drug regimens. More than 50% of organ transplant recipients develop BCCs and SCCs, and these skin cancers are the most common types of malignancies arising in these patients. The important contributory role of UVR for the formation of these skin cancers in immunosuppressed individuals is highlighted by the observation that nonwhite transplant recipients develop these skin cancers far less often than white transplant recipients. Rates of BCC and SCC increase with the duration and degree of immunosuppression. Transplant recipients ideally should be screened prior to organ transplantation, be monitored closely thereafter, and adhere to rigorous photoprotection measures, including the use of sunscreens and protective clothing as well as sun avoidance. Notably, immunosuppressive drugs that target the mTOR pathway, such as sirolimus and everolimus, may reduce the risk of NMSC in organ transplant recipients compared to that associated with the use of calcineurin inhibitors (cyclosporine and tacrolimus). The latter may contribute to NMSC formation not only through their immunosuppressive effects but also through suppression of p53-dependent cancer cell senescence pathways independent of host immunity.

Whereas the immunosuppressive effects of UVR contribute to skin cancer, UVR can also exacerbate autoimmune and inflammatory diseases of the skin, including systemic lupus erythematosus (SLE). It has been proposed that in SLE UVR-induced damage to DNA may promote autoantibody formation.

PHOTOSENSITIVITY DISEASES

The diagnosis of photosensitivity requires elicitation of a careful history to define the duration of signs and symptoms, the length of time between exposure to sunlight and the development of subjective symptoms and visible changes in the skin. The age of onset can also be a helpful diagnostic clue. For example, the acute photosensitivity of erythropoietic protoporphyria (EPP) almost always begins in infancy or early childhood, whereas the chronic photosensitivity of porphyria cutanea tarda (PCT) typically begins in the fourth and fifth decades of life. A patient's history of exposure to topical and systemic drugs and chemicals may provide important diagnostic clues. Many classes of drugs can cause photosensitivity on the basis of either phototoxicity or photoallergy.

Examination of the skin may offer important clues. Anatomic areas that are naturally protected from direct sunlight, such as the hairy scalp, the upper eyelids, the retroauricular areas, and the infranasal and submental regions, may be spared, whereas exposed areas show characteristic features of the pathologic process. These anatomic localization patterns are often helpful, but not infallible, in making the diagnosis. For example, airborne contact sensitizers that are blown onto the skin may produce dermatitis that can be difficult to distinguish from photosensitivity despite the fact that such material may trigger skin reactivity in areas shielded from direct sunlight.

Many dermatologic conditions may be caused or aggravated by sunlight (**Table 61-2**). The role of light in evoking these responses may be dependent on genetic abnormalities ranging from well-described defects in DNA repair that occur in xeroderma pigmentosum to the inherited abnormalities in heme synthesis that characterize the porphyrias.

TABLE 61-2 Classification of Photosensitivity Diseases

TYPE	DISEASE
Genetic	Erythropoietic porphyria Erythropoietic protoporphyria Porphyria cutanea tarda—familial Variegate porphyria Hepatoerythropoietic porphyria Albinism Xeroderma pigmentosum Rothmund-Thomson syndrome Bloom syndrome Cockayne syndrome Kindler syndrome Phenylketonuria
Metabolic	Porphyria cutanea tarda—sporadic Hartnup disease Kwashiorkor Pellagra Carcinoid syndrome
Phototoxic	
Internal	Drugs
External	Drugs, plants, food
Photoallergic	
Immediate	Solar urticaria
Delayed	Drug photoallergy Persistent light reaction/chronic actinic dermatitis
Neoplastic and degenerative	Photoaging Actinic keratosis Melanoma and nonmelanoma skin cancer
Idiopathic	Polymorphous light eruption Hydroa aestivale Actinic prurigo
Photoaggravated	Lupus erythematosus Systemic Subacute cutaneous Discoid Dermatomyositis Herpes simplex Lichen planus actinicus Acne vulgaris (aestivale)

Polymorphous Light Eruption The most common type of photosensitivity disease is *polymorphous light eruption* (PMLE). Many affected individuals may never seek medical attention because the condition is often transient, becoming manifest in the spring with initial sun exposure but then subsiding spontaneously with continuing exposure, a phenomenon known as "hardening." The major manifestations of PMLE include (often intensely) pruritic erythematous papules that may coalesce into plaques in a patchy distribution on exposed areas of the trunk and forearms. The face is usually less affected. Whereas the morphologic skin findings remain similar for each patient with subsequent recurrences, significant interindividual variations in skin findings are characteristic (hence the term *polymorphous*).

A skin biopsy and phototest procedures in which skin is exposed to multiple erythemal doses of UV-A and UV-B may aid in the diagnosis. The action spectrum for PMLE is usually within these portions of the solar spectrum.

Whereas the treatment of an acute flare of PMLE may require topical or systemic glucocorticoids, approaches to preventing PMLE are important and include the use of high-SPF broad-spectrum sunscreens as well as the induction of "hardening" by the cautious administration of artificial UV-B (broad-band or narrow-band) and/or UV-A radiation or the use of psoralen plus UV-A (PUVA) photochemotherapy for ~4 weeks before initial sun exposure. Such prophylactic phototherapy or photochemotherapy at the beginning of spring may prevent the occurrence of PMLE throughout the summer.

Actinic prurigo is a photo-induced pruritic eruption that shares similarities with PMLE and often occurs in the spring; however, it can persist throughout the summer and extend into the winter months.

Phototoxicity and Photoallergy These photosensitivity disorders are related to the topical or systemic administration of drugs and other chemicals that can act as chromophores. Both reactions require the absorption of energy by a drug or chemical with consequent production of an excited-state photosensitizer that can transfer its absorbed energy to a bystander molecule or to molecular oxygen, thereby generating tissue-destructive chemical species, including ROS.

Phototoxicity is a nonimmunologic reaction that can be caused by a broad range of drugs and chemicals, some of which are listed in **Table 61-3**. The usual clinical manifestations include erythema

TABLE 61-3 Drugs That May Cause a Phototoxic Reaction

DRUG	TOPICAL	SYSTEMIC
Amiodarone		+
Dacarbazine		+
Fluoroquinolones		+
5-Fluorouracil	+	+
Furosemide		+
Nalidixic acid		+
Phenothiazines		+
Psoralens	+	+
Retinoids	+/–	+
Sulfonamides		+
Sulfonylureas		+
Tetracyclines		+
Thiazides		+
Vinblastine		+

resembling a sunburn reaction that quickly desquamates, or "peels," within several days. In addition, edema, vesicles, and bullae may occur. A common phototoxic reaction that occurs after contact with plant-derived furocoumarins and exposure to UV-A radiation is called phytophotodermatitis.

Photoallergy is much less common and is distinct in that it is an immunopathologic process. The excited-state photosensitizer may create highly unstable haptenic free radicals that bind covalently to macromolecules to form a functional antigen (photoallergen) capable of evoking a delayed-type hypersensitivity response. Most photoallergic reactions are initiated by UV-A rather than UV-B exposure. Some drugs and chemicals that can produce photoallergy are listed in **Table 61-4**. The clinical manifestations typically differ from those of phototoxicity in that an intensely pruritic eczematous dermatitis tends to predominate and evolves into lichenified, thickened, "leathery" changes in sun-exposed areas. A small subset (perhaps 5–10%) of patients with photoallergy may develop a persistent exquisite hypersensitivity to light even when the offending drug or chemical is identified and eliminated, a condition known as *persistent light reaction.*

An uncommon type of persistent photosensitivity is known as *chronic actinic dermatitis.* The affected patients are typically elderly men with a long history of preexisting allergic contact dermatitis or photosensitivity. Common photoallergens associated with this condition are sunscreen ingredients and plant photoallergens. These individuals are usually exquisitely sensitive to UV-B, UV-A, and visible wavelengths.

Phototoxicity and photoallergy often can be diagnostically confirmed by phototest procedures. In patients with suspected phototoxicity,

TABLE 61-4 Drugs That May Cause a Photoallergic Reaction

DRUG	TOPICAL	SYSTEMIC
6-Methylcoumarin	+	
Aminobenzoic acid and esters	+	
Bithionol	+	
Chlorpromazine		+
Diclofenac		+
Fluoroquinolones		+
Halogenated salicylanilides	+	
Hypericin (St. John's wort)	+	+
Musk ambrette	+	
Piroxicam		+
Promethazine		+
Sulfonamides		+
Sulfonylureas		+

determining the minimal erythemal dose (MED) while the patient is exposed to a suspected agent and then repeating the MED after discontinuation of the agent may provide a clue to the causative drug or chemical. Photopatch testing can be performed to confirm the diagnosis of photoallergy. In this simple variant of ordinary patch testing, a series of known photoallergens is applied to the skin in duplicate, and one set is irradiated with a suberythemal dose of UV-A. The development of eczematous changes at sites exposed to sensitizer and light is a positive result. The characteristic abnormality in patients with persistent light reaction is a diminished threshold to erythema evoked by UV-B. Patients with chronic actinic dermatitis usually manifest a broad spectrum of UV hyperresponsiveness and require meticulous photoprotection, including avoidance of sun exposure, use of high-SPF (>30) sunscreens, and, in severe cases, systemic immunosuppression, such as with azathioprine.

The management of drug photosensitivity involves first and foremost the elimination of exposure to the chemical agents responsible for the reaction and the minimization of sun exposure. The acute symptoms of phototoxicity may be ameliorated by cool moist compresses, topical glucocorticoids, and systemically administered NSAIDs. In severely affected individuals, a tapered course of systemic glucocorticoids may be useful. Judicious use of analgesics may be necessary.

Photoallergic reactions require a similar management approach. Furthermore, patients with persistent light reaction and chronic actinic dermatitis must be meticulously protected against light exposure. In selected patients to whom chronic systemic high-dose glucocorticoids pose unacceptable risks, it may be necessary to employ an immunosuppressive drug such as azathioprine, cyclophosphamide, cyclosporine, or mycophenolate mofetil.

Porphyria The porphyrias (**Chap. 416**) are a group of diseases that have in common inherited or acquired derangements in the synthesis of heme. Heme is an iron-chelated tetrapyrrole or porphyrin, and only the nonmetal chelated porphyrins are potent photosensitizers that absorb light intensely in both the short (400–410 nm) and the long (580–650 nm) portions of the visible spectrum.

Heme cannot be reutilized and must be synthesized continuously. The two body compartments with the largest capacity for its production are the bone marrow and the liver. Accordingly, the porphyrias originate in one or the other of these organs, with an end result of excessive endogenous production of potent photosensitizing porphyrins. The porphyrins circulate in the bloodstream and diffuse into the skin, where they absorb solar energy, become photoexcited, generate ROS, and evoke cutaneous photosensitivity. The mechanism of porphyrin photosensitization is known to be photodynamic, or oxygen-dependent, and is mediated by ROS such as singlet oxygen and superoxide anions.

The group of cutaneous porphyrias can be classified as causing either (1) chronic blistering photosensitivity or (2) acute nonblistering photosensitivity. Chronic cutaneous porphyrias include PCT, congenital erythropoietic porphyria (CEP), hepatoerythropoietic porphyria (HEP), hereditary coproporphyria (HCP), and variegate porphyria (VP). CEP, HEP, and PCT manifest only with cutaneous symptoms, while HCP and VP have acute neurovisceral symptoms in addition to the skin photosensitivity. Acute cutaneous nonblistering porphyrias include EPP and X-linked protoporphyria (XLP). Representative examples of chronic and acute cutaneous porphyrias are discussed below.

Porphyria cutanea tarda (PCT) is the most common type of porphyria and is associated with decreased activity of the heme pathway enzyme uroporphyrinogen decarboxylase (UROD) to <20% of normal. Increased iron and various acquired factors (e.g., alcohol consumption, estrogens, smoking, hepatitis C or HIV infection) can reduce UROD activity. There are two basic types of PCT: (1) the sporadic or acquired type, generally seen in individuals ingesting ethanol or receiving estrogens; and (2) the inherited type, in which there is autosomal dominant transmission of deficient enzyme activity (resulting in heterozygosity for UROD with a reduction to 50% of UROD enzymatic activity and, thus, predisposing the individual to PCT). Both forms are associated with increased hepatic iron stores.

In both types of PCT, the predominant feature is chronic photosensitivity characterized by increased fragility of sun-exposed skin, particularly areas subject to repeated trauma such as the dorsa of the hands, the forearms, the face, and the ears. The predominant skin lesions are vesicles and bullae that rupture, producing moist erosions (often with a hemorrhagic base) that heal slowly, with crusting and purplish discoloration of the affected skin. Hypertrichosis, mottled pigmentary change, and scleroderma-like induration are associated features. The diagnosis can be confirmed biochemically by measurement of urinary porphyrin excretion, plasma porphyrin assay, and assay of erythrocyte and/or hepatic UROD. Multiple mutations of the *UROD* gene have been identified in human populations. Some patients with PCT have associated mutations in the *HFE* gene, which is linked to hemochromatosis and leads to increased iron absorption by reducing hepcidin expression; these mutations could contribute to the iron overload precipitating PCT, although iron status as measured by serum ferritin, iron levels, and transferrin saturation is no different from that in PCT patients without *HFE* mutations.

Treatment of PCT consists of repeated phlebotomies to diminish the excessive hepatic iron stores and/or intermittent (twice weekly) low doses of orally administered hydroxychloroquine. This treatment is highly effective for PCT but not suited for treatment of other porphyrias. Long-term remission of the disease can often be achieved if the patient eliminates exposure to porphyrinogenic agents, such as ethanol or estrogens, and avoids sun exposure.

Erythropoietic protoporphyria (EPP) is an acute nonblistering cutaneous porphyria, originates in the bone marrow, and is due to genetic mutations that in most cases decrease the activity of the mitochondrial enzyme ferrochelatase. The major clinical features include acute photosensitivity characterized by painful burning and stinging of exposed skin that often develops during or just after sun exposure. There may be associated skin swelling and, after repeated episodes, a waxlike scarring.

Detection of increased plasma protoporphyrin (PROTO) helps distinguish EPP from lead poisoning and iron-deficiency anemia, in both of which erythrocyte PROTO levels are elevated in the absence of cutaneous photosensitivity. This can be explained by the fact that metal-chelated PROTO is not a photosensitizer.

Rigorous sunlight protection is essential in the management of EPP. Notably, the U.S. Food and Drug Administration (FDA) has approved a synthetic peptide analogue of α-MSH, afamelanotide, in patients with EPP. This drug increases skin pigmentation through melanogenesis, and patients receiving it tolerate sun exposure without pain for longer periods of time and have an improved quality of life as compared to untreated patients. Interestingly, initial studies suggest that afamelanotide may also be beneficial when combined with narrow-band UV-B in the treatment of patients with vitiligo (in patients with skin phototypes IV–VI). Some studies reported that patients with EPP had a moderate increase in tolerance to sunlight after taking oral β-carotene, which may provide this effect by quenching oxygen free radicals.

An algorithm for managing patients with photosensitivity is presented in **Fig. 61-1**.

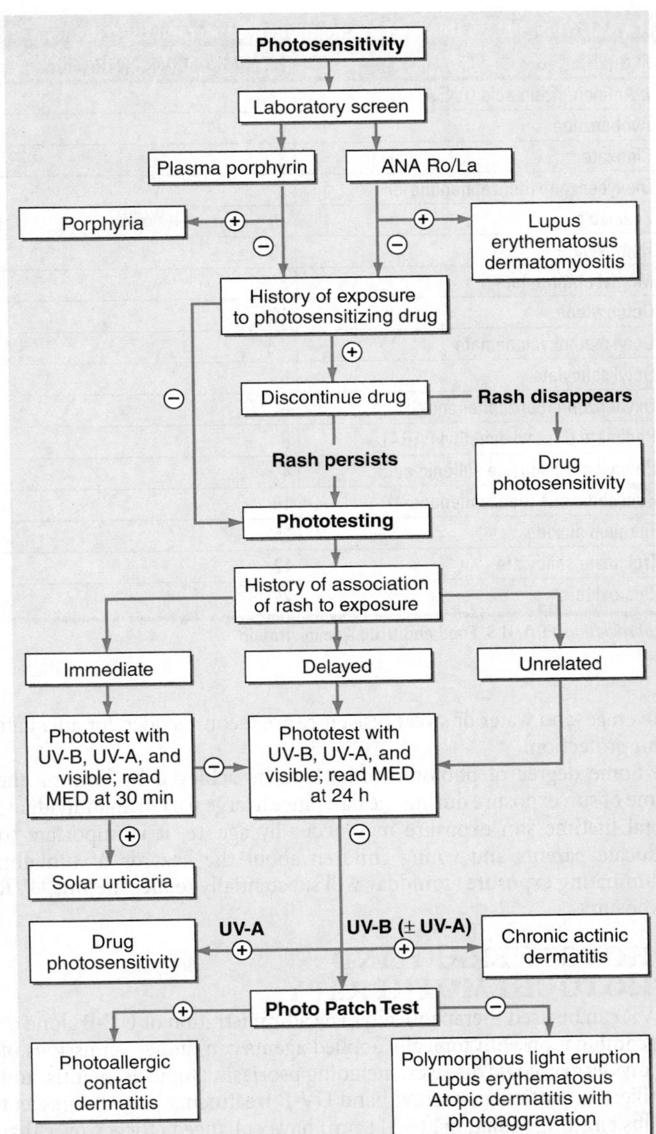

FIGURE 61-1 Algorithm for the diagnosis of a patient with photosensitivity. ANA, antinuclear antibody; MED, minimal erythemal dose; UV-A and UV-B, ultraviolet spectrum segments including wavelengths of 320–400 nm and 290–320 nm, respectively.

PHOTOPROTECTION

Since photosensitivity of the skin results from exposure to sunlight, it follows that absolute avoidance of sunlight will eliminate these disorders. However, contemporary lifestyles make this approach impractical for most individuals. Thus, better approaches to photoprotection have been sought. Natural photoprotection is provided by structural proteins in the epidermis, particularly keratins and melanin. The amount of melanin and its distribution in cells are genetically regulated, and individuals of darker complexion (skin types IV–VI) are at decreased risk for the development of acute sunburn and cutaneous malignancy. Other forms of photoprotection include clothing and sunscreens. Clothing constructed of tightly woven sun-protective fabrics, irrespective of color, affords substantial protection. Wide-brimmed hats, long sleeves, and trousers all reduce direct exposure.

Sunscreens are now considered over-the-counter drugs, and a monograph from the FDA has recognized category I ingredients as safe and effective. Those ingredients are listed in **Table 61-5**. Sunscreens are rated for their photoprotective effect by their sun protection factor (SPF). The SPF is simply a ratio of the time required to produce sunburn erythema with and without sunscreen application. The SPF of most sunscreens reflects protection from UV-B but not from UV-A. The FDA monograph stipulates that sunscreens must be rated on a scale ranging from minimal (SPF ≥2 and <12) to moderate (SPF ≥12 and <30) to high (SPF ≥30, labeled as 30+).

Broad-spectrum sunscreens contain both UV-B–absorbing and UV-A–absorbing chemicals (organic filters). These chemicals absorb UVR and transfer the absorbed energy to surrounding cells. Among these sunscreen ingredients, cinnamates, PABA derivatives, and salicylates absorb UV-B. Benzophenones or ecamsule (terephthalylidene dicamphor sulfonic acid) offer protection against UV-B and UV-A2, whereas avobenzone protects mainly against UV-A1. In contrast, physical UV blockers (zinc oxide and titanium dioxide) absorb or reflect UVR and offer broad-spectrum protection against UV-B and UV-A. In addition to light absorption, a critical determinant of the sustained photoprotective effect of sunscreens is their water resistance. Sunscreen products with an SPF of 30 or higher, broad-spectrum

TABLE 61-5 FDA Category I Monographed Sunscreen Ingredients

INGREDIENTS	MAXIMUM CONCENTRATION, %
p-Aminobenzoic acid (PABA)	15
Avobenzone	3
Cinoxate	3
Dioxybenzone (benzophenone-8)	3
Ecamsule	15
Homosalate	15
Methyl anthranilate	5
Octocrylene	10
Octyl methoxycinnamate	7.5
Octyl salicylate	5
Oxybenzone (benzophenone-3)	6
Padimate O (octyl dimethyl PABA)	8
Phenylbenzimidazole sulfonic acid	4
Sulisobenzone (benzophenone-4)	10
Titanium dioxide	25
Trolamine salicylate	12
Zinc oxide	25

Abbreviation: FDA, U.S. Food and Drug Administration.

coverage, and water or sweat resistance are recommended for adequate sun protection.

Some degree of photoprotection can be achieved by limiting the time of sun exposure during the day. Since a large part of an individual's total lifetime sun exposure may occur by age 18, it is important to educate parents and young children about the hazards of sunlight. Eliminating exposure at midday will substantially reduce lifetime UVR exposure.

PHOTOTHERAPY AND PHOTOCHEMOTHERAPY

UVR can be used therapeutically. The administration of UV-B alone or in combination with topically applied agents can induce remissions of many dermatologic diseases, including psoriasis, atopic dermatitis, and vitiligo. In particular, narrow-band UV-B treatments (with fluorescent bulbs emitting radiation at ~311 nm) have enhanced efficacy over that obtained with broad-band UV-B in the treatment of psoriasis.

Photochemotherapy in which topically applied or systemically administered psoralens are combined with UV-A (PUVA) is effective in treating psoriasis and the early stages of cutaneous T-cell lymphoma and vitiligo. Psoralens are tricyclic furocoumarins that, when intercalated into DNA and exposed to UV-A, form adducts with pyrimidine bases and eventually form DNA cross-links. These structural changes are thought to decrease DNA synthesis and to be related to the amelioration of psoriasis. Why PUVA photochemotherapy is effective in cutaneous T-cell lymphoma is only partially understood, but it has been shown to induce apoptosis of atypical T lymphocyte populations in the skin. Consequently, direct treatment of circulating atypical lymphocytes by extracorporeal photochemotherapy (photopheresis) has been used in Sézary syndrome as well as in other severe systemic diseases with circulating atypical lymphocytes, such as graft-versus-host disease.

In addition to its effects on DNA, PUVA photochemotherapy stimulates epidermal thickening and melanin synthesis; the latter property, together with its anti-inflammatory effects, provides the rationale for use of PUVA in the depigmenting disease vitiligo. Oral 8-methoxypsoralen and UV-A appear to be most effective in this regard, but as many as 100 treatments extending over 12–18 months may be required for satisfactory repigmentation.

Not surprisingly, the major side effects of long-term UV-B phototherapy and PUVA photochemotherapy mimic those seen in individuals with chronic sun exposure. Despite these risks, the therapeutic index of these modalities continues to be excellent. It is important to choose the most appropriate phototherapeutic approach for a specific dermatologic disease. For example, narrow-band UV-B has been reported in several studies to be as effective as PUVA photochemotherapy in the treatment of psoriasis but to pose a lower risk of skin cancer development than PUVA.

■ FURTHER READING

BERNARD JJ et al: Photoimmunology: How ultraviolet radiation affects the immune system. Nat Rev Immunol 11:688, 2019.

FELL GL et al: Skin beta-endorphin mediates addiction to UV light. Cell 157:1527, 2014.

HARMS PW et al: The biology and treatment of Merkel cell carcinoma: Current understanding and research priorities. Nat Rev Clin Oncol 15:763, 2018.

JANSEN R et al: Photoprotection: Part II. Sunscreen: Development, efficacy, and controversies. J Am Acad Dermatol 69:867, 2013.

LO JA et al: The melanoma revolution: From UV carcinogenesis to a new era in therapeutics. Science 346:945, 2014.

MARTINCORENA I et al: Tumor evolution. High burden and pervasive positive selection of somatic mutations in normal human skin. Science 348:880, 2015.

SANCHEZ-DANES A et al: Defining the clonal dynamics leading to mouse skin tumour initiation. Nature 536:298, 2016.

Section 9 Hematologic Alterations

62 Interpreting Peripheral Blood Smears

Dan L. Longo

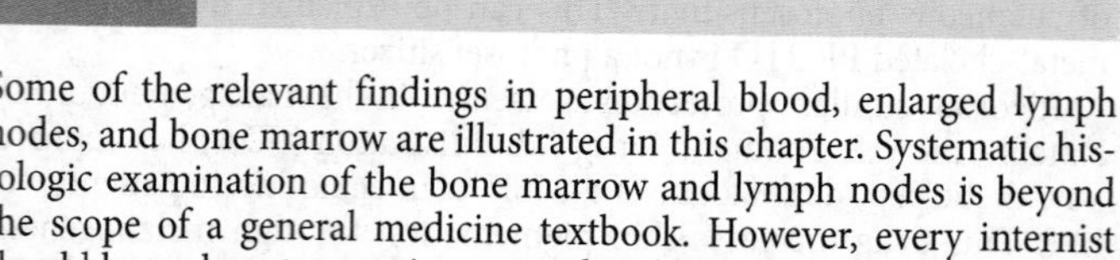

Some of the relevant findings in peripheral blood, enlarged lymph nodes, and bone marrow are illustrated in this chapter. Systematic histologic examination of the bone marrow and lymph nodes is beyond the scope of a general medicine textbook. However, every internist should know how to examine a peripheral blood smear.

The examination of a peripheral blood smear is one of the most informative exercises a physician can perform. Although advances in automated technology have made the examination of a peripheral blood smear by a physician seem less important, the technology is not a completely satisfactory replacement for a blood smear interpretation by a trained medical professional who also knows the patient's clinical history, family history, social history, and physical findings. It is useful to ask the laboratory to generate a Wright's-stained peripheral blood smear and examine it.

The best place to examine blood cell morphology is the feathered edge of the blood smear where red cells lie in a single layer, side by side, just barely touching one another but not overlapping. The author's approach is to look at the smallest cellular elements, the platelets, first and work his way up in size to red cells and then white cells.

Using an oil immersion lens that magnifies the cells 100-fold, one counts the platelets in five to six fields, averages the number per field, and multiplies by 20,000 to get a rough estimate of the platelet count. The platelets are usually 1–2 μm in diameter and have a blue granulated appearance. There is usually 1 platelet for every 20 or so red cells. Of course, the automated counter is much more accurate, but gross disparities between the automated and manual counts should be assessed. Large platelets may be a sign of rapid platelet turnover, as young platelets are often larger than old ones; alternatively, certain rare inherited syndromes can produce large platelets. If the platelet count is low, the absence of large (young) platelets may be an indicator of marrow production problems. Platelet clumping visible on the smear can be associated with falsely low automated platelet counts. Clumping may be caused by the anticoagulant into which the blood is drawn. Similarly, neutrophil fragmentation can be a source of falsely elevated automated platelet counts. The absence of platelet granules may be an artifact of the handling of the blood or may indicate marrow disease or a rare congenital anomaly, gray platelet syndrome. Elevated platelet counts usually signify a myeloproliferative disorder or a reaction to systemic inflammation.

Next one examines the red blood cells. One can gauge their size by comparing the red cell to the nucleus of a small lymphocyte. Both are normally about 8-μm wide. Red cells that are smaller than the small lymphocyte nucleus may be microcytic; those larger than the small lymphocyte nucleus may be macrocytic. Macrocytic cells also tend to be more oval than spherical in shape and are sometimes called macroovalocytes. The automated mean corpuscular volume (MCV) can assist in making a classification. However, some patients may have both iron and vitamin B_{12} deficiency, which will produce an MCV in the normal range but wide variation in red cell size. When the red cells vary greatly in size, *anisocytosis* is said to be present. When the red cells vary greatly in shape, *poikilocytosis* is said to be present. The electronic cell counter provides an independent assessment of variability in red cell size. It measures the range of red cell volumes and reports the results as "red cell distribution width" (RDW). This value is calculated from the MCV; thus, cell width is not being measured but cell volume is. The term is derived from the curve displaying the frequency of cells at each volume, also called the distribution. The width of red cell volume distribution curve is what determines the RDW. The RDW is calculated as follows: RDW = (standard deviation of MCV ÷ mean MCV) × 100. In the presence of morphologic anisocytosis, RDW (normally 11–14%) increases to 15–18%. The RDW is useful in at least two clinical settings. In patients with microcytic anemia, the differential diagnosis is generally between iron deficiency and thalassemia. In thalassemia, the small red cells are generally of uniform size with a normal small RDW. In iron deficiency, the size variability and the RDW are large. In addition, a large RDW can suggest a dimorphic anemia when a chronic atrophic gastritis can produce both vitamin B_{12} malabsorption to produce macrocytic anemia and blood loss to produce iron deficiency. In such settings, RDW is also large. An elevated RDW also has been reported as a risk factor for all-cause mortality in population-based studies, a finding that is unexplained currently.

After red cell size is assessed, one examines the hemoglobin content of the cells. They are either normal in color (*normochromic*) or pale in color (*hypochromic*). They are never "hyperchromic." If more than the normal amount of hemoglobin is made, the cells get larger—they do not become darker. In addition to hemoglobin content, the red cells are examined for inclusions. Red cell inclusions are the following:

1. *Basophilic stippling*—diffuse fine or coarse blue dots in the red cell usually representing RNA residue—especially common in lead poisoning
2. *Howell-Jolly bodies*—dense blue circular inclusions that represent nuclear remnants—their presence implies defective splenic function
3. *Nuclei*—red cells may be released or pushed out of the marrow prematurely before nuclear extrusion—often implies a myelophthisic process or a vigorous narrow response to anemia, usually hemolytic anemia
4. *Parasites*—red cell parasites include malaria and babesia **(Chap. A6)**
5. *Polychromatophilia*—the red cell cytoplasm has a bluish hue, reflecting the persistence of ribosomes still actively making hemoglobin in a young red cell

Vital stains are necessary to see precipitated hemoglobin called *Heinz bodies*.

Red cells can take on a variety of different shapes. All abnormally shaped red cells are *poikilocytes*. Small red cells without the central pallor are *spherocytes*; they can be seen in hereditary spherocytosis, hemolytic anemias of other causes, and clostridial sepsis. *Dacrocytes* are teardrop-shaped cells that can be seen in hemolytic anemias, severe iron deficiency, thalassemias, myelofibrosis, and myelodysplastic syndromes. *Schistocytes* are helmet-shaped cells that reflect microangiopathic hemolytic anemia or fragmentation on an artificial heart valve. *Echinocytes* are spiculated red cells with the spikes evenly spaced; they can represent an artifact of abnormal drying of the blood smear or reflect changes in stored blood. They also can be seen in renal failure and malnutrition and are often reversible. *Acanthocytes* are spiculated red cells with the spikes irregularly distributed. This process tends to be irreversible and reflects underlying renal disease, abetalipoproteinemia, or splenectomy. *Elliptocytes* are elliptical-shaped red cells that can reflect an inherited defect in the red cell membrane, but they also are seen in iron deficiency, myelodysplastic syndromes, megaloblastic anemia, and thalassemias. *Stomatocytes* are red cells in which the area of central pallor takes on the morphology of a slit instead of the usual round shape. Stomatocytes can indicate an inherited red cell membrane defect and also can be seen in alcoholism. *Target cells* have an area of central pallor that contains a dense center, or bull's eye. These cells are seen classically in thalassemia, but they are also present in iron deficiency, cholestatic liver disease, and some hemoglobinopathies. They also can be generated artifactually by improper slide making.

One last feature of the red cells to assess before moving to the white blood cells is the distribution of the red cells on the smear. In most individuals, the cells lie side by side in a single layer. Some patients have red cell clumping (called *agglutination*) in which the red cells pile upon one another; it is seen in certain paraproteinemias and autoimmune hemolytic anemias. Another abnormal distribution involves red cells lying in single cell rows on top of one another like stacks of coins. This is called *rouleaux formation* and reflects abnormal serum protein levels.

Finally, one examines the white blood cells. Three types of granulocytes are usually present: neutrophils, eosinophils, and basophils, in decreasing frequency. Neutrophils are generally the most abundant white cell. They are round, are 10–14 μm wide, and contain a lobulated nucleus with two to five lobes connected by a thin chromatin thread. Bands are immature neutrophils that have not completed nuclear condensation and have a U-shaped nucleus. Bands reflect a left shift in neutrophil maturation in an effort to make more cells more rapidly. Neutrophils can provide clues to a variety of conditions. Vacuolated neutrophils may be a sign of bacterial sepsis. The presence of 1- to 2-μm blue cytoplasmic inclusions, called *Döhle bodies*, can reflect infections, burns, or other inflammatory states. If the neutrophil granules are larger than normal and stain a darker blue, "toxic granulations" are said to be present, and they also suggest a systemic inflammation. The presence of neutrophils with more than five nuclear lobes suggests megaloblastic anemia. Large misshapen granules may reflect the inherited Chédiak-Higashi syndrome.

Eosinophils are slightly larger than neutrophils, have bilobed nuclei, and contain large red granules. Diseases of eosinophils are associated with too many of them rather than any morphologic or qualitative change. They normally total less than one-thirtieth the number of neutrophils. Basophils are even more rare than eosinophils in the blood. They have large dark blue granules and may be increased as part of chronic myeloid leukemia.

Lymphocytes can be present in several morphologic forms. Most common in healthy individuals are small lymphocytes with a small dark nucleus and scarce cytoplasm. In the presence of viral infections, more of the lymphocytes are larger, about the size of neutrophils, with abundant cytoplasm and a less condensed nuclear chromatin. These cells are called *reactive lymphocytes*. About 1% of lymphocytes are larger and contain blue granules in a light blue cytoplasm; they are called *large granular lymphocytes*. In chronic lymphoid leukemia, the small lymphocytes are increased in number, and many of them are ruptured in making the blood smear, leaving a smudge of nuclear material without a surrounding cytoplasm or cell membrane; they are called *smudge cells* and are rare in the absence of chronic lymphoid leukemia.

Monocytes are the largest white blood cells, ranging from 15 to 22 μm in diameter. The nucleus can take on a variety of shapes but usually appears to be folded; the cytoplasm is gray.

Abnormal cells may appear in the blood. Most often, the abnormal cells originate from neoplasms of bone marrow–derived cells, including lymphoid cells, myeloid cells, and occasionally red cells. More rarely, other types of tumors can get access to the bloodstream, and rare

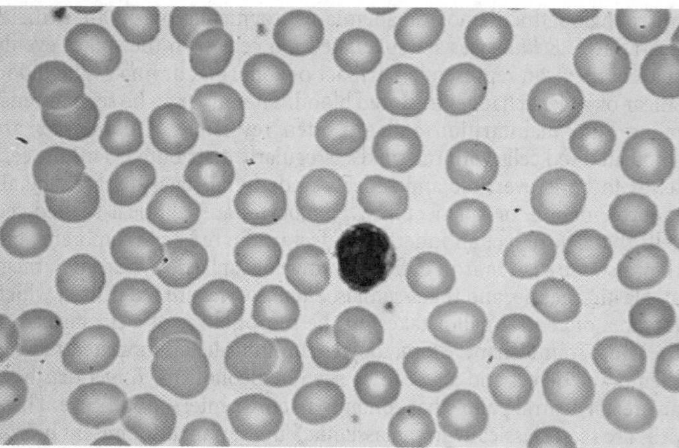

FIGURE 62-1 Normal peripheral blood smear. Small lymphocyte in center of field. Note that the diameter of the red blood cell is similar to the diameter of the small lymphocyte nucleus. *(Source: From M Lichtman et al (eds). Williams Hematology, 7th ed. New York, McGraw-Hill, 2005; RS Hillman, KA Ault, Hematology in General Practice, 4th ed. New York, McGraw-Hill, 2005.)*

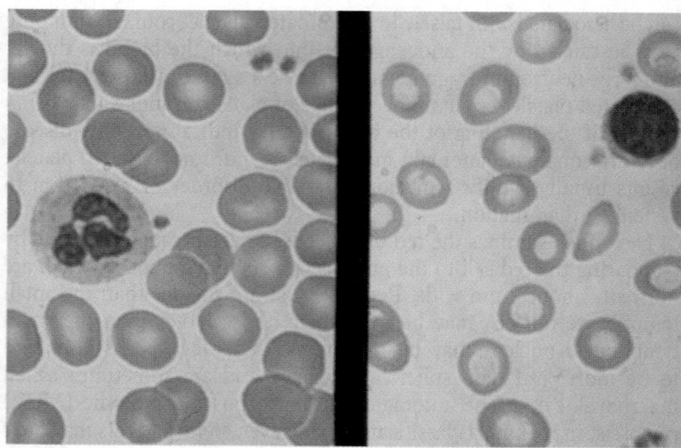

FIGURE 62-4 Iron deficiency anemia next to normal red blood cells. Microcytes (*right panel*) are smaller than normal red blood cells (cell diameter <7 μm) and may or may not be poorly hemoglobinized (hypochromic). *(Source: From M Lichtman et al (eds). Williams Hematology, 7th ed. New York, McGraw-Hill, 2005; RS Hillman, KA Ault, Hematology in General Practice, 4th ed. New York, McGraw-Hill, 2005.)*

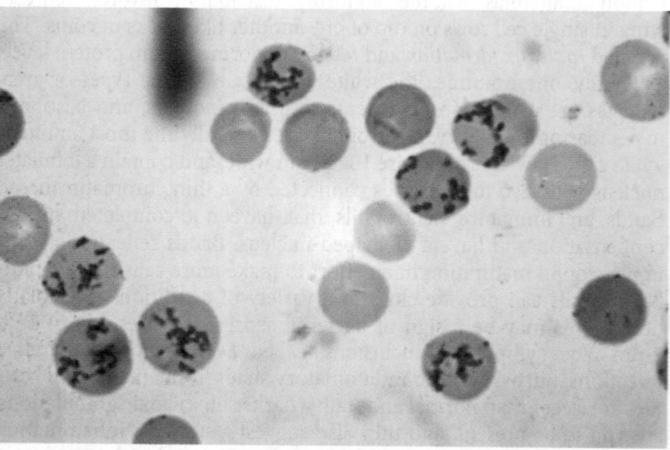

FIGURE 62-2 Reticulocyte count preparation. This new methylene blue–stained blood smear shows large numbers of heavily stained reticulocytes (the cells containing the dark blue–staining RNA precipitates). *(Source: From M Lichtman et al (eds): Williams Hematology, 7th ed. New York, McGraw-Hill, 2005; RS Hillman, KA Ault: Hematology in General Practice, 4th ed. New York, McGraw-Hill, 2005.)*

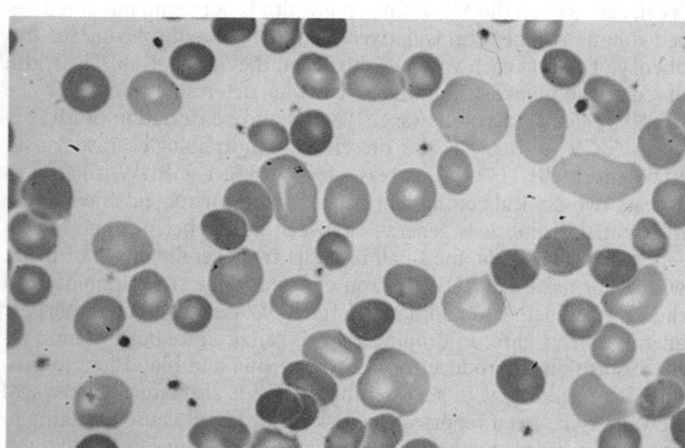

FIGURE 62-5 Polychromatophilia. Note large red cells with light purple coloring. *(Source: From M Lichtman et al (eds): Williams Hematology, 7th ed. New York, McGraw-Hill, 2005; RS Hillman, KA Ault: Hematology in General Practice, 4th ed. New York, McGraw-Hill, 2005.)*

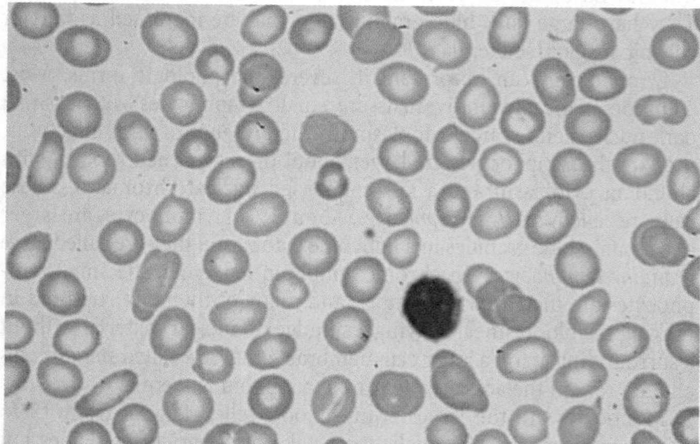

FIGURE 62-3 Hypochromic microcytic anemia of iron deficiency. Small lymphocyte in field helps assess the red blood cell size. *(Source: From M Lichtman et al (eds): Williams Hematology, 7th ed. New York, McGraw-Hill, 2005; RS Hillman, KA Ault: Hematology in General Practice, 4th ed. New York, McGraw-Hill, 2005.)*

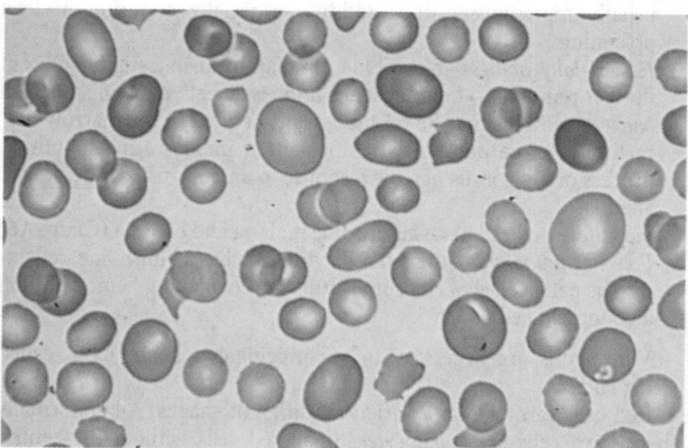

FIGURE 62-6 Macrocytosis. These cells are both larger than normal (mean corpuscular volume >100) and somewhat oval in shape. Some morphologists call these cells macroovalocytes. *(Source: From M Lichtman et al (eds): Williams Hematology, 7th ed. New York, McGraw-Hill, 2005; RS Hillman, KA Ault: Hematology in General Practice, 4th ed. New York, McGraw-Hill, 2005.)*

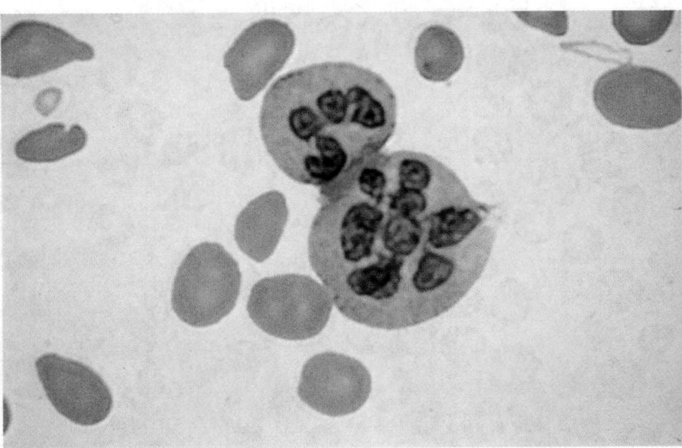

FIGURE 62-7 Hypersegmented neutrophils. Hypersegmented neutrophils (multilobed polymorphonuclear leukocytes) are larger than normal neutrophils with five or more segmented nuclear lobes. They are commonly seen with folic acid or vitamin B_{12} deficiency. *(Source: From M Lichtman et al (eds): Williams Hematology, 7th ed. New York, McGraw-Hill, 2005; RS Hillman, KA Ault: Hematology in General Practice, 4th ed. New York, McGraw-Hill, 2005.)*

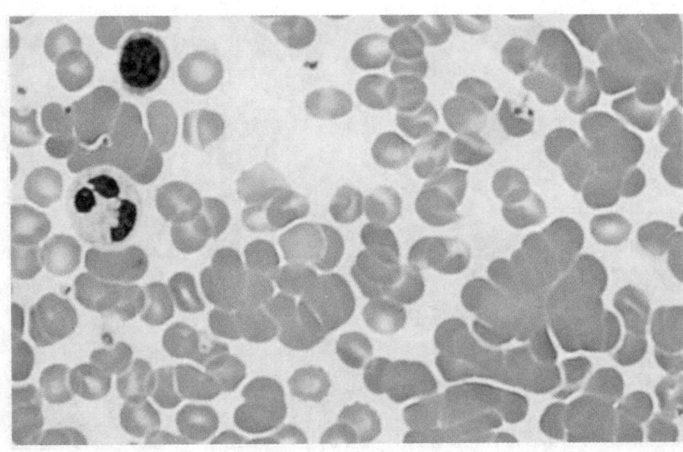

FIGURE 62-10 Red cell agglutination. Small lymphocyte and segmented neutrophil in upper left center. Note irregular collections of aggregated red cells. *(Source: From M Lichtman et al (eds): Williams Hematology, 7th ed. New York, McGraw-Hill, 2005; RS Hillman, KA Ault: Hematology in General Practice, 4th ed. New York, McGraw-Hill, 2005.)*

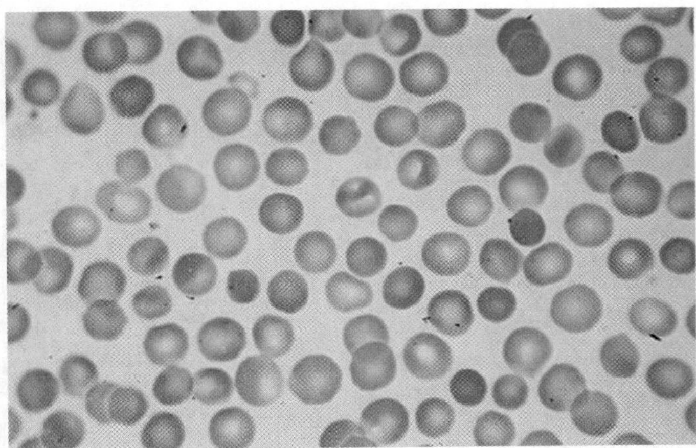

FIGURE 62-8 Spherocytosis. Note small hyperchromatic cells without the usual clear area in the center. *(Source: From M Lichtman et al (eds): Williams Hematology, 7th ed. New York, McGraw-Hill, 2005; RS Hillman, KA Ault: Hematology in General Practice, 4th ed. New York, McGraw-Hill, 2005.)*

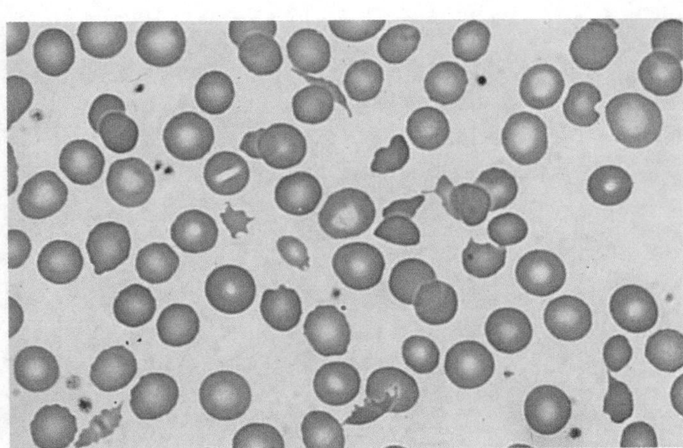

FIGURE 62-11 Fragmented red cells. Heart valve hemolysis. *(Source: From M Lichtman et al (eds): Williams Hematology, 7th ed. New York, McGraw-Hill, 2005; RS Hillman, KA Ault: Hematology in General Practice, 4th ed. New York, McGraw-Hill, 2005.)*

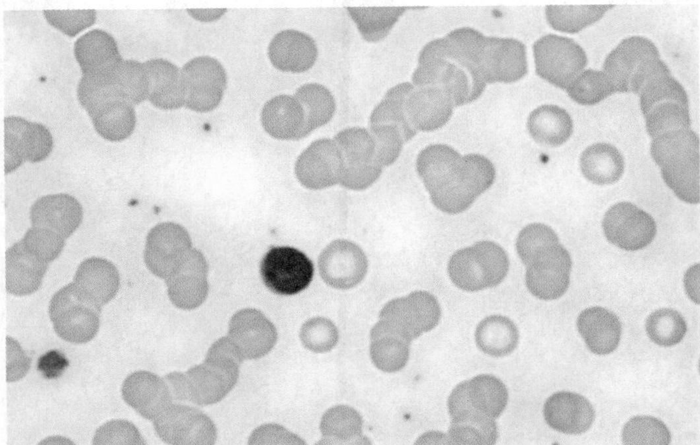

FIGURE 62-9 Rouleaux formation. Small lymphocyte in center of field. These red cells align themselves in stacks and are related to increased serum protein levels. *(Source: From M Lichtman et al (eds): Williams Hematology, 7th ed. New York, McGraw-Hill, 2005; RS Hillman, KA Ault: Hematology in General Practice, 4th ed. New York, McGraw-Hill, 2005.)*

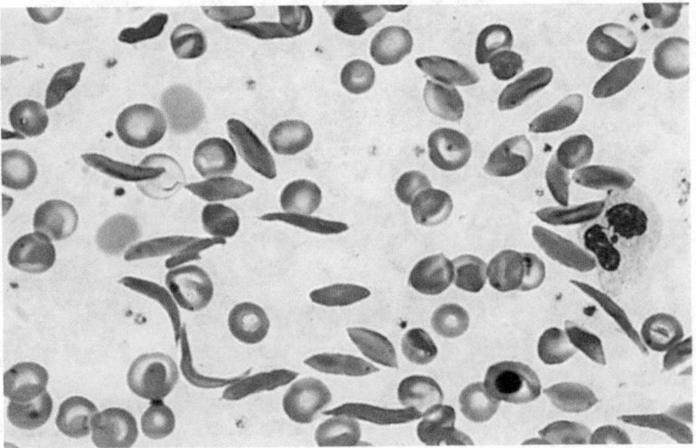

FIGURE 62-12 Sickle cells. Homozygous sickle cell disease. A nucleated red cell and neutrophil are also in the field. *(Source: From M Lichtman et al (eds): Williams Hematology, 7th ed. New York, McGraw-Hill, 2005; RS Hillman, KA Ault: Hematology in General Practice, 4th ed. New York, McGraw-Hill, 2005.)*

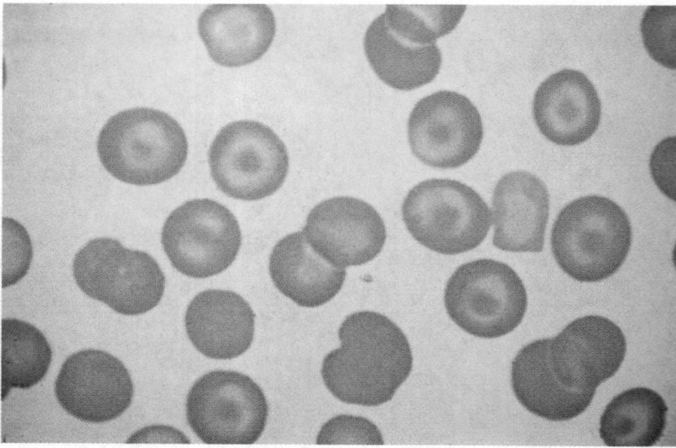

FIGURE 62-13 Target cells. Target cells are recognized by the bull's-eye appearance of the cell. Small numbers of target cells are seen with liver disease and thalassemia. Larger numbers are typical of hemoglobin C disease. *(Source: From M Lichtman et al (eds): Williams Hematology, 7th ed. New York, McGraw-Hill, 2005; RS Hillman, KA Ault: Hematology in General Practice, 4th ed. New York, McGraw-Hill, 2005.)*

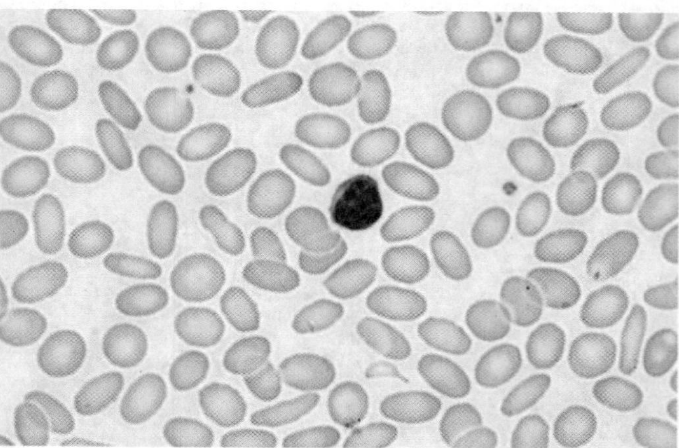

FIGURE 62-14 Elliptocytosis. Small lymphocyte in center of field. Elliptical shape of red cells related to weakened membrane structure, usually due to mutations in spectrin. *(Source: From M Lichtman et al (eds): Williams Hematology, 7th ed. New York, McGraw-Hill, 2005; RS Hillman, KA Ault: Hematology in General Practice, 4th ed. New York, McGraw-Hill, 2005.)*

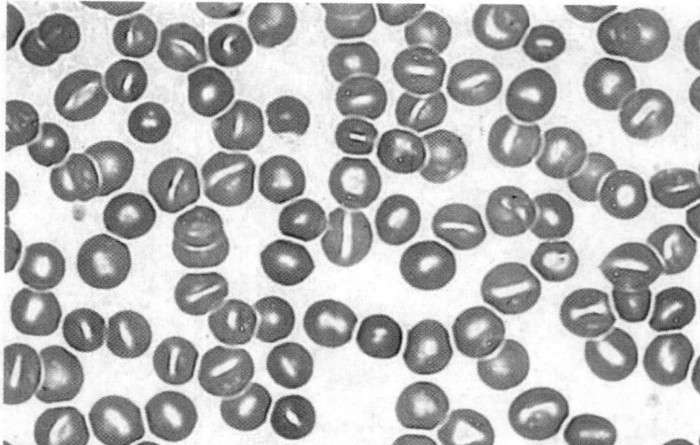

FIGURE 62-15 Stomatocytosis. Red cells characterized by a wide transverse slit or stoma. This often is seen as an artifact in a dehydrated blood smear. These cells can be seen in hemolytic anemias and in conditions in which the red cell is overhydrated or dehydrated. *(Source: From M Lichtman et al (eds): Williams Hematology, 7th ed. New York, McGraw-Hill, 2005; RS Hillman, KA Ault: Hematology in General Practice, 4th ed. New York, McGraw-Hill, 2005.)*

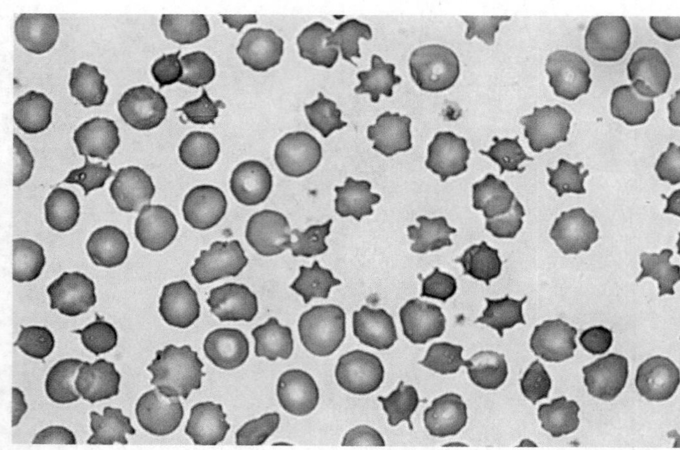

FIGURE 62-16 Acanthocytosis. Spiculated red cells are of two types: *acanthocytes* are contracted dense cells with irregular membrane projections that vary in length and width; *echinocytes* have small, uniform, and evenly spaced membrane projections. Acanthocytes are present in severe liver disease, in patients with abetalipoproteinemia, and in rare patients with McLeod blood group. Echinocytes are found in patients with severe uremia, in glycolytic red cell enzyme defects, and in microangiopathic hemolytic anemia. *(Source: From M Lichtman et al (eds): Williams Hematology, 7th ed. New York, McGraw-Hill, 2005; RS Hillman, KA Ault: Hematology in General Practice, 4th ed. New York, McGraw-Hill, 2005.)*

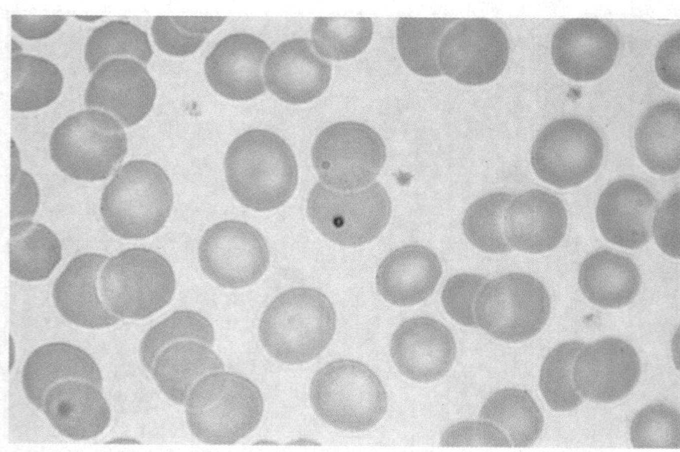

FIGURE 62-17 Howell-Jolly bodies. Howell-Jolly bodies are tiny nuclear remnants that normally are removed by the spleen. They appear in the blood after splenectomy (defect in removal) and with maturation/dysplastic disorders (excess production). *(Source: From M Lichtman et al (eds): Williams Hematology, 7th ed. New York, McGraw-Hill, 2005; RS Hillman, KA Ault: Hematology in General Practice, 4th ed. New York, McGraw-Hill, 2005.)*

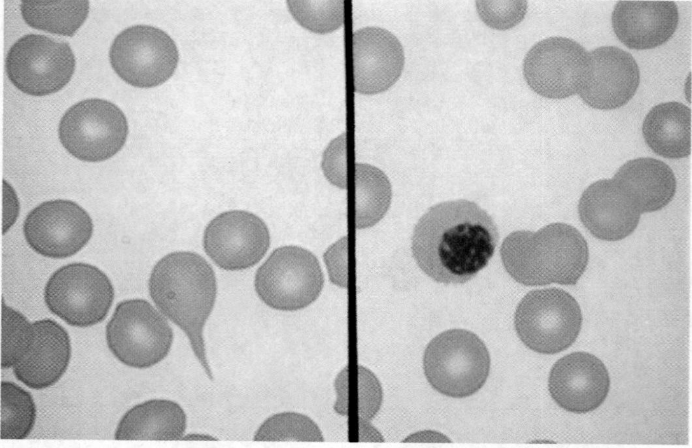

FIGURE 62-18 Teardrop cells and nucleated red blood cells characteristic of myelofibrosis. A teardrop-shaped red blood cell (*left panel*) and a nucleated red blood cell (*right panel*) as typically seen with myelofibrosis and extramedullary hematopoiesis. *(Source: From M Lichtman et al (eds): Williams Hematology, 7th ed. New York, McGraw-Hill, 2005; RS Hillman, KA Ault: Hematology in General Practice, 4th ed. New York, McGraw-Hill, 2005.)*

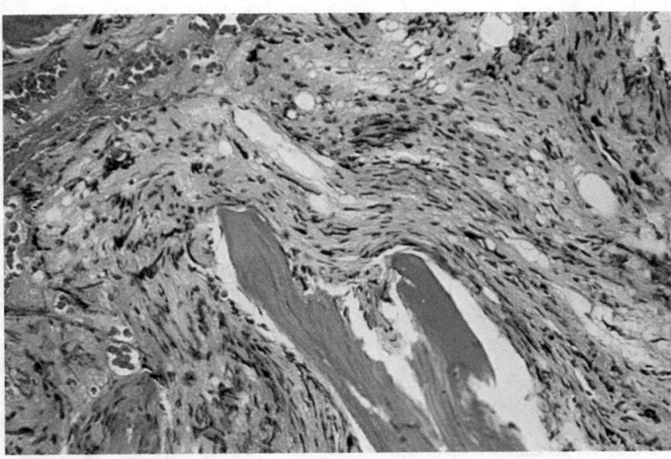

FIGURE 62-19 Myelofibrosis of the bone marrow. Total replacement of marrow precursors and fat cells by a dense infiltrate of reticulin fibers and collagen (hematoxylin and eosin stain). *(Source: From M Lichtman et al (eds): Williams Hematology, 7th ed. New York, McGraw-Hill, 2005; RS Hillman, KA Ault: Hematology in General Practice, 4th ed. New York, McGraw-Hill, 2005.)*

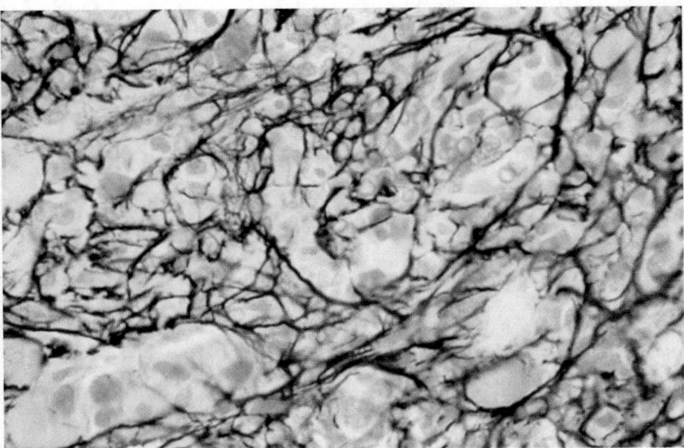

FIGURE 62-20 Reticulin stain of marrow myelofibrosis. Silver stain of a myelofibrotic marrow showing an increase in reticulin fibers (black-staining threads). *(Source: From M Lichtman et al (eds): Williams Hematology, 7th ed. New York, McGraw-Hill, 2005; RS Hillman, KA Ault: Hematology in General Practice, 4th ed. New York, McGraw-Hill, 2005.)*

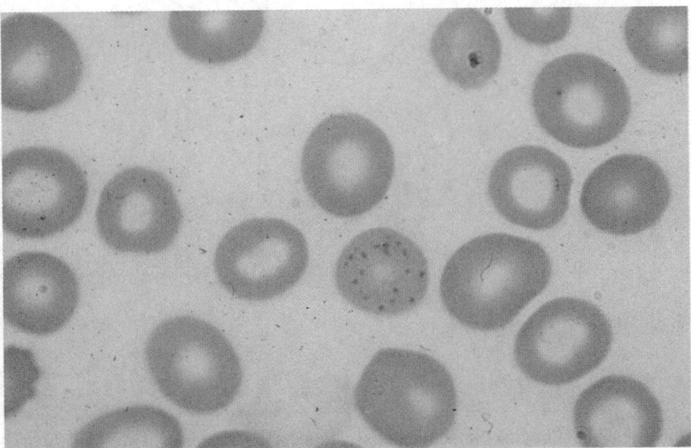

FIGURE 62-21 Stippled red cell in lead poisoning. Mild hypochromia. Coarsely stippled red cell. *(Source: From M Lichtman et al (eds): Williams Hematology, 7th ed. New York, McGraw-Hill, 2005; RS Hillman, KA Ault: Hematology in General Practice, 4th ed. New York, McGraw-Hill, 2005.)*

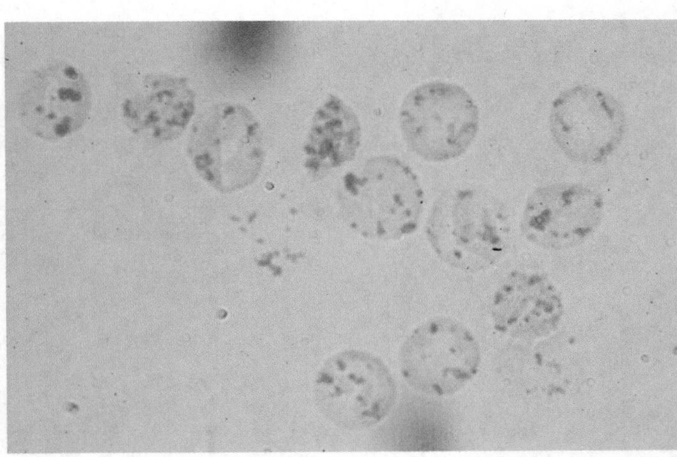

FIGURE 62-22 Heinz bodies. Blood mixed with hypotonic solution of crystal violet. The stained material is precipitates of denatured hemoglobin within cells. *(Source: From M Lichtman et al (eds): Williams Hematology, 7th ed. New York, McGraw-Hill, 2005; RS Hillman, KA Ault: Hematology in General Practice, 4th ed. New York, McGraw-Hill, 2005.)*

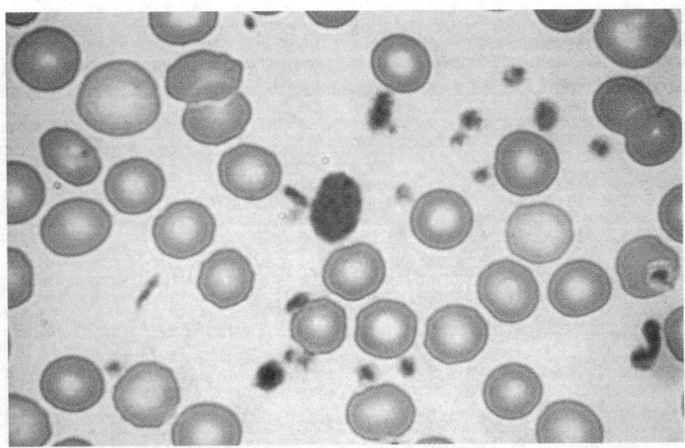

FIGURE 62-23 Giant platelets. Giant platelets, together with a marked increase in the platelet count, are seen in myeloproliferative disorders, especially primary thrombocythemia. *(Source: From M Lichtman et al (eds): Williams Hematology, 7th ed. New York, McGraw-Hill, 2005; RS Hillman, KA Ault: Hematology in General Practice, 4th ed. New York, McGraw-Hill, 2005.)*

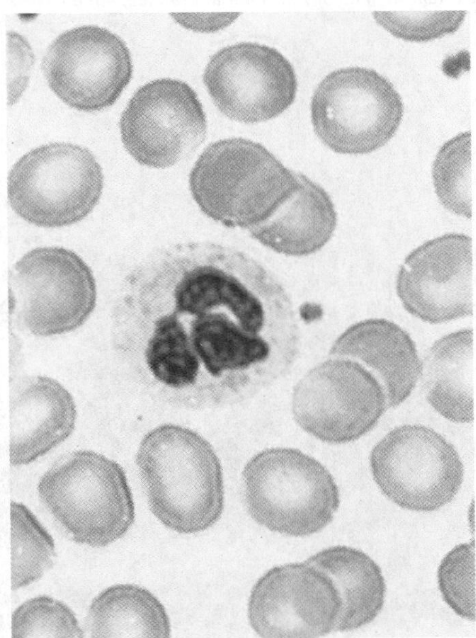

FIGURE 62-24 Normal granulocytes. The normal granulocyte has a segmented nucleus with heavy, clumped chromatin; fine neutrophilic granules are dispersed throughout the cytoplasm. *(Source: From M Lichtman et al (eds): Williams Hematology, 7th ed. New York, McGraw-Hill, 2005; RS Hillman, KA Ault: Hematology in General Practice, 4th ed. New York, McGraw-Hill, 2005.)*

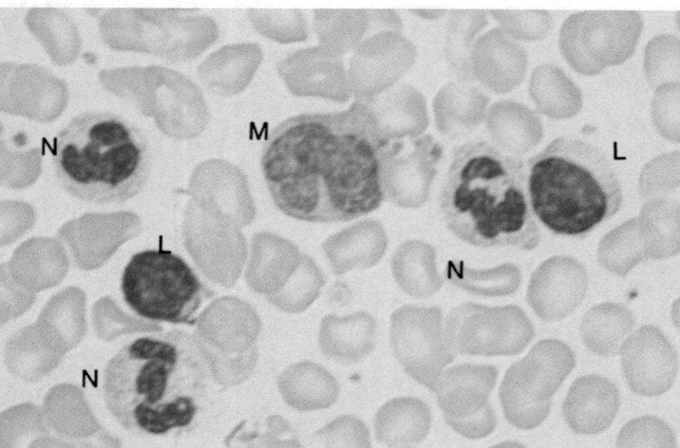

FIGURE 62-25 Normal monocytes. The film was prepared from the buffy coat of the blood from a normal donor. L, lymphocyte; M, monocyte; N, neutrophil. *(Source: From M Lichtman et al (eds): Williams Hematology, 7th ed. New York, McGraw-Hill, 2005; RS Hillman, KA Ault: Hematology in General Practice, 4th ed. New York, McGraw-Hill, 2005.)*

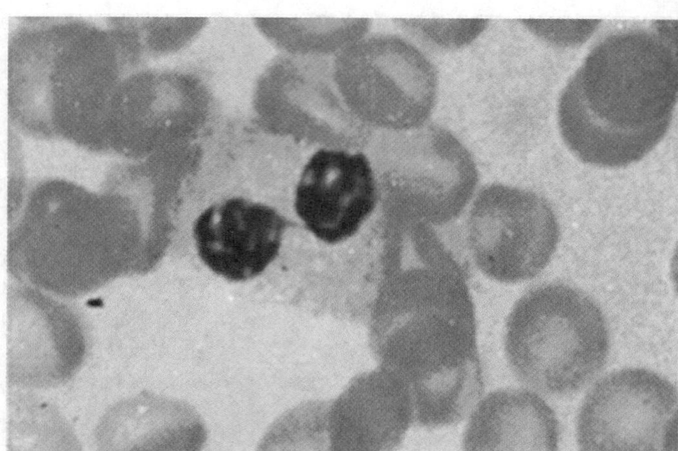

FIGURE 62-28 Pelger-Hüet anomaly. In this benign disorder, the majority of granulocytes are bilobed. The nucleus frequently has a spectacle-like, or "pince-nez," configuration. *(Source: From M Lichtman et al (eds): Williams Hematology, 7th ed. New York, McGraw-Hill, 2005; RS Hillman, KA Ault: Hematology in General Practice, 4th ed. New York, McGraw-Hill, 2005.)*

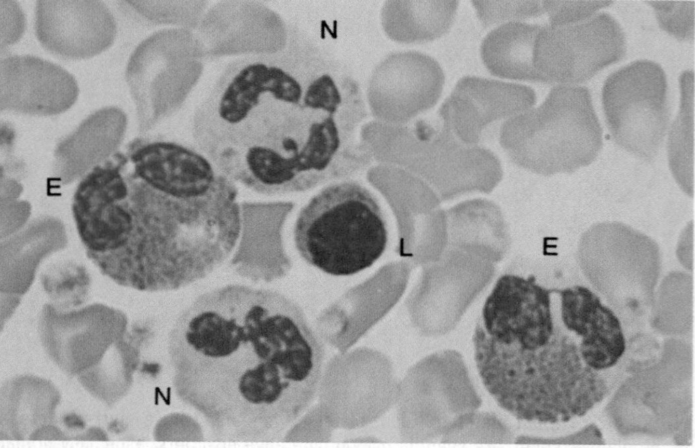

FIGURE 62-26 Normal eosinophils. The film was prepared from the buffy coat of the blood from a normal donor. E, eosinophil; L, lymphocyte; N, neutrophil. *(Source: From M Lichtman et al (eds): Williams Hematology, 7th ed. New York, McGraw-Hill, 2005; RS Hillman, KA Ault: Hematology in General Practice, 4th ed. New York, McGraw-Hill, 2005.)*

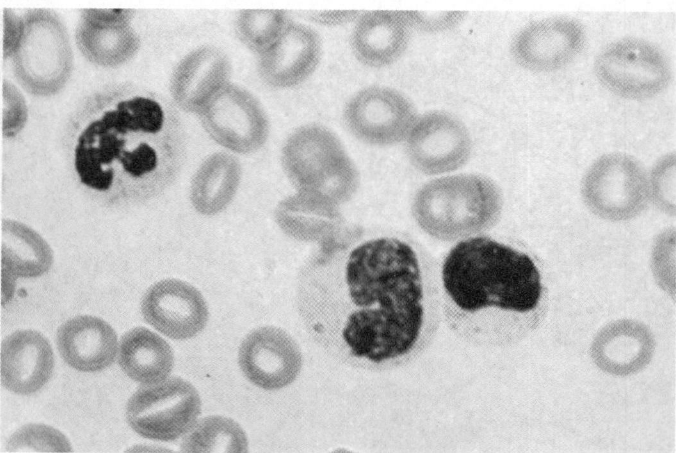

FIGURE 62-29 Döhle body. Neutrophil band with Döhle body. The neutrophil with a sausage-shaped nucleus in the center of the field is a band form. Döhle bodies are discrete, blue-staining nongranular areas found in the periphery of the cytoplasm of the neutrophil in infections and other toxic states. They represent aggregates of rough endoplasmic reticulum. *(Source: From M Lichtman et al (eds): Williams Hematology, 7th ed. New York, McGraw-Hill, 2005; RS Hillman, KA Ault: Hematology in General Practice, 4th ed. New York, McGraw-Hill, 2005.)*

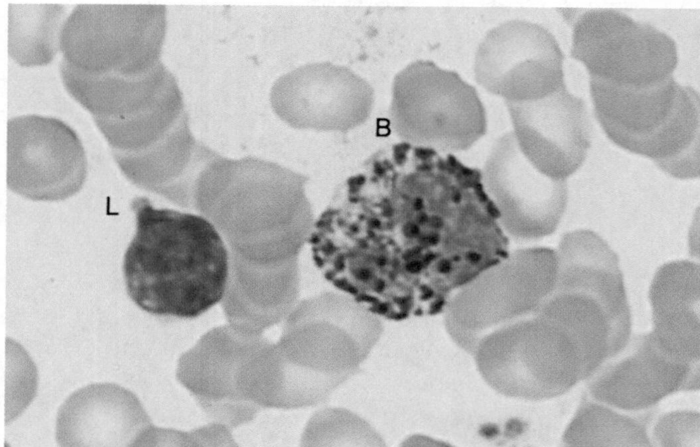

FIGURE 62-27 Normal basophil. The film was prepared from the buffy coat of the blood from a normal donor. B, basophil; L, lymphocyte. *(Source: From M Lichtman et al (eds): Williams Hematology, 7th ed. New York, McGraw-Hill, 2005; RS Hillman, KA Ault: Hematology in General Practice, 4th ed. New York, McGraw-Hill, 2005.)*

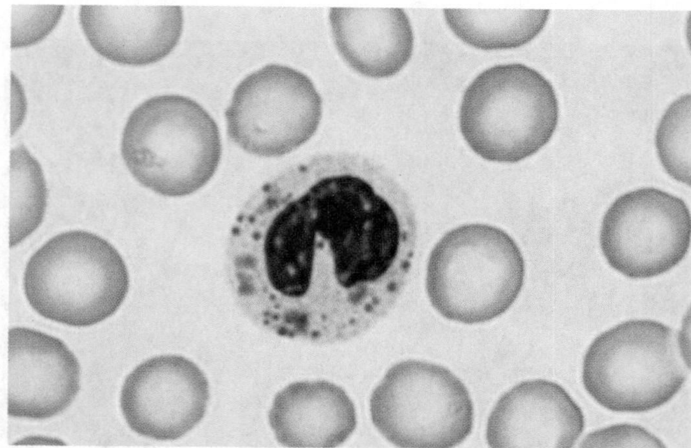

FIGURE 62-30 Chédiak-Higashi disease. Note giant granules in neutrophil. *(Source: From M Lichtman et al (eds): Williams Hematology, 7th ed. New York, McGraw-Hill, 2005; RS Hillman, KA Ault: Hematology in General Practice, 4th ed. New York, McGraw-Hill, 2005.)*

epithelial malignant cells may be identified. The chances of seeing such abnormal cells are increased by examining blood smears made from buffy coats, the layer of cells that is visible on top of sedimenting red cells when blood is left in the test tube for an hour. Smears made from finger sticks may include rare endothelial cells.

ACKNOWLEDGMENT

Figures in this chapter were borrowed from Williams Hematology, 7th edition, M Lichtman et al (eds). New York, McGraw-Hill, 2005; Hematology in General Practice, 4th edition, RS Hillman, KA Ault. New York, McGraw-Hill, 2005.

63 Anemia and Polycythemia

John W. Adamson, Dan L. Longo

HEMATOPOIESIS AND THE PHYSIOLOGIC BASIS OF RED CELL PRODUCTION

Hematopoiesis is the process by which the formed elements of blood are produced. The process is regulated through a series of steps beginning with the hematopoietic stem cell. Stem cells are capable of producing red cells, all classes of granulocytes, monocytes, platelets, and the cells of the immune system. The precise molecular mechanism by which the stem cell becomes committed to a given lineage is not fully defined. However, experiments in mice suggest that erythroid cells come from a common erythroid/megakaryocyte progenitor that does not develop in the absence of expression of the GATA-1 and FOG-1 (friend of GATA-1) transcription factors (**Chap. 96**). Following lineage commitment, hematopoietic progenitor and precursor cells come increasingly under the regulatory influence of growth factors and hormones. For red cell production, erythropoietin (EPO) is the primary regulatory hormone. EPO is required for the maintenance of committed erythroid progenitor cells that, in the absence of the hormone, undergo programmed cell death (*apoptosis*). The regulated process of red cell production is *erythropoiesis*, and its key elements are illustrated in **Fig. 63-1**.

In the bone marrow, the first morphologically recognizable erythroid precursor is the pronormoblast. This cell can undergo four to five cell divisions, which result in the production of 16–32 mature red cells. With increased EPO production, or the administration of EPO as a drug, early progenitor cell numbers are amplified and, in turn, give rise to increased numbers of erythrocytes. The regulation of EPO production itself is linked to tissue oxygenation.

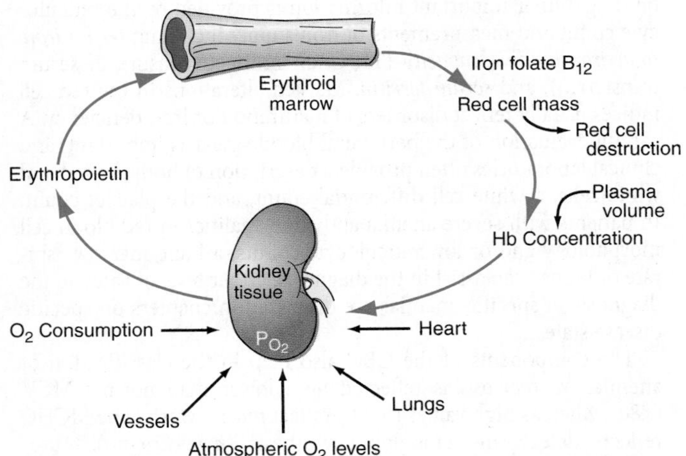

FIGURE 63-1 The physiologic regulation of red cell production by tissue oxygen tension. Hb, hemoglobin.

In mammals, O_2 is transported to tissues bound to the hemoglobin contained within circulating red cells. The mature red cell is 8 μm in diameter, anucleate, discoid in shape, and extremely pliable in order to traverse the microcirculation successfully; its membrane integrity is maintained by the intracellular generation of ATP. Normal red cell production results in the daily replacement of 0.8–1% of all circulating red cells in the body, since the average red cell lives 100–120 days. The organ responsible for red cell production is called the *erythron*. The erythron is a dynamic organ made up of a rapidly proliferating pool of marrow erythroid precursor cells and a large mass of mature circulating red blood cells. The size of the red cell mass reflects the balance of red cell production and destruction. The physiologic basis of red cell production and destruction provides an understanding of the mechanisms that can lead to anemia.

The physiologic regulator of red cell production, the glycoprotein hormone EPO, is produced and released by peritubular capillary lining cells within the kidney. These cells are highly specialized epithelial-like cells. A small amount of EPO is produced by hepatocytes. The fundamental stimulus for EPO production is the availability of O_2 for tissue metabolic needs. Key to EPO gene regulation is hypoxia-inducible factor (HIF)-1α. In the presence of O_2, HIF-1α is hydroxylated at a key proline, allowing HIF-1α to be ubiquitinated and degraded via the proteasome pathway. If O_2 becomes limiting, this critical hydroxylation step does not occur, allowing HIF-1α to partner with other proteins, translocate to the nucleus, and upregulate the expression of the EPO gene, among others.

Impaired O_2 delivery to the kidney can result from a decreased red cell mass (*anemia*), impaired O_2 loading of the hemoglobin molecule or a high O_2 affinity mutant hemoglobin (*hypoxemia*), or, rarely, impaired blood flow to the kidney (e.g., renal artery stenosis). EPO governs the day-to-day production of red cells, and ambient levels of the hormone can be measured in the plasma by sensitive immunoassays—the normal level being 10–25 U/L. When the hemoglobin concentration falls below 100–120 g/L (10–12 g/dL), plasma EPO levels increase in proportion to the severity of the anemia (**Fig. 63-2**). In circulation, EPO has a half-clearance time of 6–9 h. EPO acts by binding to specific receptors on the surface of marrow erythroid precursors, inducing them to proliferate and to mature. With EPO stimulation, red cell production can increase four- to fivefold within a 1- to 2-week period, but only in the presence of adequate nutrients, especially iron. The functional capacity of the erythron, therefore, requires normal renal production of EPO, a functioning erythroid marrow, and an adequate supply of substrates for hemoglobin synthesis. A defect in any of these key components can lead to anemia. Generally, anemia is recognized in the laboratory when a patient's hemoglobin level or hematocrit is reduced below an expected value (the normal range).

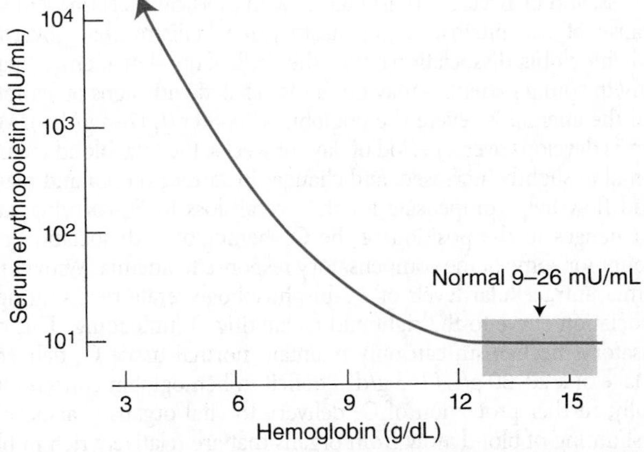

FIGURE 63-2 Erythropoietin (EPO) levels in response to anemia. When the hemoglobin level falls to 120 g/L (12 g/dL), plasma EPO levels increase logarithmically. In the presence of chronic kidney disease or chronic inflammation, EPO levels are typically lower than expected for the degree of anemia. As individuals age, the level of EPO needed to sustain normal hemoglobin levels appears to increase. *(Reproduced with permission from RS Hillman et al: Hematology in Clinical Practice, 5th ed. New York, McGraw-Hill, 2010.)*

The likelihood and severity of anemia are defined based on the deviation of the patient's hemoglobin/hematocrit from values expected for age- and sex-matched normal subjects. The hemoglobin concentration in adults has a Gaussian distribution. The normal range of hemoglobin values for adult males is 13.5–17.5 g/dL (135–175 g/L) and that for adult females is 12–15 g/dL (120–150 g/L). The World Health Organization (WHO) defines anemia as a hemoglobin level <13 g/dL (130 g/L) in men and <12 g/dL (120 g/L) in women. Hematocrit levels are less useful than hemoglobin levels in assessing anemia because they are calculated rather than measured directly. Suspected low hemoglobin or hematocrit values are more easily interpreted if previous values for the same patient are known for comparison.

The critical elements of erythropoiesis—EPO production, iron availability, the proliferative capacity of the bone marrow, and effective maturation of red cell precursors—are used for the initial classification of anemia (see below).

ANEMIA

CLINICAL PRESENTATION OF ANEMIA

Signs and Symptoms Anemia is most often recognized by abnormal screening laboratory tests. Patients less commonly present with advanced anemia and its attendant signs and symptoms. Acute anemia is due to blood loss or hemolysis. If blood loss is mild, enhanced O_2 delivery is achieved through changes in the O_2–hemoglobin dissociation curve mediated by a decreased pH or increased CO_2 (*Bohr effect*). With acute blood loss, hypovolemia dominates the clinical picture, and the hematocrit and hemoglobin levels do not reflect the volume of blood lost. Signs of vascular instability appear with acute losses of 10–15% of the total blood volume. In such patients, the issue is not anemia but hypotension and decreased organ perfusion. When >30% of the blood volume is lost suddenly, patients are unable to compensate with the usual mechanisms of vascular contraction and changes in regional blood flow. The patient prefers to remain supine and will show postural hypotension and tachycardia. If the volume of blood lost is >40% (i.e., >2 L in the average-sized adult), signs of hypovolemic shock including confusion, dyspnea, diaphoresis, hypotension, and tachycardia appear (**Chap. 101**). Such patients have significant deficits in vital organ perfusion and require immediate volume replacement.

With acute hemolysis, the signs and symptoms depend on the mechanism that leads to red cell destruction. Intravascular hemolysis with release of free hemoglobin may be associated with acute back pain, free hemoglobin in the plasma and urine, and renal failure. Symptoms associated with more chronic or progressive anemia depend on the age of the patient and the adequacy of blood supply to critical organs. Symptoms associated with moderate anemia include fatigue, loss of stamina, breathlessness, and tachycardia (particularly with physical exertion). However, because of the intrinsic compensatory mechanisms that govern the O_2–hemoglobin dissociation curve, the gradual onset of anemia—particularly in young patients—may not be associated with signs or symptoms until the anemia is severe (hemoglobin <70–80 g/L [7–8 g/dL]). When anemia develops over a period of days or weeks, the total blood volume is normal to slightly increased, and changes in cardiac output and regional blood flow help compensate for the overall loss in O_2-carrying capacity. Changes in the position of the O_2–hemoglobin dissociation curve account for some of the compensatory response to anemia. With chronic anemia, intracellular levels of 2,3-bisphosphoglycerate rise, shifting the dissociation curve to the right and facilitating O_2 unloading. This compensatory mechanism can only maintain normal tissue O_2 delivery in the face of a 20–30 g/L (2–3 g/dL) deficit in hemoglobin concentration. Finally, further protection of O_2 delivery to vital organs is achieved by the shunting of blood away from organs that are relatively rich in blood supply, particularly the kidney, gut, and skin.

Certain disorders are commonly associated with anemia. Chronic inflammatory states (e.g., infection, rheumatoid arthritis, cancer) are associated with mild to moderate anemia, whereas lymphoproliferative disorders, such as chronic lymphocytic leukemia and certain other B-cell neoplasms, may be associated with autoimmune hemolysis.

APPROACH TO THE PATIENT

Anemia

The evaluation of the patient with anemia requires a careful history and physical examination. Nutritional history related to drugs or alcohol intake and family history of anemia should always be assessed. Certain geographic backgrounds and ethnic origins are associated with an increased likelihood of an inherited disorder of the hemoglobin molecule or intermediary metabolism. Glucose-6-phosphate dehydrogenase (G6PD) deficiency and certain hemoglobinopathies are seen more commonly in those of Middle Eastern or African origin, including blacks who have a high frequency of G6PD deficiency. Other information that may be useful includes exposure to certain toxic agents or drugs and symptoms related to other disorders commonly associated with anemia. These include symptoms and signs such as bleeding, fatigue, malaise, fever, weight loss, night sweats, and other systemic symptoms. Clues to the mechanisms of anemia may be provided on physical examination by findings of infection, blood in the stool, lymphadenopathy, splenomegaly, or petechiae. Splenomegaly and lymphadenopathy suggest an underlying lymphoproliferative disease, whereas petechiae suggest platelet dysfunction. Past laboratory measurements are helpful to determine a time of onset.

In the anemic patient, physical examination may demonstrate a forceful heartbeat, strong peripheral pulses, and a systolic "flow" murmur. The skin and mucous membranes may be pale if the hemoglobin is <8–10 g/dL (80–100 g/L). This part of the physical examination should focus on areas where vessels are close to the surface such as the mucous membranes, nail beds, and palmar creases. If the palmar creases are lighter in color than the surrounding skin when the hand is hyperextended, the hemoglobin level is usually <8 g/dL (80 g/L).

LABORATORY EVALUATION

Table 63-1 lists the tests used in the initial workup of anemia. A routine complete blood count (CBC) is required as part of the evaluation and includes the hemoglobin, hematocrit, and red cell indices: the mean cell volume (MCV) in femtoliters, mean cell hemoglobin (MCH) in picograms per cell, and mean concentration of hemoglobin per volume of red cells (MCHC) in grams per liter (non-SI: grams per deciliter). The MCH is the least useful of the indices; it tends to track with the MCV. The red cell indices are calculated as shown in **Table 63-2**, and the normal variations in the hemoglobin and hematocrit with age are shown in **Table 63-3**. A number of physiologic factors affect the CBC, including age, sex, pregnancy, smoking, and altitude. High-normal hemoglobin values may be seen in men and women who live at altitude or smoke heavily. Hemoglobin elevations due to smoking reflect normal compensation due to the displacement of O_2 by CO in hemoglobin binding. Other important information is provided by the reticulocyte count and measurements of iron supply including *serum iron, total iron-binding capacity* (TIBC; an indirect measure of serum transferrin), and *serum ferritin*. Marked alterations in the red cell indices usually reflect disorders of maturation or iron deficiency. A careful evaluation of the peripheral blood smear is important, and clinical laboratories often provide a description of both the red and white cells, a white cell differential count, and the platelet count. In patients with severe anemia and abnormalities in red blood cell morphology and/or low reticulocyte counts, a bone marrow aspirate or biopsy can assist in the diagnosis. Other tests of value in the diagnosis of specific anemias are discussed in chapters on specific disease states.

The components of the CBC also help in the classification of anemia. *Microcytosis* is reflected by a lower than normal MCV (<80), whereas high values (>100) reflect *macrocytosis*. The MCHC reflects defects in hemoglobin synthesis (*hypochromia*). Automated cell counters describe the red cell volume distribution width (RDW). The MCV (representing the peak of the distribution curve)

TABLE 63-1 Laboratory Tests in Anemia Diagnosis

I. Complete blood count (CBC)
   A. Red blood cell count
      1. Hemoglobin
      2. Hematocrit
      3. Reticulocyte count
   B. Red blood cell indices
      1. Mean cell volume (MCV)
      2. Mean cell hemoglobin (MCH)
      3. Mean cell hemoglobin concentration (MCHC)
      4. Red cell distribution width (RDW)
   C. White blood cell count
      1. Cell differential
      2. Nuclear segmentation of neutrophils
   D. Platelet count
   E. Cell morphology
      1. Cell size
      2. Hemoglobin content
      3. Anisocytosis
      4. Poikilocytosis
      5. Polychromasia
II. Iron supply studies
   A. Serum iron
   B. Total iron-binding capacity
   C. Serum ferritin
III. Marrow examination
   A. Aspirate
      1. M/E ratio[a]
      2. Cell morphology
      3. Iron stain
   B. Biopsy
      1. Cellularity
      2. Morphology

[a]M/E ratio, ratio of myeloid to erythroid precursors.

TABLE 63-2 Red Blood Cell Indices

INDEX	NORMAL VALUE
Mean cell volume (MCV) = (hematocrit × 10)/(red cell count × 10^6)	90 ± 8 fL
Mean cell hemoglobin (MCH) = (hemoglobin × 10)/(red cell count × 10^6)	30 ± 3 pg
Mean cell hemoglobin concentration = (hemoglobin × 10)/hematocrit, or MCH/MCV	33 ± 2%

TABLE 63-3 Changes in Normal Hemoglobin/Hematocrit Values with Age, Sex, and Pregnancy

AGE/SEX	HEMOGLOBIN, g/dL	HEMATOCRIT, %
At birth	17	52
Childhood	12	36
Adolescence	13	40
Adult man	16 (±2)	47 (±6)
Adult woman (menstruating)	13 (±2)	40 (±6)
Adult woman (postmenopausal)	14 (±2)	42 (±6)
During pregnancy	12 (±2)	37 (±6)

Source: From RS Hillman et al: *Hematology in Clinical Practice*, 5th ed. New York, McGraw-Hill, 2010.

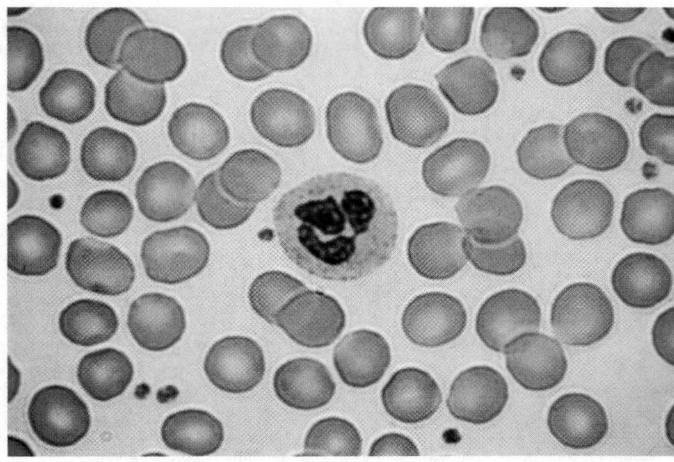

FIGURE 63-3 Normal blood smear (Wright stain). High-power field showing normal red cells, a neutrophil, and a few platelets. *(From RS Hillman et al: Hematology in Clinical Practice, 5th ed. New York, McGraw-Hill, 2010.)*

is insensitive to the appearance of small populations of macrocytes or microcytes. An experienced laboratory technician will be able to identify minor populations of large or small cells or hypochromic cells on the peripheral blood film before the red cell indices change.

Peripheral Blood Smear The peripheral blood smear provides important information about defects in red cell production (**Chap. 62**). As a complement to the red cell indices, the blood smear also reveals variations in cell size (*anisocytosis*) and shape (*poikilocytosis*). The degree of anisocytosis usually correlates with increases in the RDW or the range of cell sizes. Poikilocytosis suggests a defect in the maturation of red cell precursors in the bone marrow or fragmentation of circulating red cells. The blood smear may also reveal *polychromasia*—red cells that are slightly larger than normal and grayish blue in color on the Wright-Giemsa stain. These cells are reticulocytes that have been released prematurely from the bone marrow and their color represents residual amounts of ribosomal RNA. These cells appear in circulation in response to EPO stimulation or to architectural damage of the bone marrow (fibrosis, infiltration of the marrow by malignant cells, etc.) that results in their disordered release from the marrow. The appearance of nucleated red cells, Howell-Jolly bodies, target cells, sickle cells, and other changes may provide clues to specific disorders (**Figs. 63-3 to 63-11**).

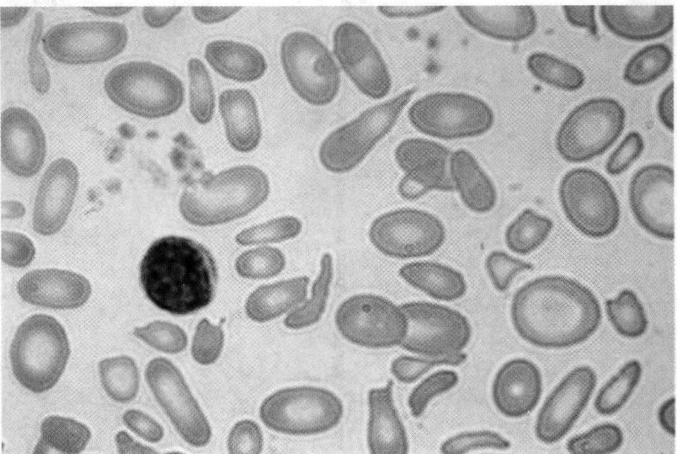

FIGURE 63-4 Severe iron-deficiency anemia. Microcytic and hypochromic red cells smaller than the nucleus of a lymphocyte associated with marked variation in size (anisocytosis) and shape (poikilocytosis). *(From RS Hillman et al: Hematology in Clinical Practice, 5th ed. New York, McGraw-Hill, 2010.)*

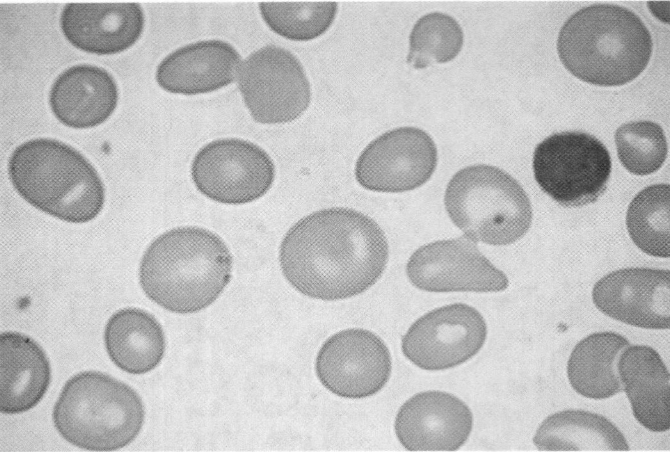

FIGURE 63-5 Macrocytosis. Red cells are larger than a small lymphocyte and well hemoglobinized. Often macrocytes are oval shaped (macro-ovalocytes). *(From RS Hillman et al: Hematology in Clinical Practice, 5th ed. New York, McGraw-Hill, 2010.)*

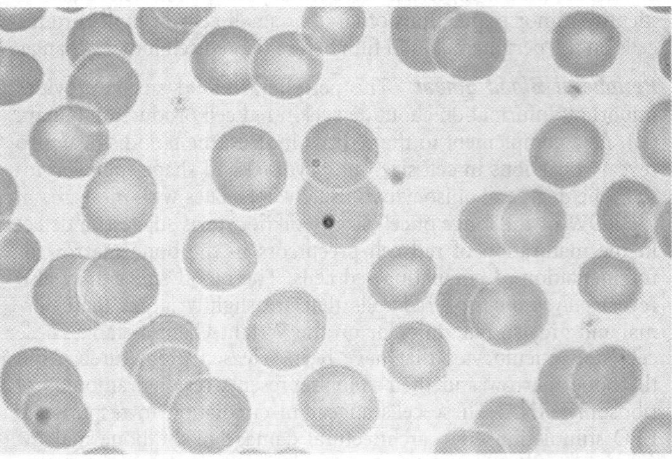

FIGURE 63-6 Howell-Jolly bodies. In the absence of a functional spleen, nuclear remnants are not culled from the red cells and remain as small homogeneously staining blue inclusions on Wright stain. *(From M Lichtman et al (eds): Williams Hematology, 7th ed. New York, McGraw-Hill, 2005; RS Hillman, KA Ault: Hematology in General Practice, 4th ed. New York, McGraw-Hill, 2005.)*

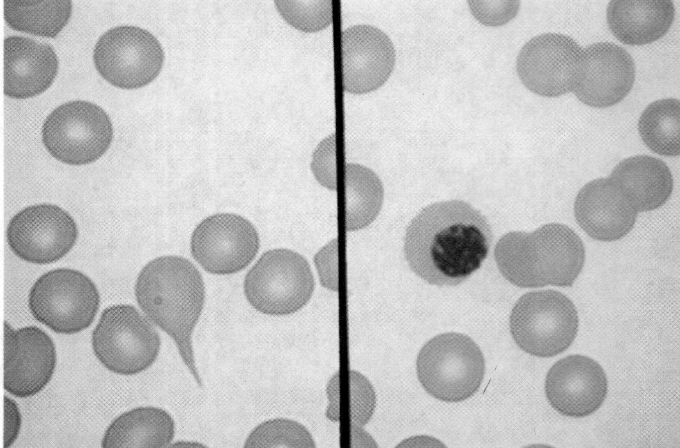

FIGURE 63-7 Red cell changes in myelofibrosis. The left panel shows a teardrop-shaped cell. The right panel shows a nucleated red cell. These forms can be seen in myelofibrosis. *(From RS Hillman et al: Hematology in Clinical Practice, 5th ed. New York, McGraw-Hill, 2010.)*

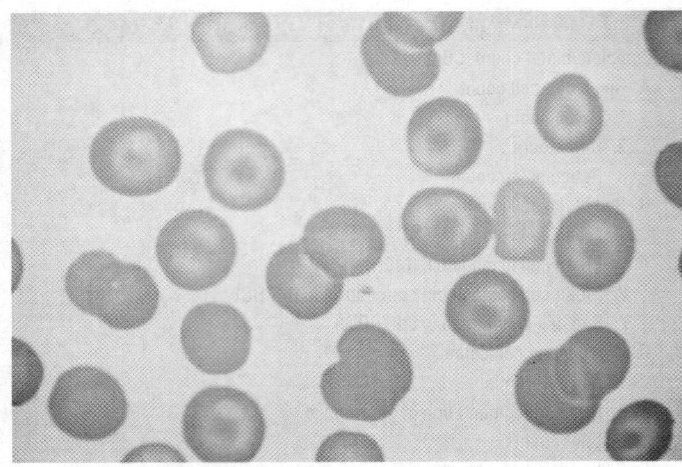

FIGURE 63-8 Target cells. Target cells have a bull's-eye appearance and are seen in thalassemia and in liver disease. *(From M Lichtman et al (eds): Williams Hematology, 7th ed. New York, McGraw-Hill, 2005; RS Hillman, KA Ault: Hematology in General Practice, 4th ed. New York, McGraw-Hill, 2005.)*

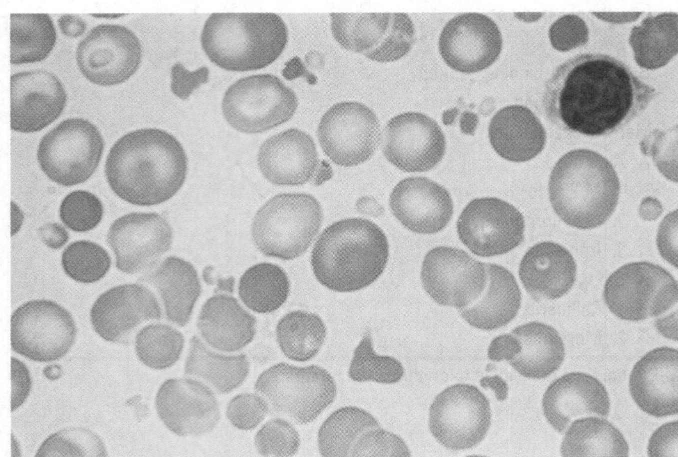

FIGURE 63-9 Red cell fragmentation. Red cells may become fragmented in the presence of foreign bodies in the circulation, such as mechanical heart valves, or in the setting of thermal injury. *(From RS Hillman et al: Hematology in Clinical Practice, 5th ed. New York, McGraw-Hill, 2010.)*

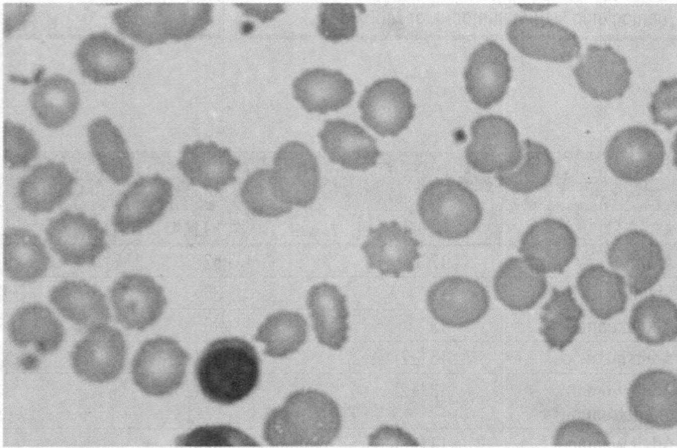

FIGURE 63-10 Uremia. The red cells in uremia may acquire numerous regularly spaced, small, spiny projections. Such cells, called burr cells or echinocytes, are readily distinguishable from irregularly spiculated acanthocytes shown in Fig. 63-11. *(From RS Hillman et al: Hematology in Clinical Practice, 5th ed. New York, McGraw-Hill, 2010.)*

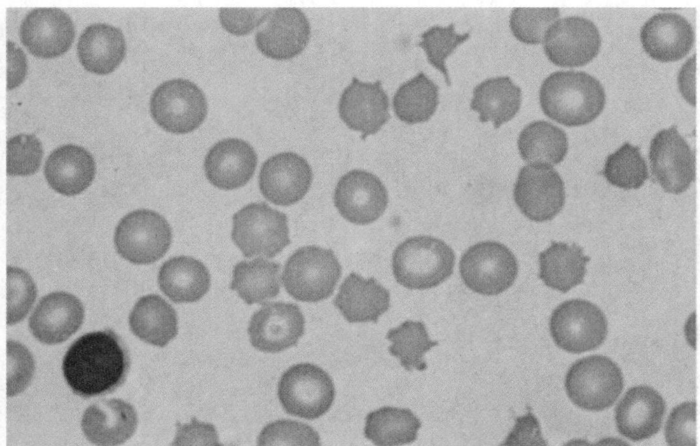

FIGURE 63-11 Spur cells. Spur cells are recognized as distorted red cells containing several irregularly distributed thorn-like projections. Cells with this morphologic abnormality are also called acanthocytes. *(From RS Hillman et al: Hematology in Clinical Practice, 5th ed. New York, McGraw-Hill, 2010.)*

Reticulocyte Count An accurate reticulocyte count is key to the initial classification of anemia. Reticulocytes are red cells that have been recently released from the bone marrow. They are identified by staining with a supravital dye that precipitates the ribosomal RNA (Fig. 63-12). These precipitates appear as blue or black punctate spots and can be counted manually or, currently, by fluorescent emission of dyes that bind to RNA. This residual RNA is metabolized over the first 24–36 h of the reticulocyte's life span in circulation. Normally, the reticulocyte count ranges from 1% to 2% and reflects the daily replacement of 0.8–1.0% of the circulating red cell population. A corrected reticulocyte percentage or the absolute number of reticulocytes provides a reliable measure of effective red cell production.

In the initial classification of anemia, the patient's reticulocyte count is compared with the expected reticulocyte response. In general, if the EPO and erythroid marrow responses to moderate anemia [hemoglobin <100 g/L (10 g/dL)] are intact, the red cell production rate increases to two to three times normal within 10 days following the onset of anemia. In the face of established anemia, a reticulocyte response less than two to three times normal indicates an inadequate marrow response.

To use the reticulocyte count to estimate marrow response, two corrections are necessary. The first correction adjusts the reticulocyte count based on the reduced number of circulating red cells. With anemia, the percentage of reticulocytes may be increased

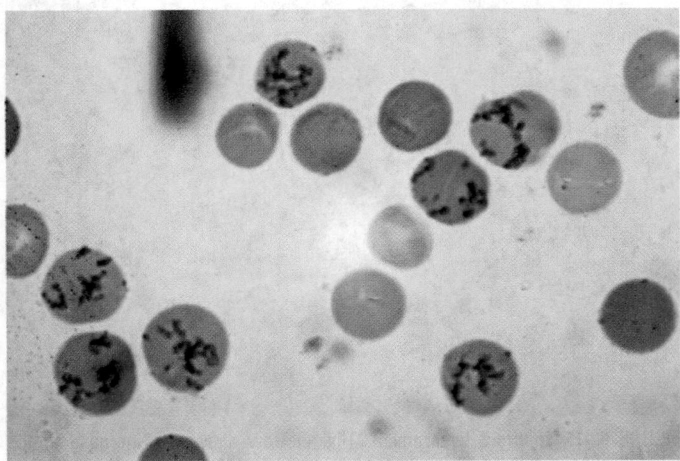

FIGURE 63-12 Reticulocytes. Methylene blue stain demonstrates residual RNA in newly made red cells. *(From RS Hillman et al: Hematology in Clinical Practice, 5th ed. New York, McGraw-Hill, 2010.)*

TABLE 63-4 Calculation of Reticulocyte Production Index

Correction #1 for Anemia:
This correction produces the corrected reticulocyte count.
In a person whose reticulocyte count is 9%, hemoglobin 7.5 g/dL, and hematocrit 23%, the absolute reticulocyte count = 9 × (7.5/15) [or × (23/45)] = 4.5%
Note. This correction is not done if the reticulocyte count is reported in absolute numbers (e.g., 50,000/μL of blood)
Correction #2 for Longer Life of Prematurely Released Reticulocytes in the Blood:
This correction produces the reticulocyte production index.
In a person whose reticulocyte count is 9%, hemoglobin 7.5 g/dL, and hematocrit 23%, the reticulocyte production index
$= 9 \times \frac{(7.5/15)(\text{hemoglobin correction})}{2(\text{maturation time correction})} = 2.25$

while the absolute number is unchanged. To correct for this effect, the reticulocyte percentage is multiplied by the ratio of the patient's hemoglobin or hematocrit to the expected hemoglobin/hematocrit for the age and sex of the patient (Table 63-4). This provides an estimate of the reticulocyte count corrected for anemia. To convert the corrected reticulocyte count to an index of marrow production, a further correction is required, depending on whether some of the reticulocytes in circulation have been released from the marrow prematurely. For this second correction, the peripheral blood smear is examined to see if there are polychromatophilic macrocytes present.

These cells, representing prematurely released reticulocytes, are referred to as "shift" cells, and the relationship between the degree of shift and the necessary shift correction factor is shown in Fig. 63-13. The correction is necessary because these prematurely released cells survive as reticulocytes in circulation for >1 day, thereby providing a falsely high estimate of daily red cell production. If polychromasia is increased, the reticulocyte count, already corrected for anemia, should be corrected again by 2 to account for the prolonged reticulocyte maturation time. The second correction factor varies from 1 to 3 depending on the severity of anemia. To simplify things, a correction of 2 is used. An appropriate correction is shown in Table 63-4. If polychromatophilic cells are not seen on

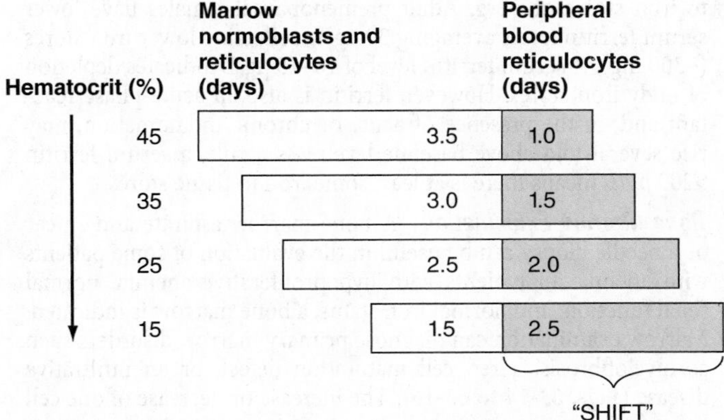

FIGURE 63-13 Correction of the reticulocyte count. To use the reticulocyte count as an indicator of effective red cell production, the reticulocyte number must be corrected based on the level of anemia and the circulating life span of the reticulocytes. Erythroid cells take ~4.5 days to mature. At a normal hemoglobin, reticulocytes are released to the circulation with ~1 day left as reticulocytes. However, with different levels of anemia, reticulocytes (and even earlier erythroid cells) may be released from the marrow prematurely. Most patients come to clinical attention with hematocrits in the mid-20s, and thus a correction factor of 2 is commonly used because the observed reticulocytes will live for 2 days in the circulation before losing their RNA.

TABLE 63-5 Normal Marrow Response to Anemia

HEMOGLOBIN	PRODUCTION INDEX	RETICULOCYTE COUNT
15 g/dL	1	50,000/μL
11 g/dL	2.0–2.5	100–150,000/μL
8 g/dL	3.0–4.0	300–400,000/μL

the blood smear, the second correction is not indicated. The now doubly corrected reticulocyte count is the *reticulocyte production index*, and it provides an estimate of marrow production relative to normal. In many hospital laboratories, the reticulocyte count is reported not only as a percentage but also in absolute numbers. If so, no correction for dilution is required. A summary of the appropriate marrow response to varying degrees of anemia is shown in Table 63-5.

Premature release of reticulocytes is normally due to increased EPO stimulation. However, if the integrity of the bone marrow release process is lost through tumor infiltration, fibrosis, or other disorders, the appearance of nucleated red cells or polychromatophilic macrocytes should still invoke the second reticulocyte correction. The shift correction should always be applied to a patient with anemia and a very high reticulocyte count to provide a true index of effective red cell production. Patients with severe chronic hemolytic anemia may increase red cell production as much as six- to sevenfold. This measure alone confirms the fact that the patient has an appropriate EPO response, a normally functioning bone marrow, and sufficient iron available to meet the demands for new red cell formation. If the reticulocyte production index is <2 in the face of established anemia, a defect in erythroid marrow proliferation or maturation must be present.

Tests of Iron Supply and Storage The laboratory measurements that reflect the availability of iron for hemoglobin synthesis include the serum iron, the TIBC, and the percent transferrin saturation. The percent transferrin saturation is derived by dividing the serum iron level (× 100) by the TIBC. The normal serum iron ranges from 9 to 27 μmol/L (50–150 μg/dL), whereas the normal TIBC is 54–64 μmol/L (300–360 μg/dL); the normal transferrin saturation ranges from 25 to 50%. A diurnal variation in the serum iron leads to a variation in the percent transferrin saturation. The serum ferritin is used to evaluate total body iron stores. Adult males have serum ferritin levels that average ~100 μg/L, corresponding to iron stores of ~1 g. Adult premenopausal females have lower serum ferritin levels averaging 30 μg/L, reflecting lower iron stores (~300 mg). A serum ferritin level of 10–15 μg/L indicates depletion of body iron stores. However, ferritin is also an acute-phase reactant and, in the presence of acute or chronic inflammation, may rise several-fold above baseline levels. As a rule, a serum ferritin >200 μg/L means there is at least some iron in tissue stores.

Bone Marrow Examination A bone marrow aspirate and smear or a needle biopsy can be useful in the evaluation of some patients with anemia. In patients with hypoproliferative anemia, normal renal function, and normal iron status, a bone marrow is indicated. Marrow examination can diagnose primary marrow disorders such as myelofibrosis, a red cell maturation defect, or an infiltrative disease (Figs. 63-14 to 63-16). The increase or decrease of one cell lineage (myeloid vs erythroid) compared to another is obtained by a differential count of nucleated cells in a bone marrow smear (the myeloid/erythroid [M/E] ratio). A patient with a hypoproliferative anemia (see below) and a reticulocyte production index <2 will demonstrate an M/E ratio of 2 or 3:1. In contrast, patients with hemolytic disease and a production index >3 will have an M/E ratio of at least 1:1. Maturation disorders are identified from the discrepancy between the M/E ratio and the reticulocyte production index (see below). Either the marrow smear or biopsy can be stained for the presence of iron stores or iron in developing red cells. The storage iron is in the form of ferritin or *hemosiderin*. On carefully prepared bone marrow smears, small ferritin granules can normally be seen under oil immersion in 20–40% of developing erythroblasts. Such cells are called *sideroblasts*.

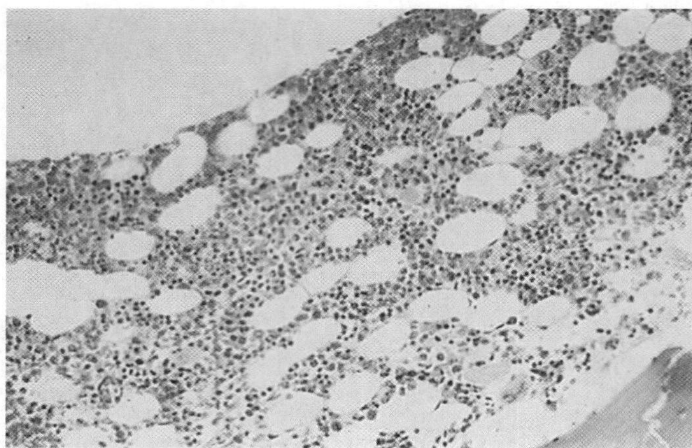

FIGURE 63-14 Normal bone marrow. This is a low-power view of a section of a normal bone marrow biopsy stained with hematoxylin and eosin (H&E). Note that the nucleated cellular elements account for ~40–50% and the fat (clear areas) accounts for ~50–60% of the area. *(From RS Hillman et al: Hematology in Clinical Practice, 5th ed. New York, McGraw-Hill, 2010.)*

OTHER LABORATORY MEASUREMENTS

Additional laboratory tests may be of value in confirming specific diagnoses. **For details of these tests and how they are applied in individual disorders, see Chaps. 97 to 101.**

DEFINITION AND CLASSIFICATION OF ANEMIA

Initial Classification of Anemia The functional classification of anemia has three major categories. These are (1) marrow production defects (*hypoproliferation*), (2) red cell maturation defects (*ineffective erythropoiesis*), and (3) decreased red cell survival (*blood loss/hemolysis*). The classification is shown in Fig. 63-17. A hypoproliferative anemia is typically seen with a low reticulocyte production index together with little or no change in red cell morphology (a normocytic, normochromic anemia) (Chap. 97). Maturation disorders typically have a slight to moderately elevated reticulocyte production index that is accompanied by either macrocytic (Chap. 99) or microcytic (Chaps. 97, 98) red cell

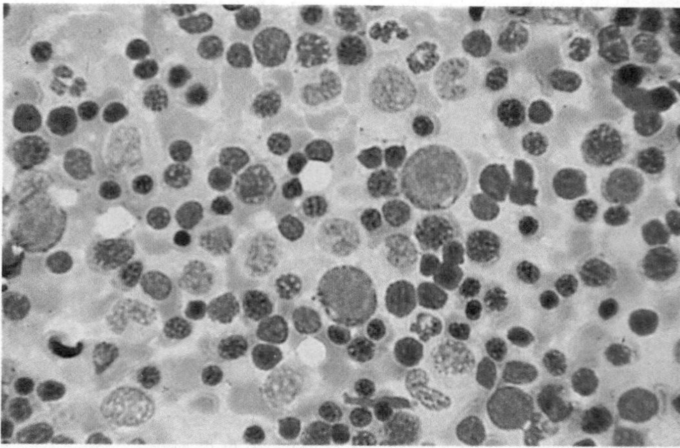

FIGURE 63-15 Erythroid hyperplasia. This marrow shows an increase in the fraction of cells in the erythroid lineage as might be seen when a normal marrow compensates for acute blood loss or hemolysis. The myeloid/erythroid (M/E) ratio is about 1:1. *(From RS Hillman et al: Hematology in Clinical Practice, 5th ed. New York, McGraw-Hill, 2010.)*

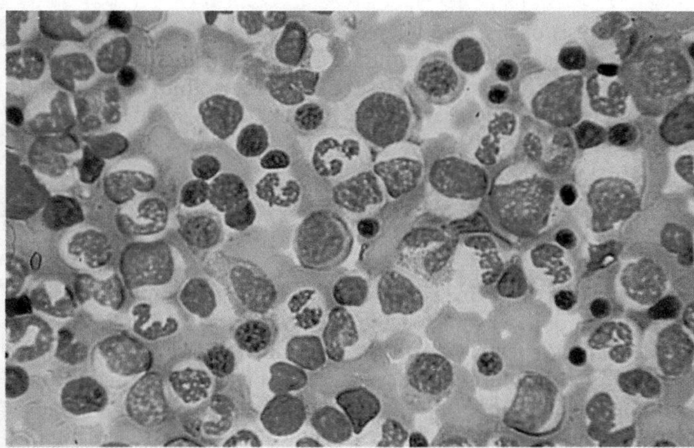

FIGURE 63-16 Myeloid hyperplasia. This marrow shows an increase in the fraction of cells in the myeloid or granulocytic lineage as might be seen in a normal marrow responding to infection. The myeloid/erythroid (M/E) ratio is >3:1. *(From RS Hillman et al: Hematology in Clinical Practice, 5th ed. New York, McGraw-Hill, 2010.)*

indices. Increased red blood cell destruction secondary to hemolysis results in an increase in the reticulocyte production index to at least three times normal **(Chap. 100)**, provided sufficient iron is available. Hemorrhagic anemia does not typically result in production indices of more than 2.0–2.5 times normal because of the limitations placed on expansion of the erythroid marrow by iron availability **(Chap. 101)**.

In the first branch point of the classification of anemia, a reticulocyte production index >2.5 indicates that hemolysis is most likely. A reticulocyte production index <2 indicates either a hypoproliferative anemia or maturation disorder. The latter two possibilities can often be distinguished by the red cell indices, by examination of the peripheral blood smear, or by a marrow examination. If the red cell indices are normal, the anemia is almost certainly hypoproliferative in nature. Maturation disorders are characterized by ineffective red cell production and a low reticulocyte production index. Bizarre red cell shapes—macrocytes or hypochromic microcytes—are seen on the peripheral blood smear. With a hypoproliferative anemia, no erythroid hyperplasia is noted in the marrow, whereas patients with ineffective red cell production have erythroid hyperplasia and an M/E ratio <1:1.

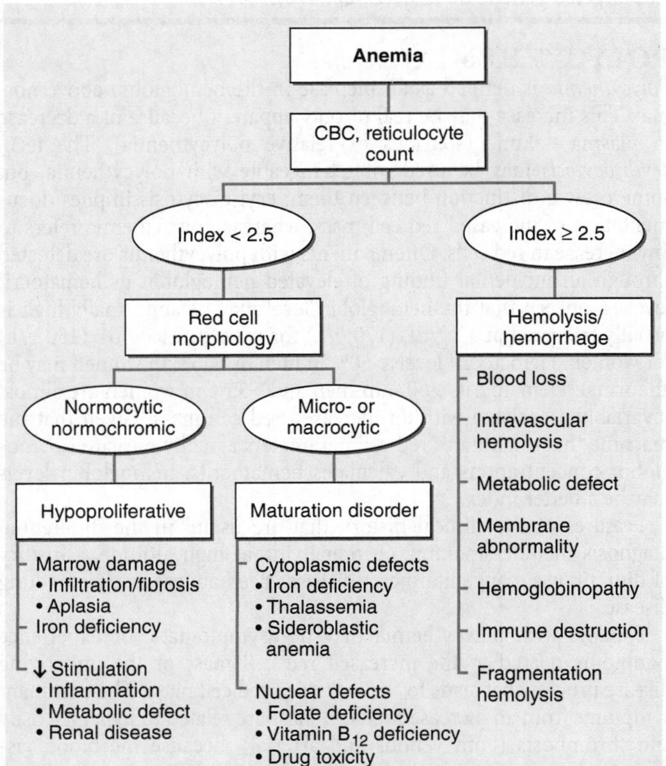

FIGURE 63-17 The physiologic classification of anemia. CBC, complete blood count.

Hypoproliferative Anemias At least 75% of all cases of anemia are hypoproliferative in nature. A hypoproliferative anemia reflects absolute or relative marrow failure in which the erythroid marrow has not proliferated appropriately for the degree of anemia. The majority of hypoproliferative anemias are due to mild to moderate iron deficiency or inflammation. A hypoproliferative anemia can result from marrow damage, iron deficiency, or inadequate EPO stimulation. The last may reflect impaired renal function, suppression of EPO production by inflammatory cytokines such as interleukin 1, or reduced tissue needs for O_2 from metabolic disease such as hypothyroidism. Only occasionally is the marrow unable to produce red cells at a normal rate, and this is most prevalent in patients with renal failure. With diabetes mellitus or myeloma, the EPO deficiency may be more marked than would be predicted by the degree of renal insufficiency. In general, hypoproliferative anemias are characterized by normocytic, normochromic red cells, although microcytic, hypochromic cells may be observed with mild iron deficiency or long-standing chronic inflammatory disease. The key laboratory tests in distinguishing between the various forms of hypoproliferative anemia include the serum iron and iron-binding capacity, evaluation of renal and thyroid function, a marrow biopsy or aspirate to detect marrow damage or infiltrative disease, and serum ferritin to assess iron stores. An iron stain of the marrow will determine the pattern of iron distribution. Patients with the anemia of acute or chronic inflammation show a distinctive pattern of serum iron (low), TIBC (normal or low), percent transferrin saturation (low), and serum ferritin (normal or high). These changes in iron values are brought about by hepcidin, the iron regulatory hormone that is produced by the liver and is increased in inflammation **(Chap. 97)**. A distinct pattern of results is noted in mild to moderate iron deficiency (low serum iron, high TIBC, low percent transferrin saturation, low serum ferritin) **(Chap. 97)**. Marrow damage by drugs, infiltrative disease such as leukemia or lymphoma, or marrow aplasia is diagnosed from the peripheral blood and bone marrow morphology. With infiltrative disease or fibrosis, a marrow biopsy is required.

Maturation Disorders The presence of anemia with an inappropriately low reticulocyte production index, macro- or microcytosis on smear, and abnormal red cell indices suggests a maturation disorder. Maturation disorders are divided into two categories: nuclear maturation defects, associated with macrocytosis, and cytoplasmic maturation defects, associated with microcytosis and hypochromia usually from defects in hemoglobin synthesis. The inappropriately low reticulocyte production index is a reflection of the ineffective erythropoiesis that results from the destruction within the marrow of developing erythroblasts. Bone marrow examination shows erythroid hyperplasia.

Nuclear maturation defects result from vitamin B_{12} or folic acid deficiency, drug damage, or myelodysplasia. Drugs that interfere with cellular DNA synthesis, such as methotrexate or alkylating agents, can produce a nuclear maturation defect. Alcohol, alone, is also capable of producing macrocytosis and a variable degree of anemia, but this is usually associated with folic acid deficiency. Measurements of folic acid and vitamin B_{12} are critical not only in identifying the specific vitamin deficiency but also because they reflect different pathogenetic mechanisms **(Chap. 99)**.

Cytoplasmic maturation defects result from severe iron deficiency or abnormalities in globin or heme synthesis. Iron deficiency occupies an unusual position in the classification of anemia. If the iron-deficiency anemia is mild to moderate, erythroid marrow proliferation is blunted and the anemia is classified as hypoproliferative. However, if the anemia is severe and prolonged, the erythroid marrow will become hyperplastic despite the inadequate iron supply, and the anemia will be classified as ineffective erythropoiesis with a cytoplasmic maturation defect. In either case, an inappropriately low reticulocyte production index, microcytosis, and a classic pattern of iron values make the diagnosis clear and easily distinguish iron deficiency from other cytoplasmic maturation defects such as the thalassemias. Defects in heme synthesis, in contrast to globin synthesis, are less common and may be acquired or inherited (**Chap. 416**). Acquired abnormalities are usually associated with myelodysplasia, may lead to either a macro- or microcytic anemia, and are frequently associated with mitochondrial iron loading. In these cases, iron is taken up by the mitochondria of the developing erythroid cell but not incorporated into heme. The iron-encrusted mitochondria surround the nucleus of the erythroid cell, forming a ring. Based on the distinctive finding of so-called ringed sideroblasts on the marrow iron stain, patients are diagnosed as having a sideroblastic anemia—almost always reflecting myelodysplasia. Again, studies of iron parameters are helpful in the differential diagnosis of these patients.

Blood Loss/Hemolytic Anemia In contrast to anemias associated with an inappropriately low reticulocyte production index, hemolysis is associated with red cell production indices ≥2.5 times normal. The stimulated erythropoiesis is reflected in the blood smear by the appearance of increased numbers of polychromatophilic macrocytes. A marrow examination is rarely indicated if the reticulocyte production index is increased appropriately. The red cell indices are typically normocytic or slightly macrocytic, reflecting the increased number of reticulocytes. Acute blood loss is not associated with an increased reticulocyte production index because of the time required to increase EPO production and, subsequently, marrow proliferation (**Chap. 101**). Subacute blood loss may be associated with modest reticulocytosis. Anemia from chronic blood loss presents more often as iron deficiency than with the picture of increased red cell production.

The evaluation of blood loss anemia is usually not difficult. Most problems arise when a patient presents with an increased red cell production index from an episode of acute blood loss that went unrecognized. The cause of the anemia and increased red cell production may not be obvious. The confirmation of a recovering state may require observations over a period of 2–3 weeks, during which the hemoglobin concentration will rise and the reticulocyte production index fall (**Chap. 101**).

Hemolytic disease, while dramatic, is among the least common forms of anemia. The ability to sustain a high reticulocyte production index reflects the ability of the erythroid marrow to compensate for hemolysis and, in the case of extravascular hemolysis, the efficient recycling of iron from the destroyed red cells to support red cell production. With intravascular hemolysis, such as paroxysmal nocturnal hemoglobinuria, the loss of iron may limit the marrow response. The level of response depends on the severity of the anemia and the nature of the underlying disease process.

Hemoglobinopathies, such as sickle cell disease and the thalassemias, present a mixed picture. The reticulocyte index may be high but is inappropriately low for the degree of marrow erythroid hyperplasia (**Chap. 98**).

Hemolytic anemias present in different ways. Some appear suddenly as an acute, self-limited episode of intravascular or extravascular hemolysis, a presentation pattern often seen in patients with autoimmune hemolysis or with inherited defects of the Embden-Meyerhof pathway or the glutathione reductase pathway. Patients with inherited disorders of the hemoglobin molecule or red cell membrane generally have a lifelong clinical history typical of the disease process. Those with chronic hemolytic disease, such as hereditary spherocytosis, may actually present not with anemia but with a complication stemming from the prolonged increase in red cell destruction such as symptomatic bilirubin gallstones or splenomegaly. Patients with chronic hemolysis are also susceptible to aplastic crises if an infectious process interrupts red cell production.

The differential diagnosis of an acute or chronic hemolytic event requires the careful integration of family history, the pattern of clinical presentation, and—whether the disease is congenital or acquired—careful examination of the peripheral blood smear. Precise diagnosis may require more specialized laboratory tests, such as hemoglobin electrophoresis or a screen for red cell enzymes. Acquired defects in red cell survival are often immunologically mediated and require a direct or indirect antiglobulin test or a cold agglutinin titer to detect the presence of hemolytic antibodies or complement-mediated red cell destruction (**Chap. 100**).

TREATMENT

Anemia

An overriding principle is to initiate treatment of mild to moderate anemia only when a specific diagnosis is made. Rarely, in the acute setting, anemia may be so severe that red cell transfusions are required before a specific diagnosis is available. Whether the anemia is of acute or gradual onset, the selection of the appropriate treatment is determined by the documented cause(s) of the anemia. Often, the cause of the anemia is multifactorial. For example, a patient with severe rheumatoid arthritis who has been taking anti-inflammatory drugs may have a hypoproliferative anemia associated with chronic inflammation as well as chronic blood loss associated with intermittent gastrointestinal bleeding. In every circumstance, it is important to evaluate the patient's iron status fully before and during the treatment of any anemia. **Transfusion is discussed in Chap. 113; iron therapy is discussed in Chap. 97; treatment of megaloblastic anemia is discussed in Chap. 99; treatment of other entities is discussed in their respective chapters (sickle cell anemia, Chap. 98; megaloblastic anemia, Chap. 99; hemolytic anemias, Chap. 100; aplastic anemia and myelodysplasia, Chap. 102).**

Therapeutic options for the treatment of anemias have expanded dramatically during the past 30 years. Blood component therapy is available and safe. Recombinant EPO as an adjunct to anemia management has transformed the lives of patients with chronic renal failure on dialysis and reduced transfusion needs of anemic cancer patients receiving chemotherapy. Eventually, patients with inherited disorders of globin synthesis or mutations in the globin gene, such as sickle cell disease, may benefit from the successful introduction of targeted genetic therapy (**Chap. 470**).

POLYCYTHEMIA

Polycythemia is defined as an increase in the hemoglobin above normal. This increase may be real or only apparent because of a decrease in plasma volume (spurious or relative polycythemia). The term *erythrocytosis* may be used interchangeably with polycythemia, but some draw a distinction between them: erythrocytosis implies documentation of increased red cell mass, whereas polycythemia refers to any increase in red cells. Often patients with polycythemia are detected through an incidental finding of elevated hemoglobin or hematocrit levels. Concern that the hemoglobin level may be abnormally high is usually triggered at 17 g/dL (170 g/L) for men and 15 g/dL (150 g/L) for women. Hematocrit levels >50% in men or >45% in women may be abnormal. Hematocrits >60% in men and >55% in women are almost invariably associated with an increased red cell mass. Given that the machine that quantitates red cell parameters actually measures hemoglobin concentrations and calculates hematocrits, hemoglobin levels may be a better index.

Features of the clinical history that are useful in the differential diagnosis include smoking, current living at high altitude, a history of diuretic use, congenital heart disease, sleep apnea, or chronic lung disease.

Patients with polycythemia may be asymptomatic or experience symptoms related to the increased red cell mass or the underlying disease process that leads to the increased red cell mass. The dominant symptoms from an increased red cell mass are related to hyperviscosity and thrombosis (both venous and arterial), because the blood viscosity increases logarithmically at hematocrits >55%. Manifestations include neurologic symptoms such as vertigo, tinnitus, headache, and visual disturbances. Hypertension is often present. Patients with *polycythemia vera* may have aquagenic pruritus, symptoms related to hepatosplenomegaly, easy bruising, epistaxis, or bleeding from the gastrointestinal tract. Peptic ulcer disease is common. Such patients also may present with digital ischemia, Budd–Chiari syndrome, or hepatic or splenic/mesenteric vein thrombosis. Patients with hypoxemia may develop cyanosis on minimal exertion or have headache, impaired mental acuity, and fatigue.

The physical examination usually reveals a ruddy complexion. Splenomegaly favors polycythemia vera as the diagnosis **(Chap. 103)**. The presence of cyanosis or evidence of a right-to-left shunt suggests congenital heart disease presenting in the adult, particularly tetralogy of Fallot or Eisenmenger's syndrome **(Chap. 269)**. Increased blood viscosity raises pulmonary artery pressure; hypoxemia can lead to increased pulmonary vascular resistance. Together, these factors can produce cor pulmonale.

Polycythemia can be spurious (related to a decrease in plasma volume; Gaisbock's syndrome), primary, or secondary in origin. The secondary causes are all mediated by EPO: either a physiologically adapted appropriate level based on tissue hypoxia (lung disease, high altitude, CO poisoning, high-affinity hemoglobinopathy) or an abnormal overproduction (renal cysts, renal artery stenosis, tumors with ectopic EPO production). A rare familial form of polycythemia is associated with normal EPO levels but hyperresponsive EPO receptors due to mutations.

APPROACH TO THE PATIENT
Polycythemia

As shown in **Fig. 63-18**, the first step is to document the presence of an increased red cell mass using the principle of isotope dilution by administering ^{51}Cr-labeled autologous red blood cells to the patient and sampling blood radioactivity over a 2-h period. If the red cell mass is normal (<36 mL/kg in men, <32 mL/kg in women), the patient has spurious or relative polycythemia. If the red cell mass is increased (>36 mL/kg in men, >32 mL/kg in women), serum EPO levels should be measured. It must be acknowledged that measurement of red cell mass is a physiologic approach to distinguishing polycythemia, and because of the use of radionuclide-labeled red cells, it is rarely performed. It is more common to measure EPO levels in a person with an elevated hemoglobin level or hematocrit. If EPO levels are low or unmeasurable, the patient most likely has polycythemia vera. A mutation in *JAK2* (Val617Phe), a key member of the cytokine intracellular signaling pathway, can be found in 90–95% of patients with polycythemia vera. Many of those without this particular *JAK2* mutation have mutations in exon 12. If EPO levels are low, check for *JAK2* mutation(s), and perform an abdominal ultrasound to assess spleen size. Tests that support the diagnosis of polycythemia vera include elevated white blood cell count, increased absolute basophil count, and thrombocytosis. In practice, many physicians order EPO levels and assessment for *JAK2* mutations at the same time.

If serum EPO levels are elevated, one needs to distinguish whether the elevation is a physiologic response to hypoxia or related to autonomous EPO production. Patients with low arterial O_2 saturation (<92%) should be further evaluated for the presence of heart or lung disease, if they are not living at high altitude. Patients with normal O_2 saturation who are smokers may have elevated EPO levels because of CO displacement of O_2. If carboxyhemoglobin (COHb) levels are high, the diagnosis is "smoker's polycythemia." Such patients should be urged to stop smoking. Those who cannot stop smoking require phlebotomy to control their polycythemia. Patients with normal O_2 saturation who do not smoke either have an abnormal hemoglobin that does not deliver O_2 to the tissues (evaluated by finding elevated O_2–hemoglobin affinity) or have a source of EPO production that is not responding to the normal feedback inhibition. Further workup is dictated by the differential diagnosis of EPO-producing neoplasms. Hepatoma, uterine leiomyoma, and renal cancer or cysts are all detectable with abdominopelvic computed tomography scans. Cerebellar hemangiomas may produce EPO, but they present with localizing neurologic signs and symptoms rather than polycythemia-related symptoms.

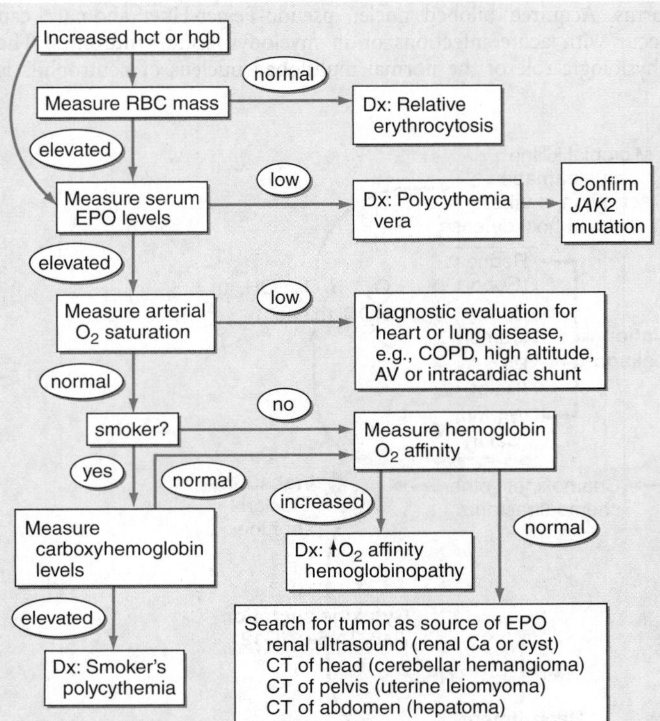

FIGURE 63-18 An approach to the differential diagnosis of patients with an elevated hemoglobin (possible polycythemia). AV, atrioventricular; Ca, calcium; COPD, chronic obstructive pulmonary disease; CT, computed tomography; EPO, erythropoietin; hct, hematocrit; hgb, hemoglobin; IVP, intravenous pyelogram; RBC, red blood cell.

FURTHER READING

HILLMAN RS et al: *Hematology in Clinical Practice*, 5th ed. New York, McGraw-Hill, 2010.

MCMULLIN MF et al: Guidelines for the diagnosis, investigation and management of polycythaemia/erythrocytosis. Br J Haematol 130:174, 2005.

SANKARAN VG, WEISS MJ: Anemia: progress in molecular mechanisms and therapies. Nat Med 21:221, 2015.

SPIVAK JL: How I manage polycythemia vera. Blood 134:341, 2019.

64 Disorders of Granulocytes and Monocytes

Steven M. Holland, John I. Gallin

Leukocytes, the major cells comprising inflammatory and immune responses, include neutrophils, T and B lymphocytes, natural killer (NK) cells, monocytes, eosinophils, and basophils. These cells have specific functions, such as antibody production by B lymphocytes or destruction of bacteria by neutrophils, but in no single infectious disease is the exact role of the cell types completely established. Thus, whereas neutrophils are classically thought to be critical to host defense against bacteria, they may also play important roles in defense against viral infections.

The blood delivers leukocytes to the various tissues from the bone marrow, where they are produced. Normal blood leukocyte counts are 4.3–10.8 × 10^9/L, with neutrophils representing 45–74% of the cells, bands 0–4%, lymphocytes 16–45%, monocytes 4–10%, eosinophils 0–7%, and basophils 0–2%. Variation among individuals and among different ethnic groups can be substantial, with lower leukocyte numbers for certain African-American ethnic groups. Lower granulocyte numbers in African-Americans are often in the 1500–2000/μL range and are generally without sequelae. The condition is termed benign ethnic neutropenia. The lower number of granulocytes is associated with null expression of the Duffy antigen receptor for cytokines (*DARC*) gene, a receptor for malarial parasites, the absence of which conveys resistance to malaria. The various leukocytes are derived from a common stem cell in the bone marrow. Three-fourths of the nucleated cells of bone marrow are committed to the production of leukocytes. Leukocyte maturation in the marrow is under the regulatory control of a number of different factors, known as colony-stimulating factors (CSFs) and interleukins (ILs). Because an alteration in the number and type of leukocytes is often associated with disease processes, total white blood cell (WBC) count (cells per μL) and differential counts are informative. This chapter focuses on neutrophils, monocytes, and eosinophils. **Lymphocytes and basophils are discussed in Chaps. 349 and 353, respectively.**

NEUTROPHILS

■ MATURATION

Important events in neutrophil life are summarized in **Fig. 64-1**. In normal humans, neutrophils are produced only in the bone marrow. The minimum number of stem cells necessary to support hematopoiesis is estimated to be 400–500 at any one time. Human blood monocytes, tissue macrophages, and stromal cells produce CSFs, hormones required for the growth of monocytes and neutrophils in the bone marrow. The hematopoietic system not only produces enough neutrophils (~1.3 × 10^{11} cells per 80-kg person per day) to carry out physiologic functions but also has a large reserve stored in the marrow, which can be mobilized in response to inflammation or infection. An increase in the number of blood neutrophils is called *neutrophilia*, and the presence of immature cells is termed a *shift to the left*. A decrease in the number of blood neutrophils is called *neutropenia*.

Neutrophils and monocytes evolve from pluripotent stem cells under the influence of cytokines and CSFs **(Fig. 64-2)**. The proliferation phase through the metamyelocyte takes about 1 week, while the maturation phase from metamyelocyte to mature neutrophil takes another week. The myeloblast is the first recognizable precursor cell and is followed by the *promyelocyte*. The promyelocyte evolves when the classic lysosomal granules, called the *primary*, or *azurophil, granules* are produced. The primary granules contain hydrolases, elastase, myeloperoxidase, cathepsin G, cationic proteins, and bactericidal/permeability-increasing protein, which is important for killing gram-negative bacteria. Azurophil granules also contain *defensins*, a family of cysteine-rich polypeptides with broad antimicrobial activity against bacteria, fungi and certain enveloped viruses. The promyelocyte divides to produce the *myelocyte*, a cell responsible for the synthesis of the *specific*, or *secondary, granules*, which contain unique (specific) constituents such as lactoferrin, vitamin B_{12}–binding protein, membrane components of the reduced nicotinamide-adenine dinucleotide phosphate (NADPH) oxidase required for hydrogen peroxide production, histaminase, and receptors for certain chemoattractants and adherence-promoting factors (CR3) as well as receptors for the basement membrane component, laminin. The secondary granules do not contain acid hydrolases and therefore are not classic lysosomes. Packaging of secondary granule contents during myelopoiesis is controlled by CCAAT/enhancer binding protein-ε. Secondary granule contents are readily released extracellularly, and their mobilization is important in modulating inflammation. During the final stages of maturation, no cell division occurs, and the cell passes through the metamyelocyte stage and then to the band neutrophil with a sausage-shaped nucleus **(Fig. 64-3)**. As the band cell matures, the nucleus assumes a lobulated configuration. The nucleus of neutrophils normally contains up to four segments **(Fig. 64-4)**. Excessive segmentation (>5 nuclear lobes) may be a manifestation of folate or vitamin B_{12} deficiency or the congenital neutropenia syndrome of warts, hypogammaglobulinemia, infections, and myelokathexis (WHIM) described below. The Pelger-Hüet anomaly **(Fig. 64-5)**, an infrequent dominant benign inherited trait caused by heterozygous mutations in the lamin B receptor, results in neutrophils with distinctive bilobed nuclei that must be distinguished from band forms. Acquired bilobed nuclei, pseudo-Pelger-Hüet anomaly, can occur with acute infections or in myelodysplastic syndromes. The physiologic role of the normal multilobed nucleus of neutrophils is

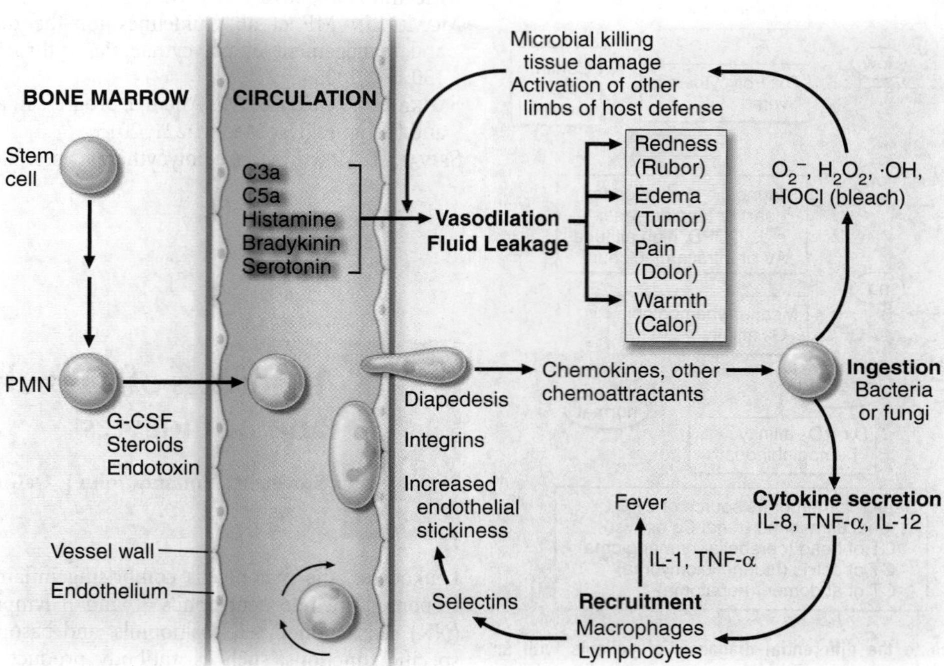

FIGURE 64-1 Schematic events in neutrophil production, recruitment, and inflammation. The four cardinal signs of inflammation (rubor, tumor, calor, dolor) are indicated, as are the interactions of neutrophils with other cells and cytokines. G-CSF, granulocyte colony-stimulating factor; IL, interleukin; PMN, polymorphonuclear leukocyte; TNF-α, tumor necrosis factor α.

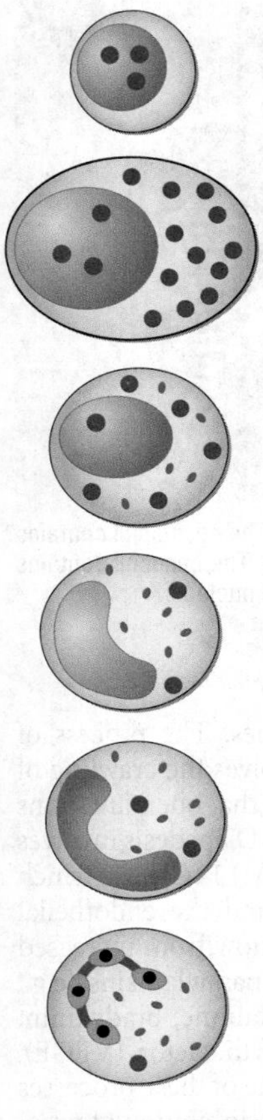

Cell	Stage	Surface Markers[a]	Characteristics
	MYELOBLAST	CD33, CD13, CD15	Prominent nucleoli
	PROMYELOCYTE	CD33, CD13, CD15	Large cell Primary granules appear
	MYELOCYTE	CD33, CD13, CD15, CD14, CD11b	Secondary granules appear
	METAMYELOCYTE	CD33, CD13, CD15, CD14, CD11b	Kidney bean–shaped nucleus
	BAND FORM	CD33, CD13, CD15, CD14, CD11b, CD10, CD16	Condensed, band–shaped nucleus
	NEUTROPHIL	CD33, CD13, CD15, CD14, CD11b, CD10, CD16	Condensed, multilobed nucleus

[a]CD = Cluster Determinant; ● Nucleolus; ● Primary granule; • Secondary granule.

FIGURE 64-2 Stages of neutrophil development shown schematically. Granulocyte colony-stimulating factor (G-CSF) and granulocyte-macrophage colony-stimulating factor (GM-CSF) are critical to this process. Identifying cellular characteristics and specific cell-surface markers are listed for each maturational stage.

unknown, but it may allow great deformation of neutrophils during migration into tissues at sites of inflammation.

In severe acute bacterial infection, prominent neutrophil cytoplasmic granules, called *toxic granulations*, are occasionally seen. Toxic granulations are immature or abnormally staining azurophil granules. Cytoplasmic inclusions, also called *Döhle bodies* (Fig. 64-3), can be seen during infection and are fragments of ribosome-rich endoplasmic reticulum. Large neutrophil vacuoles are often present in acute bacterial infection in some viral infections such as COVID-19 and probably represent pinocytosed (internalized) membrane **(Fig. 64-6)**.

Neutrophils are heterogeneous in function. Monoclonal antibodies have been developed that recognize only a subset of mature neutrophils. The meaning of neutrophil heterogeneity is not known.

The morphology of eosinophils and basophils is shown in **Fig. 64-7**.

MARROW RELEASE AND CIRCULATING COMPARTMENTS

Specific signals, including IL-1, tumor necrosis factor α (TNF-α), the CSFs, complement fragments, and chemokines, mobilize leukocytes from the bone marrow and deliver them to the blood in an unstimulated state. Under normal conditions, ~90% of the neutrophil pool is in the bone marrow, 2–3% in the circulation, and the remainder in the tissues **(Fig. 64-8)**.

The circulating pool exists in two dynamic compartments: one freely flowing and one marginated. The freely flowing pool is about one-half the neutrophils in the basal state and is composed of those cells that are in the blood and not in contact with the endothelium. Marginated leukocytes are those that are in close physical contact with the endothelium **(Fig. 64-9)**. In the pulmonary circulation, where an extensive capillary bed (~1000 capillaries per alveolus) exists, margination occurs because the capillaries are about the same size as a mature neutrophil. Therefore, neutrophil fluidity and deformability are necessary to make the transit through the pulmonary bed. Increased neutrophil rigidity and

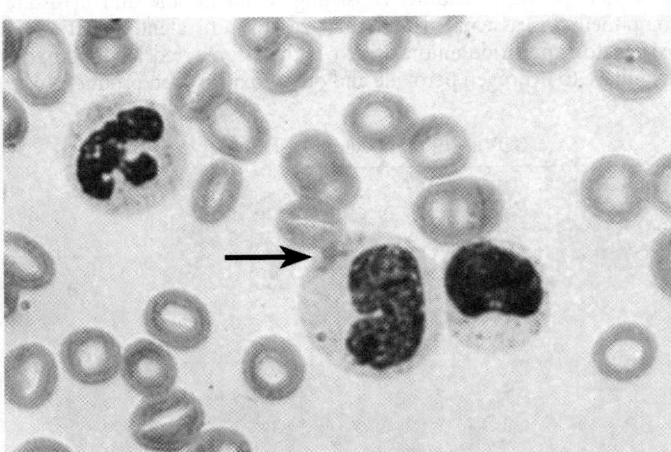

FIGURE 64-3 Neutrophil band with Döhle body. The neutrophil with a sausage-shaped nucleus in the center of the field is a band form. Döhle bodies are discrete, blue-staining, nongranular areas found in the periphery of the cytoplasm of the neutrophil in infections and other toxic states. They represent aggregates of rough endoplasmic reticulum.

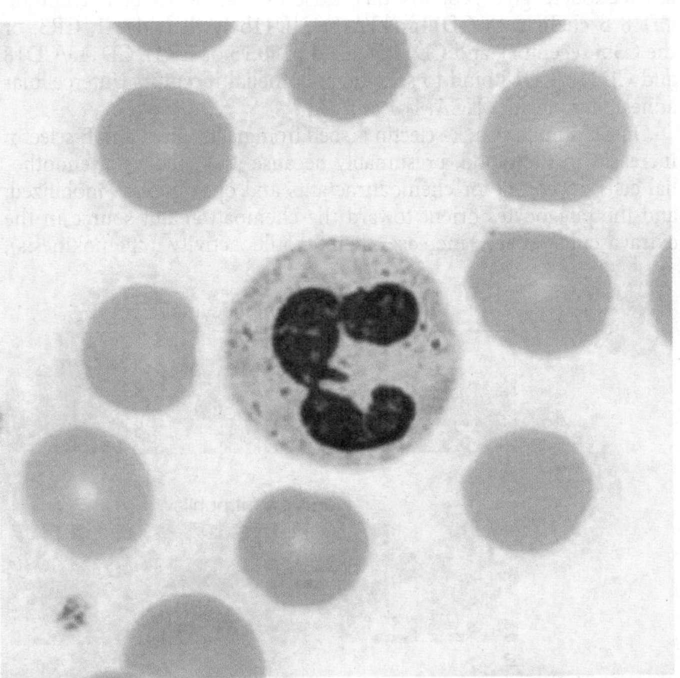

FIGURE 64-4 Normal granulocyte. The normal granulocyte has a segmented nucleus with heavy, clumped chromatin; fine neutrophilic granules are dispersed throughout the cytoplasm.

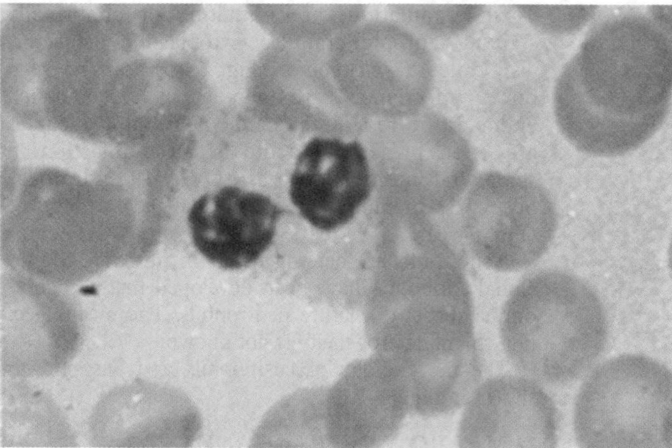

FIGURE 64-5 Pelger-Hüet anomaly. In this benign disorder, the majority of granulocytes are bilobed. The nucleus frequently has a spectacle-like, or "pince-nez," configuration. *(From M Lichtman et al (eds): Williams Hematology, 7th ed. New York, McGraw Hill, 2005; RS Hillman, KA Ault: Hematology in General Practice, 4th ed. New York, McGraw Hill, 2005.)*

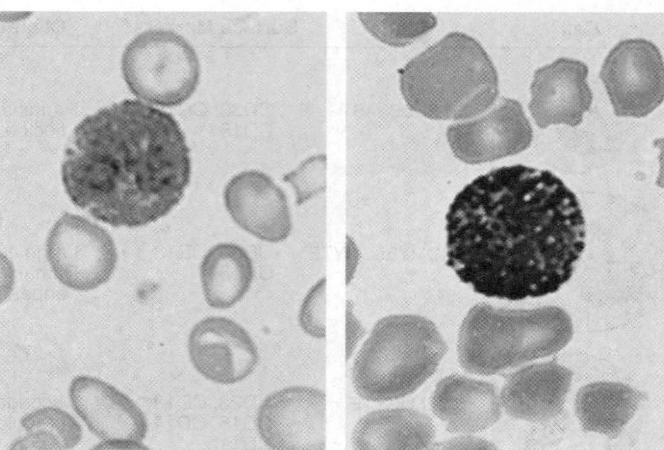

FIGURE 64-7 Normal eosinophil (*left*) and basophil (*right*). The eosinophil contains large, bright orange granules and usually a bilobed nucleus. The basophil contains large purple-black granules that fill the cell and obscure the nucleus.

decreased deformability lead to augmented neutrophil trapping and margination in the lung. In contrast, in the systemic postcapillary venules, margination is mediated by the interaction of specific cell-surface molecules called *selectins*. Selectins are glycoproteins expressed on neutrophils and endothelial cells, among others, that cause a low-affinity interaction, resulting in "rolling" of the neutrophil along the endothelial surface. On neutrophils, the molecule L-selectin (cluster determinant [CD] 62L) binds to glycosylated proteins on endothelial cells (e.g., glycosylation-dependent cell adhesion molecule [GlyCAM1] and CD34). Glycoproteins on neutrophils, most importantly sialyl-Lewis^x (SLe^x, CD15s), are targets for binding of selectins expressed on endothelial cells (E-selectin [CD62E] and P-selectin [CD62P]) and other leukocytes. In response to chemotactic stimuli from injured tissues (e.g., complement product C5a, leukotriene B_4, IL-8) or bacterial products (e.g., *N*-formylmethionylleucylphenylalanine [f-met-leu-phe]), neutrophil adhesiveness increases through mobilization of intracellular adhesion proteins stored in specific granules to the cell surface, and the cells "stick" to the endothelium through *integrins*. The integrins are leukocyte glycoproteins that exist as complexes of a common CD18 β chain with CD11a (LFA-1), CD11b (called Mac-1, CR3, or the C3bi receptor), and CD11c (called p150,95 or CR4). CD11a/CD18 and CD11b/CD18 bind to specific endothelial receptors (intercellular adhesion molecules [ICAM] 1 and 2).

On cell stimulation, L-selectin is shed from neutrophils, and E-selectin increases in the blood, presumably because it is shed from endothelial cells; receptors for chemoattractants and opsonins are mobilized; and the phagocytes orient toward the chemoattractant source in the extravascular space, increase their motile activity (chemokinesis), and migrate directionally (chemotaxis) into tissues. The process of migration into tissues is called *diapedesis* and involves the crawling of neutrophils between postcapillary endothelial cells that open junctions between adjacent cells to permit leukocyte passage. Diapedesis involves platelet/endothelial cell adhesion molecule (PECAM) 1 (CD31), which is expressed on both the emigrating leukocyte and the endothelial cells. The endothelial responses (increased blood flow from increased vasodilation and permeability) are mediated by anaphylatoxins (e.g., C3a and C5a) as well as vasodilators such as histamine, bradykinin, serotonin, nitric oxide, vascular endothelial growth factor (VEGF), and prostaglandins E and I. Cytokines regulate some of these processes (e.g., TNF-α induction of VEGF, interferon [IFN] γ inhibition of prostaglandin E).

In the healthy adult, most neutrophils leave the body by migration through the mucous membrane of the gastrointestinal tract. Normally, neutrophils spend a short time in the circulation (half-life, 6–7 h). Senescent neutrophils are cleared from the circulation by macrophages in the lung and spleen. Once in the tissues, neutrophils release enzymes, such as collagenase and elastase, which may help establish abscess cavities. Neutrophils ingest pathogenic materials that have been opsonized by IgG and C3b. Fibronectin and the tetrapeptide tuftsin also facilitate phagocytosis.

With phagocytosis comes a burst of oxygen consumption and activation of the hexose-monophosphate shunt. A membrane-associated NADPH oxidase, consisting of membrane and cytosolic components, is assembled and catalyzes the univalent reduction of oxygen to superoxide anion, which is then converted by superoxide dismutase to hydrogen peroxide and other toxic oxygen products (e.g.,

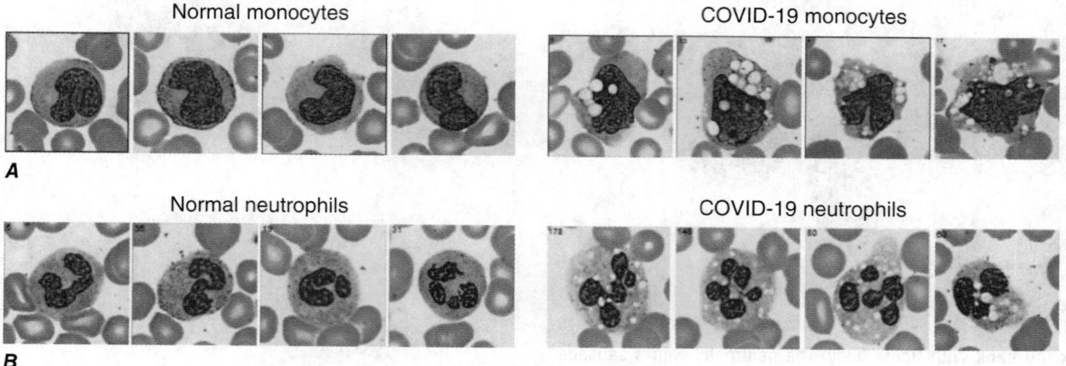

FIGURE 64-6 COVID-19: Vacuolization in peripheral blood monocytes and neutrophils of COVID-19 patients. Peripheral blood smear showing vacuolization in (***A***) monocytes and (***B***) neutrophils from hospitalized hypoxemic COVID-19 patients relative to healthy volunteers. Increased vacuoles were noted in ~80% of monocytes and ~50% of neutrophils in each COVID-19 patient throughout their hospitalization.

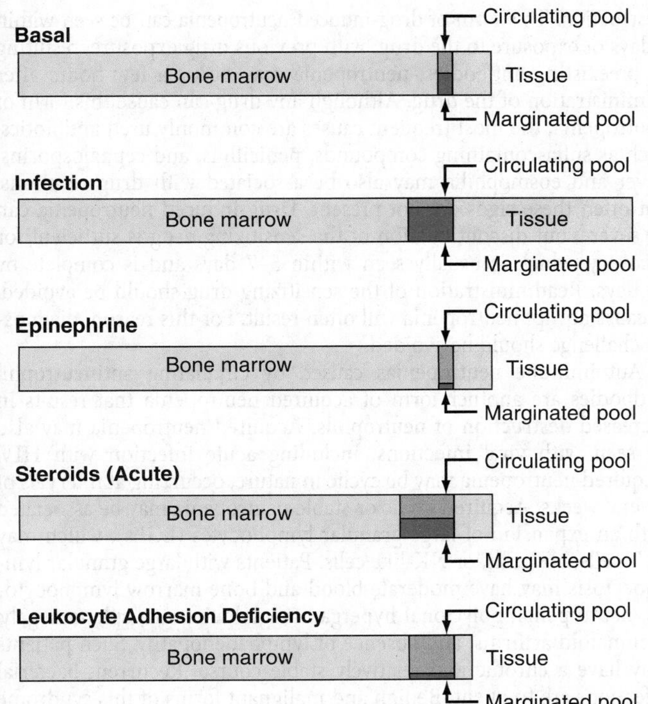

FIGURE 64-8 Schematic neutrophil distribution and kinetics between the different anatomic and functional pools.

hydroxyl radical). Hydrogen peroxide + chloride + neutrophil myeloperoxidase generates hypochlorous acid (bleach), hypochlorite, and chlorine. These products oxidize and halogenate microorganisms and tumor cells and, when uncontrolled, can damage host tissue. Strongly cationic proteins, defensins, elastase, cathepsins, and probably nitric oxide also participate in microbial killing. Lactoferrin chelates iron, an important growth factor for microorganisms, especially fungi. Other enzymes, such as lysozyme and acid proteases, help digest microbial debris. After 1–4 days in tissues, neutrophils die. The apoptosis of neutrophils is also cytokine-regulated; granulocyte colony-stimulating factor (G-CSF) and IFN-γ prolong their life span. Neutrophil extracellular traps (NETs) consisting of a DNA scaffold decorated with neutrophil-granule derived proteins, such as enzymatically active proteases and antimicrobial peptides, have been described recently and are thought to be formed as a defense mechanism to immobilize invading microorganisms. Under certain conditions, such as in delayed-type hypersensitivity, monocyte accumulation occurs within 6–12 h of initiation of inflammation. Neutrophils, monocytes, microorganisms in various states of digestion, and altered local tissue cells make up the inflammatory exudate, pus. Myeloperoxidase confers the characteristic green color to pus and may participate in turning off the inflammatory process by inactivating chemoattractants and immobilizing phagocytic cells.

Neutrophils respond to certain cytokines (IFN-γ, granulocyte-macrophage colony-stimulating factor [GM-CSF], IL-8) and produce cytokines and chemotactic signals (TNF-α, IL-8, macrophage inflammatory protein [MIP] 1) that modulate the inflammatory response. In the presence of fibrinogen, f-met-leu-phe or leukotriene B_4 IL-8 production by neutrophils is induced, providing autocrine amplification of inflammation. *Chemokines* (*chemo*attractant cyto*kines*) are small proteins produced by many different cell types, including endothelial cells, fibroblasts, epithelial cells, neutrophils, and monocytes, that regulate neutrophil, monocyte, eosinophil, and lymphocyte recruitment and activation. Chemokines transduce their signals through heterotrimeric G protein–linked receptors that have seven cell membrane–spanning domains, the same type of cell-surface receptor that mediates the response to the classic chemoattractants f-met-leu-phe and C5a. Four major groups of chemokines are recognized based on the cysteine structure near the N terminus: C, CC, CXC, and CXXXC. The CXC cytokines such as IL-8 mainly attract neutrophils; CC chemokines such as MIP-1 attract lymphocytes, monocytes, eosinophils, and basophils; the C chemokine lymphotactin is T-cell tropic; the CXXXC chemokine fractalkine attracts neutrophils, monocytes, and T cells. These molecules and their receptors not only regulate the trafficking and activation of inflammatory cells, but specific chemokine receptors also serve as co-receptors for HIV infection (**Chap. 202**), while others have roles in other viral infections (e.g., West Nile virus), susceptibility and response to *Candida*, and atherogenesis.

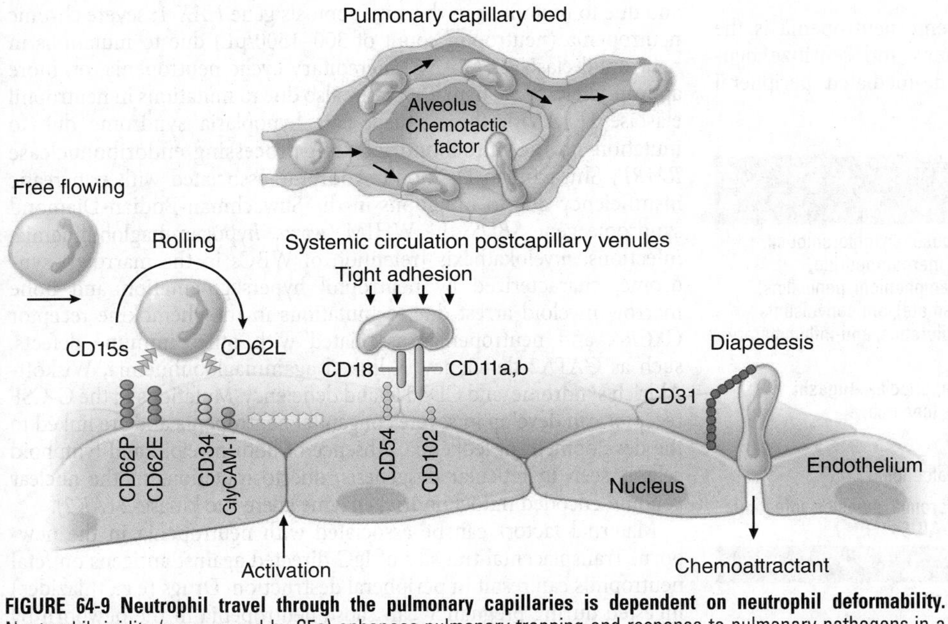

FIGURE 64-9 Neutrophil travel through the pulmonary capillaries is dependent on neutrophil deformability. Neutrophil rigidity (e.g., caused by C5a) enhances pulmonary trapping and response to pulmonary pathogens in a way that is not so dependent on cell-surface receptors. Intraalveolar chemotactic factors, such as those caused by certain bacteria (e.g., *Streptococcus pneumoniae*), lead to diapedesis of neutrophils from the pulmonary capillaries into the alveolar space. Neutrophil interaction with the endothelium of the systemic postcapillary venules is dependent on molecules of attachment. The neutrophil "rolls" along the endothelium using selectins: neutrophil CD15s (sialyl-Lewis[x]) binds to CD62E (E-selectin) and CD62P (P-selectin) on endothelial cells; CD62L (L-selectin) on neutrophils binds to CD34 and other molecules (e.g., GlyCAM-1) expressed on endothelium. Chemokines or other activation factors stimulate integrin-mediated "tight adhesion": CD11a/CD18 (LFA-1) and CD11b/CD18 (Mac-1, CR3) bind to CD54 (ICAM-1) and CD102 (ICAM-2) on the endothelium. Diapedesis occurs between endothelial cells: CD31 (PECAM-1) expressed by the emigrating neutrophil interacts with CD31 expressed at the endothelial cell-cell junction. CD, cluster determinant; GlyCAM, glycosylation-dependent cell adhesion molecule; ICAM, intercellular adhesion molecule; PECAM, platelet/endothelial cell adhesion molecule.

■ NEUTROPHIL ABNORMALITIES

Defects in the neutrophil life cycle can lead to dysfunction and compromised host defenses. When inflammation is severely depressed the clinical result is often recurrent, severe bacterial and fungal infections. Aphthous ulcers of mucous membranes (gray ulcers without pus) and gingivitis and periodontal disease suggest a phagocytic cell disorder. Patients with congenital phagocyte defects can have infections within the first few days of life. Skin, ear, upper and lower respiratory tract, and bone infections are common. Sepsis and meningitis are rare. In some disorders, the frequency of infection is variable, and patients can go for months or even years without major infection. Aggressive management of these congenital diseases, including hematopoietic stem cell transplantation and gene therapy, has extended the life span of patients well into adulthood.

Neutropenia The consequences of absent neutrophils are dramatic. Susceptibility to infectious diseases increases sharply when neutrophil counts fall to <1000 cells/μL. When the absolute neutrophil count (ANC; band forms and mature neutrophils combined) falls to <500 cells/μL, control of endogenous microbial flora (e.g., mouth, gut) is impaired; when the ANC is <200/μL, the local inflammatory process is absent. Neutropenia can be due to depressed production, increased peripheral destruction, or excessive peripheral pooling. A falling neutrophil count or a significant decrease in the number of neutrophils below steady-state levels, together with a failure to increase neutrophil counts in the setting of infection or other challenge, requires investigation. Acute neutropenia, such as that caused by cancer chemotherapy, is more likely to be associated with increased risk of infection than chronic neutropenia (months to years) that reverses in response to infection or carefully controlled administration of endotoxin (see "Laboratory Diagnosis and Management," below).

Some causes of inherited and acquired neutropenia are listed in **Table 64-1**. The most common neutropenias are iatrogenic, resulting from the use of cytotoxic or immunosuppressive therapies for malignancy or control of autoimmune disorders. These drugs cause neutropenia because they result in decreased production of rapidly growing progenitor (stem) cells of the marrow. Certain antibiotics such as chloramphenicol, trimethoprim-sulfamethoxazole, flucytosine, vidarabine, and the antiretroviral drug zidovudine may cause neutropenia by inhibiting proliferation of myeloid precursors. Azathioprine and 6-mercaptopurine are metabolized by the enzyme thiopurine methyltransferase (TMPT); hypofunctional polymorphisms that are found in 11% of whites can lead to accumulation of 6-thioguanine and profound marrow toxicity. The marrow suppression is generally dose-related and dependent on continued administration of the drug. Cessation of the offending agent and recombinant human G-CSF usually reverse these forms of neutropenia.

Another important mechanism for iatrogenic neutropenia is the effect of drugs that serve as immune haptens and sensitize neutrophils or neutrophil precursors to immune-mediated peripheral destruction. This form of drug-induced neutropenia can be seen within 7 days of exposure to the drug; with previous drug exposure, resulting in preexisting antibodies, neutropenia may occur a few hours after administration of the drug. Although any drug can cause this form of neutropenia, the most frequent causes are commonly used antibiotics, such as sulfa-containing compounds, penicillins, and cephalosporins. Fever and eosinophilia may also be associated with drug reactions, but often these signs are not present. Drug-induced neutropenia can be severe, but discontinuation of the sensitizing drug is sufficient for recovery, which is usually seen within 5–7 days and is complete by 10 days. Readministration of the sensitizing drug should be avoided, because abrupt neutropenia will often result. For this reason, diagnostic challenge should be avoided.

Autoimmune neutropenias caused by circulating antineutrophil antibodies are another form of acquired neutropenia that results in increased destruction of neutrophils. Acquired neutropenia may also be seen with viral infections, including acute infection with HIV. Acquired neutropenia may be cyclic in nature, occurring at intervals of several weeks. Acquired cyclic or stable neutropenia may be associated with an expansion of large granular lymphocytes (LGLs), which may be T cells, NK cells, or NK-like cells. Patients with large granular lymphocytosis may have moderate blood and bone marrow lymphocytosis, neutropenia, polyclonal hypergammaglobulinemia, splenomegaly, rheumatoid arthritis, and absence of lymphadenopathy. Such patients may have a chronic and relatively stable course. Recurrent bacterial infections are frequent. Benign and malignant forms of this syndrome occur. In some patients, a spontaneous regression has occurred even after 11 years, suggesting an immunoregulatory defect as the basis for at least one form of the disorder. Glucocorticoids, cyclosporine, methotrexate, and monoclonals are commonly used to manage these cytopenias.

Hereditary Neutropenias Hereditary neutropenias are rare and may manifest in early childhood as a profound constant neutropenia or agranulocytosis. Congenital forms of neutropenia include Kostmann's syndrome (neutrophil count <100/μL), which is often fatal and due to mutations in the antiapoptosis gene *HAX-1*; severe chronic neutropenia (neutrophil count of 300–1500/μL) due to mutations in neutrophil elastase (*ELANE*); hereditary cyclic neutropenia, or, more appropriately, cyclic hematopoiesis, also due to mutations in neutrophil elastase (*ELANE*); the cartilage-hair hypoplasia syndrome due to mutations in the mitochondrial RNA-processing endoribonuclease *RMRP*; Shwachman-Diamond syndrome associated with pancreatic insufficiency due to mutations in the Shwachman-Bodian-Diamond syndrome gene *SBDS*; the WHIM (*w*arts, *h*ypogammaglobulinemia, *i*nfections, *m*yelokathexis [retention of WBCs in the marrow]) syndrome, characterized by neutrophil hypersegmentation and bone marrow myeloid arrest due to mutations in the chemokine receptor *CXCR4*; and neutropenias associated with other immune defects, such as GATA2 deficiency, X-linked agammaglobulinemia, Wiskott-Aldrich syndrome, and CD40 ligand deficiency. Mutations in the G-CSF receptor can develop in severe congenital neutropenia and are linked to the development of leukemia. Absence of both myeloid and lymphoid cells is seen in reticular dysgenesis, due to mutations in the nuclear genome-encoded mitochondrial enzyme adenylate kinase-2 (*AK2*).

Maternal factors can be associated with neutropenia in the newborn. Transplacental transfer of IgG directed against antigens on fetal neutrophils can result in peripheral destruction. Drugs (e.g., thiazides) ingested during pregnancy can cause neutropenia in the newborn by either depressed production or peripheral destruction.

In Felty's syndrome—the triad of rheumatoid arthritis, splenomegaly, and neutropenia (**Chap. 358**)—spleen-produced antibodies can shorten neutrophil life span, while large granular lymphocytes can attack marrow neutrophil precursors. Splenectomy may increase the neutrophil count in Felty's syndrome and lower serum neutrophil-binding IgG. Some Felty's syndrome patients also have autoantibodies to G-CSF, while others have increased numbers of LGLs. Splenomegaly with peripheral trapping and destruction of neutrophils is also seen in lysosomal storage diseases and commonly in portal hypertension.

TABLE 64-1 Causes of Neutropenia

Decreased Production
Drug-induced—alkylating agents (nitrogen mustard, busulfan, chlorambucil, cyclophosphamide); antimetabolites (methotrexate, 6-mercaptopurine, 5-flucytosine); noncytotoxic agents (antibiotics [chloramphenicol, penicillins, sulfonamides], phenothiazines, tranquilizers [meprobamate], anticonvulsants [carbamazepine], antipsychotics [clozapine], certain diuretics, anti-inflammatory agents, antithyroid drugs, many others)
Hematologic diseases—idiopathic, cyclic neutropenia, Chédiak -Higashi syndrome, aplastic anemia, infantile genetic disorders (see text)
Tumor invasion, myelofibrosis
Nutritional deficiency—vitamin B_{12}, folate (especially alcoholics)
Infection—tuberculosis, typhoid fever, brucellosis, tularemia, measles, infectious mononucleosis, malaria, viral hepatitis, leishmaniasis, AIDS
Peripheral Destruction
Antineutrophil antibodies and/or splenic or lung trapping
Autoimmune disorders—Felty's syndrome, rheumatoid arthritis, lupus erythematosus
Drugs as haptens—aminopyrine, α-methyldopa, phenylbutazone, mercurial diuretics, some phenothiazines
Granulomatosis with polyangiitis (Wegener's)
Peripheral Pooling (Transient Neutropenia)
Overwhelming bacterial infection (acute endotoxemia)
Hemodialysis
Cardiopulmonary bypass

TABLE 64-2 Causes of Neutrophilia

Increased Production
Idiopathic
Drug-induced—glucocorticoids, G-CSF
Infection—bacterial, fungal, sometimes viral
Inflammation—thermal injury, tissue necrosis, myocardial and pulmonary infarction, hypersensitivity states, collagen vascular diseases
Myeloproliferative diseases—myelocytic leukemia, myeloid metaplasia, polycythemia vera
Increased Marrow Release
Glucocorticoids
Acute infection (endotoxin)
Inflammation—thermal injury
Decreased or Defective Margination
Drugs—epinephrine, glucocorticoids, nonsteroidal anti-inflammatory agents
Stress, excitement, vigorous exercise
Leukocyte adhesion deficiency type 1 (CD18); leukocyte adhesion deficiency type 2 (selectin ligand, CD15s); leukocyte adhesion deficiency type 3 (FERMT3)
Miscellaneous
Metabolic disorders—ketoacidosis, acute renal failure, eclampsia, acute poisoning
Drugs—lithium
Other—metastatic carcinoma, acute hemorrhage or hemolysis

Abbreviation: G-CSF, granulocyte colony-stimulating factor.

Neutrophilia Neutrophilia results from increased neutrophil production, increased marrow release, or defective margination (**Table 64-2**). The most important acute cause of neutrophilia is infection. Neutrophilia from acute infection represents both increased production and increased marrow release. Increased production is also associated with chronic inflammation and certain myeloproliferative diseases. Increased marrow release and mobilization of the marginated leukocyte pool are induced by glucocorticoids. Release of epinephrine, as with vigorous exercise, excitement, or stress, will demarginate neutrophils in the spleen and lungs and double the neutrophil count in minutes. Cigarette smoking can elevate neutrophil counts above the normal range. Leukocytosis with cell counts of 10,000–25,000/μL occurs in response to infection and other forms of acute inflammation and results from both release of the marginated pool and mobilization of marrow reserves. Persistent neutrophilia with cell counts of ≥30,000–50,000/μL is called a *leukemoid reaction*, a term often used to distinguish this degree of neutrophilia from leukemia. In a leukemoid reaction, the circulating neutrophils are usually mature and not clonally derived.

Abnormal Neutrophil Function Inherited and acquired abnormalities of phagocyte function are listed in **Table 64-3**. The resulting diseases are best considered in terms of the functional defects of adherence, chemotaxis, and microbicidal activity. The distinguishing features of the important inherited disorders of phagocyte function are shown in **Table 64-4**.

DISORDERS OF ADHESION Three main types of leukocyte adhesion deficiency (LAD) have been described. All are autosomal recessive and result in the inability of neutrophils to exit the circulation to sites of infection, leading to leukocytosis and increased susceptibility to infection (Fig. 64-9). Patients with LAD 1 have mutations in *CD18*, the common component of the integrins LFA-1, Mac-1, and p150,95, leading to a defect in tight adhesion between neutrophils and the endothelium. The heterodimer formed by CD18/CD11b (Mac-1) is also the receptor for the complement-derived opsonin C3bi (CR3). The *CD18* gene is located on distal chromosome 21q. The severity of the defect determines the severity of clinical disease. Complete lack of expression of the leukocyte integrins results in a severe phenotype in which inflammatory stimuli do not increase the expression of leukocyte integrins on neutrophils or activated T and B cells. Neutrophils (and monocytes) from patients with LAD 1 adhere poorly to endothelial cells and protein-coated surfaces and exhibit defective spreading, aggregation, and chemotaxis. The inability of neutrophils to exit the vasculature to the tissue deprives the tissue macrophage of its expected neutrophil ingestion, leading to macrophage production of IL-23, which induces T-cell production of IL-17, a potent proinflammatory cytokine. These processes conspire to drive inflammation in LAD 1. Patients with LAD 1 have recurrent bacterial infections involving the skin, oral and genital mucosa, and respiratory and intestinal tracts; persistent leukocytosis (resting neutrophil counts of 15,000–20,000/μL) because cells do not marginate; and, in severe cases, a history of delayed separation of the umbilical stump. Infections, especially of the skin, may become necrotic with progressively enlarging borders, slow healing, and development of dysplastic scars. The most common bacteria are *Staphylococcus aureus* and enteric gram-negative bacteria. LAD 2 is caused by an abnormality of fucosylation of SLe^x (CD15s), the ligand on neutrophils that interacts with selectins on endothelial cells and is responsible for neutrophil rolling along the endothelium. Infection susceptibility in LAD 2 appears to be less severe than in LAD 1. LAD 2 is also known as *congenital disorder of glycosylation IIc* (CDGIIc) due to mutation in a GDP-fucose transporter (*SLC35C1*). LAD 3 is characterized by infection susceptibility, leukocytosis, and petechial hemorrhage due to impaired integrin activation caused by mutations in the gene *FERMT3*.

DISORDERS OF NEUTROPHIL GRANULES The most common neutrophil defect is myeloperoxidase deficiency, a primary granule defect inherited as an autosomal recessive trait; the incidence is ~1 in 2000 persons. Isolated myeloperoxidase deficiency is not associated with

TABLE 64-3 Types of Granulocyte and Monocyte Disorders

	CAUSE OF INDICATED DYSFUNCTION		
FUNCTION	**DRUG-INDUCED**	**ACQUIRED**	**INHERITED**
Adherence-aggregation	Aspirin, colchicine, alcohol, glucocorticoids, ibuprofen, piroxicam	Neonatal state, hemodialysis	Leukocyte adhesion deficiency types 1, 2, and 3
Deformability		Leukemia, neonatal state, diabetes mellitus, immature neutrophils	
Chemokinesis-chemotaxis	Glucocorticoids (high dose), auranofin, colchicine (weak effect), phenylbutazone, naproxen, indomethacin, interleukin 2	Thermal injury, malignancy, malnutrition, periodontal disease, neonatal state, systemic lupus erythematosus, rheumatoid arthritis, diabetes mellitus, sepsis, influenza virus infection, herpes simplex virus infection, acrodermatitis enteropathica, AIDS	Chédiak-Higashi syndrome, neutrophil-specific granule deficiency, hyper IgE–recurrent infection (Job's) syndrome (in some patients), Down's syndrome, α-mannosidase deficiency, leukocyte adhesion deficiencies, Wiskott-Aldrich syndrome
Microbicidal activity	Colchicine, cyclophosphamide, glucocorticoids (high dose), TNF-α-blocking antibodies	Leukemia, aplastic anemia, certain neutropenias, tuftsin deficiency, thermal injury, sepsis, neonatal state, diabetes mellitus, malnutrition, AIDS	Chédiak-Higashi syndrome, neutrophil-specific granule deficiency, chronic granulomatous disease, defects in IFNγ/IL-12 axis

Abbreviations: IFNγ, interferon γ; IL, interleukin; TNF-α, tumor necrosis factor alpha.

TABLE 64-4 Inherited Disorders of Phagocyte Function: Differential Features

CLINICAL MANIFESTATIONS	CELLULAR OR MOLECULAR DEFECTS	DIAGNOSIS
Chronic Granulomatous Diseases (70% X-Linked, 30% Autosomal Recessive)		
Severe infections of skin, ears, lungs, liver, and bone with catalase-positive microorganisms such as *Staphylococcus aureus, Burkholderia cepacia* complex, *Aspergillus* spp., *Chromobacterium violaceum*; often hard to culture organism; excessive inflammation with granulomas, frequent lymph node suppuration; granulomas can obstruct GI or GU tracts; gingivitis, aphthous ulcers, seborrheic dermatitis	No respiratory burst due to the lack of one of five NADPH oxidase subunits in neutrophils, monocytes, and eosinophils	DHR or NBT test; no superoxide and H_2O_2 production by neutrophils; immunoblot for NADPH oxidase components; genetic detection
Chédiak-Higashi Syndrome (Autosomal Recessive)		
Recurrent pyogenic infections, especially with *S. aureus*; many patients get lymphoma-like illness during adolescence; periodontal disease; partial oculocutaneous albinism, nystagmus, progressive peripheral neuropathy, cognitive impairment in some patients	Reduced chemotaxis and phagolysosome fusion, increased respiratory burst activity, defective egress from marrow, abnormal skin window; defect in *CHS1*	Giant primary granules in neutrophils and other granule-bearing cells (Wright's stain); genetic detection
Specific Granule Deficiency (Autosomal Recessive and Dominant)		
Recurrent infections of skin, ears, and sinopulmonary tract; delayed wound healing; decreased inflammation; bleeding diathesis	Abnormal chemotaxis, impaired respiratory burst and bacterial killing, failure to upregulate chemotactic and adhesion receptors with stimulation, defect in transcription of granule proteins; defect in *CEBPE* or *SMARCD2*	Lack of secondary (specific) granules in neutrophils (Wright's stain), no neutrophil-specific granule contents (i.e., lactoferrin), no defensins, platelet α granule abnormality; genetic detection
Myeloperoxidase Deficiency (Autosomal Recessive)		
Clinically normal except in patients with underlying disease such as diabetes mellitus; then candidiasis or other fungal infections	No myeloperoxidase due to pre- and posttranslational defects in myeloperoxidase deficiency	No peroxidase in neutrophils; genetic detection
Leukocyte Adhesion Deficiency		
Type 1: Delayed separation of umbilical cord, sustained neutrophilia, recurrent infections of skin and mucosa, gingivitis, periodontal disease	Impaired phagocyte adherence, aggregation, spreading, chemotaxis, phagocytosis of C3bi-coated particles; defective production of CD18 subunit common to leukocyte integrins	Reduced phagocyte surface expression of the CD18-containing integrins with monoclonal antibodies against LFA-1 (CD18/CD11a), Mac-1 or CR3 (CD18/CD11b), p150,95 (CD18/CD11c); genetic detection
Type 2: Cognitive impairment, short stature, Bombay (hh) blood phenotype, recurrent infections, neutrophilia	Impaired phagocyte rolling along endothelium; due to defects in fucose transporter	Reduced phagocyte surface expression of Sialyl-Lewis^x, with monoclonal antibodies against CD15s; genetic detection
Type 3: Petechial hemorrhage, recurrent infections	Impaired signaling for integrin activation resulting in impaired adhesion due to mutation in *FERMT3*	Reduced signaling for adhesion through integrins; genetic detection
Phagocyte Activation Defects (X-Linked and Autosomal Recessive)		
NEMO deficiency: mild hypohidrotic ectodermal dysplasia; broad-based immune defect: pyogenic and encapsulated bacteria, viruses, *Pneumocystis*, mycobacteria; X-linked	Impaired phagocyte activation by IL-1, IL-18, TLR, CD40L, TNF-α leading to problems with inflammation and antibody production	Poor in vitro response to endotoxin; impaired NF-κB activation; genetic detection
IRAK4 and MyD88 deficiency: susceptibility to pyogenic bacteria such as staphylococci, streptococci, clostridia; resistant to *Candida*; autosomal recessive	Impaired phagocyte activation by endotoxin through TLR and other pathways; TNF-α signaling preserved	Poor in vitro response to endotoxin; lack of NF-κB activation by endotoxin; genetic detection
Hyper IgE–Recurrent Infection Syndrome (Autosomal Dominant) (Job's Syndrome)		
Eczematoid or pruritic dermatitis, "cold" skin abscesses, recurrent pneumonias with *S. aureus* with bronchopleural fistulae and cyst formation, mild eosinophilia, mucocutaneous candidiasis, characteristic facies, restrictive lung disease, scoliosis, delayed primary dental deciduation	Reduced chemotaxis in some patients, reduced memory T and B cells; mutation in *STAT3*	Somatic and immune features involving lungs, skeleton, and immune system; serum IgE >2000 IU/mL; genetic testing
DOCK8 deficiency (autosomal recessive), severe eczema, atopic dermatitis, cutaneous abscesses, HSV, HPV, and molluscum infections, severe allergies, cancer	Impaired T-cell proliferation to mitogens; mutation in *DOCK8*	Severe allergies, viral infections, high IgE, eosinophilia, low IgM, progressive lymphopenia, genetic detection
Mycobacterial Susceptibility (Autosomal Dominant and Recessive Forms)		
Severe extrapulmonary or disseminated infections with bacille Calmette-Guérin (BCG), nontuberculous mycobacteria, salmonella, histoplasmosis, coccidioidomycosis, poor granuloma formation	Inability to kill intracellular organisms due to low IFN-γ production or response; mutations in IFN-γ receptors, IL-12 receptors, IL-12 p40, *STAT1, NEMO, ISG15, GATA2*	Abnormally low or very high levels of IFN-γ receptor 1; functional assays of cytokine production and response; genetic detection
GATA2 Deficiency (Autosomal Dominant)		
Persistent or disseminated warts, disseminated mycobacterial disease, low monocytes, NK cells, B cells; hypoplastic myelodysplasia, leukemia, cytogenetic abnormalities, pulmonary alveolar proteinosis	Impaired macrophage activity, cytopenias; mutations in *GATA2*	Profound circulating monocytopenia, NK and B-cell cytopenias; genetic detection

Abbreviations: C/EBPε, CCAAT/enhancer binding protein-ε; DHR, dihydrorhodamine (oxidation test); DOCK8, dedicator of cytokinesis 8; GI, gastrointestinal; GU, genitourinary; HPV, human papillomavirus; HSV, herpes simplex virus; IFN, interferon; IL, interleukin; IRAK4, IL-1 receptor–associated kinase 4; LFA-1, leukocyte function–associated antigen 1; MyD88, myeloid differentiation primary response gene 88; NADPH, nicotinamide–adenine dinucleotide phosphate; NBT, nitroblue tetrazolium (dye test); NEMO, NF-κB essential modulator; NF-κB, nuclear factor-κB; NK, natural killer; STAT1–3, signal transducer and activator of transcription 1–3; TLR, Toll-like receptor; TNF, tumor necrosis factor.

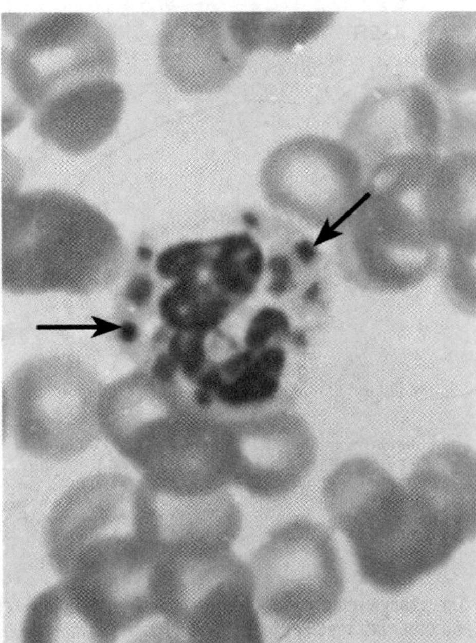

FIGURE 64-10 Chédiak-Higashi syndrome. The granulocytes contain huge cytoplasmic granules formed from aggregation and fusion of azurophilic and specific granules. Large abnormal granules are found in other granule-containing cells throughout the body.

clinically compromised defenses, presumably because other defense systems such as hydrogen peroxide generation are amplified. Microbicidal activity of neutrophils is delayed but not absent. Myeloperoxidase deficiency may make other acquired host defense defects more serious, and patients with myeloperoxidase deficiency and diabetes are more susceptible to *Candida* infections. An acquired form of myeloperoxidase deficiency occurs in myelomonocytic leukemia and acute myeloid leukemia.

Chédiak-Higashi syndrome (CHS) is a rare disease with autosomal recessive inheritance due to defects in the lysosomal transport protein LYST, encoded by the gene *CHS1* at 1q42. This protein is required for normal packaging and disbursement of granules. Neutrophils (and all cells containing lysosomes) from patients with CHS characteristically have large granules (**Fig. 64-10**), making it a systemic disease. Patients with CHS have nystagmus, partial oculocutaneous albinism, and an increased number of infections resulting from many bacterial agents. Some CHS patients develop an "accelerated phase" in childhood with a hemophagocytic syndrome and an aggressive lymphoma requiring bone marrow transplantation. CHS neutrophils and monocytes have impaired chemotaxis and abnormal rates of microbial killing due to slow rates of fusion of the lysosomal granules with phagosomes. NK cell function is also impaired. CHS patients may develop a severe disabling peripheral neuropathy in adulthood.

Specific granule deficiency is a rare autosomal recessive disease in which the production of secondary granules and their contents, as well as the primary granule component defensins, is defective. The defect in killing leads to severe bacterial infections. One type of specific granule deficiency is due to a mutation in the CCAAT/enhancer binding protein-ε, a regulator of expression of granule components. A dominant mutation in *C/EBP-ε* has also been described. Another form is caused by mutations in *SMARCD2*.

CHRONIC GRANULOMATOUS DISEASE Chronic granulomatous disease (CGD) is a group of disorders of granulocyte and monocyte oxidative metabolism due to a defect in the enzyme NADPH oxidase also called NOX2. Although CGD is rare, with an incidence of ~1 in 200,000 individuals, it is an important model of defective neutrophil oxidative metabolism. In about two-thirds of patients, CGD is inherited as an X-linked recessive trait; the remainder inherit their disease in autosomal recessive patterns. Mutations in the genes for the six proteins that allow assembly at the plasma membrane of NOX2 account for all patients with CGD. Two proteins (a 91-kDa protein, abnormal in X-linked CGD, and a 22-kDa protein, absent in one form of autosomal recessive CGD) form the heterodimer cytochrome b-558 in the plasma membrane. The protein essential for reactive oxidant signaling (EROS) is encoded by *CYBC1*, which is required to transport the 91- and 22-kDa proteins to the endoplasmic reticulum. Three other proteins (40, 47, and 67 kDa, abnormal in the other autosomal recessive forms of CGD) are cytoplasmic in origin and interact with the cytochrome after cell activation to form the NADPH oxidase, required for hydrogen peroxide production. Leukocytes from patients with CGD have severely diminished hydrogen peroxide production. The genes involved in each of the defects have been cloned and sequenced and the chromosome locations identified. Patients with CGD characteristically have increased numbers of infections due to catalase-positive microorganisms (organisms that destroy their own hydrogen peroxide) such as *S. aureus*, *Serratia marsescens*, *Burkholderia cepacia* complex, *Nocardia* and *Aspergillus* species. When patients with CGD become infected, they often have extensive inflammatory reactions, and suppuration is common despite the administration of appropriate antibiotics. Aphthous ulcers and chronic inflammation of the nares are often present. Granulomas are frequent and can obstruct the gastrointestinal or genitourinary tracts. The excessive inflammation is due to failure to downregulate inflammation, reflecting a failure to inhibit the synthesis of, degradation of, or response to ILs or chemoattractants, leading to persistent myeloid reaction. Impaired killing of intracellular microorganisms by macrophages may lead to persistent cell-mediated immune activation and granuloma formation. Autoimmune complications such as immune thrombocytopenic purpura and juvenile idiopathic arthritis are also increased in CGD. In addition, for unexplained reasons, discoid lupus is more common in X-linked carriers. Late complications, including nodular regenerative hyperplasia and portal hypertension, are increasingly recognized in adolescent and adult patients with CGD. Interestingly, patients with CGD have been reported to be protected from atherosclerosis, suggesting an important role for NADPH oxidase (NOX2) in the pathogenesis of this inflammatory disease of arteries.

DISORDERS OF PHAGOCYTE ACTIVATION Phagocytes depend on cell-surface stimulation to induce signals that evoke multiple levels of the inflammatory response, including cytokine synthesis, chemotaxis, and antigen presentation. Mutations affecting the major pathway that signals through NF-κB have been noted in patients with a variety of infection susceptibility syndromes. If the defects are at a very late stage of signal transduction, in the protein critical for NF-κB activation known as the NF-κB essential modulator (NEMO), then affected males develop ectodermal dysplasia and severe immune deficiency with susceptibility to bacteria, fungi, mycobacteria, and viruses. If the defects in NF-κB activation are closer to the cell-surface receptors, in the proteins transducing Toll-like receptor signals, IL-1 receptor–associated kinase 4 (IRAK4), and myeloid differentiation primary response gene 88 (MyD88), then children have a marked susceptibility to pyogenic infections early in life but develop resistance to infection later.

MONONUCLEAR PHAGOCYTES

The mononuclear phagocyte system is composed of monoblasts, promonocytes, and monocytes, in addition to the structurally diverse tissue macrophages that make up what was previously referred to as the reticuloendothelial system. Macrophages are long-lived phagocytic cells capable of many of the functions of neutrophils. They are also secretory cells that participate in many immunologic and inflammatory processes distinct from neutrophils. Monocytes leave the circulation by diapedesis more slowly than neutrophils and have a half-life in the blood of 12–24 h.

Many tissue macrophages ("big eaters") arise even before hematopoiesis and take up residence in tissues. In addition, there are macrophages derived from monocytes, which may have specialized functions suited for specific anatomic locations. Macrophages are particularly abundant in capillary walls of the lung, spleen, liver, and bone marrow, where they function to remove microorganisms and other noxious elements from the blood. Alveolar macrophages, liver Kupffer cells, splenic macrophages, peritoneal macrophages, bone marrow macrophages, lymphatic macrophages, brain microglial cells, and dendritic macrophages all have specialized functions. Macrophage-secreted products include lysozyme, neutral proteases, acid hydrolases, arginase, complement components, enzyme inhibitors (plasmin, α_2-macroglobulin), binding proteins (transferrin, fibronectin, transcobalamin II), nucleosides, and cytokines (TNF-α; IL-1, 8, 12, 18). IL-1 **(Chaps. 18 and 349)** has many functions, including initiating fever in the hypothalamus, mobilizing leukocytes from the bone marrow, and activating lymphocytes and neutrophils. TNF-α is a pyrogen that duplicates many of the actions of IL-1 and plays an important role in the pathogenesis of gram-negative shock **(Chap. 304)**. TNF-α stimulates production of hydrogen peroxide and related toxic oxygen species by macrophages and neutrophils. In addition, TNF-α induces catabolic changes that contribute to the profound wasting (cachexia) associated with many chronic diseases.

Other macrophage-secreted products include reactive oxygen and nitrogen metabolites, bioactive lipids (arachidonic acid metabolites and platelet-activating factors), chemokines, CSFs, and factors stimulating fibroblast and vessel proliferation. Macrophages help regulate the replication of lymphocytes and participate in the killing of tumors, viruses, and certain bacteria (*Mycobacterium tuberculosis* and *Listeria monocytogenes*). Macrophages are key effector cells in the elimination of intracellular microorganisms. Their ability to fuse to form giant cells that coalesce into granulomas in response to some inflammatory stimuli is important in the elimination of intracellular microbes and is under the control of IFN-γ. Nitric oxide induced by IFN-γ may be an important effector against intracellular parasites, including tuberculosis and *Leishmania*.

Macrophages play an important role in the immune response **(Chap. 349)**. They process and present antigen to lymphocytes and secrete cytokines that modulate and direct lymphocyte development and function. Macrophages participate in autoimmune phenomena by removing immune complexes and other substances from the circulation. Polymorphisms in macrophage receptors for immunoglobulin (FcγRII) determine susceptibility to some infections and autoimmune diseases. In wound healing, they dispose of senescent cells, and they also contribute to atheroma development. Macrophage elastase mediates development of emphysema from cigarette smoking.

DISORDERS OF THE MONONUCLEAR PHAGOCYTE SYSTEM

Many disorders of neutrophils extend to mononuclear phagocytes. Monocytosis is associated with tuberculosis, brucellosis, subacute bacterial endocarditis, Rocky Mountain spotted fever, malaria, and visceral leishmaniasis (kala azar). Monocytosis also occurs with malignancies, leukemias, myeloproliferative syndromes, hemolytic anemias, chronic idiopathic neutropenias, and granulomatous diseases such as sarcoidosis, regional enteritis, and some collagen vascular diseases. Patients with LAD, hyperimmunoglobulin E–recurrent infection (Job's) syndrome, CHS, and CGD all have defects in the mononuclear phagocyte system.

Monocyte cytokine production or response is impaired in some patients with disseminated nontuberculous mycobacterial infection who are not infected with HIV. Genetic defects in the pathways regulated by IFN-γ and IL-12 lead to impaired killing of intracellular bacteria, mycobacteria, salmonellae, and certain viruses **(Fig. 64-11)**.

Certain viral infections impair mononuclear phagocyte function. For example, influenza virus infection causes abnormal monocyte chemotaxis. Mononuclear phagocytes can be infected by HIV using CCR5, the chemokine receptor that acts as a co-receptor with CD4 for HIV. T lymphocytes produce IFN-γ, which induces FcR expression and phagocytosis and stimulates hydrogen peroxide production by mononuclear phagocytes and neutrophils. In certain diseases, such as AIDS, IFN-γ production may be deficient, whereas in other diseases, such as T-cell lymphomas, excessive release of IFN-γ may be associated with erythrophagocytosis by splenic macrophages.

Autoinflammatory diseases are characterized by abnormal cytokine regulation, leading to excess inflammation in the absence of infection. These diseases can mimic infectious or immunodeficient syndromes.

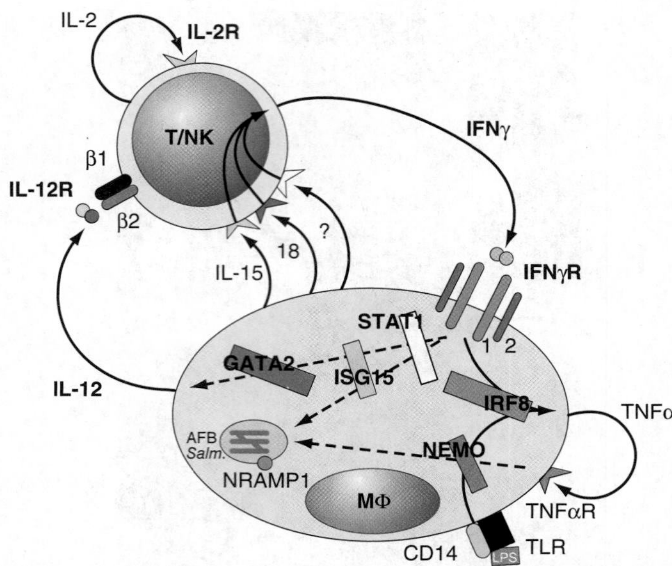

FIGURE 64-11 Lymphocyte-macrophage interactions underlying resistance to mycobacteria and other intracellular pathogens such as *Salmonella, Histoplasma,* and *Coccidioides*. Mycobacteria (and others) infect macrophages, leading to the production of IL-12, which activates T or NK cells through its receptor, leading to production of IL-2 and IFN-γ. IFN-γ acts through its receptor on macrophages to upregulate TNF-γ and IL-12 and kill intracellular pathogens. Other critical interacting molecules include signal transducer and activator of transcription 1 (STAT1), interferon regulatory factor 8 (IRF8), GATA2, and ISG15. Mutant forms of the cytokines and receptors shown in *bold type* have been found in severe cases of nontuberculous mycobacterial infection, salmonellosis, and other intracellular pathogens. AFB, acid-fast bacilli; IFN, interferon; IL, interleukin; NEMO, nuclear factor-κB essential modulator; NK, natural killer; TLR, Toll-like receptor; TNF, tumor necrosis factor.

Gain-of-function mutations in the TNF-α receptor cause TNF-α receptor–associated periodic syndrome (TRAPS), which is characterized by recurrent fever in the absence of infection, due to persistent stimulation of the TNF-α receptor **(Chap. 369)**. Diseases with abnormal IL-1 regulation leading to fever include familial Mediterranean fever due to mutations in *PYRIN*. Mutations in *cold-induced autoinflammatory syndrome 1* (*CIAS1*) lead to neonatal-onset multisystem autoinflammatory disease, familial cold urticaria, and Muckle-Wells syndrome. The syndrome of *p*yoderma gangrenosum, *a*cne, and sterile *p*yogenic *a*rthritis (PAPA syndrome) is caused by mutations in *PSTPIP1*. In contrast to these syndromes of overexpression of proinflammatory cytokines, blockade of TNF-α by the antagonists infliximab, adalimumab, certolizumab, golimumab, or etanercept has been associated with severe infections due to tuberculosis, nontuberculous mycobacteria, and fungi **(Chap. 369)**.

Monocytopenia occurs with acute infections, with stress, and after treatment with glucocorticoids. Drugs that suppress neutrophil production in the bone marrow can cause monocytopenia. Persistent severe circulating monocytopenia is seen in GATA2 deficiency, even though macrophages are found at the sites of inflammation. Monocytopenia also occurs in aplastic anemia, hairy cell leukemia, acute myeloid leukemia, and as a direct result of myelotoxic drugs.

EOSINOPHILS

Eosinophils and neutrophils share similar morphology, many lysosomal constituents, phagocytic capacity, and oxidative metabolism. Eosinophils express a specific chemoattractant receptor and respond to a specific chemokine, eotaxin, but little is known about their required role. Eosinophils are much longer lived than neutrophils, and unlike neutrophils, tissue eosinophils can recirculate. During most infections, eosinophils appear unimportant. However, in invasive helminthic infections, such as hookworm, schistosomiasis, strongyloidiasis, toxocariasis, trichinosis, filariasis, echinococcosis, and cysticercosis, the eosinophil plays a central role in host defense. Eosinophils are associated with bronchial asthma, cutaneous allergic reactions, and other hypersensitivity states.

The distinctive feature of the red-staining (Wright's stain) eosinophil granule is its crystalline core consisting of an arginine-rich protein (major basic protein) with histaminase activity, important in host defense against parasites. Eosinophil granules also contain a unique eosinophil peroxidase that catalyzes the oxidation of many substances by hydrogen peroxide and may facilitate killing of microorganisms.

Eosinophil peroxidase, in the presence of hydrogen peroxide and halide, initiates mast cell secretion in vitro and thereby promotes inflammation. Eosinophils contain cationic proteins, some of which bind to heparin and reduce its anticoagulant activity. Eosinophil-derived neurotoxin and eosinophil cationic protein are ribonucleases that can kill respiratory syncytial virus. Eosinophil cytoplasm contains Charcot-Leyden crystal protein, a hexagonal bipyramidal crystal first observed in a patient with leukemia and then in sputum of patients with asthma; this protein is lysophospholipase and may function to detoxify certain lysophospholipids.

Several factors enhance the eosinophil's function in host defense. T cell–derived factors enhance the ability of eosinophils to kill parasites. Mast cell–derived eosinophil chemotactic factor of anaphylaxis (ECFa) increases the number of eosinophil complement receptors and enhances eosinophil killing of parasites. Eosinophil CSFs (e.g., IL-5) produced by macrophages increase eosinophil production in the bone marrow and activate eosinophils to kill parasites.

■ EOSINOPHILIA

Eosinophilia is the presence of >500 eosinophils per μL of blood and is common in many settings besides parasite infection. Significant tissue eosinophilia can occur without an elevated blood count. A common cause of eosinophilia is allergic reaction to drugs (iodides, aspirin, sulfonamides, nitrofurantoin, penicillins, and cephalosporins). Allergies such as hay fever, asthma, eczema, serum sickness, allergic vasculitis, and pemphigus are associated with eosinophilia. Eosinophilia also occurs in collagen vascular diseases (e.g., rheumatoid arthritis, eosinophilic fasciitis, allergic angiitis, and periarteritis nodosa) and malignancies (e.g., Hodgkin's disease; mycosis fungoides; chronic myeloid leukemia; and cancer of the lung, stomach, pancreas, ovary, or uterus), as well as in STAT3-deficient Job's syndrome, DOCK8 deficiency (see below), and CGD. Eosinophilia is commonly present in helminthic infections. IL-5 is the dominant eosinophil growth factor. Therapeutic administration of the cytokines IL-2 or GM-CSF frequently leads to transient eosinophilia. The most dramatic hypereosinophilic syndromes are Loeffler's syndrome, tropical pulmonary eosinophilia, Loeffler's endocarditis, eosinophilic leukemia, and idiopathic hypereosinophilic syndrome (50,000–100,000/μL). IL-5 is the dominant eosinophil growth factor and can be specifically inhibited with the monoclonal antibody mepolizumab.

The idiopathic hypereosinophilic syndromes are a heterogeneous group of disorders with the common feature of prolonged eosinophilia of unknown cause and organ system dysfunction, including the heart, central nervous system, kidneys, lungs, gastrointestinal tract, and skin. The bone marrow is involved in all affected individuals, but the most severe complications involve the heart and central nervous system. Clinical manifestations and organ dysfunction are highly variable. Eosinophils are found in the involved tissues and likely cause tissue damage by local deposition of toxic eosinophil proteins such as eosinophil cationic protein and major basic protein. In the heart, the pathologic changes lead to thrombosis, endocardial fibrosis, and restrictive endomyocardiopathy. The damage to tissues in other organ systems is similar. Some cases are due to mutations involving the platelet-derived growth factor receptor, and these are extremely sensitive to the tyrosine kinase inhibitor imatinib. Glucocorticoids, hydroxyurea, and IFN-α each have been used successfully, as have therapeutic antibodies against IL-5. Cardiovascular complications are managed aggressively.

The *eosinophilia-myalgia syndrome* is a multisystem disease, with prominent cutaneous, hematologic, and visceral manifestations, that frequently evolves into a chronic course and can occasionally be fatal. The syndrome is characterized by eosinophilia (eosinophil count >1000/μL) and generalized disabling myalgias without other recognized causes. Eosinophilic fasciitis, pneumonitis, and myocarditis; neuropathy culminating in respiratory failure; and encephalopathy may occur. The disease is caused by ingesting contaminants in L-tryptophan–containing products. Eosinophils, lymphocytes, macrophages, and fibroblasts accumulate in the affected tissues, but their role in pathogenesis is unclear. Activation of eosinophils and fibroblasts and the deposition of eosinophil-derived toxic proteins in affected tissues may contribute. IL-5 and transforming growth factor β have been implicated as potential mediators. Treatment is withdrawal of products containing L-tryptophan and the administration of glucocorticoids. Most patients recover fully, remain stable, or show slow recovery, but the disease can be fatal in up to 5% of patients.

Eosinophilic neoplasms are discussed in Chap. 110.

■ EOSINOPENIA

Eosinopenia occurs with stress, such as acute bacterial infection, and after treatment with glucocorticoids. The mechanism of eosinopenia of acute bacterial infection is unknown but is independent of endogenous glucocorticoids, because it occurs in animals after total adrenalectomy. There is no known adverse effect of eosinopenia.

HYPERIMMUNOGLOBULIN E–RECURRENT INFECTION SYNDROME

The hyperimmunoglobulin E–recurrent infection syndrome, or Job's syndrome, is a rare multisystem disease in which the immune and somatic systems are affected, including neutrophils, monocytes, T cells, B cells, and osteoclasts. Autosomal *dominant* inhibitory mutations in signal transducer and activator of transcription 3 (STAT3) lead to inhibition of normal STAT signaling with broad and profound effects. Patients have characteristic facies with broad nose, kyphoscoliosis, and eczema. The primary teeth erupt normally but do not deciduate, often requiring extraction. Patients develop recurrent sinopulmonary and cutaneous infections that tend to be much less inflamed than appropriate for the degree of infection and have been referred to as "cold abscesses." Characteristically, pneumonias cavitate, leading to pneumatoceles. Coronary artery aneurysms are common, as are cerebral demyelinated plaques that accumulate with age. Importantly, IL-17–producing T cells, which are thought responsible for protection against extracellular and mucosal infections, are profoundly reduced in Job's syndrome. Despite very high IgE levels, these patients have only mildly elevated levels of allergy. An important syndrome with clinical overlap with the dominant negative STAT3 deficiency is due to autosomal recessive defects in dedicator of cytokinesis 8 (DOCK8). In DOCK8 deficiency, IgE elevation is joined to severe allergy, viral susceptibility, and increased rates of cancer. Autosomal dominant *gain-of-function* mutations in STAT3 lead to a disease characterized by onset in childhood of lymphadenopathy, autoimmune cytopenias, multiorgan autoimmunity, infections, and interstitial lung disease.

LABORATORY DIAGNOSIS AND MANAGEMENT

Initial studies of WBC and differential are essential, and careful examination of neutrophils on peripheral blood smears can diagnose Chediak-Higashi syndrome and suggest other neutrophil granule abnormalities such as specific granule deficiency. Often a bone marrow examination and serologies may be followed by either gene panel or whole exome sequencing in the cases of suspected genetic defects. Functionally, assessment of bone marrow reserves (steroid challenge test), marginated circulating pool of cells (epinephrine challenge test), and marginating ability (endotoxin challenge test) (Fig. 64-8) are also doable. In vivo assessment of inflammation is possible with a Rebuck skin window test or an in vivo skin blister assay, which measures the ability of leukocytes and inflammatory mediators to accumulate locally in the skin. In vitro tests of phagocyte aggregation, adherence, chemotaxis, phagocytosis, degranulation, and microbicidal activity (for *S. aureus*) may help pinpoint cellular or humoral lesions. Deficiencies of oxidative metabolism are detected with either the nitroblue tetrazolium (NBT) dye test or the dihydrorhodamine (DHR) oxidation test. These tests are based on the ability of products of oxidative metabolism to alter the oxidation states of reporter molecules so that they can be detected microscopically (NBT) or by flow cytometry (DHR). Qualitative studies of superoxide and hydrogen peroxide production may further define neutrophil oxidative function.

Patients with leukopenias or leukocyte dysfunction often have delayed inflammatory responses. Therefore, clinical manifestations may be minimal despite overwhelming infection, and unusual infections must always be suspected. Early signs of infection demand prompt, aggressive culturing for microorganisms, use of antibiotics, and drainage of abscesses. Prolonged courses of antibiotics are often required. In patients with CGD, prophylactic antibiotics (trimethoprim-sulfamethoxazole) and antifungals (itraconazole) markedly diminish the frequency of life-threatening infections. Glucocorticoids may relieve gastrointestinal or genitourinary tract obstruction by granulomas in patients with CGD. Although TNF-α-blocking agents may markedly relieve inflammatory bowel symptoms, extreme caution must be exercised in their use in CGD inflammatory bowel disease, because it profoundly increases these patients' already heightened susceptibility to infection. Recombinant human IFN-γ, which nonspecifically stimulates phagocytic cell function, reduces the frequency of infections in patients with CGD by 70% and reduces the severity of infection. This effect of IFN-γ in CGD is additive to the effect of prophylactic antibiotics. The recommended dose is 50 μg/m^2 subcutaneously three times weekly. IFN-γ has also been used successfully in the treatment of leprosy, nontuberculous mycobacteria, and visceral leishmaniasis.

Rigorous oral hygiene reduces but does not eliminate the discomfort of gingivitis, periodontal disease, and aphthous ulcers; chlorhexidine mouthwash and tooth brushing with a hydrogen peroxide–sodium bicarbonate paste also helps many patients. Oral antifungal agents (fluconazole, itraconazole, voriconazole, posaconazole) have reduced mucocutaneous candidiasis in patients with Job's syndrome. Androgens, glucocorticoids, lithium, and immunosuppressive therapy have been used to restore myelopoiesis in patients with neutropenia due to impaired production. Recombinant G-CSF is useful in the management of certain forms of neutropenia due to depressed neutrophil production, including those related to cancer chemotherapy. Patients with chronic neutropenia with evidence of a good bone marrow reserve need not receive prophylactic antibiotics. Patients with chronic or cyclic neutrophil counts <500/μL may benefit from prophylactic antibiotics and G-CSF during periods of neutropenia. Oral trimethoprim-sulfamethoxazole (160/800 mg) twice daily can prevent infection. Increased numbers of fungal infections are not seen in patients with CGD on this regimen. Oral quinolones such as levofloxacin and ciprofloxacin are alternatives.

In the setting of cytotoxic chemotherapy with severe, persistent lymphocyte dysfunction, trimethoprim-sulfamethoxazole prevents *Pneumocystis jiroveci* pneumonia. These patients, and patients with phagocytic cell dysfunction, should avoid heavy exposure to airborne soil, dust, or decaying matter (mulch, manure), which are often rich in *Nocardia* and the spores of *Aspergillus* and other fungi. Restriction of activities or social contact has no proven role in reducing risk of infection for phagocyte defects.

Although aggressive medical care for many patients with phagocytic disorders can allow them to go for years without a life-threatening infection, there may still be delayed effects of prolonged antimicrobials and other inflammatory complications. Cure of most congenital phagocyte defects is possible by bone marrow transplantation, and rates of success are improving **(Chap. 114)**. The identification of specific gene defects in patients with LAD 1, CGD, and other immunodeficiencies has led to gene therapy trials in a number of genetic white cell disorders.

■ FURTHER READING

Boeltz S et al: To NET or not to NET: Current opinions and state of the science regarding the formation of neutrophil extracellular traps. Cell Death Differ 26:395, 2019.

Bousfiha A et al: Human inborn errors of immunity: 2019 update of the IUIS phenotypical classification. J Clin Immunol 40:66, 2020.

Dinauer MC: Inflammatory consequences of inherited disorders affecting neutrophil function. Blood 133:2130, 2019.

Klion AD et al: Contributions of eosinophils to human health and disease. Annu Rev Pathol 15:179, 2020.

Kuhns DB: Diagnostic testing for chronic granulomatous disease. Methods Mol Biol 1982:543, 2019.

Ochoa S et al: Genetic susceptibility to fungal infection in children. Curr Opin Pediatr 32:780, 2020.

Peiseler M, Kubes P: More friend than foe: the emerging role of neutrophils in tissue repair. J Clin Invest 129:2629, 2019.

Tangye SG et al: Human inborn errors of immunity: 2019 Update on the classification from the International Union of Immunological Societies Expert Committee. J Clin Immunol 40:24, 2020.

Wu UI, Holland SM: Host susceptibility to non-tuberculous mycobacterial infections. Lancet Infect Dis 15:968, 2015.

65 Bleeding and Thrombosis

Barbara A. Konkle

The human hemostatic system provides a natural balance between procoagulant and anticoagulant forces. The procoagulant forces include platelet adhesion and aggregation and fibrin clot formation; anticoagulant forces include the natural inhibitors of coagulation and fibrinolysis. Under normal circumstances, hemostasis is regulated to promote blood flow; however, it is also prepared to clot blood rapidly to arrest blood flow and prevent exsanguination. After bleeding is successfully halted, the system remodels the damaged vessel to restore normal blood flow. The major components of the hemostatic system, which function in concert, are (1) platelets and other formed elements of blood, such as monocytes and red cells; (2) plasma proteins (the coagulation and fibrinolytic factors and inhibitors); and (3) the vessel wall.

STEPS OF NORMAL HEMOSTASIS

■ PLATELET PLUG FORMATION

On vascular injury, platelets adhere to the site of injury, usually the denuded vascular intimal surface. Platelet adhesion is mediated primarily by von Willebrand factor (VWF), a large multimeric protein present in both plasma and the extracellular matrix of the subendothelial vessel wall, which serves as the primary "molecular glue," providing sufficient strength to withstand the high levels of shear stress that would tend to detach them with the flow of blood. Platelet adhesion is also facilitated by direct binding to subendothelial collagen through specific platelet membrane collagen receptors.

Platelet adhesion results in subsequent platelet activation and aggregation. This process is enhanced and amplified by humoral mediators in plasma (e.g., epinephrine, thrombin); mediators released from activated platelets (e.g., adenosine diphosphate, serotonin); and vessel wall extracellular matrix constituents that come in contact with adherent platelets (e.g., collagen, VWF). Activated platelets undergo the release reaction, during which they secrete contents that further promote aggregation and inhibit the naturally anticoagulant endothelial cell factors. During platelet aggregation (platelet-platelet interaction), additional platelets are recruited from the circulation to the site of vascular injury, leading to the formation of an occlusive platelet thrombus. The platelet plug is anchored and stabilized by the developing fibrin mesh.

The platelet glycoprotein (Gp) IIb/IIIa ($\alpha_{IIb}\beta_3$) complex is the most abundant receptor on the platelet surface. Platelet activation converts the normally inactive Gp IIb/IIIa receptor into an active receptor, enabling binding to fibrinogen and VWF. Because the surface of each platelet has about 50,000 Gp IIb/IIIa–binding sites, numerous activated platelets recruited to the site of vascular injury can rapidly form an occlusive aggregate by means of a dense network of intercellular fibrinogen bridges.

■ FIBRIN CLOT FORMATION

Plasma coagulation proteins (*clotting factors*) normally circulate in plasma in their inactive forms. The sequence of coagulation protein reactions that culminate in the formation of fibrin was originally described as a *waterfall* or a *cascade*. Two pathways of blood coagulation have been described in the past: the so-called extrinsic, or tissue factor, pathway and the so-called intrinsic, or contact activation, pathway. We now know that coagulation is normally initiated through tissue factor (TF) exposure and activation through the classic *extrinsic pathway* but with critically important amplification through elements of the classic *intrinsic pathway*, as illustrated in **Fig. 65-1**. These reactions take place on phospholipid surfaces, usually the activated platelet surface. Coagulation testing in the laboratory can reflect other influences due to the artificial nature of the in vitro systems used (see below).

The immediate trigger for coagulation is vascular damage that exposes blood to TF that is constitutively expressed on the surfaces of subendothelial cellular components of the vessel wall, such as smooth muscle cells and fibroblasts. TF is also present in circulating microparticles, presumably shed from cells including monocytes and platelets. TF binds the serine protease factor VIIa; the complex activates factor X to factor Xa. Alternatively, the complex can indirectly activate factor X by initially converting factor IX to factor IXa, which then activates factor X. The participation of factor XI in hemostasis is not dependent on its activation by factor XIIa but rather on its positive feedback activation by thrombin. Thus, factor XIa functions in the propagation and amplification, rather than in the initiation, of the coagulation cascade. The role of factor XIIa in activation of factor XI is not fully elucidated, but studies suggest it may be a mechanism to promote thrombosis.

Factor Xa can be formed through the actions of either the TF/factor VIIa complex or factor IXa (with factor VIIIa as a cofactor) and converts prothrombin to thrombin, the pivotal protease of the coagulation system. The essential cofactor for this reaction is factor Va. Like the homologous factor VIIIa, factor Va is produced by thrombin-induced limited proteolysis of factor V. Thrombin is a multifunctional enzyme that converts soluble plasma fibrinogen to an insoluble fibrin matrix. Fibrin polymerization involves an orderly process of intermolecular associations (**Fig. 65-2**). Thrombin also activates factor XIII (fibrin-stabilizing factor) to factor XIIIa, which covalently cross-links and thereby stabilizes the fibrin clot.

The assembly of the clotting factors on activated cell membrane surfaces greatly accelerates their reaction rates and also serves to localize blood clotting to sites of vascular injury. The critical cell membrane components, acidic phospholipids, are not normally exposed on resting cell membrane surfaces. However, when platelets, monocytes, and endothelial cells are activated by vascular injury or inflammatory stimuli, the procoagulant head groups of the membrane anionic phospholipids become translocated to the surfaces of these cells or released as part of microparticles, making them available to support and promote the plasma coagulation reactions.

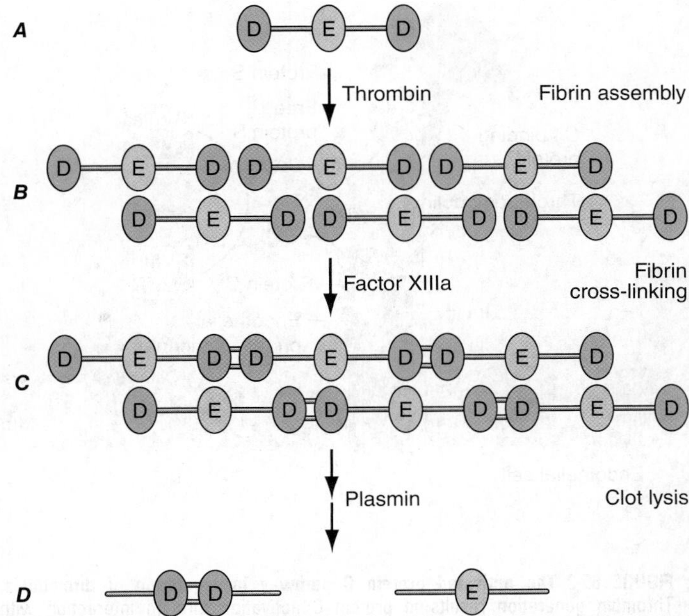

FIGURE 65-2 Fibrin formation and dissolution. (***A***) Fibrinogen is a trinodular structure consisting of two D domains and one E domain. Thrombin activation results in an ordered lateral assembly of protofibrils (***B***) with noncovalent associations. Factor XIIIa cross-links the D domains on adjacent molecules (***C***). Fibrin and fibrinogen (not shown) lysis by plasmin occurs at discrete sites and results in intermediary fibrin(ogen) degradation products (not shown). D-Dimers are the product of complete lysis of fibrin (***D***), maintaining the cross-linked D domains.

FIGURE 65-1 Coagulation is initiated by tissue factor (TF) exposure, which, with factor (F) VIIa, activates FIX and FX, which in turn, with FVIII and FV as cofactors, respectively, results in thrombin formation and subsequent conversion of fibrinogen to fibrin. Thrombin activates FXI, FVIII, and FV, amplifying the coagulation signal. Once the TF/FVIIa/FXa complex is formed, tissue factor pathway inhibitor (TFPI) inhibits the TF/FVIIa pathway, making coagulation dependent on the amplification loop through FIX/FVIII. Coagulation requires calcium (not shown) and takes place on phospholipid surfaces, usually the activated platelet membrane.

ANTITHROMBOTIC MECHANISMS

Several physiologic antithrombotic mechanisms act in concert to prevent clotting under normal circumstances. These mechanisms operate to preserve blood fluidity and to limit blood clotting to specific focal sites of vascular injury. Endothelial cells have many antithrombotic effects. They produce prostacyclin, nitric oxide, and ectoADPase/CD39, which act to inhibit platelet binding, secretion, and aggregation. Endothelial cells produce anticoagulant factors including heparan proteoglycans, TF pathway inhibitor, and thrombomodulin. They also activate fibrinolytic mechanisms through the production of tissue plasminogen activator, urokinase, plasminogen activator inhibitors, and annexin-2.

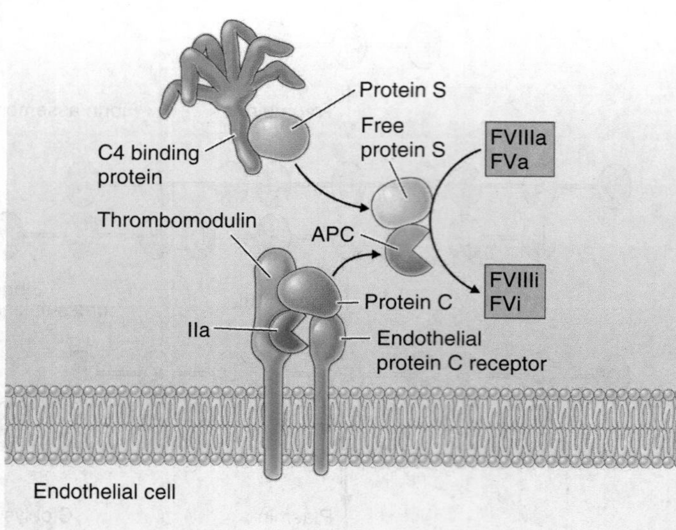

FIGURE 65-3 The activated protein C pathway in regulation of thrombosis. Thrombin generation results in protein C activation through interaction with thrombomodulin and protein C bound to the endothelial protein C receptor (EPCR). Activated protein C (APC) with free protein S converts activated factors (F) VIII and V to inactivate forms, thus in turn decreasing thrombin generation. C4BP, C4 binding protein; EC, endothelial cell; F, factor; IIa, thrombin; PC, protein C; PS, protein S; TM, thrombomodulin.

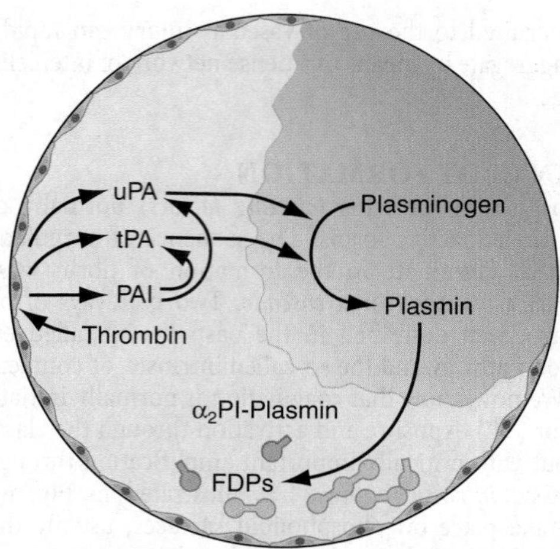

FIGURE 65-4 A schematic diagram of the fibrinolytic system. Tissue plasminogen activator (tPA) is released from endothelial cells, binds the fibrin clot, and activates plasminogen to plasmin. Release of plasminogen activator inhibitors (PAI-1 and PAI-2) inhibits tPA and urokinase (uPA). Excess fibrin is degraded by plasmin to distinct degradation products [FDPs (D-dimers)]. Any free plasmin is complexed with α_2-antiplasmin (α_2PI). PAI, plasminogen activator inhibitor; uPA, urokinase-type plasminogen activator.

Antithrombin is the major plasma protease inhibitor of thrombin and the other clotting factors in coagulation. Antithrombin neutralizes thrombin and other activated coagulation factors by forming a complex between the active site of the enzyme and the reactive center of antithrombin. The rate of formation of these inactivating complexes increases by a factor of several thousand in the presence of heparin. Antithrombin inactivation of thrombin and other activated clotting factors occurs physiologically on vascular surfaces, where glycosaminoglycans, including heparan sulfates, are present to catalyze these reactions. Inherited quantitative or qualitative deficiencies of antithrombin lead to a lifelong predisposition to venous thromboembolism.

Protein C is a plasma glycoprotein that becomes an anticoagulant when it is activated by thrombin. The thrombin-induced activation of protein C occurs physiologically on thrombomodulin, a transmembrane proteoglycan-binding site for thrombin on endothelial cell surfaces. The binding of protein C to its receptor on endothelial cells places it in proximity to the thrombin-thrombomodulin complex, thereby enhancing its activation efficiency. (**See Fig. 65-3**.) Activated protein C acts as an anticoagulant by cleaving and inactivating activated factors V and VIII. This reaction is accelerated by a cofactor, protein S, which, like protein C, is a glycoprotein that undergoes vitamin K–dependent posttranslational modification. Quantitative or qualitative deficiencies of protein C or protein S, or resistance to the action of activated protein C by a specific variant at its target cleavage site in factor Va (factor V Leiden), lead to hypercoagulable states.

Tissue factor pathway inhibitor (TFPI) is a plasma protease inhibitor that regulates the TF-induced extrinsic pathway of coagulation. TFPI inhibits the TF/factor VIIa/factor Xa complex, essentially turning off the TF/factor VIIa initiation of coagulation, which then becomes dependent on the "amplification loop" via factor XI and factor VIII activation by thrombin. TFPI is bound to lipoprotein and can also be released by heparin from endothelial cells, where it is bound to glycosaminoglycans, and from platelets. The heparin-mediated release of TFPI may play a role in the anticoagulant effects of unfractionated and low-molecular-weight heparins.

THE FIBRINOLYTIC SYSTEM

Any thrombin that escapes the inhibitory effects of the physiologic anticoagulant systems is available to convert fibrinogen to fibrin. In response, the endogenous fibrinolytic system is then activated to dispose of intravascular fibrin and thereby maintain or reestablish the patency of the circulation. Just as thrombin is the key protease enzyme of the coagulation system, plasmin is the major protease enzyme of the fibrinolytic system, acting to digest fibrin to fibrin degradation products. The general scheme of fibrinolysis and its control is shown in **Fig. 65-4**.

The plasminogen activators, tissue type plasminogen activator (tPA) and the urokinase-type plasminogen activator (uPA), cleave the Arg560-Val561 bond of plasminogen to generate the active enzyme plasmin. The lysine-binding sites of plasmin (and plasminogen) permit it to bind to fibrin, so that physiologic fibrinolysis is "fibrin specific." Both plasminogen (through its lysine-binding sites) and tPA possess specific affinity for fibrin and thereby bind selectively to clots. The assembly of a ternary complex, consisting of fibrin, plasminogen, and tPA, promotes the localized interaction between plasminogen and tPA and greatly accelerates the rate of plasminogen activation to plasmin. Moreover, partial degradation of fibrin by plasmin exposes new plasminogen and tPA-binding sites in carboxy-terminus lysine residues of fibrin fragments to enhance these reactions further. This creates a highly efficient mechanism to generate plasmin focally on the fibrin clot, which then becomes plasmin's substrate for digestion to fibrin degradation products.

Plasmin cleaves fibrin at distinct sites of the fibrin molecule, leading to the generation of characteristic fibrin fragments during the process of fibrinolysis (Fig. 65-2). The sites of plasmin cleavage of fibrin are the same as those in fibrinogen. However, when plasmin acts on covalently cross-linked fibrin, D-dimers are released; hence, D-dimers can be measured in plasma as a relatively specific test of fibrin (rather than fibrinogen) degradation. D-Dimer assays can be used as sensitive markers of blood clot formation and have been validated for clinical use to exclude the diagnosis of deep venous thrombosis (DVT) and pulmonary embolism in selected populations. D-Dimer levels increase with age. A higher cut-off value to rule out venous thromboembolism (VTE) in the elderly has been proposed but is controversial.

Physiologic regulation of fibrinolysis occurs primarily at three levels: (1) plasminogen activator inhibitors (PAIs), specifically PAI-1 and PAI-2, inhibit the physiologic plasminogen activators; (2) the thrombin-activatable fibrinolysis inhibitor (TAFI) limits fibrinolysis; and (3) α_2-antiplasmin inhibits plasmin. PAI-1 is the primary inhibitor of tPA and uPA in plasma. TAFI cleaves the N-terminal lysine residues of fibrin, which aid in localization of plasmin activity. α_2-Antiplasmin is the main inhibitor of plasmin in human plasma, inactivating any nonfibrin clot–associated plasmin.

APPROACH TO THE PATIENT

Bleeding and Thrombosis

CLINICAL PRESENTATION

Disorders of hemostasis may be either inherited or acquired. A detailed personal and family history is key in determining the chronicity of symptoms and the likelihood of the disorder being inherited, as well as providing clues to underlying conditions that have contributed to the bleeding or thrombotic state. In addition, the history can give clues as to the etiology by determining (1) the bleeding (mucosal and/or joint) or thrombosis (arterial and/or venous) site and (2) whether an underlying bleeding or clotting tendency was enhanced by another medical condition or the introduction of medications or dietary supplements.

History of Bleeding A history of bleeding is the most important predictor of bleeding risk. In evaluating a patient for a bleeding disorder, a history of at-risk situations, including the response to past surgeries, should be assessed. Does the patient have a history of spontaneous or trauma/surgery-induced bleeding? Spontaneous hemarthroses are a hallmark of moderate and severe factor VIII and IX deficiency and, in rare circumstances, of other clotting factor deficiencies. Mucosal bleeding symptoms are more suggestive of underlying platelet disorders or von Willebrand disease (VWD), termed *disorders of primary hemostasis or platelet plug formation*. Disorders affecting primary hemostasis are shown in **Table 65-1**.

A bleeding score has been validated as a tool to predict patients more likely to have type 1 VWD (International Society on Thrombosis and Haemostasis Bleeding Assessment Tool [*www.isth.org/resource/resmgr/ssc/isth-ssc_bleeding_assessment.pdf*]), and a self-administered form has been validated. This is the most useful tool in excluding the diagnosis of a bleeding disorder, thus avoiding unnecessary testing, and is recommended by 2021 guidelines for screening for VWD in primary care. Bleeding symptoms that are more common in patients with bleeding disorders include prolonged bleeding with surgery, dental procedures and extractions, and/or trauma; heavy menstrual bleeding or postpartum hemorrhage; and large bruises (often described with lumps).

Easy bruising and heavy menstrual bleeding are common complaints in patients with and without bleeding disorders. Easy bruising can also be a sign of medical conditions in which there is no identifiable coagulopathy; instead, the conditions are caused by an abnormality of blood vessels or their supporting connective tissues. In Ehlers-Danlos syndrome, there may be posttraumatic bleeding and a history of joint hyperextensibility. Cushing's syndrome, chronic steroid use, and aging result in changes in skin and subcutaneous tissue, and subcutaneous bleeding occurs in response to minor trauma. The latter has been termed *senile purpura*.

Epistaxis is a common symptom, particularly in children and in dry climates, and may not reflect an underlying bleeding disorder. However, it is the most common symptom in hereditary hemorrhagic telangiectasia and in boys with VWD. Clues that epistaxis is a symptom of an underlying bleeding disorder include lack of seasonal variation and bleeding that requires medical evaluation or treatment, including cauterization. Bleeding with eruption of primary teeth is seen in children with more severe bleeding disorders, such as moderate and severe hemophilia. It is uncommon in children with mild bleeding disorders. Patients with disorders of primary hemostasis (platelet adhesion) may have increased bleeding after dental cleanings and other procedures that involve gum manipulation.

Heavy menstrual bleeding is defined quantitatively as a loss of >80 mL of blood per cycle, based on the quantity of blood loss required to produce iron-deficiency anemia. A complaint of heavy menses is subjective and has a poor correlation with excessive blood loss. Predictors of heavy menstrual bleeding include bleeding resulting in iron-deficiency anemia or a need for blood transfusion, passage of clots >1 inch in diameter, and changing a pad or tampon more than hourly. Heavy menstrual bleeding is a common symptom in women with underlying bleeding disorders and is reported in the majority of women with VWD, factor XI deficiency, platelet function disorders, and hemophilia, including genetic carriers with borderline-normal factor levels. Women with underlying bleeding disorders are more likely to have other bleeding symptoms, including bleeding after dental extractions and postoperative and postpartum bleeding, and are much more likely to have heavy menstrual bleeding beginning at menarche than women with heavy menstrual bleeding due to other causes. Heavy menstrual bleeding may results in iron deficiency and is documented to have significant adverse effects on quality of life.

Postpartum hemorrhage is a common symptom in women with underlying bleeding disorders. In women with type 1 VWD or hemophilia A in whom levels of VWF and factor VIII usually normalize during pregnancy, postpartum hemorrhage may be delayed. Women with a history of postpartum hemorrhage may have a higher risk of recurrence with subsequent pregnancies. Women with underlying bleeding disorders are at risk for other reproductive tract bleeding, including rupture of ovarian cysts with intraabdominal hemorrhage.

Tonsillectomy is a major hemostatic challenge, because intact hemostatic mechanisms are essential to prevent excessive bleeding from the tonsillar bed. Bleeding may occur early after surgery or after approximately 7 days postoperatively, with loss of the eschar at the operative site. Similar delayed bleeding is seen after colonic polyp resection. Gastrointestinal (GI) bleeding and hematuria are usually due to underlying pathology, and procedures to identify and treat the bleeding site should be undertaken, even in patients with known bleeding disorders. VWD, particularly types 2 and 3, is associated with angiodysplasia of the bowel and GI bleeding.

Hemarthroses and spontaneous muscle hematomas are characteristic of moderate or severe congenital factor VIII or IX deficiency. They can also be seen in moderate and severe deficiencies of fibrinogen, prothrombin, and factors V, VII, and X. Spontaneous hemarthroses occur rarely in other bleeding disorders except for severe VWD, with associated factor VIII levels <5%. Muscle and soft tissue bleeds are also common in acquired factor VIII deficiency. Bleeding into a joint results in severe pain and swelling, as well as loss of function, but is rarely associated with discoloration from bruising around the joint. Life-threatening sites of bleeding

TABLE 65-1 Primary Hemostatic (Platelet Plug) Disorders

Defects of Platelet Adhesion
von Willebrand disease
Bernard-Soulier syndrome (absence or dysfunction of platelet Gp Ib-IX-V)
Defects of Platelet Aggregation
Glanzmann's thrombasthenia (absence or dysfunction of platelet glycoprotein [Gp] IIb/IIIa)
Afibrinogenemia
Defects of Platelet Secretion
Decreased cyclooxygenase activity
Drug-induced (aspirin, nonsteroidal anti-inflammatory agents, thienopyridines)
Inherited
Granule storage pool defects
Inherited
Acquired
Nonspecific inherited secretory defects
Nonspecific drug effects
Uremia
Platelet coating (e.g., paraprotein, penicillin)
Defect of Platelet Coagulant Activity
Scott's syndrome

include bleeding into the oropharynx, where bleeding can obstruct the airway, into the central nervous system, and into the retroperitoneum. Central nervous system bleeding is the major cause of bleeding-related deaths in patients with severe congenital factor deficiencies.

Prohemorrhagic Effects of Medications and Dietary Supplements Aspirin and other nonsteroidal anti-inflammatory drugs (NSAIDs) that inhibit cyclooxygenase 1 impair primary hemostasis and may exacerbate bleeding from another cause or even unmask a previously occult mild bleeding disorder such as VWD. All NSAIDs, however, can precipitate GI bleeding, which may be more severe in patients with underlying bleeding disorders. The aspirin effect on platelet function lasts for the life of the platelet; however, in individuals with typical platelet turnover, the functional defect reverts to near-normal within 2–3 days after the last dose. The effect of other NSAIDs is shorter, as the inhibitor effect is reversed when the drug is removed. Inhibitors of the ADP $P2Y_{12}$ receptor (clopidogrel, prasugrel, and ticagrelor) inhibit ADP-mediated platelet aggregation and, like NSAIDs, can precipitate or exacerbate bleeding symptoms. The risk of bleeding with these drugs is higher than with NSAIDs.

Many herbal supplements can impair hemostatic function (**Table 65-2**). Some are more convincingly associated with a bleeding risk than others. Fish oil or concentrated omega-3 fatty acid supplements impair platelet function. They alter platelet biochemistry to produce more PGI_3, a more potent platelet inhibitor than prostacyclin (PGI_2), and more thromboxane A_3, a less potent platelet activator than thromboxane A_2. In fact, diets naturally rich in omega-3 fatty acids can result in a prolonged bleeding time and abnormal platelet aggregation studies, but the actual associated bleeding risk is unclear. Vitamin E appears to inhibit protein kinase C–mediated platelet aggregation and nitric oxide production. In patients with unexplained bruising or bleeding, it is prudent to review any new medications or supplements and discontinue those that may be associated with bleeding.

Underlying Systemic Diseases That Cause or Exacerbate a Bleeding Tendency Acquired bleeding disorders are commonly secondary to, or associated with, systemic disease. The clinical evaluation of a patient with a bleeding tendency must therefore include a thorough assessment for evidence of underlying disease. Bruising or mucosal bleeding may be the presenting complaint in liver disease, severe renal impairment, hypothyroidism, paraproteinemias or amyloidosis, and conditions causing bone marrow failure. All coagulation factors are synthesized in the liver, and hepatic failure results in combined factor deficiencies. This is often compounded by thrombocytopenia and portal hypertension. Coagulation factors II, VII, IX, and X and proteins C, S, and Z are dependent on vitamin K for posttranslational modification. Although vitamin K is required in both procoagulant and anticoagulant processes, the phenotype of vitamin K deficiency or the warfarin effect on coagulation is bleeding.

The normal blood platelet count is 150,000–450,000/μL. Thrombocytopenia results from decreased production, increased destruction, and/or sequestration. Although the bleeding risk varies somewhat by the reason for the thrombocytopenia, bleeding rarely occurs in isolated thrombocytopenia at counts >50,000/μL and usually not until <10,000–20,000/μL. Coexisting coagulopathies, as is seen in liver failure or disseminated coagulation; infection; platelet-inhibitory drugs; and underlying medical conditions can all increase the risk of bleeding in the thrombocytopenic patient. Most procedures can be performed in patients with a platelet count of 50,000/μL or greater.

HISTORY OF THROMBOSIS

The risk of thrombosis, like that of bleeding, is influenced by both genetic and environmental factors. The major risk factor for arterial thrombosis is atherosclerosis, whereas for venous thrombosis, the risk factors are immobility, surgery, underlying medical conditions such as malignancy, medications such as hormonal therapy, obesity, and genetic predispositions. Factors that increase risks for venous and for both venous and arterial thromboses are shown in **Table 65-3**.

The most important point in a history related to venous thrombosis is determining whether the thrombotic event was idiopathic (meaning there was no clear precipitating factor) or was a precipitated event. In patients without underlying malignancy, having an idiopathic event is the strongest predictor of recurrence of VTE. In patients who have a vague history of thrombosis, a history of being treated with warfarin or other anticoagulants suggests a past DVT. Age is an important risk factor for venous thrombosis—the risk of DVT increases per decade, with an approximate incidence of 1/100,000 per year in early childhood to 1/200 per year among octogenarians. Family history is helpful in determining if there is a

TABLE 65-2 Herbal Supplements Associated with Increased Bleeding

Herbs with Potential Antiplatelet Activity
Ginkgo (*Ginkgo biloba L.*)
Garlic (*Allium sativum*)
Bilberry (*Vaccinium myrtillus*)
Ginger (*Gingiber officinale*)
Dong quai (*Angelica sinensis*)
Feverfew (*Tanacetum parthenium*)
Asian ginseng (*Panax ginseng*)
American ginseng (*Panax quinquefolius*)
Siberian ginseng/eleuthero (*Eleutherococcus senticosus*)
Turmeric (*Circuma longa*)
Meadowsweet (*Filipendula ulmaria*)
Willow (*Salix* spp.)
Coumarin-Containing Herbs
Motherwort (*Leonurus cardiaca*)
Chamomile (*Matricaria recutita, Chamaemelum mobile*)
Horse chestnut (*Aesculus hippocastanum*)
Red clover (*Trifolium pratense*)
Fenugreek (*Trigonella foenum-graecum*)

TABLE 65-3 Some Risk Factors for Thrombosis

VENOUS	VENOUS AND ARTERIAL
Inherited	**Inherited**
Factor V Leiden	Homocystinuria
Prothrombin G20210A	Dysfibrinogenemia
Antithrombin deficiency	**Acquired**
Protein C deficiency	Malignancy
Protein S deficiency	Antiphospholipid antibody syndrome
Acquired	Hormonal therapy
Age	Polycythemia vera
Previous thrombosis	Essential thrombocythemia
Immobilization	Paroxysmal nocturnal hemoglobinuria
Major surgery	Thrombotic thrombocytopenic purpura
Pregnancy and puerperium	Heparin-induced thrombocytopenia
Hospitalization	Disseminated intravascular coagulation
Obesity	**Unknown**[a]
Infection	Elevated factor II, VIII, IX, XI
Smoking	Elevated TAFI levels
	Low levels of TFPI

[a]Unknown whether risk is inherited or acquired.

Abbreviations: APC, activated protein C; TAFI, thrombin-activatable fibrinolysis inhibitor; TFPI, tissue factor pathway inhibitor.

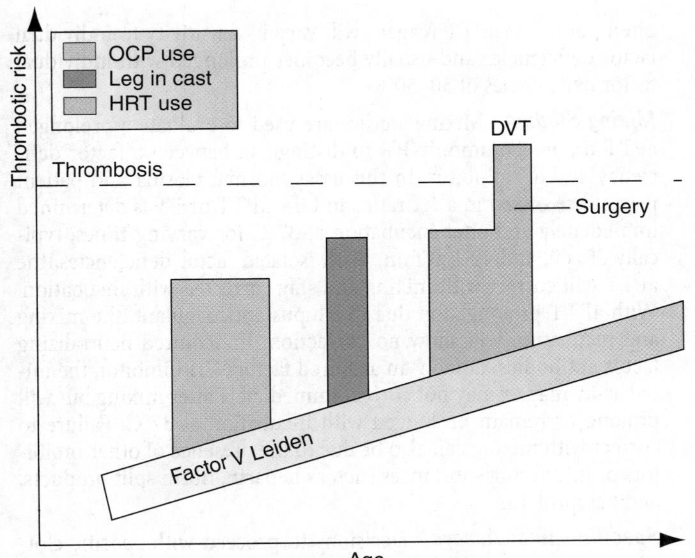

FIGURE 65-5 Thrombotic risk over time. Shown schematically is an individual's thrombotic risk over time. An underlying factor V Leiden variant provides a "theoretically" constant increased risk. The thrombotic risk increases with age and, intermittently, with oral contraceptive (OCP) or hormone replacement therapy (HRT) use; other events, like major surgery or illness, will increase the risk further. At some point, the cumulative risk may increase to the threshold for thrombosis and result in deep venous thrombosis (DVT). Note: The magnitude and duration of risk portrayed in the figure are meant for example only and may not precisely reflect the relative risk determined by clinical study. *(Sources: From BA Konkle, A Schafer, in DP Zipes et al [eds]: Braunwald's Heart Disease, 7th ed. Philadelphia, Saunders, 2005; from FR Rosendaal: Venous thrombosis: A multicausal disease. Lancet 353:1167, 1999.)*

genetic predisposition and how strong that predisposition appears to be. A genetic thrombophilia that confers a relatively small increased risk, such as being a heterozygote for the prothrombin G20210A or factor V Leiden mutation, is a minor determinant of risk in an elderly individual undergoing a high-risk surgical procedure. As illustrated in **Fig. 65-5**, a thrombotic event usually has more than one contributing factor. Predisposing factors must be carefully assessed to determine the risk of recurrent thrombosis and, with consideration of the patient's bleeding risk, determine the length of anticoagulation. Testing for inherited thrombophilias in adults should be limited to instances where results would change clinical care. Such instances are rare.

LABORATORY EVALUATION

Careful history taking and clinical examination are essential components in the assessment of bleeding and thrombotic risk. The use of laboratory tests of coagulation complements, but cannot substitute for, clinical assessment. No test exists that provides a global assessment of hemostasis. The bleeding time has been used to assess bleeding risk; however, it does not predict bleeding risk with surgery, and it is not recommended for this indication. The PFA-100, an instrument that measures platelet-dependent coagulation under flow conditions, is more sensitive and specific for VWD than the bleeding time; however, it is not sensitive enough to rule out mild bleeding disorders. PFA-100 closure times are prolonged in patients with some, but not all, inherited platelet disorders. Also, its utility in predicting bleeding risk has not been determined. Thromboelastography can be useful in guiding intraoperative transfusion and is being explored in other settings, but is not broadly applicable for the diagnosis of disorders of hemostasis and thrombosis.

For routine preoperative and preprocedure testing, an abnormal prothrombin time (PT) may detect liver disease or vitamin K deficiency that had not been previously appreciated. Studies have not confirmed the usefulness of an activated partial thromboplastin time (aPTT) in preoperative evaluations in patients with a negative bleeding history. The primary use of coagulation testing should be to confirm the presence and type of bleeding disorder in a patient with a suspicious clinical history.

Because of the nature of coagulation assays, proper sample acquisition and handling is critical to obtaining valid results. In patients with abnormal coagulation assays who have no bleeding history, repeat studies with attention to these factors frequently results in normal values. Most coagulation assays are performed in sodium citrate anticoagulated plasma that is recalcified for the assay. Because the anticoagulant is in liquid solution and needs to be added to blood in proportion to the plasma volume, incorrectly filled or inadequately mixed blood collection tubes will give erroneous results. These vacutainer tubes should be filled to >90% of the recommended fill, which is usually denoted by a line on the tube. An elevated hematocrit (>55%) can result in a false value due to a decreased plasma-to-anticoagulant ratio.

Screening Assays The most commonly used screening tests are the PT, aPTT, and platelet count. The PT assesses the factors I (fibrinogen), II (prothrombin), V, VII, and X (**Fig. 65-6**). The PT measures the time for clot formation of the citrated plasma after recalcification and addition of thromboplastin, a mixture of TF and phospholipids. The sensitivity of the assay varies by the source of thromboplastin. The relationship between defects in secondary hemostasis (fibrin formation) and coagulation test abnormalities is shown in **Table 65-4**. To adjust for this variability, the overall sensitivity of different thromboplastins to reduction of the vitamin K–dependent clotting factors II, VII, IX, and X in anticoagulation patients is expressed as the International Sensitivity Index (ISI). The international normalized ratio (INR) is determined based on the formula: $INR = (PT_{patient}/PT_{normal\ mean})^{ISI}$.

The INR was developed to assess stable anticoagulation due to reduction of vitamin K–dependent coagulation factors; it is commonly used in the evaluation of patients with liver disease. Although it does allow comparison between laboratories, reagent sensitivity as used to determine the ISI is not the same in liver disease as with warfarin anticoagulation. In addition, progressive liver failure is associated with variable changes in coagulation factors; the degree of prolongation of either the PT or the INR only roughly

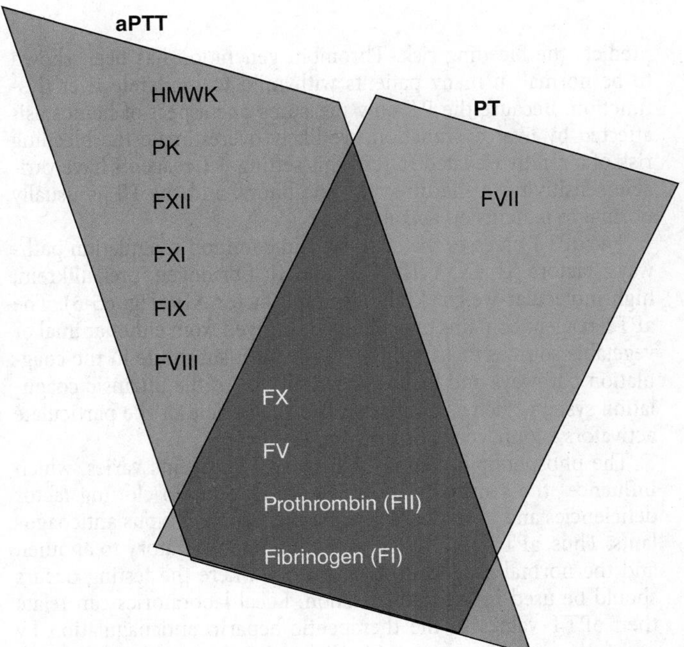

FIGURE 65-6 Coagulation factor activity tested in the activated partial thromboplastin time (aPTT) in red and prothrombin time (PT) in green, or both. F, factor; HMWK, high-molecular-weight kininogen; PK, prekallikrein.

TABLE 65-4 Hemostatic Disorders and Coagulation Test Abnormalities

Prolonged Activated Partial Thromboplastin Time (aPTT)
No clinical bleeding—↓ factor XII, high-molecular-weight kininogen, prekallikrein
Variable, but usually mild, bleeding—↓ factor XI, mild ↓ factor VIII and factor IX
Frequent, severe bleeding—severe deficiencies of factors VIII and IX
Heparin and direct thrombin inhibitors
Prolonged Prothrombin Time (PT)
Factor VII deficiency
Vitamin K deficiency—early
Warfarin anticoagulation
Direct Xa inhibitors (rivaroxaban, edoxaban, apixaban—note PT may be normal)
Prolonged aPTT and PT
Factor II, V, X, or fibrinogen deficiency
Vitamin K deficiency—late
Direct thrombin inhibitors
Prolonged Thrombin Time
Heparin or heparin-like inhibitors
Direct thrombin inhibitors (e.g., dabigatran, argatroban, bivalirudin)
Mild or no bleeding—dysfibrinogenemia
Frequent, severe bleeding—afibrinogenemia
Prolonged PT and/or aPTT Not Corrected with Mixing with Normal Plasma
Bleeding—specific factor inhibitor
No symptoms, or clotting and/or pregnancy loss—lupus anticoagulant
Disseminated intravascular coagulation
Heparin or direct thrombin inhibitor
Abnormal Clot Solubility
Factor XIII deficiency
Inhibitors or defective cross-linking
Rapid Clot Lysis
Deficiency of α_2-antiplasmin or plasminogen activator inhibitor 1
Treatment with fibrinolytic therapy

predicts the bleeding risk. Thrombin generation has been shown to be normal in many patients with mild to moderate liver dysfunction. Because the PT only measures one aspect of hemostasis affected by liver dysfunction, we likely overestimate the bleeding risk of a mildly elevated INR in this setting. PT reagents have variable sensitivity to the direct Xa inhibitors, and the PT is usually normal in patients on apixaban.

The aPTT assesses the intrinsic and common coagulation pathways; factors XI, IX, VIII, X, V, and II; fibrinogen; prekallikrein; high-molecular-weight kininogen; and factor XII (Fig. 65-6). The aPTT reagent contains phospholipids derived from either animal or vegetable sources that function as a platelet substitute in the coagulation pathways and includes an activator of the intrinsic coagulation system, such as nonparticulate ellagic acid or the particulate activators kaolin, celite, or micronized silica.

The phospholipid composition of aPTT reagents varies, which influences the sensitivity of individual reagents to clotting factor deficiencies and to inhibitors such as heparin and lupus anticoagulants. Thus, aPTT results will vary from one laboratory to another, and the normal range in the laboratory where the testing occurs should be used in the interpretation. Local laboratories can relate their aPTT values to the therapeutic heparin anticoagulation by correlating aPTT values with direct measurements of heparin activity (anti-Xa or protamine titration assays) in samples from heparinized patients, although correlation between these assays is often poor. The aPTT reagent will vary in sensitivity to individual factor deficiencies and usually becomes prolonged with individual factor deficiencies of 30–50%.

Mixing Studies Mixing studies are used to evaluate a prolonged aPTT or, less commonly PT, to distinguish between a factor deficiency and an inhibitor. In this assay, normal plasma and patient plasma are mixed in a 1:1 ratio, and the aPTT or PT is determined immediately and after incubation at 37°C for varying times, typically 30, 60, and/or 120 min. With isolated factor deficiencies, the aPTT will correct with mixing and stay corrected with incubation. With aPTT prolongation due to a lupus anticoagulant, the mixing and incubation will show no correction. In acquired neutralizing factor antibodies, notably an acquired factor VIII inhibitor, the initial assay may or may not correct immediately after mixing but will prolong or remain prolonged with incubation at 37°C. Failure to correct with mixing can also be due to the presence of other inhibitors or interfering substances such as heparin, fibrin split products, and paraproteins.

Specific Factor Assays Decisions to proceed with specific clotting factor assays will be influenced by the clinical situation and the results of coagulation screening tests. Precise diagnosis and effective management of inherited and acquired coagulation deficiencies necessitate quantitation of the relevant factors. When bleeding is severe, specific assays are urgently required to guide appropriate therapy. Individual factor assays are usually performed as modifications of the mixing study, where the patient's plasma is mixed with plasma deficient in the factor being studied. This will correct all factor deficiencies to >50%, thus making prolongation of clot formation due to a factor deficiency dependent on the factor missing from the added plasma.

Testing for Antiphospholipid Antibodies Antibodies to phospholipids (cardiolipin) or phospholipid-binding proteins (β_2-microglobulin and others) are detected by enzyme-linked immunosorbent assay (ELISA). When these antibodies interfere with phospholipid-dependent coagulation tests, they are termed *lupus anticoagulants*. The aPTT has variability sensitivity to lupus anticoagulants, depending in part on the aPTT reagents used. An assay using a sensitive reagent has been termed an *LA-PTT*. The dilute Russell viper venom test (dRVVT) is a modification of a standard test with the phospholipid reagent decreased, thus increasing the sensitivity to antibodies that interfere with the phospholipid component. These tests, however, are not specific for lupus anticoagulants, because factor deficiencies or other inhibitors will also result in prolongation. Documentation of a lupus anticoagulant requires not only prolongation of a phospholipid-dependent coagulation test but also lack of correction when mixed with normal plasma and correction with the addition of activated platelet membranes or certain phospholipids (e.g., hexagonal phase).

Other Coagulation Tests The thrombin time and the reptilase time measure fibrinogen conversion to fibrin and are prolonged when the fibrinogen level is low (usually <80–100 mg/dL) or qualitatively abnormal, as seen in inherited or acquired dysfibrinogenemias, or when fibrin/fibrinogen degradation products interfere. The thrombin time, but not the reptilase time, is prolonged in the presence of heparin. The thrombin time is markedly prolonged in the presence of the direct thrombin inhibitor, dabigatran; a dilute thrombin time can be used to assess drug activity. Measurement of anti–factor Xa plasma inhibitory activity is a test frequently used to assess low-molecular-weight heparin (LMWH) levels, as a direct measurement of unfractionated heparin (UFH) activity, or to assess activity of the direct Xa inhibitors rivaroxaban, apixaban, and edoxaban. Drug in the patient sample inhibits the enzymatic conversion of an Xa-specific chromogenic substrate to colored product by factor Xa. Standard curves are created using multiple concentrations of the specific drug and are used to calculate the concentration of anti-Xa activity in the patient plasma.

Laboratory Testing for Thrombophilia Laboratory assays to detect thrombophilic states include molecular diagnostics and immunologic and functional assays. These assays vary in their sensitivity and specificity for the condition being tested. Furthermore, acute thrombosis, acute illnesses, inflammatory conditions, pregnancy, and medications affect levels of many coagulation factors and their inhibitors. Antithrombin is decreased by heparin and in the setting of acute thrombosis. Protein C and S levels may be increased in the setting of acute thrombosis and are decreased by warfarin. Antiphospholipid antibodies are frequently transiently positive in acute illness. Testing for genetic thrombophilias should, in general, only be performed when there is a strong family history of thrombosis and results would affect clinical decision-making.

Because thrombophilia evaluations are usually performed to assess the need to extend anticoagulation, testing, if indicated, should be performed in a steady state, remote from the acute event. Functional assays, but not genetic assays, will be affected by anticoagulants including warfarin (for vitamin K–dependent proteins) and thrombin and Xa inhibitors and cannot be interpreted in patients on those drugs. In most instances, when discontinuation of anticoagulation is being considered, drugs can be stopped after the initial 3–6 months of treatment, and testing can be performed at least 3 weeks later.

Measures of Platelet Function The bleeding time was used in the past to assess bleeding risk; however, it has not been found to predict bleeding risk with surgery, and it is not recommended for use for this indication. The PFA-100 and similar instruments that measure platelet-dependent coagulation under flow conditions are generally more sensitive and specific for platelet disorders and VWD than the bleeding time; however, data are insufficient to support their use to predict bleeding risk or monitor response to therapy, and they will be normal in some patients with platelet disorders or mild VWD. When they are used in the evaluation of a patient with bleeding symptoms, abnormal results require specific testing, such as VWF assays and/or platelet aggregation studies. Because all of these "screening" assays may miss patients with mild bleeding disorders, further studies are needed to define their role in hemostasis testing.

For classic platelet aggregometry, various agonists are added to the patient's platelet-rich plasma or whole blood, and platelet aggregation is measured. Tests of platelet secretion in response to agonists can also be measured. These remain the gold standard for diagnosis of platelet function disorders. However, they are affected by many factors, including numerous medications, and the association between minor defects in these assays and bleeding risk is not clearly established.

■ FURTHER READING

Chapin JC, Hajjar KA: Fibrinolysis and the control of blood coagulation. Blood Rev 29:17, 2015.

Connors JM: Thrombophilia testing and venous thrombosis. N Engl J Med 377:12, 2017.

Connors JM: Testing and monitoring direct oral anticoagulants. Blood 132:2009, 2018.

Darzi AJ et al: Prognostic factors for VTE and bleeding in hospitalized medical patients: A systematic review and meta-analysis. Blood 135:1788, 2020.

Devreese KMJ et al: Guidance from the Scientific and Standardization Committee for lupus anticoagulant/antiphospholipid antibodies of the International Society on Thrombosis and Haemostasis Update of the guidelines for lupus anticoagulant detection and interpretation. J Thromb Haemost 18:2828, 2020.

Elbaz C, Sholzberg M: An illustrated review of bleeding assessment tools and common coagulation tests. Res Pract Thromb Haemost 4:761, 2020.

James PD et al: ASH ISTH NHF WFH 2021 guidelines on the diagnosis of von Willebrand disease. Blood Adv 5:280, 2021.

Kaufman RM et al: Platelet transfusion: A clinical practice guideline from the AABB. Ann Intern Med 162:205, 2020.

Mackie I et al: Guidelines on the laboratory aspect of assays used in haemostasis and thrombosis. Int J Lab Hem 35:1, 2013.

Moran J, Bauer KA: Managing thromboembolic risk in patients with hereditary and acquired thrombophilias. Blood 135:344, 2020.

Wagenman BL et al: The laboratory approach to inherited and acquired coagulation factor deficiencies. Clin Lab Med 29:229, 2009.

Yau JW et al: Endothelial cell control of thrombosis. BMC Cardiovasc Disord 15:130, 2015.

66 Enlargement of Lymph Nodes and Spleen

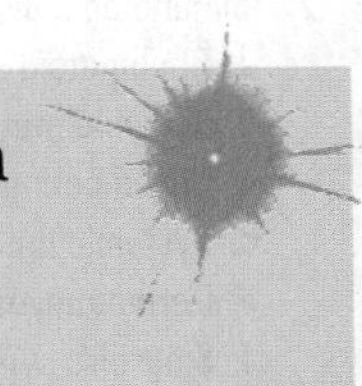

Dan L. Longo

This chapter is intended to serve as a guide to the evaluation of patients who present with enlargement of the lymph nodes (*lymphadenopathy*) or the spleen (*splenomegaly*). Lymphadenopathy is a rather common clinical finding in primary care settings, whereas palpable splenomegaly is less so.

LYMPHADENOPATHY

Lymphadenopathy may be an incidental finding in patients being examined for various reasons, or it may be a presenting sign or symptom of the patient's illness. The physician must eventually decide whether the lymphadenopathy is a normal finding or one that requires further study, up to and including biopsy. Soft, flat, submandibular nodes (<1 cm) are often palpable in healthy children and young adults; healthy adults may have palpable inguinal nodes of up to 2 cm, which are considered normal. Further evaluation of these normal nodes is not warranted. In contrast, if the physician believes the node(s) to be abnormal, then pursuit of a more precise diagnosis is needed.

APPROACH TO THE PATIENT

Lymphadenopathy

Lymphadenopathy may be a primary or secondary manifestation of numerous disorders, as shown in **Table 66-1**. Many of these disorders are infrequent causes of lymphadenopathy. In primary care practice, more than two-thirds of patients with lymphadenopathy have nonspecific causes or upper respiratory illnesses (viral or bacterial) and <1% have a malignancy. In one study, 84% of patients referred for evaluation of lymphadenopathy had a "benign" diagnosis. The remaining 16% had a malignancy (lymphoma or metastatic adenocarcinoma). Of the patients with benign lymphadenopathy, 63% had a nonspecific or reactive etiology (no causative agent found), and the remainder had a specific cause demonstrated, most commonly infectious mononucleosis, toxoplasmosis, or tuberculosis. Thus, the vast majority of patients with lymphadenopathy will have a nonspecific etiology requiring few diagnostic tests.

CLINICAL ASSESSMENT

The physician will be aided in the pursuit of an explanation for the lymphadenopathy by a careful medical history, physical examination, selected laboratory tests, and perhaps an excisional lymph node biopsy.

The *medical history* should reveal the setting in which lymphadenopathy is occurring. Symptoms such as sore throat, cough, fever, night sweats, fatigue, weight loss, or pain in the nodes should be

TABLE 66-1 Diseases Associated with Lymphadenopathy

1. Infectious diseases
   a. Viral—infectious mononucleosis syndromes (EBV, CMV), infectious hepatitis, herpes simplex, herpesvirus-6, varicella-zoster virus, rubella, measles, adenovirus, HIV, epidemic keratoconjunctivitis, vaccinia, herpesvirus-8
   b. Bacterial—streptococci, staphylococci, cat-scratch disease, brucellosis, tularemia, plague, chancroid, melioidosis, glanders, tuberculosis, atypical mycobacterial infection, primary and secondary syphilis, diphtheria, leprosy, bartonella
   c. Fungal—histoplasmosis, coccidioidomycosis, paracoccidioidomycosis
   d. Chlamydial—lymphogranuloma venereum, trachoma
   e. Parasitic—toxoplasmosis, leishmaniasis, trypanosomiasis, filariasis
   f. Rickettsial—scrub typhus, rickettsialpox, Q fever
2. Immunologic diseases
   a. Rheumatoid arthritis
   b. Juvenile rheumatoid arthritis
   c. Mixed connective tissue disease
   d. Systemic lupus erythematosus
   e. Dermatomyositis
   f. Sjögren's syndrome
   g. Serum sickness
   h. Drug hypersensitivity—diphenylhydantoin, hydralazine, allopurinol, primidone, gold, carbamazepine, etc.
   i. Angioimmunoblastic lymphadenopathy
   j. Primary biliary cirrhosis
   k. Graft-vs-host disease
   l. Silicone-associated
   m. Autoimmune lymphoproliferative syndrome
   n. IgG4-related disease
   o. Immune reconstitution inflammatory syndrome (IRIS)
3. Malignant diseases
   a. Hematologic—Hodgkin's disease, non-Hodgkin's lymphomas, acute or chronic lymphocytic leukemia, hairy cell leukemia, malignant histiocytosis, amyloidosis
   b. Metastatic—from numerous primary sites
4. Lipid storage diseases—Gaucher's, Niemann-Pick, Fabry, Tangier
5. Endocrine diseases—hyperthyroidism
6. Other disorders
   a. Castleman's disease (giant lymph node hyperplasia)
   b. Sarcoidosis
   c. Dermatopathic lymphadenitis
   d. Lymphomatoid granulomatosis
   e. Histiocytic necrotizing lymphadenitis (Kikuchi's disease)
   f. Sinus histiocytosis with massive lymphadenopathy (Rosai-Dorfman disease)
   g. Mucocutaneous lymph node syndrome (Kawasaki's disease)
   h. Histiocytosis X
   i. Familial Mediterranean fever
   j. Severe hypertriglyceridemia
   k. Vascular transformation of sinuses
   l. Inflammatory pseudotumor of lymph node
   m. Congestive heart failure

Abbreviations: CMV, cytomegalovirus; EBV, Epstein-Barr virus.

sought. The patient's age, sex, occupation, exposure to pets, sexual behavior, and use of drugs such as diphenylhydantoin are other important historic points. For example, children and young adults usually have benign (i.e., nonmalignant) disorders that account for the observed lymphadenopathy such as viral or bacterial upper respiratory infections; infectious mononucleosis; toxoplasmosis; and, in some countries, tuberculosis. In contrast, after age 50, the incidence of malignant disorders increases and that of benign disorders decreases.

The *physical examination* can provide useful clues such as the extent of lymphadenopathy (localized or generalized), size of nodes, texture, presence or absence of nodal tenderness, signs of inflammation over the node, skin lesions, and splenomegaly. A thorough ear, nose, and throat (ENT) examination is indicated in adult patients with cervical adenopathy and a history of tobacco use. Localized or regional adenopathy implies involvement of a single anatomic area. Generalized adenopathy has been defined as involvement of three or more noncontiguous lymph node areas. Many of the causes of lymphadenopathy (Table 66-1) can produce localized *or* generalized adenopathy, so this distinction is of limited utility in the differential diagnosis. Nevertheless, generalized lymphadenopathy is frequently associated with nonmalignant disorders such as infectious mononucleosis (Epstein-Barr virus [EBV] or cytomegalovirus [CMV]), toxoplasmosis, AIDS, other viral infections, systemic lupus erythematosus (SLE), and mixed connective tissue disease. Acute and chronic lymphocytic leukemias and malignant lymphomas also produce generalized adenopathy in adults.

The site of localized or regional adenopathy may provide a useful clue about the cause. Occipital adenopathy often reflects an infection of the scalp, and preauricular adenopathy accompanies conjunctival infections and cat-scratch disease. The most frequent site of regional adenopathy is the neck, and most of the causes are benign—upper respiratory infections, oral and dental lesions, infectious mononucleosis, or other viral illnesses. The chief malignant causes include metastatic cancer from head and neck, breast, lung, and thyroid primaries. Enlargement of supraclavicular and scalene nodes is always abnormal. Because these nodes drain regions of the lung and retroperitoneal space, they can reflect lymphomas, other cancers, or infectious processes arising in these areas. Virchow's node is an enlarged left supraclavicular node infiltrated with metastatic cancer from a gastrointestinal primary. Metastases to supraclavicular nodes also occur from lung, breast, testis, or ovarian cancers. Tuberculosis, sarcoidosis, and toxoplasmosis are nonneoplastic causes of supraclavicular adenopathy. Axillary adenopathy is usually due to injuries or localized infections of the ipsilateral upper extremity. Malignant causes include melanoma or lymphoma and, in women, breast cancer. Inguinal lymphadenopathy is usually secondary to infections or trauma of the lower extremities and may accompany sexually transmitted diseases such as lymphogranuloma venereum, primary syphilis, genital herpes, or chancroid. These nodes may also be involved by lymphomas and metastatic cancer from primary lesions of the rectum, genitalia, or lower extremities (melanoma).

The size and texture of the lymph node(s) and the presence of pain are useful parameters in evaluating a patient with lymphadenopathy. Nodes <1.0 cm^2 in area (1.0 cm × 1.0 cm or less) are almost always secondary to benign, nonspecific reactive causes. In one retrospective analysis of younger patients (9–25 years) who had a lymph node biopsy, a maximum diameter of >2 cm served as one discriminant for predicting that the biopsy would reveal malignant or granulomatous disease. Another study showed that a lymph node size of 2.25 cm^2 (1.5 cm × 1.5 cm) was the best size limit for distinguishing malignant or granulomatous lymphadenopathy from other causes of lymphadenopathy. Patients with node(s) $\leq$1.0 cm^2 should be observed after excluding infectious mononucleosis and/or toxoplasmosis unless there are symptoms and signs of an underlying systemic illness.

The texture of lymph nodes may be described as soft, firm, rubbery, hard, discrete, matted, tender, movable, or fixed. Tenderness is found when the capsule is stretched during rapid enlargement, usually secondary to an inflammatory process. Some malignant diseases such as acute leukemia may produce rapid enlargement and pain in the nodes. Nodes involved by lymphoma tend to be large, discrete, symmetric, rubbery, firm, mobile, and nontender. Nodes containing metastatic cancer are often hard, nontender, and nonmovable because of fixation to surrounding tissues. The coexistence of splenomegaly in the patient with lymphadenopathy implies a systemic illness such as infectious mononucleosis, lymphoma, acute or chronic leukemia, SLE, sarcoidosis, toxoplasmosis, cat-scratch disease, or other less common hematologic disorders. The patient's story should provide helpful clues about the underlying systemic illness.

Nonsuperficial presentations (thoracic or abdominal) of adenopathy are usually detected as the result of a symptom-directed diagnostic workup. Thoracic adenopathy may be detected by routine chest radiography or during the workup for superficial adenopathy. It may also be found because the patient complains of a cough or wheezing from airway compression; hoarseness from recurrent laryngeal nerve involvement; dysphagia from esophageal compression; or swelling of the neck, face, or arms secondary to compression of the superior vena cava or subclavian vein. The differential diagnosis of mediastinal and hilar adenopathy includes primary lung disorders and systemic illnesses that characteristically involve mediastinal or hilar nodes. In the young, mediastinal adenopathy is associated with infectious mononucleosis and sarcoidosis. In endemic regions, histoplasmosis can cause unilateral paratracheal lymph node involvement that mimics lymphoma. Tuberculosis can also cause unilateral adenopathy. In older patients, the differential diagnosis includes primary lung cancer (especially among smokers), lymphomas, metastatic carcinoma (usually lung), tuberculosis, fungal infection, and sarcoidosis.

Enlarged intraabdominal or retroperitoneal nodes are usually malignant. Although tuberculosis may present as mesenteric lymphadenitis, these masses usually contain lymphomas or, in young men, germ cell tumors.

LABORATORY INVESTIGATION

The laboratory investigation of patients with lymphadenopathy must be tailored to elucidate the etiology suspected from the patient's history and physical findings. One study from a family practice clinic evaluated 249 younger patients with "enlarged lymph nodes, not infected" or "lymphadenitis." No laboratory studies were obtained in 51%. When studies were performed, the most common were a complete blood count (CBC) (33%), throat culture (16%), chest x-ray (12%), or monospot test (10%). Only eight patients (3%) had a node biopsy, and half of those were normal or reactive. The CBC can provide useful data for the diagnosis of acute or chronic leukemias, EBV or CMV mononucleosis, lymphoma with a leukemic component, pyogenic infections, or immune cytopenias in illnesses such as SLE. Serologic studies may demonstrate antibodies specific to components of EBV, CMV, HIV, and other viruses; *Toxoplasma gondii*; *Brucella*; etc. If SLE is suspected, antinuclear and anti-DNA antibody studies are warranted.

The chest x-ray is usually negative, but the presence of a pulmonary infiltrate or mediastinal lymphadenopathy would suggest tuberculosis, histoplasmosis, sarcoidosis, lymphoma, primary lung cancer, or metastatic cancer and demands further investigation.

A variety of imaging techniques (CT, MRI, ultrasound, color Doppler ultrasonography) have been employed to differentiate benign from malignant lymph nodes, especially in patients with head and neck cancer. CT and MRI are comparably accurate (65–90%) in the diagnosis of metastases to cervical lymph nodes. Ultrasonography has been used to determine the long (L) axis, short (S) axis, and a ratio of long to short axis in cervical nodes. An L/S ratio of <2.0 has a sensitivity and a specificity of 95% for distinguishing benign and malignant nodes in patients with head and neck cancer. This ratio has greater specificity and sensitivity than palpation or measurement of either the long or the short axis alone.

The indications for lymph node biopsy are imprecise, yet it is a valuable diagnostic tool. The decision to biopsy may be made early in a patient's evaluation or delayed for up to 2 weeks. Prompt biopsy should occur if the patient's history and physical findings suggest a malignancy; examples include a solitary, hard, nontender cervical node in an older patient who is a chronic user of tobacco; supraclavicular adenopathy; and solitary or generalized adenopathy that is firm, movable, and suggestive of lymphoma. If a primary head and neck cancer is suspected as the basis of a solitary, hard cervical node, then a careful ENT examination should be performed. Any mucosal lesion that is suspicious for a primary neoplastic process should be biopsied first. If no mucosal lesion is detected, an excisional biopsy of the largest node should be performed. Fine-needle aspiration should not be performed as the first diagnostic procedure. Most diagnoses require more tissue than such aspiration can provide, and it often delays a definitive diagnosis. Fine-needle aspiration should be reserved for thyroid nodules and for confirmation of relapse in patients whose primary diagnosis is known. If the primary physician is uncertain about whether to proceed to biopsy, consultation with a hematologist or medical oncologist should be helpful. In primary care practices, <5% of lymphadenopathy patients will require a biopsy. That percentage will be considerably larger in referral practices, i.e., hematology, oncology, or ENT.

Two groups have reported algorithms that they claim will identify more precisely those lymphadenopathy patients who should have a biopsy. Both reports were retrospective analyses in referral practices. The first study involved patients 9–25 years of age who had a node biopsy performed. Three variables were identified that predicted those young patients with peripheral lymphadenopathy who should undergo biopsy; lymph node size >2 cm in diameter and abnormal chest x-ray had positive predictive values, whereas recent ENT symptoms had negative predictive values. The second study evaluated 220 lymphadenopathy patients in a hematology unit and identified five variables (lymph node size, location [supraclavicular or nonsupraclavicular], age [>40 years or <40 years], texture [nonhard or hard], and tenderness) that were used in a mathematical model to identify those patients requiring a biopsy. Positive predictive value was found for age >40 years, supraclavicular location, node size >2.25 cm^2, hard texture, and lack of pain or tenderness. Negative predictive value was evident for age <40 years, node size <1.0 cm^2, nonhard texture, and tender or painful nodes. Ninety-one percent of those who required biopsy were correctly classified by this model. Because both of these studies were retrospective analyses and one was limited to young patients, it is not known how useful these models would be if applied prospectively in a primary care setting.

Most lymphadenopathy patients do not require a biopsy, and at least half require no laboratory studies. If the patient's history and physical findings point to a benign cause for lymphadenopathy, careful follow-up at a 2- to 4-week interval can be employed. The patient should be instructed to return for reevaluation if there is an increase in the size of the nodes. Antibiotics are not indicated for lymphadenopathy unless strong evidence of a bacterial infection is present. Glucocorticoids should not be used to treat lymphadenopathy because their lympholytic effect obscures some diagnoses (lymphoma, leukemia, Castleman's disease) and they contribute to delayed healing or activation of underlying infections. An exception to this statement is the life-threatening pharyngeal obstruction by enlarged lymphoid tissue in Waldeyer's ring that is occasionally seen in infectious mononucleosis.

SPLENOMEGALY

■ STRUCTURE AND FUNCTION OF THE SPLEEN

The spleen is a reticuloendothelial organ that has its embryologic origin in the dorsal mesogastrium at about 5 weeks' gestation. It arises in a series of hillocks, migrates to its normal adult location in the left upper quadrant (LUQ), and is attached to the stomach via the gastrolienal ligament and to the kidney via the lienorenal ligament. When the hillocks fail to unify into a single tissue mass, accessory spleens may develop in around 20% of persons. The function of the spleen has been elusive. Galen believed it was the source of "black bile" or melancholia, and the word *hypochondria* (literally, beneath the ribs) and the idiom "to vent one's spleen" attest to the beliefs that the spleen had an important influence on the psyche and emotions. In humans, its normal physiologic roles seem to be the following:

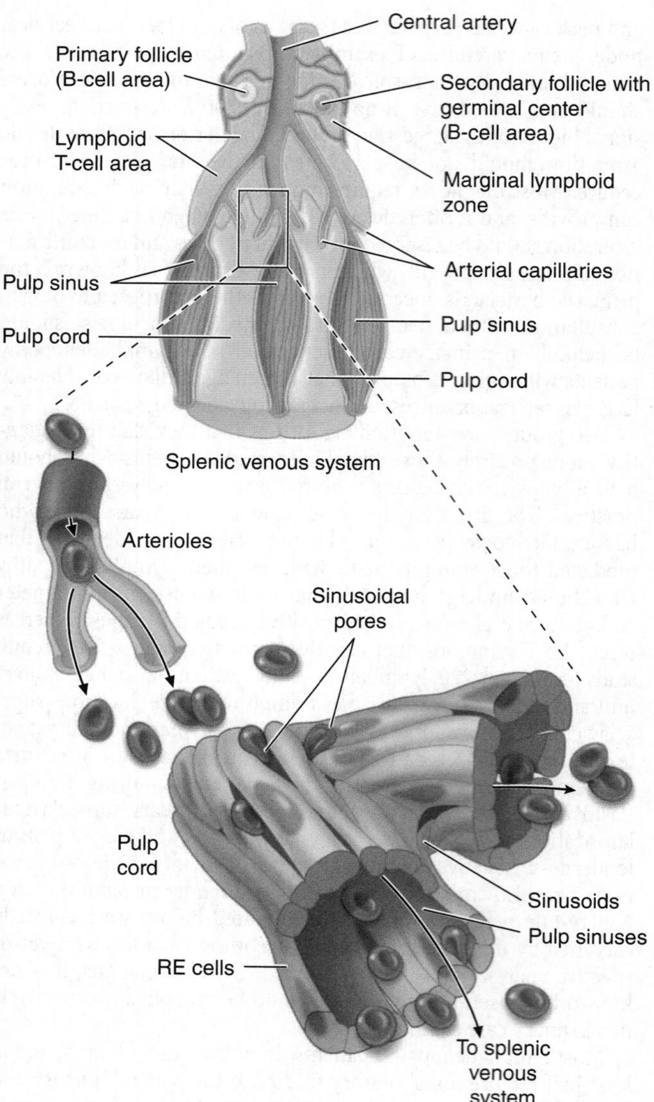

FIGURE 66-1 Schematic spleen structure. The spleen comprises many units of red and white pulp centered around small branches of the splenic artery, called *central arteries.* White pulp is lymphoid in nature and contains B-cell follicles, a marginal zone around the follicles, and T-cell–rich areas sheathing arterioles. The red pulp areas include pulp sinuses and pulp cords. The cords are dead ends. In order to regain access to the circulation, red blood cells must traverse tiny openings in the sinusoidal lining. Stiff, damaged, or old red cells cannot enter the sinuses. RE, reticuloendothelial. *(Bottom portion of figure reproduced with permission from RS Hillman, KA Ault: Hematology in Clinical Practice, 4th ed. New York, McGraw-Hill, 2005.)*

1. Maintenance of quality control over erythrocytes in the red pulp by removal of senescent and defective red blood cells. The spleen accomplishes this function through a unique organization of its parenchyma and vasculature **(Fig. 66-1)**.
2. Synthesis of antibodies in the white pulp.
3. The removal of antibody-coated bacteria and antibody-coated blood cells from the circulation.

An increase in these normal functions may result in splenomegaly.

The spleen is composed of *red pulp* and *white pulp*, which are Malpighi's terms for the red blood–filled sinuses and reticuloendothelial cell–lined cords and the white lymphoid follicles arrayed within the red pulp matrix. The spleen is in the portal circulation. The reason for this is unknown but may relate to the fact that lower blood pressure allows less rapid flow and minimizes damage to normal erythrocytes. Blood flows into the spleen at a rate of about 150 mL/min through the splenic artery, which ultimately ramifies into central arterioles. Some blood goes from the arterioles to capillaries and then to splenic veins and out of the spleen, but the majority of blood from central arterioles flows into the macrophage-lined sinuses and cords. The blood entering the sinuses reenters the circulation through the splenic venules, but the blood entering the cords is subjected to an inspection of sorts. To return to the circulation, the blood cells in the cords must squeeze through slits in the cord lining to enter the sinuses that lead to the venules. Old and damaged erythrocytes are less deformable and are retained in the cords, where they are destroyed and their components recycled. Red cell–inclusion bodies such as parasites **(Chaps. 224, 225, and A2)**, nuclear residua (Howell-Jolly bodies, **see Fig. 63-6**), or denatured hemoglobin (Heinz bodies) are pinched off in the process of passing through the slits, a process called *pitting*. The culling of dead and damaged cells and the pitting of cells with inclusions appear to occur without significant delay because the blood transit time through the spleen is only slightly slower than in other organs.

The spleen is also capable of assisting the host in adapting to its hostile environment. It has at least three adaptive functions: (1) clearance of bacteria and particulates from the blood, (2) the generation of immune responses to certain pathogens, and (3) the generation of cellular components of the blood under circumstances in which the marrow is unable to meet the needs (i.e., extramedullary hematopoiesis). The latter adaptation is a recapitulation of the blood-forming function the spleen plays during gestation. In some animals, the spleen also serves a role in the vascular adaptation to stress because it stores red blood cells (often hemoconcentrated to higher hematocrits than normal) under normal circumstances and contracts under the influence of β-adrenergic stimulation to provide the animal with an autotransfusion and improved oxygen-carrying capacity. However, the normal human spleen does not sequester or store red blood cells and does not contract in response to sympathetic stimuli. The normal human spleen contains approximately one-third of the total body platelets and a significant number of marginated neutrophils. These sequestered cells are available when needed to respond to bleeding or infection.

APPROACH TO THE PATIENT

Splenomegaly

CLINICAL ASSESSMENT

The most common *symptoms* produced by diseases involving the spleen are pain and a heavy sensation in the LUQ. Massive splenomegaly may cause early satiety. Pain may result from acute swelling of the spleen with stretching of the capsule, infarction, or inflammation of the capsule. For many years, it was believed that splenic infarction was clinically silent, which, at times, is true. However, Soma Weiss, in his classic 1942 report of the self-observations by a Harvard medical student on the clinical course of subacute bacterial endocarditis, documented that severe LUQ and pleuritic chest pain may accompany thromboembolic occlusion of splenic blood flow. Vascular occlusion, with infarction and pain, is commonly seen in children with sickle cell crises. Rupture of the spleen, from either trauma or infiltrative disease that breaks the capsule, may result in intraperitoneal bleeding, shock, and death. The rupture itself may be painless.

A palpable spleen is the major *physical sign* produced by diseases affecting the spleen and suggests enlargement of the organ. The normal spleen weighs <250 g, decreases in size with age, normally lies entirely within the rib cage, has a maximum cephalocaudad diameter of 13 cm by ultrasonography or maximum length of 12 cm and/or width of 7 cm by radionuclide scan, and is usually not palpable. However, a palpable spleen was found in 3% of 2200 asymptomatic, male, freshman college students. Follow-up at 3 years revealed that 30% of those students still had a palpable spleen without any increase in disease prevalence. Ten-year follow-up found no evidence for lymphoid malignancies. Furthermore, in some tropical countries (e.g., New Guinea), the incidence of splenomegaly may reach 60%. Thus, the presence of a palpable spleen does not always equate with presence of disease. Even when disease is present, splenomegaly may not reflect the primary disease but rather a reaction to it. For example, in patients with Hodgkin's disease, only two-thirds of the palpable spleens show involvement by the cancer.

Physical examination of the spleen uses primarily the techniques of palpation and percussion. Inspection may reveal fullness in the LUQ that descends on inspiration, a finding associated with a massively enlarged spleen. Auscultation may reveal a venous hum or friction rub.

Palpation can be accomplished by bimanual palpation, ballotment, and palpation from above (Middleton maneuver). For bimanual palpation, which is at least as reliable as the other techniques, the patient is supine with flexed knees. The examiner's left hand is placed on the lower rib cage and pulls the skin toward the costal margin, allowing the fingertips of the right hand to feel the tip of the spleen as it descends while the patient inspires slowly, smoothly, and deeply. Palpation is begun with the right hand in the left lower quadrant with gradual movement toward the left costal margin, thereby identifying the lower edge of a massively enlarged spleen. When the spleen tip is felt, the finding is recorded as centimeters below the left costal margin at some arbitrary point, i.e., 10–15 cm, from the midpoint of the umbilicus or the xiphisternal junction. This allows other examiners to compare findings or the initial examiner to determine changes in size over time. Bimanual palpation in the right lateral decubitus position adds nothing to the supine examination.

Percussion for splenic dullness is accomplished with any of three techniques described by Nixon, Castell, or Barkun:

1. *Nixon's method*: The patient is placed on the right side so that the spleen lies above the colon and stomach. Percussion begins at the lower level of pulmonary resonance in the posterior axillary line and proceeds diagonally along a perpendicular line toward the lower midanterior costal margin. The upper border of dullness is normally 6–8 cm above the costal margin. Dullness >8 cm in an adult is presumed to indicate splenic enlargement.
2. *Castell's method*: With the patient supine, percussion in the lowest intercostal space in the anterior axillary line (8th or 9th) produces a resonant note if the spleen is normal in size. This is true during expiration or full inspiration. A dull percussion note on full inspiration suggests splenomegaly.
3. *Percussion of Traube's semilunar space*: The borders of Traube's space are the sixth rib superiorly, the left midaxillary line laterally, and the left costal margin inferiorly. The patient is supine with the left arm slightly abducted. During normal breathing, this space is percussed from medial to lateral margins, yielding a normal resonant sound. A dull percussion note suggests splenomegaly.

Studies comparing methods of percussion and palpation with a standard of ultrasonography or scintigraphy have revealed sensitivity of 56–71% for palpation and 59–82% for percussion. Reproducibility among examiners is better for palpation than percussion. Both techniques are less reliable in obese patients or patients who have just eaten. Thus, the physical examination techniques of palpation and percussion are imprecise at best. It has been suggested that the examiner perform percussion first and, if positive, proceed to palpation; if the spleen is palpable, then one can be reasonably confident that splenomegaly exists. However, not all LUQ masses are enlarged spleens; gastric or colon tumors and pancreatic or renal cysts or tumors can mimic splenomegaly.

The presence of an enlarged spleen can be more precisely determined, if necessary, by liver-spleen radionuclide scan, CT, MRI, or ultrasonography. The latter technique is the current procedure of choice for routine assessment of spleen size (normal = a maximum cephalocaudad diameter of 13 cm) because it has high sensitivity and specificity and is safe, noninvasive, quick, mobile, and less costly. Equipment advances allow ultrasonography to be performed at the bedside with excellent sensitivity and specificity. Nuclear medicine scans are accurate, sensitive, and reliable but are costly, require greater time to generate data, and use immobile equipment. They have the advantage of demonstrating accessory splenic tissue. CT and MRI provide accurate determination of spleen size, but the equipment is immobile and the procedures are expensive. MRI appears to offer no advantage over CT. Changes in spleen structure such as mass lesions, infarcts, inhomogeneous infiltrates, and cysts are more readily assessed by CT, MRI, or ultrasonography. None of these techniques is very reliable in the detection of patchy infiltration (e.g., Hodgkin's disease).

DIFFERENTIAL DIAGNOSIS

Many of the diseases associated with splenomegaly are listed in **Table 66-2**. They are grouped according to the presumed basic mechanisms responsible for organ enlargement:

1. Hyperplasia or hypertrophy related to a particular splenic function such as reticuloendothelial hyperplasia (work hypertrophy) in diseases such as hereditary spherocytosis or thalassemia syndromes that require removal of large numbers of defective red blood cells; immune hyperplasia in response to systemic infection (infectious mononucleosis, subacute bacterial endocarditis) or to immunologic diseases (immune thrombocytopenia, SLE, Felty's syndrome).
2. Passive congestion due to decreased blood flow from the spleen in conditions that produce portal hypertension (cirrhosis, Budd-Chiari syndrome, congestive heart failure).
3. Infiltrative diseases of the spleen (lymphomas, metastatic cancer, amyloidosis, Gaucher's disease, myeloproliferative disorders with extramedullary hematopoiesis).

The differential diagnostic possibilities are much fewer when the spleen is "massively enlarged" or palpable >8 cm below the left costal margin or its drained weight is ≥1000 g (**Table 66-3**). The vast majority of such patients will have non-Hodgkin's lymphoma, chronic lymphocytic leukemia, hairy cell leukemia, chronic myeloid leukemia, myelofibrosis with myeloid metaplasia, or polycythemia vera.

LABORATORY ASSESSMENT

The major laboratory abnormalities accompanying splenomegaly are determined by the underlying systemic illness. Erythrocyte counts may be normal, decreased (thalassemia major syndromes, SLE, cirrhosis with portal hypertension), or increased (polycythemia vera). Granulocyte counts may be normal, decreased (Felty's syndrome, congestive splenomegaly, leukemias), or increased (infections or inflammatory disease, myeloproliferative disorders). Similarly, the platelet count may be normal, decreased when there is enhanced sequestration or destruction of platelets in an enlarged spleen (congestive splenomegaly, Gaucher's disease, immune thrombocytopenia), or increased in the myeloproliferative disorders such as polycythemia vera.

The CBC may reveal cytopenia of one or more blood cell types, which should suggest *hypersplenism*. This condition is characterized by splenomegaly, cytopenia(s), normal or hyperplastic bone marrow, and a response to splenectomy. The latter characteristic is less precise because reversal of cytopenia, particularly granulocytopenia, is sometimes not sustained after splenectomy. The cytopenias result from increased destruction of the cellular elements secondary to reduced flow of blood through enlarged and congested cords (congestive splenomegaly) or to immune-mediated mechanisms. In hypersplenism, various cell types usually have normal morphology on the peripheral blood smear, although the red cells may be spherocytic due to loss of surface area during their longer transit through the enlarged spleen. The increased marrow production of red cells should be reflected as an increased reticulocyte production index, although the value may be less than expected due to increased sequestration of reticulocytes in the spleen.

The need for additional laboratory studies is dictated by the differential diagnosis of the underlying illness of which splenomegaly is a manifestation.

TABLE 66-2 Diseases Associated with Splenomegaly Grouped by Pathogenic Mechanism

Enlargement Due to Increased Demand for Splenic Function	
Reticuloendothelial system hyperplasia (for removal of defective erythrocytes) Spherocytosis Early sickle cell anemia Ovalocytosis Thalassemia major Hemoglobinopathies Paroxysmal nocturnal hemoglobinuria Pernicious anemia Immune hyperplasia Response to infection (viral, bacterial, fungal, parasitic) Infectious mononucleosis AIDS Viral hepatitis Cytomegalovirus Subacute bacterial endocarditis Bacterial septicemia Congenital syphilis Splenic abscess Tuberculosis Histoplasmosis Malaria	Leishmaniasis Trypanosomiasis Ehrlichiosis Disordered immunoregulation Hemophagocytic lymphohistiocytosis (HLH) Rheumatoid arthritis (Felty's syndrome) Systemic lupus erythematosus Collagen vascular diseases Serum sickness Immune hemolytic anemias Immune thrombocytopenias Immune neutropenias Drug reactions Angioimmunoblastic lymphadenopathy Sarcoidosis Thyrotoxicosis (benign lymphoid hypertrophy) Interleukin 2 therapy Extramedullary hematopoiesis Myelofibrosis Marrow damage by toxins, radiation, strontium Marrow infiltration by tumors, leukemias, Gaucher's disease
Enlargement Due to Abnormal Splenic or Portal Blood Flow	
Cirrhosis Hepatic vein obstruction Portal vein obstruction, intrahepatic or extrahepatic Cavernous transformation of the portal vein Splenic vein obstruction	Splenic artery aneurysm Hepatic schistosomiasis Congestive heart failure Hepatic echinococcosis Portal hypertension (any cause including the above): "Banti's disease"
Infiltration of the Spleen	
Intracellular or extracellular depositions Amyloidosis Gaucher's disease Niemann-Pick disease Tangier disease Hurler's syndrome and other mucopolysaccharidoses Hyperlipidemias Benign and malignant cellular infiltrations Leukemias (acute, chronic, lymphoid, myeloid, monocytic) Lymphomas	Hodgkin's disease Myeloproliferative syndromes (e.g., polycythemia vera, essential thrombocytosis) Angiosarcomas Metastatic tumors (melanoma is most common) Eosinophilic granuloma Histiocytosis X Hamartomas Hemangiomas, fibromas, lymphangiomas Splenic cysts
Unknown Etiology	
Idiopathic splenomegaly Berylliosis	Iron-deficiency anemia

SPLENECTOMY

Splenectomy is infrequently performed for diagnostic purposes, especially in the absence of clinical illness or other diagnostic tests that suggest underlying disease. More often, splenectomy is performed for symptom control in patients with massive splenomegaly, for disease control in patients with traumatic splenic rupture, or for correction of cytopenias in patients with hypersplenism or immune-mediated destruction of one or more cellular blood elements. Splenectomy is necessary for staging of patients with Hodgkin's disease only in those with clinical stage I or II disease in whom radiation therapy alone is contemplated as the treatment. Noninvasive staging of the spleen in Hodgkin's disease is not a sufficiently reliable basis for treatment decisions because one-third of normal-sized spleens will be involved with Hodgkin's disease and one-third of enlarged spleens will be tumor-free. The widespread use of systemic therapy to test all stages of Hodgkin's disease has made staging laparotomy with splenectomy unnecessary. Although splenectomy in chronic myeloid leukemia (CML) does not affect the natural history of disease, removal of the massive spleen usually makes patients significantly more comfortable and simplifies their management by significantly reducing transfusion requirements.

TABLE 66-3 Diseases Associated with Massive Splenomegaly[a]

Chronic myeloid leukemia	Gaucher's disease
Lymphomas	Chronic lymphocytic leukemia
Hairy cell leukemia	Sarcoidosis
Myelofibrosis with myeloid metaplasia	Autoimmune hemolytic anemia
Polycythemia vera	Diffuse splenic hemangiomatosis

[a]The spleen extends >8 cm below left costal margin and/or weighs >1000 g.

The improvements in therapy of CML have reduced the need for splenectomy for symptom control. Splenectomy is an effective secondary or tertiary treatment for two chronic B-cell leukemias, hairy cell leukemia and prolymphocytic leukemia, and for the very rare splenic mantle cell or marginal zone lymphoma. Splenectomy in these diseases may be associated with significant tumor regression in bone marrow and other sites of disease. Similar regressions of systemic disease have been noted after splenic irradiation in some types of lymphoid tumors, especially chronic lymphocytic leukemia and prolymphocytic leukemia. This has been termed the *abscopal effect*. Such systemic tumor responses to local therapy directed at the spleen suggest that some hormone or growth factor produced by the spleen may affect tumor cell proliferation, but this conjecture is not yet substantiated. A common therapeutic indication for splenectomy is traumatic or iatrogenic splenic rupture. In a fraction of patients with splenic rupture, peritoneal seeding of splenic fragments can lead to *splenosis*—the presence of multiple rests of spleen tissue not connected to the portal circulation. This ectopic spleen tissue may cause pain or gastrointestinal obstruction, as in endometriosis. A large number of hematologic, immunologic, and congestive causes of splenomegaly can lead to destruction of one or more cellular blood elements. In the majority of such cases, splenectomy can correct the cytopenias, particularly anemia and thrombocytopenia. In a large series of patients seen in two tertiary care centers, the indication for splenectomy was diagnostic in 10% of patients, therapeutic in 44%, staging for Hodgkin's disease in 20%, and incidental to another procedure in 26%. Perhaps the only contraindication to splenectomy is the presence of marrow failure, in which the enlarged spleen is the only source of hematopoietic tissue.

Often the splenectomy is done by laparoscopy, which is associated with shorter hospital stays and faster recovery than the open procedure; however, concern has emerged that the laparoscopic approach is associated with a higher risk of postoperative portal venous system thrombosis and Budd-Chiari syndrome.

The absence of the spleen has minimal long-term effects on the hematologic profile. In the immediate postsplenectomy period, leukocytosis (up to 25,000/μL) and thrombocytosis (up to 1×10^6/μL) may develop, but within 2–3 weeks, blood cell counts and survival of each cell lineage are usually normal. The chronic manifestations of splenectomy are marked variation in size and shape of erythrocytes (anisocytosis, poikilocytosis) and the presence of Howell-Jolly bodies (nuclear remnants), Heinz bodies (denatured hemoglobin), basophilic stippling, and an occasional nucleated erythrocyte in the peripheral blood. When such erythrocyte abnormalities appear in a patient whose spleen has not been removed, one should suspect splenic infiltration by tumor that has interfered with its normal culling and pitting function.

The most serious consequence of splenectomy is increased susceptibility to bacterial infections, particularly those with capsules such as *Streptococcus pneumoniae*, *Haemophilus influenzae*, and some gram-negative enteric organisms. Patients aged <20 years are particularly susceptible to overwhelming sepsis with *S. pneumoniae*, and the overall actuarial risk of sepsis in patients who have had their spleens removed is about 7% in 10 years. The case-fatality rate for pneumococcal sepsis in splenectomized patients is 50–80%. About 25% of patients without spleens will develop a serious infection at some time in their life. The frequency is highest within the first 3 years after splenectomy. About 15% of the infections are polymicrobial, and lung, skin, and blood are the most common sites. No increased risk of viral infection has been noted in patients who have no spleen. The susceptibility to bacterial infections relates to the inability to remove opsonized bacteria from the bloodstream and a defect in making antibodies to T-cell–independent antigens such as the polysaccharide components of bacterial capsules. Pneumococcal vaccine should be administered to all patients 2 weeks before elective splenectomy. The Advisory Committee on Immunization Practices recommends that these patients receive repeat vaccination 5 years after splenectomy. Efficacy has not been proven for this group, and the recommendation discounts the possibility that administration of the vaccine may actually lower the titer of specific pneumococcal antibodies. A more effective pneumococcal conjugate vaccine that involves T cells in the response is now available (PCV13). The vaccine to *Neisseria meningitidis* should also be given to patients in whom elective splenectomy is planned. Although efficacy data for *Haemophilus influenzae* type b vaccine are not available for older children or adults, it may be given to patients who have had a splenectomy.

Splenectomized patients should be educated to consider any unexplained fever as a medical emergency. Prompt medical attention with evaluation and treatment of suspected bacteremia may be lifesaving. Routine chemoprophylaxis with oral penicillin can result in the emergence of drug-resistant strains and is not recommended.

In addition to an increased susceptibility to bacterial infections, splenectomized patients are also more susceptible to the parasitic disease babesiosis. The splenectomized patient should avoid areas where the parasite *Babesia* is endemic (e.g., Cape Cod, MA).

Surgical removal of the spleen is an obvious cause of hyposplenism. Patients with sickle cell disease often suffer from autosplenectomy as a result of splenic destruction by the numerous infarcts associated with sickle cell crises during childhood. Indeed, the presence of a palpable spleen in a patient with sickle cell disease after age 5 suggests a coexisting hemoglobinopathy, e.g., thalassemia or hemoglobin C. In addition, patients who receive splenic irradiation for a neoplastic or autoimmune disease are also functionally hyposplenic. The term *hyposplenism* is preferred to *asplenism* in referring to the physiologic consequences of splenectomy because asplenia is a rare, specific, and fatal congenital abnormality in which there is a failure of the left side of the coelomic cavity (which includes the splenic anlagen) to develop normally. Infants with asplenia have no spleens, but that is the least of their problems. The right side of the developing embryo is duplicated on the left so there is liver where the spleen should be, there are two right lungs, and the heart comprises two right atria and two right ventricles.

Acknowledgment

Patrick H. Henry, MD, friend and mentor now deceased, contributed significantly to the chapter in past editions, and much of his work remains in this chapter.

FURTHER READING

Barkun AN et al: The bedside assessment of splenic enlargement. Am J Med 91:512, 1991.

Cessford T et al: Comparing physical examination with sonographic versions of the same examination techniques for splenomegaly. J Ultrasound Med 37:1621, 2018.

Facchetti F: Tumors of the spleen. Int J Surg Pathol 18:136S, 2010.

Girard E et al: Management of splenic and pancreatic trauma. J Visc Surg 153(suppl 4):45, 2016.

Graves SA et al: Does this patient have splenomegaly? JAMA 270:2218, 1993.

Kim DK et al: Advisory committee on immunization practices reocommended immunization schedule for adults aged 19 years or older—United States, 2017. MMWR 66:136, 2017.

Kraus MD et al: The spleen as a diagnostic specimen: A review of ten years' experience at two tertiary care institutions. Cancer 91:2001, 2001.

McIntyre OR, Ebaugh FG Jr: Palpable spleens: Ten-year follow-up. Ann Intern Med 90:130, 1979.

Pangalis GA et al: Clinical approach to lymphadenopathy. Semin Oncol 20:570, 1993.

Williamson HA Jr: Lymphadenopathy in a family practice: A descriptive study of 240 cases. J Fam Pract 20:449, 1985.

67 Principles of Clinical Pharmacology

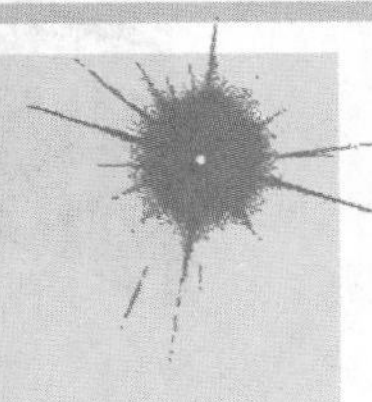

Dan M. Roden

Drugs are the cornerstone of modern therapeutics. Nevertheless, it is well recognized among health care providers and the lay community that the outcome of drug therapy varies widely among individuals. While this variability has been perceived as an unpredictable, and therefore inevitable, accompaniment of drug therapy, this is not the case.

Drugs interact with specific target molecules to produce their beneficial and adverse effects. The chain of events between administration of a drug and production of these effects in the body can be divided into two components, both of which contribute to variability in drug actions. The first component comprises the processes that determine drug delivery to, and removal from, molecular targets. The resulting description of the relationship between drug concentration and time is termed *pharmacokinetics*. The second component of variability in drug action comprises the processes that determine variability in drug actions independent of variability in drug delivery to effector drug sites. This description of the relationship between drug concentration and effect is termed *pharmacodynamics*. As discussed further below, pharmacodynamic variability can arise as a result of variability in function of the target molecule itself or of variability in the broad biologic context in which the drug-target interaction occurs to achieve drug effects. The principles described below were developed by studying small drug molecules but are equally useful in describing the effects of very large molecules, such as the therapeutic antibodies increasingly applied to autoimmune diseases and cancer.

Two important goals of clinical pharmacology are (1) to provide a description of conditions under which drug actions vary among human subjects; and (2) to determine mechanisms underlying this variability, with the goal of improving therapy with available drugs as well as pointing to mechanisms whose targeting by new drugs may be effective in the treatment of human disease. The drug development process is briefly described at the end of this chapter.

The first steps in the discipline of clinical pharmacology were empirical descriptions of the influence of disease on drug actions and of individuals or families with unusual sensitivities to adverse drug reactions (ADRs). These important descriptive findings are now being replaced by an understanding of the molecular mechanisms underlying variability in drug actions. Importantly, it is often the personal interaction of the patient with the physician or other health care provider that first identifies unusual variability in drug actions; maintained alertness to unusual drug responses continues to be a key component of improving drug safety.

One useful unifying framework is to consider that the effects of disease, drug coadministration, or familial factors in modulating drug action reflect variability in expression or function of specific genes whose products determine pharmacokinetics and pharmacodynamics. This idea forms the basis for pharmacogenomic science; a few examples are cited in this chapter, and further details are addressed in **Chap. 68**.

GLOBAL CONSIDERATIONS

It is true across all cultures and diseases that factors such as compliance, genetic variants affecting pharmacokinetics or pharmacodynamics (which themselves vary by ancestry), and drug interactions contribute to drug responses. Cost issues or cultural factors may determine the likelihood that specific drugs, drug combinations, or over-the-counter (OTC) remedies are prescribed. The broad principles of clinical pharmacology enunciated here can be used to analyze the mechanisms underlying successful or unsuccessful therapy with any drug.

INDICATIONS FOR DRUG THERAPY: RISK VERSUS BENEFIT

It is self-evident that the benefits of drug therapy should outweigh the risks. Benefits fall into broad categories: alleviation of symptoms, prevention of disease progression or complications, and prolonged life. However, establishing the balance between risk and benefit for an individual patient is not always simple. In addition to variability seen even within highly controlled drug trials, patients treated in clinical settings may display responses that were not observed in trials, sometimes due to comorbidities that were trial exclusion criteria. In addition, therapies that provide symptomatic benefits but shorten life may be entertained in patients with serious and highly symptomatic diseases such as heart failure or cancer. These considerations illustrate the continuing, highly personal nature of the relationship between the prescriber and the patient.

Adverse Effects Some adverse effects are so common and so readily associated with drug therapy that they are identified very early during clinical use of a drug. By contrast, serious ADRs may be sufficiently uncommon that they escape detection for many years after a drug begins to be widely used. The issue of how to identify rare but serious ADRs (that can profoundly affect the benefit-risk perception in an individual patient) has not been satisfactorily resolved. Potential approaches range from an increased understanding of the molecular and genetic basis of variability in drug actions to expanded postmarketing surveillance mechanisms. None of these have been completely effective, so practitioners must be continuously vigilant to the possibility that unusual symptoms may be related to specific drugs, or combinations of drugs, that their patients receive.

Therapeutic Index Beneficial and adverse reactions to drug therapy can be described by a series of dose-response relations (**Fig. 67-1**). Well-tolerated drugs demonstrate a wide margin, termed the *therapeutic ratio*, *therapeutic index*, or *therapeutic window*, between the doses required to produce a therapeutic effect and those producing toxicity. In cases where there is a similar relationship between plasma drug concentration and effects, monitoring plasma concentrations can be a highly effective aid in managing drug therapy by enabling concentrations to be maintained above the minimum required to produce an effect and below the concentration range likely to produce toxicity. Such monitoring has been widely used to guide therapy with specific agents, such as certain antiarrhythmics, anticonvulsants, and antibiotics. Many of the principles in clinical pharmacology and

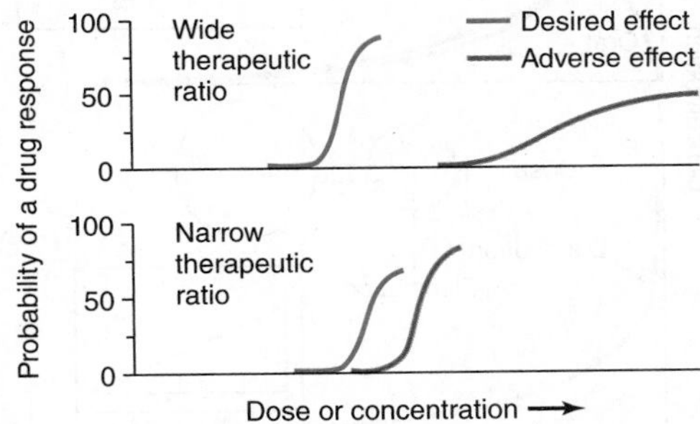

FIGURE 67-1 The concept of a therapeutic ratio. Each panel illustrates the relationship between increasing dose and cumulative probability of a desired or adverse drug effect. ***Top.*** A drug with a wide therapeutic ratio, that is, a wide separation of the two curves. ***Bottom.*** A drug with a narrow therapeutic ratio; here, the likelihood of adverse effects at therapeutic doses is increased because the curves are not well separated. Further, a steep dose-response curve for adverse effects is especially undesirable, as it implies that even small dosage increments may sharply increase the likelihood of toxicity. When there is a definable relationship between drug concentration (usually measured in plasma) and desirable and adverse effect curves, concentration may be substituted on the abscissa. Note that not all patients necessarily demonstrate a therapeutic response (or adverse effect) at any dose and that some effects (notably some adverse effects) may occur in a dose-independent fashion.

examples outlined below, which can be applied broadly to therapeutics, have been developed in these arenas.

PRINCIPLES OF PHARMACOKINETICS

The processes of absorption, distribution, metabolism, and excretion—collectively termed *drug disposition*—determine the concentration of drug delivered to target effector molecules.

ABSORPTION AND BIOAVAILABILITY

When a drug is administered orally, subcutaneously, intramuscularly, rectally, sublingually, or directly into desired sites of action, the amount of drug eventually entering the systemic circulation may be less than with the intravenous route (**Fig. 67-2A**). The fraction of drug available to the systemic circulation by other routes is termed *bioavailability*. Bioavailability may be <100% for two main reasons: (1) incomplete absorption, or (2) metabolism or elimination prior to entering the systemic circulation.

Compared to the same dose given intravenously, a nonintravenous dose will have a later and lower peak plasma concentration (**Fig. 67-2**). Drug absorption may be reduced because a drug is incompletely released from its dosage form, undergoes destruction at the site of administration, or has physicochemical properties such as insolubility that prevent complete absorption from its site of administration. Slow absorption rates are deliberately designed into "slow-release" or "sustained-release" drug formulations in order to minimize variation in plasma concentrations during the interval between doses. Therapeutic antibodies administered subcutaneously may take days to reach the systemic circulation.

"First-Pass" Effect When a drug is administered orally, it must traverse the intestinal epithelium, the portal venous system, and the liver prior to entering the systemic circulation (**Fig. 67-3**). Once a drug enters the enterocyte, it may undergo metabolism, be transported into the portal vein, or be excreted back into the intestinal lumen. Both excretion into the intestinal lumen and metabolism decrease bioavailability. Once a drug passes this enterocyte barrier, it may also be taken up into the hepatocyte, where bioavailability can be further limited by metabolism or excretion into the bile. This elimination in intestine and liver, which reduces the amount of drug delivered to the systemic circulation, is termed *presystemic elimination*, *presystemic extraction*, or *first-pass elimination*.

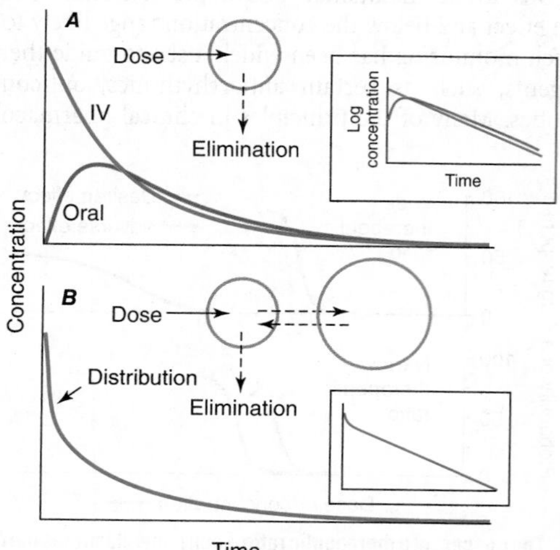

FIGURE 67-2 Idealized time-plasma concentration curves after a single dose of drug. ***A.*** The time course of drug concentration after an instantaneous intravenous (IV) bolus or an oral dose in the one-compartment model shown. The area under the time-concentration curve is clearly less with the oral drug than the IV drug, indicating incomplete bioavailability. Note that despite this incomplete bioavailability, concentration after the oral dose can be higher than after the IV dose at some time points. The inset shows that the decline of concentrations over time is linear on a log-linear plot, characteristic of first-order elimination, and that oral and IV drugs have the same elimination (parallel) time course. ***B.*** The decline of central compartment concentration when drug is distributed both to and from a peripheral compartment and eliminated from the central compartment. The rapid initial decline of concentration reflects not drug elimination but distribution.

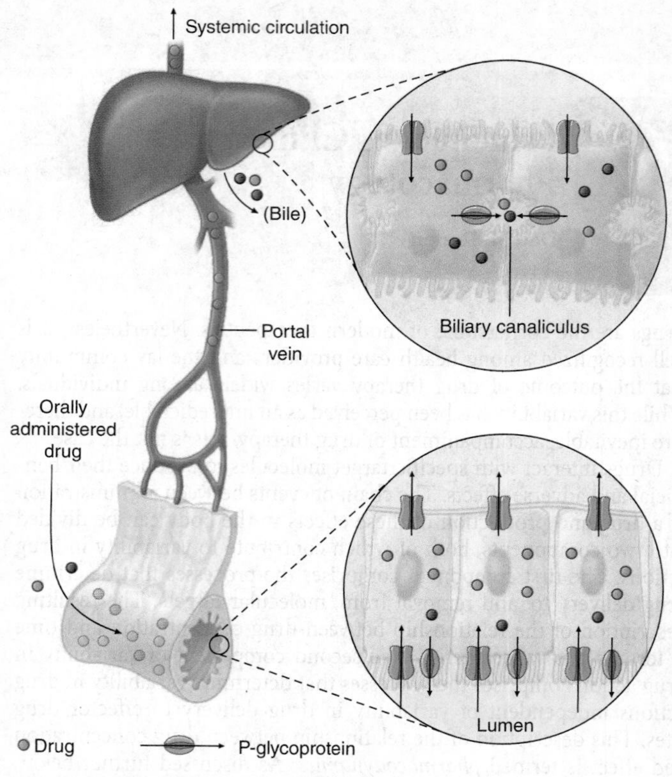

FIGURE 67-3 Mechanism of presystemic elimination. After drug enters the enterocyte, it can undergo metabolism, excretion into the intestinal lumen, or transport into the portal vein. Similarly, the hepatocyte may accomplish metabolism and biliary excretion prior to the entry of drug and metabolites to the systemic circulation. *(Adapted by permission from DM Roden, in DP Zipes, J Jalife [eds]: Cardiac Electrophysiology: From Cell to Bedside, 4th ed. Philadelphia, Saunders, 2003. Copyright 2003 with permission from Elsevier.)*

DRUG TRANSPORT

Drug movement across the membrane of any cell, including enterocytes and hepatocytes, is a combination of passive diffusion and active transport, mediated by specific drug uptake and efflux molecules. One widely studied drug transport molecule is the drug efflux pump P-glycoprotein, the product of the *ABCB1* (or *MDR1*) gene. P-glycoprotein is expressed on the apical aspect of the enterocyte and on the canalicular aspect of the hepatocyte (Fig. 67-3). In both locations, it serves as an efflux pump, limiting availability of drug to the systemic circulation. P-glycoprotein–mediated drug efflux from cerebral capillaries limits drug brain penetration and is an important component of the blood-brain barrier. Other transporters mediate uptake into cells of drugs and endogenous substrates such as vitamins or nutrients.

DRUG METABOLISM

Drug metabolism generates compounds that are usually more polar and, hence, more readily excreted than parent drug. Metabolism takes place predominantly in the liver but can occur at other sites such as kidney, intestinal epithelium, lung, and plasma. Phase I metabolism involves chemical modification, most often oxidation accomplished by members of the cytochrome P450 (CYP) monooxygenase superfamily. CYPs and other molecules that are especially important for drug metabolism are presented in **Table 67-1**, and each drug may be a substrate for one or more of these enzymes. Phase II metabolism involves conjugation of specific endogenous compounds to drugs or their metabolites. The enzymes that accomplish phase II reactions include glucuronyl-, acetyl-, sulfo-, and methyltransferases. Drug metabolites

TABLE 67-1 Molecular Pathways Mediating Drug Disposition		
ENZYME	SUBSTRATES[a]	INHIBITORS[a]
CYP3A	Calcium channel blockers	Amiodarone
	Antiarrhythmics (lidocaine, quinidine, mexiletine)	Ketoconazole, itraconazole
	HMG-CoA reductase inhibitors ("statins"; see text)	Erythromycin, clarithromycin
	Cyclosporine, tacrolimus	Ritonavir
	Indinavir, saquinavir, ritonavir	Gemfibrozil and other fibrates
CYP2D6[b]	Timolol, metoprolol, carvedilol	Quinidine (even at ultra-low doses)
	Propafenone, flecainide	Tricyclic antidepressants
	Tricyclic antidepressants	Fluoxetine, paroxetine
	Fluoxetine, paroxetine	
CYP2C9[b]	Warfarin	Amiodarone
	Phenytoin	Fluconazole
	Glipizide	Phenytoin
	Losartan	
CYP2C19[b]	Omeprazole	Omeprazole
	Mephenytoin	
	Clopidogrel	
CYP2B6[b]	Efavirenz	
Thiopurine S-methyltransferase[b]	6-Mercaptopurine, azathioprine	
N-acetyltransferase[b]	Isoniazid	
	Procainamide	
	Hydralazine	
	Some sulfonamides	
UGT1A1[b]	Irinotecan	
Pseudocholinesterase[b]	Succinylcholine	
TRANSPORTER	SUBSTRATES[a]	INHIBITORS[a]
P-glycoprotein	Digoxin	Quinidine
	HIV protease inhibitors	Amiodarone
	Many CYP3A substrates	Verapamil
		Cyclosporine
		Itraconazole
		Erythromycin
SLCO1B1[b]	Simvastatin and some other statins	

[a]Inhibitors affect the molecular pathway and thus may decrease substrate metabolism. [b]Clinically important genetic variants described; **see Chap. 68**.

Note: A listing of CYP substrates, inhibitors, and inducers is maintained at *https://drug-interactions.medicine.iu.edu/MainTable.aspx*.

may exert important pharmacologic activity, as discussed further below. Therapeutic antibodies are very slowly eliminated (allowing infrequent dosing, e.g., monthly injections), probably by lysosomal uptake and degradation.

Clinical Implications of Altered Bioavailability Some drugs undergo near-complete presystemic metabolism and thus cannot be administered orally. Nitroglycerin cannot be used orally because it is completely extracted prior to reaching the systemic circulation. The drug is, therefore, used by the sublingual, transdermal, or intravascular routes, which bypass presystemic metabolism.

Some drugs with very extensive presystemic metabolism can still be administered by the oral route, using much higher doses than those required intravenously. Thus, a typical intravenous dose of verapamil is 1–5 mg, compared to a usual single oral dose of 40–120 mg. Administration of low-dose aspirin can result in exposure of cyclooxygenase in platelets in the portal vein to the drug, but systemic sparing because of first-pass aspirin deacylation in the liver. This is an example of presystemic metabolism being exploited to therapeutic advantage.

PLASMA HALF-LIFE

Most pharmacokinetic processes, such as elimination, are first-order; that is, the rate of the process depends on the amount of drug present. Elimination can occasionally be zero-order (fixed amount eliminated per unit time), and this can be clinically important (see "Principles of Dose Selection," later in this chapter). In the simplest pharmacokinetic model (Fig. 67-2*A*), a drug bolus (D) is administered instantaneously to a central compartment, from which drug elimination occurs as a first-order process. Occasionally, central and other compartments correspond to physiologic spaces (e.g., plasma volume), whereas in other cases, they are simply mathematical functions used to describe drug disposition. The first-order nature of drug elimination leads directly to the relationship describing drug concentration (C) at any time (*t*) following the bolus:

$$C = \frac{D}{V_c} \bullet e^{(-0.69t/t_{1/2})}$$

where V_c is the volume of the compartment into which drug is delivered and $t_{1/2}$ is elimination half-life. As a consequence of this relationship, a plot of the logarithm of concentration versus time is a straight line (Fig. 67-2*A*, inset). *Half-life* is the time required for 50% of a first-order process to be completed. Thus, 50% of drug elimination is achieved after one drug-elimination half-life, 75% after two, 87.5% after three, etc. In practice, first-order processes such as elimination are near-complete after four to five half-lives.

In some cases, drug is removed from the central compartment not only by elimination but also by distribution into peripheral compartments. In this case, the plot of plasma concentration versus time after a bolus may demonstrate two (or more) exponential components **(Fig. 67-2*B*)**. In general, the initial rapid drop in drug concentration represents not elimination but drug distribution into and out of peripheral tissues (also first-order processes), while the slower component represents drug elimination; the initial precipitous decline is usually evident with administration by intravenous but not by other routes. Drug concentrations at peripheral sites are determined by a balance between drug distribution to and redistribution from those sites, as well as by elimination. Once distribution is near-complete (four to five distribution half-lives), plasma and tissue concentrations decline in parallel.

Clinical Implications of Half-Life Measurements The elimination half-life not only determines the time required for drug concentrations to fall to near-immeasurable levels after a single bolus, it is also the sole determinant of the time required for steady-state plasma concentrations to be achieved after any change in drug dosing **(Fig. 67-4)**. This applies to the initiation of chronic drug therapy (whether by multiple oral doses or by continuous intravenous infusion), a change in chronic drug dose or dosing interval, or discontinuation of drug.

Steady state describes the situation during chronic drug administration when the amount of drug administered per unit time equals drug eliminated per unit time. With a continuous intravenous infusion, plasma concentrations at steady state are stable, while with chronic oral drug administration, plasma concentrations vary during the dosing interval, but the time-concentration profile between dosing intervals is stable (Fig. 67-4).

DRUG DISTRIBUTION

In a typical 70-kg human, plasma volume is ~3 L, blood volume is ~5.5 L, and extracellular water outside the vasculature is ~20 L. The volume of distribution of drugs extensively bound to plasma proteins but not to tissue components approaches plasma volume; warfarin is an example. By contrast, for drugs highly bound to tissues, the volume of distribution can be far greater than any physiologic space. For example, the volume of distribution of digoxin and tricyclic antidepressants is hundreds

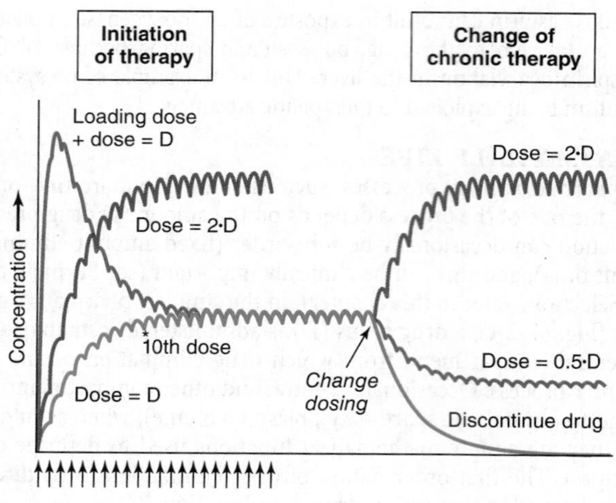

FIGURE 67-4 Drug accumulation to steady state. In this simulation, drug was administered (arrows) at intervals = 50% of the elimination half-life. Steady state is achieved during initiation of therapy after ~5 elimination half-lives, or 10 doses. A loading dose did not alter the eventual steady state achieved. A doubling of the dose resulted in a doubling of the steady state but the same time course of accumulation. Once steady state is achieved, a change in dose (increase, decrease, or drug discontinuation) results in a new steady state in ~5 elimination half-lives. *(Adapted by permission from DM Roden, in DP Zipes, J Jalife [eds]: Cardiac Electrophysiology: From Cell to Bedside, 4th ed. Philadelphia, Saunders, 2003. Copyright 2003 with permission from Elsevier.)*

of liters, obviously exceeding total-body volume. Such drugs are not readily removed by dialysis, an important consideration in overdose.

Clinical Implications of Drug Distribution In some cases, pharmacologic effects require drug distribution to peripheral sites. In this instance, the time course of drug delivery to and removal from these sites determines the time course of drug effects; anesthetic uptake into the central nervous system (CNS) is an example.

LOADING DOSES For some drugs, the indication may be so urgent that administration of "loading" dosages is required to achieve rapid elevations of drug concentration and therapeutic effects earlier than with chronic maintenance therapy (Fig. 67-4). Nevertheless, the time required for a true steady state to be achieved is still determined only by the elimination half-life.

RATE OF INTRAVENOUS DRUG ADMINISTRATION Although the simulations in Fig. 67-2 use a single intravenous bolus, this is usually inappropriate in practice because side effects related to transiently very high concentrations can result. Rather, drugs are more usually administered orally or as a slower intravenous infusion. Some drugs are so predictably lethal when infused too rapidly that special precautions should be taken to prevent accidental boluses. For example, solutions of potassium for intravenous administration >20 mEq/L should be avoided in all but the most exceptional and carefully monitored circumstances. This minimizes the possibility of cardiac arrest due to accidental increases in infusion rates of more concentrated solutions.

Transiently high drug concentrations after rapid intravenous administration can occasionally be used to advantage. The use of midazolam for intravenous sedation, for example, depends upon its rapid uptake by the brain during the distribution phase to produce sedation quickly, with subsequent egress from the brain during the redistribution of the drug as equilibrium is achieved.

Similarly, adenosine must be administered as a rapid bolus in the treatment of reentrant supraventricular tachycardias (Chap. 246) to prevent elimination by very rapid ($t_{1/2}$ of seconds) uptake into erythrocytes and endothelial cells before the drug can reach its clinical site of action, the atrioventricular node.

Clinical Implications of Altered Protein Binding Many drugs circulate in the plasma partly bound to plasma proteins. Since only unbound (free) drug can distribute to sites of pharmacologic action, drug response is related to the free rather than the total circulating plasma drug concentration. In chronic kidney or liver disease, protein binding may be decreased and thus drug actions increased. In some situations (myocardial infarction, infection, surgery), acute phase reactants transiently increase binding of some drugs and thus decrease efficacy. These changes assume the greatest clinical importance for drugs that are highly protein-bound since even a small change in protein binding can result in large changes in free drug; for example, a decrease in binding from 99 to 98% doubles the free drug concentration from 1 to 2%. For some drugs (e.g., phenytoin), monitoring free rather than total drug concentrations can be useful.

DRUG ELIMINATION

Drug elimination reduces the amount of drug in the body over time. An important approach to quantifying this reduction is to consider that drug concentrations at the beginning and end of a time period are unchanged, and that a specific volume of the body has been "cleared" of the drug during that time period. This defines clearance as volume/time. Clearance includes both drug metabolism and excretion.

Clinical Implications of Altered Clearance While elimination half-life determines the time required to achieve steady-state plasma concentration (C_{ss}), the *magnitude* of that steady state is determined by clearance (*Cl*) and dose alone. For a drug administered as an intravenous infusion, this relationship is:

$$C_{ss} = \text{dosing rate}/Cl \quad \text{or} \quad \text{dosing rate} = Cl \bullet C_{ss}$$

When a drug is administered orally, the average plasma concentration within a dosing interval ($C_{avg,ss}$) replaces C_{ss}, and the dosage (dose per unit time) must be increased if bioavailability (*F*) is <100%:

$$\text{Dose/time} = Cl \bullet C_{avg,ss}/F$$

Genetic variants, drug interactions, or diseases that reduce the activity of drug-metabolizing enzymes or excretory mechanisms lead to decreased clearance and, hence, a requirement for a downward dose adjustment to avoid toxicity. Conversely, some drug interactions and genetic variants increase the function of drug elimination pathways, and hence, increased drug dosage is necessary to maintain a therapeutic effect.

ACTIVE DRUG METABOLITES

Metabolites may produce effects similar to, overlapping with, or distinct from those of the parent drug. Accumulation of the major metabolite of procainamide, *N*-acetylprocainamide (NAPA), likely accounts for marked QT prolongation and torsades de pointes ventricular tachycardia (Chap. 252) during therapy with procainamide. Neurotoxicity during therapy with the opioid analgesic meperidine is likely due to accumulation of normeperidine, especially in renal disease.

Prodrugs are inactive compounds that require metabolism to generate active metabolites that mediate the drug effects. Examples include many angiotensin-converting enzyme (ACE) inhibitors, the angiotensin receptor blocker losartan, the antineoplastic irinotecan, the antiestrogen tamoxifen, the analgesic codeine (whose active metabolite morphine probably underlies the opioid effect during codeine administration), and the antiplatelet drug clopidogrel. Drug metabolism has also been implicated in bioactivation of procarcinogens and in the generation of reactive metabolites that mediate certain ADRs (e.g., acetaminophen hepatotoxicity, discussed below).

THE CONCEPT OF HIGH-RISK PHARMACOKINETICS

When plasma concentrations of active drug depend exclusively on a single metabolic pathway, any condition that inhibits that pathway (be it disease related, genetic, or due to a drug interaction) can lead to dramatic changes in drug concentrations and marked variability in drug action. Two mechanisms can generate highly variable drug concentrations and effects through such "high-risk pharmacokinetics." *First*, variability in bioactivation of a prodrug can lead to striking variability in drug action; examples include decreased CYP2D6 activity, which prevents analgesia by codeine, and decreased CYP2C19 activity, which reduces the antiplatelet effects of clopidogrel. The *second* setting is drug elimination that relies on a single pathway. In this case, inhibition of the elimination pathway by genetic variants or by administration of inhibiting drugs leads to marked elevation of drug concentration and, for drugs with a narrow therapeutic window, an increased likelihood of dose-related toxicity. The active S-enantiomer of the anticoagulant warfarin is eliminated by CYP2C9, and co-administration of amiodarone or phenytoin, CYP2C9 inhibitors, may therefore increase the risk of bleeding unless the dose is decreased. When drugs undergo elimination by multiple-drug metabolizing or excretory pathways, absence of one pathway (due to a genetic variant or drug interaction) is much less likely to have a large impact on drug concentrations or drug actions.

PRINCIPLES OF PHARMACODYNAMICS

Time Course of Drug Action Pharmacokinetic parameters, such as half-life and clearance, explain drug concentrations over time, but understanding the action of a drug over time (pharmacodynamics) often requires an understanding of its precise mechanism of action. Drugs act through interactions with drug targets, often in specific tissues, and with a cascade of downstream consequences. For drugs used in the urgent treatment of acute symptoms, little or no delay is anticipated (or desired) between the administration of the drug, the drug-target interaction, and the development of a clinical effect. Examples of such acute situations include vascular thrombosis, shock, or status epilepticus.

For many conditions, however, the indication for therapy is less urgent, and a delay in the onset of action clinically acceptable. Delay can be due to pharmacokinetic mechanisms such as slow elimination (resulting in slow accumulation to steady state), slow uptake into the target tissue, or slow accumulation of active metabolites. A common pharmacodynamic explanation for such a delay is the biological mechanism of action. For example, the glucocorticoid prednisolone has a plasma half-life of about 60 min. The mechanism of action, however, involves binding of the glucocorticoid receptor, translocation to the cell nucleus, and alterations in gene transcription. These downstream effects alter immune function for a much longer time frame, as evidenced by the biological half-life of 24–36 h. Other examples include proton pump inhibitors, which irreversibly bind the hydrogen/potassium adenosine triphosphatase enzyme and thus affect acid secretion for the lifetime of that enzyme, and the irreversible antiplatelet drugs, which exert effects for the duration of the life of the platelet.

Drug Effects May Be Disease Specific A drug may produce no action or a different spectrum of actions in unaffected individuals compared to patients with underlying disease. Further, concomitant disease can complicate interpretation of response to drug therapy, especially ADRs. For example, high doses of anticonvulsants such as phenytoin may cause neurologic symptoms, which may be confused with the underlying neurologic disease. Similarly, increasing dyspnea in a patient with chronic lung disease receiving amiodarone therapy could be due to the drug, underlying disease, or an intercurrent cardiopulmonary problem. As a result, alternate antiarrhythmic therapies may be preferable in patients with chronic lung disease.

While drugs interact with specific molecular receptors, drug effects may vary over time, even if stable drug and metabolite concentrations are maintained. The drug-receptor interaction occurs in a complex biologic milieu that can vary to modulate the drug effect. For example, ion channel blockade by drugs, an important anticonvulsant and antiarrhythmic effect, is often modulated by membrane potential, itself a function of factors such as extracellular potassium or local ischemia. Receptors may be up- or downregulated by disease or by the drug itself. For example, β-adrenergic blockers upregulate β-receptor density during chronic therapy. While this effect does not usually result in resistance to the therapeutic effect of the drugs, it may produce severe agonist-mediated effects (such as hypertension or tachycardia) if the blocking drug is abruptly withdrawn.

As molecular mechanisms of disease become better defined, drugs targeting those mechanisms are being introduced into practice. Antineoplastic agents targeting mutant kinases overexpressed in cancers (e.g., *BRAF* V600E in melanoma, hairy cell leukemia, and other malignancies) are revolutionizing cancer care. Ivacaftor was originally developed and marketed for patients with cystic fibrosis (CF) carrying the G551D mutation in the disease gene *CFTR* (**Chap. 291**). While the most common *CFTR* mutations causing CF generate normal chloride channels that are not correctly trafficked to the cell surface, G551D channels are trafficked normally but do not conduct chloride correctly, and ivacaftor corrects this "gating" defect. Following initial marketing for only G551D patients (5% of all CF patients), the U.S. Food and Drug Administration (FDA) approved ivacaftor for use in patients carrying other *CFTR* mutations that confer gating defects corrected by ivacaftor in vitro.

PRINCIPLES OF DOSE SELECTION

The desired goal of therapy with any drug is to maximize the likelihood of a beneficial effect while minimizing the risk of ADRs. Previous experience with the drug, in controlled clinical trials or in postmarketing use, defines the relationships between dose or plasma concentration and these dual effects (Fig. 67-1) and has important implications for initiation of drug therapy:

1. *The target drug effect should be defined when drug treatment is started.* With some drugs, the desired effect may be difficult to measure objectively, or the onset of efficacy can be delayed for weeks or months; drugs used in the treatment of cancer and psychiatric disease are examples. Sometimes a drug is used to treat a symptom, such as pain or palpitations, and here it is the patient who will report whether the selected dose is effective. In yet other settings, such as anticoagulation or hypertension, the desired response can be repeatedly and objectively assessed by simple clinical or laboratory tests.
2. *The nature of anticipated toxicity often dictates the starting dose.* If side effects are minor, it may be acceptable to start chronic therapy at a dose highly likely to achieve efficacy and down-titrate if side effects occur. However, this approach is rarely, if ever, justified if the anticipated toxicity is serious or life-threatening; in this circumstance, it is more appropriate to initiate therapy with the lowest dose that may produce a desired effect. In cancer chemotherapy, it is common practice to use maximally tolerated doses.
3. *The above considerations do not apply if these relationships between dose and effects cannot be defined.* This is especially relevant to some ADRs (discussed further below) whose development is not readily related to drug dose.
4. *If a drug dose does not achieve its desired effect, a dosage increase is justified only if toxicity is absent and the likelihood of serious toxicity is small.*

Failure of Efficacy Even assuming the diagnosis is correct and the correct drug and dose are prescribed, drugs may fail to be effective because 100% efficacy is not expected. A complete therapeutic response is often absent with antihypertensive or antidepressant drugs, and a major challenge in contemporary therapeutics is to identify patient-specific predictors of response to individual drugs. Other explanations for failure of efficacy include drug interactions, noncompliance, or unexpectedly low drug concentration due to administration of expired or degraded drug. These are situations in which measurement of plasma drug concentrations, if available, can be especially useful. Noncompliance is an especially frequent problem in the long-term treatment of diseases such as hypertension and epilepsy, occurring in ≥25% of patients in therapeutic environments in which no special effort is made to involve patients in the responsibility for their own health. Multidrug regimens with multiple doses per day are especially prone to noncompliance.

Monitoring response to therapy, by physiologic measures or by plasma concentration measurements, requires an understanding of the relationships between plasma concentration and anticipated effects. For example, measurement of QT interval is used during treatment with sotalol or dofetilide to avoid marked QT prolongation that can herald serious arrhythmias. In this setting, evaluating the electrocardiogram at the time of anticipated peak plasma concentration and effect (e.g., 1–2 h postdose at steady state) is most appropriate. Maintained high vancomycin levels carry a risk of nephrotoxicity, so dosages should be adjusted on the basis of plasma concentrations measured at trough (predose). Similarly, for dose adjustment of other drugs (e.g., anticonvulsants), concentration should be measured at its lowest during the dosing interval, just prior to a dose at steady state (Fig. 67-4), to ensure a maintained therapeutic effect.

Concentration of Drugs in Plasma as a Guide to Therapy Factors such as interactions with other drugs, disease-induced alterations in elimination and distribution, and genetic variation in drug disposition combine to yield a wide range of plasma levels in patients given the same dose. Hence, if a predictable relationship can be established between plasma drug concentration and beneficial or adverse drug effect, measurement of plasma levels can provide a valuable tool to guide selection of an optimal dose, especially when there is a narrow range between the plasma levels yielding therapeutic and adverse effects. Such therapeutic drug monitoring is commonly used with certain types of drugs including many anticonvulsants, antirejection agents, antiarrhythmics, and antibiotics. By contrast, if no such relationship can be established (e.g., if drug access to important sites of action outside plasma is highly variable), monitoring plasma concentration may not provide an accurate guide to therapy (**Fig. 67-5**).

The common situation of first-order elimination implies that average, maximum, and minimum steady-state concentrations are related linearly to the dosing rate. Accordingly, the maintenance dose may be adjusted on the basis of the ratio between the desired and measured concentrations *at steady state*; for example, if a doubling of the steady-state plasma concentration is desired, the dose should be doubled. This does not apply to drugs eliminated by zero-order kinetics (fixed amount per unit time), where small dosage increases will produce disproportionate increases in plasma concentration; examples include phenytoin and theophylline.

If an increase in dosage is needed, this is usually best achieved by increasing the drug dose and leaving the dosing interval constant (e.g., by giving 200 mg every 8 h instead of 100 mg every 8 h). However, this approach is acceptable only if the resulting maximum concentration is not toxic and the trough value does not fall below the minimum effective concentration for an undesirable period of time. Alternatively, the steady state may be changed by altering the frequency of intermittent dosing but not the size of each dose. In this case, the magnitude of the fluctuations around the average steady-state level will change—the shorter the dosing interval, the smaller the difference between peak and trough levels.

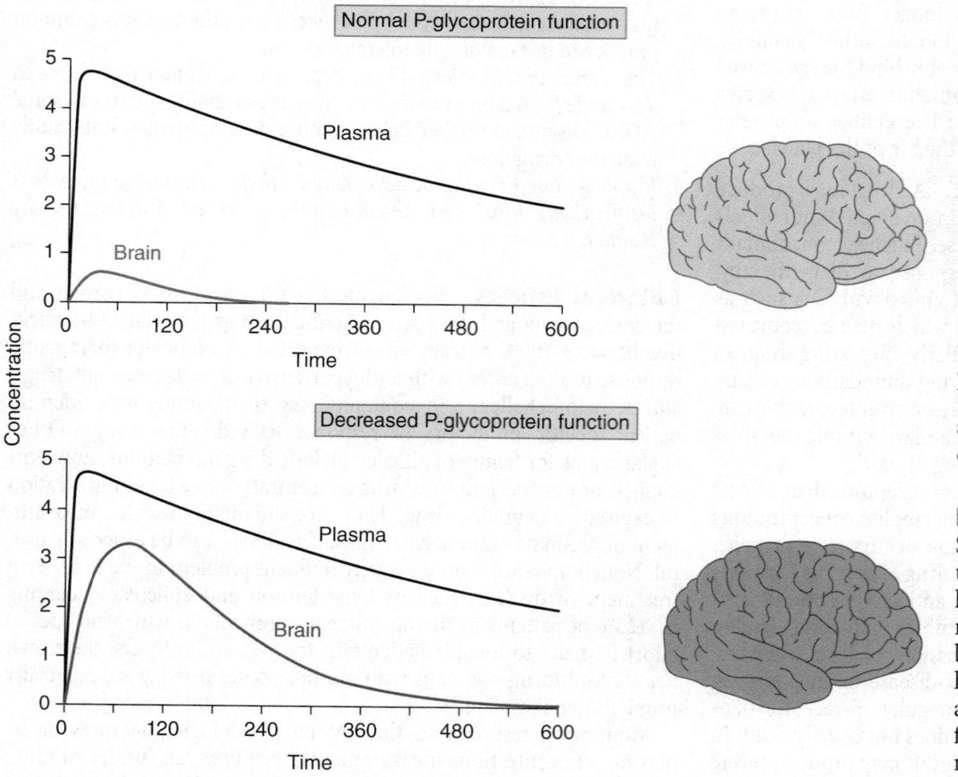

FIGURE 67-5 Drug concentrations in specific tissues may not always parallel those in plasma. For example, the efflux pump P-glycoprotein excludes drugs from the endothelium of capillaries in the brain and so constitutes a key element of the blood-brain barrier. Reduced P-glycoprotein function (e.g., due to drug interactions) can thus increase penetration of substrate drugs into the brain, even when plasma concentrations are unchanged.

EFFECTS OF DISEASE ON DRUG CONCENTRATION AND RESPONSE

RENAL DISEASE

Renal excretion of parent drug and metabolites is generally accomplished by glomerular filtration and by specific drug transporters. If a drug or its metabolites are primarily excreted through the kidneys and increased drug levels are associated with ADRs (an example of "high-risk pharmacokinetics" described above), drug dosages must be reduced in patients with renal dysfunction to avoid toxicity. The antiarrhythmics dofetilide and sotalol undergo predominant renal excretion and carry a risk of QT prolongation and arrhythmias if doses are not reduced in renal disease. In end-stage renal disease, sotalol has been given as 40 mg after dialysis (every second day), compared to the usual daily dose, 80–120 mg every 12 h. At approved doses, the anticoagulant edoxaban appears to be somewhat more effective in subjects with mild renal dysfunction, possibly reflecting higher drug levels. The narcotic analgesic meperidine undergoes extensive hepatic metabolism, so that renal failure has little effect on its plasma concentration. However, its metabolite, normeperidine, does undergo renal excretion, accumulates in renal failure, and probably accounts for the signs of CNS excitation, such as irritability, twitching, and seizures, that appear when multiple doses of meperidine are administered to patients with renal disease. Protein binding of some drugs (e.g., phenytoin) may be altered in uremia, so measuring free drug concentration may be desirable.

In non-end-stage renal disease, changes in renal drug clearance are generally proportional to those in creatinine clearance, which may be measured directly or estimated from the serum creatinine. This estimate, coupled with the knowledge of how much drug is normally excreted renally versus nonrenally, allows an estimate of the dose adjustment required. In practice, most decisions involving dosing adjustment in patients with renal failure use published recommended adjustments in dosage or dosing interval based on the severity of renal dysfunction indicated by creatinine clearance. Any such modification of dose is a first approximation and should be followed by plasma concentration data (if available) and clinical observation to further optimize therapy for the individual patient.

LIVER DISEASE

Standard tests of liver function are not useful in adjusting doses in diseases like hepatitis or cirrhosis. First-pass metabolism may decrease, leading to increased oral bioavailability as a consequence of disrupted hepatocyte function, altered liver architecture, and portacaval shunts. The oral bioavailability for high first-pass drugs such as morphine, meperidine, midazolam, and nifedipine is almost doubled in patients with cirrhosis, compared to those with normal liver function. Therefore, the size of the oral dose of such drugs should be reduced in this setting.

■ HEART FAILURE AND SHOCK

Under conditions of decreased tissue perfusion, the cardiac output is redistributed to preserve blood flow to the heart and brain at the expense of other tissues (**Chap. 257**). As a result, drugs may be distributed into a smaller volume of distribution, higher drug concentrations will be present in the plasma, and the tissues that are best perfused (the brain and heart) will be exposed to these higher concentrations, resulting in increased CNS or cardiac effects. In addition, decreased perfusion of the kidney and liver may impair drug clearance. Another consequence of severe heart failure is decreased gut perfusion, which may reduce drug absorption and thus lead to reduced or absent effects of orally administered therapies.

■ DRUG USE IN THE ELDERLY

In the elderly, multiple pathologies and medications used to treat them result in more drug interactions and ADRs. Aging also results in changes in organ function, especially of the organs involved in drug disposition. Initial doses should be less than the usual adult dosage and should be increased slowly. The number of medications, and doses per day, should be kept as low as possible.

Even in the absence of kidney disease, renal clearance may be reduced by 35–50% in elderly patients. Dosages should be adjusted on the basis of creatinine clearance. Aging also results in a decrease in the size of, and blood flow to, the liver and possibly in the activity of hepatic drug-metabolizing enzymes; accordingly, the hepatic clearance of some drugs is impaired in the elderly. As with liver disease (above), these changes are not readily predicted.

Elderly patients may display altered drug sensitivity. Examples include increased analgesic effects of opioids, increased sedation from benzodiazepines and other CNS depressants, and increased risk of bleeding while receiving anticoagulant therapy, even when clotting parameters are well controlled. Exaggerated responses to cardiovascular drugs are also common because of the impaired responsiveness of normal homeostatic mechanisms. Conversely, the elderly display decreased sensitivity to β-adrenergic receptor blockers.

ADRs are especially common in the elderly because of altered pharmacokinetics and pharmacodynamics, the frequent use of multidrug regimens, and concomitant disease. For example, use of long half-life benzodiazepines is linked to the occurrence of hip fractures in elderly patients, perhaps reflecting both a risk of falls from these drugs (due to increased sedation) and the increased incidence of osteoporosis in elderly patients. In population surveys of the noninstitutionalized elderly, as many as 10% had at least one ADR in the previous year.

■ DRUG USE IN CHILDREN

Although there are very few pediatric-specific drugs, there are many pediatric-specific drug indications (e.g., intravenous immunoglobulin and aspirin for Kawasaki disease) and ADRs (e.g., pyloric stenosis after erythromycin exposure in infants). Drug metabolism and drug response pathways mature at different rates after birth, and the relative size of various body compartments and function of various organs change during development. There is increased motivation to avoid organ toxicity, given the anticipated long post-drug-exposure life expectancy. There are few studies providing empiric evidence to guide pediatric dosing. In practice, doses are adjusted for size (weight or body surface area) as a first approximation unless age-specific data are available. As in adults, the lowest doses anticipated to achieve clinical benefit are generally prescribed, potentially followed by titration.

INTERACTIONS BETWEEN DRUGS

Drug interactions can complicate therapy by increasing or decreasing the action of a drug; interactions may be based on changes in drug disposition or in drug response in the absence of changes in drug levels (**Table 67-2**). *Interactions must be considered in the differential diagnosis of any unusual response occurring during drug therapy.* Prescribers should recognize that patients often come to them with a legacy of drugs acquired during previous medical experiences, often with multiple physicians who may not be aware of all the patient's medications. A meticulous drug history should list all medications, including agents

TABLE 67-2 Drug Interactions

MECHANISM	EXAMPLE
Pharmacokinetic Interactions Causing Decreased Drug Effect	
Decreased absorption due to drug binding in the gut	Antacids or bile acid sequestrants decrease the absorption of many drugs: Antacids/tetracyclines Cholestyramine/digoxin
Decreased solubility due to altered gastric pH	H_2 receptor blockers or proton pump inhibitors decrease solubility and absorption of weak bases: Omeprazole/ketoconazole
Induction of drug metabolism and/or drug transport: Rifampin Carbamazepine Phenytoin St. John's wort Glutethimide (also smoking, exposure to chlorinated insecticides, and chronic alcohol ingestion)	Decreased concentrations and effects of: Warfarin Quinidine Cyclosporine Losartan Oral contraceptives Methadone Dabigatran
Decreased prodrug bioactivation	Proton pump inhibitors may prevent clopidogrel bioactivation CYP2D6 inhibitors (fluoxetine, paroxetine, quinidine, and others) may prevent codeine bioactivation
Reduced delivery of drug to active sites of action	Tricyclics prevent clonidine uptake into adrenergic neurons, preventing antihypertensive effects
Pharmacokinetic Interactions Causing Increased Drug Effect	
Inhibited drug metabolism	Cimetidine (inhibits many CYPs): Warfarin Theophylline Phenytoin CYP2D6 inhibitors[a]/β blockers CYP3A inhibitors[a]: HMG-CoA reductase inhibitors Colchicine (toxicity risk) Decreased cyclosporine dose requirement
Inhibited drug transport	Amiodarone (inhibits many CYPs and P-glycoprotein): Warfarin Digoxin Dabigatran
Inhibition of drug metabolism causing accumulation of toxic metabolites	Allopurinol (xanthine oxidase inhibitor) inhibits an alternate pathway for azathioprine and 6-mercaptopurine elimination, increasing risk for toxicity
Decreased elimination due to altered renal function	Inhibitors of renal tubular transport (phenylbutazone, probenecid, salicylates) increase methotrexate toxicity
Pharmacodynamic Drug Interactions	
Combined effects on the same biologic process	Excess bleeding with combinations of antiplatelet drugs, anticoagulants, and NSAIDs Long QT–related arrhythmias with QT-prolonging antiarrhythmics plus diuretics Hyperkalemia with ACE inhibitors plus potassium Hypotension with nitrates plus sildenafil
Antagonistic effects on the same biologic process	Loss of antihypertensive drug effects with NSAIDs

[a]See Table 67-1.

Abbreviations: ACE, angiotensin-converting enzyme; CYP, cytochrome P; NSAID, nonsteroidal anti-inflammatory drug.

not often volunteered during questioning, such as OTC drugs, health food supplements, and topical agents such as eye drops. Lists of interactions are available from a number of electronic sources. While it is unrealistic to expect the practicing physician to memorize these, certain drugs consistently run the risk of generating interactions, often by inhibiting or inducing specific drug elimination pathways; these include CYP2D6, CYP3A, and P-glycoprotein inhibitors (Table 67-1) and CYP3A/P-glycoprotein inducers (Table 67-2). Accordingly, when these drugs are started or stopped, prescribers must be especially alert to the possibility of interactions.

ADVERSE DRUG REACTIONS

The beneficial effects of drugs are coupled with the inescapable risk of untoward effects. The morbidity and mortality from these ADRs often present diagnostic problems because they can involve every organ and system of the body and may be mistaken for signs of underlying disease. In addition, some surveys have suggested that drug therapy for a range of chronic conditions such as psychiatric disease or hypertension does not achieve its desired goal in up to half of treated patients; thus, the most common "adverse" drug effect may be failure of efficacy.

ADRs can be classified in two broad groups. Type A reactions result from exaggeration of an intended pharmacologic action of the drug, such as increased bleeding with anticoagulants or bone marrow suppression with some antineoplastics, and tend to be dose-dependent. Type B reactions result from toxic effects unrelated to the intended pharmacologic actions. The latter effects are often unanticipated (especially with new drugs) and frequently severe and may result from recognized (often immunologic) as well as previously undescribed mechanisms. Type B reactions may occur at low dosages and are often termed dose-independent.

Drugs may increase the frequency of an event that is common in a general population, and this may be especially difficult to recognize; an example is the increase in myocardial infarctions that was seen with the COX-2 inhibitor rofecoxib. Drugs can also cause rare and serious ADRs, such as hematologic abnormalities, arrhythmias, severe skin reactions, or hepatic or renal dysfunction. Prior to regulatory approval and marketing, new drugs are tested in relatively few patients who tend to be less sick and to have fewer concomitant diseases than those patients who subsequently receive the drug therapeutically. Because of the relatively small number of patients studied in clinical trials and the selected nature of these patients, rare ADRs are generally not detected prior to a drug's approval; indeed, if they are detected, the new drugs are generally not approved. Therefore, physicians need to be cautious in the prescription of new drugs and alert for the appearance of previously unrecognized ADRs.

Elucidating mechanisms underlying ADRs can assist development of safer compounds or allow a patient subset at especially high risk to be excluded from drug exposure. National adverse reaction reporting systems, such as those operated by the FDA (suspected ADRs can be reported online at *http://www.fda.gov/safety/medwatch/default.htm*) and the Committee on Safety of Medicines in Great Britain, can prove useful. The publication or reporting of a newly recognized ADR can in a short time stimulate many similar such reports of reactions that previously had gone unrecognized.

Occasionally, "adverse" effects may be exploited to develop an entirely new indication for a drug. Unwanted hair growth during minoxidil treatment of severely hypertensive patients led to development of the drug for hair growth. Sildenafil was initially developed as an antianginal, but its effects to alleviate erectile dysfunction not only led to a new drug indication but also to increased understanding of the role of type 5 phosphodiesterase in erectile tissue. These examples further reinforce the concept that prescribers must remain vigilant to the possibility that unusual symptoms may reflect unappreciated drug effects.

Some 25–50% of patients make errors in self-administration of prescribed medicines, and these errors can be responsible for ADRs. Similarly, patients commit errors in taking OTC drugs by not reading or following prescribing directions on the containers. Health care providers must recognize that providing directions with prescriptions does not always guarantee compliance.

In hospitals, drugs are administered in a controlled setting, and patient compliance is, in general, ensured. Errors may occur nevertheless—the wrong drug or dose may be given or the drug may be given to the wrong patient—and improved drug distribution and administration systems should help with this problem.

■ SCOPE OF THE PROBLEM

One estimate in the United Kingdom was that 6.5% of all hospital admissions are due to ADRs and that 2.3% of these patients (0.15%) died as a result. The most common culprit drugs were aspirin, nonsteroidal anti-inflammatory drugs, diuretics, warfarin, ACE inhibitors, antidepressants, opiates, digoxin, steroids, and clopidogrel. One study in the late 1990s suggested that ADRs were responsible for >100,000 in-hospital deaths in the United States, making them the fourth to sixth most common cause of in-hospital death. Another study 10 years later showed no change in this trend.

In hospital, patients receive, on average, 10 different drugs during each hospitalization. The sicker the patient, the more drugs are given, and there is a corresponding increase in the likelihood of ADRs. When <6 different drugs are given to hospitalized patients, the probability of an ADR is ~5%, but if >15 drugs are given, the probability is >40%. Serious ADRs are also well recognized with "herbal" remedies and OTC compounds; examples include kava-associated hepatotoxicity, L-tryptophan-associated eosinophilia-myalgia, and phenylpropanolamine-associated stroke, each of which has caused fatalities.

■ TOXICITY UNRELATED TO A DRUG'S PRIMARY PHARMACOLOGIC ACTIVITY

Drugs or, more commonly, reactive metabolites generated by CYPs can covalently bind to tissue macromolecules (such as proteins or DNA) to cause tissue toxicity. Because of the reactive nature of these metabolites, covalent binding often occurs close to the site of production, typically the liver.

Acetaminophen The most common cause of drug-induced hepatotoxicity is acetaminophen overdosage **(Chap. 340)**. Normally, reactive metabolites are detoxified by combining with hepatic glutathione. When glutathione becomes depleted, the metabolites bind instead to hepatic protein, with resultant hepatocyte damage. The hepatic necrosis produced by the ingestion of acetaminophen can be prevented or attenuated by the administration of substances such as *N*-acetylcysteine that reduce the binding of electrophilic metabolites to hepatic proteins. The risk of acetaminophen-related hepatic necrosis is increased in patients receiving drugs such as phenobarbital or phenytoin, which increase the rate of drug metabolism, or ethanol, which exhausts glutathione stores. Such toxicity has even occurred with therapeutic dosages, so patients at risk through these mechanisms should be warned.

Immunologic Reactions Most pharmacologic agents are haptens, small molecules with low molecular weights (<2000) that are therefore poor immunogens. Generation of an immune response to a drug therefore often requires in vivo activation and covalent linkage to protein, carbohydrate, or nucleic acid.

Drug stimulation of antibody production may mediate tissue injury by several mechanisms. The antibody may attack the drug when the drug is covalently attached to a cell and thereby destroy the cell. This occurs in penicillin-induced hemolytic anemia. Antibody-drug-antigen complexes may be passively adsorbed by a bystander cell, which is then destroyed by activation of complement; this occurs in quinine- and quinidine-induced thrombocytopenia. Heparin-induced thrombocytopenia arises when antibodies against complexes of platelet factor 4 peptide and heparin generate immune complexes that activate platelets; thus, the thrombocytopenia is accompanied by "paradoxical" thrombosis and is treated with thrombin inhibitors. Drugs or their reactive metabolites may alter a host tissue, rendering it antigenic and eliciting autoantibodies. For example, hydralazine and procainamide (or their reactive metabolites) can chemically alter nuclear material, stimulating the formation of antinuclear antibodies and occasionally causing lupus erythematosus. Drug-induced pure red cell aplasia **(Chap. 102)** is due to an immune-based drug reaction.

Serum sickness (**Chap. 352**) results from the deposition of circulating drug-antibody complexes on endothelial surfaces. Complement activation occurs, chemotactic factors are generated locally, and an inflammatory response develops at the site of complex entrapment. Arthralgias, urticaria, lymphadenopathy, glomerulonephritis, or cerebritis may result. Foreign proteins (vaccines, streptokinase, therapeutic antibodies) and antibiotics are common causes. Many drugs, particularly antimicrobial agents, ACE inhibitors, and aspirin, can elicit anaphylaxis with production of IgE, which binds to mast cell membranes. Contact with a drug antigen initiates a series of biochemical events in the mast cell and results in the release of mediators that can produce the characteristic urticaria, wheezing, flushing, rhinorrhea, and (occasionally) hypotension.

Drugs may also elicit cell-mediated immune responses. One serious reaction is Stevens-Johnson syndrome/toxic epidermal necrolysis (SJS/TEN), which can result in death due to T-cell-mediated massive skin sloughing. Another probable immune-mediated drug reaction is the DRESS (drug reaction with eosinophilia and systemic symptoms) syndrome, a rare ADR with a chronic relapsing course, often triggered by antiseizure medications and possibly arising from herpes virus reactivation. As described in **Chap. 68**, specific genetic variants appear necessary but not sufficient to elicit SJS/TEN or DRESS.

While the use of antibodies targeting immune checkpoints is dramatically improving prognosis in many cancers, these agents have also been associated with the unpredictable development of many apparently immune-related ADRs. Some, like colitis or thyroiditis, may be self-limited or medically manageable, while others, notably myocarditis, are rarer but can be rapidly fatal.

DIAGNOSIS AND TREATMENT OF ADVERSE DRUG REACTIONS

The manifestations of drug-induced diseases frequently resemble those of other diseases, and a given set of manifestations may be produced by different and dissimilar drugs. Recognition of the role of a drug or drugs in an illness depends on appreciation of the possible ADRs to drugs in any disease, on identification of the temporal relationship between drug administration and development of the illness, and on familiarity with the common manifestations of the drugs.

A suspected ADR developing after introduction of a new drug naturally implicates that drug; however, it is also important to remember that a drug interaction may be responsible. Thus, for example, a patient on a chronic stable warfarin dose may develop a bleeding complication after introduction of amiodarone; this does not reflect a direct reaction to amiodarone but rather its effect to inhibit warfarin metabolism. Many associations between particular drugs and specific reactions have been described, but there is always a "first time" for a novel association, and any drug should be suspected of causing an ADR if the clinical setting is appropriate.

Illness related to a drug's intended pharmacologic action is often more easily recognized than illness attributable to immune or other mechanisms.

For example, side effects such as cardiac arrhythmias in patients receiving digitalis, hypoglycemia in patients given insulin, or bleeding in patients receiving anticoagulants are more readily related to a specific drug than are symptoms such rash, which may be caused by many drugs or by other factors. Drug fever often escapes initial diagnosis because fever is such a common manifestation of disease.

Electronic listings of ADRs can be useful. However, exhaustive compilations often provide little sense of perspective in terms of frequency and seriousness, which can vary considerably among patients.

Eliciting a drug history from each patient is important for diagnosis. Attention must be directed to OTC drugs and herbal preparations as well as to prescription drugs. Each type can be responsible for ADRs, and adverse interactions may occur between OTC drugs and prescribed drugs. Loss of efficacy of oral contraceptives or cyclosporine with concurrent use of St. John's wort (a P-glycoprotein inducer) is an example (Table 67-2). In addition, it is common for patients to be cared for by several physicians, and duplicative, additive, antagonistic, or synergistic drug combinations may therefore be administered if the physicians are not aware of the patients' drug histories. Electronic health records (EHRs) may help mitigate this problem, but only if all treating physicians use the same EHR system. Medications stopped for inefficacy or adverse effects should be documented to avoid pointless and potentially dangerous reexposure. A frequently overlooked source of additional drug exposure is topical therapy; for example, a patient complaining of bronchospasm may not mention that an ophthalmic beta blocker is being used unless specifically asked. A history of previous ADRs in patients is common. Since these patients have shown a predisposition to drug-induced illnesses, such a history should dictate added caution in prescribing new drugs.

Laboratory studies may include demonstration of serum antibody in some persons with drug allergies involving cellular blood elements, as in agranulocytosis, hemolytic anemia, and thrombocytopenia. For example, both quinine and quinidine can produce platelet agglutination in vitro in the presence of complement and the serum from a patient who has developed thrombocytopenia following use of this drug. Biochemical abnormalities such as G6PD deficiency, serum pseudocholinesterase level, or genotyping may also be useful in diagnosis, especially after an ADR has occurred in the patient or a family member (**Chap. 68**).

Once an ADR is suspected, discontinuation of the suspected drug followed by disappearance of the reaction is presumptive evidence of a drug-induced illness. Confirming evidence may be sought by cautiously reintroducing the drug and seeing if the reaction reappears. However, that should be done only if confirmation would be useful in the future management of the patient. Because rechallenge does carry risks, it is generally avoided unless the suspected culprit drug is critical to the patient's care. When the reaction is thought to be immunologic, challenge is generally avoided. With concentration-dependent ADRs, lowering the dosage may cause the reaction to disappear, and raising it may cause the reaction to reappear. Serious immunologically mediated ADRs have been treated with high-dose steroids; other immunosuppressive agents such as rituximab, infliximab, or mycophenolate mofetil; or plasmapheresis.

If the patient is receiving many drugs when an ADR is suspected, the drugs likeliest to be responsible can usually be identified; this should include both potential culprit agents as well as drugs that alter their elimination. All drugs may be discontinued at once or, if this is not practical, discontinued one at a time, starting with the ones most suspect, and the patient observed for signs of improvement. The time needed for a concentration-dependent ADR to disappear depends on the time required for the concentration to fall below the range associated with the ADR; that, in turn, depends on the initial blood level and on the rate of elimination or metabolism of the drug. Adverse effects of drugs with long half-lives or those not directly related to serum concentration may take a considerable time to disappear.

THE DRUG DEVELOPMENT PROCESS

Drug therapy is an ancient feature of human culture. The first treatments were plant extracts discovered empirically to be effective for indications like fever, pain, or breathlessness. This symptom-based empiric approach to drug development was supplanted in the twentieth century by identification of compounds targeting more fundamental biologic processes, such as bacterial growth or elevated blood pressure. The term "magic bullet," coined by Paul Ehrlich to describe the search for effective compounds for syphilis, captures the essence of the hope that understanding basic biologic processes will lead to highly effective new therapies.

A common starting point for the development of many widely used modern therapies has been basic biologic discovery that implicates potential target molecules: examples of such target molecules include HMG-CoA reductase, a key step in cholesterol biosynthesis, or the *BRAF* V600E mutation that appears to drive the development of some malignant melanomas and other tumors. The development of compounds targeting these molecules has not only revolutionized treatment for diseases such as hypercholesterolemia or malignant melanoma, but has also revealed new biologic features of disease. Thus, for example, initial spectacular successes with vemurafenib (which targets

BRAF V600E) were followed by near-universal tumor relapse, strongly suggesting that inhibition of this pathway alone would be insufficient for tumor control. This reasoning, in turn, supports a view that many complex diseases will not lend themselves to cure by targeting a single magic bullet, but rather single drugs or combinations that attack multiple pathways whose perturbation results in disease. The use of combination therapy in settings such as hypertension, tuberculosis, HIV infection, and many cancers highlights the potential for such a "systems biology" view of drug therapy.

A common approach in contemporary drug development is to start with a high-throughput screening procedure to identify "lead" chemical(s) modulating the activity of a potential drug target. The next step is application of increasingly sophisticated medicinal chemistry-based modification of the "lead" to develop compounds with specificity for the chosen target, lack of "off-target" effects, and pharmacokinetic properties suitable for human use (e.g., consistent bioavailability, long elimination half-life, and no high-risk pharmacokinetic features). Drug evaluation in human subjects then proceeds from initial safety and tolerance (phase 1) to dose finding (phase 2) and then to large efficacy trials (phase 3). This is a very expensive process, and the vast majority of lead compounds fail at some point. Thus, new approaches to identify likely successes and failures early are needed. One idea, described further in **Chap. 68**, is to use genomic and other high-throughput profiling approaches not only to identify new drug targets but also to identify disease subsets for which drugs approved for other indications might be "repurposed," thereby avoiding the costly development process.

SUMMARY

Modern clinical pharmacology aims to replace empiricism in the use of drugs with therapy based on in-depth understanding of factors that determine an individual's response to drug treatment. Molecular pharmacology, pharmacokinetics, genetics, clinical trials, and the educated prescriber all contribute to this process. No drug response should ever be termed *idiosyncratic*; all responses have a mechanism whose understanding will help guide further therapy with that drug or successors. This rapidly expanding understanding of variability in drug actions makes the process of prescribing drugs increasingly daunting for the practitioner. However, fundamental principles should guide this process:

- The benefits of drug therapy, however defined, should always outweigh the risk.
- The smallest dosage necessary to produce the desired effect should be used.
- The number of medications and doses per day should be minimized.
- Although the literature is rapidly expanding, accessing it is becoming easier; electronic tools to search databases of literature and unbiased opinion will become increasingly commonplace.
- Genetics play a role in determining variability in drug response and may become a part of clinical practice.
- EHR and pharmacy systems will increasingly incorporate prescribing advice, such as indicated medications not used; unindicated medications being prescribed; and potential dosing errors, drug interactions, or genetically determined drug responses.
- Prescribers should be particularly wary when adding or stopping specific drugs that are especially liable to provoke interactions and adverse drug reactions.
- Prescribers should use only a limited number of drugs, with which they are thoroughly familiar.

FURTHER READING

BARRETT JS et al: Challenges and opportunities in the development of medical therapies for pediatric populations and the role of extrapolation. Clin Pharmacol Ther 103:419, 2018.

HOLFORD N: Pharmacodynamic principles and the time course of immediate drug effects. Transl Clin Pharmacol 25:157, 2017.

MACRAE CA et al: The future of cardiovascular therapeutics. Circulation 133:2610, 2016.

MUELLER KT et al: The role of clinical pharmacology across novel treatment modalities. Clin Pharmacol Ther 108:413, 2020.

SULTANA J et al: Clinical and economic burden of adverse drug reactions. J Pharmacol Pharmacother 4:S73, 2013.

ZAMEK-GLISZCZYNSKI MJ et al: Transporters in drug development: 2018 ITC recommendations for transporters of emerging clinical importance. Clin Pharmacol Ther 104:890, 2018.

68 Pharmacogenomics

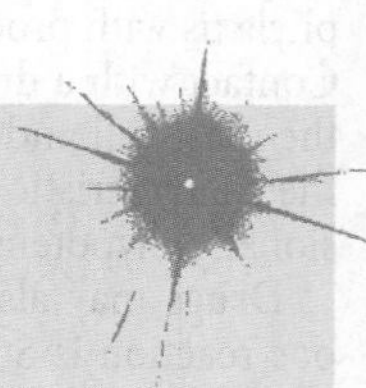

Dan M. Roden

The previous chapter discussed mechanisms underlying variability in drug action, highlighting pharmacokinetic and pharmacodynamic pathways to beneficial and adverse drug events. Work in the past several decades has defined how genetic variation can play a prominent role in modulating these pathways. Initial studies described unusual drug responses due to single genetic variants in individual subjects, defining the field of pharmacogenetics. A more recent view extends this idea to multiple genetic variants across populations, and the term "pharmacogenomics" is often used. Understanding the role of genetic variation in drug response could improve the use of current drugs, avoid drug use in those at increased risk for adverse drug reactions (ADRs), guide development of new drugs, and even be used as a lens through which to understand mechanisms of diseases themselves. This chapter will outline the principles of pharmacogenomics, the evidence as currently available that genetic factors play a role in variable drug actions, and areas of controversy and ongoing work.

PRINCIPLES OF GENETIC VARIATION AND DRUG RESPONSE (SEE ALSO CHAPS. 466 AND 467)

A goal of traditional Mendelian genetics is to identify DNA variants associated with a distinct phenotype in multiple related family members (**Chap. 467**). However, it is unusual for a drug response phenotype to be accurately measured in more than one family member, let alone across a kindred. Some clinical studies have examined drug disposition traits (such as urinary drug excretion after a fixed test dose) in twins and have, in some instances, shown greater concordance in monozygotic compared to dizygotic pairs, supporting a genetic contribution to the trait under study. However, in general, non-family-based approaches are usually used to identify and validate DNA variants contributing to variable drug actions. Both candidate gene and genome-wide studies have been used, and as with any genomic study, results require replication before they should be accepted as valid.

Types of Genetic Variants Influencing Drug Response (Table 68-1) The most common type of genetic variant is a single nucleotide polymorphism (SNP), and nonsynonymous SNPs (i.e., those that alter primary amino acid sequence encoded by a gene) are a common cause of variant function in genes regulating drug responses, often termed *pharmacogenes*. Small insertions and deletions can similarly alter protein function or lead to functionally important splice variation. Examples of synonymous coding region variants altering pharmacogene function have also been described; the postulated mechanism is an alteration in the rate of RNA translation, and hence in folding of the nascent protein. Variation in pharmacogene promoters has been described, and copy number variation (gene deletion or multiple copies of the same gene) is also well described.

Table 68-1 lists examples of individual types of genomic variation and the impact they can have on function of pharmacogenes. Multiple genotyping approaches may be needed to detect important variants; for example, SNP assays may fail to detect large gene duplications, and highly polymorphic regions (such as the major histocompatibility locus on chromosome 6 that includes multiple genes of the human leukocyte antigen [HLA] family) are currently best evaluated by sequencing.

TABLE 68-1 Examples of Genetic Variation and Ancestry

STRUCTURAL VARIANT	EXAMPLE		FUNCTIONAL EFFECT	MINOR ALLELE FREQUENCY (%)[a]		
	COMMON NAME	dbSNP		EUROPEAN	AFRICAN	EAST ASIAN
Single nucleotide polymorphism (SNP) (or single nucleotide variant, SNV)	CYP2C9*2	rs1799853	R144C: Reduction of function	12.7	2.4	b
	CYP2C9*3	rs1057910	I359L: Loss of function	6.9	1.3	3.4
	CYP2C9*8	rs7900194	R150H: Reduction of function	b	5.6	b
	CYP2C19*2	rs4244285	Splicing defect: Loss of function	14.8	18.1	31.0
	CYP2C19*3	rs4986893	Premature stop: Loss of function	b	b	6.7
	CYP2C19*17	rs12248560	Gain of function	45	45	<5
	CYP2D6*4[c]	rs3892097	Splicing defect: Loss of function	23.1	11.9	0.4
	CYP2D6*10[c]	Multiple SNPs define CYP2D6*10 (reduction of function allele):				
		rs1065852	P34S	24.9	15.1	59.1
		rs1135840	S486T			
	CYP3A5*3	rs776746	Splicing defect: Loss of function	90	33	85
	VKORC1*2	rs9923231	Promoter variant associated with decreased warfarin dose	39	11	91
	VKORC1	rs61742245	D36Y: Reduction of function, associated with increased warfarin dose	5% in East Africa, Middle East, Oceania; rare elsewhere		
	ABCB1	rs1045642	Synonymous variant; may affect mRNA stability and protein folding	47.2	79.8	62.5
Insertion/deletion	UGT1A1*28		Reduction of function promoter variant (7 TA repeats versus 6 repeats in reference allele); homozygotes have Gilbert's syndrome	31.6	39.1	14.8
Multiple variants constituting specific haplotypes	HLA-B*15:01		Predispose to immunologically mediated adverse drug reactions	b	b	5
	HLA-B*57:01			6.8	1.0	1.6
Gene deletion	CYP2D6*5		Loss of function	2.7	6	5.6
Gene duplication	CYP2D6*1xN	Duplication of normal allele	Ultra-rapid metabolizer phenotype	0.8	1.5	0.3
				Up to 3% in North Africa and the Middle East		
	CYP2D6*4xN	Duplication of loss of function allele	Extensive or poor metabolizer phenotype, depending on the opposite allele	0.3	1.4	b

Note: Allele frequencies from *https://gnomad.broadinstitute.org/* and *https://cpicpgx.org/*.
[a]Includes heterozygotes and homozygotes. [b]Allele frequency <0.05%. [c]*CYP2D6* is highly polymorphic, and multiple SNPs may be required to define a specific variant. For example, rs1065852 is present in both *4 and *10 variants. See *https://www.pharmvar.org/*.

Table 68-1 also highlights the fact that the frequency of important variation across pharmacogenes can vary strikingly by ancestry, with the result that certain ethnic groups may be at unusually high risk of displaying variant response to specific drugs.

Candidate Gene Approaches Most studies to date have used an understanding of the molecular mechanisms modulating drug action to identify candidate genes in which variants could explain variable drug responses. One very common scenario is that variable drug actions can be attributed to variability in plasma drug concentrations. When plasma drug concentrations vary widely (e.g., more than an order of magnitude), especially if their distribution is non-unimodal as in **Fig. 68-1**, variants in single genes controlling drug concentrations often contribute. In this case, the most obvious candidate genes are those responsible for drug metabolism and elimination. Other candidate genes are those encoding the target molecules with which drugs interact to produce their effects or molecules modulating that response, including those involved in disease pathogenesis.

Genome-Wide Association Studies The field has also had some success with "unbiased" approaches such as genome-wide association (GWA) **(Chap. 466)**, particularly in identifying single variants associated with high risk for certain forms of drug toxicity, and in validating the results of candidate gene studies. GWA studies have identified variants in the HLA locus that are associated with high risk for severe skin rashes during treatment with the anticonvulsant carbamazepine and hepatotoxicity with flucloxacillin, an antibiotic never marketed in the United States. A GWA study of simvastatin-associated myopathy identified a single noncoding SNP in *SLCO1B1*, encoding OATP1B1, a drug transporter known to modulate simvastatin uptake into the liver, which accounts for 60% of myopathy risk. African-American subjects are known to have higher dose requirements to achieve stable anticoagulation with warfarin, due in part to variations in *CYP2C9* and *VKORC1*, discussed below. In addition, a GWA study identified novel SNPs near *CYP2C9* that contribute to this effect in African Americans.

GENETIC VARIANTS AFFECTING PHARMACOKINETICS

Clinically important genetic variants have been described in multiple molecular pathways of drug disposition **(Table 68-2)**. A distinct multimodal distribution of drug disposition (as shown in Fig. 68-1) argues for a predominant effect of variants in a single gene in the metabolism of that substrate. Individuals with two alleles (variants) encoding for nonfunctional protein make up one group, often termed *poor metabolizers* (PM phenotype). For most genes, many variants can produce such a loss of function, and assessing whether they are on the same or different alleles (i.e., the *diplotype*) can complicate the use of genotyping in clinical practice. Furthermore, some variants produce only partial loss of function, and the presence of more than one variant may be required to define a specific allele. Individuals with one functional allele, or multiple reduction of function alleles, make up a second group (*intermediate metabolizers*) and may or may not be distinguishable from those with two functional alleles (normal metabolizers, sometimes termed *extensive metabolizers*, EMs). *Ultra-rapid metabolizers* (UMs) with especially high enzymatic activity (occasionally due

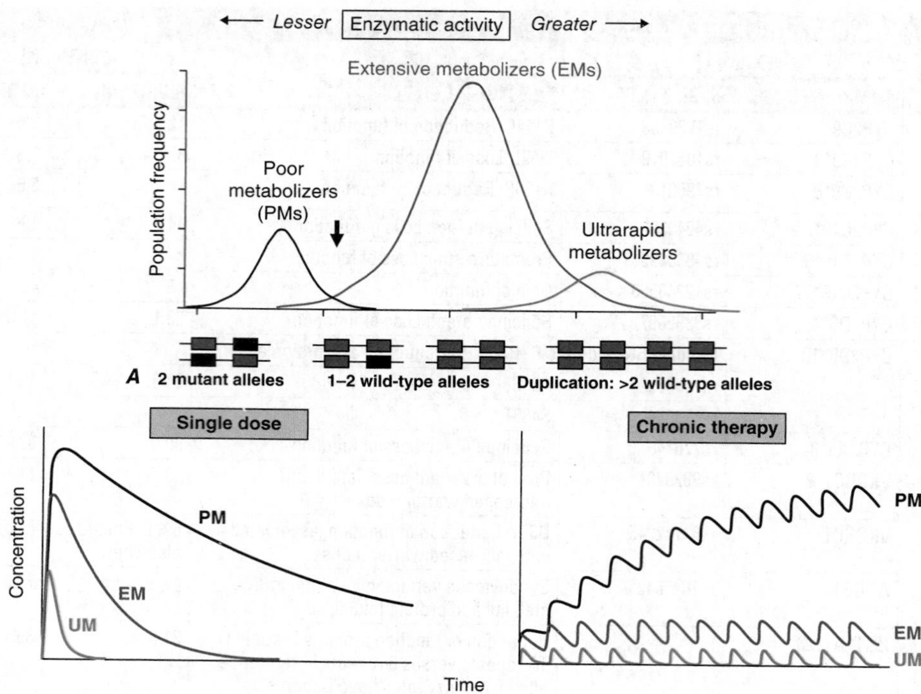

FIGURE 68-1 ***A.*** Distribution of CYP2D6 metabolic activity across a population. The heavy arrow indicates an antimode, separating poor metabolizer subjects (PMs, black), with two loss-of-function CYP2D6 alleles (black), indicated by the intron-exon structures below the chart. Individuals with one or two functional alleles are grouped together as extensive metabolizers (EMs, blue). Also shown are ultra-rapid metabolizers (UMs, red), with 2–12 functional copies of the gene, displaying the greatest enzyme activity. *(Adapted from M-L Dahl et al: J Pharmacol Exp Ther 274:516, 1995.)* ***B.*** These simulations show the predicted effects of CYP2D6 genotype on disposition of a substrate drug. With a single dose (left), there is an inverse "gene-dose" relationship between the number of active alleles and the areas under the time-concentration curves (smallest in UM subjects; highest in PM subjects); this indicates that clearance is greatest in UM subjects. In addition, elimination half-life is longest in PM subjects. The right panel shows that these single-dose differences are exaggerated during chronic therapy: steady-state concentration is much higher in PM subjects (decreased clearance), as is the time required to achieve steady state (longer elimination half-life).

TABLE 68-2 Genetic Variants and Drug Responses

GENE	DRUGS	EFFECT OF GENETIC VARIANTS[a]
Variants in Drug Metabolism Pathways		
CYP2C9	Losartan	Decreased bioactivation and effects (PMs)
	Warfarin	Decreased dose requirements; possible increased bleeding risk (PMs)
	Phenytoin	Decreased dose requirement (PMs)
CYP2C19	Omeprazole, voriconazole	Decreased effect in EMs
	Celecoxib	Exaggerated effect in PMs
	Clopidogrel	Decreased effect in PMs and IMs Consider alternate drug in PMs and alternate drug or dose increase in IMs Possible increased bleeding risk in carriers of gain-of-function variants
	Citalopram, escitalopram	Choose alternate drug in UMs; reduce dose in PMs
CYP2D6	Codeine, tamoxifen	Decreased bioactivation and drug effects in PMs
	Codeine	Respiratory depression in UMs
	Tricyclic antidepressants[b]	Increased adverse effects in PMs: Consider dose decrease Decreased therapeutic effects in UMs: Consider alternate drug
	Metoprolol, carvedilol, timolol, propafenone	Increased beta blockade in PMs
	Fluvoxamine	Reduce dose or chose alternate drug in PMs
CYP3A5	Tacrolimus, vincristine	Decreased drug concentrations and effect (CYP3A5*3 carriers)
Dihydropyrimidine dehydrogenase (*DPYD*)	Capecitabine, 5-fluorouracil, tegafur	Possible severe toxicity (PMs)
NAT2	Rifampin, isoniazid, pyrazinamide, hydralazine, procainamide	Increased risk of toxicity in PMs
Thiopurine *S*-methyltransferase (*TPMT*)	Azathioprine, 6-mercaptopurine, thioguanine	PMs: Increased risk of bone marrow aplasia EMs: Possible decreased drug action at usual dosages
Uridine diphosphate glucuronosyltransferase (*UGT1A1*)	Irinotecan	PM homozygotes: Increased risk of severe adverse effects (diarrhea, bone marrow aplasia)
	Atazanavir	High risk of hyperbilirubinemia during treatment; can result in drug discontinuation
Pseudocholinesterase (*BCHE*)	Succinylcholine and other muscle relaxants	Prolonged paralysis (autosomal recessive); diagnosis established by genotyping or by measuring serum cholinesterase activity

(Continued)

TABLE 68-2 Genetic Variants and Drug Responses (Continued)

GENE	DRUGS	EFFECT OF GENETIC VARIANTS[a]
Variants in Other Genes		
Glucose 6-phosphate dehydrogenase (*G6PD*)	Rasburicase, primaquine, chloroquine	Increased risk of hemolytic anemia in G6PD-deficient subjects
HLA-B*15:02	Carbamazepine	Carriers (1 or 2 alleles) at increased risk of SJS/TEN (mainly Asian subjects)
HLA-B*31:01	Carbamazepine	Carriers (1 or 2 alleles) at increased risk of SJS/TEN and milder skin toxicities (Caucasian and Asian subjects)
HLA-B*15:02	Phenytoin	Carriers (1 or 2 alleles) at increased risk of SJS/TEN
HLA-B*57:01	Abacavir	Carriers (1 or 2 alleles) at increased risk of SJS/TEN
HLA-B*58:01	Allopurinol	Carriers (1 or 2 alleles) at increased risk of SJS/TEN
IFNL3 (IL28B)	Interferon	Variable response in hepatitis C therapy
SLCO1B1	Simvastatin	Encodes a drug uptake transporter; variant nonsynonymous single nucleotide polymorphism increases myopathy risk especially at higher dosages
VKORC1	Warfarin	Decreased dose requirements with variant promoter haplotype Increased dose requirement in individuals with nonsynonymous loss-of-function variants
ITPA	Ribavirin	Variants modulate risk for hemolytic anemia
RYR1	General anesthetics	Variants predispose to malignant hyperthermia
CFTR	Ivacaftor, lumacaftor	Targeted therapies for cystic fibrosis indicated only in certain genotypes
Variants in Other Genomes (Infectious Agents, Tumors)		
Chemokine C-C motif receptor (CCR5)	Maraviroc	Drug effective only in HIV strains with CCR5 detectible
C-KIT	Imatinib	In gastrointestinal stromal tumors, drug indicated only with c-kit–positive cases
ALK (anaplastic lymphoma kinase)	Crizotinib	Indicated in patients with non-small cell lung cancer and ALK mutations
Her2/neu overexpression	Trastuzumab, lapatinib	Drugs indicated only with tumor overexpression
K-ras mutation	Panitumumab, cetuximab	Lack of efficacy with *KRAS* mutation
Philadelphia chromosome	Dasatinib, nilotinib, imatinib	Decreased efficacy in Philadelphia chromosome–negative chronic myelogenous leukemia

[a]Drug effect in homozygotes unless otherwise specified. [b]Many tricyclic antidepressants and selective serotonin uptake inhibitors are metabolized by CYP2D6, CYP2C19, or both, and some metabolites have pharmacologic activity. See *https://www.pharmgkb.org/view/dosing-guidelines.do*.

Abbreviations: EM, extensive metabolizer (normal enzymatic activity); IM, intermediate metabolizer (heterozygote for loss-of-function allele); PM, poor metabolizer (homozygote for reduced or loss-of-function allele); SJS/TEN, Stevens-Johnson syndrome/toxic epidermal necrolysis; UM, ultra-rapid metabolizer (enzymatic activity much greater than normal, e.g., with gene duplication, Fig. 68-1).

Further data at:

U.S. Food and Drug Administration: *http://www.fda.gov/Drugs/ScienceResearch/ResearchAreas/Pharmacogenetics/ucm083378.htm*

Pharmacogenetics Research Network/Knowledge Base: *http://www.pharmgkb.org*

The Clinical Pharmacogenomics Implementation Consortium: *https://www.pharmgkb.org/page/cpic*

Dutch Pharmacogenetics Working Group: *https://www.knmp.nl/patientenzorg/medicatiebewaking/farmacogenetica/pharmacogenetics-1/pharmacogenetics*

to gene duplication; Table 68-1 and Fig. 68-1) have also been described for some traits. Many drugs in widespread use can inhibit specific drug disposition pathways (**see Chap. 67, Table 67-1**), and so EM individuals receiving such inhibitors can respond like PM patients (*phenocopying*). Polymorphisms in genes encoding drug uptake or drug efflux transporters may be other contributors to variability in drug delivery to target sites and, hence, in drug effects.

CYP3A Members of the CYP3A family (*CYP3A4*, *CYP3A5*) metabolize the greatest number of drugs in therapeutic use. CYP3A4 activity is highly variable (up to an order of magnitude) among individuals, but nonsynonymous coding region polymorphisms (those that change the encoded amino acid) are rare. Thus, the underlying mechanism likely reflects genetic variation in regulatory regions.

Most subjects of European or Asian origin carry a polymorphism that disrupts splicing in the closely related *CYP3A5* gene. As a result, these individuals display reduced CYP3A5 activity, whereas CYP3A5 activity tends to be greater in subjects of African origin. Decreased efficacy of the antirejection agent tacrolimus in subjects of African origin has been attributed to more rapid CYP3A5-mediated elimination, and a lower risk of vincristine-associated neuropathy has been reported in CYP3A5 "expressers."

CYP2D6 CYP2D6 is second to CYP3A4 in the number of commonly used drugs that it metabolizes. CYP2D6 activity is polymorphically distributed, and 5–10% of European- and African-derived populations (but few Asians) display the PM phenotype (Fig. 68-1). Dozens of loss-of-function variants in *CYP2D6* have been described; the PM phenotype arises in individuals with two such alleles. In addition, UMs with multiple functional copies of *CYP2D6* have been identified especially in East Africa, the Middle East, and Oceania. PMs have slower elimination rates and lower clearance of substrate drugs; as a consequence (Fig. 68-1*B*), steady-state concentrations are higher and the time taken to achieve steady state is longer than in EMs (**Chap. 67**). Conversely, UMs display very low steady-state parent drug concentrations and an abbreviated time to steady state.

Codeine is biotransformed by CYP2D6 to the potent active metabolite morphine, so its effects are blunted in PMs and exaggerated in UMs. Deaths due to respiratory depression in children given codeine after tonsillectomy have been attributed to the UM trait, and the U.S. Food and Drug Administration (FDA) has revised the package insert to include a prominent "black box" warning against its use in this setting, and, in fact, forbidding its use in children less than 12 years old. In the case of drugs with beta-blocking properties metabolized by CYP2D6, greater signs of beta blockade (e.g., bronchospasm, bradycardia) have been reported in PM subjects than in EMs. This can be seen not only with orally administered beta blockers such as metoprolol and carvedilol, but also with ophthalmic timolol and with the sodium channel–blocking antiarrhythmic propafenone, a CYP2D6 substrate with beta-blocking properties. UMs may require very high dosages of nortriptyline and other tricyclic antidepressants to achieve a therapeutic effect. Tamoxifen undergoes CYP2D6-mediated biotransformation to an active metabolite, so its efficacy may be in part related to this polymorphism. In addition, the widespread use of selective serotonin reuptake inhibitors (SSRIs) to treat tamoxifen-related hot flashes may also alter the drug's effects because many SSRIs, notably fluoxetine and paroxetine, are also CYP2D6 inhibitors (Table 67-2).

CYP2C19 The PM phenotype for CYP2C19 is common (20%) among Asians and rarer (2–3%) in other populations; the frequency of the PM trait is especially high (>50%) in Oceania. The impact of polymorphic CYP2C19-mediated metabolism has been demonstrated with the proton pump inhibitor omeprazole, where ulcer cure rates with "standard" dosages were much lower in EM patients (29%) than in PMs (100%). Thus, understanding the importance of this polymorphism would have been important in developing the drug, and knowing a patient's *CYP2C19* genotype could improve therapy. CYP2C19 is responsible for bioactivation of the antiplatelet drug clopidogrel, and several large retrospective, and more recently prospective, studies have documented decreased efficacy (e.g., increased myocardial infarction after placement of coronary stents or increased stroke or transient ischemic attacks) among subjects with one or two reductions of function alleles. In addition, some studies suggest that omeprazole and possibly other proton pump inhibitors phenocopy this effect by inhibiting CYP2C19.

CYP2C9 There are common variants in *CYP2C9* that encode proteins with reduction or loss of catalytic function. These variant alleles are associated with increased rates of neurologic complications with phenytoin, hypoglycemia with glipizide, and reduced warfarin dose required to maintain stable anticoagulation. Rare patients homozygous for loss-of-function alleles may require very low warfarin dosages. Up to 50% of the variability in steady-state warfarin dose requirement is attributable to polymorphisms in *CYP2C9* and in the promoter of *VKORC1*, which encodes the warfarin target with lesser contributions by genes such as *CYP4F2* controlling vitamin K metabolism. The angiotensin receptor blocker losartan is a prodrug that is bioactivated by CYP2C9; as a result, PMs and those receiving inhibitor drugs may display little response to therapy.

DPYD Individuals homozygous for loss-of-function alleles in dihydropyrimidine dehydrogenase, encoded by *DPYD*, are at increased risk for severe toxicity when exposed to the substrate anticancer drug 5-fluorouracil (5-FU), as well as to capecitabine and tegafur, which are metabolized to 5-FU. Dose reductions have been recommended in intermediate metabolizers.

Transferase Variants Thiopurine *S*-methyltransferase (TPMT) bioinactivates the antileukemic drug 6-mercaptopurine (6-MP), and 6-MP is itself an active metabolite of the immunosuppressive azathioprine. Homozygotes for alleles encoding inactive TPMT (1/300 individuals) predictably exhibit severe and potentially fatal pancytopenia on standard doses of azathioprine or 6-MP. On the other hand, homozygotes for fully functional alleles may display less anti-inflammatory or antileukemic effect with standard doses of the drugs. GWA studies have also identified loss-of-function variants in *NUDT15* that reduce degradation of thiopurine metabolites and, thereby, also increase risk of excessive myelosuppression.

N-acetylation is accomplished by hepatic *N*-acetyl transferase (NAT), which represents the activity of two genes, *NAT1* and *NAT2*. Both enzymes transfer an acetyl group from acetyl coenzyme A to the drug; polymorphisms in *NAT2* are thought to underlie individual differences in the rate at which drugs are acetylated and thus define "rapid acetylators" and "slow acetylators." Slow acetylators make up ~50% of European and African populations but are less common among East Asians. Slow acetylators have an increased incidence of the drug-induced lupus syndrome during procainamide and hydralazine therapy and of hepatitis with isoniazid.

Individuals homozygous for a common promoter polymorphism that reduces transcription of uridine diphosphate glucuronosyltransferase (*UGT1A1*) have benign hyperbilirubinemia (Gilbert's syndrome; **Chap. 337**). This variant has also been associated with diarrhea and increased bone marrow depression with the antineoplastic prodrug irinotecan, whose active metabolite is normally detoxified by UGT1A1-mediated glucuronidation. The antiretroviral atazanavir is a UGT1A1 inhibitor, and individuals with the Gilbert's variant develop higher bilirubin levels during treatment. While this is benign, the hyperbilirubinemia can complicate clinical care because it may raise the question of whether coexistent hepatic injury is present.

Transporter Variants The risk for myotoxicity with simvastatin and possibly other statins appears increased with variants in *SLCO1B1*. Variants in *ABCB1*, encoding the drug efflux transporter P-glycoprotein, may increase digoxin toxicity. Variants in the uptake transporters *MATE1* and *MATE2* have been reported to modulate metformin's glucose-lowering activity.

GENETIC VARIANTS AFFECTING PHARMACODYNAMICS

A variant in the *VKORC1* promoter, especially common in Asian subjects (Table 68-1), reduces transcriptional activity and warfarin dose requirement. Multiple polymorphisms identified in the β_2-adrenergic receptor appear to be linked to specific drug responses in asthma and congestive heart failure, diseases in which β_2-receptor function might be expected to determine drug response. Polymorphisms in the β_2-receptor gene have also been associated with response to inhaled β_2-receptor agonists, while those in the β_1-adrenergic receptor gene have been associated with variability in heart rate slowing and blood pressure lowering. In addition, in heart failure, the arginine allele of the common β_1-adrenergic receptor gene polymorphism R389G has been associated with decreased mortality and decreased incidence of atrial fibrillation during treatment with the investigational beta blocker bucindolol.

Drugs may also interact with genetic pathways of disease to elicit or exacerbate symptoms of the underlying conditions. In the porphyrias, CYP inducers are thought to increase the activity of enzymes proximal to the deficient enzyme, exacerbating or triggering attacks (**Chap. 416**). Deficiency of glucose-6-phosphate dehydrogenase (G6PD), most often in individuals of African, Mediterranean, or South Asian descent, increases the risk of hemolytic anemia in response to the antimalarial primaquine (**Chap. 100**) and the uric acid-lowering agent rasburicase, which does not cause hemolysis in patients with normal amounts of the enzyme. Patients with mutations in *RYR1* encoding the skeletal muscle intracellular release calcium (also termed type 1 ryanodine receptor) are asymptomatic until exposed to certain general anesthetics, which can trigger the rare syndrome of malignant hyperthermia. Certain antiarrhythmics and other drugs can produce marked QT prolongation and torsades de pointes (**Chap. 246**), and in a minority of affected patients, this adverse effect represents unmasking of previously subclinical congenital long QT syndrome.

Immunologically Mediated Drug Reactions The Stevens-Johnson syndrome/toxic epidermal necrolysis (SJS/TEN) is a potentially fatal skin and systemic reaction now increasingly recognized to be linked to specific HLA alleles (Table 68-2). Cases of drug-induced hepatotoxicity and of the drug rash with eosinophilia and systemic symptoms (DRESS) syndrome have also been linked to variants in this region. The frequency of risk alleles often varies by ancestry (Table 68-1). The HLA risk alleles appear to be necessary but not sufficient to elicit these reactions. For example, HLA-B*57:01 is a risk allele for abacavir-related SJS/TEN and flucloxacillin-related hepatotoxicity. However, while 55% of abacavir-exposed subjects will develop a reaction, only 1/10,000 subjects exposed to flucloxacillin develop hepatotoxicity. Thus, a third factor, the nature of which has not yet been established, seems necessary.

Tumor and Infectious Agent Genomes The actions of drugs used to treat infectious or neoplastic disease may be modulated by variants in these nonhuman germline genomes. Genotyping tumors is a rapidly evolving approach to target therapies to underlying mechanisms and to avoid potentially toxic therapy in patients who would derive no benefit (**Chap. 71**). Trastuzumab, which potentiates anthracycline-related cardiotoxicity, is ineffective in breast cancers that do not express the Herceptin receptor. Imatinib targets a specific tyrosine kinase, BCR-Abl1, that is generated by the translocation that creates the Philadelphia chromosome typical of chronic myelogenous leukemia (CML). Imatinib is also an inhibitor of another kinase, c-kit, and the drug is remarkably effective in c-kit-driven cancer, such as gastrointestinal stromal tumors (**Chap. 71**). Vemurafenib does not inhibit wild-type *BRAF* but is active against the V600E mutant form of the kinase. Crizotinib is highly effective in non-small cell lung cancers harboring anaplastic lymphoma kinase (ALK) mutations.

■ INCORPORATING PHARMACOGENETIC INFORMATION INTO CLINICAL PRACTICE

The discovery of common variant alleles with relatively large effects on drug response raises the prospect that these variants could be used to guide therapy. Desired outcomes could be better ways of choosing likely effective drugs and dosages, or avoiding drugs that are likely to produce severe adverse drug events or be ineffective in individual subjects. Indeed, the FDA now incorporates pharmacogenetic data into package inserts meant to guide prescribing. A decision to adopt pharmacogenetically guided dosing for a given drug depends on multiple factors. The most important are the magnitude and clinical importance of the genetic effect and the strength of evidence linking genetic variation to variable drug effects (e.g., anecdote versus post-hoc analysis of clinical trial data versus randomized clinical trial [RCT]). The evidence can be strengthened if statistical arguments from clinical trial data are complemented by an understanding of underlying physiologic mechanisms. Cost versus expected benefit may also be a factor.

Point of Care Versus Preemptive Approaches Two approaches to pharmacogenetic implementation have been put in place at "early adopter" institutions and are currently being evaluated. In the first, variant-specific assays are ordered at the time of drug prescription and delivered rapidly (often within an hour or two), and the results are then used to guide therapy with that specific drug. The alternative to this "point-of-care" approach is a "preemptive" approach in which pharmacogenetic testing for large numbers of potential variants across many drugs is undertaken prior to prescription of any such drug. The data are then available in electronic health record (EHR) systems and coupled to real-time clinical decision support (CDS). When a drug whose effects are known to be influenced by pharmacogenetic variants is prescribed, the EHR system looks up whether variants likely to affect response are present; if so, CDS will alert health care providers that an alternate drug or a different dose may be required.

Challenges There are multiple challenges in putting in place either system. Assay validity and reproducibility have been issues in the past, but are less likely now. National consortia are now being put in place to develop standards for pharmacogenetic CDS. While common variants in genes such as those listed in Table 68-1 have been clearly associated with variable drug responses, the effect of rare variants, now readily discoverable by large-scale sequencing, is unknown. The extent to which a dose adjustment might be recommended may vary depending on whether zero, one, or two variant alleles are present, and whether such variants are reduction of function, loss of function, or gain of function. The Clinical Pharmacogenetics Implementation Consortium (CPIC) and the Dutch Pharmacogenetics Working Group have developed and published guidelines for multiple drug-gene pairs focusing on the question of what might be an appropriate drug dose adjustment given the availability of genetic data. These resources do not directly address the question of when or how such genetic testing should be undertaken.

Developing Evidence That Pharmacogenetic Testing Alters Drug Outcomes A major issue is whether pharmacogenetic testing affects important drug response outcomes. When the evidence is compelling, alternate therapies are not available, and there are clear recommendations for dosage adjustment in subjects with variants, there is a strong argument for deploying genetic testing as a guide to prescribing; HLA-B*57:01 testing for abacavir is an example described below. In other situations, the arguments are less compelling: the magnitude of the genetic effect may be smaller, the consequences may be less serious, alternate therapies may be available, or the drug effect may be amenable to monitoring by other approaches.

One school argues that the physiology and pharmacology are known and that RCTs are, therefore, unnecessary (and conceivably unethical). The analogy is sometimes drawn to well-recognized dose adjustment of renally excreted drugs in the presence of renal dysfunction. RCTs have not been conducted and the idea of such dose adjustment is well accepted in the medical community and recommended in FDA-approved drug labels. Others have argued that the effect of genetic variants is generally modest and variability in drug actions has many nongenetic sources, so genetic testing might provide marginal benefit at best.

Efforts to demonstrate the value of pharmacogenetic testing have met with mixed results. An RCT clearly showed that HLA-B*57:01 testing eliminates SJS/TEN due to abacavir. Similarly, regulatory authorities in some countries in Southeast Asia mandated HLA-B*15:02 testing prior to initiation of carbamazepine; however, in this case, an unfortunate outcome in some jurisdictions was that prescribers stopped using carbamazepine, often substituting phenytoin (another drug associated with SJS/TEN), so the incidence of the severe ADR was unchanged.

RCTs evaluating the effect of using pharmacogenetically guided therapy to optimize warfarin treatment have shown either no effect or a modest benefit of incorporating genetic information into prescribing the drug. Initial RCTs focused on time in therapeutic range in the first 4–12 weeks of treatment, whereas one more recent trial demonstrated that genotype-guided therapy could reduce the frequency of over-anticoagulation. Retrospective analyses of bleeding cases versus non-bleeding controls in EHRs and administrative databases have suggested a role for CYP2C9*3 or for the V433M variant in *CYP4F2* in mediating this risk.

Two large trials have randomized patients with acute coronary syndromes to newer antiplatelet therapies (ticagrelor or prasugrel) or clopidogrel if *CYP2C19* variants were absent; in one, clopidogrel was superior, and in the second, a trend in the same direction, which did not reach the prespecified endpoint, was observed.

New effective alternate therapies to warfarin and clopidogrel that appear to lack important pharmacogenetic variants have emerged. One approach to therapy, therefore, is to use pharmacogenetic testing to identify subjects in whom variants are absent and therefore standard doses of the conventional inexpensive drugs are likely to be effective and to reserve alternate more expensive therapies for subjects likely to have variant responses to warfarin or clopidogrel.

■ GENETICS AND DRUG DEVELOPMENT

Genetic tools are now being increasingly used to identify or validate new drug targets. Initial studies suggest that a new drug development program is more likely to succeed if evidence from human genetics supports the role of a possible drug target in disease pathogenesis and suggests that the risk of toxicity due to high-risk pharmacokinetics or other mechanisms is small. Furthermore, studies of the relationships between variants in genes encoding drug target molecules and a range of phenotypes (e.g., those in EHRs) are being used for drug "repurposing," identifying new indications for existing drugs.

Finding Protective Alleles Can Identify Drug Targets One example of using genetics to identify a new drug target started with the discovery that very rare gain-of-function variants in *PCSK9* are a rare cause of familial hypercholesterolemia. Subsequently, population studies showed that carriers of loss-of-function SNPs (2.5% of African Americans) had decreased low-density lipoprotein cholesterol, decreased incidence of coronary artery disease, and no deleterious consequences in other organ systems. These data triggered the development of PCSK9 monoclonal antibodies, which were marketed <10 years after the initial population studies. Other targets implicated by similar population genetic studies include HSD17B13 for prevention of chronic liver disease, SLC30A8 for the prevention of type 2 diabetes, and APOC3 for hypertriglyceridemia. Discovering rare protective alleles may require very large data sets (>100,000), such as EHR systems coupled to DNA biobanks or epidemiologic cohorts like the UK Biobank.

Cancer In cancer, tumor sequencing has identified new targets for drug development, often constitutively active kinases. A problem in this area has been the rapid emergence of drug resistance, often after extraordinary initial responses. For example, 40% of melanomas appear to be driven by the V600E mutant form of *BRAF*, and the specific inhibitor vemurafenib can produce clinically spectacular remission. However, durable responses are rare, and it is now apparent that combination therapy, often with inhibitors of the MEK pathway, can provide improved therapy. Another approach that is rapidly gaining wide use in cancer involves drugs that reverse immune system inhibition (Chap. 73). In some patients, the release of this "brake" can provide durable remissions, whereas in others, severe adverse events, including colitis, pneumonitis, and myocarditis, have been reported. Understanding the mechanisms underlying variability to these therapies is a major emerging challenge in the field.

Using Multiple Data Types The development of methods to understand associations across multiple large data sets is another approach that is being explored in drug development. For example, a GWA study of risk of rheumatoid arthritis identified multiple risk loci, and many encode proteins that are known targets for intervention in the disease. Interestingly, others encode proteins that are targets for drugs used in other conditions, such as certain cancers, raising the question of whether such drugs could be "repurposed" for rheumatoid arthritis.

While the field has, to date, focused on individual high effect size variants (that are often common in a population), newer approaches combining many (dozens to millions) common variants into polygenic risk scores to predict drug responses are also being explored. An extension of this approach is the broader issue of systems pharmacology, in which multiple sources of data are used to identify potential molecules or pathways that would be amenable to treatment, by new drugs or by existing agents, using analysis of genomic, transcriptomic, proteomic, and other large data sets. Similar approaches are being developed to predict toxicity expected from targeting specific genes or disease pathways.

SUMMARY

The science of pharmacogenomics has evolved from isolated examples of rare adverse drug actions to a more comprehensive view of the role of genetic variation in mediating the effects of most drugs. Current principles include:

- Genetic variants with an important effect on drug actions can be common, and their frequencies often vary by ancestry.
- One common mechanism is modulation of drug concentrations.
- No practitioner can be expected to remember all variants important for all drugs. Electronic data systems can now be accessed to describe this information. Ultimately, this information will be used by linking individual pharmacogenetic data to smart EHR systems.
- Incorporating genetic approaches into drug development projects holds the promise of more rapid development of targeted, safe, and effective therapies.

FURTHER READING

CHENOWETH MJ et al: Global pharmacogenomics within precision medicine: Challenges and opportunities. Clin Pharmacol Ther 107:57, 2020.

DIOGO D et al: Phenome-wide association studies across large population cohorts support drug target validation. Nat Commun 9:4285, 2018.

LUZUM JA et al: The Pharmacogenomics Research Network Translational Pharmacogenetics Program: Outcomes and metrics of pharmacogenetic implementations across diverse healthcare systems. Clin Pharmacol Ther 102:502, 2017.

OSANLOU O et al: Pharmacogenetics of adverse drug reactions. Adv Pharmacol 83:155, 2018.

RELLING MV et al: The clinical pharmacogenetics implementation consortium: 10 years later. Clin Pharmacol Ther 107:171, 2020.

RODEN DM et al: Pharmacogenomics. Lancet 394:521, 2019.

Section 1 Neoplastic Disorders

69 Approach to the Patient with Cancer

Dan L. Longo

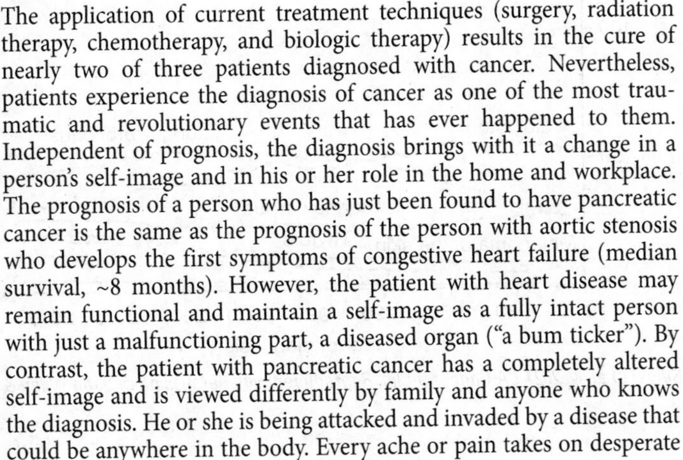

The application of current treatment techniques (surgery, radiation therapy, chemotherapy, and biologic therapy) results in the cure of nearly two of three patients diagnosed with cancer. Nevertheless, patients experience the diagnosis of cancer as one of the most traumatic and revolutionary events that has ever happened to them. Independent of prognosis, the diagnosis brings with it a change in a person's self-image and in his or her role in the home and workplace. The prognosis of a person who has just been found to have pancreatic cancer is the same as the prognosis of the person with aortic stenosis who develops the first symptoms of congestive heart failure (median survival, ~8 months). However, the patient with heart disease may remain functional and maintain a self-image as a fully intact person with just a malfunctioning part, a diseased organ ("a bum ticker"). By contrast, the patient with pancreatic cancer has a completely altered self-image and is viewed differently by family and anyone who knows the diagnosis. He or she is being attacked and invaded by a disease that could be anywhere in the body. Every ache or pain takes on desperate significance. Cancer is an exception to the coordinated interaction among cells and organs. In general, the cells of a multicellular organism are programmed for collaboration. Many diseases occur because the specialized cells fail to perform their assigned task. Cancer takes this malfunction one step further. Not only is there a failure of the cancer cell to maintain its specialized function, but it also strikes out on its own; the cancer cell competes to survive using natural mutability and natural selection to seek advantage over normal cells in a recapitulation of evolution. One consequence of the traitorous behavior of cancer cells is that the patient feels betrayed by his or her body. The cancer patient feels that he or she, and not just a body part, is diseased.

THE MAGNITUDE OF THE PROBLEM

No nationwide cancer registry exists; therefore, the incidence of cancer is estimated on the basis of the National Cancer Institute's Surveillance, Epidemiology, and End Results (SEER) database, which tabulates cancer incidence and death figures from 13 sites, accounting for about 10% of the U.S. population, and from population data from the U.S. Census Bureau. In 2021, 1.898 million new cases of invasive cancer (970,250 men and 927,910 women) were diagnosed, and 608,570 persons (319,420 men and 289,150 women) died from cancer. The percent distribution of new cancer cases and cancer deaths by site for men and women is shown in **Table 69-1**. Cancer incidence has been declining by about 2% each year since 1992. Cancer is the cause of one in four deaths in the United States.

The most significant risk factor for cancer overall is age; two-thirds of all cases were in those aged >65 years. Cancer incidence increases as the third, fourth, or fifth power of age in different sites. For the interval

TABLE 69-1 Distribution of Cancer Incidence and Deaths for 2021

MALE			FEMALE		
SITES	%	NUMBER	SITES	%	NUMBER
Cancer Incidence					
Prostate	26	248,530	Breast	30	281,550
Lung	12	119,100	Lung	13	116,660
Colorectal	8	79,520	Colorectal	8	69,980
Bladder	7	64,280	Endometrial	7	66,570
Melanoma	6	62,260	Melanoma	5	43,850
Kidney	5	48,780	Lymphoma	4	35,930
Lymphoma	5	45,630	Thyroid	3	32,130
Oral cavity	4	38,800	Pancreas	3	28,480
Leukemia	4	35,530	Kidney	3	27,300
Pancreas	3	31,950	Leukemia	3	25,560
All others	20	195,870	All others	21	199,900
All sites	100	970,250	All sites	100	927,910
Cancer Deaths					
Lung	22	69,410	Lung	22	62,470
Prostate	11	34,130	Breast	15	43.600
Colorectal	9	28,520	Colorectal	8	24,460
Pancreas	8	25,270	Pancreas	8	22,950
Liver	6	20,300	Ovary	5	14,460
Leukemia	4	13,900	Endometrial	4	12,940
Esophagus	4	12,410	Liver	3	9,930
Bladder	4	12,260	Leukemia	3	9,760
Lymphoma	4	12,170	Lymphoma	3	8,550
CNS	3	10,500	CNS	3	8,100
All others	25	80,550	All others	25	71,930
All sites	100	319,420	All sites	100	289,150

Source: From Cancer Statistics 2021, RI Seigel et al, © 2021 CA Cancer J Clin. Reproduced with permission of John Wiley & Sons Ltd.

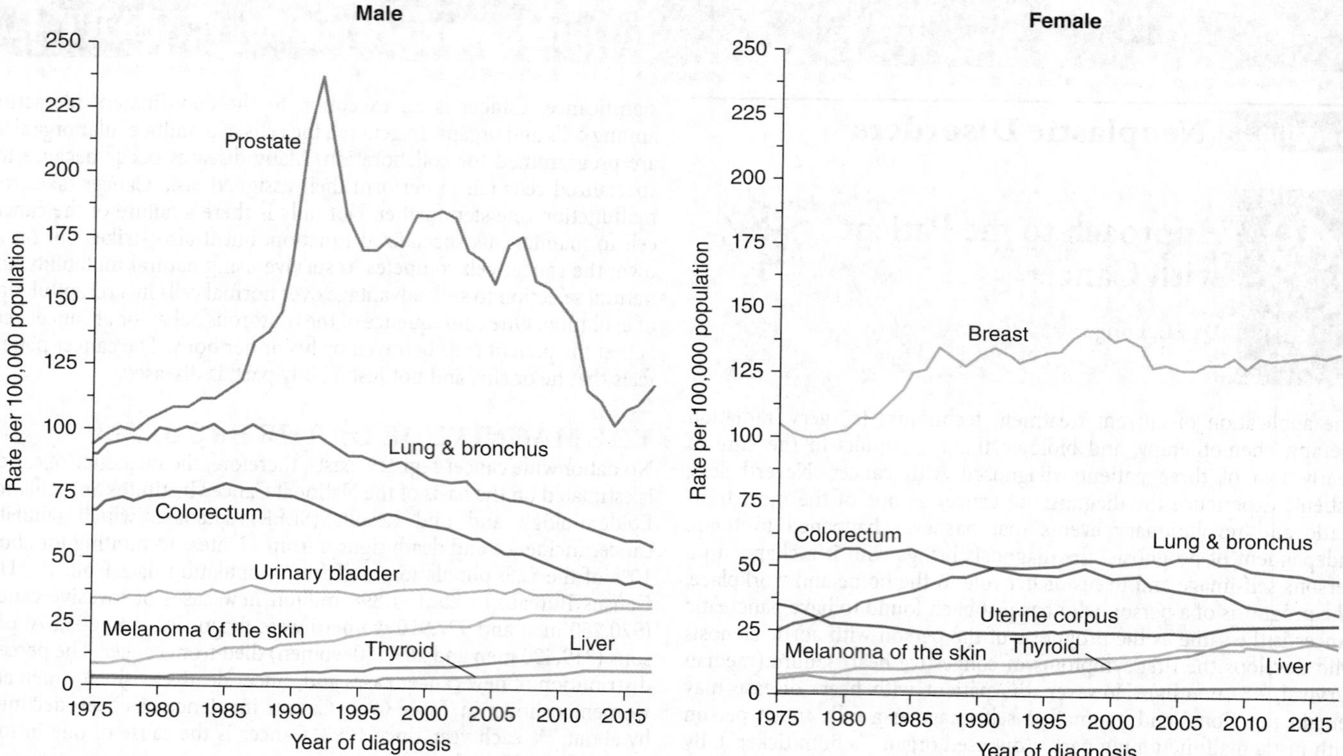

FIGURE 69-1 Trends in cancer incidence, 1975–2017. *(From Cancer Statistics 2021, Rl Seigel et al, © 2021 CA Cancer J Clin. Reproduced with permission of John Wiley & Sons Ltd.)*

between birth and age 49 years, 1 in 29 men and 1 in 19 women will develop cancer; for the interval between ages 50 and 59 years, 1 in 15 men and 1 in 17 women will develop cancer; for the interval between ages 60 and 69 years, 1 in 6 men and 1 in 10 women will develop cancer; and for people aged ≥70, 1 in 3 men and 1 in 4 women will develop cancer. Overall, men have a 40.5% risk of developing cancer at some time during their lives; women have a 38.9% lifetime risk.

Cancer is the second leading cause of death behind heart disease. Deaths from heart disease have declined 45% in the United States since 1950 and continue to decline. Cancer has overtaken heart disease as the number one cause of death in persons aged <85 years. Incidence trends over time are shown in **Fig. 69-1**. After a 70-year period of increase, cancer deaths began to decline in 1990–1991 **(Fig. 69-2)**. Between 1990 and 2010, cancer deaths decreased by 21% among men and 12.3% among women. The incidence has been steady since 2013. The magnitude of the decline is illustrated in **Fig. 69-3**. The five leading causes of cancer deaths are shown for various populations in **Table 69-2**. The 5-year survival for white patients was 39% in 1960–1963 and 68% in 2010–2016. Cancers are more often deadly in blacks; the 5-year survival was 63% for the 2010–2016 interval; however, the racial differences are narrowing over time. Incidence and mortality vary among racial and ethnic groups **(Table 69-3)**. The basis for these differences is unclear.

Advances in cancer prevention, diagnosis, and treatment since the early 1990s have averted millions of cancer deaths based on projections from the slopes of the mortality curves leading up to the 1990s **(Fig. 69-4)**.

CANCER AROUND THE WORLD

In 2018, 17 million new cancer cases and 9.5 million cancer deaths were estimated worldwide, according to estimates of GLOBOCAN 2018, developed by the International Agency for Research on Cancer (IARC). Rates are increasing worldwide. When broken down by region of the world, ~45% of cases were in Asia (which has 59.5% of the world's population), 26% in Europe (9.8% of the world's population), 14.5% in North America, 7.1% in Central/South America (the Americas, North and South, account for 13.3% of the world's population), 6% in Africa (16.9% of the world's population), and 1% in Australia/New Zealand (0.5% of the world's population) **(Fig. 69-5)**. Lung cancer is the most common cancer and the most common cause of cancer death in the world. Its incidence is highly variable, affecting only 2 per 100,000 African women but as many as 61 per 100,000 North American men. Breast cancer is the second most common cancer worldwide; however, it ranks fourth as a cause of death behind lung, stomach, and liver cancer. Among the eight most common forms of cancer, lung (2-fold), breast (3-fold), prostate (2.5-fold), and colorectal (3-fold) cancers are more common in more developed countries than in less developed countries. By contrast, liver (2-fold), cervical (2-fold), and esophageal (2- to 3-fold) cancers are more common in less developed countries. Stomach cancer incidence is similar in more and less developed countries but is much more common in Asia than North America or Africa. The most common cancers in Africa are cervical, breast, and liver cancers. It has been estimated that nine modifiable risk factors are responsible for more than one-third of cancers worldwide. These include smoking, alcohol consumption, obesity, physical inactivity, low fruit and vegetable consumption, unsafe sex, air pollution, indoor smoke from household fuels, and contaminated injections.

PATIENT MANAGEMENT

Important information is obtained from every portion of the routine history and physical examination. The duration of symptoms may reveal the chronicity of disease. The past medical history may alert the physician to the presence of underlying diseases that may affect the choice of therapy or the side effects of treatment. The social history may reveal occupational exposure to carcinogens or habits, such as smoking or alcohol consumption, that may influence the course of disease and its treatment. The family history may suggest an underlying familial cancer predisposition and point out the need to begin surveillance or other preventive therapy for unaffected siblings of the patient. The review of systems may suggest early symptoms of metastatic disease or a paraneoplastic syndrome.

DIAGNOSIS

The diagnosis of cancer relies most heavily on invasive tissue biopsy and should never be made without obtaining tissue; no noninvasive

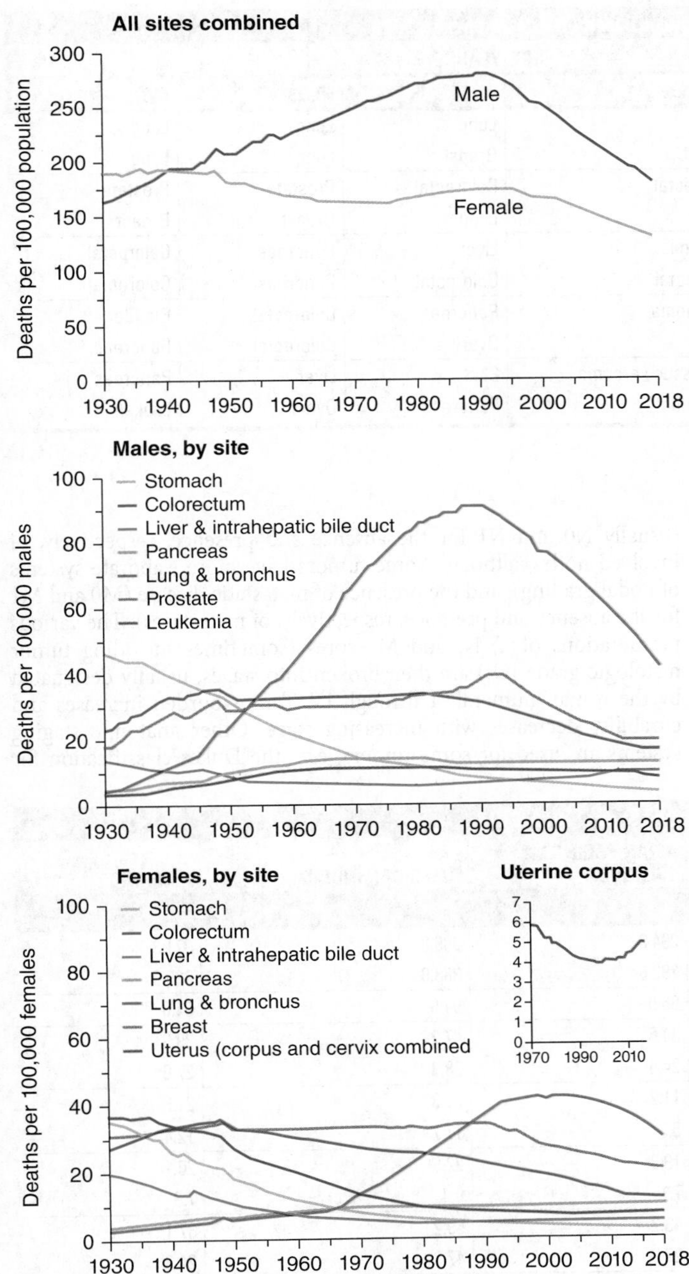

FIGURE 69-2 Trends in cancer mortality rates in men and women, 1930–2018. *(From Cancer Statistics 2021, RI Seigel et al, © 2021 CA Cancer J Clin. Reproduced with permission of John Wiley & Sons Ltd.)*

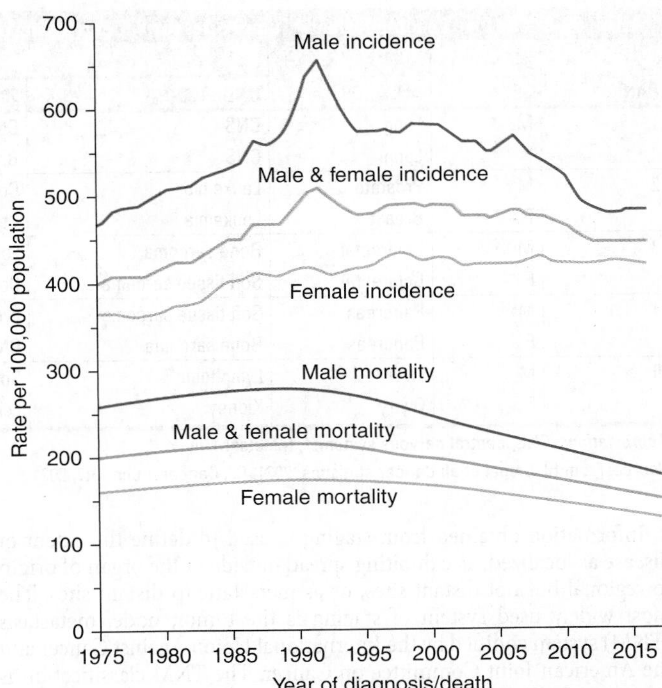

FIGURE 69-3 Trends in cancer incidence and death rates. *(From Cancer Statistics 2021, RI Seigel et al, © 2021 CA Cancer J Clin. Reproduced with permission of John Wiley & Sons Ltd.)*

diagnostic test is sufficient to define a disease process such as cancer. Although in rare clinical settings (e.g., thyroid nodules), fine-needle aspiration is an acceptable diagnostic procedure, the diagnosis generally depends on obtaining adequate tissue to permit careful evaluation of the histology of the tumor, its grade, and its invasiveness and to yield further molecular diagnostic information, such as the expression of cell-surface markers or intracellular proteins that typify a particular cancer, or the presence of a molecular marker, such as the t(8;14) translocation of Burkitt's lymphoma. Increasing evidence links the expression of certain genes with the prognosis and response to therapy **(Chaps. 71 and 72)**.

Occasionally, a patient will present with a metastatic disease process that is defined as cancer on biopsy but has no apparent primary site of disease. Efforts should be made to define the primary site based on age, sex, sites of involvement, histology and tumor markers, and personal and family history. Particular attention should be focused on ruling out the most treatable causes **(Chap. 92)**.

Once the diagnosis of cancer is made, the management of the patient is best undertaken as a multidisciplinary collaboration among the primary care physician, medical oncologists, surgical oncologists, radiation oncologists, oncology nurse specialists, pharmacists, social workers, rehabilitation medicine specialists, and a number of other consulting professionals working closely with each other and with the patient and family.

DEFINING THE EXTENT OF DISEASE AND THE PROGNOSIS

The first priority in patient management after the diagnosis of cancer is established and shared with the patient is to determine the extent of disease. The curability of a tumor usually is inversely proportional to the tumor burden. Ideally, the tumor will be diagnosed before symptoms develop or as a consequence of screening efforts **(Chap. 70)**. A very high proportion of such patients can be cured. However, most patients with cancer present with symptoms related to the cancer, caused either by mass effects of the tumor or by alterations associated with the production of cytokines or hormones by the tumor.

For most cancers, the extent of disease is evaluated by a variety of noninvasive and invasive diagnostic tests and procedures. This process is called *staging*. There are two types. *Clinical staging* is based on physical examination, radiographs, isotopic scans, computed tomography (CT) scans, and other imaging procedures; *pathologic staging* takes into account information obtained during a surgical procedure, which might include intraoperative palpation, resection of regional lymph nodes and/or tissue adjacent to the tumor, and inspection and biopsy of organs commonly involved in disease spread. Pathologic staging includes histologic examination of all tissues removed during the surgical procedure. Surgical procedures performed may include a simple lymph node biopsy or more extensive procedures such as thoracotomy, mediastinoscopy, or laparotomy. Surgical staging may occur in a separate procedure or may be done at the time of definitive surgical resection of the primary tumor. A subset of pathologic staging is the examination of tissue obtained at initial surgery that occurs after the delivery of some treatment, which is called neoadjuvant therapy. Stage of disease determined after neoadjuvant therapy is designated with the prefix y.

Knowledge of the predilection of particular tumors for spreading to adjacent or distant organs helps direct the staging evaluation.

TABLE 69-2 The Five Leading Primary Tumor Sites for Patients Dying of Cancer Based on Age and Sex in 2018

RANK	SEX	ALL AGES	AGE, YEARS				
			UNDER 20	20–39	40–59	60–79	>80
1	M	Lung	CNS	CNS	Lung	Lung	Lung
	F	Lung	CNS	Breast	Breast	Lung	Lung
2	M	Prostate	Leukemia	Colorectal	Colorectal	Prostate	Prostate
	F	Breast	Leukemia	Cervix	Lung	Breast	Breast
3	M	Colorectal	Bone sarcoma	Leukemia	Liver	Pancreas	Colorectal
	F	Colorectal	Soft tissue sarcoma	Colorectal	Colorectal	Pancreas	Colorectal
4	M	Pancreas	Soft tissue sarcoma	Lymphoma	Pancreas	Colorectal	Bladder
	F	Pancreas	Bone sarcoma	CNS	Ovary	Colorectal	Pancreas
5	M	Liver	Lymphoma	Soft tissue sarcoma	CNS	Liver	Pancreas
	F	Ovary	Kidney	Leukemia	Pancreas	Ovary	Leukemia

Abbreviations: CNS, central nervous system; F, female; M, male.
Source: From RL Siegel et al: Cancer statistics, 2021. CA Cancer J Clin 71:7, 2021.

Information obtained from staging is used to define the extent of disease as localized, as exhibiting spread outside of the organ of origin to regional but not distant sites, or as metastatic to distant sites. The most widely used system of staging is the tumor, node, metastasis (TNM) system codified by the International Union Against Cancer and the American Joint Committee on Cancer. The TNM classification is an anatomically based system that categorizes the tumor on the basis of the size of the primary tumor lesion (T1–4, where a higher number indicates a tumor of larger size), the presence of nodal involvement (usually N0 and N1 for the absence and presence, respectively, of involved nodes, although some tumors have more elaborate systems of nodal grading), and the presence of metastatic disease (M0 and M1 for the absence and presence, respectively, of metastases). The various permutations of T, N, and M scores (sometimes including tumor histologic grade [G]) are then broken into stages, usually designated by the roman numerals I through IV. Tumor burden increases and curability decreases with increasing stage. Other anatomic staging systems are used for some tumors, e.g., the Dukes classification for

TABLE 69-3 Cancer Incidence and Mortality in Racial and Ethnic Groups, United States, 2013–2018

SITE	SEX	WHITE	BLACK	ASIAN/PACIFIC ISLANDER	AMERICAN INDIAN[a]	HISPANIC
Incidence per 100,000 Population						
All	M	501.4	534.0	294.3	399.8	371.3
	F	442.2	406.6	292.6	388.8	335.5
Breast		131.6	127.3	95.6	94.9	94.8
Colorectal	M	42.6	51.6	34.6	47.2	39.9
	F	31.8	37.9	24.8	38.3	27.6
Kidney	M	23.1	26.1	11.2	31.3	21.9
	F	11.7	13.3	5.3	17.7	12.4
Liver	M	10.7	18.0	19.3	22.9	20.1
	F	3.8	5.5	7.1	9.4	7.9
Lung	M	70.8	79.8	43.2	59.2	37.1
	F	56.4	47.9	27.9	47.9	24.3
Prostate		97.7	171.6	53.8	67.7	85.6
Cervix		7.2	9.0	6.1	8.8	9.5
Deaths per 100,000 Population						
All	M	190.2	227.2	114.6	169.3	134.0
	F	137.8	154.9	84.6	120.1	94.6
Breast		20.1	28.2	11.7	14.8	13.8
Colorectal	M	16.1	23.2	11.2	18.5	14.0
	F	11.5	15.3	7.9	12.4	8.6
Kidney	M	5.5	5.5	2.5	8.3	4.9
	F	2.3	2.3	1.1	3.2	2.2
Liver	M	8.4	13.4	13.1	14.8	13.3
	F	3.6	4.9	5.4	7.0	6.0
Lung	M	49.4	57.0	28.0	38.4	23.0
	F	35.6	30.6	16.3	27.4	12.3
Prostate		17.9	38.3	8.8	18.5	15.6
Cervix		2.0	3.4	1.7	2.4	2.6

[a]Based on Indian Health Service delivery areas.
Abbreviations: F, female; M, male.
Source: From Cancer Statistics 2021, Rl Seigel et al, © 2021 CA Cancer J Clin. Reproduced with permission of John Wiley & Sons Ltd.

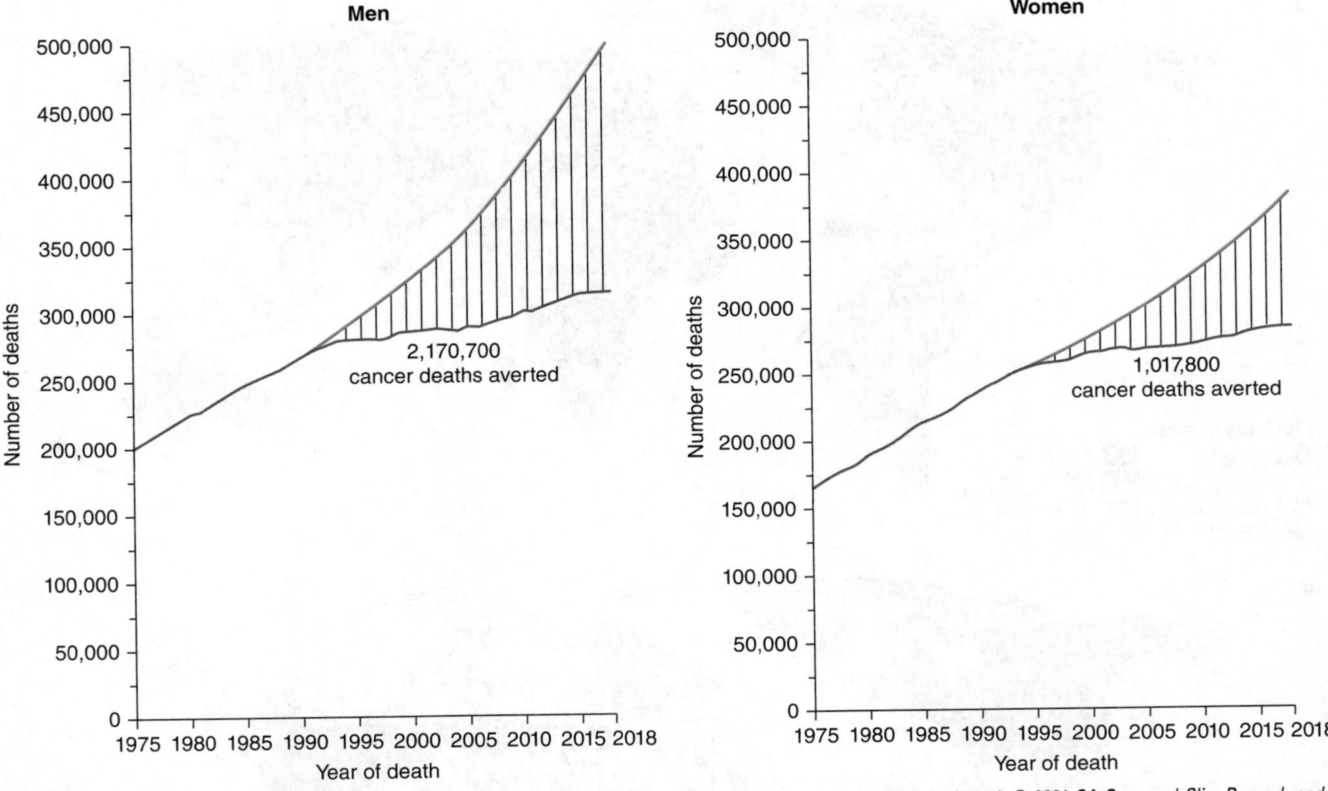

FIGURE 69-4 Cancer deaths averted in men and women since the early 1990s. *(From Cancer Statistics 2021, Rl Seigel et al, © 2021 CA Cancer J Clin. Reproduced with permission of John Wiley & Sons Ltd.)*

colorectal cancers, the International Federation of Gynecologists and Obstetricians classification for gynecologic cancers, and the Ann Arbor classification for Hodgkin's disease.

Certain tumors cannot be grouped on the basis of anatomic considerations. For example, hematopoietic tumors such as leukemia, myeloma, and lymphoma are often disseminated at presentation and do not spread like solid tumors. For these tumors, other prognostic factors have been identified (**Chaps. 104–111**).

In addition to tumor burden, a second major determinant of treatment outcome is the physiologic reserve of the patient. Patients who are bedridden before developing cancer are likely to fare worse, stage for stage, than fully active patients. Physiologic reserve is a determinant of how a patient is likely to cope with the physiologic stresses imposed by the cancer and its treatment. This factor is difficult to assess directly. Instead, surrogate markers for physiologic reserve are used, such as the patient's age or Karnofsky performance status (**Table 69-4**) or Eastern Cooperative Oncology Group (ECOG) performance status (**Table 69-5**). Older patients and those with a Karnofsky performance status <70 or ECOG performance status ≥3 have a poor prognosis unless the poor performance is a reversible consequence of the tumor.

Increasingly, biologic features of the tumor are being related to prognosis. The expression of particular oncogenes, drug-resistance genes, apoptosis-related genes, and genes involved in metastasis is being found to influence response to therapy and prognosis. The presence of selected cytogenetic abnormalities may influence survival. Tumors with higher growth fractions, as assessed by expression of proliferation-related markers such as proliferating cell nuclear antigen, behave more aggressively than tumors with lower growth fractions. Information obtained from studying the tumor itself will increasingly be used to influence treatment decisions. Host genes involved in drug metabolism can influence the safety and efficacy of particular treatments.

Enormous heterogeneity has been noted by studying tumors; we have learned that morphology is not capable of discerning certain distinct subsets of patients whose tumors have different sets of abnormalities. Tumors that look the same by light microscopy can be very different. Similarly, tumors that look quite different from one another histologically can share genetic lesions that predict responses to treatments. Furthermore, tumor cells vary enormously within a single patient even though the cells share a common origin.

MAKING A TREATMENT PLAN

From information on the extent of disease and the prognosis and in conjunction with the patient's wishes, it is determined whether the treatment approach should be curative or palliative in intent. Cooperation among the various professionals involved in cancer treatment is of the utmost importance in treatment planning. For some cancers, chemotherapy or chemotherapy plus radiation therapy delivered before the use of definitive surgical treatment (so-called neoadjuvant therapy) may improve the outcome, as seems to be the case for locally advanced breast cancer and head and neck cancers. In certain settings in which combined-modality therapy is intended, coordination among the medical oncologist, radiation oncologist, and surgeon is crucial to achieving optimal results. Sometimes the chemotherapy and radiation therapy need to be delivered sequentially, and other times concurrently. Surgical procedures may precede or follow other treatment approaches. It is best for the treatment plan either to follow a standard protocol precisely or else to be part of an ongoing clinical research protocol evaluating new treatments. Ad hoc modifications of standard protocols are likely to compromise treatment results.

The choice of treatment approaches was formerly dominated by the local culture in both the university and the practice settings. However, it is now possible to gain access electronically to standard treatment protocols and to every approved clinical research study in North America through a personal computer interface with the Internet.[1]

[1]The National Cancer Institute maintains a database called PDQ (Physician Data Query) that is accessible on the Internet under the name CancerNet at *https://www.cancer.gov/publications/pdq*. Information can be obtained through a facsimile machine using CancerFax by dialing 301-402-5874. Patient information is also provided by the National Cancer Institute in at least three formats: on the Internet via CancerNet at *www.cancer.gov*, through the CancerFax number listed above, or by calling 1-800-4-CANCER. The quality control for the information provided through these services is rigorous.

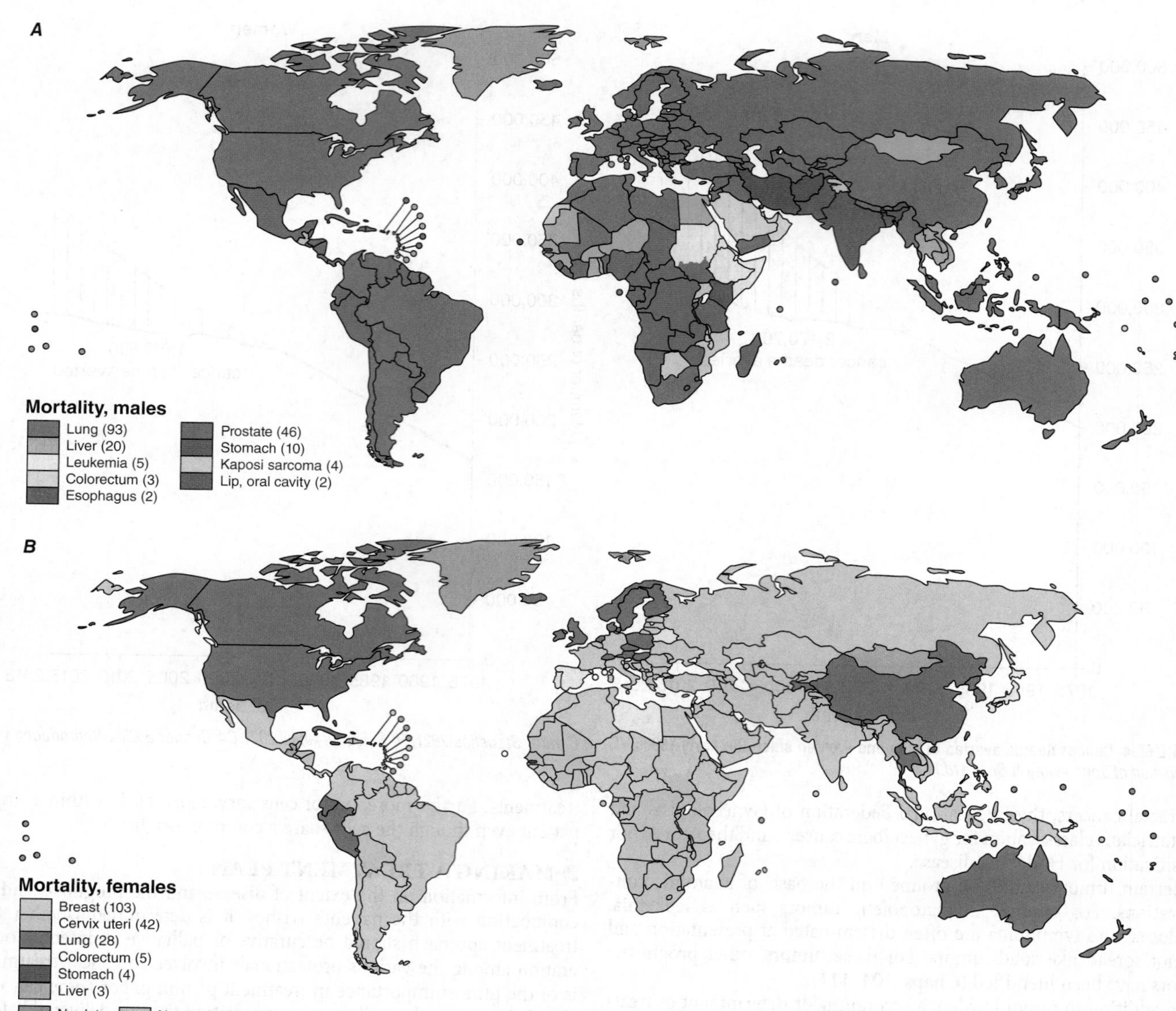

FIGURE 69-5 Global maps showing most common cause of cancer mortality by country in 2018 among (*A*) men and (*B*) women. *(Reproduced with permission from F Bray et al: Global cancer statistics 2018: GLOBOCAN estimates of incidence and mortality worldwide for 36 cancers in 185 countries. CA Cancer J Clin 68:394, 2018. Data source: Globocan 2018. Map production: IARC. World Health Organization. © WHO 2018. All rights reserved.)*

TABLE 69-4 Karnofsky Performance Index

PERFORMANCE STATUS	FUNCTIONAL CAPABILITY OF THE PATIENT
100	Normal; no complaints; no evidence of disease
90	Able to carry on normal activity; minor signs or symptoms of disease
80	Normal activity with effort; some signs or symptoms of disease
70	Cares for self; unable to carry on normal activity or do active work
60	Requires occasional assistance but is able to care for most needs
50	Requires considerable assistance and frequent medical care
40	Disabled; requires special care and assistance
30	Severely disabled; hospitalization is indicated, although death is not imminent
20	Very sick; hospitalization is necessary; active supportive treatment is necessary
10	Moribund, fatal processes progressing rapidly
0	Dead

The skilled physician also has much to offer the patient for whom curative therapy is no longer an option. Often a combination of guilt and frustration over the inability to cure the patient and the pressure of a busy schedule greatly limit the time a physician spends with a patient who is receiving only palliative care. Resist these forces. In addition

TABLE 69-5 The Eastern Cooperative Oncology Group (ECOG) Performance Scale

ECOG grade 0: Fully active, able to carry on all predisease performance without restriction
ECOG grade 1: Restricted in physically strenuous activity but ambulatory and able to carry out work of a light or sedentary nature, e.g., light housework, office work
ECOG grade 2: Ambulatory and capable of all self-care but unable to carry out any work activities. Up and about >50% of waking hours
ECOG grade 3: Capable of only limited self-care, confined to bed or chair >50% of waking hours
ECOG grade 4: Completely disabled. Cannot carry on any self-care. Totally confined to bed or chair
ECOG grade 5: Dead

Source: Reproduced with permission from MM Oken et al: Toxicity and response criteria of the Eastern Cooperative Oncology Group. Am J Clin Oncol 5:649, 1982.

to the medicines administered to alleviate symptoms (see below), it is important to remember the comfort that is provided by holding the patient's hand, continuing regular examinations, and taking time to talk.

MANAGEMENT OF DISEASE AND TREATMENT COMPLICATIONS

Because cancer therapies are toxic (**Chap. 73**), patient management involves addressing complications of both the disease and its treatment as well as the complex psychosocial problems associated with cancer. In the short term during a course of curative therapy, the patient's functional status may decline. Treatment-induced toxicity is less acceptable if the goal of therapy is palliation. The most common side effects of treatment are nausea and vomiting (see below), febrile neutropenia (**Chap. 74**), and myelosuppression (**Chap. 73**). Tools are now available to minimize the acute toxicity of cancer treatment.

New symptoms developing in the course of cancer treatment should always be assumed to be reversible until proven otherwise. The fatalistic attribution of anorexia, weight loss, and jaundice to recurrent or progressive tumor could result in a patient dying from a reversible intercurrent cholecystitis. Intestinal obstruction may be due to reversible adhesions rather than progressive tumor. Systemic infections, sometimes with unusual pathogens, may be a consequence of the immunosuppression associated with cancer therapy. Some drugs used to treat cancer or its complications (e.g., nausea) may produce central nervous system symptoms that look like metastatic disease or may mimic paraneoplastic syndromes such as the syndrome of inappropriate antidiuretic hormone. A definitive diagnosis should be pursued and may even require a repeat biopsy.

A critical component of cancer management is assessing the response to treatment. In addition to a careful physical examination in which all sites of disease are physically measured and recorded in a flow chart by date, response assessment usually requires periodic repeating of imaging tests that were abnormal at the time of staging. If imaging tests have become normal, repeat biopsy of previously involved tissue is performed to document complete response by pathologic criteria. Biopsies are not usually required if there is macroscopic residual disease. A *complete response* is defined as disappearance of all evidence of disease, and a *partial response* as >50% reduction in the sum of the products of the perpendicular diameters of all measurable lesions. The determination of partial response may also be based on a 30% decrease in the sums of the longest diameters of lesions (Response Evaluation Criteria in Solid Tumors [RECIST]). *Progressive disease* is defined as the appearance of any new lesion or an increase of >25% in the sum of the products of the perpendicular diameters of all measurable lesions (or an increase of 20% in the sums of the longest diameters by RECIST). Tumor shrinkage or growth that does not meet any of these criteria is considered *stable disease*. Some sites of involvement (e.g., bone) or patterns of involvement (e.g., lymphangitic lung or diffuse pulmonary infiltrates) are considered unmeasurable. No response is complete without biopsy documentation of their resolution, but partial responses may exclude their assessment unless clear objective progression has occurred.

For some hematologic neoplasms, flow cytometric and genetic assays may determine the presence of residual tumor cells that escape microscopic detection. In general, these techniques can reliably detect as few as 1 tumor cell among 10,000 cells. If such tests do not detect tumor cells, the patient is said to have minimal residual disease negativity, a finding generally associated with more durable remissions. Accumulating data are defining interventions in patients with minimal residual disease positivity that can extend remission duration and survival.

Tumor markers may be useful in patient management in certain tumors. Response to therapy may be difficult to gauge with certainty. However, some tumors produce or elicit the production of markers that can be measured in the serum or urine, and in a particular patient, rising and falling levels of the marker are usually associated with increasing or decreasing tumor burden, respectively. Some clinically useful tumor markers are shown in **Table 69-6**. Tumor markers are not in themselves specific enough to permit a diagnosis of malignancy to be made, but once a malignancy has been diagnosed and shown to be associated with elevated levels of a tumor marker, the marker can be used to assess response to treatment.

TABLE 69-6 Tumor Markers

TUMOR MARKERS	CANCER	NONNEOPLASTIC CONDITIONS
Hormones		
Human chorionic gonadotropin	Gestational trophoblastic disease, gonadal germ cell tumor	Pregnancy
Calcitonin	Medullary cancer of the thyroid	
Catecholamines	Pheochromocytoma	
Oncofetal Antigens		
α Fetoprotein	Hepatocellular carcinoma, gonadal germ cell tumor	Cirrhosis, hepatitis
Carcinoembryonic antigen	Adenocarcinomas of the colon, pancreas, lung, breast, ovary	Pancreatitis, hepatitis, inflammatory bowel disease, smoking
Enzymes		
Prostatic acid phosphatase	Prostate cancer	Prostatitis, prostatic hypertrophy
Neuron-specific enolase	Small-cell cancer of the lung, neuroblastoma	
Lactate dehydrogenase	Lymphoma, Ewing's sarcoma	Hepatitis, hemolytic anemia, many others
Tumor-Associated Proteins		
Prostate-specific antigen	Prostate cancer	Prostatitis, prostatic hypertrophy
Monoclonal immunoglobulin	Myeloma	Infection, MGUS
CA-125	Ovarian cancer, some lymphomas	Menstruation, peritonitis, pregnancy
CA 19-9	Colon, pancreatic, breast cancer	Pancreatitis, ulcerative colitis
CD30	Hodgkin's disease, anaplastic large-cell lymphoma	—
CD25	Hairy cell leukemia, adult T-cell leukemia/lymphoma	Hemophagocytic lymphohistiocytosis

Abbreviation: MGUS, monoclonal gammopathy of uncertain significance.

The recognition and treatment of depression are important components of management. The incidence of depression in cancer patients is ~25% overall and may be greater in patients with greater debility. This diagnosis is likely in a patient with a depressed mood (dysphoria) and/or a loss of interest in pleasure (anhedonia) for at least 2 weeks. In addition, three or more of the following symptoms are usually present: appetite change, sleep problems, psychomotor retardation or agitation, fatigue, feelings of guilt or worthlessness, inability to concentrate, and suicidal ideation. Patients with these symptoms should receive therapy. Medical therapy with a serotonin reuptake inhibitor such as fluoxetine (10–20 mg/d), sertraline (50–150 mg/d), or paroxetine (10–20 mg/d) or a tricyclic antidepressant such as amitriptyline (50–100 mg/d) or desipramine (75–150 mg/d) should be tried, allowing 4–6 weeks for response. Effective therapy should be continued at least 6 months after resolution of symptoms. If therapy is unsuccessful, other classes of antidepressants may be used. In addition to medication, psychosocial interventions such as support groups, psychotherapy, and guided imagery may be of benefit.

Many patients opt for unproven or unsound approaches to treatment when it appears that conventional medicine is unlikely to be curative. Those seeking such alternatives are often well educated and may be early in the course of their disease. Unsound approaches are usually hawked on the basis of unsubstantiated anecdotes and not only cannot help the patient but may be harmful. Physicians should strive to keep communications open and nonjudgmental, so that patients are more likely to discuss with the physician what they are actually doing. The appearance of unexpected toxicity may be an indication that a supplemental therapy is being taken.[2]

LONG-TERM FOLLOW-UP/LATE COMPLICATIONS

At the completion of treatment, sites originally involved with tumor are reassessed, usually by radiography or imaging techniques, and any persistent abnormality is biopsied. If disease persists, the multidisciplinary team discusses a new salvage treatment plan. If the patient has been rendered disease-free by the original treatment, the patient is followed regularly for disease recurrence. The optimal guidelines for follow-up care are not known. For many years, a routine practice has been to follow the patient monthly for 6–12 months, then every other month for a year, every 3 months for a year, every 4 months for a year, every 6 months for a year, and then annually. At each visit, a battery of laboratory and radiographic and imaging tests was obtained on the assumption that it is best to detect recurrent disease before it becomes symptomatic. However, where follow-up procedures have been examined, this assumption has been found to be untrue. Studies of breast cancer, melanoma, lung cancer, colon cancer, and lymphoma have all failed to support the notion that asymptomatic relapses are more readily cured by salvage therapy than symptomatic relapses. In view of the enormous cost of a full battery of diagnostic tests and their manifest lack of impact on survival, new guidelines are emerging for less frequent follow-up visits, during which the history and physical examination are the major investigations performed.

As time passes, the likelihood of recurrence of the primary cancer diminishes. For many types of cancer, survival for 5 years without recurrence is tantamount to cure. However, important medical problems can occur in patients treated for cancer and must be examined (**Chap. 95**). Some problems emerge as a consequence of the disease and some as a consequence of the treatment. An understanding of these disease- and treatment-related problems may help in their detection and management.

Despite these concerns, most patients who are cured of cancer return to normal lives.

■ SUPPORTIVE CARE

In many ways, the success of cancer therapy depends on the success of the supportive care. Failure to control the symptoms of cancer and its treatment may lead patients to abandon curative therapy. Of equal importance, supportive care is a major determinant of quality of life. Even when life cannot be prolonged, the physician must strive to preserve its quality. Quality-of-life measurements have become common endpoints of clinical research studies. Furthermore, palliative care has been shown to be cost-effective when approached in an organized fashion. A credo for oncology could be to cure sometimes, to extend life often, and to comfort always.

Pain Pain occurs with variable frequency in the cancer patient: 25–50% of patients present with pain at diagnosis, 33% have pain associated with treatment, and 75% have pain with progressive disease. The pain may have several causes. In ~70% of cases, pain is caused by the tumor itself—by invasion of bone, nerves, blood vessels, or mucous membranes or obstruction of a hollow viscus or duct. In ~20% of cases, pain is related to a surgical or invasive medical procedure, to radiation injury (mucositis, enteritis, or plexus, or spinal cord injury), or to chemotherapy injury (mucositis, peripheral neuropathy, phlebitis, steroid-induced aseptic necrosis of the femoral head). In 10% of cases, pain is unrelated to cancer or its treatment.

Assessment of pain requires the methodical investigation of the history of the pain, its location, character, temporal features, provocative and palliative factors, and intensity (**Chaps. 12 and 13**); a review of the oncologic history and past medical history as well as personal and social history; and a thorough physical examination. The patient should be given a 10-division visual analogue scale on which to indicate the severity of the pain. The clinical condition is often dynamic, making it necessary to reassess the patient frequently. Pain therapy should not be withheld while the cause of pain is being sought.

A variety of tools are available with which to address cancer pain. About 85% of patients will have pain relief from pharmacologic intervention. However, other modalities, including antitumor therapy (such as surgical relief of obstruction, radiation therapy, and strontium-89 or samarium-153 treatment for bone pain), neurostimulatory techniques, regional analgesia, or neuroablative procedures, are effective in an additional 12% or so. Thus, very few patients will have inadequate pain relief if appropriate measures are taken. **A specific approach to pain relief is detailed in Chap. 12.**

Nausea Emesis in the cancer patient is usually caused by chemotherapy (**Chap. 73**). Its severity can be predicted from the drugs used to treat the cancer. Three forms of emesis are recognized on the basis of their timing with regard to the noxious insult. *Acute emesis*, the most common variety, occurs within 24 h of treatment. *Delayed emesis* occurs 1–7 days after treatment; it is rare, but, when present, usually follows cisplatin administration. *Anticipatory emesis* occurs before administration of chemotherapy and represents a conditioned response to visual and olfactory stimuli previously associated with chemotherapy delivery.

Acute emesis is the best understood form. Stimuli that activate signals in the chemoreceptor trigger zone in the medulla, the cerebral cortex, and peripherally in the intestinal tract lead to stimulation of the vomiting center in the medulla, the motor center responsible for coordinating the secretory and muscle contraction activity that leads to emesis. Diverse receptor types participate in the process, including dopamine, serotonin, histamine, opioid, and acetylcholine receptors. The serotonin receptor antagonists ondansetron and granisetron are effective drugs against highly emetogenic agents, as are neurokinin receptor antagonists such as aprepitant and fosaprepitant (see **Chap. 73**).

As with the analgesia ladder, emesis therapy should be tailored to the situation. For mildly and moderately emetogenic agents, prochlorperazine, 5–10 mg PO or 25 mg PR, is effective. Its efficacy may be enhanced by administering the drug before the chemotherapy is delivered. Dexamethasone, 10–20 mg IV, is also effective and may enhance the efficacy of prochlorperazine. For highly emetogenic agents such as cisplatin, mechlorethamine, dacarbazine, and streptozocin, combinations of agents work best and administration should begin 6–24 h before treatment. Ondansetron, 8 mg PO every 6 h the day before therapy and IV on the day of therapy, plus dexamethasone, 20 mg IV before treatment, is an effective regimen. Addition of oral aprepitant (a substance P/neurokinin 1 receptor antagonist) to this regimen (125 mg on day 1, 80 mg on days 2 and 3) further decreases the risk of both acute and delayed vomiting. Like pain, emesis is easier to prevent than to alleviate.

Delayed emesis may be related to bowel inflammation from the therapy and can be controlled with oral dexamethasone and oral metoclopramide, a dopamine receptor antagonist that also blocks serotonin receptors at high dosages. The best strategy for preventing anticipatory emesis is to control emesis in the early cycles of therapy to prevent the conditioning from taking place. If this is unsuccessful, prophylactic antiemetics the day before treatment may help. Experimental studies are evaluating behavior modification.

Effusions Fluid may accumulate abnormally in the pleural cavity, pericardium, or peritoneum. Asymptomatic malignant effusions may not require treatment. Symptomatic effusions occurring in tumors responsive to systemic therapy usually do not require local treatment

[2]Information about unsound methods may be obtained from the National Council Against Health Fraud, Box 1276, Loma Linda, CA 92354, or from the Center for Medical Consumers and Health Care Information, 237 Thompson Street, New York, NY 10012.

but respond to the treatment for the underlying tumor. Symptomatic effusions occurring in tumors unresponsive to systemic therapy may require local treatment in patients with a life expectancy of at least 6 months.

Pleural effusions due to tumors may or may not contain malignant cells. Lung cancer, breast cancer, and lymphomas account for ~75% of malignant pleural effusions. Their exudative nature is usually gauged by an effusion/serum protein ratio of ≥0.5 or an effusion/serum lactate dehydrogenase ratio of ≥0.6. When the condition is symptomatic, thoracentesis is usually performed first. In most cases, symptomatic improvement occurs for <1 month. Chest tube drainage is required if symptoms recur within 2 weeks. Fluid is aspirated until the flow rate is <100 mL in 24 h. Then either 60 units of bleomycin or 1 g of doxycycline is infused into the chest tube in 50 mL of 5% dextrose in water; the tube is clamped; the patient is rotated on four sides, spending 15 min in each position; and, after 1–2 h, the tube is again attached to suction for another 24 h. The tube is then disconnected from suction and allowed to drain by gravity. If <100 mL drains over the next 24 h, the chest tube is pulled, and a radiograph is taken 24 h later. If the chest tube continues to drain fluid at an unacceptably high rate, sclerosis can be repeated. Bleomycin may be somewhat more effective than doxycycline but is very expensive. Doxycycline is usually the drug of first choice. If neither doxycycline nor bleomycin is effective, talc can be used.

Symptomatic pericardial effusions are usually treated by creating a pericardial window or by stripping the pericardium. If the patient's condition does not permit a surgical procedure, sclerosis can be attempted with doxycycline and/or bleomycin.

Malignant ascites is usually treated with repeated paracentesis of small volumes of fluid. If the underlying malignancy is unresponsive to systemic therapy, peritoneovenous shunts may be inserted. Despite the fear of disseminating tumor cells into the circulation, widespread metastases are an unusual complication. The major complications are occlusion, leakage, and fluid overload. Patients with severe liver disease may develop disseminated intravascular coagulation.

Nutrition Cancer and its treatment may lead to a decrease in nutrient intake of sufficient magnitude to cause weight loss and alteration of intermediary metabolism. The prevalence of this problem is difficult to estimate because of variations in the definition of cancer cachexia, but most patients with advanced cancer experience weight loss and decreased appetite. A variety of both tumor-derived factors (e.g., bombesin, adrenocorticotropic hormone) and host-derived factors (e.g., tumor necrosis factor, interleukins 1 and 6, growth hormone) contribute to the altered metabolism, and a vicious cycle is established in which protein catabolism, glucose intolerance, and lipolysis cannot be reversed by the provision of calories.

It remains controversial how to assess nutritional status and when and how to intervene. Efforts to make the assessment objective have included the use of a prognostic nutritional index based on albumin levels, triceps skinfold thickness, transferrin levels, and delayed-type hypersensitivity skin testing. However, a simpler approach has been to define the threshold for nutritional intervention as <10% unexplained body weight loss, serum transferrin level <1500 mg/L (150 mg/dL), and serum albumin <34 g/L (3.4 g/dL).

The decision is important, because it appears that cancer therapy is substantially more toxic and less effective in the face of malnutrition. Nevertheless, it remains unclear whether nutritional intervention can alter the natural history. Unless some pathology is affecting the absorptive function of the gastrointestinal tract, enteral nutrition provided orally or by tube feeding is preferred over parenteral supplementation. However, the risks associated with the tube may outweigh the benefits. Megestrol acetate, a progestational agent, has been advocated as a pharmacologic intervention to improve nutritional status. Research in this area may provide more tools in the future as cytokine-mediated mechanisms are further elucidated.

Psychosocial Support The psychosocial needs of patients vary with their situation. Patients undergoing treatment experience fear, anxiety, and depression. Self-image is often seriously compromised by deforming surgery and loss of hair. Women who receive cosmetic advice that enables them to look better also feel better. Loss of control over how one spends time can contribute to the sense of vulnerability. Juggling the demands of work and family with the demands of treatment may create enormous stresses. Sexual dysfunction is highly prevalent and needs to be discussed openly with the patient. An empathetic health care team is sensitive to the individual patient's needs and permits negotiation where such flexibility will not adversely affect the course of treatment.

Cancer survivors have other sets of difficulties. Patients may have fears associated with the termination of a treatment they associate with their continued survival. Adjustments are required to physical losses and handicaps, real and perceived. Patients may be preoccupied with minor physical problems. They perceive a decline in their job mobility and view themselves as less desirable workers. They may be victims of job and/or insurance discrimination. Patients may experience difficulty reentering their normal past life. They may feel guilty for having survived and may carry a sense of vulnerability to colds and other illnesses. Perhaps the most pervasive and threatening concern is the ever-present fear of relapse (the Damocles syndrome).

Patients in whom therapy has been unsuccessful have other problems related to the end of life.

Death and Dying The most common causes of death in patients with cancer are infection (leading to circulatory failure), respiratory failure, hepatic failure, and renal failure. Intestinal blockage may lead to inanition and starvation. Central nervous system disease may lead to seizures, coma, and central hypoventilation. About 70% of patients develop dyspnea preterminally. However, many months usually pass between the diagnosis of cancer and the occurrence of these complications, and during this period, the patient is severely affected by the possibility of death. The path of unsuccessful cancer treatment usually occurs in three phases. First, there is optimism at the hope of cure; when the tumor recurs, there is the acknowledgment of an incurable disease, and the goal of palliative therapy is embraced in the hope of being able to live with disease; finally, at the disclosure of imminent death, another adjustment in outlook takes place. The patient imagines the worst in preparation for the end of life and may go through stages of adjustment to the diagnosis. These stages include denial, isolation, anger, bargaining, depression, acceptance, and hope. Of course, patients do not all progress through all the stages or proceed through them in the same order or at the same rate. Nevertheless, developing an understanding of how the patient has been affected by the diagnosis and is coping with it is an important goal of patient management.

It is best to speak frankly with the patient and the family regarding the likely course of disease. These discussions can be difficult for the physician as well as for the patient and family. The critical features of the interaction are to reassure the patient and family that everything that can be done to provide comfort will be done. They will not be abandoned. Many patients prefer to be cared for in their homes or in a hospice setting rather than a hospital. The American College of Physicians has published a book called *Home Care Guide for Cancer: How to Care for Family and Friends at Home* that teaches an approach to successful problem-solving in home care. With appropriate planning, it should be possible to provide the patient with the necessary medical care as well as the psychological and spiritual support that will prevent the isolation and depersonalization that can attend in-hospital death.

The care of dying patients may take a toll on the physician. A "burnout" syndrome has been described that is characterized by fatigue, disengagement from patients and colleagues, and a loss of self-fulfillment. Efforts at stress reduction, maintenance of a balanced life, and setting realistic goals may combat this disorder.

End-of-Life Decisions Unfortunately, a smooth transition in treatment goals from curative to palliative may not be possible in all cases because of the occurrence of serious treatment-related complications or rapid disease progression. Vigorous and invasive medical support for a reversible disease or treatment complication is assumed to be justified. However, if the reversibility of the condition is in doubt, the patient's wishes determine the level of medical care. These wishes should be elicited before the terminal phase of illness and reviewed periodically. Information about advance directives can be obtained from the American Association of Retired Persons, 601 E Street, NW, Washington, DC 20049, 202-434-2277, or Choice in Dying, 250 West 57th Street, New York, NY 10107, 212-366-5540. Some states allow physicians to assist patients who choose to end their lives. This subject is challenging from an ethical and a medical point of view. Discussions of end-of-life decisions should be candid and involve clear informed consent, waiting periods, second opinions, and documentation. **A full discussion of end-of-life management is provided in Chap. 12.**

■ FURTHER READING

BRAY F et al: Global cancer statistics 2018: GLOBOCAN estimates of incidence and mortality worldwide for 36 cancers in 185 countries. CA Cancer J Clin 68:394, 2018.

HESKETH PJ et al: Antiemetics: ASCO guideline update. J Clin Oncol 38:2782, 2020.

KELLEY AS, MORRISON RS: Palliative care for the seriously ill. N Engl J Med 373:747, 2015.

SAMALA RV et al: Frequently asked questions about managing cancer pain: An update. Cleve Clin Med J 88:183, 2021.

SIEGEL RL et al: Cancer statistics, 2021. CA Cancer J Clin 71:7, 2021.

70 Prevention and Early Detection of Cancer

Jennifer M. Croswell, Otis W. Brawley, Barnett S. Kramer

Improved understanding of carcinogenesis has allowed cancer prevention and early detection to expand beyond identification and avoidance of carcinogens. Specific interventions to reduce cancer mortality by preventing cancer in those at risk and effective screening for early detection of cancer are the goals.

Carcinogenesis is a process that usually extends over years, a continuum of discrete tissue and cellular changes over time resulting in aberrant physiologic processes. Prevention concerns the identification and manipulation of the biologic, environmental, social, and genetic factors in the causal pathway of cancer. Examination of national epidemiologic patterns can provide indicators of the relative contributions of advances in prevention, screening, and therapy in progress against cancer, but randomized trials provide the best evidence to guide practice, especially in the healthy general population.

EDUCATION AND HEALTHFUL HABITS

Public education on the avoidance of identified risk factors for cancer and encouraging healthy habits contributes to cancer prevention. The clinician is a powerful messenger in this process. The patient-provider encounter provides an opportunity to teach patients about the hazards of smoking, influence of a healthy lifestyle and other exposures, and use of proven cancer screening methods.

■ SMOKING CESSATION

Tobacco smoking is a strong, modifiable risk factor for cardiovascular disease, pulmonary disease, and cancer. Smokers have an ~1 in 3 lifetime risk of dying prematurely from a tobacco-related cancer, cardiovascular, or pulmonary disease. Tobacco use causes more deaths from cardiovascular disease than from cancer. Lung cancer and cancers of the larynx, oropharynx, esophagus, kidney, bladder, colon, pancreas, stomach, and uterine cervix are all tobacco related.

The number of cigarettes smoked per day and the level of inhalation of cigarette smoke are correlated with risk of lung cancer mortality. Light- and low-tar cigarettes are not safer because smokers tend to inhale them more frequently and deeply.

Those who stop smoking have a 30–50% lower 10-year lung cancer mortality rate compared to those who continue smoking, despite the fact that some carcinogen-induced gene mutations persist for years after smoking cessation. Smoking cessation and avoidance would save more lives than any other public health activity.

The risk of tobacco smoke is not limited to the smoker. Environmental tobacco smoke, known as secondhand or passive smoke, is carcinogenic and associated with a variety of respiratory illnesses in exposed children.

Tobacco use prevention is a pediatric issue. More than 80% of adult American smokers began smoking before the age of 18 years. Cigarette smoking has been declining in recent years, but in recent surveys, about 8% of high school students reported smoking within the prior month. Electronic cigarettes, on the other hand, are rapidly increasing in use: approximately 28% of high school students and 11% of middle school students are current electronic cigarette users. Counseling of adolescents and young adults is critical to prevent all forms of tobacco use. A clinician's simple advice can be of benefit. Providers should query patients on tobacco use and offer smokers assistance in quitting.

Current approaches to smoking cessation recognize nicotine in tobacco as addicting **(Chap. 454)**. The smoker who is quitting goes through identifiable stages, including contemplation of quitting, an action phase in which the smoker quits, and a maintenance phase. Smokers who quit completely are more likely to be successful than those who gradually reduce the number of cigarettes smoked or change to lower-tar or lower-nicotine cigarettes. Organized cessation programs may help individual efforts. Heavy smokers may need an intensive broad-based cessation program that includes counseling, behavioral strategies, and pharmacologic adjuncts, such as nicotine replacement (gum, patches, sprays, lozenges, and inhalers), bupropion, and/or varenicline. Electronic cigarettes have been advocated as a tool to achieve smoking cessation in adults, but it is not known how effective electronic cigarettes are for this purpose. The net effects of electronic cigarettes on health are poorly studied. Absence of strict manufacturing controls of vaping material has produced serious injury.

The health risks of cigars are similar to those of cigarettes. Smoking one or two cigars daily doubles the risk for oral and esophageal cancers; smoking three or four cigars daily increases the risk of oral cancers more than eightfold and esophageal cancer fourfold. The risks of occasional use are unknown.

Smokeless tobacco also represents a substantial health risk. Chewing tobacco is a carcinogen linked to dental caries, gingivitis, oral leukoplakia, and oral cancer. The systemic effects of smokeless tobacco (including snuff) may increase risks for other cancers. Esophageal cancer is linked to carcinogens in tobacco dissolved in saliva and swallowed. The net effects of e-cigarettes on health are poorly studied.

■ PHYSICAL ACTIVITY

Physical activity is associated with a decreased risk of colon and breast cancer. A variety of mechanisms have been proposed. However, such studies are prone to confounding factors such as recall bias, association of exercise with other health-related practices, and effects of preclinical cancers on exercise habits (reverse causality).

■ DIET MODIFICATION

International epidemiologic studies suggest that diets high in fat are associated with increased risk for cancers of the breast, colon, prostate, and endometrium. Despite correlations, dietary fat has not been proven to cause cancer. Case-control and cohort epidemiologic studies give conflicting results. Diet is a highly complex exposure to many nutrients and chemicals. Low-fat diets are associated with many dietary changes beyond simple subtraction of fat. Other lifestyle factors are also associated with adherence to a low-fat diet.

In some observational studies, dietary fiber has been associated with a reduced risk of colonic polyps and invasive cancer of the colon.

Two large prospective cohort studies of >100,000 health professionals showed no association between fruit and vegetable intake and risk of cancer, however. Cancer-protective effects of increasing fiber and lowering dietary fat have not been shown in the context of a prospective clinical trial. The Polyp Prevention Trial randomly assigned 2000 elderly persons, who had polyps removed, to a low-fat, high-fiber diet versus routine diet for 4 years. No differences were noted in polyp formation.

The U.S. National Institutes of Health Women's Health Initiative, launched in 1994, was a long-term clinical trial enrolling >100,000 women age 45–69 years. It placed women into 22 intervention groups. Participants received calcium/vitamin D supplementation; hormone replacement therapy; and counseling to increase exercise, eat a low-fat diet with increased consumption of fruits, vegetables, and fiber, and cease smoking. The study showed that although dietary fat intake was lower in the diet intervention group, invasive breast cancers were not reduced over an 8-year follow-up period compared to the control group. Additionally, no reduction was seen in the incidence of colorectal cancer in the dietary intervention arm. In the aggregate, cohort studies and randomized trials suggest that reduction of red meat or processed meat consumption has a small (if any) effect on cancer incidence and mortality, although the overall evidence base is weak. Evidence does not currently establish the anticarcinogenic value of vitamin, mineral, or nutritional supplements in amounts greater than those provided by a balanced diet.

■ ENERGY BALANCE

Risk of certain cancers appears to increase modestly (relative risks generally in the 1.0–2.0 range) as body mass index (BMI) increases beyond 25 kg/m^2. A cohort study of >5 million adults included in the U.K. Clinical Practice Research Datalink (a primary care database) found that each 5 kg/m^2 increase in BMI was linearly associated with cancers of the uterus, gallbladder, kidney, cervix, thyroid, and leukemia. High BMI appears to have an inverse association with prostate and premenopausal breast cancer.

■ SUN AVOIDANCE

Nonmelanoma skin cancers (basal cell and squamous cell) are induced by cumulative exposure to ultraviolet (UV) radiation. Sunburns, especially in childhood and adolescence, may be associated with an increased risk of melanoma in adulthood. Reduction of sun exposure through use of protective clothing and changing patterns of outdoor activities can reduce skin cancer risk. Sunscreens decrease the risk of actinic keratoses, the precursor to squamous cell skin cancer, but melanoma risk may not be reduced. Sunscreens prevent burning, but they may encourage more prolonged exposure to the sun and may not filter out wavelengths of energy that cause melanoma.

Appearance-focused behavioral interventions in young women can decrease indoor tanning use and other UV exposures and may be more effective than messages about long-term cancer risks. Those who recognize themselves as being at risk tend to be more compliant with sun-avoidance recommendations. Risk factors for melanoma include a propensity to sunburn, a large number of benign melanocytic nevi, and atypical nevi.

CANCER CHEMOPREVENTION

Chemoprevention involves the use of specific natural or synthetic chemical agents to reverse, suppress, or prevent carcinogenesis before the development of invasive malignancy.

Cancer develops through an accumulation of tissue abnormalities associated with genetic and epigenetic changes, and growth regulatory pathways that are potential points of intervention to prevent cancer. The initial changes are termed *initiation*. The alteration can be inherited or acquired through the action of physical, infectious, or chemical carcinogens. Like most human diseases, cancer arises from an interaction between genetics and environmental exposures (**Table 70-1**). Influences that cause the initiated cell and its surrounding tissue microenvironment to progress through the carcinogenic process and change phenotypically are termed *promoters*. Promoters include hormones such as androgens, linked to prostate cancer, and estrogen, linked to breast and endometrial cancer. The difference between an initiator and promoter is indistinct; some components of cigarette smoke are "complete carcinogens," acting as both initiators and promoters. Cancer can be prevented or controlled through interference with the factors that cause cancer initiation, promotion, or progression. Compounds of interest in chemoprevention often have antimutagenic, hormone modulation, anti-inflammatory, antiproliferative, or proapoptotic activity (or a combination).

TABLE 70-1 Suspected Carcinogens

CARCINOGENS[a]	ASSOCIATED CANCER OR NEOPLASM
Alkylating agents	Acute myeloid leukemia, bladder cancer
Androgens	Prostate cancer
Aromatic amines (dyes)	Bladder cancer
Arsenic	Cancer of the lung, skin
Asbestos	Cancer of the lung, pleura, peritoneum
Benzene	Acute myelocytic leukemia
Chromium	Lung cancer
Diethylstilbestrol (prenatal)	Vaginal cancer (clear cell)
Epstein-Barr virus	Burkitt's lymphoma, nasal T-cell lymphoma
Estrogens	Cancer of the endometrium, liver, breast
Ethyl alcohol	Cancer of the breast, liver, esophagus, head and neck
Helicobacter pylori	Gastric cancer, gastric mucosa-associate lymphoid tissue (MALT) lymphoma
Hepatitis B or C virus	Liver cancer
Human immunodeficiency virus	Non-Hodgkin's lymphoma, Kaposi's sarcoma, squamous cell carcinomas (especially of the urogenital tract)
Human papillomavirus	Cancers of the cervix, anus, oropharynx
Human T-cell lymphotropic virus type 1 (HTLV-1)	Adult T-cell leukemia/lymphoma
Immunosuppressive agents (azathioprine, cyclosporine, glucocorticoids)	Non-Hodgkin's lymphoma
Ionizing radiation (therapeutic or diagnostic)	Breast, bladder, thyroid, soft tissue, bone, hematopoietic, and many more
Nitrogen mustard gas	Cancer of the lung, head and neck, nasal sinuses
Nickel dust	Cancer of the lung, nasal sinuses
Diesel exhaust	Lung cancer (miners)
Phenacetin	Cancer of the renal pelvis and bladder
Polycyclic hydrocarbons	Cancer of the lung, skin (especially squamous cell carcinoma of scrotal skin)
Radon gas	Lung cancer
Schistosomiasis	Bladder cancer (squamous cell)
Sunlight (ultraviolet)	Skin cancer (squamous cell and melanoma)
Tobacco (including smokeless)	Cancer of the upper aerodigestive tract, bladder
Vinyl chloride	Liver cancer (angiosarcoma)

[a]Agents that are thought to act as cancer initiators and/or promoters.

■ CHEMOPREVENTION OF CANCERS OF THE UPPER AERODIGESTIVE TRACT

Smoking causes diffuse epithelial injury in the oral cavity, neck, esophagus, and lung. Patients cured of squamous cell cancers of the lung, esophagus, oral cavity, and neck are at risk (as high as 5% per year) of developing second cancers of the upper aerodigestive tract. Cessation of cigarette smoking does not markedly decrease the cured cancer patient's risk of second malignancy, even though it does lower the cancer risk in those who have never developed a malignancy. Smoking cessation may halt the early stages of the carcinogenic process (such as metaplasia), but it may have no effect on late stages of carcinogenesis.

This "field carcinogenesis" hypothesis for upper aerodigestive tract cancer has made "cured" patients an important population for chemoprevention of second malignancies.

Persistent oral human papillomavirus (HPV) infection, particularly HPV-16, increases the risk for cancers of the oropharynx. This association exists even in the absence of other risk factors such as smoking or alcohol use (although the magnitude of increased risk appears greater than additive when HPV infection and smoking are both present). Oral HPV infection is believed to be largely sexually acquired. Although the evidence is not definitive, the use of the HPV vaccine is associated with a reduction in prevalence of oropharyngeal infection rates and may eventually reduce oropharyngeal cancer rates (unlike cancers of the cervix, no precursor lesion for oropharyngeal tumors is known).

Oral leukoplakia, a premalignant lesion commonly found in smokers, has been used as an intermediate marker of chemopreventive activity in smaller shorter-duration, randomized, placebo-controlled trials. Although therapy with high, relatively toxic doses of isotretinoin (13-*cis*-retinoic acid) causes regression of oral leukoplakia, more tolerable doses of isotretinoin have not shown benefit in the prevention of head and neck cancer.

Several large-scale trials have assessed agents in the chemoprevention of lung cancer in patients at high risk. In the α-tocopherol/β-carotene (ATBC) Lung Cancer Prevention Trial, participants were male smokers, age 50–69 years at entry. Participants had smoked an average of one pack of cigarettes per day for nearly 36 years. Participants received α-tocopherol, β-carotene, and/or placebo in a randomized, two-by-two factorial design. After median follow-up of 6 years, lung cancer incidence and mortality were statistically significantly increased in those receiving β-carotene. α-Tocopherol had no effect on lung cancer mortality. However, patients receiving α-tocopherol had a higher incidence of hemorrhagic stroke.

The β-Carotene and Retinol Efficacy Trial (CARET) involved 17,000 American smokers and workers with asbestos exposure. Entrants were randomly assigned to one of four arms and received β-carotene, retinol, and/or placebo in a two-by-two factorial design. This trial also demonstrated harm from β-carotene: a lung cancer rate of 5 per 1000 subjects per year for those taking placebo versus 6 per 1000 subjects per year for those taking β-carotene.

The ATBC and CARET results demonstrate the importance of testing chemoprevention hypotheses thoroughly before widespread implementation because the results contradict a number of observational studies.

CHEMOPREVENTION OF COLON CANCER

Many colon cancer prevention trials are based on the premise that most colorectal cancers develop from adenomatous polyps. These trials use adenoma recurrence or disappearance as a surrogate endpoint (not yet validated) for colon cancer prevention. Clinical trial results suggest that nonsteroidal anti-inflammatory drugs (NSAIDs), such as piroxicam, sulindac, and aspirin, may prevent adenoma formation or cause regression of adenomatous polyps. The mechanism of action of NSAIDs is unknown, but they are presumed to work through the cyclooxygenase pathway. A meta-analysis of four randomized controlled trials (albeit primarily designed to examine aspirin's effects on cardiovascular events) found that aspirin at doses of at least 75 mg/d resulted in a 33% relative reduction in colorectal cancer incidence after 20 years, with no clear increase in efficacy at higher doses. Based on a systematic review of evidence from randomized trials for primary prevention of cardiovascular disease, the U.S. Preventive Services Task Force concluded that the balance of benefits and harms favored initiating low-dose aspirin for colorectal cancer and cardiovascular disease prevention in adults age 50–59 if they have a 10% or greater 10-year risk of cardiovascular disease. Low-dose aspirin does not appear to benefit the elderly, however. The ASPREE trial, which compared 100 mg of daily aspirin to placebo for improvement in the composite endpoint of death, dementia, or survival in the healthy elderly, was stopped because of a lack of benefit, including cancer. Cyclooxygenase-2 (COX-2) inhibitors have been considered for colorectal cancer and polyp prevention. Trials with COX-2 inhibitors were initiated, but an increased risk of cardiovascular events in those taking the COX-2 inhibitors was noted, suggesting that these agents are not suitable for chemoprevention in the general population.

The Women's Health Initiative demonstrated that postmenopausal women taking estrogen plus progestin have a 44% lower relative risk of colorectal cancer compared to women taking placebo. Of >16,600 women randomized and followed for a median of 5.6 years, 43 invasive colorectal cancers occurred in the hormone group and 72 in the placebo group. The positive effect on colon cancer is mitigated by the modest increase in cardiovascular and breast cancer risks associated with combined estrogen plus progestin therapy.

Most case-control and cohort studies have not confirmed early reports of an association between regular statin use and a reduced risk of colorectal cancer. No randomized controlled trials have addressed this hypothesis. A meta-analysis of statin use showed no protective effect of statins on overall cancer incidence or death.

CHEMOPREVENTION OF BREAST CANCER

Tamoxifen is an antiestrogen with partial estrogen agonistic activity in some tissues, such as endometrium and bone. One of its actions is to upregulate transforming growth factor β, which decreases breast cell proliferation. In a randomized placebo-controlled prevention trial involving >13,000 pre- and postmenopausal women at high risk, tamoxifen decreased the risk of developing breast cancer by 49% (from 43.4 to 22 per 1000 women) after a median follow-up of nearly 6 years. Tamoxifen also reduced bone fractures; a small increase in risk of endometrial cancer, stroke, pulmonary emboli, and deep vein thrombosis was noted. The International Breast Cancer Intervention Study (IBIS-I) and the Italian Randomized Tamoxifen Prevention Trial also demonstrated a reduction in breast cancer incidence with tamoxifen use. A trial comparing tamoxifen with another selective estrogen receptor modulator, raloxifene, performed in postmenopausal women showed that raloxifene is comparable to tamoxifen in cancer prevention, but without the risk of endometrial cancer. Raloxifene was associated with a smaller reduction in invasive breast cancers and a trend toward more noninvasive breast cancers, but fewer thromboembolic events than tamoxifen; the drugs are similar in risks of other cancers, fractures, ischemic heart disease, and stroke. Both tamoxifen and raloxifene (the latter for postmenopausal women only) have been approved by the U.S. Food and Drug Administration (FDA) for reduction of breast cancer in women at high risk for the disease (1.66% risk at 5 years based on the Gail risk model: *http://www.cancer.gov/bcrisktool/*).

Because the aromatase inhibitors are even more effective than tamoxifen in adjuvant breast cancer therapy, it has been hypothesized that they would be more effective in breast cancer prevention. A randomized, placebo-controlled trial of exemestane reported a 65% relative reduction (from 5.5 to 1.9 per 1000 women) in the incidence of invasive breast cancer in women at elevated risk after a median follow-up of about 3 years. Common adverse effects included arthralgias, hot flashes, fatigue, and insomnia. No trial has directly compared aromatase inhibitors with selective estrogen receptor modulators for breast cancer chemoprevention.

CHEMOPREVENTION OF PROSTATE CANCER

Finasteride and dutasteride are 5-α-reductase inhibitors. They inhibit conversion of testosterone to dihydrotestosterone (DHT), a potent stimulator of prostate cell proliferation. The Prostate Cancer Prevention Trial (PCPT) randomly assigned men age 55 years or older at average risk of prostate cancer to finasteride or placebo. All men in the trial were being regularly screened with prostate-specific antigen (PSA) levels and digital rectal examination. After 7 years of therapy, the incidence of prostate cancer was 18.4% in the finasteride arm, compared with 24.4% in the placebo arm, a statistically significant difference. However, the finasteride group had more patients with tumors of Gleason score 7 and higher compared with the placebo arm (6.4 vs 5.1%). Long-term (10–15 years) follow-up did not reveal any statistically significant differences in overall or prostate cancer-specific mortality between all men in the finasteride and placebo arms or in men diagnosed with prostate cancer, but the power to detect a difference was limited.

Dutasteride has also been evaluated as a preventive agent for prostate cancer. The Reduction by Dutasteride of Prostate Cancer Events (REDUCE) trial was a randomized double-blind trial in which ~8200 men with an elevated PSA (2.5–10 ng/mL for men age 50–60 years and 3–10 ng/mL for men age 60 years or older) and negative prostate biopsy on enrollment received daily 0.5 mg of dutasteride or placebo. The trial found a statistically significant 23% relative risk reduction in the incidence of biopsy-detected prostate cancer in the dutasteride arm at 4 years of treatment (659 cases vs 858 cases, respectively). Overall, across years 1 through 4, no difference was seen between the arms in the number of tumors with a Gleason score of 7 to 10; however, during years 3 and 4, there was a statistically significant difference in tumors with Gleason score of 8 to 10 in the dutasteride arm (12 tumors vs 1 tumor, respectively).

The clinical importance of the apparent increased incidence of higher-grade tumors in the 5-α-reductase inhibitor arms of these trials likely represents an increased sensitivity of PSA and digital rectal exam for high-grade tumors in men receiving these agents due to a decrease in prostatic volume. Although the FDA acknowledged that detection bias may have accounted for the finding, a causative role for 5-α-reductase inhibitors could not be conclusively dismissed. These agents are therefore not FDA-approved for prostate cancer prevention.

Because all men in both the PCPT and REDUCE trials were being screened and because screening approximately doubles the rate of prostate cancer, it is not known if finasteride or dutasteride decreases the risk of prostate cancer in men who are not being screened or simply reduces the risk of non-life-threatening cancers detectable by screening.

Several favorable laboratory and observational studies led to the formal evaluation of selenium and α-tocopherol (vitamin E) as potential prostate cancer preventives. The Selenium and Vitamin E Cancer Prevention Trial (SELECT) assigned 35,533 men to receive 200 μg/d selenium, 400 IU/d α-tocopherol, selenium plus vitamin E, or placebo. After a median follow-up of 7 years, a trend toward an increased risk of developing prostate cancer was observed for men taking vitamin E alone as compared to the placebo arm (hazard ratio 1.17; 95% confidence interval, 1.004–1.36).

VACCINES AND CANCER PREVENTION

A number of infectious agents cause cancer. Hepatitis B and C are linked to liver cancer; some HPV strains are linked to cervical, anal, and head and neck cancer; and *Helicobacter pylori* is associated with gastric adenocarcinoma and gastric lymphoma. Vaccines to protect against these agents may therefore reduce the risk of their associated cancers.

The hepatitis B vaccine is effective in preventing hepatitis and hepatomas due to chronic hepatitis B infection.

A nonavalent vaccine (covering HPV strains 6, 11, 16, 18, 31, 33, 45, 52, and 58) is available for use in the United States. HPV types 6 and 11 cause genital papillomas. The remaining HPV types cause cervical and anal cancer; reduction in HPV types 16 and 18 alone could prevent >70% of cervical cancers worldwide. For individuals not previously infected with these HPV strains, the vaccine demonstrates high efficacy in preventing persistent strain-specific HPV infections. Studies also confirm the vaccine's ability to prevent preneoplastic lesions (cervical or anal intraepithelial neoplasia [CIN/AIN] I, II, and III). The durability of the immune response beyond 10–12 years is not currently known. The vaccine does not appear to impact preexisting infections. A two-dose schedule is currently recommended in the United States for females and males age 9–14 years; teens and young adults who start the series between 15 and 26 years are recommended to receive three doses of the vaccine. However, observational studies suggest similar efficacy with a single dose in young girls, and a large randomized trial is currently comparing one to two doses.

SURGICAL PREVENTION OF CANCER

Some organs in some individuals are at such high risk of developing cancer that surgical removal of the organ at risk may be considered. Women with severe cervical dysplasia are treated with laser or loop electrosurgical excision or conization. Colectomy may be used to prevent colon cancer in patients with familial polyposis or ulcerative colitis.

Prophylactic bilateral mastectomy may be chosen for breast cancer prevention among women with genetic predisposition to breast cancer. In a prospective series of 139 women with *BRCA1* and *BRCA2* mutations, 76 chose to undergo prophylactic mastectomy, and 63 chose close surveillance. At 3 years, no cases of breast cancer had been diagnosed in those opting for surgery, but eight patients in the surveillance group had developed breast cancer. A larger (n = 639) retrospective cohort study reported that three patients developed breast cancer after prophylactic mastectomy compared with an expected incidence of 30–53 cases. Postmastectomy breast cancer–related deaths were 81–94% lower in high-risk women compared with sister controls and 100% lower in moderate-risk women when compared with expected rates.

Prophylactic salpingo-oophorectomy may also be employed for the prevention of ovarian and breast cancers among high-risk women. A prospective cohort study evaluating the outcomes of *BRCA* mutation carriers demonstrated a statistically significant association between prophylactic salpingo-oophorectomy and a reduced incidence of ovarian or primary peritoneal cancer (36% relative risk reduction, or a 4.5% absolute difference). Studies of prophylactic oophorectomy for prevention of breast cancer in women with genetic mutations have shown relative risks of approximately 0.50; the risk reduction may be greatest for women having the procedure at younger (i.e., <50 years) ages. The observation that most high-grade serous "ovarian cancers" actually arise in the fallopian tube fimbria raises the possibility that this lethal subtype may be prevented by ovary-sparing salpingectomy.

All of the evidence concerning the use of prophylactic mastectomy and salpingo-oophorectomy for prevention of breast and ovarian cancer in high-risk women has been observational in nature; such studies are prone to a variety of biases, including case selection bias, family relationships between patients and controls, and inadequate information about hormone use. Thus, they may give an overestimate of the magnitude of benefit.

CANCER SCREENING

Screening is a means of early detection in asymptomatic individuals, with the goal of decreasing morbidity and mortality. While screening can potentially reduce disease-specific deaths and has been shown to do so in cervical, colon, lung, and breast cancer, it is also subject to a number of biases that can suggest a benefit when actually there is none. Biases can even mask net harm. Early detection does not in itself confer benefit. Cause-specific mortality, rather than survival after diagnosis, is the preferred endpoint (see below).

Because screening is done on asymptomatic, healthy persons, it should offer substantial likelihood of benefit that outweighs harm. Screening tests and their appropriate use should be carefully evaluated before their use is widely encouraged in screening programs.

A large and increasing number of genetic mutations and nucleotide polymorphisms have been associated with an increased risk of cancer. Testing for these genetic mutations could in theory define a high-risk population. However, most of the identified mutations have very low penetrance and individually provide limited predictive accuracy. The ability to predict the development of a particular cancer may someday present therapeutic options as well as ethical dilemmas. It may eventually allow for early intervention to prevent a cancer or limit its severity. People at high risk may be ideal candidates for chemoprevention and screening; however, efficacy of these interventions in the high-risk population should be investigated. Currently, persons at high risk for a particular cancer can engage in intensive screening. While this course is clinically reasonable, it is not known if it reduces mortality in these populations.

The Accuracy of Screening A screening test's accuracy or ability to discriminate disease is described by four indices: sensitivity, specificity, positive predictive value, and negative predictive value (**Table 70-2**). *Sensitivity*, also called the true-positive rate, is the proportion of persons with the disease who test positive in the screen

TABLE 70-2 Assessment of the Value of a Diagnostic Test[a]

	CONDITION PRESENT	CONDITION ABSENT
Positive test	*a*	*b*
Negative test	*c*	*d*
a = true positive		
b = false positive		
c = false negative		
d = true negative		
Sensitivity	The proportion of persons with the condition who test positive: $a/(a + c)$	
Specificity	The proportion of persons without the condition who test negative: $d/(b + d)$	
Positive predictive value (PPV)	The proportion of persons with a positive test who have the condition: $a/(a + b)$	
Negative predictive value	The proportion of persons with a negative test who do not have the condition: $d/(c + d)$	
Prevalence, sensitivity, and specificity determine PPV		
$\text{PPV} = \dfrac{\text{prevalence} \times \text{sensitivity}}{(\text{prevalence} \times \text{sensitivity}) + (1 - \text{prevalence})(1 - \text{specificity})}$		

[a]For diseases of low prevalence, such as cancer, poor specificity has a dramatic adverse effect on PPV such that only a small fraction of positive tests are true positives.

(i.e., the ability of the test to detect disease when it is present). *Specificity*, or 1 minus the false-positive rate, is the proportion of persons who do not have the disease who test negative in the screening test (i.e., the ability of a test to correctly indicate that the disease is not present). The *positive predictive value* is the proportion of persons who test positive and who actually have the disease. Similarly, *negative predictive value* is the proportion testing negative who do not have the disease. The sensitivity and specificity of a test are independent of the underlying prevalence (or risk) of the disease in the population screened, but the predictive values depend strongly on the prevalence of the disease.

Screening is most beneficial, efficient, and economical when the target disease is common in the population being screened. Specificity is at least as important to the ultimate feasibility and success of a screening test as sensitivity.

Potential Biases of Screening Tests Common biases of screening are lead time, length-biased sampling, and selection. These biases can make a screening test seem beneficial when actually it is not (or even causes net harm). Whether beneficial or not, screening can create the false impression of an epidemic by increasing the number of cancers diagnosed. It can also produce a shift in the *proportion* of patients diagnosed at an early stage (even without a reduction in absolute incidence of late-stage disease) and inflate survival statistics without reducing mortality (i.e., the number of deaths from a given cancer relative to the number of those at risk for the cancer). In such a case, the *apparent* duration of survival (measured from date of diagnosis) increases without lives being saved or life expectancy changed.

Lead-time bias occurs whether or not a test influences the natural history of the disease; the patient is merely diagnosed at an earlier date. Survival *appears* increased even if life is not prolonged. The screening test only prolongs the time the subject is aware of the disease and spends as a cancer patient.

Length-biased sampling occurs because screening tests generally can more easily detect slow-growing, less aggressive cancers than fast-growing cancers. Cancers diagnosed due to the onset of symptoms between scheduled screenings are on average more aggressive, and treatment outcomes are not as favorable. An extreme form of length bias sampling is termed *overdiagnosis*, the detection of "pseudo disease." The reservoir of some undetected slow-growing tumors is large. Many of these tumors fulfill the histologic criteria of cancer but will never become clinically significant or cause death during the patient's remaining life span. This problem is compounded by the fact that the most common cancers appear most frequently at ages when competing causes of death are more frequent.

Selection bias occurs because the population most likely to seek screening often differs from the general population to which the screening test might be applied. In general, volunteers for studies are more health conscious and likely to have a better prognosis or lower mortality rate, irrespective of the screening result. This is termed the *healthy volunteer effect.*

Potential Drawbacks of Screening Risks associated with screening include harm caused by the screening intervention itself, harm due to the further investigation of persons with positive tests (both true and false positives), and harm from the treatment of persons with a true-positive result, whether or not life is extended by treatment (e.g., even if a screening test reduces relative cause-specific mortality by 15–30%, 70–85% of those diagnosed still go on to die of the target cancer). The diagnosis and treatment of cancers that would never have caused medical problems can lead to the harm of unnecessary treatment and give patients the anxiety of a cancer diagnosis. The psychosocial impact of cancer screening can be substantial when applied to the entire population.

Assessment of Screening Tests Good clinical trial design can offset some biases of screening and demonstrate the relative risks and benefits of a screening test. A randomized controlled screening trial with cause-specific mortality as the endpoint provides the strongest support for a screening intervention. Overall mortality should also be reported to detect an adverse effect of screening and treatment on other disease outcomes (e.g., cardiovascular disease, treatment-induced cancers). In a randomized trial, two like populations are randomly established. One is given the usual standard of care (which may be no screening at all) and the other receives the screening intervention being assessed. Efficacy for the population studied is established when the group receiving the screening test has a better cause-specific mortality rate than the control group. Studies showing a reduction in the incidence of advanced-stage disease, improved survival, or a stage shift are weaker (and possibly misleading) evidence of benefit. These latter criteria are early indicators but not sufficient to establish the value of a screening test.

Although a randomized, controlled screening trial provides the strongest evidence to support a screening test, it is not perfect. Unless the trial is population-based, it does not remove the question of generalizability to the target population. Screening trials generally involve thousands of persons and last for years. Less definitive study designs are therefore often used to estimate the effectiveness of screening practices. However, every nonrandomized study design is subject to strong confounders. In descending order of strength, evidence may also be derived from the findings of internally controlled trials using intervention allocation methods other than randomization (e.g., allocation by birth date, date of clinic visit); the findings of analytic observational studies; or the results of multiple time series studies with or without the intervention.

Screening for Specific Cancers Screening for cervical, colon, and breast cancer has the potential to be beneficial for certain age groups. Depending on age and smoking history, lung cancer screening can also be beneficial in specific settings. Special surveillance of those at high risk for a specific cancer because of a family history or a genetic risk factor may be prudent, but few studies have assessed the effect on mortality. A number of organizations have considered whether or not to endorse routine use of certain screening tests. Because criteria have varied, they have arrived at different recommendations. The American Cancer Society (ACS) and the U.S. Preventive Services Task Force (USPSTF) publish screening guidelines (**Table 70-3**); the American Academy of Family Practitioners (AAFP) often follows/endorses the USPSTF recommendations; and the American College of Physicians (ACP) develops recommendations based on structured reviews of other organizations' guidelines.

TABLE 70-3 Screening Recommendations for Asymptomatic Subjects Not Known to Be at Increased Risk for the Target Condition[a]

CANCER TYPE	TEST OR PROCEDURE	USPSTF	ACS
Breast	Self-examination	"D"[b] (Not in current recommendations; from 2009)	Women, all ages: No specific recommendation
	Clinical examination	Women ≥40 years: "I" (as a stand-alone without mammography) (Not in current recommendations; from 2009)	Women, all ages: Do not recommend
	Mammography	Women 40–49 years: The decision to start screening mammography in women prior to age 50 years should be an individual one. Women who place a higher value on the potential benefit than the potential harms may choose to begin biennial screening between the ages of 40 and 49 years. ("C") Women 50–74 years: Every 2 years ("B") Women ≥75 years: "I"	Women 40–44 years: Provide the opportunity to begin annual screening Women 45–54 years: Screen annually Women ≥55 years: Transition to biennial screening or have the opportunity to continue annual screening Women ≥40 should continue screening mammography as long as their overall health is good and they have a life expectancy of 10 years or longer
	Magnetic resonance imaging (MRI)	"I" (Not in current recommendations; from 2009)	Women with >20% lifetime risk of breast cancer: Screen with MRI plus mammography annually Women with 15–20% lifetime risk of breast cancer: Discuss option of MRI plus mammography annually Women with <15% lifetime risk of breast cancer: Do not screen annually with MRI
	Tomosynthesis	Women, all ages: "I"	No specific recommendation
Cervical	Pap test (cytology)	Women <21 years: "D" Women 21–29 years: Screen with cytology alone every 3 years ("A") Women 30–65 years: Screen with cytology alone every 3 years, or with co-testing (HPV testing + cytology) every 5 years (two of three options, see HPV test below) ("A") Women >65 years, with adequate, normal prior Pap screenings: "D" Women after total hysterectomy for noncancerous causes: "D"	Women <21 years: No screening Women 21–29 years: Screen every 3 years Women 30–65 years: Screen with co-testing (HPV testing + cytology) every 5 years or cytology alone every 3 years (see HPV test below) Women >65 years: No screening following adequate negative prior screening Women after total hysterectomy for noncancerous causes: Do not screen
	HPV test	Women <30 years: Do not use HPV testing for cervical cancer screening Women 30–65 years: Screen with HPV testing alone or in combination with cytology every 5 years (two of three options, see Pap test above) ("A") Women >65 years, with adequate, normal prior Pap screenings: "D" Women after total hysterectomy for noncancerous causes: "D"	Women <30 years: Do not use HPV testing for cervical cancer screening Women 30–65 years: Preferred approach to screen with HPV and cytology co-testing every 5 years (see Pap test above) Women >65 years: No screening following adequate negative prior screening Women after total hysterectomy for noncancerous causes: Do not screen
Colorectal	Overall	Adults 50–75 years: "A" Screen for colorectal cancer; the risks and benefits of the different screening methods vary Adults 76–85 years: "C" The decision to screen should be an individual one, taking into account the patient's overall health and prior screening history	Adults ≥45–75 years: Screen for colorectal cancer with either a high-sensitivity stool-based test or a structural (visual) examination (≥45 years, qualified recommendation; ≥50 years, strong recommendation). Adults 76–85 years: Individualize screening based on patient preferences, life expectancy, health status, and prior screening history (qualified recommendation). Adults >85 years: Discourage screening (qualified recommendation). Every 5 years
	Sigmoidoscopy	Every 5 years; modeling suggests improved benefit if performed every 10 years in combination with annual FIT	Adults ≥45 years: Every 5 years
	Fecal occult blood testing (FOBT)	Every year	Adults ≥45 years: Every year
	Colonoscopy	Every 10 years	Adults ≥45 years: Every 10 years
	Fecal DNA testing	At least every 3 years	Adults ≥45 years: Every 3 years
	Fecal immunochemical testing (FIT)	Every year	Adults ≥45 years: Every year
	Computed tomography (CT) colonography	Every 5 years	Adults ≥45 years: Every 5 years

(Continued)

TABLE 70-3 Screening Recommendations for Asymptomatic Subjects Not Known to Be at Increased Risk for the Target Condition[a] (Continued)

CANCER TYPE	TEST OR PROCEDURE	USPSTF	ACS
Lung	Low-dose CT scan	Adults 55–80 years, with a ≥30 pack-year smoking history, still smoking or have quit within past 15 years: "B" Discontinue once a person has not smoked for 15 years or develops a health problem that substantially limits life expectancy or the ability to have curative lung surgery	Men and women, 55–74 years, with ≥30 pack-year smoking history, still smoking or have quit within past 15 years: Discuss benefits, limitations, and potential harms of screening; offer smoking cessation counseling where relevant; only perform screening in high-volume, high-quality lung cancer screening and treatment centers.
Ovarian	CA-125 Transvaginal ultrasound	Women, all ages: "D" Women with a high-risk hereditary cancer syndrome: No recommendation	Currently, there are no reliable screening tests for the early detection of ovarian cancer. For women at high risk of ovarian cancer, it has not been proven that using transvaginal ultrasound or serum CA-125 lowers their chances of dying from ovarian cancer.
Prostate	Prostate-specific antigen (PSA)	Men 55–69 years: The decision to undergo periodic PSA-based screening should be an individual one. Men should have an opportunity to discuss the potential benefits and harms of screening with their clinician. Clinicians should not screen men who do not express a preference for screening ("C") Men ≥70 years: "D"	Starting at age 50, men at average risk and with a life expectancy of ≥10 years should talk to a doctor about the uncertainties, risks, and potential benefits of screening. If African American or have a father or brother who had prostate cancer before age 65, men should have this talk starting at age 45. For men with more than one first-degree relative with prostate cancer diagnosed before age 65, have this talk starting at age 40. How often they are screened will depend on their PSA level.
	Digital rectal examination (DRE)	No individual recommendation	As for PSA; if men decide to be tested, they should have the PSA blood test with or without a rectal exam.
Skin	Complete skin examination by clinician or patient	Adults, all ages: "I"	No guidelines

[a]Summary of the screening procedures recommended for the general population by the USPSTF and the ACS. These recommendations refer to asymptomatic persons who are not known to have risk factors, other than age or gender, for the targeted condition. [b]USPSTF lettered recommendations are defined as follows: "A": The USPSTF recommends the service because there is high certainty that the net benefit is substantial; "B": The USPSTF recommends the service because there is high certainty that the net benefit is moderate or moderate certainty that the net benefit is moderate to substantial; "C": The USPSTF recommends selectively offering or providing this service to individual patients based on professional judgment and patient preferences; there is at least moderate certainty that the net benefit is small; "D": The USPSTF recommends against the service because there is moderate or high certainty that the service has no net benefit or that the harms outweigh the benefits; "I": The USPSTF concludes that the current evidence is insufficient to assess the balance of benefits and harms of the service.

Abbreviations: ACS, American Cancer Society; USPSTF, U.S. Preventive Services Task Force.

BREAST CANCER Breast self-examination, clinical breast examination by a caregiver, mammography, and magnetic resonance imaging (MRI) have all been variably advocated as useful screening tools.

A number of trials have suggested that annual or biennial screening with mammography in normal-risk women older than age 50 years decreases breast cancer mortality. Each trial has been criticized for design flaws. In most trials, breast cancer–related mortality rates were decreased by 15–30%. Experts disagree on whether average-risk women age 40–49 years should receive regular screening (Table 70-3). The U.K. Age Trial, the only randomized trial of breast cancer screening to specifically evaluate the impact of mammography in women age 40–49 years, found no statistically significant difference in breast cancer mortality for screened women versus controls after about 11 years of follow-up (relative risk 0.83; 95% confidence interval 0.66–1.04); however, <70% of women received screening in the intervention arm, potentially diluting the observed effect. A meta-analysis of nine large randomized trials showed an 8% relative reduction in mortality (relative risk 0.92; 95% confidence interval 0.75–1.02) from mammography screening for women age 39–49 years after 11–20 years of follow-up. This is equivalent to 3 breast cancer deaths prevented per 10,000 women >10 years (although the result is not statistically significant). At the same time, nearly half of women age 40–49 years screened annually will have false-positive mammograms necessitating further evaluation, often including biopsy. Estimates of overdiagnosis range from 10 to 50% of diagnosed invasive cancers. In the United States, widespread screening over the past several decades has not been accompanied by a reduction in incidence of metastatic breast cancer despite a large increase in early-stage disease, suggesting a substantial amount of overdiagnosis at the population level. In addition, the substantial improvements in systemic therapy have likely decreased the impact of mammography and early detection on falling breast cancer mortality rates.

Digital breast tomosynthesis is a newer method of breast cancer screening that reconstructs multiple x-ray images of the breast into superimposed "three-dimensional" slices. Although some evidence is available concerning the test characteristics of this modality, there are currently no data on its effects on health outcomes such as breast cancer–related morbidity, mortality, or overdiagnosis rates. A large randomized trial comparing standard digital mammography to tomosynthesis is in progress.

No study of breast self-examination has shown it to decrease mortality. A randomized controlled trial of approximately 266,000 women in China demonstrated no difference in breast cancer mortality between a group that received intensive breast self-exam instruction and reinforcement/reminders and controls at 10 years of follow-up. However, more benign breast lesions were discovered and more breast biopsies were performed in the self-examination arm.

Genetic screening for *BRCA1* and *BRCA2* mutations and other markers of breast cancer risk has identified a group of women at high risk for breast cancer. Unfortunately, when to begin and the optimal frequency of screening have not been defined. Mammography is less sensitive at detecting breast cancers in women carrying *BRCA1* and *BRCA2* mutations, possibly because such cancers occur in younger women, in whom mammography is known to be less sensitive. MRI screening may be more sensitive than mammography in women at high risk due to genetic predisposition or in women with very dense breast tissue, but specificity may be lower. An increase in overdiagnosis may accompany the higher sensitivity. The impact of MRI on breast cancer mortality with or without concomitant use of mammography has not been evaluated in a randomized controlled trial.

CERVICAL CANCER Screening with Papanicolaou (Pap) smears decreases cervical cancer mortality. The cervical cancer mortality rate has fallen substantially since the widespread use of the Pap smear. With the onset of sexual activity comes the risk of sexual transmission of HPV, the fundamental etiologic factor for cervical cancer. Screening guidelines recommend regular Pap testing for all women who have reached the age of 21 (before this age, even in individuals that have begun sexual activity, screening may cause more harm than benefit). The recommended interval for Pap screening is 3 years. In all cases, screening more frequently adds little benefit but leads to important harms, including unnecessary procedures and overtreatment of transient lesions. Beginning at age 30, guidelines also include HPV testing with or without Pap smear. The screening interval for women who test normal using this approach may be lengthened to 5 years.

An upper age limit at which screening ceases to be effective is not known, but women age 65 years with no abnormal results in the previous 10 years may choose to stop screening. Screening should be discontinued in women who have undergone a hysterectomy with cervical excision for noncancerous reasons.

Although the efficacy of the Pap smear in reducing cervical cancer mortality has never been directly confirmed in a randomized, controlled setting, a clustered randomized trial in India evaluated the impact of one-time cervical visual inspection and immediate colposcopy, biopsy, and/or cryotherapy (where indicated) versus counseling on cervical cancer deaths in women age 30–59 years. After 7 years of follow-up, the age-standardized rate of death due to cervical cancer was 39.6 per 100,000 person-years in the intervention group versus 56.7 per 100,000 person-years in controls.

COLORECTAL CANCER Fecal occult blood testing (FOBT), digital rectal examination (DRE), rigid and flexible sigmoidoscopy, colonoscopy, and computed tomography (CT) colonography have been considered for colorectal cancer screening. A meta-analysis of five randomized controlled trials demonstrated a 22% relative reduction in colorectal cancer mortality after two to nine rounds of biennial FOBT at 30 years of follow-up; annual screening was shown to result in a greater colorectal cancer mortality reduction in a single trial (a 32% relative reduction). However, only 2–10% of those with occult blood in the stool have cancer. The high false-positive rate of FOBT substantially increases the number of colonoscopies performed.

Fecal immunochemical tests (FITs) have higher sensitivity for colorectal cancer than FOBT tests. Limited observational evidence suggests FITs may have lower ability to detect proximal versus distal colonic tumors. Multitargeted stool DNA testing combines FIT with testing for altered DNA biomarkers in cells that are shed into the stool. Although limited evidence demonstrates that it can have a higher single-test sensitivity for colorectal cancer than FIT alone, its specificity is lower, resulting in a higher number of false-positive tests and follow-up colonoscopies. There are no studies evaluating its effects on colorectal cancer incidence, morbidity, or mortality.

A blood test for the methylated *SEPT9* gene associated with colorectal cancer is available. However, its sensitivity is low, no longitudinal data have been collected on its performance or efficacy, and it is not recommended as a first-line screening test.

Two meta-analyses of five randomized controlled trials of sigmoidoscopy found an 18% relative reduction in colorectal cancer incidence and a 28% relative reduction in colorectal cancer mortality. Participant ages ranged from 50 to 74 years, with follow-up ranging from 6 to 13 years. Diagnosis of adenomatous polyps by sigmoidoscopy should lead to evaluation of the entire colon with colonoscopy. The most efficient interval for screening sigmoidoscopy is unknown, but an interval of 5 years is often recommended. Case-control studies suggest that intervals of up to 15 years may confer benefit; the randomized U.K. trial demonstrated colorectal cancer mortality reduction with one-time screening.

One-time colonoscopy detects ~25% more advanced lesions (polyps >10 mm, villous adenomas, adenomatous polyps with high-grade dysplasia, invasive cancer) than one-time FOBT with sigmoidoscopy; comparative *programmatic* performance of the two modalities over time is not known. Perforation rates are about 4/10,000 for colonoscopy and 1/10,000 for sigmoidoscopy. Debate continues on whether colonoscopy is too expensive and invasive and whether sufficient provider capacity exists to be recommended as the preferred screening tool in standard-risk populations. Some observational studies suggest that efficacy of colonoscopy to decrease colorectal cancer mortality is primarily limited to the left side of the colon.

CT colonography, if done at expert centers, appears to have a sensitivity for polyps ≥6 mm, comparable to colonoscopy. However, the rate of extracolonic findings of abnormalities of uncertain significance that must nevertheless be worked up is high (~5–37%); the long-term cumulative radiation risk of repeated colonography screenings is also a concern.

LUNG CANCER Chest x-ray and sputum cytology have been evaluated in several randomized lung cancer screening trials. The most recent and largest (n = 154,901) of these, a component of the Prostate, Lung, Colorectal, and Ovarian (PLCO) cancer screening trial, found that, compared with usual care, annual chest x-ray did not reduce the risk of dying from lung cancer (relative risk 0.99; 95% confidence interval 0.87–1.22) after 13 years. However, it showed evidence of overdiagnosis associated with chest x-ray. Low-dose CT has also been evaluated in several randomized trials. The largest and longest of these, the National Lung Screening Trial (NLST), was a randomized controlled trial of screening for lung cancer in ~53,000 persons age 55–74 years with a 30+ pack-year smoking history. It demonstrated a statistically significant reduction of about 3 fewer deaths per 1000 people screened with CT compared to chest x-ray after 12 years. However, the harms include the potential radiation risks associated with multiple scans, the discovery of incidental findings of unclear significance, and a high rate of false-positive test results. Both incidental findings and false-positive tests can lead to invasive diagnostic procedures associated with anxiety, expense, and complications (e.g., pneumo- or hemothorax after lung biopsy). The NLST was performed at experienced screening centers, and the balance of benefits and harms may differ in the community setting at less experienced centers.

OVARIAN CANCER Adnexal palpation, transvaginal ultrasound (TVUS), and serum CA-125 assay have been considered for ovarian cancer screening. A large randomized, controlled trial has shown that an annual screening program of TVUS and CA-125 in average-risk women does not reduce deaths from ovarian cancer (relative risk 1.21; 95% confidence interval 0.99–1.48). Adnexal palpation was dropped early in the study because it did not detect any ovarian cancers that were not detected by either TVUS or CA-125. A second large randomized trial used a two-stage screening approach incorporating a risk of ovarian cancer algorithm that determined whether additional testing with CA-125 or TVUS was required. At 14 years of follow-up, there was no statistically significant reduction in ovarian cancer deaths. The risks and costs associated with the high number of false-positive results are impediments to routine use of these modalities for screening. In the PLCO trial, 10% of participants had a false-positive result from TVUS or CA-125, and one-third of these women underwent a major surgical procedure; the ratio of surgeries to screen-detected ovarian cancer was approximately 20:1. In September 2016, the FDA issued a safety communication recommending against using any screening test, including the risk of ovarian cancer algorithm, for ovarian cancer.

PROSTATE CANCER The most common prostate cancer screening modalities are digital rectal exam (DRE) and serum PSA assay. An emphasis on PSA screening has caused prostate cancer to become the most common nonskin cancer diagnosed in American males. This disease is prone to lead-time bias, length bias, and overdiagnosis, and substantial debate continues among experts as to whether screening should be offered unless the patient specifically asks to be screened. Virtually all organizations stress the importance of informing men about the uncertainty regarding screening efficacy and the associated harms. Prostate cancer screening clearly detects many asymptomatic cancers, but the ability to distinguish tumors that are lethal but still curable from those that pose little or no threat to health is limited, and randomized trials indicate that the effect of PSA screening on prostate cancer mortality across a population is, at best, small. Men older than age 50 years have a high prevalence of indolent, clinically insignificant prostate cancers (about 30–50% of men, increasing further as men age).

Two major randomized controlled trials of the impact of PSA screening on prostate cancer mortality have been published. The PLCO Cancer Screening Trial was a multicenter U.S. trial that randomized almost 77,000 men age 55–74 years to receive either annual PSA testing for 6 years or usual care. At 13 years of follow-up, no statistically significant difference in the number of prostate cancer deaths was noted between the arms (rate ratio 1.09; 95% confidence interval 0.87–1.36). More than half of men in the control arm received at least one PSA test during the trial, which may have diluted a small effect.

The European Randomized Study of Screening for Prostate Cancer (ERSPC) was a multinational study that randomized ~182,000 men between age 50 and 74 years (with a predefined "core" screening group of men age 55–69 years) to receive PSA testing or no screening. Recruitment and randomization procedures, as well as actual frequency of PSA testing, varied by country. After a median follow-up of 15.5 years, a 20% relative reduction in the risk of prostate cancer death in the screened arm was noted in the "core" screening group. The trial found that 570 men (95% confidence interval 380–1137 men) would need to be invited to screening, and 18 cases of prostate cancer detected, to avert 1 death from prostate cancer. There was an unexplained imbalance in treatment between the two study arms, with a higher proportion of men with clinically localized cancer receiving radical prostatectomy in the screening arm and receiving it at experienced referral centers.

Screening must be linked to effective therapy in order to have any benefit. Two trials conducted after the initiation of widespread PSA testing did not find a substantial decrease in prostate cancer deaths in control arms of "watchful waiting" or monitoring (i.e., no curative treatment) compared to radical prostatectomy or radiation therapy. Prostate cancer–specific survival was very good (about 99%) and nearly identical at a median follow-up of 10 years. Treatments for low-stage prostate cancer, such as surgery and radiation therapy, can cause substantial morbidity, including impotence and urinary incontinence.

SKIN CANCER Visual examination of all skin surfaces by the patient or by a health care provider is used in screening for basal and squamous cell cancers and melanoma. No prospective randomized study has been performed to look for a mortality decrease. Unfortunately, screening is associated with a substantial rate of overdiagnosis.

FURTHER READING

Fenton JJ et al: Prostate-specific antigen-based screening for prostate cancer: Evidence report and systematic review for the U.S. Preventive Services Task Force. JAMA 319:1914, 2018.

Kramer BS, Croswell JM: Cancer screening: The clash of science and intuition. Annu Rev Med 60:125, 2009.

Manson JE et al: Vitamin D supplements and prevention of cancer and cardiovascular disease. N Engl J Med 380:33, 2019.

McNeil JJ et al: Effect of aspirin on all-cause mortality in the healthy elderly. N Engl J Med 379:1519, 2018.

Melnikow J et al: Screening for cervical cancer with high-risk human papillomavirus testing: Updated evidence report and systematic review for the US Preventive Services Task Force. JAMA 320:687, 2018.

National Lung Screening Trial Research Team: Lung cancer incidence and mortality with extended follow-up in the National Lung Screening Trial. J Thorac Oncol 14:1732, 2019.

Nelson HD: Effectiveness of breast cancer screening: Systematic review and meta-analysis to update the 2009 U.S. Preventive Services Task Force recommendation. Ann Intern Med 164:244, 2016.

US Preventive Services Task Force et al: Screening for colorectal cancer: US Preventive Services Task Force recommendation. JAMA 325:1965, 2021.

Welch HG et al: Epidemiologic signatures in cancer. N Engl J Med 384:14, 2019.

Zeraatkar D et al: Effect of lower versus high red meat intake on cardiometabolic and cancer outcomes: A systematic review of randomized trials. Ann Intern Med 171:721, 2019.

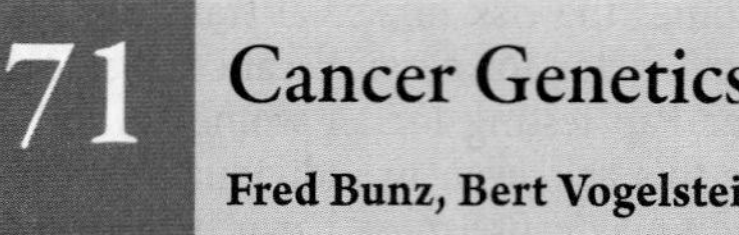
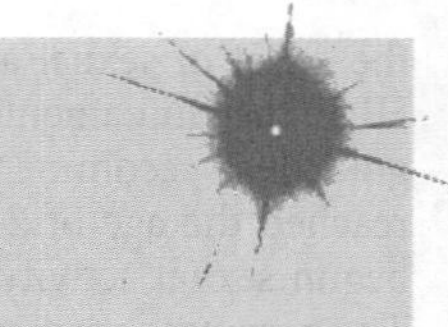

71 Cancer Genetics

Fred Bunz, Bert Vogelstein

CANCER IS A GENETIC DISEASE

Cancer arises through a series of somatic alterations in DNA that result in unrestrained cellular proliferation. Most of these alterations involve subtle sequence changes in DNA (i.e., mutations). The somatic mutations may originate as a consequence of random replication errors or exposure to carcinogens (e.g., radiation) and can be exacerbated by faulty DNA repair processes. While most cancers arise sporadically, clustering of cancers occurs in families that carry a germline mutation in a cancer gene.

HISTORICAL PERSPECTIVE

The idea that cancer progression is driven by sequential somatic mutations in specific genes has only gained general acceptance in the past 30 years. Before the advent of the microscope, cancer was believed to be composed of aggregates of mucus or other noncellular matter. By the middle of the nineteenth century, it became clear that tumors were masses of cells and that these cells arose from the normal cells of the tissue from which the cancer originated. The molecular basis for the uncontrolled proliferation of cancer cells was to remain a mystery for another century. During that time, a number of theories for the origin of cancer were postulated. The great biochemist Otto Warburg proposed the combustion theory of cancer, which stipulated that cancer was due to abnormal oxygen metabolism. Others believed that all cancers were caused by viruses and that cancer was in fact a contagious disease.

In the end, observations of cancer occurring in chimney sweeps, studies of x-rays, and the overwhelming data demonstrating cigarette smoke as a causative agent in lung cancer, together with Ames's work on chemical mutagenesis, were consistent with the idea that cancer originated through changes in DNA. However, it was not until the somatic mutations responsible for cancer were identified at the molecular level that the genetic basis of cancer was definitively established. Although the viral theory of cancer did not prove to be generally accurate (with exceptions such as human papillomaviruses, which can cause cervical and other cancers), the study of retroviruses led to the discovery of the first human *oncogenes* in the late 1970s. Oncogenes are one of the two major classes of cancer driver genes. The study of families with genetic predisposition to cancer was instrumental to the discovery of the other major class of cancer driver genes, called *tumor-suppressor genes*. Current technologies permit the sequence analysis of entire cancer genomes and provide a comprehensive view of the genetic changes that cause tumors to arise and become malignant. The field that studies the various types of mutations, as well as the consequences of these mutations in tumor cells, is now known as *cancer genetics*.

THE CLONAL ORIGIN AND MULTISTEP NATURE OF CANCER

Nearly all cancers originate from a single cell; this clonal origin is a critical discriminating feature between neoplasia and hyperplasia. Multiple cumulative mutational events are invariably required for the progression of a tumor from normal to fully malignant phenotype. The process can be seen as Darwinian microevolution in which, at each successive step, the mutated cells gain a growth advantage resulting in the expansion of a neoplastic clone (**Fig. 71-1**). Based on observations of cancer frequency increases during aging, the epidemiologists Armitage and Doll and Nordling independently proposed that cancer is a result of three discrete cellular changes. Remarkably, this early model has been validated by extensive sequencing of cancer genomes. These studies revealed that just three causal mutations are required for the development of several of the most common cancers. Overall, it is currently believed that most common solid tumors require a minimum of three mutated cancer driver genes (either oncogenes or tumor-suppressor genes) for their development. One or two mutations are

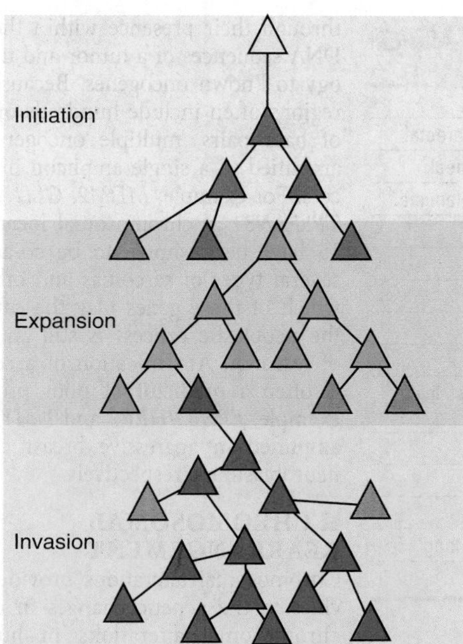

FIGURE 71-1 Multistep clonal development of malignancy. In this diagram, a series of three cumulative mutations, each with a modest growth advantage acting alone, eventually results in a malignant tumor. Note that not all such alterations result in progression. The actual number of cumulative mutations necessary to transform from the normal to the malignant state has been estimated to be three for several of the most common types of cancer. *(Adapted and modified from PC Nowell: The clonal evolution of tumor cell populations. Science 194:23, 1976.)*

sufficient for benign tumorigenesis, but not for the invasive capacity that distinguishes cancers from benign tumors. Less common tumors, such as liquid tumors (leukemias or lymphomas), sarcomas, and childhood tumors, appear to require only two driver gene alterations for malignancy. Note that a cancer driver gene is best defined as one containing a mutation that increases the selective growth advantage of the cell containing it. Normally, cell birth and cell death are in perfect equilibrium; every time a cell is born, another in the same lineage dies. Cancer driver gene mutations alter this equilibrium, so that more cells are born than die. The imbalance is often slight, so that the difference between cell birth and cell death can be less than 1%. This explains, in combination with the low rate of mutation, why tumorigenesis—the journey from a normal cell to a typical malignant, solid tumor—often takes decades.

We now know the precise nature of the genetic alterations responsible for nearly all malignancies and are beginning to understand how these alterations promote the distinct stages of tumor growth. The prototypical example is colon cancer, in which analyses of genomes from the entire spectrum of neoplastic growths—from normal colon epithelium through adenoma to carcinoma—have identified mutations that are highly characteristic of each type of lesion (**Fig. 71-2**).

TWO TYPES OF CANCER GENES: ONCOGENES AND TUMOR-SUPPRESSOR GENES

Oncogenes and tumor-suppressor genes exert their effects on tumor growth through their ability to determine cell fates, influence cell survival, and contribute to genome maintenance. The underlying molecular mechanisms can be extremely complex. While tightly regulated in normal cells, oncogenes acquire mutations that typically relieve this control and lead to increased activity of the gene products. This activating mutational event occurs in a single allele. In contrast, the normal function of tumor-suppressor genes is usually to restrain cell growth, and this function is lost in cancer. Because of the diploid nature of mammalian cells, both alleles must be inactivated for a cell to completely lose the function of a tumor-suppressor gene. Thus, it requires two genetic events to inactivate a tumor-suppressor gene mutation, while only one genetic event is required to activate an oncogene.

A subset of tumor-suppressor genes controls the ability of the cell to maintain the integrity of its genome. Cells with a deficiency in these genes acquire an increased number of mutations throughout their genomes, including those in oncogenes and tumor-suppressor genes. This "mutator" phenotype was first hypothesized by Loeb to explain how the multiple rare mutational events required for tumorigenesis can occur in the lifetime of an individual. A mutator phenotype underlies several forms of cancer, such as those associated with deficiencies in DNA mismatch repair. The great majority of cancers do not harbor repair deficiencies, and their rate of mutation is similar to that observed in normal cells. Many of these cancers, however, appear to harbor a different kind of genetic instability, affecting the loss or gains of whole chromosomes or large parts thereof (as explained in more detail below).

ONCOGENES IN HUMAN CANCER

Work by Peyton Rous in the early 1900s revealed that a chicken sarcoma could be transmitted from animal to animal in cell-free extracts, suggesting that cancer could be induced by an agent acting positively to promote tumor formation. The agent responsible for the transmission of the cancer was a retrovirus (Rous sarcoma virus [RSV]), and the oncogene responsible was identified 75 years later as *V-SRC*. Other oncogenes were also discovered through their presence in the genomes of retroviruses that are capable of causing cancers in chickens, mice, and rats. The nonmutated cellular homologues of these viral genes are called proto-oncogenes and are often targets of mutation or aberrant regulation in human cancer. Whereas many oncogenes were discovered on the basis of their presence in retroviruses, other oncogenes, particularly those involved in translocations characteristic of particular leukemias and lymphomas, were identified through genomic approaches. Investigators cloned the sequences surrounding the chromosomal translocations observed cytogenetically and identified the genes activated at the breakpoints (see below). Some of these were oncogenes previously found in retroviruses (like *ABL*, involved in chronic myeloid leukemia [CML]), whereas others were new (like *BCL2*, involved in B-cell lymphoma). In the normal cellular environment, proto-oncogenes have crucial roles in cell proliferation and

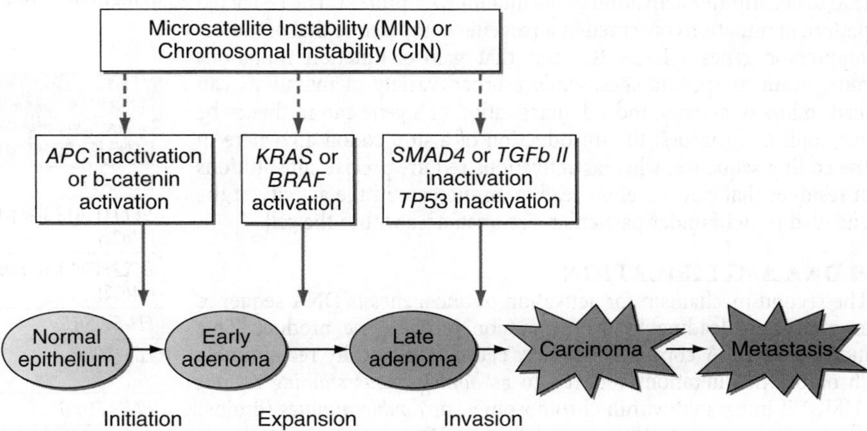

FIGURE 71-2 Progressive somatic mutational steps in the development of colon carcinoma. The accumulation of alterations in a number of different genes results in the progression from normal epithelium through adenoma to full-blown carcinoma. Genetic instability (microsatellite or chromosomal) accelerates the progression by increasing the likelihood of mutation at each step. Patients with familial polyposis are already one step into this pathway, because they inherit a germline alteration of the *APC* gene. TGF, transforming growth factor.

TABLE 71-1 Oncogenes Commonly Altered in Human Cancers

ONCOGENE	FUNCTION	ALTERATION IN CANCER	NEOPLASM
AKT1	Serine/threonine kinase	Point mutation	Skin
BRAF	Serine/threonine kinase	Point mutation	Melanoma, thyroid, colorectal
CCND1	Cell cycle progression	Amplification	Esophageal, head and neck
CTNNB1	Signal transduction	Point mutation	Colon, liver, uterine, melanoma
EGFR	Signal transduction	Point mutation	Lung
FLT3	Signal transduction	Point mutation	AML
IDH1	Chromatin modification	Point mutation	Glioma
MDM2	Inhibitor of p53	Amplification	Sarcoma, glioma
MDM4	Inhibitor of p53	Amplification	Breast
MYC	Transcription factor	Amplification	Prostate, ovarian, breast, liver, pancreatic
MYCL1	Transcription factor	Amplification	Ovarian, bladder
MYCN	Transcription factor	Amplification	Neuroblastoma
PIK3CA	Phosphoinositol-3-kinase	Point mutation	Multiple cancers
KRAS	GTPase	Point mutation	Pancreatic, colorectal, lung
NRAS	GTPase	Point mutation	Melanoma

Abbreviation: AML, acute myeloid leukemia.

differentiation. **Table 71-1** is a partial list of oncogenes known to be involved in human cancer.

The normal growth and differentiation of cells is controlled by growth factors that bind to receptors on the surface of the cell. The signals generated by the membrane receptors are transmitted inside the cells through signaling cascades involving kinases, G proteins, and other regulatory proteins. Ultimately, these signals affect the activity of transcription factors in the nucleus, which regulate the expression of genes crucial in cell proliferation, cell differentiation, and cell death. Oncogene products function at critical steps in these signaling pathways **(Chap. 72)**. Inappropriate activation of these pathways can lead to tumorigenesis.

MECHANISMS OF ONCOGENE ACTIVATION

POINT MUTATION

Point mutation (alternatively known as single nucleotide substitution) is a common mechanism of oncogene activation. For example, mutations in *KRAS* are present in >95% of pancreatic cancers and 40% of colon cancers. Activating *KRAS* mutations are less common in other cancer types, although they can occur at significant frequencies in leukemia, lung, and thyroid cancers. Remarkably—and in contrast to the diversity of mutations found in tumor-suppressor genes—most of the activated *KRAS* alleles contain point mutations in codons 12, 13, or 61. These mutations lead to constitutive activation of the mutant RAS protein. The restricted pattern of mutations observed in oncogenes compared to that of tumor-suppressor genes reflects the fact that gain-of-function mutations must occur at specific sites, while a broad variety of mutations can lead to loss of activity. Indeed, inactivation of a gene can in theory be accomplished through the introduction of a stop codon anywhere in the coding sequence, whereas activations require precise substitutions at residues that can somehow lead to an increase in the activity of the encoded protein under particular circumstances within the cell.

DNA AMPLIFICATION

The second mechanism for activation of oncogenes is DNA sequence amplification, leading to overexpression of the gene product. This increase in DNA copy number may cause cytologically recognizable chromosome alterations referred to as *homogeneous staining regions* (HSRs) if integrated within chromosomes, or *double minutes* (dmins) if extrachromosomal. With microarray and DNA sequencing technologies, the entire genome can be surveyed for gains and losses of DNA sequences, thus pinpointing chromosomal regions likely to contain genes important in the development or progression of cancer.

Numerous genes have been reported to be amplified in cancer. Several of these genes, including *NMYC* and *LMYC*, were identified through their presence within the amplified DNA sequences of a tumor and their homology to known oncogenes. Because amplified regions often include hundreds of thousands of base pairs, multiple oncogenes may be amplified in a single amplicon in some cancers. For example, *MDM2, GLI1, CDK4,* and *TPSPAN31* at chromosomal location 12q13-15 have been shown to be co-amplified in several types of sarcomas and other tumors; which of these genes play the causal role in the neoplastic process is still an active area of research. Amplification of a cellular gene is often a predictor of poor prognosis; for example, *ERBB2/HER2* and *NMYC* are often amplified in aggressive breast cancers and neuroblastoma, respectively.

CHROMOSOMAL REARRANGEMENT

Chromosomal alterations provide important clues to the genetic changes in cancer. The chromosomal alterations in human solid tumors such as carcinomas are heterogeneous and complex and occur as a result of the frequent chromosomal instability observed in these tumors (see below). In contrast, the chromosome alterations in myeloid and lymphoid tumors are often simple translocations, that is, reciprocal transfers of chromosome arms from one chromosome to another. The breakpoints of recurring chromosome abnormalities usually occur at the site of cellular oncogenes. **Table 71-2** lists representative examples of recurring chromosome alterations in malignancy and the associated gene(s) rearranged or deregulated by the chromosomal rearrangement. Translocations are often observed in liquid tumors in general and are particularly common in lymphoid tumors, probably because these cell types have the capability to rearrange their DNA to generate antigen receptors. Indeed, antigen receptor genes are commonly involved in the translocations, implying that an imperfect regulation of receptor gene rearrangement may be involved in their pathogenesis. In addition to transcription factors and signal transduction molecules, translocation may result in the overexpression of cell cycle regulatory proteins or proteins such as cyclins and of proteins that regulate cell death. Recurrent translocations have more recently been identified in solid tumors such as prostate cancers. For example, fusions between *TMPRSS2* and *ERG*, which are normally located in tandem on chromosome 21, contribute to more than one-third of all prostate cancers.

The first reproducible chromosome abnormality detected in human malignancy was the Philadelphia chromosome detected in CML.

TABLE 71-2 Representative Oncogenes at Chromosomal Translocations

GENE (CHROMOSOME)	TRANSLOCATION	MALIGNANCY
BCR-ABL	(9;22)(q34;q11)	Chronic myeloid leukemia
BCL1 (11q13.3)–*IgH* (14q32)	(11;14)(q13;q32)	Mantle cell lymphoma
BCL2 (18q21.3)–*IgH* (14q32)	(14;18)(q32;q21)	Follicular lymphoma
FLI-EWSR1	(11;22)(q24;q12)	Ewing's sarcoma
LCK-TCRB	(1;7)(p34;q35)	T-cell acute lymphocytic leukemia
PAX3-FOXO1	(2;13)(q35;q14)	Rhabdomyosarcoma
PAX8-PPARG	(2;3)(q13;p25)	Thyroid
IL21R-BCL6	(3;16)(q27;p11)	Non-Hodgkin's lymphoma
TAL1-TCTA	(1;3)(p34;p21)	Acute T-cell leukemia
TMPRSS2-ERG	Rearrangement on Chr21q22	Prostate

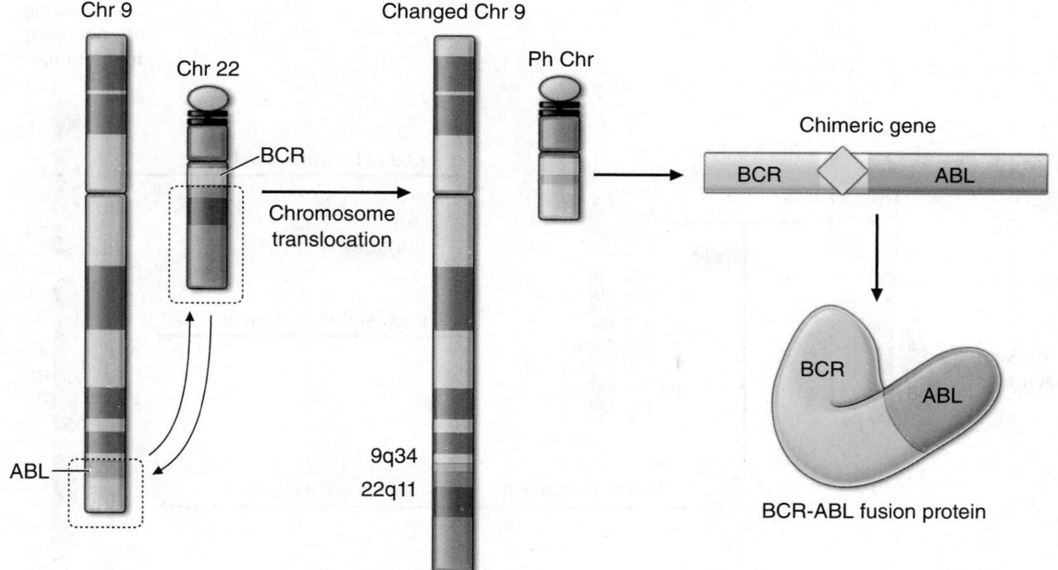

FIGURE 71-3 Specific translocation seen in chronic myeloid leukemia (CML). The Philadelphia chromosome (Ph) is derived from a reciprocal translocation between chromosomes 9 and 22 with the breakpoint joining the sequences of the *ABL* oncogene with the *BCR* gene. The fusion of these DNA sequences allows the generation of an entirely novel fusion protein with modified function.

This cytogenetic abnormality is generated by reciprocal translocation involving the *ABL* oncogene on chromosome 9, encoding a tyrosine kinase, being placed in proximity to the breakpoint cluster region (*BCR*) gene on chromosome 22. **Figure 71-3** illustrates the generation of the translocation and its protein product. The consequence of expression of the *BCR-ABL* gene product is the activation of signal transduction pathways leading to cell growth independent of normal external signals. Imatinib (marketed as Gleevec), a drug that specifically blocks the activity of Abl tyrosine kinase, has shown remarkable efficacy with little toxicity in patients with CML. The successful targeting of *BCR-ABL* by imatinib is the paradigm for molecularly targeted anticancer therapies.

CHROMOSOMAL INSTABILITY IN SOLID TUMORS

Solid tumors generally contain an abnormal number of chromosomes, a state known as aneuploidy; chromosomes from aneuploid tumors exhibit structural alterations such as translocations, deletions, and amplifications. These abnormalities reflect an underlying defect in cancer cells known as chromosomal instability. While aneuploidy is a striking cellular phenotype, chromosomal instability is manifest as only a small increase in the tendency of cells to gain, lose, or rearrange chromosomes during any given cell cycle. This intrinsically low rate of chromosome aberration implies that cancer cells become aneuploid only after many generations of clonal expansion. The molecular basis of aneuploidy remains incompletely understood. It is widely believed that defects in checkpoints, the quality-control mechanisms that halt the cell cycle if chromosomes are damaged or misaligned, contribute to chromosomal instability. This hypothesis emerged from experimental observations that the tumor suppressor p53 controls checkpoints that regulate the initiation of DNA replication and the onset of mitosis. These processes are therefore defective in many cancer cells. The mitotic spindle checkpoint, which ensures proper chromosome attachment to the mitotic spindle before allowing the sister chromatids to separate, is also altered in some cancers, irrespective of p53 status. The precise relationship between checkpoint deficiency, p53, and chromosomal instability remains unclear, but it is believed that even a subtle perturbation of the highly orchestrated process of cell division can impact the ability of a cell to faithfully replicate and segregate its complement of chromosomes. From a therapeutic standpoint, the checkpoint defects that are prevalent in cancers have been proposed as vulnerabilities that may be exploited by novel agents and combinatorial strategies.

In contrast to the genome-wide cytogenetic changes that are typical indications of an underlying chromosomal instability, more focal patterns of chromosomal rearrangement have been recurrently detected in several cancer types. A curious phenomenon known as *chromothripsis* causes dozens of distinct breakpoints that are localized on one or several chromosomes. These striking structural alterations are thought to reflect a single event in which a chromosome is fragmented and then imprecisely reassembled. While the exact process that underlies chromothripsis remains obscure and its effects on driver genes are not yet clear, a transient period of extreme instability stands in contrast to the gradual loss, gain, and rearrangement of chromosomes that are typically observed in serially cultured cancer cells.

TUMOR-SUPPRESSOR GENE INACTIVATION IN CANCER

The first functional evidence for tumor-suppressor genes came from experiments showing that fusion of mouse cancer cells with normal mouse fibroblasts led to a nontumorigenic phenotype in the fused cells. The normal role of tumor-suppressor genes is to restrain cell growth, and the function of these genes is inactivated in cancer. The three major types of somatic lesions observed in tumor-suppressor genes during tumor development are *point mutations*, small insertions and/or deletions known as *indels*, and *large deletions*. Point mutations or indels in the coding region of tumor-suppressor genes will frequently lead to truncated protein products or allele-specific loss of RNA expression by the process of *nonsense-mediated decay*. Unlike the highly recurrent point mutations that are found in critical positions of activated oncogenes, known as mutational *hotspots*, the point mutations that cause tumor-suppressor gene inactivation tend to be distributed throughout the open reading frame. Large deletions lead to the loss of a functional product and sometimes encompass the entire gene or even the entire chromosome arm, leading to loss of heterozygosity (LOH) in the tumor DNA compared to the corresponding normal tissue DNA (**Fig. 71-4**). LOH in tumor DNA often indicates the presence of a tumor-suppressor gene at a particular chromosomal location, and LOH studies have been useful in the positional cloning of many tumor-suppressor genes. The rate of LOH is increased in the presence of chromosomal instability, a relationship that would explain the selective forces leading to the high prevalence of aneuploidy in late-stage cancers.

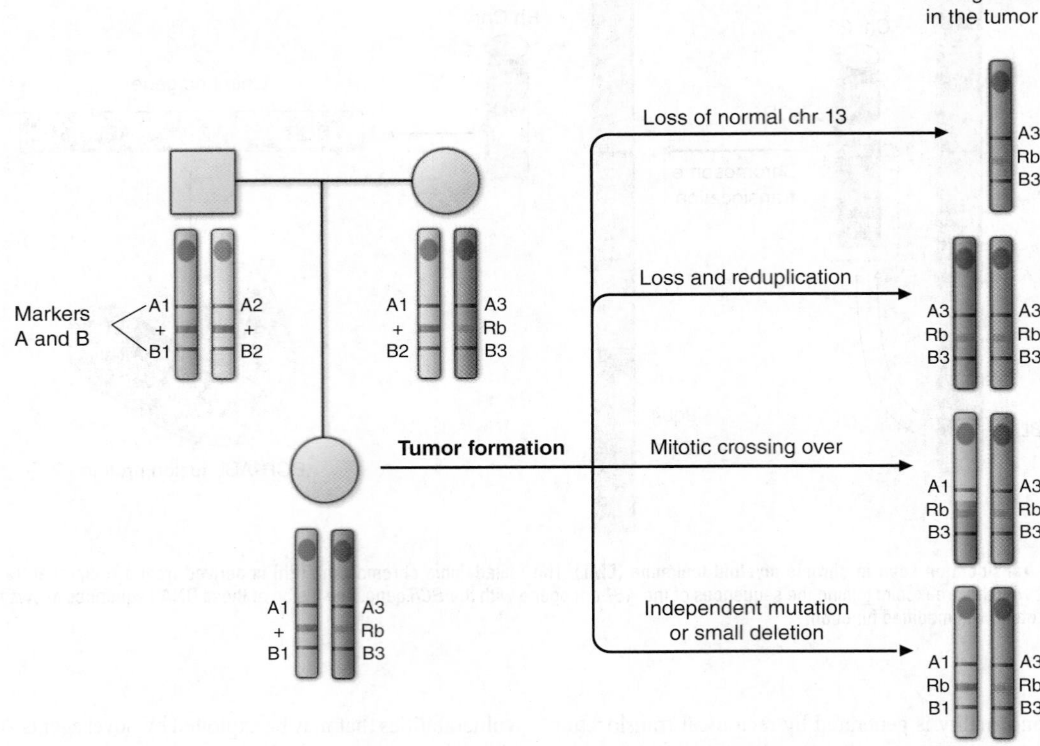

FIGURE 71-4 Diagram of possible mechanisms for tumor formation in an individual with hereditary (familial) retinoblastoma. On the left is shown the pedigree of an affected individual who has inherited the abnormal (Rb) allele from her affected mother. The normal allele is shown as a (+). The four chromosomes of her two parents are drawn to indicate their origin. Flanking the retinoblastoma locus are genetic markers (A and B) also analyzed in this family. Markers A3 and B3 are on the chromosome carrying the retinoblastoma disease gene. Tumor formation results when the normal allele, which this patient inherited from her father, is inactivated. On the right are shown four possible ways in which this could occur. In each case, the resulting chromosome 13 arrangement is shown. Note that in the first three situations, the normal allele (B1) has been lost in the tumor tissue, which is referred to as loss of heterozygosity (LOH) at this locus.

Gene silencing, an epigenetic change that leads to the loss of gene expression, occurs in conjunction with hypermethylation of the promoter and histone deacetylation, and is another mechanism of tumor-suppressor gene inactivation. An *epigenetic modification* refers to a covalent modification of chromatin, heritable by cell progeny that may involve DNA but does not involve a change in the DNA sequence. The inactivation of the second X chromosome in female cells is a physiologic example of an epigenetic silencing that prevents gene expression from the inactivated chromosome. Genomic regions of hypermethylated and hypomethylated DNA can be detected by specialized techniques, and a subset of these regional modifications has consequences on the cell's behavior.

FAMILIAL CANCER SYNDROMES

A small fraction of cancers occurs in patients with a genetic predisposition. Based on studies of inherited and sporadic forms of retinoblastoma, Knudson and others formulated a hypothesis that explains the differences between sporadic and inherited forms of the same tumor type. In inherited forms of cancer, called *cancer predisposition syndromes*, one allele of a particular tumor-suppressor gene is inherited in mutant form. This germline mutation is not sufficient to initiate a tumor, however; the other allele, inherited from the unaffected parent, must become somatically inactivated in a normal stem cell for tumorigenesis to be initiated. In sporadic (noninherited) forms of the same disease, all cells in the body start out with two normal copies of the tumor-suppressor gene. A single cell must then sequentially acquire mutations in both alleles of the tumor-suppressor gene to initiate a tumor. Thus, biallelic mutations of the same tumor-suppressor gene are required for both inherited and noninherited forms of the disease; the only difference is that individuals with the inherited form have a "head start": they already have one allele mutated, from conception, and only need one additional mutation to initiate the process (Fig. 71-4).

This distinction explains why those with inherited forms of the disease develop more cancers, at an earlier age, than the general population. It also explains why, even though every cell in an individual with a cancer predisposition syndrome has a mutant gene, only a relatively small number of tumors arise during his or her lifetime. The reason is that the vast majority of cells within such individuals are functionally normal because one of the two alleles of the tumor-suppressor gene is normal. Mutations are uncommon events, and only the rare cells that develop a mutation in the remaining normal allele will exhibit uncontrolled proliferation. The same principle applies to virtually all types of cancer predisposition syndromes, though the particular genes differ. For example, inherited mutations in *RB1*, *WT1*, *VHL*, *APC*, and *BRCA1* lead to predispositions to retinoblastomas, Wilms' tumors, renal cell carcinomas, colorectal carcinomas, and breast carcinomas, respectively (**Table 71-3**). Also note that the biallelic inactivation of any of these genes is not sufficient to develop cancer; it requires other, additional somatic alterations in other genes for the initiating cells to evolve to malignancy, as noted above.

Roughly 100 familial cancer syndromes have been reported; the great majority are very rare. Most of these syndromes exhibit an autosomal dominant pattern of inheritance, although some of those associated with DNA repair abnormalities (xeroderma pigmentosum, Fanconi's anemia, ataxia telangiectasia) are inherited in an autosomal recessive fashion. Table 71-3 shows a number of cancer predisposition syndromes and the responsible genes.

The next section examines inherited colon cancer predispositions in detail because several lessons of general importance have been derived from the study of these syndromes.

Familial adenomatous polyposis (FAP) is a dominantly inherited colon cancer syndrome caused by germline mutations in the adenomatous polyposis coli (*APC*) tumor-suppressor gene on chromosome 5. Affected individuals develop hundreds to thousands of adenomas in

TABLE 71-3 Cancer Predisposition Syndromes and Associated Genes

SYNDROME	GENE	CHROMOSOME	INHERITANCE	TUMORS
Ataxia telangiectasia	*ATM*	11q22-q23	AR	Breast
Autoimmune lymphoproliferative syndrome	*FAS* *FASL*	10q24 1q23	AD	Lymphomas
Bloom's syndrome	*BLM*	15q26.1	AR	Various
Cowden's syndrome	*PTEN*	10q23	AD	Breast, thyroid
Familial adenomatous polyposis	*APC* *MUTYH*	5q21 1p34.1	AD AR	Colorectal (early onset)
Familial melanoma	*CDKN2A*	9p21	AD	Melanoma, pancreatic
Familial Wilms' tumor	*WT1*	11p13	AD	Kidney (pediatric)
Hereditary breast/ovarian cancer	*BRCA1* *BRCA2*	17q21 13q12.3	AD	Breast, ovarian, prostate
Hereditary diffuse gastric cancer	*CDH1*	16q22	AD	Stomach
Hereditary multiple exostoses	*EXT1* *EXT2*	8q24 11p11-12	AD	Exostoses, chondrosarcoma
Hereditary retinoblastoma	*RB1*	13q14.2	AD	Retinoblastoma, osteosarcoma
Hereditary nonpolyposis colon cancer (HNPCC)	*MSH2* *MLH1* *MSH6* *PMS2*	2p16 3p21.3 2p16 7p22	AD	Colon, endometrial, ovarian, stomach, small bowel, ureter carcinoma
Hereditary papillary renal carcinoma	*MET*	7q31	AD	Papillary kidney
Juvenile polyposis syndrome	*SMAD4* *BMPR1A*	18q21	AD	Gastrointestinal, pancreatic
Li-Fraumeni syndrome	*TP53*	17p13.1	AD	Sarcoma, breast
Multiple endocrine neoplasia type 1	*MEN1*	11q13	AD	Parathyroid, endocrine, pancreas, and pituitary
Multiple endocrine neoplasia type 2a	*RET*	10q11.2	AD	Medullary thyroid carcinoma, pheochromocytoma
Neurofibromatosis type 1	*NF1*	17q11.2	AD	Neurofibroma, neurofibrosarcoma, brain
Neurofibromatosis type 2	*NF2*	22q12.2	AD	Vestibular schwannoma, meningioma, spine
Nevoid basal cell carcinoma syndrome (Gorlin's syndrome)	*PTCH1*	9q22.3	AD	Basal cell carcinoma, medulloblastoma, jaw cysts
Tuberous sclerosis	*TSC1* *TSC2*	9q34 16p13.3	AD	Angiofibroma, renal angiomyolipoma
von Hippel–Lindau disease	*VHL*	3p25-26	AD	Kidney, cerebellum, pheochromocytoma

Abbreviations: AD, autosomal dominant; AR, autosomal recessive.

the colon. In each of these adenomas, the *APC* allele inherited from the affected parent has been inactivated by virtue of a somatic mutation (Fig. 71-2). This inactivation usually occurs through a gross chromosomal event resulting in loss of all or a large part of the long arm of chromosome 5, where *APC* resides. In other cases, the remaining allele is inactivated by a subtle intragenic mutation of *APC*, which is typically a single base substitution resulting in a nonsense codon. Gross chromosomal losses occur more commonly than point mutations in normal cells, explaining why chromosomal loss rather than point mutation is the predominant mechanism underlying the inactivation of the normal allele of *APC*. The same is true for other cancer predisposition syndromes caused by other inherited tumor suppressor gene mutations; gross chromosomal events are generally responsible for inactivation of the tumor-suppressor gene allele inherited from the nonaffected parent. Several thousand adenomas form in FAP patients, and a small subset of the millions of cells within an adenoma will acquire a second mutation, leading to tumor progression, that is, a larger adenoma. A third mutation in such a larger adenoma may convert it to a carcinoma. If untreated (by colectomy), at least one of the adenomas will progress to cancer by the time patients are in their mid-40s. *APC* can be considered to be a gatekeeper for colon tumorigenesis in that in the absence of mutation of this gatekeeper (or a gene acting within the same pathway), a colorectal tumor simply cannot be initiated. **Figure 71-5** shows the germline and somatic mutations found in the *APC* gene. A negative regulator of a signaling pathway that determines cell fate during development, the APC protein provides differentiation and apoptotic cues to colonic epithelial cells as they migrate up the crypt. Defects in this process can lead to abnormal accumulation of cells that would otherwise differentiate and eventually undergo apoptosis.

In contrast to patients with FAP, patients with hereditary nonpolyposis colon cancer (HNPCC, or Lynch's syndrome) do not develop polyposis, but instead develop only one or a small number of adenomas that rapidly progress to cancer. HNPCC is due to inherited mutations in one of four DNA mismatch repair genes (Table 71-3) that are components of a repair system responsible for correcting errors in newly replicated DNA. Germline mutations in *MSH2* and *MLH1* account for more than 90% of HNPCC cases, and mutations in *MSH6* and *PMS2* account for the remainder. When a somatic mutation inactivates the remaining wild-type allele of a mismatch repair gene, the cell develops a hypermutable phenotype characterized by profound genomic instability that is most readily apparent in short repeated sequences called *microsatellites* and is sometimes called microsatellite instability (MSI). The high rate of mutation in such cells impacts all genes, including oncogenes and tumor suppressor genes, and thereby accelerates the activation of the former and the inactivation of the latter (Fig. 71-2). HNPCC can be considered a disease of tumor progression; once tumors are initiated (by an inactivating mutation of *APC* or by some other gene in the APC pathway), tumors rapidly progress because of the accelerated mutation rate. Progression from a tiny adenoma to carcinoma takes only a few years in HNPCC patients instead of the two or three decades this progression takes in patients with FAP (or in patients with sporadic colorectal tumors). Approximately half of

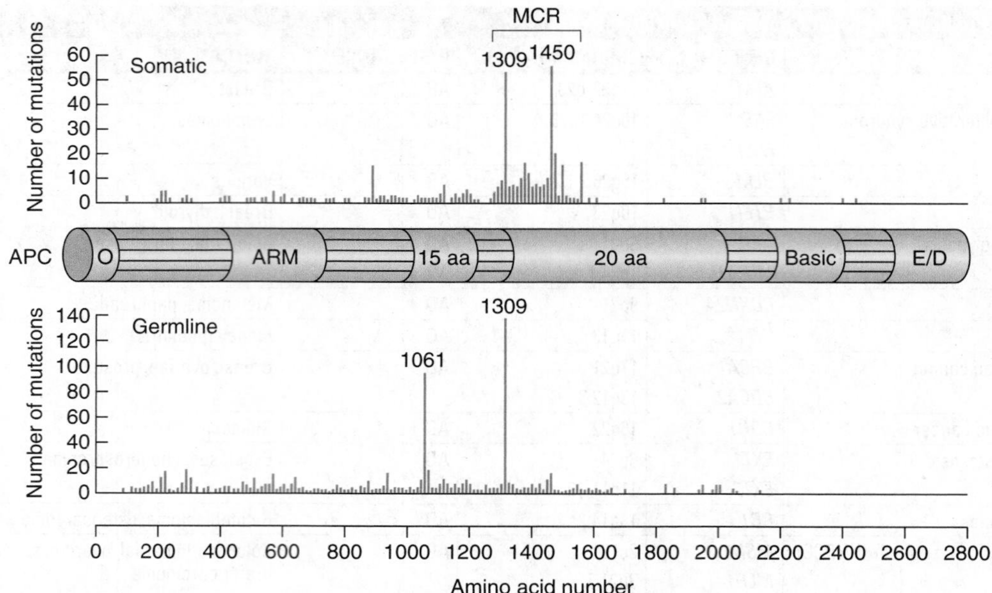

FIGURE 71-5 Germline and somatic mutations in the tumor-suppressor gene adenomatous polyposis coli (*APC*). *APC* encodes a 2843-amino-acid protein with six major domains: an oligomerization region (O), armadillo repeats (ARM), 15-amino-acid repeats (15 aa), 20-amino-acid repeats (20 aa), a basic region, and a domain involved in binding EB1 and the *Drosophila* discs large homologue (E/D). Shown are 650 somatic and 826 germline mutations representative of the mutations that occur within the *APC* gene (from the *APC* database at *www.umd.be/APC*). All known pathogenic mutations of *APC* result in the truncation of the APC protein. Germline mutations are found to be relatively evenly distributed up to codon 1600 except for two mutation hotspots surrounding amino acids 1061 and 1309, which together account for one-third of the mutations found in familial adenomatous polyposis (FAP) families.

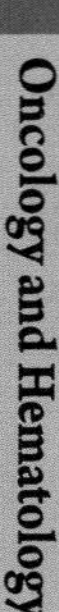

HNPCC patients develop colorectal cancers by the time they are in their mid-40s—similar to that of FAP patients. This coincidence in age of onset emphasizes that both tumor initiation (abnormal in FAP patients) and tumor progression (abnormal in HNPCC patients) are the two pillars of cancer development and are equally important for cancer development.

Another general principle is apparent from the comparison between FAP and HNPCC patients. The tumors in FAP patients, like those in patients without hereditary predisposition to cancers, exhibit chromosomal instability rather than MSI. Indeed, MSI and chromosomal instability tend to be mutually exclusive in colon cancers, suggesting that they represent alternative mechanisms for the generation of genomic instability (Fig. 71-2). Other cancer types rarely exhibit MSI. Chromosomal instability is far more prevalent than MSI among all cancer types, perhaps explaining why nearly all cancers are aneuploid.

Although most autosomal dominant inherited cancer syndromes are due to mutations in tumor-suppressor genes (Table 71-3), there are a few interesting exceptions. Multiple endocrine neoplasia type 2, a dominant disorder characterized by pituitary adenomas, medullary carcinoma of the thyroid, and (in some pedigrees) pheochromocytoma, is due to gain-of-function mutations in the proto-oncogene *RET* on chromosome 10. Similarly, gain-of-function mutations in the tyrosine kinase domain of the *MET* oncogene lead to hereditary papillary renal carcinoma. Interestingly, loss-of-function mutations in the *RET* gene cause a completely different disease, Hirschsprung's disease (aganglionic megacolon [**Chaps. 328** and **388**]).

Although the heritable forms of cancer have taught us much about the mechanisms of growth control, most forms of cancer do not follow simple Mendelian patterns of inheritance. The majority of human cancers arise in a sporadic fashion, solely as a result of somatic mutation, and in the absence of any mutations in cancer-predisposing genes in their germlines.

GENETIC TESTING FOR FAMILIAL CANCER

The discovery of cancer susceptibility genes raises the possibility of DNA testing to predict the risk of cancer in individuals of affected families. An algorithm for cancer risk assessment and decision making in high-risk families using genetic testing is shown in **Fig. 71-6**. Once a mutation is discovered in a family, subsequent testing of asymptomatic family members can be crucial in patient management. A negative gene test in these individuals can prevent years of anxiety, providing comfort in the knowledge that their cancer risk is no higher than that of the general population. On the other hand, a positive test may lead to alteration of clinical management, such as increased frequency of cancer screening and, when feasible and appropriate, prophylactic surgery. Potential negative consequences of a positive test result include psychological distress (anxiety, depression) and discrimination, although the Genetic Information Nondiscrimination Act (GINA) makes it illegal for predictive genetic information to be used to discriminate in health insurance or employment. Testing should therefore not be conducted without counseling before testing is administered and during and after disclosure of the test result.

It is now feasible to obtain high-quality sequence of all of the protein-coding DNA sequences, and even of the entire genome, in any given individual. In such studies, numerous variants in DNA sequences will inevitably be identified in every subject, but the significance of the vast majority of these DNA sequence findings will be unclear. Even mutations in tumor-suppressor genes will be difficult to interpret unless there is an obvious functional implication, such as the truncation of the open reading frame, or that particular mutation has previously been correlated with cancer in other individuals. Germline mutations associated with cancer predisposition are uncommon in individuals without a family history of cancer, though they do occur. Much more common are *variants of unknown significance* (*VUS*). VUS that are found during genetic testing cannot be used to evaluate the relative risk of cancer but may nonetheless cause anxiety because they represent a deviation from the reference allele that is established as "normal." Because of the low yield of informative mutations that modify cancer risk and the frequent identification of VUS, it is generally not appropriate to use DNA sequencing to assess cancer risk in individuals without a family history of cancer. However, there are exceptions: *testing may be appropriate in some subpopulations with a known increased risk, even without a personal family history*. For example, two mutations in the breast cancer susceptibility gene *BRCA1*, 185delAG and 5382insC, exhibit a sufficiently high frequency in the Ashkenazi

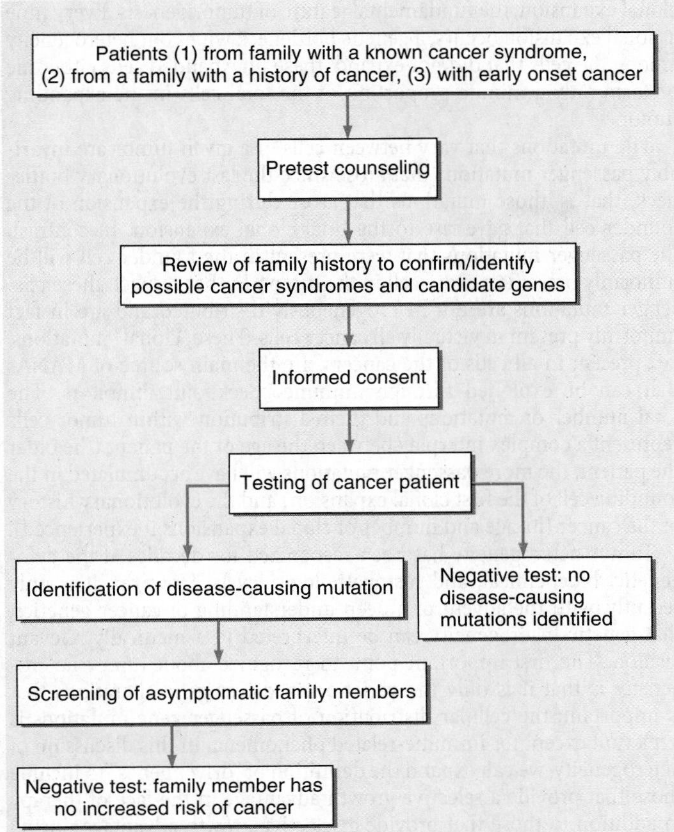

FIGURE 71-6 Algorithm for genetic testing in a family with cancer predisposition. The key step is the identification of a disease mutation in a cancer patient, which is an indication for the testing of asymptomatic family members. Asymptomatic family members who test positive may require increased screening or surgery, whereas those who test negative are at no greater risk for cancer than the general population. It should be emphasized that no molecular assay used for this sort of testing is 100% sensitive; negative results must be interpreted with this caveat in mind.

Jewish population that genetic testing based on ethnicity alone may be warranted.

It is important that genetic test results be communicated to families by trained genetic counselors. To ensure that the families clearly understand its advantages and disadvantages and the impact it may have on disease management and psyche, genetic testing should never be done *before* counseling. Significant expertise is needed to communicate the results of genetic testing to families.

VIRUSES IN HUMAN CANCER

Several human malignancies are associated with viruses. Examples include Burkitt's lymphoma (Epstein-Barr virus; **Chap. 194**), hepatocellular carcinoma (hepatitis viruses), cervical cancer (human papillomavirus [HPV]; **Chap. 198**), and T-cell leukemia (retroviruses; **Chap. 201**). There are several types of HPV, including the high-risk types 16 and 18 that are strongly associated with the development of cervical, vulvar, vaginal, penile, anal, and oropharyngeal cancer. The mechanisms of action of all these viruses involve inactivation of tumor-suppressor genes. For example, HPV proteins E6 and E7 bind to and inactivate cellular tumor suppressors p53 and pRB, respectively. This is the reason that HPV is such a potent initiator of cancer: infection with a virus is tantamount to having two of the three mutant driver genes required for cancer, that is, one viral oncogene inactivates p53 and the other inactivates Rb. Once these two inactivated gene products initiate tumorigenesis, only one additional mutant gene is required for these tumors to progress to malignancy.

CANCER GENOMES

The advent of relatively inexpensive technologies for rapid and high-throughput DNA sequencing has facilitated the comprehensive analysis of numerous genomes from many types of tumors. This unprecedented view into the genetic nature of cancer has provided remarkable insights. Most cancers do not arise in the context of a mutator phenotype, and accordingly, the number of mutations in even the most advanced cancers is relatively modest. Common solid tumors harbor 30–70 subtle mutations that are nonsynonymous (i.e., result in an amino acid change in the encoded protein). Liquid tumors such as leukemias, as well as pediatric tumors, typically have fewer than 20 mutations. The vast majority of the mutations detected in tumors are not functionally significant; they simply arose by chance in a single cell that gave rise to an expanding clone. Such mutations, which provide no selective advantage to the cell in which they occur, are known as *passenger* mutations. As noted above, only a small number of the mutations confer a selective growth advantage and thereby promote tumorigenesis. These functional mutations are known as *driver* mutations, and the genes in which they occur are called driver genes.

The frequency and distribution of driver mutations within a single tumor type can be represented as a topographical landscape. The picture that emerges from these studies reveals that most genes that are mutated in tumors are actually mutated at relatively low frequencies, as would be expected of passenger genes, whereas a small number of genes (the driver genes) are mutated in a large proportion of tumors. It appears that there are only a total of ~120 bona fide driver genes contributing to the development of solid tumors of all kinds, though other driver genes that play a role in a small fraction of cancers are still being discovered. The majority of the mutations in driver genes provide a direct selective growth advantage by altering the signaling pathways that mediate cell survival or the determination of cell fate. The remaining driver gene mutations indirectly provide a selective growth advantage by accelerating the mutation rate of proto-oncogenes and tumor-suppressor genes. That the same driver genes play a role in multiple cancer types was unexpected before their discovery and has important implications for the development of new "tumor-agnostic" therapeutic and diagnostic approaches. Moreover, the functions of all these driver genes can be organized into a small number of signaling pathways, as shown in **Table 71-4**.

As a consequence of the mutations they harbor, cancer cells invariably express mutant proteins that are only rarely found in normal cells. Some of these mutant proteins are processed and displayed on the cell surface in the context of major histocompatibility complexes, a process that would normally facilitate their recognition by the adaptive immune system. Thus, all cancers have the theoretical potential to be recognized as foreign, or "nonself," via the display of these tumor-specific antigens, known as mutation-associated neoantigens (MANAs). In fact, established tumors invariably prevent the activation of local

TABLE 71-4 Signaling Pathways Altered in Cancer

PROCESS	PATHWAY	REPRESENTATIVE DRIVER GENES
Cell survival	Cell cycle regulation/apoptosis	*RB1, BCL2*
	RAS	*KRAS, BRAF*
	PIK3CA	*PTEN, PIK3CA*
	JAK/STAT	*JAK2, FLT3*
	MAPK	*MAP3K, ERK*
	TGF-β	*BMPR1A, SMAD4*
Cell fate	Notch	*NOTCH1, FBWX7*
	Hedgehog	*PTCH1, SMO*
	WNT/APC	*APC, CTNNB1*
	Chromatin modification	*DNMT1, IDH1*
	Transcriptional regulation	*AR, KLF4*
Genome maintenance	DNA damage signaling and repair	*ATM, BRCA1*

T cells by inducing an intercellular suppressive mechanism known as an *immune checkpoint*. Therapeutic approaches to exploit this potential vulnerability by blocking immune checkpoints have elicited striking responses in patients with several types of cancer.

It was hypothesized that the potential immunogenicity of a tumor would be related to the total number of distinctive neoantigens it can express, which in turn is directly determined by the total number of mutations in the cancer genome. This does seem to be the case. Colorectal cancers that develop as a result of mismatch repair deficiency and smoking-related lung cancers, both of which characteristically harbor large numbers of mutations, exhibit more robust responses to therapeutic immune checkpoint blockade than most other tumor types. Notably, driver mutations as well as passenger mutations that result in the expression of mutant proteins can both contribute to the display of immunogenic neoantigens. Thus, the total number of coding mutations, a metric known as *mutational load*, is one of the determinants of potential immunogenicity.

■ TUMOR HETEROGENEITY

The mutant cells that compose a single tumor are not genetically identical. Rather, cells obtained from different sites on a tumor will harbor common mutations as well as mutations that are unique to each sample. Genetic heterogeneity results from the ongoing acquisition of mutations during tumor growth. Each time a genome is replicated, there is a small but quantifiable probability that a mutation will spontaneously arise as a result of a replication error and be passed on to the cellular progeny. This is true in normal cells or in tumor cells. Any randomly chosen cell from the skin of one individual will harbor hundreds of genetic alterations that distinguish it from a different randomly chosen skin cell, and the same is true for all organs of self-renewing tissues. Tumors are actually *less* genetically heterogeneous than normal tissues; any two randomly chosen cells from a tumor of an individual will have fewer differences than any two randomly chosen cells from that individual's normal tissues. The reason for this decrease in heterogeneity is clonal expansion, the fundamental feature of tumorigenesis. Every time a clonal expansion occurs, a genetic bottleneck wipes out heterogeneity among the cells that did not expand; these unexpanded cells either die or form only a minute proportion of the total cells in the expanding tumor.

The mutations that vary between cells of a given tumor are invariably passenger mutations that arose since the last evolutionary bottleneck, that is, those mutations that arose during the expansion of the founder cell that gave rise to the final clonal expansion. In contrast, the passenger mutations that were present in the founder cell will be uniformly present in every cell in the tumor. In that respect, these passenger mutations are not heterogeneously distributed and are in fact uniformly present in virtually all cancer cells. These "clonal" mutations, i.e., present in all cells of the cancers, are the main source of MANAs that can be exploited through immune checkpoint inhibitors. The total number of mutations and their distribution within tumor cells represent a complex interplay between the age of the patient (the older the patient, the more passenger mutations will have accumulated in the founding cell of the first clonal expansion) and the evolutionary history of the cancer (its age and number of clonal expansions it experienced).

Tumor heterogeneity has been recognized for decades at the cytogenetic, biochemical, and histopathologic levels. However, it is only recently, with the advent of a deep understanding of cancer genetics, that genetic heterogeneity can be interpreted in a medically relevant fashion. The first important point to recognize about tumor heterogeneity is that it is only the variation in driver gene alterations that is important; the cellular distribution of passenger gene mutations is irrelevant except for immune-related phenomena. In this discussion of heterogeneity, we can expand the definition of "driver genes" to include those that provide a selective growth advantage in the face of therapy in addition to those that provide a selective growth advantage during tumor evolution, prior to treatment.

Type I heterogeneity refers to that among tumors of the same type from different patients (**Fig. 71-7**). Though adenocarcinomas of the

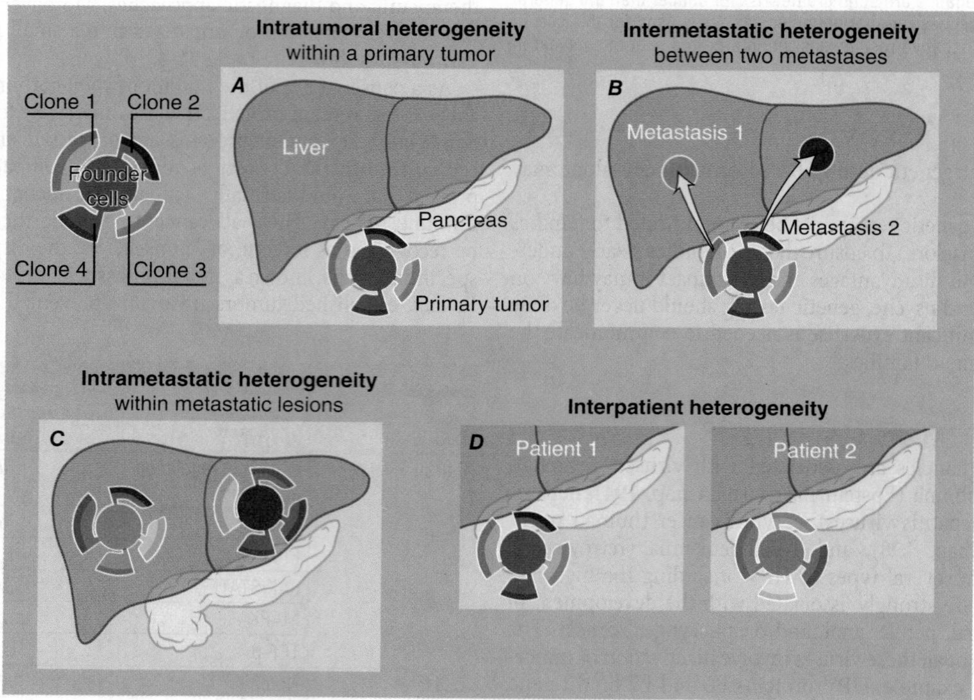

FIGURE 71-7 Four types of tumor heterogeneity. Tumor heterogeneity is the inevitable result of cell proliferation, as new mutations are introduced during clonal expansion. In a typical tumor (*upper left*), founder cells that harbor a large fraction of the total mutations give rise to subclones, which continue to evolve independently. The tumors of the founding populations are shown in the middle of each circle; the distinct subclones are shown around the periphery. ***A.*** Heterogeneity among the cells of a primary tumor is known as intratumoral heterogeneity. ***B.*** Heterogeneity among the founding cells of distinct metastatic lesions (marked as 1 and 2) that arise in the same patient is known as intermetastatic heterogeneity. ***C.*** Heterogeneity among the cells of each metastatic tumor is known as intrametastatic heterogeneity. ***D.*** Interpatient heterogeneity. The mutations in the tumors of two patients are almost completely distinct. *(From B Vogelstein et al: Cancer genome landscapes. Science 339:1546, 2013. Reprinted with permission from AAAS.)*

lung generally harbor mutations in three or more driver genes, the genes differ among the patients, and the precise mutations within the same gene can vary considerably. Type I heterogeneity is the basis for precision medicine, where the goal is to treat patients with drugs that target the proteins encoded by genetic alterations within their specific tumors. Type II heterogeneity refers to the genetic heterogeneity among different cells from the same primary tumor. Tumors continue to evolve as they grow, and different cells of the same cancer, in its original site (e.g., the pancreas), may acquire other driver gene mutations that are not shared among the other cells of the tumor. Such a mutation can result in a small clonal expansion that may or may not be important biologically. In cases in which the primary tumor can be surgically excised, such mutations are unimportant unless they give rise to type III heterogeneity (described below). The reason they are unimportant is because all primary tumor cells, whether homogeneous or not, are removed by the surgical procedure. In primary tumors that cannot be completely excised (such as most advanced brain tumors and many pancreatic ductal adenocarcinomas), heterogeneity is biomedically important because it can give rise to drug resistance, analogously to that described for type IV heterogeneity (see below). Type III heterogeneity refers to the genetic differences among the founder cells of the metastatic lesions from the same patient. For example, a patient with melanoma may have 100 different metastases distributed throughout various organs. Only if a mutant *BRAF* is present in every founder cell of every metastasis, then the patient has a chance at a complete response to a *BRAF* inhibitor. There have been several recent detailed studies of the metastases from various tumor types. Fortunately, these studies suggest there is very little, if any, type III heterogeneity among driver genes, a necessary prerequisite for the successful implementation of current and future targeted therapies. Finally, type IV heterogeneity refers to that among cells of individual metastatic lesions. As the founder cell of each metastasis expands to become detectable, it acquires mutations, a small number of which can act as "drivers" when the patient is exposed to therapeutics. This type of heterogeneity is of major clinical importance, as it has been shown to be responsible for the development of resistance in virtually all targeted therapies. The development of such resistance is a fait accompli based simply on known mutation rates and genetic resistance mechanisms. The only way to circumvent acquired resistance is to treat metastatic tumors earlier (i.e., in adjuvant setting, before much tumor expansion has occurred) or to treat with combinations of drugs for which cross-resistance is genetically impossible.

PERSONALIZED CANCER DETECTION AND TREATMENT

High-throughput DNA sequencing has led to an unprecedented understanding of cancer at the molecular level. A comprehensive mutation profile provides a molecular history of a given tumor and insights into how it arose. Because tumor cells and tumor DNA are shed into the blood and other bodily fluids, common driver mutations can be used as highly specific biomarkers for early detection. For diagnosed tumors, tumor-specific mutations can be used to estimate tumor burden, assess treatment responses, and detect recurrence.

In some cases, information regarding specific genes and pathways that are altered provides patients and physicians with options for personalized therapy. This general approach is sometimes referred to as *precision medicine.* Because tumor behavior is highly variable, even within a tumor type, personalized information-based medicine can supplement and perhaps eventually supplant histology-based tumor assessment, especially in the case of tumors that are resistant to conventional therapeutic approaches. Conversely, molecular nosology has revealed similarities in tumors of diverse histotype. The success of the precision medicine approach in any given patient depends on the presence of tumor-associated genetic alterations that are actionable (i.e., can be targeted with a specific drug). Examples of currently actionable changes include mutations in *BRAF* (targeted by the drug vemurafenib), *RET* (targeted by sunitinib and sorafenib), *ALK* rearrangements (targeted by crizotinib), and mismatch repair genes (targetable by immune checkpoint inhibitors). At present, the proportion of tumors that can be treated with such precision medicine approaches is relatively small, but future therapeutic development will hopefully change this situation. The development of new targeted agents is at present hindered by the fact that most such agents can only target activated oncogenes, while the great majority of genetic alterations in common solid tumors are those that inactivate tumor-suppressor genes. Because all drugs, whether for use in oncology or any other purpose, can only inhibit protein actions, drugs cannot be used to directly target the proteins encoded by inactivated tumor-suppressor genes; these proteins are already inactive. More information about the pathways through which tumor-suppressor genes act may provide a way around this obstacle. For example, when a tumor-suppressor gene is inactivated, some downstream component of the pathway is likely to be activated, thereby presenting a realistic target. An example of this is provided by PARP-1 inhibitors, which have been successfully used to treat patients whose tumors have inactivating mutations of genes involved in DNA repair processes, such as *BRCA1.* Patterns of global gene expression can be used to help unravel such pathways and are already being used to predict drug sensitivities and provide prognostic information in addition to that provided by DNA sequence analysis. Evaluation of proteomic and metabolomics patterns may also prove useful for this purpose.

THE FUTURE

A revolution in cancer genetics has occurred in the past 30 years. Most types of cancer are now understood at the DNA sequence level, and this accomplishment has led to an increasingly refined understanding of tumorigenesis. Cancer gene mutations have proven to be reliable biomarkers for cancer detection and monitoring as well as for informing therapeutics through precision medicine approaches. Gene-based tests are already standard of care for patients with certain tumor types, such as melanoma and colorectal and lung cancers, and the utility of these tests will undoubtedly be expanded in the coming years as new therapies and ways of predicting responses to therapies are developed. While effective treatment of advanced cancers remains difficult, the early promise shown by immune-based therapies notwithstanding, it is expected that breakthroughs in these areas will continue to emerge and be applicable to an ever-increasing number of cancers. Moreover, with the hoped-for advances in diagnostics, particularly in the earlier detection of cancers, the new and old therapies for cancer can be expected to have a much greater impact on reducing cancer deaths.

Acknowledgments

The authors gratefully acknowledge the past contributions of Pat J. Morin, Jeff Trent, and Francis Collins to earlier versions of this chapter.

FURTHER READING

Bunz F: *Principles of Cancer Genetics*, 2nd ed. Dordrecht, Springer, 2016.

Le DT et al: PD-1 Blockade in tumors with mismatch-repair deficiency. N Engl J Med 372:2509, 2015.

Vogelstein B et al: Cancer genome landscapes. Science 339:1546, 2013.

Vogelstein B, Kinzler KW: The path to cancer—three strikes and you're out. N Engl J Med 373:1895, 2015.

72 Cancer Cell Biology

Jeffrey W. Clark, Dan L. Longo

CANCER CELL BIOLOGY

Cancers are characterized by unregulated cell division, avoidance of cell death, tissue invasion, and the ability to spread to other areas of the body (metastasize). A neoplasm is *benign* when it grows in an unregulated fashion without tissue invasion or metastasizing. The presence of unregulated growth, tissue invasion, and the ability to metastasize is characteristic of *malignant* neoplasms. Cancers are named based on their origin: those derived from epithelial tissue are called *carcinomas*, those derived from mesenchymal tissues are *sarcomas*, and those derived from hematopoietic tissue are *leukemias*, *lymphomas*, and *plasma cell dyscrasias* (including *multiple myeloma*).

Cancers nearly always arise as a consequence of genetic alterations, the vast majority of which begin in a single cell and therefore are monoclonal in origin. However, because a wide variety of genetic and epigenetic changes can occur in different cells within malignant tumors over time, most cancers are characterized by marked heterogeneity in the populations of cells. In addition, extrinsic factors in the cancer environment (e.g., the stroma, infiltrating cells, various cell-to-cell interactions, spatial orientation, secreted factors, and availability of oxygen and nutrients) vary in different areas within the tumor or different metastases, compounding this heterogeneity. This heterogeneity significantly complicates the treatment of most cancers because it is likely that there are subsets of cells that will be resistant to therapy for a variety of reasons and will therefore survive and proliferate even if the majority of cells are killed.

A few cancers appear to, at least initially, be primarily driven by an alteration in a dominant gene that produces uncontrolled cell proliferation. Examples include chronic myeloid leukemia (*abl*), about half of melanomas (*braf*), Burkitt's lymphoma (c-*myc*), and subsets of lung adenocarcinomas (*egfr, alk, ros1, met, ret, braf,* and *ntrk*). Genes that can promote cell growth when altered are often called *oncogenes*. They were first identified as critical elements of viruses that cause animal tumors; it was subsequently found that the viral genes had normal counterparts with important functions in the cell and had been captured and mutated by viruses as they passed from host to host.

However, most human cancers are characterized by a multiple-step process involving many genetic abnormalities, each of which contributes to the loss of control of cell proliferation and differentiation and the acquisition of capabilities, such as tissue invasion, the ability to metastasize, and angiogenesis (development of new blood vessels required for tumor growth). These properties are not found in the normal adult cell from which the tumor is derived. Indeed, normal cells have a large number of safeguards against DNA damage (including multiple DNA repair and extensive DNA damage response mechanisms), uncontrolled proliferation, and invasion. Many cancers go through recognizable steps of progressively more abnormal phenotypes: hyperplasia, to adenoma, to dysplasia, to carcinoma in situ, to invasive cancer with the ability to metastasize (**Table 72-1**). For most cancers, these changes occur over a prolonged period of time, usually many years.

TABLE 72-1 Phenotypic Characteristics of Malignant Cells

Deregulated cell proliferation: Loss of function of negative growth regulators (tumor suppressor genes, i.e., *Rb, p53*), and increased action of positive growth regulators (oncogenes, i.e., *Ras, Myc*). Leads to aberrant cell cycle control and includes loss of normal checkpoint responses.
Failure to differentiate: Arrest at a stage before terminal differentiation. May retain stem cell properties. (Frequently observed in leukemias due to transcriptional repression of developmental programs by the gene products of chromosomal translocations.)
Loss of normal apoptosis pathways: Inactivation of p53, increases in Bcl-2 (antiapoptotic) family members. This defect enhances the survival of cells with oncogenic mutations and genetic instability and allows clonal expansion and diversification within the tumor without activation of physiologic cell death pathways.
Genetic instability: Defects in DNA repair pathways leading to either single nucleotide or oligonucleotide mutations (as in microsatellite instability, MIN) or, more commonly, chromosomal instability (CIN) leading to aneuploidy (abnormal number of chromosomes in a cell). Caused by loss of function of a number of proteins including p53, BRCA1/2, mismatch repair genes, DNA repair enzymes, and the spindle checkpoint. Leads to accumulation of a variety of mutations in different cells within the tumor and heterogeneity.
Loss of replicative senescence: Normal cells stop dividing in vitro after 25–50 population doublings. Arrest is mediated by the Rb, $p16^{INK4a}$, and p53 pathways. While most cells remain arrested, genetic and epigenetic changes in a subset of cells allow further replication, leading to telomere loss, with crisis leading to death of many cells. Cells that survive often harbor gross chromosomal abnormalities and the ability to continue to proliferate. These cells express telomerase, which maintains telomeres and is important for ongoing growth of these cells. Relevance to human in vivo cancer remains uncertain. Many human cancers express telomerase.
Nonresponsiveness to external growth-inhibiting signals: Cancer cells have lost responsiveness to signals normally present to stop proliferating when they have overgrown the niche normally occupied by the organ from which they are derived. Our understanding about this mechanism of growth regulation remains limited.
Increased angiogenesis: Due to increased gene expression of proangiogenic factors (VEGF, FGF, IL-8, angiopoietin) by tumor or stromal cells, or loss of negative regulators (endostatin, tumstatin, thrombospondin).
Invasion: Cell mobility and ability to move through extracellular matrix and into other tissues or organs. Loss of cell-cell contacts (gap junctions, cadherins) and increased production of matrix metalloproteinases (MMPs). Can take the form of epithelial-to-mesenchymal transition (EMT), with anchored epithelial cells becoming more like motile fibroblasts.
Metastasis: Spread of tumor cells to lymph nodes or distant tissue sites. Limited by the ability of tumor cells to migrate out of initial site and to survive in a foreign environment, including evading the immune system (see below).
Evasion of the immune system: Downregulation of MHC class I and II molecules; induction of T-cell tolerance; inhibition of normal dendritic cell and/or T-cell function; antigenic loss variants and clonal heterogeneity; increase in regulatory T cells.
Shift in cell metabolism: Complex changes including alterations due to tumor stress such as hypoxia and energy generation shifts from oxidative phosphorylation to aerobic glycolysis generate building blocks for malignant cell production and proliferation.

Abbreviations: FGF, fibroblast growth factor; IL, interleukin; MHC, major histocompatibility complex; VEGF, vascular endothelial growth factor.

In most organs, only primitive undifferentiated cells are capable of proliferating and cells lose the capacity to proliferate as they differentiate and acquire functional capabilities. The expansion of the primitive cells (stem cells) is linked to some functional need in the host through receptors that receive signals from the local environment or through hormonal and other influences delivered by the vascular supply. In the absence of such signals, the cells are at rest. The signals that keep the primitive cells at rest remain incompletely understood. These signals must be environmental, based on the observations that a regenerating liver stops growing when it has replaced the portion that has been surgically removed after partial hepatectomy and regenerating bone marrow stops growing when the peripheral blood counts return to normal. Cancer cells clearly have lost responsiveness to such controls and do not recognize when they have overgrown the niche normally occupied by the organ from which they are derived. A better understanding of these mechanisms of growth regulation in the context of organ homeostasis is evolving.

CANCER AS AN ORGAN THAT IGNORES ITS NICHE

The fundamental cellular defects that create a malignant neoplasm act at the cellular level, and some of these are cell autonomous. However, that is not the entire story. Cancers consist of both malignant cells as well as other cells, blood vessels, extracellular matrix, and signaling and other molecules in the cancer microenvironment. They behave as organs that have lost their specialized function and stopped responding to signals that would limit their growth in tightly regulated normal tissue homeostasis. Most human cancers usually become clinically detectable when a primary mass is approximately 1 cm in diameter—such a mass consists of about 10^9 cells. Often, patients present with tumors that are approximately 10^{10} cells. Although it varies by type of cancer and where the primary tumor and metastases are located, a lethal tumor burden is usually about 10^{12}–10^{13} cells. If all malignant cells were dividing without any cell death at the time of diagnosis, most patients would reach a lethal tumor burden in a very short time. However, human tumors grow by Gompertzian kinetics—this means that not every daughter cell produced by a cell division is actively dividing. In addition, the overall growth rate of a tumor depends on differences between growth rates of different cells within the tumor and rate of cell loss. The growth fraction of a tumor declines with time, largely due to factors in the microenvironment. The growth fraction of the first malignant cell is 100%, and by the time a patient presents for medical care, the growth fraction is estimated to be <10%, although the fraction varies between different types of cancers and even different cancers of the same type in different individuals. This fraction is often similar to the growth fraction of normal bone marrow and normal intestinal epithelium, the most highly proliferative normal tissues in the human body, a fact that may explain the dose-limiting toxicities to these tissues of agents that target dividing cells.

The implication of these data is that the tumor is slowing its own growth over time. How does it do this? The tumor cells have multiple genetic lesions that tend to promote proliferation, yet by the time the tumor is clinically detectable, its capacity for proliferation has declined. Better understanding of how a tumor slows its own growth would provide important clues for better cancer treatment. A number of factors, including those in the tumor microenvironment, are known to contribute to the decreased proliferation of tumor cells over time in vivo. Some cells are hypoxemic and have inadequate supply of nutrients and energy. Some have sustained too much genetic damage to complete the cell cycle but have lost the capacity to undergo apoptosis and therefore survive but do not proliferate. However, an important subset is not actively dividing but retains the capacity to divide and can start dividing again under certain conditions such as when the tumor mass is reduced by treatments leading to improved conditions in the tumor microenvironment favorable for cell proliferation. Just as the bone marrow increases its rate of proliferation in response to bone marrow–damaging agents, the tumor also seems to sense when tumor cell numbers have been reduced and can respond by increasing growth rate. However, the critical difference is that the marrow stops growing when it has reached its production goals, whereas tumors do not.

The ultimate structure and organization of an organ are based on a number of factors including growth, migration, elimination, and death of various cells; communication between cells to establish the correct architecture; competition between cells; and the composition of the extracellular matrix that is produced. In addition to normal cells stopping proliferation in an organ when that is appropriate, normal tissues have various mechanisms for eliminating cells both in the process of development as well as ongoing homeostasis of an organ. These include mechanical processes based on a number of factors including cell size, shape, and topology between cells that can determine cell fate as well as an active process of cell extrusion, which plays a major role in the elimination of both cells that are no longer needed by the organ and cells that are damaged and potentially dangerous (such as those with mutations that might be precursors for malignancy). The process of cell extrusion may depend on cell cycle arrest in the S phase; aberrations in this process may contribute to the metastatic process. A variety of processes, including major alterations in cell cycle control, apoptosis and other mechanisms of cell death, and uncontrolled cell signaling, all contribute to defects in appropriate cell extrusion contributing to the development of cancer.

Additional tumor cell vulnerabilities are likely to be detected when we learn more about how normal cells respond to "stop" signals from their environment, and why and how tumor cells and tissues fail to heed such signals.

■ CELL CYCLE CHECKPOINTS

The cell division cycle consists of four phases—G_1 (growth and preparation for DNA synthesis), S (DNA synthesis), G_2 (preparation to divide), and M (mitosis, cell division). Cells can also exit the cell cycle and be quiescent (G_0). Progression of a cell through the cell cycle is tightly regulated at a number of checkpoints (especially at the G_1/S boundary, the G_2/M boundary, and during M [spindle checkpoint]) by an array of genes that are targeted by specific genetic alterations in cancer. Critical proteins in these control processes that are frequently mutated or otherwise inactivated in cancers are called tumor-suppressor genes. Examples include p53 and Rb (discussed below). In the first phase, G_1, preparations are made to replicate the genetic material. The cell stops before entering the DNA synthesis phase, or S phase, to take inventory. Are we ready to replicate our DNA? Is the DNA repair machinery in place to fix any mutations that are detected? Are the DNA replicating enzymes available? Is there an adequate supply of nucleotides? Is there sufficient energy to proceed? The retinoblastoma protein, Rb, plays a central role in placing a brake on the process until the cell is ready. When the cell determines that it is prepared to move ahead, sequential activation of cyclin-dependent kinases (CDKs) results in the inactivation of the brake, Rb, by phosphorylation. Phosphorylated Rb releases the S phase–regulating transcription factor, E2F/DP1, and genes required for S-phase progression are expressed. If the cell determines that it is unready to move ahead with DNA replication, a number of inhibitors are capable of blocking the action of the CDKs, including p21Cip2/Waf1, p16Ink4a, and p27Kip1. Nearly every cancer has one or more defects in the G_1 checkpoint that permit progression to S phase despite abnormalities in DNA repair machinery or other deficiencies that would affect normal DNA synthesis.

At the end of the G_2 phase and prior to the M phase, after the cell has exactly duplicated its DNA content, a second inventory is taken at the G_2 checkpoint. Have all of the chromosomes been fully duplicated? Were all segments of DNA copied only once? Has all damaged DNA been repaired? Do we have the right number of chromosomes and the right amount of DNA? If so, the cell proceeds to prepare for division by synthesizing mitotic spindle and other proteins needed to produce two daughter cells. If DNA damage is detected, the p53 pathway is normally activated. Called the guardian of the genome, p53 is a transcription factor that is normally present in the cell in very low levels. This level is generally regulated through its rapid turnover. Normally, p53 is bound to mdm2, a ubiquitin ligase that both inhibits p53 transcriptional activation and also targets p53 for degradation in the proteasome. When DNA damage is sensed, the ATM (ataxia-telangiectasia mutated) pathway is activated; ATM phosphorylates mdm2, releasing it from its inhibitory bond to p53. p53 then stops cell cycle progression, directs the synthesis of repair enzymes, or if the damage is too great, initiates apoptosis (programmed cell death) of the cell to prevent the propagation of a damaged cell (**Fig. 72-1**).

A second method of activating p53 involves the induction of p14ARF by hyperproliferative signals from oncogenes. p14ARF competes with p53 for binding to mdm2, allowing p53 to escape the effects of mdm2 and accumulate in the cell. p53 then stops cell cycle progression by activating CDK inhibitors such as p21 and/or initiating the apoptosis pathway. Not surprisingly given its critical role in controlling cell cycle progression, mutations in the gene for p53 on chromosome 17p are among the most frequent mutations in human cancers, although percentages vary between different cancers. Most commonly these mutations are acquired in the malignant tissue in one allele and the second allele is inactivated (such as by deletion or epigenetic silencing), leaving the cell unprotected from DNA-damaging agents or activated oncogenes. Some environmental exposures produce signature mutations in p53; for example, aflatoxin exposure leads to mutation of arginine to serine at codon 249 and leads to hepatocellular carcinoma. In rare instances, p53 mutations are in the germline (Li-Fraumeni syndrome) and produce a familial cancer syndrome. Another mechanism for inactivation of p53 in malignant cells is due to alterations in regulators such as overexpression of the inhibitory mdm2 protein. Whether inactivated by mutation or inhibited by regulatory factors, absence of normal p53 function leads to chromosomal instability and accumulation of DNA

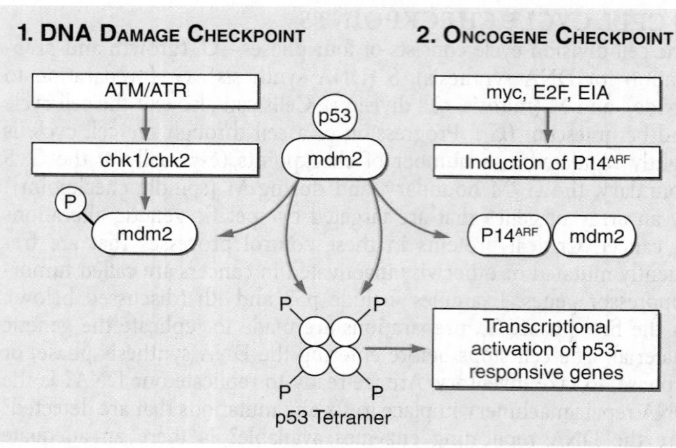

FIGURE 72-1 Induction of p53 by the DNA damage and oncogene checkpoints. In response to noxious stimuli, p53 and mdm2 are phosphorylated by the ataxia-telangiectasia mutated (ATM) and related ATR serine/threonine kinases, as well as the immediate downstream checkpoint kinases, Chk1 and Chk2. This causes dissociation of p53 from mdm2, leading to increased p53 protein levels and transcription of genes leading to cell cycle arrest ($p21^{Cip1/Waf1}$) or apoptosis (e.g., the proapoptotic Bcl-2 family members Noxa and Puma). Inducers of p53 include hypoxemia, DNA damage (caused by ultraviolet radiation, gamma irradiation, or chemotherapy), ribonucleotide depletion, and telomere shortening. A second mechanism of p53 induction is activated by oncogenes such as *Myc*, which promote aberrant G_1/S transition. This pathway is regulated by a second product of the Ink4a locus, $p14^{ARF}$ (p19 in mice), which is encoded by an *a*lternative *r*eading *f*rame (ARF) of the same stretch of DNA that codes for $p16^{Ink4a}$. Levels of ARF are upregulated by *Myc* and E2F, and ARF binds to mdm2 and rescues p53 from its inhibitory effect. This *oncogene checkpoint* leads to the death or senescence (an irreversible arrest in G_1 of the cell cycle) of renegade cells that attempt to enter S phase without appropriate physiologic signals. Senescent cells have been identified in patients whose premalignant lesions harbor activated oncogenes, for instance, dysplastic nevi that encode an activated form of BRAF (see below), demonstrating that induction of senescence is a protective mechanism that operates in humans to prevent the outgrowth of neoplastic cells.

damage including acquisition of properties that give the abnormal cell a proliferative and survival advantage. Like Rb dysfunction, most cancers have mechanisms that disable the p53 pathway. Indeed, the importance of p53 and Rb in the development of cancer is underscored by the neoplastic transformation mechanism of human papillomavirus. This virus has two main oncogenes, E6 and E7. E6 acts to increase the rapid turnover of p53, and E7 acts to inhibit Rb function; inhibition of these two targets is required for transformation of epithelial cells.

Another cell cycle checkpoint exists when the cell is undergoing division (M phase); this is the spindle checkpoint, which acts to ensure that there is proper attachment of chromosomes to the mitotic spindle before progression through the cell cycle can occur. If the spindle apparatus does not properly align the chromosomes for division, if the chromosome number is abnormal (i.e., greater or less than $4n$), or if the centromeres are not properly paired with their duplicated partners, then the cell initiates a cell death pathway to prevent the production of aneuploid progeny (having an altered number of chromosomes). Abnormalities in the spindle checkpoint facilitate the development of aneuploidy, which is frequently found in cancers. In some tumors, aneuploidy is a predominant genetic feature.

In other tumors, a defect in the cells' ability to repair errors in the DNA, such as due to mutations in genes coding for the proteins critical for mismatched DNA repair, is the primary genetic lesion. Cancer cells can have defects in any of several DNA repair pathways in addition to mismatch repair, including deficient interstrand cross-link, double-strand breaks (homologous recombination or nonhomologous end joining repair), single-strand breaks, base excision, nucleotide excision, and translesional synthesis.

In general, tumors have either defects in chromosome number or defective DNA repair pathways but not both. Defects that lead to cancer include abnormal cell cycle checkpoints, inadequate DNA repair, and failure to preserve genome integrity leading to DNA damage. These defects and the stress of the resultant increased DNA damage make cancer cells more vulnerable to additional DNA damage, which can be exploited by chemotherapy, radiation therapy, targeted therapy, and immunotherapy—the major systemic therapeutic approaches effective against cancer.

Alternatively, research is ongoing in an attempt to therapeutically restore the defects in cell cycle regulation and DNA repair that characterize cancer, although this remains a challenging problem because it is much more difficult to restore normal biologic function than to inhibit abnormal function of proteins driving cell proliferation, such as occurs with oncogenes. Newer approaches to gene editing (e.g., clustered regularly interspaced short palindromic repeats [CRISPR]) and subsequent modifications to this approach should make this more feasible.

CELLULAR SENESCENCE

The irreversible cessation of growth of normal cells while the cells remain viable has been termed cellular senescence. This was initially identified by the fact that when normal cells are placed in culture in vitro, most are not capable of sustained growth. They quickly reach a point where they either undergo cell death due to excessive DNA damage or other factors or they become senescent. Fibroblasts are an exception to this rule. When they are cultured, fibroblasts may divide 30–50 times and then they undergo what has been termed a "crisis" during which the majority of cells stop dividing (usually due to an increase in p21 expression, a CDK inhibitor). This form of senescence is termed replicative senescence. Many other cells die, and a small fraction emerge that have acquired genetic and epigenetic changes that permit their uncontrolled growth.

Among the cellular changes during in vitro propagation is telomere shortening. DNA polymerase is unable to replicate the tips of chromosomes, resulting in the loss of DNA at the specialized ends of chromosomes (called *telomeres*) with each replication cycle. At birth, human telomeres are 15- to 20-kb pairs long and are composed of tandem repeats of a six-nucleotide sequence (TTAGGG) that associate with specialized telomere-binding proteins to form a T-loop structure that protects the ends of chromosomes from being mistakenly recognized as damaged. The loss of telomeric repeats with each cell division cycle causes gradual telomere shortening, leading to growth arrest when one or more critically short telomeres trigger a p53-regulated DNA-damage checkpoint response. Cell death usually ensues when the unprotected ends of chromosomes lead to chromosome fusions or other catastrophic DNA rearrangements. Cells with certain abnormalities, such as those with nonfunctional pRb and p53, can bypass this growth arrest. *The ability to bypass telomere-based growth limitations is thought to be a critical step in the evolution of most malignancies.* This occurs by reactivation of telomerase expression in cancer cells. Telomerase is an enzyme that adds TTAGGG repeats onto the 3′ ends of chromosomes. It contains a catalytic subunit with reverse transcriptase activity (hTERT) and an RNA component that provides the template for telomere extension. Most normal somatic cells do not express sufficient telomerase to prevent telomere attrition with each cell division. Exceptions include stem cells (such as those found in hematopoietic tissues, gut and skin epithelium, and germ cells) that require extensive cell division to maintain tissue homeostasis. More than 90% of human cancers express high levels of telomerase that prevent telomere shortening to critical levels and allow indefinite cell proliferation. In vitro experiments indicate that inhibition of telomerase activity leads to tumor cell apoptosis. Major efforts are underway to develop methods to inhibit telomerase activity in cancer cells. For example, the protein component of telomerase (hTERT) may act as one of the most widely expressed tumor-associated antigens and can be targeted by vaccine approaches. However, a caveat to targeting telomerase for anticancer treatment is the potential for inhibiting its activity in certain normal cells (such as stem cells) required for maintaining the normal physiologic state.

Although most of the functions of telomerase relate to cell division, it also has several other effects including interfering with the differentiated functions of at least certain stem cells. However, the impact on differentiated function of normal nonstem cells is less clear. The picture is further complicated by the fact that rare genetic defects in the telomerase enzyme seem to cause dyskeratosis congenita (characterized by abnormalities in various rapidly dividing cells in the body including skin, nails, oral mucosa, hair, and bone marrow with increased risk for leukemia and certain other cancers). This can be associated with a number of other abnormalities including pulmonary fibrosis, bone marrow failure (aplastic anemia), or liver fibrosis. However, paradoxically, defects in nutrient absorption in the gastrointestinal tract, a site that should be highly sensitive to defective cell proliferation, are not seen. Much remains to be learned about how telomere shortening and telomere maintenance are related to human illness in general and cancer in particular.

A variety of other stresses on cells (both environmental and intrinsic including radiation, chemotherapy, reactive oxygen species, and oncogenic mutations) can also lead to senescence, primarily those that induce DNA damage similar to that seen in cells with shortened telomeres. This is termed *replicative senescence.*

SIGNAL TRANSDUCTION PATHWAYS IN CANCER CELLS

Signals that affect cell behavior come from adjacent cells, the stroma in which the cells are located, hormonal signals that originate remotely, and the cells themselves (autocrine signaling). These signals generally exert their influence on the receiving cell through activation of signal transduction pathways that have as their end result the induction of activated transcription factors that mediate a change in cell behavior or function or the acquisition of effector machinery to accomplish a new task. Although signal transduction pathways can lead to a wide variety of outcomes, many such pathways rely on cascades of signals that sequentially activate different proteins or glycoproteins and lipids or glycolipids, and the activation steps often involve the addition or removal of one or more phosphate groups on a downstream target. Other chemical changes can result from signal transduction pathways, but reversible phosphorylation and dephosphorylation play a major role. Proteins that add phosphate groups to other molecules (proteins, lipids, or nucleic acids) are called kinases. Two major classes of kinases involved in signal transduction pathways important for cancer cells are tyrosine kinases that phosphorylate tyrosine and serine/threonine kinases that phosphorylate serine/threonine either directly or indirectly. However, some kinases can phosphorylate both, such as the MEK kinases that can phosphorylate both threonine and tyrosine. Phosphatases (protein tyrosine phosphatases and protein serine/threonine phosphatases) remove the phosphate groups to reverse the kinase activity.

Various kinases play critical roles in signal transduction pathways important for malignant cells. These include a number of receptor tyrosine kinases (RTKs) as well as various protein kinases (both tyrosine and serine/threonine kinases) downstream of receptors that transmit the signals within the cell (**Fig. 72-2**). Two important signaling pathways are the RAS-RAF-MEK-ERK pathway and the phosphatidylinositol-3-kinase (PI3K) pathway (Fig. 72-2). Although pathways are depicted as distinct, there are complex interactions between pathways within cells.

Normally, kinase activity is short-lived and reversed by protein phosphatases. However, in many human cancers, RTKs or components of their downstream pathways are activated by mutation, gene amplification, or chromosomal translocations to have enhanced and/or prolonged activity. Because these pathways are important in regulating proliferation, survival, migration, and angiogenesis, they have been identified as important targets for cancer therapeutics.

Inhibition of kinase activity is effective in the treatment of a number of neoplasms. Lung cancers with mutations in the epidermal growth factor receptor are highly responsive to osimertinib as well as other inhibitors (**Table 72-2**). Inhibitors have been developed to treat lung cancers with other tyrosine kinase–activating mutations (including anaplastic lymphoma kinase [ALK], ROS1, NTRK, MET, and RET) BRAF (a serine/threonine kinase) inhibitors are highly effective in melanomas and thyroid cancers and are also used in combination with other agents for lung and colon cancers in which BRAF is mutated. Targeting the MEK protein (which phosphorylates both threonine and tyrosine residues) downstream of BRAF also has activity against BRAF mutant melanomas, and combined inhibition of BRAF and MEK is more effective than either alone with activity that extends to BRAF mutant lung cancer. Janus kinase (JAK) inhibitors are active in myeloproliferative syndromes in which JAK2 activation is a pathogenetic event. Imatinib (which targets a number of tyrosine kinases) is an effective agent in tumors that have translocations of the c-Abl and BCR gene (such as chronic myeloid leukemia), mutant c-Kit (gastrointestinal stromal cell tumors), or mutant platelet-derived growth factor receptor (PDGFRα; gastrointestinal stromal tumors). Second-generation inhibitors of BCR-Abl, dasatinib and nilotinib, are even more effective, and the third-generation agent bosutinib has activity in some patients who have progressed on other inhibitors, while the third-generation agent ponatinib has activity against the T315I mutation, which is resistant to the other agents. Although almost all tyrosine kinase inhibitors are not entirely selective for one protein, certain inhibitors have significant activity against a broad number of proteins. These include sorafenib, regorafenib, cabozantinib, sunitinib, and lenvatinib. These have shown antitumor activity in various malignancies, including renal cell cancer (RCC) (sorafenib, sunitinib, cabozantinib, lenvatinib), hepatocellular carcinoma (sorafenib, regorafenib, lenvatinib), gastrointestinal stromal tumor (GIST) (sunitinib, regorafenib), thyroid cancer (sorafenib, cabozantinib, lenvatinib), colorectal cancer (regorafenib), and pancreatic neuroendocrine tumors (sunitinib).

Inhibitors of the PI3K pathway also have been approved for cancer therapy. The PI3K family includes three classes and several isoforms within each class. Inhibitors against different isoforms have proved effective against different types of malignancies, with inhibitors of the delta isoform (either specifically or also with inhibition of other isoforms; e.g., idelalisib) having activity against lymphoid malignancies, whereas the specific inhibitor of a mutation in the alpha isoform (alpelisib) has activity against breast cancers with this mutation. Inhibitors of mammalian target of rapamycin (mTOR; which is downstream of PI3K; e.g., everolimus, temsirolimus) are active in RCC, pancreatic neuroendocrine tumors, and breast cancer. Additional inhibitors of the PI3K pathway and other phospholipid signaling pathways such as the phospholipase C-gamma pathway, which are involved in a large number of cellular processes important in cancer development and progression, are being evaluated.

The list of active agents and treatment indications is growing rapidly (Table 72-2). These agents have ushered in a new era of personalized therapy. It is becoming more common for tumor biopsies to be assessed for specific molecular changes that predict response and to have clinical decision-making guided by those results. This is now an important component of standard therapy for metastatic lung, gastroesophageal, melanoma, breast, and colorectal cancers as well as in adjuvant therapy for breast cancer.

An alternative approach to testing samples directly from tumors is to test blood for the presence of mutations or amplification in circulating tumor DNA, which has the significant advantage of being noninvasive. As cancers grow, some of the cells die and break down with release of cellular contents, including DNA, into the circulation. Sensitive methods have been developed to detect this DNA and to identify mutations and other DNA changes in the malignant cells. This has the potential advantage over tumor biopsies of sampling all of the tumor and not being limited to one site that may not be representative of the overall tumor heterogeneity. In addition to identifying potential changes that can be targeted for therapy, there is also the potential for monitoring a patient's response to therapy, identifying resistance mechanisms to therapy earlier, detecting disease recurrence before it can be detected by tumor markers or scans, monitoring bodily fluids in addition to blood, and possibly providing a means of earlier initial detection of cancer if sufficiently sensitive and specific detection methods can be developed.

However, none of these targeted therapies has yet been curative by themselves for any malignancy, although prolonged periods of disease control lasting many years frequently occur in chronic myeloid leukemia (CML), including a >80% survival rate at 10 years. The reasons for the failure to cure are not completely defined, although resistance

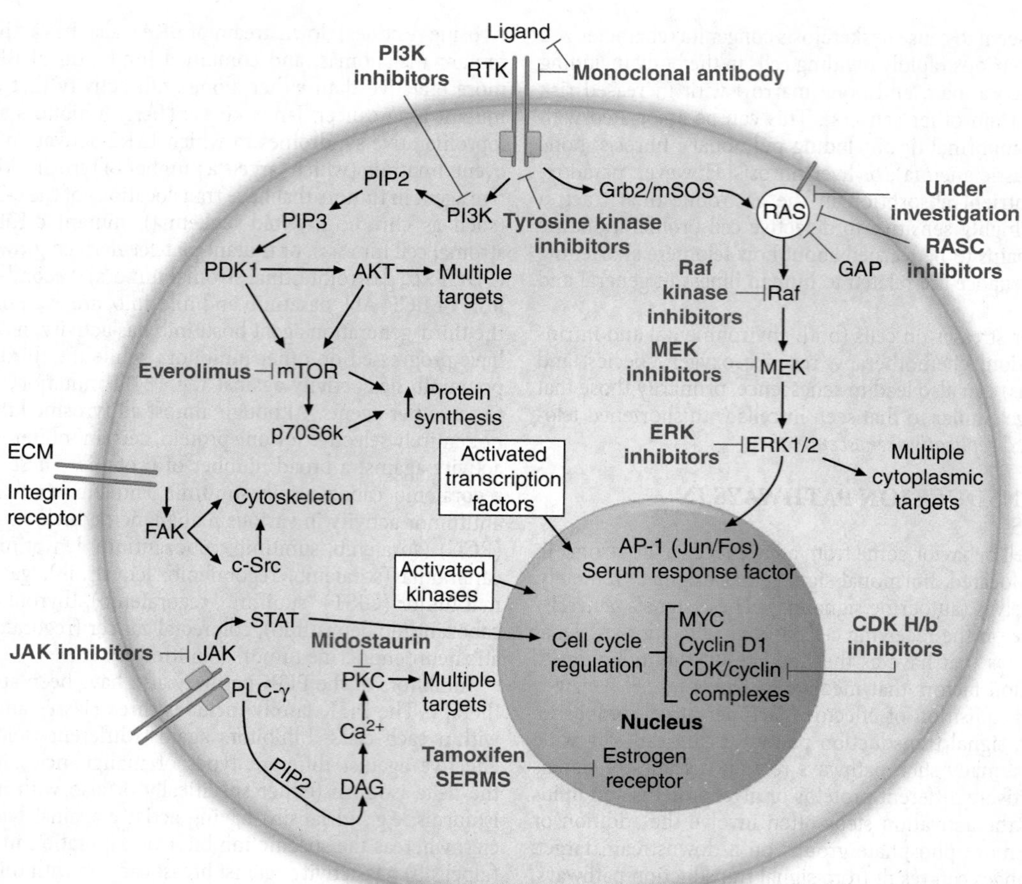

FIGURE 72-2 Therapeutic targeting of signal transduction pathways in cancer cells. Three major signal transduction pathways are activated by receptor tyrosine kinases (RTKs). *1.* The protooncogene Ras is activated by the Grb2/mSOS guanine nucleotide exchange factor, which induces an association with Raf and activation of downstream kinases (MEK and ERK1/2). *2.* Activated PI3K phosphorylates the membrane lipid PIP_2 to generate PIP_3, which acts as a membrane-docking site for a number of cellular proteins including the serine/threonine kinases PDK1 and Akt. PDK1 has numerous cellular targets, including Akt and mTOR. Akt phosphorylates target proteins that promote resistance to apoptosis and enhance cell cycle progression, while mTOR and its target p70S6K upregulate protein synthesis to potentiate cell growth. *3.* Activation of PLC-γ leads the formation of diacylglycerol (DAG) and increased intracellular calcium, with activation of multiple isoforms of PKC and other enzymes regulated by the calcium/calmodulin system. Other important signaling pathways involve non-RTKs that are activated by cytokine or integrin receptors. Janus kinases (JAK) phosphorylate STAT (signal transducer and activator of transcription) transcription factors, which translocate to the nucleus and activate target genes. Integrin receptors mediate cellular interactions with the extracellular matrix (ECM), inducing activation of FAK (focal adhesion kinase) and c-Src, which activate multiple downstream pathways, including modulation of the cell cytoskeleton. Many activated kinases and transcription factors migrate into the nucleus, where they regulate gene transcription, thus completing the path from extracellular signals, such as growth factors, to a change in cell phenotype, such as induction of differentiation or cell proliferation. The nuclear targets of these processes include transcription factors (e.g., Myc, AP-1, and serum response factor) and the cell cycle machinery (cyclin-dependent kinases [CDKs] and cyclins). Inhibitors of many of these pathways have been developed for the treatment of human cancers. Examples of inhibitors that are either approved or are currently being evaluated in clinical trials are shown in purple type.

to the treatment ultimately develops in most patients. In some tumors, resistance to kinase inhibitors is related to proliferation of cells with a mutation in the target kinase that inhibits drug binding. Many of these kinase inhibitors act as competitive inhibitors of the ATP-binding pocket. ATP is the phosphate donor in these phosphorylation reactions. For example, mutation in the critical BCR-ABL kinase in the ATP-binding pocket (such as the threonine to isoleucine change at codon 315 [T315I]) can prevent imatinib binding. Other resistance mechanisms include alterations in other signal transduction pathways to bypass the inhibited pathway. As resistance mechanisms continue to be better defined, rational strategies to overcome resistance are emerging. In addition, many kinase inhibitors are less specific for an oncogenic target than was hoped, and toxicities related to off-target inhibition of kinases limit the use of the agent at a dose that would optimally inhibit the cancer-relevant kinase.

Antibodies against protein targets more highly expressed on malignant than normal cells can also be used to deliver highly toxic compounds relatively specifically to cancer cells. Examples of protein targets for currently approved antibody-drug conjugates include CD30 for Hodgkin's and anaplastic lymphomas; HER2 on breast cancer; CD33 on acute myeloid leukemias; CD22 on B-cell acute lymphocytic and hairy cell leukemias; and CD79b on diffuse large B-cell lymphomas.

Another strategy to enhance the antitumor effects of targeted agents is to use them in rational combinations with each other as well as with chemotherapy or immunotherapy agents that kill cells in ways distinct from agents targeting specific mutant or overexpressed proteins. Combinations of trastuzumab (a monoclonal antibody that targets the HER2 receptor [member of the EGFR family]) with chemotherapy have significant activity against breast and stomach cancers that have high levels of expression of the HER2 protein. The activity of trastuzumab and chemotherapy can be enhanced further by combinations with another targeted monoclonal antibody (pertuzumab), which prevents dimerization of the HER2 receptor with other HER family members including HER3.

Although targeted therapies have not yet resulted in cures when used alone, their use in the adjuvant setting and when combined with other effective treatments has substantially increased the fraction of patients cured. For example, the addition of rituximab, an anti-CD20 antibody, to combination chemotherapy in patients with diffuse large B-cell lymphoma improves cure rates by ~15%. The addition

TABLE 72-2 Some FDA-Approved Molecularly Targeted Agents for the Treatment of Cancer

DRUG	MOLECULAR TARGET	DISEASE	MECHANISM OF ACTION
All-*trans* retinoic acid	PML-RARα oncogene	Acute promyelocytic leukemia M3 AML, t(15;17)	Inhibits transcriptional repression by PML-RARα
Imatinib	Bcr-Abl, c-Abl, c-Kit, PDGFR-α/β	Chronic myeloid leukemia, GIST	Blocks ATP binding to tyrosine kinase active site
Ripretinib	c-Kit, PDGFR-α	GIST	Inhibits tyrosine kinase activity
Dasatinib, nilotinib, ponatinib, bosutinib	Bcr-Abl (primarily)	Chronic myeloid leukemia	Blocks ATP binding to tyrosine kinase active site
Sunitinib	c-Kit, VEGFR-2, PDGFR-β, Flt-3	GIST, RCC, PNET	Inhibits activated c-Kit and PDGFR in GIST; inhibits VEGFR in RCC and probably in PNET
Sorafenib	RAF, VEGFR-2, PDGFR-α/β, Flt-3, c-Kit	RCC, hepatocellular carcinoma (HCC), differentiated thyroid cancer, desmoid	Targets VEGFR pathways in RCC and HCC. Possible activity against BRAF in thyroid cancer
Regorafenib	VEGFR1–3, TIE-2, FGFR1, KIT, RET, PDGFR	Colorectal cancer, GIST, HCC	Competitive inhibitor ATP binding site of tyrosine kinase domain multiple kinases including VEGFR
Larotrectinib, entrectinib	NTRK	Cancers with NTRK mutation	Competitive inhibitor of ATP binding site of the tyrosine kinase domain of NTRK
Axitinib	VEGFR1–3	RCC	Competitive inhibitor ATP binding site of tyrosine kinase domain VEGF receptors
Erlotinib	EGFR	NSCLC, pancreatic cancer	Competitive inhibitor of the ATP-binding site of the EGFR
Afitinib	EGFR (and other HER family)	NSCLC	Irreversible inhibitor of ATP-binding site of HER family members
Osimertinib	EGFR (T790M)	NSCLC	Inhibits EGFR mutations including T790M mutant NSCLC
Dacomitinib	EGFR	NSCLC (exon19 deletion/exon 21 L858R)	Inhibits EGFR mutant lung cancer
Erdafitinib, pemigatinib	FGFR2, FGFR3	Urothelial (erdafitinib), cholangiocarcinoma (pemigatinib)	Inhibits tyrosine kinase of FGFR
Lapatinib, tucatinib	HER2/neu	Breast cancer	Competitive inhibitor of the ATP-binding site of HER2
Crizotinib, ceritinib, alectinib, brigatinib, lorlatinib	ALK	NSCLC	Inhibitor of ALK tyrosine kinase
Crizotinib, entrectinib	ROS1	NSCLC	Inhibitor of ROS1 tyrosine kinase
Palbociclib, ribociclib, abemaciclib	CDK4/6	Breast	Inhibitor of CDK4/6
Bortezomib, carfilzomib, ixazomib	Proteasome	Multiple myeloma	Inhibits proteolytic degradation of multiple cellular proteins
Vemurafenib, dabrafenib	BRAF	Melanoma	Inhibitor of serine-threonine kinase domain of V600E mutant of BRAF
Encorafenib	MEK	CRC	Inhibits BRAFV600E mutation; used in combination with cetuximab
Trametinib, Cobimetinib	MEK	Melanoma	Inhibitor of serine-threonine kinase domain of MEK
Cabozantinib	RET, MET, VEGFR	MTC, RCC	Competitive inhibitor of ATP-binding site of tyrosine kinase domain of multiple kinases, including VEGFR2 and RET
Capmatinib	MET	NSCLC with MET exon14 deletions	
Vandetanib	RET, VEGFR, EGFR	MTC	Competitive inhibitor of ATP-binding site of tyrosine kinase domain of multiple kinases, including RET
Selpercatinib	RET	NSCLC, MTC, RET fusion thyroid cancer	Inhibitor of RET, VEGFR1, VEGFR2 tyrosine kinases
Temsirolimus	mTOR	RCC	Competitive inhibitor of mTOR serine-threonine kinase
Everolimus	mTOR	RCC, PNET	Binds to immunophilin FK binding protein-12, which forms a complex that inhibits mTOR kinase
Vorinostat, romidepsin, belinostat	HDAC	CTCL/PTL	HDAC inhibitor, epigenetic modulation
Panobinostat	HDAC	MM	HDAC inhibitor, epigenetic modulation
Ruxolitinib	JAK-1, 2	Myelofibrosis	Competitive inhibitor of tyrosine kinase
Vismodegib	Hedgehog pathway	Basel cell cancer (skin)	Inhibits smoothened in hedgehog pathway
Lenvatinib	Multikinase inhibitor (VEGFR, FGFR, PGFR-α, others)	RCC, thyroid cancer, HCC	Competitive inhibitor of ATP-binding site of tyrosine kinase domain of multiple kinases
Olaparib, rucaparib, niraparib, talazoparib	PARP	BRCA mutant ovarian, breast, prostate, pancreas cancers; not all agents approved for all cancers	Inhibits PARP and DNA repair
Venetoclax	BCL-2	CLL (with 17p deletion)	Inhibits BCL-2 and enhances apoptosis
Ibrutinib, acalabrutinib	Bruton tyrosine kinase (BTK)	CLL, MCL, MZL, SLL, WM	Inhibitor of BTK

(Continued)

TABLE 72-2 Some FDA-Approved Molecularly Targeted Agents for the Treatment of Cancer (Continued)

DRUG	MOLECULAR TARGET	DISEASE	MECHANISM OF ACTION
Ivosidenib	IDH1	AML	IDH1 inhibitor
Gilteritinib	FLT3	AML	FLT3 inhibitor
Idelalisib	PI3K-delta	CLL, SLL, FL	Inhibits PI3k-delta, preventing proliferation and inducing apoptosis
Alpelisib	PIK3CA	Breast cancer with a PIK3CA mutation	Inhibits PIK3CA
Monoclonal Antibodies Alone			
Trastuzumab	HER2/neu (ERBB2)	Breast cancer, gastric cancer	Binds HER2 on tumor cell surface and induces receptor internalization
Pertuzumab	HER2/neu (ERBB2)	Breast cancer	Binds HER2 on tumor cell surface at distinct site from trastuzumab and prevents binding to other receptors
Cetuximab	EGFR	Colon cancer, squamous cell carcinoma of the head and neck	Binds extracellular domain of EGFR and blocks binding of EGF and TGF-α; induces receptor internalization. Potentiates the efficacy of chemotherapy and radiotherapy
Panitumumab	EGFR	Colon cancer	Similar to cetuximab but fully humanized rather than chimeric
Necitumumab	EGFR	Squamous NSCLC	Binds EGFR
Rituximab	CD20	B-cell lymphomas and leukemias that express CD20	Multiple potential mechanisms, including direct induction of tumor cell apoptosis and immune mechanisms
Alemtuzumab	CD52	Chronic lymphocytic leukemia and CD52-expressing lymphoid tumors	Immune mechanisms
Bevacizumab	VEGF	Colorectal, lung cancers, RCC, glioblastoma	Inhibits angiogenesis by high-affinity binding to VEGF
Ziv-aflibercept	VEGFA, VEGFB, PLGF	Colorectal cancers	Inhibits angiogenesis by high-affinity binding to VEGFA, VEGFB, and PLGF
Ramucirumab	VEGFR	Gastric, colorectal, lung cancers	Inhibits angiogenesis by binding to VEGFR
Ipilimumab	CTLA-4	Melanoma, HCC, MSI-high colorectal cancer	Blocks CTLA-4, preventing interaction with CD80/86 and T-cell inhibition
Nivolumab, pembrolizumab	PD-1	Melanoma, head and neck cancer, NSCLC, SCLC, Hodgkin's disease, urothelial cancer, RCC, HCC, gastric cancer, MSI-high cancers, endometrial cancer	Blocks PD-1, preventing interaction with PD-L1 and T-cell inhibition
Atezolizumab, durvalumab, avelumab	PD-L1	NSCLC, urothelial cancer, SCLC (durvalumab), HCC (atezolizumab), Merkel cell cancer (avelumab)	Blocks PD-L1, preventing interaction with PD-1 and T-cell inhibition
Denosumab	Rank ligand	Breast, prostate	Inhibits Rank ligand, primary signal for bone removal
Dinutuximab	Glycolipid GD2	Neuroblastoma (pediatric)	Immune-mediated attack on GD2-expressing cells
Daratumumab	CD38	MM	Binds to CD38 on MM cells causing apoptosis by antibody-dependent or compliment-mediated cytotoxicity
Elotuzumab	SLAMF7	MM	Activating NK cells to kill MM cells
Olaratumab	PDGFRα	Soft tissue sarcomas	Blocks PDGFRα activity
Blinatumomab	CD19 and CD3	Ph-relapsed precursor B-cell ALL	Binds CD19 on ALL cells and CD3 on T cells; immune attack on CD19-expressing cells
Antibody-Chemotherapy Conjugates			
Brentuximab vedotin	CD30	Hodgkin's disease, anaplastic lymphoma	Delivery of chemotherapeutic agent (MMAE) to CD30-expressing tumor cells
Ado-trastuzumab emtansine	HER2	Breast cancer	Delivery of chemotherapeutic agent emtansine to HER2-expressing breast cancer cells
Fam-trastuzumab	HER2	Breast cancer, gastric cancer	Delivery of chemotherapeutic agent deruxtecan to HER2-expressing breast cancer cells
CAR-T Cells			
Tisagenlecleucel, axicabtagene ciloleucel	CD19	ALL (tisagenlecleucel), DLBCL/high-grade BCL (axicabtagene ciloleucel)	Targeted T cells to protein on surface of malignant cells

Abbreviations: ALL, acute lymphocytic leukemia; AML, acute myeloid leukemia; BCL, B-cell lymphoma; CAR-T, chimeric antigen receptor T cells; CLL, chronic lymphocytic leukemia; CRC, colorectal cancer; CTCL, cutaneous T-cell lymphoma; DLBCL, diffuse large B-cell lymphoma; EGFR, epidermal growth factor receptor; FDA, U.S. Food and Drug Administration; FGFR, fibroblast growth factor receptor; FL, follicular lymphoma; Flt-3, fms-like tyrosine kinase-3; GIST, gastrointestinal stromal tumor; HDAC, histone deacetylases; MCL, mantle cell lymphoma; MM, multiple myeloma; MSI, microsatellite instability; MTC, medullary thyroid cancer; mTOR, mammalian target of Rapamycin; MZL, mantle zone lymphoma; NK, natural killer; NSCLC, non-small-cell lung cancer; PARP, poly-ADP ribose polymerase; PDGFR, platelet-derived growth factor receptor; PLGF, placenta growth factor; PML-RARα, promyelocytic leukemia–retinoic acid receptor-alpha; PNET, pancreatic neuroendocrine tumors; PTL, peripheral T-cell lymphoma; RCC, renal cell cancer; t(15;17), translocation between chromosomes 15 and 17; SCLC, small-cell lung cancer; SLL, small lymphocytic lymphoma; TGF-α, transforming growth factor-alpha; VEGFR, vascular endothelial growth factor receptor; WM, Waldenström's macroglobulinemia.

of trastuzumab, antibody to HER2, to combination chemotherapy in the adjuvant treatment of HER2-positive breast cancer significantly improves overall survival.

A major effort continues to develop targeted therapies for mutations in the *ras* family of genes, which play a critical role in transmitting signals through a number of downstream signaling pathways including the MAP (mitogen-activated protein) kinase and PI3K pathways. Mutations in *ras* are the most common mutations in oncogenes in cancers (especially *kras*) but have proved to be very difficult targets for a number of reasons related to the structure of RAS proteins as well as mechanisms of activation and inactivation (active when bound to guanosine triphosphate [GTP] and inactive when bound to guanosine diphosphate [GDP]). RAS proteins are not kinases but bind directly to the BRAF serine/threonine kinase with preferential binding when RAS is in the active GTP bound state. Preliminary evidence indicates antitumor activity of agents that target one of the mutant forms of KRAS (12C) that is found in a subset of cancers. Indirect inhibition of RAS function by inhibiting farnesyl transferase, which is important for RAS binding to the membrane and is required for activation, has shown some promise against HRAS mutant head and neck cancers. Targeted therapies against a subset of proteins downstream of RAS in the MAP kinase signaling pathway (including BRAF and MAP kinase) have proven to have significant antitumor activity against V600E *BRAF* mutant melanoma, with improved efficacy when they are used in combination. However, similar activity is not seen against *ras* mutant tumors. Additional targeted therapies against other proteins downstream of RAS (including ERK, or combinations of MAP kinase inhibitors and immunotherapy) are being studied, both individually and in combination. However, at this time, there is no clinically approved approach to inhibiting RAS mutant tumors.

One of the strategies for new drug development is to take advantage of so-called oncogene addiction. This situation **(Fig. 72-3)** is created when a tumor cell develops an activating mutation in an oncogene that becomes a dominant pathway for survival and growth with reduced contributions from other pathways, even when there may be abnormalities in those pathways. This dependency on a single pathway creates a cell that is vulnerable to inhibitors of that oncogene pathway. For example, cells harboring mutations in *BRAF* are very sensitive to MEK inhibitors that inhibit downstream signaling in the BRAF pathway.

Proteins critical for transcription of other proteins essential for malignant cell survival or proliferation provide another potential target for treating cancers. The transcription factor nuclear factor (NF)-κB is a heterodimer composed of p65 and p50 subunits that associate with an inhibitor, IκB, in the cell cytoplasm. In response to growth factor or cytokine signaling, a multisubunit kinase called IKK (IκB-kinase) phosphorylates IκB and directs its degradation by the ubiquitin/proteasome system. NF-κB, free of its inhibitor, translocates to the nucleus and activates target genes, many of which promote the survival of tumor cells. One of the mechanisms by which novel drugs called *proteasome inhibitors* are thought to produce an anticancer effect is by blocking the proteolysis of IκB, thereby preventing NF-κB activation. For reasons that have not been fully elucidated, this has a differential toxicity effect on tumor, as compared to normal, cells. Although this mechanism appears to be an important aspect of the antitumor effects of proteasome inhibitors, there are other effects involving the inhibition of the degradation of multiple cellular proteins important in malignant cell survival or proliferation. Proteasome inhibitors (bortezomib, carfilzomib, ixazomib) have activity in patients with multiple myeloma, including partial and complete remissions. Inhibitors of IKK are also in development, with the hope of more selectively blocking the degradation of IκB, thus "locking" NF-κB in an inhibitory complex and rendering the cancer cell more susceptible to apoptosis-inducing agents. Many other transcription factors are activated by phosphorylation, which can be prevented by tyrosine or serine/threonine kinase inhibitors, a number of which are currently in clinical trials.

Estrogen receptors (ERs) and androgen receptors (ARs), members of the steroid hormone family of nuclear receptors, are targets of inhibition by drugs used to treat breast and prostate cancers, respectively. Selective estrogen receptor modulators (SERMs) have been developed as a treatment approach for ER-positive breast cancer. Tamoxifen, a partial agonist and antagonist of ER function, is frequently used in breast cancer and can mediate tumor regression in metastatic breast cancer and can prevent disease recurrence in the adjuvant setting. Tamoxifen binds to the ER and modulates its transcriptional activity, inhibiting activity in the breast but promoting activity in bone but unfortunately also in uterine epithelium, leading to a small increased risk of uterine cancer. Attempts have been made to develop SERMs that would have antiestrogenic effects in both breast and uterus while maintaining protective effects on bone. However, none of these to date has been an improvement over tamoxifen. Aromatase inhibitors, which

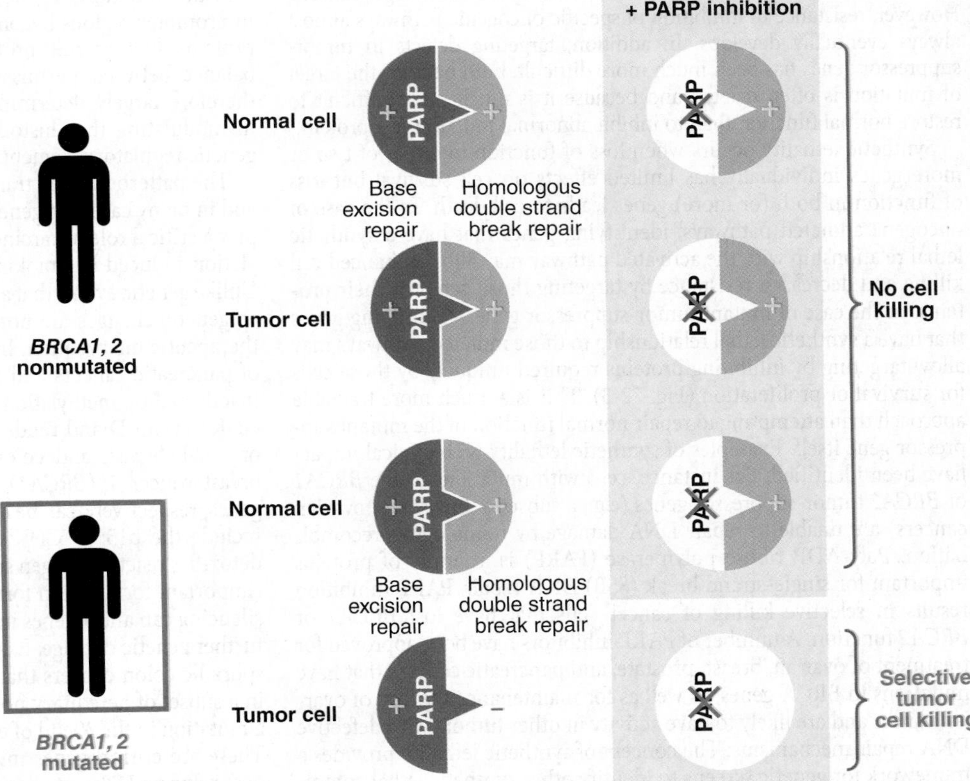

FIGURE 72-3 Synthetic lethality. Genes are said to have a synthetic lethal relationship when mutation of either gene alone is tolerated by the cell, but mutation of both genes leads to lethality, as originally noted by Bridges and later named by Dobzhansky. Thus, mutant *gene a* and *gene b* have a synthetic lethal relationship, implying that the loss of one gene makes the cell dependent on the function of the other gene. In cancer cells, loss of function of a DNA repair gene like *BRCA1*, which repairs double-strand breaks, makes the cell dependent on base excision repair mediated in part by *PARP*. If the PARP gene product is inhibited, the cell attempts to repair the break using the error-prone nonhomologous end-joining method, which results in tumor cell death. High-throughput screens can now be performed using isogenic cell line pairs in which one cell line has a defined defect in a DNA repair pathway. Compounds can be identified that selectively kill the mutant cell line; targets of these compounds have a synthetic lethal relationship to the repair pathway and are potentially important targets for future therapeutics.

block the conversion of androgens to estrogens in breast and subcutaneous fat tissues, have demonstrated improved clinical efficacy compared with tamoxifen in postmenopausal women and are often used as first-line therapy in postmenopausal patients with ER-positive disease. They are occasionally used in premenopausal patients with ER-positive disease in combination with ovarian suppression approaches such as luteinizing hormone–releasing hormone (LHRH) agonists. A number of approaches have been developed for blocking androgen stimulation of prostate cancer, including decreasing production by the testicles (e.g., orchiectomy, LHRH agonists or antagonists), directly blocking actions of androgen (a number of agents have been developed to do this), or blocking production by inhibiting the enzyme CYP17, which is central in production of androgens from cholesterol **(Chap. 79)**.

■ CANCER-SPECIFIC GENETIC CHANGES AND SYNTHETIC LETHALITY

The concepts of oncogene addiction and synthetic lethality have spurred new drug development targeting oncogene- and tumor-suppressor pathways. As discussed earlier in this chapter and outlined in Fig. 72-3, cancer cells can become dependent upon signaling pathways containing activated oncogenes; this can effect proliferation (i.e., mutated KRAS, BRAF, overexpressed MYC, or activated tyrosine kinases). Additional genetic changes in malignant cells or unique features of tumors including defects in DNA repair (e.g., loss of *BRCA1* or *BRCA2* gene function), modifications in cell cycle control (e.g., changes in protein levels or mutations in cyclins and cyclin dependent kinases), enhanced survival mechanisms (overexpression of Bcl-2 or NF-κB), altered cell metabolism (such as occurs when mutant KRAS enhances glucose uptake and aerobic glycolysis), tumor-stromal interactions, and angiogenesis (e.g., production of vascular endothelial growth factor [VEGF] in response to HIF-2α in RCC) can also be successfully exploited to relatively specifically target cancers. However, resistance to inhibition of specific oncogenic pathways almost always eventually develops. In addition, targeting defects in tumor-suppressor genes has been much more difficult, both because the target of mutation is often deleted and because it is much more difficult to restore normal function than to inhibit abnormal function of a protein.

Synthetic lethality occurs when loss of function in either of two or more genes individually has limited effects on cell survival but loss of function in both (or more) genes leads to cell death. In the case of oncogene addicted pathways, identifying genes that have a synthetic lethal relationship with the activated pathway may allow enhanced cell killing and decreased resistance by targeting those genes or their proteins. In the case of mutant tumor-suppressor genes, identifying genes that have a synthetic lethal relationship to those mutated pathways may allow targeting by inhibiting proteins required uniquely by those cells for survival or proliferation (Fig. 72-3). This is a much more tractable approach than attempting to repair normal function of the mutant suppressor gene itself. Examples of synthetic lethality with clinical impact have been identified. For instance, cells with mutations in the *BRCA1* or *BRCA2* tumor-suppressor genes (e.g., a subset of breast and ovarian cancers) are unable to repair DNA damage by homologous recombination. Poly-ADP ribose polymerase (PARP) is a family of proteins important for single-strand break (SSB) DNA repair. PARP inhibition results in selective killing of cancer cells that have lost *BRCA1* or *BRCA2* function. A number of PARP inhibitors have been approved for treatment of ovarian, breast, prostate, and pancreatic cancers that have mutations in BRCA genes, as well as for maintenance therapy of ovarian cancer and are likely to have activity in other tumors with defective DNA repair mechanisms. The concept of synthetic lethality provides a framework for genetic screens to identify other synthetic lethal combinations involving known tumor-suppressor genes and development of novel therapeutic agents to target dependent pathways. Other unique aspects of malignant tumors, including those outlined elsewhere in the chapter, may also be vulnerable to synthetic lethal interactions.

■ EPIGENETIC INFLUENCES ON CANCER GENE TRANSCRIPTION

Chromatin structure regulates the hierarchical order of sequential gene transcription that governs differentiation and tissue homeostasis. Disruption of chromatin remodeling (the process of modifying chromatin structure to control exposure of specific genes to transcriptional proteins, thereby controlling the expression of those genes) leads to aberrant gene expression that can significantly alter the biology of cells including inducing proliferation or migration of cells. *Epigenetic* changes are those that alter the pattern of gene expression that persist across at least one cell division, but are not caused by changes in the DNA code. These include alterations of chromatin structure mediated by methylation of cytosine residues of DNA (primarily in context of CpG dinucleotides in somatic cells), modification of histones by altering acetylation or methylation, or changes in higher-order chromosome structure **(Fig. 72-4)**. Appropriate control of DNA methylation is essential for normal cell function and development, and both altered methylation and hypomethylation of histones occur in cancers. Hypermethylation of DNA promoter regions is a common mechanism by which tumor-suppressor loci are epigenetically silenced in cancer cells. Thus, one allele of a tumor-suppressor gene may be inactivated by mutation or deletion, while expression of the other allele is epigenetically silenced, usually by methylation, leading to loss of gene function. Aberrant hypomethylation is also frequently found in a number of cancers consistent with the dysregulated pattern of gene transcription that is a hallmark of cancer cells, with some genes being inappropriately turned off while others are inappropriately turned on.

Acetylation of the amino terminus of the core histones H3 and H4 induces an open chromatin conformation that promotes transcription initiation. Histone acetylases are components of coactivator complexes recruited to promoter/enhancer regions by sequence-specific transcription factors during the activation of genes (Fig. 72-4). Histone deacetylases (HDACs; multiple HDACs are encoded in the human genome) are recruited to genes by transcriptional repressors and prevent the initiation of gene transcription. Methylated cytosine residues in promoter regions become associated with methyl cytosine–binding proteins that recruit protein complexes with HDAC activity. The balance between permissive and inhibitory chromatin structure is therefore largely determined by the activity of transcription factors in modulating the "histone code" and the methylation status of the genetic regulatory elements of genes.

The pattern of gene transcription is aberrant in all human cancers, and in many cases, epigenetic events are responsible. Epigenetic events play a critical role in carcinogenesis (e.g., long-lasting changes in methylation induced by smoking) and are found in premalignant lesions. Unlike genetic events that alter DNA primary structure (e.g., deletions), epigenetic changes are potentially reversible and appear amenable to therapeutic intervention. In certain human cancers, including a subset of pancreatic cancers and multiple myeloma, the $p16^{Ink4a}$ promoter is inactivated by methylation, thus permitting the unchecked activity of CDK4/cyclin D and rendering pRb nonfunctional. In sporadic forms of renal, breast, and colon cancer, the von Hippel–Lindau (*VHL*), breast cancer 1 (*BRCA1*), and serine/threonine kinase 11 (*STK11*) genes, respectively, can be epigenetically silenced. Other targeted genes include the $p15^{Ink4b}$ CDK inhibitor, glutathione-S-transferase (which detoxifies reactive oxygen species [ROS]), and the E-cadherin molecule (important for junction formation between epithelial cells). Epigenetic silencing can affect genes involved in DNA repair, thus predisposing to further genetic damage. Examples include MLH1 (mutL homologue in sporadic colon cancers that have microsatellite instability) and MSH2 in a subset of hereditary nonpolyposis colon cancer patients who have a mutation in the 3′ end of epithelial cell adhesion molecule (EPCAM). These are critical genes involved in repair of mismatched bases that occur during DNA synthesis, and their silencing can lead to mutations in the DNA.

Human leukemias often have chromosomal translocations that code for novel fusion proteins with activities that alter chromatin structure by interacting with HDACs or histone acetyl transferases (HATs). For example, the promyelocytic leukemia–retinoic acid receptor α (PML-RARα) fusion protein, generated by the t(15;17) translocation observed in most cases of acute promyelocytic leukemia (APL), binds to promoters containing retinoic acid response elements and recruits HDACs to these promoters, effectively inhibiting gene expression.

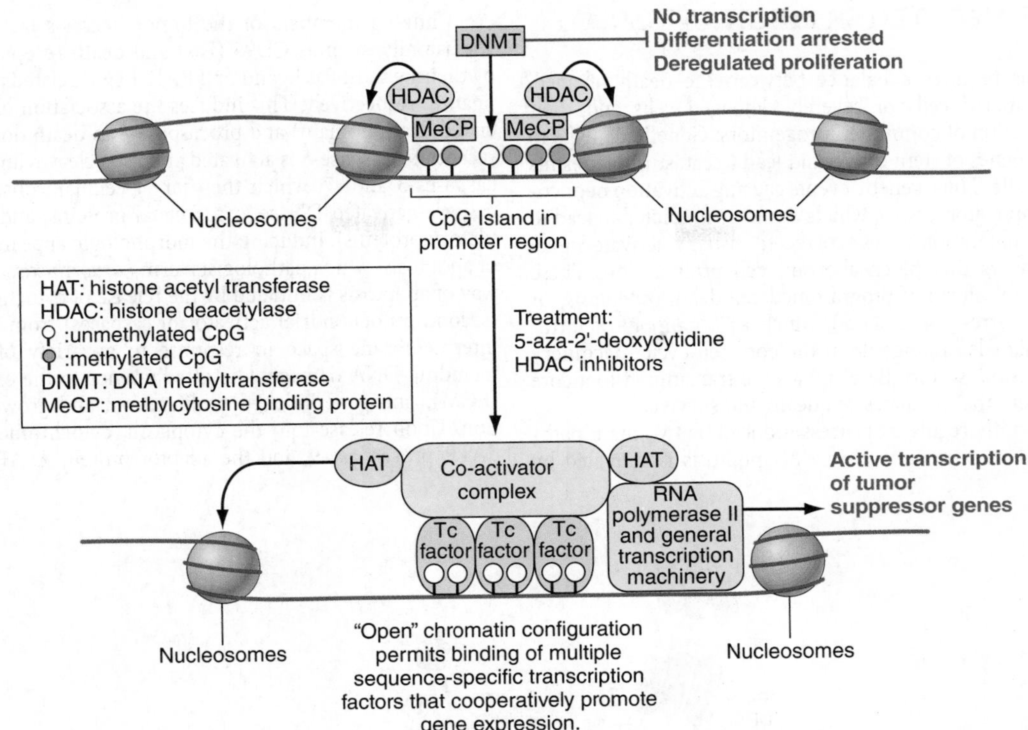

FIGURE 72-4 Epigenetic regulation of gene expression in cancer cells. Tumor-suppressor genes are often epigenetically silenced in cancer cells. In the upper portion, a CpG island within the promoter and enhancer regions of the gene has been methylated, resulting in the recruitment of methyl-cytosine binding proteins (MeCP) and complexes with histone deacetylase (HDAC) activity. Chromatin is in a condensed, nonpermissive conformation that inhibits transcription. Clinical trials are under way utilizing the combination of demethylating agents such as 5-aza-2′-deoxycytidine plus HDAC inhibitors, which together confer an open, permissive chromatin structure (*lower portion*). Transcription factors bind to specific DNA sequences in promoter regions and, through protein-protein interactions, recruit coactivator complexes containing histone acetyl transferase (HAT) activity. This enhances transcription initiation by RNA polymerase II and associated general transcription factors. The expression of the tumor-suppressor gene commences, with phenotypic changes that may include growth arrest, differentiation, or apoptosis.

This arrests differentiation at the promyelocyte stage and promotes tumor cell proliferation and survival. Treatment with pharmacologic doses of all-*trans* retinoic acid (ATRA), the ligand for RARα, results in the release of HDAC activity and the recruitment of coactivators, which overcome the differentiation block. This induced differentiation of APL cells has improved treatment of these patients but also has led to a novel treatment toxicity when newly differentiated tumor cells infiltrate the lungs. ATRA represents a treatment paradigm for the reversal of epigenetic changes in cancer. Other leukemia-associated fusion proteins, such as Tel-acute myeloid leukemia (AML1), AML1-eight-twenty-one (ETO), and the MLL fusion proteins seen in acute myeloid leukemia (AML) and acute lymphocytic leukemia, also lead to repression through the HDAC complex. Therefore, efforts are ongoing to determine the structural basis for interactions between translocation fusion proteins and chromatin-remodeling proteins and to use this information to rationally design small molecules that will disrupt specific protein-protein associations, although this has proven to be technically difficult. Several drugs that block the enzymatic activity of HDACs (HDAC inhibitors [HDACis]) are approved for cancer treatment, and others are being tested. HDACis have demonstrated sufficient antitumor activity against cutaneous T-cell lymphoma (vorinostat, romidepsin), peripheral T-cell lymphoma (romidepsin, belinostat), and multiple myeloma (panobinostat) to be approved by the U.S. Food and Drug Administration (FDA).

HDACis have also demonstrated antitumor activity in clinical studies against some solid tumors, and additional studies are ongoing. HDACis may target cancer cells via a number of mechanisms including both epigenetic modulation via histone acetylation and effects on other proteins that are acetylated. The pleiotropic effects of some HDACis include enhancement of apoptosis by upregulation of a number of proteins that enhance apoptosis including death receptors (DR4/5, FAS, and their ligands) and downregulation of proteins that inhibit apoptosis (e.g., X-linked inhibitor of apoptosis [XIAP]); upregulation of proteins that inhibit cell cycle progression (e.g., p21Cip1/Waf1); inhibition of DNA repair and generation of ROS leading to increased DNA damage; and disruption of the chaperone protein HSP90.

Efforts are also under way to modulate other epigenetic processes such as reversing the hypermethylation of CpG islands that characterizes many malignancies. Drugs that induce DNA demethylation, such as 5-aza-2-deoxycytidine, can lead to reexpression of silenced genes in cancer cells with restoration of function, and 5-aza-2-deoxycytidine is approved for use in myelodysplastic syndrome. However, 5-aza-2-deoxycytidine has limited aqueous solubility and is myelosuppressive, limiting its usefulness. Other inhibitors of DNA methyltransferases are in development. In ongoing clinical trials, inhibitors of DNA methylation are being combined with HDACis, with the idea that reversing coexisting epigenetic changes will reverse the deregulated patterns of gene transcription in cancer cells.

Epigenetic gene regulation can also occur via microRNAs or long noncoding RNAs (lncRNA). MicroRNAs (miRNA) are short (average 22 nucleotides in length) RNA molecules that silence gene expression after transcription by binding and inhibiting the translation or promoting the degradation of mRNA transcripts. It is estimated that >1000 miRNAs are encoded in the human genome. Each tissue has a distinctive repertoire of miRNA expression, and this pattern is altered in specific ways in cancers. Specific correlations between miRNA expression and tumor biology and clinical behavior are continuing to emerge. Therapies targeting miRNAs are not currently at hand but represent an ongoing area of treatment development. LncRNAs are longer than 200 nucleotides and comprise the largest group of noncoding RNAs. Some of them have been shown to play important roles in gene regulation. The potential for altering these RNAs for therapeutic benefit is an area of active investigation.

APOPTOSIS AND OTHER MECHANISMS OF CELL DEATH

Tissue homeostasis requires a balance between the death of aged, terminally differentiated cells or severely damaged cells and their renewal by proliferation of committed progenitors. Genetic damage to growth-regulating genes of stem cells could lead to catastrophic results for the host as a whole. Thus, genetic events causing activation of oncogenes or loss of tumor suppressors, which would be predicted to lead to unregulated cell proliferation unless corrected, usually activate signal transduction pathways that block aberrant cell proliferation. These pathways can lead to a form of programmed cell death (*apoptosis*) or irreversible growth arrest (*senescence*). Much as a panoply of intra- and extracellular signals impinge upon the core cell cycle machinery to regulate cell division, so too these signals are transmitted to a core enzymatic machinery that regulates cell death and survival.

Apoptosis is a tightly regulated process induced by two main pathways **(Fig. 72-5)**. The extrinsic pathway of apoptosis is activated by cross-linking members of the tumor necrosis factor (TNF) receptor superfamily, such as CD95 (Fas) and death receptors DR4 and DR5, by their ligands, Fas ligand or TRAIL (TNF-related apoptosis-inducing ligand), respectively. This induces the association of FADD (Fas-associated death domain) and procaspase-8 to death domain motifs of the receptors. Caspase-8 is activated and then cleaves and activates effector caspases-3 and -7, which then target cellular constituents (including caspase-activated DNase, cytoskeletal proteins, and a number of regulatory proteins), inducing the morphologic appearance characteristic of apoptosis, which pathologists term *karyorrhexis*. The intrinsic pathway of apoptosis is initiated by the release of cytochrome c and SMAC (second mitochondrial activator of caspases) from the mitochondrial intermembrane space in response to a variety of noxious stimuli, including DNA damage, loss of adherence to the extracellular matrix (ECM), oncogene-induced proliferation, and growth factor deprivation. Upon release into the cytoplasm, cytochrome c associates with dATP, procaspase-9, and the adaptor protein APAF-1, leading to the

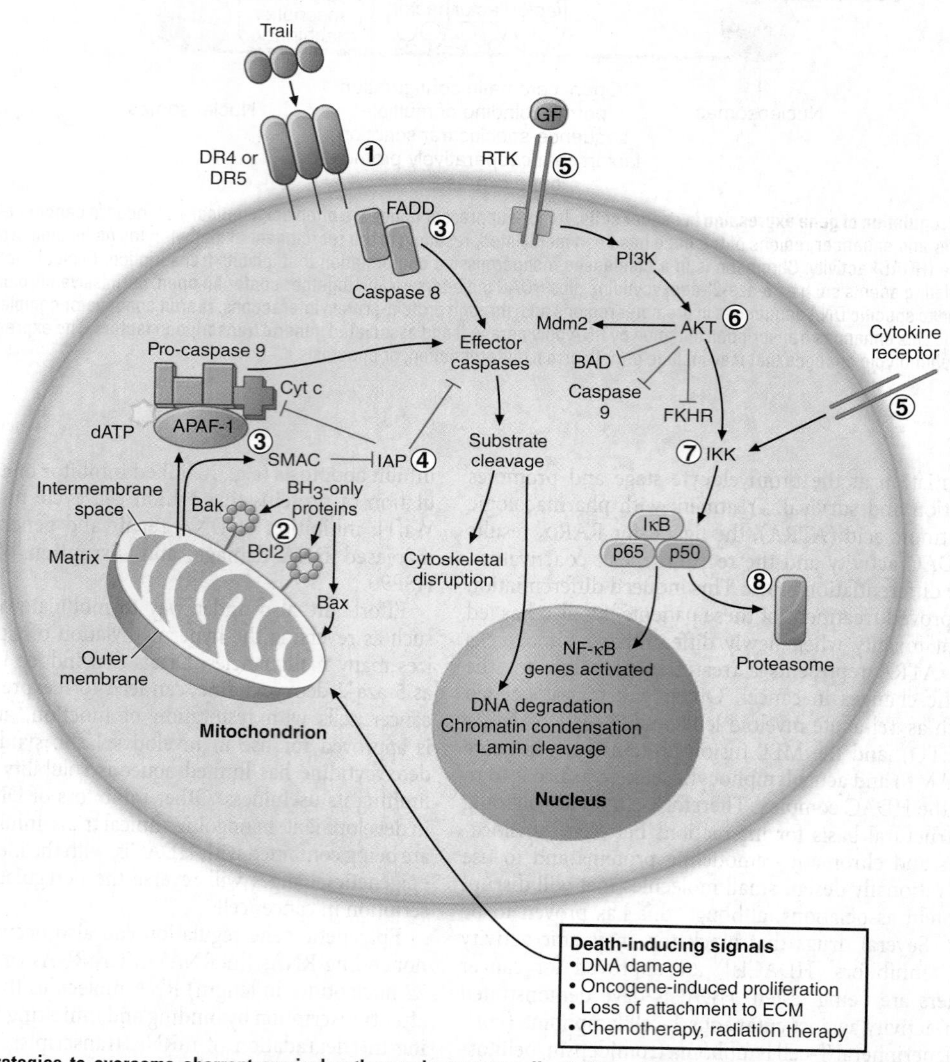

FIGURE 72-5 Therapeutic strategies to overcome aberrant survival pathways in cancer cells. *1.* The extrinsic pathway of apoptosis can be selectively induced in cancer cells by TRAIL (the ligand for death receptors 4 and 5) or by agonistic monoclonal antibodies. *2.* Inhibition of antiapoptotic Bcl-2 family members with antisense oligonucleotides or inhibitors of the BH_3-binding pocket will promote formation of Bak- or Bax-induced pores in the mitochondrial outer membrane. *3.* Epigenetic silencing of APAF-1, caspase-8, and other proteins can be overcome using demethylating agents and inhibitors of histone deacetylases. *4.* Inhibitor of apoptosis proteins (IAP) blocks activation of caspases; small-molecule inhibitors of IAP function (mimicking SMAC action) should lower the threshold for apoptosis. *5.* Signal transduction pathways originating with activation of receptor tyrosine kinase receptors (RTKs) or cytokine receptors promote survival of cancer cells by a number of mechanisms. Inhibiting receptor function with monoclonal antibodies, such as trastuzumab or cetuximab, or inhibiting kinase activity with small-molecule inhibitors can block the pathway. *6.* The Akt kinase phosphorylates many regulators of apoptosis to promote cell survival; inhibitors of Akt may render tumor cells more sensitive to apoptosis-inducing signals; however, the possibility of toxicity to normal cells may limit the therapeutic value of these agents. *7* and *8.* Activation of the transcription factor NF-κB (composed of p65 and p50 subunits) occurs when its inhibitor, IκB, is phosphorylated by IκB-kinase (IKK), with subsequent degradation of IκB by the proteasome. Inhibition of IKK activity should selectively block the activation of NF-κB target genes, many of which promote cell survival. Inhibitors of proteasome function are U.S. Food and Drug Administration approved and may work in part by preventing destruction of IκB, thus blocking NF-κB nuclear localization. NF-κB is unlikely to be the only target for proteasome inhibitors.

sequential activation of caspase-9 and effector caspases. SMAC binds to and blocks the function of inhibitor of apoptosis proteins (IAP), negative regulators of caspase activation.

The release of apoptosis-inducing proteins from the mitochondria is regulated by pro- and antiapoptotic members of the Bcl-2 family. Antiapoptotic members (e.g., Bcl-2, Bcl-XL, and Mcl-1) associate with the mitochondrial outer membrane via their carboxyl termini, exposing to the cytoplasm a hydrophobic binding pocket composed of Bcl-2 homology (BH) domains 1, 2, and 3 that is crucial for their activity. Perturbations of normal physiologic processes in specific cellular compartments lead to the activation of BH3-only proapoptotic family members (e.g., Bad, Bim, Bid, Puma, Noxa, and others) that can alter the conformation of the outer-membrane proteins Bax and Bak, which then oligomerize to form pores in the mitochondrial outer membrane resulting in cytochrome c release. If proteins comprised only by BH3 domains are sequestered by Bcl-2, Bcl-XL, or Mcl-1, pores do not form and apoptosis-inducing proteins are not released from the mitochondria. The ratio of levels of antiapoptotic Bcl-2 family members and the levels of proapoptotic BH3-only proteins at the mitochondrial membrane determines the activation state of the intrinsic pathway. The mitochondrion must therefore be recognized not only as an organelle with vital roles in intermediary metabolism and oxidative phosphorylation but also as a central regulatory structure of the apoptotic process.

The evolution of tumor cells to a more malignant phenotype requires the acquisition of genetic changes that subvert apoptosis pathways and promote cancer cell survival and resistance to anticancer therapies. However, cancer cells may be more vulnerable than normal cells to therapeutic interventions that target the apoptosis pathways that cancer cells depend upon. For instance, overexpression of Bcl-2 as a result of the t(14;18) translocation contributes to follicular lymphoma, and it is highly expressed in many lymphoid malignancies including chronic lymphocytic leukemia (CLL). Upregulation of Bcl-2 expression is also observed in other cancers including prostate, breast, and lung cancers and melanoma. Targeting of antiapoptotic Bcl-2 family members has been accomplished by the identification of several low-molecular-weight compounds that bind to the hydrophobic pockets of either Bcl-2 or Bcl-XL and block their ability to associate with death-inducing BH3-only proteins. An oral BH3 mimetic inhibitor of BCL-2, venetoclax, is approved for use in patients with refractory CLL with 17p deletion and is active in acute myeloid leukemia.

Preclinical studies targeting death receptors DR4 and -5 have demonstrated that recombinant, soluble, human TRAIL or humanized monoclonal antibodies with agonist activity against DR4 or -5 can induce apoptosis of tumor cells while sparing normal cells. The mechanisms for this selectivity may include expression of decoy receptors or elevated levels of intracellular inhibitors (such as FLIP, which competes with caspase-8 for FADD) by normal cells but not tumor cells. Synergy has been shown between TRAIL-induced apoptosis and chemotherapeutic agents in some preclinical studies. However, studies have not yet shown significant clinical activity of approaches targeting the TRAIL pathway.

Many of the signal transduction pathways perturbed in cancer promote tumor cell survival (Fig. 72-5). These include activation of the PI3K/Akt pathway, increased levels of the NF-κB transcription factor, and epigenetic silencing of genes such as *APAF-1* (apoptosis protease activating factor-1 involved in activating caspase-9 and essential for apoptosis) and *caspase-8*. Each of these pathways is a target for therapeutic agents that, in addition to affecting cancer cell proliferation or gene expression, may render cancer cells more susceptible to apoptosis, thus promoting synergy when combined with other chemotherapeutic agents.

Some tumor cells resist drug-induced apoptosis indirectly by eliminating the noxious stimulus-inducing apoptosis through expression of one or more members of the ABC (ATP-binding cassette proteins) family of ATP-dependent efflux pumps that mediate the multidrug-resistance (MDR) phenotype. The prototype member of this family, P-glycoprotein (PGP), spans the plasma membrane 12 times and has two ATP-binding sites. Hydrophobic drugs (e.g., anthracyclines and vinca alkaloids) are recognized by PGP as they enter the cell and are pumped out. Numerous clinical studies have failed to demonstrate that drug resistance can be overcome using inhibitors of PGP. However, ABC transporters have different substrate specificities, and inhibition of a single family member may not be sufficient to overcome the MDR phenotype. Efforts to reverse PGP-mediated drug resistance continue.

Cells, including cancer cells, can also undergo other mechanisms of cell death including *autophagy* (degradation of proteins and organelles by lysosomal proteases) and *necrosis* (digestion of cellular components and rupturing of the cell membrane). Necrosis usually occurs in response to external forces resulting in release of cellular components, which leads to inflammation and damage to surrounding tissues. Although necrosis was thought to be unprogrammed, evidence now suggests that at least some aspects may also be programmed. The exact role of necrosis in cancer cell death in various settings is still being determined. In addition to its role in cell death, autophagy can also serve as a homeostatic mechanism to promote survival for the cell by recycling cellular components to provide necessary energy. The mechanisms that control the balance between enhancing survival versus leading to cell death are still not fully understood. Autophagy appears to play conflicting roles in the development and survival of cancer. Early in the carcinogenic process, it can act as a tumor suppressor by preventing the cell from accumulating abnormal proteins and organelles. However, in established tumors, it may serve as a mechanism of survival for cancer cells when they are stressed by damage such as from chemotherapy. Preclinical studies have indicated that inhibition of this process can enhance the sensitivity of cancer cells to chemotherapy or radiation therapy, and ongoing trials are evaluating inhibitors of autophagy in combination with chemotherapy and/or radiation therapy. Better understanding of the factors that control the survival-promoting versus death-inducing aspects of autophagy is required in order to know how to best manipulate it for therapeutic benefit.

■ METASTASIS

The metastatic process accounts for the vast majority of deaths from solid tumors, and therefore, an understanding of this process is critical for improvements in survival from cancer. The biology of metastasis is complex and requires multiple steps. The initial step involves cell migration and invasion through the ECM. The three major features of tissue invasion are cell adhesion to the basement membrane, local proteolysis of the membrane, and movement of the cell through the rent in the membrane and the ECM. Cells that lose contact with the ECM normally undergo programmed cell death (anoikis-apoptosis induced by the loss of contact), and this process has to be suppressed in cells that metastasize. Another process important for many, but not necessarily all, metastasizing epithelial cancer cells is epithelial-mesenchymal transition (EMT). This is a process by which cells lose their epithelial properties and gain mesenchymal properties. This normally occurs during the developmental process in embryos, allowing cells to migrate to their appropriate destinations in the embryo. It also occurs in wound healing, tissue regeneration, and fibrotic reactions, but in all of these processes, cells stop proliferating when the process is complete. Malignant cells that metastasize often undergo EMT as an important step in that process but retain the capacity for unregulated proliferation. However, there is evidence that not all metastasizing cancer cells require EMT, and the exact role of EMT in different metastasizing cancer cells continues to be elucidated. Malignant cells that gain access to the circulation must then repeat those steps at a remote site, find a hospitable niche in a foreign tissue, avoid detection and elimination by host defenses including the immune system, and induce the growth of new blood vessels. Some metastatic cells occur as oligoclonal clusters, which appear to be more potent in establishing metastasis than single cells, perhaps, in part, through differential and cooperative effects in evading host defenses. The rate-limiting step for metastasis is the ability for tumor cells to survive and expand in the novel microenvironment of the metastatic site, and multiple host-tumor interactions determine the ultimate outcome (**Fig. 72-6**). Few drugs have been developed to attempt to directly target the process of metastasis, in part because the specifics of the critical steps in the process that would be potentially good targets for drugs are still being

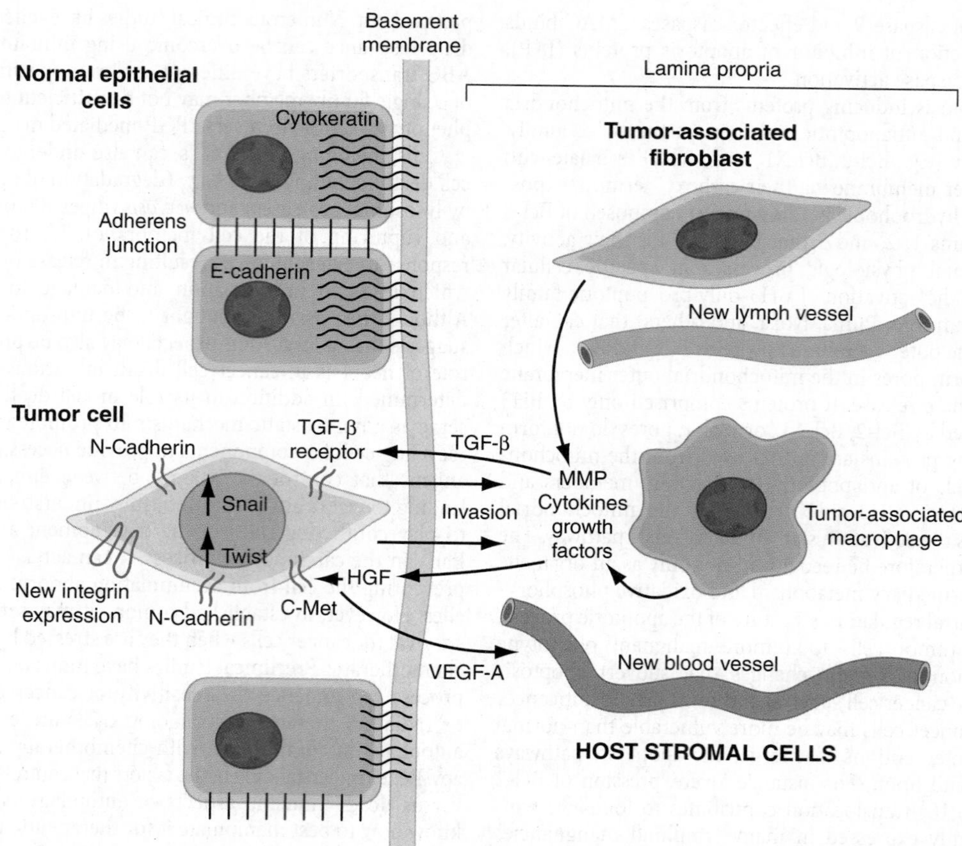

FIGURE 72-6 Oncogene signaling pathways are activated during tumor progression and promote metastatic potential. This figure shows a cancer cell that has undergone epithelial to mesenchymal transition (EMT) under the influence of several environmental signals. Critical components include activated transforming growth factor beta (TGF-β) and the hepatocyte growth factor (HGF)/c-Met pathways, as well as changes in the expression of adhesion molecules that mediate cell-cell and cell–extracellular matrix interactions. Important changes in gene expression are mediated by the Snail and Twist family of transcriptional repressors (whose expression is induced by the oncogenic pathways), leading to reduced expression of E-cadherin, a key component of adherens junctions between epithelial cells. This, in conjunction with upregulation of N-cadherin, a change in the pattern of expression of integrins (which mediate cell–extracellular matrix associations that are important for cell motility), and a switch in intermediate filament expression from cytokeratin to vimentin, results in the phenotypic change from adherent highly organized epithelial cells to motile and invasive cells with a fibroblast or mesenchymal morphology. EMT is thought to be an important step leading to metastasis in some human cancers. Host stromal cells, including tumor-associated fibroblasts and macrophages, play an important role in modulating tumor cell behavior through secretion of growth factors and proangiogenic cytokines, and matrix metalloproteinases that degrade the basement membrane. VEGF-A, -C, and -D are produced by tumor cells and stromal cells in response to hypoxemia or oncogenic signals and induce production of new blood vessels and lymphatic channels through which tumor cells metastasize to lymph nodes or tissues.

identified. However, a number of potential targets are known. HER2 can enhance the metastatic potential of breast cancer cells, and as discussed above, the monoclonal antibody trastuzumab, which targets HER2, improves survival in the adjuvant setting for HER2-positive breast cancer patients. A number of other potential targets that increase metastatic potential of cells in preclinical studies include HIF-1 and -2, transcription factors induced by hypoxia within tumors, growth factors (e.g., cMET and VEGFR), oncogenes (e.g., SRC), adhesion molecules (e.g., focal adhesion kinase [FAK]), ECM proteins (e.g., matrix metalloproteinases 1 and 2), and inflammatory molecules (e.g., COX-2).

The metastatic phenotype is likely restricted to a fraction of tumor cells (Fig. 72-6). A number of genetic and epigenetic changes are required for tumor cells to be able to metastasize, including activation of metastatic-promoting genes and inhibition of genes that suppress the metastatic ability. Given the role of microRNAs in controlling gene expression (see epigenetic section) including those critical to the metastatic process, efforts are under way to modulate these to try to inhibit metastasis. Cells with metastatic capability frequently express chemokine receptors that are likely important in the metastatic process. A number of candidate metastasis-suppressor genes have been identified, including genes coding for proteins that enhance apoptosis, suppress cell division, are involved in the interactions of cells with each other or the ECM, or suppress cell migration. The loss of function of these genes enhances metastasis. Gene expression profiling is being used to study the metastatic process and other properties of tumor cells that may predict susceptibilities.

An example of the ability of malignant cells to survive and grow in a novel microenvironment is bone metastases. Bone metastases can be extremely painful, cause fractures of weight-bearing bones, can lead to hypercalcemia, and are a major cause of morbidity for cancer patients. Osteoclasts and their monocyte-derived precursors express the surface receptor RANK (receptor activator of NF-κB), which is required for terminal differentiation and activation of osteoclasts. Osteoblasts and other stromal cells express RANK ligand (RANKL), as both a membrane-bound and soluble cytokine. Osteoprotegerin (OPG), a soluble receptor for RANKL produced by stromal cells, acts as a decoy receptor to inhibit RANK activation. The relative balance of RANKL and OPG determines the activation state of RANK on osteoclasts. Many tumors increase osteoclast activity by secretion of substances such as parathyroid hormone (PTH), PTH-related peptide, interleukin (IL) 1, or Mip1 that perturb the homeostatic balance of bone remodeling by increasing RANK signaling. One example is multiple myeloma, where tumor cell–stromal cell interactions activate osteoclasts and inhibit osteoblasts, leading to the development of multiple lytic bone lesions. Inhibition of RANKL by an antibody (denosumab) can prevent further bone destruction. Bisphosphonates are also effective inhibitors of osteoclast function that are used in the treatment of cancer patients with bone metastases.

■ CANCER STEM CELLS

Normal tissues have stem cells capable of self-renewal and repairing damaged tissue, whereas the majority of cells in normal tissues do not have this capacity. Similarly, only a small proportion of the cells within a tumor are capable of initiating colonies in vitro or forming tumors at high efficiency when injected into immunocompromised NOD/SCID mice. For example, AML and CML have a small population of cells (estimated to be <1%) that have properties of stem cells, such as unlimited self-renewal and the capacity to cause leukemia when serially transplanted in mice. These cells have an undifferentiated phenotype (Thy1–CD34+CD38– and do not express other differentiation markers) and resemble normal stem cells in many ways but are no longer under homeostatic control (**Fig. 72-7**). Solid tumors may also contain a population of stem cells. It is not yet known how often cancers may originate within a stem cell population. Cancer stem cells, like their normal counterparts, have unlimited proliferative capacity and paradoxically traverse the cell cycle at a slow rate; cancer growth occurs largely due to expansion of the stem cell pool, the unregulated proliferation of an amplifying population, and failure of apoptosis pathways (Fig. 72-7). Slow cell cycle progression and high levels of expression of antiapoptotic Bcl-2 family members and drug efflux pumps of the MDR family render cancer stem cells less vulnerable to cancer chemotherapy or radiation therapy. Implicit in the cancer stem cell hypothesis is the idea that failure to cure most human cancers is due to the fact that current therapeutic agents do not kill the stem cells. Identification and isolation of cancer stem cells will allow determination of the aberrant signaling pathways that distinguish these cells from normal tissue stem cells. These would serve as potential therapeutic targets. Evidence that cells with stem cell properties can arise from other epithelial cells within the cancer by processes such as epithelial mesenchymal transition also implies that it is essential to treat all of the cancer cells, and not just those with current stem cell–like properties, in order to eliminate the self-renewing cancer cell population. The exact nature of cancer stem cells remains an area of investigation. One of the unanswered questions is the exact origin of cancer stem cells for the different cancers.

PLASTICITY AND RESISTANCE

Cancer cells, and especially stem cells, have the capacity for significant plasticity allowing them to alter multiple aspects of cell biology in response to external factors (e.g., chemotherapy, radiation therapy, inflammation, immune response). In addition, heterogeneity between the different clones of cells within the tumor population and their interactions with each other and the tumor microenvironment provides the tumor with the capacity for significant plasticity in dealing with both internal and external stresses. Thus, a major problem in cancer therapy is that malignancies have a wide spectrum of mechanisms for both initial and adaptive resistance to treatments. These include inhibiting drug delivery to the cancer cells, blocking drug uptake and retention, increasing drug metabolism, altering levels of target proteins making them less sensitive to drugs, acquiring mutations in target proteins making them no longer sensitive to the drug, modifying metabolism and cell signaling pathways, using alternate signaling pathways, adjusting the cell replication process including mechanisms

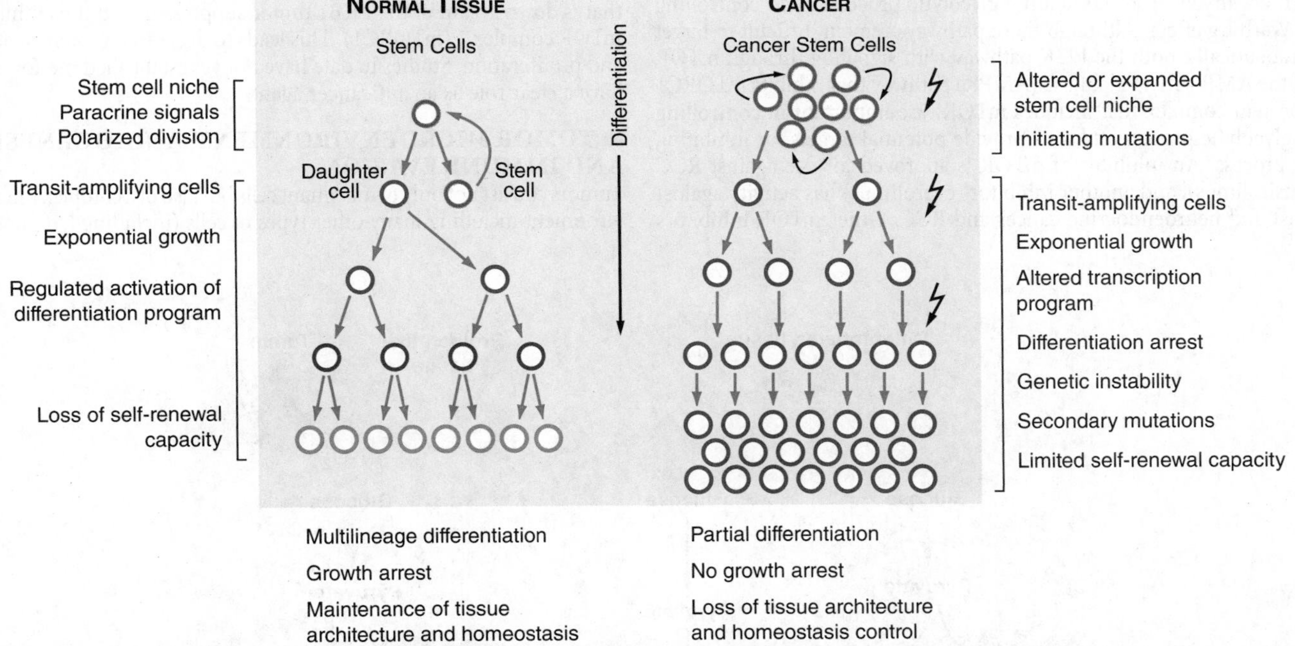

FIGURE 72-7 Cancer stem cells play a critical role in the initiation, progression, and resistance to therapy of malignant neoplasms. In normal tissues (*left*), homeostasis is maintained by asymmetric division of stem cells leading to one progeny cell that will differentiate and one cell that will maintain the stem cell pool. This occurs within highly specific niches unique to each tissue, such as in close apposition to osteoblasts in bone marrow, or at the base of crypts in the colon. Here, paracrine signals from stromal cells, such as sonic hedgehog or Notch ligands, as well as upregulation of β-catenin and telomerase, help to maintain stem cell features of unlimited self-renewal while preventing differentiation or cell death. This occurs in part through upregulation of the transcriptional repressor Bmi-1 and inhibition of the p16^{Ink4a}/Arf and p53 pathways. Daughter cells leave the stem cell niche and enter a proliferative phase (referred to as *transit-amplifying*) for a specified number of cell divisions, during which time a developmental program is activated, eventually giving rise to fully differentiated cells that have lost proliferative potential. Cell renewal equals cell death, and homeostasis is maintained. In this hierarchical system, only stem cells are long-lived. The hypothesis is that cancers harbor stem cells that make up a small fraction (i.e., 0.001–1%) of all cancer cells. These cells share several features with normal stem cells, including an undifferentiated phenotype, unlimited self-renewal potential, and a capacity for some degree of differentiation; however, due to initiating mutations (mutations are indicated by lightning bolts), they are no longer regulated by environmental cues. The cancer stem cell pool is expanded, and rapidly proliferating progeny, through additional mutations, may attain stem cell properties, although most of this population is thought to have a limited proliferative capacity. Differentiation programs are dysfunctional due to reprogramming of the pattern of gene transcription by oncogenic signaling pathways. Within the cancer transit-amplifying population, genomic instability generates aneuploidy and clonal heterogeneity as cells attain a fully malignant phenotype with metastatic potential. The cancer stem cell hypothesis has led to the idea that current cancer therapies may be effective at killing the bulk of tumor cells but do not kill tumor stem cells, leading to a regrowth of tumors that is manifested as tumor recurrence or disease progression. Research is in progress to identify unique molecular features of cancer stem cells that can lead to their direct targeting by novel therapeutic agents.

by which the cell deals with DNA damage, inhibiting apoptosis, and evading the immune system. Thus, most metastatic cancers (except those curable with chemotherapy such as germ cell tumors) eventually become resistant to the therapy being utilized. Overcoming resistance is a major area of research.

CANCER METABOLISM

One of the distinguishing characteristics of cancer cells is that they have altered metabolism as compared with normal cells in supporting survival, their high rates of proliferation, and ability to metastasize. Complicating studies evaluating metabolic differences between normal and malignant cells is that there is heterogeneity in metabolism between different cells within a cancer. Malignant cells must focus a significant fraction of their energy resources into synthesis of proteins and other molecules (building blocks required for the production of new cells) while still maintaining sufficient ATP production to survive and grow. Although normal proliferating cells also have similar needs, there are differences in how cancer cells metabolize glucose and a number of other compounds including the amino acid glutamine as compared to normal cells in part because of genetic and epigenetic changes within cancer cells but also likely due to differences in the environments of cancer and normal cells. Many cancer cells utilize aerobic glycolysis (the Warburg effect) (**Fig. 72-8**) to metabolize glucose, leading to increased lactic acid production, whereas normal cells utilize oxidative phosphorylation in mitochondria under aerobic conditions, a much more efficient process for generating ATP for energy utilization but one that does not produce the same level of building blocks needed for new cells. One consequence is increased glucose uptake and utilization by cancer cells, a fact utilized in fluorodeoxyglucose (FDG)-positron emission tomography (PET) scanning to detect tumors. A number of proteins in cancer cells, including cMYC, HIF1, RAS, p53, pRB, and AKT, are involved in modulating glycolytic processes and controlling the Warburg effect. Although these pathways remain difficult to target therapeutically, both the PI3K pathway with signaling through mTOR and the AMP-activated kinase (AMPK) pathway that inhibits mTORC1 (a protein complex that includes mTOR) are important in controlling the glycolytic process and thus provide potential targets for inhibiting this process. An inhibitor of mTOR is approved for use against RCC (temsirolimus), and another inhibitor (everolimus) has activity against breast and neuroendocrine cancer and RCC. Other mTOR inhibitors are in trials, and modulators of AMPK are being investigated. The inefficient utilization of glucose by malignant cells also leads to a need for alternative metabolic pathways for other compounds as well, one of which is glutamine. Similar to glucose, this provides both a source for structural molecules as well as energy production. Similarly to glucose, glutamine is also inefficiently utilized by cancer cells. Cancer cells can also take up nutrients released by surrounding cells and tissues, increasing the complexity of successfully therapeutically inhibiting metabolism in cancer.

Mutations in genes involved in the metabolic process occur in a number of cancers. Among the most frequently found to date are mutations in isocitrate dehydrogenases 1 and 2 (IDH1 and IDH2). These have been most commonly seen in gliomas, AMLs, and intrahepatic cholangiocarcinomas. These mutations lead to the production of an oncometabolite (2-hydroxyglutarate [2HG]) instead of the normal product α-ketoglutarate. Although the exact mechanisms of oncogenesis by 2HG are still being elucidated, α-ketoglutarate is a key cofactor for a number of dioxygenases involved in controlling DNA methylation. 2HG can act as a competitive inhibitor for α-ketoglutarate, leading to alterations in methylation status (primarily hypermethylation) of genes (leading to epigenetic changes) that can have profound effects on a number of cellular processes including differentiation. Inhibitors of mutant IDH1 and IDH2 are approved for treating IDH mutant AML and are in clinical trials for glioblastomas and cholangiocarcinomas.

Much needs to be learned about the specific differences in metabolism between cancer cells and normal cells; however, even with the currently limited state of knowledge, modulators of metabolism are being tested clinically. The first of these is the antidiabetic agent metformin, both alone and in combination with chemotherapeutic agents. Metformin inhibits gluconeogenesis and may have direct effects on tumor cells by activating AMPK, a serine/threonine protein kinase that is downstream of the LKB1 tumor suppressor, and thus inhibiting mTOR complex 1 (mTORC1). This leads to decreased protein synthesis and proliferation. Studies to date have not yet established metformin to have a clear role as an anticancer agent.

TUMOR MICROENVIRONMENT, ANGIOGENESIS, AND IMMUNE EVASION

Tumors consist not only of malignant cells but also of a complex microenvironment including many other types of cells (including lymphocytes,

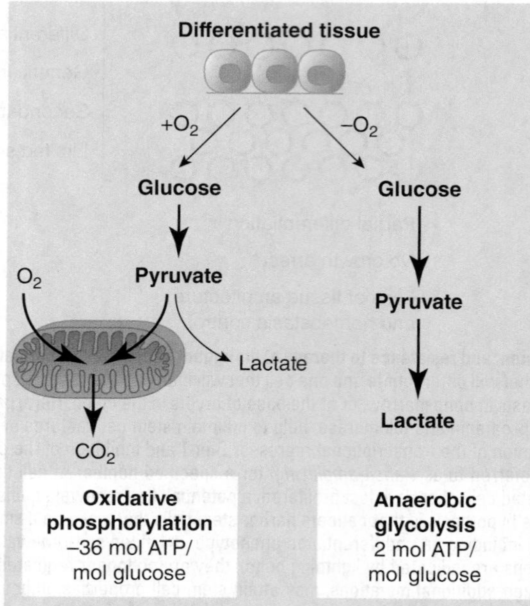

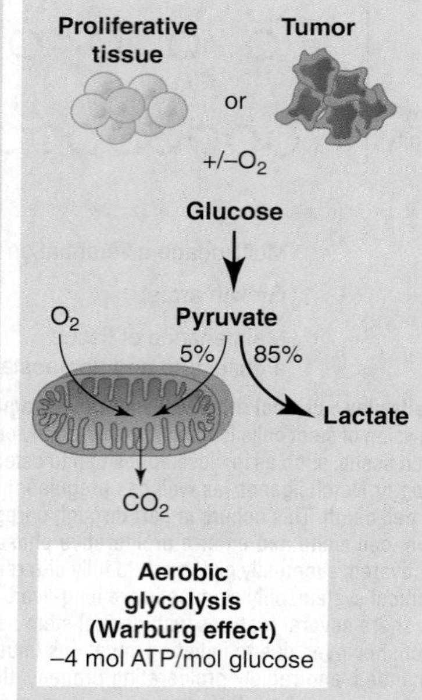

FIGURE 72-8 Warburg versus oxidative phosphorylation. In most normal tissues, the vast majority of cells are differentiated and dedicated to a particular function within the organ in which they reside. The metabolic needs are mainly for energy and not for building blocks for new cells. In these tissues, ATP is generated by oxidative phosphorylation that efficiently generates about 36 molecules of ATP for each molecule of glucose metabolized. By contrast, proliferative tumor tissues, especially in the setting of hypoxia, a typical condition within tumors, use aerobic glycolysis to generate energy for cell survival and generation of building blocks for new cells.

macrophages, myeloid cells, other inflammatory cells, fibroblasts, and fat cells), ECM, secreted factors (including growth factors and hormones), reactive oxygen and nitrogen species, mechanical factors, blood vessels, and lymphatics. This microenvironment is not static but rather is dynamic and continually evolving. Both the complexity and dynamic nature of the microenvironment enhance the difficulty of treating tumors. The microenvironment can contribute to resistance to anticancer therapies through a number of mechanisms.

■ OBESITY AND CANCER

Significant evidence links obesity and the increased risk of developing certain cancers including postmenopausal breast, colorectal, ovarian, endometrial, esophageal, gallbladder, thyroid, and kidney cancers, among others. Less certain are the mechanisms responsible for this risk. As outlined above, cancers arise in an environment with multiple factors, many of which can stimulate cell proliferation. Obesity impacts a variety of factors including hormonal factors, altered metabolism (especially adipose metabolism), and mediators of inflammatory response that all can impact the development of malignancy. Obesity is associated with a number of hormonal changes including high insulin, glucagon, and leptin levels that can stimulate growth of cells. It also leads to insulin resistance, which may contribute to cancer cell development, in part by increasing insulin-like growth factor-1 (IGF-1) levels. Obesity also leads to alterations in adipose, including fatty acid, metabolism, with production of compounds important for energy metabolism as well as for membrane function within cells that may contribute to carcinogenic process. Obesity contributes to an inflammatory environment in a variety of ways including increased levels of inflammatory proteins such as IL-6 and TNF-α. In terms of impact on survival with cancer, data primarily from breast cancer suggest that obesity is associated with decreased survival likely due, at least in part, to the impact of obesity on hormonal factors in development of certain breast cancers, although this may be limited to subsets of breast cancer patients. Some studies have suggested, paradoxically, that obesity may be associated with improved survival in some patients such as those with advanced-stage colorectal cancer. Clearly, the biology of the association between obesity and cancer and its impact on disease outcome is complex, and additional studies are necessary to better define the mechanisms involved.

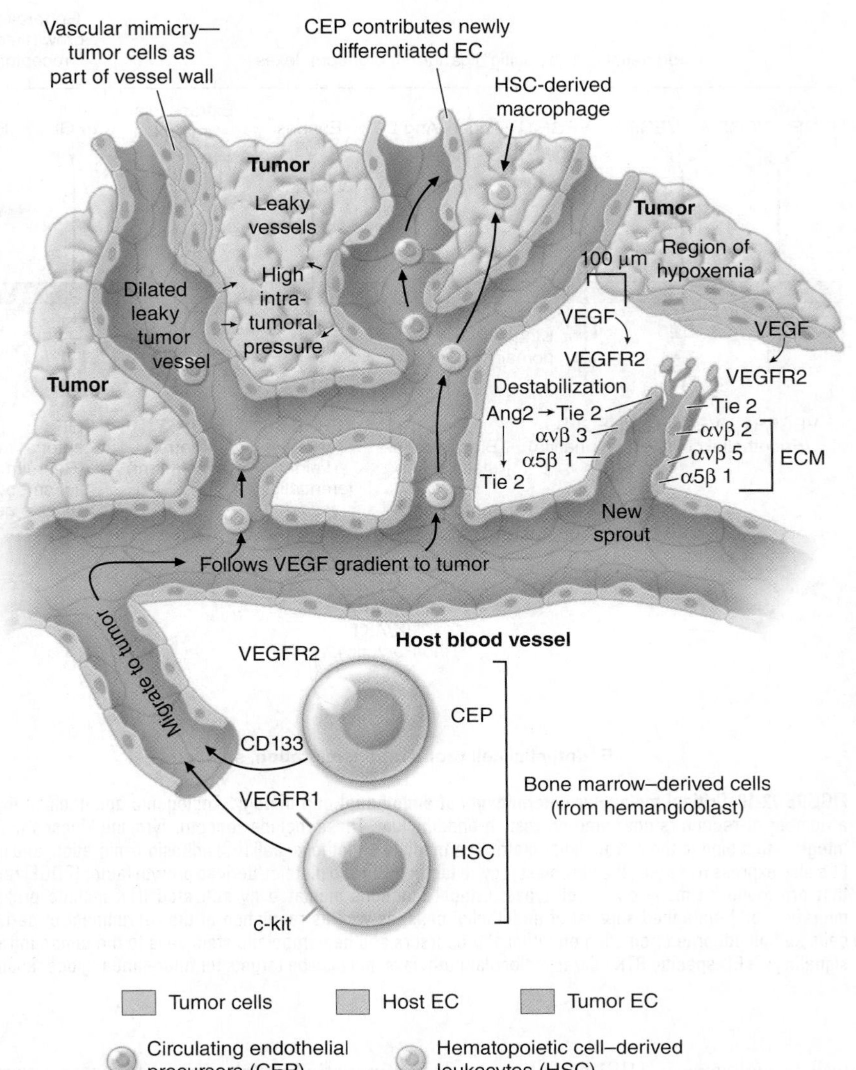

FIGURE 72-9 Tumor angiogenesis is a complex process involving many different cell types that must proliferate, migrate, invade, and differentiate in response to signals from the tumor microenvironment. Endothelial cells (ECs) sprout from host vessels in response to VEGF, bFGF, Ang2, and other proangiogenic stimuli. Sprouting is stimulated by VEGF/VEGFR2, Ang2/Tie-2, and integrin/extracellular matrix (ECM) interactions. Bone marrow–derived circulating endothelial precursors (CEPs) migrate to the tumor in response to VEGF and differentiate into ECs, while hematopoietic stem cells differentiate into leukocytes, including tumor-associated macrophages that secrete angiogenic growth factors and produce matrix metalloproteinases (MMPs) that remodel the ECM and release bound growth factors. Tumor cells themselves may directly form parts of vascular channels within tumors. The pattern of vessel formation is haphazard: vessels are tortuous, dilated, leaky, and branch in random ways. This leads to uneven blood flow within the tumor, with areas of acidosis and hypoxemia (which stimulate release of angiogenic factors) and high intratumoral pressures that inhibit delivery of therapeutic agents.

■ MECHANISMS OF TUMOR VESSEL FORMATION

One of the critical elements of tumor cell proliferation is delivery of oxygen, nutrients, and circulating factors important for growth and survival. Thus, a critical element in growth of primary tumors and formation of metastatic sites is the *angiogenic switch*: the ability of the tumor to promote the formation of new blood vessels, including the recruitment of vascular endothelial cells (ECs). The angiogenic switch is a phase in tumor development when the dynamic balance of pro- and antiangiogenic factors is tipped in favor of vessel formation by the effects of the tumor on its immediate environment. Stimuli for tumor angiogenesis include hypoxemia, inflammation, and genetic lesions in oncogenes or tumor suppressors that alter tumor cell gene expression. Angiogenesis consists of several steps, including the stimulation of ECs by growth factors, degradation of the ECM by proteases, proliferation and migration of ECs into the tumor, and the eventual formation of new capillary tubes.

Tumors use a number of mechanisms to promote vascularization, subverting normal angiogenic processes for this purpose (**Fig. 72-9**). Primary or metastatic tumor cells sometimes arise in proximity to host blood vessels and grow around these vessels, parasitizing nutrients by co-opting the local blood supply. However, most tumor blood vessels arise by the process of sprouting, in which tumors secrete trophic angiogenic molecules, the most potent being VEGFs, that induce the proliferation and migration of host ECs into the tumor. Sprouting in normal and pathogenic angiogenesis is regulated by three families of transmembrane RTKs expressed on ECs and their ligands (VEGFs, angiopoietins, ephrins; **Fig. 72-10**), which are produced by tumor cells, inflammatory cells, or stromal cells in the tumor microenvironment.

Central to the angiogenic response are hypoxia-inducible factors (HIFs; especially 1 and 2), which are transcription factors that normally, in response to hypoxia, stimulate the transcription of a large number of genes responsive to hypoxia, including genes involved in metabolism as

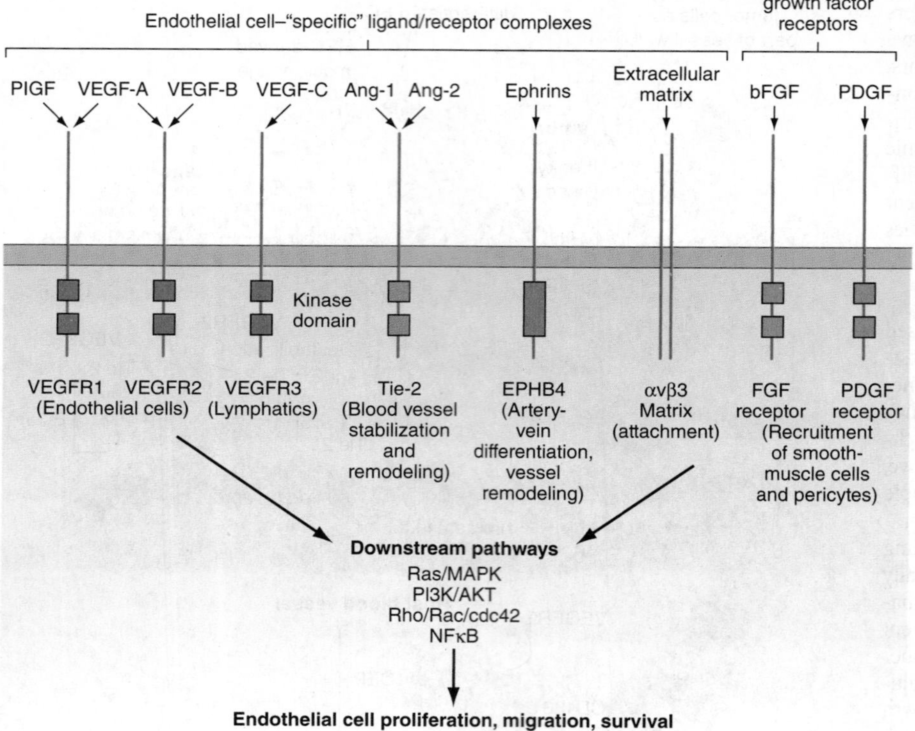

FIGURE 72-10 Critical molecular determinants of endothelial cell biology. Angiogenic endothelium expresses a number of receptors not found on resting endothelium. These include receptor tyrosine kinases (RTKs) and integrins that bind to the extracellular matrix and mediate endothelial cell (EC) adhesion, migration, and invasion. ECs also express RTKs (i.e., the fibroblast growth factor [FGF] and platelet-derived growth factor [PDGF] receptors) that are found on many other cell types. Critical functions mediated by activated RTK include proliferation, migration, and enhanced survival of endothelial cells, as well as regulation of the recruitment of perivascular cells and bloodborne circulating endothelial precursors and hematopoietic stem cells to the tumor. Intracellular signaling via EC-specific RTK utilizes molecular pathways that may be targets for future antiangiogenic therapies.

well as angiogenesis. HIF1 has a bigger role in stimulating metabolism (glycogenesis), whereas HIF2 plays a bigger role in angiogenesis. HIF protein function can also be enhanced in a number of ways in cancer not involving hypoxia, including mutations in the von Hippel–Lindau tumor suppressor gene (an E3 ubiquitin ligase that controls HIF levels by targeting it for degradation), such as occurs in some RCCs. Among the genes stimulated by HIF are VEGF and VEGF receptors. VEGFs and their receptors are required for embryonic vasculogenesis (development of new blood vessels when none preexist) and normal (wound healing, corpus luteum formation) and pathologic angiogenesis (tumor angiogenesis, inflammatory conditions such as rheumatoid arthritis). VEGF-A is a heparin-binding glycoprotein with at least four isoforms (splice variants) that regulates blood vessel formation by binding to the RTKs VEGFR1 and VEGFR2, which are expressed on all ECs in addition to a subset of hematopoietic cells (Fig. 72-9). VEGFR2 plays a more direct role in regulating EC proliferation, migration, and survival, whereas VEGFR1 appears to have more nuanced functions with a less direct role in stimulating EC processes in the normal adult (even acting as a decoy protein for VEGFA to decrease binding to VEGFR2) but with important effects during embryogenesis and on tumor angiogenesis. Tumor vessels may be more dependent on VEGFR signaling for growth and survival than normal ECs.

While VEGF signaling is a critical initiator of angiogenesis, this is a complex process regulated by additional signaling pathways (Fig. 72-10). The angiopoietin, Ang1, produced by stromal cells, binds to the EC RTK Tie-2 and promotes the interaction of ECs with the ECM and perivascular cells, such as pericytes and smooth-muscle cells, to form tight, nonleaky vessels. PDGF and basic fibroblast growth factor (bFGF) help to recruit these perivascular cells. Ang1 is required for maintaining the quiescence and stability of mature blood vessels and prevents the vascular permeability normally induced by VEGF and inflammatory cytokines.

For tumor cell–derived VEGF to initiate sprouting from host vessels, the stability conferred by the Ang1/Tie2 pathway must be perturbed; this occurs by the secretion of Ang2 by ECs that are undergoing active remodeling. Ang2 binds to Tie2 and is a competitive inhibitor of Ang1 action: under the influence of Ang2, preexisting blood vessels become more responsive to remodeling signals, with less adherence of ECs to stroma and associated perivascular cells and more responsiveness to VEGF. Therefore, Ang2 is required at early stages of tumor angiogenesis for destabilizing the vasculature by making host ECs more sensitive to angiogenic signals. In the presence of Ang2, there is no stabilization by the Ang1/Tie2 interaction, and tumor blood vessels are leaky, hemorrhagic, and have poor association of ECs with underlying stroma. Sprouting tumor ECs express high levels of the transmembrane protein ephrin-B2 and its receptor, the RTK EPH, whose signaling appears to work with the angiopoietins during vessel remodeling. During embryogenesis, EPH receptors are expressed on the endothelium of primordial venous vessels while the transmembrane ligand ephrin-B2 is expressed by cells of primordial arteries; the reciprocal expression may regulate differentiation and patterning of the vasculature.

A number of additional ubiquitously expressed host molecules play critical roles in normal and pathologic angiogenesis. Proangiogenic cytokines, chemokines, and growth factors secreted by stromal cells or inflammatory cells make important contributions to neovascularization, including bFGF, transforming growth factor-β (TGF-β), TNF-α, and IL-8. In contrast to normal endothelium, angiogenic endothelium overexpresses specific members of the integrin family of ECM-binding proteins that mediate EC adhesion, migration, and survival. Specifically, expression of integrins αvβ3, αvβ5, and α5β1 mediates spreading and migration of ECs and is required for angiogenesis induced by VEGF and bFGF, which in turn can upregulate EC integrin expression. The αvβ3 integrin physically associates with VEGFR2 in the plasma membrane and promotes signal transduction from each receptor to promote EC proliferation (via focal adhesion kinase, src, PI3K, and other pathways) and survival (by inhibition of p53 and increasing the Bcl-2/Bax expression ratio). In addition, αvβ3 forms cell-surface complexes with matrix metalloproteinases (MMPs), zinc-requiring proteases that cleave ECM proteins, leading to enhanced EC migration and the release of heparin-binding growth factors, including VEGF and bFGF. EC adhesion molecules can be upregulated (i.e., by VEGF, TNF-α) or downregulated (by TGF-β); this, together with chaotic blood flow, explains poor leukocyte-endothelial interactions in tumor blood vessels and may help tumor cells avoid immune surveillance.

Tumor blood vessels are not normal; they have chaotic architecture and blood flow. Due to an imbalance of angiogenic regulators such as VEGFs and angiopoietins (see below), tumor vessels are tortuous and dilated with an uneven diameter, excessive branching, and shunting. Tumor blood flow is variable, with areas of hypoxemia and acidosis leading to the selection of variants that are resistant to hypoxemia-induced apoptosis (often involving the loss of p53 expression). Tumor vessel walls have numerous openings, widened interendothelial junctions, and discontinuous or absent basement membrane. This contributes to the high permeability of these vessels and, together with lack of functional intratumoral lymphatics, causes increased interstitial

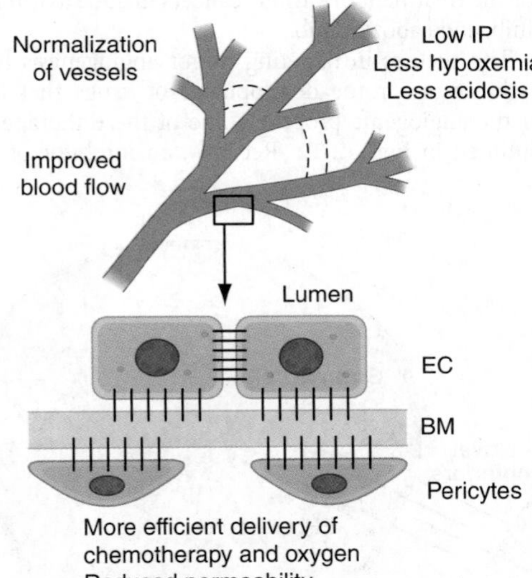

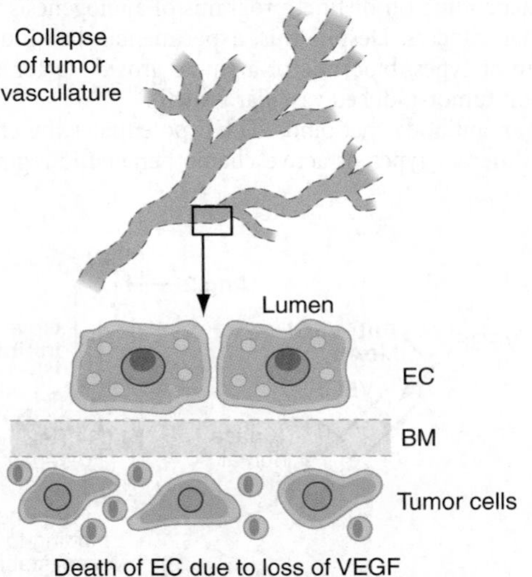

FIGURE 72-11 Normalization of tumor blood vessels due to inhibition of VEGF signaling. ***A.*** Blood vessels in normal tissues exhibit a regular hierarchical branching pattern that delivers blood to tissues in a spatially and temporally efficient manner to meet the metabolic needs of the tissue (top). At the microscopic level, tight junctions are maintained between endothelial cells (ECs), which are adherent to a thick and evenly distributed basement membrane (BM). Pericytes form a surrounding layer that provides trophic signals to the EC and helps maintain proper vessel tone. Vascular permeability is regulated, interstitial fluid pressure (IP) is low, and oxygen tension and pH are physiologic. ***B.*** Tumors have abnormal vessels with tortuous branching and dilated, irregular interconnecting branches, causing uneven blood flow with areas of hypoxemia and acidosis. This harsh environment selects genetic events that result in resistant tumor variants, such as the loss of p53. High levels of VEGF (secreted by tumor cells) disrupt gap junction communication, tight junctions, and adherens junctions between EC via src-mediated phosphorylation of proteins such as connexin 43, zonula occludens-1, VE-cadherin, and α/β-catenins. Tumor vessels have thin, irregular BM, and pericytes are sparse or absent. Together, these molecular abnormalities result in a vasculature that is permeable to serum macromolecules, leading to high tumor interstitial pressure, which can prevent the delivery of drugs to the tumor cells. This is made worse by the binding and activation of platelets at sites of exposed BM, with release of stored VEGF and microvessel clot formation, creating more abnormal blood flow and regions of hypoxemia. ***C.*** In experimental systems, treatment with bevacizumab or blocking antibodies to VEGFR2 leads to changes in the tumor vasculature that have been termed *vessel normalization.* During the first week of treatment, abnormal vessels are eliminated or pruned (dotted lines), leaving a more normal branching pattern. ECs partially regain features such as cell-cell junctions, adherence to a more normal BM, and pericyte coverage. These changes lead to a decrease in vascular permeability, reduced interstitial pressure, and a transient increase in blood flow within the tumor. Note that in murine models, this normalization period lasts only for ~5–6 days. ***D.*** After continued anti-VEGF/VEGFR therapy (which is often combined with chemo- or radiotherapy), ECs die, leading to tumor cell death (either due to direct effects of the chemotherapy or lack of blood flow).

pressure within the tumor (which also interferes with the delivery of therapeutics to the tumor; **Figs. 72-9, 72-10, and 72-11**). Tumor blood vessels have a deficit of perivascular cells such as pericytes and smooth-muscle cells that normally regulate flow in response to tissue metabolic needs.

Unlike normal blood vessels, the vascular lining of tumor vessels is not a homogeneous layer of ECs but often consists of a mosaic of ECs and tumor cells, which, because of their plasticity, can upregulate expression of genes normally only seen in ECs under hypoxic conditions. These cancer cell–derived vascular channels, which may be lined by ECM secreted by the tumor cells, are referred to as *vascular mimicry*. During tumor angiogenesis, ECs are highly proliferative and express a number of plasma membrane proteins that are characteristic of activated endothelium, including growth factor receptors and adhesion molecules such as integrins. These abnormalities in tumor vasculature provide potential differential sensitivities from normal vessels to approaches to inhibit the process, allowing for the use of antiangiogenic agents in cancer treatment.

Lymphatic vessels also exist within tumors. Development of tumor lymphatics is associated with expression of VEGFR3 and its ligands VEGF-C and VEGF-D. The role of these vessels in tumor cell metastasis to regional lymph nodes remains to be determined. However, VEGF-C levels correlate significantly with metastasis to regional lymph nodes in lung, prostate, and colorectal cancers.

ANTIANGIOGENIC THERAPY

Angiogenesis inhibitors function by targeting the critical molecular pathways involved in EC proliferation, migration, and/or survival, many of which are highly expressed in the activated endothelium in tumors. Inhibition of growth factor and adhesion-dependent signaling pathways can induce EC apoptosis with concomitant inhibition of tumor growth. Different types of tumors can use distinct combinations of molecular mechanisms to activate the angiogenic switch. Therefore, it is doubtful that a single antiangiogenic strategy will suffice for all human cancers; rather, a number of agents or combinations of agents will be needed, depending on distinct programs of angiogenesis used by different human cancers. Despite this, experimental data indicate that for some tumor types, blockade of a single growth factor (e.g., VEGF) may inhibit tumor-induced vascular growth.

Bevacizumab, an antibody that binds VEGF, potentiates the effects of a number of different types of active chemotherapeutic regimens used to treat a variety of different tumor types including colon, lung, ovarian, and cervical cancers. It also has activity in combination with interferon against RCCs and alone for glioblastomas. Other protein inhibitors of the VEGF signaling pathway approved for anticancer therapy include ramucirumab (a monoclonal antibody directed against VEGFR2, approved for use against gastric/gastroesophageal, colon, and lung cancers) and ziv-aflibercept (a recombinant protein inhibitor of VEGF, approved for colorectal cancer). Hypertension is the most common side effect of inhibitors of VEGF (or its receptors) but can be treated with antihypertensive agents and uncommonly requires discontinuation of therapy. Rare but serious potential risks include arterial thromboembolic events, including stroke and myocardial infarction, hemorrhage, bowel perforation, and inhibition of wound healing.

Several small-molecule inhibitors (SMIs) that target VEGF RTK activity but are also inhibitory to other kinases have also been approved to treat certain cancers. Sunitinib (see above and Table 72-2) has activity directed against mutant c-Kit receptors (approved for GIST), but also targets VEGFR and PDGFR, and has antitumor activity against pancreatic neuroendocrine and metastatic RCCs, presumably on the basis of its antiangiogenic activity. Similarly, sorafenib, originally developed as a Raf kinase inhibitor but with potent activity against VEGFR and PDGFR, has activity against RCC, differentiated thyroid and hepatocellular cancers, and desmoid tumors. A closely related molecule to sorafenib, regorafenib, has activity against colorectal cancer, GIST, and hepatocellular cancer. Other inhibitors of the VEGF pathway approved for the treatment of various cancers include axitinib, pazopanib, lenvatinib, and cabozantinib.

The success in targeting tumor angiogenesis has led to enhanced enthusiasm for the development of drugs that target other aspects of the angiogenic process; some of these therapeutic approaches are outlined in **Fig. 72-12**. Recently, an inhibitor of HIF2-α has shown

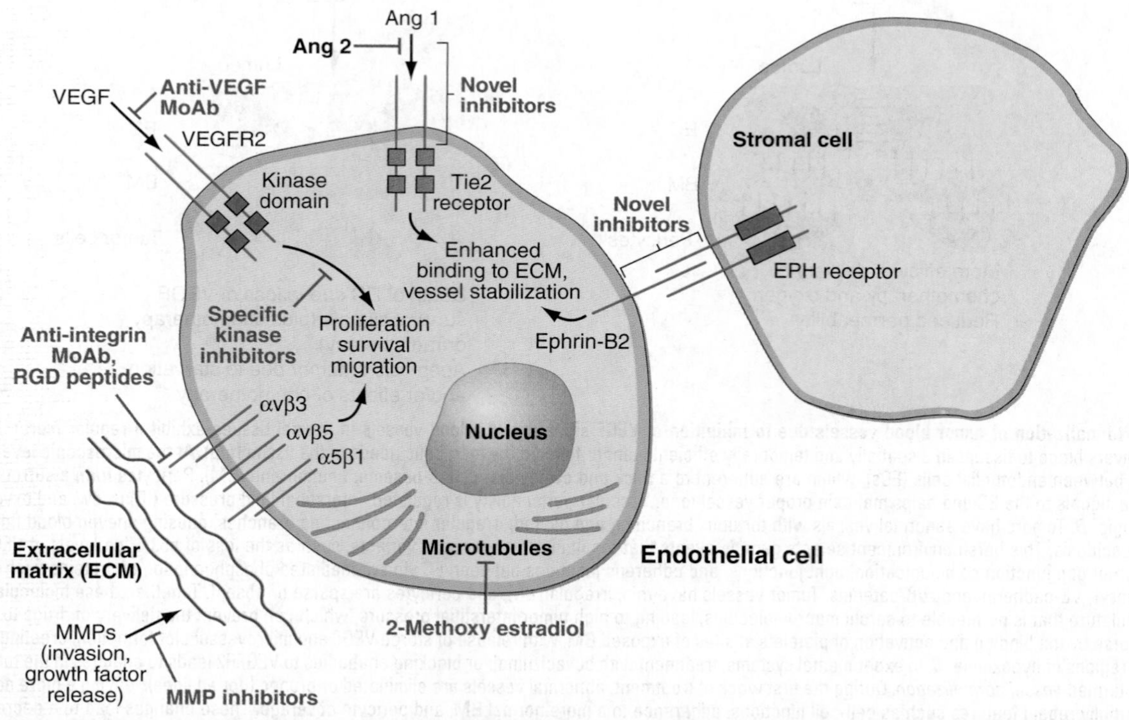

FIGURE 72-12 Knowledge of the molecular events governing tumor angiogenesis has led to a number of therapeutic strategies to block tumor blood vessel formation. The successful therapeutic targeting of VEGF and its receptors VEGFR is described in the text. Other endothelial cell–specific receptor tyrosine kinase pathways (e.g., angiopoietin/Tie2 and ephrin/EPH) are likely targets for the future. Ligation of the $\alpha_v\beta_3$ integrin is required for EC survival. Integrins are also required for EC migration and are important regulators of matrix metalloproteinase (MMP) activity, which modulates EC movement through the ECM as well as release of bound growth factors. Targeting of integrins includes development of blocking antibodies, small peptide inhibitors of integrin signaling, and arg-gly-asp–containing peptides that prevent integrin:ECM binding. Peptides derived from normal proteins by proteolytic cleavage, including endostatin and tumstatin, inhibit angiogenesis by mechanisms that include interfering with integrin function. Signal transduction pathways that are dysregulated in tumor cells indirectly regulate EC function. Inhibition of EGF-family receptors, whose signaling activity is upregulated in a number of human cancers (e.g., breast, colon, and lung cancers), results in downregulation of VEGF and IL-8, while increasing expression of the antiangiogenic protein thrombospondin-1. The Ras/MAPK, PI3K/Akt, and Src kinase pathways constitute important antitumor targets that also regulate the proliferation and survival of tumor-derived EC. The discovery that ECs from normal tissues express tissue-specific "vascular addressins" on their cell surface suggests that targeting specific EC subsets may be possible.

preliminary evidence of antitumor activity against RCC in a clinical trial. There is also evidence suggesting potential enhanced activity when anti-VEGF agents are used in combination with immunomodulators including immune checkpoint inhibitors. However, it is not yet known whether this will produce a clinically meaningful enhancement of antitumor activity.

EVASION OF THE IMMUNE SYSTEM BY CANCERS

The immune system plays a critical role in maintaining organismal integrity including by defending against pathogens as well as preventing and limiting the growth of cancers. There is a complex interaction between cancer and the host from the development of the first malignant cell to the establishment of a clinical cancer and its subsequent growth, invasion, and metastasis. The immune system plays a critical role in the prevention of cancer development. This is exemplified by the increased risk for cancer development in individuals who are significantly immunosuppressed, such as by inherited defects in mechanisms important for immune function, the immunosuppression necessary to maintain allogeneic organ transplants, and immunosuppression seen from certain infections such as human immunodeficiency virus. There are two components of the immune system. The first is innate immunity (present in the organism and not dependent on prior exposure to a specific antigen, such as those present in a pathogen or malignant cell), which tends to be general and not specific. The second is the adaptive immune component, which depends on the innate immune component for activation and provides the specificity to the response with significant expansion of cells to target the specific antigens present on the pathogen or malignant cell. Thus, while the innate process provides the first line of defense, the adaptive process is necessary for the specificity of response and providing memory to more rapidly attack cells should the pathogen infection recur or the malignant cells grow. The immune system has to be tightly regulated to allow for clearance of unwanted antigens while preventing an immune-mediated attack on the self. (See **Chap. 349** for details on the function of the immune system).

Not surprisingly, since cancers arise from normal cells within the body that have a variety of processes to prevent destruction by the immune system, they have a variety of mechanisms that allow them to evade detection and elimination by the immune system (**Fig. 72-13**). These include downregulation of cell surface proteins involved in immune recognition (including MHC proteins and tumor-specific antigens), expression of other cell surface proteins that inhibit immune function (including members of the B7 family of proteins such as PD-L1), secretion of proteins and other molecules that are immunosuppressive, recruitment and expansion of immunosuppressive cells such as regulatory T cells (which are important for maintaining tolerance against self-antigens), induction of T cell tolerance, and downregulation of death receptors (**Fig. 72.14**). Due to the marked heterogeneity of cells within a cancer, a variety of immune-suppressive mechanisms are continuously occurring and changing. In addition, the inflammatory effects of some of the immune mediator cells in the tumor microenvironment (especially tissue-associated macrophages and myeloid-derived suppressor cells) can suppress T cell responses to the tumor as well as stimulate inflammation that can enhance tumor growth.

There are marked differences in the way different malignancies respond to current immunotherapeutic approaches. For example, melanomas, RCC, Merkel cell carcinomas, cancers with defects in DNA repair associated with microsatellite instability with accumulation of gene mutations, and lymphomas respond well to current immunotherapeutic approaches, whereas pancreatic and microsatellite-stable colon cancers do not. While there is not a complete understanding of why these differences exist and there are many factors both within the cancer cells and in the microenvironment that play a role, several factors have been identified that appear to be important. These include the number of mutations present in the tumor (tumor mutational burden), presence of new or neoantigens, expression of immune checkpoint proteins (e.g., PD-L1 for anti-PD-1 or anti-PD-L1 therapy), density of tumor-infiltrating lymphocytes, and host genetic factors. One of these (PD-L1 expression by the tumor) has sufficient predictive value for certain tumors (e.g., non-small-cell lung cancer) to be used in making treatment decisions regarding the use of antibodies targeting PD-1 or PD-L1. However, neither PD-L1 expression nor any other marker can predict responsiveness of most tumors to immunotherapy. Better biomarkers that define potential responsiveness of specific cancers to immunotherapy are badly needed. A major area of research is to try to identify approaches that would convert cancers that are not responsive to immunotherapy to being responsive.

Immunotherapy approaches to treat cancer can be divided into those aimed at activating the immune response and those designed to

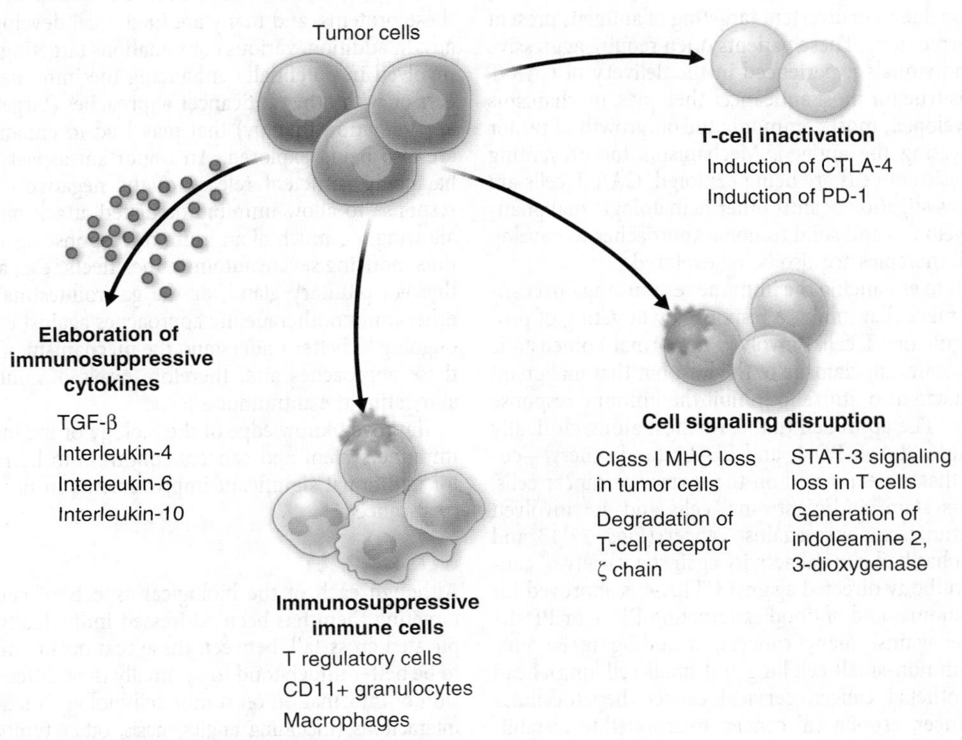

FIGURE 72-13 Tumor-host interactions that suppress the immune response to the tumor.

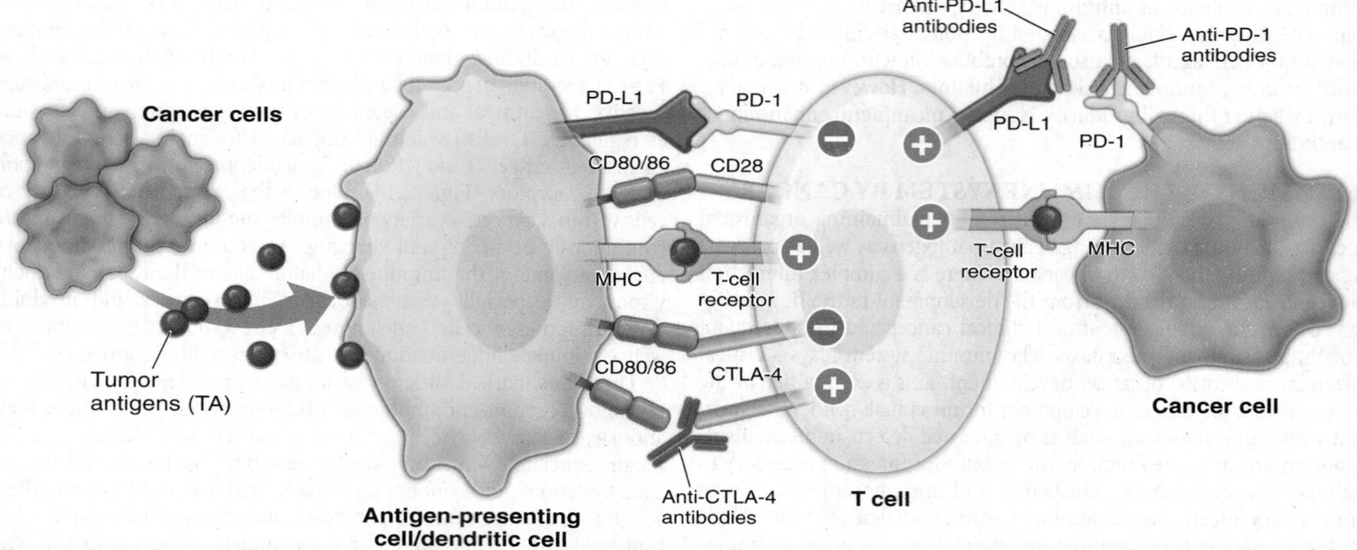

FIGURE 72-14 Inhibition of T-cell activation against cancer cells by engagement of co-inhibitory molecules including PD-1, PD-L1, and CTLA-4 and reversal of this inhibition by antibodies against these proteins. The red ovals in the T cell indicate inhibitory signals, and the green oval indicates stimulatory signals.

release the brakes that prevent an effective immune response against tumors. Approaches at activating the immune response against cancer including using immunostimulatory molecules such as interferons, IL-2, and especially monoclonal antibodies have had some success.

A more direct approach to enhance the activity of T cells directed against specific tumors involves isolating T cells from patients and re-engineering the cells to express chimeric antigen receptors (CAR-T cells) that recognize antigens present on the cells of that individual's tumor. The most commonly used approach to date has been to engineer the cells to express receptors targeting the CD19 antigen on acute lymphocytic leukemia (ALL) and diffuse large B-cell lymphoma (DLBCL) cells. These have been shown to have significant antitumor activity in the treatment of patients with ALL and DLBCL, including durable remissions in patients refractory to standard therapies, and are approved for these malignancies. However, there have also been significant issues with toxicity including cytokine release syndrome, organ toxicity felt to be due to inadvertent targeting of antigens present in the organ, and neurotoxicity. These patients often require aggressive supportive care by individuals experienced in the delivery of CAR-T cells. In addition, as is true for most anticancer therapies, mechanisms of resistance have developed, most commonly the outgrowth of tumor cells no longer expressing the antigen. Mechanisms for preventing the development of resistant cells are being explored. CAR-T cells are undergoing clinical investigation against other hematologic malignancies (e.g., multiple myeloma) and solid tumors. Approaches to develop allogeneic CAR-T-cell therapies are also being explored.

The other approach to enhancing the immune response against cancers is releasing the brakes that inhibit a response by targeting of proteins or cells (e.g., regulatory T cells) involved in normal homeostatic control to prevent autoimmune damage to the host but that malignant cells and their stroma can also utilize to inhibit the immune response directed against them. The approach that is furthest along clinically has involved targeting CTLA-4, PD-1, and PD-L1 (and others)—co-inhibitory molecules that are expressed on the surface of cancer cells, cells of the immune system, and/or stromal cells and are involved in inhibiting the immune response against cancer (Figs. 72-13 and 72-14). This approach has had clinical activity against a variety of cancers. A monoclonal antibody directed against CTLA-4 is approved for the treatment of melanoma, and antibodies targeting PD-1 or PD-L1 are approved for use against many cancers, including melanoma, RCC, lung cancer (both non-small-cell lung and small-cell lung), head and neck cancer, urothelial cancer, cervical cancer, hepatocellular carcinoma, gastric cancer, esophageal cancer, microsatellite instability (MSI)-high cancers, cancers with high tumor mutational burden (TMB), Merkel cell cancer, primary B-cell mediastinal lymphoma, and Hodgkin's lymphoma. They continue to be evaluated against other malignancies as well. The combination of anti-CTLA-4 and anti-PD-1 antibodies has been approved for treatment of a number of cancers including melanoma, RCC, lung cancer, pleural mesothelioma, and MSI-high metastatic colorectal cancers. Immune checkpoint inhibitors are being used singly, in pairs, and in combination with chemotherapy in many ongoing clinical trials. Specific determinants of response to immune checkpoint inhibitors are still being defined, but in addition to high PD-L1 expression, the presence of increased neoantigens in the tumor, such as seen in patients with MSI-high and TMB-high cancers, may be one important determinant of better responses.

A number of other proteins are involved in controlling the immune response (both ones that enhance activity [e.g., CD27 and CD40] as well as ones involved in inhibiting response [e.g., LAG3, TIM-3, TIGIT]). Antibodies have been developed to modulate function of these proteins, and many are in clinical development for cancer therapy. In addition, various combinations targeting more than one protein involved in potentially enhancing the immune response against cancers or with other anticancer approaches (targeted agents, chemotherapy, radiation therapy) that may lead to enhanced antitumor activity are also being explored. An important aspect of these approaches is balancing sufficient release of the negative control of the immune response to allow immune-mediated attack on the tumors while not allowing too much of an immune response against normal tissues and thus inducing severe autoimmune effects (e.g., against lung, liver, skin, thyroid, pituitary gland, or the gastrointestinal tract). As is true for other immunotherapeutic approaches against cancer, major efforts are ongoing to better understand the mechanism of immune toxicity from these approaches and, therefore, ways of controlling this while not abrogating the antitumor effects.

Improved knowledge of the biology of the interactions between the immune system and cancers continues to be rapid with the promise for additional significant improvements in use of immunotherapy to treat cancer.

SUMMARY

Although each of the biological aspects of cancers and examples of targeting them has been addressed individually, clearly there is complicated cross-talk between these that occurs in all cancers that needs to be better understood to optimally treat different cancers. The explosion of information on tumor cell biology, metastasis, and tumor-host interactions (including angiogenesis, other tumor-stromal interactions, and immune evasion by tumors) has ushered in a new era of rational targeted therapy for cancer. Furthermore, it has become clear that specific molecular factors detected in individual tumors (specific gene mutations, gene expression profiles, miRNA expression, overexpression of specific proteins) can be used to tailor therapy and maximize antitumor effects. Potentially of greater impact on decreasing deaths from cancer, better understanding of the biology of early cancer development and technologic development to improve sensitivity and specificity in detecting cancer-specific molecules (e.g., mutated genes) provide hope that approaches for earlier detection of cancer can be developed.

ACKNOWLEDGMENT

Robert G. Fenton contributed to this chapter in prior editions, and important material from those prior chapters has been included here.

FURTHER READING

BOUSSIOTIS VA: Molecular and biochemical aspects of the PD-1 checkpoint pathway. N Engl J Med 375:1767, 2016.

DE PALMA M et al: Microenvironmental regulation of tumour angiogenesis. Nat Rev Cancer 17:457, 2017.

DU W, ELEMENTO O: Cancer systems biology: Embracing complexity to develop better anticancer therapeutic strategies. Oncogene 34:3215, 2015.

FLEUREN ED et al: The kinome "at large" in cancer. Nat Rev Cancer 16:83, 2016.

HE S, SHARPLESS NE: Senescence in health and disease. Cell 169:1000, 2017.

LAMBERT AW et al: Emerging biological principles of metastasis. Cell 168:670, 2017.

OTTO T, SICINSKI P: Cell cycle proteins as promising targets in cancer therapy. Nat Rev Cancer 17:93, 2017.

TOMASETTI C et al: Stem cell divisions, somatic mutations, cancer etiology and cancer prevention. Science 355:1330, 2017.

VANDER HEIDEN MG, DEBERARDINIS RJ: Understanding the intersections between metabolism and cancer biology. Cell 168:657, 2017.

VOGELSTEIN B et al: Cancer genome landscapes. Science 339:1546, 2013.

73 Principles of Cancer Treatment

Edward A. Sausville, Dan L. Longo

CANCER PRESENTATION

Localized or systemic cancer is frequent in the differential diagnosis of a variety of common complaints. Affording patients the greatest opportunity for cure or meaningful prolongation of life is greatly aided by cancer diagnosis early in its natural history. The spectrum of possible cancer-related interventions to make cure possible are shown in **Table 73-1**.

DETECTION OF A CANCER

The term *cancer*, as used here, is synonymous with the term *tumor*, whose original derivation from Latin simply meant "swelling," not otherwise specified. Swelling reflects increased interstitial fluid pressure and increased cellular and stromal mass, compared to normal tissue. Leukemias, a cancer of the blood-forming tissues, presents in a disseminated form frequently without tumor masses. Tumors can also present by organ dysfunction, such as dyspnea on exertion from anemia caused by leukemia replacing normal marrow, cough from lung cancers, jaundice from tumors blocking bile ducts, or neurologic signs from gliomas. Hemorrhage frequently results from involvement

TABLE 73-1 Spectrum of Cancer-Related Interventions

Asymptomatic patient (breast, cervix, colon, some lung) screening
Consideration of cancer in a differential diagnosis
Physical examination, imaging, or endoscopy to define a possible tumor
Phlebotomy for molecular studies and circulating tumor cell characterization
Diagnosis of cancer by biopsy or removal:
Routine histology
Specialized histology: immunohistochemistry
Molecular studies
Cytogenetic studies
Staging the cancer: Where has it spread?
Treatment
Localized (surgical removal with or without local radiation therapy and/or topical therapy may be curative)
Systemic (prevent or reverse organ compromise)
Supportive care
During treatment: related to tumor effects on patient
During treatment: to counteract side effects of treatment
After treatment: to ameliorate the adverse effects of treatment
Palliative and end of life
When useful treatments are not feasible or desired

of hollow viscera, but also may reflect altered platelet number or blood coagulation. Tumors may also present with a "paraneoplastic syndrome" owing to the effects of substances they secrete. Although statistically the fraction of patients with cancer underlying a particular presenting sign or symptom may be low, the implications of missing an early-stage tumor call for vigilance in considering cancer as the basis for persistent signs or symptoms.

Evidence of a tumor's existence can come from careful physical examination, e.g., enlarged lymph nodes in lymphomas or palpable mass in a breast or soft tissue site. A mass may also be detected or confirmed by an imaging modality, such as plain x-ray, computed tomography (CT) scan, ultrasound, positron emission tomography (PET) imaging, or nuclear magnetic resonance approaches. Endoscopy may directly visualize a tumor.

ESTABLISHING A CANCER DIAGNOSIS

Once a potential tumor is defined, establishing the diagnosis is the next step in the intervention spectrum. This requires a biopsy procedure in most circumstances and pathologic confirmation that cancer is present; very rarely, where biopsy would be definitely injurious and imaging modalities are unequivocal, such as with a likely brainstem glioma, treatment might be reasonably considered based on clinical and imaging evidence without biopsy. In addition to light microscopy, biopsied tissue also allows definition of genetic abnormalities and protein expression patterns (**Table 73-2**).

The extent of specialized testing needs to be tailored to an individual patient's case. Global DNA sequencing of genes expressed in tumors has not been shown to convey conclusive advantage in terms of survival. But the aggregate "mutational burden" present in tumors and the intactness of DNA repair genes (e.g., breast cancer susceptibility 1 and 2 [*BRCA1/2*], microsatellite instability, homologous recombination pathway–associated genes) may suggest valuable treatment courses in tumors without curative potential. Testing for certain abnormalities in Table 73-2 can be the basis for use of specific U.S. Food and Drug Administration (FDA)-approved therapeutic agents.

Optimally, an *excisional biopsy* occurs, in which the entire tumor mass is removed with a margin of normal tissue surrounding it. If an excisional biopsy cannot be performed, *incisional biopsy* is the procedure of second choice: a wedge of tissue is removed, trying to include the majority of the cross-sectional diameter to minimize sampling error. Biopsy techniques that involve cutting into tumor risk facilitating the spread of the tumor, and consideration with a surgeon of whether the biopsy approach is a potential prelude to a curative surgery

TABLE 73-2 Diagnostic Biopsy: Standard-of-Care Molecular and Special Studies to Be Considered

All solid tumors:
Tumor mutational burden
Microsatellite instability DNA repair pathway intactness
Homologous recombination DNA repair pathway intactness
Breast cancer: primary and suspected metastatic
Breast cancer susceptibility 1 and 2 (*BRCA1/2*) gene mutations
Hormone receptor expression: estrogen, progesterone
HER2/neu oncoprotein
PI3KA mutation status
Lung cancer: primary and suspected metastatic
If nonsquamous non-small-cell:
Epidermal growth factor receptor (*EGFR*) mutation
ALK gene fusion
BRAF V600E mutation
Programmed cell death ligand 1 (PD-L1) expression
Colon cancer: suspected metastatic
KRAS mutation
BRAF V600E mutation
Gastrointestinal stromal tumor
KIT mutation
Melanoma
BRAF mutation
c-kit expression and *KIT* mutation if present
Pancreatic cancer
BRCA1/2 mutation
Prostate cancer
BRCA1/2 mutation
Thyroid cancer
RET gene alterations (mutations, translocations, amplification)
Gliomas
1p/19q co-deletion
Alkylguanine alkyltransferase promoter methylation
Isocitrate dehydrogenase 1 and 2 mutation
Leukemia (peripheral blood mononuclear cells and/or bone marrow)
Cytogenetics
Flow cytometry
Treatment-defining chromosomal translocations/mutations
Bcr-Abl fusion protein
t(15;17)
inversion 16
t(8;21)
FMS-associated tyrosine kinase (*FLT3*) mutation
Nucleophosmin gene mutational status
Isocitrate dehydrogenase 1 and 2 mutation
Lymphoma
Immunohistochemistry for CD20, CD30, T-cell markers
Treatment-defining chromosomal translocations:
t(14;18)
t(8;14)
Translocations involving *ALK* gene

accounting for possible diagnoses may best inform the approach taken. *Core-needle biopsy* usually obtains considerably less tissue but can provide information to plan a treatment. *Fine-needle aspiration* generally yields a suspension of cells from a mass. If positive for cancer, it may allow inception of systemic treatment, or it can provide a basis for planning a more extensive surgical procedure. It is unreliable as a sole diagnostic method to make a cancer diagnosis in most cases. A "negative" fine-needle aspiration cannot be taken as definitive evidence that a tumor is absent. In some instances, features of diagnostic imaging are sufficient to make a reliable diagnosis without obtaining tissue, usually with presence of a tumor associated circulating diagnostic marker, e.g., alpha fetoprotein in hepatocellular carcinoma.

CANCER STAGING

An essential component of correct patient management in many cancer types is defining the extent of disease to determine whether localized treatments, "combined-modality" approaches, or systemic treatments should initially be considered. Radiographic and other imaging tests can be helpful in defining the *clinical stage*; *pathologic staging* documents the histologic presence of tumor in tissue biopsies obtained through a surgical procedure. Lymph node sampling in breast cancer, melanoma, lung, head and neck, colon, and other intra-abdominal cancers may provide crucial information.

Staging systems have evolved to define a "T" component related to the size of the tumor or its invasion into local structures, an "N" component related to the number and nature of lymph node groups adjacent to the tumor with evidence of tumor spread, and an "M" component, based on the presence of local or distant metastatic sites. The various TNM components are then aggregated to stages, usually stage I to III or IV, depending on the anatomic site. The numerical stages reflect similar long-term survival outcomes of the aggregated TNM groupings in a numeric stage after treatment tailored to the stage. In general, stage I tumors are T1 (reflecting small size), N0 or N1 (reflecting no or minimal node spread), and M0 (no metastases). Such early-stage tumors are usually amenable to curative approaches with local treatments. On the other hand, stage IV tumors have metastasized to distant sites or locally invaded viscera in a nonresectable way. They are treated with palliative intent, except for those diseases with exceptional sensitivity to systemic treatments such as chemotherapy or immunotherapy. Also, the TNM staging system is not useful in diseases such as leukemia, where bone marrow infiltration is never localized, or central nervous system (CNS) tumors, where tumor histology and the extent of feasible resection are more important in driving prognosis.

CANCER TREATMENT

The goal of cancer treatment is first to eradicate the cancer; if not possible, the goal shifts to palliation: amelioration of symptoms and preservation of quality of life while striving to extend life. When cure of cancer is possible, cancer treatments may be undertaken despite the certainty of severe toxicities, and these may produce toxicity with no benefit. Conversely, when the clinical goal is palliation, careful attention to minimizing the toxicity of treatments becomes a significant goal.

Cancer treatments are divided into two main types: *local* and *systemic*. Local treatments include surgery, radiation therapy (including photodynamic therapy), and ablative approaches, including radiofrequency and thermal or cryosurgical approaches. Systemic treatments include chemotherapy (including hormonal therapy and molecular targeted therapy) and biologic therapy (including immunotherapy). The modalities are often used in combination. *Oncology*, the study of tumors including treatment approaches, is a multidisciplinary effort with surgical, radiation, and internal medicine–related areas of oncologic expertise.

Normal organs and cancers share the property of having a population of cells actively progressing through the cell cycle, with their division providing a basis for organ or tumor growth, and a population of cells not in cycle; these include *stem cells*, whose properties are being elucidated. Cancer stem cells serve as a basis for tumor initiating or repopulating cells. Tumors follow a Gompertzian growth curve (**Fig. 73-1**), with the growth fraction of a neoplasm high with small tumor burdens and declining until, at the time of diagnosis, with a tumor burden of 1–5 × 10^9 tumor cells, the growth fraction is usually 1–4% for many solid tumors. By this view, the most rapid growth rate occurs before the tumor is detectable. An alternative explanation for such growth properties may also emerge from the ability of tumors at metastatic sites to recruit circulating tumor cells from the primary tumor or other metastases. Key features of tumor growth are the ability to stimulate new supporting stroma through angiogenesis and ingrowth of fibroblasts and immune cells (**Chap. 72**).

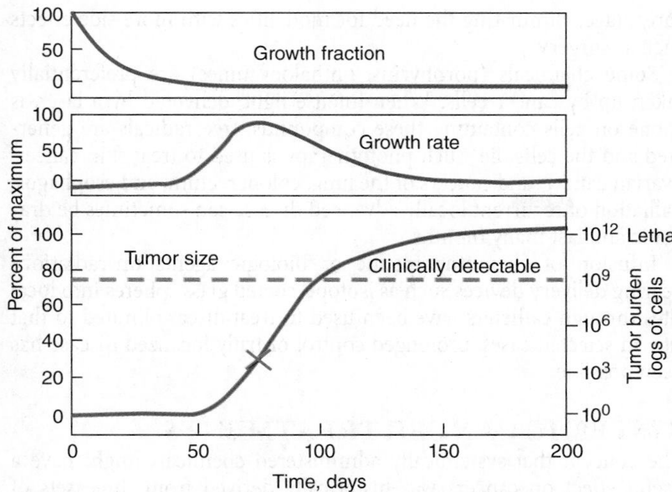

FIGURE 73-1 Gompertzian tumor growth. The growth fraction of a tumor declines exponentially over time (*top*), peaking before it is clinically detectable (*middle*). Tumor size increases slowly, goes through an exponential phase, and slows again as the tumor has limitation of nutrients or host regulatory influences occur. The maximum growth rate occurs at 1/e, the point at which the tumor is about 37% of its maximum size (*marked with an X*). Tumor becomes detectable at a burden of about 10^9 (1 cm^3) cells and kills the patient at a tumor cell burden of about 10^{12} (1 kg).

LOCALIZED CANCER TREATMENTS

■ SURGERY

Surgery is unquestionably the most effective means of treating cancer. At least 40% of cancer patients are cured by surgery. Unfortunately, a large fraction of patients with solid tumors have metastatic disease not accessible for removal. Even when cancer is not curable by surgery alone, the removal of tumor can afford local control of tumor, preserve organ function, achieve debulking that permits more effective subsequent therapy, and allow more detailed staging. Cancer surgery aiming for cure is usually planned to excise the tumor completely with an adequate margin of normal tissue (the margin varies with the tumor and the anatomy), touching the tumor as little as possible to prevent vascular and lymphatic spread, and minimizing operative risk. Such a resection is defined as an R0 resection. R1 and R2 resections, in contrast, are imprecisely defined pathologically as having microscopic or macroscopic, respectively, tumor at resection margins. Such outcomes may be the basis for reoperation to obtain optimal margins if feasible and of likely clinical utility. Extending the procedure to resect draining lymph nodes obtains prognostic information and may, in some anatomic locations, improve survival.

Laparoscopic approaches are being used for primary abdominal and pelvic tumors, although with certain tumors (e.g., uterine and cervix), controversy exists as to the desirability of laparoscopic tissue removal. Lymph node spread may be assessed using the sentinel node approach, in which the first draining lymph node is defined by injecting a dye or radioisotope into the tumor site at operation and then resecting the first node to turn blue or collect isotope. The sentinel node assessment appears to provide information without the risks (lymphedema, lymphangiosarcoma) associated with resection of all regional nodes. Advances in adjuvant chemotherapy (chemotherapy given systemically after removal of all local disease surgically without evidence of active metastatic disease) and radiation therapy following surgery have permitted a substantial decrease in the extent of primary surgery necessary to obtain the best outcomes. Thus, "lumpectomy" with radiation therapy is as effective as modified radical mastectomy for breast cancer, and limb-sparing surgery followed or preceded by adjuvant radiation therapy and chemotherapy has replaced amputation for most childhood rhabdomyosarcomas and osteosarcomas. More limited surgery spares organ function, as in larynx and bladder cancer. In some settings (e.g., bulky testicular cancer or stage III breast cancer), surgery is not the first treatment modality used. After diagnostic biopsy, chemotherapy and/or radiation therapy is delivered, followed by a surgical procedure to remove residual masses; this is called *neoadjuvant therapy*. Coordination among the surgical oncologist, radiation oncologist, and medical oncologist is crucial.

Surgery may be curative in a subset of patients with metastatic disease. Patients with limited lung metastases from osteosarcoma may be cured by resection of the lung lesions. In patients with colon cancer who have fewer than five liver metastases restricted to one lobe and no extrahepatic metastases, hepatic lobectomy may produce long-term disease-free survival in 25% of selected patients. In the setting of hormonally responsive tumors, oophorectomy may eliminate estrogen production, and orchiectomy may reduce androgen production, hormones that drive metastatic breast and all prostate cancers, respectively. In selecting a surgeon or center for primary cancer treatment, consideration must be given to the volume of cancer surgeries undertaken by the site. Studies in a variety of cancers have shown that increased annual procedure volume appears to correlate with outcome. Surgery is used in a number of ways for palliative or supportive care of the cancer patient. These include insertion and care of central venous catheters, control of pleural and pericardial effusions and ascites, caval interruption for recurrent pulmonary emboli, stabilization of cancer-weakened weight-bearing bones, and control of hemorrhage, among others. Surgical bypass of gastrointestinal, urinary tract, or biliary tree obstruction can alleviate symptoms and prolong survival. Surgical procedures may provide relief of pain or neurologic dysfunction (spinal cord decompression). Splenectomy may relieve symptoms and reverse hypersplenism. Intrathecal or intrahepatic therapy relies on surgical placement of appropriate infusion portals. Surgery may correct other treatment-related toxicities such as adhesions or strictures. Plastic and reconstructive surgery can correct the effects of disfiguring primary treatment. Surgery is also a tool valuable in the prevention of cancers in high-risk populations. Prophylactic mastectomy, colectomy, oophorectomy, and thyroidectomy are mainstays of prevention of genetic cancer syndromes.

■ RADIATION

Radiation Biology and Medicine Therapeutic radiation is ionizing, causing breaks in DNA and generation of free radicals from cell water that damage cancer cell membranes, proteins, and organelles. Radiation damage is augmented by oxygen; hypoxic cells are more resistant.

$$\text{Ionizing radiation} + H_2O \rightarrow H_2O^+ + e^-$$
$$H_2O^+ + H_2O \rightarrow H_3O^+ + OH^\bullet$$
$$OH^\bullet \rightarrow \text{cell damage}$$

X-ray and gamma-ray photons are the forms of ionizing radiation most commonly used to treat cancer. Particulate ionizing radiation using protons has also become available.

Radiation dose is quantitated based on the amount of energy absorbed by the tumor, not on radiation generated by the machine. The International System (SI) unit for radiation dose is the Gray (Gy): 1 Gy refers to 1 J/kg of tissue; 1 Gy equals 100 centigrays (cGy) of absorbed dose. A historically used unit appearing in the oncology literature, the *rad* (*r*adiation *a*bsorbed *d*ose), is defined as 100 ergs of energy absorbed per gram of tissue and is equivalent to 1 cGy. Radiation dose is measured by placing detectors at the body surface or in radiated phantoms that resemble human form and substance. The features that make a particular cell more or less sensitive to radiation involve DNA repair proteins that, in their physiologic role, protect against environmentally related DNA damage.

Localized Radiation Therapy Radiation effect is influenced by three determinants: total absorbed dose, number of fractions, and time of treatment. A typical course of radiation therapy should be described as 4500 cGy delivered to a particular target (e.g., mediastinum) over 5 weeks in 180-cGy fractions. Most curative radiation treatment programs are delivered once a day, 5 days a week, in 150- to 200-cGy fractions. Nondividing cells are more resistant than dividing cells; delivering radiation in repeated fractions is done to expose a larger number of tumor cells that have entered the division cycle. The energy of the radiation determines its ability to penetrate tissue. Low-energy x-rays (150–400 kV) scatter when they strike the body, resulting in more damage to adjacent normal tissues and less radiation delivered to the tumor. Megavoltage radiation (>1 MeV) has very low lateral scatter; this produces a skin-sparing effect, more homogeneous distribution of the radiation energy, and greater deposit of the energy in the tumor, or *target volume*. The *transit volume* includes the tissues through which the beam passes to the target volume. Computational approaches and delivery of many beams to converge on a target volume are the basis for "gamma knife" and related approaches to deliver high doses to tumor, sparing normal tissue.

Therapeutic radiation is delivered in three ways: (1) *teletherapy*, with focused beams of radiation generated at a distance and aimed at the tumor within the patient; (2) *brachytherapy*, with encapsulated sources of radiation implanted directly into or adjacent to tumor tissues; and (3) *systemic therapy*, with radionuclides administered, for example, intravenously but perhaps targeted by some means to a tumor site. Teletherapy with x-ray or gamma-ray photons is the most commonly used form of radiation therapy and also delivers particulate forms of radiation such as proton beams. The difference between photons and protons relates to volume with greatest delivery of energy: protons have a narrow range of energy deposition. Electron beams are a particulate form of radiation that, in contrast to photons and protons, have a very low tissue penetrance and are used to treat cutaneous tumors. Certain drugs used in cancer treatment may also act as radiation sensitizers. For example, compounds that incorporate into DNA (e.g., halogenated pyrimidines, cisplatin) augment radiation effects at local sites and are important adjuncts to radiation of certain tumors, e.g., squamous head and neck, uterine cervix, and rectal cancers.

Toxicity of Radiation Therapy Although radiation therapy is most often administered to a local region, systemic effects, including fatigue, anorexia, nausea, and vomiting, may develop that are related in part to the volume of tissue irradiated, dose fractionation, radiation fields, and individual susceptibility. Injured tissues release cytokines that act systemically to produce these effects. Bone is among the most radio-resistant organs, with radiation effects being manifested mainly in children through premature fusion of the epiphyseal growth plate. By contrast, the male testis, female ovary, and bone marrow are the most sensitive organs. Any bone marrow in a radiation field will be eradicated by therapeutic irradiation. Organs with less need for cell renewal, such as heart, skeletal muscle, and nerves, are more resistant to immediate radiation effects. In radiation-resistant organs, the vascular endothelium is the most sensitive component. Acute toxicities include mucositis, skin erythema (ulceration in severe cases), and bone marrow toxicity. Often these can be alleviated by periodic interruption of treatment.

Chronic toxicities are more serious. Radiation of the head and neck region produces thyroid failure; cataracts and retinal damage can lead to blindness; salivary glands stop making saliva, which leads to dental caries and poor dentition. Mediastinal irradiation increases myocardial vascular disease. Other late vascular effects include chronic constrictive pericarditis, lung fibrosis, viscus stricture, spinal cord transection, and radiation cystitis or enteritis.

A serious late toxicity is the development of second solid tumors in or adjacent to the radiation fields. Such tumors can develop in any organ or tissue and occur at a rate of ~1% per year beginning in the second decade after treatment.

OTHER LOCALIZED CANCER TREATMENTS

Endoscopy allows placement of stents to unblock viscera by mechanical means, palliating, for example, gastrointestinal or biliary obstructions. Radiofrequency ablation (RFA) refers to focused microwave nonionizing radiation to induce thermal injury within a volume of tissue. RFA can be useful in the control of metastatic lesions, particularly in liver, that may threaten biliary drainage (as one example in patients with otherwise unresectable disease). Cryosurgery uses extreme cold to sterilize lesions in certain sites, such as prostate and kidney, at a very early stage, eliminating the need for modalities with more side effects such as surgery.

Some chemicals (porphyrins, phthalocyanines) are preferentially taken up by cancer cells. When intense light, delivered by a laser, is shone on cells containing these compounds, free radicals are generated and the cells die. Such phototherapy is used to treat skin cancer; ovarian cancer; and cancers of the lung, colon, rectum, and esophagus. Palliation of recurrent locally advanced disease can sometimes be dramatic and last many months.

Infusion of chemotherapeutic or biologic agents or radiation-bearing delivery devices such as isotope-coated glass spheres into local sites through catheters have been used to treat disease limited to that site; in selected cases, prolonged control of truly localized disease has been possible.

SYSTEMIC CANCER TREATMENTS

The concept that systemically administered chemicals might have a useful effect on cancers was historically derived from three sets of observations. Paul Ehrlich in the nineteenth century observed that different dyes reacted with different cell and tissue components. He hypothesized the existence of "magic bullets" that might bind to tumors, owing to the affinity of the agent for the tumor. Observation of the toxic effects of certain mustard gas derivatives on the bone marrow during World War I suggested that smaller doses of these agents might be used to treat tumors of marrow-derived cells. Finally, the fact that tumors from hormone-responsive tissues, e.g., breast tumors, could shrink after oophorectomy led to the idea that endogenous or exogenous substances might modulate tumor growth by altering its regulatory biology. Chemicals achieving each of these goals are currently used as cancer chemotherapy agents.

Anecdotal reports of tumor regression following intratumoral injection of bacterial extracts raised the possibility of immune system–mediated tumor regression. Serotherapy of infectious disease in the preantibiotic era encouraged analogous efforts to develop vaccine- and antibody-based treatments for cancer. Administration of autologous immune cells obtained by pheresis procedures from a patient or purified from a patient's removed tumor, activated by cytokines ex vivo, achieved durable disease control in a small fraction of patients. These observations provided the rationale for more modern efforts to treat tumors using cell-mediated immunity.

Systemic cancer treatments are of three broad types. *Cytotoxic chemotherapy agents* are "small molecules" (generally with molecular mass <1500 Da) that cause major regression of experimental tumors growing in animals. These agents mainly target DNA structure or segregation of chromosomes in mitosis. *Cancer molecular target therapies* refer to small molecules designed and developed to interact with a defined macromolecule important in maintaining the malignant state. As described in **Chap. 72**, successful tumors have activated biochemical pathways that lead to uncontrolled proliferation through the action of hormone receptor proteins, oncogene products, loss of cell cycle inhibitors, or loss of cell death regulation, and have acquired the capacity to replicate chromosomes indefinitely, invade, metastasize, and evade the immune system. *Cancer biologic therapies* are most frequently macromolecules, cells, or cell extracts that have a particular target (e.g., anti-growth factor receptor, cytokine, or immunomodulatory antibodies) or may have the capacity to induce a host immune response to kill tumor cells. Most recent additions to cancer biologic therapies include genetically modified cells that directly attack tumor cells and tumor-infecting viruses that can kill tumor cells but also elicit host antitumor immune responses.

SYSTEMIC CANCER THERAPY OVERVIEW

General Principles The *therapeutic index* of any drug is the degree of separation between toxic and therapeutic doses. Really useful drugs have large therapeutic indices, and this usually occurs when the drug target is expressed in the disease-causing compartment as opposed to the normal compartment. Cytotoxic chemotherapeutic agents have the unfortunate property that their main targets, DNA and microtubules, are present in both normal and tumor tissues. Therefore, they have relatively narrow therapeutic indices. Targeted agents can also cause effects on their target in normal tissues, or "off-target" effects on unrelated targets in organs experiencing damage. Biologic therapies may elicit misdirected immune responses on normal organ function. A key activity in oncology drug development is striving to administer a dose of agent that can convey benefit with a minimal or tolerable side effect profile.

Figure 73-2 illustrates steps in cancer drug development. Following demonstration of antitumor activity in animal models, potentially useful anticancer agents are further evaluated to define an optimal schedule of administration and suitable drug formulation. Safety testing in two animal species on an analogous schedule of administration defines the starting dose for a phase 1 trial in humans, usually but not always in patients with cancer who have exhausted "standard" (already approved) treatments. The initial dose is usually one-sixth to one-tenth of the dose just causing easily reversible toxicity in the more sensitive animal species. If the agent is not intrinsically toxic, doses of drug achieving fractions of the useful concentration from model systems are studied. Escalating doses of drug are then given during the human phase 1 trial until reversible toxicity is observed or the desired drug concentration is achieved. Dose-limiting toxicity (DLT) defines a dose that conveys greater toxicity than would be acceptable in routine practice, allowing definition of a lower maximum-tolerated dose (MTD). The occurrence of toxicity is, if possible, correlated with plasma drug concentrations. The MTD or a dose just lower than the MTD is usually the dose suitable for phase 2 trials, where a fixed dose is administered to a relatively homogeneous set of patients with a particular tumor type. If no toxicity has emerged in phase 1 trials, administration of the optimal biologic dose to achieve effective drug concentrations is undertaken. A partial response (PR) historically was defined as a decrease of at least 50% in a tumor's bidimensional area obtained by imaging; more recent response criteria (e.g., Response Evaluation Criteria in Solid Tumors [RECIST]) may use a 30% decrease in aggregate unidimensional areas of target lesions. Response criteria for immunologically directed agents may allow a substantial transient increase in tumor volume as long as a patient's clinical status is stable, as these agents may evoke inflammatory responses in tumors with subsequent shrinkage or stabilization of lesions then occurring subsequently. A complete response (CR) connotes disappearance of all tumor; progression of disease signifies an increase in size of existing lesions by >25% from baseline or best response or development of new lesions; stable disease fits into none of the above categories.

In a phase 3 trial, evidence of improved overall survival or improvement in the time to progression of disease on the part of the new drug is sought in comparison to an appropriate control population. Data from the entire process are the basis for application to a regulatory agency to approve the new agent for commercial marketing.

Cancer drug clinical trials conventionally use a toxicity grading scale where grade 1 toxicities do not require treatment, grade 2 toxicities may require symptomatic treatment but are not life-threatening, grade 3 toxicities are potentially life-threatening if untreated, grade 4 toxicities are actually life-threatening, and grade 5 toxicities are those that result in the patient's death. Active efforts to quantitate effects of anticancer agents on quality of life also frequently occur in early development of oncology drugs.

Development of targeted agents may proceed differently. While phase 1–3 trials are still conducted, focus on a particular tumor type even in phase 1 may be enabled by molecular analysis to define target expression in a patient's tumor necessary for or relevant to the drug's action. Ideally, pharmacodynamic studies would also assess whether the target has been hit. The failure of a targeted therapy can be either because the drug missed the target or it hit the target but the target was not central to the tumor's growth and survival. Within the past decade, agents have been approved for clinical use not in relation to an

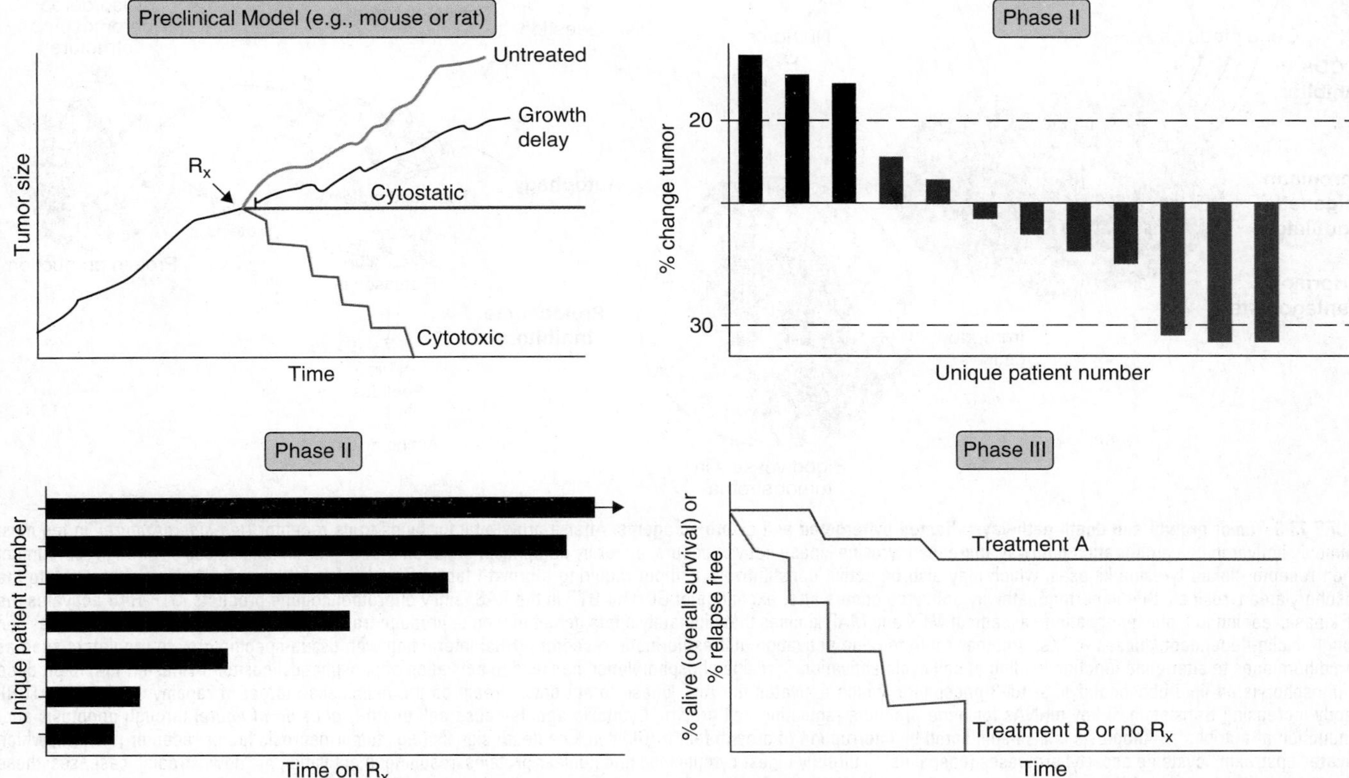

FIGURE 73-2 Steps in cancer drug discovery and development. Preclinical activity (*top left*) in animal models of cancers may be used as evidence to support the entry of the drug candidate into phase 1 trials in humans to define a correct dose and observe any clinical antitumor effect. The drug may then be advanced to phase 2 trials directed against specific cancer types, with rigorous quantitation of antitumor effects. *Waterfall plots* are a standard representation of how patients' tumor sizes change in relation to treatment, with predefined cutoffs defining progression of disease (20% increase in size) or partial response (30% decrease in size) serving as benchmarks of potential valuable effect (*top right*). *Swimmer plots* (*bottom left*) allow the delineation of patients with especially long (or short) times on treatment even without response, another basis in the former case for potential perceived clinical benefit of the treatment. *Kaplan-Meier plots* (*bottom right*) of survival indices in phase 3 comparative trials may allow definition of superiority, inferiority, or no difference of treatment effect compared to standard or no treatment.

originating organ site of disease but across all organ types possessing certain molecular or biologic features.

Useful cancer drug treatment strategies using conventional chemotherapy agents, targeted agents, hormonal treatments, or biologicals all have one of two valuable outcomes. They can induce cancer cell death, resulting in tumor shrinkage with corresponding clinical benefit evidenced by improvement in patient survival, or increase in time until the disease progresses. Another potential outcome is induction of cancer cell *differentiation* or *dormancy* with loss of tumor cell replicative potential and reacquisition of phenotypic properties resembling normal cells. Interaction of a chemotherapeutic drug with its target induces a "cascade" of further signaling steps. These signals ultimately lead to cell death by triggering an "execution phase," where proteases, nucleases, and endogenous regulators of the cell death pathway are activated (**Fig. 73-3**), or differentiation by alteration of cancer genome function.

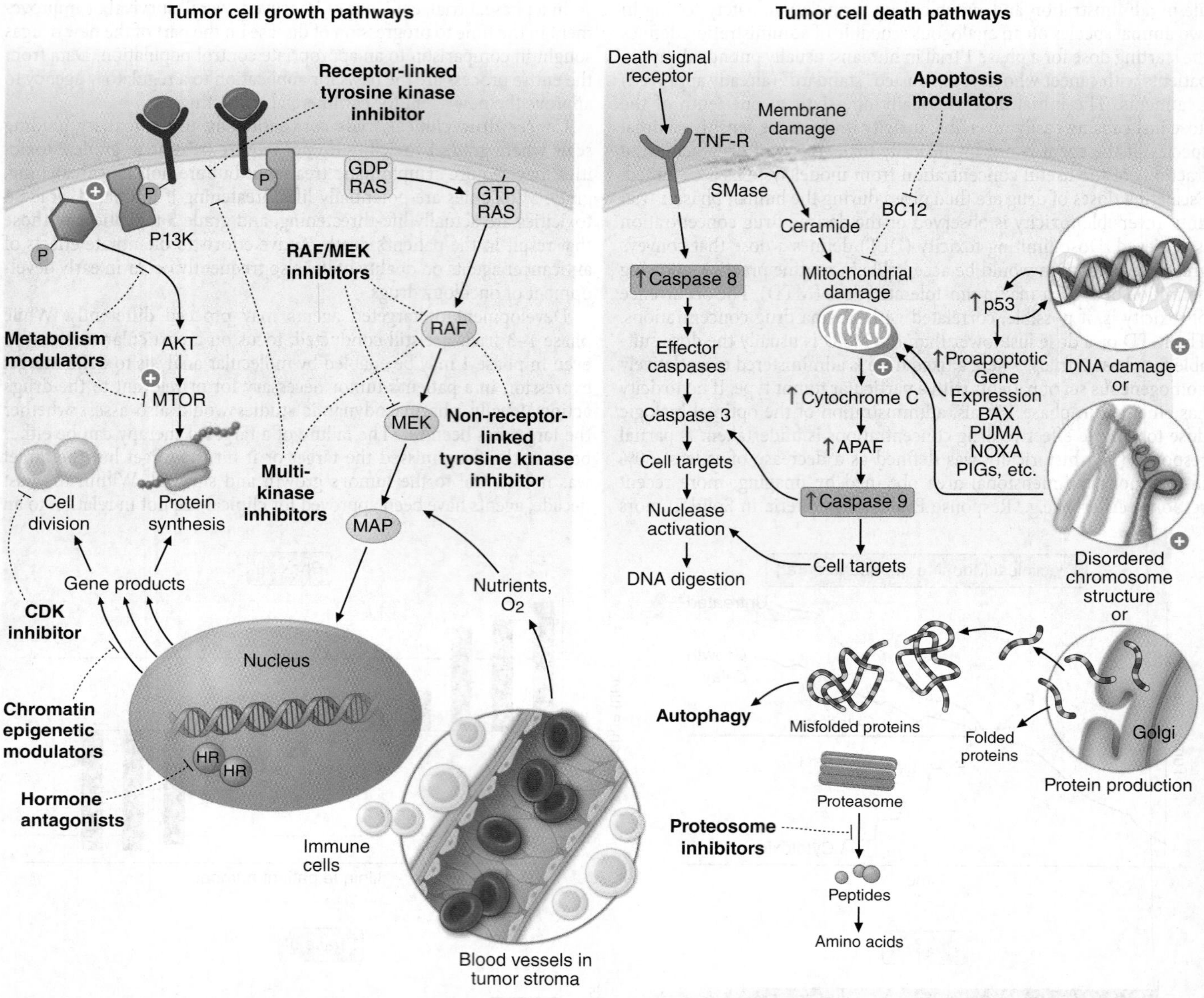

FIGURE 73-3 Tumor growth and death pathways affected by targeted and cytotoxic agents. After a growth factor binds to its receptor (*left side of figure*), in the most commonly activated cell proliferation pathway, increased tyrosine kinase activity occurs, either by autophosphorylation of receptor-linked kinases or through recruitment of non-receptor-linked tyrosine kinases, which may also be active constitutively, without requiring a growth factor. This leads to docking of "adaptor" proteins to the phosphorylated tyrosines. One important pathway activated occurs after exchange of GDP for GTP in the RAS family of protooncogene products. GTP-RAS activates the RAF kinase, leading to a phosphorylation cascade of MEK and MAP kinases that ultimately alters gene function to produce transcripts that activate cell cycle progression through cyclin-dependent kinases (CDKs). Another route to gene activation utilizes hormone receptors (HRs) interacting with tissue-specific growth regulators such as steroid hormones to alter gene function leading to cell cycle activation. Tyrosine phosphorylation can lead to activation of phosphatidylinositol-3-kinase (PI3K) to produce the phosphorylated lipid phosphatidylinositol-3-phosphate, which activates the AKT kinase to act downstream on the mammalian target of rapamycin kinase (mTOR), directly increasing translation of key mRNAs for gene products regulating cell growth. Cytotoxic agents cause cell death (*right side of figure*) through apoptosis and/or induction of autophagy. Apoptosis is also stimulated by interruption of growth factor (GF) cytokine death signals (e.g., tumor necrosis factor receptor [TNF-R]), which activate "upstream" cysteine aspartyl proteases (caspases) to directly digest cytoplasmic and nuclear proteins, resulting in activation of "downstream" caspases; these activate nucleases to cause DNA fragmentation, a hallmark of apoptosis. Chemotherapy agents that create lesions in DNA or alter mitotic spindle function activate gene function to alter mitochondrial integrity. The antiapoptotic protein BCL2 attenuates mitochondrial toxicity, whereas proapoptotic gene products such as BAX, PUMA, etc., antagonize the action of BCL2. Damaged mitochondria release cytochrome C and apoptosis-activating factor (APAF), which activate caspase 9 to cause DNA fragmentation. In addition, membrane damage with activation of sphingomyelinases results in the production of ceramides that can cause direct damage to mitochondria. Protein translation is followed by a folding process in the Golgi apparatus. Misfolded proteins are processed through the proteasome for protease digestion and recycling of amino acids. Disruption of this process can contribute to autophagy, where the cell starves for critical nutrients, or itself induce apoptosis through a distinct pathway activated by misfolded protein accumulation. Antiangiogenic agents and immune therapies work in the tumor stroma (*lower left*) on supporting elements including blood vessels and host inflammatory cells.

Targeted agents differ from chemotherapy agents in that they do not indiscriminately cause macromolecular lesions but regulate the action of macromolecules to whose function tumors have been described as "addicted" in the sense that without the pathway's continued action, the tumor cell cannot survive. In this way, targeted agents directed at such "oncogenic driver" molecules may alter the threshold for tumors driven by these molecules to undergo cell death.

Strategies in Systemic Cancer Management The past 30 years have witnessed a marked evolution in the systemic treatment of cancer not amenable to cure by locally applied treatments. Nonspecific cytotoxic agents of limited efficacy for most patients but highly active and curative in a minority disease types have been joined by targeted and biologic therapies. **Table 73-3, A** lists those tumors considered curable by conventionally available chemotherapeutic agents even when disseminated or metastatic. If a tumor is truly localized to a single site, consideration of surgery or primary radiation therapy should be given as well. Chemotherapy may be used as part of multimodality approaches to offer primary treatment to a clinically localized tumor (**Table 73-3, B**). Chemotherapy can be administered as an *adjuvant*, i.e., in addition to surgery or radiation (**Table 73-3, C**), even after all clinically apparent disease has been removed. This use of chemotherapy has curative potential in, e.g., lung, breast, and colorectal neoplasms, as it eliminates clinically unapparent tumor that may have already disseminated. *Neoadjuvant* chemotherapy refers to administration of chemotherapy before any surgery or radiation to a local tumor in an effort to enhance the effect of subsequent local treatment.

Chemotherapy is routinely used in doses that produce reversible acute side effects, primarily consisting of transient myelosuppression with or without gastrointestinal toxicity (usually nausea). "High-dose" chemotherapy regimens can produce markedly increased therapeutic effect, although at the cost of potentially life-threatening complications that require intensive support, usually in the form of hematopoietic stem cell support from the patient (*autologous*) or from donors matched for histocompatibility loci (*allogeneic*), or pharmacologic "rescue" strategies to block the effect of the high-dose chemotherapy on normal tissues. High-dose regimens have curative potential in defined clinical settings (**Table 73-3, D**).

If cure is not possible, chemotherapy may be undertaken with the goal of palliating the tumor's effect on the host (**Table 73-3, E**). In this usage, value is perceived by the demonstration of improved symptom relief, progression-free survival, or overall survival. The data result from a clinical research protocol used as a basis for FDA approval for commercial use of the agent. Patients treated with palliative intent should be aware of their diagnosis and the limitations of the proposed treatments, have access to supportive care, and have suitable "performance status," according to assessment algorithms such as the one developed by Karnofsky (see **Table 69-4**) or by the Eastern Cooperative Oncology Group (ECOG) (see **Table 69-5**). ECOG performance status (PS) 0 patients are without symptoms; PS1 patients are ambulatory but restricted in strenuous physical activity; PS2 patients are ambulatory and active 50% or more of the time but unable to work; PS3 patients are capable of limited self-care but are active <50% of the time; and PS4 patients are totally confined to bed or chair and incapable of self-care. Only PS0, PS1, and PS2 patients are generally considered suitable for palliative (noncurative) treatment. If there is curative potential, even poor-PS patients may be treated (especially if their symptoms are directly related to a cancer that may respond to treatment), but their prognosis is usually inferior to that of good-PS patients treated with similar regimens. Assessment of physiologic reserve through use of the geriatric assessment tool can be helpful, but no measure of comorbidities or physiologic reserve is considered standard.

The turn of the millennium marked the arrival of alternative strategies for cancer treatment. Prominent among these are *cancer biologic therapy*, which harnesses the use of immune system–derived reagents or strategies, and *cancer targeted therapies*, which are directed at specific molecular targets differentially expressed in malignant as opposed to normal tissues.

TABLE 73-3 Clinical Impact on Cancers with Cytotoxic Chemotherapy

A. Advanced Cancers with Possible Cure	**D. Cancers Possibly Cured with High-Dose Chemotherapy with Stem Cell Support**
Acute lymphoid and acute myeloid leukemia (pediatric/adult)	Relapsed leukemias, lymphoid and myeloid
Hodgkin's disease (pediatric/adult)	Relapsed lymphomas, Hodgkin's and non-Hodgkin's
Lymphomas—certain types (pediatric/adult)	Chronic myeloid leukemia
Germ cell neoplasms	Multiple myeloma
Embryonal carcinoma	**E. Cancers Responsive with Useful Palliation, But Not Cure, by Chemotherapy**
Teratocarcinoma	Bladder carcinoma
Seminoma or dysgerminoma	Chronic myeloid leukemia
Choriocarcinoma	Hairy cell leukemia
Gestational trophoblastic neoplasia	Chronic lymphocytic leukemia
Pediatric neoplasms	Lymphoma—certain types
Wilms' tumor	Multiple myeloma
Embryonal rhabdomyosarcoma	Gastric carcinoma
Ewing's sarcoma	Cervix carcinoma
Peripheral neuroepithelioma	Endometrial carcinoma
Neuroblastoma	Soft tissue sarcoma
Small-cell lung carcinoma	Head and neck cancer
Ovarian carcinoma	Adrenocortical carcinoma
B. Advanced Cancers Possibly Cured by Chemotherapy and Radiation	Islet cell neoplasms
Squamous carcinoma (head and neck)	Breast carcinoma
Squamous carcinoma (anus)	Colorectal carcinoma
Breast carcinoma	Renal carcinoma
Carcinoma of the uterine cervix	**F. Tumors Poorly Responsive in Advanced Stages to Chemotherapy**
Non-small-cell lung carcinoma (stage III)	Pancreatic carcinoma
Small-cell lung carcinoma	Biliary tract neoplasms
C. Cancers Possibly Cured with Chemotherapy as Adjuvant to Surgery	Thyroid carcinoma
Breast carcinoma	Carcinoma of the vulva
Colorectal carcinoma[a]	Non-small-cell lung carcinoma
Osteogenic sarcoma	Prostate carcinoma
Soft tissue sarcoma	Melanoma (subsets)
	Hepatocellular carcinoma
	Salivary gland cancer

[a]Rectum also receives radiation therapy.

CANCER BIOLOGIC THERAPY

Figure 73-4 presents the landscape of cancer biologic therapy agents and actions. The goal of biologic therapy is to manipulate the host-tumor interaction in favor of the host, potentially at an optimum biologic dose that might be different than MTD. As a class, biologic therapies may be distinguished from cytotoxic and molecularly targeted agents in that biologic therapies require activity (e.g., antigen expression or internalization) on the part of the tumor cell or on the part of the host (e.g., T-cell engagement or cytokine elaboration) to allow therapeutic effect.

Antibody-Mediated Therapeutic Approaches Figure 73-4 illustrates current antibody-based strategies in cancer treatment. The ability to grow very large quantities of high-affinity monoclonal antibodies directed at specific tumor antigens produced by animals allows the grafting of animal-derived antigen-combining sequences into human immunoglobulin genes (chimerized or humanized products) or derived de novo from mice bearing human immunoglobulin gene loci. Four general strategies have emerged using antibodies. *Antitumor cell antibodies* target tumor cells directly to inhibit intracellular functions or attract immune or stromal cells. *Bispecific tumor engaging (BiTe) antibodies* directly bind to a tumor cell and to a host immune cell. *Immunoregulatory antibodies* target antigens expressed on host

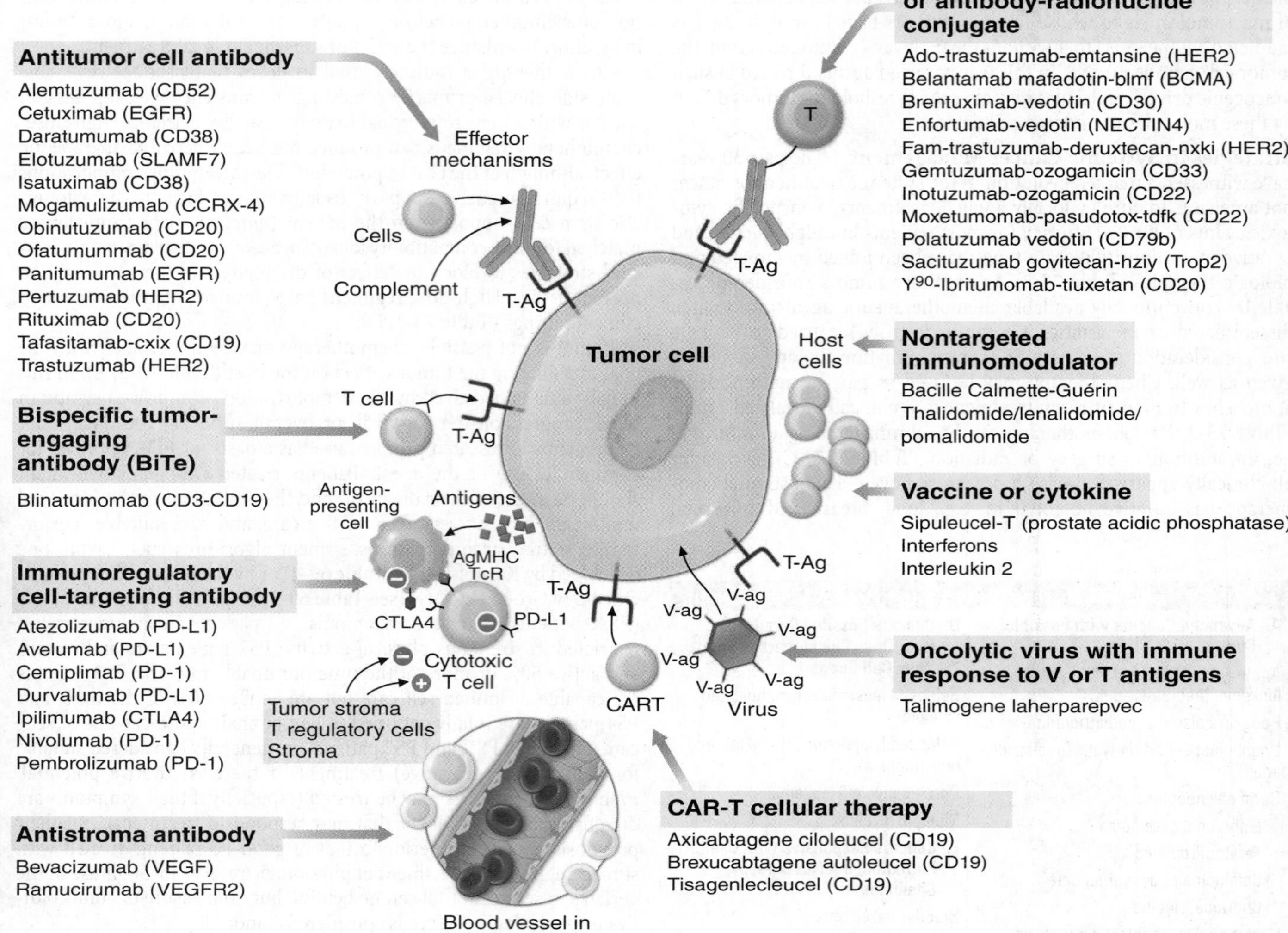

FIGURE 73-4 Immunologic treatments for cancer. Anti-tumor cell antibodies targeting antigens (T-Ag) expressed on tumor cells and indicated in parentheses for each antibody or antibody-derived construct (*upper left*) can either directly interfere with tumor cell function by, e.g., inhibiting growth-promoting pathways, or recruit host immune effector cells actively (especially through *bispecific tumor-engaging [BiTe]* strategies), Fc receptors, or cytotoxic mechanisms such as complement. Proceeding *clockwise* in the figure, *antibody conjugates* can also be engineered to deliver cytotoxic drugs, bacteria-derived toxins, or radioisotopes (T) to T-Ags (*upper right*). Relatively *nonspecific immunomodulators* include vaccines instilled directly into the tumor stroma, agents such as the "imids" that alter tumor and stromal cell cytokine production, and cytokines such as interferon or interleukin 2 (IL-2), which can affect tumor-infiltrating lymphocyte function or have direct antitumor effects. *Vaccines* targeting tumor cell antigens or live attenuated *oncolytic viruses* injected into tumors can cause tumor cell lysis with induction of a prominent host antitumor immune response to virus Ags and T-Ags. In the *left lower* portion of the figure, strategies to target stromal and immune cells include derivation of autologous T cells that are then infected with a lentivirus or other construct that targets antigens (T-Ags) expressed on tumor cells (*chimeric antigen receptor [CAR] T cells),* with the targeted antigen in parentheses. Alternatively, endogenous T cells can be activated by *immunomodulatory cell targeting antibodies.* Specifically, tumor cell–derived antigens are taken up by antigen-presenting cells (APCs), also in the stroma. Antigens are processed by the APCs to peptides presented by the major histocompatibility complex (MHC) to T-cell antigen receptors (TcRs), thus providing a positive (+) activation signal for the cytotoxic tumor cells to kill tumor cells bearing that antigen. Negative (–) signals inhibiting cytotoxic T-cell action include the CTLA4 receptor (on T cells), interacting with the B7 family of negative regulatory signals from APCs, and the PD receptor (on T cells), interacting with the PD ligand-1 (PD-L1) (–) signal coming from tumor cells expressing the PD-L1. Strategies that inhibit CTLA4 and PD-1 function are a means of stimulating cytotoxic T-cell activity to kill tumor cells. *Tumor stroma-directed antibodies* cause anti-vascular endothelial cell growth factor (VEGF)–mediated antiangiogenic and tumor interstitial pressure-modulating strategies.

immune cells to boost the host's immune response to the tumor. Finally, *antibody conjugates* link the antibody to drugs, toxins, or radioisotopes to target these "warheads" for delivery to the tumor. These will be considered with cytotoxic agents. *Stroma-directed antibodies* are currently available against tumor supporting vasculature.

ANTI-TUMOR CELL ANTIBODIES (FIG. 73-4) Humanized antibodies against the CD20 molecule expressed on B-cell lymphomas (rituximab and ofatumumab) are exemplary of antibodies that affect both signaling events driving lymphomagenesis as well as activating immune responses against B-cell neoplasms. They are used as single agents and in combination with chemotherapy and radiation in the treatment of B-cell neoplasms. Obinutuzumab is an antibody with altered glycosylation that enhances its ability to activate killer cells; it is also directed against CD20 and is of value in chronic lymphocytic leukemia.

Unintended side effects of any antibody include infusion-related hypersensitivity reactions, usually limited to the first infusion, which can be managed with glucocorticoid and/or antihistamine prophylaxis, and prolonged infusion strategies.

Anti-B-cell-directed antibodies can have the unintended effect of exacerbating immunosuppression with the emergence of increased opportunistic infections. Reactivation of latent infections may also occur; an assessment of a patient's hepatitis B and C status is conventionally done before treatment. Concomitant use of antivirals directed against hepatitis may be indicated. Patients with HIV and lymphoma need antivirals optimized to minimize interaction with anti-lymphoma treatments; consultation with infectious disease specialists is warranted. Anti-tumor cell antibodies also include approaches to activate complement and are exemplified by alemtuzumab directed against CD52; it is active in chronic lymphoid leukemia and T-cell malignancies. Tumor lysis syndrome prophylaxis may be warranted.

Epidermal growth factor receptor (EGFR)-directed antibodies (e.g., cetuximab and panitumumab) have activity in colorectal cancer refractory to chemotherapy, particularly when used to augment the activity of an additional chemotherapy program, and in the primary treatment of head and neck cancers treated with radiation therapy. Direct effects on the tumor may mediate an antiproliferative effect as well as stimulate the participation of host mechanisms involving immune cell or complement-mediated response to tumor cell–bound antibody. Anti-EGFR antibodies can cause an acneiform rash requiring topical antibiotic and glucocorticoid cream treatment; photosensitivity also occurs.

The HER2/neu receptor overexpressed on epithelial cancers, especially breast and certain gastrointestinal cancers, was initially targeted by trastuzumab, with activity in potentiating the action of chemotherapy in breast cancer as well as evidence of single-agent activity. Trastuzumab appears to interrupt intracellular signals derived from HER2/neu and to stimulate anti-tumor cell immune mechanisms. The anti-HER2 antibody pertuzumab, specifically targeting the domain of HER2/neu responsible for dimerization with other HER2 family members, is more specifically directed against HER2 signaling function and augments the action of trastuzumab. Both trastuzumab and pertuzumab can damage cardiac function, particularly in patients with prior exposure to anthracyclines, and left ventricular function should be checked pre-treatment and monitored during treatment.

The BiTe antibody blinatumomab was constructed to have an anti-CD19 antigen-combining site directed at a cancer cell as one valency with an anti-CD3 binding site as the other. This antibody can bring T cells (with their anti-CD3 activity) close to neoplastic B cells bearing the CD19 determinant. Blinatumomab is active in B-cell neoplasms such as acute lymphocytic leukemia. Unique toxicities include cytokine release syndrome (fever, hypotension, tachycardia) and neurologic deterioration manifest initially by deterioration in handwriting accuracy, which can proceed to more florid cortical dysfunction, suggesting a need for dose pausing and/or glucocorticoid use.

STROMA-DIRECTED ANTIBODIES (FIG. 73-4) The anti-vascular endothelial growth factor (VEGF) antibody bevacizumab shows some evidence of value in renal cancers, where activation of VEGF signaling occurs as part of disabled hypoxia-induced signaling in the tumor cells. When combined with chemotherapeutic agents, it may increase responses in colorectal and nonsquamous lung cancers. The mechanism for this effect may relate to improved delivery and tumor uptake of the active chemotherapeutic agent, owing to decreased tumor interstitial pressure. VEGF was originally isolated as a "tumor permeability factor" causing leakiness of tumor blood vessels. When used in gliomas, it may, by decreasing vascular permeability, allow replacement of steroids to decrease intracranial pressure. Bevacizumab is directed against VEGF, which is normally a secreted product and not attached to tumor cells. Bevacizumab has a number of side effects including hypertension, thrombosis, proteinuria, hemorrhage, and gastrointestinal perforations with or without prior surgeries; these adverse events also occur with small-molecule drugs modulating VEGFR function.

IMMUNOREGULATORY ANTIBODIES (FIG. 73-4) Purely immunoregulatory antibodies stimulate immune responses to mediate tumor-directed cytotoxicity. An understanding of the tumor-host interface has revealed that cytotoxic tumor-directed T cells are frequently inhibited by ligands upregulated in the tumor cells. The programmed death ligand 1 (PD-L1; also known as B7-homolog 1) was initially recognized as inducing T cell death through a receptor present on T cells, termed the programmed death (PD) receptor, which physiologically regulates the intensity of the immune response to any antigen. The PD family of ligands and receptors also regulates macrophage function, present in tumor stroma. These actions raised the hypothesis that antibodies directed against the PD signaling axis (both anti-PD-L1 and anti-PD) might be useful in cancer treatment by allowing reactivation of the immune response against tumors.

Ipilimumab, an antibody directed against the anti-CTLA4 (cytotoxic T lymphocyte antigen 4), which is expressed on T cells (not tumor cells), responds to signals from antigen-presenting cells (Fig. 73-4) and also downregulates the intensity of the T-cell proliferative response to antigens derived from tumor cells. Indeed, manipulation of the CTLA4 axis was the first demonstration that purely immunoregulatory antibody strategies directed at T-cell physiology could be safe and effective in the treatment of cancer. Ipilimumab, alone or in combination with PD-1-directed antibodies, is approved for treatment of metastatic melanoma and lung cancers.

Nivolumab, directed against the PD-1 receptor, or atezolizumab (anti-PD-L1) are exemplary of anti-PD-1 directed immunoregulatory antibodies, with clinical benefits in many cancers (**Table 73-4**). Pembrolizumab is approved for first-line treatment of metastatic non-small-cell lung cancer tumors that express the PD-L1 ligand. This development was a milestone in cancer therapeutics, replacing chemotherapy in this patient subset.

Importantly, the clinical observation that tumors most amenable to treatment with immunoregulatory antibodies were in sites (lung, skin, genitourinary) exposed to environmental carcinogens or occurred in patients with known mutations in DNA repair pathways stimulated specific research as to whether the "mutational burden" of tumors could predict value from anti-PD strategies. Results to date confirm this hypothesis and led to the first regulatory approvals for immunomodulating antibodies in a "tissue agnostic" fashion. Specifically, detection of deficiencies in a tumor DNA mismatch repair system or with evidence of increased tumor mutation burden is a specific indication for use of certain immunoregulatory agents, irrespective of the disease site of origin. The increased efficacy in the setting of higher tumor mutational burden is thought to be due to the presence of more proteins in the tumor structurally altered by mutation that can be recognized as foreign by the immune system.

Prominent autoimmune hepatic, endocrine, cutaneous, neurologic, and gastrointestinal adverse events can occur with the use of ipilimumab as well as the PD-1-directed antibodies. Emergency use of glucocorticoids may be required to attenuate severe toxicities. Although theoretically such glucocorticoid use can attenuate the antitumor effect, response rates do not appear to be compromised by their use to abrogate serious organ toxicity attributable to use of immunomodulatory antibodies. Importantly for the general internist, immunologic toxicities can occur late after exposure to the modulators of PD and CTLA4 action, even while the patient may have sustained control of tumor growth.

Nontargeted Immunomodulators (Fig. 73-4) Bacille Calmette-Guérin, a killed mycobacterial product, invokes a useful immune response when instilled locally into the bladder in the setting of preinvasive bladder cancers. The "imids" thalidomide, lenalidomide, and pomalidomide alter cytokine elaboration in the tumor microenvironment and have antiangiogenic actions. They are a cornerstone in the management of multiple myeloma. Thromboses (warranting consideration of prophylactic anticoagulation), gastrointestinal and neuropathic adverse events, and prominent teratogenicity can occur as a consequence of their use.

Cytokines Only interferon α (IFN-α) and interleukin 2 (IL-2) are in routine clinical use. IFN is not curative for any tumor but can induce partial responses in follicular lymphoma, hairy cell leukemia, chronic myeloid leukemia, melanoma, and Kaposi's sarcoma. It produces fever, fatigue, a flulike syndrome, malaise, myelosuppression, and depression and can induce clinically significant autoimmune disease.

IL-2 exerts its antitumor effects indirectly through augmentation of immune function. Its biologic activity is to promote the growth and activity of T cells and natural killer (NK) cells. High doses of IL-2 can produce tumor regression in certain patients with metastatic melanoma and renal cell cancer. About 2–5% of patients may experience complete remissions that are durable. Patients may require blood pressure support and intensive care to manage the toxicity. However, once

TABLE 73-4 Clinical Impact of Host T Lymphocyte–Modified Cells[a] or Host T Lymphocyte–Directed Immunoregulatory Antibodies[c]

A. Advanced Cancers with Positive Effect (at least 25% of treated patients have stable disease or progression-free survival of ≥27 weeks or better) or Frequent or Unexpected Prolonged Responders (efficacy may be limited to CD expression–dependent or PD-1 ligand–expressing subtypes)
Acute lymphoid leukemia[b]
Adrenocortical carcinoma[c]
Breast cancer, hormone receptor negative, HER2 negative (with chemotherapy)[c]
Colorectal cancer (microsatellite instability-high [MSI-H] or mismatch repair deficient, following treatment with fluoropyrimidine, oxaliplatin, and irinotecan)[c]
Cervix, squamous carcinoma[c]
Cutaneous, squamous carcinoma[c]
Diffuse large B-cell non-Hodgkin's lymphoma, not otherwise specified[a]
Diffuse large B-cell non-Hodgkin's lymphoma, primary mediastinal subtype[b]
Endometrial carcinoma (with lenvatinib, if microsatellite instability-stable [MSI-S] or mismatch repair wild-type)[c]
Esophageal squamous carcinoma
Gastric/gastroesophageal adenocarcinoma[c]
Head and neck squamous carcinoma[c]
Hepatocellular cancer (after sorafenib)[c]
Hodgkin's disease[c]
Mantle cell lymphoma[a]
Melanoma[c]
Merkel cell carcinoma[c]
MSI-H or mismatch repair–deficient solid tumors without satisfactory alternative[c]
Mycosis fungoides[c]
Multiple myeloma[a]
Non-small-cell lung carcinoma[c]
Paraganglioma/pheochromocytoma[c]
Renal cell carcinoma[c]
Small-cell lung carcinoma[c]
Solid tumors with high tumor mutational burden (TMB) (≥10 mutations/megabase) that have progressed following prior therapy without satisfactory alternative treatment[c]
Thyroid carcinoma[c]
Urothelial carcinoma[c] (including bladder, ureter)
B. Advanced Cancers with Insufficient Data to Support Host T Lymphocyte or Immunoregulatory Antibodies
Acute myeloid leukemia
Anus, squamous carcinoma
Breast cancer, hormone receptor positive
Breast cancer, hormone receptor negative, HER2 positive
Biliary tract cancers (if MSI-S or mismatch repair wild-type)
Chronic lymphocytic leukemia
Chronic myeloid leukemia
Gastrointestinal neuroendocrine/islet cell carcinoma
Glioma, all grades including glioblastoma
Germ cell neoplasms
Ovarian cancer
Osteogenic sarcoma
Pancreas adenocarcinoma
Pediatric tumors (Wilms', rhabdomyosarcoma, Ewing's, neuroblastoma, osteosarcoma)
Prostate adenocarcinoma
Salivary gland carcinoma
Soft tissue sarcoma
T-cell non-Hodgkin's lymphoma (except mycosis fungoides)
Vulva, squamous carcinoma

[a]Chimeric antigen receptor (CAR)-modified autologous T cells in relapsed or refractory cases. [b]Both CAR-modified autologous T cells or an immunoregulatory antibody. [c]T-cell directed immunoregulatory antibody strategies including anti-PD1 and/or anti-PD-L1 antibodies; or BiTe antibodies against a particular tumor cell antigen.

the agent is stopped, most of the toxicities reverse completely within 3–6 days.

T Cell–Mediated Therapies The strongest evidence that the immune system can exert clinically meaningful antitumor effects comes from allogeneic bone marrow transplantation. Adoptively transferred T cells from the donor expand in the tumor-bearing host, recognize the tumor as being foreign, and can mediate impressive antitumor effects (graft-versus-tumor effects). Three types of currently used cancer treatments take advantage of the ability of T cells to kill tumor cells.

1. *Transfer of allogeneic T cells.* This occurs in three major settings: in allogeneic bone marrow transplantation; as purified lymphocyte transfusions following bone marrow recovery after allogeneic bone marrow transplantation; and as pure lymphocyte transfusions following immunosuppressive (nonmyeloablative) therapy (also called reduced-intensity or minitransplants). In each of these settings, the effector cells are donor T cells that recognize the tumor as being foreign, probably through minor histocompatibility differences. The main risk of such therapy is the development of graft-versus-host disease because of the minimal difference between the cancer and the normal host cells. This approach has been highly effective in certain hematologic cancers refractory to chemotherapeutic strategies.
2. *Transfer of autologous T cells.* In this approach, the patient's own T cells are removed from the tumor-bearing host, manipulated in several ways in vitro, and given back to the patient. Tumor antigen–specific T cells can be developed after retroviral transduction of the desired T-cell antigen receptor and expanded to large numbers over many weeks ex vivo before administration. These chimeric antigen receptor (CAR) T cells (Fig. 73-4) have evidence of sustained value in patients with refractory hematopoietic neoplasms such as diffuse large B-cell lymphoma and mantle cell lymphoma. Prominent adverse effects include cytokine release (fever, tachycardia, hypotension) and neurologic manifestations. Clinical investigations are seeking to develop solid-tumor antigen-directed CAR strategies, as well as to utilize different immune cell populations such as NK cells to deliver the antigen receptor construct in ways that may allow "off-the-shelf" products not requiring manipulation and purification of patients' autologous cells.

   A second autologous T-cell strategy uses activation of the patient's T cells to polyclonal stimulators such as anti-CD3 and anti-CD28 after a short period ex vivo and then amplification in the host after transfer by stimulation with IL-2. Short periods removed from the patient permit the cells to overcome the tumor-induced T-cell defects, and such cells traffic and home to sites of disease better than cells that have been in culture for many weeks.
3. *Tumor vaccines aimed at boosting T-cell immunity.* Two types of vaccine approaches are currently approved. Purified autologous antigen-presenting cells can be pulsed with tumor, its membranes, or particular tumor antigens and delivered as a vaccine. Vaccine adjuvants such as granulocyte-macrophage colony-stimulating factor (GM-CSF) may be co-administered. One such vaccine, sipuleucel-T (Fig. 73-4), is approved for use in patients with hormone-independent prostate cancer. In this approach, the patient undergoes leukapheresis, wherein mononuclear cells (that include antigen-presenting cells) are removed from the patient's blood. The cells are pulsed in a laboratory with an antigenic fusion protein comprising a protein frequently expressed by prostate cancer cells, prostate acid phosphatase, fused to GM-CSF, and matured to increase their capacity to present the antigen to immune effector cells. The cells are then returned to the patient in a well-tolerated treatment. Although no objective tumor response was documented in clinical trials, median survival was increased by about 4 months.

   Another important vaccine strategy is directed at infectious agents whose action ultimately is tied to the development of human cancer. Hepatitis B vaccine in an epidemiologic sense prevents hepatocellular carcinoma, and a tetravalent human papillomavirus vaccine prevents infection by virus types currently accounting for 70% of cervical cancer. Unfortunately, these vaccines are ineffective at treating patients who have developed a virus-induced cancer.

Oncolytic Viruses (Fig. 73-4) Laboratory studies in animals have utilized viruses to destroy tumors because tumor cells lack endogenous host mechanisms, e.g., IFN elaboration or recognition strategies of viral nucleic acids, that limit virus spread. Viral infection of tumors also can stimulate a prominent host response to viral and tumor cell antigens, leading to immune effects against local tumor cells. Talimogene laherparepvec is a clinically approved attenuated herpes virus that acts to stimulate immune responses when instilled locally into melanoma deposits. Systemic effects are minimal in this application. This general strategy is being considered particularly in tumors not amenable to useful effects of currently approved immunoregulatory antibodies or in conjunction with immunoregulatory antibodies.

CANCER CYTOTOXIC THERAPY

Table 73-5 lists commonly used cytotoxic cancer chemotherapy agents and pertinent clinical aspects of their use, with particular reference to adverse effects that might be encountered by the generalist in the care of patients. The drugs were initially discovered through screening of chemicals and natural product extracts to define evidence of antitumor activity in animals or were designed with knowledge of biochemical pathways affecting nucleic acid synthesis. They may be usefully grouped into two general categories: those affecting DNA and those affecting microtubules.

As illustrated in Fig. 73-3, disruption of DNA or microtubule integrity is a major trigger of cellular apoptosis pathways. An additional factor in drug effect stems from recent observations that tumor cells have increased tolerance of specific types of DNA damage owing to defects in DNA repair pathways. This state is thought to facilitate the survival of the neoplastic clone as it experiences DNA mutations during the course of carcinogenesis. DNA-directed cytotoxic agents can interact with certain DNA repair mutations in a "synthetic lethal" fashion: the DNA repair mutation enhances lethality of the chemotherapy agent. Examples of a potential "synthetic lethal effect" will be pointed out in relation to clinical applications below.

DNA-Interactive Agents DNA replication occurs during the synthesis or S-phase of the cell cycle, with chromosome segregation of the replicated DNA in the M, or mitosis, phase. The G_1 and G_2 "gap phases" precede S and M, respectively. Chemotherapeutic agents have been divided into "phase-nonspecific" agents, which can act in any phase of the cell cycle, and "phase-specific" agents, which require the cell to be at a particular cell cycle phase to cause greatest effect.

Alkylating agents (Table 73-5) as a class are cell cycle phase–nonspecific agents. They break down, either spontaneously or after normal organ or tumor cell metabolism, to reactive intermediates that covalently modify bases in DNA. This leads to cross-linkage of DNA strands or the appearance of breaks in DNA as a result of repair efforts. Damaged DNA cannot complete normal cell division; in addition, it activates apoptosis. Alkylating agents share similar toxicities: myelosuppression, alopecia, gonadal dysfunction, mucositis, and pulmonary fibrosis. They also share the capacity to cause "second" neoplasms, particularly leukemia, years after use, particularly when used in low doses for protracted periods.

Cyclophosphamide is inactive unless metabolized by the liver to 4-hydroxy-cyclophosphamide, which decomposes into an alkylating species, as well as to chloroacetaldehyde and acrolein. The latter causes chemical cystitis; therefore, excellent hydration must be maintained while using cyclophosphamide. If severe, the cystitis may be attenuated or prevented altogether (if expected from the dose of cyclophosphamide to be used) by mesna (2-*m*ercaptoethane*s*ulfo*na*te). Liver disease impairs cyclophosphamide activation. Sporadic interstitial pneumonitis leading to pulmonary fibrosis can accompany the use of cyclophosphamide, and high doses used in conditioning regimens for bone marrow transplant can cause cardiac dysfunction. Ifosfamide is a cyclophosphamide analogue also activated in the liver, but more slowly, and it requires co-administration of mesna to prevent bladder injury. CNS effects, including somnolence, confusion, and psychosis, can follow ifosfamide use; the incidence appears related to low body surface area or decreased creatinine clearance.

Several alkylating agents are less commonly used. Bendamustine has activity in chronic lymphocytic leukemia and certain lymphomas. Busulfan can cause profound myelosuppression, alopecia, and pulmonary toxicity but is relatively "lymphocyte sparing." It is used in transplant preparation regimens. Melphalan shows variable oral bioavailability and undergoes extensive binding to albumin and α_1-acidic glycoprotein. Mucositis appears more prominently; however, it has prominent activity in multiple myeloma.

Nitrosoureas break down to carbamylating species that not only cause a distinct pattern of DNA base pair–directed reactivity but also can covalently modify proteins. They share the feature of causing relatively delayed bone marrow toxicity, which can be cumulative and long-lasting. Procarbazine is metabolized in the liver and possibly in tumor cells to yield a variety of free radical and alkylating species. In addition to myelosuppression, it causes hypnotic and other CNS effects, including vivid nightmares. It can cause a disulfiram-like syndrome on ingestion of ethanol. Dacarbazine (DTIC) is activated in the liver to yield the highly reactive methyl diazonium cation. It causes only modest myelosuppression 21–25 days after a dose but causes prominent nausea on day 1. Temozolomide is structurally related to dacarbazine but is activated by nonenzymatic hydrolysis in tumors and is bioavailable orally. Brain tumors with alkylguanine alkyl transferase deficiency are selectively susceptible to temozolomide, which alkylates the O^6 position of guanine.

Cisplatin was discovered fortuitously by observing that bacteria present in electrolysis solutions with platinum electrodes could not divide. Only the *cis* diamine configuration is active as an antitumor agent. In tumor cells, a chloride is lost from each position. The resulting positively charged species is an efficient DNA interactor, forming Pt-based cross-links. Cisplatin is administered with abundant hydration, including forced diuresis with mannitol to prevent kidney damage; even with the use of hydration, gradual decrease in kidney function is common, along with noteworthy anemia. Hypomagnesemia frequently attends cisplatin use and can lead to hypocalcemia and tetany. Other common toxicities include neurotoxocity with stocking-and-glove sensorimotor neuropathy. Hearing loss occurs in 50% of patients treated with conventional doses. Cisplatin is intensely emetogenic, requiring prophylactic antiemetics. Myelosuppression is less evident than with other alkylating agents. Chronic vascular toxicity (Raynaud's phenomenon, coronary artery disease) is a more unusual toxicity. Carboplatin displays less nephro-, oto-, and neurotoxicity. However, myelosuppression is more frequent, and because the drug is exclusively cleared through the kidney, adjustment of dose for creatinine clearance must be accomplished through use of various dosing nomograms. Oxaliplatin is a platinum analogue with noteworthy activity in colon cancers refractory to other treatments. It is prominently neurotoxic.

Trabectedin binds to DNA through the "DNA minor groove" with covalent interaction with the N2 position of certain guanines. Uniquely among the DNA interactors, this can lead to the disruption of the selective FUS-CHOP transcription factor action, important in the pathogenesis of certain liposarcomas. Transient altered liver function can occur, as well as cytopenias. Lurbinectedin is an analogue of trabectedin and also alters RNA polymerase function after binding to the minor groove of DNA, but has a distinct pharmacologic profile.

Antitumor Antibiotics and Topoisomerase Poisons Antitumor antibiotics are substances produced by bacteria that provide a chemical defense against hostile microorganisms. They bind to DNA directly and can frequently undergo electron transfer reactions to generate free radicals in close proximity to DNA, leading to DNA damage in the form of single-strand breaks or cross-links. Topoisomerase poisons include natural products or semisynthetic derivatives that modify enzymes that allow DNA to unwind during replication or transcription. These include topoisomerase I, which creates single-strand breaks that then rejoin following the passage of the other DNA strand through the break. Topoisomerase II creates double-strand breaks through which another segment of DNA duplex passes before rejoining. Owing to the role of topoisomerase I in the replication fork, topoisomerase I poisons cause lethality if the topoisomerase I–induced lesions occur in S-phase.

TABLE 73-5 Cytotoxic Chemotherapy Agents[a]

DRUG	TOXICITY	INTERACTIONS, ISSUES
Direct DNA-Interacting Agents[a]		
Alkylator		
Bendamustine	Contraindicated with prior sensitivity to polyethylene glycol 400, propylene glycol, or monothioglycerol; cytopenias, infections, cutaneous eruptions, hepatotoxicity	Monitor for tumor lysis syndrome, extravasation, anaphylaxis, and infusion reactions
Carboplatin	Marrow: platelets > WBCs; nausea, renal (high dose)	Reduce dose according to CrCl: to AUC of 5–7 mg/mL per min [AUC = dose/(CrCl + 25)]
Carmustine (BCNU)	Myeloid (delayed nadir), GI, liver (high dose), renal	Pulmonary toxicity especially after >1400 mg/m^2 cumulative dose; can be delayed in appearance
Cisplatin	Nausea, neuropathy, auditory, marrow: platelets > WBCs; renal, $\downarrow Mg^{2+}$, $\downarrow Ca^{2+}$	Maintain high urine flow; osmotic diuresis, monitor intake/output, K^+, Mg^{2+}; emetogenic—prophylaxis needed; full dose if CrCl >60 mL/min and tolerate fluid push
Chlorambucil	Common alkylator[b]	
Cyclophosphamide	Marrow (relative platelet sparing), cystitis, common alkylator[b], flulike symptoms, cardiac (high dose)	Liver metabolism required to activate to phosphoramide mustard + acrolein; mesna protects against "high-dose" bladder damage
Dacarbazine (DTIC)	Myelosuppressive, cystitis, neurologic, metabolic acidosis	Metabolic activation
Ifosfamide	Marrow, bladder, CNS	Analog of cyclophosphamide, must use concomitant mesna
Lomustine (CCNU)	Marrow (delayed nadir)	
Lurbinectedin	Marrow, hepatotoxicity, nausea, vomiting	CYP3A4
Melphalan	Marrow (delayed nadir), GI (high dose)	Decreased renal function delays clearance
Oxaliplatin	Nausea, anemia	Acute reversible neurotoxicity; chronic sensory neurotoxicity cumulative with dose; reversible laryngopharyngeal spasm
Procarbazine	Marrow, nausea, neurologic, common alkylator[b]	Liver and tissue metabolism required, disulfiram-like effect with alcohol, acts as MAOI. HBP after tyrosinase-rich foods
Temozolomide	Nausea, vomiting, headache, fatigue, constipation	Myelosuppression
Trabectedin	Neutropenia, risk of fever; thrombocytopenia; rhabdomyolysis, reversible hepatic toxicity but dose reduce with liver impairment	Unusual capillary leak risk; CYP3A4
Antitumor Antibiotics and Topoisomerase Poisons		
Bleomycin	Pulmonary, skin, Raynaud's, hypersensitivity	Monitor DLCO during treatment (inactivate by bleomycin hydrolase; decreased in lung/skin); O_2 enhances pulmonary toxicity; cisplatin-induced decrease in CrCl may increase skin/lung toxicity; reduce dose if CrCl <60 mL/min
Dactinomycin	Marrow, nausea, mucositis, vesicant, alopecia	Radiation recall
Doxorubicin and daunorubicin	Marrow, mucositis, alopecia, cardiac acute/chronic, vesicant	Heparin aggregate; coadministration increases clearance; acetaminophen, BCNU increase liver toxicity; radiation recall; dose reduce with increased bilirubin
Epirubicin	Marrow, mucositis, alopecia, cardiac acute/chronic, vesicant	Dose reduce with increased bilirubin, decreased CrCl
Etoposide (VP16-213)	Marrow (WBCs > platelet), alopecia, hypotension, hypersensitivity with rapid IV, nausea, mucositis	Hepatic metabolism and renal excretion (30%); reduce doses with liver and kidney failure; accentuate antimetabolite action
Idarubicin	Marrow, mucositis, alopecia, cardiac acute/chronic, vesicant	Dose reduce with increased bilirubin, decreased CrCl
Irinotecan	Diarrhea: "early onset" with cramping, flushing, vomiting; "late onset" after several doses; marrow, alopecia, nausea, vomiting, pulmonary	Prodrug requires enzymatic clearance to active drug SN-38; early diarrhea due to acetylcholine release, can counter with atropine; late diarrhea, use loperamide 4 mg with first stool then 2 mg q2h until 12 h without stool up to 16 mg/24 h
Mitoxantrone	Marrow, cardiac (less than doxorubicin), vesicant; blue urine, nails, and sclerae	Interacts with heparin; less alopecia, nausea than doxorubicin; radiation recall; less alopecia, nausea than doxorubicin
Topotecan	Marrow, mucositis, nausea, alopecia	Reduce dose with renal failure; rare interstitial pneumonitis
Indirectly DNA-Interacting Agents		
Antimetabolites		
Asparaginase	Decrease protein synthesis; indirect inhibition of DNA synthesis by decreased histone synthesis; clotting factors; glucose; albumin hypersensitivity; CNS; pancreatitis; hepatic	Blocks methotrexate action
Capecitabine	Diarrhea, hand-foot syndrome	Prodrug of 5-fluorouracil due to intratumoral metabolism
2-Chlorodeoxadenosine	Marrow, renal, fever	Notable use in hairy cell leukemia
Cytosine arabinoside	Marrow, mucositis, neurologic (high dose), conjunctivitis (high dose; use steroid eyedrops until 72 h after last dose), noncardiogenic pulmonary edema	Metabolized in tissues by deamination but renal excretion prominent at doses >500 mg; therefore, dose reduce in "high-dose" regimens in patients with decreased CrCl
Fludarabine phosphate	Marrow, neurologic, lung	Dose reduction with renal failure; metabolized to F-ara, converted to F-ara ATP in cells by deoxycytidine kinase
5-Fluorouracil	Marrow, mucositis, neurologic, skin changes	Toxicity enhanced by leucovorin by increasing "ternary complex" with thymidylate synthase; dihydropyrimidine dehydrogenase deficiency increases toxicity; metabolism in tissue
Gemcitabine	Marrow, nausea, hepatic, fever/"flu syndrome"	Rare pulmonary/capillary leak syndrome; rare hemolytic-uremic syndrome; rare posterior reversible encephalopathy syndrome; radiosensitization

(Continued)

TABLE 73-5 Cytotoxic Chemotherapy Agents[a] (Continued)

DRUG	TOXICITY	INTERACTIONS, ISSUES
Hydroxyurea	Marrow, nausea, mucositis, skin, rare renal, liver, lung, CNS	Decrease dose with renal failure; augments antimetabolite effect
6-Mercaptopurine (6-MP)	Marrow, liver, nausea	Variable bioavailability, metabolized by xanthine oxidase, decrease dose with allopurinol; increased toxicity with thiopurine methyltransferase deficiency
Methotrexate	Marrow, liver, lung, renal tubular, mucositis	Toxicity lessened by "rescue" with leucovorin; excreted in urine; decrease dose in renal failure; NSAIDs increase renal toxicity
Pemetrexed	Anemia; neutropenia	Supplement folate/B_{12} Caution in renal failure
Pralatrexate	Thrombocytopenia, myelosuppression, mucositis	Active in peripheral T-cell lymphoma
6-Thioguanine	Marrow, liver, nausea	Variable bioavailability; increased toxicity with thiopurine methyltransferase deficiency
Trifluridine/tipiracil	Marrow, mucositis, nausea, vomiting, unusual hand/foot syndrome.	Trifluridine directly inhibits thymidylate synthase and is incorporated into DNA; tipiracil inhibits thymidine phosphorylase, which degrades trifluridine
Antimitotic Agents		
Docetaxel	Hypersensitivity to vehicle; fluid retention syndrome; marrow; dermatologic; peripheral neuropathy; nausea infrequent; some stomatitis	Premedicate with steroids, H_1 and H_2 blockers; may require lengthened infusions to avoid hypersensitivity
Eribulin	Marrow; peripheral neuropathy; QT prolongation	Dose modify in liver and kidney impairment
Ixabepilone	Myelosuppression, neuropathy, hypersensitivity to infusion	Premedicate with steroids, H_1 and H_2 blockers; may require lengthened infusions to avoid hypersensitivity; dose modification for liver impairment; CYP3A4
Nab-paclitaxel (protein bound)	Neuropathy, anemia, marrow	Dose adjust with liver dysfunction; caution with inhibitors or inducers of either CYP2C8 or CYP3A4
Paclitaxel	Hypersensitivity to vehicle; marrow; alopecia, mucositis, peripheral neuropathy, CV conduction, infrequent nausea	Premedicate with steroids, H_1 and H_2 blockers; hepatic clearance with dose reduction with increased bilirubin; caution with inhibitors or inducers of either CYP2C8 or CYP3A4
Vinblastine	Vesicant; marrow; peripheral neuropathy (less common but similar spectrum to other vincas); hypertension, Raynaud's, ileus/constipation (use prophylactic stool softeners)	Hepatic clearance; dose reduction for bilirubin >1.5 mg/dL
Vincristine	Vesicant, marrow (less than vinblastine), neurologic, GI; ileus/constipation (use prophylactic stool softeners); SIADH; rare CV	Hepatic clearance; dose reduction for bilirubin >1.5 mg/dL
Vinorelbine	Vesicant, marrow, allergic bronchospasm (immediate), dyspnea/cough (subacute), neuropathic (less prominent but similar spectrum to other vincas)	Hepatic clearance; dose reduction for bilirubin >1.5 mg/dL

[a]All agents in this category should be regarded as potentially fetotoxic, and use during pregnancy is either contraindicated or undertaken with clear understanding of risk of fetal harm; likewise not recommended for use during lactation. [b]Common alkylator: alopecia, pulmonary, infertility, plus teratogenesis.

Abbreviations: ATP, adenosine triphosphate; AUC, area under the curve; CNS, central nervous system; CrCl, creatinine clearance; CV, cardiovascular; GI, gastrointestinal; CYP3A4, avoid concomitant strong CYP3A inhibitors and avoid concomitant strong CYP3A inducers; DLCO, diffusing capacity of carbon monoxide; F-ara, fludarabine; HBP, high blood pressure; MAOI, monoamine oxidase inhibitor; NSAID, nonsteroidal anti-inflammatory drug; SIADH, syndrome of inappropriate antidiuretic hormone secretion; WBC, white blood cells.

Doxorubicin intercalates into DNA, thereby altering DNA structure, replication, and topoisomerase II function. It can also undergo reduction of its quinone ring system, with reoxidation to form reactive oxygen radicals. It causes predictable myelosuppression, alopecia, nausea, and mucositis. In addition, it causes acute cardiotoxicity in the form of atrial and ventricular dysrhythmias, but these are rarely of clinical significance. In contrast, cumulative doses >550 mg/m^2 are associated with a 10% incidence of chronic cardiomyopathy. The incidence of cardiomyopathy appears to be related to peak serum concentration, with low-dose, frequent treatment or continuous infusions better tolerated than intermittent higher-dose exposures. Cardiotoxicity has been related to iron-catalyzed oxidation and reduction of doxorubicin in the heart. Dexrazoxane is an intracellular chelating agent that can act as a cardio-protectant. Doxorubicin's cardiotoxicity is increased when given together with trastuzumab, the anti-HER2/neu antibody. Radiation recall or interaction with concomitantly administered radiation to cause local site complications is frequent. The drug is a powerful vesicant, with necrosis of tissue apparent 4–7 days after an extravasation; therefore, it should be administered into a rapidly flowing intravenous line. Dexrazoxane also can mitigate doxorubicin extravasation. Doxorubicin is metabolized by the liver, so doses must be reduced by 50–75% in the presence of liver dysfunction. Daunorubicin is closely related to doxorubicin and is preferable to doxorubicin owing to less mucositis and colonic damage with frequent high doses used in the curative treatment of leukemia. Idarubicin is also used in leukemia treatment and may have somewhat less cardiotoxicity. Encapsulation of daunorubicin into a liposomal formulation has attenuated cardiac toxicity with antitumor activity in Kaposi's sarcoma, other sarcomas, multiple myeloma, and ovarian cancer.

Mitoxantrone is a synthetic topoisomerase II–directed agent with a mechanism similar to the anthracyclines, with less but not absent cardiotoxicity, comparing the ratio of cardiotoxic to effective doses; it is still associated with a 10% incidence of cardiotoxicity at cumulative doses of >150 mg/m^2. Etoposide binds directly to topoisomerase II and DNA in a reversible ternary complex. It stabilizes the covalent intermediate in the enzyme's action where the enzyme is covalently linked to DNA. Prominent clinical effects include myelosuppression, nausea, and transient hypotension related to the speed of administration of the agent. Etoposide is a mild vesicant but is relatively free from other large-organ toxicities.

Camptothecins target topoisomerase I. Topotecan is a camptothecin derivative approved for use in gynecologic tumors and small-cell lung cancer. Toxicity is limited to myelosuppression and mucositis. Irinotecan is a camptothecin with evidence of activity in colon carcinoma. Irinotecan is a prodrug, metabolized in the liver to SN-38, its active metabolite. Levels of SN-38 are particularly high in the setting of Gilbert's disease, characterized by defective uridine diphosphate glucuronosyl transferase (UGT) 1A1 and indirect hyperbilirubinemia, a condition that affects about 10% of the white population in the United States. In addition, irinotecan's myelosuppression is clearly influenced by the patient's genotype for UGT1As. Irinotecan causes a delayed (48–72 h) secretory diarrhea related to the toxicity of SN-38. The diarrhea can be treated effectively with loperamide or octreotide; immediate diarrhea when it occurs is responsive to atropine.

Fam-trastuzumab deruxtecan and sacituzumab govitecan are antibody-drug conjugates (Fig. 73-4) that allow specific targeting of camptothecin and SN-38, respectively, to HER2-positive and triple-negative breast cancers, respectively. Adverse events are driven by off-target effects of the chemotherapy agent and include cytopenia, nausea, vomiting, and, in the case of fam-trastuzumab deruxtecan, severe interstitial pneumonitis.

Bleomycin forms complexes with Fe^{2+} while also bound to DNA. It remains an important component of curative regimens for Hodgkin's disease and germ cell neoplasms. Oxidation of Fe^{2+} gives rise to superoxide and hydroxyl radicals, causing DNA damage. The drug causes little, if any, myelosuppression. Bleomycin is cleared rapidly, but augmented skin and pulmonary toxicity in the presence of renal failure necessitates dose reduction in renal failure. Bleomycin is not a vesicant and can be administered intravenously, intramuscularly, or subcutaneously. Common side effects include fever and chills, facial flush, and Raynaud's phenomenon. The most feared complication of bleomycin treatment is pulmonary fibrosis, which increases in incidence at >300 cumulative units administered and is minimally responsive to treatment (e.g., glucocorticoids). The earliest indicator of an adverse effect is usually a decline in the carbon monoxide diffusing capacity (DLCO) or coughing, although cessation of drug immediately upon documentation of a decrease in DLCO may not prevent further decline in pulmonary function. Bleomycin is inactivated by a bleomycin hydrolase, whose concentration is diminished in skin and lung. Because bleomycin-dependent electron transport is dependent on O_2, bleomycin toxicity may become apparent after exposure to transient very high fraction of inspired oxygen (FIO_2) even late after treatment. Thus, during surgical procedures, patients with prior exposure to bleomycin should be maintained on the lowest FIO_2 consistent with maintaining adequate tissue oxygenation.

Dactinomycin interacts directly with DNA to inhibit RNA transcription. It is important in the curative treatment of pediatric neoplasms, some of which also occur in young adults. Prominent myelosuppression, mucositis, alopecia, radiation recall, and nausea require management.

Calicheamicins are DNA-interacting antitumor antibiotics too toxic for clinical use but, when used as antibody-drug conjugates, can be useful in the treatment of CD33+ acute myeloid leukemia (gemtuzumab ozogamicin) and CD22+ acute lymphocytic leukemia (inotuzumab ozogamicin). Patients must be monitored for hypersensitivity reactions and for hepatotoxicity due to veno-occlusive disease of hepatic veins, resulting from release of the calicheamicin or metabolites in the liver.

Antimetabolites A broad definition of antimetabolites would include compounds that interfere with purine or pyrimidine synthesis. Some antimetabolites also cause DNA damage indirectly, through misincorporation into DNA. They tend to convey greatest toxicity to cells in S-phase, and the degree of toxicity increases with duration of exposure. Common toxic manifestations include stomatitis, diarrhea, and myelosuppression.

Methotrexate inhibits dihydrofolate reductase, which regenerates reduced folates from the oxidized folates produced when thymidine monophosphate is formed from deoxyuridine monophosphate. Without reduced folates, cells die a "thymine-less" death. *N*5-Tetrahydrofolate or *N*5-formyltetrahydrofolate (leucovorin) can bypass this block and rescue cells from methotrexate, which is retained in cells by polyglutamylation. Methotrexate is transported into cells by a membrane carrier, and high concentrations of drug can bypass this carrier and allow diffusion of drug directly into cells. These properties have suggested the design of "high-dose" methotrexate regimens with leucovorin rescue of normal marrow and mucosa as part of curative approaches to osteosarcoma in the adjuvant setting and hematopoietic neoplasms of children and adults. Methotrexate is cleared by the kidney via both glomerular filtration and tubular secretion, and toxicity is augmented by renal dysfunction and drugs such as salicylates, probenecid, and nonsteroidal anti-inflammatory agents that undergo tubular secretion. With normal renal function, 15 mg/m^2 leucovorin will rescue 10^{-8}–10^{-6} *M* methotrexate in 3–4 doses. However, with decreased creatinine clearance, doses of 50–100 mg/m^2 are continued until methotrexate levels are $<5 \times 10^{-8}$ *M*. In addition to bone marrow suppression and mucosal irritation, methotrexate can cause renal failure itself at high doses owing to crystallization in renal tubules; therefore, high-dose regimens require alkalinization of urine with increased flow by hydration. Methotrexate can be sequestered in third-space collections and diffuse back into the general circulation, causing prolonged myelosuppression. Less frequent adverse effects include reversible increases in transaminases and hypersensitivity-like pulmonary syndrome. Chronic low-dose methotrexate can cause hepatic fibrosis. When administered to the intrathecal space, methotrexate can cause chemical arachnoiditis and CNS dysfunction.

Pemetrexed is a folate-directed antimetabolite that inhibits the activity of several enzymes, including thymidylate synthetase (TS), dihydrofolate reductase, and glycinamide ribonucleotide formyltransferase. To avoid toxicity to normal tissues, pemetrexed is given with low-dose folate and vitamin B_{12} supplementation. Pemetrexed has notable activity against certain lung cancers and, in combination with cisplatin, also against mesotheliomas.

5-Fluorouracil (5-FU) represents an early example of "rational" drug design in that tumor cells incorporate radiolabeled uracil more efficiently into DNA than normal cells. 5-FU is metabolized in cells to 5′FdUMP, which inhibits TS. In addition, misincorporation can lead to single-strand breaks, and RNA can aberrantly incorporate FUMP. 5-FU is metabolized by dihydropyrimidine dehydrogenase, and deficiency of this enzyme can lead to excessive toxicity from 5-FU. Oral bioavailability varies unreliably, but prodrugs such as capecitabine have been developed that allow at least equivalent activity to parenteral 5-FU-based approaches. Intravenous administration of 5-FU leads to bone marrow suppression after short infusions but to stomatitis after prolonged infusions. Leucovorin augments the activity of 5-FU by promoting formation of the ternary covalent complex of 5-FU, the reduced folate, and TS. Less frequent toxicities include CNS dysfunction, with prominent cerebellar signs, and endothelial toxicity manifested by thrombosis, including pulmonary embolus and myocardial infarction. Trifluridine is a fluorinated pyrimidine that as the triphosphate is directly incorporated into DNA, evoking DNA damage, and as the monophosphate can inhibit TS. It is administered as a fixed-dose combination with tipiracil, an inhibitor of trifluridine degradation by thymidine phosphorylase.

Cytosine arabinoside (ara-C) is incorporated into DNA after formation of ara-CTP, resulting in S-phase–related toxicity. Continuous infusion schedules allow maximal efficiency, with uptake maximal at 5–7 μ*M*. Ara-C can be administered intrathecally. Adverse effects include nausea, diarrhea, stomatitis, chemical conjunctivitis, and cerebellar ataxia. Gemcitabine is a cytosine derivative that is similar to ara-C in that it is incorporated into DNA after anabolism to the triphosphate, rendering DNA susceptible to breakage and repair synthesis, which differs from that in ara-C in that gemcitabine-induced lesions are very inefficiently removed. In contrast to ara-C, gemcitabine appears to have useful activity in a variety of solid tumors, with limited nonmyelosuppressive toxicities.

6-Thioguanine and 6-mercaptopurine (6MP) are used in the treatment of acute lymphoid leukemia. Although administered orally, they display variable bioavailability. 6MP is metabolized by xanthine oxidase and therefore requires dose reduction when used with allopurinol. 6MP is also metabolized by thiopurine methyltransferase; genetic deficiency of thiopurine methyltransferase results in excessive toxicity.

Fludarabine phosphate is a prodrug of F-adenine arabinoside (F-ara-A), which in turn was designed to diminish the susceptibility of ara-A to adenosine deaminase. F-ara-A is incorporated into DNA and can cause delayed cytotoxicity even in cells with low growth fraction, including chronic lymphocytic leukemia and follicular B-cell lymphoma. CNS and peripheral nerve dysfunction and T-cell depletion leading to opportunistic infections can occur in addition to myelosuppression. 2-Chlorodeoxyadenosine is a similar compound with activity in hairy cell leukemia. Hydroxyurea inhibits ribonucleotide reductase, resulting in S-phase block. It is orally bioavailable and useful for the acute management of myeloproliferative states.

Asparaginase is a bacterial enzyme that causes breakdown of extracellular asparagine required for protein synthesis in certain leukemic cells. This effectively stops tumor cell DNA synthesis, as DNA synthesis requires concurrent protein synthesis. The outcome of asparaginase action is therefore very similar to the result of the small-molecule antimetabolites. Because asparaginase is a foreign protein, hypersensitivity reactions are common, as are effects on organs such as pancreas and liver that normally require continuing protein synthesis. This may result in decreased insulin secretion with hyperglycemia, with or without hyperamylasemia and clotting function abnormalities. Close monitoring of clotting functions should accompany use of asparaginase. Paradoxically, owing to depletion of rapidly turning over anticoagulant factors, thromboses particularly affecting the CNS may also be seen with asparaginase.

Mitotic Spindle Inhibitors Microtubules form the mitotic spindle, and in interphase cells, they are responsible for the cellular "scaffolding" along which various motile and secretory processes occur. Microtubules are composed of repeating heterodimers of α and β isoforms of the protein tubulin. Vincristine binds to the tubulin heterodimer with the result that microtubules are disaggregated. This results in the block of growing cells in M-phase, where a structurally disordered mitotic spindle apparatus is a powerful proapoptotic signal (Fig. 73-3). Vincristine is metabolized by the liver, and dose adjustment in the presence of hepatic dysfunction is required. It is a powerful vesicant, and infiltration can be treated by local heat and infiltration of hyaluronidase. At clinically used intravenous doses, neurotoxicity in the form of glove-and-stocking neuropathy is frequent. Acute neuropathic effects include jaw pain, paralytic ileus, urinary retention, and the syndrome of inappropriate antidiuretic hormone secretion. Myelosuppression is not seen at conventional doses. Vinblastine is similar to vincristine, except that it tends to be more myelotoxic, with more frequent thrombocytopenia and also mucositis and stomatitis. Vinorelbine is a vinca alkaloid that appears to have differences in resistance patterns in comparison to vincristine and vinblastine; it may be administered orally.

The taxanes include paclitaxel and docetaxel. These agents differ from the vinca alkaloids in that the taxanes stabilize microtubules against depolymerization. The "stabilized" microtubules function abnormally and are not able to undergo the normal dynamic changes of microtubule structure and function necessary for cell cycle completion. Taxanes are among the most broadly active antineoplastic agents for use in solid tumors, with evidence of activity in ovarian cancer, breast cancer, Kaposi's sarcoma, and lung tumors. They are administered intravenously, and their vehicles cause hypersensitivity reactions. Premedication with dexamethasone (8–16 mg orally or intravenously 12 and 6 h before treatment) and diphenhydramine (50 mg) and cimetidine (300 mg), both 30 min before treatment, decreases but does not eliminate the risk of hypersensitivity reactions to the paclitaxel vehicle. A protein-bound formulation of paclitaxel (called *nab-paclitaxel*) has at least equivalent antineoplastic activity and decreased risk of hypersensitivity reactions. Paclitaxel may also cause myelosuppression, neurotoxicity in the form of glove-and-stocking numbness, and paresthesia. Docetaxel causes comparable degrees of myelosuppression and neuropathy. Docetaxel uses a different vehicle that can cause fluid retention in addition to hypersensitivity reactions; dexamethasone premedication with or without antihistamines is also frequently used. Cabazitaxel is a taxane with somewhat better activity in prostate cancers than earlier generations of taxanes, perhaps due to superior delivery to sites of disease.

Epothilones represent a class of microtubule-stabilizing agents optimized for activity in taxane-resistant tumors. Ixabepilone has clear evidence of activity in breast cancers resistant to taxanes and anthracyclines such as doxorubicin. Side effects include myelosuppression and peripheral sensory neuropathy. Eribulin is a microtubule-directed agent with activity in patients who have had progression of disease on taxanes. It alters dynamics of microtubule remodeling in cells.

Ado-trastuzumab emtansine is an antibody conjugate of the HER2/neu-directed trastuzumab and a highly toxic microtubule targeted drug (emtansine), which by itself is too toxic for human use; the antibody-drug conjugate shows valuable activity in patients with breast cancer who have developed resistance to the "naked" antibody. Brentuximab vedotin is an anti-CD30 antibody drug conjugate with the distinct microtubule poison dolastatin with activity in neoplasms such as Hodgkin's lymphoma where the tumor cells frequently express CD30. Polatuzumab vedotin analogously targets CD79a in B-cell lymphomas. Enfortumab vedotin uses an antibody to NECTIN4 to target the vedotin "warhead" to urothelial neoplasms expressing that target. Belantamab mafodotin targets BCMA (B-cell maturation) expressed myeloma but using a distinct microtubule toxin, auristatin. Toxicity from these agents is driven by off-target effects of the microtubule agent and include myelosuppression and neuropathy, but belantamab mafodotin can cause ocular keratopathy, which requires monitoring.

CANCER MOLECULAR TARGETED THERAPY

Agents in this class share the characteristic that they are directed at specific cancer cell molecular targets important in the proliferation of tumors. While these agents can ultimately lead to tumor cell death, this occurs by altered regulation of a specific biochemical pathway affecting tumor cell susceptibility to apoptosis or growth arrest (Fig. 73-3).

Hormone Receptor–Directed Therapy Steroid hormone receptor–related molecules were arguably the first "molecular target" classes of anticancer drugs. When bound to their ligands, these receptors can alter gene transcription in hormone-responsive tissues. While in some cases, such as breast cancer, demonstration of the target hormone receptor is necessary for their use, in other cases such prostate cancer (androgen receptor) and lymphoid neoplasms (glucocorticoid receptor), the relevant receptor is always present in the tumor.

Glucocorticoids are generally given in "pulsed" high doses in leukemias and lymphomas, where they induce cell death in tumor cells. Cushing's syndrome and inadvertent adrenal suppression on withdrawal from high-dose glucocorticoids can be significant complications, along with infections common in immunosuppressed patients, in particular *Pneumocystis* pneumonia, which classically appears a few days after completing a course of high-dose glucocorticoids.

Tamoxifen is a partial estrogen receptor antagonist; it antagonizes in breast tumors, mirroring its effect on breast tissue, but owing to agonistic activities in vascular and uterine tissue, side effects include increased risk of thromboembolic phenomena and a small increased incidence of endometrial carcinoma, which appears after chronic use (usually >5 years). Progestational agents—including medroxyprogesterone acetate, androgens including fluoxymesterone (Halotestin), and, paradoxically, estrogens—have approximately the same degree of activity in primary hormonal treatment of breast cancers that have elevated expression of estrogen receptor protein. Estrogen itself is not used often due to prominent cardiovascular and uterotropic activity.

Aromatase refers to a family of enzymes that catalyze the formation of estrogen in various tissues, including ovary, peripheral adipose tissue, and some tumor cells. Aromatase inhibitors are of two types: irreversible steroid analogues such as exemestane and the reversible inhibitors such as anastrozole and letrozole. Anastrozole is superior to tamoxifen in the adjuvant treatment of breast cancer in postmenopausal patients with estrogen receptor–positive tumors. Letrozole treatment affords benefit following tamoxifen treatment. Adverse effects of aromatase inhibitors may include an increased risk of osteoporosis, fatigue, and altered serum lipids.

Metastatic prostate cancer is treated primarily by androgen deprivation. Orchiectomy causes responses in 80% of patients. If not accepted by the patient, testicular androgen suppression can also be induced by luteinizing hormone–releasing hormone (LHRH) agonists such as leuprolide and goserelin. These agents cause tonic stimulation of the LHRH receptor, with loss of normal pulsatile activation resulting in net decreased output of luteinizing hormone (LH) by the anterior pituitary. Therefore, as primary hormonal manipulation in prostate cancer, one can choose orchiectomy or an LHRH agonist, but not both. This pathway can also be blocked by relugolix, an oral gonadotropin-releasing hormone antagonist.

The addition of androgen receptor blockers, including flutamide or bicalutamide, is of uncertain additional benefit in extending overall response duration, although pretreatment with these agents before LHRH agonists is important to avoid a surge in testosterone after initial LH release. Enzalutamide also binds to the androgen receptor and antagonizes androgen action in a mechanistically distinct way. Somewhat analogous to inhibitors of aromatase, agents have been derived that inhibit testosterone and other androgen synthesis in the testis, adrenal gland, and prostate tissue. Abiraterone inhibits 17 α-hydroxylase/C17,20 lyase (CYP17A1) and has been shown to be active in prostate cancer patients experiencing progression despite androgen blockade.

Tumors that respond to a primary hormonal manipulation may frequently respond to second and third hormonal manipulations. Thus, breast tumors that had previously responded to tamoxifen have, on relapse, notable response rates to withdrawal of tamoxifen itself or to subsequent addition of an aromatase inhibitor or progestin. Likewise, initial treatment of prostate cancers with leuprolide plus flutamide may be followed after disease progression by response to withdrawal of flutamide. These responses may result from the removal of antagonists from mutant steroid hormone receptors that have come to depend on the presence of the antagonist as a growth-promoting influence.

Non-Receptor-Linked Tyrosine Kinase Antagonists Table 73-6 lists currently approved non–hormone receptor pathway-directed molecularly targeted chemotherapy agents, with features of their use of import to the generalist, particularly in recognizing potential drug-induced morbidities and interactions with other classes of drugs. The basis for discovery of drugs of this type was the prior knowledge of oncogene-directed pathways driving tumor growth (Fig. 73-3). In most cases, non-receptor tyrosine kinases ultimately activate signaling through the RAF/MEK/MAP kinase cascade, in common with the receptor-linked tyrosine kinases. Diagnostic demonstration of an active non-receptor tyrosine kinase may guide selection of an agent. A repeated preclinical and clinical observation in a variety of tumor types is that mutational activation of the tyrosine kinase target induces a state of "oncogene addiction" on the part of the tumor. This then is the basis for a "synthetic lethal" effect of the kinase inhibitor with respect to tumor viability.

In hematologic tumors, the prototypic agent of this type is imatinib, which targets the ATP binding site of the $p210^{bcr\text{-}abl}$ protein tyrosine kinase that is formed as the result of the chromosome 9;22 translocation producing the Philadelphia chromosome in chronic myeloid leukemia (CML). It has lesser activity in the blast phase of CML, where the cells may have acquired additional mutations in $p210^{bcr\text{-}abl}$ itself or other genetic lesions. Its side effects are relatively tolerable in most patients and include hepatic dysfunction, diarrhea, and fluid retention. Rarely, patients receiving imatinib have decreased cardiac function, which may persist after discontinuation of the drug. The quality of response to imatinib enters into the decision about when to refer patients with CML for consideration of stem cell transplant approaches. Nilotinib is a tyrosine protein kinase inhibitor with activity against $p210^{bcr\text{-}abl}$ but with increased potency and perhaps better tolerance by certain patients. Dasatinib, another inhibitor of the $p210^{bcr\text{-}abl}$ oncoproteins, also has activity against certain mutant variants of $p210^{bcr\text{-}abl}$ that are refractory to imatinib and arise during therapy or are present de novo. Dasatinib also has inhibitory action against kinases belonging to the src tyrosine protein kinase family; this activity may contribute to its effects. The T315I mutant of $p210^{bcr\text{-}abl}$ is resistant to imatinib, nilotinib, bosutinib, and dasatinib; ponatinib has activity in patients with this T315I$p210^{bcr\text{-}abl}$, but ponatinib has noteworthy associated thromboembolic toxicity. Use of this class of targeted agents is thus critically guided not only by the presence of the $p210^{bcr\text{-}abl}$ tyrosine kinase, but also by the presence of specific mutations in the ATP binding site.

Janus kinases (JAK) 1 and 2 are mutated in certain myeloproliferative states; cytopenias and infrequent arrhythmias infrequently complicate the use of ruxolitinib, the prototypic JAK inhibitor. Bruton's tyrosine kinase (BTK) is an intrinsic component of B-cell antigen receptor signaling and therefore is activate in many types of proliferating B cells. Inhibitors of BTK, including ibrutinib, acalabrutinib, and zanubritinib, have noteworthy activity in certain lymphomas. Cytopenias and cardiac arrhythmias can occur, along with propensity to infection (indeed, the BTK was discovered as deficient in congenital hypogammaglobulinemia, presenting with repeated infections in childhood). Initial use of the BTK inhibitors requires consideration of prophylaxis against tumor lysis syndrome in case of a robust lympholytic effect of the agent.

Receptor-Linked Tyrosine Kinase Antagonists Mutated *EGFR* drives a significant fraction of non-small-cell lung cancers (NSCLCs). Erlotinib and gefitinib are the prototypic EGFR antagonists that, in early clinical trials, showed evidence of responses in a small fraction of patients with NSCLC. Subsequent studies by clinical oncologists in an effort to understand the basis of these excellent responses found that the probability of response to the agents was markedly increased in patients with an activating *EGFR* mutation, and current practice now routinely profiles patients with NSCLC for the presence of sensitizing mutations of *EGFR*. Side effects were generally acceptable, consisting mostly of acneiform rash (treated with glucocorticoid creams and clindamycin gel) and diarrhea. Patients with activating mutations who initially responded to gefitinib or erlotinib but who then had progression of the disease then acquired additional mutations in the enzyme, analogous to the mutational variants responsible for imatinib resistance in CML. Subsequent generations of EGFR antagonists have activity against more uncommon mutants (osimertinib) or a biochemically irreversible mechanism (dacomitinib).

Mutated anaplastic lymphoma kinase (*ALK*) and activated *RET* oncogene likewise drive distinct fractions of NSCLCs. Crizotinib, alectinib, and lorlatinib target ALK, but have prominent adverse cardiac, metabolic, and, in the case of lorlatinib, pulmonary events. Selpercatinib targets RET in NSCLCs (and thyroid cancers) but also with the chance of cardiac and liver toxicity.

Steel factor, a blood cell precursor–related bone marrow growth factor, uses the KIT receptor tyrosine kinase. KIT and variants of the platelet-derived growth factor receptor (PDGFR) are expressed in gastrointestinal stromal sarcoma (GIST). In addition to anti-$p210^{bcr\text{-}abl}$ kinase activity, imatinib also inhibits mutants of KIT and PDGFR. Imatinib has found clinical utility in GIST, a tumor previously notable for its refractoriness to chemotherapeutic approaches. Imatinib's degree of activity varies with the specific mutational variant of KIT or PDGFR present in a particular patient's tumor.

HER2-driven breast cancers may be usefully treated with lapatinib; diarrhea and cardiac dysfunction can occur. Neratinib or tucatinib may also be useful in HER2-positive breast cancers after trastuzumab has ceased to be of value; diarrhea and liver toxicity also require monitoring and management.

Alteration of fibroblast growth factor (FGF) signaling can contribute to the growth of urothelial carcinomas and cholangiocarcinomas. Erdafitinib and pemigatinib, respectively, may be of utility with careful attention to ocular toxicity and hyperphosphatemia; the latter is an "on-target" toxicity of disrupting FGF receptor signaling in the kidney. Likewise, gilteritinib is active against the FMS-like tyrosine kinase-3 (FLT3) mutated in a fraction of poor-prognosis (treated by conventional chemotherapy) acute myeloid leukemias (AMLs). Cardiac, hepatic, gastrointestinal, and neurologic adverse events can occur, along with "differentiation" of the AML cells with cytokine elaboration and pulmonary side effects, requiring management with steroids and potentially hydroxyurea.

The neurotropic tyrosine kinase receptor (NRTK) undergoes translocation with fusion to a variety of different partners to produce a family of chimeric proteins in a small fraction of a variety of solid

TABLE 73-6 Molecularly Targeted Agents[a]

DRUG	TARGET/INDICATION	ADVERSE EVENTS	NOTES
Non-Receptor Tyrosine Kinase Antagonists			
Acalabrutinib	Bruton's tyrosine kinase; mantle cell lymphoma after one prior treatment; CLL/SLL	Cytopenias, opportunistic infections, atrial fibrillation/flutter	CYP3A4, avoid proton pump inhibitors (PPIs); stagger administration with H_2 blockers
Bosutinib	Bcr-Abl fusion protein (CML); wild-type and imatinib-resistant mutants	Myelosuppression, hepatic, QTc prolongation	CYP3A4; avoid PPIs; stagger administration with H_2 blockers
Dasatinib	Bcr-Abl fusion protein (CML/ALL); wild-type and imatinib-resistant mutants	Myelosuppression (bleeding, infection); pulmonary hypertension, CHF, fluid retention; QTc prolongation; caution with hepatic impairment	CYP3A4; avoid PPIs; stagger administration with H_2 blockers
Ibrutinib	Bruton's tyrosine kinase; CLL/SLL; mantle cell lymphoma after CD20-directed therapy; Waldenström's	Nausea, anemia, neutropenia, thrombocytopenia, fatigue, musculoskeletal pain, stomatitis, hypertension, cardiac arrhythmias, tumor lysis syndrome	CYP3A4
Imatinib	Bcr-Abl fusion protein (CML/ALL); c-kit mutants, PDGFR variants (GI stromal tumor [GIST]; eosinophilic syndromes)	Nausea, periorbital edema, rare CHF, QTc prolongation, hypothyroid	Myelosuppression not frequent in solid tumor indications; co-administration with CYP3A4 inducers/inhibitors may require dose adjustment; if need anticoagulation, no warfarin; heparinoids favored
Nilotinib	Bcr-Abl fusion protein (CML) and some imatinib-resistant variants	CHF, hepatic, QTc, electrolyte abnormalities, increased lipase, hypothyroidism	Interaction with CYP3A4-metabolized drugs; also CYP2C8, CYP2C9, CYP2D6, and CYP2B6; avoid food 2 h before and 1 h after a dose
Ponatinib	T315I mutation of Bcr-Abl fusion protein (CML)	Clotting, hepatic, CHF, pancreatitis, neuropathy, rash, arrhythmia, tumor lysis, reversible posterior leukoencephalopathy, wound healing altered	CYP3A4
Ruxolitinib	Janus kinase 1,2; intermediate- or high-risk myelofibrosis, including primary myelofibrosis, post–polycythemia vera myelofibrosis and post–essential thrombocythemia myelofibrosis	Thrombocytopenia, anemia, dizziness, headache	Adjust dose in renal and hepatic impairment, strong CYP3A4 inhibitors, or with fluconazole >200 mg doses except with GVHD
Zanubritinib	Bruton's tyrosine kinase; mantle cell lymphoma after one prior therapy	Cytopenia, cardiac arrhythmia	Avoid with CYP3A4 interacting agents
Receptor-Linked Tyrosine Kinase Antagonists			
Afatinib	First-line treatment of NSCLC with nonresistant ATP site mutation of *EGFR*	Diarrhea; rash; ocular keratitis; interstitial lung disease; hepatic failure	Dose adjustment with Pgp inhibitors
Alectinib	Anaplastic lymphoma kinase (ALK)-positive metastatic NSCLC	Hepatotoxicity; interstitial lung disease; renal impairment; bradycardia	Myalgia and CPK elevations with muscle pain, tenderness, weakness
Avapritinib	GIST unresectable or metastatic with a *PDGFRA* exon 18 mutation, including *PDGFRA* D842V mutations	Edema, nausea, fatigue, CNS effects including altered cognition, sleep and mood disorders, hallucinations	Monitor for intracranial hemorrhage; avoid CYP3A4 inducer/inhibitors
Ceritinib	ALK-positive NSCLC: advanced or metastatic	GI adverse reactions, may require dose adjustment; hepatotoxicity, hyperglycemia, interstitial lung disease (permanently discontinue); QT interval prolongation (monitor with concomitant drugs known to prolong QT)	CYP3A, CYP2C9
Crizotinib	ALK-positive NSCLC: advanced or metastatic	Interstitial pneumonitis; hepatic; QTc prolongation; bradycardia; visual loss	Avoid CYP3A4 inducer/inhibitor
Dacomitinib	Advanced or metastatic NSCLC with epidermal growth factor receptor (EGFR) exon 19 deletion or exon 21 L858R via irreversible mechanism	Diarrhea, cutaneous: hold and/or dose reduce; interstitial lung disease (permanently discontinue)	Avoid with PPIs; use locally acting antacids or H_2 receptor antagonist and administer at least 6 h before or 10 h after H_2 receptor antagonist; CYP2D6
Erdafitinib	Target FGFR; advanced or metastatic urothelial cancer with an FGFR3 or FGFR2 alteration that has progressed beyond traditional platinum-based therapies	Stomatitis, fatigue, cutaneous changes, diarrhea; uncommon central serous retinopathy; retinal detachment; therefore, monitor with ophthalmologic exams during treatment; hyperphosphatemia a pharmacodynamic effect due to FGF23/Klotho signaling disruption	CYP2C9, CYP3A4 interactors; OCT2 substrates; separate dosing by at least 6 h before or after administration of Pgp substrates
Erlotinib	First-line treatment of NSCLC with ATP site mutation of EGFR; second-line treatment of wild-type EGFR NSCLC; pancreatic cancer with gemcitabine	Rash, diarrhea, renal failure, interstitial pneumonitis, liver	Administer at least 1 h before or 2 h after meals; CYP3A4; avoid with PPIs and space dosing with antacids; can alter warfarin effect; microangiopathic hemolytic anemia especially in pancreatic cancer, rare
Gefitinib	First-line treatment of NSCLC with ATP site mutation of EGFR	Rash, diarrhea, rare interstitial pneumonitis, ocular keratitis, GI perforation	CYP3A4; avoid with PPIs; monitor warfarin effect with gefitinib. In the United States, only with prior documented benefit in second-line treatment of NSCLC if not EGFR mutated

(*Continued*)

TABLE 73-6 Molecularly Targeted Agents[a] (Continued)

DRUG	TARGET/INDICATION	ADVERSE EVENTS	NOTES
Gilteritinib	Relapsed or refractory AML with an *FLT3* mutation	Hepatotoxicity, myalgia/arthralgia, fatigue/malaise, mucositis, edema, rash, noninfectious diarrhea, dyspnea, nausea, cough, constipation, eye disorders, hypotension, vomiting, and renal impairment	Also inhibits AXL; unusual AML differentiation syndrome, requiring corticosteroids and consideration of hydroxyurea; posterior reversible encephalopathy syndrome possible (discontinue); prolonged QT interval: interrupt and/or reduce dose with a QTcF >500 ms (correct hypokalemia or hypomagnesemia prior to and during administration); pancreatitis: interrupt and/or reduce dosage; Pgp substrates; CYP3A
Lapatinib	Breast cancer: with capecitabine in HER2/neu advanced/metastatic after trastuzumab and chemotherapy; with aromatase inhibition if ER positive, HER2/neu positive	↓LVEF; liver; rash, nausea; diarrhea, palmar-plantar erythrodysesthesia	Interstitial lung disease and pneumonitis (discontinue if severe); QTc: monitor ECG and electrolytes, CYP3A4, CYP2C8, Pgp substrate interactions
Larotrectinib	Targets TRKA, TRKB, and TRKC fusion proteins; indicated in any adult or pediatric solid tumor with a neurotrophic receptor tyrosine kinase (NTRK) gene fusion without a known acquired resistance mutation, with no satisfactory alternative treatments, or that has progressed following treatment	Neurotoxicity with potential cognitive impairment; hepatotoxicity, modify dose or withhold depending on severity	CYP3A4
Lorlatinib	NSCLC: ALK-positive metastatic NSCLC that has progressed on crizotinib and at least one other ALK inhibitor; or with progression on alectinib or ceritinib as the first ALK inhibitor therapy for metastatic disease	Hyperlipidemia: initiate or increase the dose of lipid-lowering agents and withhold and resume or dose reduce based on severity; AV block: withhold and resume or dose modify; CNS effects including seizures, hallucinations, altered cognitive function, altered mood, suicidal ideation, altered speech, mental status, and sleep	Targets ALK and also anti-ROS activity but FDA label limited to ALK indications; CYP3A4 (NB severe hepatotoxicity with strong CYP3A inducers; discontinue strong CYP3A inducers for 3 plasma half-lives prior to use); interstitial lung disease (ILD): immediately withhold and consider discontinuance with suspected ILD/pneumonitis
Neratinib	Breast cancer: with capecitabine in HER2/neu advanced metastatic disease after two prior HER2/neu agents; extended adjuvant treatment after early-stage adjuvant trastuzumab	Diarrhea; nausea; vomiting; abdominal pain; increased ALT/AST	Aggressive diarrhea prophylaxis with loperamide; avoid concomitant PPI antacids; separate from administration of other antacids; avoid CYP3A4 concomitant medications
Osimertinib	First-line treatment of metastatic NSCLC with *EGFR* exon 19 deletions or exon 21 L858R mutations; *EGFR* T790M mutation–positive NSCLC, progressed on or after EGFR TKI therapy	Interstitial lung disease, QTc prolongation, cardiomyopathy, ocular keratitis	Avoid or adjust dose with strong CYP3A4 inducers
Pemigatinib	Cholangiocarcinoma: previously treated, unresectable, locally advanced or metastatic cholangiocarcinoma with a fibroblast growth factor receptor 2 (FGFR2) fusion or other rearrangement	Hyperphosphatemia as pharmacodynamic effect: adjust dose if needed; stomatitis, nausea, diarrhea.	Retinal detachment: perform ocular exam with ocular coherence tomography prior to and every 2–3 months during treatment; CYP3A4
Selpercatinib	NSCLC: advanced or metastatic and *RET* fusion positive; medullary thyroid cancer: advanced or metastatic *RET*-mutant medullary thyroid cancer; advanced or metastatic *RET* fusion–positive thyroid cancer that requires systemic therapy and that is radioactive iodine refractory (if appropriate)	Hepatotoxicity: monitor liver functions every 2 weeks during first 3 months, then monthly; hypertension, wound healing effects: withhold 1 weeks prior to surgery and at least 2 weeks after surgery; hemorrhage	QT interval prolongations: assess QTc at baseline, maintain electrolytes; avoid with QTc-prolonging drugs, avoid with antacids, but if not avoidable, take with food (with PPI) or modify administration time (with H_2 receptor antagonist or locally acting antacid); CYP3A, CYP2C8 interaction
Tucatinib	Breast cancer: with trastuzumab and capecitabine after one or more HER2/neu regimens in the metastatic setting	Diarrhea, hepatotoxicity	CYP3A4, CYP2C8 interaction
RAF/MEK Inhibitors			
Binimetinib	In combination with encorafenib, for the treatment of patients with unresectable or metastatic melanoma with a *BRAF* V600E or V600K mutation	Cardiomyopathy, venous thromboembolism; ocular, interstitial lung disease, hepatotoxicity, rhabdomyolysis	Targets MEK; dose modify with liver disease
Cobimetinib	In combination with vemurafenib for unresectable or metastatic melanoma with a *BRAF* V600E or V600K mutation	New primary malignancies, cutaneous and noncutaneous; hemorrhage, retinal vein occlusion, cardiomyopathy: evaluate LVEF before and during treatment, severe dermatologic reactions, rhabdomyolysis, hepatotoxicity, photosensitivity	CYP3A interaction

(*Continued*)

TABLE 73-6 Molecularly Targeted Agents[a] (Continued)

DRUG	TARGET/INDICATION	ADVERSE EVENTS	NOTES
Dabrafenib	*BRAF* V600E in melanoma; both alone and in combination with trametinib; may be useful in other tumors with *BRAF* V600E	As a single agent : hyperkeratosis, headache, pyrexia, arthralgia, papilloma, alopecia, and palmar-plantar erythrodysesthesia syndrome; in combination with trametinib: pyrexia, chills, fatigue, rash, nausea, vomiting, diarrhea, abdominal pain, peripheral edema, cough, headache, arthralgia, night sweats, decreased appetite, constipation, and myalgia	New primary cutaneous malignancies; hemorrhagic events as single agent; CYP3A4, CYP2C8, CYP2C19, and CYP2B6 interactions
Encorafenib	*BRAF* V600E in melanoma (in combination with binimetinib)	Uveitis, hemorrhage, QTc prolongation, fatigue, nausea, vomiting	CYP3A4 interactions; avoid with hormonal contraceptives
Trametinib	*BRAF* V600E in melanoma (both as single agent and in combination with dabrafenib)	Rash, diarrhea, lymphedema; cardiomyopathy, ocular toxicity including retinal vein occlusion, interstitial lung disease, fever, hemorrhage, venous thromboembolism, hyperglycemia	In combination with dabrafenib: second neoplasms, hemorrhage, venous thrombosis, CHF, ocular, hyperglycemia; avoid CYP3A4, CYP2C8, CYP2C9, CYP2C19, or CYP2B6 interacting drugs
Vemurafenib	*BRAF* V600E in melanoma; alone and in combination with cobimetinib; may be useful in other tumors with *BRAF* V600E	Cutaneous squamous cell carcinoma, severe rash including Stevens-Johnson, allergic hypersensitivity, QTc prolongation, hepatic, ocular, photosensitivity	Usually combined with cobimetinib in melanoma; CYP3A4, CYP1A2, and CYP2D6 interactions
Apoptosis Modulation			
Venetoclax	Targets BCL2; indicated in CLL/SLL; AML: in combination with azacitidine or decitabine or low-dose cytarabine in treatment of newly diagnosed AML in adults who are age 75 years or older or who have comorbidities that preclude use of intensive induction chemotherapy	Neutropenia; infection: withhold for grade 3 and higher	Tumor lysis syndrome (TLS): anticipate TLS, assess risk in all patients. Premedicate with anti-hyperuricemics and ensure adequate hydration, with more intensive measures (intravenous hydration, frequent monitoring, hospitalization) as overall risk increases. Immunization: No live attenuated vaccines prior to, during, or after venetoclax treatment; CYP3A, Pgp interaction; take Pgp substrates at least 6 h before venetoclax
Multikinase Inhibitors			
Axitinib	Renal cell carcinoma, second line	HBP, hemorrhage/clotting; diarrhea, other GI including GI perforation, fatigue, hand-foot syndrome, hypothyroidism, reversible posterior leukoencephalopathy, proteinuria	Targets VEGFR, PDGFR, KIT; CYP3A4/5 interaction
Brigatinib	Advanced or metastatic ALK-positive NSCLC progressed on or intolerant to crizotinib	Interstitial lung disease, bradycardia, hypertension, visual disturbances, hyperglycemia, creatine phosphokinase elevations	Targets ALK and EGFR; CYP3A interaction; hormonal contraceptives may be ineffective due to decreased exposure as CYP3A4 substrates
Cabozantinib	Medullary thyroid cancer; renal cell cancer; hepatocellular carcinoma after sorafenib	Hypertension, thrombotic events, diarrhea, fistula/GI perforation/wound healing, reversible posterior leukoencephalopathy, hemorrhage, palmar-plantar erythrodysesthesia	Targets VEGFR2, MET, AXL, RET; modify dose with CYP3A4 interactors
Capmatinib	NSCLC with MET exon 14 skipping	Interstitial lung disease, hepatic, photosensitivity	Targets MET; avoid with CYP3A4 interactors
Entrectinib	NSCLC: advanced and/or ROS1 positive; any solid tumors with an *NTRK* gene fusion without a known acquired resistance mutation, with metastasis, or in which surgical resection is likely to result in severe morbidity, or in tumors with progression following treatment or no satisfactory alternative therapy	CHF, CNS effect, skeletal fractures; hepatotoxicity: monitor liver tests, including ALT and AST, every 2 weeks during the first month of treatment, then monthly thereafter; withhold or permanently discontinue based on severity; hyperuricemia: assess serum uric acid levels prior to initiation and periodically during treatment	Targets *NTRK* gene fusion proteins; QT prolongation: assess with electrolytes at baseline and during treatment; vision disorders: withhold for new visual changes and consider ophthalmologic evaluation; CYP3A4 interaction: patients with BSA >1.50 m^2, reduce the dose of entrectinib if co-administration of moderate or strong CYP3A inhibitors and if BSA ≤1.50 m^2, avoid entrectinib; avoid with moderate and strong CYP3A inducers
Fedratinib	Intermediate-2 or high-risk primary or secondary (post-polycythemia vera or post-essential thrombocythemia) myelofibrosis	Anemia, thrombocytopenia, nausea, vomiting, diarrhea, hepatic, amylase/lipase, encephalopathy: check thiamine levels prior, replete if deficient	Targets Janus kinase 2, and FLT3, RET; CYP3A4, CYP2C19 interaction
Lenvatinib	Iodine-refractory differentiated thyroid cancer; with everolimus for renal cell carcinoma after one prior antiangiogenic; hepatocellular carcinoma; with pembrolizumab, for the treatment of advanced endometrial carcinoma that is not MSI-H or dMMR and disease progression following prior systemic therapy; candidates for curative surgery	Hypertension, cardiac dysfunction, arterial thromboembolism, hepatic, renal, proteinuria, diarrhea, fistula/GI perforation/wound healing, QTc prolongation, hypocalcemia, reversible posterior leukoencephalopathy, hemorrhage, altered thyroid	Targets VEGFR1/2/3, FGFR1/2/3/4, PDGFRα, KIT, and RET

(Continued)

TABLE 73-6 Molecularly Targeted Agents[a] (Continued)

DRUG	TARGET/INDICATION	ADVERSE EVENTS	NOTES
Midostaurin	Newly diagnosed *FLT3*-mutated AML during induction, consolidation, with daunorubicin/cytarabine-based chemotherapy; aggressive systemic mastocytosis, mast cell leukemia; systemic mastocytosis with associated hematologic malignancy	Interstitial lung disease; nausea; diarrhea	Targets mutant *FLT3*, protein kinase C, and many other protein kinases
Pazopanib	Renal cell carcinoma, soft tissue sarcoma (not GIST or adipocytic)	Fatigue, diarrhea/GI, hypertension; arterial and venous thrombosis with embolism, hemorrhage; hepatotoxicity: potentially severe/fatal; measure liver chemistries before and during treatment; GI perforation or fistula; proteinuria: monitor urine protein and interrupt treatment for 24-h urine protein ≥3 g and discontinue for repeat episodes despite dose reductions; infection: serious infections (with or without neutropenia); hypothyroidism	Targets VEGFRs, KIT, PDGFR, and FGFR; CHF ± prolonged QT intervals and torsades des pointes: monitor LVEF, ECG, and electrolytes at baseline and during treatment; reversible posterior leukoencephalopathy syndrome, interstitial lung disease/pneumonitis, thrombotic microangiopathy, including thrombotic thrombocytopenic purpura and hemolytic-uremic syndrome (permanently discontinue); CYP3A4, CYP22D6, CYP2C8 interaction; use with simvastatin increases the risk of ALT elevations and should be undertaken with caution; avoid with drugs that raise gastric pH; consider short-acting antacids in place of PPIs and H_2 receptor antagonists; separate antacid and pazopanib dosing by several hours
Pexidartinib	Indicated for tenosynovial giant cell tumor (TGCT) associated with severe morbidity or functional limitations and not amenable to improvement with surgery	Administer 1 h before or 2 h after food; can cause serious and potentially fatal liver injury; monitor liver tests prior to and during treatment and withhold, dose reduce, or permanently discontinue	Targets colony-stimulating factor-1 receptor, KIT, FLT3; avoid with agents known to cause hepatotoxicity; CYP3A, UGT interaction; avoid with PPIs; use H_2 receptor antagonists or antacids if needed
Regorafenib	Second-line colorectal cancer; GI stromal tumor	Hypertension, hemorrhage, hand-foot syndrome and other dermatologic toxicity, thromboses, GI perforations with fistula, wound healing delays	Targets VEGFR, cardiac ischemia with infarction, reversible posterior leukoencephalopathy syndrome; CYP3A4 interaction
Sorafenib	Renal cell, hepatocellular, differentiated thyroid carcinoma	Diarrhea, hemorrhage, hand-foot syndrome, other rash, hypertension, CHF, QTc prolongation, hepatic toxicity, GI perforation	Targets c-RAF more selectively than B-RAF; VEGFR; many other kinases; impaired TSH suppression in thyroid cancer; CYP3A4 interaction
Sunitinib	Renal cell carcinoma, advanced or adjuvant; pancreatic neuroendocrine tumor, GIST after imatinib	Hypertension, hemorrhagic events, GI perforation, proteinuria, leading to renal failure: interrupt treatment for 24-h urine protein ≥3 g; discontinue for repeat episodes despite dose reductions; thyroid dysfunction, hypoglycemia: check blood glucose levels and consider antidiabetic drug dose modifications; osteonecrosis of the jaw: consider preventive dentistry prior to treatment and avoid invasive dental procedures, particularly in patients receiving intravenous bisphosphonate therapy; impaired wound healing: temporary interruption prior to major surgical procedures; palmar-plantar erythrodysesthesia	Targets VEGFRs; PDGFR, RET, KIT; other protein kinases. Rare prolonged QT intervals and torsades des pointes: monitor at baseline and during treatment; maintain K, Mg levels; rare tumor lysis syndrome reported primarily in patients with RCC and GIST with high tumor burden; rare thrombotic microangiopathy, including thrombotic thrombocytopenic purpura and hemolytic-uremic syndrome (discontinue); rare necrotizing fasciitis; severe cutaneous adverse events including erythema multiforme, Stevens-Johnson syndrome (SJS), and toxic epidermal necrolysis (TEN); discontinue if these events; CYP3A4interaction
Vandetanib	Medullary thyroid cancer	Diarrhea, rash, hypertension, prolonged QTc, thromboses, fistulas, osteonecrosis, proteinuria	Targets VEGFR, RET, EGFR; CYP3A4 interaction
Cyclin-Dependent Kinase (CDK) Inhibitors			
Abemaciclib	Breast cancer: with an aromatase inhibitor as initial endocrine-based therapy for the treatment of postmenopausal HR+, HER2– advanced or metastatic breast cancer; or with fulvestrant for the treatment of women with HR+, HER2– advanced or metastatic breast cancer with disease progression following endocrine therapy; as monotherapy for the treatment of adult patients with HR+, HER2– advanced or metastatic breast cancer with disease progression following endocrine therapy and prior chemotherapy	Diarrhea, neutropenia, thrombocytopenia, hepatotoxicity, venous thromboembolism	Targets CDK4/6; avoid concomitant use of ketoconazole; CYP3A4 interaction

(*Continued*)

TABLE 73-6 Molecularly Targeted Agents[a] (Continued)

DRUG	TARGET/INDICATION	ADVERSE EVENTS	NOTES
Palbociclib	Breast cancer: HR+, HER2– advanced or metastatic breast cancer in combination with an aromatase inhibitor as initial endocrine-based therapy in postmenopausal women; or fulvestrant in women with disease progression following endocrine therapy	Neutropenia, anemia, thrombocytopenia, stomatitis, diarrhea, fatigue	Targets CDK4/6; CYP3A interaction
Ribociclib	Breast cancer: with letrozole as initial endocrine-based therapy for the treatment of postmenopausal women with HR+, HER2– advanced or metastatic breast cancer	Hepatotoxicity; neutropenia	Targets CDK4/6; unusual QT interval prolongation; drugs known to prolong QT interval should be avoided such as antiarrhythmics; CYP3A interaction
Protein Homeostasis Modulators			
Bortezomib	Multiple myeloma, mantle cell lymphoma, second line	Neuropathy, thrombocytopenia, neutropenia, nausea, diarrhea, hypotension, tumor lysis syndrome with high tumor burden; hepatic: monitor hepatic enzymes during treatment, consider interruption	Proteasome inhibitor; infiltrative pulmonary disease, reversible posterior leukoencephalopathy syndrome: consider MRI for onset of visual or neurologic symptoms and discontinue if suspected; thrombotic microangiopathy; CYP3A4 interaction
Carfilzomib	Multiple myeloma: with dexamethasone or with lenalidomide plus dexamethasone in patients with relapsed or refractory multiple myeloma who have received one to three lines of therapy, or as a single agent for the treatment of patients with relapsed or refractory multiple myeloma who have received one or more lines of therapy	Infusion reaction: premedicate with dexamethasone; thrombocytopenia; tumor lysis syndrome, with need for hydration, monitoring of metabolic parameters	Proteasome inhibitor; cardiac toxicities: including failure or ischemia, withhold and evaluate; acute renal failure: monitor serum creatinine regularly; pulmonary toxicity, including pulmonary hypertension, acute respiratory distress/failure and diffuse infiltrative pulmonary disease: withhold and evaluate promptly; dose adjust with hepatic impairment; administer after a hemodialysis procedure
Ixazomib	Multiple myeloma: with lenalidomide and dexamethasone after at least one prior therapy	Thrombocytopenia, nausea, diarrhea, peripheral neuropathy, edema, hepatotoxicity	Proteasome inhibitor; avoid with strong CYP3A4 inducers; dose adjust with hepatic or renal impairment
Selinexor	Multiple myeloma (refractory): with dexamethasone after at least four prior therapies and refractory to at least two proteasome inhibitors, at least two immunomodulatory agents, and an anti-CD38 monoclonal antibody; DLBCL (relapsed or refractory) or arising from FL after at least two lines of systemic therapy	Thrombocytopenia, neutropenia, nausea, diarrhea, hyponatremia, neurotoxicity	Targets exportin 1 and therefore decreases efficient transport of proteins from nucleus to cytoplasm, leading to cell cycle arrest
Chromatin-Modifying Epigenetic Modulators			
DNA hypomethylating agents			
Azacitidine and decitabine	AML/myelodysplastic syndrome	Marrow, nausea, liver, neurologic, myalgia	"Suicide" inhibition of DNA; methyl transferase after incorporation into DNA
Histone deacetylase inhibitors			
Belinostat	Peripheral T-cell lymphoma, relapsed or refractory	Thrombocytopenia, neutropenia, lymphopenia, anemia, infection, hepatotoxicity	Tumor lysis syndrome monitoring
Panobinostat	Multiple myeloma in combination with bortezomib and dexamethasone, in patients with multiple myeloma who have received at least two prior regimens, including bortezomib and an immunomodulatory agent.	Diarrhea, potentially severe, requiring prophylaxis; cardiac ischemic events, arrhythmias, hemorrhage, hepatotoxicity, cytopenias	CYP3A4, CYP2D6 interactions; avoid concomitant antiarrhythmic drugs/QT-prolonging drugs
Romidepsin	Cutaneous T-cell lymphoma, second line	QT prolongation, nausea, vomiting, cytopenias	Monitor QT at baseline and during treatment; monitor PT, INR with warfarin derivatives; CYP3A4 interaction
Vorinostat	Cutaneous T-cell lymphoma, second line	Fatigue, diarrhea, hyperglycemia, thrombocytopenia, embolism, GI bleeding, QT prolongation.	Monitor QT at baseline and during treatment; monitor PT, INR with warfarin derivatives

(Continued)

TABLE 73-6 Molecularly Targeted Agents[a] (Continued)

DRUG	TARGET/INDICATION	ADVERSE EVENTS	NOTES
Histone methyltransferase inhibitors			
Tazemetostat	Epithelioid sarcoma: advanced or metastatic not eligible for surgical resection; FL with *EZH2* mutation after two prior therapies or any FL that has relapsed or is refractory to alternative therapies	Fatigue, nausea, constipation	Avoid CYP3A4 inducers/inhibitors; monitor for emergence of myelodysplastic syndrome, leukemia
Metabolism Modulators: mTOR Inhibitors/PI3 Kinase Inhibitors/IDH Inhibitors			
Alpelisib	Breast cancer: with fulvestrant for postmenopausal women, and men, with HR+, HER2–, *PIK3CA*-mutated, advanced or metastatic breast cancer following progression on or after an endocrine-based treatment	Hyperglycemia: safety not established in type 1 or uncontrolled type 2 diabetes; monitor glucose levels and hemoglobin A_{1c}; optimize oral antihyperglycemics if warranted; interstitial pneumonitis: discontinue; diarrhea ≤ grade 2 frequent	Targets PI3Kα isoform; severe hypersensitivity: permanently discontinue and initiate appropriate treatment; severe cutaneous reactions including SJS, erythema multiforme (EM), and TEN: consider consultation with a dermatologist; permanently discontinue if SJS, EM, or TEN confirmed; CYP3A4, CYP2C9; avoid with BCRP inhibitors
Copanlisib	Relapsed FL patients who have received at least two prior systemic therapies; pending confirmatory trial	Infection, hyperglycemia, HBP, noninfectious pneumonitis, neutropenia, cutaneous reactions	Targets PI3Kα/δ isoforms; CYP3A4
Duvelisib	For relapsed or refractory CLL/SLL or FL; orphan drug designation for peripheral T-cell lymphoma	Neutropenia, hepatic toxicity, severe infections, diarrhea/colitis may require withholding; severe cutaneous reactions or pneumonitis in 5%	Targets PI3Kγ/δ isoforms; CYP3A
Enasidenib	Relapsed or refractory AML with an *IDH2* mutation	Nausea, vomiting, diarrhea, elevated bilirubin, and anorexia	Targets *IDH2* mutant enzyme; unusual "differentiation syndrome" reflecting leukemia response to drug, but potentially fatal if not treated; use corticosteroid therapy, hemodynamic monitoring, consider hydroxyurea until symptom resolution
Everolimus	RCC, advanced; tuberous sclerosis–associated renal angiomyolipoma and/or subependymal giant cell astrocytoma; breast cancer, HR+, resistant to anastrozole or letrozole, in combination with exemestane; pancreatic, lung, or GI neuroendocrine, NOT functional carcinoid	Fatigue, noninfectious pneumonitis, infections, severe hypersensitivity reactions, renal impairment, impaired wound healing, hyperglycemia and hyperlipidemia, myelosuppression	Targets mTOR; angioedema with patients taking concomitant ACE inhibitors may be at increased risk; stomatitis: consider dexamethasone alcohol-free mouthwash when starting treatment.; risk of reduced efficacy of vaccination: Pgp and strong CYP3A4 inhibitors: avoid concomitant use; Pgp and moderate CYP3A4 inhibitors: reduce dose; Pgp and strong CYP3A4 inducers: increase dose; geriatric patients: monitor and adjust dose for adverse reactions
Idelalisib	Relapsed CLL with rituximab; SLL, relapsed FL after two prior therapies	Hepatotoxicity, diarrhea or colitis, pneumonitis: monitor for pulmonary symptoms and bilateral interstitial infiltrates, then interrupt or discontinue; intestinal perforation: discontinue if suspected	Targets PI3Kδ isoform; CYP3A4
Ivosidenib	AML: relapsed or refractory with an *IDH1* mutation; in the United States, newly diagnosed AML with a susceptible *IDH1* mutation, in patients who are at least 75 years old or who have comorbidities that preclude the use of intensive induction chemotherapy	Fatigue, leukocytosis, arthralgia, diarrhea, dyspnea, edema, nausea, mucositis, ECG QT prolonged, rash, pyrexia, cough, and constipation	Targets *IDH1* mutant; unusual QT prolongation (check electrolytes and hold or reduce dose); Guillain-Barré syndrome (permanently discontinue); CYP3A4; monitor/avoid with increased QTc-causing drugs
Temsirolimus	RCC, second line or poor prognosis	Hypersensitivity, hepatic (adjust dose in liver dysfunction), infection, interstitial lung disease, stomatitis, thrombocytopenia, nausea, anorexia, fatigue, hyperglycemia, hyperlipidemia, poor wound healing, GI perforation, renal impairment: check before treatment and periodically	Targets mTOR; CYP3A4/5 interactions; avoid live vaccines or exposure to subjects recently vaccinated with live vaccines
Poly-ADP Ribose Polymerase (PARP) Inhibitors			
Niraparib	Maintenance treatment of adult patients with recurrent epithelial ovarian, fallopian tube, or primary peritoneal cancer who are in a complete or partial response to platinum-based chemotherapy	Cytopenias, nausea, diarrhea, fatigue	Myelodysplastic syndrome

(Continued)

TABLE 73-6 Molecularly Targeted Agents[a] (Continued)

DRUG	TARGET/INDICATION	ADVERSE EVENTS	NOTES
Olaparib	Ovarian cancer: after two or more chemotherapies with deleterious *BRCA* mutation (germline and/or somatic); maintenance therapy when in complete or partial response to platinum-based chemotherapy Breast cancer: for the treatment of adult patients with deleterious or suspected deleterious gBRCAm, HER2– metastatic breast cancer who have been treated with chemotherapy in the neoadjuvant, adjuvant, or metastatic setting; if HR+, after prior endocrine therapy or inappropriate for endocrine therapy Pancreatic cancer: maintenance treatment of adult patients with deleterious or suspected deleterious gBRCAm metastatic pancreatic adenocarcinoma whose disease has not progressed on at least 16 weeks of a first-line platinum-based chemotherapy regimen	Nausea, fatigue, anemia, thrombocytopenia, neutropenia, stomatitis, liver function abnormalities	Myelodysplastic syndrome; rare interstitial pneumonitis
Rucaparib	Ovarian/fallopian tube/primary peritoneal cancer: as with olaparib	Nausea, fatigue, anemia, thrombocytopenia, neutropenia, stomatitis, liver function abnormalities	Severe heme toxicity with emergence of myelodysplastic syndrome
Talazoparib	Ovarian/fallopian tube/primary peritoneal cancer: as with olaparib	Nausea, fatigue (including asthenia), vomiting, abdominal pain, anemia, diarrhea, neutropenia, leukopenia, decreased appetite, constipation, stomatitis, dyspnea, and thrombocytopenia	Monitor for emergence of myelodysplasia; rare interstitial pneumonitis should lead to discontinuation; avoid with strong or moderate CYP3A inhibitors, but if concomitant use cannot be avoided, reduce dose; avoid with strong or moderate CYP3A inducers
Miscellaneous			
Arsenic trioxide	APL (target PML-RARα and redox homeostasis)	↑ QT_c; hypersensitivity with vasomotor symptoms	APL differentiation syndrome (see under tretinoin)
Glasdegib	AML: in combination with low-dose cytarabine, for the treatment of newly diagnosed AML in adult patients who are ≥75 years old or who have comorbidities that preclude use of intensive induction chemotherapy	Monitor ECG and electrolytes for QTc prolongation and interrupt treatment if it occurs	Targets smoothened receptor in hedgehog pathway; CYP3A4; avoid with QTc-prolonging drugs, but if co-administration is unavoidable monitor for increased QTc
Sonidegib	Metastatic basal cell carcinoma	Muscle spasm, fatigue, transmission through semen	Targets smoothened receptor in hedgehog pathway; CYP3A4
Tagraxofusp-erzs	Blastic plasmacytoid dendritic cell neoplasm	Hypersensitivity reactions (require premedication with steroids, antihistamines); hepatotoxicity, capillary leak syndrome	Targets CD123 (IL-3 receptor) to deliver a fragment of the diphtheria toxin
Tretinoin	APL, t(15;17) positive	Cutaneous including cheilitis, skin dryness; increased intracranial pressure; hyperlipidemia, abnormal liver function tests, usually resolve	Targets PML-RARα; APL differentiation syndrome: pulmonary dysfunction/infiltrate, pleural/pericardial effusion, fever
Vismodegib	Metastatic basal cell carcinoma	GI, hair loss, fatigue, muscle spasm, dysgeusia; no blood donation for 7 months after last dose	Targets smoothened receptor in hedgehog pathway
Ziv-aflibercept	Metastatic colorectal cancer in combination with 5-fluorouracil, leucovorin, irinotecan; resistant to or has progressed following an oxaliplatin-containing regimen	Fistula formation, GI perforation, hemorrhage, thrombosis, arterial thromboembolism, proteinuria, reversible posterior leukoencephalopathy	Targets VEGF by a solubilized receptor-trapping mechanism

[a]All agents in this category should be regarded as potentially fetotoxic, and use during pregnancy is either contraindicated or undertaken with clear understanding of risk of fetal harm; likewise not recommended for use during lactation.

Abbreviations: ACE, angiotensin-converting enzyme; ALL, acute lymphocytic leukemia; ALT, alanine aminotransferase; AML, acute myeloid leukemia; APL, acute promyelocytic leukemia; AST, aspartate aminotransferase; AV, atrioventricular; BRCP, breast cancer resistance protein drug transporter; BSA, body surface area; CHF, congestive heart failure; CLL, chronic lymphocytic leukemia; CML, chronic myeloid leukemia; CNS, central nervous system; CPK, creatine phosphokinase; CYP, cytochrome p450 interactions with drugs metabolized by the indicated isoform; DLBCL, diffuse large B-cell lymphoma; dMMR, deficient mismatch repair; ECG, electrocardiogram; EGFR, epidermal growth factor receptor; ER, estrogen receptor; FDA, U.S. Food and Drug Administration; FL, follicular lymphoma; gBRCAm, germline mutated breast cancer associated protein; GI, gastrointestinal; GVHD, graft-versus-host disease; HBP, high blood pressure; MEK, mitogen activated protein kinase; HR, hormone receptor; HER2, human epidermal growth factor receptor 2; IDH, isocitrate dehydrogenase; INR, international normalized ratio; LVEF, left ventricular ejection fraction; MSI-H, microsatellite instability-high; mTOR, mammalian target of rapamycin kinase; NSCLC, non-small-cell lung cancer; PDGFR, platelet-derived growth factor receptor; Pgp, P-glycoprotein; PT, prothrombin time; QTcF, QT corrected by Frederika formula; RCC, renal cell carcinoma; SLL, small lymphocytic lymphoma; TKI, tyrosine kinase inhibitor; TSH, thyroid-stimulating hormone; UGT, uridine diphosphate glucuronosyltransferase; VEGFR, vascular endothelial growth factor receptor.

tumors. Larotrectinib and entrectinib may be quite useful in managing these tumors; indeed, these agents are exemplary of "histology agnostic" agents, where the utility of the drug is not tied to a particular histologic diagnosis, but to the possession of a specific *NRTK* gene alteration. Neurotoxicity, a long half-life of the agents, and hepatotoxic adverse events are of concern. Also, assuring that solid tumors have been appropriately screened for the existence of such sensitizing mutations can be logistically and economically challenging.

RAS/RAF/MEK Antagonists The *BRAF* V600E mutation drives a substantial fraction of melanomas and certain NSCLCs and has been detected in certain thyroid tumors, colorectal tumors, hairy cell leukemias, and unusual gliomas. BRAF inhibitors such as dabrafenib, vemurafenib, and encorafenib have activity as single agents in many such tumors but are usually most active when co-administered as "doublets" with the MEK inhibitors trametinib, cobimetinib, and binimetinib, respectively, to promote "shut down" of RAF/MEK signaling at more than pathway member. Cutaneous adverse events including generally indolent cutaneous second neoplasms and thromboembolic, cardiac, and ocular toxicity can occur.

Sotorasib is a first-in-class inhibitor of *KRAS* G12C signaling that in early clinical reports has evidence of effecting stable disease in patients with a variety of neoplasm histologies bearing that mutation, with fewer actual responses. Its initial very favorable safety profile encourages further clinical investigations alone and in combination with other agents.

Multikinase Inhibitors Agents in this class also target specific macromolecules promoting the viability of tumor cells. They are "small-molecule" ATP site-directed antagonists that inhibit more than one protein kinase and may have value in the treatment of several solid tumors. Drugs of this type with prominent activity against the VEGFR tyrosine kinase have activity in renal cell carcinoma. Sorafenib is a VEGFR antagonist also with activity against the RAF serine-threonine protein kinase, and regorafenib is a closely related drug with value in relapsed advanced colon cancer. Pazopanib also prominently targets VEGFR and has activity in renal carcinoma and soft tissue sarcomas. Sunitinib has anti-VEGFR, anti-PDGFR, and anti-KIT activity. It causes prominent responses and stabilization of disease in renal cell cancers and GISTs. Side effects for agents with anti-VEGFR activity, similar to those of the anti-VEGF antibody bevacizumab, prominently include hypertension, proteinuria, and, more rarely, bleeding and clotting disorders, perforation of scarred gastrointestinal lesions, and posterior leukoencephalopathy, probably reflecting CNS vascular damage. Also encountered are fatigue, diarrhea, and hand-foot syndrome, with erythema and desquamation of the distal extremities, in some cases requiring dose modification, particularly with sorafenib.

Other agents in this class include agents such as brigatinib (clinical activity in ALK-dependent NSCLC, but also with anti-EGFR action), entrectinib (clinical activity in NTRK fusion protein diseases, but also in *ROS*-mutated NSCLC), and fedratinib (clinical activity in myeloproliferative neoplasms, but with RET activity in addition to JAK2 and FLT3 antagonism).

Cyclin-Dependent Kinase Inhibitors Cyclin-dependent kinases (CDKs) are activated as the result of oncogene pathway activity, and CDK4 and CDK6 phosphorylate the retinoblastoma (RB) tumor-suppressor gene to allow entry into S-phase. Palbociclib, abemaciclib, and ribociclib, selective inhibitors of CDK4 and CDK6, have noteworthy activity in advanced breast cancers also expressing the estrogen receptor, usually in conjunction with continued efforts to suppress estrogen receptor signaling, and frequently in conjunction with mTOR inhibitors. Further clinical investigations in other RB intact tumors may broaden their role.

Protein Homeostasis Modulators The proteasome is a macromolecular complex that degrades misfolded proteins tagged for removal by ubiquitin ligases. Proteasome inhibitors were originally designed as potential anti-inflammatory agents owing to proteasome activity to produce inflammatory cytokines but had unexpected antiproliferative activity in a variety of cell types. Proteasome inhibitors have clinical utility in myeloma and lymphoma, where unbalanced synthesis of immunoglobulin components can accumulate after proteasome inhibitor treatment and induce apoptosis or starve cells for amino acids, inducing autophagy. Boronic acid proteasome inhibitors, including bortezomib and ixazomib, cause thrombocytopenia, gastrointestinal dysfunction, and neuropathy. Carfilzomib is a distinct chemotype with attenuated neuropathy but increased incidence of infusion reactions and cytokine release, with attendant risk of cardiopulmonary adverse events.

Exportin 1 is a nuclear membrane transport protein that is responsible for normal exit and entry of a variety of nuclear proteins. Selinexor is an inhibitor of exportin action, resulting in abnormal nuclear accumulation of, e.g., tumor-suppressor gene products or needed export of other products, e.g., oncogene products. Useful clinical activity has been seen in myeloma and diffuse large B-cell lymphomas including those arising from previously treated indolent lymphomas. Cytopenias, gastrointestinal distress, and hyponatremia are features of its clinical use.

Chromatin-Modifying Agents Gene function is altered not only by mutation of DNA structure, but also by "epigenetic" mechanisms that alter the capacity of DNA to be transcribed or interact with regulatory proteins in the nucleus including transcription factors. Initial epigenetic approaches to modulate gene expression extended from the observation that low concentrations of certain nucleosides (5′azacytidine and decitabine) caused loss of methylated cytosine in DNA, associated with gene silencing, and had clinical activity in causing differentiation of AML cells with notably less toxicity than higher concentrations. 5′Azacytidine and decitabine are misincorporated into DNA and then scavenge DNA methyl transferase to disable DNA methylation of tumor-promoting genes and thus alter their transcription.

Histone deacetylase inhibitors alter the histone protein "packing" density of chromatin and induce global changes in expression of cell cycle regulatory proteins. Vorinostat, belinostat, and romidepsin are useful in cutaneous and peripheral T-cell lymphomas; panobinostat has activity in multiple myeloma. The agents are generally well tolerated but with the potential for cytopenias. The histone methyltransferase inhibitor tazemetostat is a first-in-class inhibitor of histone methyltransferase with unique activity in epithelioid sarcoma owing to its modulation of transcriptional mechanisms unique to that tumor and, recently, in certain follicular lymphomas.

Cancer Cell Metabolism Modulators Oncogenic transformation causes a "rewiring" of cellular metabolism away from oxidative phosphorylation to glycolysis (historically defined as the "Warburg effect" of aerobic glycolysis in animal and human tumors) with attendant tolerance of hypoxia and production of metabolites important for sustaining cell proliferation. Recent clinical studies have defined clinical value from inhibitors of the cell lipid membrane localized phosphoinositide-3 (PI3) kinase and mammalian target of rapamycin (mTOR) (the latter is a kinase whose inhibition was originally discovered as the mechanism by which the immunosuppressant rapamycin, isolated from a soil bacterium, decreased T-cell proliferation). PI3 kinase is activated by numerous oncogenic tyrosine kinases to ultimately cause a cascade of metabolic alterations including increased glucose uptake and activation of mTOR isoforms, which selectively increase translation efficiency of key regulators of cell cycle progression and protein synthetic capacity.

Temsirolimus and everolimus are mTOR inhibitors with activity in renal cancers. They produce stomatitis and fatigue; some hyperlipidemia (10%) and myelosuppression (10%); and rare lung toxicity and immunosuppression in regimens used clinically. Everolimus is also useful in patients with hormone receptor–positive breast cancers displaying resistance to hormonal inhibition and in certain neuroendocrine and brain tumors, the latter arising in patients with sporadic or inherited mutations in the pathway activating mTOR. Isoform-specific PI3 kinase inhibitors are of increasing importance in breast cancers with mutated *PI3Kα* (alpelisib; hyperglycemia and cutaneous eruptions can occur) or owing to selective use of PI3Kδ by lymphoid tissues in lymphomas (idelalisib, copanlisib, and duvelisib).

Isocitrate dehydrogenase (IDH) inhibitors (ivosidenib specific for IDH1 and enasidenib specific for IDH2) have activity in tumors with IDH mutants (AML, cholangiocarcinomas) that generate the "oncometabolite" 2-hydroxyglutarate, which alters DNA and histone methyltransferase activity. The drugs thus function indirectly as epigenetic chromatin modulating agents through effects on cellular metabolism.

DNA Repair Pathway Modulators DNA repair systems act physiologically to lessen the impact of environmental genomic damaging agents and influence the susceptibility to certain chemotherapy agents. DNA repair enzyme mutations underlie inherited cancer susceptibility syndromes such as mutated *BRCA* tumor-suppressor gene–associated breast and ovarian cancers, among others.

Laboratory investigations revealed that poly-ADP ribose polymerase (PARP) acts as a synthetic lethal gene with mutations in the homologous recombination repair pathway, including the *BRCA* gene. PARP responds to detection of DNA lesions by creating chains of poly-ADP, which serve as scaffolds for the localization of DNA repair proteins still active even with mutated *BRCA* isoforms. However, without PARP activity, the scaffolds cannot form, and the DNA damage becomes lethal. This observation immediately suggested the potential utility of PARP inhibitors (e.g., olaparib) as treatments potentially useful for *BRCA*-induced tumors. Recently, PARP inhibitor utility has been extended to tumors that do not harbor *BRCA* mutations but have given evidence of responding to platinum drugs, as a way of extending the useful effect of the chemotherapy treatment. This finding underscores the likelihood that sensitivity to DNA-directed cytotoxic drugs on the part of a tumor is at least in part related to the drugs' ability to take advantage of a sensitizing effect of a tumor's endogenous DNA repair capacity.

Miscellaneous Targeted Therapies The t(15;17) chromosomal translocation is diagnostic of acute promyelocytic leukemia (APL), a subset of AML. The translocation produces a chimeric fusion protein joining the retinoic acid receptor (RAR) α to the transcription factor PML. The abnormal protein, encoding PML-RARα, blocks differentiation of the cancer cells. All-*trans*-retinoic acid (ATRA) binds to the chimeric protein, releasing the block to differentiation inducing response in APL with fewer complications from cytopenias and disordered coagulation seen with cytotoxic agents. Its use can be attended by a "differentiation syndrome" characterized by cytokine release from and organ infiltration by the tumor cells. Pulmonary function can be severely compromised but is generally responsive to glucocorticoids. Increased intracranial pressure can occur from ATRA, and headache should occasion fundoscopic exam.

Arsenic trioxide was found empirically to also be of value in treating APL, and further study revealed that it also modulates PML-RARα levels, along with decreasing the tolerance of APL cells for free radical damage, inducing apoptosis. The combination of arsenic trioxide and ATRA is productive of very high rates of complete remission in APL. Arsenic trioxide can cause lengthening of the QT interval, and careful attention to concomitant medications, Mg^{2+}, ionized Ca^{2+}, and K^+ is necessary during treatment.

The sonic hedgehog transcription factor pathway is regulated by the WNT ligands, which are active during embryonic and fetal life and in certain neoplasms. The sonic hedgehog inhibitors sonidegib and glasdegib are useful in non–surgically treatable cutaneous basal cell carcinomas and certain AMLs, respectively, where the pathway is active.

High-affinity binding to receptors on tumor cells can deliver toxins to tumor cells, exemplified by the IL-3–diphtheria toxin fusion protein tagraxofusp-erzs, targeting the IL-3 receptor (CD123) and useful in blastic plasmacytoid dendritic cell neoplasms. Capillary leak syndrome induced by the toxin component requires careful monitoring of fluid balance to avoid pulmonary dysfunction in particular. Specific receptors for cytokines and growth factors can also serve as "traps" to sequester needed growth factors. Ziv-aflibercept is not an antibody, but a solubilized VEGF receptor VEGF binding domain, and therefore may have a distinct mechanism of action from bevacizumab, but with comparable side effects.

■ SYSTEMIC RADIATION THERAPY

Systemically administered isotopes of iodide have an important role in the treatment of thyroid neoplasms, owing to the selective upregulation of the iodide transporter in the tumor cell compartment. Likewise, isotopes of samarium and radium have been found useful in the palliation of bony metastases of prostate cancer owing to their selective deposition at the tumor-bone matrix interface. Antibody-radioisotope complexes such as Y^{90}-ibritumomab-tiuxetan target CD20, are useful in treating lymphoma, or an isotope can be complexed to a ligand for which the tumor has high affinity. The latter strategy is employed by Lu^{177}-dotatate, where an analog of somatostatin brings the lutetium isotope close to tumors such as somatostatin receptor–positive gastroenteropancreatic neuroendocrine tumors.

RESISTANCE TO CANCER TREATMENTS

Resistance mechanisms to the conventional cytotoxic agents were initially characterized in the late twentieth century as defects in drug uptake, metabolism, or export by tumor cells. The *multidrug resistance* (*MDR*) gene, encoding P-glycoprotein (Pgp), is prototypic of transport proteins that efficiently excrete many drugs from tumor cells; no clinically useful modulator of this process has yet emerged. Drug-metabolizing enzymes such as cytidine deaminase are upregulated in resistant tumor cells, and this is the basis for so-called "high-dose cytarabine" regimens in the treatment of leukemia. Another resistance mechanism defined during this era involved increased expression of a drug's target, exemplified by amplification of the dihydrofolate reductase gene, in patients who had lost responsiveness to methotrexate, or mutation of topoisomerase II in tumors that relapsed after topoisomerase II modulator treatment.

A second class of resistance mechanisms involves loss of the cellular apoptotic mechanism activated after the engagement of a drug's target by the drug. This occurs in a way that is heavily influenced by the biology of the particular tumor type. For example, decreased alkylguanine alkyltransferase expression defines a subset of glioblastoma patients with the prospect of enhanced benefit from treatment with temozolomide but has no value in predicting benefit from temozolomide in epithelial neoplasms. Likewise, ovarian cancers resistant to platinating agents have decreased expression of the proapoptotic gene *BAX*.

A related class of resistance mechanisms emerged from sequencing of the targets of agents directed at oncogenic kinases, revealing mutated targets, as described previously. This relates to the phenomenon of tumor heterogeneity. Tumors harbor distinct populations of subclones that arise during the process of carcinogenesis, sharing to variable degrees mutations that may promote the growth of some subclones, but that are absent or are no longer relevant to the growth of other subclones. Really useful targeted therapies address a target present in all subclones and to which all tumor subclones require for tumor growth.

Finally, other mechanisms of resistance to targeted agents include the upregulation of alternate means of activating the pathway targeted by the agent. Thus, melanomas initially responsive to *BRAF* V600E antagonists such as vemurafenib may reactivate RAF signaling by employing variant isoforms that can bypass the drug. Likewise, inhibition of HER2/neu signaling in breast cancer cells can lead to the emergence of variants with distinct ways of activating downstream effectors such as PI3 kinase.

SUPPORTIVE CARE DURING CANCER TREATMENT

■ MYELOSUPPRESSION

Cytotoxic chemotherapeutic agents almost invariably affect bone marrow function. Titration of this effect determines the tolerated dose of the agent on a given schedule. Polymorphonuclear leukocytes (PMNs; $t_{1/2}$ = 6–8 h), platelets ($t_{1/2}$ = 5–7 days), and red blood cells (RBCs; $t_{1/2}$ = 120 days) have most, less, and least susceptibility, respectively, to usually administered cytotoxic agents. The nadir count of each cell type in response to classes of agents is characteristic. Maximal neutropenia occurs 6–14 days after conventional doses of anthracyclines, antifolates, and antimetabolites. Alkylating agents differ from each other in the timing of cytopenias. Nitrosoureas, DTIC, and procarbazine can display delayed marrow toxicity, first appearing 6 weeks after dosing.

Complications of myelosuppression result from the predictable sequelae of the missing cells' function. *Febrile neutropenia* refers to the clinical presentation of fever and <1500 granulocytes/μL. Management of febrile neutropenia is considered in **Chap. 74**. Transfusion of granulocytes has no role in the management of febrile neutropenia, owing to their exceedingly short half-life, mechanical fragility, and clinical syndromes of pulmonary compromise with leukostasis after their use. Instead, colony-stimulating factors (CSFs) are used to augment bone marrow production of PMNs. The American Society of Clinical Oncology has developed practice guidelines for the use of granulocyte CSF (G-CSF) and GM-CSF (**Table 73-7**).

TABLE 73-7 Indications for the Clinical Use of G-CSF or GM-CSF

Preventive Uses
With the first cycle of chemotherapy (so-called *primary CSF administration*)
Not needed on a routine basis
Use if the probability of febrile neutropenia is ≥20%
Use if patient has preexisting neutropenia or active infection
Age >65 years treated for lymphoma with curative intent or other tumors treated by similar regimens
Poor performance status
Extensive prior chemotherapy
Dose-dense regimens in a clinical trial or with strong evidence of benefit
With subsequent cycles if febrile neutropenia has previously occurred (so-called *secondary CSF administration*)
Not needed after short-duration neutropenia without fever
Use if patient had febrile neutropenia in previous cycle
Use if prolonged neutropenia (even without fever) delays therapy
Therapeutic Uses
Afebrile neutropenic patients
No evidence of benefit
Febrile neutropenic patients
No evidence of benefit
May feel compelled to use in the face of clinical deterioration from sepsis, pneumonia, or fungal infection, but benefit unclear
In bone marrow or peripheral blood stem cell transplantation
Use to mobilize stem cells from marrow
Use to hasten myeloid recovery
In acute myeloid leukemia
G-CSF of minor or no benefit
GM-CSF of no benefit and may be harmful
In myelodysplastic syndromes
Not routinely beneficial
Use intermittently in subset with neutropenia and recurrent infection
What Dose and Schedule Should Be Used?
G-CSF: 5 mg/kg per day subcutaneously
GM-CSF: 250 mg/m^2 per day subcutaneously
Pegfilgrastim: one dose of 6 mg 24 h after chemotherapy
When Should Therapy Begin and End?
When indicated, start 24–72 h after chemotherapy
Continue until absolute neutrophil count is 10,000/μL
Do not use concurrently with chemotherapy or radiation therapy

Abbreviations: CSF, colony-stimulating factor; G-CSF, granulocyte colony-stimulating factor; GM-CSF, granulocyte-macrophage colony-stimulating factor.

Source: From the American Society of Clinical Oncology: J Clin Oncol 24:3187, 2006.

Dangerous degrees of thrombocytopenia do not frequently complicate the management of patients with solid tumors receiving cytotoxic chemotherapy (with the possible exception of certain carboplatin-containing regimens), but they are frequent in patients with certain hematologic neoplasms where marrow is infiltrated with tumor. Severe bleeding related to thrombocytopenia occurs with increased frequency at platelet counts <20,000/μL in patients with acute leukemia and <10,000/μL in patients with solid tumors and is prevalent at counts <5000/μL.

The precise "trigger" point at which to transfuse patients has been defined as a platelet count of 10,000/μL or less in patients without medical comorbidities that may increase the risk of bleeding. This issue is important not only because of the costs of frequent transfusion but also because unnecessary platelet transfusions expose the patient to the risks of allosensitization and loss of value from subsequent transfusion, as well as the infectious and hypersensitivity risks inherent in any transfusion. Prophylactic transfusions to keep platelets >20,000/μL are reasonable in patients with leukemia who are stressed by fever or concomitant medical conditions. Careful review of medication lists to prevent exposure to nonsteroidal anti-inflammatory agents and maintenance of clotting factor levels adequate to support near-normal prothrombin and partial thromboplastin time tests are important in minimizing the risk of bleeding in the thrombocytopenic patient.

Anemia associated with chemotherapy can be managed by transfusion of packed RBCs. Transfusion is not undertaken until the hemoglobin falls to <80 g/L (8 g/dL), compromise of end-organ function occurs, or an underlying condition (e.g., coronary artery disease) calls for maintenance of hemoglobin >90 g/L (9 g/dL). Randomized trials in certain tumors have raised the possibility that erythropoietin (EPO) use may promote tumor cell survival.

NAUSEA AND VOMITING

The most common side effect of chemotherapy administration is nausea, with or without vomiting. Nausea may be acute (within 24 h of chemotherapy), delayed (>24 h), or anticipatory of the receipt of chemotherapy. Highly emetogenic drugs (risk of emesis >90%) include DTIC, cyclophosphamide at >1500 mg/m^2, and cisplatin; moderately emetogenic drugs (30–90% risk) include carboplatin, cytosine arabinoside (>1 g/m^2), ifosfamide, conventional-dose cyclophosphamide, and anthracyclines; low-risk (10–30%) agents include 5-FU, taxanes, etoposide, and bortezomib, with minimal risk (<10%) afforded by treatment with antibodies, bleomycin, busulfan, fludarabine, and vinca alkaloids.

Serotonin antagonists (5-HT_3) and neurokinin 1 (NK1) receptor antagonists are useful in "high-risk" chemotherapy regimens. The combination acts at both peripheral gastrointestinal and CNS sites that control nausea and vomiting. For example, the 5-HT_3 blocker dolasetron, 100 mg intravenously or orally; dexamethasone, 12 mg; and the NK1 antagonist aprepitant, 125 mg orally, are combined on the day of administration of severely emetogenic regimens, with repetition of dexamethasone (8 mg) and aprepitant (80 mg) on days 2 and 3 for delayed nausea. Alternate 5-HT_3 antagonists include ondansetron, given as 0.15 mg/kg intravenously for three doses just before and at 4 and 8 h after chemotherapy; palonosetron at 0.25 mg over 30 s, 30 min before chemotherapy; and granisetron, given as a single dose of 0.01 mg/kg just before chemotherapy. Emesis from moderately emetic chemotherapy regimens may be prevented with a 5-HT_3 antagonist and dexamethasone alone for patients not receiving doxorubicin and cyclophosphamide combinations; the latter combination requires the 5-HT_3/dexamethasone/aprepitant on day 1, but aprepitant alone on days 2 and 3. Emesis from low-emetic-risk regimens may be prevented with 8 mg of dexamethasone alone or with non-5-HT_3, non-NK1 antagonist approaches including the following.

Antidopaminergic phenothiazines act directly at the chemoreceptor trigger zone (CTZ) in the brainstem medulla and include prochlorperazine (Compazine), 10 mg intramuscularly or intravenously, 10–25 mg orally, or 25 mg per rectum every 4–6 h for up to four doses;

and thiethylperazine, 10 mg by potentially all of the above routes every 6 h. Haloperidol is a butyrophenone dopamine antagonist given at 1 mg intramuscularly or orally every 8 h. Metoclopramide acts on peripheral dopamine receptors to augment gastric emptying and is used in high doses for highly emetogenic regimens (1–2 mg/kg intravenously 30 min before chemotherapy and every 2 h for up to three additional doses as needed); intravenous doses of 10–20 mg every 4–6 h as needed or 50 mg orally 4 h before and 8 and 12 h after chemotherapy are used for moderately emetogenic regimens. 5-9-Tetrahydrocannabinol (Marinol) is a rather weak antiemetic compared to other available agents, but it may be useful for persisting nausea and is used orally at 10 mg every 3–4 h as needed. Olanzapine, an "atypical antipsychotic" acting at multiple neurotransmitter receptors, may be of value, most clearly in cases refractory to the measures described above. Some practice guidelines have endorsed its earlier use in adults receiving highly emetogenic chemotherapy regimens in combination with an NK1 antagonist plus an HT3 antagonist plus dexamethasone.

■ DIARRHEA

Similar to the vomiting syndromes, chemotherapy-induced diarrhea may be immediate or can occur in a delayed fashion up to 48–72 h after the drugs. Careful attention to maintained hydration and electrolyte repletion, intravenously if necessary, along with antimotility treatments such as "high-dose" loperamide (4 mg at the first occurrence of diarrhea, with 2 mg repeated every 2 h until 12 h without loose stools, not to exceed a total daily dose of 16 mg), are appropriate. Octreotide (100–150 μg), a somatostatin analogue, or intralumenally acting opiate-based preparations may be considered for patients not responding to loperamide.

■ MUCOSITIS

Irritation and inflammation of the mucous membranes (mucositis) particularly afflicting the oral and anal mucosa, but potentially involving the entire gastrointestinal tract, may accompany cytotoxic chemotherapy. Topical therapies, including anesthetics and barrier-creating preparations, may provide symptomatic relief in mild cases. Palifermin, a keratinocyte growth factor and member of the fibroblast growth factor family, is effective in preventing severe mucositis in the setting of high-dose chemotherapy with stem cell transplantation for hematologic malignancies. It may also prevent or ameliorate mucositis from radiation.

■ ALOPECIA

Chemotherapeutic agents vary widely in causing alopecia, with anthracyclines, alkylating agents, and topoisomerase inhibitors reliably causing near-total alopecia when given at therapeutic doses. Antimetabolites are more variably associated with alopecia. Psychological support and the use of cosmetic resources are to be encouraged. "Chemo caps" that reduce scalp temperature to decrease the degree of alopecia are controversial during treatment with curative intent of neoplasms, such as leukemia or lymphoma, or in adjuvant breast cancer therapy. The richly vascularized scalp can certainly harbor micrometastatic or disseminated disease.

■ GONADAL DYSFUNCTION AND PREGNANCY

All cancer treatments described in this chapter should be regarded as potentially injurious to the developing fetus and to newborns via lactation. However, there are gradations to the degree of reproductive harm. All agents tend to have increased risk of adverse outcomes when administered during the first trimester, and strategies to delay chemotherapy, if possible, until after this milestone should be considered if the pregnancy is to continue to term. Patients in their second or third trimester can be treated with most regimens for the common neoplasms afflicting women in their childbearing years, with the exception of antimetabolites, particularly antifolates, which have notable teratogenic or fetotoxic effects throughout pregnancy. The need for anticancer chemotherapy per se is infrequently a clear basis to recommend termination of a concurrent pregnancy, although each treatment strategy in this circumstance must be tailored to the individual needs of the patient.

Cessation of ovulation and azoospermia reliably result from regimens that contain alkylating agents and topoisomerase poison. The duration of these effects varies with age and sex. Sperm banking before treatment may be considered. Females experience amenorrhea with anovulation after alkylating agent therapy; egg preservation may be considered but may delay inception of urgent treatment. Recovery of normal menses is frequent if treatment is completed before age 30, but patients are unlikely to recover menses after age 35. Even those who regain menses usually experience premature menopause. Because the magnitude and extent of decreased fertility can be difficult to predict, patients should be counseled to maintain effective contraception, preferably by barrier means, during and after therapy. Resumption of efforts to conceive should be considered in the context of the patient's likely prognosis. Hormone replacement therapy should be undertaken in women who do not have a hormonally responsive tumor. For patients who have had a hormone-sensitive tumor primarily treated by a local modality, conventional practice would counsel against hormone replacement, but this issue is under investigation.

■ PALLIATIVE AND SUPPORTIVE CARE

An important perspective the primary care provider may bring to patients and their families facing incurable cancer is that, given the limited value of chemotherapeutic approaches at some point in the natural history of most metastatic cancers, *palliative care* or *hospice-based* approaches, with meticulous and ongoing attention to symptom relief and with family, psychological, and spiritual support, should receive prominent attention as a valuable therapeutic plan (**Chaps. 12** and **69**). Optimizing the quality of life rather than attempting to extend it becomes a valued intervention. Patients facing the impending progression of disease in a life-threatening way frequently choose to undertake toxic treatments of little to no potential value, and support provided by the primary caregiver in accessing palliative and hospice-based options in contrast to receiving toxic and ineffective regimens can be critical in providing a basis for patients to make sensible choices.

Late effects of cancer and its treatment are reviewed in **Chap. 95**.

■ FURTHER READING

Brown N et al: Precision medicine in non-small cell lung cancer: Current standards in pathology and biomarker interpretation. Am Soc Clin Oncol Educ Book 38:708, 2018.

Chan TA et al: Development of tumor mutation burden as an immunotherapy biomarker: Utility for the oncology clinic. Ann Oncol 30:44, 2019.

Forde PM et al: Neoadjuvant PD-1 blockade in resectable lung cancer. N Engl J Med 378:1976, 2018.

Hesketh PJ et al: Antiemetics: American Society of Clinical Oncology clinical practice update. J Clin Oncol 35:3240, 2017.

Neelapu SS et al: Chimeric antigen receptor T-cell therapy: Assessment and management of toxicities. Nat Rev Clin Oncol 15:47, 2018.

Puzanov I et al: Managing toxicities associated with immune checkpoint inhibitors: Consensus recommendations from the Society for Immunotherapy of Cancer (SITC) Toxicity Management Working Group. J Immunother Cancer 5:95, 2017.

Ribas A, Wolchok JD: Cancer immunotherapy using checkpoint blockade. Science 359:1350, 2018.

Yap TA et al: The DNA damaging revolution: PARP inhibitors and beyond. Am Soc Clin Oncol Educ Book 39:185, 2019.

74 Infections in Patients with Cancer

Robert W. Finberg*

Infections are a common cause of death and an even more common cause of morbidity in patients with a wide variety of neoplasms. Infections in cancer patients can result directly from tissue invasion by cancerous cells (either by replacement of healthy host marrow cells or by occlusion of an orifice) **(Table 74-1)** or as a result of treatment. In the era of cytotoxic chemotherapy, neutropenia as a result of chemotherapy was the major cause of infectious complications of cancer therapy. The routine use of granulocyte-stimulating cytokines has, in most cases, shortened the duration of neutropenia, and the increasing use of checkpoint inhibitors and chimeric antigen receptor (CAR) T cells has changed the field of oncology and led to better outcomes. Unfortunately, checkpoint inhibitors and immunomodulators are also associated with an increased risk of infections—particularly intracellular pathogens. An evolving approach to prevention and treatment of infectious complications of cancer has decreased infection-associated mortality rates and will probably continue to do so. This accomplishment has resulted from three major steps:

1. *Early treatment:* The practice of using early empirical antibiotics reduced mortality rates among patients with leukemia and bacteremia from 84% in 1965 to 44% in 1972. The mortality rate due to infection in febrile neutropenic patients dropped to <10% by 2013. This dramatic improvement is attributed to early intervention with appropriate antimicrobial therapy.
2. *Empirical treatment:* "Empirical" antifungal therapy has also lowered the incidence of disseminated fungal infection, with dramatic decreases in mortality rates. An antifungal agent is administered—on the basis of likely fungal infection—to neutropenic patients who, after 4–7 days of antibiotic therapy, remain febrile but have no positive cultures.
3. *Prophylaxis:* Use of antibiotics for afebrile neutropenic patients as broad-spectrum prophylaxis against infections has decreased both mortality and morbidity even further. The current approach to treatment of severely neutropenic patients (e.g., those receiving high-dose chemotherapy for leukemia or high-grade lymphoma) is based on initial prophylactic therapy at the onset of neutropenia, subsequent "empirical" antibacterial therapy targeting the organisms whose involvement is likely in light of physical findings (most often fever alone), and finally "empirical" antifungal therapy based on the known likelihood that fungal infection will become a serious issue after 4–7 days of broad-spectrum antibacterial therapy.

A physical predisposition to infection in patients with cancer (Table 74-1) can be a result of the neoplasm's production of a break in the skin. For example, a squamous cell carcinoma may cause local invasion of the epidermis, which allows bacteria to gain access to subcutaneous tissue and permits the development of cellulitis. The artificial closing of a normally patent orifice can also predispose to infection; for example, obstruction of a ureter by a tumor can cause urinary tract infection, and obstruction of the bile duct can cause cholangitis. Part of the host's normal defense against infection depends on the continuous emptying of a viscus; without emptying, a few bacteria that are present as a result of bacteremia or local transit can multiply and cause disease.

A similar problem can affect patients whose lymph node integrity has been disrupted by radical surgery, particularly patients who have had radical node dissections. A common clinical problem following radical mastectomy is the development of cellulitis (usually caused by streptococci or staphylococci) because of lymphedema and/or inadequate lymph drainage. In most cases, this problem can be addressed by local measures designed to prevent fluid accumulation and breaks in the skin, but antibiotic prophylaxis has been used in refractory cases.

A life-threatening problem common to many cancer patients is the loss of the reticuloendothelial capacity to clear microorganisms after splenectomy, which may be performed as part of the management of hairy cell leukemia, chronic lymphocytic leukemia (CLL), and chronic myelogenous leukemia (CML) as well as Hodgkin's disease. Even after curative therapy for the underlying disease, the lack of a spleen predisposes such patients to rapidly fatal infections. The loss of the spleen through trauma similarly predisposes the normal host to overwhelming infection throughout life. The splenectomized patient should be counseled about the risks of infection with certain organisms, such as the protozoan *Babesia* **(Chap. 225)** and *Capnocytophaga canimorsus*, a bacterium carried in the mouths of animals **(Chaps. 141 and 158)**. Because encapsulated bacteria (*Streptococcus pneumoniae*, *Haemophilus influenzae*, and *Neisseria meningitidis*) are the organisms most commonly associated with postsplenectomy sepsis, splenectomized persons should be vaccinated (and revaccinated; **Table 74-2** and **Chap. 123**) against the capsular polysaccharides of these organisms. Many clinicians recommend giving splenectomized patients a small supply of antibiotics effective against *S. pneumoniae*, *N. meningitidis*, and *H. influenzae* to avert rapid, overwhelming sepsis in the event that they cannot present for medical attention immediately after the onset of fever or other signs or

TABLE 74-1 Disruption of Normal Barriers in Patients with Cancer That May Predispose Them to Infections

TYPE OF DEFENSE	SPECIFIC LESION OR DEFICIENCY	CELLS INVOLVED	ORGANISM	CANCER ASSOCIATION	DISEASE
Physical barrier	Breaks in skin	Skin epithelial cells	Staphylococci, streptococci	Head and neck, squamous cell carcinoma	Cellulitis, extensive skin infection
Emptying of fluid collections	Occlusion of orifices: ureters, bile duct, colon	Luminal epithelial cells	Gram-negative bacilli	Renal, ovarian, biliary tree, metastatic diseases of many cancers	Rapid, overwhelming bacteremia; urinary tract infection
Lymphatic function	Node dissection	Lymph nodes	Staphylococci, streptococci	Breast cancer surgery	Cellulitis
Splenic clearance of microorganisms	Splenectomy	Splenic reticuloendothelial cells	*Streptococcus pneumoniae, Haemophilus influenzae, Neisseria meningitidis, Babesia, Capnocytophaga canimorsus*	Hodgkin's disease, leukemia	Rapid, overwhelming sepsis
Phagocytosis	Lack of granulocytes	Granulocytes (neutrophils)	Staphylococci, streptococci, enteric organisms, fungi	Acute myeloid and acute lymphocytic leukemias, hairy cell leukemia	Bacteremia
Humoral immunity	Lack of antibodies	B cells	*S. pneumoniae, H. influenzae, N. meningitidis*	Chronic lymphocytic leukemia, multiple myeloma	Infections with encapsulated organisms, sinusitis, pneumonia
Cellular immunity	Lack of T cells	T cells and macrophages	*Mycobacterium tuberculosis, Listeria*, herpesviruses, fungi, intracellular parasites	Hodgkin's disease, leukemia, T-cell lymphoma	Infections with intracellular bacteria, fungi, parasites; virus reactivation

*Deceased.

TABLE 74-2 Vaccination of Cancer Patients Receiving Chemotherapy[a]

VACCINE	USE IN INDICATED PATIENTS: INTENSIVE CHEMOTHERAPY	HODGKIN'S DISEASE	HEMATOPOIETIC STEM CELL TRANSPLANTATION
Diphtheria-tetanus-pertussis[b]	Primary series and boosters as necessary	No special recommendation	3 doses given 6–12 months after transplantation
Poliomyelitis[c]	Complete primary series and boosters	No special recommendation	3 doses given 6–12 months after transplantation
Haemophilus influenzae type b conjugate	Primary series and booster for children	Single dose for adults	3 doses given 6–12 months after transplantation (separated by 1 month)
Human papillomavirus (HPV)	HPV vaccine is approved for males and females 9–26 years of age. Check Centers for Disease Control and Prevention (CDC) website (*www.cdc.gov/vaccines*) for updated recommendations.	HPV vaccine is approved for males and females 9–26 years of age. Check CDC website (*www.cdc.gov/vaccines*) for updated recommendations.	HPV vaccine is approved for males and females 9–26 years of age. Check CDC website (*www.cdc.gov/vaccines*) for updated recommendations.
Hepatitis A	As indicated for normal hosts on the basis of occupation and lifestyle	As indicated for normal hosts on the basis of occupation and lifestyle	As indicated for normal hosts on the basis of occupation and lifestyle
Hepatitis B	Same as for normal hosts	As indicated for normal hosts on the basis of occupation and lifestyle	3 doses given 6–12 months after transplantation
Pneumococcal conjugate vaccine (PCV13) Pneumococcal polysaccharide vaccine (PPSV23)[d]	Finish series prior to chemotherapy if possible.	Patients with splenectomy should receive both PCV13 and PPSV23.	Three doses of PCV13, beginning 3–6 months after transplantation, are followed by a dose of PPSV23 at least 8 weeks later. A second PPSV23 dose can be given 5 years later.
Quadrivalent meningococcal vaccine[e]	Should be administered to splenectomized patients and to patients living in endemic areas, including college students in dormitories	Should be administered to splenectomized patients and to patients living in endemic areas, including college students in dormitories. An additional dose can be given after 5 years.	Should be administered to splenectomized patients and to patients living in endemic areas, including college students in dormitories. An additional dose can be given after 5 years.
Meningococcal B vaccine	See above.	See above.	See above (see *www.cdc.gov/vaccines* for updated recommendations).
Influenza	Seasonal immunization	Seasonal immunization	Seasonal immunization (A seasonal dose is recommended and can be given as early as 4 months after transplantation; if given <6 months after transplantation, an additional dose is recommended.)
Measles/mumps/rubella	Contraindicated	Contraindicated during chemotherapy	After 24 months in patients without graft-versus-host disease
Varicella-zoster virus[f]	Zoster recombinant vaccine	Zoster recombinant vaccine	Two-dose zoster recombinant vaccine recommended

[a]The latest recommendations by the Advisory Committee on Immunization Practices and the CDC guidelines can be found at *www.cdc.gov/vaccines*. [b]A single dose of TDaP (tetanus–diphtheria–acellular pertussis), followed by a booster dose of Td (tetanus–diphtheria) every 10 years, is recommended for adults. [c]Live-virus vaccine is contraindicated; inactivated vaccine should be used. [d]Two types of vaccines are used to prevent pneumococcal disease. A conjugate vaccine active against 13 serotypes (13-valent pneumococcal conjugate vaccine, or PCV13) is currently administered in three separate doses to all children. A polysaccharide vaccine active against 23 serotypes (23-valent pneumococcal polysaccharide vaccine, or PPSV23) elicits titers of antibody lower than those achieved with the conjugate vaccine, and immunity may wane more rapidly. Because the ablative chemotherapy given to recipients of hematopoietic stem cell transplants (HSCTs) eradicates immunologic memory, revaccination is recommended for all such patients. Vaccination is much more effective once immunologic reconstitution has occurred; however, because of the need to prevent serious disease, pneumococcal vaccine should be administered 6–12 months after transplantation in most cases. Because PPSV23 includes serotypes not present in PCV13, HSCT recipients should receive a dose of PPSV23 at least 8 weeks after the last dose of PCV13. Although antibody titers from PPSV23 clearly decay, experience with multiple doses of PPSV23 is limited, as are data on the safety, toxicity, or efficacy of such a regimen. For this reason, the CDC currently recommends the administration of one additional dose of PPSV23 at least 5 years after the last dose to immunocompromised patients, including transplant recipients, as well as patients with Hodgkin's disease, multiple myeloma, lymphoma, or generalized malignancies. Beyond this single additional dose, further doses are not recommended at this time. [e]Meningococcal conjugate vaccine (MenACWY) is recommended for adults ≤55 years old, and meningococcal polysaccharide vaccine (MPSV4) is recommended for those ≥56 years old. [f]Varicella vaccine is recommended for children and zoster recombinant vaccine for adults. [g]Contact the manufacturer for more information on use in children with acute lymphocytic leukemia.

symptoms of bacterial infection. A few tablets of amoxicillin/clavulanic acid (or levofloxacin if resistant strains of *S. pneumoniae* are prevalent locally) are a reasonable choice for this purpose.

The level of suspicion of infections with certain organisms depends on the type of cancer diagnosed (**Table 74-3**). Diagnosis of multiple myeloma or CLL should alert the clinician to the possibility of hypogammaglobulinemia. While immunoglobulin replacement therapy can be effective, in most cases, prophylactic antibiotics are a cheaper, more convenient method of eliminating bacterial infections in CLL patients with hypogammaglobulinemia. Patients with acute lymphocytic leukemia (ALL), patients with non-Hodgkin's lymphoma, and all cancer patients treated with high-dose glucocorticoids (or glucocorticoid-containing chemotherapy regimens) should receive antibiotic prophylaxis for *Pneumocystis* infection (Table 74-3) for the duration of their chemotherapy. In addition to exhibiting susceptibility to certain infectious organisms, patients with cancer are likely to manifest their infections in characteristic ways. For example, fever—generally a sign of infection in normal hosts—continues to be a reliable indicator in neutropenic patients. In contrast, patients receiving glucocorticoids and agents that impair T-cell function and cytokine secretion may have serious infections in the absence of fever. Similarly, neutropenic patients commonly present with cellulitis without purulence and with pneumonia without sputum or even x-ray findings (see below).

The use of monoclonal antibodies that target B and T cells as well as drugs that interfere with lymphocyte signal transduction events are associated with reactivation of latent infections. The use of infliximab and other anti-tumor necrosis factor (TNF) antibodies are associated with the development of reactivation tuberculosis. Similarly, the use of the anti-B cell antibody, retuximab, is associated with reactivation of hepatitis B and other latent viruses. Checkpoint inhibitors also predispose individuals to reactivation of intracellular pathogens, and clinicians must be aware of what viruses and other intracellular organisms

TABLE 74-3 Infections Associated with Specific Types of Cancer

CANCER	UNDERLYING IMMUNE ABNORMALITY	ORGANISM(S) CAUSING INFECTION
Multiple myeloma	Hypogammaglobulinemia	*Streptococcus pneumoniae, Haemophilus influenzae, Neisseria meningitidis*
Chronic lymphocytic leukemia	Hypogammaglobulinemia	*S. pneumoniae, H. influenzae, N. meningitidis*
Acute myeloid or lymphocytic leukemia	Granulocytopenia, skin and mucous membrane lesions	Extracellular gram-positive and gram-negative bacteria, fungi
Hodgkin's disease	Abnormal T-cell function	Intracellular pathogens (*Mycobacterium tuberculosis, Listeria, Salmonella, Cryptococcus, Mycobacterium avium*); herpesviruses
Non-Hodgkin's lymphoma and acute lymphocytic leukemia	Glucocorticoid chemotherapy, T- and B-cell dysfunction	*Pneumocystis*
Colon and rectal tumors	Local abnormalities[a]	*Streptococcus bovis* biotype 1 (bacteremia)
Hairy cell leukemia	Abnormal T-cell function	Intracellular pathogens (*M. tuberculosis, Listeria, Cryptococcus, M. avium*)

[a]The reason for this association is not well defined.

(mycobacteria, fungi, etc.) are likely to grow and pose a threat to an individual patient receiving these therapies. Like organ transplant recipients **(Chap. 143)**, patients with latent bacterial disease (like tuberculosis) and latent viral disease (like herpes simplex or zoster) should be carefully monitored for reactivation disease.

SYSTEM-SPECIFIC SYNDROMES

■ SKIN-SPECIFIC SYNDROMES

Skin lesions are common in cancer patients, and the appearance of these lesions may permit the diagnosis of systemic bacterial or fungal infection. While cellulitis caused by skin organisms such as *Streptococcus* or *Staphylococcus* is common, neutropenic patients—that is, those with <500 functional polymorphonuclear leukocytes (PMNs)/μL—and patients with impaired blood or lymphatic drainage may develop infections with unusual organisms. Innocent-looking macules or papules may be the first sign of bacterial or fungal sepsis in immunocompromised patients **(Fig. 74-1)**. In the neutropenic host, a macule progresses rapidly to ecthyma gangrenosum (see **Fig. A1-34**), a usually painless, round, necrotic lesion consisting of a central black or gray-black eschar with surrounding erythema. Ecthyma gangrenosum, which is located in nonpressure areas (as distinguished from necrotic lesions associated with lack of circulation), is often associated with *Pseudomonas aeruginosa* bacteremia **(Chap. 164)** but may be caused by other bacteria.

Candidemia **(Chap. 216)** is also associated with a variety of skin conditions (see **Fig. A1-37**) and commonly presents as a maculopapular rash. Punch biopsy of the skin may be the best method for diagnosis.

Cellulitis, an acute spreading inflammation of the skin, is most often caused by infection with group A *Streptococcus* or *Staphylococcus aureus*, virulent organisms normally found on the skin **(Chap. 129)**. Although cellulitis tends to be circumscribed in normal hosts, it may spread rapidly in neutropenic patients. A tiny break in the skin may lead to spreading cellulitis, which is characterized by pain and erythema; in the affected patients, signs of infection (e.g., purulence) are often lacking. What might be a furuncle in a normal host may require amputation because of uncontrolled infection in a patient presenting with leukemia. A dramatic response to an infection that might be trivial in a normal host can mark the first sign of leukemia. Fortunately, granulocytopenic patients are likely to be infected with certain types of organisms **(Table 74-4)**; thus, the selection of an antibiotic regimen is somewhat easier than it might otherwise be (see "Antibacterial Therapy," below). It is essential to recognize cellulitis early and to treat it aggressively. Patients who are neutropenic or who have previously

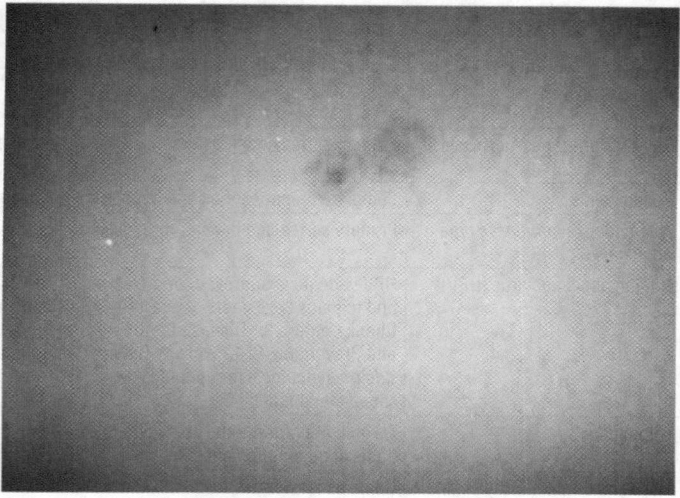

A

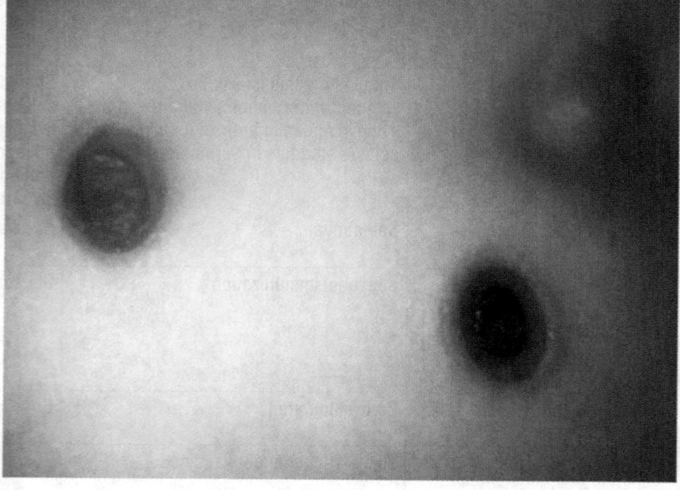

B

FIGURE 74-1 ***A.*** Papules related to *Escherichia coli* bacteremia in a patient with acute lymphocytic leukemia. ***B.*** The same lesions on the following day.

TABLE 74-4 Organisms Likely to Cause Infections in Granulocytopenic Patients

Gram-Positive Cocci	
Staphylococcus epidermidis[a]	*Staphylococcus aureus*
Viridans *Streptococcus*	*Enterococcus faecalis*
Streptococcus pneumoniae	
Gram-Negative Bacilli	
Escherichia coli	*Serratia* spp.
Klebsiella spp.	*Acinetobacter* spp.[a]
Pseudomonas aeruginosa	*Stenotrophomonas* spp.
Enterobacter spp.	*Citrobacter* spp.
Non-*aeruginosa Pseudomonas* spp.[a]	
Gram-Positive Bacilli	
Diphtheroids	JK bacillus[a]
Fungi	
Candida spp.	*Mucor/Rhizopus*
Aspergillus spp.	

[a]Often associated with intravenous catheters.

received antibiotics for other reasons may develop cellulitis with unusual organisms (e.g., *Escherichia coli*, *Pseudomonas*, or fungi). Early treatment, even of innocent-looking lesions, is essential to prevent necrosis and loss of tissue. Debridement to prevent spread may sometimes be necessary early in the course of disease, but it can often be performed after chemotherapy, when the PMN count increases.

Sweet syndrome, or *febrile neutrophilic dermatosis*, was originally described in women with elevated white blood cell (WBC) counts. The disease is characterized by the presence of leukocytes in the lower dermis, with edema of the papillary body. Ironically, this disease now is usually seen in neutropenic patients with cancer, most often in association with acute myeloid leukemia (AML) but also in association with a variety of other malignancies. Sweet syndrome usually presents as red or bluish-red papules or nodules that may coalesce and form sharply bordered plaques (see **Fig. A1-40**). The edema may suggest vesicles, but on palpation, the lesions are solid, and vesicles probably never arise in this disease. The lesions are most common on the face, neck, and arms. On the legs, they may be confused with erythema nodosum (see **Fig. A1-39**). The development of lesions is often accompanied by high fevers and an elevated erythrocyte sedimentation rate. Both the lesions and the temperature elevation respond dramatically to glucocorticoid administration. Treatment begins with high doses of glucocorticoids (prednisone, 60 mg/d) followed by tapered doses over the next 2–3 weeks.

Data indicate that *erythema multiforme* (see **Fig. A1-24**) with mucous membrane involvement is often associated with herpes simplex virus (HSV) infection and is distinct from Stevens-Johnson syndrome, which is associated with drugs and tends to have a more widespread distribution. Because cancer patients are both immunosuppressed (and therefore susceptible to herpes infections) and heavily treated with drugs (and therefore subject to Stevens-Johnson syndrome [see **Fig. A3-4**]), both of these conditions are common in this population.

Cytokines, which are used as adjuvants or primary treatments for cancer, can themselves cause characteristic rashes, further complicating the differential diagnosis. This phenomenon is a particular problem in bone marrow (stem cell) transplant recipients (**Chap. 143**), who, in addition to having the usual chemotherapy-, antibiotic-, and cytokine-induced rashes, are plagued by graft-versus-host disease.

■ CATHETER-RELATED INFECTIONS

Because intravenous (IV) catheters are commonly used in cancer chemotherapy and are prone to cause infection (**Chap. 142**), they pose a major problem in the care of patients with cancer. Some catheter-associated infections can be treated with antibiotics, whereas in others, the catheter must be removed (**Table 74-5**). If the patient has a "tunneled" catheter (which consists of an entrance site, a subcutaneous tunnel, and an exit site), a red streak over the subcutaneous part of the line (the tunnel) is grounds for immediate device removal. Failure to remove catheters under these circumstances may result in extensive cellulitis and tissue necrosis.

More common than tunnel infections are exit-site infections, often with erythema around the area where the line penetrates the skin. Most authorities (**Chap. 147**) recommend treatment (usually with vancomycin) for an exit-site infection caused by coagulase-negative *Staphylococcus*. Treatment of coagulase-positive staphylococcal infection is associated with a poorer outcome, and it is advisable to remove the catheter if possible. Similarly, most clinicians remove catheters associated with infections due to *P. aeruginosa* and *Candida* species, because such infections are difficult to treat and bloodstream infections with these organisms are likely to be deadly. Catheter infections caused by *Burkholderia cepacia*, *Stenotrophomonas* species, *Agrobacterium* species, *Acinetobacter baumannii*, *Pseudomonas* species other than *aeruginosa*, and carbapenem-resistant Enterobacteriaceae are likely to be very difficult to eradicate with antibiotics alone. Similarly, isolation of *Bacillus*, *Corynebacterium*, and *Mycobacterium* species should prompt removal of the catheter.

■ GASTROINTESTINAL TRACT–SPECIFIC SYNDROMES

Upper Gastrointestinal Tract Disease • INFECTIONS OF THE MOUTH The oral cavity is rich in aerobic and anaerobic bacteria (**Chap. 177**) that normally live in a commensal relationship with the host. The antimetabolic effects of chemotherapy cause a breakdown of mucosal host defenses, leading to ulceration of the mouth and the potential for invasion by resident bacteria. Mouth ulcerations afflict most patients receiving cytotoxic chemotherapy and have been associated with viridans streptococcal bacteremia. *Candida* infections of the mouth are very common. Fluconazole is clearly effective in the treatment of both local infections (thrush) and systemic infections (esophagitis) due to *Candida albicans*. Other azoles (e.g., voriconazole) as well as echinocandins offer similar efficacy as well as activity against the fluconazole-resistant organisms that are associated with chronic fluconazole treatment (**Chap. 216**).

Noma (*cancrum oris*), commonly seen in malnourished children, is a penetrating disease of the soft and hard tissues of the mouth and adjacent sites, with resulting necrosis and gangrene. It has a counterpart in immunocompromised patients and is thought to be due to invasion of the tissues by *Bacteroides*, *Fusobacterium*, and other normal inhabitants of the mouth. Noma is associated with debility, poor oral hygiene, and immunosuppression.

TABLE 74-5 Approach to Catheter Infections in Immunocompromised Patients

CLINICAL PRESENTATION OR ISOLATED PATHOGEN	CATHETER REMOVAL	ANTIBIOTICS	COMMENTS
Evidence of Infection, Negative Blood Cultures			
Exit-site erythema	Not necessary if infection responds to treatment	Usually, begin treatment for gram-positive cocci.	Coagulase-negative staphylococci are most common.
Tunnel-site erythema	Required	Treat for gram-positive cocci pending culture results.	Failure to remove the catheter may lead to necrosis of the involved area requiring skin grafts in the future.
Blood Culture–Positive Infections			
Coagulase-negative staphylococci	Line removal optimal but may be unnecessary if patient is clinically stable and responds to antibiotics	Usually, start with vancomycin. Linezolid, quinupristin/dalfopristin, and daptomycin are alternative agents.	If there are no contraindications to line removal, this course of action is optimal. If the line is removed, antibiotics may not be necessary.
Other gram-positive cocci (e.g., *Staphylococcus aureus*, *Enterococcus*); gram-positive rods (*Bacillus*, *Corynebacterium* spp.)	Recommended	Treat with antibiotics to which the organism is sensitive, with duration based on the clinical setting.	The incidence of metastatic infections following *S. aureus* infection and the difficulty of treating enterococcal infection make line removal the recommended course of action. In addition, gram-positive rods do not respond readily to antibiotics alone.
Gram-negative bacteria	Recommended	Use an agent to which the organism is shown to be sensitive.	Organisms like *Stenotrophomonas*, *Pseudomonas*, and *Burkholderia* are notoriously hard to treat, as are carbapenem-resistant organisms.
Fungi	Recommended	—	Fungal infections of catheters are extremely difficult to treat.

Viruses, particularly HSV, are a prominent cause of morbidity in immunocompromised patients, in whom they are associated with severe mucositis. The use of acyclovir, either prophylactically or therapeutically, is of value.

ESOPHAGEAL INFECTIONS The differential diagnosis of esophagitis (usually presenting as substernal chest pain upon swallowing) includes herpes simplex and candidiasis, both of which are readily treatable.

Lower Gastrointestinal Tract Disease Hepatic candidiasis (**Chap. 216**) results from seeding of the liver (usually from a gastrointestinal source) in neutropenic patients. It is most common among patients being treated for AML and usually presents symptomatically around the time neutropenia resolves. The characteristic picture is that of persistent fever unresponsive to antibiotics, abdominal pain and tenderness or nausea, and elevated serum levels of alkaline phosphatase in a patient with hematologic malignancy who has recently recovered from neutropenia. The diagnosis of this disease (which may present in an indolent manner and persist for several months) is based on the finding of yeasts or pseudohyphae in granulomatous lesions. Hepatic ultrasound or CT may reveal bull's-eye lesions. MRI scans reveal small lesions not visible by other imaging modalities. The pathology (a granulomatous response) and the timing (with resolution of neutropenia and an elevation in granulocyte count) suggest that the host response to *Candida* is an important component of the manifestations of disease. In many cases, although organisms are visible, cultures of biopsied material may be negative. The designation *hepatosplenic candidiasis* or *hepatic candidiasis* is a misnomer because the disease often involves the kidneys and other tissues; the term *chronic disseminated candidiasis* may be more appropriate. Because of the risk of bleeding with liver biopsy, diagnosis is often based on imaging studies (MRI, CT). Treatment should be directed to the causative agent (usually *C. albicans* but sometimes *Candida tropicalis* or other less common *Candida* species).

Typhlitis *Typhlitis* (also referred to as necrotizing colitis, neutropenic colitis, necrotizing enteropathy, ileocecal syndrome, and cecitis) is a clinical syndrome of fever and right-lower-quadrant (or generalized abdominal) tenderness in an immunosuppressed host. This syndrome is classically seen in neutropenic patients after chemotherapy with cytotoxic drugs. It may be more common among children than among adults and appears to be much more common among patients with AML or ALL than among those with other types of cancer. Physical examination reveals right-lower-quadrant tenderness, with or without rebound tenderness. Associated diarrhea (often bloody) is common, and the diagnosis can be confirmed by the finding of a thickened cecal wall on CT, MRI, or ultrasonography. Plain films may reveal a right-lower-quadrant mass, but CT with contrast or MRI is a much more sensitive means of diagnosis. Although surgery is sometimes attempted to avoid perforation from ischemia, most cases resolve with medical therapy alone. The disease is sometimes associated with positive blood cultures (which usually yield aerobic gram-negative bacilli), and therapy is recommended for a broad spectrum of bacteria (particularly gram-negative bacilli, which are likely to be found in the bowel flora).

***Clostridioides difficile*–Induced Diarrhea** Patients with cancer are predisposed to the development of *C. difficile* diarrhea (**Chap. 134**) as a consequence of chemotherapy alone. Thus, they may test positive for *C. difficile* even without receiving antibiotics. Obviously, such patients are also subject to *C. difficile*–induced diarrhea as a result of antibiotic pressure. *C. difficile* should always be considered as a possible cause of diarrhea in cancer patients who have received either chemotherapy or antibiotics. New approaches to treat *C. difficile*–induced diarrhea and to prevent *C. difficile* expansion as part of the gut microbiota may make this disease less troublesome in the future.

CENTRAL NERVOUS SYSTEM–SPECIFIC SYNDROMES

Meningitis The presentation of meningitis in patients with lymphoma or CLL and in patients receiving chemotherapy (particularly with glucocorticoids) for solid tumors suggests a diagnosis of cryptococcal or listerial infection. As noted previously, splenectomized patients are susceptible to rapid, overwhelming infection with encapsulated bacteria (including *S. pneumoniae*, *H. influenzae*, and *N. meningitidis*). Similarly, patients who are antibody-deficient (e.g., those with CLL, those who have received intensive chemotherapy, or those who have undergone bone marrow [stem cell] transplantation) are likely to have infections caused by these bacteria. Other cancer patients, however, because of their defective cellular immunity, are likely to be infected with other pathogens (Table 74-3). Central nervous system (CNS) tuberculosis should be considered, especially in patients from countries where tuberculosis is highly prevalent in the population.

Encephalitis The spectrum of disease resulting from viral encephalitis is expanded in immunocompromised patients. A predisposition to infections with intracellular organisms similar to those encountered in patients with AIDS (**Chap. 202**) is seen in cancer patients receiving (1) high-dose cytotoxic chemotherapy, (2) chemotherapy affecting T-cell function (e.g., fludarabine), or (3) antibodies that eliminate T cells (e.g., anti-CD3, alemtuzumab, anti-CD52) or cytokine activity (anti–tumor necrosis factor agents or interleukin 1 receptor antagonists). Infection with varicella-zoster virus (VZV) has been associated with encephalitis that may be caused by VZV-related vasculitis. Chronic viral infections may also be associated with dementia and encephalitic presentations. A diagnosis of progressive multifocal leukoencephalopathy (**Chap. 138**) should be considered when a patient who has received chemotherapy (rituximab in particular) presents with dementia (**Table 74-6**). Other abnormalities of the CNS that may be confused with infection include normal-pressure hydrocephalus and vasculitis resulting from CNS irradiation. It may be possible to differentiate these conditions by MRI.

Brain Masses Mass lesions of the brain most often present as headache with or without fever or neurologic abnormalities. Infections associated with mass lesions may be caused by bacteria (particularly *Nocardia*), fungi (particularly *Cryptococcus* or *Aspergillus*), or parasites (*Toxoplasma*). Epstein-Barr virus (EBV)–associated lymphoma may also present as single—or sometimes multiple—mass lesions of the brain. A biopsy may be required for a definitive diagnosis.

PULMONARY INFECTIONS

Pneumonia (**Chap. 126**) in immunocompromised patients may be difficult to diagnose because conventional methods of diagnosis depend on the presence of neutrophils. Bacterial pneumonia in neutropenic patients may present without purulent sputum—or, in fact, without any sputum at all—and may not produce physical findings suggestive of chest consolidation (rales or egophony).

In granulocytopenic patients with persistent or recurrent fever, the chest x-ray pattern may help to localize an infection and thus to determine which investigative tests and procedures should be undertaken and which therapeutic options should be considered (**Table 74-7**). In this setting, a simple chest x-ray is a screening tool; because the impaired host response results in less evidence of consolidation or infiltration, high-resolution CT is recommended for the diagnosis of pulmonary infections. The difficulties encountered in the management of pulmonary infiltrates relate in part to the difficulties of performing diagnostic

TABLE 74-6 Differential Diagnosis of Central Nervous System Infections in Patients with Cancer

	UNDERLYING PREDISPOSITION	
FINDINGS ON CT OR MRI	**PROLONGED NEUTROPENIA**	**DEFECTS IN CELLULAR IMMUNITY**[a]
Mass lesions	*Aspergillus*, *Nocardia*, or *Cryptococcus* brain abscess	Toxoplasmosis, Epstein-Barr virus lymphoma (rare)
Diffuse encephalitis	Progressive multifocal leukoencephalopathy (JC virus)	Infection with varicella-zoster virus, cytomegalovirus, herpes simplex virus, human herpesvirus type 6, JC virus, *Listeria*

[a]High-dose glucocorticoid therapy, cytotoxic chemotherapy.

TABLE 74-7 Differential Diagnosis of Chest Infiltrates in Immunocompromised Patients

	CAUSE OF PNEUMONIA	
INFILTRATE	**INFECTIOUS**	**NONINFECTIOUS**
Localized	Bacteria (including *Legionella*, mycobacteria)	Local hemorrhage or embolism, tumor
Nodular	Fungi (e.g., *Aspergillus* or *Mucor*), *Nocardia*	Recurrent tumor
Diffuse	Viruses (especially cytomegalovirus), *Chlamydia, Pneumocystis, Toxoplasma gondii*, mycobacteria	Congestive heart failure, radiation pneumonitis, drug-induced lung injury, lymphangitic spread of cancer

procedures on the patients involved. When platelet counts can be increased to adequate levels by transfusion, microscopic and microbiologic evaluation of the fluid obtained by endoscopic bronchial lavage is often diagnostic. Lavage fluid should be cultured for *Mycoplasma, Chlamydia, Legionella, Nocardia*, more common bacterial pathogens, fungi, and viruses. In addition, the possibility of *Pneumocystis* pneumonia should be considered, especially in patients with ALL or lymphoma who have not received prophylactic trimethoprim-sulfamethoxazole (TMP-SMX). The characteristics of the infiltrate may be helpful in decisions about further diagnostic and therapeutic maneuvers. Nodular infiltrates suggest fungal pneumonia (e.g., that caused by *Aspergillus* or *Mucor*). Such lesions may best be approached by visualized biopsy procedures. It is worth noting that while bacterial pneumonias classically present as lobar infiltrates in normal hosts, bacterial pneumonias in granulocytopenic hosts present with a paucity of signs, symptoms, or radiographic abnormalities; thus, the diagnosis is difficult.

Aspergillus species **(Chap. 217)** can colonize the skin and respiratory tract or cause fatal systemic illness. Although this fungus may cause aspergillomas in a previously existing cavity or may produce allergic bronchopulmonary disease in some patients, the major problem posed by this genus in neutropenic patients is invasive disease, primarily due to *Aspergillus fumigatus* or *Aspergillus flavus*. The organisms enter the host following colonization of the respiratory tract, with subsequent invasion of blood vessels. The disease is likely to present as a thrombotic or embolic event because of this ability of the fungi to invade blood vessels. The risk of infection with *Aspergillus* correlates directly with the duration of neutropenia. In prolonged neutropenia, positive surveillance cultures for nasopharyngeal colonization with *Aspergillus* may predict the development of disease.

Patients with *Aspergillus* infection often present with pleuritic chest pain and fever, which are sometimes accompanied by cough. Hemoptysis may be an ominous sign. Chest x-rays may reveal new focal infiltrates or nodules. Chest CT may reveal a characteristic halo consisting of a mass-like infiltrate surrounded by an area of low attenuation. The presence of a "crescent sign" on chest x-ray or chest CT, in which the mass progresses to central cavitation, is characteristic of invasive *Aspergillus* infection but may develop as the lesions are resolving.

In addition to causing pulmonary disease, *Aspergillus* may invade through the nose or palate, with deep sinus penetration. The appearance of a discolored area in the nasal passages or on the hard palate should prompt a search for invasive *Aspergillus*. This situation is likely to require surgical debridement. Catheter infections with *Aspergillus* usually require both removal of the catheter and antifungal therapy. Antifungal prophylaxis has led to the emergence of non-fumigatus *Aspergillus* species as well as Mucorales and *Scedosporium/Lomentospora* spp. **(Chaps. 217–219)**.

Diffuse interstitial infiltrates suggest viral, parasitic, or *Pneumocystis* pneumonia. If the patient has a diffuse interstitial pattern on chest x-ray, it may be reasonable, while considering invasive diagnostic procedures, to institute empirical treatment for *Pneumocystis* with TMP-SMX and for *Chlamydia, Mycoplasma*, and *Legionella* with a quinolone or azithromycin. Noninvasive procedures, such as staining of induced sputum smears for *Pneumocystis*, serum cryptococcal antigen tests, and urine testing for *Legionella* antigen, may be helpful. Serum galactomannan and β-D-glucan tests may be of value in diagnosing *Aspergillus* infection, but their utility is limited by their lack of sensitivity and specificity. The presence of an elevated level of β-D-glucan in the serum of a patient being treated for cancer who is not receiving prophylaxis against *Pneumocystis* suggests the diagnosis of *Pneumocystis* pneumonia. Infections with viruses that cause only upper respiratory symptoms in immunocompetent hosts, such as respiratory syncytial virus (RSV), influenza viruses, and parainfluenza viruses, may be associated with fatal pneumonitis in immunocompromised hosts. CMV reactivation occurs in cancer patients receiving chemotherapy, but CMV pneumonia is most common among hematopoietic stem cell transplant (HSCT) recipients **(Chap. 143)**. Polymerase chain reaction testing now allows rapid diagnosis of viral pneumonia, which can lead to treatment in some cases (e.g., influenza). Multiplex studies that can detect a wide array of viruses in the lung and upper respiratory tract are now available and will lead to specific diagnoses of viral pneumonias.

Bleomycin is the most common cause of chemotherapy-induced lung disease. Other causes include alkylating agents (such as cyclophosphamide, chlorambucil, and melphalan), nitrosoureas (carmustine [BCNU], lomustine [CCNU], and methyl-CCNU), busulfan, procarbazine, methotrexate, and hydroxyurea. Both infectious and noninfectious (drug- and/or radiation-induced) pneumonitis can cause fever and abnormalities on chest x-ray; thus, the differential diagnosis of an infiltrate in a patient receiving chemotherapy encompasses a broad range of conditions (Table 74-7). The treatment of radiation pneumonitis (which may respond dramatically to glucocorticoids) or drug-induced pneumonitis is different from that of infectious pneumonia, and a biopsy may be important in the diagnosis. Unfortunately, no definitive diagnosis can be made in ~30% of cases, even after bronchoscopy.

Open-lung biopsy is the gold standard of diagnostic techniques. Biopsy via a visualized thoracostomy can replace an open procedure in many cases. When a biopsy cannot be performed, empirical treatment can be undertaken; a quinolone or an erythromycin derivative (azithromycin) and TMP-SMX are used in the case of diffuse infiltrates, and an antifungal agent is administered in the case of nodular infiltrates. The risks should be weighed carefully in these cases. If inappropriate drugs are administered, empirical treatment may prove toxic or ineffective; either of these outcomes may be riskier than biopsy.

CARDIOVASCULAR INFECTIONS

Patients with Hodgkin's disease are prone to persistent infections by *Salmonella*, sometimes (and particularly often in elderly patients) affecting a vascular site. The use of IV catheters deliberately lodged in the right atrium is associated with a high incidence of bacterial endocarditis, presumably related to valve damage followed by bacteremia. Nonbacterial thrombotic endocarditis (marantic endocarditis) has been described in association with a variety of malignancies (most often solid tumors) and may follow bone marrow (stem cell) transplantation as well. The presentation of an embolic event with a new cardiac murmur suggests this diagnosis. Blood cultures are negative in this disease of unknown pathogenesis. Infective endocarditis can be a complication of cancer treatment because of the use of IV catheters that lead to bacterial infection. In addition, patients may present with infective endocarditis as an initial presentation of cancer, particularly in the case of gastrointestinal or genitourinary sources.

ENDOCRINE SYNDROMES

Infections of the endocrine system have been described in immunocompromised patients. *Candida* infection of the thyroid may be difficult to diagnose during the neutropenic period. It can be defined by indium-labeled WBC scans or gallium scans after neutrophil counts increase. CMV infection can cause adrenalitis with or without resulting adrenal insufficiency. The presentation of a sudden endocrine anomaly in an immunocompromised patient can be a sign of infection in the involved end organ.

MUSCULOSKELETAL INFECTIONS

Infection that is a consequence of vascular compromise, resulting in gangrene, can occur when a tumor restricts the blood supply to muscles, bones, or joints. The process of diagnosis and treatment of such infection is similar to that in normal hosts, with the following caveats:

1. *In terms of diagnosis*, a lack of physical findings resulting from a lack of granulocytes in the granulocytopenic patient should make the clinician more aggressive in obtaining tissue rather than more willing to rely on physical signs.
2. *In terms of therapy*, aggressive debridement of infected tissues may be required. However, it is usually difficult to operate on patients who have recently received chemotherapy, both because of a lack of platelets (which results in bleeding complications) and because of a lack of WBCs (which may lead to secondary infection). A blood culture positive for *Clostridium perfringens*—an organism commonly associated with gas gangrene—can have a number of meanings **(Chap. 154)**. *Clostridium septicum* bacteremia is associated with the presence of an underlying malignancy. Bloodstream infections with intestinal organisms such as *Streptococcus bovis* biotype 1 and *C. perfringens* may arise spontaneously from lower gastrointestinal lesions (tumor or polyps); alternatively, these lesions may be harbingers of invasive disease. The clinical setting must be considered in order to define the appropriate treatment for each case.

■ RENAL AND URETERAL INFECTIONS

Infections of the urinary tract are common among patients whose ureteral excretion is compromised (Table 74-1). *Candida*, which has a predilection for the kidney, can invade either from the bloodstream or in a retrograde manner (via the ureters or bladder) in immunocompromised patients. The presence of "fungus balls" or persistent candiduria suggests invasive disease. Persistent funguria (with *Aspergillus* as well as *Candida*) should prompt a search for a nidus of infection in the kidney.

Certain viruses are typically seen only in immunosuppressed patients. BK virus (polyomavirus hominis 1) has been documented in the urine of bone marrow transplant recipients and, like adenovirus, may be associated with hemorrhagic cystitis.

ABNORMALITIES THAT PREDISPOSE TO INFECTION

(Table 74-1)

■ THE LYMPHOID SYSTEM

It is beyond the scope of this chapter to detail how all the immunologic abnormalities that result from cancer or from chemotherapy for cancer lead to infections. Disorders of the immune system are discussed in other sections of this book. As has been noted, patients with antibody deficiency are predisposed to overwhelming infection with encapsulated bacteria (including *S. pneumoniae*, *H. influenzae*, and *N. meningitidis*). Infections that result from the lack of a functional cellular immune system are described in **Chap. 202**. It is worth mentioning, however, that patients undergoing intensive chemotherapy for any form of cancer will have not only defects due to granulocytopenia but also lymphocyte dysfunction, which may be profound. Thus, these patients—especially those receiving glucocorticoid-containing regimens or drugs that inhibit either T-cell activation (calcineurin inhibitors or drugs like fludarabine, which affect lymphocyte function) or cytokine induction—should be given prophylaxis for *Pneumocystis* pneumonia.

Patients receiving treatment that eliminates B cells (e.g., with anti-CD20 antibodies or rituximab) are especially vulnerable to intercurrent viral infections. The incidence of progressive multifocal leukoencephalopathy (caused by JC virus) is elevated among these patients.

■ THE HEMATOPOIETIC SYSTEM

Initial studies in the 1960s revealed a dramatic increase in the incidence of infections (fatal and nonfatal) among cancer patients with a granulocyte count of <500/μL. The use of prophylactic antibacterial agents has reduced the number of bacterial infections, but 35–78% of febrile neutropenic patients being treated for hematologic malignancies develop infections at some time during chemotherapy. Aerobic pathogens (both gram-positive and gram-negative) predominate in all series, but the exact organisms isolated vary from center to center. Infections with anaerobic organisms are uncommon. Geographic patterns affect the types of fungi isolated. Tuberculosis and malaria are common causes of fever in the developing world and may present in this setting as well.

Neutropenic patients are unusually susceptible to infection with a wide variety of bacteria; thus, antibiotic therapy should be initiated promptly to cover likely pathogens if infection is suspected. Indeed, early initiation of antibacterial agents is mandatory to prevent deaths. Like most immunocompromised patients, neutropenic patients are threatened by their own microbial flora, including gram-positive and gram-negative organisms found commonly on the skin and mucous membranes and in the bowel (Table 74-4). Because treatment with narrow-spectrum agents leads to infection with organisms not covered by the antibiotics used, the initial regimen should target all pathogens likely to be the initial causes of bacterial infection in neutropenic hosts. Studies performed in the 1970s suggested that administration of antimicrobial agents should be continued until neutropenia resolves—that is, the granulocyte count is sustained above 500/μL for at least 2 days. Recent studies have indicated that it is reasonable to stop antibiotics in patients who are afebrile and stable after 72 hours of treatment **(Fig. 74-2)**. Fever may not resolve prior to granulocyte recovery. In some cases, patients remain febrile after resolution of neutropenia. In these instances, the risk of sudden death from overwhelming bacteremia is greatly reduced, and the following diagnoses should be seriously considered: (1) fungal infection, (2) bacterial abscesses or undrained foci of infection, and (3) drug fever (including reactions to antimicrobial agents as well as to chemotherapy or cytokines). In the proper setting, viral infection or graft-versus-host disease should be considered. In clinical practice, antibacterial therapy is usually discontinued when the patient is no longer neutropenic and all evidence of bacterial disease has been eliminated. Antifungal agents are then discontinued if there is no evidence of fungal disease. If the patient remains febrile, a search for viral diseases or unusual pathogens is conducted while unnecessary cytokines and other drugs are systematically eliminated from the regimen.

TREATMENT

Infections in Cancer Patients

ANTIBACTERIAL THERAPY

Hundreds of antibacterial regimens have been tested for use in patients with cancer. The major risk of infection is related to the degree of neutropenia seen as a consequence of either the disease or the therapy. Many of the relevant studies have involved small populations in which the outcomes have generally been good, and most have lacked the statistical power to detect differences among the regimens studied. Each febrile neutropenic patient should be approached as a unique problem, with particular attention given to previous infections and recent antibiotic exposures. Several general guidelines are useful in the initial treatment of neutropenic patients with fever (Fig. 74-2):

1. In the initial regimen, it is necessary to use antibiotics active against both gram-negative and gram-positive bacteria (Table 74-4).
2. Monotherapy with an aminoglycoside or an antibiotic lacking good activity against gram-positive organisms (e.g., ciprofloxacin or aztreonam) is not adequate in this setting.
3. The agents used should reflect both the epidemiology and the antibiotic resistance pattern of the hospital.
4. If the pattern of resistance justifies its use, a single third-generation cephalosporin constitutes an appropriate initial regimen in many hospitals.
5. Most standard regimens are designed for patients who have not previously received prophylactic antibiotics. The development of fever in a patient who has received antibiotics affects the choice of subsequent therapy, which should target resistant organisms and organisms known to cause infections in patients being treated with the antibiotics already administered.

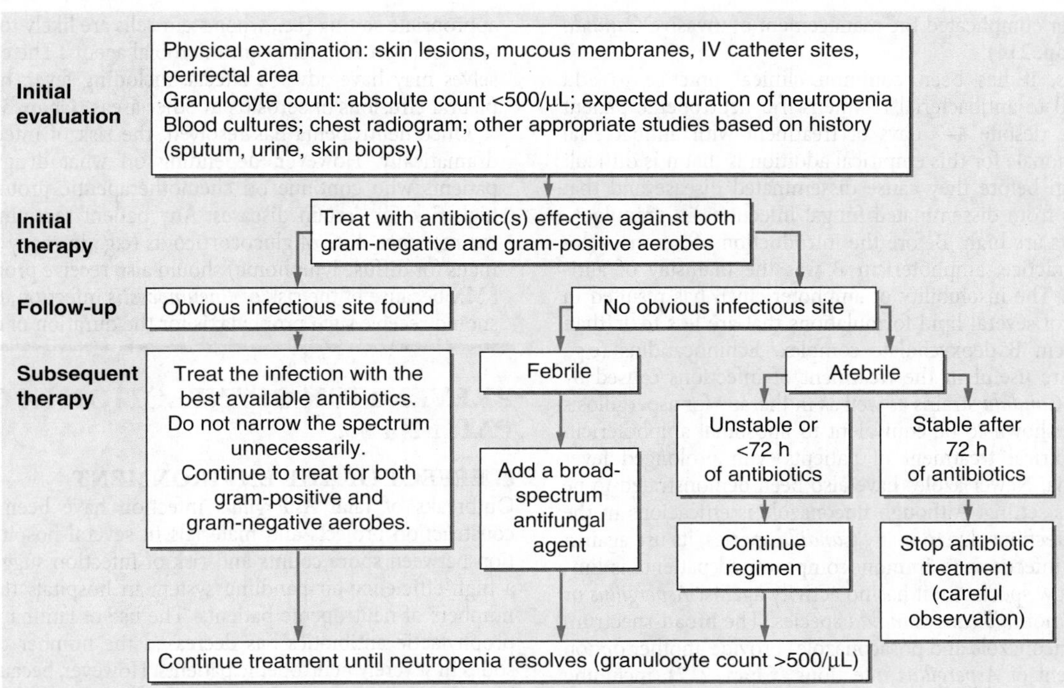
Initial evaluation
Physical examination: skin lesions, mucous membranes, IV catheter sites, perirectal area
Granulocyte count: absolute count <500/μL; expected duration of neutropenia
Blood cultures; chest radiogram; other appropriate studies based on history (sputum, urine, skin biopsy)
Initial therapy
Treat with antibiotic(s) effective against both gram-negative and gram-positive aerobes
Follow-up
Obvious infectious site found
No obvious infectious site
Subsequent therapy
Treat the infection with the best available antibiotics. Do not narrow the spectrum unnecessarily. Continue to treat for both gram-positive and gram-negative aerobes.
Febrile
Afebrile
Add a broad-spectrum antifungal agent
Unstable or <72 h of antibiotics
Stable after 72 h of antibiotics
Continue regimen
Stop antibiotic treatment (careful observation)
Continue treatment until neutropenia resolves (granulocyte count >500/μL)

FIGURE 74-2 Algorithm for the diagnosis and treatment of fever and neutropenia.

6. Randomized trials have indicated the safety of oral antibiotic regimens in the treatment of "low-risk" patients with fever and neutropenia. Outpatients who are expected to remain neutropenic for <10 days and who do not have concurrent medical problems (such as hypotension, pulmonary compromise, or abdominal pain) can be classified as low risk and treated with a broad-spectrum oral regimen.
7. Several large-scale studies indicate that prophylaxis with a fluoroquinolone (ciprofloxacin or levofloxacin) decreases morbidity and mortality rates among afebrile patients who are anticipated to have neutropenia of long duration.

Commonly used antibiotic regimens for the treatment of febrile patients in whom prolonged neutropenia (>7 days) is anticipated include (1) ceftazidime or cefepime, (2) piperacillin/tazobactam, or (3) imipenem/cilastatin or meropenem. All three regimens have shown equal efficacy in large trials. All three are active against *P. aeruginosa* and a broad spectrum of aerobic gram-positive and gram-negative organisms. Imipenem/cilastatin has been associated with an elevated rate of *C. difficile* diarrhea, and many centers reserve carbapenem antibiotics for treatment of gram-negative bacteria that produce extended-spectrum β-lactamases; these limitations make carbapenems less attractive as an initial regimen. Despite the frequent involvement of coagulase-negative staphylococci, the initial use of vancomycin or its automatic addition to the initial regimen has not resulted in improved outcomes, and the antibiotic does exert toxic effects. For these reasons, only judicious use of vancomycin is recommended—for example, when there is good reason to suspect the involvement of coagulase-negative staphylococci (e.g., the appearance of erythema at the exit site of a catheter or a positive culture for methicillin-resistant *S. aureus* or coagulase-negative staphylococci). Because the sensitivities of bacteria vary from hospital to hospital, clinicians are advised to check their local sensitivities and to be aware that resistance patterns can change quickly, necessitating a change in the approach to patients with fever and neutropenia. Similarly, infection control services should monitor for basic antibiotic resistance and for fungal infections. The appearance of a large number of *Aspergillus* infections, in particular, suggests the possibility of an environmental source that requires further investigation and remediation.

The initial antibacterial regimen should be refined on the basis of culture results (Fig. 74-2). Blood cultures are the most relevant basis for selection of therapy; surface cultures of skin and mucous membranes may be misleading. In the case of gram-positive bacteremia or another gram-positive infection, it is important that the antibiotic be optimal for the organism isolated. Once treatment with broad-spectrum antibiotics has begun, it is not desirable to discontinue all antibiotics because of the risk of failing to treat a potentially fatal bacterial infection; the addition of more and more antibacterial agents to the regimen is not appropriate unless there is a clinical or microbiologic reason to do so. Planned progressive therapy (the serial, empirical addition of one drug after another without culture data) is not efficacious in most settings and may have unfortunate consequences. Simply adding another antibiotic for fear that a gram-negative infection is present is a dubious practice. The synergy exhibited by β-lactams and aminoglycosides against certain gram-negative organisms (especially *P. aeruginosa*) provides the rationale for using two antibiotics in this setting, but recent analyses suggest that efficacy is not enhanced by the addition of aminoglycosides, while toxicity may be increased. Mere "double coverage," with the addition of a quinolone or another antibiotic that is not likely to exhibit synergy, has not been shown to be beneficial and may cause additional toxicities and side effects. Cephalosporins can cause bone marrow suppression, and vancomycin is associated with neutropenia in some healthy individuals. Furthermore, the addition of multiple cephalosporins may induce β-lactamase production by some organisms; cephalosporins and double β-lactam combinations should probably be avoided altogether in *Enterobacter* infections.

ANTIFUNGAL THERAPY

Fungal infections in cancer patients are most often associated with neutropenia. Neutropenic patients are predisposed to the development of invasive fungal infections, most commonly those due to *Candida* and *Aspergillus* species and occasionally those caused by *Mucor, Rhizopus, Fusarium, Trichosporon, Bipolaris*, and others. Invasive candidal disease is usually caused by *C. albicans* or *C. tropicalis* but can be caused by *C. krusei, C. parapsilosis*, and *C. glabrata*. The worldwide spread of *C. auris*, a species that is typically resistant to fluconazole and often resistant to amphotericin B as well, has further complicated the management of invasive *Candida* infections (**Chap. 216**).

For decades, it has been common clinical practice to add amphotericin B to antibacterial regimens if a neutropenic patient remains febrile despite 4–7 days of treatment with antibacterial agents. The rationale for this empirical addition is that it is difficult to culture fungi before they cause disseminated disease and that mortality rates from disseminated fungal infections in granulocytopenic patients are high. Before the introduction of newer azoles into clinical practice, amphotericin B was the mainstay of antifungal therapy. The insolubility of amphotericin B has resulted in the marketing of several lipid formulations that are less toxic than the amphotericin B deoxycholate complex. Echinocandins (e.g., caspofungin) are useful in the treatment of infections caused by azole-resistant *Candida* strains as well as in therapy for aspergillosis and have been shown to be equivalent to liposomal amphotericin B for the empirical treatment of patients with prolonged fever and neutropenia. Newer azoles have also been demonstrated to be effective in this setting. Although fluconazole is efficacious in the treatment of infections due to many *Candida* species, its use against serious fungal infections in immunocompromised patients is limited by its narrow spectrum: it has no activity against *Aspergillus* or against several non-*albicans Candida* species. The broad-spectrum azoles (e.g., voriconazole and posaconazole) provide another option for the treatment of *Aspergillus* infections (**Chap. 217**), including CNS infection. Clinicians should be aware that the spectrum of each azole is somewhat different and that no drug can be assumed to be efficacious against all fungi. *Aspergillus terreus* is resistant to amphotericin B. Although voriconazole is active against *Pseudallescheria boydii*, amphotericin B is not; however, voriconazole has no activity against *Mucor*. Posaconazole, which is administered orally, is useful as a prophylactic agent in patients with prolonged neutropenia. Studies in progress are assessing the use of these agents in combinations. For a full discussion of antifungal therapy, see **Chap. 211**.

ANTIVIRAL THERAPY

The availability of a variety of agents active against herpes-group viruses, including some new agents with a broader spectrum of activity, has heightened focus on the treatment of viral infections, which pose a major problem in cancer patients. Viral diseases caused by the herpes group are prominent. Serious (and sometimes fatal) infections due to HSV and VZV are well documented in patients receiving chemotherapy. CMV may also cause serious disease, but fatalities from CMV infection are more common in hematopoietic stem cell transplant recipients. The roles of human herpesvirus (HHV)-6, HHV-7, and HHV-8 (Kaposi's sarcoma–associated herpesvirus) in cancer patients are still being defined (**Chap. 195**). EBV lymphoproliferative disease (LPD) can occur in patients receiving chemotherapy but is much more common among transplant recipients (**Chap. 143**). While clinical experience is most extensive with acyclovir, which can be used therapeutically or prophylactically, a number of derivative drugs offer advantages over this agent (**Chap. 191**).

In addition to the herpes group, several respiratory viruses (especially RSV) may cause serious disease in cancer patients. Although influenza vaccination is recommended (see below), it may be ineffective in this patient population. The availability of antiviral drugs with activity against influenza viruses gives the clinician additional options for the prophylaxis and treatment of these patients (**Chaps. 191** and **200**).

The COVID-19 pandemic has affected cancer patients disproportionately. Early analyses suggest that lung cancer patients in particular are more vulnerable to serious infection with SARS-CoV-2.

OTHER THERAPEUTIC MODALITIES

A variety of cytokines, including granulocyte colony-stimulating factor and granulocyte-macrophage colony-stimulating factor, enhance granulocyte recovery after chemotherapy and consequently shorten the period of maximal vulnerability to fatal infections. Most authorities recommend their use only when neutropenia is both severe and prolonged, and they should be used only in the appropriate setting (i.e., when stem cells are likely to be responsive) and not as an adjunct to antimicrobial agents. The cytokines themselves may have adverse effects, including fever, hypoxemia, and pleural effusions or serositis in other areas (**Chap. 349**).

Once neutropenia has resolved, the risk of infection decreases dramatically. However, depending on what drugs they receive, patients who continue on chemotherapeutic protocols remain at high risk for certain diseases. Any patient receiving more than a maintenance dose of glucocorticoids (e.g., in many treatment regimens for diffuse lymphoma) should also receive prophylactic TMP-SMX because of the risk of *Pneumocystis* infection; those with ALL should receive such prophylaxis for the duration of chemotherapy.

PREVENTION OF INFECTION IN CANCER PATIENTS

EFFECT OF THE ENVIRONMENT

Outbreaks of fatal *Aspergillus* infection have been associated with construction projects and materials in several hospitals. The association between spore counts and risk of infection suggests the need for a high-efficiency air-handling system in hospitals that care for large numbers of neutropenic patients. The use of laminar-flow rooms and prophylactic antibiotics has decreased the number of infectious episodes in severely neutropenic patients. However, because of the expense of such a program and the failure to show that it dramatically affects mortality rates, most centers do not routinely use laminar flow to care for neutropenic patients. Some centers use "reverse isolation," in which health care providers and visitors to a patient who is neutropenic wear gowns and gloves. Since most of the infections these patients develop are due to organisms that colonize the patients' own skin and bowel, the validity of such schemes is dubious, and limited clinical data do not support their use. Hand washing by all staff caring for neutropenic patients should be required to prevent the spread of resistant organisms.

The presence of large numbers of bacteria (particularly *P. aeruginosa*) in certain foods, especially fresh vegetables, has led some authorities to recommend a special "low-bacteria" diet. A diet consisting of cooked and canned food is satisfactory to most neutropenic patients and does not involve elaborate disinfection or sterilization protocols. However, there are no studies to support even this type of dietary restriction. Counseling of patients to avoid leftovers, deli foods, undercooked meat, and unpasteurized dairy products is recommended since these foods have been associated with outbreaks of listerial infection.

PHYSICAL MEASURES

Although few studies address this issue, patients with cancer are predisposed to infections resulting from anatomic compromise (e.g., lymphedema resulting from node dissections after radical mastectomy). Surgeons who specialize in cancer surgery can provide specific guidelines for the care of such patients, and patients benefit from common-sense advice about how to prevent infections in vulnerable areas.

IMMUNOGLOBULIN REPLACEMENT

Many patients with multiple myeloma or CLL have immunoglobulin deficiencies as a result of their disease, and all allogeneic bone marrow transplant recipients are hypogammaglobulinemic for a period after transplantation. However, current recommendations reserve intravenous immunoglobulin replacement therapy for patients with severe, prolonged hypogammaglobulinemia (<400 mg of total IgG/dL) and a history of repeated infections. Antibiotic prophylaxis has been shown to be cheaper and is efficacious in preventing infections in most CLL patients with hypogammaglobulinemia. Routine use of immunoglobulin replacement is not recommended.

SEXUAL PRACTICES

The use of condoms is recommended for severely immunocompromised patients. Any sexual practice that results in oral exposure to feces is not recommended. Neutropenic patients should be advised to avoid any practice that results in trauma, as even microscopic cuts may result in bacterial invasion and fatal sepsis.

■ ANTIBIOTIC PROPHYLAXIS

Several studies indicate that the use of oral fluoroquinolones prevents infection and decreases mortality rates among severely neutropenic patients. Prophylaxis for *Pneumocystis* is mandatory for patients with ALL and for all cancer patients receiving glucocorticoid-containing chemotherapy regimens.

■ VACCINATION OF CANCER PATIENTS

In general, patients undergoing chemotherapy respond less well to vaccines than do normal hosts. Their greater need for vaccines thus leads to a dilemma in their management. Purified proteins and inactivated vaccines are almost never contraindicated and should be given to patients even during chemotherapy. For example, all adults should receive diphtheria–tetanus toxoid boosters at the indicated times as well as seasonal influenza vaccine. However, if possible, vaccination should not be undertaken concurrent with cytotoxic chemotherapy. If patients are expected to be receiving chemotherapy for several months and vaccination is indicated (e.g., influenza vaccination in the fall), the vaccine should be given midcycle—as far apart in time as possible from the antimetabolic agents that will prevent an immune response. The meningococcal and pneumococcal polysaccharide vaccines should be given to patients before splenectomy, if possible. The *H. influenzae* type b conjugate vaccine should be administered to all splenectomized patients.

In general, live virus (or live bacterial) vaccines should not be given to patients during intensive chemotherapy because of the risk of disseminated infection. Recommendations on vaccination are summarized in Table 74-2 (see *https://www.cdc.gov/vaccines/hcp/index.html* for updated recommendations).

■ IN MEMORIAM

Dr. Robert W. Finberg, Richard M. Haidack Distinguished Professor and Chair of Medicine, University of Massachusetts Chan Medical School (2000-2020), Professor of Medicine and Chair of Infectious Diseases, Dana Farber Cancer Institute (1996-1999), passed away on August 30, 2021. In addition to this chapter, he authored Chapter 143, "Infections in Transplant Recipients." Dr. Finberg was an internationally renowned physician-scientist and an academic leader whose career spanned four decades. A brilliant talented researcher focused on viral pathogenesis he was also a consummate clinician who attended at the bedside throughout his career. Dr. Finberg played an important role in the COVID-19 pandemic by leading clinical trials for SARS-CoV-2 vaccines and therapeutics. Warm and generous with a keen wit, he was a beloved family man, colleague and friend. As an educator and mentor he truly cared about training the next generation, as evidenced by the legacy of a very large number of trainees he leaves behind. We are indebted to Dr. Finberg for his outstanding contributions to nine editions of Harrison's Principles of Internal Medicine and to his considerable and significant contributions to the field of human health.

■ FURTHER READING

Fernández-Cruz A et al: Infective endocarditis in patients with cancer: A consequence of invasive procedures or a harbinger of neoplasm? A prospective, multicenter cohort. Medicine 96:e7913, 2017.

Friedman DZP, Schwartz IS: Emerging fungal infections: New patients, new patterns, and new pathogens. J Fungi 5:67, 2019.

Maschmeyer G et al: Infections associated with immunotherapeutic and molecular targeted agents in hematology and oncology. A position paper by the European Conference on Infections in Leukemia (ECIL). Leukemia 33:844, 2019.

Pizzo PA: Management of patients with fever and neutropenia through the arc of time. Ann Intern Med 170:389, 2019.

Zhang L et al: Clinical characteristics of COVID-19-infected cancer patients: A retrospective case study in three hospitals within Wuhan, China. Ann Oncol 31:894, 2020.

■ WEBSITE

Prevention and Treatment of Cancer-Related Infections; National Comprehensive Cancer Network Clinical Practice Guidelines in Oncology Version 2.2020 (*https://www.nccn.org*).

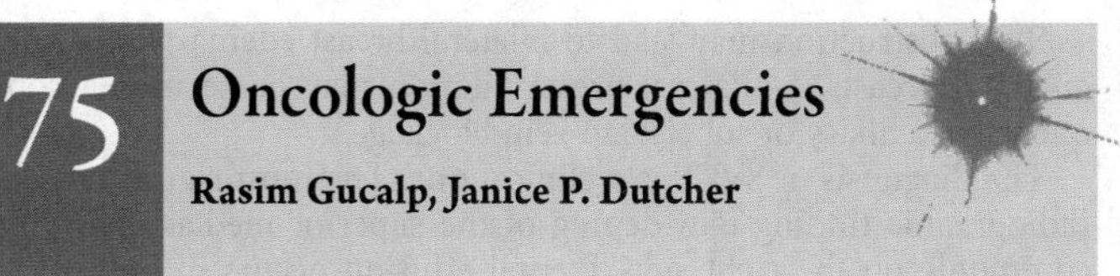

75 Oncologic Emergencies

Rasim Gucalp, Janice P. Dutcher

Emergencies in patients with cancer may be classified into three groups: pressure or obstruction caused by a space-occupying lesion, metabolic or hormonal problems (paraneoplastic syndromes, **Chap. 93**), and treatment-related complications.

STRUCTURAL-OBSTRUCTIVE ONCOLOGIC EMERGENCIES

■ SUPERIOR VENA CAVA SYNDROME

Superior vena cava syndrome (SVCS) is the clinical manifestation of superior vena cava (SVC) obstruction, with severe reduction in venous return from the head, neck, and upper extremities. Malignant tumors, such as lung cancer, lymphoma, and metastatic tumors, are responsible for the majority of SVCS cases. With the expanding use of intravascular devices (e.g., permanent central venous access catheters, pacemaker/defibrillator leads), the prevalence of benign causes of SVCS is now increasing, accounting for at least 40% of cases. Lung cancer, particularly of small-cell and squamous cell histologies, accounts for ~85% of all cases of malignant origin. In young adults, malignant lymphoma is a leading cause of SVCS. Hodgkin's lymphoma involves the mediastinum more commonly than other lymphomas but rarely causes SVCS. When SVCS is noted in a young man with a mediastinal mass, the differential diagnosis is lymphoma versus primary mediastinal germ cell tumor. Metastatic cancers to the mediastinal lymph nodes, such as testicular and breast carcinomas, account for a small proportion of cases. Other causes include benign tumors, aortic aneurysm, thyromegaly, thrombosis, and fibrosing mediastinitis from prior irradiation, histoplasmosis, or Behçet's syndrome. SVCS as the initial manifestation of Behçet's syndrome may be due to inflammation of the SVC associated with thrombosis.

Patients with SVCS usually present with neck and facial swelling (especially around the eyes), dyspnea, and cough. Other symptoms include hoarseness, tongue swelling, headaches, nasal congestion, epistaxis, hemoptysis, dysphagia, pain, dizziness, syncope, and lethargy. Bending forward or lying down may aggravate the symptoms. The characteristic physical findings are dilated neck veins; an increased number of collateral veins covering the anterior chest wall; cyanosis; and edema of the face, arms, and chest. Facial swelling and plethora are typically exacerbated when the patient is supine. More severe cases include proptosis, glossal and laryngeal edema, and obtundation. The clinical picture is milder if the obstruction is located above the azygos vein. Symptoms are usually progressive, but in some cases, they may improve as collateral circulation develops.

Signs and symptoms of cerebral and/or laryngeal edema, though rare, are associated with a poorer prognosis and require urgent evaluation. Seizures are more likely related to brain metastases than to cerebral edema from venous occlusion. Patients with small-cell lung cancer and SVCS have a higher incidence of brain metastases than those without SVCS.

Cardiorespiratory symptoms at rest, particularly with positional changes, suggest significant airway and vascular obstruction and limited physiologic reserve. Cardiac arrest or respiratory failure can occur, particularly in patients receiving sedatives or undergoing general anesthesia.

Rarely, esophageal varices may develop, particularly in the setting of SVC syndrome due to hemodialysis catheter. These are "downhill" varices based on the direction of blood flow from cephalad to caudad (in contrast to "uphill" varices associated with caudad to cephalad flow from portal hypertension). If the obstruction to the SVC is proximal to the azygous vein, varices develop in the upper one-third of the esophagus. If the obstruction involves or is distal to the azygous vein, varices occur in the entire length of the esophagus. Variceal bleeding may be a late complication of chronic SVCS.

SVC obstruction may lead to bilateral breast edema with bilateral enlarged breasts. Unilateral breast dilation may be seen as a consequence of axillary or subclavian vein blockage.

The diagnosis of SVCS is a clinical one. The most significant chest radiographic finding is widening of the superior mediastinum, most commonly on the right side. Pleural effusion occurs in only 25% of patients, often on the right side. The majority of these effusions are exudative and occasionally chylous. However, a normal chest radiograph is still compatible with the diagnosis if other characteristic findings are present. Computed tomography (CT) provides the most reliable view of the mediastinal anatomy. The diagnosis of SVCS requires diminished or absent opacification of central venous structures with prominent collateral venous circulation. Magnetic resonance imaging (MRI) is increasingly being used to diagnose SVC obstruction with a 100% sensitivity and specificity, but dyspneic SVCS patients may have difficulty remaining supine for the entire imaging process. Invasive procedures, including bronchoscopy, percutaneous needle biopsy, mediastinoscopy, and even thoracotomy, can be performed by a skilled clinician without any major risk of bleeding. Endobronchial or esophageal ultrasound-guided needle aspiration may establish the diagnosis safely. For patients with a known cancer, a detailed workup usually is not necessary, and appropriate treatment may be started after obtaining a CT scan of the thorax. For those with no history of malignancy, a detailed evaluation is essential to rule out benign causes and determine a specific diagnosis to direct the appropriate therapy.

TREATMENT

Superior Vena Cava Syndrome

The one potentially life-threatening complication of a superior mediastinal mass is tracheal obstruction. Upper airway obstruction demands emergent therapy. Diuretics with a low-salt diet, head elevation, and oxygen may produce temporary symptomatic relief. Glucocorticoids have a limited role except in the setting of mediastinal lymphoma masses.

Radiation therapy is the primary treatment for SVCS caused by non-small-cell lung cancer and other metastatic solid tumors. Chemotherapy is effective when the underlying cancer is small-cell carcinoma of the lung, lymphoma, or germ cell tumor. SVCS recurs in 10–30% of patients; it may be palliated with the use of intravascular self-expanding stents **(Fig. 75-1)**. Endovascular therapy is more frequently used first, to provide rapid relief of clinical symptoms with reduced complications. Early stenting may be necessary in patients with severe symptoms; however, the prompt increase in venous return after stenting may precipitate heart failure and pulmonary edema. Other complications of stent placement include hematoma at the insertion site, SVC perforation, stent migration in the right ventricle, stent fracture, and pulmonary embolism.

Clinical improvement occurs in most patients, although this improvement may be due to the development of adequate collateral circulation. The mortality associated with SVCS does not relate to caval obstruction but rather to the underlying cause.

SVCS AND CENTRAL VENOUS CATHETERS IN ADULTS

The use of long-term central venous catheters has become common practice in patients with cancer. Major vessel thrombosis may occur. In these cases, catheter removal should be combined with anticoagulation to prevent embolization. SVCS in this setting, if detected early, can be treated by fibrinolytic therapy without sacrificing the catheter. When managing patients with transvenous lead-related SVC syndrome, anticoagulation, local and systemic thrombolytic therapy, and surgical intervention can be effective therapy in select patients. Endovascular stenting has also been shown to be safe and promising, with minimal procedural or clinical complications. The role of anticoagulation after SVC stent placement is controversial.

PERICARDIAL EFFUSION/TAMPONADE

Malignant pericardial disease is found at autopsy in 5–10% of patients with cancer, most frequently with lung cancer, breast cancer, leukemias,

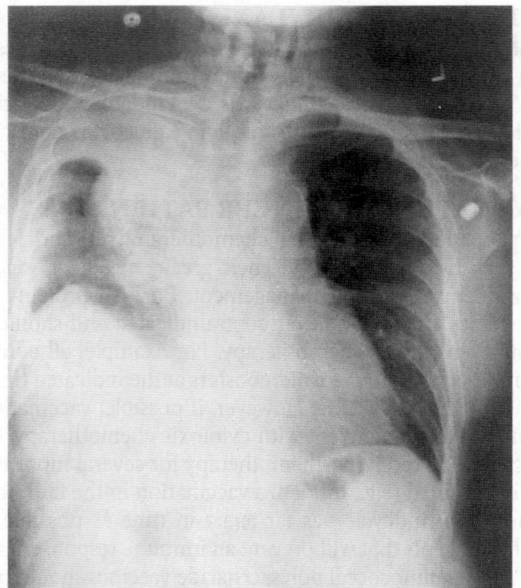
A

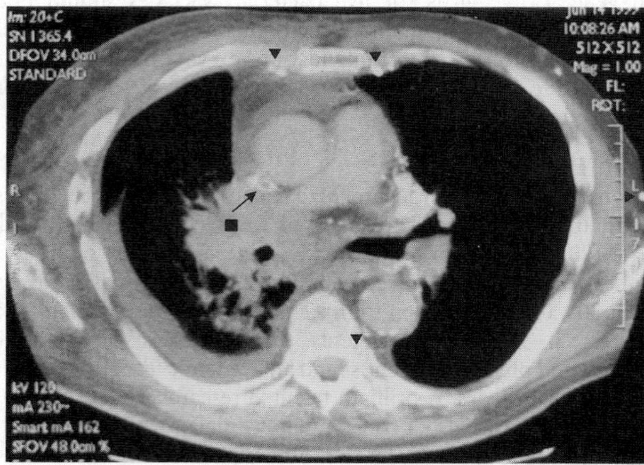
B

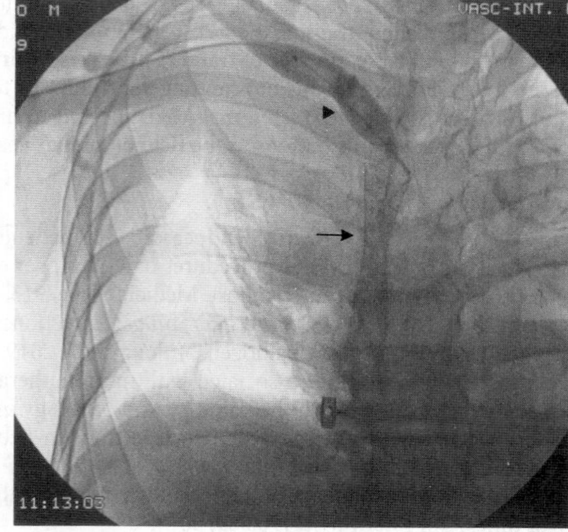

C

FIGURE 75-1 Superior vena cava syndrome (SVCS). ***A.*** Chest radiographs of a 59-year-old man with recurrent SVCS caused by non-small-cell lung cancer showing right paratracheal mass with right pleural effusion. ***B.*** Computed tomography of same patient demonstrating obstruction of the superior vena cava with thrombosis (*arrow*) by the lung cancer (*square*) and collaterals (*arrowheads*). ***C.*** Balloon angioplasty (*arrowhead*) with Wallstent (*arrow*) in same patient.

and lymphomas. Cardiac tamponade as the initial presentation of extrathoracic malignancy is rare. The origin is not malignancy in ~50% of cancer patients with symptomatic pericardial disease, but it can be related to irradiation; drug-induced pericarditis, including chemotherapeutic agents such as all-trans retinoic acid, arsenic trioxide, imatinib, and other abl kinase inhibitors; hypothyroidism; idiopathic pericarditis; infection; or autoimmune diseases. Pericardial disease has been associated with immune checkpoint inhibitors specifically in patients with advanced non-small-cell lung cancer. Two types of radiation pericarditis occur: an acute inflammatory, effusive pericarditis occurring within months of irradiation, which usually resolves spontaneously, and a chronic effusive pericarditis that may appear up to 20 years after radiation therapy and is accompanied by a thickened pericardium.

Most patients with pericardial metastasis are asymptomatic. However, the common symptoms are dyspnea, cough, chest pain, orthopnea, and weakness. Pleural effusion, sinus tachycardia, jugular venous distention, hepatomegaly, peripheral edema, and cyanosis are the most frequent physical findings. Relatively specific diagnostic findings, such as paradoxical pulse, diminished heart sounds, pulsus alternans (pulse waves alternating between those of greater and lesser amplitude with successive beats), and friction rub are less common than with nonmalignant pericardial disease. Chest radiographs and electrocardiogram (ECG) reveal abnormalities in 90% of patients, but half of these abnormalities are nonspecific. Echocardiography is the most helpful diagnostic test. Pericardial fluid may be serous, serosanguineous, or hemorrhagic, and cytologic examination of pericardial fluid is diagnostic in most patients. Measurements of tumor markers in the pericardial fluid are not helpful in the diagnosis of malignant pericardial fluid. Pericardioscopy with targeted pericardial and epicardial biopsy may differentiate neoplastic and benign pericardial disease. A combination of cytology, pericardial and epicardial biopsy, and guided pericardioscopy gives the best diagnostic yield. CT scan of chest may also reveal the presence of a concomitant thoracic neoplasm. Cancer patients with pericardial effusion containing malignant cells on cytology have a very poor survival, ~7 weeks.

TREATMENT

Pericardial Effusion/Tamponade

Pericardiocentesis with or without the introduction of sclerosing agents, the creation of a pericardial window, complete pericardial stripping, cardiac irradiation, or systemic chemotherapy are effective treatments. Acute pericardial tamponade with life-threatening hemodynamic instability requires immediate drainage of fluid. This can be quickly achieved by pericardiocentesis. The recurrence rate after percutaneous catheter drainage is ~20%. Sclerotherapy (pericardial instillation of bleomycin, mitomycin C, or tetracycline) may decrease recurrences. Alternatively, subxiphoid pericardiotomy can be performed in 45 min under local anesthesia. Thoracoscopic pericardial fenestration can be employed for benign causes; however, 60% of malignant pericardial effusions recur after this procedure. In a subset of patients, drainage of the pericardial effusion is paradoxically followed by worsening hemodynamic instability. This so-called "postoperative low cardiac output syndrome" occurs in up to 10% of patients undergoing surgical drainage and carries poor short-term survival.

INTESTINAL OBSTRUCTION

Intestinal obstruction and reobstruction are common problems in patients with advanced cancer, particularly colorectal or ovarian carcinoma. However, other cancers, such as lung or breast cancer and melanoma, can metastasize within the abdomen, leading to intestinal obstruction. Metastatic disease from colorectal, ovarian, pancreatic, gastric, and occasionally breast cancer can lead to peritoneal carcinomatosis, with infiltration of the omentum and peritoneal surface, thus limiting bowel motility. Typically, obstruction occurs at multiple sites in peritoneal carcinomatosis. Melanoma has a predilection to involve the small bowel; this involvement may be isolated, and resection may result in prolonged survival. Intestinal pseudoobstruction is caused by infiltration of the mesentery or bowel muscle by tumor, involvement of the celiac plexus, or paraneoplastic neuropathy in patients with small-cell lung cancer. Paraneoplastic neuropathy is associated with IgG antibodies reactive to neurons of the myenteric and submucosal plexuses of the jejunum and stomach. Ovarian cancer can lead to authentic luminal obstruction or to pseudoobstruction that results when circumferential invasion of a bowel segment arrests the forward progression of peristaltic contractions.

The onset of obstruction is usually insidious. Pain is the most common symptom and is usually colicky in nature. Pain can also be due to abdominal distention, tumor masses, or hepatomegaly. Vomiting can be intermittent or continuous. Patients with complete obstruction usually have constipation. Physical examination may reveal abdominal distention with tympany, ascites, visible peristalsis, high-pitched bowel sounds, and tumor masses. Erect plain abdominal films may reveal multiple air-fluid levels and dilation of the small or large bowel. Acute cecal dilation to >12–14 cm is considered a surgical emergency because of the high likelihood of rupture. CT scan is useful in defining the extent of disease and the exact nature of the obstruction and differentiating benign from malignant causes of obstruction in patients who have undergone surgery for malignancy. Malignant obstruction is suggested by a mass at the site of obstruction or prior surgery, adenopathy, or an abrupt transition zone and irregular bowel thickening at the obstruction site. Benign obstruction is more likely when CT shows mesenteric vascular changes, a large volume of ascites, or a smooth transition zone and smooth bowel thickening at the obstruction site. In challenging patients with obstructive symptoms, particularly low-grade small-bowel obstruction (SBO), CT enteroclysis often can help establish the diagnosis by providing distention of small-bowel loops. In this technique, water-soluble contrast is infused through a nasoenteric tube into the duodenum or proximal small bowel followed by CT images. The prognosis for the patient with cancer who develops intestinal obstruction is poor; median survival is 3–4 months. About 25–30% of patients are found to have intestinal obstruction due to causes other than cancer. Adhesions from previous operations are a common benign cause. Ileus induced by vinca alkaloids, narcotics, or other drugs is another reversible cause.

TREATMENT

Intestinal Obstruction

The management of intestinal obstruction in patients with advanced malignancy depends on the extent of the underlying malignancy, options for further antineoplastic therapy, estimated life expectancy, the functional status of the major organs, and the extent of the obstruction. The initial management should include surgical evaluation. Operation is not always successful and may lead to further complications with a substantial mortality rate (10–20%). Laparoscopy can diagnose and treat malignant bowel obstruction in some cases. Self-expanding metal stents placed in the gastric outlet, duodenum, proximal jejunum, colon, or rectum may palliate obstructive symptoms at those sites without major surgery. Patients known to have advanced intraabdominal malignancy should receive a prolonged course of conservative management, including nasogastric decompression. Percutaneous endoscopic or surgical gastrostomy tube placement is an option for palliation of nausea and vomiting, the so-called "venting gastrostomy." Treatment with antiemetics, antispasmodics, and analgesics may allow patients to remain outside the hospital. Octreotide may relieve obstructive symptoms through its inhibitory effect on gastrointestinal secretion. Glucocorticoids have anti-inflammatory effects and may help the resolution of bowel obstruction. They also have antiemetic effects.

URINARY OBSTRUCTION

Urinary obstruction may occur in patients with prostatic or gynecologic malignancies, particularly cervical carcinoma; metastatic disease from other primary sites such as carcinomas of the breast, stomach, lung, colon, and pancreas; or lymphomas. Radiation therapy to pelvic tumors may cause fibrosis and subsequent ureteral obstruction. Bladder outlet obstruction is usually due to prostate and cervical cancers and may lead to bilateral hydronephrosis and renal failure.

Flank pain is the most common symptom. Persistent urinary tract infection, persistent proteinuria, or hematuria in patients with cancer should raise suspicion of ureteral obstruction. Total anuria and/or anuria alternating with polyuria may occur. A slow, continuous rise in the serum creatinine level necessitates immediate evaluation. Renal ultrasound is the safest and cheapest way to identify hydronephrosis. The function of an obstructed kidney can be evaluated by a nuclear scan. CT scan can reveal the point of obstruction and identify a retroperitoneal mass or adenopathy.

TREATMENT
Urinary Obstruction

Obstruction associated with flank pain, sepsis, or fistula formation is an indication for immediate palliative urinary diversion. Internal ureteral stents can be placed under local anesthesia. Percutaneous nephrostomy offers an alternative approach for drainage. The placement of a nephrostomy is associated with a significant rate of pyelonephritis. In the case of bladder outlet obstruction due to malignancy, a suprapubic cystostomy can be used for urinary drainage. An aggressive intervention with invasive approaches to improve the obstruction should be weighed against the likelihood of antitumor response, and the ability to reverse renal insufficiency should be evaluated.

MALIGNANT BILIARY OBSTRUCTION

This common clinical problem can be caused by a primary carcinoma arising in the pancreas, ampulla of Vater, bile duct, or liver or by metastatic disease to the periductal lymph nodes or liver parenchyma. The most common metastatic tumors causing biliary obstruction are gastric, colon, breast, and lung cancers. Jaundice, light-colored stools, dark urine, pruritus, and weight loss due to malabsorption are usual symptoms. Pain and secondary infection are uncommon in malignant biliary obstruction. Ultrasound, CT scan, or percutaneous transhepatic or endoscopic retrograde cholangiography will identify the site and nature of the biliary obstruction.

TREATMENT
Malignant Biliary Obstruction

Palliative intervention is indicated only in patients with disabling pruritus resistant to medical treatment, severe malabsorption, or infection. Stenting under radiographic control, surgical bypass, or radiation therapy with or without chemotherapy may alleviate the obstruction. The choice of therapy should be based on the site of obstruction (proximal vs distal), the type of tumor (sensitive to radiotherapy, chemotherapy, or neither), and the general condition of the patient. Stenting under radiographic or endoscopic control, surgical bypass, or radiation therapy with or without chemotherapy may alleviate the obstruction. Photodynamic therapy and radiofrequency ablation are promising endoscopic therapies for malignant biliary obstruction.

Endoscopic ultrasonography-guided biliary drainage is an evolving method of biliary drainage in patients with malignant biliary obstruction, particularly in patients whom standard endoscopic retrograde cholangiopancreatography failed.

SPINAL CORD COMPRESSION

Malignant spinal cord compression (MSCC) is defined as compression of the spinal cord and/or cauda equina by an extradural tumor mass. The minimum radiologic evidence for cord compression is indentation of the theca at the level of clinical features. Spinal cord compression (SCC) occurs in 5–10% of patients with cancer. Epidural tumor is the first manifestation of malignancy in ~10% of patients. The underlying cancer is usually identified during the initial evaluation; lung cancer is the most common cause of MSCC.

Metastatic tumor involves the vertebral column more often than any other part of the bony skeleton. Lung, breast, and prostate cancers are the most frequent offenders. Multiple myeloma also has a high incidence of spine involvement. Lymphomas, melanoma, renal cell cancer, and genitourinary cancers also cause cord compression. The thoracic spine is the most common site (70%), followed by the lumbosacral spine (20%) and the cervical spine (10%). Involvement of multiple sites is most frequent in patients with breast and prostate carcinoma. Cord injury develops when metastases to the vertebral body or pedicle enlarge and compress the underlying dura. Another cause of cord compression is direct extension of a paravertebral lesion through the intervertebral foramen. These cases usually involve a lymphoma, myeloma, or pediatric neoplasm. Parenchymal spinal cord metastasis due to hematogenous spread is rare. Intramedullary metastases can be seen in lung cancer, breast cancer, renal cancer, melanoma, and lymphoma, and are frequently associated with brain metastases and leptomeningeal disease.

Expanding extradural tumors induce injury through several mechanisms. Expanding extradural tumors induce mechanical injury to axons and myelin. Compression compromises blood flow, leading to ischemia and/or infarction.

The most common initial symptom in patients with SCC is localized back pain and tenderness due to involvement of vertebrae by tumor. Pain is usually present for days or months before other neurologic findings appear. It is exacerbated by movement and by coughing or sneezing. It can be differentiated from the pain of disk disease by the fact that it worsens when the patient is supine. Radicular pain is less common than localized back pain and usually develops later. Radicular pain in the cervical or lumbosacral areas may be unilateral or bilateral. Radicular pain from the thoracic roots is often bilateral and is described by patients as a feeling of tight, band-like constriction around the thorax and abdomen. Typical cervical radicular pain radiates down the arm; in the lumbar region, the radiation is down the legs. *Lhermitte's sign*, a tingling or electric sensation down the back and upper and lower limbs upon flexing or extending the neck, may be an early sign of cord compression. Loss of bowel or bladder control may be the presenting symptom but usually occurs late in the course. Occasionally, patients present with ataxia of gait without motor and sensory involvement due to involvement of the spinocerebellar tract.

On physical examination, pain induced by straight leg raising, neck flexion, or vertebral percussion may help to determine the level of cord compression. Patients develop numbness and paresthesias in the extremities or trunk. Loss of sensibility to pinprick is as common as loss of sensibility to vibration or position. The upper limit of the zone of sensory loss is often one or two vertebrae below the site of compression. Motor findings include weakness, spasticity, and abnormal muscle stretching. An extensor plantar reflex reflects significant compression. Deep tendon reflexes may be brisk. Motor and sensory loss usually precedes sphincter disturbance. Patients with autonomic dysfunction may present with decreased anal tonus, decreased perineal sensibility, and a distended bladder. The absence of the anal wink reflex or the bulbocavernosus reflex confirms cord involvement. In doubtful cases, evaluation of postvoiding urinary residual volume can be helpful. A residual volume of >150 mL suggests bladder dysfunction. Autonomic dysfunction is an unfavorable prognostic factor. Patients with progressive neurologic symptoms should have frequent neurologic examinations and rapid therapeutic intervention. Other illnesses that may mimic cord compression include osteoporotic vertebral collapse, disk disease, pyogenic abscess or vertebral tuberculosis, radiation myelopathy, neoplastic leptomeningitis, benign tumors, epidural hematoma, and spinal lipomatosis.

Cauda equina syndrome is characterized by low back pain; diminished sensation over the buttocks, posterior-superior thighs, and perineal area in a saddle distribution; rectal and bladder dysfunction; sexual impotence; absent bulbocavernous, patellar, and Achilles'

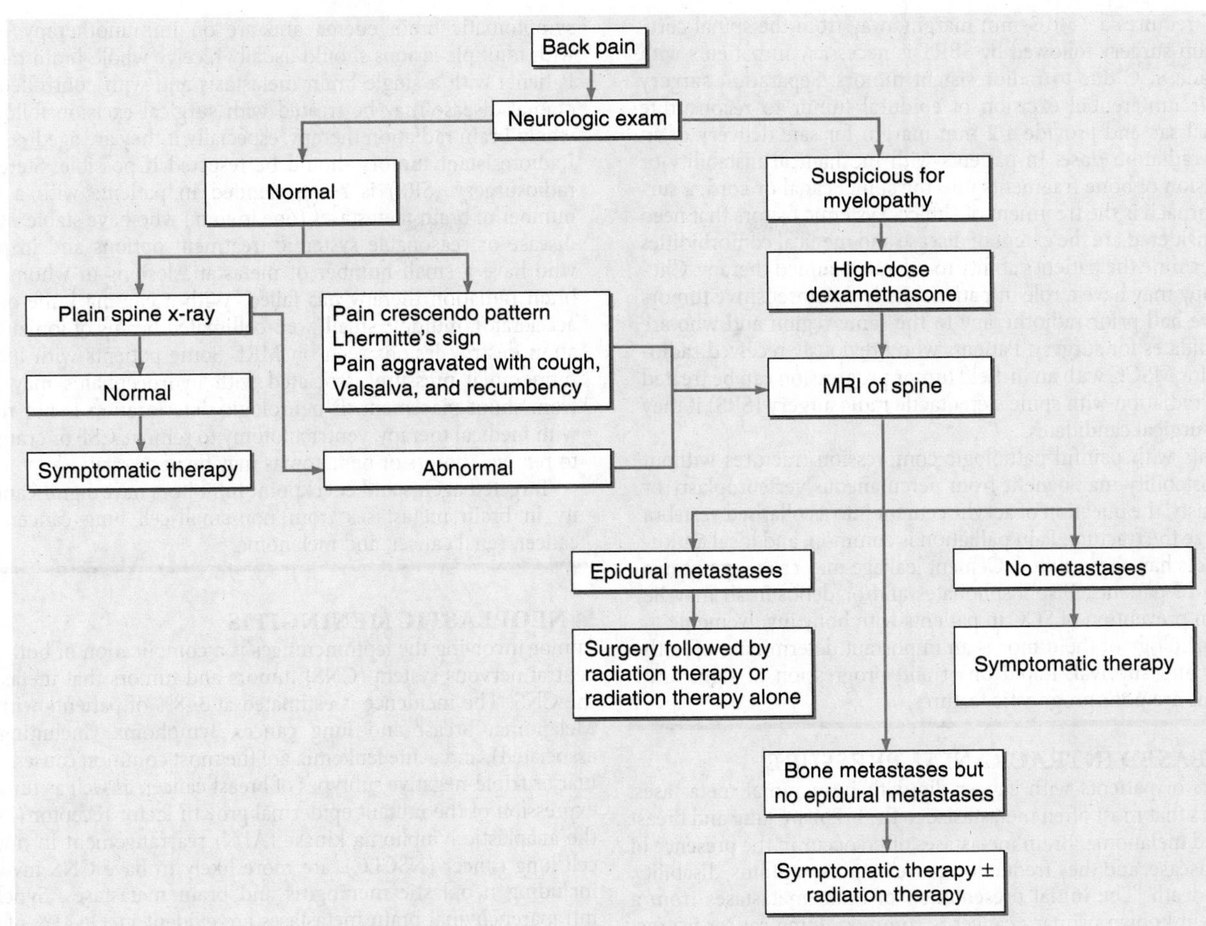

FIGURE 75-2 Management of cancer patients with back pain.

reflexes; and variable amount of lower-extremity weakness. This reflects compression of nerve roots as they form the cauda equina after leaving the spinal cord. The majority of cauda equina tumors are primary tumors of glial or nerve sheath origin; metastases are very rare.

Patients with cancer who develop back pain should be evaluated for SCC as quickly as possible (**Fig. 75-2**). Treatment is more often successful in patients who are ambulatory and still have sphincter control at the time treatment is initiated. Patients should have a neurologic examination and plain films of the spine. Those whose physical examination suggests cord compression should receive dexamethasone starting immediately and undergo MRI imaging.

Erosion of the pedicles (the "winking owl" sign) is the earliest radiologic finding of vertebral tumor in plain films; however, plain films are insensitive. Other radiographic changes include increased intrapedicular distance, vertebral destruction, lytic or sclerotic lesions, scalloped vertebral bodies, and vertebral body collapse. Vertebral collapse is not a reliable indicator of the presence of tumor; ~20% of cases of vertebral collapse, particularly those in older patients and postmenopausal women, are due not to cancer but to osteoporosis. Also, a normal appearance on plain films of the spine does not exclude the diagnosis of cancer. The role of bone scans in the detection of cord compression is not clear; this method is sensitive but less specific than spinal radiography.

The full-length image of the cord provided by MRI is the imaging procedure of choice. Multiple epidural metastases are noted in 25% of patients with cord compression, and their presence influences treatment plans. On T1-weighted images, good contrast is noted between the cord, cerebrospinal fluid (CSF), and extradural lesions. Owing to its sensitivity in demonstrating the replacement of bone marrow by tumor, MRI can show which parts of a vertebra are involved by tumor. MRI also visualizes intraspinal extradural masses compressing the cord. T2-weighted images are most useful for the demonstration of intramedullary pathology. Gadolinium-enhanced MRI can help to delineate intramedullary disease. MRI is as good as or better than myelography plus postmyelogram CT scan in detecting metastatic epidural disease with cord compression. Myelography should be reserved for patients who have poor MRIs or who cannot undergo MRI promptly. CT scan in conjunction with myelography enhances the detection of small areas of spinal destruction.

In patients with cord compression and an unknown primary tumor, a simple workup including chest radiography, mammography, measurement of prostate-specific antigen, and abdominal CT usually reveals the underlying malignancy.

TREATMENT

Spinal Cord Compression

The treatment of patients with SCC is aimed at relief of pain and restoration/preservation of neurologic function (Fig. 75-2). Management of MSCC requires a multidisciplinary approach.

Radiation therapy plus glucocorticoids is generally the initial treatment of choice for most patients with SCC. The management decision of SCC involves assessment of neurologic (N), oncologic (O), mechanical (M), and systemic factors (S). NOMS was developed by Memorial Sloan Kettering Cancer Center (MSKCC) researchers to provide an algorithm for management of SCC. The neurologic assessment is based on the degree of epidural SCC, myelopathy, and/or functional radiculopathy. Oncologic assessment involves the radiosensitivity of the tumor type. In patients with radioresistant tumors, stereotactic body radiotherapy (SBRT) is the preferred approach if radiation is appropriate. Safe delivery of SBRT requires a 2- to 3-mm margin away from the spinal cord. Separation surgery followed by SBRT is necessary in patients with high-grade SCC due to radioresistant tumors. Separation surgery is the circumferential excision of epidural tumor to reconstitute the thecal sac and provide a 2-mm margin for safe delivery of an ablative radiation dose. In patients with mechanical instability or retropulsion of bone fragments into the spinal canal or cord, a surgical approach is the treatment of choice. Systemic factors that need to be considered are the extent of disease and medical comorbidities that determine the patient's ability to tolerate planned therapy. Chemotherapy may have a role in patients with chemosensitive tumors who have had prior radiotherapy to the same region and who are not candidates for surgery. Patients who previously received radiotherapy for MSCC with an in-field tumor progression can be treated with reirradiation with spine stereotactic radiosurgery (SRS) if they are not surgical candidates.

Patients with painful pathologic compression fractures without spinal instability may benefit from percutaneous vertebroplasty or kyphoplasty, the injection of acrylic cement into a collapsed vertebra to stabilize the fracture. Pain palliation is common, and local antitumor effects have been noted. Cement leakage may cause symptoms in ~10% of patients. Bisphosphonates and/or denosumab may be helpful in prevention of SCC in patients with bony involvement.

The histology of the tumor is an important determinant of both recovery and survival. Rapid onset and progression of signs and symptoms are poor prognostic features.

INCREASED INTRACRANIAL PRESSURE

About 25% of patients with cancer die with intracranial metastases. The cancers that most often metastasize to the brain are lung and breast cancers and melanoma. Brain metastases often occur in the presence of systemic disease, and they frequently cause major symptoms, disability, and early death. The initial presentation of brain metastases from a previously unknown primary cancer is common. Lung cancer is most commonly the primary malignancy. CT scans of the chest/abdomen and MRI of the brain as the initial diagnostic studies can identify a biopsy site in most patients.

The signs and symptoms of a metastatic brain tumor are similar to those of other intracranial expanding lesions: headache, nausea, vomiting, behavioral changes, seizures, and focal, progressive neurologic changes. Occasionally the onset is abrupt, resembling a stroke, with the sudden appearance of headache, nausea, vomiting, and neurologic deficits. This picture is usually due to hemorrhage into the metastasis. Melanoma, germ cell tumors, and renal cell cancers have a particularly high incidence of intracranial bleeding. The tumor mass and surrounding edema may cause obstruction of the circulation of CSF, with resulting hydrocephalus. Patients with increased intracranial pressure may have papilledema with visual disturbances and neck stiffness. As the mass enlarges, brain tissue may be displaced through the fixed cranial openings, producing various herniation syndromes.

MRI is superior to CT scan. Gadolinium-enhanced MRI is more sensitive than CT at revealing meningeal involvement and small lesions, particularly in the brainstem or cerebellum. The MRI of the brain shows brain metastases as multiple enhancing lesions of various sizes with surrounding areas of low-density edema.

Intracranial hypertension ("pseudotumor cerebri") secondary to tretinoin therapy for acute promyelocytic leukemia has been reported as another cause of intracranial pressure in the setting of a malignancy.

TREATMENT

Increased Intracranial Pressure

Dexamethasone is the best initial treatment for all symptomatic patients with brain metastases. The current success of immunotherapy approaches for primary and metastatic brain tumors may preclude or limit glucocorticoid use since it may decrease antitumor response. Bevacizumab should be considered in patients who are unable to wean completely off of steroids as well as those who have symptomatic brain edema and are on immunotherapy. Patients with multiple lesions should usually receive whole-brain radiation. Patients with a single brain metastasis and with controlled extracranial disease may be treated with surgical excision followed by whole-brain radiation therapy, especially if they are aged <60 years. Radioresistant tumors should be resected if possible. Stereotactic radiosurgery (SRS) is recommended in patients with a limited number of brain metastases (one to four) who have stable, systemic disease or reasonable systemic treatment options and in patients who have a small number of metastatic lesions in whom whole-brain radiation therapy has failed. With a gamma knife or linear accelerator, multiple small, well-collimated beams of ionizing radiation destroy lesions seen on MRI. Some patients with increased intracranial pressure associated with hydrocephalus may benefit from shunt placement. If neurologic deterioration is not reversed with medical therapy, ventriculotomy to remove CSF or craniotomy to remove tumors or hematomas may be necessary.

Targeted agents and checkpoint inhibitors have significant activity in brain metastases from non-small-cell lung cancer, breast cancer, renal cancer, and melanoma.

NEOPLASTIC MENINGITIS

Tumor involving the leptomeninges is a complication of both primary central nervous system (CNS) tumors and tumors that metastasize to the CNS. The incidence is estimated at 3–8% of patients with cancer. Melanoma, breast and lung cancer, lymphoma (including AIDS-associated), and acute leukemia are the most common causes. The lobular or triple-negative subtypes of breast cancer, as well as tumors with expression of the mutant epidermal growth factor receptor (EGFR) or the anaplastic lymphoma kinase (ALK) rearrangement in non-small-cell lung cancer (NSCLC), are more likely to have CNS involvement including neoplastic meningitis and brain metastases. Synchronous intraparenchymal brain metastases are evident in 11–31% of patients with neoplastic meningitis. Leptomeningeal seeding is frequent in patients undergoing resection of brain metastases or receiving stereotactic radiotherapy for brain metastases.

Patients typically present with multifocal neurologic signs and symptoms, including headache, gait abnormality, mental changes, nausea, vomiting, seizures, back or radicular pain, and limb weakness. Signs include cranial nerve palsies, extremity weakness, paresthesia, and decreased deep tendon reflexes.

Diagnosis is made by demonstrating malignant cells in the CSF; however, up to 40% of patients may have false-negative CSF cytology. An elevated CSF protein level is nearly always present (except in HTLV-1–associated adult T-cell leukemia). Patients with neurologic signs and symptoms consistent with neoplastic meningitis who have a negative CSF cytology should have the spinal tap repeated at least one more time for cytologic examination. MRI findings suggestive of neoplastic meningitis include leptomeningeal, subependymal, dural, or cranial nerve enhancement; superficial cerebral lesions; intradural nodules; and communicating hydrocephalus. Spinal cord imaging by MRI is a necessary component of the evaluation of nonleukemia neoplastic meningitis because ~20% of patients have cord abnormalities, including intradural enhancing nodules that are diagnostic for leptomeningeal involvement. Cauda equina lesions are common, but lesions may be seen anywhere in the spinal canal. The value of MRI for the diagnosis of leptomeningeal disease is limited in patients with hematopoietic malignancy. Radiolabeled CSF flow studies are abnormal in up to 70% of patients with neoplastic meningitis; ventricular outlet obstruction, abnormal flow in the spinal canal, or impaired flow over the cerebral convexities may affect distribution of intrathecal chemotherapy, resulting in decreased efficacy or increased toxicity. Radiation therapy may correct CSF flow abnormalities before use of intrathecal chemotherapy. Neoplastic meningitis can also lead to intracranial hypertension and hydrocephalus. Placement of a ventriculoperitoneal shunt may effectively palliate symptoms in these patients.

The development of neoplastic meningitis usually occurs in the setting of uncontrolled cancer outside the CNS; thus, prognosis is poor (median survival 10–12 weeks). However, treatment of the neoplastic meningitis may successfully alleviate symptoms and control the CNS spread.

TREATMENT

Neoplastic Meningitis

Chemotherapy provided by either intrathecal injection or systemic routes is used to control leptomeningeal disease throughout the entire neuroaxis. Intrathecal chemotherapy, usually methotrexate, cytarabine, or thiotepa, is delivered by lumbar puncture or by an intraventricular reservoir (Ommaya). Among solid tumors, breast cancer responds best to therapy. Focal radiotherapy may have a role in bulky disease and in symptomatic or obstructive lesions. Targeted therapy such as systemically administered EGFR tyrosine kinase inhibitors (TKIs) in non-small-cell lung cancer may lead to improvement in some patients with leptomeningeal spread. Patients with neoplastic meningitis from either acute leukemia or lymphoma may be cured of their CNS disease if the systemic disease can be eliminated.

SEIZURES

Seizures occurring in a patient with cancer can be caused by the tumor itself, by metabolic disturbances, by radiation injury, by cerebral infarctions, by chemotherapy-related encephalopathies, or by CNS infections. Metastatic disease to the CNS is the most common cause of seizures in patients with cancer. However, seizures occur more frequently in primary brain tumors than in metastatic brain lesions. Seizures are a presenting symptom of CNS metastasis in 6–29% of cases. Approximately 10% of patients with CNS metastasis eventually develop seizures. Tumors that affect the frontal, temporal, and parietal lobes are more commonly associated with seizures than are occipital lesions. Both early and late seizures are uncommon in patients with posterior fossa and sellar lesions. Seizures are common in patients with CNS metastases from melanoma and low-grade primary brain tumors. Very rarely, cytotoxic drugs such as etoposide, busulfan, ifosfamide, and chlorambucil cause seizures. Treatment with bispecific antibodies and chimeric antigen receptor (CAR) T cells may also cause CNS toxicity including seizures and encephalopathy. Another cause of seizures related to drug therapy is reversible posterior leukoencephalopathy syndrome (RPLS). Chemotherapy, targeted therapy, and immunotherapies have been associated with the development of RPLS. RPLS occurs in patients undergoing allogeneic bone marrow or solid-organ transplantation. RPLS is characterized by headache, altered consciousness, generalized seizures, visual disturbances, hypertension, and symmetric posterior cerebral white matter vasogenic edema on CT/MRI. Seizures may begin focally but are typically generalized.

TREATMENT

Seizures

Patients in whom seizures due to CNS metastases have been demonstrated should receive anticonvulsive treatment with phenytoin or levetiracetam. If this is not effective, valproic acid can be added. Prophylactic anticonvulsant therapy is not recommended. In postcraniotomy patients, prophylactic antiepileptic drugs should be withdrawn during the first week after surgery. Most antiseizure medications including phenytoin induce cytochrome P450 (CYP450), which alters the metabolism of many antitumor agents, including irinotecan, taxanes, and etoposide as well as molecular targeted agents, including imatinib, gefitinib, erlotinib, tipifarnib, sorafenib, sunitinib, temsirolimus, everolimus, and vemurafenib. Levetiracetam and topiramate are anticonvulsant agents not metabolized by the hepatic CYP450 system and do not alter the metabolism of antitumor agents. They have become the preferred drugs. Surgical resection and other antitumor treatments such as radiotherapy and chemotherapy may improve seizure control.

PULMONARY AND INTRACEREBRAL LEUKOSTASIS

Hyperleukocytosis and the leukostasis syndrome associated with it are potentially fatal complications of acute leukemia (particularly myeloid leukemia) that can occur when the peripheral blast cell count is >100,000/mL. The frequency of hyperleukocytosis is 5–13% in acute myeloid leukemia (AML) and 10–30% in acute lymphoid leukemia; however, leukostasis is rare in lymphoid leukemia. At such high blast cell counts, blood viscosity is increased, blood flow is slowed by aggregates of tumor cells, and the primitive myeloid leukemic cells are capable of invading through the endothelium and causing hemorrhage. Brain and lung are most commonly affected. Patients with brain leukostasis may experience stupor, headache, dizziness, tinnitus, visual disturbances, ataxia, confusion, coma, or sudden death. On examination, papilledema, retinal vein distension, retinal hemorrhages, and focal deficit may be present. Pulmonary leukostasis may present as respiratory distress and hypoxemia and progress to respiratory failure. Chest radiographs may be normal but usually show interstitial or alveolar infiltrates. Hyperleukocytosis rarely may cause acute leg ischemia, renal vein thrombosis, myocardial ischemia, bowel infraction, and priapism. Arterial blood gas results should be interpreted cautiously. Rapid consumption of plasma oxygen by the markedly increased number of white blood cells can cause spuriously low arterial oxygen tension. Pulse oximetry is the most accurate way of assessing oxygenation in patients with hyperleukocytosis. Hydroxyurea can rapidly reduce a high blast cell count while the diagnostic workup is in progress. After the diagnosis is established, the patient should start quickly with effective induction chemotherapy. Leukapheresis should be used in patients with symptoms of hyperleukocytosis. Patients with hyperleukocytosis are also at the risk for disseminated intravascular coagulation and tumor lysis syndrome. The clinician should monitor the patient for these complications and take preventive and therapeutic actions during induction therapy. Intravascular volume depletion and unnecessary blood transfusions may increase blood viscosity and worsen the leukostasis syndrome. Leukostasis is very rarely a feature of the high white cell counts associated with chronic lymphoid or chronic myeloid leukemia.

When acute promyelocytic leukemia is treated with differentiating agents like tretinoin and arsenic trioxide, cerebral or pulmonary leukostasis may occur as tumor cells differentiate into mature neutrophils. This complication can be largely avoided by using cytotoxic chemotherapy together with the differentiating agents.

HEMOPTYSIS

Hemoptysis may be caused by nonmalignant conditions, but lung cancer accounts for a large proportion of cases. Up to 20% of patients with lung cancer have hemoptysis some time in their course. Endobronchial metastases from carcinoid tumors, breast cancer, colon cancer, kidney cancer, and melanoma may also cause hemoptysis. The volume of bleeding is often difficult to gauge. Massive hemoptysis is defined as >200–600 mL of blood produced in 24 h. However, any hemoptysis should be considered massive if it threatens life. When respiratory difficulty occurs, hemoptysis should be treated emergently. The first priorities are to maintain the airway, optimize oxygenation, and stabilize the hemodynamic status. If the bleeding side is known, the patient should be placed in a lateral decubitus position, with the bleeding side down to prevent aspiration into the unaffected lung, and given supplemental oxygen. If large-volume bleeding continues or the airway is compromised, the patient should be intubated and undergo emergency bronchoscopy. If the site of bleeding is detected, either the patient undergoes a definitive surgical procedure or the lesion is treated with a neodymium:yttrium-aluminum-garnet (Nd:YAG) laser, argon plasma coagulation, or electrocautery. In stable patients, multidetector CT angiography delineates bronchial and nonbronchial systemic arteries and identifies the source of bleeding and underlying pathology with high sensitivity. Massive hemoptysis usually originates from the high-pressure bronchial circulation. Bronchial artery embolization is considered a first-line definitive procedure for managing hemoptysis. Bronchial artery embolization may control brisk bleeding in 75–90% of patients, permitting the definitive surgical procedure to be done more safely if it is appropriate.

Embolization without definitive surgery is associated with rebleeding in 20–50% of patients. Recurrent hemoptysis usually responds to a second embolization procedure. A postembolization syndrome characterized by pleuritic pain, fever, dysphagia, and leukocytosis may occur; it lasts 5–7 days and resolves with symptomatic treatment. Bronchial or esophageal wall necrosis, myocardial infarction, and spinal cord infarction are rare complications. Surgery, as a salvage strategy, is indicated after failure of embolization and is associated with better survival when performed in a nonurgent setting.

Pulmonary hemorrhage with or without hemoptysis in hematologic malignancies is often associated with fungal infections, particularly *Aspergillus* spp. After granulocytopenia resolves, the lung infiltrates in aspergillosis may cavitate and cause massive hemoptysis. Thrombocytopenia and coagulation defects should be corrected, if possible. Surgical evaluation is recommended in patients with aspergillosis-related cavitary lesions.

Bevacizumab, an antibody to vascular endothelial growth factor (VEGF) that inhibits angiogenesis, has been associated with life-threatening hemoptysis in patients with non-small-cell lung cancer, particularly of squamous cell histology. Non-small-cell lung cancer patients with cavitary lesions or previous hemoptysis (≥2.5 mL) within the past 3 months have higher risk for pulmonary hemorrhage.

AIRWAY OBSTRUCTION

Airway obstruction refers to a blockage at the level of the mainstem bronchi or above. It may result either from intraluminal tumor growth or from extrinsic compression of the airway. The most common cause of malignant upper airway obstruction is invasion from an adjacent primary tumor, most commonly lung cancer, followed by esophageal, thyroid, and mediastinal malignancies including lymphomas. Extrathoracic primary tumors such as renal, colon, or breast cancer can cause airway obstruction through endobronchial and/or mediastinal lymph node metastases. Patients may present with dyspnea, hemoptysis, stridor, wheezing, intractable cough, postobstructive pneumonia, or hoarseness. Chest radiographs usually demonstrate obstructing lesions. CT scans reveal the extent of tumor. Cool, humidified oxygen, glucocorticoids, and ventilation with a mixture of helium and oxygen (Heliox) may provide temporary relief. If the obstruction is proximal to the larynx, a tracheostomy may be lifesaving. For more distal obstructions, particularly intrinsic lesions incompletely obstructing the airway, bronchoscopy with mechanical debulking and dilation or ablational treatments including laser treatment, photodynamic therapy, argon plasma coagulation, electrocautery, or stenting can produce immediate relief in most patients (**Fig. 75-3**). However, radiation therapy (either external-beam irradiation or brachytherapy) given together with glucocorticoids may also open the airway. Symptomatic extrinsic compression may be palliated by stenting. Patients with primary airway tumors such as squamous cell carcinoma, carcinoid tumor, adenocystic carcinoma, or non-small-cell lung cancer, if resectable, should have surgery.

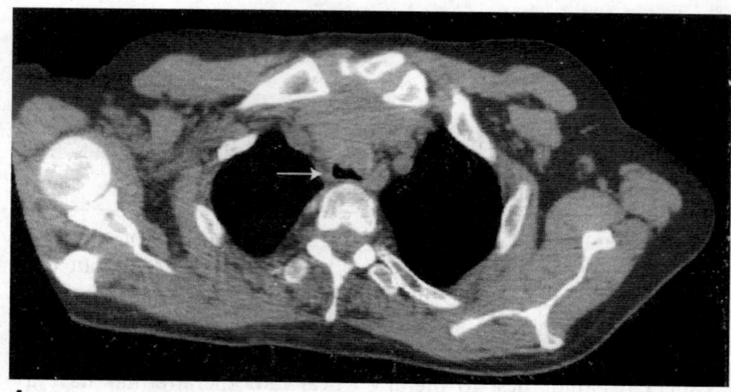

A

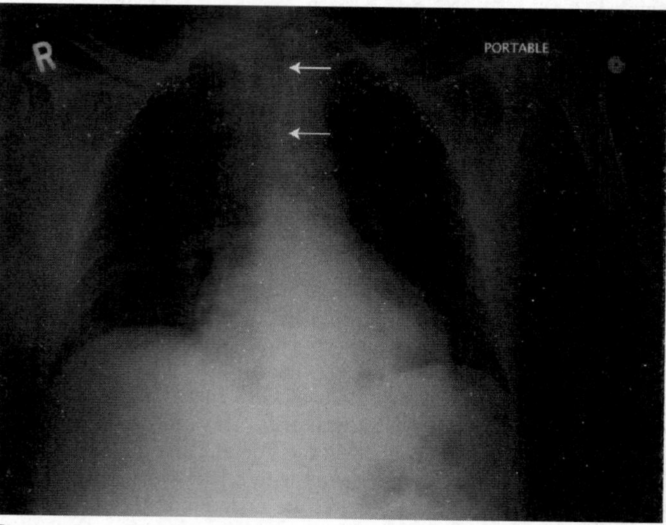

B

FIGURE 75-3 Airway obstruction. *A.* Computed tomography scan of a 62-year-old man with tracheal obstruction caused by renal carcinoma showing paratracheal mass with tracheal invasion/obstruction (*arrow*). ***B.*** Chest x-ray of same patient after stent (*arrows*) placement.

METABOLIC EMERGENCIES

HYPERCALCEMIA

Hypercalcemia is the most common paraneoplastic syndrome. Its pathogenesis and management are discussed fully in **Chaps. 93** and **410**.

SYNDROME OF INAPPROPRIATE SECRETION OF ANTIDIURETIC HORMONE

Hyponatremia is a common electrolyte abnormality in cancer patients, and syndrome of inappropriate secretion of antidiuretic hormone (SIADH) is the most common cause among patients with cancer. SIADH is discussed fully in **Chaps. 93** and **381**.

LACTIC ACIDOSIS

Lactic acidosis is a rare and potentially fatal metabolic complication of cancer. Lactic acidosis associated with sepsis and circulatory failure is a common preterminal event in many malignancies. Lactic acidosis in the absence of hypoxemia may occur in patients with leukemia, lymphoma, or solid tumors. In some cases, hypoglycemia also is present. Extensive involvement of the liver by tumor is often present. In most cases, decreased metabolism and increased production by the tumor both contribute to lactate accumulation. Tumor cell overexpression of certain glycolytic enzymes and mitochondrial dysfunction can contribute to its increased lactate production. HIV-infected patients have an increased risk of aggressive lymphoma; lactic acidosis that occurs in such patients may be related either to the rapid growth of the tumor or from toxicity of nucleoside reverse transcriptase inhibitors. Symptoms of lactic acidosis include tachypnea, tachycardia, change of mental status, and hepatomegaly. The serum level of lactic acid may reach 10–20 mmol/L (90–180 mg/dL). Treatment is aimed at the underlying disease. *The danger from lactic acidosis is from the acidosis, not the lactate.* Sodium bicarbonate should be added if acidosis is very severe or if hydrogen ion production is very rapid and uncontrolled. Other treatment options include renal replacement therapy, such as hemodialysis, and thiamine replacement. The prognosis is poor regardless of the treatment offered.

HYPOGLYCEMIA

Persistent hypoglycemia is occasionally associated with tumors other than pancreatic islet cell tumors. Usually these tumors are large; tumors of mesenchymal origin, hepatomas, or adrenocortical tumors may cause hypoglycemia. Mesenchymal tumors are usually located in the retroperitoneum or thorax. Obtundation, confusion, and behavioral aberrations occur in the postabsorptive period and may precede the diagnosis of the tumor. These tumors often secrete incompletely processed insulin-like growth factor II (IGF-II), a hormone capable of activating insulin receptors and causing hypoglycemia. Tumors secreting incompletely processed big IGF-II are characterized by an increased IGF-II to IGF-I ratio, suppressed insulin and C-peptide level, and inappropriately low growth hormone and β-hydroxybutyrate concentrations. Rarely, hypoglycemia is due to insulin secretion by a non–islet cell carcinoma. The development of hepatic dysfunction from liver metastases and increased glucose consumption by the tumor can contribute to hypoglycemia. If the tumor cannot be resected, hypoglycemia symptoms may be relieved by the administration of glucose, glucocorticoids, recombinant growth hormone, or glucagon.

Hypoglycemia can be artifactual; hyperleukocytosis from leukemia, myeloproliferative diseases, leukemoid reactions, or colony-stimulating factor treatment can increase glucose consumption in the test tube after blood is drawn, leading to pseudohypoglycemia.

■ ADRENAL INSUFFICIENCY

In patients with cancer, adrenal insufficiency may go unrecognized because the symptoms, such as nausea, vomiting, anorexia, and orthostatic hypotension, are nonspecific and may be mistakenly attributed to progressive cancer or to therapy. Primary adrenal insufficiency may develop owing to replacement of both glands by metastases (lung, breast, colon, or kidney cancer; lymphoma), to removal of both glands, or to hemorrhagic necrosis in association with sepsis or anticoagulation. Impaired adrenal steroid synthesis occurs in patients being treated for cancer with mitotane, ketoconazole, or aminoglutethimide or undergoing rapid reduction in glucocorticoid therapy. Megestrol acetate, used to manage cancer and HIV-related cachexia, may suppress plasma levels of cortisol and adrenocorticotropic hormone (ACTH). Patients taking megestrol may develop adrenal insufficiency, and even those whose adrenal dysfunction is not symptomatic may have inadequate adrenal reserve if they become seriously ill. Paradoxically, some patients may develop Cushing's syndrome and/or hyperglycemia because of the glucocorticoid-like activity of megestrol acetate. Ipilimumab, an anti-CTLA-4 antibody used for treatment of malignant melanoma, may cause autoimmunity including autoimmune-like enterocolitis, hypophysitis (leading to secondary adrenal insufficiency), hepatitis, and, rarely, primary adrenal insufficiency. Autoimmune hypophysitis may present with headache, visual field defects, and pituitary hormone deficiencies manifesting as hypopituitarism, adrenal insufficiency (including adrenal crisis), or hypothyroidism. Ipilimumab-associated hypophysitis symptoms occur at an average of 6–12 weeks after initiation of therapy. An MRI usually shows homogenous enhancement of pituitary gland. Early glucocorticoid treatment and hormone replacement are the initial treatment. The role of high-dose glucocorticoids in the treatment of hypophysitis is not clear. High-dose glucocorticoids may not improve the frequency of pituitary function recovery. Autoimmune adrenalitis can also be observed with anti-CTLA-4 antibody. Pituitary dysfunction is usually permanent, requiring long-term hormone replacement therapy. Other checkpoint inhibitors, such as monoclonal antibodies targeting programmed cell death-1 (PD-1), an inhibitory receptor expressed by T cells or one of its ligands (PD-L1), may cause hypophysitis infrequently (~1%). Autoimmune adrenalitis is more frequent with use of PD-1/PD-L1 than with CTLA-4 inhibitors, but incidence is low. Cranial irradiation for childhood brain tumors may affect the hypothalamus-pituitary-adrenal axis, resulting in secondary adrenal insufficiency. Rarely, metastatic replacement causes primary adrenal insufficiency as the first manifestation of an occult malignancy. Metastasis to the pituitary or hypothalamus is found at autopsy in up to 5% of patients with cancer, but associated secondary adrenal insufficiency is rare.

Acute adrenal insufficiency is potentially lethal. Treatment of suspected adrenal crisis is initiated after the sampling of serum cortisol and ACTH levels (**Chap. 386**).

TREATMENT-RELATED EMERGENCIES

■ TUMOR LYSIS SYNDROME

Tumor lysis syndrome (TLS) is characterized by hyperuricemia, hyperkalemia, hyperphosphatemia, and hypocalcemia and is caused by the destruction of a large number of rapidly proliferating neoplastic cells. Acidosis may also develop. Acute renal failure occurs frequently.

TLS is most often associated with the treatment of Burkitt's lymphoma, acute lymphoblastic leukemia, and other rapidly proliferating lymphomas, but it also may be seen with chronic leukemias and, rarely, with solid tumors. This syndrome has been seen in patients with chronic lymphocytic leukemia after treatment with nucleosides like fludarabine and is increased in frequency in lymphoid neoplasms treated with venetoclax, a bcl-2 antagonist. TLS has been observed with administration of glucocorticoids, hormonal agents such as letrozole and tamoxifen, and monoclonal antibodies such as rituximab, obinutuzumab, ofatumumab, and gemtuzumab. TLS usually occurs during or shortly (1–5 days) after chemotherapy. Rarely, spontaneous necrosis of malignancies causes TLS.

Hyperuricemia may be present at the time of chemotherapy. Effective treatment kills malignant cells and leads to increased serum uric acid levels from the turnover of nucleic acids. Owing to the acidic local environment, uric acid can precipitate in the tubules, medulla, and collecting ducts of the kidney, leading to renal failure. Lactic acidosis and dehydration may contribute to the precipitation of uric acid in the renal tubules. The finding of uric acid crystals in the urine is strong evidence for uric acid nephropathy. The ratio of urinary uric acid to urinary creatinine is >1 in patients with acute hyperuricemic nephropathy and <1 in patients with renal failure due to other causes. Other events may lead to renal failure in TLS. Calcium phosphate also precipitates in the interstitium and renal microvasculature, leading to nephrocalcinosis. Both types of crystals are toxic to the tubular epithelium, inducing local active inflammatory and pro-oxidative responses. Soluble uric acid may induce hemodynamic changes, with decreased renal blood flow due to vasoconstriction and impaired autoregulation (crystal-independent pathway).

Hyperphosphatemia, which can be caused by the release of intracellular phosphate pools by tumor lysis, produces a reciprocal depression in serum calcium, which causes severe neuromuscular irritability and tetany. Deposition of calcium phosphate in the kidney and hyperphosphatemia may cause renal failure. Potassium is the principal intracellular cation, and massive destruction of malignant cells may lead to hyperkalemia. Hyperkalemia in patients with renal failure may rapidly become life threatening by causing ventricular arrhythmias and sudden death.

The likelihood that TLS will occur in patients with Burkitt's lymphoma is related to the tumor burden and renal function. Hyperuricemia and high serum levels of lactate dehydrogenase (LDH >1500 U/L), both of which correlate with total tumor burden, also correlate with the risk of TLS. In patients at risk for TLS, pretreatment evaluations should include a complete blood count, serum chemistry evaluation, and urine analysis. High leukocyte and platelet counts may artificially elevate potassium levels ("pseudohyperkalemia") due to lysis of these cells after the blood is drawn. In these cases, plasma potassium instead of serum potassium should be followed. In pseudohyperkalemia, no electrocardiographic abnormalities are present. In patients with abnormal baseline renal function, the kidneys and retroperitoneal area should be evaluated by sonography and/or CT to rule out obstructive uropathy. Urine output should be watched closely.

TREATMENT

Tumor Lysis Syndrome

Recognition of risk and prevention are the most important steps in the management of this syndrome (**Fig. 75-4**). The standard preventive approach consists of allopurinol and aggressive hydration. Urinary alkalization with sodium bicarbonate is no longer recommended. It increases uric acid solubility, but a high pH decreases the solubility of xanthine, hypoxanthine, and calcium phosphate, potentially increasing the likelihood of intratubular crystallization. Intravenous allopurinol may be given in patients who cannot tolerate oral therapy. Febuxostat, a potent nonpurine selective xanthine oxidase inhibitor, is indicated for treatment of hyperuricemia. It

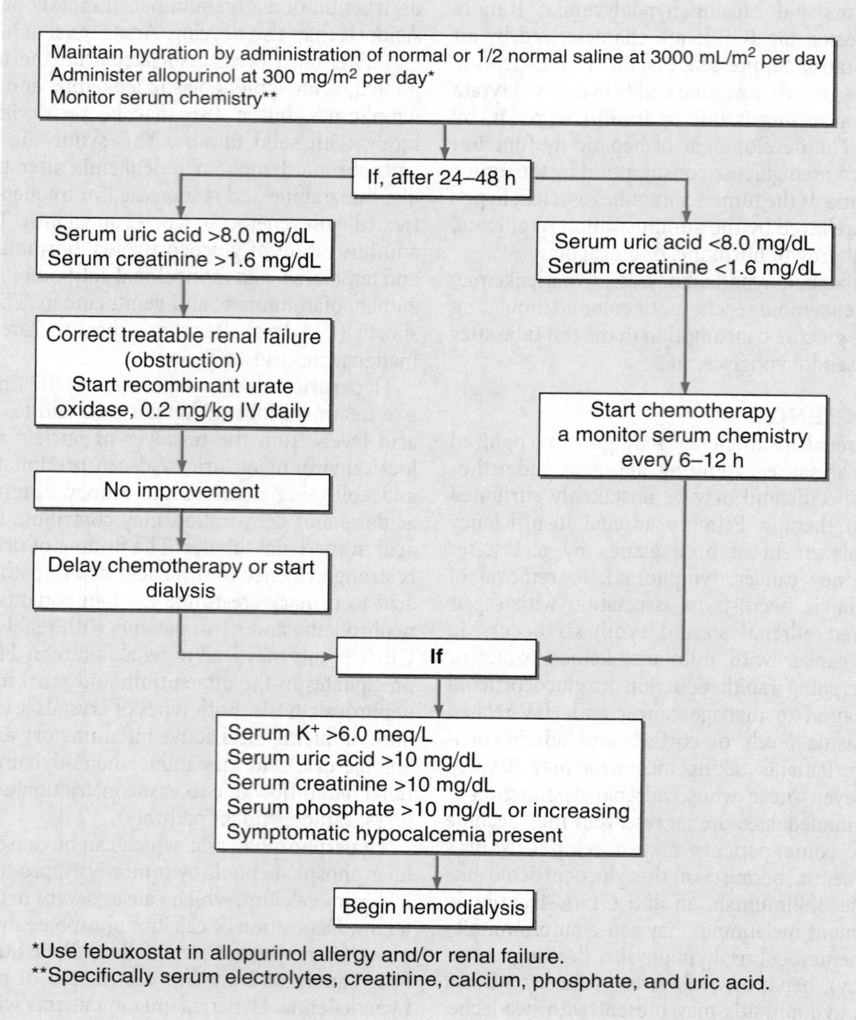
Maintain hydration by administration of normal or 1/2 normal saline at 3000 mL/m2 per day
Administer allopurinol at 300 mg/m2 per day*
Monitor serum chemistry**
If, after 24–48 h
Serum uric acid >8.0 mg/dL
Serum creatinine >1.6 mg/dL
Serum uric acid <8.0 mg/dL
Serum creatinine <1.6 mg/dL
Correct treatable renal failure (obstruction)
Start recombinant urate oxidase, 0.2 mg/kg IV daily
Start chemotherapy a monitor serum chemistry every 6–12 h
No improvement
Delay chemotherapy or start dialysis
If
Serum K+ >6.0 meq/L
Serum uric acid >10 mg/dL
Serum creatinine >10 mg/dL
Serum phosphate >10 mg/dL or increasing
Symptomatic hypocalcemia present
Begin hemodialysis
*Use febuxostat in allopurinol allergy and/or renal failure.
**Specifically serum electrolytes, creatinine, calcium, phosphate, and uric acid.

FIGURE 75-4 Management of patients at high risk for the tumor lysis syndrome.

results in fewer hypersensitivity reactions than allopurinol. Febuxostat does not require dosage adjustment in patients with mild to moderate renal impairment. Febuxostat achieved significantly superior serum uric acid control in comparison to allopurinol in patients with hematologic malignancies at intermediate to high TLS risk. In some cases, uric acid levels cannot be lowered sufficiently with the standard preventive approach. Rasburicase (recombinant urate oxidase) can be effective in these instances, particularly when renal failure is present. Urate oxidase is missing from primates and catalyzes the conversion of poorly soluble uric acid to readily soluble allantoin. Rasburicase acts rapidly, decreasing uric acid levels within hours; however, it may cause hypersensitivity reactions such as bronchospasm, hypoxemia, and hypotension. Rasburicase should also be administered to high-risk patients for TLS prophylaxis. Rasburicase is contraindicated in patients with glucose-6-phosphate dehydrogenase deficiency who are unable to break down hydrogen peroxide, an end product of the urate oxidase reaction. Rasburicase is known to cause ex vivo enzymatic degradation of uric acid in test tube at room temperature. This leads to spuriously low uric acid levels during laboratory monitoring of the patient with TLS. Samples must be cooled immediately to deactivate the urate oxidase. Despite aggressive prophylaxis, TLS and/or oliguric or anuric renal failure may occur. Renal replacement therapy is often necessary and should be considered early in the course. Hemodialysis is preferred. Hemofiltration offers a gradual, continuous method of removing cellular by-products and fluid.

HUMAN ANTIBODY INFUSION REACTIONS

The initial infusion of human or humanized antibodies (e.g., rituximab, gemtuzumab, trastuzumab, alemtuzumab, panitumumab, brentuximab vedotin, blinatumomab) is associated with fever, chills, nausea, asthenia, and headache in up to half of treated patients. Bronchospasm and hypotension occur in 1% of patients. Severe manifestations including pulmonary infiltrates, acute respiratory distress syndrome (ARDS), and cardiogenic shock occur rarely. Laboratory manifestations include elevated hepatic aminotransferase levels, thrombocytopenia, and prolongation of prothrombin time. The pathogenesis is thought to be activation of immune effector processes (cells and complement) and release of inflammatory cytokines, such as tumor necrosis factor α, interferon γ, interleukin (IL) 6, and IL-10 (cytokine release syndrome [CRS]). Although its origins are not completely understood, CRS is believed to be due to activation of a variety of cell types including monocytes/macrophages and T and B lymphocytes. Hemophagocytic lymphohistiocytosis (HLH)/macrophage activation syndrome (MAS) can develop as part of CRS and usually is a manifestation of severe CRS.

Severe CRS may require intensive support for ARDS and resistant hypotension. Emerging clinical experience at several institutions has concluded that tocilizumab is an effective treatment for severe or life-threatening CRS. Tocilizumab prevents IL-6 binding to both cell-associated and soluble IL-6 receptors and therefore inhibits both classical and trans-IL-6 signaling. Other cytokine-directed therapies, such as siltuximab, a chimeric anti-IL-6 monoclonal antibody, and anakinra, an IL-1 receptor antagonist, have been used.

Adoptive transfer of CAR-engineered T cells is a promising therapy for cancers. The most common acute toxicity of CAR T cells is CRS. CAR T cell–associated CRS may be associated with cardiac dysfunction and neurotoxicity. The management includes supportive care and tocilizumab.

Severe reactions from rituximab have occurred with high numbers (>50 × 10^9 lymphocytes) of circulating cells bearing the target antigen (CD20) and have been associated with a rapid fall in circulating tumor cells, mild electrolyte evidence of TLS, and, very rarely, death. In addition, increased liver enzymes, D-dimer, and LDH and prolongation of the prothrombin time may occur. Diphenhydramine, hydrocortisone, and acetaminophen can often prevent or suppress the infusion-related symptoms. If they occur, the infusion is stopped and restarted at half the initial infusion rate after the symptoms have abated.

HEMOLYTIC-UREMIC SYNDROME

Hemolytic-uremic syndrome (HUS) and, less commonly, thrombotic thrombocytopenic purpura (TTP) **(Chap. 317)** may rarely occur after treatment with antineoplastic drugs, including mitomycin, gemcitabine, cisplatin, bleomycin, and proteasome inhibitors, and with VEGF inhibitors. Mitomycin and gemcitabine are the most common offenders. Unlike mitomycin, there is no clear-cut relationship between the cumulative dose of gemcitabine and risk of HUS. It occurs most often in patients with gastric, lung, colorectal, pancreatic, and breast carcinoma. In one series, 35% of patients were without evident cancer at the time this syndrome appeared. Secondary HUS/TTP has also been reported as a rare but sometimes fatal complication of bone marrow transplantation.

HUS usually has its onset 4–8 weeks after the last dose of chemotherapy, but it is not rare to detect it several months later. HUS is characterized by microangiopathic hemolytic anemia, thrombocytopenia, and renal failure. Dyspnea, weakness, fatigue, oliguria, and purpura are also common initial symptoms and findings. Systemic hypertension and pulmonary edema frequently occur. Severe hypertension, pulmonary edema, and rapid worsening of hemolysis and renal function may occur after a blood or blood product transfusion. Cardiac findings include atrial arrhythmias, pericardial friction rub, and pericardial effusion. Raynaud's phenomenon is part of the syndrome in patients treated with bleomycin.

Laboratory findings include severe to moderate anemia associated with red blood cell fragmentation and numerous schistocytes on peripheral smear. Reticulocytosis, decreased plasma haptoglobin, and an LDH level document hemolysis. The serum bilirubin level is usually normal or slightly elevated. The Coombs test is negative. The white cell count is usually normal, and thrombocytopenia (<100,000/μL) is almost always present. Most patients have a normal coagulation profile, although some have mild elevations in thrombin time and in levels of fibrin degradation products. The serum creatinine level is elevated at presentation and shows a pattern of subacute worsening within weeks of the initial azotemia. The urinalysis reveals hematuria, proteinuria, and granular or hyaline casts, and circulating immune complexes may be present.

The basic pathologic lesion appears to be deposition of fibrin in the walls of capillaries and arterioles, and these deposits are similar to those seen in HUS due to other causes. These microvascular abnormalities involve mainly the kidneys and rarely occur in other organs. The pathogenesis of cancer treatment–related HUS is not completely understood, but probably the most important factor is endothelial damage. Primary forms of HUS/TTP are related to a decrease in processing of von Willebrand factor by a protease called ADAMTS13.

The case-fatality rate is high; most patients die within a few months. Optimal treatment for chemotherapy-induced HUS is debated. Immunocomplex removal through plasmapheresis, plasma exchange, immunoadsorption, or exchange transfusion, antiplatelet and anticoagulant therapies, and immunosuppression have all been employed with varying degrees of success.

The outcome with plasma exchange is generally poor, as in many other cases of secondary TTP. Rituximab is successfully used in patients with chemotherapy-induced HUS as well as in ADAMTS13-deficient TTP. Eculizumab, a complement inhibitor, is now approved by the U.S. Food and Drug Administration (FDA) and considered first line for the treatment of atypical HUS. Vaccination against *Neisseria meningitis* is mandatory before eculizumab is administered.

NEUTROPENIA AND INFECTION

These remain the most common serious complications of cancer therapy. They are covered in detail in **Chap. 74**.

PULMONARY INFILTRATES

Patients with cancer may present with dyspnea associated with diffuse interstitial infiltrates on chest radiographs. Such infiltrates may be due to progression of the underlying malignancy, treatment-related toxicities, infection, and/or unrelated diseases. The cause may be multifactorial; however, most commonly, they occur as a consequence of treatment. Infiltration of the lung by malignancy has been described in patients with leukemia, lymphoma, and breast and other solid cancers. Pulmonary lymphatics may be involved diffusely by neoplasm (pulmonary lymphangitic carcinomatosis), resulting in a diffuse increase in interstitial markings on chest radiographs. The patient is often mildly dyspneic at the onset, but pulmonary failure develops over a period of weeks. In some patients, dyspnea precedes changes on the chest radiographs and is accompanied by a nonproductive cough. This syndrome is characteristic of solid tumors. In patients with leukemia, diffuse microscopic neoplastic peribronchial and peribronchiolar infiltration is frequent but may be asymptomatic. However, some patients present with diffuse interstitial infiltrates, an alveolar capillary block syndrome, and respiratory distress. Thickening of bronchovascular bundles and prominence of peripheral arteries are CT findings suggestive of leukemic infiltration. In these situations, glucocorticoids can provide symptomatic relief, but specific chemotherapy should always be started promptly.

Several cytotoxic agents, such as bleomycin, methotrexate, busulfan, nitrosoureas, gemcitabine, mitomycin, vinorelbine, docetaxel, paclitaxel, fludarabine, pentostatin, and ifosfamide, may cause pulmonary damage. The most frequent presentations are interstitial pneumonitis, alveolitis, and pulmonary fibrosis. Some cytotoxic agents, including methotrexate and procarbazine, may cause an acute hypersensitivity reaction. Cytosine arabinoside has been associated with noncardiogenic pulmonary edema. Administration of multiple cytotoxic drugs, as well as radiotherapy and preexisting lung disease, may potentiate the pulmonary toxicity. Supplemental oxygen may potentiate the effects of drugs and radiation injury. Patients should always be managed with the lowest FIO_2 that is sufficient to maintain hemoglobin saturation.

The onset of symptoms may be insidious, with symptoms including dyspnea, nonproductive cough, and tachycardia. Patients may have bibasilar crepitant rales, end-inspiratory crackles, fever, and cyanosis. The chest radiograph generally shows an interstitial and sometimes an intraalveolar pattern that is strongest at the lung bases and may be symmetric. A small effusion may occur. Hypoxemia with decreased carbon monoxide diffusing capacity is always present. Glucocorticoids may be helpful in patients in whom pulmonary toxicity is related to radiation therapy or to chemotherapy. Treatment is otherwise supportive.

Molecular targeted agents, imatinib, erlotinib, and gefitinib are potent inhibitors of tyrosine kinases. These drugs may cause interstitial lung disease (ILD). In the case of gefitinib, preexisting fibrosis, poor performance status, and prior thoracic irradiation are independent risk factors; this complication has a high fatality rate. In Japan, incidence of ILD associated with gefitinib was ~4.5% compared to 0.5% in the United States. Temsirolimus and everolimus, both esters of rapamycin (sirolimus), are agents that block the effects of mammalian target of rapamycin (mTOR), an enzyme that has an important role in regulating the synthesis of proteins that control cell division. These agents may cause ground-glass opacities (GGO) in the lung with or without diffuse interstitial disease and lung parenchymal consolidation. Patients may be asymptomatic with only radiologic findings or may be symptomatic. Symptoms include cough, dyspnea, and/or hypoxemia, and sometimes patients present with systemic symptoms such as fever and fatigue. The incidence of everolimus-induced ILD also appears to be higher in

Japanese patients. Treatment includes dose reduction or withdrawal and, in some cases, the addition of glucocorticoids.

The FDA-approved immune checkpoint inhibitors (ICI) of the PD-1 and PD-L1 pathway, including nivolumab, pembrolizumab, durvalumab, avelumab, atezolizumab, and cemiplimab, enhance antitumor activity by blocking negative regulators of T-cell function. Immune-mediated pneumonitis is rare (10%) but may be a life-threatening complication of these drugs. Pneumonitis symptoms include cough, shortness of breath, dyspnea, and fever, and often involve only asymptomatic radiographic changes. Pneumonitis shows ground-glass patchy lesions and/or disseminated nodular infiltrates, predominantly in the lower lobes. Identifying the exact cause of a pneumonitis in a patient treated with ICIs could be challenging during the current COVID-19 outbreak (**Fig. 75-5A**). Chest CT manifestations of COVID-19 include an imaging pattern of pure GGO, consolidation, nodules, fibrous stripes, and mixed patterns, with the distribution slightly predominant in the lower lobe and peripheral areas of the lung. Treatment of immune-mediated pneumonitis includes temporary or permanent withdrawal of drug and the addition of high-dose glucocorticoids (**Fig. 75-5B**).

Radiation pneumonitis and/or fibrosis are relatively frequent side effects of thoracic radiation therapy. It may be acute or chronic. Radiation-induced lung toxicity is a function of the irradiated lung volume, dose per fraction, and radiation dose. The larger the irradiated lung field, the higher is the risk for radiation pneumonitis. The use of concurrent chemoradiation, particularly regimens including paclitaxel, increases pulmonary toxicity. Radiation pneumonitis usually develops 2–6 months after completion of radiotherapy. The clinical syndrome, which varies in severity, consists of dyspnea, cough with scanty sputum, low-grade fever, and an initial hazy infiltrate on chest radiographs. The infiltrate and tissue damage usually are confined to the radiation field. The CT scan may show GGOs, consolidation, fibrosis, atelectatic cicatrization, pleural volume loss, or pleural thickening. The patients subsequently may develop a patchy alveolar infiltrate and air bronchograms, which may progress to acute respiratory failure that is sometimes fatal. A lung biopsy may be necessary to make the diagnosis. Asymptomatic infiltrates found incidentally after radiation therapy need not be treated. However, prednisone should be administered to patients with fever or other symptoms. The dosage should be tapered slowly after the resolution of radiation pneumonitis, because abrupt withdrawal of glucocorticoids may cause an exacerbation of pneumonia. Delayed radiation fibrosis may occur years after radiation therapy and is signaled by dyspnea on exertion. Often it is mild, but it can progress to chronic respiratory failure. Therapy is supportive.

Classic radiation pneumonitis that leads to pulmonary fibrosis is due to radiation-induced production of local cytokines such as platelet-derived growth factor β, tumor necrosis factor, interleukins, and transforming growth factor β in the radiation field.

SBRT is a radiotherapy treatment method that has been applied to the treatment of stage I lung cancers in medically inoperable patients. SBRT accurately delivers a high dose of irradiation in one or few treatment fractions to an image-defined lung mass. Most of the acute changes after SBRT occur later than 3 months after treatment, and the shape of the SBRT-induced injury conforms more tightly to the tumor.

Pneumonia is a common problem in patients undergoing treatment for cancer (**Chap 74**). In patients with pulmonary infiltrates who are

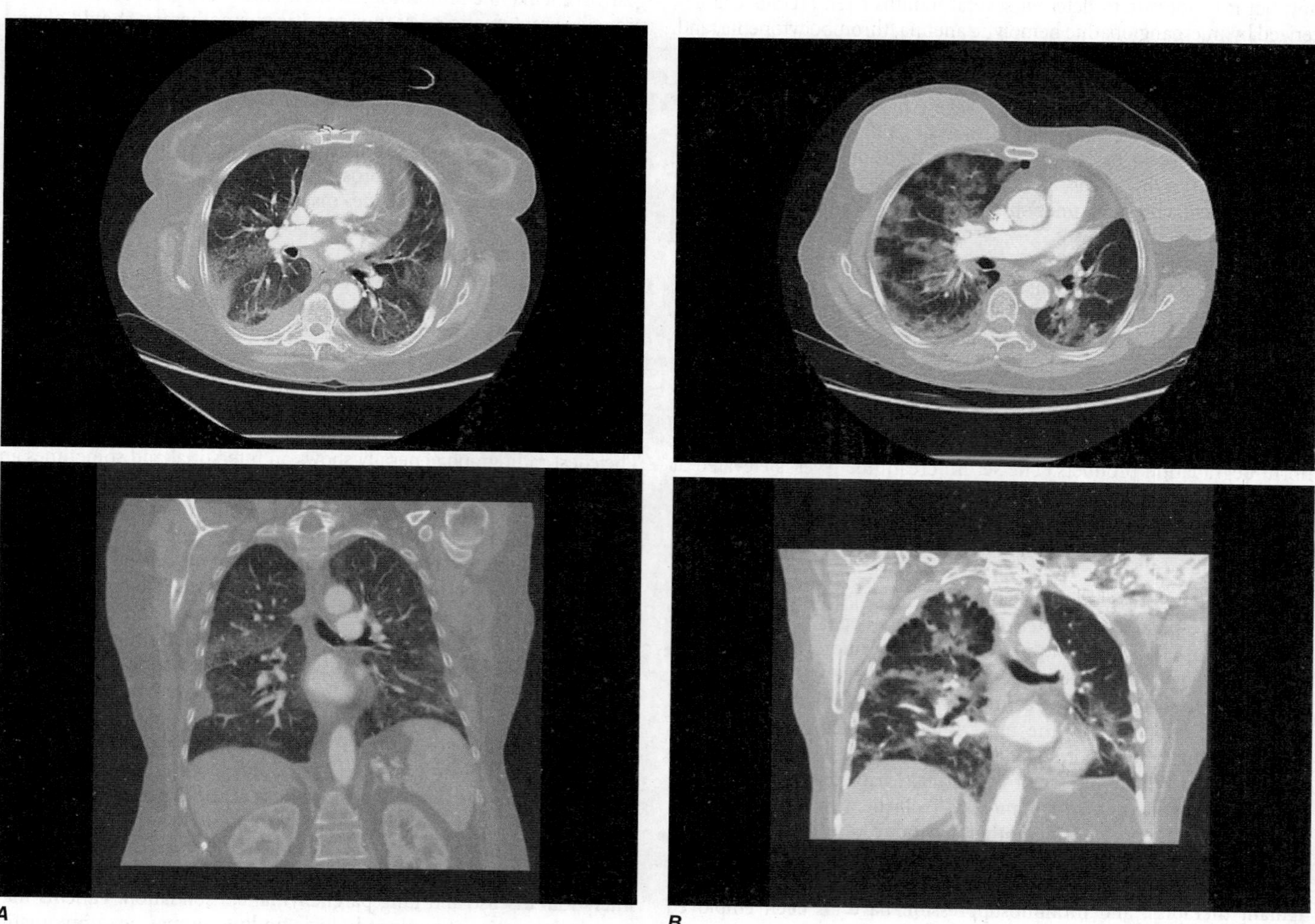

FIGURE 75-5 ***A.*** Computed tomography scan of a 63-year-old female with metastatic adenocarcinoma on nivolumab with immune check point inhibitor pneumonia showing interlobular septal thickening and diffuse ground glass opacity to nivolumab. ***B.*** Computed tomography scan of a 68-year-old female with resected adenocarcinoma of lung and COVID 19 pneumonia showing peripheral and basilar predominant patchy groundglass and consolidative opacity consistent with multifocal COVID pneumonia.

afebrile, heart failure and multiple pulmonary emboli are in the differential diagnosis.

NEUTROPENIC ENTEROCOLITIS

Neutropenic enterocolitis (typhlitis) is the inflammation and necrosis of the cecum and surrounding tissues that may complicate the treatment of acute leukemia. Nevertheless, it may involve any segment of the gastrointestinal tract including small intestine, appendix, and colon. This complication has also been seen in patients with other forms of cancer treated with taxanes, 5-fluorouracil, irinotecan, vinorelbine, cisplatin, carboplatin, and high-dose chemotherapy (**Fig. 75-6**). It also has been reported in patients with AIDS, aplastic anemia, cyclic neutropenia, idiosyncratic drug reactions involving antibiotics, and immunosuppressive therapies. The patient develops right lower quadrant abdominal pain, often with rebound tenderness and a tense, distended abdomen, in a setting of fever and neutropenia. Watery diarrhea (often containing sloughed mucosa) and bacteremia are common, and bleeding may occur. Plain abdominal films are generally of little value in the diagnosis; CT scan may show marked bowel wall thickening, particularly in the cecum, with bowel wall edema, mesenteric stranding, and ascites, and may help to differentiate neutropenic colitis from other abdominal disorders such as appendicitis, diverticulitis, and *Clostridium difficile*–associated colitis in this high-risk population. Patients with bowel wall thickness >10 mm on ultrasonogram have higher mortality rates. However, bowel wall thickening is significantly more prominent in patients with *C. difficile* colitis. Pneumatosis intestinalis is a more specific finding, seen only in those with neutropenic enterocolitis and ischemia. The combined involvement of the small and large bowel suggests a diagnosis of neutropenic enterocolitis. Rapid institution of broad-spectrum antibiotics, bowel rest, and nasogastric suction may reverse the process. Use of myeloid growth factors improved outcome significantly. Surgical intervention is reserved for severe cases of neutropenic enterocolitis with evidence of perforation, peritonitis, gangrenous bowel, or gastrointestinal hemorrhage despite correction of any coagulopathy.

C. difficile colitis is increasing in incidence. Newer strains of *C. difficile* produce ~20 times more of toxins A and B compared to previously studied strains. *C. difficile* risk is also increased with chemotherapy. Antibiotic coverage for *C. difficile* should be added if pseudomembranous colitis cannot be excluded.

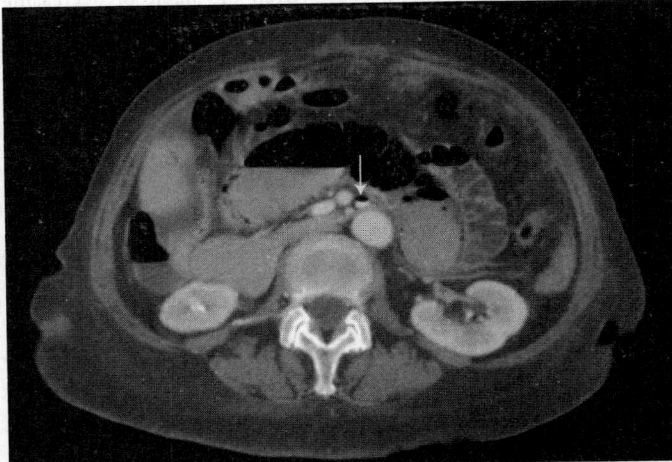

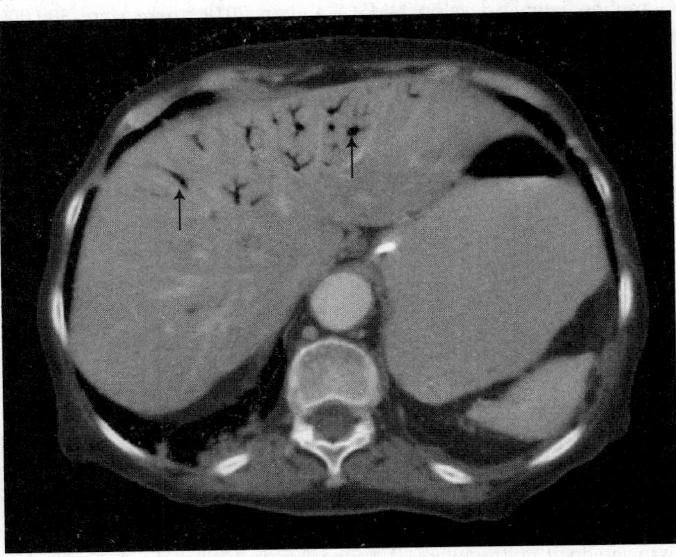

FIGURE 75-6 Abdominal computed tomography (CT) scans of a 72-year-old woman with neutropenic enterocolitis secondary to chemotherapy. ***A.*** Air in inferior mesenteric vein (*arrow*) and bowel wall with pneumatosis intestinalis. ***B.*** CT scan of upper abdomen demonstrating air in portal vein (*arrows*).

HEMORRHAGIC CYSTITIS

Hemorrhagic cystitis is characterized by diffuse bladder mucosal bleeding that develops secondary to chemotherapy (mostly cyclophosphamide or ifosfamide), radiation therapy, bone marrow transplantation (BMT), and/or opportunistic infections. Both cyclophosphamide and ifosfamide are metabolized to acrolein, which is a strong chemical irritant that is excreted in the urine. Prolonged contact or high concentrations may lead to bladder irritation and hemorrhage. Symptoms include gross hematuria, frequency, dysuria, burning, urgency, incontinence, and nocturia. The best management is prevention. Maintaining a high rate of urine flow minimizes exposure. In addition, 2-mercaptoethanesulfonate (mesna) detoxifies the metabolites and can be coadministered with the instigating drugs. Mesna usually is given three times on the day of ifosfamide administration in doses that are each 20% of the total ifosfamide dose. If hemorrhagic cystitis develops, the maintenance of a high urine flow may be sufficient supportive care. If conservative management is not effective, irrigation of the bladder with a 0.37–0.74% formalin solution for 10 min stops the bleeding in most cases. *N*-Acetylcysteine may also be an effective irrigant. Prostaglandin (carboprost) can inhibit the process. In extreme cases, ligation of the hypogastric arteries, urinary diversion, or cystectomy may be necessary.

In the BMT setting, early-onset hemorrhagic cystitis is related to drugs in the treatment regimen (e.g., cyclophosphamide), and late-onset hemorrhagic cystitis is usually due to the polyoma virus BKV or adenovirus type 11. BKV load in urine alone or in combination with acute graft-versus-host disease correlates with development of hemorrhagic cystitis. Viral causes are usually detected by polymerase chain reaction (PCR)–based diagnostic tests. Treatment of viral hemorrhagic cystitis is largely supportive, with reduction in doses of immunosuppressive agents, if possible. No antiviral therapy is approved, although cidofovir was reported to be effective in a small series. Hyperbaric oxygen therapy has been used successfully in patients with BKV-associated and cyclophosphamide-induced hemorrhagic cystitis during hematopoietic stem cell transplantation, as well as in hemorrhagic radiation cystitis that occurs in up to 5% of patients after pelvic radiation.

HYPERSENSITIVITY REACTIONS TO ANTINEOPLASTIC DRUGS

Many antineoplastic drugs may cause hypersensitivity reaction. These reactions are unpredictable and potentially life threatening. Most reactions occur during or within hours of parenteral drug administration. Taxanes, platinum compounds, asparaginase, etoposide, procarbazine, and biologic agents, including rituximab, bevacizumab, trastuzumab, gemtuzumab, cetuximab, and alemtuzumab, are more commonly associated with acute hypersensitivity reactions than are other agents. Hypersensitivity reactions to some drugs, such as taxanes, occur during the first or second dose administered. Hypersensitivity to platinum compounds occurs after prolonged exposure. Skin testing may identify patients with high risk for hypersensitivity after carboplatin exposure. Premedication with histamine H_1 and H_2 receptor antagonists and glucocorticoids reduces the incidence of hypersensitivity reaction to taxanes, particularly paclitaxel. Despite premedication, hypersensitivity reactions may still occur. In these cases, rapid desensitization in the intensive care unit setting or re-treatment may be attempted with care, but the use of alternative agents may be required. Skin testing is used to assess the involvement of IgE in the reaction. Tryptase levels measured at the time of the reaction help to explain the mechanism of the reaction and its severity. Increased tryptase levels indicate underlying mast cell activation. Candidate patients for desensitization include those who have mild to severe hypersensitivity type I, with mast cell–mediated and IgE-dependent reactions occurring during a chemotherapy infusion or shortly thereafter.

FURTHER READING

Azizi AH et al: Superior vena cava syndrome. JACC Cardiovasc Interv 13:2896, 2020.

Castells M et al: Hypersensitivity to antineoplastic agents: Mechanisms and treatment with rapid desensitization. Cancer Immunol Immunother 61:1575, 2012.

Castinetti F et al: Endocrine side-effects of new anticancer therapies: Overall monitoring and conclusions. Ann Endocrinol (Paris) 79:591, 2018.

Durani U, Hogan WJ: Emergencies in haematology: Tumour lysis syndrome. Br J Haematol 188:494, 2020.

Fajgenbaum DC, June CH: Cytokine storm. N Engl J Med 383:2255, 2020.

Gonzalez Castro LN, Milligan TA: Seizures in patients with cancer. Cancer 126:1379, 2020.

Lawton AJ et al: Assessment and management of patients with metastatic spinal cord compression: A multidisciplinary review. J Clin Oncol 37:61, 2019.

Lin AL, Avila EK: Neurologic emergencies in the patients with cancer. J Intensive Care Med 32:99, 2017.

Pellerino A et al: Neoplastic meningitis in solid tumors: From diagnosis to personalized treatments. Ther Adv Neurol Disord 11:1756286418759618, 2018.

Riaz A et al: Percutaneous management of malignant biliary disease. J Surg Oncol 120:45, 2019.

Schusler R, Meyerson SL: Pericardial disease associated with malignancy. Curr Cardiol Rep 20:92, 2018.

Thomas MR, Scully M: How I treat microangiopathic hemolytic anemia in patients with cancer. Blood 137:1310, 2021.

76 Cancer of the Skin

Brendan D. Curti, John T. Vetto, Sancy A. Leachman

MELANOMA

Pigmented lesions are among the most common findings on skin examination. The challenge for the physician is to distinguish benign lesions from cutaneous melanomas and nonmelanoma skin cancers (NMSCs). Both melanoma and NMSC are increasing in frequency, and melanoma accounts for over half of the deaths resulting from skin cancer. Melanoma is an aggressive malignancy of melanocytes, pigment-producing cells that originate from the neural crest and migrate to the skin, meninges, mucous membranes, upper esophagus, and eyes. Melanocytes in each of these locations have the potential for malignant transformation, but the vast majority of melanomas arise in the skin, often permitting detection at a time when complete surgical excision leads to cure. Cutaneous melanoma can occur in people of all ages and all colors. Examples of malignant melanoma of the skin, mucosa, eye, and nail are shown in **Fig. 76-1**.

RISK FACTORS AND EPIDEMIOLOGY

The epidemiologic patterns seen in melanoma reflect the genetic and biologic features of melanocytes and their response to environmental ultraviolet radiation (UVR). Clinical features that confer an increased risk for melanoma include: (1) vulnerability to sun damage (light/red coloration of skin, hair, or eyes; photodamaged skin; history of exposure to natural or artificial UVR; prior history of skin cancers of any type); (2) abnormal growth of melanocytes (increased absolute number of nevi, increased size of nevi, or atypical features of moles such as multiple colors, speckles, or shapes); and (3) immunosuppression (innate, functional, or drug-induced). **Table 76-1** summarizes melanoma risk factors and the relative risk associated with these factors.

The incidence and mortality rates are strongly influenced by ethnic and geographic/environmental factors, which superimpose substantial variability on melanoma rates. Specifically, the incidence of melanoma is 1/100,000 per year in populations with high skin eumelanin content and up to 27/100,000 per year in populations with low skin eumelanin. Men are affected slightly more than women (1.3:1), and the median age at diagnosis is the late fifties. Melanoma is one of the few cancer types with increasing incidence in the United States and is now the fifth leading cancer in men (60,190 new cases estimated in 2020; probability 1:28) and the sixth leading cancer in women (40,160 new cases estimated in 2020; probability 1:41). Although these rankings are based on the total number of new invasive melanoma cases (100,350 in 2020), an additional 95,710 cases of melanoma in situ are expected to occur in 2020. Given the stable or decreasing mortality (see below), it seems likely that new cases include some that represent overdiagnosis of cancers that would not progress to fatal disease.

Mortality rates begin to rise at age 55, with the greatest mortality in men age >65 years. In contrast to the increasing incidence, the mortality rates for melanoma are decreasing, though this trend appears less dramatic outside of the United States. The reasons for the decrease are not entirely clear but have been attributed in part to the recent success of melanoma therapeutics on survival. After U.S. Food and Drug Administration (FDA) approval of ipilimumab and vemurafenib in 2011, the 1-year relative survival rate increased from 42% (2008–2010) to 55% (2013–2015). The mortality rate from 2013 to 2017 dropped annually by 7% in those aged 20–64 years old and dropped 5–6% per year for individuals aged ≥65 years.

GLOBAL CONSIDERATIONS

The incidence of both nonmelanoma and melanoma skin cancers around the world has been increasing. Every year, between 2 and 3 million people develop NMSC, and in 2018, there were 300,000 cases of melanoma. A disproportionate number of cases and deaths occur in North America, Europe, Australia, and New Zealand. The highly variable incidence rates of melanoma in different populations are due to the interplay between risk factors, including host genetics and environmental factors, that distribute risk unevenly across these populations and account for the absolute risk in different ethnic groups and geographic areas.

Dark-skinned populations (such as those of India and Puerto Rico), blacks, and East Asians also develop melanoma but at rates 10–20 times lower than those in whites. Cutaneous melanomas in dark-skinned populations are more often diagnosed at a higher stage, and patients tend to have worse outcomes. Surveillance, Epidemiology, and End Results (SEER) data (2000–2004) reveal that whites have the highest incidence of melanoma at 27.2/100,000 and that the incidence drops substantially in Hispanics (4.5/100,000), Native Americans (4.1/100,000), Asians/Pacific Islanders (1.7/100,000), and blacks (1.1/100,000). In nonwhite populations, the frequency of acral (subungual, plantar, palmar) and mucosal melanomas is much higher; the incidence of melanoma in black and Hispanic populations is not associated with ultraviolet (UV) exposure. In China, about 20,000 new melanomas are reported each year, and in contrast to the United States, mortality is increasing. This may be due to the fact that in Asians and dark-skinned populations, more melanomas arise from acral and mucosal areas, which have a different biology and carry a poorer

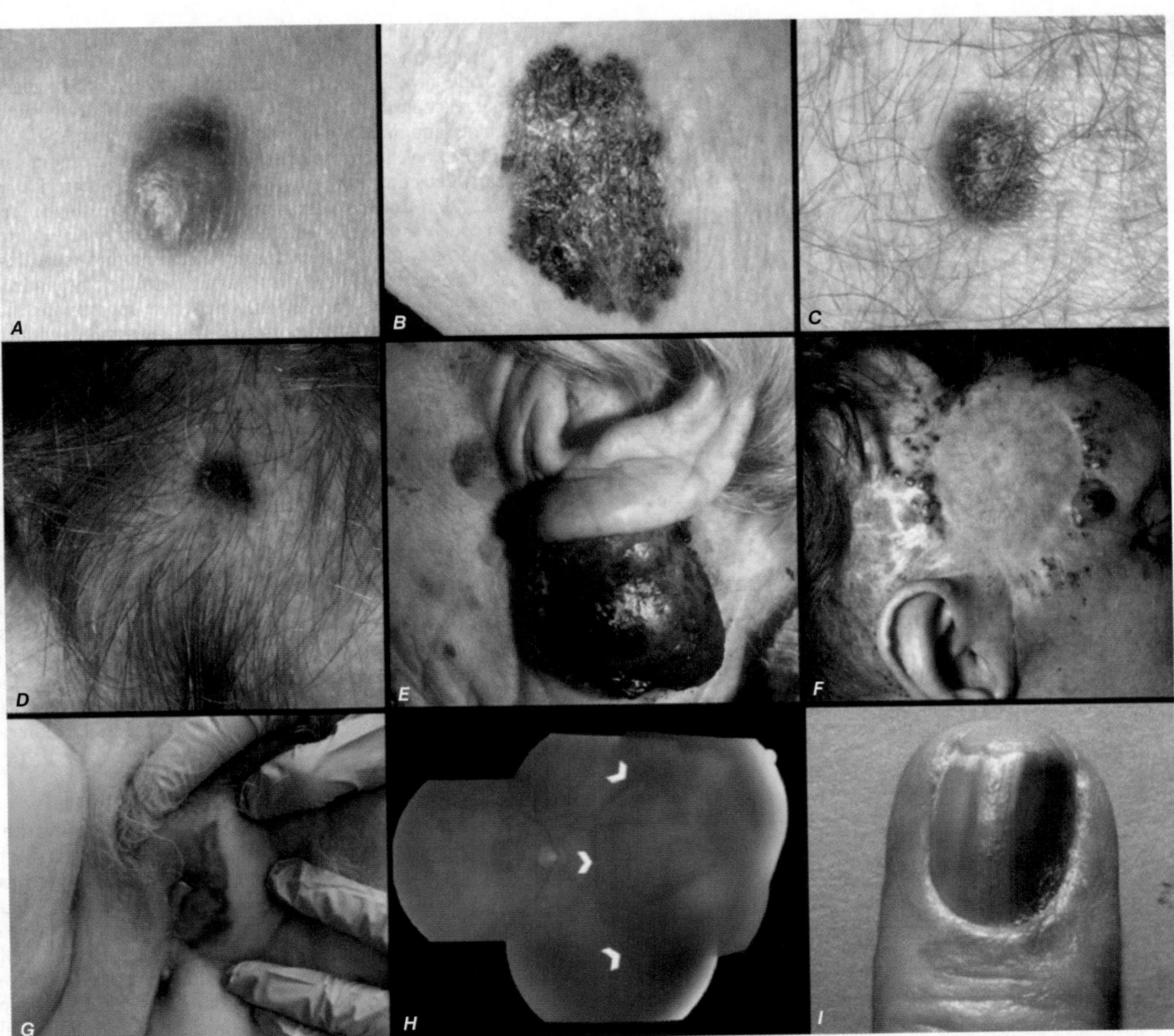

FIGURE 76-1 Types of melanoma. ***A.*** Hypomelanotic melanoma. ***B.*** Superficial spreading melanoma. ***C.*** Melanoma arising in a nevus. ***D.*** Melanoma arising in a nevus. ***E.*** Nodular melanoma. **F.** Cutaneous melanoma metastases at a surgical margin (also known as melanoma satellites when <2 cm from the primary tumor and in-transit melanoma when >2 cm). ***G.*** Mucosal melanoma arising in the vulva. ***H.*** Choroidal melanoma with tumor borders marked by arrowheads, color fundus photograph. ***I.*** Acral melanoma with Hutchinson's sign on the proximal nail fold.

prognosis than cutaneous melanomas. Little is yet known about the effects of mixed ethnicity on melanoma risk.

GENETIC SUSCEPTIBILITY TO MELANOMA

Approximately 20–40% of hereditary melanomas (0.2–2% of all melanomas) are due to germline mutations in the cell cycle regulatory gene cyclin-dependent kinase inhibitor 2A (*CDKN2A*). In fact, 70% of all cutaneous melanomas have mutations or deletions affecting the *CDKN2A* locus on chromosome 9p21. This locus encodes two distinct tumor-suppressor proteins from alternate reading frames: p16 and ARF ($p14^{ARF}$). The p16 protein inhibits CDK4/6-mediated phosphorylation and inactivation of the retinoblastoma (RB) protein, whereas ARF inhibits MDM2 ubiquitin-mediated degradation of p53. The loss of *CDKN2A* results in inactivation of two critical tumor-suppressor pathways, RB and p53, which control entry of cells into the cell cycle. Several studies have shown an increased risk of pancreatic cancer among melanoma-prone families with *CDKN2A* mutations. A second high-risk locus for melanoma susceptibility, *CDK4*, is located on chromosome 12q13 and encodes the cyclin-dependent kinase inhibited by p16. *CDK4* mutations, which also inactivate the RB pathway, are much rarer than *CDKN2A* mutations. Germline mutations in the melanoma lineage-specific oncogene microphthalmia-associated transcription factor (*MITF*), BRCA1-associated protein 1 (*BAP-1*), protection of telomeres 1 (*POT-1*), and telomerase reverse transcriptase (*TERT*) also predispose to familial melanoma with a not yet quantified high penetrance, based on families that have been tested.

The melanocortin-1 receptor (*MC1R*) gene is a moderate-risk inherited melanoma susceptibility factor. UVR stimulates the production of melanocortin (α-melanocyte-stimulating hormone [α-MSH]), the ligand for *MC1R*, which is a G-protein-coupled receptor that signals via cyclic AMP and regulates the amount and type of pigment produced by melanocytes. *MC1R* is highly polymorphic, and many among its ~80 variants result in partial or full loss of signaling and lead to the production of non-photoprotective red/yellow pheomelanins, rather than photoprotective brown/black eumelanins. The red hair color (RHC) phenotype produced by *MC1R* mutations includes lightly colored skin, red hair, freckles, increased sun sensitivity, and increased risk of melanoma. In addition to its weak UV-shielding capacity relative to eumelanin, increased pheomelanin production in patients with inactivating polymorphisms of *MC1R* also provides a UV-independent carcinogenic contribution to melanomagenesis via oxidative damage and reduced DNA damage repair.

TABLE 76-1 Melanoma Risk Factors and Relative Risk

RISK LEVEL	RISK FACTOR	RELATIVE RISK
Elevated	1 atypical nevus versus 0	1.5
	Total common nevi, 16+ versus <15	1.5
	Blue eye color versus dark	1.5
	Hazel eye color versus dark	1.5
	Green eye color versus dark	1.6
	Light brown hair versus dark	1.6
	Indoor tanning in any gender versus never	1.7
	Fitzpatrick II versus IV	1.8
	Fitzpatrick III versus IV	1.8
	History of sunburn versus no sunburn	2.0
	Blond hair versus dark	2.0
	2 atypical nevi versus 0	2.1
	Fitzpatrick I versus IV	2.1
	High density of freckles versus none	2.1
	Total common nevi 41–60 versus <15	2.2
Moderately elevated	Family history of melanoma in 1 or more first-degree relatives	1.7–3.0
	3 atypical nevi versus 0	3.0
	Total common nevi 61–80 versus <15	3.3
	Red hair versus dark	3.6
	Chronic lymphocytic leukemia	3.9
	History of actinic keratoses and/or keratinocyte carcinoma versus not	4.3
	Indoor tanning in women aged 30–39 versus never	4.3
	4 atypical nevi versus 0	4.4
High	Transplant recipient versus not	2.2–4.6
	Indoor tanning in women aged <30 versus never	6.0
	5 atypical nevi versus 0	6.4
	Total common nevi 81–120 versus <15	6.9
	Personal history of melanoma	8.2–13.4
	CDK2NA mutation carrier	14–28

Other more common, low-penetrance polymorphisms in genes related to pigmentation, nevus count, immune responses, DNA repair, metabolism, and the vitamin D receptor have small effects on melanoma susceptibility. In sum, ~50–60% of the genetic risk for hereditary melanoma can be attributed to known melanoma predisposition genes, with ~40% of the known genetic risk attributable to *CDKN2A*. The other components of inherited risk are most likely due to the presence of additional modifier genes and/or shared environmental exposures of the host.

PREVENTION AND EARLY DETECTION

Primary prevention of melanoma and NMSC is based on protection from the sun. Public health initiatives, such as the SunSmart program that started in Australia and is now operative in Europe and the United States, have demonstrated that behavioral change can decrease the incidence of NMSC and melanoma. Preventive measures should start early in life because damage from UV light begins early despite the fact that cancers develop years later. Early episodes of sun burns may be a greater risk than chronic tanning. Some individuals tan compulsively. There is greater understanding of tanning addiction and the cutaneous-neural connections that may give rise to this behavior. Compulsive tanners exhibit differences in dopamine binding and reactivity in reward pathways in the brain, such as the basal striatum, resulting in cutaneous secretion of β-endorphins after UV exposure. Identifying individuals with tanning addiction may be another prevention method. Regular use of broad-spectrum sunscreens that block UVA and UVB with a sun protection factor (SPF) of at least 30 and protective clothing should be encouraged. Physical blockers such as zinc oxide and titanium dioxide have less likelihood of being absorbed or of generating an allergic reaction than chemical sunscreens. Avoidance of sunburns, tanning beds, and midday sun exposure is recommended.

Secondary prevention comprises education and screening with the goal of early detection and can be individualized based on risk factors. A full-body skin exam is warranted in populations at higher risk for melanoma such as patients with clinically atypical moles (dysplastic nevi) and those with a personal history of melanoma. Surveillance in high-risk patients should be performed by a dermatologist and include total-body photography and dermoscopy where appropriate. Individuals with three or more primary melanomas and families with at least one invasive melanoma and two or more cases of melanoma and/or pancreatic cancer among first- or second-degree relatives on the same side of the family may benefit from genetic testing. Severely atypical nevi and melanoma in situ should be removed. Early detection of small lesions allows the use of simpler treatment modalities with higher cure rates and lower morbidity. Monthly self-screening augments provider-based screening. Patients should be taught to recognize the clinical features of melanoma and advised to report any change in a pigmented lesion. There is evidence supporting the ability of media campaigns to reduce cancer mortality in lung cancer, and results from Australia's skin cancer campaigns demonstrate improvement in attitude and behavior and a reduction in melanoma incidence. A benefit/cost analysis in Australia showed a return of $3.85 for every $1 invested. Although the U.S. Preventive Services Task Force states that there is insufficient evidence to recommend skin screening for the general population, additional research is anticipated to find best practices for skin cancer detection and prevention.

DIAGNOSIS

The goal is to identify a melanoma before it becomes invasive and life-threatening metastases have occurred. Early detection may be facilitated by applying the ABCDEs: *a*symmetry (benign lesions are usually symmetric); *b*order irregularity (most nevi have clear-cut borders); *c*olor variegation (benign lesions usually have uniform light or dark pigment); *d*iameter >6 mm (the size of a pencil eraser); and *e*volving (any change in size, shape, color, or elevation or new symptoms such as bleeding, itching, and crusting). In addition, any nevus that appears atypical and different from the rest of the nevi on that individual (an "ugly duckling") should be considered suspicious.

The entire skin surface, including the scalp and mucous membranes, as well as the nails should be examined in each patient. Bright room illumination is important, and a hand lens or dermatoscope is helpful for evaluating variation in pigment pattern. Any suspicious lesions should be biopsied, evaluated by a specialist, or recorded by chart and/or photography for follow-up. Dermoscopy employs low-level magnification of the epidermis with polarized light or water interface and permits a more precise visualization of patterns of pigmentation than is possible with the naked eye **(Fig. 76-2)**.

Biopsy Any pigmented cutaneous lesion that has changed in size or shape or has other features suggestive of malignant melanoma is a candidate for biopsy. An excisional biopsy with 1- to 3-mm margins (narrow-margin excision) is suggested. This facilitates histologic assessment of the lesion, permits accurate measurement of thickness if the lesion is melanoma, and constitutes definitive treatment if the lesion is benign. For lesions that are large or on anatomic sites where excisional biopsy may not be feasible (such as the face, hands, and feet), an incisional biopsy (partial biopsy) through the most nodular or darkest area of the lesion is acceptable. Incisional biopsy does not appear to facilitate the spread of melanoma. For suspicious lesions, every attempt should be made to preserve the ability to assess the deep and peripheral margins and to perform immunohistochemistry. Shave, saucerization, or punch biopsies are an acceptable alternative, particularly if the suspicion of malignancy is low. They should be deep enough to include the deepest component of the entire lesion, and any pigment at the base of the lesion should be removed and included with the biopsy specimen.

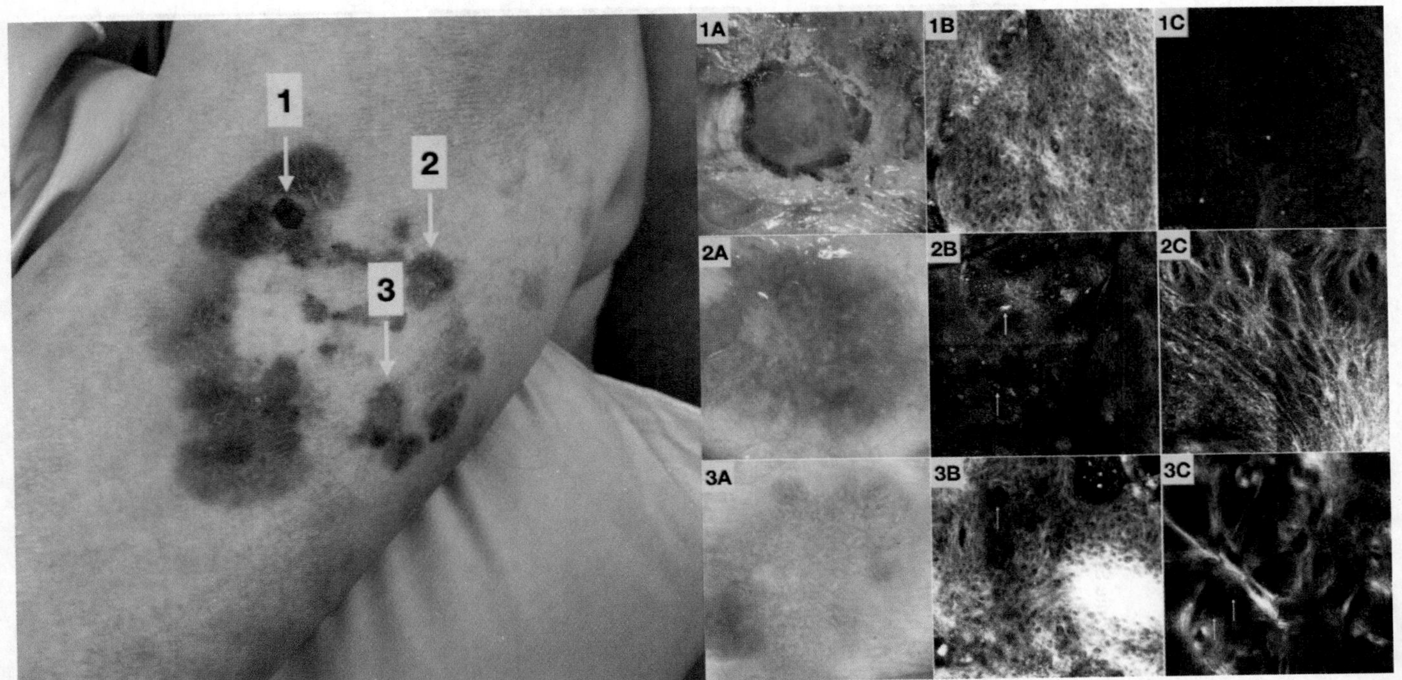

FIGURE 76-2 Clinical and confocal diagnostic findings of melanoma. ***Left panel:*** A clinical image of a large melanoma of a 60-year-old woman used to illustrate classic features of nodular melanoma (1), superficial spreading melanoma (2), and amelanotic melanoma (3). Panels ***1A***, ***2A***, and ***3A*** correspond to the dermoscopy images taken at sites 1, 2, and 3, respectively (Sklip Dermatoscope, Sklip LLC, Las Vegas, NV). Panels ***1B***, ***1C***, ***2B***, ***2C***, ***3B***, and ***3C*** are reflectance confocal microscopy images of the epidermis and upper dermis taken at sites 1, 2, and 3, respectively (Vivascope 1500 Gen 4, Caliber I.D., Rochester, NY). ***1A.*** Site 1 dermoscopy shows a pink nodule with polymorphous vessels and ulceration with active bleeding consistent with malignancy. ***1B.*** Site 1 reflectance confocal microscopy of the epidermis shows an atypical enlarged honeycombed pattern frequently seen in melanoma. ***1C.*** Site 1 reflectance confocal microscopy of the upper dermis shows cerebriform nests (*) seen in nodular melanoma. ***2A.*** Site 2 dermoscopy shows a pigmented area with an atypical, thickened network, blue-gray structures, and polymorphous vessels. ***2B.*** Site 2 reflectance confocal microscopy of the epidermis shows an irregular honeycombed pattern and pagetoid cells with nuclei (↑) typically seen in a superficial spreading melanoma. ***2C.*** Site 2 reflectance confocal microscopy of the dermoepidermal junction shows thickened junctional nests with bright reflective linear dendritic cells (*). ***3A.*** Site 3 dermoscopy shows an amelanotic area within the melanoma with milky red areas, polymorphous vessels, atypical network, and blue-gray structures classic for an amelanotic melanoma. ***3B.*** Site 3 reflectance confocal microscopy of the epidermis shows an irregular enlarged honeycombed pattern, dermal nests protruding upward into the epidermis (↑), and artefacts (*). ***3C.*** Site 3 reflectance confocal microscopy image of the dermoepidermal junction shows thickened collagen bundles (*) with atypical polymorphous vessels (↑).

Punch biopsies are more likely to clear the deep margin but more likely to be positive at the radial margins; the opposite is true for shave biopsies. The choice of biopsy type should be guided by which is most likely to remove the entire lesion for histologic evaluation.

The biopsy should be read by a pathologist experienced in pigmented lesions, and the report should include Breslow thickness, mitotic rate, presence or absence of ulceration, lymphatic invasion, regression, microsatellitosis, and the status of the peripheral and deep margins. Breslow thickness is the greatest thickness of a primary cutaneous melanoma measured on the slide from the top of the epidermal granular layer, or from the ulcer base, to the bottom of the tumor. To distinguish melanomas from benign nevi in challenging cases, fluorescence in situ hybridization with multiple probes or comparative genomic hybridization can be helpful. Gene expression profile (GEP) assays have been developed to determine prognosis and are commercially available.

CLASSIFICATION AND PATHOGENESIS

Clinical Five major types of cutaneous melanoma are described in **Table 76-2**. In *superficial spreading melanoma*, *lentigo maligna melanoma*, and *acral lentiginous melanoma*, the lesion has a period of

TABLE 76-2 Major Histologic Subtypes of Malignant Melanoma

TYPE	SITE	APPEARANCE	ASSOCIATED MUTATIONS
Lentigo maligna	Sun-exposed surfaces, particularly malar region and temple	In flat portions, brown and tan predominate, but whitish gray sometimes present; in nodules, reddish brown, bluish gray, bluish black.	*BRAF* 28% *NRAS* 15%
Superficial spreading	Any (more common on upper back and, in women, lower legs)	Brown mixed with bluish red, bluish black, reddish brown, and often whitish pink. The lesion border is often visibly and/or palpably raised.	*BRAF* 57% *NRAS* 18%
Nodular	Any	Reddish blue, purple, or bluish black; can be uniform or mixed with brown and black.	*BRAF* 47% *NRAS* 33%
Acral lentiginous	Palm, sole, nail bed, mucous membrane	In flat portions, dark brown; in raised lesions (plaques), brown-black or blue-black.	*NRAS* 25% *c-KIT* 5-10% *BRAF* 10%
Desmoplastic	Any (more common on head and neck)	Highly variable; pigmentation is frequently absent. Can mimic nodular basal cell carcinoma.	*MAPK* and *PI3K* 73% High tumor mutational burden, *BRAF* and *NRAS* uncommon

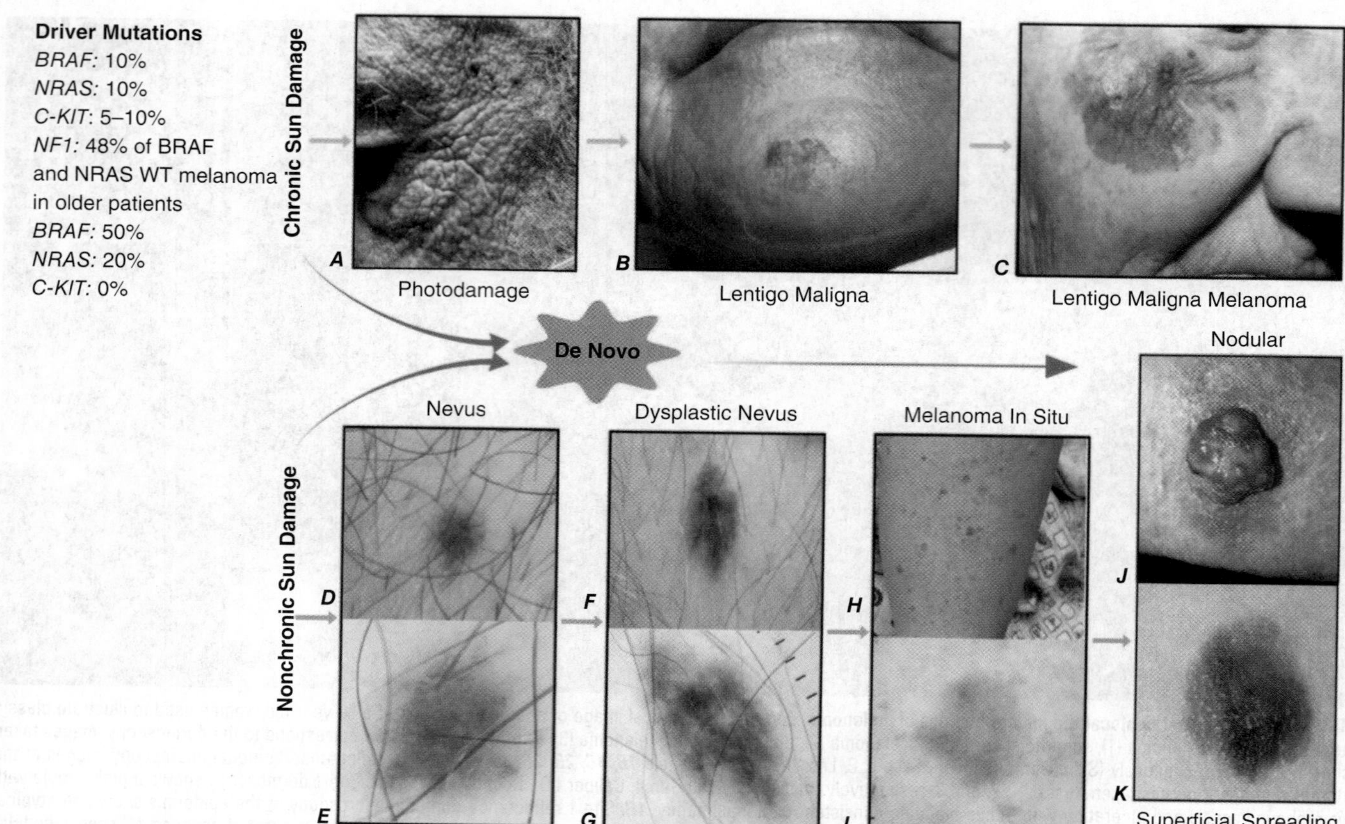

FIGURE 76-3 Cutaneous melanoma development and associated driver mutations. Chronic sun damage (***A***) predisposes to a lentigo maligna (in situ) (***B***), which can evolve into lentigo maligna melanoma (invasive) (***C***). Similarly, nonchronic sun damage can initiate melanoma de novo or in nevomelanocytes, where clinical and histologic changes of atypia may be seen prior to complete transformation. Nevi (***D, E***) can evolve into atypical lesions (***F, G***), in situ melanoma (***H, I***), and eventually invasive nodular (***J***) or superficial spreading melanomas (***K***).

superficial (radial) growth during which it increases in surface area but does not penetrate deeply and is most capable of being cured by surgical excision. Melanomas with a radial growth phase are characterized by irregular and sometimes notched borders, variation in pigment pattern, and variation in color. *Nodular melanoma* does not have a radial growth phase but usually presents with penetration deep into the skin (vertical growth phase). *Desmoplastic melanoma* is associated with a fibrotic response, neural invasion, and a greater tendency for local recurrence. Occasionally, melanomas appear clinically to be amelanotic (not pigmented), in which case the diagnosis is established microscopically after biopsy.

Although these subtypes are clinically distinct, they are primarily of historical interest because this classification has minimal prognostic value and is not part of American Joint Committee on Cancer (AJCC) staging. Characterizing the genomic and mutational profiles of melanoma has become increasingly common, informs prognosis, reflects the mechanisms of tumorigenesis, and may influence surveillance strategies and treatment.

Genomic The advent of next-generation sequencing has led to whole exome sequencing of hundreds of cutaneous melanomas derived from nonglabrous skin. This has revealed very complex genomic changes resulting from both germline (see "Genetic Susceptibility to Melanoma" above) and somatic mutations. Cutaneous melanomas have one of the highest somatic mutation rates (>10 mutations/Mb) among all cancers; the majority (76% of primary tumors and 84% of metastatic melanomas) exhibit mutations indicative of UVR exposure. The mutation rate varies based on body site; melanomas arising in chronic sun-damaged skin harbor substantially more mutations than melanomas from non-sun-damaged skin.

Melanomas can harbor thousands of mutations, but only a few are "driver" mutations that promote cell proliferation or inhibit normal pathways of apoptosis or DNA repair and confer a growth advantage to the neoplastic cell. Some of the driver mutations for cutaneous melanoma are depicted in **Fig. 76-3** along with the clinical evolution of melanoma lesions. Driver mutations are often found in combination with mutations to germline susceptibility genes such as *p16*, which affect cell cycle arrest, and *ARF*, which result in defective apoptotic responses to genotoxic damage. The altered melanocytes accumulate DNA damage and develop the malignant phenotype characterized by invasion, metastasis, and angiogenesis.

A genomic classification of cutaneous melanoma has been proposed based on the pattern of the most prevalent mutated genes, *BRAF, RAS*, and *NF1*, along with a triple wild-type (WT) in which no mutations in these three genes are found. The pattern of DNA mutations can vary with the site of origin and is independent of the histologic subtype of the tumor. An important aspect of this classification is that the mutational profile can guide therapy. The proliferative pathways affected by the mutations include the mitogen-activated protein (MAP) kinase and phosphatidylinositol 3′ kinase/AKT pathways. *RAS* and *BRAF*, members of the MAP kinase pathway, which mediate the transcription of genes involved in cell proliferation and survival, undergo somatic mutation in melanoma and thereby generate potential therapeutic targets. *NRAS* is mutated in ~20% of melanomas, and somatic activating *BRAF* mutations are found in most benign nevi and 40–50% of cutaneous melanomas. Neither mutation by itself appears to be sufficient to cause melanoma; thus, they often are accompanied by other mutations, such as *TERT*. The *BRAF* mutation is most commonly a T→A point mutation that results in a valine-to-glutamate amino acid substitution (V600E). V600E *BRAF* mutations are more common in younger patients and are present in most melanomas that arise on sites with intermittent sun exposure and are less common in melanomas from chronically sun-damaged skin (i.e., those of older patients).

Melanomas may harbor mutations in *AKT* (primarily in *AKT3*) and *PTEN* (phosphatase and tensin homolog). *AKT* can be amplified, and

PTEN may be deleted or undergo epigenetic silencing that leads to constitutive activation of the PI3K/AKT pathway and enhanced cell survival by antagonizing the intrinsic pathway of apoptosis. A loss-of-function mutation in *NF1*, which can affect both the MAP kinase and PI3K/AKT pathways, has been described in 10–15% of melanomas. In melanoma, these two signaling pathways (MAP kinase and PI3K/AKT) enhance tumorigenesis, chemoresistance, migration, and cell cycle dysregulation.

PROGNOSTIC FACTORS

The most important prognostic factors for a newly diagnosed patient are incorporated in the staging classification. The best predictor of recurrence is Breslow thickness, followed by ulceration, which together make up the T stage of the AJCC system for melanoma. The anatomic site of the primary tumor is also prognostic; favorable sites are the forearm and leg, and unfavorable sites include the scalp, hands, feet, and mucous membranes. Women with stage I or II disease have better survival than men, perhaps in part because of earlier diagnosis; women frequently have melanomas on the lower leg, where self-recognition is more likely and the prognosis is better.

Older individuals, especially men >60, have a tendency toward delayed diagnosis (and thus thicker tumors), have more head and neck and acral melanomas (which tend to have earlier vertical growth and distant metastases), and are more likely to develop melanomas in chronically UVR-damaged skin (which are more often *BRAF* wild type, with fewer options for therapy). Other important adverse factors include high mitotic rate, microscopic evidence of regression, and lymphatic/vascular invasion. Clinical features such as microsatellite lesions and/or in-transit metastases, evidence of nodal involvement, elevated serum lactate dehydrogenase (LDH), and presence and site of distant metastases all portend a higher stage and worse prognosis.

GEPs and machine-learning algorithms that associate genomic changes with clinical outcomes have been used to estimate the prognosis of melanoma. A commercially available 31-gene GEP is available that predicts for all-site (particularly distant) relapse and incorporates the increased and decreased expression, as well as the dysregulation, of genes involved in many of the cellular processes leading to melanoma progression described earlier. Although this 31-gene GEP can estimate the probability of distant relapse, it has not supplanted the prognostic estimates derived from surgical staging. It is anticipated that GEPs will be incorporated into future cutaneous melanoma management guidelines, as they have been for uveal melanoma, breast cancer, thyroid cancer, and other malignancies.

STAGING

Once the diagnosis of melanoma has been made, the tumor is staged to determine the prognosis and aid in treatment selection. The current melanoma staging criteria and estimated 10-year survival by stage are depicted in **Table 76-3**. The clinical stage is determined after the microscopic evaluation of the melanoma skin lesion and clinical and radiologic assessment. The pathologic stage also includes microscopic examination of clinically negative regional lymph nodes obtained at sentinel lymph node biopsy (SLNB), any enlarged nodes found on exam or imaging, and any suspected metastases amenable to open or image-guided biopsy.

All patients should have a complete history, with attention to symptoms that suggest metastatic disease, such as new palpable masses, malaise, weight loss, headaches, changes in vision or bowel habits, hemoptysis, and pain. The provider should look for persistent disease at the biopsy site, dermal or subcutaneous nodules that could represent satellite or in-transit metastases, and lymphadenopathy. A complete blood count, complete metabolic panel, and LDH should be performed. Although these tests rarely help uncover occult metastatic disease, a microcytic anemia would raise the possibility of bowel metastases, elevated liver function tests can suggest liver metastases, and LDH is part of the AJCC system for stage IV disease. Abnormal test results should prompt a more extensive evaluation, including computed tomography (CT) scan or a positron emission tomography (PET) scan (or CT/PET combined).

TABLE 76-3 Staging and Survival

STAGE	TNM	10-YEAR MELANOMA-SPECIFIC SURVIVAL ESTIMATE
0	TisN0M0	>99%
IA	T1aN0M0, T1bN0M0	98–96%
IB	T2aN0M0	92%
IIA	T2b-T3aN0M0	88%
IIB	T3b-T4aN0M0	81–83%
IIC	T4bN0M0	75%
IIIA	T1a-T2aN1a-2aM0	88%
IIIB	T2b-T3aN1a-N2bM0	77%
IIIC	T3b-4bN1a-N3cM0	60%
IIID	T4bN3a-N3cM0	24%
IV M1a	Any T, any N, skin, soft tissue, or distant nodal sites	50% at 5 years
IV M1b	Any T, any N, lung + any M1a sites	35–50% at 5 years
IV M1c	Any T, any N, skin, non-CNS visceral disease, any M1a or M1b sites	~25% at 5 years
IV M1d	Any T, any N, CNS metastasis + any M1a,b,c sites	<5% at 5 years

Abbreviations: CNS, central nervous system; TNM, tumor-node-metastasis.

Despite all the above considerations, >80% of patients at presentation will have disease confined to the skin and a negative history and physical examination, in which case imaging is not indicated. Although controversial, an exception is sometimes made for very-high-risk primaries (e.g., >4 mm with ulceration) in which the chance for occult distant metastases is higher than that for a positive SLNB.

TREATMENT

Melanoma

MANAGEMENT OF CLINICALLY LOCALIZED MELANOMA (STAGE I, II)

For a newly diagnosed cutaneous melanoma, wide surgical excision of the lesion with a margin of normal skin is necessary to remove all malignant cells and minimize the probability of local recurrence. The National Comprehensive Cancer Network (NCCN), based on data from six randomized trials, recommends the following radial margins for a primary melanoma: in situ, 0.5–1.0 cm; invasive up to 1 mm thick, 1 cm; >1.01–2 mm, 1–2 cm; and >2 mm, 2 cm. Smaller margins may be used for special locations such as the face, hands, feet, and genitalia due to the higher likelihood of morbidity in these regions. In all instances, however, inclusion of subcutaneous fat in the surgical specimen facilitates adequate thickness measurement and assessment of surgical margins by the pathologist. When feasible, excision should go down to fascia, with fascial resection for thick (T4) lesions. Topical imiquimod can be used to treat lentigo maligna in cosmetically sensitive locations with narrow resection margins by promoting local immune response resulting in decreased local recurrence.

SLNB is a valuable staging tool providing prognostic information to identify patients at high risk for relapse who may be candidates for adjuvant therapy. The first (sentinel) draining node(s) from the primary site is (are) located by injecting a blue dye and a gamma-emitting radioisotope around the primary site. The sentinel node(s) then is (are) identified using a handheld gamma detector brought sterilely into the operative field. The surgeon makes an incision of the area of uptake and looks for the blue-stained, "hot" node(s), which is (are) removed and subjected to histopathologic analysis with serial sectioning using hematoxylin and eosin and immunohistochemical stains (e.g., S100, HMB45, MART-1, and MelanA) to identify melanocytes.

NCCN guidelines recommend SLNB to patients with a 10% or greater chance of having tumor in the node. This includes patients with tumors >1 mm thick (T2) or T1 tumors that have ulceration (T1b). Patients with a 5–10% risk of node positivity, such as those with tumors measuring between 0.75 and 1.0 mm, transected tumors, regressed tumors, or lymphovascular invasion, should also be considered for SLNB. The NCCN does not recommend SLNB for patients with a risk of a positive SLNB ≤5% such as those with melanomas ≤0.75 mm thick and no high-risk features. In these patients, wide excision alone is the usual definitive therapy.

Patients whose SLNB is negative can either be followed or considered for a clinical trial if the primary lesion is considered high risk (i.e., stages IIB and IIC). Patients with a positive sentinel lymph node should undergo imaging (CT or PET scanning) to rule out distant metastatic disease, and if none is found (i.e., stage III), adjuvant therapy on or off a clinical study should be offered (see next section). Complete lymphadenectomy for a positive sentinel lymph node has been shown to improve relapse-free but not overall survival, and therefore, it is no longer offered routinely. This avoids the morbidity of regional node dissection in most patients. However, patients not undergoing immediate completion node dissection should have nodal bed surveillance with physical examination and ultrasound at 4- to 6-month intervals for approximately 3 years to rule out isolated nodal bed progression. Complete node dissection is therefore still offered to patients who cannot comply with follow-up and/or forgo adjuvant therapy.

MANAGEMENT OF REGIONALLY METASTATIC MELANOMA (STAGE III)

Patients with a positive sentinel lymph node, resected regional nodal macrometastases, or resected locoregional disease (e.g., recurrences in the wide excision site, within 2 cm of the site ["satellite metastases"], or >2 cm from the site ["in-transit metastases"]) are all considered as having stage III disease. Even after complete resection of stage III disease, the risk for progression to distant metastases (stage IV) may be high, and adjuvant systemic therapy should be offered. Melanomas may recur at the edge of the incision or graft, as satellite metastases, in-transit metastases, or most commonly, regional spread to a draining lymph node basin. Each of these presentations is managed surgically and, increasingly, with post-surgical adjuvant immunotherapy or targeted therapy, after which there is the possibility of long-term disease-free survival. Topical therapy with imiquimod has been useful for patients with low-volume dermal lesions. Talimogene laherparepvec is an engineered, oncolytic herpes simplex virus type 1 that is FDA approved for injection of primary or recurrent melanomas including cutaneous and subcutaneous lesions or lymph node deposits that cannot be completely removed by surgery.

Stage III patients rendered free of disease after surgery are at risk for local or distant recurrence and should be offered adjuvant therapy. Radiotherapy can reduce the risk of local recurrence after lymphadenectomy but does not influence overall survival. Patients with large nodes (>3–4 cm), four or more involved lymph nodes, or extranodal spread on microscopic examination should be considered for radiation. Systemic adjuvant therapy is indicated primarily for patients with stage III disease, but high-risk, node-negative patients (>4 mm thick or ulcerated lesions) and patients with completely resected stage IV disease also may benefit.

Current options for adjuvant therapy include anti-PD-1 (nivolumab or pembrolizumab) or targeted therapy in melanomas that express a *BRAF* V600 mutation. Both anti-PD-1 and targeted therapy have been shown to confer disease-free and overall survival benefits in stage III and stage IV melanoma (see below for further discussion). Other agents such as ipilimumab and interferon α2b (IFN-α2b) have been used in the adjuvant setting, but due to a higher percentage of immune-mediated side effects in the case of ipilimumab and limited efficacy in the case of interferon, they have been supplanted by better alternatives. Ongoing clinical trials are comparing systemic therapy before surgery (neoadjuvant) with adjuvant treatment, the optimal sequence of immunotherapy and targeted therapies, and the utility of anti-PD-1 in high-risk stage II melanoma. GEP may help to identify patients with stage II or III melanoma who are at lower risk of recurrence and could avoid the toxicity and expense of adjuvant therapy.

TREATMENT

Metastatic Disease

At diagnosis, 84% patients with melanoma will have stage I or II disease and 4% will present with metastases. Many others will develop metastases after initial therapy for locoregional disease. The probability of recurrence is related to initial stage, ranging from <5% with stage IA to >90% for subsets of patients with stage IIID disease at presentation. Patients with a history of melanoma who develop signs or symptoms suggesting recurrent disease should undergo restaging as described earlier. Distant metastases (stage IV) commonly involve skin and lymph nodes as well as viscera, bone, or the brain. The prognosis is better for patients with skin and subcutaneous metastases (M1a) than for lung (M1b) and worst for those with metastases to bone or other visceral organs (M1c) or brain (M1d). An elevated serum LDH is a poor prognostic factor and places the patient in stage M1c regardless of the metastatic sites. The 15-year survival of patients with melanoma was <10% before 2010; however, the development of targeted therapy and immunotherapy has improved disease-free and overall survival, especially for patients with M1a and M1b disease, such that currently the 15-year survival exceeds 25%. Even patients with M1c disease may have prolonged survival, and those who are progression-free for >2 years after immunotherapy or targeted therapy have a high probability of living >5 years from the onset of metastasis.

FDA-approved agents since 2011 include three immune T-cell checkpoint inhibitors (ipilimumab, nivolumab, and pembrolizumab), combination immunotherapy (ipilimumab plus nivolumab), six oral agents that target the MAP kinase pathway (the BRAF inhibitors vemurafenib, dabrafenib, and encorafenib, and the MEK inhibitors trametinib, cobimetinib, and binimetinib), and the oncolytic virus talimogene laherparepvec (**Table 76-4**).

Local modalities, such as surgery and stereotactic radiosurgery, should be considered for patients with oligometastatic disease because they may experience long-term disease-free survival after metastasectomy or ablative high-dose-per-fraction radiation. Patients with solitary metastases are the best candidates, but local modalities can also be used for patients with metastases at more than one site if a complete resection or treatment of all sites can be achieved with reasonable side effects. Patients rendered free of disease can be considered for adjuvant therapy or a clinical trial because their risk of developing additional metastases remains high. Surgery can also be used as an adjunct to systemic therapy when, for example, a few of many metastatic lesions prove resistant to

TABLE 76-4 Treatment Options for Metastatic Melanoma

Immunotherapy
Immune checkpoint blockade
Anti-PD-1: pembrolizumab or nivolumab
Anti-CTLA-4: ipilimumab
Combined ipilimumab and nivolumab
Cytokine-based immunotherapy
High-dose interleukin 2
Oncolytic virus
Talimogene laherparepvec
Targeted therapies
BRAF inhibitors: vemurafenib, dabrafenib, encorafenib
MEK inhibitors: trametinib, cobimetinib, binimetinib
Local modalities
Surgery
Stereotactic radiation

immunotherapy; it may also be helpful to obtain tumor to establish the mutational profile of the recurrent melanoma.

IMMUNOTHERAPY

Checkpoint Blockade Immunotherapies are based on an understanding of the control mechanisms of the normal immune response. Inhibitory receptors or checkpoints, including CTLA-4 and PD-1, are upregulated on T cells after engagement of the T-cell receptor by cognate tumor antigen in the context of the appropriate class I or II HLA molecules during the interaction between a T cell and antigen-presenting cell. Immune checkpoints are an absolute requirement to ensure proper regulation of a normal immune response; however, the continued expression of inhibitory receptors during chronic infection (hepatitis, HIV) and in cancer patients leads to exhausted T cells with limited potential for proliferation, cytokine production, or cytotoxicity. Checkpoint blockade with an antagonistic monoclonal antibody results in improved T-cell function and eradication of tumor cells in preclinical animal models. Ipilimumab, a fully human IgG1 antibody that binds CTLA-4 and blocks inhibitory signals, was the first drug shown in a randomized trial to improve survival in patients with metastatic melanoma. Although response rates are low (about 10%), overall survival is improved. Anti-CTLA-4 monotherapy has been supplanted by combination anti-CTLA-4 plus anti-PD-1 or anti-PD-1 monotherapy due to enhanced survival and, in the case of anti-PD-1 monotherapy, better patient tolerance, as detailed below.

Chronic T-cell activation also leads to induction of PD-1 on the surface of T cells. Expression of one of its ligands, PD-L1, on tumor cells can protect them from immune destruction. Blockade of the PD-1:PD-L1 axis by intravenous (IV) administration of anti-PD-1 or anti-PD-L1 has substantial clinical activity, including cure, in some patients with advanced melanoma and other solid tumors with significantly less toxicity than ipilimumab. The PD-1 blockers, nivolumab and pembrolizumab, have been approved to treat patients with advanced melanoma. Combination T-cell checkpoint therapy, blocking both inhibitory pathways with ipilimumab and nivolumab, leads to superior antitumor activity compared to treatment with either agent alone. Combined therapy with IV ipilimumab and nivolumab is administered in the outpatient setting every 3 weeks for four doses (induction), followed by nivolumab given every 2–4 weeks (maintenance) for up to 1 year, and is associated with an objective response rate of 56% and enhanced survival compared to ipilimumab monotherapy. There may be subsets of patients, specifically those who have >5% expression of PD-1 on T cells in a melanoma biopsy sample, who derive a similar level of clinical benefit from nivolumab monotherapy, although using PD-1 expression to select therapy remains problematic as some patients whose melanoma has no detectable PD-1 expression can still respond to immunotherapy.

T-cell checkpoint antibodies can also interfere with normal immune regulatory mechanisms, which may produce a novel spectrum of side effects. The most common immune-related adverse events were skin rash and diarrhea (sometimes severe, life-threatening colitis), but toxicity can involve almost any organ (e.g., thyroiditis, hypophysitis, hepatitis, nephritis, pneumonitis, myocarditis, neuritis). The severity and frequency of toxicity are greatest with combination T-cell checkpoint antibody therapy, followed by anti-CTLA-4 and then anti-PD-1 monotherapies. Vigilance, interruption of therapy, and early intervention with steroids or other immunosuppressive agents, such as anti–tumor necrosis factor antibodies or mycophenolate mofetil, can mitigate toxicity and prevent permanent organ damage. The management of drug-induced toxicity with immunosuppressive agents does not appear to interfere with antitumor activity, and benefit is manifest even in patients who have to discontinue immunotherapy due to immune-mediated toxicity. The use of T-cell checkpoint antibodies for metastatic melanoma has become commonplace, but there is controversy about whether all patients need combined anti-CTLA-4 and anti-PD-1, whether biomarkers can be used to select patients who may benefit from anti-PD-1 alone, and the best sequence of targeted therapy and immunotherapy in patients whose melanomas have a *BRAF* mutation. There is also a significant economic impact with any anticancer therapy, which must be placed in the context of the survival benefit.

TARGETED THERAPY

The RAS-RAF-MEK-ERK pathway delivers proliferation and survival signals from the cell surface to the cytoplasm and nucleus and is mutated in approximately 50% of melanomas. Inhibitors of BRAF and MEK can induce regression of melanomas that harbor a *BRAF* mutation. Three BRAF inhibitors, vemurafenib, dabrafenib, and encorafenib, have been approved for the treatment of patients whose stage IV melanomas harbor a mutation at position 600 in *BRAF*. Monotherapy with BRAF inhibitors has been supplanted with combined BRAF and MEK inhibition to address the rapid adaptation of the majority of melanomas that use MAP kinase pathway reactivation to facilitate growth when BRAF is inhibited. Combined therapy with BRAF and MEK inhibitors (dabrafenib and trametinib, vemurafenib with cobimetinib, or encorafenib and binimetinib) improved progression-free and overall survival compared to monotherapy with a BRAF inhibitor. Long-term results of inhibition of the MAP kinase pathway confirm that some patients achieve long intervals of disease control, yet the major limitation of both monotherapy and combined therapy appears to be the acquisition of resistance; the majority of patients relapse and eventually die. The mechanisms of resistance are diverse and reflect the genomic heterogeneity of melanoma; however, most instances involve reactivation of the MAPK pathway, often through *RAS* mutations or mutant *BRAF* amplification. Patients who develop resistance to BRAF and MEK inhibition are candidates for immunotherapy or clinical trials.

Targeted therapy is accompanied by manageable side effects that differ from those experienced during immunotherapy or chemotherapy. A class-specific side effect of BRAF inhibitor monotherapy is the development of hyperproliferative skin lesions, some of which are well-differentiated squamous cell skin cancers (SCCs) occurring in up to 25% of patients. Paradoxical activation of the MAP kinase pathway occurs from BRAF inhibitor–mediated changes in *BRAF* wild-type cells, and the activation is blocked by MEK inhibitor, which explains why these lesions occur much less frequently during combined therapy. Metastases of the treatment-induced SCCs have not been reported, and BRAF and MEK inhibitors can be continued safely following simple excision of the SCCs. Cardiac and ocular toxicities, although infrequent, can occur with BRAF and MEK inhibitors and require medical evaluation, management, and usually discontinuation of targeted therapy.

Activating mutations in the c-kit receptor tyrosine kinase are found in a minority of cutaneous melanomas with chronic sun damage but are more common in mucosal and acral lentiginous subtypes. Overall, the number of patients with *c-kit* mutations is small, but when present, they are similar to those found in gastrointestinal stromal tumors and melanomas with activating *c-kit* mutations and can have clinically meaningful responses to imatinib. The probability of objective response in patients whose melanomas harbor a *c-kit* mutation is 29%. *N-RAS* mutations occur in 15–20% of melanomas. At present, there are no effective targeted agents for these patients, but *N-RAS* inhibitors are being investigated in clinical trials.

Other systemic therapies used to treat stage IV melanoma patients include high-dose interleukin 2, which is also associated with durable remissions in some patients. Chemotherapy with dacarbazine or taxanes is infrequently used, and clinical trials remain an important option for patients with advanced melanoma.

INITIAL APPROACH TO PATIENT WITH METASTATIC DISEASE

Upon diagnosis of stage IV disease, a sample of the patient's tumor should be submitted for molecular testing to determine whether a *BRAF* or *c-kit* mutation is present. Analysis of a metastatic lesion biopsy (if possible) is preferred, but any sample will suffice because there is little discordance between primary and metastatic lesions. Treatment algorithms start with the tumor's *BRAF* status. For *BRAF* wild-type tumors, immunotherapy is recommended. For patients whose tumors harbor a *BRAF* mutation, initial therapy with either combination BRAF and MEK inhibitors or immunotherapy is acceptable. Combined therapy with BRAF and MEK inhibitors is recommended for patients with rapidly growing and symptomatic disease when a *BRAF* mutation is present. The sequence of immunotherapy and targeted therapy that confers the greatest survival benefit in patients with minimally symptomatic melanoma is not yet known, but ongoing randomized phase III trials should answer this important question. Despite improvements in therapy, the majority of patients with metastatic melanoma will not be cured, so enrollment in a clinical trial is always an important consideration, even for previously untreated patients.

Clinical trials should be considered for patients with stage IV disease who experience tumor progression despite current therapy. Many will be poor candidates for therapy because of extensive disease burden, poor performance status, or concomitant illness; thus, the timely integration of palliative care and hospice remains an important element of care.

FOLLOW-UP

Skin examination and surveillance at least once a year are recommended for all patients with melanoma. Routine blood work and imaging for patients with stage IA–IIA disease is not recommended unless symptoms are present. Surveillance diagnostic imaging can be considered in patients with stage III high-risk disease but is mainly reserved for patients with signs or symptoms of recurrent disease or to follow response to therapy. For stage-specific recommendations, please consult the NCCN guidelines (see "Further Reading").

NONMELANOMA SKIN CANCERS

NMSCs (mostly SCCs and basal cell cancer [BCC]) are the most common cancers in the United States. Although tumor registries do not routinely gather data on the incidence of NMSCs, it is estimated that the annual incidence is more than 5.3 million cases in the United States; SCCs and BCCs account for 80% and 18%, respectively. While less common, the incidence of Merkel cell carcinoma (MCC) has tripled over the past 20 years. There are now an estimated 1600 cases per year with an annual increase in incidence of 8%. While all forms of NMSCs can metastasize, MCCs do this most commonly, with sentinel lymph node positivity rates of 25% (compared to 12–19% for melanoma) and mortality rates approaching 33% at 3 years. SCCs, particularly those with high-risk features, can also metastasize and account for 2400 deaths annually.

■ PATHOPHYSIOLOGY AND ETIOLOGY

Similar to melanoma, the most significant cause of NMSCs is UVR, with a dose-response relationship between tanning bed use and the incidence of NMSC. As few as four tanning bed visits per year confers a 15% increase in BCC and an 11% increase in SCC. The risk of lip or oral SCC is increased with cigarette smoking and, like SCC of the ear, has a worse prognosis than that seen on other body sites. Human papillomaviruses and UVR may act as co-carcinogens. Inherited disorders of DNA repair, such as xeroderma pigmentosum, are associated with a greatly increased incidence of skin cancer and help to establish the link between UV-induced DNA damage, inadequate DNA repair, and skin cancer.

The genes damaged most commonly by UV in SCC include *p53* and *N-RAS*, whereas BCC is associated with damage to hedgehog signaling pathway (Hh) genes, which lead to basal cell proliferation. This is usually the result of loss of function of the tumor-suppressor patched homolog 1 (*PTCH1*), which normally inhibits the signaling of smoothened homolog (*SMO*). Two oral SMO inhibitors, vismodegib and sonidegib, have been approved by the FDA to treat advanced inoperable or metastatic BCC and locally advanced BCC that has recurred following surgery or radiotherapy, respectively. Vismodegib also reduces the incidence of BCC in patients with basal cell nevus syndrome who have *PTCH1* mutations, affirming the importance of Hh in the onset of BCC.

Immunosuppression has also been associated with the development of NMSCs; chronically immunosuppressed solid organ transplant recipients have a 65-fold increase in SCC and a 10-fold increase in BCC. The frequency of skin cancer is proportional to the level and duration of immunosuppression and the extent of sun exposure before and after transplantation. SCCs in this population are particularly aggressive, demonstrating higher rates of local recurrence, metastasis, and mortality. Tumor necrosis factor (TNF) antagonist therapy of inflammatory bowel disease and autoimmune disorders, such as rheumatoid and psoriatic arthritis, may also confer an increased risk of NMSC.

Other risk factors for NMSCs include HIV infection, ionizing radiation, thermal burn scars, *BRAF* inhibitor monotherapy, and chronic ulcerations. Albinism, xeroderma pigmentosum, Muir-Torre syndrome, Rombo's syndrome, Bazex-Dupré-Christol syndrome, dyskeratosis congenita, and basal cell nevus syndrome (Gorlin syndrome) also increase the incidence of NMSC.

Although MCC is also clearly related to UV exposure, age, and immunosuppression, this neural crest–derived cancer also appears to have a viral etiology; an oncogenic Merkel cell polyomavirus (MCPyV) is present in 80% of tumors. In patients with MCPyV-positive tumors, there is inactivation of tumor-suppressor genes, specifically the *p53* transcription factor and retinoblastoma protein (*Rb*). In addition, the viral large T antigen is expressed on tumor cells, and many patients have detectable cellular or humoral immune responses to polyoma viral proteins, although this immune response is insufficient to eradicate the malignancy.

■ CLINICAL PRESENTATION

Basal Cell Carcinoma BCC arises from epidermal basal cells. The least invasive of BCC subtypes, superficial BCC, consists of often subtle, erythematous scaling plaques that slowly enlarge and are most commonly seen on the trunk and proximal extremities (**Fig. 76-4**). This subtype may be confused with benign inflammatory dermatoses, especially nummular eczema and psoriasis or premalignant actinic keratoses. BCC also can present as a small, slowly growing, pearly nodule, often with tortuous telangiectatic vessels on its surface, rolled borders, and a central crust (nodular BCC). The occasional presence of melanin in this variant of nodular BCC (pigmented BCC) may lead to confusion with melanoma. Morpheaform (fibrosing), infiltrative, and micronodular BCC, the most invasive and potentially aggressive subtypes, manifest as solitary, flat or slightly depressed, indurated whitish, yellowish, or pink scar-like plaques. Borders are typically indistinct, and lesions can be subtle; thus, delay in treatment is common, and tumors can be more extensive than expected clinically. An archaic name for this tumor is "rodent ulcer."

Squamous Cell Carcinoma Primary *cutaneous SCC* is a malignant neoplasm of keratinizing epidermal cells that has a variable clinical course, ranging from indolent to rapid growth, with the potential to metastasize to regional and distant sites. Commonly, SCC appears as an ulcerated erythematous nodule or superficial erosion on sun-exposed skin of the head, neck, trunk, and extremities (**Fig. 76-5**). It may also appear as a banal, firm, dome-shaped papule or rough textured plaque. It is commonly mistaken for a wart or callous when the inflammatory response to the lesion is minimal. Dotted or coiled vessels are a hallmark of SCC when viewed through a dermatoscope. The margins of this tumor may be ill defined, and fixation to underlying structures may occur ("tethering").

A very rapidly growing low-grade form of SCC, called keratoacanthoma (KA), typically appears as a large dome-shaped papule with a central keratotic crater. Some KAs regress spontaneously without therapy, but because progression to metastatic SCC has been documented, KAs should be treated in the same manner as other types of cutaneous SCC. KAs occur in 15–25% of patients receiving monotherapy with a BRAF inhibitor.

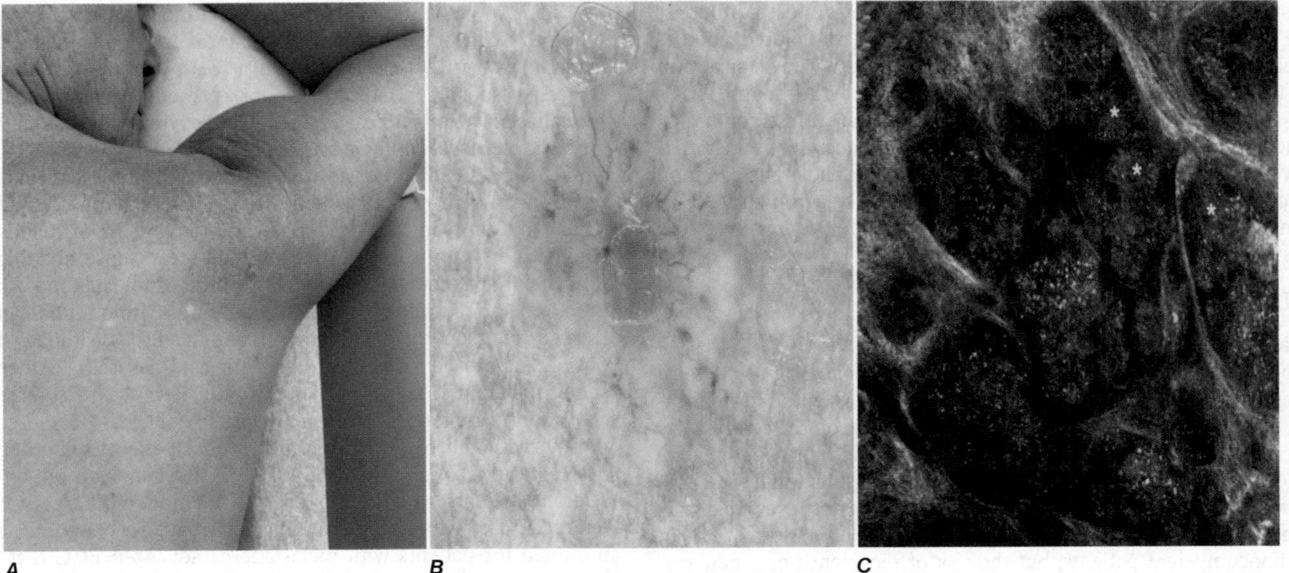

FIGURE 76-4 Clinical and confocal diagnostic findings of basal cell carcinoma. *A.* Typical basal cell carcinoma with skin-colored, slightly translucent rolled borders and a small central erosion on chronically sun-damaged skin of the lateral posterior shoulder. ***B.*** Dermoscopic image of the same lesion as in panel ***A*** clearly revealing the central erosion and classic gray, nonreticular globular structures of melanophages that characterize BCC. ***C.*** In vivo reflectance confocal microscopy of the same lesion as in panel ***A*** showing typical nests of dermal basaloid cells (*) with classic cleft formation around the nests.

Actinic keratoses and *cheilitis* (actinic keratoses on the lip), both premalignant forms of SCC, present as hyperkeratotic papules on sun-exposed areas. Malignant transformation occurs in 0.25–20% of untreated lesions. SCC in situ, also called *Bowen's disease*, is the intraepidermal form of SCC and usually presents as a scaling, erythematous plaque. SCC in situ most commonly arises on sun-damaged skin but can occur anywhere on the body. Bowen's disease occurring secondary to infection with human papillomavirus can arise on skin with minimal or no prior sun exposure, such as the buttock or posterior thigh. Treatment of premalignant and in situ lesions reduces the subsequent risk of invasive disease.

Merkel Cell Carcinoma MCC, also known as cutaneous apudoma, primary neuroendocrine carcinoma of the skin, primary small cell carcinoma of the skin, and trabecular carcinoma of the skin, arises from Merkel cells, which are neuroendocrine skin cells that act as

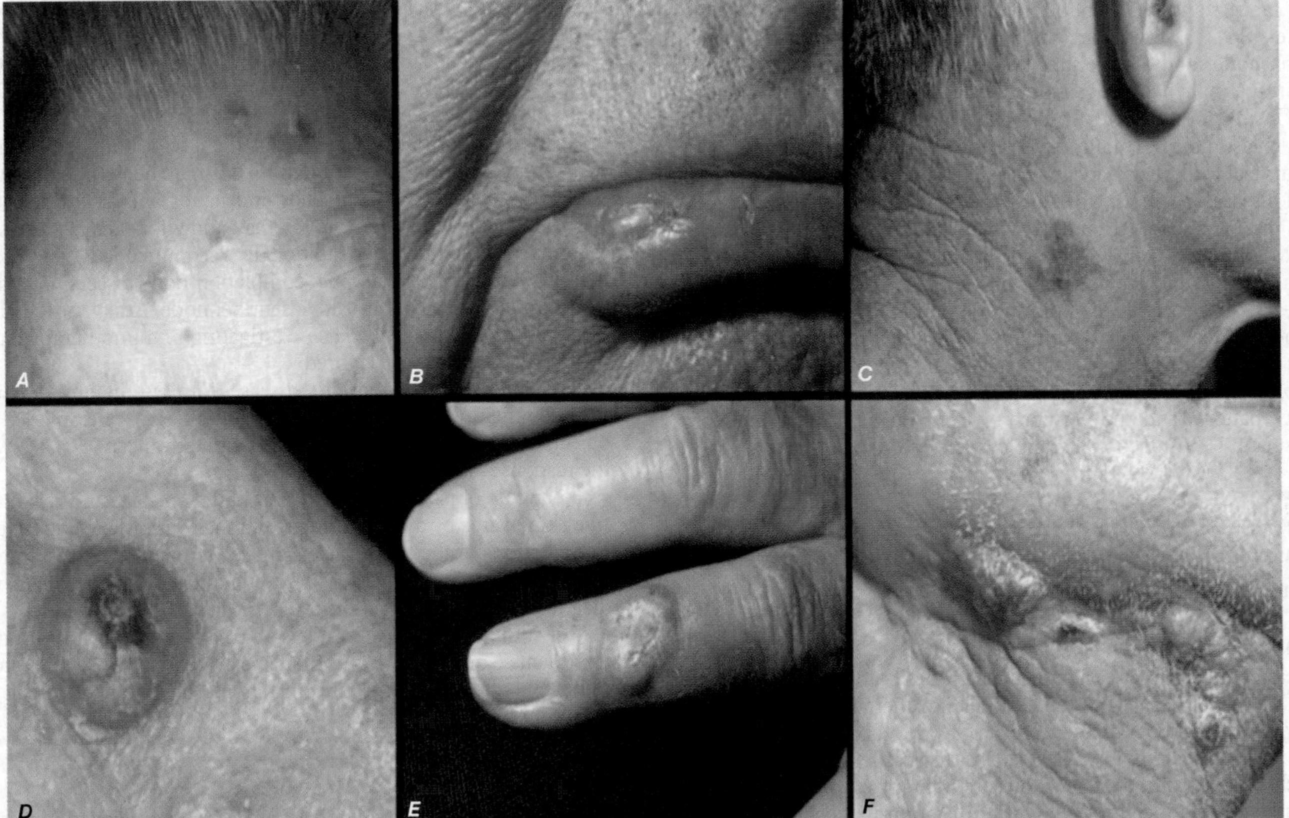

FIGURE 76-5 Progression of squamous cell carcinoma (SCC). *A.* Actinic keratoses (AKs). ***B.*** Actinic cheilitis (AK of the lip). ***C.*** Bowen's disease (SCC in situ). ***D.*** Keratoacanthoma (well-differentiated SCC). ***E.*** SCC. ***F.*** Metastatic SCC.

pressure receptors. Like other skin cancers, MCCs most commonly arise as visible skin lesions, usually as raised, flesh-colored nodules or masses; they can also be red or blue in color and vary in size from 0. 5 to >5 cm in diameter and may enlarge rapidly. Although MCCs may arise almost anywhere on the body, they are most commonly found in sun-exposed areas such as the head, neck, or extremities. They can also be found around the anus and on eyelids. The common clinical features of MCC can be summarized by the acronym AEIOU: *a*symptomatic/nontender, *e*xpand rapidly, *i*mmune suppression, *o*lder than 50 years, and *u*ltraviolet-exposed site.

■ NATURAL HISTORY

Basal Cell Carcinoma The natural history of BCC is that of a slowly enlarging, locally invasive neoplasm. The degree of local destruction and risk of recurrence vary with the size, duration, location, and histologic subtype of the tumor. Location on the central face, ears, or scalp may portend a higher risk. Small nodular, pigmented, cystic, or superficial BCCs respond well to most treatments. Large lesions and micronodular, infiltrative, and morpheaform subtypes may be more aggressive. The metastatic potential of BCC is low (0.1%) in immunocompetent patients, but the risk of recurrence or a new primary NMSC is about 40% over 5 years.

Squamous Cell Carcinoma The natural history of SCC depends on tumor and host characteristics. Tumors arising on sun-damaged skin have a lower metastatic potential than do those on non-sun-exposed areas. Cutaneous SCC metastasizes in 0.3–5.2% of individuals, most frequently to regional lymph nodes. Tumors occurring on the lower lip and ear develop regional metastases in 13 and 11% of patients, respectively, whereas the metastatic potential of SCC arising in scars, chronic ulcerations, and genital or mucosal surfaces is higher. Recurrent SCC has a 30% probability for metastatic spread. Large, poorly differentiated, deep tumors with perineural or lymphatic invasion, multifocal tumors, and those arising in immunosuppressed patients often behave aggressively.

Merkel Cell Carcinoma MCCs have clinical features of both skin cancers and neuroendocrine tumors (particularly small cell lung cancer [SCLC]); thus, they can present locally and develop spread to lymph nodes and distant sites. Molecular markers of neuroendocrine origin such as synaptophysin or chromogranin A are useful to diagnose MCC. Unlike other neuroendocrine tumors, MCCs are not associated with measurable hormone secretion or endocrine syndromes.

Survival with MCC depends on extent of disease: 90% of patients with local disease are cured, whereas 52% with nodal involvement and 10% with distant disease survive. MCC has its own tumor-node-metastasis (TNM) staging system, which incorporates tumor size (<2 cm vs. >2 cm), nodal status (which can be determined by SLNB for clinically negative nodes), and the presence of distant metastases.

Independent of stage, the prognosis of MCC is improved if the tumor cells contain virus, RB protein expression, and intratumoral CD8+ T lymphocyte infiltration, whereas p63 expression, lymphovascular infiltrative pattern, and the presence of immunosuppression (e.g., organ transplant, HIV infection, certain cancers) portend a worse prognosis.

TREATMENT

Basal Cell, Squamous Cell, and Merkle Cell Carcinoma

BASAL CELL CARCINOMA

Treatment for BCC includes electrodesiccation and curettage (ED&C), excision, cryosurgery, radiation therapy (RT), laser therapy, Mohs micrographic surgery (MMS), topical 5-fluorouracil, photodynamic therapy (PDT), and topical immunomodulators, such as imiquimod. The choice of therapy depends on tumor characteristics including depth and location, patient age, medical status, and patient preference. ED&C remains the most commonly employed treatment for superficial, minimally invasive nodular BCCs and low-risk tumors (e.g., a small tumor of a less aggressive subtype in a favorable location). Wide local excision with standard margins is usually selected for invasive, ill-defined, and more aggressive subtypes of tumors or for cosmetic reasons. MMS, a specialized type of surgical excision that provides the best method for tumor removal while preserving uninvolved tissue, is associated with cure rates >98%. It is the preferred modality for lesions that are recurrent, in high-risk or cosmetically sensitive locations (including recurrent tumors in these locations), and for which maximal tissue conservation is critical (e.g., the eyelids, lips, ears, nose, and digits). RT can cure patients not considered surgical candidates and can be used as a surgical adjunct in high-risk tumors. Imiquimod can be used to treat superficial and smaller nodular BCCs, although it is not FDA approved for nodular BCC. Topical 5-fluorouracil therapy should be limited to superficial BCC. PDT, which uses selective activation of a photoactive drug by visible light, has been used in patients with numerous tumors. Intralesional therapy (5-fluorouracil or IFN) can also be employed. Like RT, it remains an option for selected patients who cannot or will not undergo surgery. Systemic therapy with an SMO inhibitor, vismodegib or sonidegib, is indicated for patients with metastatic or advanced BCC that has recurred after local therapy and who are not candidates for surgery or RT. Targeted therapy with SMO antagonists does not cure patients with BCC but induces regression in approximately 50% of patients with a median duration of response >9 months.

SQUAMOUS CELL CARCINOMA

The principles for surgical management of SCC are the same as for BCC. Previously, advanced disease was treated with cisplatin-containing chemotherapy, intralesional 5-fluorouracil, or cetuximab. These regimens have been supplanted by cemiplimab, a monoclonal antibody targeting PD-1, which causes tumor regression in 47% of patients with advanced disease. SCC and KAs that develop in patients receiving BRAF-targeted therapy should be excised, after which BRAF therapy can be continued.

MERKEL CELL CARCINOMA

The epidemiology, clinical features, and treatments for MCC overlap those for melanoma and NMSC. Early-stage MCCs may be cured with wide local excision of the primary tumor and nodal staging with SLNB. Like SCLCs, MCC is sensitive to radiation, PD-1-directed immunotherapy, and platinum-based chemotherapy. RT is often used as postoperative adjuvant therapy at both the primary excision and SLNB sites, although its use may be withheld around sensitive areas such as the eyelids and hands and after a negative SLNB. For nonsensitive areas, RT may allow for primary excision margins smaller than the traditionally recommended 2-cm radial margins. Similar to melanoma, completion node dissection is now uncommonly used for a positive sentinel node. Adjuvant RT, close observation, and clinical trials investigating immunotherapy based on anti-PD-1 agents are favored.

For patients with metastatic disease, immunotherapy has supplanted chemotherapy. Avelumab (anti-PD-L1) therapy led to objective responses in 33% of patients with advanced MCC; 82% of the responses were durable.

Follow-up of patients with MCC is based on stage and risk. Routine skin exams by a dermatologist familiar with MCC and regular examinations of the nodal basins are recommended. A serum titer of monoclonal antibody to MCPyV should be obtained in newly diagnosed MCC patients. The test can be used to follow patients for relapse if the titer is elevated at baseline and returns to normal after treatment. Conversely, if the titer is elevated but does not return to normal after treatment, imaging should be obtained to look for occult metastases.

■ PREVENTION

The principles for prevention are those described for melanoma earlier. Unique strategies for NMSC include active surveillance for patients on immunosuppressive medications or BRAF-targeted therapy.

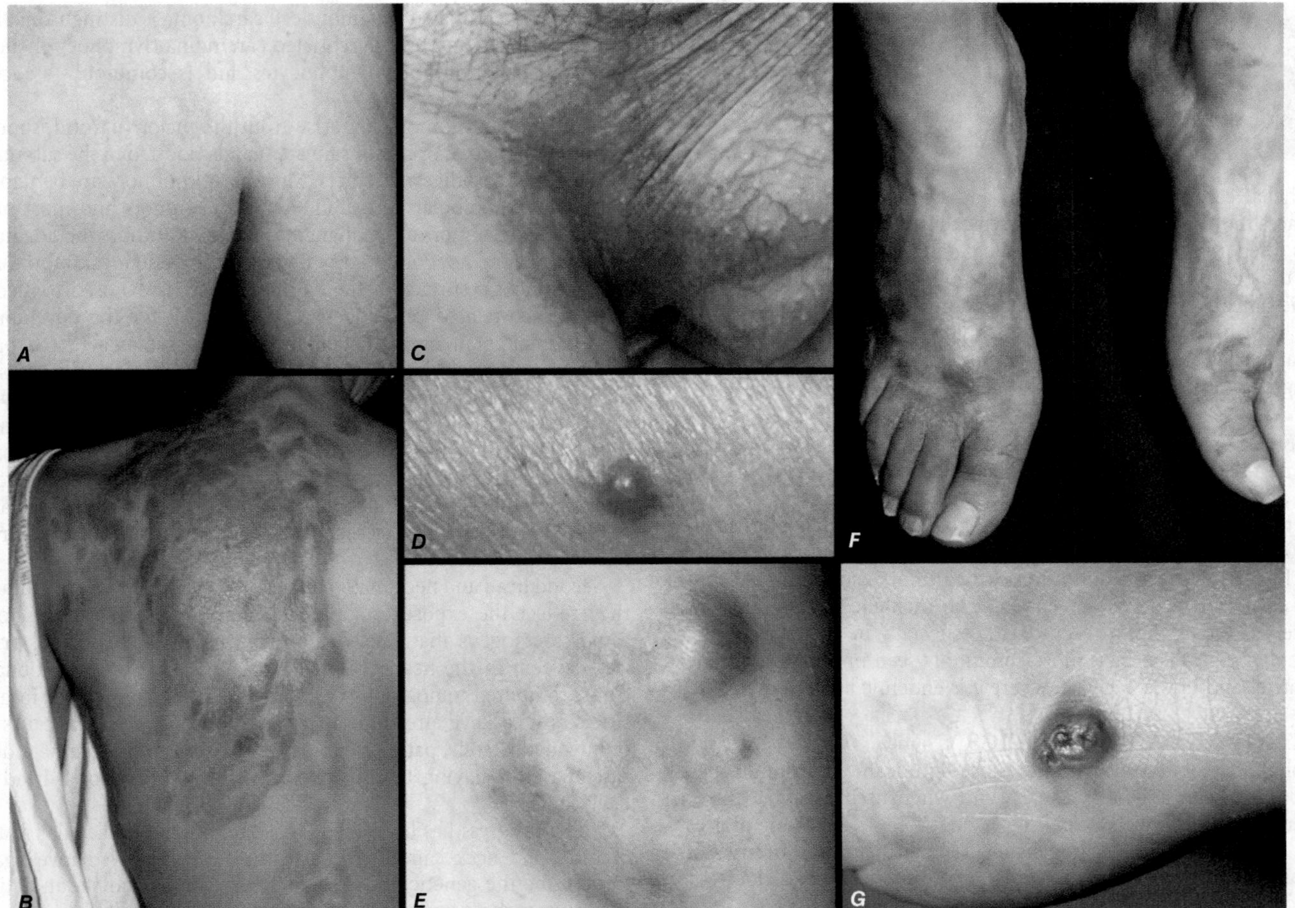

FIGURE 76-6 Other malignant cutaneous tumors. ***A.*** Patch stage mycosis fungoides (variant of cutaneous T-cell lymphoma). ***B.*** Tumor stage mycosis fungoides. ***C.*** Extramammary Paget's disease. ***D.*** Merkel cell carcinoma. ***E.*** Dermatofibrosarcoma protuberans. ***F.*** Kaposi's sarcoma. ***G.*** Kaposi's sarcoma.

Chemoprophylaxis using synthetic retinoids and immunosuppression reduction when possible may be useful in controlling new lesions and managing patients with multiple tumors. Field therapy with topical 5-fluorouracil, ingenol mebutate, or imiquimod can reduce transformation to SCC in patients with severely sun-damaged skin and numerous premalignant actinic keratoses. Older, immunosuppressed patients should be managed with the lowest doses of immunosuppression possible and encouraged to be particularly careful to minimize UV exposure. Earlier biopsy of unusual-appearing skin lesions may lead to better control of aggressive lesions.

OTHER NONMELANOMA CUTANEOUS MALIGNANCIES

Neoplasms of cutaneous adnexae and sarcomas of fibrous, mesenchymal, fatty, and vascular tissues make up the remaining 1–2% of NMSCs **(Fig. 76-6)**. Lymphomas of B- or T-cell origin can also manifest in the skin and can mimic benign conditions such as psoriasis and eczema.

Extramammary Paget's disease is an uncommon apocrine malignancy arising from stem cells of the epidermis that is characterized histologically by the presence of Paget cells. These tumors present as moist erythematous patches on anogenital or axillary skin of the elderly.

Outcomes are generally good with surgery, and 5-year disease-specific survival is 95% with localized disease. Advanced age and extensive disease at presentation confer poorer prognosis. RT or topical imiquimod can be considered for more extensive disease. Local management may be challenging because these tumors often extend far beyond clinical margins; surgical excision with MMS has the highest cure rates. Similarly, MMS is the treatment of choice in other rare cutaneous tumors with extensive subclinical extension such as *dermatofibrosarcoma protuberans.*

Kaposi's sarcoma (KS) is a soft tissue sarcoma of vascular origin that is induced by the human herpesvirus 8. The incidence of KS increased dramatically during the AIDS epidemic, but has now decreased tenfold with the institution of highly active antiretroviral therapy.

Acknowledgment

Walter Urba, MD, PhD, provided valued feedback and suggested improvements to this chapter. Clinical photos were generously provided from the OHSU Swinyer Collection (Leonard Swinyer, MD) and by Drs. Elizabeth Berry, Alexander Witkowski, Joanna Ludzik, Debbie Miller, Alison Skalet, and Justin Leitenberger. Dermoscopic images were provided by Elizabeth Berry, Alexander Witkowski, Joanna Ludzik, and Debbie Miller. Reflectance confocal microscopy images were provided by Drs. Alexander Witkowski and Joanna Ludzik.

FURTHER READING

Faries MD et al: Completion dissection or observation for sentinel-node metastasis in melanoma. N Engl J Med 376:2211, 2017.

Harms PW et al: The biology and treatment of Merkel cell carcinoma: Current understanding and research priorities. Nat Rev Clin Oncol 15:763, 2018.

Larkin J et al: Combined nivolumab and ipilimumab or monotherapy in untreated melanoma. N Engl J Med 373:23, 2015.

National Comprehensive Cancer Network: NCCN clinical practice guidelines in oncology (NCCN guidelines): Melanoma. Available from *https://www.nccn.org/professionals/physician_gls/pdf/melanoma.pdf.* Accessed May 29, 2020.

Robert C et al: Improved overall survival in melanoma with combined dabrafenib and trametinib. N Engl J Med 372:30, 2015.

Shain AH, Bastian BC: From melanocytes to melanomas. Nat Rev Cancer 16:345, 2016.

Wu YP et al: A systematic review of interventions to improve adherence to melanoma preventive behaviors for individuals at elevated risk. Prev Med 88:153, 2016.

77 Head and Neck Cancer

Everett E. Vokes

Epithelial carcinomas of the head and neck arise from the mucosal surfaces in the head and neck and typically are squamous cell in origin. This category includes tumors of the paranasal sinuses, the oral cavity, and the nasopharynx, oropharynx, hypopharynx, and larynx. Tumors of the salivary glands differ from the more common carcinomas of the head and neck in etiology, histopathology, clinical presentation, and therapy. They are rare and histologically highly heterogeneous. Thyroid malignancies are described in **Chap. 385**.

INCIDENCE AND EPIDEMIOLOGY

The number of new cases of head and neck cancers (oral cavity, pharynx, and larynx) in the United States was estimated at 65,630 in 2020, accounting for about 4% of adult malignancies; estimated deaths were 14,500. The worldwide incidence exceeds half a million cases annually. In North America and Europe, the tumors usually arise from the oral cavity, oropharynx, or larynx. The incidence of oropharyngeal cancers is increasing in recent years, especially in Western countries. Nasopharyngeal cancer is more commonly seen in the Mediterranean countries and in the Far East, where it is endemic in some areas.

ETIOLOGY AND GENETICS

Alcohol and tobacco use are the most significant environmental risk factors for head and neck cancer, and when used together, they act synergistically. Smokeless tobacco is an etiologic agent for oral cancers. Other potential carcinogens include marijuana and occupational exposures such as nickel refining, exposure to textile fibers, and woodworking.

Some head and neck cancers have a viral etiology. Epstein-Barr virus (EBV) infection is frequently associated with nasopharyngeal cancer, especially in endemic areas of the Mediterranean and Far East. EBV antibody titers can be measured to screen high-risk populations and are under investigation to monitor treatment response. Nasopharyngeal cancer has also been associated with consumption of salted fish and indoor pollution.

In Western countries, the human papillomavirus (HPV) is associated with a rising incidence of tumors arising from the oropharynx, that is, the tonsillar bed and base of tongue. Over 50% of oropharyngeal tumors are caused by HPV in the United States, and in many urban centers, this proportion is higher. HPV 16 is the dominant viral subtype, although HPV 18 and other oncogenic subtypes are seen as well. Alcohol- and tobacco-related cancers, on the other hand, have decreased in incidence. HPV-related oropharyngeal cancer frequently occurs in a younger patient population and is associated with increased numbers of sexual partners and oral sexual practices. It is associated with a better prognosis, especially for nonsmokers. Vaccination with the nine-valent HPV vaccine may prevent the disease in high-risk populations.

Dietary factors may contribute. The incidence of head and neck cancer is higher in people with the lowest consumption of fruits and vegetables. Certain vitamins, including carotenoids, may be protective if included in a balanced diet. Supplements of retinoids, such as *cis*-retinoic acid, have not been shown to prevent head and neck cancers (or lung cancer) and may increase the risk in active smokers. No specific risk factors or environmental carcinogens have been identified for salivary gland tumors.

HISTOPATHOLOGY, CARCINOGENESIS, AND MOLECULAR BIOLOGY

Squamous cell head and neck cancers are divided into well-differentiated, moderately well-differentiated, and poorly differentiated categories. Poorly differentiated tumors have a worse prognosis than well-differentiated tumors. For nasopharyngeal cancers, the less common differentiated squamous cell carcinoma is distinguished from nonkeratinizing and undifferentiated carcinoma (lymphoepithelioma) that contains infiltrating lymphocytes and is commonly associated with EBV.

Salivary gland tumors can arise from the major (parotid, submandibular, sublingual) or minor salivary glands (located in the submucosa of the upper aerodigestive tract). Most parotid tumors are benign, but half of submandibular and sublingual gland tumors and most minor salivary gland tumors are malignant. Malignant tumors include mucoepidermoid and adenoid cystic carcinomas and adenocarcinomas.

The mucosal surface of the entire pharynx is exposed to alcohol- and tobacco-related carcinogens and is at risk for the development of a premalignant or malignant lesion. Erythroplakia (a red patch) or leukoplakia (a white patch) can be histopathologically classified as hyperplasia, dysplasia, carcinoma in situ, or carcinoma. However, most head and neck cancer patients do not present with a known history of premalignant lesions. Multiple synchronous or metachronous cancers can also be observed. In fact, over time, patients with treated early-stage tobacco- and alcohol-related head and neck cancer are at greater risk of dying from a second malignancy than from a recurrence of the primary disease.

Second head and neck malignancies are usually not therapy induced; they reflect the exposure of the upper aerodigestive mucosa to the same carcinogens that caused the first cancer. These second primaries develop in the head and neck area, the lung, or the esophagus. Thus, computed tomography (CT) screening for lung cancer in heavy smokers who have already developed a head and neck cancer is recommended. Rarely, patients can develop a radiation therapy–induced sarcoma after having undergone prior radiotherapy for a head and neck cancer.

Much progress has been made in describing the molecular features of head and neck cancer. These features have allowed investigators to describe the genetic and epigenetic alterations and the mutational spectrum of these tumors. Early reports demonstrated frequent overexpression of the epidermal growth factor receptor (EGFR). Overexpression was shown to correlate with poor prognosis. However, it has not proved to be a good predictor of tumor response to EGFR inhibitors, which are active in only about 10–15% of patients as single agents. Complex genetic analyses, including those by The Cancer Genome Atlas project, have been performed. *p53* mutations are found frequently with other major affected oncogenic driver pathways including the mitotic signaling and Notch pathways and cell cycle regulation in HPV-negative tumors. HPV oncogenes act through direct inhibition of the *p53* and *RB* tumor-suppressor genes, thereby initiating the carcinogenic process. *HRAS* appears to be emerging as a potentially targetable mutation in a small patient subset. While overall mutation rates are similar in HPV-positive and carcinogen-induced tumors, the specific mutational signature of HPV-positive tumors differs, with frequent alteration of the PI3K pathway and occasional mutations in *KRAS*. Overall, these alterations affect mitogenic signaling, genetic stability, cellular proliferation, and differentiation.

CLINICAL PRESENTATION AND DIFFERENTIAL DIAGNOSIS

Most tobacco-related head and neck cancers occur in patients older than age 60 years. HPV-related malignancies are frequently diagnosed in younger patients, usually in their forties or fifties, whereas EBV-related nasopharyngeal cancer can occur at all ages, including in teenagers. The manifestations vary according to the stage and primary site of the tumor. Patients with nonspecific signs and symptoms in the head and neck area should be evaluated with a thorough otolaryngologic examination, particularly if symptoms persist longer than 2–4 weeks. Males are more frequently affected than women by head and neck cancers, including HPV-positive tumors.

Cancer of the nasopharynx typically does not cause early symptoms. However, it may cause unilateral serous otitis media due to obstruction of the eustachian tube, unilateral or bilateral nasal obstruction, or epistaxis. Advanced nasopharyngeal carcinoma causes neuropathies of the cranial nerves due to skull base involvement.

Carcinomas of the oral cavity present as nonhealing ulcers, changes in the fit of dentures, or painful lesions and masses. Tumors of the tongue base or oropharynx can cause decreased tongue mobility and alterations in speech. Cancers of the oropharynx or hypopharynx rarely cause early symptoms, but they may cause sore throat and/or otalgia. HPV-related tumors frequently present with neck lymphadenopathy as the first sign.

Hoarseness may be an early symptom of laryngeal cancer, and persistent hoarseness requires referral to a specialist for indirect laryngoscopy and/or radiographic studies. If a head and neck lesion treated initially with antibiotics does not resolve in a short period, further workup is indicated; to simply continue the antibiotic treatment may be to lose the chance of early diagnosis of a malignancy.

Advanced head and neck cancers in any location can cause severe pain, otalgia, airway obstruction, cranial neuropathies, trismus, odynophagia, dysphagia, decreased tongue mobility, fistulas, skin involvement, and massive cervical lymphadenopathy, which may be unilateral or bilateral. Some patients have enlarged lymph nodes even though no primary lesion can be detected by endoscopy or biopsy; these patients are considered to have carcinoma of unknown primary **(Fig. 77-1)**. Tonsillectomy and directed biopsies of the base of tongue can frequently identify a small primary tumor that frequently will be HPV related. If the enlarged nodes are located in the upper neck and the tumor cells are of squamous cell histology, the malignancy probably arose from a mucosal surface in the head or neck. Tumor cells in supraclavicular lymph nodes may also arise from a primary site in the chest or abdomen.

The physical examination should include inspection of all visible mucosal surfaces and palpation of the floor of the mouth and of the tongue and neck. In addition to tumors themselves, leukoplakia (a white mucosal patch) or erythroplakia (a red mucosal patch) may be observed; these "premalignant" lesions can represent hyperplasia, dysplasia, or carcinoma in situ and require biopsy. Further examination should be performed by a specialist. Additional staging procedures include CT or MRI of the head and neck to identify the extent of the disease. Patients with lymph node involvement should have CT scan of the chest and upper abdomen to screen for distant metastases. In heavy smokers, the CT scan of the chest can also serve as a screening tool to rule out a second lung primary tumor. A positron emission tomography (PET) scan can help to identify or exclude distant metastases. CT and PET scans may also be useful in evaluating response to therapy. The definitive staging procedure is an endoscopic examination under anesthesia, which may include laryngoscopy, esophagoscopy, and bronchoscopy; during this procedure, multiple biopsy samples are obtained to establish a primary diagnosis, define the extent of primary disease, and identify any additional premalignant lesions or second primaries.

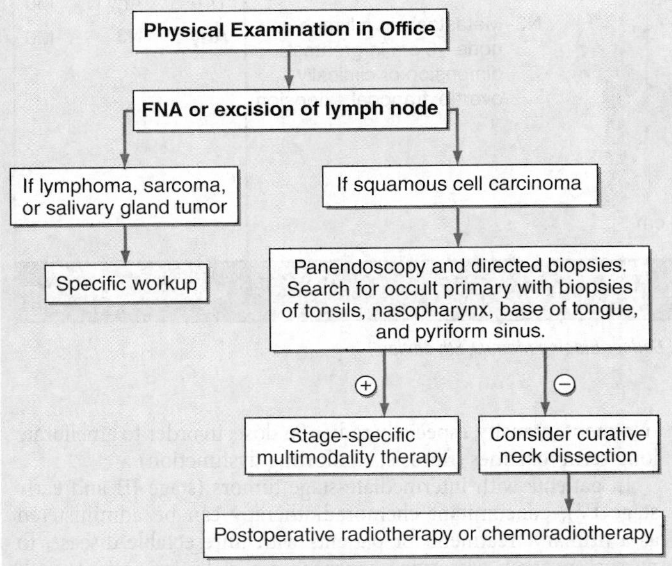

FIGURE 77-1 Evaluation of a patient with cervical adenopathy without a primary mucosal lesion; a diagnostic workup. FNA, fine-needle aspiration.

Head and neck tumors are classified according to the tumor-node-metastasis (TNM) system of the American Joint Committee on Cancer (AJCC) **(Fig. 77-2)**. This classification varies according to the specific anatomic subsite. In general, primary tumors are classified as T1 to T3 by increasing size, whereas T4 usually represents invasion of another structure such as bone, muscle, or root of tongue. Lymph nodes are staged by size, number, and location (ipsilateral vs contralateral to the primary). Distant metastases are found in <10% of patients at initial diagnosis and are more common in patients with advanced lymph node stage; microscopic involvement of the lungs, bones, or liver is more common, particularly in patients with advanced neck lymph node disease. Modern imaging techniques may increase the number of patients with clinically detectable distant metastases in the future. HPV-related oropharyngeal malignancies have consistently been shown to have a better prognosis, and in the eighth edition of the AJCC staging manual, a separate staging system that takes into account the more favorable outlook of these patients will be included. According to this system, patients with advanced nodal stage can still be considered to have an overall early stage (and associated good prognosis), especially if the patient is a nonsmoker or has limited lifelong tobacco exposure.

In patients with lymph node involvement and no visible primary, the diagnosis should be made by lymph node excision (Fig. 77-1). If the results indicate squamous cell carcinoma, a panendoscopy should be performed, with biopsy of all suspicious-appearing areas and directed biopsies of common primary sites, such as the nasopharynx, tonsil, tongue base, and pyriform sinus. HPV-positive tumors especially can have small primary tumors that spread early to locoregional lymph nodes.

TREATMENT
Head and Neck Cancer

Patients with head and neck cancer can be grossly categorized into three clinical groups: those with localized disease, those with locally or regionally advanced disease (lymph node positive), and those with recurrent and/or metastatic disease below the neck. Comorbidities associated with tobacco and alcohol abuse can affect treatment outcome and define long-term risks for patients who are cured of their disease.

LOCALIZED DISEASE

Nearly one-third of patients have localized disease, that is, T1 or T2 (stage I or stage II) lesions without detectable lymph node involvement or distant metastases. These patients are treated with curative intent by either surgery or radiation therapy. The choice of modality differs according to anatomic location and institutional expertise. Radiation therapy is often preferred for laryngeal cancer to preserve voice function, and surgery is preferred for small lesions in the oral cavity to avoid the long-term complications of radiation, such as xerostomia and osteoradionecrosis and dental decay. Randomized data have shown that a prophylactic staging neck dissection should be part of the surgical procedure to eliminate occult nodal metastatic disease. Overall 5-year survival is 60–90%. Most recurrences occur within the first 2 years following diagnosis and are usually local.

LOCALLY OR REGIONALLY ADVANCED DISEASE

Locally or regionally advanced disease—disease with a large primary tumor and/or lymph node metastases—is the stage of presentation for >50% of patients. Such patients can also be treated with curative intent, but not usually with surgery or radiation therapy alone. Combined-modality therapy, including surgery and/or radiation therapy and chemotherapy, is most successful. Chemotherapy can be administered as induction chemotherapy (chemotherapy before surgery and/or radiotherapy) or as concomitant (simultaneous)

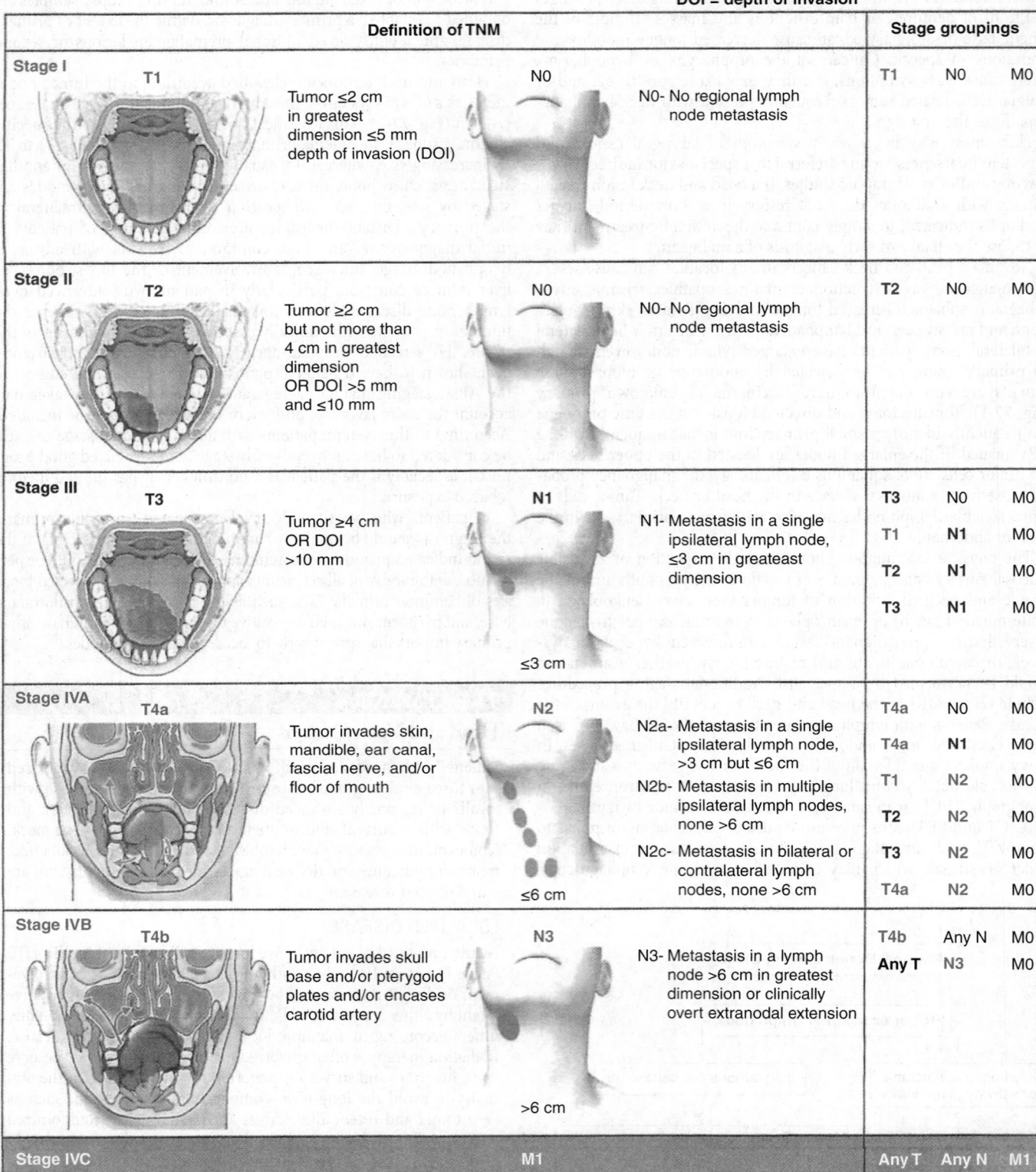

DOI = depth of invasion

Stage	Definition of TNM (T)		Definition of TNM (N)		Stage groupings		
Stage I	T1	Tumor ≤2 cm in greatest dimension ≤5 mm depth of invasion (DOI)	N0	N0- No regional lymph node metastasis	T1	N0	M0
Stage II	T2	Tumor ≥2 cm but not more than 4 cm in greatest dimension OR DOI >5 mm and ≤10 mm	N0	N0- No regional lymph node metastasis	T2	N0	M0
Stage III	T3	Tumor ≥4 cm OR DOI >10 mm	N1 (≤3 cm)	N1- Metastasis in a single ipsilateral lymph node, ≤3 cm in greateast dimension	T3	N0	M0
					T1	N1	M0
					T2	N1	M0
					T3	N1	M0
Stage IVA	T4a	Tumor invades skin, mandible, ear canal, fascial nerve, and/or floor of mouth	N2 (≤6 cm)	N2a- Metastasis in a single ipsilateral lymph node, >3 cm but ≤6 cm	T4a	N0	M0
					T4a	N1	M0
				N2b- Metastasis in multiple ipsilateral lymph nodes, none >6 cm	T1	N2	M0
					T2	N2	M0
				N2c- Metastasis in bilateral or contralateral lymph nodes, none >6 cm	T3	N2	M0
					T4a	N2	M0
Stage IVB	T4b	Tumor invades skull base and/or pterygoid plates and/or encases carotid artery	N3 (>6 cm)	N3- Metastasis in a lymph node >6 cm in greatest dimension or clinically overt extranodal extension	T4b	Any N	M0
					Any T	N3	M0
Stage IVC			M1		Any T	Any N	M1

FIGURE 77-2 Tumor-node-metastasis (TNM) staging system. *(Figure based on the AJCC Cancer Staging Manual, 8th edition.)*

chemotherapy and radiation therapy. The latter is currently most commonly used and supported by the best evidence. Five-year survival rates exceed 50% in many trials, but part of this increased survival may be due to an increasing fraction of study populations with HPV-related tumors who carry a better prognosis. HPV testing of newly diagnosed tumors should be performed for patients with oropharyngeal tumors at the time of diagnosis. Clinical trials for HPV-related tumors are focused on exploring reductions in treatment intensity, especially radiation dose, in order to ameliorate long-term toxicities (fibrosis, swallowing dysfunction).

In patients with intermediate-stage tumors (stage III and early stage IV), concomitant chemoradiotherapy can be administered as a primary treatment for patients with unresectable disease, to pursue an organ-preserving approach especially for patients with laryngeal cancer (omission of surgery), or in the postoperative setting for smaller resectable tumors with adverse prognostic features.

Induction Chemotherapy In this strategy, patients receive chemotherapy (current standard is a three-drug regimen of docetaxel, cisplatin, and fluorouracil [5-FU]) before surgery and radiation therapy. Most patients who receive three cycles show tumor reduction, and the response is clinically "complete" in up to half of patients. This "sequential" multimodality therapy allows for organ preservation in patients with laryngeal and hypopharyngeal cancer and results in higher cure rates compared with radiotherapy alone.

Concomitant Chemoradiotherapy With the concomitant strategy, chemotherapy and radiation therapy are given simultaneously rather than in sequence. Tumor recurrences from head and neck cancer develop most commonly locoregionally (in the head and neck area of the primary and draining lymph nodes). The concomitant approach is aimed at enhancing tumor cell killing by radiation therapy in the presence of chemotherapy (radiation enhancement) and is a conceptually attractive approach for bulky tumors. Toxicity (especially mucositis, grade 3 or 4, in 70–80%) is increased with concomitant chemoradiotherapy. However, meta-analyses of randomized trials document an improvement in 5-year survival of 8% with concomitant chemotherapy and radiation therapy. Cisplatin is preferentially given weekly during a course of daily radiotherapy over a 6- to 7-week course. In addition, concomitant chemoradiotherapy produces better laryngectomy-free survival (organ preservation) than radiation therapy alone in patients with advanced larynx cancer. The use of radiation therapy together with cisplatin produces improved survival in patients with advanced nasopharyngeal cancer. The outcome of HPV-related cancers seems to be especially favorable following cisplatin-based chemoradiotherapy. Trials substituting cisplatin with the EGFR inhibitor cetuximab in that patient population have shown inferior survival.

The success of concomitant chemoradiotherapy in patients with unresectable disease has led to the testing of a similar approach in patients with resected intermediate-stage disease as a postoperative therapy. Concomitant chemoradiotherapy produces a significant improvement over postoperative radiation therapy alone for patients whose tumors demonstrate higher risk features, such as extracapsular spread beyond involved lymph nodes, involvement of multiple lymph nodes, or positive margins at the primary site following surgery.

A monoclonal antibody to EGFR (cetuximab) increases survival rates when administered during radiotherapy. EGFR blockade results in radiation sensitization and has milder systemic side effects than traditional chemotherapy agents, although an acneiform skin rash is commonly observed. Nevertheless, the addition of cetuximab to current standard chemoradiotherapy regimens has failed to show further improvement in survival and is not recommended.

TREATMENT APPROACHES FOR HPV-RELATED HEAD AND NECK CANCERS

Given consistent observations of high survival rates for patients with advanced HPV-related oropharyngeal tumors using combined-modality treatment strategies, de-escalation protocols have attracted widespread interest. The goal here is to decrease the long-term morbidity resulting from high-dose radiation therapy, including extensive neck fibrosis, swallowing problems, and osteoradionecrosis of the jaw. Current studies are investigating the use of lower radiation doses, the use of induction chemotherapy and subsequent omission of chemotherapy or administration of significantly reduced chemoradiation doses in very good responders, and other strategies. In addition, interest has increased in surgical approaches using robotic surgery, which allows better visualization of the base of tongue and tonsil. While technically feasible, this approach remains investigational because a large number of patients with disease involving multiple lymph nodes will still require postoperative chemoradiotherapy, thus negating the goal of treatment de-escalation. It is expected that distinct treatment guidelines from carcinogen-induced tumors will be defined in the coming years.

RECURRENT AND/OR METASTATIC DISEASE

Five to ten percent of patients present with metastatic disease, and 30–50% of patients with locoregionally advanced disease experience recurrence, frequently outside the head and neck region. Patients with recurrent and/or metastatic disease are, with few exceptions, treated with palliative intent. Some patients may require local or regional radiation therapy for pain control, but most are given systemic therapy.

Combination chemotherapy formerly was the first-line systemic therapeutic approach to patients with recurrent disease after prior curative intent surgery and/or chemoradiotherapy or those presenting initially with metastatic disease. In particular, a combination of cisplatin with 5-FU and cetuximab (the EXTREME regimen) was frequently used.

However, immunotherapies have proven to be of value in this setting. In particular, inhibitors of the immunosuppressive lymphocyte surface receptor (PD-1) pathway have shown activity in squamous cell cancers of the head and neck. A randomized trial evaluating the PD-1 inhibitor nivolumab versus traditional chemotherapy in the second-line treatment of patients with recurrent or metastatic disease showed a significant increase in 1-year survival rates with fewer severe treatment-related toxicities. In addition, some responses were of long duration, allowing a cohort of patients to live far beyond the historical median of <1 year. The PD-1 inhibitor pembrolizumab also demonstrated activity in a similarly designed randomized trial.

Following establishment of second-line activity, pembrolizumab was compared as single-agent therapy or in combination with cisplatin and 5-FU with prior standard chemotherapy alone (cisplatin, 5-FU, and cetuximab). In this trial, overall survival was improved with pembrolizumab versus chemotherapy as well as with the combination of chemotherapy plus pembrolizumab. No statistically significant impact on progression-free survival was noted. In addition, expression of PD-L1 in the tumor tissue was shown to be of importance. Patients with tumors high in expression (PD-L1 score >20%; i.e., expression of PD-L1 on 20% of tumor cells) had a marked survival benefit with pembrolizumab as single agent, whereas patients with lower PD-L1 expression had a less impressive but still statistically significant survival benefit. However, for the group expressing lower levels of PD-L1, the combination of pembrolizumab with chemotherapy showed more substantial benefit. Current standard treatment therefore frequently consists of combination chemoimmunotherapy for patients with a low combined positive score (CPS; the fraction of tumor cells expressing PD-L1), whereas those with higher CPS scores can be treated with immunotherapy alone, especially if overall tumor burden is limited. Patients who experience progression after first-line chemoimmunotherapy or immunotherapy can then be treated with additional single-agent or combination chemotherapy.

EGFR-directed therapies, including monoclonal antibodies (e.g., cetuximab) and tyrosine kinase inhibitors (TKIs) of the EGFR signaling pathway (e.g., erlotinib or gefitinib), have single-agent activity of ~10%. Side effects are usually limited to an acneiform rash and diarrhea (for the TKIs). The addition of cetuximab to standard combination chemotherapy with cisplatin or carboplatin and 5-FU results in a significant increase in median survival. Drugs targeting specific mutations are under investigation, and patients with *HRAS* mutations have tumor shrinkage with the farnesyltransferase inhibitor tipifarnib.

COMPLICATIONS

Complications from treatment of head and neck cancer are usually correlated to the extent of surgery and exposure of normal tissue structures to radiation. Currently, the extent of surgery has been limited or completely replaced by chemotherapy and radiation therapy as the primary approach. Acute complications of radiation include mucositis and dysphagia. Long-term complications include xerostomia, loss of taste, decreased tongue mobility, second malignancies, dysphagia, and neck fibrosis. The complications of chemotherapy vary with the regimen used but usually include myelosuppression, mucositis, nausea and vomiting, and nephrotoxicity (with cisplatin).

The mucosal side effects of therapy can lead to malnutrition and dehydration. Many centers address issues of dentition before starting treatment, and some place feeding tubes to ensure control of hydration and nutrition intake. About 50% of patients develop hypothyroidism from the treatment; thus, thyroid function should be monitored.

SALIVARY GLAND TUMORS

Most benign salivary gland tumors are treated with surgical excision, and patients with invasive salivary gland tumors are treated with surgery and radiation therapy. These tumors may recur regionally; adenoid cystic carcinoma has a tendency to recur along the nerve tracks. Distant metastases may occur as late as 10–20 years after the initial diagnosis. For metastatic disease, therapy is given with palliative intent, usually chemotherapy with doxorubicin and/or cisplatin. Identification of novel agents with activity in these tumors is a high priority. It is hoped that comprehensive genomic characterization of these rare tumors will facilitate these efforts.

FURTHER READING

Agrawal N et al: Exome sequencing of head and neck squamous cell carcinoma reveals inactivating mutations in NOTCH1. Science 333:1154, 2011.

Burtness B et al: Pembrolizumab alone or with chemotherapy versus cetuximab with chemotherapy for recurrent or metastatic squamous cell carcinoma of the head and neck (KEYNOTE-048): A randomized, open-label, phase 3 study. Lancet 394:1915, 2019.

Chow LQM: Head and neck cancer. N Engl J Med 382:60, 2020.

D'Cruz AK et al: Elective versus therapeutic neck dissection in node-negative oral cancer. N Engl J Med 373:521, 2015.

Ferris RL et al: Nivolumab for recurrent squamous-cell carcinoma of the head and neck. N Engl J Med 375:1856, 2016.

Gillison ML et al: Distinct risk factor profiles for human papillomavirus type 16-positive and human papillomavirus type 16-negative head and neck cancers. J Natl Cancer Inst 100:407, 2008.

Kang H et al: Whole-exome sequencing of salivary gland mucoepidermoid carcinoma. Clin Cancer Res 23:283, 2017.

Mehanna H et al: De-escalation after DE-ESCALATE and RTOG 1016: A Head and Neck Cancer Intergroup framework for future de-escalation studies. J Clin Oncol 38:2552, 2020.

Sabatini ME et al: Human papillomavirus as a driver of head and neck cancers. Br J Cancer 122:306, 2020.

Tota JE et al: Evolution of the oropharynx cancer epidemic in the United States: Moderation of increasing incidence in younger individuals and shift in the burden to older individuals. J Clin Oncol 37:1538, 2019.

78 Neoplasms of the Lung

Leora Horn, Wade T. Iams

Lung cancer, which was rare before 1900 with fewer than 400 cases described in the medical literature, is considered a disease of modern man, killing over three times as many men as prostate cancer and nearly twice as many women as breast cancer. Although lung cancer remains the number one cause of cancer-related mortality, a decline in lung cancer deaths has emerged, attributed to improvements in testing and therapeutic strategies and a decline in tobacco usage. Tobacco consumption is the primary cause of lung cancer, a reality firmly established in the mid-twentieth century and codified with the release of the U.S. Surgeon General's 1964 report on the health effects of tobacco smoking. Following the report, cigarette use started to decline in North America and parts of Europe, and with it, so did the incidence of lung cancer. Although tobacco smoking remains the primary cause of lung cancer worldwide, approximately 60% of new lung cancers in the United States occur in former smokers (smoked ≥100 cigarettes per lifetime, quit ≥1 year), many of whom quit decades ago, or never smokers (smoked <100 cigarettes per lifetime). Moreover, one in five women and one in 12 men diagnosed with lung cancer have never smoked.

EPIDEMIOLOGY

Lung cancer is the most common cause of cancer death among American men and women. Approximately 228,000 individuals will be diagnosed with lung cancer in the United States in 2020, and >135, 000 individuals will die from the disease. Lung cancer is uncommon below age 40, with rates increasing until age 80, after which the rate tapers off. The projected lifetime probability of developing lung cancer is estimated to be ~8% among males and ~6% among females. The incidence of lung cancer varies by racial and ethnic group, with the highest age-adjusted incidence rates among African Americans. The excess in age-adjusted rates among African Americans occurs only among men, but examinations of age-specific rates show that below age 50, mortality from lung cancer is >25% higher among African American than Caucasian women. Incidence and mortality rates among Hispanics and Native and Asian Americans are ~40–50% those of whites.

RISK FACTORS

Cigarette smokers have a 10-fold or greater increased risk of developing lung cancer compared to those who have never smoked. A large-scale genomic study suggested that one genetic mutation is induced for every 15 cigarettes smoked. The risk of lung cancer is lower among persons who quit smoking than among those who continue smoking. The size of the lung cancer risk reduction increases with the length of time the person has quit smoking, although even long-term former smokers have higher risks of lung cancer than those who never smoked. Cigarette smoking has been shown to increase the risk of all major types of lung cancer. Environmental tobacco smoke (ETS) or second-hand smoke is also an established cause of lung cancer. The risk from ETS is less than from active smoking, with about a 20–30% increase in lung cancer observed among never smokers married for many years to smokers, in comparison to the 2000% increase among continuing active smokers. The impact on the development of lung cancer among users of alternate nicotine delivery devices (e-cigarettes or vaping) is undefined. While one large randomized study demonstrated the superiority of e-cigarettes compared to traditional nicotine replacement therapy in aiding smoking cessation, e-cigarette– or vaping-associated lung injury (EVALI) is an emerging phenomenon that poses risks that may counterbalance the potential benefit in helping patients reduce traditional cigarette consumption and lung cancer risk.

Although cigarette smoking is the cause of the majority of lung cancers, several other risk factors have been identified, including occupational exposure to asbestos, arsenic, bischloromethyl ether, hexavalent chromium, mustard gas, nickel (as in certain nickel-refining processes), and polycyclic aromatic hydrocarbons.

Ionizing radiation is also an established lung carcinogen, most convincingly demonstrated from studies showing increased rates of lung cancer among survivors of the atom bombs dropped on Hiroshima and Nagasaki and large excesses among workers exposed to alpha irradiation from radon in underground uranium mining. Prolonged exposure to low-level radon in homes might impart a risk of lung cancer equal to or greater than that of ETS. Prior lung diseases such as chronic bronchitis, emphysema, and tuberculosis have been linked to increased risks of lung cancer as well. The risk of lung cancer appears to be higher among individuals with low fruit and vegetable intake during adulthood. This observation led to hypotheses that specific nutrients, in particular retinoids and carotenoids, might have chemopreventative effects for lung cancer. However, randomized trials failed to validate this hypothesis.

Smoking Cessation Given the undeniable link between cigarette smoking and lung cancer, physicians must promote tobacco abstinence. Stopping tobacco use before middle age avoids >90% of the lung cancer risk attributable to tobacco. Importantly, smoking cessation can even be beneficial in individuals with an established diagnosis of lung cancer, as it is associated with improved survival, fewer side effects from therapy, and an overall improvement in quality of life. Consequently, it is important to promote smoking cessation even *after* the diagnosis of lung cancer is established.

Physicians need to understand the essential elements of smoking cessation therapy. The individual must want to stop smoking and must be willing to work hard to achieve the goal of smoking abstinence. Self-help strategies alone only marginally affect quit rates, whereas individual and combined pharmacotherapies in combination with counseling can significantly increase rates of cessation. Therapy with an antidepressant (e.g., bupropion) and nicotine replacement therapy (varenicline, a $\alpha_4\beta_2$ nicotinic acetylcholine receptor partial agonist) are approved by the U.S. Food and Drug Administration (FDA) as first-line treatments for nicotine dependence. In a randomized trial, varenicline was shown to be more efficacious than bupropion or placebo. Prolonged use of varenicline beyond the initial induction phase proved useful in maintaining smoking abstinence. Clonidine and nortriptyline are recommended as second-line treatments. A role for e-cigarettes has not been definitively established **(Chap. 454)**.

Inherited Predisposition to Lung Cancer Exposure to environmental carcinogens, such as those found in tobacco smoke, induce or facilitate the transformation from bronchoepithelial cells to a malignant phenotype. The contribution of carcinogens to transformation is modulated by polymorphic variations in genes that affect aspects of carcinogen metabolism. Certain genetic polymorphisms of the P450 enzyme system, specifically CYP1A1, and chromosome fragility are associated with the development of lung cancer. These genetic variations occur at relatively high frequency in the population, but their contribution to an individual's lung cancer risk is generally low. However, because of their population frequency, the overall impact on lung cancer risk could be high.

First-degree relatives of lung cancer probands have a two- to three-fold excess risk of lung cancer and other cancers, many of which are not smoking-related. These data suggest that specific genes and/or genetic variants may contribute to susceptibility to lung cancer. However, very few such genes have yet been identified. Individuals with inherited mutations in *RB* (patients with retinoblastoma living to adulthood) and *p53* (Li-Fraumeni syndrome) genes may develop lung cancer. Common gene variants involved in lung cancer have identified three separate loci that are associated with lung cancer (5p15, 6p21, and 15q25) and include genes that regulate acetylcholine nicotinic receptors and telomerase production. A rare germline mutation (T790M) involving the epidermal growth factor receptor (EGFR) maybe be linked to lung cancer susceptibility in never smokers. Likewise, a susceptibility locus on chromosome 6q greatly increases lung cancer risk among light and never smokers. Although progress has been made, there is a significant amount of work that remains to be done in identifying heritable risk factors for lung cancer. Currently no molecular criteria are suitable to select patients for more intense screening programs or for specific chemopreventive strategies.

PATHOLOGY

The World Health Organization (WHO) defines lung cancer as tumors arising from the respiratory epithelium (bronchi, bronchioles, and alveoli). The WHO classification system divides epithelial lung cancers into four major cell types: small-cell lung cancer (SCLC), adenocarcinoma, squamous cell carcinoma, and large-cell carcinoma; the latter three types are collectively known as non-small-cell carcinomas (NSCLCs) **(Fig. 78-1)**. Small-cell carcinomas consist of small cells with scant cytoplasm, ill-defined cell borders, finely granular nuclear chromatin, absent or inconspicuous nucleoli, and a high mitotic count. SCLC may be distinguished from NSCLC by the presence of neuroendocrine markers including CD56, neural cell adhesion molecule (NCAM), synaptophysin, and chromogranin. Adenocarcinomas possess glandular differentiation or mucin production and may show acinar, papillary, lepidic, or solid features or a mixture of these patterns. Squamous cell carcinomas of the lung are morphologically identical to extrapulmonary squamous cell carcinomas and cannot be distinguished by immunohistochemistry alone. Squamous cell tumors show keratinization and/or intercellular bridges that arise from bronchial epithelium. The tumor consists of sheets of cells rather than the three-dimensional groups of cells characteristic of adenocarcinomas. Large-cell carcinomas compose <10% of lung carcinomas. These tumors lack the cytologic and architectural features of small-cell carcinoma and glandular or squamous differentiation. Together, these four histologic types account for ~90% of all epithelial lung cancers.

All histologic types of lung cancer can develop in current and former smokers, although squamous and small-cell carcinomas are most commonly associated with tobacco use. With the decline in cigarette consumption, adenocarcinoma has become the most frequent histologic subtype of lung cancer in the United States. In lifetime never smokers or former light smokers (<10 pack-year history), women, and younger adults (<60 years), adenocarcinoma tends to be the most common form of lung cancer.

In addition to distinguishing between SCLC and NSCLC, because these tumors have quite different natural histories and therapeutic approaches (see below), it is necessary to classify whether NSCLC is squamous or nonsquamous. The classification system, developed jointly by the International Association for the Study of Lung Cancer, the American Thoracic Society, and the European Respiratory Society, provides an integrated approach to the classification of lung adenocarcinoma that includes clinical, molecular, radiographic, and pathologic information.

It is recognized that most lung cancers present in an advanced stage and are often diagnosed based on small biopsies or cytologic specimens, rendering clear histologic distinctions difficult, if not impossible. In such cases, particularly in patients with advanced-stage disease, a repeat biopsy is recommended to obtain additional tissue for further clarification. The distinction between squamous and nonsquamous lung cancer is viewed as critical to optimal therapeutic decision making, and a diagnosis of *non-small-cell carcinoma, not otherwise specified* is no longer considered acceptable. This distinction can be achieved using a single marker for adenocarcinoma (thyroid transcription factor-1 or napsin-A) plus a squamous marker (p40 or p63) and/or mucin stains. If tissue is limited and a clear morphologic pattern is evident, a diagnosis can be made without immunohistochemistry staining. In addition to determining histologic subtype, preservation of sufficient specimen material for appropriate molecular testing and PD-L1 testing necessary to help guide therapeutic decision making is recommended (see below).

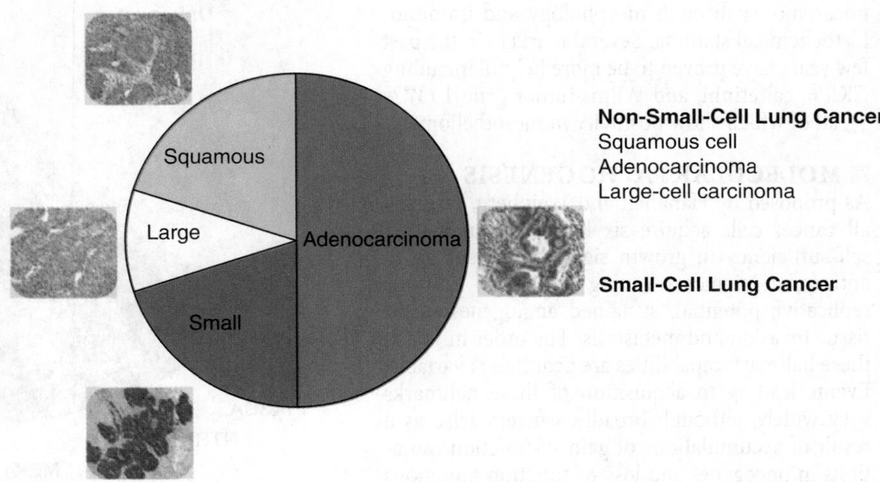

FIGURE 78-1 Histologic subsets of lung cancer.

The terms *adenocarcinoma in situ* and *minimally invasive adenocarcinoma* are now recommended for small solitary adenocarcinomas (≤3 cm) with either pure lepidic growth (term used to describe single-layered growth of atypical cuboidal cells coating the alveolar walls) or predominant lepidic growth with ≤5 mm invasion. Individuals with these entities experience 100% or near 100% 5-year disease-free survival with complete tumor resection. *Invasive adenocarcinomas*, representing more than 70–90% of surgically resected lung adenocarcinomas, are now classified by their predominant pattern: lepidic, acinar, papillary, and solid patterns. Lepidic-predominant subtype has a favorable prognosis, acinar and papillary have an intermediate prognosis, and solid-predominant has a poor prognosis. The terms *signet ring* and *clear cell adenocarcinoma* have been eliminated from the variants of invasive lung adenocarcinoma, whereas the term *micropapillary*, a subtype with a particularly poor prognosis, has been added. Because of prognostic implications, squamous cell carcinoma has also been modified to consist of keratinizing, nonkeratinizing, and basaloid, analogous to head and neck cancers.

IMMUNOHISTOCHEMISTRY

The diagnosis of lung cancer most often rests on the morphologic or cytologic features correlated with clinical and radiographic findings. Immunohistochemistry may be used to verify neuroendocrine differentiation within a tumor, with markers such as neuron-specific enolase (NSE), CD56 or NCAM, synaptophysin, chromogranin, and Leu7. Immunohistochemistry is also helpful in differentiating primary from metastatic adenocarcinomas; thyroid transcription factor-1 (TTF-1), identified in tumors of thyroid and pulmonary origin, is positive in >70% of pulmonary adenocarcinomas and is a reliable indicator of primary lung cancer, provided a thyroid primary has been excluded. A negative TTF-1, however, does not exclude the possibility of a lung primary. TTF-1 is also positive in neuroendocrine tumors of pulmonary and extrapulmonary origin. Napsin-A (Nap-A) is an aspartic protease that plays an important role in maturation of surfactant B7 and is expressed in cytoplasm of type II pneumocytes. In several studies, Nap-A has been reported in >90% of primary lung adenocarcinomas. Notably, a combination of Nap-A and TTF-1 is useful in distinguishing primary lung adenocarcinoma (Nap-A positive, TTF-1 positive) from primary lung squamous cell carcinoma (Nap-A negative, TTF-1 negative) and primary SCLC (Nap-A negative, TTF-1 positive). Cytokeratins 7 and 20 used in combination can help narrow the differential diagnosis; nonsquamous NSCLC, SCLC, and mesothelioma may stain positive for CK7 and negative for CK20, whereas squamous cell lung cancer often will be both CK7 and CK20 negative. p63 is a useful marker for the detection of NSCLCs with squamous differentiation when used in cytologic pulmonary samples. Mesothelioma can be easily identified ultrastructurally, but it has historically been difficult to differentiate from adenocarcinoma through morphology and immunohistochemical staining. Several markers in the past few years have proven to be more helpful including CK5/6, calretinin, and Wilms tumor gene-1 (*WT-1*), all of which show positivity in mesothelioma.

MOLECULAR PATHOGENESIS

As proposed by Hanahan and Weinberg, virtually all cancer cells acquire six hallmark capabilities: self-sufficiency in growth signals, insensitivity to antigrowth signals, evading apoptosis, limitless replicative potential, sustained angiogenesis, and tissue invasion and metastasis. The order in which these hallmark capabilities are acquired is variable. Events leading to acquisition of these hallmarks vary widely, although broadly, cancers arise as a result of accumulations of gain-of-function mutations in oncogenes and loss-of-function mutations in tumor-suppressor genes. Further complicating the study of lung cancer, the sequence of events that leads to disease is clearly different for the various histopathologic entities.

For cancers in general, one theory holds that a small subset of the cells within a tumor (i.e., "stem cells") are responsible for the full malignant behavior of the tumor. As part of this concept, the large bulk of the cells in a cancer are "offspring" of these cancer stem cells. While clonally related to the cancer stem cell subpopulation, most cells by themselves cannot regenerate the full malignant phenotype. The stem cell concept may explain the failure of standard medical therapies to eradicate lung cancers, even when there is a clinical complete response. Disease recurs because therapies do not eliminate the stem cell component, which may be more resistant to therapy. Precise human lung cancer stem cells have yet to be identified.

Among lung cancer histologies, adenocarcinomas have been the most extensively catalogued for recurrent genomic gains and losses as well as for somatic mutations (**Fig. 78-2, Table 78-1**). While multiple different kinds of aberrations have been found, a major class involves "driver mutations," which are mutations that occur in genes encoding signaling proteins that, when aberrant, drive initiation and maintenance of tumor cells. Importantly, driver mutations can serve as a potential Achilles' heels for tumors, if their gene products can be targeted appropriately. These genes encode cell-surface receptors consisting of an extracellular ligand-binding domain, a transmembrane structure, and an intracellular tyrosine kinase (TK) domain. The binding of ligand to receptor activates receptor dimerization and TK autophosphorylation, initiating a cascade of intracellular events, and leading to increased cell proliferation, angiogenesis, metastasis, and a decrease in apoptosis. Lung adenocarcinomas can arise when normal alveolar type II cells develop mutations in *EGFR, BRAF, MET, KRAS*, and *PIK3CA*. These same tumors display high sensitivity to small-molecule TK inhibitors (TKIs). Additional subsets of lung adenocarcinoma have been identified as defined by the presence of specific chromosomal rearrangements, resulting in the aberrant activation of the TKs *ALK, ROS1, NTRK*, and *RET*. Notably, most driver mutations in lung cancer appear to be mutually exclusive, suggesting that acquisition of one of these mutations is sufficient to drive tumorigenesis. Although driver mutations have mostly been found in adenocarcinomas, three

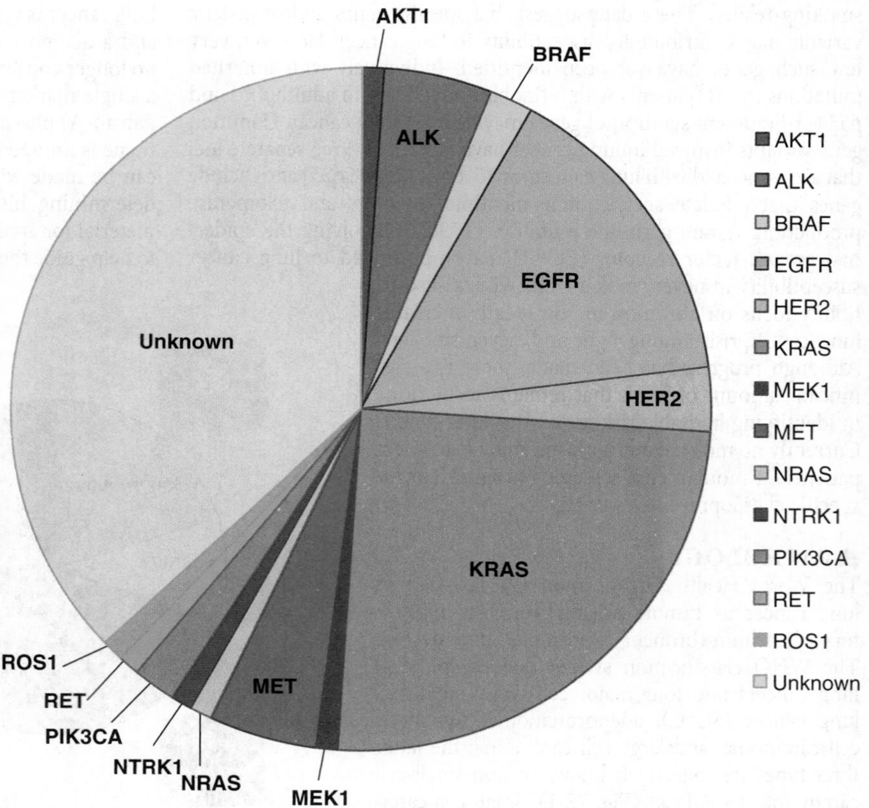

FIGURE 78-2 Driver mutations in lung adenocarcinomas.

TABLE 78-1 Driver Mutations in Non-Small-Cell Lung Cancer (NSCLC)

GENE	ALTERATION	FREQUENCY IN NSCLC	TYPICAL HISTOLOGY
AKT1	Mutation	1%	Adenocarcinoma, squamous
ALK	Rearrangement	3–7%	Adenocarcinoma
BRAF	Mutation	1–3%	Adenocarcinoma
DDR2	Mutation	~4%	Squamous
EGFR	Mutation	10–35%	Adenocarcinoma
FGFR1	Amplification	~20%	Squamous
HER2	Mutation	2–4%	Adenocarcinoma
KRAS	Mutation	15–25%	Adenocarcinoma
MEK1	Mutation	1%	Adenocarcinoma
MET	Amplification	2–4%	Adenocarcinoma
NRAS	Mutation	1%	Adenocarcinoma
NTRK	Rearrangement	1–2%	Adenocarcinoma
PIK3CA	Mutation	1–3%	Squamous
PTEN	Mutation	4–8%	Squamous
ROS1	Rearrangement	1–2%	Adenocarcinoma

potential molecular targets have been identified in squamous cell lung carcinomas: *FGFR1* amplification, *DDR2* mutations, and *PIK3CA* mutations/*PTEN* loss as well as *BRAF* and *MET* (Table 78-1).

A large number of tumor-suppressor genes have also been identified that are inactivated during the pathogenesis of lung cancer. These include *TP53*, *RB1*, *RASSF1A*, *CDKN2A/B*, *LKB1* (*STK11*), and *FHIT*. Nearly 90% of SCLCs harbor mutations in *TP53* and *RB1*. Several tumor-suppressor genes on chromosome 3p appear to be involved in nearly all lung cancers. Allelic loss of this region occurs very early in lung cancer pathogenesis, including in histologically normal smoking-damaged lung epithelium.

EARLY DETECTION AND SCREENING

In lung cancer, clinical outcome is related to the stage at diagnosis, and hence, it is generally assumed that early detection of occult tumors will lead to improved survival. Early detection is a process that involves screening tests, surveillance, diagnosis, and early treatment. Screening refers to the use of tests across a healthy population in order to identify individuals who harbor asymptomatic disease. For a screening program to be successful, the target population must have a high burden of disease; the test must be sensitive, specific, accessible, and cost effective; and effective treatment must be available that can reduce mortality. With any screening procedure, it is important to consider the possible influence of *lead-time bias* (detecting the cancer earlier without an effect on survival), *length-time bias* (indolent cancers are detected on screening and may not affect survival, whereas aggressive cancers are likely to cause symptoms earlier in patients and are less likely to be detected), and *overdiagnosis* (diagnosing cancers so slow growing that they are unlikely to cause the death of the patient).

Because a majority of lung cancer patients present with advanced disease beyond the scope of surgical resection, the value of screening for this condition is debated. Indeed, randomized controlled trials conducted in the 1960s to 1980s using screening chest x-rays (CXR), with or without sputum cytology, reported no impact on lung cancer–specific mortality in patients characterized as high risk (males age ≥45 years with a smoking history). These studies have been criticized for their design, statistical analyses, and outdated imaging modalities. In contrast to CXR, low-dose, noncontrast, thin-slice spiral chest computed tomography (LDCT) has emerged as an effective tool to screen for lung cancer. In nonrandomized studies conducted in the 1990s, LDCT scans were shown to detect more lung nodules and cancers than standard CXR in selected high-risk populations (e.g., age ≥60 years and a smoking history of ≥10 pack-years). Notably, up to 85% of the lung cancers discovered in these trials were classified as stage I disease and therefore considered potentially curable with surgical resection.

These data prompted the National Cancer Institute (NCI) to initiate the National Lung Screening Trial (NLST), a randomized study designed to determine if LDCT screening could reduce mortality from lung cancer in high-risk populations as compared with standard posterior anterior CXR. High-risk patients were defined as individuals between 55 and 74 years of age, with a ≥30 pack-year history of cigarette smoking; former smokers must have quit within the previous 15 years. Excluded from the trial were individuals with a previous lung cancer diagnosis, a history of hemoptysis, an unexplained weight loss of >15 lb in the preceding year, or a chest CT within 18 months of enrollment. A total of 53,454 persons were enrolled and randomized to annual screening yearly for 3 years (LDCT screening, n = 26,722; CXR screening, n = 26,732). Any noncalcified nodule measuring ≥4 mm in any diameter found on LDCT and CXR images with any noncalcified nodule or mass were classified as "positive." Participating radiologists had the option of not calling a final screen positive if a noncalcified nodule had been stable on the three screening examinations. Overall, 39.1% of participants in the LDCT group and 16% in the CXR group had at least one positive screening result. Of those who screened positive, the false-positive rate was 96.4% in the LDCT group and 94.5% in the CXR group. This was consistent across all three rounds. In the LDCT group, 1060 cancers were identified compared with 941 cancers in the CXR group (645 vs 572 per 100,000 person-years; relative risk [RR], 1.13; 95% confidence interval [CI], 1.03–1.23). Nearly twice as many stage IA cancers were detected in the LDCT group compared with the CXR group (40% vs 21%). The overall rates of lung cancer death were 247 and 309 deaths per 100,000 participants in the LDCT and CXR groups, respectively, representing a 20% reduction in lung cancer mortality in the LDCT-screened population (95% CI, 6.8–26.7%; $p = .004$). Compared with the CXR group, the rate of death in the LDCT group from *any* cause was reduced by 6.7% (95% CI, 1.2–13.6%; $p = .02$). The number needed to screen (NNTS) to prevent one lung cancer death was calculated to be 320.

The Nelson study was a second randomized trial comparing no screening to CT scans at baseline and in years 1, 3, and 5.5 in 13,195 men and 2594 women. Participants were 50–75 years of age and were current and former smokers with 10 years or less of cessation who smoked >15 cigarettes a day for >25 years or >10 cigarettes daily for >30 years. Participants were selected from four regions in the Netherlands or Belgium and were excluded if they were in moderate or bad self-reported health, were unable to climb two flights of stairs, had a body weight >140 kg, had a CT of the chest within the past year or a history of lung cancer <5 years ago or were still under treatment, or had current or past renal cell carcinoma, melanoma, or breast cancer. The hazard ratio for lung cancer mortality at 10 years was 0.74 (95% CI, 0.60–0.91; $p = .003$) and 0.61 (95% CI, 0.35–1.04; $p = .0543$) in men and women, respectively. These two trials have validated the use of annual CT scans for early detection of lung cancer in high-risk populations.

LDCT screening for lung cancer comes with known risks including a high rate of false-positive results, false-negative results, potential for unnecessary follow-up testing, radiation exposure, overdiagnosis, changes in anxiety level and quality of life, and substantial financial costs. By far, the biggest challenge confronting the use of CT screening is the high false-positive rate. False positives can have a substantial impact on patients through the expense and risk of unneeded further evaluation and emotional stress. The management of these patients usually consists of serial CT scans over time to see if the nodules grow, attempted fine-needle aspirates, or surgical resection. At $300 per scan (NCI estimated cost), the outlay for initial LDCT alone could run into the billions of dollars annually, an expense that only further escalates when factoring in various downstream expenditures an individual might incur in the assessment of positive findings. A formal cost-effectiveness analysis of the NLST demonstrated differences between sex, age, and current smoking status and the method of follow-up. Despite some questions, LDCT screening has been recommended for all patients meeting criteria for enrollment on NLST. When discussing the option of LDCT screening, use of absolute risks rather than relative risks is helpful because studies indicate the public can process absolute terminology more effectively than relative risk projections. A useful

TABLE 78-2 The Benefits and Harms of LDCT Screening for Lung Cancer Based on NLST Data

	LDCT	CXR
Benefits: How did CT scans help compared to CXR?		
4 in 1000 fewer died from lung cancer	13 in 1000	17 in 1000
5 in 1000 fewer died from all causes	70 in 1000	75 in 1000
Harms: What problems did CT scans cause compared to CXR?		
223 in 1000 had at least 1 false alarm	365 in 1000	142 in 1000
18 in 1000 had a false alarm leading to an invasive procedure	25 in 1000	7 in 1000
2 in 1000 had a major complication from an invasive procedure	3 in 1000	1 in 1000

Abbreviations: CXR, chest x-ray; LDCT, low-dose computed tomography; NLST, National Lung Screening Trial.

Source: From S Woloshin: Cancer screening campaigns getting past uninformative persuasion. N Engl J Med 367:1167, 2012. Copyright © (2012) Massachusetts Medical Society. Reprinted with permission from Massachusetts Medical Society.

guide has been developed by the NCI to help patients and physicians assess the benefits and harms of LDCT screening for lung cancer **(Table 78-2)**.

CLINICAL MANIFESTATIONS

Over half of all patients diagnosed with lung cancer present with locally advanced or metastatic disease at the time of diagnosis. The majority of patients present with signs, symptoms, or laboratory abnormalities that can be attributed to the primary lesion, local tumor growth, invasion or obstruction of adjacent structures, growth at distant metastatic sites, or a paraneoplastic syndrome **(Tables 78-3 and 78-4)**. The prototypical lung cancer patient is a current or former smoker of either sex, usually in the seventh decade of life. A history of chronic cough with or without hemoptysis in a current or former smoker with chronic obstructive pulmonary disease (COPD) age 40 years or older should prompt a thorough investigation for lung cancer even in the face of a normal CXR. A persistent pneumonia without constitutional symptoms and unresponsive to repeated courses of antibiotics also should prompt an evaluation for the underlying cause. Lung cancer arising in a lifetime never smoker is more common in women and East Asians. Such patients also tend to be younger than their smoking counterparts at the time of diagnosis. The clinical presentation of lung cancer in never smokers tends to mirror that of current and former smokers.

Patients with central or endobronchial growth of the primary tumor may present with cough, hemoptysis, wheeze, stridor, dyspnea, or postobstructive pneumonia. Peripheral growth of the primary tumor may cause pain from pleural or chest wall involvement, dyspnea on a restrictive basis, and symptoms of a lung abscess resulting from tumor cavitation. Regional spread of tumor in the thorax (by contiguous growth or by metastasis to regional lymph nodes) may cause tracheal obstruction, esophageal compression with dysphagia, recurrent laryngeal nerve paralysis with hoarseness, phrenic nerve palsy with elevation of the hemidiaphragm and dyspnea, and sympathetic nerve paralysis with Horner's syndrome (enophthalmos, ptosis, miosis, and anhidrosis). Malignant pleural effusions can cause pain, dyspnea, or cough. Pancoast (or superior sulcus tumor) syndromes result from local extension of a tumor growing in the apex of the lung with involvement of the eighth cervical and first and second thoracic nerves, and present with shoulder pain that characteristically radiates in the ulnar distribution of the arm, often with radiologic destruction of the first and second ribs. Often Horner's syndrome and Pancoast syndrome coexist. Other problems of regional spread include superior vena cava syndrome from vascular obstruction; pericardial and cardiac extension with resultant tamponade, arrhythmia, or cardiac failure; lymphatic obstruction with resultant pleural effusion; and lymphangitic spread through the lungs with hypoxemia and dyspnea. In addition, lung cancer can spread transbronchially, producing tumor growth along multiple alveolar surfaces with impairment of gas exchange, respiratory insufficiency, dyspnea, hypoxemia, and sputum production. Constitutional symptoms may include anorexia, weight loss, weakness, fever, and night sweats. Apart from the brevity of symptom duration, these parameters fail to clearly distinguish SCLC from NSCLC or even from neoplasms metastatic to lungs.

TABLE 78-3 Presenting Signs and Symptoms of Lung Cancer

SYMPTOM AND SIGNS	RANGE OF FREQUENCY
Cough	8–75%
Weight loss	0–68%
Dyspnea	3–60%
Chest pain	20–49%
Hemoptysis	6–35%
Bone pain	6–25%
Clubbing	0–20%
Fever	0–20%
Weakness	0–10%
Superior vena cava obstruction	0–4%
Dysphagia	0–2%
Wheezing and stridor	0–2%

Source: Reproduced with permission from MA Beckles: Initial evaluation of the patient with lung cancer. Symptoms, sign, laboratory tests, and paraneoplastic syndromes. Chest 123:97, 2003.

TABLE 78-4 Clinical Findings Suggestive of Metastatic Disease

Symptoms elicited in history	• Constitutional: weight loss >10 lb • Musculoskeletal: pain • Neurologic: headaches, syncope, seizures, extremity weakness, recent change in mental status
Signs found on physical examination	• Lymphadenopathy (>1 cm) • Hoarseness, superior vena cava syndrome • Bone tenderness • Hepatomegaly (>13 cm span) • Focal neurologic signs, papilledema • Soft-tissue mass
Routine laboratory tests	• Hematocrit, <40% in men; <35% in women • Elevated alkaline phosphatase, GGT, SGOT, and calcium levels

Abbreviations: GGT, gamma-glutamyltransferase; SGOT, serum glutamic-oxaloacetic transaminase.

Source: Reproduced with permission from GA Silvestri et al: The noninvasive staging of non-small cell lung cancer. Chest 123:147S, 2003.

Extrathoracic metastatic disease is found at autopsy in >50% of patients with squamous carcinoma, 80% of patients with adenocarcinoma and large-cell carcinoma, and >95% of patients with SCLC. Approximately one-third of patients present with symptoms as a result of distant metastases. Lung cancer metastases may occur in virtually every organ system, and the site of metastatic involvement largely determines other symptoms. Patients with brain metastases may present with headache, nausea and vomiting, seizures, or neurologic deficits. Patients with bone metastases may present with pain, pathologic fractures, or spinal cord compression. The latter may also occur with epidural metastases. Individuals with bone marrow invasion may present with cytopenias or leukoerythroblastosis. Those with liver metastases may present with hepatomegaly, right upper quadrant pain, fever, anorexia, and weight loss. Liver dysfunction and biliary obstruction are rare. Adrenal metastases are common but rarely cause pain or adrenal insufficiency unless they are large.

Paraneoplastic syndromes are common in patients with lung cancer, especially those with SCLC, and may be the presenting finding or the first sign of recurrence. In addition, paraneoplastic syndromes may mimic metastatic disease and, unless detected, lead to inappropriate palliative rather than curative treatment. Often the paraneoplastic syndrome may be relieved with successful treatment of the tumor. In some cases, the pathophysiology of the paraneoplastic syndrome is known, particularly when a hormone with biologic activity is secreted by a tumor. However, in many cases, the pathophysiology is unknown. Systemic symptoms of anorexia, cachexia, weight loss (seen in 30% of patients), fever, and suppressed immunity are paraneoplastic syndromes of unknown etiology or at least not well defined. Weight loss >10% of total body weight is considered a bad prognostic sign. Endocrine syndromes are seen in 12% of patients; hypercalcemia resulting from ectopic production of parathyroid hormone (PTH) or, more commonly, PTH-related peptide is the most common life-threatening metabolic complication of malignancy, primarily occurring with squamous cell carcinomas of the lung. Clinical symptoms include nausea, vomiting, abdominal pain, constipation, polyuria, thirst, and altered mental status.

Hyponatremia may be caused by the syndrome of inappropriate secretion of antidiuretic hormone (SIADH) or possibly atrial natriuretic peptide (ANP) **(Chap. 93)**. SIADH resolves within 1–4 weeks of initiating chemotherapy in the vast majority of cases. During this period, serum sodium can usually be managed and maintained above 128 mEq/L via fluid restriction. Demeclocycline can be a useful adjunctive measure when fluid restriction alone is insufficient. Vasopressin receptor antagonists like tolvaptan also have been used in the management of SIADH. However, the use of tolvaptan has significant limitations including liver injury and overly rapid correction of the hyponatremia, which can lead to irreversible neurologic injury. Likewise, the cost of tolvaptan may be prohibitive (as high as $300 per tablet in some areas). Of note, patients with ectopic ANP may have worsening hyponatremia if sodium intake is not concomitantly increased. Accordingly, if hyponatremia fails to improve or worsens after 3–4 days of adequate fluid restriction, plasma levels of ANP should be measured to determine the causative syndrome.

Ectopic secretion of ACTH by SCLC and pulmonary carcinoids usually results in additional electrolyte disturbances, especially hypokalemia, rather than the changes in body habitus that occur in Cushing's syndrome from a pituitary adenoma **(Chap. 93)**. Treatment with standard medications, such as metyrapone and ketoconazole, is largely ineffective due to extremely high cortisol levels. The most effective strategy for management of the Cushing's syndrome is effective treatment of the underlying SCLC. Bilateral adrenalectomy may be considered in extreme cases.

Skeletal–connective tissue syndromes include clubbing in 30% of cases (usually NSCLCs) and hypertrophic primary osteoarthropathy in 1–10% of cases (usually adenocarcinomas). Patients may develop periostitis, causing pain, tenderness, and swelling over the affected bones and a positive bone scan. Neurologic–myopathic syndromes are seen in only 1% of patients but are dramatic and include the myasthenic Eaton-Lambert syndrome and retinal blindness with SCLC, whereas peripheral neuropathies, subacute cerebellar degeneration, cortical degeneration, and polymyositis are seen with all lung cancer types. Many of these are caused by autoimmune responses such as the development of anti-voltage-gated calcium channel antibodies in Eaton-Lambert syndrome. Patients with this disorder present with proximal muscle weakness, usually in the lower extremities, occasional autonomic dysfunction, and rarely, cranial nerve symptoms or involvement of the bulbar or respiratory muscles. Depressed deep tendon reflexes are frequently present. In contrast to patients with myasthenia gravis, strength improves with serial effort. Some patients who respond to chemotherapy will have resolution of the neurologic abnormalities. Thus, chemotherapy is the initial treatment of choice. Paraneoplastic encephalomyelitis and sensory neuropathies, cerebellar degeneration, limbic encephalitis, and brainstem encephalitis occur in SCLC in association with a variety of antineuronal antibodies such as anti-Hu, anti-CRMP5, and ANNA-3. Paraneoplastic cerebellar degeneration may be associated with anti-Hu, anti-Yo, or P/Q calcium channel autoantibodies. Coagulation or thrombotic or other hematologic manifestations occur in 1–8% of patients and include migratory venous thrombophlebitis (Trousseau's syndrome), nonbacterial thrombotic (marantic) endocarditis with arterial emboli, and disseminated intravascular coagulation with hemorrhage, anemia, granulocytosis, and leukoerythroblastosis. Thrombotic disease complicating cancer is usually a poor prognostic sign. Cutaneous manifestations such as dermatomyositis and acanthosis nigricans are uncommon (1%), as are the renal manifestations of nephrotic syndrome and glomerulonephritis (≤1%).

DIAGNOSING LUNG CANCER

Tissue sampling is required to confirm a diagnosis in all patients with suspected lung cancer. In patients with suspected metastatic disease, a biopsy of a distant site of disease is preferred for tissue confirmation. Given the greater emphasis placed on molecular and PD-L1 testing for NSCLC patients, a core biopsy is preferred to ensure adequate tissue for analysis. Tumor tissue may be obtained via minimally invasive techniques such as bronchial or transbronchial biopsy during fiberoptic bronchoscopy, by fine-needle aspiration (FNA) or percutaneous biopsy using image guidance, or via endobronchial ultrasound (EBUS)-guided biopsy. Depending on the location, lymph node sampling may occur via transesophageal endoscopic ultrasound (EUS)-guided biopsy, EBUS-guided biopsy, or blind biopsy. In patients with suspected metastatic disease, a diagnosis may be confirmed by bronchoscopy, percutaneous biopsy of a soft tissue mass, lytic bone lesion, bone marrow, pleural or liver lesion, or an adequate cell block obtained from a malignant pleural effusion. In patients with a suspected malignant pleural effusion, if the initial thoracentesis is negative, a repeat thoracentesis is warranted. Although the majority of pleural effusions are due to malignant disease, particularly if they are exudative or bloody, some may be parapneumonic. In the absence of distant disease, such patients should be considered for possible curative treatment.

The diagnostic yield of any biopsy depends on several factors including location (accessibility) of the tumor, tumor size, tumor type, and technical aspects of the diagnostic procedure including the experience level of the bronchoscopist and pathologist. In general, central lesions such as squamous cell carcinomas, small-cell carcinomas, or endobronchial lesions such as carcinoid tumors are more readily diagnosed by bronchoscopic examination, whereas peripheral lesions such as adenocarcinomas and large-cell carcinomas are more amenable to transthoracic biopsy.

Sputum cytology is inexpensive and noninvasive but has a lower yield than other specimen types due to poor preservation of the cells and more variability in acquiring a good-quality specimen. The yield for sputum cytology is highest for larger and centrally located tumors such as squamous cell carcinoma and small-cell carcinoma histology. The specificity for sputum cytology averages close to 100%, although sensitivity is generally <70%. The accuracy of sputum cytology improves with increased numbers of specimens analyzed. Consequently, analysis of at least three sputum specimens is recommended. However, the quality of the specimen may not be adequate for histologic subclassification and PD-L1 and molecular testing.

STAGING LUNG CANCER

Lung cancer staging consists of two parts: first, a determination of the location of the tumor and possible metastatic sites (anatomic staging), and second, an assessment of a patient's ability to withstand various antitumor treatments (physiologic staging). All patients with lung cancer should have a complete history and physical examination, with evaluation of all other medical problems, determination of performance status, and history of weight loss. Staging with regard to a patient's potential for surgical resection is principally applicable to NSCLC.

ANATOMIC STAGING OF PATIENTS WITH LUNG CANCER

The accurate staging of patients with NSCLC is essential for determining the appropriate treatment in patients with resectable disease and for avoiding unnecessary surgical procedures in patients with advanced disease. All patients with NSCLC should undergo initial radiographic imaging with CT scan, positron emission tomography (PET), or preferably CT-PET. PET scanning attempts to identify sites of malignancy based on glucose metabolism by measuring the uptake of ^{18}F-fluorodeoxyglucose (FDG). Rapidly dividing cells, presumably in the lung tumors, will preferentially take up ^{18}F-FDG and appear as a "hot spot." To date, PET has been mostly used for staging and detection of metastases in lung cancer and in the detection of nodules >15 mm in diameter. Combined ^{18}F-FDG PET-CT imaging has been shown to improve the accuracy of staging in NSCLC compared to visual correlation of PET and CT or either study alone. CT-PET has been found to be superior in identifying pathologically enlarged mediastinal lymph nodes and extrathoracic metastases. A standardized uptake value (SUV) of >2.5 on PET is highly suspicious for malignancy. False negatives can be seen in diabetes, in lesions <8 mm, and in slow-growing tumors (e.g., carcinoid tumors or well-differentiated adenocarcinoma). False positives can be seen in certain infections and granulomatous disease (e.g., tuberculosis). Thus, PET should never be used alone to diagnose lung cancer, mediastinal involvement, or metastases. Confirmation with tissue biopsy is required. For brain metastases, magnetic resonance imaging (MRI) is the most effective method. MRI can also be useful in selected circumstances, such as superior sulcus tumors to rule out brachial plexus involvement, but in general, MRI does not play a major role in NSCLC staging.

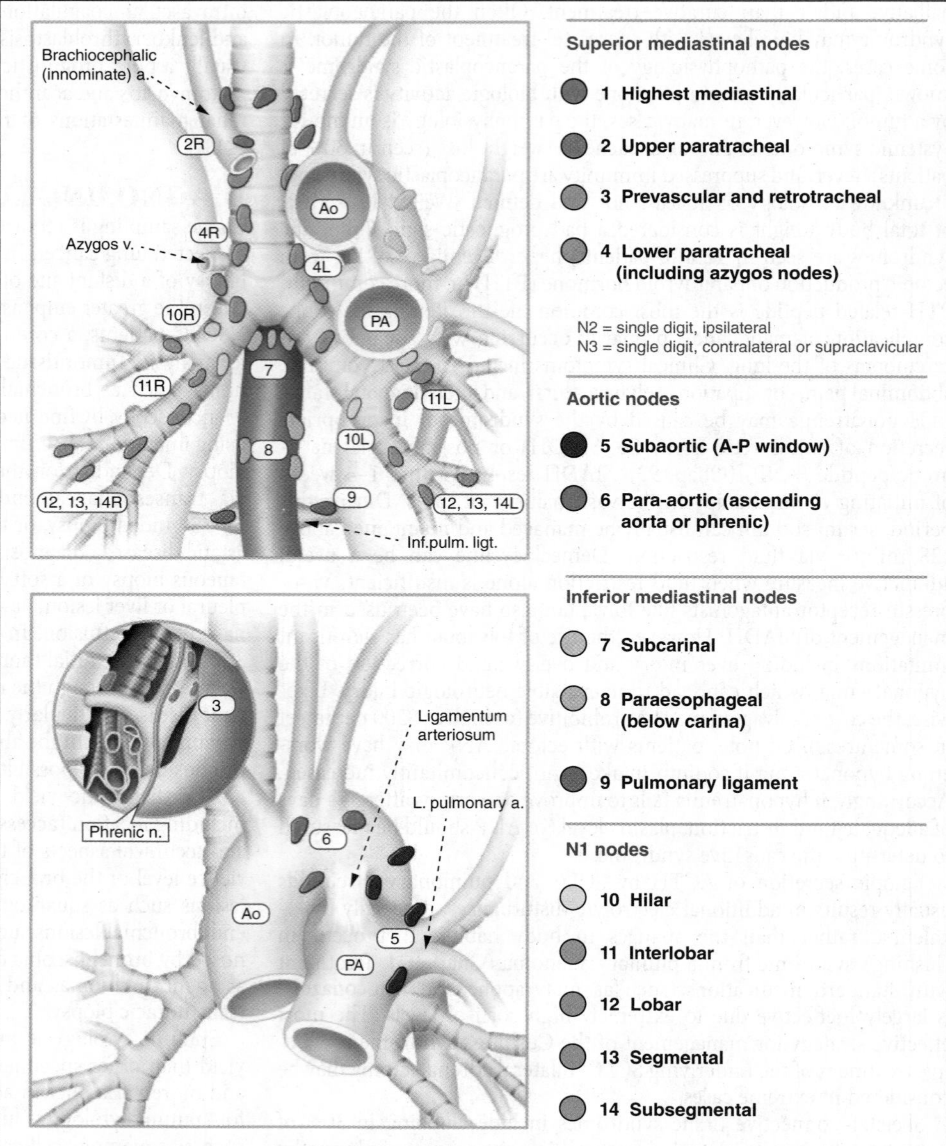

FIGURE 78-3 Lymph node stations in staging non-small-cell lung cancer. The International Association for the Study of Lung Cancer (IASLC) lymph node map, including the proposed grouping of lymph node stations into "zones" for the purposes of prognostic analyses. a., artery; Ao, aorta; Inf. pulm. ligt., inferior pulmonary ligament; n., nerve; PA, pulmonary artery; v., vein.

In patients with NSCLC, the following are contraindications to potential curative resection: extrathoracic metastases, superior vena cava syndrome, vocal cord and, in most cases, phrenic nerve paralysis, malignant pleural effusion, cardiac tamponade, tumor within 2 cm of the carina (potentially curable with combined chemoradiotherapy), metastasis to the contralateral lung, metastases to supraclavicular lymph nodes, contralateral mediastinal node metastases (potentially curable with combined chemoradiotherapy), and involvement of the main pulmonary artery. In situations where it will make a difference in treatment, abnormal scan findings require tissue confirmation of malignancy so that patients are not precluded from having potentially curative therapy.

The best predictor of metastatic disease remains a careful history and physical examination. If signs, symptoms, or findings from the physical examination suggest the presence of malignancy, then sequential imaging starting with the most appropriate study should be performed. If the findings from the clinical evaluation are negative, then imaging studies beyond CT-PET are unnecessary and the search for metastatic disease is complete. In patients in whom distant metastatic disease has been ruled out, lymph node status needs to be assessed via minimally invasive techniques such as those mentioned above and/or invasive techniques such as mediastinoscopy, mediastinotomy, thoracoscopy, or thoracotomy. Approximately one-quarter to one-half of patients diagnosed with NSCLC will have mediastinal lymph node metastases at the time of diagnosis. Lymph node sampling is recommended in all patients with enlarged nodes detected by CT or PET scan and in patients with large tumors or tumors occupying the inner third of the lung. The extent of mediastinal lymph node involvement is important in determining the appropriate treatment strategy: surgical resection followed by adjuvant chemotherapy versus combined chemoradiation followed by immunotherapy (durvalumab) (see below). A standard nomenclature for referring to the location of lymph nodes involved with lung cancer has evolved (**Fig. 78-3**).

In SCLC patients, current staging recommendations include a PET-CT scan and MRI of the brain (positive in 10% of asymptomatic patients). Bone marrow biopsies and aspirations are rarely performed now given the low incidence of isolated bone marrow metastases. Confirmation of metastatic disease, ipsilateral or contralateral lung nodules, or metastases beyond the mediastinum may be achieved by the same modalities recommended earlier for patients with NSCLC.

If a patient has signs or symptoms of spinal cord compression (pain, weakness, paralysis, urinary retention), a spinal CT or MRI scan should be performed. If metastases are evident on imaging, a neurosurgeon should be consulted for possible palliative surgical resection and/or a radiation oncologist should be consulted for palliative radiotherapy to the site of compression. If signs or symptoms of leptomeningeal disease develop at any time in a patient with lung cancer, an MRI of the brain and spinal cord should be performed, as well as a spinal tap, for detection of malignant cells. If the spinal tap is negative, a repeat spinal tap should be considered. There is currently no approved therapy for the treatment of leptomeningeal disease.

STAGING SYSTEM FOR NON-SMALL-CELL LUNG CANCER

The tumor-node-metastasis (TNM) international staging system provides useful prognostic information and is used to stage all patients with NSCLC. The various T (tumor size), N (regional node involvement), and M (presence or absence of distant metastasis) stages are combined to form different stage groups (**Tables 74-5 and 74-6**). The eighth edition of the TNM staging system went into effect in 2018. T1 tumors are divided into tumors ≤1 cm (T1a), >1 cm and ≤2 cm (T1b), and >2 cm and ≤3 cm (T1c). T2 tumors are those that are >3 cm but ≤5 cm, involve the visceral pleura or main bronchus, or are associated with atelectasis; T2a tumors are >3 cm and ≤4 cm, and T2b are >4 cm and ≤5 cm. T3 tumors are >5 cm and ≤7 cm. T3 tumors also include tumors with invasion into local structures such as the chest wall and diaphragm and with additional nodules in the same lobe. T4 tumors include tumors >7 cm or tumors of any size with invasion into mediastinum, heart, great vessels, trachea, esophagus, or spine or with multiple nodules in the ipsilateral lung. Lymph node staging depends on metastasis to ipsilateral pulmonary or hilar nodes (N1), mediastinal or subcarinal nodes (N2), or contralateral mediastinal, hilar, or supraclavicular nodes (N3). Patients with metastasis may be classified as M1a (malignant pleural or pericardial effusion, pleural nodules, or nodules in the contralateral lung), M1b (single distant metastasis to a single organ; e.g., bone, liver, adrenal, or brain metastasis), or M1c (multiple metastases to a single organ or metastases to multiple organs). The effect of stage on survival is illustrated in **Fig. 78-4**. Approximately 15% of patients have localized disease that can be treated with curative attempt (surgery or radiotherapy), about a quarter have local or regional disease that may or may not be amenable to a curative attempt, and half have metastatic disease at the time of diagnosis. In 10%, the extent of disease is undefined.

TABLE 78-5 TNM Staging System for Lung Cancer (Eighth Edition)

Primary Tumor (T)	
T1	Tumor ≤3 cm diameter, surrounded by lung or visceral pleura, without invasion more proximal than lobar bronchus
T1mi	Minimally invasive adenocarcinoma (pure lepidic pattern, <3 cm in greatest dimension and <5 mm invasion)—T1a (size <1 cm)—T1b (1 cm < size <2 cm)—T1c (2 cm < size <3 cm)
T2	Tumor >3 cm but ≤7 cm, or tumor with any of the following features: Involves main bronchus ≥2 cm distal to carina Invades visceral pleura Associated with atelectasis or obstructive pneumonitis that extends to the hilar region but does not involve the entire lung
T2a	Tumor >3 cm but ≤5 cm
T2b	Tumor >5 cm but ≤7 cm
T3	Tumor >7 cm or any of the following: Directly invades any of the following: chest wall, diaphragm, phrenic nerve, mediastinal pleura, parietal pericardium, main bronchus <2 cm from carina (without involvement of carina) Atelectasis or obstructive pneumonitis of the entire lung Separate tumor nodules in the same lobe
T4	Tumor of any size that invades the mediastinum, heart, great vessels, trachea, recurrent laryngeal nerve, esophagus, vertebral body, or carina, or with separate tumor nodules in a different ipsilateral lobe
Nodal Stage (N)	
N0	No regional lymph node metastases
N1	Metastasis in ipsilateral peribronchial and/or ipsilateral hilar lymph nodes and intrapulmonary nodes, including involvement by direct extension
N2	Metastasis in ipsilateral mediastinal and/or subcarinal lymph node(s)
N3	Metastasis in contralateral mediastinal, contralateral hilar, ipsilateral or contralateral scalene, or supraclavicular lymph node(s)
Metastases (M)	
M0	No distant metastasis
M1	Distant metastasis
M1a	Separate tumor nodule(s) in a contralateral lobe; tumor with pleural nodules or malignant pleural or pericardial effusion
M1b	Distant metastasis (in extrathoracic organs)
M1c	

Abbreviation: M1b, distant metastasis in single organ outside chest; M1c, multiple extrathoracic metastases to one or more organs; TNM, tumor-node-metastasis.

TABLE 78-6 TNM Stage Groupings, Eighth Edition

Stage IA1	T1a	N0	M0
Stage IA2	T1b	N0	M0
Stage IA3	T1c	N0	M0
Stage IB	T2a	N0	M0
Stage IIA	T2b	N0	M0
Stage IIB	T1a-T2b	N1	M0
	T3	N0	M0
Stage IIIA	T1-2b	N2	M0
	T3	N1	M0
	T4	N0/N1	M0
Stage IIIB	T1-2b	N3	M0
	T3/T4	N0/N1	M0
	T3/T4	N3	M0
Stage IVA	Any T	Any N	M1a/M1b
Stage IV B	Any T	Any N	M1c

STAGING SYSTEM FOR SMALL-CELL LUNG CANCER

In patients with SCLC, it is now recommended that both the Veterans Administration system and the American Joint Committee on Cancer/International Union Against Cancer eighth edition system (TNM) be used to classify the tumor stage. The Veterans Administration system is a distinct two-stage system dividing patients into those with limited- or extensive-stage disease. Patients with limited-stage disease (LD) have cancer that is confined to the ipsilateral hemithorax and can be encompassed within a tolerable radiation port. Thus, contralateral supraclavicular nodes, recurrent laryngeal nerve involvement, and superior vena caval obstruction can all be part of LD. Patients with extensive-stage disease (ED) have overt metastatic disease by imaging or physical examination. Cardiac tamponade, malignant pleural effusion, and bilateral pulmonary parenchymal involvement generally qualify disease as ED, because the involved organs cannot be encompassed safely or effectively within a single radiation therapy port. Sixty to 70% of patients are diagnosed with ED at presentation. The TNM staging system is preferred in the rare SCLC patient presenting with what appears to be clinical stage I disease (see above).

PHYSIOLOGIC STAGING

Patients with lung cancer often have other comorbid conditions related to smoking including cardiovascular disease and COPD. To improve their preoperative condition, correctable problems (e.g., anemia, electrolyte and fluid disorders, infections, cardiac disease, and arrhythmias) should be addressed, appropriate chest physical therapy should be instituted, and patients should be encouraged to stop smoking. Patients with a forced expiratory volume in 1 s (FEV_1) of >2 L or >80% of predicted can tolerate a pneumonectomy, and those with an FEV_1 >1.5 L have adequate reserve for a lobectomy. In patients with borderline lung function but a resectable tumor, cardiopulmonary exercise testing could be performed as part of the physiologic evaluation. This test allows an estimate of the maximal oxygen consumption (Vo_{2max}). A Vo_{2max}

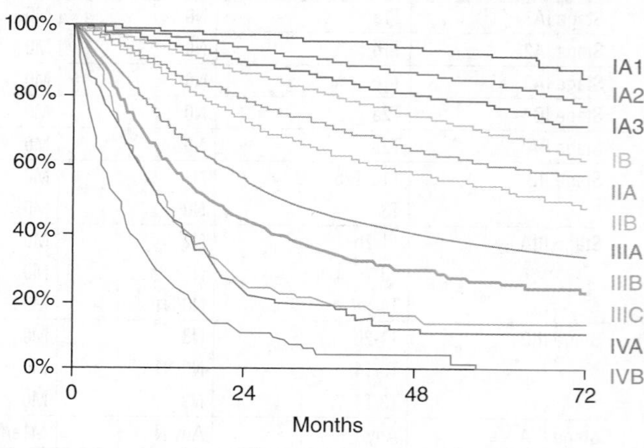

Stage	24 months	60 months
IA1	97%	92%
IA2	94%	83%
IA3	90%	77%
IB	87%	68%
IIA	79%	60%
IIB	72%	53%
IIIA	55%	36%
IIIB	44%	26%
IIIC	24%	13%
IVA	23%	10%
IVB	10%	0%

FIGURE 78-4 Influence of non-small-cell lung cancer stage on survival.

<15 mL/(kg.min) predicts for a higher risk of postoperative complications. Patients deemed unable to tolerate lobectomy or pneumonectomy from a pulmonary functional standpoint may be candidates for more limited resections, such as wedge or anatomic segmental resection, although such procedures are associated with significantly higher rates of local recurrence and a trend toward decreased overall survival. All patients should be assessed for cardiovascular risk using American College of Cardiology and American Heart Association guidelines. A myocardial infarction within the past 3 months is a contraindication to thoracic surgery because 20% of patients will die of reinfarction. An infarction in the past 6 months is a relative contraindication. Other major contraindications include uncontrolled arrhythmias, an FEV_1 of <1 L, CO_2 retention (resting Pco_2 >45 mmHg), DLco <40%, and severe pulmonary hypertension.

TREATMENT

Non-Small-Cell Lung Cancer

The overall treatment approach to patients with NSCLC is shown in **Fig. 78-5**.

OCCULT AND STAGE 0 CARCINOMAS

Patients with severe atypia on sputum cytology have an increased risk of developing lung cancer compared to those without atypia. In the uncommon circumstance where malignant cells are identified in a sputum or bronchial washing specimen but the chest imaging appears normal (TX tumor stage), the lesion must be localized. More than 90% of tumors can be localized by meticulous examination of the bronchial tree with a fiberoptic bronchoscope under general anesthesia and collection of a series of differential brushings and biopsies. Surgical resection following bronchoscopic localization has been shown to improve survival compared to no treatment. Close follow-up of these patients is indicated because of the high incidence of second primary lung cancers (5% per patient per year).

SOLITARY PULMONARY NODULE AND "GROUND-GLASS" OPACITIES

A solitary pulmonary nodule is defined as an x-ray density completely surrounded by normal aerated lung with circumscribed margins, of any shape, usually 1–6 cm in greatest diameter. The approach to a patient with a solitary pulmonary nodule is based on an estimate of the probability of cancer, determined according to the patient's smoking history, age, and characteristics on imaging (**Table 78-7**). Prior CXRs and CT scans should be obtained if available for comparison. A PET scan may be useful if the lesion is greater than 7–8 mm in diameter. If no diagnosis is apparent, Mayo investigators reported that clinical characteristics (age, cigarette smoking status, and prior cancer diagnosis) and three radiologic characteristics (nodule diameter, spiculation, and upper lobe location) were independent predictors of malignancy. At present, only two radiographic criteria are thought to predict the benign nature of a solitary pulmonary nodule: lack of growth over a period >2 years and certain characteristic patterns of calcification. Calcification alone, however, does not exclude malignancy; a dense central nidus, multiple punctuate foci, and "bull's eye" (granuloma) and "popcorn ball" (hamartoma) calcifications are highly suggestive of a benign lesion. In contrast, a relatively large lesion, lack of or asymmetric calcification, chest symptoms, associated atelectasis, pneumonitis, or growth of the lesion revealed by comparison with an old x-ray or CT scan or a positive PET scan may be suggestive of a malignant process and warrant further attempts to establish a histologic diagnosis. An algorithm for assessing these lesions is shown in **Fig. 78-6**.

Since the advent of screening CTs, small "ground-glass" opacities (GGOs) have often been observed, particularly as the increased sensitivity of CTs enables detection of smaller lesions. Many of these GGOs, when biopsied, are found to be atypical adenomatous hyperplasia (AAH), adenocarcinoma in situ (AIS), or minimally invasive adenocarcinoma (MIA). AAH is usually a nodule of <5 mm and is minimally hazy, also called nonsolid or ground glass (i.e., hazy slightly increased attenuation, no solid component, and preservation of bronchial and vascular margins). On thin-section CT, AIS is usually a nonsolid nodule and tends to be slightly more opaque than AAH. MIA is mainly solid, usually with a small (<5 mm) central solid component. However, overlap exists among the imaging features of the preinvasive and minimally invasive lesions in the lung adenocarcinoma spectrum. Lepidic adenocarcinomas are usually solid but may be nonsolid. Likewise, the small invasive adenocarcinomas also are usually solid but may exhibit a small nonsolid component.

MANAGEMENT OF STAGES I AND II NSCLC

Surgical Resection of Stage I and II NSCLC Surgical resection, ideally by an experienced thoracic surgeon, is the treatment of choice for patients with clinical stage I and II NSCLC who are able to tolerate the procedure. Operative mortality rates for patients resected by thoracic or cardiothoracic surgeons are lower compared to general surgeons. Moreover, survival rates are higher in patients who undergo resection in facilities with a high surgical volume compared to those performing fewer than 70 procedures per year, even though the higher-volume facilities often serve older and less socioeconomically advantaged populations. The improvement in survival is most evident in the immediate postoperative period. In patients with stage I NSCLC, lobectomy is superior to wedge

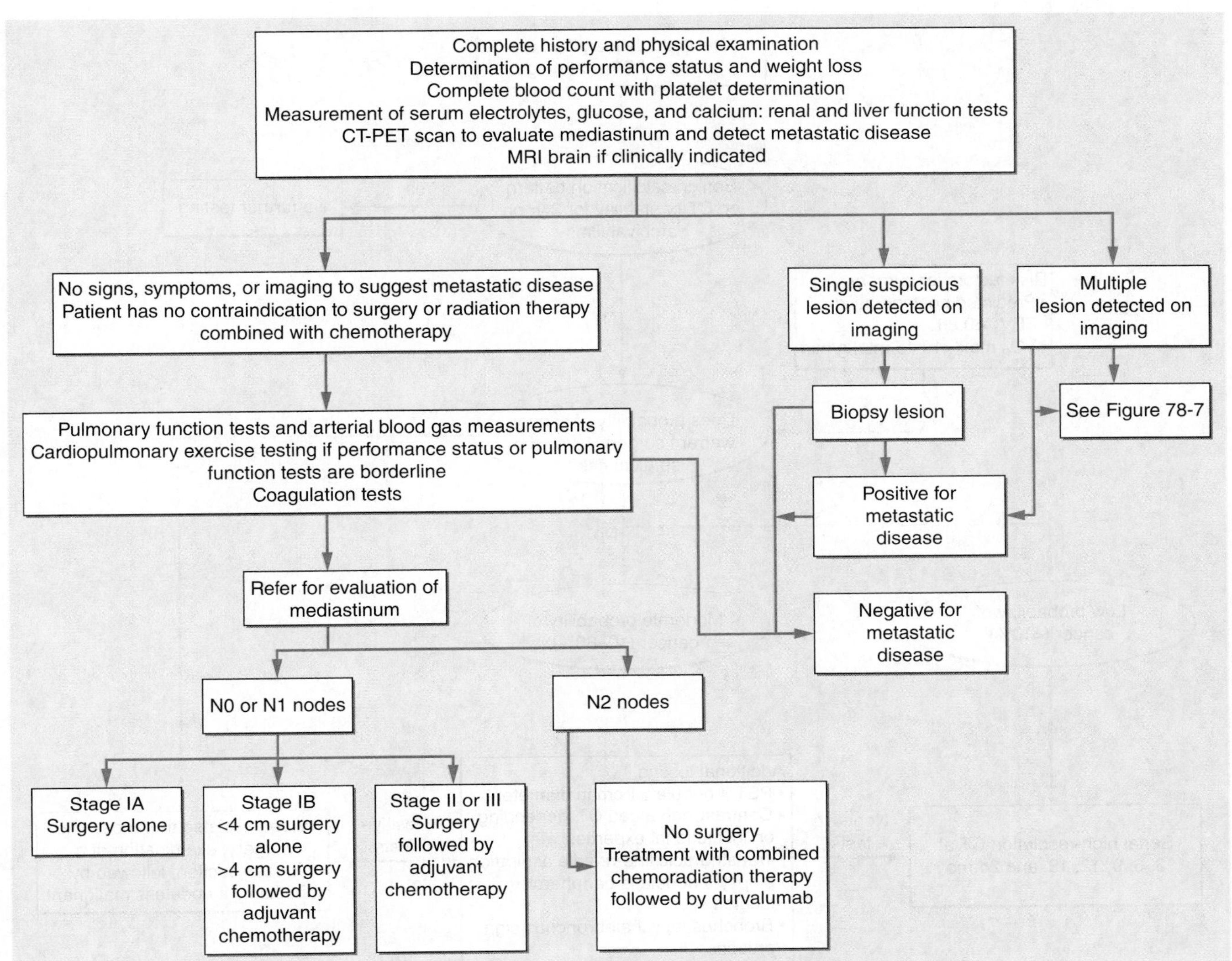

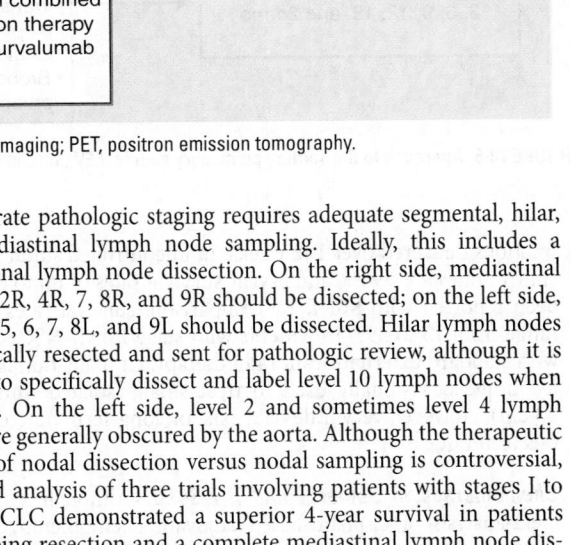

FIGURE 78-5 Algorithm for management of non-small-cell lung cancer. MRI, magnetic resonance imaging; PET, positron emission tomography.

resection with respect to rates of local recurrence. There is also a trend toward improvement in overall survival. In patients with comorbidities, compromised pulmonary reserve, and small peripheral lesions, a limited resection, wedge resection, or segmentectomy (potentially by video-assisted thoracoscopic surgery) may be reasonable surgical options. Pneumonectomy is reserved for patients with central tumors and should be performed only in patients with excellent pulmonary reserve. The 5-year survival rates are 68–92% for patients with stage I NSCLC and 53–60% for patients with stage II NSCLC.

TABLE 78-7 Assessment of Risk of Cancer in Patients with Solitary Pulmonary Nodules

	RISK		
VARIABLE	LOW	INTERMEDIATE	HIGH
Diameter (cm)	<1.5	1.5–2.2	≥2.3
Age (years)	<45	45–60	>60
Smoking status	Never smoker	Current smoker (<20 cigarettes/d)	Current smoker (>20 cigarettes/d)
Smoking cessation status	Quit ≥7 years ago or quit	Quit <7 years ago	Never quit
Characteristics of nodule margins	Smooth	Scalloped	Corona radiata or spiculated

Source: From D Ost et al: The solitary pulmonary nodule. N Engl J Med 348:2535, 2003. Copyright © (2003) Massachusetts Medical Society. Reprinted with permission from Massachusetts Medical Society.

Accurate pathologic staging requires adequate segmental, hilar, and mediastinal lymph node sampling. Ideally, this includes a mediastinal lymph node dissection. On the right side, mediastinal stations 2R, 4R, 7, 8R, and 9R should be dissected; on the left side, stations 5, 6, 7, 8L, and 9L should be dissected. Hilar lymph nodes are typically resected and sent for pathologic review, although it is helpful to specifically dissect and label level 10 lymph nodes when possible. On the left side, level 2 and sometimes level 4 lymph nodes are generally obscured by the aorta. Although the therapeutic benefit of nodal dissection versus nodal sampling is controversial, a pooled analysis of three trials involving patients with stages I to IIIA NSCLC demonstrated a superior 4-year survival in patients undergoing resection and a complete mediastinal lymph node dissection compared with lymph node sampling. Moreover, complete mediastinal lymphadenectomy added little morbidity to a pulmonary resection for lung cancer when carried out by an experienced thoracic surgeon.

Radiation Therapy in Stages I and II NSCLC There is currently no role for postoperative radiation therapy in patients following resection of stage I or II NSCLC with negative margins. However, patients with stage I and II disease who either refuse or are not suitable candidates for surgery should be considered for radiation therapy with *curative* intent. Stereotactic body radiation therapy (SBRT) is a technique used to treat patients with isolated pulmonary nodules (≤5 cm) who are not candidates for or refuse surgical resection. Treatment is typically administered in three to five

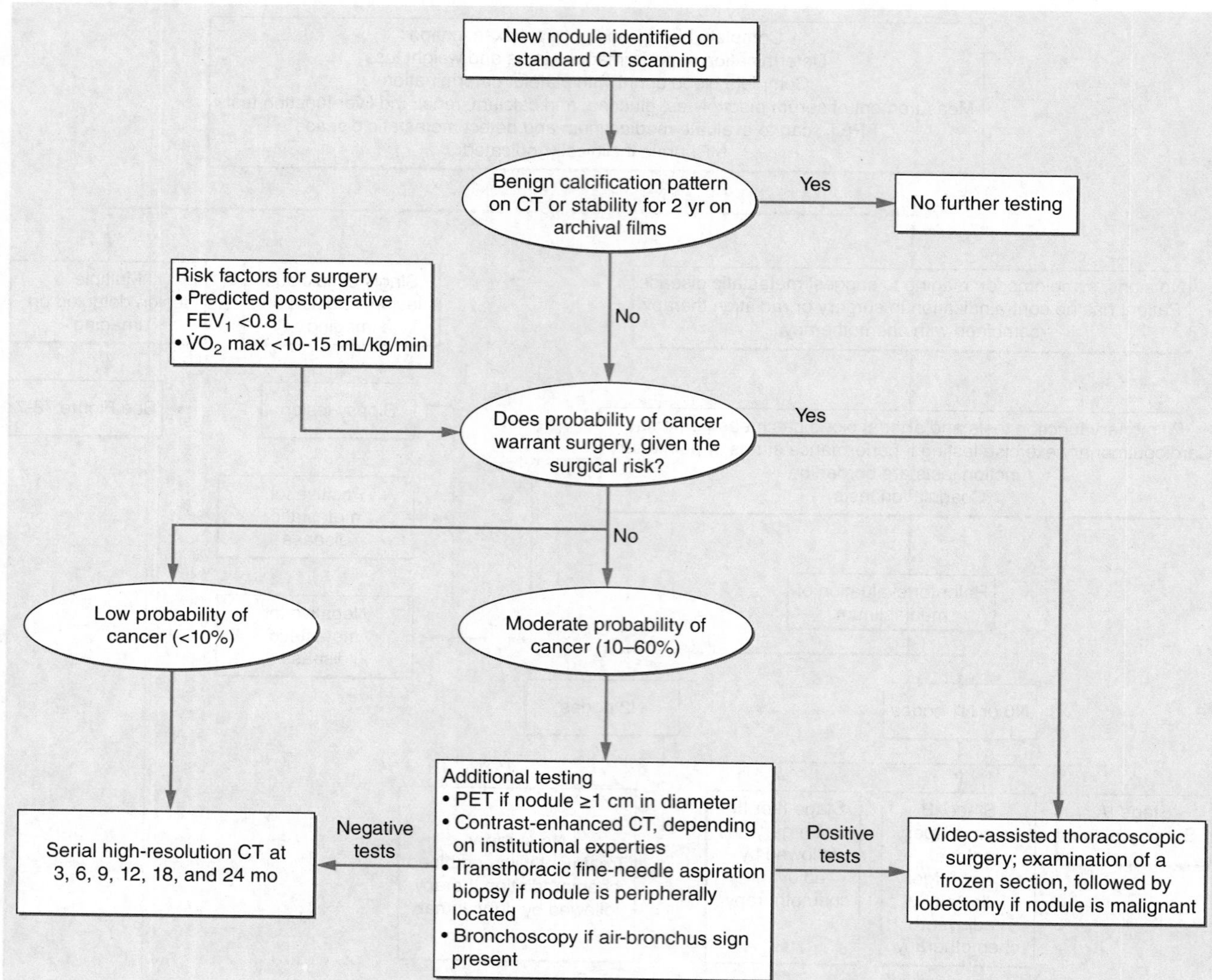

FIGURE 78-6 Approach to the solitary pulmonary nodule. FEV$_1$, forced expiratory volume in 1 s; PET, positron emission tomography.

fractions delivered over 1–2 weeks. In uncontrolled studies, disease control rates are >90%, and 5-year survival rates of up to 60% have been reported with SBRT. By comparison, survival rates typically range from 13 to 39% in patients with stage I or II NSCLC treated with standard external-beam radiotherapy. Cryoablation is another technique occasionally used to treat small, isolated tumors (i.e., ≤3 cm). However, very little data exist on long-term outcomes with this technique.

Chemotherapy in Stages I and II NSCLC Although a landmark meta-analysis of cisplatin-based adjuvant chemotherapy trials in patients with resected stages I to IIIA NSCLC (the Lung Adjuvant Cisplatin Evaluation [LACE] Study) demonstrated a 5.4% improvement in 5-year survival for adjuvant chemotherapy compared to surgery alone, the survival benefit was seemingly confined to patients with stage II or III disease (**Table 78-8**). By contrast, survival was actually worsened in stage IA patients with the application of adjuvant therapy. In stage IB, there was a modest improvement in survival of questionable clinical significance. Adjuvant chemotherapy was also detrimental in patients with poor performance status (Eastern Cooperative Oncology Group [ECOG] performance status = 2). These data suggest that adjuvant chemotherapy is best applied in patients with resected stage II or III NSCLC. There is no apparent role for adjuvant chemotherapy in patients with resected stage IA or IB NSCLC. A possible exception to the prohibition of adjuvant therapy in this setting is the stage IB patient with a resected lesion ≥4 cm. Osimertinib, an EGFR TKI, demonstrated improved disease-free survival for patients with *EGFR* mutation (exon 19 deletion or L858R)–positive NSCLC treated for 3 years following chemotherapy. However, the effect on overall survival is unknown.

As with any treatment recommendation, the risks and benefits of adjuvant chemotherapy should be considered on an individual patient basis. If a decision is made to proceed with adjuvant chemotherapy, in general, treatment should be initiated 6–12 weeks after surgery, assuming the patient has fully recovered, and should be administered for no more than four cycles. Although cisplatin-based chemotherapy is the preferred treatment regimen, carboplatin can be substituted for cisplatin in patients who are unlikely to tolerate cisplatin for reasons such as reduced renal function, presence of neuropathy, or hearing impairment. A large cooperative group trial compared cisplatin-based chemotherapy with vinorelbine, pemetrexed, gemcitabine, or docetaxel with or without antiangiogenic therapy. While adding antiangiogenic therapy to platinum-based chemotherapy offered no benefit, the trial also demonstrated no difference in survival among the four chemotherapy regimens. Therefore, no specific chemotherapy regimen is considered superior in this setting, and treatment selection may be based on cost and patient comorbidities.

Neoadjuvant chemotherapy, which is the application of chemotherapy administered *before* an attempted surgical resection, has been advocated by some experts on the assumption that such an approach will more effectively extinguish occult micrometastases compared to

TABLE 78-8 Adjuvant Chemotherapy Trials in Non-Small-Cell Lung Cancer

TRIAL	STAGE	TREATMENT	NO. OF PATIENTS	5-YEAR SURVIVAL (%)	*P*
IALT	I–III	Cisplatin-based	932	44.5	< .03
		Control	835	40.4	
BR10	IB–II	Cisplatin + vinorelbine	242	69	.03
		Control	240	54	
ANITA	IB–IIIA	Cisplatin + vinorelbine	407	60	.017
		Control	433	58	
ALPI	I–III	MVP	548	50	.49
		Control	540	45	
BLT	I–III	Cisplatin-based	192	60	.90
		Control	189	58	
CALGB	IB	Carboplatin + paclitaxel	173	59	.10
			171	57	
ECOG1505	IB > 4c – IIIA	Cisplatin – based	749	NR	.90
		Cisplatin – based + bevacizumab	752	NR	

Abbreviations: ALPI, Adjuvant Lung Cancer Project Italy; ANITA, Adjuvant Navelbine International Trialist Association; BLT, Big Lung Trial; CALGB, Cancer and Lung Cancer Group B; ECOG, Eastern Cooperative Oncology Group; IALT, International Adjuvant Lung Cancer Trial; MVP, mitomycin, vindesine, and cisplatin; NR, not reported.

postoperative chemotherapy. In addition, it is thought that preoperative chemotherapy might render an inoperable lesion resectable. A meta-analysis of 15 randomized controlled trials involving more than 2300 patients with stage I to III NSCLC suggested there may be a modest 5-year survival benefit (i.e., ~5%) that is virtually identical to the survival benefit achieved with postoperative chemotherapy. Accordingly, neoadjuvant therapy may prove useful in selected cases (see below). A decision to use neoadjuvant chemotherapy should always be made in consultation with an experienced surgeon.

All patients with resected NSCLC are at high risk of developing a second primary lung cancer or recurrence, most of which occur within 18–24 months of surgery. Thus, it is reasonable to follow these patients with periodic imaging studies. Given the results of the NLST, periodic CT scans appear to be the most appropriate screening modality. Based on the timing of most recurrences, some guidelines recommend a contrasted chest CT scan every 6 months for the first 3 years after surgery, followed by yearly CT scans of the chest without contrast thereafter.

MANAGEMENT OF STAGE III NSCLC

Management of patients with stage III NSCLC usually requires a combined-modality approach. Patients with stage IIIA disease commonly are stratified into those with "nonbulky" or "bulky" mediastinal lymph node (N2) disease. Although the definition of "bulky" N2 disease varies somewhat in the literature, the usual criteria include the size of a dominant lymph node (i.e., >2–3 cm in short-axis diameter as measured by CT), groupings of multiple smaller lymph nodes, evidence of extracapsular nodal involvement, or involvement of more than two lymph node stations. The distinction between nonbulky and bulky stage IIIA disease is mainly used to select potential candidates for *upfront* surgical resection or for resection after neoadjuvant therapy. Many aspects of therapy of patients with stage III NSCLC remain controversial, and the optimal treatment strategy has not been clearly defined. Furthermore, because stage III disease is highly heterogeneous, no single treatment approach can be recommended for all patients. Key factors guiding treatment choices include the particular combination of tumor (T) and nodal (N) disease, the ability to achieve a complete surgical resection if indicated, and the patient's overall physical condition and preferences. For example, in carefully selected patients with limited stage IIIA disease where involved mediastinal lymph nodes can be completed resected, initial surgery followed by postoperative chemotherapy (with or without radiation therapy) may be indicated. By contrast, for patients with clinically evident bulky mediastinal lymph node involvement, the standard approach to treatment is concurrent chemoradiotherapy followed by a year of immunotherapy with durvalumab or other PD-L1-directed antibody.

Absent and Nonbulky Mediastinal (N2, N3) Lymph Node Disease For the subset of stage IIIA patients initially thought to have clinical stage I or II disease (i.e., pathologic involvement of mediastinal [N2] lymph nodes is *not* detected preoperatively), surgical resection is often the treatment of choice. This is followed by adjuvant chemotherapy in patients with microscopic lymph node involvement in a resection specimen. Postoperative radiation therapy (PORT) may also have a role for those with close or positive surgical margins. Patients with tumors exceeding 7 cm in size or involving the chest wall or proximal airways within 2 cm of the carina with hilar lymph node involvement (but not N2 disease) are classified as having T3N1 stage IIIA disease. They too are best managed with surgical resection, if technically feasible, followed by adjuvant chemotherapy if completely resected. Patients with T3N0 or T3N1 disease due to the presence of satellite nodules within the same lobe as the primary tumor are also candidates for surgery, as are patients with ipsilateral nodules in another lobe and negative mediastinal nodes (IIIA, T4N0 or T4N1). Although data regarding adjuvant chemotherapy in the latter subsets of patients are limited, it is often recommended.

Patients with T4N0-1 may have involvement of the carina, superior vena cava, or a vertebral body and yet still be candidates for surgical resection in selected circumstances. The decision to proceed with an attempted resection must be made in consultation with an experienced thoracic surgeon often in association with a vascular or cardiac surgeon and an orthopedic surgeon depending on tumor location. However, if an incomplete resection is inevitable or if there is evidence of N2 involvement (stage IIIB), surgery for T4 disease is contraindicated. Most T4 lesions are best treated with concurrent chemoradiotherapy followed by durvalumab.

The role of PORT in patients with completely resected stage III NSCLC is controversial. To a large extent, the use of PORT is dictated by the presence or absence of N2 involvement and, to a lesser degree, by the biases of the treating physician. Using the Surveillance, Epidemiology, and End Results (SEER) database, a recent meta-analysis of PORT identified a significant increase in survival in patients with N2 disease but not in patients with N0 or N1 disease. An earlier analysis by the PORT Meta-analysis Trialist Group using an older database produced similar results.

Known Mediastinal (N2, N3) Lymph Node Disease When pathologic involvement of mediastinal lymph nodes is documented preoperatively, a combined-modality approach is recommended assuming the patient is a candidate for treatment with curative intent. These patients are at high risk for both local and distant recurrence if managed with resection alone. For patients with stage III disease who are not candidates for surgical resection, *concurrent* chemoradiotherapy is most commonly used as the initial treatment followed by durvalumab. Concurrent chemoradiotherapy has been shown to produce superior survival compared to *sequential* chemoradiotherapy; however, it also is associated with greater host toxicities (including fatigue, esophagitis, and neutropenia). Therefore, for patients with a good performance status, concurrent chemoradiotherapy is the preferred treatment approach, whereas sequential chemoradiotherapy may be more appropriate for patients with a performance status that is not as good. For patients who are *not* candidates for a combined-modality treatment approach, typically due to a poor performance status or a comorbidity that makes chemotherapy untenable, radiotherapy alone may provide a modest survival benefit in addition to symptom palliation.

For patients with potentially resectable N2 disease, it remains uncertain whether surgery after neoadjuvant chemoradiotherapy improves survival. In an NCI-sponsored Intergroup randomized trial comparing concurrent chemoradiotherapy alone to concurrent chemoradiotherapy followed by attempted surgical resection, no survival benefit was observed in the trimodality arm compared to the bimodality therapy. In fact, patients subjected to a pneumonectomy had a worse survival outcome. By contrast, those treated with a lobectomy appeared to have a survival advantage based on a retrospective subset analysis. Thus, in carefully selected, otherwise healthy patients with nonbulky mediastinal lymph node involvement, surgery may be a reasonable option if the primary tumor can be fully resected with a lobectomy. This is not the case if a pneumonectomy is required to achieve complete resection.

Superior Sulcus Tumors (Pancoast Tumors) Superior sulcus tumors represent a distinctive subset of stage III disease. These tumors arise in the apex of the lung and may invade the second and third ribs, the brachial plexus, the subclavian vessels, the stellate ganglion, and adjacent vertebral bodies. They also may be associated with Pancoast syndrome, characterized by pain that may arise in the shoulder or chest wall or radiate to the neck. Pain characteristically radiates to the ulnar surface of the hand. Horner's syndrome (enophthalmos, ptosis, miosis, and anhidrosis) due to invasion of the paravertebral sympathetic chain may be present as well. Patients with these tumors should undergo the same staging procedures as all patients with stage II and III NSCLC. Neoadjuvant chemotherapy or combined chemoradiotherapy followed by surgery is reserved for those without N2 involvement. This approach yields excellent survival outcomes (>50% 5-year survival in patients with an R0 resection). Patients with N2 disease are less likely to benefit from surgery and can be managed with chemoradiotherapy followed by durvalumab. Patients presenting with metastatic disease can be treated with radiation therapy (with or without chemotherapy) for symptom palliation.

MANAGEMENT OF METASTATIC NSCLC

Approximately 40% of NSCLC patients present with advanced, stage IV disease at the time of diagnosis. In addition, a significant number of patients who first presented with early-stage NSCLC will eventually relapse with distant disease. Patients who have recurrent disease have a better prognosis than those presenting with metastatic disease at the time of diagnosis. Standard medical management, the judicious use of pain medications, and the appropriate use of radiotherapy and systemic therapy—which may consist of targeted therapy, immunotherapy, and/or traditional cytotoxic chemotherapy depending on the specific diagnosis as well as PD-L1 tumor proportion score (TPS) and molecular subtype—form the cornerstone of management. Systemic therapy palliates symptoms, improves quality of life, and improves survival in patients with metastatic NSCLC, particularly in patients with good performance status. Of note, the early application of palliative care in conjunction with chemotherapy in patients with advanced NSCLC is associated with both improved survival and quality of life.

Targeted Therapies for Select Molecular Cohorts of NSCLC For a cohort of NSCLC patients, the presence of an oncogenic driver mutation allows the use of oral therapies with significant antitumor activity and improved survival compared to cytotoxic chemotherapy. These driver mutations occur in genes encoding signaling proteins that, when aberrant, promote the uncontrolled growth and metastasis of tumor cells. Importantly, driver mutations can serve as Achilles' heels for tumors, if their gene products can be targeted therapeutically with small-molecule inhibitors. All patients with advanced NSCLC should undergo molecular testing with broad panel-based testing techniques such as next-generation sequencing (NGS) to look for oncogenic drivers. Mutations, fusions, and deletions have been reported in a number of genes including *EGFR, ALK, ROS1, BRAF, RET, MET, NTRK, KRAS, PIK3CA, NRAS, AKT1*, and *MEK1* (*MAP2K1*); however, not all are considered actionable at this time. As our treatment armamentarium expands, knowledge of these mutations is critical for selection of appropriate therapy.

EGFR mutations have been detected in 10–15% of North American patients diagnosed with NSCLC. *EGFR* mutations are associated with younger age, light (<10 pack-year) and nonsmokers, and adenocarcinoma histology. Approximately 90% of these mutations are exon 19 deletions or exon 21 L858R point mutations within the EGFR TK domain, resulting in hyperactivation of both EGFR kinase activity and downstream signaling. Lung tumors that harbor activating mutations within the EGFR kinase domain display high sensitivity to small-molecule EGFR TKIs. Osimertinib, erlotinib, gefitinib, afatinib and dacomitinib are FDA-approved oral small-molecule TKIs that inhibit EGFR. Several large, international, phase 3 studies have demonstrated improved response rates and progression-free survival in patients with *EGFR* mutation–positive NSCLC treated with an EGFR TKI as compared with standard first-line chemotherapy regimens (**Table 78-9**). Osimertinib was shown in a randomized phase 3 trial to have superior progression-free and overall survival in patients with *EGFR*-mutant NSCLC compared to earlier-generation EGFR TKIs (erlotinib or gefitinib) and to chemotherapy.

Chromosomal rearrangements involving the anaplastic lymphoma kinase (*ALK*) gene on chromosome 2 have been found in ~3–7% of patients with NSCLC. *ALK* rearrangements lead to hyperactivation of the ALK TK domain. Similar to EGFR, *ALK* rearrangements are typically (but not exclusively) associated with younger age, light (<10 pack-year) and nonsmokers, and adenocarcinoma histology. Crizotinib is a first-generation ALK TKI, whereas alectinib, brigatinib and ceritinib are second-generation ALK TKIs approved as first-line treatment options for patients with lung tumors harboring *ALK* rearrangements. Both alectinib and brigatinib have been found to have superior progression-free survival to crizotinib, whereas lorlatinib, a third-generation ALK TKI, is approved in patients who progress on a second-generation ALK TKI (**Table 78-10**). *ALK* testing may be performed via fluorescence

TABLE 78-9 Phase 3 Trials of EGFR TKIs in EGFR-Positive Non-Small-Cell Lung Cancer

TRIAL	THERAPY	NO. OF PATIENTS	ORR (%)	PFS (MONTHS)
IPASS	CbP	129	47	6.3
	Gefitinib	132	71	9.3
EURTAC	CG	87	15	5.2
	Erlotinib	86	58	9.7
OPTIMAL	CG	72	36	4.6
	Erlotinib	82	83	13.1
NEJ002	CG	114	31	5.4
	Gefitinib	114	74	10.8
WJTOG3405	CD	89	31	6.3
	Gefitinib	88	62	9.2
LUX LUNG 3	CP	115	23	6.9
	Afatinib	230	56	11.1
LUX LUNG 6	CG	122	23	5.6
	Afatinib	242	67	11.0
LUX LUNG 7	Erlotinib	159	58	10.9
	Afatinib	160	73	11.0
ARCHER 1050	Gefitinib	225	72	9.2
	Dacomitinib	227	75	14.7
FLAURA	Erlotinib or Gefitinib	277	76	8.5
	Osimertinib	279	80	17.2

Abbreviations: CbP, carboplatin and paclitaxel; CD, cisplatin and docetaxel; CG, cisplatin and gemcitabine; CP, cisplatin and paclitaxel; ORR, overall response rate; PFS, progression-free survival.

TABLE 78-10 Results of Phase 3 Trials Comparing First-Line ALK Inhibitors in ALK-Positive NSCLC

TRIAL	THERAPY	NO. OF PATIENTS	ORR (%)	PFS (MONTHS)
Profile 1014	Crizotinib	172	74	10.9
	Platinum-chemotherapy	171	45	7.0
ALEX	Alectinib	152	82.9	25.7
	Crizotinib	151	75.5	10.4
J-ALEX	Alectinib	103	92	34.1
	Crizotinib	104	79	10.2
ALTA1L	Brigatinib	137	71	67% at 1 year
	Crizotinib	138	60	43% at 1 year

Abbreviations: NSCLC, non-small-cell lung cancer; ORR, overall response rate; PFS, progression-free survival.

in situ hybridization (FISH), immunohistochemistry (IHC), or NGS.

ROS1 fusions, detected by FISH or NGS, have been identified in ~1% of patients with NSCLC, and similar to *EGFR* mutations and *ALK* fusions, *ROS1* rearrangements are typically associated with younger age and light or never smoking status. Crizotinib and lorlatinib, which inhibit both ALK and ROS1 kinases, and entrectinib have been FDA approved for patients whose tumors harbor a *ROS1* fusion.

NTRK fusions occur in members of the *NTRK* gene family (*NTRK1*, *NTRK2*, *NTRK3*) and result in constitutive protein kinase activation. *NTRK* fusions are rare, occurring in <1% of patients with NSCLC. Similar to the above mutations, they more commonly occur in never smokers; however, patients with *NTRK* fusions are often older patient compared to those with *ROS1* and *ALK* alterations. Entrectinib and larotrectinib have demonstrated durable antitumor efficacy and are currently approved for *NTRK*-positive NSCLC.

MET exon 14 skipping mutations have also been identified in approximately 3–5% of patients with NSCLC. Unlike the above-mentioned mutations, *MET* exon 14 skipping mutations occur in both squamous and nonsquamous NSCLC patients and those with a history of smoking. Pharmacologic inhibition of the overactive MET pathway with capmatinib or tepotinib resulted response rates >70%, particularly in treatment-naïve NSCLC patients.

Oncogenic mutations in *BRAF* have been observed in ~2% of patients with NSCLC and, similar to *MET*, occur in both squamous and nonsquamous NSCLC and with an equal prevalence in patients with a history of smoking. This mutation is typically most targetable when it occurs at the 600th amino acid valine (V600). Combined inhibition with a BRAF and MEK inhibitor, dabrafenib plus trametinib, is a first-line or later therapeutic option in patients with *BRAF* V600–mutant NSCLC and appears to be superior to BRAF or MEK inhibition alone.

RET alterations typically occur as chromosomal rearrangements resulting in constitutive TKI activation. *RET* rearrangements may be detected by either FISH or NGS in ~1% of NSCLC patients. Analogous to capmatinib, selpercatinib has demonstrated an excellent response rate; as many as 85% of treatment-naïve NSCLC patients with *RET* alterations responded. All National Comprehensive Cancer Network–supported targetable oncogenic driver mutations and potential therapeutic options are summarized in **Fig. 78-7**.

Mutations within the *KRAS* GTPase are found in ~20% of lung adenocarcinomas. Agents targeting *KRAS* G12C are in development. Each of the other driver mutations occurs in <1–3% of lung adenocarcinomas. The great majority of the driver mutations are mutually exclusive. Most cancers have just one main driver. Defining mechanisms of acquired resistance to small-molecule inhibitors is a high research priority.

Immunotherapy Immune checkpoint inhibitors have significantly improved the quality of life and survival for a group of patients with locally advanced and metastatic NSCLC. These agents are used primarily in patients whose tumors do not express a targetable genetic lesion **(Fig. 78-8)**. Immune checkpoint inhibitors work by blocking interactions between T cells and antigen presenting cells (APCs) or tumor cells that lead to T-cell inactivation. By inhibiting this interaction, the immune system is effectively upregulated and T cells become activated against tumor cells. Several randomized studies have demonstrated superior overall survival in patients treated with pembrolizumab or atezolizumab monotherapy or nivolumab plus ipilimumab combination immunotherapy compared to chemotherapy in patients with metastatic NSCLC with PD-L1 expression in ≥50% of tumor cells (Keynote 024, IMPOWER 110) and ≥1% of tumor cells (Keynote 042, CheckMate 227) **(Table 78-11)**. The evidence supporting the use of single-agent immunotherapy in patients with tumor PD-L1 <50% remains unclear; current recommendations suggest the use of chemotherapy plus immunotherapy or immunotherapy combinations as the first-line treatment strategy in patients with metastatic NSCLC with tumor PD-L1 <50%. As discussed below, specific regimens vary by tumor histology (adenocarcinoma vs squamous cell carcinoma). Although PD-L1 has been identified as a biomarker that can predict response to immune checkpoint inhibitors, responses are observed in patients who do

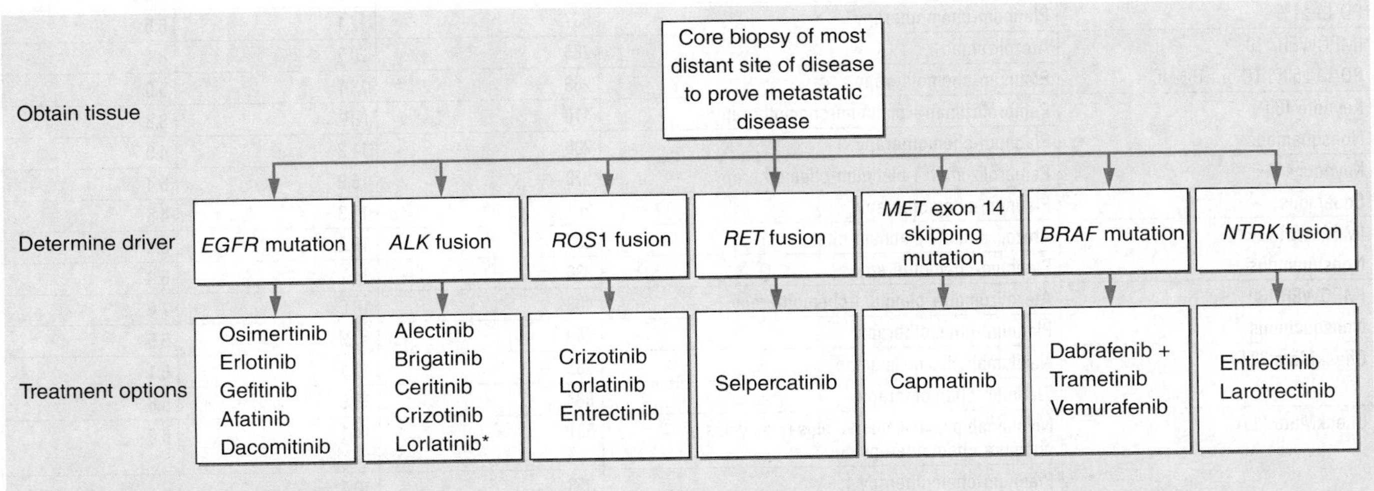

FIGURE 78-7 Approach to targeted therapy in non-small-cell lung cancer (NSCLC).

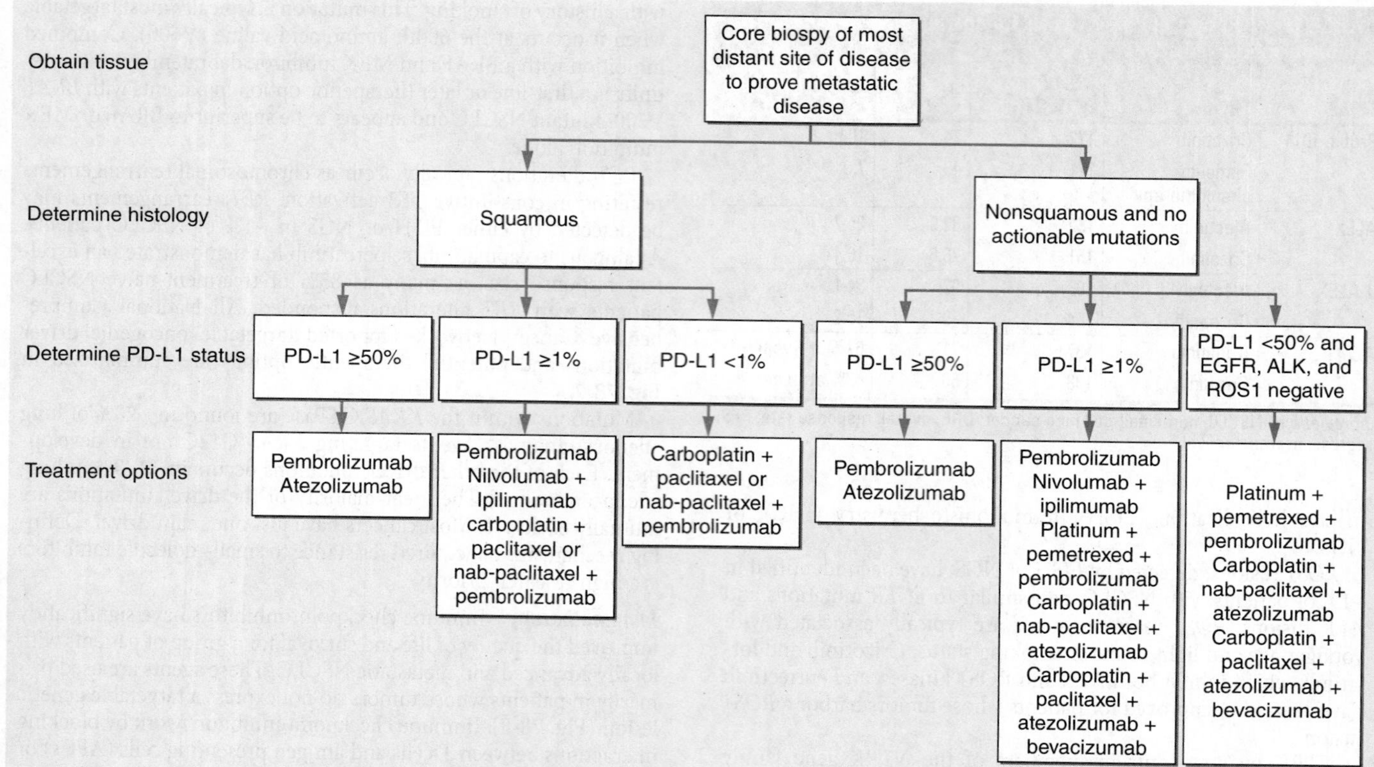

FIGURE 78-8 Approach to first-line therapy in a patient with stage IV, driver mutation–negative non-small-cell lung cancer (NSCLC).

not appear to express the biomarker, and not all PD-L1-positive patients respond to checkpoint inhibition. Importantly patients with driver mutations such as *EGFR* and *ALK* appear to derive greater benefit from targeted therapy than immunotherapy and should be treated with a TKI, even in the presence of high PD-L1 expression. Further evaluation of these agents in the neoadjuvant setting and combined with chemoradiotherapy is ongoing.

Cytotoxic Chemotherapy for Metastatic or Recurrent NSCLC Cytotoxic chemotherapy is typically used in combination with immunotherapy as the initial treatment in patients with metastatic or recurrent NSCLC only when there is no contraindication to immunotherapy. Selected chemotherapy agents perform quite differently in squamous carcinomas versus adenocarcinomas. Patients with nonsquamous NSCLC have an improved survival when

TABLE 78-11 Results of Phase 3 Trials Comparing First-Line Immunotherapy with or without Chemotherapy Versus Chemotherapy Alone in Patients with NSCLC

STUDY	THERAPY	NO. OF PATIENTS	OS (MONTHS)	PFS (MONTHS)
Keynote 024 PD-L1 ≥50%	Pembrolizumab	154	30.0	7.9
	Platinum-chemotherapy	151	14.2	3.5
Keynote 042 PD-L1 ≥1%	Pembrolizumab	637	16.7	5.4
	Platinum-chemotherapy	637	12.1	6.5
IMPOWER 110 PD-L1 ≥50% TC or ≥15% IC	Atezolizumab	286	20.2	8.1
	Platinum-chemotherapy	263	13.1	5.0
Keynote 189 Nonsquamous	Pembrolizumab + platinum-chemotherapy	410	NR	8.8
	Platinum-chemotherapy	206	11.3	4.9
Keynote 407 Squamous	Pembrolizumab + platinum-chemotherapy	278	15.9	6.4
	Platinum-chemotherapy	281	11.3	4.8
IMPOWER 150 Nonsquamous	Atezolizumab + platinum-chemotherapy	356	19.2	8.3
	Platinum-chemotherapy	336	14.7	6.8
IMPOWER 130 Nonsquamous	Atezolizumab + platinum-chemotherapy	483	18.6	7.0
	Platinum-chemotherapy	240	13.9	5.5
CheckMate 227	Nivolumab plus ipilimumab	583	17.1	5.1
	Platinum-chemotherapy	583	13.9	5.6
CheckMate-9LA	Nivolumab plus ipilimumab plus two cycles of platinum-chemotherapy	361	14.1	6.8
	Platinum-chemotherapy	358	10.7	5

Abbreviations: IC, immune cells; NR, not reported; OS, overall survival; PFS, progression-free survival; TC, tumor cells.
Note: Platinum-chemotherapy refers to first-line platinum doublet or triplet chemotherapy.

treated with cisplatin and pemetrexed compared to cisplatin and gemcitabine. By contrast, patients with squamous carcinoma have an improved survival when treated with cisplatin and gemcitabine. This survival difference is thought to be related to the differential expression between tumor types of thymidylate synthase (TS). Squamous cancers have a much higher expression of TS compared to adenocarcinomas, accounting for their lower responsiveness to pemetrexed. By contrast, the activity of gemcitabine is not impacted by the levels of TS.

Second-Line Therapy and Beyond Second-line therapy for advanced NSCLC relies on docetaxel; it improves survival compared to supportive care alone. Ramucirumab is a recombinant human IgG1 monoclonal antibody that targets VEGFR-2 and blocks the interaction of VEGF ligands and VEGFR-2. A phase 3 trial demonstrated a significant improvement in progression-free survival and overall survival when ramucirumab was combined with docetaxel as second-line therapy in patients who had progressed on platinum-based chemotherapy. Contrary to bevacizumab, ramucirumab was safe in patients with both squamous and nonsquamous NSCLC and is approved regardless of histology.

Supportive Care No discussion of the treatment strategies for patients with advanced lung cancer would be complete without a mention of supportive care. Coincident with advances in chemotherapy and targeted therapy was a pivotal study that demonstrated that the early integration of palliative care with standard treatment strategies improves both quality of life and overall survival for patients with stage IV NSCLC (**Chaps. 12 and 69**). Aggressive pain and symptom control are important components of optimal treatment of these patients.

TREATMENT

Small-Cell Lung Cancer

The overall treatment approach to patients with SCLC is shown in **Fig. 78-9**.

SURGERY FOR LIMITED-DISEASE SMALL-CELL LUNG CANCER

SCLC is a highly aggressive disease characterized by its rapid doubling time, high growth fraction, early development of disseminated disease, and dramatic response to first-line chemotherapy and radiation. In general, surgical resection is *not* routinely recommended for patients because even patients with LD-SCLC still have occult micrometastases. However, the American College of Chest Physicians Evidence-Based Clinical Practice Guidelines recommend surgical resection over nonsurgical treatment in SCLC patients with clinical stage I disease after a thorough evaluation for distant metastases and invasive mediastinal stage evaluation (grade 2C). After resection, these patients should receive platinum-based adjuvant chemotherapy (grade 1C). If the histologic diagnosis of SCLC is made in patients on review of a resected surgical specimen, such patients should receive standard SCLC chemotherapy as well.

CHEMOTHERAPY

In patients with limited-stage SCLC, concurrent chemoradiotherapy with cisplatin-etoposide for four cycles has remained standard of care for over 4 decades. Two randomized phase 3 trials have demonstrated that chemotherapy with either cisplatin or carboplatin plus either etoposide and a PD-L1 inhibitor, atezolizumab (IMPOWER 133) or durvalumab (CASPIAN), provides superior progression-free and overall survival compared to chemotherapy alone, making combination therapy the preferred choice in appropriate patients. Despite response rates to first-line therapy as high as 80%, the median survival ranges from 12 to 20 months for patients with LD and approximately 12 months for patients with ED. Regardless of disease extent, the majority of patients relapse and develop chemotherapy-resistant disease. The prognosis is especially poor for patients who relapse within the first 3 months of therapy; these patients are said to have *chemotherapy-resistant disease*. Patients are said to have *sensitive disease* if they relapse >3 months after their initial therapy and are thought to have a somewhat better overall survival. These patients also are thought to have the greatest potential benefit from second-line chemotherapy. Topotecan and

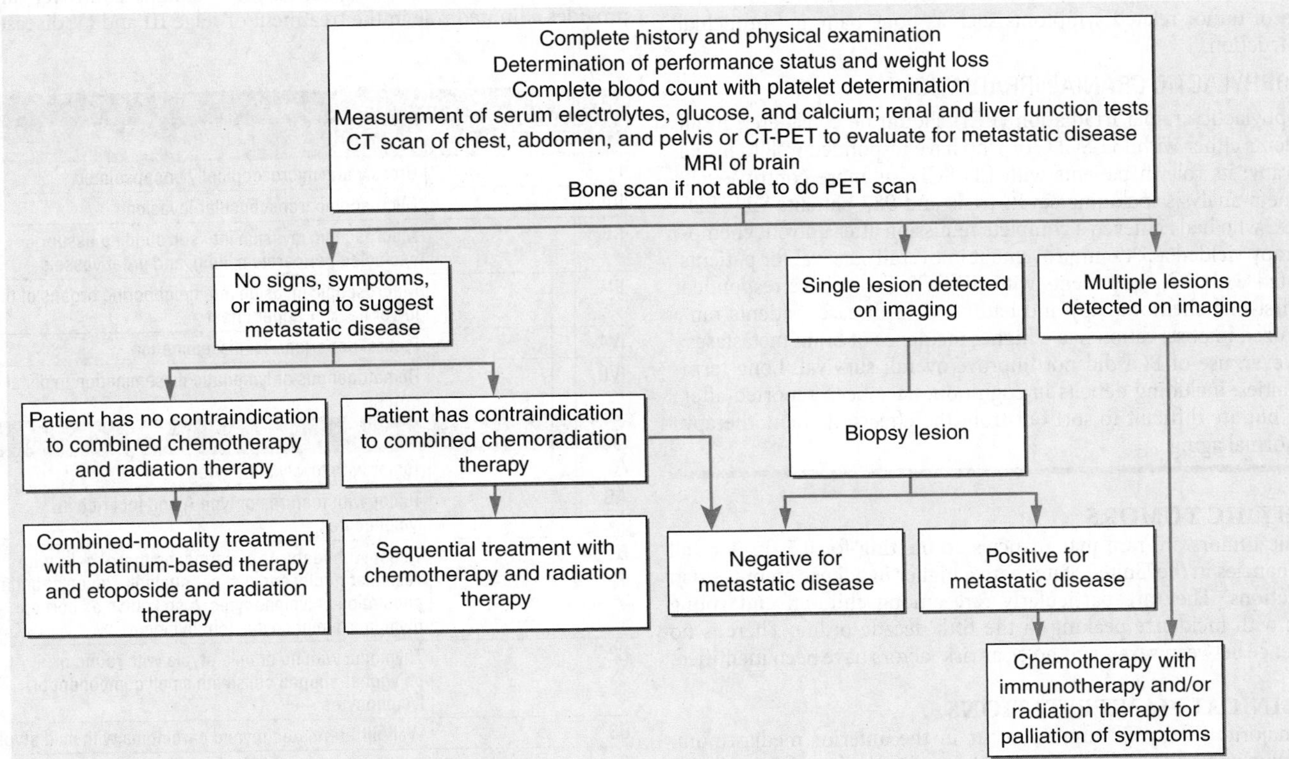

FIGURE 78-9 Algorithm for management of small-cell lung cancer. MRI, magnetic resonance imaging; PET, positron emission tomography.

lurbinectedin are FDA-approved agents for second-line therapy in patients with SCLC. Topotecan has only modest activity and can be given either intravenously or orally; it appears to have more efficacy in patients with chemotherapy-sensitive disease. Lurbinectedin has a 35% response rate and progression-free survival of 3.5 months, with a greater benefit in patients with chemotherapy-sensitive disease. Other agents with similar low levels of activity in the second-line setting include irinotecan, paclitaxel, docetaxel, vinorelbine, oral etoposide, and gemcitabine.

THORACIC RADIATION THERAPY

Thoracic radiation therapy (TRT) is a standard component of induction therapy for patients with good performance status and limited-stage SCLC. Meta-analyses indicate that chemotherapy combined with chest irradiation improves 3-year survival by ~5% as compared with chemotherapy alone. The 5-year survival rate, however, remains disappointingly low at ~10–15%. Most commonly, TRT is combined with cisplatin and etoposide chemotherapy due to a superior toxicity profile as compared to anthracycline-containing chemotherapy regimens. As observed in locally advanced NSCLC, *concurrent* chemoradiotherapy is more effective than *sequential* chemoradiation but is associated with significantly more esophagitis and hematologic toxicity. Ideally TRT should be administered with the first two cycles of chemotherapy because later application appears slightly less effective. If for reasons of fitness or availability, this regimen cannot be offered, TRT should follow induction chemotherapy. With respect to fractionation of TRT, twice-daily 1.5-Gy fractioned radiation therapy has been shown to improve survival in LD-SCLC patients but is associated with higher rates of grade 3 esophagitis and pulmonary toxicity. Although it is feasible to deliver once-daily radiation therapy doses up to 70 Gy concurrently with cisplatin-based chemotherapy, there are no data to support equivalency of this approach compared with the 45-Gy twice-daily radiotherapy dose. Therefore, the current standard regimen of a 45-Gy dose administered in 1.5-Gy fractions twice daily for 30 days is being compared with higher-dose regimens in two phase 3 trials, one in the United States and one in Europe. Patients should be carefully selected for concurrent chemoradiation therapy based on good performance status and adequate pulmonary reserve. The role of radiotherapy in ED-SCLC is largely restricted to palliation of tumor-related symptoms such as bone pain and bronchial obstruction.

PROPHYLACTIC CRANIAL IRRADIATION

Prophylactic cranial irradiation (PCI) should be considered in all patients either with LD-SCLC or who have responded well to initial therapy; its role in patients with ED-SCLC is more controversial. A meta-analysis including seven trials and 987 patients with LD-SCLC who had achieved a complete remission after upfront chemotherapy yielded a 5.4% improvement in overall survival for patients treated with PCI. In patients with ED-SCLC who have responded to first-line chemotherapy and had no CNS disease, patients randomized to observation had a higher incidence of brain metastases; however, use of PCI did not improve overall survival. Long-term toxicities, including deficits in cognition, have been reported after PCI but are difficult to sort out from the effects of chemotherapy or normal aging.

THYMIC TUMORS

Thymic tumors are rare malignancies accounting for 0.5–1.5% of all malignancies in the United States with a higher incidence among Asian populations. They are particularly rare among children and young adults with incidence peaking in the fifth decade of life. There is no difference between sexes, and no clear risk factors have been identified.

CLINICAL MANIFESTATIONS

The majority of thymic tumors occur in the anterior mediastinum. Approximately 40% of patients with mediastinal masses will be asymptomatic with an incidental finding on chest imaging. In patients presenting with an anterior mediastinal mass, if appropriate, serum β-human chorionic gonadotropin (HCG) and α fetoprotein (AFP) should be sent to rule out a germ cell tumor. A patient with a sign or symptom of thymoma or thymic carcinoma may present with chest pain, dyspnea, cough, or superior vena cava syndrome secondary to effects on adjacent organs or a paraneoplastic syndrome, most commonly myasthenia gravis, pure red cell aplasia, or hypogammaglobulinemia. More rare paraneoplastic syndromes include limbic encephalitis, aplastic anemia, hemolytic anemia, and autoimmune disease such as Sjögren's syndrome, polymyositis, rheumatoid arthritis, and ulcerative colitis, among others.

STAGING

Given the rarity of the tumor, patients with suspected thymoma should be evaluated by a multidisciplinary team including a surgeon, medical and radiation oncologist, and pathologist with experience in treating the disease. A CT scan of the chest with contrast is recommended to determine if the mass is resectable based on relationship to surrounding structures. An MRI with contrast may be performed if clinically indicated. A PET scan may be useful in the evaluation of a patient with thymic tumors, although it may be less useful in the staging of thymoma compared to thymic carcinoma. A core needle biopsy is considered standard of care for obtaining a histologic diagnosis of an anterior mediastinal tumor. This may be obtained via CT or ultrasound imaging. However, in some circumstances, a mediastinoscopy or open biopsy may be required.

Thymomas are commonly staged using the Masaoka system or the World Health Organization (WHO) staging system, as described in **Table 78-12**. WHO types A, AB, and B1 tend to be more well-differentiated, types B2 and B3 are moderately differentiated, and type C is poorly differentiated.

TREATMENT

Surgical resection is the mainstay of treatment for patients with Masaoka type I and II thymic tumors. In patients with type III and IV who have potentially resectable thymic tumors, neoadjuvant chemotherapy may be given to decrease the tumor size and allow for a resection with negative margins. Surgery remains controversial and provides a limited role in the treatment of stage III and IV disease. No

TABLE 78-12 Staging Thymic Tumors

MASAOKA STAGE	DEFINITION
I	Grossly and microscopically encapsulated
IIA	Microscopic transcapsular invasion
IIB	Macroscopic invasion into surrounding tissue excluding pericardium, lung, and great vessels
III	Macroscopic invasion into neighboring organs of the lower neck or upper chest
IVA	Pleural or pericardial dissemination
IVB	Hematogenous or lymphatic dissemination to distal organs
WHO	
A	Tumor with few lymphocytes
AB	Tumor with features of type A and foci rich in lymphocytes
B1	Tumor with features of normal epithelial cells with vesicular nuclei and distinct nucleoli and an abundant population of lymphocytes. Also known as cortical thymoma, lymphocyte-rich thymoma
B2	Thymoma with no or mild atypia with round or polygonal-shaped cells with small component of lymphocytes
B3	Well-differentiated thymic carcinoma with mild atypia
C	Thymic carcinoma with high atypia

PART 4 Oncology and Hematology

additional therapy may be required in patients with type I who have a resection with negative margins. Postoperative radiation therapy may be recommended based on extracapsular extension and the presence of positive margins in patients with type II or III thymic tumors or histologic evaluation WHO B3 and C. Radiation therapy may be beneficial in patients with locally advanced disease (type III or IV) or in patients with symptoms secondary to compression of surrounding structures. Chemotherapy with cisplatin, doxorubicin, and cyclophosphamide (CAP) remains the mainstay of therapy in the neoadjuvant and adjuvant setting as well as first-line therapy in patients with metastatic thymoma, whereas carboplatin and paclitaxel are often employed in patients with thymic carcinoma. Limited additional agents are recommended based on small phase 2 trials as second-line therapy and beyond.

COVID-19 AND LUNG CANCER

COVID-19, a respiratory tract infection caused by SARS-CoV-2, emerged in Wuhan, China, in late 2019. The rapid global spread led the WHO to declare a pandemic in early March 2020. Large retrospective data sets have shown that cancer patients, and particularly patients with lung cancer, are at increased risk of morbidity and mortality from COVID-19. The dilemma of distinguishing COVID-19 symptoms from lung cancer and radiographic diagnosis of pneumonia or pneumonitis from radiation therapy or immunotherapy versus COVID-19 pneumonia has presented a particular challenge to health care providers. Mortality as high as 35% has been reported for patients with lung cancer infected with SARS-CoV-2. Older patients (≥65 years old), patients with a worse performance status (Eastern Cooperative Oncology Group performance status ≥1), patients on glucocorticoids (≥10 mg prednisone equivalent) and anticoagulation, and patients on chemotherapy within 3 months of diagnosis appear to be particularly at risk for morality if infected. The long-term impact on lung cancer mortality due to delays in screening, diagnosis, and treatment are likely to be felt for years to come.

SUMMARY

The management of SCLC and NSCLC has undergone major change in the past decade, resulting in a reduction in lung cancer mortality. For patients with early-stage disease, advances in radiotherapy and surgical procedures as well as new systemic therapies have greatly improved prognosis in all diseases. For patients with advanced lung cancer, major progress in understanding tumor genetics and tumor immunology has led to the development of rational targets and specific inhibitors, which have documented efficacy in specific subsets of NSCLC. Furthermore, increased understanding of how to activate the immune system to drive antitumor immunity has proven to be a successful therapeutic strategy for a subset of patients with advanced lung cancer. However, only a small subset of patients responds to immune checkpoint inhibitors, and the majority of patients treated with targeted therapies or chemotherapy eventually develop resistance, which provides strong motivation for further research and enrollment of patients onto clinical trials in this rapidly evolving area.

Acknowledgment

David Johnson and Christine Lovly contributed to this chapter in the prior edition, and material from that chapter has been retained here.

FURTHER READING

Drillon et al: Selpercatinib. Available at *https://www.nejm.org/doi/full/10.1056/NEJMoa2005653.*

Drilon et al: Entrectinib. Available at *https://www.thelancet.com/journals/lanonc/article/PIIS1470-2045(19)30690-4/fulltext*

Drilon et al: Larotrectinib. Available at *https://www.nejm.org/doi/full/10.1056/NEJMoa1714448.*

Ghandi L et al: Pembrolizumab plus chemotherapy in metastatic non-small cell lung cancer. N Engl J Med 378:2078, 2018.

Goldstraw et al: The IASLC Lung Cancer Staging Project: Proposals for Revision of the TNM Stage Groupings in the Forthcoming (Eighth) Edition of the TNM Classification for Lung Cancer. JTO 11:39, 2016.

Hellmann MD et al: Nivolumab plus ipilimumab in advanced non small cell lung cancer. N Engl J Med 381:2220, 2019.

Garasino et al: COVID. Available at *https://www.sciencedirect.com/science/article/pii/S1470204520303144?via%3Dihub.*

Horn L et al: First line atezolizumab plus chemotherapy in extensive stage small-cell lung cancer. N Engl J Med 379:2220, 2018.

Li et al: Trastuzumab-Deruxtecan. Available at *https://www.nejm.org/doi/full/10.1056/NEJMoa2005653.*

Paz-Ares L et al: Pembrolizumab plus chemotherapy for squamous non-small cell lung cancer. N Engl J Med 379:2040, 2018.

Paz-Ares L et al: Durvalumab plus platinum-etoposide versus platinume toposide in first line treatment of extensive-stage small-cell lung cancer (CASPIAN): A randomised, controlled, open-label, phase 3 trial. Lancet 394:1929, 2019.

Peters S et al: Alectinib versus crizotinib in untreated ALK-positive non-small cell lung cancer. N Engl J Med 377:829, 2017.

Reck M et al: Pembrolizumab versus chemotherapy for PD-L1 positive non-small cell lung cancer. N Engl J Med 375:1823, 2016.

Soria JC et al: Osimertinib in untreated EGFR-mutated advanced nonsmall cell lung cancer. N Engl J Med 378:113, 2018.

Wolf et al: Capmatinib. Available at *https://www.nejm.org/doi/full/10.1056/NEJMoa2005653.*

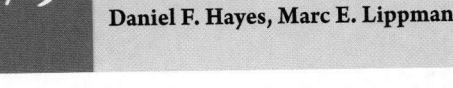

79 Breast Cancer

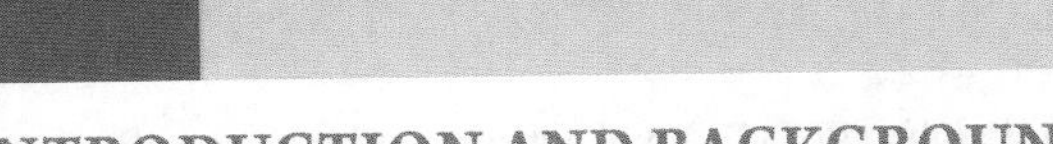

Daniel F. Hayes, Marc E. Lippman

INTRODUCTION AND BACKGROUND

CONCEPTUAL AND BIOLOGICAL ISSUES OF BREAST CANCER

Breast cancer is a malignant proliferation of epithelial cells lining the ducts or lobules of the breast. In the year 2020, approximately a quarter million cases of invasive and 61,000 cases of in situ breast cancer were diagnosed in the United States, with nearly 41,000 deaths. Epithelial malignancies of the breast are the most common cause of cancer in women (excluding skin cancer), accounting for about one-third of all cancer in women. As a result of earlier detection and improved treatments, the mortality rate from breast cancer decreased by more than one-third over the past three decades in high- and middle-income countries. This chapter does not consider rare malignancies presenting in the breast, such as sarcomas and lymphomas, but focuses on the epithelial cancers.

Breast cancer has served as a paradigm for several oncologic principles related to solid tumors. It spans a spectrum of conditions for which different clinical considerations must be made, including risk assessment, prevention, screening, evaluation of breast abnormalities, local and adjuvant systemic treatments, metastatic therapies, and survivorship issues (**Fig. 79-1**).

The unique biology of breast cancer has rendered it amenable to a variety of therapeutic "targeted" strategies based on the appreciation of differences in subtypes that reflect the need for differences in assessment and therapy. These subtypes include expression of the estrogen receptor (ER) and the human epidermal growth factor receptor type 2 (HER2), as well as germline or somatic mutations in inherited tumor suppressor genes, such as *BRCA1* and *BRCA2*. Identifiable somatic mutations in genes that appear to drive the cancer, including mammalian target of rapamycin (*mTOR*), cyclin-dependent kinase 4 and 6 (*CDK4/6*), and S-phosphatidylinositol-4,5-bisphosphate 3-kinase

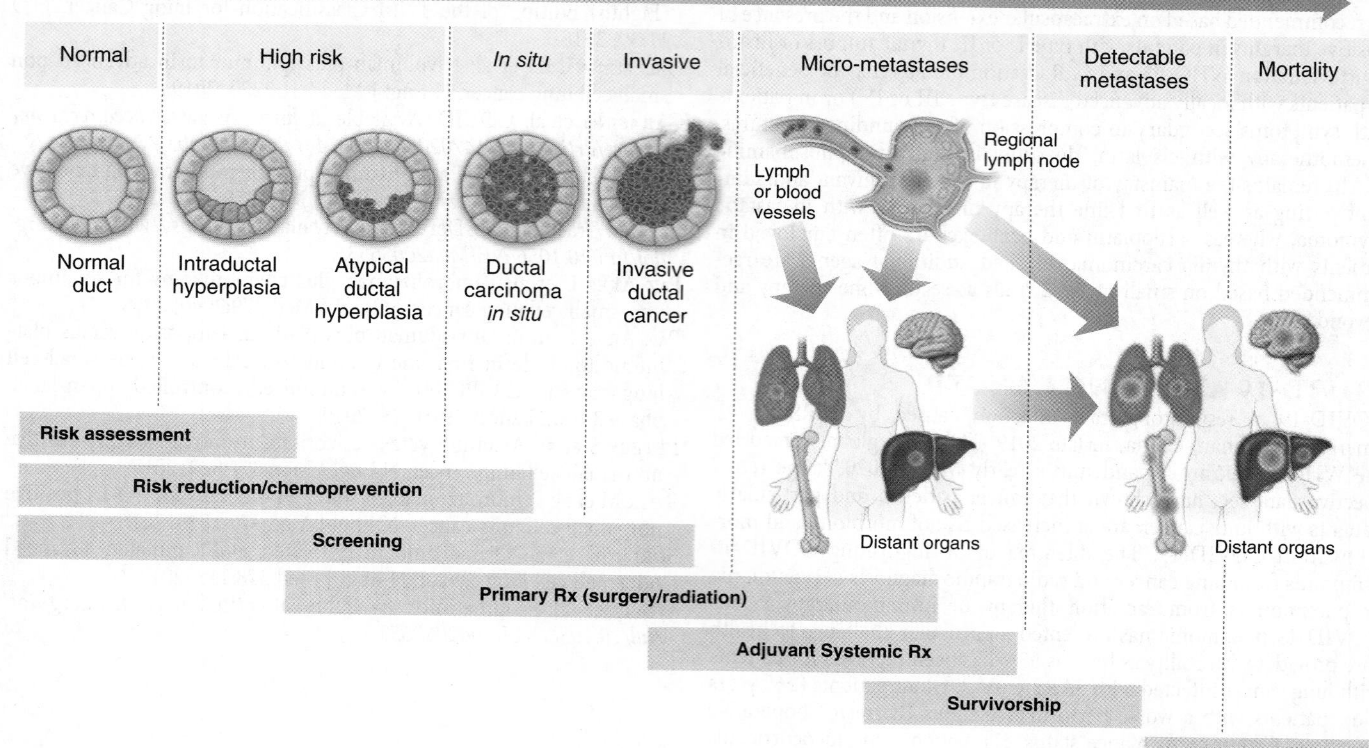

FIGURE 79-1 Breast cancer continuum conceptual model. Most breast cancers begin in epithelial cells within the lobules or ducts. They proceed through a continuum of atypia and hyperplasia to in situ malignancy to invasion into surrounding normal tissues followed by intravasation into lymph and blood channels to local lymph nodes and distant organs, culminating in distant metastases. This is a conceptual model. Not all metastatic breast cancers have progressed through these stages, and many lesions do not progress to the next.

catalytic subunit alpha (*PIK3CA*) make it susceptible to specific therapeutic interventions directed against each of these targets (**Table 79-1**). Furthermore, immune checkpoint inhibition has been applied to specific types of breast cancers.

EPIDEMIOLOGY AND RISK FACTORS

CLINICAL, HORMONAL, AND OTHER NONGENETIC RISK FACTORS

Seventy-five percent of all breast cancers occur in women aged >50 years, but breast cancer is not uncommon in women in their forties and can occur in women in their thirties and even twenties, and very rarely in adolescence.

Breast cancer is principally a sex hormone–dependent disease through increased activity of the ER and its ligands, estradiol and estrone (Fig. 79-1, Table 79-1). Indeed, the female-to-male ratio is ~150:1. Relative exposure to both endogenous and exogenous estrogens increases risk of breast cancer. Risk of developing breast cancer is higher in women with early menarche (<12 years) and late first full-term pregnancy (>35 years), and it is increased by exogenous hormone replacement therapy. Women without functioning ovaries, who experience an early menopause, or who never receive combination estrogen/progesterone replacement therapy are much less likely to develop breast cancer than those who have a normal menstrual history. Also, duration of maternal nursing correlates with substantial risk reduction independent of either parity or age at first full-term pregnancy.

Menstrual and reproductive history accounts for 70–80% of the variation in breast cancer frequency in different countries, providing insight into hormonal carcinogenesis. A woman living to age 80 years in North America has a one in nine chance of developing invasive breast cancer. Women who live in agrarian societies, especially in Asia, have traditionally had only 1/5th to 1/10th the risk of breast cancer of women in North America or Western Europe. However, Asian women who immigrate to North America or European countries during preadolescence or in adolescence have the same risk as women born in these countries. Further, with shifts from agrarian to industrialized economic systems, the incidence of breast cancer has risen dramatically in Asia, approaching that observed in Western nations.

Exogenous use of female hormones also plays a role in breast cancer incidence. The elevated risk related to oral contraceptives is quite modest if present at all. Regardless, this risk is more than balanced by avoidance of an undesired pregnancy and a substantial protective effect against ovarian epithelial and endometrial cancers.

Hormone replacement therapy (HRT) with conjugated equine estrogens plus progestins increases the risk of breast cancer; 6–7 years of HRT nearly doubles the risk of breast cancer and also increases the incidence of adverse cardiovascular events. However, it decreases the risk of bone fractures and colorectal cancer. On balance, more negative than positive events are associated with HRT. Administration of conjugated estrogens is usually combined with companion progesterone to abrogate the increased risk of endometrial cancer with estrogen alone. However, single-agent estrogen replacement therapy in women who have had hysterectomies produces no significant increase in breast cancer incidence and, if anything, reduces the risk. Thus, there are serious concerns about long-term HRT, especially in combination with progestins, in terms of cardiovascular disease and breast cancer. No comparable safety data are available for other less potent forms of estrogen replacement, such as bioequivalent estrogen found in soy, and they should not be routinely used as substitutes. Epidemiologic studies demonstrate a rapid decrease in elevated breast cancer incidence coincident with discontinuation of HRT.

HRT in women previously diagnosed with breast cancer, especially of the subtype that expresses ERs, counteracts much of the effectiveness of antineoplastic endocrine therapies and is contraindicated. Although

TABLE 79-1 Breast Cancer Molecular Features and Associated Targeted Therapies

MOLECULE	GENE THAT ENCODES MOLECULE	ABNORMALITY	CLASS OF TARGETED THERAPIES	SPECIFIC THERAPIES
Estrogen receptor (ER)	*ESR1*	Overexpression of cellular protein	Endocrine therapies	
			Estrogen ablation (surgical, chemical)	***Premenopausal*** Oophorectomy Luteinizing hormone releasing hormone (LHRH) agonists (goserelin, leuprolide) or antagonist (triptorelin) ***Postmenopausal*** Aromatase inhibitors (AIs) (anastrozole, letrozole, exemestane)
			ER antagonists	Selective estrogen receptor modulators (SERMs) (tamoxifen, toremifene, raloxifene) Selective estrogen receptor downregulators (SERDs) (fulvestrant)
Human epidermal growth factor receptor type 2 (HER2)	*c-neu/erbB2*	Overexpression of cell surface protein	Antibodies against HER2	Trastuzumab, pertuzumab, margetuximab
			Antibody-drug conjugates against HER2	Ado-trastuzumab emtansine, fam-trastuzumab deruxtecan-nxki
			Tyrosine kinase inhibitors	Lapatinib, neratinib, tucatinib
		Mutations	Tyrosine kinase inhibitors	Neratinib *(indication not FDA approved)*
Mammalian target of rapamycin (mTOR)	*MTOR*	Loss of protein suppressor of mTOR pathway, phosphatase and tensin homolog (*PTEN*)	Tyrosine kinase inhibitor	Everolimus
Cyclin-dependent kinase 4 and 6 (CDK4/6)	*CDK4, CDK6*	Loss of the protein suppressor of CDK4/6 pathway, retinoblastoma (*RB1*)	Inhibition of CDK4/6 enzyme activity	Palbociclib, ribociclib, abemociclib
Phosphatidylinositol-4,5-bisphosphate 3-kinase catalytic subunit alpha (PIK3CA)	*PIK3CA*	Mutations	Enzyme inhibition of mutated/activated PIK3CA protein	Alpelisib
BRCA1/2	*BRCA1, BRCA2*	Loss of tumor suppressor activity of BRCA1/2	Inhibition of poly (ADP-ribose) polymerase (PARP) activity and synthetic lethality	PARP inhibitors (olaparib, talazoparib)
TROP-2	*TACSTD2*	Over expression of TROP-2 cell surface protein	Antibody-drug conjugate against TROP-2	Sacituzumab govitecan
Immune checkpoints	NA	Programmed death-ligand 1 (PD-L1) suppression of immune effector cells	Inhibition of PD-L1/PD-1 suppression of immune effector cells	Atezolizumab

Abbreviations: FDA, U.S. Food and Drug Administration; NA, not applicable.

intravaginal estrogen therapy has been used for atrophic vaginitis associated with antiestrogenic endocrine therapies, it does result in some absorption and systemic estrogenic effects and should generally be avoided.

In addition to sex, age, and hormonal exposure, other risk features for breast cancer have been identified, but none with the kind of relative, attributable, or absolute risks associated with these three factors. Various differences in diets (including Asian agrarian vs modern economic) have been implicated as risk factors, although the role of diet in breast cancer etiology is controversial. Associative links exist between breast cancer risk and total caloric and fat intake, or even specific types of caloric intake, but the exact role of fat in the diet is unproven and may actually intersect with menstrual history and estrogenic exposure. Central obesity, metabolic syndrome, and type 2 diabetes mellitus are all risk factors for occurrence and recurrence of breast cancer. Moderate alcohol intake also increases the risk by an unknown mechanism. Folic acid supplementation appears to modify risk in women who use alcohol but is not additionally protective in abstainers. Recommendations favoring abstinence from alcohol must be weighed against other social pressures and the possible cardioprotective effect of moderate alcohol intake. Depression is also associated with both occurrence and recurrence of breast cancer.

Certain benign breast pathologic findings, such as atypical hyperplasia and radial scars, are associated with higher risk of subsequent breast cancers. Prior radiation is a risk factor, but principally when delivered in adolescence or early child-bearing ages. Women who have been exposed before age 30 years to radiation in the form of multiple fluoroscopies (200–300 cGy) or treatment for Hodgkin's disease (>3600 cGy) have a substantial increase in risk of breast cancer, whereas radiation exposure after age 30 years appears to have a minimal carcinogenic effect on the breast. Radioactive iodine therapy for thyroid disease is not associated with increased risk of breast cancer, whereas mediastinal radiation in younger women for lymphoma is a powerful risk factor within the radiated field.

INHERITED GERMLINE SUSCEPTIBILITY FACTORS

Family history has long been recognized as a risk factor for breast cancer. A woman with a first-degree history (mother or sister) of breast cancer has an increased relative risk of approximately 30–50% (or one-third to one-half higher) over a woman with no family history. However, family history only accounts for 10–15% of all breast cancers. Most women who develop breast cancer do not have a strong family history. For women without an identifiable inherited genetic abnormality, it is not clear whether the increased risk associated with family history is due to environmental causes or as yet unidentified genetic abnormalities.

The genetics of breast cancer require an understanding of the distinction between inherited, germline genetic differences among individuals and acquired, somatic genetic changes within cancers. The former are often called mutations but are more properly termed *single nucleotide polymorphisms* (SNPs). Some SNPs are synonymous, meaning they do not change the encoded amino acid in the affected protein product, and therefore are of no clinical significance. Some SNPs are nonsynonymous but may lead to a substituted amino acid that does not change the function of the protein, and they are likewise clinically insignificant. However, if an SNP leads to an amino acid substitution that alters the protein function or results in complete cessation of transcription or translation (a "stop" codon), it is considered deleterious and leads to higher susceptibility to developing cancer. In some cases, the significance of the SNP is unknown, and these are designated *variants of undetermined significance* (VUS).

The genes of interest serve, in the normal cell, to suppress expansion of a potentially malignant clone, either by repairing downstream randomly occurring somatic genetic abnormalities or, if not possible, by inducing programmed cell death, or apoptosis. Somatic genetic changes that are not inherited, including mutations, amplifications, insertions, deletions, translocations, and others, are responsible for the malignant behavior of a cancer, including unrestrained proliferation, as well as extravasation from one site and migration and establishment of metastases into another. As discussed below, some germline and somatic mutations can be exploited therapeutically (Table 79-1).

For most women, the increased risk associated with a family member who has had breast cancer appears to be related to both a weak, and probably multigene, germline susceptibility and similar exposure to environmental/lifestyle risk factors. Only approximately 10% of human breast cancers can be linked directly to a single inherited germline SNP. However, when one is present, the relative and absolute risks for that individual developing breast, and other, cancers in her lifetime are extraordinary.

The *BRCA1* and *BRCA2* genes, located on chromosomal loci 17q21 and 13q12, respectively, are the best characterized breast cancer susceptibility genes and have the greatest clinical importance in assessing genetic risk for breast cancer. Women who inherit mutated alleles of these genes from either parent have at least a 60–80% lifetime chance of developing breast cancer and about a 33% chance of developing ovarian cancer. The cancers that arise within a *BRCA1*-mutated patient are almost exclusively negative for ER, progesterone receptor (PgR), and HER2 (so-called "triple-negative" breast cancers). Men who carry a mutant allele of the gene have an increased incidence of breast and also prostate cancers, although the absolute risk of breast cancer in men with *BRCA2* germline SNPs is far lower than that for women who harbor them.

Overall, <1% of the general population and <5% of all patients with breast cancer harbor deleterious SNPs in *BRCA1* or *BRCA2*. Certain subgroups of women are more likely to have *BRCA1/2* mutations. The incidence is approximately 2% in women of Ashkenazi, Eastern European descent. Approximately 20% of women with triple-negative breast cancers will be positive for deleterious germline *BRCA1* SNPs, and genetic testing is warranted in most patients with triple-negative breast cancer even without a family history.

In contrast to those that arise in *BRCA1* carriers, cancers that arise in *BRCA2* contexts are more likely to be ER positive. The incidence of *BRCA2* mutations is much higher than *BRCA1* in men who develop breast cancer. However, most male breast cancer cases do not occur in *BRCA1/2*-mutated men, and the risk of breast cancer in men who do carry the *BRCA2* mutation is much lower than that in women with this genetic abnormality. Many other inherited germline mutations in known or putative tumor-suppressor genes, such as *p53* (which also accounts in part for the Li-Fraumeni familial cancer syndrome), *PTEN* (which accounts for Cowden's syndrome), and *PALB1*, have now been identified as important tumor-suppressor genes with clinical implications.

Inherited germline mutations are readily detected in blood tests of normal circulating leukocytes using so-called "panel" assays, which at present provide results from 30–45 different germline genes. However, because the rate of deleterious germline SNPS in these genes in the general population is quite low (well below 1%), germline panel genetic testing of the entire population of women is not recommended. Further, results are confounded by the presence of VUS in known tumor-suppressor genes, such as *BRCA1* and *BRCA2*, or deleterious variants or VUS in genes that are putative, but not proven, tumor-suppressor genes. Such results lead to confusion, anxiety, and inappropriate preventive strategies, such as prophylactic surgery, in individuals who may not actually be at higher risk.

Consensus guidelines on who should be tested include any woman with a family member who has been tested and found to harbor a deleterious SNP in a germline tumor-suppressor gene. Testing is indicated for any breast cancer patient with a triple-negative breast cancer, who is <40 years old, who has synchronous or metachronous contralateral breast cancers, who has a personal history of ovarian cancer, or who has a first-degree relative (mother, father, or sister) with breast or ovarian cancer. All males with breast cancer should be tested. Some guidelines suggest testing any breast cancer patient of Ashkenazi descent. Patients with these mutations should be counseled appropriately.

Some experts have recommended testing any patient diagnosed with breast cancer, both for genetic counseling but also because of the advent of effective therapies directed toward cancers that have deleterious *BRCA1/2* mutations (Table 79-1), although this strategy remains controversial. Regardless, any patient who is found to have inherited germline deleterious SNPs should receive formal genetic testing and counseling about special screening and prevention measures they might take.

PREVENTION OF BREAST CANCER

One major reason to determine risk would be to efficiently apply prevention and/or screening strategies, if either has been shown to be effective for the disease of interest. At present, although diet and exercise are certainly recommended approaches to healthy living, none has been proven to specifically decrease a woman's risk of breast cancer. Avoidance of combined estrogen/progestin HRT reduces the associated increased risk of breast cancer to that of an average woman not using HRT.

Prophylactic removal of the breasts is an effective, albeit drastic, preventive strategy. Bilateral prophylactic mastectomies reduce the risk of breast cancer incidence and mortality by >95%. Because breasts are not encapsulated organs, some normal breast tissue is always left behind, and therefore, women who elect to have prophylactic mastectomies should be counseled that they still have some risk of developing a new breast cancer. Prophylactic mastectomy is most often chosen by women with germline genetic risk, in whom there is evidence of mortality reduction. For women with average or only mildly elevated risks, such as diagnosis of a unilateral breast cancer, survival is not increased by prophylactic mastectomy, and, because of its obvious adverse effect on sexuality, cosmesis, and breast-feeding, this approach is not considered appropriate.

So-called "chemoprevention" to lower breast cancer risk can be achieved with therapies directed toward the ER/estrogen signaling pathway (Table 79-1). These include the selective estrogen receptor modulators (SERMs) as well as aromatase inhibition. The latter should only be applied in postmenopausal women, since aromatase inhibition can result in a paradoxical increase in circulating estrogen levels in women with functioning ovaries. Chemoprevention with SERMs or aromatase inhibition lowers risk of ER-positive breast cancer by approximately one-half, although it has no effect on the more lethal ER-negative breast cancers. Of interest, prophylactic bilateral oophorectomy and salpingo-oophorectomy, which are often performed in women with high genetic risk (such as those with inherited *BRCA1/2* deleterious SNPs), also reduce breast cancer in addition to ovarian cancer risk.

SCREENING FOR BREAST CANCER (FIG. 79-2)

Screening mammography results in earlier diagnosis and subsequent local and systemic therapy. Overviews of nine prospective randomized clinical trials demonstrate that screening mammography reduces breast cancer mortality by one-fifth to one-quarter in women aged ≥50 years. The relative reduction in breast cancer mortality for women between ages 40 and 50 years is similar, although the absolute numbers of women who benefit in this age group is smaller since the incidence of breast cancer is much lower in younger women. In addition to reducing breast cancer mortality, screening mammography and early detection are more likely to identify tumors at a stage more appropriate for conservative local therapy. Better technology, including digitized mammography, tomosynthesis, routine use of magnified views, and greater skill in interpretation, have all improved the accuracy of mammography. Magnetic resonance spectroscopy has higher sensitivity but lower specificity than mammography. Since none of these newer technologies has been shown to be superior to mammography in terms of mortality reduction, screening of women with standard risk by any technique other than mammography is not recommended.

The issue of screening breast imaging of any sort has been controversial. Although the prospective randomized clinical trials demonstrate a late reduction in breast cancer mortality, they do not demonstrate improvement in overall survival. Further, many authors have raised concern about diagnosis of cancers that may be biologically insignificant, raising the specter of overdiagnosis and overtreatment. Moreover, the substantial advances in both local and systemic therapies for breast cancer may have reduced the benefit of earlier diagnosis provided by screening. In contrast, in countries that have adopted widespread screening programs, nonrandomized, epidemiologic studies have demonstrated even greater magnitude reductions in breast cancer mortality than those seen in the randomized trials. Taken together, these data have led most guideline bodies to recommend annual screening for women aged 50–70 years. Many have also recommended screening for women in the 40- to 50-year-old range. For older women, caregiver and patient judgment should be used, taking into account comorbidities.

Magnetic resonance imaging (MRI) is recommended for women with particularly dense breasts, women whose first cancer was not detected by mammography, women with an axillary breast cancer presentation but no definable breast mass on physical exam or mammography, and those with high genetic risk, such as *BRCA1* or *BRCA2* carriers or those with Li-Fraumeni, Cowden's, or Bannayan-Riley-Ruvalcaba syndromes. MRI might also be considered for women with a history of radiation therapy to the chest between ages 10 and 30 years. In these women, the positive predictive value of MRI is higher because

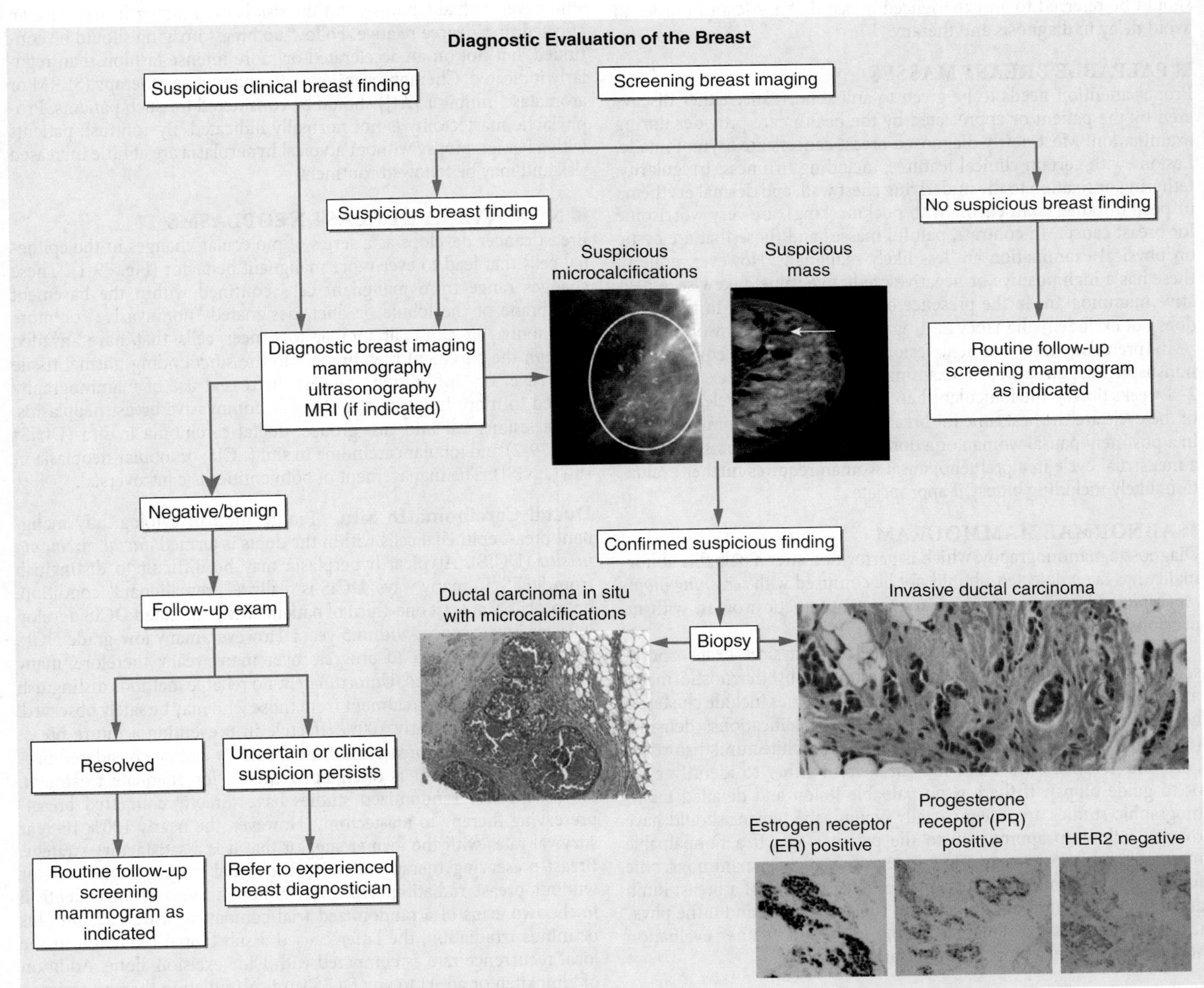

FIGURE 79-2 Evaluation and workup of breast lesions. For more extensive details, see *https://www.nccn.org/professionals/physician_gls/pdf/breast-screening.pdf*. *(Mammographic images courtesy of Drs. Mark Helvie and Colleen Neal, Department of Radiology, Michigan Medicine. Photomicrographs courtesy of Dr. Celina Kleer, Department of Pathology, Michigan Medicine.)*

of the higher incidence of cancer, and furthermore, many of them are considering prophylactic mastectomy as an alternative; therefore, the lower specificity and risk of a false-positive finding has been considered more acceptable.

Self-examination or physical breast examinations done by a health professional have poor sensitivity and specificity, and regular breast self-examination is not recommended. Nonetheless, all women should be familiar with how their breasts normally look and feel and report any changes to a health care provider right away. Because the breasts are a common site of potentially fatal malignancy in women, examination of the breast is an important part of a routine physical examination.

Screening breast imaging is not recommended for men, since it is so unusual and easily detected. It is important to note that unilateral lesions should be evaluated in the same manner as in women with an appropriately high index of suspicion.

EVALUATION OF BREAST MASSES (FIG. 79-2)

Virtually all breast cancer is diagnosed by biopsy of an abnormality detected either on a mammogram or by palpation. The presence or absence of any risk factors, such as age, family history, or menstrual history cannot be used to exclude more careful workup and, if indicated, a biopsy. Any woman with a persistent breast abnormality should be referred to an experienced breast diagnostician in order to avoid delay in diagnosis and therapy.

PALPABLE BREAST MASSES

Proper attention needs to be given to any abnormality either discovered by the patient or appreciated by the health care provider during examination. Most newly diagnosed breast cancers are asymptomatic. Lesions with certain clinical features, including firmness, irregularity, tethering or fixation to the underlying chest wall, and dermal erythema or peau d'orange (skin edema with pockmarking), are very worrisome for breast cancer. In contrast, painful masses and those that are cystic on physical examination are less likely malignant. However, none of these has a high positive or negative predictive value. Likewise, a negative mammogram in the presence of a persistent lump in the breast does not exclude malignancy and, again, deserves careful workup.

In premenopausal women, lesions that are either equivocal or nonsuspicious on physical examination should be reexamined in 2–4 weeks during the follicular phase of the menstrual cycle. Days 5–7 of the cycle are the best time for breast examination. A dominant mass in a postmenopausal woman or a dominant mass that persists through a menstrual cycle in a premenopausal woman requires further evaluation, likely including biopsy if appropriate.

ABNORMAL MAMMOGRAM

Diagnostic mammography, which is performed after a palpable abnormality has been detected, should not be confused with *screening mammography*, which is performed in an asymptomatic woman with no previously identified abnormalities.

Abnormalities that are first detected by physical exam and/or screening mammography should be evaluated by diagnostic mammography. Suspicious mammographic abnormalities include clustered, heterogeneous, linear, and branching microcalcifications; densities (especially if spiculated); and new or enlarging architectural distortion. For some lesions, ultrasound may be helpful either to identify cysts or to guide biopsy. If there is no palpable lesion and detailed mammographic studies are unequivocally benign, the patient should have routine follow-up appropriate to the patient's age. If a nonpalpable mammographic lesion has a low index of suspicion, mammographic follow-up in 3–6 months is reasonable. The presence of a breast lump and a negative mammogram does not rule out cancer, and if the physical finding persists or enlarges during follow-up, further evaluation and, if appropriate, a biopsy are indicated.

BREAST MASSES IN PREGNANCY OR LACTATION

Breast cancer develops in 1 of 3000–4000 pregnancies. The breast grows during pregnancy under the influence of estrogen, progesterone, prolactin, and human placental lactogen. After delivery and during lactation, breast tissue continues to be under the influence of unopposed prolactin. Therefore, breast examination during these times can be challenging. Nonetheless, development of a dominant mass during pregnancy or lactation should not be attributed to hormonal changes without appropriate diagnostic evaluation. Stage for stage, breast cancer in pregnant patients is no different from premenopausal breast cancer in nonpregnant patients. However, pregnant women often have more advanced disease because the significance of a breast mass was not fully considered and/or because of endogenous hormone stimulation.

PATHOLOGIC FINDINGS OF THE BREAST

BENIGN BREAST HISTOPATHOLOGY

Only ~1 in every 5–10 breast biopsies leads to a diagnosis of cancer, although the rate of positive biopsies varies in different countries and clinical settings due to variable interpretation, medico-legal considerations, and availability of mammograms. The vast majority of benign breast masses are due to fibrocystic changes, a descriptive term for small fluid-filled cysts and modest epithelial cell and fibrous tissue hyperplasia. Women with ductal or lobular cell proliferation (~30% of patients), particularly the small fraction (3%) with atypical hyperplasia, have a fourfold greater risk of developing breast cancer than women who have not had a biopsy, and the risk is even higher if they have an affected first-degree relative. Follow-up breast imaging should be continued, but not on an accelerated or more intense fashion than regularly indicated. Chemoprevention with antiestrogen therapy (SERM or aromatase inhibitor [AI]) should be considered for such patients. Prophylactic mastectomy is not normally indicated. By contrast, patients with a benign biopsy without atypical hyperplasia are at little increased risk and may be followed routinely.

NONINVASIVE BREAST NEOPLASMS

Breast cancer develops as a series of molecular changes in the epithelial cells that lead to ever more malignant behavior (Fig. 79-1). These changes range from malignant cells confined within the basement membrane of the lobule or duct, designated "noninvasive" or more commonly "in situ" carcinoma, to cancer cells that have invaded through the basement membrane into the surrounding normal tissue ("invasive" or "infiltrating" cancer). Increased use of mammography has led to more frequent diagnoses of noninvasive breast neoplasms. These lesions fall into two groups: ductal carcinoma in situ (DCIS) (Fig. 79-2) and lobular carcinoma in situ (LCIS; or lobular neoplasia in situ [LNIS]). The management of both entities is controversial.

Ductal Carcinoma In Situ Proliferation of cytologically malignant breast epithelial cells within the ducts is termed *ductal carcinoma in situ* (DCIS). Atypical hyperplasia may be difficult to distinguish from DCIS. In many ways, DCIS is really a "premalignant" condition, but probably at least one-third of patients with untreated DCIS develop invasive breast cancer within 5 years. However, many low-grade DCIS lesions do not appear to progress over many years; therefore, many patients are overtreated. Unfortunately, no reliable methods distinguish patients who require treatment from those who may be safely observed.

Mastectomy is nearly 100% effective in preventing a future breast cancer event in that breast and fundamentally can be considered prophylactic surgery, but is often not required for adequate treatment. No prospective randomized studies have directly compared breast-preserving therapy to mastectomy. However, the nearly 100% 10-year survival rates with the former suggest that it is a satisfactory strategy. Breast-preserving therapy refers to excisional surgery alone with or without breast radiation. However, although survival was identical in the two arms of a randomized trial comparing wide excision plus or minus irradiation, the latter caused a substantial reduction in the local recurrence rate as compared with wide excision alone. Addition of tamoxifen or an AI to any DCIS surgical/radiation therapy regimen further improves local control. However, in the largest trial comparing the two in DCIS, anastrozole did not improve distant disease-free or overall survival compared to tamoxifen.

Several prognostic features may help to identify patients at high risk for local recurrence after either lumpectomy alone or lumpectomy with radiation therapy and, therefore, might provide an indication for mastectomy. These include extensive disease within the breast; age <40; and cytologic features such as necrosis, poor nuclear grade, and comedo subtype with overexpression of *HER2*. In summary, it is reasonable to recommend breast-preserving surgery for patients who have a localized focus of DCIS with clear margins followed by breast irradiation and tamoxifen or anastrozole. Recently, a multifactorial gene expression assay has been shown to predict risk of recurrence in DCIS treated with breast-preserving surgery alone, but it is not clear that the in-breast risk recurrence rate in patients with low recurrence scores is sufficient to avoid radiation. The decision to irradiate such patients depends on the risk aversion to in-breast recurrence balanced against the risk associated with breast irradiation.

For patients with small, unicentric DCIS, axillary lymph node dissection is unnecessary. However, axillary sentinel lymph node (SLN) evaluation, which is discussed in greater detail below, may be indicated for widespread, larger, or poor grade DCIS or if microscopic invasion is identified on a core biopsy. In such cases, subsequent excision or mastectomy may demonstrate invasive disease on the larger specimen. Since SLN mapping is indicated in such patients, doing so at the time of excision or mastectomy avoids a further surgical procedure at a later date.

Lobular Carcinoma (Neoplasia) In Situ The presence of malignant cells within the lobules is termed *lobular carcinoma or neoplasia in situ* (LCIS). LCIS does not usually cause palpable breast masses, nor does it often induce suspicious findings on mammogram. Therefore, it usually is found as an incidental finding during pathologic examination of a breast biopsy performed for some other reason. Unlike DCIS, which is usually confined to a single area in a breast, LCIS is often spread throughout the breast, and it is frequently also found in the contralateral breast.

A diagnosis of LCIS itself does not confer a higher risk of mortality from breast cancer, but it does increase the risk of a subsequent breast cancer. Women with LCIS who do not undergo bilateral prophylactic mastectomy experience a new, invasive cancer in either breast at a rate of approximately 1% per year over at least the next 15–20 years, and probably lifelong. Therefore, LCIS is even more commonly considered a premalignant condition than DCIS, and aggressive local management seems unreasonable. Management options include careful observation with routine mammography and chemoprevention with either a SERM or an AI (for postmenopausal women) for 5 years. Beyond 5 years, such patients should be followed with subsequent annual mammography and semi-annual physical examinations. Bilateral prophylactic mastectomy is an alternative option, although it is no more effective in prolonging survival than the less aggressive approach, and it associated with substantial cosmetic, and perhaps emotional, morbidity.

INVASIVE BREAST CANCERS

Invasive breast cancers are of more concern than in situ lesions because they harbor the capacity to metastasize and cause substantial morbidity and mortality (Fig. 79-1). Eighty-five percent of invasive breast cancers are ductal in origin (Fig. 79-2), 10% are lobular or mixed ductal/lobular, and the other 5% are made up of so-called "special types" including mucinous or colloid (2.4%), tubular (1.5%), medullary (1.2%), and papillary (1%). Although not universally true, prognosis for the special types tends to be better than standard ductal or lobular cancers.

STAGING AND DIAGNOSTIC CONSIDERATIONS

Cancer staging has been traditionally based on the size of the tumor (T) and the presence or absence of regional nodal (N) and distant metastases (M). More recently, tumor grade and biological characteristics, such as expression of ER and HER2, have been incorporated into staging, making the system quite complex. Staging can be performed clinically or pathologically, before or after adjuvant systemic therapy. These are designated as a prefix before the stage as cTNM or pTNM if determined before or yTNM if determined after systemic (neoadjuvant) therapy. Although staging is an important part of the surgical evaluation and pathology reporting system, the specific elements that inform the clinician of both prognosis and likelihood of response to specific therapies have become more critical determinants of patient care than a simple stage designation. Importantly, imaging for detection of distant metastases is not needed in a patient with no signs or symptoms of widespread disease and who has a T3 or smaller tumor and fewer than four involved axillary lymph nodes, since the odds of finding distant metastases in such patients are low and the risk of false positives outweighs true-positive findings. Although finding bone marrow micrometastases or circulating tumor cells (cM0(i+)) has been associated with worse prognosis, how to integrate these into routine clinical care has not been determined, and their assessment is not recommended in patients with early-stage disease.

TREATMENT

Early-Stage Breast Cancer

GENERAL CONSIDERATIONS

Goals of Therapy The goal of therapy for breast cancer in patients who do not have obvious evidence of distant metastases (meaning outside the breast, chest wall, and regional lymph nodes) is cure, or at least substantial survival prolongation. For these patients, treatment strategies are divided into primary and systemic considerations. Primary therapies consist of surgical and radiation treatments directed toward the breast and locoregional lymph nodes. These approaches are designed to minimize the odds of locoregional recurrence while maintaining quality of life and cosmesis as much as possible by excising the cancer and sterilizing unaffected breast tissue as appropriate. Adjuvant systemic treatments, consisting of endocrine, anti-HER2, and/or chemotherapies, are given to treat micrometastases that may have already escaped to distant sites but are not yet detectable.

Prognostic and Predictive Factors All treatments for breast cancer are based on prognostic and predictive factors. Prognostic factors provide an indication of how likely a cancer will recur either locally or in distant organs in the future if a patient is not treated with the respective treatments. Predictive factors are used to determine if a given treatment is likely to work or not, assuming the patient's prognosis justifies treatment (or further treatment assuming the patient has been treated in some manner already).

Anatomic prognostic features include visual and physical examination findings of locally advanced breast cancer (T4 lesions: skin erythema ["inflammatory"] or edema ["peau d'orange"], nodules, or ulceration or tumor fixation to the chest wall). In patients without any of these findings, the most important prognostic features remain tumor size (T) and lymph node (N) status.

Biologic features, such as histologic tumor grade as well as ER, PgR, and HER2 status, are also prognostic. Indeed, gene expression patterns, or "signatures," have demonstrated that breast cancer is actually many different diseases and can be divided into a series of intrinsic subtypes. These subtypes are driven principally, although not exclusively, by expression of ER and HER2 and their respective associated pathways, as well as measures of cellular proliferation and other less important but still contributory biologic features. These intrinsic subtypes are important clinically, both in influencing natural history as well as in prognosis and therapeutic decision making. Four different intrinsic subtypes are recognized: luminal, HER2-like, basal, and claudin-low. Some, if not all, have been further divided into subgroups.

Luminal breast cancers are almost always positive for ER and negative for HER2 amplification. *Luminal A* tumors have the highest levels of ER and downstream related genes, are almost universally negative or low in HER2, are usually low grade, have low proliferative thrust, and have a generally favorable prognosis. They are most likely to respond to endocrine therapy and may appear to be less responsive to chemotherapy. *Luminal B* breast cancers tend to be PgR negative, may express HER2 but at low levels, are usually higher grade, and have higher proliferative activity than luminal A tumors. Prognosis is somewhat worse than for luminal A cancers, and although not yet proven, they may be more sensitive to chemotherapy.

HER2-amplified breast cancers exhibit co-amplification and overexpression of other genes adjacent to *HER2*. Historically, the clinical prognosis of such tumors was poor, but it has markedly improved with the introduction of targeted anti-HER2 therapies.

Basal breast cancers are mostly negative for expression of ER/PgR and HER2. Tumors of this type are often called "triple-negative" malignancies, although this is a general term, and such cancers have been further subgrouped based on other genetic abnormalities. They tend to be high grade and express cytokeratins 5/6 and 17 as well as vimentin, p63, CD10, α-smooth muscle actin, and epidermal growth factor receptor (EGFR). Patients with germline *BRCA1* mutations also usually fall within this molecular subtype.

Normal breast-like and *claudin-low* cancers have also been distinguished, but at present, these designations have failed to have clinical significance.

Over the past decade, several multiparameter tests based on gene expression have been developed to determine prognosis in patients who have node-negative, ER-positive, and HER2-negative disease. These assays have been principally used to guide decisions regarding use of adjuvant chemotherapy, as discussed below. Predictive features are usually used to guide targeted systemic therapies. These include ER for endocrine treatments and HER2 for anti-HER2 therapies, such as trastuzumab, and more recently *BRCA1/2* and *PIK3CA* mutations for poly (ADP ribose) polymerase (PARP) inhibitors and PIK3CA inhibitors, respectively.

LOCAL (PRIMARY) TREATMENTS

In the 1980s, the Halsted radical mastectomy was replaced with the less disfiguring modified radical mastectomy, in which chest wall muscles are preserved and only a sampling of axillary lymph nodes are removed. Subsequently, breast-conserving treatments, consisting of surgical excision of the primary tumor (lumpectomy, quadrantectomy, or partial mastectomy) often followed by locoregional radiation, were introduced and shown to have equal if not slightly superior outcomes to those associated with mastectomy. For women undergoing breast conservation, postlumpectomy radiation is usually indicated, although it may be less necessary in older women with ER-positive, node-negative breast cancer, since their risk of subsequent in-breast recurrence is quite low with surgery and endocrine therapy only. When lumpectomy with negative tumor margins is achieved and radiation is delivered appropriately, breast conservation is associated with a recurrence rate in the breast of ≤5%.

Not all patients are candidates for breast-conserving therapy. Contraindications include large tumor to breast ratio, inability to achieve clear margins with adequate cosmesis after extensive surgery, multifocal cancers, extensive four-quadrant DCIS, and inability to receive radiation. The latter issue arises in women with dermal autoimmune disease (such as lupus erythematosus), prior radiation to the site, and/or lack of available radiation treatment facilities. Further, although not contraindicated, breast-conserving therapy may be less cosmetically acceptable than mastectomy with reconstruction if the nipple-areolar complex is involved with cancer and must be sacrificed. This is a personal choice, and some women prefer mastectomy, especially those with high genetic risks for second breast cancers.

Enigmatically, in spite of the supporting data, only approximately one-third of women in the United States are managed by lumpectomy. It appears that many women still undergo mastectomy who could safely avoid this procedure and probably would if appropriately counseled. Most patients should consult with an experienced breast surgeon and radiation oncologist before making a final decision concerning local therapy. Indeed, a multimodality clinic in which the surgeon, radiation oncologist, medical oncologist, and other caregivers cooperate to evaluate the patient and develop a treatment plan is usually considered a major advantage by patients.

For patients who do undergo mastectomy, nipple-areolar-sparing mastectomy preserves the dermis and epidermis of the nipple but removes the major ducts from within the nipple lumen and often provides more acceptable cosmesis when combined with reconstruction. This approach is often a preferable option for patients who are having prophylactic surgery or those with cancer who are candidates for immediate reconstruction. Nipple-sparing mastectomy is contraindicated in the presence of inflammatory breast cancer, clinical involvement of the nipple-areolar complex, nipple retraction, Paget disease, bloody nipple discharge, or multicentricity. The safety of nipple-sparing mastectomy is based on retrospective, nonrandomized cohort series. In a meta-analysis of 20 studies (5594 patients), overall and disease-free survival and locoregional recurrence rates appeared similar to those of patients undergoing modified radical mastectomy.

After mastectomy, breast reconstruction is an acceptable option. Breast reconstruction can be achieved by either placement of an exogenous implant (usually silicon) or by transferring autologous tissue from another site, such as the abdomen, latissimus dorsi, or gluteal areas, to the breast. Of note, patients should be aware that a reconstructed breast is usually insensate. Risks of reconstruction include surgical complications such as infection and hemorrhage. Reconstruction does not hinder detection of future recurrences, nor is silicone implant reconstruction associated with non-cancer-related syndromes, although on occasion, these can rupture and removal is required. Breast implant–associated anaplastic large cell lymphoma is an extraordinarily rare complication of textured silicone implants. Although occasionally associated with metastatic lymphoma, it is usually confined locally and highly curable. The optimal choice of implant reconstruction should be made with an experienced breast plastic surgeon.

Postmastectomy chest wall and regional nodal radiation reduces locoregional recurrence and improves survival. It is indicated for patients with high risk of locoregional recurrence, such as those with tumors ≥5 cm, four or more positive axillary lymph nodes, or postoperative positive margins. Postmastectomy radiation is not indicated in women with cancers <2 cm, negative lymph nodes, and negative margins. It is considered for women who fall into the areas between these (2–5 cm, one to three positive nodes, or close margins) and is usually recommended if a patient has one to three involved axillary lymph nodes. Many radiation oncologists and plastic surgeons prefer postmastectomy radiation before reconstruction.

The survival of patients who have recurrence in the breast after proper treatment (adequate surgery and radiation if indicated) is somewhat worse than that of women who do not have in-breast recurrences, but it is better than those who suffer locoregional recurrence after mastectomy. Thus, locoregional recurrence is a negative prognostic variable for long-term survival but not the *cause* of distant metastasis.

Evaluation and Treatment of the Axillary Lymph Nodes SLN mapping and biopsy (SLNB) is generally the standard of care for women with localized breast cancer and clinically negative axilla. This procedure involves injecting a dye or radioactive tracer into the involved breast and, a few hours (4–24) later, undergoing resection of the axillary node containing the dye or tracer. If that lymph node is negative for tumor, more extensive axillary surgery is not required, avoiding much of the risk of postdissection lymphedema. Even in the presence of sentinel lymph node involvement, further axillary surgery may not be required for selected patients, such as older women and those with ER-positive cancers.

ADJUVANT SYSTEMIC THERAPIES

The use of adjuvant systemic therapy is based on the concept that with increasing generations of cellular replication, genetic abnormalities accumulate. These mutations occur randomly and may lead to sensitivity or resistance to therapies, but of course, the latter is of greater concern. Almost all patients with metastatic breast cancer are destined to die with, if not of, their cancer. However, treatment with the same therapies administered earlier, in the setting of micrometastatic disease only, is more effective than waiting until symptomatic, documented metastases occur and substantially improves survival. More than half of the women who would otherwise die of metastatic breast cancer remain disease-free and experience considerable survival advantage when treated with the appropriate adjuvant systemic regimen.

Prognostic and Predictive Variables Adjuvant systemic therapies are of three types: (1) chemotherapy; (2) endocrine therapy; and (3) anti-HER2 therapies. The decision of whether to apply adjuvant systemic therapy, and which type, depends on prognostic and predictive features as well as the combined judgment of the patient and caregiver.

Prognostic Factors As noted, prognostic factors help define who most likely needs, or perhaps more importantly does not need, adjuvant systemic therapy. In contrast, predictive factors help identify which therapies are likely to work, independent of prognosis (Table 79-1). The most important prognostic variables are provided by *tumor staging: tumor size (T), lymph node status (N), and detectable distant metastases (M)* (**Table 79-2**). *Histologic grading* is also important. Tumors with a poor nuclear grade (grade 3) have a higher risk of recurrence than tumors with a good nuclear grade (grade 1). Infiltrating lobular cancer, which is almost always ER positive, has roughly the same prognosis as ER-positive infiltrating ductal cancer, although the lobular subtype may be slightly worse. Lobular cancers are harder to detect on mammography and within axillary lymph nodes than ductal cancers, and when they do metastasize, they often spread to unusual sites, such as mesothelial surfaces, the ovaries, and gastrointestinal organs. Among the special types of breast cancer, pure tubular and mucinous cancers are associated with very favorable prognoses. Medullary cancers are often triple negative with poor nuclear grade, but paradoxically, they have a heavy infiltrating lymphocyte component, and they also have a favorable prognosis. However, before treatment is directed toward these types of cancers, their histology should be confirmed by an experienced breast pathologist.

Adjuvant systemic therapy may not be needed at all for patients with very small (<1 cm) tumors and negative lymph nodes. However, every patient with invasive breast cancer has some risk of subsequent distant metastases. Most patients are more likely to accept endocrine therapy for a very small potential benefit than they would accept chemotherapy for the same calculated advantage because the former is much less often associated with either life-threatening or permanently life-changing toxicities.

The greatest controversy concerns the recommendation for adjuvant *chemotherapy*. Since no established factor predicts sensitivity or resistance for this class of treatments, the decision must be made on prognosis alone. Overall, chemotherapy reduces the risk of recurrence over the 10 years subsequent to primary diagnosis by approximately one-third. For patients with T4 cancers or many positive lymph nodes, the risk of distant recurrence (and thus not being cured) in the subsequent decade is 50% or higher. Therefore, a one-third reduction of a 50% risk of recurrence means that at least 15–20% (one-third × 50%) of women will be cured who would not have been cured in the absence of adjuvant chemotherapy. The life-threatening or permanently life-changing toxicities of adjuvant chemotherapy are ~1–2%, and therefore, almost all medical oncologists would recommend adjuvant chemotherapy in this setting.

In contrast, adjuvant chemotherapy is rarely justified in most women with tumors <1 cm in size whose axillary lymph nodes are negative. However, this decision is very much influenced by the expression of ER and HER2. For example, the risk of recurrence of a patient with a small, node-negative but triple-negative breast cancer over the succeeding 10 years without any adjuvant therapy is 15%. If chemotherapy reduces this risk by approximately one-third or more, then approximately 5% or more of patients will be cured who would otherwise have died of their disease. Likewise, a patient with ER- and PgR-negative but HER2-*positive* disease has a slightly worse prognosis, with a risk of recurrence over 10 years of approximately 20%. She will benefit not only from the adjuvant chemotherapy but also from anti-HER2 therapy, so that her potential absolute benefit is even higher. Many, but not all, clinicians would recommend adjuvant chemotherapy for such patients.

On the other hand, patients with ER-positive disease have a better prognosis than those with ER-negative breast cancer, and adjuvant endocrine therapy will further reduce the odds of recurrence by approximately one-half. Therefore, the same patient in the example above (<1 cm, node negative) but who has an ER-positive and HER2-negative cancer has a lower initial risk of recurrence (~10% over 10 years). She is very likely to accept adjuvant endocrine therapy, further lowering her estimated risk of recurrence to ~5%. Even if chemotherapy reduces this residual risk by approximately one-third, no more than 1–2% (one-third × 5%) of patients will benefit. This potential benefit is approximately the same as the number of patients who will suffer life-threatening or permanently life-changing toxicities from chemotherapy. Thus, in this case, most clinicians would recommend adjuvant endocrine therapy but not chemotherapy.

Multiparameter gene expression assays have refined prognostic determination, particularly in node-negative, ER-positive, and HER2-negative breast cancers. These tests include the 21-gene Oncotype DX, the 12-gene Endopredict, the 58-gene ProSigna, and the 2-gene Breast Cancer Index. Furthermore, several investigators have reported that analysis of ER, PgR, HER2, and Ki67 by immunohistochemistry (IHC4) also provides prognostic information in this group, but the analytical validity of this assay is quite variable among different pathologists. Assuming adequate adjuvant endocrine therapy, the prognosis of such patients whose tumors have low recurrence scores, which usually identifies luminal A type cancers, with one of these assays is so good they can safely forego adjuvant chemotherapy. Indeed, the same is true for such patients with intermediate Oncotype DX recurrence scores. In contrast, those with high recurrence scores (>25) appear to have luminal B cancers, and the benefits of adjuvant chemotherapy clearly outweigh the risks.

The largest data set for directing care has been generated using the 21-gene recurrence score. However, only one of these tests should be ordered for a single patient, since they do not always give the same results, and there are no data to determine which, in the case of discordance, might be "correct." Use of these assays to determine prognosis in patients with higher anatomic stage, such as T3b/T4 lesions, or multiple positive lymph nodes, especially if more than three, is still under investigation.

Several *measures of tumor growth rate* correlate with early relapse, but their use is problematic due to analytical variability. Of these, assessment using immunohistochemical (IHC) assays for the proliferation marker Ki67 is the most widespread. However, substantial lab-to-lab variability and disagreement regarding optimal cut points exist. At present, in standard practice outside of a highly skilled laboratory, Ki67 expression is not used to make clinical decisions.

TABLE 79-2 5-Year Survival Rate for Breast Cancer by Stage

STAGE	5-YEAR SURVIVAL, %
0	99
I	92
IIA	82
IIB	65
IIIA	47
IIIB	44
IV	14

Source: Modified from data of the National Cancer Institute: Surveillance, Epidemiology, and End Results (SEER).

Predictive Factors The two most important predictive factors in breast cancer are ER and HER2 expression, and they should be performed on all primary or metastatic cancer biopsy specimens (Table 79-1). Adjuvant endocrine therapy reduces the risk of recurrence by one-half or more in patients with ER-rich cancers, whereas no detectable benefit is noted in patients with ER-poor or -negative cancers. ER is expressed as the percentage of positive cells within the cancer after IHC staining. Endocrine therapy is recommended for any patient with ≥10% positive cells, but not for those whose cancers only have 0–1% staining. The evidence supporting benefit in cases with 1–9% expression is weak, but given the potential benefit and relatively low toxicities of endocrine therapy, it is recommended for such patients with a low threshold for discontinuation if side effects are intolerable.

The HER2 protein is the target for anti-HER2-directed therapies. Adjuvant trastuzumab therapy reduces the risk of distant recurrence and death in patients with HER2-positive breast cancer by one-third or more but has no discernable effect on HER2-negative cancers. HER2 status is determined using either IHC staining for protein overexpression or fluorescent in situ hybridization (FISH) for gene amplification. IHC staining of 3+ (on a scale of 0–3+) is considered positive, whereas 0–1+ is considered negative. For cases with 2+ staining, reflex FISH analysis is recommended. FISH can either be used as the initial evaluation or for additional evaluation in IHC 2+ cases. *HER2* is considered amplified if the ratio of HER2 to centromere signal on chromosome 17 is ≥2.0. FISH is unnecessary if IHC is 3+ or 0–1+, nor is there reason for IHC testing if FISH is ≥2.0

No reliable predictive factors exist for chemotherapy in general or for specific types of chemotherapies. It has been hypothesized that chemotherapy may be more active in ER-negative and/or HER2-positive cancers. Luminal B cancers may be more chemotherapy sensitive, whereas luminal A cancers are perceived to be relatively chemotherapy resistant. At present, none of the tests for intrinsic subtype should be used to determine not to give chemotherapy to patients with poor anatomic *prognosis*, such as those with T4 or multiple positive nodes, based on *prediction* of resistance. Attempts to identify reliable predictive factors for individual classes of chemotherapeutic agents (such as anthracyclines, alkylating agents, or taxanes) have been unsuccessful. The platin salts (carboplatin, cisplatin) may have higher activity in patients with triple-negative breast cancer and perhaps in patients with HER2-positive disease. The PARP inhibitors may be more active in patients whose tumors have defects in homologous recombination DNA repair, a group that includes those with *BRCA* mutations.

Adjuvant Regimens • **Endocrine Therapy** Adjuvant endocrine therapy is indicated for nearly all patients with a diagnosis of ER-positive breast cancer and never for those with ER-negative disease. Two adjuvant endocrine therapy strategies are proven: the SERM tamoxifen or estrogen ablation. In addition to being effective in preventing new cancers and reducing the risk of locoregional recurrences in patients with DCIS, tamoxifen reduces the risk of distant recurrence and death due to invasive breast cancer by ~40% over the decade following diagnosis. It is equally effective in pre- and postmenopausal women, although it may be slightly less effective in very young (<40 years) patients. Because tamoxifen is a SERM, it has mixed ER antagonism (in the breast and brain) and agonism (in the bone, liver, and uterus). Therefore, it is active against breast cancer in the prevention, adjuvant, and metastatic settings.

Side effects of tamoxifen are predictable based on ER antagonism, including frequent hot flashes as well as vaginal discomfort/sexual dysfunction and myalgias and arthralgias. The agonistic effect results in reduction of osteopenia/osteoporosis, especially in postmenopausal women, but it increases thrombosis risk and endometrial cancers due to this effect in the liver and uterus, respectively.

Estrogen depletion can be achieved surgically in premenopausal women by oophorectomy or ovarian suppression with a gonadotropin-releasing hormone (GnRH) superagonist, such as goserelin or leuprolide, which invoke a tachyphylactic response, or a GnRH antagonist, such as triptorelin. However, women with nonfunctioning ovaries, whether induced or by natural menopause, still produce small amounts of estrogen by adrenal synthesis of estrogen precursors (testosterone, dehydroepiandrosterone [DHEA]). These are converted to estradiol and estrone by aromatase activity in peripheral fat and possibly cancer cells. In postmenopausal women, circulating estrogen can be reduced to nearly imperceptible levels with the use of oral AIs: anastrozole, letrozole, and exemestane. The three AIs are not significantly different in activity or toxicity. All are slightly more effective than tamoxifen.

Toxicities of the AIs are predictable based on very low estrogen levels. These include hot flashes, musculoskeletal symptoms, and atrophic vaginitis/sexual dysfunction. They also induce or worsen osteoporosis and fractures, although this effect can be abrogated with bone-modifying agents, such as bisphosphonates or rank ligand antagonists (denosumab).

For both tamoxifen and the AIs, musculoskeletal symptoms mimicking osteoarthritis and arthralgias can be treated with physical therapy and nonsteroidal anti-inflammatory drugs. After a brief period of washout after discontinuation, switching from one AI to another relieves this symptom in approximately a third of patients. These symptoms can also be reduced with either acupuncture or the antidepressant duloxetine. If AIs cannot be tolerated, tamoxifen is a reasonable therapy, assuming no contraindications, such as a past history of thrombosis or high risk of cerebrovascular disease. Hot flashes from either class of drugs are alleviated in approximately one-half of patients with use of one of several different antidepressant drugs.

For premenopausal women, optimal endocrine therapy depends on prognosis and patient choice. Complete estrogen depletion is slightly more effective than tamoxifen alone, but it may also be associated with more bothersome side effects, such as hot flashes, vaginal dryness, and sexual dysfunction. Complete estrogen depletion, consisting of either oophorectomy or chemical suppression of gonadotropins coupled with an AI, is indicated for women with worse prognosis, in particular node positivity. For those with more favorable prognosis, tamoxifen alone or with ovarian suppression is adequate and produces better quality of life. The AIs should not be administered to women with functioning, or dormant, ovaries, since the negative hypothalamic-pituitary feedback can result in a rebound overproduction of ovarian estrogens.

The duration of adjuvant endocrine treatment is unclear. Formerly, the standard recommendation was at least 5 years of therapy, which clearly reduces the risk of recurrence during that time and for a few years after discontinuation. However, the annual risk of distant recurrence during the subsequent 15 years is 0.5–3%, depending on the initial T and N status. Extended adjuvant endocrine therapy with either tamoxifen or an AI for at least 5 more years continues to reduce this late risk of relapse. The decision of whether to continue adjuvant endocrine therapy or not after 5 years must therefore take into consideration initial risk (T, N, grade), current side effects and potential cumulative toxicities, and the patient's perception of the relative and absolute benefits and risks.

Chemotherapy Multiple-agent adjuvant chemotherapy is more effective than single-agent chemotherapy. Although chemotherapeutic agents are usually delivered in combination, sequential single-agent chemotherapy is as effective, and may be slightly less toxic, although it requires longer total duration to deliver. Administration of four to six cycles of chemotherapy appears to be optimal; one cycle is less effective than six, but more than six cycles have generally increased toxicity without further efficacy. Importantly, although chemotherapy is combined with anti-HER2 therapy in patients with HER2-positive cancers, concurrent endocrine therapy, in particular tamoxifen, is antagonistic with chemotherapy.

Therefore, they are administered sequentially, starting the endocrine therapy after completion of chemotherapy.

Several chemotherapeutic agents have activity in the adjuvant setting. These include alkylating agents (principally cyclophosphamide), anthracyclines (doxorubicin, epirubicin), antimetabolites (5-fluoruracil [5-FU], capecitabine, methotrexate), the taxanes (paclitaxel, docetaxel), and the platinum salts (cisplatin, carboplatin). Within classes, randomized trials have failed to demonstrate superiority of one agent versus another (e.g., doxorubicin vs epirubicin, or paclitaxel vs docetaxel). Escalation above an optimal dose is not more effective. The antineoplastic advantage of more frequent scheduling for most individual agents has been demonstrated in a well-done meta-analysis. Weekly or every-other-week paclitaxel is superior to every-3-week infusion, whereas, enigmatically, the opposite is true for docetaxel. Taken together, the data support giving adjuvant chemotherapy in a dose-dense fashion.

The oldest combination regimen consists of cyclophosphamide, methotrexate, and 5-FU (CMF). Addition of an anthracycline or substitution of an anthracycline for the antimetabolites improves outcomes slightly, albeit with slightly increased risk of heart failure and secondary leukemia. Addition of a taxane to an anthracycline-based regimen further modestly reduces the chances of distant recurrence and death. Likewise, addition of an anthracycline to a taxane-based regimen is also modestly more effective than a taxane plus cyclophosphamide alone.

Which regimen is appropriate for a patient must be individualized based on prognosis, comorbid conditions, and the perspective of the patient. For example, the modest relative improvement of giving an anthracycline, cyclophosphamide, and a taxane (AC-T) may not translate to a sufficiently large absolute improvement in survival in a patient with a relatively small (T2) tumor and negative nodes, whereas that same relative reduction in death may translate to a sufficiently large absolute benefit in a patient with a worse prognosis. Therefore, the former patient might best be served with a taxane/cyclophosphamide (TC) regimen alone, while the latter might wish to accept the added risk of congestive heart failure and leukemia associated with the anthracyclines.

Neoadjuvant Chemotherapy Preoperative, or "neoadjuvant," treatment involves the administration of adjuvant systemic therapy, most commonly chemotherapy, before definitive surgery and radiation therapy. Neoadjuvant endocrine therapy for patients with ER-positive disease is usually given preoperatively for 4–6 months. However, it is generally reserved for patients for whom a reason for surgical delay exists, such as comorbid conditions.

The objective partial and complete response rates of patients with breast cancer to neoadjuvant chemotherapy range from 10 to 75% depending on the intrinsic subtype of the cancer and the regimen used. Thus, many patients will be "downstaged" by neoadjuvant chemotherapy. In this circumstance, patients with locally advanced, inoperable cancers may become candidates for surgery, and approximately 15% of patients who are not considered eligible for breast-conserving surgery may become so due to shrinkage of their cancer. However, overall survival has not been improved using this approach as compared with the same drugs given postoperatively.

Patients who achieve a pathologic complete remission (pCR) after neoadjuvant chemotherapy have a substantially improved survival compared to those who do not. It is unknown if this observation implies that the latter group did not benefit or just had a worse initial prognosis, yet still gained some benefit. Delivering more therapy to patients who do not have a pCR is appealing. However, it is possible that these patients have chemotherapy-resistant disease, and therefore, more chemotherapy may not be of value. Clearly nonchemotherapeutic strategies, such as adjuvant endocrine therapy if they have an ER-positive breast cancer and adjuvant anti-HER2 therapy if their cancer is HER2 positive, are warranted.

Adding or changing systemic therapies may benefit selected groups of patients who do not have a pCR. Approximately 6 months of a postsurgical oral fluoropyrimidine, capecitabine, reduces distant metastases in patients with triple-negative breast cancer who have residual disease after non-fluoropyrimidine-containing neoadjuvant chemotherapy. Similarly, postoperative therapy with an antibody-drug conjugate consisting of trastuzumab and the antitubulin emtansine (ado-trastuzumab emtansine) is superior to continuing unconjugated trastuzumab in patients with HER2-positive breast cancer who did not achieve pCR with preoperative chemotherapy and trastuzumab.

Chemotherapy Toxicities Chemotherapy is associated with nausea, vomiting, and alopecia in nearly 100% of patients. Nausea and vomiting are usually well controlled with modern antiemetics. Small but convincing studies have suggested that the strategy of constricting blood flow to the scalp with various means of cooling is commonly effective in sparing hair loss, without evidence of increased scalp metastases.

More importantly, chemotherapy causes potential life-threatening or life-changing toxicities in 2–3% of all treated patients. These include neutropenia and fever, with a risk of infection of ~1%, which can be prevented with appropriate use of the growth factor filgrastim. Secondary myelodysplasia and leukemia occur in ~0.5–1% of patients treated with anthracyclines as well as with high cumulative doses of cyclophosphamide, usually occurring within 2–5 years of treatment. The anthracyclines cause cumulative dose-related congestive heart failure, which occurs in ~1% of patients treated with standard four to five cycles at 60 mg/m^2. Peripheral neuropathy is the major dose-limiting and life-changing toxicity of the taxanes. Neuropathy occurs during treatment in ~15–20% of patients, and permanent, chronic neuropathy persists in 3–5%. Many patients complain of cognitive dysfunction, so-called "chemo-brain." Although occasional cases of apparent organic chemotherapeutic toxic effects on cognitive function are noted, much of this syndrome may be due to anxiety, depression, and fatigue caused by the diagnosis itself or the treatment for it. Although not always, cognitive functioning usually returns to age-adjusted baseline several months after discontinuation of therapy.

Anti-HER2 Therapy The humanized anti-HER2 monoclonal antibody trastuzumab decreases both risk of recurrence and mortality in early-stage breast cancer. Trastuzumab is optimally delivered concurrently with chemotherapy, particularly in association with a taxane. Concurrent treatment with an anthracycline is generally avoided, since the main toxicity of trastuzumab is cardiac dysfunction, which appears more often when the agent is delivered simultaneously with doxorubicin. In patients with reasonably favorable prognosis (T1 or T2, node negative), single-agent paclitaxel plus trastuzumab is an adequate regimen. The addition of a second anti-HER2 monoclonal antibody, pertuzumab, in combination with trastuzumab is modestly superior to trastuzumab alone. When given in the neoadjuvant setting, this combination results in higher pCR rates than single-agent trastuzumab. At least in patients with poor prognostic features, such as positive axillary lymph nodes, the combination significantly reduces distant metastases and perhaps mortality. As noted, neoadjuvant studies have demonstrated that postoperative ado-trastuzumab emtansine is superior to trastuzumab in patients who do not achieve a pCR.

Trastuzumab is administered intravenously weekly or every 3 weeks. Twelve months of trastuzumab therapy are optimal with no additional benefit beyond 12 months. Treatment for 6 months is more effective than no trastuzumab therapy but is inferior to 12 months. A preparation of trastuzumab for subcutaneous injection has been approved by the U.S. Food and Drug Administration.

Selected anti-HER2 tyrosine kinase inhibitors have activity against HER2-positive breast cancer, but their benefit in the adjuvant setting is limited. Lapatinib does not add to trastuzumab therapy, and single-agent adjuvant lapatinib is inferior to single-agent trastuzumab. Another anti-HER2 tyrosine kinase inhibitor, neratinib, is modestly superior to no anti-HER2 therapy. Neratinib has not been compared to trastuzumab either as a single agent or in combination.

Toxicities of Anti-HER2 Adjuvant Therapies In general, the anti-HER2 therapies are safe and effective. Occasionally patients experience allergic reactions to an initial cycle of trastuzumab, but these usually do not recur. Trastuzumab can cause cardiac muscle dysfunction, although it is rare to observe symptomatic congestive heart failure from adjuvant trastuzumab. Baseline and serial echocardiographic monitoring is indicated. Patients with a past history of cardiac abnormalities should not receive trastuzumab or should be followed and treated by a cardiologist with experience in this condition. Pertuzumab is associated with loose stools and diarrhea, which can usually be managed with antidiarrheal therapy, such as loperamide. The chemotherapy payload of ado-trastuzumab emtansine can cause thrombocytopenia and peripheral neuropathy.

Skeletal Strengthening Agents Bone-strengthening agents that are commonly used to treat osteoporosis, specifically the bisphosphonates, have some limited activity in preventing recurrent breast cancer to bone, particularly in postmenopausal women. In addition, bisphosphonate therapy also reduced breast cancer mortality in this subgroup. The benefit is not significantly associated with any specific bisphosphonate class, treatment schedule, ER status, nodal status, tumor grade, or concomitant chemotherapy. As expected, bone fractures are reduced (relative risk [RR] 0.85; 95% confidence interval [CI] 0.75–0.97; 2 $p = .02$). Joint guidelines from the American Society of Clinical Oncology and Cancer Care Ontario recommend "that, if available, zoledronic acid (4 mg intravenously every 6 months) or clodronate (1,600 mg/d orally) be considered as adjuvant therapy for postmenopausal patients with breast cancer who are deemed candidates for adjuvant systemic therapy. Further research comparing different bone-modifying agents, doses, dosing intervals, and durations is required." The rank-ligand inhibitor denosumab does not prevent relapse in bone or other sites, nor does it reduce mortality.

Novel Adjuvant Systemic Agents Other exciting adjuvant strategies are being tested (Table 79-1). These include PARP inhibitors (olaparib, talazoparib) in patients with known germline *BRCA1* or *BRCA2* mutations or those with triple-negative cancers that share similar defects in DNA repair in their etiology. Likewise, the mTOR inhibitor everolimus and the CDK4/6 inhibitors (palbociclib, ribociclib, abemociclib) are being tested in the adjuvant setting in combination with antiestrogen therapy. The remarkable results of immune checkpoint inhibitors in other cancers have led to studies of this approach in both metastatic and post-neoadjuvant chemotherapy settings. Their activity with chemotherapy in triple-negative disease appears promising.

STAGE III BREAST CANCER

Ten to 25% of patients present with so-called locally advanced or stage III breast cancer at diagnosis. Many of these cancers are technically operable (T3), whereas others, particularly cancers with chest wall involvement, inflammatory breast cancers, or cancers with large matted axillary lymph nodes (T4 or N2-3), cannot be managed with surgery initially. Neoadjuvant downstaging facilitates local therapy. Radiotherapy either to the chest wall after mastectomy or to the breast after tumor excision is almost always recommended, as is regional lymph node treatment. Adjuvant anti-HER2 and endocrine therapies are also used as appropriate. These patients should be managed in multimodality clinics to coordinate local and systemic therapies. Such approaches produce long-term disease-free survival in ~30–50% of patients.

SIMULTANEOUS NEW PRIMARY WITH DETECTABLE METASTASES

In the screening era, only a small fraction of patients (~5%) present with a new primary lesion and simultaneous metastases, detected either due to symptoms of distant disease or because they had staging scans due to locally advanced disease. Several retrospective single-institutional experiences have suggested that neoadjuvant systemic therapy followed by local therapy (breast surgery and radiation) is associated with prolonged survival. However, two prospective randomized trials have failed to demonstrate any survival benefit. Currently, local therapy for such patients is considered on a case-by-case basis depending on the response to systemic therapy and the patient's overall performance status and desires.

BREAST CANCER SURVIVORSHIP ISSUES

The odds of surviving breast cancer have increased dramatically over the past 35 years due to a combination of early detection and more effective therapies. Without these advances, >60,000 American women would have suffered breast cancer mortality in 2020, and over one-quarter million women are alive who would not have been otherwise. Coupled with the women who would have been cured even before the impressive advances of the past three decades, millions are breast cancer survivors. Thus, all clinicians, not just oncologists, need to be aware of survivorship issues in patients with previously diagnosed and treated breast cancer.

At present, no special follow-up procedures, such as serial circulating tumor biomarkers or systemic radiographic/scintigraphic imaging, are indicated in an asymptomatic patient with no physical findings of recurrence. Although randomized trials have demonstrated slightly higher incidence of detection of metastases with lead times of 3–12 months by surveillance of asymptomatic patients compared to no special follow-up, no evidence suggests that earlier detection improves overall survival. If anything, such surveillance may worsen quality of life due to higher anxiety levels associated with the testing and toxicities associated with earlier treatment in patients who were otherwise doing well at that time.

However, the risk of late metastases in breast cancer survivors is small but real, especially those who had ER-positive disease. These patients remain at risk for distant recurrence for at least 20 years after initial diagnosis, and probably lifelong. The annual risk is relentless, ranging from 0.5% per year for patients with initially negative lymph nodes and grade 1 tumors <1 cm to as high as 3% per year for those who initially had multiple positive lymph nodes. Therefore, especially in patients with prior ER-positive cancers, the physician must carefully assess and evaluate new symptoms, considering whether they might be due to the cancer, the treatment, or an unassociated condition. Judgment needs to be used to decide if blood tests or imaging are required in order to avoid missing a lesion for which appropriate treatment would improve the patient's quality of life but also to diminish overtesting, with associated inconvenience, anxieties, false-positive results, and cost. Serial echocardiography should be performed every 3 months for patients on adjuvant trastuzumab, but not after it is discontinued.

Several observations suggest that perhaps the recommendations not to do intensive surveillance in patients without signs or symptoms of recurrence might need to be reconsidered. First, the unrelenting annual incidence of long-term distant recurrence for patients with ER-positive disease demonstrates that none of these patients can ever be considered free of risk of metastases. Second, available diagnostic tests have become substantially more sophisticated in the past decade. These include the advent of liquid biopsies beyond just circulating protein markers, such as circulating tumor DNA and circulating tumor cells, as well as more sensitive and specific scintigraphic and imaging techniques, such as positron emission tomography. Finally, the identification of several highly effective targeted therapies, including new endocrine, anti-HER2, and other therapies, provides opportunities to deliver more beneficial and less toxic therapies than the few chemotherapeutic and endocrine agents that were available at the time the older randomized trials were performed (Table 79-1). Ongoing trials are addressing whether incorporating these new technologies and treatments might improve survival as opposed to waiting for emerging symptoms to initiate additional treatment strategies. At present, no clear answers are apparent.

Likewise, serial monitoring for long-term, life-threatening toxicities associated with chemotherapy, such as myelodysplastic syndromes or congestive heart failure, is not warranted since these are quite uncommon and likely to cause obvious symptoms requiring proper evaluation if they occur.

For patients on endocrine therapy, quality-of-life issues may be critical, including hot flashes, sexual difficulties, musculoskeletal complaints, and risk of osteoporosis. Although estrogen therapy, given orally, transdermally, or transvaginally, effectively reduces these side effects, careful consideration should be given for estrogen replacement therapy to these patients because it may counteract the efficacy of the endocrine therapy. Locally administered therapies are often very effective and likely less risky. Nonhormonal treatments, such as selected antidepressants for hot flashes and musculoskeletal symptoms, and counseling and water-based lubricants for sexual issues can be quite helpful. It is important to screen bone density in patients on an AI more frequently than is recommended for the average postmenopausal woman, since total estrogen depletion results in enhanced risk of osteoporosis and risk of fracture. All women should be counseled to take daily calcium and vitamin D replacement, and if osteoporosis is present or osteopenia is worsening, bone-strengthening agents should be administered.

METASTATIC DISEASE

Diagnostic Considerations (Fig. 79-3) About 15–20% of patients treated for localized breast cancer develop metastatic disease in the subsequent decade after diagnosis. Soft tissue, bone, and visceral (lung and liver) metastases each account for approximately one-third of sites of initial relapses. However, by the time of death, most patients will have bone involvement. Recurrences can appear at any time after primary therapy, but at least half occur >5 years after initial therapy, especially in patients with ER-positive disease. A variety of host factors can influence recurrence rates, including depression and central obesity, and these diseases should be managed as aggressively as possible.

For patients with no prior history of metastases, a biopsy of suspicious physical or radiographic lesions should be performed for confirmation that the lesion does represent recurrent cancer. One should not assume that an apparent abnormality is a breast cancer metastasis. Many benign conditions, such as tuberculosis, gallstones, sarcoidosis, hyperparathyroidism, or other nonmalignant diseases, can mimic a recurrent breast cancer and are of course treated much differently. Moreover, if biopsy is positive for metastases, re-evaluation of ER and HER2 is indicated, since these can differ between the primary and metastatic lesions in up to 15% of cases. Analysis for *PIK3CA* mutations should be performed if the cancer is ER positive. Predictors of immune checkpoint inhibitor susceptibility, such as PD-L1 expression, should be determined in triple-negative metastatic breast cancers (Table 79-1). Many experts are also recommending some form of next-generation sequencing of all metastatic cancers from any site, although this recommendation is controversial.

Once a recurrence/metastasis is established, some form of body imaging should be performed—either a scintigraphic bone scan and chest and abdomen CT scan or a positron emission tomography (PET)/CT scan, depending on caregiver's preference. Brain scanning (CT or MRI) is not indicated in the absence of any cognitive or neurologic signs or symptoms in most patients. However, because of increased risk of brain metastases in HER2-positive breast cancer, some experts do recommend central nervous system (CNS) imaging in such patients even in the absence of clinical indications. Regardless, body scans provide a perspective of extent of disease, which may guide therapeutic decisions, as well as the need for ancillary treatments, such as bone-modifying agents if skeletal metastases are present.

Considerations Regarding Goals of Therapy Although treatable, metastatic disease is rarely if ever cured. The median survival for all patients diagnosed with metastatic breast cancer is <3 years, but with remarkable variability depending on intrinsic subtype and treatment effects. Patients with triple-negative metastatic breast cancer have the shortest expected survival, whereas those with ER-positive disease can expect to live the longest. HER2 positivity was initially found to be a very poor prognostic factor in metastatic breast cancer, but the availability of several effective targeted treatments has improved the expected survival rates to at least those of ER-positive patients, if not better.

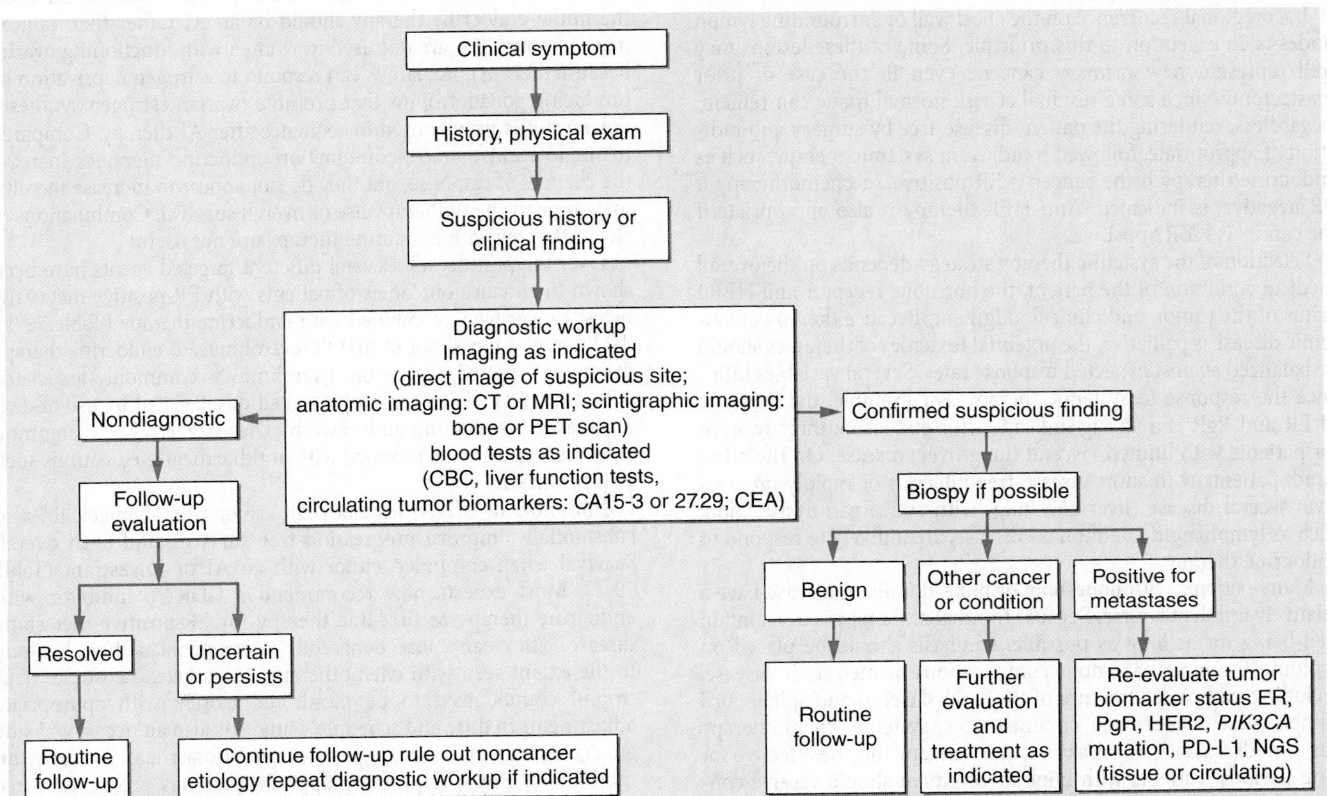

FIGURE 79-3 Evaluation of new signs or symptoms in a patient with prior history of early-stage breast cancer. See text for details. CBC, complete blood count; CEA, carcinoembryonic antigen; ER, estrogen receptor; NGS, next-generation sequencing; PET, positron emission tomography; PgR, progesterone receptor.

The overall goal of treatment of metastatic disease is palliation or, put simply, to "keep the patient feeling as well as she can for as long as she can." A secondary goal is improved survival. Overall survival has not been improved by advocating more aggressive or toxic therapies, such as high-dose or combination chemotherapy, but rather by using more selective and biologically based therapy, including endocrine or anti-HER2 therapies in patients with ER- or HER2-positive breast cancers, respectively.

Generally, a new treatment is continued until either progression or unacceptable toxicities are evident. These are both evaluated by serial history and physical examinations and periodic serologic evaluation for hematologic or hepatic abnormalities, as well as circulating tumor biomarker tests (assays for MUC1 [CA15-3 or CA27.29] and for carcinoembryonic antigen [CEA] and occasionally CA125). If all these evaluations fail to suggest progression, it is unlikely that imaging will contribute. However, if one or more of these suggest progression, whole-body imaging with whichever modality(ies) was used at baseline is indicated.

The choice of therapy requires consideration of local therapy needs, specifically surgical approaches to particularly worrisome long-bone lytic lesions or isolated CNS metastases. New back pain in patients with breast cancer should be explored aggressively on an emergent basis, usually with a spine MRI; to wait for neurologic symptoms is a potentially catastrophic error. Metastatic involvement of endocrine organs can occasionally cause profound dysfunction, including adrenal insufficiency and hypopituitarism. Similarly, obstruction of the biliary tree or other impaired organ function may be better managed with a local therapy than with a systemic approach. Radiation as an adjunct to or instead of surgery is an important consideration for particularly symptomatic disease in long or vertebral bones, locoregional recurrences, and CNS metastases. In many cases, systemic therapy can be withheld while the patient is managed with appropriate local therapy.

Aggressive local treatment, such as excision, radiation, radiofrequency ablation, or cryotherapy of metastases to the lung, liver, or other distant sites, does not improve survival. Although appealing, these strategies are associated with increased toxicity and cost and should be reserved for palliation.

Locoregional recurrence on the chest wall or surrounding lymph nodes is an exception to this principle. Some of these lesions may well represent new primary cancers, even in the case of prior mastectomy, since some residual at-risk normal tissue can remain. Regardless, rendering the patient disease-free by surgery and radiation, if appropriate, followed by adjuvant systemic therapy, such as endocrine therapy if the cancer is ER positive, or chemotherapy if ER negative, is indicated. Anti-HER therapy is also appropriate if the cancer is HER2 positive.

Selection of the systemic therapy strategy depends on the overall medical condition of the patient, the hormone receptor and HER2 status of the tumor, and clinical judgment. Because therapy of systemic disease is palliative, the potential toxicities of therapies should be balanced against expected response rates. Several variables influence the response to systemic therapy. For example, the presence of ER and PgR is a strong indication for endocrine therapy, even for patients with limited visceral (lung/liver) disease. On the other hand, patients with short disease-free intervals or rapidly progressive visceral disease (liver and lung) with end-organ dysfunction, such as lymphangitic pulmonary disease, are unlikely to respond to endocrine therapy.

Many patients with bone-only or bone-dominant disease have a relatively indolent course. Because the goal of therapy is to maintain well-being for as long as possible, emphasis should be placed on avoiding the most hazardous complications of metastatic disease, including pathologic fracture of the axial skeleton and spinal cord compression. Under such circumstances, systemic chemotherapy has a modest effect, whereas radiation therapy may be effective for long periods. Patients with bone involvement should receive concurrent bone-strengthening agents, such as bisphosphonates or the humanized monoclonal anti-RANK ligand antibody denosumab. These therapies have been proven to reduce bone pain, fractures, and hypercalcemia of malignancy.

Many patients are inappropriately treated with toxic regimens into their last days of life. Often, oncologists are unwilling to have the difficult conversations that are required with patients nearing the end of life, and not uncommonly, patients and families can pressure physicians into treatments with very little survival value. Although systemic therapy is designed to deliver palliation, formal palliative care consultation and realistic assessment of treatment expectations need to be reviewed with patients and families. We urge consideration of formal palliative care consultations for patients who have received at least two lines of therapy for metastatic disease.

SYSTEMIC TREATMENTS FOR METASTATIC BREAST CANCER

Endocrine Therapy (Table 79-1) Approximately 30–70% of patients with ER-positive breast cancer will benefit from endocrine therapy. Potential endocrine therapies are summarized in Table 79-1. Available strategies include SERMs (tamoxifen, toremifene), the AIs (anastrozole, letrozole, exemestane), and the selective estrogen receptor downregulator (SERD) fulvestrant. Additive endocrine therapies, including treatment with progestins and androgens and, enigmatically, pharmacologic doses of estrogens, are all active, but they may be associated with unacceptable side effects in many women and are rarely used. Tamoxifen withdrawal (as well as withdrawal of pharmacologic doses of estrogens) induces responses in ~15% of patients, but with the advent of so many other therapies for metastatic disease, this strategy is also rarely used in modern oncology.

The sequence of endocrine therapy is variable. Patients who respond to one endocrine therapy have at least a 50% chance of responding to a second endocrine therapy. It is not uncommon for patients to respond to two or three sequential endocrine therapies. Many, but not all, women with ER-positive breast cancer who suffer a recurrence will do so either while still taking or after recently discontinuing a prior adjuvant endocrine therapy (either tamoxifen or an AI). In most postmenopausal patients, if they have never received an AI or discontinued adjuvant AI many years before recurrence, the initial endocrine therapy should be an AI rather than tamoxifen. As noted, AIs are not used in women with functioning ovaries because their hypothalamus can respond to estrogen deprivation by producing gonadotropins that promote ovarian estrogen synthesis. Fulvestrant is usually used in sequence after AI therapy. Compared to single-agent therapy, combination endocrine therapies increase the chances of response, but they do not appear to increase the ultimate time to chemotherapy use or overall survival. Combinations of chemotherapy with endocrine therapy are not useful.

Over the past decade, several different targeted agents have been shown to enhance outcomes of patients with ER-positive metastatic breast cancer when combined with endocrine therapy (Table 79-1). Addition of an inhibitor of mTOR, everolimus, to endocrine therapy improves time to progression. Everolimus is commonly associated with mucositis, which can be prevented or alleviated by use of dexamethasone-containing mouthwash. Diarrhea is also a common side effect and can be lessened with antidiarrheal medications such as loperamide.

Inhibitors of CDK4/6 (palbociclib, ribociclib, abemaciclib) also substantially improve progression-free survival, and even overall survival when combined either with an AI or fulvestrant (Table 79-1). Most experts now recommend a CDK4/6 inhibitor with endocrine therapy as first-line therapy for ER-positive metastatic disease. They can cause dangerous neutropenia, although rarely to the extent seen with chemotherapy. Nonetheless, absolute neutrophil counts need to be monitored closely with appropriate adjustments in dose and schedule. Fatigue is also an occasional side effect, and abemaciclib frequently causes diarrhea. Similarly, an inhibitor of PIK3CA protein, alpelisib, prolongs progression-free survival in patients whose cancers harbor activating mutations of this gene. Like everolimus, it too causes mouth sores and diarrhea.

These targeted agents should not be given simultaneously but rather in sequence as appropriate.

Chemotherapy Unlike many other epithelial malignancies, breast cancer responds to multiple chemotherapeutic agents, including anthracyclines, alkylating agents, taxanes, and antimetabolites. Multiple combinations of these agents have been found to improve response rates somewhat, but they have had little effect on duration of response or survival. Unless patients have rapidly progressive visceral (lung, liver) metastases with end-organ dysfunction, single-agent chemotherapy is preferable, used in sequence as one drug fails going on to the next. Given the significant toxicity of most drugs, the use of a single-agent therapy will minimize toxicity by sparing the patient exposure to drugs that would be of little value. No method to select the drugs most efficacious for a given patient has been demonstrated to be useful.

Most oncologists use capecitabine, an anthracycline, or a taxane for first-line chemotherapy, either in a patient with ER-positive disease that is refractory to endocrine therapy or for a patient with ER-negative breast cancer. Within these general classes, one particular agent is no more preferable than another (such as doxorubicin vs epirubicin or paclitaxel vs docetaxel), and the choice has to be balanced with individual needs. Objective responses in previously treated patients may also be seen with gemcitabine, vinorelbine, and oral etoposide, as well as a newer class of agents, epothilones. Platinum-based agents have become far more widely used in both the adjuvant and advanced disease settings for some breast cancers, particularly those of the triple-negative subtype.

Anti-HER2 Therapy (Table 79-1) Initial use of a trastuzumab, either alone or with chemotherapy, improves response rate, progression-free survival, and even overall survival for women with HER2-positive disease. Indeed, anecdotal reports suggest that, on occasion, a few patients with HER2-positive metastatic breast cancer may be cured. Addition of pertuzumab to trastuzumab is more effective than trastuzumab alone. The antibody-drug conjugate, ado-trastuzumab emtansine, is effective after progression on trastuzumab. Another antibody-drug conjugate, fam-trastuzumab-deruxtecan-nxki, has been shown to be active even in patients who have progressed on multiple other anti-HER2 therapies, including ado-trastuzumab emtansine. A monoclonal antibody, margetuximab, has been engineered to specifically enhance antibody-dependent cell-mediated cytotoxicity against tumor cells overexpressing HER2. In a phase 3 trial, margetuximab plus chemotherapy improved overall survival by 1.8 months compared with trastuzumab plus chemotherapy.

Inhibitors of the HER2 tyrosine kinase domain also have activity against HER2-positive breast cancers. Lapatinib is effective when added to chemotherapy after patients progressed on trastuzumab. In addition, even after progression on trastuzumab, combination trastuzumab and lapatinib is superior to lapatinib alone. When added to oral capecitabine, neratinib is more effective than lapatinib in patients who received two or more prior anti-HER2-based regimens. In patients with heavily pretreated HER2-positive disease, including those with brain metastases, adding tucatinib to trastuzumab and capecitabine resulted in better progression-free survival and overall survival outcomes than adding placebo. Of interest, 2–3% of breast cancers that do not amplify or overexpress HER2 contain activating mutations in the gene encoding for it. Preclinical models and preliminary trials suggest that neratinib is particularly active against this mutation.

PARP Inhibitors (Table 79-1) PARP inhibitors induce synthetic lethality of cancer cells with inactive *BRCA1/2* or cancers that have *BRCA*-like biology by virtue of an ineffective homologous recombination DNA repair mechanism. Both olaparib and tolaparib have been approved for patients whose cancers have developed in the context of germline *BRCA1/2* mutations. Both agents, given as a single agent, are as effective as standard chemotherapy, but in general, they are less toxic. Unfortunately, responses are relatively short lived. PARP inhibitors are now being investigated in combination with chemotherapy and with immune checkpoint inhibitors. PARP inhibitors can cause mild nausea and occasional vomiting as well as fatigue.

Sacituzumab Govitecan (Table 79-1) An antibody-drug conjugate, sacituzumab govitecan, showed activity in a nonrandomized trial of patients with triple-negative metastatic breast cancer. Sacituzumab govitecan combines a humanized immunoglobulin G antibody targeted against TROP-2SN-38 with the active metabolite of irinotecan. In a single-arm, phase 2 trial, this agent elicited responses in one-third of such patients.

Immune Checkpoint Inhibitors (Table 79-1) These therapies permit immune effector cells to recognize and eliminate host cancer cells based on their recognition of neoantigen expression in tumor cells due to chromosomal instability and accumulated mutations. The excitement over immune checkpoint inhibitors has spread to metastatic breast cancer, especially of the triple-negative subtype. Atezolizumab in combination with nab-paclitaxel improves progression-free and perhaps overall survival, although exclusively against cancers with infiltrating immune cells that express PD-L1 (Table 79-1). The side effects of these agents can be life threatening, consisting of induction of inflammatory autoimmune responses in nearly every organ imaginable. These include thyroiditis, pneumonitis, myo- and pericarditis, esophagitis, gastritis and colitis, hepatitis, pancreatitis, hypophysitis, and dermatitis. The endocrine toxicities tend to be irreversible. Careful management should be handled by an experienced team.

Bone-Modifying Agents Bone-modifying agents, such as bisphosphonates or the anti-RANK antibody denosumab, are recommended for all patients with bone metastases. These agents substantially reduce the incidence of cancer-related skeletal events, such as bone pain, fracture, and hypercalcemia of malignancy. The bisphosphonates may cause myalgias and skeletal pain lasting a few hours to days after infusion. Both strategies have been associated with osteonecrosis of the jaw. The incidence of this complication is reduced by ensuring adequate dentition before treatment and by delivering treatment every 3 months, instead of monthly. The former has been shown to have equal efficacy.

BREAST CANCER IN PREGNANCY

As noted, breast cancer is unusual during pregnancy but does occur. Because of pregnancy-related physical breast changes, diagnosis is frequently delayed. Workup is the same as for non-pregnancy-related breast cancers, except radiographic staging should be limited or avoided, especially of the abdomen. Prognosis is similar, stage for stage, as that for age-matched women who are not pregnant. Pregnancy termination is usually not required. However, it is strongly advised that the patient be referred to a high-risk pregnancy program.

Remarkably, adjuvant chemotherapy including doxorubicin and cyclophosphamide can be safely given beyond the first trimester. Taxanes and the platinum salts may be administered safely. In contrast, anti-HER2 antibody therapies have resulted in unacceptable fetal malformations and pregnancy complications and should be avoided. Likewise, endocrine therapies should be delayed until after delivery. In general, a reasonable strategy is to deliver combination neoadjuvant chemotherapy with either concurrent or sequential single agents to permit sufficient embryogenesis followed by delivery and then breast primary therapy (surgery/radiation). Further adjuvant therapies, including additional chemotherapy and/or anti-HER2 and endocrine therapies can be delivered postoperatively. Breast feeding is discouraged, since these agents may cross into milk.

MALE BREAST CANCER

Breast cancer is ~1/150th as frequent in men as in women; ~2000 men developed breast cancer annually in the United States. Risk factors include inherited deleterious SNPs in *BRCA2*, as well as increased exposure to endogenous or exogenous estrogen. Men with Klinefelter's syndrome have two or more copies of the X chromosome and have higher levels of estrogen. Other conditions of hyperestrogenism, such as in hepatic failure and with exogenous estrogen use in transgender situations, are also associated with higher risk of male breast cancers. However, the vast majority of men who present with breast cancer have none of these conditions.

Breast cancer usually presents in men as a unilateral lump in the breast and is frequently not diagnosed promptly. Given the small amount of soft tissue and the unexpected nature of the problem, locally advanced presentations are somewhat more common. Although gynecomastia may initially be unilateral or asymmetric, any unilateral mass in a man >40 years old should be biopsied. On the other hand, bilateral symmetric breast development rarely represents breast cancer and is almost invariably due to endocrine disease or a drug effect. Nevertheless, the risk of cancer is much greater in men with gynecomastia; in such men, gross asymmetry of the breasts should arouse suspicion of cancer.

Approximately 90% of male breast cancers contain ERs, and the disease behaves similarly to that in a postmenopausal woman. When matched to female breast cancer by age and stage, its overall prognosis is identical. Male breast cancer is best managed by mastectomy and axillary lymph node dissection or SLNB, although some men prefer breast-conserving therapy. Patients with locally advanced disease or positive nodes should also be treated with irradiation. No randomized studies have evaluated adjuvant therapy for male breast cancer, but extrapolation from treatment with women suggests it is indicated. If the cancer is ER positive, which is often the case, tamoxifen is usually the agent of choice. AIs are also effective in men. Anecdotal evidence supports use of gonadotropin-releasing hormones, such as leuprolide, in combination with an AI, since testosterone is a substrate for the aromatase enzyme. The sites of relapse and spectrum of response to chemotherapeutic drugs are virtually identical for breast cancers in either sex.

FURTHER READING

Allison KH et al: Estrogen and Progesterone Receptor Testing in Breast Cancer: American Society of Clinical Oncology/College of American Pathologists Guideline Update. Arch Pathol Lab Med 2020.

Burstein HJ et al: Customizing local and systemic therapies for women with early breast cancer: the St. Gallen International Consensus Guidelines for treatment of early breast cancer 2021. Ann Oncol 32:1216, 2021.

Cardoso F et al: 3rd ESO-ESMO international consensus guidelines for Advanced Breast Cancer (ABC 3). Breast 31:244, 2017.

Dhesy-Thind S et al: Use of Adjuvant Bisphosphonates and Other Bone-Modifying Agents in Breast Cancer: A Cancer Care Ontario and American Society of Clinical Oncology Clinical Practice Guideline. J Clin Oncol 35:2062, 2017.

Harris LN et al: Use of Biomarkers to Guide Decisions on Adjuvant Systemic Therapy for Women With Early-Stage Invasive Breast Cancer: American Society of Clinical Oncology Clinical Practice Guideline. J Clin Oncol 34:1134, 2016.

Pan K et al: Breast cancer survivorship: state of the science. Breast Cancer Res Treat 168:593, 2018.

Qaseem A et al: Screening for Breast Cancer in Average-Risk Women: A Guidance Statement From the American College of Physicians. Ann Intern Med 170:547, 2019.

Samadder NJ et al: Hereditary Cancer Syndromes-A Primer on Diagnosis and Management: Part 1: Breast-Ovarian Cancer Syndromes. Mayo Clin Proc 94:1084, 2019.

Schmid P et al: Pembrolizumab for early triple-negative breast cancer. N Engl J Med 382:810, 2020.

Tutt ANJ et al: Adjuvant olaparib for patients with BRCA1- or BRCA2-mutated breast cancer. N Engl J Med 384:2394, 2021.

Visvanathan K et al: Use of Endocrine Therapy for Breast Cancer Risk Reduction: ASCO Clinical Practice Guideline Update. J Clin Oncol JCO1901472, 2019.

Wolff AC et al: Human Epidermal Growth Factor Receptor 2 Testing in Breast Cancer: American Society of Clinical Oncology/College of American Pathologists Clinical Practice Guideline Focused Update. J Clin Oncol 36:2105, 2018.

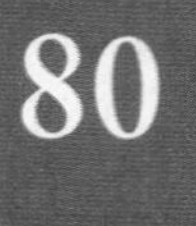

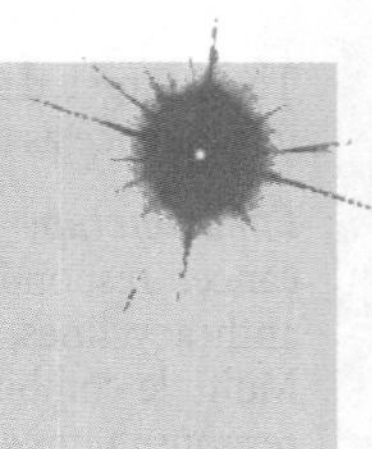

80 Upper Gastrointestinal Tract Cancers

David Kelsen

Cancers of the upper gastrointestinal tract include malignancies of the esophagus, stomach, and small bowel. Esophageal, gastroesophageal junction, and gastric cancers are among the most common of human malignancies, with 1.5 million global new cases diagnosed in 2018. In the United States, a lower risk area, it is estimated that in 2020, esophageal cancer will be diagnosed in 18,440 people and cause 16,170 deaths; for gastric cancer, 27,600 new cases will be diagnosed and 11,010 deaths will occur. Small intestine cancers are rare.

ESOPHAGEAL CANCER

INCIDENCE AND CAUSATIVE FACTORS

Two distinct forms of cancer with different epidemiologies, causative factors, and genomic profiles arise within the esophagus: squamous cell cancers, which occur more frequent in the upper and mid esophagus; and adenocarcinomas, which are almost always located in the lower esophagus and at the gastroesophageal junction. The incidence of esophageal cancer varies up to 20-fold based on geographic distribution: it is relatively uncommon in North America, but has a high incidence in Asia (especially China), the Normandy coast of France, and Middle Eastern countries such as Iran. This marked global variation is likely due to different causative factors in the development of the malignancy, leading to two different cancer types within the same tissue: squamous cell cancers are more common in high-incidence areas, usually with lower Human Development Index (HDI) scores (a measure of economic development that includes standard of living, health, and education). Overall, approximately 572,000 new cases of esophageal cancer were diagnosed globally in 2018; esophageal cancer was the seventh most common cause of malignancy and the third most common cause of cancer-related mortality, with an estimated 508,000 deaths.

The clearest high-risk factors for the squamous cell cancer subtype in Western countries are alcohol and tobacco abuse; concurrent alcohol and tobacco abuse further increases the risk. Ingestion of extremely hot substances (such as tea in Iran and mate [maté] in South America) has been proposed as a risk factor; in India, chewing the areca (betel) nut increases the risk of esophageal squamous cell cancers. Less common risk factors include chronic achalasia, radiation therapy (such as is delivered for treatment of Hodgkin's lymphoma or breast cancer), lye ingestion, and Plummer-Vinson (Patterson-Kelly) syndrome (iron deficiency anemia, glossitis, cheilosis, and the development of esophageal webs) (**Table 80-1**). Adenocarcinoma of the lower esophagus and gastroesophageal junction has been the predominant histologic subtype in the United States and Western Europe for several decades, now making up >75% of all incident cases. Risk factors for adenocarcinoma (**Table 80-2**) include chronic reflux esophagitis leading to inflammation and the development of Barrett's esophagus (the finding of glandular gastric type mucosa extending into the esophagus). Although obesity increases the risk of reflux esophagitis, a substantial number of patients with newly diagnosed adenocarcinoma of the esophagus and gastroesophageal junction are younger and fit; Barrett's esophagus may still be found in these patients. In patients with adenocarcinoma of the lower esophagus in which Barrett's esophagus is not present, the disease may arise without Barrett's esophagus, or an extensive tumor found at diagnosis may obliterate previous areas of Barrett's. Genomic alterations may be identified even before the development of frank adenocarcinoma in patients with dysplasia associated with Barrett's esophagus. These include mutations of *TP53*, a gene critical in regulating uncontrolled cell division, and aneuploidy in dysplastic regions. Risk of progression of Barrett's esophagus to cancer is about 0.4–0.5% per year. Management of Barrett's esophagus is discussed in **Chap. 323**.

TABLE 80-1 Some Etiologic Factors Associated with Squamous Cell Cancer of the Esophagus

Excess alcohol consumption
Cigarette smoking
Other ingested carcinogens
Nitrates (converted to nitrites)
Smoked opiates
Fungal toxins in pickled vegetables
Mucosal damage from physical agents
Hot tea
Lye ingestion
Radiation-induced strictures
Chronic achalasia
Host susceptibility
Esophageal web with glossitis and iron deficiency (i.e., Plummer-Vinson or Paterson-Kelly syndrome)
Congenital hyperkeratosis and pitting of the palms and soles (i.e., tylosis palmaris et plantaris)
? Dietary deficiencies of selenium, molybdenum, zinc, and vitamin A

As opposed to other gastrointestinal malignancies, such as colorectal cancer, inherited cancer susceptibility genes are rarely associated with esophagus and gastroesophageal junction cancers. An exception is the rare inherited cancer susceptibility gene driving tylosis palmaris and plantaris; a mutation in the *RHBDF2* gene is associated with an increased risk for squamous cell cancers of the esophagus. Lynch syndrome modestly increases the risk of gastric and potentially gastroesophageal junction adenocarcinomas.

■ SCREENING AND SURVEILLANCE OF HIGHER RISK GROUPS

Because of its low incidence in North America and the absence of proven blood-based biomarker for esophageal cancer assays, screening of the asymptomatic general population using, e.g., upper endoscopy is not currently recommended in the United States. Periodic endoscopy is used for surveillance of higher risk patients, such as those with Barrett's esophagus and especially with dysplasia, based on expert opinion guidelines.

■ GENOMIC ALTERATIONS

Within a tissue, subtyping has revealed substantial genomic differences between adenocarcinomas and squamous cell cancers of the esophagus. An integrated analysis involving several different genomic platforms performed by The Cancer Genome Atlas (TCGA) Research Network investigators demonstrated that esophageal squamous cell cancers more closely resembled squamous cell carcinomas of other primary sites, such as the head and neck, than adenocarcinomas arising in the esophagus. Three molecular subclasses of squamous cell cancer were identified (of note, as opposed to squamous cell cancer of the head and neck, human papillomavirus was not identified in any of the three subgroups). Among other differences, the spectrum of genomic amplifications in squamous cell cancers are substantially different than that of adenocarcinomas. In adenocarcinomas, *ERBB2* (*HER2*) was frequently amplified, as were *VEGFA* and *GATA4/6*. The genomic profile for esophageal and gastroesophageal junction adenocarcinomas was very similar to the chromosomally unstable variant of gastric adenocarcinoma, suggesting that proximal gastric and gastroesophageal junction tumors may have a similar driving factor (see below). Other studies comparing transcriptomes of adenocarcinomas and squamous cell cancers across tissues (i.e., the same tumor histology arising in different organs, such as squamous cell cancers and adenocarcinomas from the esophagus, lung, and uterine cervix) found that histologies among the different organs showed more similarity than between the different histologies within the same organ. In addition to implications regarding driving factors in the initiation and progression of cancer, these genomic alterations are important for therapeutic decisions involving systemic agents given in the neoadjuvant or postoperative adjuvant setting or for advanced metastatic disease. For esophageal cancer, genomic abnormalities that should be considered in prescribing drug-based therapy include analysis for *HER2* amplification, PD-L1 expression, and hypermutated tumors\microsatellite instability (see below).

TABLE 80-2 Some Etiologic Factors Associated with Adenocarcinoma of the Esophagus

Chronic gastroesophageal reflux
Obesity
Barrett's esophagus
Male sex
Cigarette smoking

CLINICAL FEATURES

■ PRESENTING SYMPTOMS

The most common symptoms leading to suspicion of esophageal cancer are dysphagia or odynophagia and, less frequently, hematemesis or melena. More subtle symptoms include anorexia and weight loss, and fatigue and shortness of breath if anemia from gastrointestinal bleeding is present. Because the symptoms of dysphagia or odynophagia are usually not perceived by the patient until substantial obstruction of the esophageal lumen has occurred, the large majority of patients with esophageal cancer are found with locally advanced if not metastatic disease. Patients with symptoms of dysphagia and/or odynophagia should undergo upper endoscopy (rather than a barium contrast study) to determine the presence or absence of malignancy; biopsy should be performed at the same setting to determine histology. Depending on the tumor stage, molecular diagnostic or next-generation sequencing (NGS) analysis to assist in determine potential therapies would be performed. These studies should be done on all patients with metastatic disease as it will guide therapy. NGS requires adequate tumor cellularity, which is sometimes difficult to achieve from endoscopic biopsy. Some high-volume U.S. centers routinely perform NGS on all specimens, including from the primary tumor for patients without metastatic disease.

■ STAGING

Therapeutic strategy is based on the stage of the disease using a system such as the eighth edition of the American Joint Committee on Cancer (AJCC) tumor-node-metastasis (TNM) staging system. The T stage is based on the size of the tumor and depth of penetration through the esophageal wall (which for most of its course is not covered by serosa so that invasion through the muscle layer leads directly into periesophageal tissues) (**Fig. 80-1**). Patients with regional lymph node metastases are still potentially curable. Metastatic disease is generally treated with palliative intent with rare exceptions. Because neoadjuvant (preoperative) therapy is widely employed for esophageal cancer in an effort to improve subsequent surgical outcomes, the AJCC TNM staging system includes clinical, pathologic (for patients undergoing initial surgery as first treatment), and ypTNM staging assessment for those treated with preoperative therapy. See **Table 80-3** for the TNM staging classification for gastric cancer, which is similar to esophageal cancer.

Determining tumor extent includes careful physical examination, which may reveal palpable lymphadenopathy or hepatomegaly; imaging studies including computed tomography (CT) and fluorodeoxyglucose (FDG) positron emission tomography (PET)/CT scan are used to assess for metastatic disease. If no metastatic disease is identified, endoscopic ultrasonography (EUS) is commonly performed to more definitively determine depth of penetration of the primary tumor (T) and regional lymph node involvement. For tumors of the mid and upper esophagus (5% of esophageal cancers are in the upper third of the esophagus, 20% in the middle third, and 75% in the lower third), bronchoscopy may be performed to rule out invasion of the tracheobronchial tree.

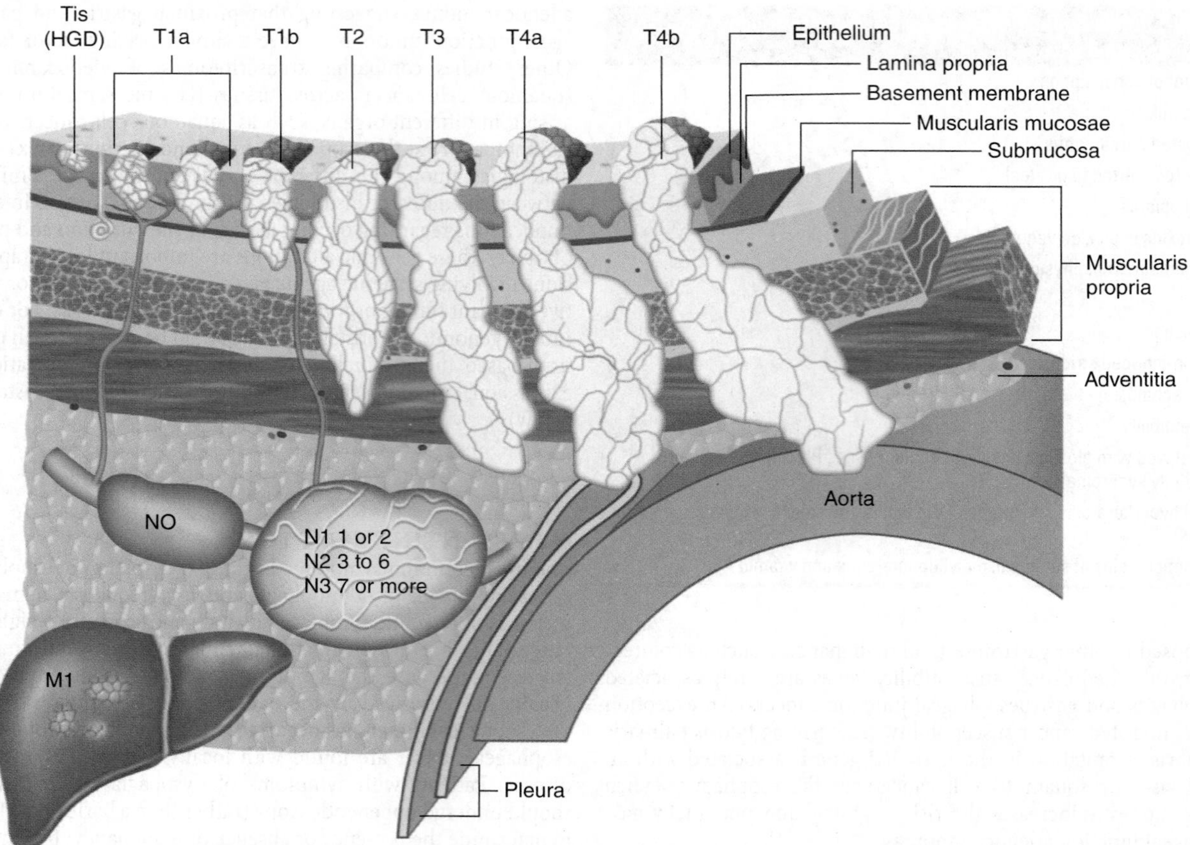

FIGURE 80-1 Patterns of spread of esophageal cancer and the basis for anatomic staging. HGD, high-grade dysplasia. *(Reproduced with permissions from TW Rice et al: Cancer of the esophagus and esophagogastric junction: An eighth edition staging primer. J Thorac Oncol 12:36, 2017.)*

TABLE 80-3 AJCC Prognostic Stage Groups for Esophageal Cancer Using cTNM (Pretreatment)

		5-YEAR SURVIVAL RATE		
TNM	**CLINICAL STAGE**	**PRESENTING AT THIS STAGE[a,b]**	**SQUAMOUS**	**ADENOCARCINOMA**
cTis, N0, M0	0	1.2%	75%	82%
cT1-2, N0, M0	I	17%	75%	78%
cT1-2, N1-3, M0	IIA	7%	53%	50%
cT3-4a, N0, M0	IIB	13%	40%	40%
cT3-4a, N1-3, M0[c]	III	31%	25%	25%
cT4b, any N, M0	IVA		17%	21%
cAny T, any N, M1	IVB	5%	10%	18%
Survival by ypTNM Staging After Neoadjuvant Chemotherapy				
		ESTIMATED 5-YEAR SURVIVAL RATE		
TNM	**yp STAGE**	**SQUAMOUS**	**ADENOCARCINOMA**	
T1-2, N0, M0 T1, N1, M0	I	46%	52%	
T3, N0-1, M0 T2, N1-2 M0 T1, N2-3, M0 T4a, N0, M0	II	34%	38%	
T4a, N1-3 M0 T4b, any N, M0 T3, N2-3, M0 T2, N3, M0	III	22%	27%	
Any T, any N, M1	IV	10%	12%	

[a]Squamous cell and adenocarcinoma histologies combined. [b]Surgical series; underestimates incidence of M1 disease at presentation. [c]Incidence includes cT4b and cNanyM0.

Sources: Adapted from TW Rice et al: CA Cancer J Clin 67:304, 2017; TW Rice et al: Dis Esophagus 29:707, 2016; and TW Rice et al: personal communication.

The finding of invasion of the trachea or bronchus rules out surgical intervention with curative intent. Regional lymph nodes may be biopsied under EUS guidance. If metastatic disease is suspected, biopsy to confirm tumor staging and to obtain adequate tissue for molecular and genomic alterations analysis should be performed. If systemic therapy is indicated as a portion of the treatment (for metastatic disease or for preoperative therapy for locally advanced cancers), serial FDG-PET/CT scans, using decrease in FDG avidity as a surrogate measure of effectiveness, are increasingly being used to guide whether the initial therapy should be continued or changed.

TREATMENT

Esophageal Cancer

Although the prognosis for patients with esophageal cancer (all stages) is still poor, a slow but steady improvement in 5-year survival has been noted. Because no effective early detection methods exist, the number of patients found to have very-early-stage cancers at the time of diagnosis has not markedly increased; the modest improvement in survival is probably a combination of somewhat improved systemic therapy as well as decreased operative morbidity and mortality when surgery is performed by high-volume surgeons at high-volume centers, as well as improvements in the delivery of external-beam radiation therapy.

For patients without evidence of metastatic disease, the goal of therapy is cure, usually by employing combined-modality therapies. Except for patients with early-stage esophageal cancer ,which might be treated by surgery alone (or for very-early-stage lesions, by endomucosal resection alone), systemic drug therapy plus external-beam radiation therapy is a standard of care option for esophageal cancers. For selected patients with gastroesophageal cancers, systemic therapy alone may be given before definitive surgical resection. For patients with squamous cell cancers of the upper and mid esophagus, combined chemotherapy plus concurrent radiation therapy is a standard of care option, with surgery reserved for patients not achieving a complete radiographic and endoscopic response. Chemotherapy plus concurrent radiation was superior to radiation therapy alone in several clinical trials. Increasingly, all systemic therapy given with curative intent is given before operation, although if surgery is the initial therapy and the patient is found to have more locally advanced cancer at pathology (e.g., regional lymph node metastasis), postoperative systemic therapy is used in the adjuvant setting. Adjuvant chemotherapy is more frequently indicated in patients with adenocarcinoma than squamous cell cancers.

For patients with metastatic disease, the goal of therapy is symptom palliation and life extension. No randomized trials of supportive care only versus systemic therapy plus best supportive care have been reported in patients with esophageal cancers. For gastric cancer (a similar histology as distal esophageal and gastroesophageal junction tumors as discussed above), clinical trials performed in the 1980s and 1990s indicated a modest improvement in 1- and 2-year survival when systemic therapy was initiated versus best supportive care only. While the cytotoxic chemotherapy regimens used for palliation have not changed dramatically over the past 10 years, subgroups of patients have been identified who benefit from therapies targeting specific genomic alterations. Approximately 20–25% of patients with adenocarcinoma of the esophagus or gastroesophageal junction are found to have amplified or overexpressed *HER2*; trastuzumab plus chemotherapy results in higher response rates and longer progression-free and overall survival compared to chemotherapy alone. Immune modulation therapy using PD-1 inhibitors is second-line palliative therapy for patients who have esophageal cancers expressing PD-L1 or having hypermutated or microsatellite-unstable genotype. Molecular diagnostic or genomic alteration analysis assays to identify these biomarkers should be performed routinely in patients with metastatic esophageal cancer to help guide therapy.

Supportive measures to improve nutrition and quality of life include placement of an endoluminal stent in the setting of high-grade obstruction; use of enteral nutrition can also be performed using a percutaneous gastrostomy. Photodynamic therapy and endoscopic laser therapy have been used to treat endoluminal obstruction.

TUMORS OF THE STOMACH

ADENOCARCINOMA OF THE STOMACH

Incidence and Causative Factors A century ago, gastric adenocarcinomas were among the most common of malignancies in the United States. Since the 1920s, the incidence of gastric cancer has steadily decreased; while the reason for this has not been definitively identified, it coincided with widespread use of refrigeration and a decreased need for food preservatives. In 2020, it is estimated that there will be 27,600 new cases of gastric cancer diagnosed in the United States; while now seen much less frequently, it remains a lethal disease, with 11,010 deaths. Globally, gastric cancer is still very common, with an overall global incidence of 1.03 million new cases per year and 780,000 deaths, making gastric cancer the third most common cause of cancer mortality. High-incidence areas, as is the case for esophageal cancers, include large Asian countries such as China, Korea, and Japan; South American countries such as Chile; and Eastern European countries.

While the number of new cases of body and distal gastric cancers has decreased in Western, high-HDI countries, the incidence of adenocarcinomas of the gastroesophageal junction has markedly increased in the same areas over the past several decades. The ingestion of high concentrations of nitrates found in dried, smoked, and salted foods may be a contributing factor. Bacteria such as *Helicobacter pylori* and ingestion of partially decayed bacterially contaminated food may lead to the generation of carcinogenic nitrites from nitrates **(Table 80-4)**. A causative factor is suspected to be chronic inflammation due to reflux of gastric contents into the esophagus, particularly in obese people. Obesity alone is not the cause, as a substantial number of these patients are fit and not overweight. Early-onset gastric cancers (gastric cancer occurring in patients under the age of 50), primarily proximal or gastroesophageal junction cancers, have also increased. A second cause of chronic inflammation, *H. pylori* infection, is a known driver in many cases of gastric cancer. While *H. pylori* is extremely common, occurring in approximately half of all humans, gastric cancer occurs in only a small subset of those infected. Higher cancer risk has been associated with certain strains of *H. pylori*; a specific human genetic predisposition has not yet been identified. Supportive evidence that *H. pylori* infection is a causative factor in the development of gastric cancer includes prospective studies demonstrating that treatment of *H. pylori* infection decreases the overall risk of gastric cancer. For example, patients with *H. pylori* infection who had at least one first-degree relative with a history of gastric cancer (increasing their own risk of stomach cancer) were randomly assigned to placebo or treatment for *H. pylori*. The group receiving *H. pylori* eradication showed a significant decrease in the incidence of gastric cancer (especially for

TABLE 80-4 Nitrate-Converting Bacteria as a Factor in the Causation of Gastric Carcinoma[a]

Exogenous sources of nitrate-converting bacteria:
Bacterially contaminated food (common in lower socioeconomic classes, who have a higher incidence of the disease; diminished by improved food preservation and refrigeration)
Helicobacter pylori infection
Endogenous factors favoring growth of nitrate-converting bacteria in the stomach:
Decreased gastric acidity
Prior gastric surgery (antrectomy) (15- to 20-year latency period)
Atrophic gastritis and/or pernicious anemia
? Prolonged exposure to histamine H_2-receptor antagonists

[a]Hypothesis: Dietary nitrates are converted to carcinogenic nitrites by bacteria.

those in whom *H. pylori* was successfully eradicated) compared to the control group. Earlier studies had demonstrated that treatment of *H. pylori* in Korean patients who had a prior very-early-stage gastric cancer decreased the incidence of a second gastric cancer. These data suggest that treatment of asymptomatic *H. pylori* gastric infection should be considered for patients who have a first-degree relative who has had gastric cancer or who themselves have a prior history of an early-stage gastric cancer.

In addition to chronic inflammatory conditions, inherited cancer susceptibility genes increase the risk of gastric cancer. These include mutations of *CDH1*, which encodes for the cell cohesion gene e-cadherin; germline *CDH1* mutations markedly increase the risk for the diffuse cell (signet cell) gastric cancer subtype (see below for discussion of histologic subtypes). Patients with an inherited deleterious *CDH1* mutation are considered for prophylactic gastrectomy. *CDH1* mutations also increase the risk for lobular breast cancer. Germline mutations in the mismatch repair pathway (Lynch syndrome) slightly increase the risk for gastric cancer. Other inherited cancer susceptibility genetic syndromes that increase the risk of gastric cancer include familial adenomatous polyposis, juvenile polyposis, and Peutz-Jeghers syndrome. Inherited cancer susceptibility genes such as *BRCA* mutations may not significantly increase risk for gastric cancer. Surveillance programs for the higher risk germline cancer susceptibility genes should be employed.

Gastric cancer stem cells originating in the bone marrow may play an important role in the development of gastric cancer. *H. pylori* may be an inciting factor for recruitment of such bone marrow gastric stem cells. If this hypothesis is confirmed, it may have important implications for therapy of gastric cancers.

Clinical Features • **SURVEILLANCE STRATEGIES** As is the case for esophageal cancer, the overwhelming majority of Western patients with gastric cancer are symptomatic at the time of diagnosis. Early detection programs, in Japan and Korea, where gastric cancer has been among the most common of malignancies (although its incidence has been decreasing), include upper endoscopy and, in Japan, upper endoscopy and serum pepsinogen; these programs have increased the number of patients found with early gastric cancer and decreased mortality rates. This strategy has not been cost effective in populations in which the incidence of gastric cancer is much lower, such as in the United States. In high-incidence areas, treatment of symptomatic *H. pylori* is a preventive measure. Exceptions to routine surveillance in the United States are asymptomatic patients with *CDH1* (and other cancer susceptibility gene) mutations who may be part of early detection programs and in whom prophylactic gastrectomy is a management option.

PRESENTING SYMPTOMS Presenting symptoms include vague upper abdominal discomfort, hematemesis or melena, anorexia and early satiety, and unexplained weight loss. For patients with esophagogastric junction cancers, dysphagia or odynophagia may be the presenting symptom. Anemia may be found due to occult bleeding. These symptoms and signs lead to upper (and if site of bleeding is uncertain, lower) endoscopy and biopsy (endoscopy has long replaced barium contrast radiography as an initial diagnostic step). Occasionally, imaging using CT performed to evaluate abdominal symptoms may identify gastric thickening or a gastric mass leading to upper endoscopy. Physical examination can reveal left supraclavicular adenopathy (Virchow's node), a periumbilical mass (Sister Mary Joseph nodule), a pelvic mass on rectal exam (Blumer's shelf), ascites, or an ovarian mass (Krukenberg tumor). More commonly, physical examination is unrevealing.

Upper endoscopy may reveal an ulcer or ulcerated mass, biopsy of which shows adenocarcinoma. For the diffuse subtype of gastric cancer, a mass or ulceration may not be seen, but rather, thickened gastric rugae may be noted. Initial biopsy may not reveal diffuse gastric cancer, which may track below the mucosal surface. In these patients, EUS may guide biopsy.

Histopathology Classification of Primary Gastric Adenocarcinomas The large majority (~85%) of gastric malignancies are adenocarcinomas or subtypes of adenocarcinoma. Other malignancies, discussed below, include neuroendocrine tumors (carcinoid tumors), primary gastric lymphomas, gastrointestinal stromal tumors (GISTs), and other rare malignancies. Using the Lauren classification, pathologists classify adenocarcinomas on the basis of histopathology as intestinal (more common) or diffuse subtype (~20%). As noted above, the diffuse subtype is associated with inherited *CDH1* mutations; in addition, in the TCGA genomic analysis of gastric cancer, approximately a third of diffuse subtype cases had somatic *CDH1* mutations. The intestinal subtype is associated with *H. pylori* infection and atopic gastritis. Histologic grade also influences the clinical course.

Genomic analysis performed by several groups has resulted in molecular classifications of gastric cancer that may, in the future, inform staging systems, provide a better understanding of the driving factors in the development of gastric cancer, and provide important information on treatment options (**Fig. 80-2**). For example, the TCGA group reported the results of a multiplatform analysis of 295 patients with previously untreated gastric cancer; both Western and Asian patients were included in the analysis. Four subtypes of gastric cancer were identified: high Epstein-Barr virus burden, microsatellite unstable with hypermutation, genomically stable (associated with the diffuse subtype), and chromosomal unstable. The Asian Cancer Research Group (ACRG), studying primary tumors from 300 Korean patients, analyzed gene expression profiles and found four subtypes: mesenchymal, microsatellite unstable, microsatellite stable with *TP53* expressed, and microsatellite unstable with *TP53* mutated. Clinical outcome was correlated with genomic subtype in both studies, with microsatellite

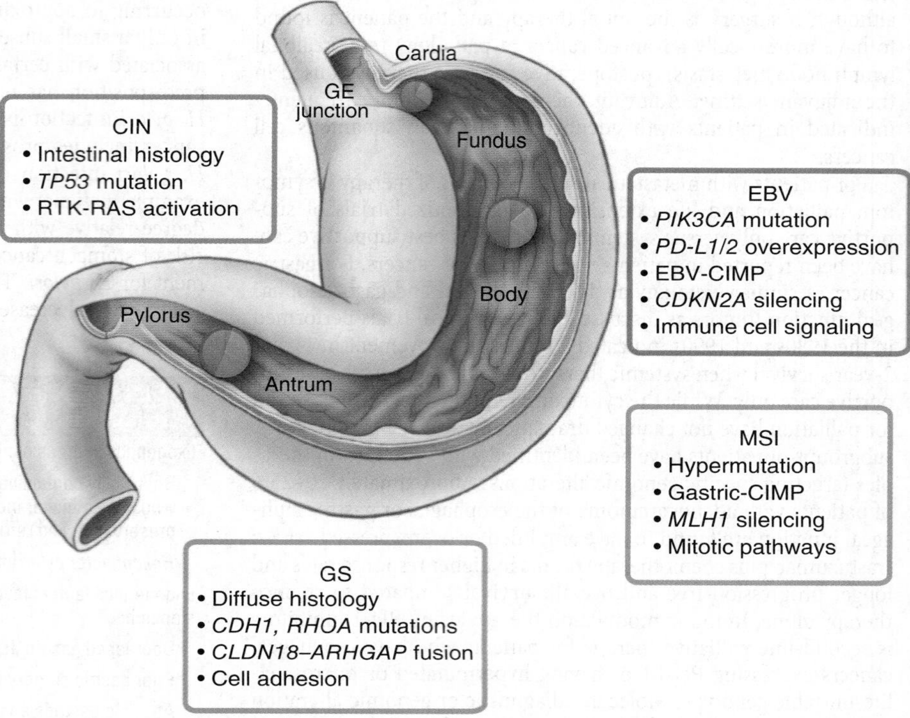

FIGURE 80-2 Molecular/genomic characterization of subtypes of gastric carcinomas. CIMP, CpG-island methylator phenotype; CIN, chromosomally unstable; EBV, Epstein-Barr virus-associated; GE, gastroesophageal; GS, genomically stable; MSI, microsatellite instability-associated.

unstable tumors having the best outcome and genomically stable (TCGA) and mesenchymal (ACRG) types the worst.

In addition to histopathology, molecular diagnostics (including NGS) are an important part of the pathology workup. The molecular subtypes have therapeutic implications; for example, ~20% of gastric cancer or gastroesophageal junction cancer patients' tumors have overexpression or amplification of *HER2*, which would lead to the addition of agents such as trastuzumab as part of systemic treatment for metastatic disease. Immune modulation therapy may be used in patients with hypermutated tumors, found by NGS or by polymerase chain reaction (PCR) for microsatellite instability (MSI). An evaluation for overexpression or amplification of *HER2*, quantification of PD-L1 by immunohistochemistry, and assessment of MSI by PCR or deficient mismatch repair protein (dMMRP) expression should be a routine part of the pathology workup of patients with metastatic gastric cancer. More controversial is whether these assays should also be routinely performed in patients with potentially operable gastric cancer because the addition of trastuzumab to neoadjuvant chemotherapy has not yet been shown to change outcome. In large-volume centers, NGS is routinely performed on pretreatment biopsies. Currently, the finding on pathologic assays of positive tumor Epstein-Barr virus (identified in 8–10% of gastric cancer patients) does not change therapeutic options.

Staging Once a diagnosis of a primary gastric adenocarcinoma is made, algorithms for clinical evaluation of stage include physical examination and imaging studies (**Fig. 80-3; Table 80-5**). Tumor-related biomarkers such as carcinoembryonic antigen (CEA) or CA19-9 may be elevated but are nonspecific (may be elevated in a number of other gastrointestinal and other site cancers). Diagnostic CT scan of the chest, abdomen, and pelvis should be performed. If metastatic

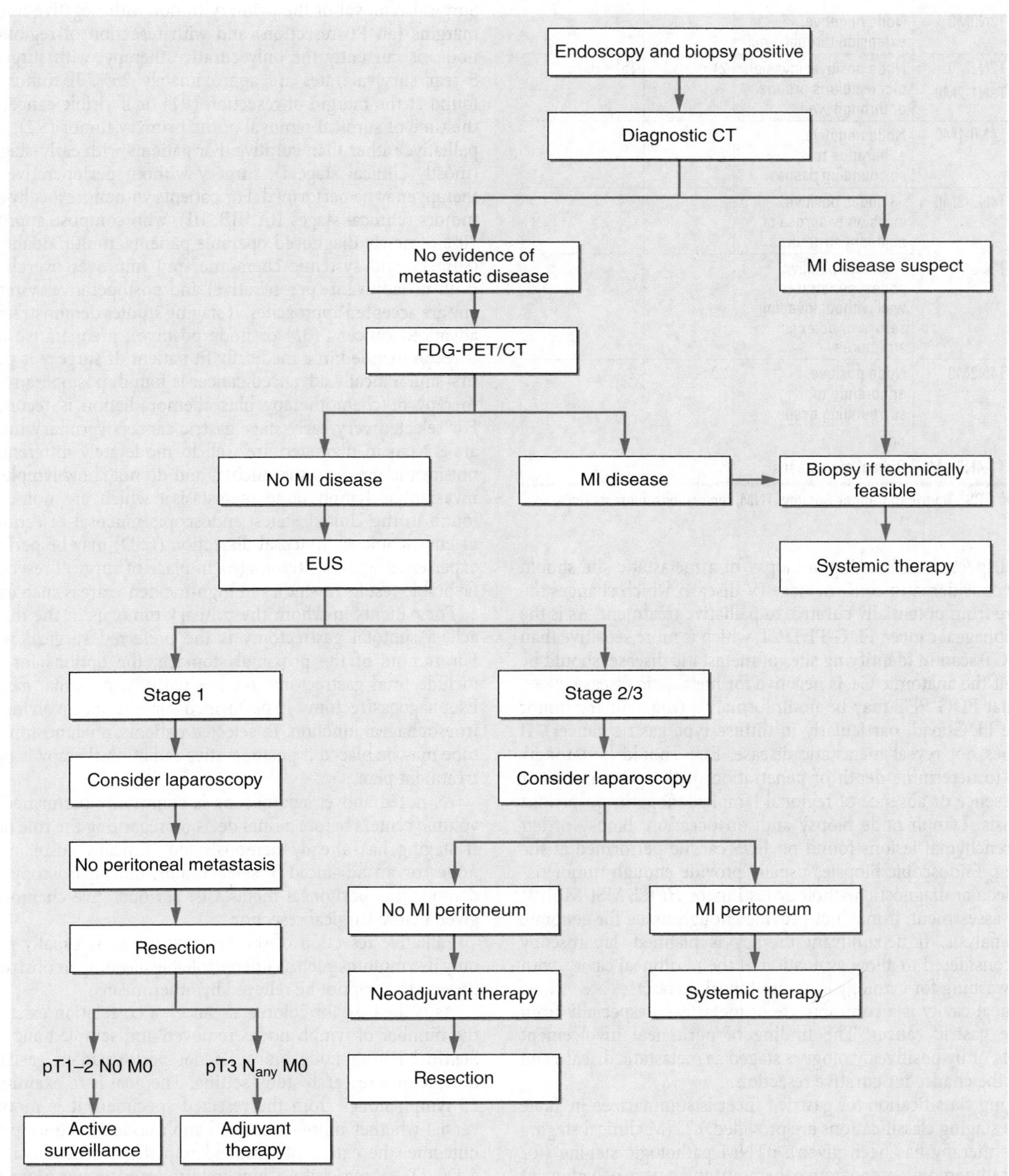

FIGURE 80-3 Staging for gastric adenocarcinoma. CT, computed tomography; EUS, endoscopic ultrasound; FDG-PET, fluorodeoxyglucose positron emission tomography.

TABLE 80-5 Staging System for Gastric Carcinoma

STAGE	TNM	FEATURES	DATA FROM ACS IN THE UNITED STATES: NO. OF CASES, %	DATA FROM ACS IN THE UNITED STATES: 5-YEAR SURVIVAL, %
0	TisN0M0	Node negative; limited to mucosa	1	90
IA	T1N0M0	Node negative; invasion of lamina propria or submucosa	7	59
IB	T2N0M0 T1N1M0	Node negative; invasion of muscularis propria	10	44
II	T1N2M0 T2N1M0	Node positive; invasion beyond mucosa but within wall	17	29
		or		
	T3N0M0	Node negative; extension through wall		
IIIA	T2N2M0 T3N1-2M0	Node positive; invasion of muscularis propria or through wall	21	15
IIIB	T4N0-1M0	Node negative; adherence to surrounding tissue	14	9
IIIC	T4N2-3M0	>3 nodes positive; invasion of serosa or adjacent structures		
	T3N3M0	7 or more positive nodes; penetrates wall without invading serosa or adjacent structures		
IV	T4N2M0	Node positive; adherence to surrounding tissue	30	3
		or		
	T1-4N0-2M1	Distant metastases		

Abbreviations: ACS, American Cancer Society; TNM, tumor-node-metastasis.

disease is suspected on imaging, a biopsy of a metastatic site should be strongly considered to confirm stage IV disease, which changes the goals of care from potentially curative to palliative treatment. As is the case for esophageal cancer, FDG-PET/CT, which is more sensitive than diagnostic CT scan in identifying sites of metastatic disease, should be performed if the anatomic CT is negative for metastatic disease. Note, however, that FDG-PET may be noninformative (the primary tumor may not be FDG-avid, particularly in diffuse-type gastric cancer). If imaging does not reveal metastatic disease, EUS should be strongly considered to determine depth of penetration of the primary tumor and the presence or absence of regional lymphadenopathy suspicious for metastasis. Lymph node biopsy and, on occasion, biopsy of left hepatic parenchymal lesions found on EUS can be performed at the same setting. Endoscopic biopsies usually provide enough tumor tissue for molecular diagnostic pathology testing for *HER2*, MSI/MMRP, and PD-L1 assessment; it may not provide enough tissue for genomic alteration analysis. If neoadjuvant therapy is planned, laparoscopy should be considered to allow evaluation of the peritoneal cavity, with peritoneal washing for cytology if no peritoneal metastases are visible. The peritoneal cavity is a common site of metastases, especially from diffuse-type gastric cancer. The finding of peritoneal involvement either visibly or by positive cytology is staged as metastatic disease and diminishes the chance for curative resection.

The staging classification for gastric cancer is summarized in Table 80-5. Three staging classifications are provided: cTNM clinical staging (before any therapy has been given), pTNM pathologic staging (for patients not undergoing preoperative therapy), and a post-neoadjuvant therapy classification staging (ypTNM). The three components take into account current standard of care options for therapy in which the AJCC prognostic stage groups from clinical staging guide therapeutic decisions. For example, after clinical evaluation, a large percentage of newly diagnosed patients will be found to have higher-stage primary cancers (penetrating through the gastric wall [T3 or T4] or lymph node–positive tumors), in which case perioperative (neoadjuvant) systemic therapy may be chosen. Pathologic examination of the resected specimen for prognostic stage classification must take into account exposure to preoperative therapies that may lead to downstaging (thus, ypTNM staging). Nomograms have been developed for predicting outcome in patients undergoing surgery as initial treatment.

TREATMENT
Gastric Cancer

POTENTIALLY CURABLE GASTRIC CANCER: SURGERY

Surgical removal of the primary tumor with negative microscopic margins (an R0 resection) and with resection of regional lymph nodes is currently the only curative therapy; with surgery alone, 5-year survival rates are approximately 25%. If tumor cells are found at the margin of resection (R1) or if visible cancer is left at the time of surgical removal of the primary tumor (R2), surgery is palliative rather than curative. For patients with early-stage tumors (mostly clinical stage I), surgery without perioperative systemic therapy may be performed. For patients with more locally advanced tumors (clinical stages IIA, IIB, III), who compose approximately 70% of newly diagnosed operable patients, multimodality therapy (surgery and systemic chemotherapy) improves overall survival. Both neoadjuvant (preoperative) and postoperative systemic therapy are accepted approaches. If staging studies demonstrate a locally advanced cancer (T3/4 or node positive), preoperative treatment is recommended in a medically fit patient. If surgery is performed first and a locally advanced cancer is found, postoperative chemotherapy or chemotherapy plus chemoradiation is recommended. For selected very-early-stage gastric cancers (primary tumors that are ≤2 cm in diameter, are well to moderately differentiated, do not invade the deep submucosa, and do not show lymphovascular invasion or lymph node metastasis), which are not commonly found in the United States, endoscopic mucosal resection (EMR) or endoscopic submucosal dissection (ESD) may be performed by experienced gastroenterologists in place of surgical resection, with favorable results in studies in high-incidence areas such as Japan.

For patients in whom the primary tumor is in the distal stomach, a subtotal gastrectomy is the preferred surgical procedure. For tumors of the proximal stomach, the options for resection include total gastrectomy or, alternatively, proximal gastrectomy. Esophagogastrectomy is performed for tumors involving the gastroesophageal junction. In selected patients, a jejunostomy feeding tube may be placed if postoperative radiation therapy is part of the treatment plan.

As noted above, laparoscopy is commonly performed at high-volume centers before a final decision regarding the role of surgery. If staging has already demonstrated clinically suspicious lymph nodes or an advanced T stage tumor, but laparoscopy does not demonstrate peritoneal metastasis, perioperative chemotherapy is given before surgical resection.

Palliative resection of the primary tumor is usually performed only if symptoms such as uncontrollable bleeding or obstruction are present that cannot be relieved by other means.

As is the case for colorectal cancer, a correlation exists between the number of lymph nodes removed and sampled and outcome. Sentinel lymph node biopsy is not performed in gastric cancer outside of a research study setting. The goal is to examine at least 15 lymph nodes from the resected specimen; it is more controversial whether more extensive lymph node resection itself affects outcome; the extent of lymphadenopathy can be classified using a D0–D3 system with a higher number meaning more extensive lymphadenopathy. In the United States, a modified D2 (D1+)

resection preserving the spleen and avoiding pancreatectomy is recommended but should be performed by experienced surgeons at high-volume centers. Japanese investigators and others have used very extensive lymph node dissections, but studies have not demonstrated an advantage for a D3 resection. Both resection of the primary tumor and its regional lymph nodes can be performed laparoscopically in appropriate patients.

In the hands of experienced surgeons, operative mortality would be anticipated to be ≤2%.

NEOADJUVANT AND POSTOPERATIVE ADJUVANT THERAPY FOR RESECTABLE GASTRIC CANCER

The large majority of potentially resectable Western gastric cancer patients have locally advanced tumors (cTNM stage IIA/B or III). Multimodality therapy using systemic chemotherapy improves 5-year survival rates by 10–15% compared to surgery alone. A widely cited study, the MAGIC clinical trial, randomly assigned patients with potentially resectable disease to receive perioperative chemotherapy or to proceed directly to surgery. Five-year overall survival for patients undergoing surgery alone was 23%; for those receiving pre- and postoperative chemotherapy, it was 36%. On the basis of this and other clinical trials, for most medically fit patients with stage cTNM II and III resectable gastric cancers, preoperative systemic chemotherapy followed by resection and, if tolerable, postoperative chemotherapy is a standard of care. Chemoradiation as given for esophageal cancers is usually used for gastroesophageal junction tumors. Preoperative chemoradiation or preoperative chemotherapy followed by chemoradiation for gastric cancer, as opposed to esophageal or gastroesophageal junction cancers, has been studied but is still an investigational approach. For patients being treated with multimodality therapy, close interactions among the surgeon, medical oncologist, and radiation oncologist are essential.

Clinical trials have compared different cytotoxic chemotherapy regimens, most of which include a platinum compound—either cisplatin or oxaliplatin. Currently, a platinum compound plus a fluorinated pyrimidine, such as fluorouracil or capecitabine, given for three to four cycles before surgery is a standard of care option. Drug combinations are favored; an example is the FOLFOX regimen, which includes fluorouracil, leucovorin, and oxaliplatin. For very fit patients, a combination of fluorouracil, oxaliplatin, and docetaxel (FLOT) may be chosen. Addition of trastuzumab to chemotherapy has not improved outcomes for patients with HER2-positive cancers. Careful monitoring of chemotherapy-related toxicities with appropriate dose modifications is important. Several clinical trials have included both preoperative and postoperative systemic therapy; a substantial number of patients will have a slow postoperative recovery and not receive postoperative treatment. Maximizing the ability to give preoperative chemotherapy is an important consideration. For patients receiving preoperative systemic chemotherapy and undergoing a D2/D1+ dissection, postoperative chemoradiation therapy has not improved outcome.

For patients in whom the primary tumor has been resected and who did not receive preoperative chemotherapy, who are found to have stage II or III cancers, or who have <15 lymph nodes found in the resected specimen, postoperative chemoradiation is a treatment option. Chemoradiation therapy may also be given for unresectable cancers in selected patients.

PALLIATIVE THERAPY FOR INCURABLE GASTRIC CANCER

Patients with clinical stage IV gastric cancers with an adequate performance status should be offered systemic drug therapies. Small clinical trials performed in the 1980s and 1990s showed a survival benefit for systemic therapy compared to best supportive care only. The cytotoxic chemotherapy regimens most commonly employed are still based on a platinum compound and a fluorinated pyrimidine (e.g., FOLFOX, as is used in the perioperative setting). However, two subgroups of gastric cancer patients have been identified who benefit from the addition of noncytotoxic agents. Those whose tumors have overexpressed or amplified *HER2* should receive HER2-targeted agents such as trastuzumab plus cytotoxic chemotherapy because a modest survival advantage has been demonstrated. Additional HER2-targeted therapy using trastuzumab-deruxtecan, a monoclonal antibody-drug conjugate, has encouraging activity in patients whose tumors were refractory to trastuzumab. For patients with MSI/dMMRP gastric cancers, PD-1 inhibitors such as pembrolizumab should be used (currently approved in the second-line setting). Immune modulation therapy using PD-1 inhibitors such as pembrolizumab or nivolumab is also approved in gastric cancer with tumor specimens having ≥1% PD-L1 expression, with modest response rates. The development of more effective immune therapies and their combination with cytotoxic chemotherapy (and in combination with trastuzumab plus chemotherapy in *HER2*-positive patients) as initial treatment are areas of active investigation.

When disease progresses after first-line treatment, other therapies include the combination of a VEGF receptor–targeted agent, ramucirumab, either alone or in combination with paclitaxel. As noted above, immune modulation therapy may cause remissions in patients whose tumors have at least 1% PD-L1 expression. PD-1 inhibitors are the preferred option for patients whose tumors are microsatellite unstable. Several other cytotoxic agents have activity in the palliative setting including irinotecan and trifluridine-tipiracil. Best results from clinical trials indicate overall survival for treated patients with stage IV disease is still only 12–15 months.

Radiation therapy using shorter regimens may be employed to palliate bleeding. For patients with advanced incurable disease, other supportive measures include placement of a duodenal stent to relieve gastric outlet obstruction; in selected patients, surgical procedures for gastric outlet obstruction may be performed. Radiation therapy might be used if not previously given. Enteral feeding using a jejunostomy tube may support nutritional needs.

GASTRIC LYMPHOMAS

Lymphomas of the stomach are an uncommon (~3%) but important subgroup of gastric malignancies. They are extranodal non-Hodgkin's lymphomas (NHL). The gastrointestinal tract is the most common site for extranodal NHL, and the stomach is the most common site within the gastrointestinal tract. The presenting symptoms are similar to those of the much more common adenocarcinoma of the stomach described above, including pain, anorexia, and bleeding. Symptoms of fever and night sweats occur in 10–15% of patients with gastric NHL. Because the treatment options are so different, obtaining adequate tissue for definitive pathologic examination is crucial in diagnosing gastric lymphomas. On occasion, this may be challenging because, similar to diffuse subtype adenocarcinoma, lymphomas may track below the mucosal surface. Multiple deep biopsies and mucosal resection may be needed to provide enough tissue for definitive pathologic assessment.

Potential driving forces in the development of gastric lymphomas include active or prior *H. pylori* infection, which is associated with mucosa-associated lymphoid tissue (MALT) subtype gastric lymphomas. MALT lymphomas may develop in nearly any organ, but the stomach is the most frequent primary site, accounting for ~35% of all MALT lymphomas. Antibacterial therapy directed against *H. pylori* can be a highly effective treatment in these patients. Other forms of NHL may involve the stomach either as primary gastric lymphoma or as a secondary site of disease, including both B-cell (e.g., mantle cell lymphoma, Burkitt's lymphoma, and follicular lymphoma) and T-cell lymphomas (e.g., enteropathy-associated T-cell lymphoma, anaplastic large-cell lymphoma, and peripheral T-cell lymphoma).

Staging is performed in a fashion similar to gastric adenocarcinoma, but the staging classification is different (see below). In addition to a contrast-enhanced diagnostic-quality CT scan of the chest, abdomen, and pelvis, an FDG-PET/CT scan may be helpful. EUS may be used to determine depth of invasion in patients in whom no evidence of metastatic disease is noted. Examination of the peripheral blood and bone marrow aspirate should be considered as part of the workup.

In all patients with gastric lymphoma, *H. pylori* infection status should be evaluated. If *H. pylori* testing is negative by histopathology, noninvasive testing by either stool antigen test or urea breath test should be used. If rituximab will be part of the treatment plan (see below), hepatitis B testing should be performed.

STAGING

The TNM staging system is not employed for gastric lymphomas. The Lugano staging system for gastrointestinal lymphomas (a modification of the Ann Arbor staging system) divides patient groups into stages I, II, and IV. Stage I tumors are limited to the gastric wall; stage II tumors have regional lymph node involvement or invasion of local structures; stage IV tumors have either more extensive lymph node involvement or have distant metastasis, including to the bone marrow or other extranodal sites.

PATHOLOGIC CLASSIFICATION

The two most common histologic subtypes of gastric lymphoma are marginal zone B-cell lymphomas (gastric marginal zone B-cell lymphomas or MALT; ~40% of newly diagnosed patients) and diffuse large B-cell lymphomas (DLBCLs; ~55%). The distinction is critical because therapeutic options are different. As part of the pathologic evaluation, for patients with *H. pylori*–positive gastric lymphomas, the finding of a t(11;18) translocation identifies a subgroup less likely to respond to *H. pylori* eradication. This translocation may be detected using PCR or fluorescent in situ hybridization (FISH); it creates a chimeric protein composed of the amino terminal of *API1* (apoptosis inhibitor) and the carboxy terminus of *MALT1*, leading to activation of nuclear factor-κB signaling.

TREATMENT
Gastric Lymphoma

Unlike adenocarcinoma of the stomach, surgical resection has no role in the treatment of primary gastric lymphoma in the absence of complications of therapy such as perforation or uncontrollable bleeding. Resection of gastric lymphoma does not improve outcome.

For patients with MALT lymphoma, eradication of *H. pylori* with antibiotics is highly effective therapy. If tests for *H. pylori* are positive and t(11;18) translocation assay is negative, one of the currently accepted antibiotic regimens for treating *H. pylori* should be the initial therapy. *H. pylori* eradication is associated with high response rates including complete remissions in the majority of patients. The time to remission may be prolonged (in some studies averaging 15–16 months); therefore, careful monitoring is important before determining that a MALT tumor is not responding to anti–*H. pylori* therapy. For patients in whom the t(11;18) translocation assay is positive, options for therapy include anti–*H. pylori* antibiotic therapy plus involved-field radiation therapy or, if radiation is contraindicated, the use of single-agent rituximab, a monoclonal antibody targeting CD20. For patients who are *H. pylori* negative, moderate-dose (24–30 Gy) involved-site radiation therapy or single-agent rituximab is a treatment option. For selected, more advanced, stage IV MALT patients who have not responded to or who have progressed after receiving anti–*H. pylori* antibiotic therapy and/or rituximab, cytotoxic chemotherapy regimens such as R-CHOP (rituximab, cyclophosphamide, doxorubicin, vincristine, and prednisolone) or rituximab and lenalidomide may be considered.

DLBCL may be a result of transformation from more indolent MALT lymphoma or may arise de novo. De novo tumors are more likely to be BCL2 and CD10 positive. MALT lymphomas that have transformed to DLBCLs are more frequently BCL2 and CD10 negative.

For patients with DLBCL, earlier stage tumors may be treated by combination chemotherapy alone or chemotherapy plus involved-field radiation therapy. For more advanced gastric DLBCL tumors, chemotherapy using R-CHOP or R-EPOCH (rituximab, etoposide, prednisolone, vincristine, cyclophosphamide, and doxorubicin) regimens is standard of care. Some reports have suggested that eradication of *H. pylori* is effective treatment for early-stage DLBCL when the patient also has *H. pylori*.

UNCOMMON TUMORS OF THE ESOPHAGUS AND STOMACH

NEUROENDOCRINE TUMORS

Neuroendocrine tumors (NETs) of the esophagus are rare, accounting for <1% of gastrointestinal NETs. They may present with dysphagia and odynophagia similar to that of more common squamous cell or adenocarcinoma of the distal esophagus and gastroesophageal junction or with more nonspecific symptoms such as substernal discomfort or burning consistent with reflux esophagitis. A potential driving factor of higher grade NET is smoking. The initial diagnostic evaluation includes upper endoscopy and biopsy. Pathology may reveal a well-differentiated grade 1 or grade 2 NET with a low metastatic potential; at the other end of the spectrum are small-cell or large-cell NETs, which are fully malignant and frequently metastasize. EUS to assess depth of penetration and presence or absence of regional lymph node metastasis is usually performed. Imaging studies include CT or FDG-PET/CT scan to assess for metastatic disease, particularly in higher grade tumors. For lower grade tumors, somatostatin analog imaging studies such as gallium-68 DOTATATE may be performed if metastatic disease is suspected. For lower grade tumors, endoscopic resection including EMR or ESD may be performed. Small-cell or large-cell NETs that are not metastatic are usually treated with chemotherapy plus external-beam radiation therapy using chemotherapy regimens similar to those employed for small- and large-cell neuroendocrine cancers of the lung **(Chap. 84)**. Systemic therapy for metastatic small- and large-cell esophagogastric NETs is also modeled on therapy for small- and large-cell thoracic NETs.

Gastric NETs (also called gastric carcinoid tumors) represent 7–9% of gastrointestinal NETs but <1% of gastric neoplasms. They are divided into three types **(Chap. 84)**. For all gastric NETs, initial evaluation includes upper endoscopy and biopsy. EUS may be helpful in assessing depth of invasion for larger tumors and for assessing regional lymph node metastases in type 3 tumors. Somatostatin analog imaging using gallium-68 DOTATATE PET/CT scanning may be performed if metastatic disease is suspected. The finding of unresectable metastatic disease that is gallium-68 DOTATATE avid not only provides staging information but also guides potential therapy using somatostatin receptor–targeted therapy.

TREATMENT
Gastric Neuroendocrine Tumors

Type 1 tumors are usually treated endoscopically with polypectomy or endomucosal resection. For larger tumors (>2 cm) or tumors invading through the muscularis or to regional lymph nodes, surgical resection is recommended. Type 2 tumors have a higher risk for regional lymph node metastasis and are usually treated surgically, although selected patients may have a combination of endoscopic resection and limited surgical resection. Type 3 tumors are not associated with elevated gastrin levels and have a higher propensity for regional lymph node metastasis and distant metastasis. Surgery is the treatment of choice for localized type 3 tumors, although EMR has been used in selected patients. Adenocarcinoma of the stomach may be found in 5–10% of type 3 tumors.

GASTROINTESTINAL STROMAL TUMORS

Gastrointestinal stromal tumors (GISTs) are rare tumors of the gastrointestinal tract associated with somatic mutations in the *cKIT* (the majority) or *PDGFRA* genes, which are both driver mutations and targets for systemic therapy for metastatic disease; in a minority of cases, neither gene is mutated. GISTs arise from Cajal cells, which bridge between the autonomic nerves to the muscle layer of the bowel. The stomach is the most frequent primary site (~50%), followed by the small bowel in about a third of cases. As endoscopy for other indications has become more widely used, otherwise asymptomatic and probably clinically insignificant small GISTs have been identified more frequently; it is not clear that the actual incidence has substantially increased. Symptoms associated with GISTs include acute gastrointestinal bleeding leading to melena and/or hematemesis. Anemia may be reflected in generalized weakness. With larger tumors, abdominal distention and pain may be presenting symptoms. At endoscopy, a nonspecific smooth bulging mass covered by normal mucosa is the most frequent finding. Initial biopsy may not reveal an epithelial neoplasm. EUS both to assess the extent of the neoplasm and to guide biopsy in order to obtain adequate tissue for histology and molecular pathology may be helpful.

Histologically, a spindle cell neoplasm is the most common subtype (~70%), with epithelioid cells making up 20%; 10% of cases are mixed histology. Immunohistochemical stains for the presence of c-kit or CD34 positivity and mutational analysis of *cKIT* and *PDGFRA* should be performed in all patients. These help to distinguish between GISTs and leiomyoma neoplasms. For nonmetastatic primary GISTs, laparoscopic surgical resection, if feasible, is the treatment of choice; because lymph node metastases are unusual, wedge or segmental resection is preferred. Endoscopic resection has been used in selected cases. Neither histology nor the presence of a *cKIT* or *PDGFRA* mutation distinguishes GISTs with clinically malignant phenotype from those that have a benign course. Higher risk tumors (larger size, higher mitotic index) may present with or develop metastatic or locally unresectable disease. For these patients, use of a c-kit tyrosine kinase inhibitor such as imatinib for tumors with *cKIT* mutations offers effective palliation. Avapritinib is used for tumors with certain *PDGFRA* mutations. However, resistance almost invariably develops, and the development of newer agents effective in tumors with secondary mutations is a high priority. For high-risk GISTs, adjuvant therapy with imatinib for 3 years improves relapse-free and overall survival.

■ SMALL-BOWEL NEOPLASMS

Although the number of new cases of small-bowel neoplasms is substantially less than that of gastric neoplasms (in 2020, there were an estimated 11,110 new cases in the United States, representing 3–4% of gastrointestinal malignancies), the spectrum of malignant tumors of the small bowel is similar and includes NETs (carcinoid), adenocarcinomas, lymphomas, and GISTs. Neuroendocrine cancers are slightly more frequent (40–45%) than adenocarcinomas (30–40%), with the remainder mostly lymphomas and ~8% GISTs. The duodenum is the most common portion of the small bowel in which malignancies develop (~50%), with ~30% occurring in the jejunum and 20% in the ileum. NETs are the most common benign and malignant tumors of the ileum. Risk factors for the development of adenocarcinoma include inflammatory bowel disease (Crohn's disease) and inherited germline mutation syndromes such as Lynch syndrome, familial adenomatous polyposis (FAP), and Peutz-Jeghers syndrome. Celiac disease is associated with a higher incidence of both small-bowel adenocarcinomas and T-cell lymphomas.

While an asymptomatic small-bowel primary adenocarcinoma might be found during surveillance in patients at high risk (such as someone with FAP), symptoms due to obstruction or bleeding (which may be occult) lead to the diagnosis of a small-bowel tumor in a substantial number of patients. Both adenocarcinoma and lymphomas might present with perforation. The development of anemia or obstructive symptoms in a patient with a germline cancer susceptibility gene mutation should lead to a high degree of suspicion for developing malignancy. Evaluation by diagnostic CT imaging may reveal an obstructing lesion. CT and/or MRI enterography can be helpful if the diagnostic CT is not informative. Endoscopy using techniques such as double balloon enteroscopy or video capsule endoscopy allows (for the former) tissue diagnosis as well as localization. Video capsule endoscopy is contraindicated in the setting of obstruction. For NETs, a gallium-68 DOTATATE scan may identify both the primary site as well as metastatic disease. Blood tumor biomarkers are nonspecific for the primary site (CEA or CA19-9 for adenocarcinoma or serum chromogranin for NET); these assays are better used to monitor response or progression of disease rather than for diagnosis.

Adenocarcinoma of the small bowel appears to be increasing in incidence. The median age for sporadic small-bowel tumors is in the seventh or eighth decade of life, but genetically predisposed patients and those with inflammatory bowel disease may be diagnosed at a much earlier age. African Americans have a higher incidence of small-bowel cancer than whites. While systemic therapies are usually modeled on agents used to treat colorectal cancer, genomic analyses have indicated that small-bowel adenocarcinoma has distinct genomic alterations compared to either colorectal or gastric cancers. Genomic alterations less frequent in small-bowel than in colorectal cancers include *TP53*, *BRAF* V600E, and *APC* mutations, whereas the rate of *KRAS* mutations is similar to colorectal cancer. Within small-bowel sites, the most striking difference is the higher rate of *ERBB2* alterations (of which a minority are amplifications) in duodenal cancers. Not surprisingly, because Lynch syndrome increases the risk of small-bowel adenocarcinoma, 15–20% of these tumors are MSI high or mismatch repair deficient; small-bowel adenocarcinoma associated with celiac disease also may have an increased rate of MSI-high tumors. MSI/MMRP status should be assessed in all patients with small-bowel adenocarcinoma. Somatic tumor genomic analysis may suggest a germline mutation, but appropriate genetic testing for a germline driver mutation should be performed in all patients with small-bowel adenocarcinoma.

Small-bowel adenocarcinoma has its own staging classification in the AJCC eighth edition.

TREATMENT
Small-Bowel Adenocarcinomas

Surgical resection with negative microscopic margins (R0), as is the case for other gastrointestinal tumors, is the best chance for cure. For duodenal adenocarcinomas, a Whipple procedure may be needed; for more distal duodenal cancers and jejunal adenocarcinomas, a segmental resection with adequate margins should be performed. Distal ileal tumors may require right hemicolectomy.

Small-bowel cancers are frequently found with locally advanced disease at the time of diagnosis. If the tumor is resectable, postoperative adjuvant systemic therapy is currently recommended for lymph node–positive patients, using regimens such as capecitabine-oxaliplatin. Benefit from adjuvant therapy has not yet been proven. Small-bowel cancers developing in patients with Lynch syndrome probably have a better prognosis; if colorectal cancer is a model, postoperative adjuvant therapy for patients with Lynch syndrome should be combination chemotherapy, not single-agent fluorinated pyrimidines. The value of immune modulation therapy is not established. For duodenal cancers, chemoradiation is considered if the resection margins are still positive.

For patients with advanced metastatic disease, in the absence of Lynch syndrome or a hypermutated tumor, similar cytotoxic regimens as deployed for gastric or colon cancers have been widely used. For tumors that are MSI high or dMMPR, immunotherapy is indicated; for tumors that are *HER2* amplified or *BRAF* mutated, targeted therapy may be useful.

■ SMALL-BOWEL GASTROINTESTINAL STROMAL TUMORS

Like small-bowel adenocarcinomas, small-bowel GISTs may present with obstruction or bleeding. Diagnostic techniques are those employed for other small-bowel neoplasms. While the pathological criteria for malignant potential are somewhat different than those used for gastric GISTs, postoperative management and treatment of metastatic disease are the same as those described above for gastric GIST.

■ CARCINOID (NEUROENDOCRINE) TUMORS OF THE SMALL BOWEL

Carcinoid tumors are the most common small-bowel neoplasms. For not yet identified reasons, the incidence of small-bowel carcinoid tumors has markedly increased over the past several decades. Although known risk factors include inherited genetic cancer susceptibility genes such as *MEN1* and neurofibromatosis 1 (*NF1*), these are unlikely to be the cause of the increase (**Chap. 84**). However, although the incidence has increased, small-bowel carcinoids are still uncommon, with an estimated incidence of approximately nine cases per million in the United States; the disease is more common in African Americans than whites.

Anatomically, the ileum is the most common part of the small bowel affected (~49%), followed by the duodenum and the jejunum. As is the case for gastric carcinoid tumors, grade is based on mitotic rate and/or Ki-67 immunohistochemistry. Histologic differentiation also uses the same criteria as in gastric carcinoid tumors.

In the absence of metastatic disease to the liver in the subgroup of patients whose tumors are functional (i.e., produce a hormone, usually serotonin; a duodenal NET may be a gastrinoma), presenting symptoms may be vague abdominal discomfort until or unless small-bowel obstruction occurs. Carcinoid syndrome may be found in patients whose tumors are diagnosed with already established hepatic metastasis. Because the liver is very efficient at clearing serotonin on first pass, carcinoid syndrome as a result of small-bowel carcinoid tumors usually does not occur in the absence of hepatic metastasis.

Clinical evaluation includes a diagnostic-quality CT or MRI of the abdomen and pelvis. For duodenal carcinoid tumors, upper endoscopy with EUS is also performed, and for jejunal or ileal carcinoid tumors, colonoscopy is performed. Small-bowel imaging may be performed by CT enterography; if an obstructing tumor is suspected, capsule endoscopy should be avoided. The diagnosis of a metastatic NET may be suspected from the radiographic appearance on CT imaging. Somatostatin analog imaging using gallium-68 DOTATATE is helpful in assessing extent of disease in patients whose tumors are somatostatin analog avid, as well as in identifying patients who may benefit from therapy targeting the somatostatin receptor. The AJCC eighth edition cancer staging manual has a specific small-bowel NET TNM stage classification.

The majority of patients present with locoregional disease, with approximately 40% having identified lymph node metastasis. Ten to 15% of patients have metastatic disease (usually to the liver) at the time of initial diagnosis.

Initial management should be surgical resection with curative intent; for patients with extensive adenopathy involving the root of the mesentery, vascular reconstruction may be required. Since small-bowel NETs may involve multiple tumors (15–30% of patients), the entire small bowel should be carefully examined. For patients with functional carcinoid tumors, somatostatin analog therapy using agents such as octreotide should be given before the induction of anesthesia to avoid a carcinoid crisis. For patients with hepatic metastasis, resection or regional therapy including ablation or hepatic artery embolization for functional tumors may provide effective palliation. Carcinoid syndrome may also be palliated by somatostatin receptor targeted therapy in the patients in whom gallium-68 DOTATATE scanning is positive (the majority of patients with carcinoid syndrome), including agents such as octreotide or lanreotide, or by peptide-directed radiation therapy using lutetium-177. Everolimus, an mTOR kinase inhibitor, has modest activity in metastatic small-bowel carcinoid tumors.

BENIGN NEOPLASMS OF THE SMALL BOWEL

As is the case for malignant small-bowel tumors, benign neoplasms of the small bowel are rare. In addition to cancers, the precursor lesion adenomas or hamartomas (from which cancers develop) may be driven by inherited cancer susceptibility genes (FAP, Lynch syndrome, Peutz-Jeghers syndrome, among others.). Other benign neoplasms include lipomas, leiomyomas, neurofibromas, and benign lymphoid nodular hyperplasia.

Patients with benign small-bowel neoplasms not associated with an inherited cancer susceptibility gene (in which case a benign tumor may be found during surveillance) are usually asymptomatic. A mass may be noted on an imaging study (usually a CT) ordered for another reason. Workup for occult or overt bleeding or intussusception of the bowel may lead to the discovery of a benign small-bowel neoplasm.

Diagnostic evaluation may include video capsule endoscopy and double balloon or push enteroscopy. In general, benign neoplasms, if found during surveillance, are removed endoscopically, if technically feasible, to decrease the risk of intussusception in Peutz-Jeghers syndrome. Mucosectomy may be used to treat bleeding hemangiomas.

FURTHER READING

Cancer Genome Atlas Research Network: Comprehensive molecular characterization of gastric adenocarcinoma. Nature 513:202, 2014.

Cancer Genome Atlas Research Network et al: Integrated genomic characterization of oesophageal carcinoma. Nature 541:169, 2017.

Choi IJ et al: *Helicobacter pylori* and prevention of gastric cancer. N Engl J Med 378:2244, 2018.

Choi IJ et al: Family history of gastric cancer and *Helicobacter pylori* treatment. N Engl J Med 382:427, 2020.

Cristescu R et al: Molecular analysis of gastric cancer identifies subtypes associated with distinct clinical outcomes. Nat Med 21:449, 2015.

Cunningham D et al: Perioperative chemotherapy versus surgery alone for resectable gastroesophageal cancer. N Engl J Med 355:11, 2006.

Goetze OT et al: Multimodal treatment in locally advanced gastric cancer. Updates Surg 70:173, 2018.

Pourmand K, Itzkowitz SH: Small bowel neoplasms and polyps. Curr Gastroenterol Rep 18:23, 2016.

Watanabe M et al: Recent progress in multidisciplinary treatment for patients with esophageal cancer. Surg Today 50:12, 2020.

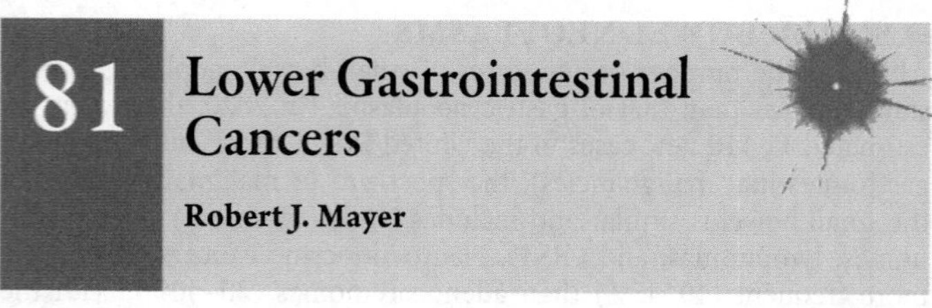

81 Lower Gastrointestinal Cancers

Robert J. Mayer

Lower gastrointestinal cancers include malignant tumors of the colon, rectum, and anus.

COLORECTAL CANCER

INCIDENCE

Cancer of the large bowel is second only to lung cancer as a cause of cancer death in the United States: 149,500 new cases were identified in 2021, and 52,980 deaths were due to colorectal cancer. The incidence rate has decreased significantly during the past 30 years in individuals 50 years of age or older, likely due in large part to enhanced and more compliantly followed screening practices. Similarly, mortality rates in the United States in this age group have decreased by more than 30%, resulting largely from early detection and improved treatment. During the same period of time, however, the incidence rate for colorectal cancer in men and women <50 years of age, having no enhanced genetic risk factor or family history for the disease, has risen by 2% each year with the presence of symptoms in this age group often being initially attributed to other causes, resulting in a more advanced disease stage at the time of diagnosis being frequently observed. A corresponding increase in mortality rates from colorectal cancer in this young adult population is now evident while, simultaneously, the trend for a decreased death rate in older individuals has continued. No distinguishing etiologic or molecular factor or clinical characteristic to account for the rising incidence of colorectal cancer in younger men and women has yet been identified with lifestyle patterns, such as diet and obesity beginning at an earlier age, having been proposed.

■ POLYPS AND MOLECULAR PATHOGENESIS

Most colorectal cancers, regardless of etiology, arise from adenomatous polyps. A polyp is a grossly visible protrusion from the mucosal surface and may be classified pathologically as a nonneoplastic hamartoma (e.g., *juvenile polyp*), a hyperplastic mucosal proliferation (*hyperplastic polyp*), or an adenomatous polyp. Only adenomas are clearly premalignant, and only a minority of adenomatous polyps evolve into cancer. Adenomatous polyps may be found in the colons of ~30% of middle-aged and ~50% of elderly people; however, <1% of polyps ever become malignant. Most polyps produce no symptoms and remain clinically undetected. Occult blood in the stool is found in <5% of patients with polyps.

A number of molecular changes are noted in adenomatous polyps and colorectal cancers that are thought to reflect a multistep process in the evolution of normal colonic mucosa to life-threatening invasive carcinoma. These developmental steps toward carcinogenesis include, but are not restricted to, point mutations in the K-*ras* proto-oncogene; hypomethylation of DNA, leading to gene activation; loss of DNA (*allelic loss*) at the site of a tumor-suppressor gene (the adenomatous polyposis coli [*APC*] gene) on the long arm of chromosome 5 (5q21); allelic loss at the site of a tumor-suppressor gene located on chromosome 18q (the deleted in colorectal cancer [*DCC*] gene); and allelic loss at chromosome 17p, associated with mutations in the *p53* tumor-suppressor gene (see Fig. 71-2). Thus, the altered proliferative pattern of the colonic mucosa, which results in progression to a polyp and then to carcinoma, may involve the mutational activation of an oncogene followed by and coupled with the loss of genes that normally suppress tumorigenesis. It remains uncertain whether the genetic aberrations always occur in a defined order. Based on this model, however, cancer is believed to develop only in those polyps in which most (if not all) of these mutational events take place.

Clinically, the probability of an adenomatous polyp becoming a cancer depends on the gross appearance of the lesion, its histologic features, and its size. Polyps may be pedunculated (stalked) or sessile (flat-based), adenomatous or serrated. Invasive cancers develop more frequently in sessile, serrated (i.e., "flat") polyps. Histologically, adenomatous polyps may be tubular, villous (i.e., papillary), or tubulovillous. Villous adenomas, most of which are sessile, become malignant more than three times as often as tubular adenomas. The likelihood that any polypoid lesion in the large bowel contains invasive cancer is related to the size of the polyp, being negligible (<2%) in lesions <1.5 cm, intermediate (2–10%) in lesions 1.5–2.5 cm, and substantial (10%) in lesions >2.5 cm in size.

Following the detection of an adenomatous polyp, the entire large bowel should be visualized endoscopically because synchronous lesions are noted in about one-third of cases. Colonoscopy should then be repeated periodically, even in the absence of a previously documented malignancy, because such patients have a 30–50% probability of developing another adenoma and are at a higher-than-average risk for developing a colorectal carcinoma. Adenomatous polyps are thought to require >5 years of growth before becoming clinically significant; colonoscopy need not be carried out more frequently than every 3 years for the vast majority of patients.

■ ETIOLOGY AND RISK FACTORS

Risk factors for the development of colorectal cancer are listed in **Table 81-1**.

TABLE 81-1 Risk Factors for the Development of Colorectal Cancer

Diet: Animal fat, obesity
Hereditary syndromes
Polyposis coli
MYH-associated polyposis
Nonpolyposis syndrome (Lynch's syndrome)
Inflammatory bowel disease
Streptococcus bovis bacteremia
Tobacco use

Diet

The etiology for most cases of large-bowel cancer appears to be related to environmental factors. The disease occurs more often in upper socioeconomic populations who live in urban areas. Mortality from colorectal cancer is directly correlated with per capita consumption of calories, meat protein, and dietary fat and oil as well as elevations in the serum cholesterol concentration and mortality from coronary artery disease. Geographic variations in incidence largely are unrelated to genetic differences because migrant groups tend to assume the large-bowel cancer incidence rates of their adopted countries. Furthermore, population groups such as Mormons and Seventh Day Adventists, whose lifestyle and dietary habits differ somewhat from those of their neighbors, have significantly lower-than-expected incidence and mortality rates for colorectal cancer. The incidence of colorectal cancer has increased in Japan since that nation has adopted a more "Western" diet. At least three hypotheses have been proposed to explain the relationship to diet, none of which is fully satisfactory.

ANIMAL FATS One hypothesis is that the ingestion of animal fats found in red meats and processed meat leads to an increased proportion of anaerobes in the gut microflora (the "microbiome"), resulting in the conversion of normal bile acids into carcinogens. This provocative hypothesis is supported by several reports of increased amounts of fecal anaerobes (*Fusobacterium nucleatum, Bacteroides fragilis*) in the stools of patients with colorectal cancer. Diets high in animal (but not vegetable) fats are also associated with high serum cholesterol, which is also associated with enhanced risk for the development of colorectal adenomas and carcinomas.

INSULIN RESISTANCE The large number of calories in Western diets coupled with physical inactivity has been associated with a higher prevalence of obesity. Obese persons develop insulin resistance with increased circulating levels of insulin, leading to higher circulating concentrations of insulin-like growth factor type I (IGF-I). This growth factor appears to stimulate proliferation of the intestinal mucosa.

FIBER Contrary to prior beliefs, the results of randomized trials and case-controlled studies have *failed* to show any value for dietary fiber or diets high in fruits and vegetables in preventing the recurrence of colorectal adenomas or the development of colorectal cancer.

The weight of epidemiologic evidence, however, implicates diet as being the major etiologic factor for colorectal cancer, particularly diets high in animal fat and in calories.

■ HEREDITARY FACTORS AND SYNDROMES

Up to 25% of patients with colorectal cancer have a family history of the disease, suggesting a hereditary predisposition. Inherited large-bowel cancers can be divided into two main groups: the well-studied but uncommon polyposis syndromes and the more common nonpolyposis syndromes **(Table 81-2)**.

Polyposis Coli

Polyposis coli (familial polyposis of the colon) is a rare condition characterized by the appearance of thousands of adenomatous polyps throughout the large bowel. It is transmitted as an autosomal dominant trait; the occasional patient with no family history probably developed the condition due to a spontaneous mutation. Polyposis coli is associated with a deletion in the long arm of chromosome 5 (including the *APC* gene) in both neoplastic (somatic mutation) and normal (germline mutation) cells. The loss of this genetic material (i.e., allelic loss) results in the absence of tumor-suppressor genes whose protein products would normally inhibit neoplastic growth. The presence of soft tissue and bony tumors, congenital hypertrophy of the retinal pigment epithelium, mesenteric desmoid tumors, and ampullary cancers in addition to the colonic polyps characterizes a subset of polyposis coli known as *Gardner's syndrome*. The appearance of malignant tumors of the central nervous system accompanying polyposis coli defines *Turcot's syndrome*. The colonic polyps in all these conditions are rarely present before puberty but are generally evident in affected individuals by age 25 years. If the polyposis is not treated surgically, colorectal cancer will develop in almost all patients aged <40 years. Polyposis coli results from a defect in the colonic mucosa, leading to an abnormal proliferative pattern and impaired DNA repair mechanisms.

TABLE 81-2 Heritable (Autosomal Dominant) Gastrointestinal Neoplasia Syndromes

SYNDROME	DISTRIBUTION OF POLYPS	HISTOLOGIC TYPE	MALIGNANT POTENTIAL	ASSOCIATED LESIONS
Familial adenomatous polyposis	Large intestine	Adenoma	Common	None
Gardner's syndrome	Large and small intestines	Adenoma	Common	Osteomas, fibromas, lipomas, epidermoid cysts, ampullary cancers, congenital hypertrophy of retinal pigment epithelium
Turcot's syndrome	Large intestine	Adenoma	Common	Brain tumors
MYH-associated polyposis	Large intestine	Adenoma	Common	None
Lynch syndrome (nonpolyposis syndrome)	Large intestine (often proximal)	Adenoma	Common	Endometrial and ovarian tumors (most frequently), gastric, genitourinary, pancreatic, biliary cancers (less frequently)
Peutz-Jeghers syndrome	Small and large intestines, stomach	Hamartoma	Rare	Mucocutaneous pigmentation; tumors of the ovary, breast, pancreas, endometrium
Juvenile polyposis	Large and small intestines, stomach	Hamartoma, rarely progressing to adenoma	Rare	Various congenital abnormalities

Once the multiple polyps are detected, patients should undergo a total colectomy. Medical therapy with nonsteroidal anti-inflammatory drugs (NSAIDs) such as sulindac and selective cyclooxygenase-2 inhibitors such as celecoxib can decrease the number and size of polyps in patients with polyposis coli; however, this effect on polyps is only temporary, and the use of NSAIDs has not been shown to reduce the risk of cancer. Colectomy remains the primary therapy/prevention. The offspring of patients with polyposis coli, who often are prepubertal when the diagnosis is made in the parent, have a 50% risk for developing this premalignant disorder and should be carefully screened by annual flexible sigmoidoscopy until age 35 years. Proctosigmoidoscopy is a sufficient screening procedure because polyps tend to be evenly distributed from cecum to anus, making more invasive and expensive techniques such as colonoscopy or barium enema unnecessary. Testing for occult blood in the stool is an inadequate screening maneuver. If a causative germline *APC* mutation has been identified in an affected family member, an alternative method for identifying carriers is testing DNA from peripheral blood mononuclear cells for the presence of the specific *APC* mutation. The detection of such a germline mutation can lead to a definitive diagnosis before the development of polyps.

MYH-Associated Polyposis MYH-associated polyposis (MAP) is a rare autosomal recessive syndrome caused by a biallelic mutation in the *MUT4H* gene. This hereditary condition may have a variable clinical presentation, resembling polyposis coli or colorectal cancer occurring in younger individuals without polyposis. Screening and colectomy guidelines for this syndrome are less clear than for polyposis coli, but annual to biennial colonoscopic surveillance is generally recommended starting at age 25–30 years.

Lynch Syndrome Lynch syndrome, previously known as hereditary nonpolyposis colon cancer, is another autosomal dominant trait. It is characterized by the presence of three or more relatives with histologically documented colorectal cancer, one of whom is a first-degree relative of the other two; one or more cases of colorectal cancer diagnosed before age 50 in the family; and colorectal cancer involving at least two generations. In contrast to polyposis coli, Lynch syndrome is associated with an unusually high frequency of cancer arising in the proximal large bowel. The median age for the appearance of an adenocarcinoma is <50 years, 10–15 years younger than the median age for the general population. Despite having a poorly differentiated, mucinous histologic appearance, the proximal colon tumors that characterize Lynch syndrome have a better prognosis than sporadic tumors from patients of similar age. Families with Lynch syndrome often include individuals with multiple primary cancers; the association of colorectal cancer with either ovarian or endometrial carcinomas is especially strong in women, and an increased appearance of gastric, small-bowel, genitourinary, pancreaticobiliary, and sebaceous skin tumors has been reported as well. It has been recommended that members of such families undergo annual or biennial colonoscopy beginning at age 25 years, with intermittent pelvic ultrasonography and endometrial biopsy for afflicted women; such a screening strategy has not yet been validated. Lynch syndrome is associated with germline mutations of several genes, particularly *hMSH2* on chromosome 2 and *hMLH1* on chromosome 3. These mutations lead to errors in DNA replication and are thought to result in DNA instability because of defective repair of DNA mismatches resulting in abnormal cell growth and tumor development. Testing tumor cells through molecular analysis of DNA for "microsatellite instability" or immunohistochemical staining for deficiency in mismatch repair proteins in patients with colorectal cancer and a positive family history for colorectal or endometrial cancer may identify probands with Lynch syndrome.

INFLAMMATORY BOWEL DISEASE

(Chap. 326) Large-bowel cancer is increased in incidence in patients with long-standing inflammatory bowel disease (IBD). Cancers develop more commonly in patients with ulcerative colitis than in those with granulomatous (i.e., Crohn's) colitis, but this impression may result in part from the occasional difficulty of differentiating these two conditions. The risk of colorectal cancer in a patient with IBD is relatively small during the initial 10 years of the disease, but then appears to increase at a rate of ~0.5–1% per year. Cancer may develop in 8–30% of patients after 25 years. The risk is higher in younger patients with pancolitis.

Cancer surveillance strategies in patients with IBD are unsatisfactory. Symptoms such as bloody diarrhea, abdominal cramping, and obstruction, which may signal the appearance of a tumor, are similar to the complaints caused by a flare-up of the underlying inflammatory disease. In patients with a history of IBD lasting ≥15 years who continue to experience exacerbations, the surgical removal of the colon can significantly reduce the risk for cancer and also eliminate the target organ for the underlying chronic gastrointestinal disorder. The value of such surveillance techniques as colonoscopy with mucosal biopsies and brushings for less symptomatic individuals with chronic IBD is uncertain. The lack of uniformity regarding the pathologic criteria that characterize dysplasia and the absence of data that such surveillance reduces the development of lethal cancers have made this costly practice an area of controversy.

OTHER HIGH-RISK CONDITIONS

***Streptococcus bovis* Bacteremia** For unknown reasons, individuals who develop endocarditis or septicemia from this fecal bacterium have a high incidence of occult colorectal tumors and, possibly, upper gastrointestinal cancers as well. Endoscopic or radiographic screening appears advisable.

Tobacco Use Cigarette smoking is linked to the development of colorectal adenomas, particularly after >35 years of tobacco use. No biologic explanation for this association has yet been proposed.

PRIMARY PREVENTION

Several orally administered compounds have been assessed as possible inhibitors of colon cancer. The most effective class of chemopreventive agents is aspirin and other NSAIDs, which are thought to suppress cell proliferation by inhibiting prostaglandin synthesis. Regular aspirin use reduces the risk of colon adenomas and carcinomas as well as death from large-bowel cancer; such use also appears to diminish the likelihood for developing additional premalignant adenomas following successful treatment for a prior colon carcinoma. This effect of aspirin on colon carcinogenesis increases with the duration and dosage of drug use. Emerging data linking adequate plasma levels of vitamin D with reduced risk of adenomatous polyps and colorectal cancer appear promising. The value of vitamin D as a form of chemoprevention is under study. Antioxidant vitamins such as ascorbic acid, tocopherols, and β-carotene are ineffective at reducing the incidence of subsequent adenomas in patients who have undergone the removal of a colon adenoma. Estrogen replacement therapy has been associated with a reduction in the risk of colorectal cancer in women, conceivably by an effect on bile acid synthesis and composition or by decreasing synthesis of IGF-I.

SCREENING

The rationale for colorectal cancer screening programs is that the removal of adenomatous polyps will prevent colorectal cancer, and that earlier detection of localized, superficial cancers in asymptomatic individuals will increase the surgical cure rate. Such screening programs are particularly important for individuals with a family history of the disease in first-degree relatives. The relative risk for developing colorectal cancer increases to 1.75 in such individuals and may be even higher if the relative was afflicted before age 60 years. The prior use of rigid proctosigmoidoscopy as a screening tool was based on the observation that 60% of early lesions are located in the rectosigmoid. For unexplained reasons, however, the proportion of large-bowel cancers arising in the rectum has been decreasing during the past several decades, with a corresponding increase in the proportion of cancers in the more proximal descending colon. As such, the potential for rigid proctosigmoidoscopy to detect a sufficient number of occult neoplasms to make the procedure cost-effective has been questioned.

Screening strategies for colorectal cancer that have been examined during the past several decades are listed in **Table 81-3**.

Many programs directed at the early detection of colorectal cancers have focused on digital rectal examinations and fecal occult blood (i.e., stool guaiac) testing. The digital examination should be part of any routine physical evaluation in adults aged >40 years, serving as a screening test for prostate cancer in men, a component of the pelvic examination in women, and an inexpensive maneuver for the detection of masses in the rectum. However, because of the proximal migration of colorectal tumors, its value as an overall screening modality for colorectal cancer has become limited. The development of the fecal occult blood test has greatly facilitated the detection of occult fecal blood. Unfortunately, even when performed optimally, the fecal occult blood test has major limitations as a screening technique. About 50% of patients with documented colorectal cancers have a negative fecal occult blood test, consistent with the intermittent bleeding pattern of these tumors. When random cohorts of asymptomatic persons have been tested, 2–4% have fecal occult blood-positive stools. Colorectal cancers have been found in <10% of these "test-positive" cases, with benign polyps being detected in an additional 20–30%. Thus, a colorectal neoplasm will not be found in most asymptomatic individuals with occult blood in their stool. Nonetheless, persons found to have fecal occult blood-positive stool routinely undergo further medical evaluation, including sigmoidoscopy and/or colonoscopy—procedures that are not only uncomfortable and expensive but also associated with a small risk for significant complications. The added cost of these studies would appear justifiable if the small number of patients found to have occult neoplasms because of fecal occult blood screening could be shown to have an improved prognosis and prolonged survival. Prospectively controlled trials have shown a statistically significant reduction in mortality rate from colorectal cancer for individuals undergoing annual stool guaiac screening. However, this benefit only emerged after >13 years of follow-up and was extremely expensive to achieve because all positive tests (most of which were falsely positive) were followed by colonoscopy. Moreover, these colonoscopic examinations quite likely provided the opportunity for cancer prevention through the removal of potentially premalignant adenomatous polyps because the eventual development of cancer was reduced by 20% in the cohort undergoing annual screening.

With the appreciation that the carcinogenic process leading to the progression of the normal bowel mucosa to an adenomatous polyp and then to a cancer is the result of a series of molecular changes, investigators have examined fecal DNA for evidence of mutations associated with such molecular changes as evidence of the occult presence of precancerous lesions or actual malignancies. Such a strategy has been tested in >4000 asymptomatic individuals whose stool was assessed for occult blood and for 21 possible mutations in fecal DNA; these study subjects also underwent colonoscopy. Although the fecal DNA strategy proved to be more effective for suggesting the presence of more advanced adenomas and cancers than did the fecal occult blood testing approach, the overall sensitivity, using colonoscopic findings as the standard, was <50%, diminishing enthusiasm for further pursuit of the fecal DNA screening strategy.

The use of imaging studies to screen for colorectal cancers has also been explored. Air contrast barium enemas had been used to identify sources of occult blood in the stool prior to the advent of fiberoptic endoscopy; the cumbersome nature of the procedure and inconvenience to patients limited its widespread adoption. The introduction of CT scanning led to the development of virtual (i.e., CT) colonography as an alternative to the growing use of endoscopic screening techniques. Virtual colonography was proposed as being equivalent in sensitivity to colonoscopy and being available in a more widespread manner because it did not require the same degree of operator expertise as fiberoptic endoscopy. However, virtual colonography requires the same cathartic preparation that has limited widespread acceptance in association with endoscopic colonoscopy, is diagnostic but not therapeutic (i.e., patients with suspicious findings must undergo a subsequent endoscopic procedure for polypectomy or biopsy), and, in the setting of general radiology practices, appears to be less sensitive as a screening technique when compared with endoscopic procedures.

With the appreciation of the inadequacy of fecal occult blood testing alone, concerns about the practicality of imaging approaches, and the wider adoption of endoscopic examinations by the primary care community, screening strategies in asymptomatic persons have changed. At present, the American Cancer Society, the American College of Gastroenterology, and the National Comprehensive Cancer Network recommend either fecal occult blood testing annually coupled with flexible sigmoidoscopy every 5 years or colonoscopy every 10 years in asymptomatic individuals with no personal or family history of polyps or colorectal cancer. In view of the emerging increase in the incidence of colorectal cancer in individuals <50 years of age, guidelines issued from these organizations have recently lowered the age at which to begin such screening from age 50 to age 45 years. The recommendation

TABLE 81-3 Screening Strategies for Colorectal Cancer
Digital rectal examination
Stool testing
• Occult blood
• Fecal DNA
Imaging
• Contrast barium enema
• Virtual (i.e., computed tomography colonography)
Endoscopy
• Flexible sigmoidoscopy
• Colonoscopy

for the inclusion of flexible sigmoidoscopy is strongly supported by the recently published results of three randomized trials performed in the United States, the United Kingdom, and Italy, involving >350,000 individuals, which consistently showed that periodic (even single) sigmoidoscopic examinations, after more than a decade of median follow-up, lead to an ~21% reduction in the development of colorectal cancer and a >25% reduction in mortality from the malignant disease. Less than 20% of participants in these studies underwent a subsequent colonoscopy. In contrast to the cathartic preparation required before colonoscopic procedures, which is only performed by highly trained specialists, flexible sigmoidoscopy requires only an enema as preparation and can be accurately performed by nonspecialty physicians or physician-extenders. The randomized screening studies using flexible sigmoidoscopy led to the estimate that ~650 individuals needed to be screened to prevent one colorectal cancer death; this contrasts with the data for mammography where the number of women needing to be screened to prevent one breast cancer death is 2500, reinforcing the efficacy of endoscopic surveillance for colorectal cancer screening. Presumably the benefit from the sigmoidoscopic screening is the result of the identification and removal of adenomatous polyps; it is intriguing that this benefit has been achieved using a technique that leaves the proximal half of the large bowel unvisualized.

It remains to be seen whether surveillance colonoscopy, which has gained increasing popularity in the United States for colorectal cancer screening, will prove to be more effective than flexible sigmoidoscopy in reducing mortality from this disease. Ongoing randomized trials being conducted in Europe are addressing this issue. Although flexible sigmoidoscopy only visualizes the distal half of the large bowel, leading to the assumption that colonoscopy represents a more informative approach, colonoscopy has been reported as being less accurate for screening the proximal rather than the distal colon, perhaps due to technical considerations but also possibly because of a greater frequency of serrated (i.e., "flat") polyps in the right colon, which are more difficult to identify. Furthermore, the vast majority of colorectal cancers that have appeared in younger adults have arisen in the left colon (i.e., distal to the splenic flexure), within the visible range of a flexible sigmoidoscopy. At present, colonoscopy performed every 10 years has been offered as an alternative to annual fecal occult blood testing with periodic (every 5 years) flexible sigmoidoscopy. Colonoscopy has been shown to be superior to double-contrast barium enema and also to have a higher sensitivity for detecting villous or dysplastic adenomas or cancers than the strategy using occult fecal blood testing and flexible sigmoidoscopy. Whether colonoscopy performed every 10 years beginning at age 45 is medically superior and economically equivalent to flexible sigmoidoscopy remains to be determined.

■ CLINICAL FEATURES

Presenting Symptoms Symptoms vary with the anatomic location of the tumor. Because stool is relatively liquid as it passes through the ileocecal valve into the right colon, cancers arising in the cecum and ascending colon may become quite large without resulting in any obstructive symptoms or noticeable alterations in bowel habits. Lesions of the right colon commonly ulcerate, leading to chronic, insidious blood loss without a change in the appearance of the stool. Consequently, patients with tumors of the ascending colon often present with symptoms such as fatigue, palpitations, and even angina pectoris and are found to have a hypochromic, microcytic anemia, indicative of iron deficiency. Because the cancers may bleed intermittently, a random fecal occult blood test may be negative. As a result, the unexplained presence of iron-deficiency anemia in any adult (with the possible exception of a premenopausal, multiparous woman) mandates a thorough endoscopic and/or radiographic visualization of the entire large bowel (**Fig. 81-1**).

Because stool becomes more formed as it passes into the transverse and descending colon, tumors arising there tend to impede the passage of stool, resulting in the development of abdominal cramping, occasional obstruction, and even perforation. Radiographs of the abdomen often reveal characteristic annular, constricting lesions ("apple-core" or "napkin-ring") (**Fig. 81-2**).

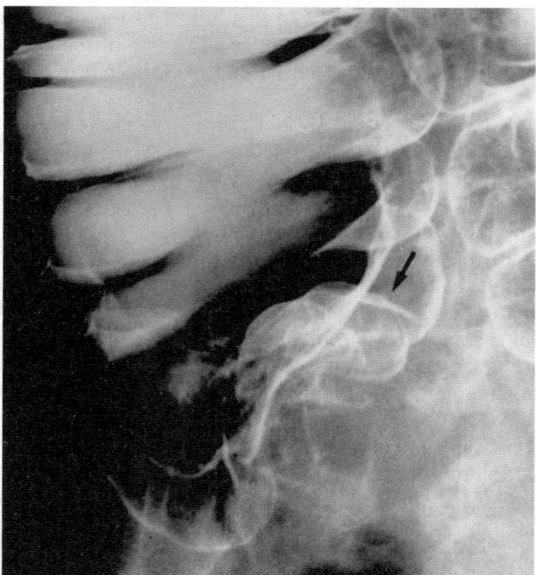

FIGURE 81-1 Double-contrast air-barium enema revealing a sessile tumor of the cecum in a patient with iron-deficiency anemia and guaiac-positive stool. The lesion at surgery was a stage II adenocarcinoma.

Cancers arising in the rectosigmoid are often associated with hematochezia, tenesmus, and narrowing of the caliber of stool; anemia is an infrequent finding. While these symptoms may lead patients and their physicians to suspect the presence of hemorrhoids, the development of rectal bleeding and/or altered bowel habits demands a prompt digital rectal examination and proctosigmoidoscopy.

Staging, Prognostic Factors, and Patterns of Spread The prognosis for individuals having colorectal cancer is related to the depth of tumor penetration into the bowel wall and the presence of both regional lymph node involvement and distant metastases. These variables are incorporated into a TNM classification method, in which T represents the depth of tumor penetration, N the presence of lymph node involvement, and M the presence or absence of distant metastases

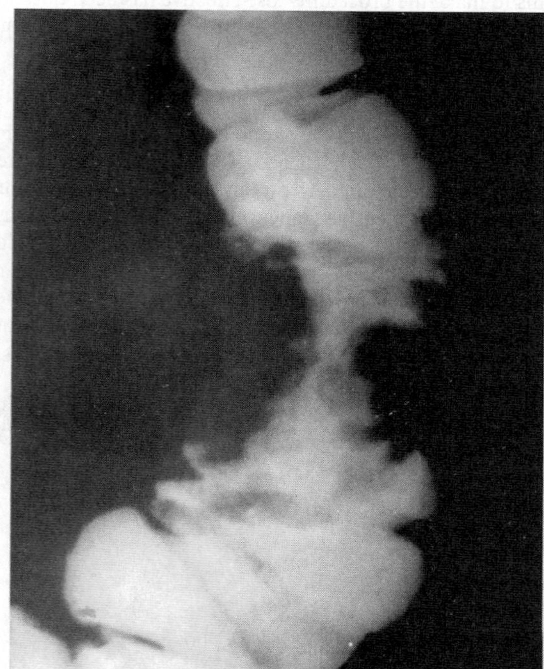

FIGURE 81-2 Annular, constricting adenocarcinoma of the descending colon. This radiographic appearance is referred to as an "apple-core" lesion and is always highly suggestive of malignancy.

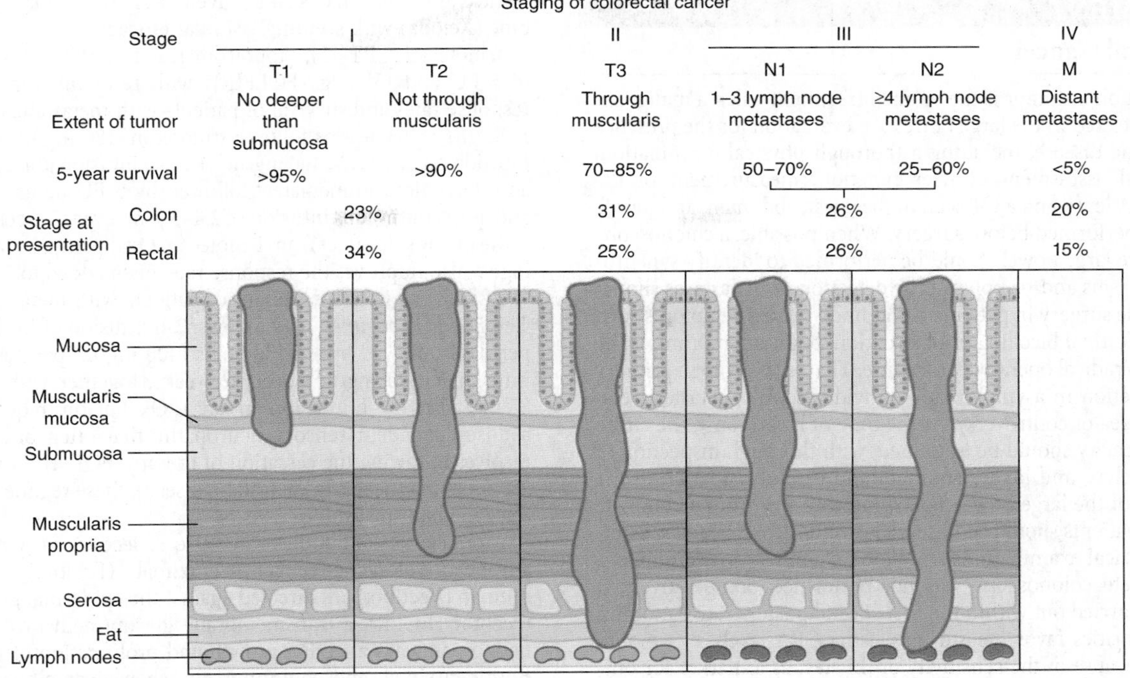

FIGURE 81-3 Staging and prognosis for patients with colorectal cancer.

(Fig. 81-3). Superficial lesions that do not involve regional lymph nodes and do not penetrate through the submucosa (T1) or the muscularis (T2) are designated as *stage I* (T1–2N0M0) disease; tumors that penetrate through the muscularis but have not spread to lymph nodes are *stage II* disease (T3-4N0M0); regional lymph node involvement defines *stage III* (TXN1-2M0) disease; and metastatic spread to sites such as liver, lung, or bone indicates *stage IV* (TXNXM1) disease. Unless gross evidence of metastatic disease is present, disease stage cannot be determined accurately before surgical resection and pathologic analysis of the operative specimens.

Most recurrences after a surgical resection of a large-bowel cancer occur within the first 4 years, making 5-year survival a fairly reliable indicator of cure. The likelihood for 5-year survival in patients with colorectal cancer is stage-related (Fig. 81-3). That likelihood has improved during the past several decades when similar surgical stages have been compared. The most plausible explanation for this improvement is more thorough intraoperative and pathologic staging. In particular, more exacting attention to pathologic detail has revealed that the prognosis following the resection of a colorectal cancer is not related merely to the presence or absence of regional lymph node involvement; rather, prognosis may be more precisely gauged by the number of involved lymph nodes (one to three lymph nodes ["N1"] vs four or more lymph nodes ["N2"]) and the number of nodes examined. A minimum of 12 sampled lymph nodes is thought necessary to accurately define tumor stage, and the more nodes examined, the better. Other predictors of a poor prognosis after a total surgical resection include tumor penetration through the bowel wall into pericolic fat, poorly differentiated histology, perforation and/or tumor adherence to adjacent organs (increasing the risk for an anatomically adjacent recurrence), and venous invasion by tumor **(Table 81-4)**. Regardless of the clinicopathologic stage, a preoperative elevation of the plasma carcinoembryonic antigen (CEA) level predicts eventual tumor recurrence. The presence of specific chromosomal aberrations, particularly a mutation in the *b-raf* gene in tumor cells, appears to predict for a higher risk for metastatic spread. Conversely, the detection of microsatellite instability in tumor tissue indicates a more favorable outcome. Tumors arising in the left colon are associated with a better prognosis than those appearing in the right colon, likely due to differences in molecular patterns. In contrast to most other cancers, the prognosis in colorectal cancer is not influenced by the size of the primary lesion when adjusted for nodal involvement and histologic differentiation.

Cancers of the large bowel generally spread to regional lymph nodes or to the liver via the portal venous circulation. The liver represents the most frequent visceral site of metastasis; it is the initial site of distant spread in one-third of recurring colorectal cancers and is involved in more than two-thirds of such patients at the time of death. In general, colorectal cancer rarely spreads to the lungs, supraclavicular lymph nodes, bone, or brain without prior spread to the liver. A major exception to this rule occurs in patients having primary tumors in the distal rectum, from which tumor cells may spread through the paravertebral venous plexus, escaping the portal venous system and thereby reaching the lungs or supraclavicular lymph nodes without hepatic involvement. The median survival after the detection of distant metastases has increased during the last 30 years from 6–9 months (hepatomegaly, abnormal liver chemistries) to 27–30 months (small liver nodule initially identified by elevated CEA level and subsequent CT scan) with increasingly effective systemic therapy improving this prognosis further.

Efforts to use gene expression profiles to identify patients at risk of recurrence or those particularly likely to benefit from adjuvant therapy have not yet yielded practice-changing results. Despite a burgeoning literature examining a host of prognostic factors, pathologic stage at diagnosis remains the best predictor of long-term prognosis. Patients with lymphovascular invasion and high preoperative CEA levels are likely to have a more aggressive clinical course.

TABLE 81-4 Predictors of Poorer Outcomes Following Total Surgical Resection of Colorectal Cancer

Tumor spread to regional lymph nodes
Number of regional lymph nodes involved
Tumor penetration through the bowel wall
Poorly differentiated histology
Perforation
Tumor adherence to adjacent organs
Venous invasion
Preoperative elevation of CEA titer (>5 ng/mL)
Specific chromosomal deletion (e.g., mutation in the *b-raf* gene)
Right-sided location of primary tumor

Abbreviation: CEA, carcinoembryonic antigen.

TREATMENT
Colorectal Cancer

Total resection of tumor is the optimal treatment when a malignant lesion is detected in the large bowel. An evaluation for the presence of metastatic disease, including a thorough physical examination, biochemical assessment of liver function, measurement of the plasma CEA level, and a CT scan of the chest, abdomen, and pelvis, should be performed before surgery. When possible, a colonoscopy of the entire large bowel should be performed to identify synchronous neoplasms and/or polyps. The detection of metastases should not preclude surgery in patients with tumor-related symptoms such as gastrointestinal bleeding or obstruction, but it often prompts the use of a less radical operative procedure. The necessity for a primary tumor resection in asymptomatic individuals with metastatic disease is an area of controversy. At the time of laparotomy, the entire peritoneal cavity should be examined, with thorough inspection of the liver, pelvis, and hemidiaphragm and careful palpation of the full length of the large bowel. Following recovery from a complete resection, patients should be observed carefully for 5 years by semiannual physical examinations and blood chemistry measurements. If a complete colonoscopy was not performed preoperatively, it should be carried out within the first several postoperative months. Some authorities favor measuring plasma CEA levels at 3-month intervals because of the sensitivity of this test as a marker for otherwise undetectable tumor recurrence. The value of periodically assessing plasma for the presence of circulating tumor DNA as a biomarker for residual or recurrent disease is under study. Subsequent endoscopic surveillance of the large bowel, probably at triennial intervals, is indicated, because patients who have been cured of one colorectal cancer have a 3–5% probability of developing an additional bowel cancer during their lifetime and a >15% risk for the development of adenomatous polyps. Anastomotic ("sutureline") recurrences are infrequent in colorectal cancer patients, provided the surgical resection margins were adequate and free of tumor. The value of periodic CT scans of the abdomen, assessing for an early, asymptomatic indication of tumor recurrence, while uncertain, has been recommended annually for the first 3 postoperative years.

Radiation therapy to the pelvis is recommended for patients with rectal cancer because it reduces the 20–25% probability of regional recurrences following complete surgical resection of stage II or III tumors, especially if they have penetrated through the serosa. This alarmingly high rate of local disease recurrence is believed to be due to the fact that the contained anatomic space within the pelvis limits the extent of the resection and because the rich lymphatic network of the pelvic side wall immediately adjacent to the rectum facilitates the early spread of malignant cells into surgically inaccessible tissue. The use of sharp rather than blunt dissection of rectal cancers (*total mesorectal excision*) appears to reduce the likelihood of local disease recurrence to ~10%. Radiation therapy, either administered pre- or postoperatively, further reduces the likelihood of pelvic recurrences but does not appear to prolong survival. Combining radiation therapy with 5-fluorouracil (5-FU)-based chemotherapy, preferably prior to surgical resection, lowers local recurrence rates and improves overall survival. Radiation therapy alone is not effective as the primary treatment of colon cancer.

Systemic therapy for patients with colorectal cancer has become more effective. 5-FU remains the backbone of treatment for this disease. Partial responses are obtained in 15–20% of patients. The probability of tumor response appears to be somewhat greater for patients with liver metastases when chemotherapy is infused directly into the hepatic artery, but intraarterial treatment is costly and toxic and does not appear to appreciably prolong survival. The concomitant administration of folinic acid (leucovorin [LV]) improves the efficacy of 5-FU in patients with advanced colorectal cancer, presumably by enhancing the binding of 5-FU to its target enzyme, thymidylate synthase. 5-FU is generally administered intravenously but may also be given orally in the form of capecitabine (Xeloda) with seemingly similar efficacy.

Irinotecan (CPT-11), a topoisomerase 1 inhibitor, has been added to 5-FU and LV (e.g., FOLFIRI) with resultant improvement in response rates and survival of patients with metastatic disease. The *FOLFIRI regimen* is as follows: irinotecan, 180 mg/m^2 as a 90-min infusion on day 1; LV, 400 mg/m^2 as a 2-h infusion during irinotecan administration; immediately followed by 5-FU bolus, 400 mg/m^2, and 46-h continuous infusion of 2.4–3 g/m^2 every 2 weeks. Diarrhea is the major side effect from irinotecan. Oxaliplatin, a platinum analogue, also improves the response rate when added to 5-FU and LV (FOLFOX) as initial treatment of patients with metastatic disease. The *FOLFOX regimen* is as follows: 2-h infusion of LV (400 mg/m^2 per day) followed by a 5-FU bolus (400 mg/m^2 per day) and 22-h infusion (1200 mg/m^2) every 2 weeks, together with oxaliplatin, 85 mg/m^2 as a 2-h infusion on day 1. Oxaliplatin frequently causes a dose-dependent sensory neuropathy that often but not always resolves following the cessation of therapy. FOLFIRI and FOLFOX are equal in efficacy. In metastatic disease, these regimens may produce median survivals of 2 years.

Monoclonal antibodies are also effective in patients with advanced colorectal cancer. Cetuximab (Erbitux) and panitumumab (Vectibix) are directed against the epidermal growth factor receptor (EGFR), a transmembrane glycoprotein involved in signaling pathways affecting growth and proliferation of tumor cells. Both cetuximab and panitumumab, when given alone, have been shown to benefit a small proportion of previously treated patients, and cetuximab appears to have therapeutic synergy with such chemotherapeutic agents as irinotecan, even in patients previously resistant to this drug; this suggests that cetuximab can reverse cellular resistance to cytotoxic chemotherapy. The antibodies are not effective in the ~65% subset of colon tumors that contain mutations in *ras* or *b-raf* genes and appear to be less likely to prove beneficial in the treatment of tumors arising from the right rather than left colon. The use of both cetuximab and panitumumab can lead to an acne-like rash, with the development and severity of the rash being correlated with the likelihood of antitumor efficacy. Inhibitors of the EGFR tyrosine kinase such as erlotinib (Tarceva) or sunitinib (Sutent) do not appear to be effective in colorectal cancer.

Bevacizumab (Avastin) is a monoclonal antibody directed against the vascular endothelial growth factor (VEGF) and is thought to act as an antiangiogenesis agent. The addition of bevacizumab to irinotecan-containing combinations and to FOLFOX appears to significantly improve the outcome observed with chemotherapy alone. The use of bevacizumab can lead to hypertension, proteinuria, and an increased likelihood of thromboembolic events.

Emerging data suggest that the use of checkpoint inhibitors (i.e., PD-1 and PD-2) as immunotherapy is more effective than chemotherapy in the subset (15%) of patients with metastatic colorectal cancer whose tumors are mismatch repair protein deficient (i.e., microsatellite unstable). Patients with solitary hepatic metastases without clinical or radiographic evidence of additional tumor involvement should be considered for partial liver resection, because such procedures are associated with 5-year survival rates of 25–30% when performed on selected individuals by experienced surgeons.

The administration of 5-FU and LV for 6 months after resection of tumor in patients with stage III disease leads to a 40% decrease in recurrence rates and 30% improvement in survival. The likelihood of recurrence has been further reduced when oxaliplatin has been combined with 5-FU and LV (e.g., FOLFOX). Reducing the duration of such oxaliplatin-containing therapy from 6 months to 3 months in patients with less invasive tumors ($T_{2-3}N_1$) has been shown to result in a similar therapeutic benefit with reduced side effects (i.e., neurotoxicity) whereas 6 months of such therapy continues to be recommended for optimally treating patients with more advanced stage III tumors (T_4 and/or N_2). Unexpectedly, the addition of irinotecan to 5-FU and LV as well as the addition of either bevacizumab or cetuximab to FOLFOX did not significantly enhance outcome.

Patients with stage II tumors do not appear to benefit appreciably from adjuvant therapy, with the use of such treatment generally restricted to those patients having biologic characteristics (e.g., perforated tumors, T4 lesions, lymphovascular invasion) that place them at higher likelihood for recurrence.

In rectal cancer, the delivery of preoperative or postoperative combined-modality therapy (5-FU or capecitabine plus radiation therapy) reduces the risk of recurrence and increases the chance of cure for patients with stage II and III tumors, with the preoperative approach being better tolerated.

CANCERS OF THE ANUS

Cancers of the anus account for 1–2% of the malignant tumors of the large bowel. Most such lesions arise in the anal canal, the anatomic area extending from the anorectal ring to a zone approximately halfway between the pectinate (or dentate) line and the anal verge. Carcinomas arising proximal to the pectinate line (i.e., in the transitional zone between the glandular mucosa of the rectum and the squamous epithelium of the distal anus) are known as *basaloid*, *cuboidal*, or *cloacogenic* tumors; about one-third of anal cancers have this histologic pattern. Malignancies arising distal to the pectinate line have squamous histology, ulcerate more frequently, and constitute ~55% of anal cancers. The prognosis for patients with basaloid and squamous cell cancers of the anus is identical when corrected for tumor size and the presence or absence of nodal spread.

The development of anal cancer is associated with infection by human papillomavirus, the same organism etiologically linked to cervical and oro-pharyngeal cancers. The virus is sexually transmitted. The infection may lead to anal warts (condyloma acuminata), which may progress to anal intraepithelial neoplasia and on to squamous cell carcinoma. The risk for anal cancer is increased among homosexual males, presumably related to anal intercourse. Anal cancer risk is increased in both men and women with AIDS, possibly because their immunosuppressed state permits more severe papillomavirus infection. Vaccination against human papilloma viruses appears to reduce the eventual risk for anal cancer. Anal cancers occur most commonly in middle-aged persons and are more frequent in women than men. At diagnosis, patients may experience bleeding, pain, sensation of a perianal mass, and pruritus.

Radical surgery (abdominal-perineal resection with lymph node sampling and a permanent colostomy) was once the treatment of choice for this tumor type. The 5-year survival rate after such a procedure was 55–70% in the absence of spread to regional lymph nodes and <20% if nodal involvement was present. An alternative therapeutic approach combining external beam radiation therapy with concomitant chemotherapy (5-FU and mitomycin C) has resulted in biopsy-proven disappearance of all tumor in >80% of patients whose initial lesion was <3 cm in size. Tumor recurrences develop in <10% of these patients, meaning that ~70% of patients with anal cancers can be cured with nonoperative treatment and without the need for a colostomy. Surgery should be reserved for the minority of individuals who are found to have residual tumor after being managed initially with radiation therapy combined with chemotherapy. The use of checkpoint immunotherapy (i.e., PD-1 inhibition) has been beneficial in some patients with recurrent disease.

■ FURTHER READING

André T et al: Pembrolizumab in microsatellite-instability-high advanced colorectal cancer. N Engl J Med 383:2207, 2020.

Colón-López V et al: Anal cancer risk among people with HIV infection in the United States. J Clin Oncol 36:68, 2018.

Dekker E et al: Colorectal cancer. Lancet 394:1467, 2019.

Grothey A et al: Duration of adjuvant chemotherapy for stage III colon cancer. N Engl J Med 378:1177, 2019.

Inadomi JM: Screening for colorectal neoplasia. N Engl J Med 376:149, 2017.

Martin D et al: Anal squamous cell carcinoma–state of the art management and future perspectives. Cancer Treat Rev 65:11, 2018.

Petrelli F et al: Prognostic survival associated with left-sided vs right-sided colon cancer. A systemic review and meta-analysis. JAMA Oncol 3:211, 2017.

Salem ME et al: Evaluation of the change of outcomes over a 10-year period in patients with stage III colon cancer: Pooled analysis of 6501 patients treated with fluorouracil, leucovorin, and oxaliplatin in the ACCENT database. Ann of Oncol 31:480, 2020.

Sclafani F et al: Systemic therapies for advanced squamous cell anal cancer. Curr Oncol Rep 20:53, 2018

Siegel RL et al: Colorectal cancer statistics 2020. CA Cancer J Clin 70:145, 2020.

82 Tumors of the Liver and Biliary Tree

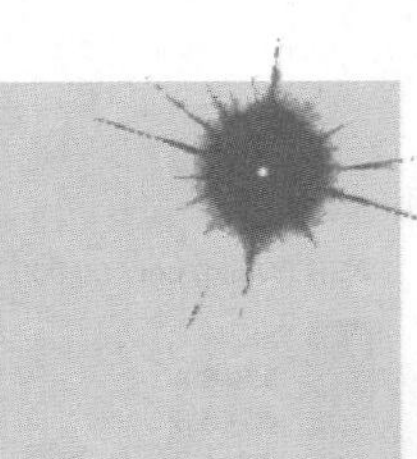

Josep M. Llovet

Liver cancer is the sixth most common cancer worldwide, the fourth leading cause of cancer-related deaths, and the leading cause of death among cirrhotic patients. Liver cancer comprises a heterogeneous group of malignant tumors with different histologic features and unfavorable prognosis that range from hepatocellular carcinoma (HCC; 85–90% cases), intrahepatic cholangiocarcinoma (iCCA; 10%), and other malignancies accounting for <1% of tumors, such as fibrolamellar HCC, mixed HCC-iCCA, epithelioid hemangiothelioma, and the pediatric cancer hepatoblastoma. The burden of liver cancer is increasing globally in almost all countries, and it is estimated to reach 1 million cases by 2025.

HEPATOCELLULAR CARCINOMA

■ EPIDEMIOLOGY AND RISK FACTORS

Overall, liver cancer accounts for 7% of all cancers (~850,000 new cases each year), and HCC represents 90% of primary liver cancers. The highest incidence rates of HCC occur in Asia and sub-Saharan Africa due to the high prevalence of hepatitis B virus (HBV) infection, with 20–35 cases per 100,000 inhabitants. Southern Europe and North America have intermediate incidence rates (10 cases per 100,000), whereas Northern and Western Europe have low incidence rates of <5 cases per 100,000 inhabitants. In the United States, liver cancer is ranked number one in terms of increased mortality during the past two decades, with an incidence of 35,000 cases per year (**Fig. 82-1**). HCC has a strong male preponderance with a male-to-female ratio estimated to be 2.5. The incidence increases with age, reaching a peak at 65–70 years old. In Chinese and in black African populations (where vertical transmission of HBV occurs), the mean age is 40–50 years. By contrast, in Japan, mean age in men is now around 75 years.

The risk factors for HCC are well established (Fig. 82-1). The main risk factor is cirrhosis—and associated chronic liver damage caused by inflammation and fibrosis—of any etiology, which underlies 80% of HCC cases worldwide and results from chronic infection by HBV or hepatitis C virus (HCV) infection, alcohol abuse, metabolic syndrome, and hemochromatosis (associated with *HFE1* gene germline mutations). Cirrhotic patients represent 1% of the human population, and one-third of them will develop HCC during their lifetime. Long-term follow-up studies have established an annual risk of HCC development of 3–8% in HBV- or HCV-infected cirrhotic patients. HCC is less common (1–3% per year) in cirrhosis associated with alcohol, nonalcoholic steatohepatitis (NASH), α_1 antitrypsin deficiency, autoimmune hepatitis, Wilson's disease, and cholestatic liver disorders. Predictors of liver cancer development among cirrhotic patients have been associated with liver disease severity (platelet count of <100,000/μL, presence

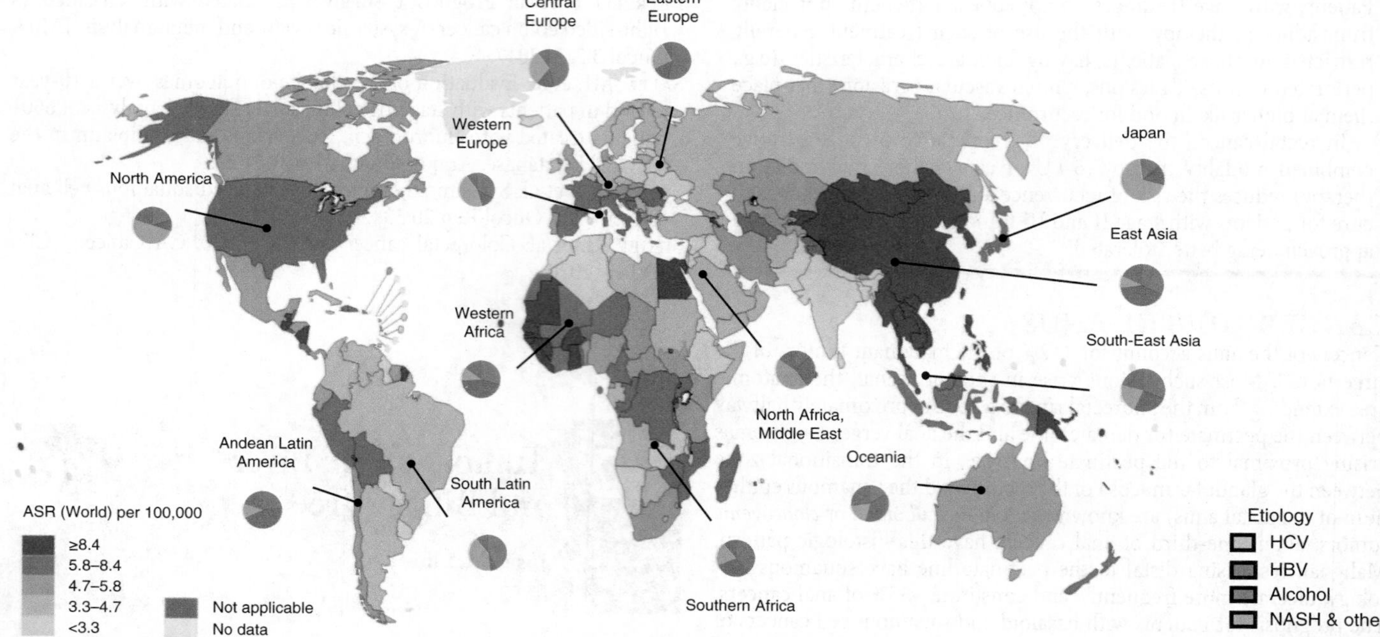

FIGURE 82-1 Distribution of hepatocellular carcinoma incidence according to geographical area and etiology. HBV, hepatitis B virus; HCV, hepatitis C virus; NASH, nonalcoholic steatohepatitis. *(Reproduced with permission from JM Llovet et al: Hepatocellular carcinoma. Nat Rev Disease Primers 6:7, 2021.)*

of portal hypertension), the degree of liver stiffness as measured by transient elastography, and liver gene signatures capturing the *cancer field effect*.

In terms of attributable risk fraction, HBV infection—a DNA virus that can cause insertional mutagenesis and affects 400 million people globally—accounts for ~60% of HCC cases in Asia and Africa and 20% in the Western world. Among patients with HBV infection, a family history of HCC, HBeAg seropositivity, high viral load, and genotype C are independent predictors of HCC development. Chronic treatments with effective antiviral HBV therapies are able to significantly decrease the risk of cancer. HCV infection—an RNA virus that affects 170 million people—is responsible for ~30% of cases and is the main cause of HCC in Europe and North America. Among patients with HCV infection, HCC occurs almost exclusively when relevant liver damage is present (either advanced fibrosis—Metavir F3 [Metavir is a scoring system for hepatic histology that grades fibrosis from 0 to 4 with higher numbers indicating more fibrosis]—or cirrhosis), particularly if associated with HCV genotype 1b. In addition, a polymorphism that activates *EGFR*, the epidermal growth factor receptor, is associated with HCV-HCC in several studies. Antiviral therapies with interferon regimens are able to prevent cirrhosis development and HCC occurrence. Direct-acting antiviral agents (DAA) induce sustained virologic response, i.e., clearance of HCV infection, in most of cases, thus resulting in 50–80% reduction in HCC risk.

Alcohol consumption and metabolic syndrome due to diabetes and obesity are responsible for ~30% of cases. NASH is becoming the leading cause of cirrhosis in developed countries and currently represents ~15–20% of HCC cases in the West. The annual incidence of HCC in NASH-related cirrhosis (1–2%/year) justifies including patients at risk in surveillance programs. Nonetheless, it has to be taken into account that 25–30% of NASH-associated HCC occurs in the absence of cirrhosis. A *PNPLA3* polymorphism is strongly associated with fatty and alcoholic chronic liver diseases and HCC occurrence. Other cofactors contributing to HCC development are tobacco and aflatoxin B1, a fungal carcinogen present in food supplies that induces *TP53* mutations. Finally, infection with adeno-associated virus 2 is associated with HCC in individuals without cirrhosis. Aside from the associations described above, genome-wide association studies have not yet confirmed polymorphisms predisposing to HCC development.

MOLECULAR PATHOGENESIS

HCC development is a complex multistep process that starts with precancerous cirrhotic nodules, so-called low-grade dysplastic nodules (LGDNs) that evolve to high-grade dysplastic nodules (HGDNs) that can transform into early-stage HCC. Molecular studies support the pivotal role of adult hepatocytes as the cell of origin, either by directly transforming to HCC or by de-differentiating into hepatocyte precursor cells. Alternatively, progenitor cells also give rise to HCC with progenitor markers.

Genomic analysis has provided a clear picture of the main drivers responsible for HCC initiation and progression. This tumor results from the accumulation of around 40–60 somatic genomic alterations per tumor, of which 4–8 are considered driver cancer genes. HCC is a prototypical inflammation-associated cancer, where immune microenvironment and oxidative stress present in chronically damaged livers play pivotal roles in inducing mutations. In preneoplastic HGDN, mutations in telomere reverse transcriptase (*TERT*) gene (20% of cases) and gains in 8q have been described. Oncogenic transformation occurs upon additional genomic hits including Wnt/β-catenin pathway activation, reexpression of fetal genes, deregulation of protein folding machinery, and the response to oxidative stress. Genomic studies and next-generation sequencing conducted during the past decade have enabled a description of the landscape of mutations, signaling pathways, and molecular classification of the disease. Nonetheless, none of these data have yet translated into actual clinical benefits for any specific molecularly based subgroups.

Molecular Drivers The landscape of mutational drivers in HCC identified by deep-genome sequencing is detailed in **Table 82-1**. The most common mutations are in the *TERT* promoter (56%), *TP53* (27%), *CTNNB1* (26%), *ARID2* (7%), *ARID1A* (6%), and *AXIN1* (5%) genes. These mutated genes participate in cell-cycle control and senescence (*TERT* and *TP53*), cell differentiation (*CTNNB1* and *AXIN1*), and chromatin remodeling (*ARID2* and *ARID1A*). Genes commonly mutated in other solid tumors such as *EGFR*, *HER2*, *PIK3CA*, *BRAF*, or *KRAS* are rarely mutated in HCC (<5%). Overall, only ~20–25% of HCCs have at least one actionable mutation. Some risk factors have been associated with specific molecular aberrations. HBV integrates into the genome of driver genes, such as the *TERT* promoter, *MLL4*, and cyclin E1 (*CCNE1*). Alcohol abuse and HCV infection have been

TABLE 82-1 Molecular Aberrations Common in Hepatocellular Carcinoma (HCC)[a]

PATHWAY	TARGET	PREVALENCE (%)
Mutations		
Telomere stability	*TERT* promoter	56
p53/cell-cycle control	*TP53*	27
	ATM	3
	RB1	3
Wnt/β-catenin signaling	*CTNNB1*	26
	AXIN1	5
Chromatin remodeling	*ARID1A*	6
	ARID2	7
	KMT2A	3
	KMT2C	3
Ras/PI3K/mTOR pathway	*RPS6KA3*	3
	TSC1/TSC2	3
Oxidative stress	*NFE2L2*	3
	KEAP1	3
High-level focal amplifications		
VEGF signaling	*VEGFA*	3
FGF signaling	*FGF19*	6
Cell-cycle control	CCND1 protein	7
Target with homozygous deletion		
TP53/cell-cycle control	*CDKN2A*	5
	TP53	4
	Retinoblastoma 1	4
Wnt/β-catenin signaling	*AXIN1*	3

[a]Recurrent mutations, focal amplifications, or homozygous deletions in HCC based on next-generation sequencing analyses.

associated with *CTNNB1* mutations. *TP53* mutations are the most frequent alterations with a specific hotspot of mutation (R249S) in patients with aflatoxin B1 exposure.

Studies assessing copy number alterations in HCCs have consistently identified: (1) high-level amplifications at 5–10% prevalence containing oncogenes in 11q13 (*CCND1* and *FGF19*) and 6p21 (*VEGFA*), *TERT* focal amplification, and homozygous deletion of *CDKN2A*; and (2) common amplifications containing *MYC* (8q gain) and *MET* genes (focal gains of 7q31). Activation of the FGF19-FGFR4 pathway mediated by epigenetic mechanisms (~20%) or high-level amplifications of 11q13 (6%) or *VEGFA* gains (high-level gains of 6p21) are also potential therapeutic targets.

Signaling Pathways Several signaling pathways have been implicated in HCC progression and dissemination. Activation of these pathways can result from structural alterations (mutations and amplifications/losses) or epigenetic modifications. In brief, (1) TERT overexpression occurs in 90% of cases, particularly related to promoter *TERT* mutations or amplifications; (2) inactivation of p53 and alterations of cell cycle are major defects in HCC, particularly in cases related to HBV infection; (3) Wnt/β-catenin pathway activation occurs in 50% of cases, either as a result of β-catenin or *AXIN1* mutation or overexpression of Frizzled receptors or inactivation of E-cadherin; (4) PI3K/PTEN/Akt/mTOR pathway is activated in 40–50% of HCCs due to mutation and focal deletion of the tuberous sclerosis complex (*TSC*)*1*/*TSC2* genes, *PTEN*, or ligand overexpression of EGF or insulin-like growth factor (IGF) upstream signals; (5) Ras MAPK signaling is activated in half of early and almost all advanced HCCs, and activation results from upstream signaling by EGF, IGF, and MET activation; (6) insulin-like growth factor receptor (IGFR) signaling is activated in 20% of cases through overexpression of the oncogenic ligand IGF2; (7) dysregulation of the c-MET receptor and its ligand HGF, critical for hepatocyte regeneration after liver injury, is a common event in advanced HCC (50%); (8) vascular endothelial growth factor (VEGF) signaling is the cornerstone of angiogenesis in HCC, along with activated angiogenic pathways such as Ang2 and FGF signaling; and (9) chromatin remodeling complexes and epigenetic regulators are frequently altered in HCC due to *ARID1A* and *ARID2* mutations.

Molecular and Immune Classes Genomic studies have revealed two molecular subclasses of HCC, each representing ~50% of patients. The proliferative subclass is enriched by activation of Ras, mTOR, and IGF signaling and *FGF19* amplification and is associated with HBV-related etiologies, overexpression of α-fetoprotein, and poor outcomes. By contrast, the so-called nonproliferative subclass contains a subtype characterized by *CTNNB1* mutations and better outcome. Another classification based on immune status has been proposed. It defines an immune HCC class in ~25% of cases characterized by immune infiltrate with expression of PD-1/PD-L1, enrichment of T cell activation, and better outcome and an immune excluded class with activation of pathways related with immune escape (i.e., Wnt signaling) or absence of T cell infiltrate. This excluded class has been proposed to be associated with resistance to immune checkpoint inhibitors, although direct translation of molecular subclasses into clinical decision making has yet to be achieved.

PREVENTION AND EARLY DETECTION

Prevention Primary prevention of HCC can be achieved by vaccination against HBV and effective treatment of HBV and HCV infection. Studies assessing the impact of universal vaccination against HBV infection have reported a significant decrease of the incidence of HCC. HBV vaccination is recommended to all newborns and high-risk groups, following World Health Organization guidelines. Vaccination is also recommended in people with risk factors for acquiring HBV infection, such as health workers, travelers to areas where HBV infection is prevalent, injection drug users, and people with multiple sex partners.

Effective antiviral treatments for patients with chronic HBV infection—achieving undetectable viral titers (circulating HBV-DNA)—reduce the risk of HCC development. Evidence of this effect is supported by one randomized trial and several cohort studies. Treatment of HCV has dramatically advanced with the new DAAs, which yield >90% sustained virologic response (SVR) rates after 12 weeks of treatment. This effect has a direct implication in reducing HCC incidence in patients with cured chronic HCV infection. Once cirrhosis is established, the incidence of HCC is lower for patients with SVR than for those with active viral disease, although they continue to have persistent HCC risk (>1% per year). Additional putative chemopreventive agents have been proposed to reduce HCC incidence in at-risk populations. Aspirin is associated with HCC cumulative incidence reduction in large studies from 8% to 4%. Similarly, compelling cohort and case-control studies demonstrated a dose-dependent relationship between coffee consumption and reduced HCC incidence. As a result, coffee consumption is recommended as a chemoprevention strategy in patients with chronic liver disease.

Surveillance The aim of surveillance is to obtain a reduction in disease-related mortality. This is usually achieved through early detection that enhances the applicability and cost-effectiveness of curative therapies. U.S. and European guidelines recommend surveillance for patients at high risk for HCC on the basis of cost-effectiveness analyses. As a general rule, high-risk populations are considered those presenting an incidence cutoff >1.5% for patients with cirrhosis and 0.2% for patients with chronic hepatitis B. However, the strength of evidence supporting surveillance is modest and is based on two randomized studies conducted in China and a meta-analysis of observational studies. Overall, these studies conclude that surveillance identifies patients with smaller tumors who are more likely to undergo curative procedures. Because of lead time bias and length time bias, it cannot be concluded that surveillance ultimately reduces HCC-related mortality.

Surveillance is recommended for cirrhotic patients due to any cause, those with HCV-related advanced fibrosis (Metavir score of F3), and patients with chronic HBV infection if Asian and aged >40 years, if African and aged >20 years, if there is a family history of HCC, or if the patient has sufficient risk by risk scores such as PAGE-B. In terms of liver dysfunction, the presence of advanced cirrhosis (Child-Pugh class C) prevents potentially curative therapies from being employed, and thus surveillance is not recommended. As an exception, patients on the waiting list for liver transplantation, regardless of liver functional status, should be screened for HCC in order to detect tumors exceeding conventional criteria and to define priority policies for transplantation. Complex scoring systems to identify at-risk populations are not yet recommended by guidelines.

Ultrasonography every 6 months, with or without serum α fetoprotein (AFP) levels, is the recommended method of surveillance. It has a sensitivity of 65–80% and a specificity of >90% for early detection. A 3-month interval does not enhance outcomes, and survival is lower with 12-month compared with 6-month intervals. A shorter follow-up interval (every 3–4 months) is recommended when a nodule of <1 cm has been detected. Computed tomography (CT) and magnetic resonance imaging (MRI) are not recommended as screening tools due to lack of data on accuracy, high cost, and possible harm (i.e., radiation with CT). Exceptionally, these techniques can be considered in patients with obesity and fatty liver, where visualization with ultrasound is difficult. Accurate tumor biomarkers for early detection need to be developed. Use of AFP levels as a stand-alone method identifies patients with HCC with 60% sensitivity but has high false-positive results. One main limitation of AFP is that only a small proportion of early tumors (~20%) present with abnormal AFP serum levels. Combining AFP with ultrasound might increase the HCC detection rate from 8–30% compared to ultrasound and depending on the performance by experienced personnel as a stand-alone method. The accuracy of other serum biomarkers proposed, such as des-γ-carboxyprothrombin (DCP) and the L3 fraction of AFP (AFP-L3), in early detection is not known.

Despite the fact that surveillance is cost-effective in HCC, the global implementation of such programs is estimated to engage ~50% of the target population in Europe and ~30% in the United States. Public health policies encouraging the implementation of such programs should lead to an increase in early tumor detection.

Diagnosis HCC is generally diagnosed at early or intermediate stages in Western countries but at advanced stages in most Asian (except Japan) and African countries. A surveillance program yields early diagnosis in 70–80% of cases. At these stages, the tumor is asymptomatic, and diagnosis can be made by noninvasive (radiologic) or invasive (biopsy) approaches. Without surveillance, HCC is discovered either as a radiologic finding or due to cancer-related symptoms. If symptoms are present, the disease is already at an advanced stage with a median life expectancy <1 year. Symptoms include malaise, weight loss, anorexia, abdominal discomfort, or signs related to advanced liver dysfunction.

NONINVASIVE (RADIOLOGIC) DIAGNOSIS Patients enrolled in a surveillance program are diagnosed by identification of a new liver nodule on abdominal ultrasound. Noninvasive diagnostic criteria can only be applied to cirrhotic patients and are based on imaging techniques obtained by four-phase multidetector CT scan (four phases are unenhanced, arterial, venous, and delayed) or dynamic contrast-enhanced MRI. A flowchart of diagnosis and recall policy recommended by U.S. and European guidelines is summarized in Fig. 82-2. Radiologic diagnosis is achieved with a high degree of confidence if the lesion is ≥1 cm in diameter and shows the *radiologic hallmarks of HCC* by one imaging technique. Using contrast-enhanced imaging techniques, the typical hallmark of HCC consists of vascular uptake of the nodule in the arterial phase with washout in the portal venous or delayed phases. This radiologic pattern captures the hypervascular nature characteristic of

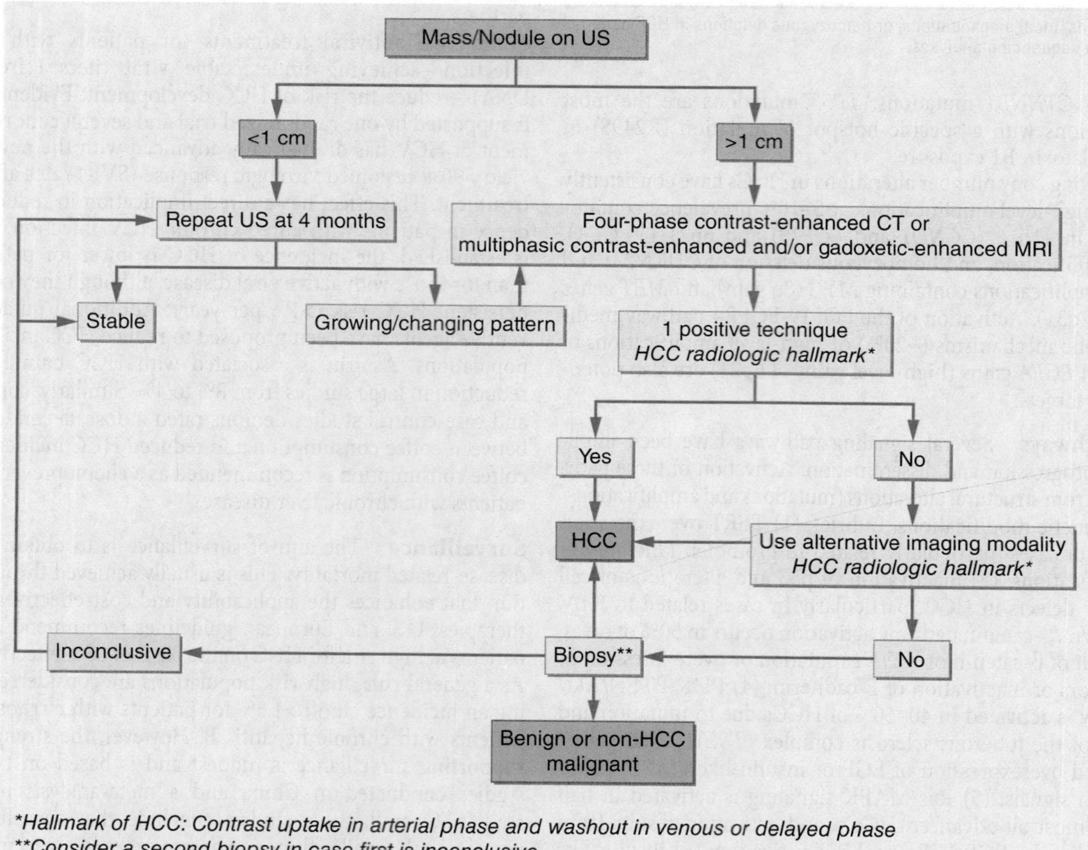

FIGURE 82-2 Recall diagnosis schedule for hepatocellular carcinoma (HCC) from the European Association for the Study of Liver Disease (EASL). ***Pink color:*** Size of the tumor at the time of detection by ultrasound (US). ***Yellow color:*** If a nodule of <1 cm is detected, repeated US at 4 months is recommended. If a nodule of >1 cm is detected, CT or MRI will be performed. Presence of *radiological hallmarks of HCC* by one imaging technique will suffice for diagnosis. This might require using one or two imaging techniques. If no diagnosis is established, then tissue biopsy would be recommended. ***Green color:*** Final diagnosis could be either HCC, benign tumor or non-HCC malignant. ***Blue color:*** If after 2 biopsies the is no conclusive diagnosis then consider follow-up with US at 4 months. *(Reproduced with permission from European Association for the Study of the Liver: EASL Clinical Practice Guidelines: Management of hepatocellular carcinoma. J Hepatology 69:182-236, 2018.)*

HCC. In these scenarios, the diagnostic specificity is ~95–100% and a biopsy is not necessary. Nodules <1 cm in size are unlikely to be HCC and would be very difficult to diagnose; thus, ultrasound follow-up at 3–4 months is recommended. MRI with liver-specific contrast agents is accepted as a diagnostic tool (Fig. 82-2). Contrast-enhanced ultrasound and angiography are less accurate for HCC diagnosis. Positron emission tomography (PET) scan performs poorly for early diagnosis. AFP levels ≥400 ng/dL are highly suspicious, but not diagnostic, of HCC according to guidelines.

The Liver Imaging Reporting and Data System (LI-RADS) has been proposed as a way of classifying radiologic findings. Essentially, nodules >10 mm visible on multiphase exams are assigned category codes reflecting their relative probability of being benign, HCC, or other hepatic malignant neoplasms. LI-RADS-1 lesions have a 0% probability of HCC, whereas lesions assigned to the LI-RADS-5 category have a 96% probability of HCC. LI-RADS-M category comprises lesions with malignant radiologic features but are not HCC malignancies in >50% of cases.

PATHOLOGIC DIAGNOSIS Pathologic diagnosis is required in two scenarios: (1) in patients without cirrhosis and (2) if imaging is not typical in at least one of two imaging techniques (CT and MRI). This occurs mainly with early-stage HCC lesions. Biopsy has not been used as the gold standard in clinical practice because of variation introduced by sampling and complications. Nonetheless, with the advent of molecular therapies and precision oncology, some guidelines advocate obtaining tissue samples in the setting of all research studies in HCC, even if radiologic criteria are met. Sensitivity of liver biopsies ranges between 70 and 90% for all tumor sizes but decreases to <50% in tumors 1–2 cm in size. The risk of complications such as tumor seeding and bleeding after liver biopsy is ~3%. Biopsies should be assessed by an expert hepatopathologist. The use of special stains may help to resolve diagnostic uncertainties. Positive staining in two of four markers (glypican 3 [GPC3], glutamine synthetase, heat shock protein 70 [HSP70], and clathrin heavy chain) is highly specific for HCC. Gene expression blueprints (glypican 3, LYVE1, and survivin) are also able to differentiate HGDNs from early HCC. Additional staining can be considered to detect progenitor cell features (K19 and EpCAM) or assess neovascularization (CD34). A negative biopsy does not eliminate the diagnosis of HCC. A second biopsy is recommended in case of inconclusive findings or if growth or change in enhancement pattern is identified during follow-up (Fig. 82-2).

TREATMENT

Overview The landscape of management of HCC has substantially changed during the past decade. Several treatments have been adopted as standard of care according to clinical practice guidelines. For early stages, resection, liver transplantation, and local ablation have substantially improved life expectancy, with median overall survival (OS) times beyond 5 years (**Fig. 82-3**). For intermediate stages, transarterial chemoembolization (TACE) has improved OS from 16 months (natural history) to 20–30 months. Finally, systemic drugs for advanced tumors (atezolizumab plus bevacizumab, sorafenib, lenvatinib, regorafenib, cabozantinib, and ramucirumab) have improved median survival times from 8 months to 19 months in first-line settings and 10 months in second-line settings. Currently, several unmet needs, such as adjuvant therapies after resection or local ablation and improving outcomes at intermediate/advanced stages with combination therapies including immunotherapies, are being addressed in the setting of phase 3 investigations (Fig. 82-3).

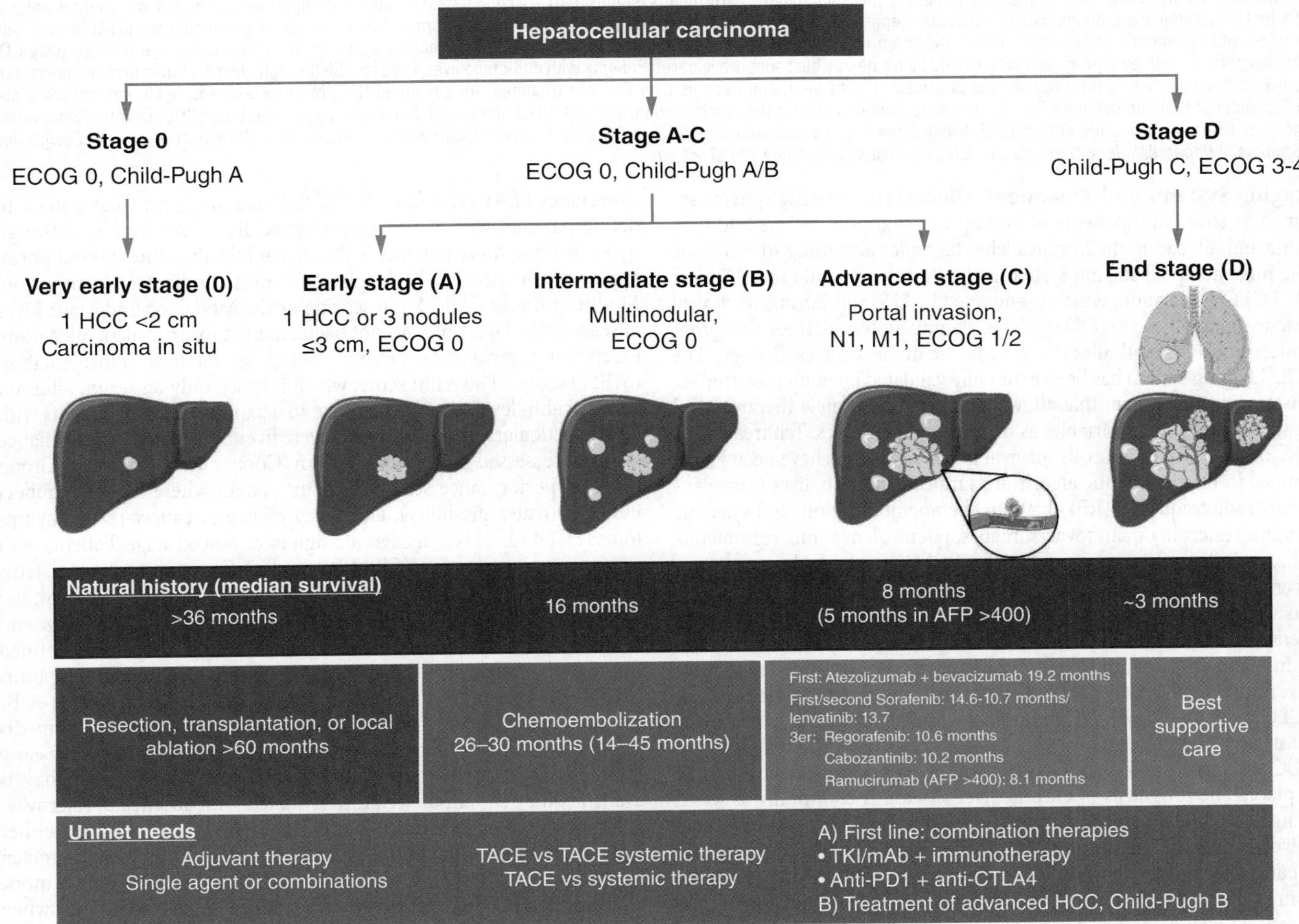

FIGURE 82-3 Natural history, impact of therapies, and unmet needs in hepatocellular carcinoma (HCC). AFP, α fetoprotein; ECOG, Eastern Cooperative Oncology Group performance status; mAb, monoclonal antibody; TACE, transarterial chemoembolization; TKI, tyrosine kinase inhibitor.

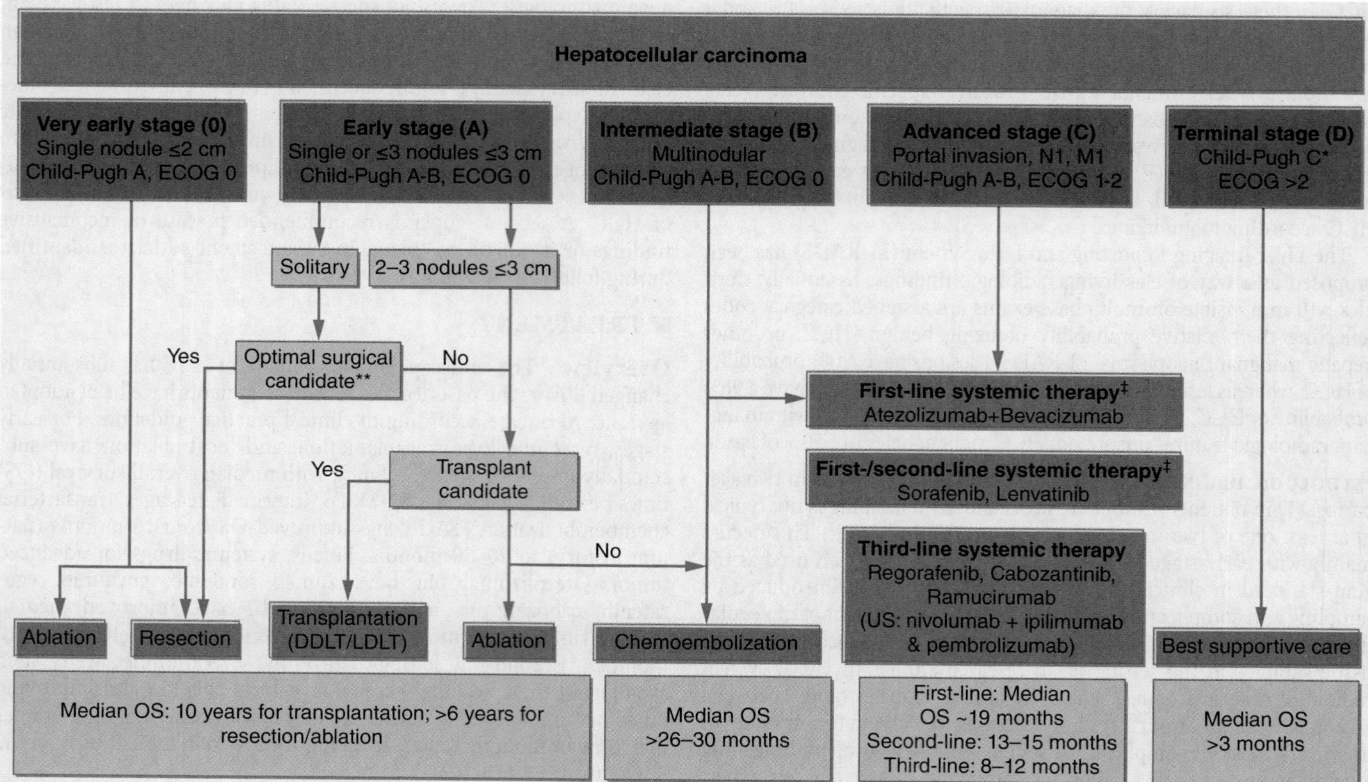

FIGURE 82-4 Staging system and therapeutic strategy. Barcelona Clinic Liver Cancer (BCLC) classification comprises five stages that select the best candidates for therapies according to evidence-based data. Patients with asymptomatic early tumors (stages 0–A) are candidates for radical therapies (resection, transplantation, or local ablation). Asymptomatic patients with multinodular hepatocellular carcinoma (HCC) (stage B) are suitable for transcatheter arterial chemoembolization (TACE), whereas patients with advanced symptomatic tumors and/or an invasive tumoral pattern (stage C) are candidates to receive systemic therapies. End-stage disease (stage D) includes patients with poor prognosis who should be treated by best supportive care. *Patients with end-stage liver disease if Child-Pugh class C should first be considered for liver transplantation. ‡Atezolizumab plus bevacizumab has been approved as new first-line treatment for advanced HCC. Nonetheless, sorafenib and lenvatinib are still considered first line options when there is a contraindication for the combination treatment. DDLT, deceased donor liver transplantation; ECOG, Eastern Cooperative Oncology Group performance status; LDLT, living donor liver transplantation; OS, overall survival. *(Reproduced with permission from JM Llovet et al: Trial Design and Endpoints in Hepatocellular Carcinoma: AASLD Consensus Conference 73:158, 2021.)*

Staging Systems and Treatment Allocation Staging systems are aimed at stratifying patients according to prognostic factors and outcome and allocating the best available therapies according to evidence. The most accepted staging system is the Barcelona Clinic Liver Cancer (BCLC) Classification, which is endorsed by U.S. and European clinical practice guidelines (**Fig. 82-4**). This staging system defines five prognostic subclasses and allocates specific treatments for each stage. The BCLC staging system has been externally validated by numerous studies. It is an evolving system that allows incorporation of new therapies and treatment-dependent variables as new evidence emerges. Ten treatments have been shown to improve survival in HCC and thus have been incorporated in the therapeutic algorithm: surgical resection, liver transplantation, radiofrequency (RF) ablation, chemoembolization, and systemic therapies (atezolizumab-bevacizumab, sorafenib, lenvatinib, regorafenib, cabozantinib, and ramucirumab). The BCLC assigns each patient to a given treatment allocation. Treatment stage migration is also applied by this scheme, meaning that if patients are not candidates for the selected therapy, the next effective therapy at more advanced stages can be given.

In HCC, three parameters are relevant for defining treatment strategy: tumor status, cancer-related symptoms, and liver dysfunction. The BCLC staging captures all three variables and allocates patients to treatments according to evidence. Since >80% of patients have two diseases, HCC and cirrhosis, a clear measurement of liver dysfunction should be in place. The prognosis of chronic liver disease is commonly assessed using the Child-Pugh score, which uses five clinical measures—total bilirubin, serum albumin, prothrombin time, ascites severity, and hepatic encephalopathy grade—to classify patients into one of three groups (A–C) of predicted survival rates. In brief, Child-Pugh class A reflects well-preserved liver function, Child-Pugh class B indicates moderate liver dysfunction with a median life expectancy of ~3 years, and Child-Pugh class C indicates severe liver dysfunction with life expectancy of ~1 year. At early BCLC stages, more granular criteria to define patients with very-well-preserved liver function (Child-Pugh hyper-A class; those patients with normal bilirubin and without portal hypertension) need to be in place to select candidates for resection. Modifications of Child-Pugh scoring or the Model for End-Stage Liver Disease (MELD) score have not been adopted for treatment allocation, except for prioritization on the waiting list for liver transplantation (MELD score). The ALBI score, which is based only on serum albumin and bilirubin levels, has been shown to accurately stratify patients with HCC, particularly those with less severe liver dysfunction. Performance status is assessed using the Eastern Cooperative Oncology Group (ECOG) performance scale (a 5-point system where higher numbers indicate greater disability), and the presence of cancer-related symptoms (ECOG 1–2) is considered a sign of advanced stage. Patients with severe liver dysfunction (Child-Pugh class C) or performance status impairment (ECOG 3–4) are offered supportive care management.

Considering all of these prognostic and predictive variables and evidence-based treatment efficacy, five BCLC stages have been defined (Fig. 82-4). Patients with liver-only neoplastic disease, no symptoms (ECOG 0), and mild to moderate liver dysfunction (Child-Pugh A-B) can be classified as very early (stage 0) or early (stage A) or intermediate (stage B) stages depending on tumor size and number. Very early HCC (BCLC 0) is defined by single tumors ≤2 cm (if pathology is available, they should be well differentiated with absence of microvascular invasion or satellites). Early HCC (BCLC A) includes either single tumors or a maximum of three nodules of ≤3 cm in diameter. Intermediate stage (BCLC B) is defined by all other liver-only tumors. Conversely, HCC is considered at advanced stages (BCLC C) when patients present with cancer-related symptoms (ECOG 1–2) or tumors with macrovascular invasion (of any type, including branch, hepatic, or portal vein), lymph node involvement, or extrahepatic spread. Finally, end-stage disease (BCLC D) is considered in cases of several impairment of quality of life/cancer-related symptoms (ECOG 3–4) or severe liver dysfunction (Child-Pugh C).

Around 40% of patients are diagnosed at stages 0 and A and, hence, are eligible for potentially curative therapies, resection, transplantation, or local ablation. These treatments provide median survival rates of 60 months and beyond, which are in sharp contrast with outcomes of 36 months reported in historical controls (Fig. 82-3, **Table 82-2**). No adjuvant therapy is recommended. Patients at intermediate stage (stage B) with preserved liver function have a documented natural history of around 16 months. These patients benefit from TACE as reported in two randomized studies and one meta-analysis and achieve an estimated survival of 25–30 months. None of the combination therapies with TACE have shown outcome advantages. Patients progressing on TACE or at advanced stage (stage C) benefit from systemic treatments. Sorafenib extends survival by ~3 months compared to placebo (from 7.9 to 10.7 months), whereas lenvatinib showed noninferiority compared to sorafenib (13.6 months vs 12.3 months, respectively). Atezolizumab (an anti-PD-L1 antibody) plus bevacizumab showed superiority compared to sorafenib (median survival 19.2 months vs 13.4 months). Three additional targeted therapies have shown improved survival compared to placebo in patients with HCC progressing on sorafenib: regorafenib, cabozantinib, and ramucirumab (only in patients with AFP >400 ng/mL). Therefore, these treatments have been adopted by guidelines and incorporated into the treatment algorithm. Patients with end-stage disease (BCLC D) should be considered for nutritional and psychological support and proper management of pain.

Although the BCLC establishes validated stages and treatment assignment according to evidence, clinical practice is not always aligned with this classification. In large cohort studies and surveys, only half of patients, or even less in Asia, are treated accordingly. Alternative staging or scoring systems have been proposed, but none of them has acquired global consensus. In contrast to BCLC, some proposed systems capture the standard of practice in Asia, such as the Hong Kong classification or the Japan Integrated Staging score. These systems capture extended indications for resection and TACE applied in clinical practice in Asia. Finally, the tumor-node-metastasis (TNM) staging system is not used in HCC since it does not incorporate the main prognostic variables related to liver function and performance status.

Due to the complexities of HCC diagnosis and management, it is recommended that patients be sent to a referral center where all the armamentarium of therapies can be offered. In principle, patient management and outcome benefit from liver cancer multidisciplinary programs that include a hepatologist, oncologist, hepatobiliary and transplant surgeons, interventional and body imaging radiologist, hepatopathologist, and specialized nurses.

SURGICAL THERAPIES

Resection Surgical resection is the first-line option for noncirrhotic patients with early-stage HCC (BCLC 0 or A) with solitary tumors (Fig. 82-4). In cirrhotic patients, ablation competes with resection for BCLC 0 tumors (<2 cm in diameter). Which treatment is better is not defined. Cost-effectiveness approaches report a benefit for local ablation with RF. For single tumors >2 cm (BCLC A), resection remains the mainstay of treatment in patients with Child-Pugh hyper-A class, i.e., those patients with normal bilirubin and absence of portal hypertension (portal hypertension is defined by hepatic venous pressure gradient ≥10 mmHg). Surrogate measures of portal hypertension are presence of esophageal varices or platelet count <100,000/μL associated with splenomegaly. Anatomic resections following the functional segments of the liver are recommended to spare uninvolved

TABLE 82-2 Summary of Key Results of Randomized and Cohort Studies in the Management of Hepatocellular Carcinoma

TREATMENT OF EARLY- AND INTERMEDIATE-STAGE HCC			
TREATMENTS	**HCC STAGE**	**TREATMENT ARMS**	**OUTCOMES (OS)**
Treatment for early HCC			
Resection	Early	Optimal (single nodule; no portal hypertension)	5 years: 50–70%
		Suboptimal (multinodular or portal hypertension)	5 years: 35–55%
Liver transplantation	Early	Milan (1 nodule <5 cm, 2–3 nodules ≤3 cm, no MVI, no EHS)	5 years: 70–80%
	Early/intermediate	Downstaged (1 nodule ≤6.5 cm, ≤3 nodules ≤4.5 cm and total diameter ≤8 cm, no MVI, no EHS)	5 years: 60–70%
Ablation	Early	RFA	Median: 50–60 months
Treatments for intermediate HCC			
Transarterial therapies	Intermediate	TACE	Median: 20–32 months

TREATMENT OF ADVANCED-STAGE HCC				
STUDY	**TREATMENT**	**MEDIAN OS, MONTHS (HR, 95% CI)**	**MEDIAN PFS, MONTHS (HR, 95% CI)**	**ORR: MRECIST/RECIST**
First-line therapies				
IMbrave150	Atezolizumab-bevacizumab	19.2 (HR 0.66, 0.52–0.85)	6.9 (HR 0.65, 0.53–0.81)	35.4%/29.8%
SHARP/REFLECT/ CheckMate-459	Sorafenib	10.7–14.6 (HR 0.69, 0.55–0.87)	3.7–3.8	2–9.2%/12.4%
REFLECT	Lenvatinib	13.6 (HR 0.92, 0.79–1.06)	7.4 (HR 0.66, 0.57–0.77)	24.1%/18.8%
Second-line therapies				
RESORCE	Regorafenib	10.6 (HR 0.63, 0.5–0.79)	3.1 (HR 0.46, 0.37–0.56)	11%/7%
CELESTIAL	Cabozantinib	10.2 (HR 0.76, 0.63–0.92)	5.2 (HR 0.44, 0.36–0.52)	NA/4%
REACH-2	Ramucirumab	8.5 (HR 0.71, 0.53–0.95)	2.8 (HR 0.45, 0.34–0.6)	NA/5%

Abbreviations: CI, confidence interval; EHS, extrahepatic spread; HCC, hepatocellular carcinoma; HR, hazard ratio; MRECIST, Modified Response Evaluation Criteria in Solid Tumors; MVI, microvascular invasion; NA, not available; NE, not evaluable; ORR, overall response rate; OS, overall survival; PFS, progression-free survival; RECIST, Response Evaluation Criteria in Solid Tumors; RFA, radiofrequency ablation; TACE, transarterial chemoembolization.

liver parenchyma and to remove satellite tumors. Predictors of recurrence are tumor size and number and presence of microsatellites or microvascular invasion at the specimen analysis. Outcomes in suboptimal candidates lead to 5-year survival rates of ~35–55%, as opposed to 60–70% for ideal candidates (Table 82-2). Macrovascular invasion, extrahepatic involvement, and liver dysfunction (Child-Pugh B-C) are major contraindications for resection.

ADJUVANT TREATMENTS Tumor recurrence represents the major complication of resection (and local ablation) and occurs in 70% of cases at 5 years. Most recurrences are intrahepatic metastases, but at least one-third are considered de novo tumors, new clones developing in the cirrhotic carcinogenic field. The type of recurrence can only be defined by molecular studies. So far, no adjuvant therapies have been proven to improve outcome or prevent recurrence after resection/ablation. Randomized trials testing adjuvant sorafenib, retinoids, chemotherapies, or chemoembolization have been negative, and thus, no adjuvant therapy recommendation has been established for patients after resection or local ablation.

Liver Transplantation Liver transplantation is the first treatment choice for cirrhotic patients with single tumors ≤5 cm and portal hypertension (including Child-Pugh B and C) or with small multinodular tumors (≤3 nodules, each ≤3 cm) (Fig. 82-4). These so-called Milan criteria have been validated over the years, and a meta-analysis reported 5- and 10-year survival rates of ~70 and ~50%, respectively, similar to outcomes achieved in non-HCC transplantation indications. Perioperative mortality rates have been reduced to <3%. Transplantation simultaneously cures the tumor and the underlying cirrhosis, and it is associated with a low risk of recurrence, around 10–15% at 5 years. No immunosuppressive regimens or antitumor therapies after transplantation have demonstrated any preventive effect on recurrence. Milan criteria are integrated in the treatment strategy (BCLC 0 and A) and have also been adopted by the United Network for Organ Sharing (UNOS) pretransplant staging for organ allocation in the United States (stage T2). Aside from size and number, conventional contraindications for organ transplantation procedures (e.g., ABO incompatibility, comorbidities) are applied in this setting.

Liver transplantation has a couple of factors, such as cost and donor availability, that limit this procedure to <5% of HCC cases. The scarcity of donors represents a major drawback of liver transplantation. Donor scarcity varies geographically, and deceased liver donation is almost zero in some Asian countries. Due to the shortage of donors, median waiting times in Western programs is ~6–12 months, leading to 20% of candidates dropping off the list due to tumor progression before receiving the procedure. Predictors of dropout are neoadjuvant treatment failure, baseline AFP >400 ng/mL, and steady increase of AFP level >15 ng/mL per month. Several strategies have been proposed to overcome this limitation. First, apply neoadjuvant therapies in patients on the waiting list. Neoadjuvant treatments such as TACE or RF ablation have been assessed in the setting of cohort and cost-effectiveness studies. In principle, the use of these therapies is recommended when the waiting time exceeds 6 months, even though impact on long-term outcome is uncertain. Second, a priority policy has been established for patients enlisted. UNOS has implemented a scoring system based on the dropout risk.

The Milan criteria are universally used as the basis for transplant eligibility, and adherence to these criteria yields good posttransplant survival. Modest expansion of Milan criteria applying the "up-to-seven" criterion (i.e., those HCCs having the number 7 as the sum of the size of the largest tumor and the number of tumors) in patients without microvascular invasion achieves competitive outcomes. These pathologically defined criteria are being used in clinical practice to predict the expected outcome after transplantation. Similarly, *downstaging to Milan criteria* is currently defined as the reduction of HCC burden by locoregional treatments to achieve Milan staging before transplantation. This strategy leads to long-term 10-year survival rates of ~50%. Since policies for enhancing organ donation have reached a ceiling during the past several years, alternatives to donation have emerged. Living donor liver transplantation represents a plausible alternative that accounts of ~5% of total transplantations performed globally. Outcomes reported are similar to those with deceased liver donors, and it is recommended as an alternative option in patients on a waiting list exceeding 6 months. The risks and benefits of this procedure should take into account both donor (death is estimated in 0.3%) and recipient, a concept known as *double equipoise*. Due to the complexity of this treatment, it must be restricted to centers of excellence in hepatobiliary surgery and transplantation.

LOCOREGIONAL THERAPIES

LOCAL ABLATION RF ablation is recommended as the primary ablative technique (Fig. 82-4). The energy generated by RF ablation (heating of tissue at 80°–100°C) induces coagulative necrosis of the tumor, producing a *safety ring* in the peritumoral tissue, which might eliminate small undetected satellites. Treatment consists of one or two sessions performed using a percutaneous approach, although in some instances, ablation with laparoscopy is needed. RF ablation is more effective in response rate and time to recurrence compared with the once-conventional percutaneous ethanol injection. HCC patients treated by RF ablation have 5-year survival rates of ~60% (Table 82-2). In tumors <2 cm, RF ablation achieves complete responses in >90% of cases with good long-term outcome and is competitive with resection in cost-effectiveness as first-line option. For BCLC A cases, RF ablation is the first-line treatment for single tumors 2–5 cm or up to three nodules, each ≤3 cm in diameter, unsuitable for surgery.

The failure rate of RF ablation increases in tumors >3 cm because of the heat loss due to perfusion-mediated tissue cooling within the area ablated. In tumors 3–5 cm in diameter, complete pathologic tumor necrosis of <50% has been reported. In particular, ~10–15% of tumors with difficult-to-treat locations, such as a subcapsular location or adjacent to the gallbladder, have a higher risk of incomplete ablation or major complications and can be approached by ethanol injection. Several approaches have been proposed to enhance the antitumor activity of RF ablation. Microwave ablation is the most widely used local image-guided technique alternative to RF. Theoretically, it provides major efficacy but higher complication rates in tumors >3 cm. Randomized trials comparing both techniques are needed. Other treatments, such as high-intensity focused ultrasound or stereotactic body radiotherapy for small tumors, have been studied in early clinical trials and are under investigation.

Chemoembolization TACE is the most widely used primary treatment for unresectable HCC worldwide and the first-line indication for patients with intermediate BCLC B stage (Fig. 82-4). Conventional chemoembolization (c-TACE) consists of the local hepatic artery administration of chemotherapy (either doxorubicin 50 mg/m^2 or cisplatin) mixed with an emulsion of lipiodol followed by obstruction of the feeding artery with sponge particles. c-TACE mainly benefits patients with liver-only disease, Child-Pugh A class or B class without ascites, good performance status (ECOG 0), and absence of branch or trunk vascular invasion. Median survival is ~20 months (compared to 16 months for pooled control arms). The best randomized phase 3 investigations have provided median survivals for TACE of 20–30 months in properly selected populations. Median objective response rates are 50–70%. In randomized studies, the treatment is either performed at a regular schedule of 0, 2, and 6 months (median number of sessions: 3) or on demand according to tumor response. TACE procedures should be stopped upon tumor progression or any other contraindication. Exceptionally, occurrence of a new small untreated nodule as the only progression feature can be considered for treatment. Around 50% of patients present with a limited postembolization syndrome of fever and abdominal pain related to ischemic injury and release of cytokines. Less than 5% of patients present with major complications (liver abscess, ischemic cholecystitis, or liver failure), and in <2% of cases, treatment-related death occurs.

Applicability of c-TACE in patients at intermediate stage is limited to half of cases, mostly as a result of the presence of liver failure (Child B or ascites or encephalopathy), technical contraindications to the procedure (i.e., impaired portal vein blood flow), or infiltrative/massive tumor burden (i.e., generally main tumor size >10 cm). Super-selective

TACE minimize the ischemic insult to nontumor tissue. According to guidelines, treatment-stage migration allows performing TACE on patients at early stages not suitable for surgical or ablative therapies. In selective studies, median survival times of 5 years have been reported in patients with single HCC treated by super-selective TACE. On the other hand, TACE performed beyond guidelines as a conventional practice in patients with advanced HCC yields poor outcomes.

Drug-eluting bead chemoembolization (DEB-TACE) differs from c-TACE in the use of more standardized embolic spheres of regular size embedded with chemotherapy. This strategy ensures drug release over a 1-week period, resulting in an enhancement of drug concentration within the tumor. DEB-TACE achieves similar antitumor activity (objective responses of ~60%) as c-TACE and is associated with significantly less systemic cytotoxic effects and better tolerance, but with no clear differences in clinical outcomes. Phase 2 and 3 studies have compared DEB-TACE with the combination of DEB-TACE plus sorafenib, orantinib, or brivanib, which are VEGF receptor inhibitors. Median survival in both arms of these international trials was 25–30 months.

Radioembolization and Other Intraarterial Therapies

Radioembolization using beads coated with yttrium-90 (Y-90)—an isotope that emits short-range β radiation—is the most promising alternative to TACE. Several phase II studies reported objective responses and overall outcome with a safe profile. Due to the lack of phase III trials, this treatment is currently not recommended in guidelines. Radioembolization requires prevention of severe lung shunting and intestinal radiation before the procedure. Around 20% of patients present with liver-related toxicity and 3% experience treatment-related death. Due to the minimally embolic effect of Y-90 microspheres, treatment can be safely used in patients with portal vein thrombosis, a setting where survival results in phase II were encouraging. However, three randomised controlled trials, including two head-to-head trials against sorafenib and one trial combining radioembolization plus sorafenib versus sorafenib alone, did not show OS endpoint superiority. Thus, these treatments are not indicated in the advanced-stage scenario.

TACE should be distinguished from other intraarterial therapies, such as chemo-lipiodolization, which involves the delivery of an emulsion of chemotherapy mixed with lipiodol; bland transcatheter embolization, where no chemotherapeutic agent is delivered; and intraarterial chemotherapy, where no embolization is performed. None of these approaches is recommended due to the lack of survival benefit.

SYSTEMIC THERAPIES

Conventional systemic chemotherapy and radiotherapy have not produced survival advantages. Randomized studies also failed to show benefit with antiestrogen therapies and vitamin D derivatives. External-beam liver-directed radiotherapy (stereotactic body radiotherapy) efficacy is currently being tested with and without sorafenib in phase III trials. In 2007, a phase III trial demonstrated survival benefits for patients with advanced-stage disease treated with sorafenib, and lenvatinib showed similar effects to sorafenib in first-line treatment. Recently, the combination of atezolizumab with bevacizumab demonstrated survival benefits in the advanced setting when compared to sorafenib and has now become the standard first-line treatment. Three additional therapies, regorafenib, cabozantinib, and ramucirumab (only in patients with AFP >400 ng/mL), have been shown to benefit patients progressing on sorafenib (Fig. 82-5).

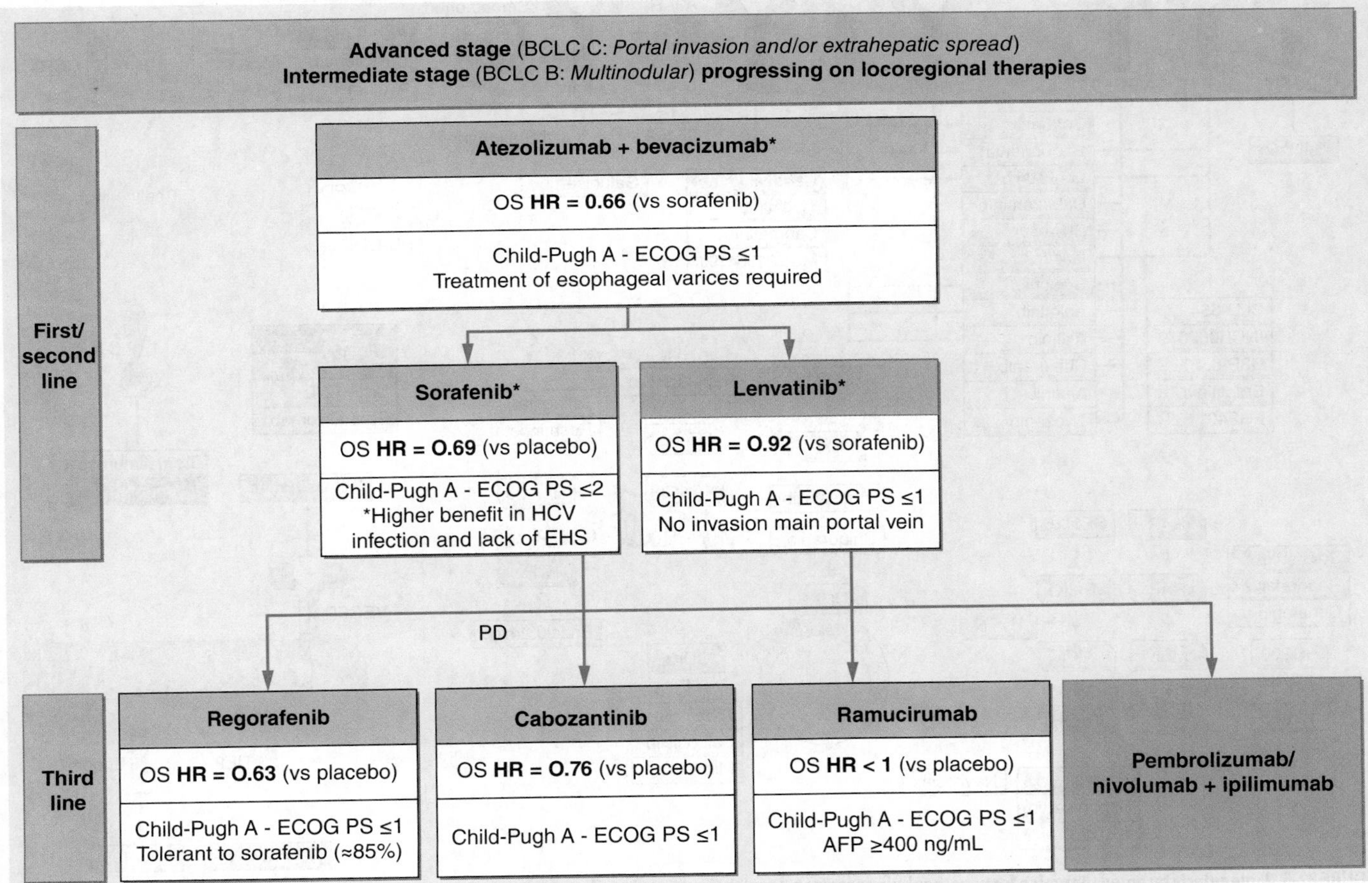

FIGURE 82-5 Treatment strategy for advanced hepatocellular carcinoma with systemic therapies. Drugs in green have positive results from phase 3 trials with a superiority design (atezolizumab plus bevacizumab, sorafenib, regorafenib, cabozantinib, and ramucirumab). Drugs in orange have positive results from phase 3 trials with a noninferiority design (lenvatinib vs sorafenib). Drugs in red have received accelerated approval from the U.S. Food and Drug Administration (FDA) based on promising efficacy results in phase 2 trials in the second-line setting (nivolumab, pembrolizumab, and nivolumab ipilimumab). Key details of the patient populations are provided. *Around 20% of patients can receive sorafenib or lenvatinib in first line due to contraindications to atezolizumab + bevacizumab. AFP, α fetoprotein; BCLC, Barcelona Clinic Liver Cancer (classification); ECOG PS, Eastern Cooperative Oncology Group performance status; EHS, extrahepatic spread; HCV, hepatitis C virus; HR, hazard ratio; mRECIST, modified Response Evaluation Criteria in Solid Tumors; OS, overall survival. *(Reproduced with permission from JM Llovet: Molecular therapies and precision medicine for hepatocellular carcinoma. Nat Rev Clin Oncol 15:599, 2018.)*

Molecular Targeted Therapies Atezolizumab (anti-PD-L1 checkpoint inhibitor) plus bevacizumab (antibody against VEGFA) has become the standard of care in first-line treatment for advanced HCC as a result of a positive phase 3 trial indicating superiority versus sorafenib in terms of survival (Fig. 82-5). Median survival with the combination was 19.2 months compared with 13.4 months for sorafenib. Combination treatment also improved progression-free survival and patient-reported quality of life outcomes. Objective response to the combination was 35.4% versus 13.9% for sorafenib. Adverse events also favored the combination (grade 3–4 adverse events, 36% vs 50% for sorafenib). The most common side effects associated with the combination were hypertension, proteinuria, and low-grade diarrhea, whereas autoimmune events were infrequent. Treatment-related adverse events leading to discontinuation of these two drugs was 15%. Upper gastrointestinal endoscopies are required before initiating the combination therapy for detection and treatment of varices to mitigate the risk of bleeding associated with bevacizumab. Thus, screening for varices is becoming standard before first-line therapy in HCC management.

Alternatively, sorafenib and lenvatinib are indicated for HCC in patients with well-preserved liver function (Child-Pugh class A) and with advanced tumors either as first-line treatment in patients with contraindications or with progression to the combination therapy (Fig. 82-5). A phase III study comparing sorafenib versus placebo showed increased survival from 7.9 months to 10.7 months (hazard ratio [HR] 0.69; 31% reduction in risk of death). Patients with HCV-related HCC achieve significantly better outcomes with sorafenib, with a median survival of 14 months. No predictive biomarkers of responsiveness to sorafenib have been identified. The recommended daily dose of sorafenib is 800 mg. Median treatment duration is about 6 months. Treatment is associated with adverse events, such as diarrhea, hand-foot skin reactions, fatigue, and hypertension. These toxicities lead to treatment discontinuation in 15% of patients and dose reduction in up to half. This therapy cannot be administered to around one-third of the targeted patients due to primary intolerance, advanced age, or liver failure (ascites or encephalopathy). Active vascular disease, either coronary or peripheral, is considered a formal contraindication.

The efficacy of sorafenib probably results from a balance between targeting cancer cells and the microenvironment by blocking up to 40 kinases, including antiangiogenic (VEGF receptor [VEGFR], platelet-derived growth factor receptor [PDGFR]) and antiproliferative drivers (serine/threonine-protein kinase B-raf [BRAF] and mast/stem cell growth factor receptor [c-Kit]) (**Fig. 82-6**). Median time to progression on sorafenib is 4–5 months in phase III trials.

Another alternative to sorafenib is the multikinase inhibitor lenvatinib; it was noninferior in a phase 3 investigation (13.6 months vs

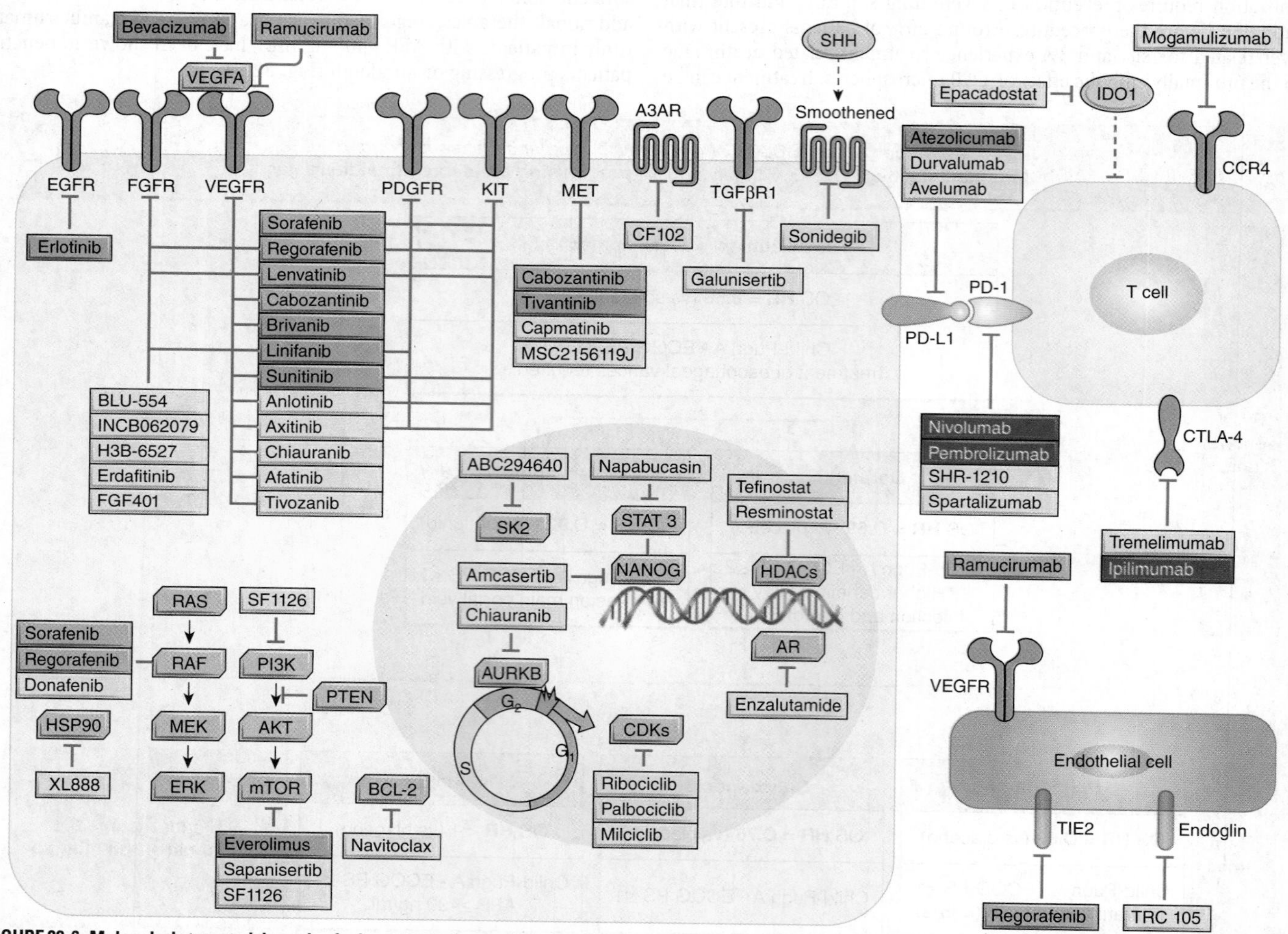

FIGURE 82-6 Molecularly targeted therapies for hepatocellular carcinoma and their target signaling pathways. Green boxes indicate drugs with positive results from phase 3 trials (atezolizumab plus bevacizumab, sorafenib, lenvatinib, regorafenib, lenvatinib, cabozantinib, and ramucirumab). Red boxes indicate drugs with negative results from phase 3 trials (everolimus, sunitinib, linifanib, erlotinib, brivanib, and tivantinib). Drugs in yellow boxes are currently in development for hepatocellular carcinoma in phase 1, 2, or 3 clinical trials. Brown boxes indicate drugs approved based on phase 2 trial data (pembrolizumab, nivolumab + ipilimumab). Dashed arrows and lines indicate indirect activities. A3AR, adenosine receptor A3; AR, androgen receptor; AURKB, aurora kinase B; BCL-2, apoptosis regulator BCL-2; CCR4, CC-chemokine receptor 4; CDKs, cyclin-dependent kinases; CTLA-4, cytotoxic T lymphocyte protein 4; HDAC, histone deacetylase; HSP90, heat shock protein 90; IDO1, indoleamine 2,3-dioxygenase 1; NANOG, homeobox protein NANOG; PD-1, programmed cell death protein 1; PD-L1, programmed cell death ligand 1; SHH, Sonic hedgehog; STAT3, signal transducer and activator of transcription 3; TIE-2, angiopoietin 1 receptor. *(Reproduced with permission from JM Llovet: Molecular therapies and precision medicine for hepatocellular carcinoma. Nat Rev Clin Oncol 15:599, 2018.)*

12.3 months; HR 0.92) (Fig. 82-5). Lenvatinib induces objective responses in 24% of cases. The main side effects are hypertension, proteinuria, asthenia, diarrhea, and weight loss. This treatment induced grade 3–4 drug-related adverse events in 55% of patients, resulting in a withdrawal rate of ~15%.

Three drugs (regorafenib, cabozantinib, and ramucirumab) have shown survival benefits versus placebo in patients progressing on sorafenib, and two additional immune-based treatments have been approved by the U.S. Food and Drug Administration (FDA) based on promising phase 2 data (pembrolizumab and nivolumab plus ipilimumab) (Fig. 82-5). The median survival of patients progressing on first-line treatment is 8 months (obtained from patients allocated to the placebo arm).

A phase III study comparing regorafenib (a more potent multikinase inhibitor than sorafenib targeting similar kinases) versus placebo in patients progressing on sorafenib reported a benefit in survival from 7.8 to 10.6 months (HR 0.62; 38% reduction in risk of death) (Fig. 82-5). Response rate was 10%. Median time on treatment was 3.5 months. Prevalence of toxicity (hand-foot reaction, fatigue, and hypertension) was higher compared with reported toxicity from sorafenib, but adverse events only led to treatment discontinuation in 10% of cases. Cabozantinib, a multikinase VEGFR inhibitor with activity against both AXL and c-MET (Fig. 82-6), improves survival compared to placebo after progression on sorafenib (10.2 months for cabozantinib vs 8.0 months in the placebo arm; HR 0.76). The most common grade 3–4 adverse events were palmar-plantar erythrodysesthesia, hypertension, increased aspartate aminotransferase level, fatigue, and diarrhea. Ramucirumab, an anti-VEGFR-2 monoclonal antibody, is the only biomarker-guided therapy in HCC based on AFP levels. The randomized, placebo-controlled, phase 3 REACH-2 study selected patients with advanced HCC in second line with baseline AFP ≥400 ng/dL. Median survival for patients treated with ramucirumab was 8.1 months, compared to 5 months for patients receiving placebo. The most common grade 3–4 adverse events were hypertension, hyponatremia, and increased aspartate aminotransferase. Patients progressing after second-line therapy and patients with BCLC D stage should receive best supportive palliative care, including management of pain, nutrition, and psychological support.

Immunotherapy and Combinations The combination of the anti-PD-L1 antibody atezolizumab with the VEGFA inhibitor bevacizumab is the first regimen to improve survival in the first-line setting compared to sorafenib. In addition, two additional treatment regimens involving immunotherapies have been approved by the FDA as second-line therapies based on phase 2 data. Single-agent checkpoint inhibitor treatments, such as nivolumab and pembrolizumab, are associated with objective responses of 15–20%, which are durable in time, generally beyond 12 months. Less than 30% of patients experience grade 3–4 treatment-related adverse events. Neither regimen hit the primary endpoint of improved survival in phase 3 investigations compared with sorafenib (nivolumab) or placebo (pembrolizumab). The median survival for nivolumab of 16.4 months in first-line treatment was not superior to the survival time of 14.7 months for sorafenib. Similarly, in the second-line setting, the median survival for pembrolizumab of 13.9 months was not superior to the median survival of 10.6 months for placebo. Emerging regimens have shown signals of efficacy, such as lenvatinib plus pembrolizumab in first-line patients with advanced HCC and the combination of an anti-CTLA-4 (ipilimumab) and anti-PD-1 (nivolumab) in second-line patients.

CHOLANGIOCARCINOMA

Cholangiocarcinoma (CCA) is classified according to its anatomic location as intrahepatic (iCCA; ~20–30%), perihilar (pCCA; ~50–60%), and distal (dCCA; ~20–30%). The latter two are also known as extrahepatic cholangiocarcinomas (eCCAs), with the second-order bile ducts acting as the separation point (**Fig. 82-7**). This classification is endorsed by the eighth edition of the *American Joint Committee on Cancer (AJCC) Staging Manual*. In addition, iCCA has been recognized as a distinct entity with specific ad hoc clinical practice guidelines. Treatment options beyond surgery are limited, and few molecular targeted therapies have been approved for its treatment. The three subtypes of CCA differ in their anatomic location, epidemiology and risk factors, cell of origin, pathogenesis, and treatment. iCCA originates from adult cholangiocytes, trans-differentiation of adult hepatocytes, and hepatic progenitor cells (cholangiocyte precursors) (**Fig. 82-8**), as opposed to HCC, which originates only from hepatic progenitor cells or adult hepatocytes. Mixed HCC-iCCA originates from hepatic progenitor cells, whereas eCCA arises from the biliary epithelium and peribiliary glands. Moreover, their mutational profiles also differ. *FGFR2* fusions and *IDH1/2* mutations mostly occur in iCCA, whereas *ERBB2/3* amplifications and *SMAD4* aberrations are characteristic of eCCA. Thus, clinical management and trials testing molecular therapies should be tailored according to each biological/anatomical subtype of CCA, as opposed to a common approach for all biliary tract cancers.

■ EPIDEMIOLOGY, RISK FACTORS, AND MOLECULAR TRAITS

CCA is the second most common liver cancer after HCC, with a 5-year survival of 10%. iCCA has globally increasing incidence and mortality rates. The incidence of iCCA varies according to exposure to risk factors, ranging from 1–2 cases per 100,000 inhabitants in Europe and North America to the highest incidence in some areas of Southeast Asia, particularly in Thailand (>80 cases per 100,000 inhabitants). The male-to-female ratio is 1.2. Overall, most cases occur with unknown risk factors. The classical risk factors for CCA development include primary sclerosing cholangitis (PSC), biliary duct cysts, hepatolithiasis, and Caroli's disease (congenital cystic dilation of the intrahepatic biliary tree). Parasitic biliary infestation with flukes (i.e., most common is *Opisthorchis viverrini* and *Clonorchis sinensis*) is a prevalent etiology in Asia that can be prevented with the antihelminth therapy praziquantel. PSC is a clear risk factor for iCCA and pCCA development, with a

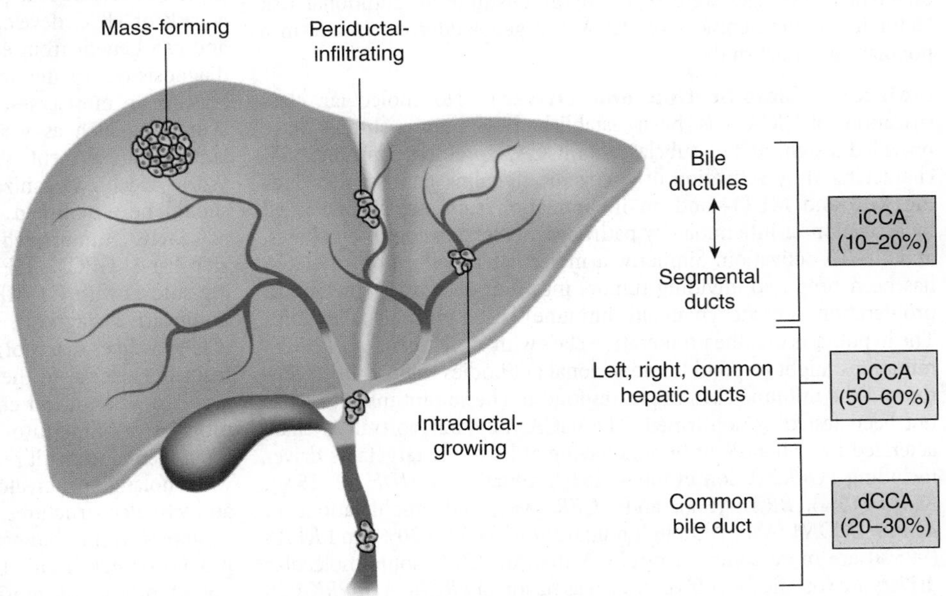

FIGURE 82-7 Anatomical classification of cholangiocarcinoma. Cholangiocarcinoma (CCA) is classified as intrahepatic (iCCA) and extrahepatic (eCCA). eCCA can be subclassified as perihilar (pCCA) and distal (dCCA). *(Reprinted with permission from JM Banales et al: Cholangiocarcinoma 2020: The next horizon in mechanisms and management. Nat Rev Gastroenterol Hepatol 17:557, 2020.)*

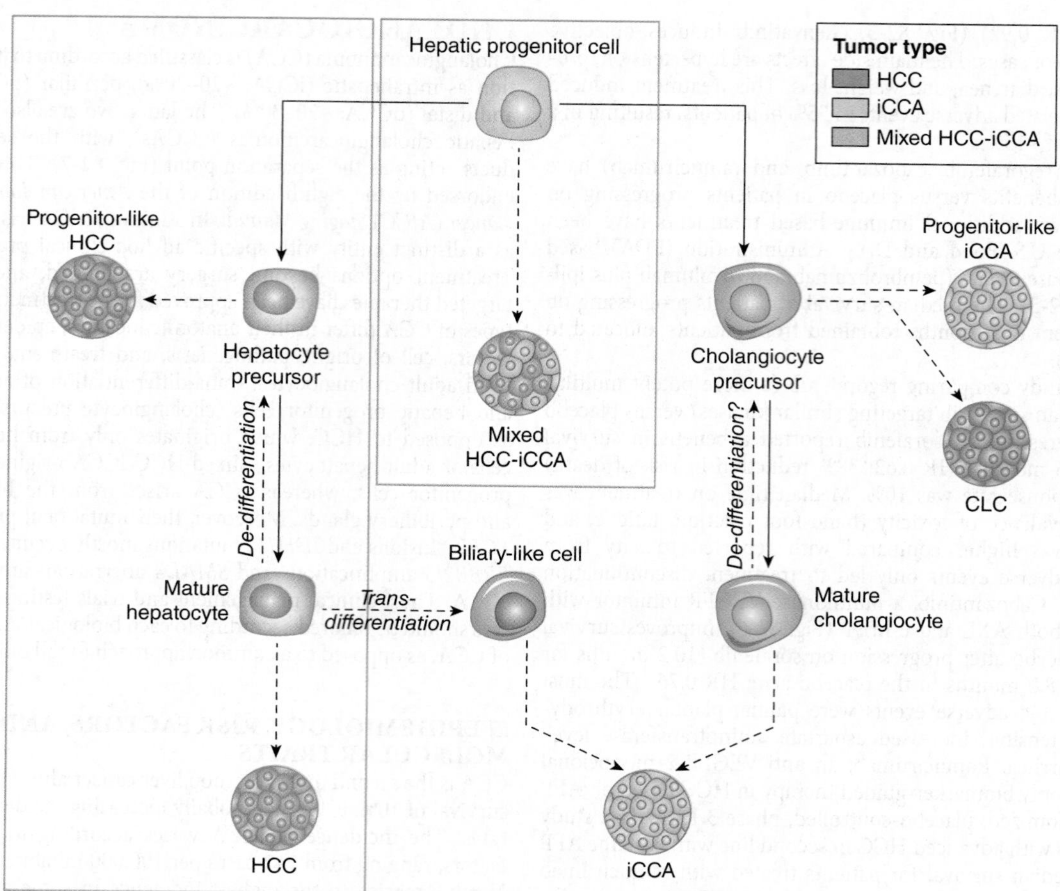

FIGURE 82-8 Cell of origin of liver cancer. Hepatocellular carcinoma (HCC) and intrahepatic cholangiocarcinoma (iCCA) can develop from the neoplastic transformation of mature hepatocytes and cholangiocytes, respectively. There is evidence showing that hepatic progenitor cells (HPCs), their intermediate states, or de-differentiated hepatocytes can originate liver cancers with progenitor-like features, including mixed HCC-iCCA (e.g., cholangiocellular carcinoma [CLC]). Mature hepatocytes can be also reprogrammed into cells that closely resemble biliary epithelial cells and induce the onset of iCCA. *(Printed with permission from ©Mount Sinai Health System.)*

lifetime incidence ranging from 5 to 10%. Surveillance in PSC patients is recommended with annual imaging techniques and CA 19-9 serum determination. Common risk factors for HCC, such as HBV and HCV infection and cirrhosis, have been associated with iCCA development. Sweetened beverages were reported to constitute an additional risk factor in the development of eCCA and gallbladder carcinoma in a population cohort study.

Molecular Classification and Drivers No molecular classification of CCA has been established. Genomic studies have provided insight on two subclasses of iCCA, a proliferation subclass—characterized by activation of oncogenic signaling pathways (including RAS and MET)—and an inflammation subclass, characterized by activation of inflammatory pathways, overexpression of cytokines, and STAT3 activation. Similarly, a molecular classification of eCCA has been proposed, dividing tumors into four categories (metabolic, proliferation, mesenchymal, and immune) based on molecular traits. The hypothesis that the proliferation class with enrichment of *ERBB2/3* mutations might respond to monoclonal antibodies against this receptor and the immune class might respond to checkpoint inhibitors has not been tested or confirmed. The iCCA mutation portrait is characterized by ~50–60% of tumors having at least one targetable driver including *FGFR2* fusion events (~25%); mutations in *IDH1/2* (15%), *KRAS* (15%), *BRAF* (5%), and *EGFR* (3%); and amplifications in *FGF19/CCDN1* (4%). Although mutations in *TP53* (~30%) and *KRAS* (~25%) are more common in eCCA than in iCCA, some molecular drivers are specific for subtypes, such as fusion of *PRKACA* or *PRKACB* for eCCA or *ERBB2* amplifications (~20%) for gallbladder cancer. Liver fluke–associated CCAs have a higher incidence of *TP53* and *SMAD4* mutations. Host genetic polymorphisms predisposing to CCA have not been established.

INTRAHEPATIC CHOLANGIOCARCINOMA

Diagnosis Diagnosis of iCCA requires pathologic confirmation. Guidelines currently do not recommend surveillance for early diagnosis because at-risk populations are ill-defined. Cirrhotic patients at risk of HCC development are enrolled in surveillance programs and can benefit from early detection of iCCA. Otherwise, incidental diagnosis occurs due to cross-sectional imaging performed for other reasons. In most cases, iCCA is diagnosed at advanced stages where symptoms such as weight loss, malaise, abdominal discomfort, or jaundice are present. Pathologic diagnosis of iCCA is based on the World Health Organization (WHO) criteria. Differential diagnosis should be established with metastatic adenocarcinoma and mixed iCCA-HCC tumors, which may require evaluation of markers such as Hep-Par-1, GPC3, HSP70, and glutamine synthetase markers. Imaging studies with CT/MRI are not accurate enough to establish iCCA noninvasive diagnosis. Dynamic CT scanning characterizes 80% of iCCAs as liver mass-forming tumors with progressive contrast uptake from the arterial to the venous/delayed phase. MRI dynamic images also show peripheral enhancement in the arterial phase followed by progressive filling in of the tumor. Atypical radiologic behavior with arterial enhancement recapitulating HCC occurs in 10% of cases. MRI with cholangiopancreatography is useful to visualize the ductal system and vascular structures. Guidelines do not recommend PET scan for diagnosis. Tumor biomarker CA 19-9 at a cutoff level of 100 U/mL has prognostic significance but lacks accuracy (sensitivity and specificity of ~60%) for early diagnosis.

Radiologic criteria are inadequate for iCCA diagnosis in cirrhotic patients. However, in noncirrhotic patients, guidelines endorse a presumed diagnosis of iCCA (i.e., venous phase contrast enhancement on dynamic CT/MRI) if resection is considered. Assessment of disease extent (venous or arterial invasion and extrahepatic disease) and resectability is best accomplished with CT and/or MRI studies. Doppler ultrasound is accurate in defining vascular invasion. Before surgery, PET scanning may be considered to rule out an occult primary or metastatic site.

Staging System The staging system for iCCA resected cases is based on the TNM staging as per the eighth edition of the AJCC/International Union Against Cancer (UICC) staging. T1 tumors are solitary without vascular invasion and can be divided into T1a or T1b if tumor size is ≤5 cm or >5 cm, respectively; T2 disease includes multiple tumors (e.g., multifocal disease, satellitosis, intrahepatic metastasis) or presence of vascular invasion (microvascular or major vascular invasion); T3 tumors perforate the visceral peritoneum; and T4 disease includes tumors involving local extrahepatic structures by direct invasion. Regional lymph node metastasis in the hilar, periduodenal, and peripancreatic nodes is considered N1 disease, while distant spread is considered M1 disease. TNM stages IA, IB, II, and IIIA overlap with T status, whereas stage IIIB includes T4N0 or N1M0 disease and stage IV includes M1 disease.

■ TREATMENT

After adopting the TNM staging system, the International Liver Cancer Association (ILCA) guidelines for management of iCCA proposed a treatment algorithm (**Fig. 82-9**), adapted and updated with the new treatment modalities accepted. Overall, most of the treatments endorsed have a modest level of evidence. Surgical resection represents the sole curative treatment option in 30–40% of patients, with a median survival of 51 months in properly selected candidates. In noncirrhotic individuals, the best candidates for resection are patients at TNM stage I–II, whereas in patients with cirrhosis, liver function should be assessed as previously described for HCC. Preoperative disease assessment should discard vascular invasion, N1, and M1. Lymphadenectomy of regional nodes is recommended given its prognostic value. The main predictors of recurrence (~50–60% at 3 years) and survival are identified at the pathologic examination, including presence of vascular invasion, lymph node metastases, and poor differentiation. A phase 3 trial (BILCAP trial) including all types of CCA in a prespecified per-protocol analysis reported improved survival with adjuvant therapy (53 months vs 36 months; adjusted HR 0.75). Based on this trial, American Society of Clinical Oncology guidelines recommend adjuvant capecitabine for a period of 6 months. Other adjuvant regimens, such as gemcitabine monotherapy or a combination of gemcitabine and oxaliplatin, did not improve OS. Liver transplantation remains controversial, and few studies have reported good outcomes for single tumors ≤2 cm.

Nonsurgical candidates have a dismal life expectancy. Overall, patients at stage III might be considered for locoregional therapies, such as chemoembolization or radioembolization, but the level of evidence is low and is mostly based on cohort studies. A meta-analysis of 14 trials testing locoregional therapies reported median survival times of 15 months. External-beam radiation therapy is not recommended as standard therapy. At more advanced stages (stage IV) in patients with an ECOG of 0–1, systemic chemotherapy with the combination of gemcitabine and cisplatin is considered the standard of practice, yielding median survival times of 11.7 months compared to 8 months

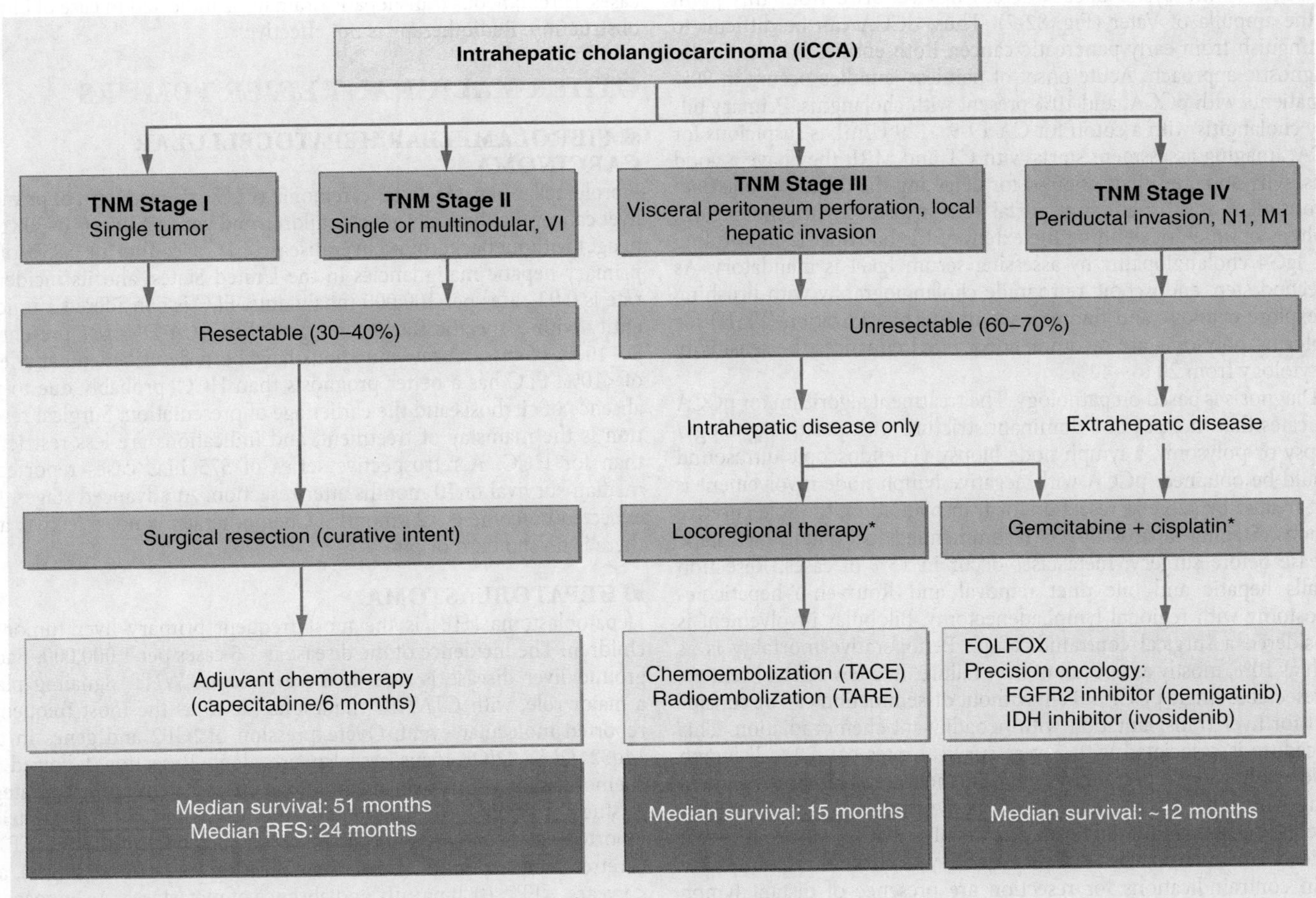

FIGURE 82-9 Staging and treatment schedule for intrahepatic cholangiocarcinoma (iCCA) proposed by the International Liver Cancer Association. FOLFOX, leucovorin, fluorouracil, and oxaliplatin; RFS, recurrence-free survival; TACE, transcatheter arterial chemoembolization; TARE, transarterial radioembolization; TNM, tumor-node-metastasis. *(Reproduced with permission from J Bridgewater et al: Guidelines for the diagnosis and management of intrahepatic cholangiocarcinoma. J Hepatol 60:1268, 2014.)*

for gemcitabine alone. This recommendation for first-line treatment of advanced tumors is based on a subgroup analysis of 80 iCCA patients included in a large randomized phase III trial (n = 410, ABC-02 Trial) of patients with advanced biliary tract tumors. In the second-line setting, a phase 3 study randomized patients who had progressed on cisplatin and gemcitabine to mFOLFOX (leucovorin, fluorouracil, and oxaliplatin) versus best supportive care. The chemotherapy regimen showed an improvement in median OS to 6.2 months (adjusted HR 0.69).

Two molecular targeted therapies have been approved in the second-line setting in iCCA patients with *IDH1/2* mutations or *FGFR2* aberrations. A phase 3 trial compared ivosidenib, an IDH-1 inhibitor, versus placebo; ivosidenib improved progression-free survival (2.7 vs 1.4 months; HR 0.37) and OS. A single-arm phase 2 study assessing pemigatinib (FGFR2 inhibitor) in iCCA patients with *FGFR2* fusions showed a median survival of 21 months and an objective response rate of 35%.

Mixed HCC-iCCA is a rare neoplasm accounting for <0.5% of all primary liver cancers. Diagnosis is based on pathology. The 2010 WHO classification defined two subtypes: the classical and the stem cell feature type. Molecular data have defined a third unique entity, cholangiocellular carcinoma, with distinct molecular traits and better outcome. Due to its low incidence, the demographic features and clinical behavior of these tumors remain ill-defined. Survival and management are similar to iCCA.

EXTRAHEPATIC CHOLANGIOCARCINOMA

Perihilar and Distal Cholangiocarcinoma The eighth edition AJCC/UICC TNM staging classification has established pCCAs as tumors that arise between the second-order bile ducts up to the insertion of the cystic duct, whereas dCCAs arise from this point to the ampulla of Vater (Fig. 82-7). Thus, dCCA can be difficult to distinguish from early pancreatic cancer. Both entities have a similar diagnostic approach. Acute onset of painless jaundice occurs in 90% of patients with pCCA, and 10% present with cholangitis. Primary biliary cholangitis with a cutoff for CA 19-9 >129 U/mL is suspicious for CCA. Imaging assessment starts with CT and MRI; they have a good sensitivity and specificity (>85%) for detecting the degree of bile duct involvement and hepatic and portal vein invasion. MRI cholangiography is optimal for defining the extent of the bile duct lesion. Ruling out IgG4 cholangiopathy by assessing serum IgG4 is mandatory. As a second step, endoscopic retrograde cholangiography with brushing to explore cytology and fluorescence in situ hybridization (FISH) for exploring polysomy are recommended. FISH enhances the sensitivity of cytology from 20 to ~40%.

Diagnosis is based on pathology. The treatment algorithm for pCCA indicates that in cases of a dominant stricture with positive cytology/biopsy or polysomy, a lymph node biopsy via endoscopic ultrasound should be obtained. pCCA with negative lymph node involvement is best treated by surgery, resection, or transplantation, the sole curative options. Staging laparoscopy is recommended to exclude metastatic disease before surgery; metastases occur in 15% of cases. Resection entails hepatic and bile duct removal and Roux-en-Y-hepaticojejunostomy with regional lymphadenectomy. Bilobular involvement is considered a surgical contraindication. Perioperative mortality is as high as 10%, mostly as a result of liver failure. In a few referral centers, unresectable single pCCA <3 cm without dissemination can be considered for liver transplantation with neoadjuvant chemoradiation. This procedure is associated with 5-year survival rates of ~70%. If lymph node involvement is present, systemic chemotherapy can be considered along with biliary tract stenting. Surgical resection (Whipple procedure) is the primary option for management of dCCA, a procedure that achieves a median survival of 2 years and 5-year survival rates of ~25%. Main contraindications for resection are presence of distant lymph node involvement, metastases, or major vascular invasion. At the pathologic examination, perineural invasion, lymph node metastasis, R0 resection (absence of residual tumor at pathologic examination), and tumor differentiation are predictors of survival. Adjuvant therapy with capecitabine for 6 months is accepted based on the BILCAP study. Consensus statements endorse first- and second-line chemotherapy strategies for unresectable eCCA similar as for iCCA. No molecular targeted therapies are available for these entities.

GALLBLADDER CANCER

Gallbladder cancer is the most common cancer of the biliary tract worldwide. The estimated cases of gallbladder cancer in the United States in 2020 were 11,980, more than CCA. The female-to-male ratio is 3:1. Cholelithiasis is the major risk factor, but <1% of patients with cholelithiasis develop this cancer. Gallbladder polyps at risk of transformation are those ≥10 mm in diameter. Early cases are discovered incidentally at routine cholecystectomy. Clinical symptoms, such as jaundice, pain, and weight loss, are associated with advanced stages. Staging of gallbladder cancer follows the TNM classification. The most accurate technique to define staging and vascular and biliary tract invasion is magnetic resonance cholangiopancreatography. CT and PET scans can be also useful for preoperative staging.

The mainstay of treatment is surgical, either simple or radical cholecystectomy (partial hepatectomy and regional lymph node dissection) for stage I or II disease, respectively. Only ~20% of patients are candidates for surgery with curative intent. Survival rates are near 80–90% at 5 years for stage I disease and range from 60 to 90% at 5 years for stage II disease. Regional nodal status and the depth of tumor invasion (T status) are the two most important prognostic factors. Adjuvant therapy with capecitabine is recommended in R0 cases. Gallbladder cancers at stage III and IV are considered unresectable. For patients with ECOG of 0–1, chemotherapy with gemcitabine and cisplatin is the standard of practice based on data from the subgroup analysis including 181 patients with gallbladder cancer in the setting of two clinical trials. Overall, median survival is 10–12 months in advanced cases. Percutaneous transhepatic drainage is indicated in case of biliary obstruction. Radiotherapy is not effective.

OTHER MALIGNANT LIVER TUMORS

FIBROLAMELLAR HEPATOCELLULAR CARCINOMA

Fibrolamellar hepatocellular carcinoma (FLC) is a rare form of primary liver cancer that typically affects children and young adults (10–30 years of age) without background liver disease. FLC accounts for 0.85% of all primary hepatic malignancies in the United States, and its incidence rate is 0.02 cases per 100,000 inhabitants. FLC is considered a unique entity with a specific fusion oncogene *PRKACA-DNAJB1* present in 80–100% of cases. A few mutations have been described, all at a level of <10%. FLC has a better prognosis than HCC, probably due to the absence of cirrhosis and the earlier age of presentation. Surgical resection is the mainstay of treatment, and indications are less restrictive than for HCC. A retrospective series of 575 FLC cases reported a median survival of 70 months after resection. At advanced stages, the expected outcome is <20 months. Chemotherapy is not effective, and there is no standard of care.

HEPATOBLASTOMA

Hepatoblastoma (HB) is the most frequent primary liver tumor in children. The incidence of the disease is 1.5 cases per 1,000,000. Background liver disease is rare in these patients. WNT signaling plays a major role, with *CTNNB1* mutations (70%) as the most frequently reported molecular event. Overexpression of IGF2 and genes in the 14q32 *DLK1/DIO3* locus are also prevalent. Resection followed by chemotherapy with doxorubicin is the mainstay treatment strategy. A study including 1605 patients randomized in eight clinical trials reported better outcome for patients with stage I–II of the PRETEXT (Pretreatment Extent of Tumor) classification (out of four stages), age <3 years, AFP >1000 ng/mL, and absence of metastases. As opposed to HCC, low AFP indicates poor prognosis. The best candidates (stage I or II with small tumors, age <3 years, and AFP >100 ng/mL) achieve 5-year disease-free survival after resection of 90%, compared with 5-year disease-free survival of 20–30% in the worst candidates (metastatic disease and AFP <100 ng/mL).

BENIGN LIVER TUMORS

The most common benign liver tumors are hemangiomas, focal nodular hyperplasia (FNH), and hepatocellular adenomas (HCA). Most benign tumors are identified incidentally by abdominal ultrasound or other imaging techniques. *Hemangiomas* are present in ~5% of the general population and are diagnosed by ultrasound, except in cirrhotic patients or oncology patients in whom contrast-enhanced imaging (contrast-enhanced ultrasound, CT, or MRI) is required. Conservative management is appropriate and follow-up is not recommended. Exceptionally, growing lesions causing symptoms by compression can be considered for resection. FNH is a benign tumor present in <2% of the population and occurs mostly in females aged 40–50 years. FNH is a polyclonal hepatocellular proliferation due to an arterial malformation. MRI has the highest diagnostic accuracy with a specificity of 100% when typical imaging features are present (homogeneous enhancement in the arterial phase with a central scar). Atypical FNH requires biopsy for diagnosis. Treatment is not recommended since these tumors do not degenerate or cause complications. In exceptional cases of expanding symptomatic lesions, surgery is the treatment of choice.

Hepatic adenomas are clonal benign proliferations resulting from single-gene driver mutations. HCAs have a low prevalence of 0.001% of the population and are frequently diagnosed in women aged 35–40 years. The female-to-male ratio is 10:1, and the main risk factors are oral contraceptives in females and use of anabolic androgenic steroids in male body builders. HCAs have the potential for hemorrhage and HCC development, particularly when >5 cm. Molecular classification of HCA is defined as follows: (1) HCA with *CTNNB1* mutations (10–20%) are at risk of HCC development and are present in men treated with androgens; (2) inflammatory adenomas (50–60%) are associated with single mutations (*Gp130*: 65%) and are more prevalent in females with obesity or diabetes; and (3) adenomas with inactivated *HNF1A*. Diagnosis is based on MRI, which correlates with molecular subtypes in 80% of cases (inflammatory and HNF-1A type). For defining HCA with *CTNNB1* mutations, biopsy is required. Upon diagnosis, discontinuation of oral contraceptives and weight loss are recommended. Resection is indicated in all cases of >5 cm, in men, or in those with *CTNNB1* mutation. For HCA <5 cm, 1-year follow-up is recommended. In case of active HCA bleeding, embolization followed by resection is the treatment of choice. The presence of multiple HCAs is common, and guidelines endorse treating them based on the size of the main nodule.

FURTHER READING

Banales J et al: Cholangiocarcinoma 2020: The next horizon in mechanisms and management. Nat Rev Gastroenterol Hepatol 17:557, 2020.

Bridgewater J et al: Guidelines for the diagnosis and management of intrahepatic cholangiocarcinoma. J Hepatol 60:1268, 2014.

EASL-EORTC Clinical Practice Guidelines: Management of hepatocellular carcinoma. J Hepatol 69:182, 2018.

Finn RS et al: Atezolizumab plus bevacizumab in unresectable hepatocellular carcinoma. N Engl J Med 382:1894, 2020.

Llovet JM et al: Sorafenib in advanced hepatocellular carcinoma. N Engl J Med 359:378, 2008.

Llovet JM et al: Molecular therapies and precision medicine for hepatocellular carcinoma. Nat Rev Clin Oncol 15:599, 2018.

Llovet JM et al: Locoregional therapies in the era of molecular and immune treatments for hepatocellular carcinoma. Nat Rev Gastroenterol Hepatol 18:293, 2021.

Llovet JM et al: Hepatocellular carcinoma. Nat Rev Dis Primers 7:6, 2021.

Marrero J et al: Diagnosis, staging, and management of hepatocellular carcinoma: 2018 practice guidance by the American Association for the Study of Liver Diseases. Hepatology 68:723, 2018.

Mazzaferro V et al: Liver transplantation for the treatment of small hepatocellular carcinomas in patients with cirrhosis. N Engl J Med 334:693, 1996.

Rizvi S et al: Cholangiocarcinoma: Evolving concepts and therapeutic strategies. Nat Rev Clin Oncol 15:95, 2018.

Schulze K et al: Exome sequencing of hepatocellular carcinomas identifies new mutational signatures and potential therapeutic targets. Nat Genet 47:505, 2015.

Villanueva A: Hepatocellular carcinoma. N Engl J Med 380:1450, 2019.

Zucman-Rossi J et al: The genetic landscape and biomarkers of hepatocellular carcinoma. Gastroenterology 149:1226, 2015.

83 Pancreatic Cancer

Daniel D. Von Hoff

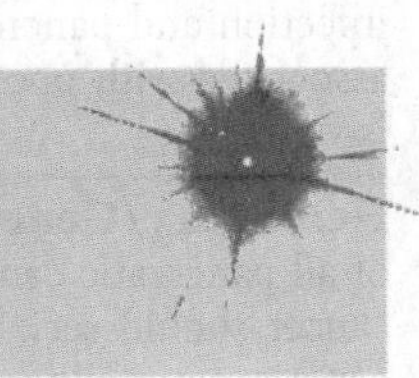

Pancreatic cancer is the third leading cause of death from cancer in the United States, with >57,000 Americans diagnosed and >47,000 dying from the disease each year. Unfortunately, pancreatic cancer is projected to be the second leading cause of death from cancer in the United States by 2030. Worldwide, pancreatic cancer is the eleventh most common cancer with 458,000 new patients diagnosed and >432,000 deaths (seventh cause of cancer deaths). Pancreatic cancer currently has the worst survival rate of any cancer with an overall 5-year survival (regardless of stage) of ~8.2%. However, that situation is changing. In particular, (1) knowledge about specific molecular subsets of the disease has become crucial to provide the best possible care for patients, and (2) the application of treatment that improves survival for patients with advanced disease used either after surgery or even earlier in the disease has improved survival.

EPIDEMIOLOGY

Pancreatic cancer accounts for 3.2% of all new cancer cases in the United States and for 7.8% of all deaths from cancer in the United States. The lifetime risk of developing pancreatic cancer is ~1.7%. The incidence of pancreatic cancer has been increasing about 1.03% per year. Pancreatic cancer is more common with increasing age and more common in men than in women. The 5-year survival rate for all stages has only increased from 3% in 1975 to 9% in 2015. The latest information from the U.S. Surveillance, Epidemiology, and End Results (SEER) database predicts that the 5-year survival for patients with localized pancreatic cancer is about 37%, 12% for those with regional disease, and 3.1% for patients with advanced metastatic disease. Pancreatic cancer is more common in developed countries (although generally it tracks with the prevalence of smoking). The incidence is highest in Western Europe and North America followed by other areas in Europe, Australia, New Zealand, and South-Central Asia. The population at greatest risk are women living in Scandinavian countries, while the lowest risk is seen for women living in middle Africa.

RISK FACTORS

Age is one of the greatest risk factors for pancreatic cancer with median age at diagnosis of 70 years (the disease is most frequently diagnosed in the 65–79 age group; for men, 65–69; for women, 75–79). The number of new cases per 100,000 persons and the number of deaths per 100,000 persons are higher for males and for blacks of both sexes. Both the number of cases and the number of deaths per 100,000 people are lower for American Indian/Alaskan natives and Asian Pacific Islanders. Both the number of cases and deaths are intermediate for the Hispanic population. People who have a non-O blood type are at higher risk of developing pancreatic cancer.

Environment The greatest risk factor for pancreatic cancer is cigarette smoking. The risk correlates with the increased number of cigarettes smoked and persists for at least 10 years after smoking cessation. About 30% of pancreatic cancer is caused by smoking. Exposure to cadmium as part of cigarette smoking or via exposure to welding, soldering, or dietary exposure has been weakly associated with an increased risk of pancreatic cancer.

Although dietary factors are often difficult to interpret, high intakes of fat or meat (particularly well-done barbequed meat) are risk factors. High intakes of citrus fruits and vegetables are associated with a decreased risk. Coffee and low-to-moderate alcohol consumption are not associated with an increased risk for pancreatic cancers, while consumption of sugary carbonated drinks has been associated with an increased risk.

Microbiome To date, no solid evidence links *Helicobacter pylori* infection and pancreatic cancer. Some data link the oral microbiome associated with poor dentition to pancreatic cancer, but the evidence is very thin.

Hereditary/Genetics Hereditary factors may account for 10–16% of all pancreatic cancers. Family members of patients with pancreatic cancer should seek participation in an early detection program with genetic counseling, definition of risk, and if appropriate, periodic MRI screening of the abdomen, although this recommendation is not yet based on research data. In addition, the identification of any pancreatic cancer–associated germline mutations could lead to specific and effective new therapeutics for patients with these abnormalities in their tumors. **Table 83-1** identifies the various germline mutations along with their familial cancer syndromes where an increased risk for pancreatic cancer is known.

Knowing the patient has a *BRCA2* or *PALB2* germline mutation or any of the above mutations should lead one to not only refer the patient's relatives to an early detection or high-risk individual clinic but also realize that for patients with a *BRCA2/PALB2* germline mutation consideration for treatment with a poly (ADP-ribose) polymerase (PARP) inhibitor should be considered (see below). Other germline mutations are under study to determine their increased risk of pancreatic cancer, including *CFTR, PRSS2, CDK4, FANCC, PALLD, APC, ATM, BMPR1A, BRCA1, EPCAM, MEN1, MLH1, MSH2, MSH6, NF1, PMS2, SMAD4, TP53, TSC1, TSC2,* and *VHL*. Some of these mutations are associated with pancreatic neuroendocrine tumors **(Chap. 84)**.

In addition to the recognized genetic syndromes, other possible familial pancreatic cancer genes have not yet been discovered. For example, a family history of pancreatic cancer is associated with a 13-fold increase in the disease. If you have one first-degree relative, the risk is increased 4.6-fold, having two first-degree relatives increases the risk 6.4-fold, and three or more first-degree relatives confers a 32-fold increased risk. The risk is also increased if a relative developed pancreatic cancer at <55 years old.

TABLE 83-1 Germline Mutations, Their Familial Cancer Syndrome, and Fold Risk of Pancreatic Cancer

GERMLINE MUTATION	FAMILIAL CANCER SYNDROME	ESTIMATED INCREASED RISK (FOLD) OF PANCREATIC CANCER
BRCA2[a]	Familial breast/ovarian cancer	2–6
PALB2 (partner and localizer of *BRCA2*)	Familial breast cancer and others	~sixfold
p16/CDKN2A	Familial atypical multiple mole melanoma (FAMMM)	15–18
STKII (*LKB1*)	Peutz-Jeghers syndrome	76–140
PRSS1 or *SPIN11*[b]	Hereditary (familial) pancreatitis	53
ATM	Ataxia-telangiectasia	Not yet established
MLH1, MSH2, MSH6, PMS2	Heredity nonpolyposis colorectal syndrome or Lynch syndrome[c]	9–30

[a]Particularly common in individuals with Ashkenazi Jewish heritage. [b]Forty percent chance of pancreatic cancer by the age of 70. [c]Very important because this is associated with microsatellite instability, which is a marker for response to an anti-PD-1/PD-L1 agent.

Other Considerations Most patients with pancreatic cancer relate that they have had developing symptoms over the past few years. Thus, early detection of the disease is possible when the index of suspicion is high.

Medical Conditions Chronic pancreatitis that is nonfamilial is also associated with an increased risk of pancreatic cancer (2.3–16.5-fold increase). Risk is also increased in people with chronic pancreatitis associated with cystic fibrosis or tropical pancreatitis.

A clear association exists between diabetes mellitus (both type 1 and type 2) and pancreatic cancer. Whether this is a causal association or whether the diabetes is the result of the cancer is not exactly clear. What is clear is that when a person presents with new-onset type 2 diabetes, they should be considered at risk for having pancreatic cancer. The excessive insulin or insulin-like growth factors associated with adult-onset diabetes and metabolic syndrome may promote pancreatic carcinogenesis.

Obesity is considered a possible risk factor for pancreatic cancer. A high body mass index (BMI) ≥30 is associated with a doubling of the risk of pancreatic cancer. Since obesity is a risk factor for diabetes, the contribution of obesity alone is unclear. Interestingly, patients with severe obesity who undergo a gastric bypass experience a reduction in the incidence of gastrointestinal (GI) cancer, including pancreatic cancer, by >30% in the first 3 years (along with a dramatic decrease in their hemoglobin A_{1c} and blood glucose). Physical inactivity also has been associated with an increased risk in pancreatic cancer.

PATHOLOGY AND MOLECULAR CONSIDERATION

Location The posterior location of the pancreas in the abdomen is likely one of the issues that leads to a late diagnosis **(Fig. 83-1*A*)**.

Pathology Cancers of the pancreas can be divided into neoplasms of the endocrine pancreas **(Chap. 84)** and tumors of the exocrine pancreas. The most common neoplasm of the exocrine pancreas and most deadly is pancreatic infiltrating ductal adenocarcinoma. These tumors arise in the head, body, or tail of the pancreas and are characterized by infiltrating desmoplastic stromal reactions **(Fig. 83-1*B*)**.

Other subtypes of nonneuroendocrine pancreatic cancers include acinar cell carcinoma (tumors of the exocrine enzyme producing cell), medullary carcinoma, adenosquamous carcinoma, and other rare subtypes. Each of these is different in behavior and in their molecular characteristics and often requires other specific types of treatment.

Molecular Characteristics The molecular characteristics of pancreatic ductal adenocarcinoma reveal four genes that are commonly mutated or inactivated (sometimes referred to as the "four horsemen"). The most common is *KRAS* (usually in codon 12). It is critical to determine the specific mutation in *KRAS* because specific mutations may indicate specific therapies that should be considered. *KRAS* mutations are seen in virtually 100% of pancreatic adenocarcinomas. In fact, with the deep sequencing now available, if a *KRAS* mutation is not detected in the patient's tumor, one should consider that the tumor is likely of a different origin (e.g., small bowel, gallbladder, or cholangiocarcinoma—all of which could require different treatments). *p16/CDKN2A* is also noted in >90% of invasive pancreatic adenocarcinomas. *TP53* and *DPC4/MADH4* are mutated in about half of these tumors. As a reference point, the *BRCA2* gene noted in Table 83-1 is mutated in 7–10% of pancreatic adenocarcinomas.

Precursor Lesions Many pancreatic adenocarcinomas seem to arise from noninvasive epithelial precursor lesions. Detection of these could allow for early diagnosis of pancreatic cancer. These pancreatic intraepithelial neoplasias (PanINs) have varying degrees of dysplasia designated as PanINs 1–3 (and constitute a progression model for pancreatic cancer). Genetic alterations become more frequent as the PanIN grade increases (e.g., grade 3). Not all PanIN lesions progress to invasive malignancy. PanINs that are ≥1 cm are called *intraductal papillary neoplasms* and are usually noninvasive. If the intraductal tumor is in a branch duct, it is usually noninvasive; however, if the intraductal tumor is in a main duct and is large and nodular, it is more likely to have malignant behavior.

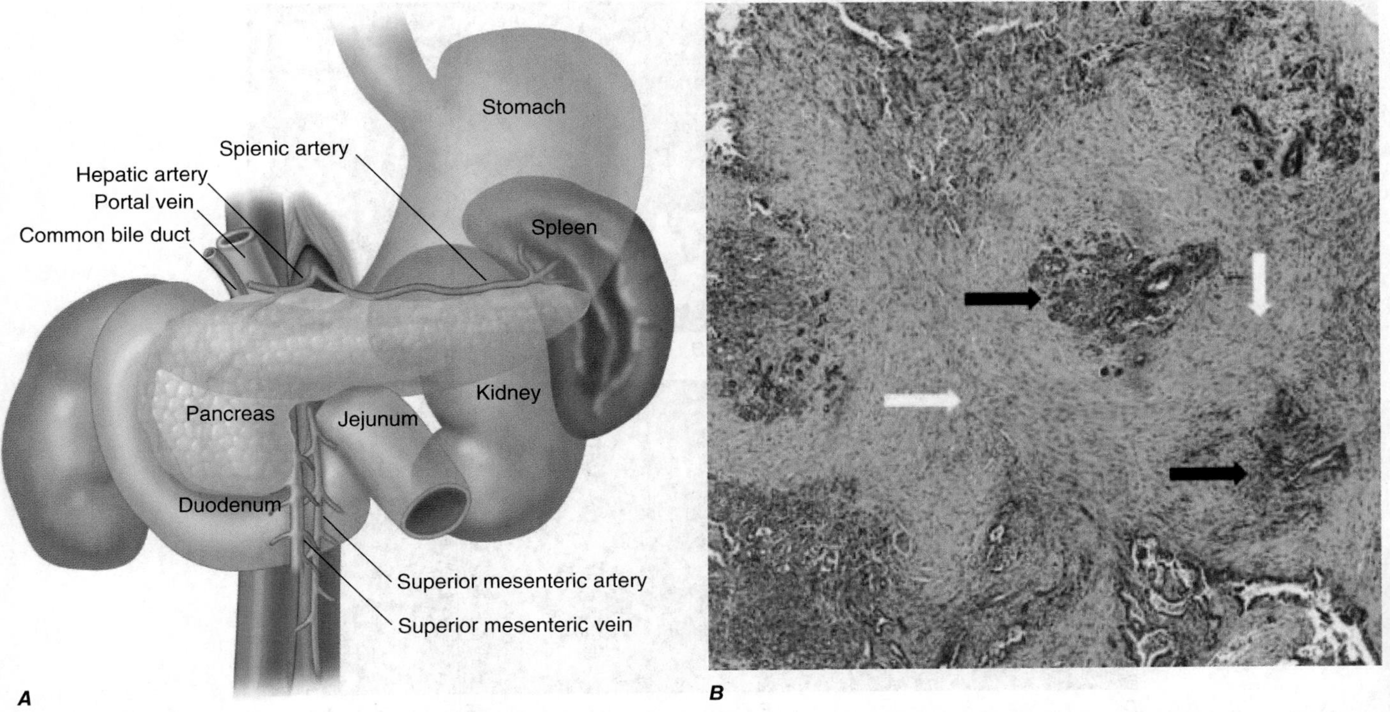

FIGURE 83-1 ***A.*** Note the relationship of the pancreas to the major vessels of the retroperitoneum. ***B.*** Ductal adenocarcinoma of the pancreas (*black arrows*), with intense stromal component (*white arrows*). *(Part A is courtesy of Mary Kay Washington, MD, PhD, Vanderbilt University. Part B is courtesy of Haiyong Han, PhD, Translational Genomics Research Institute [TGen].)*

One other pancreatic tumor is the mucinous cystic neoplasm; they may be seen as incidental findings on scans. These lesions are less likely invasive (20%) unless they are large and have nodules in them.

CLINICAL FEATURES

History and Physical The classic presentation for a patient with pancreatic cancer has been abdominal pain and weight loss with or without jaundice. The pain is midepigastric (sometimes described as a "boring-like" pain). Often the pain is in the back (due to retroperitoneal invasion of the splanchnic nerve plexus). The pain may be exacerbated by eating or lying flat. Other items of note in a history are light stool color from the absence of bile (steatorrhea also causes malodorous stools) and the onset of diabetes in the prior year. Jaundice, first detectable with a bilirubin of 2.5–3.0 mg/dL, is usually associated with tumor in the head of the pancreas. In some instances, depression is noted (with a higher subsequent number of suicides). Pruritis may be seen when the bilirubin reaches 6–8 mg/dL.

Physical signs include jaundice, signs of weight loss, a palpable gallbladder (Courvoisier's sign), hepatomegaly, an abdominal mass, and even an enlarged spleen (usually indicating a portal vein thrombosis). Migratory superficial thrombophlebitis can also be seen (Trousseau's syndrome). Signs of late disease include a lymph node palpable in the supraclavicular fossa (usually on the left where the thoracic duct enters the subclavian vein). This is clinically referred to as Virchow's node. Occasionally, one can palpate subcutaneous metastases in the periumbilical area referred to as a Sister Mary Joseph's node—named after one of the scrub nurses on the Mayo Clinic Operative Team who noted that when she prepped that area and felt those nodules, the patient often had peritoneal metastases.

The history and symptoms noted above may lead a person to see a physician; often CT and MRI scanning detects the disease before advanced disease symptoms appear.

DIAGNOSTIC WORKUP

Imaging Diagnostic imaging plays a major role in diagnosing pancreatic cancer and other intraabdominal diseases. The best technique is the use of a dual-phase contrast-enhanced spiral CT using the pancreatic cancer protocol, which allows arterial phase enhancement and portal venous phase enhancement. This special protocol can provide helpful prospective staging and assessment of resectability. **Figure 83-2** demonstrates such a CT scan (with vascular involvement). **Figure 83-3** demonstrates the use of an 18F glucose positron emission tomography (PET) scan.

Histologic Diagnosis A histologic (tissue) diagnosis is essential and should be obtained with a cutting biopsy needle (not a skinny needle with cytology). Misdiagnosis is more common based on only fine-needle aspirates. Obtaining a tissue diagnosis allows not only for accuracy but also for molecular testing for *KRAS* mutations, microsatellite instability, and other important molecular abnormalities. Those molecular abnormalities and others will be increasingly important as more targeted therapies are developed for patients with pancreatic cancer.

The core needle (16–18 gauge) biopsy can be obtained via endoscopic ultrasound-guided techniques for a tumor localized to the pancreas or, if there are liver lesions or Virchow's node, via percutaneous biopsy by interventional radiologists.

Serum Markers Before treatment, a serum sample should be obtained for levels of CA19-9, carcinoembryonic antigen (CEA), or if both are negative, for CA125 (can be positive when the CA19-9 is negative due to the patient not being a Lewis antigen secretor). These markers are not useful for staging but can be useful in following the course of pancreatic cancer.

IMPORTANT IMMEDIATE CONSIDERATIONS IN PATIENT CARE

While the patient is being evaluated and staged, one must be alert for biliary tract obstruction (and the attendant risk for sepsis from the biliary tree). A stent can be placed (plastic if temporary or metal if needed longer) to relieve the jaundice and pruritus. If surgery is being contemplated, an early surgical consultation is in order as some surgeons may want to proceed to surgery without placement of a stent. This immediate surgical approach is becoming less common as many multidisciplinary teams want consideration of use of chemotherapy

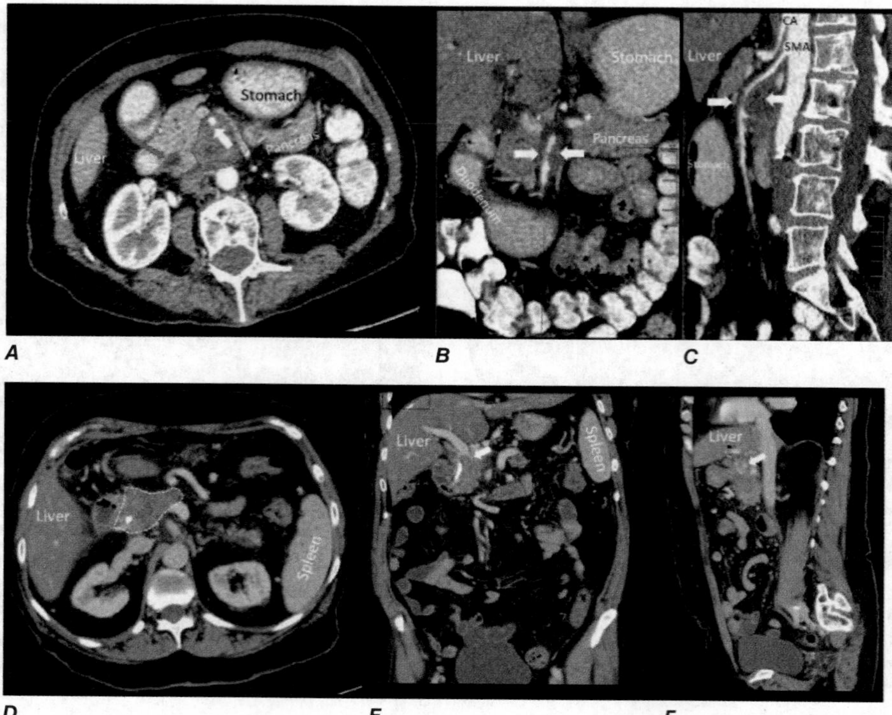

FIGURE 83-2 Selected images from contrast-enhanced CT in patients with locally advanced adenocarcinoma of the pancreas. A high-quality contrast-enhanced CT scan (arterial phase in panels ***A–C*** and portal venous phase in panels ***D–F***) is required for optimal staging of pancreas cancer. Panel ***A*** demonstrates the typical features of adenocarcinoma of the pancreas on arterial phase axial CT scans (*dotted outline*) with tumor encasement of the superior mesenteric artery (*white arrow*). Note the dilatation of the common bile duct (*red arrow*). Panels ***B*** (magnified coronal) and ***C*** (sagittal) show reconstruction of CT images into additional orthogonal planes with exquisite details to confirm the unresectable nature of the tumor due to vascular encasement. Panel ***D*** demonstrates the typical features of adenocarcinoma of the pancreas on portal venous phase axial CT scans in a different subject. The dotted line outlines a pancreas cancer lesion in the pancreatic head, which is encasing the portal splenic confluence (*dotted outline*). Panels ***E*** (*white arrow*) and ***F*** show the pinched appearance of the portal splenic confluence by tumor abutment and invasion of the superior mesenteric vein (*white arrow*) on coronal and sagittal views. Note the presence of a stent in the common bile duct (*red arrow*) to help relieve biliary obstruction caused by the tumor. CA, celiac axis; SMA, superior mesenteric artery.

with or without radiation therapy (called neoadjuvant therapy) before a patient is taken to surgery.

Patients with pancreatic cancer are often hypercoagulable and frequently have migratory thrombophlebitis (Trousseau's sign) as well as deep vein thrombosis with pulmonary emboli (a frequent cause of death). Appropriate examinations plus being alert to thromboses on the routine workup are mandatory so appropriate management can be put in place.

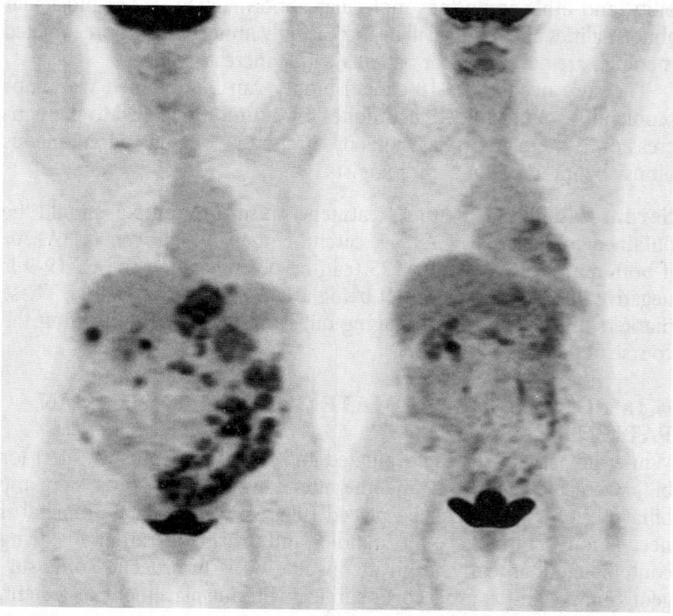

FIGURE 83-3 PET scan demonstrating metastatic disease—baseline and after 6 weeks of chemotherapy with some resolution of liver metastases.

Control of pain or of any symptoms should be pursued to help patients be as comfortable as possible for their decision-making. Sometimes simple approaches like the use of a replacement pancreatic enzyme (at good therapeutic doses) can relieve the bloating, cramping, and diarrhea. Early involvement of a palliative care team can improve a patient's quality of life and sometimes even its length.

CLINICAL STAGING

The clinical staging of pancreatic cancer according to the American Joint Commission on cancer staging is presented in **Table 83-2**.

Table 83-3 presents another clinical way to express extent of disease as well as therapeutic approaches (to be discussed later).

For proper staging, some physicians believe that a laparoscopy either before or at the time of surgery is important. If metastatic disease is found at laparoscopy, one can avoid surgery that would not be helpful because disease is already advanced.

TREATMENT

Resectable Disease

Even for patients with resectable disease, the patient should be presented to a combined-modality conference. Some clinicians feel the best approach for patients with resectable disease (as defined in Table 83-3) is surgery. Only a small percentage of patients are in this category (10–20%). Some clinicians feel neoadjuvant therapy (chemotherapy before surgery) should be given before surgery (for controlling potential micrometastatic disease and shrinking the primary tumor). The surgery for patients with tumors in the head or

TABLE 83-2 Definition of Primary Tumor (T)

T CATEGORY	T CRITERIA
TX	Primary tumor cannot be assessed
T0	No evidence of primary tumor
Tis	Carcinoma in situ This includes high-grade pancreatic intraepithelial neoplasia (PanIn-3), intraductal papillary mucinous neoplasm with high-grade dysplasia, intraductal tubulopapillary neoplasm with high-grade dysplasia, and mucinous cystic neoplasm with high-grade dysplasia
T1	Tumor ≤2 cm in greatest dimension
T1a	Tumor ≤0.5 cm in greatest dimension
T1b	Tumor >0.5 cm and <1 cm in greatest dimension
T1c	Tumor 1–2 cm in greatest dimension
T2	Tumor >2 cm and ≤4 cm in greatest dimension
T3	Tumor >4 cm in greatest dimension
T4	Tumor involves celiac axis, superior mesenteric artery, and/or common hepatic artery, regardless of size
M CATEGORY	**M CRITERIA**
M0	No distant metastasis
M1	Distant metastasis
N CATEGORY	**N CRITERIA**
NX	Regional lymph nodes cannot be assessed
N0	No regional lymph node metastases
N1	Metastasis in one to three regional lymph nodes
N2	Metastasis in four or more regional lymph nodes

AJCC Prognostic Stage Groups

WHEN T IS...	AND N IS...	AND M IS...	THEN THE STAGE GROUP IS....
Tis	N0	M0	0
T1	N0	M0	IA
T1	N1	M0	IIB
T1	N2	M0	III
T2	N0	M0	IB
T2	N1	M0	IIB
T2	N2	M0	III
T3	N0	M0	IIA
T3	N1	M0	IIB
T3	N2	M0	III
T4	Any N	M0	III
Any T	Any N	M1	IV

Source: Used with the permission of American College of Surgeons. MB Amin et al (eds): *AJCC Cancer Staging Manual*, 8th ed. Springer, 2017.

uncinate body of the pancreas is usually a pylorus-sparing pancreaticoduodenectomy (a modified Whipple procedure). For tumors in the body or tail, a distal pancreatectomy is usually performed. Clinical and pathologic findings of the resection are defined as either an R0 resection (no macroscopic or microscopic disease left after surgery) or an R1 resection, which refers to residual disease likely left behind. Patients with smaller tumors and lymph node–negative disease have a better survival (median of about 18–23 months with 5-year survival of about 20%).

TABLE 83-3 Extent of Disease and Therapeutic Approach

DESIGNATION (MEDIAN SURVIVAL)	THERAPEUTIC APPROACHES
1. Resectable (localized): (18–23 mo) • No encasement of celiac axis or superior mesenteric artery (SMA) • Patent superior mesenteric—portal veins • No extrapancreatic disease	Surgical option (or preoperative-neoadjuvant therapy first) Surgery is followed by postsurgery adjuvant therapy • Currently mFOLFIRINOX
2. Locally advanced: (6–10 mo) • Encasement of arteries • Venous occlusion (superior mesenteric vein [SMV] or portal) • No extrapancreatic disease	Either chemotherapy or chemotherapy + radiation therapy
3. Metastatic: (8.3–12.8 mo)	Systemic chemotherapy

Abbreviation: mFOLFIRINOX, modified FOLFIRINOX (folinic acid, 5-fluorouracil, irinotecan, and oxaliplatin (T Conroy et al: N Engl J Med 379:2395, 2018).

Two approaches are being explored to try to improve on this.

1. Postoperative adjuvant therapy. The standard of care is to use 24 weeks of adjuvant treatment with a modified folinic acid, 5-fluorouracil, irinotecan, and oxaliplatin (FOLFIRINOX) regimen. In the definitive clinical trial, the median survival was 54 months for the combination of modified FOLFIRINOX versus 35 months for gemcitabine alone (hazard ratio [HR] 0.64; 95% confidence interval [CI] 0.48–0.86; $p = .003$). Toxicities were manageable.
2. A newer approach is the use of neoadjuvant chemotherapy (chemotherapy given before surgery) to try to shrink the tumor and normalize the patient's serum CA19-9 level. Data suggest that patients who have borderline resectable/locally advanced disease can benefit from neoadjuvant therapy. Studies of neoadjuvant chemotherapy with or without radiation therapy are ongoing.

LOCALLY ADVANCED DISEASE (30% OF PATIENTS)

For patients with locally advanced disease, the median survival is also quite poor (6–10 months) because many of the patients die with local problems (e.g., portal vein thrombosis with bleeding varices, obstruction, sepsis). The approach has been to try to reduce the bulk of the disease with use of radiation therapy plus chemotherapy or chemotherapy alone, with the goal that the disease could become resectable. No standard therapy has been agreed upon, but experimental approaches are applying some of the treatments that show promise in advanced metastatic disease.

ADVANCED METASTATIC DISEASE (60% OF PATIENTS)

Only a few of the many phase 3 randomized trials in patients with advanced pancreatic cancer have led to meaningful increases in survival. We have learned that a regimen needs to have at least a 50% improvement in overall survival or 90% improvement in 1-year survival in a pilot phase 2 trial to predict for any degree of success in large randomized phase 3 trials.

Patients with the best chance of receiving a benefit from treatment have a good performance status (functioning up and around at least 70% of the day), have a reasonable albumin level (≥3.0 g/dL), and a neutrophil/lymphocyte ratio of ≤5.0.

Single-agent gemcitabine achieves a median survival of 6 months and a 1-year survival rate of 18%. **Table 83-4** details three combination regimens that have further improved survival modestly. Median overall survival still ranges from 6 to 11 months. However, 1-year survival is now approaching 35% for these combination regimens with some long-term 4+ year survivors.

Also of note in Table 83-4, liposomal irinotecan has U.S. Food and Drug Administration (FDA) approval in combination with 5-fluorouracil and leucovorin for patients whose tumors have progressed on gemcitabine (e.g., second-line therapy for stage IV disease) based on improved overall survival.

FOR PATIENTS WITH A SPECIFIC MOLECULAR PROFILE IN THEIR TUMOR/GERMLINE

PARP inhibitors have clinical activity against pancreatic cancers having mutations in *BRCA2, BRCA1*, or *PALB2* (i.e., defective DNA repair proteins). In addition, their tumors might be more sensitive to specific combinations of chemotherapy like gemcitabine plus cisplatin. In addition, tumors with microsatellite instability often have more mutations, and such tumors appear to have a higher response rate to immunotherapy with checkpoint inhibitors and anti-PD-1 (pembrolizumab, nivolumab) and anti-PD-L1 antibodies.

TABLE 83-4 Combination Chemotherapy Regimens That Have an Impact on Survival

STUDY DESIGN (AUTHOR/REF)	NO. OF PATIENTS	MEDIAN SURVIVAL (MONTHS)
Gemcitabine + erlotinib vs gemcitabine (Moore et al: J Clin Oncol 26:1960, 2007)	569	6.24 vs 5.91 (HR 0.82; 95% CI 0.69–0.99; *p* = .038)
FOLFIRINOX (folinic acid + 5-fluorouracil + irinotecan + oxaliplatin) vs gemcitabine (Conroy et al: N Engl J Med 364:1817, 2011)	342	11.1 vs 6.8 (HR 0.57; 95% CI 0.45–0.70; *p* <.001)
Nap-paclitaxel + gemcitabine vs gemcitabine, (Von Hoff et al: N Eng J Med 369:1691, 2013.)	861	8.5 vs 6.7 (HR 0.72; 95% CI 0.62–0.83; *p* <.001[a]
Nanoliposomal irinotecan + fluorouracil + folinic acid vs nanoliposomal irinotecan monotherapy vs fluorouracil + folinic acid (Wang-Gillam et al: Lancet 387:545, 2015)	417	6.1 vs 4.2 (HR 0.67; 95% CI 0.49-0.92; *p* = .012[b])

[a]The 2-year survival rate with this regimen is 9% and the 3+ year rate is 4%. Other studies have not reported on these parameters. [b]HR is for nanoliposomal irinotecan + 5-fluorouracil + folinic acid vs 5-fluorouracil + folinic acid.

Abbreviations: CI, confidence interval; HR, hazard ratio.

MAINTENANCE THERAPY FOR PATIENTS RESPONDING TO TREATMENT

For patients with germline *BRCA1* or *BRCA2* mutations whose disease has not progressed during a first-line platinum-based regimen, the PARP inhibitor olaparib has been shown to improve progression-free survival (7.4 vs 3.8 months; HR 0.53; 95% CI 0.35–0.82; $p = .004$) with no change in quality of life.

OTHER POTENTIAL FACTORS INFLUENCING SURVIVAL

Preclinical studies have suggested that vitamin D can inhibit the development and growth of cancer. In models of pancreatic cancer, synthetic analogues of vitamin D had an effect on both tumor cells and on the tumor microenvironment. Clinical studies are conflicting as to whether circulating levels of plasma 25-hydroxyvitamin D (25[OH]D) affect the incidence of pancreatic cancer. However, patients with prediagnostic levels of 25(OH)D that are in the normal range have a longer survival than those who have reduced levels (35% lower hazard for death).

FUTURE DIRECTIONS

Death from pancreatic cancer is often due to progressive inanition. The metabolic consequences of this cancer are being examined. The tumor can be fatal at a modest level of tumor burden based on the profound metabolic effects. Other promising areas of investigation include addressing the florid stromal reaction around the tumor cells (believed to act as a physical barrier to drug delivery and as an immune sanctuary for the tumor cells). Improvements in outcomes for pancreatic cancer would accompany earlier detection. A small decrease in the percentage of patients being diagnosed with stage IV pancreatic cancer has been noted. The reason for this encouraging sign is unknown. The 5-year survival for earlier stage patients has increased from 44.7% in 2004 to 83.7% in 2012. There is emerging evidence that the surveillance to detect *CDKN2A* mutation carriers can detect pancreatic ductal cancer at a resectable stage.

Acknowledgment

Thank you to Nicole Harkey, for assistance in the preparation of this chapter, and Drs. Elizabeth Washington, Ron Korn, and Haiyong Han and the American Joint Committee on Cancer for providing the figures and tables.

FURTHER READING

Conroy T et al: FOLFIRINOX versus gemcitabine for metastatic pancreatic cancer. N Engl J Med 364:1817, 2011.

Conroy T et al: FOLFIRINOX or gemcitabine as adjuvant therapy for pancreatic cancer. N Engl J Med 379:2395, 2018.

Golan T et al: Maintenance olaparib for germline BRCA-mutated metastatic pancreatic cancer. N Engl J Med 381:317, 2019.

Hruban RJ et al: Genetic progression in the pancreatic ducts. Am J Pathol 156:1821, 2000.

Rahib L et al: Evaluation of pancreatic cancer clinical trials and benchmarks for clinically meaningful future trials: A systemic review. JAMA Oncol 2:1209, 2016.

Rawla P et al: Epidemiology of pancreatic cancer: Global trends, etiology and risk factors. World J Oncol 10:10, 2019.

Solomon S et al: Inherited pancreatic cancer syndromes. Cancer J 18:485, 2012.

Von Hoff D et al: Increased survival in pancreatic cancer with nab-paclitaxel plus gemcitabine. N Engl J Med 369:1691, 2013.

84 Gastrointestinal Neuroendocrine Tumors

Matthew H. Kulke

Gastrointestinal (GI) neuroendocrine tumors (NETs) can be broadly grouped according to their site of origin, as either extrapancreatic NETs, historically called carcinoid tumors, or pancreatic NETs. While NETs can pursue a broad range of clinical behaviors, they classically follow a course that is more indolent than many other malignancies. NETs also have the ability to synthesize peptides, growth factors, and bioactive amines that may be ectopically secreted, giving rise to a range of unique clinical syndromes.

INCIDENCE AND PREVALENCE

The diagnosed incidence of NETs has been steadily increasing over the past several decades (**Fig. 84-1**). An analysis of data from the Surveillance, Epidemiology, and End Results (SEER) program, comprising population-based data in the United States from 1973 to 2012, showed that the incidence had increased 6.4-fold over this time period and that the estimated prevalence of patients who had been diagnosed with a NET was >170,000. This analysis also found that overall survival durations for patients with NETs had improved significantly. The increasing incidence and improved survival durations for patients with NETs likely reflect, at least in part, advances in both diagnosis and treatment. While environmental or other factors leading to an increased incidence of NETs cannot be excluded; common cancer risk factors such as tobacco or alcohol use and dietary patterns have not been clearly linked to NET development.

A minority of NETs develop in the context of autosomal inherited genetic syndromes associated with mutations in specific tumor-suppressor genes. The most common of these is multiple endocrine neoplasia type 1 (MEN 1), due to mutation and loss of function of the *menin* gene, located on chromosome 11q13 (**Chap. 388**). Patients with MEN 1 are at risk for developing pancreatic NETs as well as hyperparathyroidism and pituitary adenomas; less commonly, they may develop bronchial and thymic NETs. Other inherited syndromes associated with NETs include von Hippel–Lindau disease (VHL), von Recklinghausen's disease (neurofibromatosis type 1), and tuberous sclerosis (Bourneville's disease). Inherited mutations in the VHL gene, located on chromosome 3p25, are associated with the development of cerebellar hemangioblastomas, renal cancer, and pheochromocytomas and, less commonly, pancreatic NETs. Mutations in neurofibromin (*NF1*) are associated with neurofibromatosis (von Recklinghausen's disease); patients with neurofibromatosis are at risk of developing both pancreatic and extrapancreatic NETs. Tuberous sclerosis is caused by mutations that alter either hamartin (*TSC1*) or tuberin (*TSC2*). Both hamartin and tuberin function as inhibitors of the phosphatidylinositol 3-kinase and the mechanistic target of rapamycin (mTOR) signaling cascades, and pancreatic NETs have been reported in these patients. Rare cases of familial small intestine NETs have also been reported; in these cases, multiple synchronous tumors generally arise within the small intestine. A characteristic inherited mutation, however, has not been identified to date in the majority of these cases.

HISTOLOGIC CLASSIFICATION AND MOLECULAR FEATURES

The histologic features of NETs vary widely and are one of the most important determinants of both clinical behavior and treatment. NETs are classified based on the degree tumor differentiation (well or poorly differentiated), as assessed by a pathologist, and tumor grade (grades 1–3) (**Table 84-1**). Tumor grade closely correlates with mitotic count and Ki-67 proliferative index. Classic, well-differentiated NETs are composed of monotonous sheets of small round cells with uniform nuclei and only rare mitoses. Immunocytochemical staining for chromogranins and synaptophysin is typical. Ultrastructurally, these tumors contain electron-dense neurosecretory granules containing peptides and bioactive amines that may be ectopically secreted, giving rise to a range of clinical syndromes. These classic well-differentiated NETs have low-grade features and generally have a mitotic index of <2 mitoses per 10 high-power field (HPF) and a Ki-67 proliferative index of <3%. Less commonly, well-differentiated NETs have an intermediate histologic grade and pursue a somewhat more aggressive clinical course. These intermediate-grade tumors typically have a mitotic count of 2–20 per 10 HPF and a mitotic index of 3–20%. Well-differentiated high-grade tumors are rare and have mitotic counts that exceed 20 per 10 HPF and a Ki-67 proliferative index of >20%. Poorly

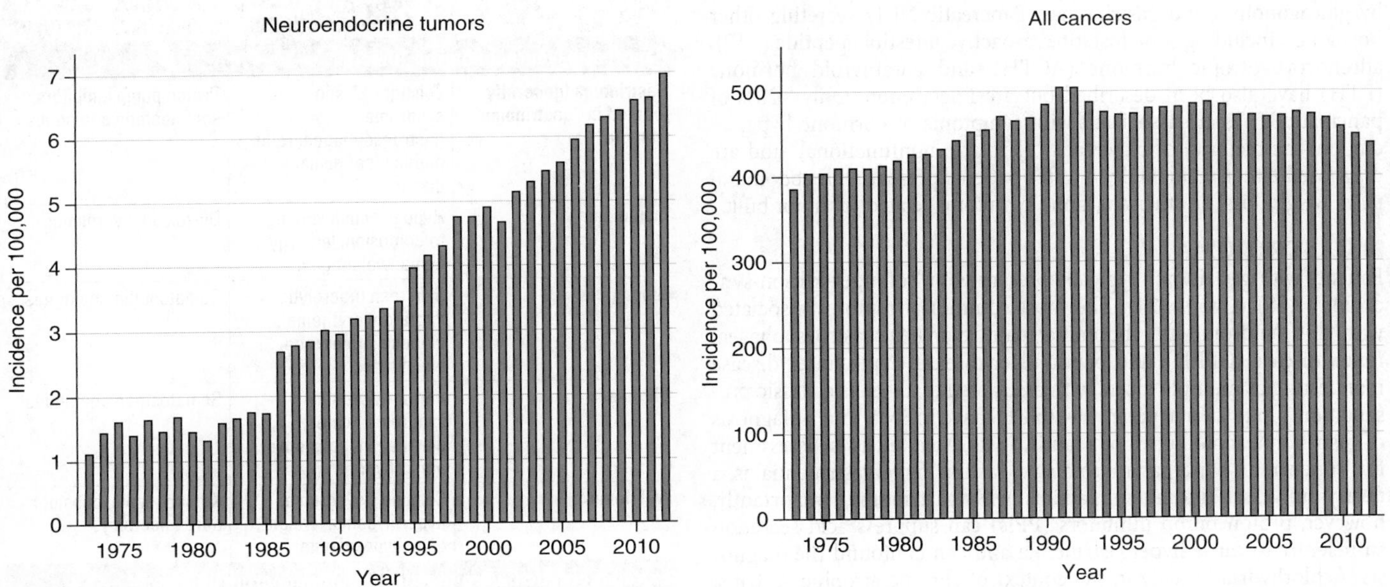

FIGURE 84-1 Incidence of neuroendocrine tumors (NETs). The incidence of neuroendocrine tumors has been increasing over the past several decades, an observation that has been attributed in part to improved diagnosis and classification. *(Adapted from A Dasari et al: Trends in the incidence, prevalence, and survival outcomes in patients with neuroendocrine tumors in the United States. JAMA Oncol 3:1335, 2017.)*

TABLE 84-1 Histologic Classification of Neuroendocrine Tumors

CLASSIFICATION	DIFFERENTIATION	GRADE	MITOTIC COUNT	KI-67
Neuroendocrine tumor	Well differentiated	Low grade (grade 1)	<2 per 10 HPF	<3%
Neuroendocrine tumor	Well differentiated	Intermediate grade (grade 2)	2–20 per 10 HPF	3–20%
Neuroendocrine tumor	Well differentiated	High grade (grade 3)	>20 per 10 HPF	>20%
Neuroendocrine carcinoma	Poorly differentiated	High grade (grade 3)	>20 per 10 HPF	>20%

Abbreviation: HPF, high-power field.

differentiated high-grade tumors form the most clinically aggressive category; prognosis and treatment for these tumors differ markedly from their well-differentiated counterparts.

Whole exome sequencing of sporadic pancreatic NETs found that the most frequently altered gene was *MEN1*, occurring in 44% of tumors. In addition, 43% of tumors had mutations in genes encoding two subunits of a transcription/chromatin remodeling complex consisting of DAXX (death-domain-associated protein) and ATRX (α-thalassemia/mental retardation syndrome X-linked). Mutations in genes associated with the mTOR pathway were identified in 15% of tumors. In contrast, recurrent mutations in extrapancreatic NETs appear to be rare. In one study that evaluated 180 small intestinal NETs using a combination of whole exome and more targeted genome-sequencing analysis, recurrent mutations were only observed in the *CDKN1B* gene (cyclin-dependent kinase inhibitor 1B [$p27^{Kip1}$]) in 8% of cases. Loss of chromosome 18 is a common finding in small-bowel NETs. Small-intestinal GI carcinoids commonly have epigenetic changes; however, the clinical significance of these alterations remains uncertain. Initial studies have suggested that well-differentiated pancreatic and extrapancreatic NETs express only low levels of the immune checkpoint markers PD-1 and PD-L1.

CLINICAL PRESENTATION AND MANAGEMENT OF LOCALIZED PANCREATIC NEUROENDOCRINE TUMORS

Pancreatic NETs have been subcategorized as either "functional," meaning associated with symptoms of hormone secretion, or nonfunctional, in which case they may be clinically silent until they cause anatomic symptoms. The clinical presentation of functional pancreatic NETs depends on the type of hormone secreted and can sometimes lead to dramatic clinical presentations (**Table 84-2**). The most common functional pancreatic NETs are insulinomas, followed in incidence by glucagonomas and gastrinomas. Pancreatic NETs secreting other hormones, including somatostatin, vasoactive intestinal peptide (VIP), adrenocorticotropic hormone (ACTH), and parathyroid hormone (PTH) have also been described but are uncommon. Only ~20% of pancreatic NETs are associated with symptoms of hormone hypersecretion; the majority of pancreatic NETs are "nonfunctional" and are diagnosed either incidentally or after patients present with abdominal pain, weight loss, or other anatomic symptoms related to tumor bulk.

■ GASTRINOMA

Patients with gastrinoma typically present with Zollinger-Ellison syndrome (ZES) (**Chap. 324**). The most common symptoms associated with this syndrome are abdominal pain, diarrhea, gastroesophageal reflux disease (GERD), and peptic ulcer disease. Peptic ulcer disease manifesting as multiple ulcers with associated diarrhea is a classic presentation. Up to 25% of patients with ZES have MEN 1, and a diagnosis of gastrinoma should prompt a family history as well as an assessment for concurrent hyperparathyroidism. Fasting hypergastrinemia is a nearly universal finding in patients with gastrinoma. Importantly, however, proton pump inhibitors (PPIs) can suppress acid secretion sufficiently to cause hypergastrinemia and can confound the diagnosis. Achlorhydria, usually in the context of chronic atrophic gastritis, will also elevate serum gastrin levels but can usually be easily distinguished from gastrinoma given the absence of other evidence of acid hypersecretion.

While often classified as pancreatic NETs, the majority of gastrinomas in fact arise in the "gastrinoma triangle," an anatomic region bounded by the duodenum, pancreas, and confluence of the cystic and common bile ducts. Most gastrinomas (50–90%) in sporadic ZES arise in the duodenum. They are frequently small and may be difficult to localize. Imaging studies generally include either CT or MRI; endoscopic ultrasound or somatostatin scintigraphy may also be helpful.

PPIs are generally highly effective in the treatment of symptoms related to gastrinoma and are considered the initial treatment of choice. Rapid resolution of both abdominal pain and diarrhea related to acid hypersecretion is common. Somatostatin analogues may also be helpful in controlling symptoms in refractory cases. Once symptoms are controlled, surgical resection is generally recommended for patients with sporadic gastrinomas, both to eliminate the cause of gastrin secretion and to decrease the risk of developing metastatic disease. The technique used for resection depends in large part on the precise location of the tumor. In some cases where preoperative imaging is not successful but a diagnosis is strongly suspected, exploratory laparotomy with intraoperative ultrasound may be undertaken. In gastrinoma patients who have underlying MEN 1, tumors are generally small and multiple; the role of routine surgery in this setting remains more controversial but generally is still recommended in patients with larger tumors measuring ≥1.5–2 cm in diameter.

■ INSULINOMA

Patients with insulinoma generally present with symptoms of hypoglycemia, which may include confusion, headache, disorientation, visual difficulties, irrational behavior, and even coma. In some cases, the diagnosis of insulinoma may not be immediately evident, and patients with

TABLE 84-2 Clinical Presentation and Management of Secretory Syndromes Associated with Neuroendocrine Tumors

	CLINICAL SYMPTOMS AND MANIFESTATIONS	TREATMENT OPTIONS TO CONTROL SECRETORY SYMPTOMS
Pancreatic Neuroendocrine Tumors		
Gastrinoma (generally located in "gastrinoma triangle")	Zollinger-Ellison syndrome: gastroesophageal reflux, peptic ulcer disease, diarrhea	Proton pump inhibitors, somatostatin analogues
Insulinoma	Hypoglycemia leading to confusion, lethargy, coma; weight gain	Diazoxide, everolimus
Glucagonoma	Skin rash (necrolytic migratory erythema), glucose intolerance, weight loss	Somatostatin analogues
VIPoma	Verner-Morrison syndrome: watery diarrhea, hypokalemia, achlorhydria	Somatostatin analogues
ACTHoma	Cushing's syndrome: hyperglycemia, weight gain, hypokalemia	Ketoconazole, consider adrenalectomy
Extrapancreatic gastrointestinal neuroendocrine tumors		
Typically in setting of advanced disease from small intestine or appendiceal primary tumors	Carcinoid syndrome: flushing, diarrhea, right-sided valvular heart disease, mesenteric fibrosis	Somatostatin analogues, telotristat ethyl

insulinoma may initially be diagnosed with psychiatric illnesses that in retrospect were hypoglycemic symptoms. The diagnosis of insulinoma is generally confirmed with elevated fasting insulin levels in conjunction with elevated proinsulin and C-peptide. Fasting hypoglycemia can also be caused by severe liver disease, alcoholism, and poor nutrition. Postprandial hypoglycemia may also occur after gastric bypass surgery. Surreptitious use of insulin or hypoglycemic agents may be difficult to distinguish from an insulinoma. Evaluation of proinsulin and C-peptide levels, both of which should be normal in patients using exogenous insulin, and measurement of sulfonylurea levels in serum or plasma are helpful in such cases.

The hypoglycemia associated with insulinomas can be severe and challenging to manage. Diazoxide has historically been used in the initial management of patients with insulinoma and results in inhibition of insulin release, though it can also be associated with side effects including sodium retention and nausea. Everolimus, in addition to its antitumor effect (see below), is highly effective in improving glycemic control in patients with insulinoma. The benefits of everolimus in this setting may be related both to induction of insulin resistance and a direct antitumor effect. While somatostatin analogues are usually effective in treating symptoms of hormone hypersecretion associated with other types of NETs, they should be used with caution in patients with insulinoma. Somatostatin analogues may suppress counterregulatory hormones, such as growth hormone (GH), glucagon, and catecholamines, and precipitously worsen hypoglycemia.

Insulinomas may be difficult to localize, as they are less consistently avid on somatostatin scintigraphy than other pancreatic NETs. Insulinomas are also generally small, with the majority measuring <2 cm in diameter. Because of their generally small size, insulinomas are best localized with endoscopic ultrasound (EUS). In the absence of metastatic disease, surgical resection is usually recommended. The primary treatment for exophytic or peripheral insulinomas is enucleation. If enucleation is not possible because of invasion or the location of the tumor within the pancreas, then pancreatoduodenectomy for tumors in the head of the pancreas or distal pancreatectomy with preservation of the spleen for smaller tumors not involving splenic vessels may be considered.

GLUCAGONOMA

Patients with glucagonoma most commonly present with a characteristic dermatitis, called necrolytic migratory erythema (**Fig. 84-2**). The rash usually involves intertriginous sites, especially in the groin or buttock, and can wax and wane. Other common presenting symptoms of glucagonoma include glucose intolerance and weight loss. The diagnosis of glucagonoma can be confirmed by demonstrating an increased plasma glucagon level, generally in excess of 1000 pg/mL. Somatostatin analogues are usually highly effective as an initial treatment to alleviate the symptoms and rash associated with glucagon hypersecretion. The majority of glucagonomas are large in size at presentation and arise in the tail of the pancreas. For patients with localized disease, distal pancreatectomy and splenectomy are recommended. A hypercoagulable state has been reported in up to 33% of patients with glucagonoma, and perioperative anticoagulation should generally be employed.

SOMATOSTATINOMA

Patients with somatostatinoma typically present with diabetes mellitus, gallbladder disease, diarrhea, and steatorrhea. Somatostatinomas occur primarily in the pancreas or duodenum, are usually large, and are commonly metastatic at presentation. They are only rarely associated with MEN 1. The diagnosis of somatostatinoma is based on the demonstration of elevated plasma somatostatin levels, and as such, the potential benefits of using somatostatin analogs as a treatment for patients with somatostatinoma is questionable. Surgery is recommended for patients with localized disease.

VIPOMA

VIPomas are associated with a distinct syndrome that has been variously called Verner-Morrison syndrome, pancreatic cholera, and WDHA syndrome (*w*atery *d*iarrhea, *h*ypokalemia, and *a*chlorhydria).

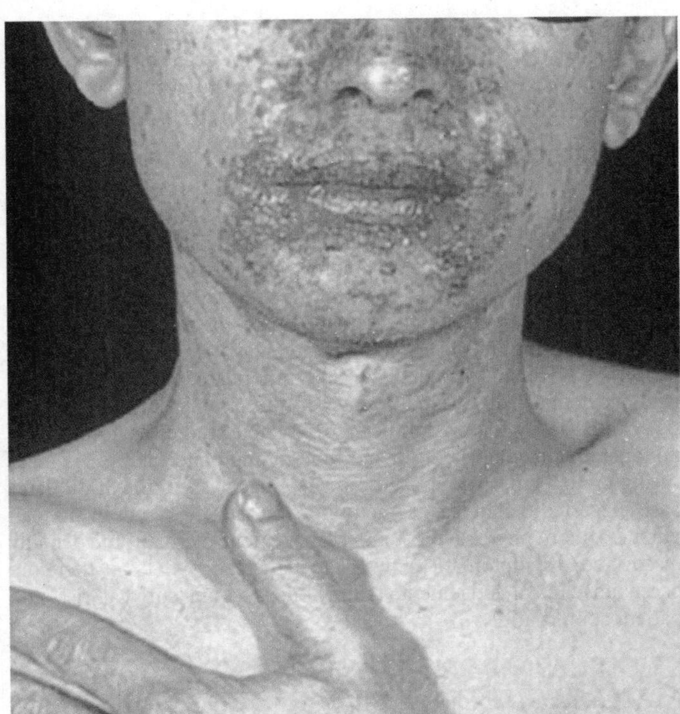

FIGURE 84-2 Glucagonoma syndrome. Patients with glucagonoma may present with a classic skin rash, necrolytic migratory erythema (shown). Other presenting symptoms include glucose intolerance and weight loss.

VIP is a 28-amino-acid peptide that mimics the effects of the cholera toxin by stimulating chloride secretion in the small intestine and increasing smooth-muscle contractility, resulting in profound diarrhea. Treatment of dehydration, hypokalemia, and electrolyte losses with fluid and electrolyte replacement is the most critical initial treatment for patients with VIPoma. VIPomas are usually solitary and arise in the pancreatic tail. Elevated plasma levels of VIP are typical but should not be the only basis of the diagnosis of VIPomas because they can occur with some diarrheal states including inflammatory bowel disease, in the setting of small bowel resection, and radiation enteritis. Chronic surreptitious use of laxatives/diuretics can be particularly difficult to detect clinically. Somatostatin analogues are usually highly effective in controlling the diarrhea; surgical resection is recommended for patients with localized disease.

OTHER SECRETORY PANCREATIC NETS

Pancreatic NETs secreting GH-releasing factor (GRF), calcitonin, ACTH, and PTH-related protein have also been described; it is also possible for pancreatic NETs to secrete more than one hormone or for the secretory profiles to evolve over time. Gastrinomas, in particular, may evolve and may be associated with secretion of ACTH, resulting in ectopic Cushing's syndrome. Tumors secreting these hormones may not be as responsive to treatment with somatostatin analogues as the more common pancreatic NETs and the associated hormonal symptoms may cause significant morbidity. As with other pancreatic NETs, patients with localized disease are generally treated with surgical resection. In patients with ACTH-secreting tumors, the associated symptoms of Cushing's syndrome can be alleviated with adrenalectomy if resection of the primary tumor is not possible or in the setting of metastatic disease.

PANCREATIC NETS ARISING IN THE SETTING OF MEN 1

Pancreatic NETs occurring in patients with MEN 1 are typically multiple and often pursue a relatively indolent course. Because of the high probability of multiple tumors, surgical resection of confirmed pancreatic NETs in patients with MEN 1 is usually undertaken with caution given the likelihood of tumors arising in the remaining pancreas if partial pancreatectomy is undertaken as well as the significant morbidities associated with total pancreatectomy. However, for symptomatic tumors or for growing tumors >2 cm in size, surgical resection may still be considered.

NONFUNCTIONING PANCREATIC NETS

As noted above, the majority of pancreatic NETs are not associated with symptoms of hormone hypersecretion and are considered "nonfunctional." As a result, they often remain clinically silent and either are diagnosed incidentally or are not diagnosed until widespread, metastatic disease is present resulting in anatomic symptoms. If they are localized at diagnosis, the general treatment recommendation is surgical resection; however, the management of small, asymptomatic pancreatic NETs is debated. Assuming tumors are low grade, patients with incidentally discovered, low-grade tumors measuring <1 cm in size can be safely followed; other retrospective studies have suggested nonoperative management for nonfunctioning pancreatic NETs measuring up to 3 cm. In contrast, however, an analysis of the SEER database suggested that at least some tumors measuring <2 cm in size can pursue a more aggressive course. Management of small, incidentally discovered, asymptomatic, low-grade pancreatic NETs is therefore based on clinical judgement, taking into account surgical risk and patient comorbidities.

CLINICAL PRESENTATION AND MANAGEMENT OF LOCALIZED EXTRAPANCREATIC GASTROINTESTINAL NEUROENDOCRINE TUMORS

Extrapancreatic GI NETs, historically called carcinoid tumors, may arise virtually anywhere in the GI tract and differ significantly in their clinical characteristics depending on their location. The most common locations for extrapancreatic NETs are the stomach, distal small intestine, appendix, and rectum.

GASTRIC NETS

Gastric NETs can be categorized into three groups: type 1 (associated with chronic atrophic gastritis); type 2 (associated with gastrinomas and ZES), and type 3 (sporadic, gastric NETs). Type 1 gastric NETs are the most common of the three types. In type 1 gastric NETs, chronic atrophic gastritis results in loss of acid secretion with consequent loss of the negative feedback loop on gastrin-producing cells in the antrum of the stomach. Pernicious anemia is also commonly associated with this condition; classic laboratory findings are a markedly elevated gastrin level and low levels of vitamin B_{12}. Unchecked gastrin secretion in these patients results in hyperplasia of the endocrine cells in the gastric fundus. A typical finding on endoscopy is diffuse endocrine cell hyperplasia with multiple gastric carcinoid tumors (**Fig. 84-3**). These tumors generally pursue a benign course and can be monitored with serial endoscopy. In cases where tumors continue to grow or become symptomatic, antrectomy to remove the source of gastrin production can result in tumor regression. Type 2 tumors are rare and usually occur in the setting of gastrinoma; as with type 1 gastric NETs, elevated gastrin levels result in diffuse gastric neuroendocrine hyperplasia and multifocal gastric NETs. Resection of the gastrinoma, removing the source of gastrin production, is the treatment of choice.

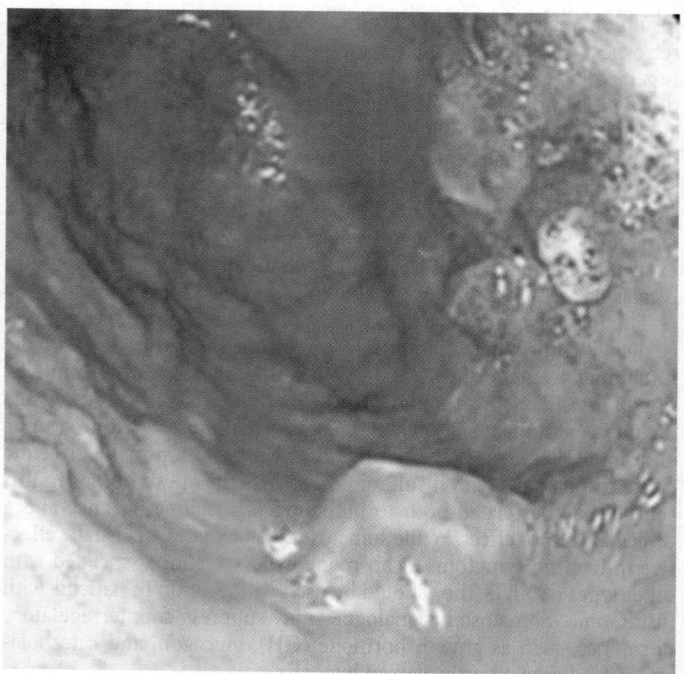

FIGURE 84-3 Multifocal gastric neuroendocrine tumor. *(Courtesy of Christopher Huang MD, Boston Medical Center.)*

In contrast to type 1 and type 2 gastric NETs, type 3 gastric NETs are generally solitary, arise in the setting of normal gastrin levels, and may pursue a far more aggressive course. For early-stage, smaller tumors, endoscopic or wedge resection may be performed. For larger tumors, partial gastrectomy with lymphadenectomy is recommended.

NETS OF THE SMALL INTESTINE

Small-bowel NETs occur most commonly in the terminal ileum and are notoriously difficult to diagnose at an early stage. One reason for this is that they arise within the muscularis, and their submucosal location makes them difficult to see during routine colonoscopy (**Fig. 84-4A**). Small-bowel NETs are also often multifocal; multifocal tumors appear to arise independently throughout the small intestine, although the mechanisms underlying this phenomenon remain uncertain.

Small-bowel NETs are often associated with desmoplasia and mesenteric fibrosis, likely as a result of fibroblast proliferation stimulated by tumor serotonin secretion. Mesenteric fibrosis frequently

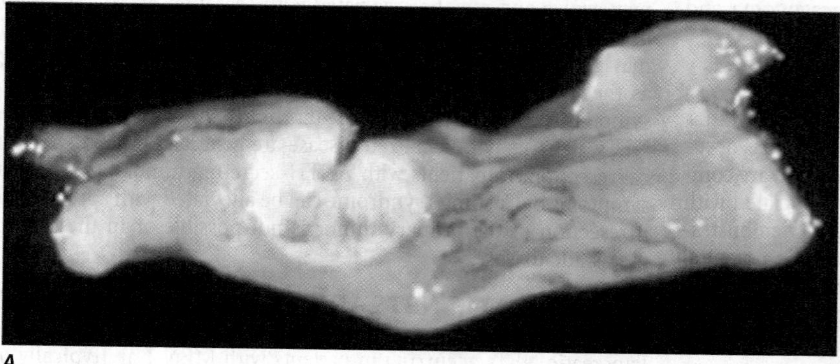

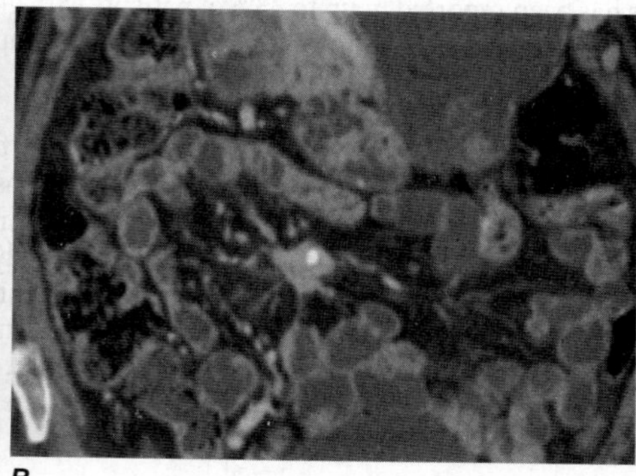

FIGURE 84-4 Small intestine neuroendocrine tumor. ***A.*** Small intestine neuroendocrine tumors arising in submucosal location. The submucosal location of small intestine neuroendocrine tumors, together with their location beyond the ileocecal valve in the terminal ileum, can make endoscopic detection challenging. ***B.*** Classic "spoke and wheel" appearance of calcified mesenteric mass associated with small intestine primary neuroendocrine tumor. Mesenteric fibrosis commonly leads to intermittent obstructive symptoms and can also lead to ischemia when the mesenteric vasculature is involved. *(Fig. B: Courtesy of Christina LeBedis MD, Boston Medical Center.)*

results in intermittent small-bowel obstruction and, in some cases, bowel ischemia due to involvement of the mesenteric vessels. Patients may experience symptoms of intermittent abdominal pain and associated diarrhea, sometimes for months or years before diagnosis, that because of the difficulty in diagnosis are often attributed to irritable bowel syndrome. One classic finding that can aid in diagnosis is that the lymph node metastases associated with small intestine NETs are usually larger than the primary tumor and may be calcified, which, together with the tethering of the small intestine caused by the associated fibrosis, results in a classic "spoke and wheel" appearance on computed tomography (**Fig. 84-4*B***).

Surgical resection of the primary tumor and associated metastases is recommended when feasible and is performed with curative intent when distant metastatic disease is not already present. Resection should also be considered in patients with metastatic disease experiencing intermittent obstruction or abdominal discomfort thought to be related to the primary tumor or associated mesenteric disease. Some have also advocated the routine resection of asymptomatic small-bowel primary tumors in patients with distant metastatic disease, with the rationale that this may be a way to prevent the future development of fibrosis and obstruction and preempt the development of unresectable disease due to tumor involvement of the mesenteric vessels. However, the available data on the benefits of resecting an asymptomatic primary tumor in this context are conflicting. Some studies have suggested that this practice results in an overall survival benefit, but the retrospective nature of these studies makes the data difficult to interpret given the high potential for selection bias in patients taken to surgery compared with those who were not. Other studies have suggested that prophylactic primary tumor resection confers no survival benefit and that surgery can be safely delayed until it is indicated based on the development of symptoms.

■ NETS OF THE APPENDIX

NETs are one of the most common tumors arising in the appendix. They are typically discovered incidentally in younger individuals undergoing appendectomy for acute appendicitis and not uncommonly are identified only at the time of pathology review. While the unexpected diagnosis of an appendiceal NET in such situations can cause considerable anxiety, in the majority of cases, the prognosis is excellent. Indeed, the clinical behavior of appendiceal NETs has been inferred from multiple large retrospective surgical series that suggest that the risk of lymph node or distant metastases from appendiceal NETs with well-differentiated histology and a tumor diameter measuring <2 cm is extremely low. In such cases, appendectomy alone is felt to be a sufficient surgical procedure.

In contrast, the risk of metastases for tumors measuring 2–3 cm is ~20–30% and is even greater for tumors measuring >3 cm. For patients with larger tumors, more formal staging studies with either cross-sectional imaging or somatostatin scintigraphy are generally recommended to assess for distant metastases, and a subsequent right colectomy to remove regional lymph nodes is performed if no distant metastases are observed. Whether right colectomy should be performed for tumors measuring <2 cm with features such as mesoappendiceal invasion or tumor origin at the appendiceal base, which in some series have suggested a poorer prognosis, remains uncertain. Additionally, tumors may arise in which neuroendocrine cells are admixed with mucin-producing cells or cells exhibiting features of frank adenocarcinoma. In such mixed neuroendocrine-adenocarcinoma tumors, sometimes termed "adenocarcinoids," treatment recommendations are generally dictated by the more aggressive component of the tumor and align with typical recommendations for colorectal adenocarcinoma.

■ RECTAL NETS

With the increased use of screening colonoscopy, the diagnosis of rectal NET has also become more common. For unclear reasons, the incidence of rectal carcinoid tumors shows geographic variation. In European studies, they compose up to 14% of all NETs, while in some Asian series (Japan, China, Korea), they compose up to 90% of all NETs. The majority of rectal NETs are small, measuring <1 cm in diameter, and have well-differentiated histology. These tumors rarely metastasize and can usually be safely removed endoscopically with subsequent endoscopic monitoring. In contrast, up to one-third of rectal NETs between 1 and 2 cm are associated with metastases, and those >2 cm, though uncommon, metastasize in >70% of patients. When identified early, these tumors generally require a surgical resection. In contrast to NETs of the appendix and small intestine, hormone secretion from rectal NETs, even when metastatic, is exceedingly rare.

CLINICAL PRESENTATION, DIAGNOSIS, AND EVALUATION OF PATIENTS WITH METASTATIC NEUROENDOCRINE TUMORS

While patients who undergo resection of localized NETs may be at risk of developing tumor recurrence or metastatic disease, postoperative treatment has not yet been shown to alter the risk of recurrence, and systemic adjuvant therapy is not recommended following resection of well-differentiated NETs, as it is for some other cancers. Whether adjuvant systemic therapy may be of benefit following resection of high-grade NETs is uncertain, and an approach utilizing platinum-based chemotherapy with or without external-beam radiation, analogous to that used in small-cell carcinoma, is sometimes considered.

The evaluation of patients with known or suspected metastatic disease generally includes both standard cross-sectional imaging such as CT or MRI and somatostatin scintigraphy. Somatostatin scintigraphy in this setting is based on the fact that >90% of NETs express somatostatin receptors. Gallium-68 (^{68}GA) dotatate, a radioligand bound to a somatostatin analogue, can be used as a nuclear medicine tracer to perform PET scanning and is highly sensitive in detecting both primary NETs and metastases (**Fig. 84-5**). Because of the sensitivity of this approach, false-positive results can occur due to somatostatin receptor expression in other tissues. Physiologic uptake in the pancreatic uncinated process is common; uptake can also occur in the setting of sarcoidosis, in meningiomas, and in thyroid goiter or thyroiditis. Standard fluorodeoxyglucose (FDG) positron emission tomography (PET) scans are often negative in well-differentiated NET due to their low metabolic activity but can show uptake in higher-grade tumors; conversely, rates of somatostatin expression tend to be lower in higher-grade tumors, and ^{68}GA dotatate scans may be negative in this setting.

The utility of blood-based tumor markers in NETs is controversial. The circulating tumor marker chromogranin A is commonly used as a screen for the presence of NETs and also to monitor for both

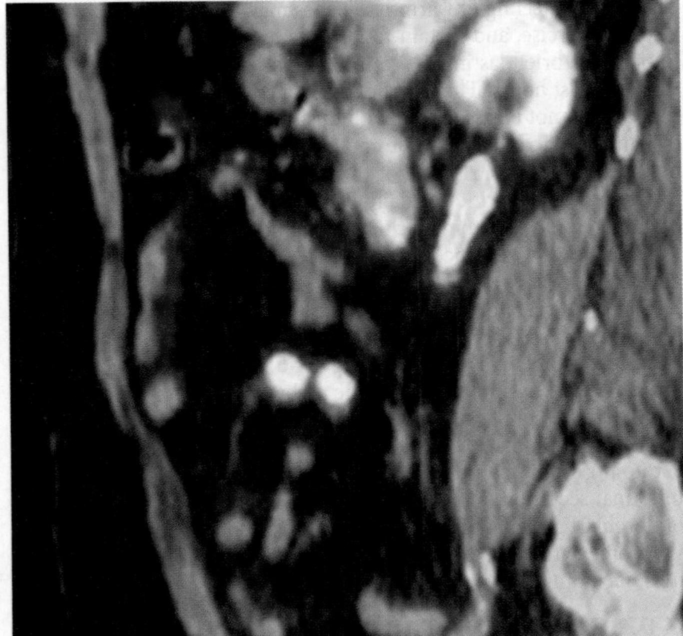

FIGURE 84-5 Gallium-68 Dotatate PET scan demonstrating a small bowel neuroendocrine tumor and associated mesenteric mass. *(Courtesy of Sara Meibom, MD, Boston Medical Center.)*

recurrence and progression of disease in patients with known metastases. While chromogranin A is elevated in patients with metastatic NETs, it is neither particularly sensitive nor specific. A broad range of different assays for chromogranin A have also posed challenges in interpreting results in a standardized fashion. Chromogranin A is often elevated in a number of nonmalignant conditions, including in patients with impaired renal function and in patients who are taking PPIs. Elevated values of chromogranin A should be interpreted with caution in patients in whom a NET is being considered but in whom a diagnosis has not been established.

The overall survival durations for patients with metastatic NETs vary significantly, depending on both the primary location of the tumor and the histologic grade. Median survival durations for patients with well-differentiated NETs have markedly increased in recent years, likely reflecting both earlier diagnoses and improved treatments. For example, in early analyses of the SEER database, the median survival for patients with advanced pancreatic NETs was ~2 years; this had increased to 4 years in a more recent analysis. Similar increases were observed in patients with advanced small intestine NETs, where the median survival for patients with well-differentiated small intestine NETs exceeds 5 years. The sometimes prolonged survival of patients with NETs can sometimes make it challenging to determine at what point to initiate treatment. In patients with symptoms of hormone secretion, decisions to initiate therapy are straightforward. In asymptomatic patients, on the other hand, observation off treatment can sometimes be appropriate. Nevertheless, the natural course of NETs is ultimately to progress, and if treatment is not initiated, close monitoring is essential to ensure patients maximize access to available treatment options over the course of their disease.

MANAGEMENT OF SYMPTOMS OF HORMONE HYPERSECRETION AND THE CARCINOID SYNDROME

Patients with advanced NETs may in some cases experience more symptoms from hormone hypersecretion than from tumor bulk. The management of hormonal symptoms associated with pancreatic NETs depends on the hormone being secreted (see above). Patients with GI NETs, particularly those with small intestine or appendiceal primaries, may develop the carcinoid syndrome. Flushing and diarrhea are the two most common symptoms associated with carcinoid syndrome. The characteristic flush is of sudden onset; it is a deep red or violaceous erythema of the upper body, especially the neck and face, often associated with a feeling of warmth. Flushes may be precipitated by stress, alcohol, exercise, and certain foods such as cheese. Flushing episodes initially are brief, lasting 2–5 min, though later in the disease course, they may last hours. The diarrhea associated with carcinoid syndrome may or may not be associated with flushing and is described as watery in nature. Diarrhea can be profound, sometimes occurring in excess of 10 times daily and is one of the symptoms that most significantly interferes with activities of daily living. Less common manifestations of the carcinoid syndrome include wheezing or asthma-like symptoms. Impaired cognitive function has also been described in particularly advanced cases.

The main secretory product implicated in the carcinoid syndrome is serotonin (5-HT). Serotonin is synthesized from tryptophan by the enzyme tryptophan hydroxylase (**Fig. 84-6**). Up to 50% of dietary tryptophan can be used in this synthetic pathway by tumor cells, resulting in inadequate supplies for conversion to niacin; hence, some patients develop symptoms of niacin deficiency and pellagra-like lesions. Serotonin has numerous biologic effects, including the stimulation of intestinal secretion, increasing intestinal motility, and the stimulation of fibroblast growth. Other secreted products contributing to carcinoid syndrome symptoms are thought to include histamines and tachykinins, including substance P.

DIAGNOSIS AND TREATMENT OF THE CARCINOID SYNDROME

While the carcinoid syndrome can develop in patients with NETs from almost any site, it is most commonly associated with appendiceal or small intestine NETs. In these patients, the syndrome usually develops only after the development of hepatic metastases or retroperitoneal lesions, allowing entry of serotonin and other vasoactive substances into the systemic circulation. While serotonin levels can be measured in plasma, such measurements are frequently highly variable. Evidence of excess serotonin secretion can be more reliably confirmed by measuring levels of the serotonin metabolite 5-hydroxyindole acetic acid (5-HIAA), commonly using a 24-h urine collection. Urine collections can be challenging, and false-positive elevations may occur if the patient is eating serotonin-rich foods (e.g., salmon, eggs). As a result, elevated levels of 5-HIAA are suggestive but not diagnostic of the carcinoid syndrome. Patients with NETs may also experience symptoms of carcinoid syndrome related to other secreted products, including histamine, absent evidence of serotonin secretion. Conversely, patients without NETs may also describe symptoms analogous to carcinoid syndrome but due to other causes. The symptoms associated with systemic mastocytosis, in particular, can be easily confused with carcinoid syndrome.

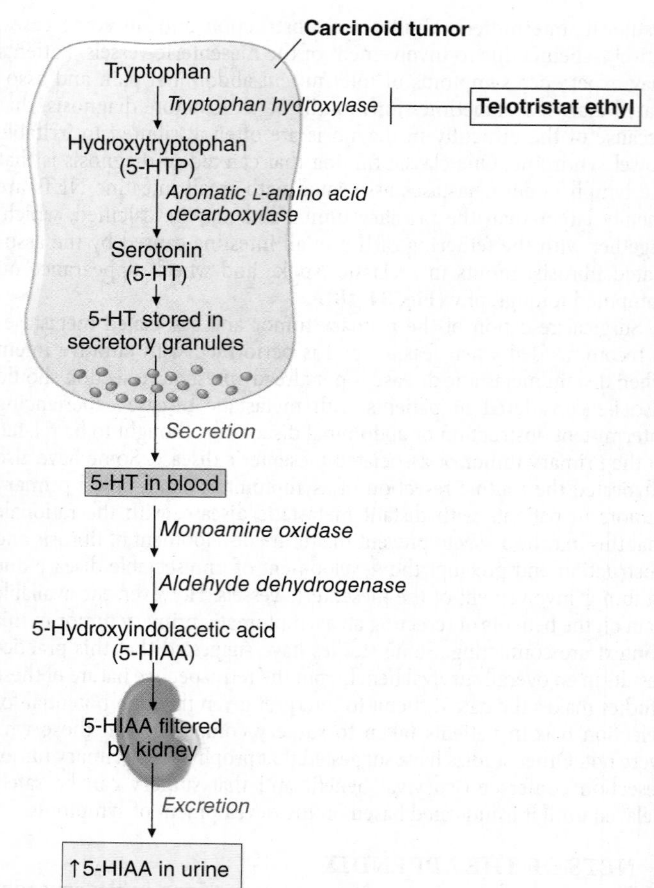

FIGURE 84-6 Serotonin synthesis and secretion in neuroendocrine tumors. Tryptophan is converted to hydroxytryptophan by tryptophan hydroxylase within the tumor cell and, subsequently, to serotonin (5-HT). Serotonin is subsequently converted to 5-hydroxyindole acetic acid (5-HIAA), which can be measured in a 24-h urine collection and can facilitate the diagnosis of carcinoid syndrome. Telotristat ethyl inhibits tryptophan hydroxylase and can be used as a treatment for carcinoid syndrome.

The symptoms of carcinoid syndrome, including diarrhea, are generally refractory to standard antidiarrheals or other traditional medications but can often be well controlled with somatostatin analogues (**Fig. 84-7**). Approximately 90% of NETs express somatostatin receptors. The presence of somatostatin receptors on NETs can be easily confirmed with uptake on somatostatin scintigraphy such as ^{68}GA dotatate PET scan; uptake on somatostatin scintigraphy is predictive of response to treatment with somatostatin analogues. Somatostatin is a 14-amino-acid peptide that inhibits the secretion of a broad range of hormones. Due to its short half-life, administration of somatostatin

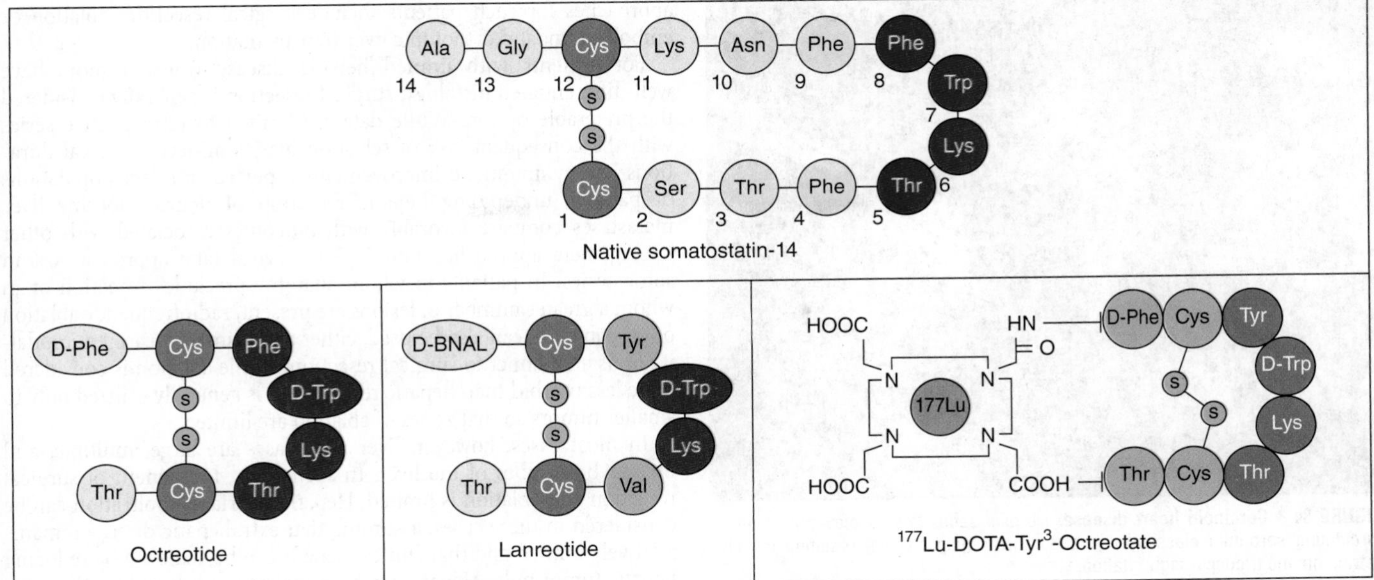

FIGURE 84-7 Somatostatin analogues. Commonly used somatostatin analogues include octreotide and lanreotide, which mirror the molecular structure of human somatostatin and bind to somatostatin receptors on neuroendocrine tumors. Somatostatin analogues inhibit tumoral hormone secretion and also have an antiproliferative effect. Radiolabeled somatostatin analogues such as ^{177}Lu-DOTA-octreotate, shown in the figure, share a similar molecular structure and are used therapeutically.

itself is not therapeutically practical. Longer-acting somatostatin analogues, including octreotide and lanreotide, share an 8-amino-acid binding domain with naturally occurring somatostatin and bind primarily to somatostatin receptor subtypes 2 and 5. Both have been shown to be effective in the treatment of carcinoid syndrome.

In an initial study, treatment of patients with octreotide 150 μg subcutaneously three times daily controlled symptoms of flushing and diarrhea in 88% of patients. A depot preparation (octreotide long-acting release [LAR]) that can be administered monthly has largely eliminated the need for daily octreotide injections and is now considered a standard approach for symptomatic treatment of advanced NETs. Lanreotide, another long-acting somatostatin analogue that is also administered monthly, appears to have similar clinical efficacy to octreotide in the treatment of metastatic NETs and the carcinoid syndrome. As described further below, both octreotide and lanreotide also share the ability to slow tumor growth, providing an additional benefit to patients.

Somatostatin analogue side effects are generally mild. Mild nausea, abdominal discomfort, bloating, and loose stools occur in up to one-third of patients during the first month or two of treatment but usually subsequently subside. Patients with persistent symptoms of bloating or loose stools may be experiencing pancreatic insufficiency associated with use of somatostatin analogues; use of pancreatic enzyme supplements can ameliorate these symptoms. Mild glucose intolerance may also occur due to inhibition of insulin secretion. One of the more significant side effects associated with somatostatin analogues is impaired gallbladder contractility, resulting in delayed gallbladder emptying, and long-term administration of somatostatin analogues has been associated with an increased risk of cholelithiasis. For this reason, patients with advanced NETs in whom surgery is planned and for whom somatostatin analogue therapy is being considered should generally also undergo prophylactic cholecystectomy.

Over time, for reasons that remain uncertain, patients receiving somatostatin analogues for symptoms of hormone secretion may become refractory to treatment. Not uncommonly, such patients experience symptom exacerbation toward the final week of each treatment cycle. Such patients may benefit from an increased frequency of administration (i.e., every 3 weeks) or use of additional short-acting octreotide for breakthrough symptoms.

The association between high levels of circulating serotonin and symptoms of the carcinoid syndrome has also led to a strategy aiming to directly inhibit serotonin synthesis (Fig. 84-6). This approach was first undertaken in the late 1960s with the drug para-chlorophenylalanine, which was reported to reduce symptoms of carcinoid syndrome but also caused significant central nervous system (CNS) side effects. Telotristat ethyl, a tryptophan hydroxylase inhibitor with minimal CNS penetration, was evaluated in a randomized trial that enrolled 135 patients with persistent carcinoid syndrome–related diarrhea while receiving somatostatin analogues. Treatment with telotristat ethyl was associated with a reduction in bowel movement frequency as well as significant decreases in urinary 5-HIAA compared to placebo. Thus, telotristat is a treatment option for patients with carcinoid syndrome who have persistent diarrhea despite treatment with somatostatin analogues.

CARCINOID CRISIS

Carcinoid crisis has been described in the setting of tumor manipulation during surgery and, less commonly, after other interventions such as hepatic artery embolization or radionuclide therapy. It may also occur as a result of exogenous administration of epinephrine or during induction of anesthesia. It is most common in patients who already have significant symptoms of carcinoid syndrome and is thought to be caused by a sudden release of biologically active compounds from the tumor. Carcinoid crisis can be life-threatening and can manifest as either profound hypotension or hypertension. Prospective studies on the prevention and management of carcinoid crisis are limited; however, somatostatin analogues should be readily available during surgical procedures, and in some cases, continuous prophylactic intravenous administration of somatostatin analogues has been utilized as a way to mitigate risk.

CARCINOID HEART DISEASE

Carcinoid heart disease occurs in approximately two-thirds of patients with the carcinoid syndrome. Carcinoid heart lesions are characterized by plaque-like, fibrous endocardial thickening that classically involves the right side of the heart and often causes retraction and fixation of the leaflets of the tricuspid and pulmonary valves (**Fig. 84-8**). The fibrosis in carcinoid heart disease is thought to be directly related to exposure of heart valve fibroblasts to high circulating levels of serotonin. Lesions similar to those observed in carcinoid heart disease were observed in patients receiving fenfluramine, a drug also known to increase serotonin signaling, as well as in patients receiving ergot-containing dopamine receptor agonists for Parkinson's disease. Metabolites of fenfluramine, as well as the dopamine receptor agonists, have high

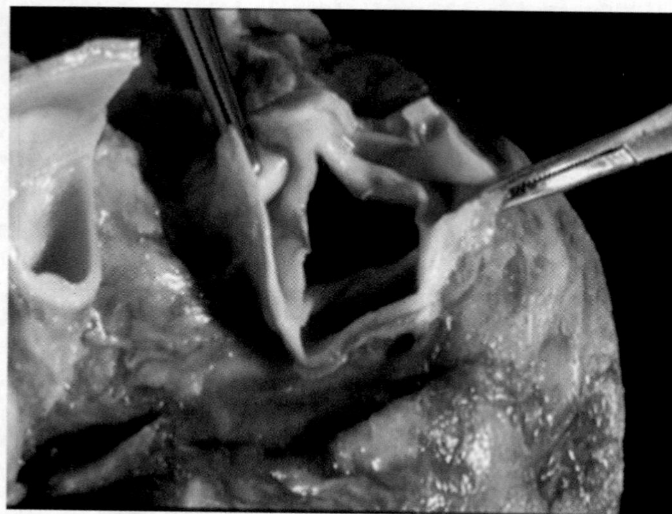

FIGURE 84-8 Carcinoid heart disease. Fibrosis secondary to elevated levels of circulating serotonin classically involves the tricuspid valve, resulting in valve retraction and tricuspid regurgitation.

affinity for serotonin receptor subtype 5-HT_{2B} receptors, whose activation is known to cause fibroblast mitogenesis and which are normally expressed in heart valve fibroblasts. These observations support the hypothesis that serotonin overproduction in patients with carcinoid syndrome mediates the valvular changes by activating 5-HT_{2B} receptors in the endocardium.

Tricuspid regurgitation is a nearly universal feature of carcinoid heart disease; tricuspid stenosis, pulmonary regurgitation, and pulmonary stenosis may also occur. Left-sided heart disease occurs in <10% of patients and has been associated with the presence of a patent foramen ovale. The preponderance of lesions in the right heart is related directly to the fact that serotonin is secreted by liver metastases or retroperitoneal tumor deposits into the venous circulation and subsequently into the right atrium and right ventricle. The lower incidence of heart disease in the left heart is postulated to be due to the fact that serotonin is metabolized in the pulmonary vasculature before entering the left atrium and ventricle. Among patients with carcinoid syndrome, patients with heart disease exhibit higher levels of serum serotonin and urinary 5-HIAA excretion than patients without heart disease. Treatment with somatostatin analogues resulting in decreased serotonin secretion does not result in regression of cardiac lesions. Reduction of serotonin levels as a result of treatment with somatostatin analogues or with the tryptophan hydroxylase inhibitor telotristat ethyl seems likely to slow progression of carcinoid heart disease but has not been formally evaluated in clinical trials.

Right-sided heart failure in patients with carcinoid heart disease may lead to significant morbidity and mortality. The development of multiple new treatments to improve overall disease control in patients with advanced NETs has led to increased interest in valvular replacement, which may result in significant clinical benefit in appropriately selected patients with carcinoid heart disease. The appropriate timing of valve replacement in such patients can be challenging given the competing desires to perform surgery before the onset of severe right-sided heart failure, which can increase surgical morbidity, and the need to achieve adequate overall tumor control. However, advanced and less invasive techniques, including catheter-based valve replacement, have made valve replacement an increasingly attractive option for patients with this condition.

HEPATIC-DIRECTED THERAPY FOR METASTATIC NETS

The liver is one of the most common sites for metastases in patients with NETs and, in some cases, is the only site of metastatic disease. Hepatic-directed therapies can often be effective as a means of controlling, if not eliminating, metastases, particularly in patients who have more indolent tumors with well-differentiated histology. Common approaches for such patients include surgical resection, ablation or embolization, and orthotopic liver transplantation.

For patients with limited hepatic disease whose tumors have well-differentiated histology, surgical resection is generally considered the preferable option. While data are limited to retrospective series with the consequent risk of selection bias, long-term survival durations and symptomatic improvements reported in select populations of patients undergoing hepatic resection of neuroendocrine liver metastases compare favorably with outcomes associated with other management approaches, and 5-year survival rates approach 90% in some series. In patients in whom anatomy precludes resection or in whom a greater number of lesions are present, radiofrequency ablation or cryoablation can also be used, either as a primary treatment modality or as an adjunct to surgical resection. While ablation is considered to be less morbid than hepatic resection, it is generally utilized only in smaller tumors so that zones of ablation are limited.

In most cases, however, liver metastases are large, multiple, and involve both lobes of the liver. In such cases, the benefit of surgical resection and ablation is limited. Hepatic arterial embolization can be considered in these cases, assuming that extrahepatic disease remains relatively limited and that clinical benefit can be achieved by reducing hepatic tumor bulk. Hepatic artery embolization is based on the principle that tumors in the liver derive most of their blood supply from the hepatic artery, whereas healthy hepatocytes derive most of their blood supply from the portal vein. Multiple different embolization techniques have been explored, ranging from the simple infusion of gel foam powder into the hepatic artery (bland embolization) to the administration of chemotherapy or chemotherapy-eluting beads into the hepatic artery (chemoembolization) or the intra-arterial administration of radioisotope-tagged microspheres (radioembolization). Limited data suggest an optimal approach to embolization, and few studies have compared these approaches directly. Tumor response rates with all of these approaches generally exceed 50%. Specific approaches are therefore often tailored to the patient, taking into account tumor location, overall tumor burden, and comorbidities. Bland embolization, for example, may be associated with less morbidity, whereas chemoembolization or radioembolization may result in longer durations of response.

The role of orthotopic liver transplantation for the treatment of NETs remains uncertain. Data from available institutional series suggest that a small number of highly selected patients may achieve long-term survival. However, 5-year overall median survival durations in most series are ~50%, and the majority of patients undergoing hepatic transplantation develop tumor recurrence. Additionally, the widespread utility of hepatic transplantation is limited by organ availability. Decisions regarding proceeding with transplantation in patients with advanced NETs are therefore highly individualized.

SYSTEMIC TREATMENT TO CONTROL TUMOR GROWTH

While hepatic-directed therapies can be effective in the management of patients with liver-predominant disease, a majority of patients will either present with or ultimately develop more widespread metastases. A number of systemic treatment options have been developed and can be effective in treating such patients. These options include treatment with traditional somatostatin analogues, peptide receptor radioligand therapy, traditional cytotoxic chemotherapy, and an increasing array of molecularly targeted therapies targeting the mTOR or vascular endothelial growth factor (VEGF) pathways **(Table 84-3)**. The choice and sequence of therapy depend in part on the type of tumor, the extent of disease, and patient symptoms and comorbidities.

■ SOMATOSTATIN ANALOGUES

While somatostatin analogues were originally developed as a treatment to reduce hormone secretion in NETs, they are also effective in slowing tumor growth. The biologic mechanisms underlying this effect remain uncertain, but clinical studies have been definitive. The first of these studies, the PROMID study, randomized patients with metastatic small-intestinal NET to receive either octreotide LAR at a

TABLE 84-3 Selected Randomized Trials of Therapeutic Agents for the Treatment of Advanced Neuroendocrine Tumors (NETs)

TUMOR TYPE	NUMBER OF PATIENTS	PROGRESSION-FREE SURVIVAL
Pancreatic and extrapancreatic NET		
Lanreotide vs placebo (CLARINET)	204	65 vs 33% at 2 years ($p < .001$)
Pancreatic NET		
Everolimus vs placebo (RADIANT 3)	410	11 months vs 4.6 months ($p < .001$)
Sunitinib vs placebo	171	11.4 months vs 5.5 months ($p < .001$)
Surufatinib vs placebo	264	10.9 months vs 3.7 months ($p = .001$)
Temozolomide/capecitabine vs temozolomide	144	22.7 months vs 14.4 months ($p = .021$)
Extrapancreatic NET		
Octreotide vs placebo (PROMID)	85	14.3 months vs 6 months[a]
Everolimus + octreotide vs octreotide (RADIANT 2)	429	16.4 months vs 11.3 months
Everolimus vs placebo (RADIANT 4)	302	11 months vs 3.9 months
Surufatinib vs placebo	198	9.2 months vs 3.8 months ($p < .0001$)
Pazopanib vs placebo	171	11.6 months vs 8.5 months ($p < .0005$)
177-Lutetium dotatate vs octreotide (NETTER 1)	230	65.2 vs 10.8% at 20 months ($p < .001$)

[a]Time to tumor progression.

dose of 30 mg monthly or placebo. The median time to tumor progression in patients receiving octreotide was 14 months compared to only 6 months for patients receiving placebo. Because the study was limited to patients with small-intestinal NET, the generalizability of these results to patients with NETs of other origins, including pancreatic NET, was initially uncertain. This question was ultimately addressed by the phase 3 CLARINET trial, which compared lanreotide, a somatostatin analogue that is similar to octreotide in its somatostatin receptor–binding affinities, to placebo in 204 patients with a range of advanced well- or moderately differentiated gastroenteropancreatic NETs. Progression-free survival duration at 2 years was 65% in patients receiving lanreotide and 33% in patients receiving placebo, a difference that was statistically significant. One unusual aspect of the PROMID and CLARINET studies is the difference in progression-free survival durations in the placebo arms of the studies, which has been attributed to differences in patient selection. Either octreotide or lanreotide is currently considered an acceptable option for control of tumor growth in patients with advanced NETs.

Whether treatment with somatostatin analogues also increases overall survival in patients with advanced NETs has not been demonstrated, although a correlation between progression-free survival and overall survival in patients with advanced NETs treated with single-agent somatostatin analogue therapy has been shown. The timing of initiation of somatostatin analogues in patients with advanced NETs remains uncertain. The variable clinical course of NETs means that tumors can remain indolent for years even without treatment. For patients with asymptomatic, small-volume disease, observation alone may be an appropriate initial option. However, for patients with a larger disease burden, evidence of disease progression, or symptomatic disease, somatostatin analogues are generally used as an initial systemic treatment due to their ease of use and tolerability.

PEPTIDE RECEPTOR RADIOLIGAND THERAPY

Peptide receptor radioligand therapy employs the systemic administration of radiolabeled somatostatin analogues and is a treatment option for patients who require more aggressive treatment due to progression on traditional somatostatin analogues or other therapies (Fig. 84-7). Peptide receptor radioligand therapy may also be considered as an initial treatment in patients with significant symptoms or tumor burden. With this approach, a radioligand is coupled to a somatostatin analogue, using the somatostatin analogue to target the tumor. When bound to the tumor cell, the radioligand is then internalized, resulting in cell death. Due to its mechanism of action, peptide receptor radioligand therapy is only considered in patients whose tumors demonstrate uptake on somatostatin scintigraphy.

Several different radioligands have been evaluated, the most successful of which have been yttrium (^{90}Y) and lutetium (^{177}Lu). These two ligands differ from one another in terms of their particle energy and tissue penetration; of the two, ^{90}Y-DOTA-TOC emits higher-energy β particles and has deeper tissue penetration. ^{90}Y-DOTA-TOC (^{90}Y-dotatoc) has been evaluated in numerous series with overall tumor responses reported in approximately one-third of patients. Enthusiasm for this approach, however, has been tempered due to concerns about side effects including both renal and hematologic toxicity.

^{177}Lu-DOTA-octreotate emits both β particles and lower-energy γ particles and, in most studies, has been associated with less toxicity than ^{90}Y-DOTA-TOC. Initial single-center studies with ^{177}Lu-DOTA-octreotate showed promising antitumor activity, and based on these studies, a randomized trial of ^{177}Lu-dotatate in midgut GI NETs was undertaken. In this study (NETTER-1), 229 patients with inoperable, somatostatin receptor–positive midgut NETs were randomly assigned to receive either four doses of ^{177}Lu-dotatate administered intravenously every 8 weeks or treatment with high-dose octreotide LAR (60 mg) every 4 weeks. Treatment with ^{177}Lu-dotatate was associated with objective tumor responses in 18% of patients and also was associated with a significant improvement in progression-free survival: progression-free survival at month 20 was 10.8% for octreotide LAR alone and 65.2% in the ^{177}Lu-dotatate group. Subsequent analyses have also suggested improved overall survival associated with ^{177}Lu-dotatate treatment, as well as improvements in quality of life across a number of parameters, including global health status, overall physical functioning, fatigue, pain, and diarrhea.

The renal clearance of radiopeptides, including ^{177}Lu-DOTA-octreotate, poses a risk of renal toxicity. The renal toxicity can be mitigated with the coadministration of intravenous amino acids during treatment. The most common adverse event among patients receiving ^{177}Lu-dotatate in the NETTER-1 study was nausea, most likely related to the amino acid infusions rather than to the radioisotope itself. Mild thrombocytopenia and leukopenia were also reported.

One limitation of the NETTER-1 study was its restriction to patients with advanced small intestine NETs. However, longer-term safety data as well as data supporting the efficacy of ^{177}Lu-dotatate in a broader range of gastroenteropancreatic NETs are available from large institutional series that include >1000 patients. Long-term toxicities from these series have included rare cases of acute leukemia and myelodysplastic syndrome, presumably associated with radiation exposure. Nevertheless, these studies generally support both the efficacy and safety of ^{177}Lu-dotatate as a treatment for patients with a range of somatostatin receptor–positive NETs.

ALKYLATING AGENTS

While the efficacy of traditional cytotoxic chemotherapy appears to be minimal in most extrapancreatic GI NETs, alkylating agents have a clear role in the treatment of advanced pancreatic NETs. Streptozocin-based combination therapy was historically used as treatment standard in such patients but has largely fallen out of favor due to both toxicity concerns and a cumbersome administration schedule. Temozolomide is an orally administered alkylating agent that has largely replaced streptozocin as a backbone in combination regimens used for the treatment of pancreatic NETs.

Initial studies evaluating temozolomide in combination with a range of different agents showed that temozolomide-based combination therapy was associated with tumor responses in 24–70% of patients. One of the most active combination regimens appeared to be temozolomide and capecitabine. This combination was subsequently compared to temozolomide alone in a prospective randomized study undertaken by the Eastern Cooperative Oncology Group that enrolled 144 patients with advanced pancreatic NETs. The overall response rates in the two arms were relatively similar; 33% of patients who received the combination of temozolomide and capecitabine experienced objective tumor responses as compared to 28% of the patients who received temozolomide as a single agent. However, progression-free survival was significantly longer in the combination arm (22.7 vs 14.4 months). Based on these results, the combination of temozolomide and capecitabine is now the preferred chemotherapy combination for advanced pancreatic NETs.

The reason that some pancreatic NETs respond to alkylating agents while others do not is uncertain. In patients with glioblastoma, methylation of the promoter region for methylguanine DNA methyltransferase (MGMT) is associated with decreased MGMT protein expression and is highly associated with temozolomide responsiveness. MGMT is an enzyme that is responsible for repairing DNA damage induced by alkylating agents. Reduced levels of MGMT presumably impair the ability of tumor cells to repair their DNA in response to treatment and enhance the cytotoxicity of temozolomide. Several retrospective studies have suggested that lack of MGMT expression in pancreatic NET may be associated with responsiveness to temozolomide-based therapy; however, this finding has not yet been prospectively validated.

SMALL-MOLECULE TYROSINE KINASE INHIBITORS

The highly vascular nature of NETs combined with observations in preclinical models that disruption of signaling pathways associated with VEGF inhibits neuroendocrine cell growth prompted a number of clinical trials evaluating therapeutic agents that inhibit the VEGF pathway in both pancreatic and extrapancreatic NETs. The VEGF pathway is activated through the binding of VEGF to its cell surface receptor, which initiates an intracellular signaling cascade that promotes angiogenesis as well as cell growth, proliferation, and survival. Clinical trials of VEGF pathway inhibitors in NETs have included a number of small-molecule tyrosine kinase inhibitors that, while they differ to some extent in specificity, all have in common the property targeting VEGFR2, the receptor isoform most strongly implicated in promoting angiogenesis.

Sunitinib, a multitargeted tyrosine kinase inhibitor that inhibits a range of growth factor receptors including VEGFR2, was one of the first agents in this class found to have activity in pancreatic NETs. In an initial phase 2 trial, sunitinib was administered to 109 patients with either pancreatic or extrapancreatic NET. Of 61 patients with pancreatic NET enrolled in the study, 11 had evidence of an objective tumor response. Based on these observations, sunitinib was evaluated in an international, randomized trial in which continuous administration of sunitinib (37.5 mg daily) was compared with placebo in 171 patients with advanced, progressive pancreatic NET. The median progression-free survival was significantly longer in patients treated with sunitinib compared with patients treated with placebo (11.4 vs 5.5 months). Common side effects associated with sunitinib included hypertension, proteinuria, and fatigue.

A second VEGFR-targeted tyrosine kinase inhibitor, surufatinib, has been evaluated in a randomized trial in which 264 patients with advanced pancreatic NETs from 21 centers in China were randomized to receive either surufatinib, administered at a dose of 300 mg daily, or placebo. Patients receiving surufatinib experienced a median progression-free survival duration of 10.9 months, as compared to 3.7 months in patients receiving placebo, closely mirroring the results of the earlier sunitinib study. Other small-molecular tyrosine kinase inhibitors have been evaluated in smaller, single-arm studies and have shown activity in pancreatic NETs, including sorafenib, cabozantinib, pazopanib, and axitinib.

Small-molecule tyrosine kinase inhibitors targeting the VEGF pathway have also been evaluated in patients with advanced nonpancreatic GI NET. In most of these studies, objective tumor response rates are lower than those seen in pancreatic NET, though many of these initial studies also revealed low rates of tumor progression and encouraging progression-free survival durations, suggesting that these agents had antitumor activity. Pazopanib was compared to placebo in a randomized study undertaken by the ALLIANCE cooperative group, which enrolled 171 patients with nonpancreatic NETs. Patients treated with pazopanib in this study had a superior progression-free survival compared to those who received placebo (11.6 vs 8.5 months), a difference that was statistically significant. Surufatinib was used in a randomized study of 198 patients with extrapancreatic NETs; the median progression-free survival was 9.2 months in patients receiving surufatinib and 3.8 months in those receiving placebo, a statistically significant difference. These studies suggest that VEGF-targeted tyrosine kinase inhibitors have antitumor activity in extrapancreatic and pancreatic NETs.

mTOR INHIBITORS

mTOR is an intracellular protein kinase that has been implicated in the regulation of a number of processes regulating cell growth in both normal and malignant cells. It functions as a downstream component of the PI3-AKT-mTOR pathway. This pathway is negatively regulated by the tuberous sclerosis complex, comprising TSC1 and TSC2. An association between the development of pancreatic NETs and inherited mutations in *TSC2* in patients with tuberous sclerosis complex was a contributing factor to initial interest in exploring mTOR inhibition as a therapeutic approach in this setting.

Following initial evidence of antitumor activity associated with everolimus (10 mg daily) in an international, multicenter, phase 2 trial of 160 patients, everolimus monotherapy (10 mg daily) was compared with best supportive care alone in the RADIANT-3 trial that enrolled 410 patients with advanced progressing pancreatic NET. While overall objective responses were uncommon, treatment with everolimus was associated with a significant prolongation in median progression-free survival (11.0 vs 4.6 months) compared to placebo, supporting its use as a standard treatment to control tumor growth in patients with advanced pancreatic NET. Common toxicities associated with everolimus are generally mild and can include stomatitis and rash; a more severe but less common side effect is pneumonitis.

Everolimus was also associated with promising activity in early phase 2 studies enrolling patients extrapancreatic NET. The first large randomized study evaluating everolimus was the RADIANT 2 trial; 429 patients with advanced GI NETs were randomly assigned to receive octreotide LAR (30 mg intramuscularly every 28 days) with or without everolimus (10 mg daily). Treatment with everolimus in this study was associated with an improvement in median progression-free survival (16.4 vs 11.3 months), but the difference in this study was of only borderline statistical significance. A second study, the RADIANT 4 study, enrolled 302 patients with advanced NETs of either GI (excluding pancreatic) or lung origin, randomizing them to receive either everolimus or placebo. In this study, treatment with octreotide was not required. As in the RADIANT 3 study, objective tumor responses were uncommon; however, median progression-free survival in patients who received everolimus was significantly longer than in those who received placebo (11 vs 3.9 months). Based on the results of this study, everolimus is considered a standard treatment for control of tumor growth in extrapancreatic NETs.

OTHER SYSTEMIC TREATMENTS FOR CONTROL OF TUMOR GROWTH

Interferon α has been used as a treatment for advanced NETs for several decades. With the development of newer approaches, its routine use has diminished. The use of interferon α was based primarily on observations in large, retrospective series where low-dose interferon α was reported to both reduce symptoms of hormonal hypersecretion and slow tumor progression. Interferon can be myelosuppressive, requiring dose titration, and in some patients can induce both fatigue and depression. Antitumor activity has also been reported with oxaliplatin-based chemotherapy regimens. A combined analysis of two phase 2 trials examining oxaliplatin-fluoropyrimidine chemotherapy plus bevacizumab in advanced NET suggested antitumor activity for these regimens; the benefit appeared to be greatest in patients with intermediate-grade rather than low-grade tumors.

SYSTEMIC THERAPY FOR HIGH-GRADE NEUROENDOCRINE CARCINOMA

High-grade NETs are relatively uncommon; their clinical behavior is fundamentally different from well-differentiated NETs in that these tumors pursue an aggressive clinical course. Systemic chemotherapy for advanced high-grade neuroendocrine carcinoma has historically followed a paradigm analogous to that used for small-cell carcinoma of the lung, with combinations of either cisplatin or carboplatin administered together with etoposide generally considered the preferred first-line approach. One of the most important elements in determining the optimal chemotherapeutic approach is assessing the Ki-67 proliferative index. A large retrospective series that evaluated 252 patients with high-grade neuroendocrine carcinoma found that the activity of platinum-based therapy was greatest in patients who had a Ki-67 proliferative index of 55% or higher; in these patients, the overall tumor response rate was 42%. In contrast, the overall response rate in patients in whom the Ki-67 proliferative index was <55% was only 15%. As in small-cell carcinoma of the lung, immune checkpoint inhibitors also appear to have some activity in high-grade neuroendocrine carcinoma. While minimal activity has been noted in well-differentiated NETs, a combination of ipilimumab and nivolumab was associated with an overall tumor response rate of 42% in an initial phase 2 trial enrolling 19 patients with high-grade neuroendocrine carcinoma.

Acknowledgement

Dr. Robert Jensen contributed this chapter in previous editions, and some material from his chapter is retained here.

FURTHER READING

Caplin ME et al: Lanreotide in metastatic enteropancreatic neuroendocrine tumors. N Engl J Med 371:224, 2014.

Dasari A et al: Trends in the incidence, prevalence, and survival outcomes for patients with neuroendocrine tumors in the United States. JAMA Oncol 3:1336, 2017.

Kulke MH et al: Telotristat ethyl, a tryptophan hydroxylase inhibitor for the treatment of carcinoid syndrome. J Clin Oncol 35:14, 2017.

Raymond E et al: Sunitinib malate for the treatment of pancreatic neuroendocrine tumors. N Engl J Med 364:501, 2011.

Rindi G et al: A common classification framework for neuroendocrine neoplasms: An International Agency for Research on Cancer (IARC) and World Health Organization (WHO) expert consensus proposal. Mod Pathol 31:1770, 2018.

Scarpa A et al: Whole genome landscape of pancreatic neuroendocrine tumors. Nature 543:65, 2017.

Strosberg J et al: Phase 3 trial of 177 Lu-dotatate for midgut neuroendocrine tumors. N Engl J Med 376:125, 2017.

Yao JC et al: Everolimus for advanced pancreatic neuroendocrine tumors. N Engl J Med 364:514, 2011.

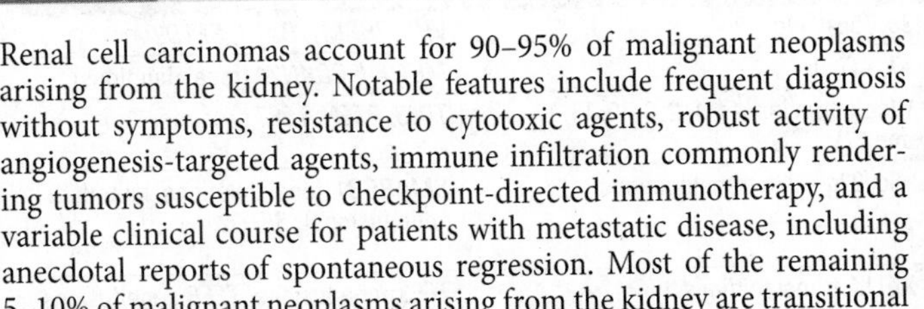

85 Renal Cell Carcinoma

Robert J. Motzer, Martin H. Voss

Renal cell carcinomas account for 90–95% of malignant neoplasms arising from the kidney. Notable features include frequent diagnosis without symptoms, resistance to cytotoxic agents, robust activity of angiogenesis-targeted agents, immune infiltration commonly rendering tumors susceptible to checkpoint-directed immunotherapy, and a variable clinical course for patients with metastatic disease, including anecdotal reports of spontaneous regression. Most of the remaining 5–10% of malignant neoplasms arising from the kidney are transitional cell carcinomas (urothelial carcinomas) originating in the lining of the renal pelvis. See **Chap. 86** for transitional cell carcinomas.

EPIDEMIOLOGY

The incidence of cancers of the kidney and renal pelvis rose for three decades, reached a plateau of approximately 64,000 cases annually in the United States between 2012 and 2018, but has since increased to approximately 76,000 cases annually, resulting in close to 14,000 deaths per year. It is the eighth most common cancer overall in the United States, the sixth most common in males, and the eighth most common in females; the male-to-female ratio is 2:1. Although this malignancy may be diagnosed at any age, it is uncommon in those under 45 years, and incidence peaks between the ages of 55 and 75 years. Many factors have been investigated as possible contributing causes; associations include cigarette smoking, obesity, and hypertension. Risk is also increased for patients with polycystic kidney disease that has been complicated by chronic renal failure.

Most cases of renal cell carcinoma (RCC) are sporadic, although familial forms have been reported (**Table 85-1**). One well established example includes clear cell RCC arising in the context of von Hippel-Lindau (VHL) syndrome, an autosomal dominant disorder. Genetic studies identified the *VHL* gene on the short arm of chromosome 3. Individuals with VHL syndrome have an estimated lifetime risk of developing clear cell RCC of around 70%. Other *VHL*-associated neoplasms include retinal hemangioma, hemangioblastoma of the spinal cord and cerebellum, pheochromocytoma, and neuroendocrine tumors and cysts. Birt-Hogg-Dubé syndrome is a rare human autosomal dominant genetic disorder characterized by fibrofolliculomas (benign tumors arising in hair follicles), pulmonary cysts, and renal cell carcinomas of varying histologies, most commonly the chromophobe type, occurring in about a third of patients. This disorder is associated with mutations in the *FLCN* gene, which codes for folliculin. Other hereditary syndromes are summarized in Table 85-1.

PATHOLOGY AND GENETICS

Renal cell malignancies represent a heterogeneous group of tumors with distinct histopathologic, genetic, and clinical features (**Table 85-2**). Categories include clear cell carcinoma (70% of cases), papillary tumors (10–15%), chromophobe tumors (≤5%), renal medullary carcinoma (<1%), translocation carcinoma (<5%), and other less common variants. Papillary tumors can be bilateral and multifocal. Chromophobe tumors tend to have a more indolent clinical course. Translocation-associated RCC, rare in adult patients, is the predominant histology in children. Renal medullary carcinoma is rare, very aggressive, and associated with sickle cell trait. Tumors that do not meet criteria for defined variants are generally referred to as "unclassified" with variable clinical courses.

Clear cell tumors, the predominant histology, are found in >80% of patients who develop metastases and arise from the epithelial cells of the proximal tubules. Loss of chromosome 3p is uniformly seen as the earliest event in the development of these cancers. This leads to loss of heterozygosity for a number of relevant 3p genes, including *VHL*, *PBRM1*, *BAP1*, and *SETD2*, which can be functionally lost through secondary events in the remaining allele. *VHL* encodes a tumor suppressor protein that is involved in regulating the transcription of vascular endothelial growth factor (VEGF) and a number of other effectors through ubiquitination of hypoxia-inducible factors (HIF). Inactivation of *VHL*, through upregulation of VEGF signaling, promotes tumor angiogenesis and growth, ultimately rendering clear cell RCC cells susceptible to antiangiogenesis therapy.

Large-scale sequencing efforts have helped elucidate recurrent patterns of genomic evolution that correlate with distinct clinical phenotypes, e.g., varying levels of aggressiveness or specific patterns of metastatic spread. For example, early loss of chromosome 9p appears to confer a high risk for early metastatic dissemination and correlates with poor cancer-specific survival.

A growing number of other RCC variants are well defined (see Table 85-2 for examples). For instance, up to 15% of RCCs are of the papillary subtype, with several subtypes that can be distinguished either by light microscopy or tumor genomics. For example, activating mutations in the *MET* oncogene or gain of chromosome 7 (where *MET* is located) are hallmark events of type 1 papillary RCC and considered

TABLE 85-1 Hereditary Renal Cell Tumors

SYNDROME	CHROMOSOME(S)	GENE	PROTEIN	KIDNEY TUMOR TYPE	ADDITIONAL CLINICAL FINDINGS
von Hippel-Lindau syndrome	3p25	*VHL*	von Hippel-Lindau protein	Clear cell	Hemangioblastoma of the retina and central nervous system; pheochromocytoma; pancreatic and renal cysts; neuroendocrine tumors
Hereditary papillary RCC	7p31	*MET*	MET	Papillary (type I)	Bilateral and multifocal kidney tumors
Hereditary leiomyomatosis and RCC (HLRCC syndrome)	1q42	*FH*	Fumarate hydratase	Papillary (non-type I)	Leiomyoma; uterine leiomyoma/ leiomyosarcoma
Birt-Hogg-Dubé syndrome	17p11	*FLCN*	Folliculin	Chromophobe; oncocytoma	Facial fibrofolliculoma; pulmonary cysts
Tuberous sclerosis	9q34 16p13	*TSC1* *TSC2*	Hamartin Tuberin	Angiomyolipomas; lymphangioleiomyomatosis; rare RCC with variety of histologic appearances	Angiofibroma, subungual fibroma; cardiac rhabdomyoma; adenomatous small intestine polyps; pulmonary and renal cysts; cortical tuber; subependymal giant cell astrocytomas
BAP1 tumor predisposition syndrome	3p21	*BAP1*	BAP1	Clear cell	Atypical Spitz tumors; uveal melanoma; cutaneous melanoma; basal cell carcinoma; malignant mesothelioma

Abbreviation: RCC, renal cell carcinoma.

actionable via targeted MET inhibitors. Tumors of the less common chromophobe subtype originate from the distal nephron. They are in part driven by changes in mitochondrial gene function and typically characterized by aneuploidy with common loss of an entire chromosome copy for chromosomes 1, 2, 6, 10, 13, and 17.

CLINICAL PRESENTATION

Presenting signs and symptoms may include hematuria, flank or abdominal pain, and a palpable mass. Other symptoms are fever, weight loss, anemia, and a varicocele. Tumors are, however, commonly detected as an incidental finding on a radiograph. Widespread use of radiologic cross-sectional imaging (computed tomography [CT], magnetic resonance imaging [MRI]) contributes to earlier detection of renal masses during evaluation for other medical conditions. The increasing number of incidentally discovered low-stage tumors has contributed to an improved 5-year survival for patients with RCC and increased use of nephron-sparing surgery (partial nephrectomy). A spectrum of paraneoplastic syndromes has been associated with these malignancies, including erythrocytosis, hypercalcemia, nonmetastatic hepatic dysfunction (Stauffer's syndrome), and acquired dysfibrinogenemia. Erythrocytosis is noted at presentation in only about 3% of patients. Anemia, commonly a sign of more advanced disease, is more common. Kidney cancer was called the "internist's tumor" since it was often discovered from the initial presentation of a paraneoplastic syndrome. This was more common before the era of modern imaging, as was initial presentation by the classic triad of hematuria, flank pain, and a palpable abdominal mass.

The standard evaluation of patients with suspected renal tumors includes a CT scan of the abdomen and pelvis, chest radiograph, and urine analysis. If metastatic disease is suspected from the chest radiograph, a CT of the chest is warranted. MRI is useful in evaluating the inferior vena cava in cases of suspected tumor involvement or invasion by thrombus, or when intravenous contrast administration given with CT is prohibited by impaired renal function. In clinical practice, any solid renal masses should be considered malignant until proven otherwise; a definitive diagnosis is required. If no metastases are demonstrated, surgery is indicated, even if the renal vein or inferior vena cava is invaded. In small tumors (particularly those of clear cell variant) the risk of impending metastatic spread is lower and surgery can potentially be delayed. In that setting, a needle biopsy should be performed to confirm the underlying histology, and radiographic surveillance is indicated until the time of surgery. The differential diagnosis of a renal mass includes cysts, benign neoplasms (adenoma, angiomyolipoma, oncocytoma), inflammatory lesions (pyelonephritis or abscesses), and other malignancies originating in the kidney such as transitional cell carcinoma of the renal pelvis, sarcoma, lymphoma, and Wilms' tumor or metastases from cancers originating in other organs. All of these are less common causes of renal masses than is RCC. The most common sites of distant metastases are the lungs, lymph nodes, liver, bone, and brain. These tumors may follow an unpredictable and protracted clinical course.

STAGING AND PROGNOSIS

Staging is based on the American Joint Committee on Cancer (AJCC) staging system (**Fig. 85-1**). Stage I tumors are ≤7 cm in greatest diameter and confined to the kidney, stage II tumors are >7 cm and confined to the kidney, stage III tumors extend through the renal capsule but are confined to Gerota's fascia, grossly infiltrate the renal vein, or involve regional lymph nodes (N1), and stage IV disease includes tumors that have invaded adjacent organs or involve nonregional lymph nodes or distant metastases. Sixty-five percent of patients present with stage I or II disease, 15–20% with stage III, and 15–20% with stage IV. The 5-year survival rate is currently 75% across all RCCs, but varies greatly by stage.

TABLE 85-2 Classification of Malignant Epithelial Neoplasms Arising from the Kidney

CARCINOMA TYPE	CHARACTERISTIC GROWTH PATTERN	CHROMOSOMAL EVENTS	GENES WITH RECURRENT SOMATIC ALTERATIONS
Clear cell	Acinar or sarcomatoid	3p–, 5q+, 14q–, 9p–	*VHL, PBRM1, BAP1, SETD2*
Papillary	Papillary or sarcomatoid	+7, +17, 9p–	*MET, FH, CDKN2A* (focal deletions)
Chromophobe	Solid, tubular, or sarcomatoid	Whole arm losses (1, 2, 6, 10, 13, 17, and 21)	*TP53, PTEN, TERT* promotor
Renal medullary carcinoma	Varying growth patterns, including cribriform, reticular, sarcomatoid, adenoid, and microcystic	+8q, 22q–, 22q translocations	*SMARCB1* (focal deletions, mutations, gene fusions), *SETD2*
MITF translocation[a]	Mimicking clear cell and papillary variants	Xp11.2 translocations; t(6;11) translocations	*TFE3* gene fusions, *TFEB* gene fusions

[a]Microphthalmia transcription factor gene family.

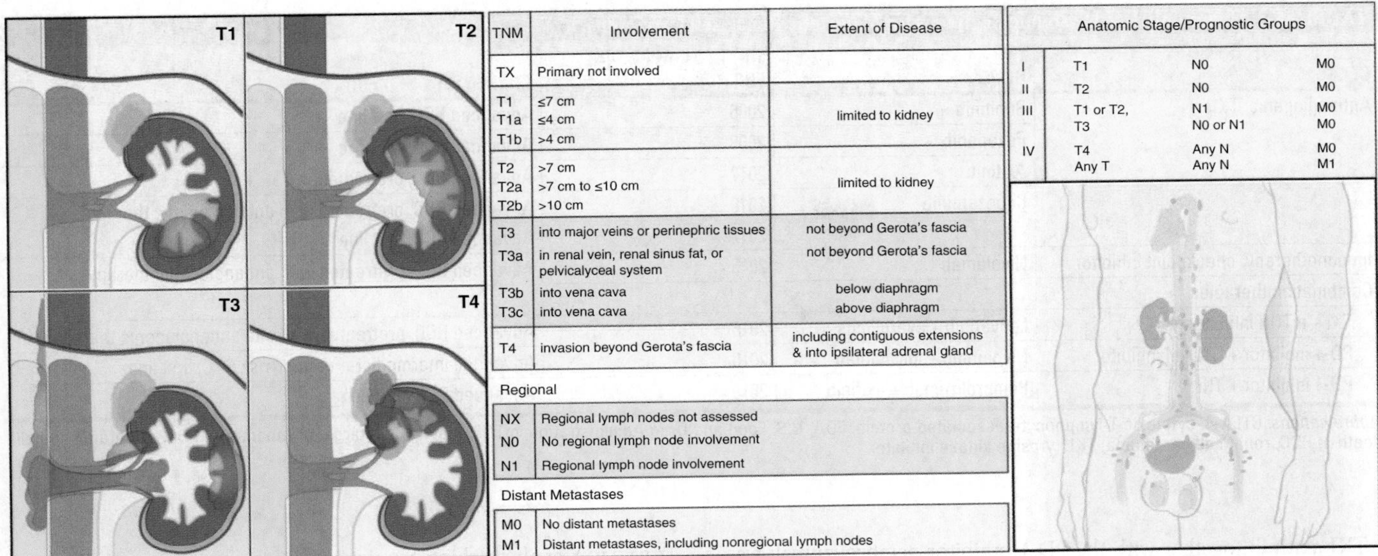

TNM	Involvement	Extent of Disease
TX	Primary not involved	
T1 T1a T1b	≤7 cm ≤4 cm >4 cm	limited to kidney
T2 T2a T2b	>7 cm >7 cm to ≤10 cm >10 cm	limited to kidney
T3	into major veins or perinephric tissues	not beyond Gerota's fascia
T3a	in renal vein, renal sinus fat, or pelvicalyceal system	not beyond Gerota's fascia
T3b	into vena cava	below diaphragm
T3c	into vena cava	above diaphragm
T4	invasion beyond Gerota's fascia	including contiguous extensions & into ipsilateral adrenal gland

Regional

NX	Regional lymph nodes not assessed
N0	No regional lymph node involvement
N1	Regional lymph node involvement

Distant Metastases

M0	No distant metastases
M1	Distant metastases, including nonregional lymph nodes

Anatomic Stage/Prognostic Groups			
I	T1	N0	M0
II	T2	N0	M0
III	T1 or T2, T3	N1 N0 or N1	M0 M0
IV	T4 Any T	Any N Any N	M0 M1

FIGURE 85-1 Renal cell carcinoma staging. TNM, tumor-node-metastasis.

Prognostic risk models are helpful for counseling patients diagnosed with metastatic disease and for anticipating survival rates when designing a clinical trial. A widely used prognostic model for advanced disease, the International Metastatic RCC Database Consortium (IMDC) risk model, incorporates six factors shown to correlate with worse survival: poor performance status, low hemoglobin concentration, high serum calcium, high neutrophil levels, high platelet levels, and <1-year interval from diagnosis to systemic treatment. Patients with zero risk factors had significantly longer median survival (43 months) than patients with one or two risk factors (22.5 months) and those with three to six risk factors (8 months) when treated with first-line angiogenesis inhibitors (see below).

TREATMENT

Renal Cell Carcinoma

LOCALIZED TUMOR

The standard management for stage I or II tumors and selected cases of stage III disease is radical or partial nephrectomy. A radical nephrectomy involves en bloc removal of Gerota's fascia and its contents, including the kidney, and commonly the ipsilateral adrenal gland and regional lymph nodes that appear abnormal on imaging or intraoperatively. Open, laparoscopic, or robotic surgical techniques may be used. The role of a template lymphadenectomy in patients without apparent lymphadenopathy is controversial. Extension into the renal vein or inferior vena cava (stage III disease) does not preclude resection, which would then include thrombectomy.

Nephron-sparing approaches, i.e., open or laparoscopic partial nephrectomy, may be appropriate depending on the size and location of the tumor. This approach is particularly relevant for patients with solitary kidneys, bilateral tumors, or chronic renal insufficiency but can also be applied electively to resect small masses for patients with normal kidney function. Radical nephrectomy carries a greater risk for chronic kidney disease and cardiovascular morbidity and mortality.

Adjuvant systemic therapies, including cytokines and targeted agents, have been studied in randomized clinical trials, largely with negative results, and the standard of care remains active surveillance after nephrectomy.

METASTATIC DISEASE

Surgery has a limited role for patients with metastatic disease. Long-term survival may occur in patients who relapse with a solitary site that is removed (metastasectomy). Nephrectomy despite presence of metastases (cytoreductive nephrectomy) is considered for carefully selected patients with stage IV disease. One indication for this approach can be to alleviate pain or hemorrhage of a primary tumor.

Radiation therapy is used for palliation of bone or brain metastases. The type of radiotherapy most commonly used is external-beam therapy, including stereotactic radiosurgery and other forms of image-guided radiotherapy.

Systemic therapy is the mainstay of care for metastatic disease. The timing of initiating such treatment should be carefully considered; some patients are asymptomatic at diagnosis, and with indolent behavior, it may be best to document progression before initiating treatment.

Metastatic RCC is refractory to cytotoxic chemotherapy. Patients are treated with molecularly targeted agents, including targeted immunotherapies. Treatments are continued with noncurative intent while tolerated and until disease progression is evident on cross-sectional imaging. Outcomes for patients with metastatic disease improved when increased understanding of underlying biology led to the successful development of several tyrosine kinase inhibitors (TKIs) targeting proangiogenic signaling through the VEGF receptors as well as allosteric inhibitors of mammalian target of rapamycin (mTOR) signaling. Serial large-scale randomized trials demonstrated that such agents, typically orally available, could be administered sequentially and in combination. Pivotal studies, by design, defined a dedicated space for each regimen in treatment-naïve or pretreated patients **(Table 85-3)**.

Targeted immunotherapies were introduced after VEGF- and mTOR-directed agents had established standards of care in the first- and second-line setting. Nivolumab, a checkpoint inhibitor targeting PD-1, was compared to the mTOR inhibitor everolimus in a randomized trial in patients who had progressed on prior TKI therapy, challenging the standard approach in pretreated patients. Nivolumab demonstrated superior overall survival, positioning it as the new second-line agent of choice. Subsequently, immunotherapy combination regimens demonstrated efficacy in randomized trials conducted in treatment-naïve patients. In separate studies, two doublets demonstrated survival benefit over standard sunitinib therapy and changed the standard of care for untreated metastatic clear cell RCC: nivolumab in combination with the CTLA-4-directed checkpoint inhibitor ipilimumab proved superior to sunitinib in patients with high-risk features per the IMDC model, achieving complete radiographic disappearance of cancer in >10% of patients treated with the combination. In a second trial, the combination of the

TABLE 85-3 Commonly Used Systemic Regimens for Metastatic Renal Cell Carcinoma

CLASS	DRUG	FIRST FDA APPROVAL FOR RCC	CURRENTLY USED FOR
Antiangiogenic: TKIs	Sunitinib	2006	Advanced RCC, first line
	Pazopanib	2009	Advanced RCC, first line
	Axitinib	2012	Advanced RCC, pretreated
	Cabozantinib	2016	Advanced RCC, pretreated with antiangiogenic therapy
		2017	Advanced RCC, first line
Immunotherapy: checkpoint inhibitor	Nivolumab	2015	Advanced RCC, pretreated with antiangiogenic therapy
Combination therapies			
TKI + mTOR inhibitor	Lenvatinib + everolimus	2016	Advanced RCC, pretreated with one antiangiogenic therapy
PD-1 inhibitor + CTLA-4 inhibitor	Nivolumab + ipilimumab	2018	Advanced intermediate- or poor-risk RCC, first line
PD-1 inhibitor + TKI	Pembrolizumab + axitinib	2019	Advanced RCC, first line

Abbreviations: CTLA-4, cytotoxic T-lymphocyte-associated protein; FDA, U.S. Food and Drug Administration; mTOR, mammalian target of rapamycin; PD-1, programmed cell death-1; RCC, renal cell carcinoma; TKI, tyrosine kinase inhibitor.

TKI axitinib together with the PD-1 inhibitor pembrolizumab was superior to sunitinib alone in all-comers with untreated metastatic RCC, again with high response rates across all IMDC risk groups. In both trials, responses were long-lasting, with improved time to disease progression and longer overall survival for combination regimens. Additional trials are ongoing to fortify the new standard of combination therapy in the first line.

With an ever-growing number of approved options directed toward different molecular targets, biomarkers are urgently needed to help individualize therapeutic choices and to gain insight as to whether and why treatments are working. Although a multitude of candidate biomarkers have been investigated for their predictive value in metastatic RCC, none have been validated for clinical use to date.

Projected overall survival in patients starting systemic therapies for newly diagnosed metastatic disease has tripled over the past 15–20 years; this can largely be attributed to the successful drug developments discussed here.

GLOBAL CONSIDERATIONS

Worldwide, over 400,000 patients are diagnosed each year with malignant tumors arising from the kidney, resulting in >175,000 deaths annually. Kidney cancer is the 10th most common cancer in men and the 15th most common cancer in women. Higher incidence is observed in developed countries, including the United States, Canada, Europe, Australia, New Zealand, and Uruguay. Relatively low rates are reported in Southeast Asia and Africa. The incidence of kidney cancer has been steadily increasing over the past four decades. Mortality trends have stabilized in Europe and the United States, but not in less developed countries. This is likely related to differences in access to optimal therapies. Treatment guidelines for both localized and metastatic renal cancer are similar between U.S. and European documents and contingent on the access to adequate health care and availability of targeted drugs to treat metastases.

FURTHER READING

Choueiri TK, Motzer RJ: Systemic therapy for metastatic renal cell carcinoma. N Engl J Med 376:354, 2017.

Moch H et al: The 2016 WHO classification of tumours of the urinary system and male genital organs—Part A: renal, penile, and testicular tumours. Eur Urol 70:93, 2016.

Motzer RJ et al: Nivolumab plus ipilimumab versus sunitinib in advanced renal-cell carcinoma. N Engl J Med 378:1277, 2018.

Motzer RJ et al: Molecular subsets in renal cancer determine outcome to checkpoint and angiogenesis blockade. Cancer Cell 38:803, 2020.

Rini BI et al: Pembrolizumab plus axitinib versus sunitinib for advanced renal-cell carcinoma. N Engl J Med 380:1116, 2019.

Sanchez A et al: Current management of small renal masses, including patient selection, renal tumor biopsy, active surveillance, and thermal ablation. J Clin Oncol 36:3591, 2018.

Turajlic S et al: Tracking cancer evolution reveals constrained routes to metastases: TRACERx Renal. Cell 173:581, 2018.

Wong MCS et al: Incidence and mortality of kidney cancer: Temporal patterns and global trends in 39 countries. Sci Rep 7:15698, 2017.

86 Cancer of the Bladder and Urinary Tract

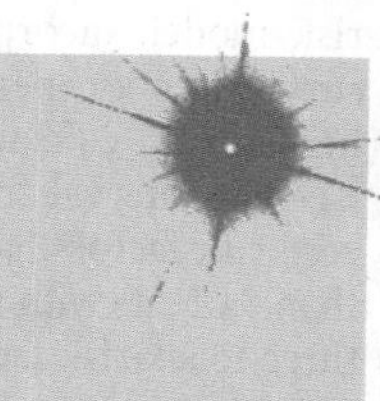

Noah M. Hahn

GLOBAL CONSIDERATIONS

Within the United States, urothelial carcinomas of the bladder and urinary tract are most closely related to tobacco smoking history. However, within developing countries, water supplies contaminated with arsenic or schistosomiasis parasites also are major carcinogenic contributors.

INTRODUCTION

Cancers of the urinary tract including the bladder, renal pelvis, ureter, and urethra occur frequently, and they represent the second most common class of genitourinary cancers. Bladder cancer alone represents the sixth most common cancer diagnosis annually in the United States with 81,400 new cases and 17,980 deaths every year. Because cancers of the renal pelvis are often lumped in with all kidney cancers, the true incidence and mortality from nonbladder urinary tract cancers are less precise. While less frequent than bladder cancer, an additional 20,000 new cases and 5000 deaths are estimated every year. An accelerated understanding of the molecular underpinnings of bladder and urinary tract cancer biology has led to a significant increase in urothelial cancer clinical trials resulting in U.S. Food and Drug Administration (FDA) approval of multiple new therapeutic agents since 2016 with more expected to follow. This chapter reviews the established, current, and emerging evidence that serves as the basis for the rapidly evolving standards of care for patients with bladder and urinary tract cancers.

CLINICAL EPIDEMIOLOGY AND RISK FACTORS

Bladder cancer typically affects older patients with a median age at diagnosis of 73 years. Males are four times more frequently affected than females. Similarly, bladder cancer is more common in Caucasians than in Asian patients. Inheritable germline genetic risk factors have been identified in up to one-seventh of patients with bladder or urinary tract cancers. However, a singular germline genetic alteration has not been observed in a majority of these cases, and the impact of germline genetic alterations on family members of urothelial cancer patients is uncertain. Patients with defects in mismatch repair genes leading to microsatellite instability (*MLH1, MSH2, MSH6*, etc.) as part of the familial cancer Lynch syndrome are at particular risk of upper urinary tract cancers of the renal pelvis and ureter. Additionally, patients with Cowden disease (*PTEN* mutations) or retinoblastoma (*RB1* mutations) are at increased risk for developing bladder cancer.

Historically, associations have existed between environmental toxic exposures and higher rates of developing bladder cancer. Carcinogenic agents associated with increased risk of bladder cancer have included the aromatic amines benzidine and beta-naphthylamine that can be present in industrial dyes as well as arsenic that can be found in some drinking water supplies in underdeveloped countries. Other chemicals in the leather, paint, rubber, textiles, and printing industries have been associated with bladder cancer. Associations with exposures to hair dyes and hair sprays in workers in the hairstyling field have been suggested. Additionally, concern has been raised regarding use of the antidiabetic medication, pioglitazone, and bladder cancer risk. Extensive reviews and meta-analyses have produced differing conclusions. The data suggest a small risk of bladder cancer from long-term pioglitazone use, which has led to inclusion of bladder cancer risk within the pioglitazone prescribing information. An association between chronic inflammatory states and the development of squamous bladder cancer clearly exists in underdeveloped countries in patients chronically infected with the parasitic disease schistosomiasis and in paraplegic patients with chronic indwelling catheters. Above and beyond each of these associations, however, smoking of tobacco products (cigarettes, cigars, pipes, etc.) remains the overwhelming leading risk factor for development of bladder cancer. Among new bladder cancer diagnoses, 90% of cases occur in current or former smokers. Toxicologists have estimated that >70 confirmed carcinogenic toxins are present within tobacco smoke. It is estimated that one-third of bladder cancer cases could be prevented through simple modification of lifestyle choices, in particular cessation of smoking.

■ CLINICAL PRESENTATION AND DIAGNOSTIC WORKUP

Occasionally, patients will present with flank pain in association with an upper tract renal pelvis or ureter cancer or due to hydronephrosis in association with a bladder tumor obstructing the orifice of the ureter within the bladder. Only in rare cases do patients present with significant cachexia and widespread metastatic disease. For most patients, painless hematuria (either gross or microscopic) represents the initial manifestation of an underlying urinary tract cancer. In females, hematuria due to malignancy can often be mistaken for a urinary tract infection or menstrual bleeding. While treatment with antibiotics is warranted if a concurrent urinary tract infection is noted on initial urinalysis, persistent hematuria requires further workup. Painless hematuria in males is almost always abnormal and should be worked up. Initial investigations in patients of either sex should include urine cytology and visual examination of the bladder by cystoscopy. Cytology is successful in identifying cancer in only 50% of individuals with high-grade bladder cancers. In addition to urine cytology, radiographic evaluation of the kidneys and upper urinary tract by CT urogram should be performed. Because of the increased sensitivity and reduced IV contrast loads, CT urograms have largely replaced IV pyelograms as the preferred upper urinary tract imaging modality. A magnetic resonance (MR) urogram may be substituted in patients with poor renal function. Additional diagnostic testing of the urine to assess for cancer-associated chromosomal changes by fluorescent in situ hybridization, increased levels of nuclear mitotic proteins, increased bladder tumor–associated antigens, or higher levels of staining on cells shed by the bladder may identify some cancers missed by traditional cytology testing. However, they may also produce abnormal results in patients who do not have cancer. For now, these adjunct molecular tests are primarily utilized in detecting recurrent cancer in patients with a prior diagnosis of urinary tract cancer. Small tumors, particularly flat noninvasive tumors of the bladder, may be detected at higher rates with the use of blue light cystoscopy or narrow-band imaging cystoscopy. Both blue light and narrow-band imaging cystoscopies are now used routinely in the monitoring of patients with bladder cancer. For patients with no bladder abnormalities in whom upper tract tumors are suspected, visualization of the upper urinary tracts and renal pelvises should be performed by ureteroscopy or retrograde pyelography.

In all patients with abnormalities noted in the bladder or upper urinary tracts, complete endoscopic resection for histologic diagnosis and staging should be performed when possible via either transurethral resection of bladder tumor (TURBT) or endoscopic resection of upper tract tumors.

■ HISTOLOGY

Urothelial carcinoma, often called transitional cell carcinoma in the past, is the most common urinary tract cancer histology and is observed in ~90% of cases. Squamous, glandular, micropapillary, plasmacytoid, sarcomatoid, and other variant features can often be found in portions of urothelial carcinoma tumors; however, pure variant histologies are rare. The presence of some variant histologies including micropapillary and plasmacytoid has been associated with worse surgical outcomes compared to urothelial carcinoma. Nonurothelial variant histologies including squamous cell carcinoma, adenocarcinoma, small-cell carcinoma, and carcinosarcoma collectively account for ≤10% of urinary tract tumors. Examples of traditional urothelial carcinoma and some of the variant histologies are shown in **Fig. 86-1**.

■ MOLECULAR BIOLOGY

Clinically, urothelial carcinoma of the bladder displays a biphasic phenotype characterized by (1) low-grade papillary tumors that frequently recur but rarely invade or metastasize and (2) high-grade sometimes flat tumors that invade early leading to lethal metastatic disease. In both of these phenotypes, loss of portions of chromosomes 9q and 9p by loss of heterozygosity is an early molecular event, whose exact significance is not clear. Potential candidate regulatory genes in these genomic regions include *CDNK2A*, a cyclin-dependent kinase inhibitor, and *TSC1*, a gene encoding hamartin mutated in tuberous sclerosis. Early investigations have demonstrated that low-grade tumors are characterized by alterations in the *RAS/RAF* signaling pathway with activating *FGFR3* mutations or gene fusions present in 60–80% of patients. In contrast, the high-grade invasive phenotype is notable for early deleterious mutations in *TP53* and *RB1*, alterations in *CDH1* (E-cadherin), and increased expression of *VEGFR2*. In urothelial carcinoma of the renal pelvis and ureter, 10–20% of cases may be associated with Lynch syndrome hereditary defects in the *MLH1, MSH2*, or *MSH6* mismatch repair genes, leading to microsatellite instability and frequent DNA mutations. Testing for germline mutations in these genes is recommended in patients with upper urinary tract urothelial carcinoma under the age of 60 at diagnosis, with a first-degree relative with a Lynch syndrome–associated cancer diagnosed under the age of 50, or with two first-degree relatives with a Lynch syndrome–associated cancer regardless of the age at diagnosis.

As genomic analysis technologies have improved, so has our understanding of the molecular biology unique to urothelial carcinoma. In 2017, the full bladder cancer results of The Cancer Genome Atlas (TCGA) project were published. This effort comprehensively analyzed gene mutations, fusions, expression, copy number variations, methylation, and microRNA across the genome of patients with bladder urothelial carcinoma treated with surgery. Key findings from this effort include (1) genomic alterations in genes (e.g., *FGFR3, EGFR, ERBB2, ERBB3, PIK3CA, TSC1*, etc.) targetable by currently approved drugs or drugs in development in 71% of patients; (2) genomic alterations in chromatin-modifying genes (*KMT2D, KDM6A, KMT2C, EP300, CREBBP*, etc.) in the majority of patients; (3) hypermethylation with epigenetic silencing of gene expression in one-fourth of patients; and (4) the identification by RNA sequencing of five distinct intrinsic molecular subtypes (luminal papillary, luminal infiltrated, luminal, basal squamous, and neuronal) closely resembling luminal and basal subclassifications of breast cancers. These bladder TCGA findings have led to clinical trial designs enriching for patients with specific

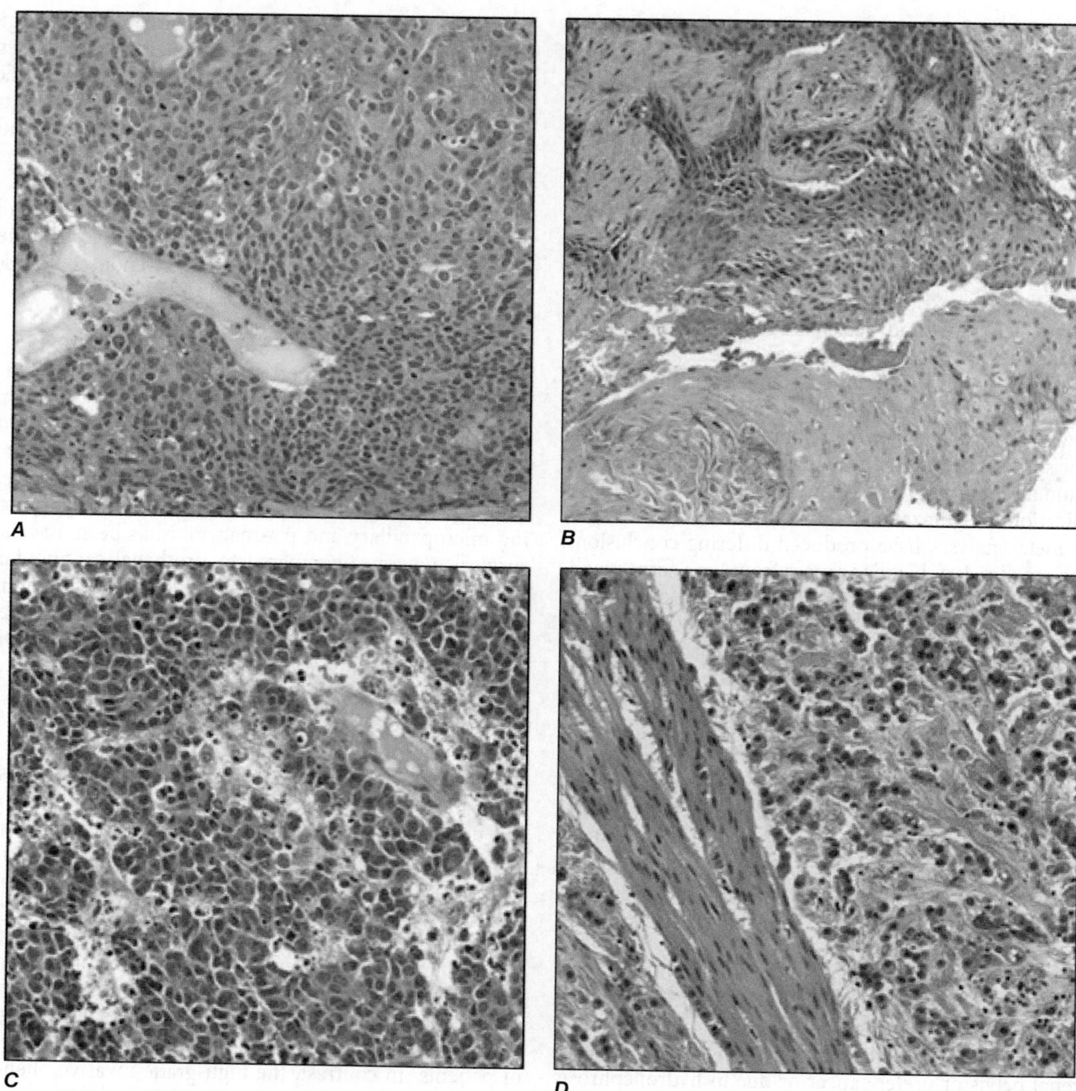

FIGURE 86-1 Bladder and urinary tract cancer histologies. ***A.*** Urothelial carcinoma. ***B.*** Squamous cell carcinoma. ***C.*** Small-cell carcinoma. ***D.*** Plasmacytoid variant. *(Courtesy of Alex Baras, MD, PhD, Johns Hopkins University Department of Pathology.)*

gene mutation profiles as well as interrogation of candidate biomarkers according to intrinsic molecular subtypes.

STAGING AND OUTCOMES BY STAGE

The staging of bladder cancer is dependent on the depth of invasion within the bladder wall, involvement of lymph nodes, and spread to surrounding and distant organs as depicted in **Fig. 86-2**. Approximately 75% of bladder cancer presents with non–muscle-invasive bladder cancer (NMIBC), 18% with disease invading into or through the muscular wall of the bladder, and only 3% presenting with metastatic spread to distant organs. NMIBC is defined by tumors that involve only the immediate epithelial layer of cells (carcinoma in situ [CIS] and Ta) or that only penetrate into the connective tissue below the urothelium (T1) but not into the muscular layer known as the *muscularis propria*. Muscle-invasive bladder cancer (MIBC) is defined by tumors that invade into the muscularis propria (T2), through the muscularis propria to involve the surrounding serosa (T3), or into immediately adjacent pelvic organs such as the rectum, prostate, vagina, or cervix (T4). Lymph node staging is classified according to involvement of a solitary node within the true pelvis (N1), two nodes involved in the true pelvis (N2), or involvement of the common iliac nodes (N3). Any disease that has spread beyond the common iliac nodes is considered metastatic (M1). The staging of bladder cancer is driven primarily by the T stage of the tumor, with stages 0a–II defined entirely by the T stage in the absence of nodal or metastatic disease. Involvement of regional lymph nodes in the true pelvis or along the common iliac artery qualifies as stage III disease, whereas involvement of any distant metastases qualifies as stage IV disease. Clinical outcomes of patients with bladder cancer correlate closely with staging at diagnosis with 5-year overall survival rates of 70–90% for disease confined to the bladder (stage I–II), 36–50% for disease that penetrates through the bladder or has spread to regional lymph nodes (stage III), and only 5% for disease extending to metastatic sites (stage IV).

TREATMENT APPROACHES

Early-Stage Disease For NMIBC, removal of all visible tumors by TURBT in the operating room is considered the mainstay of surgical treatment. Risk of recurrence can be classified as low, intermediate, or high depending on the presence of features summarized in **Table 86-1**. For patients with low-risk disease, meta-analyses have demonstrated a 12% reduction in early relapses when a single chemotherapy treatment of mitomycin C, epirubicin, or gemcitabine was instilled directly into the bladder (intravesical therapy) within 24 hours of the TURBT. For patients with intermediate- or high-risk tumors, weekly intravesical instillations for 6 consecutive weeks of the attenuated mycobacterium strain known as *Bacille Calmette-Guérin* (BCG) reduce the risk of recurrence at 12 months from 56 to 29%. In addition, BCG treatment has been shown to decrease the rate of progression to MIBC by 27%. Intravesical

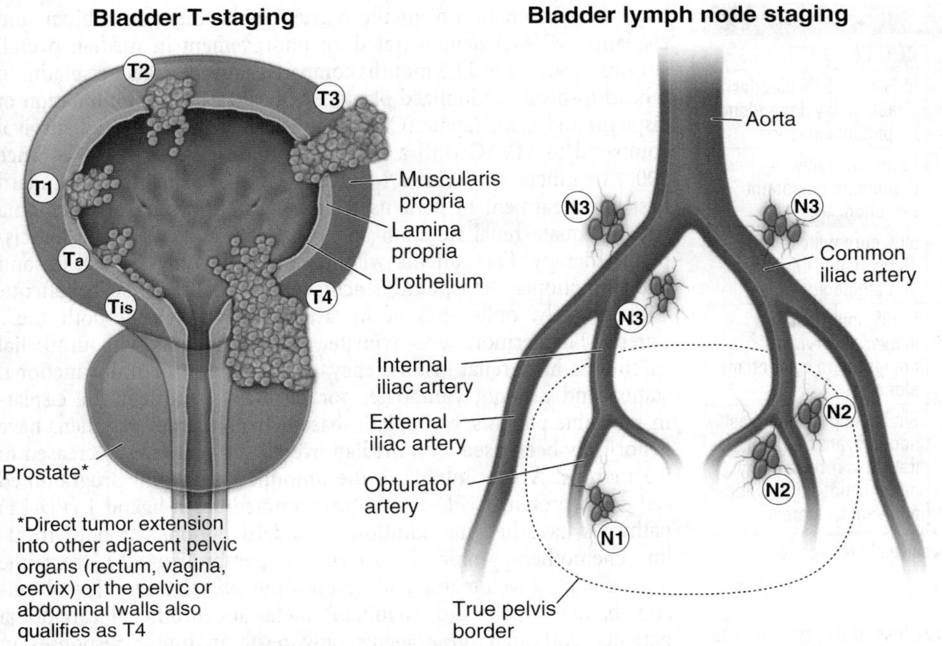

Bladder T-staging

Bladder lymph node staging

*Direct tumor extension into other adjacent pelvic organs (rectum, vagina, cervix) or the pelvic or abdominal walls also qualifies as T4

Bladder cancer prognosis according to stage

T	N	M	Stage	5-yr survival
Tis/Ta	N0	M0	0is/0a	96%
T1	N0	M0	1	90%
T2	N0	M0	2	70%
T3	N0	M0	3	50%
T1-T4	N1-N3	M0	3	36%
Any T	Any N	M1	4	5%

N1 - Cancer spread to 1 lymph node in the true pelvis

N2 - Cancer spread to 2 lymph nodes in the true pelvis

N3 - Cancer spread to lymph nodes along the common iliac artery

FIGURE 86-2 Bladder cancer staging and prognosis. TNM, tumor-node-metastasis.

BCG is generally well tolerated. Side effects can include dysuria, urinary frequency, bladder spasms, hematuria, and, in rare cases (<5%), a systemic inflammatory response that can mimic disseminated BCG infection. Following a 6-week induction BCG schedule, additional maintenance BCG treatments given according to the Southwest Oncology Group schedule further reduce the risk of recurrent NMIBC compared to induction BCG alone. In patients with NMIBC that recurs long after initial BCG treatment, a repeat course of BCG can be considered. For patients with recurrence after a second adequate course of BCG or with relapsed NMIBC within 6 months of initial BCG exposure, surgical removal of the entire bladder by cystectomy is recommended due to the high risk of progression to MIBC and potentially metastatic disease. For patients who are not fit enough for or who refuse cystectomy, non-BCG alternative intravesical agents (mitomycin C, gemcitabine, docetaxel, valrubicin) or systemically administered agents that inhibit the PD-1/PD-L1 immune checkpoint pathway (pembrolizumab) can achieve durable tumor responses in a small fraction of patients.

TABLE 86-1 Non-Muscle-Invasive Bladder Cancer Recurrence Risk Groups

RISK GROUP	CHARACTERISTICS
Low risk	Initial tumor, solitary tumor, low grade, <3 cm, no CIS
Intermediate risk	All tumors not defined in the two adjacent categories (between the category of low and high risk)
High risk	Any of the following: • T1 tumor • High-grade • CIS • Multiple and recurrent and large (>3 cm) Ta low-grade tumors (all conditions must be met for this point on Ta low-grade tumors)

Abbreviation: CIS, carcinoma in situ.

Upper Tract Disease In patients with urothelial carcinoma of the renal pelvis or ureter, endoscopic tissue acquisition and staging are more challenging than primary tumors located in the bladder. Tumors possessing all of the following are considered low risk: solitary tumor, low grade, size <1 cm, and no invasive component on imaging. Low-risk tumors can successfully be treated by laser ureteroscopic ablation or surgical resection and reanastomosis of the remaining ureter ends in tumors that cannot be successfully eradicated endoscopically.

Muscle-Invasive Disease In patients with urothelial carcinoma of the bladder that invades into or through the muscularis propria but with no evidence of metastatic spread, more aggressive therapy options summarized in **Table 86-2** are required to achieve cure. In carefully selected patients with no evidence of CIS or hydronephrosis, bladder-sparing combined-modality therapy with concurrent chemotherapy and radiation can achieve cure in ~65% of patients. Various chemotherapy regimens have been utilized in combination with radiation including cisplatin, carboplatin, 5-fluorouracil, mitomycin C, paclitaxel, and gemcitabine. It is important to note that a maximal debulking of all visible tumor by TURBT is required prior to initiation of combined-modality therapy. In patients who achieve a complete response to combined-modality therapy, regular cystoscopic monitoring of the bladder is required with salvage cystectomy offered to patients who develop MIBC in follow-up.

In a similar fashion, bladder-sparing partial cystectomy can be performed in a very small subset of MIBC patients. The ideal patient for partial cystectomy is the patient with a solitary, clinical T2 urothelial carcinoma in the dome of the bladder. In such patients, the tumor and immediate surrounding urothelium can be resected with reconstruction of the remaining bladder to maintain near physiologic urinary function.

In the majority of patients, however, resection of the entire bladder is required. In males, a cystoprostatectomy with removal of the bladder, prostate, and pelvic lymph nodes is performed, whereas in females, an anterior exenteration with removal of the bladder, uterus, ovaries, cervix, and pelvic lymph nodes is performed. With the bladder removed, three options exist to reroute the urine outflow. In an ileostomy, the bilateral ureters are connected to a portion of ileum that is brought through an incision in the abdominal wall to create a stoma that drains urine into an affixed bag outside of the body. In a continent urinary reservoir or "Indiana pouch," the ureters are connected to a portion of ileum that has been separated on both ends from the rest of the small-bowel transit to form a urinary reservoir. The remaining small bowel is reanastomosed, and the urinary reservoir is brought up just beneath the abdominal wall muscles with patients catheterizing the urinary reservoir several times per day via a small stoma tract. Last, in a neobladder, the same urinary reservoir described previously is brought down into the pelvis and is anastomosed to the remaining urethra to provide the opportunity to the patient to void urine through the urethra. The choice of which urinary reconstruction to perform is affected not only by patient choice but also by anatomic tumor considerations and

TABLE 86-2 Treatment Approaches to MIBC Patients

TREATMENT	PATIENT SELECTION	CLINICAL OUTCOMES
Bladder-sparing chemoradiation	No CIS, no hydronephrosis, maximal TURBT required	65% cure, 55% bladder intact, highly dependent on patient selection
Bladder-sparing partial cystectomy	Solitary tumors in dome of bladder are ideal	Variable, highly dependent on patient selection
Cystectomy	Any MIBC patient	50% cure with surgery alone, highly dependent on pathologic stage
Neoadjuvant cisplatin-based chemotherapy	Cisplatin-eligible MIBC patients	5–10% improvement in overall survival compared to cystectomy alone
Adjuvant cisplatin-based chemotherapy	Cisplatin-eligible high-risk postcystectomy MIBC patients (pT3-4, N+)	Similar improvement as neoadjuvant treatment, data less robust, many patients not suitable for adjuvant treatment

Abbreviations: CIS, carcinoma in situ; MIBC, muscle-invasive bladder cancer; TURBT, transurethral resection of bladder tumor.

urologist experience with each procedure. Regardless of the type of surgery performed, all patients undergo a significant catabolic change in their metabolism following removal of the bladder. While many MIBC patients are affected by weight loss preoperatively, it is not uncommon for postcystectomy patients to lose an additional 10–15 lb in the first month postoperatively. In addition, patients can experience long-term nutritional changes such as low B_{12} levels due to alterations in small-bowel physiology caused by all of the urinary diversion options.

Despite aggressive surgery, only half of patients undergoing cystectomy are cured by surgery alone. Therefore, many clinical trials have investigated the role of systemic chemotherapy before (neoadjuvant) or after (adjuvant) surgery. Meta-analyses have shown a 5–10% absolute overall survival advantage when combination chemotherapy regimens utilizing cisplatin have been used before surgery. A similar benefit exists with cisplatin-based combination chemotherapy given after surgery. However, the data in the adjuvant setting are based on smaller, older trials. Furthermore, in the postoperative setting, some patients may not recover sufficiently from their surgery within a time frame optimal for chemotherapy administration. Importantly, non–cisplatin-containing chemotherapy regimens have proven inferior to cisplatin-containing regimens. Therefore, if patients are not suitable candidates for cisplatin administration due to poor functional status or comorbidities (e.g., poor renal function), patients should proceed directly to surgery and forego neoadjuvant therapy.

For patients with high-risk urothelial carcinoma of the upper urinary tract, resection of the kidney and ureter (including the ureter bladder cuff) by nephroureterectomy is preferred. Segmental ureterectomy may be appropriate in patients with decreased renal function in which nephron-sparing outcomes are critical to prevent the need for dialysis. Similarly, in CIS patients, administration of BCG therapy via a nephrostomy tube can be considered to preserve intact renal function. The use of cisplatin-based neoadjuvant chemotherapy has been associated with a pathologic complete response at surgery of 14% in upper tract urothelial carcinoma patients. Similarly, in the post-nephroureterectomy setting, adjuvant platinum-based chemotherapy (carboplatin or cisplatin) reduced recurrence rates by 55% compared to surgery alone. The use of perioperative chemotherapy either before or after surgery is now recommended for upper tract urothelial carcinoma patients in national guidelines.

Metastatic Disease For patients with metastatic urothelial carcinoma regardless of primary tumor origin, systemic chemotherapy is the most established standard of care. In a randomized phase 3 clinical trial, the combination of methotrexate, vinblastine, doxorubicin, and cisplatin (MVAC) demonstrated an improvement in median overall survival from 8.2 to 12.5 months compared to single-agent cisplatin. In a head-to-head randomized phase 3 clinical trial, the combination of cisplatin and gemcitabine (CG) demonstrated similar overall survival compared to MVAC with a more favorable side effect profile. Since 2000, treatment with either MVAC or CG has remained a standard first-line treatment of patients with metastatic urothelial carcinoma with adequate renal function and functional status suitable for cisplatin therapy. For patients with lymph node–only metastases and good functional status, cure is achieved in 15–20% of such patients. Unfortunately, only ~5% of metastatic patients fulfill both these criteria. Furthermore, approximately half of patients with urothelial carcinoma have renal insufficiency, comorbidities, or frail functional status, and are not candidates for cisplatin treatment. In cisplatin-ineligible patients, carboplatin-based chemotherapy regimens have historically been used with median overall survival rates decreased to 9.3 months. Agents inhibiting the immune checkpoint programmed cell death protein 1 (PD-1) and programmed death ligand 1 (PD-L1) pathways have become additional standard options for both front-line chemotherapy-naive (atezolizumab, pembrolizumab), front-line maintenance (avelumab), and second-line postplatinum (pembrolizumab, nivolumab, and avelumab) metastatic urothelial carcinoma patients. Although these agents only result in tumor responses in 10–30% of patients, they have been approved due to their improved safety profiles compared to traditional chemotherapy options and the prolonged durability of some tumor responses. These agents aim to reactivate a patient's own immune system to recognize and eliminate their cancer. As such, their unique side effect profile is characterized by immune-related toxicities that are rare but can be severe and may include colitis, pneumonitis, hepatitis, nephritis, myocarditis, rash, hypothyroidism, Guillain-Barré syndrome, idiopathic thrombocytopenia purpura, and adrenal insufficiency.

In patients with activating tumor fibroblast growth factor 2 or 3 (*FGFR2/3*) mutations or fusions with progressive disease following platinum-based therapy, the oral FGFR tyrosine kinase inhibitor erdafitinib is another standard option resulting in tumor responses in 32% of patients with a median duration of response of 5.4 months. Additionally, the nectin-4–targeting antibody-drug conjugate enfortumab vedotin provides an additional standard option for patients with progression after both platinum-based therapy and PD-1/PD-L1 immune checkpoint therapy independent of tumor mutation status. Tumor responses are observed in 44% of patients, including patients with liver metastases, with a median response duration of 7.6 months. Additional novel urothelial carcinoma therapeutics are under ongoing investigation.

FURTHER READING

American Cancer Society: *Cancer Facts & Figures 2020*. Atlanta, GA: Available from *https://www.cancer.org/cancer/bladder-cancer/detection-diagnosis-staging/survival-rates.html*.

Carlo MI et al: Cancer susceptibility mutations in patients with urothelial malignancies. J Clin Oncol 38:5, 2020.

Howlader N et al: SEER Cancer Statistics Review, 1975-2017. Available from *https://seer.cancer.gov/csr/1975_2017/*. Based on November 2019 SEER data submission, posted to the SEER website, April 2020.

Kamat AM et al: Bladder cancer. Lancet 388:2796, 2016.

Knowles MA et al: Molecular biology of bladder cancer: New insights into pathogenesis and clinical diversity. Nat Rev Cancer 15:25, 2015.

Robertson AG et al: Comprehensive molecular characterization of muscle-invasive bladder cancer. Cell 171:3, 2017.

Santopietro AL et al: Advances in the management of urothelial carcinoma: is immunotherapy the answer? Expert Opin Pharmacother 22:1743, 2021.

Siegel RL et al: Cancer statistics, 2020. CA Cancer J Clin 70:1, 2020.

87 Benign and Malignant Diseases of the Prostate

Howard I. Scher, James A. Eastham

Benign and malignant changes in the prostate increase with age. Autopsies of men in the eighth decade of life show hyperplastic changes in >90% and malignant changes in >70% of individuals. The high prevalence of these diseases among the elderly, who often have competing causes of morbidity and mortality, mandates a risk-adapted approach to diagnosis and treatment. This can be achieved by considering these diseases as a series of states. Each state represents a distinct clinical milestone for which therapy(ies) may be recommended based on disease extent, current symptoms, the risk of developing symptoms, or the risk of death from disease in relation to death from other causes within a given time frame. For benign proliferative disorders, symptoms of bladder outlet obstruction and potential complications including urinary retention and urinary tract infection are weighed against the side effects and complications of medical or surgical intervention. For prostate malignancies, the likelihood that a clinically significant cancer is present in the gland and the concomitant risk of symptoms or death from cancer are balanced against the morbidities of the recommended treatments and preexisting comorbidities.

ANATOMY AND PATHOLOGY

The prostate is in the pelvis and is adjacent to the rectum, the bladder, the periprostatic and dorsal vein complexes, the neurovascular bundles that are responsible for erectile function, and the urinary sphincter that is responsible for passive urinary control. The prostate is composed of branching tubuloalveolar glands arranged in lobules surrounded by fibromuscular stroma. The acinar unit includes an epithelial compartment made up of epithelial, basal, and neuroendocrine cells separated by a basement membrane and a stromal compartment that includes fibroblasts and smooth-muscle cells. Prostate-specific antigen (PSA) and prostatic acid phosphatase (PAP) are produced in the epithelial cells. Both prostate epithelial cells and stromal cells express androgen receptors (ARs) and depend on androgens for growth. Testosterone, the major circulating androgen, is converted by the enzyme 5α-reductase to dihydrotestosterone in the gland.

The periurethral portion of the gland increases in size during puberty and after the age of 55 years due to the growth of nonmalignant cells in the transition zone of the prostate that surrounds the urethra. Most cancers develop in the peripheral zone, and cancers in this location may be palpated during a digital rectal examination (DRE).

PROSTATE CANCER

The American Cancer Society's estimates for prostate cancer in the United States for 2021 are ~248,530 new prostate cancer cases and ~34,130 deaths from prostate cancer. The absolute number of prostate cancer deaths has decreased in the past 10 years, attributed by some to the widespread use of PSA-based detection strategies. However, the paradox of management is that although 1 in 8 men will eventually be diagnosed with prostate cancer and the disease remains the second leading cause of cancer deaths in men, only 1 man in 41 with prostate cancer will die of his disease.

■ EPIDEMIOLOGY

Epidemiologic studies show that the risk of being diagnosed with prostate cancer increases 2.5-fold if one first-degree relative is affected and fivefold if two or more are affected. Current estimates are that 40% of early-onset and 5–10% of all prostate cancers are hereditary. Prostate cancer affects ethnic groups differently. Matched for age, African-American males have a higher incidence and present at a more advanced stage with higher-grade, more aggressive cancers. Genome-wide association studies (GWAS) have identified >40 prostate cancer susceptibility loci that are estimated to explain up to 25% of prostate cancer risk. Among the genes implicated in variations in incidence and outcome are single-nucleotide polymorphisms (SNPs) in the vitamin D receptor in African Americans and variants in the AR, CYP3A4, both involved in the deactivation of testosterone, as well as CYP17, which is involved in steroid biosynthesis. One early change is hypermethylation of the GSTP1 gene promoter, which leads to loss of function of a gene that detoxifies carcinogens. The finding that many prostate cancers develop adjacent to a lesion termed *proliferative inflammatory atrophy* (PIA) suggests a role for inflammation.

The prevalence of autopsy-detected cancers is similar around the world, while the incidence of clinical disease varies. Thus, environmental and dietary factors may play a role in prostate cancer growth and progression. High consumption of dietary fats, such as α-linoleic acid or polycyclic aromatic hydrocarbons that form when red meats are cooked, is believed to increase risk. Like breast cancer in Asian women, the risk of prostate cancer in Asian men increases when they move to Western environments. Protective factors include consumption of the isoflavonoid genistein (which inhibits 5α-reductase), cruciferous vegetables with isothiocyanate sulforaphane, lycopene found in tomatoes, and inhibitors of cholesterol biosynthesis (e.g., statin drugs). Not smoking, regular exercise, and maintaining a healthy body weight may reduce the risk of progression.

■ DIAGNOSIS AND TREATMENT BY CLINICAL STATE

The prostate cancer continuum—from the appearance of a preneoplastic and invasive lesion that is localized to the gland, to a metastatic lesion causing symptoms and, ultimately, mortality—can span decades. To limit overdiagnosis of clinically insignificant cancers and for disease management in general, competing risks are considered in the context of a series of clinical states (**Fig. 87-1**). The states are defined operationally based on whether or not a cancer diagnosis has been established and, for those with a diagnosis, the state of the primary tumor (treated vs untreated), whether or not metastases are detectable on imaging studies, and the measured level of testosterone in the blood. With this approach, an individual resides in only one state and remains in that state until he has progressed. At each assessment, the decision to offer treatment and the specific form of treatment are based on the presence or absence of cancer-related symptoms, and if absent, the risk posed by the cancer relative to competing causes of morbidity and mortality that may be present in that individual. It follows that the more advanced the disease, the greater is the need for treatment.

For those without a cancer diagnosis, the decision to undergo testing to detect a cancer is based on the individual's estimated life expectancy and, separately, the probability that a clinically significant cancer may be present. For those with a prostate cancer diagnosis, the clinical states model considers the probability of developing symptoms or dying from the disease. Thus, a patient with a localized tumor that has been surgically removed remains in the state of localized disease if the PSA remains undetectable. The time within a state then becomes a measure of the efficacy of an intervention, though the effect may not be assessable for years. Because many men with active cancer are not at risk for developing metastases, symptoms, or death, the clinical states model allows a distinction between *cure*—the elimination of all cancer cells, the primary therapeutic objective of treatment for most cancers—and *cancer control*, by which the tempo of the illness is determined to be so slow or has been altered by treatment to the point where it is unlikely to cause symptoms, to metastasize, or to shorten a patient's life expectancy. Importantly, from a patient standpoint, both outcomes can be considered equivalent therapeutically assuming the patient has not experienced symptoms of the disease or the treatment needed to control it. Even when a recurrence is documented, immediate therapy is not always necessary. Rather, as at the time of diagnosis, the need for intervention is based on the tempo of the illness as it unfolds in the individual, relative to the risk-to-benefit ratio of the intervention being considered.

■ NO CANCER DIAGNOSIS

Prevention No agent is currently approved for the prevention of prostate cancer. The results from several large double-blind,

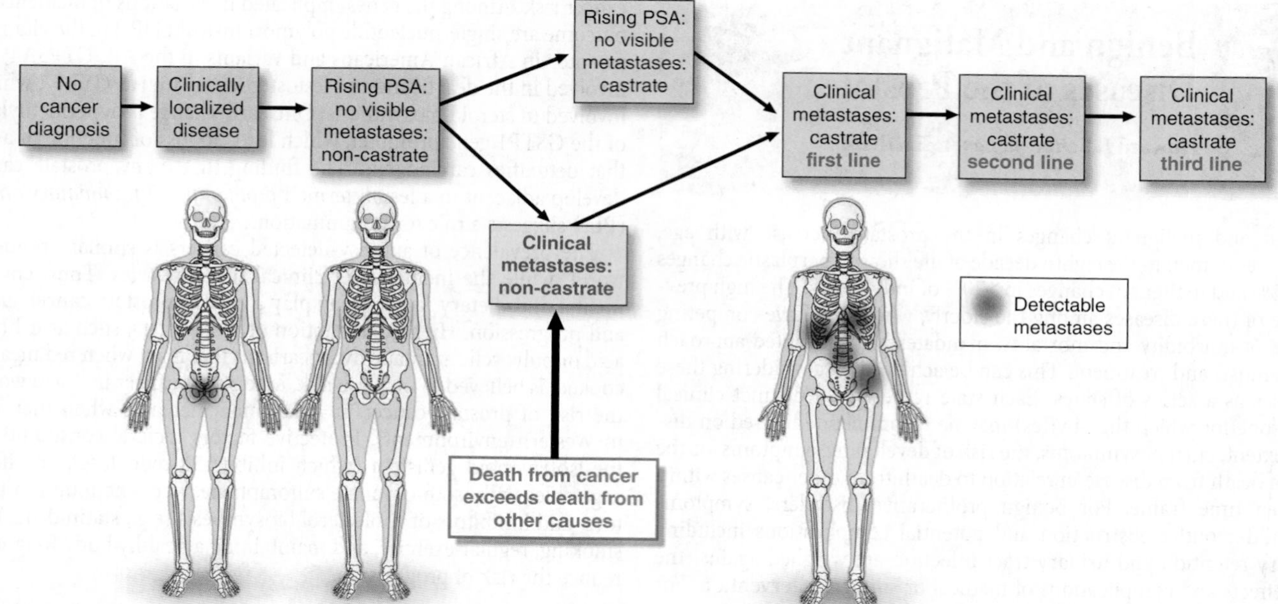

FIGURE 87-1 Clinical states of prostate cancer. PSA, prostate-specific antigen.

randomized chemoprevention trials have established 5α-reductase inhibitors (5ARIs) as the predominant therapy to reduce the future risk of a prostate cancer diagnosis. The Prostate Cancer Prevention Trial (PCPT), in which men aged >55 years received placebo or the 5ARI finasteride, which inhibits the type 1 isoform, showed a 25% (95% confidence interval 19–31%) reduction in prostate cancer incidence from 24% with placebo to 18% with finasteride. In REDUCE (Reduction by Dutasteride of Prostate Cancer Events trial), a reduction in incidence from 25% with placebo to 20% with dutasteride was found (p = .001). Dutasteride inhibits both the type 1 and type 2 5ARI isoforms. While both studies met their endpoint, there was concern that most of the cancers that were "prevented" were low risk. Neither drug is approved for prostate cancer prevention. In comparison, the Selenium and Vitamin E Cancer Prevention Trial (SELECT), which enrolled African-American men aged ≥50 years and others aged ≥55 years, showed no difference in cancer incidence in patients receiving vitamin E (4.6%) or selenium (4.9%) alone or in combination (4.6%) relative to placebo (4.4%). A similar lack of benefit for vitamin E, vitamin C, and selenium was seen in the Physicians Health Study II.

Early Detection and Diagnosis The decision to pursue a diagnosis of prostate cancer must balance the benefit from detecting and treating clinically significant cancers that, left untreated, would adversely affect a patient's quality and duration of life, against the morbidity associated with the overdiagnosis and overtreatment of clinically insignificant cancers that are highly prevalent in the general population. The balance is best approached through shared decision-making between the patient and physician. Considerations for whether to pursue a diagnosis include symptoms, an abnormal DRE, or more typically, a change in or an elevated serum PSA. Genetic risk is also considered.

PHYSICAL EXAMINATION The DRE focuses on prostate size, consistency, and abnormalities within or beyond the gland. Many cancers occur in the peripheral zone and may be palpated on DRE. Carcinomas are characteristically hard, nodular, and irregular, while induration may also be due to benign prostatic hyperplasia (BPH) or calculi. Overall, 20–25% of men with an abnormal DRE have prostate cancer.

PROSTATE-SPECIFIC ANTIGEN PSA (kallikrein-related peptidase 3; *KLK3*) is a kallikrein-related serine protease that causes liquefaction of seminal coagulum. It is produced by both nonmalignant and malignant epithelial cells and, as such, is prostate-specific, not prostate cancer–specific. Serum levels of PSA may increase from prostatitis, BPH, or prostate cancer. Serum levels are not significantly affected by the DRE. PSA circulating in the blood is inactive and mainly occurs as a complex with the protease inhibitor α_1-antichymotrypsin and as free (unbound) PSA forms. The formation of complexes between PSA, α_2-macroglobulin, or other protease inhibitors is less significant. Free PSA is rapidly eliminated from the blood by glomerular filtration with an estimated half-life of 12–18 h. Elimination of PSA bound to α_1-antichymotrypsin is slow (estimated half-life of 1–2 weeks) as it, too, is largely cleared by the kidneys. Levels should be undetectable after about 6 weeks if the prostate has been completely removed (radical prostatectomy).

PSA testing was approved by the U.S. Food and Drug Administration (FDA) in 1994 for early detection of prostate cancer, and the widespread use of the test has played a significant role in the proportion of men diagnosed with early-stage cancers: >70–80% of newly diagnosed cancers are clinically organ confined. The level of PSA in blood is strongly associated with the risk and outcome of prostate cancer. A single PSA measured at age 60 is associated (area under the curve [AUC] of 0.90) with lifetime risk of death from prostate cancer. Most (90%) prostate cancer deaths occur among men with PSA levels in the top quartile (>2 ng/mL), although only a minority of men with PSA >2 ng/mL will develop lethal prostate cancer. Despite this and mortality rate reductions reported from large randomized prostate cancer screening trials, routine use of the test remains controversial.

In 2012, the U.S. Preventive Services Task Force (USPSTF) published a review of the evidence for PSA-based screening for prostate cancer and made a clear recommendation against screening. By giving a grade of "D" in the recommendation statement that was based on this review, the USPSTF concluded that "there is moderate or high certainty that this service has no net benefit or that the harms outweigh the benefits." In 2013, the American Urological Association (AUA) updated their consensus statement regarding prostate cancer screening. They concluded that the quality of evidence for the benefits of screening was moderate for men aged 55–69 years. For men outside this age range, evidence was lacking for benefit, but the harms of screening, including overdiagnosis and overtreatment, remained. The AUA recommends shared decision-making for men aged 55–69 years considering PSA-based screening, a target age group for whom benefits may outweigh harms. Outside this age range, PSA-based screening as a routine was not recommended. The entire guideline is available at *http://www.auanet.org/guidelines/early-detection-of-prostate-cancer-(2013-reviewed-and-validity-confirmed-2015)*. As of 2017, the USPSTF has issued a revised recommendation with a grade of "C" for PSA-based prostate cancer screening for men aged 55–69. Now they recommend shared decision-making for men between the ages of 55 and 69 and do not recommend screening for men aged 70 or greater, roughly in agreement with the 2013 AUA guideline. The USPSTF also notes that the increased use of active surveillance (observation with selective delayed treatment) for low-risk prostate cancer has reduced the risks of screening.

We believe that implementation of the following three guidelines will further improve PSA screening outcomes in the United States and will have a greater practical impact on men's health than the USPSTF and AUA recommendations that are based almost solely on age. First, avoid PSA tests in men with little to gain. There is no rationale for recommending PSA screening in asymptomatic men with a short life expectancy. Hence, men over the age of 75 should only be tested in special circumstances, such as a higher than median PSA measured before age 70 or excellent overall health. In addition, because a baseline PSA is a strong predictor of the future risk of lethal prostate cancer, men with low PSAs, for example <1 ng/mL, can undergo testing less frequently, perhaps every 5 years, with screening possibly ending at age 60 if the PSA remains at ≤1 ng/mL. Men with PSAs that are above an age median but below biopsy thresholds can be counseled about their elevated risk and actively encouraged to return for regular screening and more comprehensive risk assessment. Second, do not treat those who do not need treatment. High proportions of men with screen-detected prostate cancer do not need immediate treatment and can be managed by active surveillance. Third, refer men who do need treatment to high-volume centers. Although it is clearly not feasible to restrict treatment exclusively to high-volume centers, shifting treatment trends so that more patients are treated at such centers by high-volume providers will improve cancer control and decrease complications. The goal of prostate cancer screening should be to maximize the benefits of PSA testing and minimize its harms. Following the three rules outlined here should continue to improve the ratio of harms to benefits from PSA screening.

The PSA criteria used to recommend a diagnostic prostate biopsy have evolved over time. However, based on the commonly used cut point for prostate biopsy (a total PSA ≥4 ng/mL), most men with a PSA elevation do not have histologic evidence of prostate cancer at biopsy. In addition, many men with PSA levels below this cut point harbor cancer cells in their prostate. Information from the Prostate Cancer Prevention Trial demonstrates that there is no PSA below which the risk of prostate cancer is zero. Thus, the PSA level establishes the likelihood that a man will harbor cancer if he undergoes a prostate biopsy. The goal is to increase the sensitivity of the test for younger men harboring clinically significant cancers that may cause symptoms and shorten survival and to reduce the frequency of detecting cancers of low malignant potential in elderly men more likely to die of other causes. Patients with symptomatic bacterial prostatitis should have a course of antibiotics before biopsy. However, the routine use of antibiotics in an asymptomatic man with an elevated PSA level is strongly discouraged.

SECOND-LINE SCREENING TESTS Several tests have been developed to better stratify men with an elevated PSA test into those more or less likely to have clinically significant prostate cancer. The 4Kscore® Test (OPKO Lab, Nashville, TN) measures four prostate-specific kallikreins (total PSA, free PSA, intact PSA, and human kallikrein 2). The results are combined with clinical information in an algorithm that estimates an individual's percent risk of having an aggressive prostate cancer should that individual opt for a prostate biopsy. The 4Kscore test has also been shown to identify the likelihood that an individual will develop aggressive prostate cancer, defined as high-grade prostate cancer pathology and/or poor prostate cancer clinical outcomes, within 20 years.

The Prostate Health Index (PHI™, Innovative Diagnostic Laboratory, Richmond, VA) is a blood test that estimates the risk of having prostate cancer. The PHI test is a combination of free PSA, total PSA, and the [−2]proPSA isoform of free PSA. These three tests are combined in a formula that calculates the PHI score. The PHI score is a better predictor of prostate cancer than the total PSA test alone or the free PSA test alone. Urine-based testing measuring exosomes (ExoDx Prostate Test) or mRNA levels of prostate cancer–related genes (SelectMDx) is also available.

PROSTATE BIOPSY A diagnosis of cancer is established by an image-guided needle biopsy. Direct visualization by transrectal ultrasound (TRUS), magnetic resonance imaging (MRI), or fusion of the ultrasound and MRI images ensures that all areas of the gland, including suspicious areas, are sampled. Contemporary schemas advise an extended-pattern 12-core biopsy that includes sampling from the peripheral zone as well as a lesion-directed palpable nodule or suspicious image-guided sampling. Because a prostate biopsy is subject to sampling error, men with an abnormal PSA and negative biopsy are frequently advised to undergo additional testing, which may include a 4Kscore test, PHI, prostate MRI, and/or repeat biopsy.

PATHOLOGY Each core of the biopsy is examined for the presence of cancer, and the amount of cancer is quantified based on the length of the cancer within the core and the percentage of the core involved. Of the cancers identified, >95% are adenocarcinomas; the rest are squamous or transitional cell tumors or, rarely, carcinosarcomas or small-cell histologies. Metastases to the prostate are rare, but in some cases, colon cancers or transitional cell tumors of the bladder invade the gland by direct extension.

When prostate cancer is diagnosed, a measure of histologic aggressiveness is assigned using the *Gleason grading system*, in which the dominant and secondary glandular histologic patterns are scored from 1 (well differentiated) to 5 (undifferentiated) and summed to give a total score of 2–10 for each tumor. The most poorly differentiated area of tumor (i.e., the area with the highest histologic grade) often determines biologic behavior. The presence or absence of perineural invasion and extracapsular spread is also recorded.

Over the years, the Gleason grading system has undergone several changes. Currently, Gleason total scores of 2–5 are no longer assigned, and in practice, the lowest total score is now assigned a 6, although the scale continues to range from 2 to 10. This leads to a logical yet incorrect assumption on the part of patients that their Gleason 6 cancer is in the middle of the scale, triggering the fear that their cancer is serious and the assumption that treatment is necessary despite Gleason score 6 being favorable risk. To address these issues, a new five-grade group system has been developed:

Grade group 1 (Gleason score ≤6)
Grade group 2 (Gleason score 3+4 = 7)
Grade group 3 (Gleason score 4+3 = 7)
Grade group 4 (Gleason score 4+4 = 8)
Grade group 5 (Gleason scores 9 and 10)

The new system simplifies the grading of prostate cancer, appropriately classifying the lowest risk as grade group 1 (rather than Gleason score 6), and accurately predicts prognosis.

PROSTATE CANCER STAGING The TNM (tumor, node, metastasis) staging system includes categories for cancers that are identified solely on the basis of an abnormal PSA (T1c), those that are palpable but clinically confined to the gland (T2), and those that have extended outside the gland (T3 and T4) (**Table 87-1, Fig. 87-2**). DRE alone is inaccurate in determining the extent of disease within the gland, the presence or absence of capsular invasion, involvement of seminal vesicles, and extension of disease to lymph nodes. Because of the inadequacy of DRE for staging, the TNM staging system was modified to include the results of imaging. Unfortunately, no single test has been proven to accurately indicate the stage or the presence of organ-confined disease, seminal vesicle involvement, or lymph node spread.

TRUS is the imaging technique most frequently used to assess the primary tumor, but its chief use is directing prostate biopsies, not staging. No TRUS finding consistently indicates cancer with certainty. Computed tomography (CT) lacks sensitivity and specificity to detect extraprostatic extension and is inferior to MRI in visualization of lymph nodes. In general, MRI is superior to CT to detect cancers in the prostate, to assess local disease extent, and fused with ultrasound imaging, to guide sites to biopsy within the gland. MRI is also useful for the planning of surgery and radiation therapy.

Radionuclide bone scans (bone scintigraphy) are used to evaluate spread to osseous sites. This test is sensitive but relatively nonspecific

TABLE 87-1 TNM Classification

TNM (tumor, node, metastasis) Staging System for Prostate Cancer[a]	
Tx	Primary tumor cannot be assessed
T0	No evidence of primary tumor
Localized Disease	
T1	Clinically inapparent tumor, neither palpable nor visible by imaging
T1a	Tumor incidental histologic finding in ≤5% of resected tissue; not palpable
T1b	Tumor incidental histologic finding in >5% of resected tissue
T1c	Tumor identified by needle biopsy (e.g., because of elevated PSA)
T2	Tumor confined within prostate[b]
T2a	Tumor involves half of one lobe or less
T2b	Tumor involves more than one half of one lobe, not both lobes
T2c	Tumor involves both lobes
Local Extension	
T3	Tumor extends through the prostate capsule[c]
T3a	Extracapsular extension (unilateral or bilateral)
T3b	Tumor invades seminal vesicles
T4	Tumor is fixed or invades adjacent structures other than seminal vesicles such as external sphincter, rectum, bladder, levator muscles, and/or pelvic wall
Metastatic Disease	
N1	Positive regional lymph nodes
M1	Distant metastases

[a]Revised from SB Edge et al (eds): *AJCC Cancer Staging Manual*, 7th ed. New York, Springer, 2010. [b]Tumor found in one or both lobes by needle biopsy, but not palpable or reliably visible by imaging, is classified as T1c. [c]Invasion into the prostatic apex or into (but not beyond) the prostatic capsule is classified not as T3 but as T2.
Abbreviation: PSA, prostate-specific antigen.

because it does not detect the cancer itself, only reaction of the bone to the presence of the cancer itself. Consequently, areas of increased uptake are not always related to metastatic disease. Healing fractures, arthritis, Paget's disease, and other conditions will also cause abnormal uptake. True-positive bone scans are uncommon when the PSA is <10 ng/mL unless the tumor is high-grade.

TREATMENT

Prostate Cancer

CLINICALLY LOCALIZED PROSTATE CANCER

Patients with clinically localized disease are managed by radical prostatectomy, radiation therapy, or active surveillance. Choice of therapy requires the consideration of several factors: the presence of symptoms, the probability that the untreated tumor will adversely affect the quality or duration of survival and thus require treatment, and the probability that the tumor can be cured by single-modality therapy directed to the prostate versus requiring both local and systemic therapy to achieve cure.

There is no clear evidence for the superiority of any one form of local therapy relative to another. This is due to the lack of prospective randomized trials, referral bias and physician bias, variation in the experience of the treating teams, and differences in trial endpoints and the definitions of cancer control. Often, PSA relapse-free survival is used because an effect on metastatic progression or survival may not be apparent for years. For many patients, however, a PSA recurrence does not necessarily mean that the disease will cause symptoms or shorten survival. After radical surgery to remove all prostate tissue, PSA should become undetectable in the blood within 6 weeks. If PSA remains or becomes detectable after radical prostatectomy, the patient is considered to have persistent or recurrent disease. After radiation therapy, in contrast, PSA does not become undetectable because the remaining nonmalignant elements of the gland continue to produce PSA even if all cancer cells have been eliminated. Similarly, cancer control is not well defined for a patient managed by active surveillance because PSA levels may continue to rise in the absence of therapy. Other outcomes are time to objective progression (local or systemic), cancer-specific survival, and overall survival; however, these outcomes may take years to assess.

The more extensive the local disease, the higher the probability of regional lymph node involvement (even when imaging studies are normal), the lower the probability of local control, and the higher the probability of relapse and the development of metastases. More important is that within the categories of clinical stage T1, T2, and T3 disease are cancers with a range of prognoses. Some T3 tumors are curable with therapy directed solely at the prostate, and some T1 lesions have a high probability of systemic relapse that requires the integration of local and systemic therapy to achieve cure. For T1c cancers, stage alone is inadequate to predict outcome and select treatment; other factors must be considered.

To better assess risk and guide treatment selection, many groups have developed prognostic models or nomograms that use a combination of the initial clinical T stage, biopsy Gleason score, the number of biopsy cores in which cancer is detected, and baseline PSA. Some use discrete cut points (PSA <10 or ≥10 ng/mL; Gleason score of ≤6, 7, or ≥8); others employ nomograms that use PSA and Gleason score as continuous variables. More than 100 nomograms have been reported to predict (1) the probability that a clinically significant cancer is present, (2) disease extent (organ-confined vs non–organ-confined, node-negative or -positive), or (3) the probability of treatment success for specific local therapies using pretreatment variables. Considerable controversy exists over what constitutes "high risk" based on a predicted probability of success or failure. In these situations, nomograms and predictive models can only go so far. Exactly what probability of success or failure would lead a physician to recommend and a patient to seek alternative

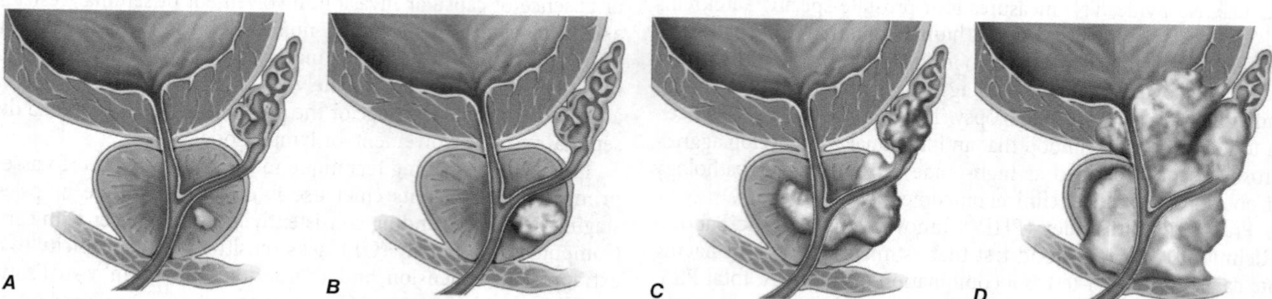

FIGURE 87-2 T stages of prostate cancer. ***A.*** T1—Clinically inapparent tumor, neither palpable nor visible by imaging. ***B.*** T2—Tumor confined within prostate. ***C.*** T3—Tumor extends through prostate capsule and may invade the seminal vesicles. ***D.*** T4—Tumor is fixed or invades adjacent structures. Eighty percent of patients present with local disease (T1 and T2), which is associated with a 5-year survival rate of 100%. An additional 12% of patients present with regional disease (T3 and T4 without metastases), which is also associated with a 100% survival rate after 5 years. Four percent of patients present with distant disease (T4 with metastases), which is associated with a 30% 5-year survival rate. (Three percent of patients are ungraded.) *(Reproduced with permission from MSKCC, data from AJCC, http://seer.cancer.gov/statfacts/html/prost.html. © 2010 Memorial Sloan-Kettering Cancer Center Medical Graphics.)*

approaches is controversial. As an example, it may be appropriate to recommend radical surgery for a younger patient with a low probability of cure. Nomograms are being refined continually to incorporate additional clinical parameters, biologic determinants, and year of treatment, which can also affect outcomes, making treatment decisions a dynamic process.

Radical Prostatectomy The goal of radical prostatectomy is to excise the cancer completely with a clear margin, to maintain continence by preserving the external sphincter, and to preserve potency by sparing the autonomic nerves in the neurovascular bundle. The procedure is advised for patients with a life expectancy of 10 years or more and is performed via a retropubic or perineal approach or via a minimally invasive robotic-assisted or hand-held laparoscopic approach. Outcomes can be predicted using postoperative nomograms that consider pretreatment factors and the pathologic findings at surgery. PSA failure is usually defined as a value >0.1 or 0.2 ng/mL. Specific criteria to guide the choice of one approach over another are lacking. Minimally invasive approaches offer the advantage of a shorter hospital stay and reduced blood loss. Rates of cancer control, recovery of continence, and recovery of erectile function are comparable. The individual surgeon, rather than the surgical approach used, is most important in determining outcomes after surgery.

Neoadjuvant hormonal treatment with gonadotropin-releasing hormone (GnRH) agonists/antagonists alone has also been explored to improve the outcomes of surgery for high-risk patients using a variety of definitions. The results of several large trials testing 3 or 8 months of androgen depletion before surgery showed that serum PSA levels decreased by 96%, prostate volumes decreased by 34%, and margin positivity rates decreased from 41–17%. Unfortunately, these findings have not been shown to improve PSA relapse–free survival.

Factors associated with incontinence following radical prostatectomy include older age and urethral length, which impacts the ability to preserve the urethra beyond the apex and the distal sphincter. The skill and experience of the surgeon are also factors.

The likelihood of recovery of erectile function is associated with younger age, quality of erections before surgery, and the absence of damage to the neurovascular bundles. In general, erectile function begins to return ~6 months after surgery if neurovascular tissue has been preserved. Potency is reduced by half if at least one neurovascular bundle is sacrificed. Overall, with the availability of drugs such as sildenafil, intraurethral inserts of alprostadil, and intracavernosal injections of vasodilators, many patients recover satisfactory sexual function.

Radiation Therapy Radiation therapy is given by external beam, by radioactive sources implanted into the gland, or by a combination of the two techniques.

External beam radiation therapy Contemporary external beam intensity-modulated radiation therapy (IMRT) permits shaping of the dose and allows the delivery of higher doses to the prostate and a dramatic reduction in normal tissue exposure compared with three-dimensional conformal treatment alone. These advances have enabled the safe administration of doses >80 Gy and resulted in higher local control rates and fewer side effects.

Cancer control after radiation therapy has been defined by various criteria, including a decline in PSA to <0.5 or 1 ng/mL, "nonrising" PSA values, and a negative biopsy of the prostate 2 years after completion of treatment. The current standard definition of biochemical failure (the Phoenix definition) is a rise in PSA by ≥2 ng/mL higher than the lowest PSA achieved. Radiation dose is critical to the eradication of prostate cancer. In a representative study, a PSA nadir of <1.0 ng/mL was achieved in 90% of patients receiving 81.0 Gy versus 76% and 56% of those receiving 70.2 and 64.8 Gy, respectively. Positive biopsy rates at 2.5 years were 4% for those treated with 81 Gy versus 27% and 36% for those receiving 75.6 and 70.2 Gy, respectively.

Hypofractionation schedules, utilizing fewer treatments of higher radiation doses, have been evaluated and shown to provide good cancer control rates based on posttreatment biopsies showing no evidence of cancer, with no apparent increase in treatment-related morbidity. Hypofractionated treatments can range from as few as 5 treatments to upward of 26 treatments, both regimens representing substantial reductions in treatment length.

Multiple clinical trials have evaluated the use of androgen deprivation therapy (ADT) in combination with radiation. In patients with unfavorable intermediate-risk prostate cancer, short-course ADT (6 months), when combined with external beam radiotherapy, has demonstrated significant improvements in overall survival. In patients with high-risk disease, longer courses of ADT (18–36 months) have proven superior to shorter courses and represent the current standard of care when combined with radiotherapy.

The Prostate Testing for Cancer and Treatment (ProtecT) trial investigated the effects of active monitoring, radical prostatectomy, and radical radiotherapy with hormones on patient-reported outcomes in men diagnosed with low- and intermediate-risk prostate cancer (~75% with Gleason score 6 or grade group 1 cancer). Patient-reported outcomes among 1643 men who completed questionnaires before diagnosis, at 6 and 12 months, and annually thereafter were compared. Of the three treatments, prostatectomy had the greatest negative effect on sexual function and urinary continence, and although there was some recovery, these outcomes remained worse in the prostatectomy group than in the other groups throughout the trial. The negative effect of radiotherapy on sexual function was greatest at 6 months, but sexual function then recovered somewhat and was stable thereafter; radiotherapy had little effect on urinary continence. Sexual and urinary function declined gradually in the active-monitoring group. Bowel function was worse in the radiotherapy group at 6 months than in the other groups but then recovered somewhat, except for the increasing frequency of bloody stools; bowel function was unchanged in the other groups. Urinary voiding and nocturia were worse in the radiotherapy group at 6 months but then mostly recovered and were like the other groups after 12 months. Effects on quality of life mirrored the reported changes in function. No significant differences were observed among the groups in measures of anxiety, depression, or general health-related or cancer-related quality of life.

Brachytherapy Brachytherapy is the direct implantation of radioactive sources (seeds) into the prostate. It is based on the principle that the deposition of radiation energy in tissues decreases as a function of the square of the distance from the source (**Chap. 73**). The goal is to deliver intensive irradiation to the prostate, minimizing the exposure of the surrounding tissues. The current standard technique achieves a more homogeneous dose distribution by placing seeds according to a customized template based on imaging assessment of the cancer and computer-optimized dosimetry. The implantation is performed transperineally as an outpatient procedure with real-time imaging.

Improvements in brachytherapy techniques have resulted in fewer complications and a marked reduction in local failure rates. In a series of 197 patients followed for a median of 3 years, 5-year actuarial PSA relapse–free survival for patients with pretherapy PSA levels of 0–4, 4–10, and >10 ng/mL were 98, 90, and 89%, respectively. In a separate report of 201 patients who underwent posttreatment biopsies, 80% were negative, 17% were indeterminate, and 3% were positive. The results did not change with longer follow-up. Brachytherapy is well tolerated, although most patients experience urinary frequency and urgency that can persist for several months. Higher complication rates are observed in patients who have undergone a prior transurethral resection of the prostate (TURP), while those with obstructive symptoms at baseline are at a higher risk for retention and persistent voiding symptoms. Proctitis has been reported in <2% of patients.

Active surveillance With the advent of PSA testing, many patients are diagnosed with low-risk prostate cancers that may not pose a threat to either the quantity or quality of man's life. Active surveillance, described previously as *watchful waiting* or *deferred therapy*, evolved from (1) studies that evaluated predominantly elderly men with well-differentiated tumors who remained untreated and demonstrated no clinically significant progression for protracted periods, (2) recognition of the contrast between incidence and disease-specific mortality, (3) the high prevalence of autopsy cancers, and (4) an effort to reduce overtreatment and treatment-related side effects. In practice, active surveillance is the treatment recommended to patients with cancers of low aggressiveness that can be safely monitored at fixed intervals with DREs, PSA measurements, imaging (usually prostate MRI), and repeat prostate biopsies as indicated until histopathologic or serologic changes correlative of progression warrant treatment with curative intent.

Case selection is critical, and determining the clinical parameters predictive of cancer aggressiveness that can be used to reliably select men most likely to benefit from active surveillance is an area of intense study. One set of criteria includes men with clinical T1c tumors that are biopsy Gleason grade 6 (grade group 1) involving three or fewer cores, with each core having <50% involvement by tumor, and a PSA density of <0.15. Nomograms to help predict which patients can safely be managed by active surveillance continue to be refined, and as their predictive accuracy improves, it can be anticipated that more patients will be candidates.

RISING PSA AFTER DEFINITIVE LOCAL THERAPY

Patients in this state include those in whom the sole manifestation of disease is a rising PSA after surgery and/or radiation therapy. There is no evidence of disease on imaging studies. For these patients, the central issue is whether the rise in PSA results from persistent disease in the primary site, systemic disease, or both. In theory, disease in the primary site may still be curable by additional local treatment.

The decision to recommend radiation therapy after prostatectomy is guided by the pathologic findings at surgery, the timing of PSA failure, and the PSA level at the time of failure. Traditional imaging (MRI, CT, and radionucleotide bone scans), especially at low levels of PSA, are typically uninformative. New positron emission tomography (PET) tracers such as C-11 choline, F-18 fluciclovine, and F-18 or Ga-68 prostate-specific membrane antigen (PSMA) that directly image the cancer are more sensitive and can detect low-volume disease in the prostate bed or other sites to better inform the decision to recommend additional local therapies. All are FDA approved. Detection rates, both in and outside the prostate bed, correlate with the absolute level of PSA. Factors that predict for response to salvage radiation therapy are a positive surgical margin, lower Gleason score in the radical prostatectomy specimen, long interval from surgery to PSA failure, slow PSA doubling time, and low (<0.5 ng/mL) PSA value at the time of radiation treatment. For patients with a rising PSA after radiation therapy, salvage local therapy can be considered if the disease was "curable" at the outset, if persistent disease has been documented by a biopsy of the prostate, and if no disease is detectable outside of the prostate bed or regional lymph nodes by imaging. Unfortunately, case selection is poorly defined in most series, and morbidities are significant. Options include salvage radical prostatectomy, salvage cryotherapy, salvage radiation therapy, and salvage high-intensity focused ultrasound.

The rise in PSA after surgery or radiation therapy may indicate subclinical or micrometastatic disease with or without local recurrence. In these cases, the need for treatment depends, in part, on the estimated probability that the patient will show evidence of metastatic disease on a scan and in what time frame. That immediate therapy is not always required was shown in a series where patients who developed a rising PSA after radical prostatectomy received no systemic therapy until metastatic disease was documented. Overall, the median time to metastatic progression was 8 years, and 63% of the patients with rising PSA values remained free of metastases at 5 years. Factors associated with progression included the Gleason score of the radical prostatectomy specimen, time to recurrence after surgery, and PSA doubling time. For those with Gleason score ≥8, the probability of metastatic progression was 37, 51, and 71% at 3, 5, and 7 years, respectively. If the time to recurrence was <2 years and PSA doubling time was long (>10 months), the proportions with metastatic disease at the same time intervals were 23, 32, and 53%, versus 47, 69, and 79% if the doubling time was short (<10 months). PSA doubling times are also prognostic for survival. In one series, all patients who succumbed to disease had PSA doubling times of ≤3 months. Most physicians advise treatment when PSA doubling times are ≤12 months. A difficulty with predicting the risk of metastatic spread, symptoms, or death from disease in the rising PSA state is that most patients receive some form of therapy before the development of metastases. Nevertheless, predictive models continue to be refined.

METASTATIC DISEASE: NONCASTRATE

The state of *noncastrate metastatic disease* includes men with metastases visible on an imaging study at the time of diagnosis or after local therapy(ies) who have testosterone levels >150 ng/dL. Symptoms of metastatic disease include pain from osseous spread, although many patients are asymptomatic despite extensive spread. Less common are symptoms related to marrow infiltration by tumor (myelophthisis), coagulopathy, or spinal cord compression. Standard treatment is to deplete or lower androgens via ADT by medical or surgical means, the latter being the least acceptable to patients. A less frequently used approach is to block androgen binding to the AR with antiandrogens. More than 90% of male hormones originate in the testes; <10% are synthesized in the adrenal gland (**Fig. 87-3**).

Testosterone-Lowering Agents Medical therapies that lower testosterone levels include the GnRH agonists/antagonists, pure GnRH antagonists, 17,20-lyase inhibitors, CYP17 inhibitors, and estrogens such as diethylstilbestrol (DES). The latter are rarely utilized due to the risk of vascular complications that include fluid retention, phlebitis, emboli, and stroke. GnRH agonists/antagonists, such as leuprolide acetate and goserelin acetate, initially produce a rise in luteinizing hormone and follicle-stimulating hormone followed by a downregulation of receptors in the pituitary gland, which effects a chemical castration. Regulatory approval was based on randomized trials showing reduced cardiovascular toxicities relative to DES, with equivalent potency. The initial rise in testosterone may result in a clinical flare of the disease, and as such, these agents are relatively contraindicated in men with significant obstructive symptoms, cancer-related pain, or spinal cord compromise, events that do not occur with GnRH antagonists such as degarelix, given by injection, or relugolix, given orally, that rapidly achieve castrate levels of testosterone. AR antagonists that block testosterone binding to the receptor are also used to prevent flare.

Agents that lower testosterone are associated with an androgen-deprivation syndrome that includes hot flushes, weakness, fatigue, loss of muscle mass, anemia, changes in cognition and personality, and depression. Changes in lipids, obesity, insulin resistance, and an increased risk of diabetes and cardiovascular disease are also seen, along with a decrease in bone density that worsens over time and results in an increased risk of clinical fractures. This is a particular concern in men with preexisting osteopenia that results from hypogonadism that may be worsened with steroid or alcohol use and significantly underappreciated. Baseline fracture risk can be assessed using the FRAX scale, and to minimize fracture risk, patients are advised to take calcium and vitamin D supplementation, along with a bisphosphonate, RANK-ligand inhibitor (denosumab), or toremifene.

Antiandrogens Nonsteroidal first-generation antiandrogens such bicalutamide and nilutamide have largely been replaced by the more potent next-generation agents (enzalutamide, apalutamide, and darolutamide) that do not lower serum androgen levels and result in fewer hot flushes, less of an effect on libido, less muscle wasting, fewer personality changes, and less bone loss relative to testosterone-lowering therapies. However, over time, testosterone

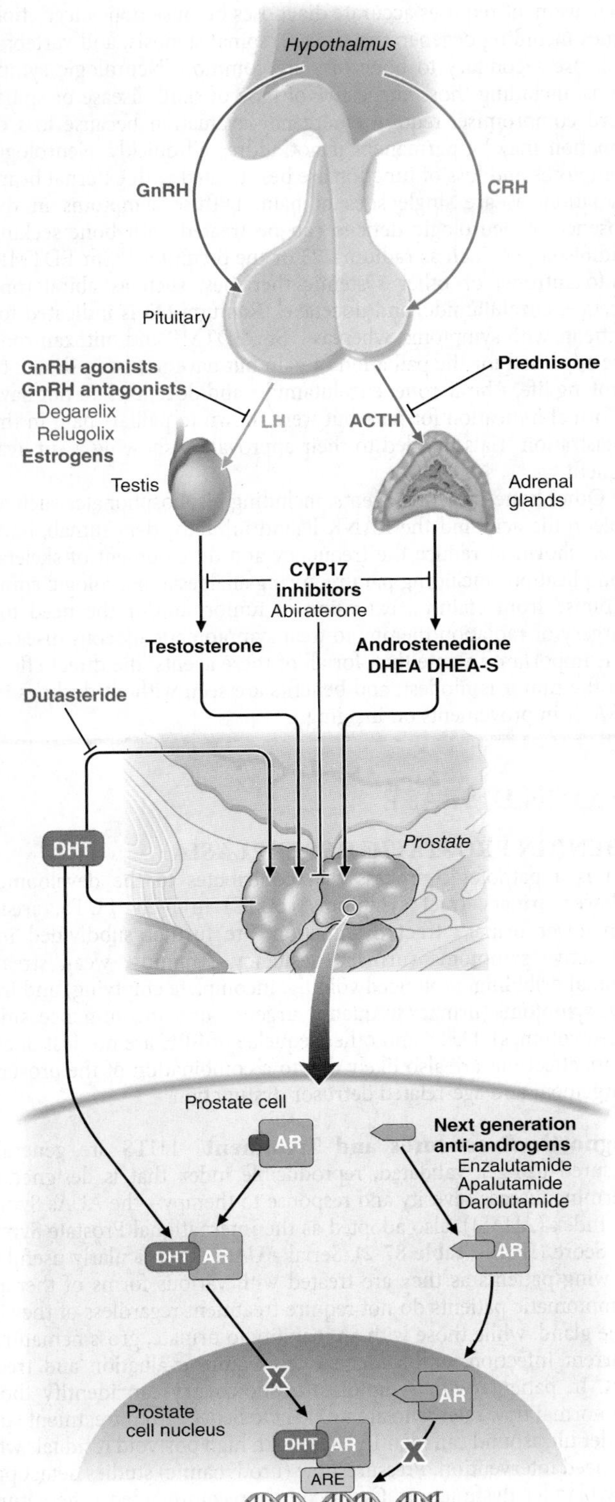

FIGURE 87-3 Sites of action of different hormone therapies.

levels increase and are converted to estrogen, which can result in mastalgia and gynecomastia that limits long-term use but can be prevented in part by tamoxifen or prophylactic breast irradiation.

Most reported randomized trials suggest that the cancer-specific outcomes are inferior when antiandrogens are used alone. Bicalutamide, even at a dose of 150 mg (three times the approved dose for use in combination in GnRH agonists), resulted in a shorter time to progression and inferior survival compared with surgical castration for patients with established metastatic disease.

Improving on the outcomes with ADT alone was a focus of the field for decades. One approach was to combine a first-generation antiandrogen (flutamide, bicalutamide, or nilutamide) with a GnRH analogue or surgical orchiectomy; however, this approach did not improve outcomes, and current use is largely limited to the first 2–4 weeks of treatment to protect against flare.

Practice standards changed when an improvement in time to progression and overall survival was shown when ADT was combined with docetaxel, the first systemic therapy shown to prolong life in metastatic castration-resistant prostate cancer (mCRPC) approved in 2004, relative to ADT alone. The greatest benefit was seen for patients with "high-volume" disease defined as the presence of ≥4 lesions on radionuclide bone scan or visceral disease. For abiraterone acetate and prednisone, benefit was seen across disease states ranging from high-risk localized to metastatic disease. Longer progression-free and overall survival times have been noted in separate phase 3 trials comparing ADT with abiraterone, a CYP17 inhibitor that blocks androgen synthesis, and ADT with the AR antagonists enzalutamide and apalutamide versus the ADT standard, further changing the standards of care.

Intermittent Androgen Deprivation Therapy (IADT) One way to reduce the side effects of androgen depletion is to administer antiandrogens on an intermittent basis. This was proposed as a way to prevent the selection of cells that are resistant to androgen depletion. The hypothesis is that by allowing endogenous testosterone levels to rise, the cells that survive androgen depletion will induce a normal differentiation pathway. In this way, the surviving cells that are allowed to proliferate in the presence of androgen will retain sensitivity to subsequent androgen depletion. Applied in the clinic, androgen depletion is continued for 2–6 months beyond the point of maximal response. Once treatment is stopped, endogenous testosterone levels increase, and the symptoms associated with hormone treatment abate. PSA levels also begin to rise, and at some level, treatment is restarted. With this approach, multiple cycles of regression and proliferation have been documented in individual patients. Unknown is whether the intermittent approach increases, decreases, or does not change the overall duration of sensitivity to androgen depletion. The approach is safe, but long-term data are needed to assess the course in men with low PSA levels. A trial to address this question is ongoing.

Outcomes of Androgen Deprivation The anti–prostate cancer effects of the various androgen depletion strategies are similar, and the clinical course is predictable: an initial response, a period of stability in which tumor cells are dormant and nonproliferative, followed after a variable period of time by a rise in PSA and regrowth that is visible on a scan as a castration-resistant lesion. Androgen depletion is not curative because cells that survive castration are present when the disease is first diagnosed. Considered by disease manifestation, PSA levels return to normal in 60–70% of patients, and measurable disease regression occurs in 50%; improvements in bone scan occur in 25% of cases, but the majority remain stable. Duration of survival is inversely proportional to disease extent at the time androgen depletion is first started and the nadir level of PSA at 6 months. Patients with nadir values above a certain threshold have markedly inferior survival times and should be considered for alternative approaches.

An unresolved question remains on how early systemic therapies should be offered to patients: in the adjuvant setting after surgery or radiation treatment of the primary tumor; at the time that a PSA recurrence is documented; or wait until metastatic disease or symptoms of disease are manifest? Trials in support of early therapy have been largely underpowered relative to the reported benefit or have been criticized on methodologic grounds. One that showed a survival benefit for patients treated with radiation therapy and 3 years of ADT, relative to radiation alone, was criticized for the poor outcomes of the control group. Another showing a survival benefit for patients with positive lymph nodes who were randomized to immediate medical or surgical castration compared with observation ($p = .02$) was criticized because the confidence intervals around the 5- and 8-year survival distributions for the two groups overlapped.

METASTATIC DISEASE: CASTRATE

Castration-resistant prostate cancer (CRPC), disease that progresses while the measured levels of testosterone in the blood are 50 ng/mL or lower, can produce some of the most feared complications of the disease and is lethal for most men. The most common manifestation is a rising PSA, frequently co-occurring with progression in bone. Nodal and/or visceral spread is less frequent. Symptoms may or may not be present. The bone- and PSA-dominant pattern limits the ability to assess treatment effects reliably because traditional bone imaging is inaccurate and no PSA-based outcome has been shown to be a true surrogate for survival, and accordingly, favorable changes with either can be used to support regulatory approvals. Critical for management is that therapeutic objectives be based on the manifestations of the disease in the individual at the time a change in therapy is being considered. As such, for the patient with symptomatic bone disease, relief of pain can be more clinically relevant than lowering the PSA. Naturally, for all patients, the central focus is delaying or preventing disease progression, symptoms, and death from disease.

Through 2010, docetaxel was the only FDA-approved life-prolonging therapy for CRPC. Since then, our understanding of the biology of the disease has increased significantly, which in turn has led to improved therapies. In particular, it is now recognized that the majority of mCRPCs continue to express the AR and remain AR signaling dependent, and upward of 50% of cases harbor a series of oncogenic changes including overexpression, splice variants lacking the ligand binding domain and that stimulate growth independent of the ligand, and upregulation of the enzymes in the androgen biosynthesis pathway, leading to an increase in intratumoral androgens. These oncogenic changes have been successfully targeted with the next-generation antiandrogens enzalutamide, apalutamide, and darolutamide and the CYP17 inhibitor abiraterone acetate (given in combination with prednisone), all of which have been proven to prolong life and are FDA approved for use in CRPC in both the pre- and postchemotherapy setting.

Large-scale molecular profiling efforts have led to a biologically based disease taxonomy that continues to evolve and showed a markedly higher than expected frequency of germline and somatic *BRCA2* alterations, along with other genes in the DNA damage repair pathway that have been targeted successfully with poly-ADP ribose polymerase (PARP) inhibitors of which two, olaparib and rucaparib, are FDA approved, and one, niraparib, has achieved a breakthrough designation. Also approved is the checkpoint inhibitor pembrolizumab for tumors with high microsatellite instability (MSI) scores, an alteration found in 2–3% of prostate cancers for which a dedicated prostate cancer trial would never have been conducted.

Other classes of therapy are approved based on a demonstrated survival benefits include the biologic agent sipuleucel-T, the second-generation taxane cabazitaxel, and the α-emitting bone-targeting radiopharmaceutical radium-223. Approval is also anticipated for PSMA-directed radionuclide therapy based on the survival benefit of Lu-177 PSMA in the phase 3 VISION trial relative to best supportive care alone. Overall, an intense focus of current CRPC research is to understand the optimal sequence in which to utilize these agents to maximize benefit for the individual patient. Most of these agents are also being tested earlier in the course of the disease when tumor burdens are lower and the disease less heterogeneous. The result has been an increase in the frequency of late-state tumors that have undergone a lineage transformation from epithelial to neuroendocrine phenotypes and are highly resistant to available therapies.

Pain Management Pain secondary to osseous metastases is one of the most feared complications of the disease and a major cause of morbidity, worsened by the narcotics needed to control symptoms. Management requires accurate diagnoses because noncancer etiologies including degenerative disease, spinal stenosis, and vertebral collapse secondary to bone loss are common. Neurologic symptoms, including those suggestive of base of skull disease or spinal cord compromise, require emergency evaluation because loss of function may be permanent if not addressed quickly. Neurologic symptoms and loss of function are best treated with external beam radiation, as are single sites of pain. Diffuse symptoms in the absence of neurologic deficits can be treated with bone-seeking radioisotopes, such as radium-223 or the β emitter ^{153}Sm-EDTMP; mitoxantrone; or other systemic therapies, such as abiraterone acetate, enzalutamide, and docetaxel. Radium-223 is indicated for patients with symptoms, whereas ^{153}Sm-EDTMP and mitoxantrone are approved for the palliation of pain but have not been shown to prolong life. Abiraterone, enzalutamide, and docetaxel do not have a formal indication for pain but were shown to palliate pain in the registration trials that led to their approval by showing a survival benefit.

Other bone-targeting agents, including bisphosphonates such as zoledronic acid and the RANK-ligand inhibitor denosumab, have been shown to reduce the frequency and development of skeletal complications including pain requiring analgesia, neurologic compromise from epidural extension of tumor, and/or the need for surgery or radiation therapy to treat symptomatic osseous disease. It is important to note that, for all of these agents, the direct effect on the tumor is modest, and benefits are seen without declines in PSA or improvements on imaging.

BENIGN DISEASE

BENIGN PROSTATIC HYPERPLASIA

BPH is a pathologic process that contributes to the development of lower urinary tract symptoms (LUTS) in men. LUTS, arising from lower urinary tract dysfunction, are further subdivided into obstructive symptoms (urinary hesitancy, straining, weak stream, terminal dribbling, prolonged voiding, incomplete emptying) and irritative symptoms (urinary frequency, urgency, urge incontinence, small voided volumes). LUTS and other sequelae of BPH are not just due to a mass effect but are also likely due to a combination of the prostatic enlargement and age-related detrusor dysfunction.

Diagnostic Procedures and Treatment LUTS are generally measured using a validated, reproducible index that is designed to determine disease severity and response to therapy—the AUA's Symptom Index (AUASI), also adopted as the International Prostate Symptom Score (IPSS) (**Table 87-2**). Serial AUASI is particularly useful in following patients as they are treated with various forms of therapy. Asymptomatic patients do not require treatment regardless of the size of the gland, while those with an inability to urinate, gross hematuria, recurrent infection, or bladder stones require evaluation and treatment. In patients with symptoms, uroflowmetry can identify those with normal flow rates who are unlikely to benefit from treatment, and bladder ultrasound can identify those with high postvoid residuals who may need intervention. Pressure-flow (urodynamic) studies detect primary bladder dysfunction. Cystoscopy is recommended if hematuria is documented and to assess the urinary outflow tract before surgery. Imaging of the upper tracts is advised for patients with hematuria, a history of calculi, or prior urinary tract problems.

Symptomatic relief is the most common reason men seek treatment for BPH, and therefore, symptomatic relief is usually the goal of therapy for BPH. α-Adrenergic receptor antagonists are thought to treat the dynamic aspect of BPH by reducing sympathetic tone of the bladder outlet, thereby decreasing resistance and improving urinary flow. 5ARIs are thought to treat the static aspect of BPH by reducing prostate volume and having a similar, albeit delayed effect. 5ARIs have also proven beneficial in the prevention of BPH progression, as measured by prostate volume, the risk of developing acute urinary retention, and the risk of having BPH-related surgery. The use of an alpha-adrenergic

TABLE 87-2 AUA Symptom Index

QUESTIONS TO BE ANSWERED	AUA SYMPTOM SCORE (CIRCLE 1 NUMBER ON EACH LINE)					
	NOT AT ALL	LESS THAN 1 TIME IN 5	LESS THAN HALF THE TIME	ABOUT HALF THE TIME	MORE THAN HALF THE TIME	ALMOST ALWAYS
Over the past month, how often have you had a sensation of not emptying your bladder completely after you finished urinating?	0+	1	2	3	4	5
Over the past month, how often have you had to urinate again less than 2 h after you finished urinating?	0	1	2	3	4	5
Over the past month, how often have you found you stopped and started again several times when you urinated?	0	1	2	3	4	5
Over the past month, how often have you found it difficult to postpone urination?	0	1	2	3	4	5
Over the past month, how often have you had a weak urinary stream?	0	1	2	3	4	5
Over the past month, how often have you had to push or strain to begin urination?	0	1	2	3	4	5
Over the past month, how many times did you most typically get up to urinate from the time you went to bed at night until the time you got up in the morning?	(None)	(1 time)	(2 times)	(3 times)	(4 times)	(5 times)
Sum of 7 circled numbers (AUA Symptom Score): ____						

Abbreviation: AUA, American Urological Association.
Source: Reproduced with permission from MJ Barry et al: The American Urological Association symptom index for benign prostatic hyperplasia. The Measurement Committee of the American Urological Association. J Urol 148:1549, 1992.

receptor antagonist and a 5ARI as combination therapy seeks to provide symptomatic relief while preventing progression of BPH.

Another class of medications that has shown improvement in LUTS secondary to BPH is phosphodiesterase-5 (PDE5) inhibitors, used currently in the treatment of erectile dysfunction. All four of the PDE5 inhibitors available in the United States—sildenafil, vardenafil, tadalafil, and avanafil—appear to be effective in the treatment of LUTS secondary to BPH. The use of PDE5 inhibitors is not without controversy, however, given the fact that short-acting phosphodiesterase inhibitors such as sildenafil need to be dosed separately from alpha blockers such as tamsulosin because of potential hypotensive effects.

Symptoms due to BPH often coexist with symptoms due to overactive bladder, and the most common pharmacologic agents for the treatment of overactive bladder symptoms are anticholinergics. This has led to multiple studies evaluating the efficacy of anticholinergics for the treatment of LUTS secondary to BPH.

Surgical therapy is now considered second-line therapy and is usually reserved for patients after a trial of medical therapy. The goal of surgical therapy is to reduce the size of the prostate, effectively reducing resistance to urine flow. Surgical approaches include TURP, transurethral incision, or removal of the gland via a retropubic, suprapubic, or perineal approach. Also used are transurethral ultrasound-guided laser-induced prostatectomy (TULIP), stents, and hyperthermia.

■ FURTHER READING

Barry MJ, Simmons LH: Prevention of prostate cancer morbidity and mortality: Primary prevention and early detection. Med Clin North Am 101:787, 2017.

Battaglia A et al: Novel insights into the management of oligometastatic prostate cancer: A comprehensive review. Eur Urol Oncol 2:174, 2019.

Buyyounouski MK et al: Prostate cancer—major changes in the American Joint Committee on Cancer eighth edition cancer staging manual. CA Cancer J Clin 67:245, 2017.

Calais J et al: ^{18}F-fluciclovine PET-CT and ^{68}Ga-PSMA-11 PET-CT in patients with early biochemical recurrence after prostatectomy: A prospective, single-centre, single-arm, comparative imaging trial. Lancet Oncol 20:1286, 2019.

De Vries KC et al: Hypofractionated versus conventionally fractionated radiation therapy for patients with intermediate- or high-risk, localized, prostate cancer: 7-year outcomes from the randomized, multicenter, open-label, phase 3 HYPRO trial. Int J Radiat Oncol Biol Phys 106:108, 2020.

Hussain M et al: Survival with olaparib in metastatic castration-resistant prostate cancer. N Engl J Med 383:2345, 2020.

Jairath NK et al: A systematic review of the evidence for the decipher genomic classifier in prostate cancer. Eur Urol 79:374, 2021.

Merseburger AS et al: Genomic testing in patients with metastatic castration-resistant prostate cancer: A pragmatic guide for clinicians. Eur Urol 79:519, 2021.

Shore ND et al: Oral relugolix for androgen-deprivation therapy in advanced prostate cancer. N Engl J Med 382:2187, 2020.

Virgo KS et al: Initial management of noncastrate advanced, recurrent, or metastatic prostate cancer: ASCO guideline update. J Clin Oncol 39:1274, 2021.

Yamada Y et al: Clinical and biological features of neuroendocrine prostate cancer. Curr Oncol Rep 23:15, 2021.

88 Testicular Cancer

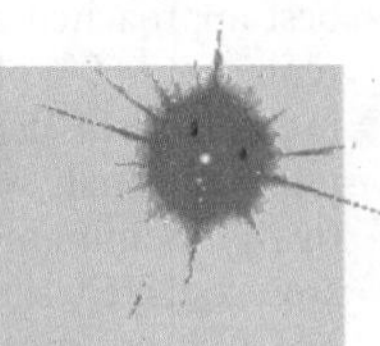

David J. Vaughn

Testicular germ cell tumors (GCTs) represent 95% of all testicular neoplasms. Non-GCTs of the testis are much less common. Approximately 5% of GCTs arise in extragonadal locations including the mediastinum, retroperitoneum, and pineal gland. Treatment for testicular GCTs is determined by pathology and stage. The development of effective chemotherapy for this disease represents a landmark achievement in oncology. About 95% of newly diagnosed patients with testicular GCTs will be cured. For this reason, testicular cancer has been called "a model for a curable neoplasm."

INCIDENCE

In 2021, ~9500 cases of testicular GCTs will be diagnosed in the United States, with <450 deaths. These tumors are diagnosed most commonly in men between 20 and 40 years. The incidence of GCTs is increasing in men age 50 years and older.

GLOBAL CONSIDERATIONS

The incidence of testicular GCTs appears to be increasing worldwide. The disease has the highest incidence in Scandinavia, Western Europe, and Australia/New Zealand. Africa and Asia have the lowest incidence. The incidence in the United States and the United Kingdom is intermediate. While there does not appear to be a distinct biology related to geography, several countries have reported a migration to earlier stage disease in part related to public awareness and earlier diagnosis.

EPIDEMIOLOGY

GCTs are predominantly seen in young Caucasian men. The disease is much less commonly seen in African Americans. Testicular GCTs have an estimated heritability of almost 50%. Interestingly, the risk of GCT is higher in male siblings than in offspring of the patient. Although epidemiologic studies have been performed attempting to identify a relationship with environmental exposures, no conclusive causal links have been established.

Risk Factors The strongest risk factors for testicular GCT include a prior history of the disease, cryptorchidism, and a history of testicular germ cell neoplasia in situ (GCNIS). Patients with a prior history of testicular GCT have a 2% risk of developing a contralateral GCT. These are more commonly metachronous than synchronous. Men with cryptorchidism have approximately a four- to sixfold increased risk of developing testicular GCT. Orchidopexy before puberty decreases but does not eliminate this risk. Interestingly, the contralateral descended testis is also at risk for this disease. Men undergoing infertility evaluation in which a testicular biopsy demonstrates GCNIS have a significant risk of developing GCT. Although scrotal ultrasound of patients with testicular GCT may demonstrate testicular microcalcifications that may be related to GCNIS, the significance of testicular microcalcifications in the general population is unclear.

BIOLOGY

The primordial germ cell is the cell of origin for GCTs. Most malignant GCTs arise from GCNIS. The molecular events that result in the development of GCNIS and subsequent malignant GCT have not been fully determined. However, genetic analysis of GCTs has demonstrated an excess copy number of isochromosome 12p (i[12p]) in most cases. Several genome-wide association studies have identified multiple independent loci associated with testicular GCT risk. The strongest of these is the *KITLG* (KIT ligand) locus on chromosome 12. These loci contribute significantly to the heritable risk of this disease.

PATHOLOGY

GCTs are either seminomas or nonseminomas. For a tumor to be considered a seminoma, it must be 100% seminoma. Any mixed GCT is best approached as a nonseminomatous GCT (NSGCT). Seminomas represent ~50% of cases. Seminomas arise most commonly in patients in the fourth decade of life. Seminomas may contain syncytiotrophoblastic cells, which may secrete β human chorionic gonadotropin (hCG). Seminomas do not secrete α fetoprotein (AFP). Seminomas are exquisitely sensitive to both chemotherapy and radiation therapy. NSGCTs are most commonly diagnosed in the third decade of life. The histologic subtypes include embryonal carcinoma, yolk sac tumor, choriocarcinoma, and teratoma. Embryonal carcinoma is the most undifferentiated NSGCT subtype with the potential to differentiate into the other subtypes. Embryonal carcinoma may secrete AFP, hCG, both, or neither. Yolk sac tumor often secretes AFP. Choriocarcinoma is an aggressive subtype, often secreting hCG at very high levels. These NSGCT subtypes are all considered chemotherapy sensitive. Teratoma is composed of somatic cell types that are derived from two or more germinal layers (endoderm, mesoderm, and ectoderm). Teratomas are classified as mature, in which cell types resemble normal adult somatic tissue; immature, in which cell types resemble fetal somatic tissue; and malignant, in which the cell types have undergone malignant transformation into the malignant counterpart of the somatic tissue. Teratomas are chemotherapy resistant and must be approached surgically.

INITIAL PRESENTATION

Signs and Symptoms Although a painless testicular mass is pathognomonic of a GCT, most patients present with testicular swelling, firmness, discomfort, or a combination of these. The differential diagnosis may include epididymitis or orchitis and a trial of antibacterials may be considered. Patients with retroperitoneal metastases may complain of back or flank pain. Patients may have cough, shortness of breath, or hemoptysis as a result of lung metastases. In patients with elevation of serum hCG, gynecomastia may be present. Diagnostic delay is not uncommon and may be associated with a more advanced stage at diagnosis.

Physical Examination Careful examination of the affected testis and the contralateral normal testis should be performed. Many tumors will have a hard consistency to palpation. Some patients may show testicular atrophy. Evaluation for supraclavicular lymphadenopathy, gynecomastia, and abdominal mass should be performed. Inguinal lymphadenopathy is rare. Most patients with lung metastases will have normal auscultation of the lungs.

Diagnostic Testing If a firm testicular mass is identified, a scrotal ultrasound should be performed. Patients with suspected epididymitis or orchitis who do not respond to antibiotics should also undergo scrotal ultrasound. Scrotal ultrasound should include both testicles. On ultrasound, a testicular GCT is hypoechoic and may be multifocal. A solid mass identified on ultrasound should be considered malignant until otherwise proven. Transscrotal aspiration or biopsy of a testicular mass should never be performed. Such scrotal violation may result in tumor seeding of the scrotum or inguinal lymph nodes.

Serum Tumor Markers Serum AFP, hCG, and lactate dehydrogenase (LDH) should be measured in patients suspected of testicular GCT. AFP is elevated in ~60–70% of patients who present with NSGCTs. Seminomas never secrete AFP. A patient with a seminoma with elevation of AFP should be approached as having an NSGCT. The half-life of AFP is 5–7 days. A falsely elevated AFP may be seen in patients with hepatic disease or a condition called hereditary persistence of AFP, in which patients may have baseline AFP levels that are mildly elevated. hCG may be elevated in both NSGCTs as well as seminomas. Patients with choriocarcinoma may have markedly elevated levels of hCG. The half-life for hCG is 24–36 h. False-positive elevation of hCG may be seen secondary to hypogonadism, marijuana use, or as a result of interfering substances measured by the assay. LDH is a nonspecific marker for GCT. Its principal use is to help in the assessment of the risk classification of a patient with metastatic disease. Although elevation of serum tumor markers supports the diagnosis of a testicular GCT, it should be remembered that most patients with seminoma and up to a third of patients with NSGCTs do not have elevated levels. Serum microRNA (miR)-371a-3 has been identified as a promising biomarker for GCT, and validation studies are ongoing.

INITIAL MANAGEMENT

Inguinal Orchiectomy Prompt referral to urology should be performed if a testicular GCT is suspected. The initial treatment for most patients suspected of having a testicular GCT is radical inguinal orchiectomy with removal of the testicle and spermatic cord to the level of the internal inguinal ring. In patients who present with metastatic disease and the diagnosis of GCT is certain, orchiectomy may be deferred until completion of chemotherapy. Although some institutions perform testis-sparing surgery in select patients, the gold standard remains radical inguinal orchiectomy. Pathologic examination of the entire testicle is important, since testicular GCTs may be multifocal. Given the rarity of this cancer, review by an experienced pathologist is essential for accurate tumor classification. Serum tumor markers should be obtained before and after orchiectomy.

Staging The staging of testicular GCT is based on an understanding of the pattern of spread. The initial spread is by the lymphatic route to the retroperitoneal lymph nodes. A left-sided testicular GCT spreads first to the primary landing zone of left paraaortic lymph nodes inferior to the left renal vessels. A right-sided testicular GCT spreads first to the primary landing zone of the aortocaval nodes inferior to the right renal vessels. Nodal metastases may extend into the iliac regions. If scrotal violation occurred, inguinal lymph node metastases may be seen. Subsequent lymphatic spread is to the retrocrural, mediastinal, and supraclavicular lymph nodes. Hematogenous spread to the lung is the next most common site of metastasis. Metastases to the liver, bone, and brain are less commonly seen. Patients with newly diagnosed testicular GCTs should undergo computed tomography (CT) scan of the abdomen and pelvis. Chest x-ray should be performed. CT scan of the chest is performed if retroperitoneal metastases are present or if lung nodules are identified on chest x-ray. Bone scan and magnetic resonance imaging (MRI) of the brain are not routinely performed unless clinically indicated. Positron emission tomography (PET) has little role in the initial staging of testicular GCTs.

The American Joint Committee on Cancer tumor-node-metastasis (TNM) staging classification is used. There are three main stages of testicular GCT. Stage I is limited to the testis; stage II involves the retroperitoneal lymph nodes; and stage III includes lymph node involvement beyond the retroperitoneum and/or distant metastatic disease.

STAGE-BASED MANAGEMENT

Treatment of testicular GCT is based on two factors: (1) whether the tumor is seminoma or NSGCT and (2) the stage of the patient. This is summarized in **Fig. 88-1**.

Stage I • SEMINOMA About 70% of newly diagnosed patients with seminoma present with stage I disease. This is defined as no evidence of metastatic disease on imaging of the chest, abdomen, and pelvis. Approximately 15% of patients with stage I seminoma have metastatic disease at the microscopic level, usually in the retroperitoneum. Historically, patients with stage I seminoma were treated with a course of adjuvant radiation therapy to the paraaortic lymph nodes. While still an option, this is not usually performed because of concerns for late radiation-induced secondary malignancies. Active surveillance is the most common approach elected by these patients following orchiectomy. With active surveillance, interval physical examination and CT scan of the abdomen are performed. For the 15% of patients who develop metastatic disease during active surveillance, treatment with definitive radiation therapy or chemotherapy is curative in nearly all. A third option for clinical stage I seminoma is adjuvant chemotherapy with carboplatin monotherapy for one or two cycles. While effective in decreasing the risk of recurrence, it should be remembered that most patients are cured by orchiectomy alone, and therefore, the additional treatment is unnecessary. In addition, long-term data on toxicity are not available.

NSGCTs About 40% of newly diagnosed patients with NSGCTs present with stage I disease. Because NSGCTs have an increased potential for invasion and metastasis, spread to the retroperitoneum and beyond is more common than with seminoma. If pre-orchiectomy serum tumor markers are elevated, these must normalize after orchiectomy to be considered stage I. Patients with persistently elevated or rising serum tumor markers after orchiectomy have stage IS disease and should be treated with cisplatin-based chemotherapy. If the tumor is limited to testis without lymphovascular invasion, the risk of recurrence is approximately 20%. However, if the tumor has high-risk features including lymphovascular invasion, invasion of the spermatic cord, or invasion of the scrotum, the risk of recurrence is ~50% or higher. Historically, a prophylactic retroperitoneal lymph node dissection (RPLND) was performed. This surgery is not only diagnostic but also therapeutic. In fact, most patients who undergo prophylactic RPLND will never require chemotherapy. While still an option, this approach subjects many patients to unnecessary major abdominal surgery. RPLND is also associated with a small risk of retrograde ejaculation due to nerve injury, and nerve-sparing techniques have been developed. Active surveillance is frequently performed especially for patients without lymphovascular invasion. Most patients who relapse will be treated with cisplatin-based chemotherapy and achieve cure rates approaching 100%. Active surveillance can also be employed for patients with higher risk features, although the risk of progression is significantly higher. For this reason, some advocate adjuvant cisplatin-based chemotherapy with BEP (bleomycin, etoposide, cisplatin) for one cycle for these patients. Other centers favor a prophylactic RPLND. Almost all patients who present with stage I NSGCTs will achieve cure.

Stage II • SEMINOMA Approximately 15–20% of newly diagnosed patients with seminoma present with stage II disease. Patients are subgrouped into IIA, IIB, or IIC based on the size of the retroperitoneal nodes (≤2 cm, >2 to 5 cm, or >5 cm, respectively). Patients with stage IIA disease are usually treated with "dogleg" radiation therapy (referring to the shape of the radiation field), which includes the paraaortic and ipsilateral iliac nodes. Cisplatin-based chemotherapy may also be considered. Stage IIB disease is treated with cisplatin-based chemotherapy or, in select patients, radiation therapy. Most patients treated with radiation therapy who relapse will subsequently be cured with cisplatin-based chemotherapy. For patients with stage IIC disease, cisplatin-based chemotherapy should be used.

NSGCTs Approximately 15% of newly diagnosed patients with NSGCTs present with clinical stage II disease. Patients with stage IIA disease may be treated with primary RPLND. Alternatively, these patients may be treated with cisplatin-based chemotherapy. Patients with stage IIB and IIC disease are best initially managed with cisplatin-based chemotherapy.

Stage III Patients who present with stage III GCT (seminoma or NSGCT) are treated with cisplatin-based chemotherapy. These patients are classified into good-, intermediate-, or poor-risk categories using the International Germ Cell Consensus Classification system, which is based on clinical factors including histology, site of primary, the presence of nonpulmonary visceral metastatic disease, and the level of postorchiectomy serum tumor markers (**Table 88-1**). Most patients with stage III GCT present with good-risk disease; >90% will be cured. The remainder present with intermediate-risk or poor-risk disease, associated with 5-year survival rates of ~80% and 50%, respectively. Select patients with rapidly progressive metastatic disease and life-threatening symptoms such as hemoptysis in whom there is a high clinical suspicion of GCT should emergently initiate cisplatin-based chemotherapy, even without a tissue diagnosis.

Chemotherapy The development of cisplatin-based chemotherapy represents an important advance in cancer medicine. Through a series of carefully performed clinical trials with the aim of maximizing cure while minimizing the extent of treatment, the chemotherapy approach to the treatment of these patients has been standardized. Patients with good-risk metastatic GCT are treated with either three cycles of BEP or four cycles of etoposide and cisplatin (EP). Patients with intermediate- and poor-risk metastatic disease are treated with either four cycles of BEP or four cycles of etoposide, ifosfamide, and cisplatin (VIP). Maintaining dose and schedule is important, as dose modifications and delays have been associated with inferior outcomes. Serum tumor markers should be monitored throughout treatment and should normalize during or after treatment. Cisplatin-based chemotherapy is associated with myelosuppression, nausea and vomiting, and alopecia. Cisplatin may result in nephrotoxicity, ototoxicity, and peripheral neuropathy. Bleomycin may result in pulmonary toxicity, and risk factors for this include age >40, renal failure, tobacco use, and the cumulative dose of bleomycin received. For patients at increased risk of bleomycin-induced pneumonitis, non-bleomycin-containing regimens as noted above may be given. Cisplatin-based chemotherapy is also associated with sterility. Approximately 30% of newly diagnosed testicular GCT patients have severe oligospermia or azoospermia. For the remainder with normal baseline spermatogenesis who receive cisplatin-based chemotherapy, all will be azoospermic at the completion of therapy. Approximately 80% of these patients will recover spermatogenesis over a period of several years. For this reason, prechemotherapy sperm banking should be offered to all patients treated with chemotherapy.

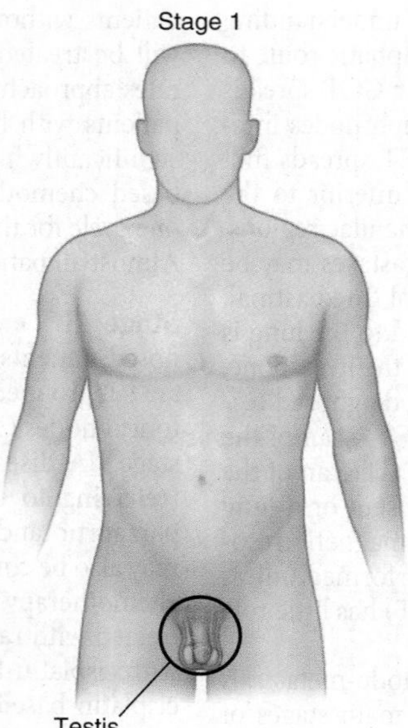

	Seminoma	NSGCT
Stage IA Testis only, no lymphovascular invasion	Active surveillance; or, Adjuvant carboplatin x 1 or 2 cycles; or, Adjuvant para-aortic RT	Active surveillance; or, Nerve-sparing RPLND; or Adjuvant BEP x 1 cycle
Stage IB Testis only, with lymphovascular invasion or invasion of spermatic cord or scrotum	Active surveillance; or, Adjuvant carboplatin x 1 or 2 cycles; or, Adjuvant para-aortic RT	Active surveillance; or, Adjuvant BEP x 1 cycle; or Nerve-sparing RPLND
Stage IS Elevated serum tumor markers post-orchiectomy	BEP x 3 cycles; or, EP x 4 cycles	BEP x 3 cycles; or, EP x 4 cycles

A

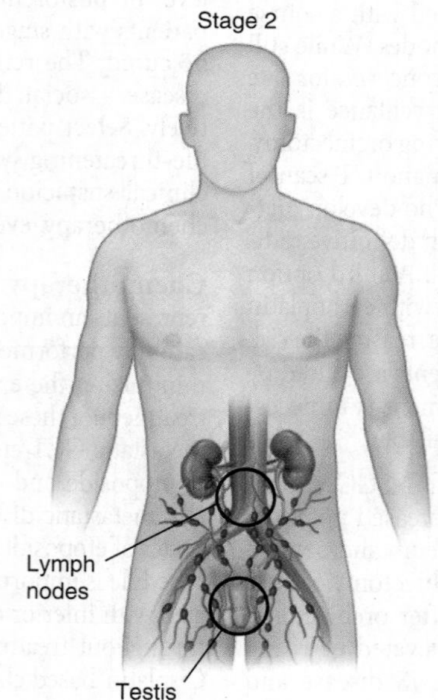

	Seminoma	NSGCT
Stage IIA N1: nodes ≤ 2 cm	Para-aortic and ipsilateral iliac RT; or, BEP x 3 cycles or EP x 4 cycles	Nerve-sparing RPLND; or, BEP x 3 cycles or EP x 4 cycles
Stage IIB N2: nodes > 2 to 5 cm	BEP x 3 cycles or EP x 4 cycles; or, Para-aortic and ipsilateral iliac RT	BEP x 3 cycles or EP x 4 cycles +/− postchemotherapy RPLND
Stage IIC N3: nodes > 5 cm	BEP x 3 cycles or EP x 4 cycles	BEP x 3 cycles or EP x 4 cycles +/− postchemotherapy RPLND

B

FIGURE 88-1 Stage-based management of testicular germ cell tumor.

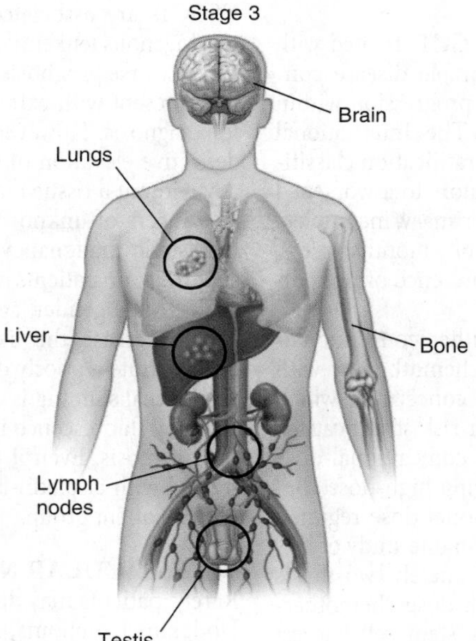

	Seminoma	NSGCT
Stage IIIA (good-risk)	BEP x 3 cycles; or, EP x 4 cycles	BEP x 3 cycles; or, EP x 4 cycles; +/– Postchemotherapy surgery
Stage IIIB (intermediate-risk)	BEP x 4 cycles; or, VIP x 4 cycles	BEP x 4 cycles; or, VIP x 4 cycles +/– Postchemotherapy surgery
Stage IIIC (poor-risk)	N/A	BEP x 4 cycles; or, VIP x 4 cycles +/– Postchemotherapy surgery

Abbreviations: BEP, bleomycin, etoposide, cisplatin; EP, etoposide, cisplatin; N/A, not applicable; NSGCT, nonseminomatous germ cell tumor; RPLND, retroperitoneal lymph node dissection; RT, radiation therapy; VIP, etoposide, ifosfamide, cisplatin.

C

FIGURE 88-1 (Continued)

TABLE 88-1 International Germ Cell Consensus Classification System

RISK GROUP	SEMINOMA	NSGCT
Good	Any primary site; and normal AFP, any hCG, any LDH; and nonpulmonary visceral metastases absent	Gonadal or retroperitoneal primary; and nonpulmonary visceral metastases absent; and AFP <1000 ng/mL; and hCG <5000 mIU/mL; and LDH <1.5 × ULN
Intermediate	Any primary site; and normal AFP, any hCG, any LDH; and nonpulmonary visceral metastases present	Gonadal or retroperitoneal primary; and nonpulmonary visceral metastases absent; and one of the following: AFP 1000–10,000 ng/mL hCG 5000–50,000 mIU/mL LDH 1.5–10 × ULN
Poor	N/A	Mediastinal primary; or nonpulmonary visceral metastases present; or one of the following: AFP >10,000 ng/mL hCG >50,000 mIU/mL LDH >10 × ULN

Abbreviations: AFP, α fetoprotein; hCG, human chorionic gonadotropin; LDH, lactate dehydrogenase; N/A, not applicable; NSGCT, nonseminomatous germ cell tumor; ULN, upper limit normal. Nonpulmonary visceral metastases include liver, bone, and brain.

Source: Reproduced with permission from International Germ Cell Cancer Collaborative Group: International Germ-Cell Consensus Classification: A prognostic factor based staging system for metastatic germ cell tumors. J Clin Oncol 15:594, 1997.

Postchemotherapy Surgery Upon completion of cisplatin-based chemotherapy, many patients with normalized serum tumor markers will have radiographic evidence of residual masses. In approximately half of patients with NSGCT, the residual mass is composed of necrosis and/or fibrosis. About 40% will have residual teratoma and only 10% will have residual viable nonteratomatous GCT. Unfortunately, radiographic imaging cannot accurately differentiate between these entities. For this reason, NSGCT patients with residual masses after chemotherapy undergo resection of all sites of disease. This most commonly includes a postchemotherapy RPLND. However, thoracotomy and neck dissection are required in some patients. If the patients are found to have residual necrosis or teratoma, no additional therapy is required. However, for patients with residual viable nonteratomatous GCT, two additional cycles of chemotherapy are frequently administered. It should be noted that in most centers, patients with minimal residual tumors defined as retroperitoneal lymph nodes of ≤1 cm will forego postchemotherapy RPLND. Patients who experience normalization of serum tumor markers with first-line chemotherapy but have enlarging tumors, most often cystic masses in the retroperitoneum, may have "growing teratoma syndrome." These patients are best approached with surgery.

For patients with metastatic seminoma, most residual masses are necrotic and do not harbor viable tumor. Patients with residual masses of 3 cm or less may be observed without surgery. For patients with residual masses >3 cm, fluorodeoxyglucose (FDG)-PET may be used to distinguish necrosis from viable seminoma and identify patients who should be considered for postchemotherapy surgery or short interval imaging.

RELAPSED DISEASE

Approximately 20–30% of patients with metastatic GCTs treated with cisplatin-based chemotherapy will not achieve durable disease control. Most of these patients will experience disease progression within 2 years following completion of chemotherapy. The International Prognostic Factors Study Group developed a risk stratification classification system for patients in first relapse. Contributors to a worsened prognosis include NSGCT histology, extragonadal primary, incomplete response to first-line chemotherapy, time to relapse of 3 months or less, level of serum tumor markers at relapse, and the presence of nonpulmonary visceral metastatic disease.

Patients in first relapse may be treated with either conventional-dose salvage chemotherapy or high-dose salvage chemotherapy with autologous stem cell rescue. There is controversy concerning which approach is optimal. Some institutions advocate for risk stratification, with more favorable prognosis patients receiving conventional-dose chemotherapy and worse prognosis patients receiving high-dose chemotherapy. The most commonly utilized conventional-dose regimen includes paclitaxel, ifosfamide, and cisplatin (TIP). In one study of TIP in patients with more favorable-risk disease, approximately two-thirds experienced 2-year progression-free survival. High-dose chemotherapy consists of initial salvage therapy followed by stem cell harvest and then two or three cycles of high-dose carboplatin and etoposide (CE) with stem cell rescue. The largest series of patients treated with high-dose chemotherapy was reported by researchers at Indiana University where this approach is considered standard for most patients in first relapse regardless of risk classification. In their study, ~70% of patients in first relapse achieved durable progression-free survival. A large retrospective analysis has compared conventional-dose salvage chemotherapy to high-dose salvage chemotherapy in patients in first relapse. This study reports a more favorable outcome with high-dose salvage chemotherapy across nearly all risk groups. However, given the retrospective nature of this study and the controversy concerning optimal approaches, an international randomized trial comparing conventional-dose chemotherapy (TIP) to high-dose chemotherapy with autologous stem cell rescue (TI-CE) is underway.

Some patients who experience disease progression after conventional-dose salvage chemotherapy may successfully be treated with high-dose salvage chemotherapy with autologous stem cell rescue. Patients with disease progression after high-dose salvage chemotherapy may be treated with subsequent chemotherapy regimens that include gemcitabine/oxaliplatin, gemcitabine/paclitaxel, epirubicin/cisplatin, and oral etoposide. While these patients may benefit from third-line chemotherapy, few will achieve durable disease control. Select patients with relapsed but resectable disease may be candidates for salvage or so-called "desperation" surgery. Studies of molecularly targeted agents and immune checkpoint inhibitors in this population have to date been generally disappointing.

Patients who experience disease progression >2 years after chemotherapy are considered to have "late relapse." Late relapse appears to have a different biology than early relapse. These patients tend to have more chemotherapy-resistant disease. Patients with late relapse usually have NSGCT with elevation of serum AFP. Many of these patients experience recurrence in the retroperitoneum many years after first-line chemotherapy, and this likely represents residual retroperitoneal disease that was not controlled after first-line therapy. These patients are best approached with salvage surgery.

EXTRAGONADAL GCTS

Approximately 5% of patients who present with GCTs have extragonadal primaries. These mainly originate in the mediastinum or retroperitoneum. Patients suspected of extragonadal GCT should undergo scrotal ultrasound to exclude a gonadal primary. Extragonadal seminomas have a similar excellent prognosis as their gonadal counterparts and are approached the same. Mediastinal NSGCTs are classified as poor risk and are treated with either four cycles of BEP or four cycles of VIP. These patients frequently require postchemotherapy thoracic surgery for residual disease. For this reason, some advocate avoiding bleomycin in this patient population. Klinefelter's syndrome is associated with an increased risk of mediastinal NSGCTs. Rarely, mediastinal NSGCTs are associated with hematologic disorders including acute myelogenous leukemia. NSGCTs arising in the retroperitoneum do not have a worse prognosis than their gonadal counterparts. Many patients who present with extragonadal GCTs will undergo core needle biopsy for diagnosis. However, select patients with extragonadal tumors and definitive elevation of serum tumor markers may initiate chemotherapy without a tissue diagnosis.

Cancers of unknown primary are defined as histologically proven metastatic malignancy in which the primary site is not obvious. A subgroup of patients with cancer of unknown primary have occult GCTs. Male gender, age <65 years, midline tumors, and nonsmoking status increase the likelihood of this presentation. Pathology may demonstrate a poorly differentiated malignant neoplasm. Immunohistochemical staining is used to exclude lymphoma. Tumor may be analyzed by fluorescence in situ hybridization for i(12p), which confirms the diagnosis. Even if the diagnosis is not certain, patients should be treated with cisplatin-based chemotherapy, which will cure up to 20% of this patient group.

TESTICULAR NON–GERM CELL TUMORS

Rarely, patients may develop testicular non-GCTs. These include non-Hodgkin's lymphoma, most commonly occurring in men over the age of 50; sex cord stromal tumors including Leydig cell tumors and Sertoli cell tumors; mesothelioma of the tunica vaginalis; and paratesticular sarcoma. Metastasis to the testis is rare, most commonly occurring in patients with advanced prostate cancer and melanoma.

SURVIVORSHIP AND LATE EFFECTS

Because most patients with testicular GCT will experience long-term survival, survivorship care is important. Since many of these patients will be followed by primary care physicians, an understanding of the physical, psychological, and social late effects is important. Late effects are defined as health problems that occur months or years after a disease is diagnosed or after treatment has ended. Late effects may be related to the underlying cancer or to the treatment the patient received. In long-term survivors of testicular GCT, increased cardiovascular risk and increased secondary malignancies have been reported. Patients treated with cisplatin-based chemotherapy have an increased risk of hypertension, hyperlipidemia, metabolic syndrome, and cardiovascular events. Patients treated with high cumulative doses of etoposide (e.g., patients who receive standard chemotherapy, relapse, and then receive salvage high-dose chemotherapy) may experience up to a 1–2% risk of developing acute myelogenous leukemia, typically 2–3 years after completing therapy and associated with an 11q23 translocation. Patients treated with radiation therapy, cisplatin-based chemotherapy, or both have an increased risk of developing secondary solid malignancies.

FURTHER READING

Einhorn LH et al: High-dose chemotherapy and stem-cell rescue for metastatic germ cell tumors. N Engl J Med 357:340, 2007.

Feldman DR et al: Medical treatment of advanced testicular cancer. JAMA 299:272, 2008.

Fung C et al: Testicular cancer survivorship. J Natl Compr Canc Netw 17:1557, 2019.

Hanna NH, Einhorn LH: Testicular cancer-discoveries and updates. N Engl J Med 371:2005, 2014.

International Prognostic Factors Study Group et al: Prognostic factors in patients with metastatic germ cell tumors who experienced treatment failure with cisplatin-based first-line chemotherapy. J Clin Oncol 28:4906, 2010.

Kollmansberger C et al: Patterns of relapse in patients with clinical stage 1 testicular cancer managed with active surveillance. J Clin Oncol 33:51, 2015.

Lorch A et al: Conventional-dose versus high-dose chemotherapy as first salvage treatment in male patients with metastatic germ cell tumors: Evidence from a large international database. J Clin Oncol 29:2178, 2011.

Pluta J et al: Identification of 22 novel susceptibility loci associated with testicular germ cell tumors. Nat Commun 12:4487, 2021.

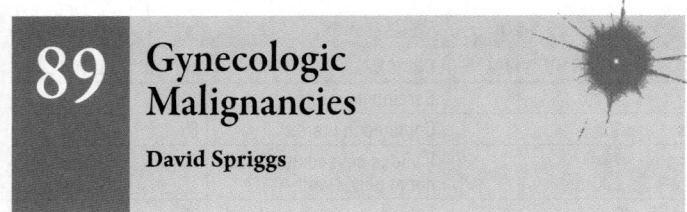

89 Gynecologic Malignancies

David Spriggs

OVARIAN CANCER

INCIDENCE AND PATHOLOGY

Ovarian cancer remains a leading cause of cancer deaths in American women, ranking behind lung, breast, colon, and pancreatic cancers. The ovary is responsible for hormone and egg production. Between menarche (11–13 years) and menopause (45–55 years), the ovary is responsible for follicle maturation associated with egg maturation, ovulation, and cyclical sex steroid hormone production. These complex biologic functions are linked to stromal and germ cells within the ovary. Cells of the ovary can be broadly grouped into stromal cells and ovarian germ cells and the enveloping epithelial cells. Malignancies arising in each group include multiple histologic variants, each with unique neoplastic behaviors. Epithelial tumors are the most common histologic variant of ovarian neoplasms; they may be benign (50%), frankly malignant (33%), or of borderline malignancy of low malignant potential (16%). In adnexal masses detected by imaging or physical exam, age influences risk of malignancy; tumors in younger women are more likely benign. In the malignant group, the most common tumors are epithelial. In the group of the ovarian epithelial malignancies are the serous tumors (60–70%), mucinous tumors (10%), endometrioid tumors (10–15%), and clear cell tumors (10–15%) tumors. The distribution of histologic types varies in different parts of the world. The less common stromal tumors arise from the ancillary, supportive cells such as steroid hormone–producing cells and likewise have different phenotypes and clinical presentations. Most stromal tumors do not produce estrogen, but ectopic hormone production can be seen in certain subtypes. Tumors arising in the ovarian germ cell lineage are generally similar in biology and behavior to testicular tumors in males, although their intraperitoneal location alters some metastatic behaviors (**Chap. 88**). Ovarian tissue may also host metastatic tumors arising from breast, colon, gastric, and pancreatic primaries. Bilateral ovarian masses from metastatic mucin-secreting gastrointestinal cancers are termed *Krukenberg tumors*. A survey of other potential primaries is commonly required during the diagnostic workup of ovarian masses.

OVARIAN CANCER OF EPITHELIAL ORIGIN

Epidemiology An American woman has approximately a 1 in 72 lifetime risk (1.6%) of developing ovarian cancer, with the majority of affected women developing epithelial tumors. In 2021 in the United States, ~21,500 cases of ovarian cancer are expected to be diagnosed, with >14,000 deaths. Sporadic (not familial) epithelial tumors of the ovary have a peak incidence in women in their fifties and sixties, although age at presentation ranges from the third decade to the eighties and nineties. Ovarian cancer risk has been linked to an interactive mixture of epidemiologic, environmental, and genetic factors. Nulliparity, obesity, diet, infertility treatments, and possibly hormone replacement therapy have all been linked to an increase in risk. Protective factors include the use of oral contraceptives, multiparity, tubal ligation, aspirin use, and breast-feeding. Other epidemiologic factors such as the historical use of perineal talc agents remain controversial. The mechanisms underlying the various protective factors are largely unknown, but theories include suppression of ovulation, modulation of gonadotropins and progestins, and perhaps reduction of ovarian inflammation and damage associated with the repair of the ovarian cortex associated with ovulation.

Genetics and Pathogenesis Ovarian cancers are divided into type 1 cancers and the more aggressive type 2 variant. The type 1 cancers are characterized by low-grade histology and generally indolent behavior. These tumors include the low malignant potential tumors, low-grade endometrial and mucinous histologies, and clear cell cancers (which are more aggressive). Genetic alterations in type 1 cancers include mutations in *KRAS, BRAF, PTEN*, and *PIK3CA*. In contrast, studies have implicated serial genetic changes in the fallopian tube as the actual site of origin for most type 2, high-grade serous epithelial ovarian cancers. These aggressive tumors are more common and linked to losses in *TP53* and defective DNA repair. Carcinoma in situ has been identified in the tubal epithelium with early losses in *TP53* and the *BRCA1/BRCA2* gene function characterizing early tubal intraepithelial cancers. Following these early genetic events, additional mutations in these transformed cells lead to tumor cell shedding, metastasis, and invasion. These type 2, poorly differentiated, serous cancer cells can then spread to the ovaries and the peritoneal cavity, aided by the ovarian cancer cell's affinity for mesothelin-expressing cells.

Type 2 serous ovarian cancer is classically a disease characterized by widespread amplifications and deletions rather than single-gene point mutations or common gene fusions. In the Tumor Genome Atlas, loss of tumor-suppressor gene *TP53* function is present in >95% of serous ovarian cancers. Damage to homologous DNA repair genes, especially *BRCA1* and *BRCA2*, is also common in these tumors. Low prevalence but statistically recurrent somatic mutations in seven other genes including *NF1, RB1*, and *CDK12* were also seen. The most common heritable abnormality linked to ovarian cancer is a germline mutation in either *BRCA1* (chromosome 17q12–21) or *BRCA2* (chromosome 13q12–13). These genes are essential parts of the homologous DNA repair machinery for double-stranded DNA break repair. Individuals inheriting a single copy of a mutant allele have an increased lifetime risk of breast (46–87% for *BRCA1*; 38–84% for *BRCA2*) and ovarian cancer (39–63% for *BRCA1*; 16.5–27% for *BRCA2*). Many of these women have a family history that includes multiple cases of breast and/or ovarian cancer of at an early age. Male breast cancer, pancreatic cancer, and prostate cancer are also linked to familial *BRCA2* mutations. The most common malignancy in women carrying germline *BRCA1/2* mutations is breast carcinoma, although women harboring germline *BRCA1* mutations also have a marked increased risk of developing ovarian malignancies in their forties and fifties. Women harboring a mutation in *BRCA2* have a lower penetrance of ovarian cancer with onset typically in their fifties or sixties. Other uncommon germline mutation of other genes encoding proteins linked to homologous DNA repair (e.g., *PALB2*) can also contribute to cancer risk, although the frequency of mutation and magnitude of risk increment are much lower and not well defined. Screening studies, even in the mutated *BRCA1/2* families, suggest that any of the available screening techniques, including structured, serial evaluation of the CA-125 serum marker and transvaginal ultrasound, remain insufficient to reliably detect early-stage ovarian cancer in prospective testing. Germline *BRCA1/2* testing is recommended for *all* incident epithelial ovarian cancers to detect probands for therapeutic intervention and identify relatives at risk. Women with these high-risk germline mutations are advised to undergo prophylactic removal of fallopian tubes and ovaries after completing childbearing, ideally before age 40. Early prophylactic salpingo-oophorectomy is highly protective. Salpingo-oophorectomy also appears to protect these women from subsequent breast cancer (risk reduction 50%). Prophylactic salpingectomy is almost certainly a key part of any surgical prophylaxis strategy for ovarian cancer prevention, but the benefits of isolated oophorectomy on either ovarian or breast cancer risk have not yet been clearly defined. Although less common, ovarian cancer is also another familial form of cancer (along with colorectal and endometrial cancer) that may develop in women with type II Lynch syndrome caused by mutations in one of the DNA mismatch repair genes (*MSH2, MLH1, MLH6, PMS1, PMS2*). Ovarian cancer may appear in women younger than 50 years of age in this syndrome.

Neoplasms of the ovary tend to be painless unless they undergo torsion. Nonspecific gastrointestinal symptoms like bloating and early satiety are common at presentation, probably related to compression of local organs or due to symptoms from metastatic disease. Women with ovarian tumors also may have an increased incidence of symptoms including pelvic discomfort, bloating, and perhaps changes in urinary or bowel pattern. Unfortunately, all of these symptoms are common in

TABLE 89-1 Staging and Survival in Gynecologic Malignancies

STAGE	OVARIAN	5-YEAR SURVIVAL, %	ENDOMETRIAL	5-YEAR SURVIVAL, %	CERVIX	5-YEAR SURVIVAL, %
0	—		—		Carcinoma in situ	100
I	Confined to ovary	88–95	Confined to corpus	>90	Confined to uterus	85
II	Confined to pelvic organs	70–80	Involves corpus and cervix	~75	Invades beyond uterus but not to pelvic wall	65
III	Intra-abdominal spread to omentum, diaphragm, or lymph nodes	20–40	Extends outside the uterus but not outside the true pelvis	45–60	Extends to pelvic wall and/or lower third of vagina, or hydronephrosis	35
IV	Spread outside abdominal cavity, parenchymal spread, and pleural effusion cytology	17	Extends outside the true pelvis or involves the bladder or rectum	~20	Invades mucosa of bladder or rectum or extends beyond the true pelvis	7

primary care and are frequently dismissed by either the woman or her health care team until later stages of disease. The pathogenic factors and timing of spread beyond the ovary are still not well understood. The most common symptoms at presentation of advanced disease include a period of progressive complaints of nausea, early satiety, bloating, indigestion, constipation, and abdominal pain. Signs include the rapid increase in abdominal girth due to the accumulation of ascites that typically alerts the patient and her physician that the concurrent gastrointestinal symptoms are likely associated with malignant pathology. Radiologic evaluation typically demonstrates a complex adnexal mass with ascites, carcinomatosis, and pelvic, para-aortic and mesenteric adenopathy in advanced disease. Positron emission tomography (PET) scans are generally not required. Laboratory evaluation often demonstrates a markedly elevated CA-125, a shed mucin component (MUC16) associated with, but not specific for, ovarian cancer. Ovarian cancers are divided into four stages, with stage I tumors confined to the ovary, stage II malignancies confined to the pelvis, and stage III confined to the peritoneal cavity and retroperitoneal nodes **(Table 89-1)**. These three stages are subdivided, with the most common presentation, stage IIIC, defined as tumors with bulky intraperitoneal disease or positive lymph node involvement. About 70% of women present with stage III disease. Stage IV disease includes women with parenchymal metastases (liver, lung, spleen) or, alternatively, abdominal wall or pleural disease. The 30% of patients not presenting with stage III disease are roughly evenly distributed among the other stages.

Screening Ovarian cancer is a highly lethal condition. It is curable in early stages but seldom curable in advanced stages; hence, screening continues to be of considerable interest. Early-stage tumors often secrete excessive amounts of normal proteins that can be measured in the serum such as CA-125, mesothelin, and HE-4. Nevertheless, the incidence of ovarian cancer in the middle-aged female population is very low, with only ~1 in 2000 women between the ages of 50 and 60 carrying an asymptomatic and undetected tumor. Thus, effective screening techniques must be both sensitive and highly specific to minimize the number of false positives. Panels of serum markers have not improved on CA-125 alone, nor have risk assessment strategies using algorithms with multiple CA-125 measurements over time. No other screening strategies have been any more successful to date. Some large studies have suggested that low-specificity screening might even worsen mortality in the screened population. Screening for ovarian cancer is currently not recommended outside of a clinical trial, but large ongoing clinical trials are studying algorithmic detection by serial sampling strategies.

TREATMENT

Ovarian Cancer

Epithelial ovarian cancer can be divided into distinct "disease states" for the purpose of treatment selection, as shown in **Fig. 89-1**. Surgery by a skilled gynecologic oncologist remains the preferred initial therapy for ovarian cancer. However, the amount of residual visible cancer at the end of a primary operation is strongly predictive of outcome and is paired with histology, grade, and stage to determine prognosis and treatment. In women presenting with a localized ovarian mass, the principal diagnostic and therapeutic maneuver is abdominal surgery to determine if the tumor is benign or malignant. In the event that the tumor is malignant, the surgical specimen will determine if the tumor arises in the ovary or is a site of metastatic disease. Metastatic disease to the ovary can be seen from primary tumors of the colon, appendix, stomach (Krukenberg tumors), and breast. Needle biopsy is contraindicated to avoid malignant contamination of the peritoneal cavity with malignant cells. Typically, women undergo laparoscopic evaluation and unilateral salpingo-oophorectomy for diagnostic purposes. If pathology reveals a primary ovarian malignancy or the laparoscopy proves disseminated disease is present, then the procedure should be followed by a total hysterectomy, removal of the remaining tube and ovary, omentectomy, and pelvic node sampling along with biopsies of the peritoneal cavity and diaphragms. This extensive surgical procedure is performed because ~30% of tumors that, by visual inspection, appear to be confined to the ovary have already disseminated to the peritoneal cavity and/or surrounding lymph nodes. As with axillary dissections in breast cancer, node sampling is diagnostic, but full lymphadenectomy appears to provide little or no additional therapeutic advantage over nodal sampling. The target outcome of an ovarian cancer surgery is always an R0 resection, with no visible residual cancer. The less favorable "optimal resection" (no disease >1 cm in size) is still clinically useful, and the prognosis of those patients is much better than that of patients who are left with >1 cm of disease at the end of surgery. These "suboptimally debulked" patients derive very little benefit from their surgery. If a suboptimal debulking is anticipated, the surgery should be delayed until after several cycles of neoadjuvant chemotherapy. Such "interval debulking" surgery achieves similar results to primary surgery with diminished surgical morbidity and more timely chemotherapy. Patients without gross residual disease after resection have a median survival in excess of 60 months, compared to 28–42 months for those left with macroscopic tumor or those undergoing interval debulking, regardless of treatment strategy.

After appropriate surgical treatment, primary chemotherapy will consist of combination treatment with paclitaxel and carboplatin. Primary chemotherapy can be delivered intravenously, or alternatively, some therapy can be directly administered into the peritoneal cavity via an indwelling catheter. Some, but not all, randomized studies have demonstrated improved survival with intraperitoneal (IP) therapy. The IP approach is technically more difficult and is increasingly replaced by carboplatin and paclitaxel, which appears to offer similar results.

With optimal debulking surgery and platinum-based chemotherapy (usually carboplatin dosed to an area under the curve [AUC] of 6.0 plus paclitaxel 175 mg/m^2 by 3-h infusion in monthly cycles), 70% of women who present with advanced-stage tumors show tumor reduction, and 40–50% experience a complete remission with normalization of their CA-125, CT scans, and physical

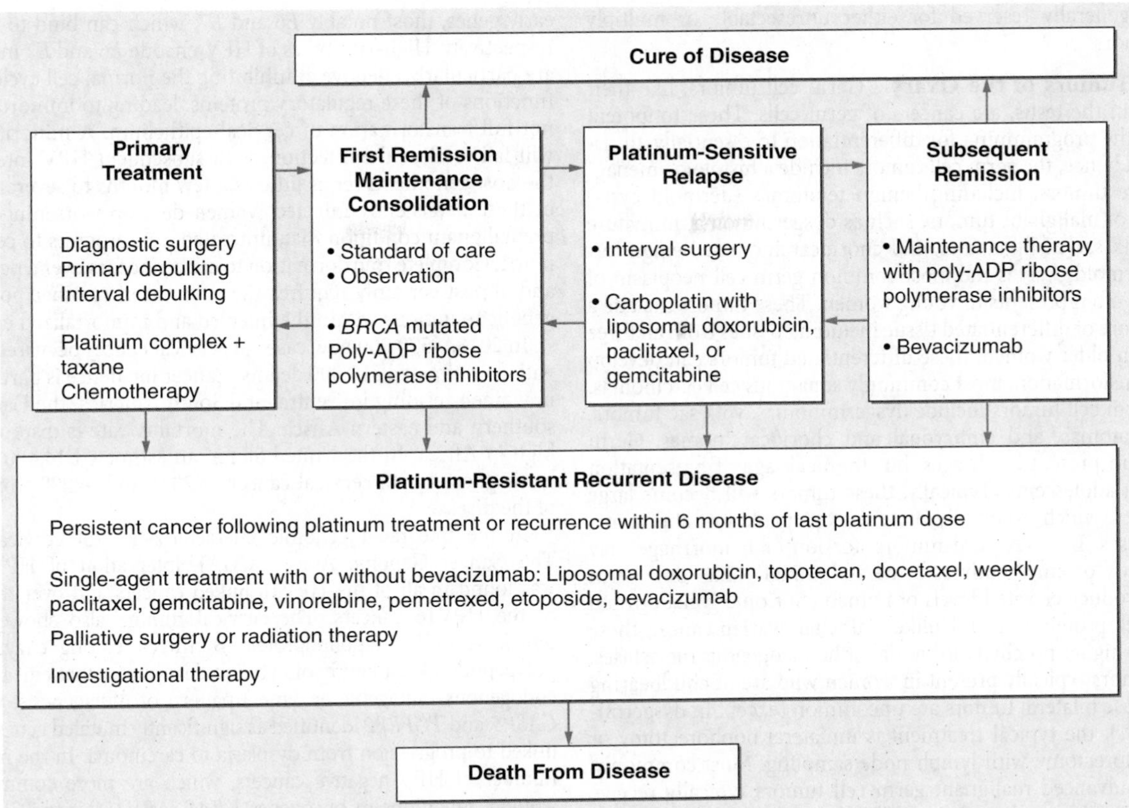

FIGURE 89-1 Disease states model of epithelial ovarian cancer and its treatment. Each box represents a relatively homogenous group of patients who share a palette of potential treatment choices and have a similar prognosis. The *arrows* indicate that a single patient may move from one state to another during the course of her illness, and the choice of treatments will become different in her new disease state.

examination. Poly-ADP ribose polymerase inhibitors (PARPi) such as niriparib or olaparib, when administered at the completion of intravenous chemotherapy, appear to substantially delay recurrence and probably provide survival advantages as well. In the majority of patients, disease still recurs within 1–4 years from the completion of their primary therapy. CA-125 levels often increase as a first sign of relapse, and CT scan findings are confirmatory. Recurrent disease is often successfully managed for years, but rarely cured, with a variety of chemotherapeutic agents. Additional surgical therapy does not appear to extend survival in randomized trials. Patients with a treatment-free interval are often best treated with additional platinum doublets, combining carboplatin with liposomal doxorubicin, gemcitabine, or a taxane. Eventually all women who experience relapse develop chemotherapy-refractory disease. Refractory ascites, poor bowel motility, and obstruction or tumor-infiltrated aperistaltic bowel are all common premorbid events. Limited surgery to relieve intestinal obstruction, localized radiation therapy to relieve pressure or pain from masses, or palliative chemotherapy may be helpful. Agents with >15% response rates include gemcitabine, topotecan, liposomal doxorubicin, and bevacizumab. Five-year survival correlates with the stage of disease: stage I, 90–95%; stage II, 70–80%; stage III, 25–40%; stage IV, 10–15% (Table 89-1). Prognosis is also influenced by histologic grade: 5-year survival is 88% for well-differentiated tumors, 58% for moderately differentiated tumors, and 27% for poorly differentiated tumors. Histologic type has less influence on outcome.

UNCOMMON OVARIAN TUMORS

Low Malignant Potential Tumors (Borderline Tumors) These type 1 tumors are found in younger women (age 30–50 years) and indolent in behavior, and few of these patients will succumb to their tumors (10-year survival may approach 98%), although recurrence is not uncommon. Certain features, such as micropapillary histology and microinvasion, are linked to more aggressive behavior. Tumors of low malignant potential should be carefully distinguished from grade 1 serous carcinomas. Borderline tumor patients are managed primarily by surgery; chemotherapy and radiation therapy do not substantially alter survival.

Stromal Tumors Approximately 7% of ovarian neoplasms are stromal tumors, with ~1800 cases expected each year in the United States. Ovarian stromal tumors or sex cord tumors are most common in women in their fifties or sixties, but tumors can present at any age. These tumors arise from the mesenchymal components of the ovary, including both steroid-producing cells and fibroblasts. Most of these tumors are indolent tumors with limited metastatic potential and present as unilateral solid masses. These tumors primarily are discovered by the detection of an abdominal mass, sometimes with abdominal pain due to ovarian torsion, intratumoral hemorrhage, or rupture. Rarely, stromal tumors can produce estrogen and present with breast tenderness as well as precocious puberty in children, menstrual disturbances in reproductively active women, or postmenopausal bleeding. In some women, estrogen-associated secondary malignancies, such as endometrial or breast cancer, may present as synchronous malignancies. Sertoli-Leydig tumors often present with hirsutism and virilization due to increased production of androgens. Hormonally inert tumors include fibromas, which present as solitary masses often in association with ascites and occasionally hydrothorax, also known as Meigs's syndrome. A subset of these tumors present in individuals with a variety of inherited disorders that predispose them to mesenchymal neoplasia including Ollier's disease (juvenile granulosa cell tumors) and Peutz-Jeghers syndrome (ovarian sex cord tumors). The treatment of these tumors is almost exclusively by surgical resection, without adjuvant chemotherapy. Chemotherapy with carboplatin and paclitaxel is generally reserved for either unresectable or multiply recurrent tumors.

Germ Cell Tumors of the Ovary Germ cell tumors, like their counterparts in the testis, are cancers of germ cells. These totipotent cells contain the programming for differentiation to essentially all tissue types, and hence, the germ cell tumors include a histologic menagerie of bizarre tumors, including benign teratomas (dermoid cysts) and a variety of malignant tumors, such as dysgerminoma, immature teratomas, yolk sac malignancies, and choriocarcinomas. Benign teratoma (or dermoid cyst) is the most common germ cell neoplasm of the ovary and often presents in young women. These tumors include a complex mixture of differentiated tissue including tissues from all three germ layers. In older women, these differentiated tumors can develop malignant transformation, most commonly squamous cell carcinomas. Malignant germ cell tumors include dysgerminomas, yolk sac tumors, immature teratomas, and embryonal and choriocarcinomas. Germ cell tumors can present at all ages, but the peak age of presentation tends to be in adolescents. Typically, these tumors will become large ovarian masses, which eventually present as palpable low abdominal or pelvic masses. Like sex cord tumors, torsion or hemorrhage may present urgently or emergently as acute abdominal pain. Some germ cell tumors produce elevated levels of human chorionic gonadotropin (hCG) or α-fetoprotein (AFP). Unlike epithelial ovarian cancer, these tumors have a higher proclivity for nodal or hematogenous metastases. Germ cell tumors typically present in women who are of childbearing age, and because bilateral tumors are uncommon (except in dysgerminoma, 10–15%), the typical treatment is unilateral oophorectomy or salpingo-oophorectomy with lymph node sampling. Most commonly, women with advanced malignant germ cell tumors typically receive bleomycin, etoposide, and cisplatin (BEP) chemotherapy, in an analogous fashion to the treatment of testicular cancers. In the majority of these women, even those with advanced-stage disease, cure is expected. Dysgerminoma is the ovarian counterpart of testicular seminoma and is highly curable. Although the tumor is highly radiation-sensitive, radiation produces infertility in many patients. BEP chemotherapy is as effective or more so without causing infertility.

FALLOPIAN TUBE CANCER

Transport of the egg to the uterus occurs through the fallopian tube, with the distal ends of these tubes composed of fimbriae that drape about the ovarian surface and capture the egg as it erupts from the ovarian cortex. As described above, the majority of type 2 ovarian cancers are now thought to arise from the tubal epithelium. As might be expected, fallopian tube malignancies are typically of serous histology and share the same biology and recommended treatment as serous ovarian cancer. These tumors often present as clinically isolated adnexal masses, but like ovarian cancer, these tumors spread relatively early throughout the peritoneal cavity. Fallopian tubal cancers have a natural history and treatment that are essentially identical to ovarian cancer (Table 89-1).

CERVICAL CANCER

ETIOLOGY AND GENETICS

Cervical cancer is the second most common and the most lethal malignancy in women worldwide. Infection with high-risk strains of human papillomavirus (HPV) is the primary neoplastic-initiating event in the vast majority of women with invasive cervical cancer. This double-stranded DNA virus infects epithelium near the transformation zone of the cervix where underlying columnar epithelium becomes squamous epithelium. More than 60 types of HPV are known, with ~20 types having the ability to generate high-grade dysplasia and malignancy. HPV16 and 18 are the types most frequently associated with high-grade dysplasia, but types 31, 33, 35, 52, and 58 are also considered to be high-risk variants. The large majority of sexually active adults are exposed to HPV, and most women clear the infection without specific intervention. The 8-kb HPV genome encodes seven early genes, most notably *E6* and *E7*, which can bind to *RB* and *p53*, respectively. High-risk types of HPV encode *E6* and *E7* molecules that are particularly effective at inhibiting the normal cell cycle checkpoint functions of these regulatory proteins, leading to immortalization but not full transformation of cervical epithelium. A minority of women will fail to clear the infection, with subsequent HPV integration into the host genome. Over as little as a few months to several years, some of these persistently infected women develop worsening dysplasia, a premalignant condition that, untreated, can progress to cervical carcinoma. Complete transformation to cancer occurs over a period of years and almost certainly requires the acquisition of other poorly defined genetic mutations within the infected and immortalized epithelium.

In 2018, ~570,000 new cases of cervical cancer occurred worldwide, with an estimated 311,000 deaths. Cancer incidence is particularly high in women residing in Central and South America, the Caribbean, and southern and eastern Africa. The mortality rate is disproportionately high in Africa. In the United States, an estimated 14,480 women will be diagnosed with cervical cancer in 2021 and ~4290 women will die of the disease.

In the integrated genomic characterization of cervical cancer by The Cancer Genome Atlas (TCGA), integration of HPV sequences was found in all of the HPV18-linked cancers and over three-quarters of the HPV16 cancers. The cervical tumors also showed a characteristic APOBEC (apolipoprotein B mRNA editing enzyme, catalytic polypeptide-like; a family of cytidine deaminases that edit DNA and are endogenous mutagenic enzymes) pattern of mutagenesis, with *ERBB3*, *CASP8*, and *TGFRB2* identified as significantly mutated genes presumably linked to progression from dysplasia to carcinoma. In the much smaller number of HPV-negative cancers, which are more common in older women, mutations in oncogenes *KRAS*, *ARID1A*, and *PTEN* were frequently seen. The clinical behavior of these cancers is likely to be different.

HPV INFECTION AND PREVENTION

The Pap smear is the primary detection method for asymptomatic preinvasive cervical dysplasia of squamous epithelial lining during a gynecologic exam. Because the delay between dysplasia and frank cervical cancer is years long, annual (or longer) screening and prevention strategies that detect precancerous dysplasia and carcinoma in situ can be implemented successfully. Annual or biannual cervical scraping for cytology (Pap smear) is highly effective in reducing the incidence of cervical cancer by early detection and subsequent surgical treatment of premalignant disease. The incorporation of HPV testing by polymerase chain reaction (PCR) or other molecular techniques increases the sensitivity of detecting cervical pathology but at the cost of lower sensitivity in that it identifies many women with transient infections who require no specific medical intervention. Unfortunately, both the collection of a Pap smear and its cytologic evaluation require infrastructure beyond the means of many middle- and low-income countries. High-throughput, low-technology prevention strategies and point-of-care testing are needed to identify and treat women bearing high-risk cervical dysplasia to prevent cancer development.

A primary prevention strategy relies on HPV vaccines. Currently approved vaccines include the recombinant proteins to the late proteins, L1 and L2 of HPV16 and 18, as well as other, less common cancer-causing isotypes 11, 31, 33, 45, 52, and 58. Vaccination of girls aged 11–13 years with two injections (1 year apart) before the initiation of sexual activity dramatically reduces the rate of high-risk HPV infection and subsequent dysplasia. Vaccination of both boys and girls is increasingly considered to reduce the risk of HPV-induced cancers of the pharynx. Partial protection is also provided against other HPV types, although vaccinated women are still at risk for HPV infection and still benefit from standard Pap smear screening.

CLINICAL PRESENTATIONS

Risk Factors Clinical risk factors include many HPV infection–linked features: a high number of sexual partners, early age of first intercourse, and history of venereal disease. Smoking is a cofactor;

heavy smokers have a higher risk of dysplasia with HPV infection. HIV infection, especially when associated with low CD4+ T-cell counts, is associated with a higher rate of high-grade dysplasia and likely a shorter latency period between infection and invasive disease. Histologically, the majority of cervical malignancies are squamous cell carcinomas associated with HPV, but adenocarcinomas are also HPV related, and both arise in the transitional zone of the endocervical canal; the lesions in the canal or cervical glands may not be seen by visual inspection of the cervix and can be missed by Pap smear screening. Less common malignancies, such as vulvar cancer, anal cancer, and pharyngeal cancer, are also linked to HPV infection.

Diagnosis of Cervical Cancer Early cancer of the cervix is asymptomatic, and this biology underlies the recommendations for routine gynecologic care. Larger, invasive carcinomas often have symptoms or signs including postcoital spotting or intermenstrual cycle bleeding or menometrorrhagia. Foul-smelling or persistent yellow discharge may also be present. Symptoms such as pelvic or sacral pain suggest lateral extension into the pelvic nerve plexus by either the primary tumor or a pelvic node metastasis and indicate advanced-stage disease. Likewise, flank pain from hydronephrosis from ureteral compression or deep-venous thrombosis from iliac vessel compression suggests either extensive nodal disease or direct extension of the primary tumor to the pelvic sidewall. The most common finding upon physical exam is a visible tumor on the cervix, but deeper tumors in the cervical os and glands should be considered. Larger tumors may be identified by inspection and biopsied directly. Staging of cervical cancer is performed by clinical exam. Stage I cervical tumors are confined to the cervix, whereas stage II tumors extend into the upper vagina or paracervical soft tissue (**Fig. 89-2**). Stage III tumors extend to the lower vagina or the pelvic sidewalls, whereas stage IV tumors invade the bladder or rectum or have spread to distant sites. While radiographic studies are not part of the formal clinical staging of cervical cancer, treatment planning requires them for appropriate therapy. CT can detect hydronephrosis indicative of pelvic sidewall disease but is not accurate at evaluating other pelvic structures. MRI is more accurate at estimating uterine extension and paracervical extension of disease into soft tissues typically bordered by broad and cardinal ligaments that support the uterus in the central pelvis. Very small stage I cervical tumors can be treated with a variety of surgical procedures, but minimally invasive surgery has inferior outcome compared to standard open hysterectomy. In young women desiring to maintain fertility, radical trachelectomy removes the cervix with subsequent anastomosis of the upper vagina to the uterine corpus; however, subsequent pregnancies may be more problematic. Patients with large stage I cervical tumors (4 cm) confined to the cervix and all stage II to IV patients are treated with radiation therapy in combination with cisplatin-based chemotherapy. This multimodality treatment can offer the patient with advanced-stage disease a 40–80% chance of cure depending on the clinical circumstances. Platinum agents (cisplatin or carboplatin) combined with paclitaxel and bevacizumab are generally considered as the best palliative choice for metastatic cervical cancer patients. Secondary chemotherapy confers minimal improvement in most patients. Immunotherapy with immune checkpoint inhibitors or adoptive T-cell therapies are promising avenues for improved outcomes in recurrent, unresectable cancers of the cervix.

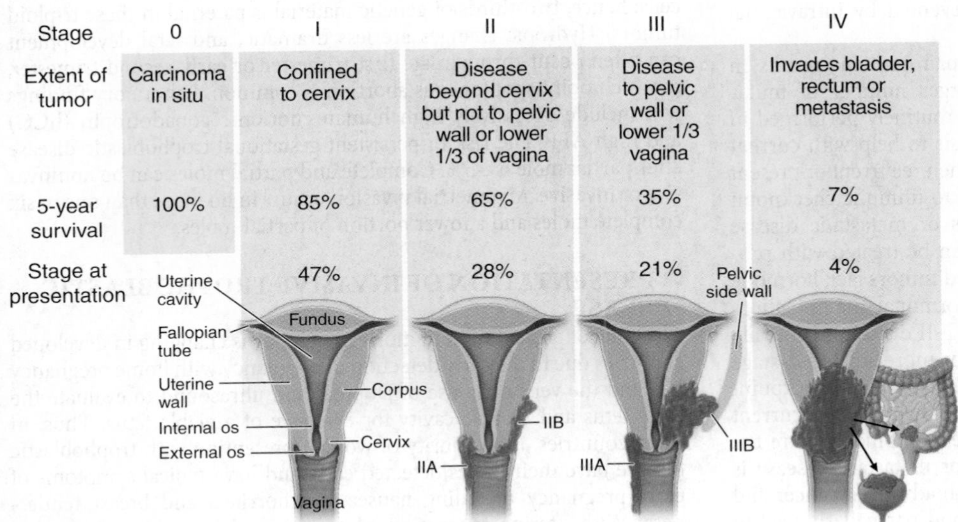

FIGURE 89-2 Anatomic display of the stages of cervix cancer defined by location, extent of tumor, frequency of presentation, and 5-year survival.

UTERINE CANCER

■ EPIDEMIOLOGY

Several different tumor types arise in the uterine corpus. Most tumors arise in the glandular lining and are endometrial adenocarcinomas. Benign (leiomyomas) and malignant tumors (leiomyosarcomas) can also arise in the uterine smooth muscle and have very different clinical features. The endometrioid histologic subtype is the most common gynecologic malignancy in the United States. In 2021, the American Cancer Society predicted that 66,570 new cancers of the uterine corpus in 2021 with 12,940 resulting deaths. Development of these tumors is a multistep process, with estrogen playing an important early role in driving endometrial gland proliferation. Relative overexposure to this class of hormones is the principal risk factor for the subsequent development of endometrioid tumors. In contrast, progestins drive glandular maturation and are protective. Hence, women with high endogenous or pharmacologic exposure to estrogens, especially if unopposed by progesterone, are at higher risk for endometrial cancer. Obese women, women treated with postmenopausal estrogens, or women with estrogen-producing tumors are at higher risk for endometrial cancer. In addition, long-term treatment with tamoxifen, which has antiestrogenic effects in breast tissue but can show weak estrogenic effects in uterine epithelium, is associated with an increased risk of endometrial cancer.

Genetics Women with a germline mutation in one of a series of DNA mismatch repair genes associated with the Lynch syndrome, also known as hereditary nonpolyposis colon cancer (HNPCC) syndrome, are at increased risk for endometrioid endometrial carcinoma. These individuals have germline mutations in *MSH2*, *MLH1*, and, in rare cases, *PMS1* and *PMS2*. Individuals who carry these mutations typically have a family history of cancer and are at markedly increased risk for colon cancer and modestly increased risk for ovarian cancer and a variety of other tumors. Middle-aged women with HNPCC carry a 4% annual risk of endometrial cancer and a relative overall risk of ~200-fold as compared to age-matched women without HNPCC. In sporadic cancers, secondary events such as mutation of the *PI3K* gene or the loss of the *PTEN* tumor-suppressor gene likely serve as secondary genetic "hits" in the carcinogenesis related to estrogenic excess. The molecular events that underlie less common endometrial cancers such as clear cell and papillary serous tumors of the uterine corpus are not well understood.

PATHOLOGY

Approximately 75–80% of endometrial cancers are adenocarcinomas and have been characterized as type 1 (estrogen-linked) endometrial cancers and type 2 cancers that have less clear associations with estrogens (clear cell cancers, serous cancers, and mucinous cancers). Endometrial serous cancers show *TP53* loss of function and behave clinically more like ovarian cancers with high risk for systemic recurrence. Prognosis for endometrial cancer depends on stage, histologic grade, and depth of myometrial invasion.

CLINICAL PRESENTATION

The majority of women with tumors of the uterine corpus present with postmenopausal vaginal bleeding due to shedding of the malignant endometrial lining. Premenopausal women often will present with atypical bleeding between typical menstrual cycles. These signs typically bring a woman to the attention of a health care professional, and the majority of women present with early-stage disease in which the tumor is confined to the uterine corpus and, consequently, have a high cure rate. Diagnosis is typically established by endometrial biopsy. Type 1 tumors may spread to pelvic or para-aortic lymph nodes and are generally subjected to sentinel lymph node biopsy at the time of primary surgery. Serous tumors tend to have patterns of spread much more reminiscent of ovarian cancer, and patients may present with omental/peritoneal disease and sometimes ascites. Some women with endometrial cancer have a history of endometriosis. Some women presenting with uterine sarcomas will present with pelvic pain. Uterine sarcomas (carcinosarcomas and leiomyosarcomas) commonly are found by detection of symptomatic large pelvic masses that may or may not be associated with dysfunctional bleeding.

TREATMENT

Uterine Cancer

Most women with endometrial cancer have disease that is localized to the uterus (75% are stage I, Table 89-1), and definitive treatment typically involves a hysterectomy with removal of the ovaries and fallopian tubes. The resection of lymph nodes does not improve outcome, but sentinel node resection provides important staging and prognostic information. Node involvement defines stage IIIC disease. Tumor grade and depth of invasion are the two key prognostic variables in early-stage tumors, and women with low-grade and/or minimally invasive tumors (<50% myometrial penetration) are typically observed after definitive surgical therapy. Patients with high-grade tumors or tumors that are deeply invasive (stage IB) are at higher risk for pelvic recurrence or recurrence at the vaginal cuff, which is typically prevented by intravaginal brachytherapy.

The loss of one or more mismatch repair proteins results in microsatellite instability (MSI) with a larger number of mutations in the tumor. MSI testing should be routinely performed in endometrial cancers at the time of diagnosis to help with current and future treatment plans. MSI cancers, when recurrent or present at an advanced stage, are likely to respond to immune checkpoint therapy. Women with regional metastases or metastatic disease (3% of patients) with low-grade tumors can be treated with progesterone or tamoxifen. Poorly differentiated tumors lack hormone receptors and are typically resistant to hormonal manipulation. The role of adjuvant chemotherapy in stage I–II disease is generally restricted to serous endometrial cancers. For more advanced-stage cancers (stage III–IV), chemotherapy and/or immune checkpoint blockade are administered because of the higher rates of recurrent systemic disease. Carboplatin and paclitaxel combinations are the current standard of care. Chemotherapy for metastatic disease is delivered with palliative intent. Patients with advanced cancer and known mismatch repair deficits may respond particularly well to immunotherapy with antagonists of the PD-1/PD-L1 axis. Lenvatinib and pembrolizumab (even for microsatellite-stable tumors) have become the most common second-line treatments, although survival data are not yet available. Other potentially active treatments include bevacizumab, mTOR inhibitors (e.g., temsirolimus), and anthracyclines. Carcinosarcomas of the uterus (also called Müllerian tumors) contain both mesenchymal and epithelial components but will often respond to paclitaxel and platinum complex therapy. Other uterine sarcomas require an entirely different approach and need histology-specific consideration. The most common are the leiomyosarcomas of the uterus, which are treated with docetaxel/gemcitabine at recurrence but do not appear to benefit from adjuvant therapy. Ifosfamide/doxorubicin and trabectedin can have some benefit in refractory disease.

GESTATIONAL TROPHOBLASTIC TUMORS

Gestational trophoblastic diseases represent a spectrum of neoplasia from benign hydatidiform mole to choriocarcinoma due to persistent trophoblastic disease associated most commonly with molar pregnancy but occasionally seen after normal gestation. The most common presentations of trophoblastic tumors are partial and complete molar pregnancies. These represent approximately 1 in 1500 conceptions in developed Western countries. The incidence widely varies globally, with areas in Southeast Asia having a much higher incidence of molar pregnancy. Regions with high molar pregnancy rates are often associated with diets low in carotene and animal fats.

RISK FACTORS

Trophoblastic tumors result from the outgrowth or persistence of placental tissue. They arise most commonly in the uterus but can also arise in other sites such as the fallopian tubes due to ectopic pregnancy. Risk factors include poorly defined dietary and environmental factors as well as conceptions at the extremes of reproductive age, with the incidence particularly high in females conceiving at younger than age 16 or older than age 50. In older women, the incidence of molar pregnancy might be as high as one in three, likely due to increased risk of abnormal fertilization of the aged ova. Most trophoblastic neoplasms are associated with complete moles, diploid tumors with all genetic material from the paternal donor (known as uniparental disomy). This is thought to occur when a single sperm fertilizes an enucleate egg that subsequently duplicates the paternal DNA. Trophoblastic proliferation occurs with exuberant villous stroma. If pseudopregnancy extends out past the 12th week, fluid progressively accumulates within the stroma, leading to "hydropic changes." Fetal development does not occur in complete moles.

Partial moles arise from the fertilization of an egg with two sperm cells; hence, two-thirds of genetic material is paternal in these triploid tumors. Hydropic changes are less dramatic, and fetal development can often occur through late first trimester or early second trimester, at which point spontaneous abortion is common. Laboratory findings will include excessively high human chorionic gonadotropin (hCG) and high AFP. The risk of persistent gestational trophoblastic disease after partial mole is ~5%. Complete and partial moles can be noninvasive or invasive. Myometrial invasion occurs in no more than one in six complete moles and a lower portion of partial moles.

PRESENTATION OF INVASIVE TROPHOBLASTIC DISEASE

The clinical presentation of molar pregnancy is changing in developed countries due to the early detection of pregnancy with home pregnancy kits and the very early use of Doppler and ultrasound to evaluate the early fetus and uterine cavity for evidence of a viable fetus. Thus, in these countries, the majority of women presenting with trophoblastic disease have their moles detected early and have typical symptoms of early pregnancy including nausea, amenorrhea, and breast tenderness. With uterine evacuation of early complete and partial moles, most women experience spontaneous remission of their disease as monitored by serial serum β-hCG levels. These women require no chemotherapy. Patients with persistent elevation of β-hCG or rising β-hCG after uterine evacuation have persistent or actively growing gestational trophoblastic disease and require therapy. Most series suggest that between 15 and 25% of women will have evidence of persistent gestational trophoblastic disease after molar evacuation.

In women who lack access to prenatal care, presenting symptoms can be life-threatening, including the development of preeclampsia or even eclampsia. Hyperthyroidism can also be seen with very high β-hCG values. Evacuation of large moles can be associated with life-threatening complications including uterine perforation, volume loss, high-output cardiac failure, and adult respiratory distress syndrome (ARDS).

For women with evidence of rising β-hCG or radiologic confirmation of metastatic or persistent regional disease, prognosis can be estimated through a variety of scoring algorithms that identify women at low, intermediate, and high risk for requiring multiagent chemotherapy. In general, women with widely metastatic nonpulmonary disease, very elevated β-hCG, and prior normal antecedent term pregnancy are considered at high risk and typically require multiagent chemotherapy at an expert center for cure. Even very advanced gestational trophoblastic disease is almost uniformly curable when managed by an expert in this rare malignancy.

TREATMENT

Invasive Trophoblastic Disease

Management of invasive trophoblastic disease should be 100% curative, and complex patients should be managed by clinicians experienced in this disease. The management for a persistent and rising β-hCG after evacuation of a molar conception is typically chemotherapy, although surgery can play an important role for chemotherapy-resistant disease that is isolated in the uterus (especially if childbearing is complete) or to control hemorrhage. For women wishing to maintain fertility or with metastatic disease, the preferred treatment is chemotherapy. Trophoblastic disease is exquisitely sensitive to chemotherapy, and guided by serial serum β-hCG testing, successful, curative treatment is the rule. Single-agent treatment with dactinomycin or methotrexate cures 90% of women with low-risk disease. Patients with high-risk disease (very high β-hCG levels, presentation ≥4 months after pregnancy, brain or liver metastases, failure of methotrexate therapy) are typically treated with multiagent chemotherapy (etoposide, methotrexate, and dactinomycin, alternating with cyclophosphamide and vincristine [EMA-CO]), which is typically curative even in women with extensive metastatic disease. A regimen of cisplatin and etoposide alternating with etoposide/methotrexate/dactinomycin is used for the highest-risk patients. In the highest-risk patients with liver, lung, and brain metastases, hemorrhage from the rich tumor vasculature is a major risk during chemotherapy initiation. Cured women may become pregnant again without evidence of increased fetal or maternal complications.

FURTHER READING

Green AK et al: A review of immune checkpoint blockade therapy in endometrial cancer. Am Soc Clin Oncol Educ Book 40:1, 2020.

Longo DL: Personalized medicine for primary treatment of serous ovarian cancer. N Engl J Med 381:2471, 2019.

Lu KH, Broaddus RR: Endometrial cancer. N Engl J Med 383:2053, 2020.

Menon U et al: Ovarian cancer population screening and mortality after long-term follow-up in the UK Collaborative Trial of Ovarian Cancer Screening (UKCTOCS): A randomised controlled trial. Lancet 397:2182, 2021.

Ramirez PT et al: Minimally invasive versus abdominal radical hysterectomy for cervical cancer. N Engl J Med 379:1895, 2018.

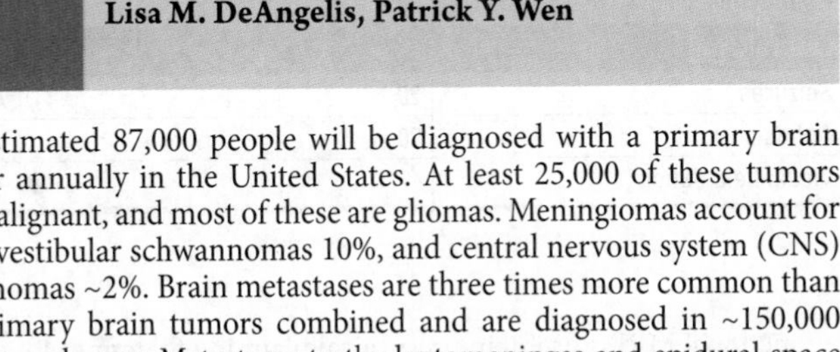

90 Primary and Metastatic Tumors of the Nervous System

Lisa M. DeAngelis, Patrick Y. Wen

An estimated 87,000 people will be diagnosed with a primary brain tumor annually in the United States. At least 25,000 of these tumors are malignant, and most of these are gliomas. Meningiomas account for 35%, vestibular schwannomas 10%, and central nervous system (CNS) lymphomas ~2%. Brain metastases are three times more common than all primary brain tumors combined and are diagnosed in ~150,000 people each year. Metastases to the leptomeninges and epidural space of the spinal cord each occur in ~3–5% of patients with systemic cancer and are also a major cause of neurologic disability.

APPROACH TO THE PATIENT

Primary and Metastatic Tumors of the Nervous System

CLINICAL FEATURES

Brain tumors of any type can present with a variety of symptoms and signs that fall into two categories: general and focal; patients often have a combination of the two (**Table 90-1**). General symptoms include headache, with or without nausea or vomiting, cognitive difficulties, personality change, and gait disorder. These symptoms arise when the enlarging tumor and its surrounding edema cause an increase in intracranial pressure or compression of cerebrospinal fluid (CSF) circulation leading to hydrocephalus. The classic brain tumor headache predominates in the morning and improves during the day, but this pattern is seen in a minority of patients. Headaches are often holocephalic but can be ipsilateral to the side of a tumor. Occasionally, headaches have features of a typical migraine with unilateral throbbing pain associated with visual scotoma. Personality changes may include apathy and withdrawal from social situations, mimicking depression. Focal or lateralizing findings include hemiparesis, aphasia, or visual field defect. Lateralizing symptoms are typically subacute and progressive; language difficulties may be mistaken for confusion. Seizures are common, occurring in ~25% of patients with brain metastases or malignant gliomas, and are the presenting symptom in up to 90% of patients with a low-grade glioma. All seizures arising from a brain tumor will have a focal onset whether or not it is apparent clinically.

NEUROIMAGING

Cranial magnetic resonance imaging (MRI) is the preferred diagnostic test for any patient suspected of having a brain tumor and should be performed with gadolinium contrast administration. Computed tomography (CT) scan should be reserved for those patients unable to undergo MRI. Malignant brain tumors—whether primary or metastatic—typically enhance with gadolinium, have central areas of necrosis, and are surrounded by edema of the neighboring white matter. Low-grade gliomas usually do not enhance with gadolinium and are best appreciated on fluid-attenuated inversion recovery (FLAIR) MRI sequences. Meningiomas have a typical appearance on MRI because they are dural-based enhancing tumors with a dural tail and compress but do not invade the brain. Dural metastases or a dural lymphoma can have a similar appearance. Imaging is characteristic for many primary and metastatic tumors and sometimes will suffice to establish a diagnosis when the location precludes surgical intervention (e.g., brainstem glioma).

TABLE 90-1 Symptoms and Signs at Presentation of Brain Tumors

	HIGH-GRADE GLIOMA (%)	LOW-GRADE GLIOMA (%)	MENINGIOMA (%)	METASTASES (%)
Generalized				
Impaired cognitive function	50	10	30	60
Hemiparesis	40	10	36	60
Headache	50	40	37	50
Lateralizing				
Seizures	20	70+	17	18
Aphasia	20	<5	—	18
Visual field deficit	—	—	—	7

Functional MRI is useful in presurgical planning to define eloquent sensory, motor, or language cortex. Positron emission tomography (PET) is useful in determining the metabolic activity of the lesions seen on MRI; MR perfusion and spectroscopy can provide information on blood flow or tissue composition. These techniques may help distinguish tumor progression from tissue necrosis due to treatment with radiation and chemotherapy. Neuroimaging is the only test necessary to diagnose a brain tumor. Laboratory tests are rarely useful, although patients with metastatic disease may have elevation of a serum tumor marker (e.g., β human chorionic gonadotropin [β-hCG] from testicular cancer). Additional testing such as cerebral angiogram, electroencephalogram (EEG), or lumbar puncture is rarely indicated or helpful.

TREATMENT

Brain Tumors

Therapy of any intracranial malignancy requires both symptomatic and definitive treatments. Definitive treatment is based on the specific tumor type and includes surgery, radiotherapy, and chemotherapy. However, symptomatic treatments apply to brain tumors of any type. Most high-grade malignancies are accompanied by substantial surrounding edema, which contributes to neurologic disability and raised intracranial pressure. Glucocorticoids are highly effective at reducing perilesional edema and improving neurologic function, often within hours of administration. Dexamethasone has been the glucocorticoid of choice because of its relatively low mineralocorticoid activity; initial doses are 8–12 mg/d. Glucocorticoids rapidly ameliorate symptoms and signs, but their long-term use causes substantial toxicity including insomnia, weight gain, diabetes mellitus, steroid myopathy, and personality changes. Consequently, a taper is indicated as definitive treatment is administered and the patient improves.

Patients with brain tumors who present with seizures require antiepileptic drug therapy. Prophylactic antiepileptic drugs are used in the perioperative setting, but there is no role for extended use in patients who have not had a seizure. The agents of choice are those drugs that do not induce the hepatic microsomal enzyme system. These include levetiracetam, topiramate, lamotrigine, valproic acid, and lacosamide (**Chap. 425**). Other drugs, such as phenytoin and carbamazepine, are used less frequently because they are potent enzyme inducers that can interfere with both glucocorticoid and chemotherapy metabolism. Venous thromboembolic disease occurs in 20–30% of patients with high-grade gliomas or brain metastases. Prophylactic anticoagulants should be used during hospitalization and in nonambulatory patients. Those who have had either a deep vein thrombosis or a pulmonary embolus can receive therapeutic doses of anticoagulation safely and without increasing the risk for hemorrhage into the tumor. Inferior vena cava filters are reserved for patients with absolute contraindications to anticoagulation such as recent craniotomy.

PRIMARY BRAIN TUMORS

EPIDEMIOLOGY

No etiology has been identified for most primary brain tumors. The only established risk factors are exposure to ionizing radiation (meningiomas, gliomas, and schwannomas) and immunosuppression (primary CNS lymphoma). There is no proven evidence for any association with exposure to electromagnetic fields including cellular telephones, head injury, foods containing *N*-nitroso compounds, or occupational risk factors. A small minority of patients have a family history of brain tumors. Some of these familial cases are associated with genetic syndromes (**Table 90-2**).

MOLECULAR PATHOGENESIS

As with other neoplasms, brain tumors arise as a result of a multistep process driven by the sequential acquisition of genetic alterations. These include loss of tumor-suppressor genes (e.g., *p53*, cyclin-dependent kinase inhibitor 2A and 2B [*CDKN2A/B*], and phosphatase and tensin homolog on chromosome 10 [*PTEN*]) and amplification and overexpression of protooncogenes such as the epidermal growth factor receptor (*EGFR*) and platelet-derived growth factor receptors (*PDGFR*). The accumulation of these genetic abnormalities results in uncontrolled cell growth and tumor formation. Many brain tumors, including glioblastomas, are characterized by significant molecular heterogeneity, which contributes to the difficulty in developing effective therapies.

Important progress has been made in understanding the molecular pathogenesis of several types of brain tumors, including glioblastoma and medulloblastoma, allowing them to be separated into different subtypes with different prognoses. This has led the World Health Organization (WHO) to issue an update on the classification of CNS tumors in 2016 that for the first time incorporates molecular parameters in addition to traditional histology into the diagnosis of brain tumors.

INTRINSIC "MALIGNANT" TUMORS

DIFFUSE GLIOMAS

Gliomas are the most common type of malignant primary brain tumor and are derived, based on their presumed lineage, into astrocytomas and oligodendrogliomas. These tumors are classified based on two highly recurrent molecular alterations, isocitrate dehydrogenase (*IDH*) mutations and 1p/19q codeletion, in addition to more conventional histopathologic parameters. Most lower-grade astrocytomas have *IDH* mutations but intact 1p/19q and often mutations in *ATRX* and *p53*. Oligodendrogliomas usually have *IDH* mutations and codeletion of 1p/19q. A minority of astrocytomas and oligodendrogliomas that lack *IDH* mutations (20–30%) have a worse prognosis.

Diffuse gliomas can present rarely as widespread infiltration of the brain tissue without a focal mass. Such tumors usually present with cognitive problems, and the MRI demonstrates confluent, typically nonenhancing areas of increased signal on FLAIR sequences without significant mass effect. Formerly known as gliomatosis cerebri, these lesions are now categorized by the pathology identified on biopsy, but they can be diagnostically challenging when the nature of the imaging

TABLE 90-2 Genetic Syndromes Associated with Primary Brain Tumors

SYNDROME	INHERITANCE	GENE/PROTEIN	ASSOCIATED TUMORS
Cowden's syndrome	AD	Mutations of *PTEN* (ch10p23)	Dysplastic cerebellar gangliocytoma (Lhermitte-Duclos disease), meningioma, astrocytoma Breast, endometrial, thyroid cancer, trichilemmomas
Familial schwannomatosis	Sporadic Hereditary	Mutations in *INI1/SNF5* (ch22q11)	Schwannomas, gliomas
Gardner's syndrome	AD	Mutations in *APC* (ch5q21)	Medulloblastoma, glioblastoma, craniopharyngioma Familial polyposis, multiple osteomas, skin and soft tissue tumors
Gorlin syndrome (basal cell nevus syndrome)	AD	Mutations in *Patched 1* gene (ch9q22.3)	Medulloblastomas Basal cell carcinoma
Li-Fraumeni syndrome	AD	Mutations in *p53* (ch17p13.1)	Gliomas, medulloblastomas Sarcomas, breast cancer, leukemias, others
Lynch syndrome	AD	Mutations in *MSH2, MSH1, MSH6, PMS2*	Glioblastoma and other gliomas Gastrointestinal, endometrial, and other cancers
Multiple endocrine neoplasia 1 (Wermer's syndrome)	AD	Mutations in *Menin* (ch11q13)	Pituitary adenoma, malignant schwannomas Parathyroid and pancreatic islet cell tumors
NF1	AD	Mutations in *NF1*/neurofibromin (ch17q12-22)	Schwannomas, astrocytomas, optic nerve gliomas, meningiomas Neurofibromas, neurofibrosarcomas, others
NF2	AD	Mutations in *NF2*/merlin (ch22q12)	Bilateral vestibular schwannomas, astrocytomas, multiple meningiomas, ependymomas
TSC (Bourneville disease)	AD	Mutations in *TSC1/TSC2* (ch9q34/16)	Subependymal giant cell astrocytoma, ependymomas, glioma, ganglioneuroma, hamartoma
Turcot syndrome	AD AR	Mutations in *APC*[a] (ch5) hMLH1 (ch3p21)	Gliomas, medulloblastomas Adenomatous colon polyps, adenocarcinoma
VHL	AD	Mutations in *VHL* gene (ch3p25)	Hemangioblastomas Retinal angiomas, renal cell carcinoma, pheochromocytoma, pancreatic tumors and cysts, endolymphatic sac tumors of the middle ear

[a]Various DNA mismatch repair gene mutations may cause a similar clinical phenotype, also referred to as Turcot syndrome, in which there is a predisposition to nonpolyposis colon cancer and brain tumors.

Abbreviations: AD, autosomal dominant; APC, adenomatous polyposis coli; AR, autosomal recessive; ch, chromosome; NF, neurofibromatosis; PTEN, phosphatase and tensin homologue; TSC, tuberous sclerosis complex; VHL, von Hippel-Lindau.

abnormalities is unclear. Often diagnosis is delayed until the patient develops worsening deficits or there is clear progression on imaging. Treatment is then determined by the pathology.

ASTROCYTOMAS

These are infiltrative tumors with a presumptive glial cell of origin. The WHO classifies astrocytomas into four prognostic grades based on histologic features: grade I (pilocytic astrocytoma, subependymal giant cell astrocytoma); grade II (astrocytoma); grade III (anaplastic astrocytoma); and grade IV (glioblastoma). Grades I and II are considered low-grade, and grades III and IV high-grade, astrocytomas.

Low-Grade Astrocytoma • GRADE I ASTROCYTOMAS Pilocytic astrocytomas (WHO grade I) are the most common tumor of childhood. They occur typically in the cerebellum but may also be found elsewhere in the neuraxis, including the optic nerves and brainstem. Frequently they appear as cystic lesions with an enhancing mural nodule. Often they have *BRAF* fusions or mutations. These are well-demarcated lesions that are potentially curable if they can be resected completely. Giant cell subependymal astrocytomas are usually found in the ventricular wall of patients with tuberous sclerosis. They often do not require intervention but can be treated surgically or with inhibitors of the mammalian target of rapamycin (mTOR).

GRADE II ASTROCYTOMAS These are infiltrative tumors that usually present with seizures in young adults. They appear as nonenhancing tumors with increased T2/FLAIR signal (**Fig. 90-1**). If feasible, patients should undergo maximal surgical resection, although complete resection is rarely possible because of the invasive nature of the tumor. In patients at higher risk for recurrence (subtotal resection or above the age of 40 years), there is evidence that radiation therapy (RT) followed by PCV (procarbazine, cyclohexylchloroethylnitrosourea [CCNU], and vincristine) chemotherapy may possibly be of benefit. The tumor transforms to a malignant astrocytoma in most patients, leading to variable survival with a median of ~5–10 years.

High-Grade Astrocytoma • GRADE III (ANAPLASTIC) ASTROCYTOMA These account for ~15–20% of high-grade

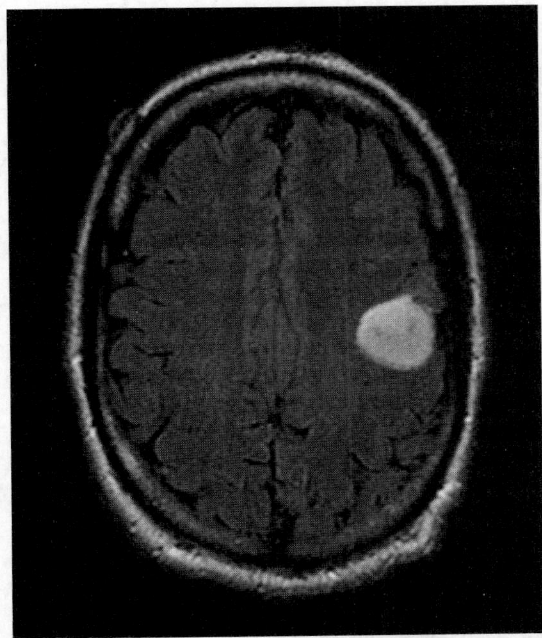

FIGURE 90-1 Fluid-attenuated inversion recovery (FLAIR) MRI of a left frontal low-grade astrocytoma. This lesion did not enhance.

astrocytomas. They generally present in the fourth and fifth decades of life as variably enhancing tumors. Treatment is the same as for glioblastoma, consisting of maximal safe surgical resection followed by RT and adjuvant temozolomide alone or RT with concurrent and adjuvant temozolomide.

GRADE IV ASTROCYTOMA (GLIOBLASTOMA) Glioblastoma accounts for the majority of high-grade astrocytomas. Approximately 10% of glioblastomas have *IDH* mutations. These tend to arise from lower-grade tumors (secondary glioblastomas) and have a better prognosis. In the next update of the WHO classification, the term glioblastoma will be restricted to tumors without *IDH* mutations. Glioblastomas with *IDH* mutations have a different biology and better prognosis and will be termed astrocytomas, *IDH*-mutant, grade 4. In addition, astrocytomas without the classic histologic features of glioblastoma (necrosis and endothelial proliferation) but that have the molecular features of glioblastoma (epidermal growth factor amplification, combined with whole chromosome 7 gain and 10 loss, or telomerase reverse transcriptase [*TERT*] promoter mutations) will also be considered glioblastomas.

Glioblastomas are the most common malignant primary brain tumor, with >12,000 cases diagnosed each year in the United States. Patients usually present in the sixth and seventh decades of life with headache, seizures, or focal neurologic deficits. The tumors appear as ring-enhancing masses with central necrosis and surrounding edema (**Fig. 90-2**). These are highly infiltrative tumors, and the areas of increased T2/FLAIR signal surrounding the main tumor mass contain invading tumor cells. Treatment involves maximal surgical resection followed by partial-field external-beam RT (6000 cGy in thirty 200-cGy fractions) with concomitant temozolomide, followed by 6 months of adjuvant temozolomide. With this regimen, median survival is increased to 14.6–18 months compared to only 12 months with RT alone, and 5-year survival is ~10%. Efforts to increase the dose of RT locally using brachytherapy or stereotactic radiosurgery (SRS) have failed to improve the outcome and these treatments are not used. Patients whose tumor contains the DNA repair enzyme O^6-methylguanine-DNA methyltransferase (MGMT) are relatively resistant to temozolomide and have a worse prognosis compared to those whose tumors contain low levels of MGMT as a result of silencing of the *MGMT* gene by promoter hypermethylation. Implantation of biodegradable polymers containing carmustine chemotherapy into the tumor bed after resection of the tumor or addition of tumor treating fields (scalp electrodes delivering low-intensity electric currents) produces a modest improvement in survival.

FIGURE 90-2 Postgadolinium T1 MRI of a large cystic left frontal glioblastoma.

For elderly patients aged >65–70 years, a hypofractionated RT regimen of 40 Gy over 3 weeks with temozolomide is well tolerated and likely leads to similar outcomes as the 6-week standard RT regimen.

Despite optimal therapy, glioblastomas invariably recur. Treatment options for recurrent disease may include reoperation, re-irradiation with bevacizumab, and alternate chemotherapeutic regimens. Bevacizumab, a humanized vascular endothelial growth factor (VEGF) monoclonal antibody, has activity in recurrent glioblastoma, increasing progression-free survival but not overall survival and reducing peritumoral edema and glucocorticoid use (**Fig. 90-3**). Immune checkpoint inhibitors have been successful in a variety of solid tumors but have failed to demonstrate substantial activity in glioblastoma. A recent phase III trial comparing bevacizumab with nivolumab in recurrent glioblastoma demonstrated an identical median overall survival of 9.8–10 months in the two arms, with similar toxicities. Treatment decisions for patients with recurrent glioblastoma must be made on an individual basis, taking into consideration such factors as previous therapy, time to relapse, performance status, and quality of life. Whenever feasible, patients should be enrolled in clinical trials. Novel therapies

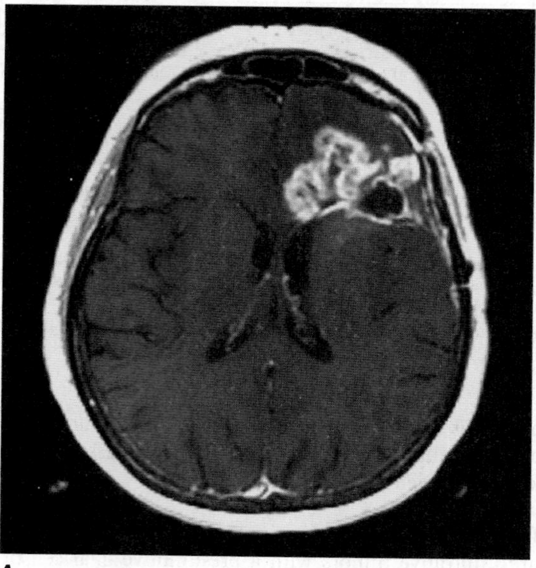

A

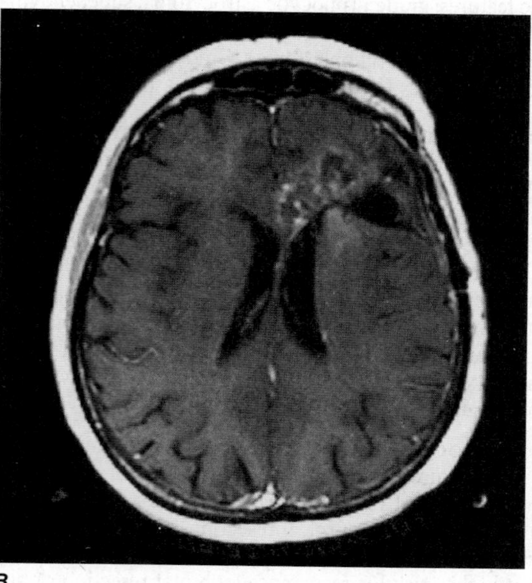

B

FIGURE 90-3 Postgadolinium T1 MRI of a recurrent glioblastoma before (***A***) and after (***B***) administration of bevacizumab. Note the decreased enhancement and mass effect.

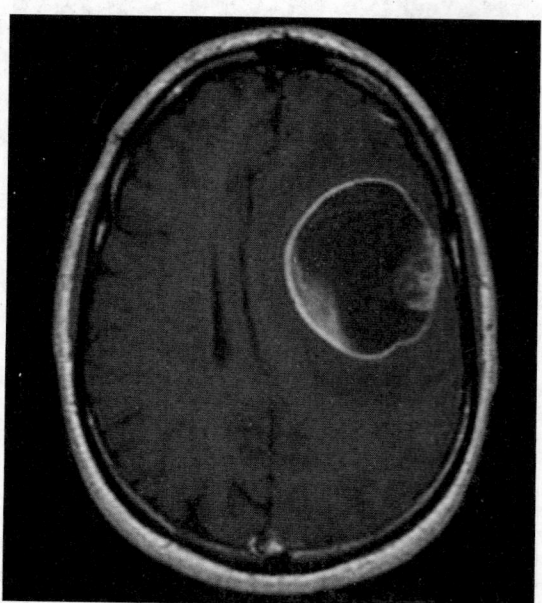

undergoing evaluation in patients with glioblastoma include targeted molecular agents directed at receptor tyrosine kinases and signal transduction pathways; immunotherapy using vaccines, novel checkpoint inhibitors, or chimeric antigen receptor (CAR) T cells; oncolytic viruses; antiangiogenic agents; chemotherapeutic agents that cross the blood-brain barrier more effectively than currently available drugs; and infusion of radiolabeled drugs and targeted toxins into the tumor and surrounding brain by means of convection-enhanced delivery.

The most important adverse prognostic factors in patients with glioblastomas are older age, absence of *IDH* mutations, unmethylated MGMT promoter, poor Karnofsky performance status, and unresectable tumor.

Gliosarcomas are a variant of glioblastoma containing both an astrocytic and a sarcomatous component and are treated in the same way as glioblastomas.

■ OLIGODENDROGLIOMA

Oligodendrogliomas account for ~15–20% of gliomas. They are characterized by codeletion of 1p/19q and have *IDH* mutations. Oligodendrogliomas are classified by the WHO into oligodendrogliomas (grade II) or anaplastic oligodendrogliomas (AOs) (grade III). Oligodendrogliomas have distinctive pathologic features such as perinuclear clearing—giving rise to a "fried-egg" appearance—and a reticular pattern of blood vessel growth. Some tumors have both an oligodendroglial as well as an astrocytic component. With molecular testing, it is now clear that almost all of these mixed tumors (oligoastrocytomas) are genetically either astrocytomas or oligodendrogliomas. As a result, the diagnosis of oligoastrocytoma is now rarely made unless molecular testing is not available.

Grade II oligodendrogliomas are generally more responsive to therapy and have a better prognosis than pure astrocytic tumors. These tumors present similarly to grade II astrocytomas in young adults. The tumors are nonenhancing and often partially calcified. They should be treated with surgery and, in patients with residual disease or aged >40 years, RT and chemotherapy. Patients with oligodendrogliomas have a median survival in excess of 10 years.

AOs present in the fourth and fifth decades as variably enhancing tumors. They are more responsive to therapy than grade III astrocytomas. Treatment involves maximal safe resection followed by RT and PCV or temozolomide chemotherapy. Median survival of patients with AO is in excess of 10 years.

■ EPENDYMOMAS

Ependymomas are tumors derived from ependymal cells that line the ventricular surface. They account for ~5% of childhood tumors, frequently arise from the wall of the fourth ventricle in the posterior fossa, are associated with *RELA* fusions, and are classified as type A and B ependymoma subtypes. Although adults can have intracranial ependymomas, they occur more commonly in the spine, especially in the filum terminale of the spinal cord where they have a myxopapillary histology. Ependymomas that can be completely resected are potentially curable. Partially resected ependymomas will recur and require irradiation. The less common anaplastic ependymoma is more aggressive and is treated with resection and RT; chemotherapy has limited efficacy. Subependymomas are slow-growing benign lesions arising in the wall of ventricles that often do not require treatment.

■ OTHER LESS COMMON GLIOMAS

Gangliogliomas and pleomorphic xanthoastrocytomas occur in young adults. They behave as more indolent forms of grade I gliomas and are usually treated with surgery. Frequently they will have *BRAF* V600E mutations. Brainstem gliomas usually occur in children or young adults and often have *H3K27M* mutations. Despite treatment with RT and chemotherapy, the prognosis is poor, with a median survival of only 1 year.

■ PRIMARY CENTRAL NERVOUS SYSTEM LYMPHOMA

Primary central nervous system lymphoma (PCNSL) is a rare non-Hodgkin's lymphoma accounting for <3% of primary brain tumors. For unclear reasons, its incidence is increasing, particularly in immunocompetent, older individuals.

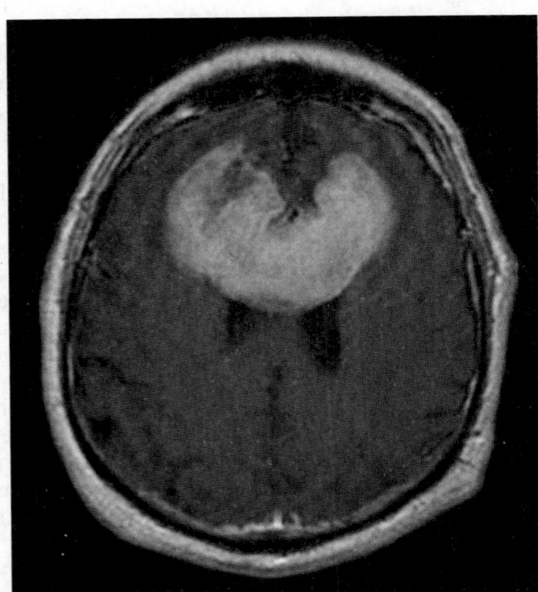

FIGURE 90-4 Postgadolinium T1 MRI demonstrating a large bifrontal primary central nervous system lymphoma (PCNSL). The periventricular location and diffuse enhancement pattern are characteristic of lymphoma.

PCNSL in immunocompetent patients is usually a diffuse large B-cell lymphoma. Immunocompromised patients, especially those infected with the human immunodeficiency virus (HIV) or organ transplant recipients, are at risk for PCNSL that is typically large cell with immunoblastic and more aggressive features. Epstein-Barr virus (EBV) plays an important role in the pathogenesis of PCNSL in this population. These patients are usually severely immunocompromised, with CD4 counts of <50/mL.

Immunocompetent patients with PCNSL are older (median 60 years) than those with HIV-related PCNSL (median 31 years). PCNSL usually presents as a mass lesion, with neuropsychiatric symptoms, lateralizing signs, or seizures. Ocular and leptomeningeal involvement each occur in 15–20% of patients, and involvement of these compartments may be asymptomatic. Rarely, it may present as isolated ocular lymphoma or as primary leptomeningeal lymphoma. When restricted to the leptomeninges, it may present as a subacute or chronic meningitis that causes progressive cranial and spinal nerve dysfunction. CSF cytologic examination or flow cytometry is required to establish the diagnosis.

On contrast-enhanced MRI, PCNSL usually appears as a densely enhancing tumor (**Fig. 90-4**). Immunocompetent patients have solitary lesions more often than immunosuppressed patients. Frequently there is involvement of the basal ganglia, corpus callosum, or periventricular region. Stereotactic biopsy is necessary to obtain a histologic diagnosis. Whenever possible, glucocorticoids should be withheld until after the biopsy has been obtained because they have a cytolytic effect on lymphoma cells and may lead to nondiagnostic tissue. In addition, patients should be tested for HIV, and the extent of disease should be assessed by performing PET or CT of the body, MRI of the spine, CSF analysis, and slit-lamp examination of the eye. Bone marrow biopsy and testicular ultrasound are occasionally performed.

TREATMENT

Primary Central Nervous System Lymphoma

PCNSL is more sensitive to glucocorticoids, chemotherapy, and RT than other primary brain tumors. Durable complete responses and long-term survival are possible with these treatments. High-dose methotrexate, a folate antagonist that interrupts DNA synthesis, produces response rates ranging from 35 to 80% and median survival of up to 50 months. The combination of methotrexate with other chemotherapeutic agents such as cytarabine increases the response rate to 70–100%. The addition of whole-brain RT (WBRT) to methotrexate-based chemotherapy prolongs progression-free survival but not overall survival, but it is associated with delayed neurotoxicity, especially in patients aged >60 years. As a result, full-dose RT is frequently omitted, but there may be a role for reduced-dose RT. The anti-CD20 monoclonal antibody rituximab is often incorporated into the chemotherapy regimen, although there are studies questioning its benefit. For some patients, high-dose chemotherapy with autologous stem cell rescue may offer the best chance of preventing relapse. At least 50% of patients will eventually develop recurrent disease. Treatment options include RT for patients who have not had prior irradiation, retreatment with methotrexate, as well as other chemotherapeutic agents such as temozolomide and pemetrexed. High-dose chemotherapy with autologous stem cell rescue may be appropriate in selected patients with relapsed disease. Bruton's tyrosine kinase (BTK) inhibitors such as ibrutinib, immunomodulatory drugs such as pomalidomide and lenalidomide, and immune checkpoint inhibitors have shown promising preliminary activity and are being evaluated in clinical trials, as are CAR T cells.

PCNSL IN IMMUNOCOMPROMISED PATIENTS

PCNSL in immunocompromised patients often produces multiple ring-enhancing lesions that can be difficult to differentiate from metastases or infections such as toxoplasmosis. The diagnosis is usually established by examination of the CSF for cytology and EBV DNA; toxoplasmosis serologic testing; brain PET imaging for hypermetabolism of the lesions, which, although nonspecific, can be consistent with tumor; and, if necessary, brain biopsy. Since the advent of highly active antiretroviral drugs, the incidence of HIV-related PCNSL has declined. These patients are preferably treated with high-dose methotrexate-based regimens and initiation of highly active antiretroviral therapy; WBRT is reserved for those who cannot tolerate systemic chemotherapy. In organ transplant recipients, reduction of immunosuppression may improve outcome.

MEDULLOBLASTOMAS

Medulloblastomas are the most common malignant brain tumor of childhood, accounting for ~20% of all primary CNS tumors among children. They arise from granule cell progenitors or from multipotent progenitors from the ventricular zone. Approximately 5% of children with medulloblastoma have an inherited syndrome, such as Gorlin, Turcot, or Li-Fraumeni, which predisposes to the development of medulloblastoma. Histologically, medulloblastomas are highly cellular tumors with abundant dark staining, round nuclei, and rosette formation (Homer-Wright rosettes). In the 2016 WHO pathologic classification, they have been divided into four molecular subgroups: (1) WNT-activated (primarily affects children and has the best outcome); (2) SHH-activated (affects adults, infants, and children, with the younger patients having the better outcome and adults doing poorly); (3) non-WNT/non-SHH, group 3 (frequently has disseminated CNS disease at diagnosis and has the worst outcome); and (4) non-WNT/non-SHH, group 4 (30% have metastases at diagnosis, but 5-year progression-free survival is 95%). Regardless of subtype, patients present with headache, ataxia, and signs of brainstem involvement. On MRI, they appear as densely enhancing tumors in the posterior fossa, sometimes associated with hydrocephalus. Treatment involves maximal surgical resection, craniospinal irradiation, and chemotherapy with agents such as cisplatin, lomustine, cyclophosphamide, and vincristine. Approximately 70% of patients overall have long-term survival but usually at the cost of significant neurocognitive impairment. A major goal of current research is to improve survival while minimizing long-term complications, and clinical trials are now being designed for specific molecular subgroups.

PINEAL REGION TUMORS

A large variety of tumors can arise in the region of the pineal gland. These typically present with headache, visual symptoms, and hydrocephalus. Patients may have Parinaud's syndrome characterized by impaired upgaze and accommodation. Some pineal tumors such as pineocytomas and benign teratomas can be treated by surgical resection. Germinomas respond to irradiation, whereas pineoblastomas and nongerminomatous germ cell tumors require craniospinal radiation and chemotherapy.

EXTRINSIC "BENIGN" TUMORS

MENINGIOMAS

Meningiomas are diagnosed with increasing frequency as more people undergo neuroimaging for various indications. They are now the most common primary brain tumor, accounting for ~35% of the total. Their incidence increases with age. They tend to be more common in women and in patients with neurofibromatosis type 2 (NF2). They also occur more commonly in patients with a history of cranial irradiation.

Meningiomas arise from the dura mater and are composed of neoplastic meningothelial (arachnoidal cap) cells. They are most commonly located over the cerebral convexities, especially adjacent to the sagittal sinus, but they can also occur in the skull base and along the dorsum of the spinal cord. Meningiomas are classified by the WHO into three histologic grades of increasing aggressiveness: grade I (benign), grade II (atypical), and grade III (malignant).

Many meningiomas are found incidentally following neuroimaging for unrelated reasons. They can also present with headaches, seizures, or focal neurologic deficits. On imaging studies, they have a characteristic appearance usually of a densely enhancing extra-axial tumor arising from the dura (**Fig. 90-5**). Typically they have a dural tail, consisting of thickened, enhanced dura extending like a tail from the mass. The main differential diagnosis of meningioma is a dural metastasis.

If the meningioma is small and asymptomatic, no intervention is necessary and the lesion can be observed with serial MRI studies. Larger, symptomatic lesions should be resected. If complete resection is achieved, the patient is cured. Incompletely resected tumors tend to recur, although the rate of recurrence can be very slow with grade I tumors. Tumors that cannot be resected, or can only be partially removed, may benefit from external-beam RT or SRS. These treatments may also be helpful in patients whose tumor has recurred after surgery. Hormonal therapy and chemotherapy are currently unproven.

Rarer tumors that resemble meningiomas include hemangiopericytomas and solitary fibrous tumors. Since they share similar molecular alterations (*NAB2-STAT6* fusion), the 2016 WHO classification introduced the combined term *solitary fibrous tumor/hemangiopericytoma* for this entity. These tumors are treated with surgery and RT but have a higher propensity to recur locally or metastasize systemically.

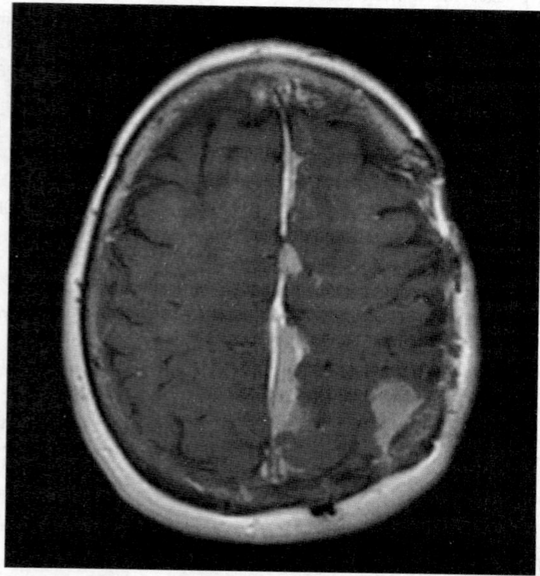

FIGURE 90-5 Postgadolinium T1 MRI demonstrating multiple meningiomas along the falx and left parietal cortex.

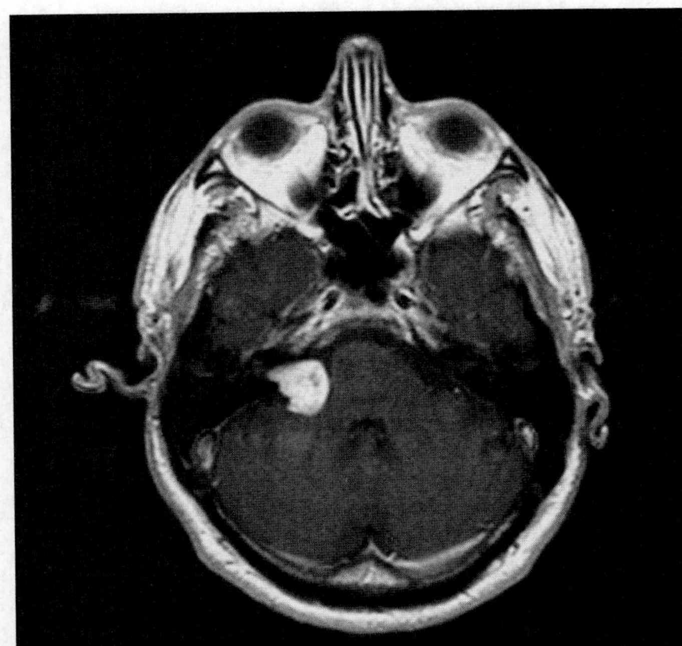

FIGURE 90-6 Postgadolinium MRI of a right vestibular schwannoma. The tumor can be seen to involve the internal auditory canal.

■ SCHWANNOMAS

These are generally benign tumors arising from the Schwann cells of cranial and spinal nerve roots. The most common schwannomas, termed *vestibular schwannomas* or *acoustic neuromas*, arise from the vestibular portion of the eighth cranial nerve and account for ~9% of primary brain tumors. Patients with NF2 have a high incidence of vestibular schwannomas that are frequently bilateral. Schwannomas arising from other cranial nerves, such as the trigeminal nerve (cranial nerve V), occur with much lower frequency. Neurofibromatosis type 1 (NF1) is associated with an increased incidence of schwannomas of the spinal nerve roots.

Vestibular schwannomas may be found incidentally on neuroimaging or present with progressive unilateral hearing loss, dizziness, tinnitus, or, less commonly, symptoms resulting from compression of the brainstem and cerebellum. On MRI, they appear as densely enhancing lesions, enlarging the internal auditory canal and often extending into the cerebellopontine angle (**Fig. 90-6**). The differential diagnosis includes meningioma. Very small, asymptomatic lesions can be observed with serial MRIs. Larger lesions should be treated with surgery or SRS. The optimal treatment will depend on the size of the tumor, symptoms, and the patient's preference. In patients with small vestibular schwannomas and relatively intact hearing, early surgical intervention increases the chance of preserving hearing.

■ PITUITARY TUMORS

These are discussed in detail in **Chap. 380**.

■ CRANIOPHARYNGIOMAS

Craniopharyngiomas are rare, usually suprasellar, partially calcified, solid, or mixed solid-cystic benign tumors that arise from remnants of Rathke's pouch. They have a bimodal distribution, occurring predominantly in children but also between the ages of 55 and 65 years. They present with headaches, visual impairment, and impaired growth in children and hypopituitarism in adults. Treatment involves surgery, RT, or a combination of the two. The papillary subtype of craniopharyngiomas often has *BRAF* V600E mutations and can be treated with RAF/MEK inhibitors.

■ OTHER BENIGN TUMORS

Dysembryoplastic Neuroepithelial Tumors (DNTs) These are benign, supratentorial tumors, usually in the temporal lobe. They typically occur in children and young adults with a long-standing history of seizures. Surgical resection is curative.

Epidermoid Cysts These consist of squamous epithelium surrounding a keratin-filled cyst. They are usually found in the cerebellopontine angle and the intrasellar and suprasellar regions. They may present with headaches, cranial nerve abnormalities, seizures, or hydrocephalus. MRI demonstrates an extra-axial lesion with characteristics that are similar to CSF but have restricted diffusion. Treatment involves surgical resection.

Dermoid Cysts Like epidermoid cysts, dermoid cysts arise from epithelial cells that are retained during closure of the neural tube. They contain both epidermal and dermal structures such as hair follicles, sweat glands, and sebaceous glands. Unlike epidermoid cysts, these tumors usually have a midline location. They occur most frequently in the posterior fossa, especially the vermis, fourth ventricle, and suprasellar cistern. On MRI, dermoid cysts resemble lipomas, demonstrating T1 hyperintensity and variable signal on T2. Symptomatic dermoid cysts can be treated with surgery.

Colloid Cysts These usually arise in the anterior third ventricle and may present with headaches, hydrocephalus, and, very rarely, sudden death. Surgical resection is curative, or a third ventriculostomy may relieve the obstructive hydrocephalus and be sufficient therapy.

NEUROCUTANEOUS SYNDROMES (PHAKOMATOSES)

A number of genetic disorders are characterized by cutaneous lesions and an increased risk of brain tumors. Most of these disorders have an autosomal dominant inheritance with variable penetrance.

■ NEUROFIBROMATOSIS TYPE 1 (von RECKLINGHAUSEN'S DISEASE)

NF1 is an autosomal dominant disorder with variable penetrance and an incidence of ~1 in 2600–3000. Approximately one-half of cases are familial; the remainder are caused by new mutations arising in patients with unaffected parents. The *NF1* gene is located on chromosome 17q11.2 and encodes neurofibromin, a guanosine triphosphatase (GTPase) activating protein (GAP) that is a negative regulator of the RAS–mitogen-activated protein (MAP) kinase signaling pathway, which includes the downstream kinase MEK. It is a classic tumor suppressor, and biallelic loss can result in a variety of nervous system tumors including neurofibromas, plexiform neurofibromas, optic nerve gliomas, astrocytomas, and meningiomas. In addition to neurofibromas, which appear as multiple, soft, rubbery cutaneous tumors, other cutaneous manifestations of NF1 include café-au-lait spots and axillary freckling. NF1 is also associated with hamartomas of the iris termed Lisch nodules, pheochromocytomas, pseudoarthrosis of the tibia, scoliosis, epilepsy, and mental retardation. The MEK inhibitor selumetinib has activity against inoperable plexiform neurofibromas and is the only treatment that targets the dysregulated signaling pathway.

■ NEUROFIBROMATOSIS TYPE 2

NF2 is less common than NF1, with an incidence of 1 in 25,000–40,000. It is an autosomal dominant disorder with full penetrance. As with NF1, approximately one-half of cases arise from new mutations. The *NF2* gene on 22q encodes a cytoskeletal protein, merlin (moesin, ezrin, radixin-like protein), that functions as a tumor suppressor. NF2 is characterized by bilateral vestibular schwannomas in >90% of patients, multiple meningiomas, and spinal ependymomas and astrocytomas. Treatment of bilateral vestibular schwannomas can be challenging because the goal is to preserve hearing for as long as possible. These patients may also have diffuse schwannomatosis that may affect the cranial, spinal, or peripheral nerves; posterior subcapsular lens opacities; and retinal hamartomas.

■ TUBEROUS SCLEROSIS (BOURNEVILLE DISEASE)

This is an autosomal dominant disorder with an incidence of ~1 in 5000–10,000 live births. It is caused by mutations in either the *TSC1* gene, which maps to chromosome 9q34 and encodes a protein termed hamartin, or the *TSC2* gene, which maps to chromosome 16p13.3 and encodes the protein tuberin. Hamartin forms a complex with tuberin, which inhibits cellular signaling through mTOR, and acts as a negative regulator of the cell cycle. Patients with tuberous sclerosis may have seizures, mental retardation, adenoma sebaceum (facial angiofibromas), shagreen patch, hypomelanotic macules, periungual fibromas, renal angiomyolipomas, and cardiac rhabdomyomas. These patients have an increased incidence of subependymal nodules, cortical tubers, and subependymal giant cell astrocytomas (SEGAs). Patients frequently require anticonvulsants for seizures. SEGAs do not always require therapeutic intervention, but the most effective therapy is with the mTOR inhibitors sirolimus or everolimus, which often decrease seizures as well as SEGA size.

TUMORS METASTATIC TO THE BRAIN

Brain metastases arise from hematogenous spread and frequently originate from a lung primary or are associated with pulmonary metastases. Most metastases develop at the gray matter–white matter junction in the watershed distribution of the brain where intravascular tumor cells lodge in terminal arterioles. The distribution of metastases in the brain approximates the proportion of blood flow such that ~85% of all metastases are supratentorial and 15% occur in the posterior fossa. The most common sources of brain metastases are lung and breast carcinomas; melanoma has the greatest propensity to metastasize to the brain, being found in 80% of patients at autopsy (**Table 90-3**). Other tumor types such as ovarian and esophageal carcinoma rarely metastasize to the brain. Prostate and breast cancers also have a propensity to metastasize to the dura and can mimic meningioma. Leptomeningeal metastases are common from hematologic malignancies and also breast and lung cancers. Spinal cord compression primarily arises in patients with prostate and breast cancer, tumors with a strong propensity to metastasize to the axial skeleton.

DIAGNOSIS OF METASTASES

Brain metastases are best visualized on MRI, where they usually appear as well-circumscribed lesions (**Fig. 90-7**). The amount of perilesional edema can be highly variable, with large lesions causing minimal edema and sometimes very small lesions causing extensive edema. Enhancement may be in a ring pattern or diffuse. Occasionally, intracranial metastases will hemorrhage; melanoma, thyroid, and kidney cancer have the greatest propensity to hemorrhage, but the most common cause of a hemorrhagic metastasis is lung cancer because it accounts for the majority of brain metastases. The radiographic appearance of brain metastasis is nonspecific, and similar-appearing lesions can occur with infection including brain abscesses, demyelinating lesions, sarcoidosis, radiation necrosis in a previously treated patient, or a primary brain tumor that may be a second malignancy in a patient with systemic cancer. Biopsy is rarely necessary for diagnosis because imaging alone in the appropriate clinical situation usually suffices. However, in ~10% of patients, a systemic cancer may present with a brain metastasis, and if there is not an easily accessible systemic site to biopsy, a brain lesion must be removed for diagnostic purposes.

TABLE 90-3 Frequency of Nervous System Metastases by Common Primary Tumors

	BRAIN (%)	LM (%)	ESCC (%)
Lung	41	17	15
Breast	19	57	22
Melanoma	10	12	4
Prostate	1	1	10
GIT	7	—	5
Renal	3	2	7
Lymphoma	<1	10	10
Sarcoma	7	1	9
Other	11	—	18

Abbreviations: ESCC, epidural spinal cord compression; GIT, gastrointestinal tract; LM, leptomeningeal metastases.

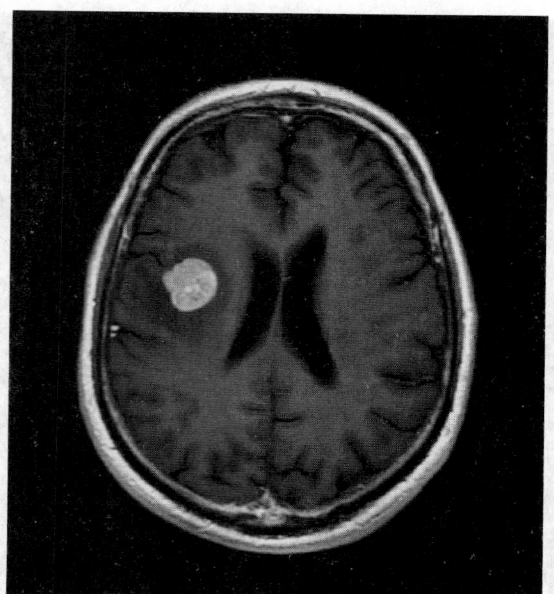

A

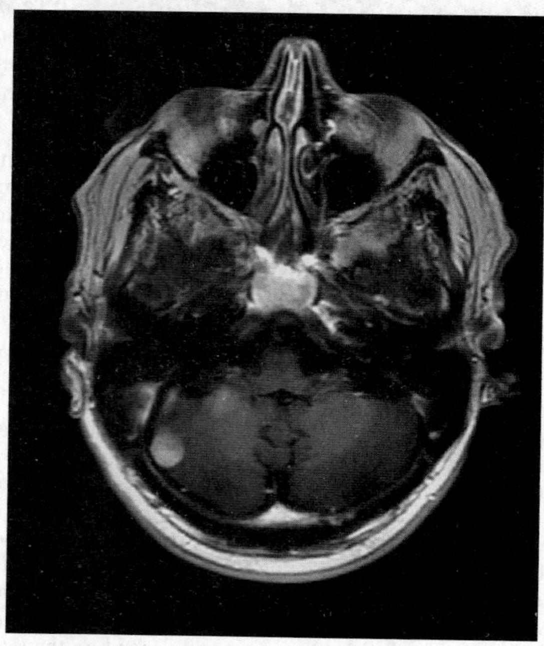

B

FIGURE 90-7 Postgadolinium T1 MRI of multiple brain metastases from non-small-cell lung cancer involving the right frontal (***A***) and right cerebellar (***B***) hemispheres. Note the diffuse enhancement pattern and absence of central necrosis.

TREATMENT

Tumors Metastatic to the Brain

DEFINITIVE TREATMENT

The number and location of brain metastases often determine the therapeutic options. The patient's overall condition and current or potential control of systemic disease are also major determinants. Brain metastases are single in approximately one-half of patients and multiple in the other half.

RADIATION THERAPY

The standard treatment for brain metastases has previously been WBRT usually administered to a total dose of 3000 cGy in 10 fractions. This affords rapid palliation, and ~80% of patients improve with glucocorticoids and RT. However, it is not curative, is associated with neurocognitive toxicity, and produces median survival of only 4–6 months. Recent data demonstrate that hippocampal avoidance during WBRT preserves cognitive function without increasing the risk of an intracranial relapse. If feasible, SRS has become the primary radiation oncology approach to brain metastases. It can be delivered through a variety of equally effective techniques including the gamma knife, linear accelerator, proton beam, or CyberKnife, all of which can deliver highly focused doses of RT, usually in a single fraction. SRS can effectively sterilize the visible lesions and afford local disease control in 80–90% of patients. Some patients have been cured of their brain metastases using SRS, whereas this is distinctly rare with WBRT. Traditionally SRS was used only for patients with 1–3 metastases, but recent data suggest that SRS can effectively treat up to 10 lesions. It is, however, confined to lesions of ≤3 cm and is most effective in metastases of ≤1 cm. The addition of WBRT to SRS improves disease control in the nervous system but does not prolong survival and thus is rarely employed.

SURGERY

Randomized controlled trials have demonstrated that surgical extirpation of a single brain metastasis followed by WBRT is superior to WBRT alone. Removal of two lesions or a single symptomatic mass, particularly if compressing the ventricular system, can also be useful. This is particularly important in patients who have highly radioresistant lesions such as renal carcinoma. Surgical resection can produce rapid amelioration of symptoms, improve control of edema, and result in prolonged survival. WBRT administered after complete resection of a brain metastasis improves disease control but does not prolong survival. Some centers administer focal RT or even SRS to a resected cavity, especially if there is concern that tumor has been left behind, but most avoid postoperative WBRT because of its cognitive effects.

CHEMOTHERAPY

Chemotherapy is becoming increasingly useful for brain metastases. Metastases from tumor types that are highly chemosensitive, such as germ cell tumors or small-cell lung cancer, may respond to chemotherapeutic regimens chosen according to the underlying malignancy. Increasingly, data demonstrate responsiveness of brain metastases to chemotherapy including targeted therapeutics, such as for patients with lung cancer harboring *EGFR* mutations that sensitize them to EGFR inhibitors. Immunotherapy is also effective against those primary tumors that are sensitive to this approach, such as melanoma. Antiangiogenic agents such as bevacizumab are effective in the treatment of CNS metastases in those primary tumors for which it is approved.

LEPTOMENINGEAL METASTASES

Leptomeningeal metastases are also described as carcinomatous meningitis, meningeal carcinomatosis, or, in the case of specific tumors, leukemic or lymphomatous meningitis. Among the hematologic malignancies, acute leukemias most commonly metastasize to the subarachnoid space, followed in frequency by aggressive diffuse lymphomas. Among solid tumors, breast and lung carcinomas and melanoma most frequently spread in this fashion. Tumor cells reach the subarachnoid space via the arterial circulation or occasionally through retrograde flow in venous systems that drain metastases along the bony spine or cranium. In addition, leptomeningeal metastases may develop as a direct consequence of prior brain metastases and occur in almost 40% of patients who have a metastasis resected from the cerebellum.

■ CLINICAL FEATURES

Leptomeningeal metastases are characterized by multilevel symptoms and signs along the neuraxis. Combinations of lumbar and cervical radiculopathies, cranial neuropathies, seizures, confusion, and encephalopathy from hydrocephalus or raised intracranial pressure can be present. Focal deficits such as hemiparesis or aphasia are rarely due to leptomeningeal metastases unless there is direct brain infiltration. New-onset limb pain in patients with breast cancer, lung cancer, or melanoma should prompt consideration of leptomeningeal spread.

■ LABORATORY AND IMAGING DIAGNOSIS

Leptomeningeal metastases are particularly challenging to diagnose because identification of tumor cells in the subarachnoid compartment may be elusive. MRI can be definitive when there are clear tumor nodules adherent to the cauda equina or spinal cord, enhancing cranial nerves, or subarachnoid enhancement on brain imaging (**Fig. 90-8**).

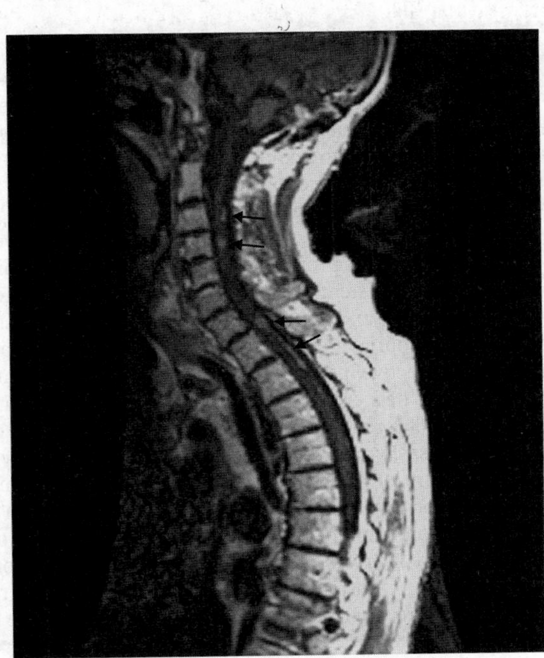

A

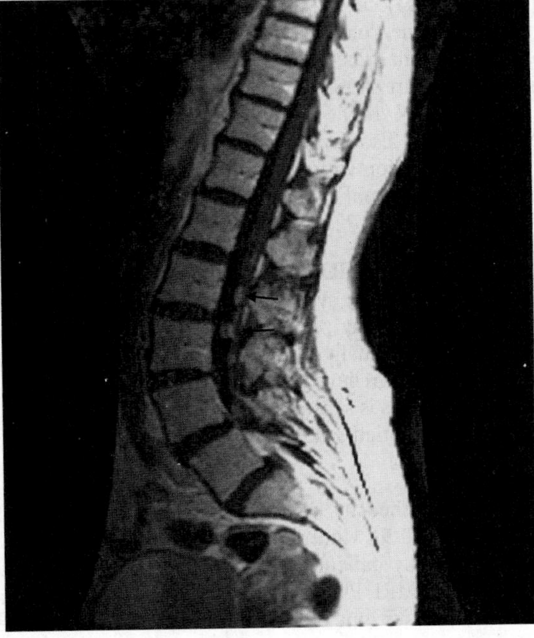

B

FIGURE 90-8 Postgadolinium MRI images of extensive leptomeningeal metastases from breast cancer. Nodules along the dorsal surface of the spinal cord (***A***) and cauda equina (***B***) are seen.

Imaging is diagnostic in ~75% of patients and is more often positive in patients with solid tumors. Demonstration of tumor cells in the CSF is definitive and often considered the gold standard. However, CSF cytologic examination is positive in only 50% of patients on the first lumbar puncture and still misses 10% after three CSF samples. New technologies, such as rare cell capture, enhance identification of tumor cells in the CSF; molecular profiling of the CSF can also identify tumor-specific mutations, indicating malignancy in the leptomeninges. CSF cytologic examination is most useful in hematologic malignancies, especially when combined with flow cytometry to identify a clonal population. Accompanying CSF abnormalities include an elevated protein concentration and an elevated white blood cell count; hypoglycorrhachia is noted in <25% of patients but is useful when present. Identification of tumor markers may be helpful in some solid tumors.

TREATMENT

Leptomeningeal Metastases

The treatment of leptomeningeal metastasis is palliative because there is no curative therapy. RT to the symptomatically involved areas, such as skull base for cranial neuropathy, can relieve pain and sometimes improve function. Craniospinal irradiation (CSI) is avoided because it has significant toxicity with myelosuppression and gastrointestinal irritation as well as limited effectiveness. However, recent data on proton beam CSI suggest better disease control with fewer systemic toxicities. Systemic chemotherapy, targeted therapeutics, and immunotherapy have all demonstrated efficacy in the appropriate setting. Alternatively, intrathecal chemotherapy can be effective, particularly in hematologic malignancies. This is optimally delivered through an intraventricular cannula (Ommaya reservoir) rather than by lumbar puncture. Few drugs can be delivered safely into the subarachnoid space, and they have a limited spectrum of antitumor activity, perhaps accounting for the relatively poor response to this approach, particularly in solid tumors. In addition, impaired CSF flow dynamics can compromise intrathecal drug delivery. Surgery has a limited role in leptomeningeal metastasis. A ventriculoperitoneal shunt can relieve raised intracranial pressure; once placed, intrathecal drug cannot be used.

EPIDURAL METASTASIS

Epidural metastasis occurs in 3–5% of patients with a systemic malignancy and causes neurologic compromise by compressing the spinal cord or cauda equina. The most common cancers that metastasize to the epidural space are those malignancies that spread to bone, such as breast and prostate. Lymphoma can cause bone involvement and compression, but it can also invade an intervertebral foramen and cause spinal cord compression without bone destruction. The thoracic spine is affected most commonly, followed by the lumbar and then cervical spine.

CLINICAL FEATURES

Back pain is the presenting symptom of epidural metastasis in virtually all patients; the pain may precede neurologic findings by weeks or months. The pain is usually exacerbated by lying down; by contrast, arthritic pain is often relieved by recumbency. Leg weakness is seen in ~50% of patients, as is sensory dysfunction. Sphincter problems are present in ~25% of patients at diagnosis.

DIAGNOSIS

Diagnosis is established by imaging, preferably with an MRI of the entire spine (**Fig. 90-9**). Contrast is not required to identify bony or epidural lesions. Any patient with cancer who has severe back pain should undergo an MRI. Plain films, bone scans, or even CT scans may show bone metastases, but only MRI can reliably delineate epidural tumor. For patients unable to have an MRI, CT myelography should be performed to outline the epidural space. The differential diagnosis of epidural tumor includes epidural abscess, acute or chronic hematomas, epidural lipomatosis, and, rarely, extramedullary hematopoiesis.

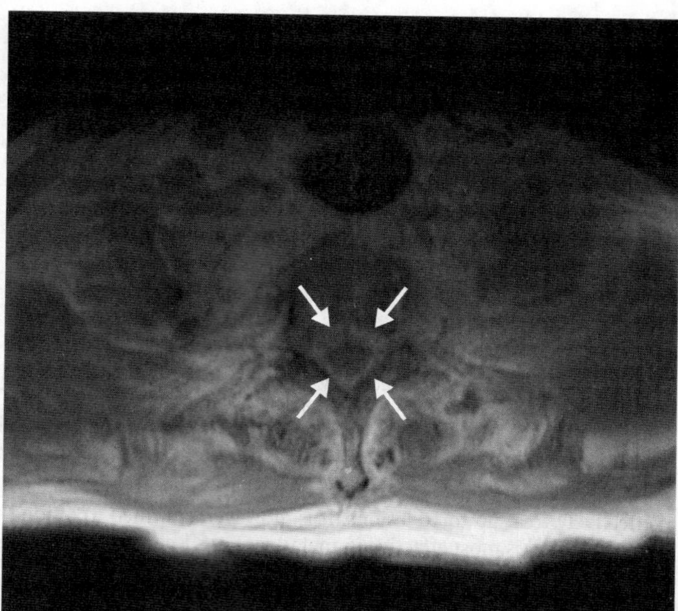

FIGURE 90-9 Postgadolinium T1 MRI showing circumferential epidural tumor around the thoracic spinal cord from esophageal cancer.

TREATMENT

Epidural Metastasis

Epidural metastasis requires immediate treatment. A randomized controlled trial demonstrated the superiority of surgical resection followed by RT compared to RT alone. However, patients must be able to tolerate surgery, and the surgical procedure of choice is a complete removal of the mass, which is typically anterior to the spinal canal, necessitating an extensive approach and resection. Otherwise, RT is the mainstay of treatment and can be used for patients with radiosensitive tumors, such as lymphoma, or for those unable to undergo surgery. SRS is increasingly being used, especially for radioresistant tumor types or for re-irradiation. Chemotherapy is rarely used for epidural metastasis unless the patient has minimal to no neurologic deficit and a highly chemosensitive tumor such as lymphoma or germinoma. Patients generally fare well if treated before there is a severe neurologic deficit. Recovery from paraparesis is better after surgery than with RT alone, but survival is often short due to widespread metastatic tumor.

NEUROLOGIC TOXICITY OF THERAPY

TOXICITY FROM RADIOTHERAPY

RT can cause a variety of toxicities in the CNS. These are usually described based on their relationship in time to the administration of RT: acute (occurring within days of RT), early delayed (months), or late delayed (years). In general, the acute and early delayed syndromes resolve and do not result in persistent deficits, whereas the late delayed toxicities are usually permanent and sometimes progressive.

Acute Toxicity Acute cerebral toxicity may occur during RT to the brain. RT can cause a transient disruption of the blood-brain barrier, resulting in edema and elevated intracranial pressure. This is usually manifest as headache, lethargy, nausea, and vomiting and can be both prevented and treated with the administration of glucocorticoids. There is no acute RT toxicity that affects the spinal cord.

Early Delayed Toxicity Early delayed toxicity is usually apparent weeks to months after completion of cranial irradiation and is likely due to focal demyelination. Clinically it may be asymptomatic or take the form of worsening or reappearance of a preexisting neurologic deficit. At times, a contrast-enhancing lesion can be seen on MRI/CT that can mimic the tumor for which the patient received the RT. For patients with a malignant glioma, this has been described as "pseudoprogression" because it mimics tumor recurrence on MRI, but it represents inflammation and necrotic debris engendered by effective therapy. This is seen with increased frequency when chemotherapy, particularly temozolomide, is given concurrently with RT. Pseudoprogression can resolve on its own or, if very symptomatic, may require glucocorticoids, resection, or bevacizumab.

In the spinal cord, early delayed RT toxicity is manifest as a Lhermitte symptom with paresthesias of the limbs or along the spine when the patient flexes the neck. Although frightening, it is benign, resolves on its own, and does not portend more serious problems.

Late Delayed Toxicity Late delayed toxicities are the most serious because they are often irreversible and cause severe neurologic deficits. In the brain, late toxicities can take several forms, the most common of which include radiation necrosis and leukoencephalopathy. Radiation necrosis is a focal mass of necrotic tissue that is contrast enhancing on CT/MRI and may be associated with significant edema. This may appear identical to pseudoprogression but is seen months to years after RT and is always symptomatic. Clinical symptoms and signs include seizures and findings referable to the location of the necrotic mass. The necrosis is caused by the effect of RT on cerebral vasculature with fibrinoid necrosis and occlusion of blood vessels. It can mimic tumor radiographically, but unlike tumor, it is typically hypometabolic on a PET scan and has reduced perfusion on perfusion MR sequences. It may require resection for diagnosis and treatment unless it can be managed with glucocorticoids. There are reports of improvement with hyperbaric oxygen or bevacizumab, but symptomatic benefit does not always accompany radiographic improvement.

Leukoencephalopathy is seen most commonly after WBRT as opposed to focal RT. On T2 or FLAIR MR sequences, there is diffusely increased signal seen throughout the hemispheric white matter, often bilaterally and symmetrically. There tends to be a periventricular predominance that may be associated with atrophy and ventricular enlargement. Clinically, patients develop cognitive impairment, a gait disorder, and later urinary incontinence, all of which can progress over time. These symptoms mimic those of normal pressure hydrocephalus, and placement of a ventriculoperitoneal shunt can improve function in some patients but does not reverse the deficits completely. Increased age is a risk factor for leukoencephalopathy but not for radiation necrosis. Necrosis appears to depend on an unidentified predisposition.

Other late neurologic toxicities include endocrine dysfunction if the pituitary or hypothalamus was included in the RT port. An RT-induced neoplasm can occur many years after therapeutic RT for either a prior CNS or a head and neck tumor; accurate diagnosis requires surgical resection or biopsy. In addition, RT causes accelerated atherosclerosis, which can cause stroke either from intracranial vascular disease or carotid plaque from neck irradiation.

The peripheral nervous system is relatively resistant to RT toxicities. Peripheral nerves are rarely affected by RT, but the plexus is more vulnerable. Plexopathy develops more commonly in the brachial than in the lumbosacral distribution. It must be differentiated from tumor progression in the plexus, which is usually visualized by CT/MRI or PET scan demonstrating tumor infiltrating the region. Clinically, tumor progression is usually painful, whereas RT-induced plexopathy is painless. Radiation plexopathy is also more commonly associated with lymphedema and myokymia of the affected limb. Sensory loss and weakness are seen in both.

TOXICITY FROM CHEMOTHERAPY

Neurotoxicity is second to myelosuppression as the dose-limiting toxicity of chemotherapeutic agents (**Table 90-4**). Chemotherapy causes peripheral neuropathy from many commonly used agents, and the type of neuropathy can vary depending on the drug. Vincristine causes paresthesias but little sensory loss and is associated with motor dysfunction, autonomic impairment (frequently ileus), and, rarely, cranial nerve compromise. Cisplatin causes large-fiber sensory loss resulting in sensory ataxia but little cutaneous sensory loss and no weakness.

TABLE 90-4 Neurologic Signs Caused by Agents Commonly Used in Patients with Cancer

Acute encephalopathy (delirium)	Seizures
Methotrexate (high-dose IV, IT)	Methotrexate
Cisplatin	Etoposide (high-dose)
Vincristine	Cisplatin
Asparaginase	Vincristine
Procarbazine	Asparaginase
5-Fluorouracil (± levamisole)	Nitrogen mustard
Cytarabine (high-dose)	Carmustine
Nitrosoureas (high-dose or arterial)	Dacarbazine (intraarterial or high-dose)
Ifosfamide	
Etoposide (high-dose)	Busulfan (high-dose)
Bevacizumab (PRES)	Myelopathy (IT drugs)
Chronic encephalopathy (dementia)	Methotrexate
Methotrexate	Cytarabine
Carmustine	Thiotepa
Cytarabine	Peripheral neuropathy
Fludarabine	Vinca alkaloids
Visual loss	Cisplatin
Tamoxifen	Procarbazine
Gallium nitrate	Etoposide
Cisplatin	Teniposide
Fludarabine	Cytarabine
Cerebellar dysfunction/ataxia	Taxanes
5-Fluorouracil (± levamisole)	Suramin
Cytarabine	Bortezomib
Procarbazine	

Abbreviations: IT, intrathecal; IV, intravenous; PRES, posterior reversible encephalopathy syndrome.

The taxanes also cause a predominately sensory neuropathy. Agents such as bortezomib and thalidomide also cause neuropathy. Sometimes a severe neuropathy emerges after multiple neurotoxic agents have been used together or in sequence.

Encephalopathy and seizures are common toxicities from chemotherapeutic drugs. Ifosfamide can cause a severe encephalopathy, which is reversible with discontinuation of the drug and the use of methylene blue for severely affected patients. Fludarabine also causes a severe global encephalopathy that may be permanent. Bevacizumab and other anti-VEGF agents can cause posterior reversible encephalopathy syndrome. Cisplatin can cause hearing loss and less frequently vestibular dysfunction. Immunotherapy with monoclonal antibodies such as ipilimumab or nivolumab can cause an autoimmune hypophysitis, Guillain-Barré syndrome, or an autoimmune encephalitis.

FURTHER READING

Achrol AS et al: Brain metastases. Nat Rev Dis Primers 5:5, 2019.

Barzilai O et al: Predictors of quality of life improvement after surgery for metastatic tumors of the spine: Prospective cohort study. Spine J 18:1109, 2018.

Brown PD et al: Hippocampal avoidance during whole-brain radiotherapy plus memantine for patients with brain metastases: Phase III trial NRG oncology CC001. J Clin Oncol 38:1019, 2020.

Buckner JC et al: Radiation plus procarbazine, CCNU, and vincristine in low-grade glioma. N Engl J Med 374:1344, 2016.

Cancer Genome Atlas Research Network et al: Comprehensive, integrative genomic analysis of diffuse lower-grade gliomas. N Engl J Med 372:2481, 2015.

Cheng H, Perez-Soler R: Leptomeningeal metastases in non-small-cell lung cancer. Lancet Oncol 19:e43, 2018.

Grommes C et al: Comprehensive approach to diagnosis and treatment of newly diagnosed primary CNS lymphoma. Neuro Oncol 21:296, 2019.

Gross AM et al: Selumetinib in children with inoperable plexiform neurofibromas. N Engl J Med 382:1430, 2020.

Louis DN et al: The 2016 World Health Organization classification of tumors of the central nervous system: A summary. Acta Neuropathol 131:803, 2016.

McEwen AE et al: Beyond the hood: CSF-derived cfDNA for diagnosis and characterization of CNS tumors. Front Cell Dev Biol 8:45, 2020.

McGranahan T et al: Current state of immunotherapy for treatment of glioblastoma. Curr Treat Options Oncol 20:24, 2019.

Omuro A et al: R-MVP followed by high-dose chemotherapy with TBC and autologous stem-cell transplant for newly diagnosed primary CNS lymphoma. Blood 125:1403, 2015.

Ramaswamy V et al: Risk stratification of childhood medulloblastoma in the molecular era: The current consensus. Acta Neuropathol 131:821, 2016.

Reardon DA et al: Effect of nivolumab vs bevacizumab in patients with recurrent glioblastoma: The CheckMate 143 phase 3 randomized clinical trial. JAMA Oncol 6:1003, 2020.

Rishi A, Yu HHM: Current treatment of melanoma brain metastasis. Curr Treat Options Oncol 21:45, 2020.

Schiff D et al: Recent developments and future directions in adult lower-grade gliomas: Society for Neuro-Oncology (SNO) and European Association of Neuro-Oncology (EANO) consensus. Neuro Oncol 21:837, 2019.

Tsakonas G et al: Management of brain metastasized non-small cell lung cancer (NSCLC)—From local treatment to new systemic therapies. Cancer Treat Rev 54:122, 2017.

Wen PY et al: Glioblastoma in adults: A Society for Neuro-Oncology (SNO) and European Society of Neuro-Oncology (EANO) consensus review on current management and future directions. Neuro Oncol 22:1073, 2020.

Yamada Y et al: The impact of histology and delivered dose on local control of spinal metastases treated with stereotactic radiosurgery. Neurosurg Focus 42:E6, 2017.

91 Soft Tissue and Bone Sarcomas and Bone Metastases

Shreyaskumar R. Patel

Sarcomas are rare (<1% of all malignancies) mesenchymal neoplasms that arise in bone and soft tissues. These tumors are usually of mesodermal origin, although a few are derived from neuroectoderm, and they are biologically distinct from the more common epithelial malignancies. Sarcomas affect all age groups; 15% are found in children <15 years of age, and 40% occur after age 55 years. Sarcomas are one of the most common solid tumors of childhood and are the fifth most common cause of cancer deaths in children. Sarcomas may be divided into two groups, those derived from bone and those derived from soft tissues.

SOFT TISSUE SARCOMAS

Soft tissues include muscles, tendons, fat, fibrous tissue, synovial tissue, vessels, and nerves. Approximately 60% of soft tissue sarcomas arise in the extremities, with the lower extremities involved three times as often as the upper extremities. Thirty percent arise in the trunk, with the retroperitoneum accounting for 40% of all trunk lesions. The remaining 10% arise in the head and neck.

INCIDENCE

Approximately 13,130 new cases of soft tissue sarcomas occurred in the United States in 2020. The annual age-adjusted incidence is 3 per 100,000 population, but the incidence varies with age. Soft tissue sarcomas constitute 0.7% of all cancers in the general population and 6.5% of all cancers in children.

EPIDEMIOLOGY

Malignant transformation of a benign soft tissue tumor is extremely rare, with the exception that malignant peripheral nerve sheath tumors (neurofibrosarcoma, malignant schwannoma) can arise from neurofibromas in patients with neurofibromatosis. Several etiologic factors have been implicated in soft tissue sarcomas.

Environmental Factors Trauma or previous injury is rarely involved, but sarcomas can arise in scar tissue resulting from a prior operation, burn, fracture, or foreign body implantation. Chemical carcinogens such as polycyclic hydrocarbons, asbestos, and dioxin may be involved in the pathogenesis.

Iatrogenic Factors Sarcomas in bone or soft tissues occur in patients who are treated with radiation therapy. The tumor nearly always arises in the irradiated field. The risk increases with time.

Viruses Kaposi's sarcoma (KS) in patients with HIV type 1, classic KS, and KS in HIV-negative homosexual men is caused by human herpesvirus (HHV) 8 (**Chap. 195**). No other sarcomas are associated with viruses.

Immunologic Factors Congenital or acquired immunodeficiency, including therapeutic immunosuppression, increases the risk of sarcoma.

GENETIC CONSIDERATIONS

Li-Fraumeni syndrome is a familial cancer syndrome in which affected individuals have germline abnormalities of the tumor-suppressor gene *p53* and an increased incidence of soft tissue sarcomas and other malignancies, including breast cancer, osteosarcoma, brain tumor, leukemia, and adrenal carcinoma (**Chap. 71**). Neurofibromatosis 1 (NF-1, peripheral form, von Recklinghausen's disease) is characterized by multiple neurofibromas and café-au-lait spots. Neurofibromas occasionally undergo malignant degeneration to become malignant peripheral nerve sheath tumors. The gene for *NF1* is located in the pericentromeric region of chromosome 17 and encodes neurofibromin, a tumor-suppressor protein with guanosine 5′-triphosphate (GTP)ase-activating activity that inhibits ras function (**Chap. 90**). Germline mutation of the *RB1* locus (chromosome 13q14) in patients with inherited retinoblastoma is associated with the development of osteosarcoma in those who survive the retinoblastoma and of soft tissue sarcomas unrelated to radiation therapy. Other soft tissue tumors, including desmoid tumors, lipomas, leiomyomas, neuroblastomas, and paragangliomas, occasionally show a familial predisposition.

Ninety percent of synovial sarcomas contain a characteristic chromosomal translocation t(X;18)(p11;q11) involving a nuclear transcription factor on chromosome 18 called *SYT* and two breakpoints on X. Patients with translocations to the second X breakpoint (*SSX2*) may have longer survival than those with translocations involving *SSX1*.

Insulin-like growth factor (IGF) type II is produced by some sarcomas and may act as an autocrine growth factor and as a motility factor that promotes metastatic spread. IGF-II stimulates growth through IGF-I receptors, but its effects on motility are through different receptors. If secreted in large amounts, IGF-II may produce hypoglycemia (**Chaps. 93** and **406**). A large international sarcoma kindred study including 1162 patients and 6545 Caucasian controls revealed that about half the patients with sarcoma have putatively pathogenic monogenic and polygenic variation in previously reported and new cancer genes, some of them representing therapeutically actionable targets. These patients were diagnosed with sarcoma at an earlier age compared to controls.

CLASSIFICATION

Approximately 20 different groups of sarcomas are recognized on the basis of the pattern of differentiation toward normal tissue. For example, rhabdomyosarcoma shows evidence of skeletal muscle fibers with cross-striations; leiomyosarcomas contain interlacing fascicles of spindle cells resembling smooth muscle; and liposarcomas contain adipocytes. When precise characterization of the group is not possible, the tumors are called *unclassified sarcomas*. All of the primary bone sarcomas can also arise from soft tissues (e.g., extraskeletal osteosarcoma). The entity *malignant fibrous histiocytoma* (MFH) includes many tumors previously classified as fibrosarcomas or as pleomorphic variants of other sarcomas and is characterized by a mixture of spindle (fibrous) cells and round (histiocytic) cells arranged in a storiform pattern with frequent giant cells and areas of pleomorphism. As immunohistochemical suggestion of differentiation, particularly myogenic differentiation, may be found in a significant fraction of these patients, many are now characterized as poorly differentiated leiomyosarcomas, and the terms *undifferentiated pleomorphic sarcoma* (UPS) and *myxofibrosarcoma* are replacing MFH and myxoid MFH.

For purposes of treatment, most soft tissue sarcomas can be considered together. However, some specific tumors have distinct features. For example, *liposarcoma* can have a spectrum of behaviors. Pleomorphic liposarcomas and dedifferentiated liposarcomas behave like other high-grade sarcomas; in contrast, well-differentiated liposarcomas (better termed *atypical lipomatous tumors*) lack metastatic potential, and myxoid liposarcomas metastasize infrequently, but, when they do, they have a predilection for unusual metastatic sites containing fat, such as the retroperitoneum, mediastinum, and subcutaneous tissue. Rhabdomyosarcomas, Ewing's sarcoma, and other small-cell sarcomas tend to be more aggressive and are more responsive to chemotherapy than other soft tissue sarcomas.

Gastrointestinal stromal tumors (GISTs), previously classified as gastrointestinal leiomyosarcomas, are now recognized as a distinct entity within soft tissue sarcomas. Its cell of origin resembles the interstitial cell of Cajal, which controls peristalsis. The majority of malignant GISTs have activating mutations of the c-*kit* gene that result in ligand-independent phosphorylation and activation of the KIT receptor tyrosine kinase, leading to tumorigenesis. Approximately 5–10% of tumors will have a mutation in the platelet-derived growth factor receptor α (*PDGFRA*). GISTs that are wild type for both *KIT* and *PDGFRA* mutations may show mutations in *SDH* B, C, or D and may be driven by the IGF-I pathway.

DIAGNOSIS

The most common presentation is an asymptomatic mass. Mechanical symptoms referable to pressure, traction, or entrapment of nerves or muscles may be present. All new and persistent or growing masses should be biopsied, either by a small incision or by a cutting needle (core-needle biopsy) placed so that it can be encompassed in the subsequent excision without compromising a definitive resection. Lymph node metastases occur in 5%, except in synovial and epithelioid sarcomas, clear-cell sarcoma (melanoma of the soft parts), angiosarcoma, and rhabdomyosarcoma, where nodal spread may be seen in 17%. The pulmonary parenchyma is the most common site of metastases. Exceptions are GISTs, which metastasize to the liver; myxoid liposarcomas, which seek fatty tissue; and clear cell sarcomas, which may metastasize to bones. Central nervous system metastases are rare, except in alveolar soft part sarcoma.

Radiographic Evaluation Imaging of the primary tumor is best with plain radiographs and magnetic resonance imaging (MRI) for tumors of the extremities or head and neck and by computed tomography (CT) for tumors of the chest, abdomen, or retroperitoneal cavity. A radiograph and CT scan of the chest are important for the detection of lung metastases. Other imaging studies may be indicated, depending on the symptoms, signs, or histology.

STAGING AND PROGNOSIS

The histologic grade and size of the primary tumor are the most important prognostic factors. The current American Joint Committee on Cancer (AJCC) staging system is shown in **Table 91-1**. Prognosis is related to the stage. Cure is common in the absence of metastatic disease, but a small number of patients with metastases can also be cured. Historically, most patients with stage IV disease used to die within 12 months, but with availability of multiple lines of treatments, median survival in second-line and beyond ranges from 13 to 14 months, and some patients may live with stable or slowly progressive disease for many years.

TABLE 91-1 American Joint Commission on Cancer Staging System for Sarcomas, Eighth Edition

T1	Tumor ≤5 cm in greatest dimension
T2	Tumor >5 cm and ≤10 cm in greatest dimension
T3	Tumor >10 cm and ≤15 cm in greatest dimension
T4	Tumor >15 cm in greatest dimension
N0	No regional lymph node metastasis or unknown lymph node status
N1	Regional lymph node metastasis
M0	No distant metastasis
M1	Distant metastasis
Stage Groups	
Stage IA	T1; N0; M0; G1
Stage IB	T2, T3, T4; N0; M0; G1
Stage II	T1; N0; M0; G2/3
Stage IIIA	T1A, T2; N0; M0; G2/3
Stage IIIB	T3, T4; N0; M0; G2/3
Stage IV	Any T; N1; M0; any G Any T; any N; M1; any G

TREATMENT

Soft Tissue Sarcomas

AJCC stage I patients are adequately treated with surgery alone. Stage II patients are considered for adjuvant radiation therapy. Stage III patients may benefit from neoadjuvant or adjuvant chemotherapy. Stage IV patients are managed primarily with systemic therapy, with or without other modalities.

SURGERY

Soft tissue sarcomas tend to grow along fascial planes, with the surrounding soft tissues compressed to form a pseudocapsule that gives the sarcoma the appearance of a well-encapsulated lesion. This is invariably deceptive because "shelling out," or marginal excision, of such lesions results in a 50–90% probability of local recurrence. Wide excision with a negative margin, incorporating the biopsy site, is the standard surgical procedure for local disease. The adjuvant use of radiation therapy and/or chemotherapy improves the local control rate and permits the use of limb-sparing surgery with a local control rate (85–90%) comparable to that achieved by radical excisions and amputations. Limb-sparing approaches are indicated except when negative margins are not obtainable, when the risks of radiation are prohibitive, or when neurovascular structures are involved so that resection will result in serious functional consequences to the limb.

RADIATION THERAPY

External-beam radiation therapy is an adjuvant to limb-sparing surgery for improved local control. Preoperative radiation therapy allows the use of smaller fields and smaller doses but results in a higher rate of wound complications. Postoperative radiation therapy must be given to larger fields, because the entire surgical bed must be encompassed, and in higher doses to compensate for hypoxia in the operated field. This results in a higher rate of late complications. Brachytherapy or interstitial therapy, in which the radiation source is inserted into the tumor bed, is comparable in efficacy (except in low-grade lesions), less time consuming, and less expensive.

With the advent of stereotactic body radiotherapy (SBRT), the role of radiation therapy in oligometastatic disease in various visceral sites is being investigated and evolving.

ADJUVANT CHEMOTHERAPY

Chemotherapy is the mainstay of treatment for Ewing's sarcomas/primitive neuroectodermal tumors (PNETs) and rhabdomyosarcomas. Meta-analysis of 14 randomized trials in non-small-cell sarcomas revealed a significant improvement in local control and disease-free survival in favor of doxorubicin-based chemotherapy. Overall survival improvement was 4% for all sites and 7% for the extremity site. An updated meta-analysis including four additional trials with doxorubicin and ifosfamide combination reported a statistically significant 6% survival advantage in favor of chemotherapy. A chemotherapy regimen including an anthracycline and ifosfamide with growth factor support improved overall survival by 19% for high-risk (high-grade, ≥5 cm primary, or locally recurrent) extremity soft tissue sarcomas. Long-term follow-up of a trial evaluating neoadjuvant use of the same combination confirms survival advantage and reports a 10-year survival of 61%. A more contemporary randomized trial compared the standard anthracycline and ifosfamide combination to specific histology-tailored chemotherapy as an active control and confirmed superiority of the standard regimen.

ADVANCED DISEASE

Metastatic soft tissue sarcomas are largely incurable, but up to 20% of patients who achieve a complete response become long-term survivors. The therapeutic intent, therefore, is to produce a complete remission with chemotherapy (<10%) and/or surgery (30–40%). Surgical resection of metastases, whenever possible, is an integral part of the management. Some patients benefit from repeated surgical excision of metastases. The two most active chemotherapeutic agents are doxorubicin and ifosfamide. These drugs show a steep dose-response relationship in sarcomas. Gemcitabine with or without docetaxel has become an established second-line regimen and is particularly active in patients with UPS and leiomyosarcomas. Dacarbazine also has some modest activity. Taxanes have selective activity in angiosarcomas, and vincristine, etoposide, and irinotecan are effective in rhabdomyosarcomas and Ewing's sarcomas. Pazopanib, an inhibitor of the vascular endothelial growth factor, platelet-derived growth factor (PDGF), and c-kit, is now approved for patients with advanced soft tissue sarcomas excluding liposarcomas after failure of chemotherapy. Two additional chemotherapy drugs have gained approval from the U.S. Food and Drug Administration (FDA). Trabectedin was compared to dacarbazine in a large phase 3 randomized study in advanced leiomyosarcomas and liposarcomas after failure of an anthracycline and resulted in significant improvement in progression-free survival. Eribulin was also tested in a similar trial and showed improvement in survival, predominantly in the liposarcoma subgroup, and is therefore now approved for that subset. Tazemetostat, an EZH2 inhibitor, is now approved for use in metastatic epithelioid sarcomas characterized by loss of tumor-suppressor gene *INI1*, resulting in activation of the EZH2 pathway. Imatinib targets KIT and PDGF tyrosine kinase activity and is standard therapy for advanced/metastatic GISTs and dermatofibrosarcoma protuberans. Imatinib is also indicated as adjuvant therapy for completely resected primary GISTs. Three years of adjuvant imatinib appear to be superior to 1 year of therapy for high-risk GISTs, although the optimal treatment duration remains unknown. Sunitinib and regorafenib are approved for second- and third-line use, respectively, in metastatic GIST after failure of or intolerance to imatinib. Ripretinib, an inhibitor of c-kit and PDGFRA, was approved for fourth-line use in metastatic GIST based on a placebo-controlled randomized trial reporting an improved median progression-free and overall survival. Avapritinib also received approval for use in the specific molecular subset of *PDGFRA* D842V–mutant metastatic GIST.

BONE SARCOMAS

■ INCIDENCE AND EPIDEMIOLOGY

Bone sarcomas are rarer than soft tissue sarcomas; they accounted for only 0.2% of all new malignancies and 3600 new cases in the United States in 2020. Several benign bone lesions have the potential for malignant transformation. Enchondromas and osteochondromas can transform into chondrosarcoma; fibrous dysplasia, bone infarcts, and Paget's disease of bone can transform into either UPS or osteosarcoma.

■ CLASSIFICATION

Benign Tumors The common benign bone tumors include enchondroma, osteochondroma, chondroblastoma, and chondromyxoid fibroma, of cartilage origin; osteoid osteoma and osteoblastoma, of bone origin; fibroma and desmoplastic fibroma, of fibrous tissue origin; hemangioma, of vascular origin; and giant cell tumor, of unknown origin.

Malignant Tumors The most common malignant tumors of bone are plasma cell tumors **(Chap. 111)**. The four most common malignant nonhematopoietic bone tumors are osteosarcoma, chondrosarcoma, Ewing's sarcoma, and UPS. Rare malignant tumors include chordoma (of notochordal origin), malignant giant cell tumor, adamantinoma (of unknown origin), and hemangioendothelioma (of vascular origin).

Musculoskeletal Tumor Society Staging System Sarcomas of bone are staged according to the Musculoskeletal Tumor Society staging system based on grade and compartmental localization. A Roman numeral reflects the tumor grade: stage I is low grade, stage II is high grade, and stage III includes tumors of any grade that have lymph node or distant metastases. In addition, the tumor is given a letter reflecting its compartmental localization. Tumors designated A are intracompartmental (i.e., confined to the same soft tissue compartment as the initial tumor), and tumors designated B are extracompartmental (i.e., extending into the adjacent soft tissue compartment or into bone). The tumor-node-metastasis (TNM) staging system is shown in **Table 91-2**.

TABLE 91-2 Staging System for Bone Sarcomas

Primary tumor (T)	TX	Primary tumor cannot be assessed
	T0	No evidence of primary tumor
	T1	Tumor ≤8 cm in greatest dimension
	T2	Tumor >8 cm in greatest dimension
	T3	Discontinuous tumors in the primary bone site
Regional lymph nodes (N)	NX	Regional lymph nodes cannot be assessed
	N0	No regional lymph node metastasis
	N1	Regional lymph node metastasis
Distant metastasis (M)	MX	Distant metastasis cannot be assessed
	M0	No distant metastasis
	M1	Distant metastasis
	M1a	Lung
	M1b	Other distant sites
Histologic grade (G)	GX	Grade cannot be assessed
	G1	Well differentiated—low grade
	G2	Moderately differentiated—low grade
	G3	Poorly differentiated—high grade
	G4	Undifferentiated—high grade (Ewing's is always classed G4)

Stage Grouping				
Stage IA	T1	N0	M0	G1,2 low grade
Stage IB	T2	N0	M0	G1,2 low grade
Stage IIA	T1	N0	M0	G3,4 high grade
Stage IIB	T2	N0	M0	G3,4 high grade
Stage III	T3	N0	M0	Any G
Stage IVA	Any T	N0	M1a	Any G
Stage IVB	Any T	N1	Any M	Any G
	Any T	Any N	M1b	Any G

■ OSTEOSARCOMA

Osteosarcoma, accounting for almost 45% of all bone sarcomas, is a spindle cell neoplasm that produces osteoid (unmineralized bone) or bone. Approximately 60% of all osteosarcomas occur in children and adolescents in the second decade of life, and ~10% occur in the third decade of life. Osteosarcomas in the fifth and sixth decades of life are frequently secondary to either radiation therapy or transformation in a preexisting benign condition, such as Paget's disease. Males are affected 1.5–2 times as often as females. Osteosarcoma has a predilection for metaphyses of long bones; the most common sites of involvement are the distal femur, proximal tibia, and proximal humerus. The classification of osteosarcoma is complex, but 75% of osteosarcomas fall into the "classic" category, which includes osteoblastic, chondroblastic, and fibroblastic osteosarcomas. The remaining 25% are classified as "variants" on the basis of (1) clinical characteristics, as in the case of osteosarcoma of the jaw, postradiation osteosarcoma, or Paget's osteosarcoma; (2) morphologic characteristics, as in the case of telangiectatic osteosarcoma, small-cell osteosarcoma, or epithelioid osteosarcoma; or (3) location, as in parosteal or periosteal osteosarcoma. Diagnosis usually requires a synthesis of clinical, radiologic, and pathologic features. Patients typically present with pain and swelling of the affected area. A plain radiograph reveals a destructive lesion with a moth-eaten appearance, a spiculated periosteal reaction (sunburst appearance), and a cuff of periosteal new bone formation at the margin of the soft tissue mass (Codman's triangle). A CT scan of the primary tumor is best for defining bone destruction and the pattern of calcification, whereas MRI is better for defining intramedullary and soft tissue extension. A chest radiograph and CT scan are used to detect lung metastases. Metastases to the bony skeleton should be imaged by a bone scan or by fluorodeoxyglucose positron emission tomography (FDG-PET). Almost all osteosarcomas are hypervascular and PET-avid. Pathologic diagnosis is established either with a core-needle biopsy, where feasible, or with an open biopsy with an appropriately placed incision that does not compromise future limb-sparing resection. Most osteosarcomas are high grade. The most important predictive factor for long-term survival is response to chemotherapy. Preoperative chemotherapy followed by limb-sparing surgery (which can be accomplished in >80% of patients) followed by postoperative chemotherapy is standard management. The effective drugs are doxorubicin, ifosfamide, cisplatin, and high-dose methotrexate with leucovorin rescue. The various combinations of these agents that have been used have all been about equally successful. Long-term survival rates in extremity osteosarcoma range from 60 to 80%. Osteosarcoma is radioresistant; radiation therapy has no role in the routine management. UPS is considered a part of the spectrum of osteosarcoma and is managed similarly. A randomized trial has shown improved progression-free survival with regorafenib compared to placebo.

■ CHONDROSARCOMA

Chondrosarcoma, which constitutes ~20–25% of all bone sarcomas, is a tumor of adulthood and old age with a peak incidence in the fourth to sixth decades of life. It has a predilection for the flat bones, especially the shoulder and pelvic girdles, but can also affect the diaphyseal portions of long bones. Chondrosarcomas can arise de novo or as a malignant transformation of an enchondroma or, rarely, of the cartilaginous cap of an osteochondroma. Chondrosarcomas have an indolent natural history and typically present as pain and swelling. Radiographically, the lesion may have a lobular appearance with mottled or punctate or annular calcification of the cartilaginous matrix. It is difficult to distinguish low-grade chondrosarcoma from benign lesions by x-ray or histologic examination. The diagnosis is therefore influenced by clinical history and physical examination. A new onset of pain, signs of inflammation, and progressive increase in the size of the mass suggest malignancy. The histologic classification is complex, but most tumors fall within the classic category. Like other bone sarcomas, high-grade chondrosarcomas spread to the lungs. Most chondrosarcomas are resistant to chemotherapy, and surgical resection of primary or recurrent tumors, including pulmonary metastases, is the mainstay of therapy with the exception of two histologic variants. Dedifferentiated chondrosarcoma has a high-grade osteosarcoma or a malignant fibrous histiocytoma component that responds to chemotherapy. Mesenchymal chondrosarcoma, a rare variant composed of a small-cell element, also is responsive to systemic chemotherapy and is treated like Ewing's sarcoma.

■ EWING'S SARCOMA

Ewing's sarcoma, which constitutes ~10–15% of all bone sarcomas, is common in adolescence and has a peak incidence in the second decade of life. It typically involves the diaphyseal region of long bones and also has an affinity for flat bones. The plain radiograph may show a characteristic "onion peel" periosteal reaction with a generous soft tissue mass, which is better demonstrated by CT or MRI. This mass is composed of sheets of monotonous, small, round, blue cells and can be confused with lymphoma, embryonal rhabdomyosarcoma, and small-cell carcinoma. The presence of p30/32, the product of the *mic-2* gene (which maps to the pseudoautosomal region of the X and Y chromosomes), is a cell-surface marker for Ewing's sarcoma (and other members of the Ewing family of tumors, previously also called PNETs). Most PNETs arise in soft tissues; they include peripheral neuroepithelioma, Askin's tumor (chest wall), and esthesioneuroblastoma. Glycogen-filled cytoplasm detected by staining with periodic acid–Schiff is also characteristic of Ewing's sarcoma cells. The classic cytogenetic abnormality associated with this disease is a reciprocal translocation of the long arms of chromosomes 11 and 22, t(11;22), which creates a chimeric gene product of unknown function with components from the *fli-1* gene on chromosome 11 and *ews* on chromosome 22. This disease is very aggressive, and it is therefore considered a systemic disease. Common sites of metastases are lung, bones, and bone marrow. Systemic chemotherapy is the mainstay of therapy, often being used before surgery. Doxorubicin, cyclophosphamide or ifosfamide, etoposide, vincristine, and dactinomycin are active drugs. Topotecan or irinotecan in combination with an alkylating agent is often used in relapsed patients. Local treatment for the primary tumor includes surgical resection, usually with limb salvage or radiation therapy. Patients with lesions below the elbow and below the mid-calf have a 5-year survival rate of 80% with effective treatment. Ewing's sarcoma at first presentation is a curable tumor, even in the presence of obvious metastatic disease, especially in children <11 years old.

TUMORS METASTATIC TO BONE

Bone is a common site of metastasis for carcinomas of the prostate, breast, lung, kidney, bladder, and thyroid and for lymphomas and sarcomas. Prostate, breast, and lung primaries account for 80% of all bone metastases. Metastatic tumors of bone are more common than primary bone tumors. Tumors usually spread to bone hematogenously, but local invasion from soft tissue masses also occurs. In descending order of frequency, the sites most often involved are the vertebrae, proximal femur, pelvis, ribs, sternum, proximal humerus, and skull. Bone metastases may be asymptomatic or may produce pain, swelling, nerve root or spinal cord compression, pathologic fracture, or myelophthisis (replacement of the marrow). Symptoms of hypercalcemia may be noted in cases of bony destruction.

Pain is the most frequent symptom. It usually develops gradually over weeks, is usually localized, and often is more severe at night. When patients with back pain develop neurologic signs or symptoms, emergency evaluation for spinal cord compression is indicated **(Chap. 75)**. Bone metastases exert a major adverse effect on quality of life in cancer patients.

Cancer in the bone may produce osteolysis, osteogenesis, or both. Osteolytic lesions result when the tumor produces substances that can directly elicit bone resorption (vitamin D–like steroids, prostaglandins, or parathyroid hormone–related peptide) or cytokines that can induce the formation of osteoclasts (interleukin 1 and tumor necrosis factor). Osteoblastic lesions result when the tumor produces cytokines that activate osteoblasts. In general, purely osteolytic lesions are best detected by plain radiography, but they may not be apparent until they are >1 cm. These lesions are more commonly associated with hypercalcemia and with the excretion of hydroxyproline-containing peptides indicative of matrix destruction. When osteoblastic activity is prominent, the lesions may be readily detected using radionuclide bone scanning (which is sensitive to new bone formation), and the radiographic appearance may show increased bone density or sclerosis. Osteoblastic lesions are associated with higher serum levels of alkaline phosphatase and, if extensive, may produce hypocalcemia. Although some tumors may produce mainly osteolytic lesions (e.g., kidney cancer) and others mainly osteoblastic lesions (e.g., prostate cancer), most metastatic lesions produce both types of lesion and may go through stages where one or the other predominates.

In older patients, particularly women, it may be necessary to distinguish metastatic disease of the spine from osteoporosis. In osteoporosis, the cortical bone may be preserved, whereas cortical bone destruction is usually noted with metastatic cancer.

TREATMENT

Metastatic Bone Disease

Treatment of metastatic bone disease depends on the underlying malignancy and the symptoms. Some metastatic bone tumors are curable (lymphoma, Hodgkin's disease), and others are treated with palliative intent. Pain may be relieved by local radiation therapy. Hormonally responsive tumors are responsive to hormone inhibition (antiandrogens for prostate cancer, antiestrogens for breast cancer). Strontium-89, samarium-153, and radium-223 are bone-seeking radionuclides that can exert antitumor effects and relieve symptoms. Denosumab, a monoclonal antibody that binds to RANK ligand, inhibits osteoclastic activity and increases bone mineral density. Bisphosphonates such as pamidronate may relieve pain and inhibit bone resorption, thereby maintaining bone mineral density and reducing risk of fractures in patients with osteolytic metastases from breast cancer and multiple myeloma. Careful monitoring of serum electrolytes and creatinine is recommended. Monthly administration prevents bone-related clinical events and may reduce the incidence of bone metastases in women with breast cancer. When the integrity of a weight-bearing bone is threatened by an expanding metastatic lesion that is refractory to radiation therapy, prophylactic internal fixation is indicated. Overall survival is related to the prognosis of the underlying tumor. Bone pain at the end of life is particularly common; an adequate pain relief regimen including sufficient amounts of narcotic analgesics is required. The management of hypercalcemia is discussed in **Chap. 410**.

■ FURTHER READING

ALVAREZ RA et al: Optimization of the therapeutic approach to patients with sarcoma: Delphi consensus. Sarcoma 2019:4351308, 2019.

BALLINGER ML et al: Monogenic and polygenic determinants of sarcoma risk: An international genetic study. Lancet Oncol 17:1261, 2016.

DEMETRI GD et al: Efficacy and safety of Trabectedin or DTIC in patients with metastatic liposarcoma and leiomyosarcoma following failure of conventional chemotherapy: Results of a phase III randomized multicenter clinical trial. J Clin Oncol 34:786, 2016.

GRONCHI A et al: Short, full-dose adjuvant chemotherapy (CT) in high-risk adult soft tissue sarcomas (STS): Long-term follow-up of a randomized clinical trial from the Italian Sarcoma Group and the Spanish Sarcoma Group. Ann Oncol 27:1, 2016.

MEYER M, SEETHARAM M: First-line therapy for metastatic soft tissue sarcoma. Curr Treat Options Oncol 20:6, 2019.

PASQUALI S, GRONCHI A: Neoadjuvant chemotherapy in soft tissue sarcomas: Latest evidence and clinical implications. Ther Adv Med Oncol 9:415, 2017.

RATAN R, PATEL SR: Chemotherapy for soft tissue sarcoma. Cancer 122:2952, 2016.

SCHOFFSKI P et al: Eribulin versus dacarbazine in previously treated patients with advanced liposarcoma or leiomyosarcoma: A randomised, open-label, multicentre, phase 3 trial. Lancet 387:1629, 2016.

WAGNER MJ et al: Chemotherapy for bone sarcoma in adults. J Oncol Pract 12:208, 2016.

92 Carcinoma of Unknown Primary

Kanwal Raghav, James L. Abbruzzese, Gauri R. Varadhachary

Carcinoma (or cancer) of unknown primary (CUP) is a biopsy-proven malignancy for which the anatomic site of origin remains unidentified after a standardized detailed diagnostic evaluation. CUP is one of the 10 most frequently diagnosed cancers globally, accounting for 3–5% of all malignancies. Most investigators limit CUP to epithelial or undifferentiated cancers and do not include lymphomas, metastatic melanomas, and metastatic sarcomas because these cancers have specific histology and stage-based management guidelines, even in the absence of a primary site. CUP can occur in patients of all age groups including adolescents and young adults.

The emergence of sophisticated imaging, robust immunohistochemistry (IHC), and genomic and proteomic tools has challenged the "unknown" designation. Additionally, effective targeted therapies in several cancers and tissue agnostic biomarker-driven therapies have endorsed a change in paradigm from empiricism to a personalized approach to CUP management. The reasons cancers present as CUP remain unclear. One hypothesis is that the primary tumor either regresses after seeding the metastasis or remains so small that it is not detected. It is possible that CUP falls on the continuum of cancer presentation where the primary has been contained or eliminated by the natural body defenses, including the immune system. Alternatively, CUP may represent a specific malignant event that results in an increase in metastatic spread or survival relative to the primary. Whether the CUP metastases truly define a clone that is genetically and phenotypically unique to this diagnosis remains to be determined.

Since liver is a common site of CUP presentation, intrahepatic cholangiocarcinoma (ICC) can be often misdiagnosed as CUP. Of note, the incidence of ICC is increasing, whereas at the same time, that of CUP is declining. Improvements in diagnostic technologies including next-generation sequencing and other molecular techniques and awareness among clinicians to differentiate the two are possibly contributing to an increased recognition and incidence of ICC.

CUP BIOLOGY

Studies looking for unique signature abnormalities in CUP tumors have not been positive. Abnormalities in chromosomes 1 and 12 and other complex cytogenetic abnormalities have been reported. Aneuploidy has been described in 70% of CUP patients with metastatic adenocarcinoma or undifferentiated carcinoma. The overexpression of various genes, including *RAS*, *BCL2* (40%), *HER2* (11%), and *P53* (26–53%), has been identified in CUP samples, but they are found in many other malignancies and have no effect on response to therapy or survival. The extent of angiogenesis in CUP relative to that in metastases from known primaries has also been evaluated, but no consistent findings have emerged. Although current comprehensive genomic profiling efforts may help identify targeted therapeutic approaches to improve outcomes for this disease as discussed below, they have failed thus far to reveal a distinct molecular signature. More comprehensive and integrated multiomic efforts are needed to provide insights into CUP biology through recognition of molecular aberrations that especially drive metastatic growth.

APPROACH TO THE PATIENT

Carcinoma (or Cancer) of Unknown Primary

Initial CUP evaluation has two goals: search for the primary tumor based on pathologic evaluation of the metastases and determine the extent of disease. Focused evaluation directed by clinicopathologic cues allows for judicious and efficient use of diagnostic tests. Obtaining a thorough medical history from CUP patients is essential, including paying particular attention to previous surgeries, removed lesions, and family medical history to assess potential hereditary cancers. Adequate physical examination, including a digital rectal examination in men and breast and pelvic examinations in women, should be performed based on clinical presentation. Finally, all patients with CUP, in the absence of contraindication, must undergo a computed tomographic (CT) scan of chest, abdomen and pelvis as a part of their standard work-up.

ROLE OF SERUM TUMOR MARKERS AND CYTOGENETICS

Most tumor markers, including carcinoembryonic antigen (CEA), CA-125, CA 19-9, and CA 15-3, when elevated, are nonspecific and not helpful in determining the primary site. Men who present with adenocarcinoma and predominant osteoblastic metastasis should undergo a prostate-specific antigen (PSA) test. In patients with undifferentiated or poorly differentiated carcinoma (especially with a midline tumor), elevated β-human chorionic gonadotropin (β-hCG) and α fetoprotein (AFP) levels suggest the possibility of an extragonadal germ cell (testicular) tumor. With the availability of advanced immunohistochemistry (IHC), cytogenetic studies are rarely needed.

ROLE OF IMAGING STUDIES

In the absence of contraindications, a baseline IV contrast computed tomography (CT) scan of the chest, abdomen, and pelvis is the standard of care. This helps to search for the primary tumor, evaluate the extent of disease, and select the most accessible biopsy site. With precise imaging and reporting, latent primary cancers, defined as appearance of a new primary cancer after a latent period of several months to years, is uncommon and seen in ≤5% of CUP patients, usually in patients with very indolent presentations and/or highly responsive metastatic cancers that allows a latent primary to emerge (grow) over time.

Mammography should be performed in all women who present with metastatic adenocarcinoma, specifically in those with isolated axillary lymphadenopathy. Magnetic resonance imaging (MRI) of the breast can be considered in patients with axillary adenopathy and suspected occult primary breast carcinoma following a negative mammography and ultrasound. The results of these imaging modalities can influence surgical management; a negative MRI of the breast predicts a low tumor yield at mastectomy.

A conventional workup for a squamous cell carcinoma and cervical CUP (neck lymphadenopathy with no known primary tumor) includes a CT scan or MRI and invasive studies, including indirect and direct laryngoscopy, bronchoscopy, and upper endoscopy. Ipsilateral (or bilateral) staging tonsillectomy has been recommended for these patients. 18-Fluorodeoxyglucose positron emission tomography (18-FDG-PET) scans are useful in this patient population and may help guide the biopsy; determine the extent of disease; facilitate the appropriate treatment, including planning radiation fields; and help with disease surveillance. A smaller radiation field encompassing the metastatic adenopathy decreases the risk of chronic xerostomia. Several studies have evaluated the utility of PET in patients with squamous cervical CUP, and head and neck primary tumors were identified in ~21–30%.

The diagnostic contribution of PET to the evaluation of other CUP presentations (outside of the neck adenopathy indication) remains controversial and is not routinely recommended. PET-CT can be helpful for patients with bone metastases and those deemed candidates for aggressive multimodality therapy (surgical intervention/radiation) such as patients with solitary metastatic disease because the identification of disease in addition to the solitary metastatic site may affect treatment planning.

Invasive studies, including upper endoscopy, colonoscopy, and bronchoscopy, should be limited to symptomatic patients or those with laboratory, imaging, or pathologic abnormalities that suggest that these techniques will result in a high yield in finding a primary cancer.

ROLE OF PATHOLOGIC STUDIES

A detailed pathologic examination of the most accessible biopsied tissue specimen is mandatory in CUP patients. Pathologic evaluation typically consists of hematoxylin and eosin stains and IHC tests. The importance of adequate tissue acquisition cannot be overemphasized in CUP. In addition to pathologic evaluation, tissue is also needed for tests of biomarkers of targeted agents, immunotherapy, and clinical trials.

Light Microscopy Evaluation Adequate tissue obtained preferably by excisional biopsy or core needle biopsy (instead of only a fine-needle aspiration) is stained with hematoxylin and eosin and subjected to light microscopic examination. On light microscopy, 60–65% of CUP is adenocarcinoma, and 5% is squamous cell carcinoma. The remaining 30–35% is poorly differentiated adenocarcinoma, poorly differentiated carcinoma, or poorly differentiated neoplasm. A small percentage of lesions are diagnosed as neuroendocrine cancers (2%), mixed tumors (adenosquamous or sarcomatoid carcinomas), or undifferentiated neoplasms (**Table 92-1**).

Role of IHC Analysis IHC stains are peroxidase-labeled antibodies against specific tumor antigens that are used to define tumor lineage. The number of available IHC stains is ever-increasing. However, a tiered and uniform approach to tissue evaluation in the CUP setting is lacking. For CUP cases, more is not necessarily better, and IHC stains should be used in conjunction with the patient's clinical presentation and imaging studies to select the best therapy. Communication between the clinician and pathologist is essential. No stain is 100% sensitive or specific, and under-/overinterpretation should be avoided. Poor differentiation, even in known primary tumors, decreases sensitivity of hallmark IHC markers. PSA and thyroglobulin tissue markers, which are positive in prostate and thyroid cancer, respectively, are the most specific of the current marker panel. However, these cancers rarely present as CUP, so the yield of these tests may be low. **Figure 92-1** delineates a simple algorithm for immunohistochemical staining in CUP cases. **Table 92-2** lists additional tests that may be useful to further define the tumor lineage. A more comprehensive algorithm may improve the diagnostic accuracy but can make the process complex and increase cost. With the use of IHC markers, electron microscopic analysis, which is time-consuming and expensive, is rarely needed.

There are >20 subtypes of cytokeratin (CK) intermediate filaments with different molecular weights and differential expression in various cell types and cancers. Monoclonal antibodies to specific CK subtypes have been used to help classify tumors according to their site of origin; commonly used CK stains in adenocarcinoma CUP are CK7 and CK20. CK7 is found in tumors of the lung, ovary, endometrium, breast, and upper gastrointestinal tract including pancreaticobiliary cancers, whereas CK20 is normally expressed in the gastrointestinal epithelium, urothelium, and Merkel cells. The nuclear CDX-2 transcription factor, which is the product of a homeobox gene necessary for intestinal organogenesis, is often used to aid in the diagnosis of gastrointestinal adenocarcinomas. However, CDX-2 positivity can be seen with enteric or mucinous differentiation in tumors from diverse primary sites (e.g., mucinous ovarian cancers).

Thyroid transcription factor 1 (TTF-1) nuclear staining is frequently positive in lung and thyroid cancers. Approximately 68% of adenocarcinomas and 25% of squamous cell lung cancers stain positive for TTF-1, which helps differentiate a lung primary tumor from metastatic

TABLE 92-1 Major Histologies in Carcinoma of Unknown Primary

HISTOLOGY	PROPORTION, %
Well to moderately differentiated adenocarcinoma	60
Squamous cell cancer	5
Poorly differentiated adenocarcinoma, poorly differentiated carcinoma	30
Neuroendocrine	2
Undifferentiated malignancy	3

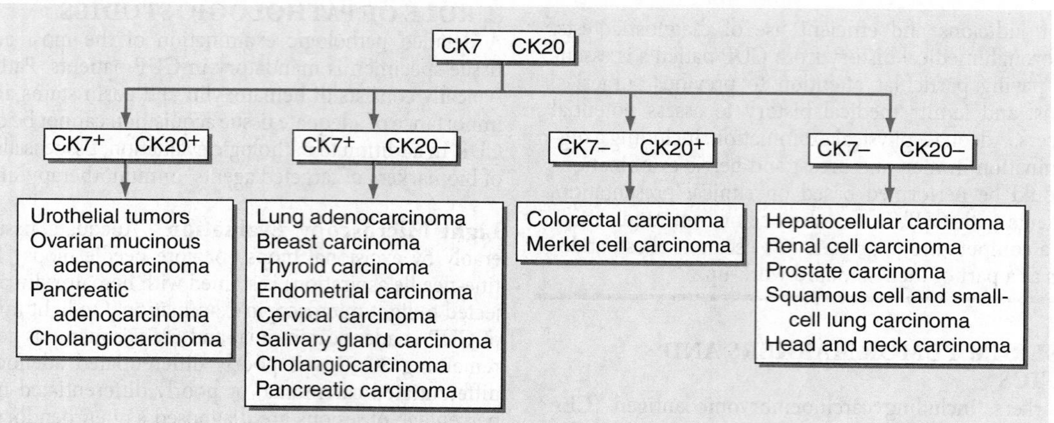

FIGURE 92-1 Approach to cytokeratin (CK7 and CK20) markers used in adenocarcinoma of unknown primary.

adenocarcinoma in a pleural effusion, the mediastinum, or the lung parenchyma.

Gross cystic disease fibrous protein-15 (GCDFP-15), a 15-kDa monomer protein, is a marker of apocrine differentiation that is detected in 62–72% of breast carcinomas. GATA3 is being increasingly used in the CUP setting when there is concern for a breast primary and can be particularly useful as a marker for metastatic breast carcinoma, especially triple-negative and metaplastic carcinomas, which lack specific endocrine markers of mammary origin. UROIII, high-molecular-weight cytokeratin, thrombomodulin, and CK20 are the markers used to diagnose lesions of urothelial origin.

TABLE 92-2 Select Immunohistochemical Stains Useful in the Diagnosis of CUP

LIKELY PRIMARY PROFILE	COMMONLY CONSIDERED IHC TO ASSIST IN DIFFERENTIAL DIAGNOSIS OF CUP[a]
Breast	ER, GCDFP-15, mammaglobin, HER2/neu, GATA3
Ovarian/mullerian	ER, WT1, CK7, PAX8, PAX2
Lung adenocarcinoma	TTF-1; nuclear staining, napsin A, SP-A1
Germ cell	β-hCG, AFP, OCT3/4, CKIT, CD30 (embryonal), SALL4
Prostate	PSA, α-methylacyl CoA racemase/P504S (AMACR/P504S), P501S (prostein), PSMA, NKX3-1
Intestinal	CK7, CK20, CDX-2, CEA
Neuroendocrine	Chromogranin, synaptophysin, CD56
Sarcoma	Desmin (desmoid tumors), factor VIII (angiosarcomas), CD31, smooth muscle actin (leiomyosarcoma), MyoD1 (rhabdomyosarcoma)
Renal	RCC, CD10, PAX8, CD10
Hepatocellular carcinoma	Hep Par-1, Arg-1, glypican-3
Melanoma	S100, SOX-10, vimentin, HMB-45, tyrosinase, melan-A
Urothelial	CK7, CK20, thrombomodulin, uroplakin III
Mesothelioma	Calretinin, WT1, D2-40, mesothelin
Lymphoma	LCA, CD3, CD4, CD5, CD20, CD45
SCC	p63, p40 (lung SCC), CK5/6

[a]Patterns emerging from coexpression of stains are better than individual stains to suggest putative primary site. Even with optimization, no IHC panel is 100% sensitive or specific (e.g., ovarian mucinous carcinoma can exhibit positivity with intestinal markers).

Abbreviations: AFP, α fetoprotein; Arg-1, arginase-1; β-hCG, β-human chorionic gonadotropin; CEA, carcinoembryonic antigen; CUP, carcinoma of unknown primary; ER, estrogen receptor; GCDFP-15, gross cystic disease fibrous protein-15; IHC, immunohistochemistry; LCA, leukocyte common antigen; PSA, prostate-specific antigen; PSMA, prostate-specific membrane antigen; SCC, squamous cell carcinoma; SP-A1, surfactant protein A precursor; TTF, thyroid transcription factor; WT, Wilms' tumor.

IHC performs the best when used in groups that give rise to patterns that are strongly indicative of certain profiles. For example, the TTF-1/CK7+ and CK20+/CDX-2+/CK7− phenotypes have been reported as very suggestive of lung and lower gastrointestinal cancer profiles, respectively. Despite their practical utility, these patterns have not been validated prospectively in CUP patients. IHC is not without its limitations; several factors affect tissue antigenicity (antigen retrieval, specimen processing, and fixation), interpretation of stains in tumor (nuclear, cytoplasmic, membrane) versus normal tissue, inter- and intraobserver variability, variable performance of different antibodies said to recognize the same antigen, and tissue heterogeneity and inadequacy (given small biopsy sizes). Communication with the pathologist is critical to determine if additional tissue will be beneficial in the pathologic evaluation. Pathologic features should not always supersede clinical or radiologic findings when considering testing for biomarkers of therapeutic response (e.g., epidermal growth factor receptor [EGFR], *ALK* mutations, human epidermal growth factor receptor 2 [HER-2]).

Role of Cancer Classifier Molecular Profiling In the absence of a known primary, developing therapeutic strategies for CUP is challenging. The current diagnostic yield with imaging and immunochemistry is ~20–30% for CUP patients. To reduce diagnostic uncertainty, sophisticated molecular analytics have been applied to CUP samples. These include gene expression profiling, messenger RNA (mRNA), microRNA, and epigenetic profiling to classify the CUP cancer.

Gene expression profiles are most commonly generated using quantitative reverse transcriptase polymerase chain reaction (RT-PCR) or DNA microarray. Neural network programs are then used to develop predictive algorithms from the gene expression profiles. Typically, a training set of gene profiles from known cancers (preferably from metastatic sites) is used to train the software. Comprehensive gene expression databases that have become available for common malignancies are then applied to CUP samples, and the program can then be used to predict the putative origin of a CUP sample.

mRNA- or microRNA-based tissue of origin cancer classifier assays have also been studied in prospective and retrospective CUP trials. More recently, a classifier based on microarray DNA methylation signatures has been studied and validated in known cancers. The DNA methylation profiling predicted a primary cancer in 87% of the 216 CUP patients.

Despite the sophistication of the cancer classifier molecular assays, most of the CUP studies have evaluated assay *performance*, although the challenge with validating the accuracy of an assay for CUP is that, by definition, the primary cancer diagnosis cannot be verified. Thus, current estimates of tissue of origin test accuracy have relied on indirect metrics, including comparison with pathology/IHC, clinical presentation, appearance of latent primaries, and autopsies. Using these measures, the assays suggest a plausible primary in ~70–80% of patients studied. Three outcomes-based studies have been performed. First, a single-arm study reported a median survival of 12.5 months for patients who received assay-directed site-specific therapy. Second, a phase 2 trial of site-specific therapy, including molecularly targeted therapy, based on predicted tumor site from an algorithm using gene expression and alteration profile showed a 1-year survival of 53.1%. However, a randomized clinical trial evaluating site-specific therapy directed by gene expression profiling versus empirical chemotherapy with paclitaxel and carboplatin failed to show a significant improvement in 1-year survival (44% vs 55%, p = .264) with this approach. Firm conclusions of therapeutic impact cannot be drawn from these studies given the sample size, design, statistical biases, confounding variables including use of subsequent lines of (empiric) therapy, and heterogeneity of the CUP cancers. Additional studies are needed to better understand the clinical impact of tissue of origin profiling tools and how these assays complement IHC and help guide therapy.

Role of Next-Generation Sequencing A significant push is being made toward personalized medicine across all cancer types with the goal of identifying driver mutation(s) in a patient who can be treated with targeted agents independent of the site of origin. A retrospective study of 200 CUP tumor specimens reported on genomic alterations using the hybrid capture–based FoundationOne assay. The authors reported that a large number of CUP samples (85%) harbored at least one clinically relevant genomic alteration with the potential to influence and personalize therapy. The mean number of genomic alterations was 4.2 per tumor, and the most common genetic alterations included *TP53* (55%), *KRAS* (20%), *CDKN2A* (19%), and *ARID1A* (11%). The adenocarcinoma CUP tumors were more frequently driven by genetic alterations in the receptor tyrosine kinase (RTK)/Ras/mitogen-activated protein kinase (MAPK) signaling pathway than nonadenocarcinoma CUP tumors. Although, druggable genetic lesions seen in CUP are comparable to those in defined large entities, whether molecularly stratified approaches for CUP will successfully improve outcomes remains to be seen and clinical trials are needed. In a single-arm phase 2 study of 97 patients with molecularly targeted therapy, five patients were found to have targetable *EGFR* mutations. Of these, four patients were treated with afatinib, an anti-EGFR drug, and two patients achieved a progression-free survival of >6 months. The emerging role of assays looking for circulating tumor cells, so-called liquid biopsies, within known tumor types has stirred interest in their potential utility in CUP.

Ongoing histology and cellular-context agnostic prospective clinical trials are studying the presence of actionable mutations and matching patients to the right targeted drug. Should this approach eventually be appropriately validated, CUP would be a natural fit for genomic alteration (GA)-based targeted therapy independent of tumor site. Immune checkpoint inhibitors (pembrolizumab) for microsatellite instability high (MSI-H) or deficient mismatch repair (dMMR) tumors and NTRK inhibitors for *NTRK* fusion–positive tumors can help a small minority of CUP patients.

TREATMENT

Carcinoma (or Cancer) of Unknown Primary

GENERAL CONSIDERATIONS

The treatment of CUP continues to evolve, albeit slowly. The median survival of most patients with disseminated CUP is ~6–10 months. Systemic chemotherapy is the primary treatment modality in most patients with disseminated disease, but the careful integration of surgery, radiation therapy, and even periods of observation is important in the overall management of this condition (**Figs. 92-2** and **92-3**). Prognostic factors include performance status, site and number of metastases, response to chemotherapy, and serum lactate dehydrogenase (LDH) levels. Culine and colleagues developed a prognostic model using performance status and serum LDH levels, which allowed the assignment of patients into two subgroups with divergent outcomes. Raghav and colleagues developed a prognostic nomogram to provide individualized survival estimates for patients with CUP based on baseline gender, ECOG performance status, histology, number of metastatic

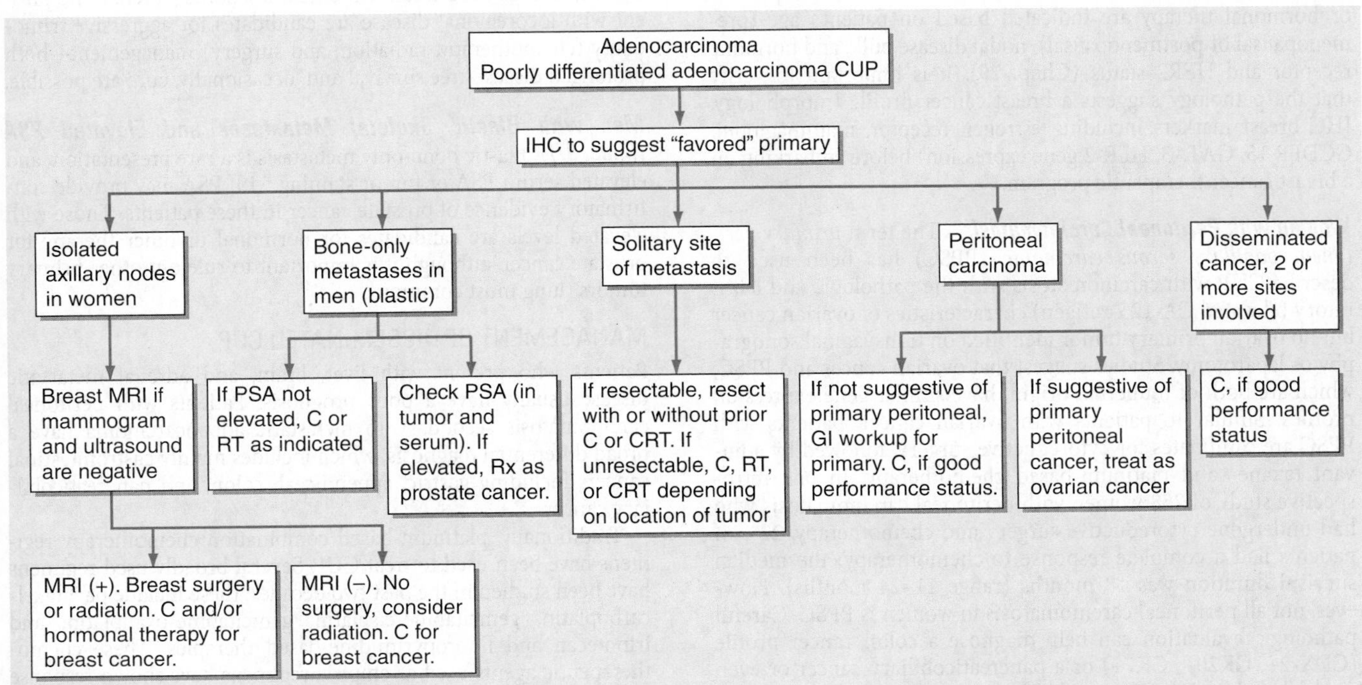

FIGURE 92-2 Treatment algorithm for adenocarcinoma and poorly differentiated adenocarcinoma of unknown primary (CUP). C, chemotherapy; CRT, chemoradiation; GI, gastrointestinal; IHC, immunohistochemistry; MRI, magnetic resonance imaging; PSA, prostate-specific antigen; RT, radiation.

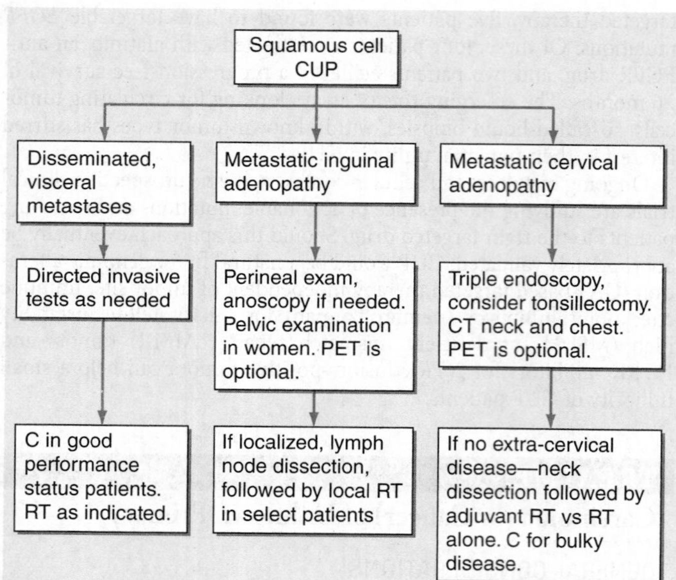

FIGURE 92-3 Treatment algorithm for squamous cell carcinoma of unknown primary (CUP). C, chemotherapy; CT, computed tomography; PET, positron emission tomography; RT, radiation.

sites and neutrophil-lymphocyte ratio. Future prospective trials using this prognostic model are warranted. Clinically, some CUP diagnoses fall into a favorable prognostic subset. Others, including those with disseminated CUP, have a more unfavorable prognosis.

TREATMENT OF FAVORABLE CUP SUBSETS

Women with Isolated Axillary Adenopathy Women with isolated axillary adenopathy with adenocarcinoma or carcinoma are usually treated for stage II or III breast cancer based on pathologic findings. These patients should undergo a breast MRI if mammogram and ultrasound are negative. Radiation therapy to the ipsilateral breast is indicated if the MRI of the breast is positive. Chemotherapy and/or hormonal therapy are indicated based on patient's age (premenopausal or postmenopausal), nodal disease bulk, and hormone receptor and HER2 status (**Chap. 79**). It is important to verify that the pathology suggests a breast cancer profile (morphology, IHC breast markers including estrogen receptor, mammaglobin, GCDFP-15, GATA3, HER-2 gene expression) before embarking on a breast cancer therapeutic program.

Women with Peritoneal Carcinomatosis The term *primary peritoneal papillary serous carcinoma* (PPSC) has been used to describe CUP with carcinomatosis with the pathologic and laboratory (elevated CA-125 antigen) characteristics of ovarian cancer but no ovarian primary tumor identified on transvaginal sonography or laparotomy. Studies suggest that ovarian cancer and PPSC, which are both of müllerian origin, have similar gene expression profiles. Similar to patients with ovarian cancer, patients with PPSC are candidates for cytoreductive surgery, followed by adjuvant taxane- and platinum-based chemotherapy. In one retrospective study of 258 women with peritoneal carcinomatosis who had undergone cytoreductive surgery and chemotherapy, 22% of patients had a complete response to chemotherapy; the median survival duration was 18 months (range 11–24 months). However, not all peritoneal carcinomatosis in women is PPSC. Careful pathologic evaluation can help diagnose a colon cancer profile (CDX-2+, CK20+, CK7–) or a pancreaticobiliary cancer or even a mislabeled peritoneal mesothelioma (calretinin, D2-40 positive; BerEp4, MOC-31 negative).

Poorly Differentiated Carcinoma with Midline Adenopathy (Chap. 88) Men with poorly differentiated or undifferentiated carcinoma who present with midline adenopathy should be evaluated for extragonadal germ cell malignancy. If diagnosed and treated as such, they often experience a good response to treatment with platinum-based combination chemotherapy. Response rates of >50% have been noted, and long-term survival rates of 10–15% have been reported. Older patients, especially smokers, who present with mediastinal adenopathy are more likely to have a lung or head and neck cancer profile.

Neuroendocrine Cancer (Chap. 84) Low-grade neuroendocrine tumor (NET) often has an indolent course, and treatment decisions are based on symptoms and tumor bulk. Urine 5-HIAA and serum chromogranin may be elevated and can be followed as markers. Often the patient is treated with somatostatin analogues alone for hormone-related symptoms (diarrhea, flushing, nausea). Specific local therapies or systemic therapy would only be indicated if the patient is symptomatic with local pain secondary to significant growth of the metastasis or the hormone-related symptoms are not controlled with endocrine therapy. Novel therapy options have demonstrated benefit in patients with low-grade NET, including sunitinib (which targets the vascular endothelial growth factor pathway), everolimus (which inhibits the mammalian target of rapamycin), and lutetium-177 dotatate (a somatostatin peptide receptor radioligand). Patients with high-grade NET are treated with platinum-based doublet therapy; 20–25% show a complete response, and up to 10% patients with limited/oligo presentations survive for >5 years. Some degree of neuroendocrine differentiation can be seen in diverse poorly differentiated carcinomas.

Squamous Cell Carcinoma Presenting as Neck Adenopathy Patients with early-stage squamous cell carcinoma involving the cervical lymph nodes are candidates for node dissection and radiation therapy, which can result in long-term survival. The role of chemotherapy in these patients is undefined, although chemoradiation therapy or induction chemotherapy is often used and is beneficial in bulky N2/N3 lymph node disease.

Solitary Metastatic Sites Patients with solitary metastases can also experience good treatment outcomes. Some patients who present with locoregional disease are candidates for aggressive trimodality (chemotherapy, radiation, and surgery) management—both prolonged disease-free survival and, occasionally, cure are possible.

Men with Blastic Skeletal Metastases and Elevated PSA (Chap. 87) Blastic bone-only metastasis is a rare presentation, and elevated serum PSA or tumor staining with PSA may provide confirmatory evidence of prostate cancer in these patients. Those with elevated levels are candidates for hormonal or other therapy for prostate cancer, although it is important to rule out other primary tumors (lung most common).

MANAGEMENT OF DISSEMINATED CUP

Patients who present with liver, brain, and adrenal metastatic disease usually have a poor prognosis. Patients with peritoneal carcinomatosis secondary to metastatic adenocarcinoma have a broad differential diagnosis, which includes mainly gastrointestinal cancers including gastric, appendiceal, colon, and pancreaticobiliary cancers.

Traditionally, platinum-based combination chemotherapy regimens have been used to treat CUP. Several broadly used regimens have been studied in the past two decades; these include paclitaxel-carboplatin, gemcitabine-cisplatin, gemcitabine-oxaliplatin, and irinotecan and fluoropyrimidine-based therapies. These chemotherapeutic agents used as empiric regimens have shown response rates of 25–40%, and their use obtains median survival times of 6–13 months.

Outside of favorable subsets, there is a small group of patients with a "definitive" IHC profile. These patients usually have a single diagnosis based on their clinicopathologic presentation and are often treated for the putative primary tumor. This does not guarantee a response, although it increases the probability of response when select drugs are chosen from a class of drugs known to be effective in that cancer type. Efforts should be made to search for biomarkers of response to tumor-agnostic effective therapies such as immunotherapy for MSI-H/dMMR tumors. Patients who do not fall into those categories are candidates for broad-spectrum platinum-based regimens, clinical trials, and additional trial-based genomic and proteomic tests. Today, we do not have many effective drugs for several CUP cancer profiles, and treatments overlap for some cancers. Immunotherapy has been an area of active interest due to robust and durable responses in cancers with known primaries and has shown some activity in CUP. However, biomarkers of response and immune-sensitive subsets need to be defined within CUP.

SUMMARY

Patients with CUP should undergo a directed diagnostic search for the primary tumor on the basis of clinical and pathologic data. Subsets of patients have prognostically favorable disease, as defined by clinical or histologic criteria, and may substantially benefit from aggressive treatment; in these patients, prolonged survival can be expected. However, for most patients who present with advanced CUP, the prognosis remains poor with early resistance to available cytotoxic therapy. The current focus has shifted away from empirical chemotherapeutic trials to understanding the metastatic phenotype, tissue of origin profiling in select patients, and next-generation sequencing to identify actionable mutations in CUP patients. As novel therapies evolve in cancers with known primaries, investigations to assess their value in CUP will likely have an impact on management of CUP patients.

FURTHER READING

Fizazi K et al: Cancers of unknown primary site: ESMO Clinical Practice Guidelines for diagnosis, treatment and follow-up. Ann Oncol 26(Suppl 5):v133, 2015.

Gatalica Z et al: Comprehensive analysis of cancers of unknown primary for the biomarkers of response to immune checkpoint blockade therapy. Eur J Cancer 94:179, 2018.

Hayashi H et al: Randomized phase II trial comparing site-specific treatment based on gene expression profiling with carboplatin and paclitaxel for patients with cancer of unknown primary site. J Clin Oncol 37:570, 2019.

Hayashi H et al: Site-specific and targeted therapy based on molecular profiling by next-generation sequencing for cancer of unknown primary site: A nonrandomized phase 2 clinical trial. JAMA Oncol 6:1, 2020.

National Comprehensive Cancer Network: Occult Primary (Cancer of Unknown Primary) version 2.2017, October 2016. *http://www.nccn.org/professionals/physician_gls/pdf/occult.pdf.*

Raghav K et al: Cancer of unknown primary in adolescents and young adults: Clinicopathological features, prognostic factors and survival outcomes. PLoS One 11:e0154985, 2016.

Raghav K et al: Defining a distinct immunotherapy eligible subset of patients with cancer of unknown primary using gene expression profiling with the 92-gene assay. Oncologist 25:e1807, 2020.

Raghav K et al: Development and validation of a novel nomogram for individualized prediction of survival in cancer of unknown primary. Clin Cancer Res 27:3414, 2021.

Ross JS et al: Comprehensive genomic profiling of carcinoma of unknown primary site: New routes to targeted therapies. JAMA Oncol 1:40, 2015.

Varadhachary GR, Raber MN: Cancer of unknown primary site. N Engl J Med 371:757, 2014.

93 Paraneoplastic Syndromes: Endocrinologic/Hematologic

J. Larry Jameson, Dan L. Longo

Neoplastic cells can produce a variety of substances that can alter the physiology of hormonal, hematologic, dermatologic, rheumatologic, renal, and neurologic systems. *Paraneoplastic syndromes* refer to the disorders that accompany benign or malignant tumors but are not directly related to mass effects or invasion. Tumors of neuroendocrine origin, such as small-cell lung carcinoma (SCLC) and carcinoids are common causes of paraneoplastic syndromes, but they have been associated with many types of tumors that produce peptide hormones, cytokines, and growth factors and induce the production of antibodies. Studies of the prevalence of paraneoplastic syndromes indicate that they are more common than is generally appreciated. The signs, symptoms, and metabolic alterations associated with paraneoplastic disorders are easily overlooked in the context of a malignancy and its treatment. Consequently, atypical clinical manifestations in a patient with cancer should prompt consideration of a paraneoplastic syndrome. The most common hormonal and hematologic syndromes associated with underlying neoplasia will be discussed here.

ENDOCRINE PARANEOPLASTIC SYNDROMES

Etiology Hormones can be produced from eutopic or ectopic sources. *Eutopic* refers to the expression of a hormone from its normal tissue of origin, whereas *ectopic* refers to hormone production from an atypical tissue source. For example, adrenocorticotropic hormone (ACTH) is expressed eutopically by the corticotrope cells of the anterior pituitary, but it can be expressed ectopically in SCLC. Many hormones are produced at low levels from tissues other than the classic endocrine source. Thus, ectopic expression is often a quantitative change rather than an absolute change in tissue expression. Nevertheless, the term *ectopic expression* is firmly entrenched and conveys the abnormal physiology associated with hormone production by neoplastic cells. In addition to high levels of hormones, ectopic expression is often characterized by abnormal regulation of hormone production (e.g., defective feedback control in ectopic ACTH) and peptide processing (resulting in large, unprocessed precursor peptide such as proopiomelanocortin [POMC]).

Many different molecular mechanisms can cause ectopic hormone production. In rare instances, genetic rearrangements account for aberrant hormone expression. For example, translocation of the parathyroid hormone (*PTH*) gene can result in high levels of PTH expression in tissues other than the parathyroid gland because the genetic rearrangement brings the *PTH* gene under the control of atypical regulatory elements. A related phenomenon is well documented in many forms of leukemia and lymphoma, in which somatic genetic rearrangements confer a growth advantage and alter cellular differentiation and function. Although genetic rearrangements cause selected cases of ectopic hormone production, this mechanism is rare, as many tumors are associated with excessive production of numerous peptides. Cellular dedifferentiation probably underlies most cases of ectopic hormone production. Many cancers are poorly differentiated, and certain tumor products, such as human chorionic gonadotropin (hCG), PTH-related protein (PTHrP), and α fetoprotein, are characteristic of gene expression at earlier developmental stages. In contrast, the propensity of certain cancers to produce particular hormones (e.g., squamous cell carcinomas produce PTHrP) suggests that dedifferentiation is partial or that selective pathways are derepressed. These expression profiles probably reflect epigenetic modifications that alter transcriptional repression, microRNA expression, and other pathways that govern cell differentiation.

In SCLC, the pathway of differentiation has been relatively well defined. The neuroendocrine phenotype is dictated in part by the basic-helix-loop-helix (bHLH) transcription factor human achaete-scute homologue 1 (hASH1), which is expressed at abnormally high levels in SCLC associated with ectopic ACTH. The abnormal expression of hASH1 and other developmental transcription factors appears to provide a link between cell proliferation and differentiation.

Ectopic hormone production might be considered merely epiphenomenon associated with cancer if it did not cause clinical manifestations. Excessive and unregulated production of hormones such as ACTH, PTHrP, and vasopressin can lead to substantial morbidity and complicate the cancer treatment plan. Moreover, the paraneoplastic endocrinopathies may be a presenting clinical feature of underlying malignancy and prompt the search for an unrecognized tumor.

A large number of paraneoplastic endocrine syndromes have been described, linking overproduction of particular hormones with specific types of tumors. However, certain recurring syndromes emerge from this group (**Table 93-1**). The most common paraneoplastic endocrine syndromes include hypercalcemia from overproduction of PTHrP and other factors, hyponatremia from excess vasopressin, and Cushing's syndrome from ectopic ACTH.

■ HYPERCALCEMIA CAUSED BY ECTOPIC PRODUCTION OF PTHRP

(See also **Chap. 410**)

Etiology Humoral hypercalcemia of malignancy (HHM) occurs in up to 20% of patients with cancer. HHM is most common in cancers of the lung, head and neck, skin, esophagus, breast, and genitourinary tract and in multiple myeloma and lymphomas, as well as metastases associated with these, and other cancers. There are several distinct humoral causes of HHM, but it is caused most commonly by overproduction of PTHrP. In addition to acting as a circulating humoral factor, bone metastases (e.g., breast, multiple myeloma) may produce PTHrP and other chemokines, leading to local osteolysis and hypercalcemia. PTHrP may also affect the initiation and progression of tumors by acting through pro-survival and chemokine pathways.

PTHrP is structurally related to PTH and binds to the PTH receptor, explaining the similar biochemical features of HHM and hyperparathyroidism. PTHrP plays a key physiologic role in skeletal development and regulates cellular proliferation and differentiation in other tissues, including skin, bone marrow, breast, and hair follicles. The mechanism of PTHrP induction in malignancy is incompletely understood; however, tumor-bearing tissues commonly associated with HHM normally produce PTHrP during development or cell renewal. PTHrP expression is stimulated by hedgehog pathways and Gli transcription factors that are active in many malignancies. Transforming growth factor β (TGF-β), which is produced by many tumors, also stimulates PTHrP. Mutations in certain oncogenes, such as *Ras*, also can activate PTHrP expression, as does loss of the tumor suppressor, p53. In addition to its role in HHM, the PTHrP pathway may also provide a potential target for therapeutic intervention to impede cancer growth.

TABLE 93-1 Paraneoplastic Syndromes Caused by Ectopic Hormone Production

PARANEOPLASTIC SYNDROME	ECTOPIC HORMONE	TYPICAL TUMOR TYPES[a]
Common		
Hypercalcemia of malignancy	Parathyroid hormone–related protein (PTHrP)	Squamous cell (head and neck, lung, skin), breast, genitourinary, gastrointestinal; osteolytic metastases
	1,25-Dihydroxyvitamin D	Lymphomas
	Parathyroid hormone (PTH) (rare)	Lung, ovary
	Prostaglandin E_2 (PGE_2) (rare)	Renal, lung
Syndrome of inappropriate antidiuretic hormone secretion (SIADH)	Vasopressin	Lung (squamous, small cell), gastrointestinal, genitourinary, ovary
Cushing's syndrome	Adrenocorticotropic hormone (ACTH)	Lung (small cell, bronchial carcinoid, adenocarcinoma, squamous), thymus, pancreatic islet, medullary thyroid carcinoma, pheochromocytoma
	Corticotropin-releasing hormone (CRH) (rare)	Pancreatic islet, carcinoid, lung, prostate
	Ectopic expression of gastric inhibitory peptide (GIP), luteinizing hormone (LH)/human chorionic gonadotropin (hCG), other G protein–coupled receptors (rare)	Macronodular adrenal hyperplasia
Less Common		
Non–islet cell hypoglycemia	Insulin-like growth factor type II (IGF-II)	Mesenchymal tumors, sarcomas, adrenal, hepatic, gastrointestinal, kidney, prostate
	Insulin (rare)	Cervix (small-cell carcinoma)
Male feminization	hCG[b]	Testis (embryonal, seminomas), germinomas, choriocarcinoma, lung, hepatic, pancreatic islet
Diarrhea or intestinal hypermotility	Calcitonin[c]	Lung, colon, breast, medullary thyroid carcinoma
	Vasoactive intestinal peptide (VIP)	Pancreas, pheochromocytoma, esophagus
Rare		
Oncogenic osteomalacia	Fibroblast growth factor 23 (FGF23) or phosphatonin	Hemangiopericytomas, osteoblastomas, fibromas, sarcomas, giant cell tumors, prostate, lung
Acromegaly	Growth hormone–releasing hormone (GHRH)	Pancreatic islet, bronchial, and other carcinoids
	Growth hormone (GH)	Lung, pancreatic islet
Hyperthyroidism	Thyroid-stimulating hormone (TSH)	Hydatidiform mole, embryonal tumors, struma ovarii
Hypertension	Renin	Juxtaglomerular tumors, kidney, lung, pancreas, ovary
Consumptive hypothyroidism	Type 3 deiodinase	Hepatic and other hemangiomas

[a]Only the most common tumor types are listed. For most ectopic hormone syndromes, an extensive list of tumors has been reported to produce one or more hormones. [b]hCG is produced eutopically by trophoblastic tumors. Certain tumors produce disproportionate amounts of the hCG α or hCG β subunit. High levels of hCG rarely cause hyperthyroidism because of weak binding to the TSH receptor. [c]Calcitonin is produced eutopically by medullary thyroid carcinoma and is used as a tumor marker.

Another relatively common cause of HHM is excess production of 1,25-dihydroxyvitamin D. Like granulomatous disorders associated with hypercalcemia, lymphomas can produce an enzyme that converts 25-hydroxyvitamin D to the more active 1,25-dihydroxyvitamin D, leading to enhanced gastrointestinal calcium absorption. Other causes of HHM include tumor-mediated production of osteolytic cytokines and inflammatory mediators.

Clinical Manifestations The typical presentation of HHM is a patient with a known malignancy who is found to be hypercalcemic on routine laboratory tests. Less often, hypercalcemia is the initial presenting feature of malignancy. Particularly when calcium levels are markedly increased (>3.5 mmol/L [>14 mg/dL]), patients may experience fatigue, mental status changes, polyuria, dehydration, or symptoms of nephrolithiasis. Hypercalcemia can shorten ST segments and QT intervals, as well as bundle branch blocks and bradyarrhythmias.

Diagnosis Features that favor HHM, as opposed to primary hyperparathyroidism, include known malignancy, recent onset of hypercalcemia, and very high serum calcium levels. Like hyperparathyroidism, hypercalcemia caused by PTHrP is accompanied by hypercalciuria and hypophosphatemia. Patients with HHM typically have metabolic alkalosis rather than hyperchloremic acidosis, as is seen in hyperparathyroidism. Measurement of PTH is useful to exclude primary hyperparathyroidism; the PTH level should be suppressed in HHM. An elevated PTHrP level confirms the diagnosis, and it is increased in ~80% of hypercalcemic patients with cancer. 1,25-Dihydroxyvitamin D levels may be increased in patients with lymphoma.

TREATMENT
Humoral Hypercalcemia of Malignancy

The management of HHM begins with removal of excess calcium in the diet, medications, or IV solutions. Saline rehydration (typically 200–500 mL/h) is used to dilute serum calcium and promote calciuresis; exercise caution in patients with cardiac, hepatic, or renal insufficiency. Forced diuresis with furosemide (20–80 mg IV in escalating doses) or other loop diuretics can enhance calcium excretion but provides relatively little value except in life-threatening hypercalcemia. When used, loop diuretics should be administered only after complete rehydration and with careful monitoring of fluid balance. Oral phosphorus (e.g., 250 mg Neutra-Phos 3–4 times daily) should be given until serum phosphorus is >1 mmol/L (>3 mg/dL). Bisphosphonates such as pamidronate (60–90 mg IV), zoledronate (4–8 mg IV), and etidronate (7.5 mg/kg per day PO for 3–7 consecutive days) can reduce serum calcium within 1–2 days and suppress calcium release for several weeks. Bisphosphonate infusions can be repeated, or oral bisphosphonates can be used for chronic treatment. Denosumab (120 mg SC weekly for 4 weeks and then monthly) can be used in patients who do not respond adequately to bisphosphonates. It acts as a decoy receptor for RANK ligand to mitigate stimulation of osteoclasts. Cinacalcet (30 mg PO bid to 90 mg PO qid) stimulates calcium-sensing receptors to suppress PTH secretion and is therefore applicable in parathyroid carcinoma and rare cases of ectopic PTH-producing tumors. Hypercalcemia associated with lymphomas, multiple myeloma, or leukemia may respond to glucocorticoid treatment (e.g., prednisone 40–100 mg PO in four divided doses). Dialysis should be considered in severe hypercalcemia when saline hydration and bisphosphonate treatments are not possible or are too slow in onset. Previously used agents such as calcitonin and mithramycin have little utility now that bisphosphonates and other agents are available.

■ ECTOPIC VASOPRESSIN: TUMOR-ASSOCIATED SYNDROME OF INAPPROPRIATE ANTIDIURETIC HORMONE

(See also **Chap. 53**)

Etiology Vasopressin is an antidiuretic hormone normally produced by the posterior pituitary gland. Ectopic vasopressin production by tumors is a common cause of the syndrome of inappropriate antidiuretic hormone (SIADH), occurring in at least half of patients with SCLC. SIADH also can be caused by a number of nonneoplastic conditions, including central nervous system (CNS) trauma, infections, and medications (**Chap. 381**). Compensatory responses to SIADH, such as decreased thirst, may mitigate the development of hyponatremia. However, with prolonged production of excessive vasopressin, the osmostat controlling thirst and hypothalamic vasopressin secretion may become reset. In addition, intake of free water, orally or intravenously, can quickly worsen hyponatremia because of reduced renal diuresis.

Tumors with neuroendocrine features, such as SCLC and carcinoids, are the most common sources of ectopic vasopressin production, but it also occurs in other forms of lung cancer and with CNS lesions, head and neck cancer, and genitourinary, gastrointestinal, and ovarian cancers. The mechanism of activation of the vasopressin gene in these tumors is unknown, but the frequent concomitant expression of the adjacent oxytocin gene suggests derepression of this locus.

Clinical Manifestations Most patients with ectopic vasopressin secretion are asymptomatic and are identified because of the presence of hyponatremia on routine chemistry testing. Symptoms may include weakness, lethargy, nausea, confusion, depressed mental status, and seizures. The severity of symptoms reflects the rapidity of onset as well as the severity of hyponatremia. Hyponatremia usually develops slowly but may be exacerbated by the administration of IV fluids or the institution of new medications.

Diagnosis The diagnostic features of ectopic vasopressin production are the same as those of other causes of SIADH (**Chaps. 53** and **381**). Hyponatremia and reduced serum osmolality occur in the setting of an inappropriately normal or increased urine osmolality. Urine sodium excretion is normal or increased unless volume depletion is present. Other causes of hyponatremia should be excluded, including renal, adrenal, or thyroid insufficiency. Physiologic sources of vasopressin stimulation (CNS lesions, pulmonary disease, nausea), adaptive circulatory mechanisms (hypotension, heart failure, hepatic cirrhosis), and medications, including many chemotherapeutic agents, also should be considered as possible causes of hyponatremia. Vasopressin measurements are not usually necessary to make the diagnosis.

TREATMENT
Ectopic Vasopressin: Tumor-Associated SIADH

Most patients with ectopic vasopressin production develop hyponatremia over several weeks or months. The disorder should be corrected gradually unless mental status is altered or there is risk of seizures. Rapid correction can cause brain dehydration and central pontine myelinolysis. Treatment of the underlying malignancy may reduce ectopic vasopressin production, but this response is slow if it occurs at all. Fluid restriction to less than urine output, plus insensible losses, is often sufficient to correct hyponatremia partially. However, strict monitoring of the amount and types of liquids consumed or administered intravenously is required for fluid restriction to be effective. Salt tablets and saline are not helpful unless volume depletion is also present. Demeclocycline (150–300 mg orally 3–4 times daily) can be used to inhibit vasopressin action on the renal distal tubule, but its onset of action is relatively slow (1–2 weeks). The vaptan class of drugs acts by inhibiting vasopressin receptors (V_{1A}, V_{1B}, V_2) in the renal collecting ducts. Conivaptan, a nonpeptide V_2-receptor antagonist, can be administered either PO (20–120 mg bid) or IV (10–40 mg) and is particularly effective when used in combination with fluid restriction in euvolemic hyponatremia. Tolvaptan (15 mg PO daily) is another vasopressin antagonist. The dose can be increased to 30–60 mg/d based on response. Severe hyponatremia (Na <115 meq/L) or mental status changes may require treatment with hypertonic (3%) or normal saline infusion together with furosemide to enhance free water clearance. The rate of sodium correction should be slow (0.5–1 meq/L per hour) to prevent rapid fluid shifts and the possible development of central pontine myelinolysis.

CUSHING'S SYNDROME CAUSED BY ECTOPIC ACTH PRODUCTION

(See also **Chap. 386**)

Etiology Ectopic ACTH production accounts for 10–20% of cases of Cushing's syndrome. The syndrome is particularly common in neuroendocrine tumors. SCLC is the most common cause of ectopic ACTH, followed by bronchial and thymic carcinoids, islet cell tumors, other carcinoids, and pheochromocytomas. Ectopic ACTH production is caused by increased expression of the proopiomelanocortin (*POMC*) gene, which encodes ACTH, along with melanocyte-stimulating hormone (MSH), β lipotropin, and several other peptides. In many tumors, there is abundant but aberrant expression of the *POMC* gene from an internal promoter, proximal to the third exon, which encodes ACTH. However, because this product lacks the signal sequence necessary for protein processing, it is not secreted. Increased production of ACTH arises instead from less abundant, but unregulated, *POMC* expression from the same promoter site used in the pituitary. Because tumors lack many of the enzymes needed to process the POMC polypeptide, it is typically released as multiple large, biologically inactive fragments along with relatively small amounts of fully processed, active ACTH.

Rarely, corticotropin-releasing hormone (CRH) is produced by pancreatic islet cell tumors, SCLC, medullary thyroid cancer, carcinoids, or prostate cancer. When levels are high enough, CRH can cause pituitary corticotrope hyperplasia and Cushing's syndrome. Tumors that produce CRH sometimes also produce ACTH, raising the possibility of a paracrine mechanism for ACTH production.

A distinct mechanism for ACTH-independent Cushing's syndrome involves ectopic expression of various G protein–coupled receptors in adrenal nodules. Ectopic expression of the gastric inhibitory peptide (GIP) receptor is the best-characterized example of this mechanism. In this case, meals induce GIP secretion, which inappropriately stimulates adrenal growth and glucocorticoid production.

Clinical Manifestations The clinical features of hypercortisolemia are detected in only a fraction of patients with documented ectopic ACTH production. Patients with ectopic ACTH syndrome generally exhibit less marked weight gain and centripetal fat redistribution, probably because the exposure to excess glucocorticoids is relatively brief and because cachexia reduces the propensity for weight gain and fat deposition. The ectopic ACTH syndrome is associated with several clinical features that distinguish it from other causes of Cushing's syndrome (e.g., pituitary adenomas, adrenal adenomas, iatrogenic glucocorticoid excess). The metabolic manifestations of ectopic ACTH syndrome are dominated by fluid retention and hypertension, hypokalemia, metabolic alkalosis, glucose intolerance, and occasionally steroid psychosis. The very high ACTH levels often cause increased pigmentation, reflecting increased activity of MSH derived from the POMC precursor peptide. The extraordinarily high glucocorticoid levels in patients with ectopic sources of ACTH can lead to marked skin fragility and easy bruising. In addition, the high cortisol levels often overwhelm the renal 11β-hydroxysteroid dehydrogenase type II enzyme, which normally inactivates cortisol and prevents it from binding to renal mineralocorticoid receptors. Consequently, in addition to the excess mineralocorticoids produced by ACTH stimulation of the adrenal gland, high levels of cortisol exert activity through the mineralocorticoid receptor, leading to severe hypokalemia.

Diagnosis The diagnosis of ectopic ACTH syndrome is usually not difficult in the setting of a known malignancy. Urine-free cortisol levels fluctuate but are typically greater than two to four times normal, and the plasma ACTH level is usually >22 pmol/L (>100 pg/mL). A suppressed ACTH level excludes this diagnosis and indicates an ACTH-independent cause of Cushing's syndrome (e.g., adrenal or exogenous glucocorticoid). In contrast to pituitary sources of ACTH, most ectopic sources of ACTH do not respond to glucocorticoid suppression. Therefore, high-dose dexamethasone (8 mg PO) suppresses 8:00 A.M. serum cortisol (50% decrease from baseline) in ~80% of pituitary ACTH-producing adenomas but fails to suppress ectopic ACTH in ~90% of cases. Bronchial and other carcinoids are well-documented exceptions to these general guidelines, as these ectopic sources of ACTH may exhibit feedback regulation indistinguishable from pituitary adenomas, including suppression by high-dose dexamethasone, and ACTH responsiveness to adrenal blockade with metyrapone. If necessary, petrosal sinus catheterization can be used to evaluate a patient with ACTH-dependent Cushing's syndrome when the source of ACTH is unclear. After CRH stimulation, a 3:1 petrosal sinus:peripheral ACTH ratio strongly suggests a pituitary ACTH source. Imaging studies (computed tomography or magnetic resonance imaging) are also useful in the evaluation of suspected carcinoid lesions, allowing biopsy and characterization of hormone production using special stains. If available, positron emission tomography or octreotide scanning may identify some sources of ACTH production.

TREATMENT

Cushing's Syndrome Caused by Ectopic ACTH Production

The morbidity associated with the ectopic ACTH syndrome can be substantial. Patients may experience depression or personality changes because of extreme cortisol excess. Metabolic derangements, including diabetes mellitus and hypokalemia, can worsen fatigue. Poor wound healing and predisposition to infections can complicate the surgical management of tumors, and opportunistic infections caused by organisms such as *Pneumocystis carinii* and mycoses are often the cause of death in patients with ectopic ACTH production. These patients have increased risk of venous thromboembolism reflecting the combination of malignancy and altered coagulation factor profiles. Depending on prognosis and treatment plans for the underlying malignancy, measures to reduce cortisol levels are often indicated. Treatment of the underlying malignancy may reduce ACTH levels but is rarely sufficient to reduce cortisol levels to normal. Adrenalectomy is not practical for most of these patients but should be considered during surgery for the malignancy or if the underlying tumor is not resectable and the prognosis is otherwise favorable (e.g., carcinoid). Medical therapy with ketoconazole (300–600 mg PO bid), metyrapone (250–500 mg PO every 6 h), mitotane (3–6 g PO in four divided doses, tapered to maintain low cortisol production), etomidate (0.1–0.3 mg/kg/h IV), or other agents that block steroid synthesis or action is often the most practical strategy for managing the hypercortisolism associated with ectopic ACTH production. Glucocorticoid replacement should be provided to prevent adrenal insufficiency (**Chap. 386**). Unfortunately, many patients eventually progress despite medical blockade. Mifepristone (200–1000 mg PO qd) inhibits both glucocorticoid and progesterone receptors, has rapid onset of action, and improves glucose intolerance and hypertension in a subset of patients. ACTH-neutralizing antibodies and ACTH receptor blockers are under investigation, as are selective inhibitors of the glucocorticoid receptor.

TUMOR-INDUCED HYPOGLYCEMIA CAUSED BY EXCESS PRODUCTION OF INSULIN-LIKE GROWTH FACTOR TYPE II

(See also **Chap. 406**) Mesenchymal tumors, hemangiopericytomas, hepatocellular tumors, adrenal carcinomas, and a variety of other large tumors have been reported to produce excessive amounts of insulin-like growth factor type II (IGF-II) precursor, which binds weakly to insulin receptors and more strongly to IGF-I receptors, leading to insulin-like actions. The gene encoding IGF-II resides on chromosome 11p15, a locus that is normally imprinted (that is, expression is exclusively from a single parental allele). Biallelic expression of the IGF-II gene occurs in a subset of tumors, suggesting loss of methylation and loss of imprinting as a mechanism for gene induction. In addition to increased IGF-II production, IGF-II bioavailability is increased due to complex alterations in circulating binding proteins. Increased IGF-II suppresses growth hormone (GH) and insulin, resulting in reduced IGF binding protein 3 (IGFBP-3), IGF-I, and acid-labile subunit (ALS). The reduction in ALS and IGFBP-3, which normally sequester IGF-II, causes it to be displaced to a small circulating complex that has greater access to insulin target tissues. For this reason, circulating IGF-II levels may not be markedly increased despite causing hypoglycemia. In addition to IGF-II–mediated hypoglycemia, tumors may occupy enough of the liver to impair gluconeogenesis.

In most cases, a tumor causing hypoglycemia is clinically apparent (usually >10 cm in size), and hypoglycemia develops in association with fasting. As with other causes of hypoglycemia, patients may present with sweating, tremors, palpitations, confusion, seizures, or coma. The diagnosis is made by documenting low serum glucose and suppressed insulin levels in association with symptoms of hypoglycemia. Serum IGF-II levels may not be increased (IGF-II assays may not detect IGF-II precursors), but an elevated IGF-II/IGF-I ratio greater than 10:1 is suggestive. Increased IGF-II mRNA expression is found in most of these tumors. Any medications associated with hypoglycemia should be eliminated. Treatment of the underlying malignancy, if possible, may reduce the predisposition to hypoglycemia. Frequent meals and IV glucose, especially during sleep or fasting, are often necessary to prevent hypoglycemia. Glucagon and glucocorticoids have also been used to enhance glucose production. Antibodies that inhibit IGF-II action are under development.

■ HUMAN CHORIONIC GONADOTROPIN

hCG is composed of α and β subunits and can be produced as intact hormone, which is biologically active, or as uncombined biologically inert subunits. Ectopic production of intact hCG occurs most often in association with testicular embryonal tumors, germ cell tumors, extragonadal germinomas, lung cancer, hepatoma, and pancreatic islet tumors. Eutopic production of hCG occurs with trophoblastic malignancies. hCG α subunit production is particularly common in lung cancer and pancreatic islet cancer. In men, high hCG levels stimulate steroidogenesis and aromatase activity in testicular Leydig cells, resulting in increased estrogen production and the development of gynecomastia. Precocious puberty in boys or gynecomastia in men should prompt measurement of hCG and consideration of a testicular tumor or another source of ectopic hCG production. Most women are asymptomatic. hCG is easily measured. Treatment should be directed at the underlying malignancy.

■ ONCOGENIC OSTEOMALACIA

Hypophosphatemic oncogenic osteomalacia, also called tumor-induced osteomalacia (TIO), is caused by excessive production of fibroblast growth factor 23 (FGF23), previously referred to as phosphotonin. Oncogenic osteomalacia is characterized by markedly reduced serum phosphorus and renal phosphate wasting, leading to muscle weakness, bone pain, and osteomalacia. Serum calcium and PTH levels are normal. FGF23 inhibits the renal conversion of 25-hydroxyvitamin D to 1,25-dihydroxyvitamin D, resulting in low levels of 1,25-dihydroxyvitamin D. Oncogenic osteomalacia is usually caused by benign mesenchymal tumors, such as hemangiopericytomas, fibromas, and giant cell tumors, often of the skeletal extremities or head. It has also been described in sarcomas and in patients with prostate or lung cancer. Resection of the tumor reverses the disorder, confirming its humoral basis. FGF23 levels are increased in some, but not all, patients with osteogenic osteomalacia. FGF23 forms a ternary complex with the klotho protein and renal FGF receptors to reduce renal phosphate reabsorption. Treatment involves removal of the tumor, if possible, and supplementation with phosphate and vitamin D. Octreotide treatment reduces phosphate wasting in some patients with tumors that express somatostatin receptor subtype 2. Octreotide scans may also be useful in detecting these tumors. The calcium-sensing receptor agonist, cinacalcet, has been effective in some patients, apparently by reducing PTH-mediated phosphaturia. FGF receptor inhibitors hold promise as future therapies targeted either to pathways that stimulate FGR23 production (e.g., FGFR1) or inhibit its action (e.g., FGF23 receptor).

■ CONSUMPTIVE HYPOTHYROIDISM

Newborns with hepatic hemangiomas can develop a rare form of hypothyroidism caused by overexpression of type 3 deiodinase (D3), an enzyme that degrades and inactivates thyroxine (T_4) and triiodothyronine (T_3). The very high expression of D3 and consumption of thyroid hormones apparently outstrip the thyroid gland's rate of hormone production. The disorder is characterized by low T_4, low T_3, high TSH, and markedly elevated reverse T_3 (rT_3), reflecting the degradation of T_4 to rT_3. In addition to treating the underlying hemangioma (rarely other tumor types), patients are treated with L-thyroxine replacement, titrated to normalize TSH. Steroids and propranolol may provide benefit, perhaps by inhibiting growth factor pathways thought to stimulate D3 production.

HEMATOLOGIC SYNDROMES

The elevation of granulocyte, platelet, and eosinophil counts in most patients with myeloproliferative disorders is caused by the proliferation of the myeloid elements due to the underlying disease rather than to a paraneoplastic syndrome. The paraneoplastic hematologic syndromes in patients with solid tumors are less well characterized than are the endocrine syndromes because the ectopic hormone(s) or cytokines responsible have not been identified in most of these tumors (**Table 93-2**). The extent of the paraneoplastic syndromes parallels the course of the cancer. With very rare exception, red cell, white cell or platelet numbers are self-limited and not associated with symptomatic abnormalities. In some circumstances, elevations in platelet counts can be a marker that influences prognosis. By far, the most consequential hematologic abnormality in cancer patients is hypercoagulability.

■ ERYTHROCYTOSIS

Ectopic production of erythropoietin by cancer cells causes most paraneoplastic erythrocytosis. The ectopically produced erythropoietin stimulates the production of red blood cells (RBCs) in the bone marrow and raises the hematocrit. Other lymphokines and hormones produced by cancer cells may stimulate erythropoietin release but have not been proved to cause erythrocytosis.

Most patients with erythrocytosis have an elevated hematocrit (>52% in men, >48% in women) that is detected on a routine blood

TABLE 93-2 Paraneoplastic Hematologic Syndromes

SYNDROME	PROTEINS	CANCERS TYPICALLY ASSOCIATED WITH SYNDROME
Erythrocytosis	Erythropoietin	Renal cancers, hepatocarcinoma, cerebellar hemangioblastomas
Granulocytosis	G-CSF, GM-CSF, IL-6	Lung cancer, gastrointestinal cancer, ovarian cancer, genitourinary cancer, Hodgkin's disease
Thrombocytosis	IL-6	Lung cancer, gastrointestinal cancer, breast cancer, ovarian cancer, lymphoma
Eosinophilia	IL-5	Lymphoma, leukemia, lung cancer
Thrombophlebitis	Unknown	Lung cancer, pancreatic cancer, gastrointestinal cancer, breast cancer, genitourinary cancer, ovarian cancer, prostate cancer, lymphoma

Abbreviations: G-CSF, granulocyte colony-stimulating factor; GM-CSF, granulocyte-macrophage colony-stimulating factor; IL, interleukin.

count. Approximately 3% of patients with renal cell cancer, 10% of patients with hepatoma, and 15% of patients with cerebellar hemangioblastomas have erythrocytosis. In most cases, the erythrocytosis is asymptomatic.

Patients with erythrocytosis due to a renal cell cancer, hepatoma, or CNS cancer should have measurement of red cell mass. If the red cell mass is elevated, the serum erythropoietin level should be measured. Patients with a cancer that has been associated with erythrocytosis, elevated erythropoietin levels, and no other explanation for erythrocytosis (e.g., hemoglobinopathy that causes increased O_2 affinity; **Chaps. 63** and **98**) have the paraneoplastic syndrome.

TREATMENT
Erythrocytosis

Successful resection of the cancer usually resolves the erythrocytosis. If the tumor cannot be resected or treated effectively with radiation therapy or chemotherapy, phlebotomy may control any symptoms or risk related to erythrocytosis.

■ GRANULOCYTOSIS

Approximately 30% of patients with solid tumors have granulocytosis (granulocyte count >8000/μL). In about half of patients with granulocytosis and cancer, the granulocytosis has an identifiable nonparaneoplastic etiology (e.g., infection, tumor necrosis, glucocorticoid administration). The other patients have proteins in urine and serum that stimulate the growth of bone marrow cells. Tumors and tumor cell lines from patients with lung, ovarian, and bladder cancers have been documented to produce granulocyte colony-stimulating factor (G-CSF), granulocyte-macrophage colony-stimulating factor (GM-CSF), and/or interleukin 6 (IL-6). However, the etiology of granulocytosis has not been characterized in most patients.

Patients with granulocytosis are nearly all asymptomatic, and the differential white blood cell count does not have a shift to immature forms of neutrophils. Granulocytosis occurs in 40% of patients with lung and gastrointestinal cancers, 20% of patients with breast cancer, 30% of patients with brain tumors and ovarian cancers, 20% of patients with Hodgkin's disease, and 10% of patients with renal cell carcinoma. Patients with advanced-stage disease are more likely to have granulocytosis than are those with early-stage disease.

Paraneoplastic granulocytosis does not require treatment. The granulocytosis resolves when the underlying cancer is treated.

■ THROMBOCYTOSIS

Some 35% of patients with thrombocytosis (platelet count >400,000/μL) have an underlying diagnosis of cancer. IL-6, a candidate molecule for the etiology of paraneoplastic thrombocytosis, stimulates the production of platelets in vitro and in vivo. Some patients with cancer and thrombocytosis have elevated levels of IL-6 in plasma. Another candidate molecule is thrombopoietin, a peptide hormone that stimulates megakaryocyte proliferation and platelet production. The etiology of thrombocytosis has not been established in most cases.

Patients with thrombocytosis are nearly all asymptomatic. Thrombocytosis is not clearly linked to thrombosis in patients with cancer. Thrombocytosis is present in 40% of patients with lung and gastrointestinal cancers; 20% of patients with breast, endometrial, and ovarian cancers; and 10% of patients with lymphoma. Patients with thrombocytosis are more likely to have advanced-stage disease and have a poorer prognosis than do patients without thrombocytosis. In ovarian cancer, IL-6 has been shown to directly promote tumor growth. Paraneoplastic thrombocytosis does not require treatment other than treatment of the underlying tumor.

■ EOSINOPHILIA

Eosinophilia is present in ~1% of patients with cancer. Tumors and tumor cell lines from patients with lymphomas or leukemia may produce IL-5, which stimulates eosinophil growth. Activation of IL-5 transcription in lymphomas and leukemias may involve translocation of the long arm of chromosome 5, to which the genes for IL-5 and other cytokines map.

Patients with eosinophilia are typically asymptomatic. Eosinophilia is present in 10% of patients with lymphoma, 3% of patients with lung cancer, and occasional patients with cervical, gastrointestinal, renal, and breast cancer. Patients with markedly elevated eosinophil counts (>5000/μL) can develop shortness of breath and wheezing. A chest radiograph may reveal diffuse pulmonary infiltrates from eosinophil infiltration and activation in the lungs.

TREATMENT
Eosinophilia

Definitive treatment is directed at the underlying malignancy. Tumors should be resected or treated with radiation or chemotherapy. In most patients who develop shortness of breath related to eosinophilia, symptoms resolve with the use of oral or inhaled glucocorticoids. IL-5 antagonists exist but have not been evaluated in this clinical setting.

■ THROMBOPHLEBITIS AND DEEP VENOUS THROMBOSIS

Deep venous thrombosis and pulmonary embolism are the most common thrombotic conditions in patients with cancer. Migratory or recurrent thrombophlebitis may be the initial manifestation of cancer. Nearly 15% of patients who develop deep venous thrombosis or pulmonary embolism have a diagnosis of cancer (**Chap. 117**). The coexistence of peripheral venous thrombosis with visceral carcinoma, particularly pancreatic cancer, is called *Trousseau's syndrome*.

Pathogenesis Patients with cancer are predisposed to thromboembolism because they are often at bed rest or immobilized, and tumors may obstruct or slow blood flow. Postoperative deep venous thrombosis is twice as common in cancer patients who undergo surgery. Chronic IV catheters also predispose to clotting. In addition, clotting may be promoted by release of procoagulants or cytokines from tumor cells or associated inflammatory cells or by platelet adhesion or aggregation. The specific molecules that promote thromboembolism have not been identified.

Chemotherapeutic agents, particularly those associated with endothelial damage, can induce venous thrombosis. The annual risk of venous thrombosis in patients with cancer receiving chemotherapy is about 11%, sixfold higher than the risk in the general population. Bleomycin, L-asparaginase, nitrogen mustard, thalidomide analogues, cisplatin-based regimens, and high doses of busulfan and carmustine are all associated with an increased risk.

In addition to cancer and its treatment causing secondary thrombosis, primary thrombophilic diseases may be associated with cancer. For example, the antiphospholipid antibody syndrome is associated with a wide range of pathologic manifestations (**Chap. 357**). About 20% of patients with this syndrome have cancers. Among patients with cancer and antiphospholipid antibodies, 35–45% develop thrombosis.

Clinical Manifestations Patients with cancer who develop deep venous thrombosis usually develop swelling or pain in the leg, and physical examination reveals tenderness, warmth, and redness. Patients who present with pulmonary embolism develop dyspnea, chest pain, and syncope, and physical examination shows tachycardia, cyanosis, and hypotension. Some 5% of patients with no history of cancer who have a diagnosis of deep venous thrombosis or pulmonary embolism will have a diagnosis of cancer within 1 year. The most common cancers associated with thromboembolic episodes include lung, pancreatic, gastrointestinal, breast, ovarian, and genitourinary cancers; lymphomas; and brain tumors. Patients with cancer who undergo surgical procedures requiring general anesthesia have a 20–30% risk of deep venous thrombosis.

Diagnosis The diagnosis of deep venous thrombosis in patients with cancer is made by impedance plethysmography or bilateral compression ultrasonography of the leg veins. Patients with a noncompressible venous segment have deep venous thrombosis. If compression ultrasonography is normal and there is a high clinical suspicion for deep venous thrombosis, venography should be done to look for a luminal filling defect. Elevation of D-dimer is not as predictive of deep venous thrombosis in patients with cancer as it is in patients without cancer; elevations are seen in people over age 65 years without concomitant evidence of thrombosis, probably as a consequence of increased thrombin deposition and turnover in aging.

Patients with symptoms and signs suggesting a pulmonary embolism should be evaluated with a chest radiograph, electrocardiogram, arterial blood gas analysis, and ventilation-perfusion scan. Patients with mismatched segmental perfusion defects have a pulmonary embolus. Patients with equivocal ventilation-perfusion findings should be evaluated as described above for deep venous thrombosis in their legs. If deep venous thrombosis is detected, they should be anticoagulated. If deep venous thrombosis is not detected, they should be considered for a pulmonary angiogram.

Patients without a diagnosis of cancer who present with an initial episode of thrombophlebitis or pulmonary embolus need no additional tests for cancer other than a careful history and physical examination. In light of the many possible primary sites, diagnostic testing in asymptomatic patients is wasteful. However, if the clot is refractory to standard treatment or is in an unusual site, or if the thrombophlebitis is migratory or recurrent, efforts to find an underlying cancer are indicated.

TREATMENT

Thrombophlebitis and Deep Venous Thrombosis

Patients with cancer and a diagnosis of deep venous thrombosis or pulmonary embolism should be treated initially with IV unfractionated heparin or low-molecular-weight heparin for at least 5 days, and warfarin should be started within 1 or 2 days. The warfarin dose should be adjusted so that the international normalized ratio (INR) is 2–3. Patients with proximal deep venous thrombosis and a relative contraindication to heparin anticoagulation (hemorrhagic brain metastases or pericardial effusion) should be considered for placement of a filter in the inferior vena cava (Greenfield filter) to prevent pulmonary embolism. Warfarin should be administered for 3–6 months. An alternative approach is to use low-molecular-weight heparin for 6 months. The new oral anticoagulants (factor Xa and thrombin inhibitors) are attractive because they do not require close monitoring of the prothrombin time and are not affected by dietary factors. Oral apixaban (10 mg bid for 7 days followed by 5 mg bid for 6 months) is noninferior to dalteparin in the treatment of cancer patients who develop deep vein thrombosis or pulmonary embolism. Patients with cancer who undergo a major surgical procedure should be considered for heparin prophylaxis or pneumatic boots. Breast cancer patients undergoing chemotherapy and patients with implanted catheters should be considered for prophylaxis. Guidelines recommend that hospitalized patients with cancer and patients receiving a thalidomide analogue receive prophylaxis with low-molecular-weight heparin or low-dose aspirin. Use of prophylaxis routinely during chemotherapy is controversial. Risk is affected by type of cancer, type of therapy, blood counts, and body mass index (all taken into account in the Khorana risk score; **Table 93-3**). Studies of Khorana high-risk patients with cancer using rivaroxaban and apixaban as clot prophylaxis have resulted in a 50% reduction in risk with a level of bleeding of about 5%. However, prophylaxis is not routinely recommended by the American Society of Clinical Oncology.

TABLE 93-3 Khorana Risk Score for Venous Thromboembolism in Cancer Patients

PATIENT CHARACTERISTICS	RISK SCORE POINTS
Site of cancer	
Very high risk (stomach, pancreas)	2
High risk (lung, lymphoma, gynecologic, genitourinary excluding prostate)	1
Prechemotherapy platelet count ≥350,000/μL	1
Hemoglobin level <10 g/dL or use of red cell growth factors	1
Prechemotherapy leukocyte count >11,000/μL	1
BMI ≥35 kg/m²	1

RISK SCORE (POINTS)	RISK CATEGORY	RATES OF sVTE ACCORDING TO SCORES (%)
0	Low	0.3–0.8
1–2	Intermediate	1.8–2.0
≥3	High	6.7–7.1

Abbreviations: BMI, body mass index; sVTE, symptomatic venous thromboembolism.

Source: AJ Muñoz Martín et al: Clinical guide SEOM on venous thromboembolism in cancer patients. Clin Transl Oncol 16:1079, 2014.

MISCELLANEOUS REMOTE EFFECTS OF CANCER

Patients with cancer can develop paraneoplastic autoimmune disorders (e.g., thrombocytopenia) and dysfunction of organs not directly invaded or involved with the cancer (rheumatologic and renal abnormalities are among the most frequent). The pathogenesis of these disorders is undefined, but often, the conditions reverse if the tumor is removed or successfully treated.

Cutaneous paraneoplastic syndromes are discussed in **Chap. 58**. Neurologic paraneoplastic syndromes are discussed in **Chap. 94**.

■ FURTHER READING

Agnelli G et al: Apixaban for the treatment of venous thromboembolism associated with cancer. N Engl J Med 382:1599, 2020.

Asonitis N et al: Diagnosis, pathophysiology and management of hypercalcemia in malignancy: A review of the literature. Horm Metab Res 51:770, 2019.

Catani MV et al: The "Janus face" of platelets in cancer. Int J Mol Sci 21:788, 2020.

Dynkevich Y et al: Tumors, IGF-2, and hypoglycemia: insights from the clinic, the laboratory, and the historical archive. Endocr Rev 34:798, 2013.

Ellison DH, Berl T: The syndrome of inappropriate antidiuresis. N Engl J Med 356:2064, 2007.

Feelders RA et al: Advances in the medical treatment of Cushing's syndrome. Lancet Diabetes Endocrinol 7:300, 2019.

Hartley IR et al: Targeted FGFR blockade for the treatment of tumor-induced osteomalacia. N Engl J Med 383:14, 2020.

Isidori AM et al: The ectopic adrenocorticotropin syndrome: Clinical features, diagnosis, management and long-term follow-up. J Clin Endocrinol Metab 91:371, 2006.

Lin RJ et al: Paraneoplastic thrombocytosis: The secrets of tumor self-promotion. Blood 124:184, 2014.

Pelosof LC, Gerber DE: Paraneoplastic syndromes: An approach to diagnosis and treatment. Mayo Clin Proc 85:838, 2010.

Workeneh BT et al: Hyponatremia in the cancer patient. Kidney Int 98:870, 2020.

94 Paraneoplastic Neurologic Syndromes and Autoimmune Encephalitis

Josep Dalmau, Myrna R. Rosenfeld, Francesc Graus

Paraneoplastic neurologic disorders (PNDs) are cancer-related syndromes that can affect any part of the nervous system **(Table 94-1)**. They are caused by mechanisms other than metastasis or by any of the complications of cancer such as coagulopathy, stroke, metabolic and nutritional conditions, infections, and side effects of cancer therapy. In 60% of patients, the neurologic symptoms precede the cancer diagnosis. Clinically disabling PNDs occur in 0.5–1% of all cancer patients, but they affect 2–3% of patients with neuroblastoma or small-cell lung cancer (SCLC) and 30–50% of patients with thymoma.

PATHOGENESIS

Most PNDs are mediated by immune responses triggered by neuronal proteins ectopically expressed by tumors (e.g., SCLC and other cancers) or as a result of altered immunologic responses caused by some types of tumors such as thymomas or lymphomas. In PNDs of the central nervous system (CNS), many antibody-associated immune responses have been identified **(Table 94-2)**. These antibodies react with neurons and the patient's tumor, and their detection in serum or cerebrospinal fluid (CSF) usually predicts the presence of cancer. When the antigens are intracellular, most syndromes are associated with extensive infiltrates of CD4+ and CD8+ T cells, microglial activation, gliosis, and variable neuronal loss. The infiltrating T cells are often in close contact with neurons undergoing degeneration, suggesting a primary pathogenic role. T-cell–mediated cytotoxicity may contribute directly to cell death in these PNDs and probably underlies the resistance of many of these conditions to therapy.

In contrast to the predominant role of cytotoxic T-cell mechanisms in PND associated with antibodies against intracellular antigens, those associated with antibodies to antigens expressed on the neuronal cell surface of the CNS or at the neuromuscular junction are mediated by direct antibody effects on the target antigens and are more responsive to immunotherapy **(Table 94-3, Fig. 94-1)**. These disorders occur with and without a cancer association and may affect children and young adults. Some disorders are triggered by viral encephalitis such as herpes simplex virus encephalitis or Japanese encephalitis, leading to autoimmune encephalitis.

In patients with cancer, the use of immune checkpoint inhibitors is associated in rare instances with immune-related adverse events accompanied by neuronal antibodies, which are indistinguishable from paraneoplastic neurologic syndromes.

Other PNDs are likely immune-mediated, although their antigens are unknown. The best example is opsoclonus-myoclonus syndrome associated with neuroblastoma or SCLC. For still other PNDs, the cause remains quite obscure. These include, among others, several neuropathies that occur in the terminal stages of cancer and a number of neuropathies associated with plasma cell dyscrasias or lymphoma without evidence of tumor infiltration or deposits of immunoglobulin, cryoglobulin, or amyloid.

TABLE 94-1 Paraneoplastic Syndromes of the Nervous System

CLASSIC SYNDROMES: USUALLY OCCUR WITH CANCER ASSOCIATION	NONCLASSIC SYNDROMES: MAY OCCUR WITH AND WITHOUT CANCER ASSOCIATION
Encephalomyelitis	Brainstem encephalitis
Limbic encephalitis	Stiff-person syndrome
Cerebellar degeneration (adults)	Progressive encephalomyelitis with rigidity and myoclonus
Opsoclonus-myoclonus	Necrotizing myelopathy
Subacute sensory neuronopathy	Motor neuron disease
Gastrointestinal paresis or pseudo-obstruction	Guillain-Barré syndrome
Dermatomyositis (adults)	Subacute and chronic mixed sensory-motor neuropathies
Lambert-Eaton myasthenic syndrome	Neuropathy associated with plasma cell dyscrasias and lymphoma
Cancer- or melanoma-associated retinopathy	Vasculitis of nerve
	Pure autonomic neuropathy
	Acute necrotizing myopathy
	Polymyositis
	Optic neuropathy
	BDUMP
	Peripheral nerve hyperexcitability (neuromyotonia)
	Myasthenia gravis

Abbreviation: BDUMP, bilateral diffuse uveal melanocytic proliferation.

TABLE 94-2 Antibodies to Intracellular Antigens, Syndromes, and Associated Cancers

ANTIBODY	ASSOCIATED NEUROLOGIC SYNDROME(S)	TUMORS
Anti-Hu (ANNA1)	Encephalomyelitis, subacute sensory neuronopathy	SCLC
Anti-Yo (PCA1)	Cerebellar degeneration	Ovary, breast
Anti-Ri (ANNA2)	Cerebellar degeneration, opsoclonus, brainstem encephalitis	Breast, gynecologic, SCLC
Anti-CRMP5 (CV2)	Encephalomyelitis, chorea, optic neuritis, uveitis, peripheral neuropathy	SCLC, thymoma, other
Anti-Ma proteins	Limbic, hypothalamic, brainstem encephalitis	Testicular (Ma2), other (Ma)
Anti-Kelch-like protein 11	Brainstem encephalitis, ataxia, hearing loss, diplopia	Seminoma, germ-cell tumor, teratoma
Anti-amphiphysin[a]	Stiff-person syndrome, encephalomyelitis	Breast, SCLC
Recoverin, bipolar cell antibodies, others[b]	Cancer-associated retinopathy (CAR), melanoma-associated retinopathy (MAR)	SCLC (CAR), melanoma (MAR)
Anti-GAD	Stiff-person, cerebellar syndromes, limbic encephalitis	Infrequent tumor association (thymoma and several cancers)

[a]Amphiphysin is likely exposed to the cell surface during synaptic vesicle endocytosis. [b]A variety of target antigens have been identified.

Abbreviations: CRMP, collapsin response-mediator protein; SCLC, small-cell lung cancer.

APPROACH TO THE PATIENT

Paraneoplastic Neurologic Disorders

Three key concepts are important for the diagnosis and management of PNDs. First, it is common for symptoms to appear before the presence of a tumor is known; second, the neurologic syndrome usually develops rapidly, producing severe deficits in a short period of time; and third, there is evidence that prompt tumor control improves the neurologic outcome. Therefore, the major concern of the physician is to recognize a disorder promptly as paraneoplastic and to identify and treat the tumor.

PND OF THE CENTRAL NERVOUS SYSTEM AND DORSAL ROOT GANGLIA

When symptoms involve brain, spinal cord, or dorsal root ganglia, the suspicion of PND is usually based on a combination of clinical, radiologic, and CSF findings. Presence of antineuronal antibodies

TABLE 94-3 Antibodies to Cell Surface or Synaptic Antigens, Syndromes, and Associated Tumors

ANTIBODY	NEUROLOGIC SYNDROME	TUMOR TYPE WHEN ASSOCIATED
Anti-NMDAR[a]	Anti-NMDAR encephalitis	Teratoma in young women (children and men rarely have tumors)
Anti-AMPAR[a]	Limbic encephalitis with relapses	SCLC, thymoma, breast, in ~70% of the patients
Anti-GluK2[a]	Encephalitis, cerebellar ataxia, cerebellitis	No tumor, rarely teratoma
Anti-$GABA_AR$[a]	Encephalitis with prominent seizures and status epilepticus	Thymoma in ~30% of the patients
Anti-$GABA_BR$[b]	Limbic encephalitis with early and prominent seizures	SCLC in ~50% of the patients
Glycine receptor[a]	PERM, stiff-person syndrome	Rarely, thymoma, lung, Hodgkin's
Anti-mGluR5[a]	Autoimmune encephalitis without distinctive features	Hodgkin's lymphoma, or no tumor
Anti-dopamine-2R[b]	Basal ganglia encephalitis	No cancer association
Anti-LGI1[a,c]	Limbic encephalitis, hyponatremia, faciobrachial dystonic seizures	Rarely thymoma
Anti-Caspr2[a,c]	Limbic encephalitis, ataxia, peripheral nerve hyperexcitability, neuropathy, Morvan's syndrome	~20% thymoma. In cases of Morvan syndrome: ~40% thymoma
Anti-DPPX[a]	Agitation, myoclonus, tremor, seizures, hyperekplexia, encephalomyelitis with rigidity	No cancer, but frequent diarrhea or cachexia suggesting paraneoplasia
Anti-neurexin 3α[b]	Autoimmune encephalitis without distinctive features	No cancer association
IgLON5[a]	NREM and REM sleep disorder, brainstem dysfunction, movement disorder, obstructive sleep apnea, stridor	No tumor association
Anti-mGluR1[a]	Cerebellar syndrome	Hodgkin's lymphoma, or no tumor
Anti-mGluR2	Cerebellar syndrome	Small-cell neuroendocrine tumor, rhabdomyosarcoma
Anti-Tr (DNER)	Cerebellar syndrome	Hodgkin's lymphoma, or no tumor
Anti-Sez6l2	Cerebellar ataxia, postural instability, frequent falls, dysarthria, extrapyramidal symptoms	No cancer association
Anti-MOG	ADEM, optic neuritis, myelitis, cortical encephalitis	No cancer association
Anti-AChR (muscle)[a]	Myasthenia gravis	Thymoma
Anti-AChR (neuronal)[a]	Autonomic ganglionopathy	SCLC
Anti-VGCC[a]	LEMS, cerebellar degeneration	SCLC

[a]A direct pathogenic role of these antibodies has been demonstrated in cultured neurons or animal models. [b]These antibodies are strongly suspected to be pathogenic. [c]Previously named voltage-gated potassium channel antibodies (VGKC); currently included under the term VGKC-complex proteins. Of note, the significance of antibodies to VGKC-complex proteins other than LGI1 and Caspr2 is uncertain (the antigens are unknown, and the response to immunotherapy is variable)

Abbreviations: AChR, acetylcholine receptor; ADEM, acute disseminated encephalomyelitis, AMPAR, α-amino-3-hydroxy-5-methylisoxazole-4-propionic acid receptor; Caspr2, contactin-associated protein-like 2; DNER, delta/notch-like epidermal growth factor-related receptor; DPPX, dipeptidyl-peptidase-like protein-6; $GABA_BR$, γ-aminobutyric acid B receptor; GAD, glutamic acid decarboxylase; GluK2, glutamate receptor ionotropic kainate 2; mGluR, metabotropic glutamate receptor; LEMS, Lambert-Eaton myasthenic syndrome; LGI1, leucine-rich glioma-inactivated 1; MOG, myelin oligodendrocyte glycoprotein; NMDAR, *N*-methyl-D-aspartate receptor; NREM, non-rapid eye movement; PERM, progressive encephalomyelitis with rigidity and myoclonus; REM, rapid eye movement; SCLC, small-cell lung cancer; Sez6l2, Seizure-related 6 homolog like 2; VGCC, voltage-gated calcium channel.

(Tables 94-2 and 94-3) may help in the diagnosis, but only 60–70% of PNDs of the CNS and <20% of those involving the peripheral nervous system have neuronal or neuromuscular junction antibodies that can be used as diagnostic tests.

Magnetic resonance imaging (MRI) and CSF studies are important to rule out neurologic complications due to the direct spread of cancer, particularly metastatic and leptomeningeal disease. In most PNDs, the MRI findings are nonspecific. Paraneoplastic limbic encephalitis is usually associated with characteristic MRI abnormalities in the mesial temporal lobes (see below), but similar findings can occur with other disorders (e.g., nonparaneoplastic autoimmune limbic encephalitis and human herpesvirus type 6 [HHV-6] encephalitis) (**Fig. 94-2*A***). The CSF profile of patients with PND of the CNS or dorsal root ganglia typically consists of mild to moderate pleocytosis (<200 mononuclear cells, predominantly lymphocytes), an increase in the protein concentration, and a variable presence of oligoclonal bands. There are no specific electrophysiologic tests that are diagnostic of PND. Moreover, a biopsy of the affected tissue is often difficult to obtain, and although useful to rule out other disorders (e.g., metastasis), the pathologic findings are not specific for PND.

PND OF NERVE AND MUSCLE

If symptoms involve peripheral nerve, neuromuscular junction, or muscle, the diagnosis of a specific PND is usually established on clinical, electrophysiologic, and pathologic grounds. The clinical history, accompanying symptoms (e.g., anorexia, weight loss), and type of syndrome dictate the studies and degree of effort needed to demonstrate a neoplasm. For example, the frequent association of Lambert-Eaton myasthenic syndrome (LEMS) with SCLC should lead to a chest and abdomen computed tomography (CT) or body positron emission tomography (PET) scan and, if negative, periodic tumor screening for at least 3 years after the neurologic diagnosis. In contrast, the weak association of polymyositis with cancer calls into question the need for repeated cancer screenings in this situation. Serum and urine immunofixation studies should be considered in patients with peripheral neuropathy of unknown cause; detection of a monoclonal gammopathy suggests the need for additional studies to uncover a B-cell or plasma-cell malignancy. In paraneoplastic neuropathies, diagnostically useful antineuronal antibodies are limited to CRMP5 (CV2) and Hu (ANNA1).

For any type of PND, if antineuronal antibodies are negative, the diagnosis relies on the demonstration of cancer and the exclusion of other cancer-related or independent neurologic disorders. Combined CT and PET scans often uncover tumors undetected by other tests. For germ cell tumors of the testis and teratomas of the ovary, ultrasound (testicular, transvaginal, or pelvic) and MRI or CT of the abdomen and pelvis may reveal tumors undetectable by PET.

SPECIFIC PARANEOPLASTIC NEUROLOGIC SYNDROMES

PARANEOPLASTIC ENCEPHALOMYELITIS AND FOCAL ENCEPHALITIS WITH ANTIBODIES AGAINST INTRACELLULAR NEURONAL PROTEINS

The term *encephalomyelitis* describes an inflammatory process with multifocal involvement of the nervous system, including brain, brainstem, cerebellum, and spinal cord. It is often associated with dorsal root ganglia and autonomic dysfunction. For any given patient, the clinical manifestations are determined by the areas predominantly involved, but pathologic studies almost always reveal abnormalities beyond the symptomatic regions. Several clinicopathologic syndromes may occur alone or in combination: (1) *cortical encephalitis*, which may present as "epilepsia partialis continua"; (2) *limbic encephalitis*, characterized by confusion, depression, agitation, anxiety, severe deficit forming new memories ("short-term memory deficit"), and temporal lobe or generalized seizures (the MRI usually shows unilateral or bilateral medial temporal lobe abnormalities, best seen with T2 and fluid-attenuated

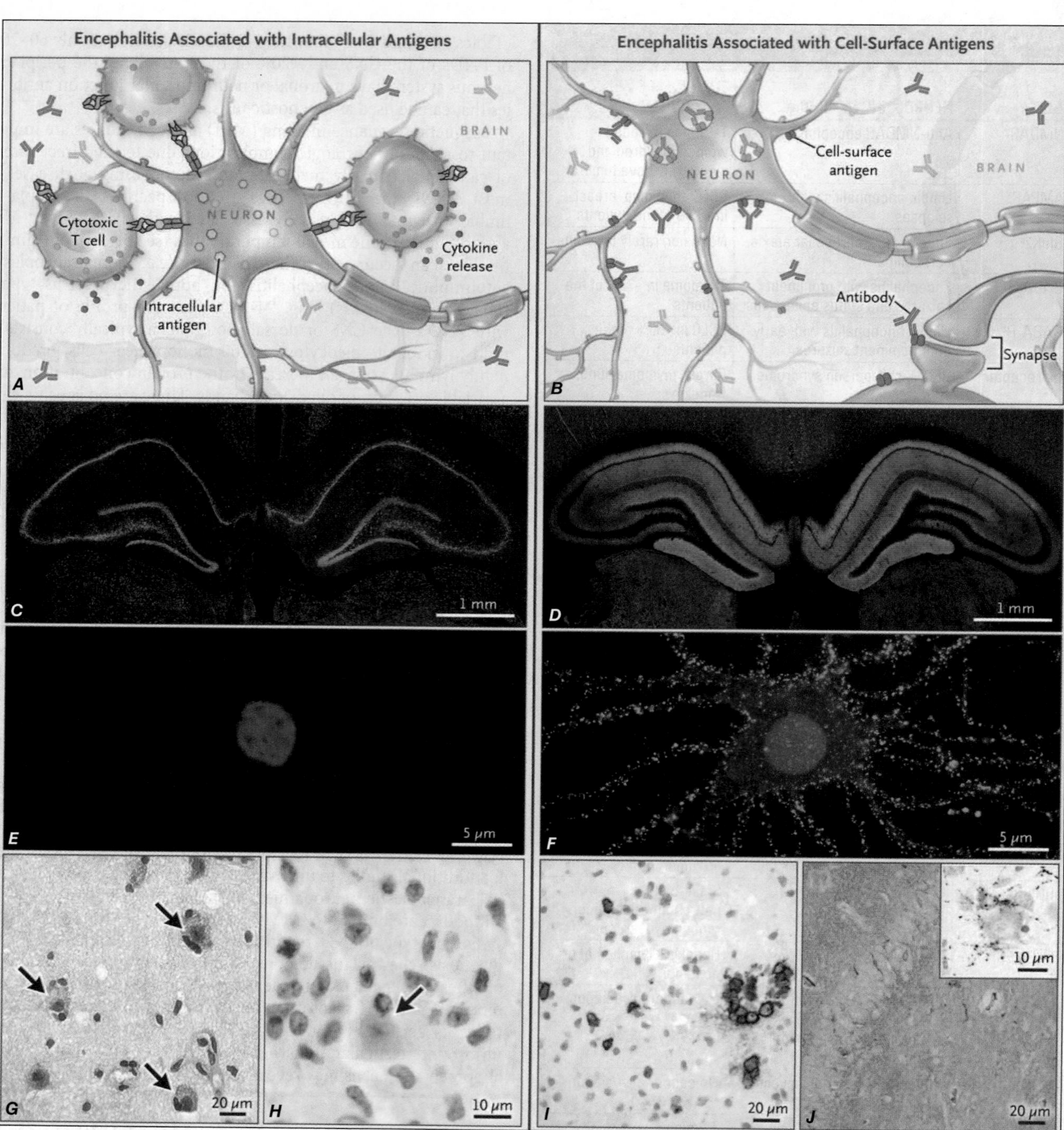

FIGURE 94-1 Antibody reactivity and pathologic findings in patients with antibodies against intracellular antigens compared with those of patients with antibodies against neuronal surface antigens. In encephalitis associated with antibodies against intracellular antigens, the antibodies cannot reach the intracellular epitopes and cytotoxic T-cell mechanisms are predominantly involved (***A***), whereas in encephalitis with antibodies against surface antigens, the antibodies have access to the epitopes and can potentially alter the structure and function of the antigen (***B***). The Hu antibodies (***C, E***) are shown here to exemplify the group of antibodies against intracellular antigens, and the NMDAR antibodies (***D, F***) are shown to exemplify the group of antibodies against cell-surface antigens. In rodent brain immunofluorescence with tissue permeabilized to allow entry of antibodies, the Hu antibodies produce a discrete pattern of cellular immunolabeling (***C***), whereas the NMDAR antibodies produce a pattern of neuropil-like immunolabeling (***D***). In contrast, with live cultured neurons, only the NMDAR antibodies have access to the target antigen showing intense immunolabeling (***F***), whereas the Hu antibodies cannot reach the intracellular antigen showing no immunolabeling (***E***). In autopsy studies, patients with encephalitis associated with antibodies to intracellular antigens (Hu or other) have extensive neuronal loss and inflammatory infiltrates (not shown); the T cells show direct contact with neurons (arrows in ***G***) likely contributing to neuronal degeneration via perforin and granzyme mechanisms (arrow in ***H***). In contrast, patients with antibodies against cell-surface antigens (NMDAR shown here, and probably applicable to other antigens) have moderate brain inflammatory infiltrates along with plasma cells (brown cells in ***I***), deposits of IgG (diffuse brown staining in ***J***), and microglial proliferation (inset in ***J***), without evidence of predominant T-cell–mediated neuronal loss (not shown). All human tissue sections (***G-J***) were obtained from hippocampus. *(From J Dalmau: Antibody mediated encephalitis. N Engl J Med 378:840, 2018. Copyright © 2018 Massachusetts Medical Society. Reprinted with permission.)*

inversion recovery [FLAIR] sequences); (3) *brainstem encephalitis,* resulting in eye movement disorders (nystagmus, opsoclonus, supranuclear or nuclear paresis), cranial nerve paresis, dysarthria, dysphagia, unsteady gait, and central autonomic dysfunction; (4) *cerebellar gait and limb ataxia*; (5) *myelitis,* which may cause lower or upper motor neuron symptoms, myoclonus, muscle rigidity, spasms, sensory deficits, and sphincter dysfunction; and (6) *autonomic dysfunction* as a result of involvement of the neuraxis at multiple levels, including hypothalamus, brainstem, and autonomic nerves (see Paraneoplastic Peripheral Neuropathies, below). Cardiac arrhythmias, postural

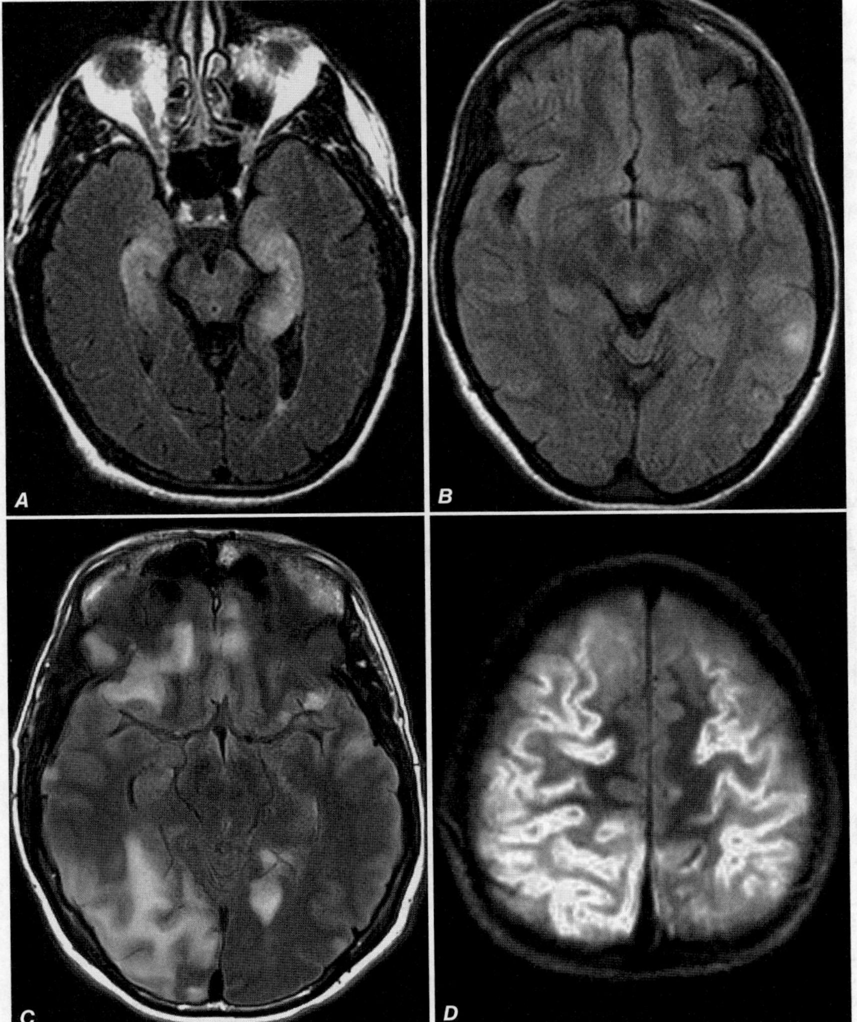

FIGURE 94-2 Brain MRI findings in paraneoplastic and autoimmune encephalitis. Representative MRI studies of patients with several types of autoimmune encephalitides. ***A.*** Limbic encephalitis (LE) may result from several different immune responses (Hu, Ma2, AMPAR, $GABA_BR$, LGI1, Caspr2) and typically manifests with unilateral or bilateral medial temporal lobe increased FLAIR signal. ***B.*** Anti-NMDAR encephalitis often occurs with normal MRI findings or mild FLAIR signal abnormalities. ***C.*** In contrast, anti-$GABA_AR$ encephalitis usually occurs with multiple cortical-subcortical increased FLAIR signal changes. ***D.*** Cortical encephalitis can occur in patients with myelin oligodendrocyte glycoprotein (MOG) antibodies, as shown in this T2-weighted MRI image from a 3-year-old boy who presented with extensive cortical abnormalities with mild enhancement (not shown here) suggesting cortical necrosis. *(Panels A-C from J Dalmau: Antibody mediated encephalitis. N Engl J Med 378:840, 2018. Copyright © 2018 Massachusetts Medical Society. Reprinted with permission. Panel D from T Armangue: Associations of paediatric demyelinating and encephalitic syndromes with myelin oligodendrocyte glycoprotein antibodies: A multicentre observational study. Lancet Neurol 19:234, 2020.)*

hypotension, and central hypoventilation can be the cause of death in patients with encephalomyelitis.

Paraneoplastic encephalomyelitis and focal encephalitis are usually associated with SCLC, but many other cancers have been implicated. Patients with SCLC and these syndromes usually have Hu antibodies in serum and CSF. CRMP5 antibodies occur less frequently; some of these patients may develop chorea, uveitis, or optic neuritis. Antibodies to Ma proteins are associated with limbic, hypothalamic, and brainstem encephalitis and occasionally with cerebellar symptoms; some patients develop hypersomnia, cataplexy, and severe hypokinesia. MRI abnormalities are frequent, including those described with limbic encephalitis and variable involvement of the hypothalamus, basal ganglia, or upper brainstem. Kelch-like protein 11 antibodies are predominantly associated with brainstem encephalitis and seminomas, germ cell tumors, and teratomas. Amphiphysin antibodies usually are associated with paraneoplastic stiff-person syndrome, but in some patients, they can occur with paraneoplastic encephalomyelitis or isolated myelitis. The oncologic associations of these antibodies are shown in Table 94-2.

Most types of paraneoplastic encephalitis and encephalomyelitis in which the antigens are intracellular respond poorly to treatment. Stabilization of symptoms or partial neurologic improvement may occur, particularly if there is a satisfactory response of the tumor to treatment. Controlled trials of therapy are lacking, but many reports and the opinion of experts suggest that therapies aimed to remove the antibodies against intracellular antigens, such as intravenous immunoglobulin (IVIg) or plasma exchange, usually fail. The main concern should be to treat the tumor and consider immunotherapies aimed at cytotoxic T-cell responses. Approximately 30% of patients with anti-Ma2-associated encephalitis respond to treatment of the tumor (usually a germ cell neoplasm of the testis) and immunotherapy.

■ ENCEPHALITIDES WITH ANTIBODIES TO CELL-SURFACE OR SYNAPTIC PROTEINS (TABLE 94-3)

These disorders are important for four reasons: (1) they can occur with and without tumor association; less frequently, they develop after a viral encephalitis (herpes simplex or Japanese encephalitis); (2) some syndromes predominate in young individuals and children; (3) despite the severity of the symptoms, patients usually respond to treatment of the tumor, if found, and immunotherapy (e.g., glucocorticoids, IVIg, plasma exchange, rituximab, or cyclophosphamide); and (4) for many of these disorders, the antibody pathogenicity has been demonstrated in models using cultures of neurons or passive transfer of patients' antibodies to animals (**Fig. 94-3**).

Encephalitis with N*-methyl-*D*-aspartate (NMDA) receptor antibodies* usually occurs in young women and children, but men and older patients of both sexes can be affected. The disorder has a characteristic pattern of symptom progression that often includes a prodrome resembling a viral process, followed in a few days by the onset of severe psychiatric symptoms, sleep dysfunction (usually insomnia), reduced verbal output, memory loss, seizures, decreased level of consciousness, abnormal movements (orofacial, limb, and trunk dyskinesias, dystonic postures), autonomic instability, and frequent hypoventilation. Monosymptomatic episodes, such as pure psychosis, occur in about 5% of patients. Clinical relapses occur in 12–24% of patients (12% during the first 2 years after initial presentation). Most patients have intrathecal synthesis of antibodies, likely by infiltrating plasma cells in brain and meninges (**Fig. 94-1*I***). In about 65% of patients, the brain MRI is normal; in the other 35%, it shows FLAIR abnormalities that can affect cortical and subcortical regions, usually mild and transient, and rarely the presence of contrast enhancement (**Fig. 94-2*B***). The syndrome may be misdiagnosed as a viral or idiopathic encephalitis, neuroleptic malignant syndrome, or encephalitis lethargica, and some patients are initially evaluated by psychiatrists with the suspicion of acute psychosis as the presentation of a primary psychiatric disease. The detection of an associated teratoma is dependent on age and gender: 46% of female patients 12 years or older have uni- or bilateral ovarian teratomas, whereas <7% of girls younger than 12 have a teratoma (**Fig. 94-4*A***). In young male patients, the detection of a tumor is rare. Patients older than 45 years are more frequently male; about 20% of these patients have tumors (e.g., cancer of the breast, ovary, or lung). Prompt diagnosis and treatment with immunotherapy (and tumor removal when it applies) improve outcome. Overall, about 85–90% of patients have substantial neurologic improvement or full recovery.

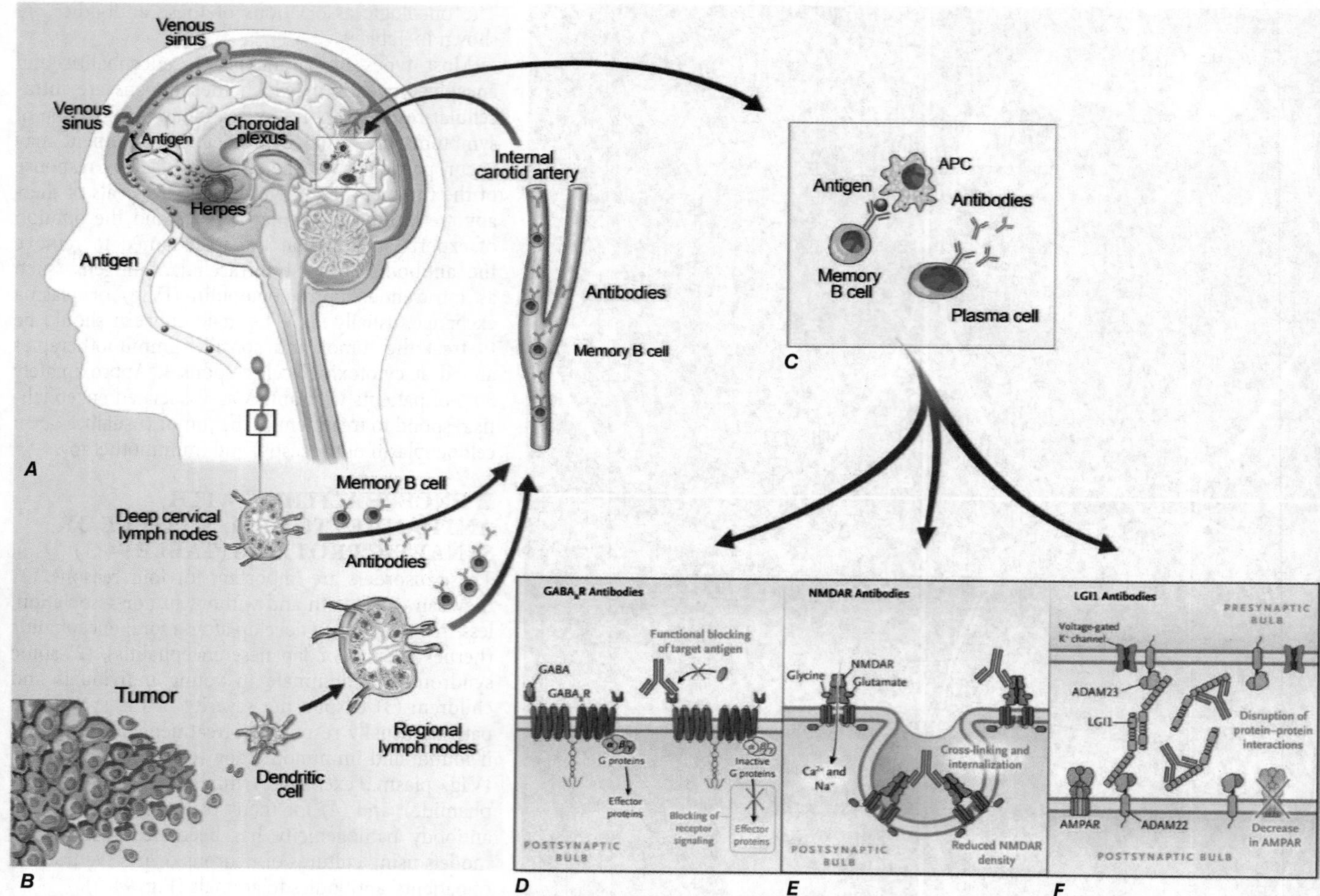

FIGURE 94-3 Proposed mechanisms of disease and functional interactions of autoantibodies with neuronal proteins. The graph shows a multistep process that results in antibody-mediated neuronal dysfunction; some of the steps have been demonstrated in reported studies, whereas others are based on proposed hypotheses. Two well-known triggers of autoimmune encephalitides are represented: herpes simplex encephalitis (***A***) and systemic tumors (***B***); the genetic susceptibility of some autoimmune encephalitides and unknown immunologic triggers are not depicted. It is postulated that antigens released by viral-induced neuronal destruction or apoptotic tumor cells are loaded into antigen-presenting cells (APCs; dendritic cells) and transported to regional lymph nodes. In the lymph nodes, naïve B cells exposed to the processed antigens, with cooperation of CD4+ T cells, become antigen-experienced and differentiate into antibody-producing plasma cells. After entering the brain, memory B cells undergo restimulation, antigen-driven affinity maturation, clonal expansion, and differentiation into antibody-producing plasma cells (***C***). The contribution of systemically produced antibodies to the pool of antibodies present in the brain is unclear and may depend on systemic antibody titers and integrity of the blood-brain barrier. Based on experimental models with cultured neurons, the presence of antibodies in the brain may lead to neuronal dysfunction by different mechanisms, including functional blocking of the target antigen (GABA$_B$R antibodies; ***D***), receptor crosslinking and internalization (NMDAR antibodies; ***E***), and disruption of protein-protein interaction, leading to downstream effects on receptors (LGI1 leading to a decrease of Kv1 potassium channels and AMPAR; ***F***). These mechanisms are influenced by the type of antibodies; for example, whereas IgG1 antibodies frequently crosslink and internalize the target antigen, IgG4 antibodies are less effective at crosslinking the target and more often alter protein-protein interactions. *(Panels D-F J Dalmau: Antibody mediated encephalitis. N Engl J Med 378:840, 2018. Copyright © 2018 Massachusetts Medical Society. Reprinted with permission.)*

Deficits of attention, memory, and executive functions may recover slowly over many months, sometimes a few years.

Approximately 25% of patients with herpes simplex encephalitis develop a form of autoimmune encephalitis that usually is associated with abnormal movements (choreoathetosis after herpes simplex encephalitis) in children and with cognitive and psychiatric symptoms in adults. This disorder develops a few weeks after the viral infection has resolved, is associated with new synthesis of antibodies against the NMDA receptor and other neuronal cell surface proteins, and is usually less responsive to immunotherapy than anti-NMDA receptor encephalitis (idiopathic or teratoma-associated).

Encephalitis with α-amino-3-hydroxy-5-methylisoxazole-4-propionic acid (AMPA) receptor antibodies affects middle-aged women, who develop acute limbic dysfunction or, less frequently, prominent psychiatric symptoms; 70% of patients have an underlying tumor in the lung, breast, or thymus (**Fig. 94-4*B***). In about 50% of cases, the brain MRI shows typical features of limbic encephalitis (similar to Fig. 94-2*A*). Neurologic relapses may occur; these also respond to immunotherapy and are not necessarily associated with tumor recurrence.

Encephalitis with GluK2 antibodies can affect children and adults and is associated with rapidly progressive encephalopathy with cerebellar ataxia or cerebellitis. Symptoms of encephalopathy may include impairment of memory and level of consciousness and motor alterations such as dyskinesias, choreoathetosis, bradykinesia, and spastic paraparesis. Some patients develop intracranial hypertension. In one patient, the symptoms were associated with teratoma.

Encephalitis with γ-aminobutyric acid type A (GABA$_A$) receptor antibodies may affect children and adults and is associated with prominent seizures and status epilepticus often requiring a pharmacologically induced coma. In approximately 80% of patients, the brain MRI shows multifocal, asynchronous, cortical-subcortical T2/FLAIR abnormalities predominantly involving temporal and frontal lobes, but also basal ganglia and other regions (**Fig. 94-2*C***). Most patients do not have an underlying tumor, but some, usually of Japanese ethnicity, may have thymoma.

Encephalitis with GABA$_B$ receptor antibodies is usually associated with limbic encephalitis and seizures. In >50% of cases, the MRI shows increased medial temporal lobe FLAIR changes characteristic of limbic encephalitis (similar to Fig. 94-2*A*). In rare instances, patients

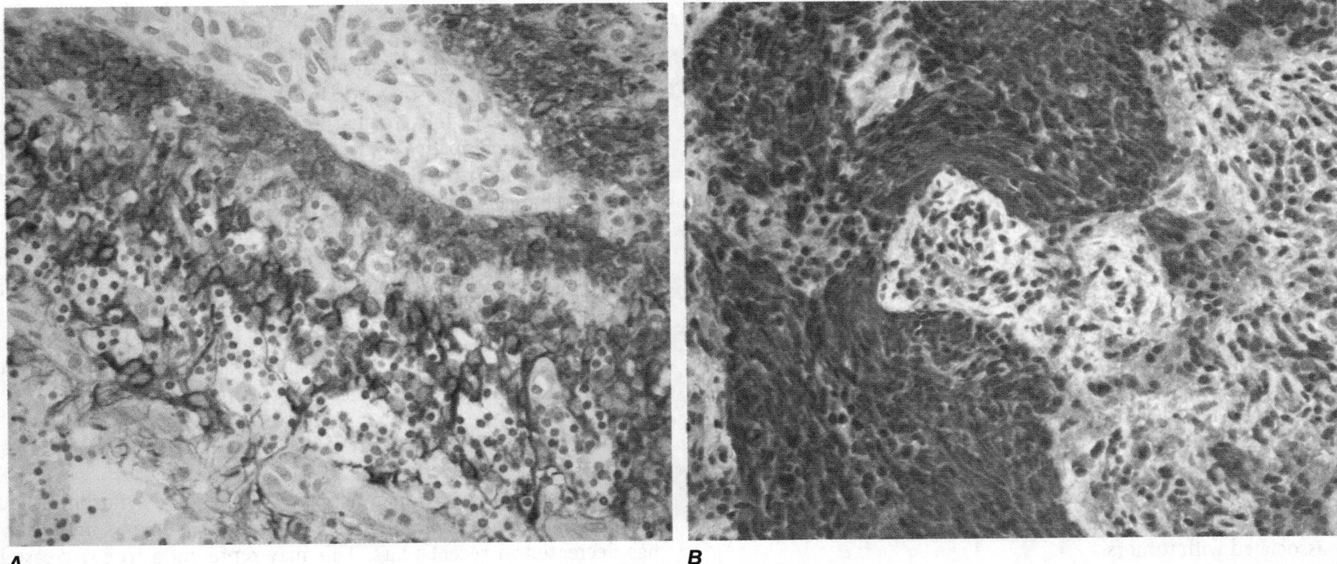

FIGURE 94-4 Immunopathological studies in tumors of patients with autoimmune encephalitis. ***A.*** Neurons and neuronal processes (brown cells; stained with MAP2) in the teratoma of a patient with anti-NMDA receptor encephalitis; these neurons express NMDA receptors (not shown). ***B.*** Lung cancer from a patient with anti–α-amino-3-hydroxy-5-methylisoxazole-4-propionic acid (AMPA) receptor encephalitis showing expression of AMPA receptors by the neoplastic cells (brown cells). *(Panel B from M Lai et al: AMPA receptor antibodies in limbic encephalitis alter synaptic receptor location. Ann Neurol 65:424, 2009.)*

develop cerebellar symptoms and opsoclonus. Fifty percent of patients have SCLC or a neuroendocrine tumor of the lung. Patients may have additional antibodies to glutamic acid decarboxylase (GAD), which are of unclear significance. Other antibodies to nonneuronal proteins are often found in these patients as well as in patients with AMPA receptor antibodies, indicating a general tendency to autoimmunity.

Encephalitis with glycine receptor (GlyR) antibodies usually manifests with a syndrome characterized by progressive encephalomyelitis with rigidity and myoclonus (PERM) or stiff-person spectrum of symptoms. The disease usually occurs in adults and rarely in children. About 20% of adult patients have a concurrent underlying tumor (thymoma, B-cell lymphoma, breast or lung cancer) or past history of cancer (thymoma, breast, Hodgkin lymphoma, melanoma).

Encephalitis with metabotropic glutamate receptor 5 (mGluR5) antibodies is characterized by nonspecific clinical features of encephalitis (confusion, agitation, memory loss, delusions, paranoid ideation, hallucinations, psychosis, or seizures) without distinctive MRI changes and frequent association with Hodgkin's lymphoma (Ophelia syndrome). The encephalitis is highly responsive to immunotherapy and treatment of the tumor.

Encephalitis with antibodies against dopamine-2 receptor has been reported in children with basal ganglia encephalitis manifesting with abnormal movements (coarse tremor, parkinsonism, chorea, oculogyric crises) along with psychiatric features, lethargy, drowsiness, brainstem dysfunction, or ataxia. The disorder is extremely rare and is not associated with cancer.

Encephalitis with leucine-rich glioma-inactivated 1 (LGI1) antibodies predominates in patients older than 50 years (65% male) and frequently presents with short-term memory loss and seizures (limbic encephalopathy), along with hyponatremia and sleep dysfunction. The MRI often shows increased FLAIR signal in one or both medial temporal lobes. In about 40% of patients, these symptoms are preceded by faciobrachial dystonic seizures, which consist of sudden, short-lasting, mainly distal muscle contractions involving the arm, face, or leg. These are unilateral but can independently affect both sides and occur multiple times during the day or night. About 15% of patients present with rapidly progressive cognitive decline, resembling a rapidly progressive dementia. Less than 5% of patients have thymoma. An association with the human leukocyte antigen (HLA) haplotypes DRB1*07:01, DQB1*02:02, DQA1*02:01, and DRB4 has been identified in nonparaneoplastic cases. All symptoms, including faciobrachial dystonic seizures, respond to immunotherapy, although about two-thirds of patients are left with memory or cognitive deficits.

Encephalitis with contactin-associated protein-like 2 (Caspr2) antibodies predominates in patients older than 50 years and is associated with a form of encephalitis with three or more of the following core symptoms: encephalopathy, cerebellar symptoms, peripheral nervous system hyperexcitability, dysautonomia, insomnia, neuropathic pain, and weight loss. Patients with Morvan's syndrome, which includes clinical features of encephalitis (confusion, hallucinations, prominent sleep dysfunction, or "agrypnia excitata"), autonomic alterations, and peripheral nerve hyperexcitability or neuromyotonia, usually have Caspr2 antibodies. About 20% of patients with Caspr2 antibody–associated syndromes have thymoma; this percentage is higher (~40%) in patients with Morvan's syndrome. An association of Caspr2 antibody–associated syndromes with HLA DRB1*11.01 has been reported.

Encephalitis with dipeptidyl-peptidase-like protein-6 (DPPX) antibodies is usually preceded or develops concurrently with diarrhea, other gastrointestinal symptoms, and substantial loss of weight that often suggest the presence of a gastrointestinal disease. Neurologic symptoms include agitation, hallucinations, paranoid delusions, and features of CNS hyperexcitability such as tremor, myoclonus, nystagmus, seizures, or hyperekplexia. Some patients develop a clinical picture similar to progressive encephalomyelitis with rigidity and myoclonus. The few patients reported with an associated tumor all had B-cell neoplasms.

Encephalitis with antibodies against neurexin 3 alpha does not have distinctive clinical features; the experience is limited, and the disorder does not appear to be associated with cancer.

Anti-IgLON5 disease is a chronic or subacute encephalopathy that characteristically is associated with rapid eye movement (REM) and non-REM (NREM) parasomnia that may be preceded or accompanied by bulbar symptoms, gait abnormalities, movement disorders (chorea, distal myoclonus, tremor, dystonia, or spasms), oculomotor dysfunction, and, in less than half of cases, cognitive decline. The median age of the patients is in the early 60s, and men and women are equally affected. The sleep disorder is characterized by abnormal sleep initiation with undifferentiated NREM sleep associated with frequent vocalizations and quasi-purposeful movements. Examination of the CSF and MRI is unrevealing or demonstrates minor changes of unclear clinical relevance. It is not associated with cancer but shows a strong association with HLA-DRB1*10:01 and HLA-DQB1*05:01. The response to immunotherapy is poor. Neuropathologic studies often show a neuronal tauopathy predominantly involving the hypothalamus and tegmentum of the brainstem.

With the exception of patients with anti-IgLON5 disease, who rarely respond to treatment, most patients with autoimmune or paraneoplastic encephalopathies associated with antibodies against cell-surface or synaptic proteins respond to immunotherapy and treatment of the tumor (if appropriate). Although there are no specific standardized treatment protocols, the most frequent approach consists of progressive escalation of immunotherapy using first a combination of glucocorticoids, IVIg, and plasma exchange, and then, if there is no response, rituximab or cyclophosphamide.

Encephalitis with myelin oligodendrocyte glycoprotein (MOG) antibodies can present with a clinical picture suggestive of autoimmune encephalitis related to neuronal antibodies. Most patients with MOG antibody–associated syndromes are children and young adults who present with optic neuritis, myelitis, or acute disseminated encephalomyelitis (ADEM). About 85% of patients with these syndromes respond to immunotherapy, although relapses occur in about 30% of cases. Besides these syndromes, there is a small group of adults and children that present with unilateral or bilateral cortical encephalitis, and their response to treatment is variable. In children, two phenotypes of poor prognosis include ADEM-like relapses progressing to leukodystrophy-like features and extensive cortical encephalitis evolving to atrophy (**Fig. 94-2*D***). In general, MOG antibody syndromes are not associated with tumors.

PARANEOPLASTIC CEREBELLAR DEGENERATION

This disorder is often preceded by a prodrome that may include dizziness, oscillopsia, blurry or double vision, nausea, and vomiting. A few days or weeks later, patients develop dysarthria, gait and limb ataxia, and variable dysphagia. The examination usually shows downbeating nystagmus and, rarely, opsoclonus. Brainstem dysfunction, upgoing toes, or a mild neuropathy may occur. Early in the course, MRI studies are usually normal; later, the MRI reveals cerebellar atrophy. The disorder results from extensive degeneration of Purkinje cells, with variable involvement of other cerebellar cortical neurons, deep cerebellar nuclei, and spinocerebellar tracts. The tumors more frequently involved are SCLC, cancer of the breast and ovary, and Hodgkin's lymphoma.

Anti-Yo (PCA1) antibodies in patients with breast or gynecologic cancers typically are associated with prominent or pure cerebellar degeneration. A variable degree of cerebellar dysfunction can be associated with virtually any of the antibodies and PND of the CNS shown in Table 94-2. A number of single case reports have described neurologic improvement after tumor removal, plasma exchange, IVIg, cyclophosphamide, rituximab, or glucocorticoids. However, most patients with paraneoplastic cerebellar degeneration and any of the antibodies shown in Table 94-2 do not improve with treatment.

A cerebellar syndrome can also occur with antibodies against cell-surface or synaptic proteins, including P/Q-type voltage-gated calcium channels (VGCC), Tr (DNER), mGluR2, or Sez6l2 (Table 94-3). The frequency and type of tumor association vary with the type of antibody. The cerebellar syndrome of patients with mGluR1 antibodies is highly responsive to treatment of the tumor and immunotherapy, whereas the syndrome of patients with Tr or VGCC antibodies is less treatment responsive. The experience with mGluR2 and Sez6l2 is limited to a few patients, but mGluR2 antibody–associated cerebellar symptoms seem to be highly responsive to treatment. Patients with GluK2 antibodies can present with cerebellitis and posterior fossa edema with compression of the 4th ventricle; the syndrome is potentially treatable with immunotherapy.

PARANEOPLASTIC OPSOCLONUS-MYOCLONUS SYNDROME

Opsoclonus is a disorder of eye movement characterized by involuntary, chaotic saccades that occur in all directions of gaze; it is frequently associated with myoclonus and ataxia. Opsoclonus-myoclonus may be cancer-related or idiopathic. When the cause is paraneoplastic, the tumors involved are usually cancer of the lung and breast in adults, neuroblastoma in children, and ovarian teratoma in adolescents and young women. The pathologic substrate of opsoclonus-myoclonus is unclear, but studies suggest that disinhibition of the fastigial nucleus of the cerebellum is involved. Most patients do not have antineuronal antibodies. A small subset of patients with ataxia, opsoclonus, and other eye-movement disorders develop Ri antibodies; these patients may also develop muscle rigidity, laryngeal spasms, and autonomic dysfunction. The tumors most frequently involved in anti-Ri-associated syndromes are breast, ovarian, and lung cancers. If the tumor is not successfully treated, the syndrome in adults often progresses to encephalopathy, coma, and death. In addition to treating the tumor, symptoms may respond to immunotherapy (glucocorticoids, plasma exchange, and/or IVIg).

At least 50% of children with opsoclonus-myoclonus have an underlying neuroblastoma. Hypotonia, ataxia, behavioral changes, and irritability are frequent accompanying symptoms. Neurologic symptoms often improve with treatment of the tumor and glucocorticoids, adrenocorticotropic hormone (ACTH), plasma exchange, IVIg, rituximab, or cyclophosphamide. Many patients are left with psychomotor retardation and behavioral and sleep problems.

PARANEOPLASTIC SYNDROMES OF THE SPINAL CORD

The number of reports of paraneoplastic spinal cord syndromes, such as *subacute motor neuronopathy* and *acute necrotizing myelopathy*, has decreased in recent years. This may represent a true decrease in incidence, due to improved and prompt oncologic interventions, or the identification of nonparaneoplastic etiologies. Some patients with cancer or lymphoma develop *upper* or *lower motor neuron dysfunction* or both, resembling amyotrophic lateral sclerosis. It is unclear whether these disorders have a paraneoplastic etiology or simply coincide with the presence of cancer.

Paraneoplastic myelitis may present with upper or lower motor neuron symptoms, segmental myoclonus, sensory deficits, sphincter dysfunction, and neurogenic pruritus and can be the first manifestation of encephalomyelitis. The spine MRI usually shows longitudinally extensive, symmetric tract or gray matter abnormalities in the spinal cord. It is mainly associated with breast and lung carcinomas and with CRMP5 or amphiphysin antibodies. The prognosis is poor. *Neuromyelitis optica (NMO) with aquaporin 4 antibodies* may occur in rare instances as a paraneoplastic manifestation of a cancer. NMO is discussed in detail in **Chap. 445**.

PARANEOPLASTIC STIFF-PERSON SYNDROME

This disorder is characterized by progressive muscle rigidity, stiffness, and painful spasms triggered by auditory, sensory, or emotional stimuli. Rigidity mainly involves the lower trunk and legs, but it can affect the upper extremities and neck. Sometimes, only one extremity is affected (*stiff-limb syndrome*). Symptoms improve with sleep and general anesthetics. Electrophysiologic studies demonstrate continuous motor unit activity. The associated antibodies target proteins (GAD, amphiphysin) involved in the function of inhibitory synapses using γ-aminobutyric acid (GABA) or glycine as neurotransmitters. The presence of amphiphysin antibodies usually indicates a paraneoplastic etiology related to SCLC and breast cancer. By contrast, GAD antibodies may occur in some cancer patients but are much more frequently present in the nonparaneoplastic disorder. GlyR antibodies may occur in some patients with stiff-person syndrome; these antibodies are more frequently detectable in patients with PERM (**Fig. 94-5**).

Optimal treatment of stiff-person syndrome requires therapy of the underlying tumor, glucocorticoids, and symptomatic use of drugs that enhance GABA-ergic transmission (diazepam, baclofen, sodium valproate, tiagabine, vigabatrin). IVIg and plasma exchange are transiently effective in some patients, and there are reports of responses to rituximab in patients who did not respond to other treatments.

PARANEOPLASTIC SENSORY NEURONOPATHY OR DORSAL ROOT GANGLIONOPATHY

This syndrome is characterized by sensory deficits that may be symmetric or asymmetric, painful dysesthesias, radicular pain, and decreased or absent reflexes. All modalities of sensation and any part of the body including face and trunk can be involved. Special senses such as taste and hearing can also be affected. Electrophysiologic studies show decreased or absent sensory nerve potentials with normal or

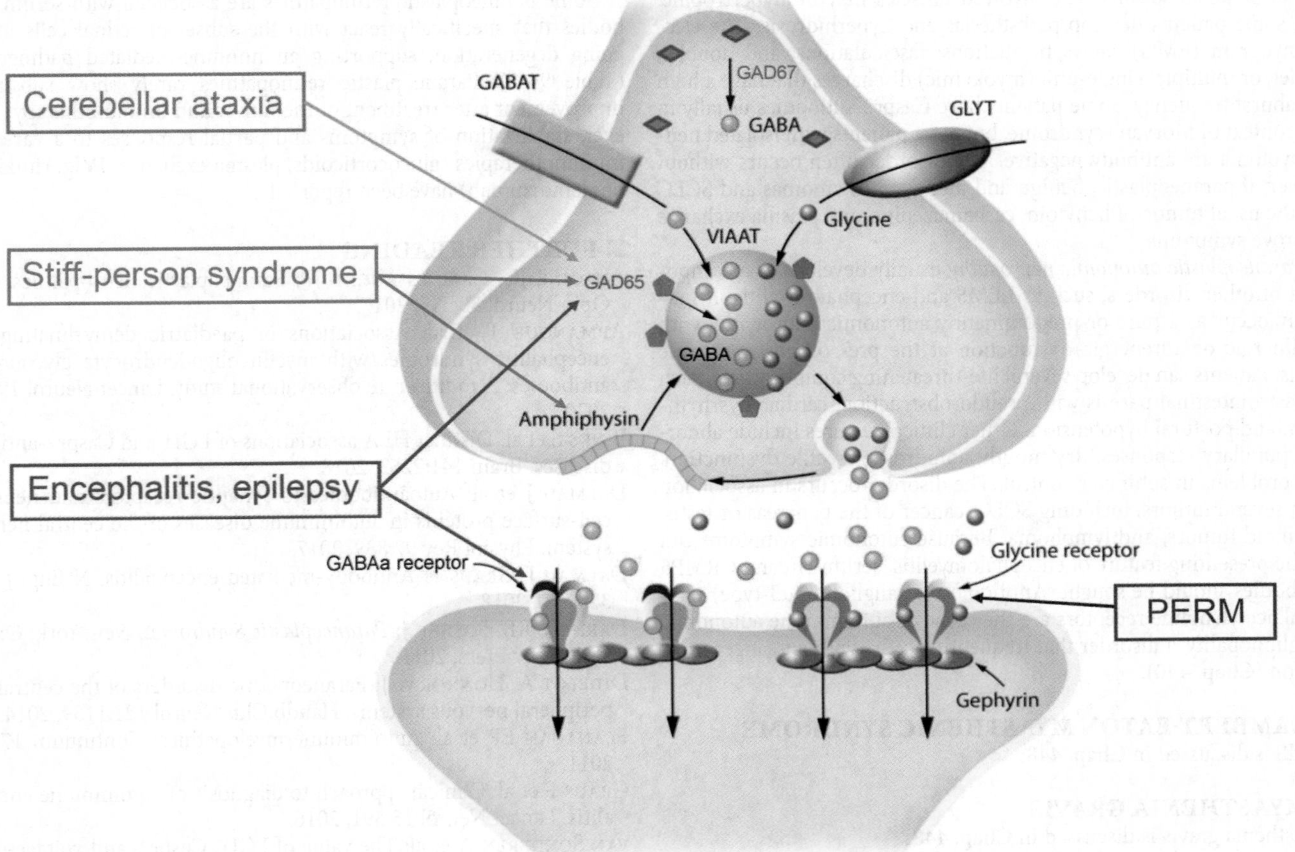

FIGURE 94-5 Schematic representation of an inhibitory synapse showing the main autoimmune targets (GAD, amphiphysin, GABA receptor, and glycine receptor) and the corresponding neurologic disorders. GAD antibodies predominantly occur in stiff-person syndrome (SPS), cerebellar ataxia, and epilepsy, sometimes in the setting of encephalitis. Amphiphysin antibodies are markers of paraneoplastic SPS and breast cancer, GlyR antibodies often associate with progressive encephalomyelitis with rigidity and myoclonus (PERM), and $GABA_A$ receptor antibodies occur in a form of autoimmune encephalitis that is frequently associated with refractory seizures and status epilepticus. *(Modified from F Graus et al: Nat Rev Neurol 16:353, 2020.)*

near-normal motor conduction velocities. Symptoms result from an inflammatory, likely immune-mediated, process that targets the dorsal root ganglia, causing neuronal loss and secondary degeneration of the posterior columns of the spinal cord. The dorsal and, less frequently, the anterior nerve roots and peripheral nerves may also be involved. This disorder often precedes or is associated with encephalomyelitis and autonomic dysfunction and has the same immunologic and oncologic associations (Hu antibodies, SCLC).

As with anti-Hu-associated encephalomyelitis, the therapeutic approach focuses on prompt treatment of the tumor and cytotoxic T-cell–mediated mechanisms. Glucocorticoids occasionally produce clinical stabilization or improvement. The benefit of IVIg and plasma exchange is not proven.

PARANEOPLASTIC PERIPHERAL NEUROPATHIES

These disorders may develop any time during the course of the neoplastic disease. Neuropathies occurring at late stages of cancer or lymphoma usually cause mild to moderate sensorimotor deficits due to axonal degeneration of unclear etiology. These neuropathies are often masked by concurrent neurotoxicity from chemotherapy and other cancer therapies. In contrast, the neuropathies that develop in the early stages of cancer frequently show a rapid progression, sometimes with a relapsing and remitting course, and evidence of inflammatory infiltrates and axonal loss or demyelination. If demyelinating features predominate **(Chaps. 446** and **447)**, IVIg, plasma exchange, or glucocorticoids may improve symptoms. Occasionally, CRMP5 antibodies are present; detection of anti-Hu suggests concurrent dorsal root ganglionitis.

Guillain-Barré syndrome **(Chap. 447)** and *brachial plexitis* **(Chap. 446)** have occasionally been reported in patients with Hodgkin's lymphoma, but there is no clear evidence of a paraneoplastic association.

Diseases associated with monoclonal gammopathies such as multiple myeloma, osteosclerotic myeloma, cryoglobulinemia, amyloidosis, Waldenström's macroglobulinemia, or POEMS (polyneuropathy, organomegaly, endocrinopathy, M-protein spike, and skin manifestations) syndrome, among others, may cause neuropathy by a variety of mechanisms, including compression of roots and plexuses by metastasis to vertebral bodies and pelvis, by deposits of amyloid in peripheral nerves, or through a direct interaction of the abnormal immunoglobulin with peripheral nerve antigens. In other patients, the mechanisms underlying the neuropathy remain unknown and paraneoplastic immune-mediated mechanisms have not been ruled out. Neuropathies more often occur with IgM gammopathies followed by IgG and IgA. The phenotype of the neuropathy and likelihood of improvement with successful treatment of the gammopathy are dependent on the underlying hematologic disorder **(Chap. 447)**.

Vasculitis of the nerve and muscle causes a painful symmetric or asymmetric distal axonal sensorimotor neuropathy with variable proximal weakness. It predominantly affects elderly men and is associated with an elevated erythrocyte sedimentation rate and increased CSF protein concentration. SCLC and lymphoma are the primary tumors involved. Glucocorticoids and cyclophosphamide often result in neurologic improvement.

Peripheral nerve hyperexcitability (*neuromyotonia,* or *Isaacs' syndrome*) is characterized by spontaneous and continuous muscle fiber activity of peripheral nerve origin. Clinical features include cramps, muscle twitching (fasciculations or myokymia), stiffness, delayed muscle relaxation (pseudomyotonia), and spontaneous or evoked carpal or pedal spasms. The involved muscles may be hypertrophic, and some patients develop paresthesias and hyperhidrosis. The electromyogram (EMG) shows fibrillations; fasciculations; and doublet, triplet, or multiplet single-unit (myokymic) discharges that have a high intraburst frequency. Some patients have Caspr2 antibodies usually in the context of Morvan's syndrome, but most patients with isolated neuromyotonia are antibody negative. The disorder often occurs without cancer; if paraneoplastic, benign and malignant thymomas and SCLC are the usual tumors. Phenytoin, carbamazepine, and plasma exchange improve symptoms.

Paraneoplastic autonomic neuropathy usually develops as a component of other disorders, such as LEMS and encephalomyelitis. It may rarely occur as a pure or predominantly autonomic neuropathy with cholinergic or adrenergic dysfunction at the pre- or postganglionic levels. Patients can develop several life-threatening complications, such as gastrointestinal paresis with pseudo-obstruction, cardiac dysrhythmias, and postural hypotension. Other clinical features include abnormal pupillary responses, dry mouth, anhidrosis, erectile dysfunction, and problems in sphincter control. The disorder occurs in association with several tumors, including SCLC, cancer of the pancreas or testis, carcinoid tumors, and lymphoma. Because autonomic symptoms can be the presenting feature of encephalomyelitis, serum Hu and CRMP5 antibodies should be sought. Antibodies to ganglionic (α3-type) neuronal acetylcholine receptors are the cause of autoimmune autonomic ganglionopathy, a disorder that frequently occurs without cancer association (**Chap. 440**).

LAMBERT-EATON MYASTHENIC SYNDROME

LEMS is discussed in **Chap. 448**.

MYASTHENIA GRAVIS

Myasthenia gravis is discussed in **Chap. 448**.

POLYMYOSITIS-DERMATOMYOSITIS

Polymyositis and dermatomyositis are discussed in detail in **Chap. 365**.

IMMUNE-MEDIATED NECROTIZING MYOPATHY

Patients with this syndrome develop myalgias and rapid progression of weakness involving the extremities, neck, pharyngeal, respiratory, and sometimes cardiac muscles. Serum muscle enzymes are elevated, and muscle biopsy shows extensive necrosis with minimal or absent inflammation and sometimes deposits of complement. The disorder may occur without cancer association (sometimes as a result of statin exposure, connective tissue disease, or HIV) or with cancer association. Patients with antibodies against 3-hydroxy-3-methylglutaryl-coenzyme A reductase (HMGCR) and seronegative patients are more likely to have an underlying cancer than those with antibodies against signal recognition particle. No specific type of cancer has been found to be predominant. Successful treatment of the tumor and aggressive immunotherapy (steroids, IVIg, and steroid-sparing immunosuppressants) may lead to complete or substantial recovery. Immune-mediated necrotizing myopathy is discussed in **Chap. 365**.

PARANEOPLASTIC VISUAL SYNDROMES

This group of disorders involves the retina and, less frequently, the uvea and optic nerves. The term *cancer-associated retinopathy* is used to describe paraneoplastic cone and rod dysfunction characterized by photosensitivity, progressive loss of vision and color perception, central or ring scotomas, night blindness, and attenuation of photopic and scotopic responses in the electroretinogram (ERG). The most commonly associated tumor is SCLC. Melanoma-associated retinopathy affects patients with metastatic cutaneous melanoma. Patients develop acute onset of night blindness and shimmering, flickering, or pulsating photopsias that often progress to visual loss. The ERG shows reduced b-waves with normal dark adapted a-waves. Paraneoplastic optic neuritis and uveitis can develop in association with encephalomyelitis. Patients with paraneoplastic uveitis and optic neuritis may harbor CRMP5 antibodies.

Some paraneoplastic retinopathies are associated with serum antibodies that specifically react with the subset of retinal cells undergoing degeneration, supporting an immune-mediated pathogenesis (Table 94-2). Paraneoplastic retinopathies rarely show substantial improvement after treatment of the tumor and immunotherapy; however, stabilization of symptoms and partial responses to a variety of immunotherapies (glucocorticoids, plasma exchange, IVIg, rituximab, or alemtuzumab) have been reported.

FURTHER READING

Antoine JC, Camdessanché JP: Paraneoplastic neuropathies. Curr Opin Neurol 30:513, 2017.

Armangue T et al: Associations of paediatric demyelinating and encephalitic syndromes with myelin oligodendrocyte glycoprotein antibodies: A multicentre observational study. Lancet Neurol 19:234, 2020.

Binks S et al: Distinct HLA associations of LGI1 and Caspr2-antibody diseases. Brain 141:2263, 2018.

Dalmau J et al: Autoantibodies to synaptic receptors and neuronal cell-surface proteins in autoimmune diseases of the central nervous system. Physiol Rev 97:839, 2017.

Dalmau J, Graus F: Antibody-mediated encephalitis. N Engl J Med 378:840, 2018.

Darnell RB, Posner J: *Paraneoplastic Syndromes*. New York, Oxford University Press, 2011.

Didelot A, Honnorat J: Paraneoplastic disorders of the central and peripheral nervous systems. Handb Clin Neurol 121:1159, 2014.

Flanagan EP et al: Autoimmune myelopathies. Continuum 17:776, 2011.

Graus F et al: Clinical approach to diagnosis of autoimmune encephalitis. Lancet Neurol 15:391, 2016.

van Sonderen A et al: The value of LGI1, Caspr2, and voltage-gated potassium channel antibodies in encephalitis. Nat Rev Neurol 13:290, 2017.

95 Cancer Survivorship and the Long-Term Impact of Cancer and Its Treatment

Mark Roschewski, Dan L. Longo

The impact of cancer extends well past initial diagnosis. Patients are significantly affected by cancer and treatment-related toxicities often extending beyond the initial treatment period. Adult survivors of childhood, adolescent, and young adult cancer face special health consequences of cancer treatment related to premature physiologic aging and frailty. More than 40% of these patients will experience a severe, disabling, or life-threatening condition or die of a chronic condition. Long-term effects include toxicities that emerge during therapy and continue beyond treatment, while late effects include toxicities that may not emerge for months or years after treatment. Significant improvements in cancer treatments have enabled more people to survive once-deadly diseases, leading to more cancer survivors subjected to the potential long-term impact of cancer treatment (**Table 95-1** lists potential long-term and late effects of cancer therapy by organ system). The direct causality of emerging treatments may not be immediately evident, and pharmacovigilance remains critical after treatments first become approved.

TABLE 95-1 Organ Systems at Risk for Long-Term and Late Effects of Cancer Treatment

ORGAN SYSTEM	LONG-TERM EFFECTS	LATE EFFECTS
Cardiovascular	Congestive heart failure	Congestive heart failure
	Arrhythmias	Arrhythmias
	Pericardial disease	Coronary artery disease
	Myocarditis	Peripheral vascular disease
	Hypertension	Cardiac valvular disease
Pulmonary	Pneumonitis	Pulmonary fibrosis
		Radiation recall pneumonitis
Immunologic	Opportunistic infections	Second malignancies
	Autoimmune disease	Myelodysplasia
		Recurrent infections
		Autoimmune disease
Endocrine	Fractures	Gonadal dysfunction/infertility
	Hypopituitarism	Premature ovarian insufficiency
	Avascular necrosis	Sarcopenia
	Diabetes insipidus	Diabetes
		Osteoporosis
		Thyroid disorders
Neurologic	Peripheral sensorimotor neuropathy	Cognitive impairment
	Myelopathy	
	Hearing loss	
Gastrointestinal	Malabsorption	Chronic diarrhea
	Colitis	Small bowel obstruction
	Chronic liver disease	Gastrointestinal stricture
Genitourinary	Chronic renal failure	Hemorrhagic cystitis
		Ureteral stricture
Psychological	Anxiety	Mood disorders
	Depression	Posttraumatic stress disorder
		Sexual dysfunction
		Substance abuse disorders
		Financial hardship
		Psychosocial dysfunction

In the United States, the number of cancer survivors may increase from 17 million to nearly 26 million by the year 2040, and the number of patients who survive at least 5 years after initial diagnosis is expected to increase by 35% over the next decade. Improvements in cancer treatments for children and adolescents have led to modern 5-year survival rates of approximately 80% or greater. Despite the magnitude of the growing problem, the core issues related to cancer survivorship remain understudied and the research is often concentrated in highly prevalent cancers. Most studies are observational and descriptive with fewer studies focused on the prevention and treatment of complications. Cancer survivorship remains an area that is ripe for further discovery; a deeper understanding of the biological basis and/or the influence of genetics on host susceptibility and the long-term effects of cancer therapy is needed.

Our primary understanding of the long-term impact of cancer treatment originated from survivors of childhood malignancies who are often cured after treatment with a combination of chemotherapy, radiation, and surgery. Treatment paradigms for cancer continuously evolve, however, and newer treatments including targeted agents and immunotherapy have introduced unique long-term effects, particularly when these agents are administered indefinitely (**Table 95-2** lists the potential long-term effects of specific cancer treatments). Improvements in the tolerability of cancer therapy and in supportive care have allowed a greater number of patients with comorbid conditions and advanced age to receive treatment, which has increased the rate of chronic morbidity. Approximately 60% of current cancer survivors are older than age 65. Indeed, the cause-specific mortality following initial treatment of Hodgkin lymphoma includes nearly 40% of deaths attributed to nonlymphoma causes. Indeed, more patients diagnosed with Hodgkin lymphoma die from treatment-related late toxicity than from Hodgkin lymphoma. Individuals aged 60–74 have a disproportionate excess of deaths related to heart disease, lung disease, infections, and adverse effects of drugs. The complexities of cancer survivorship and the importance of longitudinal care of cancer patients are recognized as vital components to comprehensive cancer care, and model systems have been specifically developed for this purpose. Still, the primary goal of cancer therapy remains long-term disease control, and the treating physician must maintain proper perspective when considering these relative risks. The fear of long-term complications should not prevent the application of effective cancer treatment, particularly when delivered with curative intent. In a sense, managing long-term effects is a privilege only afforded those fortunate enough to overcome the initial threat to life represented by the cancer diagnosis.

CARDIOVASCULAR DYSFUNCTION

The excess risks of cardiovascular disease after anthracycline chemotherapy and radiation that involves the mediastinum are well characterized and include arrhythmias, cardiac ischemia, congestive heart failure (CHF), pericardial disease, myocarditis, and peripheral vascular disease. It is estimated that one in eight childhood cancer survivors will experience a life-threatening cardiovascular event within 30 years after initial exposure, and cardiovascular disease is the most common cause of noncancer death in this population. Newer targeted agents and immunotherapy have introduced additional cardiovascular risks that extend into older populations as well. A new discipline of cardio-oncology has been developed to better characterize individuals at high risk for treatment-related cardiac toxicities, develop surveillance strategies, and improve the management of long-term effects.

Radiation therapy that includes the heart can cause interstitial myocardial fibrosis, acute and chronic pericarditis, valvular disease, and accelerated premature atherosclerotic coronary artery disease. Repeated or high (>6000 cGy) radiation doses are associated with greater risk, as is concomitant cardiotoxic cancer chemotherapy exposure. Symptoms of acute pericarditis peak about 9 months after treatment and include dyspnea, chest pain, and fever. Chronic constrictive pericarditis may develop 5–10 years following radiation therapy. Cardiac valvular disease includes aortic insufficiency from fibrosis or papillary muscle dysfunction resulting in mitral regurgitation. Extensive radiation fields are associated with accelerated coronary artery disease and peripheral vascular disease and a markedly increased risk of fatal myocardial infarction or thromboembolic stroke. Three-dimensional conformal techniques and newer particles including proton beams may more precisely target the tumor and spare normal tissue, but these are not widely available and the degree to which they will decrease long-term cardiovascular effects is unknown. In recognition of the risks of radiation, careful planning procedures are performed before treatment designed to limit the field of radiation to the greatest extent possible.

The myocardial toxicity of anthracyclines is dose-dependent and is associated with the pathognomonic finding of myofibrillar dropout on endomyocardial biopsy. Anthracycline cardiotoxicity occurs through a root mechanism of chemical free radical damage. Fe^{3+}-doxorubicin complexes damage DNA, nuclear and cytoplasmic membranes, and mitochondria. These cardiotoxic effects may also be mediated by topoisomerase IIB. Approximately 5% of patients receiving >450–550 mg/m^2 total dose of doxorubicin will develop CHF, but it can also develop at substantially lower doses in some patients. Anthracycline-related CHF is often irreversible and carries a high mortality rate, making prevention crucial. Genome-wide association studies have identified multiple genetic polymorphisms associated with a higher risk of cardiotoxicity, but our ability to risk-stratify is limited. The risk of cardiac failure appears to be related to the route of administration, and regimens that use continuous infusion of doxorubicin or liposomally encapsulated doxorubicin are associated with less cardiotoxicity. Baseline assessment of cardiac function with multigated acquisition scan (MUGA) or

TABLE 95-2 Long-Term Effects of Cancer Treatment by Type of Therapy

THERAPY TYPE	LONG-TERM EFFECT
Radiation	Second malignancies
	Coronary artery disease
	Pericardial disease
	Peripheral vascular disease
	Cardiac valvular disease
	Neurocognitive impairment
	Hypopituitarism and infertility
	Hypothyroidism and reduced bone density
	Gastrointestinal stricture
	Hepatic venoocclusive disease
Chemotherapy and Hormonal Agents	
Anthrayclines, trastuzumab, cyclophosphamide	Congestive heart failure
Bleomycin, oxaliplatin, 5-fluorouracil	Pulmonary fibrosis
Nitrosoureas, methotrexate, fludarabine, brentuximab	Pneumonitis
Alkylating agents, anthracyclines, tamoxifen, bendamustine, platinum agents	Second malignancies/myelodysplasia
Bendamustine, alkylating agents, anthracyclines	Immune dysfunction and recurrent infections
Alkylating agents	Infertility
Cyclophosphamide, Ifosfamide	Hemorrhagic cystitis
Platinum agents	Renal tubular dysfunction
Vinca alkaloids, taxanes, platinum agents	Neuropathy
Cytarabine	Ataxia
Aromatase inhibitors	Vasomotor symptoms
Antiandrogens	Sexual dysfunction
Immunotherapy Agents	
Immune checkpoint inhibitors	Autoimmune conditions/autoimmune hepatitis
Immune checkpoint inhibitors	Pericarditis and fulminant myocarditis
CAR-T therapy	Congestive heart failure
CAR-T therapy	Arrhythmias
CAR-T therapy, bi-specific monoclonal antibodies, immune checkpoint inhibitors	Peripheral neuropathy
CAR-T therapy, bi-specific monoclonal antibodies	B-cell aplasia
Targeted Agents	
Immunomodulatory agents	Second cancers/leukemia
Proteasome inhibitors	Peripheral neuropathy
Anti-CD20 agents, immunomodulatory agents	Neutropenia
BTK inhibitors, ALK inhibitors	Atrial and ventricular arrhythmias
PI3K inhibitors, CDK inhibitors	Hepatitis, colitis
Gemtuzumab	Sinusoidal obstruction syndrome
EGFR inhibitors, anti-VEGF agents, BCR-ABL inhibtors, MEK inhibitors, proteasome inhibitors	Congestive heart failure
BCR-ABL inhibitors	Pleural effusions, pancreatitis
BCR-ABL inhibitors, PI3K inhibitors, BTK inhibitors, immunomodulatory agents, EGFR inhibitors	Chronic diarrhea
BCR-ABL inhibitors	Impaired growth and stature
Anti-VEGF agents, BCR-ABL inhibitors	Thyroid dysfunction
PI3K inhibitors, mTOR inhibitors, BRAF inhibitors	Hyperglycemia
FLT3 inhibitors, anti-VEGF agents, PI3K inhibitors	Systemic hypertension
Anti-VEGF agents, BCR-ABL inhibitors	Pulmonary hypertension

Abbreviation: CAR-T, chimeric antigen receptor T cell.

transthoracic echocardiograms is commonly performed, and a patient who develops symptoms suggestive of CHF should be tested immediately while therapy is held. Periodic surveillance testing during therapy is often done in asymptomatic patients with preexisting risk factors.

Trastuzumab is a monoclonal antibody targeting human epidermal growth factor receptor 2 (HER2) that is also associated with CHF. It is used in combination with chemotherapy as both adjuvant therapy and as treatment of metastatic breast cancer, and it is sometimes combined with anthracyclines, which is believed to result in additive or possibly synergistic toxicity. In contrast to anthracyclines, cardiotoxicity is not dose related, is usually reversible, is not associated with pathologic changes on cardiac myofibrils, and has a different biochemical mechanism inhibiting intrinsic cardiac repair mechanisms. Monitoring for cardiac toxicity is typically performed every three or four doses using functional cardiac testing, and treatment is interrupted when ejection fractions significantly decline from baseline. Other potentially cardiotoxic chemotherapy agents include phosphoramide mustards (cyclophosphamide) at high doses and ifosfamide.

Small-molecule inhibitors, including tyrosine kinase inhibitors, are novel classes of molecularly targeted anticancer agents that have become routinely applicable across a variety of malignancies. Although the overall tolerability of these drugs is often better than chemotherapy, they are frequently administered indefinitely, which introduces new notions of cumulative long-term effects. These agents also carry risks of cardiovascular toxicities including CHF, atrial and ventricular arrhythmias, prolongation of the QT interval, and pulmonary and systemic hypertension. New anticancer agents often become available for use on accelerated approvals before a full understanding of the long-term toxicity profile is known. Two illustrative examples of this are lapatinib and ponatinib, which both had their approvals updated with black box cardiovascular toxicity warnings a median of 4 years after initial drug approval. Other small-molecule inhibitors that have been associated with CHF include bosutinib, dasatinib, nilotinib, pazopanib, axitinib, trametinib, sunitinib, carfilzomib, and sorafenib. Systemic hypertension is commonly associated with agents targeting vascular endothelial growth factor or its receptors (e.g., bevacizumab, cabozantinib, lenvatinib, nintedanib), ponatinib (an Abl inhibitor), and trametinib (a MEK inhibitor), whereas dasatinib (an Abl inhibitor) has a well-documented association with pulmonary hypertension. Ibrutinib (a BTK inhibitor) has been associated with atrial fibrillation as well as ventricular arrythmias. As more of these small-molecule inhibitors become approved for use and their indications broaden, additional monitoring for long-term and late effects should be incorporated into the routine surveillance of oncologists, cardiologists, and primary care providers.

Immunotherapy agents have also emerged as effective anticancer therapies that have substantially improved clinical outcomes in a variety of cancers. Immune checkpoint inhibitors have been associated with a number of important cardiovascular toxicities including pericardial disease, vasculitis, and fulminant myocarditis. The mechanism of these toxicities is T cell mediated, and the toxicities often respond to early institution of glucocorticoids, but they can be severe or fatal if not recognized promptly. Combinations of multiple immune checkpoint inhibitors increase the risk of these immune-related toxicities, and no clear pattern of which patients are most susceptible has emerged. Chimeric antigen receptor T-cell (CAR-T) therapies are associated with cytokine release syndromes (CRS), which can be severe and associated with arrhythmias or decompensated heart failure. Interleukin 6 receptor blockers may decrease these risks, and supportive care guidelines recommend early institution of these agents in severe CRS.

The management of treatment-associated cardiovascular disease is essentially the same as for cardiac disease unrelated to cancer treatment. Discontinuation of the offending agent is the first step. Diuretics, fluid and sodium restriction, and antiarrhythmic agents are often useful for acute symptoms. Afterload reduction with angiotensin-converting enzyme inhibitors or β-adrenergic blockers may improve systolic function over time, and digitalis may improve symptoms. Routine screening for asymptomatic systolic dysfunction is currently recommended for survivors at high risk for cardiomyopathy including those with an anthracycline exposure ≥250 mg/m^2, ≥35 Gy of chest radiation, or combined therapy with both anthracyclines and radiation. Echocardiography is the recommended screening modality, and surveillance should begin no later than 2 years after exposure and should be repeated a minimum of every 5 years thereafter.

PULMONARY DYSFUNCTION

Radiation-induced lung injury presents in early phases as acute pneumonitis at 4 weeks following treatment, but it can evolve into pulmonary fibrosis in late phases. Risk factors for radiation pneumonitis include advanced age, smoking, poor performance status, preexisting compromised pulmonary function, and radiation volume and dose. It occurs most commonly in patients with lung cancer, mediastinal lymphoma, and breast cancer, and the incidence is decreasing due to advances in radiation delivery techniques. The dose "threshold" is thought to be in the range of 5–20 Gy. Hypoxemia and dyspnea on exertion are characteristic, and the severity of symptoms may be out of proportion to the lung volume irradiated. Fine, high-pitched "Velcro rales" may be an accompanying physical finding, and fever, cough, and pleuritic chest pain are common symptoms. The diffusion capacity of the lungs for carbon dioxide (DL_{CO}) is the most sensitive measure of pulmonary functional impairment, and ground-glass infiltrates often correspond with relatively sharp edges to the irradiated volume, although the pneumonitis may progress beyond the field and even occasionally involve the contralateral unirradiated lung. The mechanism of lung injury is a direct effect of radiation that leads to increased capillary permeability and pulmonary edema. Damage to type I and II pneumocytes leads to surfactant loss and the transudation of serum proteins into the alveoli. Cytokines including tumor necrosis factor α are released from the damaged lung cells and attract inflammatory cells to the alveoli and interstitial space. The late phases of injury are caused by reactive oxygen species that stimulate collagen production and lead to fibrosis but do not occur in all cases. Transforming growth factor β (TGF-β) is particularly important in stimulating collagen synthesis and may represent a therapeutic target to prevent pulmonary fibrosis.

Bleomycin generates activated free radical oxygen species and causes pneumonitis associated with a radiographic or interstitial ground-glass appearance diffusely throughout both lungs, often worse in the lower lobes. A nonproductive cough with or without fever may be an early sign. This toxicity is dose-related and dose-limiting. The DL_{CO} is a sensitive measure of toxicity and recovery, and a baseline value is generally obtained for future comparison before administering bleomycin therapy. Doses are reduced or stopped if the baseline DL_{CO} falls 25% or more. Additive or synergistic risk factors include age, prior lung disease, and concomitant use of other chemotherapy, lung irradiation, and high concentrations of inspired oxygen. Other chemotherapeutic agents notable for pulmonary toxicity include mitomycin, nitrosoureas, doxorubicin with radiation, gemcitabine combined with weekly docetaxel, methotrexate, and fludarabine. High-dose alkylating agents, cyclophosphamide, ifosfamide, and melphalan are frequently used in the hematopoietic stem cell transplant setting, often with whole-body radiation. This therapy may result in severe pulmonary fibrosis and/or pulmonary venoocclusive disease.

Radiation-induced lung injury and chemotherapy-induced pneumonitis are generally glucocorticoid responsive, except in the case of nitrosoureas. Prednisone 1 mg/kg is often used to control acute symptoms and prevent pulmonary dysfunction with a slow taper over 12 weeks. Prolonged glucocorticoid therapy requires gastrointestinal protection with proton pump inhibitors, management of hyperglycemia, heightened infection management, and prevention or treatment of steroid-induced osteoporosis. Antibiotics, bronchodilators, oxygen in only lowest necessary doses, and diuretics may all play an important role in management of pneumonitis, and consultation with a pulmonologist should be routinely undertaken. Relapses can occur after an initial response to glucocorticoids and may respond to agents such as azathioprine or cyclosporine. Amifostine is a free radical scavenger and radioprotective agent that reduces the rate of pneumonitis, but it is associated with severe nausea and hypotension that limit its use. No effective therapy exists for pulmonary fibrosis, and the treatment is primarily supportive with supplemental oxygen. Targeted anti-inflammatory agents are being tested to reduce the incidence of pulmonary fibrosis, but they remain experimental.

Pulmonary toxicity resulting from targeted anticancer agents including small-molecule inhibitors and immunotherapy agents is uncommon but can be potentially life-threatening and often lead to drug discontinuation. Noninfectious pneumonitis is associated with cough, dyspnea, and infiltrates on chest imaging and has been reported to be associated with sunitinib, sorafenib, epidermal growth factor receptor (EGFR) inhibitors (cetuximab, afatinib), crizotinib (ALK inhibitor), phosphoinositide 3-kinase (PI3K) inhibitors (idelalisib, copanlisib), and mammalian target of rapamycin (mTOR) inhibitors (everolimus, temsirolimus). The antibody-drug conjugate brentuximab vedotin may also cause severe pulmonary toxicity when used in combination with other chemotherapy agents, particularly bleomycin. The onset of drug-induced pneumonitis can be rapid, and prompt use of glucocorticoids is important once infectious causes are excluded. Severe pneumonitis is typically a reason to discontinue the offending drug permanently.

IMMUNE SYSTEM DYSFUNCTION

A significant risk of most anticancer treatment is hematologic toxicity with cumulative effects on the host immune system leading to a higher risk of second malignancies and impaired long-term immune health. Second malignancies in cancer survivors are a major cause of death, and survivors of childhood cancers have a twofold increased risk of solid tumors beyond the age of 40 years compared to the general population. The induction of second malignancies is governed by the complex interplay of age, sex, environmental exposures, genetic susceptibility, and specific cancer treatments. Often, the events that led to the primary cancer remain, and a risk of a second malignancy persists. Patients with a history of lung cancer remain at increased risk of other cancers that are associated with tobacco use including esophageal, head and neck, kidney, and bladder cancers. Patients with breast cancer are at increased risk of breast cancer in the opposite breast. Patients with Hodgkin lymphoma are at risk for other B-cell non-Hodgkin lymphomas. Genetic cancer syndromes (e.g., multiple endocrine neoplasia or Li-Fraumeni, Lynch's, Cowden's, and Gardner's syndromes) are examples of genetically based second malignancies of specific types. Cancer treatment itself does not appear to be responsible for the risk of these secondary malignancies. Genetic disorders that result in DNA repair deficiencies including ataxia-telangiectasia, Bloom's syndrome, and Fanconi's anemia greatly increase the lifetime risk of cancers as well as the risks associated with DNA-damaging agents. Importantly, the risk of treatment-related second malignancies is at least additive and often synergistic with combined chemotherapy and radiation therapy, and hence for such combined-therapy treatment approaches, it is important to establish the necessity of each component in the treatment program. These patients require indefinite surveillance and prophylactic surgery in some cases.

Patients receiving radiation have an increasing and lifelong risk of second malignancies that is 1–2% in the second decade following treatment but increases to >25% after 25 years. The risk of second malignancies from radiation is dose-dependent and often occurs within or near the treatment field. Common radiation-related solid tumors include central nervous system (CNS), breast, lung, thyroid, skin, and bone cancers and sarcomas, which are often aggressive and have a poor prognosis. An example of an organ-, age-, and sex-dependent radiation-induced secondary malignancy is breast cancer, in which the risk is small with radiation in women aged older than 30 years but increases about twentyfold over baseline in women aged younger than 30 years. A 25-year-old woman treated with mantle radiation for Hodgkin lymphoma has a 29% actuarial risk of developing breast cancer by age 55.

Chemotherapy is significantly associated with two fatal second malignancies: acute leukemia and myelodysplastic syndromes. Two types of secondary leukemia have been described; in patients treated with chronic alkylating agents (especially combined with radiation therapy), acute myeloid leukemia is associated with deletions in chromosome 5 or 7 and complex karyotypes and often is preceded by myelodysplasia. The lifetime risk is about 1–5%, is increased by radiation therapy, and increases with age. The incidence of these leukemias peaks at 5–8 years, with risk returning close to baseline at 10 years. The other type of acute myeloid leukemia is related to therapy with topoisomerase inhibitors, is associated with chromosome 11q23 translocations, has an incidence of <1%, generally occurs 1.5–3 years after treatment, and is rarely preceded by myelodysplasia. Both of these acute myeloid leukemias are largely refractory to treatment and have a high mortality. The development of myelodysplastic syndromes is increased following chemotherapy, and these cases are often associated with leukemic progression and a dismal prognosis. A fraction of the population develops clonal hematopoiesis not related to prior cancer treatment, and the percentage increases with age. In such patients, the hematopoietic stem cells carry mutations that are associated with myeloid malignancy despite normal blood counts. It is thought that the presence of these genetic lesions may predispose patients to develop myeloid malignancies, but evidence is greater that clonal hematopoiesis increases the risk of lymphoma and atherosclerotic heart disease.

Other cytotoxic agents are associated with long-term alterations in immunity beyond the initial treatment period and neutrophil recovery. Bendamustine has significant effects on both B-cell and T-cell subpopulations that can persist for years, and long-term studies of lymphoma patients treated with bendamustine-based regimens show higher rates of death from second malignancies compared to other chemotherapy regimens. Purine analogues like cladribine and pentostatin also produce long-term T-cell suppression. The risk of solid tumors is also increased after chemotherapy, and alkylating agents increase the risk of thyroid, lung, breast, and bladder cancers and sarcomas. Cyclophosphamide increases the risk of both sarcoma and breast cancer in a dose-dependent manner. Other chemotherapy agents, including procarbazine and platinum agents, have been associated with gastrointestinal malignancies. Treatment of breast cancer with tamoxifen for 5 years or longer is associated with a 1–2% risk of endometrial cancer. Surveillance is generally effective at finding these cancers at an early stage. The risk of mortality from tamoxifen-induced endometrial cancer is low compared to the benefit of tamoxifen as adjuvant therapy for breast cancer. Treatment of multiple myeloma with the immunomodulatory agent lenalidomide is associated with a significantly increased risk of second hematologic malignancies including lymphomas and leukemias. These risks are highest after prior use of the alkylating agent melphalan.

Given the high risk of second malignancies in cancer survivors, patients need indefinite surveillance. Guidelines for breast cancer surveillance in survivors exposed to chest radiation recommend that patients be screened with mammograms and/or breast MRI beginning at age 25 years or 8 years after treatment, whichever occurs later. Any organ in the treatment field is susceptible to developing a cancer; e.g., radiation to the chest may increase the risk of gastric or esophageal cancer. Patients exposed to abdominal or pelvic radiation should have annual colonoscopies starting at age 35 years or 10 years after exposure. For patients treated with neck radiation, no formal surveillance is recommended, but fine-needle aspiration should be performed on any palpable thyroid nodules and thyroid-stimulating hormone (TSH) levels should be monitored periodically.

Combination chemotherapy is also associated with impaired immune health and increases the risk of opportunistic infections, autoimmune complications, and impaired host protection from infections. Survivors of lymphoma have elevated risks of developing autoimmune hemolytic anemia, viral or fungal pneumonias, meningitis, or other infections, and these risks remain high decades after treatment. Agents or treatment regimens that result in significant T-cell depletion, including antithymocyte globulin or antibodies targeting cell surface proteins on T cells, increase the risk of Epstein-Barr virus–associated B-cell lymphoproliferative disorders. Discontinuing immunosuppressive therapy, if possible, is often associated with complete disease regression. Anti-CD20 monoclonal antibodies, CAR-T therapy, bi-specific monoclonal antibodies targeting both B cells and T cells, and immune checkpoint inhibitors have all been associated with long-term B-cell aplasia that often requires intravenous immunoglobulin replacement and persistent vigilance for recurrent sinopulmonary infections. Rituximab and immunomodulatory agents have both been associated with late-onset neutropenia that can occur months after exposure to the drug and often requires growth factor support. Given these risks of impaired immune system function, all cancer survivors should undergo annual influenza vaccination and should be considered for pneumococcal vaccination depending on age and immune health status.

REPRODUCTIVE AND ENDOCRINE DYSFUNCTION

Endocrine complications are prevalent in childhood cancer survivors. Nearly half of all survivors will have at least one hormonal disorder in their lifetime, and these most commonly present as late effects. Radiation to the head, neck, or pelvis is associated with the greatest risk of endocrine dysfunction. Testicles and ovaries in prepubertal patients are sensitive to radiation damage in a dose-related fashion;

spermatogenesis is affected by low doses of radiation, and complete azoospermia occurs at 600–700 cGy. Leydig cell dysfunction, in contrast, occurs at <2000 cGy, and hence, endocrine function is lost at much higher radiation doses than spermatogenesis. Erectile dysfunction occurs in up to 80% of men treated with external-beam radiation therapy for prostate cancer. Sildenafil may be useful in reversing erectile dysfunction. Ovarian function damage with radiation is age-related and occurs at doses of 150–500 cGy. Hormone replacement therapy is often contraindicated (as in estrogen receptor–positive breast cancer). Attention must be paid to maintenance of bone mass with calcium and vitamin D supplements and oral bisphosphonates, and bone mass should be monitored using bone density determinations. Paroxetine, clonidine, pregabalin, and other drugs may be useful in symptomatically controlling hot flashes. Long-term survivors of childhood cancer who have received cranial radiation may have altered leptin biology and growth hormone deficiency, leading to obesity and reduced strength, exercise tolerance, and bone density. Radiation therapy to the neck may lead to hypothyroidism, Graves' disease, thyroiditis, and thyroid malignancies. TSH is followed routinely in such patients to prevent hypothyroidism and to suppress persistently elevated levels of TSH, which may cause or drive thyroid cancer. Cranial radiation may also be associated with an array of endocrine abnormalities with disruption of normal pituitary-hypothalamic axis function, and a high index of suspicion needs to be maintained to identify and treat this toxicity. Efforts to eliminate unnecessary radiation such as prophylactic CNS irradiation may decrease some of the late endocrine effects. Patients who have received abdominal radiation should receive annual screens for obesity and diabetes mellitus with heigh and weight measurements along with a hemoglobin A_{1C} at least every 2 years.

Alkylating agents are the chemotherapy agents associated with the highest rates of male and female infertility, which is directly dependent on age, dose, and duration of treatment. The age at treatment is an important determinant of fertility outcome, with prepubertal patients having the highest tolerance. Ovarian failure is age related, and females who resume menses after treatment are still at increased risk for premature menopause. Males generally have reversible azoospermia during lower intensity alkylator chemotherapy, and long-term infertility is associated with doses of cyclophosphamide >9 g/m^2 and with high-intensity therapy, such as that used in hematopoietic stem cell transplantation. All patients should be counseled on the potential impact on future reproduction, and timely referral for established interventions such as sperm cryopreservation, oocyte preservation, and embryo preservation should be offered when feasible and appropriate. Assisted reproductive technologies can be helpful to couples with chemotherapy-induced infertility.

Combination chemotherapy can impair bone health, and older patients may be more susceptible to these effects. Due to the combined risk of age-related osteoporosis and the effect of therapy, the risk of fractures in patients over the age of 70 years may be as high as 5–10% within a few years of finishing therapy. The risk of low bone mineral density is highest in certain high-risk groups including survivors of pediatric acute lymphoblastic leukemia and CNS tumors and those who have undergone hematopoietic stem cell transplant.

Immune checkpoint inhibitors that target CTLA-4 and PD-1 have led to serious chronic toxicities including the breaking of self-tolerance and the autoimmune destruction of certain endocrine organs, particularly the thyroid and adenohypophysis (anterior pituitary). Hypophysitis is more commonly reported in association with CTLA-4 inhibitors, whereas thyroid dysfunction is more common with PD-1 inhibitors. Most immune-related toxicities occur within 8–12 weeks of starting treatment, but they can occur at any time during treatment or even after therapy has stopped. Patients with autoimmune thyroiditis or hypophysitis require lifelong hormone replacement, and early recognition is important.

Tyrosine kinase inhibitors such as imatinib have been associated with growth deceleration in children, particularly when treatment is initiated before puberty. The mechanism is postulated to be related to disruptions in growth hormone signaling or inhibition of the insulin-like growth factor 1 (IGFR-1) receptor. Other BCR-ABL inhibitors, including nilotinib and dasatinib, have been associated with both hyper- and hypothyroidism. Endocrine effects that have been reported to be associated with other tyrosine kinase inhibitors include alterations in bone remodeling, reduced calcium and vitamin D levels, thyroid dysfunction, gonadal dysfunction, adrenal dysfunction, altered glucose metabolism, and secondary hyperparathyroidism. Thyroid function tests should be monitored periodically while patients are on these targeted agents, and replacement hormones and/or vitamins should be prescribed as necessary.

NEUROLOGIC DYSFUNCTION

Neurologic dysfunction from cancer treatment is increasing in both incidence and severity as a result of improved supportive care that enables more aggressive regimens, an expanded number of older patients receiving treatment, extended durations of therapy, and longer periods of cancer survivorship. Direct effects on myelin, glial cells, and neurons have all been implicated, with alterations in cellular cytoskeleton, axonal transport, and cellular metabolism as potential mechanisms. Telomere shortening that occurs with normal aging may be accelerated by radiation. Survivors of CNS tumors are at the greatest risk of late-onset neurocognitive impairment that includes impaired intelligence and slower processing speeds along with deficits in executive function, memory, and attention. These toxicities are reported after treatment with both radiation and chemotherapy in childhood survivors.

Acute radiation CNS toxicity occurs within weeks and is characterized by nausea, drowsiness, hypersomnia, and ataxia, which typically recover over time. Early delayed toxicity occurring weeks to 3 months following therapy is associated with similar symptoms as acute toxicity and is pathologically associated with reversible demyelination. Chronic, late radiation injury occurs 9 months to up to 10 years following therapy, and dysfunction increases over time. Radiation-associated spinal cord injury (myelopathy) is highly dose-dependent and rarely occurs with modern radiation therapy. An early, self-limited form involving electric sensations down the spine on neck flexion (Lhermitte's sign) is seen 6–12 weeks after treatment and generally resolves over weeks. Peripheral nerve toxicity is quite rare owing to relative radiation resistance. Diffuse radiation injury is associated with global CNS neurologic dysfunction and diffuse white matter changes on computed tomography (CT) or MRI. Pathologically, small vessel changes are prominent and focal necrosis is common. Necrotizing encephalopathy is the most severe form of radiation injury and almost always is associated with concurrent use of chemotherapy, notably methotrexate. Prophylactic cranial irradiation in both childhood and adult leukemias/lymphomas has largely been abandoned due to the acute and long-term effects of therapy. Glucocorticoids may be symptomatically useful for acute toxicities but do not alter the course. Psychostimulants such as methylphenidate may improve attention and executive functioning in childhood survivors.

In children and adolescent cancers, younger age, higher cranial irradiation dose, larger brain volumes irradiated, and longer treatment times are associated with worse neurocognitive outcomes. In adult cancers, patients over the age of 60 who receive whole-brain radiation therapy are at high risk for neurocognitive impairment after therapy. Genetic polymorphisms may be associated with an increased risk of neurocognitive problems, and emerging evidence suggests polymorphisms in the folate pathway, oxidative stress genes, and enzymes that regulate both catecholamines and deamination of amines are associated with individual risk.

Vinca alkaloids produce a characteristic "stocking-glove" neuropathy with numbness and tingling advancing to loss of motor function, which is highly dose related. Distal sensorimotor polyneuropathy prominently involves loss of deep tendon reflexes with initially loss of pain and temperature sensation, followed by proprioceptive and vibratory loss. This requires careful patient history and physical examination by experienced oncologists to decide when the drug must be stopped or reduced to prevent permanent damage. Milder toxicity often slowly completely resolves after treatment discontinuation. Vinca alkaloids may sometimes be associated with jaw claudication, hoarseness, autonomic neuropathy, ileus, cranial nerve palsies, and, in severe cases, encephalopathy, seizures, and coma. Cisplatin is associated with sensorimotor neuropathy and hearing loss, especially at doses >400 mg/m^2, requiring audiometry in patients with preexisting hearing compromise. Carboplatin is often substituted in such cases given its lesser effect on hearing. Many of the agents that target kinase enzymes in tumor cells and 5-fluorouracil congeners produce dysesthesias and painful hands and feet known as hand-foot syndrome or palmar-plantar erythrodysesthesia. Symptoms usually abate when the agent is stopped. Methotrexate alone may cause acute leukoencephalopathy characterized by somnolence and confusion that is often reversible. Acute toxicity is dose-related, especially at doses >3 g/m^2, with younger patients being at greater risk. Subacute methotrexate toxicity occurs weeks after therapy and is often ameliorated with glucocorticoid therapy. Chronic methotrexate toxicity (leukoencephalopathy) develops months or years after treatment and is characterized clinically as progressive loss of cognitive function and focal neurologic signs, which are irreversible, promoted by synchronous or metachronous radiation therapy, and more pronounced at a younger age. Neurocognitive decline following chemotherapy alone occurs notably in breast cancer patients receiving adjuvant chemotherapy with anthracyclines, taxanes, or cyclophosphamide; this has been referred to as "chemo brain." It is clinically associated with impaired memory, learning, attention, and speed of information processing. There is no clear mechanistic explanation for its cause and no clearly effective therapy, although regular exercise is associated with improved symptoms. Most symptoms improve within a year of therapy, but symptoms can persist in 10–20% of patients for extended periods of time.

Newer molecularly targeted agents and immunotherapy have also been associated with neurologic dysfunction and may exacerbate persistent neuropathy from prior therapy. Proteasome inhibitors are associated with neuropathic pain and motor neuropathy that can occur immediately or be delayed in onset. The proposed mechanism is through enhanced oxidative stress on neural cells. Subcutaneous administration of these agents is associated with less peripheral neuropathy than intravenous infusions. Immunotherapy agents such as CAR-T therapies and bi-specific monoclonal antibodies targeting both T cells and B cells are associated with significant acute neurotoxicity including confusion, encephalopathy, seizures, and cerebellar symptoms. These symptoms are hypothesized to be related to the CRS associated with these therapies and often are time limited. However, a minority of patients treated with these agents will have persistent central and neurologic dysfunction for which management is mainly supportive. Glucocorticoids may be useful in the short term, but treatment with interleukin 6 receptor antagonists that are effective for decreasing the severity of CRS is largely ineffective at preventing neurologic toxicities. Progressive multifocal leukoencephalopathy (PML) is a rare but serious brain infection that is caused by the JC virus and has been reported as a rare complication of treatment with rituximab, ibrutinib, and PI3K inhibitors. The inflammatory response to the virus presents as unifocal or multifocal hyperintense lesions involving the subcortical white matter that are best seen on T2/fluid-attenuated inversion recovery (FLAIR) images on MRI. Treatment is supportive and includes removal of the offending agent. Other targeted agents that may be associated with neurologic dysfunction when given for extended durations of treatment include dasatinib, thalidomide, and lenalidomide.

Antibody-drug conjugates (ADCs) are novel therapies in which a monoclonal antibody targeted to a tumor antigen is attached to a potent anticancer agent via a chemical linker. Often, these agents are associated with significant central and peripheral neurotoxicity, as has been described with agents such as brentuximab vedotin and pertuzumab. These neuropathies often emerge during treatment similar to those seen with chemotherapy and are dose-dependent. Early recognition of treatment-emergent neuropathy induced by ADCs mandates dose interruption or modification to less frequent dosing schedules in order for patients to remain on therapy. Immune checkpoint inhibitors have been associated with autoimmune complications and unique neurologic manifestations such as optic neuritis that may be reversible after glucocorticoids.

HEPATIC AND GASTROINTESTINAL DYSFUNCTION

Long-term hepatic damage from standard chemotherapy regimens is rare. Long-term methotrexate or high-dose chemotherapy alone or with radiation therapy, for example, in preparative regimens for bone marrow transplantation, may result in venoocclusive disease of the liver. This potentially lethal complication classically presents with anicteric ascites, elevated alkaline phosphatase, and hepatosplenomegaly. Pathologically, there is venous congestion, epithelial cell proliferation, and hepatocyte atrophy progressing to frank fibrosis. Frequent monitoring of liver function tests during any chemotherapy is necessary to avoid both idiosyncratic and expected toxicities. Certain nucleoside drugs have been associated with hepatic dysfunction; however, this complication is rare in oncology. Hepatic radiation damage depends on dose, volume, fractionation, preexisting liver disease, and synchronous or metachronous chemotherapy. In general, radiation doses to the liver >1500 cGy can produce hepatic dysfunction with a steep dose-injury curve. Radiation-induced liver disease closely mimics hepatic venoocclusive disease.

Novel targeted agents including immunotherapy agents have introduced a number of gastrointestinal toxicities that can occur late in the course of treatment including hepatitis, colitis, malabsorption, and chronic diarrhea. Early signs of serious liver injury should lead to discontinuation of the offending agent as the effect does not appear to be dose-related and dose reductions do not reliably reduce further liver injury. The mechanisms for colitis or hepatitis associated with these targeted agents are not completely understood but are hypothesized to be T cell–mediated, and the risk is highest when used in targeted agent combinations. Diarrhea with or without severe colitis can be associated with virtually all targeted agents including PI3K inhibitors, BCR-ABL inhibitors, BTK inhibitors, EGFR inhibitors, MEK inhibitors, CDK inhibitors, and immunomodulatory agents. Even if the diarrhea is not severe, the impact associated with indefinite treatment greatly interferes with the quality of life and often leads to discontinuation of targeted therapy if not managed effectively. Immunomodulatory agents including lenalidomide are associated with late onset of diarrhea that is caused by bile acid malabsorption and often responds to bile acid sequestrants. Immune checkpoint inhibitors are associated with colitis and hepatitis that may be responsive to prompt initiation of glucocorticoids that may require a long taper for resolution.

RENAL AND BLADDER DYSFUNCTION

Cisplatin produces reversible decrements in renal function but may also produce severe irreversible toxicity in the presence of renal disease and may predispose to accentuated damage with subsequent renal insults. Cyclophosphamide and ifosfamide are prodrugs primarily activated in the liver with cleavage products (acrolein) that can produce hemorrhagic cystitis. This can be prevented with the free radical scavenger MESNA (mercaptoethane sulfonate), which is required for ifosfamide administration. Hemorrhagic cystitis caused by these agents may predispose to bladder cancer.

Targeted agents generally do not carry significant acute nephrotoxic risks, but a number of agents, including PI3K inhibitors, anti-VEGF agents, and FLT3 inhibitors, are associated with systemic hypertension, which can lead to late effects or a progressive decline in renal function. Renal dysfunction following immunotherapy is uncommon, but acute interstitial nephritis can occur. Similar to other immune-related toxicities, this acute toxicity requires prompt use of glucocorticoids to avoid long-term effects on renal function.

PSYCHOLOGICAL DYSFUNCTION AND SOCIOECONOMIC IMPACT OF SURVIVORSHIP

The diagnosis and treatment of cancer can introduce long-term and late psychological effects that continue throughout life. Cancer survivors are at increased risk for anxiety, depression, attention problems, and posttraumatic stress syndromes. Many cancer patients experience intrusive or debilitating concerns about cancer recurrence following successful therapy. In addition, these patients may experience socioeconomic stressors that affect employment, insurance, relationships and lead to financial and/or sexual difficulties. Survivors of childhood cancers are less likely to graduate from college or gain full-time employment than their peers and are more likely to engage in risky health behaviors such as substance abuse and excessive alcohol use. The long-term psychosocial effects of treatment are greatest in patients who undergo CNS-directed therapies including radiation and intensive combination chemotherapy regimens. Oncologists should ask about and address these issues explicitly with patients and provide appropriate counseling or support systems. The overall risk of suicidal ideation and suicide is low but is greater in cancer patients and survivors than age-matched controls. Tailored cognitive-behavioral therapy may improve the anxiety and posttraumatic stress associated with cancer survivorship.

CANCER SURVIVORSHIP CARE PLANS

Survivorship starts at the time of diagnosis and continues indefinitely. Many guidelines recommend that every patient be provided with a survivorship care plan unique to their situation, but the evidence that these improve health outcomes is limited and sufficient resources to implement recommendations are often lacking. Focused surveillance plans for late effects are critical for early detection and implementation of interventions but also must include risk stratification to avoid unnecessary surveillance testing that wastes resources and leads to overdiagnosis and/or psychological distress. Survivorship care has traditionally been performed by oncologists, but the scope of the problem mandates that primary care physicians, midlevel providers, and preventive medicine specialists be trained in the follow-up of treated cancer patients in remission. All former cancer patients should undergo surveillance for recurrence and second malignancies and be monitored for long-term effects of treatment; however, as a practical matter, nearly all recurrences are detected because of symptoms. Health promotion and disease prevention with age- and sex-specific routine screening tests (e.g., colonoscopy, Pap smears, mammography, human papillomavirus vaccination, dual-energy x-ray absorptiometry scans) should be a focus of survivorship care along with psychosocial well-being. Annual mammography should start no later than 10 years after breast radiation. Patients receiving radiation fields encompassing thyroid tissue should have regular thyroid examinations and TSH testing. Localized pain or palpable abnormality in a previously radiated field should prompt radiographic evaluation. Patients treated with alkylating agents or topoisomerase inhibitors should have a complete blood count every 6–12 months, and cytopenias, abnormal cells on peripheral smear, or macrocytosis should be evaluated with bone marrow biopsy and aspirate and include cytogenetics, flow cytometry, or fluorescence in situ hybridization (FISH) studies as appropriate.

As the population of cancer survivors increases and patients live longer, cancer survivorship has become increasingly important, and the Institute of Medicine and National Research Council have published a monograph entitled *From Cancer Patient to Cancer Survivor: Lost in Transition.* The monograph proposes a plan that would inform clinicians caring for cancer survivors of the complete details of patients' previous treatments, complications thereof, signs and symptoms of late effects, and recommended screening and follow-up procedures.

OUTLOOK

Survivorship care is one of the most challenging problems facing oncologists today. The challenge is to develop cancer treatments that utilize the most effective combination of surgery, chemotherapy, radiation, targeted agents, or immunotherapy that is required to cure disease or effect long-term disease control with the least amount of toxicity. As cancer treatments continue to improve, the need for cancer care increases due to more cancer survivors with increasing life expectancy. Clearly, much work remains to elucidate the pathophysiology of cancer treatment–related effects and identification of patient characteristics associated with an increased vulnerability to adverse effects. Clinical management strategies focused on the clinical management of acute toxicities and prevention of long-term effects after therapy are necessary. Finally, research initiatives should recognize that as treatment paradigms continue to evolve, the nature and biologic basis for toxicities will change. Advances in genomic medicine may add depth to our understanding of toxicities and allow for more personalized surveillance strategies. Longitudinal monitoring of the health of cancer survivors is required since the incidence of late effects of treatment does not appear to plateau over time.

ACKNOWLEDGMENT

We would like to acknowledge the contribution of Carl E. Freter who coauthored a previous version of this chapter; material from his chapter was retained in this version.

FURTHER READING

Armenian SH et al: Cardiovascular disease in survivors of childhood cancer: Insights into epidemiology, pathophysiology, and prevention. J Clin Oncol 36:2135, 2018.

Brinkman TM et al: Psychological symptoms, social outcomes, socioeconomic attainment, and health behaviors among survivors of childhood cancer: Current state of the literature. J Clin Oncol 36:2190, 2018.

Chao C et al: Chronic comorbidities among survivors of adolescent and young adult cancer. J Clin Oncol 38:3161, 2020.

Chemaitilly W et al: Endocrine late effects in childhood cancer survivors. J Clin Oncol 36:2153, 2018.

Chow EJ et al: New agents, emerging late effects, and the development of precision durvivorship. J Clin Oncol 36:2231, 2018.

Rowland JH et al: Survivorship science at the NIH: Lessons learned from grants funded in fiscal year 2016. J Natl Cancer Inst 111:109, 2019.

Shapiro CL: Cancer survivorship. N Engl J Med 379:2438, 2018.

Shapiro CL et al: ReCAP: ASCO core curriculum for cancer survivorship education. J Oncol Pract 12:e08, 2016.

Shree T et al: Impaired immune health in survivors of diffuse large B-cell lymphoma. J Clin Oncol 38:1664, 2020.

Turcotte LM et al: Risk, risk factors, and surveillance of subsequent malignant neoplasms in survivors of childhood cancer: A review. J Clin Oncol 36:2145, 2018.

Section 2 Hematopoietic Disorders

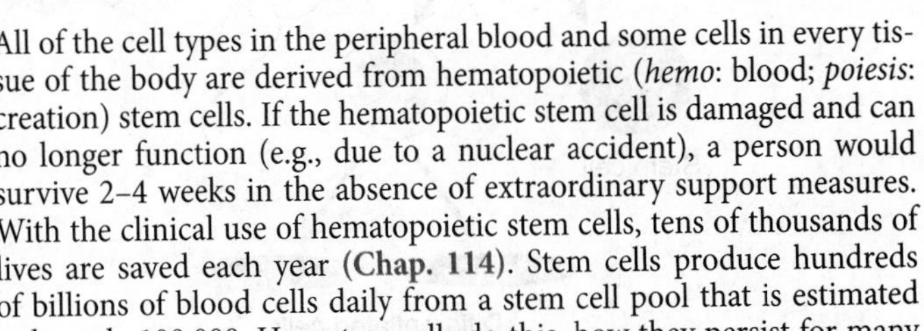

96 Hematopoietic Stem Cells

David T. Scadden, Dan L. Longo

All of the cell types in the peripheral blood and some cells in every tissue of the body are derived from hematopoietic (*hemo*: blood; *poiesis*: creation) stem cells. If the hematopoietic stem cell is damaged and can no longer function (e.g., due to a nuclear accident), a person would survive 2–4 weeks in the absence of extraordinary support measures. With the clinical use of hematopoietic stem cells, tens of thousands of lives are saved each year (**Chap. 114**). Stem cells produce hundreds of billions of blood cells daily from a stem cell pool that is estimated to be only 100,000. How stem cells do this, how they persist for many decades despite the production demands, and how they may be better used in clinical care are important issues in medicine.

The study of blood cell production has become a paradigm for how other tissues may be organized and regulated. Basic research in hematopoiesis includes defining stepwise molecular changes accompanying functional changes in maturing cells, aggregating cells into functional subgroups, and demonstrating hematopoietic stem cell regulation by a specialized microenvironment; these concepts are worked out in hematology and offer models for other tissues. Moreover, these concepts may not be restricted to normal tissue function but extend to malignancy. Stem cells are rare cells among a heterogeneous population of cell types, and their behavior is assessed mainly in experimental animal models involving reconstitution of hematopoiesis. Thus, much of what we know about stem cells is imprecise and based on inferences from genetically manipulated animals.

CARDINAL FUNCTIONS OF HEMATOPOIETIC STEM CELLS

All stem cell types have two cardinal functions: self-renewal and differentiation (**Fig. 96-1**). Stem cells exist to generate, maintain, and repair tissues. They function successfully if they can replace a wide variety of shorter-lived mature cells over prolonged periods. The process of self-renewal (see below) assures that a stem cell population can be sustained over time. Without self-renewal, the stem cell pool would become exhausted and tissue maintenance would not be possible. The process of differentiation leads to production of the effectors of tissue function: mature cells. Without proper differentiation, the integrity of tissue function would be compromised and organ failure or neoplasia would ensue.

In the blood, mature cells have variable average life spans, ranging from hours for mature neutrophils to a few months for red blood cells to many years for memory lymphocytes. However, the stem cell pool is the central, durable source of all blood and immune cells, maintaining a capacity to produce a broad range of cells from a single cell source, yet keeping itself vigorous over decades of life. As an individual stem cell divides, it has the capacity to accomplish one of three division outcomes: two stem cells, two cells destined for differentiation, or one stem cell and one differentiating cell. The former two outcomes are the result of symmetric cell division, whereas the latter indicates a different outcome for the two daughter cells—an event termed asymmetric cell division. The relative balance for these types of outcomes may change during development and under particular kinds of demands on the stem cell pool.

DEVELOPMENTAL BIOLOGY OF HEMATOPOIETIC STEM CELLS

During development, blood cells are produced at different sites. Initially, the yolk sac provides oxygen-carrying red blood cells and many of the macrophage-like cells that are resident in tissues: cells like microglia in the brain. The placenta and several sites of intraembryonic blood cell production then become involved in sequential order. These move from the genital ridge at a site where the aorta, gonadal tissue, and mesonephros are emerging to the fetal liver and then, in the second trimester, to the bone marrow and spleen. As the location of stem cells changes, the cells they produce also change. The yolk sac provides red cells expressing embryonic hemoglobins and tissue-resident macrophages. Intraembryonic sites of hematopoiesis generate stem cells, red cells, platelets, and the circulating cells of innate immunity. The production of the cells of adaptive immunity occurs then as well but becomes robust as the thymus forms and the bone marrow is colonized in the second trimester. Stem cell proliferation remains high, even in the bone marrow, until shortly after birth, when it appears to dramatically decline. The cells in the bone marrow are thought to arrive by the bloodborne transit of cells from the fetal liver after calcification of the long bones has begun. The presence of stem cells in the circulation is not unique to a time window in development, however, as hematopoietic stem cells circulate throughout life. The time that stem cells spend freely circulating appears to be brief (measured in minutes in the mouse), but the stem cells that do circulate are functional and can be used for transplantation. The number of stem cells that circulate can be increased in a number of ways to facilitate harvest and transfer to the same or a different host.

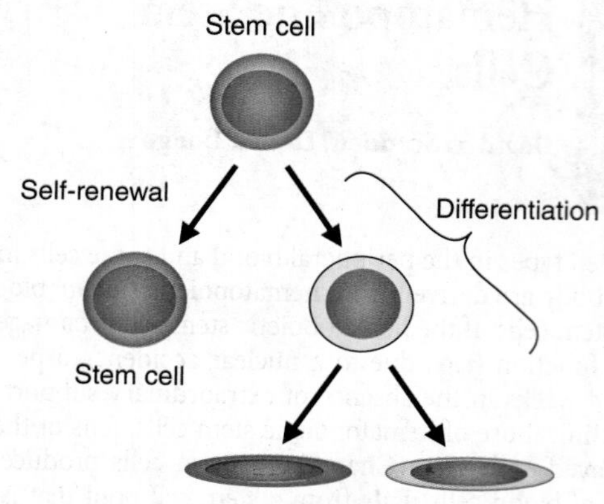

FIGURE 96-1 Signature characteristics of the stem cell. Stem cells have two essential features: the capacity to differentiate into a variety of mature cell types and the capacity for self-renewal. Intrinsic factors associated with self-renewal include expression of *Bmi-1, Gfi-1, PTEN, STAT5, Tel/Atv6, p21, p18, MCL-1, Mel-18, RAE28,* and *HoxB4*. Extrinsic signals for self-renewal include Notch, Wnt, SHH, angiogenin, and Tie2/Ang-1. Based mainly on murine studies, hematopoietic stem cells express the following cell surface molecules: CD34, Thy-1 (CD90), c-Kit receptor (CD117), CD133, CD164, and c-Mpl (CD110, also known as the thrombopoietin receptor).

MOBILITY OF HEMATOPOIETIC STEM CELLS

Cells entering and exiting the bone marrow do so through a series of molecular interactions. Circulating stem cells (through CD162 and CD44) engage the lectins (carbohydrate binding proteins) P- and E-selectin on the endothelial surface to slow the movement of the cells to a rolling phenotype. Stem cell integrins are then activated and accomplish firm adhesion between the stem cell and vessel wall, with a particularly important role for stem cell VCAM-1 engaging endothelial VLA-4. The chemokine CXCL12 (SDF1) interacting with stem cell CXCR4 receptors and ionic calcium interacting with the calcium-sensing receptor appear to be important in the process of stem cells getting from the circulation to where they engraft in the bone marrow. This is particularly true in the developmental move from fetal liver to bone marrow.

In the adult, the role for CXCR4 is in retention of stem cells in the bone marrow as well as getting them there. Interrupting that retention process through specific molecular blockers of the CXCR4/CXCL12 interaction, cleavage of CXCL12, or downregulation of the CXCR4 receptor can result in the release of stem cells into the circulation. This process is an increasingly important aspect of recovering stem cells for therapeutic use as it has permitted the harvesting process to be done by leukapheresis rather than bone marrow punctures in the operating room. Granulocyte colony-stimulating factor and plerixafor, a macrocyclic compound that can block CXCR4, are both used clinically to mobilize marrow hematopoietic stem cells for transplant. Refining our knowledge of how stem cells get into and out of the bone marrow may improve our ability to obtain stem cells and make them more efficient at finding their way to the specific sites for blood cell production, the so-called stem cell niche.

HEMATOPOIETIC STEM CELL MICROENVIRONMENT

The concept of a specialized microenvironment, or stem cell niche, was first proposed to explain why cells derived from the bone marrow of one animal could be used in transplantation and again be found in the bone marrow of the recipient. This niche is more than just a housing site for stem cells, however. It is an anatomic location where regulatory signals are provided that allow the stem cells to thrive, to expand if needed, and to provide varying amounts of descendant daughter cells. In addition, unregulated growth of stem cells may be problematic based on their undifferentiated state and self-renewal capacity. Thus, the niche must also regulate the number of stem cells produced. In this manner, the niche has the dual function of serving as a site of nurture but imposing limits for stem cells: in effect, acting as both a nutritive and constraining home.

The niche for blood stem cells changes with each of the sites of blood production during development, but for most of human life, it is located in the bone marrow. Within the bone marrow, the perivascular space particularly in regions of trabecular bone serves as a niche. The mesenchymal and endothelial cells of the marrow microvessels produce kit ligand and CXCL12, both known to be important for hematopoietic stem cells. Other cell types, such as sympathetic neurons, nonmyelinating Schwann cells, macrophages, megakaryocytes, osteoclasts, and osteoblasts, have been shown to regulate stem cells, some by direct and others by indirect effects. Extracellular matrix proteins like osteopontin and heparan sulfates also affect stem cell function. The endosteal region appears to be particularly important for transplanted cells, in part because many of the mesenchymal cells and sinusoidal blood vessels of the central marrow are disrupted by the conditioning regimens used to prepare a patient for transplantation. The functioning of the niche as a supportive context for stem cells is of obvious importance for maintaining hematopoiesis and in transplantation. An active area of study involves determining whether the niche is altered in disease as experimental models have shown that mutations in niche cells can lead to myeloid malignancies. It logically follows that targeting of niche functions is a potential therapeutic strategy for both malignant and normal hematopoiesis.

■ EXCESS CAPACITY OF HEMATOPOIETIC STEM CELLS

In the absence of disease, one never runs out of hematopoietic stem cells. Indeed, serial transplantation studies in mice suggest that sufficient stem cells are present to reconstitute several animals in succession, with each animal having normal blood cell production. The fact that allogeneic stem cell transplant recipients also never run out of blood cells in their life span, which can extend for decades, argues that even the limiting numbers of stem cells provided to them are sufficient. How stem cells respond to different conditions to increase or decrease their mature cell production remains poorly understood. Clearly, negative feedback mechanisms affect the level of production of most of the cells, leading to the normal tightly regulated blood cell counts. However, many of the regulatory mechanisms that govern production of more mature progenitor cells do not apply or apply differently to stem cells. Similarly, most of the molecules shown to be able to change the size of the stem cell pool have little effect on more mature blood cells. For example, the growth factor erythropoietin, which stimulates red blood cell production from precursor cells, has no effect on stem cells. Similarly, granulocyte colony-stimulating factor drives the rapid proliferation of granulocyte precursors but has little or no effect on the cell cycling of stem cells. Rather, it changes the location of stem cells by indirect means, altering molecules such as CXCL12 that tether stem cells to their niche. Molecules shown to be important for altering the proliferation, self-renewal, or survival of stem cells, such as cyclin-dependent kinase inhibitors, transcription factors like Bmi-1, microRNA-processing enzymes like Dicer, or even metabolic regulators like pyruvate kinase isoforms, have little or different effects on progenitor cells. Hematopoietic stem cells have governing mechanisms that are distinct from the cells they generate.

■ HEMATOPOIETIC STEM CELL DIFFERENTIATION

Hematopoietic stem cells sit at the base of a branching hierarchy of cells culminating in the many mature cell types that compose the blood and immune system (**Fig. 96-2**). The maturation steps leading to terminally differentiated and functional blood cells take place both as a consequence of intrinsic changes in gene expression and niche-directed and cytokine-directed changes in the cells. Our knowledge of the details remains incomplete. As stem cells mature to progenitors, precursors, and, finally, mature effector cells, they undergo a series of functional changes. These include the obvious acquisition of functions defining mature blood cells, such as phagocytic capacity or hemoglobin synthesis. They also include the progressive loss of plasticity (i.e., the ability to become other cell types). For example, the myeloid progenitor can make all cells in the myeloid series but none in the lymphoid series. As common myeloid progenitors mature, they become precursors for either monocytes and granulocytes or erythrocytes and megakaryocytes, but not both. Some amount of reversibility of this process may exist early in the differentiation cascade, but that is lost beyond a distinct stage in normal physiologic conditions. With genetic interventions, however, blood cells, like other somatic cells, can be reprogrammed to become a variety of cell types.

As cells differentiate, they may also lose proliferative capacity (**Fig. 96-3**). Mature granulocytes are incapable of proliferation and only increase in number by increased production from precursors. The exceptions to the rule are some tissue-resident macrophages, which appear capable of proliferation, and lymphoid cells. Lymphoid cells retain the capacity to proliferate but have linked their proliferation to the recognition of particular proteins or peptides by specific antigen receptors on their surface. Like many tissues with short-lived mature cells such as the skin and intestine, blood cell proliferation is largely accomplished by a more immature progenitor population. In general, cells within the highly proliferative progenitor cell compartment are also relatively short-lived, making their way through the differentiation process in a defined molecular program involving the sequential activation of particular sets of genes. For any particular cell type, the differentiation program is difficult to speed up. The time it takes for hematopoietic progenitors to become mature cells is ~10–14 days in humans, evident clinically by the interval between cytotoxic chemotherapy and blood count recovery in patients.

Although hematopoietic stem cells are generally thought to have the capacity to form all cells of the blood, it is becoming clear that individual stem cells may not be equal in their differentiation potential. That is, some stem cells are "biased" to become mature cells of a particular type. In addition, the general concept of cells having a binary choice of lymphoid or myeloid differentiation is not entirely accurate. A cell population with limited megakaryocytic and erythroid or myeloid (monocyte and granulocyte) and lymphoid potential is now added to the commitment steps stem cells may undergo.

■ SELF-RENEWAL

The hematopoietic stem cell must balance its three potential fates: apoptosis, self-renewal, and differentiation. The proliferation of cells is generally not associated with the ability to undergo a self-renewing division except among memory T and B cells and among stem cells. Self-renewal capacity has generally been regarded as giving way to differentiation as the only option after cell division when cells leave the stem cell compartment, unless they become memory lymphocytes. However, emerging data suggest that some myeloid committed progenitors may also have self-renewing potential in vivo, providing long-term production of cells. Stem cells all have self-renewing capacity by definition, and they have an additional feature characterizing their proliferation machinery. Stem cells in many mature adult tissues are heterogeneous with some being deeply quiescent, serving as a deep reserve, whereas others are more proliferative and replenish the short-lived progenitor population. In the hematopoietic system, stem cells are generally cytokine-resistant, remaining dormant even when cytokines drive bone marrow progenitors to proliferation rates measured in hours. Stem cells, in contrast, are thought to divide at far longer intervals, measured in months to years, for the most quiescent cells. This quiescence is difficult to overcome in vitro, limiting the ability to effectively expand human hematopoietic stem cells. The process may be controlled by particularly high levels of cyclin-dependent kinase inhibitors like p57 or CDKN1c that restrict entry of stem cells into the cell cycle, blocking the G_1-S transition. Exogenous signals from the niche also appear to enforce quiescence, including angiogenin, interleukin 18, and perhaps angiopoietin 1.

The regulation of stem cell proliferation also appears to change with age. Both cell intrinsic features like the cyclin-dependent kinase inhibitor p16INK4a and bone marrow microenvironment features like declining sympathetic innervation are implicated in age-related stem cell changes. Either lowering expression of p16INK4a or stimulating beta-3 adrenergic receptors in older animals improves stem cell cycling and capacity to reconstitute hematopoiesis in adoptive hosts, making them similar to younger animals. Mature cell numbers are unaffected. Therefore, molecular events governing the specific functions of stem cells are being gradually made clear and offer the potential of new

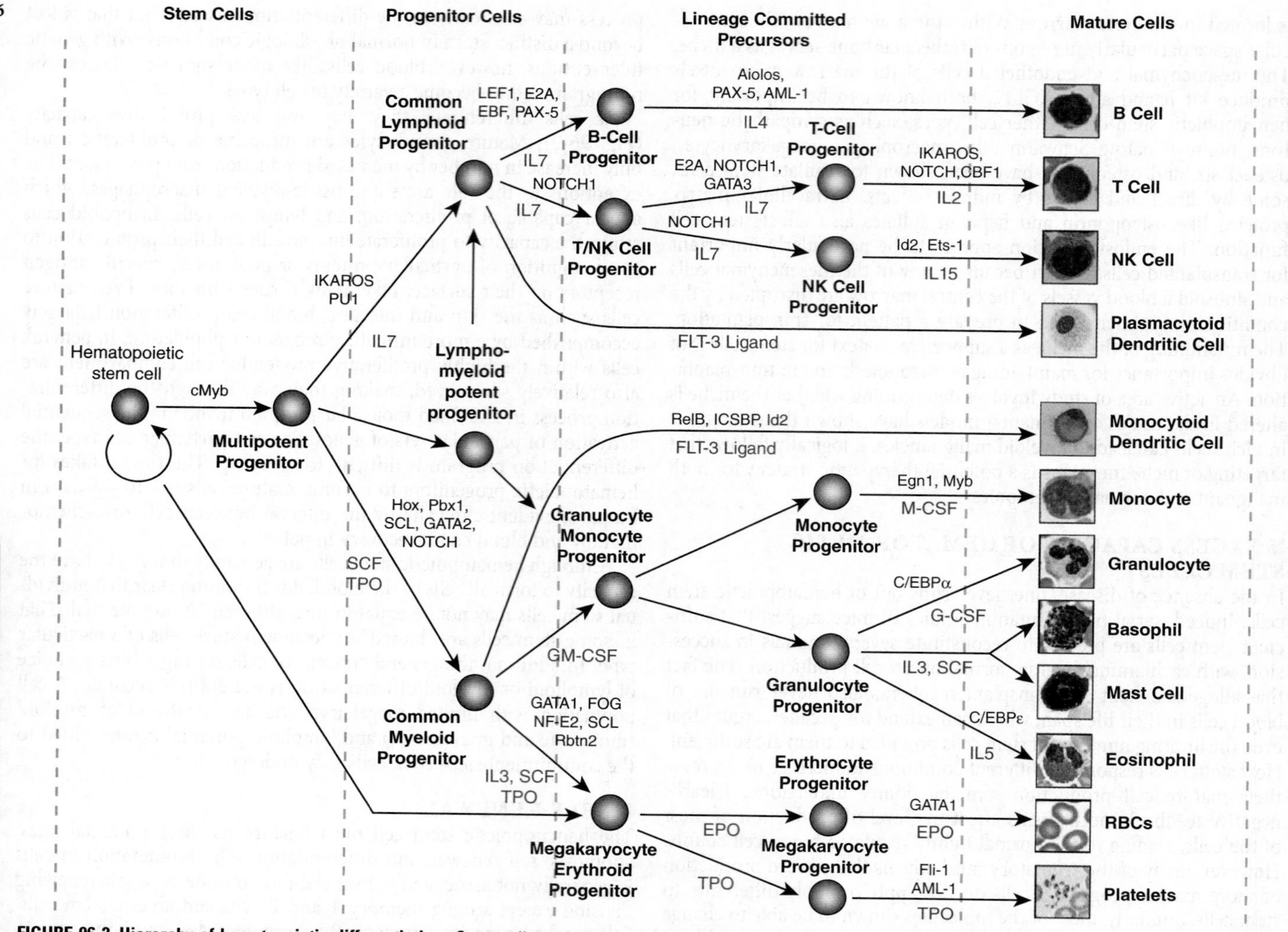

Stem Cells
Progenitor Cells
Lineage Committed Precursors
Mature Cells
Hematopoietic stem cell
cMyb
Multipotent Progenitor
IKAROS
PU1
IL7
Common Lymphoid Progenitor
LEF1, E2A, EBF, PAX-5
B-Cell Progenitor
Aiolos, PAX-5, AML-1
IL4
B Cell
IL7
NOTCH1
IL7
T/NK Cell Progenitor
E2A, NOTCH1, GATA3
IL7
T-Cell Progenitor
IKAROS, NOTCH,CBF1
IL2
T Cell
NOTCH1
IL7
NK Cell Progenitor
Id2, Ets-1
IL15
NK Cell
FLT-3 Ligand
Plasmacytoid Dendritic Cell
Lympho-myeloid potent progenitor
RelB, ICSBP, Id2
FLT-3 Ligand
Monocytoid Dendritic Cell
Hox, Pbx1, SCL, GATA2, NOTCH
Granulocyte Monocyte Progenitor
Monocyte Progenitor
Egn1, Myb
M-CSF
Monocyte
C/EBPα
G-CSF
Granulocyte
Basophil
SCF
TPO
GM-CSF
Granulocyte Progenitor
IL3, SCF
Mast Cell
Common Myeloid Progenitor
GATA1, FOG
NFE2, SCL
Rbtn2
C/EBPε
IL5
Eosinophil
IL3, SCF
TPO
Erythrocyte Progenitor
GATA1
EPO
EPO
RBCs
Megakaryocyte Erythroid Progenitor
Megakaryocyte Progenitor
TPO
Fli-1
AML-1
TPO
Platelets

FIGURE 96-2 Hierarchy of hematopoietic differentiation. *Stem cells* are multipotent cells that are the source of all descendant cells and have the capacity to provide either long-term (measured in years) or short-term (measured in months) cell production. *Progenitor cells* have a more limited spectrum of cells they can produce and are generally a shorter-lived, highly proliferative population also known as transient amplifying cells. *Precursor cells* are cells committed to a single blood cell lineage but with a continued ability to proliferate; they do not have all the features of a fully mature cell. *Mature cells* are the terminally differentiated product of the differentiation process and are the effector cells of specific activities of the blood and immune system. Progress through the pathways is mediated by alterations in gene expression. The regulation of the differentiation by soluble factors and cell-cell communications within the bone marrow niche are still being defined. The transcription factors that characterize particular cell transitions are illustrated on the *arrows*; the soluble factors that contribute to the differentiation process are in *blue*. This picture is a simplification of the process. Active research is revealing multiple discrete cell types in the maturation of B cells and T cells and has identified cells that are biased toward one lineage or another (rather than uncommitted) in their differentiation. EPO, erythropoietin; RBC, red blood cell; SCF, stem cell factor; TPO, thrombopoietin.

Stem
Progenitor
Precursor
Mature
Differentiation state
More
Less
Self-renewal ability
Proliferation activity
Lymphoid exception (memory B and T cells)

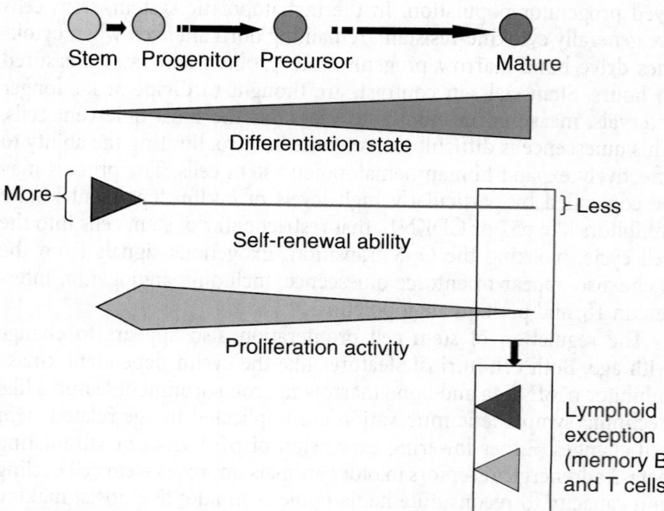

FIGURE 96-3 Relative function of cells in the hematopoietic hierarchy. The boxes represent distinct functional features of cells in the myeloid (*upper box*) versus lymphoid (*lower box*) lineages.

therapeutic approaches to changing stem cell functions. One critical stem cell function that remains poorly defined is the molecular regulation of self-renewal.

For medicine, self-renewal is perhaps the most important function of stem cells because it is critical in regulating the number of stem cells. Stem cell number is a key limiting parameter for both autologous and allogeneic stem cell transplantation. Were we to have the ability to use fewer stem cells or expand limited numbers of stem cells ex vivo, it might be possible to reduce the morbidity and expense of stem cell harvests, enable use of other stem cell sources, and improve the potential for gene-modified stem cell transplant. For example, umbilical cord blood is a rich source of stem cells but generally has an inadequate number of stem cells for use in transplantation in adults. These cells have two advantages over other stem cell sources: there is a lower incidence of graft-versus-host disease, and cord blood banks have representation of populations underrepresented in adult donor registries. Hematopoietic reconstitution from cord blood is slow, however, in part due to cell number. Expansion might improve this; however, advances in haploidentical donor cell transplantation have reduced cord blood use.

Gene-modified stem cells are increasingly being tested and have been found to offer great promise for genetic blood diseases like congenital immunodeficiencies and hemoglobinopathies such as sickle cell disease. However, the complexity and cost of modifying enough stem cells for transplantation is problematic. Expanding a small number of gene-modified stem cells may mitigate that issue. Therefore, understanding self-renewal offers the potential to facilitate development of an important new area of stem cell–based medicine. Some limited understanding of self-renewal exists and, intriguingly, implicates gene products that are associated with the chromatin state, a high-order organization of chromosomal DNA that influences transcription. These include members of the polycomb family, a group of zinc finger–containing transcriptional regulators that interact with the chromatin structure, contributing to the accessibility of groups of genes for transcription. One member, Bmi-1, is important in enabling hematopoietic stem cell self-renewal through modification of cell cycle regulators such as the cyclin-dependent kinase inhibitors. In the absence of Bmi-1 or of the transcriptional regulator, Gfi-1, hematopoietic stem cells decline in number and function. In contrast, dysregulation of Bmi-1 has been associated with leukemia; it may promote leukemic stem cell self-renewal when it is overexpressed. The same is true for the polycomb gene, *Asxl1*, that is commonly mutated in myelodysplasia and leukemia. Other transcription regulators have also been associated with self-renewal, particularly homeobox, or "hox," genes. These transcription factors are named for their ability to govern large numbers of genes, including those determining body patterning in invertebrates. HoxB4 is capable of inducing extensive self-renewal of stem cells through its DNA-binding motif. Other members of the hox family of genes have been noted to affect normal stem cells, but they are also associated with leukemia. Epigenetic modifiers such as the DNA methyl transferase DNMT3a or the dioxygenase involved in DNA demethylation, Tet2, also play a role in stem cell regulation. Like *Asxl1*, mutations of these genes are associated with clonal outgrowth of stem cells bearing the mutations. These mutations are not sufficient for malignancy, but they enable clones bearing them to gain dominance and predispose cells to malignant transformation. They are often referred to as "founder mutations" because myelodysplastic and leukemic cells appear to evolve from them by DNA sequencing analysis.

CANCER IS SIMILAR TO AN ORGAN WITH SELF-RENEWING CAPACITY

The relationship of stem cells to cancer is an important dimension of adult stem cell biology. Cancer may share principles of organization with normal tissues. Cancer cells are heterogeneous even within a given patient and may have a hierarchical organization of cells with a base of stem-like cells capable of the signature stem cell features: self-renewal and differentiation. These stem-like cells might be the basis for perpetuation of the tumor and represent a slowly dividing, rare population with distinct regulatory mechanisms, including a relationship with a specialized microenvironment. A subpopulation of self-renewing cells has been defined for some, but not all, cancers. These include myeloid leukemias where founder mutations appear to enable clones of cells to expand. With additional mutations, these can serve as the initiating or stem cells of a cancer, and eliminating them may be necessary for curing the patient. Understanding the hierarchical cell organization within cancers and whether eliminating cancer stem cell equivalents can improve cure rates is an area of active investigation.

Does the concept of cancer stem cells provide insight into the cellular origin of cancer? The fact that some cells within a cancer have stem cell–like properties does not necessarily mean that the cancer arose in the stem cell itself. Rather, more mature cells could have acquired the self-renewal characteristics of stem cells. Any single genetic event is unlikely to be sufficient to enable full transformation of a normal cell to a frankly malignant one. Rather, cancer is a multistep process, and for the multiple steps to accumulate, the cell of origin must be able to persist for prolonged periods. It must also be able to generate large numbers of daughter cells. The normal stem cell has these properties and, by virtue of its having intrinsic self-renewal capability, may be more readily converted to a malignant phenotype. This hypothesis has been tested experimentally in the hematopoietic system. Taking advantage of the cell-surface markers that distinguish hematopoietic cells of varying maturity, stem cells, progenitors, precursors, and mature cells can be isolated. Powerful transforming gene constructs were placed in these cells, and it was found that the cell with the greatest potential to produce a malignancy was dependent on the transforming gene. In some cases, it was the stem cell, but in others, the progenitor cell functioned to initiate and perpetuate the cancer. This shows that cells can acquire stem cell–like properties in malignancy.

WHAT ELSE CAN HEMATOPOIETIC STEM CELLS DO?

Some experimental data have suggested that hematopoietic stem cells or other bone marrow cells are capable of playing a role in healing the vascular and tissue damage associated with stroke and myocardial infarction. These data are controversial, and the applicability of a stem cell approach to nonhematopoietic conditions remains experimental. However, reprogramming technology offers the potential for using readily obtained hematopoietic cells as a source for cells with other capabilities. Active areas of investigation are to use reprogrammed cells to generate mature lymphoid cells for immuno-oncology applications or red cells and platelets to overcome dependency on blood donors.

STEM CELLS AS TARGETS OF GENE THERAPY

Tools to alter gene sequence, expression, and regulation are becoming increasingly feasible. The hematopoietic stem cell is a target for a wide range of interventions. Lentiviral, retroviral, and adenoviral vectors are being used to replace defective genes (e.g., in primary immunodeficiency diseases). Antisense technology is being applied to block gene expression (e.g., blocking the Bcl11a repression of fetal globin expression in sickle cell disease and thalassemia). CRISPR/Cas technology is being applied to repair abnormal gene sequences. Precision genetic manipulations are expanding, and the hematopoietic system is central to it.

In sum, the stem cell has tremendous healing capacity and is essential for life. However, if dysregulated, it can threaten the life it maintains. Understanding how stem cells function, the signals that modify their behavior, and the tissue niches that modulate stem cell responses to injury and disease is critical for more effectively developing stem cell–based medicines.

■ FURTHER READING

Adelman ER, Figueroa ME: Human hematopoiesis: Aging and leukemogenic risk. Curr Opin Hematol 1:57, 2021.

Baryawno N et al: A cellular taxonomy of the bone marrow stroma in homeostasis and leukemia. Cell 7:1915, 2019.

Ito Y et al: Turbulence activates platelet biogenesis to enable clinical scale ex vivo production. Cell 3:636, 2018.

Rodriguez-Fraticelli AE, Camargo F: Systems analysis of hematopoiesis using single-cell lineage tracing. Curr Opin Hematol 1:18, 2021.

97 Iron Deficiency and Other Hypoproliferative Anemias

John W. Adamson

Anemias associated with normocytic and normochromic red cells and an inappropriately low reticulocyte response (reticulocyte index <2–2.5) are *hypoproliferative anemias*. This category includes early iron deficiency (before hypochromic microcytic red cells develop), acute and chronic inflammation (including many malignancies), renal disease, hypometabolic states such as protein malnutrition and endocrine

TABLE 97-1 Body Iron Distribution

	IRON CONTENT, mg	
	ADULT MALE, 80 kg	ADULT FEMALE, 60 kg
Hemoglobin	2500	1700
Myoglobin/enzymes	500	300
Transferrin iron	3	3
Iron stores	600–1000	0–300

deficiencies, and anemias from marrow damage. Marrow damage states are discussed in **Chap. 102**.

Hypoproliferative anemias are the most common anemias, and in the clinic, iron deficiency anemia is the most common of these followed by the anemia of inflammation. The anemia of inflammation, similar to iron deficiency, is related in part to abnormal iron metabolism. The anemias associated with renal disease, inflammation, cancer, and hypometabolic states are characterized by a suboptimal erythropoietin response to the anemia.

IRON METABOLISM

Iron is a critical element in the function of all cells, although the amount of iron required by individual tissues varies during development. At the same time, the body must protect itself from free iron, which is highly toxic in that it participates in chemical reactions that generate free radicals such as singlet O_2 or OH^-. Consequently, elaborate mechanisms have evolved that allow iron to be made available for physiologic functions while at the same time conserving this element and handling it in such a way that toxicity is avoided.

The major role of iron in mammals is to carry O_2 as part of hemoglobin. O_2 is also bound by myoglobin in muscle. Iron is a critical element in iron-containing enzymes, including the cytochrome system in mitochondria. Iron distribution in the body is shown in **Table 97-1**. Without iron, cells lose their capacity for electron transport and energy metabolism. In erythroid cells, hemoglobin synthesis is impaired, resulting in anemia and reduced O_2 delivery to tissue.

■ THE IRON CYCLE IN HUMANS

Figure 97-1 outlines the major pathways of internal iron exchange in humans. Iron absorbed from the diet or released from stores circulates in the plasma bound to *transferrin*, the iron transport protein. Transferrin is a bilobed glycoprotein with two iron-binding sites. Transferrin that carries iron exists in two forms—*monoferric* (one iron atom) or *diferric* (two iron atoms). The turnover (half-clearance time) of transferrin-bound iron is very rapid—typically 60–90 min. Because almost all of the iron transported by transferrin is delivered to the erythroid marrow, the clearance time of transferrin-bound iron from the circulation is affected most by the plasma iron level and the erythroid marrow activity. When erythropoiesis is markedly stimulated, the pool of erythroid cells requiring iron increases, and the clearance time of iron from the circulation decreases. The half-clearance time of iron in the presence of iron deficiency is as short as 10–15 min. With suppression of erythropoiesis, the plasma iron level typically increases, and the half-clearance time may be prolonged to several hours. Normally, the iron bound to transferrin turns over 6–8 times per day. Assuming a normal plasma iron level of 80–100 μg/dL, the amount of iron passing through the transferrin pool is 20–24 mg/day.

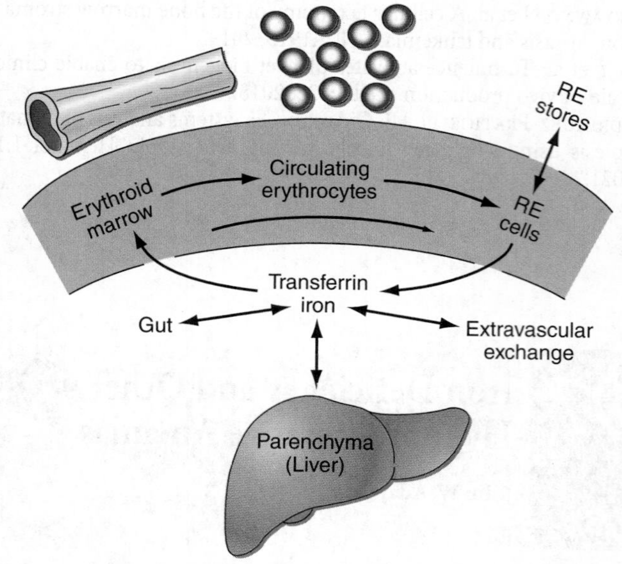

FIGURE 97-1 Internal iron exchange. Normally 80% of iron passing through the plasma transferrin pool is recycled from senescent red cells. Absorption of ~1 mg/d is required from the diet in men, and 1.4 mg/d in women to maintain homeostasis. As long as transferrin saturation is maintained between 20 and 60% and erythropoiesis is not increased, use of iron stores is not required. However, in the event of blood loss, dietary iron deficiency, or inadequate iron absorption, up to 40 mg/d of iron can be mobilized from stores. RE, reticuloendothelial.

The iron-transferrin complex circulates in the plasma until it interacts with specific *transferrin receptors* on the surface of marrow erythroid cells. Diferric transferrin has the highest affinity for transferrin receptors; apotransferrin (not carrying iron) has very little affinity. Although transferrin receptors are found on cells in many tissues within the body—and all cells at some time during development will display transferrin receptors—the cell having the greatest number of receptors (300,000–400,000/cell) is the developing erythroblast.

Once the iron-bearing transferrin interacts with its receptor, the complex is internalized via clathrin-coated pits and transported to an acidic endosome, where the iron is released at the low pH. The iron is then made available for heme synthesis while the transferrin-receptor complex is recycled to the surface of the cell, where the bulk of the transferrin is released back into circulation and the transferrin receptor re-anchors into the cell membrane. At this point, a certain amount of the transferrin receptor protein may be released into circulation and can be measured as soluble transferrin receptor protein. Within the erythroid cell, iron in excess of the amount needed for hemoglobin synthesis binds to a storage protein, *apoferritin*, forming *ferritin*. This mechanism of iron exchange also takes place in other cells of the body expressing transferrin receptors, especially liver parenchymal cells where the iron can be incorporated into heme-containing enzymes or stored. The iron incorporated into hemoglobin subsequently enters the circulation as new red cells are released from the bone marrow. The iron is then part of the red cell mass and will not become available for reutilization until the red cell dies.

In a normal individual, the average red cell life span is 120 days. Thus, 0.8–1% of red cells are replaced each day. At the end of its life span, the red cell is recognized as senescent by the cells of the *reticuloendothelial (RE) system*, and the red cell undergoes phagocytosis. Once within the RE cell, the ingested hemoglobin is broken down, the globin and other proteins are returned to the amino acid pool, and the iron is shuttled back to the surface of the RE cell, where it is presented to circulating transferrin via the iron export channel, ferroportin. It is the efficient and highly conserved recycling of iron from senescent red cells that supports steady-state (and even accelerated) erythropoiesis.

Because each milliliter of red cells contains 1 mg of elemental iron, the amount of iron needed to replace those red cells lost through senescence amounts to 20 mg/d (assuming an adult with a red cell mass of 2 L). Any additional iron required for daily red cell production comes from the diet. Normally, an adult male will need to absorb at least 1 mg of elemental iron daily to meet needs, while females in the childbearing years will need to absorb an average of 1.4 mg/d. However, to achieve a maximum proliferative erythroid marrow response to anemia, additional iron must be available. With markedly stimulated erythropoiesis, demands for iron are increased by as much as six- to eightfold. With extravascular hemolytic anemia, the rate of red cell destruction is increased, but the iron recovered from the red cells is efficiently reutilized for hemoglobin synthesis. In contrast, with intravascular hemolysis or blood loss anemia, the rate of red cell production is limited by the amount of iron that can be mobilized from stores. Typically, the rate of mobilization under these circumstances will not support red cell production more than 2.5 times normal. If the delivery of iron to the stimulated marrow is suboptimal, the marrow's proliferative response is blunted, and hemoglobin synthesis is impaired. The result is a hypoproliferative marrow accompanied by microcytic, hypochromic anemia.

Whereas blood loss or hemolysis places a demand on the iron supply, inflammatory conditions interfere with iron release from stores and can result in a rapid decrease in the serum iron (see below).

NUTRITIONAL IRON BALANCE

The balance of iron in humans is tightly controlled and designed to conserve iron for reutilization. There is no regulated excretory pathway for iron, and the only mechanisms by which iron is lost are blood loss (via gastrointestinal bleeding, menses, or other forms of bleeding) and the loss of epithelial cells from the skin, gut, and genitourinary tract. Normally, the only route by which iron comes into the body is via absorption from food or from medicinal iron taken orally. Iron may also enter the body through red cell transfusions or injection of iron complexes. The margin between the amount of iron available for absorption and the requirement for iron in growing infants and the adult female is narrow; this accounts for the great prevalence of iron deficiency worldwide—currently estimated at more than one billion people.

The amount of iron required from the diet to replace losses averages ~10% of body iron content a year in men and 15% in women of childbearing age. Dietary iron content is closely related to total caloric intake (~6 mg of elemental iron per 1000 calories). Iron bioavailability is affected by the nature of the foodstuff, with heme iron (e.g., red meat) being most readily absorbed. In the United States, the average iron intake in an adult male is 15 mg/d with 6% absorption; for the average female, the intake is 11 mg/d with 12% absorption. An individual with iron deficiency can increase iron absorption to ~20% of the iron present in a meat-containing diet but only 5–10% of the iron in a vegetarian diet. As a result, one-third of the female population in the United States has virtually no iron stores. Vegetarians are at an additional disadvantage because certain foodstuffs that include phytates and phosphates reduce iron absorption by ~50%. When ionizable iron salts are given together with food, the amount of iron absorbed is reduced. When the percentage of iron absorbed from individual food items is compared with the percentage for an equivalent amount of ferrous salt, iron in vegetables is only about one-twentieth as available, egg iron one-eighth, liver iron one-half, and heme iron one-half to two-thirds.

Infants, children, and adolescents may be unable to maintain normal iron balance because of the demands of body growth and lower dietary intake of iron. During the last two trimesters of pregnancy, daily iron requirements increase to 5–6 mg, and iron supplements are strongly recommended for pregnant women in developed countries.

Iron absorption takes place largely in the duodenum and proximal small intestine and is a carefully regulated process. For absorption, iron must be taken up by the luminal cell. That process is facilitated by the acidic contents of the stomach, which maintains the iron in solution. At the brush border of the absorptive cell, the ferric iron is converted to the ferrous form by a ferrireductase. Transport across the membrane is accomplished by divalent metal transporter type 1 (DMT-1, also known as natural resistance macrophage-associated protein type 2 [Nramp 2] or DCT-1). DMT-1 is a general cation transporter. Once inside the gut cell, iron may be stored as ferritin or transported through the cell to be released at the basolateral surface to plasma transferrin through the membrane-embedded iron exporter, ferroportin. The function of ferroportin is negatively regulated by hepcidin, the principal iron regulatory hormone. In the process of release, iron interacts with another ferroxidase, hephaestin, which oxidizes the iron to the ferric form for transferrin binding. Hephaestin is similar to ceruloplasmin, the copper-carrying protein.

Iron absorption is influenced by a number of physiologic states. Erythroid hyperplasia stimulates iron absorption even in the face of normal or increased iron stores, and hepcidin levels are inappropriately low. Thus, patients with anemias associated with high levels of ineffective erythropoiesis absorb excess amounts of dietary iron. The molecular mechanism underlying this is the production of erythroferrone (ERFE) by developing erythroblasts. ERFE suppresses hepcidin production, and over time, this may lead to iron overload and tissue damage. In iron deficiency, hepcidin levels are also low and iron is much more efficiently absorbed; the contrary is true in states of secondary iron overload. The normal individual can reduce iron absorption in situations of excessive intake or medicinal iron intake; however, while the percentage of iron absorbed goes down, the absolute amount goes up. This accounts for the acute iron toxicity occasionally seen when children ingest large numbers of iron tablets. Under these circumstances, the amount of iron absorbed exceeds the transferrin binding capacity of the plasma, resulting in free iron that affects critical organs such as cardiac muscle cells.

IRON-DEFICIENCY ANEMIA

Iron deficiency is one of the most prevalent forms of malnutrition. Globally, 50% of anemia is attributable to iron deficiency and accounts for approximately nearly a million deaths annually worldwide. Africa and parts of Asia bear 71% of the global mortality burden; North America represents only 1.4% of the total morbidity and mortality associated with iron deficiency.

STAGES OF IRON DEFICIENCY

The progression to iron deficiency can be divided into three stages (Fig. 97-2). The first stage is *negative iron balance*, in which the demands for (or losses of) iron exceed the body's ability to absorb iron from the diet. This stage results from a number of physiologic mechanisms, including blood loss, pregnancy (in which the demands for red cell production by the fetus outstrip the mother's ability to provide iron), rapid growth spurts in the adolescent, or inadequate dietary iron intake. Blood loss in excess of 10–20 mL of red cells per day is greater than the amount of iron that the gut can absorb from a normal diet. Under these circumstances, the iron deficit must be made up by mobilization of iron from RE storage sites. During this period, iron stores—reflected by the serum ferritin level or the appearance of stainable iron on bone marrow aspirations—decrease. As long as iron stores are present and can be mobilized, the serum iron, total iron-binding

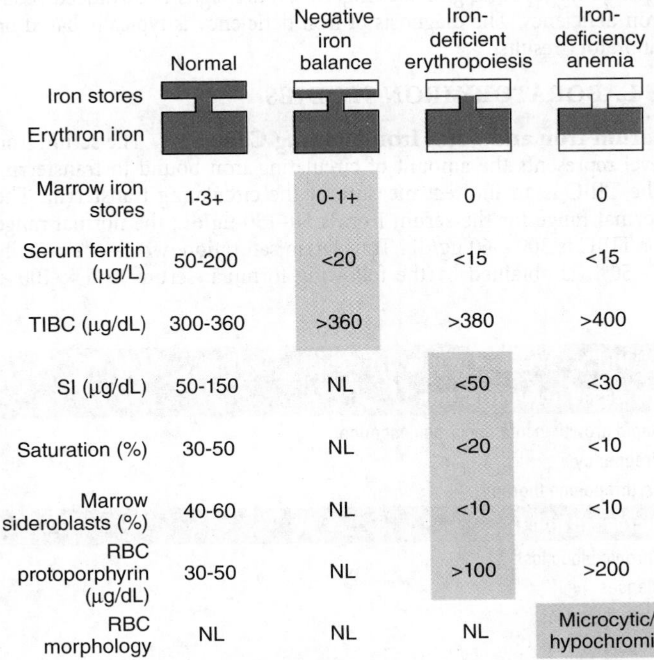

Normal
Negative iron balance
Iron-deficient erythropoiesis
Iron-deficiency anemia
Iron stores
Erythron iron
Marrow iron stores: 1-3+ | 0-1+ | 0 | 0
Serum ferritin (μg/L): 50-200 | <20 | <15 | <15
TIBC (μg/dL): 300-360 | >360 | >380 | >400
SI (μg/dL): 50-150 | NL | <50 | <30
Saturation (%): 30-50 | NL | <20 | <10
Marrow sideroblasts (%): 40-60 | NL | <10 | <10
RBC protoporphyrin (μg/dL): 30-50 | NL | >100 | >200
RBC morphology: NL | NL | NL | Microcytic/hypochromic

FIGURE 97-2 Laboratory studies in the evolution of iron deficiency. Measurements of marrow iron stores, serum ferritin, and total iron-binding capacity (TIBC) are sensitive to early iron-store depletion. Iron-deficient erythropoiesis is recognized from additional abnormalities in the serum iron (SI), percent transferrin saturation, the pattern of marrow sideroblasts, and the red blood cell (RBC) protoporphyrin level. Patients with iron-deficiency anemia demonstrate all the same abnormalities plus hypochromic microcytic anemia. *(Based on RS Hillman, CA Finch: The Red Cell Manual, 7th ed. Philadelphia, F.A. Davis and Co, 1996.)*

capacity (TIBC), and red cell protoporphyrin levels remain within normal limits. At this stage, red cell morphology and indices are normal.

When iron stores become depleted, the serum iron begins to fall. Gradually, the TIBC increases, as do red cell protoporphyrin levels. By definition, marrow iron stores are absent when the serum ferritin level is <15 μg/L. As long as the serum iron remains within the normal range, hemoglobin synthesis is unaffected despite the dwindling iron stores. Once the transferrin saturation falls to 15–20%, hemoglobin synthesis becomes impaired. This is a period of *iron-deficient erythropoiesis*. Careful evaluation of the peripheral blood smear reveals the first appearance of microcytic cells, and if the laboratory technology is available, one finds hypochromic reticulocytes in circulation. Gradually, the hemoglobin begins to fall, reflecting *iron-deficiency anemia*. The transferrin saturation at this point is <10–15%.

When moderate anemia is present (hemoglobin 10–13 g/dL), the bone marrow remains hypoproliferative. With more severe anemia (hemoglobin 7–8 g/dL), hypochromia and microcytosis become more prominent, target cells and misshapen red cells (poikilocytes) appear on the blood smear as cigar- or pencil-shaped forms, and the erythroid marrow becomes increasingly ineffective. Consequently, with severe prolonged iron-deficiency anemia, erythroid hyperplasia of the marrow develops, rather than hypoproliferation.

■ CAUSES OF IRON DEFICIENCY

Conditions that increase demand for iron, increase iron loss, or decrease iron intake or absorption can produce iron deficiency (**Table 97-2**).

■ CLINICAL PRESENTATION OF IRON DEFICIENCY

Certain clinical conditions carry an increased likelihood of iron deficiency. Pregnancy, adolescence, periods of rapid growth, and an intermittent history of blood loss of any kind should alert the clinician to possible iron deficiency. A cardinal rule is that the appearance of iron deficiency in an adult male or postmenopausal female means gastrointestinal blood loss until proven otherwise. Signs related to iron deficiency depend on the severity and chronicity of the anemia in addition to the usual signs of anemia—fatigue, pallor, and reduced exercise capacity. *Cheilosis* (fissures at the corners of the mouth) and *koilonychia* (spooning of the fingernails) are signs of advanced tissue iron deficiency. The diagnosis of iron deficiency is typically based on laboratory results.

■ LABORATORY IRON STUDIES

Serum Iron and Total Iron-Binding Capacity The serum iron level represents the amount of circulating iron bound to transferrin. The TIBC is an indirect measure of the circulating transferrin. The normal range for the serum iron is 50–150 μg/dL; the normal range for TIBC is 300–360 μg/dL. Transferrin saturation, which is normally 25–50%, is obtained by the following formula: serum iron × 100 ÷

TABLE 97-2 Causes of Iron Deficiency

Increased Demand for Iron
Rapid growth in infancy or adolescence
Pregnancy
Erythropoietin therapy
Increased Iron Loss
Chronic blood loss
Menses
Acute blood loss
Blood donation
Phlebotomy as treatment for polycythemia vera
Decreased Iron Intake or Absorption
Inadequate diet
Malabsorption from disease (sprue, Crohn's disease)
Malabsorption from surgery (gastrectomy and some forms of bariatric surgery)
Acute or chronic inflammation

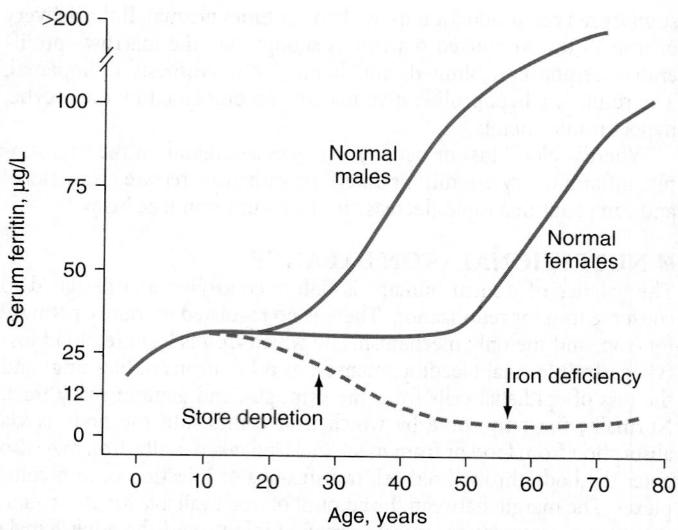

FIGURE 97-3 Serum ferritin levels as a function of sex and age. Iron store depletion and iron deficiency are accompanied by a decrease in serum ferritin level below 20 μg/L. *(Reproduced with permission from RS Hillman: Hematology in Clinical Practice, 5th ed. New York, McGraw-Hill, 2011.)*

TIBC. Iron-deficiency states are associated with saturation levels <20%. There is a diurnal variation in the serum iron. A transferrin saturation >50% indicates that a disproportionate amount of the iron bound to transferrin is being delivered to nonerythroid tissues. If this persists for an extended time, tissue iron overload may occur.

Serum Ferritin Free iron is toxic to cells, and the body has established an elaborate set of protective mechanisms to bind iron in various tissue compartments. Within cells, iron is stored complexed to protein as ferritin or hemosiderin. Apoferritin binds to free ferrous iron and stores it in the ferric state. As ferritin accumulates within cells of the RE system, protein aggregates are formed as hemosiderin. Iron in ferritin or hemosiderin can be extracted for release by the RE cells, although hemosiderin is less readily available. Under steady-state conditions, the serum ferritin level correlates with total body iron stores; thus, the serum ferritin level is the most convenient laboratory test to estimate iron stores. The normal value for ferritin varies according to the age and gender of the individual (**Fig. 97-3**). Adult males have serum ferritin values averaging 100 μg/L, while adult females have levels averaging 30 μg/L. As iron stores are depleted, the serum ferritin falls to <15 μg/L. Such levels are diagnostic of absent body iron stores.

Evaluation of Bone Marrow Iron Stores Although RE iron stores can be estimated from the iron stain of a bone marrow aspirate or biopsy, the measurement of serum ferritin has largely supplanted these procedures for determination of storage iron (**Table 97-3**). The serum ferritin level is a better indicator of iron overload than the marrow iron stain. However, in addition to storage iron, the marrow iron stain provides information about the effective delivery of iron to developing erythroblasts. Normally, when the marrow smear is stained for iron, 20–40% of developing erythroblasts—called *sideroblasts*—will have visible ferritin granules in their cytoplasm. This represents iron in excess of that needed for hemoglobin synthesis. In states in which

TABLE 97-3 Iron Store Measurements

IRON STORES	MARROW IRON STAIN, 0–4+	SERUM FERRITIN, μg/L
0	0	<15
1–300 mg	Trace to 1+	15–30
300–800 mg	2+	30–60
800–1000 mg	3+	60–150
1–2 g	4+	>150
Iron overload	—	>500–1000

release of iron from storage sites is blocked, RE iron will be detectable, and there will be few or no sideroblasts. In the myelodysplastic syndromes, mitochondrial dysfunction can occur, and accumulation of iron in mitochondria appears in a necklace fashion around the nucleus of the erythroblast. Such cells are referred to as *ring sideroblasts.*

Red Cell Protoporphyrin Levels Protoporphyrin is an intermediate in the pathway to heme synthesis. Under conditions in which heme synthesis is impaired, protoporphyrin accumulates within the red cell. This reflects an inadequate iron supply to erythroid precursors to support hemoglobin synthesis. Normal values are <30 μg/dL of red cells. In iron deficiency, values >100 μg/dL are seen. The most common causes of increased red cell protoporphyrin levels are absolute or relative iron deficiency and lead poisoning.

Serum Levels of Transferrin Receptor Protein Because erythroid cells have the highest numbers of transferrin receptors of any cell in the body, and because transferrin receptor protein (TRP) is released by cells into the circulation, serum levels of TRP reflect the total erythroid marrow mass. Another condition in which TRP levels are elevated is absolute iron deficiency. Normal values are 4–9 μg/L determined by immunoassay. This laboratory test is becoming increasingly available and, along with the serum ferritin, has been proposed to distinguish between iron deficiency and the anemia of inflammation (see below).

DIFFERENTIAL DIAGNOSIS

Other than iron deficiency, only three conditions need to be considered in the differential diagnosis of a hypochromic microcytic anemia **(Table 97-4)**. The first is an inherited defect in globin chain synthesis: the thalassemias. These are differentiated from iron deficiency most readily by serum iron values; normal or increased serum iron levels and transferrin saturation are characteristic of the thalassemias. In addition, the red blood cell distribution width (RDW) index is generally normal in thalassemia and elevated in iron deficiency.

The second condition is the anemia of inflammation (AI; also referred to as the anemia of chronic disease) with inadequate iron supply to the erythroid marrow. The distinction between true iron-deficiency anemia and AI is among the most common diagnostic problems encountered by clinicians (see below). Usually, AI is normocytic and normochromic. The iron values usually make the differential diagnosis clear, as the ferritin level is normal or increased and the percent transferrin saturation and TIBC are typically below normal.

Finally, the myelodysplastic syndromes represent the third and least common condition. Occasionally, patients with myelodysplasia have impaired hemoglobin synthesis with mitochondrial dysfunction, resulting in impaired iron incorporation into heme. The iron values again reveal normal stores and more than an adequate supply to the marrow, despite the microcytosis and hypochromia.

TREATMENT

Iron-Deficiency Anemia

The severity and cause of iron-deficiency anemia will determine the appropriate approach to treatment. As an example, symptomatic elderly patients with severe iron-deficiency anemia and cardiovascular instability may require red cell transfusions. Younger individuals who have compensated for their anemia can be treated more conservatively with iron replacement. The foremost issue for the latter patient is the precise identification of the cause of the iron deficiency.

For the majority of cases of iron deficiency (pregnant women, growing children and adolescents, patients with infrequent episodes of bleeding, and those with inadequate dietary intake of iron), oral iron therapy will suffice. For patients with unusual blood loss or malabsorption, specific diagnostic tests and appropriate therapy take priority. Once the diagnosis of iron-deficiency anemia and its cause is made, there are three major therapeutic approaches.

RED CELL TRANSFUSION

Transfusion therapy is reserved for individuals who have symptoms of anemia, cardiovascular instability, and continued and excessive blood loss from whatever source and who require immediate intervention. The management of these patients is less related to the iron deficiency than it is to the consequences of the severe anemia. Not only do transfusions correct the anemia acutely, but the transfused red cells provide a source of iron for reutilization, assuming they are not lost through continued bleeding. Transfusion therapy will stabilize the patient while other options are reviewed.

ORAL IRON THERAPY

In the asymptomatic patient with established iron-deficiency anemia and an intact gastrointestinal tract, treatment with oral iron is usually adequate. Encouraging dietary intake of iron-rich foods is also useful. Such foods include oysters, kidney beans, beef liver, tofu, beef (chuck roast, lean ground beef), turkey leg, whole-wheat bread, tuna, eggs, shrimp, peanut butter, leg of lamb, brown rice, raisin bran (whole grain–enriched cereals), lentils, and beans. Multiple preparations of oral iron supplements are available, ranging from simple iron salts to complex iron compounds designed for sustained release throughout the small intestine **(Table 97-5)**. Although the various preparations contain different amounts of iron, they are generally all absorbed well and are effective in treatment. Some come with other compounds designed to enhance iron absorption, such as ascorbic acid. It is not clear whether the benefits of such compounds justify their costs. Typically, for iron replacement therapy, up to 200 mg of elemental iron per day is given, usually

TABLE 97-5 Oral Iron Preparations

GENERIC NAME	TABLET (IRON CONTENT), mg	ELIXIR (IRON CONTENT), mg IN 5 mL
Ferrous sulfate	325 (65) 195 (39)	300 (60) 90 (18)
Extended release	525 (105)	
Ferrous fumarate	325 (107) 195 (64)	 100 (33)
Ferrous gluconate	325 (39)	300 (35)
Polysaccharide iron	150 (150) 50 (50)	100 (100)

TABLE 97-4 Diagnosis of Microcytic Anemia

TESTS	IRON DEFICIENCY	INFLAMMATION	THALASSEMIA	SIDEROBLASTIC ANEMIA
Smear	Micro/hypo	Normal micro/hypo	Micro/hypo with targeting	Variable
Serum iron (μg/dL)	<30	<50	Normal to high	Normal to high
TIBC (μg/dL)	>360	<300	Normal	Normal
Percent saturation	<10	10–20	30–80	30–80
Ferritin (μg/L)	<15	30–200	50–300	50–300
Hemoglobin pattern on electrophoresis	Normal	Normal	Abnormal with β thalassemia; can be normal with α thalassemia	Normal

Abbreviation: TIBC, total iron-binding capacity.

as three or four iron tablets (each containing 50–65 mg elemental iron) given over the course of the day. Ideally, oral iron preparations should be taken on an empty stomach, since food may inhibit iron absorption. Some patients with gastric disease or prior gastric surgery require special treatment with iron solutions because the retention capacity of the stomach may be reduced. The retention capacity is necessary for dissolving the shell of the iron tablet before the release of iron. A dose of 200 mg of elemental iron per day should result in the absorption of iron up to 50 mg/d. This supports a red cell production level of two to three times normal in an individual with a normally functioning marrow and appropriate erythropoietin (EPO) stimulus. However, as the hemoglobin level rises, EPO stimulation decreases, and the amount of iron absorbed is reduced. The goal of therapy in individuals with iron-deficiency anemia is not only to repair the anemia, but also to provide stores of at least 0.5–1 g of iron. Sustained treatment for a period of 6–12 months after correction of the anemia will be necessary to achieve this.

Of the complications of oral iron therapy, gastrointestinal distress is the most prominent and is seen in at least 15–20% of patients. Abdominal pain, nausea, vomiting, or constipation may lead to noncompliance. Although small doses of iron or iron preparations with delayed release may help somewhat, the gastrointestinal side effects are a major impediment to the effective treatment of a number of patients.

The response to iron therapy varies, depending on the EPO stimulus and the rate of absorption. Typically, the reticulocyte count should begin to increase within 4–7 days after initiation of therapy and peak at 1–1½ weeks. The absence of a response may be due to poor absorption, noncompliance (which is common), or a confounding diagnosis. A useful test in the clinic to determine the patient's ability to absorb iron is the *iron tolerance test*. Two iron tablets are given to the patient on an empty stomach, and the serum iron is measured serially over the subsequent 2–3 h. Normal absorption will result in an increase in the serum iron of at least 100 μg/dL. If iron deficiency persists despite adequate treatment, it may be necessary to switch to parenteral iron therapy.

PARENTERAL IRON THERAPY

Intravenous iron can be given to patients who are unable to tolerate oral iron; whose needs are relatively acute; or who need iron on an ongoing basis, usually due to persistent gastrointestinal or menstrual blood loss. Parenteral iron use has been increasing rapidly over the past several years with the recognition that recombinant EPO therapy induces a large demand for iron—a demand that frequently cannot be met through the physiologic release of iron from RE sources or oral iron absorption. The safety of parenteral iron has been a concern largely driven by the high adverse reaction rate to high-molecular-weight iron dextran. The newer iron complexes that are available, such as ferumoxytol (Feraheme), sodium ferric gluconate (Ferrlecit), iron sucrose (Venofer), low-molecular-weight (LMW) iron dextran (InFed), ferric derisomaltose (Monoferric), and ferric carboxymaltose (Injectafer), have much lower rates of adverse effects. Ferumoxytol delivers 510 mg of iron per infusion; ferric gluconate 125 mg per infusion; LMW iron dextran up to 1500 mg per infusion; ferric carboxymaltose 750 mg per infusion; ferric derisomaltose 1000 mg per infusion; and iron sucrose 200 mg per infusion.

Parenteral iron is used in two ways: one is to administer the total dose of iron required to correct the hemoglobin deficit and provide the patient with at least 500 mg of iron stores; the second is to give repeated small doses of parenteral iron over a protracted period. The latter approach is common in dialysis centers, where it is not unusual for 100 mg of elemental iron to be given weekly for 10 weeks to augment the response to recombinant EPO therapy. The amount of iron needed by an individual patient is calculated by the following formula:

$$\text{Body weight (kg)} \times 2.3 \times (15 - \text{patient's hemoglobin, g/dL}) + 500 \text{ or } 1000 \text{ mg (for stores)}$$

In administering any intravenous iron preparation, anaphylaxis is a concern. Anaphylaxis is much rarer with the newer preparations. The factors that have correlated with an anaphylactic-like reaction include a history of multiple allergies or a prior allergic reaction to an iron preparation. Generalized symptoms appearing several days after the infusion of a large dose of iron can include arthralgias, skin rash, and low-grade fever. These may be dose-related, but they do not preclude the further use of parenteral iron in the patient. To date, patients with sensitivity to one iron preparation have been safely treated with other parenteral iron preparations. If a large dose of LMW iron dextran is to be given (>100 mg), the iron preparation should be diluted in 5% dextrose in water or 0.9% NaCl solution. The iron solution can then be infused over a 60- to 90-min period (for larger doses) or at a rate convenient for the attending nurse or physician. Although a test dose (25 mg) of parenteral LMW iron dextran is recommended, in reality, a slow infusion of a larger dose of parenteral iron solution will afford the same kind of early warning as a separately injected test dose. Early in the infusion of iron, if chest pain, wheezing, a fall in blood pressure, or other systemic symptoms occur, the infusion of iron should be stopped immediately.

OTHER HYPOPROLIFERATIVE ANEMIAS

In addition to mild to moderate iron-deficiency anemia, the hypoproliferative anemias can be divided into four categories: (1) chronic inflammation, (2) renal disease, (3) endocrine and nutritional deficiencies (hypometabolic states), and (4) marrow damage (**Chap. 102**). With chronic inflammation, renal disease, or hypometabolism, endogenous EPO production is inadequate for the degree of anemia observed. For the anemia of chronic inflammation, the erythroid marrow also responds inadequately to stimulation, due in part to defective *iron reutilization*. As a result of the lack of adequate EPO stimulation, an examination of the peripheral blood smear will disclose only an occasional polychromatophilic ("shift") reticulocyte. In cases of iron deficiency or marrow damage, appropriate elevations in endogenous EPO levels are typically found, and shift reticulocytes will be present on the blood smear.

ANEMIA OF ACUTE AND CHRONIC INFLAMMATION/INFECTION (AI)

AI, which encompasses inflammation, infection, tissue injury, and conditions (e.g., cancer) associated with the release of proinflammatory cytokines, is one of the most common forms of anemia seen clinically. It is the most important anemia in the differential diagnosis of iron deficiency because many of the features of the anemia are brought about by inadequate iron delivery to the marrow, despite the presence of normal or increased iron stores. This is reflected by a low serum iron, increased red cell protoporphyrin, a hypoproliferative marrow, transferrin saturation in the range of 15–20%, and a normal or increased serum ferritin. The serum ferritin values are often the most distinguishing features between true iron-deficiency anemia and the iron-restricted erythropoiesis associated with inflammation. Typically, serum ferritin values increase threefold over basal levels in the face of inflammation. These changes are due to the effects of inflammatory cytokines and hepcidin, the key iron regulatory hormone, acting at several levels of erythropoiesis (**Fig. 97-4**).

Interleukin 1 (IL-1) directly decreases EPO production in response to anemia. IL-1, acting through accessory cell release of interferon γ (IFN-γ), suppresses the response of the erythroid marrow to EPO—an effect that can be overcome by EPO administration in vitro and in vivo. In addition, tumor necrosis factor (TNF), acting through the release of IFN-β by marrow stromal cells, also suppresses the response to EPO. Hepcidin, made by the liver, is increased in inflammation via an IL-6–mediated pathway, and acts to suppress iron absorption and iron release from storage sites. The overall result is a chronic hypoproliferative anemia with classic changes in iron metabolism. The anemia is further compounded by a mild to moderate shortening in red cell survival.

With chronic inflammation, the primary disease will determine the severity and characteristics of the anemia. For example, many

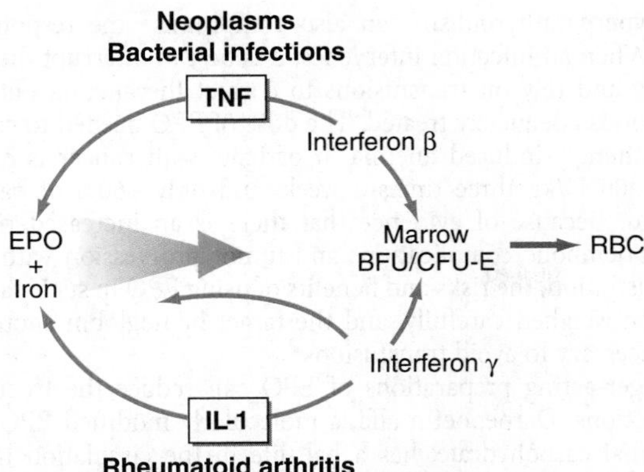

FIGURE 97-4 Suppression of erythropoiesis by inflammatory cytokines. Through the release of tumor necrosis factor (TNF) and interferon β (IFN-β), neoplasms and bacterial infections suppress erythropoietin (EPO) production and the proliferation of erythroid progenitors (erythroid burst-forming units and erythroid colony-forming units [BFU/CFU-E]). The mediators in patients with vasculitis and rheumatoid arthritis include interleukin 1 (IL-1) and IFN-γ. The *red arrows* indicate sites of inflammatory cytokine inhibitory effects. RBC, red blood cell.

patients with cancer also have anemia that is typically normocytic and normochromic. In contrast, patients with long-standing active rheumatoid arthritis or chronic infections such as tuberculosis will have a microcytic, hypochromic anemia. In both cases, the bone marrow is hypoproliferative, but the differences in red cell indices reflect differences in the availability of iron for hemoglobin synthesis. Occasionally, conditions associated with chronic inflammation are also associated with chronic blood loss. Under these circumstances, the measurement of soluble transferrin receptor protein may be necessary to rule out absolute iron deficiency. However, the administration of iron in this case will correct the iron-deficiency component of the anemia and leave the inflammatory component unaffected.

The anemia associated with acute infection or inflammation is typically mild but becomes more pronounced over time. Acute infection can produce a decrease in hemoglobin levels of 2–3 g/dL within 1 or 2 days; this is largely related to the hemolysis of red cells near the end of their natural life span. The fever and cytokines released exert a selective pressure against cells with more limited capacity to maintain the red cell membrane. In most individuals, the mild anemia is reasonably well tolerated, and symptoms, if present, are associated with the underlying disease. Occasionally, in patients with preexisting cardiac disease, moderate anemia (hemoglobin 10–11 g/dL) may be associated with angina, exercise intolerance, and shortness of breath. The erythropoietic profile that distinguishes the anemia of inflammation from the other causes of hypoproliferative anemias is shown in Table 97-6.

ANEMIA OF CHRONIC KIDNEY DISEASE (CKD)

Progressive CKD is usually associated with a moderate to severe hypoproliferative anemia; the level of the anemia correlates with the stage of CKD. Red cells are typically normocytic and normochromic, and reticulocytes are decreased. The anemia is primarily due to a failure of EPO production by the diseased kidney and a reduction in red cell survival. In certain forms of acute renal failure, the correlation between the anemia and renal function is weaker. Patients with the hemolytic-uremic syndrome increase erythropoiesis in response to the hemolysis, despite renal failure. Polycystic kidney disease also shows a smaller degree of EPO deficiency for a given level of renal failure. By contrast, patients with diabetes or myeloma have more severe EPO deficiency for a given level of renal failure.

Assessment of iron status provides information to distinguish the anemia of CKD from the other forms of hypoproliferative anemia (Table 97-6) and to guide management. Patients with the anemia of CKD usually present with normal serum iron, TIBC, and ferritin levels. However, those maintained on chronic hemodialysis may develop iron deficiency from blood loss through the dialysis procedure. Iron must be replenished in these patients to ensure an adequate response to EPO therapy (see below).

ANEMIA IN HYPOMETABOLIC STATES

Patients who are starving, particularly for protein, and those with a variety of endocrine disorders that produce lower metabolic rates, may develop a mild to moderate hypoproliferative anemia. The release of EPO from the kidney is sensitive to the need for O_2, not just O_2 levels. Thus, EPO production is triggered at lower levels of blood O_2 content in disease states (e.g., hypothyroidism and starvation) where metabolic activity, and thus O_2 demand, is decreased.

Endocrine Deficiency States The difference in the levels of hemoglobin between men and women is related to the effects of androgen and estrogen on erythropoiesis. Testosterone and anabolic steroids augment erythropoiesis; castration and estrogen administration to males decrease erythropoiesis. Patients who are hypothyroid or have deficits in pituitary hormones also may develop a mild anemia. Pathogenesis may be complicated by other nutritional deficiencies because iron and folic acid absorption can be affected by these disorders. Usually, correction of the hormone deficiency reverses the anemia.

Anemia may be more severe in Addison's disease, depending on the level of thyroid and androgen hormone dysfunction; however, anemia may be masked by decreases in plasma volume. Once such patients are given cortisol and volume replacement, the hemoglobin level may fall rapidly. Mild anemia complicating hyperparathyroidism may be due to decreased EPO production as a consequence of the renal effects of hypercalcemia or to impaired proliferation of erythroid progenitors.

Protein Starvation Decreased dietary intake of protein may lead to mild to moderate hypoproliferative anemia; this form of anemia may be prevalent in the elderly. The anemia can be more severe in patients with a greater degree of starvation. In marasmus, where patients are both protein- and calorie-deficient, the release of EPO is impaired in proportion to the reduction in metabolic rate; however, the degree of anemia may be masked by volume depletion and becomes apparent after refeeding. Deficiencies in other nutrients (iron, folate) may also complicate the clinical picture but may not be apparent at diagnosis. Changes in the erythrocyte indices on refeeding should prompt evaluation of iron, folate, and B_{12} status.

Anemia in Liver Disease A mild hypoproliferative anemia may develop in patients with chronic liver disease from nearly any cause. The peripheral blood smear may show spur cells and stomatocytes

TABLE 97-6 Diagnosis of Hypoproliferative Anemias

TESTS	IRON DEFICIENCY	INFLAMMATION	RENAL DISEASE	HYPOMETABOLIC STATES
Anemia	Mild to severe	Mild	Mild to severe	Mild
MCV (fL)	60–90	80–90	90	90
Morphology	Normo-microcytic	Normocytic	Normocytic	Normocytic
SI (μg/dL)	<30	<50	Normal	Normal
TIBC (μg/dL)	>360	<300	Normal	Normal
Saturation (%)	<10	10–20	Normal	Normal
Serum ferritin (μg/L)	<15	30–200	115–150	Normal
Iron stores	0	2–4+	1–4+	Normal

Abbreviations: MCV, mean corpuscular volume; SI, serum iron; TIBC, total iron-binding capacity.

from the accumulation of excess cholesterol in the membrane from a deficiency of lecithin-cholesterol acyltransferase. Red cell survival is shortened, and the production of EPO is inadequate to compensate. In alcoholic liver disease, nutritional deficiencies are common and complicate the management. Folate deficiency from inadequate intake, as well as iron deficiency from blood loss and inadequate intake, can alter the red cell indices.

ANEMIA IN AGING

Anemia is common in people over age 65 years. It has been estimated to affect ~11% of community-living older adults and up to 40% of nursing home residents. In at least one-third of these anemic people, a cause for the anemia is not found. Patients with the unexplained anemia of aging do not have nutrient deficiency or renal dysfunction, and although older people can have an increase in systemic inflammatory cytokines (the inflammation of aging), the levels are not high enough to mimic the anemia of chronic inflammation. If hepcidin levels are elevated at all, they are minimally so.

Investigations into the cause(s) of this form of anemia have noted that EPO levels are generally in the normal range, that is, they are inappropriately low for the hemoglobin level. In general, in older people who maintain a normal hemoglobin level, EPO levels increase with age. This compensatory increase to maintain normal oxygen delivery seems to be due to a relative resistance to EPO stimulation; studies of red cell life span in older people have not noted a decrease in red cell survival. More data on the mechanism are needed.

The importance of this unexplained anemia of aging is that low hemoglobin levels are associated with increases in falls, hospitalizations, development of frailty, and mortality. It is not clear whether reversing the anemia would influence these increased risks. Anecdotal evidence suggests that this form of anemia is responsive to exogenous EPO.

TREATMENT

Hypoproliferative Anemias

Many patients with hypoproliferative anemias experience recovery of normal hemoglobin levels when the underlying disease is appropriately treated. For those in whom such reversals are not possible—such as patients with end-stage kidney disease, cancer, and chronic inflammatory diseases—symptomatic anemia requires treatment. The two major forms of treatment are transfusions and EPO.

TRANSFUSIONS

Thresholds for transfusion should be determined based on the patient's symptoms. In general, patients without serious underlying cardiovascular or pulmonary disease can tolerate hemoglobin levels above 7–8 g/dL and do not require intervention until the hemoglobin falls below that level. Patients with more physiologic compromise may need to have their hemoglobin levels kept above 11 g/dL. Usually, a unit of packed red cells increases the hemoglobin level by 1 g/dL. Transfusions are associated with certain infectious risks **(Chap. 113)**, and chronic transfusions can produce iron overload. Importantly, the liberal use of blood has been associated with increased morbidity and mortality, particularly in the intensive care setting. Therefore, in the absence of documented tissue hypoxia, a conservative approach to the use of red cell transfusions is preferable.

ERYTHROPOIETIN

EPO is particularly useful in anemias in which endogenous EPO levels are inappropriately low, such as CKD or AI. Iron status must be evaluated and iron replaced to obtain optimal effects from EPO. In patients with CKD, the usual dose of EPO is 50–150 U/kg three times a week intravenously. Hemoglobin levels of 10–12 g/dL are usually reached within 4–6 weeks if iron levels are adequate; 90% of these patients respond. Once a target hemoglobin level is achieved, the EPO dose can be decreased. A decrease in hemoglobin level occurring in the face of EPO therapy usually signifies the development of an infection or iron depletion. Aluminum toxicity and hyperparathyroidism can also compromise the response to EPO. When an infection intervenes, it is best to interrupt the EPO therapy and rely on transfusions to correct the anemia until the infection is adequately treated. The dose of EPO needed to correct chemotherapy-induced anemia in patients with cancer is higher, up to 300 U/kg three times a week, and only ~60% of patients respond. Because of evidence that there is an increased risk of thromboembolic complications and tumor progression with EPO administration, the risks and benefits of using EPO in such patients must be weighed carefully, and the target hemoglobin should be that necessary to avoid transfusions.

Longer-acting preparations of EPO can reduce the frequency of injections. Darbepoetin alfa, a molecularly modified EPO with additional carbohydrate, has a half-life in the circulation that is three to four times longer than recombinant human EPO, permitting weekly or every other week dosing.

Orally bioavailable EPO mimetics such as roxadustat (usual dose 50 mg PO thrice weekly) that act to increase the biological half-life of active hypoxia-inducible factor (HIF) are demonstrating activity to increase hemoglobin levels in patients with chronic renal disease and other settings.

FURTHER READING

Andrews N: Forging a field. The golden age of iron biology. Blood 112:219, 2008.

Auerbach M, Adamson J: How we diagnose and treat iron deficiency anemia. Am J Hematol 91:31, 2016.

Drüeke T, Parfrey P: Summary of the KDIGO guideline on anemia and comment: Reading between the (guide)line(s). Kidney Int 82:952, 2012.

Ganz T: Anemia of inflammation. N Engl J Med 381:1149, 2019.

Kautz L et al: Identification of erythroferrone as an erythroid regulator of iron metabolism. Nat Genet 46:678, 2014.

Krayenbuehl P-A et al: Intravenous iron for the treatment of fatigue in non-anemic, premenopausal woman with low serum ferritin concentration. Blood 118:3222, 2011.

Punnonen K et al: Serum transferrin receptor and its ratio to serum ferritin in the diagnosis of iron deficiency. Blood 89:1052; 1997.

98 Disorders of Hemoglobin

Martin H. Steinberg

Hemoglobinopathies affect the amino acid sequence of globin; thalassemia is a disorder of reduced globin biosynthesis. Together, these disorders of the hemoglobin molecule are our most common Mendelian genetic diseases. They are responsible for most cases of hemolytic anemia. Sickle cell disease and the hemoglobin E (HbE)–associated syndromes are the most prevalent hemoglobinopathies; β and α thalassemia are the most prevalent thalassemias. In addition to these common disorders of hemoglobin, rare globin mutations can cause hemoglobin instability, increased or decreased affinity of hemoglobin for oxygen (O_2), and oxidized hemoglobin reducing O_2 transport. O_2 transport by hemoglobin can also be reduced by exposure to carbon monoxide (CO) and some oxidizing agents **(Table 98-1)**.

Phenotypic diversity among hemoglobin disorders is enormous. Mutations can be asymptomatic, for example in heterozygous carriers of sickle hemoglobin (HbS) and thalassemia, or cause intrauterine death as when all α-globin genes are deleted. Impressive gains in understanding the biological basis of hemoglobinopathies and thalassemia have led to novel therapeutics with the promise of improved patient outcomes.

TABLE 98-1 Disorders of Hemoglobin
I. **Hemoglobinopathies**—hemoglobin variants with amino acid sequence variants that alter the physical, chemical, or functional properties of hemoglobin
A. Common variants with unusual properties
1. HbS—polymerization
2. HbE—reduced biosynthesis
3. HbC—hemoglobin-membrane interaction
B. Altered oxygen affinity
1. High affinity—erythrocytosis
2. Low affinity—cyanosis, anemia
C. Hemoglobins that oxidize readily
1. Unstable hemoglobins—hemolytic anemia, jaundice
2. M hemoglobins—methemoglobinemia, cyanosis
II. **Thalassemias**—defective biosynthesis of globin chains
A. α Thalassemias
B. β Thalassemias
C. Complex thalassemias
III. **Hereditary persistence of fetal hemoglobin**—persistence of higher than normal levels of HbF into adult life
A. Deletions within the *HBB* cluster—15–30% HbF in heterozygotes, pancellular
B. Point mutations in *HBG2/1* promoters—5–30% HbF in heterozygotes; pancellular or heterocellular
IV. **Acquired hemoglobinopathies**
A. Methemoglobin due to toxic exposures
B. Sulfhemoglobin due to toxic exposures
C. Carboxyhemoglobin
D. HbH in erythroleukemia
E. Elevated HbF in myelodysplasia

HEMOGLOBIN

Easy access to erythrocytes to study hemoglobin structure and function, reticulocytes to examine hemoglobin biosynthesis, and leukocyte DNA to define the mutations of hemoglobin and the availability of hematopoietic stem and progenitor cells from blood and bone marrow have placed hemoglobin disorders in the forefront of molecular medicine. A review of the biology of hemoglobin provides the background for understanding the pathophysiology of its many genetic and acquired disorders and approaches to their treatment.

DEVELOPMENTAL BIOLOGY

Successive waves of erythropoiesis beginning in the yolk sac, moving to the fetal liver and bone marrow, and culminating in the adult marrow direct the synthesis of different hemoglobin molecules that result from sequential activation and silencing of the globin genes (**Fig. 98-1**).

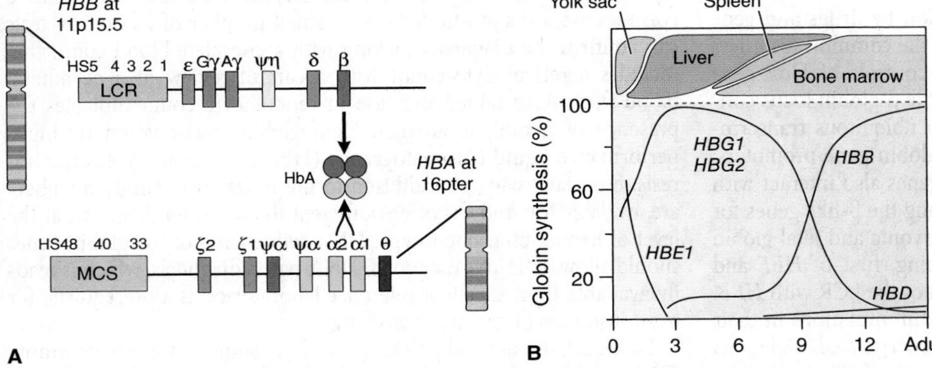

FIGURE 98-1 Globin gene clusters and their hemoglobin products during gestation. ***A.*** The order of globin genes in the β- and α-globin gene clusters along with their upstream enhancers, the locus control region (LCR) and multispecies conserved sequences (MCS). Normal hemoglobin tetramers contain two α-globin chains and two non-α-globin chains. In the example shown, this is adult HbA. ***B.*** Sites of erythropoiesis and globin synthesized from the yolk sac and the early embryo (months 1–3), the fetus (months 3–9), after delivery (months 9–12), and afterward (adult).

Hemoglobin is a tetramer of two pairs of unlike globin polypeptide chains, each chain containing a tetrapyrrole heme group. O_2 binds to heme as erythrocytes traverse the lungs and is released in the tissues. Heme is nestled within a protective pocket of each globin subunit.

GLOBIN GENE CLUSTERS

Globin is encoded in two nonallelic gene clusters. The β-globin gene cluster is on the short arm of chromosome 11 (11p15.4); the α-globin gene cluster is on chromosome 16 (16p13.3) (Fig. 98-1). The β-globin gene cluster contains an embryonic ε-globin gene (*HBE*), two nearly identical fetal γ-globin genes (*HBG2, HBG1*) a major adult β-globin gene (*HBB*), and a minor adult δ-globin gene (*HBD*). The α-globin gene cluster contains an embryonic ζ-globin gene (*HBZ*) and duplicated α-globin genes (*HBA2, HBA1*) with identical proteins. Embryonic hemoglobins include Gower I ($\zeta_2\varepsilon_2$), Gower II ($\alpha_2\varepsilon_2$), Portland I ($\zeta_2\gamma_2$), and Portland II ($\zeta_2\beta_2$). Fetal hemoglobin (HbF, $\alpha_2\gamma_2$) production begins at 6–8 weeks' gestation, peaks during mid-gestation, then falls to <1% of total hemoglobin during the first 6 months of extrauterine life. Adult hemoglobin A (HbA; $\alpha_2\beta_2$) production follows a pattern reciprocal to that of HbF. The hemoglobin composition of normal adults is >95% HbA, ~1% HbF, and 2–3% HbA_2 ($\alpha_2\delta_2$). In adults, HbF and HbA_2 have little functional significance because of their low concentrations, although they can be diagnostically important. Hemoglobin is also subject to posttranslational modifications, the most important being the nonenzymatic glycosylation of HbA forming the adduct HbA_{1c}, which is of diagnostic utility in the management of diabetes mellitus.

HEMOGLOBIN STRUCTURE

All globin polypeptides have similar but not identical primary structures. α-Globins contain 141 amino acids, and β-like globins have 146 amino acids. This primary structure dictates, according to the constraints of protein folding, the secondary structure of globin into α-helical sections joined by small nonhelical stretches. Each globin chain folds into a tertiary conformation known as the globin fold, whereby charged amino acid residues face the exterior of the molecules and uncharged residues face the hydrophobic interior. The iron-containing tetrapyrrole heme moiety is protected from oxidation and located between two of the helical segments; O_2 loading and unloading occur when heme iron is in its reduced ferrous form. Globin gene mutations affecting critical heme-binding amino acid residues allows iron to be oxidized, forming methemoglobin, which has high O_2 affinity and does not release O_2 in tissues. Dimers of α- and non-α-globin chains reversibly assemble into tetramers, forming a quaternary structure.

HEMOGLOBIN FUNCTION

Hemoglobin transports O_2 from lungs to tissues and carbon dioxide (CO_2) from tissues to lungs and is a nitrate reductase that releases nitric oxide (NO) from nitrite to promote vasodilation. Oxygen binding is defined by the sigmoidal shape of the hemoglobin-O_2 dissociation curve. P_{50} is a point on this curve that indicates the partial pressure of O_2 where hemoglobin is half saturated (**Fig. 98-2**). The P_{50} is influenced by the binding of 2,3-bisphosphoglycerate, a product of glycolysis, in the central cavity of hemoglobin, and by pH and temperature. Normal P_{50} is ~26 mmHg; low P_{50} indicates that hemoglobin has high O_2 affinity, decreasing O_2 delivery to tissues; high P_{50} indicates that hemoglobin has low O_2 affinity, releasing more O_2 to tissues. The conformation of hemoglobin fully saturated with O_2 is known as the R or relaxed state; desaturated hemoglobin is in the T or tense state. The transition between T and R states occurs when two or three O_2 molecules are bound. Cooperativity describes the progressively more rapid binding of O_2 once the first molecule

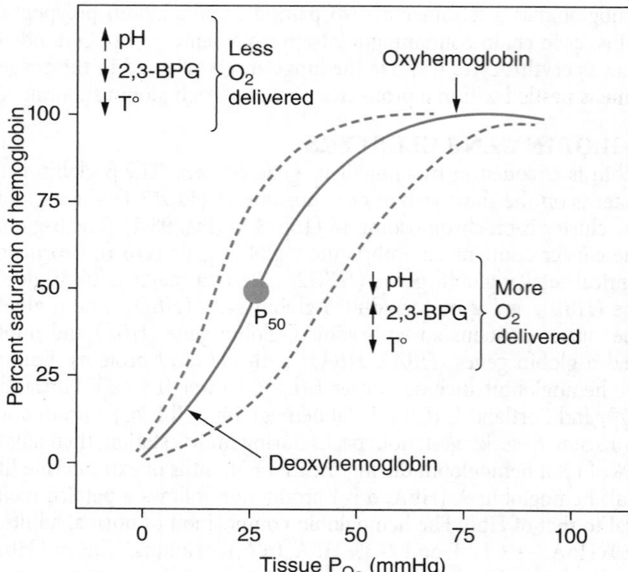

FIGURE 98-2 Hemoglobin-oxygen dissociation curve. The hemoglobin tetramer can bind up to four molecules of oxygen (O_2) in the iron-containing sites of the heme molecules. As O_2 is bound, 2,3-bisphosphoglycerate (2,3-BPG) and carbon dioxide (CO_2) are expelled. Salt bridges are broken, and each of the globin molecules changes its conformation to facilitate O_2 binding. O_2 release to the tissues is the reverse process, with salt bridges being formed and 2,3-BPG and CO_2 bound. Deoxyhemoglobin does not bind O_2 efficiently until the cell returns to conditions of higher pH, the most important modulator of O_2 affinity (Bohr effect). When acid is produced in the tissues, the dissociation curve shifts to the right, facilitating O_2 release and CO_2 binding. Alkalosis has the opposite effect, reducing O_2 delivery.

is bound. Hemoglobin variants that decrease P_{50} are characterized by isolated erythrocytosis as compensation for hypoxia; variants with increased P_{50} sometimes are accompanied by cyanosis and anemia as hemoglobin becomes unsaturated and O_2 delivery is enhanced. Mutations of residues critical for heme binding, R-T transitions, or tetramer stability cause hemoglobinopathies characterized by hemolytic anemia, methemoglobinemia, erythrocytosis and cyanosis.

GLOBIN GENE SWITCHING

The sequential activation and inactivation of globin genes during development shown in Fig. 98-1 is called "hemoglobin switching." Transcription factors along with epigenetic elements such as DNA methyltransferases and demethylases, interact with enhancers "upstream" of the β-globin gene cluster that contact globin gene promoters, silencing the embryonic and fetal genes. Activation of fetal globin gene repressors during development allows expression of the adult genes. Developmental factors such as RNA-binding factors and microRNAs also impact hemoglobin switching.

β-Globin Gene Switching HbF reactivation by drugs and gene therapy is a prime therapeutic goal for treating the common disorders of hemoglobin, meriting a discussion of the controls of HbF gene silencing. An upstream super-enhancer called the β-globin locus control region (LCR) binds erythroid-specific and ubiquitous transcription factors. The LCR interacts directly with globin gene promoters; transcription factors that silence and activate genes also interact with elements of the globin genes. Competition among the β-like genes for the LCR and autonomous silencing of the embryonic and fetal globin genes depends on transcription factors. Silencing, first of *HBE* and then of *HBG2* and *HBG1*, favors the interaction of the LCR with *HBB*. When *HBG2* or *HBG1* is upregulated by rare point mutations in their promoters, expression of the linked *HBB* is downregulated. Deletions of the *HBB* promoter remove competition for the LCR, increasing the expression of *HBG2*, *HBG1*, and *HBD*. The transcription factors BCL11A (2p16) and ZBTB7A (19p13) silence the HbF genes; BCL11A binds to the HbF gene promoters, repressing them and silencing transcription; ZBTB7A binds upstream of BCL11A with similar repressive effects. This accounts for the bulk of the switch from HbF to HbA. Mutations in these binding sites abolish the normal silencing of the HbF genes, leading to one type of the benign condition called hereditary persistence of fetal hemoglobin (HPFH). Disruption of the *BCL11A* regulatory elements or the binding sites for BCL11A by gene editing is a prime therapeutic target for HbF induction.

α-Globin Gene Switching A less complex switch takes place in the α-globin gene cluster where a regulatory locus of four elements termed R1–R4 is present within introns of the gene *NPRL3* that is upstream of *HBA2*. A developmental switch from embryonic ζ- to adult α-globin gene expression occurs at about 6 weeks' gestation.

Modulation of HbF Level Variations in three quantitative trait loci (QTL), *BCL11A*, *MYB* (6q23), and a locus linked to the *HBB* cluster, account for a major portion of HbF variation among normal individuals and patients with sickle cell anemia and β thalassemia. BCL11A, a zinc finger protein that represses HbF genes, binds TGACCA motifs, the most important at position –115 in the promoter of each γ-globin gene. ZBTB7A binds 85 nucleotides upstream of these BCL11A binding sites; its binding also represses γ-globin gene transcription. When binding of either BCL11A or ZBTB7A is disrupted, silencing of *HBG2* and *HBG1* is abrogated. The unique impact of *BCL11A* variants on HbF in sickle cell anemia and β thalassemia is due their large effect and the high frequency of the variant allele associated with increased HbF.

The *MYB* gene is essential for hematopoiesis and erythroid differentiation. *MYB* inhibits HbF expression directly by activation of *KLF1* and other repressors and indirectly through alteration of the kinetics of erythroid differentiation.

The third QTL is marked by a common variant 158 nucleotides upstream of the transcription start site of *HBG2* and could be a binding site for an uncharacterized HbF repressor. Haplotypes associated with the *HBB* cluster have been defined by single nucleotide polymorphisms (SNPs) among these genes. Sickle cell anemia patients with the Senegal and Arab-Indian HbS gene-associated haplotypes have higher HbF levels than patients with other haplotypes. These two haplotypes have the common–158 C-T variant in the *HBG2* promoter.

DIAGNOSIS OF HEMOGLOBIN DISORDERS

α-Globin gene mutations are expressed in the embryo and fetus and persist throughout life; HbF mutations are expressed in the fetus and in the first months of life, vanishing from notice afterward; δ-globin gene mutations are innocuous and usually not detected; β-globin gene mutations can become clinically apparent after the synthesis of HbF dwindles to stable adult levels.

With rare exceptions, all disorders of hemoglobin are autosomal recessive or co-dominant disorders; a family history of anemia, a common feature of most symptomatic hemoglobinopathies and thalassemias, is often present. In addition to pallor and jaundice, splenomegaly is often present. In sickle cell disease, acute painful vasoocclusive episodes are a diagnostic feature. A small number of laboratory tests can confirm the diagnosis starting with a complete blood count that includes a reticulocyte count with a careful review of a peripheral blood film. A sustained increase in reticulocyte count indicates the presence of hemolytic anemia. Hemoglobin fractionation by high-performance liquid chromatography (HPLC) or capillary electrophoresis, especially when, in addition to the index case, family members are available for study, is often sufficient to confirm a diagnosis at the level of hemoglobin phenotype. DNA sequencing of the globin genes should allow definitive diagnosis. DNA-based diagnosis, which is readily available from excellent reference laboratories, is a prerequisite for most instances of genetic counseling.

Sickle cell disease and β thalassemia have some features in common. They are caused by mutations in the β-globin gene; both are chronic hemolytic anemias sharing complications associated with hemolysis such as venous thrombosis, leg ulcers, and pulmonary hypertension; and they can be cured by hematopoietic stem cell transplantation. Key differences are that only HbS polymerizes and that ineffective erythropoiesis is a prominent feature of β thalassemia and responsible for its severe anemia. Both diseases could be cured by inducing sufficiently high levels of HbF; in sickle cell disease, HbF prevents the polymerization of HbS; in β thalassemia, sufficient HbF compensates for the deficit of HbA.

SICKLE CELL DISEASE

Sickle cell disease is a clinical and hematologic phenotype caused by an assortment of genotypes (**Table 98-2**). Sickle cell anemia, defined as homozygosity for the sickle hemoglobin mutation ($\alpha_2\beta^S_2$; glutamic acid [E] 7 valine [V] GAG-GTG), is the most common of these genotypes, followed by HbSC disease or compound heterozygosity for HbS and HbC ($\alpha_2\beta^C_2$; E 7 lysine [K] GAG-AAG) genes. Many different thalassemia mutations contribute to the HbS-β thalassemias. The compound heterozygous genotypes are less common than HbS homozygotes; as a rule, their symptoms develop later in life and are less severe. HbS has also been described with many other variant hemoglobins. Few of these genotypes, other than HbSO^{Arab}, HbSE, and HbSD^{Punjab} are symptomatic.

ORIGIN, SPREAD, AND EPIDEMIOLOGY

HbS originated in Africa between 7000 and 22,000 years ago, reaching high frequencies because of the increased genetic fitness of heterozygotes under selective pressure from *Plasmodium falciparum*. The HbS gene became associated with five common β-globin gene haplotypes: Benin, Bantu, Senegal, Cameroon, and Arab-Indian. These haplotypes have a loose association with the severity of disease because each haplotype has a different average level of HbF. In some regions of Africa, India, and the Middle East, nearly half the population have sickle cell trait. Nigeria alone has ~150,000 newborns each year with sickle cell anemia, about one-third of the world's total newborns; most die before age 5. Coerced and free population movement have spread the HbS gene throughout the world. The HbS carrier, or sickle cell trait, prevalence is 2–15% in emigrant populations; ~100,000 patients in the United States have sickle cell disease; their death in childhood is rare, with the median age of death in the fifth or sixth decade.

PATHOPHYSIOLOGY

Pathophysiologic features of sickle cell disease are summarized in **Fig. 98-3**. HbS is physiologically similar to HbA in most respects except it polymerizes when deoxygenated. Contacts between one of the β^7 valine residues of deoxyHbS and specific amino acid residues of β- and α-globin culminate in fascicles of hemoglobin that injure the sickle erythrocyte. A delay occurs between the initiation of polymerization and the accumulation of sufficient polymer to damage the cell. It is unclear how much polymer is needed for cell injury, but it is clear that polymer leads directly and indirectly to the multiple abnormalities of the sickle erythrocyte that generate the pathophysiology of disease. Prominent among these abnormalities are HbS polymer penetration of the membrane causing vesiculation with membrane microparticle release; increased activity of the Gardos, K/CL cotransport, and P_{sickle} channels that dehydrate the cell, increasing mean corpuscular sickle hemoglobin concentration (MC[HbS]C), reducing cellular deformability, and increasing the polymerization potential of HbS; translocation of amino phospholipids such as phosphatidylserine to the outer leaflet of the membrane; and oxidation of erythrocyte contents. These and other abnormalities lead to the formation of irreversibly sickled cells (ISCs), which are sickle erythrocytes that are forever deformed because of permanent membrane damage regardless of whether HbS remains polymerized. Damaged sickle erythrocytes are responsible for initiating the vasoocclusive, hemolytic, and inflammatory features of the disease shown in Fig. 98-3.

DIAGNOSIS

Although sickle cell disease can appear in any ethnic group, most often it is present in people of African, Middle Eastern, Mediterranean, and

TABLE 98-2 Common Sickle Hemoglobinopathies

GENOTYPE	CLINICAL ABNORMALITIES	HEMOGLOBIN LEVEL, g/L (g/dL)/MCV, fL	HEMOGLOBIN FRACTIONS (%)
Sickle cell trait (HbAS)	8% of African Americans; hematuria, papillary necrosis, hyposthenuria, increased incidence of chronic kidney disease; 2–4 times increased VTE risk; ? stroke; splenic infarction at altitude; rhabdomyolysis	Normal	HbA: 60–70 HbS: 30–40 Percent HbS dependent on presence or absence of α thalassemia
Sickle cell anemia (HbSS)	Vasoocclusion related: pain, acute chest syndrome, osteonecrosis, splenic infarction Hemolysis related: stroke, pulmonary and systemic vasculopathy, nephropathy, leg ulceration gallstones, priapism, leg ulcers	70–100 (7–10)/80–100	HbS: >75 HbF: 2–25 HbA_2: 3–4
HbS-β^0 thalassemia	Rate of complications similar to HbSS	80–100 (8–11)/60–85	HbS: >75 HbF: 2–15 HbA_2: 5–6
HbS-β^+ thalassemia	Rate of complications about half the rate of HbSS depending on percent HbA	100–140 (10–14)/70–80	HbS: 60–90 HbA: 5–40 HbF: 1–10 HbA_2: 5–6
Hemoglobin SC disease (HbSC)	Nearly asymptomatic to severe disease; about half the rate of complications as HbSS. Increased risk of retinopathy	100–140 (10–14)/70–100	HbS: 50 HbC: 50
HbSE	Resembles clinically HbS-β^+ thalassemia; symptoms delayed; often Asian/Indian ancestry	90–130 (9–13)/65–75	HbS: 65 HbE: 35 HbF: 1-5
HbSS-α thalassemia	Present in 30% of HbSS; phenocopies HbS-β^0 thalassemia; similar to HbSS but with fewer strokes and leg ulcers and less pulmonary vascular and renal disease	80–100 (8–11)/60–85	HbS: >75 HbF: 2–15 HbA_2: 4–5
HbS-HPFH	Most common genotype is due to large *HBB* deletions and is asymptomatic	110–140 (11–14)/70–80	HbS: 70 HbF: 20–30 HbA_2: 1–2

Note: Laboratory values are averages in untreated adults.

Abbreviation: VTE, venous thromboembolism.

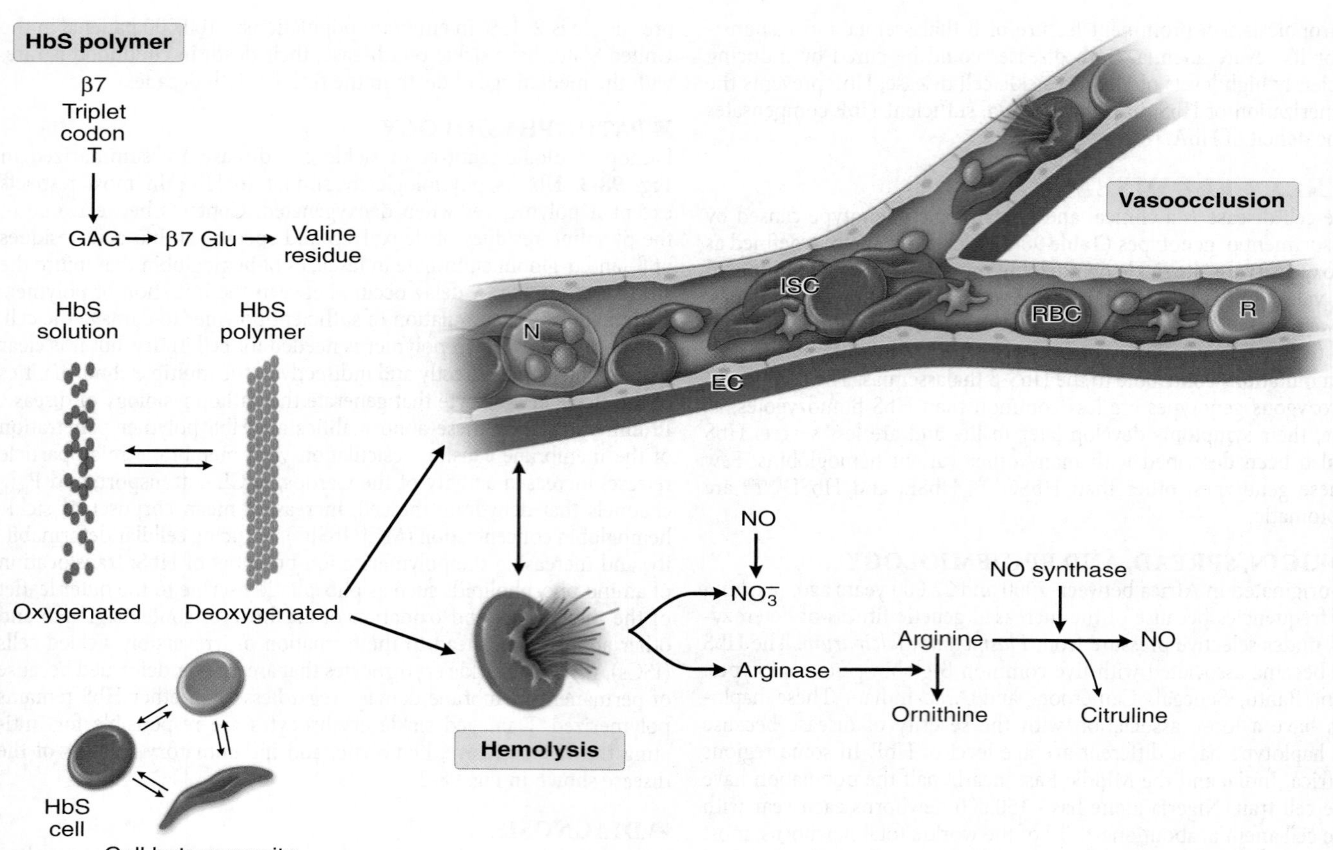

FIGURE 98-3 Pathophysiology of sickle cell disease. HbS is in solution when oxygenated but reversibly polymerizes when deoxygenated. Polymerization is dependent on the 30th power of hemoglobin concentration. In the sickle cell, this means that small changes in hemoglobin concentration or cell hydration can have large effects on polymerization. Polymerization begins seconds to minutes following deoxygenation. Erythrocyte deformation, or sickling, is initially reversible, but after an undetermined number of cell sickling events, the cell becomes irreversibly deformed. These are known as irreversibly sickled cells (ISCs). Their membrane is permanently damaged, although depending on their oxygen (O_2) content, HbS could be in solution. Sickle erythrocytes lead to the clinical and laboratory phenotypes of disease. Sickle cells interact with endothelial cells and other blood cells, occluding flow in small and sometimes large vessels and causing the many complications thought to be a result of vasoocclusion. Sickle cells also live <20 days (normal ~120 days) hemolyzing intra- and extravascularly. Intravascular hemolysis depletes haptoglobin and hemopexin while liberating heme, arginase, and other danger-associated molecular patterns (DAMPs) into the blood. This scavenges nitric oxide (NO), activates platelets and endothelium, reduces antioxidant activity, causes vasoconstriction, and is proinflammatory.

Indian descent. The chief presenting symptom is pain that might be an arthritis-like hand-foot syndrome in young children or the typical acute painful episode in older children and adults. In HbSC disease and HbS-β^+ thalassemia, acute vasoocclusive episodes occur less often and complications develop later in life; rarely, patients with these genotypes are asymptomatic. The key elements of laboratory diagnosis are outlined in Table 98-2 showing typical hematologic findings and hemoglobin fractions. **Figure 98-4** displays HPLC profiles and blood films in typical patients with sickle cell trait, sickle cell anemia, and HbSC disease. Clinical and basic laboratory diagnosis is sufficient for general management and counseling; genetic counseling and family planning usually require DNA-based diagnosis.

■ COMPLICATIONS

Complications of sickle cell disease can be grouped into those that likely are a consequence of sickle vasoocclusion and ones that appeared to be triggered by intravascular hemolysis. Although there is a relationship between these two limbs of pathophysiology, complications associated with vasoocclusion seem to respond best to induction of HbF. Some complications of disease are presented in **Table 98-3**. Early and effective treatment with hydroxyurea and the integration into management of new treatments discussed below should change this profile.

Acute Painful Episodes Characterized by unprovoked severe pain in extremities or torso that is often symmetrical and stereotypical for each patient and usually requires treatment with strong opioids in the emergency department, acute painful episodes are the most common acute events in sickle cell disease. They are the chief cause of concern for patients, most of whom have them at some time in their life. Their frequency varies; most patients have one to two episodes a year; some rarely have them; others are hardly ever without them. Acute painful episodes last days to weeks. Complicating the diagnosis and management of the acute pain episode, pain in sickle cell disease can be chronic from complications such as osteonecrosis, osteoporosis, or leg ulcers; chronic and acute pain can overlap; and pain can also be induced by opioid treatment of pain. Diary studies have shown that most of the time patients have some degree of pain that does not reach the intensity of the acute episode. Most patients use oral opioid analgesics for control of this pain. Reliable patients can be given a reasonable supply of oral opioids on a monthly basis.

No diagnostic test can confirm or refute the presence of an acute pain episode; often a 1 to 2 g/dL decrease in hemoglobin level and a modest increase in the leukocyte count are noted during the painful episode. Drastic decreases in hemoglobin and platelet levels with more extreme leukocytosis can portend development of severe acute chest syndrome or multiorgan failure. Acute painful episodes have little to do with the presence of ISCs in the blood or the reticulocyte count. The most anemic patients seem to have the least pain. It is unusual for a cause of acute painful episodes to be identified. Physical examination is not often useful diagnostically. Some patients will have pain on

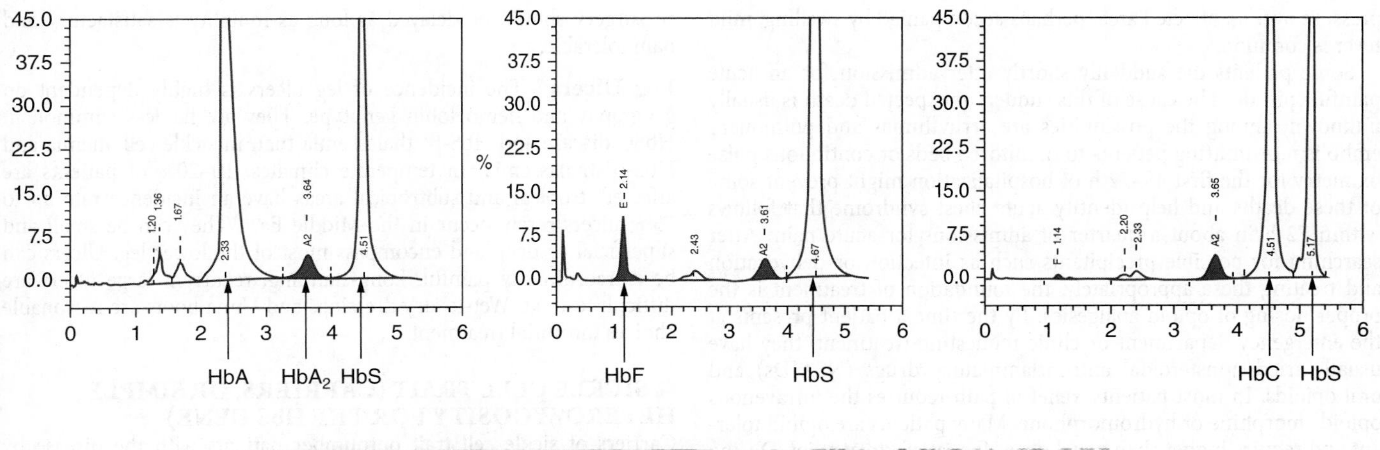

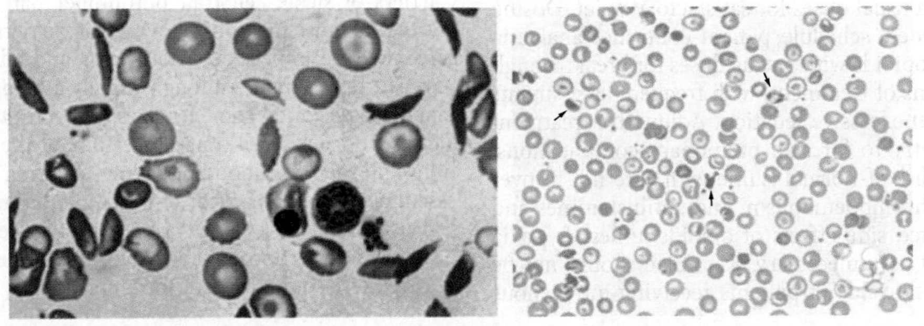

FIGURE 98-4 Diagnosis of sickle cell disease. ***A.*** From *left to right*, high-performance liquid chromatography separation in sickle cell trait, sickle cell anemia, and HbSC disease. Beneath each chromatogram, the individual protein peaks are identified. ***B.*** *Left:* Dense, elongated, and pointed cells are the irreversibly sickled cells characteristic of the sickle cell anemia and sickle cell-β⁰ thalassemia. Target cells and nucleated red cells are also present. *Right:* Target cells, cells with squared ends of HbC crystals, cells folded like tacos, and contracted microspherocytes are typical of HbSC disease. *(Source: B [right]: Reproduced with permission from American Society of Hematology.)*

TABLE 98-3 Complications of Sickle Cell Disease

COMPLICATION	INCIDENCE, DIAGNOSIS, AND FEATURES	TREATMENT
Priapism	~30% of males; can be episodic and short duration (stuttering); severe episodes can cause impotence; associated with markers of hemolysis	Many unproven therapies including α-adrenergic agonists, stilbesterol; consult urology for therapy, which is time-critical
Stroke and silent infarction	10–15% of all cases; infarction in early childhood into adulthood; hemorrhagic in adults; neurocognitive abnormalities in adults even without apparent stroke; associated with markers of hemolysis	Transcranial Doppler screening in children aged 2–16; transfusion for at-risk patients; hydroxyurea
Gallstones/surgery	~40% of patients; bilirubin levels and stones related to polymorphisms of *UGT1A*; in surgery requiring general anesthesia, simple preoperative transfusion to a hemoglobin of 10 g/dL is recommended	If asymptomatic, usually let be; otherwise, laparoscopic cholecystectomy
Hepatic disease	>80% of patients have hepatomegaly; intrahepatic cholestasis can have bilirubin ~100 mg/dL; viral hepatitis, iron overload, RBC sequestration, extrahepatic cholestasis also contribute	Exchange transfusion for intrahepatic cholestasis; transplant for end-stage liver failure
Nephropathy	~30% of adults age >30 years; hyperfiltration in children, renal failure in adults; early albuminuria, later nephrotic-range proteinuria; associated with markers of hemolysis	Screen for microalbuminuria by age 10 years; avoid NSAIDs; use ACE inhibitors or receptor antagonists for albuminuria; erythropoietin for symptomatic anemia; dialysis or transplant for renal failure
Lung/pulmonary hypertension	Restrictive disease; asthma common; 5–10% have pulmonary hypertension by right heart catheterization; 30% have increased TRV that portends poor prognosis; associated with markers of hemolysis	Consult expert pulmonologist; screen yearly by echocardiography measurement of TRV
Retinopathy	30% in HbSC disease, 3% in HbSS,[a] develops in peripheral retina; vitreous hemorrhage and retinal detachment can cause blindness	Screen annually starting at age 10 tears with fluorescein angiography; laser photocoagulation for proliferative disease
Acute anemic episodes	B19 parvovirus infection, folic acid deficiency, splenic sequestration, delayed hemolytic transfusion reaction with destruction of transfused and sometimes autologous red cells	RBC transfusion if symptomatic; splenectomy if more than one or two episodes of sequestration; anti-parvovirus IgM positive in acute infection, IgG in past infection
Multiorgan failure	Can accompany severe acute chest syndrome; often confused with sepsis and can coexist with sepsis; CNS, liver, muscle, lung, kidney affected	Exchange transfusion, ICU support
Pregnancy	Screening both partners for hemoglobin disorders with risk counseling is critical component of family planning.	All pregnancies are "high risk"; transfuse if sickle cell events increase, if previous miscarriage, multiple fetuses

[a]Sickle cell anemia (HbSS).

Abbreviations: ACE, angiotensin-converting enzyme; CNS, central nervous system; ICU, intensive care unit; NSAIDs, nonsteroidal anti-inflammatory drugs; TRV, tricuspid regurgitant jet velocity.

pressure over an affected area, perhaps accompanied by swelling; mild fever is common.

Some patients die suddenly shortly after admission for an acute painful episode. The cause of this sudden unexpected death is usually unknown; among the possibilities are arrhythmias and pulmonary embolism. Admitting patients to monitored beds or continuous pulse oximetry for the first 48–72 h of hospitalization might prevent some of these deaths and help identify acute chest syndrome that follows within 72 h in about a quarter of admissions for acute pain. After searching for possible precipitants such as infection or dehydration and treating these appropriately, the foundation of treatment is the proper dosing of opioid analgesics. By the time a patient presents at the emergency department or clinic requesting treatment, they have usually tried nonsteroidal anti-inflammatory drugs (NSAIDs) and oral opioids. In most patients, relief of pain requires the intravenous opioids morphine or hydromorphone. Many patients are opioid tolerant and require higher than usual doses for satisfactory relief. Dosing should not be on an "as-needed" schedule; patient-controlled analgesia or a frequent fixed dose of opioids with rescue doses for breakthrough pain are the preferred means of treatment, with frequent assessments to ensure pain relief without excessive sedation. Adjunctive treatment includes incentive spirometry to forestall pulmonary complications, maintaining hydration with half-normal saline with care not to overhydrate, prophylaxis for thromboembolism, and antihistamines and laxatives to counter expected side effects of opioids; unless hypoxia is present, supplemental O_2 is unnecessary. Ketorolac should not be used, and NSAIDs have little value in patients receiving intravenous opioids.

Acute Chest Syndrome This pneumonia-like illness is the second most frequent acute sickle cell–related event. It occurs in >50% of patients, often more than once. Acute chest syndrome can be mild, especially in children, in whom it can result from viral infection, or devastating, where multiple lobes of the lung are affected with severe hypoxia, multiorgan failure, and death. Chest pain, cough, fever, and hypoxia and a pulmonary infiltrate on chest x-ray are the major diagnostic criteria. The etiology includes in situ thrombosis, emboli, any type of infection, and postoperative hypoventilation. Management in adults is dictated by the severity of the episode. Patients who are hypoxic and febrile are often admitted directly to the intensive care unit. Antibiotics are almost always used in febrile patients even though a causative bacterium is not often cultured. Supplemental O_2 is given for an O_2 saturation <95%. Overhydration and excessive opioids can compound dyspnea and hypoxia. Hypoxic patients who are febrile with leukocytosis and have more than a trivial infiltrate on x-ray are transfused. In the more severely ill patient, exchange transfusion is the preferred modality. When hemoglobin level or symptoms indicate the need for transfusion of the severely ill patient and hours are needed to arrange red cell exchange, simple or top-up transfusion should be started first. Simple transfusions also suffice for less severely affected patients. Most patients survive acute chest syndrome, but in the most severe cases, often caused by embolization of necrotic bone marrow, death can be rapid even with prompt and proper treatment. Thrombocytopenia, leukocyte counts in excess of 20,000/dL, and rapidly developing acute anemia often portend severe acute chest syndrome with the possibility of acute respiratory distress syndrome and multiorgan failure. Many adults have chronic lung disease that could be a sequela of acute chest syndrome, and asthma is very common in patients with sickle cell disease.

Osteonecrosis This painful and sometimes crippling complication that most often affects hips bilaterally occurs in about half of all patients with sickle cell anemia and is also common in HbSC disease; shoulders are less often affected. Beginning with chronic pain that can become severe, loss of function is often the final stage, especially in the hips. MRI can detect the earliest stages, whereas x-ray is less sensitive. Physical therapy and NSAIDs provide some relief; unfortunately, oral opioids are sometimes required. Joint replacement can restore lost mobility and relieve pain, but the life span of prosthetic joints is finite so surgery should be delayed as long as mobility is satisfactory and pain tolerable.

Leg Ulcers The incidence of leg ulcers is highly dependent on geography and hemoglobin genotype. They are far less common in HbSC disease and HbS-β^+ thalassemia than in sickle cell anemia and HbS-β^0 thalassemia. In temperate climates, 10–20% of patients are affected; tropical and subtropical areas have an incidence rate up to 75%; ulcers rarely occur in the Middle East. They can be small and superficial or deep and encompass most of the lower leg. Ulcers can be extraordinarily painful. Long-standing, recurrent large ulcers are difficult to treat. Wet-to-dry dressings and Unna boots are reasonable choices for initial treatment.

■ SICKLE CELL TRAIT (CARRIERS, OR SIMPLE HETEROZYGOSITY FOR THE HbS GENE)

Carriers of sickle cell trait outnumber patients with the disease by 25 to 1. Counseling and follow-up of carriers detected by cord blood screening are imperfect. Adolescents and adults can forget that they have sickle cell trait. Although usually a benign condition with a normal life expectancy, some features of this trait are shown in Table 98-2. Counseling sickle cell trait carriers about the small risks of complications and their likelihood of having offspring with sickle cell disease is essential. Counseling prior to participation in sports is also important because of the risk, albeit a very small one, of sudden death from heat-related exertional rhabdomyolysis. Optimal hydration before and during exercise can prevent most episodes of heat-related illness.

■ TREATMENT, SCREENING, COUNSELING, AND ANTENATAL DIAGNOSIS

Patients should, if possible, be referred to a sickle cell center for initial consultation, follow-up, and institution of therapy. Cooperation among primary care providers, hematologists, and other specialists can provide the best preventive care and management of complications. The frequency at which a patient is seen depends on their therapeutic regimen.

Remarkable changes in the treatment landscape have occurred with the promise of even greater benefits from new curative approaches based on gene therapy. The following discussion focuses on treatment to prevent the complications of disease.

Hydroxyurea Hydroxyurea is the standard of care for all patients with sickle cell anemia and HbS-β^0 thalassemia. It is recommended for patients of all ages regardless of symptoms and should be started in the first year of life. The major mechanism of action of hydroxyurea is to induce high levels of HbF. Hydroxyurea increases HbF unevenly in the red cell population (heterocellularly), so some cells have greater protection from HbS polymerization than others. Although often employed in symptomatic patients with HbSC disease, its benefits in this genotype are understudied. In adults, where the average HbF is ~5%, the increase in HbF is often modest. Nevertheless, pain and acute chest syndrome are reduced by about half, hemoglobin concentration increases by ~1 g/dL, and after 17.5 years of follow-up, mortality was reduced by 49%. In contrast, all children respond robustly to hydroxyurea. When started at <1 year of age at a dose of ~27 mg/kg, HbF levels were 33.3 ± 9.1% and hemoglobin concentration was 10.1 ± 1.3 g/dL. Acute events were markedly reduced with little toxicity. Based on these and other studies in high- and low-resource countries, unless there is a contraindication, hydroxyurea is standard of care for all patients starting in the first year of life at a dose of ~20 mg/kg and titrated to the maximal tolerated dose based on neutrophil and platelet counts.

Voxelotor Voxelotor increases the affinity of the hemoglobin molecule for O_2 (decreases the P_{50}). Voxelotor, 1500 mg daily, was associated with a 1-g/dL increase in hemoglobin concentration in 59% of patients with a reduction in the biomarkers of hemolysis. Although vasoocclusive events were not significantly reduced in the initial report of efficacy, further analysis after a longer observation period suggested that patients achieving the highest hemoglobin had the fewest acute vasoocclusive events. Voxelotor increases hemoglobin-oxygen affinity in all erythrocytes (pancellularly), and this should provide an increment in polymerization inhibition beyond hydroxyurea. Many questions remain about the long-term effects of voxelotor. Less hemolysis reduces the propensity for stroke, nephropathy, pulmonary hypertension, leg ulcers, and priapism. Will voxelotor be accompanied by these long-term benefits? Could the high O_2 affinity of a modified hemoglobin be harmful for some patients? The answers to these important questions require further study.

Crizanlizumab Downstream effects of HbS polymerization include adhesive interactions among endothelial cells, leukocytes, platelets, and erythrocytes. P-selectin is one molecule involved in these interactions; blocking selectins prevents sickle cell–endothelial adhesion. A P-selectin-blocking monoclonal antibody given intravenously every month reduced acute painful episodes by ~45%, a reduction similar to that seen with hydroxyurea. There were no effects on hemolysis.

L-Glutamine The mechanism of action of this agent, presumed to be the reduction of oxidative stress in sickle erythrocytes, is unsettled. In a phase 3 clinical trial, compared with a placebo, L-glutamine was associated with a 25% reduction in painful episodes and 33% reduction in hospitalization.

There is little consensus regarding how recently approved drugs should be integrated into treatment with hydroxyurea. The effects of voxelotor and crizanlizumab appear to be additive to those of hydroxyurea. Voxelotor can be added to hydroxyurea if the benefits of hydroxyurea alone are insufficient, as they are in most adults. If both hydroxyurea and voxelotor are taken at effective doses and acute vasoocclusive complications continue, crizanlizumab could then be added. The dropout rates in the crizanlizumab and L-glutamine trials was ~35% so adherence to these therapeutics could be problematic.

Transfusion Transfusions are overutilized and underutilized. Major indications for transfusion include severe symptomatic anemia; treatment and prevention of stroke; increasing hemoglobin level to ~10 g/dL before surgery requiring general anesthesia; and acute chest syndrome with hypoxia or multiple lobe involvement. Sometimes transfusions are given during pregnancy when there is a history of complications or fetal loss. Transfusions should usually be avoided in acute pain episodes and for repair of stable chronic anemia. There is a preference for automated red cell exchange transfusion in acute stroke, severe acute chest syndrome, or multiorgan failure or when chronic transfusions are planned. Recent guidelines formulated by experts recommended extended red cell antigen profiling, if possible before the first transfusion, and antigen matching for Rh (C, E or C/c, E/e) and K antigens in addition to ABO/RhD. Complications of transfusion include hyperviscosity, alloimmunization (which occurred in 18.6% of patients transfused between 1979 and 1984 and 27.3% of patients transfused between 2001 and 2011), iron overload, delayed hemolytic transfusion reactions, and hyperhemolysis.

Stem Cell Transplantation Given the excellent results of human leukocyte antigen (HLA)–identical related donor transplants, which have an event-free survival of >95%, this option might be extended to all patients with a suitable donor. Unfortunately, only 15% of patients have a fully matched donor. New approaches to haploidentical transplants are improving event-free survival in these patients.

Preventive Measures and Screening Cord blood screening for sickle cell disease is done in many countries and all 50 states. Affected patients are then directed to clinics that can initiate early preventive care. In childhood, transcranial Doppler screening beginning at age 2 years and repeated annually until age 16 years, prophylactic penicillin (125 mg for children younger than 3 years; 250 mg for children 3 years and older) twice daily until age 5 years, and vaccination with pneumococcal vaccines are the main measures to prevent stroke and invasive pneumococcal infection. Folic acid, 1 mg daily, is given to prevent megaloblastic erythropoiesis; it is probably unnecessary in people with nutritious diets.

All women planning pregnancy should be screened for disorders of hemoglobin by blood counts, erythrocyte indices, and HPLC analysis of hemoglobin. Individuals with HbS or β thalassemia trait should have their partners tested. Only then is it possible to know the risks of a fetus having sickle cell disease (Table 98-2). Antenatal diagnosis using chorionic villus sampling is widely available.

Emerging Treatments Gene therapy has curative potential and requires neither matched donors nor immunosuppression. Autologous hematopoietic CD34+ stem cells are mobilized and modified ex vivo to produce an antisickling globin. These cells are reinfused following myeloablative conditioning. Phase 1/2 clinical trials have used lentivirus transduction of CD34+ cells with an antisickling β-globin or have interfered with the HbF-suppressive effects of BCL11A using CRISPR/Cas, zinc finger nucleases, or shRNA. These approaches have resulted in HbF or antisickling hemoglobin levels of nearly 50%, reduced hemolysis, total hemoglobin levels of >11 g/dL, and resolution of acute vasoocclusive events. It is too early to know their long-term safety or cure rate.

THALASSEMIA

Thalassemia is caused by reduced accumulation of either α- or β-globin chains causing a relative excess of the unaffected chain. Unbalanced globin synthesis is the hallmark of thalassemia and the proximate cause of its pathophysiology; unpaired globin chains damage the developing erythroblast. Like the HbS mutation and many other red cell traits, thalassemia reached polymorphic levels in tropical and subtropical populations because heterozygotes are protected from *Plasmodium falciparum* infection. Estimates are that 1–5% of the world's population carries a thalassemia mutation; in some locales, most people have a thalassemia mutation. These mutations can affect any globin gene, but clinically, β and α thalassemia are the most important. With nearly 500 unique thalassemia-causing mutations *(www.globin.bx.psu.edu)* that can interact with each other and with hemoglobinopathies, thalassemia syndromes are remarkably diverse. Where resources permit and the mutation is known, genetic counseling can be provided and antenatal diagnosis is possible.

HbE (β^{27} glu-lys) is a common variant whose biosynthesis is reduced because the site of the mutation alters its mRNA processing. Its reduced biosynthesis leads to a deficit of β^E-globin chains and features of β thalassemia. Hemoglobin Constant Spring is caused by a mutation of the termination codon of *HBA2* that leads to the synthesis of an elongated α-globin chain that is unstable and suboptimally synthesized. This variant therefore behaves as an α thalassemia variant.

β THALASSEMIA

EPIDEMIOLOGY

Once known as Mediterranean anemia, because of the concentration of cases in Italy, Greece, and other countries bordering the Mediterranean Sea, or as Cooley's anemia after the physician first describing cases, β thalassemia is common in most areas of the world where malaria was endemic. Effective programs of screening, counseling, and antenatal diagnosis have reduced the birth of new cases from the Mediterranean region. The bulk of new patients now are of Asian, Middle Eastern, and Indian origin. About 40,000 β thalassemia patients are born yearly. In the United States there are ~1000 cases of severe β thalassemia.

CLASSIFICATION

β^0 Thalassemia mutations totally prevent the accumulation of any globin from the affected gene; β^+ thalassemia mutations cause minor or extreme reductions in β-globin synthesis. β Thalassemia major and β thalassemia intermedia are now categorized as transfusion-dependent and non-transfusion-dependent based on the number and frequency of transfusions required to sustain a good quality of life.

Pathophysiology Single nucleotide changes are the most common β thalassemia mutations, but gene deletions also occur. A partial listing of the classes of mutations causing β thalassemia include mutations in the promoter elements affecting gene transcription causing mild and sometimes silent β^+ thalassemia; mutations in the junctions between exons and introns that affect mRNA processing causing β^0 and β^+ thalassemia; introduction of alternative splice sites into introns or exons usually causing β^+ thalassemia; 3′ end-processing sequence mutations preventing RNA polyadenylation leading to mild or silent β^+ thalassemia; mutations preventing initiation of translation causing β^0 thalassemia; and introduction of stop codons that prematurely terminate translation (nonsense mutations) producing reading frameshifts and resulting in truncated globin mRNA and β^0 thalassemia.

In β thalassemia, the deficit in β-globin chain synthesis allows α-globin chains to accumulate in excess. Without a non-α-globin chain partner in dimer and tetramer formation, unpaired α-globin chains are unstable, cannot form a tetramer, and precipitate within the developing erythroblast, causing membrane lipid oxidation and damage. The predominant cause of anemia is intramedullary destruction of erythroid precursors, known as ineffective erythropoiesis. Reduced deformability and phosphatidyl serine exposure also cause extra- and intravascular hemolysis of those erythrocytes that gain entrance into the circulation. In poorly treated β thalassemia, severe anemia leads to bone marrow expansion; hepatosplenomegaly; iron accumulation in liver, heart, and endocrine organs; pulmonary hypertension; and thromboembolic disease.

Frightening pictures of children with severe β thalassemia permeate the literature. These examples of near-terminal disease should be relegated to history because treatment with transfusion and iron chelation can prevent their occurrence and hematopoietic stem cell transplantation can "cure" patients who have suitable donors.

DIAGNOSIS

Heterozygous β thalassemia, also known as β thalassemia trait and β thalassemia minor, has mild or no anemia but microcytic/hypochromic erythrocytes with minimal or no increase in reticulocyte count. After recognizing these hematologic abnormalities and excluding iron deficiency, finding an elevated level of HbA_2 and perhaps HbF by HPLC is sufficient to establish this diagnosis. The hematologic characteristics of this heterozygous carrier state are listed in **Table 98-4**. Sometimes, the spleen is enlarged. Before genetic counseling and antenatal diagnosis are considered after carrier identification by red cell indices and quantitation of HbA_2, the thalassemia-causing mutation should be identified. This is the key to preventing homozygotes or compound heterozygotes with transfusion-dependent thalassemia.

The more severe forms of β thalassemia are hemolytic anemias with hypochromia, microcytosis, reticulocytosis, marked anisocytosis, and poikilocytosis with variable numbers of circulating nucleated red cells (**Fig. 98-5**).

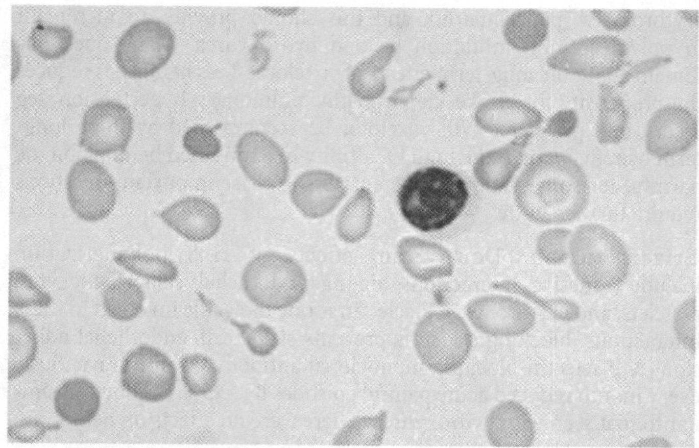

FIGURE 98-5 β Thalassemia intermedia. Target cells and marked variation in cell size and shape but with general hypochromia and microcytosis characterize the blood film. A lymphocyte is shown for size comparison.

COMPLICATIONS

Complications of severe β thalassemia are many. They are a consequence of chronic hemolytic anemia, chronic transfusion, and iron loading. Increased iron absorption is especially common in non-transfusion-dependent thalassemia. Most complications, listed in **Table 98-5**, develop because of either inadequate blood transfusion and/or poor iron chelation and iron loading. Even when chelation is optimized, some complications attributable to iron toxicity will develop. Many complications have complex and multifactorial etiologies. Iron stores are estimated by serum ferritin levels; MRI is the most widespread means of noninvasively measuring iron accumulation in liver and heart.

MANAGEMENT, SCREENING, COUNSELING, AND ANTENATAL DIAGNOSIS

Heterozygote screening and counseling couples at risk for affected fetuses, with antenatal diagnosis, if needed, is an effective preventive approach. Severe thalassemia should be dealt with in specialized

TABLE 98-4 β Thalassemias

CLASSIFICATION	HEMOGLOBIN (g/dL)/ MCV (fL)	HEMOGLOBIN FRACTIONS (%)	CLINICAL FEATURES
β Thalassemia trait	100–140 (10–14)/60–80	HbA: 94 HbF: 1–2 HbA_2: 4–6	Heterozygosity for β^+ or β^0 thalassemia mutations; "silent" carriers can have normal HbA_2 and red cell indices.
Non-transfusion-dependent β thalassemia (thalassemia intermedia)	70–120 (7–12)/65–80	HbA: 60–90 HbF: 10–40 HbA_2: 4–6	Defined by infrequent or no transfusion requirement; caused by many different genotypes including homozygosity for "mild" β^+ mutations, combinations of β and α thalassemia, homozygous β thalassemia with high HbF producing capacity, and many others. Iron loading, thromboembolic disease, and pulmonary hypertension are major clinical events.
Transfusion-dependent β thalassemia (thalassemia major)	20–40 (2–4)/50–80	HbA: 0–5 HbF: 90–100 HbA_2: 2–5	Caused by many different genotypes including homozygosity and compound heterozygosity for β^0 and β^+ mutations, combinations of β and α thalassemia; transplantation curative; iron chelation required.
HbE-β thalassemia	50–80 (5–8)/60–70	HbE: 50–70 HbF: 30–50	Common in SE Asian populations; in some parts of the word, the most prevalent severe thalassemia; in HbE-β^0 thalassemia, only HbE and HbF are found; in HbE-β^+ thalassemia, HbA is present. Transfusion dependence depends in part on the thalassemia mutation.
δβ Thalassemia and hemoglobin Lepore	110–120 (11–12)/65–75	HbA: 70 HbF: 7–13 HbA_2: 2	Rare; deletions removing the δ- and β-globin genes cause δβ thalassemia; Lepore hemoglobins are fusion globin chains; values are for heterozygotes; homozygotes have 100% HbF with hemoglobin 10–11 g/dL.
Gene deletion HPFH	120–140 (12–14)/75–85	HbA: 70 HbF: 15–30 HbA_2: 2	Rare; large deletions removing the δ- and β-globin genes; values are for heterozygotes; homozygotes, who are asymptomatic, have 100% HbF without anemia.

Note: Laboratory results are averages in adults.

TABLE 98-5 Complications of β Thalassemia

COMPLICATION	INCIDENCE, DIAGNOSIS, AND FEATURES
Growth retardation	Most often a feature of delayed or inadequate transfusions but can occur in well-transfused children.
Delayed puberty; secondary amenorrhea	50% and 25%, respectively.
Splenomegaly	Can trap 1–40% of red blood cell volume; increases plasma volume, worsening heart failure. Splenectomy indicated when transfusion requirement to maintain ideal hemoglobin increases. Prophylactic penicillin after splenectomy.
Heart	Due to chronic anemia, heightened sensitivity to iron toxicity, thromboembolic pulmonary hypertension, other causes. Progresses through stages to congestive failure and arrhythmias. Assessed by T2* on MRI. The available chelating agents might have differential effects on different measures of cardiac function and can be used in combination.
Leg ulcers	Common in thalassemia intermedia.
Hepatic disease	Fibrosis progressing to cirrhosis is related to hepatic iron concentration that can be monitored by MRI. Hepatitis also plays a role.
Lung disease/ pulmonary hypertension	Fibrosis, chronic thromboembolic disease, restrictive pathophysiology, intravascular hemolysis, and reduced nitric oxide bioavailability
Thromboembolism	Multifactorial etiology including platelet activation, red cell–endothelial interactions, thrombocytosis; endothelial activation; splenectomy.
Endocrinopathies	Diabetes, hypothyroidism, hypoparathyroidism, adrenal insufficiency; hypogonadism; hypothalamic-pituitary axis might be especially sensitive to iron.
Bone disease	Caused by bone marrow expansion, severe iron loading, hypogonadism; osteoporosis in ~50% of patients, even those well treated. Extramedullary hematopoietic masses are a feature of thalassemia intermedia.
Infections	Transfusion associated; linked to iron overload (*Yersinia*); malaria.

centers where these and other services are available and managed by a team led by a hematologist experienced with this disease with help from endocrinologists, cardiologists, transfusion medicine specialists, and social services.

Transfusion and Iron Chelation Transfusion every 2–4 weeks with a goal pretransfusion hemoglobin concentration of 9–10.5 g/dL, coupled with oral iron chelation to prevent the accumulation of excess toxic iron that accompanies transfusion, has prevented the development of cardiomyopathy and endocrinopathies while extending life to at least 50 years. When to begin transfusions, whether partial exchange transfusion is preferable to simple transfusion, and the choice of blood product require consultation with experts. To be effective, transfusions and iron chelation must be started early, be uninterrupted, and continue lifelong. Older patients who did not have the advantage of effective chelation are more likely to develop multiple disease-related morbidities such as osteoporosis, endocrinopathies, liver disease, and renal failure. Two orally effective chelating agents, deferasirox and deferiprone, and one intravenous chelator, deferoxamine, are available.

Hematopoietic Stem Cell Transplantation There is consensus that patients with available donors should be offered transplantation because of the difficulty of lifelong transfusion and chelation and its imperfect efficacy. Quality of life in successfully transplanted patients exceeds that in patients treated with transfusion and chelation. Transplantation from matched sibling donors is curative in >80% of all cases. Unfortunately, only a third of patients have matched donors. The best results are in the youngest patients who have been effectively chelated and received fewer transfusions. Graft failure, graft rejection, graft-versus-host disease, and a mortality of 5–20% depending on risk factors are the major drawbacks of this procedure. Results of haploidentical and unrelated donor transplants are improving but lag those of matched sibling donors.

Improving Ineffective Erythropoiesis Luspatercept, a fusion protein containing the extracellular domain of human activin type IIB receptor and the Fc domain of human IgG, was recently approved for treatment of transfusion-dependent thalassemia. By binding transforming growth factor β superfamily ligands and reducing Smad2/3 signaling, luspatercept enhances late-stage erythropoiesis. Given subcutaneously, 1 mg/kg every 3 weeks, it was associated with a 33% reduction in transfusion requirements.

Gene Therapy Lentiviral mediated gene therapy using autologous CD34+ hematopoietic stem cells has been approved in Europe for some patients with transfusion-dependent thalassemia who lack a matched donor. In a clinical trial with a median follow-up of 26 months, where patients received autologous CD34+ cells transduced with a lentiviral vector containing a modified HbA, transfusions were reduced or eliminated and hemoglobin levels stabilized between 8.2 and 13.7 g/dL. However, the results were dependent on the β thalassemia mutation, and although transfusion independence was achieved, some features of disease such as ineffective erythropoiesis were not eliminated. The initial results of CRISPR/Cas editing to downregulate *BCL11A* in β thalassemia have eliminated the need for transfusion and normalized hemoglobin levels (see Sickle Cell Disease).

α THALASSEMIA

In some respects the obverse of β thalassemia, clinically consequential α thalassemia is less common than severe β thalassemia. α Thalassemia is most often found in Asian populations and is usually caused by deletion of α-globin genes rather than point mutations.

EPIDEMIOLOGY

Carriers of the most common α thalassemia chromosomes (**Table 98-6**) are found in 5–80% of people from tropical and subtropical regions of Africa, the Middle East, India, Southern China, and Melanesia. About 30% of African Americans carry the common $-\alpha^{3.7}$ chromosome that contains a single functional α-globin gene. HbH disease, the chief clinically important α thalassemia, is most prevalent in Southern China and Southeast Asia. Estimates are that in Thailand ~3500 patients with severe α thalassemia are born yearly. Pregnancies affected by hemoglobin (Hb) Bart's hydrops fetalis occur mainly in Southern China and Southeastern Asia.

CLASSIFICATION

Each normal chromosome 16 contains two α-globin genes; normal diploid individuals have four α-globin genes. A classification of inherited α thalassemia, as summarized in Table 98-6, is based on the number of functional α-globin genes. If one or two α-globin genes are missing or poorly expressed, these people have α thalassemia trait. Their hematologic abnormalities are almost always trivial. HbH disease is usually caused by deletion or malfunction of three α-globin genes. Hb Bart's hydrops fetalis fetuses have no normally functioning α-globin genes. Hundreds of different sized deletions and rarer point mutations affect the production of α globin and the magnitude of imbalanced globin synthesis. Because of this mutational complexity, many different variations of the common α thalassemia syndromes are found.

PATHOPHYSIOLOGY

Reduced accumulation of α-globin leaves non-α-globins unpaired and unable to participate in the formation of functional hemoglobin tetramers. In the fetus, absent or reduced synthesis of α-globin allows unpaired γ-globin chains, which are usually part of the HbF tetramer, to form γ_4 or Hb Bart's; in adults, when γ-globin synthesis is mostly silenced, unpaired β-globin chains, lacking a suitable partner to form HbA, tetramerize as β_4 or HbH. Both Hb Bart's and HbH have very high O_2 affinity and do not unload O_2 in tissues; HbH is also unstable. Severe anemia in Hb Bart's hydrops fetalis is a result of absent normal

TABLE 98-6 α Thalassemias

CLASSIFICATION	α-GLOBIN GENE ARRANGEMENT	HEMOGLOBIN LEVEL, g/L (g/dL)/MCV (fL)	CLINICAL FEATURES
α Thalassemia trait	–α/αα –α/–α – –/αα $\alpha^T\alpha/\alpha\alpha$	120–150 (12–15)/65–80	The chromosome with one deleted α gene (–α/) is called α^+ thalassemia (α thalassemia-2); the chromosome with both deleted α genes is α^0 thalassemia (α thalassemia-1); non–gene deletion α thalassemias (α^T) often have a more severe phenotype.
Hemoglobin H disease	– –/–α $\alpha^T\alpha$/– – $\alpha^T\alpha/\alpha^T\alpha$	50–120 (5–12)/60–70	Mild to moderate anemia depending on genotype; non–gene deletion forms of α thalassemia can produce severe HbH disease.
Hb Bart's hydrops fetalis	––/––		Fatal in utero or at birth with rare survivors. Hydrops can also result from combinations of gene deletion and non–gene deletion α thalassemia.
α Thalassemia/intellectual disability syndromes (ATR-16) (ATR-X)	– –/αα or – –/–α in ATR-16 αα/αα in ATR-X		ATR-16: Large deletions and rearrangements in chr16p. ATR-X: No α-globin gene deletion or mutation, *ATRX* mutations, X-linked.
α Thalassemia with myelodysplasia (ATMDS)	αα/αα		Mutations in *ATRX*; striking male predominance. Hematologic findings of HbH disease.

Note: Laboratory values are averages in adults. αα/ denotes the chromosome with two intact α-globin genes; –α/ chromosome with one α-globin gene deleted; – –/ chromosome with both α-globin genes deleted; α^T represents non–gene deletion α thalassemia caused by point mutations. The –α/ chromosome, referred to as α^+ or α thalassemia-2, most often has a deletion of 3.7 kb of DNA ($-\alpha^{3.7}$) or 4.2 kb of DNA ($-\alpha^{4.2}$) that leaves but a single α-globin gene intact. The chromosome where both α-globin genes are deleted (– – –/) is called α^0 thalassemia or α thalassemia-1. These chromosomes are caused by different-sized deletions that are usually named after their regions of highest frequency such as -SEA, -MED, -FI, and -THAI.

hemoglobin and ineffective erythropoiesis; in HbH disease, unstable HbH leads to oxidative membrane damage with extravascular hemolysis in the spleen and ineffective erythropoiesis.

■ DIAGNOSIS

Microcytosis/hypochromia with nearly normal hemoglobin concentrations, in the absence of iron deficiency and the increased level of HbA_2 that is diagnostic of β thalassemia, is sufficient for a presumptive diagnosis of α thalassemia trait. When genetic counseling is needed and antenatal diagnosis contemplated, the molecular basis of the presumed α thalassemia is required. HbH disease, which is usually due to compound heterozygosity for one chromosome with both α-globin genes deleted and one chromosome with only a single α-globin gene, is defined by the hematologic findings shown in Table 98-6 along with varying levels of reticulocytosis. At birth, when hemoglobin is separated by HPLC, 20–30% Hb Bart's is present; in adults, traces to 40% HbH are present along with residual Hb Bart's in some cases. HbH inclusions can be induced in some red cells after incubation and staining with brilliant cresyl blue. Hemoglobin composition in Hb Bart's hydrops fetalis is predominantly Hb Bart's with some Hb Portland if the deletion removing α-globin genes preserves the ζ-globin gene.

■ COMPLICATIONS

HbH disease is very heterogeneous because of the different combinations of genotypes that can cause this phenotype. Generally, when non–gene deletion mutants, such as Hb Constant Spring, contribute to the genotype, the disease is more severe. In the most common – –/–α genotype, mean hemoglobin in adults is ~11 g/dL Hepatosplenomegaly, jaundice, thalassemic bone changes in the face, and growth impairment are seen 20–50% of cases, depending on the underlying genotype. Iron loading occurs but is not the severe problem it is in β thalassemia. Pregnancy in these patients should be considered high risk and managed accordingly. Mothers of infants with Hb Bart's hydrops fetalis have a history of stillbirth and develop preeclampsia, polyhydramnios, and antepartum hemorrhage and have difficult labor and delivery. Intrauterine transfusion of the fetus is possible.

■ MANAGEMENT, SCREENING, COUNSELING, AND ANTENATAL DIAGNOSIS

When planning families, couples from regions where α thalassemia is common who have red cell indices that suggest the possibility of carrying an α thalassemia gene should have genetic counseling based on DNA analysis of their globin genes. Iron should be avoided in non-iron-deficient individuals with α thalassemia trait and microcytosis. Transfusions are not usually needed in HbH disease. Nevertheless, depending on the genotype of disease, transfusions might be necessary especially when anemia becomes more severe, for example, with acute anemic episodes or pregnancy. Iron stores should be checked periodically by measuring serum ferritin or MRI; chelation does not appear to be needed.

Hb Bart's hydrops fetalis is best prevented by screening couples at risk and antenatal diagnosis. Intrauterine therapy and perinatal intensive care have permitted survival of some infants with Hb Bart's hydrops fetalis. As growth retardation affects ~40% and neurodevelopmental delay is present in 20% of survivors, prevention is the best approach.

OTHER HEMOGLOBINOPATHIES OF CLINICAL IMPORTANCE (TABLE 98-7)

Thirteen-hundred mutations affecting hemoglobin structure have been described *(www.globin.bx.psu.edu)*. Most are clinically silent. HbC and HbE are common. HbC is found in people of African descent and HbE in South China and Southeast Asia. Heterozygotes for HbC and HbE are clinically well. Even individuals homozygous for these mutations, where the variant hemoglobin comprises >90% of the hemolysate, are clinically well with very mild anemia and microcytosis. The major importance of these variants is the interaction of HbC with HbS and HbE with β thalassemia, as outlined in Tables 98-2 and 98-4. A definitive diagnosis for all rare variants depends on DNA analysis.

Unexpected low O_2 saturation by pulse oximetry (SpO_2) with normal O_2 saturation of arterial blood is occasionally seen in rare hemoglobin variants with clinical phenotypes. Asymptomatic patients with unexpectedly low SpO_2 should not be subjected to unneeded cardiopulmonary investigations in search of the cause of their "hypoxemia" until the existence of a hemoglobin variant is excluded.

■ M HEMOGLOBINS

M (met) hemoglobins are characterized by oxidation of the heme-iron from its ferrous (Fe^{++}) to ferric (Fe^{+++}) form. The major clinical feature of these disorders is cyanosis that is asymptomatic. Nine M hemoglobin variants have been described. In seven, the mutation involves histidine residues that interact with heme. Asymptomatic slate gray/brownish pseudocyanosis is the main clinical finding. Spectrophotometric recording of the visible spectrum of the hemolysate is

TABLE 98-7 HbC, HbE, and Rare Hemoglobinopathies

CLASSIFICATION	CLINICAL ABNORMALITIES	HEMOGLOBIN LEVEL, g/L (g/dL)/MCV, fL	HEMOGLOBIN FRACTIONS (%)
HbC trait	2% of African Americans; target cells; no disease	Normal	HbC: 30–40 HbA_2: 2–3
HbC disease	Target cells; HbC crystals; mild reticulocytosis; splenomegaly	100–130 (10–13)/60–70	HbC: >95 HbF: 2–4 HbA_2: 2–3
HbE trait	50% incidence in some Asian populations; a few target cells; clinically normal	120–140 (12–14)/80–90	HbE: 27–31[b] HbF: 1 HbA_2: 3
HbE disease	No hemolysis; 20–80% target cells; no splenomegaly	100–120 (10–12)/65–75	HbE: 85–95 HbF: 3–7 HbA_2: 3
High O_2 affinity hemoglobins	Isolated erythrocytosis; often familial; no splenomegaly; no *JAK2*^{V617F} mutation	150–200 (15–20)	Variants in α- and β-globin genes; patients are heterozygotes; ~25–50% variant
Low O_2 affinity hemoglobins	Asymptomatic mild anemia; cyanosis	100–140 (10–14)	~50% variant
Unstable hemoglobins	Pigmenturia; hemolysis; reticulocytosis; splenomegaly	90–140 (9–14)/70–90	20–35% variant; rare hyperunstable variants can be undetectable and have the phenotype of thalassemia
M hemoglobins	Some have mild hemolysis; few symptoms	100–140 (10–14)/80–90	20–50% variant depending on gene affected

Note: Laboratory values are averages in adults. As noted for HbAS, the amount of HbC and HbE in heterozygotes depends on the number of α-globin genes.

diagnostic. To distinguish M hemoglobins from methemoglobinemia due to drugs or cytochrome b5 reductase (*CYB5R3*) deficiency, potassium cyanide (KCN) can be added to the hemolysate; methemoglobin-containing blood will turn red, but KCN has no effect on M hemoglobin. Treatment is not needed.

UNSTABLE HEMOGLOBINS

Sometimes referred to as congenital Heinz body hemolytic anemias, some mutations result in a hemoglobin tetramer that is unstable and precipitates intracellularly. Such variants are rare and often a result of a new mutation that affects the tertiary or quaternary structure of the molecule. The most common class of mutations introduce a proline residue in the α helix or a polar amino acid into the interion of the molecule. Heinz bodies are intraerythrocytic precipitates that are detectable as dark globular aggregates after staining with a dye such as brilliant cresyl blue. Three unstable hemoglobins are the most common of these rare variants. Hemoglobin Köln (β^{99} val-met) has been found in multiple families, Hb Hasharon (α^{47} asp-his) is found in Ashkenazi Jews, and Hb Zurich (β^{63} his-arg) is susceptible to oxidant drug-induced hemolysis. Unstable variants present with nonspherocytic hemolytic anemia, but presentation is highly variable. The associated disease is usually mild and does not require transfusion. Heating blood to 50°C or incubation with isopropanol precipitates unstable hemoglobins but must be done with careful controls. Some variants can be detected by HPLC.

HEMOGLOBINS WITH HIGH OXYGEN AFFINITY AND LOW OXYGEN AFFINITY

Rare mutations in areas involved in the R-T transition, at critical interfaces between globin chains of the tetramer that reduce the affinity for 2,3-bisphosphoglycerate, or present in the heme pocket account for most of these variants. High O_2 affinity hemoglobins outnumber low O_2 affinity variants by two to one. Isolated erythrocytosis in the absence of splenomegaly suggests the presence of a high O_2 affinity hemoglobin. High O_2 affinity hemoglobin variants shift the hemoglobin-O_2 dissociation curve leftward, causing a low P_{50} and thereby stimulating erythropoiesis. Many of these variants are due to new mutations. The clinical course is benign, and phlebotomy because of erythrocytosis is usually not required. Early diagnosis is important to forestall unnecessary diagnostic procedures and therapeutics such as cardiac catheterization to exclude congenital heart disease or treatment for polycythemia vera. Low O_2 affinity variants often present with cyanosis. Their hemoglobin-O_2 dissociation curve is right-shifted with high P_{50}. HPLC might reveal the presence of a hemoglobin variant. Treatment is often not necessary.

ACQUIRED DISORDERS OF HEMOGLOBIN

CO binds hemoglobin with high affinity forming carboxyhemoglobin. Carboxyhemoglobin levels can be accurately measured by co-oximetry of arterial blood. Standard pulse oximeters cannot accurately make this measurement. Some newly developed pulse oximeters are able to measure both carboxyhemoglobin and methemoglobin. Bound CO inhibits the transport of O_2; the hemoglobin-O_2 binding curve is left-shifted. Acute and chronic CO intoxication, caused by occupational exposure and other sources of incomplete combustion of hydrocarbons, presents with headache, altered mental status, and other constitutional symptoms. High-flow O_2 via facemask is the preferred treatment; criteria have been developed to guide the use of hyperbaric O_2.

Acquired methemoglobinemia and methemoglobinemia due to deficiency of *CYB5R3* are more common than the M hemoglobins. *CYB5R3* is required for the reduction of methemoglobin by NADH. Affected individuals with "toxic" methemoglobinemia can be cyanotic and symptomatic. As in carboxyhemoglobinemia, O_2 transport is reduced and reflected by the left-shift in the hemoglobin-O_2 binding curve. *CYB5R3* deficiency usually affects only erythrocytes (type I), causing a mild disorder; when all cells are affected (type II), a severe disease results. Intravenous methylene blue is the preferred treatment in symptomatic patients with acquired methemoglobinemia and 40–60% methemoglobin. The usual dose is 1–2 mg/kg. Alternative treatment with ascorbic acid is preferable in people who are glucose-6-phosphate dehydrogenase deficient. Methylene blue interferes with co-oximetry, reducing the value of co-oximetry for monitoring treatment.

Many drugs and chemicals can induce methemoglobin in the absence of *CYB5R3* deficiency. Dapsone and topical anesthetics such as benzocaine are the most common offending agents.

FURTHER READING

Chakravorty S, Dick MC: Antenatal screening for haemoglobinopathies: Current status, barriers and ethics. Br J Haematol 187:431, 2019.

Kato GL et al: Sickle cell disease. Nat Rev Dis Primers 4:18010, 2018.

Leonard A et al: Curative options for sickle cell disease: Haploidentical stem cell transplantation or gene therapy? Br J Haematol 189:408, 2020.

Markham A: Luspatercept: First approval. Drugs 80:85, 2020.

Nardo-Marino A et al: Emerging therapies in sickle cell disease. Br J Haematol 190:149, 2020.

Orkin SH, Bauer DE: Emerging genetic therapy for sickle cell disease. Annu Rev Med 70:257, 2019.

Pinto VM et al: Management of the aging beta-thalassemia transfusion-dependent population: The Italian experience. Blood Rev 38:100594, 2019.

Steinberg MH: Fetal hemoglobin in sickle cell anemia. Blood 136:2392, 2020.

Steinberg MH: Treating sickle cell anemia: A new era dawns. Am J Hematol 95:338, 2020.

Thein SL, Howard J: How I treat the older adult with sickle cell disease. Blood 132:1750, 2018.

Taher AT et al: Beta-thalassemia. N Engl J Med 384:727, 2021.

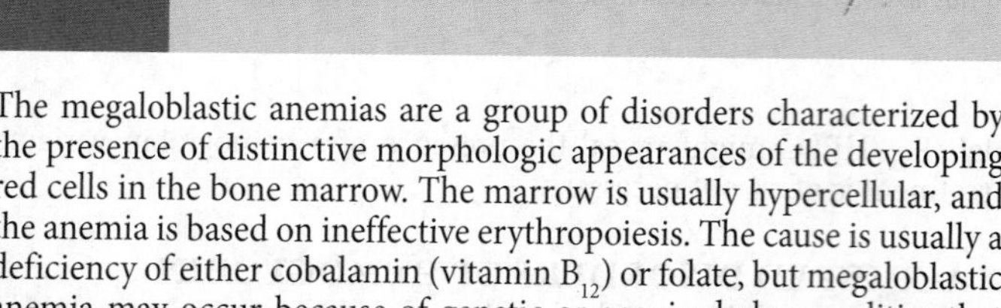

99 Megaloblastic Anemias

A. Victor Hoffbrand

The megaloblastic anemias are a group of disorders characterized by the presence of distinctive morphologic appearances of the developing red cells in the bone marrow. The marrow is usually hypercellular, and the anemia is based on ineffective erythropoiesis. The cause is usually a deficiency of either cobalamin (vitamin B_{12}) or folate, but megaloblastic anemia may occur because of genetic or acquired abnormalities that affect the metabolism of these vitamins or because of defects in DNA synthesis not related to cobalamin or folate (**Table 99-1**).

COBALAMIN

Cobalamin (vitamin B_{12}) exists in a number of different chemical forms. All have a cobalt atom at the center of a corrin ring. In nature, the vitamin is mainly in the 2-deoxyadenosyl (ado) form, which is located in mitochondria. It is the cofactor for the enzyme L-methylmalonyl coenzyme A (CoA) mutase. The other major natural cobalamin is methylcobalamin, the form in human plasma and in cell cytoplasm. It is the cofactor for methionine synthase. Minor amounts of hydroxocobalamin are also present to which methyl- and adocobalamin are converted rapidly by exposure to light.

DIETARY SOURCES AND REQUIREMENTS

Cobalamin is synthesized solely by microorganisms. Ruminants obtain cobalamin from the foregut, but the only source for humans is food of animal origin, for example, meat, fish, and dairy products. Vegetables, fruits, and other foods of nonanimal origin are free from cobalamin unless they are contaminated by bacteria. A normal Western diet contains 5–30 μg of cobalamin daily. Adult daily losses (mainly in the urine and feces) are 1–3 μg (~0.1% of body stores), and because the body does not have the ability to degrade cobalamin, daily requirements are also about 1–3 μg. Body stores are of the order of 2–3 mg, sufficient for 3–4 years if supplies are completely cut off.

TABLE 99-1 Causes of Megaloblastic Anemia

Cobalamin deficiency or abnormalities of cobalamin metabolism **(see Tables 99-3, 99-4)**
Folate deficiency or abnormalities of folate metabolism **(see Table 99-5)**
Therapy with antifolate drugs (e.g., methotrexate)
Independent of either cobalamin or folate deficiency and refractory to cobalamin and folate therapy:
Some cases of acute myeloid leukemia, myelodysplasia
Therapy with drugs interfering with synthesis of DNA (e.g., cytosine arabinoside, hydroxyurea, 6-mercaptopurine, azidothymidine [AZT])
Orotic aciduria (responds to uridine)
Thiamine-responsive

ABSORPTION

Two mechanisms exist for cobalamin absorption. One is passive, occurring equally through buccal, duodenal, and ileal mucosa; it is rapid but extremely inefficient, with <1% of an oral dose being absorbed by this process. The normal physiologic mechanism is active; it occurs through the ileum and is efficient for small (a few micrograms) oral doses of cobalamin, and it is mediated by gastric intrinsic factor (IF). Dietary cobalamin is released from protein complexes by enzymes in the stomach, duodenum, and jejunum; it combines rapidly with a salivary glycoprotein that belongs to the family of cobalamin-binding proteins known as haptocorrins (HCs). In the intestine, the HC is digested by pancreatic trypsin and the cobalamin is transferred to IF.

IF (gene at chromosome 11q13) is produced in the gastric parietal cells of the fundus and body of the stomach, and its secretion parallels that of hydrochloric acid. Normally, a vast excess of IF is available. The IF-cobalamin complex passes to the ileum, where IF attaches to a specific receptor (cubilin) on the microvillus membrane of the enterocytes. Cubilin also is present in yolk sac and renal proximal tubular epithelium. Cubilin appears to traffic by means of amnionless (AMN), an endocytic receptor protein that directs sublocalization and endocytosis of cubilin with its ligand IF-cobalamin complex. The cobalamin-IF complex enters the ileal cell, where IF is destroyed. After a delay of about 6 h, the cobalamin appears in portal blood attached to transcobalamin (TC) II.

Between 0.5 and 5 μg of cobalamin enter the bile each day. This binds to IF, and a major portion of biliary cobalamin normally is reabsorbed together with cobalamin derived from sloughed intestinal cells. Because of the appreciable amount of cobalamin undergoing enterohepatic circulation, cobalamin deficiency develops more rapidly in individuals who malabsorb cobalamin than it does in vegans, in whom reabsorption of biliary cobalamin is intact.

TRANSPORT

Two main cobalamin transport proteins exist in human plasma; they both bind cobalamin—one molecule for one molecule. One HC, also known as TC I, is closely related to other cobalamin-binding HCs in milk, gastric juice, bile, saliva, and other fluids. The gene *TCNL* is at chromosome 11q11-q12.3. These HCs differ from each other only in the carbohydrate moiety of the molecule. TC I is derived primarily from the specific granules in neutrophils. Normally, it is about two-thirds saturated with cobalamin, which it binds tightly. TC I does not enhance cobalamin entry into tissues. Glycoprotein receptors on liver cells are involved in the removal of TC I from plasma, and TC I may play a role in the transport of cobalamin analogues (which it binds more effectively than IF) to the liver for excretion in bile.

The other major cobalamin transport protein in plasma is transcobalamin, also known as TC II. The gene is on chromosome 22q11-q13.1. As for IF and HC, there are nine exons. The three proteins are likely to have a common ancestral origin. TC II is synthesized by liver and by other tissues, including macrophages, ileum, and vascular endothelium. It normally carries only 20–60 ng of cobalamin per liter of plasma and readily gives up cobalamin to marrow, placenta, and other tissues, which it enters by receptor-mediated endocytosis involving the TC II receptor and megalin (encoded by the *LRP-2* gene). The TC II cobalamin is internalized by endocytosis via clathrin-coated pits; the complex is degraded, but the receptor probably is recycled to the cell membrane as is the case for transferrin. Export of "free" cobalamin is via the ATP-binding cassette drug transporter alias multidrug resistance protein 1.

FOLATE

DIETARY FOLATE

Folic (pteroylglutamic) acid is a yellow, crystalline, water-soluble substance. It is the parent compound of a large family of natural folate compounds, which differ from it in three respects: (1) they are partly or

TABLE 99-2 Biochemical Reactions of Folate Coenzymes

REACTION	COENZYME FORM OF FOLATE INVOLVED	SINGLE CARBON UNIT TRANSFERRED	IMPORTANCE
Formate activation	THF	–CHO	Generation of 10-formyl-THF
Purine synthesis			
Formation of glycinamide ribonucleotide	5,10-Methylene-THF	–CHO	Formation of purines needed for DNA, RNA synthesis, but reactions probably not rate-limiting
Formylation of aminoimidazole carboxamide ribonucleotide (AICAR)	10-Formyl (CHO)THF		
Pyrimidine synthesis			
Methylation of deoxyuridine monophosphate (dUMP) to thymidine monophosphate (dTMP)	5,10-Methylene-THF	$-CH_3$	Rate limiting in DNA synthesis Oxidizes THF to DHF Some breakdown of folate at the C-9–N-10 bond
Amino acid interconversion			
Serine-glycine interconversion	THF	$=CH_2$	Entry of single carbon units into active pool
Homocysteine to methionine	5-Methyl(M)THF	$-CH_3$	Demethylation of 5-MTHF to THF; also requires cobalamin, flavine adenine dinucleotide, ATP, and adenosylmethionine
Forminoglutamic acid to glutamic acid in histidine catabolism	THF	–HN–CH=	

Abbreviations: DHF, dihydrofolate; THF, tetrahydrofolate.

completely reduced to dihydrofolate (DHF) or tetrahydrofolate (THF) derivatives, (2) they usually contain a single carbon unit (**Table 99-2**), and (3) 70–90% of natural folates are folate-polyglutamates.

Most foods contain some folate. The highest concentrations are found in liver, yeast, spinach, other greens, and nuts (>100 μg/100 g). The total folate content of an average Western diet is ~250 μg daily, but the amount varies widely according to the type of food eaten and the method of cooking. Folate is easily destroyed by heating, particularly in large volumes of water. Total-body folate in the adult is ~10 mg, with the liver containing the largest store. Daily adult requirements are ~100 μg, and so stores are sufficient for only 3–4 months in normal adults, and severe folate deficiency may develop rapidly.

ABSORPTION

Folates are absorbed rapidly from the upper small intestine. The absorption of folate polyglutamates is less efficient than that of monoglutamates; on average, ~50% of food folate is absorbed. Polyglutamate forms are hydrolyzed to the monoglutamate derivatives either in the lumen of the intestine or within the mucosa. All dietary folates are converted to 5-methyl-THF (5-MTHF) within the small intestinal mucosa before entering portal plasma. The monoglutamates are actively transported across the enterocyte by a proton-coupled folate transporter (PCFT, SCL46A1). This is situated at the apical brush border and is most active at pH 5.5, which is about the pH of the duodenal and jejunal surface. Genetic mutations of this protein underlie hereditary malabsorption of folate (see below). Pteroylglutamic acid at doses >400 μg is absorbed largely unchanged and converted to natural folates in the liver. Lower doses are converted to 5-MTHF during absorption through the intestine.

About 60–90 μg of folate enter the bile each day and are excreted into the small intestine. Loss of this folate, together with the folate of sloughed intestinal cells, accelerates the speed with which folate deficiency develops in malabsorption conditions.

TRANSPORT

Folate is transported in plasma; about one-third is loosely bound to albumin, and two-thirds are unbound. In all body fluids (plasma, cerebrospinal fluid, milk, bile), folate is largely, if not entirely, 5-MTHF in the monoglutamate form. Three types of folate-binding protein are involved. A reduced folate transporter (RFC, SLC19A1) is the major route of delivery of plasma folate (5-MTHF) to cells. Two folate receptors, FR2 and FR3 embedded in the cell membrane by a glycosyl phosphatidylinositol anchor, transport folate into the cell via receptor-mediated endocytosis. The third protein, proton-coupled folate transporter (PCFT), transports folate at low pH from the vesicle to the cell cytoplasm. The reduced folate transporter also mediates uptake of methotrexate by cells.

BIOCHEMICAL FUNCTIONS

Folates (as the intracellular polyglutamate derivatives) act as coenzymes in the transfer of single-carbon units (**Fig. 99-1** and Table 99-2). Two of these reactions are involved in purine synthesis and one in pyrimidine synthesis necessary for DNA and RNA replication. Folate is also a coenzyme for methionine synthesis, in which methylcobalamin is also involved and in which THF is regenerated. THF is the acceptor of single carbon units newly entering the active pool via conversion of serine to glycine. Methionine, the other product of the methionine synthase reaction, is the precursor for *S*-adenosylmethionine (SAM), the universal methyl donor involved in >100 methyltransferase reactions (Fig. 99-1).

During thymidylate synthesis, 5,10-methylene-THF is oxidized to DHF. The enzyme DHF reductase converts this to THF. The drugs methotrexate, pyrimethamine, and (mainly in bacteria) trimethoprim inhibit DHF reductase and so prevent formation of active THF coenzymes from DHF. A small fraction of the folate coenzyme is not recycled during thymidylate synthesis but is degraded at the C9-N10 bond.

BIOCHEMICAL BASIS OF MEGALOBLASTIC ANEMIA

The common feature of all megaloblastic anemias is a defect in DNA synthesis that affects rapidly dividing cells in the bone marrow. All conditions that give rise to megaloblastic changes have in common a disparity in the rate of synthesis or availability of the four immediate precursors of DNA: the deoxyribonucleoside triphosphates (dNTPs)—dA(adenine)TP and dG(guanine)TP (purines), dT(thymine)TP, and dC(cytosine)TP (pyrimidines). In deficiencies of either folate or cobalamin, there is failure to convert deoxyuridine monophosphate (dUMP) to deoxythymidine monophosphate (dTMP), the precursor of dTTP (Fig. 99-1). This is the case because folate is needed as the coenzyme 5,10-methylene-THF polyglutamate for conversion of dUMP to dTMP; the availability of 5,10-methylene-THF is reduced in either cobalamin or folate deficiency. DNA replication from multiple origins along the chromosome is slower than normal during mitosis, and there is failure of joining up the incomplete replicons with resulting single-stranded DNA breaks. An alternative theory for megaloblastic anemia in cobalamin or folate deficiency is misincorporation of uracil into DNA because of the accumulation of deoxyuridine triphosphate (dUTP) at

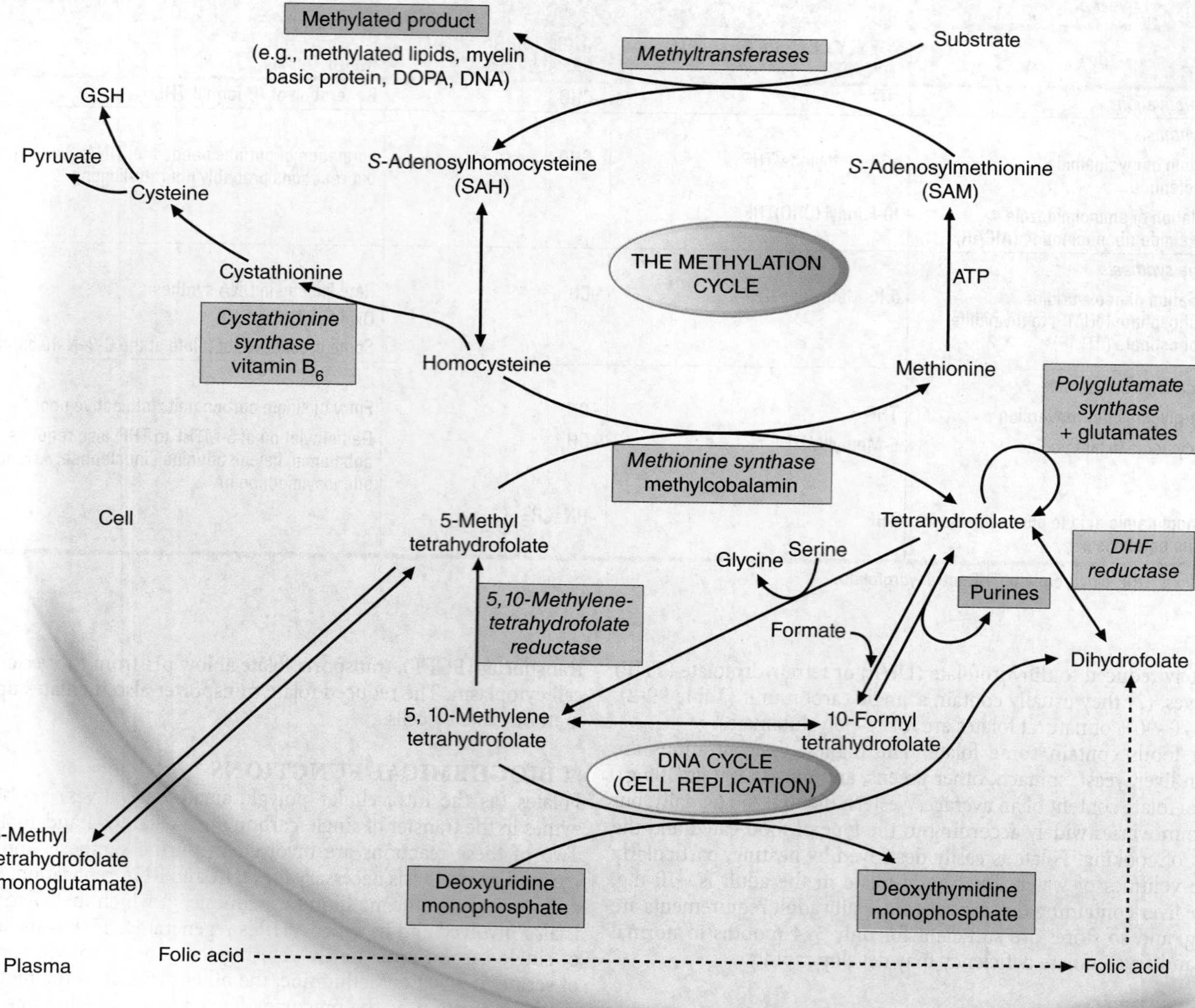

FIGURE 99-1 The role of folates in DNA synthesis and in formation of *S*-adenosylmethionine (SAM), which is involved in numerous methylation reactions. DHF, dihydrofolate; GSH, glutathione. *(Reproduced with permission from AV Hoffbrand et al [eds]: Postgraduate Haematology, 5th ed. Oxford, UK, Blackwell Publishing, 2005.)*

the DNA replication fork as a consequence of the block in conversion of dUMP to dTMP.

■ COBALAMIN-FOLATE RELATIONS

Folate is required for many reactions in mammalian tissues. Only two reactions in the body are known to require cobalamin. Methylmalonyl-CoA isomerization requires adocobalamin, and the methylation of homocysteine to methionine requires both methylcobalamin and 5-MTHF (Fig. 99-1). This reaction is the first step in the pathway by which 5-MTHF, which enters bone marrow and other cells from plasma, is converted into all the intracellular folate coenzymes. The coenzymes are all polyglutamated (the larger size aiding retention in the cell), but the enzyme folate polyglutamate synthase can use only THF, not MTHF, as substrate. In cobalamin deficiency, MTHF accumulates in plasma, and intracellular folate concentrations fall due to failure of formation of THF, the substrate on which folate polyglutamates are built. This has been termed *THF starvation*, or the *methylfolate trap*.

This theory explains the abnormalities of folate metabolism that occur in cobalamin deficiency (high serum folate, low cell folate, positive purine precursor aminoimidazole carboxamide ribonucleotide [AICAR] excretion; Table 99-2) and also why the anemia of cobalamin deficiency responds to folic acid in large doses.

CLINICAL FEATURES

Many symptomless patients are detected through the finding of a raised mean corpuscular volume (MCV) on a routine blood count. The main clinical features in more severe cases are those of anemia. Anorexia is usually marked, and there may be weight loss, diarrhea, or constipation. Glossitis, angular cheilosis, a mild fever in more severely anemic patients, jaundice (unconjugated), and reversible melanin skin hyperpigmentation also may occur with a deficiency of either folate or cobalamin. Thrombocytopenia sometimes leads to bruising, and this may be aggravated by vitamin C deficiency or alcohol in malnourished patients. The anemia and low leukocyte count may predispose to infections, particularly of the respiratory and urinary tracts. Cobalamin deficiency has also been associated in a few studies with impaired bactericidal function of phagocytes and with osteoporosis.

Neurologic Manifestations Vitamin B_{12} is needed for the myelination of the central nervous system. Its deficiency may cause a bilateral peripheral neuropathy or degeneration (demyelination) of the cervical and thoracic posterior and lateral (pyramidal) tracts of the spinal cord and, less frequently, of the cranial nerves and of the white matter of the brain. Optic atrophy and cerebral symptoms including dementia, depression, psychotic symptoms, and cognitive impairment may be prominent. There may also be anosmia and loss of taste. MRI may show the "spongy" degeneration of the cord.

The patient, more frequently male, typically presents with paresthesias, muscle weakness, or difficulty in walking but sometimes may present with dementia, psychotic disturbances, or visual impairment. There is usually loss of proprioception and vibration sensation with positive Romberg and Lhermitte signs. Gait may be ataxic with spasticity (hyperreflexia). Autonomic nervous dysfunction can result in postural hypotension, impotence, and incontinence.

Long-term nutritional cobalamin deficiency in infancy leads to poor brain development and impaired intellectual development. In infancy, there may be feeding difficulties, lethargy, and coma. Convulsions and myoclonus have been described. An important clinical problem is the nonanemic patient with neurologic or psychiatric abnormalities and a low or borderline serum cobalamin level. In such patients, it is necessary to try to establish whether there is significant cobalamin deficiency, for example, by careful examination of the blood film, tests for pernicious anemia (PA) by serum gastrin level and for antibodies to IF or parietal cells, along with serum methylmalonic acid (MMA) measurement if available. A trial of cobalamin therapy for at least 3 months will usually also be needed to determine whether the symptoms improve.

The biochemical basis for cobalamin neuropathy remains obscure. Its occurrence in the absence of methylmalonic aciduria in TC II deficiency suggests that the neuropathy is related to the defect in homocysteine-methionine conversion. Accumulation of *S*-adenosylhomocysteine in the brain, resulting in inhibition of transmethylation reactions, has been suggested. Folate deficiency has been suggested to cause organic nervous disease, but this is uncertain, although methotrexate injected into the cerebrospinal fluid may cause brain or spinal cord damage.

Psychiatric disturbance as discussed above is common in both folate and cobalamin deficiencies. This, like the neuropathy, has been attributed to a failure of the synthesis of SAM, which is needed in methylation of biogenic amines (e.g., dopamine) as well as that of proteins, phospholipids, and neurotransmitters in the brain (Fig. 99-1). Associations between lower serum folate or cobalamin levels and higher homocysteine levels and the development of decreased cognitive function and dementia in Alzheimer's disease have been reported. A meta-analysis of randomized, placebo-controlled trials of homocysteine-lowering B-vitamin supplementation of individuals with and without cognitive impairment, however, showed that supplementation with vitamin B_{12}, vitamin B_6, and folic acid alone or in combination did not improve cognitive function. Some studies done in China suggest some cognitive improvement with supplements of both vitamins. It is unknown whether prolonged treatment with these B vitamins can reduce the risk of dementia in later life.

GENERAL TISSUE EFFECTS OF COBALAMIN AND FOLATE DEFICIENCIES

Epithelial Surfaces After the marrow, the next most frequently affected tissues are the epithelial cell surfaces of the mouth (with glossitis), stomach, and small intestine and the respiratory, urinary, and female genital tracts. The cells show macrocytosis, with increased numbers of multinucleate and dying cells. The deficiencies may cause cervical smear abnormalities.

Complications of Pregnancy The gonads are also affected, and infertility is common in both men and women with severe deficiency of either vitamin. Maternal folate deficiency has been implicated as a cause of prematurity, and both folate deficiency and cobalamin deficiency have been implicated in recurrent fetal loss and neural tube defects, as discussed below.

Neural Tube Defects Folic acid supplements at the time of conception and in the first 12 weeks of pregnancy reduce by ~70% the incidence of neural tube defects (NTDs) (anencephaly, meningomyelocele, encephalocele, and spina bifida) in the fetus. Most of this protective effect can be achieved by taking folic acid, 0.4 mg daily, at the time of conception.

The incidence of cleft palate and harelip also can be reduced by prophylactic folic acid. There is no clear simple relationship between maternal folate status and these fetal abnormalities, although overall, the lower the maternal folate, the greater is the risk to the fetus. NTDs also can be caused by antifolate and antiepileptic drugs.

An underlying maternal folate metabolic abnormality has also been postulated. One abnormality has been identified: reduced activity of the enzyme 5,10-methylene-THF reductase (MTHFR) (Fig. 99-1) caused by a common C677T polymorphism in the *MTHFR* gene. In one study, the prevalence of this polymorphism was found to be higher than in controls in the parents of NTD fetuses and in the fetuses themselves: homozygosity for the TT mutation was found in 13% of cases compared with 5% of control subjects. The polymorphism codes for a thermolabile form of MTHFR. The homozygous state results in a lower mean serum and red cell folate level compared with control subjects, as well as significantly higher serum homocysteine levels. Tests for mutations in other enzymes possibly associated with NTDs, for example, methionine synthase and serine–glycine hydroxymethylase, have been negative. Serum vitamin B_{12} levels are also lower in the sera of mothers of NTD infants than in controls. In addition, maternal TC II receptor polymorphisms are associated with increased risk of NTD births. However, no studies show that dietary fortification with vitamin B_{12} reduces the incidence of NTDs.

Cardiovascular Disease Children with severe homocystinuria (blood levels ≥100 μmol/L) due to deficiency of one of three enzymes (methionine synthase, MTHFR, or cystathionine synthase; Fig. 99-1) have vascular disease, for example, ischemic heart disease, cerebrovascular disease, or pulmonary embolus, as teenagers or in young adulthood. Lesser degrees of raised serum homocysteine and low levels of serum folate and homozygous inherited mutations of *MTHFR* have been found to be associated with cerebrovascular, peripheral vascular, and coronary heart disease and with deep vein thrombosis. Prospective randomized trials of lowering homocysteine levels with supplements of folic acid, vitamin B_{12}, and vitamin B_6 against placebo over a 5-year period in patients with vascular disease or diabetes have not, however, shown a reduction of first event fatal or nonfatal myocardial infarction, nor have these supplements reduced the risk of recurrent cardiovascular disease after an acute myocardial infarct. Meta-analysis showed an 18% reduction in strokes. The benefit for stroke prevention has been confirmed by a large (>20,000 subjects) randomized prospective study in hypertensive subjects in China. This showed a significant reduction in the first incidence of stroke in subjects receiving enalapril and folic acid compared to enalapril alone. The effect was especially marked in the subjects commencing the prospective trial with the lowest serum folate levels. Venous thrombosis has been reported to be more frequent in folate-deficient or vitamin B_{12}–deficient subjects than in controls and to occur at unusual sites such as cerebral venous sinuses. This tendency was ascribed to raised plasma homocysteine levels in folate or vitamin B_{12} deficiency.

Malignancy Prophylactic folic acid in pregnancy has been found in some but not all studies to reduce the subsequent incidence of acute lymphoblastic leukemia (ALL) in childhood. A significant negative association has also been found with the *MTHFR* C677T polymorphism and leukemias with mixed lineage leukemia (MLL) translocations, but a positive association was found with hyperdiploidy in infants with ALL or acute myeloid leukemia or with childhood ALL. A second polymorphism in the *MTHFR* gene, A1298C, is also strongly associated with hyperdiploid leukemia. Various positive and negative associations are noted between polymorphisms in folate-dependent enzymes and the incidence of adult ALL. The C677T polymorphism is thought to lead to increased thymidine pools and "better quality" of DNA synthesis by shunting one-carbon groups toward thymidine and purine synthesis. This may explain its reported association with a lower risk for colorectal cancer. Most but not all studies suggest that prophylactic folic acid also protects against colon adenomas. Other tumors that have been associated with folate polymorphisms or status include follicular lymphoma, breast cancer, and gastric cancer. A meta-analysis of 50,000 individuals given folic acid (0.5–40 mg daily) or placebo in cardiovascular or colon adenoma prevention trials found that folic acid supplementation did not significantly increase or decrease the overall incidence of cancer or of any site-specific cancer during a weighted average scheduled treatment duration of 5.7 years. Because folic acid may "feed" tumors, it probably should be avoided in those with established tumors unless there is severe megaloblastic anemia due to folate deficiency.

HEMATOLOGIC FINDINGS

PERIPHERAL BLOOD

Oval macrocytes, usually with considerable anisocytosis and poikilocytosis, are the main feature (**Fig. 99-2*A***). The MCV is usually >100 fL unless a cause of microcytosis (e.g., iron deficiency or thalassemia trait) is present. Some of the neutrophils are hypersegmented (more than five nuclear lobes). There may be leukopenia due to a reduction in granulocytes and lymphocytes, but this is usually $>1.5 \times 10^9$/L; the platelet count may be moderately reduced, rarely to $<40 \times 10^9$/L. The severity of all these changes parallels the degree of anemia. In a nonanemic patient, the presence of a few macrocytes and hypersegmented neutrophils in the peripheral blood may be the only indication of the underlying disorder.

BONE MARROW

In a severely anemic patient, the marrow is hypercellular with an accumulation of primitive cells due to selective death by apoptosis of more mature forms. The erythroblast nucleus maintains a primitive appearance despite maturation and hemoglobinization of the cytoplasm. The cells are larger than normoblasts, and an increased number of cells with eccentric lobulated nuclei or nuclear fragments may be present (**Fig. 99-2*B***). Giant and abnormally shaped metamyelocytes and enlarged hyperpolyploid megakaryocytes are characteristic. In severe cases, the accumulation of primitive cells may mimic acute myeloid leukemia, whereas in less anemic patients, the changes in the marrow may be difficult to recognize. The terms *intermediate*, *mild*, and *early* have been used. The term *megaloblastoid* does not mean mildly megaloblastic. It is used to describe cells with both immature-appearing nuclei and defective hemoglobinization and is usually seen in myelodysplasia.

CHROMOSOMES

Bone marrow cells, transformed lymphocytes, and other proliferating cells in the body show a variety of changes, including random breaks, reduced contraction, spreading of the centromere, and exaggeration of secondary chromosomal constrictions and overprominent satellites. Similar abnormalities may be produced by antimetabolite drugs (e.g., cytosine arabinoside, hydroxyurea, and methotrexate) that interfere with either DNA replication or folate metabolism and that also cause megaloblastic appearances.

INEFFECTIVE HEMATOPOIESIS

Unconjugated bilirubin accumulates in plasma due to the death of nucleated red cells in the marrow (ineffective erythropoiesis). Other evidence for this includes raised urine urobilinogen, reduced haptoglobins and positive urine hemosiderin, and a raised serum lactate dehydrogenase. A weakly positive direct antiglobulin test due to complement can lead to a false diagnosis of autoimmune hemolytic anemia.

CAUSES OF COBALAMIN DEFICIENCY

Cobalamin deficiency is usually due to malabsorption. The only other cause is inadequate dietary intake.

INADEQUATE DIETARY INTAKE

Adults Dietary cobalamin deficiency arises in vegans who omit meat, fish, eggs, cheese, and other animal products from their diet. The largest group in the world consists of Hindus, and it is likely that many millions of Indians are at risk of deficiency of cobalamin on a nutritional basis. Subnormal serum cobalamin levels are found in up to 50% of randomly selected, young, adult Indian vegans, but the deficiency usually does not progress to megaloblastic anemia since the diet of most vegans is not totally lacking in cobalamin and the enterohepatic circulation of cobalamin is intact. Dietary cobalamin deficiency may also arise rarely in nonvegetarian individuals who exist on grossly inadequate diets because of poverty or psychiatric disturbance.

Infants Cobalamin deficiency has been described in infants born to severely cobalamin-deficient mothers. These infants develop megaloblastic anemia at about 3–6 months of age, presumably because they are born with low stores of cobalamin and because they are fed breast milk with low cobalamin content. The babies have also shown growth retardation, impaired psychomotor development, and other neurologic sequelae. MRI shows delayed myelination and atrophy.

GASTRIC CAUSES OF COBALAMIN MALABSORPTION

See **Tables 99-3** and **99-4**.

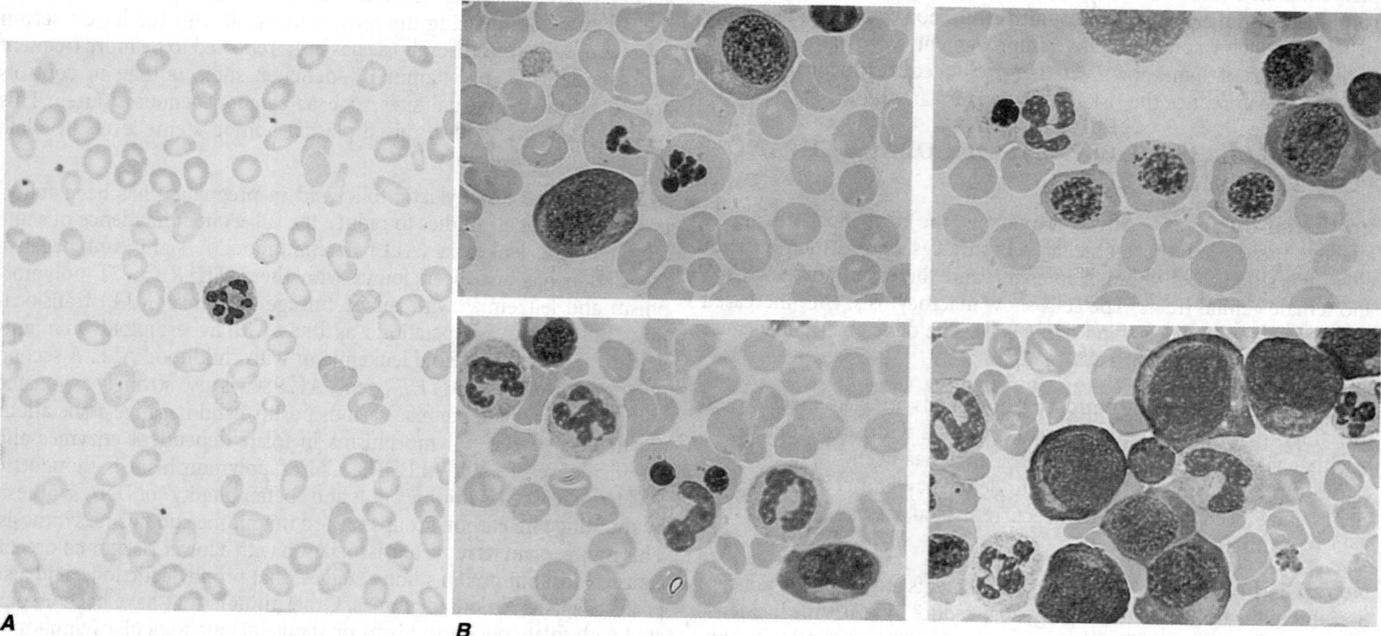

FIGURE 99-2 ***A.*** The peripheral blood in severe megaloblastic anemia. ***B.*** The bone marrow in severe megaloblastic anemia. *(Reprinted from AV Hoffbrand et al [eds]: Postgraduate Haematology, 5th ed. Oxford, UK, Blackwell Publishing, 2005; with permission.)*

TABLE 99-3 Causes of Cobalamin Deficiency Sufficiently Severe to Cause Megaloblastic Anemia

NUTRITIONAL	VEGANS
Malabsorption	Pernicious anemia
Gastric causes	Congenital absence of intrinsic factor or functional abnormality
	Total or partial gastrectomy
Intestinal causes	Intestinal stagnant loop syndrome: jejunal diverticulosis, ileocolic fistula, anatomic blind loop, intestinal stricture, etc.
	Ileal resection and Crohn's disease
	Selective malabsorption with proteinuria
	Tropical sprue
	Transcobalamin II deficiency
	Fish tapeworm

Formerly, the pathogenesis of B_{12} malabsorption was distinguishable based on the results of a Schilling test in which a radioactive form of B_{12} was administered orally and its appearance in the urine was a sign of absorption. Radioactive B_{12} is no longer available, and Schilling tests are no longer performed. Other approaches to the differential diagnosis of B_{12} malabsorption are now employed.

Pernicious Anemia PA may be defined as a severe lack of IF due to gastric atrophy. It is a common disease in northern Europeans but occurs in all countries and ethnic groups. It is more frequent in people of African than Asian ancestry. The overall incidence is about 120 per 100,000 population in the United Kingdom (UK). The ratio of incidence in men and women among whites is ~1:1.6, and the median age of onset is 70–80 years, with only 10% of patients being <40 years of age. However, in some ethnic groups, notably blacks and Latin Americans, the age at onset of PA is generally lower. The disease occurs more commonly than by chance in close relatives and in persons with other organ-specific autoimmune diseases, for example, thyroid diseases, vitiligo, hypoparathyroidism, type 1 diabetes, and Addison's disease. It is also associated with hypogammaglobulinemia, premature graying or blue eyes, and persons of blood group A. An association with human leukocyte antigen (HLA) 3 has been reported in some but not all series and, in those with endocrine disease, with HLA-B8, -B_{12}, and -BW15. Life expectancy is normal in women once regular treatment has begun. Men had a slightly subnormal life expectancy as a result of a higher incidence of carcinoma of the stomach than in control subjects, but current data on their life expectancy are unavailable. Gastric output of hydrochloric acid, pepsin, and IF is severely reduced. The serum gastrin level is raised, and serum pepsinogen I levels are low.

TABLE 99-4 Malabsorption of Cobalamin May Occur in the Following Conditions but Is Not Usually Sufficiently Severe and Prolonged to Cause Megaloblastic Anemia

Gastric causes
Simple atrophic gastritis (food cobalamin malabsorption)
Zollinger-Ellison syndrome
Gastric bypass or bariatric surgery
Use of proton pump inhibitors
Intestinal causes
Gluten-induced enteropathy
Severe pancreatitis
HIV infection
Radiotherapy
Graft-versus-host disease
Deficiencies of cobalamin, folate, protein, ?riboflavin, ?nicotinic acid
Therapy with colchicine, para-aminosalicylate, neomycin, slow-release potassium chloride, anticonvulsant drugs, metformin,[a] cytotoxic drugs
Alcohol

[a]It is now thought that metformin lowers serum vitamin B_{12} level by lowering the level of transcobalamin I.

Gastric Biopsy A single endoscopic examination is recommended if PA is diagnosed. Gastric biopsy usually shows atrophy of all layers of the body and fundus, with loss of glandular elements, an absence of parietal and chief cells and replacement by mucous cells, a mixed inflammatory cell infiltrate, and perhaps intestinal metaplasia. The infiltrate of plasma cells and lymphocytes contains an excess of CD4 cells. These are directed against gastric H/K-ATPase. The antral mucosa is usually well preserved. *Helicobacter pylori* infection occurs infrequently in PA, but it has been suggested that *H. pylori* gastritis occurs at an early phase of atrophic gastritis and presents in younger patients as iron-deficiency anemia but in older patients as PA. *H. pylori* is suggested to stimulate an autoimmune process directed against parietal cells, with the *H. pylori* infection then being gradually replaced, in some individuals, by an autoimmune process.

Serum Antibodies Two types of IF immunoglobulin G antibody may be found in the sera of patients with PA. The "blocking," or type I, antibody prevents the combination of IF and cobalamin, whereas the "binding," or type II, antibody prevents attachment of IF to ileal mucosa. Type I occurs in the sera of ~55% of patients, and type II in 35%. IF antibodies cross the placenta and may cause temporary IF deficiency in a newborn infant. Patients with PA also show cell-mediated immunity to IF. Type I antibody has been detected rarely in the sera of patients without PA but with thyrotoxicosis, myxedema, Hashimoto's disease, or diabetes mellitus and in relatives of PA patients. IF antibodies also have been detected in gastric juice in ~80% of PA patients. These gastric antibodies may reduce absorption of dietary cobalamin by combining with small amounts of remaining IF.

Parietal cell antibody is present in the sera of almost 90% of adult patients with PA but is frequently present in other subjects. Thus, it occurs in as many as 16% of randomly selected female subjects age >60 years. The parietal cell antibody is directed against the α and β subunits of the gastric proton pump (H^+, K^+-ATPase).

JUVENILE PERNICIOUS ANEMIA

This usually occurs in older children and resembles PA of adults. Gastric atrophy, achlorhydria, and serum IF antibodies are all present, although parietal cell antibodies are usually absent. About one-half of these patients show an associated endocrinopathy such as autoimmune thyroiditis, Addison's disease, or hypoparathyroidism; in some, mucocutaneous candidiasis occurs.

CONGENITAL INTRINSIC FACTOR DEFICIENCY OR FUNCTIONAL ABNORMALITY

An affected child usually presents with megaloblastic anemia in the first to third year of life; a few have presented as late as the second decade. The child usually has no demonstrable IF but has a normal gastric mucosa and normal secretion of acid. The inheritance is autosomal recessive. Parietal cell and IF antibodies are absent. Variants have been described in which the child is born with IF that can be detected immunologically but is unstable or functionally inactive, unable to bind cobalamin or to facilitate its uptake by ileal receptors.

GASTRECTOMY

After total gastrectomy, cobalamin deficiency is inevitable, and prophylactic cobalamin therapy should be commenced immediately after the operation. After partial gastrectomy, 10–15% of patients also develop this deficiency. The exact incidence and time of onset are most influenced by the size of the resection and the preexisting size of cobalamin body stores.

FOOD COBALAMIN MALABSORPTION

Failure of release of cobalamin from binding proteins in food is believed to be responsible for this condition, which is more common in the elderly. It is associated with low serum cobalamin levels, with or without raised serum levels of MMA and homocysteine. Typically, these patients have normal cobalamin absorption, as measured with crystalline cobalamin, but show malabsorption when a modified test using food-bound cobalamin is used. It is usually due to mild forms of atrophic gastritis or therapy with proton pump inhibitors. Bariatric surgery is likely to be an increasing cause of this form of B_{12} malabsorption and deficiency. The frequency of progression to severe cobalamin deficiency and the reasons for this progression are not clear.

INTESTINAL CAUSES OF COBALAMIN MALABSORPTION

Intestinal Stagnant Loop Syndrome Malabsorption of cobalamin occurs in a variety of intestinal lesions in which there is colonization of the upper small intestine by fecal organisms. This may occur in patients with jejunal diverticulosis, enteroanastomosis, or an intestinal stricture or fistula or with an anatomic blind loop due to Crohn's disease, tuberculosis, or an operative procedure.

Ileal Resection Removal of ≥1.2 m of terminal ileum causes malabsorption of cobalamin. In some patients after ileal resection, particularly if the ileocecal valve is incompetent, colonic bacteria may contribute further to the onset of cobalamin deficiency.

Selective Malabsorption of Cobalamin with Proteinuria (Imerslund's Syndrome; Imerslund-Gräsbeck Syndrome; Congenital Cobalamin Malabsorption; Autosomal Recessive Megaloblastic Anemia; MGA1) This autosomal recessive disease is the most common cause of megaloblastic anemia due to cobalamin deficiency in infancy in Western countries. More than 200 cases have been reported with familial clusters in Finland, Norway, the Middle East, and North Africa. The patients secrete normal amounts of IF and gastric acid but are unable to absorb cobalamin. In Finland, impaired synthesis, processing, or ligand binding of cubilin due to inherited mutations is found. In Norway, mutation of the gene for *AMN* has been reported. Other tests of intestinal absorption are normal. Over 90% of these patients show nonspecific proteinuria, but renal function is otherwise normal, and renal biopsy has not shown any consistent renal defect. A few have shown aminoaciduria and congenital renal abnormalities, such as duplication of the renal pelvis.

Tropical Sprue Nearly all patients with acute and subacute tropical sprue show malabsorption of cobalamin; this may persist as the principal abnormality in the chronic form of the disease, when the patient may present with megaloblastic anemia or neuropathy due to cobalamin deficiency. Absorption of cobalamin usually improves after antibiotic therapy and, in the early stages, folic acid therapy.

Fish Tapeworm Infestation The fish tapeworm (*Diphyllobothrium latum*) lives in the small intestine of humans and accumulates cobalamin from food, rendering the cobalamin unavailable for absorption. Individuals acquire the worm by eating raw or partly cooked fish. Infestation is common around the lakes of Scandinavia, Germany, Japan, North America, and Russia. Megaloblastic anemia or cobalamin neuropathy occurs only in those with a heavy infestation.

Gluten-Induced Enteropathy Malabsorption of cobalamin occurs in ~30% of untreated patients (presumably those in whom the disease extends to the ileum). Cobalamin deficiency is not severe in these patients and is corrected with a gluten-free diet.

Severe Chronic Pancreatitis In this condition, lack of trypsin is thought to cause dietary cobalamin attached to gastric non-IF (R) binder to be unavailable for absorption. It also has been proposed that in pancreatitis, the concentration of calcium ions in the ileum falls below the level needed to maintain normal cobalamin absorption.

HIV Infection Serum cobalamin levels tend to fall in patients with HIV infection and are subnormal in 10–35% of those with AIDS. Malabsorption of cobalamin not corrected by IF has been shown in some, but not all, patients with subnormal serum cobalamin levels. Cobalamin deficiency sufficiently severe to cause megaloblastic anemia or neuropathy is rare.

Zollinger-Ellison Syndrome Malabsorption of cobalamin has been reported in the Zollinger-Ellison syndrome. It is thought that there is a failure to release cobalamin from R-binding protein due to inactivation of pancreatic trypsin by high acidity, as well as interference with IF binding of cobalamin.

Radiotherapy Both total-body irradiation and local radiotherapy to the ileum (e.g., as a complication of radiotherapy for carcinoma of the cervix) may cause malabsorption of cobalamin.

Graft-versus-Host Disease This commonly affects the small intestine. Malabsorption of cobalamin due to abnormal gut flora, as well as damage to ileal mucosa, is common.

Drugs The drugs that have been reported to cause malabsorption of cobalamin are listed in Table 99-4. However, megaloblastic anemia due to these drugs is rare. It has been suggested that metformin lowers serum B_{12} by lowering TC I level rather than causing malabsorption of B_{12}.

ABNORMALITIES OF COBALAMIN METABOLISM

Congenital Transcobalamin II Deficiency or Abnormality Infants with TC II deficiency usually present with megaloblastic anemia within a few weeks of birth. Serum cobalamin and folate levels are normal, but the anemia responds to massive (e.g., 1 mg three times weekly) injections of cobalamin. Some cases show neurologic complications. The protein may be present but functionally inert. Genetic abnormalities found include mutations of an intraexonic cryptic splice site, extensive deletion, single nucleotide deletion, nonsense mutation, and an RNA editing defect. Malabsorption of cobalamin occurs in all cases, and serum immunoglobulins are usually reduced. Failure to institute adequate cobalamin therapy or treatment with folic acid may lead to neurologic damage.

Congenital Methylmalonic Acidemia and Aciduria Infants with this abnormality are ill from birth with vomiting, failure to thrive, severe metabolic acidosis, ketosis, and mental retardation. Anemia, if present, is normocytic and normoblastic. The condition may be due to a functional defect in either mitochondrial methylmalonyl-CoA mutase or its cofactor adocobalamin. Mutations in the methylmalonyl-CoA mutase are not responsive or are only poorly responsive to treatment with cobalamin. A proportion of infants with failure of adocobalamin synthesis respond to cobalamin in large doses. Some children have combined methylmalonic aciduria and homocystinuria due to defective formation of both cobalamin coenzymes. This usually presents in the first year of life with feeding difficulties, developmental delay, microcephaly, seizures, hypotonia, and megaloblastic anemia.

Acquired Abnormality of Cobalamin Metabolism: Nitrous Oxide Inhalation Nitrous oxide (N_2O) irreversibly oxidizes methylcobalamin to an inactive precursor; this inactivates methionine synthase. Megaloblastic anemia has occurred in patients undergoing prolonged N_2O anesthesia (e.g., in intensive care units). A neuropathy resembling cobalamin neuropathy has been described in dentists and anesthetists who are exposed repeatedly to N_2O. Methylmalonic aciduria does not occur as adocobalamin is not inactivated by N_2O.

CAUSES OF FOLATE DEFICIENCY

(Table 99-5)

NUTRITIONAL

Dietary folate deficiency is common. Indeed, in most patients with folate deficiency, a nutritional element is present. Certain individuals are particularly prone to have diets containing inadequate amounts of folate (Table 99-5). In the United States and other countries where fortification of the diet with folic acid has been adopted, the prevalence of folate deficiency has dropped dramatically and is now almost restricted to high-risk groups with increased folate needs. Nutritional folate deficiency occurs in kwashiorkor and scurvy and in infants with repeated infections or those who are fed solely on goats' milk, which has a low folate content.

TABLE 99-5 Causes of Folate Deficiency

Dietary[a]
Particularly in: old age, infancy, poverty, alcoholism, chronic invalids, and the psychiatrically disturbed; may be associated with scurvy or kwashiorkor
Malabsorption
Major causes of deficiency
Tropical sprue, gluten-induced enteropathy in children and adults, and in association with dermatitis herpetiformis, specific malabsorption of folate, intestinal megaloblastosis caused by severe cobalamin or folate deficiency
Minor causes of deficiency
Extensive jejunal resection, Crohn's disease, partial gastrectomy, congestive heart failure, Whipple's disease, scleroderma, amyloid, diabetic enteropathy, systemic bacterial infection, lymphoma, sulfasalazine (Salazopyrin)
Excess utilization or loss
Physiologic
Pregnancy and lactation, prematurity
Pathologic
Hematologic diseases: chronic hemolytic anemias, sickle cell anemia, thalassemia major, myelofibrosis
Malignant diseases: carcinoma, lymphoma, leukemia, myeloma
Inflammatory diseases: tuberculosis, Crohn's disease, psoriasis, exfoliative dermatitis, malaria
Metabolic disease: homocystinuria
Excess urinary loss: congestive heart failure, active liver disease
Hemodialysis, peritoneal dialysis
Antifolate drugs[b]
Anticonvulsant drugs (phenytoin, primidone, barbiturates), sulfasalazine
Nitrofurantoin, tetracycline, antituberculosis (less well documented)
Mixed causes
Liver diseases, alcoholism, intensive care units

[a]In severely folate-deficient patients with causes other than those listed under Dietary, poor dietary intake is often present. [b]Drugs inhibiting dihydrofolate reductase are discussed in the text.

MALABSORPTION

Malabsorption of dietary folate occurs in tropical sprue and in gluten-induced enteropathy. In the rare congenital recessive syndrome of selective malabsorption of folate due to mutation of the PCFT, there is an associated defect of folate transport into the cerebrospinal fluid, and these patients show megaloblastic anemia, which responds to physiologic doses of folic acid given parenterally but not orally. They also show mental retardation, convulsions, and other central nervous system abnormalities. Minor degrees of malabsorption may also occur after jejunal resection or partial gastrectomy, in Crohn's disease, and in systemic infections, but in these conditions, if severe deficiency occurs, it is usually largely due to poor nutrition. Malabsorption of folate has been described in patients receiving sulfasalazine (Salazopyrin), cholestyramine, and triamterene.

EXCESS UTILIZATION OR LOSS

Pregnancy Folate requirements are increased by 200–300 μg to ~400 μg daily in a normal pregnancy, partly because of transfer of the vitamin to the fetus but mainly because of increased folate catabolism due to cleavage of folate coenzymes in rapidly proliferating tissues. Megaloblastic anemia due to this deficiency is prevented by prophylactic folic acid therapy. It occurred in 0.5% of pregnancies in the UK and other Western countries before prophylaxis with folic acid, but the incidence is much higher in countries where the general nutritional status is poor.

Prematurity A newborn infant, whether full term or premature, has higher serum and red cell folate concentrations than does an adult. However, a newborn infant's demand for folate has been estimated to be up to 10 times that of adults on a weight basis, and the neonatal folate level falls rapidly to the lowest values at about 6 weeks of age. The falls are steepest and are liable to reach subnormal levels in premature babies, a number of whom develop megaloblastic anemia responsive to folic acid at about 4–6 weeks of age. This occurs particularly in the smallest babies (<1500 g birth weight) and those who have feeding difficulties or infections or have undergone multiple exchange transfusions. In these babies, prophylactic folic acid should be given.

Hematologic Disorders Folate deficiency frequently occurs in chronic hemolytic anemia, particularly in sickle cell disease, autoimmune hemolytic anemia, and congenital spherocytosis. In these and other conditions of increased cell turnover (e.g., myelofibrosis, malignancies), folate deficiency arises because it is not completely reutilized after performing coenzyme functions.

Inflammatory Conditions Chronic inflammatory diseases such as tuberculosis, rheumatoid arthritis, Crohn's disease, psoriasis, exfoliative dermatitis, bacterial endocarditis, and chronic bacterial infections cause deficiency by reducing the appetite and increasing the demand for folate. Systemic infections also may cause malabsorption of folate. Severe deficiency is virtually confined to the patients with the most active disease and the poorest diet.

Homocystinuria This is a rare metabolic defect in the conversion of homocysteine to cystathionine. Folate deficiency occurring in most of these patients may be due to excessive utilization because of compensatory increased conversion of homocysteine to methionine.

Long-Term Dialysis Because folate is only loosely bound to plasma proteins, it is easily removed from plasma by dialysis. In patients with anorexia, vomiting, infections, and hemolysis, folate stores are particularly likely to become depleted. Routine folate prophylaxis is now given.

Congestive Heart Failure and Liver Disease Excess urinary folate losses of >100 μg per day may occur in some of these patients. The explanation appears to be release of folate from damaged liver cells.

ANTIFOLATE DRUGS

A large number of epileptics who are receiving long-term therapy with phenytoin or primidone, with or without barbiturates, develop low serum and red cell folate levels. The exact mechanism is unclear. Alcohol may also be a folate antagonist, as patients who are drinking spirits may develop megaloblastic anemia that will respond to normal quantities of dietary folate or to physiologic doses of folic acid only if alcohol is withdrawn. Macrocytosis of red cells is associated with chronic alcohol intake even when folate levels are normal. Inadequate folate intake is the major factor in the development of deficiency in spirit-drinking alcoholics. Beer is relatively folate-rich in some countries, depending on the technique used for brewing.

The drugs that inhibit DHF reductase include methotrexate, pyrimethamine, and trimethoprim. Methotrexate has the most powerful action against the human enzyme, whereas trimethoprim is most active against the bacterial enzyme and is likely to cause megaloblastic anemia only when used in conjunction with sulfamethoxazole in patients with preexisting folate or cobalamin deficiency. The activity of pyrimethamine is intermediate. The antidote to these drugs is folinic acid (5-formyl-THF).

CONGENITAL ABNORMALITIES OF FOLATE METABOLISM

Some infants with congenital defects of folate enzymes (e.g., cyclohydrolase or methionine synthase) have had megaloblastic anemia.

DIAGNOSIS OF COBALAMIN AND FOLATE DEFICIENCIES

The diagnosis of cobalamin or folate deficiency has traditionally depended on the recognition of the relevant abnormalities in the peripheral blood and analysis of the blood levels of the vitamins.

COBALAMIN DEFICIENCY

Serum Cobalamin This is measured by an automated enzyme-linked immunosorbent assay (ELISA) or competitive-binding luminescence assay (CBLA). Normal serum levels range from 118–148 pmol/L (160–200 ng/L) to ~738 pmol/L (1000 ng/L). In patients with megaloblastic anemia due to cobalamin deficiency, the level is usually <74 pmol/L (100 ng/L). In general, the more severe the deficiency, the lower is the serum cobalamin level. In patients with spinal cord damage due to the deficiency, levels are very low even in the absence of anemia. Values between 74 and 148 pmol/L (100 and 200 ng/L) are regarded as borderline. They may occur, for instance, in pregnancy, in patients with megaloblastic anemia due to folate deficiency. They may also be due to heterozygous, homozygous, or compound heterozygous mutations of the gene *TCN1* that codes for HC (TC I). There is then no clinical or hematologic abnormality. The serum cobalamin level is sufficiently robust, cost-effective, and most convenient to rule out cobalamin deficiency in the vast majority of patients suspected of having this problem. However, problems have arisen with commercial CBLA assays involving IF in PA patients with intrinsic antibodies in serum. These antibodies may cause false normal serum vitamin B_{12} levels in up to 50% of cases tested. Where clinical indications of PA are strong, a normal serum vitamin B_{12} does not rule out the diagnosis. Serum MMA levels will be elevated in untreated PA (see below).

Folate deficiency, TC I (HC) deficiency, oral contraceptives, and multiple myeloma have all been associated with low serum B_{12} levels that do not indicate B_{12} deficiency. On the other hand, high serum B_{12} levels are usually due to raised serum TC I levels and can be due to the presence of liver, renal, or myeloproliferative diseases or to cancer of the breast, colon, or liver.

Serum Methylmalonate and Homocysteine In patients with cobalamin deficiency sufficient to cause anemia or neuropathy, the serum MMA level is raised. Sensitive methods for measuring MMA and homocysteine in serum have been introduced and recommended for the early diagnosis of cobalamin deficiency, even in the absence of hematologic abnormalities or subnormal levels of serum cobalamin. Serum MMA levels fluctuate, however, in patients with renal failure. Mildly elevated serum MMA and/or homocysteine levels occur in up to 30% of apparently healthy volunteers, with serum cobalamin levels up to 258 pmol/L (350 ng/L) and normal serum folate levels; 15% of elderly subjects, even with cobalamin levels >258 pmol/L (>350 ng/L), have this pattern of raised metabolite levels. These findings bring into question the exact cutoff points for normal MMA and homocysteine levels. It is also unclear at present whether these mildly raised metabolite levels have clinical consequences.

Serum homocysteine is raised in both early cobalamin and folate deficiency but may be raised in other conditions, for example, chronic renal disease, alcoholism, smoking, pyridoxine deficiency, hypothyroidism, and therapy with steroids, cyclosporine, and other drugs. Levels are also higher in serum than in plasma, in men than in premenopausal women, in women taking hormone replacement therapy or in oral contraceptive users, and in elderly persons and patients with several inborn errors of metabolism affecting enzymes in transsulfuration pathways of homocysteine metabolism. Thus, homocysteine levels must be carefully interpreted for diagnosis of cobalamin or folate deficiency.

Tests for the Cause of Cobalamin Deficiency Only vegans, strict vegetarians, or people living on a totally inadequate diet will become vitamin B_{12} deficient because of inadequate intake. Studies of cobalamin absorption once were widely used, but difficulty in obtaining radioactive cobalamin and ensuring that IF preparations are free of viruses has made these tests obsolete. Tests to diagnose PA include serum gastrin, which is raised; serum pepsinogen I, which is low in PA (90–92%) but also in other conditions; and gastric endoscopy. Tests for IF and parietal cell antibodies are also used, as well as tests for individual intestinal diseases.

Patients with atrophic gastritis may also have sufficient occult gastrointestinal blood loss to have iron deficiency as well as vitamin B_{12} deficiency. Iron deficiency may blunt the development of macrocytosis when iron deficiency and B_{12} deficiency coexist. Iron deficiency is much more common than B_{12} deficiency, and in people older than age 60 years, B_{12} deficiency may accompany iron deficiency in 15–20% of cases. Thus, patients diagnosed with iron-deficiency anemia should have B_{12} levels assessed, and those diagnosed with B_{12} deficiency should have their iron status assessed.

FOLATE DEFICIENCY

Serum Folate This is also measured by an ELISA technique. In most laboratories, the normal range is from 11 nmol/L (2 μg/L) to ~82 nmol/L (15 μg/L). The serum folate level is low in all folate-deficient patients. It also reflects recent diet. Because of this, serum folate may be low before there is hematologic or biochemical evidence of deficiency. Serum folate rises in severe cobalamin deficiency because of the block in conversion of MTHF to THF inside cells; raised levels have also been reported in the intestinal stagnant loop syndrome due to absorption of bacterially synthesized folate.

Red Cell Folate The red cell folate assay is a valuable test of body folate stores. It is less affected than the serum assay by recent diet and traces of hemolysis. In normal adults, concentrations range from 880 to 3520 μmol/L (160–640 μg/L) of packed red cells. Subnormal levels occur in patients with megaloblastic anemia due to folate deficiency but also in nearly two-thirds of patients with severe cobalamin deficiency. False-normal results may occur if a folate-deficient patient has received a recent blood transfusion or if a patient has a raised reticulocyte count. Serum homocysteine assay is discussed earlier.

Tests for the Cause of Folate Deficiency The diet history is important. Tests for transglutaminase antibodies are performed to confirm or exclude celiac disease. If positive, duodenal biopsy is needed. An underlying disease causing increased folate breakdown should also be excluded.

TREATMENT

Cobalamin and Folate Deficiency

It is usually possible to establish which of the two deficiencies, folate or cobalamin, is the cause of the anemia and to treat only with the appropriate vitamin. In patients who enter the hospital severely ill, however, it may be necessary to treat with both vitamins in large doses once blood samples have been taken for cobalamin and folate assays and a bone marrow biopsy has been performed (if deemed necessary). Transfusion is usually unnecessary and inadvisable. If it is essential, packed red cells should be given slowly, one or two units only, with the usual treatment for heart failure if present. Potassium supplements have been recommended to obviate the danger of the hypokalemia but are not necessary. Occasionally, an excessive rise in platelets occurs after 1–2 weeks of therapy. Antiplatelet therapy, for example, aspirin, should be considered if the platelet count rises to >800 × 10^9/L.

COBALAMIN DEFICIENCY

It is usually necessary to treat patients who have developed cobalamin deficiency with lifelong regular cobalamin injections. In the UK, the form used is hydroxocobalamin; in the United States, cyanocobalamin. In a few instances, the underlying cause of cobalamin deficiency can be permanently corrected, for example, fish tapeworm, tropical sprue, or an intestinal stagnant loop that is amenable to surgery. The indications for starting cobalamin therapy are a well-documented megaloblastic anemia or other hematologic abnormalities and neuropathy due to the deficiency. Patients with borderline serum cobalamin levels but no hematologic or other abnormality may be followed to make sure that the cobalamin deficiency does not progress (see below). If malabsorption of cobalamin or rises in serum MMA levels have been demonstrated, however, these patients also should be given regular maintenance cobalamin therapy. Cobalamin should be given routinely to all patients who have had a total gastrectomy or ileal resection. Patients who have undergone gastric reduction for control of obesity or who are receiving long-term treatment with proton pump inhibitors should be screened and, if necessary, given cobalamin replacement.

Replenishment of body stores should be complete with six 1000-μg IM injections of hydroxocobalamin given at 3- to 7-day intervals. More frequent doses are usually used in patients with cobalamin neuropathy, but there is no evidence that they produce a better response. Allergic reactions are rare and may require desensitization or antihistamine or glucocorticoid cover. For maintenance therapy, 1000 μg hydroxocobalamin IM once every 3 months is satisfactory. Because of the poorer retention of cyanocobalamin, protocols generally use higher and more frequent doses, for example, 1000 μg IM, monthly, for maintenance treatment.

Because a small fraction of cobalamin can be absorbed passively through mucous membranes even when there is complete failure of physiologic IF-dependent absorption, large daily oral doses (1000–2000 μg) of cyanocobalamin are used in PA for replacement (especially in Canada and Sweden) and maintenance of normal cobalamin status in, for example, food malabsorption of cobalamin. Sublingual therapy has also been proposed for those in whom injections are difficult because of a bleeding tendency and who may not tolerate oral therapy. If oral therapy is used, it is important to monitor compliance, particularly with elderly, forgetful patients. This author prefers parenteral therapy for initial treatment, particularly in severe anemia or if a neuropathy is present, and for maintenance in PA. Oral B_{12} therapy even with low doses of 50 μg daily may have a larger role in treating food malabsorption of B_{12}.

For treatment of patients with subnormal serum vitamin B_{12} levels with a normal MCV and no hypersegmentation of neutrophils, a negative IF antibody test in the absence of tests of B_{12} absorption is problematic. Some (perhaps 15%) cases may be due to TC I (HC) deficiency. Homocysteine and/or MMA measurements may help, but in the absence of these tests and with otherwise normal gastrointestinal function, repeat serum B_{12} assay after 6–12 months may help one decide whether to start cobalamin therapy.

Vitamin B_{12} injections are used in a wide variety of diseases, often neurologic, despite normal serum B_{12} and folate levels and a normal blood count and in the absence of randomized, double-blind, controlled trials. These conditions include multiple sclerosis and chronic fatigue syndrome/myalgic encephalomyelitis (ME). It seems probable that any benefit is due to the placebo effect of a usually painless, pink injection. In ME, oral B_{12} therapy, despite providing equally large amounts of B_{12}, has not been beneficial, supporting the view of the effect of the injections being placebo only.

FOLATE DEFICIENCY

Oral doses of 5–15 mg of folic acid daily are satisfactory, as sufficient folate is absorbed from these extremely large doses even in patients with severe malabsorption. The length of time therapy must be continued depends on the underlying disease. It is customary to continue therapy for about 4 months, when all folate-deficient red cells will have been eliminated and replaced by new folate-replete populations.

Before large doses of folic acid are given, cobalamin deficiency must be excluded and, if present, corrected; otherwise, cobalamin neuropathy may develop despite a response of the anemia of cobalamin deficiency to folate therapy. Studies in the United States, however, suggest that there is no increase in the proportion of individuals with low serum cobalamin levels and no anemia since food fortification with folic acid, but it is unknown if there has been a change in incidence of cobalamin neuropathy.

Long-term folic acid therapy is required when the underlying cause of the deficiency cannot be corrected and the deficiency is likely to recur, for example, in chronic dialysis or hemolytic anemias. It may also be necessary in gluten-induced enteropathy that does not respond to a gluten-free diet. Where mild but chronic folate deficiency occurs, it is preferable to encourage improvement in the diet after correcting the deficiency with a short course of folic acid. In any patient receiving long-term folic acid therapy, it is important to measure the serum cobalamin level at regular (e.g., once-yearly) intervals to exclude the coincidental development of cobalamin deficiency.

Folinic Acid (5-Formyl-THF) This is a stable form of fully reduced folate. It is given orally or parenterally to overcome the toxic effects of methotrexate or other DHF reductase inhibitors, for example, trimethoprim or cotrimoxazole.

PROPHYLACTIC FOLIC ACID

Prophylactic folic acid is used in chronic dialysis patients and in parenteral feeds. Prophylactic folic acid has been used to reduce homocysteine levels to prevent cardiovascular disease and for cognitive function in the elderly, but there are no firm data to show any benefit.

Pregnancy In over 70 countries (but none in Europe), food is fortified with folic acid (in grain or flour) to reduce the risk of NTDs. Nevertheless, folic acid, 400 μg daily, should be given as a supplement before and throughout pregnancy to prevent megaloblastic anemia and reduce the incidence of NTDs, even in countries with fortification of the diet. The levels of fortification provide up to 400 μg daily on average in Chile, but in most countries, it is nearer to 200 μg, so periconceptual folic acid is still needed. Most if not all the folic acid used in fortification and eaten over three meals a day will be converted during absorption to methyltetrahydrofolate. This compound will not correct the anemia in B_{12} deficiency. Studies in early pregnancy show significant lack of compliance with the folic acid supplements, emphasizing the benefit of food fortification. Supplemental folic acid reduces the incidence of birth defects in babies born to diabetic mothers. In women who have had a previous fetus with an NTD, a dose of 5 mg daily is recommended when pregnancy is contemplated and throughout the subsequent pregnancy.

Infancy and Childhood The incidence of folate deficiency is so high in the smallest premature babies during the first 6 weeks of life that folic acid (e.g., 1 mg daily) should be given routinely to those weighing <1500 g at birth and to larger premature babies who require exchange transfusions or develop feeding difficulties, infections, or vomiting and diarrhea.

The World Health Organization currently recommends routine supplementation with iron and folic acid in children in countries where iron deficiency is common and child mortality, largely due to infectious diseases, is high. However, some studies suggest that in areas where malaria rates are high, this approach may increase the incidence of severe illness and death. Even where malaria is rare, there appears to be no survival benefit.

MEGALOBLASTIC ANEMIA NOT DUE TO COBALAMIN OR FOLATE DEFICIENCY OR ALTERED METABOLISM

This may occur with many antimetabolic drugs (e.g., hydroxyurea, cytosine arabinoside, 6-mercaptopurine) that inhibit DNA replication. Antiviral nucleoside analogues used in treatment of HIV infection may also cause macrocytosis and megaloblastic marrow changes. In the rare disease orotic aciduria, two consecutive enzymes in purine synthesis are defective. The condition responds to therapy with uridine, which bypasses the block. In thiamine-responsive megaloblastic anemia, there is a genetic defect in the high-affinity thiamine transport (*SLC19A2*) gene. This causes defective RNA ribose synthesis through impaired activity of transketolase, a thiamine-dependent enzyme in the pentose cycle. This leads to reduced nucleic acid production. It may be associated with diabetes mellitus and deafness and the presence of many ringed sideroblasts in the marrow. The explanation is unclear for megaloblastic changes in the marrow in some patients with acute myeloid leukemia and myelodysplasia.

FURTHER READING

Berry RJ: Lack of historical evidence to support folic acid exacerbation of the neuropathy caused by vitamin B12 deficiency. Am J Clin Nutr 110:554, 2019.

Bunn HF: Vitamin B12 and pernicious anemia: The dawn of molecular medicine. N Engl J Med 370:773, 2014.

Del Bo C et al: Effect of two different sublingual dosages of vitamin B12 on cobalamin nutritional status in vegans and vegetarians with a marginal deficiency: A randomized controlled trial. Clin Nutr 38:575, 2019.

Green R: Vitamin B12 deficiency from the perspective of a practicing hematologist. Blood 129:2603, 2017.

Green R et al: Vitamin B12 deficiency. Nat Rev Dis Primers 3:17040, 2017.

Hesdorffer CS, Longo DL: Drug-induced megaloblastic anemia. N Engl J Med 373:1649, 2015.

Ma F et al: Effects of folic acid and vitamin B12 lone and in combination on cognitive function and inflammatory factors in the elderly with mild cognitive impairment: A single blind experimental design. Curr Alzheimer Res 16: 622, 2019.

Miller JW: Proton pump inhibitors, H2-receptor antagonists, metformin, and vitamin B-12 deficiency: Clinical implications. Adv Nutr 9:511S, 2018.

O'Connor DMA et al: Plasma concentrations of vitamin B12 (B12) and folate and global cognitive function in an older population: cross-sectional findings from the Irish Longitudinal Study on Ageing (TILDA). Br J Nutr 124:602, 2020.

Rogers LM et al: Global folate status in women of reproductive age: A systematic review with emphasis on methodological issues. Ann N Y Acad Sci 1431:35, 2018.

Salinas M et al: High frequency of anti-parietal cell antibody (APCA) and intrinsic factor blocking antibody (IFBA) in individuals with severe vitamin B12 deficiency: An observational study in primary care patients. Clin Chem Lab Med 58:424, 2020.

Zaric BL et al: Homocysteine and hyperhomocysteinaemia. Curr Med Chem 26:2948, 2019.

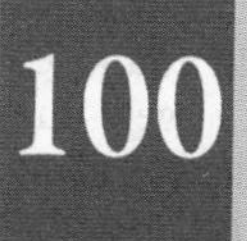

100 Hemolytic Anemias

Lucio Luzzatto, Lucia De Franceschi

DEFINITIONS

A finite life span is a distinct characteristic of red cells. Hence, a logical, time-honored classification of anemias is in three groups: (1) decreased production of red cells, (2) increased destruction of red cells, and (3) acute blood loss. Decreased production is covered in **Chaps. 97, 98,** and **102**; acute blood loss in **Chap. 101**; increased destruction is covered in this chapter.

All patients who are anemic as a result of either increased destruction of red cells or acute blood loss have one important element in common: the anemia results from overconsumption of red cells from the peripheral blood, whereas the supply of cells from the bone marrow is normal (indeed, it is usually increased). However, with blood loss, as in acute hemorrhage, the red cells are physically lost *from* the body itself; this is fundamentally different from destruction of red cells *within* the body, as in hemolytic anemias (HAs).

With respect to primary etiology, HAs may be *inherited* or *acquired*; from a clinical point of view, they may be more *acute* or more *chronic*, and they may vary from mild to very severe; the site of hemolysis may be predominantly *intravascular* or *extravascular*. With respect to mechanisms, HAs may be due to *intracorpuscular* causes or to *extracorpuscular* causes (**Table 100-1**). But before reviewing the individual types of HA, it is appropriate to consider what general features they have in common, in terms of clinical aspects and pathophysiology.

TABLE 100-1 Classification of Hemolytic Anemias[a]

	INTRACORPUSCULAR DEFECTS	EXTRACORPUSCULAR FACTORS
Inherited	Hemoglobinopathies Enzymopathies Membrane-cytoskeletal defects	Familial (atypical) hemolytic-uremic syndrome
Acquired	Paroxysmal nocturnal hemoglobinuria (PNH)	Mechanical destruction (microangiopathic) Toxic agents Drugs Infectious Autoimmune

[a]Hereditary causes correlate with intracorpuscular defects because these defects are due to inherited mutations; the one exception is PNH because the defect is due to an acquired somatic mutation. Conversely, acquired causes correlate with extracorpuscular factors because mostly these factors are exogenous; the one exception is familial hemolytic-uremic syndrome (HUS; often referred to as atypical HUS) because here an inherited abnormality permits complement activation triggered by exogenous factors, to become excessive, with bouts of production of membrane attack complex capable of destroying normal red cells. Interestingly, in both PNH and aHUS hemolysis is complement-mediated.

GENERAL CLINICAL AND LABORATORY FEATURES

The clinical presentation of a patient with anemia is greatly influenced in the first place by whether the onset is abrupt or gradual and HAs are no exception. A patient with autoimmune HA or with favism may be a medical emergency, whereas a patient with mild hereditary spherocytosis (HS) or with cold agglutinin disease (CAD) may be diagnosed after years. This is due in large measure to the remarkable ability of the body to adapt to anemia when it is slowly progressing **(Chap. 63)**.

What differentiates HAs from other anemias is that the patient has signs and symptoms arising directly from hemolysis **(Table 100-2)**. At the clinical level, the main sign is *jaundice*; in addition, the patient may report discoloration of the urine. In many cases of HA, the spleen is enlarged because it is a preferential site of hemolysis; and in some cases, the liver may be enlarged as well. In all severe congenital forms of HA, there may also be skeletal changes due to overactivity of the bone marrow: they are never as severe as in thalassemia major because there is less ineffective erythropoiesis, or none at all.

The laboratory features of HA are related to (i) hemolysis per se, and (ii) the erythropoietic response of the bone marrow. In most cases hemolysis is largely extravascular, and it produces an increase in unconjugated bilirubin and aspartate aminotransferase (AST) in the serum; urobilinogen will be increased in both urine and stool. If hemolysis is mainly intravascular, the telltale sign is hemoglobinuria (often associated with hemosiderinuria); in the serum there is free hemoglobin, lactate dehydrogenase (LDH) is increased, and haptoglobin is reduced. In contrast, the serum bilirubin level may be normal

TABLE 100-2 Features Common to Most Patients with a Hemolytic Disorder

General examination	Jaundice, pallor
Other physical findings	Spleen may be enlarged; bossing of skull in severe congenital cases
Hemoglobin level	From normal to severely reduced
MCV, MCH	Usually increased
Reticulocytes	Usually increased
Bilirubin	Almost always increased (mostly unconjugated)
LDH	Increased (up to 10× normal with intravascular hemolysis)
Haptoglobin	Reduced to absent if hemolysis is at least in part intravascular

Abbreviations: LDH, lactate dehydrogenase; MCH, mean corpuscular hemoglobin; MCV, mean corpuscular volume.

or only mildly elevated. The main sign of the erythropoietic response by the bone marrow is an increase in reticulocytes (a test all too often neglected in the initial workup of a patient with anemia). Usually the increase will be reflected in both the percentage of reticulocytes (the more commonly quoted figure) and in the absolute reticulocyte count (the more definitive parameter). The increased number of reticulocytes is associated with an increased mean corpuscular volume (MCV) in the blood count. On the blood smear, this is reflected in the presence of macrocytes; there is also polychromasia, and sometimes one sees nucleated red cells. In most cases, a bone marrow aspirate is not necessary in the diagnostic workup; if it is done, it will show erythroid hyperplasia. In practice, once an HA is suspected, specific tests will usually be required for a definitive diagnosis of a specific type of HA.

GENERAL PATHOPHYSIOLOGY

The mature red cell is the product of a developmental pathway that brings the phenomenon of differentiation to an extreme. An orderly sequence of events produces synchronous changes, whereby the gradual accumulation of a huge amount of hemoglobin in the cytoplasm (to a final level of 340 g/L, i.e., about 5 m*M*) goes hand in hand with the gradual loss of cellular organelles and of biosynthetic abilities. In the end, the erythroid cell undergoes a process that has features of apoptosis, including nuclear pyknosis and eventually extrusion of the nucleus. However, the final result is more altruistic than suicidal; the cytoplasmic body, instead of disintegrating, is now able to provide oxygen to all cells in the human organism for some remaining 120 days of the red cell life span.

As a result of this unique process of differentiation and maturation, intermediary metabolism is drastically curtailed in mature red cells (**Fig. 100-1**); for instance, cytochrome-mediated oxidative phosphorylation has been lost with the loss of mitochondria (through a process of physiologic autophagy); therefore, there is no backup to anaerobic glycolysis, which in the red cell is the only provider of adenosine triphosphate (ATP). Also, the capacity of making protein has been lost with the loss of ribosomes. This places the cell's limited metabolic apparatus at risk, because if any protein component deteriorates, it cannot be replaced, as it would be in most other cells; and in fact, the activity of most enzymes gradually decreases as red cells age. At the same time, during their long time in circulation, various red cell components inevitably accumulate damage and become physically denser. The anion exchanger known as band 3 is the most abundant protein in the red cell membrane (Fig. 100-2 and Table 100-3), with about 1.2 million molecules per red cell. As red cells age and become denser, probability is increased that a region of the band 3 molecule becomes exposed on the cell surface and contributes to creating an antigenic site recognizable by low-avidity naturally occurring anti-band 3 IgG antibodies. This process might be enhanced by the clustering of band 3 molecules favored by the antibody itself and by the binding of hemichromes arising from hemoglobin degradation. Senescent red cells thus become opsonized, and this is the signal for phagocytosis by macrophages in the spleen, in the liver, and elsewhere. This process may become accelerated in various ways in HA.

Another consequence of the relative simplicity of red cells is that they have a limited range of ways to manifest distress under hardship; in essence, any sort of metabolic failure will eventually lead either to structural damage to the membrane or to failure of the cation pump. In either case, the life span of the red cell is reduced, which is the definition of a *hemolytic disorder*. If the rate of red cell destruction exceeds the capacity of the bone marrow to produce more red cells, the hemolytic disorder will manifest as HA.

Thus, the essential pathophysiologic process common to all HAs is an increased red cell turnover; in many HAs, this is due at least in part to an acceleration of the senescence process described above. The gold standard for proving that the life span of red cells is reduced (compared to the normal value of about 120 days) is a *red cell survival* study, which can be carried out by labeling the red cells with ^{51}Cr and measuring the fall in radioactivity over several days or weeks (this classic test can now be replaced by a methodology using the nonradioactive isotope ^{15}N). If the hemolytic event is transient, it does not usually cause any long-term

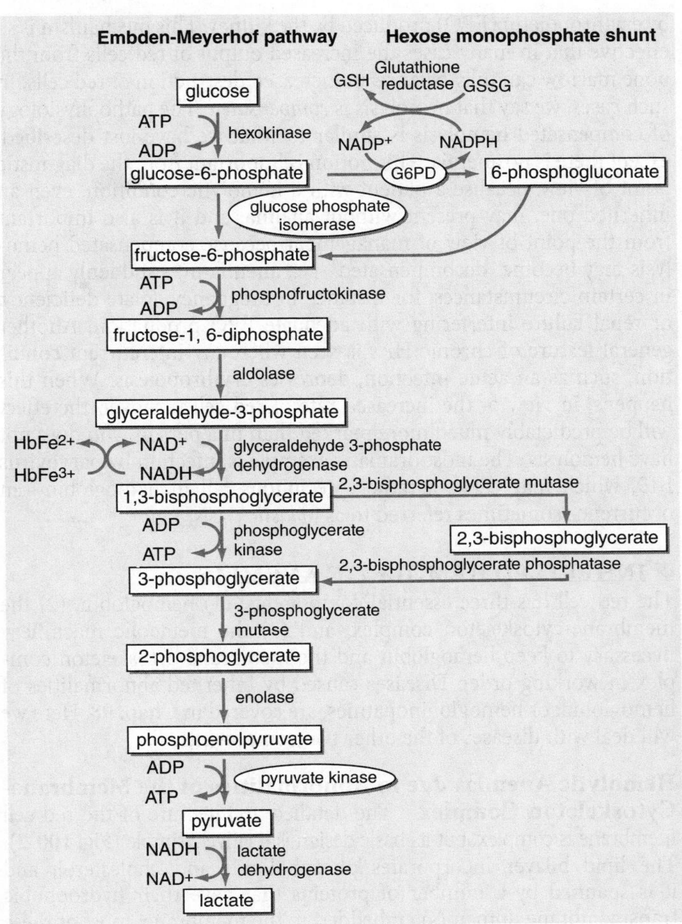

FIGURE 100-1 Red blood cell (RBC) metabolism. The Embden-Meyerhof pathway (glycolysis) generates ATP required for cation transport and for membrane maintenance. The generation of NADH maintains hemoglobin iron in a reduced state. The hexose monophosphate shunt generates NADPH that is used to reduce glutathione, which protects the red cell against oxidant stress; the 6-phosphogluconate, after decarboxylation, can be recycled via pentose sugars to glycolysis. Regulation of the 2,3-bisphosphoglycerate level is a critical determinant of oxygen affinity of hemoglobin. Enzyme deficiency states in order of prevalence: glucose-6-phosphate dehydrogenase (G6PD) > pyruvate kinase > glucose-6-phosphate isomerase > rare deficiencies of other enzymes in the pathway. The more common enzyme deficiencies are encircled.

consequences, except for an increased requirement for erythropoietic factors, particularly folic acid. However, if hemolysis is recurrent or persistent, the increased bilirubin production favors the formation of gallstones. If a considerable proportion of hemolysis takes place in the spleen, as is often the case, splenomegaly may become increasingly a feature, and hypersplenism may develop, with consequent neutropenia and/or thrombocytopenia.

The increased red cell turnover has important consequences. In normal subjects, the iron from effete red cells is very efficiently recycled by the body; however, with chronic intravascular hemolysis, the persistent hemoglobinuria will cause considerable iron loss, needing replacement. With chronic extravascular hemolysis, the opposite problem, iron overload, is more common, especially if the patient needs frequent blood transfusions. Even without blood transfusion, when erythropoiesis is massively increased, the release of erythroferrone from erythroid cells suppresses hepcidin, causing increased iron absorption. In the long run, in the absence of iron-chelation therapy, iron overload will cause secondary hemochromatosis; this will cause damage particularly to the liver, eventually leading to cirrhosis; and to the heart muscle, eventually causing heart failure.

Compensated Hemolysis versus Hemolytic Anemia Red cell destruction is a potent stimulus for erythropoiesis, which is mediated by erythropoietin (EPO) produced by the kidney. This mechanism is so effective that in many cases the increased output of red cells from the bone marrow can fully balance an increased destruction of red cells. In such cases, we say that hemolysis is *compensated*. The pathophysiology of compensated hemolysis is similar to what we have just described, except there is no anemia. This notion is important from the diagnostic point of view, because a patient with a hemolytic condition, even an inherited one, may present without anemia; and it is also important from the point of view of management because compensated hemolysis may become "decompensated," i.e., anemia may suddenly appear in certain circumstances, for instance in pregnancy, folate deficiency, or renal failure interfering with adequate EPO production. Another general feature of chronic HAs is seen when any intercurrent condition, such as an acute infection, depresses erythropoiesis. When this happens, in view of the increased rate of red cell turnover, the effect will be predictably much more marked than in a person who does not have hemolysis. The most dramatic example is infection by parvovirus B19, which may cause a rather precipitous fall in hemoglobin—an occurrence sometimes referred to as *aplastic crisis*.

INHERITED HEMOLYTIC ANEMIAS

The red cell has three essential components: (1) hemoglobin, (2) the membrane-cytoskeleton complex, and (3) the metabolic machinery necessary to keep hemoglobin and the membrane-cytoskeleton complex in working order. Diseases caused by inherited abnormalities of hemoglobin, or hemoglobinopathies, are covered in **Chap. 98**. Here we will deal with diseases of the other two components.

Hemolytic Anemias due to Abnormalities of the Membrane-Cytoskeleton Complex The detailed architecture of the red cell membrane is complex, but its basic design is relatively simple (**Fig. 100-2**). The lipid bilayer incorporates phospholipids and cholesterol, and it is spanned by a number of proteins that have their hydrophobic transmembrane domain(s) embedded in the membrane; most of these proteins also extend to both the outside (extracellular domains) and the inside of the cell (cytoplasmic domains). Other proteins are tethered to the membrane through a glycosylphosphatidylinositol (GPI) anchor; these have only an extracellular domain. Membrane proteins include energy-dependent ion transporters, ion channels, receptors for complement components, and receptors for other ligands. The most abundant red cell membrane proteins are glycophorins and the so-called band 3, an anion transporter that is an integral membrane protein. The extracellular domains of many of these proteins are heavily glycosylated, and they carry antigenic determinants that correspond to blood groups. Underneath the membrane, and tangential to it, is a network of other proteins that make up the cytoskeleton. The main cytoskeletal protein is the spectrin tetramer, consisting of a head-to-head association of two α-spectrin-β-spectrin heterodimers. The cytoskeleton is linked to the membrane through the *ankyrin complex* (that includes also band 4.2) and the *junctional complex* (that includes adducin and band 4.1) (Fig. 100-2). These multiprotein complexes make membrane and cytoskeleton intimately connected to each other, thus supporting membrane stability and at the same time providing the erythrocyte with the important property of deformability.

The membrane-cytoskeleton complex has essentially three functions: It is an envelope for the red cell cytoplasm; it maintains the normal red cell shape; it provides cross-membrane transport of electrolytes and of metabolites such as glucose and amino acids. In the membrane-cytoskeleton complex, the individual components are so intimately associated with each other that an abnormality of almost any of them will be disturbing or disruptive, causing mechanical instability of the membrane and/or reduced red cell deformability, ultimately causing hemolysis. These abnormalities are almost invariably inherited mutations; thus diseases of the membrane-cytoskeleton complex belong to the category of inherited HAs. Before the red cells lyse, they often exhibit more or less specific changes that alter the normal biconcave disk shape. Thus, the majority of the diseases in this group have been known for over a century as hereditary spherocytosis (HS) and hereditary elliptocytosis (HE). More recently a third morphologic entity, whereby on a blood smear the round-shaped central pallor of a red cell is replaced by a linear-shaped central pale area, has earned the name *stomatocytosis*: because this abnormal shape is related to abnormalities of channel molecules, the underlying disorders are also referred to as channelopathies. From an understanding of the molecular basis of these disorders, it has emerged (**Table 100-3**) that, although these disorders are predominantly monogenic, no one-to-one correlation exists between a certain gene and a certain disorder. Rather, what has been regarded as a single disorder (e.g., HS) can arise through mutation of one of several genes; conversely, what have been regarded as different disorders can arise through different mutations of the very same gene (**Fig. 100-3**).

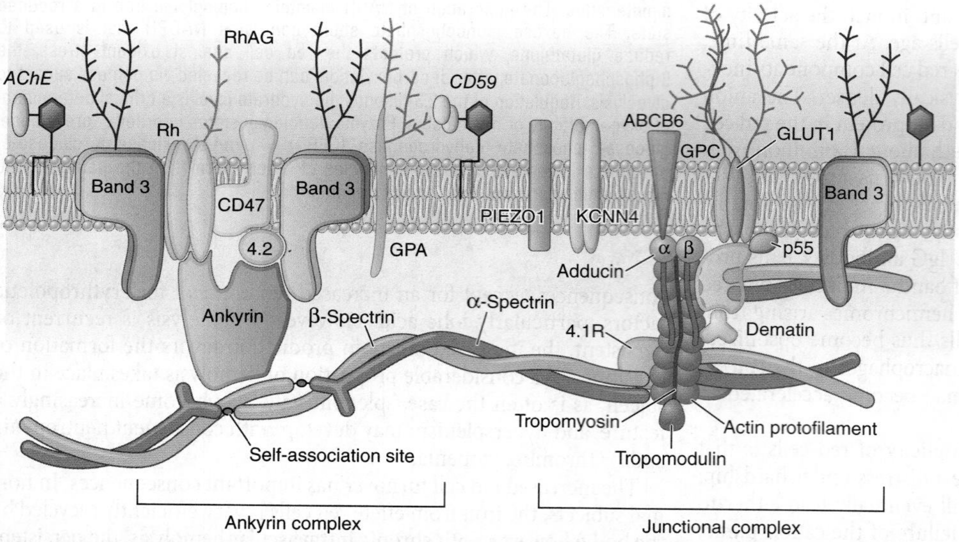

FIGURE 100-2 The red cell membrane and cytoskeleton. Within the membrane lipid bilayer several integral membrane proteins are shown: band 3 (anion exchanger 1 [AE1]) is the most abundant. *PIEZO1* is a mechanoreceptor, *KCNN4*, a Ca^{2+} activated K^{+} channel, and *ABCB6* is an ion channel: they are important in the regulation of the red cell volume. Other proteins, e.g., acetylcholinesterase (AChE) and the two complement-regulatory proteins CD59 and CD55, are tethered to the membrane through the glycosylphosphatidylinositol (GPI) anchor: in these cases the entire polypeptide chain is extracellular. Many of the membrane proteins bear polypeptide and/or carbohydrate red cell antigens. Underneath the membrane, the α–β spectrin dimers, that associate head-to-head into tetramers, together with actin and other proteins, form most of the cytoskeleton. The *ankyrin complex*, that also involves the band 4.2 protein, and the *junctional complex*, that involves the band 4.1 protein and dematin, connect the membrane to the cytoskeleton. The ankyrin complex provides mainly radial (also called vertical) connections; the junctional complex provides mainly tangential (also called horizontal) connections: pathogenic changes in the former can cause spherocytosis, whereas pathogenic changes in the latter can cause elliptocytosis; pathogenic changes in spectrin can cause either. Branched lines symbolize carbohydrate moiety of proteins. The various molecules are obviously not drawn to the same scale. Additional explanations are found in the text. *(Reproduced with permission from N Young et al: Clinical Hematology. Philadelphia, Elsevier, 2006.)*

HEREDITARY SPHEROCYTOSIS This is most common among this group of HAs, with an estimated prevalence of 1:2000–1:5000 in populations of European ancestry. Its identification is credited to Minkowksy and Chauffard, who, at the end of the nineteenth century, reported families who had spherocytes in their peripheral blood (**Fig. 100-4A**). In vitro studies revealed that the red cells were abnormally susceptible to lysis in hypotonic media; indeed, the presence of

TABLE 100-3 Inherited Diseases of the Red Cell Membrane-Cytoskeleton Complex

GENE	CHROMOSOMAL LOCATION	PROTEIN PRODUCED	DISEASE(S) WITH CERTAIN MUTATIONS (INHERITANCE)	COMMENTS
SPTA1	1q22-q23	α-Spectrin	HS (recessive)	Rare
			HE (dominant)	Mutations of this gene account for about 65% of HE. More severe forms may be due to coexistence of an otherwise silent mutant allele.
SPTB	14q23-q24.1	β-Spectrin	HS (dominant)	Rare
			HE (dominant)	Mutations of this gene account for about 30% of HE, including some severe forms.
ANK1	8p11.2	Ankyrin	HS (dominant)	May account for majority of HS.
SLC4A1	17q21	Band 3; also known as AE (anion exchanger) or AE1	HS (dominant)	Mutations of this gene may account for about 25% of HS.
			Southeast Asia ovalocytosis (dominant)	Polymorphic mutation (deletion of nine amino acids); in heterozygotes clinically asymptomatic and protective against *Plasmodium falciparum.*
			Stomatocytosis (cryohydrocytosis)	Certain specific missense mutations shift protein function from anion exchanger to cation conductance.
EPB41	1p33-p34.2	Band 4.1	HE (dominant)	Mutations of this gene account for about 5% of HE, mostly with prominent morphology but little/no hemolysis in heterozygotes; severe hemolysis in homozygotes.
EPB42	15q15-q21	Band 4.2	HS (recessive)	Mutations of this gene account for about 3% of HS.
RHAG	6p21.1-p11	Rhesus-associated glycoprotein	Chronic nonspherocytic hemolytic anemia (recessive)	Very rare; associated with total loss of all Rh antigens. One specific mutation in this gene entails loss of stomatin from the cell membrane, causing overhydrated stomatocytosis.
PIEZO1	16q23-q24	PIEZO1 (mechanosensitive ion channel component 1 channel)	Dehydrated hereditary stomatocytosis (dominant)	Also known as xerocytosis with pseudohyperkalemia. Patients may present with perinatal edema.
KCNN4	19q13.31	KCNN4 Intermediate conductance calcium-activated potassium channel protein 4 (Gardos channel)	Dehydrated hereditary stomatocytosis (dominant)	Clinical presentation similar to that of *PIEZO1* mutants.
ABCB6	2q35-q36	ATP-binding cassette subfamily B member 6	Familial pseudohyperkalemia (dominant)	Increased potassium leakage upon storage in blood bank condition: this can cause hyperkalemia in the recipient. ABCB6 mutation is present in 0.3% of blood donors.
SLC2A1	1p34.2	GLUT1 glucose transporter	Overhydrated hereditary stomatocytosis	Associated with serious neurological manifestations.

Note: PIEZO1, KCNN4, ABCB6, and *GLUT1* are channel molecules; conditions associated with mutations in the respective genes are appropriately named channelopathies.

Abbreviations: HE, hereditary elliptocytosis; HS, hereditary spherocytosis.

osmotic fragility became the main diagnostic test for HS. Today we know that HS, thus defined, is genetically heterogeneous; i.e., it can arise from a variety of mutations in one of several genes (Table 100-3). It has been also recognized that the inheritance of HS is not always autosomal dominant (with the patient being heterozygous); indeed, some of the most severe forms are instead autosomal recessive (with the patient being homozygous).

Clinical Presentation and Diagnosis The spectrum of clinical severity of HS is broad. Severe cases may present in infancy with severe anemia, whereas mild cases may present in young adults or even later in life. The main clinical findings are jaundice, an enlarged spleen, and often gallstones; indeed, it may be the finding of gallstones in a young person that triggers diagnostic investigations.

The variability in clinical manifestations that is observed among patients with HS is largely due to the different underlying molecular lesions (Table 100-3). Not only are mutations of several genes involved, even different mutations of the same gene can give very different clinical manifestations. In milder cases, hemolysis is often compensated (see above), but changes in clinical expression may be seen even in the same patient because intercurrent conditions (e.g., pregnancy, infection) may cause decompensation. The anemia is usually normocytic with the characteristic morphology that gives the disease its name. An increased mean corpuscular hemoglobin concentration (MCHC >34) and increased red cell distribution width (RDW >14%) associated with normal or slightly decreased MCV on an ordinary blood count report should raise the suspicion of HS. The spleen plays a key role in HS through a dual mechanism. On one hand, like in many other HAs, the spleen itself is a major site of destruction; on the other hand, because the red cells in HS are less deformable, transit through the splenic circulation makes them more prone to vesiculate, thus accelerating their demise.

When there is a family history, it is usually easy to make a diagnosis based on features of HA and typical red cell morphology. However, family history may be negative for at least two reasons. First, the patient may have a de novo mutation, i.e., a mutation that has taken place in a germ cell of one of the patient's parents or early after zygote formation. Second, the patient may have a recessive form of HS (Table 100-3). In such cases, more extensive laboratory investigations are required, including osmotic fragility, the acid glycerol lysis test, the eosin-5'-maleimide (EMA)–binding test, and SDS-gel electrophoresis of membrane proteins; these tests are usually carried out in laboratories with special expertise in this area. Sometimes a definitive diagnosis can be obtained only by molecular studies demonstrating a mutation in one of the genes underlying HS (Table 100-3).

TREATMENT

Hereditary Spherocytosis

We do not have a causal treatment for HS; i.e., no way has yet been found to correct the basic defect in the membrane-cytoskeleton structure. Given the special role of the spleen in HS (see above),

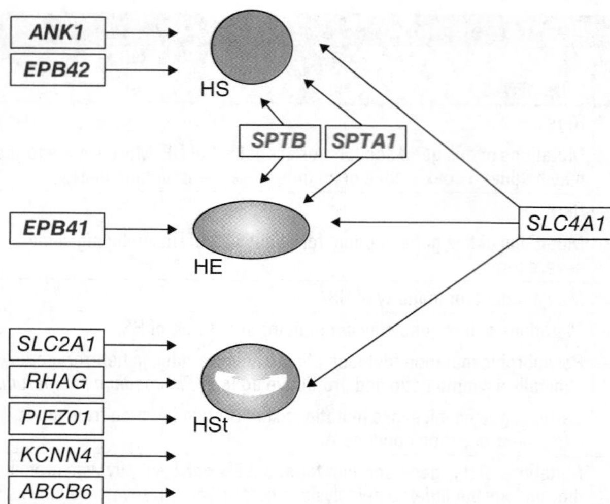

FIGURE 100-3 Hereditary spherocytosis (HS), hereditary elliptocytosis (HE), and hereditary stomatocytosis (HSt) are three morphologically distinct forms of congenital hemolytic anemia. It has emerged that each one can arise from mutation of one of several genes and that different mutations of the same gene can give one or another form. (See also Table 100-3.) Genes encoding membrane proteins are in *black*; genes encoding cytoskeleton proteins are in *green*; genes encoding proteins in the junctional and ankyrin complexes are in *purple*.

splenectomy is often beneficial. Current recommendations are to proceed with splenectomy at the age of 4–6 years in severe cases, to delay splenectomy until puberty in moderate cases, and to avoid splenectomy in mild cases. Partial splenectomy can be considered in certain cases; and it is helpful to know about the outcome of splenectomy in the patient's affected relatives. Before splenectomy, vaccination against encapsulated bacteria (*Neisseria meningitidis* and *Streptococcus pneumonia)* is imperative; penicillin prophylaxis after splenectomy is controversial. Along with splenectomy, cholecystectomy should not be carried out automatically; but it should be carried out, usually by the laparoscopic approach, whenever it is clinically indicated.

HEREDITARY ELLIPTOCYTOSIS HE is at least as heterogeneous as HS, both from the genetic point of view (Table 100-3, Fig. 100-3) and from the clinical point of view. The global incidence of HE is 1:2000–4000 subjects. Again, it is the shape of the red cells (**Fig. 100-4*B***) that gives the name to the condition, but there is no direct correlation between the elliptocytic morphology and clinical severity. In fact, some mild or even asymptomatic cases may have nearly 100% elliptocytes (or ovalocytes). Indeed, the diagnosis of HE is generally incidental, because hemolysis may be compensated and there may be no anemia, although this may become evident in the course of infection. One particular in-frame deletion of nine amino acids in the *SLC4A1* gene encoding band 3 underlies the so-called Southeast Asia ovalocytosis (SAO): it is not a disease, but rather a polymorphism with a frequency of up to 5–7% in certain populations (e.g., Papua New Guinea, Indonesia, Malaysia, Philippines), presumably as a result of malaria selection; it is asymptomatic in heterozygotes and probably lethal in homozygotes. The cases of HE with the most severe HA are those with biallelic mutations of one of the genes involved (see Fig. 100-3), and these are said to have pyropoikilocytosis (HPP): here the instability of the cytoskeleton protein network may result from decreased tetramerization of spectrin dimers. The red cell volume is decreased (MCV: 50–60 fL), and all kinds of bizarre poikilocytes are seen on the blood smear (**Fig. 100-4*C***). HPP patients have splenomegaly and often benefit from splenectomy.

Channelopathies These rare conditions (see Fig. 100-3) are characterized by abnormalities in red cell ion content and alteration of erythrocyte volume. Cation leak can cause hyperkalemia; in some cases, this leak is accelerated in the cold (the resulting spuriously high serum K^+ is then referred to as pseudo-hyperkalemia). The less rare form, dehydrated stomatocytosis (DHS; also referred to as xerocytosis) is a (usually compensated) macrocytic hemolytic disorder, with increased MCHC (generally higher than 36 g/dL) associated with mild jaundice. Mutations in either *PIEZO1*, encoding an ion channel activated by

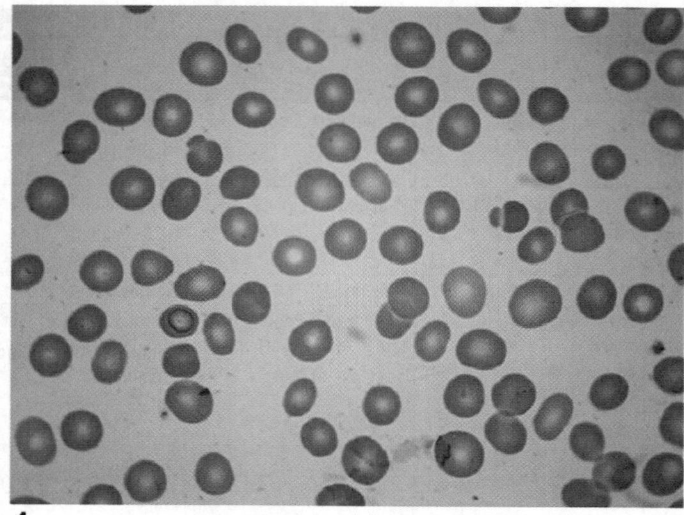
A

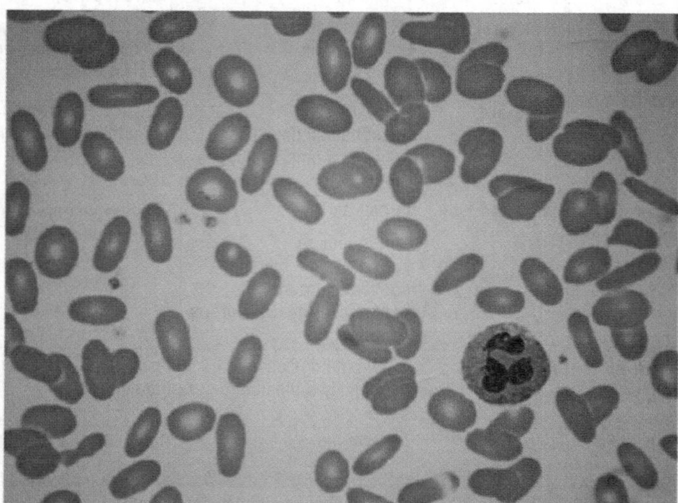
B

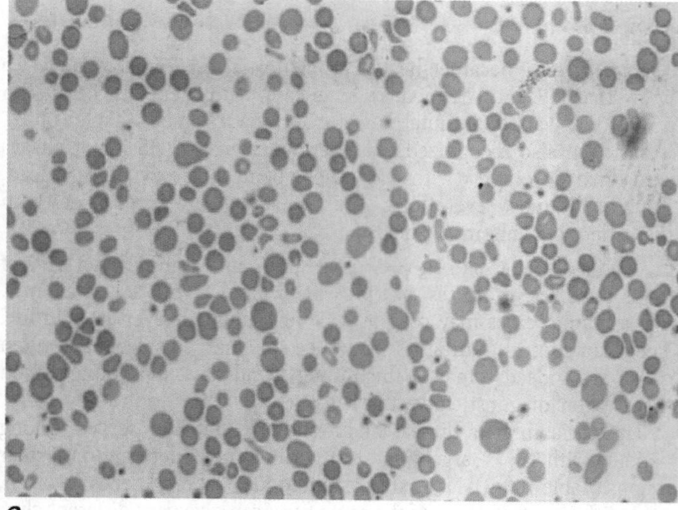
C

FIGURE 100-4 Peripheral blood smear from patients with membrane-cytoskeleton abnormalities. ***A.*** Hereditary spherocytosis. ***B.*** Hereditary elliptocytosis, heterozygote. ***C.*** Pyropoikilocytosis, with both alleles of the α-spectrin gene mutated.

pressure (mechanoreceptor), or in *KCCN4*, encoding the Ca^{2+} activated K^+ channel (Gardos channel) have been recognized to cause DHS (see Table 100-3).

Another form is overhydrated stomatocytosis (OHS): this too is macrocytic (MCV >110 fL), but the MCHC is low (<30 g/dL). The underlying mutation is in the Rhesus gene *RHAG*, which encodes an ammonia channel. Yet other patients with stomatocytosis (Table 100-3) have mutations in *SLC4A1* (encoding band 3) and *SLC2A1* (encoding the glucose transporter GLUT1). Mutations of the latter are responsible for *cryohydrocytosis*, a channelopathy in which the red cells swell and burst when they are cooled. In vivo hemolysis can vary from relatively mild to quite severe. Familial hyperkalemia has been recently linked to mutations in *ABCB6*, resulting in abnormal cation leak with extracellular release of a large amount of K+ (hyperkaliemia). Mutations in *ABCB6* have been identified in almost 0.3% of blood donors. However, splenectomy is contraindicated in stomatocytosis due to the significant proportion of severe thromboembolic complications observed in splenectomized DHS patients.

A specialized technique to measure erythrocyte deformability through laser diffraction analysis is *ektacytometry*: this has been used extensively in order to investigate membrane-cytoskeleton abnormalities. For diagnostic purposes, systematic sequencing of a panel of genes in patients' DNA is a powerful approach already in use and destined to be used increasingly.

Enzyme Abnormalities When an important defect in a component of the membrane-cytoskeleton complex is present, hemolysis is a direct consequence of the fact that the very structure of the red cell is compromised. Instead, when one of the enzymes is defective, the consequences will depend on the precise role of that enzyme in the metabolic machinery of the red cell. This machinery has two main functions: (1) to provide energy in the form of ATP, and (2) to prevent oxidative damage to hemoglobin and to other proteins by providing sufficient reductive potential; the key molecule for this is NADPH.

ABNORMALITIES OF THE GLYCOLYTIC PATHWAY Because red cells, in the course of their differentiation, have sacrificed not only their nucleus and their ribosomes but also their mitochondria, they rely exclusively on the anaerobic portion of the glycolytic pathway for producing ATP, most of which is required by the red cell for cation transport against a concentration gradient across the membrane. If this fails due to a defect of any of the enzymes of the glycolytic pathway (**Table 100-4**), the result will be hemolytic disease.

Pyruvate Kinase Deficiency Abnormalities of the glycolytic pathway are all inherited and all rare. Among them, deficiency of pyruvate kinase (PK) is the least rare, with an estimated prevalence in most populations of 1:10,000. However, recently, a polymorphic PK mutation (E277K) was found in some African populations with heterozygote frequencies of 1–7%, suggesting that this may be another malaria-related polymorphism. HA secondary to PK deficiency is an autosomal recessive disease (**Fig. 100-5**).

The clinical picture of homozygous (or biallelic) PK deficiency is that of an HA that often presents in the newborn with neonatal jaundice, requiring nearly always phototherapy and frequently exchange transfusion; the jaundice persists, and it is often associated with reticulocytosis. The anemia is of variable severity; sometimes it is so severe as to require regular blood transfusion treatment, whereas sometimes it is mild, bordering on a nearly compensated hemolytic disorder. As a result, the diagnosis may be delayed: in some cases, it is made, for instance, in a young woman during her first pregnancy, when the anemia may get worse. The delay in diagnosis may be caused in part by the fact that the anemia is often remarkably well tolerated because

TABLE 100-4 Red Cell Enzyme Abnormalities Causing Hemolysis

	ENZYME (ACRONYM)	GENE SYMBOL; CHROMOSOMAL LOCATION	PREVALENCE OF ENZYME DEFICIENCY (RANK)	CLINICAL MANIFESTATIONS EXTRA-RED CELL	COMMENTS
Glycolytic Pathway					
	Hexokinase (HK)	*HK1*; 10q22	Very rare		May benefit from splenectomy; BMT[c]
	Glucose 6-phosphate isomerase (G6PI)	*GPI*; 19q31.1	Rare (4); at least 60 cases reported[a]	NM, CNS	May benefit from splenectomy
	Phosphofructokinase (PFK)[b]	*PFKM*; 12q13	Very rare	Myopathy; myoglobinuria	
	Aldolase	*ALDOA*; 16q22-24	Very rare	Myopathy	
	Triose phosphate isomerase (TPI)	*TPI1*; 12p13.31	Very rare	CNS (severe), NM	
	Glyceraldehyde 3-phosphate dehydrogenase (GAPD)	*GAPDH*; 12p13.31	Very rare	Myopathy	
	Bisphosphoglycerate mutase (BPGM)	*BPGM*; 7q33	Very rare		Erythrocytosis rather than hemolysis; some of the rare mutations are in the enzyme active site
	Phosphoglycerate kinase (PGK)	*PGK1*; Xq21.1	Very rare	CNS, NM	May benefit from splenectomy; BMT[c]
	Pyruvate kinase (PK)	*PKLR*; 1q22	Rare (2)[a]		May benefit from splenectomy; BMT[c]
Redox					
	Glucose 6-phosphate dehydrogenase (G6PD)	*G6PD*; Xq28	Common (1)[a]	Very rarely granulocytes	In almost all cases, only AHA from exogenous trigger
	Glutathione synthase	*GSS*; 20q11.22	Very rare	CNS	
	Glutathione reductase	*GSR*; 8p12	Very rare	Cataracts	AHA from exogenous trigger (favism)
	γ-Glutamylcysteine synthase	*GCLC*; 6p12.1	Very rare	CNS	Mutations affect catalytic subunit
	Cytochrome b5 reductase	*CYB5R3*; 22q13.2	Rare	CNS	Methemoglobinemia rather than hemolysis
Nucleotide Metabolism					
	Adenylate kinase (AK)	*AK1*; 9q34.11	Very rare	CNS	May benefit from splenectomy
	Pyrimidine 5′ nucleotidase (P5N)	*NTSC3A*; 7p14.3	Rare (3)[a]		May benefit from splenectomy

[a]The numbers from (1) to (4) indicate the ranking order of these enzymopathies in terms of frequency. [b]PFK deficiency is associated with increased glycogen in muscle, and it is also known as glycogen storage disease type VII or Tarui's disease. [c]Occasional report of successful treatment of the hematologic manifestations by BMT.

Abbreviations: AHA, acquired hemolytic anemia; BMT, bone marrow transplantation; CNS, central nervous system; NM, neuromuscular.

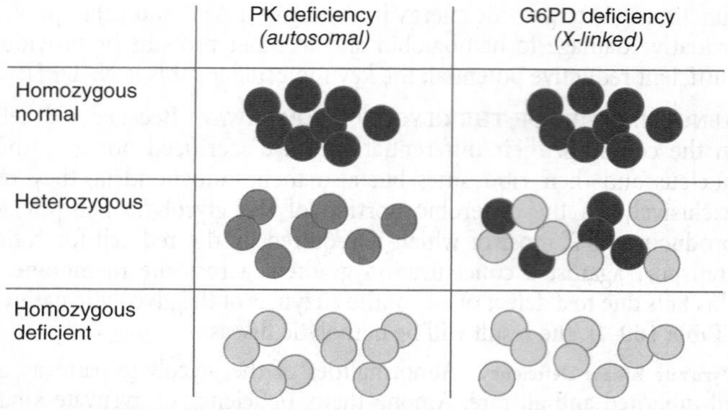

PK deficiency (autosomal)
G6PD deficiency (X-linked)
Homozygous normal
Heterozygous
Homozygous deficient

FIGURE 100-5 Different phenotypes of heterozygotes for red cell enzymopathies. In a heterozygote for deficiency of PK, encoded by an autosomal gene (see Table 100-4), the level of enzyme is about one-half of normal in all red cells. Because this level of enzyme is sufficient, there are no clinical consequences, i.e., PK deficiency is recessive. In a heterozygote for deficiency of G6PD, encoded by an X-linked gene, the situation is quite different: X-chromosome inactivation generates red cell mosaicism, whereby some red cells are entirely normal and others are G6PD deficient. Therefore, G6PD deficiency is expressed in heterozygotes: it is not recessive.

the metabolic block at the last step in glycolysis causes an increase in 2,3-bisphosphoglycerate (or DPG; Fig. 100-1), a major effector of the hemoglobin-oxygen dissociation curve; thus the oxygen delivery to the tissues is enhanced, a remarkable compensatory feat.

TREATMENT
Pyruvate Kinase Deficiency

The management of PK deficiency is mainly supportive. In view of the marked increase in red cell turnover, oral folic acid supplements should be given constantly. Blood transfusion should be used as necessary, and iron chelation may be required even in some patients who, though not receiving blood transfusion, may be developing iron overload (see "General Pathophysiology" above). About one-half of patients sooner or later undergo splenectomy, which usually provides a modest but significant increase in hemoglobin (paradoxically, often reticulocytes also increase considerably). Cholecystectomy may also be required. Some patients with severe disease have received bone marrow transplantation (BMT) from an HLA-identical PK-normal sibling. Prenatal diagnosis has been carried out in a mother who had already had an affected child. A clinical trial of a small molecule that is a specific PK ligand and may increase the stability and/or catalytic efficiency of mutant PK is currently ongoing. Rescue of inherited PK deficiency through lentiviral-mediated human PK gene transfer has been successful in mice. An oral small molecule allosteric activator of PK called *mitapivat* raised hemoglobin levels in about half of PK deficient patients in a small phase 2 study.

Other Glycolytic Enzyme Abnormalities All of these defects are rare to very rare (Table 100-4), and most of them cause HA with varying degrees of severity. It is not unusual for the presentation to be in the guise of severe neonatal jaundice, which may require exchange transfusion; if the anemia is less severe, it may present later in life, or it may even remain asymptomatic and be detected incidentally when a blood count is done for unrelated reasons. The spleen is often enlarged. When other systemic manifestations occur, they can involve the central nervous system (sometimes entailing severe mental retardation, particularly in the case of triose phosphate isomerase deficiency), the neuromuscular system, or both (see Table 100-4). This is not altogether surprising if we consider that these are housekeeping genes, i.e., expressed in all tissues. The diagnosis of HA is usually not difficult, thanks to the triad of normo-macrocytic anemia, reticulocytosis, and hyperbilirubinemia. Enzymopathies should be considered in the differential diagnosis of any chronic Coombs-negative HA. Unlike with membrane disorders, in most cases of glycolytic enzymopathies, morphologic abnormalities are conspicuous by their absence. A definitive diagnosis can be made only by demonstrating the deficiency of an individual enzyme by quantitative assays; these are carried out in only a few specialized laboratories. If a particular molecular abnormality is already known in the family, then one could test directly for that defect at the DNA level, thus bypassing the need for enzyme assays. Of course the time may be getting nearer when a patient will present with her or his exome already sequenced, and we will need to concentrate on which genes to look up within the file. The principles for the management of these conditions are similar as for PK deficiency. In isolated cases of glycolytic enzyme abnormalities, BMT has been carried out successfully, although unfortunately nonhematologic manifestations, if any, are not reversed.

ABNORMALITIES OF REDOX METABOLISM • Glucose-6-phosphate Dehydrogenase (G6PD) Deficiency G6PD is a housekeeping enzyme critical in the redox metabolism of all aerobic cells (Fig. 100-1). In red cells, its role is even more critical because it is the only source of NADPH, which directly and via glutathione (GSH) defends these cells against oxidative stress (**Fig. 100-6**). G6PD deficiency-related HA is a prime example of an HA due to interaction between an intracorpuscular cause and an extracorpuscular cause: indeed, in the vast majority of cases hemolysis is triggered by an exogenous agent. Although the G6PD activity is decreased in most tissues of G6PD-deficient subjects, in other cells the decrease is much less pronounced than in red cells, and it does not seem to impact on clinical expression.

GENETIC CONSIDERATIONS

The G6PD gene is X-linked, and this has important implications. First, because males have only one G6PD gene (i.e., they are hemizygous for this gene), they must be either normal or G6PD deficient. By contrast, females, who have two G6PD genes, can be either normal or deficient (homozygous) or intermediate (heterozygous). Second, as a result of the phenomenon of X chromosome inactivation, heterozygous females are genetic mosaics (see Fig. 100-5), with a highly variable ratio of G6PD-normal to G6PD-deficient cells and an equally variable degree of clinical expression; some heterozygotes can be just as affected as hemizygous males. The enzymatically active form of G6PD is either a dimer or a tetramer of a single protein subunit of 514 amino acids. G6PD-deficient subjects have been found invariably to have mutations in the coding region of the G6PD gene. Almost all of the 230 different mutations known are single missense point mutations, entailing single amino acid replacements in the G6PD protein. In most cases, these mutations cause G6PD deficiency by decreasing the in vivo stability of the protein; thus the physiologic decrease in G6PD activity that takes place with red cell aging is greatly accelerated. In some cases, an amino acid replacement can also affect the catalytic function of the enzyme.

Among these mutations, those underlying chronic nonspherocytic hemolytic anemia (CNSHA; see below) are a discrete subset. This much more severe clinical phenotype can be ascribed in some cases to adverse qualitative changes (for instance, a decreased affinity for the substrate glucose-6-phosphate) or simply to the fact that the enzyme deficit is more extreme because of a more severe instability of the enzyme. For instance, a cluster of mutations map at or near the dimer interface, and clearly they compromise severely the formation of the dimer.

Epidemiology G6PD deficiency is widely distributed in tropical and subtropical parts of the world (Africa, Southern Europe, the Middle East, Southeast Asia, and Oceania) (**Fig. 100-7**) and wherever people from those areas have migrated. A conservative estimate is that at least 500 million people have a G6PD deficiency gene. In several of these areas, the frequency of a G6PD deficiency gene may be as high as 20% or more. It would be quite extraordinary for a trait that causes significant pathology to spread widely and reach high frequencies in many populations without conferring some biologic advantage. Indeed, G6PD is one of the best-characterized examples of genetic polymorphisms in the human species. Clinical field studies and in

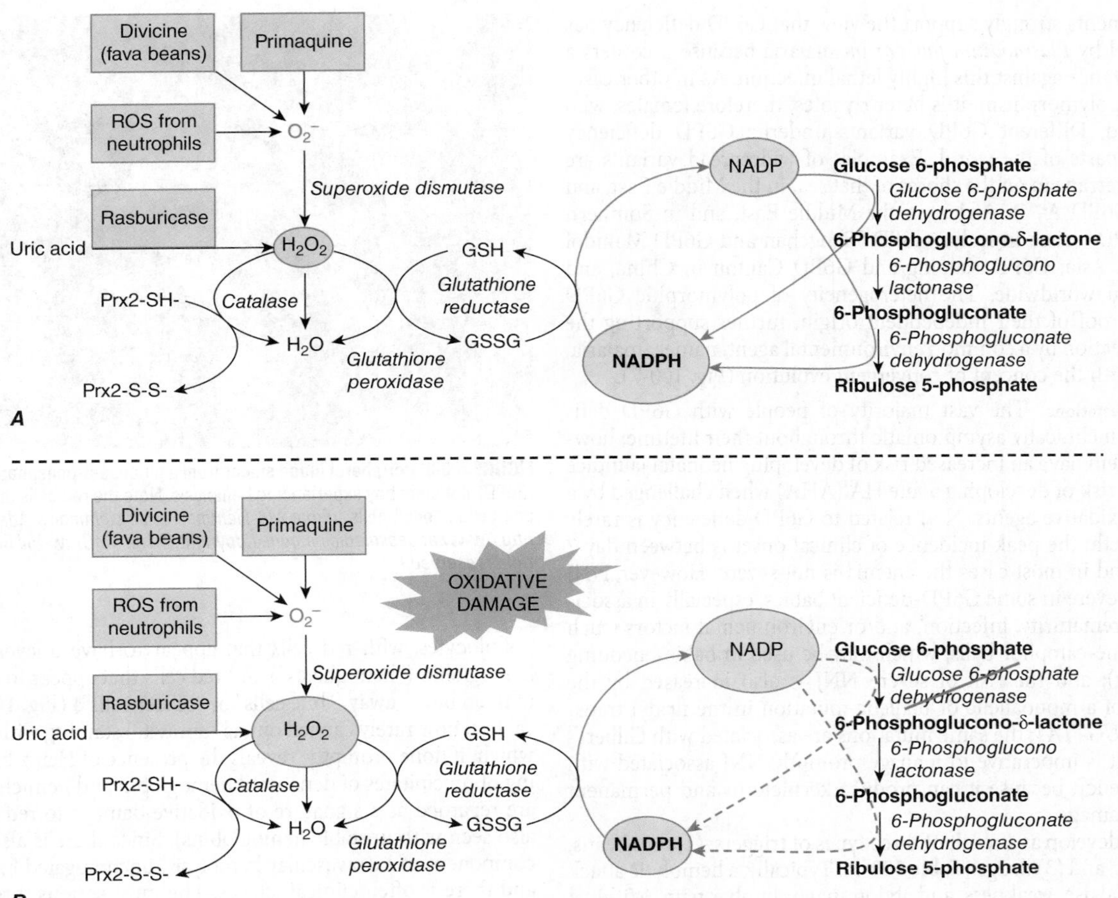

FIGURE 100-6 The role of G6PD in protecting red cells from oxidative damage. ***A.*** In G6PD-normal red cells, G6PD and 6-phosphogluconate dehydrogenase—two of the enzymes of the pentose phosphate pathway—provide ample supply of NADPH, which in turn regenerates GSH when this is oxidized by reactive oxygen species (e.g., O_2^- and H_2O_2). Thus when O_2^- (meant here to represent itself and other reactive oxygen species or ROS) is produced by pro-oxidant compounds such as primaquine, or the glucosides in fava beans (divicine), or the oxidative burst of neutrophils, these ROS are rapidly neutralized; similarly, when rasburicase administered to degrade uric acid produces an equimolar amount of hydrogen peroxide, this is rapidly degraded by the combined action of glutathione peroxidase, catalase, and Prx2 (peroxiredoxin-2: all three mechanisms are NADPH dependent). ***B.*** In G6PD-deficient red cells, where the enzyme activity is reduced, NADPH production is limited, and it may not be sufficient to cope with the excess ROS generated by pro-oxidant compounds, and the consequent excess hydrogen peroxide. This diagram also explains why a defect in glutathione reductase has very similar consequences to G6PD deficiency.

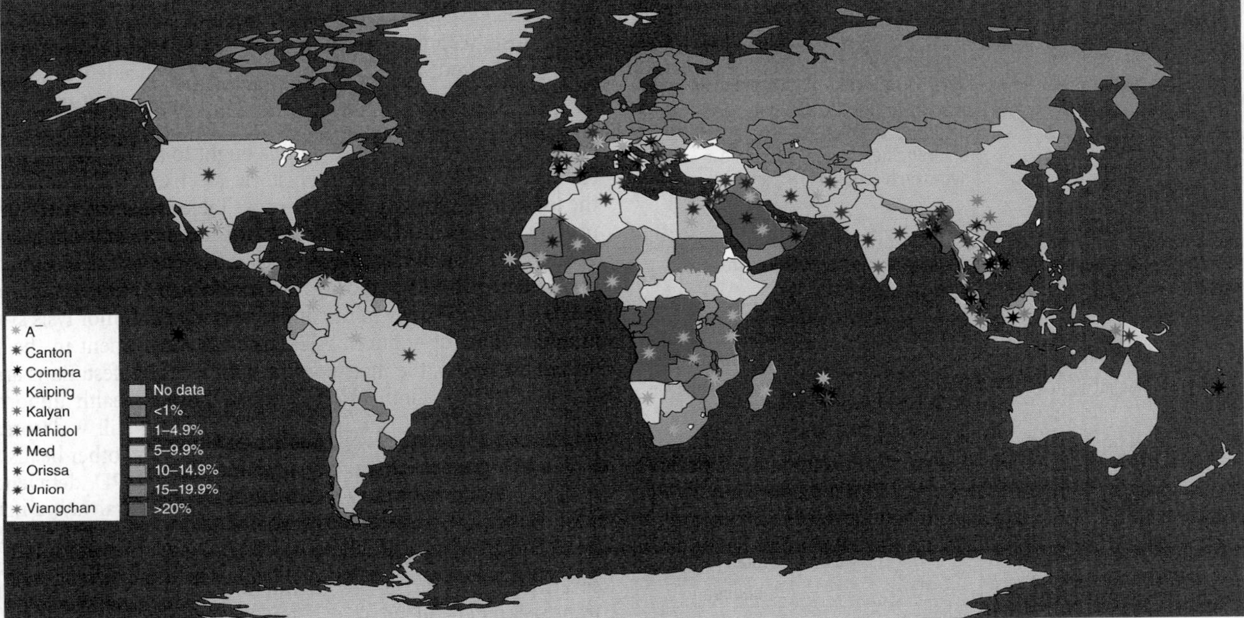

FIGURE 100-7 Epidemiology of G6PD deficiency throughout the world. Each country on the map is shaded in a color based on the best estimate of the mean frequency of G6PD deficiency allele(s) in that country (this is the same as the frequency of G6PD deficient males). The small panel on the left gives the key to color shadings corresponding to each country. The larger panel gives a color-coded list of ten common G6PD variants associated with G6PD deficiency: asterisk-shaped symbols in the corresponding colors are shown in the countries where these variants have been observed (for graphic reasons symbols could not be inserted in all countries). *(Republished with permission of American Society of Hematology, from Glucose-6-phosphate dehydrogenase deficiency, L Luzzatto et al. 136:1225, 2020 permission conveyed through Copyright Clearance Center, Inc.)*

vitro experiments strongly support the view that G6PD deficiency has been selected by *Plasmodium falciparum* malaria because it confers a relative resistance against this highly lethal infection. As in other cases of balanced polymorphism, it is heterozygotes, therefore females, who are protected. Different G6PD variants underlie G6PD deficiency in different parts of the world. Examples of widespread variants are G6PD Mediterranean on the shores of that sea, in the Middle East, and elsewhere; G6PD A– in Africa, in the Middle East, and in Southern Europe; G6PD Orissa in India; G6PD Viangchan and G6PD Mahidol in Southeast Asia; G6PD Kaiping and G6PD Canton in China; and G6PD Union worldwide. The heterogeneity of polymorphic G6PD variants is proof of their independent origin, further supporting the notion of selection by a common environmental agent, namely malaria, in keeping with the concept of convergent evolution (Fig. 100-7).

Clinical Manifestations The vast majority of people with G6PD deficiency remain clinically asymptomatic throughout their lifetime; however, all of them have an increased risk of developing neonatal jaundice (NNJ) and a risk of developing acute HA (AHA) when challenged by a number of oxidative agents. NNJ related to G6PD deficiency is rarely present at birth; the peak incidence of clinical onset is between day 2 and day 3, and in most cases the anemia is not severe. However, NNJ can be very severe in some G6PD-deficient babies, especially in association with prematurity, infection, and/or environmental factors (such as naphthalene-camphor balls, which may be used in babies' bedding and clothing); and the risk of severe NNJ is also increased by the coexistence of a monoallelic or biallelic mutation in the uridyl transferase gene (*UGT1A1*; the same mutations are associated with Gilbert's syndrome). It is imperative to manage promptly NNJ associated with G6PD deficiency, because it can produce kernicterus and permanent neurologic damage.

AHA can develop as a result of three types of triggers: (1) fava beans, (2) infections, and (3) drugs (**Table 100-5**). Typically, a hemolytic attack starts with malaise, weakness, and abdominal or lumbar pain. Within a timeframe of several hours to 2–3 days, the patient develops jaundice and often dark urine. The onset can be extremely abrupt, especially with favism in children. The anemia is moderate to extremely severe, usually normocytic and normochromic, and due partly to intravascular hemolysis; hence, it is associated with hemoglobinemia, hemoglobinuria, high LDH, and low or absent plasma haptoglobin. The blood film shows anisocytosis, polychromasia, and spherocytes; in addition, the most typical feature of G6PD deficiency is the presence of bizarre poikilocytes, with red cells that appear to have unevenly distributed hemoglobin ("hemighosts") and red cells that appear to have had parts of them bitten away ("bite cells" or "blister cells") (**Fig. 100-8**). A classical test, now rarely carried out, is supravital staining with methyl violet, which, if done promptly, reveals the presence of Heinz bodies (consisting of precipitates of denatured hemoglobin and hemichromes), which are regarded as a signature of oxidative damage to red cells (they are also seen with unstable hemoglobins). Since there is also a substantial component of extravascular hemolysis, unconjugated bilirubin is high and there is often clinical icterus. The most serious threat from AHA in adults is the development of acute renal failure (this is exceedingly rare in children). Once the threat of acute anemia is over and in the absence of comorbidity, full recovery from AHA associated with G6PD deficiency is the rule.

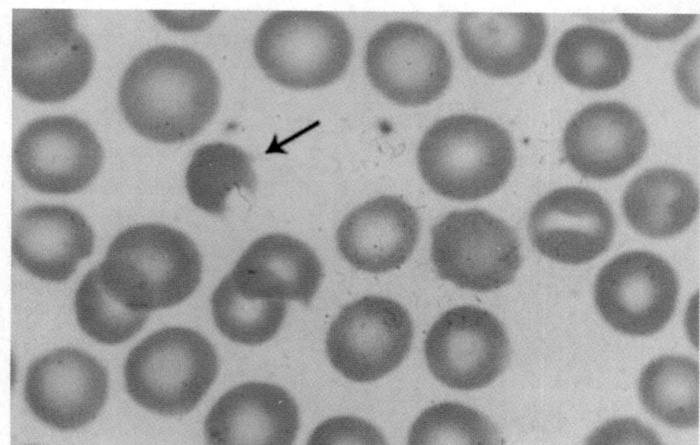

FIGURE 100-8 Peripheral blood smear from a glucose-6-phosphate dehydrogenase (G6PD)-deficient boy experiencing hemolysis. Note the red cells that are misshapen and called "bite" cells. *(From MA Lichtman et al: Lichtman's Atlas of Hematology: http://www.accessmedicine.com. Copyright © The McGraw-Hill Companies, Inc. All rights reserved.)*

TABLE 100-5 Drugs That Carry Risk of Clinical Hemolysis in Persons with Glucose 6-Phosphate Dehydrogenase Deficiency

	DEFINITE RISK	POSSIBLE RISK	DOUBTFUL RISK
Antimalarials	Primaquine	Chloroquine; hydroxychloroquine	Quinine
	Dapsone/chlorproguanil[a]		
Sulphonamides/sulphones	Dapsone	Sulfamethoxazole	Sulfisoxazole
		Sulfasalazine	
		Sulfadimidine	Sulfadiazine
Antibacterial/antibiotics	Cotrimoxazole	Ciprofloxacin	Chloramphenicol
	Nalidixic acid	Norfloxacin	*p*-Aminosalicylic acid
	Nitrofurantoin		
	Niridazole		
Antipyretic/analgesics	Acetanilide	Acetylsalicylic acid high dose (>3 g/d)	
	Phenazopyridine		Acetaminophen
			Phenacetin
Other	Rasburicase	Vitamin K analogues	Doxorubicin
	Naphthalene		
	Methylene blue	Ascorbic acid (>1 g)	Probenecid

[a]Marketed as Lapdap from 2003 to 2008.

It was primaquine (PQ)-induced AHA that led to the discovery of G6PD deficiency, but this drug has not been very prominent subsequently because it is not necessary for the treatment of life-threatening *P. falciparum* malaria. Today there is a revival in the use of PQ for two reasons. First, it is the only effective agent for eliminating the gametocytes of *P. falciparum* (thus preventing further transmission): a small single dose (0.25 mg/kg) is required, and it is safe for G6PD-deficient persons. Second, a 14-day course of PQ is needed for eliminating the hypnozoites of *Plasmodium vivax* (thus preventing endogenous relapse). In countries aiming to eliminate malaria, there may be a call for mass administration of PQ; this ought to be associated with G6PD testing. At the other end of the historic spectrum, the latest additions to the list of potentially hemolytic drugs (Table 100-5) are rasburicase and pegloticase; again G6PD testing ought to be made mandatory before giving either of these drugs, because fatal cases have been reported upon using one of these drugs, which generate hydrogen peroxide, in newborns with kidney injury and in adults with tumor lysis syndrome.

Although drug-induced AHA has been prominent in the study of G6PD deficiency, the most common clinical manifestations are in fact NNJ and favism, both of which are of public health importance in many populations. Contrary to beliefs that are still widespread, fava bean pollen inhalation does not cause favism, and other beans are safe.

A very small minority of subjects with G6PD deficiency have CNSHA of variable severity. The patient is nearly always a male, usually with a history of NNJ, who may present with anemia, unexplained jaundice, or gallstones later in life. The spleen may be enlarged. The severity of anemia ranges in different patients from borderline to transfusion dependent. The anemia is usually normo-macrocytic, with reticulocytosis. Bilirubin and LDH are increased. Although hemolysis is, by definition, chronic in these patients, they are also vulnerable to acute oxidative damage, and therefore the same agents that can cause AHA in people with the ordinary type of G6PD deficiency will cause severe exacerbations in people with CNSHA associated with G6PD deficiency. In some cases of CNSHA, the deficiency of G6PD is so severe in granulocytes that it limits their capacity to produce an oxidative burst, with consequent increased susceptibility to some bacterial infections.

Laboratory Diagnosis The suspicion of G6PD deficiency can be confirmed by semiquantitative methods often referred to as screening tests, which are suitable for population studies and can correctly classify male subjects, in the steady state, as G6PD normal or G6PD deficient. However, in clinical practice, a diagnostic test is usually needed when the patient has had a hemolytic attack: whereby the oldest, most G6PD-deficient red cells have been selectively destroyed, and young red cells, having higher G6PD activity, are being released into the circulation. Under these conditions, only a quantitative test can give a definitive result. In males, this test will identify normal hemizygotes and G6PD-deficient hemizygotes; among females, some heterozygotes will be missed, but those who are at most risk of hemolysis will be identified. Of course, G6PD deficiency also can be diagnosed by DNA testing. Currently easy-to-use "point of care" tests for G6PD deficiency are becoming available, geared especially to the prospect of mass administration of PQ or of the newly introduced derivative tafenoquine.

TREATMENT

G6PD Deficiency

The AHA of G6PD deficiency is largely preventable by avoiding exposure to triggering factors of previously screened subjects. Of course, the practicability and cost-effectiveness of screening depend on the prevalence of G6PD deficiency in each individual community. Favism is entirely preventable in G6PD-deficient subjects by not eating fava beans. Drug-induced hemolysis can be prevented by testing for G6PD deficiency before prescribing; in many cases one can use alternative drugs. When AHA develops and once its cause is recognized, no specific treatment is needed in most cases. However, if the anemia is severe, it may be a medical emergency, especially in children, requiring immediate action, including blood transfusion. This has been the case with an antimalarial drug combination containing dapsone (called Lapdap, introduced in 2003) that has caused severe acute hemolytic episodes in children with malaria in several African countries; after a few years, the drug was taken off the market. If there is acute renal failure, hemodialysis may be necessary, but if there is no previous kidney disease, recovery is the rule. The management of NNJ associated with G6PD deficiency is no different from that of NNJ due to other causes.

In cases with CNSHA, if the anemia is not severe, regular folic acid supplements and regular hematologic surveillance will suffice. It will be important to avoid exposure to potentially hemolytic drugs, and blood transfusion may be indicated when exacerbations occur, mostly in concomitance with intercurrent infection. In rare patients, regular blood transfusions may be required, in which case appropriate iron chelation should be instituted. Unlike in HS, there is no evidence of selective red cell destruction in the spleen; however, in practice, splenectomy has proven beneficial in severe cases.

Other Abnormalities of the Redox System As mentioned previously, GSH is a key player in the defense against oxidative stress. Inherited defects of GSH metabolism are exceedingly rare, but each one can give rise to chronic HA (Table 100-4). A rare, peculiar, and severe but usually self-limited HA occurring in the first month of life, called *infantile poikilocytosis*, may be associated with deficiency of glutathione peroxidase (GSHPX) due not to an inherited abnormality, but to transient nutritional deficiency of selenium, an element essential for the activity of GSHPX.

PYRIMIDINE 5'-NUCLEOTIDASE (P5N) DEFICIENCY P5N is a key enzyme in the catabolism of nucleotides arising from the degradation of nucleic acids that takes place in the final stages of erythroid cell maturation. How exactly its deficiency causes HA is not well understood, but a highly distinctive feature of this condition is a morphologic abnormality of the red cells known as *basophilic stippling*. The condition is rare, but it probably ranks third in frequency among red cell enzyme defects (after G6PD deficiency and PK deficiency). The anemia is lifelong, of variable severity, and may benefit from splenectomy.

Familial (Atypical) Hemolytic-Uremic Syndrome (aHUS) This term is used to designate a group of rare disorders, mostly affecting children, characterized by microangiopathic HA with presence of fragmented erythrocytes in the peripheral blood smear, thrombocytopenia (usually mild), and acute renal failure. (The word *atypical* in this phrase should be consigned to history: it was introduced originally to distinguish this condition from the hemolytic-uremic syndrome [HUS] caused by infection with *Escherichia coli* producing the Shiga toxin, regarded as *typical*.) The genetic basis of atypical HUS (aHUS) has been elucidated. Studies of >100 families have revealed that those family members who developed HUS had mutations in any one of several genes encoding complement regulatory proteins: complement factor H (*CFH*), CD46 or membrane cofactor protein (*MCP*), complement factor I (*CFI*), complement component C3, complement factor B (*CFB*), thrombomodulin, and others. Thus, whereas all other inherited HAs are due to intrinsic red cell abnormalities, this group is unique in that hemolysis results from an inherited defect external to red cells (Table 100-1). Because the regulation of the complement cascade has considerable redundancy, in the steady state any of the above abnormalities can be tolerated. However, when an intercurrent infection or some other trigger briskly activates complement the deficiency of one of the complement regulators becomes critical. Endothelial cells get damaged, especially in the kidney; at the same time, and partly as a result of this, there will be brisk hemolysis (thus, the more common Shiga toxin–related HUS (**Chap. 166**) can be regarded as a phenocopy of aHUS). aHUS is a severe disease, with up to 15% mortality in the acute phase and up to 50% of cases progressing to end-stage renal disease (ESRD). Not infrequently, aHUS undergoes spontaneous remission. Because it is an inherited abnormality, it is not surprising that, given renewed exposure to a trigger, the syndrome will tend to recur; when it does, the prognosis is always serious. The traditional treatment has been plasma exchange, which will supply the deficient complement regulator. This has changed since the introduction of the anti-C5 complement inhibitor eculizumab (see "Paroxysmal Nocturnal Hemoglobinuria") was found to greatly ameliorate the microangiopathic picture, with improvement in platelet counts and in renal function, thus abrogating the need for plasma exchange, which is not always effective and not free of complications. Because the basis of aHUS is genetic, and relapses are always possible even after complete remission, there is a rationale for continuing eculizumab indefinitely, especially in order to prevent ESRD. Patients who relapsed after discontinuing eculizumab have responded again. Discontinuation of eculizumab might be reasonable especially in patients heterozygous for a MCP mutation. However, there is no evidence base at the moment for balancing the pros and cons of lifetime eculizumab (a very expensive drug).

ACQUIRED HEMOLYTIC ANEMIA

Mechanical Destruction of Red Cells Although red cells are characterized by the remarkable deformability that enables them to squeeze through capillaries narrower than themselves for thousands of times in their lifetime, there are at least two situations in which they succumb to shear, if not to wear and tear; the result is intravascular hemolysis, resulting in hemoglobinuria (**Table 100-6**). One situation is acute and self-inflicted, *march hemoglobinuria*. Why sometimes a marathon runner may develop this complication, whereas on another occasion, this does not happen, we do not know (perhaps her or his footwear needs attention). A similar syndrome may develop after prolonged barefoot ritual dancing or intense playing of bongo drums. The other situation is chronic and iatrogenic (it has been called *microangiopathic hemolytic anemia*). It takes place in patients with prosthetic heart valves, especially when paraprosthetic regurgitation is present. If the hemolysis consequent on mechanical trauma to the red cells is mild, and if the supply of iron is adequate, the loss may be largely

TABLE 100-6 Diseases and Clinical Situations in Which Hemolysis Is Largely Intravascular

	ONSET/TIME COURSE	MAIN MECHANISM	APPROPRIATE DIAGNOSTIC PROCEDURE	COMMENTS
Mismatched blood transfusion	Abrupt	Nearly always ABO incompatibility	Repeat cross-match	
Paroxysmal nocturnal hemoglobinuria (PNH)	Chronic with acute exacerbations	Complement (C)-mediated destruction of CD59(–) red cells	Flow cytometry to display a CD59(–) red cell population	Exacerbations due to C activation through any pathway
Paroxysmal cold hemoglobinuria (PCH)	Acute	Immune lysis of normal red cells	Test for Donath-Landsteiner antibody	Often triggered by viral infection
Septicemia	Very acute	Exotoxins produced by *Clostridium perfringens*	Blood cultures	Other organisms may be responsible
Microangiopathic	Acute or chronic	Red cell fragmentation	Red cell morphology on blood smear	Different causes ranging from endothelial damage to hemangioma to leaky prosthetic heart valve
March hemoglobinuria	Abrupt	Mechanical destruction	Targeted history taking	Has been reported after extreme ritual dancing
Favism	Acute	Destruction of older fraction of G6PD-deficient red cells	G6PD assay	Triggered by ingestion of large dish of fava beans[a]

[a]The trigger of acute hemolytic anemia, often with hemoglobinuria, can be infection or a drug (see Table 100-5) rather than fava beans. Hemoglobinuria may or may not be reported by patient; but it is often macroscopic, i.e., recognizable by simple inspection of urine.

Abbreviation: G6PD, glucose 6-phosphate dehydrogenase.

compensated; if more than mild anemia develops, reintervention to correct regurgitation may be required.

Infection By far the most frequent infectious cause of HA in endemic areas is malaria **(Chap. 224)**. In other parts of the world, the most frequent direct cause is probably Shiga toxin–producing *E. coli* O157:H7, now recognized as the main etiologic agent of HUS, which is more common in children than in adults **(Chap. 161)**. Life-threatening intravascular hemolysis, due to a toxin with lecithinase activity, occurs with *Clostridium perfringens* sepsis, particularly following open wounds, septic abortion, or as a disastrous accident due to a contaminated blood unit. Rarely, and if at all in children, HA is seen with sepsis or endocarditis from a variety of organisms. In addition, bacterial and viral infections can cause HA by indirect mechanisms (see Table 100-6).

Immune Hemolytic Anemias These can arise through at least two distinct mechanisms. First, when an antibody directed against a certain molecule (e.g., a drug) reacts with that molecule, red cells may get caught in the reaction (the so-called innocent bystander mechanism: see section below on Hemolytic Anemia from Toxic Agents and Drugs), whereby they are damaged or destroyed. Second, and more frequently, a true autoantibody is directed against a red cell antigen, i.e., a molecule present on the surface of red cells. Autoimmune hemolytic anemias have been originally classified into two types, depending on the thermal amplitude of the autoantibodies involved: this classification is valid, because the two types have different pathophysiological and clinical features.

AUTOIMMUNE HEMOLYTIC ANEMIA, WARM TYPE (WAIHA: FOR SIMPLICITY WE WILL USE THE ACRONYM AIHA) This type has an estimated incidence in the United States of about 1–3:100,000 per year, and a prevalence of 17:100,000. AIHA can be serious since even with appropriate management the mortality is of the order of 5–10%.

Clinical Features and Diagnosis The onset is often abrupt and can be dramatic. The hemoglobin level may drop, within days, to as low as 4 g/dL; the massive red cell removal will produce jaundice, and sometimes the spleen is enlarged. When this triad is present, the suspicion of AIHA must be high. The reticulocyte count is typically elevated, except when erythroid precursors are also targeted by the autoantibody attack. LDH may also be elevated. In some cases, AIHA can be associated, on first presentation or subsequently, with autoimmune thrombocytopenia. This double autoimmune condition, referred to as Evans syndrome, may be a manifestation of common variable immune deficiency, and in children it may suggest one of several primary immune deficiency syndromes. Evans syndrome signals high-risk disease. Other predictors of the outcome and of the probability of relapse of AIHA are severe anemia (Hb <6 g/dL), certain characteristics of the antibody, acute renal failure, and infection.

There are few situations in hematology where one laboratory test is as informative as the direct antiglobulin test developed in 1945 by R. R. A. Coombs and known since then by this name. The currently recommended version of this test uses in the first instance a "broad-spectrum" reagent, i.e., one that will detect not only immunoglobulins (Ig) but also complement (C) components (usually C3 fragments) bound to the surface of the patient's red cells. If the test is positive (and barring special circumstances such as previous blood transfusion), it is practically diagnostic of AIHA, and one can then determine, by using specific reagents, whether Ig or C or both are implicated. The sensitivity of the Coombs test varies depending on the techniques that are used: in general, the test is positive if there are an average of at least 400 molecules of Ig and/or C on each red cell; but with more advanced techniques involving flow cytometry analysis or enzyme-linked radiolabeled tests allowing the detection of ~30–40 antibody molecules per erythrocyte, the sensitivity can be pushed to as low as 30–40 molecules per red cell. Therefore liaison with a specialized laboratory is desirable; a dual direct antiglobulin test has also been developed. In the past the diagnosis of "Coombs-negative AIHA" was regarded as a last resort, but it is important to know that a patient with this label may have severe AIHA, because if the antibody is powerful (high affinity/avidity), few molecules may be sufficient to opsonize red cells. Based on the Coombs test findings as well as on the thermal characteristics and the antigenic specificities of the autoantibodies **(Table 100-7)**, AIHA has been classified into subtypes.

In AIHA the autoantibody reacts best at 37°C and it is usually Rhesus-specific (sometimes specifically anti-e). The main mechanism of hemolysis in AIHA is that the Fc portion of the IgG antibody bound to red cells is recognized by the Fc receptor of macrophages: this will trigger erythrophagocytosis wherever macrophages are abundant, i.e., in the liver, in the bone marrow, but especially in red pulp of the spleen (see **Fig. 100-9**) that, also because of its special anatomy, is often the predominant site of red cell destruction.

AIHA may be seen in isolation (and it is then called *idiopathic*) or as secondary to other disorders such as systemic autoimmune disorders (systemic lupus erythematosus [SLE]: sometimes AIHA may be the first manifestation that leads to a diagnosis of SLE) or lymphoproliferative disorders (Table 100-7). Like all autoimmune diseases, AIHA must arise from a dysregulation of immunity. It is therefore not surprising that it is increasingly being recognized in chronic lymphocytic leukemia (CLL), whether treated or untreated; after BMT; and after solid organ transplantation entailing immunosuppressive treatment. Recently, warm antibody AIHA has also occurred as a side effect of the use of immune checkpoint inhibitors, such as nivolumab, in patients with various types of cancer.

TABLE 100-7 Classification of Acquired Immune Hemolytic Anemias

	TYPE OF ANTIBODY	
CLINICAL SETTING	COLD, MOSTLY IgM, OPTIMAL TEMPERATURE 4°C–30°C	WARM, MOSTLY IgG, OPTIMAL TEMPERATURE 37°C; OR MIXED
Primary	CAD	AIHA (idiopathic)
Secondary to viral infection	EBV CMV Other	Parvovirus B19 HIV HCV EBV Viral vaccines
Secondary to other infection	Mycoplasma infection: paroxysmal cold hemoglobinuria	Babesia
Secondary to/associated with other disease	CAD in: Waldenström's disease Lymphoma	AIHA in: SLE, scleroderma, RA CLL Lymphoproliferative disorders Multiple myeloma Other malignancy Chronic inflammatory disorders (e.g., IBD) Thyroiditis (including Hashimoto) After allogeneic HSCT Common variable immunodeficiency After immune checkpoint modulating drugs
Secondary to drugs: drug-induced immune hemolytic anemia	Small minority (e.g., with lenalidomide)	Majority: currently most common culprit drugs are cefotetan, ceftriaxone, piperacillin, methyldopa, fludarabine
	Drug-dependent: antibody destroys red cells only when drug present (e.g., rarely penicillin)	
	Drug-independent: antibody can destroy red cells even when drug no longer present (e.g., methyldopa)	
Associated with	Pregnancy	

Abbreviations: AIHA, autoimmune hemolytic anemia; CAD, cold agglutinin disease; CLL, chronic lymphocytic leukemia; CMV, cytomegalovirus; EBV, Epstein-Barr virus; HCV, hepatitis C virus; HIV, human immunodeficiency virus; HSCT, hematopoietic stem cell transplantation; IBD, inflammatory bowel disease; SLE, systemic lupus erythematosus; RA: rheumatoid arthritis.

TREATMENT

Warm Antibody Autoimmune Hemolytic Anemia

Severe acute AIHA can be a medical emergency. The immediate treatment almost invariably includes transfusion of red cells. This may pose a special problem because many or all of the blood units cross-matched may be incompatible. In these cases, it is often correct, if paradoxical, to transfuse ABO-matched but incompatible blood: the rationale being that the transfused red cells will be destroyed no less—but no more—than the patient's own red cells, and in the meantime the patient stays alive. A situation like this requires close liaison and understanding between the clinical unit treating the patient and the blood transfusion/serology lab. Whenever the anemia is not immediately life-threatening, blood transfusion should be withheld (because compatibility problems may increase with each unit of blood transfused), and medical treatment started immediately with prednisone (1 mg/kg per day), which will produce a remission promptly in at least one-half of patients. Rituximab (anti-CD20), previously regarded as second-line treatment, is increasingly being used at a relatively low dose (100 mg/week × 4), together with prednisone as part of first-line treatment. It is especially encouraging that this approach seems to reduce the rate of relapse, a common occurrence in AIHA.

For patients who do relapse or are refractory to medical treatment, additional therapeutic strategies are now available. Splenectomy does not cure the disease, but it can produce significant benefit by removing a major site of hemolysis, thus improving the anemia and/or reducing the need for other therapies (e.g., the dose of prednisone); of course, splenectomy is not free of risk, as it entails increased risk of sepsis and of thrombosis. The response rate to splenectomy and to rituximab are similar. Since the introduction of rituximab, azathioprine, cyclophosphamide, cyclosporine, mycophenolate and intravenous immunoglobulin have become second- or third-line agents. In very rare severe refractory cases, one may have to consider a high dose of cyclophosphamide (50 mg/kg/d for 4 days) followed by a myelo-stimulating agent to support bone marrow or the anti-CD52 agent, alemtuzumab. When severe anemia is associated with reticulocytopenia, the use of erythropoietin may help to reduce or avoid the requirement for transfusion of red cells.

PAROXYSMAL COLD HEMOGLOBINURIA (PCH) PCH is a rare form of AIHA occurring mostly in children, usually triggered by a viral infection, usually self-limited, and characterized by the so-called Donath-Landsteiner antibody. In vitro, this antibody has unique serologic features; it has usually anti-P specificity and it binds to red cells only at a low temperature (optimally at 4°C), but when the temperature is shifted to 37°C, lysis of red cells takes place in the presence of complement. Consequently, in vivo there is intravascular hemolysis, resulting in hemoglobinuria. Clinically the differential diagnosis must include other causes of hemoglobinuria (Table 100-6), but the presence of the Donath-Landsteiner antibody will prove PCH. Active supportive treatment, including blood transfusion, may be needed to control the anemia; subsequently, recovery is the rule.

COLD AGGLUTININ DISEASE This designation indicates the other main type of AIHA, which has quite different features when compared with wAIHA. First, cold agglutinin disease (CAD) is a chronic and more frequently indolent condition—in contrast to the abrupt onset of warm antibody AIHA. Second, the term *cold* refers to the fact that the autoantibody involved reacts with red cells poorly or not at all at 37°C, whereas it reacts strongly at lower temperatures. As a result, hemolysis is more prominent the more the body is exposed to the cold. Third, the antibody is produced by a clone of autoreactive B lymphocytes. Sometimes the antibody concentration in the serum is high enough to show up as a spike in plasma protein electrophoresis, thus qualifying CAD as an IgM monoclonal gammopathy; however, it differs from Waldenström macroglobulinemia by not having the characteristic *MYD88* mutation (see **Chap. 111**): there is instead, in the B-cell clone of a majority of CAD patients, a somatic mutation in the *KMT2D* gene, encoding a lysine histone methylase that seems to favor proliferation. The antibody produced by the B-cell clone is IgM; usually it has an anti-I specificity (the I antigen is present on the red cells of almost everybody), and it may have a very high titer (1:100,000 or more has been observed). IgM, when bound to red cells, is a powerful activator of the complement cascade, with ultimate formation of the membrane attack complex (see Fig. 100-9): this will directly cause destruction of red cells (*intravascular hemolysis:* indeed, CAD patients may present with hemoglobinuria). In addition, once complement is activated C3b will bind to red cells that, thus opsonized, will be destroyed by macrophages (*extravascular hemolysis*); unlike in AIHA, there is no predominance of the spleen in this process.

In mild forms of CAD, avoidance of exposure to cold may be all that is needed to enable the patient to have a reasonably comfortable quality of life; but in more severe forms, the management of CAD is not easy. Plasma exchange will remove antibodies and is, therefore, in theory, a rational approach in severe cases. However, the management of CAD has changed significantly with the advent of the anti-CD20 antibody rituximab: up to 60% of patients respond. If remission is followed by relapse, a new course of rituximab may be again effective, and remissions may be more durable with a rituximab-fludarabine combination, in particular in CAD associated with lymphoproliferative disorders. Therefore, even

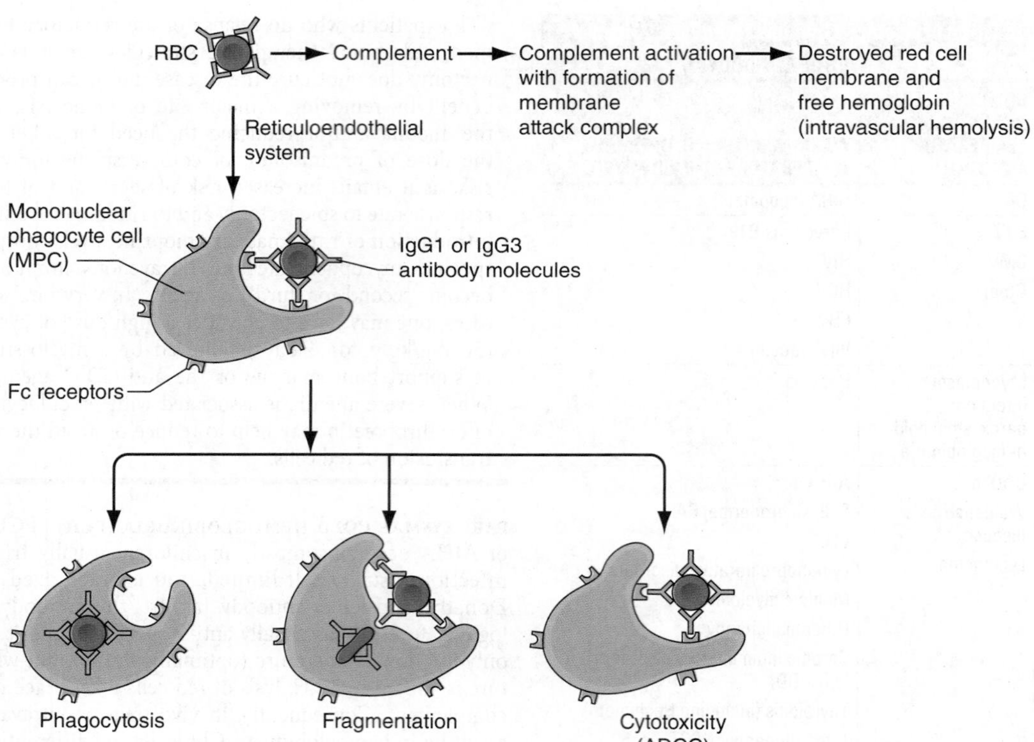

FIGURE 100-9 Mechanism of antibody-mediated immune destruction of red blood cells (RBCs). The three bottom images illustrate three different modalities of extravascular hemolysis. ADCC, antibody-dependent cell-mediated cytotoxicity. *(Reproduced with permission from N Young et al: Clinical Hematology. Philadelphia, Elsevier, 2006.)*

in the absence of a formal trial, rituximab has become de facto first-line treatment: especially since previously used immunosuppressive/cytotoxic agents, although they can reduce the antibody titer, have limited clinical efficacy and, in view of the chronic nature of CAD, their side effects may prove unacceptable. Unlike in AIHA, prednisone and splenectomy are ineffective. In the management of CAD in relapse, there is an emerging role for the B-cell receptor inhibitors venetoclax and ibrutinib, as well as for the proteasome inhibitor bortezomib. A different approach targeting complement inhibitors has been also explored by using eculizumab (anti-C5) or sutimlimab (anti-C1s): a limitation of this approach is that hemolysis will be curbed only for as long as these agents are administered.

In terms of supportive treatment, blood transfusion may be helpful—in spite of the fact that red cells from the donor, being I-positive, will survive no longer than those of the patient: both the blood bag and the patient's extremities must be kept warm during transfusion.

Hemolytic Anemia from Toxic Agents and Drugs A number of chemicals with oxidative potential, whether medicinal or not, can cause hemolysis even in people who are not G6PD deficient (for which, see above). Examples are hyperbaric oxygen (or 100% oxygen), nitrates, chlorates, methylene blue, dapsone, cisplatin, and numerous aromatic (cyclic) compounds. Other chemicals may be hemolytic through nonoxidative, largely unknown mechanisms; examples include arsine, stibine, copper, and lead. The HA caused by lead poisoning is characterized by basophilic stippling; it is in fact a phenocopy of that seen in P5N deficiency (see above), suggesting it is mediated at least in part by lead inhibiting this enzyme.

In these cases, hemolysis appears to be mediated by a direct chemical action on red cells. But drugs can cause hemolysis through at least two other mechanisms. (1) A drug can behave as a hapten and induce antibody production; in rare subjects, this happens, for instance, with penicillin. Upon a subsequent exposure, red cells are caught, as innocent bystanders, in the reaction between penicillin and antipenicillin antibodies. Hemolysis will subside as soon as penicillin administration is stopped. (2) A drug can trigger, perhaps through mimicry, the production of an antibody against a red cell antigen. The best-known example is methyldopa, an antihypertensive agent no longer in use, which in a small fraction of patients stimulated the production of the Rhesus antibody anti-e. In patients who have this antigen, the anti-e is a true autoantibody, which then causes true AIHA (see above). Usually this will gradually subside once methyldopa is discontinued.

Severe intravascular hemolysis can be caused by the venom of certain snakes (cobras and vipers), and HA can also follow spider bites.

Paroxysmal Nocturnal Hemoglobinuria (PNH) PNH is an acquired chronic HA characterized by persistent intravascular hemolysis with occasional or frequent recurrent exacerbations. In addition to (i) hemolysis, there may be (ii) pancytopenia and (iii) a distinct tendency to venous thrombosis. This triad makes PNH a truly unique clinical condition; however, when not all of these three features are manifest on presentation, the diagnosis is often delayed, although it can always be made by appropriate laboratory investigations (see below).

PNH is encountered in all populations throughout the world, but it is a rare disease, with an estimated prevalence of ~5 per million (it may be somewhat less rare in Southeast Asia and in the Far East). PNH has about the same frequency in men and women. PNH is not inherited, and it has never been reported as a congenital disease, but it can present in small children or as late as in the seventies, although most patients are young adults.

CLINICAL FEATURES When seeking medical attention, the patient may report that one morning, she or he "passed blood instead of urine." This distressing or frightening event may be regarded as the classic presentation; however, more frequently, this symptom is not noticed or not reported. Indeed, the patient often presents simply as a problem in the differential diagnosis of anemia, whether symptomatic or discovered incidentally. Sometimes the anemia is associated from the outset with neutropenia, thrombocytopenia, or both, thus signaling an element of bone marrow failure (see below). Some patients may present with recurrent attacks of severe abdominal pain eventually found to be related to thrombosis in abdominal veins, or attributable to NO depletion associated with intravascular hemolysis. When thrombosis affects the hepatic vein, it may produce acute hepatomegaly and ascites, i.e., a full-fledged Budd-Chiari syndrome, which, in the absence of liver disease, ought to raise the suspicion of PNH.

The natural history of PNH can extend over decades. In the past, with supportive treatment only, the median survival was estimated to be about 10–20 years, with the most common cause of death being venous thrombosis, followed by infection secondary to severe neutropenia and hemorrhage secondary to severe thrombocytopenia. Rarely (estimated 1–2% of all cases), PNH may terminate in acute myeloid leukemia. On the other hand, full spontaneous recovery from PNH has been documented, albeit rarely.

LABORATORY INVESTIGATIONS AND DIAGNOSIS The most consistent blood finding is anemia, which may range from mild to moderate to very severe. The anemia is usually normo-macrocytic, with unremarkable red cell morphology. If the MCV is high, it is usually largely accounted for by reticulocytosis, which may be quite marked (up to 20%, or up to 400,000/μL). The anemia may become microcytic if the patient is allowed to become iron-deficient as a result of chronic iron loss through hemoglobinuria. Unconjugated bilirubin is mildly or moderately elevated; LDH is typically markedly elevated (values in the thousands are common); and haptoglobin is usually undetectable. All of these findings make the diagnosis of HA compelling. Hemoglobinuria may be overt in a random urine sample; if it is not, it may be helpful to obtain serial urine samples (Fig. 100-9) because hemoglobinuria can vary dramatically from day to day and even from hour to hour. The bone marrow is usually cellular, with marked to massive erythroid hyperplasia, often with mild to moderate dyserythropoietic features (these overlap with those seen in myelodysplastic syndromes, but PNH remains a separate entity). At some stage of the disease, the marrow may become hypocellular or even frankly aplastic (see below).

The definitive diagnosis of PNH must be based on the demonstration that a substantial proportion of the patient's red cells have an increased susceptibility to complement (C), due to the deficiency on their surface of proteins (particularly CD59 and CD55) that normally protect the red cells from activated C. The sucrose hemolysis test is unreliable; in contrast, the acidified serum (Ham) test is highly reliable but is carried out only in a few laboratories. The gold standard today is flow cytometry, which can be carried out on granulocytes as well as on red cells and has a very high sensitivity. In PNH, characteristically, one sees a bimodal distribution of cells, with a discrete population that is CD59 and CD55 negative. Although very small populations of CD59(–) cells are of interest in terms of pathophysiology (particularly of aplastic anemia [AA]), no patient should be diagnosed with PNH unless the proportion is substantial: in first approximation at least 5% of the total red cells and at least 20% of the total granulocytes.

PATHOPHYSIOLOGY Hemolysis in PNH is mainly intravascular and is due to an intrinsic abnormality of the red cell, which makes it exquisitely sensitive to activated C, whether C is activated through the alternative pathway or through an antigen-antibody reaction (classic pathway). The former mechanism is mainly responsible for chronic hemolysis in PNH; the latter explains why the hemolysis can be dramatically exacerbated in the course of a viral or bacterial infection. Hypersusceptibility to C is due to deficiency in the red cell membrane of several protective proteins (**Fig. 100-10**), among which CD59 is the most important because it is able to hinder the insertion into the membrane of C9 polymers (the so-called membrane attack complex, or MAC). The molecular basis for the deficiency of these proteins has been pinpointed not to a defect in any of the respective genes, but rather to the shortage of a unique glycolipid molecule, GPI (Fig. 100-2), which, through a peptide bond, anchors these proteins to the surface membrane of cells. The shortage of GPI is due in turn to a somatic mutation in an X-linked gene, called *PIGA*, required for an early step in GPI biosynthesis. As a result, the patient's marrow is a mosaic of mutant and nonmutant cells, and the peripheral blood always contains both GPI-negative (PNH) cells and GPI-positive (non-PNH) cells: in most cases the former prevail. Thrombosis is one of the most immediately life-threatening complications of PNH, and yet one of the least understood in its pathogenesis. It could be that deficiency of CD59 on the PNH platelet causes inappropriate platelet activation; however, other mechanisms are possible. In very rare cases PNH can be caused by biallelic mutations of the *PIGT* gene, in the absence of a *PIGA* mutation. In these cases, because GPI is produced but cannot bind to proteins, the clinical picture is further complicated by the coexistence of a chronic inflammatory state.

BONE MARROW FAILURE (BMF) AND RELATIONSHIP BETWEEN PNH AND APLASTIC ANEMIA (AA) It is not unusual that patients with firmly established PNH have a previous history of AA, sometimes well documented; indeed, BMF preceding overt PNH is probably the rule rather than the exception. On the other hand, sometimes a patient with PNH becomes less hemolytic and more pancytopenic and ultimately has the clinical picture of AA. The relationship between PNH and AA manifested in the clinical course of patients may reflect a close link in pathogenesis. AA is thought to be an organ-specific autoimmune disease, in which T cells cause damage to hematopoietic stem cells via an as yet unidentified molecular target. The same may be true of PNH, and in this condition the target might be the GPI molecule itself. This would explain why GPI-negative (PNH) stem cells are spared; *PIGA* mutations can be demonstrated in normal people. Thus, PNH results from the combined action of two factors: failure of normal hematopoiesis and massive expansion of a PNH clone. There is evidence from mouse models that PNH stem cells do not expand on their own, and there is evidence from human patients that expansion is associated with negative selection against GPI-positive cells by GPI-specific T cells. Thus, PNH is a prime example of a clonal disease that is not malignant.

TREATMENT

Paroxysmal Nocturnal Hemoglobinuria

Until some 15 years ago there were essentially two treatment options for PNH: either allogeneic BMT, providing a definitive cure at the cost of nonnegligible risks; or continued supportive treatment for what, unlike other acquired HAs, may be a lifelong condition. A major advance has been the introduction in 2007 of a humanized monoclonal antibody, eculizumab, which binds to the complement component C5 near the site that, when cleaved, will trigger the distal part of the complement cascade leading to formation of the MAC. With C5 blocked by anti-C5, the patient is relieved of intravascular hemolysis and of its attendant consequences, including hemoglobinuria; with a substantial decrease in the rate of thrombosis. In the majority of those patients who needed regular blood transfusion, the transfusion requirement is either abolished or significantly reduced. For many PNH patients, eculizumab has meant a real improvement in the quality of life, as well as a decrease in complications, particularly thrombosis. At the same time, it is important to know that in patients on eculizumab the PNH red cells, now protected from being lysed through the MAC, do still bind C3 fragments and thus become opsonized. Therefore, hemolysis continues, but it is now extravascular. The extent to which this happens depends in part on a genetic polymorphism of the complement receptor CR1. Those patients who, on eculizumab, are still receiving blood transfusion are at risk of iron overload. Based on its half-life, eculizumab must be administered intravenously every 14 days. Ravulizumab, a long-lived anti-C5 derivative of eculizumab, is administered at 8-week rather than 2-week intervals: it provides similar benefit with obvious practical advantage.

Eculizumab and ravulizumab are very expensive and for this reason not accessible to patients in many parts of the world. Therefore, the management of PNH by supportive treatment is still very important. Folic acid supplements (at least 3 mg/d) are mandatory; the serum iron should be checked periodically, and iron supplements should be administered as appropriate. Transfusion of white cell-free red cells should be used whenever necessary, which, for some patients, means quite frequently. Long-term glucocorticoids are not indicated because there is no evidence that they have any effect on chronic hemolysis; in fact, they are contraindicated

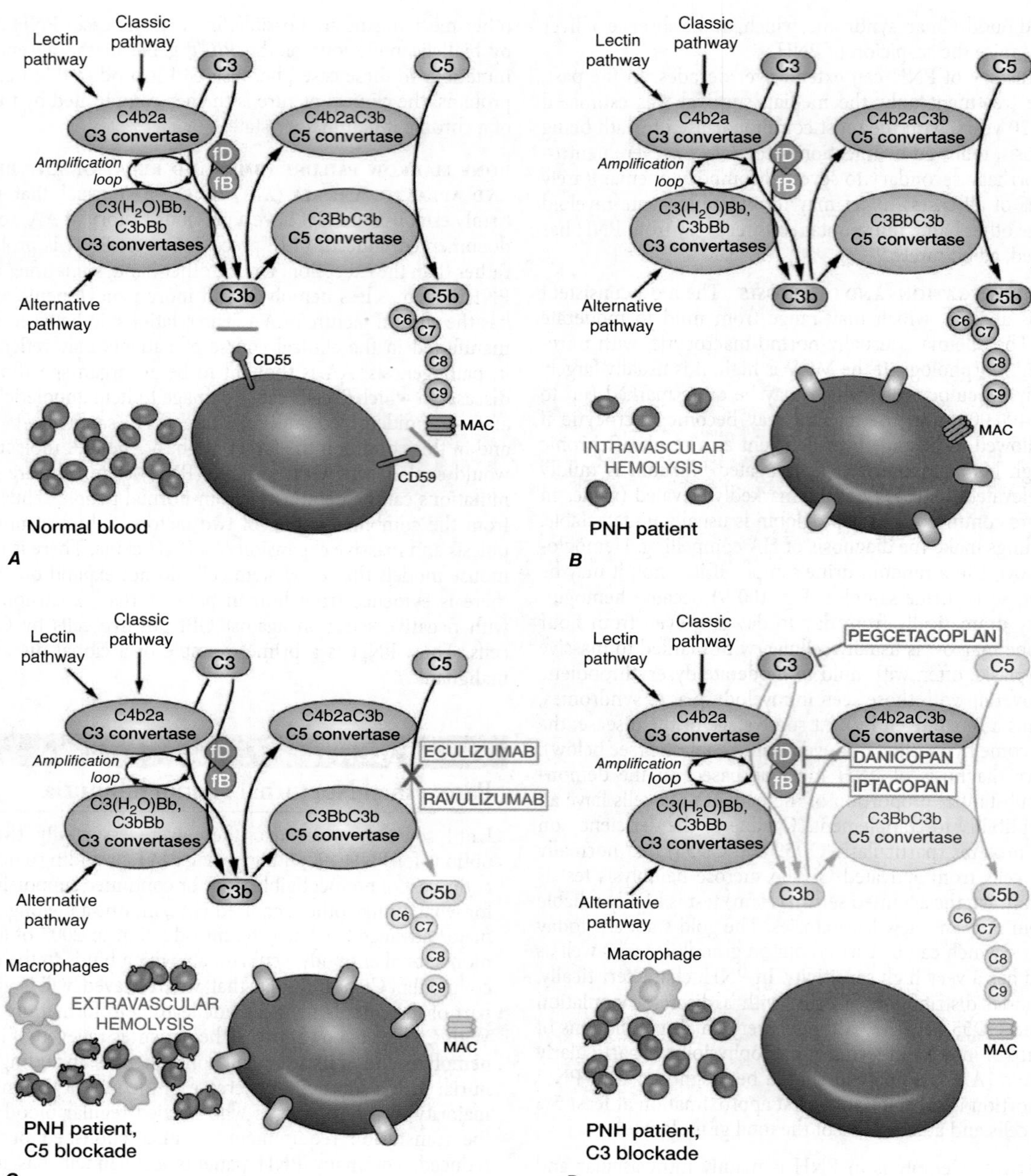

FIGURE 100-10 The complement cascade and the fate of red cells. ***A.*** In normal blood, when complement is activated, red cells are protected from lysis in several ways: primarily by the 2 glycosylphosphatidylinositol (GPI)-linked surface proteins CD55 (prevents binding of C3 fragments) and CD59 (prevents the membrane attack complex [MAC] from inserting into the membrane). ***B.*** PNH red cells are deficient in CD55 and CD59 because the GPI biosynthetic pathway is blocked as a result of a PIGA mutation; therefore, C3 fragments, particularly C3d, bind to their surface, and the red cells are rapidly lysed by the action of the MAC. ***C.*** With drugs (monoclonal antibodies) that bind to C5 and prevent it splitting into C5a and C5b, the entire distal pathway from C5 onward is blocked, MAC is not formed, and IVH is abrogated. However, red cells opsonized by C3d will be destroyed in the spleen and elsewhere; this drug-induced EVH varies in severity between patients. The Coombs test, which is characteristically negative in PNH, becomes positive (provided that a "broad spectrum" or an anticomplement reagent is used). ***D.*** With a drug that targets C3, C3b formation is inhibited, and the distal pathway is not triggered by C3b. Therefore, again, no MAC is formed (abrogating IVH), and, at the same time, opsonization of red cells by C3d is prevented, so that EVH is also curbed. The same is largely true for drugs that target factor B or factor D, although C3b can still be formed through the classical pathway. *(Reproduced with permission from L Luzzatto: Control of hemolysis in patients with PNH. Blood 138:1909, 2021.)*

because their side effects are considerable. A short course of prednisone may be useful when an inflammatory process exacerbates hemolysis. Any patient who has had venous thrombosis or who has a genetically determined thrombophilic state in addition to PNH should be on regular anticoagulant prophylaxis. With thrombotic complications that do not resolve otherwise, thrombolytic treatment with tissue plasminogen activator may be indicated.

Where anti-C5 therapy is available the proportion of PNH patients receiving BMT has decreased significantly. However, when an HLA-identical sibling is available, BMT should be taken into consideration for any young patient with severe PNH; and for patients with the so-called PNH-AA syndrome, since eculizumab has no effect on BMF. For these patients immunosuppressive treatment with antithymocyte globulin and cyclosporine A may be an alternative, and it may be compatible with concurrent administration of eculizumab.

In view of persistent extravascular hemolysis, and sometimes persistent blood transfusion requirement in PNH patients on C5 blockade therapy, there has been great stimulus to developing agents that may inhibit complement activation more upstream. Several compounds that inhibit either the convertase function of C3 or plasma factors required for this function are currently in clinical trials (**see Fig. 100-11**).

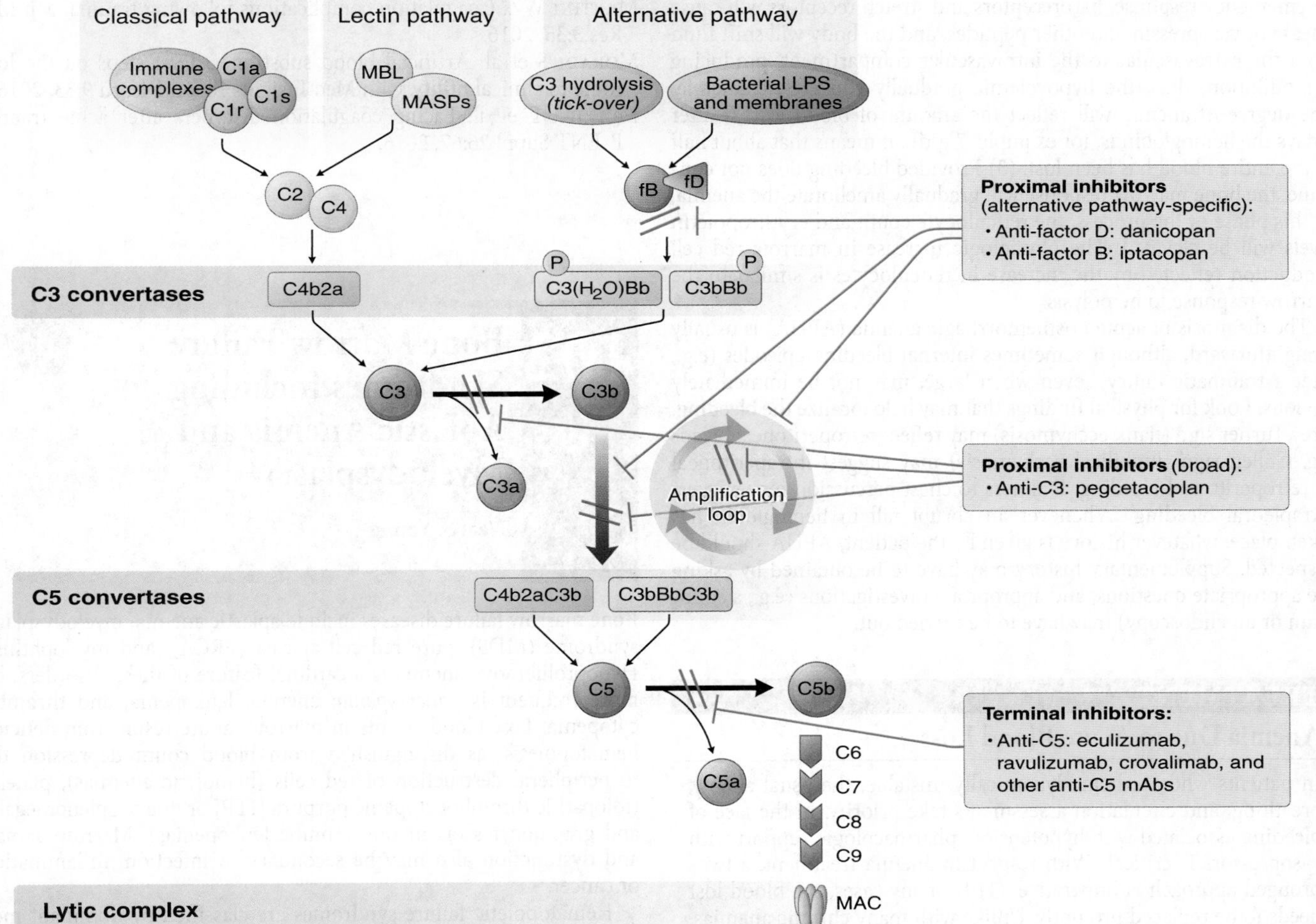

FIGURE 100-11 Monoclonal antibodies and small molecules in use or in development for the management of PNH and other complement-related disorders. Complement components are indicated by C followed by a number. MBL stands for mannose-binding lectin; MASP1 for mannose-binding lectin-associated serine protease 1. P is properdin. Of the inhibitors shown on the right, only eculizumab and ravulizumab, which bind to C5 and are therefore inhibitors of the distal pathway, are already licensed drugs: both effectively abrogate MAC formation but they do not interfere with the formation of either the C3 convertase or the C5 convertase: in contrast, this can be achieved with the upstream inhibitors danicopan, iptacopan, and pegcetacoplan.

FURTHER READING

Barcellini W et al: The changing landscape of autoimmune hemolytic anemia. Front Immunol 11:1, 2020.

Brodsky RA: Warm autoimmune hemolytic anemia. N Engl J Med 381:647-654, 2019.

Dacie J: *The Haemolytic Anaemias*. London, Churchill Livingstone, volumes 1-5, 1985-1999.

De Franceschi L et al: Acute hemolysis by hydroxycloroquine was observed in G6PD-deficient patient with severe COVD-19 related lung injury. Eur J Intern Med 77:136, 2020.

Grace RF et al: Clinical spectrum of pyruvate kinase deficiency: Data from the Pyruvate Kinase Deficiency Natural History Study. Blood 131:2183, 2018.

Iolascon A et al: Advances in understanding the pathogenesis of red cell membrane disorders. Br J Haematol 187:13, 2019.

Loirat C et al: An international consensus approach to the management of atypical hemolytic uremic syndrome in children. Pediatr Nephrol 31:15, 2016.

Luzzatto L, Karadimitris A: Paroxysmal nocturnal haemoglobinuria (PNH): Novel therapies for an ancient disease. Br J Haematol 191:579, 2020.

Luzzatto L et al: Glucose-6-phosphate dehydrogenase deficiency. Blood 136:1225, 2020.

Uyoga S et al: Glucose-6-phosphate dehydrogenase deficiency and the risk of malaria and other diseases in children on the coast of Kenya: A case-control and a cohort study. Lancet Haematology 2:e437, 2015.

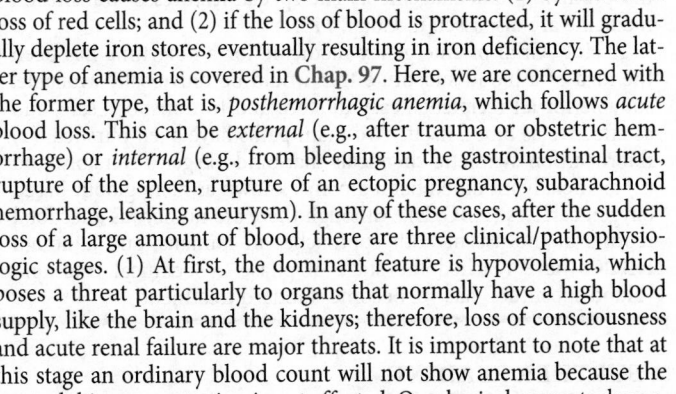

101 Anemia Due to Acute Blood Loss

Dan L. Longo

Blood loss causes anemia by two main mechanisms: (1) by the direct loss of red cells; and (2) if the loss of blood is protracted, it will gradually deplete iron stores, eventually resulting in iron deficiency. The latter type of anemia is covered in **Chap. 97**. Here, we are concerned with the former type, that is, *posthemorrhagic anemia*, which follows *acute* blood loss. This can be *external* (e.g., after trauma or obstetric hemorrhage) or *internal* (e.g., from bleeding in the gastrointestinal tract, rupture of the spleen, rupture of an ectopic pregnancy, subarachnoid hemorrhage, leaking aneurysm). In any of these cases, after the sudden loss of a large amount of blood, there are three clinical/pathophysiologic stages. (1) At first, the dominant feature is hypovolemia, which poses a threat particularly to organs that normally have a high blood supply, like the brain and the kidneys; therefore, loss of consciousness and acute renal failure are major threats. It is important to note that at this stage an ordinary blood count will not show anemia because the hemoglobin concentration is not affected. On physical exam, tachycardia, tachypnea, decreased pulse pressure, cold skin that appears pale and mottled, and decreased urine output may be noted. (2) Next, as an emergency response, baroreceptors and stretch receptors will cause release of vasopressin and other peptides, and the body will shift fluid from the extravascular to the intravascular compartment, producing hemodilution; thus, the hypovolemia gradually converts to anemia. The degree of anemia will reflect the amount of blood lost. If after 3 days the hemoglobin is, for example, 7 g/dL, it means that about half of the entire blood has been lost. (3) Provided bleeding does not continue, the bone marrow response will gradually ameliorate the anemia. In this phase of the process, the reticulocyte count and erythropoietin levels will be elevated. The physiologic increase in marrow red cell production reflected by the increase in reticulocytes is similar to the marrow response to hemolysis.

The diagnosis of acute posthemorrhagic anemia (APHA) is usually straightforward, although sometimes internal bleeding episodes (e.g., after a traumatic injury), even when large, may not be immediately obvious. Look for physical findings that may help localize the bleeding. Grey Turner sign (flank ecchymosis) may reflect retroperitoneal bleeding. Cullen sign (umbilical ecchymosis) may suggest intraperitoneal or retroperitoneal bleeding. Dullness to chest percussion may suggest intrapleural bleeding. Whenever an abrupt fall in hemoglobin has taken place, whatever history is given by the patient, APHA should be suspected. Supplementary history may have to be obtained by asking the appropriate questions, and appropriate investigations (e.g., a sonogram or an endoscopy) may have to be carried out.

TREATMENT

Anemia Due to Acute Blood Loss

In patients who are hemodynamically unstable, the usual airway, breathing, and circulation assessments take priority. In the face of bleeding associated with hypotension, pharmacologic support with vasopressors is critical. With respect to anemia treatment, a two-pronged approach is imperative. (1) In many cases, the blood lost needs to be replaced promptly. Unlike with many chronic anemias, when finding and correcting the cause of the anemia is the first priority and blood transfusion may not be even necessary because the body is adapted to the anemia, with acute blood loss, the reverse is true; because the body is not adapted to the anemia, blood transfusion takes priority. (2) While the emergency is being confronted, it is imperative to stop the hemorrhage and to eliminate its source.

In an acute hemorrhage situation, plasma may be preferred to saline for volume expansion since dilution of clotting factors with crystalloid may interfere with hemostasis.

A special type of APHA is blood loss during and immediately after surgery, which can be substantial (e.g., up to 2 L in the case of a radical prostatectomy). Of course with elective surgical procedures, the patient's own stored blood may be available (through preoperative autologous blood donation), and in any case, blood loss ought to have been carefully monitored/measured. The fact that this blood loss is iatrogenic dictates that ever more effort should be invested in optimizing its management. The special features of transfusion medicine are discussed in **Chap. 113**.

A Holy Grail of emergency medicine for a long time has been the idea of a blood substitute that would be universally available, suitable for all recipients, easy to store and to transport, safe, and as effective as blood itself. Two main paths have been pursued: (1) fluorocarbon synthetic chemicals that bind oxygen reversibly, and (2) artificially modified hemoglobins, known as hemoglobin-based oxygen carriers (HBOCs). Although there are numerous anecdotal reports of the use of both approaches in humans, and although HBOCs have reached the stage of phase 2–3 clinical trials, no "blood substitute" has yet become standard treatment.

FURTHER READING

Haldar R et al: Artificial blood: A futuristic dimension of modern day transfusion sciences. Cardiovasc Hematol Agents Med Chem 17:11, 2019.

Martini WZ: Coagulation complications following trauma. Mil Med Res 3:35, 2016.

Moradi S et al: Artificial blood substitutes: First steps on the long route to clinical utility. Clin Med Insights Blood Disord 9:33, 2016.

Mullier F et al: Facing coagulation disorders after acute trauma. B-ENT Suppl 26:67, 2016.

102 Bone Marrow Failure Syndromes Including Aplastic Anemia and Myelodysplasia

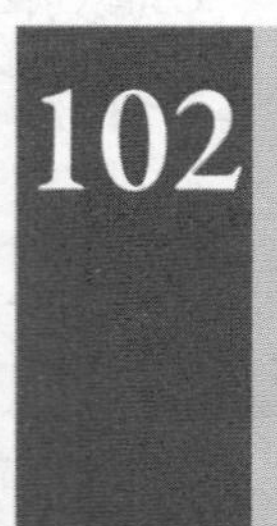

Neal S. Young

Bone marrow failure diseases include aplastic anemia, myelodysplastic syndrome (MDS), pure red cell aplasia (PRCA), and myelophthisis. Hypoproliferative anemia is a cardinal feature of these disorders, but more frequent is *pancytopenia*: anemia, leukopenia, and thrombocytopenia. Low blood counts in marrow failure result from deficient hematopoiesis, as distinguished from blood count depression due to peripheral destruction of red cells (hemolytic anemias), platelets (idiopathic thrombocytopenic purpura [ITP] or due to splenomegaly), and granulocytes (as in the immune leukopenias). Marrow damage and dysfunction also may be secondary to infection, inflammation, or cancer.

Hematopoietic failure syndromes are classified by dominant morphologic features of the bone marrow (**Table 102-1**). Although practical distinction among these syndromes usually is clear from the marrow pathology, some processes are so closely related that the diagnosis may be complex. Separation between aplastic anemia and hypocellular MDS can be particularly difficult. Mutations on genomic screens may be etiologic or interpreted as risk factors. Patients may seem to suffer from two or three related diseases simultaneously, or one diagnosis may appear to evolve into another. Many of these syndromes share an immune-mediated mechanism of marrow destruction and some element of genomic instability resulting in a higher rate of malignant transformation.

It is important that the internist and general practitioner recognize the marrow failure syndromes because quality of life and ultimate prognosis may be poor if the patient is untreated; effective therapies are often available but sufficiently complicated in their choice and delivery so as to warrant the care of a hematologist or oncologist. While the identification of pathogenic mutations on genomic screen, often on testing ordered by the internist and pediatrician, has revolutionized the diagnosis of the marrow failure syndromes, these results often require the interpretation of the hematologist and oncologist.

APLASTIC ANEMIA

DEFINITION

Aplastic anemia is pancytopenia with bone marrow hypocellularity. Acquired aplastic anemia is distinguished from iatrogenic aplasia, from marrow hypocellularity after intensive cytotoxic chemotherapy for cancer, and from usually accidental physical and chemical injury, as in radiation poisoning. Aplastic anemia can also be constitutional. Genetic diseases such as Fanconi anemia and dyskeratosis congenita usually (but not always) present in early childhood and have typical physical anomalies. Telomere diseases (see **Chap. 469**) and hematologic manifestations of mutations in genes such as *GATA2, RUNX1*, and *MPL* can present as marrow failure in normal-appearing adults.

TABLE 102-1 Differential Diagnosis of Pancytopenia

Pancytopenia with Hypocellular Bone Marrow	
Acquired aplastic anemia	
Constitutional aplastic anemia (Fanconi anemia, dyskeratosis congenita, and others)	
Hypocellular myelodysplastic syndrome	
Rare aleukemic leukemia	
Some acute lymphoid leukemia	
Rare lymphomas of bone marrow	
Copper deficiency	
Pancytopenia with Cellular Bone Marrow	
Primary bone marrow diseases	Secondary to systemic diseases
Myelodysplastic syndromes	Systemic lupus erythematosus
Paroxysmal nocturnal hemoglobinuria (PNH)	Hypersplenism
Myelofibrosis	B_{12}, folate deficiency
Aleukemic leukemia	Copper deficiency
Myelophthisis	Alcohol
Bone marrow lymphoma	HIV infection
Hairy cell leukemia	Brucellosis
	Sarcoidosis
	Tuberculosis
	Leishmaniasis
	Sepsis
Hypocellular Bone Marrow ± Pancytopenia	
Q fever	
Legionnaires' disease	
Anorexia nervosa, starvation	
Mycobacterium	

Acquired aplastic anemia is often stereotypical in its manifestations, with the abrupt onset of low blood counts in a previously well young adult; seronegative hepatitis or a course of an incriminated medical drug may precede the onset. The diagnosis in these instances is uncomplicated. Sometimes blood count depression is moderate or incomplete, resulting in anemia, leukopenia, and thrombocytopenia in some combination. Aplastic anemia is related to both paroxysmal nocturnal hemoglobinuria (PNH; **Chap. 100**) and to MDS, and a clear distinction among these disorders may not be possible.

■ EPIDEMIOLOGY

The incidence of acquired aplastic anemia in Europe and Israel is two cases per million persons annually. In Thailand and China, rates of five to seven per million have been established. Men and women are affected with equal frequency, but the age distribution is biphasic, with the major peak in the teens and twenties and a second rise in older adults.

■ ETIOLOGY

The origins of aplastic anemia have been inferred from several recurring clinical associations (**Table 102-2**); unfortunately, these relationships are not reliable in an individual patient and may not be etiologic. In addition, although most cases of aplastic anemia are idiopathic, little other than history separates these cases from those with a presumed etiology such as a drug exposure.

Radiation Marrow aplasia is a major acute sequela of radiation. Radiation damages DNA; tissues dependent on active mitosis are particularly susceptible. Nuclear accidents involve not only power plant workers but also employees of hospitals, laboratories, and industry (food sterilization, metal radiography, etc.), as well as innocents exposed to stolen, misplaced, or misused sources. Whereas the radiation dose can be approximated from the rate and degree of decline in blood counts, dosimetry by reconstruction of the exposure can help to estimate the patient's prognosis and also to protect medical personnel

TABLE 102-2 Classification of Aplastic Anemia and Single Cytopenias

ACQUIRED	INHERITED/CONSTITUTIONAL
Aplastic Anemia	
Secondary	Fanconi anemia
Radiation	Dyskeratosis congenita/telomere disease
Drugs and chemicals	Shwachman-Diamond syndrome
Regular effects	Familial aplastic anemia/leukemia predisposition syndromes: *GATA2, RUNX1, CTLA4*, and others
Idiosyncratic reactions	
Viruses	
Epstein-Barr virus (infectious mononucleosis)	Nonhematologic syndromes (Down, Dubowitz, Seckel)
Hepatitis (non-A, non-B, non-C hepatitis)	
Parvovirus B19 (transient aplastic crisis, pure red cell aplasia [PRCA])	
HIV-1 (AIDS)	
Immune diseases	
Eosinophilic fasciitis	
Hypoimmunoglobulinemia	
Large granular lymphocytosis (LGL)	
Thymoma/thymic carcinoma	
Graft-versus-host disease in immunodeficiency	
Paroxysmal nocturnal hemoglobinuria (PNH)	
Pregnancy	
Idiopathic (immune)	
Cytopenias	
PRCA (see Table 102-4)	Congenital PRCA (Diamond-Blackfan anemia)
Neutropenia/agranulocytosis	
Idiopathic	Kostmann syndrome
Drugs, toxins	Shwachman-Diamond syndrome
LGL	Reticular dysgenesis
Pure white cell aplasia (+/− thymoma)	
Thrombocytopenia	
Drugs, toxins	Amegakaryocytic thrombocytopenia
Acquired amegakaryocytic thrombocytopenia	Thrombocytopenia with absent radii
	Other rare germline mutations

from contact with radioactive tissue and excreta. MDS and leukemia, but probably not aplastic anemia, are late effects of radiation.

Chemicals Benzene is a notorious cause of bone marrow failure: epidemiologic, clinical, and laboratory data link benzene to aplastic anemia, acute leukemia, and blood and marrow abnormalities. For leukemia, incidence is correlated with cumulative exposure, but susceptibility must also be important because only a minority of even heavily exposed workers develop myelotoxicity. The employment history is important, especially in industries where benzene is used for a secondary purpose, usually as a solvent. Benzene-related blood diseases have declined with regulation of industrial exposure. Although benzene is no longer generally available as a household solvent, exposure to its metabolites occurs in the normal diet and in the environment. The association between marrow failure and other chemicals is much less well substantiated. Further, there is scant direct evidence of marrow failure as a late effect of exposure, even to benzene.

Drugs (Table 102-3) Many chemotherapeutic drugs have marrow suppression as a major toxicity; effects are dose dependent and will

TABLE 102-3 Some Drugs and Chemicals Associated with Aplastic Anemia

Agents that regularly produce marrow depression as major toxicity in commonly used doses or normal exposures:
Cytotoxic drugs used in cancer chemotherapy: *alkylating agents, antimetabolites, antimitotics*, some antibiotics
Agents that frequently but not inevitably produce marrow aplasia:
Benzene
Agents associated with aplastic anemia but with a relatively low probability:
Chloramphenicol
Insecticides
Antiprotozoals: *quinacrine* and chloroquine, mepacrine
Nonsteroidal anti-inflammatory drugs (including *phenylbutazone*, indomethacin, ibuprofen, sulindac, aspirin)
Anticonvulsants (*hydantoins, carbamazepine*, phenacemide, felbamate)
Heavy metals (*gold*, arsenic, bismuth, mercury)
Sulfonamides: some antibiotics, antithyroid drugs (methimazole, methylthiouracil, propylthiouracil), antidiabetes drugs (tolbutamide, chlorpropamide), carbonic anhydrase inhibitors (acetazolamide and methazolamide)
Antihistamines (*cimetidine*, chlorpheniramine)
D-Penicillamine
Estrogens (in pregnancy and in high doses in animals)
Agents whose association with aplastic anemia is more tenuous:
Other antibiotics (streptomycin, tetracycline, methicillin, mebendazole, trimethoprim/sulfamethoxazole, flucytosine)
Sedatives and tranquilizers (chlorpromazine, prochlorperazine, piperacetazine, chlordiazepoxide, meprobamate, methyprylon)
Allopurinol
Methyldopa
Quinidine
Lithium
Guanidine
Potassium perchlorate
Thiocyanate
Carbimazole

Note: Terms set in italics show the most consistent association with aplastic anemia.

occur in all recipients. In contrast, idiosyncratic reactions to a large and diverse group of drugs may lead to aplastic anemia without a clear dose-response relationship. A large international study in Europe in the 1980s quantitated drug relationships, especially for nonsteroidal analgesics, sulfonamides, thyrostatic drugs, some psychotropics, penicillamine, allopurinol, and gold. Association does not equal causation: a drug may have been used to treat the first symptoms of bone marrow failure (antibiotics for fever or a preceding viral illness) or provoked the first symptom of a preexisting disease (petechiae by nonsteroidal anti-inflammatory agents administered to the thrombocytopenic patient). In the context of total drug use, idiosyncratic reactions, although individually devastating, are rare events. Risk estimates are usually lower when determined in population-based studies. Furthermore, the low absolute risk is also made more obvious: even a 10- or 20-fold increase in risk translates, in a rare disease, to just a handful of drug-induced aplastic anemia cases among hundreds of thousands of exposed persons.

Infections Transient, mild blood count depression is frequent in the course of many viral and bacterial infections. Aplastic anemia can rarely follow infectious mononucleosis. Parvovirus B19 does not usually cause generalized bone marrow failure.

Immunologic Diseases Aplasia is a major consequence and the inevitable cause of death in *transfusion-associated graft-versus-host disease* (GVHD) that can occur after infusion of nonirradiated blood products to an immunodeficient recipient. Aplastic anemia is strongly associated with the rare collagen vascular syndrome eosinophilic fasciitis that is characterized by painful induration of subcutaneous tissues (**Chap. 360**). Thymoma and hypoimmunoglobulinemia are occasional associations with aplastic anemia. Pancytopenia with marrow hypoplasia can also occur in systemic lupus erythematosus (SLE).

Hepatitis Posthepatitis marrow failure accounts for ~5% of etiologies in most series. Patients are usually young men who have recovered from a bout of liver inflammation 1–2 months earlier; the subsequent pancytopenia is very severe. The hepatitis is seronegative (non-A, non-B, non-C); intensive laboratory efforts including deep sequencing have not disclosed an infectious agent, and the hepatitis is presumed to be immune-mediated. Fulminant liver failure in childhood can follow seronegative hepatitis, and marrow failure occurs at a high rate in these patients.

Pregnancy Aplastic anemia very rarely may occur and recur during pregnancy and resolve with delivery or with spontaneous or induced abortion.

Paroxysmal Nocturnal Hemoglobinuria An acquired mutation in the *PIG-A* gene in a hematopoietic stem cell is required for the development of PNH, but *PIG-A* mutations probably occur commonly in normal individuals. If the PIG-A mutant stem cell proliferates, the result is a clone of progeny deficient in glycosylphosphatidylinositol-linked cell surface membrane proteins (**Chap. 100**). Small clones of deficient cells can be detected by sensitive flow cytometry tests in one-half or more of patients with aplastic anemia at the time of presentation. Functional studies of bone marrow from PNH patients, even those with mainly hemolytic manifestations, show evidence of defective hematopoiesis. Patients with an initial clinical diagnosis of PNH, especially younger individuals, may later develop frank marrow aplasia and pancytopenia; patients with an initial diagnosis of aplastic anemia may suffer later from hemolytic PNH years after recovery of blood counts.

Constitutional Syndromes Fanconi anemia, an autosomal recessive disorder, manifests as congenital developmental anomalies, progressive pancytopenia, and an increased risk of malignancy. Chromosomes in Fanconi anemia are susceptible to DNA cross-linking agents, the basis for a diagnostic assay. Patients with Fanconi anemia typically have short stature, café au lait spots, and anomalies involving the thumb, radius, and genitourinary tract. At least 17 different genetic defects (all but one with an identified gene) have been defined; the most common, type A Fanconi anemia, is due to a mutation in *FANCA*. Most of the Fanconi anemia gene products form a protein complex that activates FANCD2 by monoubiquitination to play a role in the cellular response to DNA damage and especially interstrand cross-linking.

Diamond-Blackfan anemia (see below) and Shwachman-Diamond syndrome are ribosomopathies, genetic defects in ribosome assembly that are tissue specific. In Shwachman-Diamond syndrome, presentation is early in life with neutropenia, pancreatic insufficiency, and malabsorption; most patients have compound heterozygous mutations in *SBDS*.

In the telomeropathies, inherited genetic defects alter telomere repair or one of the shelterin protein components of the telomere. The pediatric syndrome dyskeratosis congenita is characterized by the triad of mucous membrane leukoplasia, dystrophic nails, reticular hyperpigmentation, and early development of aplastic anemia (**Chap. 469**). Dyskeratosis congenita is due to mutations in genes of the telomere repair complex, which acts to maintain telomere length in replicating cells: the X-linked variety is due to mutations in the *DKC1* (*dyskerin*) gene; the more unusual autosomal dominant type is due to mutation in *TERC*, which encodes an RNA template. Rarely, mutations can also occur in genes such as *TNF2* that encode shelterin proteins, which bind telomere DNA.

Mutations in *TERC* and *TERT*, which encodes the catalytic reverse transcriptase telomerase, have subtle and milder effects on hematopoietic function, and presentation in adults is not unusual. It manifests as moderate aplastic anemia, which can be chronic and not progressive, and isolated macrocytic anemia or thrombocytopenia. Physical anomalies are usually not present, but early hair graying is a clue to the diagnosis. A detailed personal and family history may disclose pulmonary fibrosis and hepatic cirrhosis. Variable penetrance means that *TERT* and *TERC* mutations represent risk factors for marrow failure, as family members with the same mutations may have normal or only slight hematologic abnormalities but more subtle evidence of (compensated) hematopoietic insufficiency. Measurement of telomere length of peripheral blood leukocytes is a commercially available functional test.

■ PATHOPHYSIOLOGY

Bone marrow failure results from severe damage to the hematopoietic cell compartment. In aplastic anemia, replacement of the bone marrow by fat is apparent in the morphology of the biopsy specimen (**Fig. 102-1**) and magnetic resonance imaging (MRI) of the spine. Cells bearing the CD34 antigen, a marker of early hematopoietic cells, are greatly diminished, and in functional studies, committed and primitive progenitor cells are virtually absent; in vitro assays have suggested that the stem cell pool is reduced to ≤1% of normal in severe disease at the time of presentation.

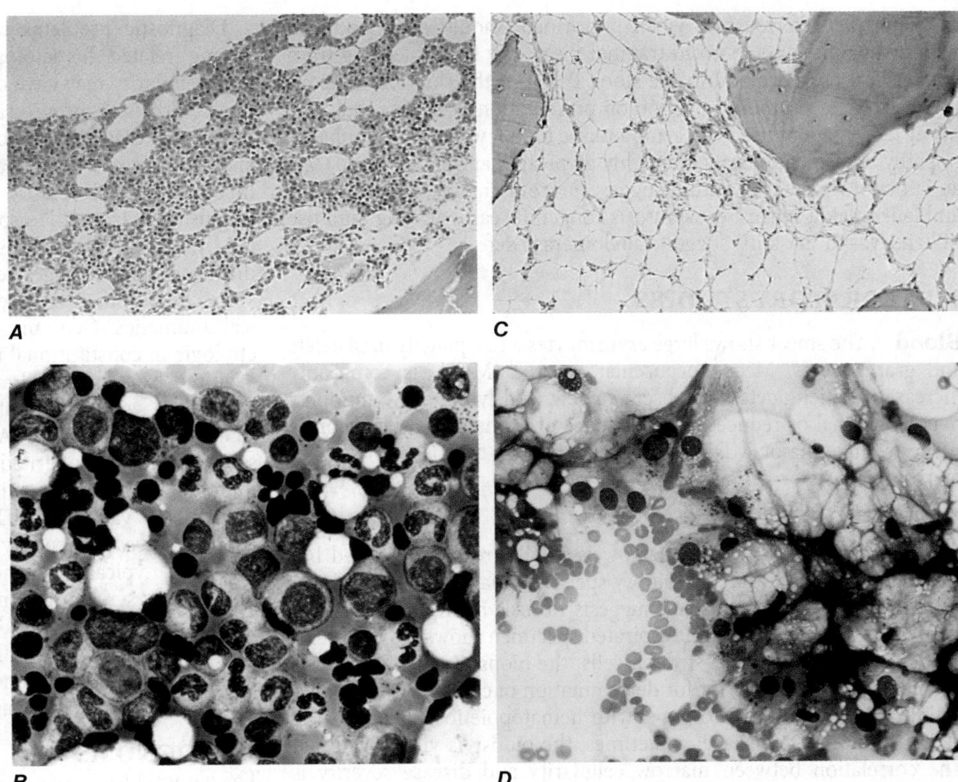

FIGURE 102-1 Normal and aplastic bone marrow. ***A.*** Normal bone marrow biopsy. ***B.*** Normal bone marrow aspirate smear. The marrow is normally 30–70% cellular, and there is a heterogeneous mix of myeloid, erythroid, and lymphoid cells. ***C.*** Aplastic anemia biopsy. ***D.*** Marrow smear in aplastic anemia. The marrow shows replacement of hematopoietic tissue by fat and only residual stromal and lymphoid cells.

Constitutional Genetic Syndromes

An intrinsic stem cell defect exists for the constitutional aplastic anemias: in a critical DNA repair pathway in Fanconi anemia, manifested in the laboratory as chromosome damage and cell death on exposure to certain chemical agents. In the telomeropathies, inability to repair telomeres or to protect chromosome ends is the result of mutations in genes of the telomerase complex or the shelterin proteins; telomere defects limit the cell's capacity to proliferate. Mutations in the *GATA* and *RUNX* genes affect signal transduction and transcriptional regulation in hematopoietic gene networks.

Chemical and Drug Injury Extrinsic damage to the marrow follows massive physical or chemical insults such as high doses of radiation and toxic chemicals. For the more common idiosyncratic reaction to modest doses of medical drugs, altered drug metabolism has been invoked as a mechanism. The metabolic pathways of many drugs and chemicals, especially if they are polar and have limited water solubility, involve enzymatic degradation to highly reactive electrophilic compounds; these intermediates are toxic because of their propensity to bind to cellular macromolecules. For example, derivative hydroquinones and quinolones are responsible for benzene-induced tissue injury. Excessive generation of toxic intermediates or failure to detoxify the intermediates may be genetically determined and apparent only on specific drug challenge; the complexity and specificity of the pathways imply multiple susceptibility loci and would provide an explanation for the rarity of idiosyncratic drug reactions.

Immune-Mediated Stem Cell Destruction The recovery of marrow function in some patients prepared for bone marrow transplantation with antilymphocyte globulin first suggested that aplastic anemia might be immune mediated. Laboratory data, including animal models, support an important role for the immune system in aplastic anemia. Blood and bone marrow cells of patients can suppress normal hematopoietic progenitor cell growth, and removal of T cells from aplastic anemia bone marrow improves hematopoiesis in vitro. Increased numbers of activated cytotoxic T-cell clones usually decline with successful immunosuppressive therapy; type 1 cytokines are implicated; and interferon γ (IFN-γ) induces Fas expression on CD34 cells, leading to apoptotic cell death. Hematopoietic stem cells that have lost human leukocyte antigen (HLA) expression may be selectively expanded. The rarity of aplastic anemia despite common exposures (medicines, seronegative hepatitis) suggests that genetically determined features of the immune response can convert a normal physiologic response into a sustained abnormal autoimmune process, including polymorphisms in histocompatibility antigens, cytokine genes, and genes that regulate T-cell polarization (maturation toward helper or cytotoxic phenotypes) and effector function.

■ CLINICAL FEATURES

History Aplastic anemia can appear abruptly or insidiously. Bleeding is the most common early symptom; a complaint of days to weeks of easy bruising, oozing from the gums, nose bleeds, heavy menstrual flow, and sometimes petechiae will have been noticed. With thrombocytopenia, massive hemorrhage is unusual, but small amounts of bleeding in the central nervous system can result in catastrophic intracranial or retinal hemorrhage. Symptoms of anemia are also frequent, including lassitude, weakness, shortness of breath, and a pounding sensation in the ears. Infection is an unusual first symptom in aplastic anemia (unlike in agranulocytosis, where pharyngitis, anorectal infection, or frank sepsis occurs early). Patients often feel and look remarkably well despite drastically reduced blood counts. Systemic complaints and weight loss should point to other etiologies of pancytopenia. Prior medical drug use, chemical exposure, and preceding viral illnesses must often be elicited with directed questioning. A family history of hematologic diseases or blood abnormalities, of pulmonary or liver fibrosis, or of early hair graying points to a telomeropathy; a family history of unusual infections and warts points to *GATA2* deficiency.

Physical Examination Petechiae and ecchymoses are typical, and retinal hemorrhages may be present. Pelvic and rectal examinations can often be deferred but, when performed, should be undertaken with great gentleness to avoid trauma; these may show bleeding from the cervical os and blood in the stool. Pallor of the skin and mucous membranes is common. Infection on presentation is unusual but may occur if the patient has been symptomatic for a few weeks. Lymphadenopathy and splenomegaly are highly atypical of aplastic anemia. Café au lait spots and short stature suggest Fanconi anemia; peculiar nails and leukoplakia suggest dyskeratosis congenita; early graying (and use of hair dyes to mask it!) suggests a telomerase defect.

■ LABORATORY STUDIES

Blood The smear shows large erythrocytes and a paucity of platelets and granulocytes. Mean corpuscular volume (MCV) is commonly increased. Reticulocytes are absent or few, and lymphocyte numbers may be normal or reduced. The presence of immature myeloid forms suggests leukemia or MDS; nucleated red blood cells (RBCs) suggest marrow fibrosis or tumor invasion; abnormal platelets suggest either peripheral destruction or MDS.

Bone Marrow The bone marrow is usually readily aspirated but dilute on smear, and the fatty biopsy specimen may be grossly pale on withdrawal; a "dry tap" instead suggests fibrosis or myelophthisis. In severe aplasia, the smear of the aspirated specimen shows only red cells, residual lymphocytes, and stromal cells; the biopsy (which should be >1 cm in length) is superior for determination of cellularity and shows mainly fat under the microscope, with hematopoietic cells occupying <25% of the marrow space; sometimes, the biopsy is virtually all fat. The correlation between marrow cellularity and disease severity is imperfect; patients with moderate disease by blood counts can have empty iliac crest biopsies, whereas "hot spots" of hematopoiesis may be seen in severe cases. Residual hematopoietic cells should have normal morphology, except for mildly megaloblastic erythropoiesis; megakaryocytes are greatly reduced and usually absent. Granulomas may indicate an infectious etiology of the marrow failure.

Ancillary Studies Chromosome breakage studies of peripheral blood using diepoxybutane or mitomycin C should be performed on children and younger adults to exclude Fanconi anemia. Very short telomere length strongly suggests the presence of a telomerase or shelterin mutation, which can be pursued by family studies and nucleotide sequencing. Chromosome studies of bone marrow cells are often revealing in MDS but should be negative in typical aplastic anemia. Flow cytometry offers a sensitive diagnostic test for PNH. Serologic studies may show evidence of recent viral infection, such as Epstein-Barr virus and HIV. Posthepatitis aplastic anemia is seronegative.

Genomics Next-generation sequencing allows for large number of genes to be tested for the presence of pathogenic mutations. Panels are available commercially and in certified academic laboratories. While expensive, they are very useful and sometimes critical in establishing the correct diagnosis. Germline gene panels examine 50 or more genes etiologic in constitutional bone marrow failure, including many for which functional assays (described above) are not available. A germline panel should be considered for all children and those adults with suggestive clinical features or family histories. Somatic mutations are sought when MDS is suspected. Myeloid neoplasm gene panels can query about 100 genes that are recurrently mutated in MDS and acute myeloid leukemia (AML). Pathogenic mutations in spliceosome genes and genes in the cohesion family are frequent in MDS and unexpected in aplastic anemia.

■ DIAGNOSIS

The diagnosis of aplastic anemia is usually straightforward, based on the combination of pancytopenia with a fatty bone marrow. Aplastic anemia is a disease of the young and should be a leading diagnosis in the pancytopenic adolescent or young adult. When pancytopenia is secondary, the primary diagnosis is usually obvious from either history or physical examination: the massive spleen of alcoholic cirrhosis, the history of metastatic cancer or SLE, or miliary tuberculosis on chest radiograph (Table 102-1).

Diagnostic problems can occur with atypical presentations and among related hematologic diseases. Patients with bone marrow hypocellularity may have depression of only one or two of three blood lines, with later progression to pancytopenia. The most important differential diagnoses are between acquired and constitutional aplastic anemia, and between aplastic anemia and MDS. The bone marrow in constitutional aplastic anemia is usually morphologically indistinguishable from the aspirate in acquired disease (an exception is *GATA2* deficiency with its characteristic megakaryocyte atypia). The diagnosis can be suggested by family history, abnormal blood counts since childhood, or the presence of associated, sometimes subtle physical anomalies. Genomic testing for pathogenic mutations in genes etiologic in constitutional marrow failure syndromes can discriminate acquired from inherited aplastic anemia (but results may not return for several weeks, a problem in the severely pancytopenic patient). Acute myeloid leukemia (AML) and MDS in a pedigree should prompt screening for an inherited predispositon syndrome, such as RUNX1 mutations. Aplastic anemia may be difficult to distinguish from the hypocellular variety of MDS: MDS is favored by finding morphologic abnormalities, particularly of megakaryocytes and myeloid precursor cells, and typical cytogenetic abnormalities and somatic mutations on genomic screening of myeloid neoplasm genes (see above). There remains an unclear boundary between immune aplastic anemia and low-risk MDS: patients with deletion of 13q and 20q may respond well to immunosuppression, and mutations in genes such as *DNMT3A* and *ASXL1* occur in both diseases.

■ PROGNOSIS

The natural history of severe aplastic anemia is rapid deterioration and death. Historically, provision first of RBCs and later of platelet transfusions and effective antibiotics were of some benefit, but few patients show spontaneous recovery. The major prognostic determinant is the blood count. Severe disease historically has been defined by the presence of two of three parameters: absolute neutrophil count <500/μL, platelet count <20,000/μL, and corrected reticulocyte count <1% (or absolute reticulocyte count <60,000/μL). In the era of effective immunosuppressive therapies, absolute numbers of reticulocytes (>25,000/μL) and lymphocytes (>1000/μL) may be better predictors of response to treatment and long-term outcome.

Other prognostic factors include the presence of a PNH clone, short telomeres on presentation, and somatically mutated white cells. Even small PNH clones may indicate an immune pathophysiology and responsiveness to immunosuppressive therapies. Telomere shortening in most patients likely reflects stem cell reserve, regenerative stress, and susceptibility to chromosomal instability. Collectively, the presence of mutations in the same myeloid neoplasia genes that are mutated in clonal hematopoiesis of indeterminate potential (*ASXL1*, *DNMT3A*) is associated with worse prognosis and clonal evolution.

TREATMENT

Aplastic Anemia

Severe acquired aplastic anemia can be cured by replacement of the absent hematopoietic cells (and the immune system) by stem cell transplant, or it can be ameliorated by suppression of the immune system to allow recovery of the patient's residual bone marrow function. Glucocorticoids are not of value as primary therapy. Suspect exposures to drugs or chemicals should be discontinued; however, spontaneous recovery of severe blood count depression is rare, and a waiting period before beginning treatment may not be advisable unless the blood counts are only modestly depressed.

HEMATOPOIETIC STEM CELL TRANSPLANTATION

This is the first choice for the younger patient with a fully histocompatible sibling donor (**Chap. 114**). HLA typing should be ordered as soon as the diagnosis of aplastic anemia is established in a child or younger adult. In transplant candidates, transfusion of blood from family members should be avoided so as to prevent sensitization to histocompatibility antigens. In general, limited numbers of blood products probably do not greatly affect outcome, especially when blood products are depleted of leukocytes. For allogeneic transplant from fully matched siblings, long-term survival rates for children are ~90%. Transplant morbidity and mortality are increased among adults, due to the higher risk of chronic GVHD and infections. Nevertheless, transplant should be considered early in all but the most elderly, including from alternative donors.

Most patients do not have a suitable sibling donor. Occasionally, a full phenotypic match can be found within the family and serve as well. Matched unrelated donors in large registries are available for the majority of Caucasian patients. With high-resolution matching at HLA, outcomes are similar to those with sibling donors, although complications (mainly GVHD and infection) are more frequent. Cord blood also can be a source of stem cells, especially for children. Matched unrelated donor transplants are often considered as initial treatment in children and as salvage therapy for adults after failed immunosuppression. Transplantation from an HLA haploidentical family donor is increasingly popular, as a donor is almost always quickly available. There is large experience in China, where lymphocyte depletion is usually performed before donor cell infusion. Posttransplant cyclophosphamide appears effective in preventing GVHD. Transplant protocols for marrow failure now usually do not include radiation in order to avoid late occurrence of cancer.

IMMUNOSUPPRESSION

The standard regimen of antithymocyte globulin (ATG) in combination with cyclosporine induces hematologic recovery (independence from transfusion and a leukocyte count adequate to prevent infection) in 60–70% of patients. Children do especially well, whereas older adult patients can suffer complications due to the presence of comorbidities. An early robust hematologic response correlates with long-term survival. Improvement in granulocyte number is generally apparent within 2 months of treatment. Most recovered patients continue to have some degree of blood count depression, the MCV remains elevated, and bone marrow cellularity returns toward normal very slowly if at all. Relapse (recurrent pancytopenia) is frequent, often occurring as cyclosporine is tapered or discontinued; most, but not all, patients respond to reinstitution of immunosuppression, but some responders become dependent on continued cyclosporine administration. "Clonal evolution," isolated chromosomal abnormalities or the development of MDS, with typical cytogenetic aberrations and abnormal marrow morphology, occurs in ~15% of treated patients over a decade following initiation of ATG, usually but not invariably associated with a return of pancytopenia, and some patients develop leukemia. A laboratory diagnosis of PNH can generally be made at the time of presentation of aplastic anemia by flow cytometry; recovered patients may have frank hemolysis if the PNH clone expands. Bone marrow examinations should be performed if there is an unfavorable change in blood counts.

Horse ATG is administered as intravenous infusions and requires hospitalization. Rabbit ATG is much less effective, perhaps because it reduces T-regulatory cell numbers in patients. Serum sickness, a flulike illness with a characteristic cutaneous eruption and arthralgia, may develop ~10 days after initiating treatment. Methylprednisolone is administered with ATG to ameliorate the immune consequences of heterologous protein infusion. (Excessive or extended glucocorticoid therapy is associated with avascular joint necrosis.) Cyclosporine is administered orally at an initial high dose, with subsequent adjustment according to blood levels. Its most important side effects are nephrotoxicity, hypertension, and seizures.

Most patients with aplastic anemia lack a suitable marrow donor, and immunosuppression is the treatment of choice. Overall survival is equivalent with transplantation and immunosuppression. However, successful transplant cures marrow failure, whereas patients who recover adequate blood counts after immunosuppression remain at risk of relapse and malignant evolution. Increasing age and the severity of neutropenia are the most important factors weighing in the decision between transplant and immunosuppression in adults who have a matched family donor: older patients do better with ATG and cyclosporine, whereas transplant is preferred if neutropenia is profound.

ELTROMBOPAG

Hematopoietic growth factors (HGFs) such as erythropoietin (EPO) and granulocyte colony-stimulating factor (G-CSF) are not effective in aplastic anemia, probably because endogenous blood levels in patients are extremely high. Circulating thrombopoietin is also elevated, but a thrombopoietin mimetic showed unexpected activity in refractory disease, producing robust, trilineage, and usually durable hematologic responses. Likely the mechanism of action of thrombopoietin mimetics is stimulation of the hematopoietic stem cell, but iron chelation and increased regulatory T cells are also possibly beneficial effects. Eltrombopag added to first-line immunosuppression with horse ATG markedly increased overall and complete response rates, to about 80% and 50%, respectively. Eltrombopag is approved by the U.S. Food and Drug Administration (FDA) as monotherapy for refractory aplastic anemia and in combination with horse ATG and cyclosporine as initial therapy.

Transplant from a suitable donor is preferred in the young patient, whereas immunosuppression is preferred in the older adult. Even heavily transfused and infected patients in whom immunosuppression has failed can be salvaged by stem cell transplant later.

ANDROGENS

The effectiveness of androgens has not been verified in controlled trials, but occasional patients will respond or even demonstrate blood count dependence on continued therapy. Sex hormones upregulate telomerase gene activity in vitro, which is possibly also their mechanism of action in improving marrow function. For patients with moderate disease, especially if a telomere gene defect is present, a 3- to 4-month trial may improve all blood counts **(Chap. 470)**.

SUPPORTIVE CARE

Meticulous medical attention is required so that the patient may survive to benefit from definitive therapy or, having failed treatment, to maintain a reasonable existence in the face of pancytopenia. First and most important, infection in the presence of severe neutropenia must be aggressively treated by prompt institution of parenteral, broad-spectrum antibiotics. Therapy is empirical and must not await results of culture, although specific foci of infection such as oropharyngeal or anorectal abscesses, pneumonia, sinusitis, and typhlitis (necrotizing colitis) should be sought on physical examination and with radiographic studies. When indwelling plastic catheters become contaminated, vancomycin should be added. Persistent or recrudescent fever implies fungal disease: *Candida* and *Aspergillus* are common, especially after several courses of antibacterial antibiotics. A major reason for the improved prognosis in aplastic anemia has been the development of better antifungal drugs and the timely institution of such therapy when infection is suspected. Granulocyte transfusions can be effective when bacterial or fungal infection is progressive or refractory to antibiotics. Hand washing, the single best method of preventing the spread of infection, remains a neglected practice. Nonabsorbed antibiotics for gut decontamination are poorly tolerated and unproven, nor does reverse isolation reduce mortality from infections.

Both platelet and erythrocyte numbers can be maintained by transfusion. Alloimmunization historically limited the usefulness of platelet transfusions and is now minimized by several strategies, including use of single donors to reduce exposure and physical or chemical methods to diminish leukocytes in the product; HLA-matched platelets are usually effective in patients refractory to random donor products. Inhibitors of fibrinolysis such as aminocaproic acid have not been shown to relieve mucosal oozing; the use of low-dose glucocorticoids to induce "vascular stability" is unproven and not recommended. With prophylactic platelet transfusions, the goal is to maintain the platelet count >10,000/μL (oozing from the gut increases sharply at counts <5000/μL). Menstruation should be suppressed either by oral estrogens or nasal follicle-stimulating hormone/luteinizing hormone antagonists. Aspirin and other nonsteroidal anti-inflammatory agents must be avoided in the presence of thrombocytopenia.

RBCs should be transfused so as to allow patient a normal level of activity, usually at a hemoglobin value of 70 g/L (90 g/L if there is underlying cardiac or pulmonary disease); a regimen of 2 units every 2 weeks will replace normal losses in a patient without a functioning bone marrow. In chronic anemia, the iron chelators deferoxamine and deferasirox should be added at approximately the fiftieth transfusion to avoid secondary hemochromatosis.

PURE RED CELL APLASIA

Other more restricted forms of marrow failure occur, in which only a single cell type is affected and the marrow shows corresponding absence or decreased numbers of specific precursor cells: aregenerative anemia as in PRCA (see below), thrombocytopenia with amegakaryocytosis **(Chap. 115)**, and neutropenia without marrow myeloid cells in agranulocytosis **(Chap. 64)**. In general, and in contrast to aplastic anemia and MDS, the unaffected lineages appear quantitatively and qualitatively normal. Agranulocytosis, the most frequent of these syndromes, is usually a complication of medical drug use, either by a mechanism of direct chemical toxicity or by immune destruction. Agranulocytosis has an incidence similar to aplastic anemia (but geographically more frequent in Europe than in Asia); in contrast to aplastic anemia, agranulocytosis is more prevalent among older adults and in women. Agranulocytosis should resolve with discontinuation of exposure, but significant mortality is attached to neutropenia in the older and often previously unwell patient. Both pure white cell aplasia (agranulocytosis without incriminating drug exposure) and amegakaryocytic thrombocytopenia are exceedingly rare and, like PRCA, appear to be due to a destructive immune response. In all of the single-lineage failure syndromes, progression to pancytopenia or leukemia is unusual.

■ DEFINITION AND DIFFERENTIAL DIAGNOSIS

PRCA is characterized by anemia, reticulocytopenia, and absent or rare erythroid precursor cells in the bone marrow. The classification of PRCA is shown in **Table 102-4**. In adults, PRCA is acquired. An identical syndrome can occur constitutionally: Diamond-Blackfan anemia, or congenital PRCA, is diagnosed at birth or in early childhood and often responds to glucocorticoid treatment; mutations in ribosome protein genes are etiologic. Temporary red cell failure occurs in transient aplastic crisis of hemolytic anemias due to acute parvovirus infection **(Chap. 197)** and in transient erythroblastopenia of childhood, which occurs in normal children.

■ CLINICAL ASSOCIATIONS AND ETIOLOGY

PRCA has important associations with immune system diseases. A minority of cases occur with a thymoma. More frequently, red cell aplasia can be the major manifestation of large granular lymphocytosis or complicates chronic lymphocytic leukemia. Some patients may be hypogammaglobulinemic. A ribosomal protein gene is deleted in the 5q- syndrome, such that the MDS may manifest as an acquired red cell aplasia. Occasionally (as compared to agranulocytosis), PRCA can be due to an idiosyncratic drug reaction. Subcutaneous administration of EPO has provoked PRCA mediated by neutralizing antibodies to the hormone. PRCA due to antibodies to blood group antigens (isoagglutins) is a complication of allogeneic stem cell transplant. For most PRCAs, T-cell inhibition is probably the prevalent immune mechanism.

■ PERSISTENT PARVOVIRUS B19 INFECTION

Chronic parvovirus infection is a treatable cause of red cell aplasia. This common virus causes a benign exanthem of childhood (fifth disease) and a polyarthralgia/arthritis syndrome in adults. In patients with underlying hemolysis (or any condition that increases demand for RBC production), parvovirus infection can cause a transient aplastic crisis and an abrupt but temporary worsening of the anemia due to failed erythropoiesis. In normal individuals, acute infection is resolved by production of neutralizing antibodies to the virus, but in the setting of congenital, acquired, or iatrogenic immunodeficiency, persistent viral infection may occur. The bone marrow shows red cell aplasia and the presence of giant pronormoblasts **(Fig. 102-2)**, which is the cytopathic sign of B19 parvovirus infection. Viral tropism for human erythroid progenitor cells is due to its use of erythrocyte P antigen as a cellular receptor for entry. Direct cytotoxicity of virus causes anemia if demands on erythrocyte production are high; in normal individuals, the temporary cessation of red cell production is not clinically apparent, and skin and joint symptoms are mediated by immune complex deposition.

TABLE 102-4 Classification of Pure Red Cell Aplasia

Self-limited
Transient erythroblastopenia of childhood
Transient aplastic crisis of hemolysis (acute B19 parvovirus infection)
Fetal red blood cell aplasia
Nonimmune hydrops fetalis (in utero B19 parvovirus infection)
Constitutional pure red cell aplasia
Congenital pure red cell aplasia (Diamond-Blackfan anemia)
Acquired pure red cell aplasia
MDS (5q- syndrome)
Cancer
Thymoma
Lymphoid malignancies (and more rarely other hematologic diseases)
Paraneoplastic to solid tumors
Connective tissue disorders with immunologic abnormalities
Systemic lupus erythematosus, juvenile rheumatoid arthritis, rheumatoid arthritis
Multiple endocrine gland insufficiency
Viruses
Persistent B19 parvovirus, hepatitis, adult T-cell leukemia virus, Epstein-Barr virus
Pregnancy
Drugs
Especially phenytoin, azathioprine, chloramphenicol, procainamide, isoniazid
Antibodies to erythropoietin
Idiopathic (immune)

TREATMENT

Pure Red Cell Aplasia

History, physical examination, and routine laboratory studies may disclose an underlying disease or a drug exposure. Thymoma should be sought by radiographic procedures; tumor excision is indicated, but anemia does not necessarily improve with surgery. The diagnosis of parvovirus infection requires detection of viral DNA sequences in the blood (IgG and IgM antibodies are commonly absent). The presence of erythroid colonies has been considered predictive of response to immunosuppressive therapy in idiopathic PRCA.

Red cell aplasia is compatible with long-term survival with supportive care alone: a combination of erythrocyte transfusions and iron chelation. For persistent B19 parvovirus infection, almost all patients respond to intravenous immunoglobulin therapy. The majority of patients with acquired PRCA respond favorably to immunosuppression: glucocorticoids, cyclosporine, ATG, azathioprine, and cyclophosphamide are effective.

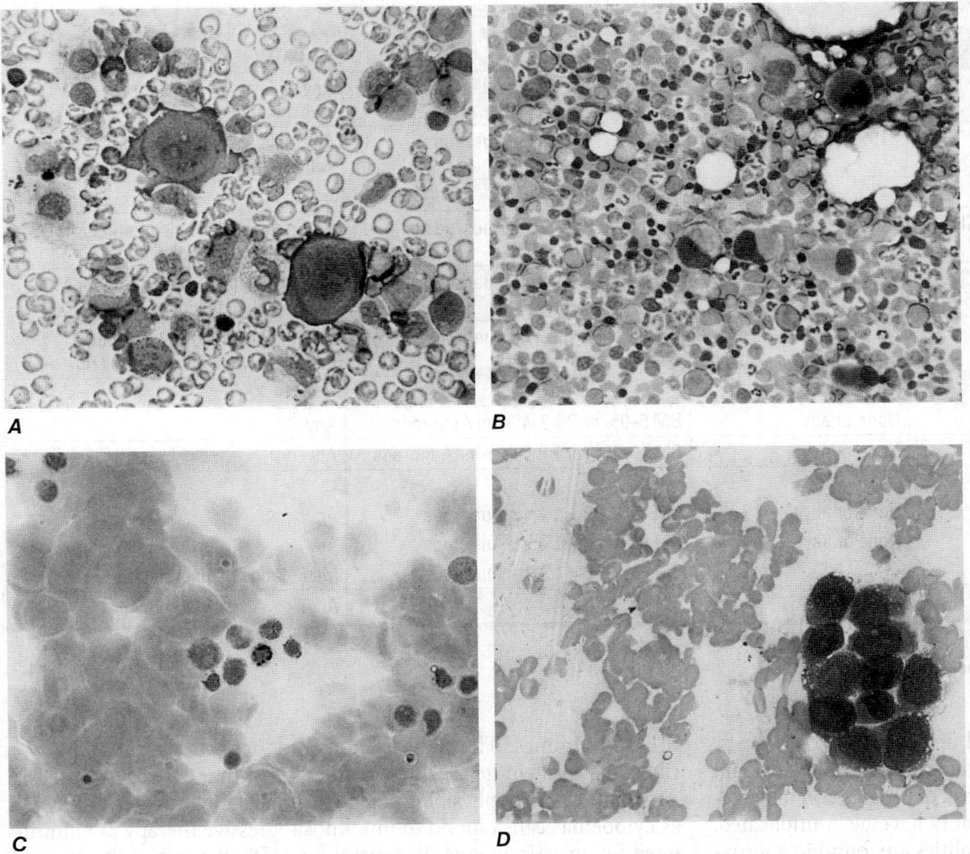

FIGURE 102-2 Pathognomonic cells in marrow failure syndromes. ***A.*** Giant pronormoblast, the cytopathic effect of B19 parvovirus infection of the erythroid progenitor cell. ***B.*** Uninuclear megakaryocyte and microblastic erythroid precursors typical of the 5q– myelodysplasia syndrome. ***C.*** Ringed sideroblast showing perinuclear iron granules. ***D.*** Tumor cells present on a touch preparation made from the marrow biopsy of a patient with metastatic carcinoma.

MYELODYSPLASTIC SYNDROMES

DEFINITION

The MDS are a heterogeneous group of hematologic disorders characterized by both (1) cytopenias due to bone marrow failure and (2) a high risk of development of AML. Anemia due to ineffective erythropoiesis, often with thrombocytopenia and neutropenia, occurs with dysmorphic (abnormal appearing) and usually cellular bone marrow, or with specific chromosome abnormalities or acquired mutations. In patients with "low-risk" MDS, marrow failure dominates the clinical course. In other patients, myeloblasts are present at diagnosis, chromosomes are abnormal, and the "high risk" is due to leukemic progression. MDS may be fatal due, most often, to complications of pancytopenia or to progression to leukemia, but a large proportion of patients will die of concurrent disease, the comorbidities typical in an elderly population. A useful nosology of these often-confusing entities was first developed by the French-American-British Cooperative Group in 1983. Five subtypes were defined then: refractory anemia (RA), refractory anemia with ringed sideroblasts (RARS), refractory anemia with excess blasts (RAEB), refractory anemia with excess blasts in transformation (RAEB-t), and chronic myelomonocytic leukemia (CMML). The World Health Organization (WHO) classification (2002) recognized that the distinction between RAEB-t and AML was arbitrary, grouped them together as acute leukemia, and clarified that CMML behaves as a myeloproliferative disease. The current WHO classification of 2016 is more refined but also more complicated (**Table 102-5**): blast percentage remains critical in defining MDS categories; erythroid predominant leukemias are now largely regarded as MDS; defining cytogenetic abnormalities are reaffirmed; and a single somatic mutation, in *SF3B1*, is now a feature of sideroblastic anemias. Identification of somatically mutated genes and their correlation with clinical outcomes will be increasingly important in defining classification, prognosis, and targeting therapy.

The diagnosis of MDS can be a challenge, even for the expert, because sometimes subtle clinical and pathologic features must be distinguished, and precise diagnostic categorization requires a hematopathologist knowledgeable in the latest classification scheme. Unfortunately, agreement among pathologists on morphologic features and classification is imperfect; changes in the appearance of megakaryocytes are more reliable than loss of granules in neutrophil precursors or dyserythropoiesis. Further, dysplastic changes can be observed in normal individuals, and they can occur with vitamin deficiencies and as drug effects. Genomic testing is increasingly routine and can be difficult to interpret, as in differences between somatic and germline mutations, pathogenic mutations versus those of unknown significance (clonal hematopoiesis increases in frequency with age and involves genetic changes that may be clinically silent or convey an increased risk of hematologic malignancy), and clone size and changes over time. It is important that the internist and primary care physician be sufficiently familiar with MDS to expedite referral to a hematologist because many new therapies are now available to improve hematopoietic function and the judicious use of supportive care can improve the patient's quality of life.

EPIDEMIOLOGY

MDS is a disease of the elderly; the mean age at onset is older than 70 years. There is a slight male predominance. MDS is a relatively common form of bone marrow failure, with reported incidence rates of 35 to >100 per million persons in the general population and 120 to >500 per million in older adults. Estimates of incidence in the United States range from 30,000 to 40,000 new cases annually and a prevalence of 60,000–120,000 in the population. Rates of MDS have increased over time due to better recognition of the syndrome by physicians and an aging population.

MDS is rare in children, in whom it often has a constitutional genetic basis that can be identified on genomic screens of myeloid cancer predisposition panels.

Secondary or therapy-related MDS, usually related to previous iatrogenic exposure to alkylating agents and other chemotherapy as well as radiation, is not age related.

ETIOLOGY AND PATHOPHYSIOLOGY

MDS is associated with environmental exposures such as radiation and benzene; other risk factors have been reported inconsistently. Secondary, therapy-related MDS occurs as a late toxicity of cancer treatment; radiation and the radiomimetic alkylating agents such as busulfan, nitrosourea, or procarbazine (with a latent period of 5–7 years); or the DNA topoisomerase inhibitors (2-year latency). Acquired aplastic anemia, Fanconi anemia, and other constitutional marrow failure diseases can evolve into MDS; occasionally, MDS in adults is recognized as due to germline *GATA2*, *RUNX1*, or telomere gene mutations. The typical MDS patient does not have a suggestive environmental exposure history or a preceding hematologic disease. MDS is a disease of aging, consistent with accumulation of mutations within a hematopoietic stem cell in an aging marrow environment.

TABLE 102-5 World Health Organization (WHO) Classification of Myelodysplastic Syndromes (MDS)/Neoplasms

NAME	RING SIDEROBLASTS	MYELOBLASTS	KARYOTYPE
MDS with single lineage dysplasia (MDS-SLD)	<15% (<5%)[a]	BM <5%, PB <1%, no Auer rods	Any, unless fulfills all criteria for MDS with isolated del(5q)
MDS with multilineage dysplasia (MDS-MLD)	<15% (<5%)[a]	BM <5%, PB <1%, no Auer rods	Any, unless fulfills all criteria for MDS with isolated del(5q)
MDS with ring sideroblasts (MDS-RS)			
MDS-RS with single lineage dysplasia (MDS-RS-SLD)	≥15% / ≥5%[a]	BM <5%, PB <1%, no Auer rods	Any, unless fulfills all criteria for MDS with isolated del(5q)
MDS-RS with multilineage dysplasia (MDS-RS-MLD)	≥15% / ≥5%[a]	BM <5%, PB <1%, no Auer rods	Any, unless fulfills all criteria for MDS with isolated del(5q)
MDS with isolated del(5q)	None or any	BM <5%, PB <1%, no Auer rods	del(5q) alone or with 1 additional abnormality except −7 or del(7q)
MDS with excess blasts (MDS-EB)			
MDS-EB-1	None or any	BM 5–9% or PB 2–4%, no Auer rods	Any
MDS-EB-2	None or any	BM 10–19% or PB 5–19% or Auer rods	Any
MDS, unclassifiable (MDS-U)			
• with 1% blood blasts	None or any	BM <5%, PB = 1%, no Auer rods	Any
• with single lineage dysplasia and pancytopenia	None or any	BM <5%, PB = 1%, no Auer rods	Any
• based on defining cytogenetic abnormality	<15%	BM <5%, PB = 1%, no Auer rods	MDS-defining abnormality
Refractory cytopenia of childhood	None	BM <5%, PB <2%	Any

[a]If *SF3B1* mutation is present.

Abbreviations: BM, bone marrow; PB, peripheral blood.

MDS is a clonal hematopoietic stem cell disorder characterized by disordered cell proliferation, impaired differentiation, and aberrant hematopoiesis, resulting in cytopenias and risk of progression to leukemia. Both chromosomal and genetic instability have been implicated; both are aging-related. Cytogenetic abnormalities are found in approximately one-half of patients, and some of the same specific lesions are also seen in leukemia; aneuploidy (chromosome loss or gain) is more frequent than translocations. Accelerated telomere attrition may destabilize the genome in marrow failure and predispose to acquisition of chromosomal lesions. Cytogenetic abnormalities are not random (loss of all or part of 5, 7, and 20, trisomy of 8) and may be related to etiology (11q23 following topoisomerase II inhibitors). The type and number of cytogenetic abnormalities strongly correlate with the probability of leukemic transformation and survival.

Genomics has illuminated the role of specific mutations and distinct molecular pathways in the pathophysiology of MDS. Somatic mutations in about 100 genes, which are recurrently present in myeloid neoplasms and are acquired in about 100 genes, are arise in the abnormal marrow cells (and are absent in the germline). Many of the same genes are mutated in AML and in MDS, whereas others are distinctive in subtypes of MDS. A prominent example is *SF3B1*, in which mutations strongly associate with sideroblastic anemia. Some mutations correlate with prognosis: spliceosome defects (like *SF3B1*) correlate with favorable outcome, and mutations in *EZH2*, *TP53*, *RUNX1*, and *ASXL1* with poor outcome. Correlation and exclusion in the pattern of mutations indicate a functional genomic architecture. Driver genes mutated early are consistent with normal blood counts and marrow morphology, but these expanded clones of cells containing them are susceptible to malignant transformation with the acquisition of additional mutations. Deep sequencing results in patients whose MDS evolved to AML have shown clonal succession, with founder clones acquiring additional mutations to produce clonal dominance. Mutations and cytogenetic abnormalities are not independent: *TP53* mutations associate with complex cytogenetic abnormalities and *TET2* mutations with normal cytogenetics. The prevalence of abnormal cells by morphology underestimates bone marrow involvement by MDS clones, as cells normal in appearance are derived from the abnormal clones. Presenting and evolving hematologic manifestations result from the accumulation of multiple genetic lesions: loss of tumor-suppressor genes, activating oncogene, epigenetic pathways that affect mRNA processing and methylation status, or other harmful alterations. Pathophysiology has been linked to mutations and chromosome abnormalities in some specific MDS syndromes. The 5q− deletion leads to heterozygous loss of a ribosomal protein gene which mimics constitutional red cell aplasia. An immune pathophysiology may be important in lower risk MDS, as cytopenias can respond to immunosuppressive therapy as administered for aplastic anemia. In general for MDS, the role of the immune system and its cells and cytokines; the role of the hematopoietic stem cell niche, the microenvironment, and cell–cell interactions; the fate of normal cells in the Darwinian competitive environment of the dysplastic marrow; and how mutant cells produce marrow failure in MDS are still not completely understood.

CLINICAL FEATURES

Anemia dominates the early course. Most symptomatic patients complain of the gradual onset of fatigue and weakness, dyspnea, and pallor, but at least one-half of patients are asymptomatic, and their MDS is discovered only incidentally on routine blood counts. Previous chemotherapy or radiation exposure is an important historic fact. Fever and weight loss are more often features of a myeloproliferative rather than myelodysplastic process. MDS in childhood is rare and, when diagnosed, implicates an underlying genetic disease. Children with Down syndrome are susceptible to MDS as well as leukemia. A family history may indicate a hereditary form of sideroblastic anemia, Fanconi anemia, or a telomeropathy. Inherited *GATA2* mutations, as in the MonoMAC syndrome (with increased susceptibility to viral, mycobacterial, and fungal infections, as well as deficient numbers of monocytes, natural killer cells, and B lymphocytes), predispose to MDS. Germline *RUNX1* mutations also confer a high risk of MDS and leukemia, often preceded by years of modest thrombocytopenia. A family history is important in all MDS patients, as constitutional mutations may not result in manifest disease until adulthood.

The physical examination in MDS is remarkable for signs of anemia; approximately 20% of patients have splenomegaly. Some unusual skin lesions, including Sweet's syndrome (febrile neutrophilic dermatosis), occur with MDS. Accompanying autoimmune syndromes are not infrequent. In the younger patient, stereotypical anomalies point to a constitutional syndrome (short stature, abnormal thumbs in Fanconi anemia; early graying in the telomeropathies; cutaneous warts in *GATA2* deficiency).

LABORATORY STUDIES

Blood Anemia is present in most cases, either alone or as part of bi- or pancytopenia; isolated neutropenia or thrombocytopenia is more unusual. Macrocytosis is common, as in most marrow failure disease. Platelets also are large and lack granules. In functional studies, they may show marked abnormalities, and patients may have bleeding symptoms despite seemingly adequate numbers. Neutrophils are hypogranulated; have hyposegmented, ringed, or abnormally segmented nuclei; contain Döhle bodies; and may be functionally deficient. Circulating myeloblasts usually correlate with marrow blast numbers, and their quantity is important for classification and prognosis. The total white blood cell count (WBC) is usually normal or low, except in CMML. As in aplastic anemia, MDS can be associated with a clonal population of PNH cells. Genetic testing is commercially available for constitutional syndromes.

Bone Marrow The bone marrow is usually normal or hypercellular, but in about 20% of cases, it is sufficiently hypocellular to lead to confusion with aplastic anemia. No single characteristic feature of marrow morphology distinguishes MDS, but the following are commonly observed: dyserythropoietic changes (especially nuclear abnormalities) and ringed sideroblasts in the erythroid lineage; hypogranulation and hyposegmentation in granulocytic precursors, with an increase in myeloblasts; and megakaryocytes showing reduced numbers of or disorganized nuclei. Megaloblastic nuclei and defective hemoglobinization in the erythroid lineage are common. Prognosis strongly correlates with the proportion of marrow blasts, which should be enumerated manually on the marrow smear and by flow cytometry of an aspirate. Flow cytometry can also reveal characteristically aberrant hematopoietic differentiation. Cytogenetics and fluorescent in situ hybridization can identify chromosomal abnormalities.

DIFFERENTIAL DIAGNOSIS

Deficiencies of vitamin B_{12} or folate should be excluded by appropriate blood tests; vitamin B_6 deficiency can be assessed by a therapeutic trial of pyridoxine if the bone marrow shows ringed sideroblasts. Copper deficiency can lead to cytopenias and dysplastic marrows of varying cellularity. Marrow dysplasia can be observed in acute viral infections, drug reactions, or chemical toxicity but should be transient. More difficult are the distinctions between hypocellular MDS and aplasia or between RA with excess blasts and acute leukemia: the WHO considers 20% blasts in the marrow as the criterion that separates AML from MDS. In young patients, underlying, predisposing genetic diseases should be considered and appropriate genomic testing performed (see above).

PROGNOSIS

The median survival varies greatly from years for patients with 5q− or sideroblastic anemia to a few months in RA with excess blasts or severe pancytopenia associated with monosomy 7. The International Prognostic Scoring System (IPSS), revised in 2012 **(Table 102-6)**, assists in making predictions. Even "lower-risk" MDS has significant morbidity and mortality. More refined (and also more complicated) prognostic scoring systems can separate those with intermediate-1 risk who have relatively poor prognoses. Prognostic systems have been developed based on survival from diagnosis, but prognosis changes over time, and hazard ratios for survival and leukemic transformation converge over time among risk categories, consistent with dynamic changes in clonal architecture.

Most patients die as a result of complications of pancytopenia and not due to leukemic transformation; perhaps one-third succumb to diseases unrelated to their MDS. Precipitous worsening of pancytopenia, acquisition of new chromosomal abnormalities on serial cytogenetic determination, increase in the number of blasts, and marrow fibrosis are all poor prognostic indicators. The outlook in therapy-related MDS, regardless of type, is extremely poor, and most patients progress within a few months to refractory AML.

TABLE 102-6 Revised International Prognostic Scoring System (IPSS-R)

1. New marrow blast categories
   ≤2%, >2%–<5%, 5–10%, >10–30%
2. Refined cytogenetic abnormalities and risk groups
   16 (vs 6) specific abnormalities, 5 (vs 3) subgroups[a]
3. Evaluation of depth of cytopenias[b]
   Clinically and statistically relevant cut points used
4. Inclusion of differentiating features
   Age, performance status, serum ferritin, LDH; β_2-microglobulin
5. Prognostic model with 5 (vs 4) risk categories
   Improved predictive power

[a]Good, normal, −Y, del(5q), del (20q); poor, complex (≥3 abnormalities) or chromosome 7 abnormalities; intermediate, all other abnormalities. [b]Cytopenias at baseline, cut points: hemoglobin <80, 80–<100, or ≥100 g/L; platelet count <50, 50–100, or ≥100,000/μL, and absolute neutrophil count <800 versus ≥800/μL.

Abbreviation: LDH, lactate dehydrogenase.

TREATMENT

Myelodysplasia

Historically, therapy of MDS has been unsatisfactory, but several drugs may not only improve blood counts but also delay onset of leukemia and improve survival. The choice of therapy for an individual patient, administration of treatment, and management of toxicities are complicated and require hematologic expertise.

Only hematopoietic stem cell transplantation offers cure of MDS. The survival rate in selected patient cohorts is ~50% at 3 years but improving. Results using unrelated matched donors are similar to those with siblings, and patients in their fifties and older have been successfully transplanted. Nevertheless, treatment-related mortality and morbidity increase with recipient age. The transplant conundrum is that the high-risk patient (by IPSS score and presence of monosomal karyotype), for whom the procedure is most obviously indicated, has a high probability of a poor outcome from transplant-related mortality or disease relapse, whereas the low-risk patient, who is more likely to tolerate transplant, also may do well for years with less aggressive therapies. In practice, only a small proportion of MDS patients undergo transplantation.

MDS has been regarded as particularly refractory to cytotoxic chemotherapy regimens, and as in AML in the older adult, drug toxicity is frequent and often fatal, and remissions, if achieved, are brief. Low doses of cytotoxic drugs have been administered for their "differentiation" potential, and from this experience, drug therapies have emerged based on pyrimidine analogues. These drugs are classified as epigenetic modulators, believed to act through a demethylating mechanism to alter gene regulation and allow differentiation to mature blood cells from the abnormal MDS stem cell. The hypomethylating agents azacitidine and decitabine are frequently used in bone marrow failure clinics. Azacitidine improves blood counts and survival in MDS, compared to best supportive care. Azacitidine is usually administered subcutaneously, daily for 7 days, at 4-week intervals, for at least four cycles before assessing for response. Overall, generally improved blood counts with a decrease in transfusion requirements occurred in ~50% of patients in published trials. Response is dependent on continued drug administration, and most patients eventually become refractory to drug intervention and experience recurrent cytopenias or progression to AML. Decitabine is closely related to azacitidine; 30–50% of patients show responses in blood counts, with a duration of response of almost a year. Decitabine is usually administered by continuous intravenous infusion in regimens of varying doses and durations of 3–10 days in repeating cycles. The major toxicity of azacitidine and decitabine is myelosuppression, leading to worsening blood counts. Hypomethylating agents are frequently used in the high-risk patient who is not a candidate for stem cell transplant. In the lower risk patient, they are also effective, but alternative therapies should be considered.

Lenalidomide, a thalidomide derivative with a more favorable toxicity profile, is particularly effective in reversing anemia in MDS patients with 5q− syndrome; not only do a high proportion of these patients become transfusion independent with normal or near-normal hemoglobin levels, but their cytogenetics also become normal. The drug has many biologic activities, and it is unclear which is critical for clinical efficacy. Lenalidomide is administered orally. Most patients will improve within 3 months of initiating therapy. Toxicities include myelosuppression (worsening thrombocytopenia and neutropenia, necessitating blood count monitoring) and an increased risk of deep vein thrombosis and pulmonary embolism.

Immunosuppression also may produce sustained independence from transfusion and improve survival. ATG, cyclosporine, and the anti-CD52 monoclonal antibody alemtuzumab are especially effective in younger MDS patients (<60 years old) with more favorable IPSS. In a consortium retrospective review, about 50% of patients with mainly refractory anemia responded to ATG, usually combined with cyclosporine, particularly patients with hypocellular marrow.

HGFs can improve blood counts but, as in most other marrow failure states, have been most beneficial to patients with the least severe pancytopenia. EPO alone or in combination with G-CSF can improve hemoglobin levels, particularly in those with low serum EPO levels who have no or a modest need for transfusions. Survival may be enhanced by EPO and amelioration of anemia. G-CSF treatment alone failed to improve survival in a controlled trial. Thrombopoietin mimetics appear to improve platelet counts in some MDS patients, with no clear evidence that they increase the rate of leukemic transformation.

New drugs for MDS are entering the clinic or are in late development. Luspatercept, which affects transforming growth factor β–mediated suppression of erythropoiesis, has been approved by the FDA for anemia in MDS. Novel targeted therapies in trials include inhibitors of hypoxia-inducible factor and spliceosome genes, drugs that act to restore TP53 activity, and venetoclax, an inhibitor of the bcl2 protein that increases programmed cell death (and is approved for use or employed off-label in other hematologic malignancies).

The same principles of supportive care described for aplastic anemia apply to MDS. Many patients will be anemic for years. RBC transfusion support should be accompanied by iron chelation to prevent secondary hemochromatosis.

MYELOPHTHISIC ANEMIAS

Fibrosis of the bone marrow (see **Fig. 100-2**), usually accompanied by a characteristic blood smear picture called *leukoerythroblastosis*, can occur as a primary hematologic disease, called *myelofibrosis* or *myeloid metaplasia* (**Chap. 103**), and as a secondary process, called *myelophthisis*. Myelophthisis, or secondary myelofibrosis, is reactive. Fibrosis can be a response to invading tumor cells, usually an epithelial cancer of breast, lung, or prostate origin or neuroblastoma. Marrow fibrosis may occur with infection of mycobacteria (both *Mycobacterium tuberculosis* and *Mycobacterium avium*), fungi, or HIV and in sarcoidosis. Intracellular lipid deposition in Gaucher disease and obliteration of the marrow space related to absence of osteoclast remodeling in congenital osteopetrosis also can produce fibrosis. Secondary myelofibrosis is a late consequence of radiation therapy or treatment with radiomimetic drugs. Usually the infectious or malignant underlying processes are obvious. Marrow fibrosis can also be a feature of a variety of hematologic syndromes, especially chronic myeloid leukemia, multiple myeloma, lymphomas, myeloma, and hairy cell leukemia.

The pathophysiology has three distinct features: proliferation of fibroblasts in the marrow space (myelofibrosis); the extension of hematopoiesis into the long bones and into extramedullary sites, usually the spleen, liver, and lymph nodes (myeloid metaplasia); and ineffective erythropoiesis. The etiology of the fibrosis is unknown but most likely involves dysregulated production of growth factors: platelet-derived growth factor and transforming growth factor β have been implicated. Abnormal regulation of other hematopoietins would lead to localization of blood-producing cells in nonhematopoietic tissues and uncoupling of the usually balanced processes of stem cell proliferation and differentiation. Myelofibrosis is remarkable for pancytopenia despite very large numbers of circulating hematopoietic progenitor cells.

Anemia is dominant in secondary myelofibrosis, usually normocytic and normochromic. The diagnosis is suggested by the characteristic leukoerythroblastic smear (see **Fig. 100-1**). Erythrocyte morphology is highly abnormal, with circulating nucleated RBCs, teardrops, and shape distortions. WBC numbers are often elevated, sometimes mimicking a leukemoid reaction, with circulating myelocytes, promyelocytes, and myeloblasts. Platelets may be abundant and are often of giant size. Inability to aspirate the bone marrow, the characteristic "dry tap," can allow a presumptive diagnosis in the appropriate setting before the biopsy is decalcified.

The course of secondary myelofibrosis is determined by its etiology, usually a metastatic tumor or an advanced hematologic malignancy. Treatable causes must be excluded, especially tuberculosis and fungus. Transfusion support can relieve symptoms.

FURTHER READING

Arber DA et al: The 2016 revision to the World Health Organization (WHO) classification of myeloid neoplasms and acute leukemia. Blood 127:2391, 2016.

Attalah E et al: Comparison of patient age groups in transplantation for myelodysplastic syndrome: The Medicare coverage with evidence development study. JAMA Oncol 6:486, 2020.

DeZern AE et al: Haplotidentical BMT for severe aplastic anemia with intensive GVHD prophylaxis including posttransplant cyclophosfamide. Blood Adv 4: 1770, 2020.

Greenberg PL et al: Revised international prognostic scoring system for myelodysplastic syndromes. Blood 120:2454, 2012.

Mustjoki S, Young NS: Somatic mutations in "benign" disease. N Engl J Med 384:2039, 2021.

Ogawa S: Genetics of MDS. Blood 133:1049, 2019.

Platzbecker U: Treatment of MDS. Blood 133:1096, 2019.

Sallman DA, List AF: The central role of inflammatory signaling in the pathogenesis of myelodysplastic syndromes. Blood 133:1039, 2019.

Townsley DM et al: Eltrombopag added to standard immunosuppression for aplastic anemia. N Engl J Med 376:1540, 2017.

Yoshizato T et al: Somatic mutations and clonal hematopoiesis in aplastic anemia. N Engl J Med 373:35, 2015.

Young NS: Aplastic anemia. N Engl J Med 379:1643, 2018.

103 Polycythemia Vera and Other Myeloproliferative Neoplasms

Jerry L. Spivak

The World Health Organization (WHO) classification of the chronic myeloproliferative neoplasms (MPNs) includes eight disorders, some of which are rare or poorly characterized (**Table 103-1**) but all of which share an origin in a hematopoietic cell; overproduction of one or more of the formed elements of the blood without significant dysplasia; and a predilection to extramedullary hematopoiesis, myelofibrosis, and transformation at varying rates to acute leukemia. Within this broad classification, however, significant phenotypic heterogeneity exists. Some diseases such as chronic myelogenous leukemia (CML), chronic neutrophilic leukemia (CNL), and chronic eosinophilic leukemia (CEL) express primarily a myeloid phenotype, whereas in other diseases, such as polycythemia vera (PV), primary myelofibrosis (PMF), and essential thrombocytosis (ET), erythroid or megakaryocytic

TABLE 103-1 World Health Organization Classification of Chronic Myeloproliferative Neoplasms

Chronic myeloid leukemia, *BCR-ABL*–positive
Chronic neutrophilic leukemia
Chronic eosinophilic leukemia, not otherwise specified
Polycythemia vera
Primary myelofibrosis
Essential thrombocytosis
Mastocytosis
Myeloproliferative neoplasms, unclassifiable

hyperplasia predominates. The latter three disorders, in contrast to the former three, also appear capable of transforming into each other.

Such phenotypic heterogeneity has a genetic basis; CML is the consequence of the balanced translocation between chromosomes 9 and 22 (t[9;22][q34;11]); CNL has been associated with a t(15;19) translocation; and CEL occurs with a deletion or balanced translocations involving the *PDGFRα* gene. By contrast, PV, PMF, and ET are characterized by driver mutations that directly or indirectly constitutively activate JAK2, a tyrosine kinase essential for the function of the erythropoietin and thrombopoietin receptors and also utilized by the granulocyte colony-stimulating factor receptor. This important distinction is reflected in the natural histories of CML, CNL, and CEL, which are usually measured in years, with a high rate of leukemic transformation. The natural histories of PV, PMF, and ET, by contrast, are usually measured in decades, and transformation to acute leukemia is uncommon in the absence of chemotherapy. This chapter focuses only on PV, PMF, and ET because their clinical features and driver mutation overlap are substantial, although their disease duration varies.

The other chronic MPNs will be discussed in **Chaps. 105** and **110**.

POLYCYTHEMIA VERA

PV is a clonal hematopoietic stem cell disorder in which phenotypically normal red cells, granulocytes, and platelets accumulate in the absence of a recognizable physiologic stimulus. The most common of the MPNs, PV occurs in 2.5 per 100,000 persons, sparing no adult age group and increasing with age to rates >10/100,000. Familial transmission is infrequent, and women under age 50 predominate among sporadic cases.

ETIOLOGY

Nonrandom chromosome abnormalities such as deletion 20q and deletion 13q or trisomy 9 occur in up to 30% of untreated PV patients, but unlike CML, no consistent cytogenetic abnormality has been associated with the disorder. However, a mutation in the autoinhibitory pseudokinase domain of the tyrosine kinase JAK2 that replaces valine with phenylalanine (V617F), causing constitutive kinase activation, has a central role in PV pathogenesis.

JAK2 is a member of an evolutionarily well-conserved, nonreceptor tyrosine kinase family and serves as the cognate tyrosine kinase for the erythropoietin and thrombopoietin receptors. It also functions as an obligate chaperone for these receptors in the Golgi apparatus and is responsible for their cell-surface expression. The conformational change induced in the erythropoietin and thrombopoietin receptors following binding to their respective cognate ligands, erythropoietin or thrombopoietin, leads to JAK2 autophosphorylation, receptor phosphorylation, and phosphorylation of proteins involved in cell proliferation, differentiation, and resistance to apoptosis. Transgenic animals lacking *JAK2* die as embryos from severe anemia. Constitutive activation of JAK2, on the other hand, explains the erythropoietin hypersensitivity, erythropoietin-independent erythroid colony formation, rapid terminal differentiation, increased Bcl-X_L expression, and apoptosis resistance in the absence of erythropoietin that characterize the in vitro behavior of PV erythroid progenitor cells.

More than 95% of PV patients express this mutation, as do ~50% of PMF and ET patients. Importantly, the *JAK2* gene is located on the short arm of chromosome 9, and loss of heterozygosity on chromosome 9p involving the segment containing the *JAK2* locus over time due to mitotic recombination (uniparental disomy) is the most common cytogenetic abnormality in PV. Loss of heterozygosity in this region leads to homozygosity for *JAK2* V617F and occurs in ~60% of PV patients and to a lesser extent in PMF but is rare in ET. Most PV patients who do not express *JAK2* V617F express a mutation in exon 12 of the gene and are not clinically different from those who do, with the exception of a higher frequency of isolated erythrocytosis, nor do *JAK2* V617F heterozygotes differ clinically from homozygotes. Importantly, the predisposition to acquire *JAK2* mutations appears to be associated with a specific *JAK2* gene haplotype, GGCC. *JAK2* V617F is the basis for many of the phenotypic and biochemical characteristics of PV such as increased blood cell production and increased inflammatory cytokine production; however, it cannot solely account for the entire PV phenotype and is probably not the initiating lesion in any of the MPNs. First, PV patients with the same phenotype and documented clonal disease can have mutations in *LNK*, a JAK2 inhibitor, or rarely, calreticulin (*CALR*), an ER chaperone. Second, ET and PMF patients have the same mutation but different clinical phenotypes. Third, familial PV can occur without the mutation, even when other members of the same family express it. Fourth, inhibition of *JAK2* V617F–expressing hematopoietic progenitor cells by the nonspecific JAK1/2 kinase inhibitor, ruxolitinib, does not affect the behavior of the involved hematopoietic stem cells. Finally, in some *JAK2* V617F–positive PV or ET patients, acute leukemia can occur in a *JAK2* V617F–negative progenitor cell, suggesting the presence of an ancestral precursor cell.

CLINICAL FEATURES

Although PV is a panmyelopathy, isolated thrombocytosis, leukocytosis, or splenomegaly may be its initial presenting manifestation, but most often, the disorder is first recognized by the incidental discovery of a high hemoglobin, hematocrit, or red cell count. With the exception of aquagenic pruritus, or erythromelalgia, no symptoms distinguish PV from other causes of erythrocytosis.

Uncontrolled erythrocytosis causes hyperviscosity, leading to neurologic symptoms such as vertigo, tinnitus, headache, visual disturbances, and transient ischemic attacks (TIAs). Systolic hypertension is also a feature of the red cell mass elevation. In some patients, venous or arterial thrombosis may be the presenting manifestation of PV. Any vessel can be affected, but cerebral, cardiac, and mesenteric vessels are most commonly involved. Hepatic venous thrombosis (Budd-Chiari syndrome) is particularly common in young women and may be catastrophic if sudden and complete obstruction of the hepatic vein occurs. Indeed, PV should be suspected in any patient who develops hepatic vein thrombosis, since this is the only type of thrombosis associated with *JAK2* V617F expression. Digital ischemia, easy bruising, epistaxis, acid-peptic disease, or gastrointestinal hemorrhage may occur due to vascular stasis or thrombocytosis. In the latter instance, absorption and proteolysis of high-molecular-weight von Willebrand multimers by the large platelet mass cause acquired von Willebrand's disease. Erythema, burning, and pain in the extremities, a symptom complex known as erythromelalgia, is another complication of thrombocytosis in PV due to increased platelet stickiness. Given the large turnover of hematopoietic cells, hyperuricemia with secondary gout, uric acid stones, and symptoms due to hypermetabolism can also complicate the disorder.

DIAGNOSIS

When PV presents with erythrocytosis in combination with leukocytosis, thrombocytosis, or splenomegaly or any combination of these, the diagnosis is apparent. However, when patients present with an elevated hemoglobin, hematocrit, or red cell count alone, the diagnostic evaluation is more complex because of the many diagnostic possibilities (**Table 103-2**). Furthermore, unless the hemoglobin level is ≥20 g/dL (hematocrit ≥60%), it is not possible to distinguish true erythrocytosis from disorders causing plasma volume contraction. This is because uniquely in PV, in contrast to other causes of true erythrocytosis, there is expansion of the plasma volume, which can mask the elevated red cell mass, particularly in women; thus, red cell mass and plasma

TABLE 103-2 Causes of Erythrocytosis

Relative Erythrocytosis	
Hemoconcentration secondary to dehydration, diuretics, ethanol abuse, androgens, or tobacco abuse	
Absolute Erythrocytosis	
Hypoxia	**Tumors**
Carbon monoxide intoxication	Hypernephroma
High-oxygen-affinity hemoglobins	Hepatoma
High altitude	Cerebellar hemangioblastoma
Pulmonary disease	Uterine myoma
Right-to-left cardiac or vascular shunts	Adrenal tumors
Sleep apnea syndrome	Meningioma
Hepatopulmonary syndrome	Pheochromocytoma
Renal Disease	**Drugs**
Renal artery stenosis	Androgens
Focal sclerosing or membranous glomerulonephritis	Recombinant erythropoietin
Postrenal transplantation	**Familial (with normal hemoglobin function)**
Renal cysts	Erythropoietin receptor mutations
Bartter's syndrome	*VHL* mutations (Chuvash polycythemia)
	2,3-*BPG* mutation
	PHD2 and *HIF2α* mutations
	Polycythemia vera

Abbreviations: 2,3-BPG, 2,3-bisphosphoglycerate; VHL, von Hippel-Lindau.

volume determinations are necessary to establish the presence of an absolute erythrocytosis and distinguish this from relative erythrocytosis due to a reduction in plasma volume alone (also known as *stress* or *spurious erythrocytosis* or *Gaisböck's syndrome*). **Figure 63-18** illustrates a diagnostic algorithm for the evaluation of suspected erythrocytosis. Assay for *JAK2* mutations in the presence of a normal arterial oxygen saturation provides an alternative diagnostic approach to erythrocytosis when red cell mass and plasma volume determinations are not available; a normal serum erythropoietin level does not exclude the presence of PV, but an elevated erythropoietin level is more consistent with a secondary cause for the erythrocytosis.

Other laboratory studies that may aid in diagnosis include the red cell count, mean corpuscular volume, and red cell distribution width (RDW), particularly when the hematocrit or hemoglobin levels are less than 60% or 20 g/dL, respectively. Only three situations cause microcytic erythrocytosis: β-thalassemia trait, hypoxic erythrocytosis, and PV. With β-thalassemia trait, the RDW is usually normal, whereas with hypoxic erythrocytosis and PV, the RDW may be elevated due to associated iron deficiency. Today, however, the assay for *JAK2* V617F has superseded other tests for establishing the diagnosis of PV. Of course, in patients with associated acid-peptic disease, occult gastrointestinal bleeding may lead to a presentation with hypochromic, microcytic anemia, masking the presence of PV.

A bone marrow aspirate and biopsy provide no specific diagnostic information because these may be normal or indistinguishable from ET or PMF. Similarly, no specific cytogenetic abnormality is associated with the disease, and the absence of a cytogenetic marker does not exclude the diagnosis.

COMPLICATIONS

Many of the clinical complications of PV relate directly to the increase in blood viscosity associated with red cell mass elevation and indirectly to the increased turnover of red cells, leukocytes, and platelets with the attendant increase in uric acid and inflammatory cytokine production. The latter appears to be responsible for constitutional symptoms. Peptic ulcer disease can also be due to *Helicobacter pylori* infection, the incidence of which is increased in PV, while the pruritus associated with this disorder may be a consequence of mast cell activation by *JAK2* V617F. A sudden increase in spleen size can be associated with painful splenic infarction. Myelofibrosis appears to be part of the natural history of the disease but is a reactive, reversible process that does not itself impede hematopoiesis and by itself has no prognostic significance. In ~15% of patients, however, myelofibrosis is associated with hematopoietic stem cell failure, manifested by substantial extramedullary hematopoiesis in the liver and spleen and transfusion-dependent anemia. The organomegaly can cause significant mechanical discomfort, portal hypertension, and progressive cachexia. Although the incidence of acute myeloid leukemia is increased in PV, the incidence of acute leukemia in patients not exposed to chemotherapy or radiation therapy is low. Interestingly, chemotherapy, including hydroxyurea, has been associated with acute leukemia in *JAK2* V617F–negative stem cells in some PV patients. *Erythromelalgia* is a curious syndrome of unknown etiology associated with thrombocytosis, primarily involving the lower extremities and usually manifested by erythema, warmth, and pain of the affected appendage and occasionally digital infarction. It occurs with a variable frequency and is usually responsive to salicylates. Some of the central nervous system symptoms observed in patients with PV, such as ocular migraine, appear to represent a variant of erythromelalgia.

Left uncontrolled, erythrocytosis can lead to thrombosis involving vital organs such as the liver, heart, brain, or lungs. Patients with massive splenomegaly are particularly prone to thrombotic events because the associated increase in plasma volume masks the true extent of the red cell mass elevation measured by the hematocrit or hemoglobin level. A "normal" hematocrit or hemoglobin level in a PV patient with massive splenomegaly should be considered indicative of an elevated red cell mass until proven otherwise.

TREATMENT

Polycythemia Vera

PV is generally an indolent disorder, the clinical course of which is measured in decades, and its management should reflect its tempo. Thrombosis due to erythrocytosis is the most significant complication and often the presenting manifestation; maintenance of the hemoglobin level at ≤140 g/L (14 g/dL; hematocrit <45%) in men and ≤120 g/L (12 g/dL; hematocrit <42%) in women is mandatory to avoid thrombotic complications. Phlebotomy serves initially to reduce hyperviscosity by reducing the red cell mass to normal while further expanding the plasma volume. Periodic phlebotomies thereafter serve to maintain the red cell mass within the normal range and induce a state of iron deficiency that prevents accelerated reexpansion of the red cell mass. In most PV patients, once an iron-deficient state is achieved, phlebotomy is usually only required at 3-month intervals. Neither phlebotomy nor iron deficiency increases the platelet count relative to the effect of the disease itself, and neither thrombocytosis nor leukocytosis is correlated with thrombosis in PV, in contrast to the strong correlation between erythrocytosis and thrombosis. The use of salicylates to prevent thrombosis in PV patients is not only potentially harmful if the red cell mass is not controlled by phlebotomy but also an unproven remedy, particularly in patients over age 70.

Anticoagulation is indicated when a thrombosis has occurred, and the newer oral anticoagulants may be preferable to a vitamin K antagonist since they do not require monitoring. Asymptomatic hyperuricemia (<10 mg/dL) requires no therapy, but allopurinol should be administered to avoid further elevation of the uric acid when chemotherapy is used to reduce splenomegaly or leukocytosis or to treat pruritus. Generalized pruritus intractable to antihistamines or antidepressants such as doxepin can be a major problem in PV; the JAK1/2 inhibitor ruxolitinib, pegylated interferon α (IFN-α), psoralens with ultraviolet light in the A range (PUVA) therapy, and hydroxyurea are other methods of palliation. Asymptomatic thrombocytosis requires no therapy unless the platelet count is sufficiently high to cause bleeding due to acquired von Willebrand's disease, but bleeding in this situation is not usually spontaneous and is responsive to tranexamic acid or ε-aminocaproic acid. Symptomatic splenomegaly can be treated with either ruxolitinib or pegylated IFN-α. Pegylated IFN-α has the advantage over recombinant IFN-α of being better tolerated and requiring only weekly administration and produced complete hematologic and molecular remissions in ~20% of PV patients; its role in this disorder is currently under investigation. Anagrelide, a phosphodiesterase inhibitor, can reduce the platelet count and, if tolerated, is preferable to hydroxyurea because it lacks marrow toxicity and is also protective against venous thrombosis while hydroxyurea is not.

A reduction in platelet number may be necessary for the treatment of erythromelalgia or ocular migraine if salicylates are not effective or if the platelet count is sufficiently high to increase the risk of hemorrhage but only to the degree that symptoms are alleviated. Alkylating agents and radioactive sodium phosphate (^{32}P) are leukemogenic in PV, and their use should be avoided. If a cytotoxic agent must be used, hydroxyurea is preferred, but this drug does not prevent either thrombosis or myelofibrosis in PV, is itself leukemogenic, and should be used for as short a time as possible. Previously, PV patients with massive splenomegaly unresponsive to reduction by chemotherapy or interferon required splenectomy. However, with the introduction of the nonspecific JAK2 inhibitor ruxolitinib, it has been possible in the majority of patients with PV complicated by myelofibrosis and myeloid metaplasia to reduce spleen size while at the same time alleviating constitutional symptoms and pruritus due to cytokine release and reducing the phlebotomy requirement. However, in contrast to PMF, these patients have a more chronic course. In contrast to other malignancies, PV patients have a low rate of mutation accumulation, and the acquisition of deleterious mutations such as *TP*53 mutations as detected by next-generation sequencing is usually associated with leukemic transformation. Since hydroxyurea antagonizes *TP53* and also causes del17p, leading to *TP53* haploinsufficiency, its use should be constrained in PV.

Ruxolitinib has also been demonstrated in a phase 3 clinical trial to be effective in PV patients without myelofibrosis who are intolerant or refractory to hydroxyurea or best available supportive therapy. In some patients with end-stage disease, pulmonary hypertension may develop due to fibrosis or extramedullary hematopoiesis. A role for bone marrow transplantation, either allogeneic or haploidentical, in PV has not been defined.

Most patients with PV can live long lives without functional impairment when their red cell mass is effectively managed with phlebotomy alone. Chemotherapy is never indicated to control the red cell mass in PV, but when venous access is an issue, ruxolitinib or pegylated interferon is the preferred therapy.

PRIMARY MYELOFIBROSIS

Chronic PMF (other designations include *idiopathic myelofibrosis*, *agnogenic myeloid metaplasia*, or *myelofibrosis with myeloid metaplasia*) is a clonal hematopoietic stem cell disorder associated with mutations in *JAK2, MPL*, or *CALR* and characterized by marrow fibrosis, extramedullary hematopoiesis, and splenomegaly. PMF is the least common MPN, and establishing its diagnosis in the absence of a specific clonal marker is difficult because myelofibrosis and splenomegaly are also features of both PV and CML. Furthermore, myelofibrosis and splenomegaly also occur in a variety of benign and malignant disorders (**Table 103-3**), many of which are amenable to specific therapies not effective in PMF. In contrast to the other MPNs and so-called acute or malignant myelofibrosis, which can occur at any age, PMF primarily afflicts men in their sixth decade or later.

ETIOLOGY

Nonrandom chromosome abnormalities such as 9p, 20q−, 13q−, trisomy 8 or 9, or partial trisomy 1q are common in PMF, but no cytogenetic abnormality specific to the disease has been identified. *JAK2* V617F is present in ~55% of PMF patients, and mutations in the thrombopoietin receptor, *MPL*, occur in ~4%. Most of the rest have mutations in the calreticulin gene (*CALR*) that alter the carboxy-terminal portion of the protein, permitting it to bind and activate MPL.

TABLE 103-3 Disorders Causing Myelofibrosis

MALIGNANT	NONMALIGNANT
Acute leukemia (lymphocytic, myelogenous, megakaryocytic)	HIV infection
Chronic myeloid leukemia	Hyperparathyroidism
Hairy cell leukemia	Renal osteodystrophy
Hodgkin's disease	Systemic lupus erythematosus
Primary myelofibrosis	Tuberculosis
Lymphoma	Vitamin D deficiency
Multiple myeloma	Thorium dioxide exposure
Myelodysplasia	Gray platelet syndrome
Metastatic carcinoma	
Polycythemia vera	
Systemic mastocytosis	

The degree of myelofibrosis and the extent of extramedullary hematopoiesis are not related. Fibrosis in this disorder is associated with overproduction of transforming growth factor β and tissue inhibitors of metalloproteinases, while osteosclerosis is associated with overproduction of osteoprotegerin, an osteoclast inhibitor. Marrow angiogenesis occurs due to increased production of vascular endothelial growth factor. Importantly, fibroblasts in PMF are polyclonal and not part of the neoplastic clone but can be induced by it to produce inflammatory cytokines.

CLINICAL FEATURES

No signs or symptoms are specific for PMF. Many patients are asymptomatic at presentation, and the disease is often detected by the discovery of splenic enlargement and/or abnormal blood counts during a routine examination. In contrast to its companion MPN, night sweats, fatigue, and weight loss are common presenting complaints. A blood smear will show the characteristic features of extramedullary hematopoiesis: teardrop-shaped red cells, nucleated red cells, myelocytes, and promyelocytes; myeloblasts may also be present (**Fig. 103-1**). Anemia, usually mild initially, is common, whereas the leukocyte and platelet counts are either normal or increased, but either can be depressed. Mild hepatomegaly may accompany the splenomegaly but is unusual in its absence; isolated lymphadenopathy should suggest another diagnosis. Both serum lactate dehydrogenase and alkaline phosphatase levels can be elevated. Marrow is usually inaspirable due to the myelofibrosis (**Fig. 103-2**), and bone x-rays may reveal osteosclerosis. Exuberant extramedullary hematopoiesis can cause ascites; portal, pulmonary, or

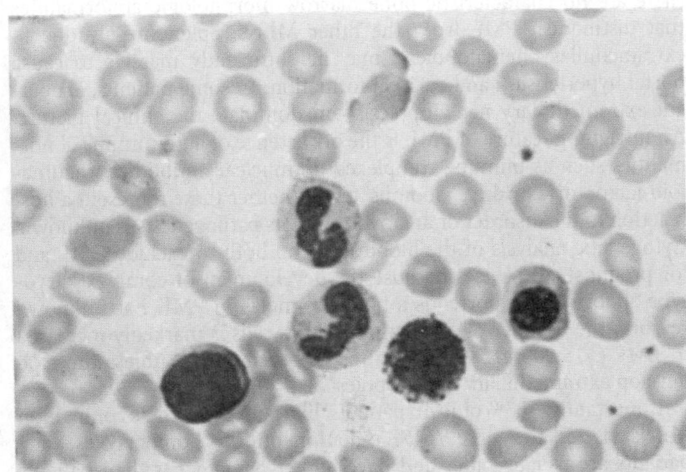

FIGURE 103-1 Teardrop-shaped red blood cells indicative of membrane damage from passage through the spleen, a nucleated red blood cell, and immature myeloid cells indicative of extramedullary hematopoiesis are noted. This peripheral blood smear is related to any cause of extramedullary hematopoiesis.

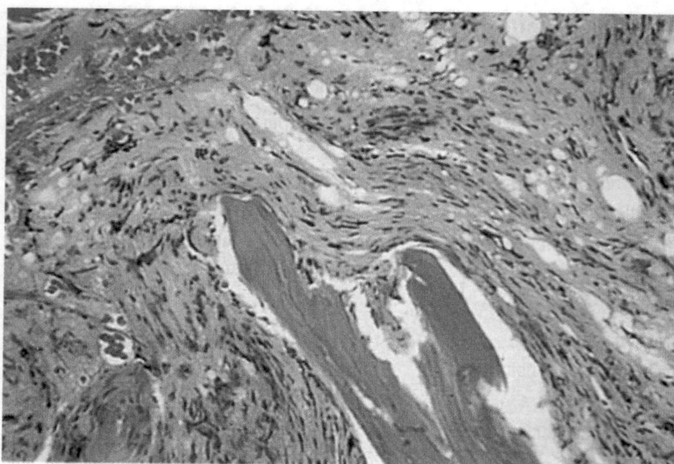

FIGURE 103-2 This marrow section shows the marrow cavity replaced by fibrous tissue composed of reticulin fibers and collagen. When this fibrosis is due to a primary hematologic process, it is called *myelofibrosis*. When the fibrosis is secondary to a tumor or a granulomatous process, it is called *myelophthisis*.

intracranial hypertension; intestinal or ureteral obstruction; pericardial tamponade; spinal cord compression; or skin nodules. Splenic enlargement can be sufficiently rapid to cause splenic infarction with fever and pleuritic chest pain. Hyperuricemia and secondary gout may ensue.

DIAGNOSIS

While the clinical picture described above is characteristic of PMF, all of these clinical features can be observed in PV or CML. Massive splenomegaly commonly masks erythrocytosis in PV, and reports of intraabdominal thrombosis in PMF most likely represent instances of unrecognized PV. In some PMF patients, erythrocytosis has developed during the course of the disease. Furthermore, because many other disorders have features that overlap with PMF but respond to distinctly different therapies, the diagnosis of PMF is one of exclusion, which requires that the disorders listed in Table 103-3 be ruled out.

The presence of teardrop-shaped red cells, nucleated red cells, myelocytes, and promyelocytes establishes the presence of extramedullary hematopoiesis, while the presence of leukocytosis, thrombocytosis with large and bizarre platelets, and circulating myelocytes suggests the presence of an MPN as opposed to a secondary form of myelofibrosis (Table 103-3). Marrow is usually inaspirable due to increased marrow reticulin, but marrow biopsy will reveal a hypercellular marrow with trilineage hyperplasia and, in particular, increased numbers of megakaryocytes in clusters and with large, dysplastic nuclei. However, there are no characteristic bone marrow morphologic abnormalities that distinguish PMF from the other MPNs. Splenomegaly due to extramedullary hematopoiesis may be sufficiently massive to cause portal hypertension and variceal formation. In some patients, exuberant extramedullary hematopoiesis can dominate the clinical picture. An intriguing feature of PMF is the occurrence of autoimmune abnormalities such as immune complexes, antinuclear antibodies, rheumatoid factor, or a positive Coombs' test. Whether these represent a host reaction to the disorder or are involved in its pathogenesis is unknown. Cytogenetic analysis of the blood is useful both to exclude CML and for prognostic purposes because the development of complex karyotype abnormalities portends a poor prognosis in PMF. For unknown reasons, the number of circulating CD34+ cells is markedly increased in PMF (>15,000/μL) compared to the other MPNs, unless they too develop extramedullary hematopoiesis.

Importantly, ~55% of PMF patients, like patients with its companion MPNs, express the *JAK2* V617F mutation, often as homozygotes. Such patients are usually older and have higher hematocrits than patients with *MPL* (4%) or *CALR* (36%) mutations; PMF patients expressing an *MPL* mutation tend to be more anemic and have lower leukocyte counts than *JAK2* V617F–positive patients. Somatic mutations (due to deletions [type 1] or insertions [type 2]) in exon 9 of *CALR* have been found in a majority of patients with PMF who lack mutations in either *JAK2* or *MPL*. In some studies, type 1 mutations, the most common *CALR* mutation in PMF, had a survival advantage compared to *JAK2* or *MPL* mutations but not with respect to leukemic transformation. PMF patients who lack a known MPN driver mutation appear to have the worst prognosis.

TABLE 103-4 Three Current Scoring Systems for Estimating Prognosis in PMF Patients

RISK FACTOR	IPSS (2009)[a]	DIPSS (2010)[b]	DIPSS PLUS (2011)[c]
Anemia (<10 g/dL)	X	X	X
Leukocytosis (>25,000/μL)	X	X	X
Peripheral blood blasts (≥1%)	X	X	X
Constitutional symptoms	X	X	X
Age (>65 years)	X	X	X
Unfavorable karyotype			X
Platelet count (<100,000/μL)			X
Transfusion dependence			X

[a]Blood 113:2895, 2009. [b]Blood 115:1703, 2010. [c]J Clin Oncol 29:392, 2011.

Note: The Dynamic International Prognostic Scoring System (DIPSS) was developed to determine if the International Prognostic Scoring System (IPSS) risk factors identified as important for survival at the time of primary myelofibrosis (PMF) diagnosis could also be used for risk stratification following their acquisition during the course of the disease. One point is assigned to each risk factor for IPSS scoring. For DIPSS, the same is true, but anemia is assigned 2 points. The DIPSS Plus scoring system represents recognition that the addition of unfavorable karyotype, thrombocytopenia, and transfusion dependence improved the DIPSS risk stratification system for which additional points are assigned (Table 103-5). More recent studies suggest that mutational analysis of the *ASXL1, EZH2, SRSF2,* and *IDH1/2* genes further improves risk stratification for survival and leukemic transformation (Leukemia 27:1861, 2013), as can cytogenetic abnormalities (Leukemia 32:1631, 2018). These prognostic scoring systems are not accurate for risk assessment in polycythemia vera or essential thrombocytosis patients who have developed myelofibrosis (Haematologica 99:e55, 2014).

COMPLICATIONS

Survival in PMF varies according to specific risk factors at diagnosis (**Tables 103-4** and **103-5**) but is shorter than in PV and ET patients. The natural history of PMF is one of increasing marrow failure with transfusion-dependent anemia and increasing organomegaly due to extramedullary hematopoiesis. As with CML, PMF can evolve from a chronic to an accelerated phase with constitutional symptoms and increasing marrow failure. About 10% of patients spontaneously transform to an aggressive form of acute leukemia for which therapy is usually ineffective. Additional important prognostic factors for disease acceleration during the course of PMF include the presence of complex cytogenetic abnormalities, thrombocytopenia, and transfusion-dependent anemia. Mutations in the *ASXL1, EZH2, SRSF2,* and *IDH1/2* genes have been identified as risk factors for early death or transformation to acute leukemia, as have complex cytogenetic abnormalities, and have proved to be more useful for PMF risk assessment than clinical scoring systems.

TABLE 103-5 IPSS and DIPSS Risk Stratification Systems

RISK CATEGORIES[a]	NUMBER OF RISK FACTORS		
	IPSS	DIPSS	DIPSS PLUS
Low	0	0	0
Intermediate-1	1	1–2	1
Intermediate-2	2	3–4	2–3
High	≥3	>4	4–6

[a]The corresponding survival curves for each risk category can be found in the references cited in the footnotes of Table 103-4.

Abbreviations: DIPSS, Dynamic International Prognostic Scoring System; IPSS, International Prognostic Scoring System.

TREATMENT
Primary Myelofibrosis

No specific therapy exists for PMF. The causes for anemia are multifarious and include ineffective erythropoiesis uncompensated by splenic extramedullary hematopoiesis, hemodilution due to splenomegaly, splenic sequestration, blood loss secondary to thrombocytopenia or portal hypertension, folic acid deficiency, systemic inflammation, and autoimmune hemolysis. Neither recombinant erythropoietin nor androgens such as danazol have proven to be consistently effective as therapy for anemia. Erythropoietin may worsen splenomegaly and will be ineffective if the serum erythropoietin level is >125 mU/L. Given the inflammatory milieu that characterizes PMF, glucocorticoids can ameliorate anemia as well as constitutional symptoms such as fever, chills, night sweats, anorexia, and weight loss, and combining these with low-dose thalidomide has proved effective as well. Thrombocytopenia can be due to impaired marrow function, splenic sequestration, or autoimmune destruction and may also respond to low-dose thalidomide and prednisone.

Splenomegaly is by far the most distressing and intractable problem for PMF patients, causing abdominal pain, portal hypertension, easy satiety, and cachexia, whereas surgical removal of a massive spleen is associated with significant postoperative complications including mesenteric venous thrombosis, hemorrhage, rebound leukocytosis and thrombocytosis, and hepatic extramedullary hematopoiesis with no amelioration of either anemia or thrombocytopenia when present. For unexplained reasons, splenectomy also increases the risk of blastic transformation.

Splenic irradiation is, at best, temporarily palliative and associated with a significant risk of neutropenia, infection, and subsequent operative hemorrhage if splenectomy is attempted. Allopurinol can control significant hyperuricemia, and bone pain can be alleviated by local irradiation. Pegylated IFN-α can ameliorate fibrosis in early PMF, but in advanced disease, it may exacerbate the bone marrow failure. The JAK2 inhibitor ruxolitinib has proved effective in reducing splenomegaly and alleviating constitutional symptoms in a majority of advanced PMF patients while possibly prolonging survival, although it usually does not significantly influence the *JAK2* V617F neutrophil allele burden. Although anemia and thrombocytopenia are its major side effects, these are dose-dependent, and with time, anemia stabilizes and thrombocytopenia may improve. Fedratinib, a new tyrosine kinase inhibitor with anti-FLT3 activity, has proved useful in patients with disease refractory to ruxolitinib.

In some patients, hypomethylating agents such as azacytidine or decitabine in combination with high-dose ruxolitinib have been used to control the disease or prepare patients for bone marrow transplantation. Transformation to acute leukemia in PMF, like PV or ET, is usually refractory to treatment.

Allogeneic bone marrow transplantation is the only curative treatment for PMF and should be considered in younger patients and older patients with high-risk disease; nonmyeloablative conditioning regimens permit hematopoietic cell transplantation to be extended to older individuals.

ESSENTIAL THROMBOCYTOSIS

ET (other designations include *essential thrombocythemia*, *idiopathic thrombocytosis*, *primary thrombocytosis*, and *hemorrhagic thrombocythemia*) is a clonal hematopoietic stem cell disorder associated with mutations in *JAK2* (V617F), *MPL*, or *CALR* and manifested clinically by overproduction of platelets without a definable cause. ET has an incidence of 1–2/100,000 and a distinct female predominance. Canonical MPN driver mutations distinguish 90% of ET patients from the more common nonclonal, reactive forms of thrombocytosis **(Table 103-6)**; mutation-negative ET patients may have either uncommon *MPL* mutations, *JAK2* V617F expression limited to the platelets, or a hereditary form of thrombocytosis. Once considered a disease of the elderly and responsible for significant morbidity due to hemorrhage or thrombosis, it is now clear that ET can occur at any age in adults and often without symptoms or disturbances of hemostasis. There is an unexplained female predominance in contrast to PMF or the reactive forms of thrombocytosis where no sex difference exists. Because no specific clonal marker is available, clinical and laboratory criteria have been proposed to distinguish ET from other MPNs, which may also present with initially with isolated thrombocytosis but have differing prognoses and therapies (Table 103-6). These criteria are useful in identifying disorders such as CML, PV, PMF, or myelodysplasia, which can masquerade as ET. Furthermore, as with "idiopathic" erythrocytosis, nonclonal benign forms of thrombocytosis exist (e.g., hereditary overproduction of thrombopoietin and those with noncanonical *JAK2* driver mutations) that are not widely recognized because we currently lack diagnostic assays. Approximately 50% of ET patients express *JAK2* V617F, 30% *CALR* (both type 1 and type 2), and 8% *MPL* mutations. ET patients lacking a canonical MPN driver mutation usually have a benign prognosis.

TABLE 103-6 Causes of Thrombocytosis

Tissue inflammation: collagen vascular disease, inflammatory bowel disease	Hemorrhage
Malignancy	Iron-deficiency anemia
Infection	Surgery
Myeloproliferative disorders: polycythemia vera, primary myelofibrosis, essential thrombocytosis, chronic myelogenous leukemia	Rebound: Correction of vitamin B_{12} or folate deficiency, post-ethanol abuse
Myelodysplastic disorders: 5q– syndrome, idiopathic refractory sideroblastic anemia	Hemolysis
Postsplenectomy or hyposplenism	Familial: Thrombopoietin overproduction, *JAK2* or *MPL* mutations

ETIOLOGY

Megakaryocytopoiesis and platelet production depend on thrombopoietin and its receptor MPL. As in the case of early erythroid and myeloid progenitor cells, early megakaryocytic progenitors require the presence of interleukin 3 (IL-3) and stem cell factor for optimal proliferation in addition to thrombopoietin. Their subsequent terminal development is also enhanced by the chemokine stromal cell-derived factor 1 (SDF-1). Interestingly, terminal megakaryocyte maturation and platelet production do not require thrombopoietin.

Megakaryocytes are unique among hematopoietic progenitor cells because reduplication of their genome is endomitotic rather than mitotic and promoted by thrombopoietin. Unlike erythropoietin, thrombopoietin is produced primarily in the liver but has important functions in the bone marrow where it functions to maintain hematopoietic stem cells quiescent in their endosteal niches; once released from their niches, thrombopoietin promotes the proliferation of these cells in the sinusoidal niche. Like plasma erythropoietin and its target erythroblasts, an inverse correlation exists between the platelet count and plasma thrombopoietin. However, unlike erythropoietin, thrombopoietin is only constitutively produced and the plasma thrombopoietin level is controlled by the size of the platelet and megakaryocyte progenitor cell pools. Also, in contrast to erythropoietin, but like its myeloid counterparts, granulocyte and granulocyte-macrophage colony-stimulating factors, thrombopoietin not only enhances the proliferation of its target cells but also enhances the reactivity of their end-stage product, the platelet. Paradoxically, in the three MPNs, expression of the thrombopoietin receptor, MPL, is impaired and plasma thrombopoietin is increased despite the increased number of megakaryocytes and platelets.

The clonal nature of ET was established by analysis of glucose-6-phosphate dehydrogenase isoenzyme expression in patients hemizygous for this gene. Although thrombocytosis is its principal manifestation, like the other MPNs, a hematopoietic stem cell is involved in ET. Furthermore, a number of families have been described in which ET was inherited, in one instance as an autosomal dominant trait. In addition to ET, PMF and PV have also been observed in such kindreds.

CLINICAL FEATURES

Clinically, ET is most often identified incidentally when a platelet count is obtained during the course of a routine medical evaluation. Occasionally, review of previous blood counts will reveal that an elevated platelet count was present but overlooked for many years. No symptoms or signs are specific for ET, but these patients can have hemorrhagic and thrombotic tendencies expressed as easy bruising for the former and microvascular occlusive events for the latter such as erythromelalgia, ocular migraine, or a TIA. Physical examination is generally unremarkable. Splenomegaly is indicative of another MPN, in particular PV, PMF, or CML.

Anemia is unusual, but a mild neutrophilic leukocytosis is not. The blood smear is most remarkable for the number of platelets present, some of which may be very large. The large mass of circulating platelets may prevent the accurate measurement of serum potassium due to release of platelet potassium upon blood clotting. This type of hyperkalemia is a test tube artifact and not associated with electrocardiographic abnormalities. Similarly, arterial oxygen measurements can be inaccurate unless thrombocythemic blood is collected on ice. The prothrombin and partial thromboplastin times are normal, whereas abnormalities of platelet function such as a prolonged bleeding time and impaired platelet aggregation can be present. However, despite much study, no platelet function abnormality is characteristic of ET, and no platelet function test predicts the risk of clinically significant bleeding or thrombosis.

The elevated platelet count may hinder marrow aspiration, but marrow biopsy usually reveals megakaryocyte hypertrophy and hyperplasia, as well as an overall increase in marrow cellularity. If marrow reticulin is increased, another diagnosis should be considered. The absence of stainable iron demands an explanation because iron deficiency alone can cause thrombocytosis, and absent marrow iron in the presence of marrow hypercellularity is a feature of PV.

Nonrandom cytogenetic abnormalities occur in ET but are uncommon, and no specific or consistent abnormality is notable, even those involving chromosomes 3 and 1, where the genes for thrombopoietin and its receptor, MPL, respectively, are located.

DIAGNOSIS

Thrombocytosis is encountered in a broad variety of clinical disorders (Table 103-6), in many of which inflammatory cytokine production is increased. The absolute level of the platelet count is not a useful diagnostic aid for distinguishing between benign and clonal causes of thrombocytosis. About 50% of ET patients express the *JAK2* V617F mutation. When *JAK2* V617F is absent, cytogenetic evaluation is mandatory to determine if the thrombocytosis is due to CML or a myelodysplastic disorder such as the 5q– syndrome or sideroblastic anemia. Because the *BCR-ABL* translocation can be present in the absence of the Ph chromosome, and because the *BCR-ABL* reverse transcriptase polymerase chain reaction is associated with false-positive results, fluorescence in situ hybridization (FISH) analysis for *BCR-ABL* is the preferred assay in patients with thrombocytosis in whom a cytogenetic study for the Ph chromosome is negative. *CALR* mutations (type 1 or type 2) are present in 30% and *MPL* mutations are present in 8% of ET patients who do not have a *JAK2* mutation. Anemia and ringed sideroblasts are not features of ET, but they are features of idiopathic refractory sideroblastic anemia, and in some of these patients, the thrombocytosis occurs in association with expression of *JAK2* V617F, *CALR*, or an *MPL* mutation. Significant splenomegaly should suggest the presence of another MPN, and in this setting, a red cell mass determination should be performed because splenomegaly can mask the presence of erythrocytosis. Importantly, what appears to be ET can evolve into PV (usually in women with *JAK2* V617F) or PMF (usually in men with type 1 *CALR* mutations) after a period of many years due to clonal evolution or succession. There is sufficient overlap of the *JAK2* V617F neutrophil allele burden between ET and PV that this cannot be used as a distinguishing diagnostic feature with the exception that, in ET, the quantitative *JAK2* V617F neutrophil allele is never greater than 50%; only a red cell mass and plasma volume determination can distinguish PV from ET, and importantly in this regard, 64% of *JAK2* V617F–positive ET patients in one study actually were found to have PV when red cell mass and plasma volume determinations were performed. Claims that ET and PV form a biological continuum are unfounded as these disorders have different gene expression profiles and different natural histories.

COMPLICATIONS

Perhaps no other condition in clinical medicine has caused otherwise astute physicians to intervene inappropriately more often than thrombocytosis, particularly if the platelet count is >1 × 10^6/μL. It is commonly believed that a high platelet count causes thrombosis; however, no controlled clinical study has ever established this association, and in patients younger than age 60 years, the incidence of thrombosis was not greater in patients with thrombocytosis than in age-matched controls, and tobacco use appears to be the most important risk factor for thrombosis in ET patients.

To the contrary, very high platelet counts are associated primarily with hemorrhage due to acquired von Willebrand's disease. This is not meant to imply that an elevated platelet count cannot cause symptoms in an ET patient, but rather that the focus should be on the patient, not the platelet count. For example, some of the most dramatic neurologic problems in ET are migraine-related and respond only to lowering of the platelet count, whereas other symptoms such as erythromelalgia respond simply to platelet cyclooxygenase-1 inhibitors such as aspirin or ibuprofen, without a reduction in platelet number. Still others may represent an interaction between an atherosclerotic vascular system and a high platelet count, and others may have no relationship to the platelet count whatsoever. Recognition that PV can present with thrombocytosis alone as well as the discovery of previously unrecognized causes of hypercoagulability (**Chaps. 116 and 117**) make the older literature on the complications of thrombocytosis unreliable.

TREATMENT

Essential Thrombocytosis

Survival of ET patients is not different than the general population regardless of their driver mutation. An elevated platelet count in an asymptomatic patient without cardiovascular risk factors or tobacco use requires no therapy. Indeed, before any therapy is initiated in a patient with thrombocytosis, the cause of symptoms must be clearly identified as due to the elevated platelet count. When the platelet count rises above 1 × 10^6/μL, a substantial quantity of high-molecular-weight von Willebrand multimers are removed from the circulation and destroyed by the enlarged platelet mass, resulting in an acquired form of von Willebrand's disease. This can be identified by a reduction in ristocetin cofactor activity. In this situation, aspirin could promote hemorrhage. Bleeding in this situation is rarely spontaneous and usually responds to tranexamic acid or ε-aminocaproic acid, which can be given prophylactically before and after elective surgery.

Plateletpheresis is at best a temporary and inefficient remedy that is rarely required. Importantly, ET patients treated with ^{32}P or alkylating agents are at risk of developing acute leukemia without any proof of benefit; combining either therapy with hydroxyurea increases this risk. If platelet reduction is deemed necessary on the basis of symptoms refractory to salicylates alone, pegylated IFN-α, the quinazoline derivative anagrelide, or hydroxyurea can be used to reduce the platelet count, but none of these is uniformly effective or without significant side effects. Hydroxyurea and aspirin were more effective than anagrelide and aspirin for prevention of TIA because hydroxyurea is a nitric oxide donor, but they were not more effective for the prevention of other types of arterial thrombosis and actually less effective for venous thrombosis. The risk of gastrointestinal bleeding is also higher when aspirin is combined with anagrelide. Normalizing the platelet count does not prevent either arterial or venous thrombosis. Pegylated interferon can produce a complete molecular remission in some ET patients, but a role for it or ruxolitinib in ET management has not yet been established.

As more clinical experience is acquired, ET appears more benign than previously thought. Evolution to acute leukemia is more likely to be a consequence of therapy than of the disease itself. In managing patients with thrombocytosis, the physician's first obligation is to do no harm.

FURTHER READING

Alvarez-Larran A et al: Antiplatelet therapy versus observation in low-risk essential thrombocythemia with CALR mutation. Haematologica 101:926, 2016.

Asher S et al: Current and future therapies for myelofibrosis. Blood Rev 42:100715, 2020.

Passamonti F et al: A clinical-molecular prognostic model to predict survival in patients with post polycythemia vera and post essential thrombocythemia myelofibrosis. Leukemia 31:2726, 2017.

Spivak JL: How I treat polycythemia vera. Blood 134:341, 2019.

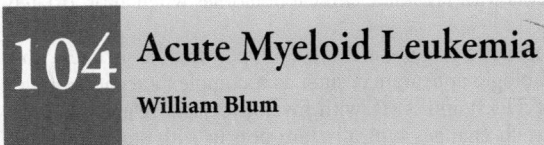

104 Acute Myeloid Leukemia

William Blum

INCIDENCE

Acute myeloid leukemia (AML) is a neoplasm characterized by infiltration of the blood, bone marrow, and other tissues by proliferative, clonal, poorly differentiated cells of the hematopoietic system. These leukemias comprise a spectrum of malignancies that untreated are uniformly fatal. In 2020, the estimated number of new AML cases in the United States was 19,940. AML is the diagnosis in 1.3% of all cancer cases and 31% of all new acute leukemias but causes 62% of leukemic deaths. AML is the most common acute leukemia in older patients, with a median age at diagnosis of 67 years. Long-term survival is infrequent; U.S. registry data report that only 27% of patients survive 5 years.

ETIOLOGY

Most cases of AML are idiopathic. Genetic predisposition, radiation, chemical/other occupational exposures, and drugs have been implicated in the development of AML, but AML cases with established etiology are relatively rare. No direct evidence suggests a viral etiology. Genome sequencing studies suggest that most cases of AML arise from a limited number of mutations that accumulate with advancing age. Indeed, genome sequencing is providing paradigm-shifting advances in our understanding of leukemogenesis. The Cancer Genome Atlas (TCGA) and other databases demonstrate that blood cells from up to 5–6% of normal individuals aged >70 years contain potentially "premalignant" mutations that are associated with clonal expansion.

Use of the term *premalignant* to describe these lesions is not precisely accurate; rather, these mutations represent clonal hematopoiesis of *indeterminate* potential (CHIP; sometimes called age-related clonal hematopoiesis). The genes most commonly altered include the epigenetic regulators *DNMT3A*, *TET2*, and *ASXL1*.

Study of CHIP is important because CHIP has relevance not just to blood cancer evolution but also other medical conditions. Clonal expansion driven by the acquisition of new mutations is associated with a 10-fold increase in risk for developing a hematologic malignancy (compared to matched patients without CHIP), but it is clear that additional "hits" must occur to drive toward leukemia. We do not yet fully understand why or how these secondary lesions occur. Patients with CHIP also have increased risk of cardiovascular mortality that is not fully explained. The link between these two seemingly unrelated issues (cardiovascular and hematologic malignancy) may lie in understanding the interactions between circulating clonally expanded blood cells and vascular endothelium. A "proinflammatory" state caused by clonal, infiltrating monocytes leads to accelerated atherosclerotic plaque development and altered cardiac remodeling. Similar phenomena may occur in the marrow and blood—altered relationships between hematopoietic stem cells with the marrow microenvironment along with altered immune surveillance. Both increase the likelihood that a clone may survive, acquire additional mutations, and then further expand eventually to leukemia. Whether early identification of CHIP in patients will provide therapeutic opportunities for patients remains to be seen. Certainly, modifying cardiovascular risk in patients with CHIP seems prudent, but development of mutation-directed therapies to eliminate problematic clones to prevent leukemia is likely to be more elusive.

Genetic Predisposition Myeloid neoplasms typically occur sporadically in adults; inherited predisposition is rare. Yet, it is clear that myeloid neoplasms with germline predisposition represent an important and growing subset of disease. Germline mutations associated with increased risk of developing a myeloid neoplasm include *CEBPA*, *DDX41*, *RUNX1*, *ANKRD26*, *ETV6*, and *GATA2* (**Table 104-1**). Likewise, myeloid neoplasms with germline predisposition are a feature of several well-described clinical syndromes, including bone marrow failure disorders (e.g., Fanconi anemia, Shwachman-Diamond syndrome, Diamond-Blackfan anemia) and telomere biology disorders (e.g., dyskeratosis congenita). As new mutations and associations are added to a rapidly growing list, it is increasingly clear that genetic predisposition plays a larger role than has been previously understood.

Several genetic syndromes with somatic cell chromosome aneuploidy, such as Down syndrome with trisomy 21, are associated with an increased incidence of AML. Down syndrome–associated AML in young children (<4 years) is typically of the acute megakaryocytic subtype and is associated with mutation in the *GATA1* gene. Such

TABLE 104-1 WHO 2016 Classification of Myeloid Neoplasms with Germline Predisposition

CLASSIFICATION[a]
Myeloid neoplasms with germline predisposition without a preexisting disorder or organ dysfunction
Acute myeloid leukemia with germline *CEBPA* mutation
Myeloid neoplasms with germline *DDX41* mutation[b]
Myeloid neoplasms with germline predisposition and preexisting platelet disorders
Myeloid neoplasms with germline *RUNX1* mutation[b]
Myeloid neoplasms with germline *ANKRD26* mutation[b]
Myeloid neoplasms with germline *ETV6* mutation[b]
Myeloid neoplasms with germline predisposition and other organ dysfunction
Myeloid neoplasms with germline *GATA2* mutation
Myeloid neoplasms associated with bone marrow failure syndromes
Myeloid neoplasms associated with telomere biology disorders
Myeloid neoplasms associated with Noonan syndrome
Myeloid neoplasms associated with Down syndrome[b]

[a]Recognition of familial myeloid neoplasms requires that physicians take a thorough patient and family history to assess for typical signs and symptoms of known syndromes, including data on malignancies and previous bleeding episodes. Molecular genetic diagnostics is guided by a detailed patient and family history. Diagnostics should be performed in close collaboration with a genetic counselor; patients with a suspected heritable myeloid neoplasm, who test negative for known predisposition genes, should ideally be entered on a research study to facilitate new syndrome discovery. [b]Lymphoid neoplasms also reported.

Source: Reproduced with permission from L Peterson et al: Myeloid neoplasms with germline predisposition, in *World Health Organization Classification of Tumours of Haematopoietic and Lymphoid Tissues,* 4th revised ed. Geneva, Switzerland: World Health Organization, 2017.

patients have excellent clinical outcomes but require dose modification of chemotherapy due to high treatment-related toxicities. Inherited diseases with defective DNA repair (e.g., Fanconi anemia, Bloom syndrome, and ataxia-telangiectasia) are also associated with AML. Each syndrome is associated with unique clinical features and atypical toxicities with chemotherapy, requiring expert care. Congenital neutropenia (Kostmann syndrome), due to mutations in the genes encoding the granulocyte colony-stimulating factor receptor and neutrophil elastase, is another disorder that may evolve into AML.

Chemical, Radiation, and Other Exposures Anticancer drugs are the leading cause of therapy-associated AML. Alkylating agent–associated leukemias occur on average 4–6 years after exposure, and affected individuals often have multilineage dysplasia and monosomy/aberrations in chromosomes 5 and 7. Topoisomerase II inhibitor–associated leukemias occur 1–3 years after exposure, and affected individuals often have AML with monocytic features and aberrations involving chromosome 11q23. Exposure to ionizing radiation, benzene, chloramphenicol, phenylbutazone, and other drugs can uncommonly result in bone marrow failure that may evolve into AML.

CLASSIFICATION

The current categorization of AML uses the World Health Organization (WHO) classification (**Table 104-2**), which defines biologically distinct groups based on cytogenetic and molecular abnormalities in addition to clinical features and light microscope morphology. Myeloid neoplasms with germline predisposition, as introduced above, are included as a new and important feature of this classification (Table 104-1).

TABLE 104-2 WHO 2016 Classification of Acute Myeloid Leukemia and Related Neoplasms

Acute myeloid leukemia (AML) with recurrent genetic abnormalities
AML with t(8;21)(q22;q22); *RUNX1-RUNX1T1*
AML with inv(16)(p13.1q22) or t(16;16)(p13.1;q22); *CBFB-MYH11*
Acute promyelocytic leukemia with *PML-RARA*
AML with t(9;11)(p21.3;q23.3); *MLLT3-KMT2A*
AML with t(6;9)(p23;q34.1); *DEK-NUP214*
AML with inv(3)(q21.3q26.2) or t(3;3)(q21.3;q26.2); *GATA2, MECOM*
AML (megakaryoblastic) with t(1;22)(p13.3;q13.3); *RBM15-MKL1*
Provisional entity: AML with BCR-ABL1
AML with mutated *NPM1*
AML with biallelic mutations of *CEBPA*
Provisional entity: AML with mutated RUNX1
AML with myelodysplasia-related changes
Therapy-related myeloid neoplasms
AML, not otherwise specified (NOS)
AML with minimal differentiation
AML without maturation
AML with maturation
Acute myelomonocytic leukemia
Acute monoblastic/monocytic leukemia
Pure erythroid leukemia
Acute megakaryoblastic leukemia
Acute basophilic leukemia
Acute panmyelosis with myelofibrosis
Myeloid sarcoma
Myeloid proliferations related to Down syndrome
Transient abnormal myelopoiesis (TAM)
Myeloid leukemia associated with Down syndrome

Note: Marrow blast count of ≥20% is required, except for AML with the recurrent genetic abnormalities t(15;17), t(8;21), inv(16), or t(16;16).

Source: Adapted from DA Arber et al: Acute myeloid leukaemia (AML) with recurrent genetic abnormalities, in *World Health Organization Classification of Tumours of Haematopoietic and Lymphoid Tissues*, 4th revised ed. Geneva, Switzerland: World Health Organization; 2017.

The WHO classification enables the identification of subsets of disease that may be treated differently (now or in the future) and enhances recognition of the molecular basis of disease from the time of diagnosis. Marrow (or blood) blast count of ≥20% is required to establish the diagnosis of AML, except for AML with the recurrent genetic abnormalities t(15;17), t(8;21), inv(16), or t(16;16).

Clinical Features Even with advances in molecular biology, recognizing clinical features remains important in understanding AML. For example, therapy-related AML is a distinct entity that develops following prior chemotherapy (e.g., alkylating agents, topoisomerase II inhibitors) or ionizing radiation. AML with myelodysplasia-related changes is recognized in part on morphology but also on a medical history of an antecedent myelodysplastic syndrome (MDS) or myelodysplastic/myeloproliferative neoplasm. These clinical features contribute to AML prognosis and are therefore in the WHO classification.

Genetic Findings Subtypes of AML are recognized due to the presence or absence of specific, recurrent cytogenetic, and/or genetic abnormalities. For example, the diagnosis of *acute promyelocytic leukemia* (APL) is based on the presence of either the t(15;17)(q22;q12) cytogenetic rearrangement or the *PML-RARA* fusion product of the translocation. Similarly, core binding factor (CBF) AML is designated based on the presence of t(8;21)(q22;q22), inv(16)(p13.1q22), or t(16;16)(p13.1;q22) or the respective fusion products *RUNX1-RUNX1T1* and *CBFB-MYH11*. Each of these three groups identifies patients with favorable clinical outcomes when appropriately treated.

Several cytogenetic or genetic AML subtypes often associate with a specific morphologic appearance, such as a complex karyotype (and/or mutation of *TP53*) and AML with myelodysplasia-related changes. Patients with such changes typically fare poorly with standard treatments. However, only one abnormality is invariably associated with specific morphologic features: t(15;17)(q22;q12) or the molecular fusion *PML-RARA* with APL. Other cytogenetic and genetic findings may be commonly, but not always, associated with a morphologic description, highlighting the necessity of genetic and cytogenetic testing for precise diagnosis. Several chromosomal abnormalities often associate primarily with one morphologic/immunophenotypic group. Examples include inv(16)(p13.1q22) with AML with abnormal bone marrow eosinophils; t(8;21)(q22;q22) with slender Auer rods, expression of CD19, and increased normal eosinophils; and t(9;11)(p22;q23) and other translocations involving 11q23 with monocytic features. Mutation of nucleophosmin (nucleolar phosphoprotein B23, numatrin, *NPM1*), especially when co-occurring with mutation of fms-related tyrosine kinase 3 (*FLT3*), often presents with "cup-shaped" nuclear morphology. Recurring chromosomal abnormalities in AML may also be loosely associated with specific clinical characteristics. More commonly associated with younger age are t(8;21) and t(15;17), and with older age, del(5q), del(7q), and mutated *TP53*. Myeloid sarcomas are associated with t(8;21); disseminated intravascular coagulation (DIC) is associated with t(15;17). 11q23 aberrations and monocytic leukemia are associated with extramedullary sites of involvement at presentation, especially gingival hypertrophy. High leukocyte count is commonly observed with *NPM1* or *FLT3* mutation.

The WHO classification also incorporates molecular abnormalities by recognizing fusion genes or specific genetic mutations with a role in leukemogenesis. As a classic example, t(15;17) results in the fusion gene *PML-RARA* that encodes a chimeric protein, promyelocytic leukemia (Pml)–retinoic acid receptor α (Rarα), which is formed by the fusion of the retinoic acid receptor α (*RARA*) gene from chromosome 17 and the promyelocytic leukemia (*PML*) gene from chromosome 15. Unique clinical therapy with retinoic acid and arsenic trioxide has revolutionized the care of APL patients (see "Treatment of Acute Promyelocytic Leukemia" section). Similar examples of molecular subtypes included in the category of AML with recurrent genetic abnormalities are those characterized by the leukemogenic fusion genes *RUNX1-RUNX1T1* and *CBFB-MYH11* and the so-called CBF AML subtypes noted cytogenetically as t(8;21), inv(16), or t(16;16). Additional fusions are *MLLT3-KMT2A* and *DEK-NUP214*, resulting from t(9;11) and t(6;9)(p23;q34), respectively, among others.

The WHO classification of AML continues to expand as knowledge of specific genetic or cytogenetic aberrations grows. Several AML subtypes are defined by the presence of genetic mutations rather than chromosomal aberrations. For example, *AML with mutated NPM1* and *AML with biallelic mutated CEBPA*, respectively, are associated with more favorable clinical outcome, though the presence of coexisting mutation in *FLT3* affects *NPM1* prognostic impact. Activating mutations of *FLT3* are present in ~30% of adult AML patients, primarily due to internal tandem duplications (ITDs) in the juxtamembrane domain that have negative prognostic impact. In contrast, point mutations of the activating loop of the kinase (called tyrosine kinase domain [TKD] mutations) have uncertain prognostic impact. Aberrant activation of the *FLT3*-encoded protein provides increased proliferation and antiapoptotic signals to the myeloid progenitor cell. *FLT3*-ITD, the more common of the *FLT3* mutations, occurs preferentially in patients with cytogenetically normal AML (CN-AML). The importance of identifying *FLT3*-ITD at diagnosis relates to the fact that it is not only useful as a prognosticator but also may predict response to specific treatment such as a tyrosine kinase inhibitor (TKI). Several TKIs targeting FLT3 are either approved for AML (e.g., midostaurin, only in first-line therapy in combination with chemotherapy; gilteritinib, in relapse as monotherapy) or currently in clinical investigation (e.g., quizartinib, crenolanib, sorafenib, and others). The *FLT3* allelic ratio (of the number of mutated alleles to wild-type alleles) provides information beyond the mere presence or absence of the mutation. Several mutational scenarios, such as one mutated gene and one wild-type gene or one mutated gene with no (deleted) wild-type gene, and the ratio of malignant to nonmalignant cells in the sample affect the ratio. The allelic ratio affects the prognostic impact of the *FLT3*-ITD mutation; patients with *FLT3*-ITD "low" allelic ratio (<0.5) fare better. Accordingly, mutated *NPM1* without *FLT3*-ITD or with *FLT3*-ITD^{low} is viewed as favorable risk by the European LeukemiaNet (ELN) risk stratification schema **(Table 104-3)**. Conversely, *FLT3*-ITD^{high} has an adverse prognostic impact; patients with both mutated *NPM1* and *FLT3*-ITD with an allelic ratio >0.5 are intermediate risk by ELN stratification. Involving a different tyrosine kinase, AML with *BCR-ABL1* fusion is a new WHO provisional entity to recognize rare cases that may benefit from *BCR-ABL* TKI therapy (Table 104-2).

Immunophenotypic Findings The immunophenotype of human leukemia cells can be studied by multiparameter flow cytometry after the cells are labeled with monoclonal antibodies to cell-surface antigens. This can be important in quickly distinguishing AML from acute lymphoblastic leukemia and for identifying some subtypes of AML. For example, AML with minimal differentiation, characterized by immature morphology and no lineage-specific cytochemical reactions, may be diagnosed by flow-cytometric demonstration of the myeloid-specific antigens cluster designation (CD) 13 and/or 117. Similarly, acute megakaryoblastic leukemia can often be diagnosed only by expression of the platelet-specific antigens CD41 and/or CD61. Although flow cytometry is widely used, and in some cases essential for the diagnosis of AML, it has only a supportive role in establishing the different subtypes of AML through the WHO classification. Increasingly, multiparameter flow cytometry is used for the measurement of measurable residual disease (MRD) after remission is achieved.

PROGNOSTIC FACTORS

Several factors predict outcome of AML patients treated with chemotherapy; they should be used for risk stratification and treatment guidance.

Chromosome and molecular investigations performed at diagnosis currently provide the most important prognostic information. WHO has categorized patients as having favorable, intermediate, or adverse risk based on the presence of structural and/or numerical chromosomal or genetic aberrations. Patients with t(15;17) have a very good prognosis (~85% cured), and those with t(8;21) and inv(16) have a good prognosis (~55% cured), whereas those with no cytogenetic abnormality have an intermediate outcome risk (~40% cured). Patients with a *TP53* mutation, complex karyotype, t(6;9), inv(3), or −7 have a very poor prognosis. Another cytogenetic subgroup, the monosomal karyotype, has been suggested to adversely influence the outcome of AML patients other than those with t(15;17), t(8;21), or inv(16) or t(16;16). The monosomal karyotype subgroup is defined by the presence of at least two autosomal monosomies (loss of chromosomes other than Y or X) or a single autosomal monosomy with additional structural abnormalities.

For patients lacking prognostic cytogenetic abnormalities, i.e., those with CN-AML, testing for several mutated genes can help to risk-stratify. In addition to *NPM1* mutation and *FLT3*-ITD as described above, biallelic *CEBPA* mutations have prognostic value. Such mutations predict favorable outcome. Given the proven prognostic importance of *NPM1*, *CEBPA*, and *FLT3*, molecular assessment of these genes at diagnosis has been incorporated into AML management guidelines by the National Comprehensive Cancer Network (NCCN) and the ELN. The same markers help to define genetic groups in the ELN standardized reporting system, which is based on both cytogenetic and molecular abnormalities and is used for comparing clinical features/treatment response among subsets of patients reported across different clinical studies (Table 104-3). These genetic groups should be used for risk stratification and treatment guidance.

TABLE 104-3 2017 European LeukemiaNet Risk Stratification by Genetics for Acute Myeloid Leukemia (AML)[a]

RISK CATEGORY[b]	GENETIC ABNORMALITY
Favorable	t(8;21)(q22;q22); *RUNX1-RUNX1T1*
	inv(16)(p13.1q22) or t(16;16)(p13.1;q22); *CBFB-MYH11*
	Mutated *NPM1* without *FLT3*-ITD or with *FLT3*-ITD$^{low(c)}$
	Biallelic mutated *CEBPA*
Intermediate	Mutated *NPM1* and *FLT3*-ITD$^{high(c)}$
	Wild-type *NPM1* without *FLT3*-ITD or with *FLT3*-ITD$^{low(c)}$ (w/o adverse-risk genetic lesions)
	t(9;11)(p21.3;q23.3); *MLLT3-KMT2A*[d]
	Cytogenetic abnormalities not classified as favorable or adverse
Adverse	t(6;9)(p23;q34.1); *DEK-NUP214*
	t(v;11q23.3); *KMT2A* rearranged
	t(9;22)(q34.1;q11.2); *BCR-ABL1*
	inv(3)(q21.3q26.2) or t(3;3)(q21.3;q26.2); *GATA2, MECOM(EVI1)*
	−5 or del(5q); −7; −17/abn(17p)
	Complex karyotype,[e] monosomal karyotype[f]
	Wild type *NPM1* and *FLT3*-ITD$^{high(c)}$
	Mutated *RUNX1*[g]
	Mutated *ASXL1*[g]
	Mutated *TP53*[h]

[a]This table excludes acute promyelocytic leukemia. Frequencies, response rates, and outcome measures should be reported by risk category and, if sufficient numbers are available, by specific genetic lesions indicated. [b]Prognostic impact of a marker is treatment-dependent and may change with new therapies. [c]Low, low allelic ratio (<0.5); high, high allelic ratio (≥0.5); semiquantitative assessment of *FLT3*-ITD allelic ratio (using DNA fragment analysis) is determined as ratio of the area under the curve (AUC) "*FLT3*-ITD" divided by AUC "*FLT3*-wild type"; recent studies indicate that acute myeloid leukemia with *NPM1* mutation and *FLT3*-ITD low allelic ratio may also have a more favorable prognosis and patients should not routinely be assigned to allogeneic hematopoietic cell transplantation. [d]The presence of t(9;11)(p21.3;q23.3) takes precedence over rare, concurrent adverse-risk gene mutations. [e]Three or more unrelated chromosome abnormalities in the absence of one of the World Health Organization–designated recurring translocations or inversions, i.e., t(8;21), inv(16) or t(16;16), t(9;11), t(v;11)(v;q23.3), t(6;9), inv(3), or t(3;3); AML with *BCR-ABL1*. [f]Defined by the presence of one single monosomy (excluding loss of X or Y) in association with at least one additional monosomy or structural chromosome abnormality (excluding core binding factor AML). [g]These markers should not be used as an adverse prognostic marker if they co-occur with favorable-risk AML subtypes. [h]*TP53* mutations are significantly associated with AML with complex and monosomal karyotype.

Source: Republished with permission of American Society of Hematology, from Diagnosis and management of acute myeloid leukemia in adults: 2017 recommendations from an international expert panel, Döhner H et al. 129:424, 2017; permission conveyed through Copyright Clearance Center, Inc.

TABLE 104-4 Molecular Prognostic Markers in AML[a]

GENE SYMBOL	GENE LOCATION	PROGNOSTIC IMPACT
Genes Included in the WHO Classification and ELN Reporting System		
NPM1 mutations	5q35.1	Favorable
CEBPA mutations	19q13.1	Favorable
FLT3-ITD	13q12	Depends on allelic ratio and *NPM1* mutational status
Genes Encoding Receptor Tyrosine Kinases		
KIT mutation	4q12	Adverse
FLT3-TKD	13q12	Unclear
Genes Encoding Transcription Factors		
RUNX1 mutations	21q22.12	Adverse
WT1 mutations	11p13	Adverse
Genes Encoding Epigenetic Modifiers		
ASXL1 mutations	20q11.21	Adverse
DNMT3A mutations	2p23.3	Adverse
IDH mutations (*IDH1* and *IDH2*)	2q34 & 15q26.1	Adverse
KMT2A-PTD	11q23	Adverse
TET2 mutations	4q24	Adverse
Deregulated Genes		
BAALC overexpression	8q22.3	Adverse
ERG overexpression	21q22.3	Adverse
MN1 overexpression	22q12.1	Adverse
EVI1 overexpression	3q26.2	Adverse
Deregulated MicroRNAs		
miR-155 overexpression	21q21.3	Adverse
miR-3151 overexpression	8q22.3	Adverse
miR-181a overexpression	1q32.1 and 9q33.3	Favorable

[a]This table excludes acute promyelocytic leukemia.

Abbreviations: AML, acute myeloid leukemia; ELN, European LeukemiaNet; ITD, internal tandem duplication; PTD, partial tandem duplication; TKD, tyrosine kinase domain; WHO, World Health Organization.

In addition to *NPM1, CEBPA* , *FLT3,* and *TP53* mutations, molecular aberrations in other genes may be routinely used for prognostication (**Table 104-4**). Among these mutated genes are those encoding receptor tyrosine kinases (*KIT*), transcription factors (*RUNX1* and *WT1*), and epigenetic modifiers (*ASXL1, DNMT3A*, isocitrate dehydrogenase 1 [*IDH1*], *IDH2, KMT2A* [also known as *MLL*], and *TET2*). Although *KIT* mutations are almost exclusively present in CBF AML and impact adversely the outcome, the remaining markers have been reported primarily in CN-AML. Mutations of *ASXL1* and *RUNX1* are associated with adverse outcome, independent of other prognostic factors. However, for some of these mutations, data remain unclear on the prognostic impact due to conflicting reports (e.g., *TET2, IDH1, IDH2*). Increasingly, novel drugs that inhibit/modulate aberrant pathways activated by some of these genes (especially *FLT3, IDH1,* and *IDH2*) have been remarkably effective in subsets of disease, leading to U.S. Food and Drug Administration approvals (see section on treatment of AML).

In addition to gene mutations, deregulation of the expression levels of coding genes and of short noncoding RNAs (microRNAs) also provides prognostic information (Table 104-4). Overexpression of genes such as *BAALC, ERG, MN1,* and MDS1 and EVI1 complex locus (*MECOM*; also known as *EVI1*) predict poor outcome, especially in CN-AML. Similarly, deregulated expression levels of microRNAs, naturally occurring noncoding RNAs that regulate the expression of proteins via degradation or translational inhibition of their target coding RNAs, have also been associated with prognosis in AML. Overexpression of *miR-155* and *miR-3151* predicts unfavorable outcome in CN-AML, whereas overexpression of *miR-181a* predicts favorable outcome both in CN-AML and cytogenetically abnormal AML.

Because prognostic molecular markers in AML are not mutually exclusive and often occur concurrently (>80% patients have at least two or more prognostic gene mutations), the likelihood that distinct marker combinations may be more informative than single markers is increasingly clear.

Epigenetic changes (e.g., DNA methylation and/or posttranslational histone modification) and microRNAs are often involved in deregulation of genes involved in hematopoiesis, contribute to leukemogenesis, and may associate with the previously discussed prognostic gene mutations. These changes have been shown to provide biologic insights into leukemogenic mechanisms and provide independent prognostic information. Therapeutic progress based on advances in understanding the role of epigenetic changes in AML is currently unfolding. For example, in patients with mutations of *IDH1* or *IDH2*, novel active enzymes produced from these respective mutations hijack the citric acid cycle, leading to production of a novel "oncometabolite," 2-hydroxyglutarate, which disrupts a myriad of epigenetic processes. Pharmacologic inhibition of these aberrant enzymes can reverse these leukemogenic activities.

In addition to cytogenetic and molecular aberrations, several other factors are associated with outcome in AML. Age at diagnosis is one of the most important risk factors. Advancing age is associated with a poor prognosis for two reasons: (1) its influence on the ability to survive induction therapy due to coexisting medical comorbidities, and (2) with each successive decade of age, a greater proportion of patients have intrinsically more resistant disease. A prolonged symptomatic interval with cytopenias preceding AML diagnosis or a history of antecedent hematologic disorders including MDS or myeloproliferative neoplasms is often found in older patients. Cytopenia is a clinical feature associated with a lower complete remission (CR) rate and shorter survival time. The CR rate is lower in patients who have had anemia, leukopenia, and/or thrombocytopenia for >3 months before the diagnosis of AML, when compared to those without such a history. Responsiveness to chemotherapy declines as the duration of the antecedent disorder increases. Likewise, AML developing after treatment with cytotoxic agents for other malignancies is usually difficult to treat successfully. In addition, older patients less frequently harbor favorable cytogenetic abnormalities (i.e., t[8;21], inv[16], and t[16;16]) and more frequently harbor adverse cytogenetic (e.g., complex and monosomal karyotypes) and/or molecular (e.g., *ASXL1, TP53*) abnormalities.

Other factors independently associated with worse outcome are a poor performance status that influences ability to survive induction therapy and a high presenting leukocyte count that in some series is an adverse prognostic factor for attaining a CR. Among patients with hyperleukocytosis (>100,000/μL), early central nervous system bleeding and pulmonary leukostasis contribute to poor outcomes.

Following administration of therapy, achievement of CR is associated with better outcome and longer survival. CR is defined after examination of both blood and bone marrow and essentially represents eradication of detectable leukemia *and* restoration of normal hematopoiesis. The blood neutrophil count must be ≥1000/μL and the platelet count ≥100,000/μL. Hemoglobin concentration is not considered in determining CR. Circulating blasts should be absent. Although rare blasts may be detected in the blood during marrow regeneration, they should disappear on successive studies. At CR, the bone marrow should contain <5% blasts, and Auer rods should be absent. Extramedullary leukemia should not be present.

CLINICAL PRESENTATION

Symptoms Patients with AML usually present with nonspecific symptoms that begin gradually, or abruptly, and are the consequence of anemia, leukocytosis, leukopenia/leukocyte dysfunction, or thrombocytopenia. Nearly half have symptoms for ≤3 months before the leukemia is diagnosed.

Fatigue is a frequent first symptom among AML patients. Anorexia and weight loss are common. Fever with or without an identifiable infection is the initial symptom in ~10% of patients. Signs of abnormal hemostasis (bleeding, easy bruising) are common. Bone pain, lymphadenopathy, nonspecific cough, headache, or diaphoresis may also occur.

Rarely, patients may present with symptoms from a myeloid sarcoma (a tumor mass consisting of myeloid blasts occurring at anatomic sites other than bone marrow). Sites involved are most commonly the skin, lymph node, gastrointestinal tract, soft tissue, and testis. This rare presentation, often characterized by chromosome aberrations (e.g., monosomy 7, trisomy 8, 11q23 rearrangement, inv[16], trisomy 4, t[8;21]), may precede or coincide with blood and/or marrow involvement by AML. Patients who present with isolated myeloid sarcoma typically develop blood and/or marrow involvement quickly thereafter and cannot be cured with local therapy (radiation or surgery) alone.

Physical Findings Fever, infection, and hemorrhage are often found at the time of diagnosis; splenomegaly, hepatomegaly, lymphadenopathy, and "bone pain" may also be present less commonly. Hemorrhagic complications are most commonly and, classically, found in APL. APL patients often present with DIC-associated minor hemorrhage but may have significant gastrointestinal bleeding, intrapulmonary hemorrhage, or intracranial hemorrhage. Likewise, thrombosis is another less frequent but well recognized clinical feature of DIC in APL. Bleeding associated with coagulopathy may also occur in monocytic AML and with extreme degrees of leukocytosis or thrombocytopenia in other morphologic subtypes. Retinal hemorrhages are detected in 15% of patients. Infiltration of the gingiva, skin, soft tissues, or meninges with leukemic blasts at diagnosis is characteristic of the monocytic subtypes and those with 11q23 chromosomal abnormalities.

Hematologic Findings Anemia is usually present at diagnosis, although it is not typically severe. The anemia is usually normocytic normochromic. Decreased erythropoiesis in the setting of AML often results in a reduced reticulocyte count, and red blood cell (RBC) survival is decreased by accelerated destruction. Active blood loss may rarely contribute to the anemia.

The median presenting leukocyte count is ~15,000/μL. Lower presenting leukocyte counts are more typical of older patients and those with antecedent hematologic disorders. Between 25 and 40% of patients have counts <5000/μL, and 20% have counts >100,000/μL. Fewer than 5% have no detectable leukemic cells in the blood. In AML, the cytoplasm often contains primary (nonspecific) granules, and the nucleus shows fine, lacy chromatin with one or more nucleoli characteristic of immature cells. Abnormal rod-shaped granules called Auer rods are not uniformly present, but when they are, AML is virtually certain (**Fig. 104-1**).

Platelet counts <100,000/μL are found at diagnosis in ~75% of patients, and ~25% have counts <25,000/μL. Both morphologic and functional platelet abnormalities can be observed, including large and bizarre shapes with abnormal granulation and inability of platelets to aggregate or adhere normally to one another.

Pretreatment Evaluation Once the diagnosis of AML is suspected, thorough evaluation and initiation of appropriate therapy should follow. In addition to clarifying the subtype of leukemia, initial studies should evaluate the overall functional integrity of the major organ systems, including the cardiovascular, pulmonary, hepatic, and

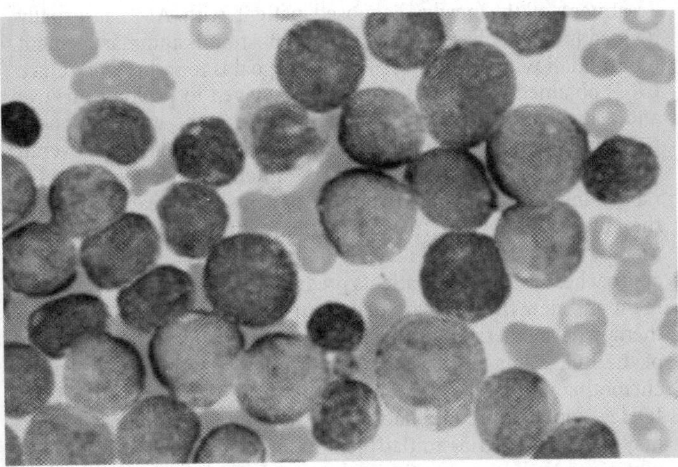

A

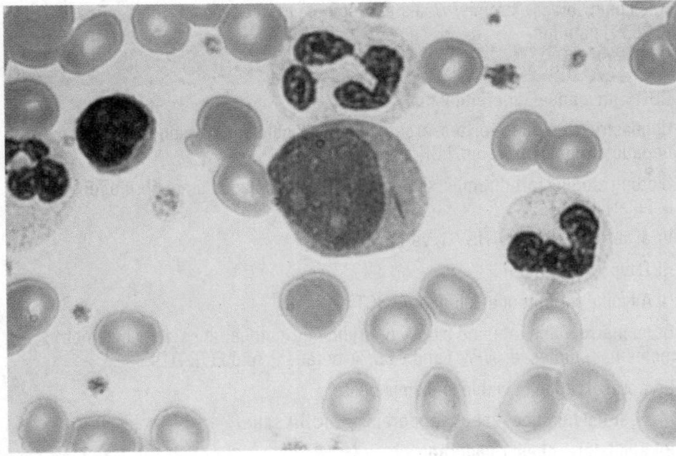

B

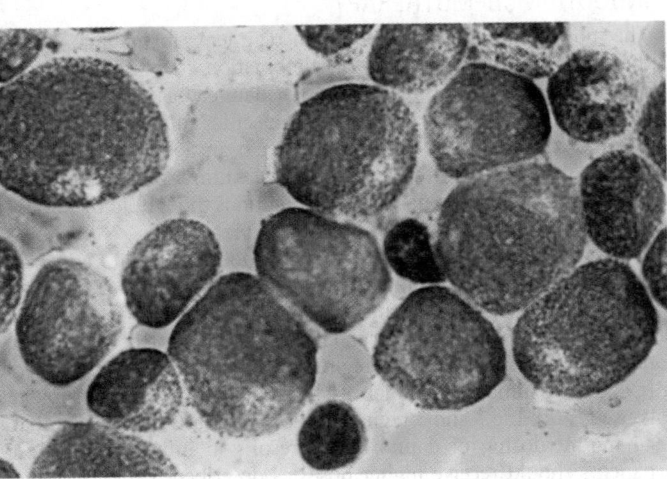

C

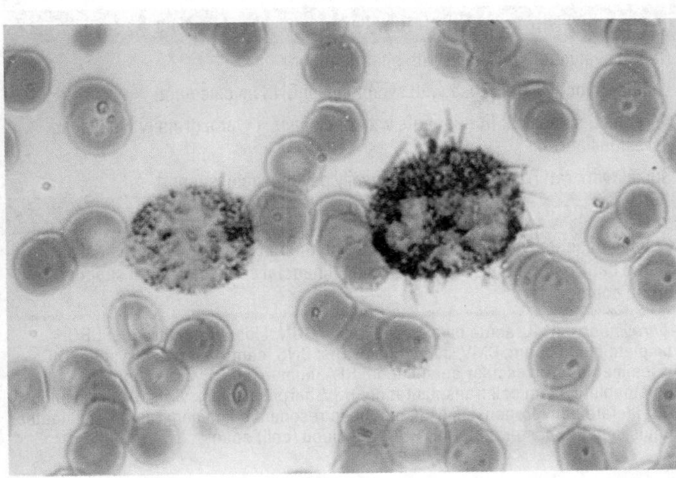

D

FIGURE 104-1 Morphology of acute myeloid leukemia (AML) cells. ***A.*** Uniform population of primitive myeloblasts with immature chromatin, nucleoli in some cells, and primary cytoplasmic granules. ***B.*** Leukemic myeloblast containing an Auer rod. ***C.*** Promyelocytic leukemia cells with prominent cytoplasmic primary granules. ***D.*** Peroxidase stain shows dark blue color characteristic of peroxidase in granules in AML.

TABLE 104-5 Initial Diagnostic Evaluation and Management of Adult Patients with AML

History
Increasing fatigue or decreased exercise tolerance (anemia)
Excess bleeding or bleeding from unusual sites (DIC, thrombocytopenia)
Fevers or recurrent infections (neutropenia)
Headache, vision changes, nonfocal neurologic abnormalities (CNS leukemia or bleed)
Early satiety (splenomegaly)
Family history of AML (Fanconi, Bloom, or Kostmann syndromes or ataxia-telangiectasia)
History of cancer (exposure to alkylating agents, radiation, topoisomerase II inhibitors)
Occupational exposures (radiation, benzene, petroleum products, paint, smoking, pesticides)
Physical Examination
Performance status (prognostic factor)
Ecchymosis and oozing from IV sites (DIC, possible acute promyelocytic leukemia)
Fever and tachycardia (signs of infection)
Papilledema, retinal infiltrates, cranial nerve abnormalities (CNS leukemia)
Poor dentition, dental abscesses
Gum hypertrophy (leukemic infiltration, most common in monocytic leukemia)
Skin infiltration or nodules (leukemia infiltration, most common in monocytic leukemia)
Lymphadenopathy, splenomegaly, hepatomegaly
Back pain, lower extremity weakness (spinal granulocytic sarcoma, most likely in t[8;21] patients)
Laboratory and Radiologic Studies
CBC with manual differential cell count
Chemistry tests (electrolytes, creatinine, BUN, calcium, phosphorus, uric acid, hepatic enzymes, bilirubin, LDH, amylase, lipase)
Clotting studies (prothrombin time, partial thromboplastin time, fibrinogen, D-dimer)
Viral serologies (CMV, HSV-1, varicella-zoster)
RBC type and screen
HLA typing for potential allogeneic HCT
Bone marrow aspirate and biopsy (morphology, cytogenetics, flow cytometry, molecular studies for *NPM1* and *CEBPA* mutations and *FLT3*-ITD)
Cryopreservation of viable leukemia cells
Myocardial function (echocardiogram or MUGA scan)
PA and lateral chest radiograph
Placement of central venous access device
Interventions for Specific Patients
Dental evaluation (for those with poor dentition)
Lumbar puncture (for those with symptoms of CNS involvement)
Screening spine MRI (for patients with back pain, lower extremity weakness, paresthesias)
Social work referral for patient and family psychosocial support
Counseling for All Patients
Provide patients with information regarding their disease and genetic risks, sperm banking or menstrual suppression, financial counseling, and support group contact

Abbreviations: AML, acute myeloid leukemia; BUN, blood urea nitrogen; CBC, complete blood count; CMV, cytomegalovirus; CNS, central nervous system; DIC, disseminated intravascular coagulation; HLA, human leukocyte antigen; HCT, hematopoietic stem cell transplantation; HSV, herpes simplex virus; IV, intravenous; LDH, lactate dehydrogenase; MRI, magnetic resonance imaging; MUGA, multigated acquisition; PA, posteroanterior; RBC, red blood (cell) count.

renal systems (**Table 104-5**). Factors that have prognostic significance, either for achieving CR or for CR duration, should also be assessed before initiating treatment including cytogenetics and molecular markers. Leukemic cells should be obtained from all patients and cryopreserved for future investigational testing as well as potential future use as new diagnostics and therapeutics become available. All patients should be evaluated for infection. During the ongoing global pandemic, testing for the presence of the novel coronavirus, SARS-COV2, is recommended before initiation of chemotherapy.

Most patients are anemic and thrombocytopenic at presentation. Replacement of the appropriate blood components, if necessary, should begin promptly. Because qualitative platelet dysfunction or the presence of an infection may increase the likelihood of bleeding, evidence of hemorrhage justifies the immediate use of platelet transfusion, even if the platelet count is only moderately decreased.

About 50% of patients have a mild to moderate elevation of serum uric acid at presentation. Only 10% have marked elevations, but renal precipitation of uric acid and the nephropathy that may result is a serious but uncommon complication. The initiation of chemotherapy may aggravate hyperuricemia, and patients are usually started immediately on allopurinol and hydration at diagnosis. Rasburicase (recombinant uric oxidase) is also useful for treating uric acid nephropathy and often can normalize the serum uric acid level within hours with a single dose of treatment, although its expense suggests that limiting its use to patients with severe hyperuricemia and/or kidney injury may be prudent. The presence of high concentrations of lysozyme, a marker for monocytic differentiation, may be etiologic in renal tubular dysfunction for a minority of patients.

TREATMENT

Acute Myeloid Leukemia

Treatment of the newly diagnosed patient with AML is usually divided into two phases, induction and postremission management (consolidation) (**Fig. 104-2**). The initial goal is to induce CR. Once CR is obtained, further therapy must be given to prolong survival and achieve cure. The initial induction treatment and subsequent postremission therapy are chosen based on the patient's age, overall fitness, and cytogenetic/molecular risk. Intensive therapy with cytarabine and anthracycline in younger patients (<60 years) increases the cure rate of AML. In older patients, the benefit of intensive therapy is controversial in all but favorable-risk patients; novel approaches for selecting patients predicted to be responsive to treatment and new therapies are being pursued. Additional options for therapy have emerged for older AML patients such as the addition of the BCL2 antagonist venetoclax to one of several low-intensity chemotherapies. Likewise, novel oral drugs targeting IDH1 or IDH2, alone or in combination with low-intensity chemotherapy, may be considered as initial therapy for older patients who have mutations in those respective pathways.

INDUCTION CHEMOTHERAPY

The most commonly used induction regimens (for patients other than those with APL) consist of combination chemotherapy with cytarabine and an anthracycline (e.g., daunorubicin, idarubicin). Cytarabine is a cell cycle S-phase–specific antimetabolite that becomes phosphorylated intracellularly to an active triphosphate form that interferes with DNA synthesis. Anthracyclines are DNA intercalators. Their primary mode of action is thought to be inhibition of topoisomerase II, leading to DNA breaks.

In adults, cytarabine used at standard dose (100–200 mg/m^2) is administered as a continuous intravenous infusion for 7 days. With cytarabine, anthracycline therapy generally consists of daunorubicin (60–90 mg/m^2) or idarubicin (12 mg/m^2) intravenously on days 1, 2, and 3 (the 7 and 3 regimen). Other agents can be added (e.g., gemtuzumab ozogamicin) when 60 mg/m^2 of daunorubicin is used. With the 7 and 3 regimen, it is now clearly established that 45 mg/m^2 dosing of daunorubicin results in inferior outcomes; patients should receive higher doses as described. Patients failing remission after one induction are offered reinduction with the same (or slightly modified) therapy. The CD33-targeting immunoconjugate gemtuzumab ozogamicin may be added to induction therapy for subsets of patients, especially those with CBF AML.

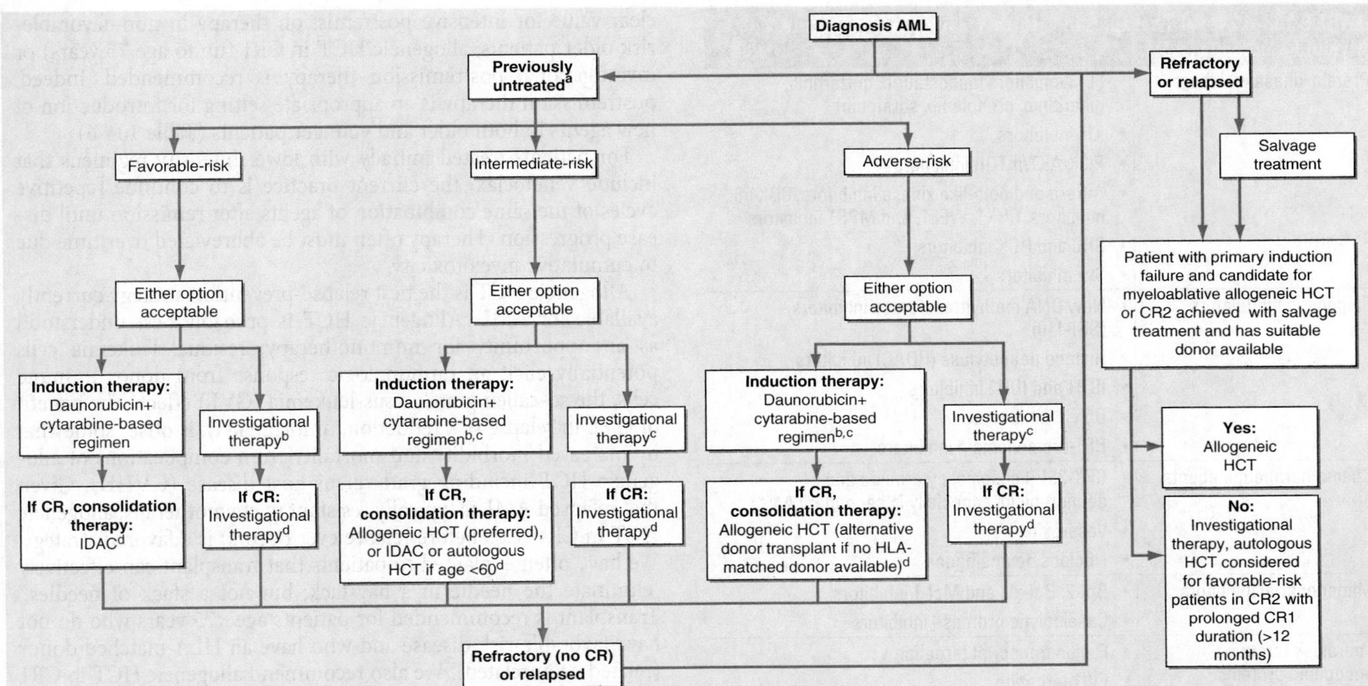

FIGURE 104-2 Algorithm for the therapy of newly diagnosed acute myeloid leukemia (AML). [a]Risk stratification according to the European LeukemiaNet (see Table 104-3). [b]Younger patients (<60–65 years) should routinely be offered investigational therapy on a backbone of standard chemotherapy for induction and consolidation. [c]Older patients, especially those >65 years or with adverse risk disease, or those who are unfit for intensive anthracycline + cytarabine regimens, may be considered for investigational therapy alone or in combination with lower intensity chemotherapy (azacitidine, decitabine, cytarabine), or lower intensity chemotherapy in combination with venetoclax. [d]Investigational therapy as maintenance should be considered if available (after consolidation for younger patients and older patients with favorable-risk disease, and for all other older patients after induction).

Allogeneic hematopoietic cell transplantation (HCT) is a consideration for all eligible patients in first complete remission (CR) with non–favorable-risk disease and highly recommended for older patients (60–75 years) and those with adverse risk.

For all forms of AML in fit patients, except acute promyelocytic leukemia (APL), standard induction therapy includes a regimen based on a 7-day continuous infusion of cytarabine (100–200 mg/m^2/d) and a 3-day course of daunorubicin (60–90 mg/m^2/d) with or without additional drugs. Idarubicin (12 mg/m^2/d) can be used in place of daunorubicin (not shown). The value of postremission/consolidation therapy for older patients (>60 years) who do not have favorable-risk disease is uncertain. Patients who achieve CR undergo postremission consolidation therapy, including sequential courses of intermediate-dose cytarabine, allogeneic HCT, autologous HCT, or novel therapies, based on their predicted risk of relapse (i.e., risk-stratified therapy). Patients receiving induction of lower intensity chemotherapy with venetoclax (or investigational therapy) typically receive repetitive cycles of same on an attenuated schedule, if necessary due to myelotoxicity, after achieving remission. Patients with APL (see text for treatment) usually receive tretinoin and arsenic trioxide–based regimens with or without anthracycline-based chemotherapy and possibly maintenance with tretinoin. HLA, human leukocyte antigen; IDAC, intermediate-dose cytarabine.

In older patients (age ≥60–65 years), the outcome with conventional intensive therapy is generally poor due to a higher frequency of resistant disease and increased rate of treatment-related mortality. This is especially true in patients with prior hematologic disorders (MDS or myeloproliferative neoplasms), therapy-related AML, or cytogenetic and genetic abnormalities that adversely influence clinical outcome. Patients still fare far better with treatment than with supportive care only. Conventional therapy for fit older patients is similar to that for younger patients: the 7 and 3 regimen with standard-dose cytarabine and idarubicin (12 mg/m^2), or daunorubicin (60 mg/m^2). For patients aged >65 years, high-dose daunorubicin (90 mg/m^2) has increased toxicity and is not recommended. A novel liposomal preparation of cytarabine and daunorubicin in a fixed molar ratio may instead be administered to fit patients with AML with myelodysplasia-related changes or arising from MDS. Older patients and those unable to receive intensive therapy due to medical comorbidity may receive repetitive cycles of lower intensity therapy with a hypomethylating agent (HMA; decitabine or azacitidine) or low-dose cytarabine, in combination with daily venetoclax. As noted, targeted IDH1- or IDH2-directed therapy is another consideration. All patients should be considered for clinical trials. Investigational therapy remains the best option for many older patients but especially those with adverse-risk features. **(Table 104-6).**

With the 7 and 3 regimen, 60–80% of younger and 33–60% of older patients (among those who are candidates for intensive therapy) with primary AML achieve CR. Response rates around 60% have been similarly reported with the combination of HMA plus venetoclax in older or infirm patient groups. Of patients who do not achieve CR, most have drug-resistant leukemia. Induction death is more frequent with advancing age and medical comorbidity. Patients with refractory disease after induction should be considered for salvage treatments, preferably on clinical trials. Planning for the possibility of allogeneic hematopoietic stem cell transplantation (HCT) for all eligible patients under age 75 years is part of optimal initial AML care. Typically, allogeneic HCT is performed for patients in CR but at risk for relapse, but fit younger patients with primary refractory disease (not in remission after initial induction) have ~15–20% cure rates with allogeneic HCT (after myeloablative conditioning). For this reason, early planning for possible future allogeneic HCT (including human leukocyte antigen [HLA] typing, donor search, etc.) should be part of the initial approach for most AML patients.

POSTREMISSION THERAPY

Induction of a durable first CR (CR1) is critical to long-term survival in AML. However, without further therapy, virtually all CR patients will eventually relapse. Thus, postremission therapy is designed to eradicate residual (typically undetectable) leukemic cells to prevent relapse and prolong survival. As with induction, the type of postremission therapy in AML is selected for each individual patient based on age, fitness, and cytogenetic/molecular risk.

TABLE 104-6 Novel Therapies in Clinical Development in Acute Myeloid Leukemia (AML)

Protein kinase inhibitors	• FLT3 inhibitors (midostaurin, quizartinib, gilteritinib, crenolanib, sorafenib) • KIT inhibitors • PI3K/AKT/mTOR inhibitors • Aurora and polo-like kinase inhibitors, CDK4/6 inhibitors, CHK1, WEE1, and MPS1 inhibitors • SRC and HCK inhibitors • Syk inhibitors
Epigenetic modulators	• New DNA methyltransferase inhibitors (SGI-110) • Histone deacetylase (HDAC) inhibitors • IDH1 and IDH2 inhibitors • DOT1L inhibitors • BET-bromodomain inhibitors
Chemotherapeutic agents	• CPX-351 (liposomal cytarabine and daunorubicin, especially in secondary AML) • Vosaroxin • Nucleoside analogues
Mitochondrial inhibitors	• Bcl-2, Bcl-xL, and Mcl-1 inhibitors • Caseinolytic protease inhibitors
Therapies targeting oncogenic proteins	• Fusion transcript targeting • EVI1 targeting • NPM1 targeting • Hedgehog inhibitors (glasdegib)
Antibodies and immunotherapies	• Monoclonal antibodies against CD33, CD44, CD47, CD123, CLEC12A • Immunoconjugates (e.g., gemtuzumab ozogamicin, SGN33A) • Bispecific T-cell engagers (BiTEs) and dual affinity retargeting molecules (DARTs) • Chimeric antigen receptor (CAR) T cells or genetically engineered T-cell receptor (TCR) T cells • Immune checkpoint inhibitors (PD-1/PD-L1, CTLA-4) • Vaccines (e.g., WT1)
Therapies targeting AML environment	• CXCR4 and CXCL12 antagonists • Antiangiogenic therapies

Source: Republished with permission of American Society of Hematology, from Diagnosis and management of acute myeloid leukemia in adults: 2017 recommendations from an international expert panel, Döhner H et al. 129:424, 2017; permission conveyed through Copyright Clearance Center, Inc.

The choice between consolidation with chemotherapy or with transplantation is complex and based on age, risk, and practical considerations. In younger patients receiving chemotherapy, postremission therapy with intermediate- or high-dose cytarabine for two to four cycles is standard practice. Higher doses of cytarabine during postremission therapy appear more effective than standard doses (such as are used in induction) for those who do not have adverse-risk genetics. Recent studies suggest that the long-standing practice of high-dose cytarabine (3 g/m^2, every 12 h on days 1, 3, and 5) may not improve survival over intermediate-dose cytarabine (IDAC; 1–1.5 g/m^2) for such patients. Thus, the ELN has recommended IDAC at 1–1.5 g/m^2, every 12 h, on days 1–3, as the optimal postremission chemotherapy approach for favorable- and intermediate-risk younger patients, for two to four cycles. While high-dose cytarabine may not be necessary, it is important to note that younger, favorable-risk patients have worse outcomes when doses <1 g/m^2 are used. In contrast to favorable-risk patients, intermediate- or adverse-risk patients should proceed with allogeneic HCT in CR1 when feasible (see transplant discussion below). Because older patients have increased toxicities with higher doses of cytarabine, ELN recommends relatively attenuated cytarabine doses (0.5–1 g/m^2, every 12 h, on days 1–3) in favorable-risk older patients. There is no clear value for intensive postremission therapy in non–favorable-risk older patients; allogeneic HCT in CR1 (up to age 75 years) or investigational postremission therapy is recommended. Indeed, postremission therapy is an appropriate setting for introduction of new agents in both older and younger patients (Table 104-6).

For patients treated initially with lower intensity regimens that include venetoclax, the current practice is to continue repetitive cycles of the same combination of agents after remission until disease progression. Therapy often must be abbreviated over time due to cumulative myelotoxicity.

Allogeneic HCT is the best relapse-prevention strategy currently available for AML. Allogeneic HCT is probably best understood as an opportunity for immunotherapy; residual leukemia cells potentially elicit an immunologic response from donor immune cells, the so-called graft-versus-leukemia (GVL) effect. The benefit of GVL in relapse risk reduction, unfortunately, is offset somewhat by increased morbidity and mortality from complications of allogeneic HCT including graft-versus-host disease (GVHD). Given that relapsed AML is typically resistant to chemotherapy, allogeneic HCT in CR1 (e.g., before relapse ever occurs) is a favored strategy. We have often explained to patients that transplant can effectively "eliminate the needle in a haystack, but not a stack of needles." Transplant is recommended for patients age <75 years who do not have favorable-risk disease and who have an HLA-matched donor (related or unrelated). We also recommend allogeneic HCT in CR1 for patients with intermediate-risk disease (Table 104-3). However, considerable debate exists regarding whether allogeneic HCT in CR1 is a requirement for younger patients with intermediate-risk AML, as one large series from the Medical Research Council reported that such patients have similar outcomes if transplanted only after relapse (and achievement of CR2), sparing some the long-term morbidity of transplantation. That said, allogeneic HCT is generally recommended as soon as possible after CR1 is achieved unless the patient is in a favorable-risk group. Increasingly, patients without HLA-matched donors are considered for alternative donor transplants (e.g., HLA-mismatched unrelated, haploidentical related, and umbilical cord blood) even in CR1. More effective and safe methods of in vivo T-cell depletion (i.e., posttransplant cyclophosphamide following mismatched transplantation) have broadened the availability of potential allogeneic HCT donors. Now, virtually any patient with a healthy parent or child (i.e., haploidentical) has an available donor suitable for allogeneic HCT if desired. Long-term outcomes with conventional chemotherapy for older patients are dismal; transplantation for such patients is expanding. Even for older patients, nonrandomized data demonstrate curative potential for older patients in CR1 treated with reduced-intensity conditioning regimens and allogeneic HCT.

Trials comparing allogeneic HCT with intensive chemotherapy or autologous HCT have shown improved duration of remission with allogeneic HCT. However, the relapse risk reduction observed with allogeneic HCT is partially offset by the increase in fatal treatment-related toxicity (GVHD, organ toxicity). Despite this, there is no debate that patients with adverse-risk AML have improved long-term survival with early allogeneic HCT. Alternatively, high-dose chemotherapy with autologous HCT rescue is another postremission approach in non–adverse-risk subsets. Autologous HCT patients receive their own stem cells (collected during remission and cryopreserved), following administration of myeloablative chemotherapy. The toxicity is relatively low with autologous HCT (5% mortality rate), but the relapse rate is higher than with allogeneic HCT due to the absence of the GVL effect. Favorable- and intermediate-risk patients may benefit from autologous HCT more so than adverse-risk patients. Practically speaking, however, autologous HCT in AML patients is less frequently employed currently due to enhanced relapse risk reduction seen with allogeneic HCT and the growing availability of HLA-mismatched donors (in novel transplantation approaches).

Prognostic factors help to select the appropriate postremission therapy in patients in CR1. Our approach includes allogeneic HCT in CR1 for patients without favorable cytogenetics or genotype. Patients with adverse-risk disease should proceed to allogeneic HCT at CR1 if possible. The decision for allogeneic HCT for younger intermediate-risk patients is complex and individualized as described above; we recommend it when an HLA-matched donor is available. Subsets of patients may benefit from targeted therapy given during remission; emerging data demonstrate survival benefit from incorporation of the FLT3 inhibitor midostaurin, for example, into induction and postremission therapies for patients with *FLT3*-mutated AML. Allogeneic transplantation in CR1 is still recommended for these patients.

For patients in morphologic CR, measurement of MRD remains a very important and challenging research area. Cytogenetics are a mainstay of disease assessment, and persistence of abnormal karyotype (in spite of morphologic CR) is clearly associated with poor clinical outcomes. Immunophenotyping to detect minute populations of blasts or sensitive molecular assays (e.g., reverse transcriptase polymerase chain reaction [RT-PCR]) to detect AML-associated molecular abnormalities (e.g., *NPM1*, *RUNX1/RUNX1T1* and *CBFB/MYH11* transcripts, *PML/RARA*) can be performed to assess whether MRD is present at sequential time points during or after treatment. Whether emerging next-generation sequencing or serial quantitative assessment using flow or RT-PCR, performed during remission, can effectively direct successful subsequent therapy and improve clinical outcome remains to be determined. Currently, no consensus exists for the optimal MRD measurement technique or its application, although it is increasingly employed in clinical practice. Data suggest that MRD measurement can in some settings be a reliable discriminator between patients who will continue in CR or relapse, but whether subsequent therapy (i.e., allogeneic HCT or additional therapy) can effectively eradicate disease in such patients is not yet clear. However, in the subset of patients with APL, serial RT-PCR (for the *PML/RARA* transcript) is a very useful and reliable tool to detect early relapse and to direct initiation of reinduction therapy prior to onset of overt relapse. Critical in the general understanding of MRD in all disease subsets is the recognition that even patients with undetectable levels of MRD remain at risk for leukemic relapse.

SUPPORTIVE CARE

Measures geared to supporting patients through several weeks of neutropenia and thrombocytopenia are critical to successful AML therapy. Patients with AML should be treated in centers expert in providing supportive care. Multi-lumen central venous catheters should be inserted as soon as newly diagnosed AML patients have been stabilized. They should be used thereafter for administration of intravenous medications/chemotherapy and transfusions, as well as for blood drawing instead of venipuncture during prolonged periods of myelosuppression.

Adequate and prompt blood bank support is critical to therapy of AML. Platelet transfusions should be given as needed to maintain a platelet count ≥10,000/μL. The platelet count should be kept at higher levels in febrile patients and during episodes of active bleeding or DIC. Patients with poor posttransfusion platelet count increments may benefit from administration of ABO-matched platelets or platelets from HLA-matched donors. RBC transfusions should be considered to keep the hemoglobin level >70–80 g/L (7–8 g/dL) in the absence of active bleeding, DIC, or congestive heart failure, which require higher hemoglobin levels. Blood products leukodepleted by filtration should be used to avert or delay alloimmunization as well as febrile reactions. Blood products may also be irradiated to prevent transfusion-associated GVHD. Cytomegalovirus (CMV)-negative blood products should be used for CMV-seronegative patients who are potential candidates for allogeneic HCT; fortunately, white blood cell filtration is quite effective at reducing CMV exposure as well.

Neutropenia (neutrophils <500/μL or <1000/μL and predicted to decline to <500/μL over the next 48 h) can be part of the initial presentation and/or a side effect of the chemotherapy treatment in AML patients. Thus, infectious complications remain the major cause of morbidity and death during induction and postremission chemotherapy for AML. Antibacterial (i.e., quinolones) and antifungal (i.e., posaconazole) prophylaxis, especially in conjunction with regimens that cause mucositis, is beneficial. For patients who are herpes simplex virus or varicella-zoster seropositive, antiviral prophylaxis should be initiated (e.g., acyclovir, valacyclovir).

Fever develops in most patients with AML, but infections are documented in only half of febrile patients. Early initiation of empirical broad-spectrum antibacterial and antifungal antibiotics has significantly reduced the number of patients dying of infectious complications (**Chap. 74**). An antibiotic regimen adequate to treat gram-negative organisms should be instituted at the onset of fever in a neutropenic patient after clinical evaluation, including a detailed physical examination with inspection of the indwelling catheter exit site and a perirectal examination (for perirectal abscess), as well as procurement of cultures and radiographs aimed at documenting the source of fever. Specific antibiotic regimens should be based on institutional antibiotic sensitivity data obtained from where the patient is being treated. Acceptable regimens for empiric antibiotic therapy include monotherapy with imipenem-cilastatin, meropenem, piperacillin/tazobactam, or an extended-spectrum antipseudomonal cephalosporin (cefepime or ceftazidime). The combination of an aminoglycoside with an antipseudomonal penicillin (e.g., piperacillin) or an aminoglycoside in combination with an extended-spectrum antipseudomonal cephalosporin should be considered in complicated or resistant cases. Aminoglycosides should be avoided, if possible, in patients with renal insufficiency. Empirical vancomycin should be added in neutropenic patients with catheter-related infections, blood cultures positive for gram-positive bacteria before final identification and susceptibility testing, hypotension or shock, or known colonization with penicillin/cephalosporin-resistant pneumococci or methicillin-resistant *Staphylococcus aureus*. In special situations where decreased susceptibility to vancomycin, vancomycin-resistant organisms, or vancomycin toxicity is documented, other options including linezolid and daptomycin need to be considered.

Caspofungin (or a similar echinocandin), voriconazole, isavuconazonium, or liposomal amphotericin B should be considered for antifungal treatment if fever persists for 4–7 days following initiation of empiric antibiotic therapy. Although liposomal formulations of amphotericin B have improved the toxicity profile of this agent, use has been limited to situations with high risk of or documented mold infections, especially in those in whom an azole fails. Caspofungin has been approved for empiric antifungal treatment. Voriconazole has also been shown to be equivalent in efficacy and less toxic than amphotericin B; isavuconazonium may also be effective with fewer drug-drug interactions. Antibacterial and antifungal antibiotics should be continued until patients are no longer neutropenic, regardless of whether a specific source has been found for the fever. Unfortunately, this practice likely contributes to development of resistance and increased incidence of nosocomial infections such as *Clostridium difficile* colitis, so great care should be taken preferably in hospital-wide antibiotic surveillance and isolation strategies to reduce these complications. Recombinant hematopoietic growth factors have a limited role in AML; myeloid growth factors may be useful in the postremission setting but are not recommended in induction or for "palliative" care for patients not in remission.

TREATMENT FOR REFRACTORY OR RELAPSED AML

In patients who relapse after achieving CR, the length of first CR is predictive of response to salvage chemotherapy treatment; patients with longer first CR (>12 months) generally relapse with drug-sensitive disease and have a higher chance of attaining a CR, even with the same chemotherapeutic agents used for first remission induction. Patients with short prior CR duration are at high risk for treatment failure. Similar to patients with refractory disease, patients with relapsed disease are rarely cured by salvage chemotherapy treatments alone. Therefore, patients who eventually achieve a second CR and are eligible for allogeneic HCT should be transplanted. For patients who relapse after allogeneic HCT, no consensus for best therapy exists; outcomes in this setting are very poor.

Because achievement of a second CR with routine salvage therapies is relatively uncommon, especially in patients who relapse rapidly after achievement of first CR (<12 months), these patients and those lacking HLA-compatible donors or who are not candidates for allogeneic HCT should be considered for innovative approaches on clinical trials. Many new agents are in current testing (Table 104-6). The discovery of novel gene mutations and mechanisms of leukemogenesis that might represent actionable therapeutic targets has prompted the development of many new targeting agents. In addition to kinase inhibitors for *FLT3*-mutated AML, other compounds targeting the aberrant activity of mutant proteins (e.g., IDH1/2 inhibitors) and numerous other biologic mechanisms are being tested in clinical trials. Inhibitors of FLT3 (gilteritinib), IDH1 (ivosidenib), or IDH2 (enasidenib) are monotherapies for relapsed AML patients who have targetable mutations. Furthermore, approaches with antibodies targeting markers commonly expressed on leukemia blasts (e.g., CD33) or leukemia-initiating cells (e.g., CD123) are also under investigation. Once these compounds have demonstrated safety and activity as single agents, investigation of combinations with other molecular targeting compounds and/or chemotherapy should be pursued.

TREATMENT OF ACUTE PROMYELOCYTIC LEUKEMIA

APL is a highly curable AML subtype, and ~85% of these patients achieve long-term survival with current approaches. APL has long been shown to be responsive to cytarabine and daunorubicin, but in the past, patients who were treated with these drugs alone frequently died from DIC induced by the release of granule components by the chemotherapy-treated leukemia cells. However, the prognosis of APL patients has changed dramatically with the introduction of tretinoin (all-*trans*-retinoic acid [ATRA]), an oral drug that induces the differentiation of leukemic cells bearing the t(15;17), where disruption of the *RARA* gene encoding a retinoid acid receptor occurs. ATRA decreases the frequency of DIC but often produces another complication called the APL (differentiation) syndrome. Occurring within the first 3 weeks of treatment, it is characterized by fever, fluid retention, dyspnea, chest pain, pulmonary infiltrates, pleural and pericardial effusions, and hypoxemia. The syndrome is related to adhesion of differentiated neoplastic cells to the pulmonary vasculature endothelium. Glucocorticoids, chemotherapy for cytoreduction, and/or supportive measures can be effective for management of the APL syndrome. Temporary discontinuation of ATRA is necessary in cases of severe APL syndrome (i.e., patients developing renal failure or requiring admission to the intensive care unit due to respiratory distress). The mortality rate of this syndrome is ~10%. APL syndrome may also occur, less commonly, with arsenic trioxide (ATO) in APL.

In adults with low-risk APL (low leukocyte count at presentation), ATRA (45 mg/m^2/d) plus ATO (0.15 mg/kg/d) was recently compared to ATRA plus concurrent idarubicin chemotherapy. ATRA/ATO was superior and is the new standard of care for such patients. CR rates in low-risk disease approach 100%, with excellent long-term survival. Notably, patients with high-risk APL (defined as leukocyte count >10,000/μL) must be uniquely treated, as they require immediate cytoreduction with chemotherapy due to life-threatening APL syndrome and rapidly rising leukocyte count after initiation of ATRA. High-risk patients are at increased risk for induction death due to this syndrome as well as increased frequency of hemorrhagic complications (related to DIC).

Assessment of residual disease by RT-PCR amplification of the t(15;17) chimeric gene product *PML-RARA* following the final cycle of treatment is important. Disappearance of the signal is associated with long-term disease-free survival; its persistence or reemergence invariably predicts relapse. Sequential monitoring of RT-PCR for *PML-RARA* is now considered standard for postremission monitoring of APL, at least in high-risk patients.

Patients in molecular, cytogenetic, or clinical relapse should be salvaged with ATO with or without ATRA; in patients who were treated with ATRA plus chemotherapy in the front-line setting, ATO-based therapy at relapse produces meaningful responses in up to 85% of patients. Although experience with relapsed APL in patients who received ATO during initial induction is limited (given that few relapses occur in low-risk patients and widespread use of ATO during first-line therapy is relatively new), ATO remains the preferred reinduction therapy for patients who relapse, although the duration of prior remission should be a factor in this choice. Achievement of CR2 should be followed by consolidation with autologous HCT (for patients who achieve RT-PCR-negative status). In the minority who do not achieve negative RT-PCR or who relapse again, allogeneic HCT may still be potentially curative.

ACKNOWLEDGEMENT

Clara Bloomfield, an important contributor to the field and to this chapter in past editions, passed away since the publication of the 20th edition. Material from prior versions of this chapter on which she was an author have been retained here.

FURTHER READING

ARBER DA et al: Acute myeloid leukaemia (AML) with recurrent genetic abnormalities, in *World Health Organization Classification of Tumours of Haematopoietic and Lymphoid Tissues*, 4th revised ed. Geneva, Switzerland: World Health Organization; 2016.

DINARDO CD et al: Venetoclax combined with decitabine or azacitidine in treatment-naive, elderly patients with acute myeloid leukemia. Blood 133:7, 2019.

DÖHNER H et al: Diagnosis and management of acute myeloid leukemia in adults: 2017 recommendations from an international expert panel, on behalf of the European LeukemiaNet. Blood 129:424, 2017.

JAISWAL S, EBERT BL: Clonal hematopoiesis in human aging and disease. Science 366:eaan4673, 2019.

JONGEN-LAVRENIC M et al: Molecular minimal residual disease in acute myeloid leukemia. N Engl J Med 378:1189, 2018.

LO-COCO F et al: Retinoic acid and arsenic trioxide for acute promyelocytic leukemia. N Engl J Med 369:111, 2013.

PAPAEMMANUIL E et al: Genomic classification and prognosis in acute myeloid leukemia. N Engl J Med 374:2209, 2016.

PERL AE et al: Gilteritinib or chemotherapy for relapsed or refractory FLT3-mutated AML. N Engl J Med 381:1728, 2019.

POLLYEA DA et al: Enasidenib, an inhibitor of mutant IDH2 proteins, induces durable remissions in older patients with newly diagnosed acute myeloid leukemia. Leukemia 33:2575, 2019.

ROBOZ GJ et al: Ivosidenib induces deep durable remissions in patients with newly diagnosed IDH1-mutant acute myeloid leukemia. Blood 135:463, 2020.

STONE RM et al: Midostaurin plus chemotherapy for acute myeloid leukemia with a FLT3 mutation. N Engl J Med 377:454, 2017.

105 Chronic Myeloid Leukemia

Hagop Kantarjian, Elias Jabbour, Jorge Cortes

Chronic myeloid leukemia (CML) is a clonal hematopoietic myeloproliferative stem cell neoplasm. The disease is driven by the *BCR/ABL1* chimeric gene that codes for a constitutively active tyrosine kinase, resulting from a reciprocal balanced translocation between the long arms of chromosomes 9 and 22, t(9;22)(q34.1;q11.2), known as the

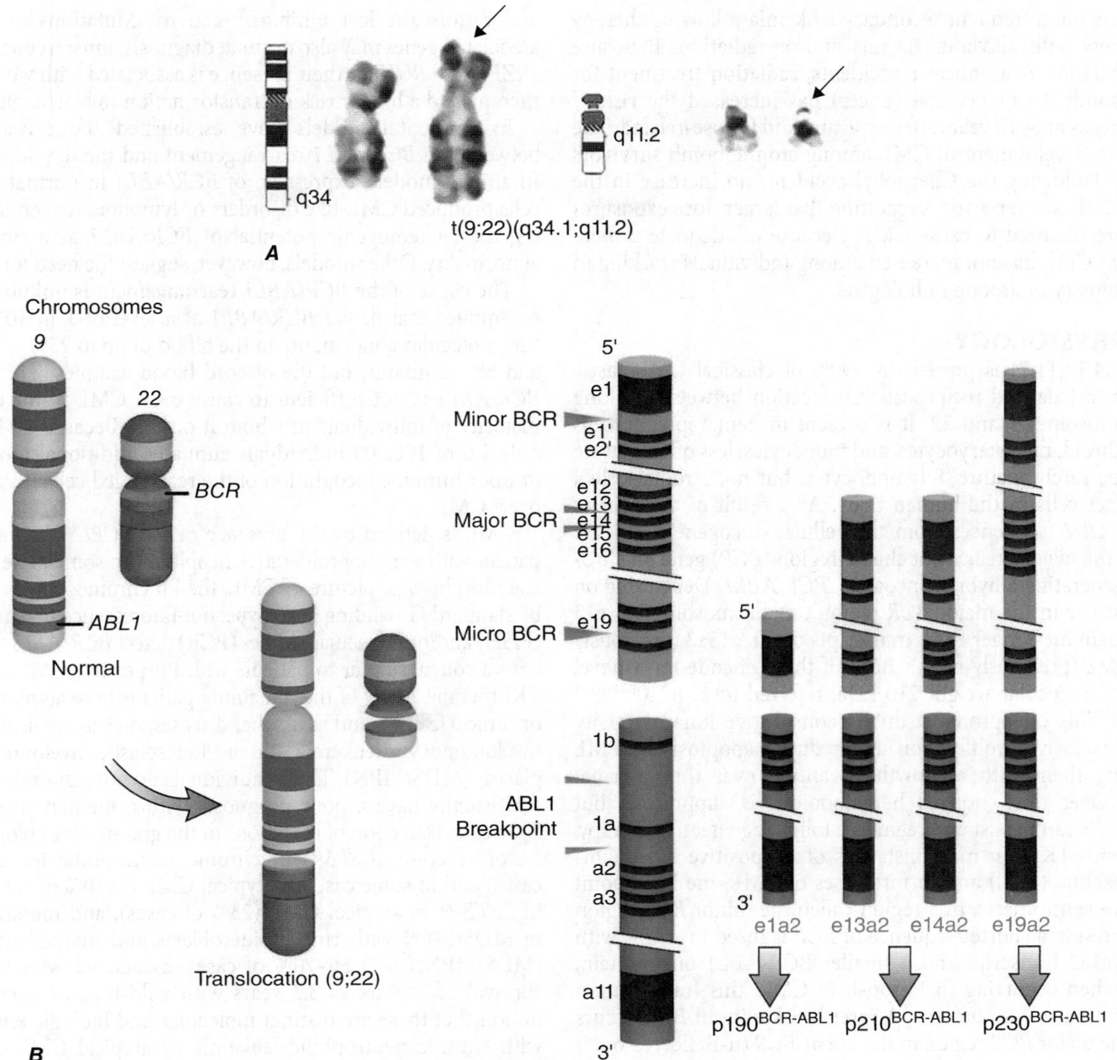

FIGURE 105-1 ***A.*** The Philadelphia (Ph) chromosome cytogenetic abnormality. ***B.*** Breakpoints in the long arms of chromosome 9 (*ABL1* locus) and chromosome 22 (*BCR* regions) result in at least three different BCR-ABL1 oncoprotein messages, p210$^{BCR-ABL1}$ (most common message in chronic myeloid leukemia [CML]), p190$^{BCR-ABL1}$ (present in two-thirds of patients with Ph-positive acute lymphoblastic leukemia; rare in CML), and p230$^{BCR-ABL1}$ (rare in CML and associated with an indolent course). Other rearrangements (e.g., e14a3, e14a3) are less common. *(© 2013 The University of Texas MD Anderson Cancer Center.)*

Philadelphia chromosome (Ph) (Fig. 105-1). Untreated, the course of CML is typically biphasic or triphasic, with an early indolent or chronic phase, followed often by an accelerated phase and a terminal blastic phase. Before the era of BCR-ABL1 tyrosine kinase inhibitors (TKIs), the median survival in CML was 3–7 years, and the 10-year survival rate was 30% or less. Introduced into standard CML therapy in 2000, TKIs have revolutionized the treatment, natural history, and prognosis of CML. Today, the estimated 10-year survival rate with imatinib mesylate, the first BCR-ABL1 TKI approved, is greater than 85% and approaches that of the general population. Allogeneic stem cell transplantation (SCT), a curative approach but one that involves more risks, is now offered as second- or third-line therapy after failure of TKIs.

INCIDENCE AND EPIDEMIOLOGY

CML accounts for ~15% of all cases of leukemia. There is a slight male predominance (male-to-female ratio 1.6:1). The median age at diagnosis is 55–65 years. It is uncommon in children; only 3% of patients with CML are younger than 20 years, although in recent years, a higher proportion of young patients are diagnosed. The incidence of CML increases gradually with age, with a steeper increase after the age of 40–50 years. The annual incidence of CML is 1.6 cases per 100,000 individuals. In the United States, this translates into about 8500–9000 new cases per year. The incidence of CML has not changed over several decades. By extrapolation, the worldwide annual incidence of CML is about 200,000 cases. With a median survival of 3–6 years before 2000, the disease prevalence in the United States was ~30,000 cases. With TKI therapy, the annual mortality has been reduced from 10–20% to about 2%. Therefore, the prevalence of CML is expected to continue to increase. Based on an estimated annual mortality of 2% and an incidence of 8500 cases per year, the plateau prevalence of CML is estimated to be reached at ~425,000 in the United Stated (8500 × 100/2) by about 2040, with full TKI optimal treatment penetration. The worldwide prevalence will depend on the treatment penetration of TKIs and their effect on reduction of worldwide annual mortality. Ideally, with full TKI treatment penetration, the worldwide prevalence should plateau at 35 times the incidence, or ~9–10 million patients. These estimates are all based on extrapolations from the incidence and prevalence of CML in the United States, as well as an estimated annual mortality of 2% with modern TKI therapy; they could vary considerably if the estimates were to change.

ETIOLOGY

There are no familial associations in CML. The risk of developing CML is not increased in monozygotic twins or in relatives of patients with CML. No etiologic agents are incriminated, and no associations exist with exposures to benzene or other toxins, fertilizers, insecticides, or viruses. CML is not a frequent secondary leukemia following therapy of other cancers with alkylating agents and/or radiation. Exposure to ionizing radiation (e.g., nuclear accidents, radiation treatment for ankylosing spondylitis or cervical cancer) has increased the risk of CML, which peaks at 5–10 years after exposure and is dose-related. The median time to development of CML among atomic bomb survivors was 6.3 years. Following the Chernobyl accident, no increase in the incidence of CML was reported, suggesting that larger dose exposures of radiation are required to cause CML. Because of adequate protection, the risk of CML has not increased among individuals working in the nuclear industry or among radiologists.

PATHOPHYSIOLOGY

The t(9;22)(q34.1;q11.2) is present in >90% of classical CML cases. It results from a balanced reciprocal translocation between the long arms of chromosomes 9 and 22. It is present in hematopoietic cells (myeloid, erythroid, megakaryocytes, and monocytes; less often mature B lymphocytes; rarely mature T lymphocytes, but not stromal cells), but not in other cells in the human body. As a result of the genetic translocation, DNA sequences from the cellular oncogene *ABL1* are juxtaposed to the major breakpoint cluster region (*BCR*) gene on chromosome 22, generating a hybrid oncogene, *BCR/ABL1*. Depending on the breakpoint site in the major *BCR* region on chromosome 22 (e13 or e14), two main messenger RNA transcripts occur, e13a2 (previously b2a2) and e14a2 (previously b3a2). Both of them encode for a novel oncoprotein of molecular weight 210 kDa, referred to as p210$^{BCR-ABL1}$ (Fig. 105-1*B*). This oncoprotein exhibits constitutive kinase activity that leads to excessive proliferation and reduced apoptosis of CML cells, endowing them with a growth advantage over their normal counterparts. Over time, normal hematopoiesis is suppressed, but normal stem cells can persist and reemerge following effective therapy, for example with TKIs. In most instances of Ph-positive acute lymphoblastic leukemia (ALL) and in rare cases of CML, the breakpoint in *BCR* is more centromeric, in a region called the minor *BCR* region (*mBCR*). As a result, a shorter sequence of *BCR* is fused to *ABL1*, with a consequent e1a2 transcript and a smaller BCR-ABL1 oncoprotein, p190$^{BCR-ABL1}$. When occurring in Ph-positive CML, this translocation is associated with a worse outcome. A rarer breakpoint in *BCR* occurs telomeric to the major *BCR* region in the *micro-BCR* (μ-BCR) region. It juxtaposes a larger fragment of the *BCR* gene to *ABL1* and produces an e19a2 transcript and a larger p230$^{BCR-ABL1}$ oncoprotein (associated with a more indolent CML course). Other rearrangements (based on different breakpoints in the *ABL* region), such as e13a3 or e14a3 (also resulting in a p210$^{BCR-ABL1}$ oncoprotein), occur much less frequently. These are not readily identifiable nor quantifiable with the routine polymerase chain reaction (PCR) probes, thus producing falsely negative PCR levels on follow-up studies if not tested at diagnosis.

The constitutive activation of *BCR/ABL1* results in autophosphorylation and activation of multiple downstream pathways that affect gene transcription, apoptosis, stromal adherence, skeletal organization, and degradation of inhibitory proteins. These transduction pathways involve RAS, mitogen-activated protein (MAP) kinases, signal transducers and activators of transcription (STAT), phosphatidylinositol-3-kinase (PI3k), MYC, and others. These interactions are mostly mediated through tyrosine phosphorylation and require binding of BCR-ABL1 to adapter proteins such as GRB-2, CRK, CRK-like (CRK-L) protein, and Src homology containing proteins (SHC). Most BCR-ABL1 TKIs bind to the BCR-ABL1 ATP-binding domain, inhibiting its kinase activity, preventing the activation of transformation pathways, and inhibiting downstream signaling. As a result, proliferation of CML cells is inhibited and apoptosis induced, allowing the reemergence of normal hematopoiesis. An additional layer of complexity is related to differences in signal transduction between CML-differentiated cells and early progenitors. Beta-catenin, Wnt1, Foxo3a, transforming growth factor β, interleukin-6, PP2A, SIRT1, and others have been implicated in CML stem cell survival. ABL1 also has a myristoyl site that functions as a negative regulator of its kinase activity. This site and its negative regulatory activity are lost upon fusion with BCR. Novel ABL1 inhibitors (e.g., asciminib) bind this myristoyl site and restore the lost inhibitory activity. Mutations in other cancer-associated genes may also occur at diagnosis, most frequently in *ASXL1*, *IKZF1*, and *RUNX1*; their presence is associated with worse response to therapy and a higher risk of transformation to blastic phase.

Experimental models have established the causal relationship between the *BCR/ABL1* rearrangement and the development of CML. In animal models, expression of *BCR/ABL1* in normal hematopoietic cells produced CML-like disorders or lymphoid leukemia, demonstrating the leukemogenic potential of *BCR/ABL1* as a single oncogenic abnormality. Other models, however, suggest the need for a "second hit."

The cause of the *BCR/ABL1* rearrangement is unknown. Molecular techniques that detect *BCR/ABL1* at a level of 1 in 10^8 cells identify this molecular abnormality in the blood of up to 25% of normal adults and 5% of infants, but 0% of cord blood samples. This suggests that *BCR/ABL1* is not sufficient to cause overt CML in the overwhelming majority of individuals in whom it occurs. Because CML develops in only 1.6 of 100,000 individuals annually, additional molecular events or poor immune recognition of the rearranged cells may contribute to overt CML.

CML is defined by the presence of the *BCR/ABL1* fusion gene in a patient with a myeloproliferative neoplasm. In some patients with a typical morphologic picture of CML, the Ph chromosome is not detectable by standard G-banding karyotype, but fluorescence in situ hybridization (FISH) and/or molecular studies (PCR) detect *BCR/ABL1*. These patients have a course similar to patients with Ph-positive CML and respond to TKI therapy. Many of the remaining patients have atypical morphologic or clinical features and have other diseases, such as atypical CML, chronic myelomonocytic leukemia, and myelodysplastic/myeloproliferative neoplasms (MDS/MPN). These individuals do not respond to TKI therapy and usually have a poor prognosis with a median survival of about 2–3 years. Detection of mutations in the granulocyte colony-stimulating factor receptor (*CSF3R*) in chronic neutrophilic leukemia (80% of cases) and in some cases of atypical CML (5–10% of cases), mutations in *SETBP1* in atypical CML (25% of cases), and mutations in *SF3B1* in MDS/MPN with ringed sideroblasts and marked thrombocytosis (MDS/MPN-RS-T; 50–70% of cases, associated with longer median survival of 7 years vs 3.3 years with wild-type *SF3B1*) supports the notion that these are distinct molecular and biologic entities. Patients with chronic neutrophilic leukemia or atypical CML whose disease is associated with *CSF3R* mutation may respond well to ruxolitinib (a JAK2 inhibitor) therapy (complete response in 50–60% of such patients).

The events associated with the transition of CML from a chronic to accelerated-blastic phase are poorly understood. Characteristic chromosomal abnormalities such as a double Ph, trisomy 8, isochromosome 17 or deletion of 17p (loss of *TP53*), 20q−, translocations involving 3q26, and others may be seen with disease acceleration. Molecular events associated with transformation include mutations in *TP53*, retinoblastoma 1 (*RB1*), myeloid transcriptions factors like *RUNX1*, and cell cycle regulators like *p16*. A plethora of other mutations or functional abnormalities have been implicated in blastic transformation, but no unifying theme has emerged other than the fact that *BCR/ABL1* itself induces genetic instability that favors the acquisition of additional molecular defects and eventually results in blastic transformation. One critical effect of TKIs is to stabilize the CML genome, leading to a reduced transformation rate. In particular, the previously observed sudden blastic transformations (i.e., abrupt transformation to blastic phase in a patient who had been in cytogenetic response) have become uncommon, occurring rarely in younger patients in the first 1–2 years of TKI therapy (usually sudden lymphoid blastic transformations). Sudden transformations beyond the third year of TKI therapy are rare in patients who continue on TKI therapy. Moreover, the course of CML is now frequently more indolent in patients treated with TKI, even without cytogenetic response, compared to previous experience with hydroxyurea/busulfan, suggesting a definite clinical benefit of continued inhibition of the kinase activity.

Among patients developing resistance to TKIs, several resistance mechanisms have been observed. The most clinically relevant one is the development of *ABL1* kinase domain mutations that may prevent the binding of TKIs to the catalytic site (ATP-binding site) of the kinase or maintain the kinase activity despite the presence of a TKI. More than 100 *ABL1* kinase domain mutations have now been described, many of which confer relative or absolute resistance to imatinib. Consequently, second-generation (i.e., dasatinib, nilotinib, bosutinib) and third-generation (ponatinib) TKIs were developed, the latter with significant efficacy against T315I, a "gatekeeper" mutation that prevents binding of and causes resistance to all other currently available TKIs. Asciminib, olverembatinib (HQP1351) and other novel TKIs under development are also active against the T315I mutation.

CLINICAL PRESENTATION

The presenting signs and symptoms in CML depend on the availability of and access to health care, including physical examinations and screening tests. In the United States, because of the wider access to health care screening and physical examinations, 50–60% of patients are diagnosed on routine blood tests and have minimal symptoms at presentation, such as fatigue. In geographic locations where access to health care is more limited, patients often present with high CML burden including splenomegaly, anemia, and related symptoms (abdominal pain, weight loss, fatigue), associated with a higher frequency of high-risk CML. Presenting findings in patients diagnosed in the United States are shown in **Table 105-1**.

Symptoms Most patients with CML (90%) present in the indolent or chronic phase. Depending on the timing of diagnosis, patients are often asymptomatic (if the diagnosis is discovered during health care screening tests). Common symptoms, when present, are manifestations of anemia and splenomegaly. These may include fatigue, malaise, weight loss (if high leukemia burden), or early satiety and left upper quadrant pain or masses (from splenomegaly). Less common presenting findings include thrombotic or hyperviscosity-related events from severe leukocytosis or thrombocytosis. These include priapism, cardiovascular complications, myocardial infarction, venous thrombosis, visual disturbances, dyspnea and pulmonary insufficiency, drowsiness, loss of coordination, confusion, or cerebrovascular accidents.

TABLE 105-1 Presenting Signs and Symptoms of Newly Diagnosed Philadelphia Chromosome–Positive Chronic Myeloid Leukemia in Chronic Phase

PARAMETER	PERCENTAGE
Age ≥60 years (median)	40–50 (55–65)
Female gender	35–45
Splenomegaly	30
Hepatomegaly	5–10
Lymphadenopathy	5
Other extramedullary disease	2
Hemoglobin <10 g/dL	10–15
Platelets	
>450 × 10⁹ cells/L	30–35
<100 × 10⁹ cells/L	3–5
White blood cells ≥50 × 10⁹ cells/L	35–40
Marrow	
≥5% blasts	5
≥5% basophils	10–15
Peripheral blood	
≥3% blasts	8–10
≥7% basophils	10
Cytogenetic clonal evolution other than the Philadelphia chromosome	4–5
Sokal risk	
Low	60–65
Intermediate	25–30
High	10

Manifestations of bleeding diatheses include retinal hemorrhages, gastrointestinal bleeding, and others. Patients who present with, or progress to, the accelerated or blastic phases frequently have additional symptoms including unexplained fever, significant weight loss, severe fatigue, bone and joint pain, bleeding and thrombotic events, and infections.

Physical Findings Splenomegaly is the most common physical finding, occurring in 20–70% of patients depending on health care screening frequency. Other less common findings include hepatomegaly (5–10%), lymphadenopathy (5–10%), and extramedullary disease (skin or subcutaneous lesions). The latter indicates CML transformation if a biopsy confirms predominance of blasts. Other physical findings are manifestations of complications of high tumor burden described earlier (e.g., cardiovascular, cerebrovascular, bleeding). High basophil counts may be associated with histamine overproduction causing pruritus, diarrhea, flushing, and even gastrointestinal ulcers.

Hematologic and Marrow Findings In untreated CML, leukocytosis ranging from 10–500 × 10^9/L is common. The peripheral blood differential shows left-shifted hematopoiesis with predominance of neutrophils and the presence of bands, myelocytes, metamyelocytes, promyelocytes, and blasts (usually ≤5%). Basophils and/or eosinophils are frequently increased. Thrombocytosis is common, but thrombocytopenia is rare and, when present, suggests a worse prognosis, disease acceleration, or an unrelated etiology. Anemia is present in one-third of patients. Cyclic oscillations of counts are noted in 10–20% of patients without treatment. Biochemical abnormalities include a low leukocyte alkaline phosphatase score and high levels of vitamin B_{12}, uric acid, lactic dehydrogenase, and lysozyme. The presence of unexplained and sustained leukocytosis, with or without splenomegaly, should lead to a marrow examination and cytogenetic analysis.

The bone marrow is hypercellular with marked myeloid hyperplasia and a high myeloid-to-erythroid ratio of 15–20:1. Marrow blasts are typically 5% or less; when higher, they carry a worse prognosis or represent transformation to accelerated phase (if they are ≥15%). Increased reticulin fibrosis (detected with silver stain) is common, with 30–40% of patients demonstrating grade 3–4 reticulin fibrosis. This was considered adverse in the pre-TKI era. With TKI therapy, reticulin fibrosis resolves in most patients and is not an indicator of poor prognosis. Collagen fibrosis (Wright-Giemsa stain) is rare at diagnosis. Disease progression with a "spent phase" of myelofibrosis (myelophthisis, or burnt-out marrow) was a relatively common end-stage CML condition with busulfan therapy (20–30%); it is extremely rare now with TKI therapy.

Cytogenetic and Molecular Findings The diagnosis of CML is straightforward and depends on documenting the t(9;22) (q34.1;q11.2), which is identified by G-banding in 90% of cases. This is known as the Philadelphia chromosome (initially identified in Philadelphia as a minute chromosome, later identified to be chromosome 22) (Fig. 105-1). Some patients (~10%) may have complex translocations (complex variant Ph) involving three or more chromosomes including chromosomes 9 and 22 and one or more additional chromosomes. Others may have a "masked Ph," involving translocations between chromosome 9 and a chromosome other than 22 (but molecularly showing the *BCR/ABL1* rearrangement; known as simple variant Ph). The prognosis of these patients and their response to TKI therapy are similar to those in patients with Ph. About 5–10% of patients may have additional chromosomal abnormalities (ACAs) in the Ph-positive cells at diagnosis. These usually involve trisomy 8, a double Ph, isochromosome 17 or 17p deletion, 20q–, or others. This is referred to as cytogenetic clonal evolution and was historically a sign of adverse prognosis, particularly when trisomy 8, double Ph, or chromosome 17 abnormalities were noted. A less common abnormality involving chromosome 3q26.2 occurs with disease progression and carries a poor prognosis.

Techniques such as FISH and PCR are now used to aid in the diagnosis of CML. They are more sensitive to estimate the CML burden in patients on TKI therapy. They can be done on peripheral blood and thus are more convenient to patients. Patients with CML at diagnosis should have a FISH analysis to quantify the percentage of Ph-positive cells, if FISH is used to replace marrow cytogenetic analysis in monitoring response to therapy. FISH will not detect additional chromosomal abnormalities (clonal evolution); thus, a cytogenetic analysis is recommended at the time of diagnosis. In addition, 10–15% of patients may develop chromosomal abnormalities in Ph-negative metaphases after responding to TKIs. These abnormalities may carry a worse prognosis but are not detected by FISH unless already identified and FISH is used to follow them. Molecular studies at diagnosis are important to document the type and presence of *BCR-ABL1* transcripts to avoid spurious "undetectable" *BCR-ABL1* transcripts on follow-up studies, with the false impression of a complete molecular response. The presence of the Philadelphia chromosome with "negative" PCR with standard methodology should prompt investigation of atypical transcripts.

Both FISH and PCR studies can be falsely positive at low levels or falsely negative because of technical issues. Therefore, a diagnosis of CML must always rely on a marrow analysis with routine cytogenetics. The diagnostic bone marrow confirms the presence of the Ph chromosome, detects clonal evolution, and quantifies the percentage of marrow blasts and basophils. In 10% of patients, the percentage of marrow blasts and basophils can be significantly higher than in the peripheral blood, conferring poorer prognosis or even representing disease transformation.

Monitoring patients on TKI therapy by cytogenetics, FISH, and PCR has become an important standard practice to assess response to therapy, emphasize compliance, evaluate possible treatment resistance, identify the need to change TKI therapy, and determine the need to assess for kinase domain mutations. Because of the decreasing reliance of bone marrow aspirations to monitor response, equivalence has been established to correlate cytogenetic results with PCR values. These are not absolute correlations but provide adequate guidance. A partial cytogenetic response is defined as the presence of 35% or less Ph-positive metaphases by routine cytogenetic analysis. This is roughly equivalent to *BCR-ABL1* transcripts by the International Scale (IS) of 10% or less. A complete cytogenetic response refers to the absence of Ph-positive metaphases (0% Ph positivity). This is approximately equivalent to *BCR-ABL1* transcripts (IS) of 1% or less. A major molecular response (MMR or MR3) refers to *BCR-ABL1* transcripts (IS) ≤0.1%, or roughly a 3-log or greater reduction of *BCR-ABL1* transcripts from a standardized baseline. MR4 refers to *BCR-ABL1* transcripts (IS) ≤0.01%, and MR4.5 (deep molecular response) refers to *BCR-ABL1* transcripts (IS) ≤0.0032%, roughly equivalent to a 4.5-log reduction or greater of transcripts.

Findings in CML Transformation Progression of CML is usually associated with leukocytosis resistant to therapy, increasing anemia, fever and constitutional symptoms, and increased blasts and basophils in the peripheral blood or marrow. Criteria of accelerated-phase CML, historically associated with median survival of <1.5 years, include the presence of 15% or more peripheral blasts, 30% or more peripheral blasts plus promyelocytes, 20% or more peripheral basophils, cytogenetic clonal evolution (presence of chromosomal abnormalities in addition to Ph), and thrombocytopenia $<100 \times 10^9$/L (unrelated to therapy). About 5–10% of patients present with de novo accelerated phase or blastic phase. The prognosis of de novo accelerated phase with TKI therapy has improved significantly, with an estimated 8-year survival rate of 75%. The median survival of accelerated phase evolving from chronic phase has also improved from a historical median survival of 18 months to an estimated 4-year survival rate of 70% on TKI therapy. Therefore, the criteria for accelerated-phase CML should be revisited because most clinical criteria defining accelerated phase have lost much of their prognostic significance. Blastic-phase CML is defined by the presence of 30% or more peripheral or marrow blasts or the presence of sheets of blasts in extramedullary disease (usually skin, soft tissues, or lytic bone lesions). Blastic-phase CML is commonly myeloid (60%) but can present uncommonly as erythroid, promyelocytic, monocytic, or megakaryocytic. Lymphoid blastic phase occurs in about 25% of patients. Lymphoblasts are terminal deoxynucleotide transferase positive and peroxidase negative (although occasionally with low positivity up to 3–5%) and express lymphoid markers (CD10, CD19, CD20, CD22). However, they also often express myeloid markers (50–80%), resulting in diagnostic challenges. Proper immunophenotypic diagnosis is important because lymphoid blastic-phase CML is quite responsive to anti-ALL-type chemotherapy (e.g., hyper-CVAD [cyclophosphamide, vincristine, doxorubicin, and dexamethasone]) in combination with TKIs (complete response rate 70%; median survival 3 years; high rates of bridging to allogeneic SCT and possible cure).

PROGNOSIS AND CML COURSE

Before the imatinib era, the annual mortality in CML was 10% in the first 2 years and 15–20% thereafter. The median survival in CML was 3–7 years (with hydroxyurea-busulfan and interferon α). Without a curative option of allogeneic SCT, the course of CML was toward transformation to, and death from, accelerated or blastic phases for most patients as the rate of complete cytogenetic response with interferon was low. Even apparent disease stability was unpredictable, with some patients demonstrating sudden transformation to a blastic phase. With imatinib therapy, the annual mortality in CML has decreased to 1–2% in the first 20 years of observation. More than half of the deaths are from conditions other than CML, such as old age, comorbidities, accidents, suicides, other cancers, and other medical conditions (e.g., infections, surgical procedures). The estimated 10-year survival rate is 86%, or 92% if only CML-related deaths are considered (**Fig. 105-2**). The course of CML has also become quite predictable. In the first 2 years of TKI therapy, rare sudden transformations are still reported (1–2%), usually lymphoid blastic transformations that respond to combinations of chemotherapy and TKIs followed by allogeneic SCT. These may be explained by the intrinsic mechanisms of sudden transformation already existing in the CML clones before the start of therapy that were not amenable to TKI inhibition, in particular imatinib. Second-generation TKIs (nilotinib, dasatinib, bosutinib) used as frontline therapy have reduced the incidence of transformation in the first 2–3 years from 6–8% with imatinib to 2–5% with second-generation TKIs. Disease transformation to accelerated or blastic phase is rare with continued TKI therapy, estimated at <1% annually in years 4–10 of follow-up on the original imatinib trials. Patients usually develop resistance in the form of cytogenetic resistance or relapse, followed by hematologic relapse and subsequent transformation, rather than the previously feared sudden transformations without the warning signals of cytogenetic-hematologic relapse.

Before the imatinib era, several pretreatment prognostic factors predicted for worse outcome in CML and have been incorporated into prognostic models and staging systems. These have included older age, significant splenomegaly, anemia, thrombocytopenia or thrombocytosis, high percentages of blasts and basophils (and/or eosinophils), marrow fibrosis, interstitial deletions in the long arm of chromosome 9, clonal evolution, and others. Different risk models and staging systems, derived from multivariate analyses, were proposed to define different risk groups. As with the introduction of cisplatin into testicular cancer therapy, the introduction of TKIs into CML therapy has decreased or, in some instances, eliminated the prognostic impact of most of these prognostic factors and the significance of the CML models (e.g., Sokal, Hasford, European Treatment and Outcome Study [EUTOS]). Treatment-related prognostic factors have emerged as the most important prognostic factors in the era of imatinib therapy. Achievement of complete cytogenetic response has become the major therapeutic endpoint and is the only endpoint associated with improvement in survival. Achievement of MMR or MR3 is associated with decreased risk of events (relapse) and CML transformation but has not been associated with survival prolongation among patients with complete cytogenetic response. This may be due to the survival benefit conferred by the achievement of complete cytogenetic response, which approximates normal life expectancy, and to the efficacy of salvage TKI therapies, which are and should be implemented at the first evidence of cytogenetic relapse. Achievement of undetectable *BCR-ABL1* transcripts (complete molecular response [CMR]) or deep molecular response (DMR; defined as MR4 or MR4.5), particularly when sustained (>2–5 years), may offer the possibility of treatment-free remission and may

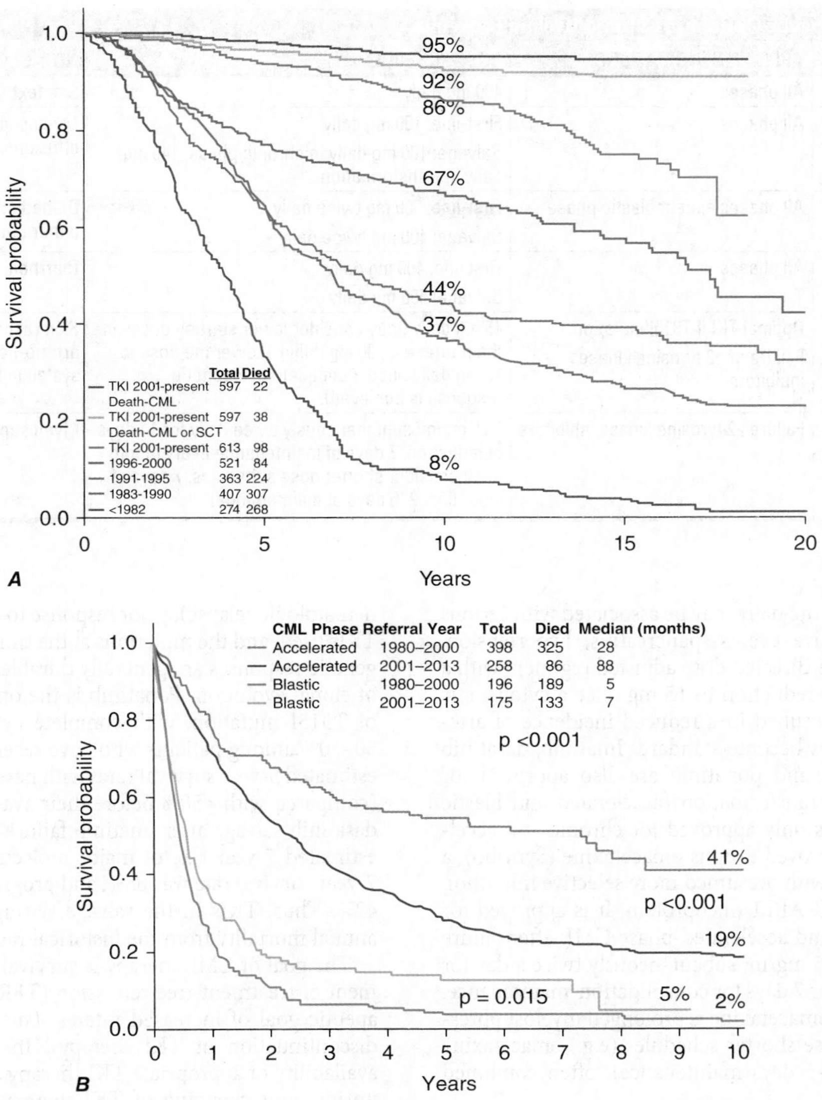

FIGURE 105-2 ***A.*** Survival in newly diagnosed chronic-phase chronic myeloid leukemia (CML) by era of therapy (MD Anderson Cancer Center experience from 1965 to present). Top blue curve is survival with tyrosine kinase inhibitors (TKIs), accounting for only CML-related deaths. The orange curve (second from top) accounts for deaths related to CML or CML treatment complications (e.g., deaths following allogeneic stem cell transplant [SCT]). The red curve (third from top) is survival including all deaths regardless of causality (old age, car accidents, suicide, gun shots, second cancers, complications of unrelated surgeries, infections, others). The difference in the denominators, 613 minus 597 cases, is because 16 deaths were from unknown/undocumented causes (outside MD Anderson and no good tracking for cause of death). ***B.*** Survival in patients with accelerated- and blastic-phase CML referred to MD Anderson Cancer Center by era of therapy, demonstrating the significant survival benefit in the TKI era in accelerated-phase CML but the modest benefit in blastic-phase CML. Referred cases included de novo and post-chronic-phase transformations.

allow temporary therapy interruption in women pursuing pregnancy. The lack of achievement of MMR or DMR should not be considered as "failure" of a particular TKI therapy and/or an indication to change the TKI or to consider allogeneic SCT.

Long-term updates of randomized trials suggest that second-generation TKIs and imatinib are similarly effective in lower-risk CML; second-generation TKIs may offer a therapeutic advantage among patients with high-risk CML.

TREATMENT

Chronic Myeloid Leukemia

Since 2001, six drugs have been approved by the U.S. Food and Drug Administration (FDA) for the treatment of CML. These include five oral TKIs: imatinib (Gleevec, Glivec), nilotinib (Tasigna), dasatinib (Sprycel), bosutinib (Bosulif), and ponatinib (Iclusig). Dasatinib, nilotinib, and bosutinib are referred to as second-generation TKIs; ponatinib is referred to as a third-generation TKI. Nilotinib is similar in structure to imatinib but 30 times more potent. Dasatinib and bosutinib inhibit the SRC family of kinases in addition to ABL1, with dasatinib reported to be 300 times more potent and bosutinib 30–50 times more potent than imatinib. In contrast to all other TKIs, bosutinib has no activity against c-Kit or platelet-derived growth factor receptor (PDGFR). Ponatinib is highly effective against wild-type and mutant *BCR/ABL1* clones. It is also the only available BCR-ABL1 TKI active against T315I, a gatekeeper mutation resistant to the other four ATP-competitive TKIs **(Table 105-2)**. Ponatinib also inhibits vascular endothelial growth factor receptor (VEGFR), which may be at least partly responsible for the high incidence of hypertension observed with this agent (Table 105-2). Imatinib 400 mg orally daily, nilotinib 300 mg orally twice a day (on an empty stomach), dasatinib 100 mg orally daily, and bosutinib 400 mg orally daily are approved for frontline therapy of CML. Dasatinib 50 mg orally daily is as effective in frontline therapy as 100 mg daily, and significantly less toxic. All four are also approved for salvage therapy (nilotinib 400 mg twice daily; bosutinib 500 mg daily; others at the same dose as frontline therapy), in addition to ponatinib

TABLE 105-2 Medical Therapeutic Options in Chronic Myeloid Leukemia

AGENT (BRAND NAME)	APPROVED INDICATIONS	DOSE SCHEDULE	NOTABLE TOXICITIES
Imatinib mesylate (Gleevec)	All phases	400 mg daily	See text
Dasatinib (Sprycel)	All phases	First-line: 100 mg daily Salvage: 100 mg daily in chronic phase; 140 mg daily in transformation	Myelosuppression; pleural and pericardial effusions; pulmonary hypertension
Nilotinib (Tasigna)	All phases except blastic phase	First-line: 300 mg twice daily Salvage: 400 mg twice daily	Diabetes; arterio-occlusive disease; pancreatitis
Bosutinib (Bosulif)	All phases	First line: 400 mg daily Salvage: 500 mg daily	Diarrhea; liver toxicity; renal dysfunction
Ponatinib (Iclusig)	Optimal TKI if T315I mutation Failure of ≥2 tyrosine kinase inhibitors	45 mg daily (may consider lower starting doses in the future, e.g., 30 mg daily). (Lower the dose to 15 mg daily once a complete cytogenetic response is achieved).	Skin rashes (10–20%); pancreatitis (5%); arterio-occlusive disease (10–20%); systemic hypertension (10–15%)
Omacetaxine mepesuccinate (Synribo)	Failure ≥2 tyrosine kinase inhibitors	1.25 mg/m² subcutaneously twice daily for 14 days of induction; 7 days of maintenance every month (may consider shorter dose schedules, 7 days of induction, 2–5 days of maintenance)	Myelosuppression

(45 mg daily). Ponatinib 45 mg daily may be associated with serious side effects: arterio-occlusive events, pancreatitis, hypertension, and skin rashes. A response-directed dose adjusted regimen, with a starting dose of 45 mg and reduction to 15 mg once a cytogenetic response is achieved, has resulted in a reduced incidence of arterio-occlusive events and has become standard. Imatinib, dasatinib (140 mg daily), bosutinib, and ponatinib are also approved for the treatment of CML in transformation (accelerated and blastic phase), whereas nilotinib is only approved for chronic and accelerated phase. The sixth approved drug is omacetaxine (Synribo), a protein synthesis inhibitor with presumed more selective inhibition of the synthesis of the BCR-ABL1 oncoprotein. It is approved for the treatment of chronic- and accelerated-phase CML after failure of two or more TKIs, at 1.25 mg/m² subcutaneously twice a day for 14 days for induction and for 7 days for consolidation-maintenance. The main adverse event of omacetaxine is prolonged myelosuppression; thus, many experts use shorter schedules (e.g., omacetaxine 5–7 days induction and 2–5 days maintenance), often combined with a TKI (Table 105-2).

Imatinib, dasatinib, bosutinib, and nilotinib are all acceptable frontline therapies in CML. The long-term results of imatinib are very favorable. The 10-year follow-up results show a cumulative complete cytogenetic response rate (occurring at least once) of 83%, with 60–65% of patients being in complete cytogenetic response at 5-year follow-up. The estimated 10-year survival rate is ~85%. Among patients continuing on imatinib, the annual rate of transformation to accelerated-blastic phase in years 4–8 is <1%. In three randomized studies, one comparing nilotinib 300 mg twice daily or 400 mg twice daily with imatinib (ENESTnd), another comparing dasatinib 100 mg daily with imatinib (DASISION), and a third comparing bosutinib 400 mg daily with imatinib (BFORE), the second-generation TKIs were associated with better outcomes in early surrogate endpoints, including higher rates of complete cytogenetic responses (85–87% vs 77–82%), MMRs (5-year rates 76–77% vs 60–64%), and MR4.5 (5-year rates 42–53% vs 31–33%), with lower rates of transformation to accelerated and blastic phase (2–5% vs 7%). However, no study has shown a survival benefit with second-generation TKIs. This may be because the rate of complete cytogenetic response is ultimately similarly high with imatinib versus second-generation TKIs, and also because sequential therapy with TKIs (following close observation and treatment change at progression) provides highly effective therapy for most patients; this ensures adequate long-term outcome despite relapse or intolerance after initial therapy.

Salvage therapy in chronic phase with dasatinib, nilotinib, bosutinib, or ponatinib is associated with complete cytogenetic response rates of 30–60%, depending on the salvage status (cytogenetic vs hematologic relapse), prior response to other TKIs, number of prior TKIs used, and the mutations at the time of relapse. Complete cytogenetic responses are generally durable, particularly in the absence of clonal evolution. Ponatinib is the only TKI active in the setting of T315I mutation, with complete cytogenetic response rates of 50–70% among patients who have received two or more TKIs. The estimated 5-year survival rates with new TKIs as salvage are 70–75% (compared with <50% before their availability). For example, with dasatinib salvage after imatinib failure in chronic-phase CML, the estimated 7-year rate of major molecular was 46%, the estimated 7-year survival rate was 65%, and progression-free survival rate was 42%. Thus, TKIs in the salvage setting have already reduced the annual mortality from the historical rate of 10–15% to ≤5%.

The goal of CML therapy is survival prolongation. The achievement of treatment-free remission (TFR) status has become a therapeutic goal of increased interest (sustained DMR or CMR after discontinuation of TKI therapy). In current practice, with the availability of appropriate TKI therapy and with compliance, monitoring, and changing of TKI therapy as indicated by response/resistance and side effects, patients can have a near-normal life expectancy, with a "relative" survival similar to that of the general population. Therefore, in standard practice, achievement and maintenance of a complete cytogenetic response are the aims of therapy, because complete cytogenetic response is the only outcome associated with survival prolongation. Lack of achievement of an MMR (protects against events; associated with longer event-free survival) or of DMR (offers the potential of treatment discontinuation and of TFR) should not be considered indications to change TKI therapy or to consider allogeneic SCT. A general practice rule is to continue the particular TKI chosen at the most tolerable dose schedule not associated with grade 3–4 side effects or with bothersome chronic side effects, for as long as possible, until either cytogenetic relapse or the persistence of unacceptable side effects. These two factors (i.e., cytogenetic relapse and intolerable side effects) are the indicators of "failure" of a particular TKI therapy. A second emerging general practice rule is that patients with CML should always receive daily TKI therapy throughout their lifetime (chronic, transformation), either alone (chronic) or in combinations (possibly for those in transformation, although combinations not formally approved), except perhaps in situations of "molecular cure" (TFR; elective discontinuation of TKI if DMR sustained for >2 to 5 years, followed by close monitoring) or after allogeneic SCT with undetectable disease.

Because of the increasing prevalence of CML (cost of TKI therapy) and the emerging evidence of possible organ toxicities with long-term use (e.g., renal with imatinib and bosutinib; arterio-occlusive with nilotinib, dasatinib, and ponatinib), a goal of therapy of increasing interest in CML is to achieve eradication of the disease (molecular "cure" or TFR) that is prolonged and durable, with recovery of nonneoplastic, nonclonal hematopoiesis off TKI therapy. The first step toward this aim is to obtain the highest rates of DMR lasting for at least 2 or more years. This is currently achievable in about 25–30% of patients treated with imatinib and in 40–45% of patients treated with second-generation TKIs. Approximately 50–60% of those who meet these criteria and discontinue therapy remain free from therapy and in DMR-MMR. As a result, TFR rates are estimated to be about 15–20% after imatinib therapy and 25–30% after second-generation TKIs.

Recommendations provided by the National Comprehensive Cancer Network (NCCN) and by the European LeukemiaNet (ELN) propose optimal/expected, suboptimal/warning, and failure response scenarios at different time points of TKI treatment duration. Unfortunately, they may have been misinterpreted in current practice because oncologists often report that their aim of treatment is the achievement of MMR and disease eradication. Significantly, a substantial proportion of oncologists consider a change of TKI therapy in a patient in complete cytogenetic response if they note loss of MMR (increase of *BCR-ABL1* transcripts [IS] from ≤0.1% to >0.1%). This perception may be the result of confusion regarding the aims of the NCCN and ELN guidelines, which have been updated often as a result of maturing data and have multiple treatment endpoint considerations. Although such endpoints may have been suggested as possible criteria for failure or suboptimal response, it is important to emphasize that no randomized study has yet shown that a change of TKI treatment in patients with complete cytogenetic response because of a loss of MMR, versus changing at the time of cytogenetic relapse, improves survival or other long-term outcomes. This is likely because of the high efficacy of salvage TKI therapy at the time of cytogenetic relapse.

Side effects of TKIs are generally mild to moderate, although with long-term TKI therapy, they could affect the patient's quality of life. Serious side effects occur in <5–10% of patients. With imatinib therapy, common mild to moderate side effects include fluid retention, weight gain, nausea, diarrhea, skin rashes, periorbital edema, bone or muscle aches, fatigue, and others (rates of 10–20%). In general, second-generation TKIs are associated with lower rates of these bothersome adverse events. However, dasatinib 100 mg daily is associated with higher rates of myelosuppression (20–30%), particularly thrombocytopenia, with pleural (10–25%) or pericardial effusions (≤5%), and with pulmonary hypertension (<5%). A lower dose of dasatinib (50 mg daily instead of 100 mg daily) used in frontline CML therapy has resulted in similar efficacy and a lower incidence of serious side effects (pleural effusions <5%, myelosuppression <10%). Nilotinib is associated with higher rates of hyperglycemia (10–20%), pruritus and skin rashes, hyperbilirubinemia (typically among patients with Gilbert's syndrome and mostly of no clinical consequences), and headaches. Nilotinib is also associated with occasional instances of pancreatitis (<5%). Nilotinib 300–400 mg twice daily is associated with a 10-year cumulative incidence of cardiovascular complications of 15–25%. Bosutinib is associated with higher rates of liver toxicity, renal dysfunction, and early and self-limited gastrointestinal adverse events, particularly diarrhea (70–85%). Occasionally, the gastrointestinal symptoms mimic chronic severe enterocolitis, which reverses with treatment discontinuation. Ponatinib 45 mg daily is associated with higher rates of serious skin rashes (10–15%), pancreatitis (10%), elevations of amylase/lipase (10%), and systemic hypertension (50–60%; severe in 20%). Arterio-occlusive events (cardiovascular, cerebrovascular, and peripheral arterial) have been reported with most TKIs. The incidence appears to be highest with ponatinib, but both nilotinib and dasatinib are associated with these events at an incidence significantly higher than imatinib. Among the TKIs, bosutinib is associated with the lowest incidence of cardiovascular events. Nilotinib and dasatinib may cause prolongation of the QTc interval; therefore, they should be evaluated cautiously in patients with prolonged QTc interval on electrocardiogram (>470–480 ms), and drugs given for other medical conditions should have relatively smaller or no effects on QTc. These side effects can often be dose-dependent and are generally reversible with treatment interruptions and dose reductions. Dose reductions can be individualized. However, the lowest estimated effective doses of TKIs (from different studies and treatment practices) are imatinib 100–200 mg daily; nilotinib 150 mg twice daily or 200 mg daily; dasatinib 20 mg daily; bosutinib 200–300 mg daily; and ponatinib 15 mg daily.

With long-term follow-up, rare but clinically relevant serious toxicities are emerging. Renal dysfunction and occasionally renal failure (creatinine elevations >2–3 mg/dL) are observed in 2–3% of patients, more frequently with imatinib and bosutinib than other TKIs, and usually reverse with TKI discontinuation and/or dose reduction. Rarely, patients may develop TKI-related peripheral neuropathy or even central neurotoxicities that are misdiagnosed as dementia or Alzheimer's disease; they may reverse slowly after TKI discontinuation. Pulmonary hypertension has been reported with dasatinib (<1–2%) and should be considered in a patient with shortness of breath and a normal chest x-ray (echocardiogram with emphasis on measurement of pulmonary artery pressure). This may be reversible with dasatinib discontinuation and occasionally the use of sildenafil citrate. Systemic hypertension has been observed more often with ponatinib. Hyperglycemia and occasionally diabetes have been noted more frequently with nilotinib. Finally, mid- and small-vessel arterio-occlusive and vasospastic events have been reported at low but significant rates with nilotinib and ponatinib and should be considered possibly TKI-related and represent indications to interrupt or reduce the dose of the TKI. These events include angina, coronary artery disease, myocardial infarction, peripheral arterial occlusive disease, transient ischemic attacks, cerebral vascular accidents, Raynaud's phenomenon, and accelerated atherosclerosis. Although these events are uncommon (<5%) (10-year cumulative rates of 15% with nilotinib 300 mg BID and 20–25% with 400 mg BID, compared with <5% with imatinib), they are clinically significant for the patient's long-term prognosis and occur at significantly higher rates than in the general population, particularly among patients with other risk factors for such events. Serious arterio-occlusive and vasospastic events are more common with ponatinib 45 mg daily (5-year rates 20%).

Discontinuation of TKIs and Treatment-Free Remissions Several studies have confirmed that TKI discontinuation among patients who achieve DMR (MR4.5) for longer than 2–3 years can result in TFR rates of 40–60%. Discontinuation of TKI therapy after 5+ years of CMR is associated with TFR rates of 70–80% or greater. Since the incidence of durable MR4.5 (*BCR-ABL* transcripts [IS] ≤0.0032%) is 30–60%, ~15–30% of all patients with CML on TKI therapy may achieve TFR. This approach is ready for community practice provided it is done under optimal conditions. These include the following: patients must have low or intermediate Sokal risk CML in first chronic phase (no evidence or history of transformation), with history of quantifiable *BCR-ABL1* transcripts (e13a2, e14a2), on long-term TKI therapy (5–8+ years), with documented DMR for >2–3 years (assessed every 6 months during this time span and with a PCR with adequate sensitivity), and should be monitored at referral centers that offer rigorous testing of residual CML disease. Patients must also be compliant to frequent monitoring (PCR studies every 1–2 months for the first 6 months, then every 2 months until 2 years and every 3–6 months thereafter).

ALLOGENEIC STEM CELL TRANSPLANT

Allogeneic SCT, a curative modality in CML, is associated with long-term survival rates of 40–60% when implemented in chronic phase. It is associated with early (1-year) mortality rates of 5–30%. Although the 5- to 10-year survival rates were reported to be ~50–60% (and considered as cure rates), ~10–15% of patients die in the subsequent 1–2 decades from subtle long-term complications of the transplant (rather than from CML relapse). These are related to chronic graft-versus-host disease (GVHD), organ dysfunction, development of second cancers, occasional late relapses, and hazard ratios for mortality higher than in the normal population. Other significant morbidities include infertility, chronic immune-mediated complications, cataracts, hip necrosis, and other morbidities affecting quality of life. The cure and early mortality rates in chronic-phase CML are also associated with several factors: patient age, duration of chronic phase, whether the donor is related or unrelated, degree of matching, preparative regimen, and others. In accelerated-phase CML, the cure rates with allogeneic SCT are 30–50%, depending on the definition of accelerated disease. Patients with clonal evolution as the only criterion have cure rates of up to 40–50%. Patients undergoing allogeneic SCT in second chronic phase have cure rates of 40–50%. The cure rates with allogeneic SCT in blastic-phase CML are ≤20%. Post–allogeneic SCT strategies are now implemented in the setting of molecular or cytogenetic relapse or in hematologic relapse/transformation. These include the use of TKIs for prevention or treatment of relapse, donor lymphocyte infusions, and second allogeneic SCTs, among others. TKIs appear to be highly successful at reinducing cytogenetic/molecular remissions in the setting of cytogenetic or molecular relapse after allogeneic SCT.

Choice and Timing of Allogeneic SCT Allogeneic SCT was considered first-line CML therapy before 2000. The maturing positive experience with TKIs has now relegated its use to after first-line TKI failures. An important question is the optimal timing and sequence of TKIs and allogeneic SCT (whether allogeneic SCT should be used as second- or third-line therapy). Among patients who present with or evolve to blastic phase, combinations of chemotherapy and TKIs should be used to induce remission, followed by allogeneic SCT as soon as possible. The same applies to patients who evolve from chronic to accelerated phase. Patients with de novo accelerated-phase CML may do well with long-term TKI therapy (estimated 8-year survival rate 75%); the timing of allogeneic SCT depends on their optimal response to TKI (achievement of complete cytogenetic response). Among patients who relapse in chronic phase, the treatment sequence depends on several factors: (1) patient age and availability of appropriate donors; (2) risk of allogeneic SCT; (3) presence or absence of clonal evolution and mutations; (4) patient's prior history and comorbidities; and (5) patient and physician preferences (**Table 105-3**). Patients with T315I mutations at relapse should be offered ponatinib and considered for allogeneic SCT particularly if in blastic phase and perhaps also in accelerated phase (because of the short follow-up with ponatinib). Patients with mutations involving Y253H, E255K/V, and F359V/C/I respond better to dasatinib or bosutinib. Patients with mutations involving V299L, T315A, and F317L/F/I/C respond better to nilotinib. Comorbidities such as diabetes, hypertension, pulmonary hypertension, chronic lung disease, cardiac conditions, and pancreatitis may influence the choice for or against a particular TKI. Patients with clonal evolution, unfavorable mutations, or lack of major/complete cytogenetic response within 1 year of salvage TKI therapy have short remission durations and should consider allogeneic SCT as more urgent in the setting of salvage. Patients without clonal evolution or mutations at relapse and who achieve a complete cytogenetic response with TKI salvage have long-lasting complete remissions and may delay the option of allogeneic SCT to third-line therapy. Finally, older patients (age 65–70 years or older) and those with high risk of mortality with allogeneic SCT may forgo this curative option for several years of disease control in chronic phase with or without cytogenetic response (Table 105-3). In emerging nations, where generic imatinib is now available at the annual price of $400–3000, frontline imatinib is a cost-effective therapy. However, second-line therapy with allogeneic SCT, a one-time curative option with a cost of $20,000–100,000, may be considered (in preference to second-generation TKIs—annual cost above $40,000–100,000) as a more cost-effective national health care strategy in CML. Table 105-3 summarizes a general guidance to the choice of TKIs versus allogeneic SCT.

TABLE 105-3 General Suggestions Regarding the Use of Tyrosine Kinase Inhibitors (TKIs) and Allogeneic Stem Cell Transplantation (SCT) in Chronic Myeloid Leukemia (CML)

CML PHASE	USE OF TKI	CONSIDERATION OF ALLOGENEIC SCT
Accelerated or blastic	Interim therapy to achieve minimal CML burden	As soon as possible (exception: de novo accelerated phase)
T315I mutation	Ponatinib to achieve minimal CML burden	Depends on longer term follow-up results of ponatinib efficacy
Imatinib failure in chronic phase; no clonal evolution, no mutations, good initial response; no T315I	Second-line TKIs long term	Third-line after second-line TKI failures
Clonal evolution or mutations, or no cytogenetic response to second-line TKI	Interim therapy with alternative second-generation TKI or ponatinib to achieve minimal CML burden	Second-line
Older patients (≥65–70 years) after imatinib failure in chronic phase	Salvage TKIs as longer-term therapy	May forgo allogeneic SCT in favor of good quality of life and survival in chronic phase
Imatinib failure; emerging nation	—	Second-line: curative, one-time cost $20,000–100,000 (vs >$40,000–100,000/year with TKI)

Note: Mutations involving Y253H, E255K/V, or F359V/C/I: prefer dasatinib or bosutinib. Mutations involving V299L, T315A, or F317L/F/I/C: prefer nilotinib.

MONITORING THERAPY IN CML

Achievement of complete cytogenetic response by 12 months of imatinib therapy and its persistence later, the only consistent prognostic factor associated with prolonged survival, is now the main therapeutic endpoint in CML. Failure to achieve a complete cytogenetic response by 12 months or occurrence of later cytogenetic or hematologic relapse is considered as treatment failure and an indication to change therapy. Because salvage therapy with other TKIs may re-establish good outcome, it is important to ensure patient compliance to continued TKI therapy and change therapy when cytogenetic relapse is confirmed unless this is related to nonadherence. Patients on frontline imatinib therapy should be closely monitored until documentation of complete cytogenetic response, at which time they can be monitored every 6 months with peripheral blood PCR, or more frequently (e.g., every 3 months), if there are concerns about changes in *BCR-ABL1* transcripts. Cytogenetic relapse on imatinib is an indication of treatment failure and need to change TKI therapy. Mutational analysis in this instance helps in the selection of the next TKI and identifies mutations in 30–50% of patients. Mutational studies by standard Sanger sequencing (which is the technique currently available in most clinical laboratories) in patients in complete cytogenetic response (in whom there may be concerns of increasing *BCR-ABL1* transcripts) identify mutations in ≤5% and are therefore not indicated. Earlier response has been identified as a prognostic factor for long-term outcome, including achievement of partial cytogenetic response (*BCR-ABL1* transcripts ≤10%) by 3–6 months of therapy. Failure to achieve such a response has been associated with significantly worse survival.

The use of second-generation TKIs (dasatinib, bosutinib, nilotinib) as frontline therapy changed the monitoring approach slightly. Patients are expected to achieve major cytogenetic response (or *BCR-ABL1* transcripts ≤10%) by 3–6 months of therapy. Failure to do so is associated with worse event-free survival, transformation rates, and survival. However, the 3- to 5-year estimated survival among such patients is still high, ~80–90%, which is better than what would be anticipated if such patients were offered allogeneic SCT at that time. Changes of therapy for patients with "slow" response have not been proven to be of long-term benefit compared to changes when more obvious signs of resistance appear. Thus, slow response to therapy is considered a warning signal, but it is not known whether changing therapy to other TKIs at that time would improve longer-term outcome.

TREATMENT OF ACCELERATED AND BLASTIC PHASES

Patients in accelerated or blastic phase may receive therapy with TKIs, preferably second- or third-generation TKIs (dasatinib, nilotinib, bosutinib, ponatinib), alone or in combination with chemotherapy, to reduce the CML burden, before undergoing allogeneic SCT. Response rates (major hematologic) with single-agent TKIs range from 30 to 50% in accelerated phase and from 20 to 30% in blastic phase. Cytogenetic responses, particularly complete cytogenetic responses, are uncommon (10–30%) and transient in blastic phase. Studies of TKIs in combination with chemotherapy show that combined TKI-chemotherapy strategies increase the response rates and their durability and improve survival. This is particularly true in CML lymphoid blastic phase, where the combination of anti-ALL chemotherapy with TKIs results in complete response rates of 70% and median survival times of 3 years (compared with historical response rates of 40–50% and median survival times of 12–18 months). This allows many patients to undergo allogeneic SCT in a state of minimal CML burden or second chronic phase, which are associated with higher probability of long-term survival. In CML nonlymphoid blastic phase, anti–acute myeloid leukemia chemotherapy combined with TKIs results in CR rates of 30–50% and median survival times of 9–12 months (compared with historical response rates of 20–30% and median survival times of 3–5 months). In accelerated phase, response to single TKIs is significant in conditions where "softer" accelerated phase criteria are considered (e.g., clonal evolution alone, thrombocytosis alone, significant splenomegaly or resistance to hydroxyurea, but without evidence of high blast and basophil percentages). In accelerated phase, combinations frequently include TKIs with low-intensity chemotherapy such as low-dose cytarabine, decitabine, interferon α, hydroxyurea, or others.

OTHER TREATMENTS AND SPECIAL THERAPEUTIC CONSIDERATIONS

Interferon α Interferon α is considered in combination with TKIs (an investigational approach), sometimes after CML failure on TKIs, occasionally in patients during pregnancy, or as part of investigational strategies with TKIs to eradicate residual molecular disease.

Chemotherapeutic Agents Hydroxyurea remains a safe and effective agent (at daily doses of 0.5–10 g) to reduce initial CML burden, as a temporary measure in between definitive therapies, or in combination with TKIs to sustain complete hematologic or cytogenetic responses. Busulfan is often used in allogeneic SCT preparative regimens. Because of its side effects (delayed myelosuppression, Addison-like disease, pulmonary and cardiac fibrosis, myelofibrosis), it is now rarely used in the chronic management of CML. Low-dose cytarabine, decitabine, anthracyclines, 6-mercaptopurine, 6-thioguanine, thiotepa, anagrelide, and other agents are sometimes useful in different CML settings to control the disease burden.

Others Splenectomy is now seldom considered to alleviate symptoms of massive splenomegaly and/or hypersplenism. Splenic irradiation is rarely used, if at all, because of the postirradiation adhesions and complications. Leukapheresis is occasionally used in patients presenting with extreme leukocytosis and leukostatic complications. Single doses of high-dose cytarabine or high doses of hydroxyurea, with tumor lysis management, may be as effective and less cumbersome.

Special Considerations Women with CML who become pregnant should discontinue TKI therapy immediately. Among 125 babies delivered to women with CML who discontinued imatinib therapy as soon as the pregnancy was known, three babies were born with neurologic, skeletal, and renal malformations, suggesting the teratogenicity of imatinib known from animal studies. A similar experience has been reported with dasatinib, where the incidence of malformations was reported to be higher, 10–12%. There are no or little data with other TKIs. Control of CML during pregnancy can be managed with leukapheresis for severe symptomatic leukocytosis in the first trimester and with hydroxyurea subsequently until delivery. There are reports of successful pregnancies and deliveries of normal babies with interferon α therapy and registry studies in essential thrombocytosis of its safety, but interferon α has side effects that may be troublesome during pregnancy, can be antiangiogenic, and may increase the risk of spontaneous abortions.

Approximately 10–15% of patients on TKI therapy may develop chromosomal abnormalities in the Ph-negative cells. These may involve loss of chromosome Y, trisomy 8, 20q−, chromosome 5 or 7 abnormalities, and others. Most chromosomal abnormalities disappear spontaneously and may be indicative of the genetic instability of the hematopoietic stem cells that predisposes the patient to develop CML in the first place. Rarely (in <1% of instances), abnormalities involving chromosomes 5 or 7 may be truly clonal and evolve into myelodysplastic syndrome or acute myeloid leukemia. This is thought to be part of the natural course of patients in whom CML was suppressed and who live long enough to develop other hematologic malignancies.

GLOBAL ASPECTS OF CML

Routine physical examinations and blood tests in the United States and advanced countries result in early detection of CML in most patients. About 50–70% of patients with CML are diagnosed incidentally, and high-risk CML as defined by prognostic models (e.g., Sokal risk groups) is found in only 10% of patients. This is not the same situation in emerging nations where most patients are diagnosed following evaluation for symptoms and many present with high tumor burden, such as massive splenomegaly, and advanced phases of CML (high-risk CML documented in 20–30%). Therefore, the prognosis of such patients on TKI therapy may be worse than the published experience.

The high cost of TKI therapies (annual costs of $90,000–140,000 in the United States; lower but variable in the rest of the world) makes the general affordability of such treatments difficult. Although TKI treatment penetration is high in nations where cost of therapy is not an issue (e.g., Sweden, European Union), it may be less so in other nations, even in advanced ones like the United States, where out-of-pocket expenses may be prohibitive to a subset of patients. Although the estimated 10-year survival in CML is >85% in single-institution studies (e.g., MD Anderson Cancer Center), in national studies in countries with TKI affordability (Sweden) (**Figs.** 105-2 and **105-3**) or in clinical trials (where all patients have access to TKIs throughout their care), the estimated 10-year survival worldwide, even 16 years after the introduction of TKI therapies, is likely to be <50%. The Surveillance, Epidemiology, and End Results (SEER) data from the United States report an estimated 5-year survival rate of 60% in the era of TKIs. It appears that the treatment penetration of imatinib and other TKIs into CML therapy worldwide is still not optimal.

The current high cost of TKI therapies poses two additional considerations. The first are the treatment pathways and guidelines in nations where TKIs may not be affordable by patients or the health care system. In these conditions, there are trends of pathways advocating allogeneic SCT as frontline or second-line therapy (i.e., after imatinib failure; as a onetime cost of $20,000–100,000) despite the associated mortality and morbidities. The second is the choice of frontline TKI therapy. Imatinib is now available in generic forms at affordable costs ($400–10,000 per

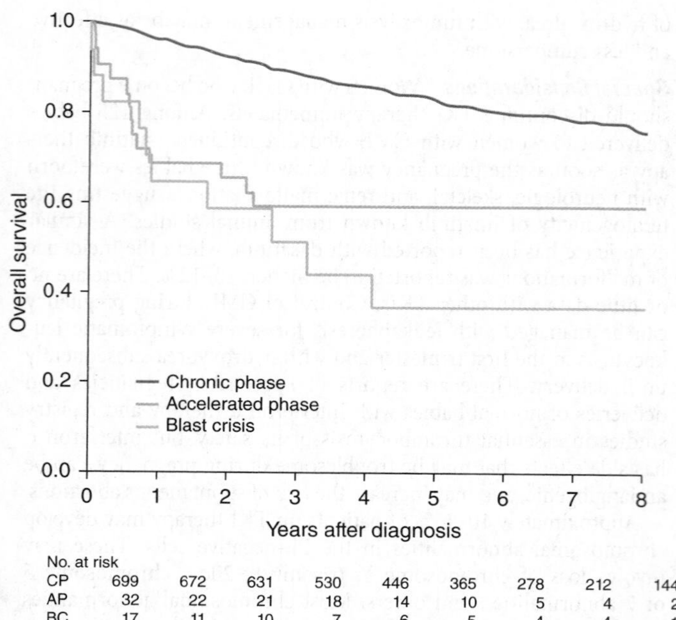

FIGURE 105-3 Survival in chronic (CP), accelerated (AP), and blastic crisis (BC) phases of chronic myeloid leukemia (CML) in the population-based Swedish national registry study. The accelerated- and blastic-phase cases are de novo presentations. The favorable outcome with de novo blastic phase may be due to use of 20% blasts or more to define blastic phase. *(With permission from Dr. Martin Hoglund, Swedish CML Registry, 2013.)*

year). Dasatinib is available in generic forms in many geographies. Safe and effective generic TKIs may become preferred frontline and salvage therapies in CML, precluding the necessity of an allogeneic SCT in first salvage in poorer nations.

FURTHER READING

Cortes JE et al: Final 5-year study results of DASISION: The dasatinib versus imatinib study in treatment-naïve chronic myeloid leukemia patients trial. J Clin Oncol 34:2333, 2016.

Cortes JE et al: Bosutinib versus imatinib for newly diagnosed chronic myeloid leukemia: Results from the randomized BFORE Trial. J Clin Oncol 36:231, 2018.

Cortes JE et al: Ponatinib efficacy and safety in Philadelphia chromosome-positive leukemia: Final 5-year results of the phase 2 PACE trial. Blood 132:393, 2018.

Hochhaus A et al: Long-term outcomes of imatinib treatment for chronic myeloid leukemia. N Engl J Med 376:917, 2017.

Hochhaus A et al: European LeukemiaNet 2020 recommendations for treating chronic myeloid leukemia. Leukemia 34:966, 2020.

Jabbour E, Kantarjian H: Chronic myeloid leukemia: 2020 update on diagnosis, therapy and monitoring. Am J Hematol 95:691, 2020.

Kantarjian H et al: Long-term outcomes with frontline nilotinib versus imatinib in newly diagnosed chronic myeloid leukemia in chronic phase: ENESTnd 10-year analysis. Leukemia 35:440, 2021.

Naqvi K et al: Long-term follow-up of lower dose dasatinib (50 mg daily) as frontline therapy in newly diagnosed chronic-phase chronic myeloid leukemia. Cancer 126:67, 2020.

Sasaki K et al: Conditional survival in patients with chronic myeloid leukemia in chronic phase in the era of tyrosine kinase inhibitors. Cancer 122:238, 2016.

Saussele S et al: Discontinuation of tyrosine kinase inhibitor therapy in chronic myeloid leukaemia (EURO-SKI): A prespecified interim analysis of a prospective, multicentre, non-randomised trial. Lancet Oncol 19:747, 2018.

Shih YT et al: Treatment value of second-generation BCR-ABL1 tyrosine kinase inhibitors compared with imatinib to achieve treatment-free remission in patients with chronic myeloid leukaemia: A modelling study. Lancet Haematol 6:e398, 2019.

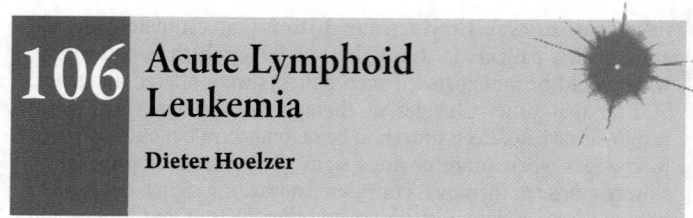

106 Acute Lymphoid Leukemia

Dieter Hoelzer

In acute lymphoblastic leukemia (ALL), the malignant clone arises from hematopoietic progenitors in the bone marrow or lymphatic system resulting in an increase of immature nonfunctioning leukemic cells. Infiltration of bone marrow leads to anemia, granulocytopenia, and thrombocytopenia with the clinical manifestations of fatigue, weakness, infection, and hemorrhage. These symptoms are more often the reason a patient first seeks medical advice rather than consequences of tumor bulk, such as lymph node enlargement, hepatosplenomegaly caused by leukemic infiltration, or symptoms of the central nervous system (meningeosis leukemica).

INCIDENCE AND AGE

ALL is the most frequent neoplastic disease in children with an early peak at the age of 3–4 years. The incidence in adults ranges from 0.7 to 1.8/100 000 per year, being somewhat higher in adolescents and young adults (AYAs), decreasing in adults, but increasing again in elderly people. Thus, Philadelphia chromosome–positive ALL (Ph+ ALL; *BCR/ABL* translocation) is observed in half of elderly B-lineage patients. The frequency of immunologic, cytogenetic, and genetic subtypes changes substantially with age.

ETIOLOGY

The etiology of acute leukemias is unknown. Internal and external factors influence the incidence of leukemia. Exposure to ionizing radiation or to chemicals, including prior chemotherapy, is associated with an increased risk of developing leukemia, more often observed in acute myeloid leukemia (AML). However, increasingly, secondary ALLs have been observed, particularly after cytostatic treatment with alkylating agents and topoisomerase inhibitors as treatment for primary tumors, most often for AML, myelodysplastic syndromes, or breast cancer.

CONGENITAL DISORDERS

Patients with some rare congenital chromosomal abnormalities have a higher risk of development of acute leukemia (e.g., Klinefelter's syndrome, Fanconi's anemia, Bloom's syndrome, ataxia-telangiectasia, and neurofibromatosis). Those with Down's syndrome have a twentyfold increased incidence of leukemia; ALL is increased in childhood and AML at an older age.

INFECTIOUS AGENTS

No direct evidence implicates viruses as a major cause of human acute leukemia. However, viruses are involved in the pathogenesis of two lymphoid neoplasias. In the endemic African type of Burkitt's lymphoma, the Epstein-Barr virus, a DNA virus of the herpes family, has been implicated as a potential causative agent (see **Chap. 194**). Endemic infection with human T-cell leukemia virus I in Japan and the Caribbean has been shown to be an etiologic agent for rare cases of adult T-cell leukemia/lymphoma (see **Chap. 201**).

DIAGNOSIS AND CLASSIFICATION

The diagnosis of acute leukemia is first made by examination of the peripheral blood and bone marrow. For further classification of the leukemic blast cells, cytochemical stains, immunologic markers, and cytogenetic and molecular analysis are required. The immunologic markers are still the major criteria to subdivide into B-cell lineage or T-cell lineage ALL leukemias.

PERIPHERAL BLOOD

Peripheral blood counts and a differential count from a Wright-Giemsa–stained blood smear are essential at the time of presentation. The white blood cell (WBC) count in ~40% of ALL patients is reduced or normal (**Table 106-1**). Only 16% of patients have a WBC above

TABLE 106-1 Laboratory Values at Diagnosis of Acute Lymphoblastic Leukemia (ALL)

		ALL
NO.		1273*
Initial white blood cell count (× 10⁹/L)	<10	41%
	10–50	31%
	>50–100	28%
	>100	16%
Neutrophils (× 10⁹/L)	<50–100	12%
	<100,000	16%
Platelets (× 10⁹/L)	<20	22%
	21–40	22%
	41–100	29%
	>100	27%
Hemoglobin (g/dL)	<7	20%
	7–9	33%
	>9	47%
Leukemic blasts in peripheral blood	0%	8%
	25–75%	34%
	>75%	36%
Leukemic blasts in bone marrow	<50%	4%
	51–90%	25%
	>90%	71%

Source: Data from three consecutive German Multicenter Trials for Adult ALL (GMALL).

100 × 10^5/L. It is noteworthy that in 8% of ALL patients, no circulating leukemic blast cells were observed. Thus, in the frequently used automatic blood cell counting, the diagnosis may not be detected.

Peripheral blood characteristically shows anemia, thrombocytopenia, and neutropenia. Nearly one-third of patients have hemoglobin levels <7–8 g/dL. A platelet count below the critical number of 20 × 10^9/L and neutropenia (neutrophils <0.5 × 10^9/L), which is associated with a higher risk of infection, are each noted in one-fifth of adults with ALL.

BONE MARROW EXAMINATION

Bone marrow aspirates/biopsies are important to assess immunologic, cytogenetic, and genomic markers. Direct smears from the bone marrow are essential to confirm the diagnosis of acute leukemia and to distinguish between AML and ALL. The bone marrow is usually heavily packed with leukemic blast cells with >90% in ~70% of patients, and thus, the normal hemopoietic elements are greatly reduced or absent. A biopsy of the bone marrow will further demonstrate marked hypercellularity with replacement of fat spaces, normal elements, and occasionally increased fibrosis.

LUMBAR PUNCTURE

The examination of the cerebrospinal fluid is an essential routine diagnostic measure for ALL. Central nervous system (CNS) leukemia is diagnosed if ≥5 cells/μL or leukemic blast cells were observed by morphology in cerebrospinal fluid. Opinions differ as to when the first lumbar puncture should be done—i.e., either delay lumbar puncture until remission is achieved to avoid seeding of the CNS with leukemic blast cells from the peripheral blood during the spinal tap, or perform the lumbar puncture before treatment starts, since early recognition of CNS disease will lead to immediate CNS-specific therapy. Lumbar puncture is restricted to patients with an adequate platelet count (>20 × 10^9/L) and without manifest clinical hemorrhages. To eliminate potentially transferred blast cells, patients should receive intrathecal methotrexate at the first lumbar puncture.

MORPHOLOGIC SUBTYPES IN ALL

The French-American-British (FAB) classification distinguished three subgroups. L1 and L2 morphology has no clinical consequences. Only the L3 morphology, observed in up to 5% of adult patients, is indicative for mature B-cell lineage ALL (B-ALL) **(see Chap. 62)**.

IMMUNOLOGIC SUBTYPES

A series of monoclonal antibodies is employed to identify antigens expressed on the surface of leukemic cells, corresponding to the pathways of normal B-cell differentiation (see **Fig. 108-2**). The aim of the immunologic classification is to subdivide ALLs according to the presence or absence of B-cell or T-cell markers. A marker is considered positive if >20% of the cells are stained with the monoclonal antibody.

There are different immunologic classifications, such as that of the European Group for the Immunological Characterization of Leukemias (EGIL), with clear therapeutic implications. **Table 106-2** gives a simplified correlation of immunologic subtypes, cytogenetics and molecular aberrations, and clinical characteristics.

B-Cell Lineage ALL (B-ALL) More than 70% of adult ALLs are of B-cell origin, and the most frequent immunologic subtype, common ALL, is characterized by the presence of the ALL antigen CD10 without markers of relatively mature B cells such as cytoplasmic or surface membrane immunoglobulins. Pre-B-ALL (early B-ALL) is characterized by the expression of cytoplasmic immunoglobulin, which is negative in common ALL, but otherwise is identical with respect to all other cell markers. Pro-B-ALL corresponds to early B-cell differentiation and was formerly termed non-T-, non-B-ALL or null ALL because neither T-cell nor B-cell features could be demonstrated. This subtype is HLA-DR, terminal deoxynucleotidyl transferase, and CD19 positive and composes ~12% of adult ALLs. Mature B-ALL is seen in 3–4% of adults and is also known as Burkitt's leukemia. In mature B-ALL, blast cells express surface antigens of mature B cells, including the sIgM.

T-Cell Lineage ALL (T-ALL) Approximately 25% of adult ALLs are of T-cell lineage. All cases express the T-cell antigen CD7 and cytoplasmatic CD3 (CyCD3) or surface CD3. According to their phase of T-cell differentiation, they may express other T-cell antigens (e.g., the E-rosette receptor CD2 and/or the cortical thymocyte antigen CD1a). Early pro/pre-T-ALL (also termed early T precursor ALL [ETP-ALL]), cortical or thymic T-ALL, and mature T-ALL can be distinguished with these markers. ETP-ALL is characterized by lack of CD1a and CD8, weak CD5 expression, and at least one myeloid/stem cell marker.

Biphenotypic or Mixed Leukemias Biphenotypic leukemias are defined as those expressing markers of both lymphoid and myeloid lineages on the same leukemic cells. Bilineage leukemias are those with two populations of blast cells with either lymphoid or myeloid antigens. It is not clear whether these patients should receive an ALL or AML treatment protocol. In pediatric studies, starting with a pediatric ALL protocol seemed preferable, which was then followed by AML consolidation elements.

CYTOGENETIC AND MOLECULAR ANALYSIS

Cytogenetic and molecular analyses should be performed in all cases in ALL. They are important to define ALL subtypes, can identify independent prognostic markers of disease-free survival, and may determine specific targeted therapies.

The diagnostic techniques for ALL are standard cytogenetics, fluorescence in situ hybridization, and reverse transcriptase polymerase chain reaction. These methods allow the detection of Ph+ ALL, with the chromosomal translocation t(9;22)(q34;q11) and the detection of the corresponding *BCR-ABL1* gene rearrangement. Further ALL entities that have been identified are t(4;11)(q21;q23)/*MLL-AFA4*, abn11q23/*MLL*, and t(1;19)(q23;p13)/*PBX-E2A*.

Gene expression profiling, single nucleotide polymorphism array analysis, array-comparative genomic hybridization, and next-generation sequencing recognize the newly defined ALL entities: ETP-ALL and Ph-like ALL.

Ph-like ALL, also known as *BCR-ABL1*-like ALL, is characterized by genetic lesions similar to Ph+ ALL, associated with *IKZF1* (Ikaros) gene deletion, *CLRF2* (gene for cytokine-like receptor-2) overexpression, and tyrosine kinase activating rearrangements involving *ABL1*, *JAK2*, *PDGFRB*, and several other genes; however, it is *BCR-ABL1* negative. The frequency is 10% in children and 25–30% in young adults but does not increase further with age like Ph+ ALL. Treatment based on the underlying genetic lesion with BCR-ABL inhibitors

TABLE 106-2 Immunologic, Cytogenetic, Molecular, and Clinical Characteristics of Adult Acute Lymphoblastic Leukemia (ALL)

SUBTYPES	MARKER	INCIDENCE	FREQUENT CYTOGENETIC ABERRATIONS	GENETIC ABERRATIONS AND FUSION TRANSCRIPTS	CLINICAL CHARACTERISTICS	RELAPSE KINETICS AND LOCALIZATION
B-lineage ALL (B-ALL)	**HLA-DR+, TdT+, CD19+, and/or CD79a+, and/or CD22+**	**76%**				
Pro B-ALL	No additional differentiation markers Frequent myeloid coexpression (>50%) CD10–	12%	t(4;11)(q21;q23)	70% *ALL1-AF4* (20% Flt3 in MLL+)	High WBC (>100,000/μL) (26%)	Mainly BM (>90%)
Common ALL	CD10+	49%	t(9;22)(q34;q11) del(6q)	33% *BCR-ABL* with 54% *IKFZ1* del >25% *CDKN2A/B*	Higher age >50 years (24%)	Mainly BM (>90%) Prolonged relapse kinetics (up to 5–7 years)
Pre-B-ALL	CD10±, cyIg+	11%	t(9;22)(q34;q11) t(1;19)(q23;p13)	4% t(1;19)/*PBX-E2A*		
Mature B-ALL	CD10±, sIg+	4%	t(8;14)(q24;q32) t(2;8)(p12;q24) t(8;22)(q24;q11)		Higher age >55 years (27%) Frequent organ involvement (32%) and CNS involvement (13%)	Frequent CNS (10%) Short relapse kinetics (up to 1–1.5 years)
T-lineage ALL (T-ALL)	**cyCD3 or sCD3**	**24%**	t(10;14)(q24;q11) t(11;14)(p13;q11)	50% *NOTCH1B* 33% *HOX11b* 5% *HOX11L2b* 4% *NUP213-ABL1*	Younger age (90% <50 years) Frequent mediastinal tumors (60%) Frequent CNS involvement (8%) High WBC (>50/μL) (46%)	Frequent CNS (up to 10%) Extramedullary (6%) Intermediate relapse kinetics (up to 3–4 years) When relapsed, fast progression
Early Pro/ Pre T-ALL	No additional differentiation markers, mostly CD2–	6%				
Cortical T-ALL	CD1a+, sCD3±	12%				
Mature T-ALL	sCD3+, CD1a–	6%				

Abbreviations: BM, bone marrow; CNS, central nervous system; WBC, white blood cells.

(e.g., dasatinib) or JAK2 inhibitors (e.g., ruxolitinib) has so far had limited success in adults.

MINIMAL RESIDUAL DISEASE

Minimal residual disease (MRD) is the detection of residual leukemic cells that are not recognizable by light microscopy. Methods for determining MRD are based on the detection of leukemia-specific aberrant immunophenotypes by flow cytometry, the evaluation of leukemia-specific rearranged immunoglobulin or T-cell receptor sequences by real-time quantitative polymerase chain reaction, or the detection of fusion genes associated with chromosomal abnormalities (e.g., *BCR-ABL, MLL-AF4*). The detection limit with these methods is 10^{-3}–10^{-5} (0.1–0.001%). With new techniques such as next-generation sequencing (NGS) or digital droplet polymerase chain reaction (ddPCR), the sensitivity may increase to 10^{-5}–10^{-6}. The phenotypic aberrations are unique to each patient with ALL and can be detected in up to 95% of individuals. Collection of bone marrow at diagnosis for identification of patients' individual markers is essential for follow-up of MRD.

MOLECULAR RESPONSE AFTER INDUCTION THERAPY AND IMPACT ON OUTCOME

Achievement of molecular complete response/molecular remission is the most relevant independent prognostic factor for disease-free survival and overall survival in pediatric and adult ALL **(Table 106-3)**. Patients with molecular complete remission after induction therapy had significantly superior outcomes in several studies, with a disease-free survival rate of ~70% compared to <40% for MRD-positive patients. Patients with molecular failure after induction should proceed to a targeted therapy to reduce the tumor load, followed by allogeneic stem cell transplantation (SCT), if possible.

PROGNOSTIC FACTORS, RISK STRATIFICATION, AND MRD

The aim of identification of prognostic parameters at diagnosis, which include age, white blood cell count, immunophenotype, and cytogenetic and genetic aberrations, is to stratify patients into risk groups: standard-risk patients are patients without any risk factor, and high-risk patients are those with one or more risk factors. High-risk patients are most often candidates for SCT in first complete remission (CR). MRD is thus the most important prognostic factor during therapy **(Fig. 106-1)**; 20–30% of adult ALL patients who are MRD negative after induction will relapse. Potential reasons include loss of sensitivity, evolution of leukemic subclones, and extramedullary origin of disease. If the MRD status of a patient is not available, risk stratification should rely on clinical and laboratory risk factors evaluated at diagnosis.

TABLE 106-3 Response Parameters According to Minimal Residual Disease (MRD)

TERMINOLOGY	DEFINITION
Complete hematologic remission (CHR)	Leukemic cells not detectable by light microscopy (<5% blast cells in bone marrow [BM])
Complete molecular remission/MRD negativity	Patient in complete remission, MRD not detectable, ≤0.01% = ≤1 leukemia cell in 10,000 BM cells
Molecular failure/MRD positivity	Patient in complete hematologic remission, but not in molecular complete remission >0.01%
Molecular relapse/MRD positivity	Patient still in complete remission, had prior molecular complete remission, leukemic blast cells in BM not detectable (<5%)
Hematologic relapse	>5% blast cells in BM/blood

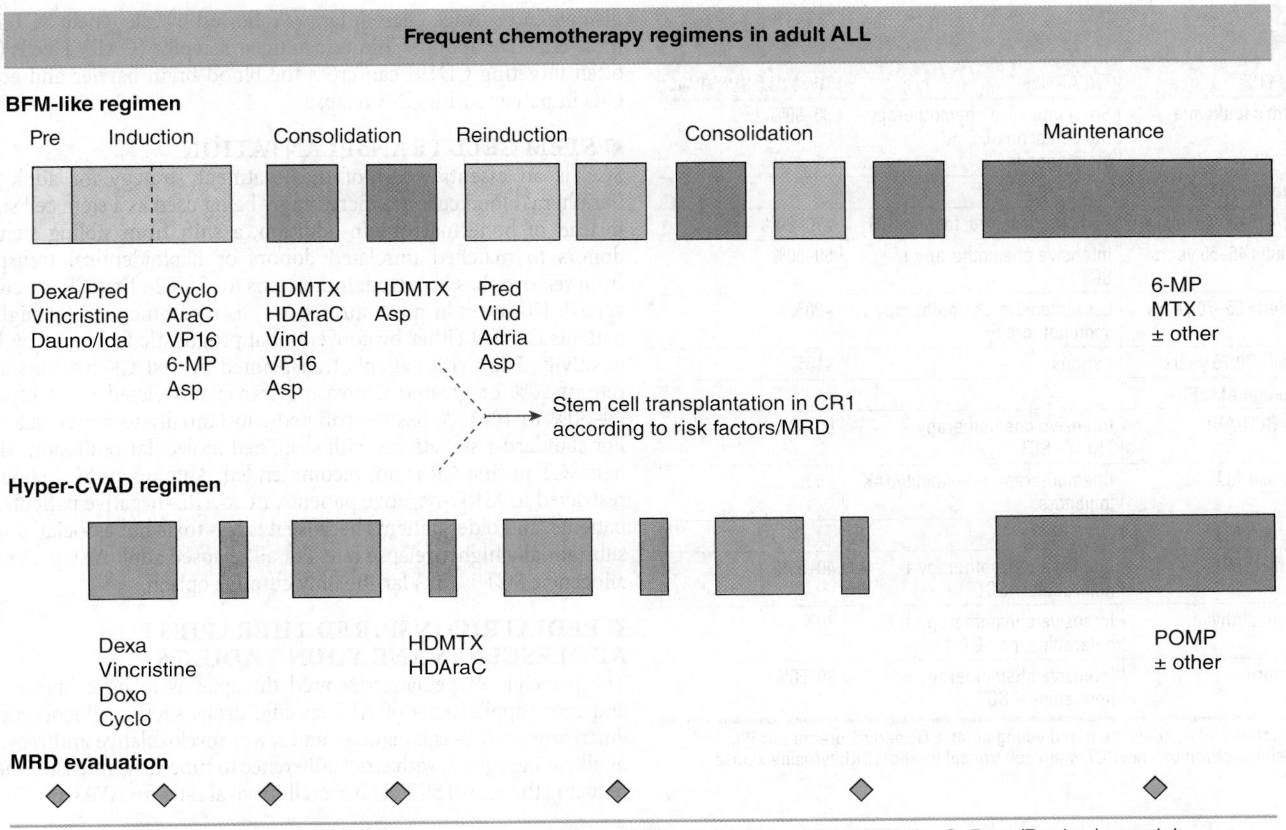

FIGURE 106-1 A schematic treatment algorithm in acute lymphoblastic leukemia (ALL). 6-MP, 6-mercaptopurine; Adria, Adriamycin (doxorubicin); AraC, cytarabine; Asp, asparaginase; BFM, Berlin-Frankfurt-Münster; CNS, central nervous system; CR1, first complete remission; Cyclo, cyclophosphamide; Dauno, daunorubicin; Dexa, dexamethasone; Doxo, doxorubicin; HD, high-dose; Hyper-CVAD, hyperfractionated cyclophosphamide, vincristine, doxorubicin, and dexamethasone; Ida, idarubicin; MRD, minimal residual disease; MTX, methotrexate; POMP, mercaptopurine, vincristine, methotrexate, and prednisolone; Pred, prednisolone; Vind, vindesine; VP16, etoposide.

TREATMENT PRINCIPLES

Treatment of ALL consists usually of pre-phase therapy, induction therapy, consolidation cycles, and maintenance treatment. Treatment should start immediately when the diagnosis of ALL is established.

Pre-Phase Therapy Pre-phase therapy consisting of glucocorticoids (prednisone 20–60 mg/d or dexamethasone 6–16 mg/d, both IV or PO) alone or in combination with another drug (e.g., vincristine, cyclophosphamide) is usually given for ~5–7 days. It allows safe tumor reduction to avoid tumor lysis syndrome, to initiate supportive therapy, such as substitution of platelets/erythrocytes, or to treat infections. The time required for pre-phase therapy will also allow time to obtain results of the diagnostic workup (e.g., cytogenetics, molecular genetics).

Induction Therapy The goal of induction therapy is the achievement of a CR or, even better, a molecular CR. With current regimens, the CR rate has increased to 80–90% and is higher for standard-risk patients (>90%) and lower for high-risk patients (~60%).

Induction regimens are centered around vincristine, glucocorticoids, and anthracyclines with or without cyclophosphamide or cytarabine. L-Asparaginase is the only ALL-specific drug and is now more intensively used in adults. Pegylated asparaginase has the advantage of a significantly longer period of asparagine depletion. Dexamethasone is often preferred to prednisone because it penetrates the blood-brain barrier and also acts on resting leukemic blast cells.

Two chemotherapy regimens are widespread (Fig. 106-1). One is patterned after the pediatric BFM (Berlin-Frankfurt-Münster) protocol, which is mostly used in European adult ALL trials. Another approach is to repeat two different alternating intensive chemotherapy cycles, identical for induction and consolidation, for eight cycles, such as Hyper-CVAD (hyperfractionated cyclophosphamide, vincristine, doxorubicin, and dexamethasone) protocol, which is preferentially used in the United States but also in many other parts of the world.

Postremission Consolidation Usual protocols use six to eight courses and often contain systemic high-dose (HD) therapy to reach sufficient drug levels in sanctuary sites such as the CNS. Most often HD methotrexate (1–1.5 g/m^2 and up to 3–5 g/m^2) and/or HD cytarabine (4–12 doses at 1–3 g/m^2) are administered.

Maintenance Therapy Maintenance therapy, a strategy transferred from childhood ALL, is mandatory. It consists of 6-mercaptopurine and methotrexate plus intrathecal therapy. The potential effect of further intensification cycles during maintenance remains unclear. The duration of maintenance therapy for T-ALL and B-ALL is 2–2.5 years, except for Burkitt's leukemia, for which it is not required. In Ph+ ALL, patients also require maintenance therapy that should include a tyrosine kinase inhibitor (TKI), most likely the TKI that has been used during induction and consolidation therapy. It is also standard to give a TKI after allogeneic SCT. The duration of maintenance therapy with a TKI is also 2–2.5 years and should be guided by MRD evaluation. TKI use is often interrupted or switched to another TKI if toxicity occurs.

TREATMENT OF ALL PATIENTS ACCORDING TO AGE

The outcome of ALL is strictly related to the age of a patient, with cure rates of ~90% in children, decreasing to <10% in elderly or frail

TABLE 106-4 Best Results in Recent Studies for Adult Acute Lymphoblastic Leukemia (ALL)

SUBTYPE	TREATMENT	OVERALL SURVIVAL
Burkitt's leukemia	Short intensive chemotherapy + rituximab; no SCT; no maintenance	80–90%
B-lineage ALL, Ph–		
AYA 15–35/45 years	Pediatric inspired, few/no SCT	≥70–80%
Adults 45–55 years	Intensive chemotherapy +/– SCT	50–60%
Elderly 55–70 years	Less intensive chemotherapy + immunotherapy	~30%
Frail >70/75 years	Various	≤10%
B-lineage ALL, Ph+		
Ph BCR-ABL	Intensive chemotherapy + TKI +/– SCT	60–70%
Ph-like ALL	Chemotherapy + dasatinib/JAK inhibitors	≤50%
T-lineage ALL		
Early (ETP)	Intensive chemotherapy + nelarabine + SCT	40–50%
Cortical/thymic	Intensive chemotherapy + nelarabine, no SCT	70%
Mature	Intensive chemotherapy + nelarabine + SCT	30–50%

Abbreviations: AYA, adolescent and young adult; ETP, early T precursor; Ph, Philadelphia chromosome; SCT, stem cell transplantation; TKI, tyrosine kinase inhibitor.

patients. Thus, age-adapted protocols have emerged, where the age limits are directed by the hematologic and nonhematologic toxicities. **Table 106-4** provides a summary of the best results obtained in adult ALL according to ALL subtype, age, and treatment. Molecular CRs are often durable. The major risk of relapse is in the first 2 years; thereafter, relapse is much less likely.

PROPHYLAXIS AND TREATMENT OF CENTRAL NERVOUS SYSTEM LEUKEMIA

Prophylactic CNS therapy in ALL is essential in order to prevent CNS leukemia and to avoid spread of leukemic cells from the CNS back to the periphery. Treatment options include intrathecal therapy, systemic HD chemotherapy, and cranial radiation therapy (CRT). Intrathecal therapy mostly consists of methotrexate as a single drug or in combination with cytosine arabinoside (AC) with or without glucocorticoids. The route of intrathecal therapy application is generally lumbar puncture. Systemic HD chemotherapy may comprise HDAC or HD methotrexate since both drugs reach cytotoxic drug levels in the CSF and show effectiveness in overt CNS leukemia. CRT (18–24 Gy in 12 fractions over 16 days) is also effective as preventive treatment of CNS leukemia. Using combined modalities for CNS prophylaxis, the CNS relapse rate has decreased to 2–5%.

Particular attention to CNS prophylaxis is required for targeted therapies. In Ph+ ALL, not all TKIs cross the blood-brain barrier equally. Dasatinib and probably ponatinib do cross the blood-brain barrier, whereas imatinib and nilotinib do not. In addition to immunotherapy, intrathecal therapy is required because most antibodies do not enter the CNS.

CNS involvement at diagnosis is observed in 5–10% of adult patients and is higher in mature B-ALL (up to 10–15%) and T-ALL (up to 10%). Treatment consists of the standard chemotherapy with additional intrathecal applications 3–5 times per week until blast cells are cleared in the spinal fluid. Patients with initial CNS involvement have a similar overall survival as CNS-negative patients.

Relapse in CNS is usually accompanied by bone marrow involvement, and if blast cells are not seen morphologically, MRD as a sign of discrete infiltration is positive in nearly all cases. CNS relapse requires local as well as systemic therapy. The outcome after CNS relapse is dismal, and salvage chemotherapy followed by allogeneic SCT is the most effective option. Chimeric antigen receptor (CAR) T cells (most often targeting CD19) can cross the blood-brain barrier and achieve CRs in patients with CNS relapse.

STEM CELL TRANSPLANTATION

SCT is an essential part of the treatment strategy for adult ALL. Peripheral blood cells are increasingly being used as a stem cell source, instead of bone marrow. In addition, a shift from sibling stem cell donors to matched unrelated donors or haploidentical transplants from relatives has occurred. Indications for SCT in first CR are controversial. However, in most studies, SCT is recommended for high-risk patients defined either by conventional prognostic factors or by MRD positivity. High-risk patients transplanted in first CR have a survival rate of 50% or greater; decreasing transplant-related mortality from 20–30% to 10–15% has contributed substantially to better outcomes. For standard-risk patients with sustained molecular remission, allogeneic SCT in first CR is not recommended. Autologous SCT should be restricted to MRD-negative patients, *BCR-ABL*–negative patients, Ph+ patients, and older patients because it is less toxic but associated with a substantially higher relapse rate. For all relapsed adult ALL patients, an allogeneic SCT is thus far the only curative option.

PEDIATRIC-INSPIRED THERAPIES FOR ADOLESCENTS AND YOUNG ADULTS

The principle of pediatric-inspired therapies is to have higher doses and more applications of ALL-specific drugs such as glucocorticoids, vincristine, and L-asparaginase and fewer myeloablative anthracyclines or alkylating agents, with strict adherence to time-dose intensity, thereby reducing the role of SCT. The overall survival rates for AYAs are 70–80%.

ADULT ALL

The treatment results for adult ALL patients have greatly improved with more intensive chemotherapy, optimized SCT, and better supportive care. In several recent multicenter prospective trials, the overall survival rate for standard-risk patients was >70% with chemotherapy alone, and for high-risk patients, the overall survival rate has increased from 20–30% to >50%.

ELDERLY ALL

Palliative treatment regimens for elderly patients have failed, with CR rates of ~40%, a high early death rate of 24%, and a poor overall survival of only a few months. Intensive chemotherapy has also failed, with a higher CR rate of 56%, but still an early death rate of 23%, and only moderate improvement of overall survival to 14 months. Specific elderly ALL protocols with less intensive therapy based on glucocorticoids, vincristine, and asparaginase, largely avoiding anthracyclines and alkylating agents, have improved outcomes. The early treatment-related death rate decreased to <10%, CR rates improved to ~90%, and overall survival of ~30 months was noted.

Frail patients above the age of 70–75 years have very poor survival of <10%. Hopefully, this will improve with ongoing targeted therapies with either TKIs in Ph+ ALL or immunotherapies.

TARGETED THERAPIES

Substantial progress in adult ALL has been made in the past decade by the introduction of new targeted therapies, including TKIs and immunotherapeutic approaches (**Table 106-5**).

TYROSINE KINASE INHIBITORS IN PHILADELPHIA-POSITIVE ALL

Patients with Ph+ ALL constitute ~25% of adult B-ALL patients, with the frequency increasing to ~50% among elderly patients. In the pre-imatinib era, CR rates were 60–70%; survival with chemotherapy was ~10%, and after allogeneic SCT, it was ~30%. With the first-generation TKI imatinib, CR rates increased to 80–90%, the rate of *BCR-ABL* negativity increased from 5 to 50%, and the 5- to 10-year overall survival improved to 50–70%.

Faster and deeper molecular responses are achieved with second-generation TKIs (dasatinib, nilotinib), and these responses apparently

TABLE 106-5 Targeted Therapies in Adult Acute Lymphoblastic Leukemia (ALL)

Tyrosine Kinase Inhibitors (TKIs)
Ph/BCR-ABL+ ALL
TKIs
Imatinib, dasatinib, nilotinib, bosutinib, ponatinib
Ph/BCR-ABL-like ALL
ABL1, ABL2: dasatinib; JAK2: ruxolitinib
Immunologic Approaches
Antibodies directed leukemia surface antigens
Monovalent antibodies
Bivalent antibodies against the tumor and CD3 (e.g., blinatumomab)
Adoptive cellular therapy
T cells engineered to kill leukemic cells
Checkpoint Inhibitors

translate into a survival benefit. The third-generation TKI ponatinib is also effective in tumors bearing mutations (particularly T315I) that convey resistance to earlier-generation TKIs.

Treating adult Ph+ ALL with an allogeneic SCT in first CR is still a good treatment option for adult patients, with a 5-year overall survival of 60–70%. In elderly patients, when low-intensity chemotherapy was combined with dasatinib, the CR rate was >90%. In a next step, by combining mini-chemotherapy with a TKI and adding immunotherapy with inotuzumab (an anti-CD22 antibody), the CR rate was >90% and the overall survival improved further. A pilot experience with a chemotherapy-free regimen composed of dexamethasone, the TKI dasatinib, and the bispecific antibody blinatumomab (anti-CD19 and anti-CD3) demonstrated a CR rate of 98% and 2-year overall and disease-free survival rates of 95% and 88%, respectively. Blinatumomab eliminates Ph+ leukemic cells with resistant mutations.

IMMUNOTHERAPEUTIC APPROACHES

Treatments involving monoclonal antibodies or activated T cells are currently changing the treatment paradigm of ALL. The prerequisite is that B-lineage blast cells express a variety of specific antigens, such as CD19, CD20, and CD22 (**Table 106-6**) that are targetable with a wide variety of monoclonal antibodies. A new treatment principle is the activation of the patient's T cells to destroy their CD19+ leukemic blasts.

Anti-CD20 The anti-CD20 monoclonal antibody rituximab has improved the outcome of patients with de novo Burkitt's leukemia/

TABLE 106-6 Expression of Antigens in B-Cell Lineage Acute Lymphoblastic Leukemia (ALL) for Potential Antibody Therapy

SURFACE ANTIGEN	ALL SUBTYPES	EXPRESSION ON LBC[a]	MONOCLONAL ANTIBODY
CD20	Burkitt's lymphoma/ leukemia	86–100%	Rituximab
	B-precursor	30–40%	Ofatumumab
CD22	B-precursor	93–98%	Inotuzumab
	Mature B-ALL	~100%	Epratuzumab
			Moxetumomab pasudotox
CD19	B-precursor	95–<100%	T cell–activating therapies
	Mature B-ALL	94–<100%	Blinatumomab
			Bispecific CD3/CD19
			Chimeric antigen receptor modified T cells (CAR T cells)

[a]Defined as ≥20% positive blast cells.

Abbreviation: LBC, leukemic blast count.

Source: Republished with permission of American Society of Hematology, from D Hoelzer: Novel antibody-based therapies for acute lymphoblastic leukemia. 2011: 243, 2011: permission conveyed through Copyright Clearance Center, Inc.

lymphoma. With repeated short cycles of intensive chemotherapy combined with rituximab, the overall survival increased to >80%. Rituximab is now included in most B-ALL regimens and is given at the usual dose of 375 mg/m² on day –1 before chemotherapy for at least eight or more cycles. This leads to a significant increase in MRD negativity and improved survival.

Anti-CD22 Monoclonal antibodies directed against CD22 are linked to cytotoxic agents, such as calicheamicin (inotuzumab ozogamicin), or to plant or bacterial toxins (epratuzumab). In a randomized trial of relapsed or refractory ALL patients, the CR rate was 66% and significantly superior to the CR rate with standard chemotherapy. Inotuzumab is now included in first-line therapy for Ph+ and Ph– patients.

Anti-CD19 Targeting CD19 is of great interest because this antigen is highly expressed in all B-lineage cells, most likely including early lymphoid precursor cells. A new promising approach is the bispecific antibody blinatumomab, which combines single-chain antibodies to CD19 and CD3, such that T cells lyse the CD19-bearing B cells.

Blinatumomab is particularly effective in MRD-positive patients, with a 70–80% conversion to MRD negativity, translating into improved overall survival; ~25% of MRD-negative patients survived without any further treatment. Blinatumomab has also moved to frontline therapy.

CAR-T Cells The adoptive transfer of CAR-modified T cells directed against CD19 is a promising approach for the treatment of CD19+ childhood or adult ALL. In the first three larger studies in adults with relapsed or refractory ALL, the CR rate ranged from 67 to 91% with MRD negativity in 60–81% of the patients who achieved CR. Overall survival is 50% or more at ≥2 years, which is remarkable for these heavily pretreated patients. CAR-T cells are also effective in CNS leukemia and in other extramedullary sites. CAR-T cell therapy in relapsed or refractory ALL was first considered as a bridge to allogeneic SCT, applied in 10–50% of patients, but the necessity for an allogeneic SCT after CAR-T cells is unclear. CAR-T cell therapies are also moving to the frontline. CD19-negative relapses after CAR-T cell therapy or blinatumomab due to downregulation of CD19 expression are a relevant obstacle.

Toxicities of Immunotherapies The anti-CD22 agent inotuzumab ozogamicin is associated with hepatotoxicity, including veno-occlusive disease, particularly after allogeneic SCT, but can be managed by reduced dosing and limitation of cycles. For anti-CD19 therapies, cytokine release syndrome and severe neurotoxicity are the most prominent toxicities and often require intensive care unit care (more so after CAR-T cells than blinatumomab). Management of these complications has improved with early recognition. Because toxic death after immunotherapies is very low compared to intensive chemotherapy or allogeneic SCT, immunotherapies are now increasingly included in frontline therapy.

TREATMENT OF T-ALL

Immunotherapy for T-ALL is still not available and intensive chemotherapy is still the mainstay in combination with the T cell–specific drug nelarabine. Currently, γ-secretase targeting *NOTCH1*, checkpoint inhibitors such as bortezomib and venetoclax, and HDAC inhibitors are being explored.

CONCLUSION AND FUTURE DIRECTIONS

Cytogenetic and molecular analysis at diagnosis allows identification of ALL subentities, requiring different treatment options. Evaluation of MRD is the most important parameter for treatment decisions. The greatest progress has been achieved by targeted therapies, such as TKIs for Ph+ ALL and new immunotherapeutic approaches. This will lead to further improved outcome of adult ALL patients, 50% of whom are already surviving 5–10 years and are most likely cured. New options and advances, such as low-intensity chemotherapy, reduction of SCT, incorporation of targeted therapies, and reduction of toxicities, will improve the quality of life of patients and lead to individualized approaches for each patient.

FURTHER READING

BROWN P et al: Effect of postreinduction therapy consolidation with blinatumomab vs chemotherapy on disease-free survival in children, adolescents, and young adults with first relapse of B-cell acute lymphoblastic leukemia A randomized clinical trial. JAMA 325:833, 2021.

FOA R et al: Dasatinib-blinatumomab for Ph-positive acute lymphoblastic leukemia in adults. N Engl J Med 383:1613, 2020.

FREY NV et al: Optimizing chimeric antigen receptor T-cell therapy for adults with acute lymphoblastic leukemia. J Clin Oncol 38:415, 2020.

HOELZER D et al: Improved outcome of adult Burkitt lymphoma/leukemia with rituximab and chemotherapy: report of a large prospective multicenter trial. Blood 124: 3870, 2014.

HOELZER D et al: Acute lymphoblastic leukaemia in adult patients: ESMO Clinical Practice Guidelines for diagnosis, treatment and follow-up. Ann Oncol 27(suppl 5):v69, 2016.

IACOBUCCI I, MULLIGHAN C: Genetic basis of acute lymphoblastic leukemia. J Clin Oncol 35:975, 2017.

KANTARJIAN HM et al: Inotuzumab ozogamicin versus standard therapy for acute lymphoblastic leukemia. N Engl J Med 375:740, 2016.

ROBERTS KG et al: Targetable kinase-activating lesions in Ph-like acute lymphoblastic leukemia. N Engl J Med 371:1005, 2014.

107 Chronic Lymphocytic Leukemia

Jennifer A. Woyach, John C. Byrd

Chronic lymphocytic leukemia (CLL) is a monoclonal proliferation of mature B lymphocytes defined by an absolute number of malignant cells in the blood (5×10^9/mL). The presence of malignant B cells under this count in the blood without nodal, spleen, or liver involvement and absent cytopenias is a precursor of this disease called *monoclonal B cell lymphocytosis* (MBL) with ~1–2% chance per year of progressing to overt CLL. CLL is a heterogeneous disease in terms of natural history, with some patients presenting asymptomatically and never requiring therapy, whereas others present with symptomatic disease, require multiple lines of therapy, and eventually die of their disease. Over the past 10–15 years, the understanding of CLL origin and biology has grown exponentially, leading first to more refined disease definition, prognostic markers, and, subsequently, introduction of novel therapies that have significantly changed the natural history of this disease. In this chapter, we review the epidemiology, biology, and management of CLL, with a focus on new knowledge that is currently changing standards of care.

EPIDEMIOLOGY

CLL is primarily a disease of older adults, with a median age at diagnosis of 71 and an age-adjusted incidence of 4.5/100,000 people in the United States. The prevalence of CLL has increased over the past decades due to improvements in therapy for this disease and also survival of older patients from other medical ailments. In 1980, the 5-year overall survival of patients was 69%, and this increased to 87.9% in 2007 and is likely even higher today. The male-to-female ratio is 2:1; however, as patients age, the ratio becomes more even, and over the age of 80, the incidence is equal between men and women. The disease is most common in Caucasians, less common in Hispanic and African Americans, and rare in the Asian population.

Unlike many other malignancies, there have been no definitive links between CLL and exposures. Indeed, CLL is one of the only types of leukemia not linked to radiation exposure. Agent Orange exposure has been implicated, and CLL is thus a service-connected condition for those who were exposed to Agent Orange in the Vietnam conflict.

CLL is one of the most familial-associated malignancies, and the first-degree relative of a CLL patient has an 8.5-fold elevated risk of developing CLL than the general population. MBL is also more common in families with two first-degree relatives having CLL, further supporting a genetic predisposition of this disease. Despite this, specific genes conferring risk in the familial setting outside of specific families have been difficult to identify. In genome-wide association studies (GWAS), ~30 single nucleotide polymorphisms have been identified, which is estimated to account for 19% of the familial risk of CLL. Genes involved in apoptosis, telomere function, B-cell receptor (BCR) activation, and B-cell differentiation have all been implicated in GWAS. Variants in shelterin complex proteins involved in telomere maintenance such as POT1 have been identified in a small number of families.

BIOLOGY AND PATHOPHYSIOLOGY

CELL OF ORIGIN

The cell of origin in CLL has not definitively been established. The morphology, immunophenotype, and gene expression pattern of CLL cells are that of a mature B cell (**Fig. 107-1**), and so it has been presumed that the initiating cell is a mature lymphocyte, perhaps memory B cells. However, many facets of CLL biology do not support this idea, including antigen-binding characteristics of CLL cells and the presence of stereotyped BCRs. Other possibilities include a stepwise process including a series of transforming events at various stages of B-cell development, potentially including de-differentiation of more mature cells. The self-renewing, multipotent hematopoietic stem cell (HSC) might also be the originating cell of CLL, postulated based on transplant studies in mice showing clonal leukemic cell development with different characteristics from donor leukemia after transplantation of HSCs. More work will be required to elucidate the origins of CLL.

B-CELL RECEPTOR SIGNALING IN CLL

Perhaps the most important advancement in CLL biology is the understanding of the role of BCR signaling in the disease. CLL has distinct BCR signaling as compared to normal B cells, which is characterized by low-level IgM expression, variable response to antigen stimulation, and tonic activation of antiapoptotic signaling pathways that promote tumor survival. CLL cells by gene expression profiling share many features with antigen-activated mature B cells, suggesting a role for activation of BCR signaling in the disease pathogenesis. Tissue-based microarrays have revealed upregulation of BCR pathway genes in the lymph nodes and bone marrow compared to the peripheral blood, suggesting a particular importance of this pathway in microenvironmental homing.

Fitting with the role of BCR signaling in CLL, one of the most influential prognostic factors identified in this disease is the mutational status of the immunoglobulin heavy chain variable (IGHV) region. During normal B-cell maturation, the variable regions of the

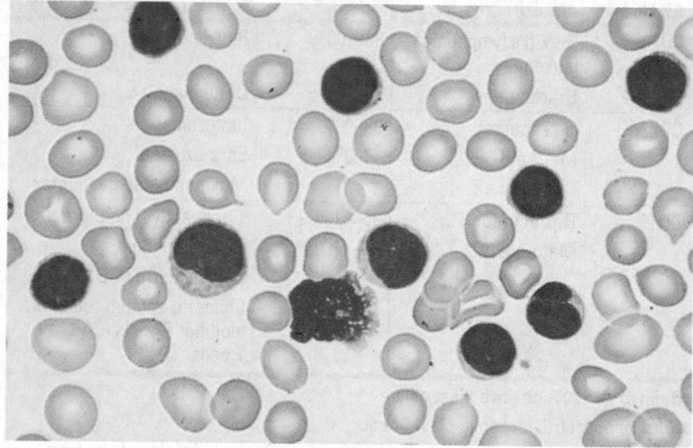

FIGURE 107-1 Chronic lymphoid leukemia in the peripheral blood. *(From M Lichtman et al [eds]: Williams Hematology, 7th ed. New York, McGraw-Hill, 2005.)*

immunoglobulin heavy chain undergo somatic hypermutation. In CLL, ~60% of patients have IGHV that is ≥2% mutated from germline. This may indicate a more mature, postgerminal center progenitor, and is typically associated with a more indolent disease course. Conversely, ~40% of patients will have IGHV <2% mutated from germline, which is associated with more rapid progression of disease and short survival prior to the era of therapeutics that target BCR. Unfavorable biologic properties including enhanced telomerase activity, overexpression of activation-induced cytidine deaminase, increased nuclear factor-κB (NF-κB) activity, high-risk genomic mutations (e.g., *NOTCH1*, *SF3B1*, *TP53*, *ATM*), and clonal evolution are also associated with IGHV unmutated disease.

Because IGHV sequencing was initially cumbersome to perform, a number of surrogate factors have been identified; however, none yet have been shown to be equal or superior to IGHV sequencing. The most prevalent of these surrogate markers are Zap-70 expression, *ZAP-70* methylation, and surface CD38 expression. Zap-70 protein is a normal intracellular T-cell signaling protein that is aberrantly expressed in most IGHV unmutated CLL cells. CD38 is a marker that is also more highly expressed on the surface of IGHV unmutated CLL cells. Both of these prognostic factors are widely used but limited in their applicability. Zap-70 protein status is difficult to measure by flow cytometry and has low reproducibility. Measurement of methylation status of the *ZAP-70* promoter is much more precise but not widely available. CD38 expression is easier to measure by flow cytometry but not as highly predictive of outcomes and can change during the course of disease.

CYTOGENETIC ABNORMALITIES

Besides IGHV mutational status, recurrent cytogenetic abnormalities are the most robust prognostic factor clinically available in CLL. These abnormalities are typically identified by fluorescent in situ hybridization (FISH) analysis; however, stimulated metaphase karyotype has a role as well. The most well-characterized abnormalities include del(13)(q14.3), trisomy 12, del(11)(q22.3), and del(17)(p13.1) (**Fig. 107-2**). The presence of sole del(13)(q14.3) is associated with more indolent disease, prolonged survival, and good response to traditional therapies. Usually, this abnormality is not seen on banded karyotype analysis, and when present on karyotype, it indicates a larger deletion involving the retinoblastoma gene, which negates the favorable prognosis associated with this marker. Trisomy 12 has a more intermediate prognosis. The del(11)(q23.3) results in deletion of the *ATM* gene and is associated with bulky lymphadenopathy and aggressive disease in young patients, with inferior prognosis, and more rapid progression to symptomatic disease. The del(17)(p13.1) results in loss of one allele of the tumor suppressor TP53 and is associated with the poorest prognosis in CLL with rapid disease progression, poor response to traditional therapies, and shorter survival. Other abnormalities have been shown to be important in smaller studies but are not routinely performed at all centers. Finally, complex karyotype (three or more abnormalities) on stimulated metaphase karyotype analysis has significant adverse impact on time to treatment and overall survival, with data indicating that increasing complexity is even more deleterious to response and survival.

Clonal evolution, or acquisition of cytogenetic or molecular abnormalities, is common in CLL, especially in patients with IGHV unmutated CLL. Because the tumor cytogenetics can change over time, it is recommended that FISH, with or without cytogenetics, is checked before every line of therapy, mostly to evaluate acquisition of del(17)(p13.1).

GENE MUTATIONS AND MIR ALTERATIONS

Compared with many other malignancies, the genome in CLL is relatively simple, with an average CLL genome carrying ~20 nonsynonymous alterations and ~5 structural abnormalities. And, unlike many other hematologic malignancies, there is no unifying genetic lesion, and most recurrent genetic driving mutations exist at frequencies of <5%. Whole genome and whole exome sequencing have identified the most common mutations in CLL to be in *SF3B1*, *NOTCH1*, *MYD88*, *ATM*, and *TP53* (**Table 107-1**). Most of the identified mutations in these genes are common among different malignancies, and with the exception of *MYD88*, they are generally identified with much higher frequency in IGHV unmutated disease.

NOTCH1 mutations are present in ~15% of CLL patients and are commonly associated with trisomy 12. Although multiple different mutations are seen, most are located within the PEST (proline, glutamic acid, serine, and threonine) domain and result in constitutive NOTCH signaling. *NOTCH1* mutations have been associated with lower sensitivity to CD20 antibody therapy and increased risk of transformation to aggressive diffuse large B-cell lymphoma (DLBCL; Richter's transformation), although its relevance in the era of targeted therapies is less clear. *SF3B1* is a component of the RNA spliceosome and is mutated in 10–15% of CLL cases. Mutations appear to be associated with

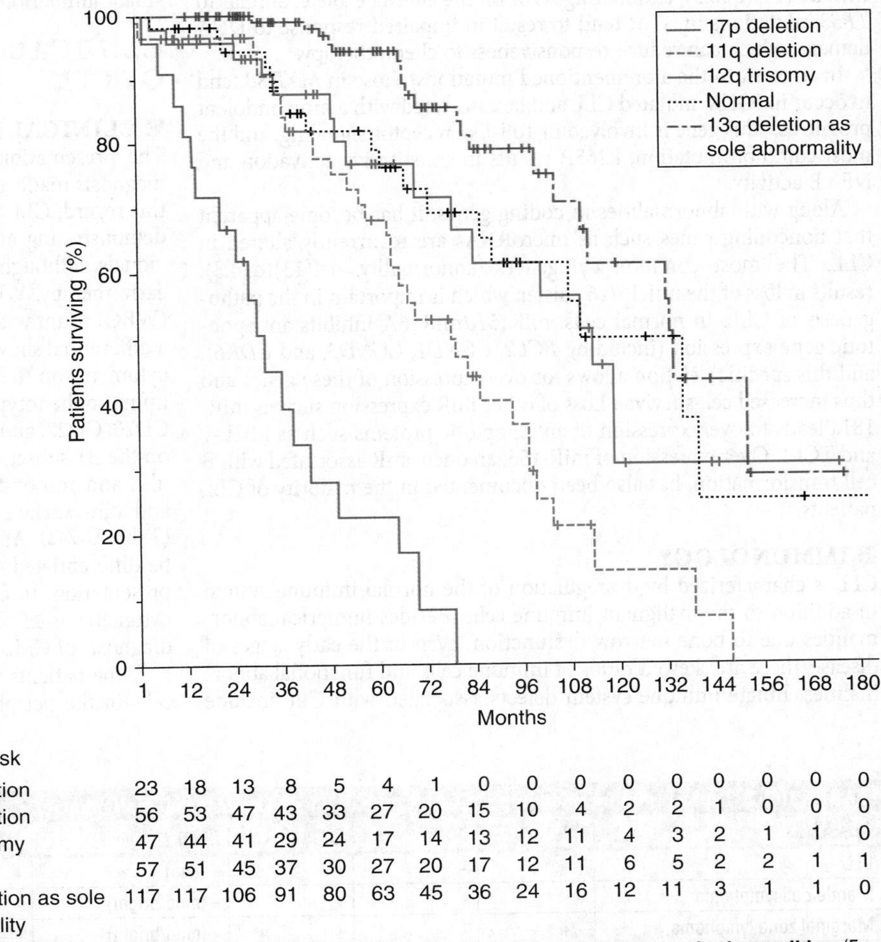

No. AT Risk																
17p deletion	23	18	13	8	5	4	1	0	0	0	0	0	0	0	0	0
11q deletion	56	53	47	43	33	27	20	15	10	4	2	2	1	0	0	0
12q trisomy	47	44	41	29	24	17	14	13	12	11	4	3	2	1	1	0
Normal	57	51	45	37	30	27	20	17	12	11	6	5	2	2	1	1
13q deletion as sole abnormality	117	117	106	91	80	63	45	36	24	16	12	11	3	1	1	0

FIGURE 107-2 Outcomes among chronic lymphocytic leukemia patients with various cytogenetic abnormalities. *(From H Döhner et al: Genomic aberrations and survival in chronic lymphocytic leukemia. N Engl J Med 343:1910, 2000. Copyright © (2000) Massachusetts Medical Society. Reprinted with permission from Massachusetts Medical Society.)*

TABLE 107-1 Recurrent Mutations in CLL

GENE	FREQUENCY OF MUTATIONS (%)
SF3B1	8–14
TP53	5–13
NOTCH1	10–13
MYD88	4–8
ATM	8–11
BIRC3	<5
XPO1	<5
FBXW7	<5
POT1	<5
BRAF	<5
EGR2	<5
IKZF3	<5

Abbreviation: CLL, chronic lymphocytic leukemia.

intermediate-risk disease, and, functionally, *SF3B1* may be important in the response to DNA damage.

Mutations of the tumor suppressor *TP53* are found in ~5% of CLL patients with previously untreated early-stage disease and up to 40% with later stages. Seventy percent of the time, these mutations coexist with del(17)(p13.1), effectively eliminating TP53 function. As expected, and consistent with other malignancies, *TP53* mutations are associated with a poor prognosis and expected lack of response to DNA-damaging therapies.

ATM mutations, which are heterogeneous and occur throughout the gene, occur in 10–15% of CLL patients. *ATM* mutations often coexist with del(11)(q22.3), eliminating *ATM* on the alternate allele. Similar to *TP53*, mutations in *ATM* tend to result in impaired response to DNA damage, which can reduce responsiveness to chemotherapy.

In contrast to the aforementioned mutations, those in *MYD88* tend to occur in IGHV mutated CLL and be associated with a more indolent prognosis. This gene is involved in Toll-like receptor signaling, and the most common mutation, L265P, results in constitutive activation and NF-κB activity.

Along with abnormalities in coding genes, it has become apparent that noncoding genes such as microRNAs are recurrently altered in CLL. The most common cytogenetic abnormality, del(13)(q14.3), results in loss of the miR15/16 cluster, which is important in the pathogenesis of CLL. In normal cells, miR15A/miR16A inhibits antiapoptotic gene expression (including *BCL2, CCND1, CCND3*, and *CDK6*), and this specific deletion allows for overexpression of these genes and thus increased cell survival. Loss of other miR expression such as miR-181a leads to overexpression of antiapoptotic proteins such as MCL-1 and TCL1. Overexpression of miR-155, an onco-miR associated with B cell transformation, has also been documented in the majority of CLL patients.

■ IMMUNOLOGY

CLL is characterized by dysregulation of the normal immune system in addition to the malignant immune cells. Besides numerical abnormalities due to bone marrow dysfunction, even in the early stages of disease, there are skewed ratios of immune cells and functional abnormalities. Innate immune system defects associated with CLL include reduced complement proteins and activity, qualitative neutrophil defects, and functional defects of natural killer cells.

More focus has been placed on the impairments in the adaptive immune system in this disease. Within the CD4+ T-cell compartment, a qualitative defect is noted similar to chronic antigen stimulation inducing a phenotype of T-cell exhaustion typical of what is seen in chronic viral infections such as hepatitis. This has been demonstrated to lead to impaired T-cell cytotoxic capacity and reduced proliferative ability. Additionally, there are physical changes in the T-cell cytoskeleton that cause impaired immune synapse formation with antigen presenting cells. In addition to a lack of capacity to respond to pathogens, the T-cell defect in CLL also likely leads to tumor cell tolerance. During the course of the disease, the polarization of the CD4+ T cells shifts from a Th1 (cytotoxic) phenotype to a Th2 phenotype, which leads to expansion of immunosuppressive cytokines such as interleukin 10 (IL-10). Additionally, in the later stage of disease, T regulatory cells are expanded, which contributes to an immunosuppressive phenotype.

Other components of the immune microenvironment are altered as well to form a more supportive environment for the malignant cells. M2 monocytes have been shown to differentiate into a type of tumor-associated macrophage known as a *nurse-like cell* in CLL. These cells promote survival by secreting chemokines and cytokines that increase migration and activation.

The humoral immune system in CLL is also dysregulated, as is expected for a malignancy that results in very few normal B cells. Hypogammaglobulinemia is very common and affects all subclasses of immunoglobulins, occurring in ~85% of patients at some time in their disease course, and is more common as disease progresses. A correlation between low IgG and IgA and infection risk has been established, but isolated IgM reduction does not seem to be associated with excess infection risk. Also, CLL cells can secrete monoclonal IgM or IgG in a small number of cases, and this can correlate with disease progression.

CLINICAL PRESENTATION AND DIAGNOSIS OF CLL

■ CLINICAL PRESENTATION AND DIAGNOSIS

The presentation of CLL most commonly occurs as an incidental diagnosis made at the time of medical evaluation for another cause. In this regard, CLL is most commonly diagnosed on routine blood work demonstrating an elevated lymphocyte count in asymptomatic individuals, although some patients present with symptoms and require early therapy. When noting either an elevated total white blood cell (WBC) count with lymphocytic predominance or a normal WBC with a differential showing a lymphocytosis, the next step is to perform flow cytometry on the peripheral blood. In CLL, this will reveal the typical immunophenotype that includes the typical B cell markers CD19, CD20, CD22, and CD23; the T-cell marker CD5 (CD5 is also expressed on the B1 subset of B cells that typically has unmutated immunoglobulin and responds to antigens independent of cognate T cell help); and dim surface immunoglobulin of either kappa or lambda type (**Table 107-2**). Atypical phenotypes can be seen as well and usually can be differentiated on the basis of morphology, cytogenetics, or clinical presentation. In cases in which the clonal B cell count based on flow cytometry is $\geq 5 \times 10^9$/L, no further workup is needed to confirm the diagnosis of CLL.

Some patients will present with a small clonal proliferation of CLL cells in the peripheral blood but will also have lymphadenopathy or

TABLE 107-2 Typical Immunophenotype of CLL Compared with Other B Cell Malignancies

DISEASE	CD5	CD10	CD19	CD20	CD23	CYCLIN D1	SURFACE IG
CLL	+	–	+	+ (dim)	+	–	+ (dim)
Mantle cell lymphoma	+	–	+	+ (mod/bright)	–	+	+ (mod/bright)
Marginal zone lymphoma	–/+	–	+	+ (mod/bright)	–/+	–	+ (mod/bright)
Follicular lymphoma	–	+	+	+	+	–	

Abbreviation: CLL, chronic lymphocytic leukemia.

splenomegaly. In these cases, the likely diagnosis is small lymphocytic lymphoma (SLL), a semantic designation from CLL that denotes a primarily tissue-based disease rather than bone marrow/blood-based disease. The genetic and molecular features of SLL are identical to those of CLL. The retention of the cells in tissues may be related to the expression of a particular adhesion molecule. Thus, SLL patients are managed identically to CLL patients, and often in the later stages of disease, these patients will have blood and bone marrow involvement as well.

MONOCLONAL B-CELL LYMPHOCYTOSIS

Patients who do not meet the diagnostic criteria for CLL based on quantification of clonal B cells in the peripheral blood and who do not have associated signs of CLL including lymphadenopathy, organomegaly, or cytopenias have a disorder known as monoclonal B-cell lymphocytosis (MBL), which is now thought to precede every case of CLL. Analogous to monoclonal gammopathy of uncertain significance (MGUS) in myeloma, not all MBL progresses to CLL. MBL is initially characterized by a CLL-like immunophenotype in ~75% of cases but can also be atypical (CD23 negative or bright CD20) or CD5 negative. More relevant for prognosis is characterization by count, with low-count MBL defining those patients with $<0.5 \times 10^9$ clonal B cells/L, and high-count MBL defining those with $>0.5 \times 10^9$ but $<5 \times 10^9$/L. Patients with low-count MBL have a negligible rate of progression to CLL, whereas those with high count progress to overt CLL at a rate of 1–2% per year, warranting continued monitoring. Population-based studies have estimated the prevalence of MBL to be up to ~12% in the general population, where it is most common in elderly men. It is especially common in first-degree relatives of CLL patients, where the frequency is ~18%.

Although the risk of MBL progression is relatively low, it has become apparent that patients still experience complications that suggest an immune dysfunction in MBL that is similar to that seen with CLL. Rates of serious infections requiring hospitalization appear to be significantly increased in MBL, similar to the rates seen in CLL. In a case-control study, patients with MBL had a 16% chance of hospitalization over a 4-year time period, compared with 18.4% in patients with newly diagnosed CLL. Secondary cancers also appear to be increased in MBL. These data suggest that monitoring for patients with MBL should focus on vaccinations and age-appropriate cancer screening, as the probability of complications appears to be higher than the risk of progression in most of these patients. Follow-up for patients with MBL can occur with the primary care physician as this does not represent a malignancy, whereas CLL is mostly comanaged with both a primary care physician and a hematologist.

COMPLICATIONS OF CLL

A significant amount of morbidity and mortality related to CLL is due to complications of the disease. In general, complications besides disease progression include infections, secondary cancers, autoimmune complications, and transformation to a more aggressive clonally related lymphoma.

INFECTIONS

Infections are a leading cause of both disease-related morbidity and death in patients with CLL, with ~30–50% of deaths in CLL patients attributed to infection. Owing to the immune dysfunction associated with the disease, patients are at risk for both typical and atypical infections. Besides this baseline risk of infections, most CLL therapies can increase infection risk. For many nucleoside analogue–based chemotherapy regimens used in CLL, prophylaxis for *Pneumocystis* pneumonia is indicated for at least 6 months following therapy to allow recovery of functional T cells. Viral prophylaxis is also indicated for many chemotherapy regimens and for patients with a history of varicella-zoster to diminish reactivation and morbidity from this virus.

Because of the abnormalities in cellular and humoral immunity, vaccine responses in CLL are limited in many patients, especially in the later stages of disease. In one study, one dose of 13-valent pneumococcal vaccine produced an adequate immune response in only 58% of patients compared with 100% in age-matched controls. Despite the known limitations, vaccination against influenza and pneumococcal pneumonia is recommended in CLL. The recombinant zoster vaccine has approximately a 60% response in previously untreated CLL, is safe, and should be considered for this patient group. In contrast, live vaccines should be avoided in the setting of CLL because of the small risk of viral reactivation with an immunocompromised host.

As discussed earlier, hypogammaglobulinemia is common in CLL and can be associated with significant risk for infections, primarily of mucocutaneous etiology such as sinusitis and bronchitis. In addition, women can have frequent urinary tract infections. While administration of prophylactic intravenous immunoglobulin (IVIg) has not been shown to improve survival, it has been shown to reduce the number of minor or moderate bacterial infections and thus is indicated in patients with hypogammaglobulinemia who suffer from recurrent infections or have pulmonary bronchiectasis. We also administer at least one dose of immunoglobulin to CLL patients who develop influenza with coexisting hypogammaglobulinemia to diminish risk of postinfluenza pneumococcal pneumonia. IVIg is also indicated in patients who have been hospitalized for a serious infection and in those whose IgG level is <300–500 mg/dL.

SECONDARY MALIGNANCIES

Multiple population-based studies have shown that patients with CLL are at an elevated risk to develop other cancers, with a rate up to three times that of the general population, even in the absence of cytotoxic chemotherapy. The most common types of cancers seen in CLL are skin, prostate, and breast cancers, although other cancers are seen as well. Skin cancers are particularly common, with a rate that is 8- to 15-fold higher than in the general population, and may behave more aggressively. All CLL patients should be counseled on the use of sunscreen while outdoors and should undergo preventative skin examinations.

In one single-center study, older age at CLL diagnosis, male sex, high β_2-microglobulin, high lactate dehydrogenase (LDH), and chronic kidney disease were associated with excess risk of other cancers; other CLL-specific risk factors have not shown association with other cancer risk.

While cancer risk is higher, no specific recommendations for increased cancer screening in CLL patients have been validated. Age- and sex-appropriate screenings should be recommended.

Conflicting data exist regarding the risk of cancers following CLL-specific therapy. Chemoimmunotherapy, in particular alkylator-containing regimens, seems to be associated with an increased risk for secondary cancers. Secondary cancers are also seen in the setting of targeted therapies. Bruton tyrosine kinase (BTK) inhibitors appear to have a secondary cancer risk similar to what is seen in the CLL population in general, but potentially a higher rate of nonmelanoma skin cancers. With short follow-up, the risk of secondary cancers appears to be slightly higher with venetoclax-based regimens than chlorambucil-based chemoimmunotherapy, and further evaluation of this trend is ongoing.

AUTOIMMUNE COMPLICATIONS

Autoimmune complications are frequent in CLL. Most commonly, these include autoimmune cytopenias, but autoimmune complications of other organs including glomerulonephritis, vasculitis, and neuropathies have also been reported. Of the autoimmune cytopenias, the most common is autoimmune hemolytic anemia (AIHA), which is an antibody-mediated destruction of autologous red blood cells (RBCs). Second most common is immune thrombocytopenia (ITP), which shares some features with AIHA and has a similar mechanism targeting platelets. These two syndromes may occur in isolation, occur sequentially in the same patient, or present in combination as Evan's syndrome. Pure red cell aplasia (PRCA) and autoimmune granulocytopenia (AIG) are comparatively rare and can occur alone or in combination with other autoimmune cytopenias. It is difficult to tease out whether autoimmune cytopenias lead to worse prognosis in CLL because of various complicating factors. However, it is clear that these can lead to significant morbidity, both due to the process itself and due to therapies required for management.

AIHA usually presents as an isolated anemia with an elevated reticulocyte count and features of hemolysis including elevated bilirubin and LDH and low haptoglobin. Detection of a warm IgG antibody on the surface of RBCs with a Coombs test can help solidify the diagnosis, although Coombs-negative cases can occur. Immediate therapy is almost always necessary and consists of transfusion and immunosuppression. Glucocorticoids are often used for initial therapy, although in most cases, additional treatment is needed due to either poor response or recurrence with taper of glucocorticoid dosing. Rituximab can be successful, and therapy directed toward the underlying CLL is often effective in more resistant cases. Transfusion of blood in cases of robust AIHA must be initiated with caution as transfusion reactions can be seen due to poorly matched blood, but should be pursued in those with severe, symptomatic anemia. Death from uncontrolled AIHA can occur in the absence of appropriate supportive care (**Chap. 100**).

ITP can be more difficult to diagnose as it may be difficult to differentiate from progression of disease due to the lack of laboratory tests that identify platelet destruction from this mechanism. Signs that point toward ITP include isolated thrombocytopenia and rapid decline in platelet levels in the absence of an alternative etiology. A bone marrow biopsy showing normal or increased megakaryocytes can be used to confirm the diagnosis but is often not necessary. In CLL, treatment for ITP is usually instituted when platelet levels drop to 20,000–30,000 or if evidence of bleeding complications or need for invasive procedures develops. Like AIHA, initial therapy consists of glucocorticoids and IVIg, with rituximab also being an effective method to induce long-term remissions. Also, the thrombopoietin receptor agonists romiplostim and eltrombopag are effective in secondary ITP. In many cases, ITP can be successfully treated without treating the underlying CLL. In cases in which anemia or thrombocytopenia appears, it is important to investigate the mechanism because the approach to therapy of autoimmune cytopenias in CLL differs from cytopenias due to marrow replacement (**Chap. 115**).

■ RICHTER'S TRANSFORMATION

One of the most devastating complications of CLL is Richter's transformation, which is transformation of CLL to an aggressive lymphoma, most commonly DLBCL. The World Health Organization also recognizes Hodgkin's lymphoma (HL) as a variant of Richter's transformation; other aggressive lymphomas are rarely identified. Some older series have included prolymphocytic transformation in this category, although this has much less prognostic impact on long-term outcome. The prevalence of Richter's transformation is difficult to estimate based on previous studies, but one prospective observational study estimated a rate of 0.5% per year for DLBCL and 0.05% per year for HL. Risk factors for development include bulky lymphadenopathy, *NOTCH1* mutations, del(17)(p13.1), and a specific stereotyped IGHV usage. Lymphomas arising in the setting of CLL can either be clonally related or unrelated to the initial CLL, with prognosis significantly better for clonally unrelated lymphomas. In addition, patients with Hodgkin's transformation have improved outcome, particularly in the absence of prior fludarabine treatment. B-cell prolymphocytic leukemia (PLL) arising from CLL is currently classified as Richter's transformation as well; however, clinical features and therapy are quite different, so these two should be differentiated for therapeutic purposes.

Clinical signs of Richter's transformation include rapid progression in adenopathy, often in a specific area, and constitutional symptoms including fatigue, night sweats, fever, and weight loss. LDH is usually high. In suspected cases, the first step is ^{18}FDG-PET/CT (fluorodeoxyglucose–positron emission tomography combined with computed tomography) scan to localize an area for biopsy. Standardized uptake values (SUVs) <5 are consistent with CLL and can rule out Richter's transformation in many cases. SUVs >5 are suspicious for Richter's transformation, with SUVs ≥10 being very concerning. Excisional biopsy is the preferred mode of diagnosis, and fine-needle aspiration should be discouraged.

Therapy for DLBCL Richter's transformation usually involves combination chemoimmunotherapy (e.g., R-CHOP [rituximab, cyclophosphamide, doxorubicin, vincristine, and prednisolone], dose-adjusted EPOCH-R [etoposide, prednisone, vincristine, cyclophosphamide, doxorubicin, and rituximab]; **Chap. 108**). Outcomes may be poor with median survivals of 6–16 months in most series for clonally related Richter's versus ~5 years for clonally unrelated. For fit patients who achieve a response with therapy, stem cell transplantation has the possibility to induce long-term remissions and should be explored. In addition, chimeric antigen receptor T-cell (CAR-T) therapy has shown promising results in small groups of patients and remains an area of active clinical investigation. Patients with Hodgkin's disease can be treated according to the algorithm for this disease, with many individuals being cured.

WORKUP OF CLL AND APPROACH TO THERAPY

■ WORKUP AND STAGING

Workup of a patient with a new diagnosis of CLL based on typical immunophenotyping includes a detailed history of infectious disease; family history of CLL; and careful physical examination with attention to the lymph nodes, spleen, and liver. In patients desiring to know the expected natural history of their CLL, prognostic testing using FISH and stimulated karyotype and sequencing for *TP53* and *IGHV* mutation status can be performed. Imaging with CT scan is usually not necessary unless there are symptoms and concern for intraabdominal nodes out of proportion to peripheral nodes. Bone marrow biopsy is not undertaken until therapy is initiated except in cases of unexplained cytopenias.

■ STAGING

There are two widely used staging systems in CLL. The Rai staging system is used more commonly in the United States, whereas the Binet system is more commonly used in Europe. Both characterize CLL on the basis of disease bulk and marrow failure (**Table 107-3**). Both rely on physical examination and laboratory studies and do not require imaging or bone marrow analysis. While the initial staging systems could reliably predict survival in CLL, with the changes in therapy since the original description of the stages, the impact of initial stage on survival is not as clear. Cytogenetic and genomic testing can help refine outcomes of these staging tests. An international collaboration integrated both clinical and genomic staging to better predict outcome at diagnosis and time of initial treatment, which led to development of the CLL International Prognostic Index (**Table 107-4**). This index has been shown to be useful in prediction of both time to first treatment and outcome with chemoimmunotherapy. Validation in the setting of novel targeted therapies has not occurred.

■ CRITERIA FOR THE INITIATION OF THERAPY

Currently, a watchful waiting strategy is used for most patients with CLL, with therapy reserved for patients with symptomatic disease. This recommendation is based on multiple trials showing no survival advantage with earlier therapy, although this question continues to be a focus of active investigation.

With the exception of patients participating on early intervention studies in CLL, disease-related symptoms that require the initiation of therapy are outlined in **Table 107-5**. Except for the rare patient who

TABLE 107-3 Staging of CLL

Rai Staging System	
Low risk (stage 0)	Lymphocytosis only
Intermediate risk (stage I/II)	Lymphocytosis with lymphadenopathy, with or without splenomegaly or hepatomegaly
High risk (stage III/IV)	Lymphocytosis with anemia or thrombocytopenia due to bone marrow involvement
Binet Staging System	
A	<3 areas of lymphadenopathy
B	≥3 areas of lymphadenopathy
C	Hemoglobin ≤10 g/dL and/or platelets <100,000/μL

Abbreviation: CLL, chronic lymphocytic leukemia.

TABLE 107-4 CLL International Prognostic Index

Risk Score

VARIABLE	ADVERSE FACTOR	RISK SCORE
TP53 status	Deleted or mutated	4
IGHV mutational status	Unmutated	2
β_2-microglobulin concentration	>3.5 mg/L	2
Clinical stage	Rai I–IV or Binet B–C	1
Age	>65 years	1

Implications of Risk Score

RISK SCORE	RISK CLASSIFICATION	5-YEAR SURVIVAL (TRAINING SET DATA)
0–1	Low	93.2%
2–3	Intermediate	79.3%
4–6	High	63.3%
7–10	Very high	23.3%

Abbreviation: CLL, chronic lymphocytic leukemia.

presents with disease requiring urgent therapy, most times, these symptoms can be monitored over short periods to determine relatedness to CLL and need for therapy.

INITIAL THERAPY FOR CLL

Over the past decade, the initial therapy of CLL has dramatically changed. Whereas chemoimmunotherapy was once standard for all patients, now most patients are treated with oral therapies targeted against BTK or BCL2 with or without a CD20 monoclonal antibody. This continues to be an area of active investigation, with standards of care shifting rapidly. The major classes of these therapies are outlined here.

BTK Inhibitors BTK is an attractive target in CLL because, unlike other kinases in the BCR pathway, BTK does not have natural redundancy and is relatively selective for B cells, so inhibition leads to a predominant B cell–specific phenotype. The first-in-class BTK inhibitor is ibrutinib, which is relatively selective for BTK but also inhibits a number of structurally similar kinases. As initial therapy, ibrutinib was initially compared with chlorambucil (RESONATE 2 study), and there was an 84% lower risk of progression or death with ibrutinib, with 70% of ibrutinib-treated patients alive and progression-free at 5 years. Subsequent studies compared ibrutinib alone or with the anti-CD20 antibody rituximab to standard chemoimmunotherapy with fludarabine plus cyclophosphamide plus rituximab (FCR) in younger patients (<70 years; E1912 study) or bendamustine plus rituximab (BR) in older patients (≥65 years; A041202 study). In younger patients, ibrutinib plus rituximab (IR) showed increased progression-free survival (PFS) and overall survival (OS) when compared with FCR, with a 3-year PFS of 89% for IR compared with 71% for FCR. In older patients, ibrutinib alone as well as with rituximab showed superior PFS compared with BR, with 24-month PFS rates of 88% for IR, 87% for ibrutinib alone, and 74% for BR. IR was not superior to ibrutinib alone, and OS was not different in this trial at 24 months. Side effects distinct to ibrutinib include arthralgias/myalgias, rash, diarrhea, dyspepsia, increased risk of bleeding (particularly when on anticoagulation therapy or with surgery), hypertension, and atrial fibrillation.

The second-generation BTK inhibitor acalabrutinib is more specific for BTK than ibrutinib and consequentially shows better tolerability, with less incidence of atrial fibrillation, myalgias/arthralgias, and skin and nail changes than reported with ibrutinib. In the frontline setting, acalabrutinib and acalabrutinib plus obinutuzumab were compared with chlorambucil plus obinutuzumab. Both acalabrutinib alone and acalabrutinib with obinutuzumab showed superior 30-month PFS compared with chlorambucil plus obinutuzumab (82%, 90%, and 34%, respectively), with improved PFS for acalabrutinib plus obinutuzumab compared with acalabrutinib alone in an unplanned post hoc analysis.

TABLE 107-5 Criteria for the Initiation of Therapy

Symptoms Indicating Need for Therapy in CLL
Evidence of progressive marrow failure (worsening of anemia or thrombocytopenia not due to autoimmune destruction)
Massive (≥6 cm below costal margin), progressive, or symptomatic splenomegaly
Massive (≥10 cm), progressive, or symptomatic lymphadenopathy
Progressive lymphocytosis with an increase of ≥50% over a 2-month period or lymphocyte doubling time <6 months
Autoimmune anemia or thrombocytopenia not responsive to standard therapy
Symptomatic or functional extranodal involvement
Constitutional symptoms (one or more of the following: unintentional weight loss ≥10% over 6 months, significant fatigue, fevers ≥100.5°C for 2+ weeks without infection, night sweats for >1 month without infection)

Abbreviation: CLL, chronic lymphocytic leukemia.

BCL2 Inhibitor Venetoclax is an orally bioavailable, selective inhibitor of the antiapoptotic protein BCL2, which is upregulated in CLL. Unlike with BTK inhibitors, where many phase 3 studies support benefit over chemoimmunotherapy, only one study has been published with venetoclax. The CLL14 study compared venetoclax plus obinutuzumab (VO) to chlorambucil plus obinutuzumab in previously untreated patients with coexisting medical conditions. Unlike BTK inhibitors, which are administered continuously until disease progression, VO treatment is given for a 1-year fixed duration. At 3 years of follow-up, PFS was 82% in the VO group compared with 50% in the chlorambucil plus obinutuzumab group. No difference has been observed in OS with this follow-up. Side effects associated with venetoclax include tumor lysis syndrome, neutropenia, and nausea.

PI3K Inhibitors Inhibitors of PI3K delta have been studied in CLL due to the specificity of the delta isoform for B lymphocytes. Two agents, idelalisib and duvelisib, are approved for use in relapsed CLL, but trials of idelalisib in frontline CLL demonstrated toxicity that precluded further development in this area. Toxicities seen with idelalisib and duvelisib include pneumonitis, diarrhea/colitis, and transaminitis. More recently, a second-generation PI3K delta inhibitor umbralisib was combined with the anti-CD20 antibody ublituximab in the frontline setting and compared with chlorambucil plus obinutuzumab. Twenty-four-month PFS was 61% for ublituximab plus umbralisib compared with 40% with chlorambucil plus obinutuzumab. PI3K inhibitor–specific toxicities appear to be lower with umbralisib compared with idelalisib and duvelisib, but comparative trials are lacking. As outcome with this combination appears inferior to that with BTK inhibitors or BCL2 inhibitors, it is unlikely this treatment will be used in CLL outside of rare circumstances where other classes of drugs are contraindicated.

Chemoimmunotherapy For the most part, targeted therapy has supplanted chemoimmunotherapy in CLL. However, long-term follow-up of studies of FCR has demonstrated that a subset of patients treated with this regimen can have durable responses over 10 years, with a likely cure of CLL. This group is composed almost exclusively of patients with mutated *IGHV* and favorable cytogenetics. However, despite the efficacy of this regimen, short- and long-term toxicities limit its adaptability to many patients with *IGHV* mutated disease. Short-term toxicities are mostly related to myelosuppression and include neutropenia and infection. Long-term cytopenias are less common, but they do occur. Also, there is about a 3–5% risk of therapy-related myeloid neoplasm with this regimen that is almost always fatal. In the E1912 study of FCR versus IR, at follow-up, there was no difference in PFS or OS between FCR and IR for patients with mutated *IGHV*, suggesting that there may remain a place for this regimen in clinical practice. In addition, current studies are focused on limiting chemotherapy and/or adding novel agents in efforts to achieve cure but limit toxicity.

THERAPY OF RELAPSED CLL

Currently, the mainstays of treatment for relapsed CLL are the same classes as initial therapy. The optimal sequencing of targeted agents in

TABLE 107-6 Response Criteria in CLL

	LYMPHOCYTE COUNT	LYMPH NODES[a]	SPLEEN/LIVER SIZE[b]	BONE MARROW[c]	PERIPHERAL BLOOD COUNTS
CR	<4000/μL	None >1.5 cm	Not palpable	Normocellular, <30% lymphocytes, no B lymphoid nodules	• Platelet count >100,000/μL • Hemoglobin >11 g/dL • Neutrophils >1500/μL
PR	Decrease ≥50% from baseline	Decrease ≥50% from baseline	Decrease ≥50% from baseline	Infiltrate ≤50% of baseline	One of the following: • Platelet count >100,000/μL or ≥50% from baseline • Hemoglobin >11 g/dL or ≥50% from baseline • Neutrophils >1500/μL or ≥50% from baseline
Stable disease	Not meeting CR/PR/PD criteria	Not meeting CR/PR/PD criteria	Not meeting CR/PR/PD criteria	Not meeting CR/PR/PD criteria	Not meeting CR/PR/PD criteria
PD	Increase ≥50%	Increase ≥50%	Increase ≥50%		• Platelet count ≤50% of baseline due to CLL • Hemoglobin decrease >2 g/dL due to CLL

[a]Refers to sum of the products of multiple lymph nodes evaluated by CT scan. [b]Based on physical examination. [c]Bone marrow only required to confirm CR.
Abbreviations: CLL, chronic lymphocytic leukemia; CR, complete response; PD, progressive disease; PR, partial response.

CLL has not been established; however, the available data suggest that the sequence of either BTK inhibitor and then BCL2 inhibitor or the reverse are both acceptable. In a trial of venetoclax for patients who had relapsed after ibrutinib therapy, the overall response rate (ORR) was 65% with a median PFS of ~2 years in a very heavily pretreated patient population. Retrospective data of BTK inhibitor given after venetoclax suggests that this sequence is effective as well, with an ORR of 84% and median PFS of 32 months. PI3K inhibitors also have activity in relapsed CLL; however, activity following both BTK and BCL2 inhibitors is likely minimal. In addition, many new agents are in development in CLL including novel oral targeted therapies, antibodies, and immune-based treatments.

Immune Therapies Immune therapies in CLL are currently focused in the relapsed setting and include allogenic stem cell transplantation, CAR-T therapy, and oral immunomodulatory agents such as lenalidomide.

Stem cell transplantation is a curative approach to CLL. Because most CLL patients are older and many have significant comorbidities, myeloablative transplantations incur extensive morbidity and mortality, making them prohibitive in many individuals. Reduced-intensity conditioning (RIC) allogeneic transplantations have been successfully incorporated into the treatment of patients up to ~75 years in age but still have a ≥50% frequency of chronic graft-versus-host disease. This is still considered a standard treatment in CLL but has fallen out of favor with the introduction of well-tolerated novel agents, as well as clinical trials of CAR-T cells. CD19 CAR-T cell trials have not been as successful in CLL as they have been in other B cell malignancies due to the immunosuppression associated with the disease. Many current trials are focused on optimizing CD19 CAR-T cells by adding agents such as BTK inhibitors or PI3K inhibitors or modifying the CAR-T structure, and other studies are testing different targets outside of CD19. In addition, recent studies have shown that natural killer (NK) cell CAR cells also can induce clinical response in CLL patients. This area remains a focus of intense investigation in CLL.

ASSESSING RESPONSE TO THERAPY AND MINIMAL RESIDUAL DISEASE IN CLL

Following the completion of therapy or during therapy for indefinite targeted agents, response is initially assessed using physical examination and laboratory studies (**Table 107-6**). If residual disease is not detected using these methodologies, CT scans are used to assess response. Bone marrow biopsies with flow cytometry are indicated if no disease is detected to confirm complete response.

It has been established in various malignancies that complete tumor eradication is associated with longer survival. In CLL, if no malignant cells can be detected in the bone marrow down to a level of 1 CLL cell in 10^4 leukocytes (0.01%), the patient is said to be negative for minimal residual disease (MRD). Following combination chemoimmunotherapy, eradication of MRD correlates with long-term survival and potentially cure in a subset of patients receiving FCR chemoimmunotherapy. Undetectable MRD in blood or bone marrow is also associated with improvement in PFS in venetoclax-based regimens. However, eradication of MRD has not been shown to be a meaningful endpoint with BTK or PI3K inhibitors as monotherapy. Higher sensitivity of 1 CLL in 10^6 leukocytes (0.0001%) can be obtained using next-generation sequencing methods such as ClonoSeq. This technique is currently available in clinical practice, although at this point, there are no data confirming that increased sensitivity is clinically meaningful, and studies are underway to support the need for this higher sensitivity with novel combination approaches of BTK/BCL2 inhibitor regimens.

CONCLUSION

CLL is treated only when it becomes symptomatic. At the time of therapy, FCR chemoimmunotherapy in a small subset of young patients with very-good-risk CLL is potentially curative. In the majority of patients with symptomatic CLL, targeted therapy directed at BTK or BCL2 can produce durable remissions and allow patients many years of disease-free survival.

FURTHER READING

Burger JA: Treatment of chronic lymphocytic leukemia. N Engl J Med 383:460, 2020.

Fischer K et al: Venetoclax and obinutuzumab in patients with CLL and coexisting conditions. N Engl J Med 380:2225, 2019.

Hallek M et al: iwCLL guidelines for diagnosis, indications for treatment, response assessment, and supportive management of CLL. Blood 131:2745, 2018.

Oakes CC et al: DNA methylation dynamics during B cell maturation underlie a continuum of disease phenotypes in chronic lymphocytic leukemia. Nat Genet 48:253, 2016.

Puente XS et al: Whole-genome sequencing identifies recurrent mutations in chronic lymphocytic leukaemia. Nature 475:101, 2011.

Shanafelt TD et al: Ibrutinib-rituximab or chemoimmunotherapy for chronic lymphocytic leukemia. N Engl J Med 38:432, 2019.

Sharman JP et al: Acalabrutinib with or without obinutuzumab versus chlorambucil and obinutuzumab for treatment-naïve chronic lymphocytic leukemia (ELEVATE TN): A randomized, controlled, phase 3 trial. Lancet 395:1278, 2020.

Thompson PA et al: Fludarabine, cyclophosphamide, and rituximab treatment achieves long-term disease-free survival in IGHV-mutated chronic lymphocytic leukemia. Blood 127:303, 2016.

Woyach JA et al: Ibrutinib regimens versus chemoimmunotherapy in older patients with untreated CLL. N Engl J Med 380:1680, 2018.

108 Non-Hodgkin's Lymphoma

Caron A. Jacobson, Dan L. Longo

Non-Hodgkin's lymphomas (NHL) are cancers of mature B, T, and natural killer (NK) cells. They were distinguished from Hodgkin's lymphoma (HL) upon recognition of the Reed-Sternberg (RS) cell and differ from HL with respect to their biologic and clinical characteristics. Whereas ~80–85% of patients with HL will be cured of their lymphoma by chemotherapy with or without radiotherapy, the prognosis and natural history of NHL tends to be more variable. NHL can be classified as either a mature B-NHL or a mature T/NK-NHL depending on whether the cancerous lymphocyte is a B, T, or NK cell, respectively. Within each category are lymphomas that grow quickly and behave aggressively, as well as lymphomas that are more indolent, or slow growing, in nature. For a list of the World Health Organization (WHO) classification of lymphoid neoplasms, see **Table 108-1**.

EPIDEMIOLOGY AND ETIOLOGY

In 2020, >77,000 new cases of NHL were diagnosed in the United States, ~4% of all new cancers in both males and females, making it the seventh most common cause of cancer-related death in both women and men. The incidence is nearly 10 times the incidence of HL. There is a slight male-to-female predominance and a higher incidence for Caucasians than for African Americans. The incidence rises steadily with age, especially after age 40, but lymphomas are also among the most common malignancies in adolescent and young adult patients. The incidence of NHL has nearly doubled over the past 20–40 years and continues to rise by 1.5–2% each year. Patients with both primary and secondary immunodeficiency states are predisposed to developing NHL. These include patients with HIV infection, patients who have undergone organ transplantation, and patients with inherited immune deficiencies and autoimmune conditions. The 5-year survival rates for NHL are 72% for Caucasians and 63% for African Americans.

TABLE 108-1 WHO Classification of Lymphoid Malignancies

B CELL	T CELL
Mature (peripheral) B-cell neoplasms	Mature (peripheral) T-cell neoplasms
Lymphoplasmacytic lymphoma (Waldenström's macroglobulinemia)	T-cell granular lymphocytic leukemia
Hairy cell leukemia	Adult T-cell leukemia/lymphoma (HTLV-1+)
Splenic marginal zone B-cell lymphoma	Extranodal NK/T-cell lymphoma, nasal type
Extranodal marginal zone B-cell lymphoma of MALT type	Enteropathy-associated T-cell lymphoma
Nodal marginal zone B-cell lymphoma	Hepatosplenic T-cell lymphoma
Follicular lymphoma	Subcutaneous panniculitis-like T-cell lymphoma
Mantle cell lymphoma	Mycosis fungoides
Diffuse large B-cell lymphoma (including subtypes)	Sezary syndrome
High-grade B-cell lymphoma with MYC and BCL2 and/or BCL6 rearrangements	Peripheral T-cell lymphoma NOS
	Angioimmunoblastic T-cell lymphoma
High-grade B-cell lymphoma NOS	Anaplastic large-cell lymphoma, ALK+
Burkitt's lymphoma/Burkitt's cell leukemia	Anaplastic large-cell lymphoma, ALK–
Primary mediastinal large B-cell lymphoma	
Plasmablastic lymphoma	
Primary effusion lymphoma	
HHV8+ DLBCL NOS	
Intravascular large B-cell lymphoma	
ALK+ large B-cell lymphoma	

Abbreviations: DLBCL, diffuse large B-cell lymphoma; HHV, human herpesvirus; HTLV, human T-cell lymphotropic virus; MALT, mucosa-associated lymphoid tissue; NK, natural killer; NOS, not otherwise specified; WHO, World Health Organization.

Source: Adapted from SH Swerdlow et al: *WHO Classification of Tumours of Haematopoietic and Lymphoid Tissues*, 5th ed. IARC, 2016.

The incidence of NHL and the patterns of expression of the various subtypes differ geographically and across age groups. T-cell lymphomas are more common in Asia than in Western countries, whereas certain subtypes of B-cell lymphomas such as follicular lymphoma (FL) are more common in Western countries. A specific subtype of NHL known as the angiocentric nasal T/NK cell lymphoma has a striking geographic occurrence, being most frequent in southern Asia and parts of Latin America. Another subtype of NHL associated with infection by human T-cell lymphotropic virus (HTLV) 1 is seen particularly in southern Japan and the Caribbean. Likewise, there are differences in the age-dependent incidence of NHL by histologic subtype, with aggressive lymphomas like diffuse large B-cell lymphoma (DLBCL) and Burkitt's lymphoma (BL) being the most common entities in children, and DLBCL and indolent lymphomas including FL being the most common forms in adults. The relative frequencies of the various types of lymphoid malignancies, including HL, plasma cell disorders, and lymphoid leukemias, is shown in **Fig. 108-1**.

A number of environmental factors have been implicated in the occurrence of NHL, including infectious agents, chemical exposures, and medical treatments. Several studies have demonstrated an association between exposure to agricultural chemicals and an increased incidence of NHL. Patients treated for HL can develop NHL; it is unclear whether this is a consequence of the HL or its treatment, especially radiation.

Several NHLs are associated with infectious agents (**Table 108-2**). Epstein-Barr virus (EBV) is associated with the development of BL in Central Africa and the occurrence of aggressive NHL in immunosuppressed patients in Western countries. The majority of primary central nervous system (CNS) lymphomas are associated with EBV. EBV infection is strongly associated with the occurrence of extranodal nasal NK/T-cell lymphomas in Asia and South America. HTLV-1 infects T cells and leads directly to the development of adult T-cell lymphoma (ATL) in a small percentage of patients infected as babies through ingestion of breast milk of infected mothers. The median age of patients with ATL is ~56 years; thus, HTLV-1 demonstrates a long latency from infection to oncogenesis (**Chap. 201**). Infection with HIV predisposes to the development of aggressive, B-cell NHL. This may be through overexpression of interleukin 6 by infected macrophages. Infection of the stomach by the bacterium *Helicobacter pylori* induces the development of gastric mucosa-associated lymphoid tissue (MALT) lymphomas. This association is supported by evidence that patients treated with antibiotics to eradicate *H. pylori* have regression of their MALT lymphoma. The bacterium does not transform lymphocytes to produce the lymphoma; instead, a vigorous immune response is made to the bacterium, and the chronic antigenic stimulation leads to the neoplasia. MALT lymphomas of the skin may be related to *Borrelia* sp. infections in Europe, those of the eyes to *Chlamydophila psittaci*, and those of the small intestine to *Campylobacter jejuni*. Chronic hepatitis C virus infection has been associated with the development of lymphoplasmacytic lymphoma and splenic marginal zone lymphoma (MZL). Human herpesvirus 8 is associated with primary effusion lymphoma in HIV-infected persons and multicentric Castleman's disease, a diffuse lymphadenopathy associated with systemic symptoms of fever, malaise, and weight loss.

In addition to infectious agents, a number of other diseases or exposures may predispose to developing lymphoma (**Table 108-3**). Diseases of inherited and acquired immunodeficiency as well as autoimmune diseases are associated with an increased incidence of lymphoma. The association between immunosuppression and induction of NHLs is compelling because if the immunosuppression can be reversed, a percentage of these lymphomas regress spontaneously. The incidence of NHL is nearly a hundredfold increased for patients undergoing organ transplantation necessitating chronic immunosuppression and is greatest in the first year posttransplant. About 30% of these arise as

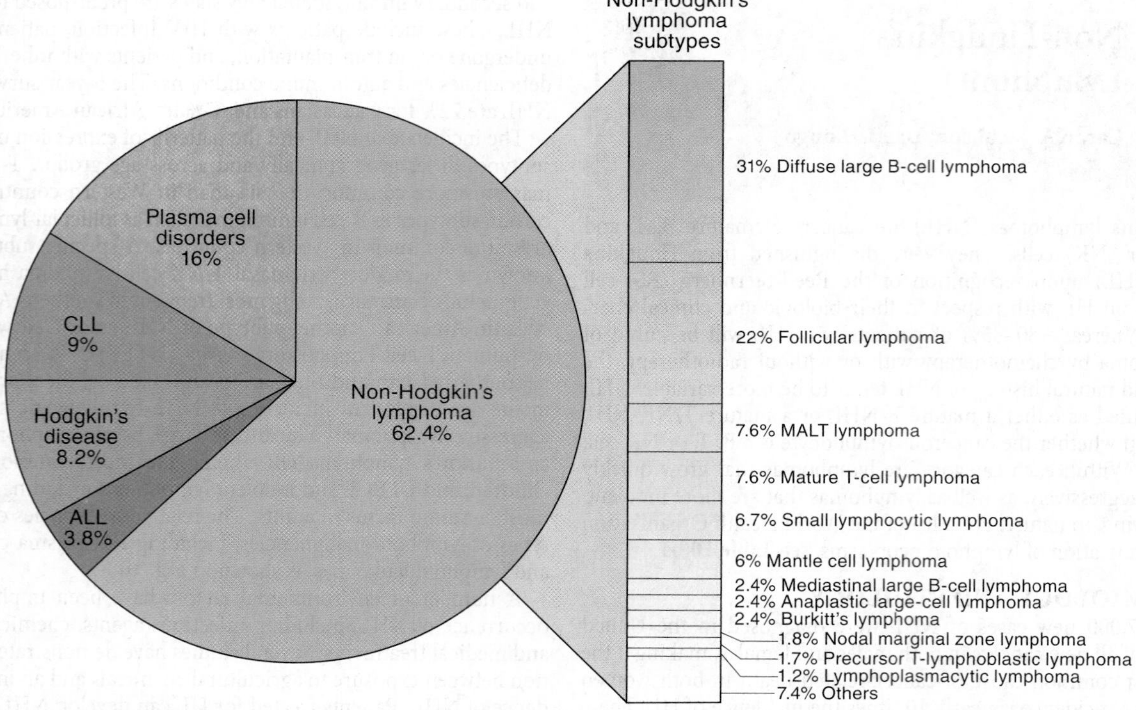

FIGURE 108-1 Relative frequency of lymphoid malignancies. ALL, acute lymphoid leukemia; CLL, chronic lymphocytic leukemia; MALT, mucosa-associated lymphoid tissue.

a polyclonal B-cell proliferation that evolves into a clonal B cell malignancy. The NHLs that occur in the context of immunosuppression or immunodeficiency, including HIV infection, are frequently associated with EBV. Histologically, DLBCLs are most frequently associated with immunosuppression and autoimmune diseases, although almost all histologies can be seen, especially MALT lymphomas in the context of autoimmune diseases such as Sjögren's syndrome and Hashimoto's thyroiditis. The rare inherited immunodeficiency diseases X-linked lymphoproliferative syndrome, Wiskott-Aldrich syndrome, Chédiak-Higashi syndrome, ataxia-telangiectasia, and common variable immunodeficiency syndrome are complicated by highly aggressive lymphomas. The elevated incidence of lymphoma in iatrogenic immunosuppression, AIDS, and autoimmune disease argues strongly for immune dysregulation contributing in the pathogenesis of some lymphomas. An increased risk of NHL has been observed in first-degree relatives with NHL, HL, or chronic lymphocytic leukemia (CLL). In large database studies, ~9% of patients with lymphoma or CLL have a first-degree relative with a lymphoproliferative disorder.

TABLE 108-2 Infectious Agents Associated with the Development of Lymphoid Malignancies

INFECTIOUS AGENT	LYMPHOID MALIGNANCY
Epstein-Barr virus	Burkitt's lymphoma
	Post–organ transplant lymphoma
	Primary CNS diffuse large B-cell lymphoma
	Hodgkin's lymphoma
	Extranodal NK/T-cell lymphoma, nasal type
HTLV-1	Adult T-cell leukemia/lymphoma
HIV	Diffuse large B-cell lymphoma
	Burkitt's lymphoma
Hepatitis C virus	Lymphoplasmacytic lymphoma
Helicobacter pylori	Gastric MALT lymphoma
Human herpesvirus 8	Primary effusion lymphoma
	Multicentric Castleman's disease

Abbreviations: CNS, central nervous system; HIV, human immunodeficiency virus; HTLV, human T-cell lymphotropic virus; MALT, mucosa-associated lymphoid tissue; NK, natural killer.

IMMUNOLOGY

All lymphoid cells are derived from a common hematopoietic progenitor that gives rise to lymphoid, myeloid, erythroid, monocyte, and megakaryocyte lineages. Through the ordered and sequential activation of a series of transcription factors, the cell first becomes committed to the lymphoid lineage and then gives rise to B and T cells.

About 90% of all lymphomas are of B cell origin. A cell becomes committed to B cell development when it expresses the master B lineage transcription factor PAX5, which ultimately results in a transcriptional program that leads to the rearrangement of its immunoglobulin genes, which involves chromosomal recombination as well as somatic hypermutation to create an immunoglobulin gene that is unique to that B cell. The sequence of cellular changes, including changes in cell-surface phenotype that characterizes normal B cell development, is shown in **Fig. 108-2.** Most B-cell lymphomas arise following the process of immunoglobulin gene recombination and somatic hypermutation, which leads to class switching and affinity maturation of the mature immunoglobulin, respectively, suggesting that it is the error-prone nature of these genetic events that contributes to oncogenesis. Certainly the frequency of chromosomal translocations that result in the activation of an oncogene or the inactivation of a tumor-suppressor gene in B-cell NHL may be the result of these normal cellular processes gone awry (see below). In addition, the key roles of the transcription factors MYC and BCL6 and the antiapoptotic protein BCL2 in the

TABLE 108-3 Diseases or Exposures Associated with Increased Risk of Development of Malignant Lymphoma

Inherited immunodeficiency disease	Autoimmune disease
Klinefelter's syndrome	Sjögren's syndrome
Chédiak-Higashi syndrome	Celiac sprue
Ataxia-telangiectasia syndrome	Rheumatoid arthritis and systemic lupus erythematosus
Wiskott-Aldrich syndrome	
Common variable immunodeficiency disease	Chemical or drug exposures
	Phenytoin
Acquired immunodeficiency diseases	Dioxin, phenoxy herbicides
Iatrogenic immunosuppression	Radiation
HIV-1 infection	Prior chemotherapy and radiation therapy
Acquired hypogammaglobulinemia	

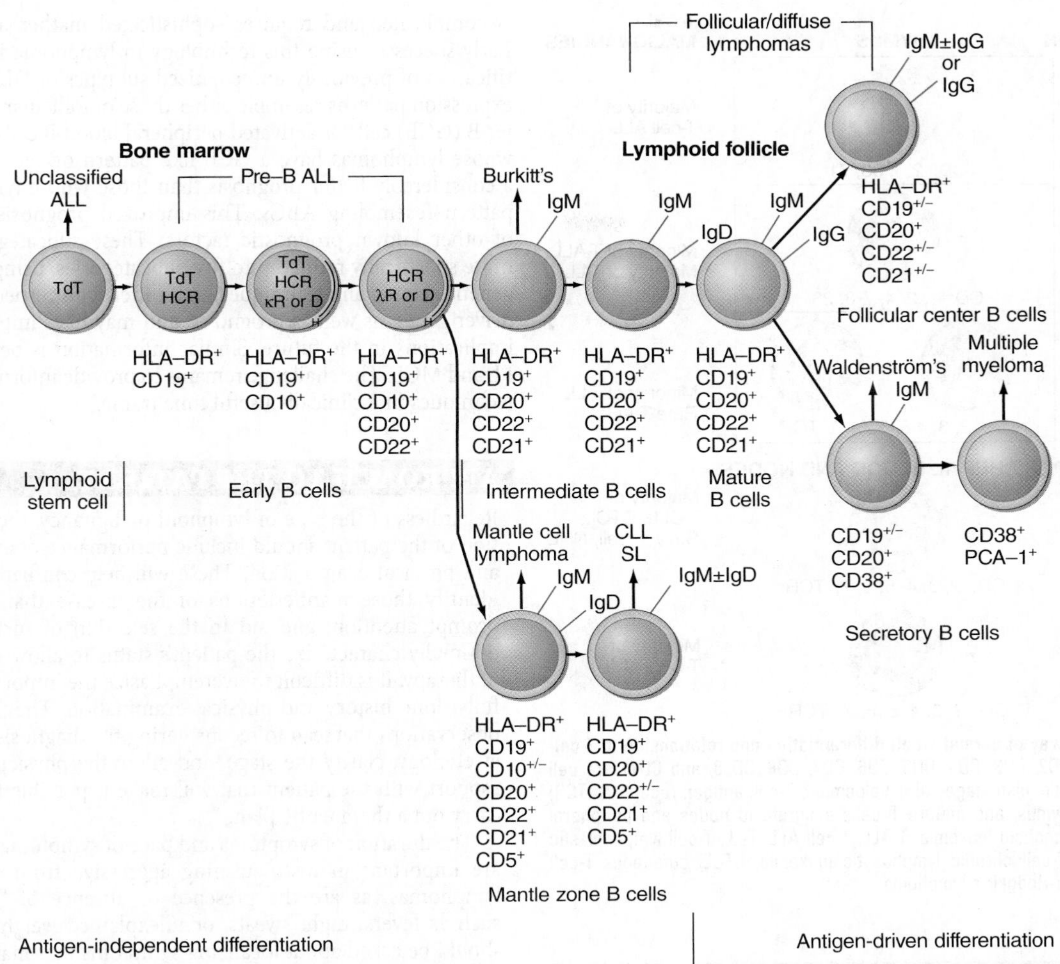

FIGURE 108-2 Pathway of normal B-cell differentiation and relationship to B-cell lymphomas. HLA-DR, CD10, CD19, CD20, CD21, CD22, CD5, and CD38 are cell markers used to distinguish stages of development. Terminal transferase (TdT) is a cellular enzyme. Immunoglobulin heavy chain gene rearrangement (HCR) and light chain gene rearrangement or deletion (κR or D, λR or D) occur early in B-cell development. The approximate normal stage of differentiation associated with particular lymphomas is shown. ALL, acute lymphoid leukemia; CLL, chronic lymphocytic leukemia; SL, small lymphocytic lymphoma.

process of B cell development explain why the genes encoding these proteins are commonly mutated in B-cell lymphomas.

A cell becomes committed to T-cell differentiation upon migration to the thymus and rearrangement of T-cell receptor (TCR) genes. This requires the expression of the T-cell master regulatory transcription factor, NOTCH-1. As in B cells, the development of the mature TCR involves the rearrangement and recombination of the TCR loci, which is error-prone and potentially oncogenic. The sequence of the events that characterize T-cell development is depicted in **Fig. 108-3**.

Although lymphoid malignancies often retain the cell-surface phenotype of lymphoid cells at particular stages of differentiation, this information is of little clinical or prognostic consequence. The so-called stage of differentiation of a malignant lymphoma does not predict its natural history. The antigen footprint, or immunophenotype, of the cell, however, is valuable diagnostically as it allows for the distinguishing of specific NHL subtypes. It can be detected by flow cytometry of single-cell suspension from blood, bone marrow, body fluid, or disaggregated tissue using fluorescently labeled antibodies against these antigens or by immunohistochemical staining of paraffin-embedded tissue sections with enzyme-linked antibodies against these antigens followed by a colorimetric reaction.

As already mentioned, malignancies of lymphoid cells are associated with recurring genetic abnormalities including chromosomal translocations and genetic mutations that may in part be the result of aberrant immunoglobulin or TCR development. While specific genetic abnormalities have not been identified for all subtypes of lymphoid malignancies, it is presumed that they exist. As previously discussed, B cells are even more susceptible to acquiring mutations during their maturation in germinal centers; the generation of antibody of higher affinity requires the introduction of mutations into the variable region genes in the germinal centers. Given this, other nonimmunoglobulin genes, e.g., *bcl-6*, may acquire mutations as well. Likewise, many lymphomas contain balanced chromosomal translocations involving the antigen receptor genes; immunoglobulin genes on chromosomes 2, 14, and 22 in B cells; and T-cell antigen receptor genes on chromosomes 7 and 14 in T cells. The rearrangement of chromosome segments to generate mature antigen receptors must create a site of vulnerability to aberrant recombination. Examples of this type of event include the (8;14)(q24;q32) translocation in BL, involving the *MYC* proto-oncogene and the IgH gene; the (14;18)(q32;q32) translocation in FL, involving the *BCL2* proto-oncogene and the IgH gene; and the (11;14)(q13;q32) translocation in mantle cell lymphoma (MCL), involving the gene encoding cyclin D1 (*CCDN1*) and the IgH gene. Less commonly, chromosomal translocations produce fusion genes that encode chimeric oncogenic proteins. Examples of this include the (2;5)(p23;q35) translocation involving the *ALK* and *NPM1* genes in anaplastic large-cell lymphoma (ALCL) and the t(11;18)(q21;q21) translocation involving the *API2* and *MLT* genes in MALT lymphoma. **Table 108-4** presents the most common translocations and associated oncogenes for various subtypes of lymphoid malignancies.

Gene profiling using array technology allows the simultaneous assessment of the expression of thousands of genes. This technology provides the possibility to identify new genes with pathologic importance in lymphomas, the identification of patterns of gene expression with diagnostic and/or prognostic significance, and the identification of new therapeutic targets. Recognition of patterns of gene expression

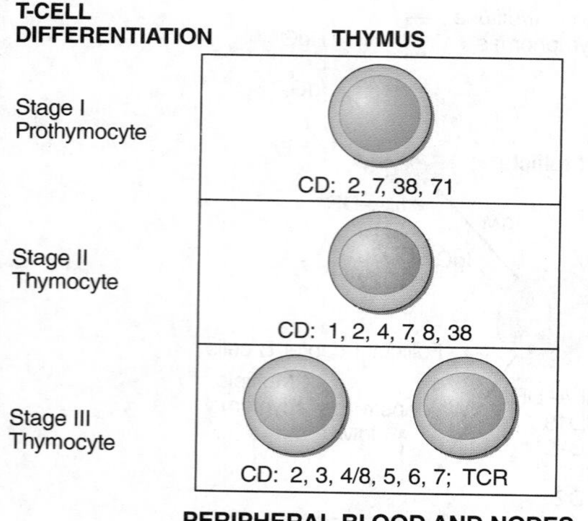

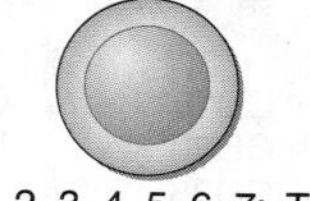
Mature T Helper Cell
CD: 2, 3, 4, 5, 6, 7; TCR
Majority of T-CLL, CTCL, Sezary Cell, NHL

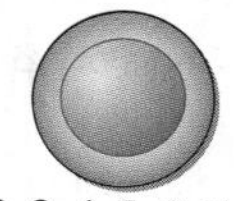

FIGURE 108-3 Pathway of normal T-cell differentiation and relationship to T-cell lymphomas. CD1, CD2, CD3, CD4, CD5, CD6, CD7, CD8, CD38, and CD71 are cell markers used to distinguish stages of development. T-cell antigen receptors (TCR) rearrange in the thymus, and mature T cells emigrate to nodes and peripheral blood. ALL, acute lymphoid leukemia; T-ALL, T-cell ALL; T-LL, T-cell lymphoblastic lymphoma; T-CLL, T-cell chronic lymphocytic leukemia; CTCL, cutaneous T-cell lymphoma; NHL, non-Hodgkin's lymphoma.

TABLE 108-4 Genetic Features of B- and T-Cell Lymphomas

GENETIC FEATURE	GENES	LYMPHOMA
t(8;14) t(2;8) t(8;22)	*MYC/IgH* *MYC/Igκ* *MYC/Ig λ*	Burkitt's lymphoma
t(11;14)	*BCL1 (CCND1)/IgH*	Mantle cell lymphoma; multiple myeloma
t(14;18) t(3;14)	*BCL2/IgH* *BCL6/IgH*	Follicular lymphoma, diffuse large B-cell lymphoma (DLBCL)
t(11;18) t(1;14) t(14;18) t(3;14)	*API2/MALT1* *BCL10/IgH* *MALT1/IgH* *FOXP1/IgH*	MALT lymphoma
Trisomy 3 7q21 deletion	Unknown *CDK6*	Splenic marginal zone lymphoma
t(9;14) 6q21 deletion	*PAX5/IgH* Unknown	Lymphoplasmacytic lymphoma
inv(14) t(14;14)	*TCRα/TCL1*	Peripheral T-cell lymphoma, NOS; T-PLL
t(2;5) t(1;2) t(2;3) t(2;17) inv(2)	*NPM1/ALK* *TPM3/ALK* *TFG/ALK* *CTLC/ALK* *ATIC/ALK*	Anaplastic large-cell lymphoma (ALCL)
Trisomy 3 Trisomy 5	Unknown Unknown	Angioimmunoblastic T-cell lymphoma
Isochromosome 7q	Unknown	Hepatosplenic T-cell lymphoma

Abbreviations: MALT, mucosa-associated lymphoid tissue; NOS, not otherwise specified; T-PLL, T-cell prolymphocytic leukemia.

is complicated and requires sophisticated mathematical techniques. Early successes using this technology in lymphoma include the identification of previously unrecognized subtypes of DLBCL whose gene expression patterns resemble either those of follicular or germinal center B (GCB) cells or activated peripheral blood B cells (ABC). Patients whose lymphomas have a GCB-like pattern of gene expression have a considerably better prognosis than those whose lymphomas have a pattern resembling ABCs. This improved prognosis is independent of other known prognostic factors. These subcategories have been more specifically refined into five subcategories, using more advanced genetic sequencing techniques, that differ with respect to biology and driver genes, as well as prognosis, and may have important treatment implications in the future. Similar information is being generated in FL and MCL. The challenge remains to provide information from such techniques in a clinically useful time frame.

APPROACH TO THE PATIENT

Regardless of the type of lymphoid malignancy, the initial evaluation of the patient should include performance of a careful history and physical examination. These will help confirm the diagnosis, identify those manifestations of the disease that might require prompt attention, and aid in the selection of further studies to optimally characterize the patient's status to allow the best choice of therapy. It is difficult to overemphasize the importance of a carefully done history and physical examination. They might provide observations that lead to reconsidering the diagnosis, provide hints at etiology, clarify the stage, and allow the physician to establish rapport with the patient that will make it possible to develop and carry out a therapeutic plan.

The duration of symptoms and pace of symptomatic progression are important in distinguishing aggressive from more indolent lymphomas, as are the presence or absence of "B" symptoms, such as fevers, night sweats, or unexplained weight loss. Patients should be asked about localizing symptoms that may point toward lymphomatous involvement of specific sites, such as the chest, abdomen, or CNS. Comorbid diagnoses that may impact therapy or monitoring on therapy should be reviewed and acknowledged, including a history of diabetes or congestive heart failure. A physical examination should pay close attention to all the peripherally accessible sites of lymph nodes; the liver and spleen size; Waldeyer's ring; whether there is a pleural or pericardial effusion or abdominal ascites; whether there is an abdominal, testicular, or breast mass; and whether there is cutaneous involvement because all of these findings may influence further evaluation and disease management.

Laboratory studies should include a complete blood count, routine chemistries, liver function tests, and serum protein electrophoresis to document the presence of circulating monoclonal paraproteins. The serum β_2-microglobulin level and serum lactate dehydrogenase (LDH) are important independent prognostic factors in NHL. Staging of certain diseases may involve a bone marrow biopsy; results of other laboratory and staging studies may also warrant a marrow evaluation. A lumbar puncture for evaluation of lymphomatous involvement may be indicated in the setting of concerning neurologic signs or symptoms or diseases that are high risk for CNS involvement. The latter may include disease involving the paranasal sinuses, testes, breast, kidneys, adrenal glands, and epidural space, as well as highly aggressive histologies like BL. Since HIV and hepatitis B and C infection can be risk factors for developing NHL, and since treatment for some NHLs can result in the potentially life-threatening reactivation of hepatitis B, patients with a new diagnosis of NHL should be screened for these viruses as well.

Lymphoma histology and clinical presentation dictate which imaging studies should be ordered. Chest, abdominal, and pelvic computed tomography (CT) scans are essential for accurate staging to assess lymphadenopathy for indolent lymphomas, whereas positron emission tomography (PET) using ^{18}F-fluorodeoxyglucose

TABLE 108-5 Staging Evaluation for Non-Hodgkin's Lymphoma

Physical examination
Documentation of B symptoms
Laboratory evaluation
- Complete blood counts
- Liver function tests
- Uric acid
- Calcium
- Serum protein electrophoresis
- Serum β_2-microglobulin

Chest radiograph
CT scan of abdomen, pelvis, and usually chest
Bone marrow biopsy
Lumbar puncture in lymphoblastic, Burkitt's, and diffuse large B cell lymphoma with positive marrow biopsy
Gallium scan (SPECT) or PET scan in large-cell lymphoma

Abbreviations: CT, computed tomography; PET, positron emission tomography; SPECT, single-photon emission computed tomography.

TABLE 108-7 International Prognostic Index for NHL

Five Clinical Risk Factors

Age ≥60 years
Serum lactate dehydrogenase levels elevated
Performance status ≥2 (ECOG) or ≤70 (Karnofsky)
Ann Arbor stage III or IV
>1 site of extranodal involvement

For Diffuse Large B Cell Lymphoma	
0, 1 factor = low risk	35% of cases; 5-year survival, 73%
2 factors = low-intermediate risk	27% of cases; 5-year survival, 51%
3 factors = high-intermediate risk	22% of cases; 5-year survival, 43%
4, 5 factors = high risk	16% of cases; 5-year survival, 26%
For Diffuse Large B Cell Lymphoma Treated With R-CHOP	
0 factor = good	10% of cases; 4-year survival, 94%
1, 2 factors = intermediate	45% of cases; 4-year survival, 80%
3, 4, 5 factors = poor	45% of cases; 4-year survival, 53%

Abbreviations: ECOG, Eastern Cooperative Oncology Group; NHL, non-Hodgkin's lymphoma; R-CHOP, rituximab, cyclophosphamide, doxorubicin, vincristine, prednisone.

(FDG-PET) is useful for aggressive lymphomas, including BL, DLBCL, plasmablastic lymphoma, and the aggressive T-cell NHLs. FDG-PET is highly sensitive for detecting both nodal and extranodal sites involved by NHL. The intensity of FDG avidity, or standardized uptake value (SUV), correlates with histologic aggressiveness, and may be useful in cases when disease transformation of an indolent lymphoma to a diffuse aggressive lymphoma is suspected. PET scanning can also differentiate between treated disease and active disease at the end of therapy in patients with residual masses on CT scans. Consensus recommendations regarding PET scanning were published as a result of an International Harmonization Project and state that PET should only be used for DLBCL and HL, that scanning during therapy should only be done as part of clinical trials, and that the end-of-treatment scan should not be done before 3 weeks but preferably 6–8 weeks after chemotherapy and 8–12 weeks after radiation or chemoradiotherapy. There is no evidence that long-term follow-up should include PET scanning. More recently, though, PET scan results at the end of therapy for FL have been associated with prognosis, with patients with residual PET-avid disease at the end of treatment having a poorer prognosis than those who are PET negative, and so it may be used for this prognostic purpose. Finally, magnetic resonance imaging (MRI) is useful in detecting bone, bone marrow, and CNS disease in the brain and spinal cord. The staging evaluation is outlined in **Table 108-5**.

The Ann Arbor staging system developed in 1971 for HL was adapted for staging NHLs (**Table 108-6**). This staging system focuses on the number of tumor sites (nodal and extranodal), location, and the presence or absence of systemic, or B, symptoms. Table 108-6 summarizes the essential features of the Ann Arbor system.

This anatomic based system is less useful in NHL, which disseminates widely, not in an ordered stepwise fashion. A majority of patients with NHL have advanced-stage disease at diagnosis. Apart from early-stage disease limited to a radiation field where local therapy with radiation is an option, all other disease is treated the same regardless of stage. Histology and clinical parameters at presentation are more important than stage with respect to prognosis. The International Prognostic Index (IPI) is perhaps the best predictor of outcome (**Table 108-7**). The IPI was developed based on the analysis of >2000 patients with aggressive NHLs treated with an anthracycline-containing regimen. Age (≤60 vs >60), serum LDH (≤ normal vs > normal), performance status (0 or 1 vs 2–4), stage (I or II vs III or IV), and extranodal involvement (<1 site vs >1 site) were identified as independently prognostic for overall survival (OS). A point is awarded for each risk factor and then summed, defining four risk groups: low (0 or 1); low-intermediate (2); high-intermediate (3); and high (4–5). The 5-year OS rates for patients with scores of 0 to 1, 2, 3, and 4–5 were 73, 51, 43, and 26%, respectively. The age-adjusted IPI separates patients ≤60 from patients >60. For the age-adjusted IPI, only stage, LDH, and performance status were important. Younger patients with 0, 1, 2, or 3 risk factors had 5-year survival rates of 83, 69, 46, and 32%, compared to 56, 44, 37, and 21% for older patients. When factoring in the introduction and clinical benefit of rituximab, the 4-year progression-free survival rates are 94, 80, and 53% for 0 and 1, 2, or 3 or more risk factors, respectively.

The Follicular Lymphoma International Prognostic Index (FLIPI) is a similar predictive model for FL, derived from the analysis of >4000 patients. Age >60, stage III/IV disease, the presence of >4 nodal sites, an elevated serum LDH concentration, and a hemoglobin <12 were identified as independent prognostic variables, and summation of each variable identified three risk groups. The median 10-year survival rates for patients with zero to one (low risk), two (intermediate risk), or three or more (high risk) of these adverse factors were 71, 51, and 36%, respectively. Similar disease-specific IPIs have been developed for MCL and peripheral T-cell lymphoma (PTCL) as well. These prognostic indices take into account the proliferative index and cell-surface markers, respectively.

Finally, as mentioned previously, gene expression profiling has identified DLBCLs with differential prognoses: GCB and ABC, where GCB-like DLBCL is associated with a significantly better

TABLE 108-6 Ann Arbor Staging for Lymphoma[a]

STAGE	DESCRIPTION
I	Involvement of a single lymph node region (I) or single extranodal site (IE)
II	Involvement of two or more lymph node regions or lymphatic structures on the same side of the diaphragm alone (II) or with involvement of limited, contiguous, extralymphatic organ or tissue (IIE)
III	Involvement of lymph node regions on both sides of the diaphragm (III), which may include the spleen (IIIS), or limited, contiguous, extralymphatic organ or tissue (IIIE), or both (IIIES)
IV	Diffuse or disseminated foci of involvement of one or more extralymphatic organs or tissues, with or without associated lymphatic involvement

[a]All stages are further subdivided according to the absence (A) or presence (B) of systemic B symptoms including fevers, night sweats, and/or weight loss (>10% of body weight over 6 months prior to diagnosis).

OS. A more readily accessible immunohistochemical algorithm has been developed, based on the presence of absence of CD10, BCL6, and MUM1 that correlates closely with gene expression profiles and can differentiate the majority of GCB from non-GCB-like DLBCL. These profiles have prognostic importance but, to date, do not alter treatment recommendations for the primary treatment of DLBCL. Current clinical trials do stratify by DLBCL subtype, and it appears that agents like the Bruton tyrosine kinase (BTK) inhibitor ibrutinib and lenalidomide are most active in non-GCB DLBCL in the relapsed setting. Treatment may then be differentiated by these subtypes in the future.

CLINICAL FEATURES, TREATMENT, AND PROGNOSIS OF SPECIFIC NHL

MATURE B-CELL NEOPLASMS

B-cell NHLs can be characterized into two broad groups—those that behave aggressively, require immediate or urgent treatment with combination chemotherapy regimens, and are potentially curable; and those that are more indolent in nature, can be observed and treated only when they cause symptoms or signs of organ function impairment, are very responsive to therapy, but are not ultimately curable in the vast majority of cases. Among the aggressive diseases, the most common are NHL and DLBCL, and the most rapidly prolific are NHL and BL. FL is the second most common NHL and the most common indolent NHL. Other indolent NHLs include MZL, lymphoplasmacytic lymphoma (LPL), and hairy cell leukemia (HCL). MCL is an intermediate-grade lymphoma that shares some characteristics with the aggressive lymphomas (fairly urgent need for treatment and aggressive upfront combination chemotherapy regimens), but like the indolent lymphomas, it is not readily curable with conventional-dose therapies.

Burkitt's Lymphoma Burkitt's lymphoma/leukemia (BL) is a rare disease in adults in the United States, making up <1% of NHL, but it makes up ~30% of childhood NHL. It is one of the fastest growing neoplasms, with a doubling time of <24 h. In general, it is a pediatric tumor that has three major clinical presentations. The endemic (African) form presents as a jaw or facial bone tumor that spreads to extranodal sites including ovary, testis, kidney, breast, and especially the bone marrow and meninges. The nonendemic form has an abdominal presentation with massive disease, ascites, and renal, testis, and/or ovarian involvement and, like the endemic form, also spreads to the bone marrow and CNS. Immunodeficiency-related cases more often involve lymph nodes and may present as acute leukemia. BL has a male predominance and is typically seen in patients <35 years of age.

On biopsy, there is a monotonous infiltration of medium-sized cells with round nuclei, multiple nucleoli, and basophilic cytoplasm with vacuoles. The proliferation rate is ~100%, and tingible body macrophages give rise to the classic "starry sky" appearance of this tumor (**Fig. 108-4**). Tumor cells are positive for B-cell antigens CD19 and CD20 and surface immunoglobulin. They are also uniformly positive for CD10 and BCL6 but negative for BCL2. Endemic BLs are EBV positive, whereas the majority of nonendemic BLs are EBV negative. BL is associated with a translocation involving MYC on chromosome 8q24 in >95% of the cases. The most common partners are chromosomes 14, 2, or 22, rearrangements that produce fusions of MYC with either the IgH (80%), kappa (15%), or lambda (5%) light chain genes, respectively.

While exquisitely chemosensitive, it is imperative that treatment for BL be initiated quickly given the rapid doubling time and high morbidity of this disease. There are several effective intensive combination chemotherapy regimens, all of which incorporate high doses of cyclophosphamide. Prophylactic therapy to the CNS is mandatory. Cure can be expected in 80–90% of patients when treated promptly and correctly. Dose-adjusted EPOCH-R (rituximab, infusional etoposide/vincristine/doxorubicin, cyclophosphamide, prednisone) is highly effective. Salvage therapy has been generally ineffective in patients whose disease progresses after upfront therapy, emphasizing the importance of the initial treatment approach and referral to a tertiary cancer center with experience treating this disease.

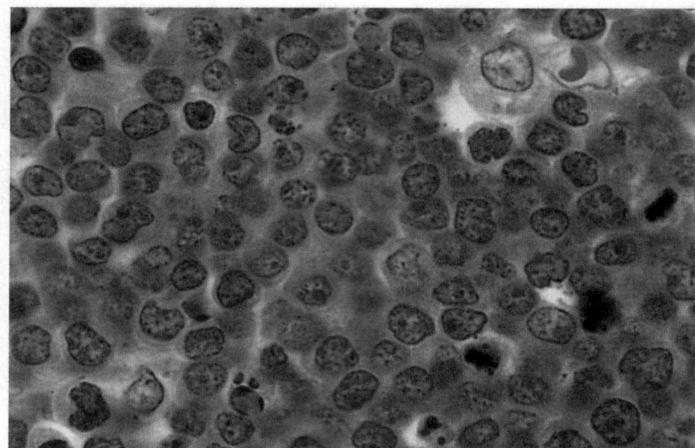

FIGURE 108-4 Burkitt's lymphoma. The neoplastic cells are homogeneous, medium-sized B cells with frequent mitotic figures, a morphologic correlate of high growth fraction. Reactive macrophages are scattered through the tumor, and their pale cytoplasm in a background of blue-staining tumor cells gives the tumor a so-called starry sky appearance.

Diffuse Large B-Cell Lymphoma DLBCL is the most common histologic subtype of NHL diagnosed, representing about one-third of all cases. Previously felt to be "one disease," it is now recognized as a heterogeneous collection of multiple entities. It is slightly more common in Caucasians and men, and the median age at diagnosis is 64. The relative risk (RR) of DLBCL is higher among people with affected first-degree relatives (RR 3.5-fold), and patients with congenital or acquired immunodeficiency, patients on immunosuppression, and patients with autoimmune disorders also have a higher risk of developing DLBCL, often EBV-related. The majority of patients present with advanced-stage disease, with only 30–40% of patients having stage I or II disease; ~40% of patients will have "B" symptoms, and 50% of patients will have an elevated LDH. Up to 40% of patients will have involvement of non–lymph node sites including bone marrow, CNS, gastrointestinal tract, thyroid, liver, and skin. Patients with extensive bone marrow involvement or involvement of the testes, breast, kidney, adrenal gland, paranasal sinus, or epidural space are at increased risk of CNS dissemination.

The tumor consists of a diffuse proliferation of large, atypical lymphocytes with a high proliferative index (**Fig. 108-5**). These cells typically express the B-cell antigens CD19, CD20, and CD79a. Expression of CD10 and BCL6 is consistent with the tumor cell being of germinal center origin (GCB), while the expression of MUM1 corresponds with

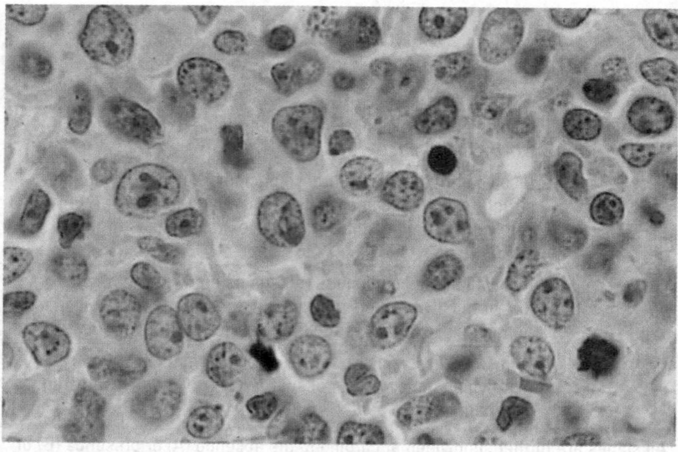

FIGURE 108-5 Diffuse large B-cell lymphoma. The neoplastic cells are heterogeneous but predominantly large cells with vesicular chromatin and prominent nucleoli.

the non–germinal center or activated B cell (ABC) subtype. BCL2 is overexpressed in anywhere from 25 to 80% of DLBCLs, whereas BCL6 is positive in more than two-thirds of cases, either as the result of translocations, gain of copy number, or promoter mutations. MYC is rearranged in 10% of DLBCLs, and ~20% of MYC-rearranged cases have concurrent BCL2 or BCL6 rearrangements, a combination referred to as "double-hit lymphoma." These double-hit lymphomas are associated with an extremely poor prognosis with a median OS of only 12–18 months. Amplification and/or overexpression of MYC independent of rearrangements or amplification have also been described and are also associated with a poor, albeit better, prognosis.

Combination chemotherapy offers potentially curative therapy for DLBCL, regardless of the stage. The addition of the anti-CD20 antibody rituximab to cyclophosphamide, doxorubicin, vincristine, and prednisone (R-CHOP) improved survival beyond CHOP alone and is the standard first-line chemotherapy for this disease. For patients with early-stage disease localized to a radiation field, treatment options include full-course chemotherapy with R-CHOP every 3 weeks for six cycles or abbreviated chemotherapy for three to four cycles followed by involved field radiotherapy. For advanced-stage DLBCL, therapy is with a full course of chemotherapy. On average, ~60–65% of patients with DLBCL can be expected to be cured with this approach, and the likelihood of cure is predicted by the IPI, gene expression profile cell of origin, and/or MYC cytogenetics and expression. Several studies have investigated alternative anthracycline-containing chemotherapy regimens and/or consolidation autologous stem cell transplantation in first remission for higher-risk disease without improvement over R-CHOP alone. Dose-adjusted R-EPOCH is one such regimen. Although this regimen did not appear to be better than R-CHOP for DLBCL in one multicenter clinical trial, it is often used to treat primary mediastinal large B-cell lymphoma and double-hit DLBCL based on results from phase 2 and retrospective studies, respectively. CNS prophylaxis with either intrathecal chemotherapy or high-dose systemic methotrexate and leucovorin rescue should be considered for patients with high risk of CNS dissemination. This includes patients with primary testicular involvement and breast involvement, as well as patients with several IPI risk factors and diffuse bone marrow involvement, renal involvement, or adrenal involvement. The use of CNS prophylaxis for disease involving the paranasal sinuses or the epidural space is less clear but may be considered.

Over one-third of patients will either have primary refractory disease or disease that relapses after first-line chemotherapy. These patients may still be cured with salvage chemotherapy regimens followed by autologous stem cell transplantation. However, patients with a poor performance status or advanced age who are not candidates for such an approach are often managed with palliative intentions. Radiation to symptomatic areas of disease can be transiently helpful. Less intensive chemotherapy with drugs like gemcitabine, cytarabine, or bendamustine can help control disease and symptoms for a limited period of time. These patients should be referred for clinical trials when applicable. For patients in whom more aggressive therapy is an option, treatment is with combination chemotherapy using various combinations of drugs primarily in order to identify patients with chemosensitive disease. Patients with chemosensitive disease have the greatest likelihood of benefiting from high-dose chemotherapy and autologous stem cell transplant, which improves response duration and survival over salvage chemotherapy alone and leads to long-term disease-free survival in ~40–50% of patients. For patients with chemorefractory disease, chimeric antigen receptor T cells (CAR-T cells) offer a potentially curative option. For this therapy, T cells are collected from a patient and are then genetically modified to express a receptor that will bind to a surface antigen expressed on the patient's own tumor cells. In the case of B cell malignancies, CD19 has been targeted most commonly. After infusion, autologous CAR-T cells home to sites of disease and also persist over time. The CARs consist of an extracellular antigen recognition domain (typically a single chain Fv variable fragment from a monoclonal antibody) linked via a transmembrane domain to an intracellular signaling domain (usually the CD3ζ endodomain), resulting in the redirection of T cell specificity toward target antigen-positive cells, and one or more costimulatory domains including CD28, 4-1BB, or OX40 to enhance cytokine secretion and effector cell expansion and prevent activation-induced apoptosis and immune suppression by tumor-related metabolites. Anti-CD19 CAR-T cells have been approved for the treatment of relapsed/refractory DLBCL following two prior systemic therapies. This would include patients with chemotherapy-insensitive disease following second-line salvage chemotherapy for whom autologous stem cell transplant is not an option or patients who relapse after autologous stem cell transplant. In this setting, the response rate of CAR-T cells is >80%, with >50% of patients achieving a complete response. These responses appear to be durable, with 40% of patients in remission at long-term follow-up.

Targeting CD19 with the monoclonal antibody tafasitamab in combination with lenalidomide also yielded high response rates and prolonged response durability, leading to approval of this regimen in relapsed disease. Reports of ongoing studies exploring bispecific antibodies that target CD20 on malignant B cells while also binding CD3 on T cells, thereby activating T cells to attack the malignant B cell, have been very promising in both aggressive and indolent B-cell NHL. The antibody-drug conjugate polatuzumab vedotin, which combines an anti-CD79b antibody with the microtubule toxin monomethyl aurostatin E (MMAE), was approved for the treatment of relapsed/refractory DLBCL in combination with bendamustine and rituximab based on the results of a randomized clinical trial against bendamustine and rituximab alone. The oral drug selinexor, a selective inhibitor of nuclear export, has modest activity in relapsed DLBCL as a single agent and is approved for this indication. These drugs, along with drugs such as lenalidomide alone or ibrutinib, should be viewed as a bridge to allogeneic stem cell transplant for eligible patients in whom curative therapy is the goal because they are unlikely to lead to durable or permanent remissions.

Other large B-cell lymphomas include intravascular large B-cell lymphoma, T-cell/histiocyte–rich large B-cell lymphoma, EBV-positive DLBCL of the elderly, and ALK-positive large B-cell lymphoma. Patients with the latter two diseases tend to have a poor prognosis, whereas the addition of rituximab to CHOP chemotherapy has dramatically improved outcomes with intravascular large B-cell lymphoma, and the outcomes in T-cell/histiocyte–rich large B-cell lymphoma are similar to DLBCL. R-CHOP remains the treatment of choice for each of these lymphomas.

Follicular Lymphoma FLs are the second leading NHL diagnosis in the United States and Europe and make up 22% of NHLs worldwide and at least 30% of NHLs diagnosed in the United States. This type of lymphoma can be diagnosed accurately on morphologic findings alone and has been the diagnosis in the majority of patients in therapeutic trials for "low-grade" lymphoma in the past.

Evaluation of an adequate biopsy by an expert hematopathologist is sufficient to make a diagnosis of FL. The tumor is composed of small cleaved and large cells in varying proportions organized in a follicular pattern of growth (**Fig. 108-6**). Confirmation of B-cell immunophenotype (monoclonal immunoglobulin light chain, CD19, CD20, CD10, and BCL6 positive, and CD5 and CD23 negative) and the existence of the t(14;18) and abnormal expression of BCL2 protein are confirmatory. While >85% of FLs will harbor a t(14;18) and overexpress the antiapoptotic protein BCL2, this genetic event is necessary but not sufficient for malignant transformation of the B lymphocytes, and multiple genetic events are required for the development of FL. Studies have identified the most common recurrent genetic events in FL, and they included mutations in several epigenetic modifying genes, including *MLL2, EZH2, CREBBP*, and *EP300*. The major differential diagnosis is between lymphoma and reactive follicular hyperplasia. The coexistence of DLBCL must be considered. Patients with FL are often subclassified, or graded, into those with predominantly small cells, those with a mixture of small and large cells, and those with predominantly large cells. The WHO classification adopted grading from I to III based on the number of centroblasts, or large cells, counted per high-power field (hpf): grade I, from 0 to 5 centroblasts/hpf; grade II, from 6 to 15 centroblasts/hpf; and grade III, >15 centroblasts/hpf. Grade III has

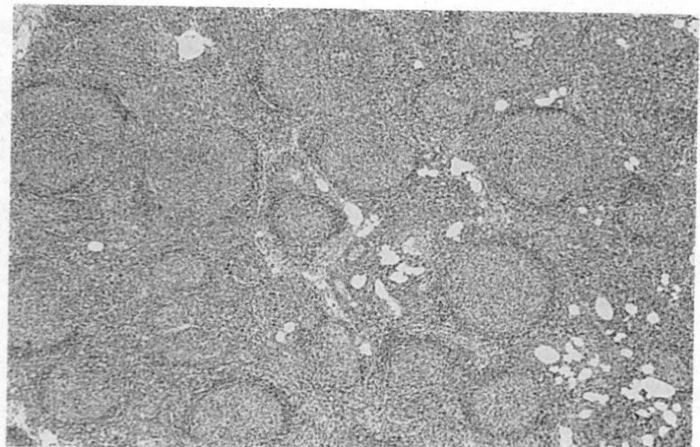

FIGURE 108-6 Follicular lymphoma. The normal nodal architecture is effaced by nodular expansions of tumor cells. Nodules vary in size and contain predominantly small lymphocytes with cleaved nuclei along with variable numbers of larger cells with vesicular chromatin and prominent nucleoli.

been subdivided into grade IIIa, in which centrocytes predominate, and grade IIIb, in which there are sheets of centroblasts. While this distinction cannot be made simply or very reproducibly, these subdivisions do have prognostic significance. Patients with FL with predominantly large cells have a higher proliferative fraction, progress more rapidly, and have a shorter OS with simple chemotherapy regimens. Grade IIIb FL is an aggressive disease and considered most similar to DLBCL and treated as such with curative intent.

The most common presentation for FL is with new, painless lymphadenopathy. Multiple sites of lymphoid involvement are typical, and unusual sites such as epitrochlear nodes are sometimes seen. However, essentially any organ can be involved, and extranodal presentations do occur. Most patients do not have an elevated LDH or fevers, night sweats, or weight loss, although histologic transformation to DLBCL does occur at a rate of ~3% per year and can be associated with these signs or symptoms. As discussed previously, prognosis is best predicted by the FLIPI. Staging is typically done with CT scans of the chest, abdomen, and pelvis, as well as the neck if neck disease is suspected, although PET/CT scans can be helpful in cases where disease transformation is suspected, as transformed disease will be more FDG avid than indolent disease, or for confirmation of early-stage disease, where definitive local therapy with radiation may be considered.

Although FL is highly sensitive to chemotherapy and radiotherapy, these therapies are usually not ultimately curative, except in the setting of early-stage disease. If the disease can be encompassed in a radiation field, involved field radiotherapy at a dose of 24–30 Gy may be curative, with 5-, 10-, and 15-year freedom from treatment failure rates of 72, 46, and 39%, and overall 5-, 10-, and 15-year survival rates of 93, 75, and 62%, respectively. If radiation therapy would not be tolerated or if a patient prefers not to receive radiation, observation is a reasonable alternative with a median time to treatment not reached at 7 years of follow-up in one study. Many of these patients are diagnosed incidentally or at a time when their lymphoma is not causing symptoms or signs of organ function impairment. Numerous studies have shown that treating patients with asymptomatic disease does not improve survival compared with a program of close observation, with treatment reserved for symptomatic disease progression or organ dysfunction. Thus, asymptomatic patients should be observed.

When treatment is indicated, there are a variety of treatment options, including the use of the monoclonal antibody against CD20, rituximab, alone or in combination with chemotherapy. Treatment decisions are often determined by the indication for treatment and/or by the volume of disease being treated. For patients requiring therapy for inflammatory or autoimmune phenomenon thought to be driven by FL, or for patients with low-volume disease, single-agent rituximab is associated with a response rate of ~70% and a median response duration of >2 years. This response duration is improved with the addition of maintenance rituximab following a favorable response to rituximab induction therapy. For patients with a larger volume of disease at the time of treatment initiation, the addition of rituximab to chemotherapy regimens such as CHOP or cyclophosphamide, vincristine, and prednisone (CVP) has improved survival in this disease. The combination of bendamustine and rituximab (BR) has been compared to R-CHOP and results in longer response duration and less toxicity. Thus, BR has become the standard of care for the first-line therapy of medium- to high-volume FL. Similarly, the addition of maintenance rituximab following a good response to R-CHOP or R-CVP improves response duration when used in newly treated FL patients. A newer anti-CD20 antibody, obinutuzumab, has been tested in combination with chemotherapy in a randomized trial against rituximab plus chemotherapy in previously untreated FL. The obinutuzumab combinations resulted in improvements in minimal residual disease (MRD) negativity as well as progression-free survival at the expense of more infection and infusion reactions. Based on these results, both rituximab plus chemotherapy and obinutuzumab plus chemotherapy are options for untreated FL in need of treatment. The superiority of one over the other has not been established.

In patients with FL, the disease nearly always recurs following therapy, after which retreatment is again reserved for symptomatic disease or disease interfering with organ function. Single-agent rituximab or alternative chemotherapy regimens, with both rituximab and obinutuzumab, can again be employed. Both autologous and allogeneic hematopoietic stem cell transplantations yield high complete response rates in patients with relapsed FL, and long-term remissions can occur in 40 and 60% of patients, respectively. The latter is associated with considerable treatment-related morbidity and mortality and so is usually reserved for patients with multiply relapsed FL that is no longer responsive to chemotherapy. More targeted oral therapies like lenalidomide and the PI3 kinase inhibitors idelalisib, duvelisib, and copanlisib are active in both untreated and relapsed FL. Inhibitors of one of the most commonly mutated genes in FL, *EZH2*, have activity in both *EZH2* mutated as well as unmutated lymphomas, and one, tazemetostat, is approved for this indication. Anti-CD19–directed CAR-T cell therapies are also being tested in FL, with complete responses seen in >80% of patients with multiply relapsed disease, and with many of those responses proving durable, albeit with limited follow-up. Longer follow-up is needed to determine if this may be a definitive treatment strategy for a subset of relapsed FL patients. On average, most patients will live with FL for 15–20 years, a number that is increasing given our improved understanding of the genetics and microenvironment of FL and the increasing number of drugs and therapies being tested in this disease. However, in addition to a high-risk FLIPI, patients who do not have a complete metabolic response by PET/CT scanning to their primary therapy and patients who relapse within 2 years of the completion of their primary chemotherapy tend to do poorly with chemotherapy.

Patients with FL have a high rate of histologic transformation to DLBCL (~3% per year). This is recognized ~40% of the time during the course of the illness by repeat biopsy and is present in almost all patients at autopsy. This transformation is usually heralded by rapid growth of lymph nodes—often localized—and the development of systemic symptoms such as fevers, sweats, and weight loss. When this happens in patients who have had previously untreated FL, treatment with R-CHOP chemotherapy, as for DLBCL, can be curative for the aggressive component while the FL may eventually recur. In patients with previously treated FL that transforms to DLBCL, prognosis is poor, and successful therapy with an aggressive combination chemotherapy regimen should be consolidated with an autologous stem cell transplant. Finally, as discussed previously, grade IIIb FL is more similar to DLBCL than it is to FL and should be treated as such.

Marginal Zone Lymphoma The second most common indolent B-cell NHL is MZL. There are three main types: splenic MZL, extranodal MZL of MALT, and nodal MZL.

Nodal MZL most closely resembles FL clinically, and much of the way we manage and treat it is based on studies done in FL. Tumor biopsies in this disease show parafollicular and perivascular infiltration by monocytoid-appearing atypical lymphocytes with folded nuclear contours that are positive for CD19, CD20, and CD79a but negative for CD10 and largely negative for CD5. Some cases can have plasmacytoid differentiation and can be associated with a monoclonal expression of kappa or lambda light chains and with small monoclonal immunoglobulin spikes. Treatment is often similar to that of FL, with the exception that the BTK inhibitor ibrutinib is highly active in this disease, while largely disappointing in FL, and is a good treatment option for relapsed nodal MZL as well as other MZL subtypes.

Splenic MZL is largely a disease of older Caucasian patients; infection with hepatitis C is a risk factor for this disease, and treatment of hepatitis C can result in regression of the lymphoma. Patients present with a lymphocytosis with or without cytopenias and splenomegaly. Bone marrow involvement is common. Diagnosis can be made by flow cytometry of the peripheral blood; malignant lymphocytes will be positive for surface immunoglobulin, CD19, and CD20 and will generally lack CD5 and CD10. On peripheral smear, they have small nuclei and abundant cytoplasm with "shaggy" or villous projections. It can be differentiated from HCL by the absence of CD25, CD103, and annexin A1. Recurrent cytogenetic abnormalities include trisomy 3 and abnormalities of chromosome 7q. Therapy is indicated for symptomatic disease or significant cytopenias. Splenectomy is reasonable for selected patients with excellent relief of symptoms and cytopenias. Splenectomy is associated with an overall response rate of 85% and estimated progression-free survival and OS rates at 5 years of 58 and 77%, respectively. Single-agent rituximab can improve splenomegaly and cytopenias in >90% of patients. In a study of induction with weekly rituximab followed by maintenance, the response rate was 95%, with overall and progression-free survival rates at 5 years of 92 and 73%, respectively. Other options for therapy at relapse are similar to those used for FL and include retreatment with rituximab, alkylating agents, and purine analogues in combination with rituximab. The survival rate of patients is in excess of 70% at 10 years.

MALT lymphoma is an MZL lymphoma of extranodal tissue, most commonly the stomach, but other common sites include the skin, salivary glands, lung, small bowel, ocular adnexa, breasts, bladder, thyroid, dura, and synovium. It is associated with states of chronic inflammation due to either autoimmune diseases like Sjögren's syndrome or Hashimoto's thyroiditis or chronic infections with organisms like *H. pylori* (gastric), *Borrelia burgdorferi* (skin), *C. psittaci* (conjunctiva), *C. jejuni* (intestines), and hepatitis C virus. The essential pathologic feature of MALT lymphoma is the presence of lymphoepithelial lesions, which result from invasion of mucosal glands and crypts by the neoplastic lymphocytes. These cells are positive for CD19, CD20, and CD79a and negative for CD5 and CD10. Recurrent cytogenetic abnormalities include t(11;18), t(14;18), t(1;14), t(3;14), and trisomy 8. The t(11;18) is most common, occurring in up to 50% of MALT lymphomas. It results in the fusion of the apoptosis inhibitor 2 (*API2*) gene and the *MALT1* gene, resulting in activation of nuclear factor-κB (NF-κB). Unlike other indolent B-cell lymphomas, MALT lymphomas present most commonly with stage I or II disease. In these cases, radiation therapy may be curative. Alternatively, patients may respond to antibiotics for the associated underlying infection. Treatment of symptomatic or organ-impairing relapsed, refractory, or advanced-stage disease is similar to approaches used in FL with chemotherapy, immunotherapy, or chemoimmunotherapy.

Lymphoplasmacytic Lymphoma About 1% of all NHLs will be LPLs, which are indolent B-cell NHLs with lymphoplasmacytic differentiation, most commonly associated with a monoclonal IgM paraprotein. Nearly all patients will have stage IV disease at diagnosis with bone marrow involvement. Patients with high levels of circulating IgM paraproteins constitute a specific entity known as Waldenström's macroglobulinemia and can have symptoms due to hyperviscosity as a result of the circulating IgM. Activating mutations in MYD88, an adaptor protein that is involved in signaling downstream of the Ig receptor leading to NF-κB activation, are present in >90% of cases. Tumor biopsies are notable for proliferation of small lymphocytes, lymphoplasmacytic cells, and plasma cells, and malignant lymphocytes are positive for CD19, CD20, and surface IgM but generally negative for CD5 and CD10. Like the other indolent NHLs, treatment is indicated for disease that causes symptoms or interferes with organ function; hyperviscosity related to elevated serum IgM and paraneoplastic neuropathy are additional indications for therapy. Single-agent rituximab may be useful for low-volume disease but can be associated with a transient rise in serum IgM concentrations that can cause or exacerbate hyperviscosity. Chemoimmunotherapy with regimens such as BR and rituximab, cyclophosphamide, and dexamethasone is active, as are myeloma therapies such as bortezomib. Ibrutinib in combination with rituximab is highly active in this disease and is an option for both previously untreated and relapsed disease. Given that 85% of IgM remains intravascular, acute relief of hyperviscosity symptoms can be obtained by plasmapheresis. For recurrent disease, one can often use agents that were previously used. For patients with more refractory LPL, the mammalian target of rapamycin (mTOR) inhibitor everolimus and the oral BTK ibrutinib are active. Selected patients with relapsed disease are considered for high-dose therapy with autologous or allogeneic stem cell transplantation. The results seen are similar to those of other indolent lymphomas.

Mantle Cell Lymphoma MCL composes ~6% of NHLs. It is an intermediate-grade lymphoma that, like the indolent B-cell NHLs, is not curable with conventional therapies but, like the aggressive lymphomas, often requires more aggressive chemoimmunotherapy regimens with or without an autologous stem cell transplant to achieve a reasonable response duration. This therapy is not curative, however, and median survival with this disease is on the order of 5–10 years. An exception to this is a more indolent SOX11 variant that often presents with circulating disease with splenomegaly but without significant lymphadenopathy and with a low Ki67 (<10%). This subset behaves more like the indolent B-cell NHLs and can be observed until treatment is indicated by symptoms or organ function impairment. Similarly, there is a blastic variant with a high Ki67 index that is associated with a poor prognosis and a median OS of only 18 months. For other patients, prognosis is best predicted by the biologic MCL International Prognostic Index (MIPI), which factors in age, performance status, LDH, white blood cell count, and Ki67 expression to determine a risk group. This disease is more common in men, and the average age of diagnosis is 63. MCLs with a mutation in *TP53* or a complex karyotype are particularly high risk as well. Over two-thirds of patients will have stage IV disease, mostly with bone marrow and peripheral blood involvement, at the time of diagnosis. Another common extranodal site of involvement is the gastrointestinal tract, where diffuse lymphomatous polyposis may be seen.

The pathognomonic cytogenetic finding in MCL is t(11;14), which brings the gene for the cell cycle control protein cyclin D1 under the control of the immunoglobulin heavy chain gene promoter on chromosome 14. This translocation is present in >90% of cases. The remaining cases usually overexpress cyclin D2, cyclin D3, or cyclin E. Tumor cells also are positive for B cell markers CD19 and CD20, as well as CD5. They usually lack CD10 and CD23.

Therapies for MCL are evolving. Patients with localized disease might be treated with combination chemotherapy followed by radiotherapy; however, these patients are exceedingly rare. Similarly, patients with the indolent variant can be observed until disease progresses to cause symptoms or signs of organ function impairment. For the usual presentation with disseminated disease, standard lymphoma treatments like R-CHOP have been unsatisfactory, with the minority of patients achieving complete remission. The addition of high-dose cytarabine to an R-CHOP–like backbone with or without consolidation autologous stem cell transplantation in first remission has improved progression-free survival, but it has not elicited cures in this disease. These include the Nordic regimens and R-HyperCVAD (rituximab, cyclophosphamide, vincristine, doxorubicin, dexamethasone, cytarabine, and methotrexate). BR has activity in this disease and is more effective and better tolerated than R-CHOP. Newer studies with short follow-up suggest that strategies that combine BR with cytarabine with or without autologous stem cell transplant may be effective and well tolerated. Maintenance rituximab, following a good response to induction chemotherapy or after autologous stem cell transplant, also improves outcomes over observation alone. For relapsed disease, the BTK inhibitors ibrutinib and acalabrutinib have single-agent activity with a response rate of almost 70% but a response duration of only 18 months. These drugs are being explored in combination with chemotherapy as well as with the BCL2 antagonist venetoclax. Anti-CD19–directed CAR-T cell therapies are approved for the treatment of relapsed/refractory MCL; two-thirds of patients who had progressed after chemoimmunotherapy (with or without an autologous stem cell transplant) and BTK inhibition have achieved complete responses, many of which are durable through limited follow-up. As in FL, longer follow-up is needed to determine if some of these patients may be cured, which would make this the only curative therapy for this disease outside of an allogeneic stem cell transplantation. Drugs such as lenalidomide, venetoclax, bortezomib, and temsirolimus can similarly induce transient partial responses. Appropriate patients who respond to salvage therapy, with the exception of CAR-T cell therapy, should be considered for allogeneic stem cell transplant, which can lead to long-term disease-free survival in 30–50% of patients.

MATURE (PERIPHERAL) T CELL DISORDERS

Mature T cell disorders include cutaneous lymphomas, such as mycosis fungoides, and the PTCLs, some of which are distinguished based on specific clinical presentations or contexts or by molecular or biologic features, but many of which fall into the category of PTCL not otherwise specified (NOS). T-cell NHLs are significantly rarer than B-cell NHLs, and as such, our understanding of their biology is less advanced and our therapies are less well developed. While some T-cell lymphomas, like mycosis fungoides, can behave indolently and some, like ALK-positive ALCL, can be cured with chemotherapy, the majority are associated with a poor prognosis. The advent of genomic technologies is enhancing our ability to understand the genetic and biologic basis of these neoplasms.

Mycosis Fungoides Mycosis fungoides is also known as cutaneous T-cell lymphoma. This lymphoma is more often seen by dermatologists than internists. The median age of onset is in the mid-fifties, and the disease is more common in males and in blacks.

Mycosis fungoides is an indolent lymphoma, with patients often having several years of eczematous or dermatitic skin lesions before the diagnosis is finally established. The skin lesions progress from patch stage to plaque stage to cutaneous tumors. Early in the disease, biopsies are often difficult to interpret, and the diagnosis may only become apparent by observing the patient over time. Adenopathy may reflect involvement with mycosis fungoides or be read as dermatopathic change. In advanced stages, the lymphoma can spread to lymph nodes and visceral organs. Patients with this lymphoma may develop generalized erythroderma and circulating tumor cells, called *Sézary's syndrome*.

Rare patients with localized early-stage mycosis fungoides can be cured with radiotherapy, often total-skin electron beam irradiation. More advanced disease has been treated with topical glucocorticoids, topical nitrogen mustard, phototherapy, psoralen with ultraviolet A (PUVA), extracorporeal photopheresis, retinoids (bexarotene), electron beam radiation, interferon, antibodies, fusion toxins, histone deacetylase inhibitors, brentuximab (for CD30+ disease), and systemic cytotoxic therapy. Mogamulizumab, an anti-CCR4 antibody, has activity in this disease and has been approved by the U.S. Food and Drug Administration for this indication. Unfortunately, these treatments are palliative.

Peripheral T-Cell Lymphoma, Not Otherwise Specified PTCLs include a number of entities, which constitute 15% of all NHLs in adults. PTCL NOS, which composes 6% of all NHLs, is the term used for cases that are not other entities defined in the WHO classification. Named varieties include ALCL, angioimmunoblastic T-cell lymphoma (AITL), hepatosplenic T-cell lymphoma, enteropathy-associated T-cell lymphoma, and subcutaneous panniculitis T-cell lymphoma. PTCL NOS is a disease of older individuals, with a median age at presentation of 65, and the majority of patients will have advanced-stage disease at diagnosis, with involvement of the bone marrow, liver, spleen, and skin being common. Associated "B" symptoms and pruritis are also common. These lymphomas can be associated with a reactive eosinophilia as well as hemophagocytic syndrome. The IPI has been applied to PTCL NOS and provides some assessment of outcomes, but even the low-risk group has a median OS of just >2 years.

This diagnostic category is a collection of heterogeneous lymphomas that vary widely and lack typical findings of other specific PTCL subgroups. Because of this heterogeneity, histology, immunophenotype, and genetics are variable. Often lymph nodes are effaced by atypical lymphoid cells of various sizes, sometimes associated with vascular proliferation or an infiltrate of eosinophils and/or macrophages. As most of these lymphomas behave aggressively, note is often made of mitotic and apoptotic figures as well as geographic necrosis. The cells often are positive for CD3, and the majority of PTCL NOS is positive for CD4 rather than CD8, but some are negative for both markers. There can be loss of more mature T-cell markers like CD5 and CD7, and this is associated with a more aggressive course. There are some recurrent translocations, including t(7;14), t(11;14), inv(14), and t(14;14), all of which involve the TCR genes.

The most common primary therapy for PTCL NOS involves a CHOP-like chemotherapy backbone—either CHOP alone or CHOP in combination with etoposide (CHOEP). The latter may provide the most benefit to younger patients and patients with more favorable disease risk factors. Brentuximab in combination with cyclophosphamide, doxorubicin, and prednisone (CHP) has been tested in a randomized clinical trial against CHOP in CD30+ T-cell lymphomas; progression-free survival was improved with the brentuximab-containing arm, and this was most pronounced for patients with ALCL (see below). Autologous stem cell transplant has been investigated for patients in their first remission and does seem to improve progression-free survival in certain contexts. Drugs such as gemcitabine, bendamustine, and pralatrexate have activity in relapsed disease, as do the histone deacetylase inhibitors romidepsin and belinostat. The PI3 kinase inhibitor duvelisib is being investigated in these diseases with early signals of activity. All of these agents are associated with transient responses in a minority of patients. Patients should be considered for clinical trials. For patients who do achieve remission, reduced-intensity allogeneic stem cell transplantation can yield long-term nonrelapse survival rates of ~40–50%.

Angioimmunoblastic T-Cell Lymphoma AITL constitutes ~20% of T-cell NHLs and ~4% of all NHLs diagnosed. Patients present with a variety of signs and symptoms, most often including lymphadenopathy, hepatosplenomegaly, "B" symptoms, rash, polyarthritis, and hemolytic anemia. Over 80% of patients have advanced-stage disease at diagnosis, and bone marrow involvement is common. Polyclonal hypergammaglobulinemia is common, as are elevated LDH, eosinophilia, a positive Coombs test, and opportunistic infections.

On biopsy, lymph nodes are effaced by a polymorphous infiltrate of lymphocytes, ranging in size and shape, and of immunoblasts. The neoplastic lymphocytes are positive for CD3 as well as CXCL13, PD-1, CD10, and BCL6, most closely resembling CD4-positive follicular helper T cells. There is an expanded follicular dendritic cell network surrounding tumor cells. Scattered immunoblasts are often EBV positive and may give rise to secondary EBV-positive B-cell lymphomas at a later time. Genetic analysis of this disease has revealed recurrent mutations in *TET2* (76%), *DNMT3* (33%), and *IDH2* (20%).

There is a subset of AITL that can remit with immunosuppression with agents like glucocorticoids or methotrexate. Most patients, however, will need combination chemotherapy with regimens like those used in PTCL NOS. Median response duration is short, and median OS is only 15–36 months. Treatment of relapsed disease is similar to that of relapsed PTCL NOS.

Anaplastic Large-Cell Lymphoma ALCL is the next most common T-cell lymphoma after AITL but is more common in children, accounting for up to 10% of pediatric lymphomas. Approximately 40–60% of cases harbor t(2;5), which fuses a portion of the nucleolar protein nucleophosmin-1 (*NPM1*) gene to a part of the anaplastic lymphoma kinase (*ALK*) gene, the product of which has constitutive tyrosine kinase activity. These patients have a much more favorable prognosis compared to ALK-negative ALCL, akin to that of DLBCL. There is an additional, more indolent and favorable subtype that occurs in the breast tissue of patients with breast implants, and there is a cutaneous variant. In general, this is a disease that is more common in men. ALK-positive disease is a disease of younger patients, with a median age at diagnosis of 34 years, whereas the median age at diagnosis of ALK-negative patients is 58. With the exception of the cutaneous variant and the variant associated with breast implants, most patients present with rapidly growing lymphadenopathy with or without extranodal involvement; "B" symptoms are common.

Most cases of ALCL involve large atypical lymphocytes with horseshoe-shaped nuclei with prominent nucleoli ("hallmark" cells). Tumor cells tend to be localized within the lymph node sinuses, and almost all are positive for CD30 but negative for CD15. A majority will also express CD3, CD25, CD43, and CD4. ALK-rearranged ALCL can be diagnosed by fluorescence in situ hybridization (FISH) cytogenetics for t(2;5) or by immunohistochemical staining for ALK.

ALCL is generally treated with CHOP, although like PTCL NOS, CHOEP may benefit younger patients, particularly with ALK-positive disease. Overall, ALCL has a better prognosis than PTCL, and this is particularly true for ALK-positive disease, which has an 8-year OS rate of 82%, versus 49% for ALK-negative disease. Relapsed ALK-positive ALCL is treated similarly to relapsed DLBCL, with salvage combination chemotherapy to identify chemotherapy sensitivity followed by autologous stem cell transplant. For patients with chemotherapy-insensitive disease or for ALK-negative disease, the conjugated anti-CD30 antibody to MMAE brentuximab is highly active, with a response rate of 86% and a complete response rate of 57%. As mentioned earlier, brentuximab in combination with CHP chemotherapy is an approved frontline regimen for the treatment of CD30+ T-cell lymphomas, including ALCL. The ALK inhibitors, including crizotinib, are active in refractory ALK-positive ALCL with excellent outcomes.

Other PTCL Subtypes Enteropathy-associated T-cell lymphoma, hepatosplenic T-cell lymphoma, and subcutaneous panniculitis-like T-cell lymphoma are other less common PTCL subtypes. *Enteropathy-type intestinal T-cell lymphoma* is a rare disorder. Type I occurs in patients with a history of gluten-sensitive enteropathy and is associated with HLADQA1*0501, DQB1*0201; a gluten-free diet can prevent the development of this lymphoma. Type II is not associated with celiac disease and may be a separate disease entity. Patients are frequently cachectic and sometimes present with intestinal perforation. The prognosis is poor, with a median survival of 10 months. Therapy is often with combination chemotherapy, including high-dose methotrexate, and autologous stem cell transplant in first remission.

Hepatosplenic γδ T-cell lymphoma is a systemic illness that presents with sinusoidal infiltration of the liver, spleen, and bone marrow by malignant T cells. Tumor masses generally do not occur. The disease is associated with systemic symptoms and is often difficult to diagnose. Recurrent genetic events include isochromosome 7q and trisomy 8. Treatment outcome is poor, but regimens that include ifosfamide, such as ifosfamide, carboplatin, and etoposide (ICE) or ifosfamide, etoposide, and cytarabine (IVAC), are associated with better outcomes in small series of patients. Responding patients should be considered for allogeneic stem cell transplantation.

Subcutaneous panniculitis-like T-cell lymphoma is a rare disorder that is often confused with panniculitis. Patients present with multiple subcutaneous nodules, which progress and can ulcerate.

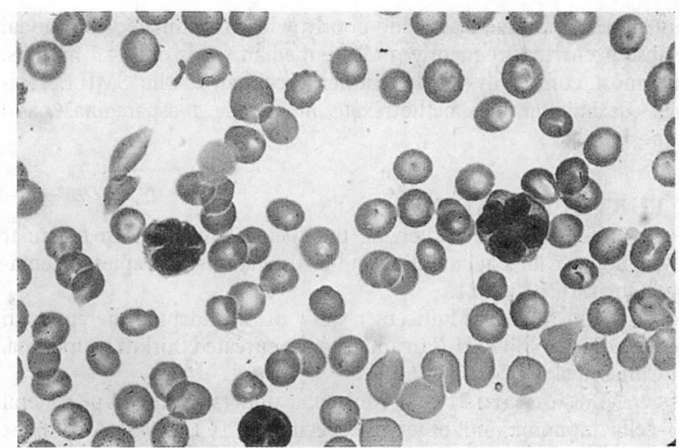

FIGURE 108-7 Adult T-cell leukemia/lymphoma. Peripheral blood smear showing leukemia cells with typical "flower-shaped" nucleus.

There is a more indolent form that tends to express α/β TCRs and can be managed with immune suppression, whereas lymphomas that express γ/δ TCRs are more aggressive and are associated with a worse prognosis and coincident hemophagocytic syndrome. This is a disease of young men in their fifth and sixth decades of life. Patients with aggressive disease are managed with multiagent chemotherapy, and responding patients should be considered for allogeneic stem cell transplantation.

Adult T-Cell Leukemia/Lymphoma Adult T-cell leukemia/lymphoma (ATLL) is a disease that is most prevalent in Japan and the Caribbean basin. It is a neoplasm that is driven by HTLV-1, often contracted through the breast milk of infected mothers. The average age at diagnosis is 60, so there is a long latency between viral infection and viral transformation, and only 4% of infected patients will develop the disease. This suggests that HTLV-1 may not be sufficient to cause the malignant phenotype. There are four disease variants: acute (60% of patients), lymphomatous (20% of patients), chronic (15% of patients), and smoldering (5% of patients); prognosis varies across these groups, with median survival times of 6, 10, and 24 months, and not yet reached, respectively. Presentation depends on the subtype, but most commonly, patients present with circulating disease and bone marrow involvement, hypercalcemia, lytic bone lesions, lymphadenopathy, hepatosplenomegaly, skin lesions, and opportunistic infections.

The pathognomonic finding is the malignant "flower cell" that is positive for CD4 and CD25, as well as CD2, CD3, and CD5 but lacking CD7 (**Fig. 108-7**). Combination chemotherapy is generally used, but for patients fortunate enough to respond, response durations are very short. Other active agents in this disease include the antiretroviral agent zidovudine, interferon α, and arsenic. In any patients who do respond to therapy, allogeneic stem cell transplant should be considered.

Extranodal NK/T-Cell Lymphoma, Nasal Type Extranodal NK/T-cell lymphoma, nasal type, is a lymphoma that is associated with EBV infection in nearly all cases and more common in Asia and native populations in Peru. It usually presents with a mass and obstructive symptoms in the upper aerodigestive tract with occasional extranodal sites, but over two-thirds of patients will have localized disease. It is more common in men, and the median age at diagnosis is 60. This disease has its own prognostic score, which takes into account the presence or absence of "B" symptoms, disease stage, whether LDH is elevated, and whether there is lymph node involvement. EBV viral load at diagnosis and at the end of therapy is also predictive.

Treatment for early-stage disease is usually with combined-modality therapy of chemotherapy (commonly using etoposide, ifosfamide, cisplatin, and dexamethasone) and intensity-modulated radiation therapy (50–55 Gy), and patients with localized disease involving the nasal passages do quite well, with 3-year OS of ~85%. Patients with more advanced-stage disease do poorly, with disseminated extranodal relapse occurring frequently, and the median OS is only 4.3 months. The most commonly used treatment regimen is the SMILE regimen (dexamethasone, methotrexate, ifosfamide, L-asparaginase, and etoposide).

FURTHER READING

HANEL W, EPPERLA N: Evolving therapeutic landscape in follicular lymphoma: a look at emerging and investigational therapies. J Hematol Oncol 14:104, 2021.

ROSCHEWSKI M et al: Multicenter study of risk-adapted therapy with dose-adjusted EPOCH-R in adults with untreated Burkitt lymphoma. J Clin Oncol 38:2519, 2020.

SAKATA-YANAGIMOTO M et al: Molecular understanding of peripheral T-cell lymphomas, not otherwise specified (PTCL, NOS): A complex disease category. J Clin Exp Hematop 61:61, 2021.

SILKENSTEDT E, DREYLING M: Mantle cell lymphoma–advances in molecular biology, prognostication, and treatment approaches. Hematol Oncol 39 Suppl 1:31, 2021.

109 Hodgkin's Lymphoma

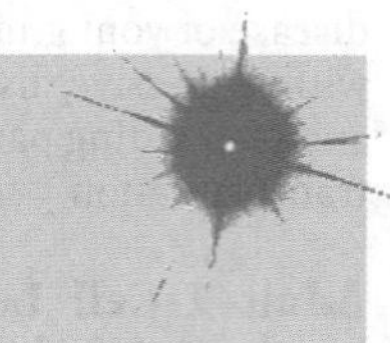

Caron A. Jacobson, Dan L. Longo

Hodgkin's lymphoma (HL) is a malignancy of mature B lymphocytes. It represents ~10% of all lymphomas diagnosed each year. The majority of HL diagnoses are classical HL (cHL), but there is a second subtype of HL, nodular lymphocyte-predominant HL (NLPHL). While this diagnosis does resemble cHL morphologically in certain respects, there is some evidence that it is more related to the indolent B-cell non-Hodgkin's lymphomas (NHLs) biologically than it is to cHL. The majority of this chapter will be specific to cHL, with a discussion of NLPHL at the end.

cHL is one of the success stories of modern oncology. Until the advent of extended-field radiotherapy in the mid-twentieth century, it was a highly fatal disease of young people. Radiation therapy cured some patients with early-stage disease, and the introduction of multiagent chemotherapy in the 1970s resulted in further improved cure rates, both for patients with early- and advanced-stage disease. Cure rates now are >85%. The new challenge in the treatment of HL is late therapy-related toxicity, including a high rate of secondary malignancies and cardiovascular disease. Current clinical trials are aimed at minimizing this risk while preserving efficacy.

EPIDEMIOLOGY AND ETIOLOGY

HL is of B-cell origin. The incidence of HL appears fairly stable, with 8480 new cases diagnosed in 2020 in the United States. HL is more common in whites than in blacks and more common in males than in females. A bimodal distribution of age at diagnosis has been observed, with one peak incidence occurring in patients in their twenties and the other in those in their eighties. Some of the late age peak may be attributed to confusion among entities with similar appearance such as anaplastic large-cell lymphoma and T-cell/histiocyte–rich B-cell lymphoma. There are four distinct subtypes of cHL that are differentiated based on their histopathologic features (**Table 109-1**): nodular sclerosis, mixed cellularity, lymphocyte-rich, and lymphocyte-depleted. Patients in the younger age groups diagnosed in the United States largely have the nodular sclerosing subtype of HL. Elderly patients, patients infected with HIV, and patients in developing countries more commonly have mixed-cellularity HL or lymphocyte-depleted HL. Together, nodular sclerosis and mixed-cellularity types account for nearly 95% of cases. Infection by HIV is a risk factor for developing HL. In addition, an association between infection by Epstein-Barr virus (EBV) and HL has been suggested. A monoclonal or oligoclonal proliferation of EBV-infected cells in 20–40% of the patients with HL has led to proposals for this virus having an etiologic role in HL. However, the matter is not settled definitively. Viral oncogenesis appears to play a greater role in HIV-related cHL: EBV can be detected in nearly all cases of HIV-associated cHL, compared to only one-third of cases of non–HIV-associated cHL. Reed-Sternberg (HRS) cells are the malignant cells in HL. HRS cells in HIV-associated cHL express the EBV-transforming protein latent membrane protein 1 (LMP-1), and the EBV genomes from multiple disease sites in the same HIV-associated cHL patient are episomal and clonal, suggesting that EBV is directly involved in early lymphomagenesis.

TABLE 109-1 World Health Organization Classification of Hodgkin's Lymphoma

Nodular lymphocyte-predominant Hodgkin's lymphoma
Classical Hodgkin's lymphoma
Nodular sclerosis
Lymphocyte-rich
Mixed cellularity
Lymphocyte-depleted

Histologically, the HRS cell is diagnostic of cHL (**Fig. 109-1**). These cells are large cells with abundant cytoplasm with bilobed and/or multiple nuclei. By immunohistochemistry, they are often PAX-5 positive but have low to no expression of other B-cell antigens like CD19 and CD20. They express CD15 and CD30 in 85 and 100% of cases, respectively. These cells, though, comprise <1% of the tumor cellularity, with the majority of the tumor made up of a surrounding inflammatory infiltrate of polyclonal lymphocytes, eosinophils, neutrophils, macrophages, plasma cells, fibroblasts, and collagen. The HRS cell interacts with its microenvironment via cell-cell contact and elaboration of growth factors and cytokines, which results in a surrounding cellular milieu that protects it from host immune attack. The surrounding environmental cells likewise support the HRS cells via cell-cell signaling and cytokine production, which provides signals that promote proliferation and survival of the HRS cell itself. Interestingly, 97% of HRS cells in cHL harbor genetic aberrations in the PD-L1 locus on chromosome 9p24.1, resulting in overexpression of PD-L1, the ligand for the inhibitory PD-1 receptor on immune cells. This is one mechanism whereby the HRS cell may be able to avoid immune destruction in its inflammatory microenvironment and may contribute to the generalized immune suppression in HL patients.

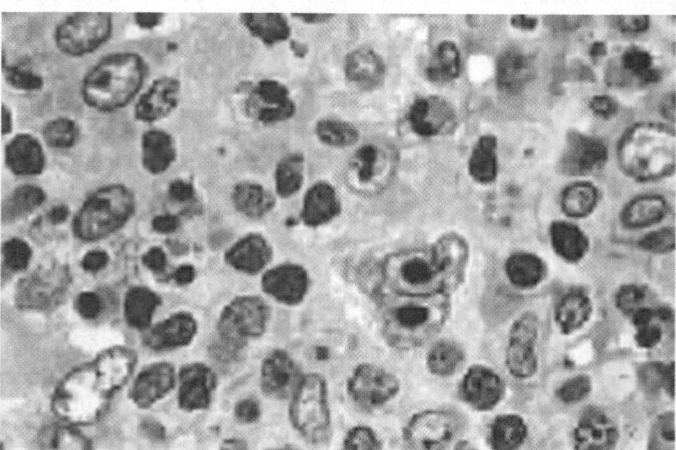

FIGURE 109-1 Hodgkin's disease: A classic Reed-Sternberg (RS) cell is present near the center of the field. RS cells are large cells with a bilobed nucleus and prominent nucleoli surrounded by a pleiomorphic cellular infiltrate. *(From DL Kasper: Harrison's Principles of Internal Medicine, 16th ed. New York, NY: McGraw-Hill; 2005, Fig. 97-11, p. 654.)*

APPROACH TO THE PATIENT
Classical Hodgkin's Lymphoma

Most patients with cHL present with palpable lymphadenopathy that is nontender; in most patients, these lymph nodes are in the neck, supraclavicular area, and axilla. More than half of the patients will have mediastinal adenopathy at diagnosis, and this is sometimes the initial manifestation. Subdiaphragmatic presentation of cHL is unusual and more common in older males. One-third of patients present with fevers, night sweats, and/or weight loss, or "B" symptoms. Occasionally, HL can present as a fever of unknown origin. This is more common in older patients who are found to have mixed-cellularity HL in an abdominal site. Rarely, the fevers persist for days to weeks, followed by afebrile intervals and then recurrence of the fever. This pattern is known as *Pel-Ebstein* fever. HL can occasionally present with unusual manifestations. These include severe and unexplained itching, cutaneous disorders such as erythema nodosum and ichthyosiform atrophy, paraneoplastic cerebellar degeneration and other distant effects on the CNS, nephrotic syndrome, immune hemolytic anemia and thrombocytopenia, hypercalcemia, and pain in lymph nodes on alcohol ingestion.

Evaluation of patients with HL will typically begin with a careful history and physical examination. Patients should be asked about the presence or absence of "B" symptoms. Comorbid diagnoses that may impact therapy should be reviewed, including a history of pulmonary disease and congestive heart failure given the use of chemotherapy drugs that can cause both lung and heart toxicity. A physical examination should pay attention to the peripherally accessible sites of lymph nodes and to the liver and spleen size. Laboratory evaluation should include a complete blood count with differential; erythrocyte sedimentation rate (ESR); chemistry studies reflecting major organ function including serum albumin; and HIV and hepatitis virus testing. A positron emission tomography (PET)/computed tomography (CT) scan is used for staging and is more accurate than a bone marrow biopsy for evaluation of bone marrow involvement as the bone marrow involvement in cHL tends to be patchy and therefore potentially missed on a unilateral bone marrow biopsy. The initial evaluation of a patient with HL or NHL is similar. In both situations, the determination of an accurate anatomic stage is an important part of the evaluation. Staging is done using the Ann Arbor staging system (**Table 109-2**).

TABLE 109-2 The Ann Arbor Staging System for Hodgkin's Lymphoma

STAGE	DEFINITION
I	Involvement of a single lymph node region or lymphoid structure (e.g., spleen, thymus, Waldeyer's ring)
II	Involvement of two or more lymph node regions on the same side of the diaphragm (the mediastinum is a single site; hilar lymph nodes should be considered "lateralized" and, when involved on both sides, constitute stage II disease)
III	Involvement of lymph node regions or lymphoid structures on both sides of the diaphragm
III_1	Subdiaphragmatic involvement limited to spleen, splenic hilar nodes, celiac nodes, or portal nodes
III_2	Subdiaphragmatic involvement includes paraaortic, iliac, or mesenteric nodes plus structures in III_1
IV	Involvement of extranodal site(s) beyond that designated as "E"
	More than one extranodal deposit at any location
	Any involvement of liver or bone marrow
A	No symptoms
B	Unexplained weight loss of >10% of the body weight during the 6 months before staging investigation
	Unexplained, persistent, or recurrent fever with temperatures >38°C during the previous month
	Recurrent drenching night sweats during the previous month
E	Localized, solitary involvement of extralymphatic tissue, excluding liver and bone marrow

The diagnosis of HL is established by review of an adequate biopsy specimen by an expert hematopathologist. HL is a tumor characterized by rare neoplastic cells of B-cell origin (immunoglobulin genes are rearranged but not expressed) in a tumor mass that is largely polyclonal inflammatory infiltrate, probably a reaction to cytokines produced by the tumor cells. The differential diagnosis of a lymph node biopsy suspicious for HL includes inflammatory processes, mononucleosis, NHL, phenytoin-induced adenopathy, and nonlymphomatous malignancies.

Staging for cHL is anatomically based given the propensity of the disease to march from one lymph node group to the next group, often contiguous to the first. Staging is important for selecting therapy of appropriate intensity, but the outcome of optimal therapy for all the stages is excellent. Patients are stratified based on whether they have early-stage disease (stage I or II) or advanced-stage disease (stage III or IV). Patients with early-stage disease have a better prognosis overall but are further classified as favorable or unfavorable based on a variety of factors. These factors vary from study to study but include bulky disease, number of lymph node areas involved, an elevated ESR (>30 if "B" symptoms are present; >50 if "B" symptoms are absent), and age. Prognosis in advanced-stage disease is best predicted by the International Prognostic Score (IPS), which ascribes 1 point for male sex, older age (>45 years), stage IV disease, serum albumin <4 g/dL, hemoglobin <10.5 g/dL, white blood cell count ≥15,000/μL, and a lymphocyte count <600/μL and/or <8% of white blood cell count. Five-year progression-free survival ranges from 88% for patients with no risk factors to 62% for patients with four or more factors, but very few patients have multiple risk factors.

TREATMENT
Classical Hodgkin's Lymphoma

The overwhelming majority of patients with HL will be cured with either chemotherapy alone or a combination of chemotherapy and radiation therapy. It has long been appreciated that patients with advanced-stage disease do not benefit from the addition of radiation therapy to chemotherapy and are thus treated with chemotherapy alone. For early-stage disease, however, treatment with combined-modality therapy has been associated with a small decrease in risk of relapse but with an increased risk of late toxicity including secondary malignancies, thyroid disease, and premature cardiovascular disease and stroke resulting in minimal or no improvement in long-term survival. Much of this risk can be attributed to radiation therapy. Thus, investigation into the treatment of early-stage HL at present is aimed at trying to maximize treatment outcome without using radiotherapy. This is an area of controversy in the treatment of HL.

EARLY-STAGE DISEASE

The most common chemotherapy regimen used to treat HL in the United States is ABVD (doxorubicin, bleomycin, vinblastine, and dacarbazine). This regimen is given every other week, with each cycle including two treatments. In patients with low-risk, or favorable, disease, the use of four to six cycles of ABVD alone, without radiation therapy, results in progression-free and overall survival rates of 88–92% and 97–100%, respectively, at 5–7 years. This may be associated with a slightly increased risk of relapse when compared with abbreviated chemotherapy (ABVD for four cycles) followed by involved field radiation therapy (30 Gy), but with no difference in overall survival owing to the excellent salvage strategies used for relapsed HL and to the late toxicities seen following radiation therapy to the chest. German studies have examined a very abbreviated chemotherapy regimen (ABVD for two cycles) and low-dose radiation (20 Gy) for particularly good-risk disease with two or fewer lymph node areas involved and found that this was equally effective to standard combined-modality therapy of ABVD for four cycles and 30 Gy of radiation. However, long-term follow-up is not yet available to assess the impact of the lower radiotherapy dose on late toxicities. Finally, the use of an early interim PET/CT scan can aid decisions regarding the duration and extent of therapy. In one study, a negative PET/CT scan after three cycles of ABVD predicted for excellent outcomes with no additional therapy; in another, a negative PET/CT scan after two cycles of ABVD predicted for good outcomes with two additional cycles of ABVD alone, without radiation therapy.

For unfavorable-risk disease, the omission of radiation therapy following chemotherapy is associated with a more significant increased risk of relapse compared to favorable-risk disease, but again with no change in overall survival. For these patients, treatment options would include ABVD for four cycles followed by involved field radiation therapy or ABVD alone for six cycles. Treatment decisions are often based on the extent of the radiation field and the unfavorable risk factor, with patients with nonbulky disease being candidates for chemotherapy alone if radiation would be contraindicated for another reason. Combined modality therapy has typically been used for patients with bulky disease, although patients with bulky disease who have a negative PET/CT scan after chemotherapy may not benefit from additional radiation therapy.

Alternative chemotherapy regimens to ABVD have been developed and include the Stanford V regimen and escalated BEACOPP (bleomycin, etoposide, doxorubicin, cyclophosphamide, vincristine, procarbazine, and prednisone). Neither of these regimens has resulted in improved outcomes in patients with early-stage disease.

ADVANCED-STAGE DISEASE

Patients with advanced-stage disease do not benefit from the addition of radiation therapy after a complete response to chemotherapy alone and should be treated with chemotherapy alone. The most common regimen used in the United States is ABVD for six cycles. Again, Stanford V and escalated BEACOPP have been evaluated in advanced-stage disease and are not associated with an improvement in overall survival but are associated with increased toxicity. The small fraction of patients who do not achieve complete remission with chemotherapy alone (partial responders with persistent PET scan positivity account for <10% of patients) may benefit from the addition of involved field radiotherapy.

Newer drugs have been developed for the treatment of relapsed HL (see "Relapsed Disease," below). These include the antibody-drug conjugate brentuximab vedotin, which is an antibody against CD30 conjugated to the microtubule inhibitor monomethyl auristatin E (MMAE). This drug has been combined with doxorubicin, bleomycin, and dacarbazine in early-phase studies for advanced-stage HL with favorable efficacy compared to historical controls. Eschelon-1, a randomized trial of doxorubicin, vinblastine, and dacarbazine (AVD) plus brentuximab compared to ABVD, was a positive study in that it demonstrated an improvement in progression-free survival for AVD plus brentuximab, especially among younger patients, patients from North America, and patients with higher risk disease. Drugs that target the PD-1/PD-L1 axis have been developed in an attempt to boost the host immune recognition of tumors. This was particularly attractive in HL given the overexpression of PD-L1 on the HRS cell surface. In the setting of relapsed disease, these drugs, which include pembrolizumab and nivolumab, have very high response rates and are associated with durable responses. These are now being tested in conjunction with chemotherapy both as salvage therapy for relapsed disease and in previously untreated patients, including in a multicenter randomized trial against AVD plus brentuximab as initial therapy for advanced-stage disease.

RELAPSED DISEASE

Patients who relapse after primary therapy of HL can frequently still be cured. Patients who relapse after an effective chemotherapy regimen are usually not curable with subsequent chemotherapy administered at standard doses. Alternative salvage chemotherapy administered at standard doses, then, is given in order to document sensitivity to chemotherapy and to achieve maximum reduction of tumor mass. For patients who respond completely or nearly so, autologous stem cell transplantation can cure over half of patients. Standard salvage chemotherapy regimens include ICE (ifosfamide, carboplatin, and etoposide) and GND (gemcitabine, vinorelbine, and doxorubicin). Newer combinations, including brentuximab with either chemotherapy or immune checkpoint inhibitors such as nivolumab, have also been tested with promising early results. For patients with early-stage disease who do not respond sufficiently to salvage chemotherapy, radiation therapy can be very effective to achieve a remission; whether to consolidate such a remission with an autologous stem cell transplant is debated. For patients with advanced-stage disease in whom salvage chemotherapy fails, the antibody-drug conjugate brentuximab vedotin, a CD30-directed antibody linked to the microtubule toxin MMAE, is active and can be tried as a bridge to allogeneic transplant. It is also used as a maintenance therapy following successful autologous stem cell transplantation based on results of a randomized trial versus observation. The anti-PD-1 immune checkpoint inhibitors, nivolumab and pembrolizumab, have efficacy in relapsed HL, and many responses are durable. Increasingly, there is an appreciation that use of checkpoint inhibitors restores the HRS cell's sensitivity to chemotherapy by unknown mechanisms; autologous stem cell transplantation may be a potentially curative option for patients who had previously been felt to have chemotherapy-resistant disease. Finally, anti-CD30 chimeric antigen receptor (CAR) T-cell therapy has been tested in multiply relapsed cHL with promising early results; these products are now being tested in multicenter phase 2 clinical trials.

Two other options may be useful in the setting of disease relapse after ABVD chemotherapy. Alkylating agent–based combinations such as ChlVPP (chlorambucil, vincristine, prednisone, and procarbazine) may be active in patients with disease resistant to ABVD. In addition, relapse following bone marrow transplant can be responsive to weekly low-dose single-agent vinblastine.

SURVIVORSHIP

Because of the very high cure rate in patients with HL, long-term complications have become a major focus for clinical research. In fact, in some series of patients with early-stage disease, more patients died from late complications of therapy than from HL itself. This is particularly true in patients with localized disease. The most serious late side effects include second malignancies and cardiac injury. Patients are at risk for the development of acute leukemia in the first 10 years after treatment with combination chemotherapy regimens that contain alkylating agents plus radiation therapy. The risk for development of acute leukemia is greater after MOPP-like (mechlorethamine, vincristine, procarbazine, and prednisone) and BEACOPP-like regimens than with ABVD. The risk of development of acute leukemia after treatment for HL is also related to the number of exposures to potentially leukemogenic agents (i.e., multiple treatments after relapse) and the age of the patient being treated, with those aged >60 years at particularly high risk. The development of carcinomas as a complication of treatment for HL is a major problem. These tumors usually occur ≥10 years after treatment and are associated with use of radiotherapy. For this reason, young women treated with thoracic radiotherapy for HL should institute screening mammograms 5–10 years after treatment, and all patients who receive thoracic radiotherapy for HL should be discouraged from smoking. Mediastinal radiation also accelerates coronary artery disease, and patients should be encouraged to minimize risk factors for coronary artery disease such as smoking and elevated cholesterol levels. Cervical radiation therapy increases the risk of carotid atherosclerosis and stroke and thyroid disease, including cancer.

A number of other late side effects from the treatment of HL are well known. Patients who receive thoracic radiotherapy are at very high risk for the eventual development of hypothyroidism and should be observed for this complication; intermittent measurement of thyrotropin should be made to identify the condition before it becomes symptomatic. Lhermitte's syndrome occurs in ~15% of patients who receive thoracic radiotherapy. This syndrome is manifested by an "electric shock" sensation into the lower extremities on flexion of the neck. Because of the young age at which HL is often diagnosed, infertility is a concern for patients undergoing treatment for HL. Chemotherapy regimens containing alkylating agents induce permanent infertility in nearly all men. The risk of permanent infertility in women treated with alkylating agent–containing chemotherapy is age-related, with younger women more likely to recover fertility. Infertility is very rare after treatment with ABVD.

NODULAR LYMPHOCYTE-PREDOMINANT HODGKIN'S LYMPHOMA

NLPHL is now recognized as an entity distinct from cHL. Previous classification systems recognized that biopsies from a small subset of patients diagnosed as having HL contained a predominance of small lymphocytes and rare Reed-Sternberg–like cells; tumors had a nodular growth pattern and a clinical course that varied from that of patients with cHL. This is an unusual clinical entity and represents <5% of cases of HL and defines NLPHL.

NLPHL has a number of characteristics that suggest its relationship to NHL, rather than cHL, however. The HRS-like cell, or L&H (lymphocyte and histiocyte) or "popcorn" cell, is a clonal proliferation of B-cells that are positive for B-cell markers CD45, CD79a, CD20, CD19, and BCL2. They do not express two markers normally found on HRS cells, CD30 and CD15. This lymphoma tends to have a chronic, relapsing course and sometimes transforms to diffuse large B-cell lymphoma, including a specific subtype of diffuse large B-cell lymphoma known as T-cell/histiocyte–rich B-cell lymphoma, which shares an immunophenotype with the L&H cell. This natural history most closely resembles that of the indolent B-cell NHLs outlined in **Chaps. 108** and **110**.

Patients with NLPHL are more commonly male (75%). Like cHL, the age distribution of patients with this disease has two peaks, but unlike cHL, these peaks include children and adults ages 30–40 years, respectively. The majority of patients diagnosed have stage I or II disease (75%), with a minority having advanced-stage disease at diagnosis. "B" symptoms are uncommon.

Patients with early-stage disease at diagnosis should be treated with definitive radiotherapy. This is associated with a 15-year nonrelapse survival rate of 82%. The treatment of patients with advanced-stage NLPHL is controversial. Some clinicians favor no treatment of asymptomatic disease and merely close follow-up, akin to the indolent B-cell NHLs. For patients who need therapy due to symptoms or signs of organ function impairment, both cHL regimens and B-cell NHL regimens have been used, including ABVD and R-CHOP (rituximab, cyclophosphamide, doxorubicin, vincristine, and prednisone). A single-institution experience with R-CHOP resulted in a 100% response rate in a small group of patients without a single relapse with 42 months of follow-up. Although this is short follow-up for an indolent disease, some believe R-CHOP may be curative in this disease and advocate treating patients with advanced-stage disease at diagnosis, regardless of symptoms or organ function.

FURTHER READING

Chen R et al: Pembrolizumab in relapsed or refractory Hodgkin lymphoma: 2-year follow-up of KEYNOTE-087. Blood 134:1144, 2019.

Gillessen S et al: Intensified treatment of patients with early stage, unfavourable Hodgkin lymphoma: Long-term follow-up of a randomised, international phase 3 trial of the German Hodgkin Study Group (GHSG HD14). Lancet Haematol 8:e278, 2021.

Moskowitz CH et al: Five-year PFS from the AETHERA trial of brentuximab vedotin for Hodgkin lymphoma at high risk of progression or relapse. Blood 132:2639, 2018.

Rashidi A et al: Allogeneic hematopoietic stem cell transplantation in Hodgkin lymphoma: A systemic review and meta-analysis. Bone Marrow Transplant 51:521, 2016.

Straus DJ et al: CALGB 50604: Risk-adapted treatment of non-bulky early-stage Hodgkin lymphoma based on interim PET. Blood 132:1013, 2018.

Straus DJ et al: Brentuximab vedotin with chemotherapy for stage III or IV classical Hodgkin lymphoma (ECHELON-1): 5-year update of an international, open-label, randomised, phase 3 trial. Lancet Haematol 8:e410, 2021.

110 Less Common Lymphoid and Myeloid Malignancies

Ayalew Tefferi, Dan L. Longo

The most common lymphoid malignancies are discussed in **Chaps. 106, 107, 108, 109**, and **111**, myeloid leukemias in **Chaps. 104** and **105**, myelodysplastic syndromes (MDS) in **Chap. 102**, and myeloproliferative syndromes in **Chap. 103**. This chapter will focus on the more unusual forms of hematologic malignancy. The diseases discussed here are listed in **Table 110-1**. Each of these entities accounts for <1% of hematologic neoplasms.

RARE LYMPHOID MALIGNANCIES

All the lymphoid tumors discussed here are mature B-cell or T-cell natural killer (NK) cell neoplasms.

MATURE B-CELL NEOPLASMS

B-Cell Prolymphocytic Leukemia (B-PLL) This is a malignancy of medium-sized (about twice the size of a normal small

TABLE 110-1 Unusual Lymphoid and Myeloid Malignancies

Lymphoid
Mature B-cell neoplasms
B-cell prolymphocytic leukemia
Splenic marginal zone lymphoma
Hairy cell leukemia
Nodal marginal zone B-cell lymphoma
Mediastinal large B-cell lymphoma
Intravascular large B-cell lymphoma
Primary effusion lymphoma
Lymphomatoid granulomatosis
Mature T-cell and natural killer (NK) cell neoplasms
T-cell prolymphocytic leukemia
T-cell large granular lymphocytic leukemia
Aggressive NK cell leukemia
Extranodal NK/T-cell lymphoma, nasal type
Enteropathy-type T-cell lymphoma
Hepatosplenic T-cell lymphoma
Subcutaneous panniculitis-like T-cell lymphoma
Blastic NK cell lymphoma
Primary cutaneous CD30+ T-cell lymphoma
Angioimmunoblastic T-cell lymphoma
Myeloid
Chronic neutrophilic leukemia
Chronic eosinophilic leukemia/hypereosinophilic syndrome
Histiocytic and Dendritic Cell Neoplasms
Histiocytic sarcoma
Langerhans cell histiocytosis
Langerhans cell sarcoma
Interdigitating dendritic cell sarcoma
Follicular dendritic cell sarcoma
Mast Cells
Mastocytosis
Cutaneous mastocytosis
Systemic mastocytosis
Mast cell sarcoma
Extracutaneous mastocytoma

lymphocyte), round lymphocytes with a prominent nucleolus and light blue cytoplasm on Wright's stain. It predominantly affects the blood, bone marrow (BM), and spleen and usually does not cause adenopathy. The median age of affected patients is 70 years, and men are more often affected than women (male-to-female ratio is 1.6). This entity is distinct from chronic lymphoid leukemia (CLL) and does not develop as a consequence of that disease.

Clinical presentation is generally from symptoms of splenomegaly or incidental detection of an elevated white blood cell (WBC) count. The clinical course can be rapid. The cells express surface IgM (with or without IgD) and typical B-cell markers (CD19, CD20, CD22). CD23 is absent, and about one-third of cases express CD5. The CD5 expression along with the presence of the t(11;14) translocation in 20% of cases leads to confusion in distinguishing B-PLL from the leukemic form of mantle cell lymphoma. No reliable criteria for the distinction have emerged, and gene expression studies suggest a close relationship between mantle cell lymphoma and B-PLL and significant differences with CLL. About half of patients have mutation or loss of p53, and deletions have been noted in 11q23 and 13q14. Nucleoside analogues like fludarabine and cladribine and combination chemotherapy (cyclophosphamide, doxorubicin, vincristine, and prednisone [CHOP]) have produced responses. CHOP plus rituximab may be more effective than CHOP alone, but the disease is sufficiently rare that large series have not been reported. Splenectomy can produce palliation of symptoms but appears to have little or no impact on the course of the disease. BM transplantation may be curative. Imatinib may also have activity.

Splenic Marginal Zone Lymphoma (SMZL) This tumor of mainly small lymphocytes originates in the marginal zone of the spleen white pulp, grows to efface the germinal centers and mantle, and invades the red pulp. Splenic hilar nodes, BM, and peripheral blood (PB) may be involved. The circulating tumor cells have short surface villi and are called villous lymphocytes. **Table 110-2** shows differences in tumor cells of a number of neoplasms of small lymphocytes that aid in the differential diagnosis. SMZL cells express surface immunoglobulin and CD20 but are negative for CD5, CD10, CD43, and CD103. Lack of CD5 distinguishes SMZL from CLL, and lack of CD103 separates SMZL from hairy cell leukemia.

The median age of patients with SMZL is mid-fifties, and men and women are equally represented. Patients present with incidental or symptomatic splenomegaly or incidental detection of lymphocytosis in the PB with villous lymphocytes. Autoimmune anemia or thrombocytopenia may be present. The immunoglobulin produced by these cells contains somatic mutations that reflect transit through a germinal center, and ongoing mutations suggest that the mutation machinery has remained active. About 40% of patients have either deletions or translocations involving 7q21, the site of the *FLNC* gene (filamin Cγ, involved in cross-linking actin filaments in the cytoplasm). *NOTCH2* mutations are seen in 25% of patients. Chromosome 8p deletions may also be noted. The genetic lesions typically found in extranodal marginal zone lymphomas (e.g., trisomy 3 and t[11;18]) are uncommon in SMZL.

The clinical course of disease is generally indolent with median survivals exceeding 10 years. Patients with elevated lactate dehydrogenase (LDH) levels, anemia, and hypoalbuminemia generally have a poorer prognosis. Long remissions can be seen after splenectomy. Rituximab, ibrutinib, and PI3 kinase inhibitors are also active. A small fraction of patients undergo histologic progression to diffuse large B-cell lymphoma with a concomitant change to a more aggressive natural history. Experience with combination chemotherapy in SMZL is limited.

TABLE 110-2 Immunophenotype of Tumors of Small Lymphocytes

	CD5	CD20	CD43	CD10	CD103	sIG	CYCLIN D1
Follicular lymphoma	neg	pos	pos	pos	neg	pos	neg
Chronic lymphoid leukemia	pos	pos	pos	neg	neg	pos	neg
B-cell prolymphocytic leukemia	pos	pos	pos	neg	neg	pos	pos
Mantle cell lymphoma	pos	pos	pos	neg	neg	pos	pos
Splenic marginal zone lymphoma	neg	pos	neg	neg	neg	pos	neg
Hairy cell leukemia	neg	pos	?	neg	pos	pos	neg

Abbreviations: neg, negative; pos, positive.

TABLE 110-3 Differential Diagnosis of "Dry Tap"—Inability to Aspirate Bone Marrow

Dry taps occur in about 4% of attempts and are associated with:	
Metastatic carcinoma infiltration	17%
Chronic myeloid leukemia	15%
Myelofibrosis	14%
Hairy cell leukemia	10%
Acute leukemia	10%
Lymphomas, Hodgkin's disease	9%
Normal marrow	Rare

Hairy Cell Leukemia Hairy cell leukemia is a tumor of small lymphocytes with oval nuclei, abundant cytoplasm, and distinctive membrane projections (hairy cells). Patients have splenomegaly and diffuse BM involvement. While some circulating cells are noted, the clinical picture is dominated by symptoms from the enlarged spleen and pancytopenia. The mechanism of the pancytopenia is not completely clear and may be mediated by both inhibitory cytokines and marrow replacement. The marrow has an increased level of reticulin fibers; indeed, hairy cell leukemia is a common cause of inability to aspirate BM or so-called "dry tap" (**Table 110-3**). Monocytopenia is profound and may explain a predisposition to atypical mycobacterial infection that is observed clinically. The tumor cells have strong expression of CD22, CD25, and CD103; soluble CD25 level in serum is an excellent tumor marker for disease activity. The cells also express tartrate-resistant acid phosphatase. The immunoglobulin genes are rearranged and mutated, indicating the influence of a germinal center. No specific cytogenetic abnormality has been found, but most cases contain the activating *BRAF* mutation V600E.

The median age of affected patients is mid-fifties, and the male-to-female ratio is 5:1. Treatment options are numerous. Splenectomy is often associated with prolonged remission. Nucleosides including cladribine and deoxycoformycin are highly active but are also associated with further immunosuppression and can increase the risk of certain opportunistic infections. However, after brief courses of these agents, patients usually obtain very durable remissions during which immune function spontaneously recovers. Interferon α is also an effective therapy but is not as effective as nucleosides. Chemotherapy-refractory patients have responded to vemurafenib, a BRAF inhibitor. Vemurafenib does not appear to be curative, but responses can be maintained with chronic treatment. More durable remissions occur when rituximab is added to vemurafenib.

Nodal Marginal Zone B Cell Lymphoma This rare node-based disease bears an uncertain relationship with extranodal marginal zone lymphomas, which are often mucosa-associated and are called mucosa-associated lymphoid tissue (MALT) lymphomas, and SMZLs. Patients may have localized or generalized adenopathy. The neoplastic cell is a marginal zone B cell with monocytoid features and has been called monocytoid B cell lymphoma in the past. Up to one-third of the patients may have extranodal involvement, and involvement of the lymph nodes can be secondary to the spread of a mucosal primary lesion. In authentic nodal primaries, the cytogenetic abnormalities associated with MALT lymphomas (trisomy 3 and t[11;18]) are very rare. The clinical course is indolent. Patients often respond to combination chemotherapy, although remissions have not been durable. Few patients have received CHOP plus rituximab, which is likely to be an effective approach to management.

Mediastinal (Thymic) Large B-Cell Lymphoma This entity was originally considered a subset of diffuse large B-cell lymphoma; however, additional study has identified it as a distinct entity with its own characteristic clinical, genetic, and immunophenotypic features. This is a disease that can be bulky in size but usually remains confined to the mediastinum. It can be locally aggressive, including progressing to produce a superior vena cava obstruction syndrome or pericardial effusion. About one-third of patients develop pleural effusions, and in 5–10% of cases, disease can disseminate widely to kidney, adrenal, liver, skin, and even brain. The disease affects women more often than men (male-to-female ratio is 1:2–3), and the median age is 35–40 years.

The tumor is composed of sheets of large cells with abundant cytoplasm accompanied by variable, but often abundant, fibrosis. It is distinguished from nodular sclerosing Hodgkin's disease by the paucity of normal lymphoid cells and the absence of lacunar variants of Reed-Sternberg cells. However, more than one-third of the genes that are expressed to a greater extent in primary mediastinal large B-cell lymphoma than in usual diffuse large B-cell lymphoma are also overexpressed in Hodgkin's disease, suggesting a possible pathogenetic relationship between the two entities that affect the same anatomic site. Tumor cells may overexpress *MAL*. The genome of tumor cells is characterized by frequent chromosomal gains and losses. The tumor cells in mediastinal large B-cell lymphoma express CD20, but surface immunoglobulin and human leukocyte antigen (HLA) class I and class II molecules may be absent or incompletely expressed. Expression of lower levels of class II HLA identifies a subset with poorer prognosis. The cells are CD5 and CD10 negative but may show light staining with anti-CD30. The cells are CD45 positive, unlike cells of classical Hodgkin's disease.

Methotrexate, leucovorin, doxorubicin, cyclophosphamide, vincristine, prednisone, and bleomycin (MACOP-B) and rituximab plus CHOP are effective treatments, achieving 5-year survival of 75–87%. Dose-adjusted therapy with prednisone, etoposide, vincristine, cyclophosphamide, and doxorubicin (EPOCH) plus rituximab has produced 5-year survival of 97%. A role for mediastinal radiation therapy has not been definitively demonstrated, but it is frequently used, especially in patients whose mediastinal area remains positron emission tomography–avid after 4–6 cycles of chemotherapy.

Intravascular Large B-Cell Lymphoma This is an extremely rare form of diffuse large B-cell lymphoma characterized by the presence of lymphoma in the lumen of small vessels, particularly capillaries. It is also known as malignant angioendotheliomatosis or angiotropic large-cell lymphoma. It is sufficiently rare that no consistent picture has emerged to define a clinical syndrome or its epidemiologic and genetic features. It is thought to remain inside vessels because of a defect in adhesion molecules and homing mechanisms, an idea supported by scant data suggesting absence of expression of β-1 integrin and ICAM-1. Patients commonly present with symptoms of small-vessel occlusion, skin lesions, or neurologic symptoms. The tumor cell clusters can promote thrombus formation. A subset of patients have tumors with *MYD88* or *CD79B* mutations. In general, the clinical course is aggressive and the disease is poorly responsive to therapy. Often a diagnosis is not made until very late in the course of the disease or at autopsy.

Primary Effusion Lymphoma This entity is another variant of diffuse large B-cell lymphoma that presents with pleural effusions, usually without apparent tumor mass lesions. It is most common in the setting of immune deficiency disease, especially AIDS, and is caused by human herpes virus 8 (HHV-8)/Kaposi's sarcoma herpes virus (KSHV). It is also known as *body cavity–based lymphoma*. Some patients have been previously diagnosed with Kaposi's sarcoma. It can also occur in the absence of immunodeficiency in elderly men of Mediterranean heritage, similar to Kaposi's sarcoma but even less common.

The malignant effusions contain cells positive for HHV-8/KSHV, and many are also co-infected with Epstein-Barr virus. The cells are large with large nuclei and prominent nucleoli that can be confused with Reed-Sternberg cells. The cells express CD20 and CD79a (immunoglobulin-signaling molecule), although they often do not express immunoglobulin. Some cases aberrantly express T-cell markers such as CD3 or rearranged T-cell receptor genes. No characteristic genetic lesions have been reported, but gains in chromosome 12 and X material have been seen, similar to other HIV-associated lymphomas. The clinical course is generally characterized by rapid progression and death within 6 months. CHOP plus lenalidomide or bortezomib may produce responses. Highly active antiretroviral therapy for HIV should be maintained during treatment.

Lymphomatoid Granulomatosis This is an angiocentric, angiodestructive lymphoproliferative disease comprised by neoplastic Epstein-Barr virus–infected monoclonal B cells accompanied and outnumbered by a polyclonal reactive T-cell infiltrate. The disease is graded based on histologic features such as cell number and atypia in the B cells. It is most often confused with extranodal NK/T-cell lymphoma, nasal type, which can also be angiodestructive and is Epstein-Barr virus–related. The disease usually presents in adults (males > females) as a pulmonary infiltrate. Involvement is often entirely extranodal and can include kidney (32%), liver (29%), skin (25%), and brain (25%). The disease often but not always occurs in the setting of immune deficiency.

The disease can be remitting and relapsing in nature or can be rapidly progressive. The course is usually predicted by the histologic grade. The disease is highly responsive to combination chemotherapy and is curable in most cases. Some investigators have claimed that low-grade disease (grade I and II) can be treated with interferon α.

■ MATURE T-CELL AND NK CELL NEOPLASMS

T-Cell Prolymphocytic Leukemia This is an aggressive leukemia of medium-sized prolymphocytes involving the blood, marrow, nodes, liver, spleen, and skin. It accounts for 1–2% of all small lymphocytic leukemias. Most patients present with elevated WBC count (often >100,000/μL), hepatosplenomegaly, and adenopathy. Skin involvement occurs in 20%. The diagnosis is made from PB smear, which shows cells about 25% larger than those in small lymphocytes, with cytoplasmic blebs and nuclei that may be indented. The cells express T-cell markers like CD2, CD3, and CD7; two-thirds of patients have cells that are CD4+ and CD8–, and 25% have cells that are CD4+ and CD8+. T-cell receptor β chains are clonally rearranged. In 80% of patients, inversion of chromosome 14 occurs between q11 and q32. Ten percent have t(14;14) translocations that bring the T-cell receptor alpha/beta gene locus into juxtaposition with oncogenes *TCL1* and *TCL1b* at 14q32.1. Chromosome 8 abnormalities are also common. Deletions in the *ATM* gene are also noted. Activating *JAK3* mutations have also been reported.

The course of the disease is generally rapid, with median survival of about 12 months. Responses have been seen with the anti-CD52 antibody alemtuzumab, nucleoside analogues, and CHOP chemotherapy. Histone deacetylase inhibitors like vorinostat and romidepsin may also have activity. Small numbers of patients with T-cell prolymphocytic leukemia have also been treated with high-dose therapy, and allogeneic BM transplantation after remission has been achieved with alemtuzumab or conventional-dose therapy.

T-Cell Large Granular Lymphocytic Leukemia T-cell large granular lymphocytic (LGL) leukemia is characterized by increases in the number of LGLs in the PB (2000–20,000/μL) often accompanied by severe neutropenia, with or without concomitant anemia. Patients may have splenomegaly and frequently have evidence of systemic autoimmune disease, including rheumatoid arthritis, hypergammaglobulinemia, autoantibodies, and circulating immune complexes. BM involvement is mainly interstitial in pattern, with <50% lymphocytes on differential count. Usually the cells express CD3, T-cell receptors, and CD8; NK-like variants may be CD3–. The leukemic cells often express Fas and Fas ligand.

The course of the disease is generally indolent and dominated by the neutropenia. Paradoxically, immunosuppressive therapy with cyclosporine, methotrexate, or cyclophosphamide plus glucocorticoids can produce an increase in granulocyte counts. Nucleosides have been used anecdotally. Occasionally the disease can accelerate to a more aggressive clinical course.

Aggressive NK Cell Leukemia NK neoplasms are very rare, and they may follow a range of clinical courses from very indolent to highly aggressive. They are more common in Asians than whites, and the cells frequently harbor a clonal Epstein-Barr virus episome. The PB white count is usually not greatly elevated, but abnormal large lymphoid cells with granular cytoplasm are noted. The aggressive form is characterized by symptoms of fever and laboratory abnormalities of pancytopenia. Hepatosplenomegaly is common; node involvement is less common. Patients may have hemophagocytosis, coagulopathy, or multiorgan failure. Serum levels of Fas ligand are elevated.

The cells express CD2 and CD56 and do not have rearranged T-cell receptor genes. Deletions involving chromosome 6 are common. The disease can be rapidly progressive. Some forms of NK neoplasms are more indolent. They tend to be discovered incidentally with LGL lymphocytosis and do not manifest the fever and hepatosplenomegaly characteristic of the aggressive leukemia. The cells are also CD2 and CD56 positive, but they do not contain clonal forms of Epstein-Barr virus and are not accompanied by pancytopenia or autoimmune disease.

Extranodal NK/T-Cell Lymphoma, Nasal Type Like lymphomatoid granulomatosis, extranodal NK/T-cell lymphoma tends to be an angiocentric and angiodestructive lesion, but the malignant cells are not B cells. In most cases, they are CD56+ Epstein-Barr virus–infected cells; occasionally, they are CD56–Epstein-Barr virus–infected cytotoxic T cells. They are most commonly found in the nasal cavity. Historically, this illness was called lethal midline granuloma, polymorphic reticulosis, and angiocentric immunoproliferative lesion. This form of lymphoma is prevalent in Asia, Mexico, and Central and South America; it affects males more commonly than females. When it spreads beyond the nasal cavity, it may affect soft tissue, the gastrointestinal tract, or the testis. In some cases, hemophagocytic syndrome (HPS) may influence the clinical picture. Patients may have B symptoms. Many of the systemic manifestations of disease are related to the production of cytokines by the tumor cells and the cells responding to their signals. Deletions and inversions of chromosome 6 are common.

Many patients with extranodal NK/T-cell lymphoma, nasal type, have excellent antitumor responses with combination chemotherapy regimens, particularly those with localized disease. Radiation therapy is often used after completion of chemotherapy. Four risk factors have been defined, including B symptoms, advanced stage, elevated LDH, and regional lymph node involvement. Patient survival is linked to the number of risk factors: 5-year survival is 81% for zero risk factors, 64% for one risk factor, 32% for two risk factors, and 7% for three or four risk factors. Combination regimens without anthracyclines have been touted as superior to CHOP, but data are sparse. High-dose therapy with stem cell transplantation has been used, but its role is unclear.

Enteropathy-Type T-Cell Lymphoma Enteropathy-type T-cell lymphoma is a rare complication of longstanding celiac disease. It most commonly occurs in the jejunum or the ileum. In adults, the lymphoma may be diagnosed at the same time as celiac disease, but the suspicion is that the celiac disease was a longstanding precursor to the development of lymphoma. The tumor usually presents as multiple ulcerating mucosal masses, but may also produce a dominant exophytic mass or multiple ulcerations. The tumor expresses CD3 and CD7 nearly always and may or may not express CD8. The normal-appearing lymphocytes in the adjacent mucosa often have a similar phenotype to the tumor. Most patients have the HLA genotype associated with celiac disease, HLA DQA1*0501 or DQB1*0201.

The prognosis of this form of lymphoma is typically poor (median survival is 7 months), but some patients have a good response to CHOP chemotherapy. Patients who respond can develop bowel perforation from responding tumor. If the tumor responds to treatment, recurrence may develop elsewhere in the celiac disease–affected small bowel.

Hepatosplenic T-Cell Lymphoma Hepatosplenic T-cell lymphoma is a malignancy derived from T cells expressing the gamma/delta T-cell antigen receptor that affects mainly the liver and fills the sinusoids with medium-size lymphoid cells. When the spleen is involved, dominantly the red pulp is infiltrated. It is a disease of young people, especially young people with an underlying immunodeficiency or with an autoimmune disease that demands immunosuppressive therapy. The use of thiopurine and infliximab is particularly common in the history of patients with this disease. The cells are CD3+ and usually CD4– and CD8–. The cells may contain isochromosome 7q, often together with trisomy 8. The lymphoma has an aggressive natural history. Combination chemotherapy may induce remissions, but most patients relapse. Median survival is about 2 years. The tumor does not appear to respond to reversal of immunosuppressive therapy.

Subcutaneous Panniculitis-Like T-Cell Lymphoma Subcutaneous panniculitis-like T-cell lymphoma involves multiple subcutaneous collections of neoplastic T cells that are usually cytotoxic cells in phenotype (i.e., contain perforin and granzyme B and express CD3 and CD8). The rearranged T-cell receptor is usually alpha/beta-derived, but occasionally, the gamma/delta receptors are involved, particularly in the setting of immunosuppression. The cells are negative for Epstein-Barr virus. Patients may have an HPS in addition to the skin infiltration; fever and hepatosplenomegaly may also be present. Nodes are generally not involved. Patients frequently respond to combination chemotherapy, including CHOP. When the disease is progressive, the HPS can be a component of a fulminant downhill course. Effective therapy can reverse the HPS.

Blastic NK Cell Lymphoma The neoplastic cells express NK cell markers, especially CD56, and are CD3 negative. They are large blastic-appearing cells and may produce a leukemia picture, but the dominant site of involvement is the skin. Morphologically, the cells are similar to the neoplastic cells in acute lymphoid and myeloid leukemia. No characteristic chromosomal abnormalities have been described. The clinical course is rapid, and the disease is largely unresponsive to typical lymphoma treatments.

Primary Cutaneous CD30+ T-Cell Lymphoma This tumor involves the skin and is composed of cells that appear similar to the cells of anaplastic T-cell lymphoma. Among cutaneous T-cell tumors, ~25% are CD30+ anaplastic lymphomas. If dissemination to lymph nodes occurs, it is difficult to distinguish between the cutaneous and systemic forms of the disease. The tumor cells are often CD4+, and the cells contain granules that are positive for granzyme B and perforin in 70% of cases. The typical t(2;5) of anaplastic T-cell lymphoma is absent; indeed, its presence should prompt a closer look for systemic involvement and a switch to a diagnosis of anaplastic T-cell lymphoma. This form of lymphoma has sporadically been noted as a rare complication of silicone or saline breast implants. The natural history of breast implant–associated lymphoma is generally indolent. Cutaneous CD30+ T-cell lymphoma often responds to therapy. The anti-CD30 immunotoxin conjugate brentuximab vedotin is active. Radiation therapy can be effective, and surgery can also produce long-term disease control. Five-year survival exceeds 90%.

Angioimmunoblastic T-Cell Lymphoma Angioimmunoblastic T-cell lymphoma is a systemic disease that accounts for ~15% of all T-cell lymphomas. Patients frequently have fever, advanced stage, diffuse adenopathy, hepatosplenomegaly, skin rash, polyclonal hypergammaglobulinemia, and a wide range of autoantibodies including cold agglutinins, rheumatoid factor, and circulating immune complexes. Patients may have edema, arthritis, pleural effusions, and ascites. The nodes contain a polymorphous infiltrate of neoplastic T cells and nonneoplastic inflammatory cells together with proliferation of high endothelial venules and follicular dendritic cells (FDCs). The most common chromosomal abnormalities are trisomy 3, trisomy 5, and an extra X chromosome. Aggressive combination chemotherapy can induce regressions. The underlying immune defects make conventional lymphoma treatments more likely to produce infectious complications.

RARE MYELOID MALIGNANCIES

The World Health Organization (WHO) system uses PB counts and smear analysis, BM morphology, and cytogenetic and molecular genetic tests in order to classify myeloid malignancies into several major categories (**Table 110-4**). Among them, acute myeloid leukemia (AML) is discussed in **Chap. 104**, myelodysplastic syndromes (MDS) in **Chap. 102**, chronic myeloid leukemia (CML) in **Chap. 105**, and *JAK2* mutation–enriched myeloproliferative neoplasms (MPNs) in **Chap. 103**. In this chapter, we focus on the rest (listed in Table 110-4) including chronic neutrophilic leukemia (CNL); atypical CML, *BCR-ABL1* negative (aCML); chronic myelomonocytic leukemia (CMML); juvenile myelomonocytic leukemia (JMML); chronic eosinophilic leukemia, not otherwise specified (CEL-NOS); mastocytosis; MPN, unclassifiable (MPN-U); MDS/MPN, unclassifiable (MDS/MPN-U); MDS/MPN with ring sideroblasts and thrombocytosis (MDS/MPN-RS-T); and myeloid/lymphoid neoplasms with eosinophilia and rearrangements of *PDGFRA*, *PDGFRB*, or *FGFR1* or with *PCM1-JAK2*. This chapter also includes histiocytic and dendritic cell neoplasms, transient myeloproliferative disorders, and a broader discussion on primary eosinophilic disorders including hypereosinophilic syndrome (HES).

■ CHRONIC NEUTROPHILIC LEUKEMIA

CNL is a clonal proliferation of mature neutrophils with few or no circulating immature granulocytes. In 2013, CNL was described to be associated with activating mutations of the gene (*CSF3R*) encoding for the receptor for granulocyte colony-stimulating factor (G-CSF), also known as colony-stimulating factor 3 (CSF3). Patients with CNL might be asymptomatic at presentation but also display constitutional symptoms, splenomegaly, anemia, and thrombocytopenia. Median survival is approximately 2 years and causes of death include leukemic transformation, progressive disease associated with severe cytopenias and marked treatment-refractory leukocytosis. The true incidence of CNL is not known due to diagnostic uncertainty with >200 currently reported cases. Median age at diagnosis is approximately 67 years with a slight male preponderance in gender distribution.

TABLE 110-4 World Health Organization Classification of Myeloid Malignancies

1. Acute myeloid leukemia (AML) and related precursor neoplasms
2. Myeloproliferative neoplasms (MPN)
2.1. Chronic myeloid leukemia (CML), *BCR-ABL1* positive
2.2. *JAK2* mutation–enriched MPN
2.2.1. Polycythemia vera
2.2.2. Primary myelofibrosis
2.2.3. Essential thrombocythemia
2.3. Chronic neutrophilic leukemia (CNL)
2.4. Chronic eosinophilic leukemia, not otherwise specified (CEL-NOS)
2.5. Myeloproliferative neoplasm, unclassifiable (MPN-U)
3. Myelodysplastic syndromes (MDS)
3.1. MDS with single lineage dysplasia
3.2. MDS with ring sideroblasts (MDS-RS)
3.3. MDS with multilineage dysplasia
3.4. MDS with excess blasts
3.5. MDS with isolated del(5q)
3.6. MDS, unclassifiable (MDS-U)
3.7. *Provisional entity: Refractory cytopenia of childhood*
4. MDS/MPN overlap
4.1. Chronic myelomonocytic leukemia (CMML)
4.2. Atypical chronic myeloid leukemia (aCML), *BCR-ABL1* negative
4.3. Juvenile myelomonocytic leukemia (JMML)
4.4. MDS/MPN with ring sideroblasts and thrombocytosis (MDS/MPN-RS-T)
4.5. MDS/MPN, unclassifiable (MDS/MPN-U)
5. Mastocytosis
6. Myeloid/lymphoid neoplasms with eosinophilia and rearrangement of *PDGFRA, PDGFRB,* or *FGFR1* or with *PCM1-JAK2*
6.1. Myeloid/lymphoid neoplasms with *PDGFRA* rearrangement
6.2. Myeloid/lymphoid neoplasms with *PDGFRB* rearrangement
6.3. Myeloid/lymphoid neoplasms with *FGFR1* rearrangement
6.4. *Provisional entity: Myeloid/lymphoid neoplasms with PCM1-JAK2 translocation*
7. Myeloid neoplasms with germline predisposition

Pathogenesis CSF3 is the main growth factor for granulocyte proliferation and differentiation. Accordingly, recombinant CSF3 is used for the treatment of severe neutropenia, including severe congenital neutropenia (SCN). Some patients with SCN acquire *CSF3R* mutations, and the frequency of such mutations is significantly higher (~80%) in patients who experience leukemic transformation. SCN-associated *CSF3R* mutations occur in the region of the gene coding for the cytoplasmic domain of CSF3R and result in truncation of the C-terminal-negative regulatory domain. In 2013, Maxson et al described a different class of *CSF3R* mutations in ~ 90% of patients with CNL; these were mostly membrane proximal, the most frequent being a C-to-T substitution at nucleotide 1853 (T618I). In a subsequent confirmatory study, *CSF3R* mutations were found to be specific to WHO-defined CNL. About 40% of the T618I-mutated cases also harbored *SETBP1* mutations. *CSF3R* T618I has been shown to induce lethal myeloproliferative disorder in a mouse model and in vitro sensitivity to JAK inhibition.

Diagnosis Diagnosis of CNL requires exclusion of the more common causes of neutrophilia including infections and inflammatory processes. In addition, one should be mindful of the association between some forms of metastatic cancer or plasma cell neoplasms with secondary neutrophilia. Neoplastic neutrophilia also occurs in other *BCR-ABL1*-negative myeloid malignancies including aCML and CMML. Accordingly, the WHO diagnostic criteria for CNL are designed to exclude the possibilities of both secondary/reactive neutrophilia and leukocytosis associated with myeloid malignancies other than CNL (**Table 110-5**): leukocytosis ($\geq 25 \times 10^9$/L), ≥80% segmented/band neutrophils, <10% immature myeloid cells, <1% circulating blasts, and absence of dysgranulopoiesis or monocytosis (monocyte count $<1 \times 10^9$/L). BM in CNL is hypercellular and displays increased number and percentage of neutrophils with a very high myeloid-to-erythroid ratio and minimal left shift, myeloid dysplasia, or reticulin fibrosis.

The recent discovery of *CSF3R* mutations (see above) and their almost invariable association with WHO-defined CNL has allowed its incorporation in the WHO diagnostic criteria (Table 110-5). In practical terms, the presence of a membrane proximal *CSF3R* mutation in a patient with predominantly neutrophilic granulocytosis should be sufficient for the diagnosis of CNL, regardless of the degree of leukocytosis. Unfortunately, several exclusionary criteria still need to be met for diagnosing CNL in the absence of *CSF3R* mutations (Table 110-5).

Treatment Current treatment in CNL is largely palliative and suboptimal in its efficacy. Several drugs alone or in combination have been tried, and none have shown remarkable efficacy. As such, allogeneic hematopoietic stem cell transplant (AHSCT) is reasonable to consider in the presence of symptomatic disease, especially in younger patients. Otherwise, cytoreductive therapy with hydroxyurea is probably as good as anything, and a more intensive combination chemotherapy may not have additional value. However, response to hydroxyurea therapy is often transient, and some have successfully used interferon α as an alternative drug. Response to treatment with ruxolitinib (a JAK1 and JAK2 inhibitor) has been reported in several case reports, but as is the case with hydroxyurea treatment, the response was often incomplete and temporary. In a recently reported phase 2 study of ruxolitinib in 44 patients with CNL or aCML, 21 patients had CNL (76% harbored *CSF3R* mutations), of whom only 4 (20%) experienced complete or partial response according to conventional response criteria.

TABLE 110-5 2016 World Health Organization (WHO) Diagnostic Criteria for Chronic Neutrophilic Leukemia (CNL), Atypical Chronic Myeloid Leukemia, *BCR-ABL1*-Negative (aCML), and Chronic Myelomonocytic Leukemia (CMML)

VARIABLES	CNL	aCML	CMML
PB leukocyte count	≥25 × 10^9/L	Granulocytosis	
PB segmented neutrophils/bands	≥80%		
PB immature granulocytes[a]	<10%	≥10%	
PB blast count	<1%	<20%	<20%
PB monocyte count	<1 × 10^9/L	No or minimal monocytosis	≥1 × 10^9/L Persistent and lasting for at least 3 months
Dysgranulopoiesis	No	Yes	
PB basophil percentage		<2%	
PB monocyte percentage		<10%	≥10%
BM	Hypercellular ↑Neutrophils, number and % <5% blasts Normal neutrophilic maturation	Hypercellular ↑Granulocyte proliferation Granulocytic dysplasia ± erythroid/ megakaryocyte Dysplasia <20% blasts	Dysplasia in ≥1 myeloid lineages or Clonal cytogenetic/molecular abnormality <20% blasts or promonocytes
BCR-ABL1	No	No	No
PDGFRA, PDGFRB, FGFR1, or *PCM1-JAK2* rearrangement	No	No	No
CSF3R T618I or other activating *CSF3R* mutation or persistent neutrophilia, splenomegaly, and no identifiable cause of reactive neutrophilia	Yes		
PB and BM blasts/promonocytes		<20%	<20%
Evidence for other MPN: CML, PV, ET, or PMF	No	No	No
Evidence for reactive leukocytosis[b] or monocytosis	No		No

[a]Immature granulocytes include myeloblasts, promyelocytes, myelocytes, and metamyelocytes. [b]Causes of reactive neutrophilia include plasma cell neoplasms, solid tumor, infections, and inflammatory processes.

Abbreviations: BM, bone marrow; CML, chronic myeloid leukemia; ET, essential thrombocythemia; MPN, myeloproliferative neoplasms; PB, peripheral blood; PMF, primary myelofibrosis; PV, polycythemia vera.

■ ATYPICAL CHRONIC MYELOID LEUKEMIA

"Atypical chronic myeloid leukemia, *BCR-ABL1* negative (aCML)" is formally classified under the MDS/MPN category of myeloid malignancies and is characterized by left-shifted granulocytosis and dysgranulopoiesis. The differential diagnosis of aCML includes CML, which is distinguished by the presence of *BCR-ABL1*; CNL, which is distinguished by the absence of dysgranulopoiesis and presence of *CSF3R* mutations; and CMML, which is distinguished by the presence of monocytosis (absolute monocyte count ≥1 × 10^9/L). The WHO diagnostic criteria for aCML are listed in Table 110-5 and include granulocytosis; dysgranulopoiesis; ≥10% immature granulocytes; <20% PB or BM myeloblasts; <10% PB monocytes; <2% basophils; absence of otherwise specific mutations such as *BCR-ABL1, PDGFRA, PDGFRB, FGFR1*, or *PCM1-JAK2*; and not meeting WHO criteria for CML, primary myelofibrosis (PMF), polycythemia vera (PV), or essential thrombocytopenia (ET). The BM in aCML is hypercellular with granulocyte proliferation and dysplasia with or without erythroid or megakaryocytic dysplasia.

The molecular pathogenesis of aCML is incompletely understood; about a fourth of patients express *SETBP1* mutations, which are, however, also found in several other myeloid malignancies, including CNL and CMML. *SETBP1* mutations in aCML are prognostically detrimental and mostly located between codons 858 and 871; similar mutations are seen with Schinzel-Giedion syndrome (a congenital disease with severe developmental delay and various physical stigmata including midface retraction, large forehead, and macroglossia). More recently, a somatic missense mutation in ethanolamine kinase 1 (*ETNK1* N244S) was described in 9% of patients with aCML but was also seen in 14% of patients with CMML, 6% of patients with mastocytosis (especially in association with eosinophilia), and rarely in other MPNs.

In a series of 55 patients with WHO-defined aCML, median age at diagnosis was 62 years with female preponderance (57%); splenomegaly was reported in 54% of the patients, red cell transfusion requirement in 65%, abnormal karyotype in 20% (20q− and trisomy 8 being the most frequent), and leukemic transformation in 40%. Median survival was 25 months. Outcome was worse in patients with marked leukocytosis, transfusion requirement, and increased immature cells in the PB. In a more recent Mayo Clinic study of 25 molecularly annotated and strictly WHO-defined aCML patients, median age was 70 years and 84% were male. Cytogenetic abnormalities were seen in 36% and gene mutations in 100%. Mutational frequencies were as follows: *ASXL1* 28%, *TET2* 16%, *NRAS* 16%, *SETBP1* 12%, *RUNX1* 12%, *ETNK1* 8%, and *PTPN11* 4%. Median survival was 10.8 months, and at last follow-up (median 11 months), 17 deaths (68%) and 2 leukemic transformations (8%) were documented. In multivariable analysis, advanced age, low hemoglobin, and *TET2* mutations were shown to carry independent prognostic significance; other mutations, including *ASXL1* and *SETBP1*, lacked prognostic significance. Conventional chemotherapy is largely ineffective in the treatment of aCML. Similarly, treatment response to the JAK1/2 inhibitor ruxolitinib has not been impressive. However, a favorable experience with autologous stem cell transplantation (ASCT) was reported in nine patients; after a median follow-up of 55 months, the majority of the patients remained in complete remission.

■ CHRONIC MYELOMONOCYTIC LEUKEMIA

CMML is classified under the WHO category of MDS/MPN and is defined by an absolute monocyte count (AMC) of ≥1 × 10^9/L in the PB and accounting for ≥10% of the leukocyte count. Median age at diagnosis ranges from 65 to 75 years, and there is a 2:1 male predominance.

Clinical presentation is variable and depends on whether the disease presents with MDS-like or MPN-like phenotype; the former is associated with cytopenias and the latter with splenomegaly and features of myeloproliferation such as fatigue, night sweats, weight loss, and cachexia. About 20% of patients with CMML experience serositis involving the joints (arthritis), pericardium (pericarditis and pericardial effusion), pleura (pleural effusion), or peritoneum (ascites).

Pathogenesis Almost all patients with CMML harbor somatic mutations involving epigenetic regulator genes (e.g., *ASXL1*, *TET2*), spliceosome pathway genes (e.g., *SRSF2*), DNA damage response genes (e.g., *TP53*), and tyrosine kinases/transcription factors (e.g., *KRAS*, *NRAS*, *CBL*, and *RUNX1*). However, none of these mutations are specific to CMML, and their precise pathogenetic contribution is unclear. Clonal cytogenetic abnormalities are seen in about a third of patients with CMML and include trisomy 8 and abnormalities of chromosome 7. More recent studies have demonstrated the presence of BM dendritic cell aggregates suggesting systemic immune dysregulation and distinct phenotypic features of monocytes in CMML.

Diagnosis Reactive monocytosis is uncommon but has been reported in association with certain infections and inflammatory conditions. Clonal (i.e., neoplastic) monocytosis defines CMML but is also seen with JMML and AML with monocytic differentiation. The WHO diagnostic criteria for CMML are listed in Table 110-5 and include persistent PB monocyte count of ≥1 × 10^9/L with monocyte percentage of ≥10%; absence of *BCR-ABL1*, *PDGFRA*, *PDGFRB*, *FGFR1*, or *PCM1-JAK2* rearrangements; not meeting WHO criteria for CML, PV, ET, or PMF; <20% blasts and promonocytes in the PB and BM; and dysplasia involving one or more myeloid lineages or, in the absence of dysplasia, presence of an acquired clonal cytogenetic or molecular genetic abnormality or nonreactive monocytosis lasting for at least 3 months.

The BM in CMML is hypercellular with granulocytic and monocytic proliferation. Dysplasia is often present and may involve one, two, or all myeloid lineages. On immunophenotyping, the abnormal cells often express myelomonocytic antigens such as CD13 and CD33, with variable expression of CD14, CD68, CD64, and CD163. Monocytic-derived cells are almost always positive for the cytochemical nonspecific esterases (e.g., butyrate esterase), while normal granulocytic precursors are positive for lysozyme and chloroacetate esterase. In CMML, it is common to have a hybrid cytochemical staining pattern with cells expressing both chloroacetate and butyrate esterases simultaneously (dual esterase staining). Monocytosis can be associated with reactive as well as other myeloid neoplasms. Based on flow cytometric expression of CD14/CD16, monocytes can be classified into classical MO1 (CD14+/CD16–), intermediate MO2 (CD14+/CD16+), and nonclassical MO3 (CD14–/CD16+) fractions, with MO1 constituting the major monocyte population (85%) in healthy conditions. Recent studies have suggested characteristic increase in classical monocytes in CMML patients, distinguishing them from other causes of reactive and clonal monocytosis.

Prognosis A recent meta-analysis showed median survival of 1.5 years in CMML. Numerous prognostic systems have attempted to better define and stratify the natural history of CMML. One of these, the Mayo prognostic model, assigns one point each to the following four independent prognostic variables: AMC >10 × 10^9/L, presence of circulating immature cells, hemoglobin <10 g/dL, and platelet count <100,000/mL. This model stratified patients into three risk groups: low (0 points), intermediate (1 point), and high (≥2 points), translating to median survival of 32, 18, and 10 months, respectively. Another prognostic model referred to as the CMML-specific prognostic scoring system (CPSS) identified four variables as being prognostic for both overall survival and leukemia-free survival: French-American-British (FAB) and WHO CMML subtypes, red blood cell transfusion dependency, and the Spanish cytogenetic risk stratification system. A French study incorporated *ASXL1* mutational status in 312 CMML patients; in a multivariable model, independent predictors of poor survival were WBC >15 × 10^9/L (3 points), *ASXL1* mutations (2 points), age >65 years (2 points), platelet count <100,000/mL (2 points), and hemoglobin <10 g/dL in females and <11 g/dL in males (2 points). This model stratified patients into three groups: low (0–4 points), intermediate (5–7 points), and high risk (8–12 points), with median survivals of not reached and 38.5 and 14.4 months, respectively. More recent studies have highlighted the adverse prognostic effect of *ASXL1* and *DNMT3A* mutations in CMML. To further clarify the prognostic relevance of *ASXL1* mutations, an international collaborative cohort of 466 CMML patients was analyzed. In multivariable analysis, *ASXL1* mutations, AMC >10 × 10^9/L, hemoglobin <10 g/dL, platelets <100 × 10^9/L, and circulating immature myeloid cells were independently predictive of shortened overall survival. More recently, the aforementioned CPSS model was updated to include molecular abnormalities including *ASXL1*, *RUNX1*, *NRAS*, and *SETBP1* mutations (CPSS-Mol). In a report of 171 patients with blast phase CMML (median age 71 years), treatment included best supportive care in 25%, hypomethylating agent therapy in 10%, AML-like induction chemotherapy in 38%, AML-like induction chemotherapy followed by AHSCT in 15%, upfront AHSCT in 2%, and clinical trials in 11%. After a median follow-up of 4.4 months, 141 deaths (82%) were recorded. Median overall survival was 6 months with 1-, 3-, and 5-year survival rates of 25%, 9%, and 6%, respectively.

Treatment Current treatment in CMML consists of hydroxyurea and supportive care, including red cell transfusions and use of erythropoiesis-stimulating agents (ESAs). The value of hydroxyurea was reinforced by a randomized trial against oral etoposide. No other single or combination chemotherapy has been shown to be superior to hydroxyurea. AHSCT is a viable treatment option for transplant-eligible patients with poor prognostic features. Given the MDS/MPN overlap phenotype and the presence of MDS-like genetic/methylation abnormalities in CMML, hypomethylating agents such as 5-azacitidine and decitabine have been used with limited efficacy; in a recent study using decitabine in CMML, overall response rate was 48% with 17% complete remissions and median survival of 17 months. The experience with 5-azacytidine was somewhat similar. In a recent Mayo Clinic report, among 406 consecutive CMML patients (age ≤75 years at diagnosis) seen between January 1990 and December 2018, 70 (17%) underwent AHSCT (median age 58 years) including 46 (66%) in chronic phase and 24 (34%) in blast phase. At a median follow-up of 70 months, there were 22 deaths (31%) in the chronic phase transplant group, 11 (24%) from disease relapse and 9 (20%) from nonrelapse mortality. Posttransplant median survival was 67 months in the chronic phase and 16 months in the blast phase (p <.01) transplant groups; 5-year survival rates were 51% and 19%, respectively.

JUVENILE MYELOMONOCYTIC LEUKEMIA

JMML is primarily a disease of early childhood and is included, along with CMML, in the MDS/MPN WHO category. Both CMML and JMML feature leukocytosis, monocytosis, and hepatosplenomegaly. Additional characteristic features in JMML include thrombocytopenia and elevated fetal hemoglobin. Myeloid progenitors in JMML display granulocyte-macrophage colony-stimulating factor (GM-CSF) hypersensitivity that has been attributed to dysregulated RAS/MAPK signaling. The latter is believed to result from mutually exclusive mutations involving *RAS*, *PTPN11*, and *NF1*. A third of patients with JMML that is not associated with Noonan syndrome carry *PTPN11* mutations, whereas the incidence of *NF1* in patients without neurofibromatosis type 1 (NF1) and *RAS* mutations is ~15% each. In general, ~85% of JMML cases have one of the classical RAS pathway mutations (*PTPN11*, *NRAS*, *KRAS*, *NF1*, or *CBL*); in addition, a myriad of other mutations, such as *ASXL1*, *RUNX1*, *SETBP1*, *JAK3*, and *CUX1*, have recently been reported. Drug therapy is relatively ineffective in JMML, and the treatment of choice is AHSCT, which results in a 5-year survival of approximately 50%.

The 2016 revised WHO diagnostic criteria for JMML require the presence of PB monocyte count ≥1 × 10^9/L, <20% blasts in blood or BM, splenomegaly, and absence of *BCR-ABL1*. Diagnosis also requires the presence of one of the following: somatic mutation of *PTPN11*,

KRAS, or *NRAS*; clinical diagnosis of NF1 or *NF1* mutation; germline mutation of *CBL*; and loss of heterozygosity. Diagnosis of JMML can still be considered without the aforementioned genetic features in the presence of monosomy 7 or any other cytogenetic abnormality or in the presence of two of the following: increased hemoglobin F, presence of myeloid or erythroid precursors in the PB, GM-CSF hypersensitivity in colony assay, and hyperphosphorylation of STAT5.

MDS/MPN, UNCLASSIFIABLE (MDS/MPN-U)

The WHO classifies patients with morphologic and laboratory features that resemble both MDS and MPN as "MDS/MPN overlap." This category includes CMML, aCML, and JMML, which have been discussed above. In addition, MDS/MPN includes a fourth category referred to as MDS/MPN, unclassifiable (MDS/MPN-U). Diagnosis of MDS/MPN-U requires the presence of both MDS and MPN features that are not adequate to classify patients as CMML, aCML, or JMML. MDS/MPN also includes the provisional category of refractory anemia with ring sideroblasts and thrombocytosis (RARS-T); the 2016 revision of the WHO classification document has changed the term *RARS-T* to *MDS/MPN-RS-T*.

In a representative study of 85 patients with MDS/MPN-U, median age was 70 years and 72% were male. Splenomegaly at presentation was present in 33%, thrombocytosis in 13%, leukocytosis in 18%, *JAK2* mutations in 30%, and abnormal karyotype in 51%; the most frequent cytogenetic abnormality was trisomy 8. Median survival was 12.4 months and favorably affected by thrombocytosis. Treatment with hypomethylating agents, immunomodulators, or AHSCT did not appear to favorably affect survival.

MDS/MPN WITH RING SIDEROBLASTS AND THROMBOCYTOSIS (MDS/MPN-RS-T)

MDS/MPN-RS-T is classified in the MDS/MPN category because it shares dysplastic features with MDS-RS and myeloproliferative features with ET. The 2016 revised WHO diagnostic criteria for MDS/MPN-RS-T includes anemia associated with erythroid lineage dysplasia, presence of ≥15% ring sideroblasts, blast count of <5% in BM and <1% in the PB, platelet count of ≥450 × 10^9/L, and absence of *BCR-ABL1, PDGFRA, PDGFRB, FGFR1*, or *PCM1-JAK2* mutations or t(3;3)(q21;q26), inv(3)(q21q26), or del(5q). These new diagnostic criteria also require the absence of history of MPN, MDS, or other type of MDS/MPN and also either the presence of *SF3B1* mutation or absence of exposure to cytotoxic or other treatment that could be blamed for the morphologic abnormalities.

In a recent study, 111 patients with MDS/MPN-RS-T were compared with 33 patients with RARS. The frequency of *SF3B1* mutations in MDS/MPN-RS-T-T (87%) was similar to that in MDS-RS (85%). *JAK2* V617F mutation was detected in 49% of MDS/MPN-RS-T patients (including 48% of those mutated for *SF3B1*) but none of those with MDS-RS. In MDS/MPN-RS-T, *SF3B1* mutations were more frequent in females (95%) than in males (77%), and mean ring sideroblast counts were higher in *SF3B1*-mutated patients. Median overall survival was 6.9 years in *SF3B1* mutated cases versus 3.3 years in unmutated cases. Six-year survival was 67% in *JAK2* mutated cases versus 32% in unmutated cases. Multivariable analysis identified younger age and *JAK2* and *SF3B1* mutations as favorable factors. Predictors of poor survival in MDS/MPN-RS-T include anemia, abnormal karyotype, and presence of *ASXL1* or *SETBP1* mutations. Interestingly, the presence of *SF3B1* mutations in MDS/MPN-RS-T was recently shown to be associated with increased risk of thrombosis. Several case reports have suggested that treatment with lenalidomide might induce red cell transfusion independency and complete remissions in MDS/MPN-RS-T. Most recently, luspatercept, a recombinant fusion protein that binds transforming growth factor β superfamily ligands to reduce SMAD signaling, has also been shown to benefit some patients with MDS-RS-T; in a recently published phase 3 trial involving 229 patients with transfusion-dependent very-low- to intermediate-risk MDS-RS-T, transfusion independence for ≥8 weeks was achieved in 38% of the patients receiving luspatercept versus 13% of patients in the placebo group (p <.01).

MYELOPROLIFERATIVE NEOPLASM, UNCLASSIFIABLE (MPN-U)

The category of MPN-U includes MPN-like neoplasms that cannot be clearly classified as one of the other seven subcategories of MPN (Table 110-4). Examples include patients presenting with unusual thrombosis or unexplained organomegaly with normal blood counts but found to carry MPN-characteristic mutations such as *JAK2* and *CALR* or display BM morphology that is consistent with MPN. It is possible that some cases of MPN-U represent earlier disease stages in PV or ET, which however fail to meet the threshold hemoglobin levels or platelet counts that are required per WHO diagnostic criteria. Specific treatment interventions might not be necessary in asymptomatic patients with MPN-U, whereas patients with arterial thrombotic complications might require cytoreductive and aspirin therapy and those with venous thrombosis might require systemic anticoagulation.

MYELOID NEOPLASMS WITH GERMLINE PREDISPOSITION

The 2016 WHO revision on the classification of myeloid neoplasms added a section referred to as "myeloid neoplasms with germline predisposition" and that includes cases of AML, MDS, and MDS/MPN that arise in the setting of a germline predisposition mutation, such as *CEBPA, DDX41, RUNX1, ANKRD26, ETV6*, or *GATA2*. This particular category of diseases also includes myeloid neoplasms that arise in the background of BM failure syndromes, Down syndrome, Noonan syndrome, neurofibromatosis, and telomeropathies.

TRANSIENT MYELOPROLIFERATIVE DISORDER (TMD)

TMD, also referred to as transient abnormal myelopoiesis (TAM), constitutes an often but not always transient phenomenon of abnormal megakaryoblast proliferation, which occurs in ~10% of infants with Down syndrome. TMD is usually recognized at birth and either undergoes spontaneous regression (75% of cases) or progresses to acute megakaryoblastic leukemia (AMKL) (25% of cases). Almost all patients with TMD and TMD-derived AMKL display somatic *GATA1* mutations. TMD-associated *GATA1* mutations constitute exon 2 insertions, deletions, or missense mutations, affecting the N-terminal transactivation domain of GATA-1, and result in loss of full-length (50-kD) GATA-1 and its replacement with a shorter isoform (40-kD) that retains friend of GATA-1 (FOG-1) binding. In contrast, inherited forms of exon 2 *GATA1* mutations produce a phenotype with anemia, whereas exon 4 mutations that affect the N-terminal, FOG-1-interactive domain produce familial dyserythropoietic anemia with thrombocytopenia or X-linked macrothrombocytopenia.

PRIMARY EOSINOPHILIA

Eosinophilia refers to a PB absolute eosinophil count (AEC) that is above the upper normal limit of the reference range. The term *hypereosinophilia* is used when the AEC is >1500 × 10^9/L. Eosinophilia is operationally classified into secondary (nonneoplastic proliferation of eosinophils) and primary (proliferation of eosinophils that is either neoplastic or otherwise unexplained). Secondary eosinophilia is by far the most frequent cause of eosinophilia and is often associated with infections, especially those related to tissue-invasive helminths, allergic/vasculitic diseases, drugs, and metastatic cancer. Primary eosinophilia is the focus of this chapter and is considered when a cause for secondary eosinophilia is not readily apparent.

Primary eosinophilia is classified as clonal or idiopathic. Diagnosis of clonal eosinophilia requires morphologic, cytogenetic, or molecular evidence of a myeloid neoplasm. Idiopathic eosinophilia is considered when both secondary and clonal eosinophilias have been ruled out as a possibility. HES is a subcategory of idiopathic eosinophilia with persistent AEC of ≥1.5 × 10^9/L and associated with eosinophil-mediated organ damage (**Table 110-6**). An HES-like disorder that is associated with clonal or phenotypically abnormal T cells is referred to as lymphocytic variant hypereosinophilia (Table 110-6).

Clonal Eosinophilia Examples of clonal eosinophilia include eosinophilia associated with AML, MDS, CML, mastocytosis, and MDS/

PART 4 Oncology and Hematology

TABLE 110-6 Primary Eosinophilia Classification

VARIABLES	EOSINOPHILIA ASSOCIATED WITH *PDGFRA, PDGFRB, FGFR1,* OR *PCM1-JAK2* ABNORMALITY	CHRONIC EOSINOPHILIA NOT OTHERWISE SPECIFIED (CEL-NOS)	LYMPHOCYTIC VARIANT HYPEREOSINOPHILIA	HYPEREOSINOPHILIC SYNDROME
Absolute eosinophil count	$>600 \times 10^9$/L	$>1500 \times 10^9$/L	$>1500 \times 10^9$/L	$>1500 \times 10^9$/L
Peripheral blood blasts >2%	Yes or no	Yes or no	No	No
Bone marrow blasts >5%	Yes or no	Yes or No	No	No
Abnormal karyotype	Yes or no	Yes or no	No	No
PDGFRA, PDGFRB, FGFR1, or *PCM1-JAK2* abnormality	Yes	No	No	No
BCR-ABL1	No	No	No	No
Abnormal T lymphocyte phenotype or clonal T-cell clones	No	No	Yes	No
Eosinophil-mediated tissue damage	Yes or no	Yes or no	Yes or no	Yes

MPN overlap. Myeloid neoplasm–associated eosinophilia also includes the WHO MPN subcategory of chronic eosinophilic leukemia, not otherwise specified (CEL-NOS) and the WHO myeloid malignancy subcategory referred to as myeloid/lymphoid neoplasms with eosinophilia and rearrangement of platelet-derived growth factor receptor (*PDGFR*) α/β or fibroblast growth factor receptor 1 (*FGFR1*) or with *PCM1-JAK2* (Table 110-4).

The diagnostic workup for clonal eosinophilia that is not associated with morphologically overt myeloid malignancy should start with PB mutation screening for *FIP1L1-PDGFRA* and *PDGFRB* mutations using fluorescence in situ hybridization (FISH) or reverse transcription polymerase chain reaction. This is crucial since such eosinophilia is easily treated with imatinib. If mutation screening is negative, a BM examination with cytogenetic studies is indicated. In this regard, one must first pay attention to the presence or absence of 5q33, 4q12, 8p11.2, or t(8;9)(p22;p24.1) translocations, which, if present, would suggest *PDGFRB*-, *PDGFRA*-, or *FGFR1*-rearranged or *PCM1-JAK2*-associated clonal eosinophilia, respectively. The presence of 5q33 or 4q12 translocations predicts favorable response to treatment with imatinib mesylate and presence of t(8;9)(p22;p24.1) predicts a transient response to ruxolitinib, whereas 8p11.2 translocations are associated with aggressive myeloid malignancies that are refractory to current drug therapy.

Chronic Eosinophilic Leukemia, Not Otherwise Specified (CEL-NOS) CEL-NOS is a subset of clonal eosinophilia that is neither molecularly defined nor classified as an alternative clinicopathologically assigned myeloid malignancy. We prefer to use the term strictly in patients with an HES phenotype who also display either a clonal cytogenetic/molecular abnormality or excess blasts in the BM or PB. The WHO defines CEL-NOS as the presence of $\geq 1.5 \times 10^9$/L AEC that is accompanied by either the presence of myeloblast excess (either >2% in the PB or 5–19% in the BM) or evidence of myeloid clonality.

In a recent Mayo Clinic survey of 1416 patients with PB eosinophilia evaluated between 2008 and 2019, 17 patients (1.2%) fulfilled the WHO 2016 criteria for CEL-NOS. Median age was 63 years (range 25–92 years) with the vast majority of patients (88%) presenting with systemic symptoms. Organ involvement was a prominent feature, and involved organs included spleen, cardiac and pulmonary organs, and distal esophagus. Laboratory abnormalities included anemia, leukocytosis, and eosinophilia (median eosinophil count of 6.4×10^9/L; range 2.0–53.1). The most common BM abnormalities included abnormal eosinophils, abnormal and increased megakaryocytes, and fibrosis (18%). Cytogenetic abnormalities occurred in 88% of patients and included trisomy 8, complex karyotype, 13q–, 20q–, and chromosome 1 abnormalities. All seven patients with next-generation sequencing studies harbored one or more mutations, including *ASXL1* (43%) and *IDH1* (29%). Half of patients treated with hydroxyurea-based regimens responded with a persistent decline in eosinophil count for a median duration of 18 months. One-third of patients treated with prednisone responded, with a median duration of response of 13 months. Three patients were treated with imatinib, of whom two had normalization of eosinophil count. At a median follow-up of 13 months, nine patients had died including three patients who underwent leukemic transformation.

***PDGFR* Mutated Eosinophilia** Both platelet-derived growth factor receptors α (*PDGFRA* located on chromosome 4q12) and β (*PDGFRB* located on chromosome 5q31-q32) are involved in MPN-relevant activating mutations. Clinical phenotype in both instances includes prominent blood eosinophilia and excellent response to imatinib therapy. In regard to *PDGFRA* mutations, the most popular is *FIP1L1-PDGFRA*, a karyotypically occult del(4)(q12), that was described in 2003 as an imatinib-sensitive activating mutation. Functional studies have demonstrated transforming properties in cell lines and the induction of MPN in mice. Cloning of the *FIP1L1-PDGFRA* fusion gene identified a novel molecular mechanism for generating this constitutively active fusion tyrosine kinase, wherein a ~800-kb interstitial deletion within 4q12 fuses the 5′ portion of *FIP1L1* to the 3′ portion of *PDGFRA*. *FIP1L1-PDGFRA* occurs in a very small subset of patients who present with the phenotypic features of either systemic mastocytosis (SM) or HES, but the presence of the mutation reliably predicts complete hematologic and molecular response to imatinib therapy.

In a recent retrospective survey of 151 patients with *FIP1L1-PDGFRA*–associated eosinophilia (143 males; mean age at diagnosis 49 years), organopathy involved the spleen (44%), skin (32%), lungs (30%), heart (19%), and central nervous system (9%); none of 31 patients initially treated with corticosteroids achieved complete hematologic remission, whereas all 148 patients treated with imatinib achieved complete hematologic responses and also molecular responses, when evaluated. Treatment discontinuation was documented in 46 patients followed by a 57% relapse rate; the 1-, 5-, and 10-year overall survival rates in imatinib-treated patients were 99%, 95%, and 84%, respectively. Other studies have confirmed the possibility of treatment-free remissions in some patients after imatinib discontinuation. Infrequent occurrence of *FIP1L1-PDGFRA* mutated acute myeloid leukemia associated with eosinophilia has also been shown to respond to low-dose imatinib therapy (100 mg/d).

The association between eosinophilic myeloid malignancies and *PDGFRB* rearrangement was first characterized and published in 1994 where fusion of the tyrosine kinase encoding region of *PDGFRB* to the *ets*-like gene *ETV6* (*ETV6-PDGFRB*, t[5;12][q33;p13]) was demonstrated. The fusion protein was transforming to cell lines and resulted in constitutive activation of PDGFRB signaling. Since then, several other *PDGFRB* fusion transcripts with similar disease phenotypes have been described, and cell line transformation and MPD induction in mice have been demonstrated. Imatinib therapy was shown to be effective when employed.

***FGFR1* Mutated Eosinophilia** The 8p11 myeloproliferative syndrome (EMS) (also known as human stem cell leukemic/lymphoma syndrome) constitutes a clinical phenotype with features of both lymphoma and eosinophilic MPN and is characterized by a fusion mutation that involves the gene for fibroblast growth factor receptor-1 (*FGFR1*), which is located on chromosome 8p11. In EMS, both myeloid and lymphoid lineage cells exhibit the 8p11 translocation, thus demonstrating the stem cell origin of the disease. The disease features several 8p11-linked chromosome translocations, and some of the corresponding fusion *FGFR1* mutants have been shown to transform cell lines and induce EMS- or CML-like disease in mice depending on the specific *FGFR1* partner gene (*ZNF198* or *BCR*, respectively). Consistent with this laboratory observation, some patients with *BCR-FGFR1* mutation manifest a more indolent CML-like disease. The mechanism of *FGFR1* activation in EMS is similar to that seen with *PDGFRB*-associated MPD; the tyrosine kinase domain of *FGFR1* is juxtaposed to a dimerization domain from the partner gene. EMS is aggressive and requires combination chemotherapy followed by ASCT.

***PCM1-JAK2*–Associated Myeloid/Lymphoid Neoplasm with Eosinophilia** The 2016 revised WHO document includes a provisional entity under myeloid/lymphoid neoplasms with eosinophilia referred to as "myeloid/lymphoid neoplasms with *PCM1-JAK2*." The entity is characterized by the t(8;9)(p22;p24.1) cytogenetic abnormality and a phenotype that displays marked male predominance, hepatosplenomegaly, eosinophilia, and morphologic features similar to MPN, MDS, or MDS/MPN. Current drug therapy for *PCM1-JAK2*–associated disease is suboptimal, although some affected patients have displayed transient responses to ruxolitinib therapy.

Hypereosinophilic Syndrome Blood eosinophilia that is neither secondary nor clonal is operationally labeled as being "idiopathic." HES is a subcategory of idiopathic eosinophilia with persistent increase of the AEC to $\geq 1.5 \times 10^9$/L and presence of eosinophil-mediated organ damage, including cardiomyopathy, gastroenteritis, cutaneous lesions, sinusitis, pneumonitis, neuritis, and vasculitis. In addition, some patients manifest thromboembolic complications, hepatosplenomegaly, and either cytopenia or cytosis.

BM histologic and cytogenetic/molecular studies should be examined before a working diagnosis of HES is made. Additional blood studies that are currently recommended during the evaluation of HES include serum tryptase (an increased level suggests mastocytosis and warrants molecular studies to detect *FIP1L1-PDGFRA*), T-cell immunophenotyping, and T-cell receptor antigen gene rearrangement analysis (a positive test suggests an underlying clonal or phenotypically abnormal T-cell disorder). In addition, initial evaluation in HES should include echocardiogram and measurement of serum troponin levels to screen for myocardial involvement by the disease.

Initial evaluation of the patient with eosinophilia should include tests that facilitate assessment of target organ damage: complete blood count, chest x-ray, echocardiogram, and serum troponin level. Increased level of serum cardiac troponin has been shown to correlate with the presence of cardiomyopathy in HES. Typical echocardiographic findings in HES include ventricular apical thrombus, posterior mitral leaflet or tricuspid valve abnormality, endocardial thickening, dilated left ventricle, and pericardial effusion.

In a recent Mayo Clinic study of 98 consecutive patients with idiopathic eosinophilia, including HES, median age was 53 years (55% males) and overt organ involvement was seen in >80% of the cases, including 54% involving organs other than the skin. The frequencies of cardiac involvement, hepatosplenomegaly, and increased serum tryptase and interleukin 5 (IL-5) levels were 8%, 4%, 24%, and 31%, respectively. The study also revealed that 11% of the affected patients harbored pathogenetic mutations including *TET2*, *ASXL1*, and *KIT*; the presence of such mutations did not appear to influence phenotype, and the number of informative cases was too small to assess prognostic relevance. Instead, the study identified anemia and presence of cardiac involvement or hepatosplenomegaly as risk factors for survival.

Corticosteroids are the cornerstone of therapy in HES. Treatment with oral prednisone is usually started at 1 mg/kg/d and continued for 1–2 weeks before the dose is tapered slowly over the ensuing 2–3 months. If symptoms recur at a prednisone dose level of >10 mg/d, either hydroxyurea or interferon α is used as a steroid-sparing agent. In patients who fail usual therapy as outlined above, mepolizumab or alemtuzumab might be considered. Mepolizumab is a monoclonal antibody that targets IL-5, which is a well-recognized survival factor for eosinophils. Alemtuzumab targets the CD52 antigen, which has been shown to be expressed by eosinophils but not by neutrophils. In a recently reported, placebo-controlled, phase 3 study, HES patients received subcutaneous mepolizumab (300 mg) every 4 weeks, in addition to their preprotocol therapy, and experienced significantly fewer disease flare ups or treatment discontinuations (28 vs 56% for placebo), without excess adverse events. Mepolizumab was approved by the U.S. Food and Drug Administration (FDA) for use in HES on September 25, 2020. In a smaller phase 2 study, benralizumab (monoclonal antibody targeting the receptor for IL-5; 30 mg given subcutaneously every 4 weeks) was also shown to reduce eosinophil count more efficiently compared to placebo (90 vs 30%).

MASTOCYTOSIS

Mast cell disease (MCD) is defined as tissue infiltration by morphologically and immunophenotypically abnormal mast cells. MCD is classified into two broad categories: cutaneous mastocytosis (CM) and systemic mastocytosis (SM). MCD in adults is usually systemic, and the clinical course can be either indolent or aggressive, depending on the respective absence or presence of impaired organ function. Symptoms and signs of MCD include urticaria pigmentosa, mast cell mediator release symptoms (e.g., headache, flushing, lightheadedness, syncope, anaphylaxis, pruritus, urticaria, angioedema, nausea, diarrhea, abdominal cramps), and organ damage (lytic bone lesions, osteoporosis, hepatosplenomegaly, cytopenia). Aggressive SM can be associated with another myeloid malignancy, including MPN, MDS, or MDS/MPN overlap (e.g., CMML), or present as overt mast cell leukemia. In general, life expectancy is near normal in indolent SM but significantly shortened in aggressive SM.

Diagnosis of SM is based on BM examination that shows clusters of morphologically abnormal, spindle-shaped mast cells that are best evaluated by the use of immunohistochemical stains that are specific to mast cells (tryptase, CD117). In addition, mast cell immunophenotyping reveals aberrant CD25 expression by neoplastic mast cells. Other laboratory findings in SM include increased levels of serum tryptase, histamine and urine histamine metabolites, and prostaglandins. SM is associated with *KIT* mutations, usually *KIT* D816V, in the majority of patients. Accordingly, mutation screening for *KIT* D816V is diagnostically useful. However, the ability to detect *KIT* D816V depends on assay sensitivity and mast cell content of the test sample. The 2016 WHO classification of mastocytosis includes (1) CM, (2) SM, and (3) mast cell sarcoma (MCS). SM is further classified into (1) indolent SM (ISM), (2) smoldering SM (SSM), (3) SM with an associated hematologic neoplasm (SM-AHN), (4) aggressive SM (ASM), and (5) mast cell leukemia (MCL).

In a recent Mayo Clinic study of 580 patients (median age 55 years; range 18–88 years) with SM, morphologic subcategories were indolent/smoldering in 291 patients (50%) and advanced in 289 patients (50%), including SM-AHN in 199, ASM in 85, and MCL in 5. Multivariable analysis of clinical variables identified age >60 years, advanced SM, thrombocytopenia $<150 \times 10^9$/L, anemia below sex-adjusted normal, and increased alkaline phosphatase as independent risk factors for survival. In addition, *ASXL1*, *RUNX1*, and *NRAS* mutations were also independently associated with inferior survival. Combined clinical, cytogenetic, and molecular risk factor analysis confirmed the independent prognostic contribution of adverse mutations, advanced SM, thrombocytopenia, increased alkaline phosphatase, and age >60 years. These data were subsequently used to develop clinical and hybrid clinical-molecular risk models. The clinical risk model uses six readily accessible risk variables including age >60 years, platelet count $<150 \times 10^9$/L, anemia, hypoalbuminemia, increased alkaline phosphatase, and morphologic classification as advanced SM. Accordingly, median survival times were not reached, 148, 65, 31, 18, and 5 months in the presence of ≤1, 2, 3, 4, 5, and 6 of these risk factors, respectively.

Both ISM and ASM patients might experience mast cell mediator release symptoms, which are usually managed by both H_1 and H_2 histamine receptor blockers as well as cromolyn sodium. In addition, patients with propensity to vasodilatory shock should wear a medical alert bracelet and carry an Epi-Pen self-injector for self-administration of subcutaneous epinephrine. Urticaria pigmentosa shows variable response to both topical and systemic corticosteroid therapy. Cytoreductive therapy is not recommended for ISM, and instead, such patients are managed with use of H_1 and H_2 blockers, leukotriene antagonists, sodium cromolyn, phototherapy, topical steroids, and osteoporosis prevention with diphosphonates including alendronate and pamidronate. In ASM, either interferon α or cladribine is considered first-line therapy and benefits the majority of patients. Cladribine is administered by 2-h infusion (5 mg/m^2) daily for 5 days, repeated monthly for 4–6 cycles; expected overall response is ~ 50%, including major response in ~38%. In contrast, imatinib is ineffective in the treatment of *PDGFR* unmutated SM. A controlled study of patients with ISM or SSM demonstrated marginal value of masitinib (oral tyrosine kinase inhibitor that inhibits KIT and LYN), with a reported cumulative symptomatic response rate of 18.7% versus 7.4% for placebo. Treatment responses were more impressive in another study that used the multikinase inhibitor midostaurin in patients with the more aggressive forms of SM, with 45% of the patients achieving major response. Most recently, equally impressive responses were seen with the use of another kinase inhibitor, avapritinib (specifically targets *KIT* D816V), in both ISM and ASM; however, significant drug-related toxicity, including intracranial bleed, cognitive impairment, and moderate to severe cytopenias, has been observed.

DENDRITIC AND HISTIOCYTIC NEOPLASMS

Dendritic cell (DC) and histiocyte/macrophage neoplasms are extremely rare. DCs are antigen-presenting cells, whereas histiocytes/macrophages are antigen-processing. BM myeloid stem cells (CD34+) give rise to monocyte (CD14+, CD68+, CD11c+, CD1a–) and DC (CD14–, CD11c+/–, CD1a+/–) precursors. Monocyte precursors, in turn, give rise to macrophages (CD14+, CD68+, CD11c+, CD163+, lysozyme+) and interstitial DCs (CD68+, CD1a–). DC precursors give rise to Langerhans cell DCs (Birbeck granules, CD1a+, S100+, langerin+) and plasmacytoid DCs (CD68+, CD123+). Follicular DCs (CD21+, CD23+, CD35+) originate from mesenchymal stem cells. Dendritic and histiocytic neoplasms are operationally classified into macrophage/histiocyte-related and DC-related. The former includes histiocytic sarcoma/malignant histiocytosis, and the latter includes Langerhans cell histiocytosis, Langerhans cell sarcoma, interdigitating DC sarcoma, and follicular DC sarcoma.

Histiocytic Sarcoma/Malignant Histiocytosis Histiocytic sarcoma represents malignant proliferation of mature tissue histiocytes and is often localized. Median age at diagnosis is estimated at 46 years with slight male predilection. Some patients might have history of lymphoma, MDS, or germ cell tumors at time of disease presentation. The three typical disease sites are lymph nodes, skin, and gastrointestinal system. Patients may or may not have systemic symptoms including fever and weight loss, and other symptoms include hepatosplenomegaly, lytic bone lesions, and pancytopenia. Immunophenotype includes presence of histiocytic markers (CD68, lysozyme, CD11c, CD14) and absence of myeloid or lymphoid markers. Prognosis is poor and treatment often ineffective. The term *malignant histiocytosis* (MH) refers to a disseminated disease and systemic symptoms. Lymphoma-like treatment induces complete remissions in some patients, and median survival is estimated at 2 years.

Langerhans Cell Histiocytosis Langerhans cells (LCs) are specialized DCs that reside in mucocutaneous tissue and, upon activation, become specialized for antigen presentation to T cells. LC histiocytosis (LCH; also known as histiocytosis X) represents neoplastic proliferation of LCs (S100+, CD1a+, and Birbeck granules on electron microscopy). LCH incidence is estimated at 5 per million, and the disease typically affects children with a male predilection. Presentation can be either unifocal (eosinophilic granuloma) or multifocal. The former usually affects bones and less frequently lymph nodes, skin, and lung, whereas the latter is more disseminated. Unifocal disease often affects older children and adults, whereas multisystem disease affects infants. LCH of the lung in adults is characterized by bilateral nodules. Prognosis depends on organs involved. Only 10% of patients progress from unifocal to multiorgan disease. LCH of the lung might improve upon cessation of smoking. Approximately 55% of patients with LCH harbor *BRAF* V600E gain-of-function mutations, which indicates high-risk disease and resistance to first-line therapy; however, responses to targeted therapy with vemurafenib have been reported. Other forms of treatment for LCH include combination chemotherapy and MEK inhibitors in *BRAF* wild-type disease with other MAPK pathway mutations. Unfortunately, such targeted therapy has not secured long-lasting, treatment-free remissions.

Langerhans Cell Sarcoma Langerhans cell sarcoma (LCS) also represents neoplastic proliferation of LCs with overtly malignant morphology. The disease can present de novo or progress from antecedent LCH. There is a female predilection, and median age at diagnosis is estimated at 41 years. Immunophenotype is similar to that seen in LCH, and liver, spleen, lung, and bone are the usual sites of disease. Prognosis is poor and treatment generally ineffective.

Interdigitating Dendritic Cell Sarcoma Interdigitating DC sarcoma (IDCS), also known as reticulum cell sarcoma, represents neoplastic proliferation of IDCs. The disease is extremely rare and affects elderly adults with no sex predilection. Typical presentation is asymptomatic solitary lymphadenopathy. Immunophenotype includes S100 positivity and negativity for vimentin and CD1a. Prognosis ranges from benign local disease to widespread lethal disease.

Follicular Dendritic Cell Sarcoma FDCs reside in B-cell follicles and present antigen to B cells. FDC neoplasms (FDCNs) are usually localized and often affect adults. FDCN might be associated with Castleman's disease in 10–20% of cases, and increased incidence in schizophrenia has been reported. Cervical lymph nodes are the most frequent site of involvement in FDCN, and other sites include maxillary, mediastinal, and retroperitoneal lymph nodes; oral cavity; gastrointestinal system; skin; and breasts. Sites of metastasis include lung and liver. Immunophenotype includes CD21, CD35, and CD23. Clinical course is typically indolent, and treatment includes surgical excision followed by regional radiotherapy and sometimes systemic chemotherapy.

Hemophagocytic Syndrome Hemophagocytic syndrome (HPS), also known as hemophagocytic lymphohistiocytosis (HLH), represents nonneoplastic proliferation and activation of macrophages that induce cytokine-mediated BM suppression and features of intense phagocytosis in BM and liver. HPS may result from genetic (primary) or acquired (secondary) disorders of macrophages. The former entail genetically determined inability to regulate macrophage proliferation and activation and might include alterations in familial HLH genes (*PRF1*, *UNC13D*, *STXBP2*, and *STX11*), granule/pigment abnormality genes (*RAB27A*, *LYST*, and *AP3B1*), or X-linked lymphoproliferative disease genes (*SH2D1A* and *XIAP*). Acquired HPS is often precipitated by viral infections, most notably Epstein-Barr virus. HPS might also accompany certain malignancies such as T-cell lymphoma and autoimmune diseases. Clinical presentation includes fever, severe constitutional symptoms, enlarged lymph nodes, hepatosplenomegaly, neurologic dysfunction, and abnormalities in multiple organ function tests. Diagnosis is accomplished by either detection of HLH-related mutations or meeting five of the following eight conventional criteria: (1) hemophagocytosis in the BM/spleen/lymph nodes; (2) serum ferritin ≥500 μg/L; (3) hypofibrinogenemia (fibrinogen ≤1.5 g/L) or hypertriglyceridemia (triglycerides ≥3 mmol/L); (4) low NK cell activity; (5) elevated soluble IL-2 receptor (CD25) ≥2400 U/mL; (6) bi- or tricytopenia (platelets $<100 \times 10^9$/L, hemoglobin <9 g/dL, absolute neutrophil count $<1 \times 10^9$/L); (7) splenomegaly palpable >3 cm below left costal margin; and (8) fever. Clinical course is often fulminant and fatal. Current therapeutic approaches for primary or secondary HLH include the so-called "HLH-94 protocol," which consists of weekly treatments with etoposide and dexamethasone, stem cell transplantation, emapalumab (a monoclonal antibody that binds and neutralizes interferon γ), and the JAK1/2 inhibitor ruxolitinib. Emapalumab was FDA approved in

November 2018 for use in pediatric and adult patients with primary HLH with refractory or progressive disease.

FURTHER READING

ALLEN CE et al: The coming of age of Langerhans cell histiocytosis. Nat Immunol 21:1, 2020.

DAO KT et al: Efficacy of ruxolitinib in patients with chronic neutrophilic leukemia and atypical chronic myeloid leukemia. J Clin Oncol 38:1006, 2020.

MAURER M et al: Results from PIONEER: A randomized, double-blind, placebo-controlled, phase 2 study of avapritinib in patients with indolent systemic mastocytosis (ISM). Oncol Res Treat 43:77, 2020.

PATNAIK MM, TEFFERI A: Chronic myelomonocytic leukemia: 2020 update on diagnosis, risk stratification and management. Am J Hematol 95:97, 2020.

ROUFOSSE F et al: Efficacy and safety of mepolizumab in hypereosinophilic syndrome: A phase III, randomized, placebo-controlled trial. J Allergy Clin Immunol 146:1397, 2020.

SUKSWAI N et al: Diffuse large B-cell lymphoma variants: An update. Pathology 52:53, 2020.

SWERDLOW SH et al: The 2016 revision of the World Health Organization classification of lymphoid neoplasms. Blood 127:2375, 2016.

SZUBER N et al: Chronic neutrophilic leukemia: 2020 update on diagnosis, molecular genetics, prognosis, and management. Am J Hematol 95:212, 2020.

VALLURUPALLI M, BERLINER N: Emapalumab for the treatment of relapsed/refractory hemophagocytic lymphohistiocytosis. Blood 134:1783, 2019.

111 Plasma Cell Disorders

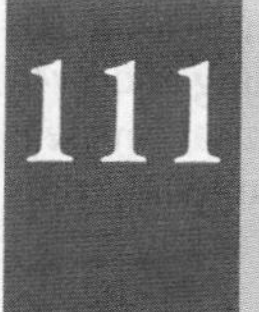

Nikhil C. Munshi, Dan L. Longo, Kenneth C. Anderson

The *plasma cell disorders* are monoclonal neoplasms related to each other by virtue of their development from common progenitors in the late B-lymphocyte lineage. Multiple myeloma (MM), Waldenström's macroglobulinemia, primary amyloidosis (**Chap. 112**), and the heavy chain diseases comprise this group and may be designated by a variety of synonyms such as *monoclonal gammopathies, paraproteinemias, plasma cell dyscrasias*, and *dysproteinemias*. Mature B lymphocytes destined to produce IgG bear surface immunoglobulin molecules of both μ and γ heavy chain isotypes with both isotypes having identical idiotypes (variable regions). Under normal circumstances, maturation to antibody-secreting plasma cells and their proliferation is stimulated by exposure to the antigen for which the surface immunoglobulin is specific; however, in the plasma cell disorders, the control over this process is lost. The clinical manifestations of all the plasma cell disorders relate to the expansion of the neoplastic cells, to the secretion of cell products (immunoglobulin molecules or subunits, lymphokines), and to some extent to the host's response to the tumor. Normal development of B lymphocytes is discussed in **Chap. 349** and depicted in **Fig. 108-2**.

Three categories of structural variation are present among immunoglobulin molecules that form antigenic determinants, and these are used to classify immunoglobulins. *Isotypes* are those determinants that distinguish among the main classes of antibodies of a given species and are the same in all normal individuals of that species. Therefore, isotypic determinants are, by definition, recognized by antibodies from a distinct species (heterologous sera) but not by antibodies from the same species (homologous sera). There are five heavy chain isotypes (M, G, A, D, E) and two light chain isotypes (κ, λ). *Allotypes* are distinct determinants that reflect regular small differences between individuals of the same species in the amino acid sequences of otherwise similar immunoglobulins. These differences are determined by allelic genes; by definition, they are detected by antibodies made in the same species. *Idiotypes* are the third category of antigenic determinants. They are unique to the molecules produced by a given clone of antibody-producing cells. Idiotypes are formed by the unique structure of the antigen-binding portion of the molecule.

Antibody molecules (**Fig. 111-1**) are composed of two heavy chains (~50,000 molecular weight [mol wt]) and two light chains (~25,000 mol wt). Each chain has a constant portion (limited amino acid sequence variability) and a variable region (extensive sequence variability). The light and heavy chains are linked by disulfide bonds and are aligned so that their variable regions are adjacent to one another. This variable region forms the antigen recognition site of the antibody molecule; its unique structural features form idiotypes that are reliable markers for a particular clone of cells because each antibody is formed and secreted by a single clone. Because of the mechanics of the gene rearrangements necessary to specify the immunoglobulin variable regions (VDJ joining for the heavy chain, VJ joining for the light chain), a particular clone rearranges only one of the two chromosomes to produce an immunoglobulin molecule of only one light chain isotype and only one allotype (allelic exclusion) (Fig. 111-1). After exposure to antigen, the variable region may become associated with a new heavy chain isotype (class switch). Each clone of cells performs these sequential gene arrangements in a unique way. This results in each clone producing a unique immunoglobulin molecule. In most plasma cells, light chains are synthesized in slight excess, secreted as free light chains, and cleared by the kidney, but <10 mg of such light chains is excreted per day.

Electrophoretic analysis permits separation of components of the serum proteins (**Fig. 111-2**). The immunoglobulins move heterogeneously in an electric field and form a broad peak in the gamma region, which is usually increased in the sera of patients with plasma cell tumors. There is a sharp spike in this region called an *M component* (M for monoclonal). Less commonly, the M component may appear in the β_2 or α_2 globulin region. The monoclonal antibody must be present at a concentration of at least 5 g/L (0.5 g/dL) to be accurately quantitated by this method. This corresponds to ~10^9 cells producing the antibody. Confirmation of the type of immunoglobulin and that it is truly monoclonal is determined by immunoelectrophoresis that reveals a single heavy and/or light chain type. Hence, immunoelectrophoresis and electrophoresis provide qualitative and quantitative assessment of the M component, respectively. Once the presence of an M component has been confirmed, the amount of M component in the serum is a reliable measure of the tumor burden, making M component an excellent tumor marker to manage therapy, yet it is not specific enough to be used to screen asymptomatic patients. In addition to the plasma cell disorders, M components may be detected in other lymphoid neoplasms such as chronic lymphocytic leukemia (CLL) and lymphomas of B- or T-cell origin; nonlymphoid neoplasms such as chronic myeloid leukemia, breast cancer, and colon cancer; a variety of nonneoplastic conditions such as cirrhosis, sarcoidosis, parasitic diseases, Gaucher's disease, and pyoderma gangrenosum; and a number of autoimmune conditions, including rheumatoid arthritis, myasthenia gravis, and cold agglutinin disease. Monoclonal proteins are also observed in immunosuppressed patients after organ transplant and, rarely, allogeneic transplant. At least two very rare skin diseases—lichen myxedematosus (also known as papular mucinosis) and necrobiotic xanthogranuloma—are associated with a monoclonal gammopathy. In papular mucinosis, highly cationic IgG is deposited in the dermis of patients. This organ specificity may reflect the specificity of the antibody for some antigenic component of the dermis. Necrobiotic xanthogranuloma is a histiocytic infiltration of the skin, usually of the face, that produces red or yellow nodules that can enlarge to plaques. Approximately 10% progress to myeloma. Five percent of patients with sensory motor neuropathy also have a monoclonal paraprotein.

The nature of the M component is variable in plasma cell disorders. It may be an intact antibody molecule of any heavy chain subclass, or it may be an altered antibody or fragment. Isolated light or heavy chains may be produced. In some plasma cell tumors such as extramedullary

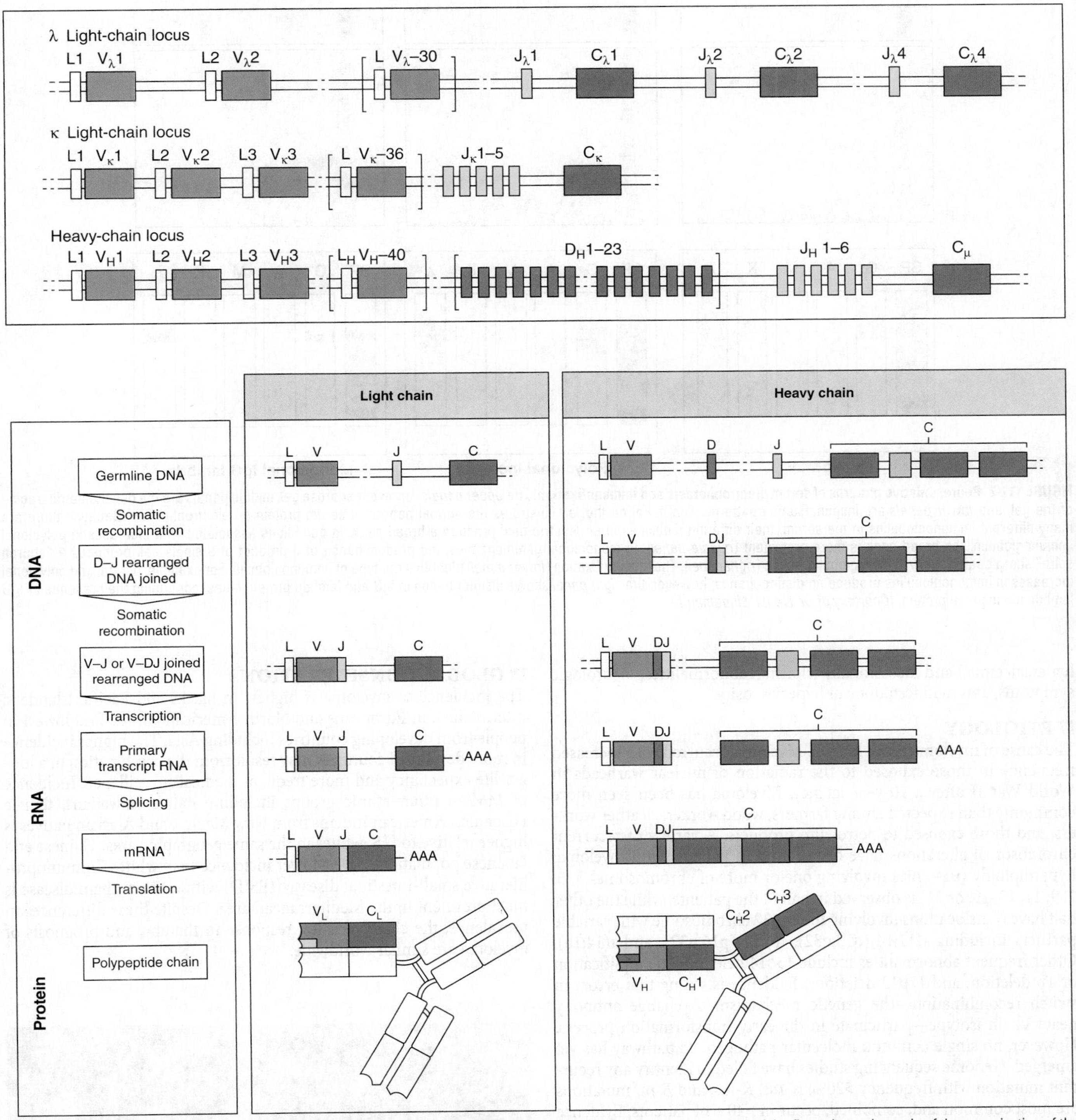

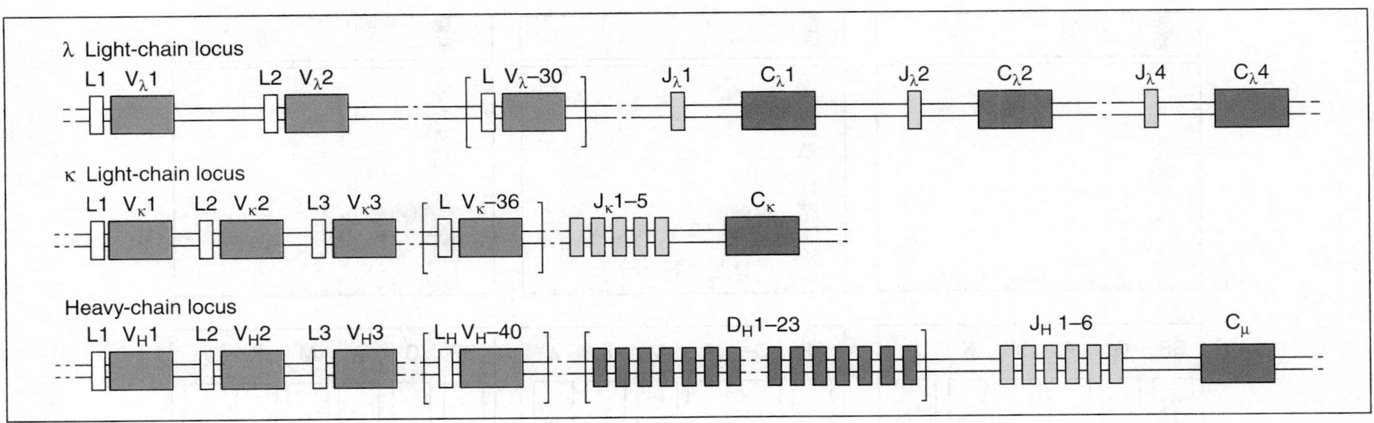

FIGURE 111-1 Immunoglobulin genetics and the relationship of gene segments to the antibody protein. The *top* portion of the figure is a schematic of the organization of the immunoglobulin genes, λ on chromosome 22, κ on chromosome 2, and the heavy chain locus on chromosome 14. The heavy chain locus is >2 megabases, and some of the D region gene segments are only a few bases long, so the figure depicts the schematic relationship among the segments, not their actual size. The *bottom* portion of the figure outlines the steps in going from the noncontiguous germline gene segments to an intact antibody molecule. Two recombination events juxtapose the V-D-J (or V-J for light chains) segments. The rearranged gene is transcribed, and RNA splicing cuts out intervening sequences to produce an mRNA, which is then translated into an antibody light or heavy chain. The sites on the antibody that bind to antigen (the so-called CDR3 regions) are encoded by D and J segments for heavy chains and the J segments for light chains. *(From Janeway's Immunobiology, 9th ed by Kenneth Murphy and Casey Weaver. Copyright © 2017 by Garland Science, Taylor & Francis Group, LLC. Used by permission of W. W. Norton & Company, Inc.)*

or solitary bone plasmacytomas, less than one-third of patients will have an M component. In ~20% of myelomas, only light chains are produced and, in most cases, are secreted in the urine as Bence Jones proteins. The frequency of myelomas of a particular heavy chain class is roughly proportional to the serum concentration, and therefore, IgG myelomas are more common than IgA and IgD myelomas. In ~1% of patients with myeloma, biclonal or triclonal gammopathy is observed.

MULTIPLE MYELOMA

■ DEFINITION

MM represents a malignant proliferation of plasma cells derived from a single clone. The tumor, its products, and the host response to it result in a number of organ dysfunctions and symptoms, including bone pain or fracture, renal failure, susceptibility to infection, anemia,

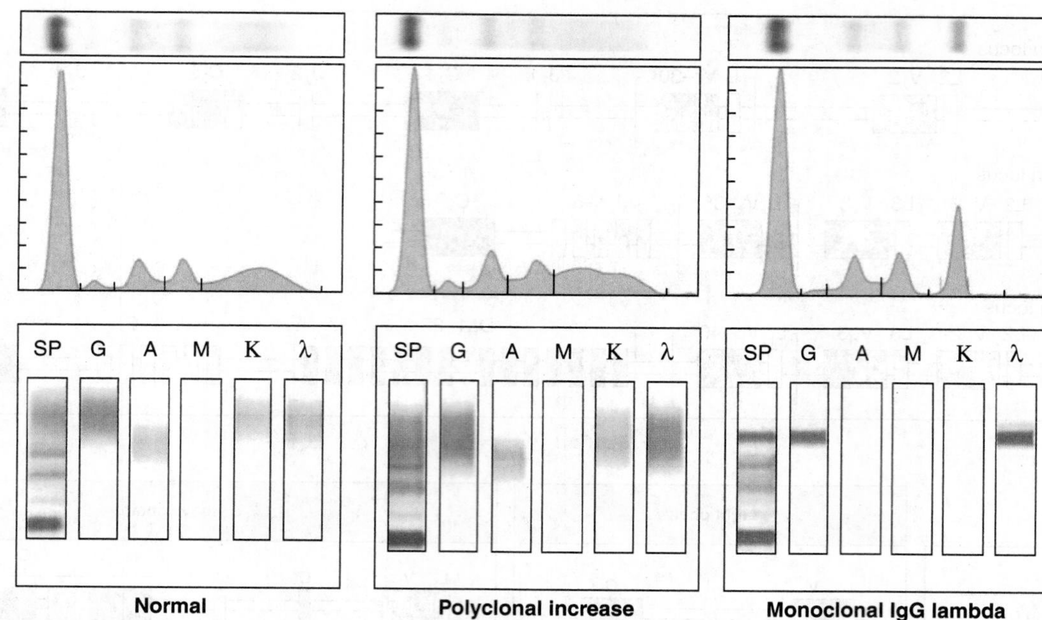

FIGURE 111-2 Representative patterns of serum electrophoresis and immunofixation. The *upper panels* represent agarose gel, middle panels are the densitometric tracing of the gel, and *lower panels* are immunofixation patterns. The panel on the *left* illustrates the normal pattern of serum protein on electrophoresis. Because there are many different immunoglobulins in the serum, their differing mobilities in an electric field produce a broad peak. In conditions associated with increases in polyclonal immunoglobulin, the broad peak is more prominent (*middle panel*). In monoclonal gammopathies, the predominance of a product of a single cell produces a "church spire" sharp peak, usually in the γ globulin region (*right panel*). The immunofixation (*lower panel*) identifies the type of immunoglobulin. For example, normal and polyclonal increases in immunoglobulins produce no distinct bands; however, the *right panel* shows distinct bands in IgG and lambda protein lanes, confirming the presence of IgG lambda monoclonal protein. *(Courtesy of Dr. Neal I. Lindeman.)*

hypercalcemia, and occasionally clotting abnormalities, neurologic symptoms, and manifestations of hyperviscosity.

ETIOLOGY

The cause of myeloma is not known. Myeloma occurred with increased frequency in those exposed to the radiation of nuclear warheads in World War II after a 20-year latency. Myeloma has been seen more commonly than expected among farmers, wood workers, leather workers, and those exposed to petroleum products. A variety of recurrent chromosomal alterations have been found in patients with myeloma: hyperdiploidy (trisomies involving one or more of chromosomes 3, 5, 7, 9, 11, 15, 19, or 21) is observed in half of the patients, while the other half have translocations involving the 14q32 chromosome with variable partners including t(11;14)(q13;q32), t(4;14)(p16;q32), and t(14;16). Other frequent abnormalities include 13q14 deletion, 1q amplification or 1p deletion, and 17p13 deletions. Evidence is strong that errors in switch recombination—the genetic mechanism to change antibody heavy chain isotype—participate in the early transformation process. However, no single common molecular pathogenetic pathway has yet emerged. Genome sequencing studies have failed to identify any recurrent mutation with frequency >20%; *N-ras*, *K-ras*, and *B-raf* mutations are most common and, combined, occur in >40% of patients. Evidence of complex clusters of subclonal variants is present at diagnosis, and additional mutations are acquired over time, indicative of genomic evolution that may drive disease progression. Interleukin (IL) 6 may play a role in driving myeloma cell proliferation. It remains difficult to distinguish benign from malignant plasma cells based on morphologic criteria in all but a few cases **(Fig. 111-3)**.

INCIDENCE AND PREVALENCE

In 2021 in the United States, 34,920 new cases of myeloma were estimated to be diagnosed, and 12,410 people were estimated to die from the disease. Myeloma increases in incidence with age. The median age at diagnosis is 69 years; it is uncommon under age 40. Males are more commonly affected than females, and blacks have nearly twice the incidence of whites. In 2018, myeloma accounted for 1.8% of all malignancies, with incidence rates per 100,000 of 6.1 in whites and 13.6 in blacks.

GLOBAL CONSIDERATIONS

The incidence of myeloma is highest in blacks and Pacific Islanders; intermediate in Europeans and North American whites; and lowest in people from developing countries including Asia. The higher incidence in more developed countries may result from the combination of a longer life expectancy and more frequent medical surveillance. Incidence of MM in other ethnic groups including native Hawaiians, female Hispanics, American Indians from New Mexico, and Alaskan natives is higher relative to U.S. whites in the same geographic area. Chinese and Japanese populations have a lower incidence than whites. Immunoproliferative small-intestinal disease (IPSID) with α heavy chain disease is most prevalent in the Mediterranean area. Despite these differences in prevalence, the characteristics, response to therapy, and prognosis of myeloma are similar worldwide.

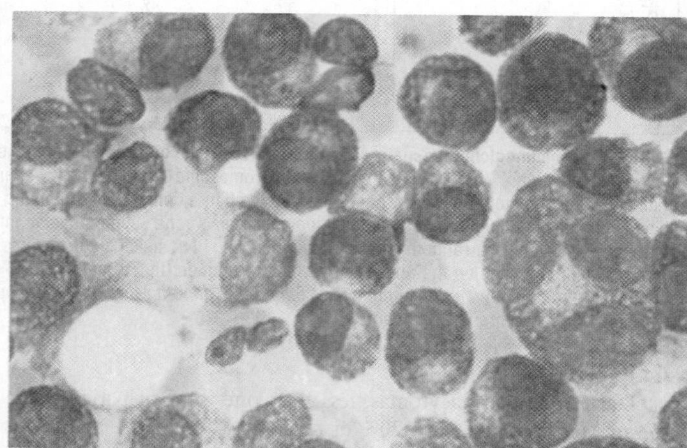

FIGURE 111-3 Multiple myeloma (marrow). The cells bear characteristic morphologic features of plasma cells: round or oval cells with an eccentric nucleus composed of coarsely clumped chromatin, a densely basophilic cytoplasm, and a perinuclear clear zone containing the Golgi apparatus. Binucleate and multinucleate malignant plasma cells can be seen.

■ PATHOGENESIS AND CLINICAL MANIFESTATIONS

MM cells bind via cell-surface adhesion molecules to bone marrow stromal cells (BMSCs) and extracellular matrix (ECM), which triggers MM cell growth, survival, drug resistance, and migration in the bone marrow milieu (**Fig. 111-4**). These effects are due both to direct MM cell–BMSC binding via adhesion molecules and to induction of various cytokines, including IL-6, insulin-like growth factor type 1 (IGF-1), vascular endothelial growth factor (VEGF), and stromal cell–derived growth factor (SDF)-1a. Growth, drug resistance, and migration are mediated via Ras/Raf/mitogen-activated protein kinase, PI3K/Akt, and protein kinase C signaling cascades, respectively. Other cellular elements in the bone marrow microenvironment also significantly impact MM cell growth and survival. The major myeloma supporting interactions are with endothelial cells and osteoclasts. Immune cells such as plasmacytoid dendritic cells (pDC), myeloid-derived suppressor cells (MDSC), and T helper 17 (T_H17) cells are increased in number and support myeloma growth, while antimyeloma immune responses, especially T helper and cytotoxic cells, B cells, and natural killer T cells, are suppressed.

Bone pain is the most common symptom in myeloma, affecting nearly 70% of patients. Persistent localized pain usually signifies a pathologic fracture. The bone lesions of myeloma are caused by the proliferation of tumor cells, activation of osteoclasts that destroy bone, and suppression of osteoblasts that form new bone. The increased osteoclast activity is mediated by osteoclast activating factors (OAFs) produced by the myeloma cells (mediated by several cytokines, including IL-1, lymphotoxin, vascular endothelial growth factor [VEGF], receptor activator of nuclear factor-κB [RANK] ligand, macrophage inhibitory factor [MIP]-1α, and tumor necrosis factor [TNF]). The bone lesions are lytic in nature (**Fig. 111-5**) and are rarely associated with osteoblastic new bone formation due to their suppression by dickhoff-1 (DKK-1) produced by myeloma cells. Therefore, radioisotopic bone scanning is less useful in diagnosis than is plain radiography. The bony lysis results in substantial mobilization of calcium from bone, and serious acute and chronic complications of hypercalcemia may dominate the clinical picture (see below). Localized bone lesions may cause the collapse of vertebrae, leading to spinal cord compression. The next most common clinical problem in patients with myeloma is susceptibility to bacterial infections. The most common infections are pneumonias and pyelonephritis, and the most frequent pathogens are *Streptococcus pneumoniae, Staphylococcus aureus*, and *Klebsiella pneumoniae* in the lungs and *Escherichia coli* and other gram-negative organisms in the urinary tract. In ~25% of patients, recurrent infections are the presenting features, and >75% of patients will have a serious infection at some time in their course. The susceptibility to infection has several contributing causes. First, patients with myeloma have diffuse hypogammaglobulinemia if the M component is excluded. The hypogammaglobulinemia is related to both decreased production and increased destruction of normal antibodies. The large M component results in fractional catabolic rates of 8–16% instead of the normal 2%. Moreover, some patients generate a population of circulating regulatory cells in response to their myeloma that can suppress normal antibody synthesis. These patients have very poor antibody responses, especially to polysaccharide antigens such as those on bacterial cell walls. Various abnormalities in T-cell function are also observed including decreased T_H1 response, increase in T_H17 cells producing

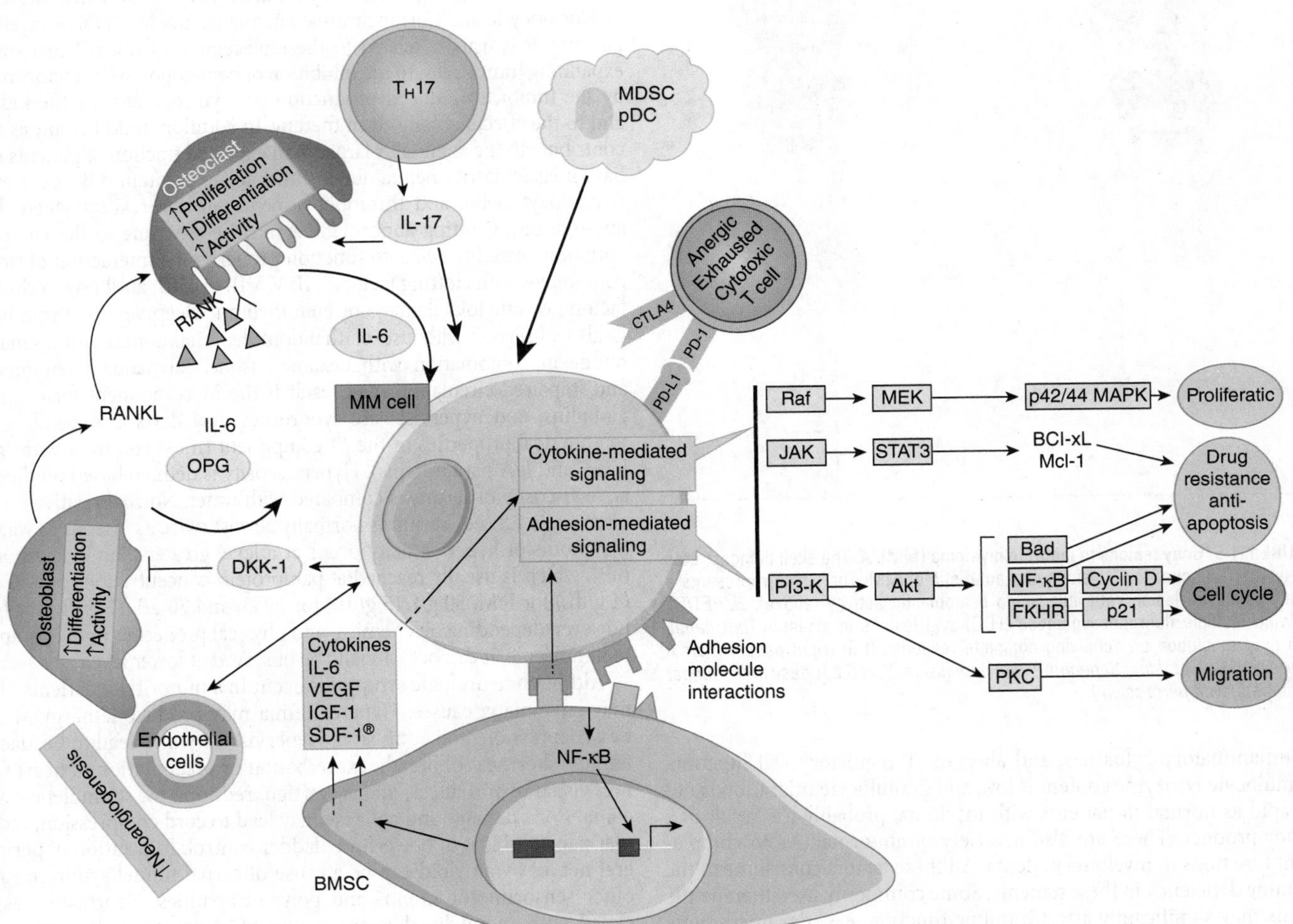

FIGURE 111-4 Pathogenesis of multiple myeloma. Multiple myeloma (MM) cells interact with bone marrow stromal cells (BMSCs) and extracellular matrix proteins via adhesion molecules, triggering adhesion-mediated signaling as well as cytokine production. This triggers cytokine-mediated signaling that provides growth, survival, and antiapoptotic effects as well as development of drug resistance. Additional bidirectional interactions lead to inhibition of osteoblast and increase in osteoclast activity which leads to bone-related issues in myeloma. Similar interactions with immune microenvironment lead to augmentation of tumor promoting immune responses and suppression of tumor protective immune responses, overall allowing myeloma cell growth. *(Adapted from G Bianchi, NC Munshi: Blood 125: 3049, 2015.)*

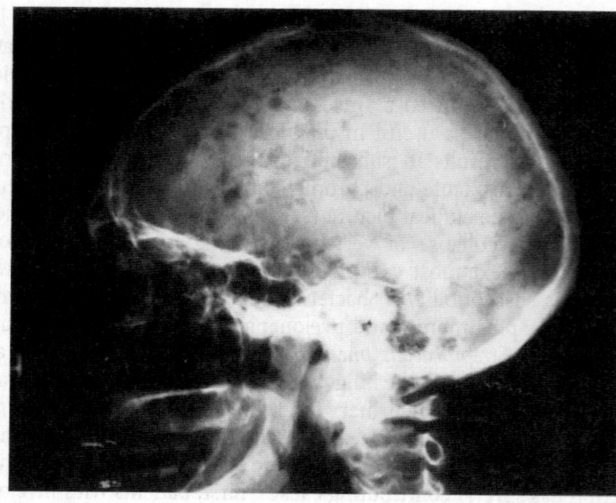

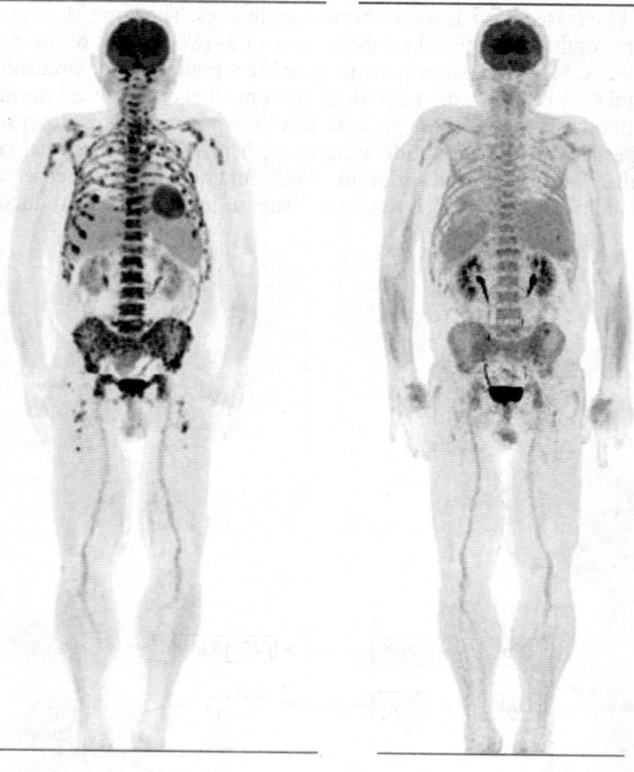

FIGURE 111-5 Bony lesions in multiple myeloma (MM). ***A.*** The skull demonstrates the typical "punched out" lesions characteristic of MM. The lesion represents a purely osteolytic lesion with little or no osteoblastic activity (above). ***B.*** PET/CT showing multiple fluorodeoxyglucose (FDG)-avid lesions in skeleton (*left panel*) with their resolution on achieving complete response (CR) (*right panel*). *(Part A courtesy of Dr. Geraldine Schechter; with permission. Part B courtesy of Dr. Sundar Jagannath; with permission.)*

proinflammatory cytokines, and aberrant T regulatory cell function. Granulocyte lysozyme content is low, and granulocyte migration is not as rapid as normal in patients with myeloma, probably the result of a tumor product. There are also a variety of abnormalities in complement functions in myeloma patients. All these factors contribute to the immune deficiency in these patients. Some commonly used therapeutic agents may significantly affect immune function; e.g., dexamethasone suppresses immune responses and increases susceptibility to bacterial and fungal infection, B-cell maturation antigen (BCMA)–targeting chimeric antigen receptor T (CAR-T) cells can eliminate plasma cells inducing hypogammaglobulinemia, and bortezomib predisposes to herpesvirus reactivation.

Renal failure occurs in nearly 25% of myeloma patients, and some renal pathology is noted in >50%. Of many contributing factors, hypercalcemia is the most common cause of renal failure. Glomerular deposits of amyloid, hyperuricemia, recurrent infections, frequent use of nonsteroidal anti-inflammatory agents for pain control, use of iodinated contrast dye for imaging, bisphosphonate use, and occasional infiltration of the kidney by myeloma cells all may contribute to renal dysfunction. However, tubular damage associated with the excretion of light chains is almost always present. Normally, light chains are filtered, reabsorbed in the tubules, and catabolized. With the increase in the amount of light chains presented to the tubule, the tubular cells become overloaded with these proteins, and tubular damage results either directly from light chain toxic effects or indirectly from the release of intracellular lysosomal enzymes. The earliest manifestation of this tubular damage is the adult Fanconi's syndrome (a type 2 proximal renal tubular acidosis), with loss of glucose and amino acids, as well as defects in the ability of the kidney to acidify and concentrate the urine. The proteinuria is not accompanied by hypertension, and the protein is nearly all light chains. Generally, very little albumin is in the urine because glomerular function is usually normal. When the glomeruli are involved, nonselective proteinuria is also observed. Patients with myeloma also have a decreased anion gap [i.e., $Na^+ - (Cl^- + HCO_3^-)$] because the M component is cationic, resulting in retention of chloride. This is often accompanied by hyponatremia that is felt to be artificial (pseudohyponatremia) because each volume of serum has less water as a result of the increased protein. Renal dysfunction due to light chain deposition disease, light chain cast nephropathy, and amyloidosis is partially reversible with effective therapy. Myeloma patients are susceptible to developing acute renal failure if they become dehydrated.

Normocytic and normochromic anemia occurs in ~80% of myeloma patients. It is usually related to the replacement of normal marrow by expanding tumor cells, to the inhibition of hematopoiesis by factors made by the tumor, to reduced production of erythropoietin by the kidney, and to the effects of long-term therapy. In addition, mild hemolysis may contribute to the anemia. A larger than expected fraction of patients may have megaloblastic anemia due to either folate or vitamin B_{12} deficiency. Granulocytopenia and thrombocytopenia are rare except when therapy-induced. Clotting abnormalities may be seen due to the failure of antibody-coated platelets to function properly; the interaction of the M component with clotting factors I, II, V, VII, or VIII; antibody to clotting factors; or amyloid damage of endothelium. Deep venous thrombosis is also observed with use of thalidomide, lenalidomide, or pomalidomide in combination with dexamethasone. Raynaud's phenomenon and impaired circulation may result if the M component forms cryoglobulins, and hyperviscosity syndromes may develop depending on the physical properties of the M component (most common with IgM, IgG3, and IgA paraproteins). Hyperviscosity is defined based on the relative viscosity of serum as compared with water. Normal relative serum viscosity is 1.8 (i.e., serum is normally almost twice as viscous as water). Symptoms of hyperviscosity occur at a level greater than 4 centipoises (cP), which is usually reached at paraprotein concentrations of ~40 g/L (4 g/dL) for IgM, 50 g/L (5 g/dL) for IgG3, and 70 g/L (7 g/dL) for IgA; however, depending on chemical and physical properties of the paraprotein molecule, it can occasionally be observed at lower levels.

Although neurologic symptoms occur in a minority of patients, they may have many causes. Hypercalcemia may produce lethargy, weakness, depression, and confusion. Hyperviscosity may lead to headache, fatigue, shortness of breath, exacerbation or precipitation of heart failure, visual disturbances, ataxia, vertigo, retinopathy, somnolence, and coma. Bony damage and collapse may lead to cord compression, radicular pain, and loss of bowel and bladder control. Infiltration of peripheral nerves by amyloid can be a cause of carpal tunnel syndrome and other sensorimotor mono- and polyneuropathies. Neuropathy associated with monoclonal gammopathy of undetermined significance (MGUS) and myeloma is more frequently sensory than motor neuropathy and is associated with IgM more than other isotypes. In >50% of patients with neuropathy, the IgM monoclonal protein is directed against myelin-associated globulin (MAG). Sensory neuropathy is also a side effect of therapy, specifically thalidomide and bortezomib.

Many of the clinical features of myeloma, e.g., cord compression, pathologic fractures, hyperviscosity, sepsis, and hypercalcemia, can present as medical emergencies. Despite the widespread distribution of plasma cells in the body, tumor expansion is dominantly within bone and bone marrow and, for reasons unknown, rarely causes enlargement of spleen, lymph nodes, or gut-associated lymphatic tissue.

DIAGNOSIS AND STAGING

The diagnosis of myeloma requires marrow plasmacytosis (>10%), a serum and/or urine M component, and at least one of the myeloma-defining events detailed in **Table 111-1**. Bone marrow plasma cells are CD138+ and either monoclonal kappa or lambda light chain positive. The most important differential diagnosis in patients with myeloma involves their separation from individuals with MGUS or smoldering multiple myeloma (SMM). MGUS is vastly more common than myeloma, occurring in 1% of the population aged >50 years and in up to 10% of individuals aged >75 years. The diagnostic criteria for MGUS, SMM, and myeloma are described in Table 111-1. Although ~1% of patients per year with MGUS go on to develop myeloma, all cases of myeloma are preceded by MGUS. Non-IgG subtype, abnormal kappa/lambda free light chain ratio, and serum M protein >15 g/L (1.5 g/dL) are associated with higher incidence of progression of MGUS to myeloma. Absence of all three features predicts a 5% chance of progression, whereas higher-risk MGUS with the presence of all three features predicts a 60% chance of progression over 20 years. The features responsible for higher risk of progression from SMM to MM are bone marrow plasmacytosis >10%, abnormal kappa/lambda free light chain ratio, and serum M protein >30 g/L (3 g/dL). Patients with only one of these three features have a 25% chance of progression to MM in 5 years, whereas patients with high-risk SMM with all three features have a 76% chance of progression. Two important variants of myeloma are solitary bone plasmacytoma and solitary extramedullary plasmacytoma. These lesions are associated with an M component in <30% of the cases, they may affect younger individuals, and both are associated

TABLE 111-1 Diagnostic Criteria for Multiple Myeloma, Myeloma Variants, and Monoclonal Gammopathy of Undetermined Significance

Monoclonal Gammopathy of Undetermined Significance (MGUS)
Serum monoclonal protein (non-IgM type) <30 g/L
Clonal bone marrow plasma cells <10%[a]
Absence of myeloma-defining events or amyloidosis that can be attributed to the plasma cell proliferative disorder
Smoldering Multiple Myeloma (Asymptomatic Myeloma)
Both criteria must be met:
• Serum monoclonal protein (IgG or IgA) ≥30 g/L or urinary monoclonal protein ≥500 mg per 24 h and/or clonal bone marrow plasma cells 10–60%
• Absence of myeloma-defining events or amyloidosis
Symptomatic Multiple Myeloma
Clonal bone marrow plasma cells or biopsy-proven bony or extramedullary plasmacytoma[a] and any one or more of the following myeloma-defining events:
• Evidence of one or more indicators of end-organ damage that can be attributed to the underlying plasma cell proliferative disorder, specifically:
• Hypercalcemia: serum calcium >0.25 mmol/L (>1 mg/dL) higher than the upper limit of normal or >2.75 mmol/L (>11 mg/dL)
• Renal insufficiency: creatinine clearance <40 mL/min[b] or serum creatinine >177 μmol/L (>2 mg/dL)
• Anemia: hemoglobin value of >20 g/L below the lower limit of normal, or a hemoglobin value <100 g/L
• Bone lesions: one or more osteolytic lesions on skeletal radiography, CT, or PET-CT[c]
• Any one or more of the following biomarkers of malignancy:
• Clonal bone marrow plasma cell percentage[a] ≥60%
• Involved: uninvolved serum free light chain ratio[d] ≥100
• >1 focal lesion on MRI studies[e]
Nonsecretory Myeloma
No M protein in serum and/or urine with immunofixation[f]
Bone marrow clonal plasmacytosis ≥10% or plasmacytoma[a]
Myeloma-related organ or tissue impairment (end-organ damage, as described above)
Solitary Plasmacytoma
Biopsy-proven solitary lesion of bone or soft tissue with evidence of clonal plasma cells
Normal bone marrow with no evidence of clonal plasma cells[a]
Normal skeletal survey and MRI (or CT) of spine and pelvis (except for the primary solitary lesion)
Absence of end-organ damage such as hypercalcemia, renal insufficiency, anemia, or bone lesions (CRAB) that can be attributed to a lymphoplasma cell proliferative disorder
POEMS Syndrome
All of the following four criteria must be met:
1. Polyneuropathy
2. Monoclonal plasma cell proliferative disorder
3. Any one of the following: (a) sclerotic bone lesions; (b) Castleman's disease; (c) elevated levels of vascular endothelial growth factor (VEGF)
4. Any one of the following: (a) organomegaly (splenomegaly, hepatomegaly, or lymphadenopathy); (b) extravascular volume overload (edema, pleural effusion, or ascites); (c) endocrinopathy (adrenal, thyroid, pituitary, gonadal, parathyroid, and pancreatic); (d) skin changes (hyperpigmentation, hypertrichosis, glomeruloid hemangiomata, plethora, acrocyanosis, flushing, and white nails); (e) papilledema; (f) thrombocytosis/polycythemia[g]

[a]Clonality should be established by showing κ/λ light chain restriction on flow cytometry, immunohistochemistry, or immunofluorescence. Bone marrow plasma cell percentage should preferably be estimated from a core biopsy specimen; in case of a disparity between the aspirate and core biopsy, the highest value should be used. [b]Measured or estimated by validated equations. [c]If bone marrow has <10% clonal plasma cells, more than one bone lesion is required to distinguish from solitary plasmacytoma with minimal marrow involvement. [d]These values are based on the serum Freelite assay (The Binding Site Group, Birmingham, United Kingdom). The involved free light chain must be ≥100 mg/L. [e]Each focal lesion must be ≥5 mm in size. [f]A small M component may sometimes be present. [g]These features should have no other attributable causes and have temporal relation with each other.

Abbreviations: PET-CT, ^{18}F-fluorodeoxyglucose positron emission tomography with computed tomography; POEMS, polyneuropathy, organomegaly, endocrinopathy, M-protein, and skin changes.

with median survivals of ≥10 years. Solitary bone plasmacytoma is a single lytic bone lesion without marrow plasmacytosis. Extramedullary plasmacytomas usually involve the submucosal lymphoid tissue of the nasopharynx or paranasal sinuses without marrow plasmacytosis. Both tumors are highly responsive to local radiation therapy. If an M component is present, it should disappear after treatment. Solitary bone plasmacytomas may recur in other bony sites or evolve into myeloma. Extramedullary plasmacytomas rarely recur or progress.

Serum protein electrophoresis and measurement of serum immunoglobulins and free light chains are useful for detecting and characterizing M spikes, supplemented by immunoelectrophoresis, which is especially sensitive for identifying low concentrations of M components not detectable by protein electrophoresis. A 24-h urine specimen is necessary to quantitate Bence Jones protein (immunoglobulin light chain) excretion. The serum M component will be IgG in 53% of patients, IgA in 25%, and IgD in 1%; 20% of patients will have only light chains in serum and urine. Dipsticks for detecting proteinuria are not reliable at identifying light chains, and the heat test for detecting Bence Jones protein is falsely negative in ~50% of patients with light chain myeloma. Fewer than 1% of patients have no identifiable M component; these patients usually have light chain myeloma in which renal catabolism has made the light chains undetectable in the urine. In most of these patients, light chains can now be detected by serum free light chain assay. IgD myeloma may also present with light chain disease. About two-thirds of patients with serum M components also have urinary light chains. The light chain isotype may have an impact on disease behavior. Whether this is due to some genetically important determinant of cell proliferation or because lambda light chains are more likely to cause renal damage and form amyloid than are kappa light chains is unclear. The heavy chain isotype may have an impact on patient management as well. About half of patients with IgM paraproteins develop hyperviscosity compared with only 2–4% of patients with IgA and IgG M components. Among IgG myelomas, it is the IgG3 subclass that has the highest tendency to form both concentration- and temperature-dependent aggregates, leading to hyperviscosity and cold agglutination at lower serum concentrations. A standard workup directed at detecting monoclonal plasma cells and myeloma-defining events as well as prognosis is detailed in **Table 111-2**.

A complete blood count with differential may reveal anemia. Erythrocyte sedimentation rate is elevated. Rare patients (~1%) may have plasma cell leukemia with >2000 plasma cells/μL. This may be seen in disproportionate frequency in IgD (12%) and IgE (25%) myelomas. Serum calcium, urea nitrogen, creatinine, and uric acid levels may be elevated. Serum alkaline phosphatase is usually normal even with extensive bone involvement because of the absence of osteoblastic activity. It is also important to quantitate serum β_2-microglobulin and albumin (see below).

Chest and bone radiographs may reveal lytic lesions or diffuse osteopenia. Magnetic resonance imaging (MRI) offers a sensitive means to document extent of bone marrow infiltration and cord or root compression in patients with pain syndromes. ^{18}F-fluorodeoxyglucose (^{18}F-FDG) positron emission tomography (PET)/computed tomography (CT) is a valuable tool to assess bone damage and detect extramedullary sites of the disease (Fig. 111-5). The use of ^{18}F-FDG PET/CT is recommended to distinguish between smoldering and active MM and to confirm a suspected diagnosis of solitary plasmacytoma. It is also a valuable tool to evaluate response in patients with oligo- or nonsecretory myeloma.

PROGNOSIS

Serum β_2-microglobulin is the single most powerful predictor of survival and can substitute for staging. β_2-Microglobulin is the light chain of the class I major histocompatibility antigens (HLA-A, -B, -C) on the surface of every cell. Combination of serum β_2-microglobulin and albumin levels forms the basis for a three-stage International Staging System (ISS) (**Table 111-3**) that predicts survival. With the use of high-dose therapy and the newer agents, the Durie-Salmon staging system is unable to predict outcome and is no longer used. High labeling index, circulating plasma cells, performance status, and high levels of lactate dehydrogenase are also associated with poor prognosis.

TABLE 111-2 Standard Investigative Workup in Multiple Myeloma (MM)

Investigations to Evaluate for Clonal Plasma Cells
Bone marrow aspirate and biopsy (fine-needle aspiration of plasmacytoma if indicated)
• Histology
• Clonality by kappa/lambda immunostaining by flow cytometry or immunohistochemistry
Investigations to Evaluate Clonal Paraprotein
Serum protein electrophoresis and immunofixation
Quantitative serum immunoglobulin levels (IgG, IgA, and IgM)
24-h urine protein electrophoresis and immunofixation
Serum free light chain and ratio
Immunofixation for IgD or IgE in select cases
Investigation to Evaluate End-Organ Damage
Hemogram to assess for anemia
Chemistry panel for renal function and calcium
Skeletal survey to evaluate bone lesions
PET/CT or MRI if smoldering MM or solitary plasmacytoma with no other MDE or extramedullary disease
Investigation for Risk Stratification
β_2-Microglobulin and serum albumin for ISS stage
Fluorescent in situ hybridization for hyperdipoidy, del17p, t(4;14); t(11;14), t(14;16), t(14;20), amp1q34, and del13 on bone marrow sample
LDH
Specialized Investigation in Selected Cases
Abdominal fat pad for amyloid
Serum viscosity if IgM component or high IgA levels or serum M component >7 g/dL
Myd88 and *CXCR4* mutation analysis if IgM component

Abbreviations: ISS, International Staging System; LDH, lactate dehydrogenase; MRI, magnetic resonance imaging; PET/CT, positron emission tomography/computed tomography.

Other factors that may influence prognosis are detection of any cytogenetic abnormalities including hypodiploidy by karyotype, fluorescent in situ hybridization (FISH)–identified chromosome 17p deletion, and translocations t(4;14), (14;16), and t(14;20) and 1q34 amplification. Chromosome 13q deletion, previously thought to predict poor outcome, is not a predictor following the use of newer agents. The ISS system incorporating the cytogenetic changes (Revised ISS) is the most widely used method for assessing prognosis (Table 111-3). Microarray profiling has formed the basis for RNA-based prognostic staging systems. Genome sequencing efforts have allowed for characterization of critical genes, pathways, and clonal heterogeneity in myeloma. The median number of mutations per transcribed genome in myeloma is ~58, and within the whole genome, it is >7000. A very heterogeneous mutational landscape with no unifying mutation has been observed. The most frequently mutated genes are *KRAS* and *NRAS* (~20% each), followed by *TP53, DIS3, FAM46C*, and *BRAF*, all mutated in 5–10% of patients. All other mutations were observed in <5% of the patients. These results are now being applied to develop new targeted personalized therapies in myeloma.

TREATMENT

Multiple Myeloma

MGUS, SMM, AND SOLITARY PLASMACYTOMA

No specific intervention is indicated for patients with MGUS. Follow-up once a year or less frequently is adequate except in higher-risk MGUS, where serum protein electrophoresis, complete blood count, creatinine, and calcium should be repeated every 6 months. A patient with MGUS and severe polyneuropathy is considered for therapeutic intervention if a causal relationship can be

TABLE 111-3 Risk Stratification in Myeloma

CHROMOSOMAL ABNORMALITIES (CA)		
METHOD	STANDARD RISK (80%) (EXPECTED SURVIVAL 6–7+ YEARS)	HIGH RISK (20%) (EXPECTED SURVIVAL 2–3 YEARS)
Karyotype	No chromosomal aberration	Any abnormality on conventional karyotype
FISH	t(11;14) del(13)	del(17p) t(4:14) t(14:16) t(14;20) amp 1q34
INTERNATIONAL STAGING SYSTEM (ISS)		
	STAGE	MEDIAN SURVIVAL, MONTHS
β_2M <3.5, alb ≥3.5	I (28%)[a]	62
β_2M <3.5, alb <3.5 *or* β_2M = 3.5–5.5	II (39%)	44
β_2M >5.5	III (33%)	29
REVISED INTERNATIONAL STAGING SYSTEM (R-ISS)		
Stage I: ISS stage 1; standard risk for CA and normal LDH		
Stage II: Patients not meeting criteria for stage I or stage III		
Stage III: ISS stage III and either high risk for CA *or* high LDH		
Other features suggesting high-risk disease: De novo plasma cell leukemia Extramedullary disease Elevated LDH High-risk gene expression profile		

[a]Percentage of patients presenting at each stage.

Abbreviations: β_2M, serum β_2-microglobulin in mg/L; alb, serum albumin in g/dL; FISH, fluorescent in situ hybridization; LDH, lactate dehydrogenase.

assumed, especially in the absence of any other potential causes for neuropathy. Therapy can include plasmapheresis and occasionally rituximab in patients with IgM MGUS or myeloma-like therapy in those with IgG or IgA disease. A subset of patients with MGUS develop renal dysfunction usually based on renal damage from the monoclonal antibody. The damage may affect the glomeruli, tubules, or vessels. No consensus exists on management, but lowering the level of the monoclonal antibody with bortezomib has had some advocates.

About 10% of patients have SMM and will have an indolent course demonstrating only slow progression of disease over many years. For patients with SMM, no specific therapeutic intervention is indicated, although early intervention with lenalidomide and dexamethasone may prevent progression from high-risk SMM to active MM. At present, patients with SMM only require antitumor therapy when myeloma-defining events are identified.

Patients with solitary bone plasmacytomas and extramedullary plasmacytomas may be expected to enjoy prolonged disease-free survival after local radiation therapy at a dose of ~40 Gy. Occult marrow involvement may occur at low incidence in patients with solitary bone plasmacytoma. Such patients are usually identified because their serum M component falls slowly or disappears initially after local therapy, only to return after a few months. These patients respond well to systemic therapy.

SYMPTOMATIC MM

Patients with symptomatic myeloma require therapeutic intervention. In general, such therapy has two purposes: (1) systemic therapy to control myeloma; and (2) supportive care to control symptoms of the disease, its complications, and adverse effects of therapy. Therapy can significantly prolong survival and improve the quality of life for myeloma patients.

The therapy of myeloma includes an initial induction regimen followed by consolidation and/or maintenance therapy and, on subsequent progression, management of relapsed disease. All agents available for use at various stages of the therapy and their doses, schedules, and combinations are detailed in **Table 111-4**. Therapy is partly dictated by the patient's age and comorbidities, which may affect a patient's ability to undergo high-dose therapy and transplantation (**Fig. 111-6**).

Three important classes of agents approved for treatment of newly diagnosed MM are immunomodulatory agents, proteasome inhibitors, and targeted antibodies. Thalidomide, when combined with dexamethasone, achieved responses in two-thirds of newly diagnosed MM patients. Subsequently, lenalidomide, an immunomodulatory derivative of thalidomide, and bortezomib, a proteasome inhibitor, have each been combined with dexamethasone with high response rates (>80%) in newly diagnosed patients with MM. Importantly, their lower toxicity profile with improved efficacy has made them the preferred agents for induction therapy. Efforts to improve the depth and frequency of response have involved using three-drug regimens. The combination of lenalidomide with a proteasome inhibitor (bortezomib or carfilzomib) and dexamethasone achieves close to a 100% response rate and a >30% complete response (CR) rate, making this combination one of the preferred induction regimens in transplant-eligible patients. Other similar three-drug combinations (bortezomib, thalidomide, and dexamethasone or bortezomib, cyclophosphamide, and dexamethasone) also achieve >90% response rate. Addition of a fourth agent, daratumumab, an anti-CD38 antibody, is providing even deeper responses. Usually between four and six cycles of these combination regimens are utilized to achieve initial deep cytoreduction before consideration of high-dose therapy with autologous stem cell transplantation.

In patients who are not transplant candidates due to physiologic age >70 years, significant cardiopulmonary problems, or other comorbid illnesses, the same two- or three-drug combinations described above are considered standard of care as induction therapy with age- and frailty-guided dose and schedule modifications. Modified lenalidomide-bortezomib-dexamethasone (RVD lite) combination achieves high overall response rate (86%) and CR (32%). Intermittent pulses of melphalan, an alkylating agent, with prednisone (MP) are combined with novel agents to achieve superior response and survival outcomes. In patients >65 years old, combining thalidomide with MP (MPT) obtains higher response rates and overall survival compared with MP alone. Similarly, significantly improved response (71 vs 35%) and overall survival (3-year survival 72 vs 59%) were observed with the combination of bortezomib and MP compared with MP alone. Continuous use of the lenalidomide and dexamethasone combination appears to be superior to the MPT regimen, and its combination with the anti-CD38 antibody daratumumab provides even higher overall response (92.9%) and CR rates (46.7%) and improved survival; the combination of lenalidomide, dexamethasone, and daratumumab is a standard-of-care regimen for older adults with myeloma.

HIGH-DOSE THERAPY WITH AUTOLOGOUS STEM CELL TRANSPLANTATION

High-dose therapy (HDT) and consolidation/maintenance are standard practice in the majority of eligible patients. In patients who are transplant candidates, alkylating agents such as melphalan should be avoided because they damage stem cells and compromise the ability to collect stem cells. Similarly, in patients receiving lenalidomide, stem cells should be collected within 6 months because the continued use of lenalidomide may compromise the ability to collect adequate numbers of stem cells. Randomized studies comparing standard-dose therapy to high-dose melphalan therapy with hematopoietic stem cell support have shown that HDT can achieve higher overall response rates, with up to 25–40% additional CRs and prolonged progression-free and overall survival; however, few, if any, patients are cured. Although two successive HDTs (tandem

TABLE 111-4 Standard Therapeutic Agents in Myeloma

CLASS	AGENT	STANDARD DOSAGE AND ADMINISTRATION	COMBINATION	MYELOMA INDICATION
Immunomodulatory drugs (IMiD)	Thalidomide (T)	Oral 50–200 mg qd	TD, VTD	Newly diagnosed and relapsed
	Lenalidomide (R)	Oral 5–25 mg daily × 21 days q 4 weeks	RD, RVD, DaRD, ERD, KRD, IRD	Newly diagnosed, maintenance, and relapsed
	Pomalidomide (P)	Oral 2–4 mg daily × 21 days q 4 weeks	PD	Relapsed
Proteasome inhibitors (PI)	Bortezomib (V)	IV or SC 1.3 mg/m² days 1, 4, 8, 11 OR days 1, 8, 15	VD, VTD, VRD, DaVD, VCD	Newly diagnosed and relapsed
	Carfilzomib (K)	IV 20–56 mg/m² days 1, 2, 8, 9, 15, 16 q 4 weeks	KD, KRD, KPD, Da KD, Da KRD, IsaKD	Newly diagnosed and relapsed
	Ixazomib (I)	Oral 4 mg days 1, 8, 15	IRD	Relapsed
Antibodies	Daratumumab (Da)	IV 16 mg/kg per week for 8 weeks then every 2 weeks for 16 weeks and then every 4 weeks thereafter	Dara, DaRD, DaVD, DaPD, DaKD	Newly diagnosed, maintenance, and relapsed
	Elotuzumab (E)	IV 10 mg/kg days 1, 8, 15, and 22 for first two cycles, then on days 1 and 15; along with RD	ERD, EPD	Relapsed
	Isatuximab (Isa)	IV 10 mg/kg weekly for 4 weeks and then every 2 weeks	IsaPD, IsaKD	Relapsed
	Belantamab mafodotin	IV 2.5 mg/kg once every 3 weeks		Relapsed or refractory - 4 prior lines of therapy
Selective inhibitor of nuclear export (SINE)	Selinexor (S)	Oral 80 mg on days 1 and 3 of each week	SVD	Relapsed
Histone deacetylase inhibitor	Panobinostat (Pa)	Oral 20 mg once every other day for 3 doses/week for 2 weeks every 21 days	PaVD	Relapsed
Alkylating agents	Melphalan (M)	Oral 0.25 mg/kg per day for 4 days (with P) every 4–6 weeks	MP, MPT, MPR, MPV, DaMPV, high-dose M	Newly diagnosed and relapsed conditioning
	Cyclophosphamide (C)	IV—300–500 mg/m² weekly × 2 q 4 weeks Oral—50 mg qd × 21 days	VCD	Newly diagnosed and relapsed
	Bendamustine (B)	IV 70–90 mg days 1, 2 OR days 1, 8 q 4 weeks	BD or BVD	Relapsed
	Melflufen (Me)	IV 40 mg day 1 (with D 40 mg on days 1, 8, 15, and 22) q 28 days	MeD	Relapsed or refractory - 4 prior lines of therapy
Cellular therapy	Idecabtagene vicleucel (Ide-cel)	IV 450 × 10⁶ cells	None	Relapsed or refractory - 4 prior lines of therapy with prior exposure to PI, IMiD, and anti-CD38 antibody
Glucocorticoid	Dexamethasone (D)	Oral 10–40 mg q week		All stages
	Prednisone (P)	Oral 1 mg/kg		

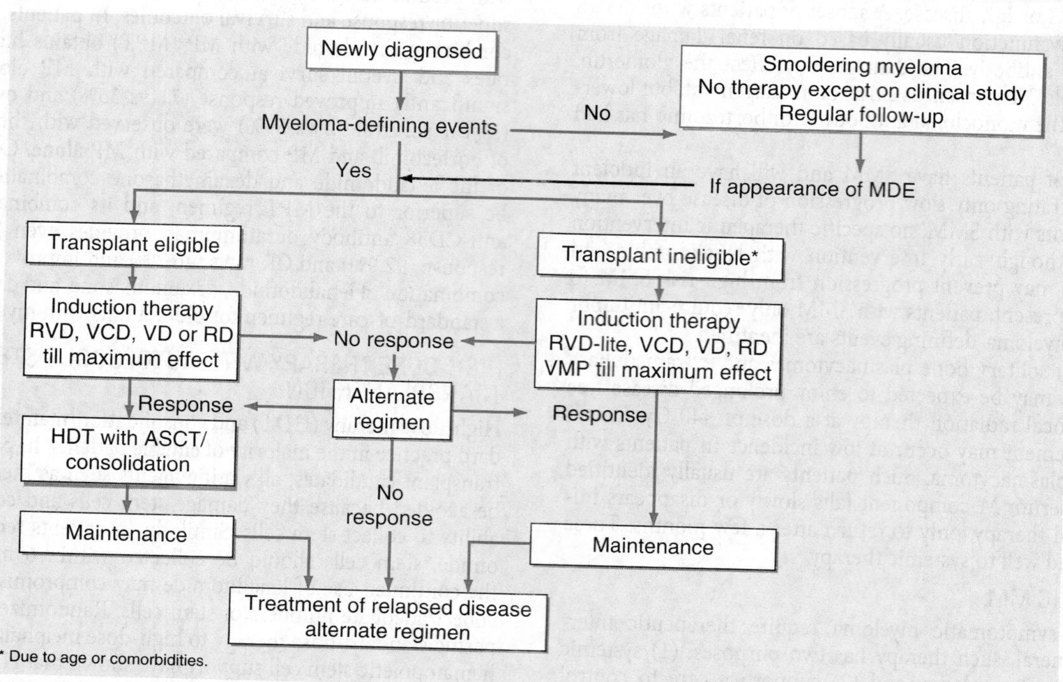

FIGURE 111-6 Treatment algorithm for multiple myeloma. C, cyclophosphamide; D, dexamethasone; M, melphalan; P, prednisone; R, lenalidomide; RVD-lite, weekly regimen; V, bortezomib. *Alternate regimen* indicates combinations including daratumumab, elotuzumab, panobinostat, carfilzomib, ixazomib, pomalidomide, or other agents. ASCT, autologous stem cell transplantation; HDT, high-dose therapy; MDE, myeloma-defining events.

transplantations) are more effective than single HDT, the benefit is only observed in the subset of patients who do not achieve a complete or very good partial response to the first transplantation, which is a rare subset. Moreover, a randomized study failed to show any significant difference in overall survival between early transplantation after induction therapy versus delayed transplantation at relapse. These data allow an option to delay transplantation, especially with the availability of newer agents and combinations. Allogeneic transplantations may also produce high response rates, but with significant toxicities. Nonmyeloablative allogeneic transplantation can reduce toxicity but is recommended only under the auspices of a clinical trial to exploit an immune graft-versus-myeloma effect while avoiding attendant toxicity.

Maintenance therapy prolongs remissions following standard-dose regimens as well as HDT. Two phase 3 studies have demonstrated improved progression-free survival, and one study showed prolonged overall survival in patients receiving lenalidomide compared to placebo as maintenance therapy after HDT. In non-transplant candidates, two phase 3 studies showed prolonged progression-free survival with lenalidomide maintenance after MP plus lenalidomide or lenalidomide plus dexamethasone induction therapy. Although concern arises regarding an increased incidence of second primary malignancies in patients receiving lenalidomide maintenance, its benefits in reducing the risk of progressive disease and death from myeloma far outweigh the small increased risk of second cancers. In patients with high-risk cytogenetics, lenalidomide and bortezomib or an oral proteasome inhibitor, ixazomib, show promise as maintenance combination therapy after transplantation.

RELAPSED DISEASE

Relapsed myeloma can be treated with a number of agents including lenalidomide and/or bortezomib, if previously not used. The second-generation proteasome inhibitor carfilzomib and immunomodulatory agent pomalidomide have shown efficacy in relapsed and refractory MM, even MM refractory to lenalidomide and bortezomib. An oral proteasome inhibitor, ixazomib, has also been approved in combination with lenalidomide and dexamethasone as an all-oral regimen for relapsed MM. Three antibodies are approved for treatment of relapsed MM. Daratumumab targeting CD38 achieves high response rates and improved progression-free survival as a single agent with further improvement in response and survival when added to bortezomib and dexamethasone or lenalidomide and dexamethasone. A formulation of daratumumab for subcutaneous administration provides decreased toxicity and improved convenience. Isatuximab, another antibody targeting CD38, achieves high response rates and improved progression-free survival in combination with pomalidomide or carfilzomib and dexamethasone. Elotuzumab, which targets SLAMF7, has shown significant activity in combination with lenalidomide and dexamethasone in relapsed/refractory myeloma but not as a single agent. Panobinostat, a histone deacetylase inhibitor, in combination with bortezomib and dexamethasone has been approved for treatment of relapsed refractory myeloma based on superior response and progression-free survival compared to bortezomib and dexamethasone alone. Two additional newer agents have unique mechanisms of action: selinexor is a first-in-class exportin inhibitor that blocks export of proteins from the cell nucleus, and melflufen is an alkylating agent conjugated to a peptide to improve specific delivery to myeloma cells that express aminopeptidase required for cleaving of the peptide to deliver the drug intracellularly in myeloma cells. Both agents have been approved based on their effectiveness in relapsed/refractory myeloma. Another therapeutic focus has been to target BCMA, which is exclusively expressed on normal plasma cells and myeloma cells. An anti-BCMA antibody-drug conjugate, belantamab, targets BCMA and delivers auristatin to the tumor cells and achieves responses in relapsed/refractory myeloma. The drug has a unique ophthalmologic toxicity that requires close monitoring. Finally, a cellular therapy approved for myeloma is an anti-BCMA CAR transduced T cell (idecabtagene vicleucel [Ide-cel]), which is approved beyond fourth-line therapy. In patients with advanced myeloma with a median of six prior lines of treatment, 73% of patients receiving Ide-cel responded, and a CR rate of 33% was observed. Cytokine release syndrome and neurotoxicity remain primary toxicities requiring close monitoring and aggressive management. BCMA is also the target for a number of investigational agents including other CAR-T cell approaches as well as bispecific antibodies combining anti-BCMA with anti-CD3 antibody. Incorporation of the large number of active agents at various stages of treatment, including in newly diagnosed patients, is improving survival as well as quality of life.

THERAPY ENDPOINT

Improvement in the serum M component may lag behind the symptomatic improvement due to longer serum half-life (~3 weeks) of the immunoglobulin. The fall in M component depends on the rate of tumor kill and the fractional catabolic rate of immunoglobulin. Serum and urine light chains with a functional half-life of ~6 h may fall much quicker within the first week of treatment. Because urine light chain levels may relate to renal tubular function, they are not a reliable measure of tumor cell kill in patients with renal dysfunction. Achieving CR, defined as disappearance of serum and urine monoclonal protein with normal bone marrow by light microscopy, has been a standard goal of therapy. However, sequencing or multicolor flow cytometry–based assessment of minimal residual disease (MRD) in bone marrow to measure the presence of one myeloma cell in a million cells is being considered as an important new endpoint, especially in newly diagnosed patients. Absence of MRD at this sensitivity predicts for both longer progression-free survival and longer overall survival. Although patients may not achieve complete remission, clinical responses may last for long periods of time in small numbers of patients.

The median overall survival of patients with myeloma is 8+ years, with subsets of younger patients surviving >10 years. The major causes of death are progressive myeloma, renal failure, sepsis, or therapy-related myelodysplasia. Nearly a quarter of patients die of myocardial infarction, chronic lung disease, diabetes, or stroke, which are all intercurrent illnesses related more to the age of the patient group than to the tumor.

SUPPORTIVE THERAPY

Herpes zoster prophylaxis is indicated if bortezomib is used, and neuropathy attendant to bortezomib can be decreased both by its subcutaneous administration and by administration on a weekly schedule. Lenalidomide use requires prophylaxis for deep-vein thrombosis (DVT) with either aspirin or, if patients are at a greater risk of DVT, warfarin, low-molecular-weight heparin, or direct-acting anticoagulants. Patients receiving anti-BCMA CAR-T cell therapy may need supplementation with intravenous γ globulin due to induction of prolonged hypogammaglobulinemia.

Supportive care directed at the anticipated complications of the disease may be as important as primary antitumor therapy. Hypercalcemia generally responds well to bisphosphonates, glucocorticoid therapy, hydration, and natriuresis and rarely requires calcitonin as well. Bisphosphonates (e.g., pamidronate 90 mg or zoledronate 4 mg initially once a month for 12–24 months and later every 2–3 months) reduce osteoclastic bone resorption and preserve performance status and quality of life, decrease bone-related complications, and may also have antitumor effects. Osteonecrosis of the jaw and renal dysfunction can occur in a minority of patients receiving bisphosphonate therapy. Denosumab is an alternative agent administered intravenously at 120 mg monthly and achieves a similar level of effect as bisphosphonates to prevent bone-related complications in myeloma. Treatments aimed at strengthening the skeleton such as fluorides, calcium, and vitamin D, with or without androgens, have been suggested but are not of proven efficacy. Kyphoplasty or vertebroplasty should be considered in patients with painful collapsed vertebra. Iatrogenic worsening of renal function may be prevented by maintaining a high fluid intake to prevent dehydration and enhance excretion of light chains and calcium. In the event of acute renal failure, plasmapheresis is ~10 times more effective at clearing light chains than peritoneal dialysis; however, its role in reversing renal failure remains controversial. Importantly, reducing the protein load by effective antitumor therapy with agents such as bortezomib may result in improvement in renal function in over half of the patients. Use of lenalidomide in renal failure is possible but requires dose modification because it is renally excreted. Urinary tract infections should be watched for and treated early. Plasmapheresis may be the treatment of choice for hyperviscosity syndromes. Although the pneumococcus is a dreaded pathogen in myeloma patients, pneumococcal polysaccharide vaccines may not elicit an antibody response. The pneumococcal conjugate vaccines are more protective. Prophylactic administration of intravenous γ globulin preparations is used in the setting of recurrent serious infections. Chronic oral antibiotic prophylaxis is not warranted. Patients developing neurologic symptoms in the lower extremities, severe localized back pain, or problems with bowel and bladder control may need emergency MRI and local radiation therapy and glucocorticoids if cord compression is identified. In patients in whom neurologic deficit is increasing or substantial, emergent surgical decompression may be necessary. Most bone lesions respond to analgesics and systemic therapy, but certain painful lesions may respond more promptly to localized radiation. The anemia associated with myeloma may respond to erythropoietin along with hematinics (iron, folate, cobalamin). The pathogenesis of the anemia should be established and specific therapy instituted, whenever possible.

WALDENSTRÖM'S MACROGLOBULINEMIA

In 1948, Waldenström described a malignancy of lymphoplasmacytoid cells that secreted IgM. In contrast to myeloma, the disease was associated with lymphadenopathy and hepatosplenomegaly, but the major clinical manifestation was hyperviscosity syndrome. The disease resembles the related diseases CLL, myeloma, and lymphocytic lymphoma. It originates from a post–germinal center B cell that has undergone somatic mutations and antigenic selection in the lymphoid follicle and has the characteristics of an IgM-bearing memory B cell. Waldenström's macroglobulinemia (WM) and IgM myeloma follow a similar clinical course, but therapeutic options are different. The diagnosis of IgM myeloma is usually reserved for patients with lytic bone lesions and predominant infiltration with CD138+ plasma cells in the bone marrow. Such patients are at greater risk of pathologic fractures than patients with WM.

A familial occurrence is common in WM, but its molecular bases are yet unclear. A distinct *MYD88* L265P somatic mutation is present in >90% of patients with WM and the majority of IgM MGUS. Other commonly occurring mutations include *CXCR4* (30–40%), *ARID1A* (17%), and *CD79B* (8–15%). Presence of *MYD88* mutation status is now used as a diagnostic test to discriminate WM from marginal zone lymphomas (MZLs), IgM-secreting myeloma, and CLL with plasmacytic differentiation. This mutation also explains the molecular pathogenesis of the disease with involvement of Toll-like receptor (TLR) and interleukin 1 receptor (IL-1R) signaling leading to activation of IL-1R–associated kinase (IRAK) 4 and IRAK1 followed by nuclear factor-κB (NF-κB) activation. *MYD88* mutation also triggers Bruton's tyrosine kinase (BTK) and hemopoietic cell kinase (HCK)-mediated growth and survival signaling, which are now important therapeutic targets in WM. *CXCR4* mutations induce AKT and extracellular regulated kinase 1/2 (ERK1/2) signaling. This pathway can lead to development of drug resistance in the presence of its ligand CXCL12.

The disease is similar to myeloma in being slightly more common in men and occurring with increased incidence with increasing age (median age 64 years). The IgM in some patients with macroglobulinemia may have specificity for myelin-associated glycoprotein (MAG), a protein that has been associated with demyelinating disease of the peripheral nervous system and may be lost earlier and to a greater extent than the better-known myelin basic protein in patients with multiple sclerosis. Sometimes patients with macroglobulinemia develop a peripheral neuropathy, and half of these patients are positive for anti-MAG antibody. The neuropathy may precede the appearance of the neoplasm. The whole process may begin with a viral infection that may elicit an antibody response that cross-reacts with a normal tissue component.

Like myeloma, the disease involves the bone marrow, but unlike myeloma, it does not cause bone lesions or hypercalcemia. Bone marrow shows >10% infiltration with lymphoplasmacytic cells (surface IgM+, CD19+, CD20+, and CD22+, rarely CD5+, but CD10– and CD23–) with an increase in number of mast cells. Like myeloma, an M component is present in the serum in excess of 30 g/L (3 g/dL), but unlike myeloma, the size of the IgM paraprotein results in little renal excretion, and only ~20% of patients excrete light chains. Therefore, renal disease is not common. The light chain isotype is kappa in 80% of the cases. Patients present with weakness, fatigue, and recurrent infections similar to myeloma patients, but epistaxis, visual disturbances, and neurologic symptoms such as peripheral neuropathy, dizziness, headache, and transient paresis are much more common in macroglobulinemia. Presence of *MYD88* and *CXCR4* mutations also affects disease presentation. Presence of *CXCR4* mutations is associated with higher bone marrow disease burden and higher incidence of hyperviscosity. Patients with wild-type *MYD88* show lower bone marrow disease burden.

Physical examination reveals adenopathy and hepatosplenomegaly, and ophthalmoscopic examination may reveal vascular segmentation and dilation of the retinal veins characteristic of hyperviscosity states. Patients may have a normocytic, normochromic anemia, but rouleaux formation and a positive Coombs test are much more common than in myeloma. Malignant lymphocytes are usually present in the peripheral blood. About 10% of macroglobulins are cryoglobulins. These are pure M components and are not the mixed cryoglobulins seen in rheumatoid arthritis and other autoimmune diseases. Mixed cryoglobulins are composed of IgM or IgA complexed with IgG, for which they are specific. In both cases, Raynaud's phenomenon and serious vascular symptoms precipitated by the cold may occur, but mixed cryoglobulins are not commonly associated with malignancy. Patients suspected of having a cryoglobulin based on history and physical examination should have their blood drawn into a warm syringe and delivered to the laboratory in a container of warm water to avoid errors in quantitating the cryoglobulin.

TREATMENT

Waldenström's Macroglobulinemia

A diagnosis of WM requires lymphoplasmacytic infiltrate of any level in the bone marrow and an IgM monoclonal paraprotein of any size. Treatment is usually not initiated unless the disease is symptomatic or increasing anemia, hyperviscosity, lymphadenopathy, or hepatosplenomegaly is present. Control of serious hyperviscosity symptoms such as an altered state of consciousness or paresis can be achieved acutely by plasmapheresis because 80% of the IgM paraprotein is intravascular. The median survival of affected individuals is ~50 months. However, many patients with WM have indolent disease that does not require therapy. Pretreatment parameters including older age, male sex, general symptoms, and cytopenias define a high-risk population. BTK inhibitors (ibrutinib), alkylating drugs (bendamustine and cyclophosphamide), and proteasome inhibitors (bortezomib, carfilzomib, and ixazomib), alone or more frequently in combination with rituximab, are considered as first-line therapy for symptomatic patients with WM. Ibrutinib targets the constitutively activated BTK. In patients with one prior line of therapy, the overall response to ibrutinib was 91%. Best responses to ibrutinib are observed in patients with mutated *MYD88* and wild-type *CXCR4* status, while delayed and lower response rates to ibrutinib are observed in patients with mutated *CXCR4*. At first relapse, in patients with an initial durable response, either the previous regimen or another primary therapy regimen can be used. The therapeutic choice is dependent upon the genomic features, drug availability, and the patient's clinical profile.

Rituximab can produce an IgM flare, so either plasmapheresis should be used before rituximab or its use should be initially withheld in patients with high IgM levels. Fludarabine (25 mg/m^2 per d for 5 days every 4 weeks) and cladribine (0.1 mg/kg per d for 7 days every 4 weeks) are also highly effective single agents. With identification of the *MYD88* mutation, novel BTK inhibitors (acalabrutinib, zanubrutinib, and tirabrutinib), inhibitors targeting IRAK1/4, and the BCL2 antagonist venetoclax are being explored for the treatment of WM. Although HDT plus autologous transplantation is an option, its use has declined due to the availability of other effective agents.

POEMS SYNDROME

The features of this syndrome are *p*olyneuropathy, *o*rganomegaly, *e*ndocrinopathy, *M*-protein, and *s*kin changes (POEMS). Diagnostic criteria are described in Table 111-1. Patients usually have a severe, progressive sensorimotor polyneuropathy associated with sclerotic bone lesions from myeloma. Polyneuropathy occurs in ~1.4% of myelomas, but the POEMS syndrome is only a rare subset of that group. Unlike typical myeloma, hepatomegaly and lymphadenopathy occur in about two-thirds of patients, and splenomegaly is seen in one-third. The lymphadenopathy frequently resembles Castleman's disease histologically, a condition that has been linked to IL-6 overproduction. The endocrine manifestations include amenorrhea in women and impotence and gynecomastia in men. Hyperprolactinemia due to loss of normal inhibitory control by the hypothalamus may be associated with other central nervous system manifestations such as papilledema and elevated cerebrospinal fluid pressure and protein. Type 2 diabetes mellitus occurs in about one-third of patients. Hypothyroidism and adrenal insufficiency are occasionally noted. Skin changes are diverse: hyperpigmentation, hypertrichosis, skin thickening, and digital clubbing. Other manifestations include peripheral edema, ascites, pleural effusions, fever, and thrombocytosis. Not all the components of POEMS syndrome may be present initially.

The pathogenesis of the disease is unclear, but high circulating levels of the proinflammatory cytokines IL-1, IL-6, VEGF, and TNF have been documented, and levels of the inhibitory cytokine transforming growth factor β are lower than expected. Treatment of the myeloma may result in an improvement in the other disease manifestations.

Patients are often treated similarly to those with myeloma. Plasmapheresis does not appear to be of benefit in POEMS syndrome. Patients presenting with isolated sclerotic lesions may have resolution of neuropathic symptoms after local therapy for plasmacytoma with radiotherapy. Similar to MM, novel agents and HDT with autologous stem cell transplantation have been pursued in selected patients and have been associated with prolonged progression-free survival.

HEAVY CHAIN DISEASES

The heavy chain diseases are rare lymphoplasmacytic malignancies. Their clinical manifestations vary with the heavy chain isotype. Patients have absence of light chain and secrete a defective heavy chain that usually has an intact Fc fragment and a deletion in the Fd region. Gamma, alpha, and mu heavy chain diseases have been described, but no reports of delta or epsilon heavy chain diseases have appeared. Molecular biologic analysis of these tumors has revealed structural genetic defects that may account for the aberrant chain secreted.

GAMMA HEAVY CHAIN DISEASE (FRANKLIN'S DISEASE)

This disease affects individuals of widely different age groups and countries of origin. It is characterized by lymphadenopathy, fever, anemia, malaise, hepatosplenomegaly, and weakness. It is frequently associated with autoimmune diseases, especially rheumatoid arthritis. Its most distinctive symptom is palatal edema, resulting from involvement of nodes in Waldeyer's ring, and this may progress to produce respiratory compromise. The diagnosis depends on the demonstration of an anomalous serum M component (often <20 g/L [<2 g/dL]) that reacts with anti-IgG but not anti–light chain reagents. The M component is typically present in both serum and urine. Most of the paraproteins have been of the γ_1 subclass, but other subclasses have been seen. The patients may have thrombocytopenia, eosinophilia, and nondiagnostic bone marrow that may show increased numbers of lymphocytes or plasma cells that do not stain for light chain. Patients usually have a rapid downhill course and die of infection; however, some patients have survived 5 years with chemotherapy. Therapy is indicated when symptomatic and involves chemotherapeutic combinations used in low-grade lymphoma. Rituximab has also been reported to show efficacy.

ALPHA HEAVY CHAIN DISEASE (SELIGMANN'S DISEASE)

This is the most common of the heavy chain diseases. It is closely related to a malignancy known as Mediterranean lymphoma, a disease that affects young persons in parts of the world where intestinal parasites are common, such as the Mediterranean, Asia, and South America. The disease is characterized by an infiltration of the lamina propria of the small intestine with lymphoplasmacytoid cells that secrete truncated alpha chains. Demonstrating alpha heavy chains is difficult because the alpha chains tend to polymerize and appear as a smear instead of a sharp peak on electrophoretic profiles. Despite the polymerization, hyperviscosity is not a common problem in alpha heavy chain disease. Without J chain–facilitated dimerization, viscosity does not increase dramatically. Light chains are absent from serum and urine. The patients present with chronic diarrhea, weight loss, and malabsorption and have extensive mesenteric and paraaortic adenopathy. Respiratory tract involvement occurs rarely. Patients may vary widely in their clinical course. Some may develop diffuse aggressive histologies of malignant lymphoma. Chemotherapy may produce long-term remissions. Rare patients appear to have responded to antibiotic therapy, raising the question of the etiologic role of antigenic stimulation, perhaps by some chronic intestinal infection. Chemotherapy plus antibiotics may be more effective than chemotherapy alone. IPSID is recognized as an infectious pathogen–associated human lymphoma associated with *Campylobacter jejuni*. It involves mainly the proximal small intestine, resulting in malabsorption, diarrhea, and abdominal pain. IPSID is associated with excessive plasma cell differentiation and produces truncated alpha heavy chain proteins lacking the light chains as well as the first constant domain. Early-stage IPSID responds to antibiotics (30–70% complete remission). Most untreated IPSID patients progress to lymphoplasmacytic and immunoblastic lymphoma. Patients not responding to antibiotic therapy are considered for treatment with combination chemotherapy used to treat low-grade lymphoma.

MU HEAVY CHAIN DISEASE

The secretion of isolated mu heavy chains into the serum appears to occur in a very rare subset of patients with CLL. The only features that may distinguish patients with mu heavy chain disease are the presence of vacuoles in the malignant lymphocytes and the excretion of kappa light chains in the urine. The diagnosis requires ultracentrifugation or gel filtration to confirm the nonreactivity of the paraprotein with the light chain reagents because some intact macroglobulins fail to interact with these serums. The tumor cells seem to have a defect in the assembly of light and heavy chains because they appear to contain both in their cytoplasm. Such patients are not treated differently from other patients with CLL (Chap. 107).

FURTHER READING

Attal M et al: IFM 2009 study. Lenalidomide, bortezomib, and dexamethasone with transplantation for myeloma. N Engl J Med 376:1311, 2017.

Corre J et al: Risk factors in multiple myeloma: is it time for a revision? Blood 137:16, 2021.

Hideshima T, Anderson KC: Signaling pathway mediating myeloma cell growth and survival. Cancers (Basel) 13:216, 2021.

HILLENGASS J et al: International myeloma working group consensus recommendations on imaging in monoclonal plasma cell disorders. Lancet Oncol 20:e302, 2019.

HUNTER ZR et al: Genomics, signaling, and treatment of Waldenström macroglobulinemia. J Clin Oncol 35:994, 2017.

KUMAR S et al: International Myeloma Working Group consensus criteria for response and minimal residual disease assessment in multiple myeloma. Lancet Oncol 17:e328, 2016.

MOREAU P et al: Treatment of relapsed and refractory multiple myeloma: Recommendations from the International Myeloma Working Group. Lancet Oncol. 22:e105, 2021.

RAJKUMAR SV et al: International Myeloma Working Group updated criteria for the diagnosis of multiple myeloma. Lancet Oncol 15:e538, 2014.

ROBIOU DU PONT S et al: Genomics of multiple myeloma. J Clin Oncol 35:963, 2017.

TERPOS E et al: Treatment of multiple myeloma-related bone disease: Recommendations from the Bone Working Group of the International Myeloma Working Group. Lancet Oncol 22:e119, 2021.

112 Amyloidosis

John L. Berk, Vaishali Sanchorawala

GENERAL PRINCIPLES

Amyloidosis is the term for a group of protein misfolding disorders characterized by the extracellular deposition of insoluble polymeric protein fibrils in tissues and organs. A robust cellular machinery exists to chaperone proteins during the process of synthesis and secretion, to ensure that they achieve correct tertiary conformation and function, and to eliminate proteins that misfold. However, genetic mutation, incorrect processing, and other factors may favor misfolding, with consequent loss of normal protein function and intracellular or extracellular aggregation. Many diseases, ranging from cystic fibrosis to Alzheimer's disease, are now known to involve protein misfolding. In the amyloidoses, the aggregates are typically extracellular, and the misfolded protein subunits assume a common antiparallel, β-pleated sheet–rich structural conformation that leads to the formation of higher-order oligomers and then fibrils with unique staining properties. The term *amyloid* was coined around 1854 by the pathologist Rudolf Virchow, who thought that these deposits resembled starch (Latin *amylum*) under the microscope.

Amyloid diseases, defined by the biochemical nature of the protein composing the fibril deposits, are classified according to whether they are systemic or localized, whether they are acquired or inherited, and their clinical patterns (**Table 112-1**). The standard nomenclature is *AX*, where *A* indicates amyloidosis and *X* represents the protein present in the fibril. This chapter focuses primarily on the systemic forms. *AL* refers to amyloid composed of immunoglobulin light chains (LCs); this disorder, formerly termed *primary systemic amyloidosis*, arises from a clonal B-cell or plasma cell disorder and can be associated with myeloma or lymphoma. *ATTR*, the most prevalent of the *familial amyloidoses*, refers to amyloid derived from wild-type or mutated transthyretin (TTR), the transport protein for thyroid hormone and retinol-binding protein. *AA* amyloid is composed of the acute-phase reactant protein serum amyloid A (SAA) and occurs in the setting of chronic inflammatory or infectious diseases; for this reason, this type was formerly known as *secondary amyloidosis*. *A*β_2*M* amyloid results from misfolded β_2-microglobulin, occurring in individuals with long-standing renal disease who have undergone dialysis, typically for years. *Aβ*, the most common form of localized amyloidosis, is found in the brain of patients with Alzheimer's disease after abnormal proteolytic processing and aggregation of polypeptides derived from the amyloid precursor protein.

Diagnosis and treatment of the amyloidoses rest upon the histopathologic identification of amyloid deposits and immunohistochemical, biochemical, or genetic determination of amyloid type (**Fig. 112-1**). In the systemic amyloidoses, the clinically involved

TABLE 112-1 Amyloid Precursor Proteins and Their Clinical Syndromes

DESIGNATION	PRECURSOR	CLINICAL SYNDROME	CLINICAL INVOLVEMENT
Systemic Amyloidoses			
AL	Immunoglobulin light chain	Primary or myeloma-associated[a]	Any
AH	Immunoglobulin heavy chain	Rare variant of primary or myeloma-associated	Any
AA	Serum amyloid A protein	Secondary; reactive[b]	Renal, heart, other
Aβ_2M	β_2-Microglobulin	Hemodialysis-associated	Synovial tissue, bone
ATTR	Transthyretin	Familial (mutant) Age-related (wild type)	Cardiac, peripheral and autonomic nerves, soft tissues, spine, bladder
AApoAI	Apolipoprotein AI	Familial	Hepatic, renal
AApoAII	Apolipoprotein AII	Familial	Renal
AGel	Gelsolin	Familial	Cornea, cranial nerves, skin, renal
AFib	Fibrinogen Aα	Familial	Renal, vascular
ALys	Lysozyme	Familial	Renal, hepatic
ALECT2	Leukocyte chemotactic factor 2	Undefined	Renal
Localized Amyloidoses			
Aβ	Amyloid β protein	Alzheimer's disease; Down's syndrome	Central nervous system
ACys	Cystatin C	Cerebral amyloid angiopathy	Central nervous system, vascular
APrP	Prion protein	Spongiform encephalopathies	Central nervous system
AIAPP	Islet amyloid polypeptide (amylin)	Diabetes-associated	Pancreas
ACal	Calcitonin	Medullary carcinoma of the thyroid	Thyroid
AANF	Atrial natriuretic factor	Atrial fibrillation	Cardiac atria
APro	Prolactin	Endocrinopathy	Pituitary
ASgI	Semenogelin I	Age-related; incidental autopsy or biopsy finding	Seminal vesicles

[a]Localized AL deposits can occur in skin, conjunctiva, urinary bladder, and the tracheobronchial tree. [b]Secondary to chronic inflammation or infection or to a hereditary periodic fever syndrome such as familial Mediterranean fever.

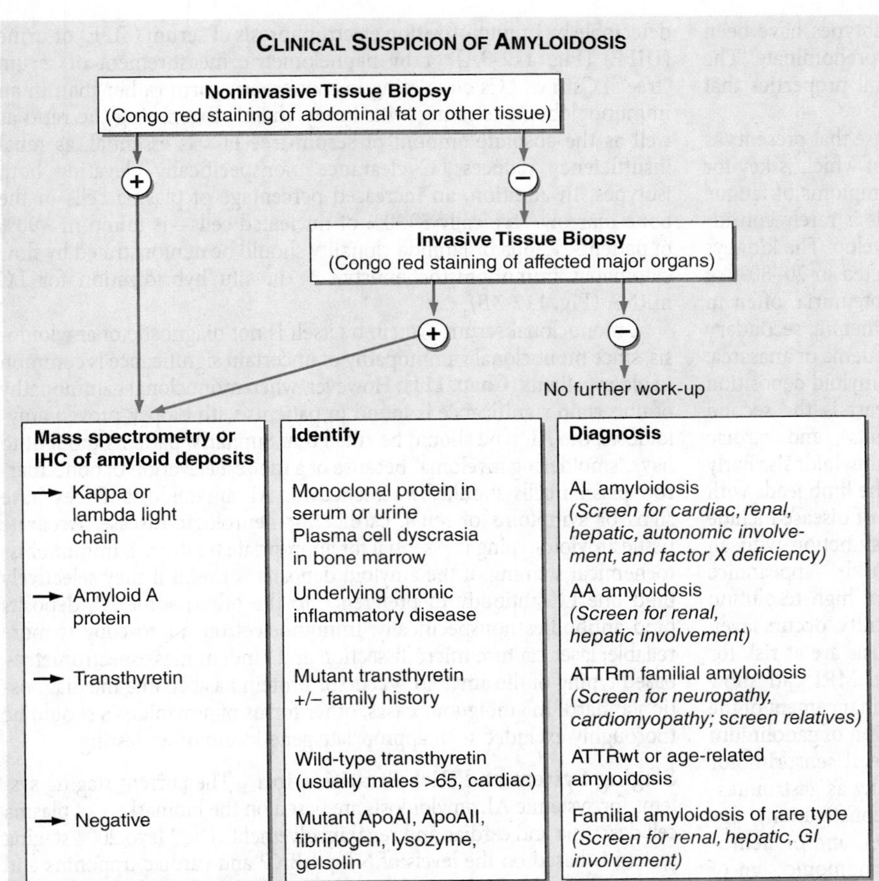

FIGURE 112-1 Algorithm for the diagnosis of amyloidosis and determination of type. Clinical suspicion: unexplained nephropathy, cardiomyopathy, neuropathy, enteropathy, arthropathy, and macroglossia. ApoAI, apolipoprotein AI; ApoAII, apolipoprotein AII; GI, gastrointestinal; IHC, immunohistochemistry.

organs can be biopsied, but amyloid deposits may be found in any tissue of the body. Historically, blood vessels of the gingiva or rectal mucosa were often examined, but the most easily accessible tissue—positive in more than 80% of patients with systemic amyloidosis—is abdominal fat. After local anesthesia, fat is aspirated with a 16-gauge needle from the subcutaneous layer of the abdominal wall. Fat globules expelled onto a glass slide can be stained for amyloid, thus avoiding a surgical procedure. If this material is negative, more invasive biopsies of the kidney, heart, liver, tongue, or gastrointestinal tract can be considered in patients in whom amyloidosis is suspected. The regular β-sheet structure of amyloid deposits exhibits a unique "apple green" birefringence by polarized light microscopy when stained with Congo red dye; other regular protein structures (e.g., collagen) appear white under these conditions. The 10-nm-diameter fibrils can also be visualized by electron microscopy of paraformaldehyde-fixed tissue. Once amyloid is found, the precursor protein type must be determined by immunohistochemistry, immunoelectron microscopy, or extraction and biochemical analysis employing mass spectrometry; gene sequencing is used to identify mutants causing hereditary amyloidosis. The patient's history, physical findings, and clinical presentation, including age and ethnic origin, organ system involvement, underlying diseases, and family history, may provide helpful clues as to the type of amyloidosis. However, there can be considerable overlap in clinical presentations, and accurate typing is essential to guide appropriate therapy.

The mechanisms of fibril formation and tissue toxicity remain controversial. The "amyloid hypothesis," as it is currently understood, proposes that precursor proteins undergo a process of reversible unfolding or misfolding; misfolded proteins form oligomeric aggregates, higher-order polymers, and then fibrils that deposit in tissues. Accumulating evidence suggests that the oligomeric intermediates may constitute the most toxic species. Oligomers are more capable than large fibrils of interacting with cells and inducing formation of reactive oxygen species and stress signaling. Ultimately, the fibrillar tissue deposits are likely to interfere with normal organ function. A more sophisticated understanding of the mechanisms leading to amyloid formation and cell and tissue dysfunction will continue to provide new targets for therapies.

The clinical syndromes of the amyloidoses are associated with relatively nonspecific alterations in routine laboratory tests. Blood counts are usually normal, although the erythrocyte sedimentation rate is frequently elevated. Patients with glomerular kidney involvement generally have proteinuria, often in the nephrotic range, leading to hypoalbuminemia that may be severe; patients with serum albumin levels <2 g/dL generally have pedal edema or anasarca. Amyloid cardiomyopathy is characterized by concentric ventricular hypertrophy and diastolic dysfunction associated with elevation of brain natriuretic peptide (BNP) or *N*-terminal pro–brain natriuretic peptide (NT-proBNP) as well as troponin. These cardiac biomarkers can be used for disease staging, prognostication, and disease activity monitoring in patients with AL amyloidosis. Notably, renal insufficiency can falsely elevate levels of these biomarkers. Recently, biomarkers of cardiac remodeling—that is, matrix metalloproteinases and tissue inhibitors of metalloproteinases—have been found to be altered in the serum of patients with amyloid cardiomyopathy. Electrocardiographic and echocardiographic features of amyloid cardiomyopathy are described below. Patients with liver involvement, even when advanced, usually develop cholestasis with an elevated alkaline phosphatase concentration with minimal alteration of the aminotransferases and preservation of synthetic function. In AL amyloidosis, endocrine organs may be infiltrated with fibrils, and hypothyroidism, hypoadrenalism, or even hypopituitarism can occur. Although none of these findings is specific for amyloidosis, the presence of abnormalities in multiple organ systems should raise suspicions of the diagnosis.

AL AMYLOIDOSIS

Etiology and Incidence AL amyloidosis is most frequently caused by a clonal expansion of bone marrow plasma cells that secrete a monoclonal immunoglobulin LC depositing as amyloid fibrils in tissues. Whether the clonal plasma cells produce a LC that misfolds and leads to AL amyloidosis or an LC that folds properly, allowing the cells to inexorably expand over time and develop into multiple myeloma **(Chap. 111)**, may depend upon primary sequence of the clonal LC or other genetic or epigenetic factors. AL amyloidosis can occur with multiple myeloma or other B lymphoproliferative diseases, including non-Hodgkin's lymphoma **(Chap. 108)** and Waldenström's macroglobulinemia **(Chap. 111)**. AL amyloidosis is the most common type of systemic amyloidosis diagnosed in North America. Its incidence has been estimated at 4.5 cases/100,000 population; however, ascertainment continues to be inadequate, and the true incidence may be much higher. AL amyloidosis, like other plasma cell disorders, usually occurs after age 40 and is often progressive and fatal if untreated.

Pathology and Clinical Features Amyloid deposits are usually widespread in AL amyloidosis and can be present in the interstitium of any organ outside the central nervous system. The amyloid fibril deposits are composed of full-length 23-kDa monoclonal immunoglobulin LCs as well as fragments. Accessory molecules co-deposited with LC fibrils (as well as with other amyloid fibrils) include serum amyloid P component, apolipoproteins e and A-IV, glycosaminoglycans, and metal ions. Although all kappa and lambda LC subtypes have been identified in AL amyloid fibrils, lambda subtypes predominate. The lambda 6 subtype appears to have unique structural properties that predispose it to fibril formation, often in the kidney.

AL amyloidosis is often a rapidly progressive disease that presents as a pleiotropic set of clinical syndromes, recognition of which is key for initiation of the appropriate workup. Nonspecific symptoms of fatigue and weight loss are common; however, the diagnosis is rarely considered until symptoms referable to a specific organ develop. The kidneys are the most frequently involved organ and are affected in 70–80% of patients. Renal amyloidosis usually manifests as proteinuria, often in the nephrotic range and associated with hypoalbuminemia, secondary hypercholesterolemia and hypertriglyceridemia, and edema or anasarca. In some patients, interstitial rather than glomerular amyloid deposition can produce azotemia without proteinuria. The heart is the second most commonly affected organ (50–60% of patients), and cardiac involvement is the leading cause of death from AL amyloidosis. Early on, the electrocardiogram may show low voltage in the limb leads with a pseudo-infarct pattern. Echocardiographic features of disease include concentrically thickened ventricles and diastolic dysfunction with an abnormal global longitudinal strain pattern; a "sparkly" appearance has been described but is often not seen with modern high-resolution echocardiographic techniques. Poor atrial contractility occurs even in sinus rhythm, and patients with cardiac amyloidosis are at risk for development of atrial thrombi and stroke. Cardiac MRI can show increased wall thickness, and characteristic delayed enhancement of the subendocardium has been described following injection of gadolinium contrast. Nervous system symptoms include peripheral sensorimotor neuropathy and/or autonomic dysfunction manifesting as gastrointestinal motility disturbances (early satiety, diarrhea, constipation), dry eyes and mouth, impotence, orthostatic hypotension, and/or neurogenic bladder. Macroglossia (**Fig. 112-2*A***), a pathognomonic sign of AL amyloidosis, is seen in only ~10% of patients. Liver involvement causes cholestasis and hepatomegaly. The spleen is frequently involved, and there may be functional hyposplenism in the absence of significant splenomegaly. Many patients experience "easy bruising" due to amyloid deposits in capillaries or deficiency of clotting factor X due to binding to amyloid fibrils; cutaneous ecchymoses appear, particularly around the eyes, producing another uncommon but pathognomonic finding, the "raccoon-eye" sign (**Fig. 112-2*B***). Other findings include nail dystrophy (**Fig. 112-2*C***), alopecia, and amyloid arthropathy with thickening of synovial membranes in the wrists and shoulders. The presence of a multisystemic illness or general fatigue along with any of these clinical syndromes should prompt a workup for amyloidosis.

Diagnosis Identification of an underlying clonal plasma cell or B lymphoproliferative process and a clonal LC are key to the diagnosis of AL amyloidosis. Serum protein electrophoresis and urine protein electrophoresis, although of value in multiple myeloma, are *not* useful screening tests if AL amyloidosis is suspected because the clonal LC or whole immunoglobulin often is not present in sufficient amounts to produce a monoclonal "M-spike" in the serum or LC (Bence Jones) protein in the urine. However, more than 90% of patients with AL amyloidosis have serum or urine monoclonal LC or whole immunoglobulin detectable by immunofixation electrophoresis of serum (SIFE) or urine (UIFE) (**Fig. 112-3*A***) or by nephelometric measurement of serum "free" LCs (i.e., LCs circulating in monomeric form rather than in an immunoglobulin tetramer with heavy chain). Examining the ratio as well as the absolute amount of serum-free LCs is essential, as renal insufficiency reduces LC clearance, nonspecifically elevating both isotypes. In addition, an increased percentage of plasma cells in the bone marrow—typically 5–30% of nucleated cells—is found in ~90% of patients. Kappa or lambda clonality should be demonstrated by flow cytometry, immunohistochemistry, or in situ hybridization for LC mRNA (**Fig. 112-3*B***).

A monoclonal serum protein by itself is not diagnostic of amyloidosis, since monoclonal gammopathy of uncertain significance is common in older patients (**Chap. 111**). However, when monoclonal gammopathy of uncertain significance is found in patients with biopsy-proven amyloidosis, the AL type should be ruled out. Similarly, patients thought to have "smoldering myeloma" because of a modest elevation of bone-marrow plasma cells should be screened for AL amyloidosis if they have signs or symptoms of renal, cardiac, or neurologic disease. Accurate tissue amyloid typing is essential for appropriate treatment. Immunohistochemical staining of the amyloid deposits is useful if they selectively bind one LC antibody in preference to the other; some AL deposits bind antibodies nonspecifically. Immunoelectron microscopy is more reliable; laser capture microdissection and tandem mass spectrometry–based typing of the amyloid precursor protein has become the diagnostic standard. In ambiguous cases, other forms of amyloidosis should be thoroughly excluded with appropriate genetic and other testing.

Staging System and Risk Stratification The current staging systems for systemic AL amyloidosis are based on the biomarkers of plasma cell dyscrasia and cardiac and renal involvement. The Mayo 2004 staging system is based on the levels of NT-proBNP and cardiac troponins and was modified by European investigators to identify and classify very-high-risk patients. This cardiac staging system is the most widely used to determine patient management. This staging system was modified (Mayo 2012) to include clonal burden, assessed by dFLC (difference between involved and uninvolved circulating free light chain) concentration, which has independent ability to predict survival. Boston University investigators introduced a staging system incorporating BNP and troponin I that also is able to predict survival. Patients with AL amyloidosis with a very low (<50 mg/L) dFLC level have a significantly better outcome irrespective of cardiac stage. A renal staging system based on 24-h urine protein excretion and estimated glomerular filtration rate (eGFR) predicting the progression to dialysis at 2 years has also been developed and validated. Several other biomarkers have been shown to predict outcomes and survival but have not been incorporated in staging systems yet.

TREATMENT

AL Amyloidosis

Extensive multisystemic involvement typifies AL amyloidosis, and the median survival period without treatment is usually only ~1–2 years from the time of diagnosis. Current therapies target the

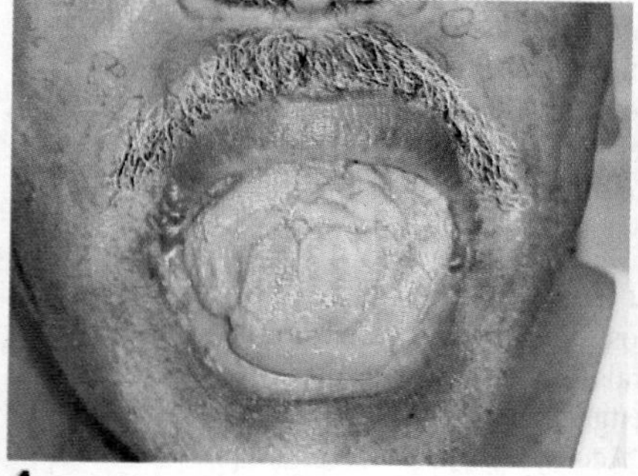
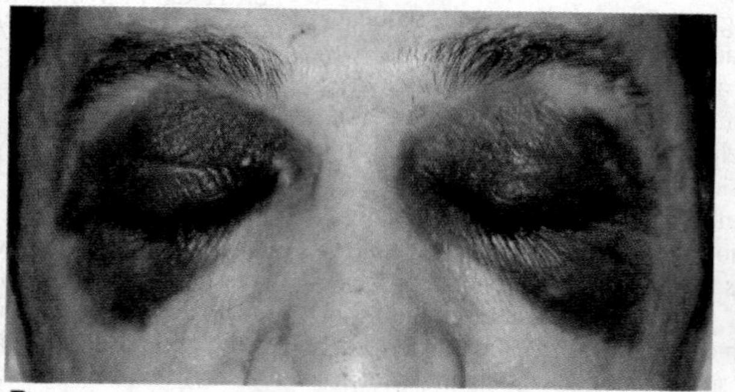
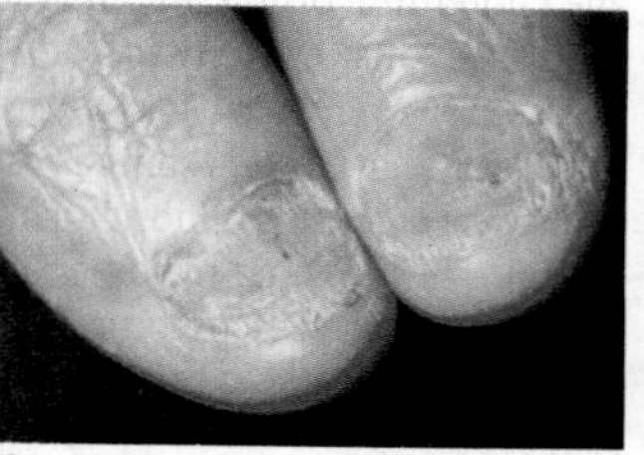

FIGURE 112-2 Clinical signs of AL amyloidosis. ***A.*** Macroglossia. ***B.*** Periorbital ecchymoses. ***C.*** Fingernail dystrophy.

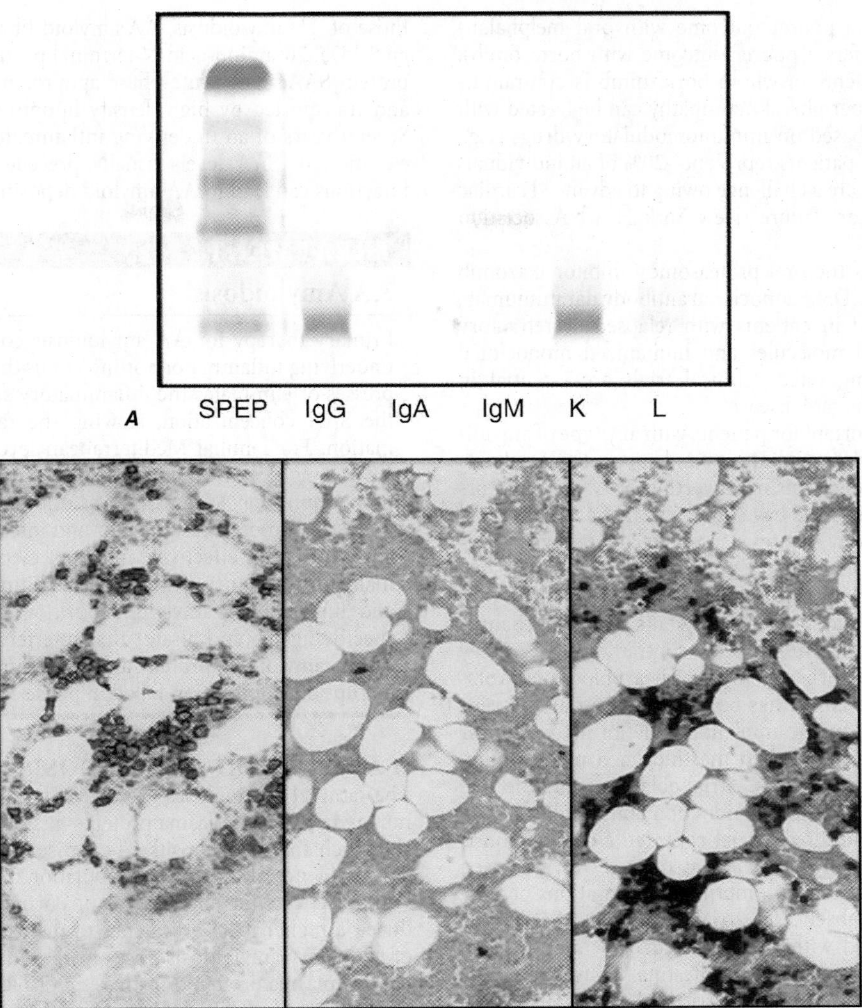

FIGURE 112-3 Laboratory features of AL amyloidosis. ***A.*** Serum immunofixation electrophoresis reveals an IgGκ monoclonal protein in this example; serum protein electrophoresis is often normal. ***B.*** Bone marrow biopsy sections stained by immunohistochemistry with antibody to CD138 (syndecan, highly expressed on plasma cells) (*left*) or by in situ hybridization with fluorescein-tagged probes (Ventana Medical Systems) binding to κ mRNA (*center*) and λ mRNA (*right*) in plasma cells. *(Photomicrograph courtesy of C. O'Hara; with permission.)*

clonal bone marrow plasma cells, using approaches employed for multiple myeloma. Treatment with oral melphalan and prednisone can decrease the plasma cell burden but rarely leads to complete hematologic remission, meaningful organ responses, or improved survival and is no longer widely used. The substitution of dexamethasone for prednisone produces a higher response rate and more durable remissions, although dexamethasone is not always well tolerated by patients with significant edema or cardiac disease. High-dose intravenous (IV) melphalan followed by autologous stem cell transplantation (HDM/SCT) produces complete hematologic responses in ~40% of treated patients, as determined by loss of clonal plasma cells in the bone marrow and disappearance of the amyloidogenic monoclonal LC, as determined by SIFE/UIFE and free LC quantitation. Six to 12 months after achieving a hematologic response, improvements in organ function and quality of life may occur. Hematologic responses appear to be more durable after HDM/SCT than in multiple myeloma, with remissions continuing in some patients beyond 15 years without additional treatment. Unfortunately, only ~20–30% of all AL amyloidosis patients are suitable for aggressive treatment, and even at specialized treatment centers, transplantation-related mortality rates are higher than those for other hematologic diseases because of impaired organ function at initial presentation. Amyloid cardiomyopathy, poor nutritional and performance status, and multiorgan disease contribute to excess morbidity and mortality. A bleeding diathesis resulting from adsorption of clotting factor X to amyloid fibrils also increases mortality rates; however, this syndrome occurs in only 5–10% of patients. A randomized multicenter trial conducted in France compared oral melphalan and dexamethasone with HDM/SCT and failed to show a benefit of dose-intensive treatment, although the transplantation-related mortality rate in this study was very high. It has become clear that careful selection of patients and expert peritransplantation management are essential in reducing transplantation-related mortality.

For patients with AL amyloidosis and impaired cardiac function or arrhythmias due to involvement of the myocardium, the median survival period is only ~6 months without treatment. In these patients, cardiac transplantation can be performed and followed by HDM/SCT to eliminate the noxious LC clone and prevent amyloid deposition in the transplanted heart or other organs.

The best therapy for those who are transplant ineligible varies between centers and countries. A regimen of oral chemotherapy with melphalan and dexamethasone (MDex) had been the standard for patients not eligible for HDM/SCT for more than a decade. Regimens using bortezomib (a proteasome inhibitor) are now considered the standard of care in most patients with AL amyloidosis not eligible for SCT. There is a fine balance between chosen treatment regimens and toxicities, and patient characteristics should be considered when choosing a regimen; for example, treatment with bortezomib plus MDex can overcome the effects of both gain of 1q21 (which confers a poorer outcome with oral melphalan) and t(11;14) (which confers a poorer outcome with bortezomib). Transplant-ineligible patients in whom bortezomib is contraindicated due to preexisting peripheral neuropathy can be treated with MDex or combinations based on immunomodulatory drugs (e.g., lenalidomide). High-risk patients represent ~20% of all individuals with AL amyloidosis and are a challenge owing to advanced cardiac stage (IIIb) or severe heart failure (New York Heart Association class III or IV).

Newer agents, such as the oral proteasome inhibitor ixazomib and the humanized anti-CD38 monoclonal antibody daratumumab, have also been evaluated in patients with relapsed or refractory disease. Anti-fibril small molecules and humanized monoclonal antibodies are also being tested. Clinical trials are essential in improving therapy for this rare disease.

Supportive care is important for patients with any type of amyloidosis. For nephrotic syndrome, diuretics and supportive stockings can ameliorate edema; angiotensin-converting enzyme inhibitors should be used with caution and have not been shown to slow renal disease progression. Effective diuresis can be facilitated with albumin infusions to raise intravascular oncotic pressure. Congestive heart failure due to amyloid cardiomyopathy is best treated with diuretics; it is important to note that digitalis, calcium channel blockers, and beta blockers are relatively contraindicated as they can interact with amyloid fibrils and produce heart block and worsening heart failure. Amiodarone has been used for atrial and ventricular arrhythmias. Automatic implantable defibrillators appear to have reduced effectiveness due to the thickened myocardium, but they may benefit some patients. Atrial ablation is an effective approach for atrial fibrillation. For conduction abnormalities, ventricular pacing may be indicated. Atrial contractile dysfunction is common in amyloid cardiomyopathy and associated with increased thromboembolic complications, prompting considerations of anticoagulation even in the absence of atrial fibrillation. Autonomic neuropathy can be treated with α agonists such as midodrine to support postural blood pressure; gastrointestinal dysfunction may respond to motility or bulk agents. Nutritional supplementation, either oral or parenteral, is also important.

In localized AL amyloidosis, amyloid deposits can be produced by clonal plasma cells infiltrating local sites in the airways, bladder, skin, or lymph nodes (Table 112-1). These deposits may respond to surgical intervention or elimination of the responsible plasma cell clone by low-dose radiation therapy (typically only 20 Gy); systemic treatment generally is not appropriate. Patients should be referred to a center familiar with management of these rare manifestations of amyloidosis.

AA AMYLOIDOSIS

Etiology and Incidence AA amyloidosis can occur in association with almost any chronic inflammatory state (e.g., rheumatoid arthritis, inflammatory bowel disease, ankylosing spondylitis, familial Mediterranean fever **[Chap. 369]**, or other periodic fever syndromes) or chronic infections such as tuberculosis, osteomyelitis, or subacute bacterial endocarditis. In the United States and Europe, AA amyloidosis has become less common, occurring in fewer than 2% of patients with these diseases, presumably because of advances in anti-inflammatory and antimicrobial therapies. It has also been described in association with Castleman's disease, lymphomas, and renal cell carcinoma, emphasizing the diagnostic importance of CT scanning to look for such tumors as well as serologic and microbiologic studies. In up to 30% of patients, AA amyloidosis can also be seen without any identifiable underlying disease. AA is the most frequent systemic amyloidosis that occurs in children.

Pathology and Clinical Features Organ involvement in AA amyloidosis usually begins in the kidneys. Hepatomegaly, splenomegaly, and autonomic neuropathy can also occur as the disease progresses; cardiomyopathy is a late manifestation in ~25% of patients. The symptoms and signs of AA disease cannot be reliably distinguished from those of AL amyloidosis. AA amyloid fibrils are usually composed of an 8-kDa, 76-amino-acid *N*-terminal portion of the 12-kDa precursor protein SAA. This acute-phase apoprotein is synthesized in the liver and transported by high-density lipoprotein (HDL3) in the plasma. Several years of an underlying inflammatory disease causing chronic elevation of SAA levels usually precede fibril formation, although infections can lead to AA amyloid deposition more rapidly.

TREATMENT

AA Amyloidosis

Primary therapy for AA amyloidosis consists of treatment of the underlying inflammatory or infectious disease. Treatment that suppresses or eliminates the inflammatory state or infection decreases the SAA concentration, slowing the rate of amyloid fibril formation. For familial Mediterranean fever, colchicine at a dose of 1.2–1.8 mg/d is the standard treatment. However, colchicine has not been helpful for AA amyloidosis of other causes or for other amyloidoses. Tumor necrosis factor and interleukin 1 and interleukin 6 antagonists can effectively interrupt cytokine signaling that drives many inflammatory syndromes, inhibiting hepatic SAA production and limiting AA amyloid deposition. Development of a fibril-specific agent (eprodisate) that interferes with the interaction of serum amyloid A protein and glycosaminoglycans to prevent or disrupt fibril formation failed in phase 3 trials.

ATTR AND AF AMYLOIDOSIS

The familial amyloidoses are autosomal dominant diseases in which mutated or variant plasma proteins misfold or aggregate to form beta-sheet rich amyloid deposits. These diseases are rare, with an estimated case incidence of <1/100,000 population in the United States, although founder effects in remote areas of Portugal, Sweden, and Japan produced a higher local prevalence of disease. The most prevalent form of hereditary amyloidosis arises from mutation of the abundant liver-derived plasma protein transthyretin (TTR, also known as *prealbumin*) and is termed hATTR amyloid. More than 130 TTR mutations typically conferring one-amino-acid substitutions have been described, with most inducing clinical ATTR amyloid disease. Toxic TTR oligomers and ATTR amyloid deposits target peripheral and autonomic nervous systems and the heart. One TTR variant, V122I, occurs in nearly 4% of the African-American and Afro-Caribbean populations and is associated with late-onset cardiac amyloidosis. The actual incidence and penetrance of disease in the African-American population is the subject of ongoing research, but considerations of V122I ATTR amyloidosis is warranted in African-American patients who present with concentric cardiac hypertrophy and evidence of diastolic heart failure, particularly in the absence of a history of hypertension or valvular disease. Other familial amyloidoses, caused by variant apolipoproteins AI or AII, gelsolin, fibrinogen Aα, or lysozyme, are reported with lower prevalence worldwide. New amyloidogenic serum proteins continue to be identified periodically, including leukocyte chemotactic factor LECT2, which is a cause of renal amyloidosis in Hispanic and Pakistani populations. Although the clustering of ALECT2 cases suggests heritability, no LECT2 gene-coding sequence variations have been identified.

Normal (wild-type) transthyretin can also misfold and aggregate to form ATTR amyloid, typically expressed in men beginning in the seventh decade with increasing prevalence with age. Formerly termed senile systemic amyloidosis, ATTRwt amyloid is reported at autopsy in 25% of hearts from patients who are 80 years and older. Although it is unclear why a wild-type protein becomes amyloidogenic, aging inefficiencies of intracellular quality-assurance mechanisms (termed the unfolded protein response) likely predispose to secretion of proteins prone to misaggregation. Due to the numbers of aging men globally, ATTRwt is the most prevalent and rapidly growing form of amyloidosis in the world today.

Clinical Features and Diagnosis hATTR amyloidosis has a varied presentation predicted by the specific TTR mutation. Consequently, kindreds typically express similar disease timing and clinical course. Apparent sporadic presentations (no recognized family history) often reflect incomplete penetrance of the TTR mutation and not a spontaneous event. hATTR amyloidosis presents as familial amyloidotic polyneuropathy (nerve damage) or familial amyloidotic cardiomyopathy (heart damage). Peripheral neuropathy begins as a length-dependent small-fiber sensorimotor neuropathy first exhibited in the feet with ascending progression to the upper extremities. Autonomic neuropathy manifests as smooth muscle dysmotility (dysphagia, diarrhea, urinary retention), vascular dysregulation (orthostatic hypotension, erectile dysfunction), and anhidrosis. Soft tissue disease (carpal tunnel syndrome, tendonopathy, and spinal stenosis) commonly precedes nerve or heart manifestations of disease by 1–2 decades, particularly in ATTRwt amyloid patients who frequently report bicipital, patellar, or Achilles tendon rupture. Less common expressions of hATTR include vitreous opacities and leptomeningeal amyloid deposition from variant protein produced by the retinal epithelium and choroid plexus, respectively. ATTR amyloid involvement of the heart is clinically better tolerated than AL amyloid cardiomyopathy as reflected by the time from heart failure presentation to death in untreated cases of ATTR (median 42–48 months) versus AL (median 6 months) amyloidosis and the dramatically greater burden of disease by echocardiographic measures at symptomatic presentation.

Typical syndromes associated with other forms of AF disease include renal amyloidosis with mutant fibrinogen, lysozyme, or apolipoproteins; hepatic amyloidosis with apolipoprotein AI; and amyloidosis of cranial neuropathy with corneal lattice dystrophy pathognomonic of gelsolin amyloidosis. Patients with AF amyloidosis can present with clinical syndromes that mimic those of patients with AL disease. Rarely, AF carriers can develop AL disease or AF patients may have monoclonal gammopathy without AL. Thus, it is important to screen both for plasma cell disorders and for mutations in patients with amyloidosis. Although mass spectrometry often detects amino acid sequence variations, it is not designed to definitively identify specific protein variations; DNA sequencing is the diagnostic standard for AF mutations.

TREATMENT

ATTR Amyloidosis

Untreated, the survival period after onset of ATTR disease is 5–15 years. At present, three therapeutic strategies are used for ATTR amyloidosis: (1) orthotopic liver transplantation (OLT) to replace the factory of the mutated protein (only applicable to hATTR); (2) stabilization of circulating TTR tetramers, preventing TTR monomer release and amyloid fibril formation; and (3) TTR gene silencing (RNA interference or anti-sense oligonucleotide agents), suppressing hepatic TTR production to eliminate ATTR fibril formation. After 30 years of experience, OLT is largely limited to patients with hATTR amyloid and early peripheral neuropathy (V30M ATTR), as most patients with non-V30M TTR mutations suffer post-transplant progressive amyloid disease due to wild-type TTR from the allograft liver depositing on preexisting amyloid present in the heart and nerves. TTR tetramer stabilization successfully inhibits progressive ATTR amyloid nerve and heart disease as demonstrated by a phase 3 randomized controlled trial—the Diflunisal Trial (hATTR)—and the Transthyretin Amyloidosis Cardiomyopathy Clinical Trial (ATTR-ACT), respectively. Diflunisal, a repurposed generic nonsteroidal anti-inflammatory, and tafamidis, a proprietary thyroxine mimetic, bind TTR tetramers at the thyroxine binding site, minimizing release of the amyloidogenic TTR monomer and slowing progression of nerve and heart disease. Tafamidis, the first U.S. Food and Drug Administration–approved treatment for ATTR amyloid cardiomyopathy, extends survival and slows the decline in walking capacities and quality of life but does not appear to induce improvement in heart thickening or function. TTR gene silencers more reliably stop neurologic disease progression and, in 35–60% of treated patients with hATTR amyloid, improve sensory nerve deficits, a novel finding. Further, preliminary data suggest TTR gene silencers may promote heart remodeling and improve systolic function.

The therapeutic future of ATTR amyloid patients is bright. Phase 3 randomized controlled clinical trials examining the safety and effectiveness of TTR gene silencers in patients with ATTR amyloid cardiomyopathy are underway, as are studies to determine the impact of second-generation TTR gene silencers on ATTR amyloid neuropathy and cardiomyopathy. TTR gene editing to prevent mRNA production or correct DNA mutations is the next frontier. Finally, as survival improves for patients with ATTR amyloid, therapies that cross the blood-brain barrier to address leptomeningeal (brain) and vitreous (eye) amyloid deposition arising from the choroid plexus and retinal epithelium, respectively, will be challenges to achieve.

Aβ_2M AMYLOIDOSIS

Aβ_2M amyloid is composed of β_2-microglobulin, the invariant chain of class I human leukocyte antigens, and produces rheumatologic manifestations in patients undergoing long-term hemodialysis and, rarely, in patients with a hereditary form of disease. β_2-Microglobulin is excreted by the kidney, and levels become elevated in end-stage renal disease. The molecular mass of β_2M is 11.8 kDa—above the cutoff of some dialysis membranes. The incidence of this disease appears to be declining with the use of newer membranes in high-flow dialysis techniques. Aβ_2M amyloidosis usually presents as carpal tunnel syndrome, persistent joint effusions, spondyloarthropathy, or cystic bone lesions. Carpal tunnel syndrome is often the first symptom. In the past, persistent joint effusions accompanied by mild discomfort were found in up to 50% of patients who had undergone dialysis for >12 years. Involvement is bilateral, and large joints (shoulders, knees, wrists, and hips) are most frequently affected. The synovial fluid is noninflammatory, and β_2M amyloid can be found if the sediment is stained with Congo red. Although less common, visceral β_2M amyloid deposits do occasionally occur in the gastrointestinal tract, heart, tendons, and subcutaneous tissues of the buttocks. There are no proven specific therapies for Aβ_2M amyloidosis, but cessation of dialysis after renal allografting may lead to symptomatic improvement.

THERAPEUTIC FRONTIERS

To date, treatment strategies have focused on limiting formation of amyloidogenic proteins. Disruption of existing amyloid by targeting ubiquitous components of the tissue deposits offers theoretical means to improving major end-organ function; however, clinical trial validation remains elusive.

SUMMARY

A diagnosis of amyloidosis should be considered in patients with unexplained nephropathy, cardiomyopathy (particularly with diastolic dysfunction), neuropathy (either peripheral or autonomic), enteropathy, or the pathognomonic soft tissue findings of macroglossia or periorbital ecchymoses. Pathologic identification of amyloid fibrils can be made with Congo red staining of aspirated abdominal fat or of an involved-organ biopsy specimen. Accurate typing by a combination of immunologic, biochemical, and genetic testing is essential in selecting appropriate therapy (Fig. 112-1). Systemic amyloidosis should be considered a treatable condition, as anti–plasma cell chemotherapy is highly effective in AL disease and targeted therapies are being developed for AA and ATTR disease. The combination of precursor and end-organ amyloid therapeutics potentially provide not only disease control but also functional and quality of life improvements for patients with amyloidosis. Tertiary referral centers can provide specialized diagnostic techniques and access to clinical trials for patients with these rare diseases.

FURTHER READING

Adams D et al: Patisiran, an RNAi therapeutic, for hereditary transthyretin amyloidosis. N Engl J Med 379:11, 2018.

Benson MD et al: Inotersen treatment for patients with hereditary transthyretin amyloidosis. N Engl J Med 379:22, 2018.

Maurer MS et al: Expert consensus recommendations for the suspicion and diagnosis of transthyretin cardiac amyloidosis. Circ Heart Fail 12:e006075, 2019.

Maurer MS et al: Tafamidis treatment for patients with transthyretin amyloid cardiomyopathy. N Engl J Med 379:1007, 2018.

Merlini G et al: Systemic immunoglobulin light chain amyloidosis. Nat Rev Dis Primers 4:38, 2018.

Sanchorawala V: High dose melphalan and autologous peripheral blood stem cell transplantation in AL amyloidosis. Hematol Oncol Clin North Am 28:1131, 2014.

Sarosiek S, Sanchorawala V: Treatment options for relapsed/refractory systemic light-chain (AL) amyloidosis: Current perspectives. J Blood Med 10:373, 2019.

113 Transfusion Therapy and Biology

Pierre Tiberghien, Olivier Garraud, Jacques Chiaroni

Transfusion encompasses the use of blood components (BCs) to prevent or treat anemia, hemorrhage, and bleeding disorders. Occasionally, BCs may be used to treat infection or relapse of malignant blood diseases after allogeneic hematopoietic transplantation. BCs comprise mainly red blood cell concentrates (RBCCs), platelet concentrates (PCs), and plasma for transfusion use (as opposed to plasma for fractionation into medicinal products such as albumin and immunoglobulin). Alongside transfusion safety, ensuring BC quality, assessing in vivo efficacy, and promoting evidence-based transfusion practices are critical aspects of transfusion medicine.

Blood collection and donor medicine do not fall within the scope of this chapter. Although the processes used are particularly safe, blood donations can cause adverse reactions, among which are fainting reactions and iron deficiency. These risks require preventive approaches and appropriate treatment when needed.

BLOOD COMPONENTS

BC collection and manufacturing processes are described in **Table 113-1**. Most common BCs are collected as whole blood or directly as components by apheresis. The vast majority of BCs are homologous. Autologous BCs, sometimes collected ahead of planned surgery, are now exceptional as they present little to no evidence-based advantage over homologous BCs. Nevertheless, such donation may still be of benefit in the presence of a rare blood group phenotype.

All BCs comply with common quality and performance standards and guidelines. Quality assurance encompasses well-defined processing steps and stringent BC quality controls as defined by health authorities. Tracing of all manufacturing steps as well as hemovigilance-based reporting of adverse events and incidents associated with blood collection, BC processing, and transfusion are highly recommended.

With the obvious exception of granulocyte concentrates and mononuclear cells, the majority of BCs are now leukocyte-reduced, and universal prestorage leukocyte reduction has been recommended. These BCs contain <1–5.10^{6} donor leukocytes and are associated with reduced incidence febrile nonhemolytic transfusion reactions (FNHTRs), infections with intracellular pathogens such as cytomegalovirus (CMV), alloimmunization, and immunomodulation.

BCs may undergo additional processing steps. These may include irradiation to prevent graft-versus-host disease (GVHD) in immunosuppressed patients, pathogen reduction to further reduce the risk of transfusion-transmitted infections, plasma reduction in patients with severe allergic reactions to BCs, or the manufacturing of pediatric units for young children and neonates.

BC constituents undergo centrifugation and filtration and are placed in contact with needles, plastic tubing and bags, as well anticoagulant molecules and various additive solutions. BCs are subjected to gas exchanges that are significantly different from aerobic breathing and are maintained at temperatures that are not physiologic, such as 22°C or 4°C. Any of these elements may contribute to so-called "storage lesions" that may occur at any time during BC processing and storage. Some of these lesions have proven to be reversible in the recipient after transfusion, while others may be irreversible. The clinical impacts of such lesions are under investigation. Storage lesions may also account for a number of adverse transfusion reactions, although there is currently no consensus on this issue.

Furthermore, plasma present in BCs contains donor antibodies (Abs). When directed toward antigens (Ags) present in the recipient, such as blood group or tissue (human leukocyte antigen [HLA]) Ags, such Abs may result in adverse events. RBCCs bring only a limited amount of donor plasma (10–30 mL), unlike PCs and obviously plasma. The use of platelet additive solution can replace two-thirds of plasma in PCs, while still leaving the equivalent of one plasma unit of 200 mL per transfused PC.

BLOOD GROUP ANTIGENS AND ANTIBODIES

Red blood cells, as well as other blood constituents such as platelets and neutrophils, express allogeneic determinants. Transfusion may therefore result in alloimmunization and the production of Abs directed against allogeneic determinants. These alloantibodies (alloAbs) comprise anti-red blood cell (RBC) Abs, anti-HLA, anti-human platelet Ag (HPA) Abs, and anti-human neutrophil Ag (HNA) Abs. Anti-RBC immunization may result in hemolysis, while anti-HLA or anti-HPA Abs may result in other transfusion complications such as fever and platelet transfusion refractoriness. Furthermore, anti-HLA and anti-HNA immunization in the donor may result in a severe lung disorder called transfusion-related acute lung injury (TRALI). The Abs against red cell Ags may be IgM or IgG immunoglobulin classes. Some IgG or IgM can activate complement, and some IgG, crossing the placental barrier, may induce hemolytic disease of the fetus and newborn.

Erythrocyte blood groups refer to antigenic molecules that are expressed on the surface of RBC and other cells, genetically transmitted, and recognized by specific Abs. The polymorphism of such molecules explains their immunizing potential in situations such as transfusion, pregnancy, and transplantation. Blood groups can also interact with the environment and with infectious pathogens, leading to individual susceptibilities. For example, malaria is less severe in type O than non-O patients. Conversely, group O is associated with increased susceptibility to *Helicobacter pylori*. Currently, ~380 different blood group Ags have been described, classified within ~43 different systems. Blood group Ags belong to two broad categories based on their biochemical nature: carbohydrate blood groups and protein blood groups. RBC Ags may be the target of autoantibodies (autoAbs) generating autoimmune hemolytic anemia. Some of them, mostly IgG, are active at 37°C, called "warm autoAbs ," and are most often directed against Rh Ags, while others, most often IgM, are active at 4°C, called "cold autoAbs," and may be directed against ABO, I, I, P, and other Ags.

Carbohydrate blood groups are headed by the **ABO system** which comprises two main Ags, A and B, encoded by two alleles, which are the *A* and *B* alleles, respectively. In addition to these active alleles, there is an inactive allele: *O*. Depending on the genotype, four different phenotypes are produced (**Table 113-2**). Other carbohydrate systems (H, P1PK, Lewis, I, and GLOB) share many characteristics with the ABO system. The main common feature is biochemical. Indeed, given their carbohydrate nature, Ags of the ABO system are considered to be "secondary products" of genes. The *A* allele encodes the A enzyme, which binds the A-type sugar (GalNac) A to the H substrate (expressed by action of the H enzyme encoded by the *H* allele, which happens to be inactive in the Bombay phenotype); sugars are attached to protein substrates on the surface of the RBC and so forth.

TABLE 113-1 Blood Components: Collection and Manufacturing Processes

BLOOD COLLECTION	INITIAL PROCESSING	BLOOD COMPONENT	ADDITIONAL COMPONENT PROCESSING (OPTIONAL TO MANDATORY)	RATIONALE	VOLUME AND CONTENT	STORAGE CONDITIONS AND DURATION
Whole blood	Separation into RBCCs and platelet-rich plasma (PRP) by slow centrifugation, followed by high-speed centrifugation of the PRP to yield one unit of platelets (most often subsequently pooled) and one unit of plasma. *Or* Separation into a PRBC, a plasma, and a "buffy coat" containing leukocytes and platelets by high-speed centrifugation, followed by pooling and slow-speed centrifugation of the buffy coat to produce a pooled platelet unit. Alternatively, the buffy coat may undergo high-speed centrifugation to produce a granulocyte unit that will be subsequently pooled.	RBCC from whole blood or from apheresis	Deleukocytation to <1–5.10^6 leukocytes per unit: initial whole blood filtration or RBC elective filtration (highly recommended; mandatory in several international jurisdictions)	Reduction of posttransfusion fever and chills Reduction of intracellular pathogens (including CMV infections) Reduction of alloimmunization	250–300 mL (including additive solution, no more than 40–50 mL of plasma) Hemoglobin: 22–40 g/dL Hematocrit: 50–70% Hemolysis ≤0.8% at issuing	4 +/– 2°C Duration depends on the additive solution: 25–42 days; some solutions aim to extend shelf life to 56 days After irradiation: 24 h After plasma reduction: 24 h to 10 days depending on reduction methodology
			Irradiation: X-ray or gamma, ~25–35 Gy; most often units no older than 28 days after collection	GVHD prevention in immunosuppressed patients or intrafamilial transfusions		
			Plasma reduction	Prevention of allergic reactions in patients with prior severe reactions	Lesser volume, 10% reduction in RBC content	
			Pediatric preparation	Adjustment to low-weight recipients	Adjusted content	
			Cryopreservation (glycerol)	Most often to ensure availability of RBCCs with a rare blood group for immunized "public-negative" recipients or recipients with complex alloimmunizations[a]	Same Hb content Hematocrit: 40–80% Glycerol ≤1 g	N2 or –80°C electric freeze drying N2: unlimited; –80°C: 30 years 7 days after thawing in suitable additive solutions, 24 h if no additive solution
		Platelets from whole blood (individual units or pools of 4–6 units of ABO identical units) or from apheresis	Suspension in a platelet additive solution (PAS)	Reduction of posttransfusion fever and chills Plasma orientation toward fractionation	From 100 to 700 mL ≥2.10^{11} platelets Ph ≥6.4	At 20–24°C and under permanent motion: 3–7 days *Or* At 4°C without motion: up to 14–21 days (experimental) If irradiated: <24 h
			Deleukocytation (<1–5.10^6 leukocytes per unit): initial whole blood filtration or platelet elective filtration (highly recommended, mandatory in several international jurisdictions)	Reduction of posttransfusion fever and chills Reduction of intracellular pathogens (including CMV infections) Reduction of alloimmunization		
			Pathogen reduction: Most often nucleic acid cross-linker and/or UV illumination	Reduction of transfusion-transmitted infections Prevention of GVHD		
Apheresis	Various apheresis devices allow for the collection of BCs either as individual BCs such as plasma or platelets (possibly double, such as double RBCC) or combined BCs, such as platelets and plasma, or RBCC, platelets, and plasma.		Volume reduction	Prevention of allergic reactions in patients with prior severe reactions		
			Irradiation: X-ray or gamma, ~25–35 Gy; in general, on bags no older than 3 days after collection	Prevention of GVHD		
			Pediatric	Volume and content adjustment		

(*Continued*)

TABLE 113-1 Blood Components: Collection and Manufacturing Processes (Continued)

BLOOD COLLECTION	INITIAL PROCESSING	BLOOD COMPONENT	ADDITIONAL COMPONENT PROCESSING (OPTIONAL TO MANDATORY)	RATIONALE	VOLUME AND CONTENT	STORAGE CONDITIONS AND DURATION
			Cryopreservation (DMSO)	To ensure continuous availability in remote locations To ensure availability of platelets with rare HPA groups		6 h after thawing (depending on cryopreservation procedure, may be resuspended in plasma)
		Plasma from whole blood or from apheresis	Cryopreservation at −18°C (most often)	Shelf life extension	200–300 mL Coagulation factors, including fibrinogen (≥2 g/L), factor VIII (≥0.5 IU/mL), protein C and S, antithrombin	1–2 years if cryopreserved Up to 28 days if kept unfrozen
			Deleukocytation (<1–5.10^6 leukocytes per product): Initial whole blood filtration and/or plasma elective filtration	Reduction of posttransfusion fever and chills Reduction of intracellular pathogens (including CMV) Reduction of alloimmunization		
			Pathogen reduction: Nucleic acid cross-linker and/or UV illumination or solvent detergent treatment (most often on pooled products)	Reduction of transfusion-transmitted infections		
			Lyophilization	To facilitate transportation and storage, as well as immediate availability, in remote locations		
		Granulocyte concentrates from whole blood (pools of up to x ABO identical units) or from apheresis[b]	Irradiation (mandatory)	Prevention of GVHD	≤650 mL ≤2.10^{10} granulocytes	Room temperature ≤24 h after the end of collection
		Whole blood	Deleukocytation with a platelet-sparing device	Reduction of posttransfusion fever and chills Reduction of intracellular pathogens (including CMV) Reduction of alloimmunization	~520 mL (including additive solution)	At 2–4°C Up to 25 days
		Peripheral blood mononuclear cells (apheresis)	May undergo cryopreservation (N2)	Increased practicability Repeated administration	Number of cells adjusted for a predetermined number of T lymphocytes 10^5–10^7 CD3+ cells/recipient kg	N2: unlimited Never frozen or thawed: <6 h
		Cryoprecipitate (collected after thawing and centrifugation of plasma)	Resuspension in plasma (10–15 mL) and cryopreservation	N/A	Cold-insoluble plasma proteins (fibrinogen, factor VIII, von Willebrand factor)	12 months After thawing, may be stored at 20–24°C for up to 6 h

[a]Antigen frequency below 1 to 4% (1/1000) of the population and contraindication for using regular blood units, depending on country-specific regulations. [b]Granulocyte collection by apheresis requires donor pre-administration of steroids and/or hematopoietic growth factor and exposure to heparin and HES during the apheresis procedure.

Abbreviations: BC, blood component; CMV, cytomegalovirus; DMSO, dimethyl sulfoxide; GVHD, graft-versus-host disease; Hb, hemoglobin; HPA, human platelet antigen; N2, nitrogen gas; N/A, not applicable; RBC, red blood cell; RBCC, red blood cell concentrate; UV, ultraviolet.

TABLE 113-2 ABO Blood Groups and Antibodies: Transfusion Compatibility

GENOTYPE(S)	ENZYME(S)/IMMUNODOMINANT SUGAR(S)	PHENOTYPE	NATURAL ANTIBODIES	TRANSFUSION COMPATIBILITY REQUIREMENTS		
				RBCC	PC[a]	PLASMA
A/A or A/0	"A" transferase/N-acetylgalactosamine (GalNac)	A	Anti-B	A or 0	A, 0[b], B[b], or AB[b]	A or A,B
B/B or B/0	"B" transferase/galactose (Gal)	B	Anti-A	B or 0	B, 0, A[b], or AB[b]	B or A,B
A/B	"A" transferase and "B" transferase GalNac and Gal	A,B	None	A,B or A or B or 0	A,B, 0[b], or A[b] or B[b]	A,B
0/0	Inactive Unconverted H antigen	0	Anti-A and Anti-B	0	0, A, B, or A,B	A or B or A,B or 0

[a]Order of priority. [b]Without high-titer anti-A and/or anti-B antibody.

Abbreviations: PC, platelet concentrate; RBCC, red blood cell concentrate.

Carbohydrate Ags are ubiquitously distributed in the body. The ABO Ags, expressed on endothelial cells, are genuine "tissue" groups and may be involved in graft rejection. These Ags are not specific to humans but are shared by many species including viruses and bacteria. The presence of A and B Ags in the environment and, in particular, on the bacteria of the microbiota explains the synthesis of so-called "natural" or "regular" Abs, aside from any transfusion or pregnancy. Such Abs have a major hemolytic capacity as they bind complement and activate its cascade up to the membrane attack complex. This imposes donor-recipient stringent compatibility rules for RBCCs and whole blood transfusion and, albeit less stringently, for plasma and PC transfusion.

Protein blood groups are headed by the **Rh system** (formerly termed "Rhesus" or "Rh") for RBCs **(Table 113-3)**. As these Ags are specific to humans, the occurrence of immunization can only occur upon allogeneic stimulation. The elicited Abs are called "immune" and "irregular" because their appearance following immunization is inconstant. These Abs directed against Ags of RBC groups other than ABO must be detected before RBCC cell transfusion or transplantation and during pregnancy. Of the 43 RBC group systems described, five

TABLE 113-3 Red Blood Cell (RBC) Group Systems and Antibodies: Clinical Significance and Transfusion Recommendations

ISBT NO./ SYSTEM	SYMBOL/ GENE(S)	ANTIGENS (NO.)	MAIN ANTIBODIES (ANTI-)	HEMOLYSIS CHARACTERISTICS		RBCC TRANSFUSION RECOMMENDATIONS
				TRANSFUSION	HDFN	
1/ABO	ABO/*ABO*	4	A, B	None to severe; immediate and/or delayed	None to moderate (rarely severe)	Ab-negative RBCC
2/MNS	MNS/*GYPA, GYPB, (GYPE)*	49	M	None (except in extremely rare cases if active at 37°C)	None (except in extremely rare cases if active at 37°C)	Compatible RBCC (negative DAT at 37°C) Ag-negative red cells in the case of sickle cell disease
			N	None (may be clinically significant in the case of the rare N–S–s–U– phenotype)	None	Compatible RBCC (negative IAT at 37°C) Ag-negative RBCC in the case of N–S–s–U– phenotype
			S, s	None to moderate (rare)	None to severe (rare)	Ag-negative RBCC
			U	Mild to severe	Mild to severe (one reported case requiring an intrauterine transfusion)	Ag-negative RBCC
3/P1PK	P1PK/*A4GALT*	3	P1	None to moderate; delayed (rare)	None	Compatible RBCC (negative DAT at 37°C)
			P1, Pk, P (Tj[a])	None to severe	None to severe	Ag-negative RBCC
4/Rh	RH/*RHD, RHCE*	55	D, C, E, c, e	Mild to severe; immediate or delayed	Mild to severe	Ag-negative RBCC
6 /Kell	KEL/*KEL*	36	K	Mild to severe; delayed	Mild to severe (rare)	Ag-negative RBCC
7/Lewis	LE/*FUT3*	6	Le[a], Le[b]	None (rare cases of hemolytic reactions)	None	Compatible RBCC (negative DIAT at 37°C)
8/Duffy	FY/*ACKR1*	5	Fy[a], Fy[b]	Mild to severe (rare); immediate/delayed	Mild to severe (rare)	Ag-negative RBCC
			Fy3, Fy5	Mild to moderate; immediate (rare)/ delayed	Mild (rare) (no data for anti-Fy5)	Ag-negative RBCC
9/Kidd	JK/*SLC14A1*	3	Jk[a], Jk[b]	None to severe; immediate or delayed	Mild to moderate (rare)	Ag-negative RBCC
			Jk3	None to severe; immediate or delayed	None to mild	Ag-negative RBCC
18/H	H/*FUT1*	1	H (Bombay)	None to severe; immediate/delayed	Not none	Ag-negative RBCC
20/Globoside	GLOB/ *B3GALNT1*	2	P	None to severe	None to mild	Ag-negative RBCC

Abbreviations: Ab, antibody; Ag, antigen; DAT, direct antiglobulin test (Direct Coombs test); HDFN, hemolytic disease of the fetus and newborn; IAT, indirect antiglobulin test (Indirect Coombs test); ISBT, International Society of Blood Transfusion; RBCC, red blood cell concentrate.

(Rh, Kell, Duffy, Kidd, and MNS) are routinely investigated due to the clinical significance of Abs and their frequency. Testing for all five types ensures routine transfusion compatibility of 95%.

The Rh system comprises nearly 56 Ags, the most immunogenic of which is the RhD Ag (RH1). The Rh system has two *RH*D* and *RH*CE* genes located on chromosome 1. The *RH*D* gene codes for the RhD protein expressing the D Ag (RH1) present in 85%, 93%, and >99% of individuals of Caucasian, African, and Asian ancestry, respectively. The *RH*CE* gene codes for RhCE proteins expressing C (RH2) and/or c (RH4), and E (RH3) and/or e (RH4) Ags. The presence of the D Ag confers Rh "positivity," while its absence confers Rh negativity. The *RH*D* and *RH*CE* genes determine eight main haplotypes (*DCe, DcE, Dce, DCE, dce, dCe, dcE,* and *dCE*) whose frequencies differ considerably among different geographical populations. The high diversity of the Rh Ags includes weak or partial expression. Identifying individuals (especially young females of childbearing potential and multitransfused patients) with a weak or partial RhD Ag is important to adequately select RhD-positive or -negative RBCs. Molecular biology is now routinely applied to resolve such situations.

The **Kell system** comprises 36 Ags, one of which is routinely determined: the K antigen (KEL1); 9% and 2% of individuals of Caucasian and African ancestry are K positive (KEL:1), respectively, whereas 91% and 98%, respectively, are K negative (KEL:–1). The immunogenicity of Kell is third behind the ABO and Rh systems. The Kell protein is linked to another blood group protein called Kx. The rare absence of this protein (controlled by a gene on X) is associated with a weak KEL Ag, acanthocytosis, shortened RBC survival, and a progressive form of muscular dystrophy that includes cardiac defects. This rare condition is called the McLeod phenotype.

The **Duffy system** (FY) comprises five Ags, two of which are routinely tested: the Fy^a Ag (FY1), coded by the Fy^a allele, and the Fy^b Ag (FY2), coded by the Fy^b allele. Depending on the combination of alleles, three common phenotypes are expected: Fy (a+b+), which has the two alleles Fy^a and Fy^b; Fy (a+b–), which has only the Fy^a allele in a double dose; and Fy (a–b+), which has only a double dose of the *Fyb* allele. A particular phenotype characterized by the absence of the Fy^a and Fy^b Ags, the Fy(a–b–) phenotype, is exclusive (with some exceptions) to individuals of African ancestry where it can reach frequencies of 70–100% depending on the population. It is linked to the presence of a double dose of a silent *FY*0* allele. This distribution may be related to the fact that the Fy Ags serve as receptors for *Plasmodium vivax* and therefore the Fy(a–b–) phenotype. However, these individuals may develop Abs against two high-frequency Ags (FY3 and FY5) after transfusion or pregnancy. They may also have low granulocyte counts that come to the attention of physicians, but the condition is not associated with any disease.

The **Kidd system** (JK) comprises three Ags, two of which are routinely tested: the Jk^a Ag (JK1), coded by the Jk^a allele, and the Jk^b Ag (JK2), coded by the Jk^b allele. Depending on the combinations of alleles, three common phenotypes are seen: Jk(a+b+) displaying the two alleles Jk^a and Jk^b, Jk(a+b–) displaying only the Jk^a allele in a double dose, and Jk(a–b+) displaying only a double dose of the Jk^b allele. A particular phenotype is characterized by the absence of the Jk^a and Jk^b Ags: the Jk(a–b–) phenotype found in Polynesian populations. It is linked to the presence of a double dose of a silent *JK*0* allele. These people may develop Abs against the high-frequency anti-JK3 Ag after transfusion or pregnancy.

The **MNS system** comprises 49 Ags, four of which are routinely tested. Two genes (*GYPA, GYPB*) encode two pairs of so-called "antithetical" Ags. The M (MNS1) and N (MNS2) pair Ags encoded by the *M* and *N* alleles, respectively, are branched on the glycophorin A molecule. Their combination will determine whether or not they are present. M+ and N+ subjects have both alleles; an M+, N– subject is homozygous for the *M* allele; and an M–, N+ subject is homozygous for the *N* allele. The same holds true for the other pair of Ags, S (MNS3) and s (MNS4) expressed on glycophorin B. Therefore, an M+, N–, S–, s+ subject (in international nomenclature, this is written as MNS:1,–2,–3,5) will be homozygous for the *M* and s alleles. A rare phenotype, S–s–, found exclusively in individuals of African ancestry, can develop an Ab against the high-frequency U Ag (MNS:5) after transfusion or pregnancy.

■ RARE RBC PHENOTYPES

Some patients present with rare genotype/phenotype assortments and their RBCs display so-called private Ags or, conversely, lack public Ags (i.e., widely shared Ags) toward which the patient may develop an immune response when exposed to these Ags. Public-negative immunized individuals are virtually impossible to transfuse using conventional blood bank resources and require access to designated blood banks that have access to rare blood programs. Their primary responsibility is to identify and collect blood from donors exhibiting particular Ag displays on their RBCs or platelets that are uncommon in the given jurisdiction. Specific ethnic populations may be targeted, as some may display genotype specificities, such as the Bombay group in southwestern Indians. Several hemoglobinopathies, such as sickle cell disease, are more common in individuals of African ancestry. Such patients may display RBC phenotypes that are uncommon in countries in the Northern Hemisphere, resulting in difficulties adequately identifying donors to match the need, as a last resort, for highly valued cryopreserved BCs.

CLINICAL INDICATIONS AND EFFICACY ASSESSMENT OF BLOOD COMPONENTS

BCs are life-saving therapies but also scarce resources. Furthermore, transfusion may result in well-identified adverse reactions as well as more ill-defined adverse events, including inflammation and therapeutic inefficacy. As highlighted in so-called patient blood management programs, transfusion should be considered within a multidisciplinary approach that includes optimization of hematopoiesis, minimization of blood loss during surgical interventions, and optimization of tolerance to anemia. Clinical indications of BCs as well as means to assess therapeutic efficacy are detailed in **Table 113-4**.

ADVERSE REACTIONS TO BLOOD COMPONENTS

Adverse reactions to transfused BCs are most commonly non-life-threatening, although serious reactions can present with mild symptoms and signs. Transfused patients should be closely monitored for warning signs suggestive of adverse reactions, as described in **Table 113-5**. When an adverse reaction is suspected, the transfusion must be stopped while the recipient's clinical status is assessed and supportive care is initiated as needed. An average of 35 transfusion-associated fatalities with possible to definite imputability were reported yearly to the U.S. Food and Drug Administration (FDA) between 2014 and 2018 among ~14 million transfused BCs. Most frequent causes of death were transfusion-associated circulatory overload (TACO) (32%), followed by TRALI (26%), hemolysis (18%), and sepsis (14%).

Adverse reactions to BCs may result in immune and nonimmune mechanisms. Immune-mediated reactions are often due to recipient or donor alloimmunization and the presence of preformed recipient or donor Abs. Nonimmune causes of reactions are from the physical or chemical properties of BCs or from pathogens present in the BC.

■ IMMUNE-MEDIATED ADVERSE REACTIONS

Hemolytic Transfusion Adverse Reactions Immune-mediated acute hemolysis occurs when the recipient preformed Abs lyse transfused donor RBCs and may occur during or 24 h after transfusion. The anti-A or anti-B Abs are responsible for the majority of the most severe reactions, which can be fatal. However, alloAbs directed against other RBC Ags (i.e., Rh, Kell, and Duffy) are also responsible for severe hemolytic reactions. Such dramatic reactions are usually caused by a failure in product or patient identification, erroneous blood grouping, or unidentified anti-RBC alloimmunization in the recipient. Hemolysis, most often of lesser severity, may also occur upon tranfusion of BCs containing incompatible plasma with a large amount of alloAbs directed against the recipient's RBCs. This may typically occur after

TABLE 113-4 Blood Components: Clinical Use

COMPONENT		THERAPEUTIC INDICATION	GOAL	DONOR/RECIPIENT COMPATIBILITY	DOSAGE	EFFICACY EVALUATION
Red blood cell concentrate (RBCC)	Transfusion	Anemia and/or tissue ischemia (treatment or prevention) Hb below a given threshold (to be considered in relation with clinical symptoms): <7 g/dL for patients hemodynamically stable, except for patients undergoing orthopedic surgery, cardiac surgery, or with preexisting cardiovascular disease (<8 g/dL) as well as for patients with acute coronary disease (<9–10 g/dL). Such thresholds do not apply to neonates and patients with severe thrombocytopenia and chronic transfusion-dependent anemia. Not recommended: nutritional anemia (iron, vitamin B_{12}, or folate deficiency)	Improve systemic and tissue oxygenation	ABO compatible (cellular) and ABO identical when achievable. RhD compatibility is required in young and childbearing females, and whenever possible if multitransfused RhC/c/E/e; Kell-compatible RBCCs are required in frequently transfused patients. Additional compatibility may be required depending on the clinical setting and screening results.	1 unit at a time (250–350 mL, including additive solution), repeated per clinical status and Hb level	Reduction of anemia-related symptoms, clinical improvement Increased Hb (+1 g/dL) and hematocrit (+3%)
	RBC exchange	Anemia/sickle cell crisis in hemoglobinopathies (sickle cell disease, thalassemia)	Replace altered RBCs with donor RBCs and compensate for hemolysis, prevention of sickle cell occlusive crisis		25–30 mL/kg	Sickle cell disease: reduced percentage of HbS
Platelet concentrates (PCs) (from pooled whole blood–derived platelets or single donor apheresis), maintained at room temperature (most often) or at 4°C		Thrombocytopenia-related bleeding disorders: treatment (cold or room temperature PC) or prevention (room temperature PC) Platelet level below a given threshold: ≤5000/μL in the absence of fever or infection, ≤10,000/μL to 20,000/μL if fever or infection; ≤50,000/μL if surgery, DIC, endoscopy, invasive procedures; ≤80,000/μL if neurosurgery or eye surgery Acute hypovolemic coagulopathy (see below) Not recommended: immune thrombocytopenia, thrombotic microangiopathy, heparin-induced thrombocytopenia	Correct impaired primary hemostasis, including vessel healing Cold stored platelets, despite lower in vivo survival, have maintained and possibly improved hemostatic capacity compared with room temperature stored platelets	ABO identical preferable; if not, ABO compatible (cellular) with low-titer anti-A/B Ab; RhD compatible preferred in premenopausal women HLA compatible (negative lymphocyte crossmatch) or HLA identical in case of refractoriness related to the presence of anti-HLA Ab HPA compatible in thrombocytopenic neonates to HPA immunized mother (fetal neonatal alloimmune thrombocytopenia)	$0.5–0.7 \times 10^{10}$ platelets/kg (apheresis or pooled whole blood–derived PCs)	Prevention and/or resolution of bleeding Corrected count increment[a] $\geq 10 \times 10^9$/L within 1 h and $\geq 7.5 \times 10^9$/L within 24 h after transfusion (not applicable to cold/cryopreserved platelets)
Plasma (thawed frozen, never frozen and maintained at 4°C or at room temperature, freeze-dried)	Transfusion	Coagulation factor–related bleeding disorders Acute hypovolemic coagulopathy (see below)	Correct impaired hemostasis by providing missing elements of coagulation or fibrinolysis cascade, as well as elements to heal injured vessel endothelium	ABO compatible (plasma)	10–15 mL/kg	Reduced bleeding disorder
		Infectious disease treatment (convalescent plasma containing pathogen-specific Abs): Argentina hemorrhagic fever, viral respiratory infections (experimental)	Provide Abs against relevant pathogens		Not determined	Infection resolution
	Plasma exchange (plasma or combined plasma and albumin)	Pathogenic Ab removal and supplementation of lacking enzyme (e.g., thrombotic thrombocytopenic microangiopathy or Guillain-Barre syndrome) Pathogenic Ab removal (e.g., anti-HLA Ab prior to kidney transplantation)	Deplete pathogenic elements in the blood (auto-antibodies such as anti-ADAMTS-13 Ab in case of TTP, excess cholesterol, etc.); plasma may also bring anti-inflammatory and/or immunomodulatory factors such as immunoglobulin	ABO compatible (plasma)	45–60 mL/kg	Improved disease-specific symptomatology (i.e., apyrexia and platelet recovery in case of TTP) Reduced antibody levels (e.g., anti-HLA antibodies prior to organ transplantation)

(Continued)

TABLE 113-4 Blood Components: Clinical Use (Continued)

COMPONENT	THERAPEUTIC INDICATION	GOAL	DONOR/RECIPIENT COMPATIBILITY	DOSAGE	EFFICACY EVALUATION
Whole blood	Acute hypovolemic coagulopathy requiring massive transfusion	Balanced provision of blood components maintained at 4°C and without an additive solution and related dilution	ABO-identical or group O with low-titer anti-A/B Ab	Repeated per clinical status	Normovolemia; bleeding resolution
Multicomponent (RBCC, PC, and plasma)	Acute hypovolemic coagulopathy requiring massive transfusion	Appropriate ratio is under investigation; a ratio of 1 RBCC/1 plasma/0.25 PC (platelet content of a whole blood) is currently favored	Standard RBCC, PC, and plasma compatibility	1 RBCC/1 plasma/0.25 PC ratio, repeated per clinical status	Normovolemia; bleeding resolution
Granulocyte concentrates (apheresis or a pool of whole blood–derived granulocytes)	Severe refractory bacterial or fungal infection in patients with neutropenia (<100/µl) or with dysfunctional granulocytes (CGD) (mainly soft tissues and lung). Neutropenia can be acquired (chemotherapy) or congenital. Usefulness of granulocyte transfusions is debated. Formal proof of efficacy is lacking.	Correct impaired granulocyte function in relation to granulocytopenia or granulocyte dysfunction	ABO compatible	$1–2 \times 10^{10}$, repeated per clinical status	Infection resolution (or stabilization until recovery from neutropenia)
Donor mononuclear cells	Relapse of malignant hemopathy after allogeneic hematopoietic cell transplantation	Graft-versus-leukemia effect (and graft enhancement effect)	N/A	$10^5–10^7$ T lymphocytes/kg	Disease specific (remission)
Cryoprecipitate	Acute bleeding coagulopathy, type II (dysfunctional factor) or type III (absent factor) Von Willebrand disease, hemophilia A in the absence of factor VIII concentrates	Provision of fibrinogen, factor VIII, von Willebrand factor, and factor XIII	ABO compatibility is not required	10–15 mL/unit, pool of 4–5 units	Increased plasma fibrinogen (0.3–1 g/L)

[a]CCI calculation:

$$\text{CCI} = \frac{\text{Postransfusion count } (/\mu\text{L}) - \text{pretransfusion count } (/\mu\text{L})}{\text{Number of platelets transfused} \times 10^{11}} \times \text{Body surface area (m}^2\text{)}$$

Abbreviations: Ab, antibody; CCI, corrected count increment; CGD, chronic granulomatous disease; DIC, disseminated intravascular coagulation; Hb, hemoglobin; HLA, human leukocyte antigen; N/A, not applicable; RBC, red blood cell; TTP, thrombotic thrombocytopenic purpura.

TABLE 113-5 Transfusion Adverse Reactions: Main Warning Signs

Fever (≥38°C)	+1–2°C within 4 h	FNHTR Anti-HLA immunization and cognate Ag in the blood product TRALI (with dyspnea at the forefront)
	+1–2°C within 15 min +/–: • Chills • Dyspnea • Hypotension • Digestive disorders • Disseminated intravascular coagulation • Hemoglobinuria >2°C or ≥39°C	Transfusion-transmitted bacterial infection Hemolysis
Hypotension (≥30 mmHg decrease in systolic blood pressure)		Hemolytic shock Anaphylactic shock Septic shock TRALI (with dyspnea at the forefront)
Dyspnea		TRALI (within 6 h of transfusion) TACO (within 6 h of transfusion) Severe allergy (immediate; within 4 h)
Hemoglobinuria		Intravascular hemolysis • Immunologic • Mechanical • Toxic • Thermic
Rash	<2/3 of the body within 2–3 h	Minor allergy
	>2/3 of the body during or within 2–3 h	Severe allergy
	>2/3 of the body within 5 min Associated with dyspnea and shock	Anaphylaxis
Icterus		Delayed hemolysis
New alloantibody		Alloimmunization
Rash, diarrhea, and fever occurring 2 days to 6 weeks after transfusion		GVHD
Gum bleeding, purpura 5–12 days after transfusion		Posttransfusion purpura
Cardiac, hepatic, and/or renal insufficiency in frequently transfused patients		Posttransfusion iron overload
Top-down investigation after a blood donor is subsequently found to be infected Bottom-up investigation after another recipient of a same blood donation is found to be infected Infectious symptoms within 6 months		Transfusion-transmitted infection

Abbreviations: Ag, antigen; FNHTR, febrile nonhemolytic transfusion reaction; GVHD, graft-versus-host disease; HLA, human leukocyte antigen; TACO, transfusion-associated circulatory overload; TRALI, transfusion-related acute lung injury.

transfusion of a PC containing ABO-incompatible plasma. Estimated frequencies of acute and chronic hemolytic adverse reactions are 1–10 and 5–40 per 10^5 transfused BCs, respectively.

Mechanisms of transfusion hemolytic reactions are described in **Figure 113-1.**

Prevention of hemolytic reactions relies on **pretransfusion testing** of potential recipients. Testing will include determination of the ABO RhD phenotype (and anti-ABO Abs) as well as additional typing for the other main Rh Ags (CcEe): K Ag of the Kell system and, more rarely, Duffy, Kidd and Ss Ags, depending on the clinical setting. These determinations are most often performed by serology. However, molecular typing is increasingly being used to predict RBC phenotype and facilitate the selection of a compatible component. Special care must be taken to verify the patient's identity and apply adequate tube labeling. A double ABO determination performed separately may be considered, especially in the absence of a systematic crossmatch.

Testing will also include the screening and identification of alloAbs directed against RBC Ags other than ABO. This screen is performed by mixing patient serum with type O RBCs expressing Ags from most blood group systems and whose extended phenotype is known. The specificity of the alloAb is identified by correlating the presence or absence of Ag with the induced—or not—agglutination. Special attention should be paid to patients receiving monoclonal Ab treatment that may bind to erythrocytes in vivo (such as anti-CD38 IgG treatment for multiple myeloma) and therefore interfere with alloAb screening. Such interference may be offset by sample dithiothreitol pretreatment.

Crossmatching between the recipient plasma/serum and the sample of selected RBCs may be performed, especially when the recipient is alloimmunized against RBC or is frequently transfused, as well as in specific clinical settings such as sickle cell disease, even if the Ab screening is negative.

The selection of a compatible BC should take into account pretransfusion testing as well as the recipient's clinical status. In the case of D (Rh1)-negative patients, every attempt must be made to provide Rh-negative BC to prevent anti-D alloimmunization. In an emergency situation, D-positive RBCC can be safely transfused to a D-negative patient who lacks anti-D. However, an estimated 20–22% of RBCC recipients will become alloimmunized and produce anti-D Abs after transfusion with D-positive RBCs (this frequency is higher in healthy individuals). Such alloimmunization can occur after PC transfusion, although at a much lower frequency (~1%). Whenever possible, females with childbearing potential (to include prepubertal girls) should be transfused with D- and K (KEL1)-compatible RBCCs and D-compatible PCs to prevent alloimmunization and protect a future fetus/newborn from an alloimmune-mediated hemolytic disease. D-negative females with childbearing potential who are transfused

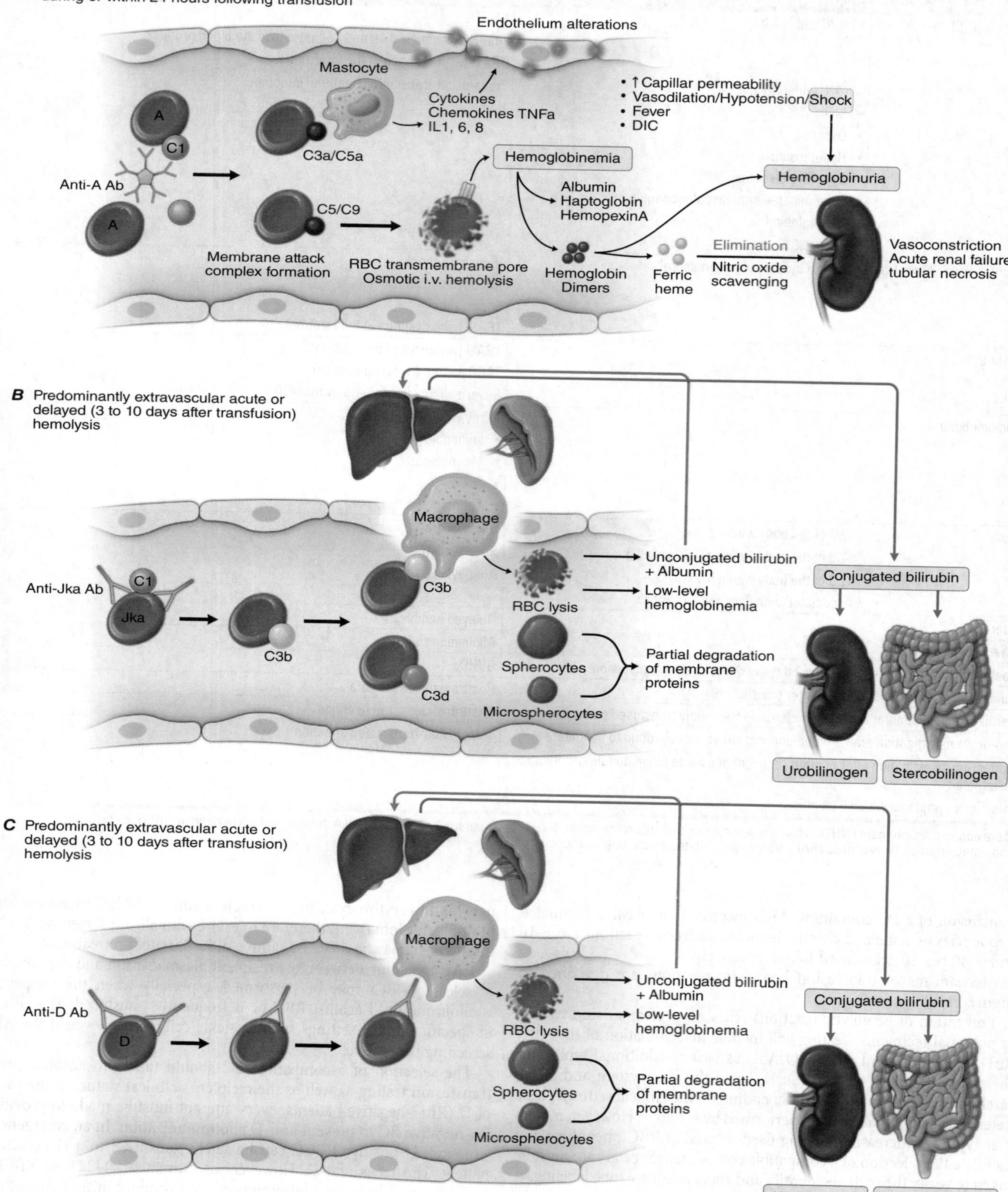

FIGURE 113-1 Mechanisms of transfusion hemolytic reactions. ***A.*** Acute responses will involve preexisting antibodies (Abs), naturally occurring anti-A/anti-B IgM or IgG directed against other RBC Ab and resulting from prior sensitization. Upon interaction with cognate antigen (Ag) on transfused red blood cells (RBCs), recipient allogeneic Ab (alloAb), mostly natural anti-A/anti-B IgM, may fix and activate complement up to C5/C9. Formation of membrane attack complex (MAC) will create pores in transfused RBCs with resulting intravascular hemolysis, release of toxic moieties including free hemoglobin responsible for end-organ damage including renal failure, and tissue factors contributing to occurrence of disseminated intravascular coagulation (DIC). ***B.*** Alternatively, complement activation may be incomplete, as typically observed in a delayed hemolytic transfusion reaction involving neoformed allogeneic IgG. In such cases, complement activation up to C3 results in C3b-mediated opsonization of RBCs, extravascular hemolysis, and clearance through immunophagocytosis. Anemia and jaundice will be the primary clinical manifestations. ***C.*** Lastly, alloAb may not fix complement while ensuring antibody-dependent cellular cytotoxicity (ADCC)–mediated phagocytosis of targeted RBC. *(Adapted from SR Panch et al: Hemolytic transfusion reactions. N Engl J Med 381:150, 2019.)*

with BCs containing Rh-positive RBCs should receive anti-D Ig to prevent allosensitization.

Hemolysis, most often of lesser severity, may also occur after transfer of alloAbs directed against the recipient's RBC Ags. Such ABO "plasmatic" incompatibility, called "minor ABO incompatibility," will occur mainly with PC transfusions, where platelets are suspended in ~100–300 mL of plasma (depending on whether part of the plasma is substituted by additive solution). BCs containing plasma with high-titer anti-A/B Ab may induce a hemolytic reaction. When the transfusion of ABO-identical (vs ABO-compatible) PCs is feasible, PCs provided by donors with low-titer anti-A/B only should be preferred. "High-titer" PCs should be restricted to group O recipients. While there is no universal definition of high-titer Abs, a threshold titer of 1/64 (as assessed by hemagglutination) may be appropriate. It should be noted that the use of an additive solution in PCs substantially mitigates this risk. Lastly, ABO plasmatic incompatibility can lead to the formation of immune complexes with soluble A and/or B Ags and ensuing inflammation and platelet activation.

Acute hemolytic reactions may present with hypotension, tachypnea, tachycardia, fever (+1–2°C), chills, chest and back pain, hemoglobinuria, and hemoglobinemia. In the most severe cases, DIC, acute renal failure, shock, and death may occur.

Delayed hemolytic reactions, with icterus and persisting or worsening anemia as the main clinical manifestations, result from an anamnestic response. Such reactions may occur in patients previously sensitized to RBC Ags who have a negative alloAb screen at the time of transfusion due to low Ab levels. The alloAb is detectable 1–2 weeks after the transfusion.

Diagnosis of transfusion-associated hemolysis relies on persistent and/or worsening anemia, depleted plasma haptoglobin levels, hemoglobinemia and hemoglobinuria, as well as elevated plasma lactate dehydrogenase and unconjugated bilirubin. The direct antiglobulin test (DAT, or direct Coombs test) that detects immunoglobulin, and possibly complement (C3d), on the surface of the recipient's RBC will most often be positive (**Fig. 113-2**). Similarly, a positive indirect antiglobulin test (IAT, or indirect Coombs test) that detects anti-RBC alloAb in the serum will also be positive. An elution of the Ab on the surface of the RBC may allow for the identification of the culprit alloAb.

The management of an immune-mediated acute hemolytic transfusion reaction is mainly supportive. Prompt interruption of the transfusion, biological workup, and a thorough clerical check to prevent a possible second misidentified transfusion are crucial initial steps. Vigorous hydration with isotonic saline and diuretics to maintain urine output is recommended. Although often self-limiting, acute hemolysis may also require forced alkaline diuresis, correction of electrolyte abnormalities, and pressor support as needed. In patients with DIC and severe bleeding, PC, plasma, and cryoprecipitate or fibrinogen may be required. When transfusion of incompatible RBCCs is unavoidable, prophylaxis with steroids (100 mg of hydrocortisone) just before the transfusion and repeated 24 h later and polyvalent immunoglobulin

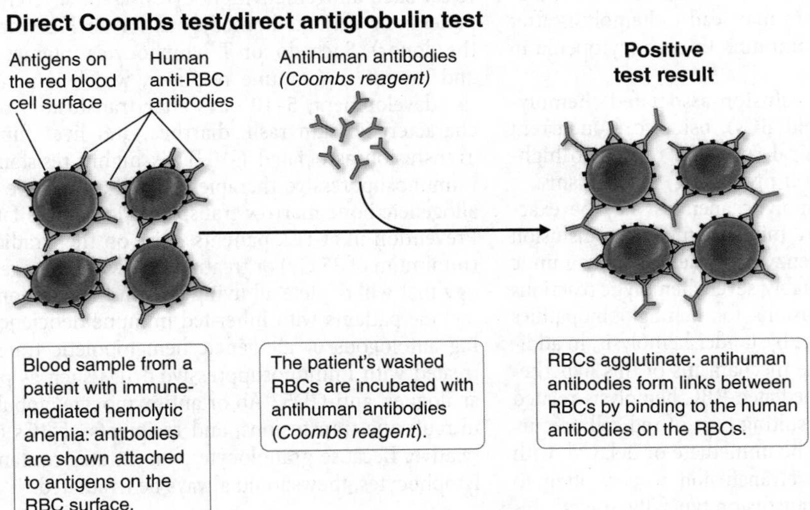
Direct Coombs test/direct antiglobulin test
Antigens on the red blood cell surface
Human anti-RBC antibodies
Antihuman antibodies (Coombs reagent)
Positive test result
Blood sample from a patient with immune-mediated hemolytic anemia: antibodies are shown attached to antigens on the RBC surface.
The patient's washed RBCs are incubated with antihuman antibodies (Coombs reagent).
RBCs agglutinate: antihuman antibodies form links between RBCs by binding to the human antibodies on the RBCs.

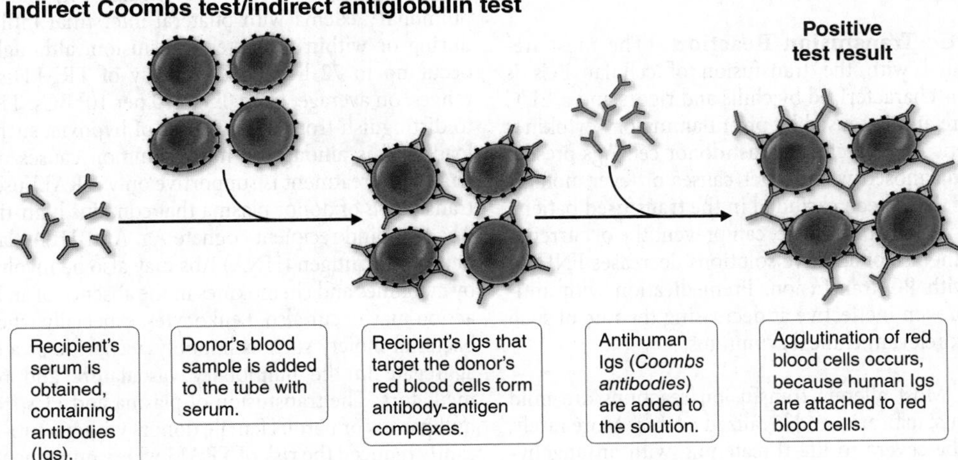
Indirect Coombs test/indirect antiglobulin test
Positive test result
Recipient's serum is obtained, containing antibodies (Igs).
Donor's blood sample is added to the tube with serum.
Recipient's Igs that target the donor's red blood cells form antibody-antigen complexes.
Antihuman Igs (Coombs antibodies) are added to the solution.
Agglutination of red blood cells occurs, because human Igs are attached to red blood cells.

FIGURE 113-2 Direct and indirect Coombs test. The direct Coombs (antiglobulin) test detects the presence of antibodies (or complement) on the surface of erythrocytes. The indirect Coombs (antiglobulin) test detects antibodies in the serum that may bind to donor erythrocytes. Igs, immunoglobulins; RBC, red blood cell. *(Adapted from http://upload.wikimedia.org/wikipedia/commons/1/1c/coombs_test_schematic.png.)*

(1.2–2.0 g/kg per day over 2–3 days, initiated just before the transfusion) have been successfully used to prevent or minimize acute and delayed hemolysis.

Immune-mediated hemolysis may also occur after allogeneic hematopoietic transplantation (most often involving a peripheral blood stem cell graft) or, more seldomly, solid organ transplantation. Minor ABO incompatibility, with subsequent red cell destruction in the recipient, is the most common cause of clinically significant hemolysis in such cases. Viable donor B lymphocytes, called "passenger lymphocytes," transferred passively with the graft, may produce alloAbs (including anti-D or anti-A1 in an A2 donor) that target recipient red cells. Such hemolysis has been reported to develop 5–14 days after transplantation. Reduced-intensity conditioning regimens and cyclosporine as prophylaxis against GVHD or rejection have been associated with increased risk. Transfusing RBCs compatible with the graft donor and the use of GVHD prophylaxis able to target B cells (e.g., methotrexate) have significantly reduced the incidence of passenger lymphocyte syndrome. Allogeneic hematopoietic transplantation may also result in acute hemolysis due to incompatible donor-derived red cell (and precursor) destruction by the recipient alloAbs (i.e., major ABO incompatibility). Prolonged pure red cell aplasia may occur in such a situation. Graft deserythrocytation will reduce the risk of early acute hemolysis.

Polyvalent immunoglobulin may contain high titers of anti-A (mostly) and/or anti-B Abs and induce acute hemolysis, most often of limited severity. Such hemolysis is particularly described in group A or A,B children receiving high-dose immunoglobulin, notably for Kawasaki's disease, as well as in adults treated for thrombotic thrombocytopenic purpura. A similar mechanism may lead to hemolysis after anti-D immunoglobulin treatment for immune thrombocytopenia in RhD-positive patients.

Nonimmune mechanisms of transfusion-associated hemolysis include thermal (overheated or cold BCs), osmotic (concurrent hypo-osmotic perfusion), and mechanical (pressure related to high-flow transfusion filtering during cell saver processing) mechanisms.

Autoimmune and drug-induced hemolytic anemias may be exacerbated by transfusion and can therefore mimic hemolytic transfusion reactions. Transfusion of RBCs with enzymatic defects may mimic immune-mediated hemolysis as well. Notably, severe hemolytic reactions in patients receiving long-term transfusions for hemoglobinopathies (mainly sickle cell disease) can precipitate bystander hemolysis, in addition to clearing transfused red cells. The mechanisms of this hyperhemolytic transfusion reaction may be a mediated RBC hemolysis-related systemic inflammatory response and resulting lysis of red cell precursors by macrophages. This process may be immediate or delayed, with hemoglobin levels falling below the pretransfusion values, often to life-threatening levels. Further RBCC transfusion typically exacerbates ongoing hemolysis, with the exogenous (transfused) allogeneic Ags probably triggering further nonspecific hemolysis.

Febrile Nonhemolytic Transfusion Reaction The most frequent reaction associated with the transfusion of cellular BCs is FNHTR. This reaction is characterized by chills and rigors and a ≥1°C rise in body temperature and is caused by proinflammatory cytokines in the BC or by recipient Abs directed against donor cell Ags present in the BC. FNHTR is diagnosed when other causes of fever, notably infection and hemolysis, have been excluded in the transfused patient. Leukocyte reduction, especially prestorage, can prevent the occurrence of FNHTR. Moreover, the use of additive solutions decreases FNHTR frequency associated with PC transfusion. Premedication with antipyretics has generally proven ineffective at decreasing the rate of such reactions and may mask relevant clinical symptoms.

Allergic Reactions Most allergic transfusion reactions are mild and include rash, pruritus, urticaria, and localized edema. More rarely, allergic reactions may be severe to life-threatening with an anaphylactic reaction that can involve bronchospasm, respiratory distress, hypotension, nausea, vomiting, and shock. Frequencies of mild and severe allergic reactions are ~100 and ~5 per 105 BCs, respectively. Allergic reactions are related to plasma proteins found in transfused components. Mild reactions may be treated by temporarily stopping the transfusion and administering antihistamine drugs. Patients with a history of allergic transfusion reaction may be premedicated with an antihistamine, although there is no consensus on this issue. Cellular components can be washed to remove residual plasma for extremely sensitized patients. Most of the allergic presentation may not depend on preformed Abs and may be attributable to soluble mediators triggering histamine and serotonin release from platelets and leukocytes. An anaphylactic reaction may occur after the transfusion of only a few milliliters of the BC. Treatment includes stopping the transfusion, maintaining vascular access, and administering adrenaline (0.3–0.5 mg subcutaneously). Additional treatment with steroids, antihistamine drugs, and bronchodilators may also be required.

Patients who are IgA deficient (<1% of the population) may be sensitized to this immunoglobulin isotype and may be at risk of anaphylactic reactions associated with plasma transfusion. As a precaution, individuals with severe IgA deficiency should therefore receive, where available, IgA-deficient plasma and washed cellular BCs. Patients who have anaphylactic or repeated allergic reactions to BCs should be tested for IgA deficiency. It should be noted that the importance, or even the reality, of such a transfusion-related allergic risk is currently debated.

Graft-Versus-Host Disease GVHD is an extremely rare adverse reaction caused by transfusion, although it is a frequent complication of allogeneic hematopoietic transplantation. Transfusion-related GVHD is mediated by engrafted donor T lymphocytes in a recipient unable to reject such allogenic lymphocytes (as in severely immunosuppressed patients or patients homozygous for an HLA haplotype shared with the donor). Such donor T lymphocytes interact with host HLA Ags and mount an immune response, which is manifested clinically by the development, 5–10 days after transfusion, of cytopenia, fever, a characteristic skin rash, diarrhea, and liver function abnormalities. Transfusion-associated GVHD is highly resistant to treatment with immunosuppressive therapies as well as ablative therapy followed by allogeneic bone marrow transplantation and is fatal in >90% of cases. Prevention in at-risk patients relies on the irradiation of cellular BCs (minimum of 25 Gy) or treating BCs with pathogen reduction technology that will deplete all living cells in the component. At-risk patients include patients with inherited immune deficiency, patients undergoing autologous or allogeneic hematopoietic transplantation, patients treated with immunosuppressive drugs such as purine or pyrimidine analogues, anti-CD52 Ab or antithymocyte globulin, fetuses receiving intrauterine transfusions, and recipients of BCs provided by a blood relative. Because granulocyte concentrates contain a large number of lymphocytes, they should always be irradiated.

Transfusion-Related Acute Lung Injury TRALI is characterized by the occurrence or worsening of hypoxia and noncardiogenic pulmonary edema with bilateral interstitial infiltrates on chest x-ray during or within 6 h after transfusion, although delayed cases may occur up to 72 h later. Frequency of TRALI is BC dependent and ranges, on average, from 0.5 to 10 per 10^5 BCs. TRALI may be difficult to distinguish from other causes of hypoxia, such as circulatory overload, and is among the most common causes of transfusion-related fatalities. Treatment is supportive only. TRALI usually results from the transfusion of donor plasma that contains high-titer anti-HLA class II Abs that bind recipient cognate Ag. Anti-HLA class I and anti–human neutrophil antigen (HNA) Abs may also be involved. TRALI mediated by cytokines and chemokines in the absence of an HLA-mediated interaction may occur also. Leukocytes, especially when primed by either a bacterial moiety such as lipopolysaccharide or a cytokine/chemokine, aggregate in the pulmonary vasculature and release inflammatory mediators. The transfusion of plasma and PCs from male donors and nulliparous or parous female donors without anti-HLA Abs has significantly reduced the risk of TRALI where implemented. Recipient factors associated with an increased risk of TRALI include smoking, chronic alcohol use, shock, liver surgery (transplantation), cancer surgery, mechanical ventilation, and positive fluid balance.

Posttransfusion Purpura This rare reaction (~1/10^5 BCs) is defined as a thrombocytopenia-related bleeding disorder developing 5–12 days after PC (and more rarely RBCC) transfusion, predominantly in women. Platelet-specific alloAbs are found in the recipient, most frequently anti-HPA-1a in HPA-1a-negative alloimmunized individuals. The delayed thrombocytopenia is due to a secondary increased production of alloAbs. The mechanisms for the destruction of the patient's own platelets remain unclear. Management is mostly supportive but may require polyvalent immunoglobulin, steroids, or plasma exchange. Additional platelet transfusions may worsen the thrombocytopenia or be associated with poor increments. Prevention of recurrence includes use of washed BCs or BCs from HPA-compatible donors.

Alloimmunization/Platelet Refractoriness A recipient may become alloimmunized to a number of Ags on cellular blood elements and plasma proteins. AlloAbs to RBC Ags are detected during pretransfusion testing, and their presence may delay finding Ag-negative crossmatch-compatible products for transfusion. Women of childbearing age who are sensitized to RBC Ags (i.e., D, c, E, Kell, or Duffy) are at risk of bearing a fetus with hemolytic disease of the fetus or newborn. Ag matching is the only pretransfusion selection test to prevent RBC alloimmunization, which is found to occur with a frequency of ~100/10^5 RBCC transfusions. Alloimmunization to Ags on leukocytes and platelets, most often anti-HLA Abs, can result in refractoriness to PC transfusions (as defined by a low increase in platelet count after transfusion). Once alloimmunization has developed, HLA-compatible (crossmatched) PCs should be preferred if available. If not, repeated PCs at shortened intervals may be considered. Use of leukocyte-reduced cellular BCs will reduce the incidence of immunization. Transfusion refractoriness may also result from an anti-HPA alloimmunization, although less commonly. Recipient factors associated with platelet refractoriness include fever, splenomegaly, bleeding, DIC, and medications such as amphotericin B. Notably, cold-stored (and cryopreserved) PCs have been found to have preserved hemostatic function in acutely bleeding patients despite poor platelet increments.

Immunomodulation Transfusion of allogeneic blood may be associated with immunosuppression, as evidenced early on by the beneficial effect of pretransplant transfusion on kidney graft survival. The intensity of such an effect is debated and, if present, is most probably attenuated by the use of leukoreduced BCs. Transfusion-related immunomodulation is indeed thought to be mainly mediated by donor leukocytes, whether transfused to the recipient or undergoing apoptosis during storage. However, leukoreduced RBCCs or PCs still release immunomodulatory mediators during storage. These mediators, along with the transfused RBCs or platelets, may exert various, possibly opposing, immune effects in vivo, including immunosuppression and inflammation.

NONIMMUNOLOGIC TRANSFUSION ADVERSE REACTIONS

Fluid Overload TACO is a common and underrecognized transfusion adverse reaction. Estimated frequencies vary from ~10 to 1000 per 10^5 BCs. TACO is now the main cause of death from transfusion since the TRALI risk has been mitigated. Risk factors include older age, renal failure, preexisting fluid overload, cardiac dysfunction, administration of a large volume of BCs, and an excessive rate of transfusion in relation to the patient's hemodynamic tolerance. TACO results in dyspnea, hypoxia, bilateral and predominantly alveolar infiltrates on chest x-ray, frequent systolic hypertension, and elevated brain natriuretic peptide. Fever may also exist. Prevention involves identifying at-risk patients, close monitoring, a slow transfusion rate (1 RBCC over 3–4 h), and use of diuretics in hemodynamically stable patients with a history of TACO. Treatment requires stopping the transfusion and administrating oxygen and diuretics.

Massive Transfusion-Associated Reactions/Electrolyte and Cold Toxicity Reactions Reactions related to massive transfusion, i.e., transfusion of 50% of the patient's total blood volume over 3 h or >5–10 units of RBCCs (plus associated BCs), include citrate toxicity, hypothermia, hyperkalemia, and dilutional coagulopathy. Citrate, which is commonly used to anticoagulate BCs, chelates calcium. Hypocalcemia, manifested by circumoral paresthesia, and changes in cardiac function may result from multiple rapid transfusions. Although citrate is quickly metabolized to bicarbonate, calcium infusion (through a separate line) may be required. Rapid transfusion of BCs still at 4°C can result in hypothermia and cardiac dysrhythmias. Use of an inline warmer will prevent this complication. RBC leakage during storage, longer storage, and irradiation increase the concentration of potassium in the unit. Neonates and patients with renal failure or other comorbidities (e.g., hyperglycemia or hypocalcemia) are at risk of hyperkalemia and resulting acute cardiac toxicity. Treatment includes insulin, glucose, calcium gluconate, and furosemide, and prevention includes the use of washed or plasma-reduced RBCCs or a storage age of <7–10 days and the avoidance of RBCCs stored for >24 h after irradiation.

Iron Overload Each unit of RBCs contains 200–250 mg of iron. In frequently transfused recipients, iron accumulation that is left untreated will affect endocrine, hepatic, and cardiac function. Death may occur from cardiac failure or arrhythmia. Iron overload can be assessed by means of serum ferritin measurements, magnetic resonance imaging, and liver biopsy. Prevention and treatment of this frequently underreported transfusion adverse event rely on careful monitoring and iron chelation.

Hypotensive Reactions Acute hypotensive transfusion reactions are defined as an abrupt drop in blood pressure of >30 mmHg early after the start of transfusion and resolving quickly once the transfusion is stopped, without further intervention. Respiratory, gastrointestinal, or mild allergic reactions may also be present. Estimated frequency is 1–10/10^5 BCs. These reactions may result from the generation of vasoactive kinins in the BCs and are more likely to occur in hypertensive patients taking angiotensin-converting enzyme (ACE) inhibitors who are therefore less able to metabolize bradykinin. Upon resolution, the same blood product should not be restarted. Switching from an ACE inhibitor to an alternative drug should be considered for patients requiring further transfusions.

Adverse Transfusion Reactions of Uncertain Imputability Necrotizing enterocolitis, which is common in preterm and very-low-birth-weight neonates, has been infrequently described with close temporal association with RBC transfusion. However, the causality of any association remains to be further ascertained, as does the efficacy of withholding feeds during transfusion to prevent such a complication. Posterior reversible encephalopathy syndrome is a rare syndrome characterized by acute reversible neurologic symptoms related to subcortical vasogenic brain edema. It has been described within 10 days after RBCC transfusion, mainly in women with severe (and long-standing) anemia. The prognosis is most often favorable, although irreversible neurologic disturbance has been described. Prevention may include avoiding rapid correction of chronic severe anemia. Again, causality remains to be established.

INFECTIOUS ADVERSE REACTIONS

Donor screening involves the selection of healthy donors without high-risk lifestyles, medical conditions, or exposure to transmissible pathogens. Tests are performed on donated blood to detect the presence of infectious agents by testing for relevant Abs or by directly detecting infectious agents most often by nucleic acid amplification testing. The increasing sensitivity of testing methods has progressively narrowed the "window" period early on after infection during which a low-titer undetectable virus may be present in the blood and result in a transfusion-transmitted infection.

Transfusion-transmitted bacterial infection remains a significant concern, notably with PCs stored at room temperature, which allows for bacterial proliferation and results in an increased risk during storage. However, some gram-negative bacteria such as *Yersinia* can grow

TABLE 113-6 Infectious Transfusion Adverse Events

PATHOGEN		DONATION PREVALENCE (/10⁴ BLOOD DONATIONS)	PREVENTION MEASURES (IN ADDITION TO DONOR DEFERRAL)	INFECTION PREVALENCE IN RECIPIENTS (/10⁶ BLOOD PRODUCTS TRANSFUSED)
Bacteria	Pyogenic bacteria	PC: 10–20	Asepsis, diversion of the initial 10–30 ml of blood, bacterial detection, pathogen reduction (for PC)	Sepsis: PC: 5–30; with bacterial detection: 2–20; with pathogen reduction: <0.5 RBCC: <0.2
	Treponema pallidum (syphilis)	~1[a]	Serology[b,c]	<0.1
Virus	HIV-1/2	~0.1	Serology, NAT (+/− p24 Ag)[b,c]	0.1–1[d]
	HBV	~0.5	Serology, NAT[b,c]	<0.5 (3 without NAT)[d]
	HCV	0.2–1.2	Serology, NAT[b,c]	<0.1–1[d]
	HTLV-1/2	0.05–0.1[a]	Serology, BC deleukocytation[b,c]	0.1–0.3[d]
	HEV	0–10 (in endemic regions)	NAT	Endemic regions: <0.1 with NAT; a transmission rate from infected donors of ~50% has been reported
	CMV	Undetermined	Serology, BC deleukocytation[b,c]	<0.1 in deleukocyted BCs
	Parvovirus B19	~0.5 with viral DNA >10⁶ IU/mL,[e] up to 100 overall	NAT	Most adults are immune to parvovirus B19; up to 0.12% in seronegative adults has been reported
	West Nile virus	Up to 3 in high season endemic regions[a]	NAT[b]	High season endemic regions: <1 with NAT
Parasite	*Plasmodium* (Malaria)	~4 (40–50 in donors from endemic regions)[a]	Serology (NAT may be soon available)	<0.1 in non endemic regions
	Babesia	~90 (in endemic regions)[a]	Serology (NAT implementation is underway)	ND (0.04% donors may be within the serology window period)
	Trypanosoma cruzi (Chagas disease)	~0.14 in donors/mothers from endemic regions[a]	Serology	ND

[a]As assessed based on seropositivity, i.e., including a varying percentage of individuals not harboring the pathogen in their blood. [b]Prevention measures may also include pathogen reduction (for PC and plasma), [c]Prevention measures may also include a quarantine of the (cryopreserved) BC pending a negative serology on a subsequent donation (for plasma), [d]Estimated residual risk. [e]Transfusion risk deemed as absent below this threshold.

Note. Other pathogens associated with transfusion-transmitted infections at a very low frequency include arboviruses other than West Nile (dengue, Zika virus), hepatitis A, human herpesvirus-8, Japanese encephalitis virus, tick-borne encephalitis virus complex, and the prion responsible for variant Creutzfeldt-Jakob disease (4 cases in the United Kingdom, in the context of the bovine spongiform encephalopathy epidemic, before implementation of systematic deleukocytation).

Abbreviations: Ag, antigen; BC, blood component; CMV, cytomegalovirus; HBV, hepatitis B virus; HCV, hepatitis C virus; HEV, hepatitis E virus; HTLV, human T-cell leukemia virus; NAT, nucleic acid detection test; ND, not determined; PC platelet concentrate; RBCC, red blood cell concentrate.

at 4°C and therefore may be implicated in infections related to RBCC transfusion. Recipients of contaminated BCs may develop abrupt (during transfusion and up to several hours after) fever and chills, which can deteriorate to septic shock, DIC, and death. Endotoxin formed within the BC may be implicated. After sampling for bacterial culture, broad-spectrum antibiotics should be promptly initiated.

Pathogen reduction of platelets and plasma, and perhaps soon of RBCs as well, offers an additional means of reducing transfusion infection risks. Although effective for a wide range of pathogens, such processes are most often ineffective for bacterial spores and nonenveloped viruses such as hepatitis A virus (HAV), parvovirus B19, and hepatitis E virus (HEV). Postdonation information provided by the donor (i.e., fever occurring within 24 h after donation) may allow the involved blood products to be quarantined and provide an additional safety measure.

Transfusion-transmitted infections are increasingly rare. However, new or previously unidentified infectious risks may occur, as highlighted by the emergence of the transfusion-associated West Nile virus infection and babesiosis in early 2000 in the United States, as well as transfusion-associated hepatitis E in early 2010 in Europe. Such occurrences require active surveillance programs and the appropriate implementation of mitigation measures such as additional testing, pathogen reduction, and travel-related deferral criteria. Along with West Nile virus, a number of other arbovirus-related infections possibly transmissible by blood transfusion are endemic or involved in large epidemic outbreaks. Despite being possibly present in the blood at asymptomatic phases of the disease, documented cases of transfusion-transmitted infections involving these arboviruses have been very rare (Zika), without a discernible clinical impact (Dengue), or absent (Chikungunya). Route of infection (i.e., intravenous vs mosquito bite), pathogen dose, ability to survive in the BC, storage temperature and duration, recipient immune status, and ongoing treatments may all impact the ability of a pathogen in the donor to induce a disease in the recipient. Estimated frequencies of transfusion-relevant infections in donors and of transfusion-transmitted infections are reported in **Table 113-6**. Such frequencies depend heavily on variables such as local epidemiology, donor deferral rules, risk reduction measures, and data reporting, and may vary considerably.

ALTERNATIVES AND PERSPECTIVES

In addition to promoting appropriate transfusion indications, patient blood management programs have highlighted a number of transfusion-sparing strategies, such as the treatment of anemia and/or iron deficiency before surgery, minimization of blood loss, and optimization of patient red cell mass. Erythropoietin stimulates erythrocyte production in patients with anemia from chronic renal failure and other conditions, thus avoiding or reducing the need for transfusion. Thrombopoietin receptor agonists has been shown to reduce platelet transfusion needs resulting from chemotherapy-induced thrombopenia. Gene therapy approaches in patients with sickle cell or major thalassemia offer the potential of dramatically reducing their transfusion needs. Stem cell–derived blood cells such as RBCs or platelets may in the future become a suitable alternative to rare blood donors.

Importantly, issues surrounding transfusion safety have evolved significantly and now fully encompass transfusion efficacy. New means of assessing transfusion efficacy are needed. Large-scale biological and population-based databases pertaining to blood donors and transfused patients will also be instrumental in assessing and understanding the basis of transfusion efficacy. Optimal transfusion care may soon require consideration of new criteria in relation to donor, blood product, and/or recipient characteristics.

Acknowledgments

The authors are indebted to Jeffery S. Dzieczkowski and Kenneth C. Anderson, who co-authored the chapter in the previous edition and expertly paved the way for this chapter.

FURTHER READING

Carson JL et al: Indications for and adverse effects of red-cell transfusion. N Engl J Med 377:1261, 2017.

Delaney M et al: Transfusion reactions: Prevention, diagnosis, and treatment. Lancet 388:2825, 2016.

Panch SR et al: Hemolytic transfusion reactions. N Engl J Med 381:150, 2019.

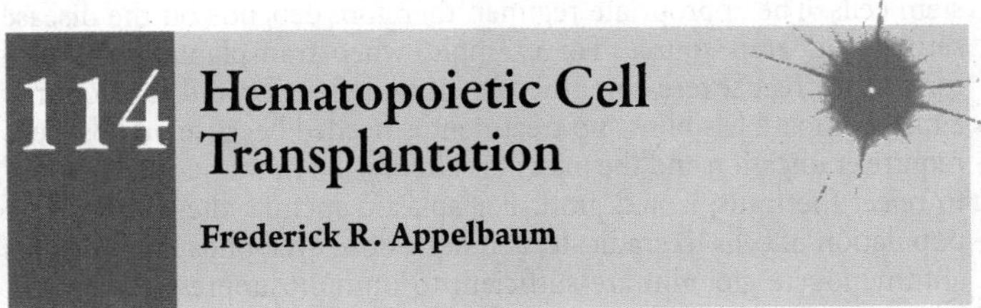

114 Hematopoietic Cell Transplantation

Frederick R. Appelbaum

Bone marrow transplantation was the original term used to describe the collection and transplantation of hematopoietic stem cells, but with the demonstration that peripheral blood and umbilical cord blood are also useful sources of stem cells, *hematopoietic cell transplantation* has become the preferred generic term for this process. Hematopoietic cell transplantation is used to treat patients with an abnormal but nonmalignant lymphohematopoietic system by replacing it with one from a normal donor. Hematopoietic cell transplantation is also used to treat malignancy by allowing the administration of higher doses of myelosuppressive therapy than would otherwise be possible and, in the setting of allogeneic Hematopoietic cell transplantation, by conferring an immunologic graft-versus-tumor effect. The use of hematopoietic cell transplantation is increasing, as it becomes safer and applicable to more diseases and as donor availability expands.

The Center for International Blood and Marrow Transplant Research (*http://www.cibmtr.org*) estimates that worldwide about 100,000 transplants were performed in 2020. The frequency of transplantation varied widely from country to country, with a close association of transplant rates with gross national income (GNI) per capita. However, even among countries with similar GNIs per capita, there are substantial differences between countries and regions regarding the frequency of transplantation, disease indications, and choice of donor type.

THE HEMATOPOIETIC STEM CELL

Several features of the hematopoietic stem cell make transplantation clinically feasible, including its remarkable regenerative capacity, its ability to home to the marrow space following intravenous injection, and the ability of the stem cell to be cryopreserved **(Chap. 96)**. Transplantation of a single stem cell can replace the entire lymphohematopoietic system of an adult mouse. In humans, transplantation of a small percentage of a donor's bone marrow volume regularly results in complete and sustained replacement of the recipient's entire lymphohematopoietic system, including all red cells, granulocytes, B and T lymphocytes, and platelets, as well as cells comprising the fixed macrophage population, including Kupffer cells of the liver, pulmonary alveolar macrophages, osteoclasts, and Langerhans cells of the skin. The ability of the hematopoietic stem cell to home to the marrow following intravenous injection is mediated, in part, by an interaction between CXCL12, also known as stromal cell–derived factor 1, produced by marrow stromal cells and the alpha-chemokine receptor CXCR4 found on stem cells. Homing is also influenced by the interaction of cell-surface molecules, termed *selectins*, including E- and L-selectin, on bone marrow endothelial cells with ligands, termed *integrins*, such as VLA-4, on early hematopoietic cells. Human hematopoietic stem cells can survive freezing and thawing with little, if any, damage, making it possible to remove and store a portion of the patient's own bone marrow for later reinfusion following treatment of the patient with high-dose myelotoxic therapy.

CATEGORIES OF HEMATOPOIETIC CELL TRANSPLANTATION

Hematopoietic cell transplantation can be described according to the relationship between the patient and the donor and by the anatomic source of stem cells. In ~1% of cases, patients have identical twins who can serve as donors. With the use of syngeneic donors, there is no risk of graft-versus-host disease (GVHD), and unlike the use of autologous marrow, there is no risk that the stem cells are contaminated with tumor cells.

Allogeneic transplantation involves a donor and a recipient who are not genetically identical. Following allogeneic transplantation, immune cells transplanted with the stem cells or developing from them can react against the patient, causing GVHD. Alternatively, if the immunosuppressive preparative regimen used to treat the patient before transplant is inadequate, immunocompetent cells of the patient can cause graft rejection. The risks of these complications are greatly influenced by the degree of matching between donor and recipient for human leukocyte antigen (HLA) molecules encoded by genes of the major histocompatibility complex.

HLA molecules are responsible for binding antigenic proteins and presenting them to T cells. The antigens presented by HLA molecules may derive from exogenous sources (e.g., during active infections) or may be endogenous proteins. If individuals are not HLA-matched, T cells from one individual will react strongly to the mismatched HLA, or "major antigens," of the second. Even if the individuals are HLA-matched, the T cells of the donor may react to differing endogenous or "minor antigens" presented by the HLA of the recipient. Reactions to minor antigens tend to be less vigorous. The genes of major relevance to transplantation include HLA-A, -B, -C, and -D; they are closely linked and therefore tend to be inherited as haplotypes, with only rare crossovers between them. Thus, the odds that any one full sibling will match a patient are one in four, and the probability that the patient has an HLA-identical sibling is $1 - (0.75)n$, where n equals the number of siblings.

With conventional techniques, the risk of graft rejection is 1–3%, and the risk of severe, life-threatening acute GVHD is ~15% following transplantation between HLA-identical siblings. The incidence of graft rejection and GVHD increases progressively with the use of family member donors mismatched for one, two, or three antigens. Although survival following a one-antigen mismatched transplant is not markedly altered, survival following two- or three-antigen mismatched transplants is reduced. Newer approaches to GVHD prophylaxis, including the use of posttransplant high-dose cyclophosphamide, make transplantation between donor/recipient pairs who share only one HLA haplotype possible. Since the formation of the National Marrow Donor Program and other registries, HLA-matched unrelated donors can be identified for many patients. The genes encoding HLA antigens are highly polymorphic, and thus the odds of any two unrelated individuals being HLA identical are extremely low, somewhat less than 1 in 10,000. However, by recruiting >30 million volunteer donors, HLA-matched donors can be found for ~60% of patients for whom a search is initiated, with higher rates among whites and lower rates among minorities and patients of mixed race. It takes, on average, 3–4 months to complete a search and schedule and initiate an unrelated donor transplant. With improvements in HLA typing and supportive care measures, survival following matched unrelated donor transplantation is essentially the same as that seen with HLA-matched siblings.

Allogeneic hematopoietic cell transplantation can be carried out across ABO blood barriers by removing isoagglutinins and/or incompatible red blood cells from the donor graft. However, depending on the direction of the mismatch, hemolysis of donor cells by persistent isoagglutinins in the host, or hemolysis of recipient red cells by isoagglutinins in the graft or developing from it may occur despite appropriate manipulation of the donor cell product.

Autologous transplantation involves the removal and storage of the patient's own stem cells with subsequent reinfusion after the patient receives high-dose myeloablative therapy. Unlike allogeneic transplantation, there is no risk of GVHD or graft rejection with autologous transplantation. On the other hand, autologous transplantation lacks a graft-versus-tumor (GVT) effect, and the autologous stem cell product can be contaminated with tumor cells, which could lead to relapse. A variety of techniques have been developed to "purge" autologous products of tumor cells, but no prospective randomized trials have shown that any approach decreases relapse rates or improves disease-free or overall survival.

Bone marrow aspirated from the posterior and anterior iliac crests initially was the source of hematopoietic stem cells for transplantation. Typically, anywhere from 1.5 to 5 × 10^8 nucleated marrow cells per kilogram are collected for allogeneic transplantation. Several studies have found improved survival following both matched sibling and unrelated transplantation by transplanting higher numbers of bone marrow cells.

Hematopoietic stem cells circulate in the peripheral blood but in very low concentrations. Following the administration of a myeloid growth factor such as granulocyte colony-stimulating factor (G-CSF) and during recovery from intensive chemotherapy, the concentration of hematopoietic progenitor cells in blood, as measured either by colony-forming units or expression of the CD34 antigen, increases markedly. This makes it possible to harvest adequate numbers of stem cells from the peripheral blood for transplantation. Donors are typically treated with 4 or 5 days of hematopoietic growth factor, following which stem cells are collected in one or two 4-h pheresis sessions. In the autologous setting, transplantation of >2.5 × 10^6 CD34 cells per kilogram, a number that can be collected in most circumstances, leads to rapid and sustained engraftment in virtually all cases. In the 5–10% of patients who fail to mobilize enough CD34+ cells with growth factor alone, the addition of plerixafor, an antagonist of CXCR4, may be useful. Blocking CXCR4 allows more stem cells to escape the marrow. When compared to the use of autologous marrow, use of peripheral blood stem cells results in more rapid hematopoietic recovery. Although this more rapid recovery diminishes the morbidity rate of transplantation, no studies show improved survival.

In the setting of allogeneic transplantation, the use of growth factor–mobilized peripheral blood stem cells also results in faster engraftment than seen with marrow but at the cost of more chronic GVHD because of donor T-cell contamination. With matched sibling donors, the increased chronic GVHD is more than balanced by reductions in relapse rates and nonrelapse mortality rates, resulting in improved overall survival. However, in the setting of matched unrelated donor transplantation, use of peripheral blood results in more chronic GVHD without a compensatory survival advantage, favoring the use of bone marrow.

Umbilical cord blood contains a high concentration of hematopoietic progenitor cells, allowing for its use as a source of stem cells for transplantation. Cord blood transplantation from family members has been used when the immediate need for transplantation precludes waiting the 9 or so months generally required for the baby to mature to the point of donating marrow. Use of cord blood results in slower peripheral count recovery than seen with marrow but a lower incidence of GVHD, perhaps reflecting the low number of T cells in cord blood. Multiple cord blood banks have been developed to harvest and store cord blood for possible transplantation to unrelated patients from material that would otherwise be discarded. Currently >800,000 units are cryopreserved and available for use. The advantages of unrelated cord blood are rapid availability and decreased immune reactivity allowing for the use of partially matched units, which is of particular importance for those without matched unrelated donors. The risks of graft failure and transplant-related mortality are related to the dose of cord blood cells per kilogram, which previously limited the application of single cord blood transplantation to pediatric and smaller adult patients. Subsequent trials have found that for patients without suitable single cord units, the use of double cord transplants diminishes the risk of graft failure and early mortality even though only one of the donors ultimately engrafts. Given the similar survival rates seen with cord blood, matched unrelated, and haploidentical family member donors, a source of allogeneic stem cells can now be found for almost every patient in need (**Table 114-1**).

TABLE 114-1 Probability of Identifying a Donor Based on Stem Cell Source and Patient Ethnicity

	UNRELATED ADULT %		UNRELATED CORD %	HAPLOIDENTICAL
Ethnicity	8/8[a]	7/8[a]	≥4/6[b]	
Caucasian	75	90	>95	95
Hispanic	35	75	95	95
Black	18	70	90	95

[a]Matching for HLA-A, -B, -C, and DRB1. [b]Matching for HLA-A, -B, and DRB1.

THE TRANSPLANT PREPARATIVE REGIMEN

The treatment regimen administered to patients immediately preceding transplantation is designed to eradicate the patient's underlying disease and, in the setting of allogeneic transplantation, immunosuppress the patient adequately to prevent rejection of the transplanted stem cells. The appropriate regimen therefore depends on the disease setting and graft source. For example, when transplantation is performed to treat severe combined immunodeficiency and the donor is a histocompatible sibling, no treatment is needed because no host cells require eradication and the patient is already too immune-incompetent to reject the transplanted graft. For aplastic anemia, there is no large population of cells to eradicate, and high-dose cyclophosphamide plus antithymocyte globulin are sufficient to immunosuppress the patient adequately to accept the marrow graft. In the setting of thalassemia and sickle cell anemia, high-dose busulfan is frequently added to cyclophosphamide to eradicate hyperplastic host hematopoiesis. A variety of different regimens have been developed to treat malignant diseases. Most regimens include agents with high activity against the tumor in question at conventional doses and with myelosuppression as their predominant dose-limiting toxicity. Therefore, these regimens commonly include busulfan, cyclophosphamide, melphalan, thiotepa, carmustine, etoposide, and total-body irradiation in various combinations.

Although high-dose treatment regimens were the initial approach to transplantation for malignancies, the realization that much of the antitumor effect of transplantation derives from an immunologically mediated GVT response led investigators to ask if reduced-intensity conditioning regimens might be effective and more tolerable. Evidence for a GVT effect comes from studies showing that posttransplant relapse rates are lowest in patients who develop acute and chronic GVHD, higher in those without GVHD, and higher still in recipients of T cell–depleted allogeneic or syngeneic marrow. The demonstration that complete remissions can be obtained in many patients who have relapsed after transplant by simply administering viable lymphocytes from the original donor further strengthens the argument for a potent GVT effect. Accordingly, a variety of alternative regimens have been studied, ranging from nonmyeloablative, which are the very minimum required to achieve engraftment (e.g., fludarabine plus 200 cGy total-body irradiation) and would cause only transient myelosuppression if no transplant were performed, to so-called reduced-intensity regimens, which would cause significant but not necessarily fatal myelosuppression in the absence of transplantation (e.g., fludarabine plus melphalan). Studies to date document that engraftment can be readily achieved with less toxicity than seen with conventional transplantation. Complete sustained responses have been documented in many patients, particularly those with more indolent hematologic malignancies. In general, relapse rates are higher following reduced-intensity conditioning, but transplant-related mortality is lower, favoring the use of reduced-intensity conditioning in patients with significant comorbidities. High-dose regimens are favored in those felt able to tolerate the treatment, particularly if patients have any evidence of measurable disease at the time of transplantation.

THE TRANSPLANT PROCEDURE

Marrow is usually collected from the donor's posterior and sometimes anterior iliac crests, with the donor under general or spinal anesthesia. Typically, 10–15 mL/kg of marrow is aspirated, placed in heparinized media, and filtered through 0.3- and 0.2-mm screens to remove fat and bony spicules. The collected marrow may undergo further processing depending on the clinical situation, such as the removal of red cells to prevent hemolysis in ABO-incompatible transplants, the removal of donor T cells to prevent GVHD, or attempts to remove possible contaminating tumor cells in autologous transplantation. Marrow donation is safe, with only very rare complications reported.

Peripheral blood stem cells are collected by leukapheresis after the donor has been treated with hematopoietic growth factors or, in the setting of autologous transplantation, sometimes after treatment with a combination of chemotherapy and growth factors. Stem cells for transplantation are infused through a large-bore central venous catheter. Such infusions are usually well tolerated, although occasionally patients develop fever, cough, or shortness of breath. These symptoms typically resolve with slowing of the infusion. When the stem cell product has been cryopreserved using dimethyl sulfoxide, patients sometimes experience short-lived nausea or vomiting due to the taste (and smell) of the cryoprotectant.

ENGRAFTMENT AND IMMUNE RECONSTITUTION

Peripheral blood counts reach their nadir several days to a week after transplant as a consequence of the preparative regimen; then cells produced by the transplanted stem cells begin to appear in the peripheral blood. The rate of recovery depends on the source of stem cells and use of posttransplant growth factors. If marrow is the source, recovery to 100 granulocytes/μL occurs on average by day 16 and to 500/μL by day 22. Use of G-CSF–mobilized peripheral blood stem cells speeds the rate of recovery by ~1 week compared to marrow, whereas engraftment following cord blood transplantation is typically delayed by ~1 week. Use of a myeloid growth factor after transplant accelerates recovery by 3–5 days. Platelet counts usually recover shortly after granulocytes.

While granulocytes and other components of innate immunity recover rapidly after hematopoietic cell transplantation, adaptive immunity, which consists of cellular (T cell) and humoral (B cell) immunity, may take 1–2 years to fully recover. Survival and peripheral expansion of infused donor T cells is the dominant mechanism for T cell recovery in the first months after hematopoietic cell transplantation and results in mostly CD8+ T cells with a limited repertoire. After several months, de novo generation of donor derived CD4+ and CD8+ T cells becomes dominant providing a more diverse T-cell repertoire. B-cell counts recover by 6 months after autologous hematopoietic cell transplantation and 9 months after allogeneic hematopoietic cell transplantation. In general, immune recovery occurs more rapidly after autologous than allogeneic hematopoietic cell transplantation and after receipt of unmodified grafts compared to the setting of in vivo or ex vivo T-cell depletion.

Following allogeneic transplantation, engraftment can be documented using fluorescence in situ hybridization of sex chromosomes if donor and recipient are sex-mismatched or by analysis of short tandem repeat polymorphisms after DNA amplification.

COMPLICATIONS FOLLOWING HEMATOPOIETIC CELL TRANSPLANTATION

Early Direct Chemoradiotoxicities The transplant preparative regimen may cause a spectrum of acute toxicities that vary according to intensity of the regimen and the specific agents used but frequently include nausea, vomiting, and mild skin erythema (**Fig. 114-1**). High-dose cyclophosphamide can result in hemorrhagic cystitis, which can usually be prevented by bladder irrigation or with the sulfhydryl compound mercaptoethanesulfonate (MESNA). Most high-dose preparative regimens will result in oral mucositis, which typically develops 5–7 days after transplant and often requires narcotic analgesia. Use of a patient-controlled analgesic pump provides the greatest patient satisfaction and results in a lower cumulative dose of narcotic. Keratinocyte growth factor (palifermin) can shorten the duration of mucositis by several days following autologous transplantation. Patients begin losing their hair 5–6 days after transplant and by 1 week are usually profoundly pancytopenic.

Depending on the intensity of the conditioning regimen, 3–10% of patients will develop sinusoidal obstruction syndrome (SOS) of the liver (formerly called venoocclusive disease), a syndrome that results from direct cytotoxic injury to hepatic-venular and sinusoidal endothelium, with subsequent deposition of fibrin and the development of a local hypercoagulable state. This chain of events leads to the clinical symptoms of tender hepatomegaly, ascites, jaundice, and fluid retention. These symptoms can develop any time during the first month after transplant, with the peak incidence at day 16. Predisposing factors include prior exposure to intensive chemotherapy, pretransplant hepatitis of any cause, and use of more intense conditioning regimens. The mortality rate of sinusoidal obstruction syndrome is ~30%, with progressive hepatic failure culminating in a terminal hepatorenal syndrome. Treatment of severe SOS with defibrotide, a polydeoxyribonucleotide, reduces mortality.

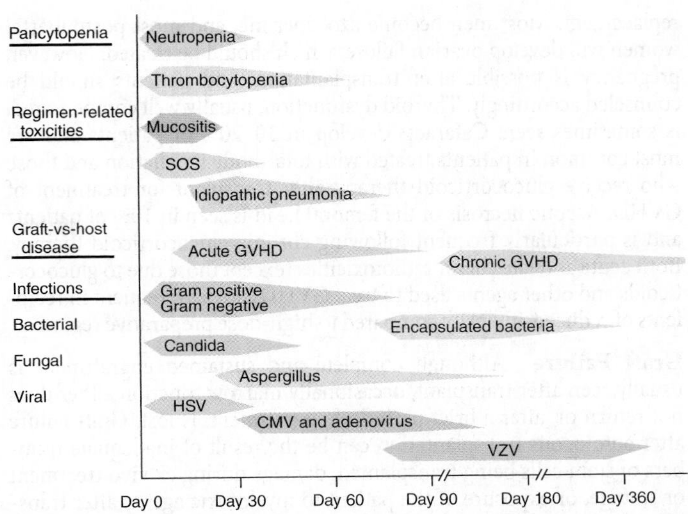

FIGURE 114-1 Major syndromes complicating marrow transplantation. CMV, cytomegalovirus; GVHD, graft-versus-host disease; HSV, herpes simplex virus; SOS, sinusoidal obstructive syndrome (formerly venoocclusive disease); VZV, varicella-zoster virus. The size of the shaded area roughly reflects the period of risk of the complication.

Although most pneumonias developing early after transplant are caused by infectious agents, in a small percentage of patients, a diffuse interstitial pneumonia will develop that is a result of direct toxicity of high-dose preparative regimens. Bronchoalveolar lavage usually shows alveolar hemorrhage, and biopsies are typically characterized by diffuse alveolar damage, although some cases may have a more clearly interstitial pattern. High-dose glucocorticoids or antitumor necrosis factor therapies are sometimes used as treatment, although randomized trials proving their utility have not been reported.

Transplant-associated thrombotic microangiopathy is seen in 5–10% of patients, appearing on average about 1 month after transplant. The syndrome is characterized by presence of schistocytes on peripheral smear, elevated lactate dehydrogenase, thrombocytopenia, and acute kidney injury and is the result of endothelial injury and complement activation. Since calcineurin inhibitors are thought to contribute to the pathogenesis of the syndrome, changing immunosuppressive regimens is sometimes effective. Patients sometimes respond to eculizumab.

Late Direct Chemoradiotoxicities Two categories of chronic pulmonary disease occur in patients >3 months after hematopoietic cell transplantation. Cryptogenic organizing pneumonia is a restrictive lung disease characterized by dry cough, shortness of breath, and chest imaging showing a diffuse, fluffy infiltrate. Biopsy shows granulation tissue within alveolar spaces and small airways and no infectious agents. The disease responds well to corticosteroids and is entirely reversible. Bronchiolitis obliterans is an obstructive disease presenting with cough, progressive dyspnea, and radiologic evidence of air trapping. Pathology shows collagen and granulation tissue in and around bronchial structures and eventually obliteration of small airways. The disease is usually associated with chronic GVHD, and although it may respond to increasing immunosuppression, complete reversal is uncommon.

Other late complications of the preparative regimen include decreased growth velocity in children and delayed development of secondary sex characteristics. These complications can be partly ameliorated with the use of appropriate growth and sex hormone replacement. Most men become azoospermic, and most postpubertal women will develop ovarian failure, which should be treated. However, pregnancy is possible after transplantation, and patients should be counseled accordingly. Thyroid dysfunction, usually well compensated, is sometimes seen. Cataracts develop in 10–20% of patients and are most common in patients treated with total-body irradiation and those who receive glucocorticoid therapy after transplant for treatment of GVHD. Aseptic necrosis of the femoral head is seen in 10% of patients and is particularly frequent following chronic glucocorticoid therapy. Both acute and late chemoradiotoxicities (except those due to glucocorticoids and other agents used to treat GVHD) are less frequent in recipients of reduced-intensity compared to high-dose preparative regimens.

Graft Failure Although complete and sustained engraftment is usually seen after transplant, occasionally marrow function either does not return or, after a brief period of engraftment, is lost. Graft failure after autologous transplantation can be the result of inadequate numbers of stem cells being transplanted, damage during ex vivo treatment or storage, or exposure of the patient to myelotoxic agents after transplant. Infections with cytomegalovirus (CMV) or human herpesvirus type 6 have also been associated with loss of marrow function. Graft failure after allogeneic transplantation can also be due to immunologic rejection of the graft by immunocompetent host cells. Such rejection is generally thought to be mostly T-cell mediated, but the presence pre-hematopoietic cell transplantation of donor-specific HLA antibodies in the patient is associated with poor engraftment, leading to the recommendation for screening for donor-directed anti-HLA antibodies in recipients prior to transplant. Immunologically based graft rejection is more common following use of less immunosuppressive preparative regimens, in recipients of T cell–depleted stem cell products, and in patients receiving grafts from HLA-mismatched donors or cord blood.

Treatment of graft failure involves removing all potentially myelotoxic agents from the patient's regimen and attempting a short trial of a myeloid growth factor. Persistence of lymphocytes of host origin in allogeneic transplant recipients with graft failure indicates immunologic rejection. Reinfusion of donor stem cells in such patients is usually unsuccessful unless preceded by a second immunosuppressive preparative regimen. Standard high-dose preparative regimens are tolerated poorly if administered within 100 days of a first transplant because of cumulative toxicities. However, reduced-intensity conditioning regimens have been effective in some cases.

Graft-Versus-Host Disease Acute GVHD occurs within the first 3 months after allogeneic transplant with a peak onset around 4 weeks and is characterized by an erythematous maculopapular rash; by persistent anorexia or diarrhea, or both; and by liver disease with increased serum levels of bilirubin, alanine and aspartate aminotransferase, and alkaline phosphatase. Because many conditions can mimic acute GVHD, the diagnosis usually requires skin, liver, or endoscopic biopsy for confirmation. In all these organs, endothelial damage and lymphocytic infiltrates are seen. In skin, the epidermis and hair follicles are damaged; in liver, the small bile ducts show segmental disruption; and in intestines, destruction of the crypts and mucosal ulceration may be noted. A commonly used rating system for acute GVHD is shown in **Table 114-2**. Grade I acute GVHD is of little clinical significance, does not affect the likelihood of survival, and does not require treatment. In contrast, grades II to IV GVHD are associated with significant symptoms and a poorer probability of survival and require aggressive therapy. The incidence of acute GVHD is higher in recipients of stem cells from mismatched or unrelated donors, in older patients, and in patients unable to receive full doses of drugs used to prevent the disease.

Currently, the standard approach to GVHD prevention is the administration of a calcineurin inhibitor (cyclosporine or tacrolimus) combined with an antimetabolite (methotrexate or mycophenolate mofetil) following transplantation. The addition of anti–T-cell immune globulin (ATG) may further reduce the incidence of GVHD but has not been shown to improve survival. Other approaches being tested in phase 3 studies include the addition of sirolimus to the standard two-drug regimen, the removal of subsets or all T cells from the stem cell inoculum, and the use of cyclophosphamide administered several days after transplant in an effort to deplete activated alloreactive T cells.

Despite prophylaxis, significant acute GVHD will develop in ~30% of recipients of stem cells from matched siblings. Factors associated with a greater risk of acute GVHD include HLA-mismatching between recipient and donor, patient and donor age, use of more intense preparative regimens, and use of multiparous women as donors. Presumably, multiparous women have more alloreactivity based on carriage of genetically disparate fetuses. Disruption of the intestinal microbiota leading to loss of diversity and overgrowth by a single taxon is associated with a higher risk of GVHD and transplant-associated mortality. Biomarkers, including ST2, REG32, and TNF R1, have been identified that predict the severity of acute GVHD. The disease is usually treated with prednisone at a daily dose of 1–2 mg/kg. Patients in whom the acute GVHD fails to respond to prednisone sometimes respond to the oral JAK2 inhibitor ruxolitinib.

Chronic GVHD occurs most commonly between 3 months and 2 years after allogeneic transplant, developing in 20–50% of recipients. The disease is more common in older patients, with the use of peripheral blood rather than marrow as the stem cell source, in recipients of mismatched or unrelated stem cells, and in those with a preceding episode of acute GVHD. The disease resembles an autoimmune disorder with malar rash, sicca syndrome, arthritis, obliterative bronchiolitis, and bile duct degeneration with cholestasis. Mild chronic GVHD can sometimes be managed using local therapies (topical glucocorticoids to skin and cyclosporine eye drops). More severe disease requires systemic therapy usually with prednisone alone or in combination with cyclosporine. Ibrutinib is sometimes effective in patients whose disease does not respond to initial therapy. Mortality rates from chronic GVHD average around 15%, but range from 5 to 50% depending on severity. In most patients, chronic GVHD resolves, but it may require 1–3 years of immunosuppressive treatment before these agents can be withdrawn without the disease recurring. Because patients with chronic GVHD are susceptible to significant infection, they should receive prophylactic trimethoprim-sulfamethoxazole, and all suspected infections should be investigated and treated aggressively.

Although onset before or after 3 months after transplant is often used to discriminate between acute and chronic GVHD, occasional patients will develop signs and symptoms of acute GVHD after 3 months (late-onset acute GVHD), whereas others will exhibit signs

TABLE 114-2 Clinical Staging and Grading of Acute Graft-versus-Host Disease

CLINICAL STAGE	SKIN	LIVER—BILIRUBIN, λmol/L (mg/dL)	GUT
1	Rash <25% body surface	34–51 (2–3)	Diarrhea 500–1000 mL/d
2	Rash 25–50% body surface	51–103 (3–6)	Diarrhea 1000–1500 mL/d
3	Generalized erythroderma	103–257 (6–15)	Diarrhea >1500 mL/d
4	Desquamation and bullae	>257 (>15)	Ileus
OVERALL CLINICAL GRADE	**SKIN STAGE**	**LIVER STAGE**	**GUT STAGE**
I	1–2	0	0
II	1–3	1	1
III	1–3	2–3	2–3
IV	2–4	2–4	2–4

and symptoms of both acute and chronic GVHD (overlap syndrome). There are as yet no data to suggest that these patients should be treated differently than those with classic acute or chronic GVHD.

From 3 to 5% of patients will develop an autoimmune disorder following allogeneic hematopoietic cell transplantation, most commonly autoimmune hemolytic anemia or idiopathic thrombocytopenic purpura. Unrelated donor source and chronic GVHD are risk factors, but autoimmune disorders have been reported in patients with no obvious GVHD. Treatment is with prednisone, cyclosporine, or rituximab.

Infection Posttransplant patients, particularly recipients of allogeneic transplantation, require unique approaches to the problem of infection. Early after transplantation, patients are profoundly neutropenic, and because the risk of bacterial infection is so great, most centers place patients on broad-spectrum antibiotics once the granulocyte count falls to <500/μL. Prophylaxis against fungal infections reduces rates of infection and improves overall survival. Fluconazole is often used for patients with standard risk, while prophylaxis with mold active agents (voriconazole or posaconazole) should be considered for patients at higher risk, such as those with a prior fungal infection. Patients seropositive for herpes simplex should receive acyclovir prophylaxis. One approach to infection prophylaxis is shown in **Table 114-3**. Despite these prophylactic measures, most patients will develop fever and signs of infection after transplant. The management of patients who become febrile despite bacterial and fungal prophylaxis is a difficult challenge and is guided by individual aspects of the patient and by the institution's experience.

The general problem of infection in the immunocompromised host is discussed in **Chap. 143**.

Once patients engraft, the incidence of bacterial infection diminishes; however, patients, particularly allogeneic transplant recipients, remain at significant risk of infection. During the period from engraftment until about 3 months after transplant, the most common causes of infection are gram-positive bacteria, fungi (particularly *Aspergillus*), and viruses including CMV. CMV disease, which in the past was frequently seen and often fatal, can be prevented in seronegative patients transplanted from seronegative donors by the use of either seronegative blood products or products from which the white blood cells have been removed. In seropositive patients or patients transplanted from seropositive donors, either prophylaxis or preemptive therapy is used. Letermovir administered over the first 3 months after transplant is effective as prophylaxis. An alternative approach is to monitor blood of patients after transplant using polymerase chain reaction assays for viral DNA and to treat reactivation preemptively with ganciclovir before clinical disease develops. Foscarnet is effective for some patients who develop CMV antigenemia or infection despite the use of ganciclovir or who cannot tolerate the drug, but it can be associated with severe electrolyte wasting.

Pneumocystis jirovecii pneumonia, once seen in 5–10% of patients, can be prevented by treating patients with oral trimethoprim-sulfamethoxazole for 1 week before transplant and resuming the treatment once patients engraft.

TABLE 114-3 Approach to Infection Prophylaxis in Allogeneic Transplant Recipients

ORGANISM	AGENT	APPROACH
Bacterial	Levofloxacin	750 mg PO or IV daily
Fungal	Fluconazole	400 mg PO qd to day 75 posttransplant
Pneumocystis jirovecii	Trimethoprim-sulfamethoxazole	1 double-strength tablet PO bid 2 days/week until day 180 or off immunosuppression
Viral		
Herpes simplex	Acyclovir	800 mg PO bid to day 30
Varicella-zoster	Acyclovir	800 mg PO bid to day 365
Cytomegalovirus	Ganciclovir	5 mg/kg IV bid for 7 days, then 5 (mg/kg)/d 5 days/week to day 100

Respiratory viruses that cause community-acquired infections, including respiratory syncytial virus (RSV), parainfluenza virus, influenza virus, and metapneumovirus, can be life threatening or fatal in the posttransplant patient. Protection of patients from infected visitors and staff by avoiding such contacts is critical. Neuraminidase inhibitors are effective for influenza infections. Inhaled ribavirin is sometimes used for RSV.

The risk of infection diminishes considerably beyond 3 months after transplant unless chronic GVHD requiring continuous immunosuppression develops. Most transplant centers recommend continuing trimethoprim-sulfamethoxazole prophylaxis while patients are receiving any immunosuppressive drugs and also recommend careful monitoring for late CMV reactivation. In addition, many centers recommend prophylaxis against varicella-zoster, using acyclovir for 1 year after transplant. Patients should be revaccinated against tetanus, diphtheria, *Haemophilus influenzae*, polio, and pneumococcal pneumonia starting at 12 months after transplant and against measles, mumps, and rubella (MMR), varicella-zoster virus, and possibly pertussis at 24 months.

TREATMENT

Nonmalignant Diseases

Evidence-based indications for hematopoietic cell transplantation have been published by several organizations and are guided not only by disease-related factors but also by patient comorbidities, socioeconomic issues, caregiver and donor availability, and patient preference.

IMMUNODEFICIENCY DISORDERS

By replacing abnormal stem cells with cells from a normal donor, hematopoietic cell transplantation can cure patients of a variety of immunodeficiency disorders including severe combined immunodeficiency, Wiskott-Aldrich syndrome, and Chédiak-Higashi syndrome. The widest experience is with severe combined immunodeficiency disease, where cure rates of 90% can be expected with HLA-identical donors and success rates of 50–70% have been reported using haplotype-mismatched parents as donors **(Table 114-4)**.

APLASTIC ANEMIA

Transplantation from matched siblings after a preparative regimen of high-dose cyclophosphamide and antithymocyte globulin cures up to 90% of patients age <40 years with severe aplastic anemia. Results in older patients and in recipients of mismatched family member or unrelated marrow are less favorable; therefore, a trial of immunosuppressive therapy is generally recommended for such patients before considering transplantation. Transplantation is effective in all forms of aplastic anemia including, for example, the syndromes associated with paroxysmal nocturnal hemoglobinuria and Fanconi's anemia. Patients with Fanconi's anemia are abnormally sensitive to the toxic effects of alkylating agents, and so less intensive preparative regimens are used in their treatment **(Chap. 102)**.

HEMOGLOBINOPATHIES

Marrow transplantation from an HLA-identical sibling following a preparative regimen of busulfan and cyclophosphamide can cure 80–90% of patients with thalassemia major. The best outcomes can be expected if patients are transplanted before they develop hepatomegaly or portal fibrosis and if they have been given adequate iron chelation therapy. Among such patients, the probabilities of 5-year survival and disease-free survival are 95 and 90%, respectively. Although prolonged survival can be achieved with aggressive chelation therapy, transplantation is the only curative treatment for thalassemia. Transplantation is potentially curative for patients with sickle cell anemia. Two-year survival and disease-free survival rates of 95 and 85%, respectively, have been reported following matched sibling or cord blood transplantation. Decisions about patient selection and the timing of transplantation remain difficult, but transplantation is a reasonable option for children and young

TABLE 114-4 Estimated 5-Year Survival Rates Following Transplantation[a]

DISEASE	ALLOGENEIC, %	AUTOLOGOUS, %
Severe combined immunodeficiency	90	N/A
Aplastic anemia	90	N/A
Thalassemia	90	N/A
Acute myeloid leukemia		
First remission	55–60	50
Second remission	40	30
Acute lymphocytic leukemia		
First remission	50	40
Second remission	40	30
Chronic myeloid leukemia		
Chronic phase	70	ID
Accelerated phase	40	ID
Blast crisis	15	ID
Chronic lymphocytic leukemia	50	ID
Myelodysplasia	45	ID
Multiple myeloma—initial therapy	N/A	60
Non-Hodgkin's lymphoma		
First relapse/second remission	40	40
Hodgkin's disease		
First relapse/second remission	40	50

[a]These estimates are generally based on data reported by the International Bone Marrow Transplant Registry. The analysis has not been reviewed by their Advisory Committee.

Abbreviations: ID, insufficient data; N/A, not applicable.

adults who have suffered complications of sickle cell anemia including stroke, recurrent vasoocclusive pain, sickle cell lung disease, or sickle nephropathy (**Chap. 98**).

OTHER NONMALIGNANT DISEASES

Theoretically, hematopoietic cell transplantation should be able to cure any disease that results from an inborn error of the lymphohematopoietic system. Transplantation has been used successfully to treat congenital disorders of white blood cells such as Kostmann's syndrome, chronic granulomatous disease, and leukocyte adhesion deficiency. Congenital anemias such as Blackfan-Diamond anemia can also be cured with transplantation. Since the penetrance of some congenital marrow failure states is variable, potential family member donors should be carefully screened before use to assure they are not affected. Infantile malignant osteopetrosis is due to an inability of the osteoclast to resorb bone, and because osteoclasts derive from the marrow, transplantation can cure this rare inherited disorder.

Hematopoietic cell transplantation has been used as treatment for a number of storage diseases caused by enzymatic deficiencies, such as Gaucher's disease, Hurler's syndrome, Hunter's syndrome, and infantile metachromatic leukodystrophy. Transplantation for these diseases has not been uniformly successful, but treatment early in the course of these diseases, before irreversible damage to extramedullary organs has occurred, increases the chance for success.

Transplantation is being explored as a treatment for severe acquired autoimmune disorders. These trials are based on studies demonstrating that transplantation can reverse autoimmune disorders in animal models and on the observation that occasional patients with coexisting autoimmune disorders and hematologic malignancies have been cured of both with transplantation. A prospective randomized trial found that patients with severe scleroderma have improved event-free and overall survival if treated with hematopoietic cell transplantation.

ACUTE LEUKEMIA

Allogeneic hematopoietic cell transplantation cures 15–20% of patients who do not achieve complete response after induction chemotherapy for acute myeloid leukemia (AML) and is the only form of therapy that can cure such patients. Thus, all patients with AML who are possible transplant candidates should have their HLA type determined soon after diagnosis to enable hematopoietic cell transplantation for those who fail to enter remission. Cure rates of 30–35% are seen when patients are transplanted in second remission or in first relapse. The best results with allogeneic transplantation are achieved when applied during first remission, with disease-free survival rates averaging 55–60%. Meta-analyses of studies comparing matched related donor transplantation to chemotherapy for adult AML patients age <60 years show a survival advantage with transplantation. This advantage is greatest for those with unfavorable-risk AML and is lost in those with favorable-risk disease. While hematopoietic cell transplantation can be performed in patients up to age 75 and possibly beyond, prospective trials comparing hematopoietic cell transplantation with chemotherapy are lacking for older patients. The role of autologous transplantation in the treatment of AML is less well defined. The rates of disease recurrence with autologous transplantation are higher than those seen after allogeneic transplantation, and cure rates are somewhat less.

Similar to patients with AML, adults with acute lymphocytic leukemia who do not achieve a complete response to induction chemotherapy can be cured in 15–20% of cases with immediate transplantation. Cure rates improve to 30–50% in second remission, and therefore, transplantation can be recommended for adults who have persistent disease after induction chemotherapy or who subsequently relapse. Transplantation in first remission results in cure rates of about 55%. Transplantation appears to offer a survival advantage over chemotherapy for patients with high-risk disease as defined by molecular profiling. Debate continues about whether adults with standard-risk disease should be transplanted in first remission or whether transplantation should be reserved until relapse. Autologous transplantation is associated with a higher relapse rate but a somewhat lower risk of nonrelapse mortality when compared to allogeneic transplantation. There is no obvious role of autologous transplantation for acute lymphocytic leukemia in first remission, and for second-remission patients, most experts recommend use of allogeneic stem cells if an appropriate donor is available.

CHRONIC LEUKEMIA

Allogeneic hematopoietic cell transplantation is indicated for patients with chronic myeloid leukemia (CML) who are in chronic phase but have failed therapy with two or more tyrosine kinase inhibitors. In such patients, cure rates of 70% can be expected. Hematopoietic cell transplantation is also recommended for patients with CML who present or progress to accelerated phase or blast crisis, although lower cure rates are seen in such patients (**Chap. 105**).

Although allogeneic transplantation can cure patients with chronic lymphocytic leukemia (CLL), it has not been extensively studied because of the chronic nature of the disease, the age profile of patients, and more recently, the availability of multiple effective therapies. In those cases where it was studied, complete remissions were achieved in the majority of patients, with disease-free survival rates of ~50% at 3 years, despite the advanced stage of the disease at the time of transplant.

MYELODYSPLASIA AND MYELOPROLIFERATIVE DISORDERS

Between 20 and 65% of patients with myelodysplasia appear to be cured with allogeneic transplantation. Results are better among younger patients and those with less advanced disease. However, patients with early-stage myelodysplasia can live for extended periods without intervention, and so transplantation is generally reserved for patients with an International Prognostic Scoring System (IPSS) score of Int-2 or higher, or for selected patients with an IPSS score of Int-1 who have other poor prognostic features

(Chap. 102). Allogeneic hematopoietic cell transplantation can cure patients with primary myelofibrosis or myelofibrosis secondary to polycythemia vera or essential thrombocythemia, with 5-year progression-free survival rates in excess of 65% being reported. It may require many months for the fibrosis to resolve.

LYMPHOMA

Patients with disseminated intermediate- or high-grade non-Hodgkin's lymphoma who have not been cured by first-line chemotherapy and are transplanted in first relapse or second remission can still be cured in 40–50% of cases. This represents a clear advantage over results obtained with conventional-dose salvage chemotherapy. It is unsettled whether patients with high-risk disease benefit from transplantation in first remission. Most experts favor the use of autologous rather than allogeneic transplantation for patients with intermediate- or high-grade non-Hodgkin's lymphoma, because fewer complications occur with this approach and survival appears equivalent. Although autologous transplantation results in high response rates in patients with recurrent disseminated indolent non-Hodgkin's lymphoma, the availability of newer agents for this category of patient leaves the role of transplantation unsettled. Reduced-intensity conditioning regimens followed by allogeneic transplantation result in high rates of complete and enduring complete responses in patients with recurrent indolent lymphomas.

The role of transplantation in Hodgkin's disease is similar to that in intermediate- and high-grade non-Hodgkin's lymphoma. With transplantation, 5-year disease-free survival is 20–30% in patients who never achieve a first remission with standard chemotherapy and up to 70% for those transplanted in second remission. Transplantation has no defined role in first remission in Hodgkin's disease.

MYELOMA

Patients with myeloma whose disease progresses after first-line therapy can sometimes benefit from allogeneic or autologous transplantation. Prospective randomized studies demonstrate that the inclusion of autologous transplantation as part of initial therapy results in improved disease-free survival and overall survival. Further benefit is seen with the use of lenalidomide maintenance therapy following transplantation. The use of autologous transplantation followed by nonmyeloablative allogeneic transplantation has yielded mixed results.

SOLID TUMORS

Patients with testicular cancer in whom first-line platinum-containing chemotherapy has failed can still be cured in ~50% of cases if treated with high-dose chemotherapy with autologous stem cell support, an outcome better than that seen with low-dose salvage chemotherapy. The use of high-dose chemotherapy with autologous stem cell support is being studied for several other solid tumors, including neuroblastoma and pediatric sarcomas. As in most other settings, the best results were obtained in patients with limited amounts of disease and in whom the remaining tumor remains sensitive to conventional-dose chemotherapy. Few randomized trials of transplantation in these diseases have been completed.

POSTTRANSPLANT RELAPSE

Patients who relapse following autologous transplantation sometimes respond to further chemotherapy and may be candidates for possible allogeneic transplantation, particularly if the remission following the initial autologous transplant was long. Several options are available for patients who relapse following allogeneic transplantation. Treatment with infusions of unirradiated donor lymphocytes results in complete responses in as many as 75% of patients with chronic myeloid leukemia, 40% with myelodysplasia, 25% with AML, and 15% with myeloma. Major complications of donor lymphocyte infusions include transient myelosuppression and the development of GVHD. These complications depend on the number of donor lymphocytes given and the schedule of infusions, with less GVHD seen with lower dose, fractionated schedules.

■ FURTHER READING

Hourigan CS et al: Impact of conditioning intensity of allogeneic transplantation for acute myeloid leukemia with genomic evidence of residual disease. J Clin Oncol 38:1273, 2020.

Jagasia M et al: Ruxolitinib for the treatment of steroid-refractory acute GVHD (REACH1): A multicenter, open-label phase 2 trial. Blood 135:1739, 2020.

Majhail NS et al: Indications for autologous and allogeneic hematopoietic cell transplantation: Guidelines from the American Society for Blood and Marrow Transplantation. Biol Blood Marrow Transplant 21:1863, 2015.

Marty FM et al: Letermovir prophylaxis for vytomegalovirus in hematopoietic-cell transplantation. N Engl J Med 377:2433, 2017.

McDonald GB et al: Survival, nonrelapse mortality, and relapse-related mortality after allogeneic hematopoietic cell transplantation: Comparing 2003-2007 versus 2013-2017 cohorts. Ann Intern Med 172:229, 2020.

Miklos D et al: Ibrutinib for chronic graft-versus-host disease after failure of prior therapy. Blood 130:2243, 2017.

Peled JU et al: Microbiota as predictor of mortality in allogeneic hematopoietic-cell transplantation. N Engl J Med 382:822, 2020.

Sullivan KM et al: Myeloablative autologous stem-cell transplantation for severe scleroderma. N Engl J Med 378:35, 2018.

Zeiser R, Blazar BR: Acute graft-versus-host disease - biologic process, prevention, and therapy. N Engl J Med 377:2167, 2017.

Zeiser R, Blazar BR: Pathophysiology of chronic graft-versus-host disease and therapeutic targets. N Engl J Med 377:2565, 2017.

Section 3 Disorders of Hemostasis

115 Disorders of Platelets and Vessel Wall

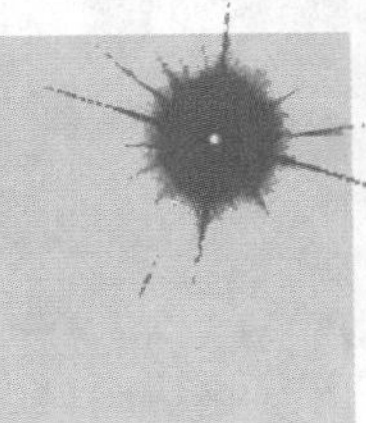

Barbara A. Konkle

Hemostasis is a dynamic process in which the platelet and the blood vessel wall play key roles. Platelets are activated upon adhesion to von Willebrand factor (VWF) and collagen in the exposed subendothelium after injury. Platelet activation is also mediated through shear forces imposed by blood flow itself, particularly in areas where the vessel wall is diseased, and is also affected by the inflammatory state of the endothelium. The activated platelet surface provides the major physiologic site for coagulation factor activation, which results in further platelet activation and fibrin formation. Genetic and acquired influences on the platelet and vessel wall, as well as on the coagulation and fibrinolytic systems, determine whether normal hemostasis or bleeding or clotting symptoms will result.

THE PLATELET

Platelets are released from the megakaryocyte, likely under the influence of flow in the capillary sinuses. The normal blood platelet count is 150,000–450,000/μL. The major regulator of platelet production is the hormone thrombopoietin (TPO), which is synthesized in the liver and other organs. Synthesis is increased with inflammation and specifically by interleukin 6. TPO binds to its receptor on platelets and megakaryocytes, by which it is removed from the circulation. Thus, a reduction in platelet and megakaryocyte mass increases the level of TPO, which then stimulates platelet production. Platelets circulate with an average life span of 7–10 days. Approximately one-third of the platelets reside in the spleen, and this number increases in proportion to splenic size, although the platelet count rarely decreases to <40,000/μL as the spleen enlarges. Platelets are physiologically very active, but are anucleate, and thus have limited capacity to synthesize new proteins.

Normal vascular endothelium contributes to preventing thrombosis by inhibiting platelet function (**Chap. 65**). When vascular endothelium is injured, these inhibitory effects are overcome, and platelets adhere to the exposed intimal surface primarily through VWF, a large multimeric protein present in both plasma and in the extracellular matrix of the subendothelial vessel wall. Platelet adhesion results in the generation of intracellular signals that lead to activation of the platelet glycoprotein (Gp) IIb/IIIa ($\alpha_{IIb}\beta_3$) receptor and resultant platelet aggregation.

Activated platelets undergo release of their granule contents, which include nucleotides, adhesive proteins, growth factors, and procoagulants that serve to promote platelet aggregation and blood clot formation and influence the environment of the forming clot. During platelet aggregation, additional platelets are recruited to the site of injury, leading to the formation of an occlusive platelet thrombus. The platelet plug is stabilized by the fibrin mesh that develops simultaneously as the product of the coagulation cascade.

THE VESSEL WALL

Endothelial cells line the surface of the entire circulatory tree, totaling 1–6 × 10^{13} cells, enough to cover a surface area equivalent to about six tennis courts. The endothelium is physiologically active, controlling vascular permeability, flow of biologically active molecules and nutrients, blood cell interactions with the vessel wall, the inflammatory response, and angiogenesis.

The endothelium normally presents an antithrombotic surface (**Chap. 65**) but rapidly becomes prothrombotic when stimulated, which promotes coagulation, inhibits fibrinolysis, and activates platelets. In many cases, endothelium-derived vasodilators are also platelet inhibitors (e.g., nitric oxide), and conversely, endothelium-derived vasoconstrictors (e.g., endothelin) can also be platelet activators. The net effect of vasodilation and inhibition of platelet function is to promote blood fluidity, whereas the net effect of vasoconstriction and platelet activation is to promote thrombosis. Thus, blood fluidity and hemostasis are regulated by the balance of antithrombotic/prothrombotic and vasodilatory/vasoconstrictor properties of endothelial cells.

DISORDERS OF PLATELETS

THROMBOCYTOPENIA

Thrombocytopenia results from one or more of three processes: (1) decreased bone marrow production; (2) sequestration, usually in an enlarged spleen; and/or (3) increased platelet destruction. Disorders of production may be either inherited or acquired. In evaluating a patient with thrombocytopenia, a key step is to review the peripheral blood smear and to first rule out "pseudothrombocytopenia," particularly in a patient without an apparent cause for the thrombocytopenia. Pseudothrombocytopenia (**Fig. 115-1*B***) is an in vitro artifact resulting from platelet agglutination via antibodies (usually IgG, but also IgM and IgA) when the calcium content is decreased by blood collection in ethylenediamine tetraacetic (EDTA) (the anticoagulant present in tubes [purple top] used to collect blood for complete blood counts [CBCs]). If a low platelet count is obtained in EDTA-anticoagulated blood, a blood smear should be evaluated and a platelet count determined in blood collected into sodium citrate (blue top tube) or heparin (green

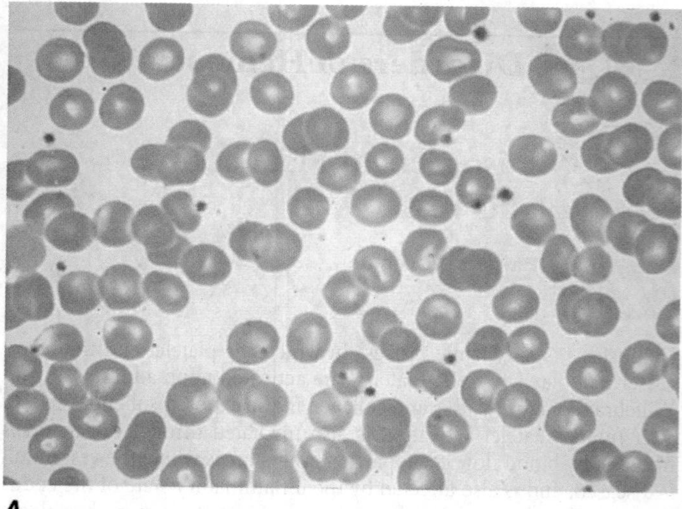

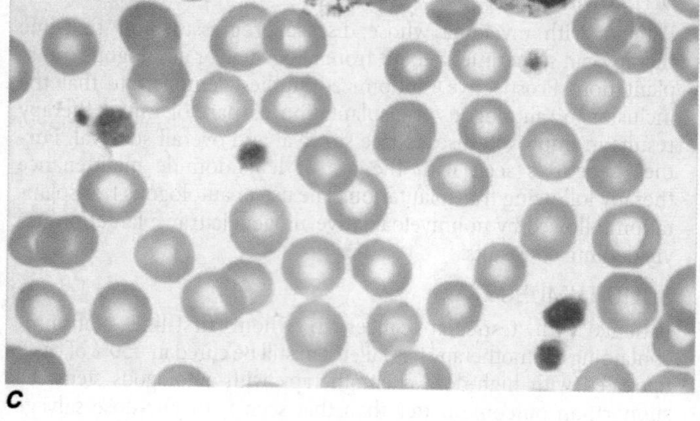

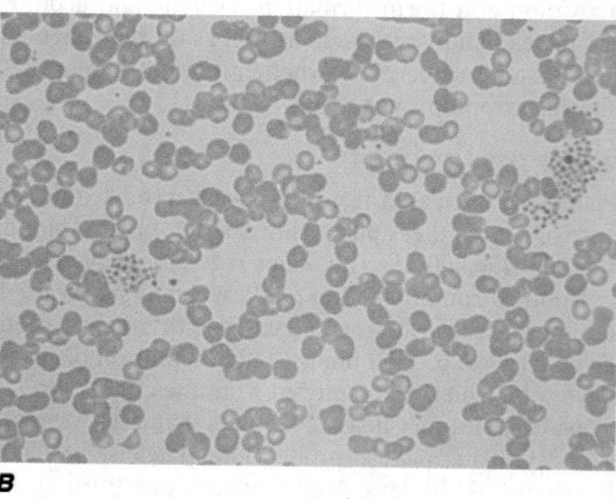

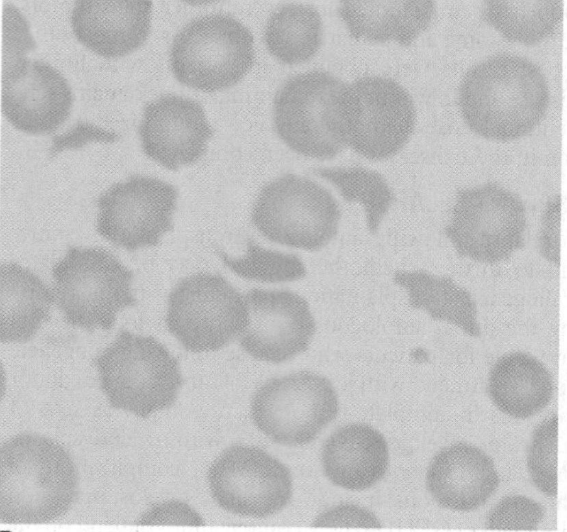

FIGURE 115-1 Photomicrographs of peripheral blood smears. *A.* Normal peripheral blood. ***B.*** Platelet clumping in pseudothrombocytopenia. ***C.*** Abnormal large platelet in autosomal dominant macrothrombocytopenia. ***D.*** Schistocytes and decreased platelets in microangiopathic hemolytic anemia.

top tube), or a smear of freshly obtained unanticoagulated blood, such as from a finger stick, can be examined.

APPROACH TO THE PATIENT

Thrombocytopenia

The history and physical examination, results of the CBC, and review of the peripheral blood smear are all critical components in the initial evaluation of thrombocytopenic patients (**Fig. 115-2**). The overall health of the patient and whether he or she is receiving drug treatment will influence the differential diagnosis. A healthy young adult with thrombocytopenia will have a much more limited differential diagnosis than an ill hospitalized patient who is receiving multiple medications. Except in unusual inherited disorders, decreased platelet production usually results from bone marrow disorders that also affect red blood cell (RBC) and/or white blood cell (WBC) production. Because myelodysplasia can present with isolated thrombocytopenia, the bone marrow should be examined in patients presenting with isolated thrombocytopenia who are older than 60 years of age or who do not respond to initial therapy. While inherited thrombocytopenia is rare, any prior platelet counts should be retrieved and a family history regarding thrombocytopenia obtained. A careful history of drug ingestion should be obtained, including nonprescription and herbal remedies, because drugs are the most common cause of thrombocytopenia.

The physical examination can document an enlarged spleen, evidence of chronic liver disease, and other underlying disorders. Mild to moderate splenomegaly may be difficult to appreciate in many individuals due to body habitus and/or obesity but can be easily assessed by abdominal ultrasound. A platelet count of approximately 5000–10,000 is required to maintain vascular integrity in the microcirculation. When the count is markedly decreased, petechiae first appear in areas of increased venous pressure, the ankles and feet in an ambulatory patient. Petechiae are pinpoint, nonblanching hemorrhages and are usually a sign of a decreased platelet number and not platelet dysfunction. Wet purpura, blood blisters that form on the oral mucosa, are thought to denote an increased risk of life-threatening hemorrhage in the thrombocytopenic patient. Excessive bruising is seen in disorders of both platelet number and function.

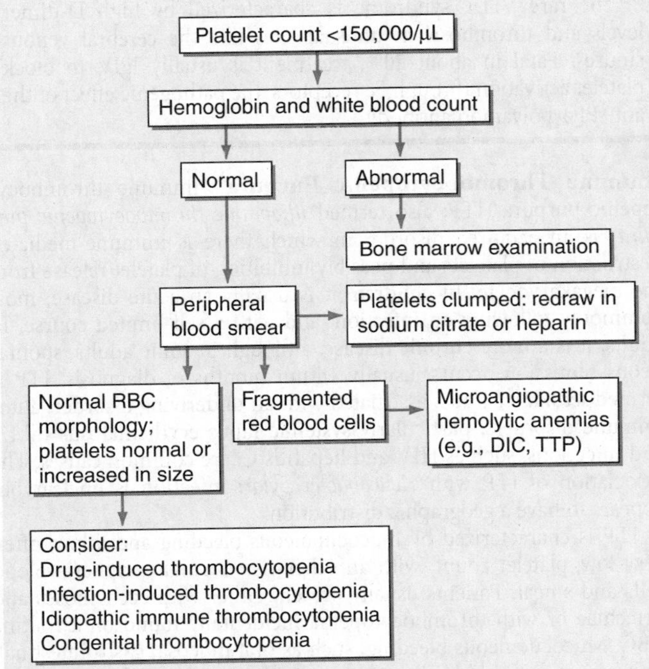

FIGURE 115-2 Algorithm for evaluating the thrombocytopenic patient. DIC, disseminated intravascular coagulation; RBC, red blood cell; TTP, thrombotic thrombocytopenic purpura.

Infection-Induced Thrombocytopenia Many viral and bacterial infections result in thrombocytopenia and are the most common noniatrogenic cause of thrombocytopenia. This may or may not be associated with laboratory evidence of disseminated intravascular coagulation (DIC), which is most commonly seen in patients with systemic infections with gram-negative bacteria and is seen in patients ill with COVID-19. Infections can affect both platelet production and platelet survival. In addition, immune mechanisms can be at work, as in infectious mononucleosis and early HIV infection. Late in HIV infection, pancytopenia and decreased and dysplastic platelet production are more common. Immune-mediated thrombocytopenia in children usually follows a viral infection and almost always resolves spontaneously. This association of infection with immune thrombocytopenic purpura is less clear in adults.

Drug-Induced Thrombocytopenia Many drugs have been associated with thrombocytopenia. A predictable decrease in platelet count occurs after treatment with many chemotherapeutic drugs due to bone marrow suppression (**Chap. 73**). Drugs that cause isolated thrombocytopenia and have been confirmed with positive laboratory testing are listed in **Table 115-1**, but all drugs should be suspect in a patient with thrombocytopenia without an apparent cause and should be stopped, or substituted, if possible. Although not as well studied, herbal and over-the-counter preparations may also result in thrombocytopenia and should be discontinued in patients who are thrombocytopenic.

Classic drug-dependent antibodies are antibodies that react with specific platelet surface antigens and result in thrombocytopenia only when the drug is present. Many drugs are capable of inducing these antibodies, but for some reason, they are more common with quinine and sulfonamides. Drug-dependent antibody binding can be demonstrated by laboratory assays, showing antibody binding in the presence of, but not without, the drug present in the assay. The thrombocytopenia typically occurs after a period of initial exposure (median length 21 days), or upon reexposure, and usually resolves in 7–10 days after drug withdrawal. The thrombocytopenia caused by the platelet Gp IIb/IIIa inhibitory drugs, such as abciximab, differs in that it may occur within 24 h of initial exposure. This appears to be due to the presence

TABLE 115-1 Drugs Reported as Definitely or Probably Causing Isolated Thrombocytopenia[a]

Abciximab	Mirtazapine
Acetaminophen	Naproxen
Amiodarone	Oxaliplatin
Amlodipine	Penicillin
Ampicillin	Phenytoin
Carbamazepine	Piperacillin
Ceftriaxone	Quinidine
Cephamandole	Quinine
Ciprofloxacin	Ranitidine
Diazepam	Rosiglitazone
Eptifibatide	Roxifiban
Furosemide	Sulfisoxazole
Gold	Suramin
Haloperidol	Tirofiban
Heparin	Tranilast
Ibuprofen	Trimethoprim/sulfamethoxazole
Lorazepam	Vancomycin

[a]Based on scoring requiring a compatible clinical picture and positive laboratory testing.

Source: Adapted from DM Arnold et al: J Thromb Hemost 11:169, 2013.

of naturally occurring antibodies that cross-react with the drug bound to the platelet.

Heparin-Induced Thrombocytopenia Drug-induced thrombocytopenia due to heparin differs from that seen with other drugs in two major ways. (1) The thrombocytopenia is not usually severe, with nadir counts rarely <20,000/μL. (2) Heparin-induced thrombocytopenia (HIT) is not associated with bleeding and, in fact, markedly increases the risk of thrombosis. The pathogenesis of HIT is complex. It results from antibody formation to a complex of the platelet-specific protein platelet factor 4 (PF4) and heparin or other glycosaminoglycans. The anti-heparin/PF4 antibody can activate platelets through the FcγRIIa receptor and also activate monocytes, endothelial cells, and coagulation proteins. Many patients exposed to heparin develop antibodies to heparin/PF4 but do not appear to have adverse consequences. A fraction of those who develop antibodies will develop HIT, and a portion of those (up to 50%) will develop thrombosis (HITT).

HIT can occur after exposure to low-molecular-weight heparin (LMWH) as well as unfractionated heparin (UFH), although it is more common with the latter. Most patients develop HIT after exposure to heparin for 5–14 days **(Fig. 115-3)**. It occurs before 5 days in those who were exposed to heparin in the prior few weeks or months (<~100 days) and have circulating anti-heparin/PF4 antibodies. Rarely, thrombocytopenia and thrombosis begin several days after all heparin has been stopped (termed *delayed-onset HIT*), and more rarely, spontaneous HIT, or autoimmune HIT syndrome, occurs where there is no history of heparin exposure and termed *vaccine-induced immune thrombocytopenia and thrombosis* (VITT). A syndrome similar to spontaneous HIT has been described rarely post-COVID-19 vaccination mainly with the ChAdOx1-S/nCoV-19 vaccine. The "4T's" have been recommended to be used in a diagnostic algorithm for HIT: *t*hrombocytopenia, *t*iming of platelet count drop, *t*hrombosis and other sequelae such as localized skin reactions, and o*t*her causes of thrombocytopenia not evident. Application of the 4T scoring system is very useful in excluding a diagnosis of HIT but will result in overdiagnosis of HIT in situations where thrombocytopenia and thrombosis due to other etiologies are common, such as in the intensive care unit. Alternative scoring systems have been recommended, including for patients after cardiopulmonary bypass.

LABORATORY TESTING FOR HIT Because of the prevalence of antiheparin antibodies without clinical disease, testing should be done in individuals who are at intermediate or high risk based on clinical pretest assessment. HIT (anti-heparin/PF4) antibodies can be detected using two types of assays. The most widely available is an enzyme-linked immunoassay (ELISA) with PF4/polyanion complex as the antigen. Because many patients develop antibodies but do not develop clinical HIT, the test has a low specificity for the diagnosis of HIT. This is especially true in patients who have undergone surgery requiring cardiopulmonary bypass, where approximately 50% of patients develop these antibodies postoperatively. IgG-specific ELISAs increase specificity but may decrease sensitivity. The other assay is a platelet activation assay, most commonly the serotonin release assay, which measures the ability of the patient's serum to activate platelets in the presence of heparin in a concentration-dependent manner. This test has lower sensitivity but higher specificity than the ELISA. However, HIT remains a clinical diagnosis.

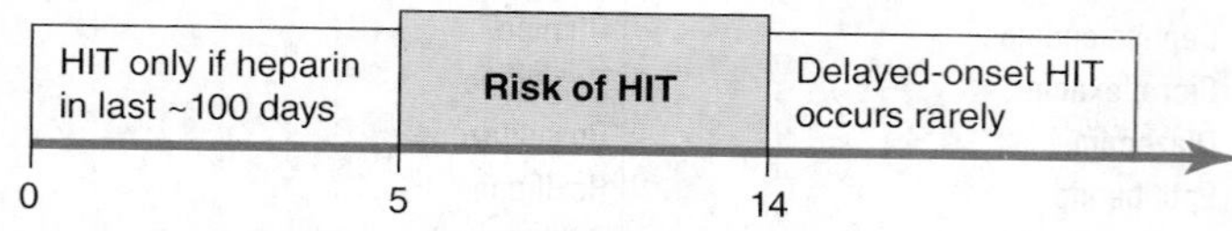

FIGURE 115-3 Time course of heparin-induced thrombocytopenia (HIT) development after heparin exposure. The timing of development after heparin exposure is a critical factor in determining the likelihood of HIT in a patient. HIT occurs early after heparin exposure in the presence of preexisting heparin/platelet factor 4 (PF4) antibodies, which disappear from circulation by ~100 days following a prior exposure. Rarely, HIT may occur later after heparin exposure (termed delayed-onset HIT). In this setting, heparin/PF4 antibody testing is usually markedly positive. HIT can occur after exposure to either unfractionated (UFH) or low-molecular-weight heparin (LMWH).

TREATMENT
Heparin-Induced Thrombocytopenia

Early recognition is key in treatment of HIT, with prompt discontinuation of heparin and use of alternative anticoagulants if bleeding risk does not outweigh thrombotic risk. Thrombosis is a common complication of HIT, even after heparin discontinuation, and can occur in both the venous and arterial systems. In patients diagnosed with HIT, imaging studies to evaluate the patient for thrombosis (at least lower extremity duplex Doppler imaging) are recommended. Patients requiring anticoagulation should be switched from heparin to an alternative anticoagulant. The direct thrombin inhibitor (DTI) argatroban is effective in HITT. The DTI bivalirudin and the antithrombin-binding pentasaccharide fondaparinux are also effective but not approved by the U.S. Food and Drug Administration (FDA) for this indication. Direct oral anticoagulants (DOACs) are being used for treatment, although they are not FDA approved for this indication. Studies in small numbers of patients suggest their use in this setting may be a viable option. HIT antibodies cross-react with LMWH, and these drugs should not be used in the treatment of HIT.

Because of the high rate of thrombosis in patients with HIT, anticoagulation should be considered, even in the absence of thrombosis. In patients with thrombosis, anticoagulation is continued for 3–6 months, but in patients without thrombosis, the duration of anticoagulation is less well defined. An increased risk of thrombosis is present for at least 1 month after diagnosis; however, most thromboses occur early, and whether thrombosis occurs later if the patient is initially anticoagulated is unknown. Options include continuing anticoagulation until a few days after platelet recovery or for 1 month. Introduction of warfarin alone in the setting of HIT or HITT may precipitate thrombosis, particularly venous gangrene, presumably due to clotting activation and severely reduced levels of proteins C and S. Warfarin therapy, if started, should be overlapped with a DTI or fondaparinux and started after resolution of the thrombocytopenia and lessening of the prothrombotic state. Evidence for use of an oral direct Xa inhibitor in this setting is growing.

The rare VITT syndrome is characterized by high D-dimer levels and thrombosis in unusual sites like the cerebral venous sinuses. Fatal in about 20%, treatment is usually IgIV to block platelet activation through Fc receptors, the pathogenic effect of the anti-PF4-polyanion antibody.

Immune Thrombocytopenic Purpura Immune thrombocytopenic purpura (ITP; also termed *idiopathic thrombocytopenic purpura*) is an acquired disorder in which there is immune-mediated destruction of platelets and possibly inhibition of platelet release from the megakaryocyte. In children, it is usually an acute disease, most commonly following an infection, and with a self-limited course. In adults, it is a more chronic disease, although in some adults, spontaneous remission occurs, usually within months of diagnosis. ITP is termed *secondary* if it is associated with an underlying disorder; autoimmune disorders, particularly systemic lupus erythematosus (SLE), and infections, such as HIV and hepatitis C, are common causes. The association of ITP with *Helicobacter pylori* infection is unclear but appears to have a geographic distribution.

ITP is characterized by mucocutaneous bleeding and a low, often very low, platelet count, with an otherwise normal peripheral blood cells and smear. Patients usually present either with ecchymoses and petechiae or with thrombocytopenia incidentally found on a routine CBC. Mucocutaneous bleeding, such as oral mucosa, gastrointestinal, or heavy menstrual bleeding, may be present. Rarely, life-threatening, including central nervous system, bleeding can occur. Wet purpura (blood blisters in the mouth) and retinal hemorrhages may herald life-threatening bleeding.

LABORATORY TESTING IN ITP Laboratory testing for antibodies (serologic testing) is usually not helpful due to the low sensitivity and specificity of the current tests. Bone marrow examination can be reserved for those who have other signs or laboratory abnormalities not explained by ITP or in patients who do not respond to initial therapy. The peripheral blood smear may show large platelets, with otherwise normal morphology. Depending on the bleeding history, iron-deficiency anemia may be present.

Laboratory testing is performed to evaluate for secondary causes of ITP and should include testing for HIV infection and hepatitis C (and other infections if indicated). Serologic testing for SLE, serum protein electrophoresis, immunoglobulin levels to potentially detect hypogammaglobulinemia, selective testing for IgA deficiency or monoclonal gammopathies, and testing for *H. pylori* infection should be considered, depending on the clinical circumstance. If anemia is present, direct antiglobulin testing (Coombs' test) should be performed to rule out combined autoimmune hemolytic anemia with ITP (Evans' syndrome).

TREATMENT

Immune Thrombocytopenic Purpura

The treatment of ITP uses drugs that decrease reticuloendothelial uptake of the antibody-bound platelet, decrease antibody production, and/or increase platelet production. The diagnosis of ITP does not necessarily mean that treatment must be instituted. Patients with platelet counts >30,000/μL appear not to have increased mortality related to the thrombocytopenia.

Initial treatment in patients without significant bleeding symptoms, severe thrombocytopenia (<5000/μL), or signs of impending bleeding (e.g., retinal hemorrhage or large oral mucosal hemorrhages) can be instituted as an outpatient using single agents. Traditionally, this has been prednisone at 1 mg/kg or a 4-day course of dexamethasone, 40 mg/d, although Rh_0(D) immune globulin therapy (WinRho SDF), at 50–75 μg/kg, is also being used in this setting. Rh_0(D) immune globulin must be used only in Rh-positive patients because the mechanism of action is production of limited hemolysis, with antibody-coated cells "saturating" the Fc receptors, inhibiting Fc receptor function. Monitoring patients for 8 h after infusion is now advised by the FDA because of the rare complication of severe intravascular hemolysis. Intravenous gamma globulin (IVIgG), which is pooled, primarily IgG antibodies, also blocks the Fc receptor system, but appears to work primarily through different mechanism(s). IVIgG has more efficacy than anti-Rh_0(D) in postsplenectomized patients. IVIgG is dosed at 1–2 g/kg total, given over 1–5 days. Side effects are usually related to the volume of infusion and infrequently include aseptic meningitis and renal failure. All immunoglobulin preparations are derived from human plasma and undergo treatment for viral inactivation.

For patients with severe ITP and/or symptoms of bleeding, hospital admission is required, and combined-modality therapy is given using high-dose glucocorticoids with IVIgG or anti-Rh_0(D) therapy and, as needed, additional immunosuppressive agents. Rituximab, an anti-CD20 (B cell) antibody, has shown efficacy in the treatment of refractory ITP, although long-lasting remission only occurs in approximately 30% of patients.

TPO receptor agonists, one administered subcutaneously (romiplostim) and another orally (eltrombopag), are effective in raising platelet counts in patients with ITP and are recommended for patients who relapse or who are unresponsive to at least one other therapy.

Other immunosuppressive drugs have also been tested. The combination of glucocorticoids with mycophenolate mofetil (500 mg PO bid, increasing to 1000 mg PO bid as tolerated) appears to be more effective than glucocorticoids alone.

Splenectomy has been used for treatment of patients who relapse after glucocorticoids are tapered and remains a treatment option. However, with the recognition that ITP will resolve spontaneously in some adult patients, observation, if the platelet count is high enough, or intermittent treatment with anti-Rh_0(D) or IVIgG, or initiation of treatment with a TPO receptor agonist may be a reasonable approach to see if the ITP will resolve, prior to splenectomy or other therapies. Vaccination against encapsulated organisms (especially pneumococcus, but also meningococcus and *Haemophilus influenzae*, depending on patient age and potential exposure) is recommended before splenectomy. Accessory spleens are a very rare cause of relapse.

Inherited Thrombocytopenia Thrombocytopenia is rarely inherited, either as an isolated finding or as part of a syndrome, and may be inherited in an autosomal dominant, autosomal recessive, or X-linked pattern. Many forms of autosomal dominant macrothrombocytopenia are now known to be associated with variants in the non-muscle myosin heavy chain *MYH9* gene. Interestingly, these include the May-Hegglin anomaly, and Sebastian, Epstein's, and Fechtner syndromes, all of which have distinct distinguishing features. A common feature of these disorders is large platelets (Fig. 115-1*C*). Autosomal recessive disorders include congenital amegakaryocytic thrombocytopenia, thrombocytopenia with absent radii, and Bernard-Soulier syndrome. The latter is primarily a functional platelet disorder due to absence of Gp Ib-IX-V, the VWF adhesion receptor. X-linked disorders include Wiskott-Aldrich syndrome and a dyshematopoietic syndrome resulting from a mutation in *GATA-1*, an important transcriptional regulator of hematopoiesis.

THROMBOTIC THROMBOCYTOPENIC PURPURA AND HEMOLYTIC-UREMIC SYNDROME

Thrombotic thrombocytopenic microangiopathies are a group of disorders characterized by microangiopathic hemolytic anemia (MAHA) defined by thrombocytopenia and fragmented RBCs (Fig. 115-1*D*) on peripheral blood smear, laboratory evidence of hemolysis (elevated lactate dehydrogenase [LDH] and unconjugated bilirubin and decreased haptoglobin), and microvascular thrombosis. They include thrombotic thrombocytopenic purpura (TTP) and hemolytic-uremic syndrome (HUS), as well as syndromes complicating bone marrow transplantation, certain medications and infections, pregnancy, and vasculitis. In DIC, although thrombocytopenia and microangiopathy are seen, a coagulopathy predominates, with consumption of clotting factors and fibrinogen resulting in an elevated prothrombin time (PT) and often activated partial thromboplastin time (aPTT). The PT and aPTT are characteristically normal in TTP or HUS.

Thrombotic Thrombocytopenic Purpura TTP was first described in 1924 by Eli Moschcowitz and characterized by a pentad of findings that include microangiopathic hemolytic anemia, thrombocytopenia, renal failure, neurologic findings, and fever. The full-blown syndrome is less commonly seen now, probably due to earlier diagnosis. The introduction of treatment with plasma exchange markedly improved the prognosis in patients, with a decrease in mortality from 85–100% to 10–30%.

The pathogenesis of inherited (Upshaw-Schulman syndrome) and idiopathic TTP (ITTP) is related to a deficiency of, or antibodies to, the metalloprotease ADAMTS13, which cleaves VWF. VWF is normally secreted as ultra-large multimers, which are then cleaved by ADAMTS13. The persistence of ultra-large VWF molecules is thought to contribute to pathogenic platelet adhesion and aggregation (**Fig. 115-4**). This defect alone, however, is not sufficient to result in TTP because individuals with a congenital absence of ADAMTS13 develop TTP only episodically, including during first pregnancy. The level of ADAMTS13 activity, as well as antibodies to ADAMTS13, can be detected by laboratory assays, which play a critical role in the differential diagnosis of MAHA. ADAMTS13 activity levels of <10% are diagnostic of TTP.

Idiopathic TTP appears to be more common in women than in men. No geographic or racial distribution has been defined. TTP is more common in patients with HIV infection and in pregnant women. Medication-related MAHA may be secondary to antibody formation (ticlopidine and possibly clopidogrel) or direct endothelial toxicity (cyclosporine, mitomycin C, tacrolimus, quinine), although this is not always so clear, and fear of withholding treatment, as well as lack of

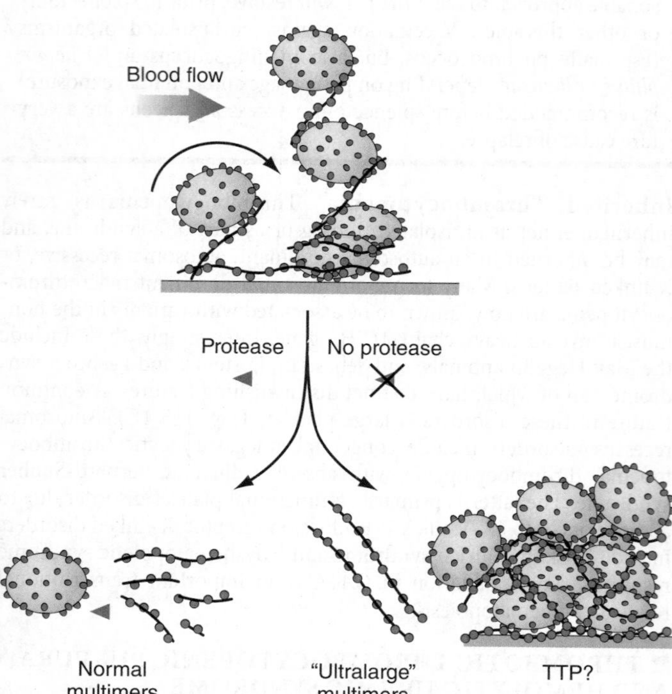

FIGURE 115-4 Pathogenesis of thrombotic thrombocytopenic purpura (TTP). Normally the ultra-high-molecular-weight multimers of von Willebrand factor (VWF) produced by the endothelial cells are processed into smaller multimers by a plasma metalloproteinase called ADAMTS13. In TTP, the activity of the protease is inhibited, and the ultra-high-molecular-weight multimers of VWF initiate platelet aggregation and thrombosis.

other treatment alternatives, may result in initial application of plasma exchange. However, withdrawal, or reduction in dose, of endothelial toxic agents usually decreases the microangiopathy.

TREATMENT

Thrombotic Thrombocytopenic Purpura

TTP is a devastating disease if not diagnosed and treated promptly. In patients presenting with new thrombocytopenia, with or without evidence of renal insufficiency and other elements of classic TTP, laboratory data (PT, aPTT, CBC with platelet count and peripheral smear, ADAMTS13 activity, LDH, bilirubin, haptoglobin, direct antiglobulin assay) should be obtained to rule out DIC and to evaluate for evidence of MAHA.

Therapeutic plasma exchange (TPE) remains the mainstay of treatment of TTP. TPE is continued until the platelet count is normal and signs of hemolysis are resolved for at least 2 days. Although never evaluated in clinical trials, the use of glucocorticoids seems a reasonable approach but should only be used as an adjunct to plasma exchange. The addition of rituximab to initial therapy decreases duration of TPE and relapses. Caplacizumab, an anti-VWF nanobody, decreases mortality and burden of care when used in patients with ADAMTS13 <10% or with high clinical probability of disease. Guidelines from the International Society of Thrombosis and Hemostasis recommend starting caplacizumab and rituximab only in individuals with diagnostic ADAMTS13 levels (usually <10%) and, additionally for rituximab, in patients with evidence of an inhibitor, given potential side effects and costs.

Patients with persistently low ADAMTS13 have a greater risk of ongoing sequelae including stroke. There is a significant relapse rate; in patients treated with TPE, 25–45% of patients relapse within 30 days of initial "remission," and 12–40% of patients have late relapses. Relapses are more frequent in patients with severe ADAMTS13 deficiency at presentation. Treatment of patients with TTP relapses should be initiated before confirmatory laboratory assays are available.

Hemolytic-Uremic Syndrome HUS is a syndrome characterized by acute renal failure, microangiopathic hemolytic anemia, and thrombocytopenia. It is seen preceded by an episode of diarrhea, often hemorrhagic in nature, predominantly in children. *Escherichia coli* O157:H7 is the most frequent, although not only, etiologic serotype. HUS not associated with diarrhea is more heterogeneous in presentation and course. Atypical HUS (aHUS) is usually due to genetic defects in complement genes or antibodies directed against complementary regulatory proteins that result in chronic complement activation. Laboratory testing for DNA variants in complement regulatory genes is available, although assigning pathogenicity to variants remains challenging. Currently, a commercially available functional assay is not available that is diagnostic of the disease.

TREATMENT

Hemolytic-Uremic Syndrome

Treatment of HUS is primarily supportive. In HUS associated with diarrhea, many (~40%) children require at least some period of support with dialysis; however, the overall mortality is <5%. In HUS not associated with diarrhea, the mortality is higher, approximately 26%. Plasma infusion or plasma exchange has not been shown to alter the overall course in HUS or aHUS, except in patients with antibodies to factor H. ADAMTS13 levels are generally reported to be normal in HUS, although occasionally they have been reported to be decreased. In patients with aHUS, eculizumab, a humanized monoclonal antibody against C5 that blocks terminal complement, has efficacy in resolution of aHUS and improving or preserving renal function. Patients with aHUS may initially be treated with plasma exchange, until the ADAMTS13 level is returned and the diagnosis is more clear, since aHUS remains a diagnosis of exclusion. However, plasma exchange has not been shown to affect clinical outcomes in aHUS.

■ THROMBOCYTOSIS

Thrombocytosis is almost always due to (1) iron deficiency; (2) inflammation, cancer, or infection (reactive thrombocytosis); or (3) an underlying myeloproliferative process (essential thrombocythemia or polycythemia vera) **(Chap. 103)** or, rarely, the 5q– myelodysplastic process **(Chap. 102)**. Patients presenting with an elevated platelet count should be evaluated for underlying inflammation and malignancy, and iron deficiency should be ruled out. Thrombocytosis in response to acute or chronic inflammation has not been clearly associated with an increased thrombotic risk. In fact, patients with markedly elevated platelet counts (>1.5 million), usually seen in the setting of a myeloproliferative disorder, have an increased risk of bleeding. This appears to be due, at least in part, to acquired von Willebrand disease (VWD) due to platelet-VWF binding and removal from the circulation.

■ QUALITATIVE DISORDERS OF PLATELET FUNCTION

Inherited Disorders of Platelet Function Inherited platelet function disorders are thought to be relatively rare, although the prevalence of mild disorders of platelet function is unclear, in part because our testing for such disorders is suboptimal. Rare qualitative disorders include the autosomal recessive disorders Glanzmann's thrombasthenia (absence of the platelet Gp IIb/IIIa receptor) and Bernard-Soulier syndrome (absence of the platelet Gp Ib-IX-V receptor). Both are inherited in an autosomal recessive fashion and present with bleeding symptoms in childhood.

Platelet storage pool disorder (SPD) is the classic autosomal dominant qualitative platelet disorder. This results from abnormalities of platelet granule formation. It is also seen as a part of inherited disorders of granule formation, such as Hermansky-Pudlak syndrome. Bleeding symptoms in SPD are variable but often are mild. The most common inherited disorders of platelet function prevent normal secretion of granule content and are termed *secretion defects*. An increasing number of genetic variants are being found in patients with these disorders, although assigning pathogenicity remains challenging.

TREATMENT

Inherited Disorders of Platelet Dysfunction

Bleeding symptoms or prevention of bleeding in patients with severe platelet dysfunction frequently requires platelet transfusion. Care must be taken to limit the risk of alloimmunization by limiting exposure and using HLA-matched single donor platelets for transfusion when needed. rFVIIa is FDA approved in Glanzmann's thrombasthenia and Bernard Soulier syndrome where use can avoid platelet alloimmunization and anti-receptor antibody formation. Platelet disorders associated with milder bleeding symptoms frequently respond to desmopressin (1-deamino-8-D-arginine vasopressin [DDAVP]). DDAVP increases plasma VWF and factor VIII levels; it may also have a direct effect on platelet function. Particularly for mucosal bleeding symptoms, antifibrinolytic therapy (tranexamic acid or ε-aminocaproic acid) is used alone or in conjunction with DDAVP or platelet therapy.

Acquired Disorders of Platelet Function Acquired platelet dysfunction is common, usually due to medications, either intentionally as with antiplatelet therapy or unintentionally as with high-dose penicillins. Acquired platelet dysfunction occurs in uremia. This is likely multifactorial, but the resultant effect is defective adhesion and activation. The platelet defect is improved most by dialysis but may also be improved by increasing the hematocrit to 27–32%, giving DDAVP (0.3 μg/kg), or use of conjugated estrogens. Platelet dysfunction also occurs with cardiopulmonary bypass due to the effect of the artificial circuit on platelets, and bleeding symptoms respond to platelet transfusion. Platelet dysfunction seen with underlying hematologic disorders can result from nonspecific interference by circulating paraproteins or intrinsic platelet defects in myeloproliferative and myelodysplastic syndromes.

VON WILLEBRAND DISEASE

VWD is the most common inherited bleeding disorder, with prevalence of symptomatic disease of 1 in 1000 to 1 in 10,000 individuals. VWF serves two roles: (1) as the major adhesion molecule that tethers the platelet to the exposed subendothelium; and (2) as the binding protein for factor VIII (FVIII), resulting in significant prolongation of the FVIII half-life in circulation. The platelet-adhesive function of VWF is critically dependent on the presence of large VWF multimers, whereas FVIII binding is not. Most of the symptoms of VWD are "platelet-like" except in more severe VWD when the FVIII is low enough to produce symptoms similar to those found in FVIII deficiency (hemophilia A).

VWD has been classified into three major types, with four subtypes of type 2 (**Table 115-2**). By far, the most common type of VWD is type 1 disease, with a parallel decrease in VWF protein, VWF function, and FVIII levels, accounting for at least 80% of cases. In type 1 VWD, patients have predominantly mucosal bleeding symptoms, although postoperative bleeding can also be seen. Bleeding symptoms are uncommon in infancy and usually manifest later in childhood with excessive bruising and epistaxis. Because these symptoms occur commonly in childhood, the clinician should particularly note bruising at sites unlikely to be traumatized and/or prolonged epistaxis requiring medical attention. Heavy menstrual bleeding is a common manifestation of VWD. Menstrual bleeding resulting in anemia should warrant an evaluation for VWD and, if negative, functional platelet disorders. Type 1 VWD may first manifest with dental extractions, particularly wisdom tooth extraction, or tonsillectomy.

Not all patients with low VWF levels have bleeding symptoms. Whether patients bleed or not will depend on the overall hemostatic balance they have inherited, along with environmental influences and the type of hemostatic challenges they experience. Although the inheritance of VWD is autosomal, many factors modulate both VWF levels and bleeding symptoms. These have not all been defined, but include blood type, thyroid hormone status, race, stress, exercise, hormonal (both endogenous and exogenous) influences, and modulators of VWF clearance. Patients with type O blood have VWF protein levels of approximately one-half those of patients with AB blood type, and in fact, the normal range for patients with type O blood overlaps that which has been considered diagnostic for VWD. Patients with mildly decreased VWF levels should be diagnosed with VWD only in the setting of bleeding symptoms and/or a family history of VWD.

TABLE 115-2 Laboratory Diagnosis of von Willebrand Disease (VWD)

TYPE	aPTT	VWF ANTIGEN	VWF ACTIVITY	FVIII ACTIVITY	MULTIMER
1	Nl or ↑	↓	↓	↓	Normal distribution, decreased in quantity
2A	Nl or ↑	↓	↓↓	↓	Loss of high- and intermediate-MW multimers
2B[a]	Nl or ↑	↓	↓↓	↓	Loss of high-MW multimers
2M	Nl or ↑	↓	↓↓	↓	Normal distribution, decreased in quantity
2N	↑↑	Nl or ↓[b]	Nl or ↓[b]	↓↓	Normal distribution
3	↑↑	↓↓	↓↓	↓↓	Absent

[a]Usually also decreased platelet count. [b]For type 2N, in the homozygous state, factor VIII is very low; in the heterozygous state, it is only seen in conjunction with type 1 VWD.

Abbreviations: aPTT, activated partial thromboplastin time; F, factor; MW, molecular weight; Nl, normal; VWF, von Willebrand factor.

Patients with type 2 VWD have functional defects; thus, the VWF antigen measurement is significantly higher than the test of function. For types 2A, 2B, and 2M VWD, platelet-binding and/or collagen-binding VWF activity is decreased. In type 2A VWD, the impaired function is due either to increased susceptibility to cleavage by ADAMTS13, resulting in loss of intermediate- and high-molecular-weight multimers, or to decreased production of these multimers by the cell. Type 2B VWD results from gain-of-function DNA variants that result in increased ADAMTS13 cleavage and binding of VWF to platelets in circulation, with subsequent clearance of this complex by the reticuloendothelial system. The resulting VWF in the patients' plasma lacks the highest molecular-weight multimers, and the platelet count is usually modestly reduced. Type 2M occurs as a consequence of a group of DNA variants that cause dysfunction but do not affect multimer structure.

Type 2N VWD is due to variants in the *VWF* gene that affect binding of FVIII. As FVIII is stabilized by binding to VWF, the FVIII in patients with type 2N VWD has a very short half-life, and the FVIII level is markedly decreased. This is sometimes termed *autosomal hemophilia*. Type 3 VWD, or severe VWD, describes patients with virtually no VWF protein and usually FVIII levels <10%. Patients experience mucosal and joint bleeding, surgery-related bleeding, and other bleeding symptoms. Some patients with type 3 VWD, particularly those with large VWF gene deletions, are at risk of developing antibodies to infused VWF.

Acquired VWD or von Willebrand syndrome is most commonly seen in patients with underlying lymphoproliferative disorders, including monoclonal gammopathies of underdetermined significance (MGUS), multiple myeloma, and Waldenström's macroglobulinemia. It is seen most commonly in the setting of MGUS and should be suspected in patients, particularly elderly patients, with a new onset of severe mucosal bleeding symptoms. Laboratory evidence of acquired VWD is found in some patients with cardiac valvular disease. Heyde's syndrome (aortic stenosis with gastrointestinal bleeding) is attributed to the presence of angiodysplasia of the gastrointestinal tract in patients with aortic stenosis. The shear stress on blood passing through the stenotic aortic valve appears to unfold VWF, making it susceptible to proteolysis. Consequently, large multimer forms are lost, leading to an acquired type 2 VWD, but return when the stenotic valve is replaced.

TREATMENT
Von Willebrand Disease

The mainstay of treatment for type 1 VWD is DDAVP (desmopressin), which results in release of VWF and FVIII from endothelial stores. DDAVP can be given intravenously, by high-concentration intranasal spray (1.5 mg/mL), or when a concentrated form is available, by subcutaneous injection. The peak activity when given intravenously is approximately 30 min, whereas it is 2 h when given intranasally. The usual dose is 0.3 μg/kg intravenously or two squirts (one in each nostril) for patients >50 kg (one squirt for those <50 kg). It is recommended that patients with VWD be tested with DDAVP to assess their response before using it. In patients who respond well (increase in laboratory values of two- to fourfold), it can be used for procedures with minor to moderate risk of bleeding. Depending on the procedure, additional doses may be needed; it is usually given every 12–24 h. Less frequent dosing may result in less tachyphylaxis, which occurs when synthesis cannot compensate for the released stores. The major side effect of DDAVP is hyponatremia due to decreased free water clearance. This occurs most commonly in the very young and the very old, but fluid restriction should be advised for all patients for the 24 h following each dose.

Some patients with types 2A VWD respond to DDAVP such that it can be used for minor procedures. For the other subtypes, for type 3 disease, and for major procedures requiring longer periods of normal hemostasis, VWF replacement can be given. Virally inactivated VWF-plasma-derived and recombinant factor concentrates are safer than cryoprecipitate as the replacement product.

Antifibrinolytic therapy using either tranexamic acid (TXA) or ε-aminocaproic acid is an important therapy, either alone or in an adjunctive capacity, particularly for the prevention or treatment of mucosal bleeding. These agents are particularly useful in treatment of heavy menstrual bleeding (TXA 1300 mg every 8 h) and postpartum hemorrhage, as prophylaxis for dental procedures, and with DDAVP or factor concentrate for dental extractions, tonsillectomies, and prostate procedures. Antifibrinolytic agents are contraindicated in the setting of upper urinary tract bleeding due to the risk of ureteral obstruction.

DISORDERS OF THE VESSEL WALL

The vessel wall is an integral part of hemostasis, and separation of a fluid phase is artificial, particularly in disorders such as TTP or HIT that clearly involve the endothelium as well. Inflammation localized to the vessel wall, such as vasculitis, and inherited connective tissue disorders are abnormalities inherent to the vessel wall.

Metabolic and Inflammatory Disorders Acute febrile illnesses may result in vascular damage. This can result from immune complexes containing viral antigens or the viruses themselves. Certain pathogens, such as the rickettsiae causing Rocky Mountain spotted fever, replicate in endothelial cells and damage them. SARS-CoV-2 also infects endothelial cells, resulting in activation and damage contributing to COVID-19 pathogenicity. Vascular purpura may occur in patients with polyclonal gammopathies but more commonly occurs in those with monoclonal gammopathies, including Waldenström's macroglobulinemia, multiple myeloma, and cryoglobulinemia. Patients with mixed cryoglobulinemia develop a more extensive maculopapular rash due to immune complex–mediated damage to the vessel wall.

Patients with scurvy (vitamin C deficiency) develop painful episodes of perifollicular skin bleeding as well as more systemic bleeding symptoms. Vitamin C is needed to synthesize hydroxyproline, an essential constituent of collagen. Patients with Cushing's syndrome or on chronic glucocorticoid therapy develop skin bleeding and easy bruising due to atrophy of supporting connective tissue. A similar phenomenon is seen with aging, where following minor trauma, blood spreads superficially under the epidermis. This has been termed *senile purpura*. It is most common on skin that has been previously damaged by sun exposure.

Henoch-Schönlein, or anaphylactoid, purpura is a distinct, self-limited type of vasculitis that occurs in children and young adults. Patients have an acute inflammatory reaction with IgA and complement components in capillaries, mesangial tissues, and small arterioles leading to increased vascular permeability and localized hemorrhage. The syndrome is often preceded by an upper respiratory infection, commonly with streptococcal pharyngitis, or is triggered by drug or food allergies. Patients develop a purpuric rash on the extensor surfaces of the arms and legs, usually accompanied by polyarthralgias or arthritis, abdominal pain, and hematuria from focal glomerulonephritis. All coagulation tests are normal, but renal impairment may occur. Glucocorticoids can provide symptomatic relief but do not alter the course of the illness.

Inherited Disorders of the Vessel Wall Patients with inherited disorders of the connective tissue matrix, such as Marfan's syndrome, Ehlers-Danlos syndrome, and pseudoxanthoma elasticum, frequently report easy bruising. Inherited vascular abnormalities can result in increased bleeding. This is notably seen in hereditary hemorrhagic telangiectasia (HHT, or Osler-Weber-Rendu disease), a disorder where abnormal telangiectatic capillaries result in frequent bleeding episodes, primarily from the nose and gastrointestinal tract. Arteriovenous malformation (AVM) in the lung, brain, and liver may also occur in HHT. The telangiectasia can often be visualized on the oral and nasal mucosa. Signs and symptoms develop over time. Epistaxis begins, on average, at the age of 12 and occurs in >95% of affected individuals by middle age. Approximately 25% have gastrointestinal bleeding usually beginning after the age of 50. HHT is caused by pathogenic DNA variants in number of genes involved in the TGFβ/BMP signaling cascade.

FURTHER READING

Boender J et al: A diagnostic approach to mild bleeding disorders. J Thromb Haemost 14:1507, 2016.

Greinacher A et al: Thrombotic thrombocytopenia after ChAdOx1 nCov-19 vaccination. N Engl J Med 384:2092, 2021.

Gresele P et al: Diagnosis of inherited platelet function disorders: Guidance from the SSC of the ISTH. J Thromb Haemost 13:314, 2015.

Hogan M, Berger JS: Heparin-induced thrombocytopenia. Review of incidence, diagnosis and management. Vasc Med 25:160, 2020.

Hunt BJ: Bleeding and coagulopathies in critical care. N Engl J Med 370:847, 2014.

James PD et al: ASH ISTH NHF WFH 2021 guidelines on the diagnosis of von Willebrand disease. Blood Adv 5:280, 2021.

Jokiranta TS: HUS and atypical HUS. Blood 129:2847, 2017.

Leebeek FWG, Eikenboom JCJ: von Willebrand's disease. N Engl J Med 375:2067, 2016.

Skeith L et al: A practical approach to evaluating postoperative thrombocytopenia. Blood Adv 4:776, 2020.

Vayne C et al: Pathophysiology and diagnosis of drug-induced immune thrombocytopenia. J Clin Med 9:2212, 2020.

Zheng XL et al: ISTH guidelines for the diagnosis of thrombotic thrombocytopenic purpura. J Thromb Hemost 18:2486, 2020.

116 Coagulation Disorders

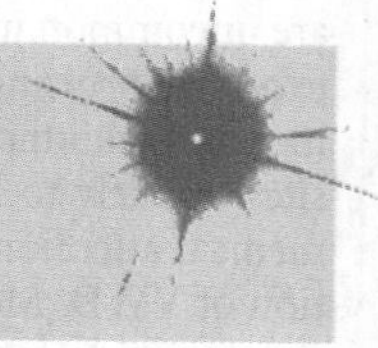

Jean M. Connors

Deficiencies of coagulation factors have been recognized for centuries. Patients with genetic deficiencies of plasma coagulation factors exhibit lifelong recurrent bleeding episodes into joints, muscles, and closed spaces, either spontaneously or following an injury. The most common inherited factor deficiencies are the hemophilias, X-linked diseases caused by deficiency of factor (F) VIII (hemophilia A) or FIX

TABLE 116-1 Genetic and Laboratory Characteristics of Inherited Coagulation Disorders

CLOTTING FACTOR DEFICIENCY	INHERITANCE	PREVALENCE IN GENERAL POPULATION	LABORATORY ABNORMALITY[a]			MINIMUM HEMOSTATIC LEVELS	TREATMENT	PLASMA HALF-LIFE
			aPTT	PT	TT			
Fibrinogen	AR	1 in 1,000,000	+	+	+	100 mg/dL	Cryoprecipitate	2–4 d
Prothrombin	AR	1 in 2,000,000	+	+	–	20%–30%	FFP/PCC	3–4 d
Factor V	AR	1 in 1,000,000	+/–	+/–	–	15%–20%	FFP[c]	36 h
Factor VII	AR	1 in 500,000	–	+	–	15%–20%	FFP/PCC	4–6 h
Factor VIII	X-linked	1 in 5000	+	–	–	30%	FVIII concentrates	8–12 h
Factor IX	X-linked	1 in 30,000	+	–	–	30%	FIX concentrates	18–24 h
Factor X	AR	1 in 1,000,000	+/–	+/–	–	15%–20%	FFP/PCC	40–60 h
Factor XI	AR	1 in 1,000,000	+	–	–	15%–20%	FFP	40–70 h
Factor XII	AR	ND	+	–	–	b	b	60 h
HK	AR	ND	+	–	–	b	b	150 h
Prekallikrein	AR	ND	+	–	–	b	b	35 h
Factor XIII	AR	1 in 2,000,000	–	–	+/–	2%–5%	Cryoprecipitate/FXIII concentrates	11–14 d

[a]Values within normal range (–) or prolonged (+). [b]No risk for bleeding; treatment is not indicated. [c]Since platelets contain FV, platelet transfusion can be used as therapy.

Abbreviations: aPTT, activated partial thromboplastin time; AR, autosomal recessive; FFP, fresh-frozen plasma; HK, high-molecular-weight kininogen; ND, not determined; PCC, prothrombin complex concentrates; PT, prothrombin time; TT, thrombin time.

(hemophilia B). Rare congenital bleeding disorders due to deficiencies of other factors, including FII (prothrombin), FV, FVII, FX, FXI, FXIII, and fibrinogen, are commonly inherited in an autosomal recessive manner **(Table 116-1)**. Disease phenotype often correlates with the level of factor activity. While patients can have a congenital deficiency of FXII accompanied by a significant prolongation in the activated partial thromboplastin time (aPTT), FXII deficiency is not accompanied by a bleeding phenotype, likely due to redundant paths to activation of the intrinsic pathway of the coagulation cascade, including direct activation of FXI by thrombin generated through the extrinsic pathway **(Fig. 116-1)**. Advances in characterization of the molecular basis of clotting factor deficiencies have contributed to better understanding of the disease phenotypes allowing the development of more targeted therapeutic approaches, including the use of small molecules, recombinant proteins, or cell- and gene-based therapies.

The two most commonly used tests of hemostasis, the prothrombin time (PT) and the aPTT, were designed to perform the first screen for clotting factor deficiency (Fig. 116-1). An isolated prolonged PT suggests FVII deficiency, whereas a prolonged aPTT indicates an intrinsic pathway factor deficiency, most commonly hemophilia A or B (FVIII or FIX, respectively) or FXI deficiency (Fig. 116-1). The prolongation of both PT and aPTT suggests a deficiency of FV, FX, FII, or fibrinogen abnormalities. A mixing study, in which the addition of normal pooled plasma to the patient's plasma, will correct a prolonged aPTT or PT due to a factor deficiency, and is the next step in determining if there is a coagulation factor deficiency. If the clotting time does not correct, it suggests the presence of an inhibitor, an antibody to a specific factor; however, a mixing study will also detect the presence of anticoagulants. Many labs have testing methods for detecting inhibitors that neutralize anticoagulants. If the mixing study corrects with normal plasma, individual factor activity assays are performed to determine which factor is deficient.

Acquired deficiencies of plasma coagulation factors are more frequent than congenital disorders; the most common disorders include hemorrhagic diathesis of liver disease, disseminated intravascular coagulation (DIC), and vitamin K deficiency. In these disorders, blood coagulation is hampered by the deficiency of more than one clotting factor, and the bleeding episodes are the result of perturbation of both primary (e.g., platelet and vessel wall interactions) and secondary (coagulation) hemostasis.

The development of alloantibodies to coagulation plasma proteins, clinically termed *inhibitors*, is a relatively rare disease that often affects hemophilia A or B and FXI-deficient patients on repetitive exposure to the missing protein to control bleeding episodes. Inhibitory autoantibodies also occur among subjects without genetic deficiency of clotting factors and although rare can be seen in the postpartum setting, as a manifestation of underlying autoimmune or neoplastic disease, or idiopathically. Rare cases of acquired inhibitors to thrombin or FV have been reported in patients receiving topical bovine thrombin preparation as a local hemostatic agent in complex surgeries. The results of a mixing study that does not correct with the addition of normal plasma indicate the presence of an inhibitor, requiring additional tests to identify the specificity of the inhibitor and measure its titer. Inhibitor

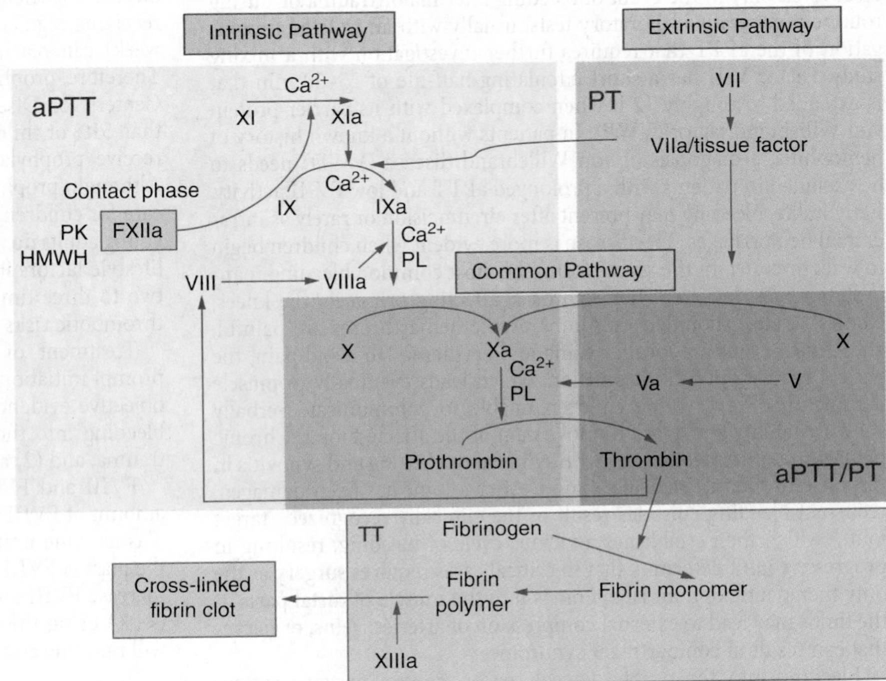

FIGURE 116-1 Coagulation cascade and laboratory assessment of clotting factor deficiency by activated partial prothrombin time (aPTT), prothrombin time (PT), thrombin time (TT), and phospholipid (PL).

detection in patients with hemophilia is of particular importance, with yearly screening performed at most hemophilia treatment centers.

The treatment of coagulation factor deficiencies in the setting of bleeding requires replacement of the deficient protein(s) using recombinant or purified plasma-derived products or fresh-frozen plasma (FFP). Prothrombin complex concentrates (PCCs) are intermediate purity plasma-derived factor concentrates initially used as sources of FVIII or FIX for hemophilia patients, but as they contain the vitamin K-dependent factors, are also used for warfarin reversal. Three-factor PCC (3F-PCC) is less frequently used now for warfarin reversal because these preparations contain low levels of FVII, requiring FFP as a source of FVII. Four-factor PCC (4F-PCC), especially the one used in the United States, contains FII, FIX, FX, higher levels of FVII than 3F-PCC, and protein S and protein C.

HEMOPHILIA A AND B

PATHOGENESIS AND CLINICAL MANIFESTATIONS

Hemophilia is an X-linked recessive hemorrhagic disease due to mutations in the *F8* gene (hemophilia A or classic hemophilia) or *F9* gene (hemophilia B). The disease affects 1 in 10,000 males worldwide, in all ethnic groups; hemophilia A represents 80% of all cases. The large size of the *F8* gene makes it more susceptible to mutation events than the smaller *F9* gene. Male subjects are clinically affected; women, who carry a single mutated gene, are generally asymptomatic. Family history of the disease is absent in ~30% of cases, and in these cases 80% of the mothers are carriers of the de novo mutated allele. More than 500 different mutations have been identified in the *F8* or *F9*. One of the most common hemophilia A mutations results from an inversion of the intron 22 sequence, and it is present in 40% of cases of severe hemophilia A. Advances in molecular diagnosis now permit precise identification of mutations, allowing accurate diagnosis of women carriers of the hemophilia gene in affected families.

Clinically, hemophilia A and hemophilia B are indistinguishable. The disease phenotype correlates with the activity of FVIII or FIX and can be classified as severe (<1%), moderate (1–5%), or mild (6–30%). In the severe and moderate forms, the disease is characterized by bleeding into the joints (hemarthrosis), soft tissues, and muscles after minor trauma or even spontaneously. Patients with mild disease experience infrequent bleeding that is usually secondary to trauma. Among those with residual FVIII or FIX activity >25% of normal, the disease is discovered only in the event of bleeding after major trauma or during routine preoperative laboratory tests, usually with an isolated prolongation of the aPTT that requires further investigation with a mixing study. Factor VIII has a short circulating half-life of 25–30 min that is extended to roughly 12 h when complexed with its carrier protein von Willebrand factor (VWF). In patients without a known history of hemophilia, a diagnosis of von Willebrand disease (VWD) needs to be excluded in patients with a prolonged aPTT and low FVIII activity. Early in life, bleeding may present after circumcision or rarely as intracranial hemorrhages. The disease is more evident when children begin to walk or crawl. In the severe form, the most common bleeding manifestations are recurrent hemarthroses, affecting primarily the knees, elbows, ankles, shoulders, and hips. Acute hemarthroses are painful, and clinical signs are local swelling and erythema. To avoid pain, the patient may adopt a fixed position, which leads eventually to muscle contractures. Very young children unable to communicate verbally show irritability and a lack of movement of the affected joint. Chronic hemarthroses are debilitating with synovial thickening and synovitis in response to the intraarticular blood. After a joint has been damaged, recurrent bleeding episodes result in the clinically recognized "target joint," which then establishes a vicious cycle of bleeding, resulting in progressive joint deformity that in critical cases requires surgery as the only therapeutic option. Hematomas into the muscle of distal parts of the limbs may lead to external compression of arteries, veins, or nerves that can result in compartment syndrome.

Bleeding into the oropharyngeal spaces, central nervous system (CNS), or retroperitoneum is life-threatening and requires immediate therapy. Retroperitoneal hemorrhages can accumulate large quantities of blood with formation of masses with calcification and inflammatory tissue reaction (pseudotumor syndrome) and also result in damage to the femoral nerve. Pseudotumors can also form in bones, especially long bones of the lower limbs. Hematuria is frequent among hemophilia patients, even in the absence of genitourinary pathology. It is often self-limited and may not require specific therapy.

TREATMENT

Hemophilia

Without treatment, severe hemophilia may limit life expectancy. Advances in the blood fractionation industry during World War II resulted in the realization that plasma could be used to treat hemophilia, but the volumes required to achieve even modest elevation of circulating factor levels limit the utility of plasma infusion as an approach to disease management. The discovery in the 1960s that the cryoprecipitate fraction of plasma was enriched for FVIII, and the eventual purification of FVIII and FIX from plasma, led to the introduction of home infusion therapy with factor concentrates in the 1970s. The availability of factor concentrates resulted in a dramatic improvement in life expectancy and in quality of life for people with severe hemophilia. However, the contamination of the blood supply with hepatitis viruses, and subsequently HIV, resulted in widespread transmission of these bloodborne infections within the hemophilia population. The introduction of viral inactivation steps in the preparation of plasma-derived products in the mid-1980s greatly reduced the risk of HIV and hepatitis; the risks were further reduced by the production of recombinant FVIII and FIX proteins in the 1990s. It is uncommon for hemophilic patients born after 1985 to have contracted either hepatitis or HIV, and for these individuals, life expectancy is ~65 years. In fact, since 1998, new infections with viral hepatitis or HIV have not been reported in hemophilia patients.

Factor replacement for hemophilia has been the mainstay of therapy for half a century; however, advances including uniquely functioning molecules and gene therapy have expanded treatment approaches. Factor replacement has been provided either in response to a bleeding episode or as prophylactic treatment. Primary prophylaxis is defined as maintaining the missing clotting factor at levels ~1% or higher on a regular basis in order to prevent bleeds, especially the onset of hemarthroses. Hemophilic boys receiving regular infusions of FVIII (3 days/week) or FIX (2 days/week) can reach puberty without detectable joint abnormalities. Therefore, prophylactic treatment has become more common. The Centers for Disease Control and Prevention reported that more than 51% of children with severe hemophilia who are aged <6 years receive prophylaxis, increasing considerably from 33% in 1995. Although prophylaxis with factor concentrates is the standard care for children and adults with severe hemophilia, teenagers and young adults do not always maintain treatment due to high cost and lifestyle factors including difficulties accessing peripheral veins for two-to-three times a week infusions, and potential infectious and thrombotic risks of long-term central vein catheters.

Treatment of hemophilia bleeds requires the following: (1) prompt initiation of factor replacement as symptoms often precede objective evidence of bleeding, especially for classic symptoms of bleeding into the joint in a reliable patient, headaches, or major trauma; and (2) avoidance of antiplatelet drugs.

FVIII and FIX are dosed in units. One unit is defined as the amount of FVIII (100 ng/mL) or FIX (5 μg/mL) in 1 mL of normal plasma. One unit of FVIII per kilogram of body weight increases the plasma FVIII level by 2%. One can calculate the dose needed to increase FVIII levels to 100% in a 70-kg severe hemophilia patient (<1%) using the simple formula below. Thus, 3500 units of FVIII will raise the circulating level to 100%.

$$\text{FVIII dose (IU)} = \text{Target FVIII levels} - \text{FVIII baseline levels} \\ \times \text{body weight (kg)} \times 0.5 \text{ unit/kg}$$

PART 4 Oncology and Hematology

The doses for FIX replacement are different from those for FVIII, because FIX recovery after infusion is usually only 50% of the predicted value. Therefore, the formula for FIX replacement is as follows:

$$\text{FIX dose (IU)} = \text{Target FIX levels} - \text{FIX baseline levels} \times \text{body weight (kg)} \times 1 \text{ unit/kg}$$

The FVIII half-life of 8–12 h requires injections twice a day to maintain therapeutic levels, whereas the FIX half-life is longer, ~24 h, so that once-a-day injection is sufficient. In specific situations such as after surgery, continuous infusion of factor may be desirable because of its safety in achieving sustained factor levels at a lower total cost.

Cryoprecipitate is enriched with FVIII protein bound to VWF (each bag contains ~80 IU of FVIII). Because of the risk of bloodborne diseases, this product should be used only in emergencies when factor concentrates are not available, although cryoprecipitate may be the only source of FVIII in developing countries.

Mild bleeds such as uncomplicated hemarthroses or superficial hematomas require achieving an initial factor level of 30–50%. Additional doses to maintain levels of 15–25% for 2 or 3 days are indicated for severe hemarthroses, especially when these episodes affect the "target joint." Large hematomas, or bleeds into deep muscles, require factor levels of 50% or even higher if the clinical symptoms do not improve, and factor replacement may be required for a period of 1 week or longer. The control of serious bleeds, including those that affect the oropharyngeal spaces, CNS, and the retroperitoneum, requires sustained protein levels of 50–100% for 7–10 days. Prophylactic replacement for surgery is aimed at achieving normal factor levels (100%) for a period of 7–10 days; replacement can then be tapered depending on the extent of the surgical wounds. Oral surgery is associated with extensive tissue damage that usually requires factor replacement for 1–3 days coupled with oral antifibrinolytic drugs.

NONTRANSFUSION THERAPY IN HEMOPHILIA

DDAVP (1-Amino-8-D-Arginine Vasopressin) DDAVP is a synthetic vasopressin analog that causes a transient rise in FVIII and VWF, but not FIX by release from stores in vascular endothelial cells. Patients with moderate or mild hemophilia A should be tested to determine if they respond to DDAVP before use. DDAVP at doses of 0.3 μg/kg body weight, over a 20-min period, is expected to raise FVIII levels by two- to threefold over baseline, peaking between 30 and 60 min after infusion. DDAVP does not improve FVIII levels in severe hemophilia A patients because no stores are available to release. Repeated dosing of DDAVP results in tachyphylaxis as storage pools are depleted. After three consecutive doses, if further therapy is indicated, exogenous FVIII is required.

Antifibrinolytic Drugs Bleeding in the gums, in the gastrointestinal tract, and during oral surgery can be treated with oral antifibrinolytic drugs such as ε-amino caproic acid (EACA) or tranexamic acid to prevent fibrin degradation by plasmin. The duration of the treatment depending on the clinical indication is 1 week or longer. Tranexamic acid is given at doses of 25 mg/kg three to four times a day. EACA treatment requires a loading dose of 200 mg/kg (maximum of 10 g) followed by 100 mg/kg per dose (maximum 30 g/d) every 6 h. These drugs are not indicated to control hematuria because of concern for forming an occlusive clot in the lumen of genitourinary tract structures.

COMPLICATIONS

Inhibitor Formation The formation of alloantibodies to FVIII or FIX is the major complication of hemophilia treatment. The prevalence of inhibitors to FVIII is estimated to be ~30% in severe hemophilia A patients and 10% among patients with nonsevere hemophilia A. Inhibitors to FIX are detected in only 3–5% of all hemophilia B patients. The high-risk group for inhibitor formation includes severe deficiency (>80% of all cases of inhibitors), familial history of inhibitor, African descent, mutations in the FVIII or FIX gene resulting in deletion of large coding regions, or gross gene rearrangements. Inhibitors usually appear early in life, at a median of 2 years of age, and after 10 cumulative days of exposure. However, intensive replacement therapy such as for major surgery, intracranial bleeding, or trauma increases the risk of inhibitor formation for patients of all ages and degree of clinical severity, such that patients require close laboratory monitoring in the weeks following these events.

The clinical diagnosis of an inhibitor is suspected when patients do not respond to factor replacement at therapeutic doses. Inhibitors increase both morbidity and mortality in hemophilia. Because early detection of an inhibitor is critical to a successful correction of the bleeding or to eradication of the antibody, most hemophilia centers perform annual screening with aPTT and mixing studies. The Bethesda assay uses a similar principle as a mixing study and defines the specificity of the inhibitor and its titer. The results are expressed in Bethesda units (BU), in which 1 BU is the amount of antibody that neutralizes 50% of the FVIII or FIX present in normal plasma after 2 h of incubation at 37°C. Clinically, inhibitor patients are classified as low responders or high responders, with response defined as increase in antibody titer; knowledge of responder type guides therapy. Therapy for inhibitor patients has two goals: the control of acute bleeding episodes and the eradication of the inhibitor. For the control of bleeding episodes, low responders, those with titer <5 BU, respond well to high doses of human FVIII (50–100 U/kg), with minimal or no increase in the inhibitor titers. However, high-responder patients, those with initial inhibitor titer >5 BU or an anamnestic response with increase in the antibody titer to >5 BU, even if low titer initially, do not respond to FVIII. The control of bleeding episodes in high-responder patients can be achieved by using concentrates enriched for prothrombin, FVII, FIX, FX (prothrombin complex concentrates [PCCs] but usually activated PCCs [aPCCs]), and recombinant activated factor VII (FVIIa) known as "bypass agents" as they activate coagulation downstream of the inhibited/absent factor or through a different pathway (Fig. 116-1). For FIX inhibitor patients, high doses of FIX can be used (<5 BU); however, allergic or anaphylactic reactions are common in FIX inhibitor patients; thus bypass products should be used to treat or prevent bleeding as well as for those cases of high titer inhibitors. For eradication of the inhibitory antibody, immunosuppression alone is not effective. The most effective strategy is immune tolerance induction (ITI) based on daily infusion of the missing protein until the inhibitor disappears, typically requiring periods >1 year, with success rates of ~60%. The management of patients with severe hemophilia and inhibitors resistant to ITI is challenging. The use of anti-CD20 monoclonal antibody (rituximab) combined with ITI was thought to be effective but while it reduces the inhibitor titers in some cases, sustained eradication is uncommon.

Other Therapeutic Approaches for Hemophilia A and B Engineered clotting factors, using fusion to polyethylene glycol (FVIII, FIX), IgG1-Fc (FVIII, FIX) or albumin (FIX) with resultant longer half-lives, have been in development, with one currently approved for use. These new-generation products (for FVIII and FIX) aim to facilitate prophylaxis by requiring fewer weekly injections to maintain circulating levels >1%, with infusion frequency decreasing from 3 to 2 days a week in hemophilia A, and notably for hemophilia B, only once-a-week injections of long-acting FIX are required. Other novel approaches to manipulating the coagulation cascade components, such as targeting the natural anticoagulants and inhibitors of activation of coagulation, are in development.

Emicizumab is an asymmetric bispecific antibody with one immunoglobulin variable chain region that binds FIXa and another that binds FX bringing them in close contact resulting in activation of FX by FIXa. FXa subsequently cleaves prothrombin to thrombin—without the need for FVIII (**Fig. 116-2**). It is effective in patients with severe hemophilia A with or without inhibitors. After initial once-a-week subcutaneous injections (an improvement

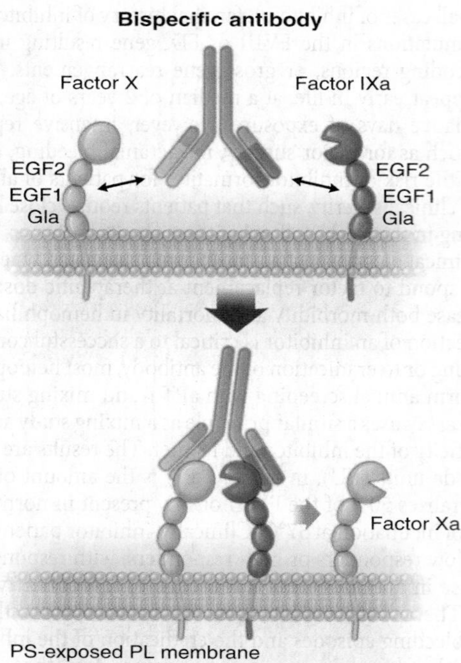

FIGURE 116-2 Mechanism of action of emicizumab. Emicizumab is a bifunctional antibody; the two binding sites recognize different protein sequences, unlike normal antibodies where both variable regions recognize the same antigen. One arm of emicizumab recognizes factor IXa and the other factor X. It functions to bring these two factors in proximity so that factor IXa can activate factor X to factor Xa, which then cleaves prothrombin to thrombin and activates the clotting cascade. *(From T Kitazawa, M Shima: Emicizumab, a humanized bispecific antibody to coagulation factors IXa and X with a factor VIIIa-cofactor activity. Int J Hematol 111:20, 2020.)*

over intravenous administration of factors) for 4 weeks, patients can be maintained with once-a-month dosing to prevent spontaneous bleeds, an overwhelmingly dramatic improvement in quality of life when compared to even the twice-weekly infusion schedule of "long-acting" FVIII compounds. Breakthrough bleeds can occur, however, and need to be carefully managed, as a small number of patients with inhibitors treated with aPCC or recombinant FVIIa developed thrombotic events or fatal thrombotic microangiopathy.

These X-linked disorders are ideally suited for gene therapy as small increases in plasma factor level will result in significant clinical improvement. FIX has been the most studied as the gene is smaller and easier to package in the viral vectors used. In one approach, the sequence of a known spontaneous FIX gain of function mutation that has marked increase in specific activity, FIX Padua, is used so that small increments in plasma level of FIX are also accompanied by even greater increase in functional activity. The larger FVIII gene has also been successfully transferred through an adeno-associated viral vector to a few patients with hemophilia A. The early results appear promising. Complications include transaminitis and loss of gene expression for a variety of reasons; no gene therapy approaches have regulatory approval yet (**Chap. 470**).

INFECTIOUS DISEASES

Hemophilia patients treated with clotting factor concentrates before the development of recombinant factors in the 1990s were almost universally infected with hepatitis C virus (HCV) and HIV. These infections are the major cause of morbidity and the second leading cause of death in these patients. Co-infection of HCV and HIV, present in almost 50% of hemophilia patients, is an aggravating factor for the evolution of liver disease as correction of both genetic and acquired (secondary to liver disease) factor deficiencies may be needed. Improvements in treatment of both HIV and HCV have altered the devastating prognosis for many infected patients. In some select cases with cirrhosis, liver transplant has been performed, which also is curative for hemophilia.

EMERGING CLINICAL PROBLEMS IN AGING HEMOPHILIA PATIENTS

The number of patients living with hemophilia well into adulthood has increased with the advances in treatments. The life expectancy of patients with severe hemophilia is now only ~10 years shorter than the general male population, and near normal in patients with mild or moderate hemophilia. The older hemophilia population has distinct needs relating to more severe arthropathy, chronic pain, and high rates of HCV and/or HIV infections.

Although mortality from coronary artery disease is lower in hemophilia patients with hypocoagulability decreasing thrombus formation, atherogenesis is not prevented. Typical cardiovascular risk factors such as age, obesity, and smoking, along with physical inactivity, hypertension, and chronic renal disease are seen in hemophilia patients as in the general population.

Management of an acute ischemic event and coronary revascularization should include collaboration among hematologists, cardiologists, and internists. Cancer due to HIV- and HCV-related malignancies is also a concern in this population, with hepatocellular carcinoma (HCC) the most common cause of death in HIV-negative patients. The recommendations for cancer screening for the general population should be the same for age-matched hemophilia patients, including routine screening for HCC. Screening for GU or GI tract neoplasms in patients with hematuria or hematochezia may be delayed. Hemophilia patients benefit from the same preventive and therapeutic approaches to minimize the risk of cardiovascular disease and malignancy as the general population.

MANAGEMENT OF CARRIERS OF HEMOPHILIA

Women carriers of hemophilia with factor levels ~50% of normal may not have an increased risk for bleeding. However, a wide range of factor activity (22–116%) due to random inactivation of the X chromosome (*lyonization*) can occur and lead to unexpected bleeding in women with low levels. The factor level of carriers should be measured to optimize perioperative management. During pregnancy, FVIII levels increase approximately two- to threefold compared to nonpregnant women, whereas the FIX increase is less pronounced. After delivery, a rapid fall in the pregnancy-induced rise of maternal clotting factor levels occurs resulting in an imminent risk of bleeding that can be prevented by infusion of factor concentrate to levels of 50–70% for 3 days for vaginal delivery and up to 5 days for cesarean delivery. In mild cases, the use of DDAVP and/or antifibrinolytic drugs is recommended.

FACTOR XI DEFICIENCY

Factor XI deficiency, also known as hemophilia C, is a rare autosomal bleeding disorder that occurs at a frequency of one in a million. However, the disease is highly prevalent among Ashkenazi and Iraqi Jewish populations, reaching a frequency of 6% heterozygotes and 0.1–0.3% homozygotes. More than 65 mutations in the FXI gene have been reported, whereas fewer mutations (two to three) are found among affected Jewish populations.

Normal FXI clotting activity levels range from 70–150 U/dL. Levels vary depending on the presence of heterozygous, homozygous, or double heterozygous mutations with levels <1 U/dL seen in the latter two. Patients with FXI levels <10% of normal have a high risk of bleeding, but the phenotype does not always correlate with FXI clotting activity. The family history is informative, with the bleeding risk based on bleeding in kindreds. Clinically, mucocutaneous hemorrhages such as bruises, gum bleeding, epistaxis, hematuria, and menorrhagia are common, especially following trauma. This hemorrhagic phenotype suggests that tissues rich in fibrinolytic activity are more susceptible to FXI deficiency. Postoperative bleeding is common but not always present, even among patients with very low FXI levels.

FXI replacement is indicated in patients with severe disease for major surgical procedures. A negative history of bleeding complications following invasive procedures does not exclude the possibility of an increased risk for hemorrhage.

TREATMENT
Factor XI Deficiency

Sources of FXI are limited to FFP in the United States, while a plasma-derived FXI concentrate is available in other countries. FFP at doses of 15–20 mL/kg to maintain trough levels ranging from 10–20% can be given every other day in the setting of bleeding or major surgery as FXI has a half-life of 40–70 h. Antifibrinolytic drugs can be used for minor bleeds and as adjunctive treatment with FXI replacement with the exception of GU tract bleeding. The development of an FXI inhibitor can be seen in 10% of severely FXI-deficient patients. Although inhibitors are not associated with spontaneous bleeding, bleeding with surgery or trauma can be severe; treatment with PCC/aPCC or recombinant activated FVII is effective.

RARE BLEEDING DISORDERS

Inherited disorders resulting from deficiencies of clotting factors other than FVIII, FIX, and FXI (Table 116-1) occur infrequently. Bleeding manifestations vary from generally asymptomatic as with dysfibrinogenemia or FVII deficiency to life-threatening as with FX or FXIII deficiency. In contrast to hemophilia, hemarthroses are rare but bleeding in the mucosal tract or after umbilical cord clamping is common. Individuals heterozygous for plasma coagulation deficiencies are often asymptomatic. The laboratory assessment for the specific deficient factor following screening with general coagulation tests (Table 116-1) identifies the diagnosis.

Replacement therapy using FFP or PCCs for deficiencies provides adequate hemostasis for bleeds or prophylactic treatment, although specific concentrates for FX and fibrinogen are available. Cryoprecipitate or FXIII concentrate is needed for FXIII deficiency. FVII deficiency, like FXI, has an increased prevalence in the Ashkenazi Jewish population and is best treated with rVIIa rather than FFP or PCCs depending on the severity of bleeding or type of surgery.

FAMILIAL MULTIPLE COAGULATION DEFICIENCIES

Several bleeding disorders are characterized by the inherited deficiency of more than one plasma coagulation factor. To date, the genetic defects in two of these diseases have been characterized, and they provide new insights into the regulation of hemostasis by gene-encoding proteins outside blood coagulation.

Combined Deficiency of FV and FVIII Patients with combined FV and FVIII deficiency exhibit ~5% of residual clotting activity of each factor, yet it is associated with a mild bleeding tendency, often following trauma. A mutation in the lectin mannose binding 1 (*LMAN1*) gene, a mannose-binding protein localized in the Golgi apparatus that functions as a chaperone for both FV and FVIII, is responsible. In other families, mutations in the multiple coagulation factor deficiency 2 (*MCFD2*) gene have been defined; this gene encodes a protein that forms a Ca^{2+} dependent complex with *LMAN1* and provides cofactor activity in the intracellular mobilization of both FV and FVIII. Replacement therapy to control or prevent bleeding consists of FFP to maintain FV levels and DDAVP or FVIII concentrate to achieve FVIII levels of 20–40%. Alternatively, platelets, which contain FV, can also be used.

Multiple Deficiencies of Vitamin K–Dependent Coagulation Factors Two enzymes involved in vitamin K metabolism have been associated with combined deficiency of all vitamin K–dependent proteins, including the procoagulant proteins prothrombin (II), VII, IX, and X and the anticoagulant proteins C and S. Vitamin K is a fat-soluble vitamin that is a cofactor for carboxylation of the gamma carbon of the glutamic acid residues in the vitamin K–dependent factors, a critical step for calcium and phospholipid binding of these proteins

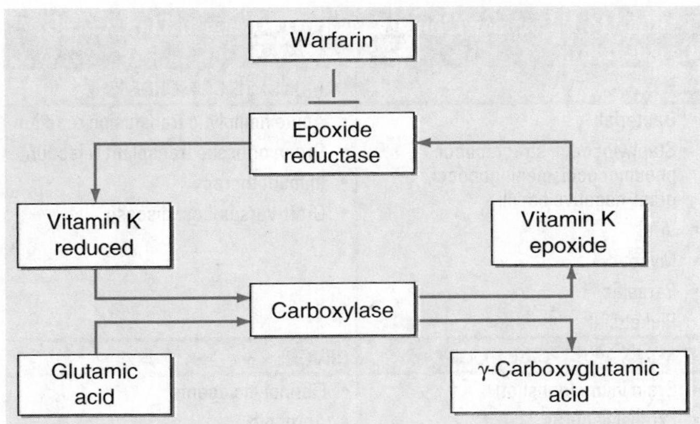

FIGURE 116-3 The vitamin K cycle. Vitamin K is a cofactor for the formation of γ-carboxyglutamic acid residues on coagulation proteins. Vitamin K–dependent γ-glutamylcarboxylase, the enzyme that catalyzes the vitamin K epoxide reductase, regenerates reduced vitamin K. Warfarin blocks the action of the reductase and competitively inhibits the effects of vitamin K.

(Fig. 116-3). The enzymes γ-glutamylcarboxylase and epoxide reductase are critical for the metabolism and regeneration of vitamin K. Mutations in the genes encoding the γ-carboxylase (GGCX) or vitamin K epoxide reductase complex 1 (VKORC1) result in defective enzymes and thus in vitamin K–dependent factors with reduced activity, varying from 1–30% of normal. Patients can have mild to severe bleeding episodes present from birth. Some patients respond to oral vitamin K1 (5–20 mg/d), or parenteral vitamin K1 at doses of 5–20 mg/week. For severe bleeding, replacement therapy with PCC may be necessary.

DISSEMINATED INTRAVASCULAR COAGULATION

In 2001, the International Society on Thrombosis and Haemostatis (ISTH) defined disseminated intravascular congestion (DIC) as "an acquired syndrome characterized by the intravascular activation of coagulation with loss of localization arising from different causes that can originate from and cause damage to the microvasculature, which if sufficiently severe, can produce organ dysfunction." Many disparate processes are associated with DIC (Table 116-2).

The most common causes are bacterial sepsis, although viral and fungal sepsis can also cause DIC, trauma, obstetric causes such as abruptio placentae or amniotic fluid embolism, and malignant disorders especially mucin-producing adenocarcinomas and acute promyelocytic leukemia. Activation of inflammatory pathways in response to infectious pathogens results in increased expression of tissue factor, activation of neutrophils and monocytes with release of cytokines and development of neutrophil extracellular traps, and release of polyphosphates that engage in cross talk with the coagulation system to cause thrombin generation; this process is known as *thrombo-inflammation*. Damage to vascular endothelial cells results in the loss of their native antithrombotic properties; such damage especially occurs with sepsis and trauma. Systemic inflammatory response syndrome (SIRS) and cytokine storm are cytokine-mediated exuberant inflammatory responses often in the setting of infection that are associated with increased mortality and DIC. Purpura fulminans is a severe form of DIC resulting in thrombosis of extensive areas of the skin; it affects predominantly young children following viral or bacterial infection, particularly those with inherited or acquired hypercoagulability due to deficiencies of the components of the protein C pathway. Neonates homozygous for protein C deficiency can develop neonatal purpura fulminans with or without thrombosis of large vessels.

The central mechanism of DIC is the uncontrolled generation of thrombin by multiple mechanisms (Fig. 116-4). Simultaneous disruption of the physiologic anticoagulant mechanisms and abnormal fibrinolysis further accelerate the process. These abnormalities contribute to systemic fibrin deposition in small and midsize vessels. The duration and intensity of the fibrin deposition can compromise

TABLE 116-2 Common Clinical Causes of Disseminated Intravascular Coagulation

SEPSIS	IMMUNOLOGIC DISORDERS
• Bacterial: Staphylococci, streptococci, pneumococci, meningococci, gram-negative bacilli • Viral • Mycotic • Parasitic • Rickettsial	• Acute hemolytic transfusion reaction • Organ or tissue transplant rejection • Immunotherapy • Graft-versus-host disease
TRAUMA AND TISSUE INJURY	**DRUGS**
• Brain injury (gunshot) • Extensive burns • Fat embolism • Rhabdomyolysis	• Fibrinolytic agents • Aprotinin • Warfarin (especially in neonates with protein C deficiency) • Prothrombin complex concentrates • Recreational drugs (amphetamines)
VASCULAR DISORDERS	**ENVENOMATION**
• Giant hemangiomas (Kasabach-Merritt syndrome) • Large vessel aneurysms (e.g., aorta)	• Snake • Insects
OBSTETRICAL COMPLICATIONS	**LIVER DISEASE**
• Abruptio placentae • Amniotic fluid embolism • Dead fetus syndrome • Septic abortion	• Fulminant hepatic failure • Cirrhosis • Fatty liver of pregnancy
CANCER	**MISCELLANEOUS**
• Adenocarcinoma (prostate, pancreas, etc.) • Hematologic malignancies (acute promyelocytic leukemia)	• Shock • Respiratory distress syndrome • Massive transfusion

the blood supply of many organs, especially the lung, kidney, liver, and brain, with consequent organ failure; for example, pulmonary microvascular thrombosis is a component of adult respiratory distress syndrome (ARDS). The sustained activation of coagulation and formation of fibrin can result in consumption of clotting factors and platelets, which in turn leads to systemic bleeding that can be aggravated by secondary hyperfibrinolysis that occurs in late stages of DIC.

Clinical manifestations of DIC are related to the magnitude of the imbalance of hemostasis, to the underlying disease, or to both. The most common clinical findings include petechiae, ecchymoses, and bleeding ranging from oozing from venipuncture sites to severe hemorrhage from the gastrointestinal tract, lung, or into the CNS. In chronic DIC, the bleeding symptoms are discrete and restricted to skin or mucosal surfaces. The hypercoagulability of DIC manifests as the occlusion of vessels in the microcirculation and resulting organ failure. Thrombosis of large vessels and cerebral embolism can also occur. Hemodynamic complications and shock are common among patients with acute DIC, due to the underlying disease, with mortality ranging from 30 to >80%.

Making the diagnosis of DIC can be difficult. The ISTH has developed a validated scoring tool to aid in the diagnosis of overt DIC with a separate tool for pregnant women. It incorporates platelet count, D-dimer level, prothrombin time (PT), and fibrinogen level, and assigns points for different levels of each with the aggregate score helping to make the diagnosis of DIC (**Table 116-3**). The peripheral smear should be assessed for schistocytes. The laboratory diagnosis of DIC should prompt a search for the underlying disease if not already apparent. In critically ill patients, these tests should be repeated over a period of 6–8 h as patients can rapidly deteriorate.

Chronic DIC Low-grade, compensated DIC can occur in clinical situations including giant hemangioma, metastatic carcinoma, or the dead fetus syndrome. Plasma levels of FDP or D-dimers are elevated. aPTT, PT, and fibrinogen values are within the normal range or high. Mild thrombocytopenia or normal platelet counts are also common findings. Red cell fragmentation is often detected but at a lower degree than in acute DIC.

Differential Diagnosis Distinguishing between DIC and severe liver disease is challenging and requires serial measurements of the laboratory parameters of DIC. Patients with severe liver disease manifest laboratory features including thrombocytopenia due to platelet sequestration, portal hypertension, or hypersplenism; decreased synthesis of coagulation factors and natural anticoagulants; and elevated levels of D-dimer. However, in contrast to DIC, these laboratory parameters in liver disease do not change rapidly.

Although microangiopathic disorders such as acquired thrombotic thrombocytopenic purpura present with acute onset accompanied by

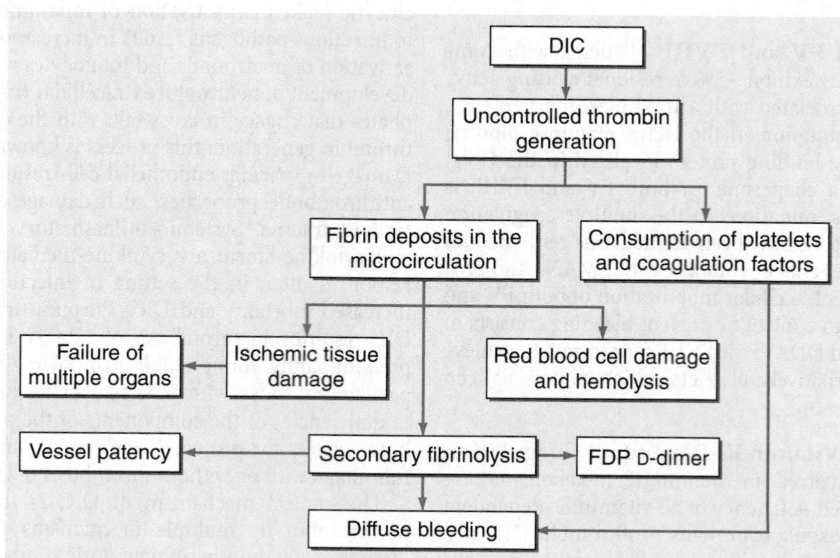

FIGURE 116-4 The pathophysiology of disseminated intravascular coagulation (DIC). Interactions between coagulation and fibrinolytic pathways result in bleeding and thrombosis in the microcirculation in patients with DIC. FDP, fibrin degradation product.

TABLE 116-3 ISTH Criteria for Overt DIC

PARAMETER	VALUE	POINTS
Platelets	>100,000 × 10⁹/L	0
	>50 – <100 × 10⁹/L	1
	<50 × 10⁹/L	2
D-dimer*	Normal	0
	Moderate increase	2
	Severe increase	3
Prothrombin time (PT) prolonged	<3 s	0
	3 – <6 s	1
	>6 s	2
Fibrinogen	>1 g/L	0
	<1 g/L	1
Total Score		**<5 Low-grade DIC**
		>5 Overt DIC

*D-dimer assays are not standardized and have different ranges of normal. Check your institution range of normal to assess degree of increase.

Note: A score of <5 suggests non-overt DIC/low-grade DIC and should be repeated every 1–2 days. A score of >5 suggests overt DIC, lab values should be repeated daily to assess critical changes. Not to be used in pregnant patients.

thrombocytopenia, red cell fragmentation, and multiorgan failure, the clinical presentation and laboratory findings such as an inhibitor to ADAMTS13 levels assist in making the microangiopathic disorder diagnosis (**Chap. 115**).

TREATMENT

Disseminated Intravascular Coagulation

The morbidity and mortality associated with DIC are primarily related to the underlying disease. Management of the underlying disease is required to control and eliminate DIC; however, support with platelets and coagulation factors may be needed until the inciting cause is under control. Many patients with overt DIC are critically ill, usually requiring management in the intensive care unit to treat shock physiology and other manifestations of the underlying illness.

MANAGEMENT OF HEMORRHAGIC SYMPTOMS

Patients with active bleeding or at high risk of bleeding during invasive procedures or after chemotherapy require transfusion support; however, transfusion solely to correct mildly to moderately abnormal coagulation parameters is not indicated. Platelet transfusion for platelet counts <10,000–20,000/μL and replacement of fibrinogen and coagulation factors with FFP, with cryoprecipitate or fibrinogen concentrate as a source of fibrinogen, are indicated with amounts determined by the degree of abnormal PT, aPTT, and fibrinogen levels, as well as severity of bleeding or bleeding risk with invasive procedures. For these situations, fibrinogen level should be maintained at >150 mg/dL and PT prolonged no more than 3 s above the upper limit of normal. Vitamin K should be given. Patients should be frequently monitored, and transfusion support adjusted as the patient's condition changes and dictates.

REPLACEMENT OF COAGULATION OR FIBRINOLYSIS INHIBITORS

Anticoagulants such as heparin, antithrombin III (ATIII), and thrombomodulin concentrates, and antifibrinolytic drugs have all been tried in the treatment of DIC. Low doses of continuous-infusion heparin (5–10 U/kg per h) may be effective in patients with low-grade DIC associated with solid tumors, acute promyelocytic leukemia, or in a setting with recognized thrombosis. Heparin is also indicated for the treatment of purpura fulminans, during the surgical resection of giant hemangiomas, and during removal of a dead fetus. In acute hemorrhagic DIC, the use of heparin is likely to aggravate bleeding. The use of heparin in patients with severe DIC, although demonstrating improved coagulation parameters, has not had a survival benefit; professional society recommendations for use vary widely. Although the use of concentrates of the serine protease inhibitors, antithrombin and thrombomodulin, for sepsis demonstrated little efficacy in all treated patients, post hoc analyses of those with sepsis and confirmed DIC suggest a survival advantage and require further study. Activated protein C treatment for septic shock was withdrawn from the market years ago as findings in clinical practice did not replicate the mortality advantage seen in the clinical trial; impact on DIC was not evaluated.

In patients who have DIC characterized by a primary hyperfibrinolytic state with concomitant severe bleeding, the administration of antifibrinolytics may be considered. However, concern for increasing the risk of thrombosis has led to consideration of concomitant use of heparin. Patients with acute promyelocytic leukemia or those with chronic DIC associated with giant hemangiomas are among the few patients who may benefit from this therapy.

■ VITAMIN K DEFICIENCY

Vitamin K–dependent proteins are a heterogeneous group, including clotting factor proteins and also proteins found in bone, lung, kidney, and placenta. Vitamin K mediates posttranslational modification of glutamate residues to γ-carboxylglutamate, a critical step for the activity of vitamin K–dependent proteins for calcium binding and proper assembly on phospholipid membranes (Fig. 116-3). Inherited mutations with decreased functional activity of the enzymes GGCX or VKORC1 (see above) result in bleeding disorders. Vitamin K in the diet is often limiting for the carboxylation reaction; thus recycling of the vitamin K by these enzymes is essential to maintain normal levels of vitamin K–dependent proteins. In adults, severe vitamin K deficiency due to low dietary intake in adults is rare but is common in association with the use of broad-spectrum antibiotics, or with disease or surgical interventions that affect the ability of the intestinal tract to absorb vitamin K, through anatomic alterations or by changing the fat content of bile salts and pancreatic enzymes in the proximal small bowel. Chronic liver diseases such as primary biliary cirrhosis also deplete vitamin K stores. Neonatal vitamin K deficiency and the resulting hemorrhagic disease of the newborn have been almost entirely eliminated by routine administration of vitamin K to all neonates. Prolongation of PT values is the most common and earliest finding in vitamin K–deficient patients due to the short half-life of FVII, and occurs before prolongation of the aPTT. Parenteral administration of 10 mg of vitamin K is sufficient to restore normal levels of clotting factor within 8–10 h. More rapid correction of the coagulopathy requires replacement with FFP or PCC, the choice depending on patient intravascular volume status and need for rapidity of correction. The reversal of excessive anticoagulant therapy with vitamin K antagonists, such as warfarin, can be achieved by minimal doses of vitamin K (1 mg orally or by intravenous injection) for asymptomatic patients. This strategy can diminish the risk of bleeding while maintaining therapeutic anticoagulation for an underlying prothrombotic state. For emergent reversal of warfarin in the setting of life-threatening bleeding or need for emergency surgery, use of 4F-PPC is the standard of care.

In patients with underlying vascular disease, vascular trauma, atrial fibrillation, and other comorbidities, re-initiation of anticoagulation needs to be carefully considered to prevent subsequent thromboembolic complications.

■ COAGULATION DISORDERS ASSOCIATED WITH LIVER FAILURE

The liver is the site of synthesis and clearance of most procoagulant and natural anticoagulant proteins and of essential components of the fibrinolytic system. Liver failure is associated with a high risk of bleeding due to deficient synthesis of procoagulant factors and enhanced fibrinolysis; hepatologists refer to this as accelerated intravascular coagulation and fibrinolysis (AICF). Thrombocytopenia is common in patients with liver disease and may be due to decreased thrombopoietin that is synthesized in the liver, congestive splenomegaly (hypersplenism), or immune-mediated shortened platelet life span

TABLE 116-4 Coagulation Disorders and Hemostasis in Liver Disease

Bleeding
Portal hypertension
Esophageal varices
Thrombocytopenia
Splenomegaly
Chronic or acute DIC
Decreased synthesis of clotting factors
Hepatocyte failure
Vitamin K deficiency
Systemic fibrinolysis
DIC
Dysfibrinogenemia
Thrombosis
Decreased synthesis of coagulation inhibitors: protein C, protein S, antithrombin
Hepatocyte failure
Vitamin K deficiency (protein C, protein S)
Failure to clear activated coagulation proteins (DIC)
Dysfibrinogenemia

Abbreviation: DIC, disseminated intravascular coagulation.

(primary biliary cirrhosis). In addition, several anatomic abnormalities secondary to underlying liver disease further increase the risk of bleeding (**Table 116-4**). Dysfibrinogenemia is a relatively common finding in patients with liver disease due to impaired fibrin polymerization. The development of DIC in patients with chronic liver disease is not uncommon and may enhance the risk for bleeding. Laboratory evaluation is mandatory for an optimal therapeutic strategy, either to control ongoing bleeding or before invasive procedures. Typically, these patients present with prolonged PT, aPTT, and TT depending on the degree of liver damage, thrombocytopenia, and normal or slight increase in D-dimer. Fibrinogen levels are low only in fulminant hepatitis, decompensated cirrhosis, advanced liver disease, or in the presence of DIC. The presence of prolonged TT and normal fibrinogen and D-dimer levels suggests dysfibrinogenemia. FVIII levels are often normal or elevated in patients with liver failure, and decreased levels suggest superimposed DIC. FV is only synthesized in the hepatocyte and is not a vitamin K–dependent protein; therefore, reduced levels of FV may be an indicator of liver failure. Normal levels of FV and low levels of FVII suggest vitamin K deficiency. Vitamin K levels may be reduced in patients with liver failure due to compromised storage in hepatocellular disease, changes in bile acids, or cholestasis that can diminish the absorption of vitamin K. Replacement with IV vitamin K may improve hemostasis.

Although treatment of bleeding with FFP was the standard approach to correcting hemostasis in patients with liver failure, the use of 4F-PCC is now favored due to lower volume, less increase in portal pressure, reduced risk of circulatory overload, and other complications associated with FFP transfusion. As in any clinical situation, treatment should not be given simply to correct laboratory abnormalities in a patient who is not bleeding or with no need for invasive procedures. Platelet concentrates are indicated when platelet counts are <10,000–20,000/μL to control bleeding or immediately before an invasive procedure if counts are <50,000/μL. Cryoprecipitate is indicated only when fibrinogen levels are <100–150 mg/mL unless the patient is bleeding in which case a higher target is used. The use of antifibrinolytic drugs as adjuncts to control bleeding in patients with liver failure is not thought to result in an increased risk of thrombosis; however, their impact on acute thrombosis propagation is not well studied.

Liver Disease and Thromboembolism Bleeding in patients with stable liver disease is often mild or even asymptomatic. However, as the disease progresses, the hemostatic balance is precarious and easily disturbed; comorbid complications such as infections and renal failure can rapidly upset this balance (**Fig. 116-5**). Past assumptions based on abnormal coagulation tests have been that patients with liver disease have a decreased risk of thrombosis; however, multiple factors contribute to hypercoagulability, including decreased levels of the natural anticoagulant proteins S and C, as well as endothelial cell changes and hemodynamic changes that result in stasis such that portal vein thrombosis is common. Patients with liver disease can also develop deep-vein thrombosis and pulmonary embolism; those with cirrhosis appear to have a 1.5- to 2-fold increase in the rate of venous thromboembolism (VTE). Patients with compensated cirrhosis do not appear to have increased bleeding with the use of VTE prophylaxis or even therapeutic dose heparin to treat acute portal vein thrombosis when carefully managed. In the outpatient setting, warfarin is avoided but low-molecular-weight heparin and direct oral anticoagulants have been safely used to treat thrombosis.

Acquired Inhibitors of Coagulation Factors An acquired inhibitor is an immune-mediated disease characterized by the presence of an autoantibody against a specific clotting factor. Almost half of patients with an acquired factor inhibitor will have an underlying autoimmune or immunoproliferative disorder, malignancy, or be peripartum. FVIII is the most common target of antibody formation and is sometimes referred to as acquired hemophilia A, but inhibitors to prothrombin (FII), FV, FIX, FX, and FXI are also reported. Acquired inhibitor to FVIII occurs predominantly in older adults (median age of 60 years) but occasionally in pregnant or postpartum women with no previous history of bleeding. Bleeding episodes occur commonly in

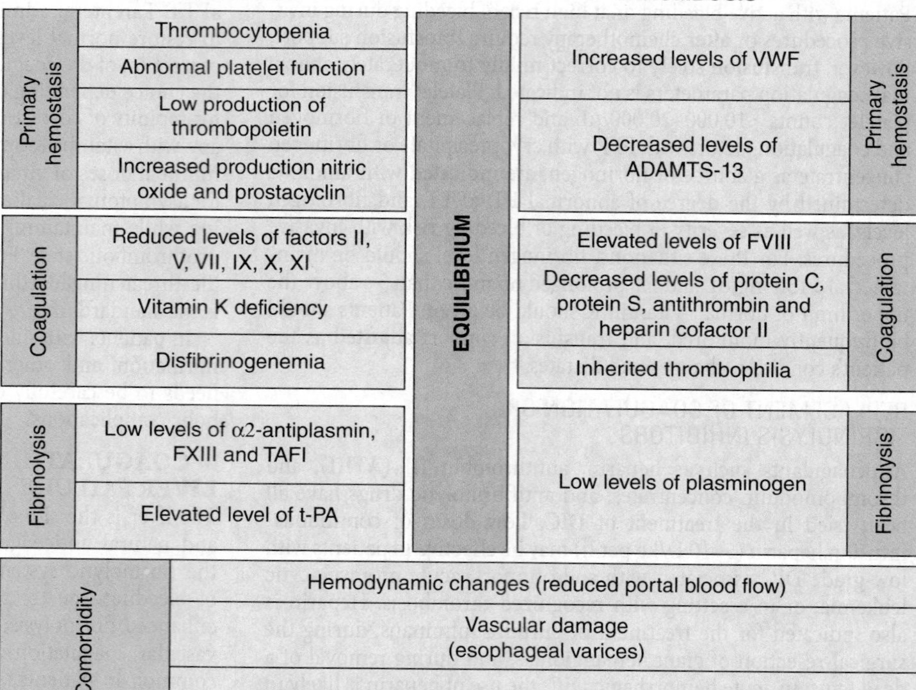

FIGURE 116-5 Balance of hemostasis in liver disease. TAFI, thrombin-activated fibrinolytic inhibitor; t-PA, tissue plasminogen activator; VWF, von Willebrand factor.

soft tissues, the gastrointestinal or urinary tracts, and skin. In contrast to hemophilia, hemarthrosis is rare in these patients. Retroperitoneal hemorrhages and other life-threatening bleeding may appear suddenly. The overall mortality in untreated patients ranges from 8–22%, and most deaths occur within the first few weeks after presentation. The diagnosis is based on the prolonged aPTT with normal PT and TT and a mixing study that does not correct with normal pooled plasma. The Bethesda assay using factor specific-deficient plasma as performed for inhibitor detection in hemophilia will confirm the diagnosis. Treatment of acquired inhibitors of coagulation factors requires control of bleeding and eradication of the inhibitor. Many patients can have life-threatening bleeding. The use of activated "bypass products" such as aPCC or recombinant FVIIa is required. The use of recombinant porcine FVIII can be effective for acquired inhibitors of FVIII. The use of emicizumab to treat acquired FVIII inhibitors has been reported and trials in this population are underway in Europe.

In contrast to hemophilia, inhibitors in nonhemophilic patients are typically responsive to immune suppression, and therapy should be initiated early for most cases. High-dose intravenous γ-globulin and anti-CD20 monoclonal antibody are reported to be effective in patients with autoantibodies to FVIII; however, no firm evidence confirms that these alternatives are superior to the first line of immunosuppressive drugs (glucocorticoids and cyclophosphamide), effective in 70% of patients. Relapse of an inhibitor to FVIII is relatively common (up to 20%) within the first 6 months following withdrawal of immunosuppression; patients should be followed up regularly for relapse.

Topical plasma-derived bovine and human thrombin are commonly used during major cardiovascular, thoracic, neurologic, and pelvic surgeries as well as in trauma patients with extensive burns. Antibody formation to the xenoantigen or its contaminant (bovine clotting protein) has the potential to cross-react with human clotting factors, particularly FV and thrombin and can result in bleeding that can be life-threatening. The development of antibodies to FV with the use of topical preparations of recombinant human thrombin has also been reported. The clinical diagnosis of these acquired coagulopathies is rare but is often complicated by the fact that the bleeding episodes may be detectable during or immediately following major surgery and could be assumed to be due to the procedure itself.

The risk of developing a cross-reacting antibody is increased by repeated exposure to topical thrombin preparations. Thus, a careful medical history of previous surgical interventions that may have occurred even decades earlier is critical to assessing risk.

The laboratory abnormalities include a combined prolongation of the aPTT and PT that often fails to improve by transfusion of FFP and vitamin K, and a mixing study that does not correct with normal pooled plasma. The specificity of the antibody is determined by the measurement of the residual activity of human FV or other suspected human clotting factor. No assays specific for bovine thrombin coagulopathy are commercially available.

No treatment guidelines have been established. Platelet transfusions have been used as a source of FV replacement for patients with FV inhibitors. FFP and vitamin K supplementation may function as coadjuvants rather than as effective treatments for the coagulopathy itself. Experience with recombinant FVIIa as a bypass agent is limited, and outcomes have been generally poor. Specific treatments to eradicate the antibodies based on immunosuppression with glucocorticoids, intravenous immunoglobulin, or serial plasmapheresis have been sporadically reported. Patients should be advised to avoid any topical thrombin sealant in the future.

The presence of lupus anticoagulant can be associated with venous or arterial thrombotic disease. However, bleeding has also been reported rarely with lupus anticoagulants due to antibodies to prothrombin, resulting in hypoprothrombinemia. Both disorders show a prolonged aPTT that does not correct on mixing. To distinguish acquired inhibitors from lupus anticoagulant, note that the dilute Russell viper venom time (dRVVT) and the hexagonal-phase phospholipids test will be negative in patients with an acquired inhibitor and positive in patients with lupus anticoagulants. Moreover, lupus anticoagulant interferes with the clotting activity of many factors (FVIII, FIX, FXI, FXII), which can be assessed in the clinical laboratory; acquired inhibitors are specific to a single factor.

Acknowledgment

Valder Arruda and Katherine High wrote this chapter in prior editions and some material from their chapter is included here.

FURTHER READING

Batty P, Lillicrap D: Advances and challenges for hemophilia gene therapy. Hum Mol Genet 28:R95, 2019.

Kitazawa T, Shima M: Emicizumab, a humanized bispecific antibody to coagulation factors IXa and X with a factor VIIIa-cofactor activity. Int J Hematol 111:20, 2020.

Levi M, Scully M: How I treat disseminated intravascular coagulation. Blood 131:845, 2018.

Menegatti M et al: Management of rare acquired bleeding disorders. Hematology Am Soc Hematol Educ Program 2019:80, 2019.

O'Leary JG et al: AGA clinical practice update: coagulation in cirrhosis. Gastroenterology 157:34, 2019.

Srivastava A et al: WFH guidelines for the management of hemophilia, 3rd edition. Haemophilia 26(Suppl 6):1, 2020.

117 Arterial and Venous Thrombosis

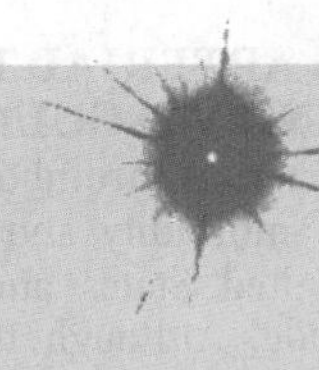

Jane E. Freedman, Joseph Loscalzo

OVERVIEW OF THROMBOSIS

GENERAL OVERVIEW

Thrombosis, the obstruction of blood flow due to the formation of clot, may result in tissue anoxia and damage, and it is a major cause of morbidity and mortality in a wide range of arterial and venous diseases and patient populations. As reported in 2020, 655,000 Americans die from heart disease each year, accounting for about 1 in 4 deaths. In 2017, coronary disease killed 365,914 people in the United States, and approximately 805,000 people experienced a heart attack and 795,000 had a stroke.

It is estimated that as many as 600,000 people each year have a pulmonary embolism or deep-venous thrombotic event, and 60,000–80,000 Americans die of these conditions annually. In the nondiseased state, physiologic hemostasis reflects a delicate interplay between factors that promote and inhibit blood clotting, favoring the former. This response is crucial as it prevents uncontrolled hemorrhage and exsanguination following injury. In specific settings, the same processes that regulate normal hemostasis can cause pathologic thrombosis, leading to arterial or venous occlusion. Importantly, many commonly used therapeutic interventions may also alter the thrombotic–hemostatic balance adversely.

Hemostasis and thrombosis primarily involve the interplay among three factors: the vessel wall, coagulation and fibrinolytic proteins, and platelets. Many prevalent acute vascular diseases are due to thrombus formation within a vessel, including myocardial infarction, thrombotic cerebrovascular events, and venous thrombosis. Although the end result is vessel occlusion and tissue ischemia, the pathophysiologic processes governing these pathologies have similarities as well as distinct differences. While many of the pathways regulating thrombus formation are similar to those that regulate hemostasis, the processes triggering or perpetuating thrombosis may be distinct and can vary in different clinical and genetic settings. In venous thrombosis, primary hypercoagulable states reflecting defects in the proteins governing coagulation and/or fibrinolysis or secondary hypercoagulable states involving abnormalities of blood vessels and blood flow or stasis lead to thrombosis. By contrast, arterial thrombosis is highly dependent on the state of the vessel wall, the platelet, and factors related to blood flow.

ARTERIAL THROMBOSIS

■ OVERVIEW OF ARTERIAL THROMBOSIS

In arterial thrombosis, platelets and abnormalities of the vessel wall typically play a key role in vessel occlusion. Arterial thrombus forms via a series of sequential steps in which platelets adhere to the vessel wall, additional platelets are recruited, and thrombin is activated (Fig. 117-1). The regulation of platelet adhesion, activation, aggregation, and recruitment will be described in detail below. In addition, while the primary function of platelets is regulation of hemostasis, our understanding of their role in other processes, such as immunity, metastasis, wound healing, and inflammation, continues to evolve.

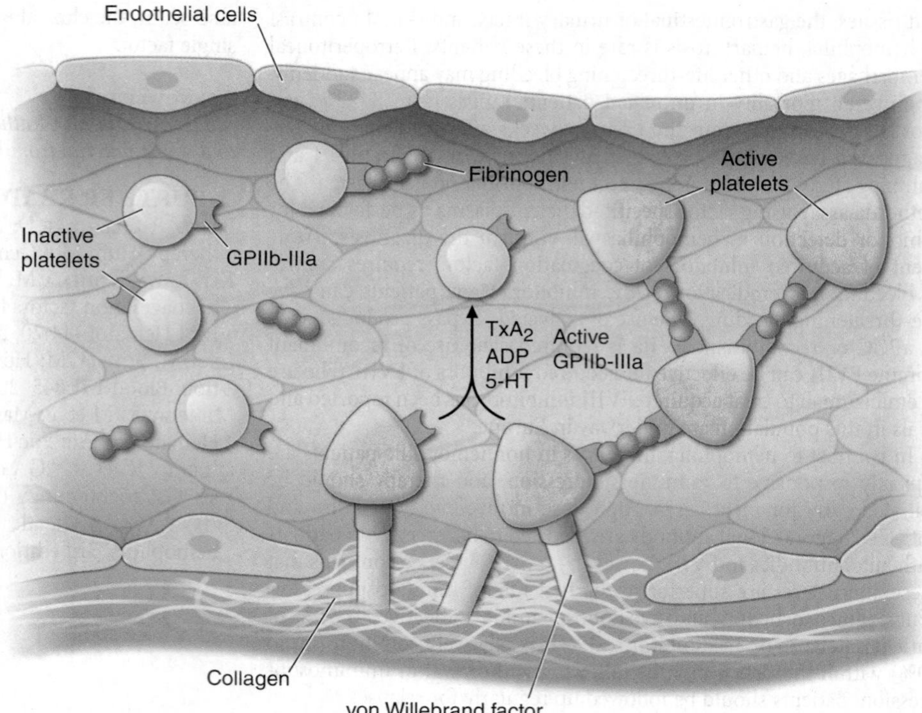

FIGURE 117-1 Platelet activation and thrombosis. Platelets circulate in an inactive form in the vasculature. Damage to the endothelium and/or external stimuli activates platelets that adhere to the exposed subendothelial von Willebrand factor and collagen. This adhesion leads to activation of the platelet, shape change, and the synthesis and release of thromboxane (TxA_2), serotonin (5-HT), and adenosine diphosphate (ADP). Platelet stimuli cause conformational change in the platelet integrin glycoprotein (GP) IIb/IIIa receptor, leading to the high-affinity binding of fibrinogen and the formation of a stable platelet thrombus.

■ ARTERIAL THROMBOSIS AND VASCULAR DISEASE

Arterial thrombosis is a major cause of morbidity and mortality both in the United States and, increasingly, worldwide. Although the rates have declined in the United States, the overall burden remains high. Overall, in 2020, heart disease was estimated to cause about 1 of every 4 deaths in the United States. In addition to the 605,000 Americans who will have a new coronary event annually, an additional 200,000 myocardial infarctions occur in those with previous heart attacks. Although the rate of strokes has fallen, each year about 795,000 people experience a new or recurrent ischemic stroke. In 2018, about 1 in 6 deaths from cardiovascular disease were due to stroke in the United States.

■ THE PLATELET

Many processes in platelets have parallels with other cell types, such as the presence of specific receptors and signaling pathways; however, unlike most cells, platelets lack a nucleus and are unable to adapt to changing biologic settings by altered gene transcription. Platelets sustain limited protein synthetic capacity from megakaryocyte-derived and intracellularly transported messenger RNA (mRNA) and microRNA (miRNA). Most of the molecules needed to respond to various stimuli, however, are maintained in storage granules and membrane compartments.

Platelets are disc-shaped, very small, anucleate cells (1–5 μm in diameter) that circulate in the blood at concentrations of 200–400,000/μL, with an average life span of 7–10 days. Platelets are derived from megakaryocytes, polyploidal hematopoietic cells found in the bone marrow. The primary regulator of platelet formation is thrombopoietin (TPO). The precise mechanism by which megakaryocytes produce and release fully formed platelets is unclear, but the process likely involves formation of proplatelets, pseudopod-like structures generated by the evagination of the cytoplasm from which platelets bud. After release into the circulation, (young, large) platelets may continue to divide. Platelet granules are synthesized in megakaryocytes before thrombopoiesis and contain an array of prothrombotic, proinflammatory, and antimicrobial mediators. The two major types of platelet granules, alpha and dense, are distinguished by their size, abundance, and content. Alpha-granules contain soluble coagulation proteins, adhesion molecules, growth factors, integrins, cytokines, and inflammatory modulators. Platelet dense-granules are smaller than alpha-granules and less abundant. Whereas alpha-granules contain proteins that may be more important in the inflammatory response, dense-granules contain high concentrations of small molecules, including adenosine diphosphate (ADP) and serotonin, that influence platelet aggregation and other related vascular processes, such as vasomotor tone.

Platelet Adhesion (See Fig. 117-1) The formation of a thrombus is initiated by the adherence of platelets to the damaged vessel wall. Damage exposes subendothelial components responsible for triggering platelet reactivity, including collagen, von Willebrand factor, fibronectin, and other adhesive proteins, such as vitronectin and thrombospondin. The hemostatic response may vary, depending on the extent of damage, the specific proteins exposed, and flow conditions. Certain proteins are expressed on the platelet surface that subsequently regulate collagen-induced platelet adhesion, particularly under flow conditions, and include glycoprotein (GP) IV, GPVI, and the integrin $\alpha_2\beta_1$. The platelet GPIb-IX-V complex adhesive receptor is central both to platelet adhesion and to the initiation of platelet activation. Damage to the blood vessel wall exposes subendothelial von Willebrand factor and collagen to the circulating blood. The GPIb-IX-V complex binds to the exposed von Willebrand factor, causing platelets to adhere (Fig. 117-1). In addition, the engagement of the GPIb-IX-V complex with ligand induces signaling pathways that lead to platelet activation. von Willebrand factor–bound GPIb-IX-V promotes a calcium-dependent conformational change in the GPIIb/IIIa receptor, transforming it from an inactive low-affinity state to an active high-affinity receptor for fibrinogen.

Platelet Activation The activation of platelets is controlled by a variety of surface receptors that regulate various functions in the activation process. Platelet receptors control many distinct processes and are stimulated by a wide variety of agonists and adhesive proteins that result in variable degrees of activation. In general terms, the stimulation of platelet receptors triggers two specific processes: (1) activation of internal signaling pathways that lead to further platelet activation and granule release, and (2) the capacity of the platelet to bind to other adhesive proteins/platelets. Both of these processes contribute to the formation of a thrombus. Stimulation of nonthrombotic receptors results in platelet adhesion or interaction with other vascular cells, including endothelial cells, neutrophils, and mononuclear cells.

Many families and subfamilies of receptors are found on platelets that regulate a variety of platelet functions. These include the seven transmembrane receptor family, which is the main agonist-stimulated receptor family. Several seven transmembrane receptors are found on platelets, including the ADP receptors, prostaglandin receptors, lipid receptors, and chemokine receptors. Receptors for thrombin comprise the major seven transmembrane receptors found on platelets. Among this last group, the first identified was the protease activation receptor 1 (PAR1). The PAR class of receptors has a distinct mechanism of activation that involves specific cleavage of the N-terminus by thrombin, which, in turn, acts as a ligand for the receptor. Other PAR receptors are present on platelets, including PAR2 (not activated by thrombin) and PAR4. Adenosine receptors are responsible for transduction of ADP-induced signaling events, which are initiated by the binding of ADP to purinergic receptors on the platelet surface. There are several distinct ADP receptors, classified as $P2X_1$, $P2Y_1$, and $P2Y_{12}$. The activation of both the $P2Y_{12}$ and $P2Y_1$ receptors is essential for ADP-induced platelet aggregation. The thienopyridine derivatives, clopidogrel and prasugrel, are clinically used inhibitors of ADP-induced platelet aggregation.

Platelet Aggregation Activation of platelets results in a rapid series of signal transduction events, including tyrosine kinase, serine/threonine kinase, and lipid kinase activation. In unstimulated platelets, the major platelet integrin GPIIb/IIIa is maintained in an inactive conformation and functions as a low-affinity adhesion receptor for fibrinogen. This integrin is unique as it is only expressed on platelets. After stimulation, the interaction between fibrinogen and GPIIb/IIIa forms intercellular connections between platelets, leading to the formation of a platelet aggregate (Fig. 117-1). A calcium-sensitive conformational change in the extracellular domain of GPIIb/IIIa enables the high-affinity binding of soluble plasma fibrinogen as a result of a complex network of inside-out signaling events. The GPIIb/IIIa receptor serves as a bidirectional conduit with GPIIb/IIIa-mediated signaling (outside-in) occurring immediately after the binding of fibrinogen. This leads to additional intracellular signaling that further stabilizes the platelet aggregate and transforms platelet aggregation from a reversible to an irreversible process (inside-out).

THE ROLE OF PLATELETS AND THROMBOSIS IN INFLAMMATION

Inflammation plays an important role during the acute thrombotic phase of acute coronary and other vascular occlusive syndromes. In the setting of acute upper respiratory infections, people are at higher risk of myocardial infarction and thrombotic stroke. Patients with acute coronary syndromes have not only increased interactions between platelets (homotypic aggregates), but also increased interactions between platelets and leukocytes (heterotypic aggregates) detectable in circulating blood. These latter aggregates form when platelets are activated, often directly by pathogens, and adhere to circulating leukocytes as part of their contribution to the immune process. Platelets bind via P-selectin (CD62P) expressed on the surface of activated platelets to the leukocyte receptor, P-selectin glycoprotein ligand 1 (PSGL-1). This association leads to increased expression of CD11b/CD18 (Mac-1) on leukocytes, which amplifies immunity but may also support further interactions with platelets partially via bivalent fibrinogen linking this integrin with its platelet surface counterpart, GPIIb/IIIa. Platelet surface P-selectin also induces the expression of tissue factor on monocytes, which promotes fibrin formation.

In addition to platelet–monocyte aggregates, the immunomodulator, soluble CD40 ligand (CD40L or CD154), also reflects a link between thrombosis and inflammation. The CD40 ligand is a trimeric transmembrane protein of the tumor necrosis factor family and, with its receptor CD40, is an important contributor to the inflammatory process leading both to thrombosis and atherosclerosis. While many immunologic and vascular cells have been found to express CD40 and/or CD40 ligand, in platelets, CD40 ligand is rapidly translocated to the surface after stimulation and is upregulated in the newly formed thrombus. The surface-expressed CD40 ligand is cleaved from the platelet to generate a soluble fragment (soluble CD40 ligand).

Links have also been established among platelets, infection, immunity, and inflammation. Bacterial and viral infections are associated with a transient increase in the risk of acute thrombotic events, such as acute myocardial infarction and stroke. In addition, platelets contribute significantly to the pathophysiology and high mortality rates of sepsis. The expression, functionality, and signaling pathways of Toll-like receptors (TLRs) have been established in platelets. Stimulation of platelet TLR2, TLR3, and TLR4 directly and indirectly activates the platelet's thrombotic and inflammatory responses, and live bacteria induce a proinflammatory response in platelets in a TLR2-dependent manner, suggesting a mechanism by which specific bacteria and bacterial components can directly activate platelet-dependent thrombosis. Additionally, viruses, such as SARS-CoV-2, HIV, hepatitis C virus, and Dengue, are also known to cause elevated levels of thrombosis, and recently, platelets have been shown to regulate immune responses to viruses via receptors TLR7 and TLR8.

Risk Factors for Arterial Thrombosis In addition to immune burden, various factors increase the risk of developing arterial thrombosis. Classically, the cardiovascular-dependent risk factors implicated in thrombosis have been hypertension, high levels of low-density lipoprotein cholesterol, and smoking. However, diabetes, pregnancy, age, and chemotherapeutic agents may also contribute to arterial thrombosis. Stillbirth and loss of multiple pregnancies may increase the risk of ischemic stroke and myocardial infarction as does hormonal replacement therapy. Systemic lupus erythematosus and rheumatoid arthritis are now well-recognized risks for thrombosis, and the former, in particular, may contribute in the pediatric population. The antiphospholipid syndrome is also another widely recognized autoimmune prothrombotic risk for arterial (and venous) thrombosis.

GENETICS OF ARTERIAL THROMBOSIS

Some studies have associated arterial thrombosis with genetic variants (**Table 117-1*A***); however, the associations have been weak and not confirmed in larger series. Platelet count and mean platelet volume have been studied by genome-wide association studies (GWAS), and this approach identified signals located to noncoding regions. Of 15 quantitative trait loci associated with mean platelet volume and platelet count, one located at 12q24 is also a risk locus for coronary artery disease.

In the area of genetic variability and platelet function, studies have primarily dealt with pharmacogenetics, the field of pharmacology dealing with the interindividual variability in drug response based on genetic determinants (**Table 117-2**). This focus has been driven by the wide variability among individuals in terms of response to antithrombotic drugs and the lack of a common explanation for this variance. The best described is the issue of "aspirin resistance," although heterogeneity for other antithrombotics (e.g., clopidogrel) has also been extensively examined. Primarily, platelet-dependent genetic determinants have been defined at the level of (1) drug effect, (2) drug compliance, and (3) drug metabolism. Many candidate platelet genes have been studied for their interaction with antiplatelet and antithrombotic agents.

Many patients have an inadequate response to the inhibitory effects of aspirin. Heritable factors contribute to the variability; however, ex vivo tests of residual platelet responsiveness after aspirin administration have not provided firm evidence for a pharmacogenetic interaction between aspirin and *COX1* or other relevant platelet receptors. As such, currently, there is no clinical indication for genotyping to optimize aspirin's antiplatelet efficiency. For the platelet P2Y12 receptor inhibitor clopidogrel, additional data suggest that genetics may affect the drug's responsiveness and utility. The responsible genetic variant appears not to be the expected P2Y12 receptor but an enzyme responsible for drug metabolism. Clopidogrel is a prodrug, and liver metabolism by specific

TABLE 117-1 Heritable Causes of Arterial and Venous Thrombosis

A. Arterial Thrombosis
Platelet Receptors
β3 and α2 integrins
P_1 A2 polymorphism
Fc(gamma)RIIA
GPIV T13254C polymorphism
GPIb
Thrombin receptor PAR1-5061 → D
Redox Enzymes
Plasma glutathione peroxidase, GPx3, promoter haplotype H2
H2 promoter haplotype
Endothelial nitric oxide synthase
−786T/C, −922A/G, −1468T/A
Paraoxonase
−107T allele, 192R allele
Homocysteine
Cystathionine β-synthase 833T → C
5,10-Methylene tetrahydrofolate reductase (MTHFR) 677C → T
B. Venous Thrombosis
Procoagulant Proteins
Fibrinogen
−455G/A, −854G/A
Prothrombin (20210G → A)
Protein C Anticoagulant Pathway
Factor V Leiden: 1691G → A (Arg506Gln)
Thrombomodulin 1481C → T (Ala455Val)
Fibrinolytic Proteins with Known Polymorphisms
Tissue plasminogen activator (tPA)
7351C/T, 20 099T/C in exon 6, 27 445T/A in intron 10
Plasminogen activator inhibitor (PAI-1)
4G/5G insertion/deletion polymorphism at position −675
Homocysteine
Cystathionine β-synthase 833T → C
5,10-MTHFR 677C → T

cytochrome P450 enzymes is required for activation. The genes encoding the CYP-dependent oxidative steps are polymorphic, and carriers of specific alleles of the CYP2C19 and CYP3A4 loci have increased platelet aggregability. Increased platelet activity has also been specifically associated with the CYP2C19*2 allele, which causes loss of platelet function in select patients. Because these are common genetic variants, this observation has been shown to be clinically relevant in large studies. In summary, although the loss-of-function polymorphism in CYP2C19 is the strongest individual variable affecting pharmacokinetics and antiplatelet response to clopidogrel, it only accounts for 5–12% of the variability in ADP-induced platelet aggregation on clopidogrel. In addition, genetic variables do not appear to contribute significantly to the clinical outcomes of patients treated with the P2Y12 receptor antagonists prasugrel or ticagrelor.

TABLE 117-2 Genetic Variation and Pharmacogenetic Responses to Platelet Inhibitors

POTENTIAL GENE ALTERED	TARGET THERAPEUTIC CLASS	SPECIFIC DRUG
P2Y1 and *P2Y12 CYP2C19, CYP3A4, CYP3A5*	ADP receptor inhibitors	Clopidogrel, prasugrel
COX1, COX2	Cyclooxygenase inhibitors	Aspirin
PIA1/A2	Receptor inhibitors	Abciximab, eptifibatide, tirofiban
INTB3, GPIbA	Glycoprotein IIb-IIIa receptor inhibitors	

VENOUS THROMBOSIS

OVERVIEW OF VENOUS THROMBOSIS

Coagulation is the process by which thrombin is activated and soluble plasma fibrinogen is converted into insoluble fibrin. These steps account for both normal hemostasis and the pathophysiologic processes influencing the development of venous thrombosis. The primary forms of venous thrombosis are deep-vein thrombosis (DVT) in the extremities and the subsequent embolization to the lungs (pulmonary embolism [PE]), referred to together as venous thromboembolic disease (VTE). Although the majority of venous thromboembolic events occur as PE or DVT of the lower extremities, up to 10% of events may occur in other vascular locations. Venous thrombosis occurs due to heritable causes (**Table 117-1*B***) and acquired causes (**Table 117-3**).

DEEP-VENOUS THROMBOSIS AND PULMONARY EMBOLISM

It is estimated that DVT or PE occurs in ~1–2 individuals per 1000 each year, resulting in 300,000–600,000 new cases of VTE each year in the United States. Approximately, 60,000–80,000 deaths are attributed to DVT or PE annually. Of new cases, up to 30% of patients die within 30 days and one-fifth suffer sudden death due to PE; 30% go on to develop recurrent VTE within 10 years. Data from the Atherosclerosis Risk in Communities (ARIC) study reported a 9% 28-day fatality rate from DVT and a 15% fatality rate from PE. PE in the setting of cancer has a 25% fatality rate. The mean incidence of first DVT in the general population is 5 per 10,000 person-years; the incidence is similar in males and females when adjusting for factors related to reproduction and birth control and increases dramatically with age from 2–3 per 10,000 person-years at 30–49 years of age to 20 per 10,000 person-years at 70–79 years of age.

OVERVIEW OF THE COAGULATION CASCADE AND ITS ROLE IN VENOUS THROMBOSIS

Coagulation is defined as the formation of fibrin by a series of linked enzymatic reactions in which each reaction product converts the subsequent inactive zymogen into an active serine protease (**Fig. 117-2**). This coordinated sequence is called the coagulation cascade and is a key mechanism for regulating hemostasis. Central to the function of the coagulation cascade is the principle of amplification: due to a series of linked enzymatic reactions, a small stimulus can lead to much greater quantities of fibrin, the end product that prevents hemorrhage at the site of vascular injury. In addition to the known risk factors relevant to hypercoagulopathy, stasis, and vascular dysfunction, newer areas of research have identified contributions from procoagulant microparticles, inflammatory cells, microvesicles, and fibrin structure.

The coagulation cascade is primarily initiated by vascular injury exposing tissue factor to blood components (Fig. 117-2). Tissue factor may also be found in bloodborne cell-derived microparticles and, under pathophysiologic conditions, in leukocytes or platelets. Plasma

TABLE 117-3 Acquired Causes of Venous Thrombosis

Surgery
Neurosurgery
Major abdominal surgery
Malignancy
Antiphospholipid syndrome
Other
Trauma
Pregnancy
Long-distance travel
Obesity
Oral contraceptives/hormone replacement
Myeloproliferative disorders
Polycythemia vera

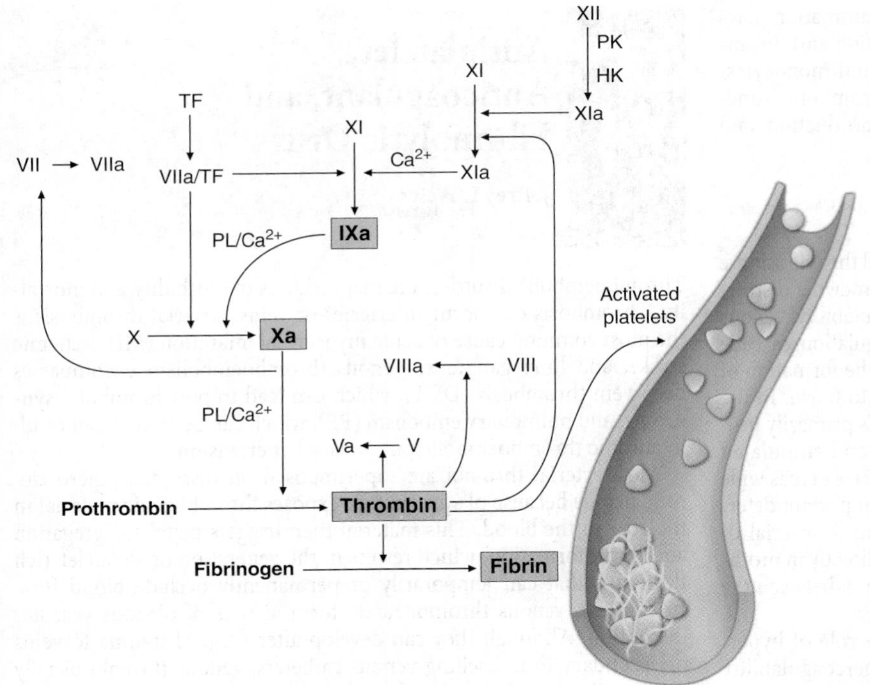

FIGURE 117-2 Summary of the coagulation pathways. Specific coagulation factors ("a" indicates activated form) are responsible for the conversion of soluble plasma fibrinogen into insoluble fibrin. This process occurs via a series of linked reactions in which the enzymatically active product subsequently converts the downstream inactive protein into an active serine protease. In addition, the activation of thrombin leads to stimulation of platelets. HK, high-molecular-weight kininogen; PK, prekallikrein; TF, tissue factor.

factor VII (FVII) is the ligand for and is activated (FVIIa) by binding to tissue factor exposed at the site of vessel damage. The binding of FVII/VIIa to tissue factor activates the downstream conversion of factor X (FX) to active FX (FXa). In an alternative reaction, the FVII/FVIIa–tissue factor complex initially converts FIX to FIXa, which then activates FX in conjunction with its cofactor factor VIII (FVIIIa). Factor Xa with its cofactor FVa converts prothrombin to thrombin, which then converts soluble plasma fibrinogen to insoluble fibrin, leading to clot or thrombus formation. Thrombin also activates FXIII to FXIIIa, a transglutaminase that covalently cross-links and stabilizes the fibrin clot. Formation of thrombi is affected by mechanisms governing fibrin structure and stability, including specific fibrinogen variants and how they alter fibrin formation, strength, and structure.

Several antithrombotic factors also regulate coagulation; these include antithrombin, tissue factor pathway inhibitor (TFPI), heparin cofactor II, and protein C/protein S. Under normal conditions, these factors limit the production of thrombin to prevent the perpetuation of coagulation and thrombus formation. Typically, after the clot has caused occlusion at the damaged site and begins to expand toward adjacent uninjured vessel segments, the anticoagulant reactions governed by the normal endothelium become pivotal in limiting the extent of this hemostatically protective clot.

RISK FACTORS FOR VENOUS THROMBOSIS

An array of different factors contributes to the risk of VTE, and it is notable that women and men of all ages, races, and ethnicities are at risk for VTE. The risk factors for venous thrombosis are primarily related to hypercoagulability, which can be genetic (Table 117-1) or acquired, or due to immobilization and venous stasis. Independent predictors for recurrence include increasing age, obesity, malignant neoplasm, and acute extremity paresis. It is estimated that 5–8% of the U.S. population has a genetic risk factor known to predispose to venous thrombosis. Often, multiple risk factors are present in a single individual. Significant risk is incurred by major orthopedic, abdominal, or neurologic surgeries. Cancer patients have an approximately fourfold increased risk of VTE as compared with the general population, and cancer patients with VTE have reduced survival. Hospitalized patients have a greatly increased risk of venous thrombosis with risk factors (increased age, male, ethnicity) and comorbid conditions, including infection, renal disease, and weight loss. Community- or hospital-acquired infection is also associated with increased risk of VTE. Supportive of this, nearly 20% of hospitalized COVID-19 patients are noted to have coagulation abnormalities as well as increased PE, DVT, and peripheral thrombotic risk. Moderate risk is promoted by prolonged bedrest, certain types of cancer, pregnancy, hormone replacement therapy or oral contraceptive use, and other sedentary conditions such as long-distance plane travel. It has been reported that the risk of developing a venous thromboembolic event doubles after air travel lasting 4 h, although the absolute risk remains low (1 in 6000). The relative risk of VTE among pregnant or postpartum women is 4.3, and the overall incidence (absolute risk) is 199.7 per 100,000 woman-years.

GENETICS OF VENOUS THROMBOSIS

(See Table 117-2) Less common causes of venous thrombosis are those due to genetic variants. These abnormalities include loss-of-function mutations of endogenous anticoagulants as well as gain-of-function mutations of procoagulant proteins. Heterozygous antithrombin deficiency and homozygosity of the factor V Leiden mutation significantly increase the risk of venous thrombosis. While homozygous protein C or protein S deficiencies are rare and may lead to fatal purpura fulminans, heterozygous deficiencies are associated with a moderate risk of thrombosis. Activated protein C impairs coagulation by proteolytic degradation of FVa. Patients resistant to the activity of activated protein C may have a point mutation in the FV gene located on chromosome 1, a mutant denoted factor V Leiden. Mildly increased risk has been attributed to elevated levels of procoagulant factors, as well as low levels of tissue factor pathway inhibitor. Polymorphisms of methylene tetrahydrofolate reductase as well as hyperhomocysteinemia have been shown to be independent risk factors for venous thrombosis, as well as arterial vascular disease; however, many of the initial descriptions of genetic variants and their associations with thromboembolism are being questioned in larger, more contemporary studies.

FIBRINOLYSIS AND THROMBOSIS

Specific abnormalities in the fibrinolytic system have been associated with enhanced thrombosis. Factors such as elevated levels of tissue plasminogen activator (tPA) and plasminogen activator inhibitor type 1 (PAI-1) have been associated with decreased fibrinolytic activity and an increased risk of arterial thrombotic disease. Specific genetic variants have been associated with decreased fibrinolytic activity, including the 4G/5G insertion/deletion polymorphism in the *PAI-1* gene. Additionally, the 311-bp Alu insertion/deletion in tPA's intron 8 has been associated with enhanced thrombosis; however, genetic abnormalities have not been associated consistently with altered function or tPA levels, raising questions about the relevant pathophysiologic mechanism. Thrombin-activatable fibrinolysis inhibitor (TAFI) is a carboxypeptidase that regulates fibrinolysis; elevated plasma TAFI levels have been associated with an increased risk of both DVT and cardiovascular disease.

The metabolic syndrome also is accompanied by altered fibrinolytic activity. This syndrome, which comprises abdominal fat (central obesity), altered glucose and insulin metabolism, dyslipidemia, and hypertension, has been associated with atherothrombosis. The mechanism for enhanced thrombosis appears to be due both to altered platelet function and to a procoagulant and hypofibrinolytic state. One of the most frequently documented prothrombotic abnormalities reported in this syndrome is an increase in plasma levels of PAI-1.

In addition to contributing to platelet function, inflammation plays a role in both coagulation-dependent thrombus formation and thrombus resolution. Both polymorphonuclear neutrophils and monocytes/macrophages contribute to multiple overlapping thrombotic functions, including fibrinolysis, chemokine and cytokine production, and phagocytosis.

THE DISTINCTION BETWEEN ARTERIAL AND VENOUS THROMBOSIS

Although there is overlap, venous thrombosis and arterial thrombosis are initiated differently, and clot formation progresses by somewhat distinct pathways. In the setting of stasis or states of hypercoagulability, venous thrombosis is activated with the initiation of the coagulation cascade primarily due to exposure of tissue factor; this leads to the formation of thrombin and the subsequent conversion of fibrinogen to fibrin. In the artery, thrombin formation also occurs, but thrombosis is primarily promoted by the adhesion of platelets to an injured vessel and stimulated by exposed extracellular matrix (Figs. 117-1 and 117-2). There is wide variation in individual responses to vascular injury, an important determinant of which is the predisposition an individual has to arterial or venous thrombosis. This concept has been supported indirectly in prothrombotic animal models in which there is poor correlation between the propensity to develop venous versus arterial thrombosis.

Despite considerable progress in understanding the role of hypercoagulable states in VTE, the contribution of hypercoagulability to arterial vascular disease is much less well understood. Although specific thrombophilic conditions, such as factor V Leiden and the prothrombin G20210A mutation, are risk factors for DVT, pulmonary embolism, and other venous thromboembolic events, their contribution to arterial thrombosis is less well defined. In fact, to the contrary, many of these thrombophilic factors have not been found to be clinically important risk factors for arterial thrombotic events, such as acute coronary syndromes.

Clinically, although the pathophysiology is distinct, arterial and venous thrombosis do share common risk factors, including age, obesity, cigarette smoking, diabetes mellitus, arterial hypertension, hyperlipidemia, and metabolic syndrome. Select genetic variants, including those of the glutathione peroxidase-3 (GPx3) gene, have also been associated with arterial and venous thrombo-occlusive disease. Importantly, arterial and venous thrombosis may both be triggered by pathophysiologic stimuli responsible for activating inflammatory and oxidative pathways.

The diagnosis and treatment of ischemic heart disease are discussed in **Chap. 273**. Stroke diagnosis and management are discussed in **Chap. 307**. The diagnosis and management of DVT and PE are discussed in **Chap. 279**.

FURTHER READING

Ackermann M et al: Pulmonary vascular endothelialitis, thrombosis, and angiogenesis in Covid-19. N Engl J Med 383:120, 2020.

Baron TH et al: Management of antithrombotic therapy in patients undergoing invasive procedures. N Engl J Med 368:2113, 2013.

Becattini C, Aegnelli G: Acute treatment of venous thromboembolism. Blood 135:305, 2020.

Engelmann B, Massberg S: Thrombosis as an intravascular effector of innate immunity. Nat Rev Immunol 13:34, 2013.

Furie B, Furie BC: Mechanisms of thrombus formation. N Engl J Med 359:938, 2008.

Koupenova M et al: Thrombosis and platelets: An update. Eur Heart J 38:785, 2017.

Mackman N: New insights into the mechanisms of venous thrombosis. J Clin Invest 122:2331, 2012.

Mozaffarian D et al: Heart disease and stroke statistics—A report from the American Heart Association 2016 update. Circulation 133:447, 2016.

Tapson VF: Acute pulmonary embolism. N Engl J Med 358:1037, 2008.

Tichelaar YI et al: Infections and inflammatory diseases as risk factors for venous thrombosis. A systematic review. Thromb Haemost 107:827, 2012.

118 Antiplatelet, Anticoagulant, and Fibrinolytic Drugs

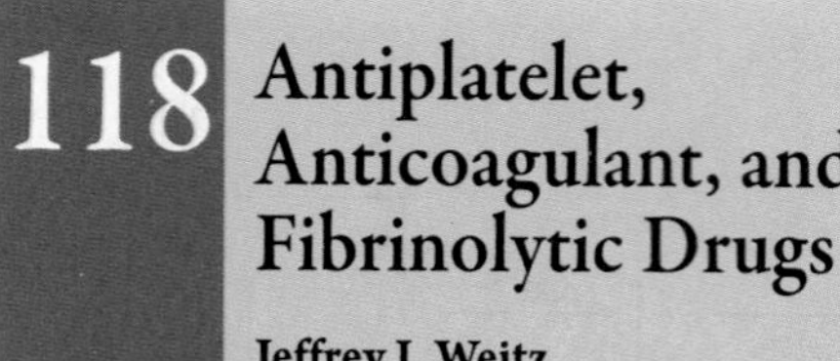

Jeffrey I. Weitz

Thromboembolic disorders are major causes of morbidity and mortality. Thrombosis can occur in arteries or veins. Arterial thrombosis is the most common cause of acute myocardial infarction (MI), ischemic stroke, and limb gangrene. Venous thromboembolism encompasses deep vein thrombosis (DVT), which can lead to postthrombotic syndrome, and pulmonary embolism (PE), which can be fatal or can result in chronic thromboembolic pulmonary hypertension.

Most arterial thrombi are superimposed on disrupted atherosclerotic plaque because plaque rupture exposes thrombogenic material in the core to the blood. This material then triggers platelet aggregation and fibrin formation, which results in the generation of a platelet-rich thrombus that can temporarily or permanently occlude blood flow. In contrast, venous thrombi rarely form at sites of obvious vascular disruption. Although they can develop after surgical trauma to veins or secondary to indwelling venous catheters, venous thrombi usually originate in the valve cusps of the deep veins of the calf or in the muscular sinuses. Sluggish blood flow reduces the oxygen supply to the avascular valve cusps. Endothelial cells lining these valve cusps become activated and express adhesion molecules on their surface. Tissue factor–bearing leukocytes and microvesicles adhere to these activated cells and induce coagulation. DNA extruded from neutrophils forms neutrophil extracellular traps (NETs) that provide a scaffold that binds platelets and promotes their activation and aggregation and activate factor XII. Local thrombus formation is exacerbated by reduced clearance of activated clotting factors because of impaired blood flow. If the thrombi extend from the calf veins into the popliteal and more proximal veins of the leg, thrombus fragments can dislodge, travel to the lungs, and produce a PE.

Arterial and venous thrombi are composed of platelets, fibrin, and trapped red blood cells, but the proportions differ. Arterial thrombi are rich in platelets because of the high shear in the injured arteries. In contrast, venous thrombi, which form under low shear conditions, contain relatively few platelets and are predominantly composed of fibrin and trapped red cells. Because of the predominance of platelets, arterial thrombi appear white, whereas venous thrombi are red in color, reflecting the trapped red cells.

Antithrombotic drugs are used for prevention and treatment of thrombosis. Targeting the components of thrombi, these agents include (1) antiplatelet drugs, (2) anticoagulants, and (3) fibrinolytic agents (**Fig. 118-1**). With the predominance of platelets in arterial thrombi, strategies to attenuate arterial thrombosis focus mainly on antiplatelet agents, although, in the acute setting, they may include anticoagulants and fibrinolytic agents. The addition of low-dose rivaroxaban, an oral factor Xa inhibitor, to dual-antiplatelet therapy reduces recurrent ischemic events and stent thrombosis in patients with acute coronary syndrome, whereas its addition to aspirin reduces the risk of major adverse coronary and limb events in patients with stable coronary or peripheral artery disease. These findings highlight the utility of combining low

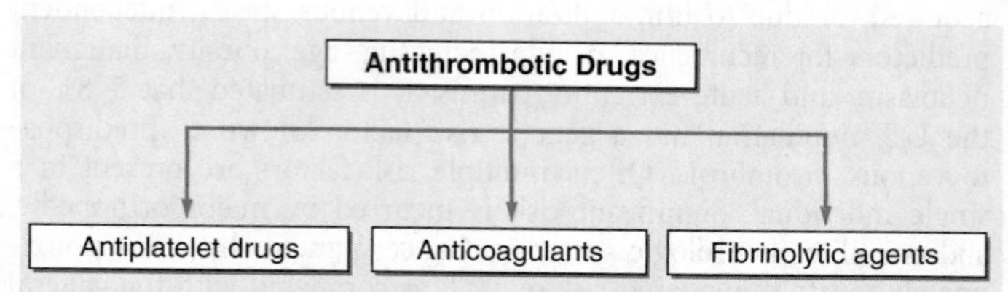

FIGURE 118-1 Classification of antithrombotic drugs.

dose anticoagulants with antiplatelet agents for secondary prevention in patients at risk for recurrent atherothrombotic events.

Anticoagulants are the mainstay of prevention and treatment of venous thromboembolism because fibrin is the predominant component of venous thrombi. Antiplatelet drugs are less effective than anticoagulants in this setting because of the limited platelet content of venous thrombi. Fibrinolytic therapy is used in selected patients with venous thromboembolism. For example, patients with massive PE can benefit from systemic or catheter-directed fibrinolytic therapy. Pharmaco-mechanical therapy also is used to restore blood flow in patients with extensive DVT involving the iliac and/or femoral veins.

ANTIPLATELET DRUGS

■ ROLE OF PLATELETS IN ARTERIAL THROMBOSIS

In healthy vasculature, circulating platelets are maintained in an inactive state by nitric oxide (NO) and prostacyclin released by endothelial cells lining the blood vessels. In addition, endothelial cells also express CD39 on their surface, a membrane-associated ecto-adenosine diphosphatase (ADPase) that degrades ADP released from activated platelets. When the vessel wall is damaged, release of these substances is impaired and subendothelial matrix is exposed. Platelets adhere to exposed collagen via $\alpha_2\beta_1$ and glycoprotein (Gp) V1 and to von Willebrand factor (VWF) via Gp Ibα and Gp IIb/IIIa ($\alpha_{IIb}\beta_3$)—receptors that are constitutively expressed on the platelet surface. Adherent platelets undergo a change in shape, secrete ADP from their dense granules, and synthesize and release thromboxane A_2. Released ADP and thromboxane A_2, which are platelet agonists, activate ambient platelets and recruit them to the site of vascular injury **(Fig. 118-2)**.

Disruption of the vessel wall also exposes tissue factor–expressing cells to the blood. Tissue factor binds factor VIIa and initiates coagulation. Activated platelets potentiate coagulation by providing a surface that binds clotting factors and supports the assembly of activation complexes that enhance thrombin generation. In addition to converting fibrinogen to fibrin, thrombin serves as a potent platelet agonist and recruits more platelets to the site of vascular injury. Thrombin also amplifies its own generation by feedback activation of factors V, VIII, and XI and solidifies the fibrin network by activating factor XIII, which then cross-links the fibrin strands.

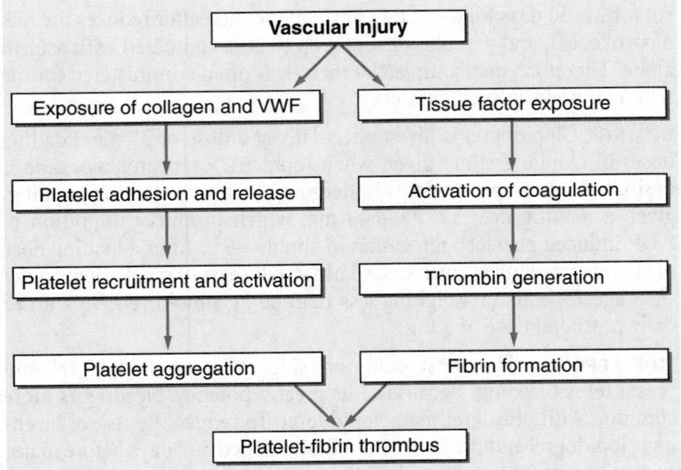

FIGURE 118-2 Coordinated role of platelets and the coagulation system in thrombogenesis. Vascular injury simultaneously triggers platelet activation and aggregation and activation of the coagulation system. Platelet activation is initiated by exposure of subendothelial collagen and von Willebrand factor (VWF), onto which platelets adhere. Adherent platelets become activated and release ADP and thromboxane A_2, platelet agonists that activate ambient platelets and recruit them to the site of injury. When platelets are activated, glycoprotein IIb/IIIa on their surface undergoes a conformational change that enables it to ligate fibrinogen and/or VWF and mediate platelet aggregation. Coagulation is triggered by tissue factor exposed at the site of injury. Tissue factor triggers thrombin generation. As a potent platelet agonist, thrombin amplifies platelet recruitment to the site of injury. Thrombin also converts fibrinogen to fibrin, and the fibrin strands then weave the platelet aggregates together to form a platelet/fibrin thrombus.

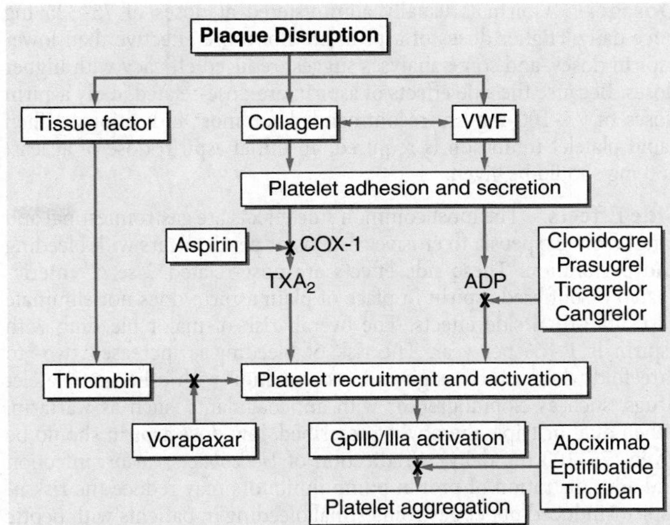

FIGURE 118-3 Site of action of antiplatelet drugs. Aspirin inhibits thromboxane A_2 (TXA_2) synthesis by irreversibly acetylating cyclooxygenase-1 (COX-1). Reduced TXA_2 release attenuates platelet activation and recruitment to the site of vascular injury. Clopidogrel and prasugrel irreversibly block $P2Y_{12}$, a key ADP receptor on the platelet surface; cangrelor and ticagrelor are reversible inhibitors of $P2Y_{12}$. Abciximab, eptifibatide, and tirofiban inhibit the final common pathway of platelet aggregation by blocking fibrinogen and von Willebrand factor binding to activated glycoprotein (Gp) IIb/IIIa. Vorapaxar inhibits thrombin-mediated platelet activation by targeting protease-activated receptor-1 (PAR-1), the major thrombin receptor on human platelets.

When platelets are activated, Gp IIb/IIIa, the most abundant receptor on the platelet surface, undergoes a conformational change that enables it to bind fibrinogen and, under high shear conditions, VWF. Divalent fibrinogen or multivalent VWF molecules bridge adjacent platelets together to form platelet aggregates. Fibrin strands, generated through the action of thrombin, then weave these aggregates together to form a platelet/fibrin mesh.

Antiplatelet drugs target various steps in this process. The commonly used drugs include aspirin, ADP receptor inhibitors, which include the thienopyridines (clopidogrel and prasugrel) as well as ticagrelor and cangrelor, dipyridamole, Gp IIb/IIIa antagonists, and vorapaxar.

■ ASPIRIN

The most widely used antiplatelet agent worldwide is aspirin. As a cheap and effective antiplatelet drug, aspirin serves as the foundation of most antiplatelet strategies.

Mechanism of Action Aspirin produces its antithrombotic effect by irreversibly acetylating and inhibiting platelet cyclooxygenase (COX)-1 **(Fig. 118-3)**, a critical enzyme in the biosynthesis of thromboxane A_2. At high doses (~1 g/d), aspirin also inhibits COX-2, an inducible COX isoform found in endothelial cells and inflammatory cells. In endothelial cells, COX-2 initiates the synthesis of prostacyclin, a potent vasodilator and inhibitor of platelet aggregation.

Indications Aspirin is widely used for secondary prevention of cardiovascular events in patients with established coronary artery, cerebral artery, or peripheral artery disease. Compared with placebo in this setting, aspirin produces a 25% reduction in the risk of cardiovascular death, MI, or stroke. Use of aspirin for primary prevention is controversial. Recent studies have questioned whether the benefits of daily aspirin for primary cardiac protection outweigh its associated risks for gastrointestinal and intracerebral hemorrhage. Consequently, aspirin is no longer recommended for primary cardiac prevention unless the baseline cardiovascular risk is at least 1% per year and 10% at 10 years and patients are at low risk for bleeding.

Dosages Aspirin is usually administered at doses of 75–325 mg once daily. Higher doses of aspirin are not more effective than lower aspirin doses, and some analyses suggest reduced efficacy with higher doses. Because the side effects of aspirin are dose-related, daily aspirin doses of 75–100 mg are recommended for most indications. When rapid platelet inhibition is required, an initial aspirin dose of at least 160 mg should be given.

Side Effects The most common side effects are gastrointestinal and range from dyspepsia to erosive gastritis or peptic ulcers with bleeding and perforation. These side effects are dose-related. Use of enteric-coated or buffered aspirin in place of plain aspirin does not eliminate gastrointestinal side effects. The overall risk of major bleeding with aspirin is 1–3% per year. The risk of bleeding is increased two- to threefold when aspirin is given in conjunction with other antiplatelet drugs, such as clopidogrel, or with anticoagulants, such as warfarin. When dual or triple therapy is prescribed, low-dose aspirin should be given (75–100 mg daily). Eradication of *Helicobacter pylori* infection and administration of proton pump inhibitors may reduce the risk of aspirin-induced upper gastrointestinal bleeding in patients with peptic ulcer disease.

Aspirin should not be administered to patients with a history of aspirin allergy characterized by bronchospasm. This problem occurs in ~0.3% of the general population but is more common in those with chronic urticaria or asthma, particularly in individuals with nasal polyps or chronic rhinitis. Hepatic and renal toxicity are observed with aspirin overdose.

Aspirin Resistance Clinical aspirin resistance is defined as the failure of aspirin to protect patients from ischemic vascular events. This is not a helpful definition because it is made after the event occurs. Furthermore, it is not realistic to expect aspirin, which only blocks thromboxane A_2–induced platelet activation, to prevent all vascular events.

Aspirin resistance has also been described biochemically as failure of the drug to produce its expected inhibitory effects on tests of platelet function, such as thromboxane A_2 synthesis or arachidonic acid-induced platelet aggregation. Potential causes of aspirin resistance include poor compliance, reduced absorption, drug-drug interaction with ibuprofen, and overexpression of COX-2. Unfortunately, the tests for aspirin resistance have not been well standardized, and there is little evidence that they identify patients at increased risk of recurrent vascular events, or that resistance can be reversed by giving higher doses of aspirin or by adding other antiplatelet drugs. Until such information is available, testing for aspirin resistance remains a research tool.

ADP RECEPTOR ANTAGONISTS

The ADP receptor antagonists include the thienopyridines (clopidogrel and prasugrel) as well as ticagrelor and cangrelor. All of these drugs target $P2Y_{12}$, the key ADP receptor on platelets.

Thienopyridines • MECHANISM OF ACTION The thienopyridines are structurally related drugs that selectively inhibit ADP-induced platelet aggregation by irreversibly blocking $P2Y_{12}$ (Fig. 118-3). Clopidogrel and prasugrel are prodrugs that require metabolic activation by the hepatic cytochrome P450 (CYP) enzyme system. Prasugrel is about 10-fold more potent than clopidogrel and has a more rapid onset of action because of better absorption and more streamlined metabolic activation.

INDICATIONS When compared with aspirin in patients with recent ischemic stroke, recent MI, or a history of peripheral arterial disease, clopidogrel reduced the risk of cardiovascular death, MI, and stroke by 8.7%. Therefore, clopidogrel is more effective than aspirin but is also more expensive. Clopidogrel and aspirin are often combined to capitalize on their capacity to block complementary pathways of platelet activation. For example, the combination of aspirin plus clopidogrel is recommended for at least 4 weeks after implantation of a bare metal stent in a coronary artery and for at least a year in those with a drug-eluting stent. Concerns about late in-stent thrombosis with drug-eluting stents have led some experts to recommend long-term use of clopidogrel plus aspirin for the latter indication.

The combination of clopidogrel and aspirin is also effective in patients with unstable angina. Thus, in 12,562 such patients, the risk of cardiovascular death, MI, or stroke was 9.3% in those randomized to the combination of clopidogrel and aspirin and 11.4% in those given aspirin alone. This 20% relative risk reduction with combination therapy was highly statistically significant. However, combining clopidogrel with aspirin increases the risk of major bleeding to about 2% per year. This bleeding risk persists even if the daily dose of aspirin is ≤100 mg. Therefore, the combination of clopidogrel and aspirin should only be used when there is a clear benefit. For example, this combination has not proven to be superior to clopidogrel alone in patients with acute ischemic stroke or to aspirin alone for primary prevention in those at risk for cardiovascular events.

Prasugrel was compared with clopidogrel in 13,608 patients with acute coronary syndromes who were scheduled to undergo percutaneous coronary intervention. The incidence of the primary efficacy endpoint, a composite of cardiovascular death, MI, or stroke, was significantly lower with prasugrel than with clopidogrel (9.9% and 12.1%, respectively), mainly reflecting a reduction in the incidence of nonfatal MI. The incidence of stent thrombosis also was significantly lower with prasugrel (1.1% and 2.4%, respectively). However, these advantages were at the expense of significantly higher rates of fatal bleeding (0.4% and 0.1%, respectively) and life-threatening bleeding (1.4% and 0.9%, respectively) with prasugrel. Because patients older than age 75 years and those with a history of prior stroke or transient ischemic attack have a particularly high risk of bleeding, prasugrel should generally be avoided in older patients, and the drug is contraindicated in those with a history of cerebrovascular disease. Caution is required if prasugrel is used in patients weighing less than 60 kg or in those with renal impairment.

When prasugrel was compared with clopidogrel in 7243 patients with unstable angina or MI without ST-segment elevation, prasugrel failed to reduce the rate of the primary efficacy endpoint, which was a composite of cardiovascular death, MI, and stroke. Because of the negative results of this study, prasugrel is reserved for patients undergoing percutaneous coronary intervention. In this setting, prasugrel is usually given in conjunction with aspirin. To reduce the risk of bleeding, the daily aspirin dose should be ≤100 mg.

For patients with noncardioembolic stroke or high-risk transient ischemic attack, the combination of clopidogrel or ticagrelor plus aspirin for 21–30 days followed by aspirin alone thereafter reduces the risk of stroke, MI, and vascular death by up to 30% compared with aspirin alone. Therefore, dual antiplatelet therapy is often administered for the first 3–4 weeks in such patients.

DOSING Clopidogrel is given once daily at a dose of 75 mg. Loading doses of clopidogrel are given when rapid ADP receptor blockade is desired. For example, patients undergoing coronary stenting are often given a loading dose of 300–600 mg, which produces inhibition of ADP-induced platelet aggregation in about 4–6 h. After a loading dose of 60 mg, prasugrel is given once daily at a dose of 10 mg. Patients older than age 75 years or weighing less than 60 kg should receive a lower daily prasugrel dose of 5 mg.

SIDE EFFECTS The most common side effect of clopidogrel and prasugrel is bleeding. Because of its greater potency, bleeding is more common with prasugrel than clopidogrel. To reduce the risk of bleeding, clopidogrel and prasugrel should be stopped 5–7 days before major surgery. In patients taking clopidogrel or prasugrel who present with serious bleeding, platelet transfusion may be helpful.

Hematologic side effects, including neutropenia, thrombocytopenia, and thrombotic thrombocytopenic purpura, are rare.

THIENOPYRIDINE RESISTANCE The capacity of clopidogrel to inhibit ADP-induced platelet aggregation varies among subjects. This variability reflects, at least in part, genetic polymorphisms in the CYP isoenzymes involved in the metabolic activation of clopidogrel. Most important of these is CYP2C19. Clopidogrel-treated patients with the loss-of-function *CYP2C19*2* allele exhibit reduced platelet inhibition compared with those with the wild-type *CYP2C19*1* allele and experience a higher rate of cardiovascular events. This is important because estimates suggest that up to 25% of whites, 30% of African Americans, and 50% of Asians carry the loss-of-function allele, which would render them resistant to clopidogrel. Even patients with the reduced function *CYP2C19*3*, **4*, or **5* alleles may derive less benefit from clopidogrel than those with the full-function *CYP2C19*1* allele. Concomitant administration of clopidogrel with proton pump inhibitors, which are inhibitors of *CYP2C19*, produces a small reduction in the inhibitory effects of clopidogrel on ADP-induced platelet aggregation. The extent to which this interaction increases the risk of cardiovascular events remains controversial.

In contrast to their effect on the metabolic activation of clopidogrel, *CYP2C19* polymorphisms appear to be less important determinants of the activation of prasugrel. Thus, no association was detected between the loss-of-function allele and decreased platelet inhibition or increased rate of cardiovascular events with prasugrel. The observation that genetic polymorphisms affecting clopidogrel absorption or metabolism influence clinical outcomes raises the possibilities that pharmacogenetic profiling may be useful to identify clopidogrel-resistant patients and that point-of-care assessment of the extent of clopidogrel-induced platelet inhibition may help detect patients at higher risk for subsequent cardiovascular events. Clinical trials designed to evaluate these possibilities have thus far been negative. Although administration of higher doses of clopidogrel can overcome a reduced response to clopidogrel, the clinical benefit of this approach is uncertain. Instead, prasugrel or ticagrelor may be better choices for these patients.

Ticagrelor As an orally active inhibitor of $P2Y_{12}$, ticagrelor differs from the thienopyridines in that ticagrelor does not require metabolic activation and it produces reversible inhibition of the ADP receptor.

MECHANISM OF ACTION Like the thienopyridines, ticagrelor inhibits $P2Y_{12}$. Because it does not require metabolic activation, ticagrelor has a more rapid onset and offset of action than clopidogrel, and it produces greater and more predictable inhibition of ADP-induced platelet aggregation than clopidogrel.

INDICATIONS Ticagrelor is indicated for the secondary prevention of atherothrombotic events in patients with an acute coronary syndrome treated medically or with percutaneous coronary intervention (PCI) with or without stent implantation or with coronary artery bypass graft (CABG) surgery. Ticagrelor also is indicated for up to 3 years for secondary prevention in patients with a prior history of MI at least one year ago who are at high risk for atherothrombotic events. For patients with acute coronary syndrome undergoing PCI, guidelines give preference to ticagrelor over clopidogrel. Guidelines give preference to ticagrelor over clopidogrel, particularly in higher risk patients.

DOSING Ticagrelor is initiated with an oral loading dose of 180 mg followed by 90 mg twice daily. The dose does not require adjustment in patients with renal impairment, but the drug should be used with caution in patients with hepatic disease and in those receiving potent inhibitors or inducers of CYP3A4 because ticagrelor is metabolized in the liver via CYP3A4. Ticagrelor is usually administered in conjunction with aspirin; the daily aspirin dose should not exceed 100 mg.

SIDE EFFECTS In addition to bleeding, the most common side effects of ticagrelor are dyspnea, which can occur in up to 15% of patients, and asymptomatic ventricular pauses. The dyspnea, which tends to occur soon after initiating ticagrelor, is usually self-limiting and mild in intensity. The mechanism responsible for this side effect is unknown.

To reduce the risk of bleeding, ticagrelor should be stopped at least 5 days before major surgery. Platelet transfusion is unlikely to be of benefit in patients with ticagrelor-related bleeding or in those requiring urgent surgery because the drug will bind to $P2Y_{12}$ on the transfused platelets. Bentracimab, an antibody fragment that binds ticagrelor and its metabolite with high affinity and rapidly reverses their platelet inhibitory effects, is under development for ticagrelor reversal prior to urgent surgery or intervention or for patients with serious bleeding.

Cangrelor Cangrelor is a rapidly acting reversible inhibitor of $P2Y_{12}$ that is administered intravenously. It has an immediate onset of action, a half-life of 3–5 min, and an offset of action within an hour. Cangrelor is licensed for use in patients undergoing percutaneous coronary intervention and produces rapid ADP receptor blockade in those who have not received pretreatment with clopidogrel, prasugrel, or ticagrelor.

Cangrelor is administered as a 30 μg/kg IV bolus prior to percutaneous coronary intervention followed by an infusion of 4 μg/kg per minute for at least 2 h or for the duration of the procedure, whichever is longer. When transitioning to oral $P2Y_{12}$ inhibitor therapy, ticagrelor can be given at a loading dose of 180 mg at any time during the cangrelor infusion or immediately after discontinuation. In contrast, loading doses of prasugrel or clopidogrel (60 and 600 mg, respectively) should only be given after cangrelor is stopped because cangrelor blocks the interaction of their active metabolites with $P2Y_{12}$.

DIPYRIDAMOLE

Dipyridamole is a relatively weak antiplatelet agent on its own, but an extended-release formulation of dipyridamole combined with low-dose aspirin, a preparation known as *Aggrenox*, is sometimes used for secondary prevention in patients with transient ischemic attacks or ischemic stroke.

Mechanism of Action By inhibiting phosphodiesterase, dipyridamole blocks the breakdown of cyclic adenosine monophosphate (AMP). Increased levels of cyclic AMP reduce intracellular calcium and inhibit platelet activation. Dipyridamole also blocks the uptake of adenosine by platelets and other cells. This produces a further increase in local cyclic AMP levels because the platelet adenosine A_2 receptor is coupled to adenylate cyclase **(Fig. 118-4)**.

Indications Dipyridamole plus aspirin was compared with aspirin or dipyridamole alone, or with placebo, in patients with an ischemic stroke or transient ischemic attack. The combination reduced the risk of stroke by 22.1% compared with aspirin and by 24.4% compared with dipyridamole. A second trial compared dipyridamole plus aspirin with aspirin alone for secondary prevention in patients with ischemic stroke. Vascular death, stroke, or MI occurred in 13% of patients given combination therapy and in 16% of those treated with aspirin alone. Another trial randomized 20,332 patients with noncardioembolic ischemic stroke to either Aggrenox or clopidogrel. The primary efficacy endpoint of recurrent stroke occurred in 9.0% of those given Aggrenox and in 8.8% of patients treated with clopidogrel. Although this difference was not statistically significant, the study failed to meet the prespecified margin to claim noninferiority of Aggrenox relative to clopidogrel. These results have dampened enthusiasm for the use of Aggrenox.

Because of its vasodilatory effects and the paucity of data supporting the use of dipyridamole in patients with symptomatic coronary artery disease, Aggrenox should not be used for stroke prevention in such patients. Clopidogrel is a better choice in this setting.

Dosing Aggrenox is given twice daily. Each capsule contains 200 mg of extended-release dipyridamole and 25 mg of aspirin.

Side Effects Because dipyridamole has vasodilatory effects, it must be used with caution in patients with coronary artery disease. Gastrointestinal complaints, headache, facial flushing, dizziness, and hypotension can also occur. These symptoms often subside with continued use of the drug.

GP IIB/IIIA RECEPTOR ANTAGONISTS

As a class, parenteral Gp IIb/IIIa receptor antagonists have a niche in patients with acute coronary syndrome. The three agents in this class are abciximab, eptifibatide, and tirofiban.

Mechanism of Action A member of the integrin family of adhesion receptors, Gp IIb/IIIa is found on the surface of platelets and megakaryocytes. With about 80,000 copies per platelet, Gp IIb/IIIa is the most abundant receptor. Consisting of a noncovalently linked heterodimer, Gp IIb/IIIa is inactive on resting platelets. When platelets

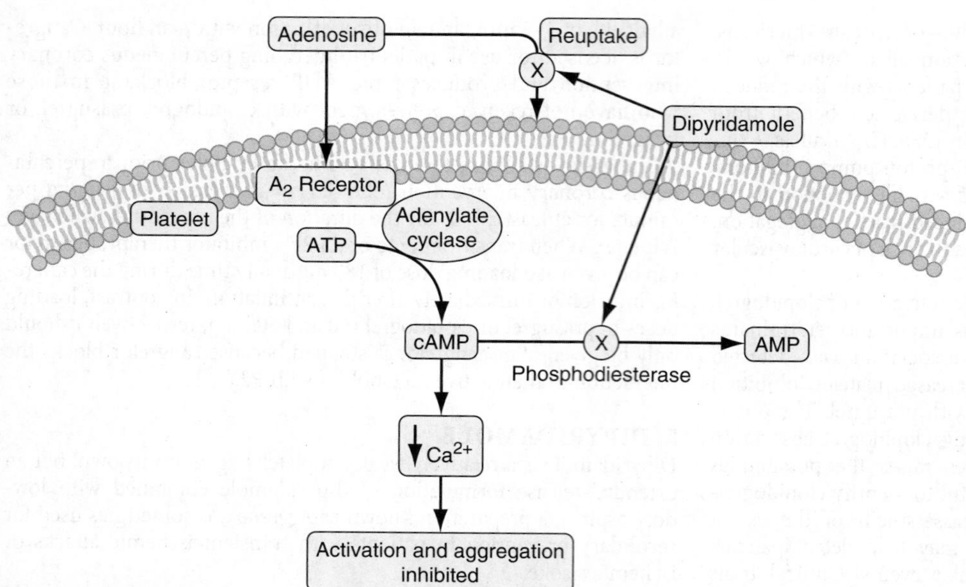

FIGURE 118-4 Mechanism of action of dipyridamole. Dipyridamole increases levels of cyclic AMP (cAMP) in platelets by (1) blocking the reuptake of adenosine and (2) inhibiting phosphodiesterase-mediated cyclic AMP degradation. By promoting calcium uptake, cyclic AMP reduces intracellular levels of calcium. This, in turn, inhibits platelet activation and aggregation.

are activated, inside-outside signal transduction pathways trigger a conformational activation of the receptor. Once activated, Gp IIb/IIIa binds adhesive molecules, such as fibrinogen and, under high shear conditions, VWF. Binding is mediated by the Arg-Gly-Asp (RGD) sequence found on the α chains of fibrinogen and on VWF, and by the Lys-Gly-Asp (KGD) sequence located within a unique dodecapeptide domain on the γ chains of fibrinogen. Once bound, fibrinogen and/or VWF bridge adjacent platelets together to induce platelet aggregation.

Although abciximab, eptifibatide, and tirofiban all target the Gp IIb/IIIa receptor, they are structurally and pharmacologically distinct (Table 118-1). Abciximab is a Fab fragment of a humanized murine monoclonal antibody directed against the activated form of Gp IIb/IIIa. Abciximab binds to the activated receptor with high affinity and blocks the binding of adhesive molecules. In contrast, eptifibatide and tirofiban are synthetic small molecules. Eptifibatide is a cyclic heptapeptide that binds Gp IIb/IIIa because it incorporates the KGD motif, whereas tirofiban is a nonpeptidic tyrosine derivative that acts as an RGD mimetic. Abciximab has a long half-life and can be detected on the surface of platelets for up to 2 weeks; eptifibatide and tirofiban have short half-lives.

Indications Abciximab and eptifibatide are used in patients undergoing percutaneous coronary interventions, particularly those who have not been pretreated with an ADP receptor antagonist. Tirofiban is used in high-risk patients with unstable angina. Eptifibatide also can be used for this indication.

TABLE 118-1 Features of Gp IIb/IIIa Antagonists

FEATURE	ABCIXIMAB	EPTIFIBATIDE	TIROFIBAN
Description	Fab fragment of humanized mouse monoclonal antibody	Cyclical KGD-containing heptapeptide	Nonpeptidic RGD mimetic
Specific for Gp IIb/IIIa	No	Yes	Yes
Plasma half-life	Short (min)	Long (2.5 h)	Long (2.0 h)
Platelet-bound half-life	Long (days)	Short (s)	Short (s)
Renal clearance	No	Yes	Yes

Abbreviation: Gp, glycoprotein.

Dosing All of the Gp IIb/IIIa antagonists are given as an IV bolus followed by an infusion. The recommended dose of abciximab is a bolus of 0.25 mg/kg followed by an infusion of 0.125 μg/kg per minute to a maximum of 10 μg/kg for 12 h. In patients undergoing percutaneous coronary intervention, eptifibatide is given as two 180 μg/kg boluses given 10 min apart, followed by an infusion of 2.0 μg/kg per minute for 18–24 h. For patients with acute coronary syndrome, the second eptifibatide bolus is withheld. Tirofiban is started at a rate of 0.4 μg/kg per minute for 30 min; the drug is then continued at a rate of 0.1 μg/kg per minute for up to 18 h. Because eptifibatide and tirofiban are cleared by the kidneys, the doses must be reduced in patients with renal insufficiency. Thus, the eptifibatide infusion is reduced to 1 μg/kg per minute in patients with a creatinine clearance below 50 mL/min, whereas the dose of tirofiban is cut in half for patients with a creatinine clearance below 30 mL/min.

Side Effects In addition to bleeding, thrombocytopenia is the most serious complication. Thrombocytopenia is immune-mediated and is caused by antibodies directed against neoantigens on Gp IIb/IIIa that are exposed upon antagonist binding. With abciximab, thrombocytopenia occurs in up to 5% of patients. Thrombocytopenia is severe in ~1% of these individuals. Thrombocytopenia is less common with the other two agents, occurring in ~1% of patients.

VORAPAXAR

An orally active PAR-1 antagonist, vorapaxar blocks thrombin-induced platelet activation. Vorapaxar has a half-life of about 200 h.

Indications When compared with placebo in 12,944 patients with acute coronary syndrome without ST-segment elevation, vorapaxar failed to significantly reduce the primary efficacy endpoint, a composite of cardiovascular death, MI, stroke, recurrent ischemia requiring rehospitalization, and urgent coronary revascularization. Moreover, vorapaxar was associated with increased rates of bleeding, including intracranial bleeding.

In a second trial, vorapaxar was compared with placebo for secondary prevention in 26,449 patients with prior MI, ischemic stroke, or peripheral arterial disease. Overall, vorapaxar reduced the risk for cardiovascular death, MI, or stroke by 13%, but doubled the risk of intracranial bleeding. In the prespecified subgroup of 17,779 patients with prior MI, however, vorapaxar reduced the risk for cardiovascular death, MI, or stroke by 20% compared with placebo (from 9.7% to 8.1%, respectively). The rate of intracranial hemorrhage was higher with vorapaxar than with placebo (0.6% and 0.4%, respectively; $p = .076$) as was the rate of moderate or severe bleeding (3.4% and 2.1%, respectively; $p < .0001$). Based on these data, vorapaxar is licensed for patients younger than 75 years with MI or peripheral artery disease who have no history of stroke, transient ischemic attack, or intracranial bleeding and weigh more than 60 kg.

Dosing Vorapaxar is given at a dose of 2.08 mg once daily.

Side Effects The major side effect is bleeding. Platelet transfusion may be of benefit for vorapaxar reversal.

ANTICOAGULANTS

There are both parenteral and oral anticoagulants. The parenteral anticoagulants include heparin, low-molecular-weight heparin (LMWH), fondaparinux (a synthetic pentasaccharide), lepirudin, desirudin, bivalirudin, and argatroban. Currently available oral anticoagulants include warfarin; dabigatran etexilate, an oral thrombin inhibitor; and rivaroxaban, apixaban, and edoxaban, which are oral factor Xa inhibitors.

PARENTERAL ANTICOAGULANTS

Heparin A sulfated polysaccharide, heparin is isolated from mammalian tissues rich in mast cells. Most commercial heparin is derived from porcine intestinal mucosa and is a polymer of alternating D-glucuronic acid and *N*-acetyl-D-glucosamine residues.

MECHANISM OF ACTION Heparin acts as an anticoagulant by activating antithrombin (previously known as antithrombin III) and accelerating the rate at which antithrombin inhibits clotting enzymes, particularly thrombin and factor Xa. Antithrombin, the obligatory plasma cofactor for heparin, is a member of the serine protease inhibitor (serpin) superfamily. Synthesized in the liver and circulating in plasma at a concentration of 2.6 ± 0.4 μM, antithrombin acts as a suicide substrate for its target enzymes.

To activate antithrombin, heparin binds to the serpin via a unique pentasaccharide sequence that is found on one-third of the chains of commercial heparin (**Fig. 118-5**). Heparin chains without this pentasaccharide sequence have little or no anticoagulant activity. Once bound to antithrombin, heparin induces a conformational change in the reactive center loop of antithrombin that renders it more readily accessible to its target proteases. This conformational change enhances the rate at which antithrombin inhibits factor Xa by at least two orders of magnitude but has little effect on the rate of thrombin inhibition. To catalyze thrombin inhibition, heparin serves as a template that binds antithrombin and thrombin simultaneously. Formation of this ternary complex brings the enzyme in close apposition to the inhibitor, thereby promoting the formation of a stable covalent thrombin-antithrombin complex.

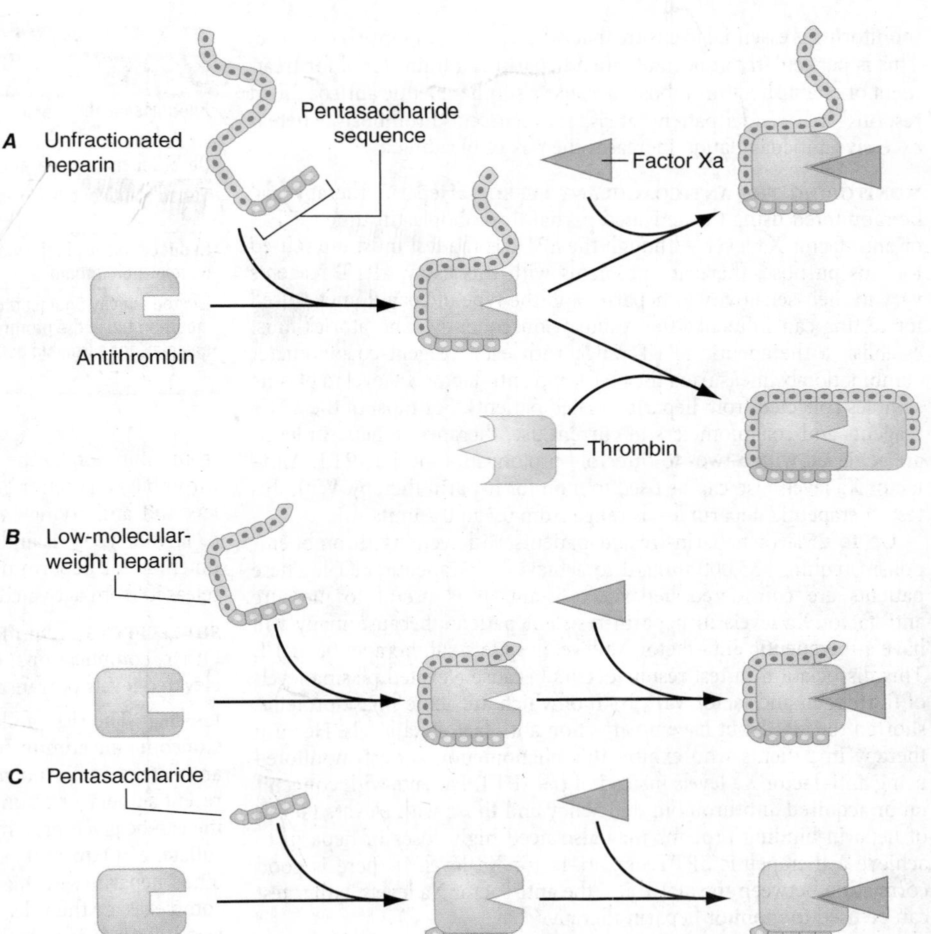

FIGURE 118-5 Mechanism of action of heparin, low-molecular-weight heparin (LMWH), and fondaparinux, a synthetic pentasaccharide. ***A.*** Heparin binds to antithrombin via its pentasaccharide sequence. This induces a conformational change in the reactive center loop of antithrombin that accelerates its interaction with factor Xa. To potentiate thrombin inhibition, heparin must simultaneously bind to antithrombin and thrombin. Only heparin chains composed of at least 18 saccharide units, which corresponds to a molecular weight of 5400, are of sufficient length to perform this bridging function. With a mean molecular weight of 15,000, all of the heparin chains are long enough to do this. ***B.*** LMWH has greater capacity to potentiate factor Xa inhibition by antithrombin than thrombin because, with a mean molecular weight of 4500–5000, at least half of the LMWH chains are too short to bridge antithrombin to thrombin. ***C.*** The pentasaccharide only accelerates factor Xa inhibition by antithrombin because the pentasaccharide is too short to bridge antithrombin to thrombin.

Only pentasaccharide-containing heparin chains composed of at least 18 saccharide units (which correspond to a molecular weight of 5400) are of sufficient length to bridge thrombin and antithrombin together. With a mean molecular weight of 15,000, and a range of 5000–30,000, almost all of the chains of unfractionated heparin are long enough to do so. Consequently, by definition, heparin has equal capacity to promote the inhibition of thrombin and factor Xa by antithrombin and is assigned an anti-factor Xa to anti-factor IIa (thrombin) ratio of 1:1.

Heparin causes the release of tissue factor pathway inhibitor (TFPI) from the endothelium. A factor Xa–dependent inhibitor of tissue factor–bound factor VIIa, TFPI may contribute to the antithrombotic activity of heparin. Longer heparin chains induce the release of more TFPI than shorter ones.

PHARMACOLOGY Heparin must be given parenterally. It is usually administered SC or by continuous IV infusion. When used for therapeutic purposes, the IV route is most often employed. If heparin is given SC for treatment of thrombosis, the dose of heparin must be high enough to overcome the limited bioavailability associated with this method of delivery.

In the circulation, heparin binds to the endothelium and to plasma proteins other than antithrombin. Heparin binding to endothelial cells explains its dose-dependent clearance. At low doses, the half-life of heparin is short because it binds rapidly to the endothelium. With higher doses of heparin, the half-life is longer because heparin is cleared more slowly once the endothelium is saturated. Clearance is mainly extra renal; heparin binds to macrophages, which internalize and depolymerize the long heparin chains and secrete shorter chains back into the circulation. Because of its dose-dependent clearance mechanism, the plasma half-life of heparin ranges from 30 to 60 min with bolus IV doses of 25 and 100 units/kg, respectively.

Once heparin enters the circulation, it binds to plasma proteins other than antithrombin, a phenomenon that reduces its anticoagulant activity. Some of the heparin-binding proteins found in plasma are acute-phase reactants whose levels are elevated in ill patients. Others, such as high-molecular-weight multimers of VWF, are released from activated platelets or endothelial cells. Activated platelets also release platelet factor 4 (PF4), a highly cationic protein that binds heparin with high affinity. The large amounts of PF4 found in the vicinity of platelet-rich arterial thrombi can neutralize the anticoagulant activity of heparin. This phenomenon may attenuate heparin's capacity to suppress thrombus growth.

Because the levels of heparin-binding proteins in plasma vary from person to person, the anticoagulant response to fixed or weight-adjusted doses of heparin is unpredictable. Consequently, coagulation monitoring is essential to ensure that a therapeutic response is obtained. This is particularly important when heparin is administered for treatment of established thrombosis because a subtherapeutic anticoagulant response may render patients at risk for recurrent thrombosis, whereas excessive anticoagulation increases the risk of bleeding.

MONITORING THE ANTICOAGULANT EFFECT Heparin therapy can be monitored using the activated partial thromboplastin time (aPTT) or anti–factor Xa level. Although the aPTT is the test most often used for this purpose, there are problems with this assay. aPTT reagents vary in their sensitivity to heparin, and the type of coagulometer used for testing can influence the results. Consequently, laboratories must establish a therapeutic aPTT range with each reagent-coagulometer combination by measuring the aPTT and anti–factor Xa level in plasma samples collected from heparin-treated patients. For most of the aPTT reagents and coagulometers in current use, therapeutic heparin levels are achieved with a two- to threefold prolongation of the aPTT. Anti–factor Xa levels also can be used to monitor heparin therapy. With this test, therapeutic heparin levels range from 0.3 to 0.7 units/mL.

Up to 25% of heparin-treated patients with venous thromboembolism require >35,000 units/d to achieve a therapeutic aPTT. These patients are considered heparin resistant. It is useful to measure anti–factor Xa levels in heparin-resistant patients because many will have a therapeutic anti–factor Xa level despite a subtherapeutic aPTT. This dissociation in test results occurs because elevated plasma levels of fibrinogen and factor VIII, both of which are acute-phase proteins, shorten the aPTT but have no effect on anti–factor Xa levels. Heparin therapy in patients who exhibit this phenomenon is best monitored using anti–factor Xa levels instead of the aPTT. Patients with congenital or acquired antithrombin deficiency and those with elevated levels of heparin-binding proteins may also need high doses of heparin to achieve a therapeutic aPTT or anti–factor Xa level. If there is good correlation between the aPTT and the anti–factor Xa levels, either test can be used to monitor heparin therapy.

DOSING For prophylaxis, heparin is usually given in fixed doses of 5000 units SC two or three times daily. With these low doses, coagulation monitoring is unnecessary. In contrast, monitoring is essential when the drug is given in therapeutic doses. Fixed-dose or weight-based heparin nomograms are used to standardize heparin dosing and to shorten the time required to achieve a therapeutic anticoagulant response. At least two heparin nomograms have been validated in patients with venous thromboembolism and reduce the time required to achieve a therapeutic aPTT. Weight-adjusted heparin nomograms have also been evaluated in patients with acute coronary syndromes. After an IV heparin bolus of 5000 units or 70 units/kg, a heparin infusion rate of 12–15 units/kg per hour is usually administered. In contrast, weight-adjusted heparin nomograms for patients with venous thromboembolism use an initial bolus of 5000 units or 80 units/kg, followed by an infusion of 18 units/kg per hour. Thus, patients with venous thromboembolism appear to require higher doses of heparin to achieve a therapeutic aPTT than do patients with acute coronary syndromes. This may reflect differences in the thrombus burden. Heparin binds to fibrin, and the amount of fibrin in patients with extensive DVT is greater than that in those with coronary thrombosis.

LIMITATIONS Heparin has pharmacokinetic and biophysical limitations (**Table 118-2**). The pharmacokinetic limitations reflect heparin's propensity to bind in a pentasaccharide-independent fashion to cells and plasma proteins. Heparin binding to endothelial cells explains its dose-dependent clearance, whereas binding to plasma proteins results in a variable anticoagulant response and can lead to heparin resistance.

The biophysical limitations of heparin reflect the inability of the heparin-antithrombin complex to inhibit factor Xa when it is incorporated into the prothrombinase complex, the complex that converts prothrombin to thrombin, and to inhibit thrombin bound to fibrin. Consequently, factor Xa bound to activated platelets within platelet-rich thrombi has the potential to generate thrombin, even in the face of heparin. Once this thrombin binds to fibrin, it too is protected from inhibition by the heparin-antithrombin complex. Clot-associated thrombin can then trigger thrombus growth by locally activating platelets and amplifying its own generation through feedback activation of factors V, VIII, and XI. Further compounding the problem is the potential for heparin neutralization by the high concentrations of PF4 released from activated platelets within the platelet-rich thrombus.

TABLE 118-2 Pharmacokinetic and Biophysical Limitations of Heparin

LIMITATIONS	MECHANISM
Poor bioavailability at low doses	Binds to endothelial cells and macrophages
Dose-dependent clearance	Binds to macrophages
Variable anticoagulant response	Binds to plasma proteins whose levels vary from patient to patient
Reduced activity in the vicinity of platelet-rich thrombi	Neutralized by platelet factor 4 released from activated platelets
Limited activity against factor Xa incorporated in the prothrombinase complex and thrombin bound to fibrin	Reduced capacity of heparin-antithrombin complex to inhibit factor Xa bound to activated platelets and thrombin bound to fibrin

SIDE EFFECTS The most common side effect of heparin is bleeding. Other complications include thrombocytopenia, osteoporosis, and elevated levels of transaminases.

Bleeding The risk of bleeding rises as the dose of heparin is increased. Concomitant administration of drugs that affect hemostasis, such as antiplatelet or fibrinolytic agents, increases the risk of bleeding, as does recent surgery or trauma. Heparin-treated patients with serious bleeding can be given protamine sulfate to neutralize the heparin. Protamine sulfate, a mixture of basic polypeptides isolated from salmon sperm, binds heparin with high affinity, and the resultant protamine-heparin complexes are then cleared. Typically, 1 mg of protamine sulfate neutralizes 100 units of heparin. Protamine sulfate is given IV. Anaphylactoid reactions to protamine sulfate can occur, and drug administration by slow IV infusion is recommended to reduce the risk.

Thrombocytopenia Heparin can cause thrombocytopenia. Heparin-induced thrombocytopenia (HIT) is an antibody-mediated process that is triggered by antibodies directed against neoantigens on PF4 that are exposed when heparin binds to this protein. These antibodies, which are usually of the IgG isotype, bind simultaneously to the heparin-PF4 complex and to platelet Fc receptors. Such binding activates the platelets and generates platelet microparticles. Circulating microparticles are prothrombotic because they express anionic phospholipids on their surface and can bind clotting factors and promote thrombin generation.

The clinical features of HIT are illustrated in **Table 118-3**. Typically, HIT occurs 5–14 days after initiation of heparin therapy, but it can manifest earlier if the patient has received heparin within the past 3 months. A platelet count <100,000/μL or a 50% decrease in the platelet count from the pretreatment value should raise the suspicion of HIT. HIT is more common in surgical patients than in medical patients and, like many autoimmune disorders, occurs more frequently in females than in males.

HIT can be associated with thrombosis, either arterial or venous. Venous thrombosis, which manifests as DVT and/or PE, is more

TABLE 118-3 Features of Heparin-Induced Thrombocytopenia

FEATURES	DETAILS
Thrombocytopenia	Platelet count of ≤100,000/μL or a decrease in platelet count of ≥50%
Timing	Platelet count falls 5–14 days after starting heparin
Type of heparin	More common with unfractionated heparin than low-molecular-weight heparin
Type of patient	More common in surgical patients and patients with cancer than general medical patients; more common in women than in men
Thrombosis	Venous thrombosis more common than arterial thrombosis

TABLE 118-4 Management of Heparin-Induced Thrombocytopenia

Stop all heparin.
Give an alternative anticoagulant, such as argatroban, bivalirudin, fondaparinux, or rivaroxaban.
Do not give platelet transfusions.
Do not give warfarin until the platelet count returns to its baseline level. If warfarin was administered, give vitamin K to restore the INR to normal.
Evaluate for thrombosis, particularly deep vein thrombosis.

Abbreviation: INR, international normalized ratio.

TABLE 118-5 Advantages of LMWH Over Heparin

ADVANTAGE	CONSEQUENCE
Better bioavailability and longer half-life after subcutaneous injection	Can be given subcutaneously once or twice daily for both prophylaxis and treatment
Dose-independent clearance	Simplified dosing
Predictable anticoagulant response	Coagulation monitoring is unnecessary in most patients
Lower risk of heparin-induced thrombocytopenia	Safer than heparin for short- or long-term administration
Lower risk of osteoporosis	Safer than heparin for extended administration

Abbreviation: LMWH, low-molecular-weight heparin.

common than arterial thrombosis. Arterial thrombosis can manifest as ischemic stroke or acute MI. Rarely, platelet-rich thrombi in the distal aorta or iliac arteries can cause critical limb ischemia.

The diagnosis of HIT is established using enzyme-linked assays to detect antibodies against heparin-PF4 complexes or with platelet activation assays. Enzyme-linked assays are sensitive but can be positive in the absence of any clinical evidence of HIT. The most specific diagnostic test for HIT is the serotonin release assay. This test is performed by quantifying serotonin release when washed platelets loaded with labeled serotonin are exposed to patient serum in the absence or presence of varying concentrations of heparin. If the patient serum contains the HIT antibody, heparin addition induces platelet activation and serotonin release.

Management of HIT is outlined in **Table 118-4**. Heparin should be stopped in patients with suspected or documented HIT, and an alternative anticoagulant should be administered to prevent or treat thrombosis. The agents most often used for this indication are parenteral direct thrombin inhibitors, such as argatroban or bivalirudin, or factor Xa inhibitors, such as fondaparinux or rivaroxaban. A HIT-like syndrome known as vaccine induced thrombotic thrombocytopenia is a rare complication after vaccination with adenovirus COVID-19 vaccines. Characterized by thrombosis and thrombocytopenia that occur 4 to 28 days after vaccination, patients can present with cerebral or splanchnic vein thrombosis as well as DVT or PE. The diagnosis is established by evidence of antibodies against PF4 and a positive serotonin release assay with added PF4. Treatment can include intravenous immunoglobulin, steroids, and plasma exchange to offset the effects of the antibodies against PF4 and anticoagulants such as argatroban, fondaprinux or rivaroxaban to treat the thrombosis.

Patients with HIT, particularly those with associated thrombosis, often have evidence of increased thrombin generation that can lead to consumption of protein C. If these patients are given warfarin without a concomitant anticoagulant that inhibits thrombin or thrombin generation, the further decrease in protein C levels induced by the vitamin K antagonist can trigger skin necrosis. To avoid this problem, patients with HIT should be treated with a direct thrombin inhibitor or with fondaparinux until the platelet count returns to normal levels. At this point, low-dose warfarin therapy can be introduced, and the parenteral anticoagulant can be discontinued when the international normalized ratio (INR) has been therapeutic for at least 2 days. Alternatively, a direct oral anticoagulant can be given.

Osteoporosis Treatment with therapeutic doses of heparin for >1 month can cause a reduction in bone density. This complication has been reported in up to 30% of patients given long-term heparin therapy, and symptomatic vertebral fractures occur in 2–3% of these individuals.

Heparin causes bone loss both by decreasing bone formation and by enhancing bone resorption. Thus, heparin affects the activity of both osteoblasts and osteoclasts.

Elevated Levels of Transaminases Therapeutic doses of heparin are frequently associated with modest elevations in the serum levels of hepatic transaminases without a concomitant increase in the level of bilirubin. The levels of transaminases rapidly return to normal when the drug is stopped. The mechanism responsible for this phenomenon is unknown.

Low-Molecular-Weight Heparin Consisting of smaller fragments of heparin, LMWH is prepared from unfractionated heparin by controlled enzymatic or chemical depolymerization. The mean molecular weight of LMWH is about 5000, one-third the mean molecular weight of unfractionated heparin. LMWH has advantages over heparin (**Table 118-5**) and has replaced heparin for most indications.

MECHANISM OF ACTION Like heparin, LMWH exerts its anticoagulant activity by activating antithrombin. With a mean molecular weight of 5000, which corresponds to about 17 saccharide units, at least half of the pentasaccharide-containing chains of LMWH are too short to bridge thrombin to antithrombin (Fig. 118-5). However, these chains retain the capacity to accelerate factor Xa inhibition by antithrombin because this activity is largely the result of the conformational changes in antithrombin evoked by pentasaccharide binding. Consequently, LMWH catalyzes factor Xa inhibition by antithrombin more than thrombin inhibition. Depending on their unique molecular weight distributions, LMWH preparations have anti–factor Xa to anti–factor IIa ratios ranging from 2:1 to 4:1.

PHARMACOLOGY Although usually given SC, LMWH also can be administered IV if a rapid anticoagulant response is needed. LMWH has pharmacokinetic advantages over heparin. These advantages reflect the fact that shorter heparin chains bind less avidly to endothelial cells, macrophages, and heparin-binding plasma proteins. Reduced binding to endothelial cells and macrophages eliminates the rapid, dose-dependent, and saturable mechanism of clearance that is a characteristic of unfractionated heparin. Instead, the clearance of LMWH is dose-independent and its plasma half-life is longer. Based on measurement of anti–factor Xa levels, LMWH has a plasma half-life of ~4 h. LMWH is cleared almost exclusively by the kidneys, and the drug can accumulate in patients with renal insufficiency.

LMWH exhibits about 90% bioavailability after SC injection. Because LMWH binds less avidly to heparin-binding proteins in plasma than heparin, LMWH produces a more predictable dose response, and resistance to LMWH is rare. With a longer half-life and more predictable anticoagulant response, LMWH can be given SC once or twice daily without coagulation monitoring, even when the drug is given in treatment doses. These properties render LMWH more convenient than unfractionated heparin. Capitalizing on this feature, studies in patients with venous thromboembolism have shown that home treatment with LMWH is as effective and safe as in-hospital treatment with continuous IV infusions of heparin. Outpatient treatment with LMWH streamlines care, reduces health care costs, and increases patient satisfaction.

MONITORING In the majority of patients, LMWH does not require coagulation monitoring. If monitoring is necessary, anti–factor Xa levels must be measured because most LMWH preparations have little effect on the aPTT. Therapeutic anti-factor Xa levels once daily and twice daily doses of LMWH range from 0.5 to 1.2 units/mL and 1.0 to 2.0 units/mL, respectively, when measured 3–4 h after drug administration. When LMWH is given in prophylactic doses, peak anti–factor Xa levels of 0.2–0.5 units/mL are desirable.

Indications for LMWH monitoring include renal impairment and obesity. LMWH monitoring in patients with a creatinine clearance of ≤30 mL/min is advisable to ensure that there is no drug accumulation.

Although weight-adjusted LMWH dosing appears to produce therapeutic anti-factor Xa levels in patients who are overweight, this approach has not been extensively evaluated in those with morbid obesity. It may also be advisable to monitor the anticoagulant activity of LMWH during pregnancy because dose requirements can change, particularly in the third trimester. Monitoring should also be considered in high-risk settings, such as in pregnant women with mechanical heart valves who are given LMWH for prevention of valve thrombosis, and when LMWH is used in treatment doses in infants or children.

DOSING The doses of LMWH recommended for prophylaxis or treatment vary depending on the LMWH preparation. For prophylaxis, once-daily SC doses of 4000–5000 units are often used, whereas doses of 2500–3000 units are given when the drug is administered twice daily. For treatment of venous thromboembolism, a dose of 150–200 units/kg is given if the drug is administered once daily. If a twice-daily regimen is used, a dose of 100 units/kg is given. In patients with unstable angina, LMWH is given SC on a twice-daily basis at a dose of 100–120 units/kg.

SIDE EFFECTS The major complication of LMWH is bleeding. Meta-analyses suggest that the risk of major bleeding is lower with LMWH than with unfractionated heparin. HIT and osteoporosis are less common with LMWH than with unfractionated heparin.

Bleeding Like the situation with heparin, bleeding with LMWH is more common in patients receiving concomitant therapy with antiplatelet or fibrinolytic drugs. Recent surgery, trauma, or underlying hemostatic defects also increase the risk of bleeding with LMWH.

Although protamine sulfate can be used as an antidote for LMWH, protamine sulfate incompletely neutralizes the anticoagulant activity of LMWH because it only binds the longer chains of LMWH. Because longer chains are responsible for catalysis of thrombin inhibition by antithrombin, protamine sulfate completely reverses the anti–factor IIa activity of LMWH. In contrast, protamine sulfate only partially reverses the anti–factor Xa activity of LMWH because the shorter pentasaccharide-containing chains of LMWH do not bind to protamine sulfate. Consequently, patients at high risk for bleeding may be more safely treated with continuous IV unfractionated heparin than with SC LMWH.

Thrombocytopenia The risk of HIT is about fivefold lower with LMWH than with heparin. LMWH binds less avidly to platelets and causes less PF4 release. Furthermore, with lower affinity for PF4 than heparin, LMWH is less likely to induce the conformational changes in PF4 that trigger the formation of HIT antibodies.

LMWH should not be used to treat HIT patients because most HIT antibodies exhibit cross-reactivity with LMWH. This in vitro cross-reactivity is not simply a laboratory phenomenon because there are case reports of thrombosis when HIT patients were switched from heparin to LMWH.

Osteoporosis Because the risk of osteoporosis is lower with LMWH than with heparin, LMWH is a better choice for extended treatment.

Fondaparinux A synthetic analogue of the antithrombin-binding pentasaccharide sequence, fondaparinux differs from LMWH in several ways (**Table 118-6**). Fondaparinux is licensed for thromboprophylaxis in general medical or surgical patients and in high-risk orthopedic patients and as an alternative to heparin or LMWH for initial treatment of patients with established venous thromboembolism. Although fondaparinux is used in Europe as an alternative to heparin or LMWH in patients with acute coronary syndrome, the drug is not licensed for this indication in the United States.

TABLE 118-6 Comparison of LMWH and Fondaparinux

FEATURES	LMWH	FONDAPARINUX
Number of saccharide units	15–17	5
Catalysis of factor Xa inhibition	Yes	Yes
Catalysis of thrombin inhibition	Yes	No
Bioavailability after subcutaneous administration (%)	90	100
Plasma half-life (h)	4	17
Renal excretion	Yes	Yes
Induces release of tissue factor pathway inhibitor	Yes	No
Neutralized by protamine sulfate	Partially	No

MECHANISM OF ACTION As a synthetic analogue of the antithrombin-binding pentasaccharide sequence found in heparin and LMWH, fondaparinux has a molecular weight of 1728. Fondaparinux binds only to antithrombin (Fig. 118-5) and is too short to bridge thrombin to antithrombin. Consequently, fondaparinux catalyzes factor Xa inhibition by antithrombin and does not enhance the rate of thrombin inhibition.

PHARMACOLOGY Fondaparinux exhibits complete bioavailability after SC injection. With no binding to endothelial cells or plasma proteins, the clearance of fondaparinux is dose independent, and its plasma half-life is 17 h. The drug is given SC once daily. Because fondaparinux is cleared unchanged via the kidneys, it is contraindicated in patients with a creatinine clearance <30 mL/min and should be used with caution in those with a creatinine clearance <50 mL/min.

Dosing Fondaparinux produces a predictable anticoagulant response after administration in fixed doses because it does not bind to plasma proteins. The drug is given at a dose of 2.5 mg once daily for prevention of venous thromboembolism. For initial treatment of established venous thromboembolism, fondaparinux is given at a dose of 7.5 mg once daily. The dose can be reduced to 5 mg once daily for those weighing <50 kg and increased to 10 mg for those >100 kg. When given in these doses, fondaparinux is as effective as heparin or LMWH for initial treatment of patients with DVT or PE and produces similar rates of bleeding.

Fondaparinux is used at a dose of 2.5 mg once daily in patients with acute coronary syndrome. When this prophylactic dose of fondaparinux was compared with treatment doses of enoxaparin in patients with non-ST-segment elevation acute coronary syndrome, there was no difference in the rate of cardiovascular death, MI, or stroke at 9 days. However, the rate of major bleeding was 50% lower with fondaparinux than with enoxaparin, a difference that likely reflects the fact that the dose of fondaparinux was lower than that of enoxaparin. In acute coronary syndrome patients who require percutaneous coronary intervention, there is a risk of catheter thrombosis with fondaparinux unless adjunctive heparin is given at the time of the procedure.

SIDE EFFECTS Fondaparinux does not cause HIT because it does not bind to PF4. In contrast to LMWH, there is no cross-reactivity of fondaparinux with HIT antibodies. Consequently, fondaparinux appears to be effective for treatment of HIT patients, although large clinical trials supporting its use are lacking.

The major side effect of fondaparinux is bleeding. Fondaparinux has no antidote. Protamine sulfate has no effect on the anticoagulant activity of fondaparinux because it fails to bind to the drug. Recombinant activated factor VII reverses the anticoagulant effects of fondaparinux in volunteers, but it is unknown whether this agent controls fondaparinux-induced bleeding.

Parenteral Direct Thrombin Inhibitors Direct thrombin inhibitors bind directly to thrombin and block its interaction with its substrates. Approved parenteral direct thrombin inhibitors include recombinant hirudins (lepirudin and desirudin), argatroban, and bivalirudin (**Table 118-7**). Lepirudin and desirudin are no longer available. Argatroban is licensed for treatment of patients with HIT, and bivalirudin is approved as an alternative to heparin in patients undergoing percutaneous coronary intervention, including those with HIT.

ARGATROBAN A univalent inhibitor that targets the active site of thrombin, argatroban is metabolized in the liver. Consequently, this drug must be used with caution in patients with hepatic insufficiency. Argatroban is not cleared via the kidneys, so this drug is safer than fondaparinux for HIT patients with renal impairment.

TABLE 118-7 Comparison of the Properties of Lepirudin, Bivalirudin, and Argatroban

	LEPIRUDIN/ DESIRUDIN	BIVALIRUDIN	ARGATROBAN
Molecular mass	7000	1980	527
Site(s) of interaction with thrombin	Active site and exosite 1	Active site and exosite 1	Active site
Renal clearance	Yes	No	No
Hepatic metabolism	No	No	Yes
Plasma half-life (min)	60 (IV) 120–180 (SC)	25	45

Argatroban is administered by continuous IV infusion and has a plasma half-life of ~45 min. The aPTT is used to monitor its anticoagulant effect, and the dose is adjusted to achieve an aPTT 1.5–3 times the baseline value, but not to exceed 100 s. Argatroban also prolongs the INR, a feature that can complicate the transitioning of patients to warfarin. This problem can be circumvented by using the levels of factor X to monitor warfarin instead of the INR. Alternatively, argatroban can be stopped for 2–3 h before INR determination.

BIVALIRUDIN A synthetic 20-amino-acid analogue of hirudin, bivalirudin is a divalent thrombin inhibitor. Thus, the N-terminus of bivalirudin interacts with the active site of thrombin, whereas its C-terminus binds to exosite 1. Bivalirudin has a plasma half-life of 25 min, the shortest half-life of all the parenteral direct thrombin inhibitors. Bivalirudin is degraded by peptidases and is partially excreted via the kidneys. When given in high doses in the cardiac catheterization laboratory, the anticoagulant activity of bivalirudin is monitored using the activated clotting time. With lower doses, its activity can be assessed using the aPTT.

Bivalirudin is licensed as an alternative to heparin in patients undergoing percutaneous coronary intervention. Bivalirudin also has been used successfully in HIT patients who require percutaneous coronary intervention or cardiac bypass surgery.

ORAL ANTICOAGULANTS

For many years, vitamin K antagonists such as warfarin were the only available oral anticoagulants. This situation changed with the introduction of the direct oral anticoagulants, which include dabigatran, rivaroxaban, apixaban, and edoxaban.

Warfarin

A water-soluble vitamin K antagonist initially developed as a rodenticide, warfarin is the coumarin derivative most often prescribed in North America. Like other vitamin K antagonists, warfarin interferes with the synthesis of the vitamin K–dependent clotting proteins, which include prothrombin (factor II) and factors VII, IX, and X. The synthesis of the vitamin K–dependent anticoagulant proteins, proteins C and S, is also reduced by vitamin K antagonists.

MECHANISM OF ACTION All of the vitamin K–dependent clotting factors possess glutamic acid residues at their N termini. A posttranslational modification adds a carboxyl group to the γ-carbon of these residues to generate γ-carboxyglutamic acid. This modification is essential for expression of the activity of these clotting factors because it permits their calcium-dependent binding to negatively charged phospholipid surfaces. The γ-carboxylation process is catalyzed by a vitamin K–dependent carboxylase. Thus, vitamin K from the diet is reduced to vitamin K hydroquinone by vitamin K reductase (**Fig. 118-6**). Vitamin K hydroquinone serves as a cofactor for the carboxylase enzyme, which in the presence of carbon dioxide replaces the hydrogen on the γ-carbon of glutamic acid residues with a carboxyl group. During this process, vitamin K hydroquinone is oxidized to vitamin K epoxide, which is then reduced to vitamin K by vitamin K epoxide reductase.

Warfarin inhibits vitamin K epoxide reductase (VKOR), thereby blocking the γ-carboxylation process. This results in the synthesis of vitamin K–dependent clotting proteins that are only partially γ-carboxylated. Warfarin acts as an anticoagulant because these

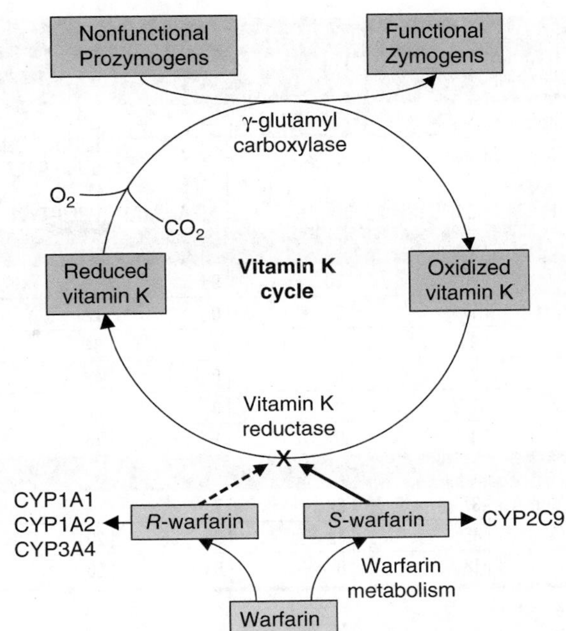

FIGURE 118-6 Mechanism of action of warfarin. A racemic mixture of *S*- and *R*-enantiomers, *S*-warfarin is most active. By blocking vitamin K epoxide reductase, warfarin inhibits the conversion of oxidized vitamin K into its reduced form. This inhibits vitamin K–dependent γ-carboxylation of factors II, VII, IX, and X because reduced vitamin K serves as a cofactor for a γ-glutamyl carboxylase that catalyzes the γ-carboxylation process, thereby converting prozymogens to zymogens capable of binding calcium and interacting with anionic phospholipid surfaces. *S*-warfarin is metabolized by CYP2C9. Common genetic polymorphisms in this enzyme can influence warfarin metabolism. Polymorphisms in the C1 subunit of vitamin K reductase (*VKORC1*) also can affect the susceptibility of the enzyme to warfarin-induced inhibition, thereby influencing warfarin dosage requirements.

partially γ-carboxylated proteins have little or no biological activity. The onset of action of warfarin is delayed until the newly synthesized clotting factors with reduced activity gradually replace their fully active counterparts.

The antithrombotic effect of warfarin depends on a reduction in the functional levels of factor X and prothrombin, clotting factors that have half-lives of 24 and 72 h, respectively. Because the antithrombotic effect of warfarin is delayed, patients with established thrombosis or at high risk for thrombosis require concomitant treatment with a rapidly acting parenteral anticoagulant, such as heparin, LMWH, or fondaparinux, for at least 5 days.

PHARMACOLOGY Warfarin is a racemic mixture of R and S isomers. Warfarin is rapidly and almost completely absorbed from the gastrointestinal tract. Levels of warfarin in the blood peak about 90 min after drug administration. Racemic warfarin has a plasma half-life of 36–42 h, and >97% of circulating warfarin is bound to albumin. Only the small fraction of unbound warfarin is biologically active.

Warfarin accumulates in the liver where the two isomers are metabolized via distinct pathways. *CYP2C9* mediates oxidative metabolism of the more active S isomer (Fig. 118-6). Two relatively common variants, *CYP2C9*2* and *CYP2C9*3*, encode an enzyme with reduced activity. Patients with these variants require lower maintenance doses of warfarin. Approximately 25% of Caucasians have at least one variant allele of *CYP2C9*2* or *CYP2C9*3*, whereas those variant alleles are less common in African Americans and Asians (**Table 118-8**). Heterozygosity for *CYP2C9*2* or *CYP2C9*3* decreases the warfarin dose requirement by 20–30% relative to that required in subjects with the wild-type *CYP2C9*1/*1* alleles, whereas homozygosity for the *CYP2C9*2* or *CYP2C9*3* alleles reduces the warfarin dose requirement by 50–70%.

Consistent with their decreased warfarin dose requirement, subjects with at least one *CYP2C9* variant allele are at increased risk for bleeding. Compared with individuals with no variant alleles, the risk of warfarin-associated bleeding is almost 2-fold higher in *CYP2C9*2* or *CYP2C9*3* carriers.

TABLE 118-8 Frequencies of *CYP2C9* Genotypes and *VKORC1* Haplotypes in Different Populations and their Effect on Warfarin Dose Requirements

GENOTYPE/ HAPLOTYPE	FREQUENCY, %			DOSE REDUCTION COMPARED WITH WILD-TYPE
	CAUCASIANS	AFRICAN AMERICANS (A/A)	ASIANS (A)	
CYP2C9				
*1/*1	70	90	95	—
*1/*2	17	2	0	22
*1/*3	9	3	4	34
*2/*2	2	0	0	43
*2/*3	1	0	0	53
*3/*3	0	0	1	76
VKORC1				
Non-A/non-A	37	82	7	—
Non-A/A	45	12	30	26
A/A	18	6	63	50

Polymorphisms in *VKORC1* also can influence the anticoagulant response to warfarin. Several genetic variations of *VKORC1* are in strong linkage disequilibrium and have been designated as non-A haplotypes. *VKORC1* variants are more prevalent than variants of *CYP2C9*. Asians have the highest prevalence of *VKORC1* variants, followed by Caucasians and African Americans (Table 118-8). Polymorphisms in *VKORC1* likely explain 30% of the variability in warfarin dose requirements. Compared with *VKORC1* non-A/non-A homozygotes, the warfarin dose requirement decreases by 25 and 50% in A haplotype heterozygotes and homozygotes, respectively. These findings prompted the U.S. Food and Drug Administration (FDA) to amend the prescribing information for warfarin to indicate that lower initiation doses should be considered for patients with *CYP2C9* and *VKORC1* genetic variants. In addition to genotype data, other pertinent patient information has been incorporated into warfarin dosing algorithms. Although such algorithms help predict suitable warfarin doses, it remains unclear whether better dose identification improves patient outcome in terms of reducing hemorrhagic complications or recurrent thrombotic events.

In addition to genetic factors, the anticoagulant effect of warfarin is influenced by diet, drugs, and various disease states. Fluctuations in dietary vitamin K intake affect the activity of warfarin. A wide variety of drugs can alter absorption, clearance, or metabolism of warfarin. Because of the variability in the anticoagulant response to warfarin, coagulation monitoring is essential to ensure that a therapeutic response is obtained.

MONITORING Warfarin therapy is most often monitored using the prothrombin time, a test that is sensitive to reductions in the levels of prothrombin, factor VII, and factor X. The test is performed by adding thromboplastin, a reagent that contains tissue factor, phospholipid, and calcium, to citrated plasma and determining the time to clot formation. Thromboplastins vary in their sensitivity to reductions in the levels of the vitamin K–dependent clotting factors. Thus, less sensitive thromboplastins will trigger the administration of higher doses of warfarin to achieve a target prothrombin time. This is problematic because higher doses of warfarin increase the risk of bleeding.

The INR was developed to circumvent many of the problems associated with the prothrombin time. To calculate the INR, the patient's prothrombin time is divided by the mean normal prothrombin time, and this ratio is then multiplied by the international sensitivity index (ISI), which is an index of the sensitivity of the thromboplastin used for prothrombin time determination to reductions in the levels of the vitamin K–dependent clotting factors. Sensitive thromboplastins have an ISI near 1.0. Most current thromboplastins have ISI values that range from 0.9 to 1.4.

Although the INR has helped to standardize anticoagulant practice, problems persist. The precision of INR determination varies depending on reagent-coagulometer combinations. This leads to variability in the INR results. Also complicating INR determination is unreliable reporting of the ISI by thromboplastin manufacturers. Furthermore, every laboratory must establish the mean normal prothrombin time with each new batch of thromboplastin reagent. To accomplish this, the prothrombin time must be measured in fresh plasma samples from at least 20 healthy volunteers using the same coagulometer that is used for patient samples.

For most indications, warfarin is administered in doses that produce a target INR of 2.0–3.0. An exception is patients with mechanical heart valves, particularly those in the mitral position or older ball and cage valves in the aortic position, where a target INR of 2.5–3.5 is recommended. Studies in atrial fibrillation demonstrate an increased risk of cardioembolic stroke when the INR falls below 1.7 and an increase in bleeding with INR values >4.5. These findings highlight the fact that vitamin K antagonists have a narrow therapeutic window. In support of this concept, a study in patients receiving long-term warfarin therapy for unprovoked venous thromboembolism demonstrated a higher rate of recurrent venous thromboembolism with a target INR of 1.5–1.9 compared with a target INR of 2.0–3.0.

DOSING Warfarin is usually started at a dose of 5–10 mg. Lower doses are used for patients with *CYP2C9* or *VKORC1* polymorphisms, which affect the pharmacodynamics or pharmacokinetics of warfarin and render patients more sensitive to the drug. The dose is then titrated to achieve the desired target INR. Because of its delayed onset of action, patients with established thrombosis or those at high risk for thrombosis are given concomitant initial treatment with a rapidly acting parenteral anticoagulant, such as heparin, LMWH, or fondaparinux. Early prolongation of the INR reflects reduction in the functional levels of factor VII. Consequently, concomitant treatment with the parenteral anticoagulant should be continued until the INR has been therapeutic for at least 2 consecutive days. A minimum 5-day course of parenteral anticoagulation is recommended to ensure that the levels of factor Xa and prothrombin have been reduced into the therapeutic range with warfarin.

Because warfarin has a narrow therapeutic window, frequent coagulation monitoring is essential to ensure that a therapeutic anticoagulant response is maintained. Even patients with stable warfarin dose requirements should have their INR determined every 3–4 weeks although there are studies suggesting that less frequent monitoring is feasible. More frequent monitoring is necessary when new medications are introduced because so many drugs enhance or reduce the anticoagulant effects of warfarin.

SIDE EFFECTS Like all anticoagulants, the major side effect of warfarin is bleeding. A rare complication is skin necrosis. Warfarin crosses the placenta and can cause fetal abnormalities. Consequently, warfarin should not be used during pregnancy.

Bleeding At least half of the bleeding complications with warfarin occur when the INR exceeds the therapeutic range. Bleeding complications may be mild, such as epistaxis or hematuria, or more severe, such as retroperitoneal or gastrointestinal bleeding. Life-threatening intracranial bleeding can also occur.

To minimize the risk of bleeding, the INR should be maintained in the therapeutic range. In asymptomatic patients whose INR is between 3.5 and 10, warfarin should be withheld until the INR returns to the therapeutic range. If the INR is over 10, oral vitamin K can be administered at a dose of 2.5–5 mg, although there is no evidence that doing so reduces the bleeding risk. Higher doses of oral vitamin K (5–10 mg) produce more rapid reversal of the INR but may render patients temporarily resistant to warfarin when the drug is restarted.

Patients with serious bleeding need more aggressive treatment. These patients should be given 5–10 mg of vitamin K by slow IV infusion. Additional vitamin K should be given until the INR is in the normal range. Treatment with vitamin K should be supplemented with four-factor prothrombin complex concentrate, which contains all four vitamin K–dependent clotting proteins. Prothrombin complex concentrate normalizes the INR more rapidly than transfusion of fresh frozen plasma.

Warfarin-treated patients who experience bleeding when their INR is in the therapeutic range require investigation into the cause of the bleeding. Those with gastrointestinal or genitourinary bleeding often have an underlying lesion.

Skin Necrosis A rare complication of warfarin, skin necrosis usually is seen 2–5 days after initiation of therapy. Well-demarcated erythematous lesions form on the thighs, buttocks, breasts, or toes. Typically, the center of the lesion becomes progressively necrotic. Examination of skin biopsies taken from the border of these lesions reveals thrombi in the microvasculature.

Warfarin-induced skin necrosis is seen in patients with congenital or acquired deficiencies of protein C or protein S. Initiation of warfarin therapy in these patients produces a precipitous fall in plasma levels of proteins C or S, thereby eliminating this important anticoagulant pathway before warfarin exerts an antithrombotic effect through lowering of the functional levels of factor X and prothrombin. The resultant procoagulant state triggers thrombosis. Why the thrombosis is localized to the microvasculature of fatty tissues is unclear.

Treatment involves discontinuation of warfarin and reversal with vitamin K, if needed. An alternative anticoagulant, such as heparin or LMWH, should be given in patients with thrombosis. Protein C concentrate can be given to protein C–deficient patients to accelerate healing of the skin lesions; fresh-frozen plasma may be of value if protein C concentrate is unavailable and for those with protein S deficiency. Occasionally, skin grafting is necessary when there is extensive skin loss.

Because of the potential for skin necrosis, patients with known protein C or protein S deficiency require overlapping treatment with a parenteral anticoagulant when initiating warfarin therapy. Warfarin should be started in low doses in these patients, and the parenteral anticoagulant should be continued until the INR is therapeutic for at least 2–3 consecutive days. Alternatively, treatment with rivaroxaban or apixaban could be given, although there is limited information about their efficacy and safety in patients with severe protein C or S deficiency.

Pregnancy Warfarin crosses the placenta and can cause fetal abnormalities or bleeding. The fetal abnormalities include a characteristic embryopathy, which consists of nasal hypoplasia and stippled epiphyses. The risk of embryopathy is highest if warfarin is given in the first trimester of pregnancy. Central nervous system abnormalities can also occur with exposure to warfarin at any time during pregnancy. Finally, maternal administration of warfarin produces an anticoagulant effect in the fetus that can cause bleeding. This is of particular concern at delivery when trauma to the head during passage through the birth canal can lead to intracranial bleeding. Because of these potential problems, warfarin is contraindicated in pregnancy, particularly in the first and third trimesters. Instead, heparin, LMWH, or fondaparinux can be given during pregnancy for prevention or treatment of thrombosis.

Warfarin does not pass into the breast milk. Consequently, warfarin can safely be given to nursing mothers.

Special Problems Patients with a lupus anticoagulant and those who need urgent or elective surgery present special challenges. Although observational studies suggested that patients with thrombosis complicating the antiphospholipid antibody syndrome required higher intensity warfarin regimens to prevent recurrent thromboembolic events, two randomized trials showed that targeting an INR of 2.0–3.0 is as effective as higher intensity treatment and produces less bleeding. Monitoring warfarin therapy can be problematic in patients with antiphospholipid antibody syndrome if the lupus anticoagulant prolongs the baseline INR; factor X levels can be used instead of the INR in such patients.

There is no need to stop warfarin before procedures associated with a low risk of bleeding; these include dental cleaning, simple dental extraction, cataract surgery, or skin biopsy. For procedures associated with a moderate or high risk of bleeding, warfarin should be stopped 5 days before the procedure to allow the INR to return to normal levels. Patients at high risk for thrombosis, such as those with mechanical heart valves, can be bridged with once- or twice-daily SC injections of LMWH when the INR falls to <2.0. The last dose of LMWH should be given 12–24 h before the procedure, depending on whether LMWH is administered twice or once daily. After the procedure, treatment with warfarin can be restarted.

Direct Oral Anticoagulants

The direct oral anticoagulants (DOACs) include dabigatran, which inhibits thrombin, and rivaroxaban, apixaban, and edoxaban, which inhibit factor Xa. These drugs have a rapid onset and offset of action and have half-lives that permit once- or twice-daily administration. Designed to produce a predictable level of anticoagulation, the DOACs are more convenient to administer than warfarin because they are given in fixed doses without routine coagulation monitoring.

MECHANISM OF ACTION The DOACs are small molecules that bind reversibly to the active site of their target enzyme. **Table 118-9** summarizes the distinct pharmacologic properties of these agents.

INDICATIONS All four DOACs are licensed for stroke prevention in patients with nonvalvular atrial fibrillation, which encompasses patients without mechanical heart valves or severe rheumatic mitral valve disease, and for treatment of venous thromboembolism (VTE). Dabigatran, rivaroxaban, and apixaban are licensed for thromboprophylaxis after elective hip or knee arthroplasty; edoxaban is only licensed for this indication in Japan. Finally, low-dose rivaroxaban is licensed for use with aspirin for secondary prevention in patients with coronary or peripheral artery disease.

DOSING For prevention of stroke in patients with nonvalvular atrial fibrillation, rivaroxaban is given at a dosage of 20 mg once daily, with a reduction to 15 mg once daily in patients with a creatinine clearance of 15–49 mL/min; dabigatran is given at a dosage of 150 mg twice daily, with a reduction to 75 mg twice daily in those with a creatinine clearance of 15–30 mL/min; apixaban is given at a dosage of 5 mg twice daily, with a reduction to 2.5 mg twice daily for patients with at least two of the "ABC" criteria (i.e., *a*ge >80 years, *b*ody weight <60 kg, and *c*reatinine >1.5 g/dL); and edoxaban is given at a dosage of 60 mg once daily for patients with a creatinine clearance of 50–95 mL/min and with a

TABLE 118-9 Comparison of the Pharmacologic Properties of the Direct Oral Anticoagulants

CHARACTERISTIC	RIVAROXABAN	APIXABAN	EDOXABAN	DABIGATRAN
Target	Factor Xa	Factor Xa	Factor Xa	Thrombin
Prodrug	No	No	No	Yes
Bioavailability	80%	60%	50%	6%
Dosing	qd (bid)	bid	qd	bid (qd)
Half-life	7–11 h	12 h	9–11 h	12–17 h
Renal excretion	33% (66%)	25%	35%	80%
Interactions	3A4/P-gp	3A4/P-gp	P-gp	P-gp

Abbreviations: bid, twice a day; P-gp, P-glycoprotein; qd., once a day.

reduction to 30 mg once daily for patients with any one of the following criteria: creatinine clearance of 15–50 mL/min, body weight of 60 kg or less, or use of potent P-glycoprotein inhibitors, such as verapamil or quinidine. At doses of 15 or 20 mg once daily, rivaroxaban must be administered with food to enhance absorption. Apixaban and edoxaban can be given with or without food. Administration of dabigatran with food may reduce dyspepsia.

For treatment of VTE, dabigatran and edoxaban are started after patients have received at least a 5-day course of treatment with a parenteral anticoagulant such as LMWH; dabigatran is given at a dose of 150 mg twice daily provided the creatinine clearance is >30 mL/min, and the dosage regimen for edoxaban is identical to that used in patients with atrial fibrillation. In contrast, rivaroxaban and apixaban can be given in all-oral regimens; rivaroxaban is started at a dose of 15 mg twice daily for 21 days and is then reduced to 20 mg once daily thereafter, whereas apixaban is started at a dose of 10 mg twice daily for 7 days and is then reduced to 5 mg twice daily thereafter. For secondary VTE prevention, the dosage of apixaban can be lowered to 2.5 mg twice daily while the dose of rivaroxaban can be lowered to 10 mg once daily, doses that have safety profiles like those of placebo and aspirin, respectively.

Thromboprophylaxis after elective hip or knee replacement surgery is started after surgery and is often continued for 30 days in patients undergoing hip replacement and for 10–14 days in patients undergoing knee replacement. Dabigatran is given at a dose of 220 mg once daily, whereas rivaroxaban and apixaban are given at doses of 10 mg once daily and 2.5 mg twice daily, respectively. In lower risk patients undergoing hip or knee replacement surgery, a 5-day course of rivaroxaban followed by a 30-day course of aspirin at a dose of 81 mg daily appears to be as effective and safe as extended thromboprophylaxis with rivaroxaban.

For secondary prevention of adverse cardiac or limb events in patients with coronary or peripheral artery disease, rivaroxaban is given at a dose of 2.5 mg twice daily on top of aspirin (81 or 100 mg once daily).

MONITORING Although designed to be administered without routine monitoring, there are situations where determination of the anticoagulant activity of the new oral anticoagulants can be helpful. These include assessment of adherence, detection of accumulation or overdose, identification of bleeding mechanisms, and determination of activity prior to surgery, intervention, or reversal. For qualitative assessment of anticoagulant activity, the prothrombin time can be used for factor Xa inhibitors and the aPTT for dabigatran. Rivaroxaban and edoxaban prolong the prothrombin time more than apixaban. In fact, because apixaban has such a limited effect on the prothrombin time, anti–factor Xa assays are needed to assess its activity. The effect of the drugs on tests of coagulation varies depending on the time that the blood is drawn relative to the timing of the last dose of the drug and the reagents used to perform the tests. Chromogenic anti–factor Xa assays and the diluted thrombin clotting time or ecarin clot time with appropriate calibrators provide quantitative assays to measure the plasma levels of the factor Xa inhibitors and dabigatran, respectively.

SIDE EFFECTS Like all anticoagulants, bleeding is the most common side effect of the DOACs. The DOACS are associated with less intracranial bleeding than warfarin, but the higher dose regimens of dabigatran, rivaroxaban, and edoxaban are associated with more gastrointestinal bleeding.

Dyspepsia occurs in up to 10% of patients treated with dabigatran; this problem improves with time and can be minimized by administering the drug with food. Dyspepsia is rare with rivaroxaban, apixaban, and edoxaban.

PERIPROCEDURAL MANAGEMENT Like warfarin, the DOACs must be stopped before procedures associated with a moderate or high risk of bleeding. The drugs should be held for 1–2 days, or longer if renal function is impaired. Assessment of residual anticoagulant activity before procedures associated with a high bleeding risk is prudent.

MANAGEMENT OF BLEEDING With minor bleeding, withholding one or two doses of drug is usually sufficient. With more serious bleeding, the approach is similar to that with warfarin, except that vitamin K administration is of no benefit; the anticoagulant and any antiplatelet drugs should be withheld, the patient should be resuscitated with fluids and blood products as necessary, and the bleeding site should be identified and managed. Coagulation testing or measurement of DOAC level will determine the extent of anticoagulation, and renal function should be assessed so that the half-life of the drug can be calculated. Timing of the last dose of anticoagulant is important; oral activated charcoal may help prevent absorption of drug administered in the past 4 h, particularly in cases of overdose. If >24 h have elapsed since the last intake, the DOAC is unlikely to be responsible for the bleeding unless there is marked impairment of renal function.

Anticoagulant reversal should be considered if bleeding continues despite supportive measures or if the bleeding is life-threatening or occurs in a critical organ (e.g., intracranial) or in a closed space (e.g., the pericardium or retroperitoneum). Idarucizumab is licensed for dabigatran reversal in such patients or in those requiring urgent surgery or intervention. A humanized antibody fragment, idarucizumab, binds dabigatran with high affinity to form an essentially irreversible complex that is cleared by the kidneys. Idarucizumab is given intravenously as a 5-g bolus and is supplied in a box containing two 50-mL vials, each containing 2.5 g of idarucizumab. Idarucizumab rapidly reverses the anticoagulant effects of dabigatran and normalizes the aPTT, diluted thrombin time, or ecarin clot time.

Andexanet alfa is available for reversal of rivaroxaban, apixaban, and edoxaban. A recombinant variant of factor Xa without catalytic activity, andexanet serves as a decoy to sequester oral factor Xa inhibitors until they are cleared from the circulation. Low- or high-dose IV andexanet regimens are used. The low-dose regimen starts with a bolus of 400 mg followed by an infusion of 4 mg/min for up to 120 min, whereas the high-dose regimen starts with a bolus of 800 mg followed by an infusion of 8 mg/min for up to 120 min. The low-dose regimen is used for reversal of doses of rivaroxaban or apixaban of 10 mg or 5 mg or less, respectively, or for any dose of rivaroxaban or apixaban if the last dose was taken >8 h prior to presentation. The high-dose regimen is used to reverse rivaroxaban or apixaban doses over 10 and 5 mg, respectively, if the last dose was taken <8 h since presentation, or for reversal if the dose of rivaroxaban or apixaban or the timing of the last dose is unknown.

Andexanet alfa is expensive and is not available in all hospitals. Because of its cost, andexanet alfa is often reserved for reversal in patients with life-threatening bleeds such intracranial hemorrhage or bleeds into a closed space such as retroperitoneal or pericardial bleeds. If andexanet is unavailable, the results of prospective cohort studies suggest that four-factor prothrombin complex concentrate (25–50 units/kg) also is effective at restoring hemostasis. If there is continued bleeding, activated prothrombin complex concentrate (50 units/kg) or recombinant factor VIIa (90 μg/kg) can be considered.

Neither andexanet alfa nor four-factor prothrombin complex concentrate has been evaluated for reversal in patients requiring urgent surgery or intervention. Furthermore, andexanet alfa not only reverses oral factor Xa inhibitors but also reverses heparin and LMWH. This could be problematic in patients who require cardiac surgery or vascular surgery, procedures where heparin is used routinely. To circumvent this problem, most surgical procedures and interventions can be undertaken without reversal, and four-factor prothrombin complex concentrate can be given if necessary. For patients requiring surgery to stop bleeding such as those with a ruptured aortic aneurysm or with bleeding secondary to polytrauma, upfront four-factor prothrombin concentrate administration can be considered.

PREGNANCY As small molecules, the DOACs pass through the placenta. Consequently, these agents are contraindicated in pregnancy, and when used by women of childbearing potential, appropriate contraception is important. The DOACs should be avoided in nursing mothers.

FIBRINOLYTIC DRUGS

■ ROLE OF FIBRINOLYTIC THERAPY

Fibrinolytic drugs are used to degrade thrombi and are administered systemically or can be delivered via catheters directly into the substance of the thrombus. Systemic delivery is used for treatment of acute MI, acute ischemic stroke, and most cases of massive PE. The goal of therapy is to produce rapid thrombus dissolution, thereby restoring blood flow. In the coronary circulation, restoration of blood flow reduces morbidity and mortality rates by limiting myocardial damage, whereas in the cerebral circulation, rapid thrombus dissolution decreases the neuronal death and brain infarction that produce irreversible brain injury. For patients with massive PE, the goal of thrombolytic therapy is to restore pulmonary artery perfusion.

Peripheral arterial thrombi and thrombi in the proximal deep veins of the leg are most often treated using catheter-directed thrombolytic therapy. Catheters with multiple side holes can be used to enhance drug delivery. In some cases, intravascular devices that fragment and extract the thrombus are used to hasten treatment. These devices can be used alone or in conjunction with fibrinolytic drugs.

■ MECHANISM OF ACTION

Currently approved fibrinolytic agents include streptokinase; acylated plasminogen streptokinase activator complex (anistreplase); urokinase; recombinant tissue-type plasminogen activator (rtPA), which is also known as alteplase or activase; and two recombinant derivatives of rtPA, tenecteplase and reteplase. All these agents act by converting plasminogen, the zymogen, to plasmin, the active enzyme (**Fig. 118-7**). Plasmin then degrades the fibrin matrix of thrombi and produces soluble fibrin degradation products.

Endogenous fibrinolysis is regulated at two levels. Plasminogen activator inhibitors, particularly the type 1 form (PAI-1), prevent excessive plasminogen activation by regulating the activity of tPA and urokinase-type plasminogen activator (uPA). Once plasmin is generated, it is regulated by plasmin inhibitors, the most important of which is α_2-antiplasmin. The plasma concentration of plasminogen is twofold higher than that of α_2-antiplasmin. Consequently, with pharmacologic doses of plasminogen activators, the concentration of plasmin that is generated can exceed that of α_2-antiplasmin. In addition to degrading fibrin, unregulated plasmin can also degrade fibrinogen and other clotting factors. This process, which is known as the *systemic lytic state*, reduces the hemostatic potential of the blood and increases the risk of bleeding.

The endogenous fibrinolytic system is geared to localize plasmin generation to the fibrin surface. Both plasminogen and tPA bind to fibrin to form a ternary complex that promotes efficient plasminogen activation. In contrast to free plasmin, plasmin generated on the fibrin surface is relatively protected from inactivation by α_2-antiplasmin, a feature that promotes fibrin dissolution. Furthermore, C-terminal lysine residues, exposed as plasmin degrades fibrin, serve as binding sites for additional plasminogen and tPA molecules. This creates a positive feedback that enhances plasmin generation. When used pharmacologically, the various plasminogen activators capitalize on these mechanisms to a lesser or greater extent.

Plasminogen activators that preferentially activate fibrin-bound plasminogen are considered fibrin-specific. In contrast, nonspecific plasminogen activators do not discriminate between fibrin-bound and circulating plasminogen. Activation of circulating plasminogen results in the generation of unopposed plasmin that can trigger the systemic lytic state. Alteplase and its derivatives are fibrin-specific plasminogen activators, whereas streptokinase, anistreplase, and urokinase are nonspecific agents.

■ STREPTOKINASE

Unlike other plasminogen activators, streptokinase is not an enzyme and does not directly convert plasminogen to plasmin. Instead, streptokinase forms a 1:1 stoichiometric complex with plasminogen. Formation of this complex induces a conformational change in plasminogen that exposes its active site (**Fig. 118-8**). The streptokinase-plasminogen complex then converts additional plasminogen to plasmin.

Streptokinase has no affinity for fibrin, and the streptokinase-plasminogen complex activates both free and fibrin-bound plasminogen. Activation of circulating plasminogen generates sufficient amounts of plasmin to overwhelm α_2-antiplasmin. Unopposed plasmin not only degrades fibrin in the occlusive thrombus but also induces a systemic lytic state.

When given systemically to patients with acute MI, streptokinase reduces mortality. For this indication, the drug is usually given as an IV infusion of 1.5 million units over 30–60 min. Patients who receive streptokinase can develop antibodies against the drug, as can patients with prior streptococcal infection. These antibodies can reduce the effectiveness of streptokinase.

Allergic reactions occur in ~5% of patients treated with streptokinase. These may manifest as a rash, fever, chills, and rigors. Although anaphylactic reactions can occur, these are rare. Transient hypotension is common with streptokinase and has been attributed to plasmin-mediated release of bradykinin from kininogen. The hypotension usually responds to leg elevation and administration of IV fluids and low doses of vasopressors, such as dopamine or norepinephrine.

■ ANISTREPLASE

To generate this drug, streptokinase is combined with equimolar amounts of Lys-plasminogen, a plasmin-cleaved form of plasminogen

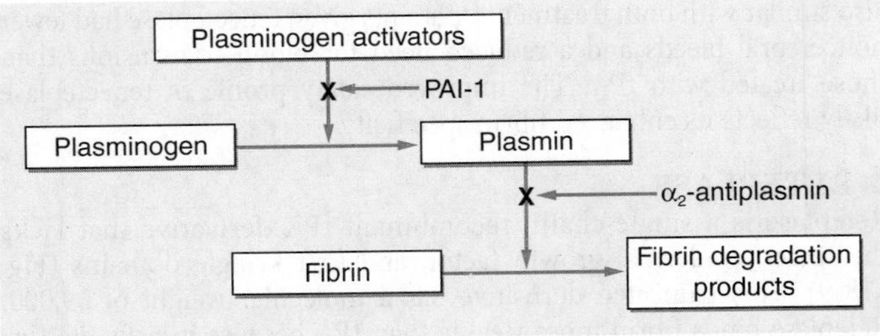

FIGURE 118-7 The fibrinolytic system and its regulation. Plasminogen activators convert plasminogen to plasmin. Plasmin then degrades fibrin into soluble fibrin degradation products. The system is regulated at two levels. Type 1 plasminogen activator inhibitor (PAI-1) regulates the plasminogen activators, whereas α_2-antiplasmin serves as the major inhibitor of plasmin.

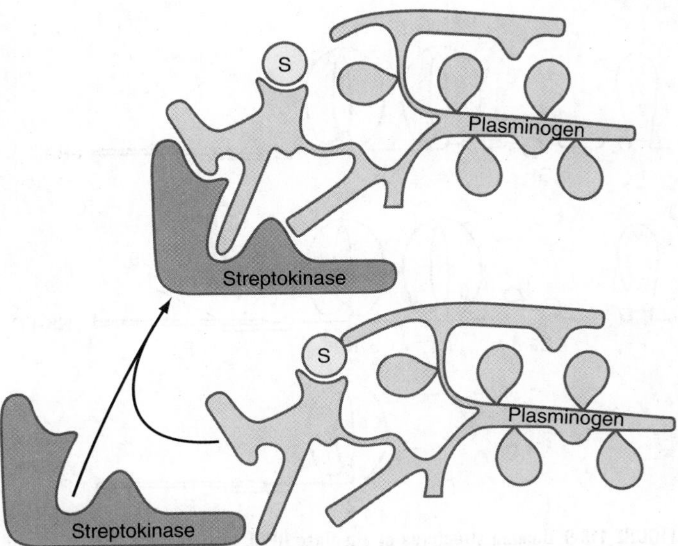

FIGURE 118-8 Mechanism of action of streptokinase. Streptokinase binds to plasminogen and induces a conformational change in plasminogen that exposes its active site. The streptokinase/plasmin(ogen) complex then serves as the activator of additional plasminogen.

with a Lys residue at its N terminal. The active site of Lys-plasminogen that is exposed upon combination with streptokinase is then masked with an anisoyl group. After IV infusion, the anisoyl group is slowly removed by deacylation, giving the complex a half-life of ~100 min. This allows drug administration via a single bolus infusion.

Although it is more convenient to administer, anistreplase offers few mechanistic advantages over streptokinase. Like streptokinase, anistreplase does not distinguish between fibrin-bound and circulating plasminogen. Consequently, it too produces a systemic lytic state. Likewise, allergic reactions and hypotension are just as frequent with anistreplase as they are with streptokinase.

When anistreplase was compared with alteplase in patients with acute MI, reperfusion was obtained more rapidly with alteplase than with anistreplase. Improved reperfusion was associated with a trend toward better clinical outcomes and reduced mortality rate with alteplase. These results and the high cost of anistreplase have dampened the enthusiasm for its use.

UROKINASE

Urokinase is a two-chain serine protease derived from cultured fetal kidney cells with a molecular weight of 34,000. Urokinase converts plasminogen to plasmin directly by cleaving the Arg560-Val561 bond. Unlike streptokinase, urokinase is not immunogenic and allergic reactions are rare. Urokinase produces a systemic lytic state because it does not discriminate between fibrin-bound and circulating plasminogen.

Despite many years of use, urokinase has never been systemically evaluated for coronary thrombolysis. Instead, urokinase is often employed for catheter-directed lysis of thrombi in the deep veins or the peripheral arteries. Because of production problems, urokinase is no longer available.

ALTEPLASE

A recombinant form of single-chain tPA, alteplase has a molecular weight of 68,000. Alteplase is rapidly converted into its two-chain form by plasmin. Although single- and two-chain forms of tPA have equivalent activity in the presence of fibrin, in its absence, single-chain tPA has tenfold lower activity.

Alteplase consists of five discrete domains (**Fig. 118-9**); the N-terminal A chain of two-chain alteplase contains four of these domains. Residues 4 through 50 make up the finger domain, a region that resembles the finger domain of fibronectin; residues 50 through 87 are homologous with epidermal growth factor, whereas residues 92 through 173 and 180 through 261, which have homology to the kringle domains of plasminogen, are designated as the first and second kringle, respectively. The fifth alteplase domain is the protease domain; it is located on the C-terminal B chain of two-chain alteplase.

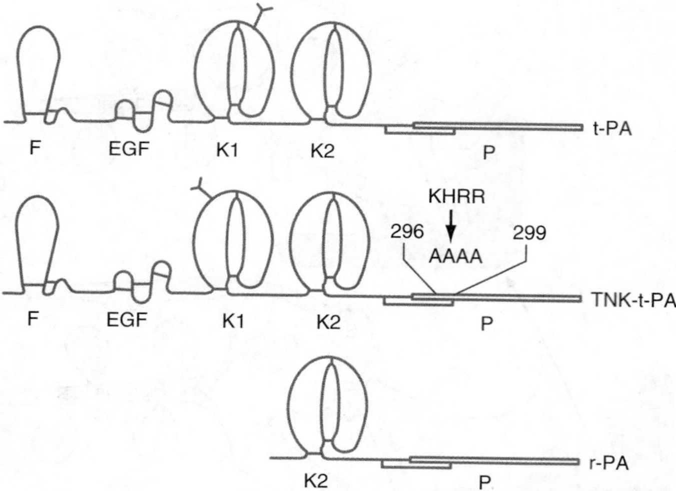

FIGURE 118-9 Domain structures of alteplase (tPA), tenecteplase (TNK-tPA), and reteplase (r-PA). The finger (F), epidermal growth factor (EGF), first and second kringles (K1 and K2, respectively), and protease (P) domains are illustrated. The glycosylation site (Y) on K1 has been repositioned in tenecteplase to endow it with a longer half-life. In addition, a tetra-alanine substitution in the protease domain renders tenecteplase resistant to type 1 plasminogen activator inhibitor (PAI-1) inhibition. Reteplase is a truncated variant that lacks the F, EGF, and K1 domains.

The interaction of alteplase with fibrin is mediated by the finger domain and, to a lesser extent, by the second kringle domain. The affinity of alteplase for fibrin is considerably higher than that for fibrinogen. Consequently, the catalytic efficiency of plasminogen activation by alteplase is two to three orders of magnitude higher in the presence of fibrin than in the presence of fibrinogen. This phenomenon helps to localize plasmin generation to the fibrin surface.

Although alteplase preferentially activates plasminogen in the presence of fibrin, alteplase is not as fibrin-selective as was first predicted. Its fibrin specificity is limited because like fibrin, (DD)E, the major soluble degradation product of cross-linked fibrin, binds alteplase and plasminogen with high affinity. Consequently, (DD)E is as potent as fibrin as a stimulator of plasminogen activation by alteplase. Whereas plasmin generated on the fibrin surface results in thrombolysis, plasmin generated on the surface of circulating (DD)E degrades fibrinogen. Fibrinogen degradation results in the accumulation of fragment X, a high-molecular-weight clottable fibrinogen degradation product. Incorporation of fragment X into hemostatic plugs formed at sites of vascular injury renders them susceptible to lysis. This phenomenon may contribute to alteplase-induced bleeding.

A trial comparing alteplase with streptokinase for treatment of patients with acute MI demonstrated significantly lower mortality with alteplase than with streptokinase, although the absolute difference was small. The greatest benefit was seen in patients age <75 years with anterior MI who presented <6 h after symptom onset.

For treatment of acute MI or acute ischemic stroke, alteplase is given as an IV infusion over 60–90 min. The total dose of alteplase usually ranges from 90 to 100 mg. Allergic reactions and hypotension are rare, and alteplase is not immunogenic.

TENECTEPLASE

Tenecteplase is a genetically engineered variant of tPA and was designed to have a longer half-life than tPA and to be resistant to inactivation by PAI-1. To prolong its half-life, a new glycosylation site was added to the first kringle domain (Fig. 118-9). Because addition of this extra carbohydrate side chain reduced fibrin affinity, the existing glycosylation site on the first kringle domain was removed. To render the molecule resistant to inhibition by PAI-1, a tetra-alanine substitution was introduced at residues 296–299 in the protease domain, the region responsible for the interaction of tPA with PAI-1.

Tenecteplase is more fibrin-specific than tPA. Although both agents bind to fibrin with similar affinity, the affinity of tenecteplase for (DD)E is significantly lower than that of tPA. Consequently, (DD)E does not stimulate systemic plasminogen activation by tenecteplase to the same extent as tPA. As a result, tenecteplase produces less fibrinogen degradation than tPA.

For coronary thrombolysis, tenecteplase is given as a single IV bolus. In a large phase III trial that enrolled >16,000 patients, the 30-day mortality rate with single-bolus tenecteplase was similar to that with accelerated-dose tPA. Although rates of intracranial hemorrhage were also similar with both treatments, patients given tenecteplase had fewer noncerebral bleeds and a reduced need for blood transfusions than those treated with tPA. The improved safety profile of tenecteplase likely reflects its enhanced fibrin specificity.

RETEPLASE

Reteplase is a single-chain, recombinant tPA derivative that lacks the finger, epidermal growth factor, and first kringle domains (Fig. 118-9). This truncated derivative has a molecular weight of 39,000. Reteplase binds fibrin more weakly than tPA because it lacks the finger domain. Because it is produced in *Escherichia coli*, reteplase is not glycosylated. This endows it with a plasma half-life longer than that of tPA. Consequently, reteplase is given as two IV boluses, which are separated by 30 min. Clinical trials have demonstrated that reteplase is at least as effective as streptokinase for treatment of acute MI, but the agent is not superior to tPA.

CONCLUSIONS AND FUTURE DIRECTIONS

Thrombosis involves a complex interplay among the vessel wall, platelets, the coagulation system, and the fibrinolytic pathways. Activation of coagulation also triggers inflammatory pathways that may exacerbate thrombosis. A better understanding of the biochemistry of blood coagulation and advances in structure-based drug design have identified new targets and resulted in the development of novel antithrombotic drugs. Well-designed clinical trials have provided detailed information on which drugs to use and when to use them. Despite these advances, however, thromboembolic disorders remain a major cause of morbidity and mortality. Therefore, the search for better and safer targets continues.

FURTHER READING

Abdelaziz HK et al: Aspirin for primary prevention of cardiovascular events. J Am Coll Cardiol 73:2915, 2019.

Alexopoulos D et al: P2Y12 inhibitors for the treatment of acute coronary syndrome patients undergoing percutaneous coronary intervention: current understanding and outcomes. Expert Rev Cardiovasc Ther 17:717, 2019.

Chan NC et al: Evolving treatments for arterial and venous thrombosis: Role of the direct oral anticoagulants. *Cir Res* 118:1409, 2016.

Greinacher A et al: Thrombotic thrombocytopenia after ChAdOx1 nCov-19 vaccination. N Engl J Med 384:2092, 2021.

Hao C et al: Low molecular weight heparins and their clinical applications. Prog Mol Biol Transl Sci 163:21, 2019.

Phipps MS, Cronin CA: Management of acute ischemic stroke. BMJ 368:l6983, 2020.

Prince M, Wenham T: Heparin-induced thrombocytopaenia. Postgrad Med J 94:453, 2018.

Rivera-Caravaca JM et al: Treatment strategies for patients with atrial fibrillation and anticoagulant-associated intracranial hemorrhage: An overview of the pharmacotherapy. Expert Opin Pharmacother 21:1867, 2020.

Satoh K et al: Recent advances in the understanding of thrombosis. Arterioscler Thromb Vasc Biol 39:e159, 2019.

Samuelson BT, Cuker A: Measurement and reversal of the direct oral anticoagulants. Blood Rev 31:77, 2017.

Scully M et al: Pathologic antibodies to platelet factor 4 after ChAdOx1 nCoV-19 vaccination. N Engl J Med 384:2202, 2021.

Steffel J et al: The COMPASS Trial: Net clinical benefit of low-dose rivaroxaban plus aspirin as compared with aspirin in patients with chronic vascular disease. Circulation 142:40, 2020.

Section 1 Basic Considerations in Infectious Diseases

119 Approach to the Patient with an Infectious Disease

Neeraj K. Surana, Dennis L. Kasper

HISTORICAL PERSPECTIVE

The origins of the field of infectious diseases are humble. The notion that communicable diseases were due to a *miasma* ("bad air") can be traced back to at least the mid-sixteenth century. Not until the work of Louis Pasteur and Robert Koch in the late nineteenth century was there credible evidence supporting the germ theory of disease—i.e., that microorganisms are the direct cause of infections. In contrast to this relatively slow start, the twentieth century saw remarkable advances in the field of infectious diseases, and the etiologic agents of numerous infectious diseases were soon identified. Furthermore, the discovery of antibiotics and the advent of vaccines against some of the most deadly and debilitating infections greatly altered the landscape of human health. Indeed, the twentieth century saw the elimination of smallpox, one of the great scourges in the history of humanity. These remarkable successes prompted Sir Frank MacFarlane Burnet, a noted immunologist and Nobel laureate, to write in a 1962 publication entitled *Natural History of Infectious Diseases*: "In many ways one can think of the middle of the twentieth century as the end of one of the most important social revolutions in history, the virtual elimination of infectious disease." Professor Burnet was not alone in this view. Robert Petersdorf, a renowned infectious disease expert and former editor of this textbook, wrote in 1978 that "even with my great personal loyalties to infectious diseases, I cannot conceive a need for 309 more [graduating trainees in infectious diseases] unless they spend their time culturing each other." Given the enormous growth of interest in the microbiome in the past 15 years, Dr. Petersdorf's statement might have been ironically clairvoyant, although he could have had no idea what was in store for humanity, with an onslaught of new, emerging, and reemerging infectious diseases.

Clearly, even with all the advances of the twentieth century, infectious diseases continue to represent a formidable challenge for patients and physicians alike. Furthermore, during the latter half of the century, several chronic diseases were demonstrated to be directly or indirectly caused by infectious microbes; perhaps the most notable examples are the associations of *Helicobacter pylori* with peptic ulcer disease and gastric carcinoma, human papillomavirus with cervical cancer, and hepatitis B and C viruses with liver cancer. In fact, ~16% of all malignancies are now known to be associated with an infectious cause. In addition, numerous emerging and reemerging infectious diseases continue to have a dire impact on global health: HIV/AIDS, SARS-CoV-2, Ebola, and Zika are but a few examples. The fear of weaponizing pathogens for bioterrorism is ever present and poses a potentially enormous threat to public health. Moreover, escalating antimicrobial resistance in clinically relevant microbes (e.g., carbapenem-resistant Enterobacteriaceae and *Acinetobacter* spp., *Candida auris*, drug-resistant *Mycobacterium tuberculosis*, and vancomycin-resistant enterococci) signifies that the administration of antimicrobial agents—once thought to be a panacea—requires appropriate stewardship. For all these reasons, infectious diseases continue to exert grim effects on individual patients as well as on international public health. Even with all the successes of the past century, physicians must be as thoughtful about infectious diseases now as they were at the beginning of the twentieth century.

GLOBAL CONSIDERATIONS

Infectious diseases remain the second leading cause of death worldwide. Although the rate of infectious disease–related deaths has decreased dramatically over the past 25 years, there were still 10.3 million such deaths in 2017 (**Fig. 119-1*A***). These deaths disproportionately affect children <1 year of age, adults older than 70 years, and persons living in low- and middle-income countries (**Fig. 119-1*B* and 119-1*C*; Chap. 474**); in 2017, ~18% of all deaths worldwide were related to infectious diseases, with a rate as high as ~58% in sub-Saharan Africa.

Given that infectious diseases are still a major cause of global mortality, understanding the local epidemiology of disease is critically important in evaluating patients. Diseases such as HIV/AIDS have decimated sub-Saharan Africa, with HIV-infected adults representing 20–23% of the total population in countries like South Africa, Botswana, and Lesotho. Moreover, drug-resistant tuberculosis is rampant throughout the former Soviet-bloc countries, India, China, and South Africa. The ready availability of this type of information allows physicians to develop appropriate differential diagnoses and treatment plans for individual patients. Programs such as the Global Burden of Disease seek to quantify human losses (e.g., deaths, disability-adjusted life-years) due to diseases by age, sex, and country over time; these data not only help inform local, national, and international health policy but can also help guide local medical decision-making.

Even though some diseases (e.g., pandemic influenza, Middle East respiratory syndrome) are seemingly geographically restricted, the increasing ease of rapid worldwide travel has raised concern about their swift spread around the globe. Indeed, human migration has historically been the source of epidemics: *Yersinia pestis* spread along trade routes in the fourteenth century, Native American populations were devastated by diseases such as smallpox and measles that were imported by European explorers in the fifteenth and sixteenth centuries, military maneuvers helped facilitate the spread of the 1918 influenza pandemic, and religious pilgrimages (e.g., the Hajj) provide the means for worldwide dissemination of diseases. The continued effects of global travel on the spread of infectious diseases are perhaps best highlighted by the SARS-CoV-2 pandemic (**Chap. 199**). Although this virus was first identified in Wuhan, China, it quickly spread across the globe and brought an abrupt end to virtually all travel and commerce throughout the world, plunging economies into a deep recession, and resulting at one point in over half the world's population living under stay-at-home orders. Not only can travelers carry person-to-person transmitted infections (e.g., influenza, HIV) anywhere in the world, but they can also introduce vector-borne infections to new geographic areas (e.g., chikungunya and Zika viruses) and contribute to the worldwide spread of multidrug-resistant organisms. The world's increasing interconnectedness has profound implications not only for the global economy but also for medicine and the spread of infectious diseases.

UNDERSTANDING THE MICROBIOTA

Normal, healthy humans are colonized with ~50 trillion bacteria as well as countless viruses, fungi, and archaea; taken together, these microorganisms outnumber human cells by ~10 times in the human body (**Chap. 471**). The major reservoir of these microbes is the gastrointestinal tract, but substantial numbers of microbes live in the female genital tract, the oral cavity, and the nasopharynx. There is increasing interest in the skin and lungs as sites where microbial colonization might be highly relevant to the biology and disease susceptibility of the host. These commensal organisms provide the host with myriad benefits, from aiding in metabolism to shaping the immune system. With regard to infectious diseases, the vast majority of infections are caused by organisms that are part of the normal microbiota (e.g., *Staphylococcus aureus*, *Streptococcus pneumoniae*, *Pseudomonas aeruginosa*), with relatively few infections due to organisms that are strictly pathogens (e.g., *Neisseria gonorrhoeae*, rabies virus). Perhaps it is not surprising that a general understanding of the microbiota is essential in the evaluation of infectious diseases.

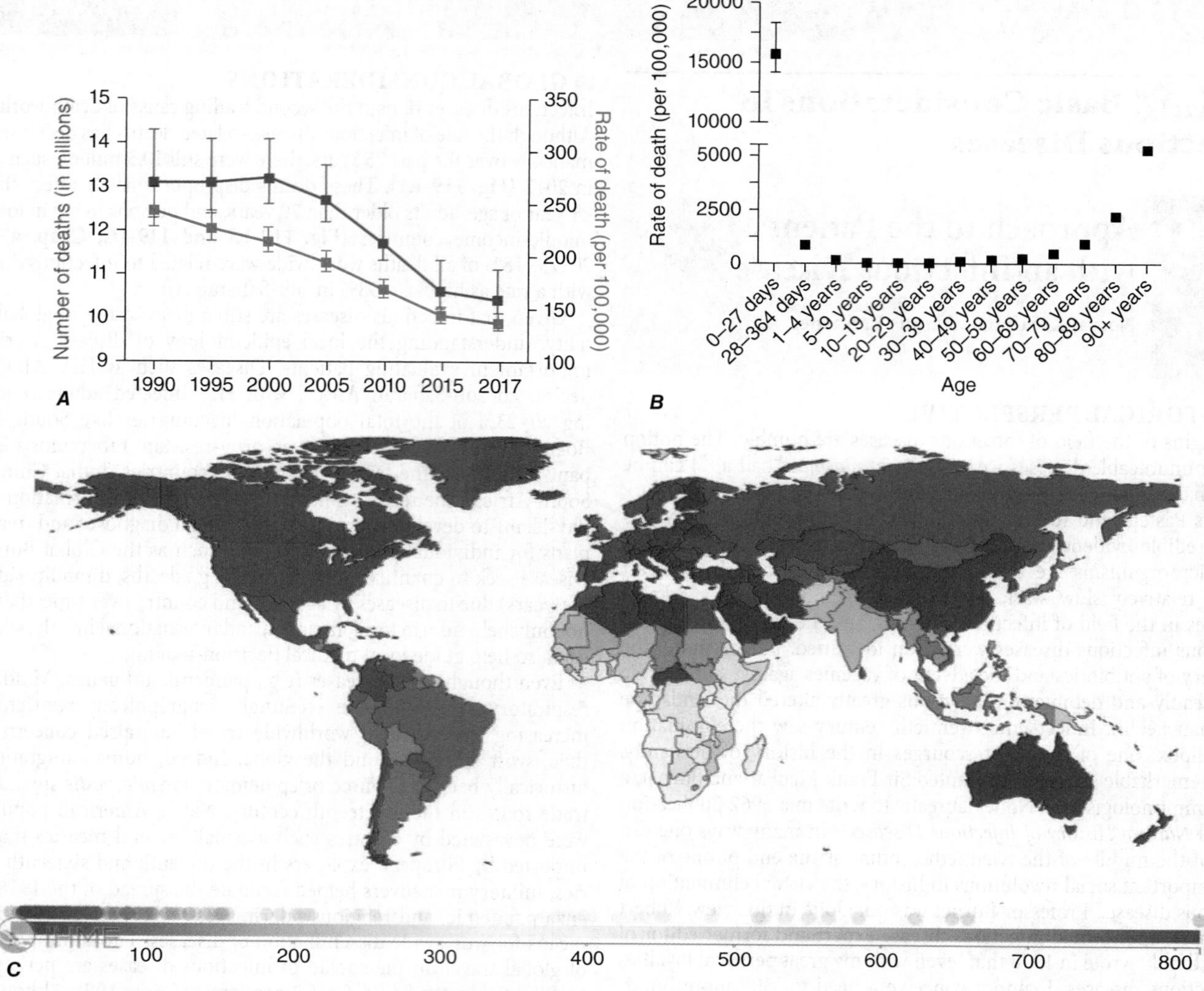

FIGURE 119-1 Magnitude of infectious disease–related deaths globally. ***A.*** The absolute number (*blue line; left axis*) and rate (*red line; right axis*) of infectious disease–related deaths throughout the world since 1990. ***B.*** Age-specific rates of infectious disease–related deaths in 2017. In both ***A*** and ***B***, the charts depict the mean estimate and 95% uncertainty intervals. ***C.*** A map depicting country-specific data for the rate of total deaths that were attributable to communicable, maternal, neonatal, and nutritional disorders in 2017. *(Source: Global Burden of Disease Study, Institute for Health Metrics and Evaluation.)*

Individuals' microbiotas have a major impact on their susceptibility to infectious diseases and even their responses to vaccines. Site-specific knowledge of the indigenous microbiota may facilitate appropriate interpretation of culture results, aid in selection of empirical antimicrobial therapy based on the likely causative agents, and provide additional impetus for rational antibiotic use to minimize the untoward effects of these drugs on the "beneficial" microbes that inhabit the body.

WHEN TO CONSIDER AN INFECTIOUS ETIOLOGY

The title of this chapter may appear to presuppose that the physician knows when a patient has an infectious disease. In reality, this chapter can serve only as a guide to the evaluation of a patient in whom an infectious disease is a possibility. Once a specific diagnosis is made, the reader should consult the subsequent chapters that deal with specific microorganisms in detail. The challenge for the physician is to recognize which patients may have an infectious disease as opposed to some other underlying disorder. This task is greatly complicated by the fact that infections have an infinite range of presentations, from acute life-threatening conditions (e.g., meningococcemia) to chronic diseases of varying severity (e.g., *H. pylori*–associated peptic ulcer disease) to no symptoms at all (e.g., latent *M. tuberculosis* infection). While it is impossible to generalize about a presentation that encompasses all infections, common findings in the history, physical examination, and basic laboratory testing often suggest that the patient either has an infectious disease or should be more closely evaluated for one. This chapter focuses on these common findings and how they may direct the ongoing evaluation of the patient.

APPROACH TO THE PATIENT

Infectious Disease

See also Chap. 122.

HISTORY

As in all of medicine, a complete and thorough history is paramount in the evaluation of a patient with a possible infectious disease. The history is critical for developing a focused differential diagnosis and for guiding the physical exam and initial diagnostic testing. Although a detailing of all the elements of a history is beyond the scope of this chapter, specific components relevant to infectious diseases require particular attention. In general, these aspects focus on two areas: (1) an exposure history that may identify microorganisms with which the patient may have come into contact and (2) host-specific factors that may predispose to the development of an infection.

***Exposure History* • History of infections or exposure to drug-resistant microbes** Information about a patient's previous infections, with the associated microbial susceptibility profiles, is very helpful in determining possible etiologic agents. Specifically, knowing whether a patient has a history of infection with drug-resistant organisms (e.g., methicillin-resistant *S. aureus*, vancomycin-resistant *Enterococcus* species, enteric organisms that produce an extended-spectrum β-lactamase or carbapenemase) or may have been exposed to drug-resistant microbes (e.g., during a recent stay in a hospital, nursing home, or long-term acute-care facility) may alter the choice of empirical antibiotics. For example, a patient presenting with sepsis who is known to have a history of invasive infection with a multidrug-resistant isolate of *P. aeruginosa* should be treated empirically with an antimicrobial regimen that will cover this strain.

Social history Although the social history taken by physicians is often limited to inquiries about a patient's alcohol and tobacco use, a complete social history can offer a number of clues to the underlying diagnosis. Knowing whether the patient has any high-risk behaviors (e.g., unsafe sexual behaviors, intravenous [IV] drug use), potential hobby-associated exposures (e.g., avid gardening, with possible *Sporothrix schenckii* exposure), or occupational exposures (e.g., increased risk for *M. tuberculosis* exposure in funeral service workers) can facilitate diagnosis. The importance of the social history is exemplified by a case in 2009 in which a laboratory researcher died of a *Y. pestis* infection acquired during his work; although this patient had visited both an outpatient clinic and an emergency department, his records at both sites failed to include his occupation—information that potentially could have led quickly to appropriate treatment and infection control measures.

Dietary habits Because certain pathogens are associated with specific dietary habits, inquiring about a patient's diet can provide insight into possible exposures. For example, Shiga toxin–producing strains of *Escherichia coli*, and *Toxoplasma gondii* are associated with the consumption of raw or undercooked meat; *Salmonella typhimurium*, *Listeria monocytogenes*, and *Mycobacterium bovis* with unpasteurized milk; *Leptospira* species, parasites, and enteric bacteria with unpurified water; and *Vibrio* species, norovirus, helminths, and protozoa with raw seafood.

Animal exposures Because animals are often important vectors of infectious diseases, patients should be asked about exposures to any animals, including contact with their own pets, visits to petting zoos, or random encounters (e.g., home rodent infestation). For example, dogs can carry ticks that serve as agents for the transmission of several infectious diseases, including Lyme disease, Rocky Mountain spotted fever, and ehrlichiosis. Cats are associated with *Bartonella henselae* infection, reptiles with *Salmonella* infection, rodents with leptospirosis, and rabbits with tularemia **(Chap. 141)**.

Travel history Attention should be paid to both international and domestic travel. Fever in a patient who has recently returned from abroad significantly broadens the differential diagnosis **(Chap. 124)**; even a remote history of international travel may reflect patients' exposure to infections with pathogens such as *M. tuberculosis* or *Strongyloides stercoralis*. Similarly, domestic travel may have exposed patients to pathogens that are not normally found in their local environment and therefore may not routinely be considered in the differential diagnosis. For example, a patient who has recently visited California or Martha's Vineyard may have been exposed to *Coccidioides immitis* or *Francisella tularensis*, respectively. Beyond simply identifying locations that a patient may have visited, the physician needs to delve deeper to learn what kinds of activities and behaviors the patient engaged in during travel (e.g., the types of food and sources of water consumed, freshwater swimming, animal exposures) and whether the patient had the necessary immunizations and/or took the necessary prophylactic medications prior to travel; these additional exposures, which the patient may not think to report without specific prompting, are as important as exposures during a patient's routine daily living.

Host-Specific Factors Because many opportunistic infections (e.g., with *Pneumocystis jirovecii*, *Aspergillus* species, or JC virus) affect primarily immunocompromised patients, it is of vital importance to determine the immune status of the patient. Defects in the immune system may be due to an underlying disease (e.g., malignancy, HIV infection, malnutrition), a medication (e.g., chemotherapy, glucocorticoids, monoclonal antibodies to components of the immune system), a treatment modality (e.g., total body irradiation, splenectomy), or a primary immunodeficiency. The type of infection for which the patient is at increased risk varies with the specific type of immune defect. In concert with determining whether a patient is immunocompromised for any reason, the physician should review the immunization record to ensure that the patient is adequately protected against vaccine-preventable diseases **(Chap. 123)**.

PHYSICAL EXAMINATION

Like the history, a thorough physical examination is crucial in evaluating patients with an infectious disease. Some elements of the physical exam (e.g., skin, lymphatics) that are often performed in a cursory manner as a result of the ever-increasing pace of medical practice may help identify the underlying diagnosis. Moreover, serial exams are critical since new findings may appear as the illness progresses. A description of all the elements of a physical exam is beyond the scope of this chapter, but the following components have particular relevance to infectious diseases.

Vital Signs Given that elevations in temperature are often a hallmark of infection, paying close attention to the temperature may be of value in diagnosing an infectious disease. The idea that 37°C (98.6°F) is the normal human body temperature dates back to the nineteenth century and was initially based on axillary measurements. Rectal temperatures more accurately reflect the core body temperature and are 0.4°C (0.7°F) and 0.8°C (1.4°F) higher than oral and axillary temperatures, respectively. This idea of a "normal" body temperature does not take into account the fact that temperatures tend to be higher later in the day, in women, and in younger people. Moreover, the average body temperature seems to have dropped ~0.03°C every decade since the early 1800s to a new normal of ~36.7°C. Although the definition of fever varies greatly throughout the medical literature, the most common definition, which is based on studies defining fever of unknown origin **(Chap. 20)**, uses a core temperature ≥38.3°C (≥101°F). Although fever is very commonly associated with infection, it is also documented in many other diseases **(Chap. 18)**. For every 1°C (1.8°F) increase in core temperature, the heart rate typically rises by 15–20 beats/min. **Table 119-1** lists infections that are associated with relative bradycardia (*Faget's sign*), where patients have a lower heart rate than might be expected for a given body temperature. Although this pulse–temperature dissociation is not highly sensitive or specific for establishing a diagnosis, it is potentially useful in low-resource settings given its ready availability and simplicity.

Lymphatics There are ~600 lymph nodes throughout the body, and infections are an important cause of lymphadenopathy. A physical examination should include evaluation of lymph nodes in multiple regions (e.g., popliteal, inguinal, epitrochlear, axillary, multiple cervical regions), with notation of the location, size (normal, <1 cm), presence or absence of tenderness, and consistency (soft, firm, or rubbery) and of whether the nodes are matted (i.e., connected and moving together). Nodes that are small and firm can also be described as "shotty," referring to the size and consistency of buckshot pellets. Of note, palpable epitrochlear nodes are always pathologic. Of patients presenting with lymphadenopathy, 75% have localized findings, and the remaining 25% have generalized lymphadenopathy (i.e., that involving more than one anatomic region). Localized lymphadenopathy in the head and neck region is

TABLE 119-1 Causes of Relative Bradycardia

Infectious Causes	
Intracellular organisms	
Gram-negative bacteria	*Salmonella typhi* *Francisella tularensis* *Brucella* spp. *Coxiella burnetii* (Q fever) *Leptospira interrogans* *Legionella pneumophila* *Mycoplasma pneumoniae*
Tick-borne organisms	*Rickettsia* spp. *Orientia tsutsugamushi* (scrub typhus) *Babesia* spp.
Other	*Corynebacterium diphtheriae* *Plasmodium* spp. (malaria)
Viruses/viral infections	Yellow fever virus Dengue virus Viral hemorrhagic fevers[a] Viral myocarditis
Noninfectious Causes	
	Drug fever Beta blocker use Central nervous system lesions Malignant lymphoma Factitious fever

[a]Primarily early in the course of infection with Marburg or Ebola virus.

found in 55% of patients, inguinal lymphadenopathy in 14%, and axillary lymphadenopathy in 5%. Determining whether the patient has generalized versus localized lymphadenopathy can help narrow the differential diagnosis, as various infections present differently.

Skin The fact that many infections have cutaneous manifestations gives the skin examination particular importance in the evaluation of patients (**Chaps. 19, 58, 129, and A1**). It is important to perform a complete skin exam, with attention to both front and back. Specific rashes are often extremely helpful in narrowing the differential diagnosis of an infection (**Chaps. 19 and A1**). In numerous anecdotal instances, patients in the intensive care unit have had "fever of unknown origin" that was actually due to unrecognized pressure ulcers. Moreover, close examination of the distal extremities for splinter hemorrhages, Janeway lesions, or Osler's nodes may yield evidence of endocarditis or other causes of septic emboli.

Foreign Bodies As previously mentioned, many infections are caused by members of the indigenous microbiota. These infections typically occur when these microbes escape their normal habitat and enter a new one. Thus, maintenance of epithelial barriers is one of the most important mechanisms in protection against infection. However, hospitalization of patients is often associated with breaches of these barriers—e.g., due to placement of IV lines, surgical drains, or tubes (e.g., endotracheal tubes and Foley catheters) that allow microorganisms to localize in sites to which they normally would not have access (**Chap. 142**). Accordingly, knowing what lines, tubes, and drains are in place is helpful in ascertaining what body sites might be infected.

DIAGNOSTIC TESTING

Laboratory and radiologic testing has advanced greatly over the past few decades and has become an important component in the evaluation of patients. The dramatic increase in the number of serologic diagnostics, antigen tests, and molecular diagnostics available to the physician has, in fact, revolutionized medical care. However, all of these tests should be viewed as adjuncts to the history and physical examination—not a replacement for them. The selection of initial tests should be based directly on the patient's history and physical exam findings. Moreover, diagnostic testing should generally be limited to those conditions that are reasonably likely and treatable, important in terms of public health considerations, and/or capable of providing a definitive diagnosis that will consequently limit other testing.

White Blood Cell (WBC) Count Elevations in the WBC count are often associated with infection, though many viral infections are associated with leukopenia. It is important to assess the WBC differential, given that different classes of microbes are associated with various leukocyte types. For example, bacteria are associated with an increase in polymorphonuclear neutrophils, often with elevated levels of earlier developmental forms such as bands; viruses are associated with an increase in lymphocytes; and certain parasites are associated with an increase in eosinophils. **Table 119-2** lists the major infectious causes of eosinophilia.

Inflammatory Markers The erythrocyte sedimentation rate (ESR) and the C-reactive protein (CRP) level are indirect and direct measures of the acute-phase response, respectively, that can be used to assess a patient's general level of inflammation. Moreover, these markers can be followed serially over time to monitor disease progress/resolution. It is noteworthy that the ESR changes relatively slowly, and its measurement more often than weekly usually is not useful; in contrast, CRP concentrations change rapidly, and daily measurements can be useful in the appropriate context. Although these markers are sensitive indicators of inflammation, neither is very specific. An extremely elevated ESR (>100 mm/h) has a 90% predictive value for a serious underlying disease (**Table 119-3**). Work is ongoing to identify other potentially useful inflammatory markers (e.g., procalcitonin, serum amyloid A protein); however, their clinical utility requires further validation.

Analysis of Cerebrospinal Fluid (CSF) Assessment of CSF is critical for patients with suspected meningitis or encephalitis. An opening pressure should always be recorded, and fluid should routinely be sent for cell counts, Gram's stain and culture, and determination of glucose and protein levels. A CSF Gram's stain typically requires $>10^5$ bacteria/mL for reliable positivity; its specificity approaches 100%. **Table 119-4** lists the typical CSF profiles for various infections. In general, CSF with lymphocytic pleocytosis and a low glucose concentration suggests either infection (e.g., with *Listeria*, *M. tuberculosis*, or a fungus) or a noninfectious disorder (e.g., neoplastic meningitis, sarcoidosis). Bacterial antigen tests of CSF (e.g., latex agglutination tests for *Haemophilus influenzae* type b, group B *Streptococcus*, *S. pneumoniae*, and *Neisseria meningitidis*) are not recommended for screening, given that these tests are no more sensitive than Gram's stain; however, these assays can be helpful in presumptively identifying organisms seen on Gram's stain. In contrast, other antigen tests (e.g., for *Cryptococcus*) and some CSF serologic testing (e.g., for *Treponema pallidum*, *Coccidioides*) are highly sensitive and are useful for select patients. In addition, polymerase chain reaction (PCR) analysis of CSF is increasingly being used for the diagnosis of bacterial (e.g., *N. meningitidis*, *S. pneumoniae*, mycobacteria) and viral (e.g., herpes simplex virus, enterovirus) infections; while these molecular tests permit rapid diagnosis with a high degree of sensitivity and specificity, they often do not allow determination of antimicrobial resistance profiles.

Cultures The mainstays of infectious disease diagnosis include the culture of infected tissue (e.g., surgical specimens) or fluid (e.g., blood, urine, sputum, pus from a wound). Samples can be sent for culture of bacteria (aerobic or anaerobic), fungi, or viruses. Ideally, specimens are collected before the administration of antimicrobial therapy; in instances where this order of events is not clinically feasible, microscopic examination of the specimen (e.g., Gram-stained or potassium hydroxide [KOH]–treated preparations) is particularly important. Culture of the organism(s) allows identification of the etiologic agent(s), determination of the antimicrobial

TABLE 119-2 Major Infectious Causes of Eosinophilia[a]

ORGAN INVOLVED	ORGANISM	EXPOSURE	GEOGRAPHIC DISTRIBUTION	DEGREE OF EOSINOPHILIA[b]
Central nervous system	*Angiostrongylus*	Raw seafood	Asia	Mild
	Gnathostoma	Raw poultry and seafood	Asia	Moderate to extreme
Eye	*Loa loa*	Insect bite	Africa	Moderate (expatriates), mild (patients living in endemic areas)
	Onchocerca	Insect bite	Africa	Mild (expatriates), moderate (patients living in endemic areas)
Lung	*Chlamydia trachomatis*	Sexual transmission	Worldwide	Mild
	Strongyloides	Soil	Tropical	Moderate (acute), mild (chronic)
	Toxocara canis/Toxocara cati[c]	Dogs, soil	Worldwide	Moderate to extreme
	Paragonimus	Crabs and crayfish	Asia	Moderate (acute), mild (chronic)
	Coccidioides immitis	Soil	Southwestern United States	Mild (acute), extreme (disseminated)
	Brugia malayi	Insect bite	Asia	Mild to moderate
	Pneumocystis jirovecii	Air	Worldwide	Mild
Liver	*Schistosoma japonicum*	Freshwater swimming	Asia	Moderate (acute), mild (chronic)
	Schistosoma mansoni	Freshwater swimming	Africa, Middle East, Latin America	Moderate (acute), mild (chronic)
	Fasciola	Watercress	Worldwide	Moderate
	Clonorchis	Raw seafood	Asia	Mild to moderate
	Opisthorchis	Raw seafood	Asia	Mild to moderate
Intestines	*Ascaris*[d]	Raw fruits and vegetables, contaminated water	Worldwide	Mild to extreme
	Hookworm	Soil	Worldwide	Mild to moderate
	Trichuris	Raw fruits and vegetables, contaminated water	Tropical	Mild
	Cystoisospora belli	Contaminated water and food	Worldwide	Mild
	Dientamoeba fragilis	Unclear; spread via fecal–oral route	Worldwide	Mild
	Capillaria	Raw seafood	Asia	Extreme
	Heterophyes	Raw seafood	Asia, Middle East	Mild
	Anisakis	Raw seafood	Worldwide	Mild
	Baylisascaris procyonis[e]	Soil	North America	Moderate to extreme
	Hymenolepis nana	Contaminated water, soil	Worldwide	Mild
Bladder	*Schistosoma haematobium*	Freshwater swimming	Africa, Middle East	Moderate (acute), mild (chronic)
Muscle	*Trichinella*	Pork	Worldwide	Moderate to extreme
Lymphatics	*Wuchereria bancrofti*[d]	Insect bite	Tropical	Moderate to extreme[f]
	Bartonella henselae	Cats	Worldwide	Mild
Other	Recovery from bacterial or viral infections	—	—	Mild
	HIV	Contaminated bodily fluid	Worldwide	Mild
	Cryptococcus neoformans	Soil	Worldwide	Moderate to extreme (disseminated)

[a]There are numerous noninfectious causes of eosinophilia, such as atopic disease, DRESS (drug reaction with eosinophilia and systemic symptoms) syndrome, and pernicious anemia, which can cause mild eosinophilia; drug hypersensitivity and serum sickness, which can cause mild to moderate eosinophilia; collagen vascular disease, which can cause moderate eosinophilia; and malignancy, Churg-Strauss syndrome, and hyper-IgE syndromes, which can cause moderate to extreme eosinophilia. [b]Mild: 500–1500 cells/μL; moderate: 1500–5000 cells/μL; extreme: >5000 cells/μL. [c]Can also affect the liver and the eyes. [d]Can also affect the lungs. [e]Can also affect the eyes and the central nervous system. [f]Levels are typically higher with pulmonary infections.

susceptibility profile, and—when there is concern about an outbreak—isolate typing. While cultures are extremely useful in the evaluation of patients, determining whether culture results are clinically meaningful or represent contamination (e.g., a non-*aureus*, non-*lugdunensis* staphylococcal species growing in a blood culture) can sometimes be challenging and requires an understanding of the patient's immune status, exposure history, and microbiota. In some cases, serial cultures to demonstrate clearance of the organism may be helpful.

Pathogen-Specific Testing Numerous pathogen-specific tests (e.g., serology, antigen testing, PCR testing) are commercially available, and many hospitals now offer some of these tests in-house to facilitate rapid turnaround that ultimately enhances patient care. The reader is directed to relevant chapters on the pathogens of interest for specific details. Some of these tests (e.g., universal PCRs) identify organisms that currently are not easily cultivable and have unclear relationships to disease, thereby complicating diagnosis. As these tests become more commonplace and the work of the Human Microbiome Project progresses, the relevance of some of these previously unrecognized bacteria to human health will likely become more apparent.

Radiology Imaging provides an important adjunct to the physical examination, allowing evaluation for lymphadenopathy in regions that are not externally accessible (e.g., mediastinum, intraabdominal sites), assessment of internal organs for evidence of infection, and facilitation of image-guided percutaneous sampling of deep spaces. The choice of imaging modality (e.g., CT, MRI, ultrasound, nuclear medicine, use of contrast) is best made in consultation with

TABLE 119-3 Causes of an Extremely Elevated Erythrocyte Sedimentation Rate (>100 mm/h)

ETIOLOGIC CATEGORY (% OF CASES)	SPECIFIC CAUSES
Infectious diseases (35–40)	Subacute bacterial endocarditis Abscesses Osteomyelitis Tuberculosis Urinary tract infection
Inflammatory diseases (15–20)	Giant cell arteritis Rheumatoid arthritis Systemic lupus erythematosus
Malignancies (15–20)	Multiple myeloma Leukemias Lymphomas Carcinomas
Other (20–35)	Drug hypersensitivity reactions (drug fever) Ischemic tissue injury/trauma Renal diseases

a radiologist to ensure that the results will address the physician's specific concerns.

TREATMENT

Physicians often must balance the need for empirical antibiotic treatment with the patient's clinical condition. When clinically feasible, it is best to obtain relevant samples (e.g., blood, CSF, tissue, purulent exudate) for culture prior to the administration of antibiotics, as antibiotic treatment often makes subsequent diagnosis more difficult. Although a general maxim for antibiotic treatment is to use a regimen with as narrow a spectrum as possible **(Chap. 144)**, empirical regimens are necessarily somewhat broad, given that a specific diagnosis has not yet been made. **Table 119-5** lists empirical antibiotic treatment regimens for commonly encountered infectious presentations. These regimens should be narrowed as appropriate once a specific diagnosis is made. In addition to antibiotics, there is sometimes a role for adjunctive therapies, such as intravenous immunoglobulin G (IVIG) pooled from healthy adults or hyperimmune globulin prepared from the blood of individuals with high titers of specific antibodies to select pathogens (e.g., cytomegalovirus, hepatitis B virus, rabies virus, vaccinia virus, *Clostridium tetani*, varicella-zoster virus, *Clostridium botulinum* toxin). Although the data suggesting efficacy are limited, IVIG is sometimes used for patients with suspected staphylococcal or streptococcal toxic shock syndrome.

INFECTION CONTROL

When evaluating a patient with a suspected infectious disease, the physician must consider what infection control methods are necessary to prevent transmission of any possible infection to other people. In 2007, the U.S. Centers for Disease Control and Prevention published guidelines for isolation precautions that are available for download at *www.cdc.gov/hicpac/2007IP/2007isolationPrecautions.html*. Persons exposed to certain pathogens (e.g., *N. meningitidis*, HIV, *Bacillus anthracis*) should receive postexposure prophylaxis to prevent disease acquisition. (See relevant chapters for details on specific pathogens.)

WHEN TO OBTAIN AN INFECTIOUS DISEASE CONSULT

At times, primary physicians need assistance with patient management from a diagnostic and/or therapeutic perspective. Multiple studies have demonstrated that an infectious disease consult is associated with improved outcomes, shorter length of hospital stay, and decreased costs for patients with various diseases. For example, in a prospective cohort study of patients with *S. aureus* bacteremia, infectious disease consultation was independently associated with a 56% reduction in 28-day mortality. In addition, infectious disease specialists provide other services (e.g., infection control, antimicrobial stewardship, management of outpatient antibiotic therapy, occupational exposure programs) that have been shown to benefit patients. Whenever such assistance would be advantageous to a patient with a possible infection, the primary physician should opt for an infectious disease consult. Specific situations that might prompt a consult include (1) difficult-to-diagnose patients with presumed infections, (2) patients who are not responding to treatment as expected, (3) patients with a complicated medical history (e.g., organ transplant recipients, patients immunosuppressed due to autoimmune or inflammatory conditions), and (4) patients with "exotic" diseases (i.e., diseases that are not typically seen within the region).

TABLE 119-4 Typical Cerebrospinal Fluid Profiles for Meningitis and Encephalitis[a]

	NORMAL	BACTERIAL MENINGITIS	VIRAL MENINGITIS	FUNGAL MENINGITIS[b]	PARASITIC MENINGITIS	TUBERCULOUS MENINGITIS	ENCEPHALITIS
WBC count (per μL)	<5	>1000	25–500	40–600	150–2000	25–100	50–500
Differential of WBC	60–70% lymphocytes, ≤30% monocytes/macrophages	↑↑PMNs (≥80%)	Predominantly lymphocytes[c]	Lymphocytes or PMNs, depending on specific organism	↑↑ Eosinophils (≥50%)[d]	Predominantly lymphocytes[c]	Predominantly lymphocytes[c]
Gram's stain	Negative	Positive (in >60% of cases)	Negative	Rarely positive	Negative	Occasionally positive[e]	Negative
Glucose (mg/dL)	40–85	<40	Normal	↓ to normal	Normal	<50 in 75% of cases	Normal
Protein (mg/dL)	15–45	>100	20–80	150–300	50–200	100–200	50–100
Opening pressure (mmH_2O)	50–180	>300	100–350	160–340	Normal	150–280	Normal to ↑
Common causes	—	*Streptococcus pneumoniae*, *Neisseria meningitidis*	Enteroviruses	*Candida*, *Cryptococcus*, and *Aspergillus* spp.	*Angiostrongylus cantonensis*, *Gnathostoma spinigerum*, *Baylisascaris procyonis*	*Mycobacterium tuberculosis*	Herpesviruses, enteroviruses, influenza virus, rabies virus

[a]Numbers indicate typical results, but actual results may vary. [b]Cerebrospinal fluid characteristics depend greatly on the specific organism. [c]Neutrophils may predominate early in the disease course. [d]Patients typically have striking eosinophilia as well. [e]Sensitivity can be increased by examination of a smear of protein coagulum (pellicle) and the use of acid-fast stains.

Abbreviations: PMNs, polymorphonuclear neutrophils; WBC, white blood cell.

TABLE 119-5 Initial Empirical Antibiotic Therapy for Common Infectious Disease Presentations[a]

CLINICAL SYNDROME	COMMON ETIOLOGIES	ANTIBIOTIC(S)	COMMENTS	SEE CHAPTER(S)
Septic shock	*Staphylococcus aureus, Streptococcus pneumoniae,* enteric gram-negative bacilli	Vancomycin, 15 mg/kg q12h[b] ***plus*** A broad-spectrum antipseudomonal β-lactam (piperacillin-tazobactam, 4.5 g q6h; imipenem, 1 g q8h; meropenem, 1 g q8h; or cefepime, 1–2 g q8–12h)	If a pseudomonal species is likely, a second antipseudomonal agent should be added.	**304**
Meningitis	*S. pneumoniae, Neisseria meningitidis*	Vancomycin, 15 mg/kg q12h[b] ***plus*** Ceftriaxone, 2 g q12h	Dexamethasone (0.15 mg/kg IV q6h for 2–4 d) should be added for patients with suspected or proven pneumococcal meningitis, with the first dose administered 10–20 min before the first dose of antibiotics.	**138** and pathogen-specific chapters
CNS abscess	*Streptococcus* spp., *Staphylococcus* spp., anaerobes, gram-negative bacilli	Vancomycin, 15 mg/kg q12h[b] ***plus*** Ceftriaxone, 2 g q12h ***plus*** Metronidazole, 500 mg q8h	—	**138**
Acute endocarditis (native valve)	*S. aureus, Streptococcus* spp., coagulase-negative staphylococci	Vancomycin, 15 mg/kg q12h[b] ***plus*** Cefepime, 2 g q8h	—	**128**
Pneumonia Community-acquired, outpatient	*S. pneumoniae, Mycoplasma pneumoniae, Haemophilus influenzae, Chlamydia pneumoniae*	No comorbidities[h]: Azithromycin, 500 mg PO × 1, then 250 mg PO qd × 4 days With comorbidities[h]: Levofloxacin, 750 mg PO qd	If MRSA is a consideration, add vancomycin (15 mg/kg q8–12h[b]) or linezolid (600 mg q12h); daptomycin should not be used in patients with pneumonia.	**126** and pathogen-specific chapters
Inpatient, non-ICU	Above plus *Legionella* spp.	A respiratory fluoroquinolone (moxifloxacin, 400 mg IV/PO qd; gemifloxacin, 320 mg PO qd; or levofloxacin, 750 mg IV/PO qd) ***or*** A β-lactam (cefotaxime, ceftriaxone, or ampicillin-sulbactam) *plus* azithromycin		
Inpatient, ICU	Above plus *S. aureus*	A β-lactam ***plus*** Azithromycin *or* a respiratory fluoroquinolone		
Hospital-acquired pneumonia[d]	*S. pneumoniae, H. influenzae, S. aureus*, gram-negative bacilli (e.g., *Pseudomonas aeruginosa, Klebsiella pneumoniae, Acinetobacter* spp.)	An antipseudomonal β-lactam (cefepime, 2 g q8h; ceftazidime, 2 g q8h; imipenem, 500 mg q6h; meropenem, 1 g q8h; or piperacillin-tazobactam, 4.5 g q6h) ***plus*** An antipseudomonal fluoroquinolone (levofloxacin, 700 mg qd, or ciprofloxacin, 400 mg q8h) *or* an aminoglycoside (amikacin, 15–20 mg/kg q24h[c]; gentamicin, 5–7 mg/kg q24h[e]; or tobramycin, 5–7 mg/kg q24h[e])	If MRSA is a consideration, add vancomycin (15 mg/kg q8–12h[b]) or linezolid (600 mg q12h); daptomycin should not be used in patients with pneumonia.	
Complicated intraabdominal infection			If MRSA is a consideration, add vancomycin (15 mg/kg q12h[b])	**132**, **177**, and pathogen-specific chapters
Mild to moderate severity	Anaerobes (*Bacteroides* spp., *Clostridium* spp.), gram-negative bacilli (*Escherichia coli*), *Streptococcus* spp.	Cefoxitin, 2 g q6h ***or*** A combination of metronidazole (500 mg q8–12h) *plus one of the following*: cefazolin (1–2 g q8h), cefuroxime (1.5 g q8h), ceftriaxone (1–2 g q12–24h), cefotaxime (1–2 g q6–8h), ciprofloxacin (400 mg q12h), levofloxacin (750 mg qd)		
High-risk patient or high degree of severity	Same as above	A carbapenem (imipenem, 500 mg q6h; meropenem, 1 g q8h; doripenem, 500 mg q8h) ***or*** Piperacillin-tazobactam, 3.375 g q6h[f] ***or*** A combination of metronidazole (500 mg q8h) *plus* an antipseudomonal cephalosporin (cefepime, 2 g q8h; ceftazidime, 2 g q8h)		

(Continued)

TABLE 119-5 Initial Empirical Antibiotic Therapy for Common Infectious Disease Presentations[a] (Continued)

CLINICAL SYNDROME	COMMON ETIOLOGIES	ANTIBIOTIC(S)	COMMENTS	SEE CHAPTER(S)
Skin and soft tissue infection	*S. aureus, Streptococcus pyogenes*	Dicloxacillin, 250–500 mg PO qid *or* Cephalexin, 250–500 mg PO qid *or* Clindamycin, 300–450 mg PO tid *or* Nafcillin/oxacillin, 1–2 g q4h	If MRSA is a consideration, clindamycin, vancomycin (15 mg/kg q12h[b]), linezolid (600 mg IV/PO q12h), or TMP-SMX (1–2 double-strength tablets PO bid[g]) can be used.	**129** and pathogen-specific chapters

[a]This table refers to immunocompetent adults with normal renal and hepatic function. All doses listed are for parenteral administration unless indicated otherwise. Local antimicrobial susceptibility profiles may influence the choice of antibiotic. Therapy should be tailored once a specific etiologic agent and its susceptibilities are identified. [b]Trough levels for vancomycin should be 15–20 μg/mL. [c]Trough levels for amikacin should be <4 μg/mL. [d]In patients with late onset (i.e., after ≥5 days of hospitalization) or risk factors for multidrug-resistant organisms. [e]Trough levels for gentamicin and tobramycin should be <1 μg/mL. [f]If *P. aeruginosa* is a concern, the dosage may be increased to 3.375 g IV q4h or 4.5 g IV q6h. [g]Data on the efficacy of TMP-SMX in skin and soft tissue infections are limited. [h]Comorbidities include chronic heart, lung, liver, or renal disease; diabetes mellitus; alcoholism; malignancy; or asplenia.

Abbreviations: CNS, central nervous system; ICU, intensive care unit; MRSA, methicillin-resistant *S. aureus*; TMP-SMX, trimethoprim-sulfamethoxazole.

PERSPECTIVE

The study of infectious diseases is really a study of host–microbial interactions and represents evolution by both the host and the microbe—an endless struggle in which microbes have generally been more creative and adaptive. Given that nearly one-fifth of deaths worldwide are still related to infectious diseases, it is clear that the war against infectious diseases has not been won. For example, a cure for HIV infection is still lacking, there have been only marginal improvements in the methods for detection and treatment of tuberculosis after more than a half century of research, new infectious disease outbreaks (e.g., viral hemorrhagic fevers, Zika, SARS-CoV-2) continue to emerge, and the threat of microbial bioterrorism remains high. The subsequent chapters in Part 5 detail—on both a syndrome and a microbe-by-microbe basis—the current state of medical knowledge about infectious diseases. At their core, all of these chapters carry a similar message: Despite numerous advances in the diagnosis, treatment, and prevention of infectious diseases, much work and research are required before anyone can confidently claim we have achieved "the virtual elimination of infectious disease." In reality, this goal will never be attained, given the rapid adaptability of microbes.

FURTHER READING

Bartlett JG: Why infectious diseases. Clin Infect Dis 59(Suppl 2):S85, 2014.

Bhatraju PK et al: Covid-19 in critically ill patients in the Seattle region: Case series. N Engl J Med 382:2012, 2020.

Khabbaz RF et al: Challenges of infectious diseases in the USA. Lancet 384:53, 2014.

Marston HD et al: Antimicrobial resistance. JAMA 316:1193, 2016.

McQuillen DP, MacIntyre AT: The value that infectious disease physicians bring to the healthcare system. J Infect Dis 216:S588, 2017.

Verghese A et al: Inadequacies of physical examination as a cause of medical errors and adverse events: A collection of vignettes. Am J Med 128:1322, 2015.

120 Molecular Mechanisms of Microbial Pathogenesis

Thomas E. Wood, Marcia B. Goldberg

Infectious diseases of humans involve intricate interactions among the infecting microbe, human tissue, and the host microbiome. The coevolution of humans and microbes has led to the presence of numerous and varied specific microbial factors that promote the disease process and a corresponding wide range of human cellular responses, both specific and nonspecific, to pathogens. Among the microbial factors that promote disease are those that alter human cells, those that inhibit host immune responses, and those that respond to the microbes that constitute the microbiota and their metabolic products. The process of infection can be divided into several stages: the encounter with and entry of the microbe into the human body (*colonization*), the attachment of the microbe in its favored niche and microbial avoidance of host defenses (*infection*), the combined deployment of microbial factors that damage human tissue and host inflammatory responses to the presence of the microbe (*disease*), and the release of the pathogen into the environment, where it can infect others (*transmission*). It is notable that for most microbial pathogens, the host inflammatory response contributes substantially to symptoms and to tissue damage. Moreover, the human microbiota (the collection of microbes that reside in and on the human body) modulates, directly or indirectly, every stage of infection (**Chap. 471**). This chapter describes the best-understood molecular and cellular mechanisms that contribute to human disease caused by bacterial pathogens.

ENTRY INTO THE HUMAN HOST

Infectious diseases occur when either a live pathogen enters the human host or a toxic pathogen product is ingested by the host, with the former being much more common than the latter.

Most bacterial infections result from entry of a pathogen into the body. Entry can occur through a break in the skin into the underlying soft tissues or at the surface of a mucous membrane of the respiratory, gastrointestinal, or genitourinary tract; the skin may also be directly infected. Entry at these sites may result in infection of the bloodstream, which may in turn lead to infection of other organ systems.

Entry into the respiratory tract occurs via respiratory droplet nuclei (airborne particles 1–5 μm in diameter) or via fomites introduced on a hand that is contaminated by contact with a contaminated inert surface (e.g., a doorknob or a faucet). Infectious droplet nuclei are generated when an individual with a communicable respiratory infection (e.g., tuberculosis, Legionnaires' disease, psittacosis, influenza, measles, chickenpox, aspergillosis, COVID-19 infection) sneezes, coughs, talks, plays a musical instrument by mouth, or sings. A cough may generate 3000 particles, whereas a sneeze may generate up to 40,000 particles; large particles may evaporate down to the 0.5- to 12-μm range, and particles that are 1.5 μm and hygroscopic increase in size as they pass through the moist nasal passages and lower respiratory tree.

Entry into the gastrointestinal tract occurs via ingestion of contaminated food or water or via person-to-person contact, typically with transfer from a contaminated hand into the mouth. Pathogens for which the infectious inoculum is large (e.g., 10^8 organisms for epidemic spread of *Vibrio cholerae*, 10^5 organisms for *Salmonella enterica* serovar Typhimurium) are generally acquired via contaminated food or water, whereas pathogens for which the infectious inoculum is small (e.g., 10^1 to 10^2 organisms for *Shigella* spp.) are more commonly acquired by person-to-person spread.

Entry into the genitourinary tract generally takes place either via colonization of the urethral meatus or vaginal introitus with fecal organisms followed by ascension of the organisms into the bladder or kidneys or via instrumentation. Pyelonephritis can also result from seeding from the bloodstream.

ESTABLISHMENT OF INFECTION

NICHE

Live Pathogens Within the human host, many bacterial pathogens display tissue tropism; the sites of infection within the human body are pathogen-specific and restricted, such that even adjacent tissues may be uninvolved. For example, group A streptococci cause pharyngitis and soft tissue infection, but rarely pneumonia. Cholera is an infection of the small intestine, but not the stomach or the colon, where *Shigella* spp. cause disease only in the rectosigmoid. Therefore, to establish infection, the pathogen must access its niche and then remain within that niche (**Table 120-1**). In the respiratory tree, the sites at which pathogens initially settle can be determined by mode of spread. Droplet nuclei reach the bronchial tree or alveoli, whereas, after contaminated hands touch the face, fomites reach the pharynx or nasal passages. Pathogens move through the gastrointestinal tract via normal intestinal motility.

Tissue association and invasion are dictated by the interaction of the bacterium with host factors, commonly glycan-decorated receptors and/or the associated extracellular matrix. The environmental conditions of the niche trigger the expression of virulence factors required for the establishment of infection; for example, bile salts in the gut stimulate the expression of *V. cholerae* adhesins and toxins and the germination of *Clostridioides difficile* spores. Bacteria commonly manipulate their particular niche environment in ways that facilitate infection. For example, the gastroduodenal pathogen *Helicobacter pylori* produces urease, which converts urea into ammonia, thereby increasing the pH of the acidic stomach environment and creating a more hospitable environment for its survival. This conversion also concomitantly alters the physiology of the gastric epithelium.

TABLE 120-1 Bacterial Pathogens, Diseases, and Niches

MOST COMMON TROPISM	BACTERIUM	DISEASE
Skin, respiratory tract, small intestine	*Bacillus anthracis*	Anthrax
Respiratory tract	*Bordetella pertussis*	Pertussis
Systemic	*Borrelia burgdorferi*	Lyme disease
Systemic	*Brucella abortus*	Brucellosis
Systemic	*Burkholderia pseudomallei*	Melioidosis
Eyes, venereal	*Chlamydia trachomatis*	Various chlamydioses, including trachoma
Colon	*Clostridioides difficile*	Colitis
Pharynx	*Corynebacterium diphtheriae*	Diphtheria
Systemic	*Coxiella burnetii*	Q fever
Colon	Enterohemorrhagic *Escherichia coli*	
Stomach	*Helicobacter pylori*	Gastritis, gastric ulcers
Respiratory tract	*Legionella pneumophila*	Legionnaires' disease
Systemic, central nervous system	*Listeria monocytogenes*	Listeriosis
Respiratory tract	*Mycobacterium tuberculosis*	Tuberculosis
Urogenital tract	*Neisseria gonorrhoeae*	Gonorrhea
Respiratory tract	*Pseudomonas aeruginosa*	
Systemic	*Salmonella enterica* serovar Typhi	Typhoid fever
Gastrointestinal tract	*Salmonella enterica* serovar Typhimurium	
Colon, rectum	*Shigella* spp.	Dysentery, shigellosis
Multiple sites	*Staphylococcus aureus*	
Soft tissue	Group A *Streptococcus*	
Small intestine	*Vibrio cholerae*	Cholera
Systemic	*Yersinia pestis*	Plague

Preformed Toxins A small number of diseases are caused by ingestion in food of preformed bacterial toxins. The most common among these are *Staphylococcus aureus* enterotoxins, which can be present in prepared foods such as dairy, meat, eggs, salads, and produce, and the *Bacillus cereus* emetic enterotoxin, which is most often found in rice or other starchy food that has been improperly refrigerated. Less common but also important is botulinum toxin produced by *Clostridium botulinum*. Preformed toxins cause disease in the small intestine (nausea and vomiting) and may cause systemic symptoms.

Although the pathogens may be killed when food is cooked, their toxins are heat stable. *S. aureus* enterotoxins can be strongly emetic. *B. cereus* produces the heat-stable peptide toxin cereulide, which acts as a potassium ionophore and induces emesis. In botulism, a flaccid paralysis caused by botulinum toxin, uptake of the toxin blocks neurotransmitter release in motor neurons, inhibiting the central nervous system and resulting in potentially fatal respiratory failure.

ATTACHMENT

Attachment of bacteria to host tissue surfaces is a prerequisite for the pathogen's establishment of an infection and is mediated by specific receptor–ligand interactions. In this context, the tissue specificity of the host cell surface receptor repertoire is a critical factor in delimiting a pathogen's niche(s). These physical associations additionally facilitate the pathogen's avoidance of host clearance mechanisms (see "Avoidance of Innate Immune Responses," below) and may contribute to formation of biofilms by the pathogen (see "Biofilms," below). Because adhesion to cellular receptors often triggers cellular signal transduction and innate immune signaling, therapeutic blocking of this interaction may in some circumstances exacerbate infection.

Adhesins Bacterial pathogens have evolved a wide range of strategies by which to attach to the diverse host cell structures they encounter. For many bacterial pathogens, ligands or adhesins for specific host receptors are known. Adhesins comprise a wide variety of surface structures, including single proteins, carbohydrates, glycoproteins, lipids, lipoproteins, and multiprotein filamentous complexes that extend several micrometers from the bacterial surface, each anchored in the outer-surface cell envelope. Most bacteria produce multiple adhesins with varying specificity, enabling the pathogen to interact with multiple receptors, including those on several distinct cell and tissue types encountered during the process of infection. These interactions are often partially redundant, are serologically variable, and contribute additively or synergistically with other binding interactions.

Common classes of adhesins are pili (also known as fimbriae), flagella, and autotransporter proteins (**Table 120-2**). Pili are hairlike extensions consisting of a polymer of the major pilin subunit capped with minor pilins that provide the adherence function of the structure. Pili are classified by type and are produced by many gram-negative bacteria and a smaller number of gram-positive bacteria. To date, efforts to prevent infection with pilus-based vaccines have been unsuccessful.

Types of pili include type I, type P, and type IV. Type I pili frequently function at mucosal surfaces. For example, they mediate the close association of uropathogenic *Escherichia coli* (UPEC) with bladder epithelial cells and the ability of this pathogen to persist, causing relapsing urinary tract infections. UPEC also produces type P pili and afimbrial adhesins. These adhesins bind sugar moieties on host surface glycoproteins, with varied specificity depending on the adhesin. The minor pilin lectins at the tip of the pili generally bind D-mannose glycans, albeit with strain specificity. For example, the type I pilus adhesin FimH of intestinal *E. coli* strains often preferentially binds

TABLE 120-2 Classes of Bacterial Adhesion Proteins and Their Host Receptors

ADHESIN	EXAMPLE	RECEPTOR
Type I pili	Fim protein, uropathogenic *Escherichia coli*	Terminal mannose of uroplakin *N*-glycan in urinary epithelial cells
Type P pili	Pap protein, uropathogenic *E. coli*	Galactose disaccharides
Type IV pili	Tfp protein, *Neisseria gonorrhoeae*	CD64, CR3, I domain–containing integrins
MSCRAMM	SdrC protein, *Staphylococcus aureus*	β-Neurexin
Opa	Opa protein, *Neisseria meningitidis*	CEACAMs[a]
Flagellum	FliC protein, *Pseudomonas aeruginosa*	Asialo-GM1 ganglioside
Autotransporter	Invasin, *Yersinia pseudotuberculosis*	β1-Integrins
Autotransporter	Ag85, *Mycobacterium tuberculosis*	Fibronectin

[a]Carcinoembryonic antigen–related cell adhesion molecules.

oligomannose, whereas the FimH of UPEC strains commonly binds monomannose. Thus, the same pilus structures in different bacterial strains can dictate adherence to distinct tissues. Type IV pili (Tfp) are widespread among gram-negative bacteria, and similar structures exist among gram-positive bacteria. These are evolutionarily related to the type II secretion system (T2SS) and, in addition to mediating adherence, allow the uptake of DNA into bacteria and the motility of bacteria on surfaces. The Tfp of *Neisseria* spp. and *V. cholerae* mediate aggregation of individual bacteria into microcolonies, which promotes colonization.

Flagella are polymeric helical filaments that propel bacteria through liquid environments by rotating about their long axis. Because flagella confer the ability to swim toward a target surface, often following a chemotactic gradient where chemical sensing influences the direction of motility, they are vital virulence factors of many pathogenic bacteria. Flagella can be localized to one end of the bacterial cell (*polar*) or distributed around the bacterial surface (*peritrichous*). Flagella are evolutionarily related to type III secretion systems (T3SSs) (see "Replicative Niche" and "Survival in the Vacuole," below) and have been shown in some instances to be responsible for the secretion of bacterial toxins. Flagella may also act as adhesins, binding to mucins of mucosal surfaces in the case of the gastrointestinal pathogens enteropathogenic *E. coli* (EPEC) and enterohemorrhagic *E. coli* (EHEC).

Autotransporter proteins comprise a subdivision of type V secretion systems (T5SSs), which are prevalent among gram-negative bacteria (**Fig. 120-1**). Extended adhesive projections anchored in the bacterial outer membrane, autotransporter proteins are pivotal virulence determinants for several human pathogens, including the filamentous hemagglutinin of *Bordetella pertussis* (the etiologic agent of whooping cough) and the IcsA adhesin and intracellular motility determinant of the *Shigella* spp. responsible for dysenteric diseases. In addition, the autotransporter proteins intimin and invasin are required for the intimate association of adhering and effacing pathogens, such as EPEC, and invasion by *Yersinia* spp., respectively. Besides these main classes of adhesins, other bacterial surface proteins are also involved in adhesion, including the Opa family of membrane proteins of *Neisseria* spp. and the gram-positive cell wall–anchored microbial surface component recognizing adhesive matrix molecules (MSCRAMMs) of *S. aureus* and various enterococci.

Receptors Carbohydrates (glycans) on the surface of and secreted by human cells play major roles in the adherence of bacterial pathogens. The surfaces of human cells are coated with glycoproteins and glycolipids, whereas the extracellular matrix (ECM) scaffold of tissues is mainly composed of secreted proteoglycans. Most mucosal surfaces are covered with a layer of mucus, which consists primarily of mucins, a family of proteins that are heavily glycosylated. Among the human enzymes involved in glycan decoration of secreted proteins is *FUT2*, for which ~20% of the human population harbors two nonfunctional alleles; the importance of human glycans in infection is highlighted by the observation that individuals who lack functional *FUT2* display increased susceptibility to certain bacterial infections, decreased susceptibility to certain viral infections, and altered susceptibility to chronic noninfectious inflammatory diseases. These data are confounded by a relative increase in secretion of sialylated glycans in individuals lacking functional *FUT2*. Glycans participate in many adhesive

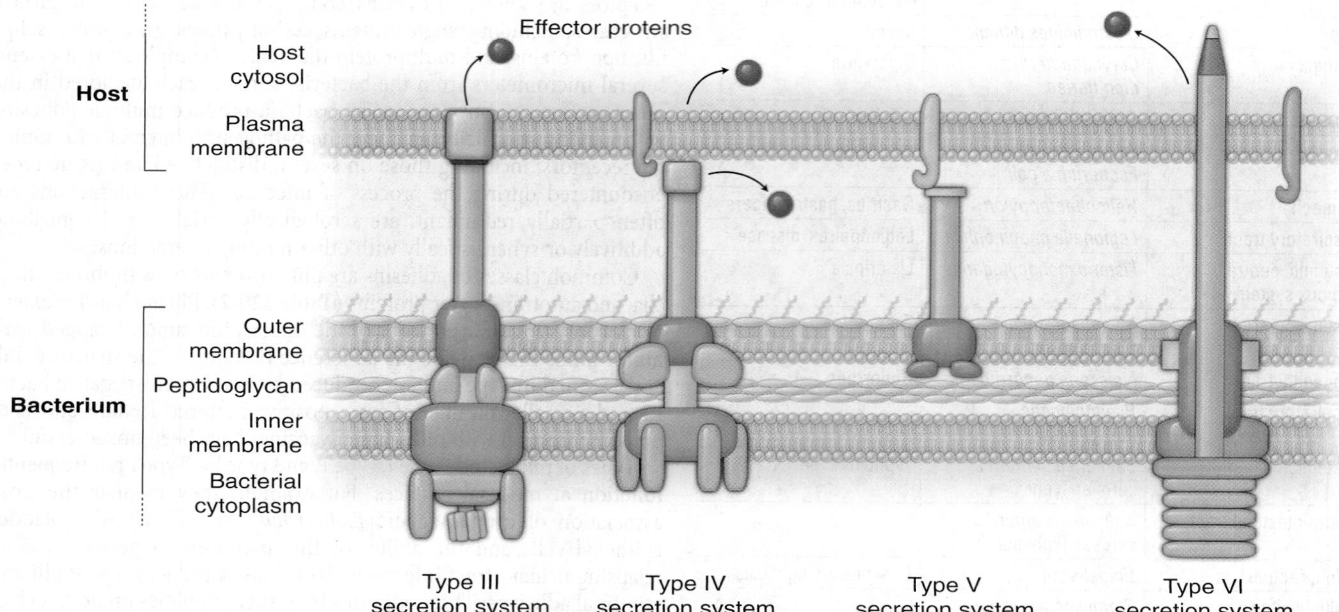

FIGURE 120-1 Major bacterial secretion systems involved in pathogenesis. Schematic of the types III, IV, V, and VI secretion systems (T3SS, T4SS, T5SS, and T6SS, respectively) of gram-negative bacteria. The T3SS, T4SS, and T6SS deliver bacterial effector proteins into host cells, whereas the T5SS participates in adhesion to the surface of cells. The architecture of the extracellular portion of the T4SS and how it translocates effector proteins remain poorly defined. Colored shapes with hooks in the host plasma membrane represent host membrane proteins that, it is thought, may participate in these processes.

interactions and serve as receptors for certain bacterial toxins. Certain bacteria enzymatically alter host glycans in a manner that enables improved access to the epithelial surface, as in the case of *V. cholerae* and the oral pathogen *Tannerella forsythia*.

The GM1 ganglioside, a glycolipid, is the receptor for cholera toxin (CTX), *Pseudomonas aeruginosa* flagella, and the *Clostridium perfringens* α toxin, whereas terminal sialic acid residues on GM1 play an important role in tropism of the gastric pathogen *H. pylori* through interactions with the bacterial membrane proteins BabA and SabA. Heparan sulfate proteoglycans and other glycosaminoglycan-conjugated proteins are commonly associated with the basolateral membranes of epithelial layers and act as ligands for the chlamydial OmcB protein and the *E. coli* cytotoxic necrotizing factor toxin; these interactions promote initial bacterial adherence in proximity to the plasma membrane and lead to engagement of additional surface molecules.

In mammals, the ECM and integrin proteins are ubiquitous. The ECM consists of laminin, vimentin, and type IV collagen, which interact via fibronectin with integrin receptors in the plasma membrane. Because of direct interaction with plasma membrane–embedded integrins, ECM alterations can result in signal transduction that directly influences immune cell behavior. Moreover, many bacterial pathogens engage integrins and the functionally related carcinoembryonic antigen–related cell adhesion molecules (CEACAMs) as host cell receptors and as triggers for their internalization into human cells (see "Mechanisms of Microbial Entry into Cells," below). The receptor for adherent-invasive *E. coli*, a pathogenic type of *E. coli*, is CEACAM6, whose levels are increased on epithelial cells in inflammatory bowel disease; adherent-invasive *E. coli* adhere at increased levels in Crohn's disease, and sites of excessive bacterial adherence display increased inflammation.

Among the many other host cell surface proteins that serve as receptors for bacterial adherence is the cystic fibrosis transmembrane conductance regulator (CFTR), a chloride channel involved in the maintenance of adequate hydration of mucosal surfaces. Mutation of the *CFTR* gene gives rise to the hereditary disease cystic fibrosis. These patients are hypersusceptible to respiratory infection because the cilia are unable to clear viscous mucus from the bronchial epithelial surface. The remarkably high frequency of cystic fibrosis (>2.5%) in Caucasian populations has been attributed to relative resistance to *Salmonella enterica* serovar Typhi infection, since *S.* Typhi adheres to CFTR via type IV pili. It has also been reported that epithelial cells utilize CFTR during internalization-mediated clearance of the extracellular pathogen *P. aeruginosa*, potentially contributing to the decreased ability of cystic fibrosis patients to clear infections by this pathogen.

REPLICATIVE NICHE

Once bacterial pathogens find their niche and associate with target host cells, they must replicate to persist. Some pathogens remain predominantly associated with the surface of epithelial cells (e.g., *Bordetella, Pseudomonas, Vibrio,* and *Clostridium* spp.), whereas others predominantly enter into cells (e.g., *Salmonella, Shigella, Francisella,* and *Listeria* spp.). Phagocytic cells actively engulf pathogens for destruction; thus extracellular bacteria must avoid or inhibit this process to remain associated with the cell surface. Many pathogens deliver cytoskeleton-disrupting proteins that perturb the phagocytic process, whereas others create structures that impede phagocytosis; examples include biofilm formation by *P. aeruginosa* and cell chaining by streptococci. In contrast, nonphagocytic cells, such as epithelial cells, may also internalize bacteria in processes that can be triggered by either the host cell (as a clearance mechanism) or the pathogen (for tissue invasion). A subpopulation of any infecting pathogen will be phagocytosed by macrophages, neutrophils, and/or dendritic cells. Many pathogens have evolved mechanisms to survive within phagocytes; for example, during colonization of the nasopharynx, *Streptococcus pneumoniae* survives within vacuoles in dendritic cells and alveolar or splenic macrophages.

Extracellular Pathogens Extracellular pathogens replicate at the surface of human cells. Many secrete enzymes that may liberate nutrients from extracellular factors and fashion a hospitable niche. For example, *V. cholerae*, an extracellular pathogen of the small intestine, secretes the mucinase vibriolysin that degrades the mucus barrier overlying intestinal epithelial cells, giving the bacterium access to the cell surface. *H. pylori*, an extracellular pathogen of the stomach, secretes a urease that converts urea into carbon dioxide and ammonia, thereby buffering the acidic pH of the stomach. *Yersinia* spp., which associates with the surface of leukocytes, delivers into these naturally phagocytic cells secreted bacterial proteins that inhibit phagocytosis. Once phagocytosed, *V. cholerae* can inhibit further phagocytosis of extracellular bacteria.

EPEC and EHEC efface the microvilli of the brush border of intestinal epithelial cells and adhere tightly to the surface of these cells. These bacteria induce formation of actin-rich pedestals at the plasma membrane, which may help prevent bacterial internalization by the epithelial cells. Epithelial polarity is important for tissue function, influencing ion flux, barrier integrity, and protein sorting. Many pathogens subvert epithelial polarity to redistribute membrane complexes in a manner that facilitates tissue penetration and dissemination and avoids internalization and subsequent cell-autonomous immune mechanisms (see "Avoidance of Innate Immune Responses," below). For certain pathogens that do not efface microvilli (e.g., *Listeria monocytogenes* and *Shigella* spp.), the basolateral compartment of the plasma membrane—rather than the mucus-covered microvillus apical surface—is the preferential site of epithelial cell invasion. Tight junctions mediate intimate associations between neighboring epithelial cells, thereby maintaining tissue barrier function; the targeted dissolution of tight junctions by pathogens facilitates bacterial penetration into the tissue.

BIOFILMS Some extracellular pathogens, including *S. aureus* and *P. aeruginosa*, establish chronic infections through the production of extracellular polymeric matrices called *biofilms*, which encase the bacteria. Biofilms commonly develop where tissue integrity has been compromised, such as in burn wounds. The biofilm matrix is composed of extracellular polysaccharides and DNA, to which the bacteria adhere. The biofilm mass protects the bacterial residents from phagocytosis while impairing the diffusion and efficacy of antibodies and administered antibiotics. Therefore, the bacteria avoid elimination and persist; meanwhile, ongoing recognition of virulence factors by the immune system may lead to massive inflammation and local tissue damage, exacerbating the infection.

Mechanisms of Microbial Entry Into Cells Essentially all bacterial pathogens that are predominantly intracellular during infection possess mechanisms for inducing internalization into human cells. Even pathogens that survive for prolonged periods in normally phagocytic cells such as macrophages (*Salmonella* spp., *L. monocytogenes*) possess mechanisms for inducing internalization into these cells.

TRIGGER MECHANISM Bacterial systems that deliver proteins into human cells are critical to many aspects of pathogenesis (Fig. 120-1). One of these systems is the type III secretion system, a specialized system that delivers proteins from the bacterial cytoplasm directly into the cytosol of eukaryotic cells. Evolutionarily conserved T3SSs are found in many gram-negative bacterial pathogens. In all cases, delivery of the proteins that are injected into the cell (*effector* proteins) has dramatic effects on the cell; for many human pathogens, these effects include the induction of bacterial uptake into the cell and the alteration of other cellular processes in ways that promote infection.

The T3SS forms an apparatus on the bacterial surface that resembles a needle and syringe, with a hollow tube down its long axis (Fig. 120-1). The base of the organelle spans the two bacterial membranes, forming a conduit from the bacterial cytoplasm, where proteins are synthesized. Anchored to the organelle base and protruding from the bacterial surface is a long needle-like structure. Upon contact of the needle tip with the plasma membrane of the eukaryotic cell, two proteins secreted through the apparatus form a pore in the plasma membrane. The tip of the needle docks onto the extracellular face of the pore, thereby forming a continuous conduit between the bacterial cytoplasm and the host cell cytosol. It is through this conduit that bacterial effector proteins are then delivered into the cell.

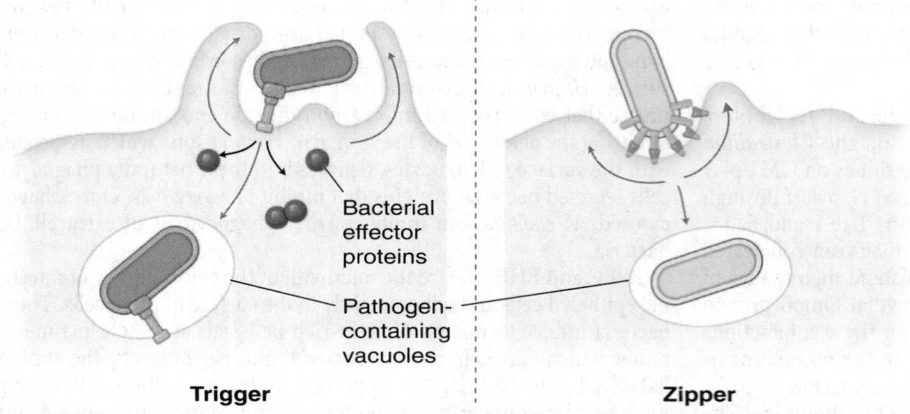

FIGURE 120-2 Common mechanisms of bacterial invasion. The mechanisms for internalization of bacteria into nonphagocytic cells are typically classified as *trigger* or *zipper* mechanisms. As examples of the trigger mechanism, *Shigella* and *Salmonella* spp. use their T3SSs to deliver into host cells effector proteins that manipulate the cytoskeleton in ways leading to the formation of cytoskeleton-supported membrane ruffles. These membrane ruffles extend and surround the pathogen, with consequent endocytosis of the bacterium. As examples of the zipper mechanism, bacterial membrane proteins of *Yersinia* and *Listeria* spp. induce clustering of host receptors. Clustering and subsequent intracellular signaling result in the uptake of the bacterium in a tightly opposed vacuole.

For those pathogens that use a T3SS to induce entry into human cells (*Salmonella*, *Shigella*, and *Chlamydia* spp.), among the first effector proteins secreted into the cell are several that activate polymerization of cellular actin immediately beneath the point where the bacterium is docked on the plasma membrane. Actin polymerization pushes outwardly against the plasma membrane, generating large ruffles of the membrane that engulf the bacterium and take it up into a membrane-bound vacuole (**Fig. 120-2**). *Shigella* spp. then escape the vacuole and reside in the host cell cytosol, whereas *Salmonella* and *Chlamydia* spp. predominantly reside within the vacuole.

ZIPPER MECHANISM Several invasive pathogens that do not utilize a T3SS for internalization enter cells using a zipper-like mechanism. In these instances, bacterial surface molecules engage with and stimulate the clustering of host cell receptors, which form close associations with the bacterium in a processive fashion until the plasma membrane is tightly opposed to and surrounding the bacterium (Fig. 120-2). For example, the *Yersinia pseudotuberculosis* invasion molecules YadA and invasin bind to β1-integrins; this binding stimulates phosphoinositide 3-kinase and protein kinase B (Akt) signaling pathways, leading to zipper-mediated entry of *Y. pseudotuberculosis* into otherwise nonphagocytic cells. In another example, *L. monocytogenes* internalins InlA and InlB engage E-cadherin and the Met receptor, activating β-catenin signaling and zipper-mediated entry of *L. monocytogenes* into otherwise nonphagocytic cells. Subpopulations of bacteria classically considered extracellular may also promote their own uptake in a similar fashion, with the lectin LecA of *P. aeruginosa* and fibronectin-binding protein of *S. aureus* performing similar functions.

SURVIVAL IN THE VACUOLE

After uptake into cells, the majority of invasive bacterial pathogens remain in a vacuole. Uptake vacuoles normally enter the endosomal pathway, acquiring host proteins that promote vesicle maturation, acidification, and degradation of contents. Many bacterial pathogens contained in these endosomes subvert this intracellular trafficking in ways that prevent endosomal maturation and block lysosomal degradation of the pathogen. A distinct subset of bacteria actively damage vacuolar membrane integrity, disrupting the vacuole and thereby escaping into the cytosol, where they replicate. For bacteria that remain in the vacuole, various bacterial effector proteins are delivered by secretion systems either into the vacuolar space or across the vacuolar membrane into the cytosol (Fig. 120-1), where these proteins manipulate host processes to the benefit of the pathogen.

TYPE III SECRETION SYSTEMS

T3SSs (Fig. 120-1) are versatile virulence systems, helping bacteria such as *P. aeruginosa* remain extracellular, but promoting both the uptake and the intracellular survival of the intracellular pathogens *S. enterica* serovar Typhimurium, *Chlamydia* spp., and *Shigella* spp. *S. enterica* serovar Typhimurium uses distinct T3SSs for the invasion and subsequent maintenance of the *Salmonella*-containing vacuole (SCV), whereas *Chlamydia* and *Shigella* each encode only one such system. The effector proteins delivered are the major determinants of the lifestyles of these pathogens; *Shigella* quickly escapes the vacuole in a T3SS-dependent manner, whereas *Chlamydia* remains in the vacuolar compartment (the *inclusion*) and uses effector proteins to hijack cellular trafficking and perturb innate immune responses. The SCV and the *Chlamydia* inclusion exhibit distinct traits: the SCV is associated with thin membranous tubules that aid nutrient acquisition, whereas the inclusion is localized at the microtubule-organizing center, which is thought to facilitate recruitment of vesicles.

TYPE IV SECRETION SYSTEMS

For other pathogens, type IV secretion systems (T4SSs, Figure 120-1)—conceptually similar, evolutionarily distinct effector protein delivery systems—are key to the ability to survive in cellular phagocytic vacuoles. These T4SSs are similar to the T3SSs described above in that they form a multiprotein apparatus that contains a continuous channel between the bacterial cytoplasm and the human cell cytosol. However, T4SSs are functionally more diverse than T3SSs, in that (1) they are present among both gram-negative and gram-positive bacteria as well as some archaea, (2) a large subset of T4SSs transport DNA in a process called conjugation, and (3) some T4SSs deliver proteins, typically toxins, into bacterial cells rather than eukaryotic cells. Not surprisingly, T4SSs also display great structural diversity.

For the human pathogens *Legionella pneumophila* (the etiologic agent of Legionnaires' disease) and *Coxiella burnetii* (the etiologic agent of Q fever), bacterial effector proteins delivered across the vacuolar membrane into the cell cytosol by a T4SS alter maturation of the vacuole in a manner that makes it hospitable for bacterial survival; the resulting vacuole is known as a *Legionella*-containing or *Coxiella*-containing vacuole (LCV or CCV, respectively). The delivered effector proteins block fusion of lysosomes with the vacuole, thereby preventing bacterial degradation by lysosomal enzymes; manipulate host vesicular trafficking pathways; and remodel intracellular membranes to alter the lipid and protein content of the vacuolar membrane. For example, the *L. pneumophila* phospholipase VipD, a T4SS substrate, reduces the levels of phosphatidylinositol 3-phosphate on the LCV, thereby preventing recruitment of the host protein Rab5 GTPase, which is involved in endosomal maturation. The mature LCV membrane contains many features that resemble cellular endoplasmic reticulum. In the case of *C. burnetii*, the vacuole displays more lysosome-like characteristics, including a relatively low pH, which induces the activation of T4SS effector delivery. The delivered bacterial effectors stimulate efficient vesicle recruitment from endosomal and autophagosomal (see "Autophagy," below) networks, massively increasing the membrane of the CCV until it occupies the majority of the cytosol. For both *L. pneumophila* and *C. burnetii*, the mature bacterium-containing vacuoles are hospitable to bacterial replication and long-term survival.

OTHER SECRETION SYSTEMS

Francisella tularensis, the etiologic agent of the zoonotic infection tularemia, is a gram-negative facultative intracellular bacterium that displays a tropism for macrophages. *F. tularensis* resides in a phagosome, the maturation of which it delays by remodeling the lipid content of the vacuolar membrane through the action of its type VI secretion system (T6SS; Fig. 120-1). *F. tularensis* then avoids destruction by lysosomal enzymes by escaping into the cytosol, where the bacteria replicate. Another pathogen that escapes into the cytosol of macrophages is the respiratory pathogen *Mycobacterium tuberculosis*. Here, the ESX-1 type VII secretion system (T7SS) is required for lysis of the phagosomal membrane. For both of these pathogens, few effectors of their cognizant secretion system have been characterized and the process of phagosomal membrane lysis remains poorly understood.

SURVIVAL IN THE CYTOSOL

All invasive bacteria initially enter cells into a vacuole (nonphagocytic cells) or a phagosome (phagocytic cells), yet, for some pathogens, residence in the vacuole or phagosome is transient. *L. monocytogenes*, *Shigella* spp., spotted fever group *Rickettsia* spp. (the etiologic agents of Rocky Mountain spotted fever, rickettsialpox, and other spotted fever diseases), and *Burkholderia pseudomallei* (the etiologic agent of melioidosis) lyse the vacuole rapidly after invasion. Infections caused by these agents are characterized by their cytosolic lifestyles, actin-based motility, and cell-to-cell spread. The gram-positive bacterium *L. monocytogenes* produces a pore-forming toxin, listeriolysin O, and phospholipases that mediate escape into the cytosol, whereas the mechanism of vacuolar escape of *Shigella* spp. is still uncertain except for a requirement for its T3SS. Once in the cytosol, bacteria readily access nutrients such as glucose and amino acids but must also evade cell-autonomous immune mechanisms, including autophagy (see "Autophagy," below). *L. monocytogenes*, *Shigella* spp., *B. pseudomallei*, and spotted fever group *Rickettsia* spp. display actin-based motility, where expression of a cell-surface protein (ActA in *L. monocytogenes*, the autotransporter IcsA in *Shigella* spp., the autotransporter BimA in *B. pseudomallei*, and RickA and Sca2 in spotted fever group *Rickettsia* spp.) recruits host factors that polymerize actin. Actin polymerization occurs at the end of the bacterium and propels the microbe through the cell cytosol. This subversion of the host cytoskeleton aids bacterial survival in the cytosol and promotes bacterial dissemination through epithelial tissues. In the case of *Shigella*, *Listeria*, and *Rickettsia*, actin-based motility pushes the bacteria into the host cell membranes to form protrusions that are subsequently taken up by the neighboring cell, resolving into a double-membrane vacuole containing the bacterium. This vacuole is lysed once more, releasing the bacteria into the cytosol, wherein they begin another round of replication. The modes of actin-based motility exhibit many similarities despite being utilized by evolutionarily diverse bacteria, indicating the importance of this virulence mechanism for cytosolic pathogens. *Burkholderia* spp., on the other hand, induce formation of multinucleated giant cells. Here, the bacteria trigger the infected host cell to fuse its membranes with adjacent cells in a T6SS-dependent manner, forming a contiguous cytoplasm.

■ NUTRIENT ACQUISITION

Regardless of the site of bacterial infection, microbes must acquire nutrients to replicate. For both extracellular and vacuolar pathogens, a global defensive strategy used by the host is the maintenance of nutrient-poor conditions. Also impacting extracellular bacteria is the microbiota, which contributes to nutritional immunity through competition for resources (**Chap. 471**). Bacterial pathogens possess an arsenal of nutrient acquisition mechanisms to overcome these challenges. For example, upon oxidative stress, to maximize nutrient uptake, several pathogens secrete metal ion-binding proteins through T4SSs (Fig. 120-1) and upregulate expression of cell surface receptors. Many bacteria manipulate the host to subvert the processes restricting nutrient availability, with intracellular bacteria commonly delivering factors that inhibit host mRNA translation and thus increase the available pool of amino acids. Pathogens within vacuoles have evolved methods of redirecting host nutrient transport to these vacuoles.

■ CELLULAR TRAFFICKING

Because the vacuolar environment is poor in nutrients, bacteria that survive in vacuoles have evolved intricate strategies for the manipulation of host processes to meet their metabolic needs. Once internalized, vacuolar pathogens modulate endosomal trafficking to prevent degradation by lysosomal compartments. Whereas cytoskeletal rearrangements are regulated by small GTPases of the Rho family, the transport of vesicles through the cell cytosol is controlled by Rab and Arf GTPases. The co-evolution of vacuole-residing bacteria with their eukaryotic hosts has promoted the acquisition of eukaryotic-like domains in many secreted bacterial effector proteins. Many of these effector proteins mimic host cellular trafficking proteins such as guanine nucleotide exchange factors (GEFs), which regulate GTPase activities, and soluble *N*-ethylmaleimide-sensitive factor attachment protein receptors (SNAREs), which control vesicle fusion with vacuolar and other membranes. These bacterial effectors cause the accumulation of host protein and lipid markers on the vacuolar membranes, thereby causing the vacuoles to resemble host compartments. Consequently, host vesicles are redirected from the endoplasmic reticulum, Golgi apparatus, and secretory pathways to the pathogen-containing vacuole, thus delivering nutrients to the vacuole. *Chlamydia* spp., which are obligate intracellular bacteria, acquire host-derived lipids in the bacterial membranes. Dissection of the modes of action of bacterial effectors has revealed novel biochemical modifications of host trafficking regulators. For example, the *L. pneumophila* T4SS secretes two effector proteins that inactivate the cellular GTPase Rab1: AnkX inactivates Rab1 by transferring to it the phospholipid phosphatidylcholine, and SidM modifies Rab1 by adding an adenosine monophosphate molecule to it. This bacterium delivers more than 300 effector proteins through its T4SS; some of these proteins (*meta-effectors*) modulate the activity of other effectors rather than host factors. The coordinated activity of the numerous effector proteins provides precise spatiotemporal control of host processes.

AVOIDANCE OF INNATE IMMUNE RESPONSES

For the host to respond to and clear an infection, it must first be capable of sensing it. The route of infection and properties of the pathogen contribute to determining the nature of the immune response. The human immune system is generally considered to consist of two arms: the innate immune system, initiated by germline-encoded sensors, and the adaptive immune system, where lymphocytes are clonally selected against specific antigens. Initial interactions of pathogens are with specific host cell types, influenced by bacterial tropism; the resulting release of danger signals and cytokines from the innate immune response shapes the later adaptive immune response.

Epithelia (e.g., in the intestinal and respiratory tracts) are commonly the first tissues that a pathogen encounters. The mucosal surfaces of these epithelia are covered in a gel-like mucus layer that contains secretory immunoglobulins, antimicrobial peptides, and commensal bacteria, which offer the first line of defense that infecting pathogens must overcome (**Chap. 471**). In the gastrointestinal tract, this barrier can be overcome through hijacking of microfold cells (M cells) in the follicle-associated epithelia. M cells sample antigens, including intact pathogenic bacteria, from the gut lumen and deliver them to the underlying gut-associated lymphoid tissue in a process known as *transcytosis*. Within the gut-associated lymphoid tissue, professional phagocytic immune cells, such as dendritic cells, macrophages, and neutrophils, engulf transcytosed material for destruction. Lysosomal degradation of pathogenic bacteria in macrophages and dendritic cells can then lead to antigen presentation, where the hydrolytic products are processed for display by the major histocompatibility complexes (MHCs). These antigen-presenting cells migrate through the lymphatic system to lymph nodes, where the adaptive immune response is stimulated through activation of B-cell and T-cell clones.

■ COMPLEMENT

Once bacteria have crossed epithelial barriers into the lamina propria, they encounter components of humoral immunity. The complement system is a complex of plasma and tissue-resident proteins that can undergo activation from their pre-protein or zymogen forms to either label pathogens for phagocytosis (*opsonization*) or lyse them directly (**Fig. 120-3**). Complement activation commences with detection of the pathogen through the binding of circulating antibodies, which are

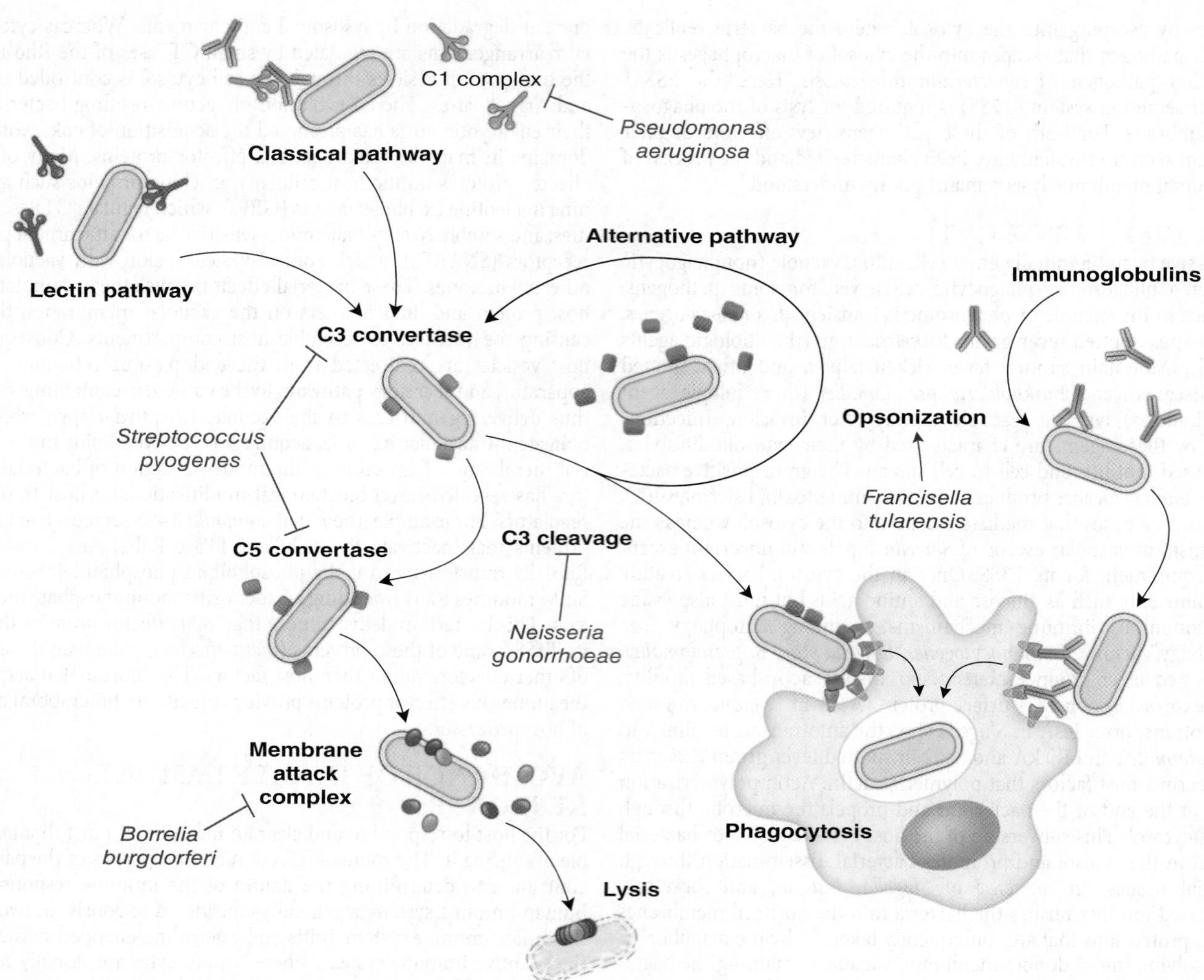

FIGURE 120-3 Overview of the complement system in bacterial infection. The *classical* and *lectin* pathways of complement activation are initiated by the binding of the C1 complex to antibodies bound to bacteria or to lectins binding carbohydrate moieties on the bacterial surface, respectively. A cascade of proteolytic cleavage generates the C3 convertase complex on the bacterial surface, which, upon activation, leads to C5 convertase formation. In the *alternative* pathway, spontaneous C3 cleavage forms alternative C3 products that lead to bacterial opsonization and to amplification of C3 convertase activation. The three complement pathways converge at the point of C3 convertase activation. In a manner similar to that seen for bacteria opsonized with circulating immunoglobulin, opsonized bacteria bind to surface receptors of phagocytes, triggering their engulfment for destruction and stimulation of the adaptive immune system. The C5 convertase, generated by conventional C3 convertase activation, recruits further complement proteins to form the membrane attack complex that directly lyses bacteria. Many bacterial pathogens inhibit specific points in the complement cascade, a selection of which are shown with blunt-ended arrows; in contrast, others, such as *Francisella* spp., promote their own opsonization and subsequent phagocytosis, enabling them to reach their intracellular replicative niche.

recognized by the C1 complex (*classical pathway*), or of lectins (*lectin pathway*) to surface carbohydrates. These pathways converge at the deposition of the C3 convertase complex on the bacterium. The *alternative pathway* is the third route of complement activation, whereby an alternative C3 convertase complex is formed either spontaneously or by the action of plasma factors, promoting amplification of the cascade. Activation of further complement components results in chemokine production, bacterial opsonization, or assembly of the membrane attack complex pore on the bacterial surface, which lyses the pathogen. Bacterial virulence factors have been described that inhibit each step of the complement pathway, highlighting the importance of this antimicrobial system to host immunity. The various strategies of bacterial interference include prevention of initial recognition by assembly of a polysaccharide capsule, modification of bacterial lipopolysaccharide (LPS), degradation of complement components, and masking of surfaces with host proteins. Streptococci employ numerous mechanisms for complement evasion and are thus a formidable foe. The streptococcal proteases ScpA and SpeB degrade many complement proteins, whereas the bacterial surface-exposed M proteins bind host proteins, including the complement inhibitor C4BP, thereby preventing C3b deposition. The thick peptidoglycan layer of gram-positive bacteria provides modest resistance to membrane attack complex–mediated lysis. Furthermore, streptococci produce a hyaluronic capsule that shields the bacterial surface from complement recognition. In comparison, *Borrelia burgdorferi*, the etiologic agent of Lyme disease, encodes a CD59-like protein that inhibits the completion of membrane attack complex assembly. Whereas many pathogens inhibit opsonization, thereby avoiding phagocytosis, other bacteria, including *Francisella* and *Yersinia* spp., promote this process, leading to uptake into the phagosomal compartment, wherein they replicate and prevent lysosomal fusion.

■ LYSOSOMES

Lysosomes are vesicular organelles of the endosomal system that contain dozens of hydrolytic and antimicrobial enzymes in a low pH environment. One such enzyme is lysozyme, which hydrolyzes the polymeric glycan chains in the bacterial cell wall peptidoglycan, resulting in bacterial lysis. In addition, release of peptidoglycan fragments stimulates other components of the innate immune system. Lysozyme is highly effective against gram-positive bacteria; however, in gram-negative bacteria, because the peptidoglycan layer lies between the outer and inner membranes, it is inaccessible to lysozyme. Gram-positive bacteria can decrease their susceptibility to lysozyme by peptidoglycan modification, such as decreased acetylation of the sugars in the glycan strand.

ANTIMICROBIAL PEPTIDES

Antimicrobial peptides, such as the positively charged defensins and cathelicidins, are concentrated in degradative compartments, where they bind the anionic surface of bacteria and perturb the integrity of the LPS of the gram-negative outer membrane and the wall teichoic acids in the gram-positive cell wall. Many bacterial pathogens modify these surfaces to reduce the net negative charge, thereby decreasing the binding of negatively charged antimicrobial peptides. In addition, *S. aureus* and the respiratory pathogen *Burkholderia cenocepacia* secrete proteases that cleave antimicrobial peptides; this action facilitates bacterial survival at mucosal surfaces and within phagosomes.

TABLE 120-3 Pattern Recognition Receptors of the Innate Immune System and Their Ligands

PATTERN RECOGNITION RECEPTOR	LIGAND OR MODE OF ACTIVATION
TLR2 (with TLR1 or TLR6)	Lipoproteins
TLR4	LPS
TLR5	Flagellin
TLR9	CpG DNA
NLRP1	Enzymatic cleavage
NLRP3	Ionic flux, mitochondrial damage
NLRP6	Lipoteichoic acid
NAIPs/NLRC4	Flagellin/T3SS
STING	Cyclic dinucleotides
NOD1 and NOD2	Peptidoglycan

OXIDATIVE BURST

Pathogens are exposed to reactive oxygen species and reactive nitrogen species produced by cells responding to infection. A well-characterized example is the neutrophil oxidative burst, where the membrane complex nicotinamide adenine dinucleotide phosphate oxidase (NADPH oxidase) produces superoxide radicals through the transfer of electrons to molecular oxygen. NADPH oxidase activation at the site of infection generates reactive oxygen species in the phagosome of neutrophils and/or in the extracellular space. Bacterial detoxification enzymes, including superoxide dismutases, peroxiredoxins, and catalases, enable bacteria to survive this oxidative burst. Many bacteria can also block the activity of NADPH oxidase; several pathogens prevent assembly of the NADPH oxidase complex by T3SS effector protein–mediated post-translational modification of small GTPases. The importance of NADPH oxidase in immune defense is highlighted clinically by the marked susceptibility to bacterial and fungal infections in patients with chronic granulomatous disease, which results from nonfunctional alleles for essential subunits of this complex.

NEUTROPHIL EXTRACELLULAR TRAPS

The oxidative burst also stimulates the release of the pro-inflammatory tumor necrosis factor α, azurophilic granules, and neutrophil extracellular traps (NETs). NETs are an extruded mesh of decondensed chromatin that are thought to ensnare pathogens, thereby restricting their spread and destroying them. Streptococci encode deoxyribonucleases (DNases) that enable pathogens to evade NETs. *S. aureus* nuclease degrades NETs; the nucleotide products of this degradation are then converted into deoxyadenosine, which functions as a potent macrophage toxin. This process showcases how bacterial pathogens may utilize antimicrobial responses to their own benefit.

PATTERN RECOGNITION RECEPTORS AND THEIR EVASION

The first line of detection of pathogens by the innate immune system is via recognition of molecular patterns that are indicative of the presence of pathogens and that distinguish self from nonself. These are the pathogen- and damage-associated molecular patterns (PAMPs and DAMPs, respectively). Recognition of these patterns enables cells to establish that an infection is occurring and to determine the nature of the pathogen, as dictated by the specific PAMP detected. Receptors for the molecular patterns include Toll-like receptors (TLRs) and pattern recognition receptors (PRRs). TLRs, transmembrane proteins at the cell surface or in the endosomal compartment, surveil the extracellular milieu, whereas other PRRs monitor threats within the cell cytosol. On phagocytic cells, TLRs may employ scavenger receptors as co-stimulatory surface receptors. TLRs recognize conserved molecules that include LPS, peptidoglycan, flagella, and nucleic acids **(Table 120-3)**. Stimulation of these receptors by ligand binding triggers assembly of supramolecular organizing centers (SMOCs), large protein complexes that are signaling platforms for all-or-nothing signal transduction via ubiquitination and phosphorylation of target proteins. Ultimately, signaling results in translocation of transcription factors, including nuclear factor-κB (NF-κB), AP-1, and interferon-regulatory factors (IRFs), into the nucleus, where they stimulate expression of cytokines, chemokines, and other immunity-related genes **(Fig. 120-4)**. Among the signaling pathways activated upon recognition of certain intracellular bacterial pathogens is the cyclic guanosine monophosphate–adenosine monophosphate synthase (cGAS) stimulator of interferon genes (STING) pathway, which was previously thought to be relevant only to recognition of intracellular viruses. In response to recognition of microbial nucleic acid, cGAS–STING activates the translocation of interferon regulatory factor 3 (IRF3) and NF-κB into the nucleus, whereupon they activate a set of interferon-regulated pro-inflammatory genes. Cytokine release alerts bystander cells and recruits immune cells from the circulation, creating a heightened immune state in the local area. The nature of the stimulus influences the type of immune response. Cytosolic ligands tend to stimulate stronger pro-inflammatory responses than extracellular ligands, a difference reflecting the higher threat perceived. Moreover, detection of cytosolic peptidoglycan, which is derived from bacteria, elicits a response distinct from that to dsRNA, which is derived from viruses.

Pathogens have evolved a plethora of strategies to avoid detection by the innate immune system. A common strategy is to mask PAMPs. For example, LPS on the surface of gram-negative bacteria contains a lipid A component that usually harbors six acyl chains. LPS that is hexa-acylated is recognized by TLR4 at the cell surface. The etiologic agent of plague, *Yersinia pestis*, produces hexa-acylated LPS in the flea vector, but, upon the organism's transmission to human hosts, the temperature shift to 37°C induces acyltransferase expression that results in production instead of tetra-acylated LPS, which does not activate the TLR4 receptor. Tetra-acylated LPS is also synthesized by the etiologic agent of tularemia, *F. tularensis*; the periodontal pathogen *Porphyromonas gingivalis*; and the gastric pathogen *H. pylori*. The flagellum of *H. pylori* is also essential for virulence, enabling the bacterium to reach the gastric epithelium after ingestion. Flagellin, the monomeric protein subunit of the flagellum, is an extracellular ligand for TLR5, but *H. pylori* bypasses flagellin recognition since its flagellin epitope is divergent from the TLR5 recognition motif. DNA in intracellular membrane compartments of the endosomal system is recognized by TLR9, which binds to CpG-containing unmethylated DNA. Because CpG motifs are usually methylated in mammalian DNA, the methylation state provides a method of discriminating self from nonself. Group A streptococci secrete the Sda1 DNase, which degrades CpG DNA, therefore reducing the immunogenicity of lysed bacteria.

Inhibition of NF-κB Signaling Upon binding to bacterial peptidoglycan, the cytosolic PRRs NOD1 and NOD2 activate NF-κB signaling, thereby priming cell immune responses. Polymorphisms in the *NOD1* and *NOD2* genes confer susceptibility to inflammatory bowel disease, an action that highlights the role of cytosolic sensing of bacterial cell wall components in immune homeostasis. The co-evolution

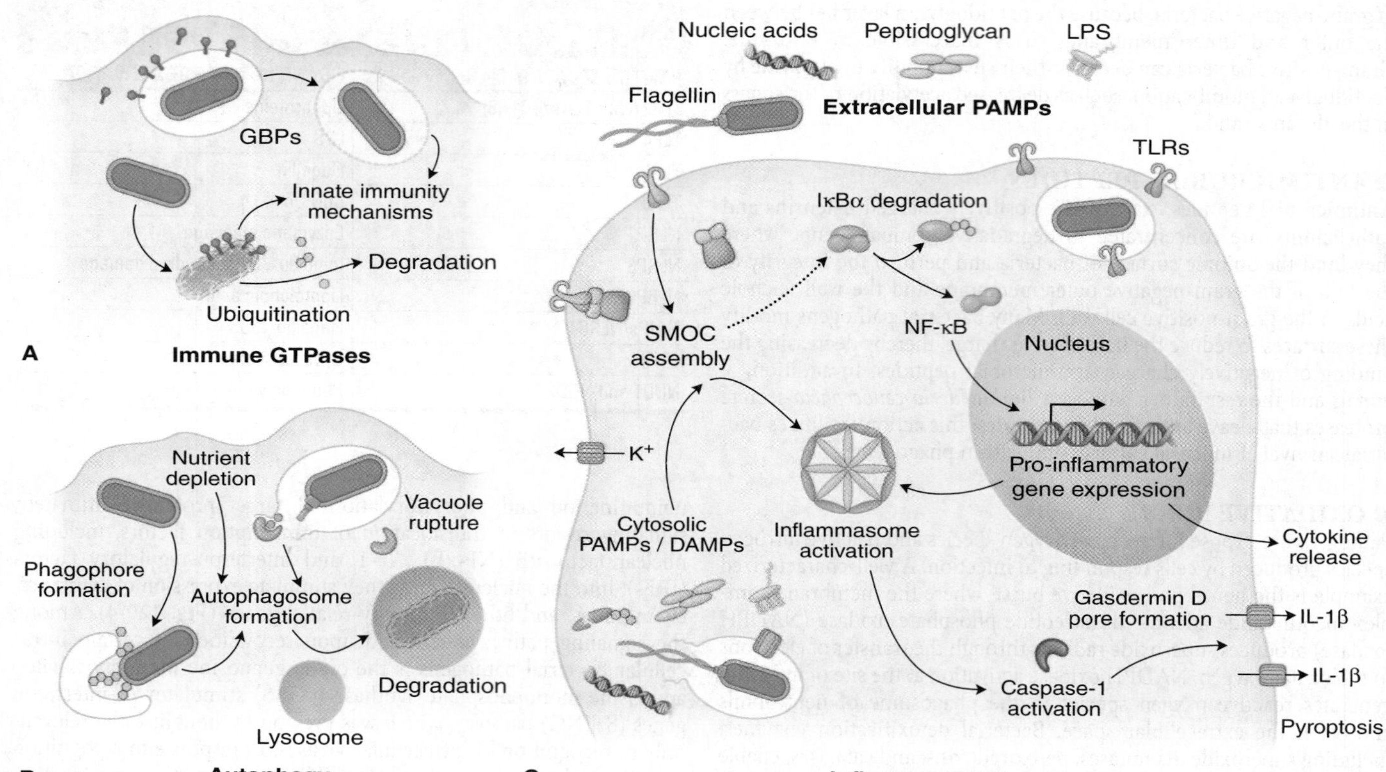

FIGURE 120-4 Overview of innate immune recognition and response to bacterial pathogens. ***A.*** Immune GTPases. Proteins of the GBP family associate with the bacterial surface, LPS shed from the bacterial surface, or pathogen-containing vacuoles, disrupting the integrity of the pathogen and leading to lysis. Labeling of intracellular pathogens with immune GTPases may instead stimulate ubiquitination of the bacterium and its destruction by cell-autonomous immune mechanisms such as autophagy. ***B.*** Autophagy. Recognition of bacterial invasion leads to host-mediated sequestration of the pathogen in an autophagosome and destruction of the pathogen upon fusion of the autophagosome with lysosomes. Bacteria may be directly labeled by ubiquitination, damaged vacuoles are recognized by the binding of galectins to exposed glycans, and/or the cellular autophagy may be induced in response to sensing starvation. ***C.*** Pattern recognition receptors and innate immune signaling. Conserved PAMPs, DAMPs, and danger signals are recognized by all cells, triggering innate immune signaling pathways and pro-inflammatory gene expression. TLRs surveil the cell surface and endosomal interior for PAMPs that include LPS, nucleic acids, and flagellin. Cytosolic PRRs, including NLRs and ALRs, recognize similar ligands as well as distinct stimuli, including dysregulation of ion homeostasis. TLR activation promotes SMOC assembly and NF-κB signaling. Under resting conditions, NF-κB is sequestered in the cytosol by IκBα, but TLR activation leads to IκBα phosphorylation, ubiquitination, and degradation, with the consequent release of NF-κB. Resultant translocation of NF-κB into the nucleus leads to pro-inflammatory gene expression and the production and release of cytokines. Stimulation of cytosolic PRRs leads to assembly of SMOCs known as inflammasomes, resulting in activation of caspases. A well-characterized example is the activation of caspase-1 by canonical and noncanonical inflammasomes, subsequent activation of the membrane pore protein GSDMD, maturation and release of pro-inflammatory cytokines IL-1β and IL-18, and pyroptotic death of the cell.

of bacterial pathogens with the host has led to the acquisition in many bacterial virulence factors of eukaryotic-like domains that enable the pathogen to hijack host signal transduction. *Ubiquitination*, a post-translational modification of eukaryotic proteins that regulates many cellular processes, is a common target among known bacterial mechanisms of host signaling inhibition. In ubiquitination, the small ubiquitin protein is covalently linked to a target protein, and additional ubiquitin molecules are added on; the consequence is branched or linear chains that signal the fate of the target. Ubiquitination-mediated target fates are degradation by the proteasome (most common), targeting to particular vesicular compartments, or signaling. The enzymes responsible for labeling targets with ubiquitin are E3 ubiquitin ligases, which transfer ubiquitin from an E2 ubiquitin–conjugating enzyme to the target protein.

A plethora of bacterial effector proteins specifically target components of the NF-κB pathway in ways that maintain repression of NF-κB-dependent pro-inflammatory genes. In doing so, these pathogens counteract activation of innate immune responses triggered by their conserved PAMPs. The translocation of NF-κB into the nucleus requires the successive phosphorylation, ubiquitination, and degradation of IκBα by the IκB kinase (IKK) complex, which in resting cells functions to inhibit NF-κB; the dissociation of the IKK complex from NF-κB enables the latter to translocate into the nucleus, where it functions as a transcriptional factor (Fig. 120-4C). The T3SS of *Shigella* spp. delivers into cells several E3 ubiquitin ligases that target components of the NF-κB pathway for degradation. The intracellular pathogens *Chlamydia trachomatis* and *B. pseudomallei* secrete bacterial deubiquitinases through T3SS and T2SS, respectively, which cleave the ubiquitin moiety from IκBα, thereby preventing its degradation, maintaining inhibited NF-κB in the cytosol, and repressing pro-inflammatory gene expression.

Other enzymatic activities of bacterial effectors can also inhibit NF-κB activation by ubiquitin-dependent processes. *L. pneumophila* delivers, via its T4SS, the MavC transglutaminase, which performs noncanonical ubiquitination of an E2 enzyme, preventing activation of the IKK complex; the *Shigella* spp. T3SS cryptic kinase OspG binds and inhibits cellular E2 ubiquitin–conjugating enzymes involved in NF-κB activation; and NleE and OspZ from EPEC and *Shigella* spp., respectively, are cysteine methyltransferases that inhibit IKK activation.

Another cellular pathway of pro-inflammatory signaling stimulated by PRRs is a phosphorylation cascade involving mitogen-activated protein kinases (MAPKs) that leads to activation of the transcription factor AP-1. The potent *Bacillus anthracis* exotoxin lethal factor exhibits metalloprotease activity that cleaves the N-terminal region of most MAPKs, thereby ablating the kinase cascade. The homologous T3SS effectors YopJ, AvrA, and VopA of *Yersinia* spp., *S. enterica* serovar Typhimurium, and *Vibrio parahaemolyticus*, respectively, acetylate key serine residues in MAPKs, which blocks their phosphorylation. Finally, OspF of *Shigella* spp. and the ortholog SpvC from *S. enterica* serovar Typhimurium are phosphothreonine lyases that irreversibly cleave phosphorylated threonine residues from MAPKs, thereby preventing their activities. *S. enterica* serovar Typhimurium also targets NF-κB directly with several T3SS metalloproteases. The broad range of effector protein mechanisms and the large number of distinct host targets underscore the need for bacterial pathogens to subvert innate immune signaling in order to establish a successful infection (Fig. 120-4).

Immune GTPases For many infectious processes, the initial interaction of the pathogen with an immune cell primes an enhanced subsequent immune response by augmenting innate immune mechanisms—for example, through upregulation of immunity-related gene expression and/or recruitment of neutrophils to the site of infection. A second stimulus then activates a more robust innate immune response that is directly geared toward clearing the pathogen or, if the threat is too great, leads to suicide of the infected cell. One set of molecules that primes cellular responses is the immune GTPases, of which the best characterized is the guanylate binding protein (GBP) family. Production of these cytosolic or membrane-associated sensors is induced by interferon signaling. GBPs target pathogen-containing vacuoles, bacterial membranes, or released fragments of bacterial membranes, such as LPS. Analogous to scavenger receptors, GBPs promote the release of PAMPs and DAMPs from these membrane structures and present the PAMP or DAMP to PRRs. For example, some GBPs extract LPS molecules from the surface of cytosolic gram-negative bacterial pathogens, and this extraction leads to activation of the noncanonical inflammasome (see below). Recruitment of GBPs to *Shigella* spp. prevents bacterial actin-based motility and promotes labeling of bacteria with ubiquitin, which targets them for degradation by the proteasome. In this case, the shigellae are able to interfere with this cellular response by secreting an E3 ubiquitin ligase effector that targets the GBPs for degradation.

Inflammasomes Whereas the extracellular environment is surveilled for signs of infection by TLRs, the cytosol is monitored by other PRRs, including members of the NOD- and AIM2-like receptor (NLR and ALR, respectively) families, which form SMOCs known as *inflammasomes*. Upon binding to ligand (for example, cytosolic wall teichoic acids and dsDNA), these PRRs oligomerize, often with the ASC scaffold protein. Oligomerization is associated with recruitment of pro-caspases, zymogens that are activated within the complexes by auto-cleavage. The cleaved forms of pro-inflammatory caspases are themselves proteases that cleave zymogen substrates. For example, caspase-1 cleaves the substrate gasdermin D (GSDMD), enabling the free amino-terminal fragment of GSDMD to assemble into a pore in the plasma membrane. Caspase-1 also cleaves and activates pro-IL-1β and pro-IL-18, releasing the mature cytokines IL-1β and IL-18, which are secreted from the cell through the GSDMD pore, and enabling cytokine signaling (Fig. 120-4). The formation of GSDMD pores also leads to lytic death of the cell, a process designated *pyroptosis* (inflammatory cell death). Pyroptosis is triggered by either of two types of inflammasomes, the canonical caspase-1 inflammasome and the noncanonical inflammasome.

The PRRs of the best characterized canonical inflammasomes are NLRP1, NLRP3, and NAIP-NLRC4. The NLRP3 inflammasome appears to be activated upon sensing of homeostatic dysregulation, including ion flux and mitochondrial damage. Thus, it may be activated by pore-forming toxins such as the phenol-soluble modulins of *S. aureus* and α-hemolysin of UPEC. NAIP-NLRC4 senses the needle protein of the T3SS and the related flagellin protein. Many pathogens have evolved mechanisms to overcome activation of the NAIP-NLRC4 inflammasome, including downregulation of flagella expression by *L. pneumophila* upon entry into cells as well as activation of pro-survival Akt signaling by the *S. enterica* serovar Typhimurium T3SS effector SopB, which reduces *nlrc4* expression during intracellular infection. In addition, caspases of the noncanonical inflammasome are directly inhibited by the binding of the T3SS effector proteins OspC3 and NleF from *Shigella* spp. and EHEC, respectively. Overall, the inhibition of inflammasomes by bacterial pathogens enables pathogens to avoid elimination by the innate immune system.

Inflammasomes have been described as organelles that assess the level of threat posed by pathogens, since they not only recognize PAMPs and DAMPs but also act as sentinels for dysregulation of host processes. Both the NOD1 and pyrin inflammasomes sense cytoskeletal perturbations by monitoring modification of small GTPases. Pyrin senses a range of covalent modifications of Rho GTPases, including glucosylation by *C. difficile* TcdB, adenylylation by *C. botulinum* C3 toxin, and deamidation by *B. cenocepacia* T6SS effector TecA. Meanwhile, recent work suggests that the NLRP1 inflammasome may act as bait for cleavage by microbial proteases or ubiquitin-targeted degradation, processes that stimulate its activation and subsequent pyroptosis. Once more, the importance of inflammasome signaling is underscored by a plethora of polymorphisms that exist in inflammasome-associated genes and that may give rise to autoinflammatory disorders or may confer high susceptibility to microbial infection.

Inhibition of Nonpyroptotic Cell Death An outcome of inflammasome activation in macrophages, and occasionally in nonphagocytic cells, is pyroptosis. This inflammatory form of cell death both destroys the pathogen residing within the cell and alerts bystander cells of the threat. Several other types of regulated (*programmed*) cell death occur, of which inflammatory necroptosis and noninflammatory apoptosis are best characterized. In *necroptosis*, activation of any of a variety of innate immune signaling pathways (interferon-γ, TLRs) leads to kinase-dependent assembly of a plasma membrane pore complex that induces cell lysis and release of DAMPs into the extracellular space, events that in turn induce an intense inflammatory response. Necroptosis has been described in bacterial pneumonia and sepsis.

In *apoptosis*, cells condense and form membranous blebs without exposing or releasing cytosolic contents into the surrounding milieu and thus without inducing inflammation in adjacent tissues. The apoptotic blebs and dead cells are disposed of by macrophages in a process known as *efferocytosis*. Apoptosis is not instigated solely upon infection; it plays a key role in development and also occurs normally in many epithelial tissues, such as the intestine, where, during normal cell turnover, epithelial cells migrate to the tips of intestinal villi, from which they extrude and detach.

Apoptosis can be initiated by intrinsic or extrinsic cellular stimuli, resulting in activation of apoptotic caspases that demolish cellular contents. The intrinsic pathway occurs through dissolution of the mitochondrial membrane potential, which commonly occurs during infection because of cellular stress or the action of bacterial toxins. The extrinsic pathway can be stimulated by interactions of cell-surface death receptors with pro-inflammatory ligands like TNF-α.

The gastrointestinal pathogens *S. enterica* serovar Typhimurium, *Yersinia enterocolitica*, and pathogenic *E. coli* inhibit signal transduction from cell-surface death receptors, thereby blocking cell death. The cell's sensing of inhibition of extrinsic apoptotic signaling leads to stimulation of alternative inflammatory cell death pathways; this scenario highlights the importance of functional redundancy of critical host immune responses. These pathogens can block signaling by modifying arginine residues of death receptor SMOCs with sugar moieties or by direct cleavage of SMOC components (Fig. 120-4).

The intracellular vacuole-residing *Chlamydia* spp. activate survival pathways through phosphoinositide 3-kinase (PI3K) and Wnt/β-catenin signaling, while simultaneously inhibiting apoptosis. T4SS effectors of vacuole-residing *L. pneumophila* and *C. burnetii* inhibit apoptosis through the sequestration of pro-apoptotic host factors. Cyclomodulins, a group of bacterial effector proteins that arrest the cell cycle, are delivered into cells by the extracellular attaching and effacing pathogens EPEC and EHEC. The EPEC and EHEC cyclomodulin Cif deamidates ubiquitin and related proteins, inactivating the host E3 ligases involved in cell cycle progression and thereby reducing epithelial turnover. The recognition by the cell of this disruption of important host cell processes triggers cell death pathways. Thus, co-evolution of bacterial pathogens with their hosts results in a tug-of-war.

Autophagy Once detection of a pathogen has been established and cytokine secretion has been triggered, nonimmune cells are able to deploy cell-autonomous immunity mechanisms to neutralize the threat. In addition to assembly of the NADPH oxidase complex and production of immune GTPases, the responses include upregulation of autophagy. Autophagy disposes of damaged organelles and recycles long-lived protein complexes through generation of double-membrane compartments (*autophagosomes*) around the cargo and delivery of the engulfed cargo to the lysosome, wherein the cargo is degraded to amino acids and other constituents. Autophagy can isolate and dispose of cytosolic pathogens. Recognition of the pathogen can be direct or can occur through the sensing of DAMPs. Here, host galectins, polysaccharide-binding molecules, participate in the recognition of pathogens and induce ubiquitination of the bacterial surface and recruitment of the host autophagy protein LC3, which triggers engulfment in autophagosomes.

The survival of intracellular bacterial pathogens is dependent on their ability to inhibit the autophagy machinery. Common mechanisms utilized by bacteria to interfere with autophagy include evasion of ubiquitination by inhibition of host E3 ligases, blocking of ubiquitination sites through decoration of surface-exposed virulence factors with host proteins, or alteration of host pathways that regulate autophagy. The cytosolic pathogen *L. monocytogenes* induces actin-based motility and cell-to-cell spread through recruitment of the host factor Arp2/3, and Arp2/3 recruitment helps mask *Listeria* surface proteins from ubiquitination. An important metabolic trigger of autophagy is intracellular depletion of amino acids, which occurs upon replication of metabolically active intracellular pathogens. The master regulator of cell metabolism is mammalian target of rapamycin (mTOR); mTOR is inactivated by intracellular starvation conditions, and its inactivation derepresses autophagy. Invasive pathogens, including *M. tuberculosis*, *S. enterica* serovar Typhimurium, and *Shigella* spp., have evolved strategies to re-activate mTOR signaling during infection, thereby evading autophagy. *S. enterica* serovar Typhimurium also secretes two effectors, SseF and SseG, that block the activation of a kinase required for autophagosome generation. Because of the ubiquity of autophagy and other cell-autonomous immunity pathways in the body, bacterial pathogens have evolved mechanisms to overcome these key host defenses regardless of cellular tropism.

Dysregulated or excessive immune responses are detrimental to the host, as in sepsis or severe COVID-19 infection, causing morbidity and sometimes death. Too weak an immune response may lead to pathogen-induced morbidity and mortality. A cellular mechanism that promotes appropriate immune responses is innate immune training, which enables cells to be primed at the transcriptional level through epigenetic modifications. Here, epigenetic alterations in chromatin structure cause stable changes in gene expression profiles. Epigenetic regulation consists of post-translational modification of histones, with alteration of their phosphorylation, acetylation, and/or methylation states—changes that influence chromatin structure and access of transcription factors to regulatory elements in the DNA. Mounting evidence indicates that the human microbiota promotes this innate immune training, modifying the methylation state of promoters of genes involved in metabolism and immunity and allowing the host to respond to infection in a well-tuned manner. Not surprisingly, pathogens also regulate host responses at the epigenetic level. *B. anthracis* and *L. pneumophila* deliver into cells histone methyltransferases that control inflammation and ribosome activity. *L. monocytogenes* listeriolysin O, the *P. aeruginosa* T3SS pore, and other plasma membrane pore-forming complexes exert epigenetic modulation through alterations in ion homeostasis, thereby manipulating the gene expression profiles of infected host cells.

INHIBITION OF ADAPTIVE IMMUNE RESPONSES

Early interactions of pathogens with host cells trigger the innate immune response, releasing cytokines that recruit additional antigen-presenting immune cells to the site of infection. To establish chronic infection, bacterial pathogens need not only to suppress the innate immune system but also to avoid elimination by the adaptive immune response. The adaptive immune system comprises clonally expanded lineages of B and T lymphocytes that have been activated by antigen-presenting cells, the best characterized of which are dendritic cells and macrophages. B cells are required for humoral immunity; genetic diseases that affect B-cell function often manifest as the inability to produce adequate antibody titers to clear extracellular bacterial infections. T cells generally mediate cell-mediated immunity, helping the host clear infected cells. The activation of T cells occurs by the presentation of processed antigen on MHC molecules of antigen-presenting cells. The activation of T cells is controlled by the specificity of MHC molecules and of their receptors. The large variety of receptors possessed by T cells enables collective recognition of a wide variety of antigens. Mutations that ablate the development of the adaptive immune system result in severe combined immunodeficiency, rendering the individual extremely vulnerable to infection.

M. tuberculosis is notorious for its ability to establish latent infections, avoiding elimination by the immune system for decades. Once phagocytosed, the pathogen induces secretion of immunosuppressive cytokines, including IL-6, IL-10, and transforming growth factor β. The result is inhibition of interferon-γ-dependent gene expression, with downregulation of MHC class II and other immune-stimulatory molecules, which inhibits induction of helper $CD4^+$ T lymphocytes. Similarly, *B. pertussis* induces dendritic cells to produce IL-10, which skews T-cell maturation into regulatory T cells, dampening the immune response. The *S. enterica* serovar Typhimurium T3SS effector protein SteD depletes MHC class II molecules from the surface of dendritic cells by the activation of the E3 ubiquitin ligase MARCH8. MARCH8 ubiquitinates MHC class II, interfering with its trafficking to the cell surface and thereby decreasing interaction with and subsequent activation of T lymphocytes.

In addition to preventing antigen-presenting cells from stimulating lymphocytes, pathogens may also directly alter B-cell and T-cell activity. The *Yersinia* T3SS effector YopH, a protein tyrosine phosphatase, dephosphorylates B-cell and T-cell receptors and thus prevents both signal transduction upon stimulation by antigen-presenting cells and lymphocyte activation. Staphylococcal toxic shock syndrome is induced by the production of superantigens by *S. aureus*. These extremely inflammatory exotoxins are potent activators of T cells, stimulating exuberant and at times fatal cytokine production. Rather than binding the specificity-determining variable regions of MHC molecules and the T-cell receptor, superantigens bind invariable regions and are therefore able to nonspecifically activate vast numbers of T cells, with a consequent cytokine storm.

BACTERIAL CYTOTOXINS

Many bacterial toxins are *cytotoxins*—toxins that trigger host cell death. The best-characterized group of bacterial cytotoxins are the AB toxins, which are defined by the presence of an active (A) subunit, which mediates the enzymatic activity of the toxin, and a binding (B) subunit, which mediates binding to the cellular receptor. This family of toxins includes Shiga toxins of *Shigella* spp. and pathogenic *E. coli*, ι toxin of *C. perfringens*, diphtheria toxin of *Corynebacterium diphtheriae*, pertussis toxin of *B. pertussis*, and CTX of *V. cholerae*. In general, upon binding to cell surface receptors, the toxin is taken up into endosomes, whereupon the A-subunit is translocated across the endosome membrane and released into the cytosol, where its toxic enzymatic activity is stimulated. CTX and pertussis toxin exhibit ADP-ribosyl transferase activity, targeting G-protein regulators of adenylate cyclases in a manner that increases cellular cyclic AMP concentrations and thereby perturbing ion homeostasis and apoptosis. Increased intracellular cyclic AMP induces chloride secretion via CFTR and inhibits sodium chloride absorption; the results are massive fluid secretion into the lumen of the small intestine and the diarrheal symptoms of cholera. Many other bacterial toxins that are not AB family toxins, including *C. perfringens* ι toxin and *P. aeruginosa* exotoxin A, display ADP-ribosyl transferase activity that targets elongation factor-2, thereby inhibiting host translation. In contrast, the *S. enterica* serovar Typhimurium protein SpvB and *C. difficile* binary toxins target actin, inhibiting normal cellular cytoskeletal rearrangements. Despite the range of enzymatic activities displayed by the bacterial toxins described above, the effects on the host cell generally fall into the few broad categories of cytoskeletal manipulation, inhibition of innate immune response signaling, and hijacking of cellular trafficking.

Pore-forming toxins are prevalent virulence factors of extracellular pathogens. They include the cholesterol-dependent cytolysins intermedilysin of *S. intermedius*, θ toxin of *C. perfringens*, anthrolysin O of *B. anthracis*, and listeriolysin O of *L. monocytogenes*. *S. aureus* produces several cytolysins, including the Panton-Valentine leucocidin; α-, β-, γ-, and δ-hemolysins; and phenol-soluble modulins. Following their release by bacteria, leukocidins and α- and γ-hemolysins form oligomeric complexes in host plasma membranes, with consequent lysis of the host cell. These pore-forming toxins have different cell-type specificities that are thought to be driven by binding of pore components with specific cell surface receptors. Phenol-soluble modulins are small peptides that, as a result of their amphipathic nature, appear to directly insert into cell membranes, such that no receptor is thought to be necessary. Lytic toxins protect *S. aureus* from phagocytosis, yet recent work has uncovered a host defense mechanism that counters cytolysins through the release of vesicles (termed *exosomes*), which act as decoys by removing cytolysins from the local environment.

TISSUE DAMAGE AND PATHOGEN DISSEMINATION

Much of the pathology associated with bacterial infection results from pro-inflammatory immune responses. Infected cells may continually signal in ways that alert the immune system, even though, as described above, many bacteria avoid elimination by cell-autonomous and immune cell–mediated mechanisms. In the intestine, tight junctions mediate intimate associations between epithelial cells that maintain tissue barrier function, linking the cytoskeletal networks of adjacent cells through intimate association of protein complexes across the cell membranes. Many intestinal pathogens perturb the integrity of the gut epithelium either by manipulating cell polarity or by disrupting intercellular junctions. *C. perfringens*, *V. cholerae*, pathogenic *E. coli*, *Shigella* spp., and *S. enterica* serovar Typhi all produce toxins in the gastrointestinal tract that disrupt tight junctions, consequently disrupting the barrier function of the tissue and facilitating access of the pathogen to deeper tissue. The RtxA multifunctional repeats-in-toxin (MARTX) toxin of *V. cholerae* causes cell rounding and barrier failure through actin-crosslinking activity, yet avoids eliciting substantial immune responses by simultaneously inactivating phospholipases and Rho GTPases. The serine protease autotransporters (SPATEs) of *Shigella* spp. and some pathogenic *E. coli* are typically secreted into the gut lumen or mucus layer, whereupon they cleave components of epithelial junctions and mucins in ways that facilitate tissue penetration. Tissue damage permits access to the underlying mucosal layers, the lymphatics, and the bloodstream; for some pathogens, this access enables seeding of other organs.

Transmission to New Hosts The host represents a replicative niche for bacterial pathogens, in which they multiply and are transmitted to new hosts. The mode of transmission is typically aligned with the mode of entry. For example, for respiratory pathogens, coughing induced by tissue damage in the lung aerosolizes the pathogen, enabling inhalation by and colonization of a new host. Similarly, gastrointestinal pathogens elicit diarrhea and are transmitted via the direct fecal–oral route or via contamination of crops or food with waste from an infected individual. The understanding of the spread of infectious diseases permits the institution of basic hygiene procedures that greatly diminish transmission rates—for example, hand washing, decontamination of communal surfaces, and adoption of social distancing measures.

Bacteriophages and Pathogen Lifestyle The reservoir of *V. cholerae* is aquatic environments. Disease is acquired through the ingestion of contaminated seawater or seafood. In regions where cholera is endemic, the disease displays seasonal peaks. This seasonality is associated with blooms of bacteria-targeting viruses (*bacteriophages*), which infect *V. cholerae* organisms, replicate, and lyse and kill the bacterial host. Bacterial lysis releases viral particles into the aquatic environment, whereupon they can infect other *V. cholerae*. Consequently, the bacteriophages regulate the abundance of pathogens, with ramifications for the epidemiology of the disease. Whether bacteriophages contribute to cyclical control of other pathogens is currently unknown.

COMPETITION WITH COMMENSAL MICROBES

In recent years, it has become clear that the host microbiota constitutes an ecosystem that contributes to host defense against infecting pathogens. This community of commensal microorganisms (bacteria, fungi, viruses) is essential for the metabolic homeostasis and immune development of the host. Furthermore, the presence of commensal organisms on external surfaces (e.g., the skin), in the nasopharynx, and in the intestinal tract provides colonization resistance against pathogens. The gut microbiota is among the densest ecosystems known. Consequently, pathogens are greatly outnumbered by flora, and, within each niche, pathogens must compete with commensals for nutrients. The importance of the microbiota is underscored by *C. difficile* infection, wherein antibiotic treatment, which eradicates components of the gut microbiota, enables *C. difficile* spores to germinate, with consequent toxin production and disease. It is notable that an effective treatment for *C. difficile* colitis is repopulation of the microbiota through fecal transplantation.

Many commensal organisms possess antibacterial systems, including bacteriocins and T6SSs. One activity of T6SSs is the delivery of toxins directly into neighboring bacteria, resulting in lysis or growth inhibition of the target. T6SSs are present in both pathogenic and commensal bacteria, and T6SS-mediated killing contributes both to the establishment of a stable gut microbial community and to colonization by invading pathogens, including *Shigella sonnei* and *V. cholerae*. In cystic fibrosis patients, upregulation of a T6SS of *P. aeruginosa* occurs; this alteration suggests a role for this system in the persistence of chronic *P. aeruginosa* infection in the cystic fibrosis lung, which is a polymicrobial environment.

SUMMARY

Bacterial pathogens display myriad mechanisms of colonization, adhesion, invasion, dissemination, and manipulation of host pathways. Infectious diseases are the result when pathogens successfully establish themselves within the host, and symptoms are usually the result of the ensuing fights between the pathogens and the immune system. The sheer diversity of virulence determinants highlights the success of the host in combating infection. Further elucidation of how bacteria cause infection will better our understanding of human biology and pathogens and will provide new opportunities for successful therapeutic intervention.

FURTHER READING

Costa TRD et al: Secretion systems in gram-negative bacteria: structural and mechanistic insights. Nat Rev Microbiol 13:343, 2015.

Evavold CL, Kagan JC: Inflammasomes: threat-assessment organelles of the innate immune system. Immunity 348:682, 2019.

Fitzgerald KA, Kagan JC: Toll-like receptors and the control of immunity. Cell 180:1044, 2020.

Galluzzi L et al: Molecular mechanisms of cell death: Recommendations of the Nomenclature Committee on Cell Death 2018. Cell Death Differ 25:486, 2018.

Lamason RL, Welch MD: Actin-based motility and cell-to-cell spread of bacterial pathogens. Curr Opin Microbiol 35:48, 2017.

Ribet D, Cossart P: How bacterial pathogens colonize their hosts and invade deeper tissues. Microbes Infect 17:173, 2015.

Santos JC, Broz P: Sensing of invading pathogens by GBPs: At the crossroads between cell-autonomous and innate immunity. J Leukoc Biol 104:729, 2018.

Stones DH, Krachler AM: Against the tide: the role of bacterial adhesion in host colonization. Biochem Soc Trans 44:1571, 2016.

Tsolis RM, Bäumler AJ: Gastrointestinal host–pathogen interaction in the age of microbiome research. Curr Opin Microbiol 53:78, 2020.

Wu YW, Li F: Bacterial interaction with host autophagy. Virulence 10:352, 2019.

121 Microbial Genomics and Infectious Disease

Roby P. Bhattacharyya, Yonatan H. Grad, Deborah T. Hung

Just as microscopy opened up the worlds of microbiology by providing a tool with which to visualize microorganisms, technological advances in genomics now provide microbiologists with powerful new methods to characterize the genetic map that underlies all microbes with unprecedented resolution, thereby illuminating their complex and dynamic interactions with each other, the environment, and human health. The field of infectious disease genomics encompasses a vast frontier of active research that is transforming the clinical practice of infectious diseases. While genetics has long played a key role in elucidating the process of infection and impacting clinical infectious diseases, the ability to extend our thinking and approaches beyond the study of single genes to an examination of the sequence, structure, and function of entire genomes allows us to identify new possibilities for research and opportunities to change clinical practice. From the development of diagnostics with unprecedented sensitivity, specificity, and speed to the design of novel public health interventions, technical and statistical genomic innovations are reshaping our understanding of the influence of the microbial world on human health and providing us with new tools to diagnose, track, and combat infection. In this chapter, we explore the application of genomics methods to microbial pathogens and the infections they cause. We discuss innovations that are driving the development of diagnostic approaches as well as the discovery of new pathogens, providing insight into novel therapeutic approaches and paradigms, and advancing methods in infectious disease epidemiology and the study of pathogen evolution that can inform infection control measures, public health responses to outbreaks, and vaccine development. We draw on examples in current practice and from the recent scientific literature as signposts that point toward ways in which the insights from pathogen genomics may influence infectious diseases in the short and long terms, and we highlight their applications to SARS-CoV-2 and COVID-19 pandemic. **Table 121-1** provides definitions for a selection of important terms used in genomics.

TABLE 121-1 Glossary of Selected Terms in Genomics

TERM	DEFINITION
Contig	A DNA sequence representing a continuous fragment of a genome, assembled from overlapping sequences; relevant for de novo assembly of sequence data that do not align to previously sequenced genomes
Genome	The entire set of heritable genetic material within an organism
Horizontal gene transfer	The transfer of genes between organisms through mechanisms other than by clonal descent, such as through transformation, conjugation, or transduction
Metagenomics	Analysis of genetic material from multiple species directly from primary samples without requiring prior culture steps
Microarray	A collection of DNA oligonucleotides ("oligos") spatially arranged on a solid surface and used to detect or quantify sequences in a sample of interest that are complementary (and therefore bind) to one or more of the arrayed oligos
Microbial genome-wide association study (GWAS)	An analytic framework to test statistical associations between microbial genotypes and phenotypes of interest, such as antibiotic resistance and virulence
Mobile genetic elements	DNA elements that can move within a genome and can be transferred between genomes through horizontal gene transfer (e.g., plasmids, bacteriophages, and transposons)
Multilocus sequence typing	A method for typing organisms based on DNA sequence fragments from a prespecified set of genes
Next-generation sequencing	High-throughput sequencing using a parallelized sequencing process that produces millions of sequences concurrently, far beyond the capacity of prior dye-terminator methods
Nucleic acid amplification test (NAAT)	A biochemical assay that evaluates for the presence of a particular string of nucleic acids through amplification by one of several methods, including polymerase and ligase chain reactions
Polymerase chain reaction (PCR)	A type of NAAT used to amplify a specific region of DNA by means of specific oligonucleotide primers and a DNA polymerase
Single-nucleotide polymorphism (SNP)	Point mutations, the number of which in different microbial isolates is a measure of their genetic distance from one another
Transcriptome	The catalog of the full set of messenger RNA (mRNA) transcripts from a cell or organism, which are typically measured by microarray or by next-generation sequencing of complementary DNA (cDNA) via a process called RNA-Seq
Whole genome sequencing (WGS)	A process that determines the full DNA sequence of an organism's genome; has been greatly facilitated by next-generation sequencing technology

MICROBIAL DIAGNOSTICS

The basic goals of a clinical microbiology laboratory are to establish the presence of a pathogen in a clinical sample, to identify the pathogen, and, when possible, to provide other information that can help guide clinical management and even affect prognosis, such as antibiotic susceptibility profiles or the presence of virulence factors. To date, clinical microbiology laboratories have largely approached these goals phenotypically by growth-based assays and biochemical testing. Bacteria, for instance, are algorithmically grouped into species by their characteristic microscopic appearance, nutrient requirements for growth, and ability to catalyze certain reactions. Antibiotic susceptibility is determined in most cases by assessing bacterial growth in the presence of antibiotic.

With the sequencing revolution paving the way to easy access of complete pathogen genomes (**Fig. 121-1**), we are now able to more systematically understand the genetic basis for these observable phenotypes. Compared with traditional growth-based methods for bacterial diagnostics that dominate the clinical microbiology laboratory, nucleic acid–based diagnostics that build on this genomic information promise improved speed, sensitivity, specificity, and breadth of information. Bridging clinical and research laboratories, adaptations of genomic technologies have begun to deliver on this promise (**Table 121-2**).

HISTORICAL LIMITATIONS AND PROGRESS THROUGH GENETIC APPROACHES

The molecular diagnostics revolution in the clinical microbiology laboratory is well under way, born of necessity in the effort to identify and characterize microbes that are refractory to traditional culture methods. Historically, diagnosis of many so-called unculturable pathogens has relied largely on serology and antigen detection. However, these methods provide only limited clinical information because of their suboptimal sensitivity and specificity, the long delays that diminish their utility for real-time patient management, and the inability to further characterize pathogens beyond identifying past exposure. Newer tests to detect pathogens based on nucleic acid content have already offered improvements in the select cases in which they have been applied.

Unlike direct pathogen detection, serologic diagnosis—measurement of the host's response to pathogen exposure—can typically be made only in retrospect, requiring both acute- and convalescent-phase serum samples. For chronic infections, distinguishing active from latent infection or identifying repeat exposure from serology alone can be difficult or impossible, depending on the syndrome. In addition, serologic diagnosis is variably sensitive, depending on the organism and the patient's immune status. For instance, tuberculosis is notoriously difficult to identify by serologic methods; tuberculin skin testing using purified protein derivative (PPD) is especially insensitive

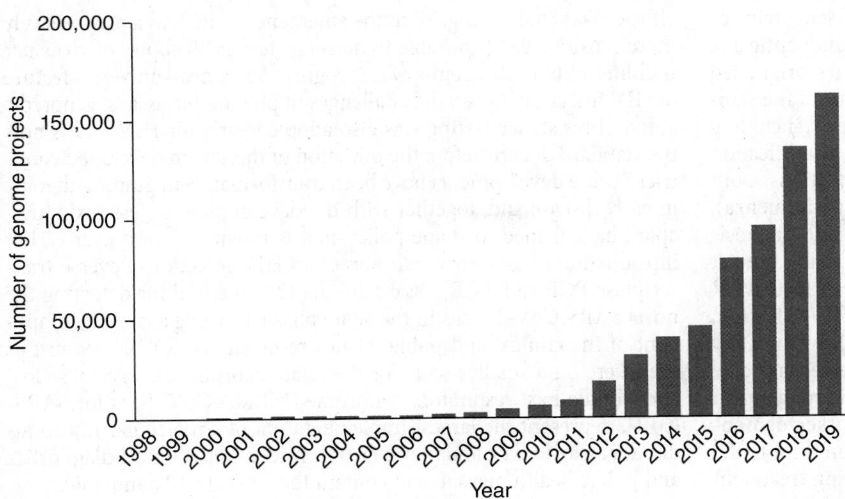

FIGURE 121-1 Bacterial genome sequencing projects submitted to the Genomes Online Database, a manually curated repository for genome and metagenome sequencing data, from 1998 to 2019. *(Data compiled from https://gold.jgi.doe.gov/statistics, accessed June 27, 2020. See S Mukherjee et al: Genomes OnLine Database (GOLD) v.7: Updates and new features. Nucleic Acids Res 47:D1, 2019.)*

in active disease and possibly cross-reactive with vaccines or other mycobacteria. Even the newer interferon γ release assays (IGRAs), which measure cytokine release from T lymphocytes in response to *Mycobacterium tuberculosis*–specific antigens in vitro, have limited sensitivity in immunodeficient hosts. Neither PPD testing nor IGRAs can distinguish latent from active infection. Serologic Lyme disease diagnostics suffer similar limitations: in patients from endemic regions, the presence of IgG antibodies to *Borrelia burgdorferi* may reflect prior exposure rather than active disease, while IgM antibodies are imperfectly sensitive and specific (50% and 80%, respectively, in early disease). The complicated nature of these tests, particularly in view of the nonspecific symptoms that may accompany Lyme disease, has had substantial implications for public perception of Lyme disease and antibiotic misuse in endemic areas. Similarly, syphilis, a chronic infection caused by *Treponema pallidum*, is notoriously difficult to stage by serology alone, requiring multiple different nontreponemal and treponemal tests (e.g., rapid protein reagin and fluorescent treponemal antibody, respectively) in conjunction with clinical suspicion. Complementing serology, antigen detection can improve sensitivity and specificity in select cases, but has been validated only for a limited set of infections. Typically, structural elements of pathogens are detected, including components of viral envelopes (e.g., hepatitis B surface antigen, HIV p24 antigen), cell surface markers in certain bacteria (e.g., *Streptococcus pneumoniae*, *Legionella pneumophila* serotype 1) or fungi (e.g., *Cryptococcus*, *Histoplasma*), and less specific fungal cell-wall components such as galactomannan and β-glucan (e.g., *Aspergillus* and some dimorphic fungi).

TABLE 121-2 Selected Clinical Applications of Infectious Disease Genomics

APPLICATION	TECHNOLOGY	NOTES/EXAMPLES
Organism Identification		
Viral detection	PCR, RT-PCR	Identification of HIV, HBV, HCV, respiratory viruses including SARS-CoV-2 and influenza, and others for diagnosis and response to therapy
TB detection	PCR	Amplification of the *rpoB* gene for species-specific identification of *Mycobacterium tuberculosis*
Pathogen detection	PCR, RT-PCR, NAAT	Multiplexed identification of dozens of viruses, bacteria, yeasts, and parasites from a variety of clinical specimens
Bacterial detection	16S ribosomal gene sequencing	Targeted amplification and sequencing of regions of the 16S rRNA gene for identification of suspected bacterial infections undiagnosed by conventional methods
Pathogen Discovery		
Bacterial pathogens	Sequencing, metagenomic assembly	Unbiased "shotgun" sequencing of isolated nucleic acid from patient samples to identify associated pathogens; proofs-of-concept: new *Bradyrhizobium* species associated with cord colitis; *Escherichia coli* O104:H4 from 2011 diarrheal outbreak in Germany; *Leptospira* species from one patient's cerebrospinal fluid; research use only at this time
Viral pathogens	Microarray, sequencing	Hybridization of clinical samples to microarrays from phylogenetically diverse known viruses identified the first SARS coronavirus and others. Direct sequencing has identified SARS-CoV-2, West Nile virus, and MERS-CoV, among others. Use is primarily in research.
Antibiotic Resistance		
MRSA detection	PCR	Detection of the *mecA* gene, the genotypic cause of methicillin resistance in *Staphylococcus aureus*
VRE detection	PCR	Detection of the *vanA* or *vanB* gene, the main genotypic causes of vancomycin resistance in *Enterococcus*
MDR-TB detection	PCR, NAAT	Detection of polymorphisms in the *rpoB* gene from *M. tuberculosis*, which account for 95% of rifampin resistance. Other probes available for *inhA* and *katG* genes can detect up to 85% of isoniazid resistance.
Carbapenemase detection	PCR	Detection of genes encoding one of several types of enzymes *(KPC, NDM, OXA-48, IMP, VIM)* that hydrolyze carbapenems, accounting for much but not all carbapenemase resistance in Enterobacteriaceae
HIV resistance detection	Targeted sequencing	Targeted sequencing of specific genes with known resistance-conferring mutations; now the standard of care prior to initial therapy in the United States and Europe
Epidemiology		
Outbreak and epidemic tracking	Sequencing	Application to tracking outbreaks and epidemics on local and international scales, including spread of carbapenemase-producing *Klebsiella*, *S. aureus*, *M. tuberculosis*, *E. coli*, *Vibrio cholerae*, Ebola virus, Zika virus, and influenza virus
Evolution and spread of pathogens	Sequencing	Sequencing collections of pathogens to shed light on pathogen dissemination, virulence factors, and antibiotic resistance determinants; innumerable examples, including *V. cholerae*, influenza virus, Ebola virus, and Zika virus

Abbreviations: HBV, hepatitis B virus; HCV, hepatitis C virus; MDR, multidrug-resistant; MERS, Middle East respiratory syndrome; MRSA, methicillin-resistant *S. aureus*; NAAT, nucleic acid amplification test; PCR, polymerase chain reaction; RT, reverse transcriptase; SARS, severe acute respiratory syndrome; TB, tuberculosis; VRE, vancomycin-resistant enterococci.

Given the impracticality of culture and the lack of sensitivity or sufficient clinical information afforded by serologic and antigenic methods, the push toward nucleic acid–based diagnostics originated in pursuit of viruses and fastidious bacteria, becoming part of the standard of care for select organisms in U.S. hospitals. Such tests, including polymerase chain reaction (PCR) and other nucleic acid amplification tests (NAATs), are now widely used for many viral infections, both chronic (e.g., HIV infection, hepatitis C) and acute (e.g., influenza). NAATs provide essential information about both the initial diagnosis and the response to therapy and in some cases genotypically predict drug resistance. Indeed, progression from antigen detection to PCR transformed our understanding of the natural course of HIV infection, with profound implications for treatment **(Fig. 121-2*A*)**. In the early years of the AIDS pandemic, p24 antigenemia was detected in acute HIV infection but then disappeared for years before emerging again with progression to AIDS **(Fig. 121-2*B*)**. Without a marker demonstrating viremia, the role of treatment during HIV infection prior to the development of clinical AIDS was uncertain, and assessing treatment efficacy was challenging. With the emergence of PCR as a progressively more sensitive test (now able to detect as few as 20 copies of virus per milliliter of blood), viremia was recognized as a near-universal feature of HIV infection. Given the challenges of phenotypic assays, genotypic antiviral resistance testing was also adopted early for HIV and is now the standard of care before the initiation of therapy in developed countries. These developments have been transformative in guiding therapy in early disease and, together with the development of less toxic therapies, have helped to shape policy that is moving toward ever-earlier introduction of antiretroviral therapy in HIV infection. Reverse transcriptase PCR (RT-PCR) assays are the core method for detecting the novel SARS-CoV-2 virus in the acute phase, forming a critical component of the clinical and public health response to COVID-19, just as they were on a smaller scale for the related coronaviruses SARS-CoV and Middle East respiratory syndrome (MERS)-CoV. Tests for SARS-CoV-2 represent the largest implementation of a molecular infectious disease assay to date and play a critical role in both clinical diagnostics and public health measures to contain the COVID-19 pandemic.

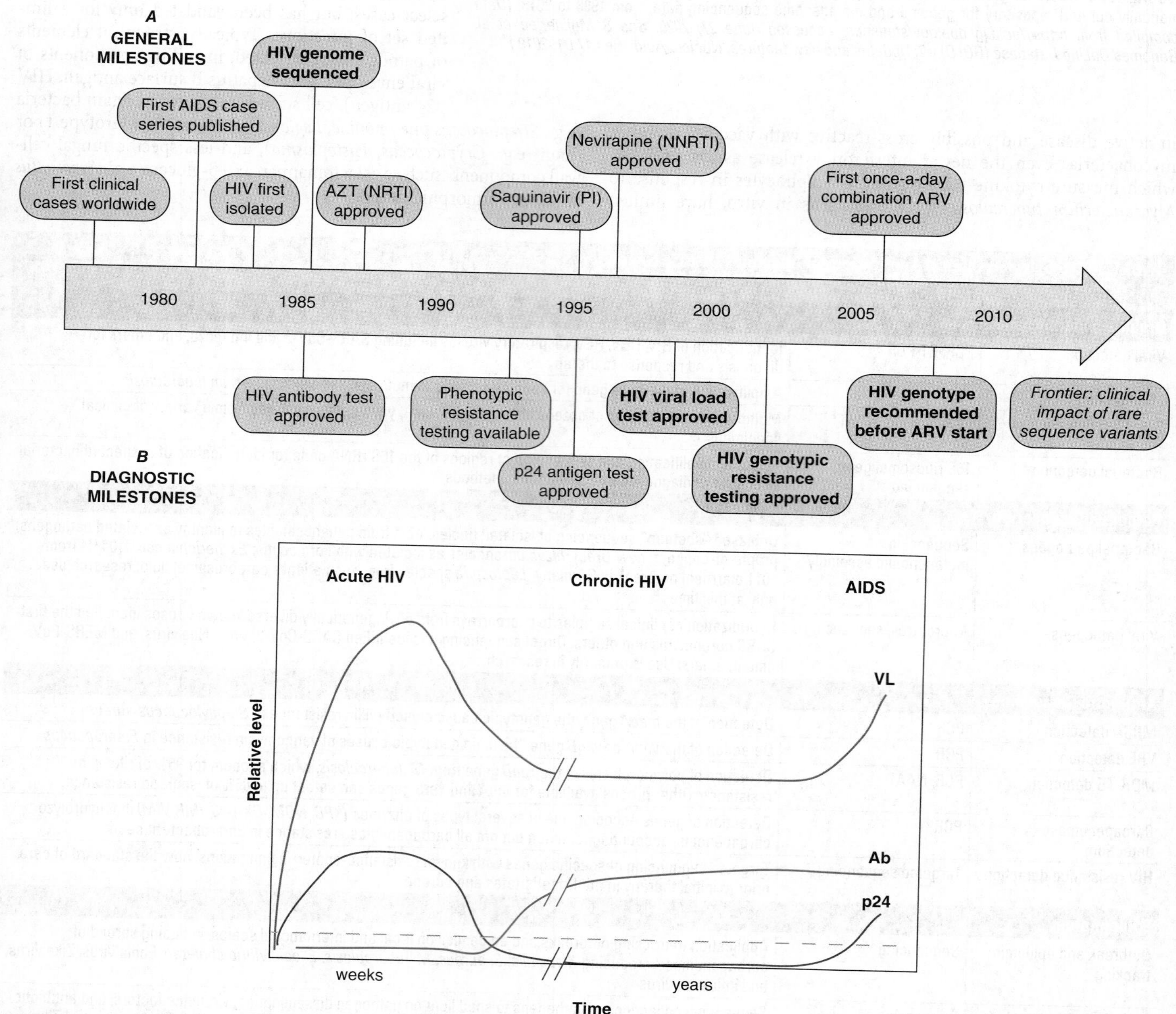

FIGURE 121-2 ***A.*** Timeline of select milestones in HIV management. Genomic advances are shown in bold type. The approvals and recommendations indicated apply to the United States. ARV, antiretroviral; AZT, zidovudine; NRTI, nucleoside reverse transcriptase (RT) inhibitor; NNRTI, nonnucleoside RT inhibitor; PI, protease inhibitor. ***B.*** Viral dynamics in the natural history of HIV infection. Three diagnostic markers are shown: HIV antibody (Ab), p24 antigen (p24), and viral load (VL). *Dashed gray line represents limit of detection. (Adapted from data in HH Fiebig et al: Dynamics of HIV viremia and antibody seroconversion in plasma donors: Implications for diagnosis and staging of primary HIV infection. AIDS 17:1871, 2003.)*

As they are for viral testing, nucleic acid–based tests have become the diagnostic tests of choice for fastidious bacteria, including the common sexually transmitted bacterial pathogens *Neisseria gonorrhoeae* and *Chlamydia trachomatis* as well as the tick-borne *Ehrlichia chaffeensis* and *Anaplasma phagocytophilum*. More recently, nucleic acid amplification–based detection has offered improved sensitivity for diagnosis of the important nosocomial pathogen *Clostridium difficile*, and NAATs have provided clinically relevant information on the presence of cytotoxins A and B as well as molecular markers of hypervirulence, such as the North American pulsotype 1 (NAP1) strain that is enriched in severe illness. The importance of genomics in selecting loci for diagnostic assays and in monitoring test sensitivity was highlighted by the emergence in Sweden of a newly recognized variant of *C. trachomatis* with a deletion that includes the gene targeted by a set of commercial NAATs. By evading detection through this deletion (and thus avoiding treatment), this strain came to be highly prevalent in some areas of Sweden. While nucleic acid–based tests remain the diagnostic approach of choice for fastidious bacteria, this example serves as a reminder of the need for careful development and ongoing monitoring of molecular diagnostics.

In contrast, for typical bacterial pathogens for which culture methods are well established, growth-based assays followed by biochemical tests still dominate in the clinical laboratory. Informed by decades of clinical microbiology, these tests have served clinicians well, yet the limitations of growth-based tests—in particular, the delays associated with waiting for growth—have left opportunities for improvements. Driven by this need, mass spectrometry–based assays that offer highly accurate organism identification within a few hours of a positive blood culture are widely adopted in clinical microbiology laboratories in well-resourced areas. Looking ahead, molecular diagnostics, greatly informed by the vast quantity of microbial genome sequences generated in recent years, offers a way forward. First, sequencing studies can readily identify key genes (or noncoding nucleic acids) that can be developed into targets for clinical assays using PCR or hybridization assay platforms. Second, sequencing itself may eventually become cheap and rapid enough to be performed routinely on clinical specimens, with consequent unbiased detection of pathogens.

One of the biggest drivers for the implementation of novel molecular technologies in the diagnosis of infectious diseases is the desire for more rapid—or even real-time—pathogen identification, ideally with antibiotic susceptibility information on those microbes for which resistance to the current anti-infective armamentarium is of concern. Such real-time tests have the potential to transform infectious disease management, impacting antibiotic stewardship in the outpatient setting, mortality risk in the critically ill (i.e., patients in whom early administration of effective antibiotics is the most significant factor in decreasing mortality risk), hospital admission, and length of hospital stay; the extent of this impact will depend on the economic forces that will help define the breadth of their deployment. On the public health level, such tests will likely play a role in improving antibiotic stewardship, thereby influencing the rise of antibiotic resistance and enabling surveillance of outbreaks by local, national, and international networks. In the United States and the United Kingdom, for example, public health agencies have shifted from pulsed-field gel electrophoresis to genome sequencing to track food-borne pathogens and identify outbreaks; in addition, these countries are rapidly expanding the routine use of genomics in identifying and characterizing other pathogens, from mycobacteria (both *M. tuberculosis* and nontuberculous mycobacteria) to *N. gonorrhoeae*. Further, international efforts to track the spread of viral diseases, including recent work on Ebola and Zika outbreaks, ongoing work on seasonal influenza, and efforts to control the SARS-CoV-2 pandemic offer opportunities for improving interventions, surveillance, and prevention efforts, ranging from more accurate selection of the influenza virus strains to include in seasonal vaccine development to improved design of trials to evaluate novel vaccines and therapies.

Technological innovations are lowering several critical barriers to the widespread adoption of genomics and other molecular methods. Specifically, for NAAT, the need for rapid thermal cycling and cold-chain storage for reagents has significantly impeded implementation in resource-limited settings. Recent efforts aim to overcome these challenges by developing isothermal amplification protocols and lyophilized reagents that do not require refrigeration or sophisticated instrumentation. For clinical sequencing, (1) the cost and speed of sequencing and analysis methods continue to fall precipitously; (2) automation and miniaturization of the preparation of a sample for sequencing promise to reduce cost and minimize the expertise needed; and (3) direct sequencing technologies that eliminate the complex molecular biology required to prepare clinical samples for sequencing are improving in accuracy and robustness. Further barriers exist, including the need for standardized pipelines to process data and present clinicians with easily interpretable and readily actionable results. However, as these advances give rise to rapid, accurate diagnostic tests, the ultimate goal is to inform a clinician in real time whether antibiotics are indicated and, if so, which will be effective. Real-time diagnostics will allow more efficient deployment of our precious antibiotic arsenal, thus improving both societal and patient-specific outcomes in much the same way that a rapid, sensitive troponin assay has transformed bedside management of chest pain.

ORGANISM IDENTIFICATION

In order to adapt nucleic acid detection to diagnostic tests and thus to identify pathogens on a wide scale, sequences must be found that are conserved enough within a species to identify the diversity of strains that may be encountered in various clinical settings, but divergent enough to distinguish one species from another. Until recently, this problem has been solved for bacteria by targeting the element of a bacterial genome that is most highly conserved within a species, the 16S ribosomal RNA (rRNA) subunit. Among many examples, this method has now been used to confirm *Mycobacterium chimaera* infections in several patients after cardiothoracic surgery, leading ultimately to recognition of a widespread outbreak. At present, 16S PCR amplification from tissue specimens can be performed by specialty laboratories, though its sensitivity and clinical utility to date have remained somewhat limited, in part because of the scarcity and relative fragility of pathogen nucleic acid in the sampled tissue, which necessitates reliable, sensitive nucleic acid amplification. As such barriers are reduced through technological advances and as the causes of culture-negative infection are clarified (perhaps in part through sequencing efforts), these tests may become both more accessible and more helpful.

With the wealth of sequencing data now available, other regions beyond 16S rRNA can be targeted for bacterial species identification. These other genomic loci can provide additional information about a clinical isolate that is relevant to patient management. For instance, detection of the presence, or potentially even the expression, of toxin genes such as *C. difficile* toxins A and B or Shiga toxin can provide clinicians with additional information that will help distinguish commensals or colonizing bacteria from pathogens and thus aid in prognostication and management as well as in diagnosis.

Beyond bacteria, one commonly used approach to PCR-based pathogen detection is so-called "syndromic panels" of multiplexed PCR to identify common causes of clinical infection syndromes, including upper respiratory infection, gastroenteritis, and meningoencephalitis. The most frequently deployed syndromic panel is the respiratory viral panel, which typically includes primer sets targeting a combination of influenza, parainfluenza, respiratory syncytial virus, adenovirus, rhinovirus, enterovirus, metapneumovirus, and common-cold coronaviruses, sometimes in conjunction with unculturable bacteria such as *Mycoplasma*, *Chlamydophila*, and *Bordetella* species. The goal of such panels is to capture common infectious causes of these syndromes in a single, standardized diagnostic test, ideally streamlining the diagnostic evaluation. The ready identification of a plausible etiologic agent may offer diagnostic clarity if judiciously used and carefully considered in the clinical context of each patient. The most dramatic recent change in PCR-based viral diagnostics has been the wide deployment of an RT-PCR assay for detection of the novel SARS-CoV-2. As noted elsewhere in this chapter, this assay has played a crucial role in patient care, triage, infection control, and epidemiology in managing the COVID-19 pandemic. One priority for the coming months is to integrate SARS-CoV-2 detection into syndromic panels for detection alongside other common respiratory pathogens to enable routine, streamlined diagnostics when appropriate.

One challenge with PCR-based assays is the relative complexity of the molecular biology and consequent need for advanced technology for implementation, including instruments and reagents. Several recent approaches have advanced the molecular biology of nucleic acid detection with the aim of increasing deployability of NAATs for use in resource-limited or even field settings. These methods couple nucleic acid detection to an enzymatic readout, enabling catalytic signal amplification. Several such approaches build on the intrinsic sensitivity, specificity, and amplification of the CRISPR (*c*lustered, *r*egularly *i*nterspaced *s*hort *p*alindromic *r*epeats) effectors Cas12a and Cas13a as nucleic acid sensors. Distinct from the famous gene editing CRISPR effector Cas9, these robust and versatile enzymes recognize short nucleic acid targets with high specificity and transduce this binding event into "collateral cleavage" of nearby nucleic acids that can be engineered to create a signal using fluorescent reporter constructs. Crucially, all of this biotechnology can be made to work in conjunction with isothermal enzymatic preamplification steps to achieve remarkable sensitivity, all robustly enough to withstand lyophilization on paper before being reconstituted in the field. Such assays are still in the early stages of development, but they have shown promise and could play a critical role in global diagnostics and surveillance.

While amplification tests such as PCR and other NAATs exemplify one approach to nucleic acid detection, other approaches exist, including detection by hybridization. Although not currently used in the clinical realm, techniques for multiplexed detection and identification of pathogens by hybridization to microarrays or in solution are being developed for other purposes. Of note, these different detection techniques require different degrees of conservation. Highly sensitive amplification methods require a high degree of sequence identity between PCR primer pairs and their short, specific target sequences; even a single base-pair mismatch (particularly near the 3′ end of the primer) may interfere with detection. In contrast, hybridization-based tests are more tolerant of mismatch and thus can be used to detect important regions that may be less precisely conserved within a species, thus potentially allowing detection of clinical isolates from a given species with greater diversity between isolates. Such assays take advantage of the predictable binding interactions of nucleic acids and do not require enzymology, broadening the range of conditions under which such assays are feasible, including directly on primary clinical specimens. The applicability of hybridization-based methods toward either DNA or RNA opens up the possibility of expression profiling, which can uncover phenotypic information from nucleic acid content.

Both PCR and hybridization methods target specific, known organisms. At the other extreme, as sequencing costs decline, metagenomic sequencing from patient samples is increasingly feasible. This shotgun sequencing approach is unbiased—i.e., is able to detect any microbial sequence, however divergent or unexpected. In one recent example, a clinical sample of cerebrospinal fluid from an immunocompromised patient with signs and symptoms of chronic meningitis was found through metagenomic sequencing and analysis to contain small amounts of *Leptospira* DNA. In light of this information, retrospective PCR testing confirmed the diagnosis of neuroleptospirosis, which had been missed prior to the sequencing result. The patient was treated with penicillin G and clinically recovered. Increasingly, efforts are under way to bring whole genome sequencing to other clinical samples, including sputum and blood, in order to more readily identify pathogens. One such assay was recently certified for clinical use in the United States—a shotgun metagenomic sequencing approach applied to cell-free DNA circulating in the bloodstream that aims to identify pathogens both in blood and other body sites, although its clinical niche remains to be defined. This new approach brings its own set of challenges, however, including the need to recognize pathogenic sequences against a background of expected host and commensal sequences and to distinguish true pathogens from either colonizers or laboratory contaminants. The burgeoning field of microbiome research is driving technology development for sequencing and analyzing complex microbial communities. Lessons from this field will inform diagnostic efforts.

■ PATHOGEN DISCOVERY

In addition to clinical diagnostic applications, novel genomic technologies, including whole genome sequencing, are being applied to clinical research specimens with a goal of identifying new pathogens in a variety of circumstances. The tremendous sensitivity and unbiased nature of sequencing is also ideal in searching clinical samples for unknown or unsuspected pathogens.

Causal inference in infectious diseases has progressed since the time of Koch, whose historical postulates provided a rigorous framework for attributing a disease to a microorganism. To modernize Koch's postulates, an organism, whether it can be cultured or not, should induce disease upon introduction into a healthy host if it is to be implicated as a causative pathogen. Current sequencing technologies are ideal for advancing this modern version of Koch's postulates because they can identify candidate causal pathogens with unprecedented sensitivity and in an unbiased way, unencumbered by limitations such as culturability. Yet, as direct sequencing on primary patient samples greatly expands our ability to recognize associations between microbes and disease states, critical thinking and experimentation will remain vital in establishing causality.

Virus discovery in particular has been greatly facilitated by new nucleic acid technology. These frontiers were first notably explored with high-density microarrays containing spatially arrayed sequences from a phylogenetically diverse collection of viruses. Despite bias toward those with homology to known viruses, novel viruses in clinical samples were successfully identified on the basis of their ability to hybridize to these prespecified sequences. This methodology famously contributed to identification of the coronavirus causing SARS. Once discovered, the SARS coronavirus was rapidly sequenced: the full genome was assembled in April 2003, <6 months after recognition of the first case.

With the advent of next-generation sequencing, unbiased pathogen discovery is now addressed through a process known as *metagenomic assembly* **(Fig. 121-3)**, largely supplanting other methods. Sequences of random nucleotide fragments can be generated from clinical specimens with no a priori knowledge of pathogen identity through a process called *shotgun sequencing*. This collection of sequences can then be computationally aligned to host (i.e., human) sequences, with aligned sequences removed and remaining sequences compared with other known genomes to detect the presence of known microorganisms. Sequence fragments that remain unaligned suggest the presence of an additional organism that cannot be matched to a known, characterized genome; these reads can be assembled into contiguous nucleic acid stretches that can be compared with known sequences to construct the genome of a potentially novel organism. Assembled genomes (or parts of genomes) can then be compared with known genomes to infer the phylogeny of new organisms and identify related classes or traits. Thus, not only can this process identify unanticipated pathogens, but it can even identify undiscovered organisms.

The emergence of COVID-19 provides a dramatic example that illustrates advances in pathogen discovery technology in the intervening 16 years since SARS-CoV was discovered: the causal coronavirus, SARS-CoV-2, was identified through metagenomic sequencing within about 1 month of the first known case and just weeks after the outbreak was first recognized. Sequencing and assembly were completed within 5 days of the discovery of the new virus, and a NAAT was released 1 day later. Given the ensuing ravages of COVID-19 and the cost of delays of even a few weeks in implementing this new diagnostic test in some locations, it is sobering to contemplate the added harm had this outbreak occurred even a decade earlier. This timeline illustrates the advancing power and speed of new diagnostic technologies, but also underscores the pressing need for continued progress.

Other early applications of sequencing on clinical samples have centered around the discovery of novel viruses, including such emerging pathogens as West Nile virus and MERS-CoV, as well as viral causes of

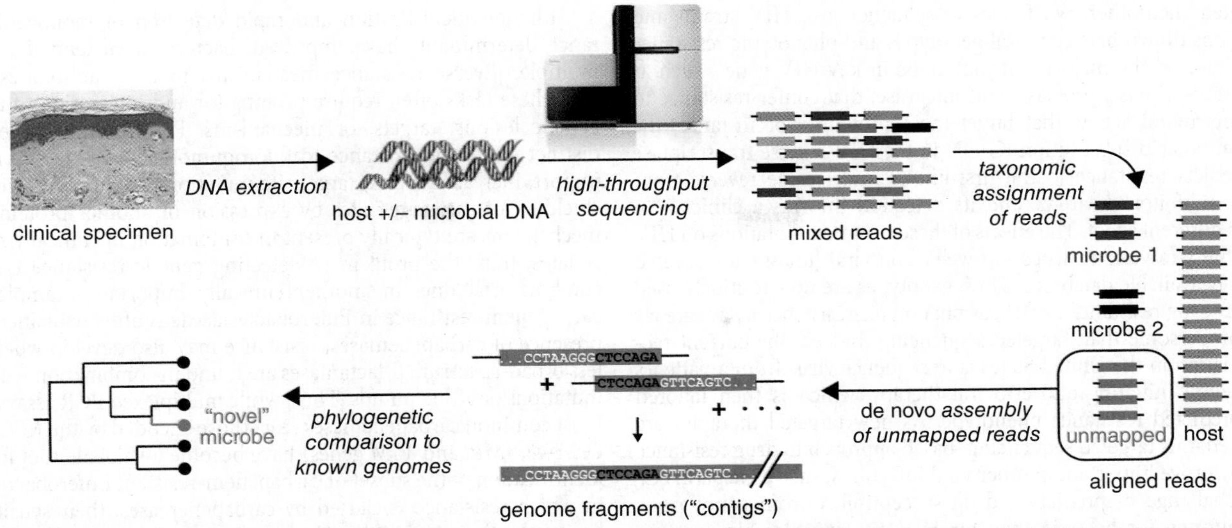

FIGURE 121-3 Workflow of metagenomic assembly for pathogen discovery. DNA is isolated from a specimen of interest (e.g., tissue, body fluid) containing a mixture of host DNA and nucleic acids from coexisting microbes, either commensal or pathogenic. All DNA (and RNA, if a reverse transcription step is added) is then sequenced, yielding a mixture of DNA sequence fragments ("reads") from the organisms present. Except for reads that do not align ("map") to any known sequence, these reads are aligned to existing reference genomes for the host or any known microbes. The unmapped reads are computationally assembled de novo into the largest contiguous stretches of DNA possible ("contigs"), representing fragments of previously unsequenced genomes. These genome fragments (contigs) are then mapped onto a phylogenetic tree based on their sequence. Some may represent known but as-yet-unsequenced organisms, while others will represent novel species. *(Figure prepared with valuable input from Dr. Ami S. Bhatt, personal communication.)*

myriad other conditions, from tropical hemorrhagic fevers to diarrhea in newborns.

As metagenomic sequencing and assembly techniques become more robust, this technology holds great promise for identifying microorganisms that are associated with clinical conditions of unknown etiology. Conventional methods already have unexpectedly linked numerous conditions with specific agents of infection—e.g., cervical and oropharyngeal cancers with human papillomavirus (HPV), Kaposi's sarcoma with human herpesvirus 8, and certain lymphomas with Epstein-Barr virus. Recently, Zika virus, first described in the 1940s, was found to be increasing in incidence as a cause of febrile syndromes, particularly in Central and South America. A concurrent increase in the incidence of microcephaly was noted that temporally and geographically matched the Zika epidemics. Zika was suspected to be neurotropic because of a previously recognized association with Guillain-Barré syndrome, but the strongest link between Zika virus and microcephaly came when the virus itself was detected by both quantitative reverse transcription PCR (RT-qPCR) and whole genome sequencing in postmortem fetal brain tissue from microcephalic infants. An argument for causality was built on the foundation of epidemiologic evidence and direct viral detection, both of which were built on nucleic acid detection and genome sequencing. Sequencing techniques offer unprecedented sensitivity and specificity for identifying foreign nucleic acid sequences that may suggest other such pathogen-associated conditions—from malignancies to inflammatory conditions to unexplained fevers or other clinical syndromes—associated with organisms from viruses to bacteria to parasites. Caution is needed, though: in the absence of the ability to fulfill Koch's postulates, sequence-based identification of a microbe from patient specimens is not, on its own, sufficient to identify a novel pathogen. The increasing sensitivity of these methods warrants greater rigor and care in defining what is "noise" and what represents a pathogen.

As sequencing-based discovery expands, microbes may be found to be associated with conditions not classically thought of as infectious, such as the link between maternal Zika virus infection and fetal microcephaly. Studies of bowel flora in laboratory animals and even humans already suggest correlations between microbe composition and various aspects of metabolic and cardiovascular health. Improved methods for pathogen detection will continue to uncover unexpected correlations between microbes and disease states, but the mere presence of a microbe does not establish causality. Fortunately, once the relatively laborious and computationally intensive metagenomic sequencing and assembly efforts have identified a pathogen, further detection can more easily be undertaken with targeted methods such as PCR or hybridization, which may be more scalable and amenable to in situ confirmation. This capacity should facilitate the additional careful investigation that will be required to progress beyond correlation and to draw causal inference.

ANTIBIOTIC RESISTANCE

At present, antibiotic resistance in bacteria and fungi is conventionally determined by isolating a single colony from a cultured clinical specimen and testing its growth in the presence of drug. The requirement for multiple growth steps in these conventional assays has several consequences. First, only culturable pathogens can be readily processed. Second, this process requires considerable infrastructure to support the sterile environment needed for culture-based testing of diverse organisms. Finally, and perhaps most significantly, even the fastest-growing organisms require 1–2 days of processing for identification and 2–3 days for determination of susceptibilities. Some slow-growing organisms take even longer; for instance, weeks must pass before drug-resistant *M. tuberculosis* can be identified by growth phenotype. Given the clinical imperative in serious illness to begin effective therapy early, this inherent delay in susceptibility determination has obvious implications for empirical antibiotic use: broad-spectrum antibiotics often must be chosen up front in situations where it is later shown that preferred narrower-spectrum drugs would have been effective or even that no antibiotics were appropriate (i.e., in viral infections). Even with this strategy, as resistant organisms become more common, the empirical choice can be incorrect, often with devastating consequences. Real-time identification of the infecting organism and information on its susceptibility profile would guide initial therapy and support judicious antibiotic use, ideally improving patient outcomes while aiding in the ever-escalating fight against antibiotic resistance by reserving the use of broad-spectrum agents for cases in which they are truly needed.

Molecular diagnostics and sequencing offer a way to accelerate detection of a pathogen's antibiotic susceptibility profile. If a genotype that confers resistance can be identified, this genotype can be targeted for molecular detection. In infectious disease, this approach has most convincingly come to fruition for HIV (Fig. 121-2*A*). (In a conceptually parallel application of genomic analysis, molecular detection of certain resistance determinants in cancers informs selection of targeted chemotherapy.) Extensive sequencing of HIV strains and correlations drawn between viral genotypes and phenotypic resistance have delineated the majority of mutations in key HIV genes, such as reverse transcriptase, protease, and integrase, that confer resistance to the antiretroviral agents that target these proteins. For instance, the single amino acid substitution K103N in the HIV reverse transcriptase gene predicts resistance to the first-line nonnucleoside reverse transcriptase inhibitor efavirenz, and its detection informs a clinician to choose a different agent. The effects of these common mutations on HIV susceptibility to various drugs—as well as on viral fitness—are curated in publicly available databases. Thus, genotypes are now routinely used to predict drug resistance in HIV, as phenotypic resistance assays are far more cumbersome than targeted sequencing. Indeed, the current recommendation in the United States is to sequence virus from a patient's blood before initiating antiretroviral therapy, which is then tailored to the predicted resistance phenotype. As new targeted therapies are introduced, this targeted sequencing–based approach to drug resistance will likely prove important in other viral infections, such as hepatitis C.

The challenge of predicting drug susceptibility from genotype is more daunting for bacteria than for HIV, yet considerable progress has been made toward sequencing-based determination of bacterial antibiotic susceptibility. Bacteria have far more complex genomes than viruses, with thousands of genes on their chromosomes (many of which can functionally interact in ways that escape a priori prediction) and the capacity to acquire many more through horizontal gene transfer of plasmids and mobile genetic elements within and between species. Thus, the task of comprehensively defining all possible genetic resistance mechanisms is orders of magnitude more complex in bacteria than in viruses, which typically have far more limited genomes. Despite these challenges, considerable progress has been made in recent years. In select cases where biological factors appear to have constrained the genotypic basis for resistance to a small, well-defined set of mutations, genotypic assays for antibiotic resistance are already being introduced into clinical practice. One important example is the detection of methicillin-resistant *Staphylococcus aureus* (MRSA). *S. aureus* is one of the most common and serious bacterial pathogens of humans, particularly in health care settings. Resistance to methicillin, the most effective class of antistaphylococcal antibiotics, has become very common, even in community-acquired strains. Vancomycin—the alternative drug to methicillin—is effective against MRSA but is measurably inferior to methicillin against methicillin-susceptible *S. aureus* (MSSA). Analysis of clinical MRSA isolates has demonstrated that the molecular basis for resistance to methicillin in essentially all cases stems from the expression of an alternative penicillin-binding protein (PBP2A) encoded by the gene *mecA*, which is found within a transferable genetic element called *mec*. This mobile cassette has spread rapidly through the *S. aureus* population via horizontal gene transfer and selection from widespread antibiotic use. Because methicillin resistance is essentially always due to the presence of the *mec* cassette, MRSA is particularly amenable to molecular detection. In recent years, a PCR test for the *mec* cassette, which saves hours to days compared with standard culture-based methods, has been approved by the U.S. Food and Drug Administration (FDA). Similar to MRSA, vancomycin-resistant enterococci (VRE) harbor one of a limited number of *van* genes found to be responsible for resistance to this important antibiotic, which occurs through alteration of the mechanism for cell wall cross-linking that vancomycin inhibits. Detection of one of these genes by PCR indicates resistance. More recently, identification of carbapenemase-encoding plasmids responsible for a significant fraction of carbapenem resistance (though not all instances) has led to multiplexed PCR assays to detect this important resistance element to this crucial antibiotic class. Finally, a PCR assay targeting the highly conserved RNA polymerase gene serves not only to detect *M. tuberculosis* directly in sputum samples but also to detect resistance to rifampin, since the determinants of resistance to this RNA polymerase inhibitor map almost exclusively to a short region of this gene. Since rifampin resistance is epidemiologically associated with, though not causal for, multidrug resistance, this assay identifies strains at high risk for multidrug resistance, enhancing its value.

Although identification and rapid detection of monogenic resistance determinants have improved, bacteria have tended to evolve multiple, diverse resistance mechanisms to most antibiotics; therefore, these tasks often require probing for and integration of multiple genetic lesions, targets, or mechanisms. For instance, at least five distinct modes of resistance to fluoroquinolones are known: reduced import, increased efflux, target site mutation, drug modification, and shielding of the target sites by expression of another protein. These mechanisms are typically present in combination in clinically resistant isolates; thus, the problem of detecting genetic resistance is often a combinatorial one. In another clinically important example, while carbapenem resistance in Enterobacteriaceae is often explained by the presence of carbapenemases, resistance may also develop when other, less broad-spectrum β-lactamases are found in combination with porin mutations or efflux pumps. Thus, while multiplexed PCR assays for the most common carbapenemases (e.g., those encoded by the *KPC*, *NDM*, *OXA-48*, *IMP*, and *VIM* genes) have become a valuable tool for rapid identification of the subset of carbapenem-resistant Enterobacteriaceae in which resistance is caused by carbapenemases, their sensitivity is limited by their inability to detect other mechanisms of carbapenem resistance. Additionally, plasmids and transposable elements, which often are enriched for antibiotic resistance determinants, may be more technically and analytically challenging to sequence, although newer long-read sequencing technologies are beginning to address these challenges. To further complicate genetic prediction, changes in gene expression (which may be detectable through mutations in promoter regions or regulatory genes without coding mutations in known resistance determinants) and even gene copy number (which may occur without changes in primary sequence) of resistance determinants play critical roles in some cases of genetic resistance. Thus, while predicting resistance when determinants are found is rapidly becoming feasible, the more clinically relevant task of predicting *susceptibility* when no known resistance determinants are found remains more difficult.

To build on early successes with the goal of advancing beyond binary detection of monogenic resistance determinants, the ultimate frontier for genetic prediction of bacterial antibiotic resistance lies in more comprehensive prediction of a resistance phenotype from sequence information—a task similar to HIV resistance prediction. Yet there is no comprehensive compendium of genetic elements conferring resistance and their pairwise and higher-order interactions with each other and with the genetic background of bacterial pathogens. Nonviral genomes are much larger than viral ones, and their abundance and diversity are such that thousands of genetic differences often exist between clinical isolates of the same species, of which perhaps only one or a few may contribute to resistance. In addition, new mechanisms may emerge in the face of antibiotic deployment or with the release of new drugs, and genetic prediction of resistance will inevitably lag behind the emergence of unforeseen mechanisms. While confident prediction of bacterial antibiotic resistance from sequencing determinants may therefore seem daunting, the vast expansion of microbial sequencing capacity (Fig. 121-1), combined with analytic methods such as microbial genome-wide association studies and machine learning algorithms, offers powerful analytical approaches to this "needle in a haystack" problem and has permitted remarkable advances in the predictive power of sequence determinants to date. Particularly in *M. tuberculosis*, where horizontal gene transfer is minimal and the pathogen is essentially restricted to human hosts so as to facilitate more representative sampling, a remarkably wide array of phenotypic resistance can be explained by known genetic determinants. Because of these biologic advantages, as well as the slow and laborious growth process that impedes traditional phenotypic assessment, whole genome sequencing has proven quite effective at predicting susceptibility profiles in this organism, to the point that the United Kingdom now routinely performs whole genome sequencing in parallel with phenotypic antibiotic susceptibility testing for *M. tuberculosis* in what some hope will be a precursor to fully whole genome sequencing–based antibiotic susceptibility testing. Even in more highly variable pathogens, with sequencing of sufficient numbers of susceptible and resistant pathogens, sequence-based prediction methods are improving in predictive accuracy, at least within the geographic region from which the test samples have been sequenced.

It is important to note that genotype-based analytical methods largely identify correlates, not necessarily surrogates or determinants, of resistance. In HIV diagnostics, surrogates (i.e., causal determinants of resistance) were found to be more reliable predictors than mere correlates in expanding sequencing-based resistance prediction to the general population. Without a mechanistic understanding of genetic resistance, a correlative relationship may be lineage-specific and less generalizable. Especially with multiple possible mechanisms of resistance to a given antibiotic and ongoing evolutionary pressure resulting in the development and acquisition of new modes of resistance, a genotypic approach to diagnosing antibiotic resistance is likely to remain challenging and to require ongoing vigilance in constantly correlating genotypic with more traditional phenotypic methods. An important corollary benefit of a genomic approach to resistance prediction, anchored in phenotypic validation, could be the systematic identification of outliers with unexplained resistance. These strains can form the basis for understanding newly emerging resistance mechanisms, which can in turn inform new drug development endeavors. Understanding resistance mechanisms may also help direct infection control efforts. For instance, the first identification of the *mcr-1* (mobilized colistin resistance) gene on a plasmid, together with other antibiotic resistance determinants, heightened concern about colistin-resistant Enterobacteriaceae identified first in China and later elsewhere because it implied rapid transmissibility of multidrug resistance. Early recognition of these potentially dangerous strains elucidated the immediate need for strict containment protocols.

In parallel with advancing sequencing technologies, progress in computational techniques, bioinformatics and statistics, and data storage as well as experimental confirmatory testing of hypotheses will be needed to advance toward the ambitious goal of a comprehensive compendium of global antibiotic resistance determinants. Open sharing and careful curation of new sequence information will be of paramount importance, as will iterative or even continuous comparison of predictions with ongoing phenotypic testing in order to assess performance and allow prediction algorithms to keep up with newly evolving or emerging resistance mechanisms.

We continuously observe the accumulation of new or unanticipated modes of resistance from ongoing evolutionary pressure caused by the widespread clinical use of antibiotics. Even with MRSA, perhaps the best-studied case of antibiotic resistance and a model of relative simplicity with a single known monogenic resistance determinant (*mecA*), a genotype-based approach to resistance detection proved imperfect. One limitation was a recall of the initial commercial genotypic resistance assay that was deployed for the identification of MRSA. A clinical isolate of *S. aureus* that emerged in Belgium expressed a variant of the *mec* cassette not detected by the assay's PCR primers. New primers were added to detect this new variant, and the assay was reapproved for use. This example illustrates the need for ongoing monitoring of any genotypic resistance assay. A second limitation is that a contradiction can occur between genotypic and phenotypic evidence for resistance. Up to 5% of MSSA strains have been reported to carry a copy of the *mecA* gene that is either nonfunctional or not expressed. Thus, the erroneous identification of these strains as MRSA by genotypic detection would lead to administration of the inferior antibiotic vancomycin rather than the preferred β-lactam therapy.

These examples illustrate one of the prime challenges of moving beyond growth-based assays: genotype is merely a proxy for the resistance phenotype that directly informs patient care. Alternative approaches currently under development attempt to circumvent the limitations of genotypic resistance testing by returning to phenotypic assays, albeit more rapid ones. One such approach is informed by genomic methods: transcriptional profiles serve as a rapid phenotypic signature for antibiotic response. Conceptually, since dying cells are transcriptionally distinct from cells fated to survive, susceptible bacteria enact different transcriptional profiles after antibiotic exposure than resistant ones, independent of the mechanism of resistance. These differences can be measured and, since transcription is one of the most rapid responses to cell stress (minutes to hours), can be used to determine whether cells are resistant or susceptible much more rapidly than is possible if growth in the presence of antibiotics is awaited (days). Like DNA, RNA can be readily detected through predictable rules governing base pairing via either amplification or hybridization-based methods. Changes in a carefully selected set of transcripts form an expression signature that can represent the total cellular response to antibiotic without requiring full characterization of the entire transcriptome. Preliminary proof-of-concept studies suggest that this approach may identify antibiotic susceptibility on the basis of transcriptional phenotype much more quickly than is possible with growth-based assays. Other rapid phenotype-based approaches to antibiotic susceptibility testing, including automated microscopy, ultrafine measurements of mass fluctuations, and others are under development as well, with the former approved for clinical use.

Because of its sensitivity in detecting even very rare nucleic acid fragments, sequencing provides an unprecedented depth of study into complex populations of cells and tissues. The strength of this depth and sensitivity applies not only to the detection of rare, novel pathogens in a sea of host signal, but also to the identification of heterogeneous pathogen subpopulations in a single host that may differ, for example, in drug resistance profiles or pathogenesis determinants. For instance, recent studies have highlighted the diversification of pathogens in chronic bacterial infections, such as *Pseudomonas* in the lungs of patients with cystic fibrosis or *M. tuberculosis* in disseminated infection, perhaps allowing for niche specialization within the host. Such diversification has long been recognized in chronic viral populations, as exemplified by HIV. Future studies will be needed to elucidate the clinical significance of these variable subpopulations, even as deep sequencing is now providing unprecedented levels of detail about majority and minority members of this population.

HOST-BASED DIAGNOSTICS

While pathogen-based diagnostics continue to be the mainstay for confirming infection, serologic testing and nonspecific biomarkers—such as erythrocyte sedimentation rate, C-reactive protein level, and even total white blood cell and neutrophil counts—have long been the basis of a strategy for measuring host responses to aid in the diagnosis of infection. Even recently identified host biomarkers of bacterial infection, such as procalcitonin, have fallen short in their versatility, with positive and negative predictive values that are thus far adequate for only a few narrow applications but inadequate for generalized clinical use. Here, too, the application of genomics is now being explored to improve upon this approach, given the previously described limitations of serologic testing and the lack of specificity of protein biomarkers identified to date. Rather than using antibody responses as a retrospective biomarker for infection, recent efforts have focused on transcriptomic analysis of the host response as a new direction with diagnostic implications for human disease.

For instance, while pathogen-based diagnostic tests to distinguish active from latent tuberculosis infection have proven elusive, recent work shows that the transcriptional profile of circulating white blood cells exhibits a differential pattern of expression of nearly 400 transcripts that distinguish active from latent tuberculosis; this expression pattern is driven in part by changes in interferon-inducible genes in the myeloid lineage. In a validation cohort, this transcriptional signature was able to distinguish patients with active versus latent disease, to distinguish tuberculosis infection from other pulmonary inflammatory states or infections, and to track responses to treatment in as little as 2 weeks, with normalization of expression toward that of patients without active disease over 6 months of effective therapy. Such a test could play an important role not only in the management of patients but also as a marker of efficacy in clinical trials of new therapeutic agents. More recently, a distilled three-transcript signature has shown promise for distinguishing active from latent tuberculosis, raising hopes of a deployable assay in the near term.

Similarly, considerable progress has been made toward identifying host transcriptional signatures in circulating blood cells that distinguish viral from bacterial causes of upper respiratory infection, with better performance characteristics than current clinical parameters or available protein biomarkers. Additional host signatures have been reported that distinguish among bacterial infection, viral infection, and inflammatory states; identify Lyme disease; identify influenza; and even distinguish between gram-positive and gram-negative bacterial infections. In some cases, results have been extended to different host populations—including adults and children, and those with varying immune function—which obviously will be critical for generalizing such an approach. Thus, profiling of host transcriptional dynamics could augment the information obtained from studies of pathogens, both enhancing diagnosis and monitoring the progression of illness and the response to therapy. The frontier of genomic applications to understand host response to infection, with the potential of identifying biomarkers or even underlying disease biology, continues to rapidly advance, incorporating novel technological and computational approaches, such as single-cell host transcriptional profiling of infected patients, to understand complex processes such as sepsis.

In this era of genome-wide association studies and attempts to move toward personalized medicine, genomic approaches are also being applied to the identification of host genetic loci and factors that contribute to infection susceptibility. Such loci will have undergone strong selection among populations in which the disease is endemic. Through identification of the beneficial genetic alleles among individuals who survive in such settings, markers for susceptibility or resistance are being discovered; these markers can be translated to diagnostic tests to identify susceptible individuals in order to implement preventive or prophylactic interventions. Further, such studies may offer mechanistic insight into the pathogenesis of infection and inform new methods of therapeutic intervention. Such beneficial genetic associations were recognized long before the advent of genomics, as in the protective effects of the negative Duffy blood group or heterozygous hemoglobin abnormalities against *Plasmodium* infection. Genomic approaches allow more systematic and widespread application of this principle to identify not only people with increased susceptibility to prevalent diseases (e.g., HIV infection, tuberculosis, and cholera) but also host factors that contribute to and thus might predict the severity of disease, including studies currently under way for COVID-19, which displays markedly variable severity that is thus far poorly understood.

THERAPEUTICS

Genomics has the potential to impact infectious disease therapeutics in two ways. By transforming the speed or type of diagnostic information that can be attained, it can influence therapeutic decision-making. Alternatively, by opening new avenues to a better understanding of pathogenesis, providing new ways to disrupt infection, and delineating new approaches to antibiotic discovery, it has the potential to facilitate the development of new therapeutic agents.

GENOMIC DIAGNOSTICS INFORMING THERAPEUTICS

Efforts at antibiotic discovery are declining, with few new agents in the pipeline and even fewer new drugs (in particular, few agents with new mechanisms of action) entering the market. This phenomenon is due in part to the lack of economic incentives for the private sector; however, it is also attributable in part to the enormous challenges involved in the discovery and development of antibiotics. Most recent efforts have focused on broad-spectrum antibiotics; the development of a chemical entity that works across an extremely diverse set of organisms (i.e., species more divergent from each other than a human is from an amoeba) is far more challenging than the development of an agent that is designed to target a single bacterial species. Nevertheless, the concept of narrow-spectrum antibiotics has heretofore been rejected because of the lack of early diagnostic information that would guide the selection of such agents. Thus, rapid diagnostics providing antibiotic susceptibility information that can guide antibiotic selection in real time has the potential to alter and simplify antibiotic strategies by allowing a paradigm shift away from broad-spectrum drugs and toward narrow-spectrum agents. Such a paradigm shift clearly would have additional implications for antibiotic resistance, helping to limit selective pressure applied to pathogens and commensal bacteria during therapy.

In yet another diagnostic paradigm with the potential to impact therapeutic interventions, genomics is opening new avenues to a better understanding not only of different host susceptibilities to infection but also of different host responses to therapy. For example, the role of glucocorticoids in tuberculous meningitis has long been debated. Recently, polymorphisms in the human genetic locus *LTA4H*, which encodes a leukotriene-modifying enzyme, were found to modulate the inflammatory response to tuberculosis. Patients with tuberculous meningitis who were homozygous for the proinflammatory *LTA4H* allele were most helped by adjunctive glucocorticoid treatment, while those who were homozygous for the anti-inflammatory allele were negatively affected by steroid treatment. Steroids have become part of the standard of care in tuberculous meningitis, but this study suggests that perhaps only a subset of patients benefit from this anti-inflammatory adjunct (while others may be harmed) and further suggests a genetic means of prospectively identifying this subset. Thus, genomic diagnostic tests may eventually approach the goal of personalized medicine, informing diagnosis, prognosis, and treatment decisions by revealing the pathogenic potential of the microbe and by detecting individualized host responses to both infection and therapy.

GENOMICS IN DRUG AND VACCINE DEVELOPMENT

Genomic technologies are dramatically changing research on host–pathogen interactions, with a goal of increasingly influencing the process of therapeutic discovery and development. Sequencing offers several possible avenues into antimicrobial therapeutic discovery. First, genome-scale molecular methods have paved the way for comprehensive identification of all essential genes encoded by a pathogen, thereby systematically identifying critical vulnerabilities within a pathogen that could be targeted therapeutically. Second, genome-scale methodologies offer rapid ways to address the mechanism of action of newly identified hits from compound screens. Whole genome sequencing offers a rapid, unbiased way to detect mutations arising in resistant mutants during selection. Similarly, transcriptional profiling can provide insights into mechanisms of action of new candidate drugs. For instance, the transcriptional signature of cell wall disruptors (e.g., β-lactams) is distinct from that of DNA-damaging agents (e.g., fluoroquinolones) or protein synthesis inhibitors (e.g., aminoglycosides). Either approach can thus suggest a mechanism of action or flag compounds for prioritization because of a potentially novel activity. In an alternative genomic strategy for determining mechanisms of action, an RNA interference approach followed by targeted sequencing was used to identify genes required for antitrypanosomal drug efficacy. This approach provided new insights into the mechanism of action of drugs that have been in use for decades for human African trypanosomiasis. Third, sequencing can readily identify the most conserved regions of a pathogen's genomes and corresponding gene products; this information is invaluable in narrowing antigen candidates in vaccine development. These surface proteins can be expressed recombinantly and tested for the ability to elicit a serologic response and protective immunity. This process, termed *reverse vaccinology*, has proved particularly useful for pathogens that are difficult to culture or poorly immunogenic. More directly, mRNA vaccines targeting conserved regions of the SARS-CoV-2 genome were developed at record speed in the face of unprecedented urgency, enabled by the rapid availability of genomic sequencing data. These vaccines proved remarkably effective in initial studies and represent a dramatic breakthrough in efforts to mitigate the pandemic. Moreover, this novel vaccine platform offers a facile way to deliver new viral antigens if needed based on genomic surveillance.

Genomics has been employed in both developing vaccines and defining their impact on microbial epidemiology and ecology. Examples include recent studies of influenza, malaria, *S. pneumoniae*, and HPV following vaccine introduction. Extensive sequencing of influenza viruses has been valuable in understanding the modest efficacy of seasonal influenza vaccination, and the combination of genomics and antigenic cartography is proving helpful in the selection of strains to include in subsequent influenza vaccines. The RTS,S/AS01 malaria vaccine was analyzed by targeted sequencing of parasites from vaccinated and control populations during a phase 3 trial conducted at 11 sites in Africa; these analyses revealed reduced vaccine efficacy against parasites with amino acid mutations in the circumsporozoite protein targeted by the vaccine. Similarly, studies of the more established pneumococcal vaccines (the 7- and 13-valent polysaccharide conjugate vaccines, PCV-7 and PCV-13) documented serotype replacement: strains targeted by the vaccine have dramatically decreased in prevalence following widespread vaccination campaigns. Given that specific serotypes of HPV (e.g., types 16 and 18) clearly are more strongly associated than others with carcinogenesis, HPV vaccines have capitalized on serotype replacement, targeting vaccine strains to specifically prevent infection with the more dangerous serotypes. Such a strategy, informed by pathogen genomics, aims to protect individuals and ideally to decrease the circulating burden of more virulent strains within society.

Large-scale gene content analysis from sequencing or expression profiling enables new research directions that provide novel insights into the interplay of pathogen and host during infection or colonization. One important goal of such research is to suggest new therapeutic approaches to disrupt this interaction in favor of the host. Indeed, one of the most immediate applications of next-generation sequencing technology has come from simply characterizing human pathogens and related commensal or environmental strains and then finding genomic correlates for pathogenicity. For instance, as *Escherichia coli* varies from a simple nonpathogenic, lab-adapted strain (K-12) to a Shiga toxin–producing enterohemorrhagic gastrointestinal pathogen (O157:H7), it displays up to a 25% difference in gene content, though it is classified as the same species. Similarly, some isolates of *Enterococcus*—a genus notorious for its increasing incidence of resistance to common antibiotics such as ampicillin, vancomycin, and aminoglycosides—also contain recently acquired genetic material comprising up to 25% of the genome on mobile genetic elements. This fact suggests that horizontal gene transfer plays an important role in the organisms' adaptation as nosocomial pathogens. On closer study, this genome expansion is associated with loss of CRISPR elements, which protect the bacterial genome from invasion by certain foreign genetic material, and may thus facilitate the acquisition of antibiotic resistance–conferring genetic elements. While loss of this regulation appears to impose a competitive disadvantage in antibiotic-free environments, these drug-resistant strains thrive in the presence of even some of the best antienterococcal therapies. In addition to insights gained from genome sequencing, extension of unbiased whole-transcriptome sequencing (RNA-Seq) efforts to bacteria is beginning to identify unexpected regulatory, noncoding RNAs in many diverse species. While the functional implications of these new transcripts are as yet largely unknown, the presence of such features—conserved across many bacterial species—implies evolutionary importance and suggests areas for future study and possible new therapeutic avenues. Transcriptomic and proteomic profiling of pathogens under various conditions that mimic colonization or infection, including existence as biofilms or in polymicrobial communities, intracellular infection models, antibiotic exposure, and nutrient starvation, has begun to reveal novel biologic features that may be targeted by the next generation of therapies. At the cutting edge of the host–pathogen interface, single-cell transcriptomic methodologies are rapidly increasing in feasibility and extent, revealing previously unknown heterogeneity in the potential outcomes of intracellular infection.

Thus, genomic studies are transforming our understanding of infection, offering evidence of virulence factors or toxins and providing insight into ongoing evolution of pathogenicity and drug resistance. One goal of such studies is to identify therapeutic agents that can disrupt the pathogenic process. There is currently much interest in the theoretical concept of antivirulence drugs that inhibit virulence factors rather than killing the pathogen outright as a means to intervene in infection. Further, with sequencing ever more accessible and efficient, ongoing large-scale studies have unprecedented statistical power to associate clinical outcomes with pathogen and host genotypes and thus to further reveal vulnerabilities in the infection process that can be targeted for disruption. Although this is just the beginning, such studies point to a tantalizing future in which the clinician is armed with genomic predictors of infection outcome and therapeutic response to guide clinical decision-making.

EPIDEMIOLOGY OF INFECTIOUS DISEASES

Epidemiologic studies of infectious diseases have several main goals: to identify and characterize outbreaks, to describe the pattern and dynamics of an infectious disease as it spreads through populations, and to identify interventions that can limit or reduce the burden of disease. One classic, paradigmatic example is John Snow's elucidation of the origin of the 1854 London cholera outbreak. Snow used careful geographic mapping of cases to determine that the likely source of the outbreak was contaminated water from the Broad Street pump, and by removing the pump handle, he aborted the outbreak. Whereas that effort was undertaken without knowledge of the causative agent of cholera, advances in microbiology and genomics have expanded the purview of epidemiology to consider not just the disease but also the pathogen, its virulence factors, and the complex relationships between microbial and host populations.

Through use of genomic tools such as high-throughput sequencing, the diversity of a microbial population can be rapidly described with unprecedented resolution, with discrimination between isolates that have single-nucleotide differences across the entire genome and advancement beyond prior approaches that relied on phenotypes (such as antibiotic susceptibility profiles) or genetic markers (such as multilocus sequence typing). The development of statistical methods grounded in molecular genetics and evolutionary theory has established analytical approaches that translate descriptions of microbial population diversity and structure into descriptions of the origin and history of pathogen spread. By linking phylogenetic reconstruction with epidemiologic and demographic data, genomic epidemiology presents the opportunity to track transmission from person to person and across demographic and geographic boundaries, to infer transmission patterns of both pathogens and sequence elements that confer phenotypes of interest, and to estimate the transmission dynamics of outbreaks.

■ TRANSMISSION NETWORKS

Whole genome sequencing of pathogen genomes can be used to infer transmission and identify point-source outbreaks. As reported in a seminal paper in 2010, a study of MRSA in a Thai hospital demonstrated the use of whole genome sequencing in reconstructing the transmission of a pathogen from patient to patient by integrating the analysis of accumulation of mutations over time with the dates and hospital locations of the infected individuals. Since then, multiple instances of the use of whole genome sequencing to define and motivate interventions aimed at interrupting transmission chains have been reported. In another MRSA outbreak in a special-care baby unit in Cambridge, United Kingdom, whole genome sequencing extended the traditional infection control analysis, which relies on typing organisms by their antibiotic susceptibilities, to sequencing of isolates from clinical samples. This approach identified an otherwise unrecognized outbreak of a specific MRSA strain that was occurring against a background of the usual pattern of infection caused by a diverse circulating population of MRSA strains. The analysis showed evidence of transmission among mothers within the special-care baby unit and in the community and demonstrated the key role of MRSA carriage in a single health care provider in the persistence of the outbreak. In yet another example, in response to the observation of 18 cases of infection by carbapenemase-producing *Klebsiella pneumoniae* over 6 months at the National Institutes of Health Clinical Research Center, genome sequencing of the isolates was used to discriminate between the possibilities that these cases represented multiple, independent introductions into the health care system or a single introduction with subsequent transmission. On the basis of network and phylogenetic analysis of genomic and epidemiologic data, the authors reconstructed the likely relationships among the isolates from patient to patient, demonstrating that the spread of resistant *Klebsiella* infection was in fact due to nosocomial transmission of a single strain. Similar approaches have elucidated the extent to which presumed nosocomial *C. difficile*, VRE, and carbapenem-resistant Enterobacteriaceae represent within-hospital transmission rather than independent acquisitions. With these demonstrations of the potential contribution of genomics to hospital infection-control efforts, an important avenue of research seeks to develop statistical methods with which to ascertain when such tools are useful and their cost-effectiveness when compared with that of current nongenomic approaches.

Genome sequencing of clinical specimens of viruses has been used to understand their epidemiologic patterns of spread. As RNA viruses use an error-prone RNA-dependent RNA polymerase, they accumulate mutations at a rapid rate, facilitating inferences about the dynamics and patterns of spread. These tools have been applied to the study of outbreaks of well-known viruses, such as recent outbreaks of yellow fever in South America and mumps in the United States, as well as recent zoonotic pathogens, such as the coronaviruses MERS-CoV and SARS-CoV. The sequencing of SARS-CoV-2 in the context of the pandemic has offered a powerful example of the contributions that genomic epidemiology can make to, and its increasingly central role in, tracking the spread of a pathogen both locally and globally and informing policy and public health decision-making.

The uncovering of unexpected transmission events by genomic epidemiology studies is motivating investigations into pathogen ecology and modes of transmission. For example, the rise in prevalence of infections with nontuberculous mycobacteria, including *Mycobacterium abscessus*, among patients with cystic fibrosis has led to speculation about the possible role of patient-to-patient transmission in the cystic fibrosis community; however, conventional typing approaches have lacked the resolution to define pathogen population structure accurately, a critical component of inferring transmission. Past infection-control guidelines discounted the possibility of acquisition of nontuberculous mycobacteria in health care settings, as no strong evidence for such transmission had been described. In whole genome sequencing studies of *M. abscessus* isolates from patients with cystic fibrosis, an analytical approach using genome sequencing, epidemiology, and Bayesian modeling revealed that, contrary to the prior belief that infections with *M. abscessus* are independently acquired, the majority of infections appear to be transmitted. Because there are often no clear epidemiologic links that place the infected patients in the same place at the same time, this finding highlights a need to explore preexisting notions of circumstances required for transmission, including the roles of fomites and aerosols, and a reconsideration of *M. abscessus* infection-control guidelines. In a clear example of the utility of whole genome sequencing for revealing unexpected transmission networks, isolates of *M. chimaera* causing infections after cardiothoracic surgery in patients in different locations were all found to be closely related. These isolates differed from one another by at most 38 pairwise single nucleotide polymorphisms out of >5 million bases; in contrast, they differed by >2900 single nucleotide polymorphisms from the nonclonally related reference isolate. Although a hospital source was initially suspected when the first of these cases were identified, this whole genome sequencing analysis strongly supported a single point-source for these geographically dispersed isolates. A subsequent investigation ultimately implicated *M. chimaera* contamination in the manufacturing chain of a temperature-control system used during cardiac bypass. Similar studies of other pathogens—particularly those that share human, other animal host, and environmental reservoirs—will continue to advance our understanding of the relative roles and prominence of sources of infection and the modes of spread through populations, thereby establishing evidence-based strategies for prevention and intervention.

As more studies aim to carefully define the origins and spread of infectious agents using the high-resolution lens of whole genome sequencing, fundamental questions arise about the diversity of infecting and colonizing microbial populations. Traditional microbiologic methods include taking a single colony from a growth plate as representative of the population. However, the more diverse the colonizing or infecting pathogen population, the less representative these individual isolates are and the greater the possibility for introducing error into whole genome sequencing–based methods while reconstructing transmission. Sequencing studies of multiple colonies of an *S. aureus* strain colonizing a single individual showed a "cloud" of diversity. What is the clinical significance of this diversity? What are the processes that generate and limit it? What amount of diversity is transmitted under different conditions and routes of transmission? How do the answers to these questions vary by infectious organism, type of infection, host, and response to treatment? More comprehensive descriptions of diversity, population dynamics, transmission bottlenecks, and the forces that shape and influence the growth and spread of microbial populations will be a critically important focus of future investigations.

ORIGINS AND DYNAMICS OF PATHOGEN SPREAD

In addition to reconstructing the transmission chains of local outbreaks, genomics-based epidemiologic methods reveal broad-scale geographic and temporal spread of pathogens. Four recent examples include the origins of cholera in Haiti, the history of HIV-1 group M, the spread of Ebola in West Africa, and the timing and nature of spread of the zoonotic COVID-19 pandemic. Cholera, a dehydrating diarrheal illness caused by infection with *Vibrio cholerae*, first spread worldwide from the Indian subcontinent in the 1800s and has since caused seven pandemics; the seventh pandemic has been ongoing since the 1960s. An investigation into the geographic patterns of cholera spread in the seventh pandemic used genome sequences from a global collection of 154 *V. cholerae* strains representing isolates from 1957 to 2010. This investigation revealed that the seventh pandemic has comprised at least three overlapping waves spreading out from the Indian subcontinent (**Fig. 121-4*A***). Further, analysis of the genome of an isolate of *V. cholerae* from the 2010 outbreak of cholera in Haiti showed it to be more closely related to isolates from South Asia than to isolates from neighboring Latin America, supporting the hypothesis that the outbreak was derived from *V. cholerae* introduced into Haiti by human travel (likely from Nepal) rather than by environmental or more geographically proximal sources. A subsequent study that dated the time to the most recent common ancestor of a population of *V. cholerae* isolates from Haiti provided further support for a single point-source introduction from Nepal. Application of similar methods that integrate pathogen genome sequences, mutation rates, geographic locations, and phylogenetic inference to HIV-1 group M dated the origin of the virus to the 1920s and the city of Kinshasa (then called Leopoldville), the capital of the Democratic Republic of the Congo (then called the Belgian Congo). This work established an understanding of how a boom in industry and a city with extensive railroad connections provide a scaffolding along which a virus can rapidly spread geographically.

Genome sequencing has proven invaluable in understanding the geographic, demographic, climatic, and administrative factors that drove, sustained, and limited the 2013–2016 Ebola outbreak that ravaged West Africa (**Fig. 121-4*B***) as well as the factors and patterns of transmission of Zika virus in the Americas and most recently the timing and origins of SARS-CoV-2 transmission in human populations. With the rapid availability of the SARS-CoV-2 viral genome sequence, data from a set of cases from early in the pandemic enabled inference of the time to the most recent common ancestor, supporting that SARS-CoV-2 entered circulation in human populations in Wuhan, China, sometime in late November to early December of 2019. Subsequently, large, coordinated sequencing networks have been able to recreate its pattern of early global spread.

These efforts illustrate the remarkable promise of genome sequencing in improving outbreak response strategies by elucidating previously hidden origins and paths of disease spread and details of the forces that shape epidemics. The combination of in-the-field sequencing with portable sequencing platforms, rapid data sharing, and rapid open analysis through sites such as *nextstrain.org* offers a paradigm by which real-time genomic epidemiology may contribute to "weather maps," enabling prediction of epidemic patterns and thus providing guidance for public health interventions to slow or control their spread.

Increasing numbers of investigations into the spread of many pathogens are contributing to a growing atlas of maps describing routes, patterns, and tempos of microbial diversification and dissemination, not just for agents of emerging infectious diseases but for common

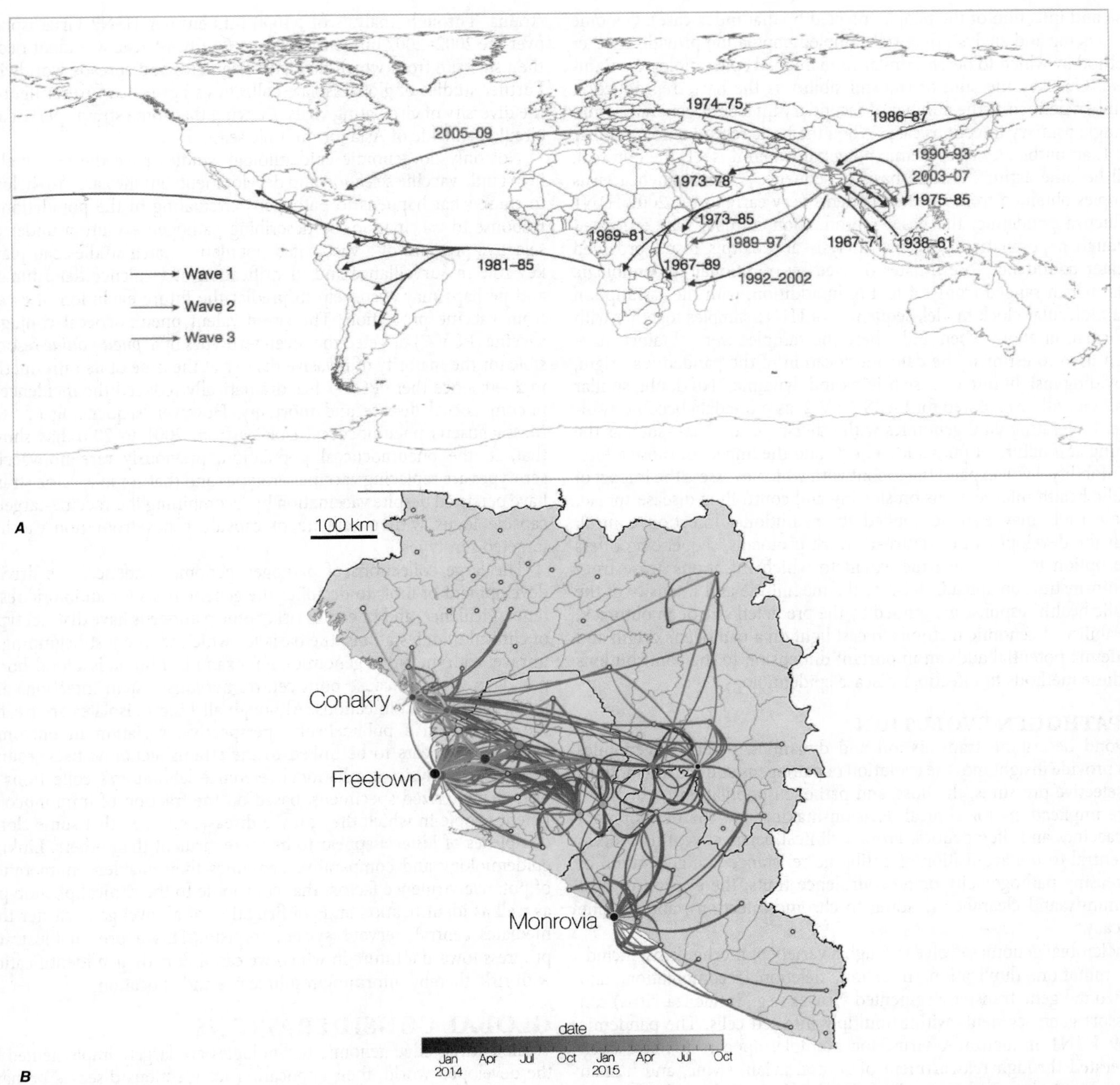

FIGURE 121-4 ***A.*** Transmission events inferred from phylogenetic reconstruction of 154 *Vibrio cholerae* isolates from the seventh cholera pandemic. Date ranges represent estimated time to the most recent common ancestor for strains transmitted from source to destination locations, based on a Bayesian model of the phylogeny. *(Reprinted by permission from the Nature Publishing Group, Nature 477:462. Evidence for several waves of global transmission in the seventh cholera pandemic, A Mutreja et al. © 2011.)* ***B.*** Inferred Ebola virus spread in West Africa (Liberia, *red*; Guinea, *green*; and Sierra Leone, *blue*) by phylogeographic methods using virus genome sequences, dates, and an evolutionary model. The lines reflect spread between population centroids of each administrative region, going from the thin end to the thick end and colored by a time scale. *(Reprinted by permission from Nature Publishing Group, Nature 544:309. Virus genomes reveal factors that spread and sustained the Ebola epidemic, G Dudas et al. © 2017.)*

pathogens as well. Such studies will create a vast amount of data that can be used to investigate the diversity and microbiologic links within distinct niches and the patterns of spread from one niche to another. The increasingly broad adoption of genome sequencing by health care and public health institutions ensures that the available catalog of genome sequences and associated epidemiologic data will grow very rapidly. For example, updating from the pulsed-field gel electrophoresis techniques that have been used to define strains of food-borne pathogens since the late 1980s, PulseNet—the U.S. Centers for Disease Control and Prevention network for monitoring these pathogens—has instituted routine genome sequencing. The COVID-19 pandemic further underscores the importance of building a new global public health infrastructure in which sequencing plays a central role to facilitate early disease discovery, rapid and close tracking of spread, and development of diagnostics and targeted effective interventions. With higher-resolution description of microbial diversity and of the dynamics of that diversity over time and across epidemiologic and demographic boundaries and evolutionary niches, we will gain even greater insights into the relationships of transmission routes and patterns of historical spread.

EPIDEMIC POTENTIAL

Defining pathogen transmissibility is a critical step in the development of public health surveillance and intervention strategies because this information can help to predict the epidemic potential of an outbreak. Transmissibility can be estimated by a variety of methods, including inference from the growth rate of an epidemic and the generation time of an infection (the mean interval between infection of an index case and infection of the people infected by that index case). Genome sequencing and analysis of a well-sampled population provide another method by which to derive similar fundamental epidemiologic parameters. One key measure of transmissibility is the basic reproduction number, defined as the number of secondary infections generated from a single primary infectious case. When the basic reproduction number is >1, an outbreak has epidemic potential; when it is <1, the outbreak will become extinct. On the basis of sequences from influenza virus samples obtained from infected patients very early in the 2009 H1N1 influenza pandemic, the basic reproduction number was estimated through a population genomic analysis at 1.2; this result provided greater confidence to estimates derived by traditional epidemiologic data, which ranged from 1.4 to 1.6. In addition, with the assumption of a molecular clock model, sequences of H1N1 samples together with information about when and where the samples were obtained have been used to estimate the date and location of the pandemic's origin, providing insight into disease origins and dynamics. No doubt, similar analyses will be explored for SARS-CoV-2, as more data become available. Integrating viral genomics with other types of data—such as the timing and nature of mitigation efforts and the impact of those efforts on mobility—will expand the toolkit with which to assess the impact of public health interventions on slowing and controlling disease spread. These tools may also be applied to institutional infection control: with the development of return-to-work protocols, sequencing offers one option to help learn the extent to which infections arose from within-institution spread. Because the magnitude and intensity of the public health response are guided by the predicted size of an outbreak, the ability of genomic methods to cast light on a pathogen's origin and epidemic potential adds an important dimension to the contributions of these methods to infectious disease epidemiology.

PATHOGEN EVOLUTION

Beyond describing transmission and dynamics, pathogen genomics can provide insight into the evolution of pathogens and the interactions of selective pressures, the host, and pathogen populations, which can have implications for clinical decision-making and the development of vaccines and therapeutics. From a clinical perspective, this process is central to the acquisition of antibiotic resistance, the generation of increasing pathogenicity or new virulence traits, the evasion of host immunity and clearance (leading to chronic infection), and vaccine efficacy.

Microbial genomes evolve through a variety of mechanisms, including mutation, duplication, insertion, deletion, recombination, and horizontal gene transfer. Segmented viruses (e.g., influenza virus) can reassort gene segments within multiply infected cells. The pandemic 2009 H1N1 influenza A virus, for example, appears to have been generated through reassortment of several avian, swine, and human influenza strains. Such potential for the evolution of novel pandemic strains has precipitated concern about the possible evolution to transmissibility of virulent strains that have been associated with high mortality rates but have not yet exhibited efficient human infectivity. Experiments with H5N1 avian influenza, for example, have defined five mutations that render it transmissible, at least in ferrets—the animal model system for human influenza. Studies that examine the genomes of pathogens collected longitudinally from individual infections have similarly demonstrated the evolution of bacteria as they adapt from colonization to invasion and to new host environments and new immune and therapeutic pressures.

The continuous antigenic evolution of seasonal influenza offers an example of how studies of pathogen evolution can impact surveillance and vaccine development. Frequent updates to the annual influenza vaccine are needed to ensure protection against the dominant strains. These updates are based on anticipating which viral populations from a pool of substantial locally and globally diverse circulating viruses will predominate in the upcoming season. Toward that end, sequencing-based studies of influenza virus dynamics have shed light on the global spread of influenza, providing concrete data on patterns of spread and helping to elucidate the origins, emergence, and circulation of novel strains. Through analysis of >1000 influenza A H3N2 virus isolates over the 2002–2007 influenza seasons, Southeast Asia was identified as the usual site from which diversity originates and spreads worldwide. Further studies of global isolate collections have shed further light on the diversity of circulating virus, showing that some strains persist and circulate outside of Asia for multiple seasons.

Not only do genomic epidemiology studies have the potential to help guide vaccine selection and development, but they are also helping to track what happens to pathogens circulating in the population in response to vaccination. By describing pathogen evolution under the selective pressure of a vaccinated population, such studies can play a key role in surveillance and identification of virulence determinants and perhaps may even help to predict the future evolution of escape from vaccine protection. The seven-valent pneumococcal conjugate vaccine (PCV-7) targeted the seven serotypes of *S. pneumoniae* responsible for the majority of invasive disease at the time of its introduction in 2000; since then, PCV-7 has dramatically reduced the incidence of pneumococcal disease and mortality. However, sequencing of >600 Massachusetts pneumococcal isolates from 2001 to 2007 has shown that, in the pneumococcal population, previously rare nonvaccine serotypes are replacing vaccine serotypes and that some vaccine strains have persisted despite vaccination by recombining the vaccine-targeted capsule locus with a cassette of capsule genes from non-vaccine-targeted serotypes.

The large collections of pathogen genome sequences are driving development of tools to decipher the genetic basis for antibiotic resistance, virulence, and infection risk. Some pathogens have distinct types of clinical manifestations, the basis for which we are just beginning to unravel with the aid of genomics. For example, *Listeria* is a food-borne pathogen that can cause both central nervous system infections and maternal/neonatal infections. Although all *Listeria* isolates are treated the same from a public health perspective, variation in outcomes exists and appears to be linked to the strains' genomic background. Molecular analysis of a national reference laboratory's collections of well-characterized specimens, based on the fraction of immunocompetent people in which they caused disease, revealed that some clonal complexes of *Listeria* appear to be more virulent than others. Linking epidemiology and comparative genomics then enabled enumeration of putative virulence factors that contribute to the clinical phenotypes as well as identification and confirmation of a novel gene cluster that mediates central nervous system tropism. This approach illustrates progress toward a future in which we can link pathogen identification with risk, thereby informing resource use and allocation.

GLOBAL CONSIDERATIONS

While cutting-edge genomic technologies are largely implemented in the developed world, their application to infectious diseases perhaps offers the biggest potential impact in less developed regions where the burden of these infections is greatest. This globalization of genomic technology and its extensions has already begun in each of the areas of focus highlighted in this chapter; it has occurred both through the application of advanced technologies to samples collected in the developing world and through the adaptation and importation of technologies directly to the developing world for on-site implementation as they become more globally accessible.

Genomic characterization of the pathogens responsible for such important global illnesses such as tuberculosis, malaria, trypanosomiasis, cholera, and most recently COVID-19, has led to insights in diagnosis, treatment, and infection control. For instance, with the increasing burden of drug-resistant tuberculosis in the developing world, a molecular diagnostic test has been developed to detect rifampin-resistant tuberculosis. The genetic basis for rifampin resistance has been well defined by targeted sequencing: characteristic mutations in the molecular target of rifampin, RNA polymerase, account for the vast majority of instances of rifampin resistance. At least in areas that can afford to implement it, a rapid, automated PCR assay that can detect both *M. tuberculosis* and a rifampin-resistant allele of RNA polymerase directly in clinical samples has been implemented in parts of Africa and Asia, transforming the recognition and management of incident tuberculosis and multidrug resistance where they are most prevalent. Since rifampin resistance frequently accompanies resistance to other antibiotics, this test can suggest the presence of multidrug-resistant *M. tuberculosis* within hours instead of weeks, without the infrastructure required for culture.

High-resolution genomic tracking of the spread of epidemics—from cholera to Ebola to Zika to COVID-19—has yielded insights into which public health measures may prove most effective in controlling local epidemics. Many genomic tracking efforts have involved close collaborations with local scientists and public health officials, and considerable investment in sequencing infrastructure in sub-Saharan Africa has made on-location epidemic tracking in the event of another such outbreak feasible. Such investment can not only enable real-time outbreak recognition and tracking but also provide the infrastructure needed to capitalize on the many other benefits of high-throughput sequencing as they are developed. The early returns of such investments are exemplified by the rapid reporting of genome sequences for SARS-CoV-2, with 55,000 viral genome sequences reported within the first 6 months of the pandemic. Overall, sequencing efforts have become cheaper and have moved closer to point-of-care with each passing year. As these technologies synergize with efforts to globalize information-technology resources, global implementation of genomic methods promises to spread state-of-the-art methods for diagnosis, treatment, and epidemic tracking of infections to areas that need these capabilities the most.

GENOMICS AND THE COVID-19 PANDEMIC

The COVID-19 pandemic, which began in 2019 and spread worldwide in 2020, resulted in hundreds of millions of documented infections and millions of deaths and serves as a prime example of the pandemic potential of infectious pathogens. It also demonstrated the central role that genomic tools now play in response to infectious outbreaks, ranging from enabling diagnostics and vaccines to tracking evolution, virulence, and transmissibility of the pathogen. The rapid discovery of SARS-CoV-2 and sequencing of its genome was complete within weeks of the recognition of the clinical syndrome. The rapid public sharing of this genome sequence led directly to two key interventions: diagnostic assay development via RT-qPCR and vaccine design. Crucially, vaccine development was informed by homology of the SARS-CoV-2 sequence to SARS and MERS coronaviruses. The dominant antigen of those viruses, the surface protein Spike, was well characterized, enabling the design of the first SARS-CoV-2 vaccines to begin the day after the genome sequence was shared. The progress of the most rapidly developed and validated vaccine in human history was unquestionably accelerated by genomic technology. WGS has also played a large role in outbreak tracking and confirmation of case clusters in institutional settings such as hospitals or congregate living facilities, in helping to distinguish reinfections from recrudescence or prolonged viral shedding, in monitoring spread through societies, and in tracking pathogen evolution, including the emergence of new variants of concern with altered transmissibility, severity, and/or partial evasion of the immune response generated to prior versions of the virus, vaccines, or monoclonal antibody therapeutics. Finally, cutting edge genomic methods including single-cell transcriptional profiling and genome-wide association studies are contributing to our understanding of the wide variability in outcomes of SARS-CoV-2 infection, ranging from asymptomatic carriage to death. Overall, just as the global response to the COVID-19 pandemic underscores the indispensable role that genomics methods have come to play in the clinical and public health management of infectious diseases, the devastating impact of this pandemic reveals the urgent need for further development and implementation of tools for disease surveillance and response.

SUMMARY

By illuminating the genetic information that encodes the most fundamental processes of life, genomic technologies are transforming many aspects of medicine. In infectious diseases, methods such as next-generation sequencing and genome-scale expression analysis offer information of unprecedented depth about individual microbes as well as microbial communities. This information is expanding our understanding of the interactions of microorganisms with each other, their human hosts, and the environment. Despite technological and financial barriers that continue to slow the widespread adoption of large-scale pathogen sequencing in clinical and public health settings, genomic methodologies have utterly transformed the research landscape in infectious disease and are beginning to make meaningful inroads into clinical settings. As even vaster amounts of data are generated, innovations in data storage, development of bioinformatics tools to manipulate the data, standardization of methods, and training of end-users in both the research and clinical realms will be required. The cost-effectiveness and applicability of whole genome sequencing, particularly in the clinic, remain to be studied, and studies of the impact of genome sequencing on patient outcomes will be needed to clarify the contexts in which these new methodologies can make the greatest contributions to patient well-being. The ongoing efforts to overcome limitations through collaboration, teaching, and reduction of financial obstacles should be applauded and expanded. With advances in genomic technologies and computational analysis, our ability to detect, characterize, treat, monitor, prevent, and control infections has advanced rapidly in recent years and will continue to do so, with the hope of heralding a new era where the clinician is better armed to combat infection and promote human health.

■ FURTHER READING

Bullman S et al: Emerging concepts and technologies for the discovery of microorganisms involved in human disease. Annu Rev Pathol 12:217, 2017.

Burnham CD et al: Diagnosing antimicrobial resistance. Nat Rev Microbiol 15:697, 2017.

Croucher NJ et al: Population genomics of post-vaccine changes in pneumococcal epidemiology. Nat Genet 45:656, 2013.

Cryptic Consortium et al: Prediction of susceptibility to first-line tuberculosis drugs by DNA sequencing. N Engl J Med 379:1403, 2018.

Dudas G et al: Virus genomes reveal factors that spread and sustained the Ebola epidemic. Nature 544:309, 2017.

Gardy JL, Loman NJ: Towards a genomics-informed, real-time, global pathogen surveillance system. Nat Rev Genet 19:9, 2018.

Grubaugh ND et al: Tracking virus outbreaks in the twenty-first century. Nat Microbiol 4:10, 2019.

Loman NJ, Pallen MJ: Twenty years of bacterial genome sequencing. Nat Rev Microbiol 13:787, 2015.

Mutreja A et al: Evidence for several waves of global transmission in the seventh cholera pandemic. Nature 477:462, 2011.

Wu Z, McGoogan JM: Characteristics of and important lessons from the coronavirus disease 2019 (COVID-19) outbreak in China. JAMA 323:1239, 2020.

122 Approach to the Acutely Ill Infected Febrile Patient

Tamar F. Barlam

The physician treating the acutely ill febrile patient must be able to recognize infections that require emergent attention. If such infections are not adequately evaluated and treated at initial presentation, the opportunity to alter an adverse outcome may be lost. In this chapter, the clinical presentations of and approach to patients with infectious disease emergencies are discussed. These infectious processes and their treatments are discussed in detail in other chapters.

APPROACH TO THE PATIENT

Acute Febrile Illness

Before the history is elicited and a physical examination is performed, an immediate assessment of the patient's general appearance can yield valuable information. The perceptive physician's subjective sense that a patient is septic or toxic often proves accurate. Visible agitation or anxiety in a febrile patient can be a harbinger of critical illness.

HISTORY

Presenting symptoms are frequently nonspecific. Detailed questions should be asked about the onset and duration of symptoms and about changes in severity or rate of progression over time. Host factors, such as extremes of age, and comorbid conditions may increase the risk of infection with certain organisms or of a more fulminant course than is usually seen. Lack of splenic function, alcoholism with significant liver disease, IV drug use, HIV infection, diabetes, malignancy, morbid obesity, organ transplantation, and chemotherapy all predispose to specific infections and frequently to increased severity. The patient should be questioned about factors that might help identify a nidus for invasive infection, such as recent upper respiratory tract infections, influenza, or varicella; prior trauma; disruption of cutaneous barriers due to lacerations, burns, surgery, body piercing, or decubiti; and the presence of foreign bodies or prosthetic devices. Travel, presence during a natural disaster such as a hurricane or tsunami, contact with pets or other animals, or activities that might result in tick or mosquito exposure can lead to diagnoses that would not otherwise be considered. Recent dietary intake, medication use, social or occupational contact with ill individuals, vaccination history, recent sexual contacts, and menstrual history may be relevant. Pregnancy might increase the risk and severity of some illnesses, such as influenza or COVID-19, or increase the risk of significant morbidity for the fetus, as in *Listeria* or Zika virus infection. A detailed review of systems should include any neurologic signs or sensorium alterations, rashes or skin lesions, and focal pain or tenderness.

PHYSICAL EXAMINATION

A complete physical examination should be performed, with special attention to several areas that are sometimes given short shrift in routine examinations such as assessment of the patient's general appearance and a detailed skin, soft tissue and neurologic evaluation.

The patient may appear either anxious and agitated or lethargic and apathetic. Fever is usually present, although elderly patients and compromised hosts (e.g., patients who are uremic or cirrhotic and those who are taking glucocorticoids or nonsteroidal anti-inflammatory drugs) may be afebrile despite serious underlying infection. Critically ill patients may be hypothermic, with a high risk of organ failure and mortality. Mortality at 30 days has been shown to decrease with increasing temperature at presentation. Measurement of blood pressure, heart rate, and respiratory rate and oxygen saturation helps determine the degree of hemodynamic and metabolic compromise. The patient's airway must be evaluated to rule out the risk of obstruction from an invasive oropharyngeal infection.

The etiologic diagnosis may become evident in the context of a thorough skin examination **(Chap. 19)**. Petechial rashes are typically seen with meningococcemia or Rocky Mountain spotted fever (RMSF; **see Fig. A1-16**); erythroderma is associated with toxic shock syndrome (TSS). On soft tissue and muscle examination, areas of erythema or duskiness, edema, and tenderness may indicate underlying necrotizing fasciitis, myositis, or myonecrosis. The neurologic examination must include a careful assessment of mental status for signs of early encephalopathy. Evidence of nuchal rigidity or focal neurologic findings should be sought.

DIAGNOSTIC WORKUP

After a quick clinical assessment, diagnostic material should be obtained rapidly and antibiotic and supportive treatment begun. Blood (for cultures; baseline complete blood count with differential; measurement of serum electrolytes, blood urea nitrogen, serum creatinine, and serum glucose; liver function tests and serum lactate; C-reactive protein, lactate dehydrogenase, and D-dimer) can be obtained at the time an IV line is placed and before antibiotics are administered. Three sets of blood cultures should be performed for patients with possible acute endocarditis. Blood smears from patients at risk for severe parasitic disease, such as malaria or babesiosis **(Chaps. 224, 225, and A2)**, must be examined for the diagnosis and quantitation of parasitemia. Blood smears may also be diagnostic in ehrlichiosis and anaplasmosis. Testing of a nasopharyngeal sample for possible COVID-19 may be indicated.

Patients with possible meningitis should have cerebrospinal fluid (CSF) drawn before the initiation of antibiotic therapy. Focal findings, depressed mental status, or papilledema should be evaluated by brain imaging prior to lumbar puncture, which, in this setting, could initiate herniation. *Antibiotics should be administered before imaging but after blood for cultures has been drawn.* If CSF cultures are negative, blood cultures will provide the diagnosis in 50–70% of cases. Molecular diagnostic techniques (e.g., broad-range 16S rRNA gene polymerase chain reaction testing for bacterial meningitis pathogens) are of increasing importance in the rapid diagnosis of life-threatening infections.

Focal abscesses necessitate immediate CT or MRI as part of an evaluation for surgical intervention. Other diagnostic procedures, such as wound cultures, should not delay the initiation of treatment for more than minutes. Once emergent evaluation, diagnostic procedures, and (if appropriate) surgical consultation (see below) have been completed, other laboratory tests can be conducted. Appropriate radiography, CT and/or MRI imaging, urinalysis, measurement of the erythrocyte sedimentation rate, C-reactive protein, and/or procalcitonin, and transthoracic or transesophageal echocardiography all may prove important.

TREATMENT

The Acutely Ill Patient

In the acutely ill patient, empirical antibiotic therapy for presumed bacterial or fungal infection is critical and should be administered without undue delay in addition to fluid resuscitation and vasopressor support as needed. Increased prevalence of antibiotic resistance in community-acquired bacteria must be considered when antibiotics are selected. **Table 122-1** lists first-line empirical regimens for infections considered in this chapter. In addition to the rapid initiation of antibiotic therapy, several of these infections require urgent surgical attention. Neurosurgical evaluation for subdural empyema, otolaryngologic surgery for possible mucormycosis, and cardiothoracic surgery for critically ill patients with acute endocarditis are as important as antibiotic therapy. For infections such as necrotizing fasciitis and clostridial myonecrosis, rapid surgical intervention supersedes other diagnostic or therapeutic maneuvers.

Adjunctive treatments may reduce morbidity and mortality rates and include dexamethasone for bacterial meningitis or IV immunoglobulin for TSS. Adjunctive therapies should usually be initiated within the first hours of treatment; however, dexamethasone for bacterial meningitis must be given before or at the time of the first dose of antibiotic. Glucocorticoids may also be harmful—e.g., when given in the setting of cerebral malaria or viral hepatitis.

SPECIFIC PRESENTATIONS

The infections considered below according to common clinical presentation can have rapidly catastrophic outcomes, and their immediate recognition and treatment can be life-saving. Recommended empirical therapeutic regimens are presented in Table 122-1.

■ SEPSIS WITHOUT AN OBVIOUS FOCUS OF PRIMARY INFECTION

Patients initially have a brief prodrome of nonspecific symptoms and signs that progresses quickly to hemodynamic instability with

TABLE 122-1 Empirical Treatment for Common Infectious Disease Emergencies[a]

CLINICAL SYNDROME	POSSIBLE ETIOLOGIES	TREATMENT	COMMENTS	SEE CHAP(S).
Sepsis without a Clear Focus				
Septic shock	*Pseudomonas* spp., gram-negative enteric bacilli, *Staphylococcus* spp., *Streptococcus* spp.	Vancomycin (15 mg/kg q12h)[b] **plus either** Piperacillin/tazobactam (4.5 g) q8h via extended infusion (EI)[c] *or* cefepime (2 g) q8h via EI	Empirical therapy should be tailored to local resistance patterns. Carbapenem or aminoglycoside antibiotics should be considered for empirical therapy when rates of multidrug-resistant gram-negative organisms are high or for patients with risk factors for resistant organisms. Adjust treatment when culture data become available.	147, 148, 161, 164, 304
Overwhelming post-splenectomy sepsis	*Streptococcus pneumoniae, Haemophilus influenzae, Neisseria meningitidis*	Ceftriaxone (2 g q12h) *plus* vancomycin (15 mg/kg q12h)[b]	If a β-lactam–sensitive strain is identified, vancomycin can be discontinued and a narrower-spectrum agent, such as penicillin, considered based on susceptibility testing.	304
Babesiosis	*Babesia microti* (U.S.), *B. divergens* (Europe)	Atovaquone (750 mg q12h) *plus* azithromycin (500 mg q24h)	Clindamycin (600 mg q8h) *plus* quinine (650 mg q8h) can be used in severe disease not responding to atovaquone and azithromycin. Treatment with doxycycline (100 mg bid) for potential co-infection with *Borrelia burgdorferi* or *Anaplasma* spp. may be prudent.	222, 225
Sepsis with Skin Findings				
Meningococcemia	*N. meningitidis*	Ceftriaxone (2 g q12h) or penicillin (4 mU q4h)	Ceftriaxone eradicates nasopharyngeal carriage of the organism. Close contacts require chemoprophylaxis with rifampin (600 mg q12h for 2 days) or ciprofloxacin (a single dose, 500 mg).	155
Rocky Mountain spotted fever (RMSF)	*Rickettsia rickettsii*	Doxycycline (100 mg bid)	If both meningococcemia and RMSF are being considered, use ceftriaxone (2 g q12h) *plus* doxycycline (100 mg bid). If RMSF is diagnosed, doxycycline is the proven superior agent.	187
Purpura fulminans	*S. pneumoniae, H. influenzae, N. meningitidis*	Ceftriaxone (2 g q12h) *plus* vancomycin (15 mg/kg q12h)[b]	If a β-lactam-sensitive strain is identified, vancomycin can be discontinued.	146, 155, 157, 304
Erythroderma: toxic shock syndrome	Group A *Streptococcus, Staphylococcus aureus*	Vancomycin (15 mg/kg q12h)[b] *plus* clindamycin (600 mg q8h)	If a penicillin- or oxacillin-sensitive strain is isolated, these agents are superior to vancomycin (penicillin, 2 mU q4h; or oxacillin, 2 g IV q4h). The site of toxigenic bacteria should be debrided; IV immunoglobulin can be used in severe cases.[d]	147, 148
Sepsis with Soft Tissue Findings				
Necrotizing fasciitis	Group A *Streptococcus*, mixed aerobic/anaerobic flora, CA-MRSA[e]	Vancomycin (15 mg/kg q12h)[b] *plus* piperacillin/tazobactam (4.5 g q8h via EI)[c] *plus* clindamycin (600 mg q8h)	Urgent surgical evaluation is critical. Empirical therapy should be tailored to local resistance patterns. For mixed aerobic/anaerobic infections, clindamycin can be discontinued. Adjust treatment when culture data become available.	129, 147, 148
Clostridial myonecrosis	*Clostridium perfringens*	Penicillin (2 mU q4h) *plus* clindamycin (600 mg q8h)	Urgent surgical evaluation is critical.	154
Neurologic Infections				
Bacterial meningitis	*S. pneumoniae, N. meningitidis*	Ceftriaxone (2 g q12h) *plus* vancomycin (15 mg/kg q12h)[b]	If a β-lactam–sensitive strain is identified, vancomycin can be discontinued. If the patient is >50 years old or has comorbid disease, add ampicillin (2 g q4h) for *Listeria* coverage. Dexamethasone (10 mg q6h for 4 days) started before, or at the time of, the first dose of antibiotic improves outcome in adults with meningitis (especially pneumococcal).	138
Brain abscess, suppurative intracranial infections	*Streptococcus* spp., *Staphylococcus* spp., anaerobes, gram-negative bacilli	Vancomycin (15 mg/kg q12h)[b] *plus* metronidazole (500 mg q8h) *plus* ceftriaxone (2 g q12h)	Urgent surgical evaluation is critical. If a penicillin- or oxacillin-sensitive strain is isolated, these agents are superior to vancomycin (penicillin, 4 mU q4h; *or* oxacillin, 2 g q4h).	138
Cerebral malaria	*Plasmodium falciparum*	Artesunate (2.4 mg/kg IV at 0, 12, and 24 h; then once daily)[f]	Avoid glucocorticoids. Until IV artesunate is available, treatment can be initiated with oral artemether-lumefantrine. Atovaquone-proguanil, quinine, and mefloquine are other options.	222, 224
Spinal epidural abscess	*Staphylococcus* spp., gram-negative bacilli	Vancomycin (15 mg/kg q12h)[b] **plus either** Piperacillin/tazobactam (4.5 g q8h via EI) *or* cefepime (2 g q8h via EI)[c]	Surgical evaluation is essential. If a penicillin- or oxacillin-sensitive strain is isolated, these agents are superior to vancomycin (penicillin, 4 mU q4h; *or* oxacillin, 2 g q4h).	442
Focal Infections				
Acute bacterial endocarditis	*S. aureus*, β-hemolytic streptococci, HACEK group,[g] *Neisseria* spp., *S. pneumoniae*	Ceftriaxone (2 g q12h) or cefepime (2 g q8h via EI)[c] *plus* vancomycin (15 mg/kg q12h)[b]	Adjust treatment when culture data become available. Surgical evaluation is essential.	128

[a]These empirical regimens include coverage for gram-positive pathogens that are resistant to β-lactam antibiotics. Local resistance patterns should be considered and may alter the need for empirical vancomycin or for expanded coverage for antibiotic-resistant gram-negative pathogens. [b]A vancomycin loading dose of 20–25 mg/kg can be considered in critically ill patients. Dosing must be adjusted based on pharmacokinetic/pharmacodynamic monitoring. [c]EI=extended infusion. β-Lactam antibiotics may exhibit unpredictable pharmacodynamics in sepsis. Prolonged or continuous infusions are often used. [d]The optimal dose of IV immunoglobulin has not been determined, but the median dose in observational studies is 2 g/kg (total dose administered for 1–5 days). [e]Community-acquired methicillin-resistant *S. aureus*. [f]In the United States, artesunate must be obtained through the Centers for Disease Control and Prevention. [g]*Haemophilus* spp., *Aggregatibacter* spp., *Cardiobacterium hominis*, *Eikenella corrodens*, and *Kingella kingae*.

hypotension, tachycardia, tachypnea, respiratory distress, and altered mental status. Disseminated intravascular coagulation (DIC) with clinical evidence of a hemorrhagic diathesis is a poor prognostic sign.

Septic Shock (See also Chap. 304) Patients with bacteremia leading to septic shock may have a primary site of infection (e.g., pneumonia, pyelonephritis, or cholangitis) that is not evident initially. Elderly patients who may have atypical presentations and often have comorbid conditions, hosts compromised by malignancy and neutropenia, and patients who have recently undergone a surgical procedure or hospitalization are at increased risk for an adverse outcome. Gram-negative bacteremia with organisms such as *Pseudomonas aeruginosa* or *Escherichia coli* and gram-positive infection with organisms such as *Staphylococcus aureus* (including methicillin-resistant *S. aureus* [MRSA]) or group A streptococci can present as intractable hypotension and multiorgan failure. Treatment can usually be initiated empirically on the basis of the presentation, host factors (**Chap. 304**), and local patterns of bacterial resistance. Outcomes are worse when antimicrobial treatment is delayed or when the responsible pathogen ultimately proves not to be susceptible to the initial regimen. The increasing prevalence of multidrug-resistant organisms makes this especially relevant. Broad-spectrum antimicrobial agents are therefore recommended and should be instituted rapidly, preferably within the first hours after presentation. Pharmacodynamics are altered in sepsis due to increased volume of distribution and renal clearance, so it is important to adequately dose antimicrobials. Risk factors for fungal infection should be assessed, as the incidence of fungal septic shock is increasing. Nonbacterial causes of shock, such as dengue virus infection, should be considered in endemic areas as mortality can increase if undiagnosed. Biomarkers such as C-reactive protein and procalcitonin have not proved reliable diagnostically or prognostically but, when measured over time, can facilitate appropriate de-escalation of therapy with improved outcomes. Glucocorticoids are often considered for patients with severe sepsis who do not respond to fluid resuscitation and vasopressor therapy, but conclusive evidence for efficacy in this setting is lacking.

Overwhelming Infection in Asplenic Patients (See also Chap. 304) Patients without splenic function are at risk for overwhelming bacterial sepsis. Asplenic adult patients succumb to sepsis at 58 times the rate of the general population. Most infections occur within the first l or 2 years, but the increased risk persists throughout life. The median interval between splenectomy and sepsis is 4–6 years, with a range of 1–19 years. In asplenia, encapsulated bacteria cause the majority of infections. Adults, who are more likely to have antibody to these organisms, are at lower risk than children. *Streptococcus pneumoniae* is the most common isolate, causing 40–70% of cases. The risk of infection with *Haemophilus influenzae* or *Neisseria meningitidis* also is greater in patients without splenic function, but reported cases are declining. Severe clinical manifestations of infections due to other organisms, such as *E. coli*, *S. aureus*, *Bordetella holmesii*, *Capnocytophaga*, *Babesia*, and *Plasmodium* species, have been described.

Babesiosis (See also Chap. 225) A history of recent travel to endemic areas raises the possibility of infection with *Babesia*. Between 1 and 4 weeks after a tick bite, the patient experiences chills, fatigue, anorexia, myalgia, arthralgia, shortness of breath, nausea, and headache; ecchymosis and/or petechiae are occasionally seen. The tick that most commonly transmits *Babesia*, *Ixodes scapularis*, also transmits *Borrelia burgdorferi* (the agent of Lyme disease) and *Anaplasma*; co-infection can occur, and may result in more severe disease. Infection with the European species *Babesia divergens* is more frequently fulminant than that due to the U.S. species *Babesia microti*. *B. divergens* causes a febrile syndrome with hemolysis, jaundice, hemoglobinemia, and renal failure and is associated with a mortality rate of >40%. Severe babesiosis is especially common in asplenic hosts but does occur in hosts with normal splenic function, particularly those >60 years of age and those with underlying immunosuppressive conditions such as HIV infection or malignancy. Complications include renal failure, acute respiratory failure, DIC, and splenic rupture.

Other Sepsis Syndromes Tularemia (**Chap. 170**) has been reported in every U.S. state except Hawaii. This disease is associated with wild rabbit, tick, horse-fly, and tabanid fly contact. It can be transmitted by arthropod bite, handling of infected animal carcasses, consumption of contaminated food and water, or inhalation. The typhoidal form can be associated with gram-negative septic shock and a mortality rate of >30%, especially in patients with underlying comorbid or immunosuppressive conditions. Plague occurs infrequently in the United States (**Chap. 171**), primarily after contact with ground squirrels, prairie dogs, or chipmunks, but is endemic in other parts of the world; >90% of all cases occur in Africa with Madagascar especially affected. The septic form is particularly rare and is associated with shock, multiorgan failure, and a 30% mortality rate. Pneumonic plague is rapidly progressive and fatal without treatment. These infections should be considered in the appropriate epidemiologic setting. The Centers for Disease Control and Prevention (CDC) lists *Francisella tularensis* and *Yersinia pestis* (the agents of tularemia and plague, respectively) along with *Bacillus anthracis* (the agent of anthrax) as important organisms that might be used for bioterrorism (**Chap. S3**).

SEPSIS WITH SKIN MANIFESTATIONS (SEE ALSO CHAP. 19)

Maculopapular rashes may reflect early meningococcal or rickettsial disease but are usually associated with nonemergent infections. Exanthems are usually viral. Primary HIV infection commonly presents with a rash that is typically maculopapular and involves the upper part of the body but can spread to the palms and soles. The patient is usually febrile and can have lymphadenopathy, severe headache, dysphagia, diarrhea, myalgias, and arthralgias. Recognition of this syndrome provides an opportunity to prevent transmission and to institute early treatment.

Petechial rashes caused by viruses are seldom associated with hypotension or a toxic appearance, although there can be exceptions (e.g., severe measles or arboviral infection). Petechial rashes limited to the distribution of the superior vena cava are rarely associated with severe disease. In other settings, petechial rashes require more urgent attention.

Meningococcemia (See also Chap. 155) Almost three-quarters of patients with *N. meningitidis* bacteremia have a rash. Meningococcemia most often affects young children (i.e., those 6 months to 5 years old). In sub-Saharan Africa, the high prevalence of serogroup A meningococcal disease has been a threat to public health for more than a century. Thousands of deaths occur annually in this area, which is known as the "meningitis belt," and large epidemic waves occur approximately every 8–12 years. Serogroups W135, X, and C also are important emerging pathogens in Africa. For example, Nigeria experienced a large serogroup C outbreak in 2016–2017 in the setting of aggressive vaccination programs against serogroup A. Outside Africa, outbreaks for the past 50 years reported in the United States and Europe are caused primarily by serogroup C (approximately 60%) followed by serogroup B (29%). In the United States, sporadic cases and outbreaks occur in day-care centers, schools (grade school through college, particularly among college freshmen living in residential halls), and army barracks. Household contacts of index cases are at 400–800 times greater risk of disease than the general population. Patients may have fever, headache, nausea, vomiting, myalgias, changes in mental status, and meningismus. However, the rapidly progressive form of disease is not usually associated with meningitis. The rash is initially pink, blanching, and maculopapular, appearing on the trunk and extremities, but then becomes hemorrhagic, forming petechiae. Petechiae are first seen at the ankles, wrists, axillae, mucosal surfaces, and palpebral and bulbar conjunctiva, with subsequent spread on the lower extremities and to the trunk. A cluster of petechiae may be seen at pressure points—e.g., where a blood pressure cuff has been inflated. In rapidly progressive meningococcemia (10–20% of cases), the petechial rash quickly becomes purpuric (**see Fig. A1-41**), and patients develop DIC, multiorgan failure, and shock; 50–60% of these patients die, and survivors often require extensive debridement or amputation of gangrenous extremities. Hypotension with petechiae for <12 h is associated with significant mortality. Cyanosis, coma, oliguria, metabolic acidosis, and elevated partial thromboplastin time also are associated with a fatal outcome. Antibiotics given in the office by the primary care provider before hospital evaluation and admission may improve prognosis; this observation suggests that early initiation of treatment may be life-saving. Meningococcal conjugate vaccines are protective against serogroups A, C, Y and W135 and are recommended for children 11–12 years of age with a booster dose at 16 years of age, and for other high-risk patients. Vaccines active against serogroup B are recommended for high-risk individuals ≥10 years of age and may be appropriate for teens and young adults (16 through 23 years of age).

Rocky Mountain Spotted Fever and Other Rickettsial Diseases (See also Chap. 187) RMSF is a tickborne disease that occurs throughout North and South America. It is caused primarily by *Rickettsia rickettsii* but can be caused by other rickettsiae (e.g., *R. parkeri, R. akari*). Up to 40% of patients do not report a history of a tick bite, but a history of travel or outdoor activity (e.g., camping in tick-infested areas) can often be ascertained. For the first 3 days, headache, fever, malaise, myalgias, nausea, vomiting, and anorexia are documented. By day 3, half of patients have skin findings. Blanching macules develop initially on the wrists and ankles and then spread over the legs and trunk. The lesions become hemorrhagic and are frequently petechial. The rash spreads to palms and soles later in the course. The centripetal spread is a classic feature of RMSF but occurs in a minority of patients. Moreover, 10–15% of patients with RMSF never develop a rash. The patient can be hypotensive and develop noncardiogenic pulmonary edema, confusion, lethargy, and encephalitis progressing to coma. The CSF contains 10–100 cells/μL, usually with a predominance of mononuclear cells. The CSF glucose level is often normal; the protein concentration may be slightly elevated. Renal and hepatic injury as well as bleeding secondary to vascular damage are noted. Delayed recognition and treatment are associated with a greater risk of death; mortality rates are 20–30% if untreated. Native Americans, Alaskan natives, Pacific Islanders, children 5–9 years of age, adults >70 years old, and persons with underlying immunosuppression are at increased risk of death as well.

Other rickettsial diseases cause significant morbidity and mortality worldwide. *Mediterranean spotted fever* caused by *Rickettsia conorii* is found in Africa, southwestern and south-central Asia, and southern Europe. Patients have fever, flu-like symptoms, and an inoculation eschar at the site of the tick bite. A maculopapular rash develops within 1–7 days, involving the palms and soles but sparing the face. Elderly patients or those with diabetes, alcoholism, uremia, or congestive heart failure are at risk for severe disease characterized by neurologic involvement, respiratory distress, and gangrene of the digits or purpura fulminans. Mortality rates associated with this severe form of disease approach 50%. *Epidemic typhus*, caused by *Rickettsia prowazekii*, is transmitted in louse-infested environments and emerges in conditions of extreme poverty, war, and natural disaster. Patients experience a sudden onset of high fevers, severe headache, cough, myalgias, and abdominal pain. A maculopapular rash develops (primarily on the trunk) in more than half of patients and can progress to petechiae and purpura. Serious signs include delirium, coma, seizures, noncardiogenic pulmonary edema, skin necrosis, and peripheral gangrene. Mortality rates approached 60% in the preantibiotic era and continue to exceed 10–15% in contemporary outbreaks. *Scrub typhus*, caused by *Orientia tsutsugamushi* (a separate genus in the family Rickettsiaceae), is transmitted by larval mites or chiggers and is one of the most common infections in southeastern Asia and the western Pacific. The organism is found in areas of heavy scrub vegetation (e.g., along riverbanks). Patients may have an inoculation eschar and may develop a maculopapular rash, lymphadenopathy, and dyspnea. Severe cases progress to pneumonia, meningoencephalitis, myocarditis, DIC, and renal failure. Mortality rates range from 1% to 70% and vary by location, increasing age, myocarditis, delirium, pneumonitis, or signs of hemorrhage.

If recognized in a timely fashion, rickettsial disease is very responsive to treatment. Doxycycline (100 mg twice daily for 3–14 days) is the treatment of choice for both adults and children. Mortality rates are higher when tetracycline-based treatment is not given.

Purpura Fulminans (See also Chaps. 155 and 304) Purpura fulminans is the cutaneous manifestation of DIC and presents as large ecchymotic areas and hemorrhagic bullae. Progression of petechiae to purpura, ecchymoses, and gangrene is associated with congestive heart failure, septic shock, acute renal failure, acidosis, hypoxia, hypotension, and death. Purpura fulminans has been associated primarily with *N. meningitidis* but, in splenectomized patients, may be associated with *S. pneumoniae, H. influenzae*, and *S. aureus*.

Ecthyma Gangrenosum Septic shock caused by *P. aeruginosa* or, less often, *Aeromonas hydrophila* or other gram-negative organisms, can be associated with ecthyma gangrenosum **(see Figs. 164-1 and A1-34)**: hemorrhagic vesicles surrounded by a rim of erythema with central necrosis and ulceration. Echthyma gangrenosum is most common among patients with neutropenia, extensive burns, and hypogammaglobulinemia.

Other Infections Associated with Rash *Vibrio vulnificus* and other noncholera *Vibrio* bacteremic infections **(Chap. 168)** can cause focal skin lesions and overwhelming sepsis in hosts with chronic liver disease, heavy alcohol consumption, iron storage disorders, diabetes, renal insufficiency, hematologic disease, or malignancy or other immunocompromising conditions. Over 95% of the cases are in the subtropical Pacific and Atlantic Oceans coastal regions in the Northern Hemisphere. After ingestion of contaminated raw shellfish (typically oysters from the Gulf Coast in U.S. cases), there is a sudden onset of malaise, chills, fever, and hypotension. The patient develops bullous or hemorrhagic skin lesions, usually on the lower extremities, and 75% of patients have leg pain. The mortality rate can be as high as 35–60%, particularly when the patient presents with hypotension. Outcomes are improved when patients are treated with fluoroquinolones with or without cephalosporins or with tetracycline-containing regimens. Other infections, caused by agents such as *Aeromonas, Klebsiella*, and *E. coli*, can cause hemorrhagic bullae and death due to overwhelming sepsis in cirrhotic patients. *Capnocytophaga canimorsus* can cause septic shock in asplenic or cirrhotic patients. Infection typically follows a dog bite. Serovars A–C appear more virulent, constituting 92% of human infections but only 7.6% of canine isolates. Patients present with fever, chills, myalgia, vomiting, diarrhea, dyspnea, confusion, and headache. Findings can include an exanthem or erythema multiforme **(see Figs. 56-9 and A1-24)**, cyanotic mottling or peripheral cyanosis, petechiae, and ecchymosis. About 30% of patients with this fulminant form die of overwhelming sepsis and DIC, and survivors may require amputation because of gangrene.

Erythroderma TSS **(Chaps. 147 and 148)** is usually associated with erythroderma. The patient presents with fever, malaise, myalgias, nausea, vomiting, diarrhea, and confusion. There is a sunburn-type rash that may be subtle and patchy but is usually diffuse and is found on the face, trunk, and extremities. Erythroderma, which desquamates after 1–2 weeks, is more common in *Staphylococcus*-associated than in *Streptococcus*-associated TSS. Hypotension develops rapidly—often within hours—after the onset of symptoms. Multiorgan failure occurs. Early renal failure may precede hypotension and distinguishes this syndrome from other septic shock syndromes. There may be no indication of a primary focal infection, although possible cutaneous or mucosal portals of entry for the organism can be ascertained when a careful history is taken. Colonization rather than overt infection of the vagina or a postoperative wound, for example, is typical with staphylococcal TSS, and the mucosal areas appear hyperemic but not infected. Streptococcal TSS is more often associated with skin or soft tissue infection (including necrotizing fasciitis), and patients are more likely to be bacteremic. TSS caused by *Clostridium sordellii* is associated with childbirth or with skin injection of black-tar heroin. The diagnosis of TSS is defined by the clinical criteria of fever, rash, hypotension, and multiorgan involvement. (Of note, fever is typically absent when TSS is caused by *C. sordellii*.) The mortality rate is 5% for menstruation-associated TSS, 10–15% for nonmenstrual TSS, 30–70% for streptococcal TSS, and up to 90% for obstetric *C. sordellii* TSS. Clindamycin improves outcomes when included in the treatment regimen. Some studies have shown that use of IV immunoglobulin is associated with improved survival as well.

Viral Hemorrhagic Fevers Viral hemorrhagic fevers (**Chaps. 209 and 210**) are zoonotic illnesses caused by viruses that reside in either animal reservoirs or arthropod vectors. These diseases occur worldwide and are restricted to areas where the host species live. They are caused by four major groups of viruses: Arenaviridae (e.g., Lassa fever in Africa), Bunyaviridae (e.g., Rift Valley fever in Africa; hantavirus hemorrhagic fever with renal syndrome in Asia; and Crimean-Congo hemorrhagic fever, which has an extensive geographic distribution), Filoviridae (e.g., Ebola and Marburg virus infections in Africa), and Flaviviridae (e.g., yellow fever in Africa and South America and dengue in Asia, Africa, and the Americas). Lassa fever and Ebola and Marburg virus infections are also transmitted from person to person. The vectors for most viral fevers are found in rural areas; dengue and yellow fever are important exceptions. After a prodrome of fever, myalgias, and malaise, patients develop evidence of vascular damage, petechiae, and local hemorrhage. Shock, multifocal hemorrhaging, and neurologic signs (e.g., seizures or coma) predict a poor prognosis. Dengue (**Chap. 209**) is the most common arboviral disease worldwide. More than half a million cases of dengue hemorrhagic fever occur each year, with at least 12,000 deaths. Patients have a triad of symptoms: hemorrhagic manifestations, evidence of plasma leakage, and platelet counts of <100,000/μL. Mortality rates are 10–20%. If dengue shock syndrome develops, mortality rates can reach 40%. Ebola infection has been associated with outbreaks with high mortality rates. The 2014 outbreak in West Africa had a mortality rate of >50%. Symptoms can appear 2–21 days after exposure, but most patients become ill within 9 days. The patient first presents with fatigue, fever, headache, and muscle pains, and the illness can progress to multiorgan failure and hemorrhaging. Careful volume-replacement therapy to maintain blood pressure and intravascular volume is key to survival in these infections. Ribavirin also may be useful against Arenaviridae and Bunyaviridae.

Other viral illnesses with rash, such as measles, can be associated with significant mortality rates. Measles continues to be responsible for more than 100,000 deaths per year, worldwide, and to cause outbreaks in populations with low vaccination rates.

SEPSIS WITH A SOFT TISSUE/MUSCLE PRIMARY FOCUS

See also Chap. 129.

Necrotizing Fasciitis This infection is characterized by extensive necrosis of the subcutaneous tissue and fascia. It may arise at a site of minimal trauma or surgical incision and may also be associated with recent varicella, childbirth, or muscle strain. The most common causes of necrotizing fasciitis are group A streptococci alone (**Chap. 148**) and a mixed facultative and anaerobic flora (**Chap. 129**); the incidence of group A streptococcal necrotizing fasciitis has been increasing for the past quarter-century. Diabetes mellitus, IV drug use, chronic liver or renal disease, and malignancy are associated risk factors. Physical findings are initially minimal compared with the severity of pain and the degree of fever. The examination is often unremarkable except for soft tissue edema and erythema. The infected area is red, hot, shiny, swollen, and exquisitely tender. In untreated infection, the overlying skin develops blue-gray patches after 36 h, and cutaneous bullae and necrosis develop after 3–5 days. Necrotizing fasciitis due to a mixed flora, but not that due to group A streptococci, can be associated with gas production. Without treatment, pain decreases because of thrombosis of the small blood vessels and destruction of the peripheral nerves—an ominous sign. The mortality rate is 15–34% overall, >70% in association with TSS, and nearly 100% without surgical intervention. With surgery, outcomes are significantly better; e.g., mortality is reduced to <40% in the setting of TSS. Necrotizing fasciitis may also be due to *Clostridium perfringens* (**Chap. 154**); in this condition, the patient is extremely toxic and the mortality rate is high. Within 48 h, rapid tissue invasion and systemic toxicity associated with hemolysis and death ensue. The distinction between this entity and clostridial myonecrosis is made by muscle biopsy. Necrotizing fasciitis caused by community-acquired MRSA also has been reported.

Clostridial Myonecrosis (See also Chap. 154) Myonecrosis is often associated with trauma or surgery but can develop spontaneously. The incubation period is usually 12–24 h long, and massive necrotizing gangrene develops within hours of onset. Systemic toxicity, shock, and death can occur within 12 h. The patient's pain and toxic appearance are out of proportion to physical findings. On examination, the patient is febrile, apathetic, tachycardic, and tachypneic and may express a feeling of impending doom. Hypotension and renal failure develop later, and hyperalertness is evident preterminally. The skin over the affected area is bronze-brown, mottled, and edematous. Bullous lesions with serosanguineous drainage and a mousy or sweet odor can develop. Crepitus can occur secondary to gas production in muscle tissue. The mortality rate is >65% for spontaneous myonecrosis, which is often associated with *Clostridium septicum* or *C. tertium* and underlying malignancy. The mortality rates associated with trunk and limb infection are 63% and 12%, respectively, and any delay in surgical treatment increases the risk of death.

NEUROLOGIC INFECTIONS WITH OR WITHOUT SEPTIC SHOCK

Bacterial Meningitis (See also Chap. 138) Bacterial meningitis is one of the most common infectious disease emergencies involving the central nervous system. Although hosts with cell-mediated immune deficiency (including transplant recipients, diabetic patients, elderly patients, and cancer patients receiving certain chemotherapeutic agents) are at particular risk for *Listeria monocytogenes* meningitis, most cases in adults are due to *S. pneumoniae* (30–60%) and *N. meningitidis* (10–35%). The classic presentation of fever, meningismus, and altered mental status is seen in only one-half to two-thirds of patients and less than one-half of adults. The elderly can present without fever or meningeal signs. Cerebral dysfunction is evidenced by confusion, delirium, and lethargy that can progress to coma. In some cases, the presentation is fulminant, with sepsis and brain edema; papilledema at presentation is unusual and suggests another diagnosis (e.g., an intracranial lesion). Focal signs, including cranial nerve palsies (IV, VI, VII), can be seen in 10–20% of cases; 50–70% of patients have bacteremia. A poor outcome is associated with coma, seizures, hypotension, a pneumococcal etiology, respiratory distress, a CSF glucose level of <0.6 mmol/L (<10 mg/dL), a CSF protein level of >2.5 g/L, a peripheral white blood cell count of <5000/μL, and a serum sodium level of <135 mmol/L. Rapid initiation of treatment is essential; the odds of an unfavorable outcome may increase by 30% for each hour that treatment is delayed. Dexamethasone is an adjunctive treatment for meningitis in adults, especially for infections caused by *S. pneumoniae*. It must be given before or with the first dose of antibiotics; otherwise, it is unlikely to improve outcomes.

Suppurative Intracranial Infections (See also Chap. 140) Suppurative intracranial infections present along with sepsis and hemodynamic instability. Rapid recognition of the toxic patient with central neurologic signs is crucial to improvement of the prognosis of these entities. Patients with diabetes or hematologic disease may be at increased risk for these infections. *Subdural empyema* arises from the paranasal sinus in 60–70% of cases. Microaerophilic streptococci and staphylococci are the predominant etiologic organisms. The patient is toxic, with fever, headache, and nuchal rigidity. Of all patients, 75% have focal signs and 6–20% die. Despite improved survival rates, 15–44% of patients are left with permanent neurologic deficits. *Septic cavernous sinus thrombosis* follows a facial or sphenoid sinus infection; 70% of cases are due to staphylococci (including MRSA), and the remainder are due primarily to aerobic or anaerobic streptococci. Fungi have been common in some series. A unilateral or retro-orbital headache progresses to a toxic appearance and fever within days. Three-quarters of patients have unilateral periorbital edema that becomes bilateral and then progresses to ptosis, proptosis, ophthalmoplegia, and papilledema. The mortality rate is as high as 30% in older studies. Recent reports indicate improved survival as high as 90% with fewer sequelae. *Septic thrombosis of the superior sagittal sinus* spreads from the ethmoid or maxillary sinuses and is caused by *S. pneumoniae*, other streptococci, and staphylococci. The fulminant course is characterized by headache, nausea, vomiting, rapid progression to confusion and coma, nuchal rigidity, and brainstem signs. If the sinus is totally thrombosed, the mortality rate exceeds 80%. Broad-spectrum antibiotics and early surgical intervention at the primary site of infection may improve outcomes. Anticoagulation or steroids are of uncertain benefit.

Brain Abscess (See also Chap. 140) Brain abscess often occurs without systemic signs. Almost half of patients are afebrile, and presentations are more consistent with a space-occupying lesion in the brain; 70% of patients have headache and/or altered mental status, 50% have focal neurologic signs, and 25% have papilledema. Abscesses can present as single or multiple lesions resulting from contiguous foci or hematogenous infection, such as endocarditis, or after surgery or trauma. The infection progresses over several days from cerebritis to an abscess with a mature capsule. More than half of infections are polymicrobial, with an etiology consisting of aerobic bacteria (primarily streptococcal species) and anaerobes. Abscesses arising hematogenously are especially apt to rupture into the ventricular space, causing a sudden and severe deterioration in clinical status and a high mortality rate. Otherwise, mortality is low (<20%) but morbidity is high (30–55%). Patients presenting with stroke and a parameningeal infectious focus, such as sinusitis or otitis, may have a brain abscess, and physicians must maintain a high level of suspicion. Prognosis worsens in patients with a fulminant course, delayed diagnosis, abscess rupture into the ventricles, multiple abscesses, or abnormal neurologic status at presentation. In one study, mortality at 1 year was 19%.

Cerebral Malaria (See also Chap. 224) This entity should be urgently considered for inhabitants of, or recent travelers to, areas endemic for malaria. Patients present with a febrile illness and lethargy or other neurologic signs. Fulminant malaria is caused by *Plasmodium falciparum* and is associated with temperatures of >40°C (>104°F), hypotension, jaundice, acute respiratory distress syndrome, and bleeding. By definition, any patient with a change in mental status or repeated seizure in the setting of fulminant malaria has cerebral malaria. In adults, this nonspecific febrile illness progresses to coma over several days; occasionally, coma occurs within hours and death within 24 h. Nuchal rigidity and photophobia are rare. On physical examination, symmetric encephalopathy is typical, and upper motor neuron dysfunction with decorticate and decerebrate posturing can be seen in advanced disease. Unrecognized infection results in a 20–30% mortality rate. Children with neurologic deficit at hospital discharge, seizure recurrence during treatment, and/or ischemic neural injury on MRI are at particular risk for neurologic and mental health sequelae.

Intracranial and Spinal Epidural Abscesses (See also Chap. 442) Spinal and intracranial epidural abscesses (SEAs and ICEAs) can result in permanent neurologic deficits, sepsis, and death. At-risk patients include those with diabetes mellitus; IV drug use; chronic alcohol abuse; recent spinal trauma, surgery, or epidural anesthesia; and other comorbid conditions, such as HIV infection. Fungal epidural abscess and meningitis can follow epidural or paraspinal glucocorticoid injections. In the United States and Canada, where early treatment of otitis and sinusitis is typical, ICEA is rare but the number of cases of SEA is on the rise. In areas with limited access to health care, SEAs and ICEAs cause significant morbidity and mortality. ICEAs typically present as fever, mental status changes, and neck pain, while SEAs often present as fever, localized spinal tenderness, and back pain. ICEAs are typically polymicrobial, whereas SEAs are most often due to hematogenous seeding, with staphylococci the most common etiologic agent. Early diagnosis and treatment, which may include surgical drainage, minimize rates of mortality and permanent neurologic sequelae. Outcomes are worse for SEA due to MRSA, for infection at a higher vertebral-body level, for impaired neurologic status on presentation, and for dorsal rather than ventral abscess location. Elderly patients and persons with renal failure, malignancy, and other comorbidities also have less favorable outcomes.

OTHER FOCAL SYNDROMES WITH A FULMINANT COURSE

Infection at virtually any primary focus (e.g., osteomyelitis, pneumonia, pyelonephritis, or cholangitis) can result in bacteremia and sepsis. Lemierre's syndrome—jugular septic thrombophlebitis caused by *Fusobacterium necrophorum*—is associated with metastatic infectious emboli (primarily to the lung but sometimes to the liver or other organs) and sepsis, with mortality rates of >15%. Fusobacterium bloodstream infections have been associated with occult gastrointestinal or genitourinary malignancy. TSS has been associated with focal infections such as septic arthritis, peritonitis, sinusitis, and wound infection. Rapid clinical deterioration and death can be associated with destruction of the primary site of infection, as is seen in endocarditis and in infections of the oropharynx (e.g., Ludwig's angina or epiglottitis, in which edema suddenly compromises the airway).

Rhinocerebral Mucormycosis (See also Chap. 218) Individuals with diabetes or immunocompromising conditions such as solid organ transplants or hematologic malignancies are at risk for invasive rhinocerebral mucormycosis. Patients present with low-grade fever, dull sinus pain, diplopia, decreased mental status, decreased ocular motion, chemosis, proptosis, dusky or necrotic nasal turbinates, and necrotic hard-palate lesions that respect the midline. Without rapid recognition, surgical intervention and antifungal therapy, the process continues on an inexorable invasive course, with mortality rates of 50–85% or greater. Uncontrolled diabetes and increasing age are negative prognostic factors.

Acute Bacterial Endocarditis (See also Chap. 128) This entity presents with a much more aggressive course than subacute endocarditis. Bacteria such as *S. aureus*, *S. pneumoniae*, *L. monocytogenes*, *Haemophilus* species, and streptococci of groups A, B, and G attack native valves. Native-valve endocarditis caused by *S. aureus* (including MRSA strains) is increasing. Mortality rates range from 10% to 40%. The host may have comorbid conditions such as underlying malignancy, diabetes mellitus, IV drug use, or alcoholism. The patient presents with fever, fatigue, and malaise <2 weeks after onset of infection. On physical examination, a changing murmur and congestive heart failure may be noted. Hemorrhagic macules on palms or soles (*Janeway lesions*) sometimes develop. Petechiae, Roth's spots, splinter hemorrhages, and splenomegaly are unusual. Rapid valvular destruction, particularly of the aortic valve, results in pulmonary edema and hypotension. Myocardial abscesses can form, eroding through the septum or into the conduction system and causing life-threatening arrhythmias or high-degree conduction block. Large friable vegetations can result in major arterial emboli, metastatic infection, or tissue infarction. Older patients with *S. aureus* endocarditis are especially likely to present with nonspecific symptoms—a circumstance that delays diagnosis and worsens prognosis. Rapid intervention is crucial for a successful outcome.

Inhalational Anthrax (See also Chap. S3) Inhalational anthrax, the most severe form of disease caused by *B. anthracis*, had not been reported in the United States for more than 25 years until the use of this organism as an agent of bioterrorism in 2001. Patients presented with malaise, fever, cough, nausea, drenching sweats, shortness of breath, and headache. Rhinorrhea was unusual. All patients had abnormal chest roentgenograms at presentation. Pulmonary infiltrates, mediastinal widening, and pleural effusions were the most common findings. Hemorrhagic meningitis was documented in 38% of these patients. Survival was more likely when antibiotics were given during the prodromal period and when multidrug regimens were used. In the absence of urgent intervention with antimicrobial agents and supportive care, inhalational anthrax progresses rapidly to hypotension, cyanosis, and death.

Viral Respiratory Tract Illness Viral respiratory tract illnesses can cause severe disease; several new syndromes have been described in the past decade. For patients who present with a respiratory illness and a relevant exposure and travel history, these viral illnesses must be considered and appropriate infection control measures instituted in addition to supportive care.

Avian and Swine Influenza (See also Chap. 200) Human cases of avian influenza have occurred primarily in Southeast Asia, particularly Vietnam (H5N1) and China (H7N9). Avian influenza should be considered in patients with severe respiratory tract illness, particularly if they have been exposed to poultry. Patients present with high fever, an influenza-like illness, and lower respiratory tract symptoms; this illness can progress rapidly to bilateral pneumonia, acute respiratory distress syndrome, multiorgan failure, and death. Younger age appears to be associated with a lower risk of complications. Early antiviral treatment with neuraminidase inhibitors should be initiated along with aggressive supportive measures. Unlike avian influenza, whose human-to-human transmission has so far been rare and has not been sustained, influenza caused by a novel swine-associated A/H1N1 virus has spread rapidly throughout the world; by 2012, 214 countries had diagnosed cases of influenza A/H1N1, with 18,449 deaths. Patients most at risk of severe disease are children <5 years of age, elderly persons, patients with underlying chronic conditions, and pregnant women. Obesity also has been identified as a risk factor for severe illness. Immunosuppression and co-infection with *S. aureus* at presentation are independent risk factors for increased mortality.

SARS, COVID-19, and MERS (See Chap. 199) Severe acute respiratory syndrome (SARS) caused by what is now labeled SARS-CoV-1 was identified in 2002 in China but has been diagnosed in several countries, primarily in Asia. Possible animal reservoirs include bats and civets. SARS-CoV-1 is characterized by efficient human transmission but relatively low mortality. It spreads from person to person via droplets; "super-spreader" airborne events have occurred. The potential SARS-CoV-1 pandemic was controlled through identification and isolation of infected patients. A 3- to 7-day prodrome characterized by fever, malaise, headache, and myalgia can progress to nonproductive cough, dyspnea, and respiratory failure. The risk of contagion is low during the prodrome. Older patients and those with diabetes mellitus, chronic hepatitis B, and other comorbidities can have less favorable outcomes.

COVID-19 caused by SARS-CoV-2 has resulted in a pandemic of historic proportion. Originally linked to cases in China, SARS-CoV-2 has spread internationally at a rapid pace. As of June 2021, cases approached 174 million worldwide with 3.7 million deaths; the United States had more than 33 million cases and ~592,000 deaths. Actual infection may exceed reported cases by 8–10 fold. The primary mode of transmission of COVID-19 is through direct person-to-person contact via respiratory droplets; transmission by the airborne route or by contact with contaminated surfaces has been documented but is much less common. Greatest risk of infection is associated with close and prolonged contact such as in household or congregate settings. Rates of secondary infection among household contacts are high, over 50% in recent studies.

Although ~80% of patients with symptomatic COVID-19 infection have mild disease such as cough, fever, gastrointestinal symptoms, and taste and smell alterations, ~5% of patients develop respiratory failure, shock, and multiorgan system failure. Patients typically have been symptomatic for 5–7 days before progression to severe pneumonia and hypoxemia. Shock, often in the setting of cardiac injury/myocarditis, arrhythmias or cardiomyopathy, and thromboembolic complications such as pulmonary emboli or stroke, can occur. Other manifestations include acute kidney or liver injury. Laboratory findings include lymphopenia, elevated lactate dehydrogenase, and often evidence of a cytokine-release type syndrome with elevated C-reactive protein, D-dimer, ferritin, and proinflammatory cytokines such as interleukin 6. Chest radiographs and CT imaging reveal diffuse ground-glass opacities. Consolidation, predominantly in the lower lobes and peripherally, is a frequent finding. Mortality rates for patients requiring intensive care and mechanical ventilation have improved significantly over the course of the pandemic but remain ≥20%. Risk factors for severe disease and poor outcomes include age ≥65 years, morbid obesity, diabetes, cardiovascular or cerebrovascular disease, hypertension, chronic obstructive lung disease, and chronic kidney disease. Severe disease and mortality is also increased in males and pregnant women.

Treatment currently includes supportive care, antiviral therapy, anti-inflammatory therapy, and anticoagulation prophylaxis or treatment. Patients with respiratory distress are hypoxemic but maintain pulmonary mechanical functioning; thus, invasive mechanical ventilation should be delayed until other interventions have been exhausted. In a meta-analysis, dexamethasone or other glucocorticoids reduced 28-day mortality in patients with severe COVID-19 disease compared with standard care: 32% and 40%, respectively (odds ratio, 0.66; 95% confidence interval, 0.53–0.82). Secondary bacterial pneumonia is uncommon in COVID-19, and antibacterial agents should not be routinely prescribed. With the availability of highly effective vaccines, prevention is the most important strategy to control COVID-19.

Middle East respiratory syndrome (MERS) is caused by a novel betacoronavirus with a likely bat reservoir and was first recognized in 2012 in Saudi Arabia. Human cases have been associated with direct and indirect contact with dromedary camels. Unlike SARS and COVID-19, MERS exhibits inefficient human transmission but carries a high mortality rate. As of 2017, >2000 cases had been confirmed, most in the Arabian Peninsula, with 35% mortality. MERS ranges from asymptomatic infection to acute respiratory distress syndrome, multiorgan failure, and death. Elderly men with comorbidities appear to be at highest risk for poor outcomes. Despite little documented human-to-human transmission in the community, nosocomial infection must be prevented by adherence to strict infection control practices. MERS is currently a low-level public health threat and is likely to remain so unless the virus mutates and its transmissibility increases.

Hantavirus Pulmonary Syndrome (See also Chap. 209) Hantavirus pulmonary syndrome has been documented in the United States since 1993 (primarily the southwestern states, west of the Mississippi River), Canada, and South America. Most cases occur in rural areas and are associated with exposure to rodents. Patients present with a nonspecific viral prodrome of fever, malaise, myalgias, nausea, vomiting, and dizziness that may progress to pulmonary edema, respiratory failure, and death. Hantavirus pulmonary syndrome causes myocardial depression and increased pulmonary vascular permeability; therefore, careful fluid resuscitation and use of pressor agents are crucial. Aggressive cardiopulmonary support during the first few hours of illness can be life-saving in this high-mortality syndrome. The early onset of thrombocytopenia may help distinguish this syndrome from other febrile illnesses in an appropriate epidemiologic setting.

***Clostridioides difficile* Infection** *C. difficile* infection (CDI) is a toxin-mediated diarrheal syndrome that is strongly associated with prior antibiotic use. Proton-pump inhibitors also have been identified as a potential risk factor for the disease. Although most cases of CDI have occurred in the health care setting, community-onset CDI is increasing. Overall, community-onset cases occur in younger patients than nosocomial cases. Patients with community-onset CDI are less likely to have a history of antibiotic or protein-pump inhibitor use. CDI is associated with significant morbidity and mortality, particularly among older patients. The CDC named *C. difficile* infection as one of the top three health threats associated with antibiotic use.

SUMMARY

Acutely ill febrile patients with the syndromes discussed in this chapter require close observation, aggressive supportive measures, and—in most cases—admission to intensive care units. The most important task of the physician is to distinguish these patients from other infected febrile patients whose illness will not progress to fulminant disease. The alert physician must recognize the acute infectious disease emergency and proceed with appropriate urgency.

FURTHER READING

Krause PJ: Human babesiosis. Int J Parasitol 49:165, 2019.

Nelson GE et al: Epidemiology of invasive Group A *Streptococcal* infections in the United States, 2005–2012. Clin Infect Dis 63:478, 2016.

Rhee C et al: Incidence and trends of sepsis in US hospitals using clinical vs claims data, 2009–2014. JAMA 318:1241, 2017.

Sterne JA et al: Association between administration of systemic corticosteroids and mortality among critically ill patients with COVID-19: A meta-analysis. JAMA 324:1330, 2020.

Theilacker C et al: Overwhelming postsplenectomy infection: A prospective multicenter cohort study. Clin Infect Dis 62:871, 2016.

Zunt JR et al: Global, regional, and national burden of meningitis, 1990–2016: A systematic analysis for the Global Burden of Disease Study 2016. Lancet Neurol 17:1061, 2018.

123 Immunization Principles and Vaccine Use

Sarah Mbaeyi, Amanda Cohn, Nancy Messonnier

Few medical interventions of the past century can rival the effect that immunization has had on longevity, economic savings, and quality of life. Seventeen diseases are now preventable through vaccines routinely administered to children and adults in the United States (**Table 123-1**), and most vaccine-preventable diseases of childhood are at historically low levels (**Table 123-2**). Health care providers deliver the vast majority of vaccines in the United States in the course of providing routine health services and therefore play an integral role in the nation's public health system.

TABLE 123-1 Diseases Preventable with Vaccines Routinely Administered in the United States to Children and/or Adults

CONDITION	TARGET POPULATION(S) FOR ROUTINE USE
Pertussis	Children, adolescents, adults
Diphtheria	Children, adolescents, adults
Tetanus	Children, adolescents, adults
Poliomyelitis	Children
Measles	Children
Mumps	Children
Rubella, congenital rubella syndrome	Children
Hepatitis B	Children and high-risk adults
Haemophilus influenzae type b infection	Children and high-risk adults
Hepatitis A	Children and high-risk adults
Influenza	Children, adolescents, adults
Varicella	Children
Pneumococcal disease	Children, older adults, and high-risk adults[a]
Serogroups A, C, W, Y meningococcal disease	Adolescents and high-risk children and adults
Serogroup B meningococcal disease	High-risk children and adults[a]
Rotavirus infection	Infants
Human papillomavirus infection, cervical and anogenital cancers	Adolescents and young adults[a]
Zoster	Older adults

[a]Others in certain age groups may be vaccinated based on shared clinical decision-making.

TABLE 123-2 Decline in Vaccine-Preventable Diseases in the United States Following Widespread Implementation of National Vaccine Recommendations

CONDITION	ANNUAL NO. OF PREVACCINE CASES (AVERAGE)	NO. OF CASES REPORTED IN 2019[a]	REDUCTION (%) IN CASES AFTER WIDESPREAD VACCINATION
Smallpox	29,005	0	100
Diphtheria	21,053	2	>99
Measles	530,217	1287	>99
Mumps	162,344	3509	98
Pertussis	200,752	15,662	92
Polio (paralytic)	16,316	0	100
Rubella	47,745	3	>99
Congenital rubella syndrome	152	0	100
Tetanus	580	19	97
Haemophilus influenzae type b infection	20,000	14[b]	>99
Hepatitis A	117,333	4000[c]	97
Hepatitis B (acute)	66,232	20,900[c]	68
Invasive pneumococcal infection: all ages	63,067	30,400[d]	52
Rotavirus hospitalizations (<3 years old)	62,500	30,625[e]	51
Varicella	4,085,120	102,128[f]	98

[a]2019 reported cases unless otherwise specified (provisional as of January 2020). [b]An additional 12 type b infections are estimated to have occurred among 243 reports of *H. influenzae* infection caused by unknown types among children <5 years of age. [c]Data from the CDC's Viral Hepatitis Surveillance, 2016. [d]Unpublished data from the CDC's Active Bacterial Core Surveillance, 2016. [e]Unpublished data from the CDC's New Vaccine Surveillance Network, 2017, U.S. rotavirus disease now has biennial pattern. [f]Unpublished data from CDC's varicella program, 2017.

Source: Adapted from SW Roush et al: JAMA 298:2155, 2007 and Morb Mortal Wkly Rep 65:924, 2017.

The COVID-19 pandemic has highlighted the importance of a strong immunization program: robust surveillance systems to detect emerging infectious disease threats; public-private partnerships to accelerate the development of novel vaccines; and systems in place to rapidly implement a vaccination program and monitor vaccine safety and effectiveness. As of July 2021, multiple COVID-19 vaccines have received authorization for emergency use in the United States and over two-thirds of adults have received at least one dose. Furthermore, the largest and most comprehensive vaccine safety program in U.S. history has demonstrated the safety of COVID-19 vaccines, and evaluations have demonstrated the vaccines to be effective against SARS-CoV-2 infections, including against severe disease that would otherwise result in hospitalization and death.

VACCINE IMPACT

Direct and Indirect Effects Immunizations against specific infectious diseases protect individuals against infection and thereby prevent symptomatic illnesses. In addition, specific vaccines may also blunt the severity of clinical illness (e.g., rotavirus vaccines and severe gastroenteritis) or reduce complications (e.g., zoster vaccines and postherpetic neuralgia). Some immunizations also reduce transmission of infectious disease agents from immunized people to others, thereby reducing the impact of infection spread. This indirect impact is known as *herd immunity*. The level of immunization in a population that is required to achieve indirect protection of unimmunized people varies substantially with the specific vaccine and disease.

Since childhood vaccines have become widely available in the United States, major declines in rates of vaccine-preventable diseases among both children and adults have become evident (Table 123-2). For example, vaccination of children <5 years of age against *Streptococcus pneumoniae* has led to not only a >90% overall reduction in invasive disease caused by the types covered by pneumococcal conjugate vaccines, but also substantial reductions in incidence among adults through herd immunity. Among children born during 1994–2013, a series of childhood vaccines targeting 13 vaccine-preventable diseases will prevent 322 million illnesses and 732,000 deaths over the course of their lifetimes and save $1.38 trillion (U.S.).

Control, Elimination, and Eradication of Vaccine-Preventable Diseases Immunization programs are associated with the goals of controlling, eliminating, or eradicating a disease. *Control* of a vaccine-preventable disease reduces poor illness outcomes and often limits the disruptive impacts associated with outbreaks of disease in communities, schools, and institutions. Control programs can also reduce absences from work for ill persons and for parents caring for sick children, decrease absences from school, and limit health care utilization associated with treatment visits.

Elimination of a disease is a more demanding goal than control, usually requiring the reduction to zero of cases in a defined geographic area but sometimes defined as reduction in the indigenous sustained transmission of an infection in a geographic area. As of 2019, the United States had eliminated indigenous transmission of measles, rubella, poliomyelitis, and diphtheria, although measles elimination status was threatened in 2019 due to imported cases into undervaccinated communities, resulting in prolonged outbreaks. Importation of pathogens from other parts of the world continues to be important, and public health efforts are intended to respond promptly to such cases in order to limit forward spread of the infectious agent.

Eradication of a disease is achieved when its elimination can be sustained without the need to continue interventions. The only vaccine-preventable disease of humans that has been globally eradicated thus far is smallpox. Although smallpox vaccine is no longer given routinely, the disease has not reemerged naturally because all chains of human transmission were interrupted through earlier vaccination efforts and humans were the only natural reservoir of the virus. Currently, a major health initiative is targeting the global eradication of polio. Two of the three wild poliovirus types (types 2 and 3) have been eradicated globally. However, type 1 continues to circulate in Afghanistan and Pakistan and outbreaks of type 2 circulating vaccine-derived poliovirus have been reported in recent years. Detection of a case of disease that has been targeted for eradication or elimination is considered a sentinel event that could permit the infectious agent to become reestablished in the community or region. Therefore, such episodes must be promptly reported to public health authorities.

Outbreak Detection and Control Clusters of cases of a vaccine-preventable disease detected in an institution, a medical practice, or a community may signal important changes in the pathogen, vaccine, or environment. Several factors can give rise to increases in vaccine-preventable disease, including (1) low rates of immunization that result in an accumulation of susceptible people (e.g., measles resurgence among vaccination abstainers); (2) changes in the infectious agent that permit it to escape vaccine-induced protection (e.g., non-vaccine-type pneumococci); (3) waning of vaccine-induced immunity (e.g., pertussis among adolescents and adults vaccinated in early childhood); and (4) point-source introductions of large inocula (e.g., food-borne exposure to hepatitis A virus). Reporting episodes of outbreak-prone diseases to public health authorities can facilitate recognition of clusters that require further interventions.

PUBLIC HEALTH REPORTING Recognition of suspected cases of diseases targeted for elimination or eradication—along with other diseases that require urgent public health interventions, such as contact tracing, administration of chemo- or immunoprophylaxis, or epidemiologic investigation for common-source exposure—is typically associated with special reporting requirements. Many diseases against which vaccines are routinely used, including measles, pertussis, *Haemophilus influenzae* type b invasive disease, and varicella, are nationally notifiable. Clinicians and laboratory staff have a responsibility to report some vaccine-preventable disease occurrences to local or state public health authorities according to specific case-definition criteria. All providers should be aware of state or city disease-reporting requirements and the best ways to contact public health authorities. A prompt response to vaccine-preventable disease outbreaks can greatly enhance the effectiveness of control measures.

GLOBAL CONSIDERATIONS Several international health initiatives currently focus on reducing vaccine-preventable diseases in regions throughout the world. The American Red Cross, the World Health Organization (WHO), the United Nations Foundation, the United Nations Children's Fund (UNICEF), and the Centers for Disease Control and Prevention (CDC) are partners in the Measles and Rubella Initiative, which targets reduction of worldwide measles deaths. During 2000–2018, global measles mortality rates declined by 73%—i.e., from an estimated 535,600 deaths in 2000 to 142,300 deaths in 2018. Rotary International, UNICEF, the CDC, and the WHO are leading partners in the global eradication of polio, an endeavor that reduced the annual number of paralytic polio cases from 350,000 in 1988 to 33 in 2018. Furthermore, there are increased global efforts to develop and introduce vaccines for emerging infectious diseases, such as Ebola virus disease and COVID-19. The GAVI Alliance and the Bill and Melinda Gates Foundation have brought substantial momentum to global efforts to reduce vaccine-preventable diseases, expanding on earlier efforts by the WHO, UNICEF, and governments in developed and developing countries.

Enhancing Immunization in Adults Although immunization has become a centerpiece of routine pediatric medical visits, it has not been as well integrated into routine health care visits for adults. This chapter focuses on immunization principles and vaccine use in adults. Accumulating evidence suggests that immunization coverage can be increased through efforts directed at consumer-, provider-, institution-, and system-level factors. The literature suggests that the application of multiple strategies is more effective at raising coverage rates than is the use of any single strategy.

RECOMMENDATIONS FOR ADULT IMMUNIZATIONS The CDC's Advisory Committee on Immunization Practices (ACIP) is the main source of recommendations for administration of vaccines approved by the U.S. Food and Drug Administration (FDA) for use in children and adults in the U.S. civilian population. The ACIP is a federal advisory committee that consists of 15 voting members (experts in fields associated with immunization) appointed by the Secretary of the U.S. Department of Health and Human Services, as well as ex officio members representing federal agencies and nonvoting representatives of various liaison organizations, including major medical societies and managed-care organizations. The ACIP recommendations, which are available at *www.cdc.gov/vaccines/hcp/acip-recs/*, are harmonized to the greatest extent possible with vaccine recommendations made by other organizations, including the American College of Physicians, American Academy of Family Physicians, American College of Obstetricians and Gynecologists, and American College of Nurse-Midwives.

ACIP makes several types of recommendations. Routine, catch-up, and risk-based recommendations are those in which everyone in a particular age or risk group are recommended to receive vaccination. Examples include recombinant zoster vaccination for adults aged ≥50 years and hepatitis B vaccination in people living with HIV. Shared clinical decision-making recommendations are individually based and informed by a decision process between the health care provider and patient. With shared clinical decision-making recommendations, the decision to vaccinate is informed by the best available evidence on who may benefit from vaccination; the individual's characteristics, values, and preferences; the health care provider's clinical discretion; and the characteristics of the vaccine being considered. Examples of shared clinical decision-making recommendations include pneumococcal conjugate vaccination of immunocompetent adults aged

≥65 years, human papillomavirus vaccination of adults aged 27–45 years, and serogroup B meningococcal vaccination of adolescents and young adults aged 16–23 years.

ADULT IMMUNIZATION SCHEDULES Immunization schedules for adults in the United States are updated annually and can be found online (*www.cdc.gov/vaccines/schedules/hcp/adult.html*). In February, the schedules are published in *American Family Physician*, *Annals of Internal Medicine*, and *Morbidity and Mortality Weekly Report* (*www.cdc.gov/mmwr*). The adult immunization schedules for 2020 are summarized in **Fig. 123-1**. Additional information and specifications are contained in the footnotes to these schedules. In the time between annual publications, additions and changes to schedules are published in *Morbidity and Mortality Weekly Report*.

IMMUNIZATION PRACTICE STANDARDS

Administering immunizations to adults involves a number of processes, such as deciding whom to vaccinate, assessing vaccine contraindications and precautions, providing vaccine information statements (VISs), ensuring appropriate storage and handling of vaccines, administering vaccines, and maintaining vaccine records. In addition, provider reporting of adverse events that follow vaccination is an essential component of the vaccine safety monitoring system. In 2014, the Standards for Adult Immunization Practice were revised to help providers take steps to ensure that their patients are fully immunized, including assessing the immunization status of patients at every clinical encounter, strongly recommending vaccines that patients need, administering vaccines or referring the patient to a vaccination provider, and documenting vaccines received by the patient.

Deciding Whom to Vaccinate Every effort should be made to ensure that adults receive all indicated vaccines as expeditiously as possible. When adults present for care, their immunization history should be assessed and recorded, and this information should be used to identify needed vaccinations according to the most current version of the adult immunization schedule. Decision-support tools incorporated into electronic health records can provide prompts for needed vaccinations. Standing orders, which are often used for routinely indicated vaccines (e.g., influenza and zoster vaccines), permit a nurse or another approved licensed practitioner to administer vaccines without a specific physician order, thus lowering barriers to adult immunization.

Assessing Contraindications and Precautions Before vaccination, all patients should be screened for contraindications and precautions. A *contraindication* is a condition that increases the risk of a serious adverse reaction to vaccination. A vaccine should not be administered when a contraindication is documented. For example, a history of an anaphylactic reaction to a dose of vaccine or to a vaccine component is a contraindication for further doses. A *precaution* is a condition that may increase the risk of an adverse event or that may compromise the ability of the vaccine to evoke immunity (e.g., administering measles vaccine to a person who has recently received a blood transfusion and may consequently have transient passive immunity to measles virus). Normally, a vaccine is not administered when a precaution is noted. However, situations may arise when the benefits of vaccination outweigh the estimated risk of an adverse event, and the provider may decide to vaccinate the patient despite the precaution.

In some cases, contraindications and precautions are temporary and may lead to mere deferral of vaccination until a later time. For example, moderate or severe acute illness with or without fever is generally considered a transient precaution to vaccination and results in postponement of vaccine administration until the acute phase has resolved; thus, the superimposition of adverse effects of vaccination on the underlying illness and the mistaken attribution of a manifestation of the underlying illness to the vaccine are avoided. Contraindications and precautions to vaccines licensed in the United States for use in adults are summarized in **Table 123-3**. It is important to recognize conditions that are *not* contraindications in order not to miss opportunities for vaccination. For example, in most cases, mild acute illness (with or without fever), a history of a mild to moderate local reaction to a previous dose of the vaccine, and breast-feeding are not contraindications to vaccination.

History of Immediate Hypersensitivity to a Vaccine Component A severe allergic reaction (e.g., anaphylaxis) to a previous dose of a vaccine or to one of its components is a contraindication to vaccination. While most vaccines have many components, substances to which individuals are most likely to have had a severe allergic reaction include egg protein, gelatin, and yeast. In addition, although natural rubber (latex) is not a vaccine component, some vaccines are supplied in vials or syringes that contain natural rubber latex. These vaccines can be identified by the product insert and should not be administered to persons who report a severe (anaphylactic) allergy to latex unless the benefit of vaccination clearly outweighs the risk for a potential allergic reaction. The much more common local or contact hypersensitivity to latex, such as to medical gloves (which contain synthetic latex that is not linked to allergic reactions), is *not* a contraindication to administration of a vaccine supplied in a vial or syringe that contains natural rubber latex.

Pregnancy Two inactivated vaccines, tetanus and diphtheria toxoids and acellular pertussis (Tdap) vaccine and inactivated influenza vaccine, are routinely recommended for pregnant women in the United States. Tdap vaccine is recommended during each pregnancy, regardless of prior vaccination status, in order to prevent pertussis in neonates. Annual influenza vaccination is recommended for all persons 6 months of age and older, including among pregnant women to protect both mother and infant. Pregnancy is not a contraindication to administration of most other inactivated vaccines when otherwise indicated or when the benefits of vaccination are judged to outweigh potential risks (e.g., serogroup B meningococcal vaccination); it is recommended that human papillomavirus (HPV) and recombinant zoster vaccination is delayed until after pregnancy. Live-virus vaccines (e.g., measles, mumps, and rubella [MMR], varicella) are contraindicated during pregnancy because of the hypothetical risk that vaccine virus replication will cause congenital infection or have other adverse effects on the fetus. Most live-virus vaccines are not secreted in breast milk; therefore, breast-feeding is not a contraindication for live-virus or other vaccines.

Immunosuppression Live-virus vaccines elicit an immune response due to replication of the attenuated (weakened) vaccine virus that is contained by the recipient's immune system. In persons with compromised immune function, enhanced replication of vaccine viruses is possible and could lead to disseminated infection with the vaccine virus. For this reason, live-virus vaccines are contraindicated for persons with severe immunosuppression, the definition of which may vary with the vaccine. Severe immunosuppression may be caused by many disease conditions, including hematologic or other malignancy. In some of these conditions, all affected persons are severely immunocompromised. In others (e.g., HIV infection), the degree to which the immune system is compromised depends on the severity of the condition, which in turn depends on the stage of disease or treatment. For example, MMR vaccine may be given to HIV-infected persons who are not severely immunocompromised. Severe immunosuppression may also be due to therapy with immunosuppressive agents, including high-dose glucocorticoids. In this situation, the dose, duration, and route of administration may influence the degree of immunosuppression.

VACCINE INFORMATION STATEMENTS

A VIS is a one-page (two-sided) information sheet produced by the CDC that informs vaccine recipients (or their parents or legal representatives) about the benefits and risks of a vaccine. VISs are mandated by the National Childhood Vaccine Injury Act (NCVIA) of 1986 and—whether the vaccine recipient is a child or an adult—must be provided for any vaccine covered by the Vaccine Injury Compensation Program. As of April 2020, vaccines that are covered by the NCVIA and that are licensed for use in adults include tetanus and diphtheria toxoids (Td), Tdap, hepatitis A, hepatitis B, HPV, inactivated influenza, live

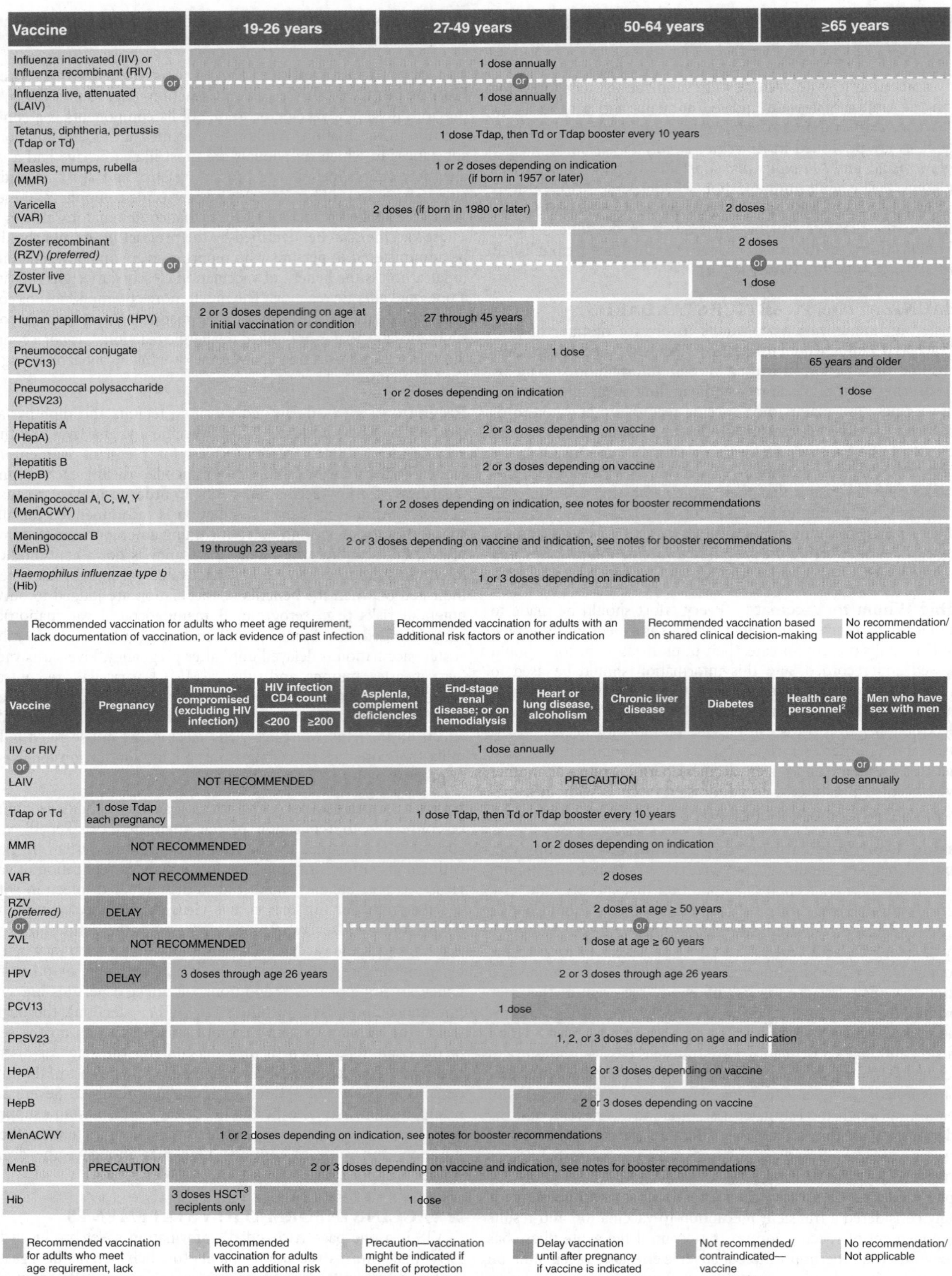

Vaccine	19-26 years	27-49 years	50-64 years	≥65 years
Influenza inactivated (IIV) or Influenza recombinant (RIV)		1 dose annually		
or		or		
Influenza live, attenuated (LAIV)		1 dose annually		
Tetanus, diphtheria, pertussis (Tdap or Td)		1 dose Tdap, then Td or Tdap booster every 10 years		
Measles, mumps, rubella (MMR)		1 or 2 doses depending on indication (if born in 1957 or later)		
Varicella (VAR)	2 doses (if born in 1980 or later)		2 doses	
Zoster recombinant (RZV) *(preferred)*			2 doses	
or			or	
Zoster live (ZVL)			1 dose	
Human papillomavirus (HPV)	2 or 3 doses depending on age at initial vaccination or condition	27 through 45 years		
Pneumococcal conjugate (PCV13)		1 dose		65 years and older
Pneumococcal polysaccharide (PPSV23)		1 or 2 doses depending on indication		1 dose
Hepatitis A (HepA)		2 or 3 doses depending on vaccine		
Hepatitis B (HepB)		2 or 3 doses depending on vaccine		
Meningococcal A, C, W, Y (MenACWY)		1 or 2 doses depending on indication, see notes for booster recommendations		
Meningococcal B (MenB)	19 through 23 years	2 or 3 doses depending on vaccine and indication, see notes for booster recommendations		
Haemophilus influenzae type b (Hib)		1 or 3 doses depending on indication		

Recommended vaccination for adults who meet age requirement, lack documentation of vaccination, or lack evidence of past infection | Recommended vaccination for adults with an additional risk factors or another indication | Recommended vaccination based on shared clinical decision-making | No recommendation/Not applicable

Vaccine	Pregnancy	Immuno-compromised (excluding HIV infection)	HIV infection CD4 count <200	HIV infection CD4 count ≥200	Asplenia, complement deficiencies	End-stage renal disease; or on hemodialysis	Heart or lung disease, alcoholism	Chronic liver disease	Diabetes	Health care personnel[2]	Men who have sex with men
IIV or RIV					1 dose annually						
or										or	
LAIV		NOT RECOMMENDED					PRECAUTION			1 dose annually	
Tdap or Td	1 dose Tdap each pregnancy				1 dose Tdap, then Td or Tdap booster every 10 years						
MMR		NOT RECOMMENDED					1 or 2 doses depending on indication				
VAR		NOT RECOMMENDED					2 doses				
RZV (preferred)	DELAY						2 doses at age ≥ 50 years				
or							or				
ZVL		NOT RECOMMENDED					1 dose at age ≥ 60 years				
HPV	DELAY	3 doses through age 26 years					2 or 3 doses through age 26 years				
PCV13					1 dose						
PPSV23							1, 2, or 3 doses depending on age and indication				
HepA							2 or 3 doses depending on vaccine				
HepB							2 or 3 doses depending on vaccine				
MenACWY			1 or 2 doses depending on indication, see notes for booster recommendations								
MenB	PRECAUTION				2 or 3 doses depending on vaccine and indication, see notes for booster recommendations						
Hib		3 doses HSCT[3] recipients only			1 dose						

Recommended vaccination for adults who meet age requirement, lack documentation of vaccination, or lack evidence of past infection | Recommended vaccination for adults with an additional risk factor or another indication | Precaution—vaccination might be indicated if benefit of protection outweighs risk of adverse reaction | Delay vaccination until after pregnancy if vaccine is indicated | Not recommended/contraindicated—vaccine should not be administered | No recommendation/Not applicable

FIGURE 123-1 Recommended adult immunization schedules, United States, 2020. Additional information, including footnotes for each vaccine, contraindications, and precautions, can be found at *https://www.cdc.gov/vaccines/schedules/hcp/imz/adult.html*. The recommendations in this schedule were approved by the Centers for Disease Control and Prevention (CDC) Advisory Committee on Immunization Practices (ACIP), the American Academy of Family Physicians (AAFP), the American College of Physicians (ACP), the American College of Obstetricians and Gynecologists (ACOG), and the American College of Nurse-Midwives (ACNM). For complete statements by the ACIP, visit *www.cdc.gov/vaccines/hcp/acip-recs/*.

TABLE 123-3 Contraindications and Precautions for Commonly Used Vaccines in Adults

VACCINE FORMULATION	CONTRAINDICATIONS AND PRECAUTIONS
All vaccines	**Contraindication** Severe allergic reaction (e.g., anaphylaxis) after a previous vaccine dose or to a vaccine component **Precaution** Moderate or severe acute illness with or without fever. Defer vaccination until illness resolves.
Td	**Precautions** GBS within 6 weeks after a previous dose of TT-containing vaccine History of Arthus-type hypersensitivity reactions after a previous dose of TD- or DT-containing vaccines (including MenACWY). Defer vaccination until at least 10 years have elapsed since the last dose. History of severe allergic reaction to dry natural rubber (latex) (certain formulations; syringe; see text)
Tdap	**Contraindication** History of encephalopathy (e.g., coma or prolonged seizures) not attributable to another identifiable cause within 7 days of administration of a vaccine with pertussis components, such as DTaP or Tdap **Precautions** GBS within 6 weeks after a previous dose of TT-containing vaccine Progressive or unstable neurologic disorder, uncontrolled seizures, or progressive encephalopathy. Defer vaccination until a treatment regimen has been established and the condition has stabilized. History of Arthus-type hypersensitivity reactions after a previous dose of TT- or DT-containing vaccines (including MenACWY). Defer vaccination until at least 10 years have elapsed since the last dose. History of severe allergic reaction to dry natural rubber (latex) (syringe; see text)
HPV	**Contraindications** History of immediate hypersensitivity to yeast **Precaution** Pregnancy (If a woman is found to be pregnant after initiation of the vaccination series, the remainder of the series should be delayed until after completion of the pregnancy. If a vaccine dose has been administered during pregnancy, no intervention is needed. Exposure to Gardasil during pregnancy should be reported to Merck at 877-888-4231.
MMR	**Contraindications** History of immediate hypersensitivity reaction to gelatin[a] or neomycin Pregnancy Known severe immunodeficiency (e.g., hematologic and solid tumors; chemotherapy; congenital immunodeficiency; long-term immunosuppressive therapy; severe immunocompromise due to HIV infection) **Precautions** Recent receipt (within 11 months) of antibody-containing blood product History of thrombocytopenia or thrombocytopenic purpura
Varicella	**Contraindications** Pregnancy Known severe immunodeficiency History of immediate hypersensitivity reaction to gelatin[a] or neomycin **Precaution** Recent receipt (within 11 months) of antibody-containing blood product
Influenza, inactivated, injectable	**Precaution**[b] History of GBS within 6 weeks after a previous influenza vaccine dose
Influenza, live attenuated nasal spray	**Contraindications**[b] Pregnancy Immunosuppression, including that caused by medications or by HIV infection; known severe immunodeficiency (e.g., hematologic and solid tumors; chemotherapy; congenital immunodeficiency; long-term immunosuppressive therapy; severe immunocompromise due to HIV infection) Close contact with severely immunosuppressed persons who require a protected environment, such as isolation in a bone marrow transplantation unit Close contact with persons with lesser degrees of immunosuppression (e.g., persons receiving chemotherapy or radiation therapy who are not being cared for in a protective environment; persons with HIV infection) is *not* a contraindication or a precaution. Health care personnel in neonatal intensive care units or oncology clinics may receive live attenuated influenza vaccine. Receipt of influenza antiviral medication within 48 h before vaccination **Precautions** History of GBS within 6 weeks of a previous influenza vaccine dose Certain chronic medical conditions, such as diabetes mellitus; chronic pulmonary disease (including asthma); chronic cardiovascular disease (except hypertension); renal, hepatic, neurologic/neuromuscular, hematologic, or metabolic disorders
Pneumococcal polysaccharide	None, other than those listed for all vaccines
Pneumococcal conjugate	None, other than those listed for all vaccines
Hepatitis A	**Contraindication** History of severe allergic reaction to dry natural rubber (latex) (syringe; see text)

(Continued)

TABLE 123-3 Contraindications and Precautions for Commonly Used Vaccines in Adults (Continued)

VACCINE FORMULATION	CONTRAINDICATIONS AND PRECAUTIONS
Hepatitis B	**Contraindications** History of immediate hypersensitivity to yeast (for Engerix-B® and Recombivax-HB®) History of severe allergic reaction to dry natural rubber (latex) (certain formulations; syringe; see text)
Meningococcal conjugate	None, other than those listed for all vaccines
Serogroup B meningococcal	**Contraindication** History of severe allergic reaction to dry natural rubber (latex) (certain formulations; syringe; see text) **Precaution** Pregnancy (vaccination may be indicated if benefits of protection outweigh risks of adverse reaction)
Zoster	**Contraindications** Pregnancy Known severe immunodeficiency (for Zostavax®) History of immediate hypersensitivity reaction to gelatin[a] or neomycin (for Zostavax®) **Precaution** Receipt of specific antiviral agents (i.e., acyclovir, famciclovir, or valacyclovir) within 24 h before vaccination (for Zostavax®)

[a]Extreme caution must be exercised in administering MMR, varicella, or live zoster vaccine to persons with a history of anaphylactic reaction to gelatin or gelatin-containing products. Before administration, skin testing for sensitivity to gelatin can be considered. However, no specific protocols for this purpose have been published. [b]History of severe allergic reaction (e.g., anaphylaxis) to egg is a labeled contraindication to the use of inactivated influenza vaccine and live attenuated influenza vaccine. However, CDC's Advisory Committee on Immunization Practices recommends that any licensed, recommended, and appropriate inactivated influenza vaccine or recombinant influenza vaccine may be administered to persons with egg allergy of any severity (*www.cdc.gov/vaccines/hcp/acip-recs/vacc-specific/flu.html*).

Abbreviations: DT, diphtheria toxoid; DTaP, diphtheria, tetanus, and pertussis; GBS, Guillain-Barré syndrome; HPV, human papillomavirus; MenACWY, quadrivalent meningococcal conjugate vaccine; MMR, measles, mumps, and rubella; Td, tetanus and diphtheria toxoids; Tdap, tetanus and diphtheria toxoids and acellular pertussis; TT, tetanus toxoid.

intranasal influenza, MMR, pneumococcal conjugate, meningococcal conjugate, serogroup B meningococcal, polio, and varicella vaccines. When combination vaccines for which no separate VIS exists are administered (e.g., hepatitis A and B combination vaccine), all relevant VISs should be provided. VISs also exist for some vaccines not covered by the NCVIA, such as pneumococcal polysaccharide, Japanese encephalitis, rabies, herpes zoster, typhoid, anthrax, and yellow fever vaccines. The use of these VISs is encouraged but is not mandated.

All current VISs are available on the Internet at two websites: the CDC's Vaccines and Immunizations site (*www.cdc.gov/vaccines/hcp/vis/*) and the Immunization Action Coalition's site (*www.immunize.org/vis/*). (The latter site also includes translations of the VISs.) VISs from these sites can be downloaded and printed.

STORAGE AND HANDLING

Injectable vaccines are packaged in multidose vials, single-dose vials, or manufacturer-filled single-dose syringes. The live attenuated nasal-spray influenza vaccine is packaged in single-dose sprayers. Oral typhoid vaccine is packaged in capsules. Some vaccines, such as MMR and varicella, come as lyophilized (freeze-dried) powders that must be reconstituted (i.e., mixed with a liquid diluent) before use. The lyophilized powder and the diluent come in separate vials. Diluents are not interchangeable but rather are specifically formulated for each type of vaccine; only the specific diluent provided by the manufacturer for each type of vaccine should be used. Once lyophilized vaccines have been reconstituted, their shelf-life is limited and they must be stored under appropriate temperature and light conditions. For example, varicella must be protected from light and administered within 30 min of reconstitution; recombinant zoster and MMR vaccines likewise must be protected from light but can be used up to 6 and 8 h after reconstitution, respectively.

Vaccines are stored either at refrigerator temperature (2–8°C) or at freezer temperature (–15°C or colder). In general, inactivated vaccines (e.g., inactivated influenza, pneumococcal polysaccharide, and meningococcal conjugate vaccines) are stored at refrigerator temperature, while vials of lyophilized-powder live-virus vaccines (e.g., varicella, live zoster, and MMR vaccines) are stored at freezer temperature. Diluents for lyophilized vaccines may be stored at refrigerator or room temperature. Live attenuated influenza vaccine—a live-virus liquid formulation administered by nasal spray—is stored at refrigerator temperature.

Vaccine storage and handling errors can result in the loss of vaccines worth millions of dollars, and administration of improperly stored vaccines may elicit inadequate immune responses in patients. To improve the standard of vaccine storage and handling practices, the CDC has published detailed guidance (available at *www.cdc.gov/vaccines/hcp/admin/storage/toolkit/storage-handling-toolkit.pdf*). For vaccine storage, the CDC recommends stand-alone units—i.e., self-contained units that either refrigerate or freeze but do not do both—as these units maintain the required temperatures better than combination refrigerator/freezer units. Dormitory-style combined refrigerator/freezer units should never be used for vaccine storage.

The temperature of refrigerators and freezers used for vaccine storage must be monitored and recorded at least twice each workday. Ideally, continuous thermometers that measure and record temperature all day and all night are used, and minimal and maximal temperatures are read and documented each workday. The CDC recommends the use of calibrated digital thermometers with a probe in thermal-buffered material; more detailed information on specifications of storage units and temperature-monitoring devices is provided at the link given above.

ADMINISTRATION OF VACCINES

Most parenteral vaccines recommended for routine administration to adults in the United States are given by either the IM or the SC route; one influenza vaccine formulation approved for use in persons 2–49 years of age is given intranasally. Some live-virus vaccines such as varicella and MMR are given SC. Most inactivated vaccines are given IM. The 23-valent pneumococcal polysaccharide vaccine may be given either IM or SC, but IM administration is preferred because it is associated with a lower risk of injection-site reactions.

Vaccines given to adults by the SC route are administered with a 5/8-inch needle into the upper outer-triceps area. Vaccines administered to adults by the IM route are injected into the deltoid muscle (**Fig. 123-2**) with a needle whose length should be selected on the basis of the recipient's sex and weight to ensure adequate penetration into the muscle. Current guidelines indicate that, for men and women weighing <152 lb (<70 kg), a 1-inch needle is sufficient; for women weighing 152–200 lb (70–90 kg) and men weighing 152–260 lb (70–118 kg), a 1- to 1.5-inch needle is needed; and for women weighing >200 lb (>90 kg) and men weighing >260 lb (>118 kg), a 1.5-inch needle is required. Additional illustrations of vaccine injection locations and techniques may be found at *www.immunize.org/catg.d/p2020.pdf.*

Aspiration, the process of pulling back on the plunger of the syringe after skin penetration but prior to injection, is not necessary because no large blood vessels are present at the recommended vaccine injection sites.

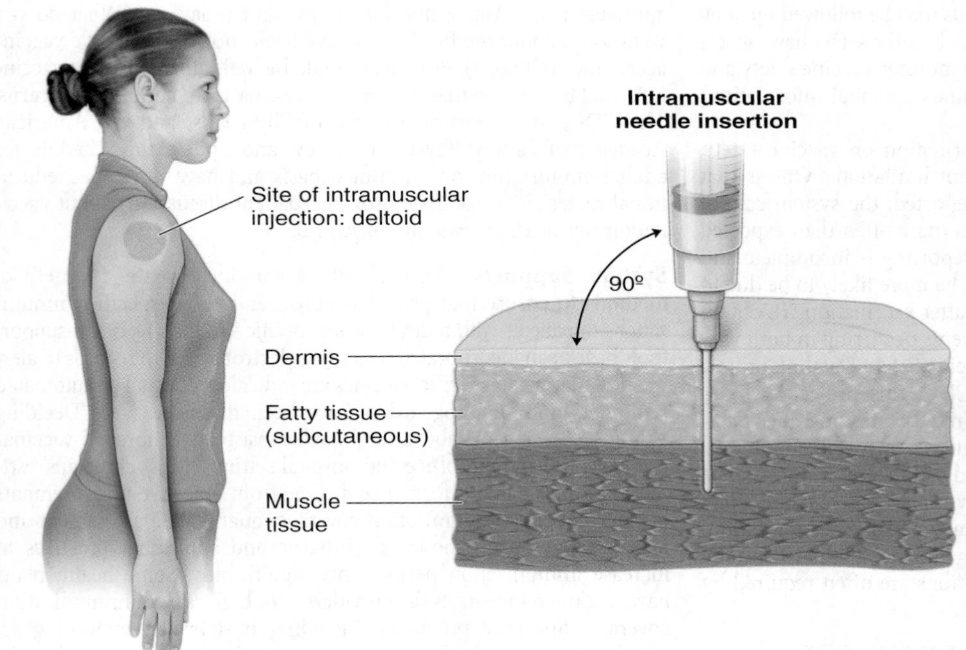

FIGURE 123-2 Technique for IM administration of vaccine.

Multiple vaccines can be administered at the same visit; indeed, administration of all needed vaccines at one visit is encouraged. Studies have shown that vaccines are as effective when administered simultaneously as they are individually, and simultaneous administration of multiple vaccines is not associated with an increased risk of adverse effects. If more than one vaccine must be administered in the same limb, the injection sites should be separated by 1–2 inches so that any local reactions can be differentiated. If a vaccine and an immune globulin preparation are administered simultaneously (e.g., Td vaccine and tetanus immune globulin), a separate anatomic site should be used for each injection.

For certain vaccines (e.g., HPV vaccine and hepatitis B vaccine), multiple doses are required for an adequate and persistent antibody response. The recommended vaccination schedule specifies the interval between doses. Many adults who receive the first dose in a multiple-dose vaccine series do not complete the series or do not receive subsequent doses within the recommended interval; this lack of adherence to protocol compromises vaccine efficacy and/or the duration of protection. Providers should implement recall systems that will prompt patients to return for subsequent doses in a vaccination series at the appropriate intervals. With the exception of oral typhoid vaccination, an interruption in the schedule does not require restarting of the entire series or the addition of extra doses.

Syncope may follow vaccination, especially in adolescents and young adults. Serious injuries, including skull fracture and cerebral hemorrhage, have occurred. Adolescents and adults should be seated or lying down during vaccination. The majority of reported syncope episodes after vaccination occur within 15 min. The ACIP recommends that vaccine providers strongly consider observing patients, particularly adolescents, with patients seated or lying down for 15 min after vaccination. If syncope develops, patients should be observed until the symptoms resolve.

Anaphylaxis is a rare complication of vaccination. All facilities providing immunizations should have an emergency kit containing aqueous epinephrine for administration in the event of a systemic anaphylactic reaction.

MAINTENANCE OF VACCINE RECORDS

All vaccines administered should be fully documented in the patient's permanent medical record. Documentation should include the date of administration, the name or common abbreviation of the vaccine, the vaccine lot number and manufacturer, the administration site, the VIS edition, the date the VIS was provided, and the name, address, and title of the person who administered the vaccine. Increasing use of two-dimensional bar codes on vaccine vials and syringes that can be scanned for data entry into compatible electronic medical records and immunization information systems may facilitate more complete and accurate recording of required information.

VACCINE SAFETY MONITORING AND ADVERSE EVENT REPORTING

Prelicensure Evaluations of Vaccine Safety Before vaccines are licensed by the FDA, they are evaluated in clinical trials with volunteers. These trials are conducted in three progressive phases. Phase 1 trials are small, usually involving <100 volunteers. Their purposes are to provide a basic evaluation of safety and to identify common adverse events. Phase 2 trials, which are larger and may involve several hundred participants, collect additional information on safety and are usually designed to evaluate immunogenicity as well. Data gained from phase 2 trials can be used to determine the composition of the vaccine, the number of doses required, and a profile of common adverse events. Vaccines that appear promising are evaluated in phase 3 trials, which typically involve several hundred to several thousand volunteers and are generally designed to demonstrate vaccine efficacy and provide additional information on vaccine safety.

Postlicensure Monitoring of Vaccine Safety After licensure, a vaccine's safety is assessed by several mechanisms. The NCVIA of 1986 requires health care providers to report certain adverse events that follow vaccination. As a mechanism for that reporting, the Vaccine Adverse Event Reporting System (VAERS) was established in 1990 and is jointly managed by the CDC and the FDA. This safety surveillance system collects reports of adverse events associated with vaccines currently licensed in the United States. *Adverse events* are defined as untoward events that occur after immunization and that might be caused by the vaccine product or vaccination process. While the VAERS was established in response to the NCVIA, any adverse event following vaccination—whether in a child or an adult, and whether or not it is believed to have actually been caused by vaccination—may be reported through the VAERS. The adverse events that health care providers are required to report are listed in the reportable-events table on the VAERS website at *vaers.hhs.gov/reportable.htm*. Approximately 30,000 VAERS reports are filed annually, with ~10–15% reporting serious events resulting in hospitalization, life-threatening illness, disability, or death.

Anyone can file a VAERS report, including health care providers, manufacturers, and vaccine recipients or their parents or guardians. VAERS reports may be submitted online or in paper form (*https://vaers.hhs.gov/reportevent.html*); additional information can be obtained by email (info@vaers.org) or phone (800-822-7967). The VAERS form asks for the following information: the type of vaccine received; the timing of vaccination; the time of onset of the adverse event; and the recipient's current illnesses or medications, history of adverse events following vaccination, and demographic characteristics (e.g., age and sex). This information is entered into a database. The individual who reported the adverse event then receives a confirmation letter by mail with a VAERS identification number that can be used if additional information is submitted later. In selected cases of serious adverse reaction, the patient's recovery status may be followed up at 60 days and 1 year after vaccination. The FDA and the CDC have access to VAERS data and use this information to monitor vaccine safety and conduct research studies. VAERS data (minus personal information) are also available to the public.

While the VAERS provides useful information on vaccine safety, this passive reporting system has important limitations. One is that events following vaccination are merely reported; the system cannot assess whether a given type of event occurs more often than expected after vaccination. A second is that event reporting is incomplete and is biased toward events that are believed to be more likely to be due to vaccination and that occur relatively soon after vaccination. To obtain more systematic information on adverse events occurring in both vaccinated and unvaccinated persons, the Vaccine Safety Datalink project was initiated in 1991. Directed by the CDC, this project includes nine managed-care organizations in the United States; member databases include information on immunizations, medical conditions, demographics, laboratory results, and medication prescriptions. The Department of Defense oversees a similar system monitoring the safety of immunizations among active-duty military personnel. In addition, postlicensure evaluations of vaccine safety may be conducted by the vaccine manufacturer. In fact, such evaluations are often required by the FDA as a condition of vaccine licensure.

CONSUMER ACCESS TO AND DEMAND FOR IMMUNIZATION

By removing barriers to the consumer or patient, providers and health care institutions can improve vaccine use. Financial barriers have traditionally been important constraints, particularly among uninsured adults. Even for insured adults, out-of-pocket costs associated with newer, more expensive adult vaccines (e.g., zoster vaccine) are an obstacle to be overcome. After influenza vaccine was included by Medicare for all beneficiaries in 1993, coverage among persons ≥65 years of age doubled (from ~30% in 1989 to >60% in 1997). Other strategies that enhance patients' access to vaccination include extended office hours (e.g., evening and weekend hours) and scheduled vaccination-only clinics where waiting times are reduced. Provision of vaccines outside the "medical home" (e.g., through occupational clinics, universities, pharmacies, and retail settings) can expand access for adults who do not make medical visits frequently. Increasing proportions of adults are being vaccinated in these settings.

Health promotion efforts aimed at increasing the demand for immunization are common. Direct-to-consumer advertising by pharmaceutical companies has been used for some newer adolescent and adult vaccines. Efforts to raise consumer demand for vaccines have not increased immunization rates unless implemented in conjunction with other strategies that target strengthening of provider practices or reduction of consumer barriers. Attitudes and beliefs related to vaccination can be considerable impediments to consumer demand. Many adults view vaccines as important for children but are less familiar with vaccinations targeting disease prevention in adults. Several vaccines are recommended for adults with certain medical risk factors, but self-identification as a high-risk individual is relatively rare. Communication research suggests that adults are motivated to get vaccines to protect their own health and many would get vaccinated to protect loved ones. Adults with chronic conditions are more likely to be aware that they need to protect their own health. Some vaccines are explicitly recommended for persons at relatively low risk of serious complications, with the goal of reducing the risk of transmission to higher-risk contacts. For example, for protection of newborns, vaccinations against influenza and pertussis are recommended for pregnant women.

STRATEGIES FOR PROVIDERS AND HEALTH CARE FACILITIES

Recommendation from the Provider Health care providers can have great influence on patients with regard to immunization. A recommendation from a doctor or nurse carries more weight than do recommendations from professional societies or endorsements by celebrities. Strong provider recommendations using a presumptive approach (e.g., "You're due for the flu shot today" vs "What do you want to do about the flu shot?") have been shown to improve vaccine acceptance **(Chap. 3)**. Providers should be well informed about vaccine risks and benefits so that they can address patients' common concerns. The CDC, the American College of Physicians, and the American Academy of Family Physicians review and update the schedule for adult immunization on an annual basis and have developed educational materials to facilitate provider–patient discussions about vaccination (*www.cdc.gov/vaccines/hcp.htm*).

System Supports Medical offices can incorporate a variety of methods to ensure that providers consistently offer specific immunizations to patients with indications for specific vaccines. Decision-support tools have been incorporated into some electronic health records to alert the provider when specific vaccines are indicated. Manual or automated reminders and standing orders have been discussed (see "Deciding Whom to Vaccinate," above) and have consistently improved vaccination coverage in both office and hospital settings. Most clinicians' estimates of their own performance diverge from objective measurements of their patients' immunization coverage; quantitative assessment and feedback have been shown in pediatric and adolescent practices to increase immunization performance significantly. Some health plans have instituted incentives for providers with high rates of immunization coverage. Specialty providers, including obstetrician–gynecologists, may be the only providers serving some high-risk patients with indications for selected vaccines (e.g., Tdap, influenza, or pneumococcal polysaccharide vaccine).

Immunization Requirements Vaccination against selected communicable diseases is required for attendance at many universities and colleges as well as for service in the U.S. military or in some occupational settings (e.g., child care, laboratory, veterinary, and health care). Immunizations are recommended and sometimes required for travel to certain countries **(Chap. 124)**.

Vaccination of Health Care Staff A particular area of focus for medical settings is vaccination of health care workers, including those with and without direct patient-care responsibilities. The Joint Commission (which accredits health care organizations), the CDC's Healthcare Infection Control Practices Advisory Committee, and the ACIP all recommend influenza vaccination of all health care personnel; recommendations also focus on requiring documentation of declination for providers who do not accept annual influenza vaccination. As part of their participation in the Centers for Medicare and Medicaid Services' Hospital Inpatient Quality Reporting program, acute-care hospitals are required to report the proportion of their health care personnel who have received seasonal influenza vaccine. Some institutions and jurisdictions have added mandates on influenza vaccination of health care workers and have expanded on earlier requirements related to vaccination or proof of immunity for hepatitis B, measles, mumps, rubella, and varicella.

VACCINATION IN NONMEDICAL SETTINGS

Receipt of vaccination in medical offices is most frequent among young children and adults ≥65 years of age. Patients in these age groups make more office visits and are more likely to receive care in a consistent "medical home" than are older children, adolescents, and nonelderly adults. Vaccination outside the medical home can expand access to those whose health care visits are limited and reduce the burden on busy clinical practices. In some locations, financial constraints related to inventory and storage requirements have led providers to stock few or no vaccines. Outside private office and hospital settings, vaccination may also occur at health department venues, workplaces, retail sites (including pharmacies and supermarkets), and schools or colleges.

When vaccines are given in nonmedical settings, it remains important for standards of immunization practice to be followed. Consumers should be provided with information on the vaccine and how to report adverse events (e.g., via provision of a VIS), and procedures should ensure that documentation of vaccine administration is forwarded to the primary care provider and the state or city public health immunization registry. Detailed documentation may be required for employment, school attendance, and travel. Personalized health records can help consumers keep track of their immunizations, and some occupational health clinics have incorporated automated immunization reports that help employees stay up-to-date with recommended vaccinations. Some pharmacy chain establishments are using automated systems to report immunization information to the state or local immunization information system.

PERFORMANCE MONITORING

Tracking of immunization coverage at national, state, institution, and practice levels can yield feedback to practitioners and programs and facilitate quality improvement. Healthcare Effectiveness Data and Information Set (HEDIS) measures related to adult immunization facilitate comparison of health plans. The CDC's National Health Interview Survey provides selected information on immunization coverage among adults and tracks progress toward achievement of Healthy People 2020 targets for immunization coverage. Vaccination coverage among adults remains suboptimal, and state-specific immunization coverage with pneumococcal polysaccharide and influenza vaccines (as measured through the CDC's Behavioral Risk Factor Surveillance System) reveals substantial geographic variation in coverage. There are persistent disparities in adult immunization coverage rates between whites and racial and ethnic minorities. In contrast, racial and economic disparities in immunization of young children have been dramatically reduced during the past 20 years. Much of this progress is attributed to the Vaccines for Children Program, which since 1994 has entitled eligible children, including those who are uninsured or underinsured, to receive free vaccines.

FUTURE TRENDS

Although most vaccines developed in the twentieth century targeted common acute infectious diseases of childhood, more recently developed vaccines prevent chronic conditions prevalent among adults. Hepatitis B vaccine prevents hepatitis B–related cirrhosis and hepatocellular carcinoma, and HPV vaccine prevents some types of cervical cancer, genital warts, and anogenital cancers and may also prevent some oropharyngeal cancers. A new herpes zoster subunit vaccine that was licensed in 2017 should substantially improve protection against zoster and postherpetic neuralgia. New targets of vaccine development and research may further broaden the definition of vaccine-preventable disease. Research is ongoing on vaccines to prevent insulin-dependent diabetes mellitus, nicotine addiction, and Alzheimer's disease. Expanding strategies for vaccine development are incorporating molecular approaches such as RNA, DNA, vector, and peptide vaccines. New technologies, such as the use of transdermal and other needle-less routes of administration, are being applied to vaccine delivery.

Acknowledgment

The authors thank Anne Schuchat, MD, and Lisa A. Jackson, MD, for their significant contributions to this chapter in the previous editions.

FURTHER READING

Centers for Disease Control and Prevention: *Epidemiology and Prevention of Vaccine-Preventable Diseases*, 13th ed. J Hamborsky et al (eds). Washington DC, Public Health Foundation, 2015.

Ezeanolue E et al: General best practice guidelines for immunization. Best practices guidance of the Advisory Committee on Immunization Practices (ACIP). Available at *www.cdc.gov/vaccines/hcp/acip-recs/general-recs/downloads/general-recs.pdf*. Accessed December 14, 2020.

McNeil MM et al: The vaccine safety datalink: Successes and challenges monitoring vaccine safety. Vaccine 32:5390, 2014.

National Vaccine Advisory Committee: Recommendations from the National Vaccine Advisory Committee: Standards for Adult Immunization Practice. Public Health Rep 129:115, 2014.

Plotkin SA et al (eds): *Plotkin's Vaccines*, 7th ed. Philadelphia, Elsevier, 2017.

Whitney CW et al: Benefits from immunization during the Vaccines for Children Program era—United States, 1994–2013. MMWR 63:352, 2014.

124 Health Recommendations for International Travel

Jesse Waggoner, Henry M. Wu

In recent decades, international travel has increased dramatically with globalization and greater access to international flights. According to the United Nations World Tourism Organization, international tourist arrivals increased 47.4% from 2010 to 2018; arrivals exceeded 1.4 billion in 2018, with the highest rate of growth in arrivals to destinations in Asia and the Pacific. In 2018, according to the United Nations Conference on Trade and Development, total global merchandise exports reached a record 19.5 trillion USD, a nearly threefold increase over the previous two decades. Although travel in 2020 dropped drastically during the COVID-19 pandemic, there has been limited recovery in 2021 and eventual resumption of pre-pandemic growth trends appears likely.

International travel has brought social, economic, and cultural benefits to the world; however, travel also widens the range of infections to which an individual may be exposed. The speed of air travel has been a major factor in the ease with which emerging infectious diseases have quickly spread worldwide in recent years. In the nineteenth century, intercontinental travel took long enough that travelers often recovered or perished from acute infections before arrival at their destinations. However, in the jet age, the time required to circumnavigate the globe has decreased to <24 hours. This duration is shorter than the incubation periods for almost all infections, increasing the likelihood that infected travelers can arrive at their destinations prior to symptom onset. Epidemics can result; examples include severe acute respiratory syndrome (SARS) in 2003, Ebola virus disease in 2014, and the COVID-19 pandemic in 2020. Furthermore, introduction of pathogens into vulnerable regions can subsequently lead to infections becoming endemic, as was observed with the reintroduction of dengue throughout much of the Americas beginning in the 1970s and the global spread of HIV infections in the 1980s.

Additional challenges include the increasing diversity of travelers. While tourism, business travel, and mission work continue to be popular, recent decades have seen increasing numbers of other types of travelers, including students, migrants, medical tourists, and persons visiting their countries of origin ("visiting friends and relatives" [VFR] travelers). Furthermore, an increasing range of individuals with risk factors for illness or injury are traveling internationally, including elderly persons, infants, pregnant women, and persons with chronic medical conditions (e.g., immunocompromising conditions). Whether practicing travel medicine, primary care, or other specialties, providers will encounter patients who travel internationally. This chapter outlines key considerations and preventive measures for international travelers, particularly those traveling to low- and middle-income countries.

EPIDEMIOLOGY OF TRAVEL-RELATED CONDITIONS

Unanticipated medical problems during travel are common. Although reported rates of travel-related morbidity and mortality vary widely by destination, traveler type, and study methodology, as many as 43–79% of travelers report developing a travel-related illness. Most illnesses are minor, with diarrhea often the most commonly reported and fewer than 1–3% of travelers reporting hospitalization. Among vaccine-preventable infections in travelers to lower-income countries, influenza is by far the most commonly reported. Typhoid and hepatitis A are reported much less often, but typically they are still reported more frequently than other infections commonly discussed in travel medicine but not frequently diagnosed, including cholera, Japanese encephalitis, meningococcal disease, rabies, poliomyelitis, and yellow fever. However, outbreaks such as the emergence of yellow fever in coastal southeastern Brazil in 2017–2018 or cholera associated with the 2010 earthquake in Haiti can result in an increased incidence of travel-associated cases. Among causes of death in travelers, studies suggest that cardiovascular events (likely associated with preexisting cardiac conditions) and injury are much more common than infections. Among United States citizens, the injuries most commonly causing deaths during international travel in 2015–2016 were motor vehicle accidents, homicide, suicide, and drowning. Stressors encountered during travel can also exacerbate or uncover psychiatric disorders, and psychological conditions such as depression and anxiety are a common reason for medical evacuation.

GENERAL APPROACH TO ADVISING INTERNATIONAL TRAVELERS

Whether advising travelers in a travel clinic or in a primary care setting, providers must cover a few key elements in a pre-travel consultation (**Table 124-1**). These include (1) a trip risk assessment based on detailed review of the itinerary and the traveler's medical profile; (2) immunizations; (3) prevention of arthropod-borne infections, including malaria chemoprophylaxis (when indicated); (4) food and water precautions and travelers' diarrhea management; and (5) prevention of injuries and other conditions associated with travel.

A detailed itinerary, including cities and areas in a country to be visited, activities, and type of accommodations, is critical for assessment of the risks of the trip and determination of the indications for specific vaccinations, malaria prophylaxis, and other preventive measures. Trip duration, sequence of countries visited, and transit stops are important considerations, especially in the assessment of immunization requirements such as those for yellow fever and polio. Numerous online resources offer recommendations for immunizations and malaria

TABLE 124-1 Overview of the Pre-Travel Consultation

CONSULTATION ELEMENT	ITEMS TO BE COVERED	INTERVENTIONS, ADVICE
Risk Assessment		
Itinerary	• Destination countries and regions • Timing • Duration of trip • Mode of travel • Accommodations • Reason for travel and anticipated activities • Altitude	• Risk assessment that considers the itinerary, traveler, and ability to implement recommended preventive measures • Shared decision-making regarding whether to travel
Traveler	• Medical history, medications • Allergies • Pregnancy status and planning • General risk tolerance	
Immunizations		
Itinerary	Recommended and required vaccinations for itinerary	• Administration of vaccines to meet recommendations and requirements • Provision of official documentation (ICVP[a]) for required immunizations
Traveler	• Immunization history • Precautions and contraindications for specific vaccines	
Malaria and Arthropod-borne Infection Prevention		
Itinerary	• Malaria and other arthropod-borne infection risk at destination • Accommodations and activities • Local malaria resistance to chemoprophylaxis drugs	• Prescription of malaria chemoprophylaxis when indicated • Arthropod-bite avoidance advice • Advice on early recognition of malaria symptoms
Traveler	• Precautions and contraindications to specific malaria chemoprophylaxis agents • Drug–drug interactions of regular medications with malaria chemoprophylaxis	
Gastrointestinal Illness		
Itinerary	• Destination hygienic standards and water quality • Source of meals (e.g., restaurants, street vendors, home-cooking)	See Figure 124-2
Traveler	• Travel style • Adventurous eating habits • Drug–drug interactions of regular medications with self-treatment antibiotics	
Other Possible Topics to Address		
	• Waterborne infection (schistosomiasis, leptospirosis) prevention • Injury and crime avoidance • Animal bite and rabies prevention • Sexually transmitted infections • Altitude illness • Venous thromboembolism • Jet lag • Motion sickness • Severe food and environmental allergies • Travel health and medical evacuation insurance • Traveler health kits and travel with medications • Mental health and cultural adaptation	

[a]ICVP, International Certificate of Vaccine Prophylaxis ("yellow card").

PART 5 Infectious Diseases

TABLE 124-2 Online Resources for Travelers and Travel Medicine Providers

SUBJECT	RESOURCES[a]
General and country-specific recommendations, clinic directories	**CDC Travelers' Health** *www.cdc.gov/travel* Country-specific immunization and malaria prevention advice, travel health notices, travel and yellow fever vaccine clinic listings **CDC Health Information for International Travel** (*Yellow Book*), available at *www.cdc.gov/travel* Comprehensive travel medicine reference covering general topics and specific infections, immunizations, special traveler populations, and common itineraries **Heading Home Healthy** *www.headinghomehealthy.org* Traveler and provider tools for trip-specific CDC recommendations **US State Department** *www.travel.state.gov* Country profiles, travel advisories, Smart Traveler Enrollment Program (STEP), traveler advice **Government of Canada Travel and Tourism** *www.travel.gc.ca* Canadian guidelines and advice for international travel **National Travel Health Network and Centre (NaTHNaC)** *www.nathnac.net* British resource for international travel and travel medicine providers **International Society of Travel Medicine** *www.istm.org* Global travel clinic directory, Pharmacist Professional Group Database on International Regulations **International Association for Medical Assistance to Travellers** *www.iamat.org* International clinic directory, advice on travel health insurance **World Health Organization** *www.who.int/travel-advice* Travel health updates, traveler advice, technical guidance **American Society of Tropical Medicine and Hygiene** *www.astmh.org* Directory for clinical specialists in tropical medicine, travel medicine, and medical parasitology
Jet lag prevention	**Jet Lag Rooster** *www.jetlagrooster.com* Online tool to create jet lag prevention plan for a specific itinerary **Entrain** *entrain.math.lsa.umich.edu* Smartphone application
For travelers with specific conditions	**American College of Obstetrics and Gynecology** *acog.org/search#q=travel&sort=relevancy* Advice for pregnant travelers **The Global Database on HIV-Specific Travel & Residence Restrictions** *www.hivtravel.org* General information for HIV-infected travelers and database on HIV-related entry restrictions **Asthma and Allergy Foundation of America** *www.aafa.org/traveling-with-asthma-allergies* Advice for traveling with asthma and allergies **FARE** *www.foodallergy.org* Resources for persons with severe food allergies, including chef card templates in several languages

[a]All websites last accessed November 7, 2020.

prophylaxis, which vary significantly among countries or even within certain countries (**Table 124-2**). The U.S. Centers for Disease Control and Prevention (CDC) travelers' health website (*www.cdc.gov/travel*) is an excellent source of comprehensive, up-to-date, country-specific recommendations on numerous topics, including immunizations, malaria chemoprophylaxis, and travel health notices for outbreaks and emerging infections. Because recommendations and requirements can change unexpectedly, providers are advised to routinely review guidance for each country prior to making recommendations.

Consideration of the traveler's medical profile is critical to recommendations for appropriate preventive measures. Key considerations include the patient's age, medical and vaccination histories, current medications, allergies (drug, food, and environmental), and pregnancy status. Although any chronic medical problem can be relevant to travel, common issues that can require particular attention include immunocompromising conditions (including HIV infection and treatment with immunosuppressive and immunomodulatory medications), cardiac and pulmonary conditions, pregnancy status, and severe allergies. Significant hepatic and renal impairment due to any etiology can affect the choice of malaria prophylaxis.

Although travel clinics with providers specializing in travel medicine—e.g., those with a Certificate in Travelers' Health issued by the International Society of Travel Medicine—are now common in many cities worldwide, many travelers do not seek pre-travel consultations, often because of an underappreciation of travel risks or a lack of awareness of the resource. Primary care providers are encouraged to routinely ask their patients about upcoming travel. Although some travel-specific vaccinations are often available only at specialized clinics, many recommended vaccines are accessible to general practitioners. Reasons to refer a patient to a travel specialist include the need for vaccines used exclusively for travel, complex itineraries or traveler medical histories, or unfamiliarity with recommended immunizations or malaria chemoprophylaxis. Because some vaccines are given as a series and all vaccines theoretically take a week or more to induce protective immunity, referral to a travel clinic at least 4–6 weeks before travel is ideal. However, when this time frame is not possible, consultations can still provide much benefit.

While the decision of whether to travel is ultimately that of the traveler, travel medicine providers play a key role in helping travelers identify the risks of a trip so that they can make an informed decision based on their personal risk tolerance. Occasionally, some situations can warrant advice against travel, including trips to areas with dangerous outbreaks or security situations or trips by a traveler who is unable to undertake critical preventive measures (e.g., travel to highly malarious areas without chemoprophylaxis). Unfortunately, travel-related vaccinations and chemoprophylactic medications can be expensive and often are not covered by health insurance. To assist travelers on a limited budget, providers can prioritize preventive measures according to degree of risk so that decisions to decline a recommendation are not based on cost alone.

IMMUNIZATIONS FOR TRAVELERS

Historically, the field of travel medicine considered immunizations as routine, recommended, or required. Because infections prevented by *routine* immunizations for children and adults are encountered worldwide, travelers should be up to date with these immunizations. *Recommended* travel vaccines in adults are those that are not included in routine schedules but that should be considered because of anticipated risks during travel. *Required* immunizations, such as yellow fever vaccination, are those that are mandated by international regulations or specific countries for entry or exit. These three categories are not mutually exclusive or fixed, as many vaccinations that originally were used exclusively for travel (e.g., hepatitis A vaccine) are now given routinely in the United States.

For entry requirements, proof of vaccination is provided on the International Certificate of Vaccination Prophylaxis (ICVP, commonly called the "yellow card") issued by travel medicine providers. When appropriate, medical waivers for required vaccinations can be granted and documented on the ICVP. While enforcement of vaccine requirements can be unpredictable, travelers without proof or medical waiver for a required immunization can be subject to entry barriers, vaccination upon arrival, quarantine, or other penalties. In some situations, a vaccine may not be routinely recommended for a specific country but is still required for entry. The most common of these situations involves yellow fever vaccination, when a traveler who has recently been in an endemic country enters certain nonendemic countries (see "Yellow Fever," below).

All vaccines that are commonly administered for travel can generally be given on the same day; however, oral typhoid vaccine should be administered at least 8 hours after oral cholera vaccine. Limited evidence on immunogenicity suggests that the response to live virus vaccines may be impaired if they are given on different days <28 days apart. For this reason, live virus vaccines (i.e., yellow fever, measles–mumps–rubella [MMR], live attenuated influenza, and varicella) should be given on the same day or spaced at least 28 days apart. If neither of these schedules is possible, the recommendation is to repeat the second vaccination after at least 28 days. **Table 124-3** outlines common immunizations for travel in adults.

IMMUNIZATIONS FOR TRAVELERS TO MOST DESTINATIONS

Hepatitis A Hepatitis A is one of the more commonly reported vaccine-preventable infections in travelers. Transmission occurs primarily through direct person-to-person contact (fecal–oral transmission) or contaminated food and water, and travel is among the most common risk factors for infection among cases reported in the United States. Travelers are at highest risk in countries with inadequate sanitation and hygienic practices; levels of hepatitis A endemicity are highest in South Asia and sub-Saharan Africa. Although hepatitis A immunization is now routinely recommended for persons with certain medical conditions and for all children in the United States, many adults have not been vaccinated. A single dose of monovalent hepatitis A vaccine is considered protective for younger, healthy adults when given prior to travel, and a booster vaccine dose given 6–18 months after the primary dose confers lifelong immunity. For persons >40 years old, immunocompromised persons, and other individuals with chronic medical conditions that might impair immune response, administration of hepatitis A immune globulin (0.1 mL/kg) at a separate site at the time of primary vaccination can be considered. No efficacy data are available to support single-dose use of hepatitis A/B combined vaccine (Twinrix) before travel.

Hepatitis B Hepatitis B is transmitted through contact with contaminated blood, blood products, or other bodily fluids. Travelers are strongly advised against high-risk activities, including tattooing, body piercing, and unprotected sexual intercourse. Even when avoiding activities that pose a high risk of exposure to hepatitis B, travelers seeking health care can be exposed through inadequate infection-control measures or blood-product screening. While all travelers may benefit from hepatitis B vaccination, ensuring immunity to hepatitis B is particularly important for long-term travelers, health care workers, and persons who have sexual encounters. Nonimmune travelers who

TABLE 124-3 Common Travel Immunizations

VACCINE	PRIMARY SERIES IN UNVACCINATED ADULTS	BOOSTER INTERVAL	PREGNANCY CONSIDERATIONS
Consider for Most Destinations			
Hepatitis A, inactivated (Havrix, Vaqta)	2 doses 6–12 months apart (Havrix); 2 doses 6–18 months apart (Vaqta)	None recommended	Limited data, generally considered safe, use if protection recommended
Hepatitis A/B combined (Twinrix)	3 doses at 0, 1, and 6 months; accelerated series: 3 doses on days 0, 7, and 21–30	Not recommended except booster at 12 months after accelerated primary series	Inadequate data
Hepatitis B, recombinant and recombinant with novel adjuvant (Heplisav-B)	Recombinant, 3 doses at 0, 1, and 6 months; recombinant with novel adjuvant, 2 doses at 0 and 1 month	Not recommended after routine vaccination schedule	Recombinant vaccine, 3-dose schedule not contraindicated; Heplisav-B, no data
Influenza, inactivated and live attenuated	1 dose	Yearly	Inactivated influenza vaccine recommended
Measles, mumps, and rubella (MMR)	2 doses (≥28 days apart)	None recommended	Contraindicated
Specific Destinations or Activities			
Typhoid, Vi capsular polysaccharide and oral live attenuated	1 dose	5 years for Vi capsular polysaccharide; 2 years for oral live attenuated	Inadequate data; use Vi polysaccharide if protection needed
Cholera, live attenuated (Vaxchora), inactivated oral (Dukoral)	1 dose (Vaxchora); 2 doses 1–6 weeks apart (Dukoral)	Undetermined for Vaxchora; 2 years for Dukoral	Inadequate data, not recommended
Japanese encephalitis, inactivated Vero cell culture–derived (IXIARO)	2 doses on days 0 and 7–28	≥1 year after primary series	Inadequate data, precaution advised against use unless risk of infection outweighs theoretical vaccine risk
Meningococcal meningitis, quadrivalent conjugate	1 dose	5 years	May be used if indicated
Poliomyelitis, inactivated	3 doses if previously unvaccinated	Single lifetime adult booster for persons who received primary series as children	May be used if indicated
Rabies, human diploid cell (HDCV), purified chick embryo cell (PCECV)	3 doses on days 0, 7, and 21 or 28[a]	None, except for postexposure prophylaxis	May be used if indicated
Yellow fever	1 dose	None routine; 10-year boosters recommended for certain groups	Precaution

[a]A two dose pre-exposure prophylaxis schedule was recommended by the CDC Advisory Committee on Immunization Practices (ACIP) in February 2021. Readers are advised to refer to the updated CDC guidance when published.

are departing too soon to complete the standard schedule for recombinant hepatitis B vaccine can consider the rapid hepatitis A/B combined vaccine (Twinrix) series or the recombinant hepatitis B vaccine with novel adjuvant (Heplisav-B).

Influenza Since seasonal influenza is one the most common vaccine-preventable infections acquired during travel, travelers should be encouraged to receive seasonal influenza vaccine when available. Because of variations in influenza seasons worldwide and year-round risk in tropical regions, influenza vaccine should be offered to unvaccinated travelers even when the influenza season has already peaked locally. Travel medicine providers can reinforce the importance of influenza immunization by emphasizing that severe illness is possible in healthy persons, and even uncomplicated infection can disrupt travel and put contacts of travelers at risk.

Measles, Mumps, and Rubella According to the World Health Organization (WHO), numbers of measles cases have increased globally in recent years, with more cases worldwide in 2019 than in any other year since 2006 (**Chap. 205**). In the past decade, countries at all income levels have had major outbreaks. Although endemic measles transmission was eliminated in the United States in 2000, cases have increased in recent years because of outbreaks initiated by infected travelers, mostly those who were unvaccinated or under-vaccinated. Unfounded vaccine hesitancy (**Chap. 3**) directed against measles vaccines is not uncommon in the United States and Europe, contributing to a recent worldwide resurgence, including outbreaks in areas that have previously eliminated transmission. Transmission events in airports and aboard aircraft have been reported, so all nonimmune travelers are potentially at risk. Travelers should have evidence of immunity to measles. For U.S. adults, acceptable criteria include (1) documented vaccination with two doses of live measles virus–containing vaccine given at least 28 days apart; (2) serologic evidence of immunity; (3) laboratory-confirmed illness; or (4) birth before 1957. Although two doses of measles virus–containing vaccine have been recommended for children in the United States since 1989, a significant number of older U.S. travelers born after 1956 may have received only one dose. In this country, the only measles vaccine available for use in adults is the combined MMR vaccine. Travelers should also have evidence of immunity to mumps and rubella; the criteria for immunity to these diseases are similar to those for measles except that a single dose of rubella virus–containing vaccine is considered adequate.

Tetanus, Diphtheria, and Pertussis Travelers should be up to date with age-appropriate tetanus, diphtheria, and pertussis vaccinations (**Chap. 123**). While the risk of tetanus and pertussis exists worldwide, diphtheria is endemic or epidemic primarily in countries without adequate levels of vaccination. Because a tetanus booster is recommended for tetanus-prone injuries if the preceding booster dose was received >5 years earlier, some experts consider an early booster (before 10 years) for travelers engaging in activities with a high risk of injury in destinations with limited access to health care.

Typhoid Fever Typhoid fever, caused by *Salmonella enterica* serotype Typhi, is transmitted through ingestion of contaminated food and water. Most cases of typhoid fever reported in the United States are diagnosed in travelers after being acquired in South Asia. Africa and Southeast Asia also are considered high risk. East Asia, South America, and the Caribbean are considered lower risk. As with other food- and waterborne infections, travelers to endemic areas are at increased risk when consuming food or drink under unhygienic conditions. The risk of typhoid fever is usually lower than the risk of travelers' diarrhea and hepatitis A; however, rising levels of antimicrobial resistance in endemic regions (particularly in South Asia) have increased the importance of prevention. Two vaccines are approved for travelers: injectable Vi capsular polysaccharide vaccine and oral live attenuated vaccine. Oral vaccine is contraindicated for immunocompromised persons, and completion of the vaccination course requires 1 week (four doses separated by 48 hours). Neither vaccine provides protection against paratyphoid fever (caused by *S. enterica* subtype A, B, or C), which is less commonly reported in U.S. travelers.

Varicella Travelers should have evidence of varicella immunity. For most U.S. travelers, this immunity can consist of documented receipt of two doses of varicella vaccine, laboratory evidence of immunity, confirmation of prior varicella or herpes zoster by a health care provider, or birth in the United States before 1980.

IMMUNIZATIONS FOR CERTAIN REGIONS OR SITUATIONS

Yellow Fever Yellow fever is endemic in much of sub-Saharan Africa and South America (**Fig. 124-1**). Requirements for yellow fever immunization are among the most common entry rules encountered by travelers. Some endemic countries require proof of immunization for all international arrivals. Other countries, including many nonendemic countries that are prone to epidemics, require proof of immunization for arriving travelers who have recently (i.e., within 10 days prior to arrival) traveled to endemic countries. Transit stops for ≥12 hours in an endemic country also can result in a requirement for proof of immunization. The United States has no requirement regarding yellow fever immunization for travelers entering the country. Country-specific recommendations and requirements for yellow fever immunization are available from the CDC Travelers' Health website (Table 124-2).

Yellow fever vaccine is available only through state-authorized official yellow fever vaccination clinics, and its administration is recorded on the ICVP. Yellow fever immunization is considered valid for entry purposes beginning 10 days after administration and extending for the lifetime of the vaccinee. Evidence indicates that a single dose of yellow fever vaccine provides most recipients with long-term protection; therefore, the previous requirement for boosting every 10 years was removed by the WHO from the International Health Regulations in 2016. Booster doses of yellow fever vaccine are still recommended after 10 years for certain individuals, including women who were pregnant during primary immunization, persons who were infected with HIV at the time of vaccination, and persons who received a hematopoietic stem cell transplant after immunization (provided they are sufficiently immunocompetent). Booster doses are also recommended for travelers who will be at particularly high risk of yellow fever during travel, including travel to areas experiencing epidemics, prolonged stays in highly endemic areas, or travel during peak transmission seasons.

All licensed yellow fever vaccines are live attenuated products. Contraindications include severe immunosuppression (e.g., during immunosuppressive or immunomodulatory therapy, in primary immunodeficiencies, or with symptomatic HIV infection or a CD4+ T lymphocyte count of <200/μL), malignant neoplasms, thymus gland disorders, and severe egg allergies. Precautions in adults include an age of ≥60 years, pregnancy, breastfeeding, and asymptomatic HIV infection with a CD4+ T lymphocyte count of 200–499/μL. Although medical waivers can be issued by yellow fever clinics, travelers must also consider the risks of traveling to endemic areas without vaccination. Common mild adverse reactions to vaccination include fevers, body aches, lymphadenopathy, localized swelling, and rash. Rare severe adverse events include anaphylaxis, neurologic complications (e.g., meningitis, encephalitis, Guillain-Barré syndrome), and yellow fever vaccine–associated viscerotropic disease (YEL-AVD). YEL-AVD is similar to yellow fever and can result in death. The risk of YEL-AVD is estimated to be ~0.3 case per 100,000 doses administered, with increased risk among immunosuppressed and elderly persons.

Poliomyelitis Although wild-type poliovirus has been eradicated from most of the world, poliomyelitis caused by circulating vaccine-derived poliovirus has been sporadically reported in numerous countries in Africa, the Middle East, and Asia where immunization rates are inadequate. For adults who have had the primary childhood polio vaccination series and are traveling to countries with reported wild-type or circulating vaccine-derived poliovirus transmission in the previous 12 months, a single booster of inactivated poliovirus vaccine before travel is recommended. This recommendation is sometimes extended to countries bordering those with poliovirus transmission when the risk of imported cases is high, especially for health care or humanitarian aid workers. Travelers who stay >4 weeks in certain countries considered high risk for exporting polio can also be subject to exit requirements for proof of recent vaccination (4 weeks to 12 months before departure). Because the list of countries with recommendations for polio booster doses is continually updated, providers should routinely review current polio booster guidance in online resources (Table 124-2).

Cholera Most cholera-endemic countries are in Africa and Asia. A notable exception is Haiti, where endemic disease resulted from the epidemic that followed the 2010 earthquake. Transmission occurs mostly through consumption of contaminated water, although contaminated food or person-to-person contact also can be responsible. The risk to travelers is extremely low when safe food and water precautions are followed. Cholera vaccination can be considered for travelers to endemic regions, particularly those visiting areas experiencing outbreaks, health care workers, or travelers who cannot adhere to strict hygienic practices. Individuals at higher risk for severe disease (e.g., those with type O blood or comorbid conditions) and those who will be in situations where access to health care will be difficult also might consider vaccination. A single-dose live attenuated oral cholera vaccine (Vaxchora) is approved for travelers in the United States and the European Union. This vaccine had an efficacy of 90% at 10 days and 80% at 3 months after administration; the duration of protection and the need for booster doses remain to be determined. Oral killed cholera vaccines are available outside the United States.

Meningococcal Disease Endemic and epidemic meningococcal disease can occur worldwide; however, immunization is primarily recommended for high-risk travelers, including those going to countries in the African "meningitis belt" during the dry season (December to June), when large-scale epidemics can take place. Travelers should receive quadrivalent meningococcal vaccine, which protects against serogroups A, C, Y, and W-135. Conjugated meningococcal vaccines are generally preferred over polysaccharide vaccines because of their increased immunogenicity and the reduced carriage of meningococci by vaccinees; in fact, the polysaccharide vaccines are no longer available in the United States. Pilgrims traveling to the Kingdom of Saudi Arabia for the Hajj and Umrah pilgrimages are required to demonstrate proof of vaccination with quadrivalent meningococcal conjugate vaccine within the preceding 5 years or with quadrivalent meningococcal polysaccharide vaccine within the preceding 3 years. Vaccination against serogroup B meningococcal disease is not recommended for travelers except in specific outbreak situations.

Japanese Encephalitis Japanese encephalitis is a potentially severe viral infection passed to humans by evening-biting mosquitoes in much of Asia and parts of the western Pacific (**Chap. 209**). Although the WHO estimates that as many as 68,000 cases occur each year in Asia, the risk to travelers from nonendemic areas is estimated to be <1 case per 1 million travelers. However, certain travelers are at increased risk, such as long-term expatriates, persons traveling in rural areas during peak transmission seasons, and those with increased outdoor exposure (particularly during the evening). Short-term travelers to urban areas appear to be at lowest risk. In addition to mosquito avoidance measures, vaccination can be considered for travelers at risk for infection. Multiple Japanese encephalitis vaccines are available

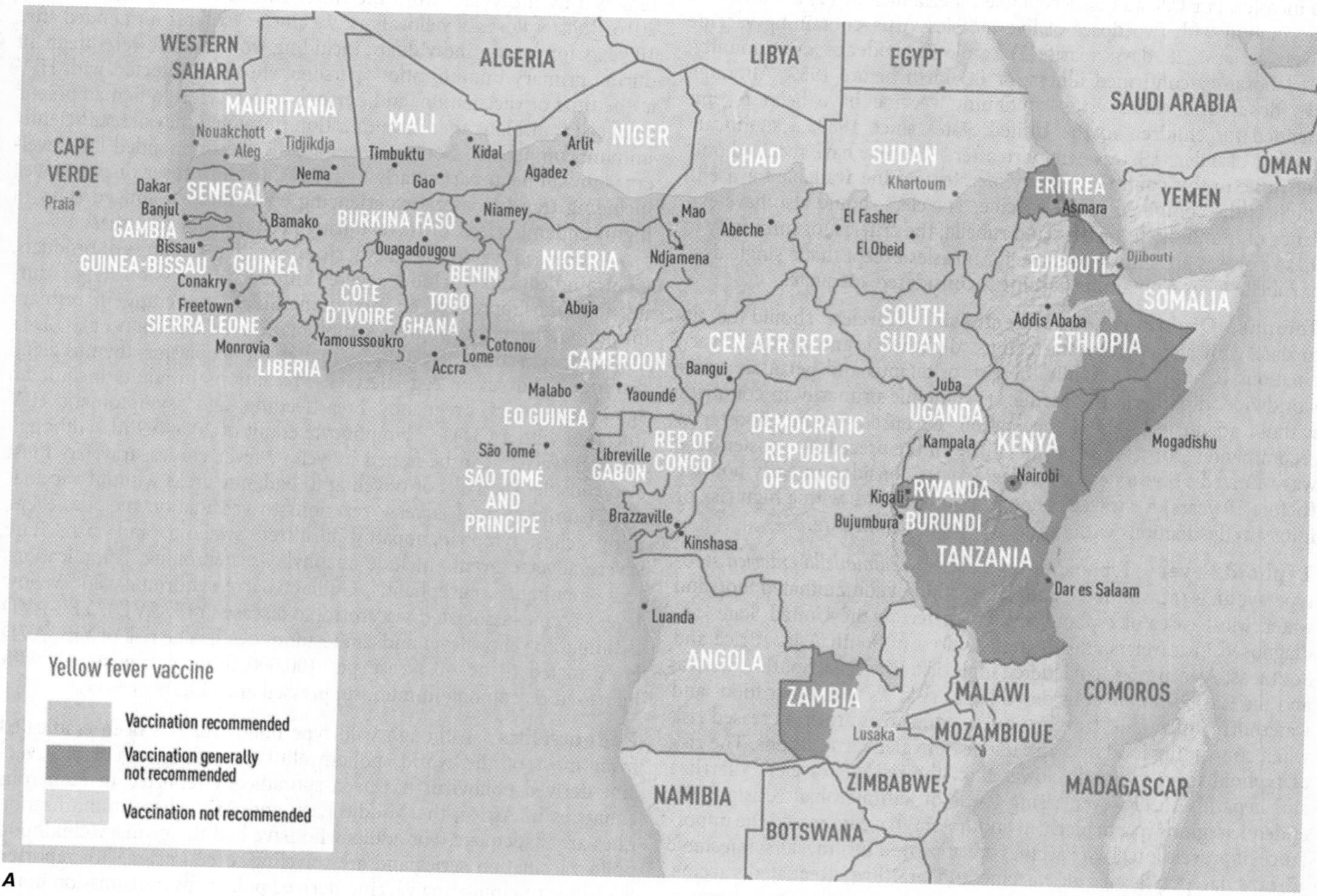

FIGURE 124-1 Yellow fever recommendations in (A) Africa and (B) the Americas. Vaccination of travelers to areas with low exposure risk (designated in green) is not routinely recommended but can be considered for travelers at increased risk due to high exposure to mosquitoes or prolonged travel. Recommendations current as of August 2018. See CDC Travelers' Health website for current recommendations. *(From GW Brunette et al [eds]: Yellow Book 2020 Health Information for International Travel. New York, Oxford Publishing Limited, 2019. Reproduced with permission of the Licensor through PLSclear.)*

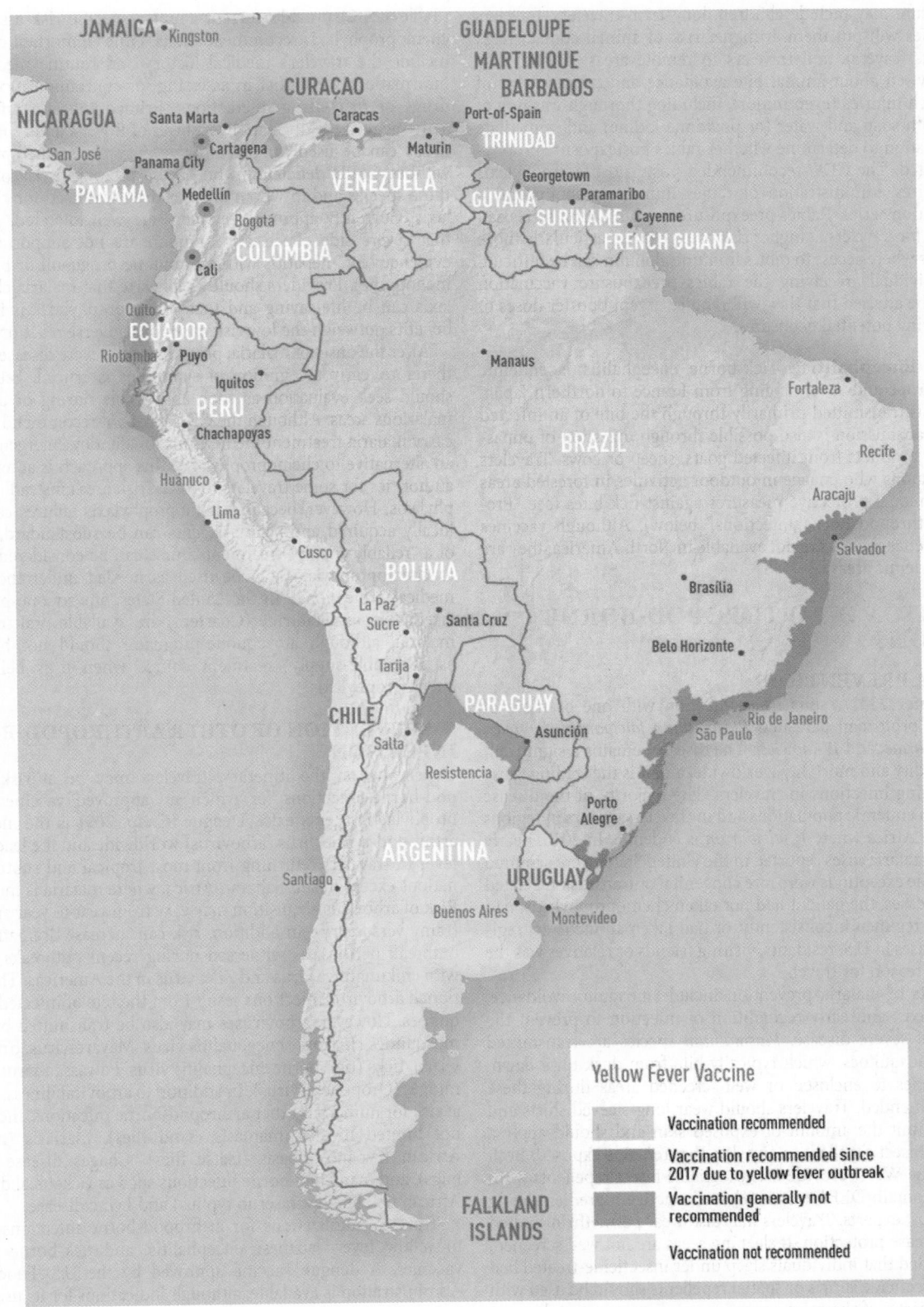

FIGURE 124-1 (Continued)

worldwide. An inactivated Vero cell culture–derived vaccine (IXIARO) is available in the United States and Europe and can be given to adults as a two-dose primary series, with doses administered 7–28 days apart.

Rabies Rabies (**Chap. 208**) is endemic to all continents except Antarctica and to numerous islands worldwide. Although many mammalian species can be infected with rabies virus, terrestrial carnivores and bats are the main reservoirs. In countries without animal control or routine pet vaccination, bites from infected dogs are often the most common source of rabies infection. Management of animal bites carrying a rabies risk is a common reason travelers seek urgent health care during or after travel. Individuals at higher risk for exposure may include children, long-term travelers, travelers whose activities will put them at higher risk of animal contact (e.g., field biologists, cavers), and travelers to remote areas. All travelers should be advised about animal bite avoidance and management of bite and scratch injuries (even minor), including thorough washing of the wound with soap and water (or povidone iodine) and immediate medical evaluation to determine whether rabies postexposure prophylaxis is indicated. The CDC-recommended postexposure prophylaxis regimen requires administration of rabies immune globulin and a rabies vaccination series. Rabies preexposure immunization series can be considered for travelers at higher risk of exposure, particularly those to destinations where access to rabies immune globulin can be difficult. However, individuals receiving the rabies preexposure vaccination series should be advised that they will require urgent booster doses of vaccine following potential exposures.

Tick-Borne Encephalitis Tick-borne encephalitis is endemic to parts of Europe and Asia, ranging from France to northern Japan. The infection is transmitted primarily through the bite of an infected *Ixodes* tick. Transmission is also possible through ingestion of unpasteurized dairy products from infected goats, sheep or cows. Travelers to endemic regions who engage in outdoor activities in forested areas should use personal protective measures against tick bites (see "Prevention of Arthropod-Borne Infections," below). Although vaccines for tick-borne encephalitis are not available in North America, they are available in endemic areas.

PREVENTION OF ARTHROPOD-BORNE INFECTIONS

MALARIA PREVENTION

Malaria **(Chapter 224)** results from infection with one or more of five species of protozoan parasites: *Plasmodium falciparum*, *P. vivax*, *P. ovale*, *P. malariae*, and *P. knowlesi*. The disease remains a significant cause of morbidity and mortality worldwide, and it is the leading cause of life-threatening infections in travelers. The majority of the disease burden, both in endemic populations and in travelers, occurs in regions of sub-Saharan Africa where *P. falciparum* is endemic. In 2016, nearly all of the 2078 malaria cases reported in the United States were acquired during travel; the exceptions were rare congenital or transfusion-related cases. In most cases, the patient had not taken chemoprophylaxis, had adhered to the regimen inconsistently, or had taken an incorrect regimen. Among cases in U.S. residents, visiting friends or relatives was the most common reason for travel.

Key elements of malaria prevention include mosquito avoidance, chemoprophylaxis, and early recognition of infection to prevent the development of severe disease. *Plasmodium* species are transmitted by *Anopheles* mosquitoes, which typically bite from dusk until dawn. Limiting activities to enclosed or well-screened areas during these hours is recommended. Travelers should wear long-sleeved shirts and long pants to limit the amount of exposed skin and should apply a recommended insect repellent to any skin that remains exposed. Both the CDC and the WHO provide lists of reliable insect repellents, with products that contain DEET (20–50%) as the active ingredient being preferred by most experts. Travelers may also wear permethrin-treated clothing to increase protection. If sleeping areas are not well screened, it is recommended that individuals sleep under insecticide-treated bed nets. Indoor insecticide sprays or spatial repellents should be used with caution; the efficacy of these measures in malaria prevention has not been proven, and there may be risks from direct inhalation.

In addition to mosquito avoidance, chemoprophylaxis to prevent symptomatic disease is recommended for travelers to higher-risk regions. Current drugs used for malaria chemoprophylaxis include atovaquone-proguanil (Malarone), chloroquine (and hydroxychloroquine), doxycycline, mefloquine, primaquine, and tafenoquine (see **Chap. 224** for detailed regimens). Chemoprophylaxis recommendations should be based on careful review of the traveler's itinerary to determine malaria risk, predominant malaria species, and drug resistance patterns. The CDC and other travel medicine resources (Table 124-2) provide current country-specific risk assessments and chemoprophylaxis recommendations. Other important considerations include the traveler's medical history and routine medications; this information is essential in assessing for contraindications to specific drugs or drug–drug interactions. Primaquine and tafenoquine are active against the dormant liver stages of *P. vivax* and *P. ovale*, and both drugs can be used for presumptive anti-relapse therapy in travelers without G6PD deficiency who have a prolonged risk of exposure to these species and in whom another drug was used for chemoprophylaxis. Currently approved regimens are well tolerated, and concerns that severe side effects are common are not supported by clinical evidence (e.g., hepatitis with atovaquone-proguanil or psychosis with mefloquine). Providers should emphasize that malaria chemoprophylaxis can be life-saving and that, when prophylaxis is indicated, the benefits outweigh the low risk of serious adverse reactions.

After the onset of malaria, progression to severe disease can be rapid; therefore, early recognition of symptoms is crucial. Febrile travelers should seek evaluation as soon as possible during or after travel to malarious areas. Although the CDC does not recommend that travelers carry malaria treatment medications for standby emergency therapy as an alternative to chemoprophylaxis, this approach is accepted by some authorities for some travelers to lower-risk areas instead of chemoprophylaxis. However, because chemoprophylaxis failures can occur and locally acquired antimalarial agents can be substandard, prescription of a "reliable-supply" treatment course can be considered (in addition to chemoprophylaxis), to be used as needed under the advice of a medical professional. In the United States, atovaquone-proguanil and artemether-lumefantrine (Coartem) are available oral treatments for malaria, although atovaquone-proguanil should not be prescribed as a reliable-supply treatment course when it is being used for chemoprophylaxis.

PREVENTION OF OTHER ARTHROPOD-BORNE INFECTIONS

Depending on the itinerary, travelers may be at risk for arthropod-borne infections for which no approved vaccines or chemoprophylactic agents exist. Dengue **(Chap. 209)** is the most common arthropod-borne virus (arbovirus) worldwide and the leading cause of fever in travelers returning from most tropical and subtropical destinations except in sub-Saharan Africa, where malaria is most common. Risk of arbovirus acquisition may vary from year to year and by season (rainy versus dry). In addition, risk can increase dramatically during outbreak periods, as witnessed during recent outbreaks of infection with chikungunya virus and Zika virus in the Americas. The aforementioned arbovirus infections result from the bite of infected *Aedes* mosquitoes. However, arboviruses may also be transmitted by non-*Aedes* mosquitoes (Japanese encephalitis virus, Mayaro virus, o'nyong-nyong virus), ticks (tick-borne encephalitis virus, Powassan virus), and biting midges (Oropouche virus). In addition to arboviral illness, travelers are at risk for numerous other arthropod-borne infections, including—but not limited to—leishmaniasis (sand flies), filariasis (mosquitoes), African trypanosomiasis (tsetse flies), Chagas disease (triatomine bugs), and many tick-borne infections such as rickettsial diseases (e.g., African tick bite fever, scrub typhus) and Lyme disease.

Travel immunizations for arthropod-borne infections are limited to yellow fever, Japanese encephalitis, and tick-borne encephalitis vaccines. A dengue vaccine approved by the U.S. Food and Drug Administration is available, although indications for its use are limited to individuals with evidence of a past dengue virus infection who reside in regions of endemicity.

Prevention of most arthropod-borne infections relies on avoidance of biting insects. Recommendations for avoiding arthropod bites in general are similar to those provided for *Anopheles* mosquito avoidance to prevent malaria. However, in contrast to malaria, many disease-transmitting arthropods bite during the day and may be encountered across a wider range of environments. Travelers at risk for tick bites can tuck pants into socks and perform daily self-inspections for attached ticks. Avoidance of sleeping in mud or thatch housing in areas endemic for Chagas disease is recommended.

GASTROINTESTINAL ILLNESS

Depending on the itinerary and season, as many as 30–70% of travelers report travelers' diarrhea (TD). Symptoms can include urgently passed loose stools, abdominal pain, fever, and vomiting, and more severe cases can result in volume depletion or bloody diarrhea (dysentery). The majority (~80%) of TD cases result from bacterial infections, with the most common pathogens being *Escherichia coli* and *Campylobacter*, *Shigella*, and *Salmonella* species. A minority of cases are caused by viruses, preformed bacterial toxins, and protozoa (most commonly *Giardia*). Although travelers may develop gastrointestinal illness during travel to any destination, TD is most likely to occur in low- and middle-income countries, where unhygienic food preparation practices constitute the greatest risk for development of disease.

Precautions Recommendations for the prevention of TD center on appropriate food and beverage selection as well as hand hygiene. Food is safest when cooked and served hot. Uncooked fruits and vegetables, unless they can be washed and peeled by the traveler, are considered risky. Dairy products should be pasteurized. Travelers are advised to drink bottled or purified water during travel and to avoid drinking beverages with ice, which may be made with water from unsafe sources. Before drinking any bottled or canned beverage, travelers should confirm that the factory seal is intact, as refilling of bottles with untreated water or questionable beverages is common. Street-side vendors can be particularly risky. Individuals traveling to more remote areas without access to bottled water can use one of a number of methods to purify water, including boiling, chemical treatments, filtration, or ultraviolet irradiation devices.

Prophylaxis For prophylaxis of TD, bismuth subsalicylate can be considered for short-term use. This medication, taken as two tablets (or 2 oz of liquid) four times daily, has been shown to decrease TD incidence by 50% in Mexico. The safety of bismuth subsalicylate prophylaxis when used for >21 days has not been established. Furthermore, the high dosing frequency of this regimen, common side effects (constipation, black tongue), and potential drug interactions (e.g., with acetazolamide or warfarin) limit its utility. Probiotics have not been proven to prevent TD, although research is ongoing. Prophylactic antibiotics generally are not recommended for TD prevention given increasing concerns about adverse reactions, colonization or infection with multidrug-resistant pathogens, and development of *Clostridium difficile* infection. However, short-term antibiotic prophylaxis (with rifaximin increasingly favored over fluoroquinolones) can be considered in rare situations for travelers at high risk for complications from TD. Oral killed cholera vaccine (Dukoral, available in Europe and Canada) shows some cross-protection against enterotoxigenic *E. coli*; however, given the wide range of TD pathogens, the protection conferred by this vaccine against TD is likely to be minimal.

Self-Treatment In general, TD is a self-limited illness, with symptoms resolving in 3–7 days for bacterial infections. Recovery times are typically shorter for infections with viral pathogens and may be prolonged for parasitic infections. For travelers who develop TD, initiation of self-treatment should be based on the patient-assessed functional impact of illness (**Fig. 124-2**). TD can be considered *mild* (not distressing and has no impact on activities), *moderate* (distressing and may interfere with planned activities), or *severe* (incapacitating or prevents participation in planned activities). All dysenteric TD is considered severe. For all levels of severity, replacement of fluid and electrolyte losses resulting from diarrhea and/or vomiting is a mainstay of treatment. In severe cases, replacement with oral rehydration solution (available over the counter) is ideal; however, milder cases can be managed with any potable liquid. In addition, for patients with mild or moderate TD, self-treatment with antimotility agents alone (e.g., loperamide) can be considered.

Antibiotic treatment can decrease the duration of TD to 1–2 days, with potential further benefits from adjunctive loperamide. However, the risks of adverse effects, drug–drug interactions, and alterations in the traveler's microbiota are increasingly recognized in patients treated with antibiotics. Consequences of an altered microbiota can include *C. difficile* colitis and acquisition of multidrug-resistant organisms. Studies have shown that international travelers, particularly those who take antibiotics during travel, are at risk for becoming colonized with multidrug-resistant organisms, including extended-spectrum β-lactamase–producing Enterobacteriaceae. Travelers colonized with multidrug-resistant organisms may be at elevated risk for drug-resistant infections (e.g., urinary tract infection). The role of travelers in the global spread of multidrug-resistant organisms is uncertain. Given these concerns, routine self-treatment with antibiotics is recommended only in severe TD. Self-treatment with antibiotics, with or without

	Counsel travelers on			
Pre-travel	• Food and water precautions • Definition of travelers' diarrhea and severity classification • Importance of oral rehydration and salt intake for all types of travelers' diarrhea • Different travelers' diarrhea treatments and possible provision of antibiotics for self-treatment • Antibiotic prophylaxis (considered only for travelers at high risk for complications from travelers' diarrhea)			
	Self-determination of travelers' diarrhea severity			
During travel	**Mild** Tolerable, not distressing, and does not interfere with planned activities	**Moderate** Distressing or interferes with activities	**Severe** Incapacitating or prevents planned activities	
			Non-dysentery	**Dysentery**
	May use: Loperamide or bismuth subsalicylates	**May use:** Loperamide or antibiotics* or loperamide and antibiotics*	**Should use:** Antibiotics* with or without loperamide	**Should use:** Antibiotics*

*Azithromycin is preferred as first line for severe diarrhea or diarrhea acquired in areas with widespread quinolone resistance including Southeast and South Asia. Quinolones and rifaximin may be considered second-line treatment in moderate diarrhea or severe diarrhea without dysentery or high fever.

FIGURE 124-2 Management of travelers' diarrhea. *(Adapted from MS Riddle et al: Guidelines for the prevention and treatment of travelers' diarrhea: A graded expert panel report. J Travel Med 24:S63, 2017.)*

antimotility agents, can be considered for moderate TD cases. Increasing quinolone resistance, most clearly documented in *Campylobacter* in Southeast and South Asia, has limited the utility of this antibiotic class for TD. The authors' preferred antibiotic regimen for TD self-treatment is azithromycin at a dose of 500 mg daily for 3 days, although a single 1000-mg dose also is effective. Rifaximin or rifamycin SV can also be considered, especially for persons unable to take other antibiotics because of drug–drug interactions. However, *Campylobacter* species are resistant to rifamycins, and their efficacy against dysentery has not been established. Treatment regimens for TD are covered in detail in **Chap. 133**. Empirical treatment of acute TD with antiprotozoal agents such as metronidazole is not recommended.

A small proportion of individuals develop prolonged symptoms (≥14 days), which may result from persistent infection (most often secondary to protozoa), secondary infection (*C. difficile*), or postinfectious irritable bowel syndrome. Antibiotic treatment for acute TD has not been proven to reduce the incidence of postinfectious irritable bowel syndrome, and patients with protracted symptoms should undergo a thorough evaluation.

PREVENTION OF OTHER TRAVEL-RELATED PROBLEMS

■ ACTIVITY-SPECIFIC INFECTION RISKS

Travelers should avoid direct contact with freshwater bodies (lakes, ponds, rivers) because of possible risks of leptospirosis and schistosomiasis. Schistosomiasis is endemic in Africa, Asia, and South America. Diving in African Rift Valley lakes (especially Lake Malawi) and rafting on the Nile River are popular activities that put travelers at risk for schistosomiasis. Appropriate footwear is important in tropical countries to prevent infection with *Strongyloides stercoralis* and hookworm as well as snakebites. Animals of all types (wild, stray, or even pets) are best avoided to minimize bite risk.

Travelers who engage in casual sex, including that with commercial sex workers, should be aware that the risk of sexually transmitted infections (**Chap. 136**) can be high, especially when barrier protections are not used. Injection drug use, tattooing, and even acupuncture in unhygienic settings can pose a high risk for blood-borne infections such as HIV infection and hepatitis B and C.

■ VENOUS THROMBOEMBOLISM

Travelers are at risk for venous thromboembolism (**Chap. 117**), particularly after long-haul flights or other extended periods of limited mobility. General precautions for prevention include ambulation during travel, calf exercises, and aisle seating. Travelers at increased risk for venous thromboembolism may benefit from graduated compression stockings. Anticoagulation may be considered for high-risk individuals.

■ ALTITUDE ILLNESS

Travelers to high-altitude destinations (>2500 m) should be counseled on altitude illness, and the prescription of medications for prophylaxis, such as acetazolamide, may be indicated (**Chap. 462**). Popular high-altitude destinations include Cusco, Peru (the usual gateway to Machu Picchu), mountains that attract climbers (e.g., Mt. Kilimanjaro), and Nepal (trekking).

■ JET LAG

Jet lag (**Chap. 31**) occurs when travel across time zones causes the traveler's circadian rhythm to become asynchronous with the local time zone. Symptoms are most significant with travel across more than three time zones and can result in poor sleep, daytime sleepiness (with poor physical and mental performance), gastrointestinal symptoms, and altered mood. Strategies to help circadian rhythms adjust to new time zones include shifting of sleep schedules prior to travel, timed light exposures after arrival, and melatonin use. Online resources to assist travelers in timing interventions to minimize jet lag are available (Table 124-2), although none has been validated in clinical trials. While caffeine use can reduce daytime drowsiness, it can also disrupt sleep. Prescription of hypnotics (e.g., zolpidem) for travel-related insomnia should generally be avoided, since adverse effects, including excessive fatigue and impaired cognition upon awakening, can be problematic during travel. When used, the lowest effective dose of a hypnotic medication should be used, and travelers should be cautioned about use during flights (when extended immobilization is problematic) or any situation when a full course of sleep is not possible. Sedative-hypnotic and anxiolytic medications are among the classes of drugs that are potentially restricted by certain countries (see "Traveling with Prescription Medications," below).

■ INJURIES

International travel presents numerous factors that contribute a higher risk of injuries and death. Travelers may face unfamiliar environments and language barriers and rely heavily on other people (e.g., tour operators) for protection. Furthermore, in low- and middle-income countries, safety protections that are typical in high-income countries are often less stringent, unenforced, or nonexistent. Travelers often exhibit increased risk-taking behaviors during travel, frequently in association with the use of alcohol. When injuries do occur, access to adequate trauma care can be limited. Motor vehicle accidents are a common cause of injury deaths in travelers. In addition to poor road conditions, traffic rules are often less strictly enforced overseas. Riding on motorbikes (especially without a helmet), on overcrowded public transit, in improperly maintained vehicles, and in vehicles without seatbelts should be avoided. Drowning prevention and crime avoidance are important safety topics. The U.S. State Department provides country-specific safety and security advice for U.S. travelers (Table 124-2).

TRAVELERS WITH PREEXISTING MEDICAL CONDITIONS

Travel is increasingly common for persons with chronic medical conditions. Risks vary depending on the condition, destination, and activities. Travelers with chronic medical conditions are encouraged to plan their trips carefully and to consult with their physicians to assess fitness for travel. Notably, cardiovascular events are a frequent cause of in-flight emergencies and death during travel. Travel across time zones and changes in diet can create challenges in conditions—e.g., diabetes mellitus—that require regulation of diet and consistent medication timing. Providers can assist travelers by providing copies of prescriptions (or medication lists), a medical problems list, and a baseline electrocardiogram.

Adverse events caused by drug–drug interactions can be difficult to manage during travel, especially in destinations with limited emergency care. Therefore, providers should review the traveler's medication list for potential drug interactions when prescribing prophylactic or self-treatment medications. Azithromycin and quinolones prescribed for travelers' diarrhea self-treatment can cause additive QT interval prolongation when used with some antidepressant and antiarrhythmic medications. Malaria prophylaxis medications can affect the international normalized ratio in patients who are taking warfarin.

■ IMMUNOCOMPROMISED TRAVELERS

An increasing number of immunocompromised persons are traveling, including organ transplant recipients, HIV-infected persons, cancer patients, persons with asplenia, and persons receiving immunosuppressive therapies (e.g., biologic agents, antimetabolites, or chronic high-dose glucocorticoids). Although each of these conditions has unique risks, general concerns include increased susceptibility to infection, decreased vaccine efficacy, and—for patients with severe immunosuppression—contraindications to live virus vaccines. Routinely recommended precautions (e.g., food and water hygiene, insect bite avoidance) are particularly important for travelers with immunocompromising conditions.

Conditions associated with severe immunocompromise that preclude use of live virus vaccines include active leukemia or lymphoma, generalized malignancy, graft-versus-host disease, HIV/AIDS (with a CD4+ count of <200 cells/μL), and congenital immunodeficiencies. Immunosuppressive therapies that preclude live virus vaccines include high-dose glucocorticoid treatment (defined as ≥20 mg of prednisone or the equivalent daily for ≥2 weeks), alkylating agent administration, antimetabolite therapy (e.g., azathioprine, methotrexate), transplant-related immunosuppression, cancer chemotherapy, radiation therapy, and treatment with biologic agents, including tumor necrosis factor blockers, checkpoint inhibitors, and lymphocyte-depleting agents. If possible, travel immunizations should be administered prior to iatrogenic immunosuppression (≥2 weeks for inactivated vaccines and ≥4 weeks for live vaccines). The duration of immunosuppression after discontinuation of immunosuppressive therapies can be prolonged, particularly for biologic agents. Travelers unable to receive a required yellow fever vaccine because of immunosuppression should be given a medical waiver if travel cannot be avoided. Providers are advised to review the detailed guidance for immunizing immunocompromised travelers provided in the CDC *Yellow Book* (Table 124-2) and other resources.

HIV-INFECTED TRAVELERS

Infection risk in HIV-infected individuals generally correlates with the level of immunosuppression (i.e., the CD4+ T-cell count). Adults with HIV infection and CD4+ counts of >500 cells/μL are generally considered to have levels of risk similar to those faced by travelers without immunocompromising conditions. Live MMR and varicella vaccines can generally be administered to HIV-infected travelers with a CD4+ count of >200 cells/μL for ≥6 months. Guidance for yellow fever immunization of HIV-infected persons is reviewed above. Oral live attenuated typhoid and live attenuated influenza vaccines should not be administered to HIV-infected persons, given the availability of polysaccharide and inactivated versions of these vaccines, respectively.

The number of countries that restrict the entry of HIV-infected persons has decreased in recent years, particularly for short-term travelers and tourists. However, HIV-infected travelers should review the policies of their destination, especially when they plan to work abroad or stay for longer terms. Resources include embassies in destination countries, the U.S. State Department, and online resources for travelers with HIV infection (Table 124-2).

PREGNANT TRAVELERS

Travel medicine providers should assess pregnancy status and the possibility of conception during travel. The pregnant traveler faces numerous unique risks. These include limited availability of emergency care for pregnancy complications, increased risk of certain infections, and exposure to specific infections that can result in pregnancy complications. Although most airlines will allow pregnant women to travel up to 36 weeks of pregnancy, the American College of Obstetrics and Gynecology recommends travel during the middle period of pregnancy (weeks 14–28), when morning sickness has improved, before mobility becomes impaired, and when the risk of spontaneous abortion or premature labor is minimal. Pregnancy-related contraindications and relative contraindications to travel are numerous and are reviewed in the CDC *Yellow Book* (Table 124-2).

Pregnant travelers are at increased risk of various infections (e.g., malaria, influenza, hepatitis E, listeriosis) and/or severity of illness when traveling. Some infections, notably Zika virus disease, toxoplasmosis, and rubella, can result in birth defects or fetal death. Pregnant travelers should contemplate the infectious risks of their destination and consider delaying travel to areas where particularly dangerous infections, such as malaria or Zika, are present. Currently, only mefloquine and chloroquine are approved for malaria chemoprophylaxis in pregnancy, and plasmodial resistance to these drugs can further limit options. Travel immunizations considered safe during pregnancy also are limited (Table 124-3). When used as directed, insect repellents registered by the Environmental Protection Agency, such as DEET, are considered safe during pregnancy.

TRAVELERS WITH SEVERE ALLERGIES

Travelers with severe allergies to food, insect stings, and environmental allergens can be at increased risk during travel, particularly in destinations without adequate emergency care. Avoidance of food allergens can be challenging, particularly when eating in restaurants or catered settings. Language barriers can present difficulties in avoiding food or medication allergies. Regional variations in culinary practices and ingredients can lead to unexpected food allergen exposure. Outdoor activities can increase the risk of stings by hymenopterous insects (bees, wasps, ants). Solo travelers can face particular challenges when experiencing severe allergies.

Providers should ensure that travelers have an emergency care plan for severe allergies and an adequate supply of emergency self-treatment, including epinephrine auto-injectors and antihistamines. It can be prudent to bring other medications, including rescue bronchodilator inhalers (for individuals with asthma) and short courses of glucocorticoids, especially for travelers who will have no immediate access to health care. Written documentation of the allergic disorder and self-treatment medications should be carried, especially when injectable medications are involved. Travelers with severe food allergies should alert restaurants and hosts. Printable food allergy alert cards in various languages are available online (Table 124-2).

OTHER PRE-TRAVEL PREPARATIONS

TRAVEL HEALTH KITS

A carefully planned travel health kit can minimize the need to seek care for self-treatable conditions. The ideal contents depend on the destination, duration, and activities during travel as well as on individual health issues. Routine and trip-specific prescription medications (e.g., malaria prophylaxis, travelers' diarrhea self-treatment antibiotics) should be carried in original labeled prescription bottles to aid in identification. A digital thermometer and typically used over-the-counter medications, such as analgesics and antipyretics, antidiarrheal medications, medications for motion sickness, antacids, laxatives, oral rehydration salts, antihistamines, and topical steroid creams, can be important. Basic first-aid items, such as gloves, bandages, tape, antibiotic ointment, and tweezers, are helpful. Critical medications should always be carried and not packed in checked luggage; however, travelers must take into account any restrictions about flying with sharp objects or liquids, particularly in their carry-on baggage.

TRAVELING WITH PRESCRIPTION MEDICATIONS

Carrying copies of prescriptions (or a signed medication list from a physician's office) is recommended. Many countries, particularly in Asia, the Middle East, and Africa, have stringent restrictions on certain drugs that are less restricted in the United States. These regulations can include controlled substances such as opioid analgesics, anxiolytics and sedatives, and medications for attention deficit hyperactivity disorder. Even some over-the-counter medications such as pseudoephedrine and diphenhydramine are restricted in certain countries. Requirements for traveling with restricted medications can include carrying copies of prescriptions or even obtaining advance approval from the destination country's health ministry. Levels of enforcement and penalties for violations vary widely. Travelers who plan to carry potentially restricted medications should contact the embassy of their destination to review policies. Travelers should carry only amounts appropriate for the duration of their itinerary. The International Society of Travel Medicine's Pharmacist Professional Group maintains a list of known policies for certain countries (Table 124-2).

Although many medications that require prescription in the United States are available over the counter overseas, the quality of locally acquired pharmaceuticals can vary. Counterfeit medications, particularly antimalarials, are common in much of the world. Whenever possible, travelers are cautioned to avoid obtaining critical medications such as malaria chemoprophylaxis during travel.

HEALTH CARE OVERSEAS AND TRAVEL HEALTH INSURANCE

Travelers should consider where they would seek urgent or emergency health care, particularly if they have chronic health conditions, are pregnant, or will participate in activities with a high risk of injury or illness (e.g., altitude sickness). International travelers should be aware that most countries do not accept routine health insurance from other countries and that such insurance is unlikely to cover out-of-pocket health care costs or to provide assistance in identifying providers overseas. Travelers are advised to review their health insurance policies before travel to assess the scope of international coverage (including emergency care, hospitalization, psychiatric care, and obstetric care, if applicable) and the availability of 24-hour physician-backed support.

For many travelers, supplemental insurance coverage of some type is prudent. *Travel insurance* usually consists of coverage for financial losses due to trip cancellation (e.g., due to unexpected illness) or lost baggage. *Supplemental travel health insurance* policies cover health care costs overseas and typically provide 24-hour support centers. *Medical evacuation (medevac) insurance* can be a part of a travel health insurance policy or a stand-alone policy and covers medical evacuation when it is determined that the local level of care is inadequate. Further information on travel health insurance is available from online resources listed in Table 124-2.

SPECIAL TRAVEL POPULATIONS

Travelers are increasingly diverse in their reasons for and types of travel, each of which poses unique risks and challenges (**Table 124-4**). A major challenge in travel medicine is presented by VFR travelers who are visiting their countries of origin. VFR travelers face increased risks for travel-related infections, as they often travel to areas not frequented by tourists, stay in local homes, and adopt local food and transportation habits. Immunity resulting from malaria infection is not long-term, but immigrants from malaria-endemic countries often incorrectly assume that they are immune. Barriers to appropriate pre-travel advice can include financial and language issues or a lack of trust in the medical system.

POST-TRAVEL MEDICAL CARE

Acute febrile illness in returning travelers can represent a potentially life-threatening illness, such as malaria, typhoid fever, or leptospirosis. Early diagnosis and treatment can be critical and potentially life-saving for many travel-related infections. Although most acute febrile illnesses have incubation periods of <14 days, infections including typhoid, malaria, leptospirosis, and acute schistosomiasis can have prolonged incubation periods. Travelers should be advised to always inform their health care providers of their travel history, even when their travel does not immediately precede illness onset. Exposure risk occurring as much as a year prior to illness onset should be considered for malaria. Providers unfamiliar with infections common to a region recently visited by an acutely ill traveler should consult with infectious disease or travel medicine specialists and/or their local public health departments.

OUTBREAKS AND EMERGING INFECTIOUS DISEASES

Emerging and re-emerging infectious diseases create challenges for international travel. During outbreaks of novel or emerging infections (e.g., the recent Ebola virus disease epidemics in western and central Africa or the emergence of Zika in the Americas in 2015–2016), information can be limited or can rapidly change. Providers counseling travelers can help them make informed decisions by carefully reviewing available travel health notices, surveillance reports, and clinical literature on infections. Individuals may be advised against travel to certain areas when risks are significant. Significant travel disruption can also occur when outbreaks of well-known infections take place in previously unaffected areas. The 2017–2018 yellow fever outbreak in southeastern Brazil included the metropolitan areas of Rio de Janeiro and São Paolo, two major travel destinations for which vaccination had not previously been recommended. This outbreak coincided with a yellow fever vaccine supply disruption in North America, resulting in significant challenges for travelers and providers.

TABLE 124-4 Risks and Prevention Strategies in Special Travel Populations

GROUP	RISKS AND CHALLENGES	PREVENTION STRATEGIES
Travelers visiting friends and relatives (VFR)	• Greater likelihood of visiting areas outside usual travel destinations • Frequent adoption of food, accommodation, and transportation habits similar to those of locals • Failure to recognize importance of travel immunizations or malaria prophylaxis • Financial or cultural barriers to seeking pre-travel advice or immunization	• Questions about planned travel during routine care visits • Prioritization of vaccines and prophylaxis for highest-risk infections when resources are limited
Budget travelers	• Financial barriers to seeking pre-travel advice or immunization • Lower quality of accommodations, transportation, and food establishments	• Prioritization of vaccines and prophylaxis for highest-risk infections when resources are limited • Education about high-risk activities (e.g., motorbike taxis)
Last-minute travelers	• Minimal advance notice for pre-travel consultations or immunizations	• Several vaccines are effective with a single dose. • Some vaccination series can be accelerated. • Some malaria chemoprophylaxis can be started 1 day prior to entering risk areas. • Consider broad immunization coverage and standing malaria chemoprophylaxis supply for aircrews or other travelers with unpredictable, last-minute trips.
Long-term travelers	• Increased risk of infection and injury due to longer duration • Increased likelihood of adopting local food, accommodation, and transportation standards • Potential need for extended supply of malaria chemoprophylaxis	• Increased emphasis on importance of certain vaccines, such as hepatitis B, rabies, typhoid, or Japanese encephalitis (in endemic areas) • Long-term malaria chemoprophylaxis
Health care workers on medical missions	• Risk of infections acquired through patient care because of inadequate infection-control standards • Potentially high prevalence of untreated transmissible infections in patients • Limited or no access to urgent postexposure prophylaxis for HIV infection and hepatitis B • Exposure to emerging infections and outbreaks	• Ensure that traveler has received recommended immunizations for health care workers. • Advise traveler to assess availability of adequate personal protective equipment and medications for HIV postexposure prophylaxis and to consider potential need to bring own supplies. • Advise traveler against working with organizations inexperienced in delivering care in the destination area.
Medical tourists	• Nosocomial infections and other complications of medical procedures overseas • Substandard accreditation, infection control, safety guidelines, drugs, and blood-product screening • Increased risk of thromboembolism following surgery	• Advise traveler on potential risks. • Direct tourist to internationally accredited facilities and providers. • Tourist should acquire a copy of medical records for providers who will provide follow-up care. • See CDC *Yellow Book* (Table 124-2) for specific resources.

Finally, the 2020 COVID-19 pandemic quickly reversed a decades-long rising trend in rates of international travel and created novel concerns about domestic and international travel. The pandemic spread particularly quickly among international travelers, facilitated by its potential for transmission from asymptomatic or mildly ill persons. To address these challenges, travelers and the travel industry are adapting to new preventive strategies, including universal face coverings and social distancing. Countries and even U.S. states have issued specific vaccination, testing, or quarantine requirements for entry, and travelers from certain high-incidence regions may be barred from entry altogether. The development of rapid testing platforms and vaccines for COVID-19 raises hope that travel will eventually return to levels seen prior to the pandemic.

■ FURTHER READING

ANGELO KM et al: What proportion of international travellers acquire a travel-related illness? A review of the literature. J Travel Med 24:1, 2017.

BRUNETTE GW et al (eds): *Yellow Book 2020 Health Information for International Travel.* New York, Oxford University Press, 2019.

KEYSTONE JS et al (eds): *Travel Medicine,* 4th ed. Edinburgh, Elsevier, 2019.

MACE KE et al: Malaria surveillance—United States, 2016. MMWR Surveill Summ 68:1, 2019.

RIDDLE MS et al: Guidelines for the prevention and treatment of travelers' diarrhea: A graded expert panel report. J Travel Med 24:S63, 2017.

125 Climate Change and Infectious Disease

Aaron S. Bernstein

The release of greenhouse gases—principally carbon dioxide—into Earth's atmosphere since the late nineteenth century has contributed to a climate unfamiliar to our species, *Homo sapiens.* This new climate has already altered the epidemiology of infectious diseases. Continued accumulation of greenhouse gases in the atmosphere will further alter the planet's climate and the incidence and severity of infections. In some cases, climate change may establish conditions favoring the emergence of infectious diseases, while in others it may render areas that are presently suitable for certain diseases unsuitable. This chapter presents the current state of knowledge regarding the known and prospective infectious-disease consequences of climate change.

OVERVIEW

The term *climate change* refers to multi-decadal alterations in temperature, precipitation, wind, humidity, and other components of weather. Over the past 2.5 million years, the earth has warmed and cooled, cycling between glacial and interglacial periods during which average global temperatures moved up and down by 4–7°C. During the last glacial period, which ended roughly 12,000 years ago, global temperatures were, on average, 5°C cooler than in the mid-twentieth century **(Fig. 125-1)**.

The present climate period, known as the Holocene, is remarkable for its stability: temperatures have largely remained within a range of 2–3°C. This stability has enabled the successful population and cultivation of much of the earth's landmass by humanity. Current climate change differs from that in the past not only because its primary cause is human activities but also because its pace is faster. The current rate of warming on Earth is unprecedented in the last 50 million years. The 5°C of warming that occurred at the end of the last ice age about 12,000 years ago took roughly 5000 years, whereas such a temperature increment may occur within the next 150 years unless the release of greenhouse gases is substantially reduced in coming decades. Climate science, although still a relatively new discipline, has provided an ever-clearer picture of how the changing chemistry of the atmosphere has influenced, and will continue to influence, the global climate.

■ GREENHOUSE GASES

Greenhouse gases **(Table 125-1 and Fig. 125-2)** are a group of gases in Earth's atmosphere that absorb infrared radiation and thus retain heat inside the atmosphere. In the absence of these gases, the earth's average temperature would be about 33°C colder. Carbon dioxide, released into the atmosphere primarily from fossil fuel combustion and deforestation, has had the greatest effect on climate since the Industrial Revolution. Of note, the Swedish scientist Svante Arrhenius suggested in the late nineteenth century that the addition of carbon dioxide to the Earth's atmosphere would increase the planet's surface temperature. Water vapor is the most abundant and a highly potent greenhouse gas but, given its short atmospheric life span and sensitivity to temperature, is not a major factor in recently observed warming.

The atmosphere, some of the aerosols suspended in it, and clouds reflect a portion of incoming solar radiation back toward space. The remainder reaches Earth's surface, where it is absorbed and some is then emitted back at the atmosphere. The earth emits energy absorbed from the sun at longer wavelengths, primarily infrared, that greenhouse gases are able to absorb. The change in wavelength that occurs as solar radiation is absorbed and re-emitted from the earth's surface is fundamental to the greenhouse effect **(Fig. 125-3)**.

■ TEMPERATURE

Climate change has become nearly synonymous with global warming, as a clear signal from rising greenhouse gas concentrations has been an increase in the mean global surface temperature of ~0.85°C since 1880. However, this mean warming belies warming that is occurring much faster in certain regions. The Arctic has warmed twice as fast overall, and winters are warming faster than summers. Nighttime minimum temperatures are also rising faster than daytime high temperatures. Each of these nuances bears upon the incidence of infectious diseases in general and vector-borne disease specifically.

A moderate projection based on the best available scientific evidence suggests that average global temperatures will warm an additional 1.4–3.1°C by 2100 compared with the period 1986–2005. Because of climate change, extreme heat waves have already become more common and are expected to be even more frequent later in this century. Besides contributing directly to morbidity and mortality in human populations, heat waves wilt crops and are expected to contribute substantially to predicted agricultural losses. For example, the 2010 heat wave in Russia, which was unprecedented in its severity, contributed to hundreds of forest fires that generated enough air pollution to kill an estimated 56,000 people and that burned 300,000 acres of crops, including roughly 25% of the nation's wheat fields. Nutritional deficiencies underlie a substantial portion of the global burden of many infectious diseases.

■ PRECIPITATION

In addition to changing temperature, the emission of greenhouse gases and the consequent increase in energy in Earth's atmosphere have influenced the planet's water cycle. Since 1950, substantial increases in the heaviest precipitation events (i.e., those above the 95th percentile) have been observed in Europe and North America. While trends over that same interval are less clear in other regions because of limited data, regions of Southeast Asia and southern South America have likely experienced increases in heavy precipitation as well. Other areas have seen greater drought, notably southern Australia and the southwestern United States.

A warmer atmosphere holds more water vapor. Specifically, air holds 6–7.5% more water vapor per degree (Celsius) of warming in the lower atmosphere. For areas that have traditionally had more precipitation on average, warming tends to promote heavier precipitation events.

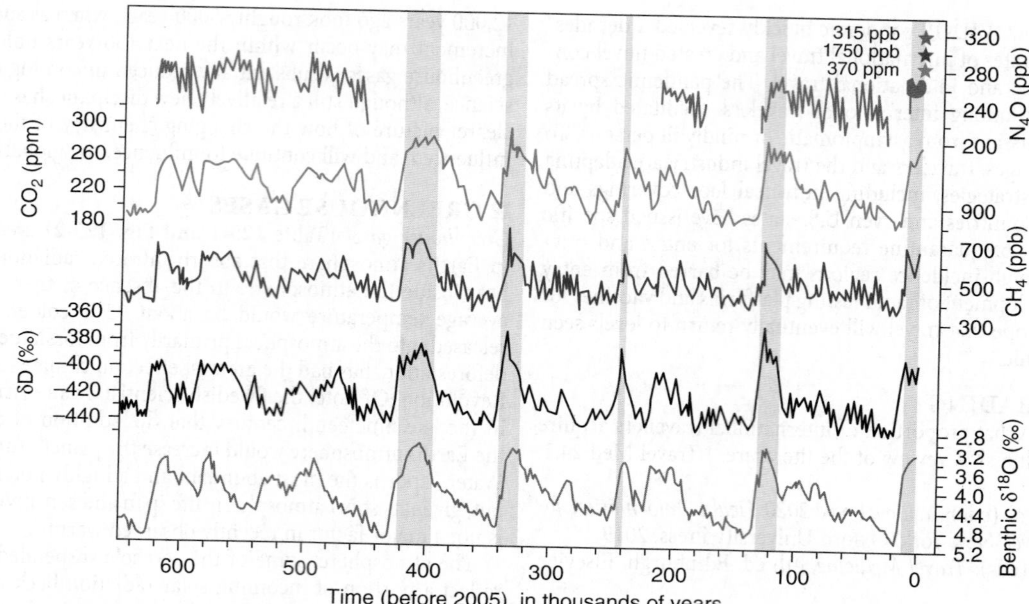

FIGURE 125-1 Overview of the earth's temperature and primary greenhouse gases over the last 600,000 years. Variations of deuterium (δD; *black*) serve as a proxy for temperature. Atmospheric concentrations of greenhouse gases—CO_2 (*red*), CH_4 (*blue*), and nitrous oxide (N_2O; *green*)—were derived from air trapped within Antarctic ice cores and from recent atmospheric measurements. *Shaded areas* indicate interglacial periods. Benthic $\delta^{18}O$ marine records (*dark gray*) are a proxy for global ice-volume fluctuations and can be compared to the ice core data. Downward trends in the benthic $\delta^{18}O$ curve reflect increasing ice volumes on land. The *stars* and *labels* indicate atmospheric concentrations as of the year 2000. CO_2 levels surpassed 400 ppm as of 2013 and are rising at a rate of 2–2.5 ppm per year. *(From Intergovernmental Panel on Climate Change Fourth Assessment Report. Working Group I. Cambridge University Press, 2007, Fig. 6.3.)*

In contrast, in regions prone to drought, warming tends to result in greater periods between rainfalls and in the risk of drought. Floods and droughts have been associated with outbreaks of waterborne infectious diseases.

HURRICANES

The world's oceans have absorbed 90% of the excess heat that greenhouse gases have kept in Earth's atmosphere since the 1960s. Ocean heat provides energy for hurricanes, and warmer years tend to have greater hurricane activity. An analysis of satellite observations from 1983 to 2005 has shown a trend toward increasing severity—albeit decreasing frequency—of Atlantic hurricanes. Modeling of future tropical cyclones suggests that their intensity may increase 2–11% by 2100 and that the average storm will bring 20% more rainfall.

SEA LEVEL RISE

Between 1901 and 2010, the global sea level rose ~200 mm, or ~1.7 mm per year on average. From 1993 to 2010, the rate of rise nearly doubled—i.e., to 3.2 mm annually. Most of this sea level rise has resulted from the thermal expansion of water. Glacial ice melt is the second greatest factor, and its contribution is accelerating. By 2100, global sea level may rise by 0.8–2 m, with an annual rate of rise of 8–16 mm at the century's end. Ice melt off Greenland and Antarctica is the largest contributor to sea level rise.

Sea level rise is not uniform. The rate of rise on the eastern seaboard of North America has been roughly double the global rate. Compounding sea level rise is the subsidence of coastal areas due to human settlement. In the absence of levee upgrades, an estimated 300 million people living near coasts worldwide will be at risk of flooding in 2050 because of the combined effects of subsidence, erosion, and sea level rise.

Along with extreme storms and overuse of coastal aquifers, rising seas also contribute to salinization of coastal groundwater. About 1 billion people rely on coastal aquifers for potable water.

EL NIÑO SOUTHERN OSCILLATION

The *El Niño Southern Oscillation* (ENSO) refers to periodic changes in water temperature in the eastern Pacific Ocean that occur roughly every 5 years. ENSO cycles have dramatic effects on weather around the globe. Warmer-than-average water temperatures in the eastern Pacific define *El Niño events* (see below), whereas cooler-than-average water temperatures define La Niña periods. Evidence is accruing that climate change may be increasing the frequency and severity of El Niño events.

TABLE 125-1 Greenhouse Gases: Sources, Sinks, and Forcings

GAS	HUMAN SOURCES	SINK[a]	RADIATIVE FORCING[b] (95% CONFIDENCE INTERVAL)
Carbon dioxide (CO_2)	Fossil fuel combustion, deforestation	Uptake by oceans (~30%), plants	1.68 (1.33–2.03)
Methane (CH_4)	Fossil fuel production, ruminant animals, decomposition in landfills	Hydroxyl radicals in the troposphere	0.97 (0.74–1.20)
Nitrous oxide (N_2O)	Fertilizer, fossil fuel combustion, biomass burning, livestock manure	Photolysis in the stratosphere	0.17 (0.14–0.23)
Halocarbons	Refrigerants, electrical insulation, aluminum production	Hydroxyl radicals in the troposphere, sunlight in the stratosphere	0.18 (0.01–0.35)

[a]In this table, a *sink* refers to the place where greenhouse gases are naturally stored or the mechanism through which they are destroyed. [b]*Radiative forcing*, measured in watts per meter squared, refers to how much an entity can alter the balance of incoming and outgoing radiation to and from Earth's atmosphere. It is measured relative to a preindustrial (i.e., 1750) baseline. Greenhouse gases have a positive "forcing"; that is, on balance, they increase the amount of radiation (and specifically infrared radiation) that is retained in Earth's atmosphere.

Sources: Intergovernmental Panel on Climate Change Fifth Assessment Report, Working Group 1, Chapter 8; American Chemical Society "Greenhouse gas sources and sinks," available at *www.acs.org/content/acs/en/climatescience/greenhousegases/sourcesandsinks.html*.

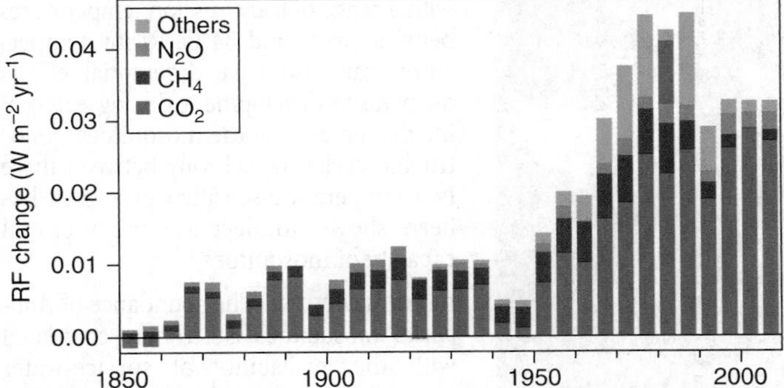

FIGURE 125-2 Acceleration of radiative forcing (RF) from release of major greenhouse gases, 1850–2011. For definition of *radiative forcing*, see footnote *b* to Table 125-1. *(From Intergovernmental Panel on Climate Change Fifth Assessment Report, Working Group 1, p. 677, Fig. 8.6.)*

El Niño events drive alterations in weather worldwide (**Fig. 125-4**) and are associated with extreme events and consequently higher rates of morbidity and mortality. Hurricane Mitch, one of the most powerful hurricanes ever observed, with winds reaching 290 km/h, dropped 1–1.8 m (3–6 feet) of rain over 72 h on parts of Honduras and Nicaragua. As a result of this storm, 11,000 people died and 2.7 million were displaced. Outbreaks of cholera, leptospirosis, and dengue occurred in the storm's aftermath.

POPULATION MIGRATION AND CONFLICT

The final common outcome of all climate-change effects is human displacement. Sea level rise, extreme heat and precipitation, droughts, and salinization of water supplies all conspire to make regions, including some inhabited by humans for millennia, uninhabitable. Among climate-change migrants in the near future may be the 8 million inhabitants of low-lying South Pacific islands that are vulnerable to sea level rise.

Climate change may also be contributing to humanitarian crises and conflicts. A severe 2011 drought in East Africa may have incited the Somali famine that resulted in 1 million refugees; mortality rates reached 7.4/10,000 in some refugee camps. Crop losses associated with the 2010 Russian heat wave led Russia to halt grain exports, causing higher grain prices on the world market and food riots in developing nations.

EFFECTS OF CLIMATE CHANGE ON INFECTIOUS DISEASE

The incidence of most, if not all, infectious diseases depends on climate. For any given infection, however, climate change is but one of many factors that determine disease epidemiology. In instances in which climate change creates conditions favorable to the spread of infections, diseases may be kept in check through interventions such as vector control or antibiotic treatment.

Detecting climate-change influence on an emerging human disease can be challenging. Research with animal pathogens, which in most instances are less well monitored and intervened upon than that with their human counterparts, has suggested how climate change may influence disease spread. For example, the life cycle of nematode parasites of caribou and musk oxen shortens as temperatures rise. As the Arctic has warmed, higher nematode burdens and consequently higher rates of morbidity and mortality have been observed. Other examples from animals, such as the spread of the protozoan parasite *Perkinsus marinus* in oysters, demonstrate how warming can enable range expansion of pathogens previously held in check by colder temperatures.

As these and other examples from studies of animals make clear, the influence of climate change on infectious diseases can be pronounced. The following sections deal with the infectious diseases for which research has explored the influence of climate change.

VECTOR-BORNE DISEASE

Because insects are cold-blooded, ambient temperature dictates their geographic distribution. With increases in temperatures (in particular, nighttime minimum temperatures), insects are freed to move poleward and up mountainsides. At the same time, as new areas become climatically suitable, current mosquito habitats may become unsuitable as a result of heat extremes.

In addition, insects tend to be sensitive to water availability. Mosquitoes that transmit malaria, dengue, and other infections may breed

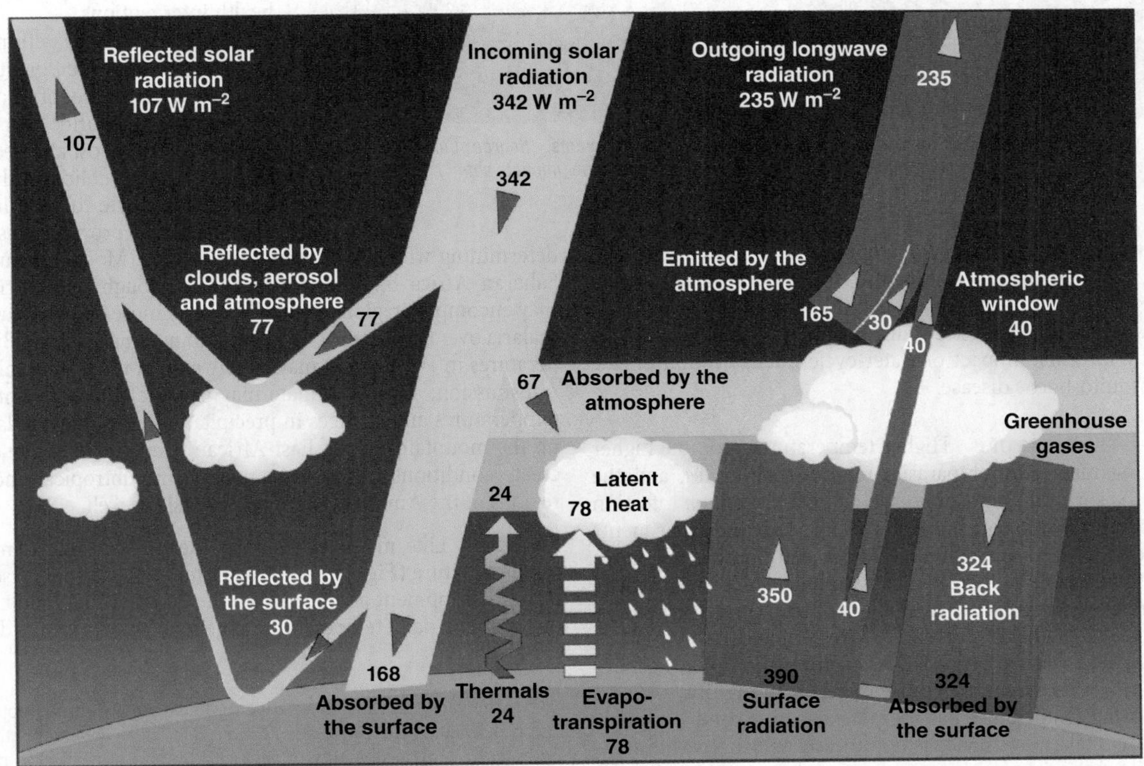

FIGURE 125-3 Earth's energy balance. *(Reproduced with permission from JT Kiehl: Earth's annual global mean energy budget. Bull Am Meteor Soc 78:197, 1997. © American Meteorological Society. Used with permission.)*

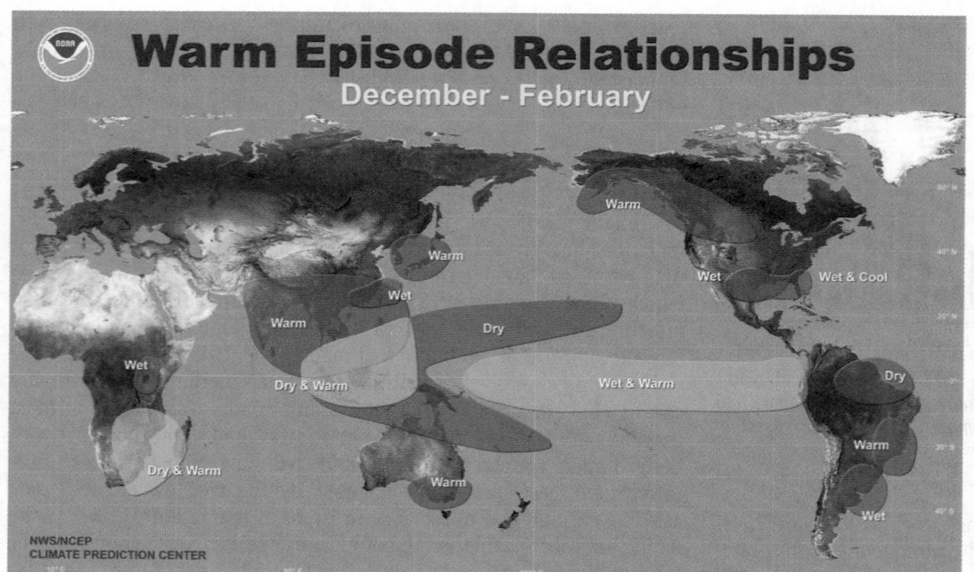

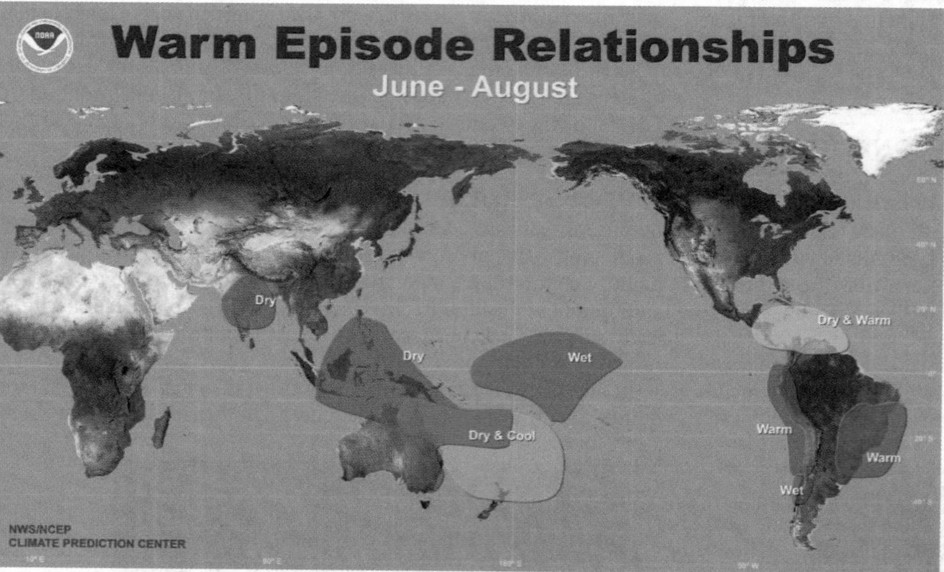

FIGURE 125-4 Characteristic weather anomalies, by season, during El Niño events. *(Source: Climate Prediction Center, https://www.cpc.ncep.noaa.gov/products/analysis_monitoring/impacts/warm_impacts.shtml.)*

in pools of water created by heavy downpours. As has been observed in the Amazon, breeding pools can also appear during periods of drought when rivers recede and leave behind stagnant pools of water for *Anopheles* mosquitoes. These circumstances have raised interest in the potentially favorable impact of water-cycle intensification on the spread of mosquito-borne disease.

Malaria • TEMPERATURE Higher temperatures promote higher mosquito-biting rates, shorter parasite reproductive cycles, and the potential for the survival of mosquito vectors of *Plasmodium* infection in locations previously too cold to sustain them. Modeling experiments have identified highland areas of East Africa and South America as perhaps most vulnerable to increased malarial incidence as a result of rising temperatures. In addition, an analysis of interannual malaria in Ecuador and Colombia has documented a greater incidence of malaria at higher altitudes in warmer years. Highland populations may be more vulnerable to malaria epidemics because they lack immunity.

Although rising temperature has the potential to expand the viable range of disease, malaria incidence is not linearly associated with temperature. While mosquitoes and parasites may adapt to a warming climate, the present optimal temperature for malaria transmission is ~25°C, with a range of transmission temperatures between 16°C and 34°C. Rising temperatures can also have differential effects on parasite development during external incubation and on the mosquitoes' gonotrophic cycle. Asynchrony between these two temperature-sensitive processes has been shown to decrease the vectorial capacity of mosquitoes.[1]

PRECIPITATION The abundance of *Anopheles* mosquitoes is strongly correlated with the availability of surface-water pools for mosquito breeding, and biting rates have been linked to soil moisture (a surrogate for breeding pools). Research in the East African highlands has documented that increased variance in rainfall over time has strengthened the association between precipitation and disease incidence. These disease-promoting effects of precipitation may be countered by the potential for extreme rainfall to flush mosquito larvae from breeding sites.

PROJECTIONS Climate models have begun to deliver output on regional scales, permitting projections of climate-suitable regions to assist national and local health authorities. Climate models speak to the temperature and precipitation ranges necessary for malaria transmission but do not account for the capacity of malaria control programs to halt the spread of disease. The global reduction in malaria distribution over the past century makes it clear that, even with climate change, malaria occurs in far fewer places today because of public health interventions.

Despite intensive efforts, malaria remains the single greatest vector-borne disease cause of morbidity and death in the world. Particularly in regions that are most affected by malaria and where the public health infrastructure is inadequate to contain it, climate modeling may provide a useful tool in determining where the disease may spread. Modeling studies in sub-Saharan Africa have suggested that, although East African nations may encompass regions that will become more climatically suitable for malaria over this century, West African nations may not. By 2100, temperatures in West Africa may largely exceed those optimal for malaria transmission, and the climate may become drier; in contrast, higher temperatures and changes in precipitation may allow malaria to move up the mountainsides of East African countries. Climate change may create conditions favorable to malaria in subtropical and temperate regions of the Americas, Europe, and Asia as well.

Dengue Like malaria epidemics, dengue fever epidemics depend on temperature (Fig. 125-5). Higher temperatures increase the rate of larval development and accelerate the emergence of adult *Aedes* mosquitoes. The daily temperature range may also influence dengue virus

[1] *rVc* is the vectorial capacity relative to the vector-to-human population ratio and is defined by the equation $rVc = a^2 b_h b_m e^{-\mu_m n}/\mu_m$ where a is the vector biting rate; b_h is the probability of vector-to-human transmission per bite; b_m is the probability of human-to-vector infection per bite; n is the duration of the extrinsic incubation period; and μ_m is the vector mortality rate.

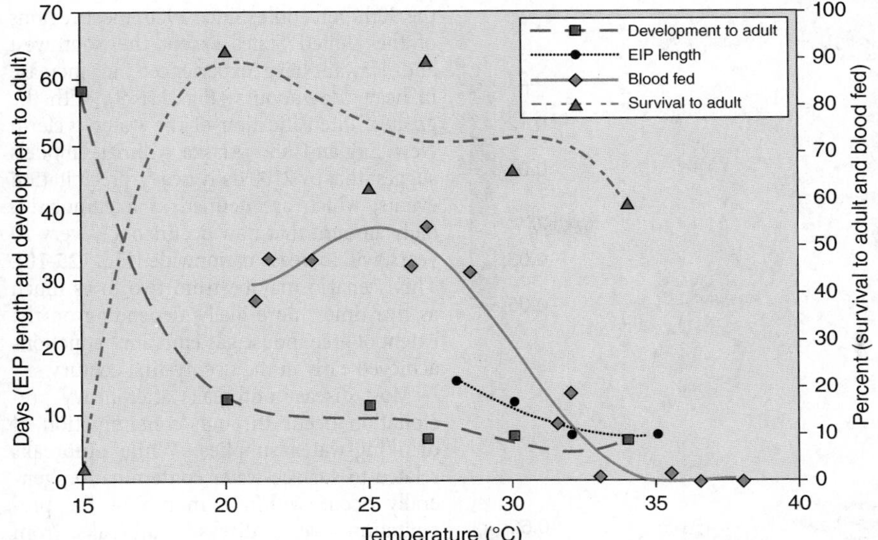

FIGURE 125-5 Effects of temperature on variables associated with dengue transmission. Shown are the number of days required for development of immature *Aedes aegypti* mosquitoes to adults, the length of the dengue virus type 2 extrinsic incubation period (EIP), the percentage of *Ae. aegypti* mosquitoes that complete a blood meal within 30 min after a blood source is made available, and the percentage of hatched *Ae. aegypti* larvae surviving to adulthood. *(Reproduced from CW Morin et al: Climate and dengue transmission: Evidence and implications. Environ Health Perspect 121:1264, 2013.)*

transmission, with a smaller range corresponding to a higher transmission potential. Temperatures <15°C or >36°C substantially reduce mosquito feeding. In a *Rhesus* model of dengue, viral replication can occur in as little as 7 days with temperatures of >32–35°C; at 30°C, replication takes ≥12 days; and replication does not reliably occur at 26°C. Research on dengue in New Caledonia has shown peak transmission at ~32°C, reflecting combined effects of a shorter extrinsic incubation period, a higher feeding frequency, and more rapid development of mosquitoes. Along with temperature, peak relative humidity is a strong predictor of dengue outbreaks.

The association between dengue epidemics and precipitation is less consistent in the peer-reviewed literature, possibly because of the mosquito vector's greater reliance on domestic breeding sites than on natural pools of water. For instance, in some studies, increased access to a piped water supply has been linked to dengue epidemics, presumably because of associated increased domestic water storage. Nonetheless, several studies have established rainfall as a predictor of the seasonal timing of dengue epidemics.

The current global distribution of dengue largely overlaps the geographic spread of *Aedes* mosquitoes (**Fig. 125-6**). The presence of *Aedes* without dengue endemicity in large regions of North and South America and Africa illustrates the relevance of variables other than climate to disease incidence. Nevertheless, coupled climatic–epidemiologic modeling suggests dramatic shifts in the relative vectorial capacity for dengue by the end of this century should little or no mitigation of greenhouse gas emissions occur (**Fig. 125-7**).

Other Arbovirus Infections Climate change may favor increased geographic spread of other arboviral diseases, including Zika virus disease, chikungunya virus disease, West Nile virus disease, and eastern equine encephalitis. Zika virus moved to the Western Hemisphere from French Polynesia around 2013 and rapidly spread in Brazil in 2016. Although air travel was essential for the delivery of the virus to the Americas, the available evidence suggests that the 2015 El Niño event provided an optimal climate for the infection to take root and spread. *Ae. aegypti* is the primary vector for Zika virus. Chikungunya virus disease emerged in Italy in 2007, having previously been mostly a disease of African nations. Climate models predict that, should competent vectors be present, conditions will be suitable for the chikungunya virus to gain a foothold in Western Europe, especially France, in the first half of the twenty-first century. In North America, areas favorable to West Nile virus outbreaks are expected to shift northward in this century. Current hotspots in North America are the California Central Valley, southwestern Arizona, southern Texas, and Louisiana, which have both compatible climates and avian reservoirs for the disease. By

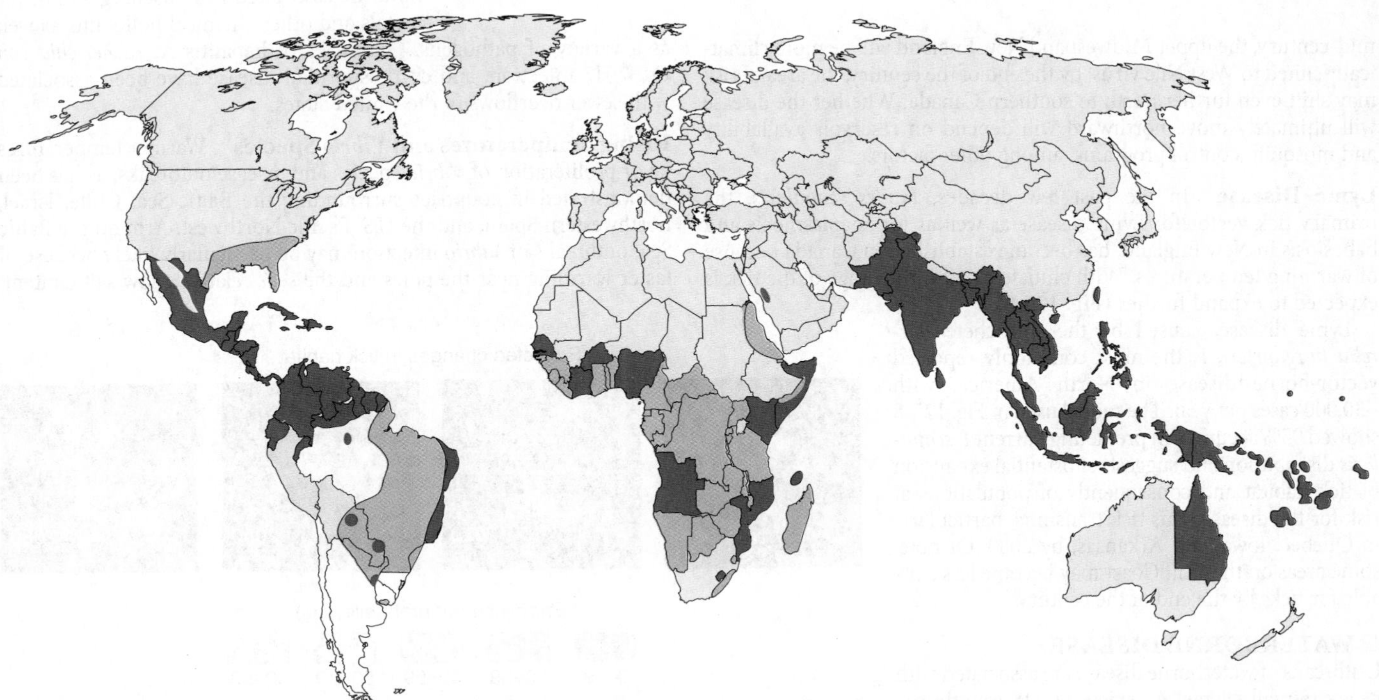

FIGURE 125-6 Distribution of *Aedes aegypti* mosquitoes (*turquoise*) and dengue fever epidemics (*red*). *(Map produced by the Agricultural Research Service of the U.S. Department of Agriculture.)*

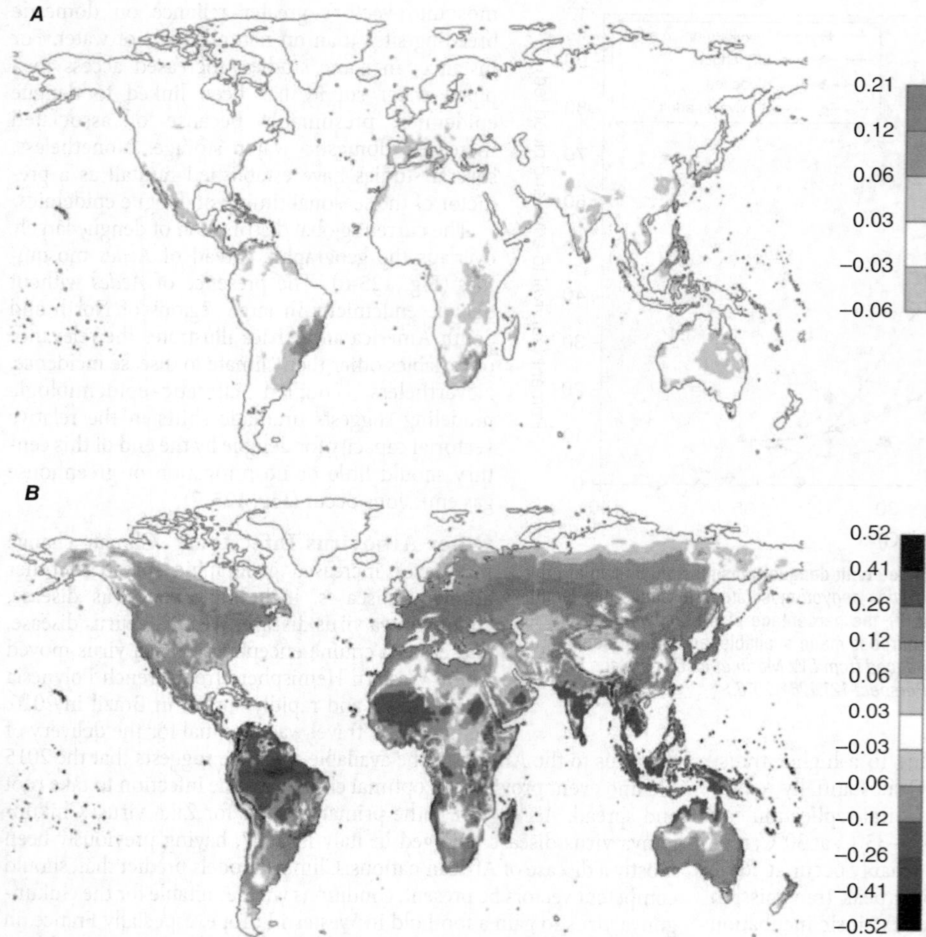

FIGURE 125-7 Trend of annually averaged global dengue epidemic potential (*rVc*). Differences in rVc are based on 30-year averages of temperature and daily temperature range. ***A.*** Differences between 1980–2009 and 1901–1930. ***B.*** Differences between 2070–2099 and 1980–2009. The mean value of rVc was averaged from five global climate models under RCP8.5, a scenario of high greenhouse-gas emission. The color bar describes the values of the rVc. *(From J Liu-Helmersson et al: Vectorial capacity of Aedes aegypti: Effects of temperature and implications for global dengue epidemic potential. PLoS One 9:e89783, 2014.)*

mid-century, the upper Midwest and New England will be more climatically suited to West Nile virus; by the end of the century, the area of risk may shift even further north to southern Canada. Whether the disease will ultimately move northward will depend on reservoir availability and mosquito control programs, among other factors.

Lyme Disease In the past few decades, *Ixodes scapularis*, the primary tick vector for Lyme disease as well as for anaplasmosis and babesiosis in New England, has become established in Canada because of warming temperatures. With climate change, the range of the tick is expected to expand further (**Fig. 125-8**).

Lyme disease, caused by the spirochete *Borrelia burgdorferi*, is the most commonly reported vector-borne disease in North America, with ~30,000 cases per year. The model used in Fig. 125-8 showed 95% accuracy in predicting current *I. scapularis* distribution and suggests substantial expansion of tick habitat and consequently of populations at risk for the diseases this tick transmits, particularly in Quebec, Iowa, and Arkansas, by 2080. Of note, some areas on the Gulf Coast may become less suitable for ticks by the end of the century.

WATERBORNE DISEASE

Outbreaks of waterborne disease are associated with heavy rainfall events. A review of 548 waterborne disease outbreaks in the United States found that 51% were preceded by precipitation levels above the 90th percentile. Since 1900, most regions of the United States except the Southwest and Hawaii have experienced an increase in heavy downpours (**Fig. 125-9**), with the greatest intensification of the water cycle in New England and Alaska. Climate models suggest that by 2100 daily heavy-precipitation events, which are defined as a cumulative daily amount that now occurs once every 20 years, will increase nationwide (**Fig. 125-10**). This scenario may be from two to as much as five times more likely, depending on the extent of greenhouse gas emission reductions achieved early in the twenty-first century.

Most disease outbreaks after heavy precipitation occur through contamination of drinking-water supplies. While outbreaks related to surface-water contamination generally occur within a month of the precipitation event, disease outbreaks from groundwater contamination tend to occur ≥2 months later. According to a review of published reports of waterborne disease outbreaks, *Vibrio* and *Leptospira* species are the pathogens most commonly involved in the wake of heavy precipitation.

Combined Sewer Systems Roughly 40 million people in the United States and millions more around the world rely on combined sewer systems in which storm water and sanitary wastewater are conveyed in the same pipe to treatment facilities. These systems were designed on the basis of the nineteenth-century climate, in which heavy downpours were less frequent than they are today. The frequency of combined sewer overflows resulting in untreated sewage discharge, usually into freshwater bodies, has been increasing in cities worldwide. Overflows are associated with discharges of heavy metals and other chemical pollutants as well as a variety of pathogens. Outbreaks of hepatitis A, *Escherichia coli* O157:H7 infection, and cryptosporidial disease have been associated with sewer overflows in the United States.

Rising Temperatures and *Vibrio* Species Warmer temperatures favor proliferation of *Vibrio* species and disease outbreaks, as has been demonstrated in countries surrounding the Baltic Sea, Chile, Israel, northwestern Spain, and the U.S. Pacific Northwest. Around the Baltic Sea, outbreaks of *Vibrio* infection may be particularly likely because of faster warming near the poles and the sea's relatively low salt content.

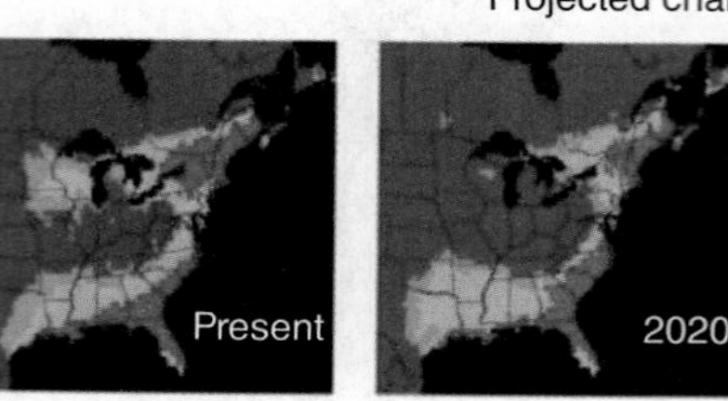

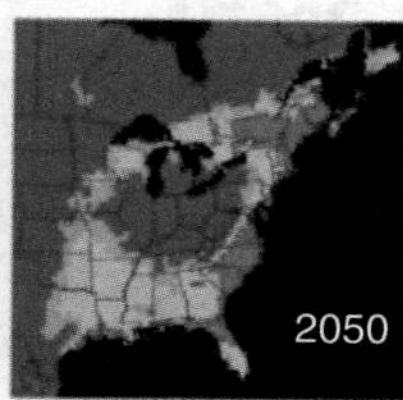

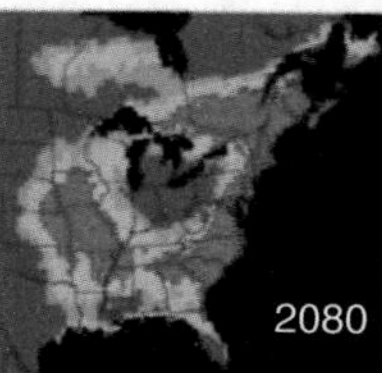

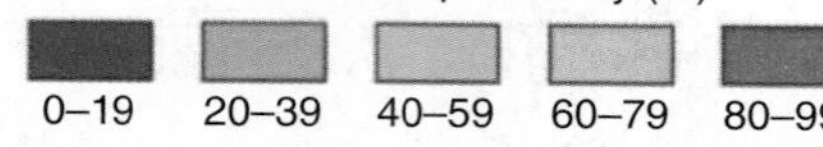

FIGURE 125-8 Present and projected probability of establishment of *Ixodes scapularis*. *(From U.S. National Climate Assessment 2014, adapted from JS Brownstein et al: Effect of climate change on Lyme disease risk in North America. Ecohealth 2:38, 2005.)*

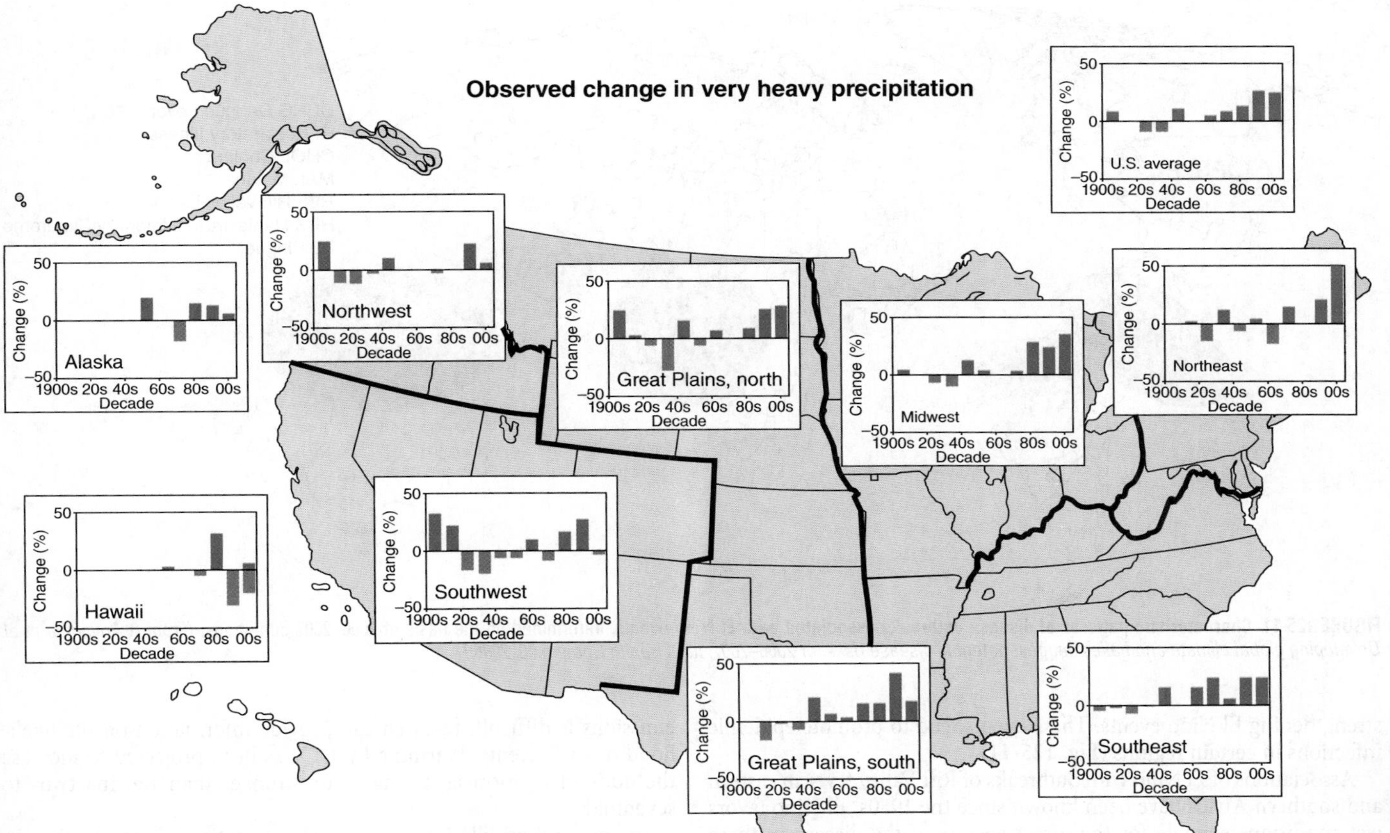

Observed change in very heavy precipitation

FIGURE 125-9 Percentage changes in the annual amount of precipitation falling in very heavy events, defined as the heaviest 1% of all daily events from 1901 to 2012 for each region. Changes are relative to a 1901–1960 average for all regions except values for Alaska and Hawaii, which are relative to the 1951–1980 average. *(From U.S. National Climate Assessment 2014, NOAA National Climate Data Center/Cooperative Institute for Climate and Satellites, North Carolina.)*

In 2004, a *Vibrio parahaemolyticus* outbreak arising from consumption of Alaskan oysters occurred. This pathogen was unknown in Alaskan oysters prior to this event and extended the known geographic range of the disease 1000 km northward.

ENSO-Related Outbreaks In the past, El Niño events were used as a model to investigate the potential for extreme weather–related infectious disease epidemics occurring in association with climate change. Recent evidence indicates that climate change itself may be

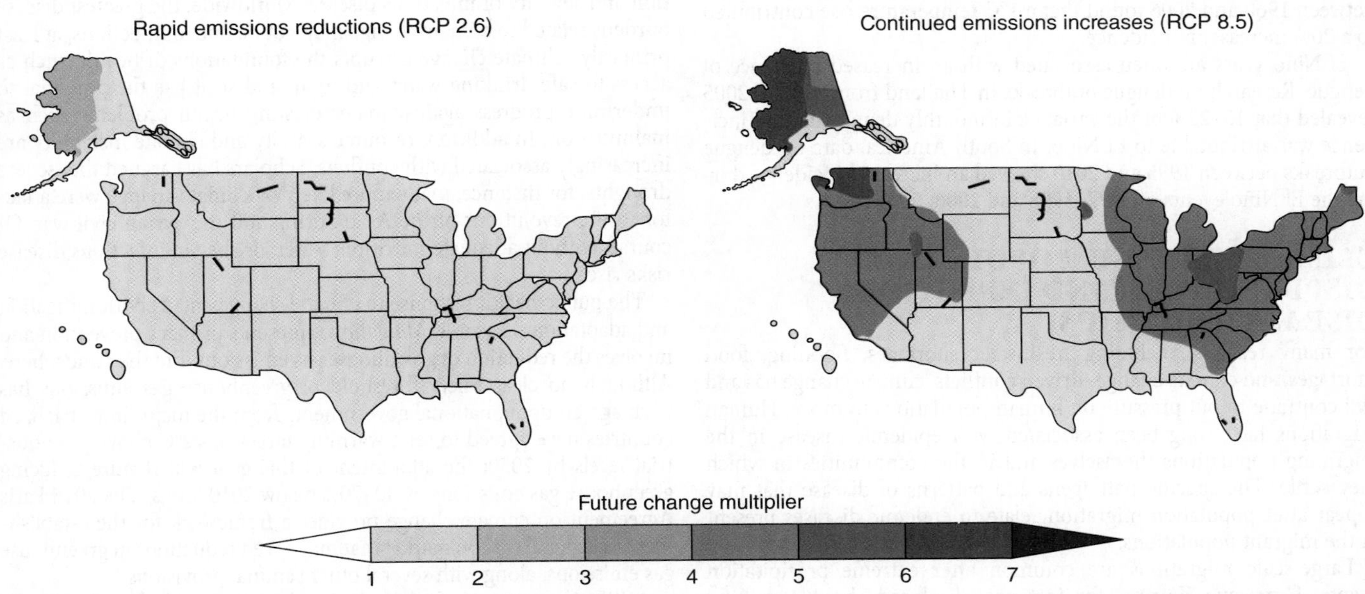

FIGURE 125-10 Increased frequency of extreme daily precipitation events (defined as a daily amount that now occurs once in 20 years) by the latter part of the twenty-first century (2081–2100) compared to the frequency in the latter part of the twentieth century (1981–2000). A representative concentration pathway (RCP) describes a plausible climate future based on a net radiative forcing (e.g., 2.6 or 8.5) in 2100. *(From U.S. National Climate Assessment 2014, NOAA National Climate Data Center/Cooperative Institute for Climate and Satellites, North Carolina.)*

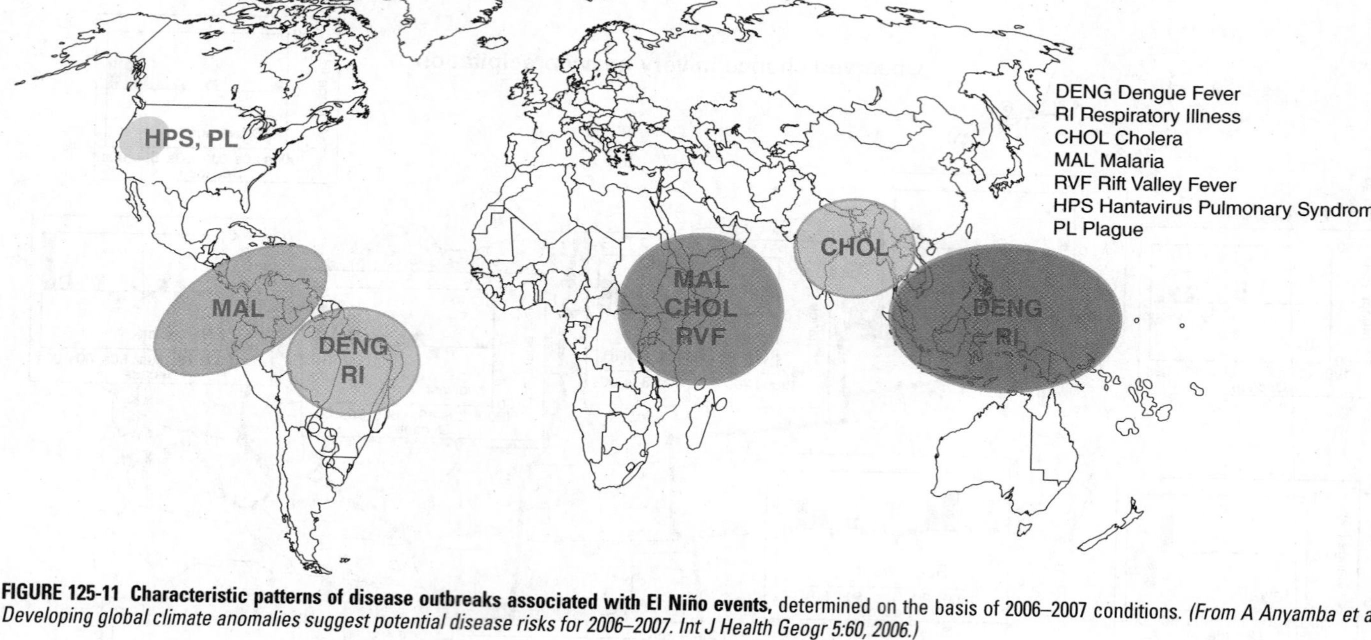

FIGURE 125-11 Characteristic patterns of disease outbreaks associated with El Niño events, determined on the basis of 2006–2007 conditions. *(From A Anyamba et al: Developing global climate anomalies suggest potential disease risks for 2006–2007. Int J Health Geogr 5:60, 2006.)*

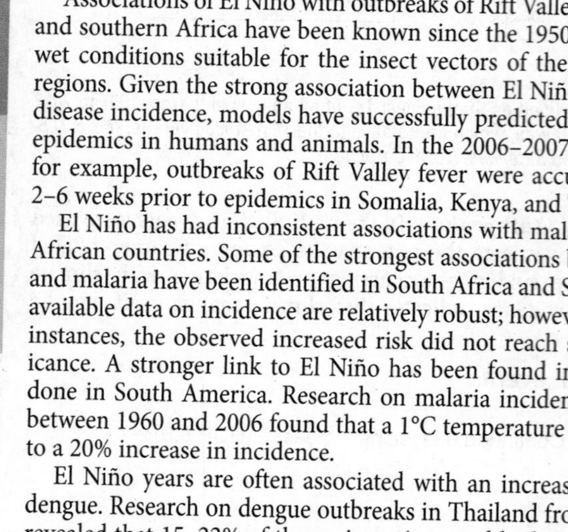

strengthening El Niño events. These events tend to promote epidemic infections in certain regions (Fig. 125-11).

Associations of El Niño with outbreaks of Rift Valley fever in eastern and southern Africa have been known since the 1950s. El Niño favors wet conditions suitable for the insect vectors of the disease in these regions. Given the strong association between El Niño conditions and disease incidence, models have successfully predicted Rift Valley fever epidemics in humans and animals. In the 2006–2007 El Niño season, for example, outbreaks of Rift Valley fever were accurately predicted 2–6 weeks prior to epidemics in Somalia, Kenya, and Tanzania.

El Niño has had inconsistent associations with malaria incidence in African countries. Some of the strongest associations between El Niño and malaria have been identified in South Africa and Swaziland, where available data on incidence are relatively robust; however, even in these instances, the observed increased risk did not reach statistical significance. A stronger link to El Niño has been found in several studies done in South America. Research on malaria incidence in Colombia between 1960 and 2006 found that a 1°C temperature rise contributed to a 20% increase in incidence.

El Niño years are often associated with an increased incidence of dengue. Research on dengue outbreaks in Thailand from 1996 to 2005 revealed that 15–22% of the variance in monthly dengue disease incidence was attributable to El Niño. In South America, data on dengue outbreaks between 1995 and 2010 showed an increased incidence during the El Niño events of 1997–1998 and 2006–2007.

CLIMATE CHANGE, POPULATION DISPLACEMENT, AND INFECTIOUS DISEASE EPIDEMICS

For many reasons, including freshwater shortages, flooding, food shortages, and climate change–driven conflicts, climate change has and will continue to put pressure on human populations to move. Human migrations have long been associated with epidemic disease in the migrating populations themselves and in the communities in which they settle. The specific pathogens and patterns of disease that may appear after population migration relate to endemic diseases present in the migrant populations.

Large-scale migrations are common after extreme precipitation events. Hurricane Katrina, for instance, displaced about 1 million people from the U.S. Gulf Coast. Among Katrina refugees, outbreaks of respiratory, diarrheal, and skin diseases were most common. While attribution of a single weather event to increased greenhouse-gas emissions is difficult, research can provide information on the likelihood of such events. Warming by 1°C has been projected to increase the odds of a storm as strong as or stronger than Katrina two- to sevenfold.

In low- and middle-income countries, infectious disease outbreaks associated with population displacement may be harder to detect and respond to. People forced to leave their homes en masse are at risk for contracting infections with any pathogen that may be present within the displaced population, including sexually transmitted diseases such as HIV, or airborne or droplet transmitted diseases such as tuberculosis and measles. Mitigation of disease risk requires overlaying of climate-related migration risk with foci of disease epidemics.

A BROADER VIEW OF CLIMATE CHANGE AND HEALTH

While climate change has far-reaching implications for the distribution and severity of infectious diseases worldwide, the greatest disease burdens related to climate change may not be due to infections, at least primarily. Climate change disrupts the foundations of health, such as access to safe drinking water and food, and so it has the potential to undermine progress against major existing health problems such as malnutrition. In addition, resource scarcity and climate instability are increasingly associated with conflicts. Scholars have argued that severe droughts, for instance, made more likely by climate change were a factor in the revolutions of the Arab Spring and the Syrian civil war. Of course, without adequate nutrition, water, or shelter, infectious disease risks rise.

The public health response to climate change entails both mitigation and adaptation measures. *Mitigation* represents primary prevention and involves the reduction of greenhouse gas emissions into the atmosphere. Although no clear safety threshold of greenhouse gas emissions has been agreed upon, national governments from the major industrialized countries have agreed to set a warming target of <2°C above preindustrial levels by 2050; the attainment of this goal will require reducing greenhouse gas emissions by 40–70% below 2010 levels. The 2016 Paris Agreement on climate change provides a framework for the establishment of a global carbon market that may speed reductions in greenhouse gas emissions, along with several other seminal provisions.

Mitigation also confers health co-benefits, including better air quality and lower incidence and severity of respiratory infections, associated with less bio- or fossil fuel combustion. Biofuel-burning cookstoves, for instance, used by some 3 billion people around the world, release air pollution that constitutes about one-fourth of the global black-carbon emissions that warm the planet and kill roughly 4 million people a year. Clean cookstoves simultaneously mitigate climate change and indoor air pollution–related mortality. Of note, evidence has shown that long-term air pollution exposure may contribute to mortality risk from COVID-19.

Climate *adaptation* is secondary prevention and seeks to reduce harms associated with sea level rise, heat waves, floods, droughts, wildfires, and other greenhouse gas–driven events. The efficacy of adaptation is constrained by the challenges inherent in predicting the precise location, duration, and severity of extreme weather events and flooding related to sea level rise, among other considerations.

■ FURTHER READING

ANYAMBA A et al: Prediction of a Rift Valley fever outbreak. Proc Natl Acad Sci USA 106:955, 2009.

CAI W et al: Increasing frequency of extreme El Niño events due to greenhouse warming. Nat Clim Change 4:111, 2014.

CAMINADE C et al: Impact of climate change on global malaria distribution. Proc Natl Acad Sci USA 111:3286, 2014.

COLÓN-GONZÁLEZ FJ et al: The effects of weather and climate change on dengue. PLoS Negl Trop Dis 7:e2503, 2013.

GETHING PW et al: Climate change and the global malaria recession. Nature 465:342, 2010.

NATIONAL CLIMATIC DATA CENTER: Mitch: The deadliest Atlantic hurricane since 1780. Available from *ftp://ftp.ncdc.noaa.gov/pub/data/extremeevents/specialreports/Hurricane-Mitch-1998.pdf.* Accessed January 13, 2017.

OGDEN NH et al: Climate change and the potential for range expansion of the Lyme disease vector *Ixodes scapularis* in Canada. Int J Parasitol 36:63, 2006.

PAAIJMANS KP et al: Temperature-dependent pre-bloodmeal period and temperature-driven asynchrony between parasite development and mosquito biting rate reduce malaria transmission intensity. PLoS One 8:e55777, 2013.

SEMENZA JC: Cascading risks of waterborne diseases from climate change. Nat Immunol 21:484, 2020.

WATTS DM et al: Effect of temperature on the vector efficiency of *Aedes aegypti* for dengue 2 virus. Am J Trop Med Hyg 36:143, 1987.

WU X et al: Exposure to air pollution and COVID-19 mortality in the United States. medRxiv 2020.04.05.20054502, 2020.

ZHOU G et al: Association between climate variability and malaria epidemics in the East African highlands. Proc Natl Acad Sci USA 101:2375, 2004.

Section 2 Clinical Syndromes: Community-Acquired Infections

126 Pneumonia

Lionel A. Mandell, Michael S. Niederman

DEFINITION

Pneumonia is an infection of the pulmonary parenchyma. Despite significant morbidity and mortality, it is often misdiagnosed, mistreated, and underestimated. Pneumonia has usually been classified as community-acquired (CAP), hospital-acquired (HAP), or ventilator-associated (VAP). A fourth category, health care–associated pneumonia (HCAP) was introduced to encompass cases caused by multidrug-resistant (MDR) pathogens typically associated with HAP and cases in unhospitalized individuals at risk of MDR infection. Unfortunately, this category has not reliably predicted infection with resistant pathogens and has been associated with increased use of broad-spectrum antibiotics, particularly those employed for treatment of methicillin-resistant *Staphylococcus aureus* (MRSA) and antipseudomonal β-lactams. Accordingly, use of the HCAP category should be discontinued. Rather than relying on a predefined subset of pneumonia cases, it is better to assess patients individually on the basis of risk factors for infection with a resistant organism. Risk factors for infection with MRSA and *Pseudomonas aeruginosa* include prior isolation of the organism, particularly from the respiratory tract during the preceding year, and/or hospitalization and treatment with an antibiotic in the previous 90 days.

Pneumonia caused by macroaspiration of oropharyngeal or gastric contents, usually referred to as aspiration pneumonia, is best thought of as a point on the continuum that includes CAP and HAP. Estimates suggest that aspiration pneumonia accounts for 5–15% of CAP cases, but reliable figures for HAP are unavailable. The airways or pulmonary parenchyma may be involved, and patients usually represent a clinical phenotype with risk factors for macroaspiration and involvement of characteristic anatomic pulmonary locations.

PATHOPHYSIOLOGY

Pneumonia is the result of the proliferation of microbial pathogens at the alveolar level and the host's response to them. Until recently, it was thought that the lungs were sterile and that pneumonia resulted from the introduction of potential pathogens into this sterile environment. Typically, this introduction occurred through microaspiration of oropharyngeal organisms into the lower respiratory tract. Overcoming of innate and adaptive immunity by such microorganisms could result in the clinical syndrome of pneumonia.

Recent use of culture-independent techniques of microbial identification has demonstrated a complex and diverse community of bacteria in the lungs that constitutes the lung microbiota. Awareness of this microbiota has prompted a rethinking of how pneumonia develops. Mechanical factors, such as the hairs and turbinates of the nares, the branching tracheobronchial tree, mucociliary clearance, and gag and cough reflexes, all play a role in host defense but are insufficient to effectively block bacterial access to the lower airways. In the absence of a sufficient barrier, microorganisms may reach the lower respiratory tract by a variety of pathways, including inhalation, microaspiration, and direct mucosal dispersion.

The constitution of the lung microbiota is determined by three factors: microbial entry into the lungs, microbial elimination, and regional growth conditions for bacteria, such as pH, oxygen tension, and temperature. The key question, however, is how a dynamic homeostasis among bacterial communities results in acute infection. Pneumonia therefore does not appear to be the result of the invasion of a sterile space by a particular microorganism but is more likely an emergent phenomenon dependent upon a number of mechanisms, including self-accelerating positive feedback loops.

A possible model for pneumonia is as follows. An inflammatory event resulting in epithelial and or endothelial injury results in the release of cytokines, chemokines, and catecholamines, some of which may selectively promote the growth of certain bacteria, such as *Streptococcus pneumoniae* and *P. aeruginosa.* This cycle of inflammation, enhanced nutrient availability, and release of potential bacterial growth factors may result in a positive feedback loop that further accelerates inflammation and the growth of particular bacteria, which may then become dominant. In cases of CAP and HAP, the trigger may be a viral infection compounded by microaspiration of oropharyngeal organisms. In cases of true aspiration pneumonia, the trigger may simply be the macroaspiration event itself.

Once triggered, innate and adaptive immune responses can ideally help contain potential pathogens and prevent the development of pneumonia. However, in the face of continuing inflammation (and especially if a positive feedback loop becomes sustainable), the process may proceed to a full-fledged pneumonia syndrome. Inflammatory mediators such as interleukin 6 and tumor necrosis factor result in fever, and chemokines such as interleukin 8 and granulocyte colony-stimulating factor increase local neutrophil numbers. Mediators released by macrophages and neutrophils may create an alveolar capillary leak resulting in impaired oxygenation, hypoxemia, and radiographic infiltrates. Moreover, some bacterial pathogens appear to interfere with the hypoxic vasoconstriction that would normally occur with fluid-filled alveoli, and this interference may result in severe hypoxemia. Decreased compliance due to capillary leak, hypoxemia, increased respiratory drive, increased secretions, and occasionally infection-related bronchospasm all lead to worsening dyspnea. If severe enough, changes in lung mechanics secondary to reductions in lung volume, compliance, and intrapulmonary shunting of blood may cause respiratory failure.

Cardiovascular events with pneumonia, particularly in the elderly and usually in association with pneumococcal pneumonia and influenza, are increasingly recognized. These events, which may be acute or whose occurrence may extend to at least 1 year, include congestive heart failure, arrhythmia, myocardial infarction, or stroke and may be caused by a variety of mechanisms, including increased myocardial load and/or destabilization of atherosclerotic plaques by inflammation. In animal models, direct myocardial invasion by pneumococci may result in scarring and impaired myocardial function and conductivity.

PATHOLOGY

Classic pneumonia evolves through a series of stages. The initial stage is edema with a proteinaceous exudate and often bacteria in the alveoli. Next is a rapid transition to the red hepatization phase. Erythrocytes in the intraalveolar exudate give this stage its name. In the third phase, gray hepatization, no new erythrocytes are extravasating, and those already present have been lysed and degraded. The neutrophil is the predominant cell, fibrin deposition is abundant, and bacteria have disappeared. This phase corresponds with the successful containment of the infection and improvement in gas exchange. In the final phase, resolution, the macrophage reappears as the dominant cell in the alveolar space and the debris of neutrophils, and bacteria and fibrin have been cleared, as has the inflammatory response.

This pattern has been described best for lobar pneumococcal pneumonia but may not apply to pneumonia of all etiologies. In VAP, respiratory bronchiolitis may precede the development of a radiologically apparent infiltrate. A bronchopneumonia pattern is most common in nosocomial pneumonias, whereas a lobar pattern is more common in bacterial CAP. Despite the radiographic appearance, viral and *Pneumocystis* pneumonias represent alveolar rather than interstitial processes.

COMMUNITY-ACQUIRED PNEUMONIA

■ ETIOLOGY

The list of potential etiologic agents of CAP includes bacteria, fungi, viruses, and protozoa. Newer viral pathogens include metapneumoviruses, the coronaviruses responsible for severe acute respiratory syndrome (SARS) and Middle East respiratory syndrome (MERS), and the recently discovered coronavirus that originated in Wuhan, China, and is designated SARS-CoV-2. First described in December 2019, SARS-CoV-2 and its associated clinical disease, COVID-19, have reached pandemic proportions and are a cause of significant morbidity and mortality. The virus and the disease are discussed in detail in **Chap. 199**.

Although most CAP cases are caused by relatively few pathogens, an accurate determination of their prevalence is difficult because laboratory testing methods are often insensitive and indirect (**Table 126-1**). Separation of potential agents into "typical" bacterial pathogens and "atypical" organisms may be helpful. The former group includes *S. pneumoniae, Haemophilus influenzae,* and, in selected patients, *S. aureus* and gram-negative bacilli such as *Klebsiella pneumoniae* and *P. aeruginosa.* The "atypical" organisms include *Mycoplasma pneumoniae, Chlamydia pneumoniae,* and *Legionella* species as well as respiratory viruses such as influenza virus, adenoviruses, human metapneumoviruses, respiratory syncytial virus, and coronaviruses. With the increasing use of pneumococcal vaccine, the incidence of pneumococcal pneumonia is decreasing. Cases due to *M. pneumoniae* and *C. pneumoniae*, however,

TABLE 126-1 Microbial Causes of Community-Acquired Pneumonia, by Site of Care

	HOSPITALIZED PATIENTS	
OUTPATIENTS	**NON-ICU**	**ICU**
Streptococcus pneumoniae	*S. pneumoniae*	*S. pneumoniae*
Mycoplasma pneumoniae	*M. pneumoniae*	*Staphylococcus aureus*
Haemophilus influenzae	*Chlamydia pneumoniae*	*Legionella* spp.
C. pneumoniae	*H. influenzae*	Gram-negative bacilli
Respiratory viruses[a]	*Legionella* spp.	*H. influenzae*
	Respiratory viruses[a]	Respiratory viruses

[a]Influenza A and B viruses, human metapneumovirus, adenoviruses, respiratory syncytial viruses, parainfluenza viruses, coronaviruses (e.g., SARS-CoV-2).

Abbreviation: ICU, intensive care unit.

appear to be increasing, especially among young adults. Viruses are recognized as increasingly important in pneumonia, and polymerase chain reaction (PCR)–based testing indicates their presence in the respiratory tract of 20–30% of healthy adults and in the same percentage of pneumonia patients, including those who are severely ill. The most common are influenza, parainfluenza, and respiratory syncytial viruses. Whether they are true etiologic pathogens, co-pathogens, or simply colonizers cannot always be determined. Atypical organisms cannot be cultured on standard media or seen on Gram's stain, but their frequency and importance have significant implications for therapy. They are intrinsically resistant to all β-lactams and require treatment with a macrolide, a fluoroquinolone, or a tetracycline. In the 10–15% of CAP cases that are polymicrobial, the etiology usually includes a combination of typical and atypical pathogens.

Earlier literature suggested that aspiration pneumonia was caused primarily by anaerobes, with or without aerobic pathogens. A shift, however, has been noted recently: if aspiration pneumonia is acquired in a community or hospital setting, the likely pathogens are those usually associated with CAP or HAP. Anaerobes may still play a role, especially in patients with poor dentition, lung abscess, necrotizing pneumonia, or empyema.

S. aureus pneumonia is known to complicate influenza virus infection. However, MRSA has been reported as a primary etiologic agent of CAP. Although cases caused by MRSA are relatively uncommon, clinicians must be aware of its potentially serious consequences, such as necrotizing pneumonia. Two factors have led to this problem: the spread of MRSA from the hospital setting to the community and the emergence of genetically distinct strains of MRSA in the community. Community-associated MRSA (CA-MRSA) strains may infect healthy individuals who have had no association with health care.

Despite a careful history, physical examination, and radiographic studies, the causative pathogen is often difficult to predict with certainty, and in more than half of cases a specific etiology is not determined. Nevertheless, epidemiologic and risk factors may suggest certain pathogens (**Table 126-2**).

■ EPIDEMIOLOGY

More than 5 million CAP cases occur annually in the United States. Along with influenza, CAP is the eighth leading cause of death in this country. CAP causes more than 55,000 deaths annually and results in more than 1.2 million hospitalizations; ~70% of patients are treated as outpatients and 30% as inpatients. The mortality rate among outpatients is usually <5% but ranges from ~12% to 40% among hospitalized patients, with the exact rate depending on whether treatment takes place in or outside the intensive care unit (ICU). In the United States, CAP is the leading cause of death from infection among patients >65 years of age. Moreover, 18% of hospitalized CAP patients are readmitted within 1 month of discharge. The overall yearly CAP cost is estimated at $17 billion. The overall incidence among adults is ~16–23 cases per 1000 persons per year, with the highest rates at the extremes of age.

The risk factors for CAP in general and for pneumococcal pneumonia in particular have implications for treatment. They include

TABLE 126-2 Epidemiologic Factors Suggesting Possible Causes of Community-Acquired Pneumonia

FACTOR	POSSIBLE PATHOGEN(S)
Alcoholism	*Streptococcus pneumoniae*, oral anaerobes, *Klebsiella pneumoniae*, *Acinetobacter* spp., *Mycobacterium tuberculosis*
COPD and/or smoking	*Haemophilus influenzae*, *Pseudomonas aeruginosa*, *Legionella* spp., *S. pneumoniae*, *Moraxella catarrhalis*, *Chlamydia pneumoniae*
Structural lung disease (e.g., bronchiectasis)	*P. aeruginosa*, *Burkholderia cepacia*, *Staphylococcus aureus*
Dementia, stroke, decreased level of consciousness	Oral anaerobes, gram-negative enteric bacteria
Lung abscess	CA-MRSA, oral anaerobes, endemic fungi, *M. tuberculosis*, atypical mycobacteria
Travel to Ohio or St. Lawrence river valley	*Histoplasma capsulatum*
Travel to southwestern United States	Hantavirus, *Coccidioides* spp.
Travel to Southeast Asia	*Burkholderia pseudomallei*, avian influenza virus
Stay in hotel or on cruise ship in previous 2 weeks	*Legionella* spp.
Local influenza activity	Influenza virus, *S. pneumoniae*, *S. aureus*
Exposure to infected humans	SARS-CoV-2
Exposure to birds	*H. capsulatum*, *Chlamydia psittaci*
Exposure to rabbits	*Francisella tularensis*
Exposure to sheep, goats, parturient cats	*Coxiella burnetii*

Abbreviations: CA-MRSA, community-acquired methicillin-resistant *Staphylococcus aureus*; COPD, chronic obstructive pulmonary disease; SARS-CoV-2, severe acute respiratory syndrome coronavirus 2.

alcoholism, asthma, immunosuppression, institutionalization, and age >70 years. In the elderly, decreased cough and gag reflexes and reduced antibody and Toll-like receptor responses increase the likelihood of pneumonia. Risk factors for pneumococcal pneumonia include dementia, seizure disorders, heart failure, cerebrovascular disease, alcoholism, tobacco smoking, chronic obstructive pulmonary disease (COPD), and HIV infection. CA-MRSA pneumonia is more likely in patients with skin colonization or infection with CA-MRSA and after viral infection. Enterobacteriaceae tend to infect patients who have recently been hospitalized or given antibiotics or who have comorbidities such as alcoholism, heart failure, or renal failure. *P. aeruginosa* is a particular problem in patients with severe structural lung disease (e.g., bronchiectasis, cystic fibrosis, or severe COPD). Risk factors for *Legionella* infection include diabetes, hematologic malignancy, cancer, severe renal disease, HIV infection, smoking, male gender, and a recent hotel stay or trip on a cruise ship.

CLINICAL MANIFESTATIONS

The clinical presentation of pneumonia can vary from indolent to fulminant and from mild to fatal in severity. Manifestations of worsening severity include both constitutional findings and those limited to the lung and associated structures. The patient is frequently febrile and/or tachycardic and may experience chills and/or sweats. Cough may be nonproductive or productive of mucoid, purulent, or blood-tinged sputum. Gross hemoptysis is suggestive of necrotizing pneumonia (e.g., that due to CA-MRSA). Depending on severity, the patient may be able to speak in full sentences or may be short of breath. With pleural involvement, the patient may experience pleuritic chest pain. Up to 20% of patients may have gastrointestinal symptoms such as nausea, vomiting, or diarrhea. Other symptoms may include fatigue, headache, myalgias, and arthralgias.

Findings on physical examination vary with the degree of pulmonary consolidation and the presence or absence of a significant pleural effusion. An increased respiratory rate and use of accessory muscles of respiration are common. Palpation may reveal increased or decreased tactile fremitus, and the percussion note can vary from dull to flat, reflecting underlying consolidated lung and pleural fluid, respectively. Crackles, bronchial breath sounds, and possibly a pleural friction rub may be heard. The clinical presentation may be less obvious in the elderly, who may initially display new-onset or worsening confusion but few other manifestations. Severely ill patients may have septic shock and evidence of organ failure. In cases of CAP, symptoms can range from almost nonexistent to severe, and chest radiographic findings are often in gravity-dependent parts of the lung.

DIAGNOSIS

When confronted with possible CAP, the physician must ask two questions: is this pneumonia, and, if so, what is the likely pathogen? The former question is answered by clinical and radiographic methods, whereas the latter requires laboratory techniques.

Clinical Diagnosis The differential diagnosis includes infectious and noninfectious entities, including acute bronchitis, exacerbations of chronic bronchitis, heart failure, and pulmonary embolism. The importance of a careful history cannot be overemphasized. The diagnosis of CAP requires a compatible history, such as cough, sputum production, fever and dyspnea, and a new infiltrate on chest radiography.

Unfortunately, the sensitivity and specificity of findings on physical examination are only 58% and 67%, respectively. Chest radiography is often necessary to differentiate CAP from other conditions. Radiographic findings may suggest increased severity (e.g., cavitation or multilobar involvement). Occasionally, radiographic results suggest an etiologic diagnosis, such as pneumatoceles in *S. aureus* infection or an upper-lobe cavitating lesion in tuberculosis. CT may be of value in suspected loculated effusion or cavitary cases or in postobstructive pneumonia caused by a tumor or foreign body. For outpatients, clinical and radiologic assessments are usually all that is required before treatment is started since most laboratory results are not available soon enough to influence initial management. In certain cases, the availability of rapid point-of-care outpatient tests can be important; for example, rapid diagnosis of influenza infection can prompt specific anti-influenza treatment and secondary prevention measures.

Etiologic Diagnosis The etiology of pneumonia usually cannot be determined solely on the basis of clinical or radiographic presentation. Data from more than 17,000 emergency department CAP cases showed an etiologic determination in only 7.6%. Except for CAP patients admitted to the ICU, no data exist to show that treatment directed at a specific pathogen is statistically superior to empirical therapy. The benefit of establishing a microbial etiology may be questioned, particularly in light of the cost of diagnostic testing. However, a number of reasons exist for attempting an etiologic diagnosis. Identification of a specific or unexpected pathogen allows narrowing of the initial empirical regimen, with a consequent decrease in antibiotic selection pressure and in the risk of resistance. Pathogens with important public safety implications, such as *Mycobacterium tuberculosis* and influenza virus, may be found. Finally, without susceptibility data, trends in resistance cannot be followed accurately, and appropriate empirical therapeutic regimens are harder to devise.

GRAM'S STAIN AND CULTURE OF SPUTUM The main purpose of the sputum Gram's stain is to ensure suitability of a specimen for culture. (To be suitable, a sputum sample must have >25 neutrophils and <10 squamous epithelial cells per low-power field.) However, staining may also identify certain pathogens (e.g., *S. pneumoniae*, *S. aureus*, and gram-negative bacteria). The sensitivity and specificity of the sputum Gram's stain and culture are highly variable. Even in cases of proven bacteremic pneumococcal pneumonia, the yield of positive cultures from sputum is ≤50%.

Many patients, particularly elderly individuals, may be unable to produce an appropriate sputum sample. Others may be taking antibiotics that interfere with culture results. Inability to produce sputum can be caused by dehydration, whose correction may result in increased sputum production and a more obvious infiltrate on chest radiography. For patients admitted to the ICU and intubated, a deep-suction aspirate or bronchoalveolar lavage sample has a high yield on culture when sent to the laboratory as soon as possible. Since pathogens in severe and mild CAP may differ (Table 126-1), the greatest benefit of staining and culturing respiratory secretions is to alert the physician to unexpected and/or resistant pathogens and to permit appropriate modification of therapy. Other stains and cultures (e.g., for *M. tuberculosis* or fungi) may be useful as well. The sputum Gram's stain and culture are recommended only for hospitalized CAP patients, particularly those with severe cases or those with risks of MRSA or *P. aeruginosa* infection.

BLOOD CULTURES The yield from blood cultures, even when samples are collected before antibiotic therapy, is disappointingly low. Only 5–14% of cultures from hospitalized CAP patients are positive, and the most common pathogen is *S. pneumoniae.* Since recommended empirical regimens all provide pneumococcal coverage, a blood culture positive for this pathogen has little, if any, effect on clinical outcome. However, susceptibility data may allow narrowing of antibiotic therapy in appropriate cases. Because of the low yield and the lack of significant impact on outcome, blood cultures are not considered *de rigueur* for all hospitalized CAP patients. Certain high-risk patients should have blood cultured, including those with neutropenia secondary to pneumonia, asplenia, complement deficiencies, chronic liver disease, or severe CAP and those at risk of MRSA or *P. aeruginosa* infection.

URINARY ANTIGEN TESTS Two commercially available tests detect pneumococcal and *Legionella* antigen in urine. The *Legionella pneumophila* test detects only serogroup 1, which accounts for most community-acquired cases of Legionnaires' disease in the United States. The sensitivity and specificity of this antigen test are 70% and 99%, respectively. The pneumococcal urine antigen test also is quite sensitive and specific (70% and >90%, respectively). Although false-positive results can be obtained for pneumococcus-colonized children, the test is generally reliable. Both tests can detect antigen even after the initiation of appropriate antibiotic therapy. Testing of urine for pneumococcal antigen can be reserved for severe cases; *Legionella* antigen can be sought in severe cases and in situations where relevant epidemiologic factors are present.

POLYMERASE CHAIN REACTION PCR tests amplify a microorganism's DNA or RNA, and multiplex PCR panels test for a number of viral and bacterial pathogens. These tests dramatically improve response times, but the contamination of respiratory specimens by upper-airway flora may make semiquantitative or quantitative assays necessary for best results. PCR of nasopharyngeal swabs has become the standard for diagnosis of respiratory viral infection. PCR can also detect the nucleic acid of *Legionella* species, *M. pneumoniae, C. pneumoniae,* and mycobacteria. The cost-effectiveness of PCR testing, however, has not been definitively established.

SEROLOGY A fourfold rise in specific IgM antibody titer between acute- and convalescent-phase serum samples is generally considered diagnostic of infection with a particular pathogen. Until recently, serologic tests were used to help identify atypical pathogens as well as selected unusual organisms such as *Coxiella burnetii.* However, these tests have fallen out of favor because of the time required to obtain a final result for the convalescent-phase sample and the difficulty of interpretation.

BIOMARKERS Two of the most commonly used markers are C-reactive protein (CRP) and procalcitonin (PCT). Levels of these acute-phase reactants increase in the presence of an inflammatory response, particularly to bacterial pathogens. Nevertheless, PCT is insufficiently accurate for use in the diagnosis of bacterial CAP, and initial serum PCT levels should not be used as a basis for withholding initial antibiotic treatment. CRP is considered even less sensitive than PCT for detecting bacterial pathogens. Thus these tests should not be used alone but, in conjunction with findings from the history, physical examination, radiography, and laboratory tests, may facilitate antibiotic stewardship and appropriate management of seriously ill CAP patients.

TREATMENT

Community-Acquired Pneumonia

SITE OF CARE

The decision to hospitalize a patient with CAP has considerable implications. The cost of inpatient management exceeds that of outpatient treatment by a factor of 20, and hospitalization accounts for most CAP-related expenditures. However, late admission to the ICU is associated with increased mortality rates. The choice can be difficult: some patients can be managed at home, while others require hospitalization. Tools that objectively assess the risk of adverse outcomes, including severe illness and death, can help to minimize unnecessary hospital admissions. The two most frequently used rules are the Pneumonia Severity Index (PSI), a prognostic model that identifies patients at low risk of dying, and the CURB-65 criteria, which yield a severity-of-illness score.

To determine the PSI, points are given for 20 variables, including age, coexisting illness, and abnormal physical and laboratory findings. On the basis of the score, patients are assigned to one of five classes with these mortality rates: class 1, 0.1%; class 2, 0.6%; class 3, 2.8%; class 4, 8.2%; and class 5, 29.2%. Use of the PSI results in lower admission rates for class 1 and class 2 patients. Class 3 patients could ideally be admitted to an observation unit pending further decisions.

The CURB-65 criteria include five variables: confusion (C); urea >7 mmol/L (U); respiratory rate ≥30/min (R); blood pressure—systolic ≤90 mmHg or diastolic ≤60 mmHg (B); and an age of ≥65 years. Patients with a score of 0 (a 30-day mortality rate of 1.5%) can be treated as outpatients. With a score of 1 or 2, the patient should be hospitalized unless the score is entirely or in part attributable to an age of ≥65 years; in such cases, hospitalization may not be necessary. Among patients with scores of ≥3, mortality rates are 22% overall; these patients may require ICU admission. The PSI has greater efficacy than CURB-65 but is more difficult to calculate.

If a patient is unable to maintain oral intake, if compliance is thought to be an issue when assessed on the basis of mental condition or living situation (e.g., cognitive impairment or homelessness), or if the patient's O_2 saturation on room air is <92%, hospitalization is necessary. If these considerations do not apply, clinical judgment in conjunction with a prediction rule should be used to determine the site of care.

Neither PSI nor CURB-65 is accurate in determining the need for ICU admission. Patients with septic shock requiring vasopressors or with acute respiratory failure requiring intubation and mechanical ventilation should be admitted directly to an ICU **(Table 126-3)**, and those with three of the nine minor criteria listed in the latter table should be admitted to an ICU or a high-level monitoring unit. Mortality rates are higher among less ill patients who were admitted

TABLE 126-3 Criteria for Severe Community-Acquired Pneumonia

Minor criteria
Respiratory rate ≥30 breaths/min
PaO_2/FiO_2 ratio ≤250
Multilobar infiltrates
Confusion/disorientation
Uremia (BUN level ≥20 mg/dL)
Leukopenia (WBC count <4000 cells/μL)
Thrombocytopenia (platelet count <100,000 cells/μL)
Hypothermia (core temperature <36°C)
Hypotension requiring aggressive fluid resuscitation
Major criteria
Respiratory failure requiring invasive mechanical ventilation
Septic shock requiring vasopressors

Abbreviations: BUN, blood urea nitrogen; PaO_2/FiO_2, arterial oxygen pressure/fraction of inspired oxygen; WBC, white blood cell.

to a medical floor but then deteriorated than among equally ill patients initially monitored in the ICU.

ANTIBIOTIC RESISTANCE

Antimicrobial resistance is a significant problem that threatens to diminish our therapeutic armamentarium. Antibiotic misuse results in increased antibiotic selection pressure that can affect resistance locally and globally by clonal dissemination. For CAP, the main resistance issues currently involve *S. pneumoniae* and CA-MRSA.

S. pneumoniae In general, pneumococcal resistance to β-lactams is acquired by (1) direct DNA incorporation and remodeling of penicillin-binding proteins through contact with closely related oral commensal bacteria (e.g., viridans group streptococci), (2) the process of natural transformation, or (3) mutation of certain genes.

The *S. pneumoniae* minimal inhibitory concentration (MIC) breakpoint cutoffs for penicillin in pneumonia are ≤2 μg/mL for susceptible, >2–4 μg/mL for intermediate, and ≥8 μg/mL for resistant. A change in susceptibility thresholds dramatically decreased the proportion of pneumococcal isolates considered nonsusceptible. For meningitis, MIC thresholds remain at the former lower levels. Fortunately, resistance to penicillin appeared to plateau even before the change in MIC thresholds. Of isolates in the United States, <20% are resistant to penicillins and <1% to cephalosporins. Risk factors for penicillin-resistant pneumococcal infection include recent antimicrobial therapy, an age of <2 or >65 years, attendance at a day-care center, recent hospitalization, and HIV infection.

In contrast to penicillin resistance, macrolide resistance is increasing in *S. pneumoniae* through several mechanisms. *Target-site modification* caused by ribosomal methylation in 23S rRNA encoded by the *ermB* gene results in high-level resistance (MIC, ≥64 μg/mL) to macrolides, lincosamides, and streptogramin B–type antibiotics. The *efflux mechanism* encoded by the *mef* gene (*M phenotype*) is usually associated with low-level resistance (MIC, 1–32 μg/mL). These two mechanisms account for ~40% and ~60%, respectively, of resistant pneumococcal isolates in the United States. High-level resistance to macrolides is more common in Europe, whereas lower-level resistance predominates in North America. The prevalence of macrolide-resistant *S. pneumoniae* exceeds 25% in some countries; in Canada the prevalence is ~22%, and in the United States it exceeds 30%. Much of this resistance is high-level, and failures of treatment may result in such cases. In these situations, a macrolide should not be used as empirical monotherapy. Estimates of the prevalence of doxycycline resistance in the United States are generally <20%.

The rate of pneumococcal resistance to fluoroquinolones (e.g., ciprofloxacin, moxifloxacin, and levofloxacin) is usually <2%. Changes can occur in one or both target sites (topoisomerases II and IV); these changes are attributable to mutations in the *gyrA* and *parC* genes, respectively. In addition, an efflux pump may play a role in pneumococcal resistance to fluoroquinolones.

Isolates resistant to drugs from three or more antimicrobial classes with different mechanisms of action are considered MDR strains. The propensity for an association of pneumococcal resistance to penicillin with reduced susceptibility to other drugs, such as macrolides, tetracyclines, and trimethoprim-sulfamethoxazole, is of concern. In the United States, 58.9% of penicillin-resistant pneumococcal blood isolates are also resistant to macrolides.

The most important risk factor for antibiotic-resistant pneumococcal infection is use of a specific antibiotic within the previous 3 months. A history of prior antibiotic treatment is a critical factor in avoiding the use of an inappropriate antibiotic.

CA-MRSA CAP due to MRSA may be caused by the classic hospital-acquired strains or by genotypically and phenotypically distinct community-acquired strains. Most infections with the former have been acquired either directly or indirectly during contact with the health care environment. However, in some hospitals, CA-MRSA strains are displacing the classic hospital-acquired strains; this change suggests that the newer community-acquired strains may be more robust.

Methicillin resistance in *S. aureus* is determined by the *mecA* gene, which encodes for resistance to all β-lactam drugs. At least five staphylococcal chromosomal cassette *mec* (SCC*mec*) types have been described. The typical hospital-acquired strain usually has a type II or III SCC*mec* element, whereas CA-MRSA has type IV. CA-MRSA isolates tend to be less resistant than the older hospital-acquired strains and are often susceptible to trimethoprim-sulfamethoxazole, clindamycin, and tetracycline in addition to vancomycin and linezolid. However, the most important distinction is that CA-MRSA strains also carry genes for superantigens such as enterotoxins B and C and Panton-Valentine leukocidin; the latter is a membrane-tropic toxin that can create cytolytic pores in neutrophils, monocytes, and macrophages.

M. pneumoniae Macrolide-resistant *M. pneumoniae* has been reported in a number of countries, including Germany (3%), Japan (30%), China (95%), and France and the United States (5–13%). *Mycoplasma* resistance to macrolides is increasing as a result of binding-site mutation in domain V of 23S rRNA.

Gram-Negative Bacilli A detailed discussion of resistance among gram-negative bacilli is beyond the scope of this chapter (**see Chap. 161**). Fluoroquinolone resistance among community isolates of *Escherichia coli* is increasing. *Enterobacter* species are typically resistant to cephalosporins, and the drugs of choice for use against these organisms are usually fluoroquinolones or carbapenems. Similarly, when infections due to bacteria producing extended-spectrum β-lactamases (ESBLs) are documented or suspected, a carbapenem should be considered.

INITIAL ANTIBIOTIC MANAGEMENT

Since the etiology of CAP is rarely known at the outset of treatment, initial therapy is usually empirical and designed to cover the likeliest pathogens. In all cases, treatment should be initiated as expeditiously as possible. New CAP treatment guidelines in the United States have been presented in a joint statement from the American Thoracic Society (ATS) and the Infectious Diseases Society of America (IDSA). These guidelines consider the likely pathogens, risk of antimicrobial resistance, severity of illness, site of care, and risk of infection with specific bacteria such as MRSA and *P. aeruginosa* (**Fig. 126-1, Tables 126-4** and **126-5**). In the figure and the tables, the antibiotics are not listed in order of preference.

The approach to treatment of aspiration pneumonia is based upon a number of factors, including site of acquisition (community

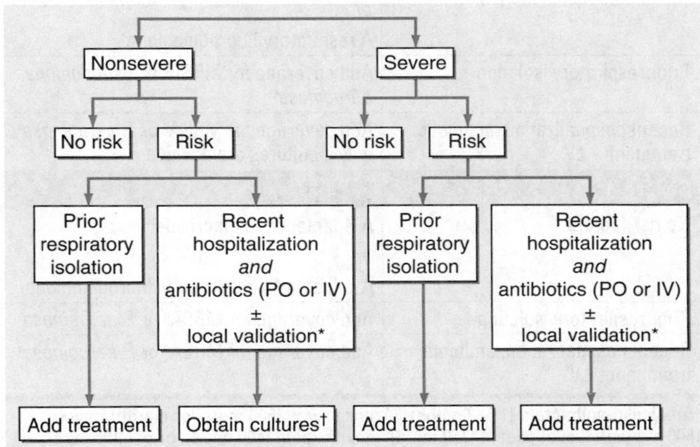

FIGURE 126-1 Algorithm for assessment of inpatient risk of infection with MRSA or *Pseudomonas aeruginosa*. Underlying lung disease (e.g., bronchiectasis or very severe COPD) are also risks for *P. aeruginosa* infection. *Local validation consists of information on local prevalence, resistance, and risk factors. †Can also use MRSA rapid nasal PCR if available.

TABLE 126-4 Initial Treatment Strategies for Outpatients with Community-Acquired Pneumonia

STATUS	STANDARD REGIMEN
No comorbidities or risk factors for antibiotic resistance[a]	Combination therapy with amoxicillin (1 g tid) + either a macrolide[b] or doxycycline (100 mg bid)
	Or
	Monotherapy with doxycycline (100 mg bid)
	Or
	Monotherapy with a macrolide[b,c]
With comorbidities[d] ± risk factors for antibiotic resistance[a]	Combination therapy with
	amoxicillin/clavulanate[e] or a cephalosporin[f] + either a macrolide[b] or doxycycline (100 mg bid)
	Or
	Monotherapy with a respiratory fluoroquinolone[g]

[a]Antibiotic treatment within the past 3 months or contact with the health care system. [b]Azithromycin (500 mg on day 1, then 250 mg/d for 4 days), clarithromycin (500 mg bid), or clarithromycin ER (1000 mg/d). [c]If local prevalence of pneumococcal resistance is <25%. [d]Including chronic heart, lung, liver, or kidney disease; diabetes mellitus; alcoholism; malignancy; or asplenia. [e]500/125 mg tid or 875/125 mg bid. [f]Cefpodoxime (200 mg bid) or cefuroxime (500 mg bid). [g]Levofloxacin (750 mg/d), moxifloxacin (400 mg/d), or gemifloxacin (320 mg/d).

vs hospital), normal or abnormal chest radiograph, and additional variables such as illness severity, state of dentition, and risk of infection with an MDR pathogen. Routine coverage of anaerobes is unnecessary unless dentition is poor or there is a lung abscess or necrotizing pneumonia.

Our approach to the treatment of CAP (Tables 126-4 and 126-5) is very similar to that proposed in the new CAP guidelines with the exceptions listed below.

Outpatients The exceptions to the CAP guidelines that we follow in treating patients are:

- We usually initiate coverage that includes atypical organisms as well as *S. pneumoniae*.
- Generally, we do not consider the risk of infection with *P. aeruginosa* or MRSA particularly significant in outpatients.
- Prior antibiotic use should include both oral and parenteral agents.

TABLE 126-5 Initial Treatment for Inpatients with or without Risk Factors for Infection with MRSA or *Pseudomonas aeruginosa*

DISEASE SEVERITY, RISK STATUS	REGIMEN
Nonsevere	
No risk factors	A β-lactam[a] + a macrolide[b]
	or
	A respiratory fluoroquinolone[c]
Prior respiratory isolation	Add coverage for MRSA[d] or *Pseudomonas aeruginosa*[e]
Recent hospitalization, antibiotic treatment, ± LV[f]	Add coverage for MRSA[d] or *P. aeruginosa*[e] only if cultures are positive
Severe	
No risk factors	A β-lactam[a] + a macrolide[b]
	or
	A β-lactam[a] + respiratory fluoroquinolone[c]
Prior respiratory isolation	Add coverage for MRSA[d] or *P. aeruginosa*[e]
Recent hospitalization, antibiotic treatment ± LV[f]	Add coverage for MRSA[d] or *P. aeruginosa*[e]

[a]Ampicillin-sulbactam (1.5–3 g q6h). [b]Azithromycin (500 mg/d) or clarithromycin (500 mg bid). [c]Levofloxacin (750 mg/d), moxifloxacin (400 mg/d), or gemifloxacin (320 mg/d). [d]Vancomycin (15 mg/kg q12h, with adjustment based on serum levels) or linezolid (600 mg q12h). [e]Piperacillin-tazobactam (4.5 g q6h), cefepime (2 g q8h), ceftazidime (2 g q8h), imipenem (500 mg q6h), meropenem (1 g q8h), or aztreonam (2 g q8h). [f]Obtain cultures. MRSA rapid nasal PCR can also be used if available.

Abbreviations: LV, local validation (local prevalence, resistance, risk factors); MRSA, methicillin-resistant *Staphylococcus aureus*.

Patients are stratified into two groups: those without comorbidity or risk factors for antibiotic resistance and those with comorbidities (e.g., chronic heart, lung, liver, or kidney disease; diabetes; alcoholism; malignancy; or asplenia) with or without risk factors for resistance (Table 126-4). As a general rule, if patients have been treated with a drug from a particular class of antibiotics within the previous 3 months, drugs from a different class should be used to minimize resistance issues.

For those without comorbidity or resistance risk factors, amoxicillin alone or doxycycline is recommended in the recent guidelines. Monotherapy with amoxicillin is based on evidence of its efficacy in the treatment of hospitalized CAP patients. This recommendation is a change from that in the 2007 IDSA/ATS CAP guidelines. As a rule, however, we usually tend to initiate treatment that includes coverage for S. *pneumoniae* as well as the atypical pathogens (Table 126-4).

Monotherapy with a macrolide is recommended in the new guidelines only if there are contraindications to amoxicillin or doxycycline and there is documented low risk of macrolide resistance (<25%). Otherwise, the treatment of outpatients is quite similar to the regimens recommended in the 2007 IDSA/ATS guidelines.

Inpatients Our exceptions to the recommendations in the CAP guidelines are:

- As a general rule, when initiating treatment for infection with *P. aeruginosa*, we use double coverage.
- The presence of all three risk factors is not required for drug resistance (recent hospitalization, recent oral or IV antibiotic treatment, ± local validation) (Fig. 126-1, Table 126-5).

The main considerations for determining initial empirical treatment of hospitalized CAP patients are clinical severity and risk factors for infection with drug-resistant pathogens such as MRSA or *P. aeruginosa*. Hospitalization alone is not now considered a significant risk factor for these pathogens. Hospitals should collect local data on MRSA and *P. aeruginosa* with regard to prevalence, risk factors for infection, and antibiotic susceptibilities. Patients can be categorized as having nonsevere or severe CAP (Table 126-3), and those in each of these categories may or may not have risk factors for MRSA or *P. aeruginosa* (Fig. 126-1). In the scenarios involving these variables in hospitalized CAP patients, empirical treatment for either of these pathogens should be added to standard therapy unless a patient's illness is considered nonsevere and the risk factors are recent hospitalization and antibiotic treatment ± local validation data (Fig. 126-1). Depending upon the patient, we may begin treatment in this situation and then de-escalate it if appropriate. In such cases, cultures should be performed but treatment usually withheld unless the culture results or the rapid nasal PCR results for MRSA are positive.

Nonsevere, No Risk Factors For patients with nonsevere infection and no risk factors, treatment should consist of either a combination of a β-lactam and a macrolide or monotherapy with a respiratory fluoroquinolone (Table 126-5). In the event of contraindications to macrolides and fluoroquinolones, a β-lactam together with doxycycline may be used. Treatment with a combination of a β-lactam and a macrolide or a fluoroquinolone alone results in lower mortality than monotherapy with a β-lactam.

Severe, No Risk Factors Patients with severe infection but no risk factors should receive combination therapy with either a β-lactam and a macrolide or a β-lactam and a respiratory fluoroquinolone (Table 126-5).

Nonsevere and Severe, with Risk Factors To date, there are no prediction rules reliably identifying patients who should be started empirically on treatment for MRSA or *P. aeruginosa*. Current risk factors for infection with these pathogens are hierarchical. Prior isolation of these organisms, especially from the respiratory tract within the previous year, is a more robust risk factor than recent hospitalization and exposure to parenteral antibiotics. For

P. aeruginosa, underlying lung disease (e.g., bronchiectasis or very severe COPD) also is an important risk factor. If MRSA or *P. aeruginosa* has been isolated previously, appropriate empirical therapy should be started in both severe and nonsevere cases (Table 126-5). We prefer linezolid over vancomycin as first-line treatment for MRSA because of its inhibition of bacterial exotoxin and its better lung penetration. If the organism is not isolated from respiratory secretions or blood and/or the nasal or bronchoalveolar lavage PCR test for MRSA is negative and the patient is improving at 48 h, treatment may be de-escalated to a standard regimen.

If, on the other hand, the risk factors are recent hospitalization and antibiotic use within the previous 3 months, appropriate samples should be obtained for culture, and, in severe cases, extended-spectrum treatment for MRSA or *P. aeruginosa* should be initiated. Depending upon the severity of infection, local data on *P. aeruginosa* resistance, and antibiotic use within the previous 90 days, single- or double-drug coverage should be used.

If two antipseudomonal agents are started, the drugs should not be from the same class. Whenever possible, assessment for possible de-escalation of therapy is urged. If the patient's illness is not severe, empirical extended treatment should be withheld until culture results are available.

Regardless of the site of care, CAP patients testing positive for influenza should be given anti-influenza treatment (e.g., oseltamivir) as well as appropriate antibacterial therapy. Physicians should be vigilant about possible superinfection with MRSA.

Although hospitalized patients have traditionally received initial therapy by the IV route, some drugs, particularly the fluoroquinolones, are very well absorbed and may be given orally from the outset to select patients. For those initially treated with IV agents, a switch to oral treatment is appropriate when the patient can ingest and absorb the drugs, is hemodynamically stable, and is showing clinical improvement. A 5-day course of treatment is usually sufficient for uncomplicated CAP, but longer treatment may be required for patients who have not stabilized clinically and for those with bacteremia, metastatic infection, or infection with a more virulent pathogen such as *P. aeruginosa* or MRSA.

ADJUNCTIVE MEASURES

In addition to appropriate antimicrobial therapy, certain adjunctive measures should be used. Adequate hydration, oxygen therapy for hypoxemia, vasopressor treatment, and assisted ventilation when necessary are critical to successful treatment. Routine use of glucocorticoids is not recommended for CAP except in patients with refractory septic shock.

FAILURE TO IMPROVE

Patients slow to respond to therapy should be reevaluated at about day 3 (sooner if their condition is worsening), with several scenarios considered. A number of noninfectious conditions mimic pneumonia, including pulmonary edema, pulmonary embolism, lung carcinoma, radiation and hypersensitivity pneumonitis, and connective tissue disease involving the lungs. If the patient truly has CAP and empirical treatment is aimed at the correct pathogen, lack of response may be explained in a number of ways. The pathogen may be resistant to the drug selected, or a sequestered focus (e.g., lung abscess or empyema) may prevent antibiotic access to the pathogen. The patient may be getting the wrong drug or the correct drug at the wrong dose or frequency of administration. Another possibility is that CAP has been diagnosed correctly but an unexpected pathogen (e.g., CA-MRSA, *M. tuberculosis*, or a fungus) is the cause. Nosocomial superinfections—both pulmonary and extrapulmonary—are other possible explanations for a hospitalized patient's failure to improve. In all cases of delayed response or worsening condition, the patient must be carefully reassessed and appropriate studies initiated, possibly including CT or bronchoscopy.

COMPLICATIONS

Complications of severe CAP include respiratory failure, shock and multiorgan failure, and exacerbation of comorbid illnesses. Three particularly noteworthy conditions are metastatic infection, lung abscess, and complicated pleural effusion. Metastatic infection (e.g., brain abscess or endocarditis) is unusual and requires a high degree of suspicion and a detailed workup for proper treatment. Lung abscess may occur in association with aspiration pneumonia or with infection caused by pathogens such as CA-MRSA, *P. aeruginosa*, or (rarely) *S. pneumoniae*. A significant pleural effusion should be tapped for both diagnostic and therapeutic purposes. If the fluid has a pH <7.2, a glucose level of <2.2 mmol/L, and a lactate dehydrogenase concentration of >1000 U/L or if bacteria are seen or cultured, drainage is needed.

FOLLOW-UP

Fever and leukocytosis usually resolve within 2–4 days in otherwise healthy patients with CAP, but physical findings may persist longer. Chest radiographic abnormalities are slowest to resolve (4–12 weeks), with the speed of clearance depending on the patient's age and underlying lung disease. Patients may be discharged from the hospital once their clinical condition, including any comorbidity, is stable. The site of residence after discharge (nursing home, home with family, home alone) is an important consideration, particularly for elderly patients. For a hospitalized patient, we generally recommend a follow-up radiograph ~4–6 weeks later. If relapse or recurrence is documented, particularly in the same lung segment, the possibility of an underlying neoplasm must be considered. For individuals managed as outpatients, routine follow-up chest radiography is not necessary if they are nonsmokers, if they are otherwise well, and if their symptoms resolved within 5–7 days.

PROGNOSIS

The prognosis depends on the patient's age, comorbidities, and site of treatment (inpatient or outpatient). Young patients without comorbidity do well and usually recover fully after ~2 weeks. Older patients and those with comorbid conditions may take several weeks longer to recover fully. The overall mortality rate for the outpatient group is <5%. For patients requiring hospitalization, overall mortality ranges from 12% to 40%, depending on the category of patient and the processes of care, particularly the timely administration of appropriate antibiotics.

PREVENTION

The main preventive measure is vaccination (**Chap. 123**). Recommendations of the Advisory Committee on Immunization Practices should be followed for influenza and pneumococcal vaccines.

A pneumococcal polysaccharide vaccine (PPSV23) and a protein conjugate pneumococcal vaccine (PCV13) are available in the United States (**Chap. 146**). The former contains capsular material from 23 pneumococcal serotypes; in the latter, capsular polysaccharide from 13 of the most common pneumococcal pathogens affecting children is linked to an immunogenic protein. PCV13 produces T-cell–dependent antigens, resulting in long-term immunologic memory. Administration of this vaccine to children has led to a decrease in the prevalence of antimicrobial-resistant pneumococci and in the incidence of invasive pneumococcal disease among both children and adults. However, vaccination can result in the replacement of vaccine with nonvaccine serotypes, as seen with serotypes 19A and 35B following introduction of the original 7-valent conjugate vaccine. PCV13 is also recommended for the elderly and for younger immunocompromised patients. Because of an increased risk of pneumococcal infection, even among patients without obstructive lung disease, smokers should be strongly encouraged to quit.

The influenza vaccine is available in an inactivated or recombinant form. During an influenza outbreak, unprotected patients at risk from complications should be vaccinated immediately and given chemoprophylaxis with either oseltamivir or zanamivir for 2 weeks—i.e., until vaccine-induced antibody levels are sufficiently high.

VENTILATOR-ASSOCIATED PNEUMONIA

Research on hospital-acquired pneumonia has focused on VAP. However, the same information and principles can also be applied to ventilated HAP and to non-ICU HAP. Approximately 70% of HAP cases are acquired outside the ICU and 30% in the ICU; the fact that 30% of all HAP patients need mechanical ventilation defines ventilated HAP as a distinct entity. In non-intubated patients with HAP, an expectorated sputum sample is used for microbiologic diagnosis, but results are confounded by frequent colonization by oral pathogens. Microbiologic information in VAP and ventilated HAP is obtained from direct access to deep lower respiratory tract samples, which provide reliable microbiologic data; however, these samples can also contain colonizing pathogens.

■ ETIOLOGY

Potential etiologic agents of VAP include both MDR and non-MDR bacterial pathogens (**Table 126-6**). The non-MDR group of "core pathogens" is nearly identical to the pathogens found in severe CAP (Table 126-1); it is not surprising that such pathogens predominate if VAP develops in the first 5–7 days of the hospital stay. However, if patients have other risk factors (particularly prior antibiotic treatment), MDR pathogens are a consideration, even early in the hospital course. The relative frequency of individual MDR pathogens can vary significantly from hospital to hospital and even between different critical care units within the same institution. Most hospitals have problems with *P. aeruginosa* and MRSA, but other MDR pathogens are often institution-specific. Less commonly, fungal and viral pathogens cause VAP, usually affecting severely immunocompromised patients. Rarely, community-associated viruses cause mini-epidemics, usually when introduced by ill health care workers.

■ EPIDEMIOLOGY

Pneumonia is a common complication among patients requiring mechanical ventilation. Prevalence estimates vary between 6 and 52 cases per 100 patients, depending on the population studied. On any given day in the ICU, an average of 10% of patients will have pneumonia—VAP in the overwhelming majority of cases, although in recent years the frequency of this infection is declining as a result of effective prevention strategies. The frequency of diagnosis is not static but changes with the duration of mechanical ventilation, with the highest hazard ratio in the first 5 days and a plateau in additional cases (1% per day) after ~2 weeks. However, the cumulative rate among patients who remain ventilated for as long as 30 days is as high as 70%. These rates often do not reflect the recurrence of VAP in the same patient. Once a ventilated patient is transferred to a chronic-care facility or to home, the incidence of pneumonia drops significantly, especially in the absence of other risk factors for pneumonia. However, in chronic ventilator units, purulent tracheobronchitis becomes a significant issue, often interfering with efforts to wean patients off mechanical ventilation (**Chap. 302**).

Three factors are critical in the pathogenesis of VAP: colonization of the oropharynx with pathogenic microorganisms, aspiration of these organisms from the oropharynx into the lower respiratory tract, and compromise of normal host defense mechanisms. Most risk factors and their corresponding prevention strategies pertain to one of these three factors (**Table 126-7**).

TABLE 126-6 Microbiologic Causes of Ventilator-Associated Pneumonia

NON-MDR PATHOGENS	MDR PATHOGENS
Streptococcus pneumoniae	*Pseudomonas aeruginosa*
Other *Streptococcus* spp.	Methicillin-resistant *S. aureus*
Haemophilus influenzae	*Acinetobacter* spp.
Methicillin-sensitive *Staphylococcus aureus*	Antibiotic-resistant Enterobacteriaceae
Antibiotic-sensitive Enterobacteriaceae	ESBL-positive strains
	Carbapenem-resistant strains
Escherichia coli	*Legionella pneumophila*
Klebsiella pneumoniae	*Burkholderia cepacia*
Proteus spp.	*Aspergillus* spp.
Enterobacter spp.	
Serratia marcescens	

Abbreviations: ESBL, extended-spectrum β-lactamase; MDR, multidrug-resistant.

TABLE 126-7 Pathogenic Mechanisms and Corresponding Prevention Strategies for Ventilator-Associated Pneumonia

PATHOGENIC MECHANISM	PREVENTION STRATEGY
Oropharyngeal colonization with pathogenic bacteria	
Elimination of normal flora, overgrowth by pathogenic bacteria	Avoidance of prolonged antibiotic courses; consider oral chlorhexidine[a]
Large-volume oropharyngeal aspiration around time of intubation	Short course of prophylactic antibiotics for comatose patients[b]
Gastroesophageal reflux	Postpyloric enteral feeding with orally placed feeding tube[a]; avoidance of high gastric residuals, prokinetic agents
Bacterial overgrowth of stomach	Avoidance of prophylactic agents that raise gastric pH[a]; selective decontamination of digestive tract with nonabsorbable antibiotics[a]
Cross-infection from other colonized patients	Hand washing, especially with alcohol-based hand rub; intensive infection control education[b]; isolation; proper cleaning of reusable equipment
Large-volume aspiration	Endotracheal intubation; rapid-sequence intubation technique; avoidance of sedation; decompression of small-bowel obstruction
Ventilator circuit humidification	Change ventilator circuits only when soiled and with new patient; drain ventilator circuit condensate away from patient; replace heat moisture exchanger every 5–7 days or if soiled or malfunctioning[a]
Microaspiration around endotracheal tube	
Endotracheal intubation	Noninvasive ventilation[b]
Prolonged duration of ventilation	Daily awakening from sedation,[b] weaning protocols[b]
Abnormal swallowing function	Early percutaneous tracheostomy[b]
Secretions pooled above endotracheal tube	Head of bed elevated[b]; continuous aspiration of subglottic secretions with specialized endotracheal tube[b]; avoidance of reintubation; minimization of sedation and patient transport; prophylactic PEEP[c] of 5–8 cm
Altered lower respiratory host defenses	Tight glycemic control[a]; lowering of hemoglobin transfusion threshold

[a]Strategies with negative randomized trials or conflicting results. [b]Strategies demonstrated to be effective in at least one randomized controlled trial. [c]Positive end-expiratory pressure.

The most obvious risk factor is the endotracheal tube, which bypasses the normal mechanical factors preventing aspiration. While the presence of an endotracheal tube may prevent large-volume aspiration, microaspiration is actually exacerbated by secretions pooling above the cuff. The endotracheal tube and the concomitant need for suctioning can damage the tracheal mucosa, thereby facilitating tracheal colonization. In addition, pathogenic bacteria can form a glycocalyx biofilm on the tube's surface that protects them from both antibiotics and host defenses. The bacteria can also be dislodged during suctioning (done preferably with a closed catheter system) and can reinoculate the trachea, or tiny fragments of a glycocalyx can embolize to distal airways, carrying bacteria with them. The ventilator circuit tubing can harbor pathogenic organisms that can wash back to the patient if manipulated too often; thus circuits are changed only when soiled and with each new patient. Heat moisture exchangers are changed every 5–7 days or if visibly soiled or malfunctioning.

In a high percentage of critically ill patients, the normal oropharyngeal flora is replaced by pathogenic microorganisms. The most important risk factors are antibiotic selection pressure, cross-infection from other infected/colonized patients or contaminated equipment, severe systemic illness, and malnutrition. Of these factors, antibiotic exposure poses the greatest risk by far. Pathogens such as *P. aeruginosa* almost never cause infection in patients without prior exposure to antibiotics. The recent emphasis on hand hygiene has lowered the cross-infection rate.

Almost all intubated patients experience microaspiration and are at least transiently colonized with pathogenic bacteria. However, only around one-third of colonized patients develop VAP. Colony counts increase to high levels, sometimes days before the development of clinical pneumonia; these increases suggest that the final step in VAP development, independent of aspiration and oropharyngeal colonization, is the overwhelming of host defenses by a large bacterial inoculum. Severely ill patients with sepsis and trauma appear to enter a state of immunoparalysis several days after admission to the ICU—a time that corresponds to the greatest risk of developing VAP. The mechanism of this immunosuppression is not clear, although hyperglycemia and frequent transfusions adversely affect the immune response.

■ CLINICAL MANIFESTATIONS

The clinical manifestations of HAP and VAP are nonspecific: fever, leukocytosis, increased respiratory secretions, and pulmonary consolidation on physical examination, along with a new or changing radiographic infiltrate. The frequency of abnormal chest radiographs before the onset of pneumonia in intubated patients and the limitations of portable radiographic technique make interpretation of radiographs more difficult than in patients who are not intubated. Other clinical features may include tachypnea, tachycardia, worsening oxygenation, and increased minute ventilation. Serial changes in oxygenation may identify pneumonia earlier than other findings and may also be a means to monitor improvement with therapy.

■ DIAGNOSIS

No single set of criteria is reliably diagnostic of pneumonia in a ventilated patient. The inability to accurately identify such patients compromises efforts to prevent and treat VAP and even calls into question estimates of the impact of VAP on mortality rates.

Application of the clinical criteria typical for CAP consistently results in overdiagnosis of VAP, largely because of (1) frequent tracheal colonization with pathogenic bacteria in patients with endotracheal tubes, (2) multiple alternative causes of radiographic infiltrates in mechanically ventilated patients, and (3) the high frequency of other sources of fever in critically ill patients. The differential diagnosis of VAP includes atypical pulmonary edema, pulmonary contusion, alveolar hemorrhage, hypersensitivity pneumonitis, acute respiratory distress syndrome, and pulmonary infarction. Findings of fever and/or leukocytosis may have alternative causes, including antibiotic-associated diarrhea, central line–associated infection, sinusitis, urinary tract infection, pancreatitis, and drug fever. Conditions mimicking pneumonia are often documented in patients in whom VAP has been ruled out by accurate diagnostic techniques. Most of these alternative diagnoses do not require antibiotic treatment; require antibiotics different from those used to treat VAP (fungal or viral pneumonia); or require some additional intervention, such as surgical drainage or catheter removal, for optimal management.

This diagnostic dilemma has led to debate and controversy about whether a quantitative-culture approach as a means of eliminating false-positive clinical diagnoses is superior to a clinical approach enhanced by principles learned from quantitative-culture studies. The most recent IDSA/ATS guidelines for HAP/VAP give a weak recommendation for a clinical approach based on semiquantitative cultures, with consideration of the availability of resources, cost, and the availability of expertise. The guidelines acknowledge that the use of a quantitative approach may result in less antibiotic use, which may be critical for antibiotic stewardship in the ICU. Therefore, the approach at each institution—or potentially for each patient—should be individualized and based on local colonization rates, local diagnostic expertise, and recent history of antibiotic therapy.

Quantitative-Culture Approach This method uses quantitative cultures of deep respiratory tract samples to distinguish colonization from true infection. The more distal in the respiratory tree the diagnostic sampling, the more specific the results and therefore the lower the threshold of growth necessary to diagnose pneumonia and exclude colonization. For example, a quantitative endotracheal aspirate yields proximal samples, and the diagnostic threshold is 10^6 cfu/mL. The protected specimen brush method, in contrast, collects distal samples and has a threshold of 10^3 cfu/mL. Conversely, sensitivity declines as more distal secretions are obtained, especially when they are collected blindly (i.e., by a technique other than bronchoscopy). Additional tests that may increase the diagnostic yield include Gram's staining, differential cell counts, staining for intracellular organisms, and detection of local protein levels elevated in response to infection.

If the quantitative approach is used, therapy decisions should be linked to culture results, with antibiotics withheld until results are available unless the patient is critically ill. Studies have documented less antibiotic use with this approach than with the clinical approach, but the results are less clear if antibiotic decisions are not directly linked to culture data. One common limitation of the quantitative approach is the use of a new and effective antibiotic agent in the 24–48 h prior to sampling, which can lead to false-negative results. With sensitive microorganisms, a single antibiotic dose can reduce colony counts below the diagnostic threshold. After 3 days, the operating characteristics of the tests improve to the point at which they are equivalent to results obtained when no prior antibiotic therapy has been given. Conversely, colony counts above the diagnostic threshold during antibiotic therapy suggest that the current antibiotics are ineffective. In addition, quantitative cultures may give results below the diagnostic threshold if samples are collected early in the course of infection or if sampling is delayed until after an effective host response has reduced bacterial counts. Ideally, a specimen should be obtained as soon as pneumonia is suspected and before antibiotic therapy is initiated or changed.

Clinical Approach The lack of specificity of a clinical diagnosis of VAP has hampered its utility, but this approach has been improved by the addition of microbiologic and other laboratory data. Tracheal aspirates generally yield at least twice as many potential pathogens as quantitative cultures, but the causative pathogen is almost always present. The absence of bacteria in Gram-stained endotracheal aspirates makes pneumonia an unlikely cause of fever or pulmonary infiltrates. These findings, coupled with a heightened awareness of the alternative diagnoses possible in patients with suspected VAP, can prevent inappropriate antibiotic overtreatment. Furthermore, the absence of an MDR pathogen in tracheal aspirate cultures eliminates the need for MDR coverage, allowing de-escalation of empirical antibiotic therapy. Similarly, with newer and more sensitive molecular diagnostic methods, a suspected MDR pathogen can be eliminated as a therapy target if test results are negative. A clinical approach that focuses on careful antimicrobial use and de-escalation of therapy after culture results become available may have an impact on the avoidance of antimicrobial overuse and the consideration of alternative sites of infection similar to that of a quantitative-culture approach.

TREATMENT

Ventilator-Associated Pneumonia

Many studies have demonstrated higher mortality rates with the delay of initially appropriate empirical antibiotic therapy. The key to appropriate antibiotic management of VAP is an appreciation of the resistance patterns of the most likely pathogens in a given patient.

ANTIBIOTIC RESISTANCE

Because of a higher risk of infection with MDR pathogens (Table 126-6), VAP is treated with antibiotics different from those used for severe CAP. Antibiotic selection pressure leads to the frequent involvement of MDR pathogens by selecting either for drug-resistant isolates of common pathogens (MRSA and Enterobacteriaceae producing ESBLs or carbapenemases) or for intrinsically resistant pathogens (*P. aeruginosa* and *Acinetobacter* species). Frequent use of β-lactam drugs, especially cephalosporins, appears to be the major risk factor for infection with MRSA and ESBL-positive strains.

P. aeruginosa can develop resistance to all routinely used antibiotics, and, even if initially sensitive, *P. aeruginosa* isolates may develop resistance during treatment. Either derepression of resistance genes or selection of resistant clones within the large bacterial inoculum associated with most pneumonias may be the cause. *Acinetobacter* species, *Stenotrophomonas maltophilia*, and *Burkholderia cepacia* are intrinsically resistant to many of the empirical antibiotic regimens employed (see below). VAP caused by these pathogens emerges during treatment of other infections, and resistance is always evident at initial diagnosis.

EMPIRICAL THERAPY

Recommended options for empirical therapy are listed in **Table 126-8.** Treatment should be started once diagnostic specimens have been obtained. The major factors in the selection of agents are the presence of risk factors for MDR pathogens and the predicted risk of death (≤15% is considered low risk). Choices among the various options listed depend on local patterns of resistance and—a very important factor—the patient's prior antibiotic exposure. Knowledge of the local hospital's—and even the specific ICU's—antibiogram and the local incidence of specific MDR pathogens (e.g., MRSA) is critical in selecting appropriate empirical therapy.

The majority of patients *without* risk factors for MDR infection can be treated with a single agent. In fact, mortality is lower with a single agent than with combination therapy for those with a low mortality risk. Unfortunately, the proportion of patients with no MDR risk factors is <10% in some ICUs and is unknown for HAP patients. The major difference from CAP is the markedly lower incidence of atypical pathogens in VAP; the exception is *Legionella*, which can be a nosocomial pathogen, especially with local epidemics due to breakdowns in the treatment of potable water in the hospital. The standard recommendation for patients *with* risk factors for MDR infection and a high mortality risk is for three antibiotics: two directed at *P. aeruginosa* and one at MRSA. However, in the absence of septic shock, a single agent may be effective for these patients, provided there is a single agent that is likely to be effective against at least 90% of the gram-negative pathogens in that ICU. Empirical combination therapy enhances the likelihood of initially appropriate therapy over that with monotherapy. A β-lactam agent provides the greatest coverage, yet even the broadest-spectrum agent—a carbapenem—still constitutes inappropriate initial therapy in up to 10–15% of cases at some centers. The emergence of carbapenem resistance at some institutions requires the addition of polymyxins to the combination-therapy options. A number of emerging agents may modify our approach to therapy. New antipseudomonal agents include ceftazidime–avibactam, ceftolozane-tazobactam, imipenem–relebactam, and plazomicin. Therapy for carbapenem-resistant Enterobacteriaceae can consist of ceftazidime–avibactam, imipenem–relebactam, or meropenem–vaborbactam, while organisms that produce metallo-β-lactamases can be treated with ceftazidime–avibactam or cefiderocol.

TABLE 126-8 Empirical Antibiotic Treatment of Hospital-Acquired and Ventilator-Associated Pneumonia

NO RISK FACTORS FOR RESISTANT GRAM-NEGATIVE PATHOGEN	RISK FACTORS FOR RESISTANT GRAM-NEGATIVE PATHOGEN[a] *(CHOOSE ONE FROM EACH COLUMN)*	
Piperacillin-tazobactam (4.5 g IV q6h)	Piperacillin-tazobactam (4.5 g IV q6h)	Amikacin (15–20 mg/kg IV q24h)
Cefepime (2 g IV q8h)	Cefepime (2 g IV q8h)	Gentamicin (5–7 mg/kg IV q24h)
Levofloxacin (750 mg IV q24h)	Ceftazidime (2 g IV q8h)	Tobramycin (5–7 mg/kg IV q24h)
	Imipenem (500 mg IV q6h)	Ciprofloxacin (400 mg IV q8h)
	Meropenem (1 g IV q8h)	Levofloxacin (750 mg IV q24h)
		Colistin (loading dose of 5 mg/kg IV followed by maintenance doses of 2.5 mg × [1.5 × CrCl + 30] IV q12h)
		Polymyxin B (2.5–3.0 mg/kg per day IV in 2 divided doses)
Risk Factors for MRSA[b] ***(Add to above)***		
Linezolid (600 mg IV q12h) *or*		
Adjusted-dose vancomycin (trough level, 15–20 mg/dL)		

[a]Prior antibiotic therapy, prior hospitalization, local antibiogram. [b]Prior antibiotic therapy, prior hospitalization, known MRSA colonization, chronic hemodialysis, local documented MRSA pneumonia rate >10% (or local rate unknown).

Abbreviations: CrCl, creatinine clearance rate; MRSA, methicillin-resistant *Staphylococcus aureus.*

SPECIFIC TREATMENT

Once an etiologic diagnosis is made, broad-spectrum empirical therapy can be modified (de-escalated) to specifically address the known pathogen. For patients with MDR risk factors, antibiotic regimens can be reduced to a single agent in most cases. Only a minority of cases require a complete course with two or three drugs. A negative tracheal-aspirate culture or growth below the threshold for quantitative cultures of samples obtained before any antibiotic change strongly suggests that antibiotics should be discontinued or that an alternative diagnosis should be pursued. Identification of other confirmed or suspected sites of infection may require ongoing antibiotic therapy, but the spectrum of pathogens (and the corresponding antibiotic choices) may be different from those for VAP. A 7- or 8-day course of therapy is just as effective as a 2-week course and is associated with less frequent emergence of antibiotic-resistant strains. Exceptions include cases in which initial therapy is inappropriate or consists of second-line antibiotics and cases caused by some more resistant organisms, such as carbapenemase-producing *Acinetobacter* species.

A major controversy regarding specific therapy for VAP concerns the need for ongoing combination treatment of *Pseudomonas* pneumonia. No randomized controlled trials have demonstrated a benefit of combination therapy with a β-lactam and an aminoglycoside, nor have subgroup analyses in other trials found a survival benefit with such a regimen. Combination therapy may have value in bacteremic infection with septic shock, but the benefit may last for only a few days. The unacceptably high rates of clinical failure and death despite combination therapy among patients with VAP caused by *P. aeruginosa* (see "Failure to Improve," below) indicate that better regimens are needed, perhaps including aerosolized antibiotics. In most cases of *Pseudomonas* pneumonia, current guidelines recommend against continuing combination therapy after the isolate's microbial susceptibility is known.

FAILURE TO IMPROVE

Treatment failure is not uncommon in VAP, especially that caused by MDR pathogens. VAP caused by MRSA is associated with a 40% clinical failure rate when treated with standard-dose vancomycin. One proposed but unproven solution is the use of high-dose individualized treatment, although the risk of renal toxicity increases with this strategy. In addition, the MIC of MRSA to vancomycin has been increasing, and a high percentage of clinical failures occur when the MIC is in the upper range of sensitivity (i.e., 1.5–2 μg/mL). Linezolid appears to be 15% more efficacious than even adjusted-dose vancomycin and is preferred in patients with renal insufficiency and those infected with high-MIC isolates of MRSA. VAP due to *Pseudomonas* has a 40–50% failure rate, no matter what the regimen. Causes of clinical failure vary with the pathogen(s) and the antibiotic(s). Inappropriate initial therapy can usually be minimized by use of the recommended combination regimen (Table 126-8). However, the emergence of β-lactam resistance during therapy is an important problem, especially in infection with *Pseudomonas* and *Enterobacter* species. Recurrent VAP caused by the same pathogen is possible because the biofilm on endotracheal tubes allows persistence and reintroduction of the microorganism. Studies of VAP caused by *Pseudomonas* show that approximately half of recurrent cases are caused by a new strain. Some studies have suggested that treatment failure may be less common with optimized β-lactam dosing and use of either prolonged or continuous infusion therapy.

Treatment failure and its cause are very difficult to determine early in the therapeutic course. Pneumonia due to superinfection, the presence of extrapulmonary infection, and drug toxicity must be considered. Serial quantitative cultures may clarify the microbiologic response, but biomarkers such as PCT are of uncertain value in this setting.

COMPLICATIONS

Apart from death, the major complication of VAP is prolongation of mechanical ventilation, with corresponding increases in the duration of ICU and hospital stay. In most studies, the common need for an additional week of mechanical ventilation resulting from VAP justifies aggressive efforts at prevention.

In rare cases, necrotizing pneumonia (e.g., due to *P. aeruginosa* or *S. aureus*) can cause significant pulmonary hemorrhage. More commonly, necrotizing infections result in the long-term complications of bronchiectasis and parenchymal scarring leading to recurrent pneumonia. Other long-term complications of pneumonia can include long-term oxygen therapy, a catabolic state in a patient already nutritionally at risk, the need for prolonged rehabilitation, and—in the elderly—an inability to return to independent function and the need for nursing home placement.

FOLLOW-UP

Clinical improvement, if it occurs, is usually evident within 48–72 h of the initiation of antimicrobial treatment, usually with an improvement in oxygenation. Because findings on chest radiography often worsen initially during treatment, they are less helpful than clinical criteria as an indicator of response to therapy.

PROGNOSIS

VAP is associated with crude mortality rates as high as 50–70%, but the real issue is attributable mortality. Many patients with VAP have underlying diseases that would result in death even if VAP did not occur. Attributable mortality exceeded 25% in one matched-cohort study, while more recent studies have suggested much lower rates. Some variability in VAP mortality rates is clearly related to the type of patient and ICU studied. VAP in trauma patients is not associated with attributable mortality, possibly because many of the patients were otherwise healthy before being injured. The causative pathogen also plays a major role. Generally, MDR pathogens are associated with significantly greater attributable mortality than non-MDR pathogens. Pneumonia caused by some pathogens (e.g., *S. maltophilia*) is simply a marker for a patient whose immune system is so compromised that death is almost inevitable.

PREVENTION (TABLE 126-7)

Because endotracheal intubation is a risk factor for VAP, the most important preventive intervention is to avoid intubation or minimize its duration. Successful noninvasive ventilation avoids many of the problems associated with endotracheal tubes. Strategies that minimize the duration of ventilation through daily holding of sedation and formal weaning protocols have also been highly effective in preventing VAP.

Unfortunately, a tradeoff in risks is sometimes necessary. Aggressive attempts to extubate early may result in reintubation(s) and increase aspiration, posing a risk of VAP. Heavy continuous sedation increases VAP risk, but self-extubation because of insufficient sedation is also a risk. The tradeoffs also apply to antibiotic therapy. Short-course antibiotic prophylaxis can decrease the risk of early-onset VAP in comatose patients requiring intubation, and data suggest that antibiotics decrease VAP rates overall. Conversely, prolonged courses of antibiotics consistently increase the risk of MDR VAP; pseudomonal VAP is rare among patients who have not recently received antibiotics.

Minimizing microaspiration around the endotracheal tube cuff also can prevent VAP. Simply elevating the head of the bed (at least 30° above horizontal, but preferably 45°) and using specially modified endotracheal tubes that allow removal of the secretions pooled above the cuff can prevent microaspiration. The risk-to-benefit ratio of transporting the patient outside the ICU for diagnostic tests or procedures should be carefully considered since VAP rates are increased among transported patients.

The role played by overgrowth of the normal bowel flora in the stomach—in the presence of elevated gastric pH—in the pathogenesis of VAP is questionable. Therefore, avoidance of agents that raise gastric pH may be relevant only in certain populations, such as liver transplant recipients and patients who have undergone other major intraabdominal procedures or who have bowel obstruction. MRSA and nonfermenters such as *P. aeruginosa* and *Acinetobacter* species are not normally part of the bowel flora but reside primarily in the nose and on the skin, respectively.

In outbreaks of VAP due to specific pathogens, the possibility of a breakdown in infection control measures (particularly contamination of reusable equipment) should be investigated. Even high rates of pathogens that are already common in a particular ICU may result from cross-infection. Education and reminders of the need for consistent hand washing and other infection-control practices can minimize this risk.

HOSPITAL-ACQUIRED PNEUMONIA

While less well studied than VAP, HAP in non-intubated patients—both inside and outside the ICU—is similar to VAP. The main differences are the higher frequency of non-MDR pathogens and the generally better underlying host immunity in non-intubated patients. The lower frequency of MDR pathogens allows monotherapy in a larger proportion of cases of HAP than of VAP. However, the bacteriology and outcome of ventilated HAP patients may be very similar to those of patients with VAP.

The only pathogens that may be more common in the non-VAP population are anaerobes because of a greater risk of macroaspiration and the lower oxygen tensions in the lower respiratory tract of these patients. Anaerobes usually contribute only to polymicrobial pneumonias, and specific therapy targeting anaerobes probably is not needed since many of the recommended antibiotics are active against anaerobes.

Diagnosis is even more difficult for HAP in the non-intubated patient than for VAP. Lower respiratory tract samples appropriate for culture are considerably more difficult to obtain from non-intubated patients. Many of the underlying diseases that predispose a patient to HAP are also associated with an inability to cough adequately. Since blood cultures are infrequently positive (<15% of cases), the majority of patients with HAP do not have culture data on which antibiotic modifications can be based, and de-escalation is less likely. Despite these difficulties, the better host defenses in non-ICU patients result in lower mortality rates than are documented for VAP and for ventilated HAP. In addition, the risk of antibiotic failure is lower in HAP.

GLOBAL IMPACT

From the available data, it is virtually impossible to accurately assess the impact of pneumonia from a global perspective. Any differences in incidence, disease burden, and costs across different age, ethnic, and racial groups are compounded by differences among countries in terms of etiologic pathogens, resistance rates, access to health-care and diagnostic facilities, and vaccine availability and use.

A standard approach with clearly defined outcome measures is needed before the impact of pneumonia can be accurately evaluated. However, simple extrapolation from U.S. data for CAP and HAP/VAP shows that pneumonia has a significant impact on quality of life, morbidity, health costs, and mortality rates and that this impact has implications for patients and for society as a whole.

Acknowledgment

The authors gratefully acknowledge the contributions of Richard Wunderink, MD, to this chapter in the previous edition.

FURTHER READING

Chastre J et al: Comparison of 8 vs 15 days of antibiotic therapy for ventilator-associated pneumonia in adults: A randomized trial. JAMA 290:2588, 2003.

DICKSON RP et al: Towards an ecology of the lung: New conceptual models of pulmonary microbiology and pneumonia pathogenesis. Lancet Respir Med 2:238, 2014.

FAGON JY et al: Invasive and noninvasive strategies for management of suspected ventilator-associated pneumonia. A randomized trial. Ann Intern Med 132:621, 2000.

JAIN S et al: Community-acquired pneumonia requiring hospitalization among U.S. adults. N Engl J Med 373:415, 2015.

KALIL AC et al: Management of adults with hospital-acquired and ventilator-associated pneumonia: 2016 clinical practice guidelines by the Infectious Diseases Society of America and the American Thoracic Society. Clin Infect Dis 63:e61, 2016.

MANDELL LA, NIEDERMAN MS: Aspiration pneumonia. N Engl J Med 380:651, 2019.

MANDELL LA et al: Infectious Diseases Society of America/American Thoracic Society consensus guidelines on the management of community-acquired pneumonia in adults. Clin Infect Dis 44(Suppl 2):S27, 2007.

METLAY JP et al: Diagnosis and treatment of adults with community-acquired pneumonia. An Official Clinical Practice Guideline of the American Thoracic Society and Infectious Diseases Society of America. Am J Respir Crit Care Med 200:e45, 2019.

SHINDO Y et al: Risk factors for drug-resistant pathogens in community-acquired and healthcare-associated pneumonia. Am J Respir Crit Care Med 188:985, 2013.

WUNDERINK RG, WATERER GW: Community-acquired pneumonia. N Engl J Med 370:541, 2014.

127 Lung Abscess

Rebecca M. Baron, Beverly W. Baron, Miriam Baron Barshak

Lung abscess represents necrosis and cavitation of the lung following microbial infection. Lung abscesses can be single or multiple but usually are marked by a single dominant cavity >2 cm in diameter.

ETIOLOGY

The low prevalence of lung abscesses makes them difficult to study in randomized controlled trials. Although the incidence of lung abscesses has decreased in the antibiotic era, they are still a source of significant morbidity and mortality.

Lung abscesses usually are characterized as either primary (~80% of cases) or secondary. *Primary* lung abscesses generally arise from aspiration, often are caused principally by anaerobic bacteria, and occur in the absence of an underlying pulmonary or systemic condition. *Secondary* lung abscesses arise in the setting of an underlying condition, such as a postobstructive process (e.g., a bronchial foreign body or tumor) or a systemic process (e.g., HIV infection or another immunocompromising condition). Lung abscesses can also be characterized as acute (<4–6 weeks in duration) or chronic (~40% of cases).

EPIDEMIOLOGY

The majority of the existing epidemiologic information involves primary lung abscesses. In general, middle-aged men are more commonly affected than middle-aged women. The major risk factor for primary lung abscesses is aspiration. Patients at particular risk for aspiration, such as those with altered mental status, alcoholism, drug overdose, seizures, bulbar dysfunction, prior cerebrovascular or cardiovascular events, or neuromuscular disease, are most commonly affected. At additional risk are patients with esophageal dysmotility or esophageal lesions (strictures or tumors) and those with gastric distention and/or gastroesophageal reflux, especially those who spend substantial time in the recumbent position.

It is widely thought that colonization of the gingival crevices by anaerobic bacteria or microaerophilic streptococci (especially in patients with gingivitis and periodontal disease), combined with a risk of aspiration, is important in the development of lung abscesses. In fact, many physicians consider it extremely rare for lung abscesses to develop in the absence of teeth as a nidus for bacterial colonization.

The importance of these risk factors in the development of lung abscesses is highlighted by a significant reduction in abscess incidence in the late 1940s that coincided with a change in oral surgical technique: beginning at that time, these operations were no longer performed with the patient in the seated position without a cuffed endotracheal tube, and the frequency of perioperative aspiration events was thus decreased. In addition, the introduction of penicillin around the same time significantly reduced the incidence of and mortality rate from lung abscess.

PATHOGENESIS

Primary Lung Abscesses The development of primary lung abscesses is thought to originate when chiefly anaerobic bacteria (as well as microaerophilic streptococci) in the gingival crevices are aspirated into the lung parenchyma in a susceptible host (**Table 127-1**). Patients who develop primary lung abscesses usually carry an overwhelming burden of aspirated material or are unable to clear the bacterial load. Pneumonitis develops initially (exacerbated in part by tissue damage caused by gastric acid); then, over a period of 7–14 days, the anaerobic bacteria produce parenchymal necrosis and cavitation whose extent depends on host–pathogen interaction (**Fig. 127-1**). Anaerobes are thought to produce more extensive tissue necrosis in polymicrobial infections in which virulence factors of the various bacteria can act synergistically to cause more significant tissue destruction.

Secondary Lung Abscesses The pathogenesis of secondary abscesses depends on the predisposing factor. For example, in cases of bronchial obstruction from malignancy or a foreign body, the obstructing lesion prevents clearance of oropharyngeal secretions, leading to abscess development. With underlying systemic conditions (e.g., immunosuppression after bone marrow or solid organ transplantation), impaired host defense mechanisms lead to increased susceptibility to the development of lung abscesses caused by a broad range of pathogens, including opportunistic organisms (Table 127-1).

Lung abscesses also arise from septic emboli, either in tricuspid valve endocarditis (often involving *Staphylococcus aureus*) or in Lemierre's syndrome, in which an infection begins in the pharynx (classically involving *Fusobacterium necrophorum*) and then spreads

TABLE 127-1 Examples of Microbial Pathogens That can Cause Lung Abscesses

CLINICAL CONDITION	PATHOGENS
Primary lung abscess (usually with risk factors for aspiration)	Anaerobes (e.g., *Peptostreptococcus* spp., *Prevotella* spp., *Bacteroides* spp., *Streptococcus milleri*), microaerophilic streptococci
Secondary lung abscess (often with underlying immunocompromise)	*Staphylococcus aureus*, gram-negative rods (e.g., *Pseudomonas aeruginosa*, Enterobacteriaceae), *Nocardia* spp., *Aspergillus* spp., Mucorales, *Cryptococcus* spp., *Legionella* spp., *Rhodococcus equi*, *Pneumocystis jirovecii*
Embolic lesions	*Staphylococcus aureus* (often from endocarditis), *Fusobacterium necrophorum* (Lemierre's syndrome; see text for details)
Endemic infections (with or without underlying immunocompromise)	*Mycobacterium tuberculosis* (as well as *Mycobacterium avium* and *Mycobacterium kansasii*), *Coccidioides* spp., *Histoplasma capsulatum*, *Blastomyces* spp., parasites (e.g., *Entamoeba histolytica*, *Paragonimus westermani*, *Strongyloides stercoralis*)
Miscellaneous conditions	Bacterial pathogen (often *S. aureus*) after influenza or another viral infection, *Actinomyces* spp.

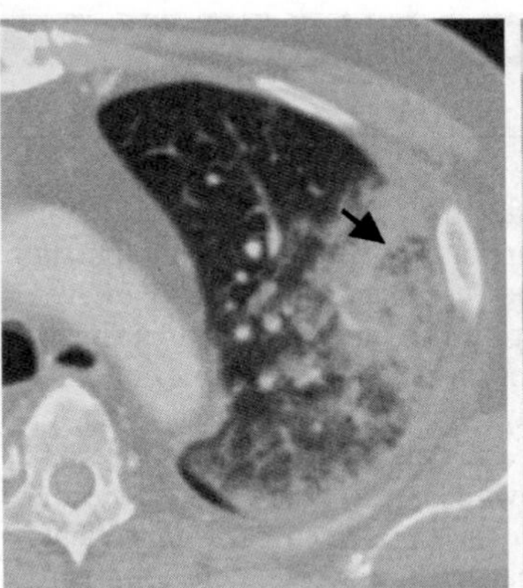

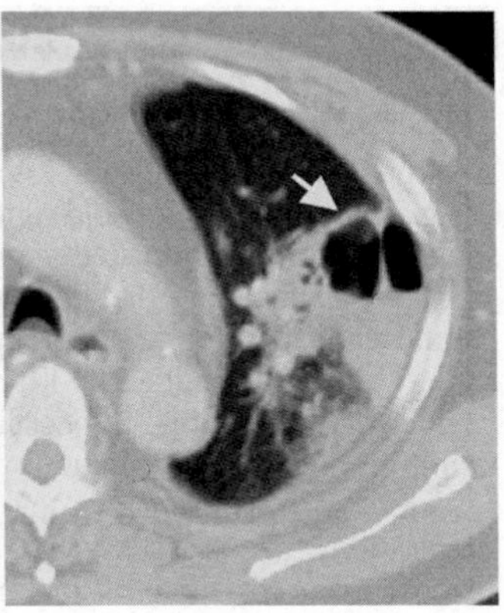

FIGURE 127-1 Representative chest CT scans demonstrating development of lung abscesses. This patient was immunocompromised by underlying lymphoma and developed severe *Pseudomonas aeruginosa* pneumonia, as represented by a left lung infiltrate with concern for central regions of necrosis (*panel **A**, black arrow*). Two weeks later, areas of cavitation with air-fluid levels were visible in this region and were consistent with the development of lung abscesses (*panel **B**, white arrow*). *(Images provided by Dr. Ritu Gill, Division of Chest Radiology, Brigham and Women's Hospital, Boston; with permission.)*

to the neck and the carotid sheath (which contains the jugular vein) to cause septic thrombophlebitis.

PATHOLOGY AND MICROBIOLOGY

Primary Lung Abscesses The dependent segments (posterior upper lobes and superior lower lobes) are the most common locations of primary lung abscesses, given the predisposition of aspirated materials to be deposited in these areas. Generally, the right lung is affected more commonly than the left because the right mainstem bronchus is less angulated.

Primary lung abscesses often are polymicrobial, primarily including anaerobic organisms as well as microaerophilic streptococci (Table 127-1). The retrieval and culture of anaerobes can be complicated by the contamination of samples with microbes from the oral cavity, the need for expeditious transport of the cultures to the laboratory, the need for early plating with special culture techniques, the prolonged time required for culture growth, and the need for collection of specimens prior to administration of antibiotics. When attention is paid to these factors, rates of recovery of specific isolates are reportedly as high as 78%.

Because it is not clear that knowing the identity of the causative anaerobic isolate alters the response to treatment of a primary lung abscess, practice has shifted away from the use of specialized techniques to obtain material for culture, such as transtracheal aspiration and bronchoalveolar lavage with protected brush specimens that allow recovery of culture material while avoiding contamination from the oral cavity. When no pathogen is isolated from a primary lung abscess (which occurs as often as 40% of the time), the abscess is termed a *nonspecific lung abscess*, and the presence of anaerobes is often presumed. A *putrid lung abscess* refers to cases with foul-smelling breath, sputum, or empyema; these manifestations are essentially diagnostic of an anaerobic lung abscess.

Secondary Lung Abscesses The location of secondary abscesses may vary with the underlying cause. The microbiology of secondary lung abscesses can encompass a broad bacterial spectrum, with infection by *Pseudomonas aeruginosa* and other gram-negative rods the most common. In addition, a broad array of pathogens can be identified in patients from certain endemic areas and in specific clinical scenarios (e.g., a significant incidence of fungal infections among immunosuppressed patients following bone marrow or solid organ transplantation). Because immunocompromised hosts and patients without the classic presentation of a primary lung abscess can be infected with a wide array of unusual organisms (Table 127-1), it is of special importance to obtain culture material in order to target therapy.

CLINICAL MANIFESTATIONS

Clinical manifestations initially may be similar to those of pneumonia, with fevers, cough, sputum production, and chest pain; a more chronic and indolent presentation that includes night sweats, fatigue, and anemia is often observed with anaerobic lung abscesses. A subset of patients with putrid lung abscesses may report discolored phlegm and foul-tasting or foul-smelling sputum. Patients with lung abscesses due to non-anaerobic organisms, such as *S. aureus*, may present with a more fulminant course characterized by high fevers and rapid progression.

Findings on physical examination may include fevers, poor dentition, and/or gingival disease as well as amphoric and/or cavernous breath sounds on lung auscultation. Additional findings may include digital clubbing and the absence of a gag reflex.

DIFFERENTIAL DIAGNOSIS

The differential diagnosis of lung abscesses is broad and includes other noninfectious processes that result in cavitary lung lesions, including lung infarction, malignancy, sequestration, cryptogenic organizing pneumonia, sarcoidosis, vasculitides and autoimmune diseases (e.g., granulomatosis with polyangiitis), lung cysts or bullae containing fluid, and septic emboli (e.g., from tricuspid valve endocarditis). Other less common entities can include pulmonary manifestations of diseases that usually present at locations other than the chest (e.g., inflammatory bowel disease, pyoderma gangrenosum).

DIAGNOSIS

Lung abscesses are documented by chest imaging. Although a chest radiograph usually detects a thick-walled cavity with an air-fluid level, CT permits better definition and may provide earlier evidence of cavitation. CT may also yield additional information regarding a possible underlying cause of lung abscess, such as malignancy, and may help distinguish a peripheral lung abscess from a pleural infection. This distinction has important implications for treatment because a pleural space infection, such as an empyema, may require urgent drainage.

As described earlier (see "Pathology and Microbiology," above), more invasive diagnostics (such as transtracheal aspiration) were traditionally undertaken for primary lung abscesses, whereas empirical therapy that includes drugs targeting anaerobic organisms currently is used more often. While sputum can be collected noninvasively for Gram's stain and culture, which may yield a pathogen, the infection is likely to be polymicrobial, and culture results may not reflect the presence of anaerobic organisms. Increasing use of molecular techniques for bacterial detection (e.g., 16S RNA gene amplification) may eventually yield increased specific pathogen identification. As stated above, many physicians consider putrid-smelling sputum to be virtually diagnostic of an anaerobic infection.

When a secondary lung abscess is present or empirical therapy fails to elicit a response, sputum and blood cultures are advised in addition to serologic studies for opportunistic pathogens (e.g., viruses and fungi causing infections in immunocompromised hosts). Additional diagnostics, such as bronchoscopy with bronchoalveolar lavage or protected brush specimen collection and CT-guided percutaneous needle aspiration, can be undertaken. Risks posed by these more invasive diagnostics include spillage of abscess contents into the other lung (with bronchoscopy) and pneumothorax and bronchopleural fistula development (with CT-guided needle aspiration). However, early diagnostics in secondary abscesses, especially in immunocompromised hosts, are particularly important because the patients involved may be especially fragile, at risk for infection with a broad array of pathogens, and therefore less likely than other patients to respond to empirical therapy.

TREATMENT

Lung Abscess

The availability of antibiotics in the 1940s and 1950s established therapy with this drug class as the primary approach to the treatment of lung abscess. Previously, surgery had been relied upon much more frequently. For many decades, penicillin was the antibiotic of choice for primary lung abscesses in light of its anaerobic coverage; however, because oral anaerobes can produce β-lactamases, clindamycin has proved superior to penicillin in clinical trials. For primary lung abscesses, the recommended regimens are (1) clindamycin (600 mg IV three times daily; then, with the disappearance of fever and clinical improvement, 300 mg PO four times daily) or (2) an IV-administered β-lactam/β-lactamase combination, followed—once the patient's condition is stable—by orally administered amoxicillin-clavulanate. This therapy should be continued until imaging demonstrates that the lung abscess has cleared or regressed to a small scar. Treatment duration may range from 3–4 weeks to as long as 14 weeks. One small study suggested that moxifloxacin (400 mg/d PO) is as effective and well tolerated as ampicillin-sulbactam. Notably, metronidazole is not effective as a single agent: it covers anaerobic organisms but not the microaerophilic streptococci that are often components of the mixed flora of primary lung abscesses.

In secondary lung abscesses, antibiotic coverage should be directed at the identified pathogen, and a prolonged course (until resolution of the abscess is documented) is often required. Treatment regimens and courses vary widely, depending on the immune state of the host and the identified pathogen. Other interventions may be necessary as well, such as relief of an obstructing lesion or treatment directed at the underlying condition predisposing the patient to lung abscess. Similarly, if the condition of patients with presumed primary lung abscess fails to improve, additional studies to rule out an underlying predisposing cause for a secondary lung abscess are indicated.

Although it can take as long as 7 days for patients receiving appropriate therapy to defervesce, as many as 10–20% of patients may not respond at all, with continued fevers and progression of the abscess cavity on imaging. An abscess >6–8 cm in diameter is less likely to respond to antibiotic therapy without additional interventions. Options for patients who do not respond to antibiotics and whose additional diagnostic studies fail to identify an additional pathogen that can be treated include surgical resection and percutaneous drainage of the abscess, especially when the patient is a poor surgical candidate. Timing of surgical intervention can be challenging; the goal is to balance the morbidity/mortality risk of a procedure with the need for definitively clearing the abscess in the setting of persistent infection that is not responsive to nonsurgical approaches. Possible complications of percutaneous drainage include bacterial contamination of the pleural space as well as pneumothorax and hemothorax.

■ COMPLICATIONS

Larger cavity size on presentation may correlate with the development of persistent cystic changes (pneumatoceles) or bronchiectasis. Additional possible complications include recurrence of abscesses despite appropriate therapy, extension to the pleural space with development of empyema, life-threatening hemoptysis, and massive aspiration of lung abscess contents.

■ PROGNOSIS AND PREVENTION

Reported mortality rates for primary abscesses have been as low as 2%, while rates for secondary abscesses are generally higher—as high as 75% in some case series. Other poor prognostic factors include age >60, the presence of aerobic bacteria, sepsis at presentation, symptom duration of >8 weeks, and abscess size >6 cm.

Mitigation of underlying risk factors may be the best approach to prevention of lung abscesses, with attention directed toward airway protection, oral hygiene, and minimized sedation with elevation of the head of the bed for patients at risk for aspiration. Prophylaxis against certain pathogens in at-risk patients (e.g., recipients of bone marrow or solid organ transplants or patients whose immune systems are significantly compromised by HIV infection) may be undertaken.

APPROACH TO THE PATIENT
Lung Abscess

For patients with a lung abscess and a low likelihood of malignancy (e.g., smokers <45 years old) and with risk factors for aspiration, it is reasonable to administer empirical treatment and then to pursue further evaluation if therapy does not elicit a response. However, some clinicians may opt for up-front cultures, even in primary lung abscesses. In patients with risk factors for malignancy or other underlying conditions (especially immunocompromised hosts) or with an atypical presentation, earlier diagnostics should be considered, such as bronchoscopy with biopsy or CT-guided needle aspiration. Bronchoscopy should be performed early in patients whose history, symptoms, or imaging findings are consistent with possible bronchial obstruction. In patients from areas endemic for tuberculosis or patients with other risk factors for tuberculosis (e.g., underlying HIV infection), induced sputum samples should be examined early in the workup to rule out this disease.

■ FURTHER READING

Bartlett JG: How important are anaerobic bacteria in aspiration pneumonia: When should they be treated and what is optimal therapy. Infect Dis Clin North Am 27:149, 2013.

Davis B, Systrom DM: Lung abscess: Pathogenesis, diagnosis, and treatment. Curr Clin Top Infect Dis 18:252, 1998.

Desai H, Agrawal A: Pulmonary emergencies: Pneumonia, acute respiratory distress syndrome, lung abscess, and empyema. Med Clin North Am 96:1127, 2012.

Duncan C et al: Understanding the lung abscess microbiome: Outcomes of percutaneous lung parenchymal abscess drainage with microbiologic correlation. Cardiovasc Intervent Radiol 40:902, 2017.

Mukae H et al: The importance of obligate anaerobes and the *Streptococcus anginosus* group in pulmonary abscess. Respiration 92:80, 2016.

Ott SR et al: Moxifloxacin vs ampicillin/sulbactam in aspiration pneumonia and primary lung abscess. Infection 36:23, 2008.

Raymond D: Surgical intervention for thoracic infections. Surg Clin North Am 94:1283, 2014.

128 Infective Endocarditis

Sara E. Cosgrove, Adolf W. Karchmer

The prototypic lesion of infective endocarditis (IE), the *vegetation* **(Fig. 128-1)**, is a mass of platelets, fibrin, microorganisms, and scant inflammatory cells. Infection most commonly involves heart valves but may also occur on the low-pressure side of a ventricular septal defect, on mural endocardium damaged by aberrant jets of blood or foreign bodies, or on intracardiac devices. The analogous process involving arteriovenous shunts, arterio-arterial shunts (patent ductus arteriosus), or a coarctation of the aorta is called *infective endarteritis*.

IE can be classified according to the temporal evolution of disease, the site of infection, the cause of infection, or the predisposing risk factor (e.g., injection drug use, health care–associated). *Acute IE* is a hectically febrile illness that rapidly damages cardiac structures, seeds extracardiac sites, and, if untreated, progresses to death within weeks. *Subacute IE* follows an indolent course; causes structural cardiac damage only slowly, if at all; rarely metastasizes; and is gradually progressive unless complicated by a major embolic event or a ruptured mycotic aneurysm.

In the United States and likely in other developed countries, the incidence of IE is estimated to be 12 cases per 100,000 population per

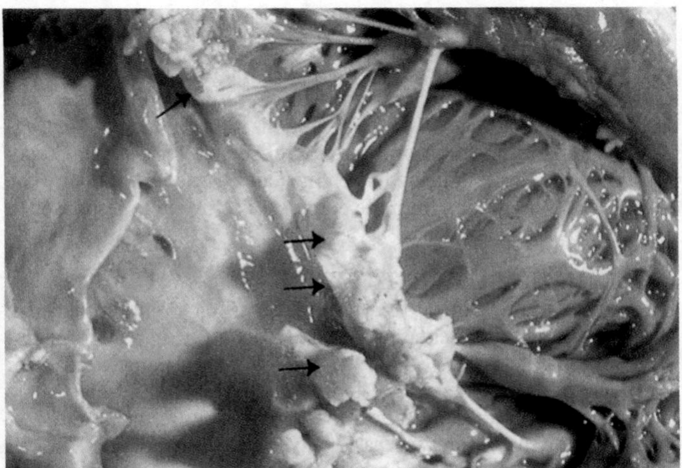

FIGURE 128-1 Vegetations (arrows) due to viridans streptococci endocarditis involving the mitral valve.

year, with progressive increases during recent decades. While congenital heart diseases remain a constant predisposition, predisposing conditions in developed countries have shifted from chronic rheumatic heart disease (still common in developing countries) to injection drug use, degenerative valve disease, and intracardiac devices. The incidence of IE is notably increased among the elderly. In developed countries, 25–35% of cases of native-valve endocarditis (NVE) are health care–associated, and 16–30% of all cases are prosthetic-valve infections (PVE). The risk of PVE is greatest during the initial year after valve replacement; gradually declines to a low, stable rate thereafter; and is greater for bioprosthetic valves than mechanical valves. The incidence of infection involving transcatheter implanted aortic valves (TAVR-PVE) per 100 patient-years (PY) is 1.4–2.8 in the first year and 0.8 in each of the ensuing 4 years. The incidence of TAVR-PVE is similar to that for surgically implanted bioprosthetic aortic valves. IE involving cardiovascular implantable electronic devices (CIED-IE)—greater on implanted defibrillators and resynchronization devices than on permanent pacemakers—occurs in 0.5–1.14 cases per 1000 recipients.

ETIOLOGY

Although many species of bacteria and fungi cause sporadic episodes of IE, a few bacterial species cause the majority of cases (**Table 128-1**). Recent large studies from developed areas identify *Staphylococcus aureus* as the most common bacterial species causing IE. The oral cavity, skin, and upper respiratory tract are the respective primary portals for viridans streptococci, staphylococci, and HACEK organisms (*Haemophilus* species, *Aggregatibacter* species, *Cardiobacterium hominis, Eikenella corrodens*, and *Kingella kingae*). *Streptococcus gallolyticus* subspecies *gallolyticus* (formerly *S. bovis* biotype 1) originates from the gastrointestinal tract and is associated with colonic polyps and tumors. Enterococci enter the bloodstream primarily from the genitourinary tract. Health care–associated IE, most commonly caused by *S. aureus*, coagulase-negative staphylococci (CoNS), and enterococci, may have either a nosocomial onset (55%) or a community onset (45%). IE complicates 8–25% of episodes of catheter-associated *S. aureus* bacteremia; the higher rates are detected in high-risk patients studied by transesophageal echocardiography (TEE) (see "Cardiac Imaging," below).

PVE arising within 2 months of valve surgery—i.e., early PVE—is generally nosocomial and is the result of intraoperative contamination of the prosthesis or a postoperative infection. This nosocomial origin is reflected in the microbial causes: *S. aureus*, CoNS, facultative gram-negative bacilli, diphtheroids, and fungi. The portals of entry and organisms causing PVE beginning >12 months after surgery—i.e., late PVE—are similar to those in community-acquired NVE. Regardless of the time of onset after surgery, at least 68–85% of CoNS strains that cause PVE are resistant to methicillin. The microbiology of TAVR-PVE, while generally similar to that of PVE, is notable for an increased frequency of enterococci. Risk factors associated with TAVR-PVE include male sex, diabetes, renal failure, and moderate postimplantation aortic valve regurgitation.

CIED-IE involves the device or the endothelium at points of device contact. Occasionally, there is concurrent aortic or mitral valve infection. One-third of cases of CIED IE present within 3 months after device implantation or manipulation, one-third between 4–12 months, and one-third >1 year. *S. aureus* and CoNS cause the majority of cases.

IE in people who inject drugs (PWID), especially that involving the tricuspid valve, is commonly caused by *S. aureus*, which is often

TABLE 128-1 Organisms Causing Major Clinical Forms of Infective Endocarditis (IE)

	PROPORTION OF CASES						
	NATIVE-VALVE IE		PROSTHETIC-VALVE IE AT INDICATED TIME OF ONSET (MONTHS) AFTER VALVE SURGERY			TAVR PVE	CIED-IE
ORGANISM(S)	COMMUNITY-ACQUIRED (*N* = 1718)	HEALTH CARE–ASSOCIATED (*N* = 1110)	<2 (*N* = 144)	>2-12 (*N* = 31)	>12 (N = 194)	(*N* = 295)	(*N* = 337)
Streptococci[b]	40	13	1	10	31	18	2
Pneumococci	2	—	—	—	—	-	—
Enterococci[c]	9	16	8	13	11	24	4
Staphylococcus aureus	28[a]	52[d]	22	13	18	23	36
Coagulase-negative staphylococci	5	11	33	35	11	20	41
Fastidious gram-negative coccobacilli (HACEK group)[e]	3	—	—	—	6	—	—
Gram-negative bacilli	1	1	13	3	6	1	6
Candida spp.	<1	1	8	13	1	1	2
Polymicrobial/miscellaneous	3	3	3	6	5	8	2
Diphtheroids	—	<1	6	—	3		1
Culture-negative	9	3	5	7	8	5	6

[a]Includes methicillin-susceptible and -resistant isolates. [b]Includes viridans streptococci; *Streptococcus gallolyticus*; other non–group A, groupable streptococci; and *Abiotrophia* and *Granulicatella* spp. (nutritionally variant, pyridoxal-requiring streptococci). [c]Primarily *E. faecalis* or nonspeciated isolates; occasionally *E. faecium* or other less likely species. [d]Methicillin resistance is common among these *S. aureus* strains. [e]Includes *Haemophilus* spp., *Aggregatibacter* spp., *Cardiobacterium hominis, Eikenella corrodens*, and *Kingella kingae*.

Abbreviations: CIED: cardiac implantable electronic device, TAVR: transcatheter aortic valve replacement.

Note: Data are compiled from multiple studies.

resistant to methicillin. Left-sided valve infections in PWID has a more varied etiology. In addition to the usual causes of IE, infection due to Enterobacterales, *Pseudomonas aeruginosa*, *Candida* species, and sporadically by unusual organisms (*Bacillus*, *Lactobacillus*, *Corynebacterium* species) is encountered. HIV infection in PWID does not significantly alter the causes of IE.

About 5–15% of patients with IE have negative blood cultures; in one-third to one-half of these cases, cultures are negative because of prior antibiotic exposure. The remainder are infected by fastidious organisms, such as some streptococci, nutritionally variant bacteria now designated *Granulicatella* and *Abiotrophia* species, HACEK organisms, *Coxiella burnetii*, and *Bartonella* species. Some fastidious organisms occur in characteristic geographic settings (e.g., *C. burnetii* and *Bartonella* species in Europe, *Brucella* species in the Middle East). *Tropheryma whipplei* causes an indolent, culture-negative, afebrile form of IE. *C. burnetii* has a predilection for prosthetic valves. *Corynebacterium* species and *Propionibacterium acnes* may involve intracardiac devices and be slow to grow in blood cultures. *Mycobacterium chimaera*, which may be difficult to recover from blood cultures unless special media is used, has caused a global outbreak of PVE and disseminated infection as a result of aerosols from contaminated heater-cooler machines used during cardiopulmonary bypass. Lastly, atrial myxoma, marantic endocarditis, and the antiphospholipid antibody syndrome may mimic culture-negative IE.

PATHOGENESIS

The undamaged endothelium is resistant to infection by most bacteria. Endothelial injury (e.g., at the site of impact of high-velocity blood jets or on the low-pressure side of a cardiac structural lesion) allows either direct infection by virulent organisms or the development of a platelet–fibrin thrombus—a condition called *nonbacterial thrombotic endocarditis* (NBTE). This thrombus serves as a site of bacterial attachment during transient bacteremia. The cardiac conditions most commonly resulting in NBTE are mitral regurgitation, aortic stenosis, aortic regurgitation, ventricular septal defects, and complex congenital heart disease. NBTE also arises as a result of a hypercoagulable state; this phenomenon gives rise to *marantic endocarditis* (uninfected vegetations seen in patients with malignancy and chronic diseases) and to bland vegetations complicating systemic lupus erythematosus and antiphospholipid antibody syndrome.

Organisms that cause IE enter the bloodstream from colonized body surfaces or sites of infection. *S. aureus* adherence to intact endothelium may be mediated by local inflammation inducing von Willebrand factor on endothelial cell surfaces with resulting adherence of both platelets and *S. aureus*. Alternatively, *S. aureus* adherence to injured endothelium may be mediated by local deposition of fibrin and circulating von Willebrand factor on exposed subendothelial tissue to which in turn *S. aureus* adhere directly. Other microorganisms in the blood adhere to NBTE. The organisms that commonly cause IE have surface adhesin molecules, collectively called microbial surface components recognizing adhesin matrix molecules (MSCRAMMs) that mediate adherence to NBTE sites or injured endothelium. Adherence is facilitated by fibronectin-binding proteins present on many gram-positive bacteria; by clumping factor (a fibrinogen- and fibrin-binding surface protein) on *S. aureus*; by fibrinogen-binding surface proteins (Fss2), collagen-binding surface protein (Ace), and Ebp pili (the latter mediating platelet adherence) on *Enterococcus faecalis*; and by glucans or FimA (a member of the family of oral mucosal adhesins) on streptococci. Fibronectin-binding proteins are required for *S. aureus* invasion of intact endothelium; thus, these surface proteins may facilitate infection of previously normal valves. If resistant to the bactericidal activity of serum and the microbicidal peptides released locally by platelets, adherent organisms proliferate to form dense microcolonies. Microorganisms also induce platelet deposition and a localized procoagulant state by eliciting tissue factor from the endothelium and, in the case of *S. aureus*, from monocytes as well. Fibrin deposition combines with platelet aggregation and microorganism proliferation to generate an infected vegetation. Organisms deep in vegetations are metabolically inactive (nongrowing) and relatively resistant to killing by antimicrobial agents. Proliferating surface organisms are shed into the bloodstream continuously.

The clinical manifestations of IE—other than constitutional symptoms, which probably result from cytokine production—arise from damage to intracardiac structures; embolization of vegetation fragments leading to infection or infarction of remote tissues; hematogenous infection of sites during bacteremia; and tissue injury due to the deposition of circulating immune complexes or immune responses to deposited bacterial antigens.

CLINICAL MANIFESTATIONS

The highly variable clinical IE syndrome spans a continuum between acute and subacute presentations. Most forms of IE share clinical and laboratory manifestations (**Table 128-2**). The causative microorganism is primarily responsible for the temporal course of IE. β-Hemolytic streptococci, *S. aureus*, and pneumococci typically result in an acute course, although *S. aureus* occasionally causes subacute disease. IE caused by *Staphylococcus lugdunensis* (a coagulase-negative species) or by enterococci may present acutely. Subacute IE is typically caused by viridans streptococci, enterococci, CoNS, and the HACEK group. IE caused by *Bartonella* species, *T. whipplei*, *C. burnetii*, or *M. chimaera* is exceptionally indolent.

In patients with subacute presentations, fever is typically low-grade rarely exceeding 39.4°C (103°F); in contrast, temperatures of 39.4°–40°C (103°–104°F) are often noted in acute IE. Fever may be blunted in patients who are elderly, are severely debilitated, or have renal failure.

Cardiac Manifestations Although heart murmurs are usually indicative of the predisposing cardiac pathology rather than of IE, valvular damage and ruptured chordae may result in new regurgitant murmurs. In acute IE involving a normal valve, murmurs may be absent initially but ultimately are detected in 85% of cases. Congestive heart failure (CHF) resulting from valve dysfunction or, occasionally, intracardiac fistulae develops in 30–40% of patients. Extension of leaflet infection into adjacent annular or myocardial tissue results in paravalvular abscesses, which in turn may cause intracardiac fistulae with new murmurs. Aortic paravalvular infection may burrow into the

TABLE 128-2 Clinical and Laboratory Features of Infective Endocarditis

FEATURE	FREQUENCY, %
Fever	80–90
Chills and sweats	40–75
Anorexia, weight loss, malaise	25–50
Myalgias, arthralgias	15–30
Back pain	7–15
Heart murmur	80–85
New/worsened regurgitant murmur	20–50
Arterial emboli	20–50
Splenomegaly	15–50
Clubbing	10–20
Neurologic manifestations	20–40
Peripheral manifestations (Osler's nodes, subungual hemorrhages, Janeway lesions, Roth's spots)	2–15
Petechiae	10–40
Laboratory manifestations	
Anemia	70–90
Leukocytosis	20–30
Microscopic hematuria	30–50
Elevated erythrocyte sedimentation rate	60–90
Elevated C-reactive protein level	>90
Rheumatoid factor	50
Circulating immune complexes	65–100
Decreased serum complement	5–40

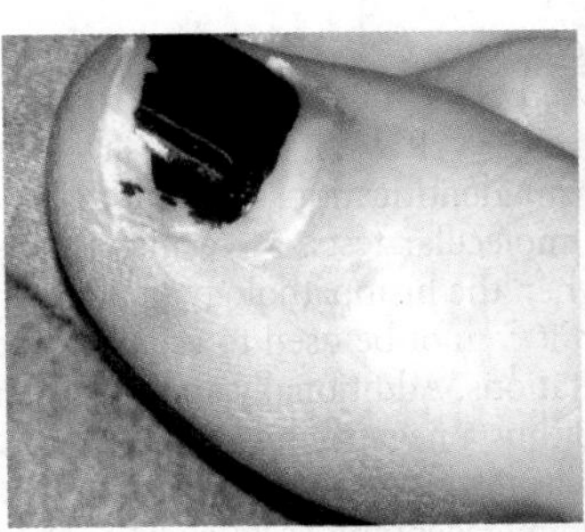

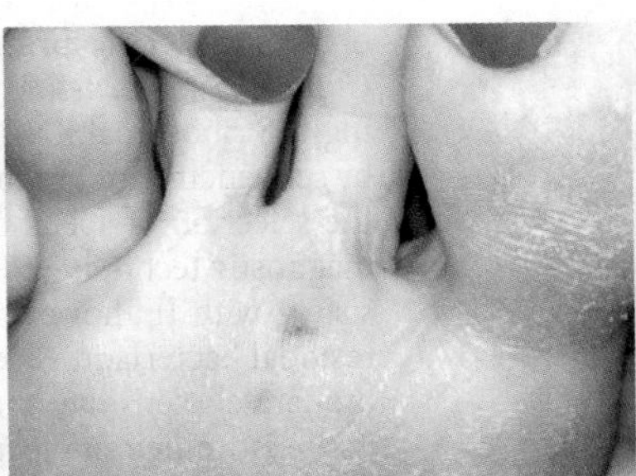

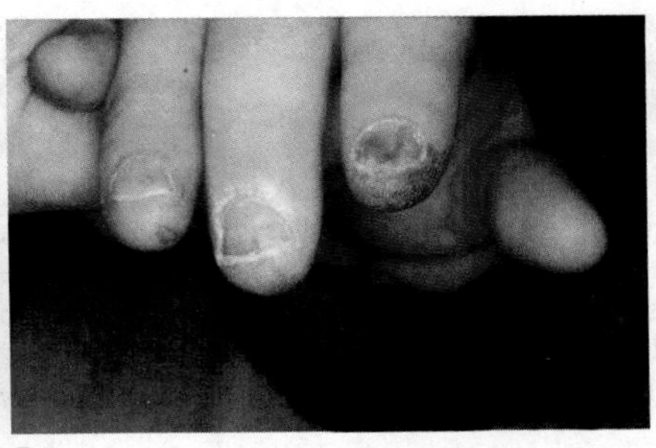

A B

FIGURE 128-2 ***A.*** Janeway lesions on the toe (*left*) and plantar surface (*right*) of the foot in subacute *Neisseria mucosa* IE. (*Images courtesy of Rachel Baden, MD.*) ***B.*** Septic emboli with hemorrhage and infarction due to acute *Staphylococcus aureus* IE.

upper ventricular septum and interrupt the conduction system, leading to varying degrees of heart block. Mitral paravalvular abscesses are more distant from the conduction system and rarely cause conduction abnormalities. Coronary artery emboli occur in 2% of patients and may result in myocardial infarction.

Noncardiac Manifestations The classic nonsuppurative peripheral manifestations of subacute IE (e.g., Janeway lesions; **Fig. 128-2A**) are related to prolonged infection; with early diagnosis and treatment, these have become infrequent. In contrast, septic embolization mimicking some of these lesions (subungual hemorrhage, Osler's nodes) is common in patients with acute *S. aureus* IE (**Fig. 128-2B**). Musculoskeletal pain usually remits promptly with treatment but must be distinguished from focal metastatic infections (e.g., spondylodiscitis), which may complicate 10–15% of cases. Hematogenously seeded focal infection occurs most often in the skin, spleen, kidneys, skeletal system, and meninges. Arterial emboli, one-half of which precede the diagnosis of IE, are clinically apparent in up to 50% of patients. *S. aureus* IE, mobile vegetations >10 mm in diameter, and infection involving the mitral valve anterior leaflet are independently associated with an increased risk of embolization. Embolic arterial occlusion causes regional pain or ischemia-induced organ dysfunction (e.g., of the kidney, spleen, bowel, extremity). Cerebrovascular emboli presenting as strokes or occasionally as encephalopathy complicate 15–35% of cases; however, evidence of clinically asymptomatic emboli is found on MRI in 30–65% of patients with left-sided IE. The frequency of stroke is 8 per 1000 patient-days during the week prior to diagnosis and decreases to 4.8 and 1.7 per 1000 patient-days during the first and second weeks of effective antimicrobial therapy, respectively. Only 3% of strokes occur after 1 week of effective therapy. Emboli occurring late during or after effective therapy do not in themselves constitute evidence of failed antimicrobial treatment.

Other neurologic complications include aseptic or purulent meningitis, intracranial hemorrhage due to hemorrhagic infarcts or ruptured mycotic aneurysms, and seizures. *Mycotic aneurysms* are focal dilations of arteries occurring at points in the artery wall that have been weakened by infection in the vasa vasorum or where septic emboli have lodged. Microabscesses in the brain and meninges occur commonly in *S. aureus* IE; intracerebral abscesses requiring surgical drainage are infrequent.

Immune complex deposition on the glomerular basement membrane causes diffuse hypocomplementemic glomerulonephritis and renal dysfunction, which typically improve with effective antimicrobial therapy. Embolic renal infarcts cause flank pain and hematuria but rarely renal dysfunction.

Manifestations with Specific Predisposing Conditions Among PWID, 35–60% of IE is limited to the tricuspid valve and presents with fever but with faint or no murmur and without peripheral manifestations. Septic pulmonary emboli, which are common with tricuspid IE, cause cough, pleuritic chest pain, nodular pulmonary infiltrates, and occasionally empyema or pyopneumothorax. Infection of the aortic or mitral valve presents with the typical clinical features of IE, including peripheral manifestations.

Health care–associated IE has typical manifestations unless associated with an intracardiac device or masked by the symptoms of concurrent illness. CIED-IE may be associated with obvious (especially within 6 months of device manipulation) or cryptic generator pocket infection, or arise through bacteremic seeding without pocket infection. Fever, sepsis, minimal murmur, and occasionally pulmonary symptoms due to septic emboli are seen. Late-onset PVE and TAVR-PVE present with typical clinical features. In early PVE, symptoms may be masked by recent surgery. In both early and late PVE, paravalvular infection is common and often results in partial valve dehiscence, regurgitant murmurs, CHF, or disruption of the conduction system.

DIAGNOSIS

Careful clinical, microbiologic, and echocardiographic evaluations should be pursued when febrile patients have IE predispositions, cardiac or noncardiac (e.g., stroke or splenic infarct) features of IE, or blood cultures yielding an IE-associated organism.

Duke Criteria The diagnosis of IE is established with certainty only when vegetations are examined histologically and microbiologically. Nevertheless, a common clinical approach utilizes a sensitive and specific diagnostic schema—the *modified Duke criteria*—based on clinical, laboratory, and echocardiographic findings commonly encountered in patients with IE (**Table 128-3**). Clinical judgment must be exercised in order to use the criteria effectively. A clinical diagnosis of definite IE requires documentation of two major criteria, of one major and three minor criteria, or of five minor criteria. IE is rejected if an alternative diagnosis is established, if symptoms resolve and do not recur with ≤4 days of antibiotic therapy, or if surgery or autopsy after ≤4 days of antimicrobial therapy yields no histologic evidence of IE. Cases not classified as definite or rejected are considered possible IE when either one major and one minor criteria or three minor criteria are fulfilled. Absent extenuating circumstances, patients with definite and possible IE are treated as having IE.

The blood culture requirement emphasizes multiple positive blood cultures over time (consistent with the continuous bacteremia characteristic of IE) and the bacterial species that commonly cause IE. To fulfill a major criterion, an organism that causes both IE and non-IE-related bacteremia (e.g., *S. aureus*, enterococci) must be recovered in multiple blood cultures and the clinical presentation be unexplained by an extracardiac focus of infection. Organisms that commonly contaminate blood cultures (e.g., diphtheroids, CoNS) must be found in repeated blood cultures to satisfy a major criterion.

Blood Cultures In patients with suspected NVE, PVE, TAVR-PVE, or CIED-IE who have not received antibiotics during the prior 2 weeks, three two-bottle blood culture sets containing the appropriate volume of blood (10 mL per bottle) should be obtained from different venipuncture sites over 1–2 hours. If the cultures remain negative after 48–72 h, two or three additional blood culture sets should be obtained, and the laboratory should be consulted for advice regarding optimal culture techniques. Pending culture results, empirical antimicrobial therapy should be withheld initially from hemodynamically and clinically stable patients with suspected subacute IE, especially

TABLE 128-3 The Modified Duke Criteria for the Clinical Diagnosis of Infective Endocarditis[a]

Major Criteria
1. Positive blood culture
Typical microorganism for infective endocarditis from two separate blood cultures
Viridans streptococci, *Streptococcus gallolyticus*, HACEK group organisms, *Staphylococcus aureus*, *or*
Community-acquired enterococci in the absence of a primary focus,
or
Persistently positive blood culture, defined as recovery of a microorganism consistent with infective endocarditis from:
Blood cultures drawn >12 h apart; *or*
All of 3 or a majority of ≥4 separate blood cultures, with first and last drawn at least 1 h apart
or
Single positive blood culture for *Coxiella burnetii* or phase I IgG antibody titer of >1:800
2. Evidence of endocardial involvement
Positive echocardiogram[b]
Oscillating intracardiac mass on valve or supporting structures or in the path of regurgitant jets or in implanted material, in the absence of an alternative anatomic explanation, *or*
Abscess, *or*
New partial dehiscence of prosthetic valve,
or
New valvular regurgitation (increase or change in preexisting murmur not sufficient)
Minor Criteria
1. Predisposition: predisposing heart conditions[c] or injection drug use
2. Fever ≥38.0°C (≥100.4°F)
3. Vascular phenomena: major arterial emboli, septic pulmonary infarcts, mycotic aneurysm, intracranial hemorrhage, conjunctival hemorrhages, Janeway lesions
4. Immunologic phenomena: glomerulonephritis, Osler's nodes, Roth's spots, rheumatoid factor
5. Microbiologic evidence: positive blood culture but not meeting major criterion, as noted previously,[d] *or* serologic evidence of active infection with an organism consistent with infective endocarditis

[a]Definite endocarditis is defined by documentation of two major criteria, of one major criterion and three minor criteria, or of five minor criteria. See text for further details. [b]Transesophageal echocardiography is required for optimal assessment of possible prosthetic valve endocarditis or complicated endocarditis. European Society of Cardiology includes finding on EKG-gated cardiac CT angiogram or FDG-PET/CT as major criteria (see text). [c]Valvular disease with stenosis or regurgitation, presence of a prosthetic valve, congenital heart disease including corrected or partially corrected conditions (except isolated atrial septal defect, repaired ventricular septal defect, or closed patent ductus arteriosus), prior endocarditis, or hypertrophic cardiomyopathy. [d]Excluding single positive cultures for coagulase-negative staphylococci and diphtheroids, which are common culture contaminants, or for organisms that do not cause endocarditis frequently, such as gram-negative bacilli.

Source: Reproduced with permission from JS Li et al: Proposed modifications to the Duke criteria for the diagnosis of infective endocarditis: Clin Infect Dis 30:633, 2000.

those who have received antibiotics within the preceding 2 weeks. The delay allows blood for additional cultures to be obtained without the confounding effect of empirical treatment. Patients with sepsis or deteriorating hemodynamics who may require urgent surgery should receive empirical treatment immediately after the initial three sets of blood cultures are obtained.

Non-Blood-Culture Tests Serologic tests can be used to implicate organisms that are difficult to recover by blood culture such as *Brucella*, *Bartonella*, *T. whipplei*, and *C. burnetii*. In vegetations recovered at surgery or by embolectomy, pathogens can be identified by culture and histopathologic examination with special stains. A sample of the vegetation should be collected using sterile technique and saved for molecular testing using polymerase chain reaction (PCR) with organism-specific primers (e.g., *C. burnetii*, *Bartonella*, *T. whipplei*, *Cutibacterium acnes*, *Mycoplasma hominis*) or broad-range PCR targeting 16S ribosomal RNA (or 28S rRNA, if fungi are suspected) followed by sequencing for organism identification. Histopathology may inform the selection of specific molecular tests. Molecular testing is a useful diagnostic technology when the histopathology of a vegetation is consistent with IE; however, it cannot be used to establish the viability of residual bacteria in vegetations. Additionally, molecular testing is only moderately sensitive and thus a negative test cannot exclude IE. When tissue is limited, molecular testing should be prioritized over culture. Next-generation (shotgun metagenomic) sequencing of pathogen DNA from serum has emerged as a novel nonculture technology capable of identifying a wide array of organisms in blood culture–negative IE.

Cardiac Imaging Echocardiography anatomically confirms and measures vegetations, detects intracardiac complications, and assesses cardiac function. Transthoracic echocardiography (TTE) is exceptionally specific; however, in 20% of patients the images are inadequate. TTE fails to detect vegetations in 20–35% of patients with definite clinical IE, missing vegetations <2 mm in diameter. It is not optimal for evaluating prosthetic valves, especially TAVR with large stents, or detecting intracardiac complications. TEE detects vegetations in >90% of patients with definite IE; nevertheless, initial studies may yield false-negative results in 6–18% of IE patients, especially in TAVR-PVE. A negative TEE, when IE is likely, does not exclude the diagnosis but rather warrants repeating the study in 7–10 days. TEE is sometimes augmented by 3-D TEE for the diagnosis of PVE and CIED-IE and for the detection of myocardial abscess, fistulae, or valve perforations.

Other imaging, if available, should be pursued when anatomic confirmation of IE is unclear, when TEE is not confirmatory or is contraindicated, and in suspected PVE. Electrocardiographic-gated multislice cardiac CT angiogram (CTA), which is comparable to TEE in detection of vegetations and possibly superior in defining paravalvular infection, may be definitive. While less sensitive than TEE or CTA in detecting intracardiac pathology in NVE or CIED-IE, 18-fluorodeoxyglucose positron emission tomography (^{18}FDG PET/CT) provides increased sensitivity in assessing suspected PVE (also TAVR-PVE), infection of ascending aorta grafts, extracardiac complications and CIED pocket infection. As a whole-body image, findings may modify therapy in 25% of NVE and PVE patients. However, ^{18}FDG-PET/CT is costly, requires preprocedure patient preparation, can have false-positive results in patients with recent cardiac surgery, and requires experienced radiographers for interpretation. Of note, the European Society of Cardiology has included findings from these imaging techniques as major criteria in a further modification of the Duke criteria.

In population-based studies and large series (using various diagnostic criteria), IE occurs frequently among patients who have monomicrobial bacteremia due to those gram-positive organisms that are commonly associated with IE. For example, 12–17% of patients with blood cultures growing *E. faecalis* have IE; 7% of patients with blood cultures growing non-β-hemolytic streptococci have IE; and 8–14% of patients with blood cultures growing *S. aureus* have IE. IE risk-prediction scoring systems have been developed to identify patients, among those with one or more positive monomicrobial blood cultures, who are at sufficient risk of IE to justify echocardiographic assessment (**Table 128-4**). Because *S. aureus* bacteremia is associated with a high prevalence of IE and a resultant high risk for mortality, echocardiographic evaluation (high-quality TTE or preferably TEE) is recommended routinely. Prediction scores suggest that with *S. aureus* bacteremia, a patient with any of the features listed in Table 128-4 incurs at least a 6% risk of IE, with risk increasing when multiple features are present. Thus, when present these findings are a strong indication for early TEE. In their absence, TTE should suffice unless other findings suggest IE. Among patients with either monomicrobial *E. faecalis* or non-β-hemolytic streptococcal bacteremia, any three of the respective listed features (Table 128-4) are associated with a significant frequency of IE. For these patients, the estimated number needed to test with TEE to detect IE is 2.4 and 3.6, respectively. While

TABLE 128-4 Features Guiding the Need for Echocardiographic Assessment in Patients with Selected Monomicrobial Bacteremia

BLOOD CULTURE ISOLATE		
S. AUREUS[a]	*E. FAECALIS*[b]	NON-β-HEMOLYTIC STREPTOCOCCI[c]
Intracardiac device	Symptoms ≥7 days	Symptoms ≥7 days
Prior endocarditis	Emboli	Greater than two positive cultures
Injection drug use	Greater than two positive cultures	One species: *S. gallolyticus, S. sanguinis, S. mutans* (not *S. anginosus*)
Cerebral/peripheral emboli	Unknown origin (no focus)	
Meningitis	Heart murmur	Heart murmur or valve disease
Preexisting valve disease	Valve disease (including prior endocarditis)	Community acquired
Persistent bacteremia (≥72 hours)		
Vertebral osteomyelitis		
Community acquisition		
Non-nosocomial health care associated		
Indeterminate or positive TTE		

Source: [a]S Tubiana et al: J Infect 72:544, 2016 and A Showler et al: JACC Cardiovasc Imaging 8:924, 2015. [b]A Berge et al: Infection 47:45, 2019. [c]T Sunnerhagen et al: Clin Infect Dis 66:693, 2018.

these predictive scoring systems need further evaluation and should be used with clinical judgment, they appear to have a high sensitivity and therefore a high negative predictive value, which allows identification of patients at low risk of IE where echocardiography, particularly TEE, can be omitted. An approach to echocardiographic evaluation of patients with suspected IE is illustrated in **Fig. 128-3**.

Other Studies Many studies that are not diagnostic—i.e., complete blood count, creatinine determination, liver function tests, chest radiography, and electrocardiography—are important in the management of patients with IE. The erythrocyte sedimentation rate, C-reactive protein level, rheumatoid factor, and circulating immune complex titer are commonly increased in IE (Table 128-2). CTA, although exposing patients to radiation and contrast dye, can be used in lieu of preoperative cardiac catheterization to assess coronary artery patency in patients at low to intermediate risk of coronary disease. Brain MRI/MRA should be obtained in patients with neurologic signs or symptoms, including unusual headache, to assess for emboli, hemorrhage, or mycotic aneurysms. The findings can support the IE diagnosis as well as provide evidence requiring changes in planned surgical treatment. Contrast-enhanced whole-body tomography to detect silent emboli in patients without localizing symptoms is not likely to enhance diagnostic accuracy and is associated with significant risk of kidney injury due to contrast media exposure.

TREATMENT

Infective Endocarditis

ANTIMICROBIAL THERAPY

To cure IE, all bacteria in the vegetation must be killed. This is difficult because local host defenses are deficient and because the bacteria are largely nongrowing and metabolically inactive and thus are less easily killed by antibiotics. Consequently, therapy must be bactericidal and prolonged. Antibiotics are generally given parenterally to achieve serum concentrations that, through passive diffusion, result in effective concentrations in the depths of the vegetation. The decision to initiate treatment empirically must balance

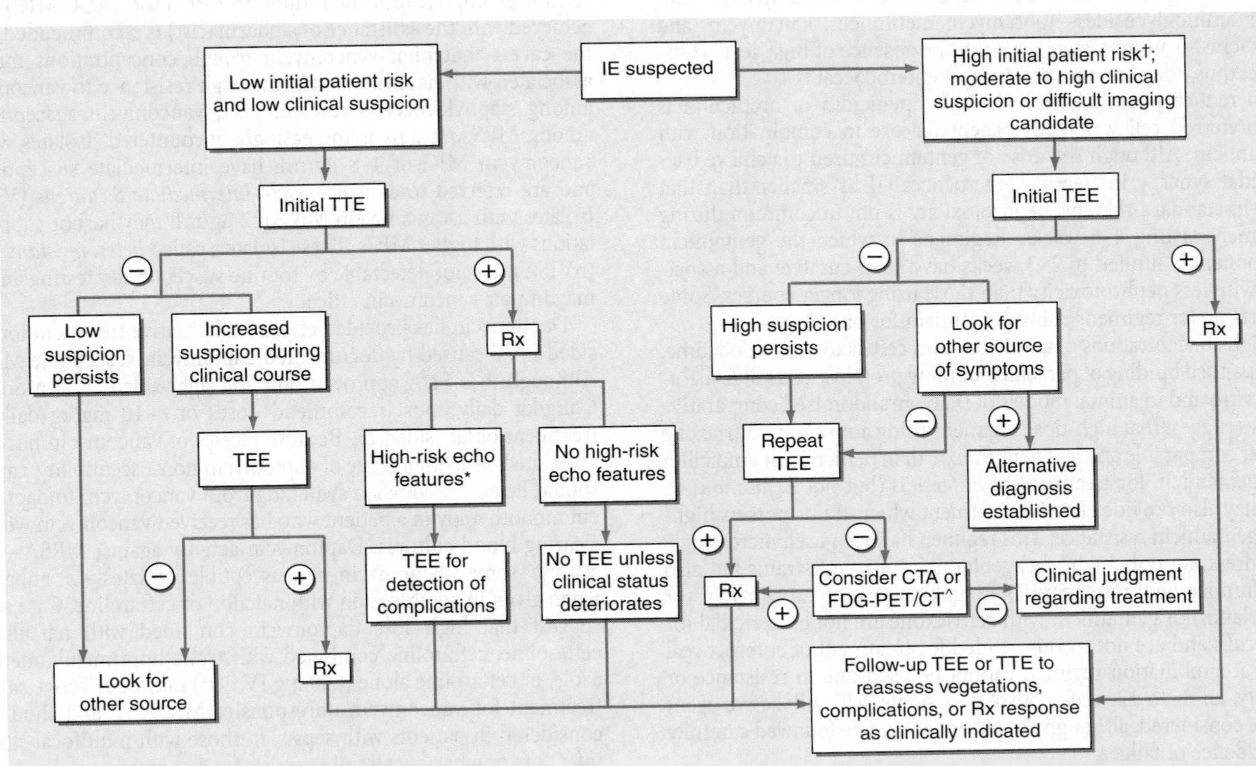

FIGURE 128-3 The diagnostic use of transesophageal and transthoracic echocardiography (TEE and TTE, respectively). †High initial patient risk for infective endocarditis (IE) or evidence of intracardiac complications (new regurgitant murmur, new electrocardiographic conduction changes, or congestive heart failure). *High-risk echocardiographic features include large vegetations, valve insufficiency, paravalvular infection, or ventricular dysfunction. Rx indicates initiation of antibiotic therapy. CTA, ECG-gated cardiac CT angiogram; FDG-PET/CT, fluorodeoxyglucose-positron emission tomography CT. ^See text for discussion of these modalities. *(Reproduced with permission from AS Bayer: Diagnosis and management of infective endocarditis and its complications. Circulation 98:2936, 1998.)*

the need to establish a microbiologic diagnosis against the potential disease progression or the need to control infection prior to urgent surgery (see "Blood Cultures," above). Infection at other sites (such as the meninges), allergies, end-organ dysfunction, interactions with concomitantly administered medications, and risks of adverse events must be considered in the selection of therapy.

The regimens recommended for the treatment of PVE (except that caused by staphylococci), although given for several weeks longer, are similar to those used to treat NVE (**Table 128-5**). Recommended antibiotic dosing and duration of therapy, which is measured from the time blood cultures become negative, should be followed unless alterations are required by end-organ dysfunction or adverse events.

Organism-Specific Therapies **•** **Streptococci** The recommended therapies for streptococcal IE are based on the minimal inhibitory concentration (MIC) of penicillin for the causative isolate (Table 128-5). The 2-week penicillin/gentamicin and ceftriaxone/gentamicin regimens should not be used to treat NVE complicated by cardiac or extracardiac abscess or PVE. Caution should be exercised in considering aminoglycoside-containing regimens in patients at increased risk for aminoglycoside toxicity (renal or eighth cranial nerve). The regimens recommended for relatively penicillin-resistant streptococci are advocated for treatment of group B, C, or G streptococcal IE. *Granulicatella*, *Abiotrophia*, and *Gemella* species are treated with the regimens for moderately penicillin-resistant streptococci, as is PVE caused by these organisms or by streptococci with a penicillin MIC of >0.1 μg/mL (Table 128-5).

Enterococci Enterococci are resistant to oxacillin, nafcillin, and the cephalosporins and are only inhibited—not killed—by the cell wall–active agents penicillin, ampicillin, teicoplanin (not available in the United States), and vancomycin. Enterococci are killed by the synergistic interaction of these cell wall–active antibiotics combined with gentamicin, unless the isolate exhibits high-level resistance to gentamicin, defined as growth of the isolate in the presence of gentamicin at ≥500 μg/mL. Bactericidal synergy with other aminoglycosides—tobramycin, netilmicin, kanamycin, and amikacin—is unpredictable even in the absence of high-level resistance; thus, they are not used to treat enterococcal IE.

To reduce potential nephrotoxicity, penicillin or ampicillin is the preferred cell wall–active agent for use in combination with gentamicin. Although the dose of gentamicin used to achieve bactericidal synergy in treating enterococcal IE is smaller than that used in standard therapy, nephrotoxicity is not uncommon during treatment lasting 4–6 weeks. Regimens in which the gentamicin component is limited to 2–3 weeks have been curative and associated with less nephrotoxicity than those using longer courses. Some experts prefer regimens using gentamicin for only 2–3 weeks.

High concentrations of ampicillin plus ceftriaxone or cefotaxime, by expanded binding of penicillin-binding proteins, also kill *E. faecalis* in vitro and in animal models of IE. Nonrandomized comparative studies suggest that high-dose regimens using ampicillin-ceftriaxone appear comparable and less nephrotoxic than penicillin or ampicillin plus gentamicin for treatment of *E. faecalis* (but not *E. faecium*) IE and may also provide effective treatment when strains possess high-level gentamicin resistance. This regimen has been used increasingly to address not only high-level gentamicin-resistant strains but also to minimize nephrotoxicity. The combinations of vancomycin (or teicoplanin) or gentamicin with ceftriaxone are not bactericidal for *E. faecalis* and are not recommended for treatment of enterococcal IE. If a combination regimen cannot be used due to resistance or toxicity, an 8- to 12-week course of a single cell wall–active agent can be considered, although the patient should be followed carefully for evidence of failure.

Treatment of IE caused by *E. faecium*, which is generally more antibiotic resistant than *E. faecalis* or may be vancomycin resistant, is not well established. Successful treatment of IE caused by vancomycin-resistant enterococci with high-dose daptomycin (10–12 mg/kg IV once daily), occasionally in combination with ampicillin, has been reported. If the isolate susceptibility allows treatment with penicillin/ampicillin plus gentamicin, this is preferred. These cases should be managed in conjunction with an infectious disease consultant.

Staphylococci Management of *S. aureus* bacteremia and IE in conjunction with infectious disease consultants has been associated with improved outcomes and is recommended. Treatment of staphylococcal IE (Table 128-5) is based on the presence of a prosthetic valve or foreign device, the native valve(s) involved (right vs left side), and the antibiotic susceptibility of the isolate. Penicillin resistance and, except in specific countries, methicillin resistance is widespread among staphylococci. Thus, empirical therapy for possible staphylococcal IE should use a regimen effective against methicillin-resistant organisms. Therapy should be revised to a β-lactam agent (preferably an antistaphylococcal penicillin) if the isolate is susceptible to methicillin. Cefazolin is generally considered an alternative β-lactam agent for the treatment of methicillin-susceptible staphylococcal (MSSA) IE. Ease of administration and reduced adverse events compared to treatment with an antistaphylococcal penicillin have prompted use of cefazolin as a primary agent in this setting. Concerns, however, have been raised about inactivation of cefazolin by type A and C staphylococcal β-lactamases (these do not hydrolyze antistaphylococcal penicillins) and resulting treatment failure in high-inoculum infections. Initiating treatment with an antistaphylococcal penicillin until there is source control and a reduced inoculum and then transition to cefazolin is advised. The addition of gentamicin to a β-lactam antibiotic or vancomycin to enhance therapy for left-sided NVE has not improved survival rates and is associated with nephrotoxicity. Most guidelines do not recommend the routine addition of gentamicin, fusidic acid, or rifampin to regimens for *S. aureus* NVE.

For treatment of NVE due to *methicillin-resistant S. aureus* (MRSA), vancomycin, dosed to achieve trough concentrations of at least 15 μg/mL, (or more precisely an area under the time concentration curve/broth microdilution MIC ratio [AUC:MIC] >400 achieved with the assistance of a pharmacist) is recommended, with the caveat that high vancomycin trough concentrations may be associated with nephrotoxicity. Although resistance to vancomycin among staphylococci is rare, reduced vancomycin susceptibility among MRSA strains is increasingly encountered. Isolates with a vancomycin MIC of 4–8 μg/mL have intermediate susceptibility and are referred to as *vancomycin-intermediate S. aureus* (VISA). Isolates with a vancomycin MIC of 2 μg/mL may harbor subpopulations with higher MICs. These isolates, called *heteroresistant VISA* (hVISA), are not detectable by routine susceptibility testing and yet may impair vancomycin efficacy.

Daptomycin has provided effective alternative treatment for left-sided NVE caused by documented daptomycin-susceptible MRSA. Although it is FDA approved only for right-sided IE at a dose of 6 mg/kg daily, most recommend doses of 8–10 mg/kg daily for treatment of left-sided IE. Because receipt of vancomycin has been associated with emergence of daptomycin nonsusceptibility, caution should be exercised when switching from vancomycin to daptomycin monotherapy in a patient who has received vancomycin without clearing blood cultures. Daptomycin activity against MRSA—even against some daptomycin-nonsusceptible isolates—is enhanced when given in combination with nafcillin or ceftaroline. Case series suggest that high-dose daptomycin combined with nafcillin or ceftaroline, ceftaroline combined with trimethoprim/sulfamethoxazole, or ceftaroline alone (600 mg IV q8h) may be effective salvage treatment for vancomycin-unresponsive MRSA IE and should be considered in patients with sepsis, in those with multifocal sites of infection, or when bacteremia persists for 4 or more days. Eradicable sources of bacteremia should always be addressed; failure of source control is a very common reason for persistent MRSA bacteremia.

MSSA IE that is uncomplicated and limited to the tricuspid or pulmonic valve can often be treated with 2 weeks of oxacillin or nafcillin (but not vancomycin). Prolonged fever (≥5 days) during

TABLE 128-5 Antibiotic Treatment for Infective Endocarditis Caused by Common Organisms[a]

ORGANISM(S)	DRUG (DOSE, DURATION)	COMMENTS
Streptococci		**For PVE 6-week regimens are preferred.**
Penicillin-susceptible streptococci, *S. gallolyticus* (MIC ≤0.12 μg/mL[b])	• Penicillin G (2–3 mU IV q4h for 4 weeks)	Can use ampicillin or amoxicillin (2 g IV q4h) if penicillin is unavailable.
	• Ceftriaxone (2 g daily as a single dose for 4 weeks)	Can use ceftriaxone in patients with non-immediate penicillin allergy.
	• Vancomycin[c] (15 mg/kg IV q12h for 4 weeks)	Use vancomycin for patients with immediate (urticarial) or severe penicillin allergy. Obtain allergy consultation for further evaluation including role of β-lactam desensitization.
	• Penicillin G (2–3 mU IV q4h) *or* ceftriaxone (2 g IV daily) for 2 weeks ***plus*** Gentamicin[d] (3 mg/kg daily IV or IM, as a single dose[e] or divided into equal doses q8h for 2 weeks)	Avoid 2-week regimen when risk of aminoglycoside toxicity is increased and in prosthetic-valve or complicated endocarditis. Can use ampicillin or amoxicillin (2 g IV q4h) if penicillin is unavailable.
Relatively penicillin-resistant streptococci, *S. gallolyticus* (MIC >0.12 μg/mL and <0.5 μg/mL[f])	• Penicillin G (4 mU IV q4h) *or* ceftriaxone (2 g IV daily) for 4 weeks ***plus*** Gentamicin[d] (3 mg/kg daily IV or IM, as a single dose[e] or divided into equal doses q8h for 2 weeks)	Can use ampicillin or amoxicillin (2 g IV q4h) if penicillin is unavailable. Penicillin alone at this dose for 6 weeks or with gentamicin during the initial 2 weeks is preferred for PVE caused by streptococci with penicillin MICs of ≤0.12 μg/mL.
	• Vancomycin[c] as noted above for 6 weeks	Use vancomycin for patients with immediate (urticarial) or severe penicillin allergy. Obtain allergy consultation for further evaluation including role of β-lactam desensitization. Ceftriaxone alone or with gentamicin can be used in patients with non-immediate β-lactam allergy.
Moderately penicillin-resistant streptococci (MIC, ≥0.5 μg/mL and <8 μg/mL[g]); *Granulicatella*, *Abiotrophia*, or *Gemella* spp.	• Penicillin G (4–5 mU IV q4h) *or* ceftriaxone (2 g IV daily) for 6 weeks ***plus*** Gentamicin[d] (3 mg/kg daily IV or IM as a single dose[e] *or* divided into equal doses q8h for 6 weeks)	Preferred for PVE caused by streptococci with penicillin MICs of >0.12 μg/mL. Can use ampicillin or amoxicillin (2 g IV q4h) if penicillin is unavailable.
	• Vancomycin[c] as noted above for 6 weeks	Regimen is preferred by some.
Enterococci[h]		**For PVE 6-week regimens are preferred.**
	• Penicillin G (4–5 mU IV q4h) *plus* gentamicin[d] (1 mg/kg IV q8h), both for 4–6 weeks	Can treat NVE for 4 weeks if symptoms last <3 months. Treat NVE with >3 months of symptoms for 6 weeks. Can abbreviate gentamicin course in some patients (see text).
	• Ampicillin (2 g IV q4h) *plus* gentamicin[d] (1 mg/kg IV q8h), both for 4–6 weeks	Can use IV amoxicillin in lieu of ampicillin (same dose). Can abbreviate gentamicin course in some patients (see text).
	• Vancomycin[c] (15 mg/kg IV q12h) *plus* gentamicin[d] (1 mg/kg IV q8h), both for 6 weeks	Use vancomycin plus gentamicin only for penicillin-allergic patients (preferable to desensitize to penicillin if immediate (urticarial) allergy; consult allergy) and for isolates resistant to penicillin/ampicillin.
	• Ampicillin (2 g IV q4h) *plus* ceftriaxone (2 g IV q12h), both for 6 weeks	Use for *E. faecalis* isolates with or without high-level resistance to gentamicin or for patients at high risk for aminoglycoside nephrotoxicity (creatinine clearance rate <50 mL/min; see text).
Staphylococci (*S. aureus* and coagulase-negative)		
MSSA infecting native valves (no foreign devices) including complicated right-sided and left-sided endocarditis.	• Nafcillin, oxacillin, *or* flucloxacillin (2 g IV q4h for 6 weeks)	Addition of gentamicin is not recommended. For uncomplicated right-sided endocarditis a 2-week course may be effective (see text).
	• Cefazolin (2 g IV q8h for 6 weeks)	Can use cefazolin regimen for patients with non-immediate penicillin allergy; see text regarding cefazolin vs antistaphylococcal penicillin as primary therapy. Addition of gentamicin not recommended.
	• Vancomycin[c] (15 mg/kg IV q12h for 6 weeks)	Only use vancomycin for patients with immediate (urticarial) or severe penicillin allergy until allergy consultation can be obtained for β-lactam desensitization evaluation; addition of gentamicin not recommended.
MRSA infecting native valves (no foreign devices)	• Vancomycin[c] (15 mg/kg IV q8–12h) or daptomycin (8–10 mg/kg daily) for 6 weeks	No role for routine use of rifampin (see text). For daptomycin treatment, see text.
MSSA infecting prosthetic valves	• Nafcillin, oxacillin, *or* flucloxacillin (2 g IV q4h for 6–8 weeks) ***plus*** Gentamicin[d] (1 mg/kg IM or IV q8h for 2 weeks) ***plus*** • Rifampin[i] (300 mg PO q8h for 6–8 weeks)	Use gentamicin during initial 2 weeks; determine gentamicin susceptibility and await blood culture clearance before initiating rifampin (see text); if patient is highly allergic to penicillin, use regimen for MRSA and obtain allergy consultation; if β-lactam allergy is of the minor non-immediate type, cefazolin can be substituted for oxacillin, nafcillin, or flucloxacillin.
MRSA infecting prosthetic valves	• Vancomycin[c] (15 mg/kg IV q12h for 6–8 weeks) ***plus*** Gentamicin[d] (1 mg/kg IM or IV q8h for 2 weeks) ***plus*** • Rifampin[i] (300 mg PO q8h for 6–8 weeks)	Use gentamicin during initial 2 weeks; determine gentamicin susceptibility and await blood culture clearance before initiating rifampin (see text). Daptomycin (8–10 mg/kg daily) could be considered as an alternative to vancomycin but data are limited.
HACEK Organisms		**For PVE 6-week regimens are preferred.**
	• Ceftriaxone (2 g/d IV as a single dose for 4 weeks)	Can use another third-generation cephalosporin at comparable dose.
	• Ampicillin/sulbactam (3 g IV q6h for 4 weeks)	Use ampicillin only if β-lactamase production can be excluded. If the isolate is susceptible, ciprofloxacin (400 mg IV q12h) can be used.

(*Continued*)

TABLE 128-5 Antibiotic Treatment for Infective Endocarditis Caused by Common Organisms[a] (Continued)

ORGANISM(S)	DRUG (DOSE, DURATION)	COMMENTS
Coxiella burnetii		
	• Doxycycline (100 mg PO q12h) *plus* hydroxychloroquine (200 mg PO q8h), both for at least 18 (native valve) or 24 (prosthetic valve) months	Follow serology to monitor response during treatment (antiphase I IgG and IgA decreased 4-fold and IgM antiphase II negative) and thereafter for relapse.
***Bartonella* spp.**		
	• Doxycycline (100 mg q12h PO) for 6 weeks ***plus*** Gentamicin (1 mg/kg IV q8h for 2 weeks)	If doxycycline is not tolerated, use azithromycin (500 mg PO daily). Some experts recommend that doxycycline be continued for 3–6 months unless all infection is resected surgically.

[a]Regimens adapted from the guidelines of the American Heart Association and the European Society of Cardiology (ESC). Doses of gentamicin, vancomycin, and daptomycin must be adjusted for reduced renal function. Ideal body weight is used to calculate doses of gentamicin and daptomycin per kilogram (men = 50 kg + 2.3 kg per inch over 5 feet; women = 45.5 kg + 2.3 kg per inch over 5 feet). [b]MIC ≤0.125 μg/mL per ESC. [c]Vancomycin dose is based on actual body weight. Adjust for trough level of 10–15 μg/mL for streptococcal and enterococcal infections and 15–20 μg/mL for staphylococcal infections (see text). [d]Aminoglycosides should not be administered as single daily doses for enterococcal endocarditis and should be introduced as part of the initial treatment. Target peak and trough serum concentrations of divided-dose gentamicin 1 h after a 20- to 30-min infusion or IM injection are ~3.5 μg/mL and ≤1 μg/mL, respectively; [e]Netilmicin (4 mg/kg qd, as a single dose) can be used in lieu of gentamicin for streptococcal infection only. [f]MIC >0.125 μg/mL and ≤2.0 μg/mL per ESC. [g]MIC >2.0 μg/mL per ESC; treat with regimen for enterococci (BSAC). [h]Antimicrobial susceptibility must be evaluated; see text. [i]Rifampin increases warfarin and dicumarol requirements for anticoagulation.

Abbreviations: MIC, minimal inhibitory concentration; MRSA, methicillin-resistant *S. aureus*; MSSA, methicillin-sensitive *S. aureus*; NVE, native-valve endocarditis; PVE, prosthetic-valve endocarditis.

therapy or multiple septic pulmonary emboli mandates standard-duration therapy. Right-sided MRSA IE is treated for at least 4 weeks with vancomycin or daptomycin (6 mg/kg daily); 2-week courses of therapy are suboptimal.

Staphylococcal PVE is treated for 6–8 weeks with a multidrug regimen (Table 128-5). To achieve long-term bacterial eradication, rifampin, which kills staphylococci embedded in biofilm adherent to foreign material, is an essential component of this regimen. Rifampin resistance can emerge during therapy. To prevent emergence of resistance, administration of rifampin should be delayed until initial therapy with two agents (gentamicin plus an antistaphylococcal penicillin or vancomycin selected on the basis of susceptibility testing) has eradicated bacteremia (reduced the inoculum). The isolate's susceptibility to gentamicin or an alternative agent as well as to rifampin should be established before rifampin treatment is begun. Possible alternatives for gentamicin include another aminoglycoside, a fluoroquinolone (chosen on the basis of susceptibility), ceftaroline, or another active agent.

Other Organisms In the absence of meningitis, IE caused by *Streptococcus pneumoniae* isolates with a penicillin MIC of ≤4 μg/mL can be treated with IV penicillin (4 million units IV every 4 h), ceftriaxone (2 g daily as a single dose or cefotaxime at a comparable dose), or vancomycin. Ceftriaxone or vancomycin is preferred for pneumococcal strains with a penicillin MIC of ≥ 2 μg/mL. If meningitis is suspected, treatment with vancomycin plus ceftriaxone—at the doses advised for meningitis—should be initiated until susceptibility results are known. Definitive therapy should then be selected on the basis of meningitis breakpoints (penicillin MIC, 0.06 μg/mL; or ceftriaxone MIC, 0.5 μg/mL). Pneumococcal NVE is treated for 4 weeks and pneumococcal PVE for 6 weeks. *P. aeruginosa* IE is treated with an antipseudomonal cephalosporin and high doses of tobramycin (8 mg/kg per day in three divided doses). IE caused by *Enterobacterales* is treated with a β-lactam antibiotic plus an aminoglycoside. Corynebacterial IE is treated with penicillin plus an aminoglycoside (if the organism is susceptible to the aminoglycoside) or with vancomycin, which is highly bactericidal for most strains. Therapy for *Candida* IE consists of a lipid formulation of amphotericin B (3–5 mg/kg IV daily) with or without flucytosine (25 mg/kg PO q6h) (if using flucytosine monitor renal function, flucytosine levels, and bone marrow function). Alternatively, a high-dose echinocandin regimen can be used. If there is valve dysfunction or PVE, early surgery is advised, as is long-term (if not indefinite) oral azole suppression. Absent valve dysfunction, medical treatment with long-term oral azole suppression may achieve results comparable to surgical treatment.

Empirical Therapy and Treatment for Culture-Negative IE In designing therapy to be administered before culture results are known or when cultures are truly negative, clinical clues to etiology (e.g., acute vs subacute presentation, NVE, early or late PVE, the patient's predispositions) as well as epidemiologic clues (region of residence, animal exposure) must be considered. Thus empirical therapy for acute IE should cover MRSA and in a PWID or for health care–associated NVE potentially antibiotic-resistant gram-negative bacilli. Treatment with vancomycin plus gentamicin or cefepime, initiated immediately after blood cultures are obtained, covers these organisms as well as many others. For empirical treatment of NVE with a subacute presentation, vancomycin plus ceftriaxone is reasonable. For blood culture–pending PVE, vancomycin, gentamicin, and cefepime should be used if the prosthetic valve has been in place for ≤1 year. Empirical therapy for late PVE (valve in place for >1 year) is similar to that for culture-negative NVE. Therapy is revised once a pathogen has been identified.

In the treatment of blood culture–negative episodes, marantic endocarditis and the antiphospholipid antibody syndrome must be considered. In the absence of prior antibiotic therapy, it is unlikely that infection due to *S. aureus*, CoNS, enterococci, or *Enterobacterales* will present with negative blood cultures; thus recommended empirical therapy targets fastidious streptococci, *Abiotrophia*, *Granulicatella*, the HACEK group, and *Bartonella* species. Pending the availability of diagnostic data, blood culture–negative subacute NVE is treated with vancomycin plus ampicillin-sulbactam (12 g every 24 h) or ceftriaxone; doxycycline (100 mg twice daily) is added for enhanced *Bartonella* coverage. If cultures are negative because of prior antibiotic administration, pathogens likely to be inhibited by the specific prior therapy should be considered.

TAVR-PVE The vast majority of these patients are treated medically with classic PVE antibiotic regimens for the given pathogen. Selection of empirical therapy pending blood culture results similarly parallels that for classic PVE but with recognition that enterococcal infection occurs with increased frequency.

CIED-IE Antimicrobial therapy for CIED IE (as well as for generator pocket and lead infection) is adjunctive to complete removal of the device. The antimicrobial selected is based on the causative organism and should be used as recommended for NVE (Table 128-5). Bacteremic CIED infection may be complicated by coincident left-sided NVE, PVE, or remote-site infection (e.g., osteomyelitis), which may require modification of antimicrobial therapy. A 4- to 6-week course of IE-targeted therapy is recommended for patients with CIED-IE and for those with bacteremia that continues after device removal. Generator pocket infection without bacteremia is treated with a 10- to 14-day course, some of which can be given orally. In the absence of another source, *S. aureus* bacteremia (and persistent CoNS bacteremia) is likely indicative of CIED-IE or valvular IE and should be investigated and managed accordingly. However, not all bloodstream infections in these patients indicate IE. If evidence suggesting CIED-IE is lacking, bloodstream infection due to gram-negative bacilli, streptococci, and enterococci species may not indicate CIED-IE and can be treated with antimicrobial therapy for the alternative diagnosis. However, in these patients relapse after antimicrobial therapy increases the likelihood of CIED-IE and warrants treatment as such. Attempted salvage of an infected CIED with antibiotics alone and long-term suppressive therapy is usually unsuccessful and should be reserved for patients whose devices cannot be removed or who refuse removal. Careful follow-up is required.

Partial Oral Antibiotic Treatment of IE Recent studies have examined the use of oral antibiotics to complete therapy in patients who have received an initial course of intravenous treatment (with or without cardiac surgery). A noninferiority, multicenter, randomized study found mortality among patients with left-sided IE caused by streptococci, enterococci, and staphylococci who received partial oral treatment comparable to that of patients who were treated intravenously for the full course of therapy (6.5% and 7.5%, respectively). Four hundred clinically stable patients (20% of the population screened) who had received at least 10 days of parenteral therapy (or at least 7 days after surgery) were enrolled. IE was caused by streptococci (49%), enterococci (24%), and MSSA (22%); no patients had MRSA. Of note, the median duration of intravenous treatment before the switch to oral agents was 16 days (interquartile range, 13–23); thus, some patients may have been effectively cured by intravenous therapy with or without surgery prior to transition to oral therapy. The results in this highly selected and monitored cohort with relatively small numbers of patients with enterococcal and *S. aureus* IE may not be generalizable to most patients with IE. Thus caution is advised before adopting this approach as standard care.

Outpatient Antimicrobial Therapy Fully compliant, clinically stable patients who are no longer bacteremic, are not febrile, and have no clinical or echocardiographic findings that suggest an impending complication may complete IV therapy as outpatients. Careful follow-up and a stable home setting are necessary, as are predictable IV access and use of antimicrobial agents that are stable in solution and less frequently associated with severe adverse effects. Recommended regimens should not be compromised to accommodate outpatient therapy.

Monitoring Antimicrobial Therapy Antibiotic-related adverse events occur in 25–40% of IE patients and commonly arise after several weeks of therapy. Blood tests to detect renal, hepatic, and hematologic toxicity should be performed periodically. Serum concentrations of aminoglycosides and vancomycin should be monitored and doses adjusted to optimize treatment and minimize toxicity.

Control of peripheral sites of infection—source control—should be addressed promptly. Blood cultures should be repeated daily until sterile in patients with IE due to *S. aureus* or difficult-to-treat organisms, rechecked if there is recrudescent fever, and performed again 4–6 weeks after therapy to document cure. Blood cultures become sterile after 2 days of appropriate therapy when infection is caused by viridans streptococci, *E. faecalis*, or HACEK organisms. In MSSA IE, β-lactam therapy results in sterile cultures in 3–5 days, whereas in MRSA IE, the duration of bacteremia is often longer with vancomycin or daptomycin treatment. MRSA bacteremia persisting despite an appropriate dosage of vancomycin or daptomycin may indicate emergence of reduced susceptibility in the infecting strain and point to a need for alternative therapy. When fever persists for 7 days despite appropriate antibiotic therapy, patients should be evaluated further for paravalvular abscess, extracardiac abscesses (spleen, kidney), or complications (embolic events). Recrudescent fever raises the possibility of these complications but also of drug reactions or complications of hospitalization. Vegetations become smaller with effective therapy; however, 3 months after cure, 50% are unchanged, and 25% each are slightly larger or smaller.

Antithrombotic Therapy Because patients with IE are at risk for hemorrhagic transformation of embolic strokes and for intracerebral hemorrhage from septic arteritis or ruptured mycotic aneurysms, initiation of antithrombotic (anticoagulant or antiplatelet) therapy requires careful consideration of the risks and benefits. Antithrombotic therapy can render such bleeding catastrophic. Neither anticoagulant nor antiplatelet therapy reduces the risk of emboli in patients with NVE, and thus such treatment is not indicated for that purpose. However, patients with IE may have coexisting conditions wherein anticoagulation is indicated. Thus, in the absence of a contraindication (i.e., no clinical or imaging evidence of a recent large embolic stroke, intracerebral hemorrhage, or mycotic aneurysm), anticoagulant therapy is given to patients who have a mechanical prosthetic valve, atrial fibrillation with either mitral stenosis or a CHA2DS2-VASc score ≥2, or deep-vein thrombophlebitis. Most experts use unfractionated or low-molecular-weight heparin for ease of reversal. Anticoagulant therapy should be reversed, at least temporarily, in most patients who have had an acute ischemic stroke or an intracerebral hemorrhage.

SURGICAL TREATMENT

The indications for cardiac surgical treatment of IE (**Table 128-6**) have been derived from observational studies and expert opinion. The strength of specific indications varies; thus the risks and benefits as well as the timing of surgery must be individualized (**Table 128-7**). These are best weighed by a team that includes cardiologists, cardiac surgeons, infectious disease physicians, and neurologists if there have been neurologic complications. Between 25% and 40% of patients with left-sided IE undergo cardiac surgery during active infection, with slightly higher surgery rates for PVE than NVE. The benefit of surgery has been assessed primarily in retrospective studies comparing populations of medically and

TABLE 128-6 Indications for Cardiac Surgical Treatment in Patients with Endocarditis

Surgery Required for Optimal Outcome
Native-valve or prosthetic-valve endocarditis
Moderate or severe congestive heart failure or shock due to valve dysfunction
Paravalvular extension of infection with abscess, fistula, or heart block
Persistent bacteremia without an extracardiac cause despite 7–10 days of optimal antimicrobial therapy
Lack of effective antimicrobial therapy (e.g., fungal [see text regarding *Candida* spp.], *Brucella*, multidrug-resistant gram-negative bacillary endocarditis)
Prosthetic-valve endocarditis
Partially dehisced unstable prosthetic valve
Paravalvular extension of infection with abscess, fistula, or heart block (see text)
Surgery To Be Strongly Considered for Improved Outcome[a]
Prosthetic-valve endocarditis
S. aureus infection with intracardiac complications
Relapse after optimal antimicrobial therapy
Native-valve endocarditis
Large (>10-mm) hypermobile vegetation, particularly with prior systemic embolus and significant valve dysfunction[b]
Very large (>30-mm) vegetation
Persistent unexplained fever (≥10 days) in blood culture–negative endocarditis
Poorly responsive or relapsed endocarditis due to highly antibiotic-resistant enterococci or gram-negative bacilli

[a]Carefully consider surgery. Multiple findings are often combined to justify surgery.
[b]In the group with an estimated low cardiac-surgery mortality risk (see text).

TABLE 128-7 Timing of Cardiac Surgical Intervention in Patients with Endocarditis

TIMING	INDICATION FOR SURGICAL INTERVENTION	
	STRONG SUPPORTING EVIDENCE	CONFLICTING EVIDENCE, BUT MAJORITY OF OPINIONS FAVOR SURGERY
Emergent (same day)	Valve dysfunction with pulmonary edema or cardiogenic shock Acute aortic regurgitation plus preclosure of mitral valve Sinus of Valsalva abscess ruptured into right heart Rupture into pericardial sac	
Urgent (within 1–2 days)	Valve obstruction by vegetation Unstable (dehisced) prosthesis Acute aortic or mitral regurgitation with heart failure (New York Heart Association class III or IV) Septal perforation Paravalvular extension of infection with or without new electrocardiographic conduction system changes Lack of effective antibiotic therapy	Vegetation diameter >10 mm plus severe but not urgent aortic or mitral valve dysfunction[a] Major embolus plus persisting large vegetation (>10 mm) Mobile vegetation >30 mm
Elective (earlier usually preferred)	Progressive paravalvular prosthetic regurgitation Valve dysfunction plus persisting infection after ≥7–10 days of antimicrobial therapy Fungal (mold) endocarditis	Staphylococcal prosthetic-valve endocarditis with intracardiac complications Early prosthetic-valve endocarditis (≤2 months after valve surgery) *Candida* spp. endocarditis (see text) Antibiotic-resistant organisms

[a]Supported by a single-institution randomized trial showing benefit from early surgery. Implementation requires clinical judgment. If surgery is elected, it must be done early (see text).

Source: Reproduced with permission from L Olaison, G Pettersson: Current best practices and guidelines: Indications for surgical intervention in infective endocarditis. Infect Dis Clin North Am 16:453, 2002.

surgically treated patients matched for the necessity of surgery, with adjustments for predictors of death (comorbidities) and the timing of surgical intervention (a correction for survival bias). Although study results vary, surgery for NVE based on current indications appears to convey a significant survival benefit (27–55%), which is greatest among those with the most pressing indications. The survival benefit becomes more apparent after ≥6 months. The effect of surgery for PVE is more nuanced, with survival benefits accruing largely to those with intracardiac complications. Of note, surgery itself carries mortality risks that may offset survival benefits in patients with lesser indications. Among patients with TAVR-PVE, 50–80% are reported to have an indication for surgical intervention—yet because of high pre-TAVR estimated operative mortality, <15% undergo surgery. Some patients with significant aortic regurgitation after medical cure of infection have undergone valve-in-valve redo-TAVR.

Indications • **Congestive Heart Failure** Moderate to severe refractory CHF caused by new or worsening valve dysfunction or intracardiac fistulae is the major indication for cardiac surgery. Surgery can relieve functional stenosis due to large vegetations or restore competence to damaged regurgitant valves by repair or replacement. At 6–12 months of follow-up of patients with left-sided NVE or PVE and moderate to severe CHF due to valve dysfunction, survival is significantly improved among those treated surgically compared with those treated medically. The survival benefit with surgery is inversely related to the severity of preoperative CHF; thus surgery should not be delayed in the face of deteriorating hemodynamics.

Paravalvular Infection This complication, which is most common with aortic valve infection, occurs in 10–15% of patients with NVE and in 45–60% of those with PVE. It is suggested clinically by persistent unexplained fever during appropriate therapy, new electrocardiographic conduction disturbances, or pericarditis. TEE with color Doppler is the test of choice to detect paravalvular abscesses (sensitivity, ≥85%). Occasionally, three-dimensional TEE, ECG-gated CTA, or ^{18}FDG-PET/CT demonstrate paravalvular infection not detected by TEE. For optimal outcome, paravalvular infection requires surgery, especially when fever persists, fistulae develop, prostheses are dehisced and unstable, or infection relapses after appropriate treatment. Cardiac rhythm must be monitored since high-grade heart block may require insertion of a pacemaker.

Uncontrolled Infection Continued positive blood cultures or otherwise unexplained persistent fevers despite optimal antibiotic therapy may reflect uncontrolled infection that warrants surgery. Surgical treatment is also advised for IE caused by organisms against which effective antimicrobial therapy is lacking (e.g., yeasts, molds, *P. aeruginosa*, other highly antibiotic-resistant bacteria, *Brucella* species).

***S. aureus* IE** The mortality rate for *S. aureus* PVE exceeds 50% with medical treatment and may be reduced with surgical treatment. Nevertheless, surgery is not routinely advised for uncomplicated *S. aureus* PVE. Rather, survival benefits are most likely in those with paravalvular infection, dysfunctional valves, and CHF. Surgical treatment of *S. aureus* NVE should be guided by the standard indications. Isolated tricuspid-valve *S. aureus* IE, even with persistent fever, rarely requires surgery.

Prevention of Systemic Emboli Persisting morbidity and/or death may result from cerebral or coronary artery emboli. Antithrombotic therapy does not prevent systemic emboli in NVE. The frequency of embolization decreases rapidly with effective antimicrobial therapy. Thus, if emboli are to be prevented through surgical intervention, surgery must occur very early. Vegetation characteristics defined echocardiographically can identify patients at high risk of embolization but do not identify those patients in whom surgery to prevent emboli will increase survival. In a small randomized trial in patients who were at low risk of surgery-related mortality and had large vegetations (>10 mm) and significant valve dysfunction, emboli were prevented by early surgery (≤48 h after diagnosis), but there was no survival benefit. Rarely is prevention of emboli the sole indication for surgery; more often this may be an additional benefit of early surgery for other indications. Valve repair, with the consequent avoidance of a prosthesis, improves the benefit-to-risk ratio of surgery performed to eliminate vegetations.

CIED-IE Removal of all hardware is recommended for patients with established CIED-IE as well as for pocket or intracardiac lead infection. Percutaneous lead extraction is preferred; if hardware remains after attempted percutaneous extraction, surgical removal should be considered. With lead vegetations >2 cm, there is a risk of a pulmonary embolism; nevertheless, the need for CIED removal surgically is unclear. Removal of the infected CIED during the initial hospitalization is associated with increased 30-day and 1-year survival rates over those attained with antibiotic therapy and device retention. The CIED, if needed, can be reimplanted at a new site after at least 10–14 days of effective antimicrobial therapy. CIEDs should be replaced when patients undergo surgery for IE.

Timing of Cardiac Surgery With life-threatening indications for surgery (valve dysfunction and severe CHF, perivalvular abscess, major prosthesis dehiscence), surgery during the initial days of therapy is associated with greater survival than later surgery. With less compelling indications, surgery may reasonably be delayed to allow further treatment as well as improvement in overall health (Table 128-7). Recrudescent IE on a newly implanted prosthetic valve follows surgery for active NVE and PVE in 2% and 6–15% of patients, respectively. These frequencies do not justify the increased mortality risk associated with delaying surgery in patients with severe heart failure, valve dysfunction, and uncontrolled infections. Delay is justified when infection and CHF are controlled with medical therapy.

Neurologic complications of IE may be exacerbated during cardiac surgery. The risk of neurologic deterioration is related to the type and severity of the preoperative neurologic complication and the interval between the complication and surgery. Non-urgent cardiac surgery should be delayed for 2–3 weeks after a large nonhemorrhagic embolic infarction and for 4 weeks after a significant cerebral hemorrhage. A ruptured mycotic aneurysm should be treated before cardiac surgery. In a non-obtunded patient with an ischemic stroke and hemorrhage excluded by imaging, cardiac surgery, if urgent, should be performed early.

Antibiotic Therapy after Cardiac Surgery Organisms have been detected on Gram stain—or their DNA has been detected by PCR—in excised valves from 45% of patients who have completed the recommended therapy for IE. However, organisms, most of which are unusual or antibiotic resistant, are rarely cultured from these valves. Detection of organisms or their DNA does not necessarily indicate antibiotic failure; in fact, relapse after surgery for active IE is uncommon. Thus, in uncomplicated NVE caused by susceptible organisms, the duration of preoperative plus postoperative treatment should equal the total duration of recommended therapy. For IE complicated by perivalvular abscess, partially treated PVE, or valves culture-positive for the original organism, a full course of therapy should be given postoperatively.

Treatment of IE in PWID PWID should be treated according to the standard guidelines for antibiotic selection and surgical intervention. Additionally, opiate use disorder (OUD) must be recognized as an ongoing predisposition for IE and treated; this includes medication-assisted therapy that is initiated during hospitalization and continued without delay upon discharge. Addressing OUD significantly increases completion of antibiotic therapy, decreases resumption of injection drug use, and decreases recurrent IE and requirement for cardiac surgery.

Extracardiac Complications Splenic abscess develops in 3–5% of patients with IE. Effective therapy requires either image-guided percutaneous drainage or splenectomy. Mycotic aneurysms occur in 2–15% of IE patients; one-half of these cases involve the cerebral arteries and present as headaches, focal neurologic symptoms, or hemorrhage. Cerebral aneurysms should be monitored by angiography. Some will resolve with effective antimicrobial therapy, but those that have leaked or persist or enlarge should be treated surgically, if possible. Extracerebral aneurysms present as local pain, a mass, local ischemia, or bleeding; these are treated surgically.

OUTCOME

IE is a heterogeneous disease that occurs in extremely heterogeneous patient populations. Adverse outcomes are associated with older age, severe comorbid conditions and diabetes, delayed diagnosis, involvement of prosthetic valves or the aortic valve, an invasive (*S. aureus*) or antibiotic-resistant (*P. aeruginosa*, yeast) pathogen, intracardiac and major neurologic complications, and health–care associated infection. Death or poor outcome often is related not to failure of antibiotic therapy but rather to the interactions of comorbidities and IE-related end-organ complications. In developed countries, overall survival rates are 80–85%; however, rates vary considerably among subpopulations of IE patients. The outcome for a given patient depends on that individual's infection, the complexity of required therapy, and preexisting comorbidities. About 85–90% of patients with NVE caused by viridans streptococci, HACEK organisms, or enterococci (susceptible to synergistic therapy) survive. For *S. aureus* NVE in patients who do not inject drugs, survival rates are 55–70%; rates are 85–90% among PWID. However, 1-year mortality rises to 20–30% among PWID if addiction is not successfully addressed. PVE beginning within 2 months after valve replacement results in mortality rates of 40–50%, whereas rates are only 10–20% in late-onset cases. In the elderly population with TAVR-PVE the in-hospital mortality is 35–50% and increases to 60–75% at 1 year. Crude survival rates after successful treatment of IE generally are 80–90% and 70–80% at 1 and 2 years, respectively.

PREVENTION

Prevention of IE has been a goal of clinical practice; however, the evidence establishing benefit from *antibiotic prophylaxis for IE* is insufficient to recommend it as a widespread standard of care. The American Heart Association and the European Society of Cardiology recommend limiting prophylactic antibiotics (**Table 128-8**) to only patients at highest risk for severe morbidity or death from IE (**Table 128-9**). The National Institute for Health and Clinical Excellence in the United Kingdom initially advised discontinuation of all antibiotic prophylaxis for IE but recently became less dogmatic, allowing clinicians to use clinical judgment in the settings outlined.

In at-risk patients, maintaining good dental hygiene is recommended and antibiotic prophylaxis is recommended only when there is manipulation of gingival tissue or the periapical region of the teeth or perforation of the oral mucosa (including with respiratory tract surgery). Recent studies suggest that severe adverse events related to amoxicillin prophylaxis are exceedingly rare; however, clindamycin prophylaxis has been associated with low but significant rates of fatal and nonfatal adverse reactions with *Clostridioides difficile* infection. Consequently, the American Heart Association now recommends against the use of clindamycin for prophylaxis. Although prophylaxis is not advised for patients undergoing gastrointestinal or genitourinary

TABLE 128-8 Antibiotic Regimens for Prophylaxis of Endocarditis in Adults with High-Risk Cardiac Lesions[a,b]

A. Standard oral regimen
Amoxicillin: 2 g PO 1 h before procedure
B. Inability to take oral medication
Ampicillin: 2 g IV or IM within 1 h before procedure
C. Penicillin allergy
1. Clarithromycin or azithromycin: 500 mg PO 1 h before procedure
2. Cephalexin[c]: 2 g PO 1 h before procedure
3. Doxycycline: 100 mg PO 1 h before procedure
D. Penicillin allergy, inability to take oral medication
Cefazolin[c] or ceftriaxone[c]: 1 g IV or IM 30 min before procedure

[a]Dosing for children: for amoxicillin, ampicillin, cephalexin, or cefadroxil, use 50 mg/kg PO; cefazolin, 25 mg/kg IV; clindamycin, 20 mg/kg PO or 25 mg/kg IV; clarithromycin, 15 mg/kg PO; and vancomycin, 20 mg/kg IV. [b]For high-risk lesions, see Table 128-9. Prophylaxis is not advised for other lesions. [c]Do not use cephalosporins in patients with immediate hypersensitivity (urticaria, angioedema, anaphylaxis) to penicillin.

Source: Table created using the guidelines published by the American Heart Association and the European Society of Cardiology (W Wilson et al: Circulation 116:1736, 2007; W Wilson et al: Circulation 143:e963, 2021; and G Habib et al: Eur Heart J 30:2369, 2009).

TABLE 128-9 High-Risk Cardiac Lesions for Which Endocarditis Prophylaxis is Advised Before Dental Procedures

Prosthetic heart valves or material
Left ventricular assist devices or implantable heart
Prior endocarditis
Unrepaired cyanotic congenital heart disease, including palliative shunts or conduits
Completely repaired congenital heart defects during the 6 months after repair
Repaired congenital heart disease with residual defects adjacent to prosthetic material
Surgical or transcatheter pulmonary artery valve or conduit placement
Valvulopathy developing after cardiac transplantation[a]

[a]Not a target population for prophylaxis according to recommendations of the European Society for Cardiology.

Source: Table created using the guidelines published by the American Heart Association and the European Society of Cardiology (W Wilson et al: Circulation 116:1736, 2007; W Wilson et al: Circulation 143:e963, 2021; and G Habib et al: Eur Heart J 30:2369, 2009).

tract procedures, genitourinary tract infections (or skin infection) should be treated before or when these sites undergo procedures.

In patients with aortic or mitral valve regurgitation or a prosthetic valve, treatment of acute Q fever for 12 months with doxycycline plus hydroxychloroquine (see Table 128-4) is highly effective in preventing *C. burnetii* IE.

■ FURTHER READING

Baddour LM et al: Infective endocarditis in adults: Diagnosis, antimicrobial therapy, and management of complications: A scientific statement for healthcare professionals from the American Heart Association. Circulation 132:1435, 2015.

Blomstrom-Lundqvist C et al: European Heart Rhythm Association (EHRA) International consensus document on how to prevent, diagnose, and treat cardiac implantable electronic device infections—endorsed by the Heart Rhythm Society (HRS), the Asia Pacific Heart Rhythm Society (APHRS), the Latin American Heart Rhythm Society (LAHRS), International Society for Cardiovascular Infectious Diseases (ISCVID) and the European Society of Clinical Microbiology and Infectious Diseases (ESCMID) in collaboration with the European Association for Cardio-Thoracic Surgery (EACTS). Eur J Cardiothorac Surg 57:e1, 2020.

Cahill TJ et al: Challenges in infective endocarditis. J Am Coll Cardiol 69:325, 2017.

Chirouze C et al: Impact of early valve surgery on outcome of *Staphylococcus aureus* prosthetic valve infective endocarditis: Analysis in the International Collaboration of Endocarditis–Prospective Cohort Study. Clin Infect Dis 60:741, 2015.

Duval X et al: Impact of systematic whole-body 18F-fluorodeoxyglucose PET/CT on the management of patients suspected of infective endocarditis: The prospective multicenter TEPvENDO study. Clin Infect Dis 73:393, 2021.

Habib G et al: 2015 ESC guidelines for the management of infective endocarditis. Eur Heart J 36:3075, 2015.

Lalani T et al: Analysis of the impact of early surgery on in-hospital mortality of native valve endocarditis: Use of propensity score and instrumental variable methods to adjust for treatment-selection bias. Circulation 121:1005, 2010.

Lalani T et al: In-hospital and 1-year mortality in patients undergoing early surgery for prosthetic valve endocarditis. JAMA Intern Med 173:1495, 2013.

Liesman RM et al: Laboratory diagnosis of infective endocarditis. J Clin Microbiol 55:2599, 2017.

Regueiro A et al: Association between transcatheter aortic valve replacement and subsequent infective endocarditis and in-hospital death. JAMA 316:1083, 2016.

Wilson W et al: Prevention of viridans group streptococcal infective endocarditis: A scientific statement from the American Heart Association. Circulation 143:e963, 2021.

129 Infections of the Skin, Muscles, and Soft Tissues

Dennis L. Stevens, Amy E. Bryant

Skin and soft tissue infections occur in all races, all ethnic groups, and all geographic locations, although some have unique geographic niches. In modern times, the frequency and severity of some skin and soft tissue infections have increased for several reasons. First, microbes are rapidly disseminated throughout the world via efficient air travel, acquiring genes for virulence factors and antibiotic resistance. Second, natural disasters, such as earthquakes, tsunamis, tornadoes, and hurricanes, appear to be increasing in frequency, and the injuries sustained during these events commonly cause major skin and soft-tissue damage that predisposes to infection. Third, trauma and casualties resulting from combat and terrorist activities can markedly damage or destroy tissues and provide both endogenous and exogenous pathogens with ready access to deeper structures. Unfortunately, because the marvels of modern medicine may not be available during human-instigated and natural disasters, primary treatment may be delayed and the likelihood of severe infection and death increased.

ANATOMIC RELATIONSHIPS: CLUES TO THE DIAGNOSIS OF SOFT TISSUE INFECTIONS

Skin and soft tissue infections have been common human afflictions for centuries. However, between 2000 and 2004, hospital admissions for these infections rose by 27%, a remarkable increase that was attributable largely to the emergence of the USA300 clone of methicillin-resistant *Staphylococcus aureus* (MRSA). This chapter provides an anatomic approach to understanding the types of soft tissue infections and the diverse microbes responsible.

Protection against infection of the epidermis depends on the mechanical barrier afforded by the stratum corneum since the epidermis itself is devoid of blood vessels (**Fig. 129-1**). Disruption of this layer by burns or bites, abrasions, foreign bodies, primary dermatologic disorders (e.g., herpes simplex, varicella, ecthyma gangrenosum), surgery, or vascular or pressure ulcer allows penetration of bacteria to the deeper structures. Similarly, the hair follicle can serve as a portal either for components of the normal flora (e.g., *Staphylococcus*) or for extrinsic bacteria (e.g., *Pseudomonas* in hot-tub folliculitis). Intracellular infection of the squamous epithelium with vesicle formation may

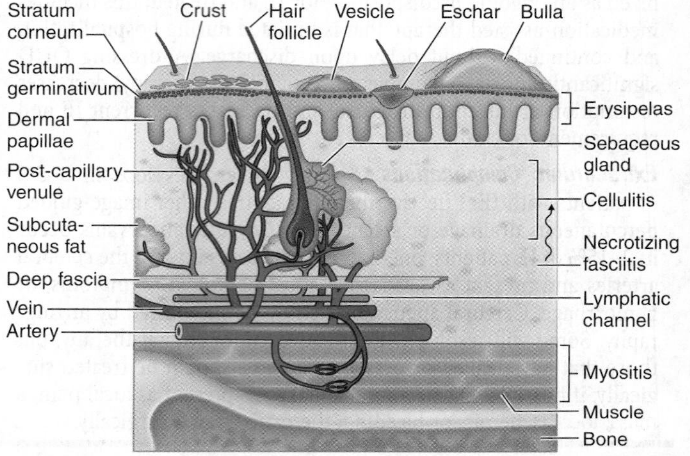

FIGURE 129-1 Structural components of the skin and soft tissues, superficial infections, and infections of the deeper structures. The rich capillary network beneath the dermal papillae plays a key role in the localization of infection and in the development of the acute inflammatory reaction.

arise from cutaneous inoculation, as in infection with herpes simplex virus (HSV) type 1; from the dermal capillary plexus, as in varicella and infections due to other viruses associated with viremia; or from cutaneous nerve roots, as in herpes zoster. Bacteria infecting the epidermis, such as *Streptococcus pyogenes*, may be translocated laterally to deeper structures via lymphatics, an event that results in the rapid superficial spread of erysipelas. Later, engorgement or obstruction of lymphatics causes flaccid edema of the epidermis, another characteristic of erysipelas.

The rich plexus of capillaries beneath the dermal papillae provides nutrition to the stratum germinativum, and physiologic responses of this plexus produce important clinical signs and symptoms. For example, infective vasculitis of the plexus results in petechiae, Osler's nodes, Janeway lesions, and palpable purpura, which, if present, are important clues to the existence of endocarditis (**Chap. 128**). In addition, metastatic infection within this plexus can result in cutaneous manifestations of disseminated fungal infection (**Chap. 216**), gonococcal infection (**Chap. 156**), *Salmonella* infection (**Chap. 165**), *Pseudomonas* infection (i.e., ecthyma gangrenosum; **Chap. 164**), meningococcemia (**Chap. 155**), and staphylococcal infection (**Chap. 147**). The plexus also provides bacteria with access to the circulation, thereby facilitating local spread or bacteremia. The postcapillary venules of this plexus are a prominent site of polymorphonuclear leukocyte sequestration, diapedesis, and chemotaxis to the site of cutaneous infection.

Amplification of these physiologic mechanisms by excessive levels of cytokines or bacterial toxins causes leukostasis, venous occlusion, and pitting edema. Edema with purple bullae, ecchymosis, and cutaneous anesthesia suggests loss of vascular integrity and necessitates exploration of the deeper structures for evidence of necrotizing fasciitis or myonecrosis. An early diagnosis requires a high level of suspicion in instances of unexplained fever and of pain and tenderness in the soft tissue, even in the absence of acute cutaneous inflammation.

Table 129-1 indicates the chapters in which the infections described below are discussed in greater detail. Many of these infections are illustrated in the chapters cited or in **Chap. A1**.

INFECTIONS ASSOCIATED WITH VESICLES

(Table 129-1) Vesicle formation due to infection is caused by viral proliferation within the epidermis. In varicella and variola, viremia precedes the onset of a diffuse centripetal rash that progresses from macules to vesicles, then to pustules, and finally to scabs over the course of 1–2 weeks. Vesicles of varicella have a "dewdrop" appearance and develop in crops randomly about the trunk, extremities, and face over 3–4 days. Herpes zoster occurs in a single dermatome; the appearance of vesicles is preceded by pain for several days. Zoster may occur in persons of any age but is most common among immunosuppressed individuals and elderly patients, whereas most cases of varicella occur in young children. Vesicles due to HSV are found on or around the lips (HSV-1) or genitals (HSV-2) but also may appear on the head and neck of young wrestlers (herpes gladiatorum) or on the digits of health care workers (herpetic whitlow). Recurrent herpes labialis (HSV-1) and herpes genitalis (HSV-2) commonly follow primary infection. Coxsackievirus A16 characteristically causes vesicles on the hands, feet, and mouth of children. Orf is caused by a DNA virus related to smallpox virus and infects the fingers of individuals who work around goats and sheep. Molluscum contagiosum virus induces flaccid vesicles on the skin of healthy and immunocompromised individuals. Although variola (smallpox) in nature was eradicated as of 1977, postmillennial terrorist events have renewed interest in this devastating infection (**Chap. S3**). Viremia beginning after an incubation period of 12 days is followed by a diffuse maculopapular rash, with rapid evolution to vesicles, pustules, and then scabs. Secondary cases can occur among close contacts.

Rickettsialpox begins after mite-bite inoculation of *Rickettsia akari* into the skin. A papule with a central vesicle evolves to form a 1- to 2.5-cm painless crusted black eschar with an erythematous halo and proximal adenopathy. While more common in the northeastern United States and Ukraine in 1940–1950, rickettsialpox has recently been described in Ohio, Arizona, and Utah. Blistering dactylitis is a painful, vesicular, localized *S. aureus* or group A streptococcal infection of the pulps of the distal digits of the hands.

INFECTIONS ASSOCIATED WITH BULLAE

(Table 129-1) Staphylococcal scalded-skin syndrome (SSSS) in neonates is caused by a toxin (exfoliatin) from phage group II *S. aureus*. SSSS must be distinguished from toxic epidermal necrolysis (TEN), which occurs primarily in adults, is drug-induced, and is associated with a higher mortality rate. Punch biopsy with frozen section is useful in making this distinction since the cleavage plane is the stratum corneum in SSSS and the stratum germinativum in TEN (Fig. 129-1). Intravenous γ-globulin is a promising treatment for TEN. Necrotizing fasciitis and gas gangrene also induce bulla formation (see "Necrotizing Fasciitis," below). Halophilic *Vibrio* infection can be as aggressive and fulminant as necrotizing fasciitis; a helpful clue in its diagnosis is a history of exposure to waters of the Gulf of Mexico or the Atlantic seaboard or (in a patient with cirrhosis) the ingestion of raw seafood. The etiologic organism (*Vibrio vulnificus*) is highly susceptible to tetracycline.

INFECTIONS ASSOCIATED WITH CRUSTED LESIONS

(Table 129-1) Impetigo contagiosa is caused by *S. pyogenes*, and bullous impetigo is due to *S. aureus*. Both skin lesions may have an early bullous stage but then appear as thick crusts with a golden-brown color. Epidemics of impetigo caused by MRSA have been reported. Streptococcal lesions are most common among children 2–5 years of age, and epidemics may occur in settings of poor hygiene, particularly among children in lower socioeconomic settings in tropical climates. It is important to recognize impetigo contagiosa because of its relationship to poststreptococcal glomerulonephritis. Rheumatic fever is not a complication of skin infection caused by *S. pyogenes*. Superficial dermatophyte infection (ringworm) can occur on any skin surface, and skin scrapings with KOH staining are diagnostic. Primary infections with dimorphic fungi such as *Blastomyces dermatitidis* and *Sporothrix schenckii* can initially present as crusted skin lesions resembling ringworm. Disseminated infection with *Coccidioides immitis* can also involve the skin, and biopsy and culture should be performed on crusted lesions when the patient is from an endemic area. Crusted nodular lesions caused by *Mycobacterium chelonee* have been described in HIV-seropositive patients. Treatment with clarithromycin looks promising.

FOLLICULITIS

(Table 129-1) Hair follicles serve as portals for a number of bacteria, although *S. aureus* is the most common cause of localized folliculitis. Sebaceous glands empty into hair follicles and ducts and, if these portals are blocked, form sebaceous cysts that may resemble staphylococcal abscesses or may become secondarily infected. Inflammation of sweat glands (hidradenitis suppurativa) also can mimic infection of hair follicles, particularly in the axillae, but new treatments with potent anti-inflammatory agents hold promise. Chronic folliculitis is uncommon except in acne vulgaris, where constituents of the normal flora (e.g., *Propionibacterium acnes*) may play a role.

Diffuse folliculitis occurs in two settings. *Hot-tub folliculitis* is caused by *Pseudomonas aeruginosa* in waters that are insufficiently chlorinated and maintained at temperatures of 37–40°C. Infection is usually self-limited, although bacteremia and shock have been reported. *Swimmer's itch* occurs when a skin surface is exposed to water infested with freshwater avian schistosomes. Warm water temperatures and alkaline pH are suitable for mollusks that serve as intermediate hosts between birds and humans. Free-swimming schistosomal cercariae readily penetrate human hair follicles or pores but quickly die and elicit a brisk allergic reaction, causing intense itching and erythema.

PAPULAR AND NODULAR LESIONS

(Table 129-1) Raised lesions of the skin occur in many different forms. *Mycobacterium marinum* infections of the skin may present as cellulitis or as raised erythematous nodules. Similar lesions caused by

TABLE 129-1 Skin and Soft Tissue Infections

LESION, CLINICAL SYNDROME	INFECTIOUS AGENT(S)	SEE ALSO CHAP(S).
Vesicles		
Smallpox	Variola virus	S3
Chickenpox	Varicella-zoster virus	193
Shingles (herpes zoster)	Varicella-zoster virus	193
Cold sores, herpetic whitlow, herpes gladiatorum	Herpes simplex virus	192
Hand-foot-and-mouth disease	Coxsackievirus A16	204
Orf	Parapoxvirus	196
Molluscum contagiosum	Molluscum contagiosum poxvirus	196
Rickettsialpox	*Rickettsia akari*	187
Blistering distal dactylitis	*Staphylococcus aureus* or *Streptococcus pyogenes*	147, 148
Bullae		
Staphylococcal scalded-skin syndrome	*S. aureus*	147
Necrotizing fasciitis	*S. pyogenes, Clostridium* spp., mixed aerobes and anaerobes	148, 154, 177
Gas gangrene	*Clostridium* spp.	154
Halophilic *Vibrio*	*Vibrio vulnificus*	168
Crusted lesions		
Bullous impetigo/ecthyma	*S. aureus*	147
Impetigo contagiosa	*S. pyogenes*	148
Ringworm	Superficial dermatophyte fungi	219
Sporotrichosis	*Sporothrix schenckii*	219
Histoplasmosis	*Histoplasma capsulatum*	212
Coccidioidomycosis	*Coccidioides immitis*	213
Blastomycosis	*Blastomyces dermatitidis*	214
Cutaneous leishmaniasis	*Leishmania* spp.	226
Cutaneous tuberculosis	*Mycobacterium tuberculosis*	178
Nocardiosis	*Nocardia asteroides*	174
Folliculitis		
Furunculosis	*S. aureus*	147
Hot-tub folliculitis	*Pseudomonas aeruginosa*	164
Swimmer's itch	*Schistosoma* spp.	234
Acne vulgaris	*Propionibacterium acnes*	57
Papular and nodular lesions		
Fish-tank or swimming-pool granuloma	*Mycobacterium marinum*	180
Creeping eruption (cutaneous larva migrans)	*Ancylostoma braziliense*	231
Dracunculiasis	*Dracunculus medinensis*	233
Cercarial dermatitis	*Schistosoma mansoni*	234
Verruca vulgaris	Human papillomaviruses 1, 2, 4	198
Condylomata acuminata (anogenital warts)	Human papillomaviruses 6, 11, 16, 18	198
Onchocerciasis nodule	*Onchocerca volvulus*	233
Cutaneous myiasis	*Dermatobia hominis*	461
Verruca peruana	*Bartonella bacilliformis*	172
Cat-scratch disease	*Bartonella henselae*	172
Lepromatous leprosy	*Mycobacterium leprae*	179
Secondary syphilis (papulosquamous and nodular lesions, condylomata lata)	*Treponema pallidum*	182
Tertiary syphilis (nodular gummatous lesions)	*T. pallidum*	182
Ulcers with or without eschars		
Anthrax	*Bacillus anthracis*	S3
Ulceroglandular tularemia	*Francisella tularensis*	170, S3
Bubonic plague	*Yersinia pestis*	171, S3
Buruli ulcer	*Mycobacterium ulcerans*	180
Leprosy	*M. leprae*	179
Cutaneous tuberculosis	*M. tuberculosis*	178
Chancroid	*Haemophilus ducreyi*	157
Primary syphilis	*T. pallidum*	182
Erysipelas	*S. pyogenes*	148
Cellulitis	*Staphylococcus* spp., *Streptococcus* spp., various other bacteria	Various
Necrotizing fasciitis		
Streptococcal gangrene	*S. pyogenes*	148
Fournier's gangrene	Mixed aerobic and anaerobic bacteria	177
Staphylococcal necrotizing fasciitis	Methicillin-resistant *S. aureus*	147
Myositis and myonecrosis		
Pyomyositis	*S. aureus*	147
Streptococcal necrotizing myositis	*S. pyogenes*	148
Gas gangrene	*Clostridium* spp.	154
Nonclostridial (crepitant) myositis	Mixed aerobic and anaerobic bacteria	177
Synergistic nonclostridial anaerobic myonecrosis	Mixed aerobic and anaerobic bacteria	177

Mycobacterium abscessus and *M. chelonei* have been described among patients undergoing cosmetic laser surgery and tattooing, respectively. Erythematous papules are early manifestations of cat-scratch disease (with lesions developing at the primary site of inoculation of *Bartonella henselae*) and bacillary angiomatosis (also caused by *B. henselae*). Raised serpiginous or linear eruptions are characteristic of cutaneous larva migrans, which is caused by burrowing larvae of dog or cat hookworms (*Ancylostoma braziliense*) and which humans acquire through contact with soil that has been contaminated with dog or cat feces. Similar burrowing raised lesions are present in dracunculiasis caused by migration of the adult female nematode *Dracunculus medinensis*. Nodules caused by *Onchocerca volvulus* measure 1–10 cm in diameter and occur mostly in persons bitten by *Simulium* flies in Africa. The nodules contain the adult worm encased in fibrous tissue. Migration of microfilariae into the eyes may result in blindness. Verruga peruana is caused by *Bartonella bacilliformis*, which is transmitted to humans by the sandfly *Phlebotomus*. This condition can take the form of single gigantic lesions (several centimeters in diameter) or multiple small lesions (several millimeters in diameter). Numerous subcutaneous nodules may also be present in cysticercosis caused by larvae of *Taenia solium*. Multiple erythematous papules develop in schistosomiasis; each represents a cercarial invasion site. Skin nodules as well as thickened subcutaneous tissue are prominent features of lepromatous leprosy. Large nodules or gummas are features of tertiary syphilis, whereas flat papulosquamous lesions are characteristic of secondary syphilis. Human papillomavirus may cause singular warts (verruca vulgaris) or multiple warts in the anogenital area (condylomata acuminata). The latter are major problems in HIV-infected individuals.

ULCERS WITH OR WITHOUT ESCHARS

(Table 129-1) Cutaneous anthrax begins as a pruritic papule, which develops within days into an ulcer with surrounding vesicles and edema and then into an enlarging ulcer with a black eschar. Cutaneous anthrax may cause chronic nonhealing ulcers with an overlying dirty-gray membrane, although lesions may also mimic psoriasis, eczema, or impetigo. Ulceroglandular tularemia may have associated ulcerated skin lesions with painful regional adenopathy. Although buboes are the major cutaneous manifestation of plague, ulcers with eschars, papules, or pustules also are present in 25% of cases.

Mycobacterium ulcerans typically causes chronic skin ulcers on the extremities of individuals living in the tropics. *Mycobacterium leprae* may be associated with cutaneous ulcerations in patients with lepromatous leprosy related to Lucio's phenomenon, in which immune-mediated destruction of tissue bearing high concentrations of *M. leprae* bacilli occurs, usually several months after initiation of effective therapy. *Mycobacterium tuberculosis* also may cause ulcerations, papules, or erythematous macular lesions of the skin in both immunocompetent and immunocompromised patients.

Decubitus ulcers are due to tissue hypoxemia secondary to pressure-induced vascular insufficiency and may become secondarily infected with components of the skin and gastrointestinal flora, including anaerobes. Ulcerative lesions on the anterior shins may be due to pyoderma gangrenosum, which must be distinguished from similar lesions of infectious etiology by histologic evaluation of biopsy sites. Ulcerated lesions on the genitals may be either painful (chancroid) or painless (primary syphilis).

ERYSIPELAS

(Table 129-1) Erysipelas is due to *S. pyogenes* and is characterized by an abrupt onset of fiery-red swelling of the face or extremities. The distinctive features of erysipelas are well-defined indurated margins, particularly along the nasolabial fold; rapid progression; and intense pain. Flaccid bullae may develop during the second or third day of illness, but extension to deeper soft tissues is rare. Treatment with penicillin is effective; swelling may progress despite appropriate treatment, although fever, pain, and the intense red color diminish. Desquamation of the involved skin occurs 5–10 days into the illness. Infants and elderly adults are most commonly afflicted, and the severity of systemic toxicity varies.

CELLULITIS

(Table 129-1) Cellulitis is an acute inflammatory condition of the skin that is characterized by localized pain, erythema, swelling, and heat. It may be caused by indigenous flora colonizing the skin and appendages (e.g., *S. aureus* and *S. pyogenes*) or by a wide variety of exogenous bacteria. Because the exogenous bacteria involved in cellulitis occupy unique niches in nature, a thorough history (including epidemiologic data) offers important clues to etiology. When there is drainage, an open wound, or an obvious portal of entry, Gram's stain and culture provide a definitive diagnosis. In the absence of these findings, the bacterial etiology of cellulitis is difficult to establish, and in some cases staphylococcal and streptococcal cellulitis may have similar features. Even with needle aspiration of the leading edge or a punch biopsy of the cellulitis tissue itself, cultures are positive in only 20% of cases. This observation suggests that relatively low numbers of bacteria may cause cellulitis and that the expanding area of erythema within the skin may be a direct effect of extracellular toxins or of the soluble mediators of inflammation elicited by the host.

Bacteria may gain access to the epidermis through cracks in the skin, abrasions, cuts, burns, insect bites, surgical incisions, and IV catheters. Cellulitis caused by *S. aureus* spreads from a central localized infection, such as an abscess, folliculitis, or an infected foreign body (e.g., a splinter, a prosthetic device, an IV catheter). MRSA is rapidly replacing methicillin-sensitive *S. aureus* (MSSA) as a cause of cellulitis in both inpatient and outpatient settings. Cellulitis caused by MSSA or MRSA is usually associated with a focal infection, such as a furuncle, a carbuncle, a surgical wound, or an abscess; the U.S. Food and Drug Administration preferentially refers to these types of infection as *purulent cellulitis*. In contrast, cellulitis due to *S. pyogenes* is a more rapidly spreading, diffuse process that is frequently associated with lymphangitis and fever and should be referred to as *nonpurulent cellulitis*. Recurrent streptococcal cellulitis of the lower extremities may be caused by organisms of group A, C, or G in association with chronic venous stasis or with saphenous venectomy for coronary artery bypass surgery. Streptococci also cause recurrent cellulitis among patients with chronic lymphedema resulting from elephantiasis, lymph node dissection, or Milroy disease. Recurrent staphylococcal cutaneous infections are more common among individuals who have eosinophilia and elevated serum levels of IgE (Job syndrome) and among nasal carriers of staphylococci. Cellulitis caused by *Streptococcus agalactiae* (group B *Streptococcus*) occurs primarily in elderly patients and those with diabetes mellitus or peripheral vascular disease. *Haemophilus influenzae* typically causes periorbital cellulitis in children in association with sinusitis, otitis media, or epiglottitis. It is unclear whether this form of cellulitis will (like meningitis) become less common as a result of the impressive efficacy of the *H. influenzae* type b vaccine.

Many other bacteria also cause cellulitis. It is fortunate that these organisms occur in such characteristic settings that a good history provides useful clues to the diagnosis. Cellulitis associated with cat bites and, to a lesser degree, with dog bites is commonly caused by *Pasteurella multocida*, although in the latter case *Staphylococcus intermedius* and *Capnocytophaga canimorsus* also must be considered. Sites of cellulitis and abscesses associated with dog bites and human bites also contain a variety of anaerobic organisms, including *Fusobacterium*, *Bacteroides*, aerobic and anaerobic streptococci, and *Eikenella corrodens*. *Pasteurella* is notoriously resistant to dicloxacillin and nafcillin but is sensitive to all other β-lactam antimicrobial agents as well as to quinolones, tetracycline, and erythromycin. Amoxicillin-clavulanate, ampicillin-sulbactam, and cefoxitin are good choices for the treatment of animal or human bite infections. *Aeromonas hydrophila* causes aggressive cellulitis and occasionally necrotizing fasciitis in tissues surrounding lacerations sustained in freshwater (lakes, rivers, and streams). This organism remains sensitive to aminoglycosides, fluoroquinolones, chloramphenicol, trimethoprim-sulfamethoxazole, and third-generation cephalosporins; it is resistant to ampicillin, however. *P. aeruginosa* causes three types of soft tissue infection: ecthyma gangrenosum in neutropenic patients, hot-tub folliculitis, and cellulitis following penetrating injury. Most commonly, *P. aeruginosa* is introduced into the deep tissues when a person steps on a nail. Treatment includes surgical inspection and drainage, particularly if the injury also involves bone or joint capsule. Choices for empirical treatment while antimicrobial susceptibility data are awaited include an aminoglycoside, a third-generation cephalosporin (ceftazidime, cefoperazone, or cefotaxime), a semisynthetic penicillin (ticarcillin, mezlocillin, or piperacillin), or a fluoroquinolone (although drugs of the last class are not indicated for the treatment of children <13 years old).

Gram-negative bacillary cellulitis, including that due to *P. aeruginosa*, is most common among hospitalized, immunocompromised hosts. Cultures and sensitivity tests are critically important in this setting because of multidrug resistance (**Chap. 164**).

The gram-positive aerobic rod *Erysipelothrix rhusiopathiae* is most often associated with fish and domestic swine and causes cellulitis primarily in bone renderers and fishmongers. *E. rhusiopathiae* remains susceptible to most β-lactam antibiotics (including penicillin), erythromycin, clindamycin, tetracycline, and cephalosporins but is resistant to sulfonamides, chloramphenicol, and vancomycin. Its resistance to vancomycin, which is unusual among gram-positive bacteria, is of potential clinical significance since this agent is sometimes used in empirical therapy for skin infection. Fish food containing the water flea *Daphnia* is sometimes contaminated with *M. marinum*, which can cause cellulitis or granulomas on skin surfaces exposed to the water in aquariums or injured in swimming pools. Rifampin plus ethambutol has been an effective therapeutic combination in some cases, although no comprehensive studies have been undertaken. In addition, some strains of *M. marinum* are susceptible to tetracycline or trimethoprim-sulfamethoxazole.

NECROTIZING FASCIITIS

(Table 129-1) Necrotizing fasciitis, formerly called *streptococcal gangrene*, may be associated with group A *Streptococcus* or mixed aerobic–anaerobic bacteria or may occur as a component of gas gangrene caused by *Clostridium perfringens*. Strains of MRSA that produce the Panton-Valentine leukocidin (PVL) toxin have been reported to cause necrotizing fasciitis. Early diagnosis may be difficult when pain or unexplained fever is the only presenting manifestation. Swelling then develops and is followed by brawny edema and tenderness. With progression, dark-red induration of the epidermis appears, along with bullae filled with blue or purple fluid. Later the skin becomes friable and takes on a bluish, maroon, or black color. By this stage, thrombosis of blood vessels in the dermal papillae (Fig. 129-1) is extensive. Extension of infection to the level of the deep fascia causes this tissue to take on a brownish-gray appearance. Rapid spread occurs along fascial planes, through venous channels and lymphatics. Patients in the later stages are toxic and frequently manifest shock and multiorgan failure.

Necrotizing fasciitis caused by mixed aerobic–anaerobic bacteria begins with a breach in the integrity of a mucous membrane barrier, such as the mucosa of the gastrointestinal or genitourinary tract. The portal can be a malignancy, a diverticulum, a hemorrhoid, an anal fissure, or a urethral tear. Other predisposing factors include peripheral vascular disease, diabetes mellitus, surgery, and penetrating injury to the abdomen. Leakage into the perineal area results in a syndrome called *Fournier's gangrene*, characterized by massive swelling of the scrotum and penis with extension into the perineum or the abdominal wall and the legs.

Necrotizing fasciitis caused by *S. pyogenes* has increased in frequency and severity since 1985. There are two distinct clinical presentations: those with no portal of entry and those with a defined portal of entry. Infections in the first category often begin deep at the site of a nonpenetrating minor trauma, such as a bruise or a muscle strain. Seeding of the site via transient bacteremia is likely, although most patients deny antecedent streptococcal infection. The affected patients present with only severe pain and fever. Late in the course, the classic signs of necrotizing fasciitis, such as purple (violaceous) bullae, skin sloughing, and progressive toxicity, develop. In infections of the second type, *S. pyogenes* may reach the deep fascia from a site of cutaneous infection or penetrating trauma. These patients have early signs of superficial skin infection with progression to necrotizing fasciitis. In either case, toxicity is severe, and renal impairment may precede the development of shock. In 20–40% of cases, myositis occurs concomitantly, and, as in gas gangrene (see below), serum creatine phosphokinase levels may be markedly elevated. Necrotizing fasciitis due to mixed aerobic–anaerobic bacteria may be associated with gas in deep tissue, but gas usually is not present when the cause is *S. pyogenes* or MRSA. Prompt surgical exploration down to the deep fascia and muscle is essential. Necrotic tissue must be surgically removed, and Gram's staining and culture of excised tissue are useful in establishing whether group A streptococci, mixed aerobic–anaerobic bacteria, MRSA, or *Clostridium* species are present (see "Treatment," below).

MYOSITIS AND MYONECROSIS

(Table 129-1) Muscle involvement can occur with viral infection (e.g., influenza, dengue, or coxsackievirus B infection) or parasitic invasion (e.g., trichinellosis, cysticercosis, or toxoplasmosis). Although myalgia develops in most of these infections, severe muscle pain is the hallmark of pleurodynia (coxsackievirus B), trichinellosis, and bacterial infection. Acute rhabdomyolysis predictably occurs with clostridial and streptococcal myositis but may also be associated with influenza virus, echovirus, coxsackievirus, Epstein-Barr virus, and *Legionella* infections.

Pyomyositis is usually due to *S. aureus*, is common in tropical areas, and generally has no known portal of entry. Cases of pyomyositis caused by MRSA producing the PVL toxin have been described among children in the United States. Muscle infection begins at the exact site of blunt trauma or muscle strain. Infection remains localized, and shock does not develop unless organisms produce toxic shock syndrome toxin 1 or certain enterotoxins and the patient lacks antibodies to the toxin produced by the infecting organisms. In contrast, *S. pyogenes* may induce primary myositis (referred to as *streptococcal necrotizing myositis*) in association with severe systemic toxicity. Myonecrosis occurs concomitantly with necrotizing fasciitis in ~50% of cases. Both are part of the streptococcal toxic shock syndrome.

Gas gangrene usually follows severe penetrating injuries that result in interruption of the blood supply and introduction of soil into wounds. Such cases of traumatic gangrene are usually caused by the clostridial species *C. perfringens*, *C. septicum*, and *C. histolyticum*. Rarely, latent or recurrent gangrene can occur years after penetrating trauma; dormant spores that reside at the site of previous injury are most likely responsible. Spontaneous nontraumatic gangrene among patients with neutropenia, gastrointestinal malignancy, diverticulosis, or recent radiation therapy to the abdomen is caused by several clostridial species, of which *C. septicum* is the most commonly involved. The tolerance of this anaerobe to oxygen probably explains why it can initiate infection spontaneously in normal tissue anywhere in the body.

Gas gangrene of the uterus, especially that due to *Clostridium sordellii*, historically occurred as a consequence of illegal or self-induced abortion and nowadays also follows spontaneous abortion, vaginal delivery, and cesarean section. *C. sordellii* has also been implicated in medically induced abortion. Postpartum *C. sordellii* infections in young, previously healthy women present as a unique clinical picture: little or no fever, lack of a purulent discharge, refractory hypotension, extensive peripheral edema and effusions, hemoconcentration, and a markedly elevated white blood cell count. The infection is almost uniformly fatal, with death ensuing rapidly. *C. sordellii* and *C. novyi* have also been associated with cutaneous injection of black tar heroin; mortality rates are lower among the affected individuals, probably because their aggressive injection-site infections are readily apparent and diagnosis is therefore prompt.

Synergistic nonclostridial anaerobic myonecrosis, also known as *necrotizing cutaneous myositis* and *synergistic necrotizing cellulitis*, is a variant of necrotizing fasciitis caused by mixed aerobic and anaerobic bacteria with the exclusion of clostridial organisms (see "Necrotizing Fasciitis," above).

DIAGNOSIS

This chapter emphasizes the physical appearance and location of lesions within the soft tissues as important diagnostic clues. Other crucial considerations in narrowing the differential diagnosis are the

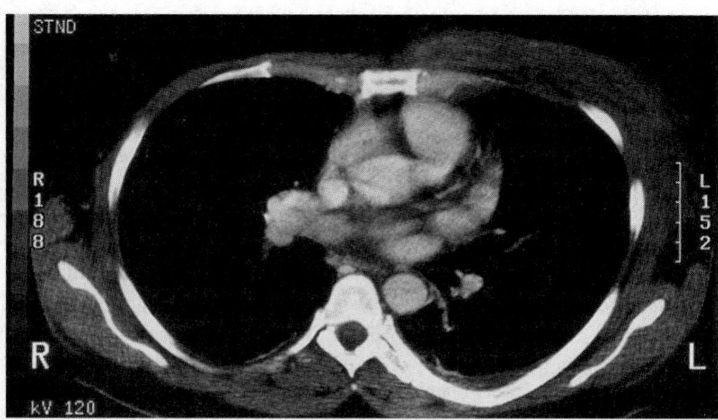

FIGURE 129-2 CT showing edema and inflammation of the left chest wall in a patient with necrotizing fasciitis and myonecrosis caused by group A *Streptococcus*.

temporal progression of the lesions as well as the patient's travel history, animal exposure or bite history, age, underlying disease status, and lifestyle. However, even the astute clinician may find it challenging to diagnose all infections of the soft tissues by history and inspection alone. Soft tissue radiography, CT (**Fig. 129-2**), and MRI may be useful in determining the depth of infection and should be performed when the patient has rapidly progressing lesions or evidence of a systemic inflammatory response syndrome. These tests are particularly valuable for defining a localized abscess or detecting gas in tissue. Unfortunately, they may reveal only soft tissue swelling and thus are not specific for fulminant infections such as necrotizing fasciitis or myonecrosis caused by group A *Streptococcus* (Fig. 129-2), where gas is not found in lesions.

Aspiration of the leading edge or punch biopsy with frozen section may be helpful if the results of imaging tests are positive, but false-negative results occur in ~80% of cases. There is some evidence that aspiration alone may be superior to injection and aspiration with normal saline. Frozen sections are especially useful in distinguishing SSSS from TEN and are quite valuable in cases of necrotizing fasciitis. Open surgical inspection, with debridement as indicated, is clearly the best way to determine the extent and severity of infection and to obtain material for Gram's staining and culture. Such an aggressive approach is important and may be lifesaving if undertaken early in the course of fulminant infections where there is evidence of systemic toxicity.

TREATMENT

Infections of the Skin, Muscles, and Soft Tissues

A full description of the treatment of all the clinical entities described herein is beyond the scope of this chapter. As a guide to the clinician in selecting appropriate treatment, the antimicrobial agents useful in the most common and the most fulminant cutaneous infections are listed in **Table 129-2**. There are several new antibiotics that have been approved by the FDA for uncomplicated skin and soft tissue infections including ceftaroline, dalbavancin, oritavancin, tedizolid, delafloxacin, and omadacycline (see "Further Reading," below).

Furuncles, carbuncles, and abscesses caused by MRSA and MSSA are common, and their treatment depends upon the size of the lesion. Furuncles <2.5 cm in diameter are usually treated with moist heat. Those that are larger (4.5 cm of erythema and induration) require surgical drainage, and the occurrence of these larger lesions in association with fever, chills, or leukocytosis requires both drainage and antibiotic treatment. Previous studies in children demonstrated that surgical drainage of abscesses (mean diameter, 3.8 cm) was as effective when used alone as when combined with trimethoprim-sulfamethoxazole treatment. However, the rate of recurrence of new lesions was lower in the group undergoing both drainage and antibiotic treatment. A more recent study in patients with predominantly MRSA localized abscesses suggested that a 7- to 10-day course of treatment with trimethoprim-sulfamethoxazole or clindamycin was associated with higher cure rates and fewer recurrences.

Early and aggressive surgical exploration is essential in cases of suspected necrotizing fasciitis, myositis, or gangrene to (1) visualize the deep structures, (2) remove necrotic tissue, (3) reduce

TABLE 129-2 Treatment of Common Infections of the Skin

DIAGNOSIS/CONDITION	PRIMARY TREATMENT	ALTERNATIVE TREATMENT	SEE ALSO CHAP(S).
Animal bite (prophylaxis or early infection)[a]	Amoxicillin–clavulanate (875/125 mg PO bid)	Doxycycline (100 mg PO bid)	141
Animal bite[a] (established infection)	Ampicillin–sulbactam (1.5–3 g IV q6h)	Clindamycin (600–900 mg IV q8h) ***plus*** Ciprofloxacin (400 mg IV q12h) *or* cefoxitin (2 g IV q6h)	141
Bacillary angiomatosis	Erythromycin (500 mg PO qid)	Doxycycline (100 mg PO bid)	172
Herpes simplex (primary genital)	Acyclovir (400 mg PO tid for 10 days)	Famciclovir (250 mg PO tid for 5–10 days) *or* valacyclovir (1000 mg PO bid for 10 days)	192
Herpes zoster (immunocompetent host >50 years of age)	Acyclovir (800 mg PO 5 times daily for 7–10 days)	Famciclovir (500 mg PO tid for 7–10 days) *or* valacyclovir (1000 mg PO tid for 7 days)	193
Cellulitis (staphylococcal or streptococcal[b,c])	Nafcillin or oxacillin (2 g IV q4–6h)	Cefazolin (1–2 g q8h) *or* ampicillin/sulbactam (1.5–3 g IV q6h) *or* erythromycin (0.5–1 g IV q6h) *or* clindamycin (600–900 mg IV q8h)	147, 148
MRSA skin infection[d]	Vancomycin (1 g IV q12h)	Linezolid (600 mg IV q12h)	147
Necrotizing fasciitis (group A streptococcal[b])	Clindamycin (600–900 mg IV q6–8h) *plus* penicillin G (4 million units IV q4h)	Clindamycin (600–900 mg IV q6–8h) *plus* a cephalosporin (first- or second-generation)	148
Necrotizing fasciitis (mixed aerobes and anaerobes)	Ampicillin (2 g IV q4h) *plus* clindamycin (600–900 mg IV q6–8h) *plus* ciprofloxacin (400 mg IV q6–8h)	Vancomycin (1 g IV q6h) *plus* metronidazole (500 mg IV q6h) *plus* ciprofloxacin (400 mg IV q6–8h)	122, 177
Gas gangrene	Clindamycin (600–900 mg IV q6–8h) *plus* penicillin G (4 million units IV q4–6h)	Clindamycin (600–900 mg IV q6–8h) *plus* cefoxitin (2 g IV q6h)	154

[a]*Pasteurella multocida*, a species commonly associated with both dog and cat bites, is resistant to cephalexin, dicloxacillin, clindamycin, and erythromycin. *Eikenella corrodens*, a bacterium commonly associated with human bites, is resistant to clindamycin, penicillinase-resistant penicillins, and metronidazole but is sensitive to trimethoprim-sulfamethoxazole and fluoroquinolones. [b]The frequency of erythromycin resistance in group A *Streptococcus* is currently ~5% in the United States but has reached 70–100% in some other countries. Most, but not all, erythromycin-resistant group A streptococci are susceptible to clindamycin. Approximately 90% of *Staphylococcus aureus* strains are sensitive to clindamycin, but resistance—both intrinsic and inducible—is increasing. [c]Severe hospital-acquired *S. aureus* infections or community-acquired *S. aureus* infections that are not responding to the β-lactam antibiotics recommended in this table may be caused by methicillin-resistant strains, requiring a switch to vancomycin, daptomycin, or linezolid. [d]Some strains of methicillin-resistant *S. aureus* (MRSA) remain sensitive to tetracycline and trimethoprim-sulfamethoxazole. Daptomycin (4 mg/kg IV q24h) or tigecycline (100-mg loading dose followed by 50 mg IV q12h) is an alternative treatment for MRSA.

compartment pressure, and (4) obtain suitable material for Gram's staining and for aerobic and anaerobic cultures. Appropriate empirical antibiotic treatment for mixed aerobic–anaerobic infections could consist of ampicillin-sulbactam, cefoxitin, or the following combination: (1) clindamycin (600–900 mg IV every 8 h) or metronidazole (500 mg every 6 h) plus (2) ampicillin or ampicillin-sulbactam (1.5–3 g IV every 6 h) plus (3) gentamicin (1–1.5 mg/kg every 8 h). Group A streptococcal and clostridial infection of the fascia and/or muscle carries a mortality rate of 20–50% with penicillin treatment. In experimental models of streptococcal and clostridial necrotizing fasciitis/myositis, clindamycin has exhibited markedly superior efficacy, but no comparative clinical trials have been performed. A retrospective study of children with invasive group A streptococcal infection demonstrated higher survival rates with clindamycin treatment than with β-lactam antibiotic therapy. Hyperbaric oxygen treatment also may be useful in gas gangrene due to clostridial species. Antibiotic treatment should be continued until all signs of systemic toxicity have resolved, all devitalized tissue has been removed, and granulation tissue has developed (**Chaps. 148, 154, and 177**).

In summary, infections of the skin and soft tissues are diverse in presentation and severity and offer a great challenge to the clinician. This chapter provides an approach to diagnosis and understanding of the pathophysiologic mechanisms involved in these infections. More in-depth information is found in chapters on specific infections.

■ FURTHER READING

Aldape MJ et al: *Clostridium sordellii* infection: Epidemiology, clinical findings, and current perspectives on diagnosis and treatment. Clin Infect Dis 43:1436, 2006.

Stevens DL, Bryant AE: Life threatening skin and soft tissue infections, in *Netter's Infectious Diseases*, EC Jong and DL Stevens (eds). Philadelphia, Elsevier, 2011, pp 94–101.

Stevens DL et al: Practice guidelines for the diagnosis and management of skin and soft tissue infections: 2014 update by the Infectious Diseases Society of America. Clin Infect Dis 59:e10, 2014. (Erratum: Clin Infect Dis 60:1448, 2015.)

Talan DA et al: Bacteriologic analysis of infected dog and cat bites. Emergency Medicine Animal Bite Infection Study Group. N Engl J Med 340:85, 1999.

Stevens DL, Bryant AE: Necrotizing infections. N Engl J Med 377:2253, 2017.

Daum RS et al: A placebo-controlled trial of antibiotics for smaller skin abscesses. N Engl J Med 376:2545, 2017.

Tirupathi R et al: Acute bacterial skin and soft tissue infections: New drugs in ID armamentarium. J Community Hosp Intern Med Perspect 9:310, 2019.

130 Infectious Arthritis

Lawrence C. Madoff,
Nongnooch Poowanawittayakom

Although *Staphylococcus aureus*, streptococci, and *Neisseria gonorrhoeae* are the most common causes of infectious arthritis, various mycobacteria, spirochetes, fungi, and viruses also infect joints (**Table 130-1**). Since acute bacterial infection can destroy articular cartilage rapidly, all inflamed joints must be evaluated without delay to exclude noninfectious processes and determine appropriate antimicrobial therapy and drainage procedures. For more detailed information on infectious arthritis caused by specific organisms, the reader is referred to the chapters on those organisms.

TABLE 130-1 Differential Diagnosis of Arthritis Syndromes

ACUTE MONARTICULAR ARTHRITIS	CHRONIC MONARTICULAR ARTHRITIS	POLYARTICULAR ARTHRITIS
Staphylococcus aureus	*Mycobacterium tuberculosis*	*Neisseria meningitidis*
Streptococcus pneumoniae	Nontuberculous mycobacteria	*N. gonorrhoeae*
β-Hemolytic streptococci	*Borrelia burgdorferi*	Nongonococcal bacterial arthritis
Gram-negative bacilli	*Treponema pallidum*	Bacterial endocarditis
Neisseria gonorrhoeae	*Candida* spp.	*Candida* spp.
Candida spp.	*Sporothrix schenckii*	Poncet's disease (tuberculous rheumatism)
Crystal-induced arthritis	*Coccidioides immitis*	Hepatitis B virus
Fracture	*Blastomyces dermatitidis*	Parvovirus B19
Hemarthrosis	*Aspergillus* spp.	HIV
Foreign body	*Cryptococcus neoformans*	Human T-lymphotropic virus type 1
Osteoarthritis	*Nocardia* spp.	Rubella virus
Ischemic necrosis	*Brucella* spp.	Arthropod-borne viruses
Monoarticular rheumatoid arthritis	Legg-Calvé-Perthes disease	Sickle cell disease flare
	Osteoarthritis	Reactive arthritis
		Serum sickness
		Acute rheumatic fever
		Inflammatory bowel disease
		Systemic lupus erythematosus
		Rheumatoid arthritis/Still's disease
		Other vasculitides
		Sarcoidosis

Acute bacterial infection typically involves a single joint or a few joints. Subacute or chronic monoarthritis or oligoarthritis suggests mycobacterial or fungal infection; episodic inflammation is seen in syphilis, Lyme disease, and the reactive arthritis that follows enteric infections and chlamydial urethritis. Acute polyarticular inflammation occurs as an immunologic reaction during the course of endocarditis, rheumatic fever, disseminated neisserial infection, and acute viral hepatitis. Viruses often infect multiple joints; however, bacterial infections generally cause mono- or oligoarthritis except in persons with underlying diseases such as rheumatoid arthritis

APPROACH TO THE PATIENT

Infectious Arthritis

Aspiration of synovial fluid—an essential element in the evaluation of potentially infected joints—can be performed without difficulty in most cases by the insertion of a large-bore needle into the site of maximal fluctuance or tenderness or by the route of easiest access. Ultrasonography or computed tomography (CT) may be used to guide aspiration of difficult-to-localize effusions of the hip and, occasionally, the shoulder and other joints. Normal synovial fluid contains <180 cells (predominantly mononuclear cells) per microliter. Synovial cell counts averaging 100,000/μL (range, 25,000–250,000/μL), with >90% neutrophils, are characteristic of acute bacterial infections. Crystal-induced, rheumatoid, and other noninfectious inflammatory arthritides usually are associated with <30,000–50,000 cells/μL; cell counts of 10,000–30,000/μL, with 50–70% neutrophils and the remainder lymphocytes, are common in mycobacterial and fungal infections. Definitive diagnosis of an infectious process relies on identification of the pathogen in stained smears of synovial fluid, isolation of the pathogen from cultures of synovial fluid and blood, or detection of microbial nucleic acids and proteins by nucleic acid amplification tests (NAATs) and immunologic techniques. Gram stain is positive in about 30–50% of cases, and synovial fluid culture is positive in >60% of nongonococcal bacterial arthritis cases. Matrix-assisted laser desorption/ionization–time of flight (MALDI-TOF) mass spectrometry is helpful in patients who have negative culture and high suspicion of infectious arthritis. Sonication of explanted prosthetic joints (placement of the material into liquid and then immersion in an ultrasound bath) increases the yield of organism detection, especially in the case of prior antibiotic use within 14 days.

ACUTE BACTERIAL ARTHRITIS

PATHOGENESIS

Bacteria enter the joint from the bloodstream; from a contiguous site of infection in bone or soft tissue; or by direct inoculation during surgery, injection, animal or human bite, or trauma. In hematogenous infection, bacteria escape from synovial capillaries, which have no limiting basement membrane, and within hours provoke neutrophilic infiltration of the synovium. Neutrophils and bacteria enter the joint space; later, bacteria adhere to articular cartilage. Degradation of cartilage begins within 48 h as a result of increased intraarticular pressure, release of proteases and cytokines from chondrocytes and synovial macrophages, and invasion of the cartilage by bacteria and inflammatory cells. Histologic studies reveal bacteria lining the synovium and cartilage as well as abscesses extending into the synovium, cartilage, and—in severe cases—subchondral bone. Synovial proliferation results in the formation of a pannus over the cartilage, and thrombosis of inflamed synovial vessels develops. Bacterial factors that appear important in the pathogenesis of infective arthritis include various surface-associated adhesins in *S. aureus* that permit adherence to cartilage and endotoxins that promote chondrocyte-mediated breakdown of cartilage.

MICROBIOLOGY

The hematogenous route of infection is the most common route in all age groups, and nearly every bacterial pathogen is capable of causing septic arthritis. In infants, group B streptococci, gram-negative enteric bacilli, and *S. aureus* are the most common pathogens. Since the advent of the *Haemophilus influenzae* vaccine, the predominant causes among children <5 years of age have been *S. aureus*, *Streptococcus pyogenes* (group A *Streptococcus*), and (in some centers) *Kingella kingae*. Among young adults and adolescents, *N. gonorrhoeae* is the most commonly implicated organism. *S. aureus* accounts for most nongonococcal isolates in adults of all ages; gram-negative bacilli, pneumococci, and β-hemolytic streptococci—particularly groups A and B but also groups C, G, and F—are involved in up to one-third of cases in older adults, especially those with underlying comorbid illnesses.

Infections after surgical procedures or penetrating injuries are due most often to *S. aureus* and occasionally to other gram-positive bacteria or gram-negative bacilli. Infections with coagulase-negative staphylococci are unusual except after the implantation of prosthetic joints or arthroscopy. Anaerobic organisms, often in association with aerobic or facultative bacteria, are found after human bites and when decubitus ulcers or intraabdominal abscesses spread into adjacent joints. Polymicrobial infections complicate traumatic injuries with extensive contamination. Bites and scratches from cats and other animals may introduce *Pasteurella multocida* or *Bartonella henselae* into joints either directly or hematogenously, and bites from humans may introduce *Eikenella corrodens* or other components of the oral flora. Penetration of a sharp object through a shoe is associated with *Pseudomonas aeruginosa* arthritis in the foot.

NONGONOCOCCAL BACTERIAL ARTHRITIS

Epidemiology Although hematogenous infections with virulent organisms such as *S. aureus*, *H. influenzae*, and pyogenic streptococci occur in healthy persons, there is an underlying host predisposition in many cases of septic arthritis. Patients with rheumatoid arthritis have the highest incidence of infective arthritis (most often secondary to *S. aureus*) because of chronically inflamed joints; glucocorticoid therapy; and frequent breakdown of rheumatoid nodules, vasculitic ulcers, and skin overlying deformed joints. Diabetes mellitus, glucocorticoid therapy, hemodialysis, and malignancy all carry an increased risk of infection with *S. aureus* and gram-negative bacilli. Tumor necrosis factor inhibitors (e.g., etanercept, infliximab), which increasingly are used for the treatment of rheumatoid arthritis, predispose to mycobacterial infections and possibly to other pyogenic bacterial infections and could be associated with septic arthritis in this population. Pneumococcal infections complicate alcoholism, deficiencies of humoral immunity, and hemoglobinopathies. Pneumococci, *Salmonella* species, and *H. influenzae* cause septic arthritis in persons infected with HIV. Persons with primary immunoglobulin deficiency are at risk for mycoplasmal arthritis, which results in permanent joint damage if tetracycline and replacement therapy with IV immunoglobulin are not administered promptly. IV drug users acquire staphylococcal and streptococcal infections from their own flora and acquire pseudomonal and other gram-negative infections from drugs and injection paraphernalia.

Clinical Manifestations Patients with acute septic arthritis usually present with joint pain aggravated by movement, joint swelling, and/or erythema. Approximately 90% of patients present with involvement of a single joint—most commonly the knee; less frequently the hip; and still less often the shoulder, wrist, or elbow. Small joints of the hands and feet are more likely to be affected after direct inoculation or a bite. Among IV drug users, infections of the spine, sacroiliac joints, and sternoclavicular joints (**Fig. 130-1**) are more common than infections of the appendicular skeleton. Polyarticular infection is most common among patients with rheumatoid arthritis and may resemble a flare of the underlying disease.

The usual presentation consists of moderate to severe pain that is uniform around the joint, effusion, muscle spasm, and decreased range of motion. Fever in the range of 38.3–38.9°C (101–102°F) and sometimes higher is common but may not be present, especially in persons with rheumatoid arthritis, renal or hepatic insufficiency, or conditions requiring immunosuppressive therapy. The inflamed, swollen joint is usually evident on examination except in the case of a deeply situated joint such as the hip, shoulder, or sacroiliac joint. Cellulitis, bursitis, and acute osteomyelitis, which may produce a similar clinical picture, should be distinguished from septic arthritis by preservation of passive range of motion and less-than-circumferential swelling. A focus of extraarticular infection, such as a boil or pneumonia, should be sought. Peripheral-blood leukocytosis with a left shift and elevation of the erythrocyte sedimentation rate or C-reactive protein level are common.

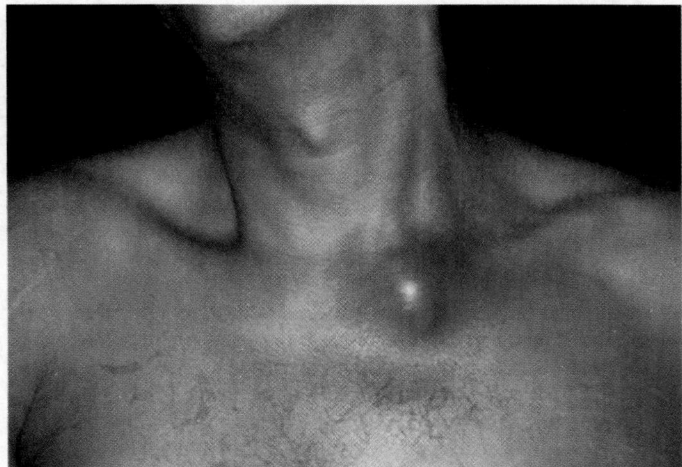

FIGURE 130-1 Acute septic arthritis of the sternoclavicular joint. A man in his forties with a history of cirrhosis presented with a new onset of fever and lower neck pain. He had no history of IV drug use or previous catheter placement. Jaundice and a painful swollen area over his left sternoclavicular joint were evident on physical examination. Cultures of blood drawn at admission grew group B *Streptococcus*. The patient recovered after treatment with IV penicillin. *(Courtesy of the late Francisco M. Marty, MD, Brigham and Women's Hospital, Boston; with permission.)*

Plain radiographs show evidence of soft tissue swelling, joint space widening, and displacement of tissue planes by the distended capsule. Narrowing of the joint space and bony erosions indicate advanced infection and a poor prognosis. Ultrasound is useful for detecting effusions in the hip, and CT or MRI can demonstrate infections of the sacroiliac joint, the sternoclavicular joint, and the spine very well.

Laboratory Findings Specimens of peripheral blood and synovial fluid should be obtained before antibiotics are administered. Blood cultures are positive in up to 50–70% of *S. aureus* infections but are less frequently positive in infections due to other organisms. The synovial fluid is turbid, serosanguineous, or frankly purulent. Gram-stained smears confirm the presence of large numbers of neutrophils. Levels of total protein and lactate dehydrogenase in synovial fluid are elevated, and the glucose level is depressed; however, these findings are not specific for infection, and measurement of these levels is not necessary for diagnosis. The synovial fluid should be examined for crystals because gout and pseudogout can resemble septic arthritis clinically, and infection and crystal-induced disease occasionally occur together. Organisms are seen on synovial fluid smears in nearly three-quarters of infections with *S. aureus* and streptococci and in 30–50% of infections due to gram-negative and other bacteria. Cultures of synovial fluid are positive in >90% of cases. Inoculation of synovial fluid into bottles containing liquid media for blood cultures increases the yield of a culture, especially if the pathogen is a fastidious organism or the patient is taking an antibiotic. Nucleic acid amplification (NAA)-based assays for bacterial DNA or MALDI-TOF, when available, can be useful for the diagnosis of partially treated or culture-negative bacterial arthritis. Inflammatory markers such as erythrocyte sedimentation rate and C-reactive protein tend to be elevated in septic arthritis but are nonspecific. Serum procalcitonin elevation is only ~50% sensitive and should not be used to rule out infectious arthritis.

TREATMENT

Nongonococcal Bacterial Arthritis

Prompt administration of systemic antibiotics and drainage of the involved joint can prevent destruction of cartilage, postinfectious degenerative arthritis, joint instability, or deformity. Once samples of blood and synovial fluid have been obtained for culture, empirical antibiotics should be directed against the bacteria visualized on smears or the pathogens that are likely in light of the patient's age and risk factors. Initial therapy should consist of IV-administered bactericidal agents; direct instillation of antibiotics into the joint is not necessary to achieve adequate levels in synovial fluid and tissue. If there are gram-positive cocci on the smear, IV vancomycin (15–20 mg/kg/dose) every 8–12 h should be started empirically. If methicillin-resistant *S. aureus* is an unlikely pathogen (e.g., when it is not widespread in the community), cefazolin (2 g every 8 h), oxacillin (2 g every 4 h), or nafcillin (2 g every 4 h) should be given.

If initial Gram's stain shows gram-negative bacilli, an IV third-generation cephalosporin such as cefotaxime (1 g every 8 h) or ceftriaxone (1–2 g every 24 h) provides adequate empirical coverage for most community-acquired infections. In addition, cefepime (2 g every 8–12 h) or ceftazidime (2 g every 8 h) should be given to IV drug users and to other patients in whom *P. aeruginosa* may be the responsible agent. Double coverage of *Pseudomonas* with cephalosporin and ciprofloxacin or aminoglycoside can be considered in severely ill patients.

Definitive therapy is based on the identity and antibiotic susceptibility of the bacteria isolated in culture. Infections due to staphylococci are treated with cefazolin, oxacillin, nafcillin, or vancomycin for 4 weeks. In patients without evidence of endocarditis, IV antibiotics can be used for at least 14 days of treatment followed by oral antibiotics to complete the treatment course. Pneumococcal and streptococcal infections due to penicillin-susceptible organisms respond to 2 weeks of therapy with penicillin G (2 million units IV every 4 h); infections caused by *H. influenzae* and by strains of *Streptococcus pneumoniae* that are resistant to penicillin are treated with cefotaxime or ceftriaxone for 2 weeks. Most enteric gram-negative infections can be cured in 3–4 weeks by a second- or third-generation cephalosporin given IV or by a fluoroquinolone such as levofloxacin (500 mg IV or PO every 24 h). *P. aeruginosa* infection should be treated for at least 2 weeks with a combination regimen composed of an aminoglycoside plus either an extended-spectrum penicillin such as piperacillin (3–4 g IV every 4 h) or an antipseudomonal cephalosporin such as ceftazidime (1–2 g IV every 8 h). If tolerated, this regimen is continued for an additional 2 weeks; alternatively, a fluoroquinolone such as ciprofloxacin (750 mg PO twice daily) is given by itself or with the penicillin or cephalosporin in place of the aminoglycoside.

Timely drainage of pus and necrotic debris from the infected joint is required for a favorable outcome. Needle aspiration of readily accessible joints such as the knee may be adequate if loculations or particulate matter in the joint does not prevent its thorough decompression. Arthroscopic drainage and lavage may be employed initially or within several days if repeated needle aspiration fails to relieve symptoms, decrease the volume of the effusion and the synovial white cell count, and clear bacteria from smears and cultures. In some cases, arthrotomy is necessary to remove loculations and debride infected synovium, cartilage, or bone. Septic arthritis of the hip is best managed with arthrotomy, particularly in young children, in whom infection threatens the viability of the femoral head. Septic joints do not require immobilization except for pain control before symptoms are alleviated by treatment. Weight bearing should be avoided until signs of inflammation have subsided, but frequent passive motion of the joint is indicated to maintain full mobility. Although addition of glucocorticoids to antibiotic treatment improves the outcome of *S. aureus* arthritis in experimental animals, no clinical trials have evaluated this approach in humans.

GONOCOCCAL ARTHRITIS

Epidemiology In the past, gonococcal arthritis **(Chap. 156)** accounted for up to 70% of episodes of infectious arthritis in persons <40 years of age in the United States. As the rates of mucosal gonorrhea have fallen in the United States, it is likely that the proportion of septic arthritis caused by *N. gonorrhoeae* has also fallen considerably. Arthritis due to *N. gonorrhoeae* is a consequence of bacteremia arising from gonococcal infection or, more frequently, from asymptomatic gonococcal mucosal colonization of the urethra, cervix, or pharynx. Women are at greatest risk during menses and during pregnancy and overall are two to three times more likely than men to develop disseminated gonococcal infection (DGI) and arthritis. Persons with complement deficiencies, especially of the terminal components, are prone to recurrent episodes of gonococcemia. Strains of gonococci that are most likely to cause DGI include those that produce transparent colonies in culture, have the type IA outer-membrane protein, or are of the AUH-auxotroph type.

Clinical Manifestations and Laboratory Findings The most common manifestation of DGI is a syndrome of fever, chills, rash, and articular symptoms. Small numbers of papules that progress to hemorrhagic pustules develop on the trunk and the extensor surfaces of the distal extremities. Migratory arthritis and tenosynovitis of the knees, hands, wrists, feet, and ankles are prominent. The cutaneous lesions and articular findings are believed to be the consequence of an immune reaction to circulating gonococci and immune-complex deposition in tissues. Thus, cultures of synovial fluid are consistently negative, and blood cultures are positive in <45% of patients. Synovial fluid may be difficult to obtain from inflamed joints and usually contains only 10,000–20,000 leukocytes/μL.

True gonococcal septic arthritis is less common than the DGI syndrome and always follows DGI, which is unrecognized in one-third of patients. A single joint such as the hip, knee, ankle, or wrist is usually involved. Synovial fluid, which contains >50,000 leukocytes/μL, can be obtained with ease; the gonococcus is evident only occasionally in Gram-stained smears, and cultures of synovial fluid are positive in <40% of cases. Blood cultures are almost always negative.

Because it is difficult to isolate gonococci from synovial fluid and blood, specimens for culture should be obtained from potentially infected mucosal sites. NAA-based urine tests also may be positive. Culture requires endocervical (in female patients) or urethral (in male patients) swab specimens. Culture is available for detection of rectal, oropharyngeal, and conjunctival gonococcal infection, but NAAT is not cleared by the U.S. Food and Drug Administration for use with these specimens. Cultures and Gram-stained smears of skin lesions are occasionally positive. All specimens for culture should be plated onto Thayer-Martin agar directly or in special transport media at the bedside and transferred promptly to the microbiology laboratory in an atmosphere of 5% CO_2. NAA-based assays are extremely sensitive in detecting gonococcal DNA in synovial fluid. A dramatic alleviation of symptoms within 12–24 h after the initiation of appropriate antibiotic therapy supports a clinical diagnosis of the DGI syndrome if cultures are negative.

TREATMENT

Gonococcal Arthritis

Initial treatment consists of ceftriaxone (1 g IV or IM every 24 h) to cover possible penicillin-resistant organisms. Once local and systemic signs are clearly resolving, a 7-day course of antibiotics may be completed with daily IM ceftriaxone given at 250 mg daily. An oral fluoroquinolone such as ciprofloxacin (500 mg twice daily) may be used if the organism is known to be susceptible. If penicillin-susceptible organisms are isolated, amoxicillin (500 mg three times daily) may be used. Suppurative arthritis usually responds to needle aspiration of involved joints and 7–14 days of antibiotic treatment. Arthroscopic lavage or arthrotomy is rarely required. Patients with DGI should be treated for *Chlamydia trachomatis* infection unless this infection is ruled out by appropriate testing. Addition of azithromycin (1 g orally as a single dose) is recommended to treat chlamydial co-infection, which is common. Sexual partners should be offered testing and presumptive treatment for gonorrhea and chlamydial infection. It is noteworthy that arthritis symptoms similar to those seen in DGI occur in meningococcemia. A dermatitis–arthritis syndrome, purulent monoarthritis, and reactive polyarthritis have been described. All respond to treatment with appropriate antibiotics.

SPIROCHETAL ARTHRITIS

LYME DISEASE

Lyme disease (**Chap. 186**) due to infection with the spirochete *Borrelia burgdorferi* causes arthritis in up to 60% of persons who are not treated. Intermittent arthralgias and myalgias—but not arthritis—occur within days or weeks of inoculation of the spirochete by the *Ixodes* tick. Later, there are three patterns of joint disease: (1) Fifty percent of untreated persons experience intermittent episodes of monoarthritis or oligoarthritis involving the knee and/or other large joints. The symptoms wax and wane without treatment over months, and each year, 10–20% of patients report loss of joint symptoms. (2) Twenty percent of untreated persons develop a pattern of waxing and waning arthralgias. (3) Ten percent of untreated patients develop chronic inflammatory synovitis that results in erosive lesions and destruction of the joint. Serologic tests for IgG antibodies to *B. burgdorferi* are positive in >90% of persons with Lyme arthritis, and an NAA-based assay detects *Borrelia* DNA in 85%.

TREATMENT

Lyme Arthritis

Lyme arthritis generally responds well to therapy. A regimen of oral doxycycline (100 mg twice daily for 28 days), oral amoxicillin (500 mg three times daily for 28 days), or parenteral ceftriaxone (2 g/d for 2–4 weeks) is recommended. Patients who do not respond to a total of 2 months of oral therapy or 1 month of parenteral therapy are unlikely to benefit from additional antibiotic therapy and are treated with anti-inflammatory agents or synovectomy. Failure of therapy is associated with host features such as the human leukocyte antigen DR4 (HLA-DR4) genotype, persistent reactivity to OspA (outer-surface protein A), and the presence of hLFA-1 (human leukocyte function–associated antigen 1), which cross-reacts with OspA.

SYPHILITIC ARTHRITIS

Articular manifestations occur in different stages of syphilis (**Chap. 182**). In early congenital syphilis, periarticular swelling and immobilization of the involved limbs (*Parrot's pseudoparalysis*) complicate osteochondritis of long bones. *Clutton's joint*, a late manifestation of congenital syphilis that typically develops between ages 8 and 15 years, is caused by chronic painless synovitis with effusions of large joints, particularly the knees and elbows. Secondary syphilis may be associated with arthralgias, with symmetric arthritis of the knees and ankles and occasionally of the shoulders and wrists, and with sacroiliitis. The arthritis follows a subacute to chronic course with a mixed mononuclear and neutrophilic synovial-fluid pleocytosis (typical cell counts, 5000–15,000/μL). Immunologic mechanisms may contribute to the arthritis, and symptoms usually improve rapidly with penicillin therapy. In tertiary syphilis, Charcot joint results from sensory loss due to tabes dorsalis. Penicillin is not helpful in this setting.

MYCOBACTERIAL ARTHRITIS

Tuberculous arthritis (**Chap. 178**) accounts for ~1% of all cases of tuberculosis and 10% of extrapulmonary cases. The most common presentation is chronic granulomatous monoarthritis. An unusual syndrome, *Poncet's disease*, is a reactive symmetric form of polyarthritis that affects persons with visceral or disseminated tuberculosis. No mycobacteria are found in the joints, and symptoms resolve with antituberculous therapy.

Unlike tuberculous osteomyelitis (**Chap. 131**), which typically involves the thoracic and lumbar spine (50% of cases), tuberculous arthritis primarily involves the large weight-bearing joints, in particular the hips, knees, and ankles, and only occasionally involves smaller non-weight-bearing joints. Progressive monoarticular swelling and pain develop over months or years, and systemic symptoms are seen in only half of all cases. Tuberculous arthritis occurs as part of a disseminated primary infection or through late reactivation, often in persons with HIV infection or other immunocompromised hosts. Coexistent active pulmonary tuberculosis is unusual.

Aspiration of the involved joint yields fluid with an average cell count of 20,000/μL, with ~50% neutrophils. Acid-fast staining of the fluid yields positive results in fewer than one-third of cases, and cultures are positive in 80%. Culture of synovial tissue taken at biopsy is positive in ~90% of cases and shows granulomatous inflammation in most. NAA methods can shorten the time to diagnosis to 1 or 2 days. Radiographs reveal peripheral erosions at the points of synovial attachment, periarticular osteopenia, and eventually joint-space narrowing. Therapy for tuberculous arthritis is the same as that for tuberculous pulmonary disease, requiring the administration of multiple agents for 6–9 months. Therapy is more prolonged in immunosuppressed individuals, such as those infected with HIV.

Various atypical mycobacteria (**Chap. 180**) found in water and soil may cause chronic indolent arthritis. Such disease results from trauma and direct inoculation associated with farming, gardening, or aquatic activities. Smaller joints, such as the digits, wrists, and knees, are usually involved. Involvement of tendon sheaths and bursae is typical. The mycobacterial species involved include *Mycobacterium marinum*, *M. avium complex*, *M. terrae*, *M. kansasii*, *M. fortuitum*, and *M. chelonae*. In persons who have HIV infection or are receiving immunosuppressive therapy, hematogenous spread to the joints has been reported for *M. kansasii*, *M. avium* complex, and *M. haemophilum*. Diagnosis usually requires biopsy and culture, and therapy is based on antimicrobial susceptibility patterns.

FUNGAL ARTHRITIS

Fungi are an unusual cause of chronic monoarticular arthritis. Granulomatous articular infection with the endemic dimorphic fungi *Coccidioides immitis*, *Blastomyces dermatitidis*, and (less commonly) *Histoplasma capsulatum* (**Fig. 130-2**) results from hematogenous seeding or direct extension from bony lesions in persons with disseminated disease. Joint involvement is an unusual complication of sporotrichosis (infection with *Sporothrix schenckii*) among gardeners and other persons who work with soil or sphagnum moss. Articular sporotrichosis is six times more common among men than among women, and alcoholics and other debilitated hosts are at risk for polyarticular infection.

Candida infection involving a single joint—usually the knee, hip, or shoulder—results from surgical procedures, intraarticular injections, or (among critically ill patients with debilitating illnesses such as diabetes mellitus or hepatic or renal insufficiency and patients receiving immunosuppressive therapy) hematogenous spread. *Candida* infections in IV drug users typically involve the spine, sacroiliac joints, or other fibrocartilaginous joints. Unusual cases of arthritis due to *Aspergillus* species, *Cryptococcus neoformans*, *Pseudallescheria boydii*, and the dematiaceous fungi also have resulted from direct inoculation or disseminated hematogenous infection in immunocompromised persons. In the United States, a 2012 national outbreak of fungal arthritis (and meningitis) caused by *Exserohilum rostratum* was linked to intraspinal and intraarticular injection of a contaminated preparation of methylprednisolone acetate.

The synovial fluid in fungal arthritis usually contains 10,000–40,000 cells/μL, with ~70% neutrophils. Stained specimens and cultures of synovial tissue often confirm the diagnosis of fungal arthritis when studies of synovial fluid give negative results. Treatment consists of drainage and lavage of the joint and systemic administration of an antifungal agent directed at a specific pathogen. The doses and duration of therapy are the same as for disseminated disease (**see Part 5, Section 16**). Intraarticular instillation of amphotericin B has been used in addition to IV therapy.

VIRAL ARTHRITIS

Viruses produce arthritis by infecting synovial tissue during systemic infection or by provoking an immunologic reaction that involves joints. As many as 50% of women report persistent arthralgias and 10% report frank arthritis within 3 days of the rash that follows natural infection with rubella virus and within 2–6 weeks after receipt of live-virus vaccine. Episodes of symmetric inflammation of fingers, wrists, and knees uncommonly recur for >1 year, but a syndrome of chronic fatigue, low-grade fever, headaches, and myalgias can persist for months or years. IV immunoglobulin has been helpful in selected cases. Self-limited monoarticular or migratory polyarthritis may develop within 2 weeks of the parotitis of mumps; this sequela is more common among men than women. Approximately 10% of children and 60% of women develop arthritis after infection with parvovirus B19. In adults, arthropathy sometimes occurs without fever or rash. Pain and stiffness, with less prominent swelling (primarily of the hands but also of the knees, wrists, and ankles), usually resolve within weeks, although a small proportion of patients develop chronic arthropathy.

About 2 weeks before the onset of jaundice, up to 10% of persons with acute hepatitis B develop an immune complex–mediated, serum sickness–like reaction with maculopapular rash, urticaria, fever, and arthralgias. Less common developments include symmetric arthritis involving the hands, wrists, elbows, or ankles and morning stiffness that resembles a flare of rheumatoid arthritis. Symptoms resolve at the time jaundice develops. Many persons with chronic hepatitis C infection report persistent arthralgia or arthritis, both in the presence and in the absence of cryoglobulinemia.

Painful arthritis involving larger joints often accompanies the fever and rash of several arthropod-borne viral infections, including those caused by Zika, chikungunya, O'nyong-nyong, Ross River, Mayaro, and Barmah Forest viruses (**Chap. 209**). Symmetric arthritis involving the hands and wrists may occur during the convalescent phase of infection with lymphocytic choriomeningitis virus. Patients infected with an enterovirus frequently report arthralgias, and echovirus has been isolated from patients with acute polyarthritis.

Several arthritis syndromes are associated with HIV infection. Reactive arthritis with painful lower-extremity oligoarthritis often follows an episode of urethritis in HIV-infected persons. HIV-associated reactive arthritis appears to be extremely common among persons with the HLA-B27 haplotype, but sacroiliac joint disease is unusual and is seen mostly in the absence of HLA-B27. Up to one-third of HIV-infected persons with psoriasis develop psoriatic arthritis. Painless monoarthropathy and persistent symmetric polyarthropathy occasionally complicate HIV infection. Chronic persistent oligoarthritis of the shoulders, wrists, hands, and knees occurs in women infected with human T-lymphotropic virus type 1. Synovial thickening, destruction of articular cartilage, and leukemic-appearing atypical lymphocytes in synovial fluid are characteristic, but progression to T-cell leukemia is unusual.

PARASITIC ARTHRITIS

Arthritis due to parasitic infection is rare. The guinea worm *Dracunculus medinensis* may cause destructive joint lesions in the lower extremities as migrating gravid female worms invade joints or cause ulcers in

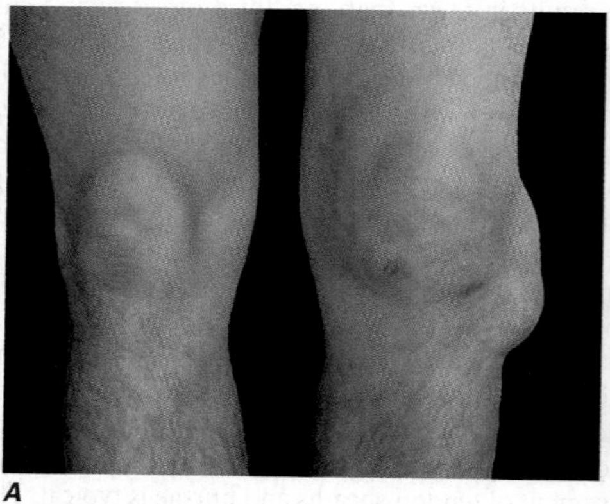
A

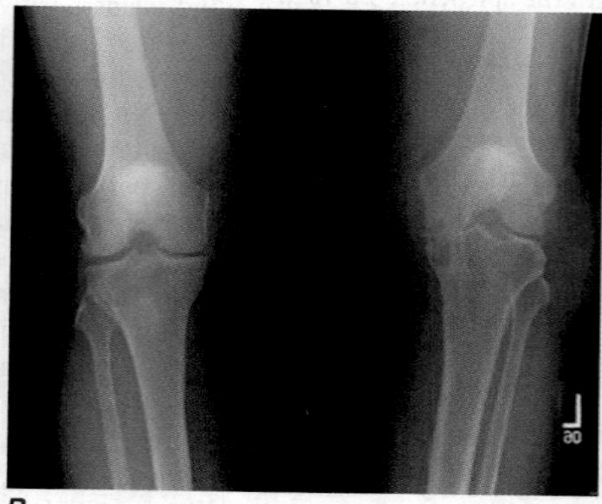
B

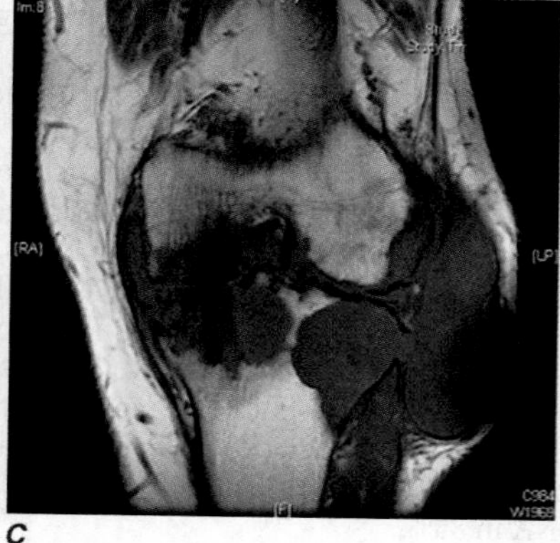

C

FIGURE 130-2 Chronic arthritis caused by *Histoplasma capsulatum* in the left knee. ***A.*** A man in his sixties from El Salvador presented with a history of progressive knee pain and difficulty walking for several years. He had undergone arthroscopy for a meniscal tear 7 years before presentation (without relief) and had received several intraarticular glucocorticoid injections. The patient developed significant deformity of the knee over time, including a large effusion in the lateral aspect. ***B.*** An x-ray of the knee showed multiple abnormalities, including severe medial femorotibial joint-space narrowing, several large subchondral cysts within the tibia and the patellofemoral compartment, a large suprapatellar joint effusion, and a large soft tissue mass projecting laterally over the knee. ***C.*** MRI further defined these abnormalities and demonstrated the cystic nature of the lateral knee abnormality. Synovial biopsies demonstrated chronic inflammation with giant cells, and cultures grew *H. capsulatum* after 3 weeks of incubation. All clinical cystic lesions and the effusion resolved after 1 year of treatment with itraconazole. The patient underwent a left total-knee replacement for definitive treatment. *(Courtesy of the late Francisco M. Marty, MD, Brigham and Women's Hospital, Boston; with permission.)*

adjacent soft tissues that become secondarily infected. Hydatid cysts infect bones in 1–2% of cases of infection with *Echinococcus granulosus*. The expanding destructive cystic lesions may spread to and destroy adjacent joints, particularly the hip and pelvis. In rare cases, chronic synovitis has been associated with the presence of schistosomal eggs in synovial biopsies. Monoarticular arthritis in children with lymphatic filariasis appears to respond to therapy with diethylcarbamazine even in the absence of microfilariae in synovial fluid. Reactive arthritis has been attributed to hookworm, *Strongyloides*, *Cryptosporidium*, and *Giardia* infection in case reports, but confirmation is required.

POSTINFECTIOUS OR REACTIVE ARTHRITIS

Reactive polyarthritis develops several weeks after ~1% of cases of nongonococcal urethritis and 2% of enteric infections, particularly those due to *Yersinia enterocolitica*, *Shigella flexneri*, *Campylobacter jejuni*, *Clostridioides difficile*, and *Salmonella* species. Only a minority of these patients have the other findings of classic reactive arthritis, including urethritis, conjunctivitis, uveitis, oral ulcers, and rash. Studies have identified microbial DNA or antigen in synovial fluid or blood, but the pathogenesis of this condition is poorly understood. The arthritis may occur several days or weeks after the infection and can be associated with dactylitis, enthesitis, or extraarticular involvement such as conjunctivitis.

Reactive arthritis is most common among young men (except after *Yersinia* infection) and has been linked to the HLA-B27 locus as a potential genetic predisposing factor. Patients report painful, asymmetric oligoarthritis that affects mainly the knees, ankles, and feet. Low back pain is common, and radiographic evidence of sacroiliitis is found in patients with long-standing disease. Most patients recover within 6 months, but prolonged recurrent disease is more common in cases that follow chlamydial urethritis. Anti-inflammatory agents help relieve symptoms, but the role of prolonged antibiotic therapy in eliminating microbial antigen from the synovium is controversial.

Migratory polyarthritis and fever constitute the usual presentation of acute rheumatic fever in adults **(Chap. 359)**. This presentation is distinct from that of poststreptococcal reactive arthritis, which also follows infections with group A *Streptococcus* but is not migratory, lasts beyond the typical 3-week maximum of acute rheumatic fever, and responds poorly to aspirin.

INFECTIONS IN PROSTHETIC JOINTS

Infection complicates 1–4% of total joint replacements. The majority of infections are acquired intraoperatively or immediately postoperatively as a result of wound breakdown or infection; less commonly, these joint infections develop later after joint replacement and are the result of hematogenous spread or direct inoculation. The presentation may be acute, with fever, pain, and local signs of inflammation, especially in infections due to *S. aureus*, pyogenic streptococci, and enteric bacilli. Alternatively, infection may persist for months or years without causing constitutional symptoms when less virulent organisms, such as coagulase-negative staphylococci or diphtheroids, are involved. Such indolent infections usually are acquired during joint implantation and are discovered during evaluation of chronic unexplained pain or after a radiograph shows loosening of the prosthesis; the erythrocyte sedimentation rate and C-reactive protein level are usually elevated in such cases.

The diagnosis is best made by needle aspiration of the joint; accidental introduction of organisms during aspiration must be avoided meticulously. Synovial fluid pleocytosis with a predominance of polymorphonuclear leukocytes is highly suggestive of infection, since other inflammatory processes uncommonly affect prosthetic joints. Culture and Gram's stain usually yield the responsible pathogen. Sonication of explanted prosthetic material can improve the yield of culture, presumably by breaking up bacterial biofilms on the surfaces of prostheses. NAAT may also improve the yield. Use of special media for unusual pathogens such as fungi, atypical mycobacteria, and *Mycoplasma* may be necessary if routine and anaerobic cultures are negative.

TREATMENT
Prosthetic Joint Infections

Treatment includes surgery and high doses of parenteral antibiotics, which are given for 4–6 weeks because bone is usually involved. In most cases, the prosthesis must be removed and replaced to cure the infection. Implantation of a new prosthesis is best delayed for several weeks or months because relapses of infection occur most commonly within this time frame. In some cases, reimplantation is not possible, and the patient must manage without a joint, with a fused joint, or even with amputation. Cure of infection without removal of the prosthesis is occasionally possible in cases that are due to streptococci or pneumococci and that lack radiologic evidence of loosening of the prosthesis. In these cases, antibiotic therapy must be initiated within several days of the onset of infection, and the joint should be drained vigorously by open arthrotomy or arthroscopically. In selected patients who prefer to avoid the high morbidity rate associated with joint removal and reimplantation, suppression of the infection with antibiotics may be a reasonable goal. A high cure rate with retention of the prosthesis has been reported when the combination of oral rifampin and another antibiotic (e.g., a quinolone, an antistaphylococcal penicillin, or vancomycin) is given for 3–6 months to persons with staphylococcal prosthetic joint infection of short duration. This approach, which is based on the ability of rifampin to kill organisms adherent to foreign material and in the stationary growth phase, requires confirmation in prospective trials.

■ PREVENTION

To avoid the disastrous consequences of infection, candidates for joint replacement should be selected with care. Rates of infection are particularly high among patients with rheumatoid arthritis, persons who have undergone previous surgery on the joint, and persons with medical conditions requiring immunosuppressive therapy. Perioperative antibiotic prophylaxis, usually with cefazolin, and measures to decrease intraoperative contamination, such as laminar flow, have lowered the rates of perioperative infection to <1% in many centers. After implantation, measures should be taken to prevent or rapidly treat extraarticular infections that might give rise to hematogenous spread to the prosthesis. The effectiveness of prophylactic antibiotics for the prevention of hematogenous infection after dental procedures has not been demonstrated; in fact, viridans streptococci and other components of the oral flora are extremely unusual causes of prosthetic joint infection. Accordingly, the American Dental Association and the American Academy of Orthopaedic Surgeons do not recommend antibiotic prophylaxis for most dental patients with total joint replacements and have stated that there is no convincing evidence to support its use. Similarly, guidelines issued by the American Urological Association and the American Academy of Orthopaedic Surgeons do not recommend the use of prophylactic antibiotics for most patients with prosthetic joints who are undergoing urologic procedures but state that prophylaxis should be considered in certain situations—e.g., for patients (especially immunocompromised patients) who are undergoing a procedure posing a relatively high risk of bacteremia (e.g., lithotripsy or surgery involving bowel segments).

■ FURTHER READING

Bardin T: Gonococcal arthritis. Best Pract Res Clin Rheumatol 17:201, 2003.

Borzio R et al: Predictors of septic arthritis in the adult population. Orthopedics 39:e657, 2016.

Franssila R, Hedman K: Infection and musculoskeletal conditions: Viral causes of arthritis. Best Pract Res Clin Rheumatol 20:1139, 2006.

Harrington JT: Mycobacterial and fungal arthritis. Curr Opin Rheumatol 10:335, 1998.

Meehan AM et al: Outcome of penicillin-susceptible streptococcal prosthetic joint infection treated with debridement and retention of the prosthesis. Clin Infect Dis 36:845, 2003.

Mohammad M et al: The role of *Staphylococcus aureus* lipoproteins in hematogenous septic arthritis. Sci Rep 10:7936, 2020.

Osmon DR et al: Diagnosis and management of prosthetic joint infection: Clinical practice guidelines by the Infectious Diseases Society of America. Clin Infect Dis 56:e1, 2013.

Ross J et al: Septic arthritis and the opioid epidemic: 1465 cases of culture-positive native joint septic arthritis from 1990–2018. Open Forum Infect Dis 7:ofaa089, 2020.

Zeller V et al: One-stage exchange arthroplasty for chronic periprosthetic hip infection: Results of a large prospective cohort study. J Bone Joint Surg Am 96:e1, 2014.

Zimmerli W et al: Prosthetic-joint infections. N Engl J Med 351:145, 2004.

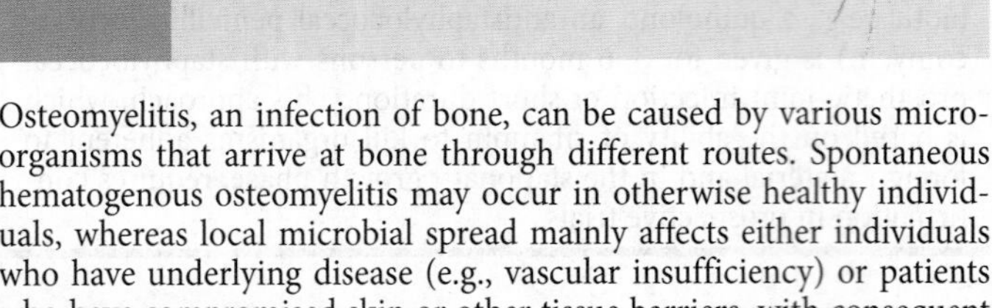

131 Osteomyelitis

Werner Zimmerli

Osteomyelitis, an infection of bone, can be caused by various microorganisms that arrive at bone through different routes. Spontaneous hematogenous osteomyelitis may occur in otherwise healthy individuals, whereas local microbial spread mainly affects either individuals who have underlying disease (e.g., vascular insufficiency) or patients who have compromised skin or other tissue barriers, with consequent exposure of bone. The latter situation typically follows surgery involving bone, such as sternotomy or orthopedic repair.

The manifestations of osteomyelitis are different in children and adults. In children, circulating microorganisms seed mainly long bones, whereas in adults, the vertebral column is the most commonly affected site.

Management of osteomyelitis differs greatly depending on whether an implant is involved. The most important aim of the management of either type of osteomyelitis is to prevent progression to chronic osteomyelitis by rapid diagnosis and prompt treatment. Device-related bone and joint infection necessitates a multidisciplinary approach requiring antibiotic therapy and, in many cases, surgical removal of the device. For most types of osteomyelitis, the optimal duration and route of antibiotic treatment has not been established in clinical trials. Therefore, the recommendations for therapy in this chapter reflect mainly expert opinions.

CLASSIFICATION

There is no generally accepted, comprehensive system for classification of osteomyelitis, primarily because of the multifaceted presentation of this infection. Different specialists are confronted with different facets of bone disease. Most often, however, general practitioners or internists are the first to encounter patients with the initial signs and symptoms of osteomyelitis. These primary care physicians should be able to recognize this disease in any of its forms. Osteomyelitis cases can be classified by various criteria, including pathogenesis, duration of infection, location of infection, and presence or absence of foreign material. The widely used Cierny-Mader staging system is useful mainly for trauma surgeons. It classifies osteomyelitis according to anatomic site, comorbidity, and radiographic findings, with stratification of long-bone osteomyelitis to optimize surgical management; this system encompasses both systemic and local factors affecting immune status, metabolism, and local vascularity.

Any of three mechanisms can underlie osteomyelitis: (1) hematogenous spread; (2) spread from a contiguous site following surgery; and (3) secondary infection in the setting of vascular insufficiency or concomitant neuropathy. Hematogenous osteomyelitis in adults typically involves the vertebral column. In only about half of patients a primary focus can be detected. The most common primary foci of infection are the urinary tract, skin/soft tissue, intravascular catheterization sites, and the endocardium. Spread from a contiguous source follows either bone trauma or surgical intervention. Wound infection leading to osteomyelitis typically occurs after cardiovascular intervention involving the sternum, orthopedic repair after open fracture, or prosthetic joint insertion. Osteomyelitis secondary to vascular insufficiency or peripheral neuropathy most often follows chronic, progressively deep skin and soft tissue infection of the foot. The most common underlying condition is diabetes. In diabetes that is poorly controlled, the *diabetic foot syndrome* is caused by skin, soft tissue, and bone ischemia combined with motor, sensory, and autonomic neuropathy.

Classification of osteomyelitis according to the duration of infection, although ill defined, is useful because the management of acute and chronic osteomyelitis differs. However, not a defined duration of infection, but the presence or absence of bone necrosis (sequesters) is crucial. Acute osteomyelitis without bone necrosis can generally be treated with antibiotics alone. In contrast, for chronic osteomyelitis antibiotic treatment should be combined with debridement surgery. Acute hematogenous or contiguous osteomyelitis evolves over a short period—i.e., a few days or weeks. In contrast, subacute or chronic osteomyelitis lasts for weeks or months before treatment is started. Typical examples of a subacute course are vertebral osteomyelitis due to tuberculosis or brucellosis and delayed implant-associated infections caused mainly by low-virulence microorganisms (coagulase-negative staphylococci, *Cutibacterium acnes*). Chronic osteomyelitis develops when insufficient therapy leads to persistence or recurrence, most often after sternal, mandibular, or foot infection.

Classification by location distinguishes among cases in the long bones, the vertebral column, and the periarticular bones. Long bones are generally involved after hematogenous seeding in children or contiguous spread following trauma or surgery. The risk of vertebral osteomyelitis in adults increases with age. Periarticular osteomyelitis, which complicates septic arthritis that has not been adequately treated, is especially common in periprosthetic joint infection.

Osteomyelitis involving a foreign device requires surgical management for cure. Even acute implant-associated infection calls for prolonged antimicrobial therapy. Therefore, identification of this type of disease is of practical importance.

VERTEBRAL OSTEOMYELITIS

PATHOGENESIS

Vertebral osteomyelitis, also referred to as *disk-space infection*, *septic diskitis*, *spondylodiskitis*, or *spinal osteomyelitis*, is the most common manifestation of hematogenous bone infection in adults. This designation reflects a pathogenic process leading to involvement of the adjacent vertebrae and the corresponding intervertebral disk. In adults, the disk is avascular. Microorganisms invade via the segmental arterial circulation in adjacent endplates and then spread into the disk. Alternative routes of infection are retrograde seeding through the prevertebral venous plexus and direct inoculation during spinal surgery, epidural infiltration, or trauma. In the setting of implant surgery, microorganisms are inoculated either during the procedure or, if wound healing is impaired, in the early postoperative period.

EPIDEMIOLOGY

Vertebral osteomyelitis occurs more often in male than in female patients (ratio, 1.5:1). Between 1995 and 2008, the incidence rate increased from 2.2 to 5.8 cases/100,000 person-years. There is a clear age-dependent increase from 0.3 case/100,000 at ages <20 years to 6.5 cases/100,000 at ages >70 years. The observed increase in reported cases during the past two decades may reflect improvements in diagnosis resulting from the broad availability of MRI technology. In addition, the fraction of cases of vertebral osteomyelitis acquired in association with health care is increasing as a consequence of comorbidity and the rising number of invasive interventions.

MICROBIOLOGY

Vertebral osteomyelitis is typically classified as pyogenic or nonpyogenic. However, this distinction is arbitrary: in "nonpyogenic" cases (tuberculous, brucellar), macroscopic pus formation (caseous necrosis, abscess) is quite common. A more accurate scheme is to classify cases as acute or subacute/chronic. Whereas the microbiologic spectrum of acute cases is similar in different parts of the world, the spectrum of subacute/chronic cases varies according to the geographic region. The great majority of cases are monomicrobial in etiology. Of episodes of acute vertebral osteomyelitis, 40–50% are caused by *Staphylococcus aureus*, 12% by streptococci, and 20% by gram-negative bacilli—mainly *Escherichia coli* (9%) and *Pseudomonas aeruginosa* (6%). Subacute vertebral osteomyelitis is typically caused by *Mycobacterium tuberculosis* or *Brucella* species in regions where these microorganisms are endemic. Osteomyelitis due to viridans streptococci also has a subacute presentation; these infections most often occur as secondary foci in patients with endocarditis. In vertebral osteomyelitis due to *Candida* species, the diagnosis is often delayed by several weeks; this etiology should be suspected in IV drug users who do not use sterile paraphernalia. In implant-associated spinal osteomyelitis, coagulase-negative staphylococci and *C. acnes*—which, in the absence of an implant, are generally considered contaminants—typically cause low-grade (chronic) infections. As an exception, coagulase-negative staphylococci can cause native spinal osteomyelitis in cases of prolonged bacteremia (e.g., in patients with infected pacemaker electrodes or implanted vascular catheters that are not promptly removed).

CLINICAL MANIFESTATIONS

The signs and symptoms of vertebral osteomyelitis are nonspecific. Only about half of patients develop fever >38°C (>100.4°F), perhaps because patients frequently use analgesic drugs. Back pain is the leading initial symptom (>85% of cases). The location of the pain corresponds to the site of infection: the cervical spine in ~10% of cases, the thoracic spine in 30%, and the lumbar spine in 60%. One exception is involvement at the thoracic level in two-thirds of cases of tuberculous osteomyelitis and at the lumbar level in only one-third. This difference is due to direct mycobacterial spread via pleural or mediastinal lymph nodes in pulmonary tuberculosis.

Neurologic deficits, such as radiculopathy, weakness, or sensory loss, are observed in about one-third of cases of vertebral osteomyelitis. Neurologic signs and symptoms are caused mostly by spinal epidural abscess. This complication starts with severe localized back pain and progresses to radicular pain, reflex changes, sensory abnormalities, motor weakness, bowel and bladder dysfunction, and paralysis.

A primary focus should always be sought but is found in only half of cases. Overall, endocarditis is identified in ~10% of patients. In osteomyelitis caused by viridans streptococci, endocarditis is the source in about half of patients.

Implant-associated spinal osteomyelitis can present as either early- or late-onset infection. Early-onset infection is diagnosed within 30 days after implant placement. *S. aureus* is the most common pathogen. Wound healing impairment and fever are the leading findings. Late-onset infection is diagnosed beyond 30 days after surgery, with low-virulence organisms such as coagulase-negative staphylococci or *C. acnes* as typical infecting agents. Fever is rare. One-quarter of patients have a sinus tract. Because of the delayed course and the lack of classic signs of infection, rapid diagnosis requires a high degree of suspicion.

DIAGNOSIS

Leukocytosis and neutrophilia have low levels of diagnostic sensitivity (only 65% and 40%, respectively). In contrast, an increased erythrocyte sedimentation rate or C-reactive protein (CRP) level has been reported in 98% and 100% of cases, respectively; thus, these tests are helpful in excluding vertebral osteomyelitis. The fraction of blood cultures that yield positive results depends heavily on whether the patient has been pretreated with antibiotics; across studies, the range is 30%–78%. In view of this low rate of positive blood culture after antibiotic treatment, such therapy should be withheld until microbial growth is proven unless the patient has sepsis syndrome. In patients with negative blood cultures, CT-guided or open biopsy is needed. Whether a CT-guided biopsy with a negative result is repeated or followed by open biopsy depends on the experience of personnel at the specific center. Bone samples should be cultured for aerobic, anaerobic, and fungal agents, with a portion of the sample sent for histopathologic study. In cases with a subacute/chronic presentation, a suggestive history, or a granuloma detected during histopathologic analysis, mycobacteria and brucellae also should be sought. When blood and tissue cultures are negative despite suggestive histopathology, nonculture techniques (eubacterial or multiplex polymerase chain reaction analysis, metagenomics) of biopsy specimens or aspirated pus should be considered. These techniques allow detection of unusual pathogens such as *Helicobacter* spp. or *Tropheryma whipplei*.

Given that signs and symptoms of osteomyelitis are nonspecific, the clinical differential diagnosis of febrile back pain is broad, including pyelonephritis, pancreatitis, and viral syndromes. In addition, multiple noninfectious pathologies of the vertebral column, such as osteoporotic fracture, seronegative spondylitis (ankylosing spondylitis, psoriasis, reactive arthritis, enteropathic arthritis), and spinal stenosis must be considered.

Imaging procedures are the most important tools not only for the diagnosis of vertebral osteomyelitis but also for the detection of pyogenic complications and alternative conditions (e.g., bone metastases or osteoporotic fractures). Plain radiography is a reasonable first step in evaluating patients without neurologic symptoms and may reveal an alternative diagnosis. Because of its low sensitivity, plain radiography generally is not helpful in acute osteomyelitis, but it can be useful in subacute or chronic cases. The gold standard is MRI, which should be performed expeditiously in patients with neurologic impairment in order to rule out a herniated disk or to detect pyogenic complications in a timely manner (**Figure 131-1, left**). Even if the pathologic findings on MRI suggest vertebral osteomyelitis, alternative diagnoses should be considered, especially when blood cultures are negative. The most common alternative diagnosis is erosive osteochondrosis. Septic bone necrosis, gouty spondylodiskitis, and erosive diskovertebral lesions (Andersson lesions) in ankylosing spondylitis may likewise mimic vertebral osteomyelitis. CT is less sensitive than MRI but may be helpful in guiding a percutaneous biopsy. Positron emission tomography (PET) with ^{18}F-fluorodeoxyglucose, which has a high degree of diagnostic accuracy, is an alternative imaging procedure when MRI is contraindicated (**Fig.131-1, right**). ^{18}F-fluorodeoxyglucose PET should be considered for patients with implants and patients in whom several foci are suspected.

TREATMENT

Vertebral Osteomyelitis

The aims of therapy for vertebral osteomyelitis are (1) elimination of the pathogen(s), (2) protection from further bone loss, (3) relief of back pain, (4) prevention of complications, and (5) stabilization, if needed.

Table 131-1 summarizes suggested antimicrobial regimens for infections attributable to the most common etiologic agents. For optimal antimicrobial therapy, identification of the infecting agent is required. Therefore, in patients without sepsis syndrome, antibiotics should not be administered until the pathogen is identified in a blood culture, a bone biopsy, or an aspirated pus collection. Traditionally, bone infections are at least initially treated by the IV route. However, the preference for the IV route is not evidence based. There are no good arguments for the assumption that IV therapy is superior to oral administration if the following requirements are met: (1) optimal antibiotic spectrum, (2) excellent bioavailability of the oral drug, (3) clinical studies confirming efficacy of the oral drug, (4) normal intestinal function, and (5) no vomiting. Indeed, in a controlled trial in patients with bone and joint infections, including vertebral osteomyelitis, oral antibiotic therapy was noninferior to intravenous therapy when used during the first 6 weeks. Nevertheless, a short initial course of parenteral therapy with a β-lactam antibiotic may lower the risk of emergence of fluoroquinolone resistance, especially if *P. aeruginosa* infection is treated with ciprofloxacin or staphylococcal infection with the combination of a fluoroquinolone plus rifampin. These suggestions are based on

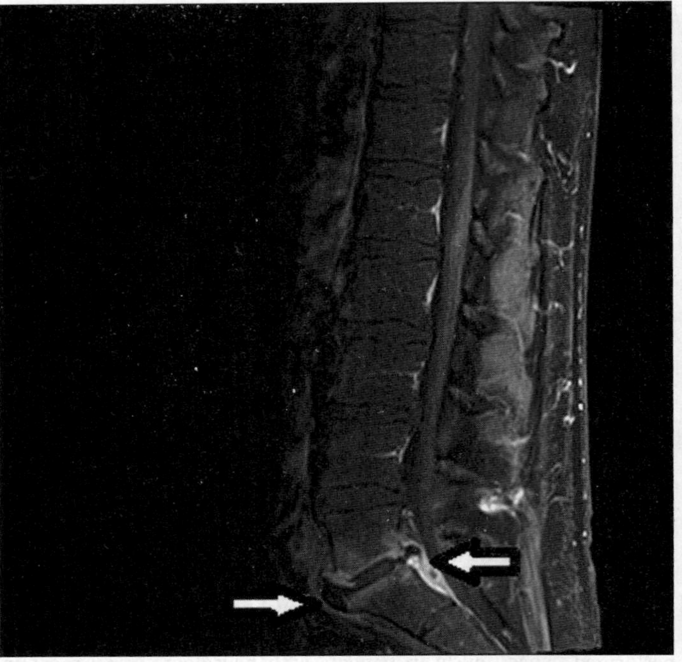

A

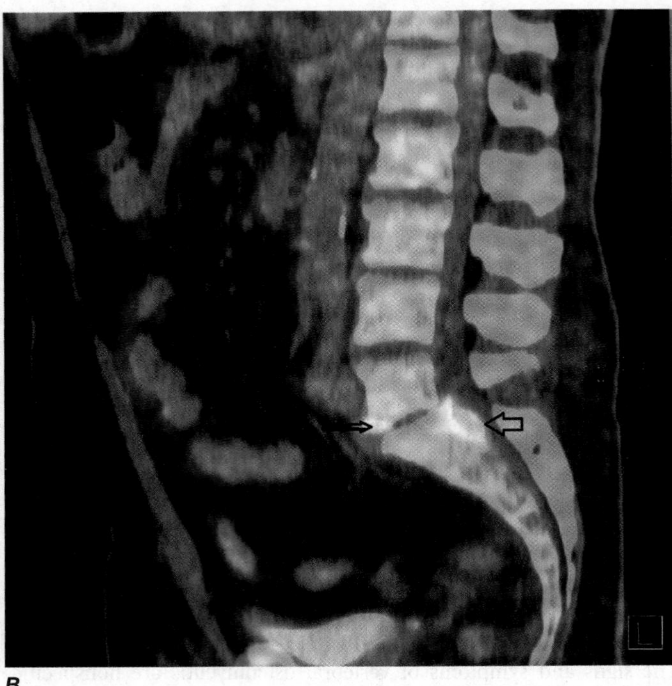

B

FIGURE 131-1 Left: MRI from a 53-year-old man suffering from prosthetic aortic valve endocarditis (*Aggregatibacter actinomycetemcomitans*). In addition, he experienced lumbar pain for 7 weeks. MRI sagittal sequence shows on T1 fat-saturated post-gadolinium image enhancement in the intervertebral disk space (*ventral arrow*) and a small epidural abscess (dorsal arrow). **Right:** PET/CT from the same patient 4 weeks earlier. PET/CT fusion shows fluorodeoxyglucose uptake at L5 ventral (*small arrow*) and dorsal of S1 (*large arrow*: epidural abscess). *(Figures courtesy of Damien Toia, MD, Kantonsspital Baselland; with permission.)*

observational studies and expert opinion. A randomized, controlled trial showed that 6 weeks of antibiotic treatment is not inferior to a 12-week course in patients with pyogenic vertebral osteomyelitis. The cure rate was 90.9% in both groups 1 year after therapy. Thus, prolonged antibiotic therapy is required only for patients with undrained abscesses and for patients with spinal implants. Treatment efficacy should be regularly monitored through inquiries about signs and symptoms (fever, pain) and assessment for signs of inflammation (elevated CRP concentrations). Follow-up MRI is appropriate only for patients with pyogenic complications since the correlation between clinical healing and improvement on MRI is very poor.

Surgical treatment generally is not needed in acute hematogenous vertebral osteomyelitis. However, it is always necessary in implant-associated spinal infection. Early infections (those occurring up to 30 days after internal stabilization) can be cured with debridement, implant retention, and a 3-month course of antibiotics (**Table 131-2**). In contrast, in late infection with a duration of >30 days, implant removal and a 6-week course of antibiotics (Table 131-1) are required for complete elimination of the infection. If implants cannot be removed, oral suppressive long-term treatment should follow the initial course of IV antibiotics. The optimal duration of suppressive therapy is unknown. However, if antibiotic therapy is discontinued after, for example, 1 year, close clinical and laboratory (CRP) follow-up is needed.

■ COMPLICATIONS

Complications should be suspected when there is persistent pain, a persistently increased CRP level, and new-onset or persistent neurologic impairment. In cases of persistent pain with or without signs of inflammation, paravertebral, epidural, or psoas abscesses must be sought. Epidural abscesses occur in 15–20% of cases. This complication is more common in the cervical column (30%) than in the lumbar spine (12%). Risk factors for severe neurologic deficit were epidural abscess, cervical and/or thoracic involvement, and *S. aureus* vertebral osteomyelitis. Persistent pain despite normalization of CRP values indicates mechanical complications such as severe osteonecrosis or spinal instability. These patients require a consult with an experienced orthopedic surgeon.

■ GLOBAL CONSIDERATIONS

The incidence rate of acute vertebral osteomyelitis is similar in different regions of the world. In contrast, subacute/chronic vertebral osteomyelitis predominates in defined regions. Cases attributable to brucellosis predominate in endemic areas such as the Middle East, Africa, Central and South America, and the Indian subcontinent. Tuberculosis is an especially frequent cause in Africa and Asia (India, Indonesia, China), where more than two-thirds of the global tuberculosis burden is reported. Thus, specific diagnostic tests are needed in patients either living in or having traveled to these regions.

OSTEOMYELITIS IN LONG BONES

■ PATHOGENESIS

Osteomyelitis in long bones is a consequence of hematogenous seeding, exogenous contamination during trauma (open fracture), or perioperative contamination during surgery involving bone. Hematogenous infection in long bones typically occurs in children. In adults, the leading pathogenic source is exogenous infection, mainly associated with internal fixation devices. For classification, the presence of a sequestrum and the status of the surrounding soft tissue are crucial for the decision as to whether a surgical intervention is required. Chronic osteomyelitis can be reactivated after a symptom-free interval of >70 years. Such recurrences are most common among elderly patients who developed *S. aureus* osteomyelitis in the preantibiotic era.

■ EPIDEMIOLOGY

In adults, most cases of long-bone osteomyelitis are posttraumatic or postsurgical; less frequently, late recurrence arises from hematogenous infections during childhood. The risk of infection depends on the type of fracture. After closed fracture, implant-associated infection occurs in fewer than 1% of patients. In contrast, after open fracture, the risk of osteomyelitis ranges from ~2% up to 30%, with the precise figure depending on the degree of tissue damage during trauma and the time between injury and admission to a specialized center.

TABLE 131-1 Antibiotic Therapy for Osteomyelitis in Adults without Implants[a]

MICROORGANISM	ANTIMICROBIAL AGENT (DOSE,[b] ROUTE)
Staphylococcus spp.	
Methicillin-susceptible	Nafcillin or oxacillin[c] (2 g IV q6h) ***followed by*** Rifampin (300–450 mg PO q12h) plus levofloxacin (750 mg PO q24h or 500 mg PO q12h)
Methicillin-resistant	Vancomycin[d] (15 mg/kg IV q12h) or daptomycin (8–10 mg/kg IV q24h) ***followed by*** Rifampin (300–450 mg PO q12h) ***plus*** Levofloxacin (750 mg PO q24h or 500 mg PO q12h) or TMP-SMX[e] (1 double-strength tablet PO q8h) or fusidic acid (500 mg PO q8h)
Streptococcus spp.	Penicillin G[c] (5 million units IV q6h) or ceftriaxone (2 g IV q24h)
Enterobacteriaceae	
Quinolone-susceptible	Ciprofloxacin (750 mg PO q24h)
Quinolone-resistant[f]	Imipenem (500 mg IV q6h) or meropenem (1–2g IV q8h)
Pseudomonas aeruginosa	Cefepime or ceftazidime (2 g IV q8h) *plus* an aminoglycoside[g] ***or*** Piperacillin-tazobactam (4.5 g IV q8h) plus an aminoglycoside[g] for 2–4 weeks ***followed by*** Ciprofloxacin[h] (750 mg PO q12h)
Anaerobes	Clindamycin (600 mg IV q6–8h) for 2–4 weeks ***followed by*** Clindamycin[i] (300 mg PO q6h)

[a]Unless otherwise indicated, the total duration of antimicrobial treatment is generally 6 weeks. [b]All dosages are for adults with normal renal function. [c]When the patient has delayed-type penicillin hypersensitivity, cefuroxime (1.5 g IV q6–8h) can be administered. When the patient has immediate-type penicillin hypersensitivity, the penicillin should be replaced by vancomycin (1 g IV q12h). [d]Target vancomycin trough level: 15–20 μg/mL. [e]Trimethoprim-sulfamethoxazole. A double-strength tablet contains 160 mg of trimethoprim and 800 mg of sulfamethoxazole. [f]Including isolates producing extended-spectrum β-lactamase. [g]The need for addition of an aminoglycoside has not yet been proven. However, this addition may decrease the risk of emergence of resistance to the β-lactam. [h]The rationale for starting ciprofloxacin treatment only after pretreatment with a β-lactam is the increased risk of emergence of quinolone resistance in the presence of a heavy bacterial load. [i]Alternatively, penicillin G (5 million units IV q6h) or ceftriaxone (2 g IV q24h) can be used against gram-positive anaerobes (e.g., *Propionibacterium acnes*), and metronidazole (500 mg IV/PO q8h) can be used against gram-negative anaerobes (e.g., *Bacteroides* spp.).

Source: From W Zimmerli: Vertebral osteomyelitis. N Engl J Med 362:1022, 2010.

MICROBIOLOGY

The spectrum of microorganisms causing hematogenous long-bone osteomyelitis does not differ from that in vertebral osteomyelitis. *S. aureus* is most commonly isolated in each type of osteomyelitis. In rare cases, mycobacteria or fungal agents such as *Cryptococcus* species, *Sporothrix schenckii*, *Blastomyces dermatitidis*, or *Coccidioides* species are found in patients who live or have traveled in endemic regions. Impaired cellular immunity (e.g., in HIV infection or after transplantation) predisposes to these etiologies. Coagulase-negative staphylococci are the second most common etiologic agents (after *S. aureus*) in implant-associated osteomyelitis. After open fracture, contiguous long-bone osteomyelitis is typically caused by gram-negative bacilli or a polymicrobial mixture of organisms.

CLINICAL MANIFESTATIONS

The leading symptoms in adults with primary or recurrent hematogenous long-bone osteomyelitis are pain and low-grade fever. Infection occasionally manifests as clinical sepsis and local signs of inflammation (erythema and swelling). After internal fixation, osteomyelitis can be classified as early (acute; <3 weeks), delayed (3–10 weeks), or late (chronic) infection. Early/acute long-bone osteomyelitis manifests as signs of surgical site infection, such as erythema and impaired wound healing. Acute implant-associated infection may also follow hematogenous seeding at any time after implantation of a device. Typical symptoms are new-onset pain and signs of sepsis. Delayed or late (chronic) infections are usually caused by low-virulence microorganisms or occur after ineffective treatment of early-onset infection. Patients may present with persisting pain, subtle local signs of inflammation, intermittent discharge of pus, or fluctuating erythema over the scar (**Fig. 131-2**).

DIAGNOSIS

The diagnostic workup for acute hematogenous long-bone osteomyelitis is similar to that for vertebral osteomyelitis. Bone remodeling and thus marker uptake are increased for at least 1 year after surgery. Therefore, the three-phase bone scan is not useful during this interval. However, in late recurrences it allows rapid diagnosis at low cost. If the results are positive, CT is required to estimate the extent of inflamed tissue and detect bone necrosis (sequesters). Implant-associated infection should be suspected if CRP values do not return to the normal range or rise after an initial decrease. Clinical and laboratory suspicion should prompt surgical exploration and sampling.

In osteomyelitis of >1 year's duration, single-photon emission CT plus conventional CT (SPECT/CT) is a good option, either with ^{99m}Tc methylene diphosphonate (^{99m}Tc-MDP)–labeled leukocytes or with labeled monoclonal antibodies to granulocytes. Surgical debridement is needed for diagnostic (biopsy culture, histology) and therapeutic reasons.

TREATMENT

Osteomyelitis in Long Bones

Treatment for acute hematogenous infection in long bones is identical to that for acute vertebral osteomyelitis (Table 131-1). The suggested duration of antibiotic therapy is 4–6 weeks. In patients with good soft tissue condition and no sequestra or implants, generally no surgical intervention is required. According to a controlled trial, oral treatment can be given, provided that a regimen with excellent oral biocompatibility is available. An initial IV course can be as short as a few days, if the microorganism and its antibiotic susceptibility is known. In recurrences of chronic osteomyelitis as well as in each type of exogenous osteomyelitis (acute, chronic, with or without an implant), a combination of surgical debridement, obliteration of dead space, and long-term antibiotic therapy is required. The length of therapy depends on the completeness of the surgical intervention (removal of sequestra, implants, and necrotic tissue).

The therapeutic aims in patients whose infections are associated with internal fixation devices are consolidation of the fracture and prevention of chronic osteomyelitis. Stable implants can be maintained except in patients with uncontrolled sepsis. Appropriate antimicrobial therapies are listed in Table 131-2. The cure rate for early staphylococcal implant-associated infections treated with a fluoroquinolone plus rifampin is >90%. Rifampin is efficacious against staphylococcal biofilms of ≤3 weeks' duration. Similarly, fluoroquinolones are active against biofilms formed by gram-negative bacilli. In these cases, a short initial course of IV therapy with a β-lactam antibiotic is suggested to minimize the risk of emergence of resistance to the oral drugs. The total duration of treatment is 3 months, and the device can be retained even after antibiotics have been discontinued. In contrast, in cases caused by rifampin-resistant staphylococci or fluoroquinolone-resistant gram-negative bacilli, all hardware should be removed after consolidation of the fracture and before discontinuation of antibiotics. These patients are treated with an oral antibiotic (suppressive therapy) as long as the hardware is retained.

TABLE 131-2 Antibiotic Therapy for Osteomyelitis Associated with Orthopedic Devices

MICROORGANISM	ANTIMICROBIAL AGENT[a] (DOSE, ROUTE)
Staphylococcus spp.	*Recommendation for initial treatment phase (2 weeks with implant)*
Methicillin-susceptible	Rifampin (450 mg PO/IV q12h[b])
	plus
	Nafcillin or oxacillin[c] (2 g IV q6h)
Methicillin-resistant	Rifampin (450 mg PO/IV q12h[b])
	plus
	Vancomycin (15 mg/kg IV q12h) or daptomycin (8–10 mg/kg IV q24h)
Staphylococcus spp.	*Recommendation after completion of initial treatment phase*
	Rifampin (450 mg PO q12h[b])
	plus
	Levofloxacin (750 mg PO q24h or 500 mg PO q12h) or ciprofloxacin (750 mg PO q12h) or fusidic acid (500 mg PO q8h) or TMP-SMX[d] (1 double-strength tablet PO q8h) or minocycline (100 mg PO q12h) or linezolid (600 mg PO q12h) or clindamycin (1200–1350 mg/d PO in 3 or 4 divided doses)
Streptococcus spp.[e]	Penicillin G[c] (18–24 million units/d IV in 6 divided doses) or ceftriaxone (2 g IV q24h) for 4 weeks
	followed by
	Amoxicillin (750–1000 mg PO q6–8h) or clindamycin (1200–1350 mg/d PO in 3 or 4 divided doses)
Enterococcus spp.[f]	
Penicillin-susceptible	Penicillin G[c] (24 million units/d IV in 6 divided doses) *or* ampicillin or amoxicillin[g] (2 g IV q4–6h)
Penicillin-resistant	Vancomycin (15 mg/kg IV q12h) or daptomycin (6–10 mg/kg IV q24h) or linezolid (600 mg IV/PO q12h)
Enterobacteriaceae	A β-lactam selected in light of in vitro susceptibility profile for 2 weeks[h]
	followed by
	Ciprofloxacin (750 mg PO q12h)
Enterobacter spp.[i] and nonfermenters[j] (e.g., *Pseudomonas aeruginosa*)	Cefepime or ceftazidime (2 g IV q8h) *or* meropenem (1–2 g IV q8h[k]) for 2–4 weeks
	followed by
	Ciprofloxacin (750 mg PO q12h)
Cutibacterium spp.	Penicillin G[c] (18–24 million units/d IV in 6 divided doses) or clindamycin (600–900 mg IV q8h) for 2–4 weeks
	followed by
	Amoxicillin (750–1000 mg PO q6–8h) or clindamycin (1200–1350 mg/d PO in 3 or 4 divided doses)
Gram-negative anaerobes (e.g., *Bacteroides* spp.)	Metronidazole (500 mg IV/PO q8h)
Mixed bacteria (without methicillin-resistant staphylococci)	Ampicillin-sulbactam (3 g IV q6h) or amoxicillin-clavulanate[l] (2.2 g IV q6h) or piperacillin-tazobactam (4.5 g IV q8h) or imipenem (500 mg IV q6h) or meropenem (1–2 g IV q8h[k]) for 2–4 weeks
	followed by
	Individualized oral regimens chosen in light of antimicrobial susceptibility

[a]Antimicrobial agents should be chosen in light of the isolate's in vitro susceptibility, the patient's drug allergies and intolerances, potential drug interactions, and contraindications to specific drugs. All dosages recommended are for adults with normal renal and hepatic function. See text for total durations of antibiotic treatment. [b]Other dosages and intervals of administration with equivalent success rates have been reported. [c]When the patient has delayed-type penicillin hypersensitivity, cefazolin (2 g IV q8h) can be administered. When the patient has immediate-type penicillin hypersensitivity, the penicillin should be replaced by vancomycin (1 g IV q12h). [d]Trimethoprim-sulfamethoxazole. A double-strength tablet contains 160 mg of trimethoprim and 800 mg of sulfamethoxazole. [e]Determination of the minimal inhibitory concentration (MIC) of penicillin is advisable. [f]Combination therapy with an aminoglycoside is optional since its superiority to monotherapy for prosthetic joint infection is unproved. When using combination therapy, monitor for signs of aminoglycoside ototoxicity and nephrotoxicity; the latter is potentiated by other nephrotoxic agents (e.g., vancomycin). [g]For patients with hypersensitivity to penicillin, see treatment options for penicillin-resistant enterococci. [h]Ciprofloxacin (PO or IV) can be administered to patients with hypersensitivity to β-lactams. [i]Ceftriaxone and ceftazidime should not be administered for treatment targeting *Enterobacter* species, even strains that test susceptible in the laboratory, but can be used against nonfermenters. Strains producing extended-spectrum β-lactamases should not be treated with any cephalosporin, including cefepime. *Enterobacter* infections can also be treated with ertapenem (1 g IV q24h); however, ertapenem is not effective against *Pseudomonas* spp. and other nonfermenters. [j]Addition of an aminoglycoside is optional. Use of two active drugs can be considered in light of the patient's clinical condition. [k]The recommended dosage is in line with the guidelines of the Infectious Diseases Society of America. In Europe, 2 g IV q8h is suggested for *P. aeruginosa* infections. [l]Not available as an IV formulation in the United States.

Source: Modified from W Zimmerli et al: N Engl J Med 351:1645, 2004. Massachusetts Medical Society.

■ COMPLICATIONS

The main complication of long-bone osteomyelitis is the persistence of infection with progression to chronic osteomyelitis. This risk is especially high after internal fixation of an open fracture and among patients with implant-associated osteomyelitis that is treated without surgical debridement. In longstanding osteomyelitis, recurrent sinus tracts result in severe damage to skin and soft tissue (Fig. 131-2). Patients who have chronic open wounds need a therapeutic approach combining orthopedic repair and plastic reconstructive surgery.

■ GLOBAL CONSIDERATIONS

In North American and Western European countries, tuberculous osteomyelitis is extremely rare, occurring mainly in very old people, HIV-infected patients, and immigrants from endemic countries. In contrast, in countries where the prevalence of tuberculosis is high (India, Indonesia, China), tuberculous osteomyelitis must routinely be considered.

PERIPROSTHETIC JOINT INFECTION

■ PATHOGENESIS

Implanted foreign material is highly susceptible to local infection due to local immunodeficiency around the device. Infection occurs by either the exogenous or the hematogenous route. More rarely, contiguous spread from adjacent sites of osteomyelitis or deep soft-tissue infection may cause periprosthetic joint infection (PJI). The fact that foreign devices are covered with host proteins such as fibronectin favors the adherence of staphylococci and the formation of a biofilm that resists phagocytosis.

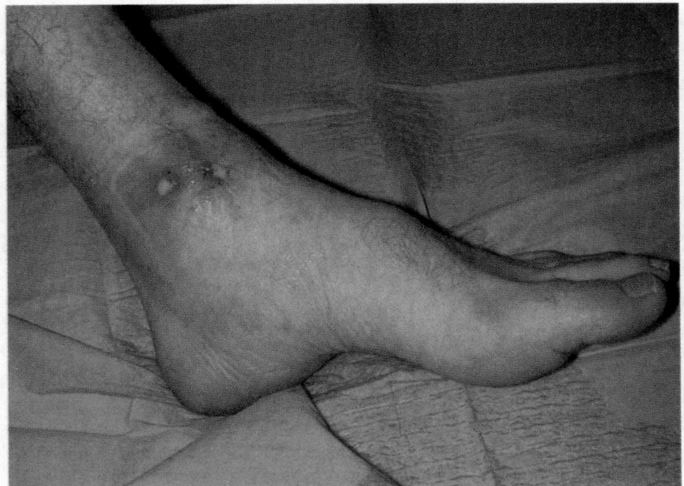

FIGURE 131-2 A 42-year-old man who had sustained a malleolar fracture 6 weeks previously had persistent pain and slight inflammation after orthopedic repair. His infection was treated with oral antibiotics without debridement surgery. This insufficient management of an implant-associated *Staphylococcus aureus* infection was complicated by a sinus tract.

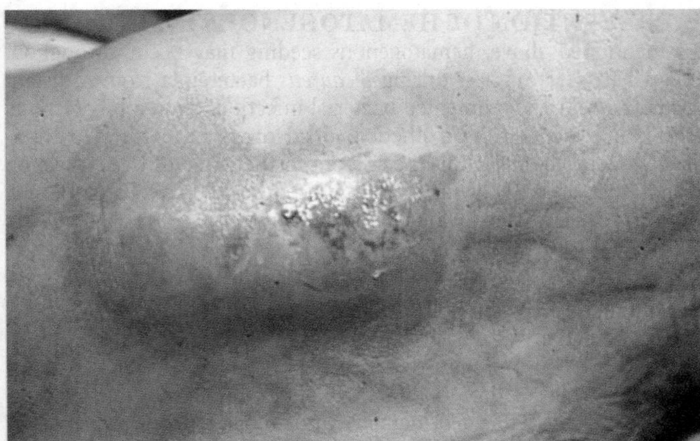

FIGURE 131-3 Acute postoperative periprosthetic joint infection of the left hip caused by group B streptococci in a 68-year-old woman.

EPIDEMIOLOGY

The risk of infection manifesting during the first 2 postoperative years varies according to the joint. It is lowest after hip and knee arthroplasty (0.3–1.5%) and highest after ankle and elbow replacement (4–10%). The risk of hematogenous PJI is highest in the early postoperative period. However, hematogenous seeding occurs throughout life, and most cases therefore develop >2 years after implantation. The rate of risk for secondary PJI during *S. aureus* bacteremia is 30–40%.

MICROBIOLOGY

About 50–70% of cases of PJI are caused by staphylococci (*S. aureus* and coagulase-negative staphylococci), 6–10% by streptococci, 4–10% by gram-negative bacilli, and the rest by various other microorganisms. In some centers, the fraction of PJI cases caused by gram-negative bacilli is much higher for unknown reasons. All microorganisms can cause PJI, including fungi and mycobacteria. *C. acnes* causes up to one-third of episodes of periprosthetic shoulder infection.

CLASSIFICATION AND CLINICAL MANIFESTATIONS

PJI is traditionally classified as early (<3 months after implantation), delayed (3–24 months after surgery), or late (>2 years after implantation). For therapeutic decision-making (see below), it is more useful to classify PJI as (1) acute hematogenous PJI with <3 weeks of symptoms, (2) early postinterventional PJI manifesting within 1 month after surgery, or (3) chronic PJI with symptom duration of >3 weeks.

Acute exogenous PJI typically presents with local signs of infection (**Fig. 131-3**). In contrast, acute hematogenous PJI is most often caused by *S. aureus* and is characterized by new-onset pain. Local inflammatory signs are rare in hip PJI but frequent in knee PJI. Fever is rare after the initial phase of bacteremia. Key findings in chronic PJI are joint effusion, local pain, implant loosening, and occasionally a sinus tract. Chronic PJI is most commonly caused by low-virulence microorganisms such as coagulase-negative staphylococci or *P. acnes*. These infections are characterized by nonspecific symptoms, such as chronic pain caused by low-grade inflammation or early loosening.

DIAGNOSIS

Blood tests such as the measurement of CRP (elevated levels, ≥10 mg/L) and erythrocyte sedimentation rate (elevated rates, ≥30 mm/h) are sensitive (91–97%) but not specific (70–78%). Synovial fluid cell counts are ~90% sensitive and specific, with threshold values of 1700 leukocytes/μL in periprosthetic knee infection and 4200 leukocytes/μL in periprosthetic hip infection. A biomarker, α-defensin, can be tested in synovial fluid; this biomarker is highly specific and therefore useful in confirming PJI. However, this test is expensive and its sensitivity is limited; therefore, it should not be used for screening. During debridement surgery, at least three but optimally six tissue samples should be obtained for culture and histopathology. If implant material (modular parts, screws, or the prosthesis) is removed, sonication of this material followed by culture and/or use of molecular methods to examine the sonicate fluid allows the detection of microorganisms in biofilms.

The three-phase bone scan is very sensitive for detecting PJI but is not specific. As mentioned above, this test does not differentiate bone remodeling from infection and therefore is not useful during at least the first year after implantation. CT and MRI detect soft tissue infection, prosthetic loosening, and bone erosion, but imaging artifacts caused by metal implants limit their use. ^{18}F-fluorodeoxyglucose PET (^{18F}-FD-PET) is an alternative method with good sensitivity but low specificity for the detection of PJI. Therefore, ^{18}F-FDG-PET/CT is useful only in excluding but not confirming PJI.

TREATMENT

Periprosthetic Joint Infection

The outcome following treatment of PJI is better when managed using a multidisciplinary approach involving an experienced orthopedic surgeon, an infectious disease specialist, a plastic reconstructive surgeon, and a microbiologist. Therefore, most patients are referred to a specialized center. In general, the goal of treatment is cure—i.e., a pain-free functional joint with complete eradication of the infecting pathogen(s). However, for patients with severe comorbidity, lifelong suppressive antimicrobial therapy may be preferred. As a rule, antimicrobial therapy without surgical intervention is not curative but merely suppressive. There are four curative surgical options: debridement and implant retention, one-stage implant exchange, two-stage implant exchange, and implant removal without replacement. Implant retention offers a good chance of infection-free survival (>80%) only if the following conditions are fulfilled: (1) acute infection, (2) stable implant, (3) pathogen susceptible to a biofilm-active antimicrobial agent (see below), and (4) skin and soft tissue in good condition.

Table 131-2 summarizes pathogen-specific antimicrobial therapy for PJI. Initial IV therapy is followed by long-term oral antibiotics. Efficacious treatment is best defined in staphylococcal implant-associated infections. Rifampin exhibits excellent activity against biofilms composed of susceptible staphylococci. Because of the risk of rapid emergence of resistance, rifampin must always be combined with another effective antibiotic. If gram-negative infections are treated with implant retention, fluoroquinolones should be used because of their activity against gram-negative biofilms.

■ PREVENTION OF HEMATOGENOUS INFECTION

As mentioned above, hematogenous seeding may occur throughout life. This risk is highest during *S. aureus* bacteremia from a distant focus. Therefore, documented bacterial infections should be promptly treated in patients with prosthetic joints. However, according to a prospective case-control study, the risk of prosthetic hip or knee infection is not increased following dental procedures. Therefore, antibiotic prophylaxis is not needed during dental work.

■ GLOBAL CONSIDERATIONS

Rifampin and fluoroquinolones are still the only antimicrobial agents with good activity against staphylococcal and gram-negative biofilms, respectively. Thus, in countries with high rates of rifampin resistance in staphylococci and/or high rates of fluoroquinolone resistance in gram-negative bacilli, debridement with implant retention generally does not yield a good cure rate.

STERNAL OSTEOMYELITIS

■ PATHOGENESIS

Sternal osteomyelitis occurs primarily after sternal surgery (with the entry of exogenous organisms) and more rarely by hematogenous seeding or contiguous extension from adjacent sites of sternocostal arthritis. Exogenous sternal osteomyelitis after open sternal surgery is also called *deep sternal-wound infection.* Exogenous infection may follow minor sternal trauma, sternal fracture, and manubriosternal septic arthritis. Tuberculous sternal osteomyelitis typically manifests during hematogenous seeding in children or as reactivated infection in adults. Reactivation is sometimes preceded by blunt trauma. In rare cases, tuberculous sternal osteomyelitis is caused by continuous infection from an infected internal mammary lymph node.

■ EPIDEMIOLOGY

The incidence of poststernotomy wound infection varies from 0.5–2%, but figures are even higher among patients with risk factors such as diabetes, obesity, chronic renal failure, emergency surgery, use of bilateral internal mammary artery grafts, and re-exploration for bleeding. Rapid diagnosis and correct management of superficial sternal wound infection prevent its progression to sternal osteomyelitis. Primary (hematogenous) sternal osteomyelitis accounts for only 0.3% of all cases of osteomyelitis. Risk factors are IV drug use, HIV infection, radiotherapy, blunt trauma, cardiopulmonary resuscitation, alcohol abuse, liver cirrhosis, and hemoglobinopathy.

■ MICROBIOLOGY

Poststernotomy osteomyelitis is generally caused by *S. aureus* (10–20% of cases), coagulase-negative staphylococci (40–60%), gram-negative bacilli (15–25%), or *C. acnes* (2–10%). Fungal infections caused by *Candida* species also play a role. The fact that ~20% of cases are polymicrobial is indicative of exogenous superinfection during therapy. Hematogenous sternal osteomyelitis is caused most commonly by *S. aureus*. Other microorganisms play a role in special populations—e.g., *P. aeruginosa* in IV drug users, *Salmonella* species in individuals with sickle cell anemia, and *M. tuberculosis* in patients from endemic areas who have previously had tuberculosis.

■ CLINICAL MANIFESTATIONS

Exogenous sternal osteomyelitis manifests as fever, increased local pain, erythema, wound discharge, and sternal instability (**Fig. 131-4**). Contiguous mediastinitis is a feared complication, occurring in ~10–30% of patients with sternal osteomyelitis. Hematogenous sternal osteomyelitis is characterized by sternal pain, swelling, and erythema. In addition, most patients have systemic signs and symptoms of sepsis.

The differential diagnosis of hematogenous sternal osteomyelitis includes immunologic processes typically presenting as systemic or multifocal inflammation of the sternum or of the sternoclavicular or sternocostal joints (e.g., SAPHO [synovitis, acne, pustulosis, hyperostosis, osteitis], vasculitis, chronic multifocal relapsing osteomyelitis).

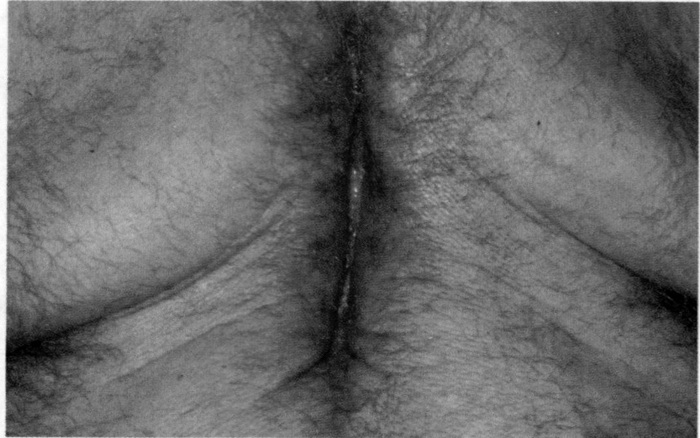

FIGURE 131-4 Sternal osteomyelitis caused by *Staphylococcus epidermidis* 5 weeks after sternotomy for aortocoronary bypass in a 72-year-old man.

■ DIAGNOSIS

In primary sternal osteomyelitis, the diagnostic workup does not differ from that in other types of hematogenous osteomyelitis (see above). When a patient has grown up in regions where tuberculosis is endemic, a specific workup for mycobacterial infection should be performed, especially if osteomyelitis had its onset after a blunt sternal trauma. In secondary sternal osteomyelitis, leukocyte counts may be normal, but the CRP level is >100 mg/L in most cases. Tissue sampling for microbiologic studies is crucial. In osteomyelitis associated with sternal wires, low-virulence microorganisms, such as coagulase-negative staphylococci, play an important role. In order to differentiate between colonization and infection, samples from at least three deep biopsies should be subjected to microbiologic examination. Superficial swab cultures are not diagnostic and may be misleading. No studies have compared the value of the various imaging modalities in suspected primary sternal osteomyelitis. However, MRI is the current gold standard for detection of each type of osteomyelitis.

TREATMENT

Sternal Osteomyelitis

In cases of deep sternal-wound infection, a combined approach using both surgery and antibiotic treatment is required. Antimicrobial therapy should be started immediately after samples have been obtained for microbiologic analyses in order to control clinical sepsis. To protect a newly inserted heart valve, initial treatment should be directed against staphylococci, with consideration of the local susceptibility pattern. In centers with a high prevalence of methicillin-resistant *S. aureus*, vancomycin or daptomycin should be added to a broad-spectrum β-lactam drug. As soon as cultures of blood and/or deep wound biopsies have confirmed the pathogen's identity and susceptibility pattern, treatment should be optimized and narrowed accordingly. Tables 131-1 and 131-2 show appropriate therapeutic choices for the most frequently identified microorganisms causing sternal osteomyelitis in the absence and presence, respectively, of an implanted device. In a recent observational study of patients with staphylococcal deep sternal-wound infection, the use of a rifampin-containing regimen was predictive of success. The optimal duration of antibiotic therapy has not been established. In acute sternal osteomyelitis without hardware, a 6-week course is the rule. In patients with remaining sternal wires, treatment duration is generally prolonged to 3 months (Table 131-2). Like other types of tuberculous bone infection, tuberculous sternal osteomyelitis is treated for 6–12 months.

Primary sternal osteomyelitis can generally be treated without surgery. In contrast, in secondary sternal osteomyelitis, debridement is always required. This procedure should be performed by a team of experienced surgeons, since mediastinitis, bone infection, and skin and soft tissue damage may need to be treated during the same intervention.

PROGNOSIS

Primary sternal osteomyelitis poses a minimal mortality risk. In contrast, the in-hospital mortality rates from secondary sternal osteomyelitis are 15–30% after sternal surgery.

GLOBAL CONSIDERATIONS

In endemic areas, microorganisms such as *M. tuberculosis*, *Salmonella* species, and *Brucella* species should be considered during sampling for microbiologic diagnosis.

FOOT OSTEOMYELITIS

PATHOGENESIS

Osteomyelitis of the foot usually occurs in patients with diabetes, peripheral arterial insufficiency, or peripheral neuropathy and after foot surgery. These entities are often linked to each other, especially in diabetic patients with late complications. However, foot osteomyelitis is also seen in patients with isolated peripheral neuropathy and can manifest as implant-associated osteomyelitis in patients without comorbidity due to a deep wound infection after foot surgery (hallux valgus surgery, arthrodesis, total ankle arthroplasty). Foot osteomyelitis is acquired almost exclusively by the exogenous route. It is a complication of deep pressure ulcers and of impaired wound healing after surgery.

EPIDEMIOLOGY

The incidence of diabetic foot infection is 30–40 cases/1000 persons with diabetes per year. The condition starts with skin and soft tissue lesions and progresses to osteomyelitis, especially in patients with risk factors. About 20–60% of patients with diabetic foot infection have confirmed osteomyelitis. Diabetic foot osteomyelitis increases the risk of amputation. With adequate management of the early stage of diabetic foot infections, the rate of amputation can be lowered.

RISK FACTORS

Risk factors for diabetic foot infection are (1) peripheral motor, sensory, and autonomic neuropathy; (2) neuro-osteoarthropathic deformities (Charcot foot; **Fig. 131-5**); (3) arterial insufficiency; (4) uncontrolled hyperglycemia; (5) disabilities such as reduced vision; and (6) maladaptive behavior.

MICROBIOLOGY

The correlation between cultures from bone biopsy and those from wound swabs or even deep soft-tissue punctures is poor. In a study of 31 patients with simultaneous sampling, the correlation between needle biopsy and bone biopsy cultures was only 24%. The correlation is better when *S. aureus* is isolated (40–50%) than when anaerobes (20–35%), gram-negative bacilli (20–30%), or coagulase-negative staphylococci (0–20%) are identified. When only bone-biopsy samples are considered, the leading pathogens are *S. aureus* (25–40%), anaerobes (5–20%), and various gram-negative bacilli (18–40%). The precise distribution depends on whether the patient has already been treated with antibiotics. Anaerobes are especially prevalent in chronic wounds. Pretreatment typically selects for *P. aeruginosa*, methicillin-resistant *S. aureus*, or enterococci.

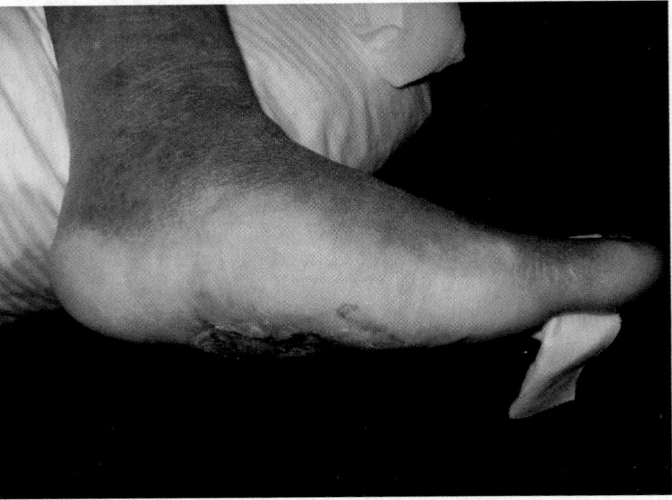

FIGURE 131-5 Neuropathic joint disease (Charcot foot) complicated by chronic foot osteomyelitis in a 78-year-old woman with diabetes mellitus complicated by severe neuropathy.

DIAGNOSIS

In many cases, foot osteomyelitis can be diagnosed clinically, without imaging procedures. Most clinicians rely on the "probe-to-bone" test, which has a positive predictive value of ~90% in populations with a high pretest probability. Thus, in a patient with diabetes who is hospitalized for a chronic deep foot ulcer, the diagnosis of foot osteomyelitis is highly probable if bone can be directly touched with a metal instrument. In a patient with a lower pretest probability, MRI should be performed because of its high sensitivity (80–100%) and specificity (80–90%). Plain radiography has a sensitivity of only 30–90% and a specificity of only 50–90%; it may be considered for follow-up of patients with confirmed diabetic foot osteomyelitis.

TREATMENT

Foot Osteomyelitis

As mentioned above, correlation between cultures of bone and those of wound swabs or wound punctures is poor. Antibiotic treatment should be based on bone culture. If no bone biopsy is performed, empirical therapy chosen in light of the most common infecting agents and the type of clinical syndrome should be given. In a controlled therapeutic trial of diabetic patients in whom no infected bone needed to be resected, the outcome of a 6-week course of antibiotics was not different from a 12-week course. Wound debridement combined with a 4- to 6-week course of antibiotics renders amputation unnecessary in about two-thirds of patients. According to the 2012 Infectious Diseases Society of America's clinical practice guideline for the diagnosis and treatment of diabetic foot infections, the following management strategies should be considered. If a foot ulcer is clinically infected, prompt empirical antimicrobial therapy may prevent progression to osteomyelitis. When the risk of methicillin-resistant *S. aureus* is considered high, an agent active against these strains (e.g., vancomycin) should be chosen. If the patient has not recently received antibiotics, the spectrum of the selected antibiotic must include gram-positive cocci (e.g., clindamycin, ampicillin-sulbactam). If the patient has received antibiotics within the past month, the spectrum of empirical antibiotics should include gram-negative bacilli (e.g., clindamycin plus a fluoroquinolone). If the patient has risk factors for *Pseudomonas* infection (previous colonization, residence in a warm climate, frequent exposure of the foot to water), an empirical antipseudomonal agent (e.g., piperacillin-tazobactam, cefepime) is indicated. If osteomyelitis is suspected either on clinical grounds (probe to bone) or on the basis of imaging procedures (MRI), bone biopsy should be performed. If infected bone is not entirely removed by surgery, the patient should be treated for 4–6 weeks in line with the identified pathogen(s) and their susceptibility. Treatment should initially be given by the IV route. Whether therapy can later be administered by the oral route depends on the bioavailability of oral drugs that cover the infecting agents. If dead bone cannot be removed, long-term therapy (at least 3 months) should be considered. In such cases, cure of osteomyelitis is usually the exception, and repetitive suppressive treatment may be needed.

GLOBAL CONSIDERATIONS

The number of multiresistant microorganisms causing diabetic foot infection is increasing. The prevalence of methicillin-resistant *S. aureus* is 5–43% in various countries. In a study of 102 patients with diabetic foot infection from India, 69% of aerobic gram-negative bacilli produced extended-spectrum β-lactamase and 43% of *S. aureus* isolates were methicillin resistant. Risk factors for multidrug-resistant microorganisms are poor glycemic control, prolonged duration of infection, and large ulcer size.

■ FURTHER READING

Depypere M et al: Pathogenesis and management of fracture-related infection. Clin Microbiol Infect 26:572, 2020.

Li H-K et al: Oral versus intravenous antibiotics for bone and joint infection. N Engl J Med 380:425, 2019.

Lipsky BA et al: 2012 Infectious Diseases Society of America clinical practice guideline for the diagnosis and treatment of diabetic foot infections. Clin Infect Dis 54:e132, 2012.

Osmon DR et al: Diagnosis and management of prosthetic joint infection: Clinical practice guidelines by the Infectious Diseases Society of America. Clin Infect Dis 56:e1, 2013.

Yusuf E et al: Current perspectives on diagnosis and management of sternal wound infections. Infect Drug Res 11:961, 2018.

Zimmerli W: Vertebral osteomyelitis. N Engl J Med 362:1022, 2010.

132 Intraabdominal Infections and Abscesses

Miriam Baron Barshak, Dennis L. Kasper

Intraperitoneal infections generally arise because a normal anatomic barrier is disrupted. This disruption may result from a variety of causes—e.g., when the appendix, a diverticulum, or an ulcer ruptures; when the bowel wall is weakened by ischemia, tumor, or inflammation (e.g., in inflammatory bowel disease); or with adjacent inflammatory processes, such as pancreatitis or pelvic inflammatory disease, in which enzymes (in the former case) or organisms (in the latter) may leak into the peritoneal cavity. Whatever the inciting event, once inflammation develops and organisms usually contained within the bowel or another organ enter the normally sterile peritoneal space, a knowable series of events takes place. Intraabdominal infections occur in two stages: peritonitis and—if the patient survives this stage and goes untreated—abscess formation. The types of microorganisms predominating in each stage of infection are responsible for the pathogenesis of disease.

PERITONITIS

Peritonitis is a life-threatening event that is often accompanied by bacteremia and sepsis syndrome **(Chap. 304)**. The peritoneal cavity is large but is divided into compartments. The upper and lower peritoneal cavities are divided by the transverse mesocolon; the greater omentum extends from the transverse mesocolon and from the lower pole of the stomach to line the lower peritoneal cavity. The pancreas, duodenum, and ascending and descending colon are located in the anterior retroperitoneal space; the kidneys, ureters, and adrenals are found in the posterior retroperitoneal space. The other organs, including the liver, stomach, gallbladder, spleen, jejunum, ileum, transverse and sigmoid colon, cecum, and appendix, are within the peritoneal cavity. The cavity is lined with a serous membrane that can serve as a conduit for fluids—a property exploited in peritoneal dialysis **(Fig. 132-1)**. A small amount of serous fluid is normally present in the peritoneal space, with a protein content (consisting mainly of albumin) of <30 g/L and <300 white blood cells (WBCs, generally mononuclear cells) per microliter. In bacterial infections, leukocyte recruitment into the infected peritoneal cavity consists of an early influx of polymorphonuclear leukocytes (PMNs) and a prolonged subsequent phase of mononuclear cell migration. The phenotype of the infiltrating leukocytes during the course of inflammation is regulated primarily by resident-cell chemokine synthesis.

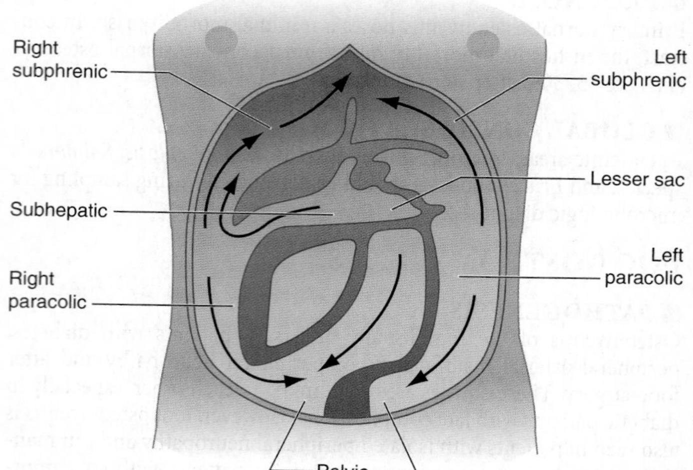

FIGURE 132-1 Diagram of the intraperitoneal spaces, showing the circulation of fluid and potential areas for abscess formation. Some compartments collect fluid or pus more often than others. These compartments include the pelvis (the lowest portion), the subphrenic spaces on the right and left sides, and Morrison's pouch, which is a posterosuperior extension of the subhepatic spaces and is the lowest part of the paravertebral groove when a patient is recumbent. The falciform ligament separating the right and left subphrenic spaces appears to act as a barrier to the spread of infection; consequently, it is unusual to find bilateral subphrenic collections. *(Republished with permission of Springer Nature, from Atlas of Infectious Diseases, vol VII: Intra-abdominal infections, hepatitis, and gastroenteritis, B Lorber et al. 1996; permission conveyed through Copyright Clearance Center, Inc.)*

■ PRIMARY (SPONTANEOUS) BACTERIAL PERITONITIS

Peritonitis is either primary (without an apparent source of contamination) or secondary. The types of organisms found and the clinical presentations of these two processes are different. In adults, primary bacterial peritonitis (PBP) occurs most commonly in conjunction with cirrhosis of the liver (frequently the result of alcoholism). However, the disease has been reported in adults with metastatic malignant disease, postnecrotic cirrhosis, chronic active hepatitis, acute viral hepatitis, congestive heart failure, systemic lupus erythematosus, and lymphedema as well as in patients with no underlying disease. Although PBP virtually always develops in patients with preexisting ascites, it is, in general, an uncommon event, occurring in ≤10% of cirrhotic patients. The cause of PBP has not been established definitively but is believed to involve hematogenous spread of organisms in a patient in whom a diseased liver and altered portal circulation result in a defect in the usual filtration function. Organisms multiply in ascites, a good medium for growth. Proteins of the complement cascade are found in peritoneal fluid, with lower levels in cirrhotic patients than in patients with ascites of other etiologies. The opsonic and phagocytic properties of PMNs are diminished in patients with advanced liver disease. Cirrhosis is associated with alterations in the gut microbiota, including an increased prevalence of potentially pathogenic bacteria such as Enterobacteriaceae. Small-intestinal bacterial overgrowth is frequently present in advanced stages of liver cirrhosis and has been linked with pathologic bacterial translocation and PBP. Factors promoting these changes in cirrhosis may include deficiencies in Paneth cell defensins, reduced intestinal motility, decreased pancreatobiliary secretions, and portal-hypertensive enteropathy.

The presentation of PBP differs from that of secondary peritonitis. The most common manifestation is fever, which is reported in up to 80% of patients. Ascites is found but virtually always predates infection. Abdominal pain, an acute onset of symptoms, and peritoneal irritation during physical examination can be helpful diagnostically, but the absence of any of these findings does not exclude this often-subtle diagnosis. Nonlocalizing symptoms (such as malaise, fatigue, or encephalopathy) without another clear etiology also should prompt consideration of PBP in a susceptible patient. It is vital to sample the peritoneal fluid of any cirrhotic patient with ascites and fever. The finding of >250 PMNs/μL is diagnostic for PBP, according to Conn. This criterion does not apply to secondary peritonitis (see below). The microbiology of PBP also is distinctive. While enteric gram-negative bacilli such as *Escherichia coli* are commonly encountered, gram-positive organisms such as streptococci, enterococci, or even pneumococci are sometimes found. In an important development, widespread use of quinolones to prevent PBP in high-risk subgroups of patients, frequent hospitalizations, and exposure to broad-spectrum antibiotics have led to a change in the etiology of infections in patients with cirrhosis, with more gram-positive bacteria and extended-spectrum β-lactamase (ESBL)–producing Enterobacteriaceae in recent years. Risk factors for multidrug-resistant infections include nosocomial origin of infection, long-term norfloxacin prophylaxis, recent infection with multiresistant bacteria, and recent use of β-lactam antibiotics. In PBP, a single organism is typically isolated; anaerobes are found less frequently in PBP than in secondary peritonitis, in which a mixed flora including anaerobes is the rule. In fact, if PBP is suspected and multiple organisms including anaerobes are recovered from the peritoneal fluid, the diagnosis must be reconsidered and a source of secondary peritonitis sought.

The diagnosis of PBP is not easy. It depends on the exclusion of a primary intraabdominal source of infection. Contrast-enhanced CT is useful in identifying an intraabdominal source for infection. It may be difficult to recover organisms from cultures of peritoneal fluid, presumably because the burden of organisms is low. However, the yield can be improved if 10 mL of peritoneal fluid is placed directly into a blood culture bottle. Because bacteremia frequently accompanies PBP, blood should be cultured simultaneously. To maximize the yield, culture samples should be collected prior to administration of antibiotics. There is interest in identifying biomarkers in ascites that may be associated with PBP. No specific radiographic studies are helpful in the diagnosis of PBP. A plain film of the abdomen would be expected to show ascites. Chest and abdominal radiography should be performed when patients have abdominal pain to exclude free air, which signals a perforation **(Fig. 132-2)**.

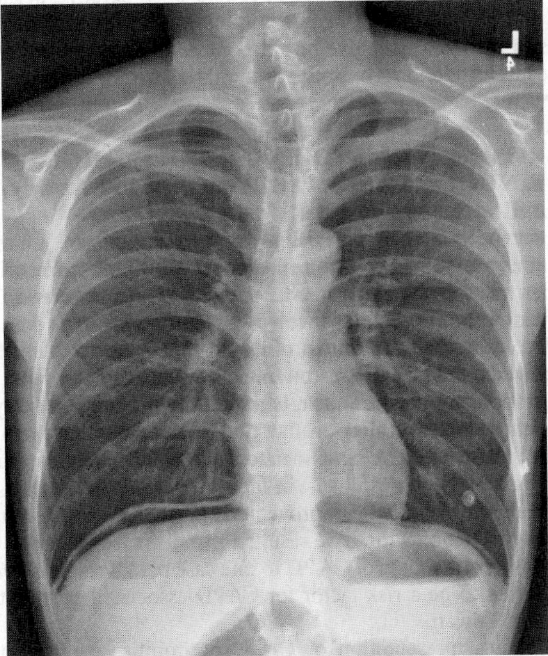

FIGURE 132-2 Pneumoperitoneum. Free air under the diaphragm on an upright chest film suggests the presence of a bowel perforation and associated peritonitis. *(Image courtesy of Dr. John Braver; with permission.)*

TREATMENT
Primary Bacterial Peritonitis

Treatment for PBP is directed at the isolate from blood or peritoneal fluid. Gram's staining of peritoneal fluid often gives negative results in PBP. Therefore, until culture results become available, therapy should cover gram-negative aerobic bacilli and gram-positive cocci. Third-generation cephalosporins such as cefotaxime (2 g q8h, administered IV) provide reasonable initial coverage in moderately ill patients. Broad-spectrum antibiotics, such as β-lactam/β-lactamase inhibitor combinations (e.g., piperacillin/tazobactam, 3.375 g q6h IV for adults with normal renal function) or ceftriaxone (2 g q24h IV), also are options. Broader empirical coverage aimed at resistant hospital-acquired gram-negative bacteria (e.g., treatment with a carbapenem or newer agents, such as ceftolozane-tazobactam or ceftazidime-avibactam) may be appropriate for nosocomially acquired PBP until culture results become available. Empirical coverage for anaerobes is not necessary. A mortality benefit from albumin (1.5 g/kg of body weight within 6 h of detection and 1.0 g/kg on day 3) has been demonstrated for patients who present with serum creatinine levels ≥1 mg/dL, blood urea nitrogen levels ≥30 mg/dL, or total bilirubin levels ≥4 mg/dL but not for patients who do not meet these criteria. After the infecting organism is identified, therapy should be narrowed to target the specific pathogen. Patients with PBP usually respond within 72 h to appropriate antibiotic therapy. Antimicrobial treatment can be administered for as little as 5 days if rapid improvement occurs and blood cultures are negative, but a course of up to 2 weeks may be required for patients with bacteremia and for those whose improvement is slow. Persistence of WBCs in the ascitic fluid after therapy should prompt a search for additional diagnoses.

Prognosis: PBP is associated with significant morbidity and mortality, perhaps reflecting the fact that PBP risk is highest among patients with advanced liver disease. In a 2018 study of hospitalized patients with PBP in the United States, in-hospital mortality was 17.6%. Another study in 2019 found that among patients at a U.S. tertiary academic center, mortality following PBP was 23% at 30 days and 37% at 90 days. The morbidity and mortality associated with PBP has led to interest in strategies for PBP prevention.

Prevention • PRIMARY PREVENTION Several observational studies and a meta-analysis raise the concern that gastric acid suppression may increase the risk of PBP. No prospective studies have yet addressed whether avoidance of such therapy may prevent PBP. Nonselective beta blockers may prevent secondary bacterial peritonitis. A 2012 guideline from the American Association for the Study of Liver Diseases recommends chronic antibiotic prophylaxis with a regimen described in the next section for patients who are at highest risk for PBP—that is, those with an ascitic-fluid total protein level <1.5 g/dL along with impaired renal function (creatinine, ≥1.2 mg/dL; blood urea nitrogen, ≥25 mg/dL; or serum sodium, ≤130 mg/dL) and/or liver failure (Child-Pugh score, ≥9; and bilirubin, ≥3 mg/dL). A 7-day course of antibiotic prophylaxis is recommended for patients with cirrhosis and gastrointestinal bleeding.

SECONDARY PREVENTION PBP has a high rate of recurrence. Up to 70% of patients experience a recurrence within 1 year. Antibiotic prophylaxis is recommended for patients with a history of PBP to reduce this rate to <20% and improve short-term survival rates. Prophylactic regimens for adults with normal renal function include fluoroquinolones (ciprofloxacin, 500 mg weekly; or norfloxacin [not available in the United States], 400 mg/d) or trimethoprim-sulfamethoxazole (one double-strength tablet daily). However, long-term administration of broad-spectrum antibiotics in this setting has been shown to increase the risk of severe staphylococcal infections. There is increased interest in using rifaximin, a broad-spectrum antibiotic that is used already for hepatic encephalopathy and is not absorbed, for PBP prophylaxis (1200 mg daily).

■ SECONDARY PERITONITIS

Secondary peritonitis develops when bacteria contaminate the peritoneum as a result of spillage from an intraabdominal viscus. The organisms found almost always constitute a mixed flora in which facultative gram-negative bacilli and anaerobes predominate, especially when the contaminating source is colonic. Early in the course of infection, when the host response is directed toward containment, exudate containing fibrin and PMNs is found. Early death in this setting is attributable to gram-negative bacillary sepsis and to potent endotoxins circulating in the bloodstream (**Chap. 304**). Gram-negative bacilli, particularly *E. coli*, are common bloodstream isolates, but *Bacteroides fragilis* bacteremia also occurs. The severity of abdominal pain and the clinical course depend on the inciting process. The organisms isolated from the peritoneum also vary with the source of the initial process and the normal flora at that site. Secondary peritonitis can result primarily from chemical irritation and/or bacterial contamination. For example, as long as the patient is not achlorhydric, a ruptured gastric ulcer will release low-pH gastric contents that will serve as a chemical irritant. The normal flora of the stomach comprises the same organisms found in the oropharynx but in lower numbers. Thus, the bacterial burden in a ruptured ulcer is negligible compared with that in a ruptured appendix. The normal flora of the colon below the ligament of Treitz contains ~10^{11} anaerobic organisms/g of feces but only 10^8 aerobes/g; therefore, anaerobic species account for 99.9% of the bacteria (**Chap. 471**). Leakage of colonic contents (pH 7–8) does not cause significant chemical peritonitis, but infection is intense because of the heavy bacterial load.

Depending on the inciting event, local symptoms may occur in secondary peritonitis—for example, epigastric pain from a ruptured gastric ulcer. In appendicitis (**Chap. 331**), the initial presenting symptoms are often vague, with periumbilical discomfort and nausea followed in a number of hours by pain more localized to the right lower quadrant. Unusual locations of the appendix (including a retrocecal position) can complicate this presentation further. Once infection has spread to the peritoneal cavity, pain increases, particularly with infection involving the parietal peritoneum, which is innervated extensively. Patients usually lie motionless, often with knees drawn up to avoid stretching the nerve fibers of the peritoneal cavity. Coughing and sneezing, which increase pressure within the peritoneal cavity, are associated with sharp pain. There may or may not be pain localized to the infected or diseased organ from which secondary peritonitis has arisen. Patients with secondary peritonitis generally have abnormal findings on abdominal examination, with marked voluntary and involuntary guarding of the anterior abdominal musculature. Later findings include tenderness, especially rebound tenderness. In addition, there may be localized findings in the area of the inciting event. In general, patients are febrile, with marked leukocytosis and a left shift of the WBCs to band forms.

While recovery of organisms from peritoneal fluid is easier in secondary than in primary peritonitis, a tap of the abdomen is rarely the procedure of choice in secondary peritonitis. An exception is in cases involving trauma, where the possibility of a hemoperitoneum may need to be excluded early. Emergent studies (such as abdominal CT) to find the source of peritoneal contamination should be undertaken if the patient is hemodynamically stable; unstable patients may require surgical intervention without prior imaging. Results of cultures from drain sites are not reliable for defining the etiology of infections.

TREATMENT

Secondary Peritonitis

Treatment for secondary peritonitis includes early administration of antibiotics aimed particularly at aerobic gram-negative bacilli and anaerobes (see below). The most appropriate regimen depends on the anticipated flora and the degree of illness. Community-acquired infections associated with mild to moderate disease can be treated with many drugs covering these organisms, including broad-spectrum β-lactam/β-lactamase inhibitor combinations (e.g., ticarcillin/clavulanate, 3.1 g q4–6h IV; or piperacillin/tazobactam, 3.375 g q6h IV) or a combination of either a fluoroquinolone (e.g., levofloxacin, 750 mg q24h IV) or a third-generation cephalosporin (e.g., ceftriaxone, 2 g q24h IV) plus metronidazole (500 mg q8h IV). Eravacycline is a newer antibiotic in the tetracycline class that has been approved by the U.S. Food and Drug Administration for treatment of complicated intraabdominal infections (1 mg/kg q12h IV). Patients in intensive care units and/or those with health care–associated infections should receive antibiotics targeting more resistant gram-negative organisms such as *Pseudomonas aeruginosa*—e.g., imipenem (500 mg q6h IV), meropenem (1 g q8h IV), higher-dose piperacillin/tazobactam (4.5 g IV q6h), or drug combinations such as cefepime (2 g IV q8h) or ceftazidime (2 g IV q8h) plus metronidazole. The role of enterococci and *Candida* species in mixed infections is controversial; however, because cephalosporin-based regimens lack activity against enterococci, ampicillin or vancomycin can be added to these regimens for enterococcal coverage in very ill patients until culture results are available. For patients known to be colonized with ampicillin-resistant, vancomycin-resistant enterococci (VRE), a VRE-active agent, such as linezolid or daptomycin, should be included. Antifungal coverage is warranted if there is growth of *Candida* species from a sterile site. Patients who are known to be colonized with highly resistant gram-negative organisms may require treatment with a newer agent such as ceftazidime/avibactam or ceftolozane/tazobactam. Secondary peritonitis usually requires both surgical intervention to address the inciting process and antibiotics to treat early bacteremia, to decrease the incidence of abscess formation and wound infection, and to prevent distant spread of infection. Although surgery is rarely indicated in PBP in adults, it may be life-saving in secondary peritonitis. Recombinant human activated protein C (APC) was considered at one time for treatment of severe sepsis from causes including secondary peritonitis but was withdrawn from the market in 2011 after it was determined that the drug was associated with an increased risk of bleeding and that evidence for its beneficial effects was inadequate. Thus APC should not be used for sepsis or septic shock outside randomized clinical trials.

Peritonitis may develop as a complication of abdominal surgeries. These infections may be accompanied by localizing pain and/or nonlocalizing signs or symptoms such as fever, malaise, anorexia, and toxicity. As a nosocomial infection, postoperative peritonitis may be associated with organisms such as staphylococci, components of the gram-negative hospital microflora, and the microbes that cause PBP and secondary peritonitis, as described above.

■ PERITONITIS IN PATIENTS UNDERGOING CONTINUOUS AMBULATORY PERITONEAL DIALYSIS

A third type of peritonitis arises in patients who are undergoing continuous ambulatory peritoneal dialysis (CAPD). Unlike PBP and secondary peritonitis, which are caused by endogenous bacteria, CAPD-associated peritonitis usually involves skin organisms. The pathogenesis of infection is similar to that of intravascular device–related infection, in which skin organisms migrate along the catheter, which both serves as an entry point and exerts the effects of a foreign body. Exit-site or tunnel infection may or may not accompany CAPD-associated peritonitis. Like PBP, CAPD-associated peritonitis is usually caused by a single organism. Peritonitis is, in fact, the most common reason for discontinuation of CAPD. Improvements in equipment design, especially the Y-set connector, have resulted in a decrease from one case of peritonitis per 9 months of CAPD to one case per 24 months. Diabetes was reported to be a risk factor for CAPD-associated peritonitis in a study from Taiwan.

The clinical presentation of CAPD peritonitis resembles that of secondary peritonitis in that diffuse pain and peritoneal signs are common. The dialysate is usually cloudy and contains >100 WBCs/μL, >50% of which are neutrophils. However, the number of cells depends in part on dwell time. According to a guideline from the International Society for Peritoneal Dialysis (2016), for patients undergoing automated peritoneal dialysis who present during their nighttime treatment and whose dwell time is much shorter than with CAPD, the clinician should use the percentage of PMNs rather than the absolute number of WBCs to diagnose peritonitis. As the normal peritoneum has very few PMNs, a proportion above 50% is strong evidence of peritonitis even if the absolute WBC count does not reach 100/μL. Meanwhile, patients undergoing automated peritoneal dialysis without a daytime exchange who present with abdominal pain may have no fluid to withdraw, in which case 1 L of dialysate should be infused and permitted to dwell a minimum of 1–2 h, then drained, examined for turbidity, and sent for cell count with differential and culture. The differential (with a shortened dwell time) may be more useful than the absolute WBC count. In equivocal cases or in patients with systemic or abdominal symptoms in whom the effluent appears clear, a second exchange is performed, with a dwell time of at least 2 h. Clinical judgment should guide initiation of therapy.

The most common organisms are *Staphylococcus* species, which accounted for ~45% of cases in one series. Historically, coagulase-negative staphylococcal species were identified most commonly in these infections, but these isolates have more recently been decreasing in frequency. *Staphylococcus aureus* is more often involved among patients who are nasal carriers of the organism than among those who are not, and this organism is the most common pathogen in overt exit-site infections. Gram-negative bacilli and fungi such as *Candida* species also are found. Vancomycin-resistant enterococci and vancomycin-intermediate *S. aureus* have been reported to produce peritonitis in CAPD patients. The finding of more than one organism in dialysate culture should prompt evaluation for secondary peritonitis. As with PBP, culture of dialysate fluid in blood culture bottles improves the yield. To facilitate diagnosis, several hundred milliliters of removed dialysis fluid should be concentrated by centrifugation before culture.

TREATMENT

CAPD Peritonitis

Empirical therapy for CAPD peritonitis should be directed at *S. aureus*, coagulase-negative *Staphylococcus*, and gram-negative bacilli until the results of cultures become available. Guidelines suggest that agents should be chosen on the basis of local experience with resistant organisms. In some centers, a first-generation cephalosporin such as cefazolin (for gram-positive bacteria) and a fluoroquinolone or a third-generation cephalosporin such as ceftazidime (for gram-negative bacteria) may be reasonable; in areas with high rates of infection with methicillin-resistant *S. aureus*, vancomycin should be used instead of cefazolin, and gram-negative coverage may need to be broadened—e.g., with an aminoglycoside, ceftazidime, cefepime, or a carbapenem. Broad coverage including vancomycin should be particularly considered for patients with septic physiology or exit-site infections. Vancomycin should also be included in the regimen if the patient has a history of colonization or infection with methicillin-resistant *S. aureus* or has a history of severe allergy to penicillins and cephalosporins. Loading doses are administered intraperitoneally; doses depend on the dialysis method and the patient's renal function. Intraperitoneal antibiotics are given either continuously (i.e., with each exchange) or intermittently (i.e., once daily, with the dose allowed to remain in the peritoneal cavity for at least 6 h). If the patient is severely ill, IV antibiotics should be added at doses appropriate for the patient's degree of renal failure. The clinical response to an empirical treatment regimen should be rapid; if the patient has not responded after 48–96 h of treatment, new samples should be collected for cell counts and cultures, and catheter removal should be considered. For patients who lack exit-site or tunnel infection, the typical duration of antibiotic treatment is 14 days. For patients with exit-site or tunnel infection, catheter removal should be considered, and a longer duration of antibiotic therapy (up to 21 days) may be appropriate. In fungal infections, the catheter should be removed immediately.

TUBERCULOUS PERITONITIS

See Chap. 178.

INTRAABDOMINAL ABSCESSES

INTRAPERITONEAL ABSCESSES

Abscess formation is common in untreated peritonitis if overt gram-negative sepsis either does not develop or develops but is not fatal. In experimental models of abscess formation, mixed aerobic and anaerobic organisms have been implanted intraperitoneally. Without therapy directed at anaerobes, animals develop intraabdominal abscesses. As in humans, these experimental abscesses may stud the peritoneal cavity, lie within the omentum or mesentery, or even develop on the surface of or within viscera such as the liver.

Pathogenesis and Immunity There is often disagreement about whether an abscess represents a disease state or a host response. In a sense, it represents both: while an abscess is an infection in which viable infecting organisms and PMNs are contained in a fibrous capsule, it is also a process by which the host confines microbes to a limited space, thereby preventing further spread of infection. In any event, abscesses do cause significant symptoms, and patients with abscesses can be quite ill. Experimental work has helped to define both the host cells and the bacterial virulence factors responsible—most notably in the case of *B. fragilis*. This organism, although accounting for only 0.5% of the normal colonic flora, is the anaerobe most frequently isolated from intraabdominal infections, is especially prominent in abscesses, and is the most common anaerobic bloodstream isolate. On clinical grounds, therefore, *B. fragilis* appears to be uniquely virulent. Moreover, *B. fragilis* acts alone to cause abscesses in animal models of intraabdominal infection, whereas most other *Bacteroides* species must act synergistically with a facultative organism to induce abscess formation.

Of the several virulence factors identified in *B. fragilis*, one is critical: the capsular polysaccharide complex found on the bacterial surface. This complex comprises at least eight distinct surface polysaccharides. Structural analysis of these polysaccharides has shown an unusual motif of oppositely charged sugars. Polysaccharides having these *zwitterionic* characteristics, such as polysaccharide A, evoke a host response in the peritoneal cavity that localizes bacteria into abscesses. *B. fragilis* and polysaccharide A have been found to adhere to primary mesothelial cells in vitro; this adherence, in turn, stimulates the production of tumor necrosis factor α and intercellular adhesion molecule 1 by peritoneal macrophages. Although abscesses characteristically contain PMNs, the process of abscess induction depends on the stimulation of T lymphocytes by these unique zwitterionic polysaccharides. The stimulated CD4+ T lymphocytes secrete leukoattractant cytokines and chemokines. The alternative pathway of complement and fibrinogen also participate in abscess formation.

While antibodies to the capsular polysaccharide complex enhance bloodstream clearance of *B. fragilis*, CD4+ T cells are critical in immunity to abscesses. When administered experimentally, *B. fragilis* polysaccharide A has immunomodulatory characteristics and stimulates CD4+ T regulatory cells via an interleukin 2–dependent mechanism to produce interleukin 10. Interleukin 10 downregulates the inflammatory response, thereby preventing abscess formation.

Clinical Presentation Of all intraabdominal abscesses, 74% are intraperitoneal or retroperitoneal and are not visceral. Most intraperitoneal abscesses result from fecal spillage from a colonic source, such as an inflamed appendix. Abscesses can also arise from other processes. They usually form within weeks of the development of peritonitis and may be found in a variety of locations from omentum to mesentery, pelvis to psoas muscles, and subphrenic space to a visceral organ such as the liver, where they may develop either on the surface of the organ or within it. Periappendiceal and diverticular abscesses occur commonly. Diverticular abscesses are least likely to rupture. Infections of the female genital tract and pancreatitis also are among the more common causative events. When abscesses occur in the female genital tract—either as a primary infection (e.g., tuboovarian abscess) or as an infection extending into the pelvic cavity or peritoneum—*B. fragilis* figures prominently among the organisms isolated. *B. fragilis* is not found in large numbers in the normal vaginal flora. For example, it is encountered less commonly in pelvic inflammatory disease and endometritis without an associated abscess. In pancreatitis with leakage of damaging pancreatic enzymes, inflammation is prominent. Therefore, clinical findings such as fever, leukocytosis, and even abdominal pain do not distinguish pancreatitis itself from complications such as pancreatic pseudocyst, pancreatic abscess (**Chap. 348**), or intraabdominal collections of pus. Especially in cases of necrotizing pancreatitis, in which the incidence of local pancreatic infection may be as high as 30%, needle aspiration under CT guidance is performed to sample fluid for culture. Traditionally, many centers have prescribed preemptive antibiotics for patients with necrotizing pancreatitis. Imipenem is frequently used for this purpose because it reaches high tissue levels in the pancreas (although it is not unique in this regard). Randomized controlled studies have not demonstrated a benefit from this practice, and many guidelines no longer recommend preemptive antibiotics for patients with acute pancreatitis. If needle aspiration yields infected fluid in the setting of acute necrotizing pancreatitis, antibiotic treatment is appropriate in conjunction with surgical and/or percutaneous drainage of infected material. Infected pseudocysts that occur remotely from acute pancreatitis are unlikely to be associated with significant amounts of necrotic tissue and may be treated with either surgical or percutaneous catheter drainage in conjunction with appropriate antibiotic therapy.

Diagnosis Scanning procedures have considerably facilitated the diagnosis of intraabdominal abscesses. Abdominal CT probably has the highest yield, although ultrasonography is particularly useful for the right upper quadrant, kidneys, and pelvis. Both indium-labeled WBCs and gallium tend to localize in abscesses and may be useful in finding a collection. Because gallium is taken up in the bowel, indium-labeled WBCs may have a slightly greater yield for abscesses near the bowel. Neither indium-labeled WBC scans nor gallium scans serve as a basis for a definitive diagnosis, however; both need to be followed by other, more specific studies, such as CT, if an area of possible abnormality is identified. PET scanning should also be considered due to its ready availability and because it provides more resolution. Abscesses contiguous with or contained within diverticula are particularly difficult to diagnose with scanning procedures. Although barium should not be injected if a perforation is suspected, a barium enema occasionally may detect a diverticular abscess not diagnosed by other procedures. If one study is negative, a second study sometimes reveals a collection. Although exploratory laparotomy has been less commonly used since the advent of CT, this procedure still must be undertaken on occasion if an abscess is strongly suspected on clinical grounds.

TREATMENT

Intraperitoneal Abscesses

An algorithm for the management of patients with intraabdominal (including intraperitoneal) abscesses by percutaneous drainage is presented in **Fig. 132-3**. Treatment of intraabdominal infections involves determination of the initial focus of infection, administration of broad-spectrum antibiotics targeting the organisms involved, and performance of a drainage procedure if one or more definitive abscesses have formed. Antimicrobial therapy, in general, is adjunctive to drainage and/or surgical correction of an underlying lesion or process in intraabdominal abscesses. Results

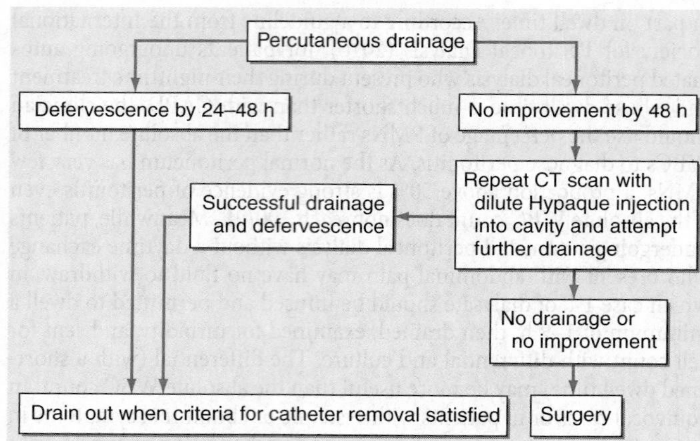

FIGURE 132-3 Algorithm for the management of patients with intraabdominal abscesses by percutaneous drainage. Antimicrobial therapy should be administered concomitantly. *(Republished with permission of Springer Nature, from Atlas of Infectious Diseases, vol VII: Intra-abdominal infections, hepatitis, and gastroenteritis, B Lorber et al. 1996; permission conveyed through Copyright Clearance Center, Inc.)*

of cultures from drain sites are not reliable for defining the etiology of infections. Unlike the intraabdominal abscesses resulting from most causes, for which drainage of some kind is generally required, abscesses associated with diverticulitis usually wall off locally after rupture of a diverticulum, so that surgical intervention is not routinely required.

A number of agents exhibit excellent activity against aerobic gram-negative bacilli. Because death in intraabdominal sepsis is linked to gram-negative bacteremia, empirical therapy for intraabdominal infection always needs to include adequate coverage of gram-negative aerobic, facultative, and anaerobic organisms. Even if anaerobes are not cultured from clinical specimens, they still must be covered by the therapeutic regimen. Empirical antibiotic therapy should be the same as that discussed above for secondary peritonitis. Most clinical treatment failures are due to failure to drain the abscess and thereby achieve source control. The appropriate duration of antibiotic treatment for abdominal abscesses depends on whether the presumptive source of the intraabdominal infection has been controlled. With adequate source control, antibiotic treatment may be limited to 4 or 5 days.

VISCERAL ABSCESSES

Liver Abscesses The liver is the organ most subject to the development of abscesses. In one study of 540 intraabdominal abscesses, 26% were visceral. Liver abscesses made up 13% of the total number, or 48% of all visceral abscesses. Liver abscesses may be solitary or multiple; they may arise from hematogenous spread of bacteria or from local spread from contiguous sites of infection within the peritoneal cavity. In the past, appendicitis with rupture and subsequent spread of infection was the most common source for a liver abscess. Currently, associated disease of the biliary tract is most common. Pylephlebitis (suppurative thrombosis of the portal vein), usually arising from infection in the pelvis but sometimes from infection elsewhere in the peritoneal cavity, is another common source for bacterial seeding of the liver.

Fever is the most common presenting sign of liver abscess. Some patients, particularly those with associated disease of the biliary tract, have symptoms and signs localized to the right upper quadrant, including pain, guarding, punch tenderness, and even rebound tenderness. Nonspecific symptoms, such as chills, anorexia, weight loss, nausea, and vomiting, also may develop. Only 50% of patients with liver abscesses, however, have hepatomegaly, right-upper-quadrant tenderness, or jaundice; thus, one-half of patients have no symptoms or signs

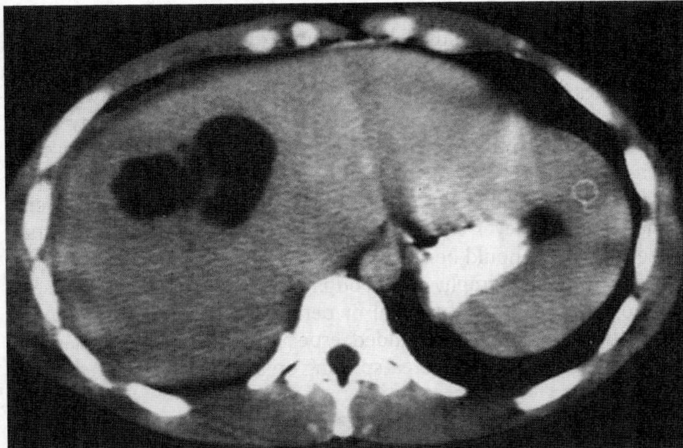

FIGURE 132-4 Multilocular liver abscess on CT scan. Multiple or multilocular abscesses are more common than solitary abscesses. *(Reprinted with permission from B Lorber [ed]: Atlas of Infectious Diseases, vol VII: Intra-abdominal Infections, Hepatitis, and Gastroenteritis. Philadelphia, Current Medicine, 1996, Fig. 1.22.)*

to direct attention to the liver. Fever of unknown origin may be the only manifestation of liver abscess, especially in the elderly. Diagnostic studies of the abdomen, especially the right upper quadrant, should be a part of any workup for fever of unknown origin. The single most reliable laboratory finding is an elevated serum concentration of alkaline phosphatase, which is documented in 70% of patients with liver abscesses. Other tests of liver function may yield normal results, but 50% of patients have elevated serum levels of bilirubin, and 48% have elevated concentrations of aspartate aminotransferase. Other laboratory findings include leukocytosis in 77% of patients, anemia (usually normochromic, normocytic) in 50%, and hypoalbuminemia in 33%. Concomitant bacteremia is found in one-third to one-half of patients. A liver abscess is sometimes suggested by chest radiography, especially if a new elevation of the right hemidiaphragm is seen; other suggestive findings include a right basilar infiltrate and a right pleural effusion.

Imaging studies are the most reliable methods for diagnosing liver abscesses. These studies include ultrasonography, CT (**Fig. 132-4**), indium-labeled WBC or gallium scan, and MRI. More than one such study may be required.

Organisms recovered from liver abscesses vary with the source. In liver infection arising from the biliary tree, enteric gram-negative aerobic bacilli and enterococci are common isolates. *Klebsiella pneumoniae* liver abscess has been well described in Southeast Asia for more than 20 years and has become an emerging syndrome in North America and elsewhere. These community-acquired infections have been linked to a virulent hypermucoviscous *K. pneumoniae* phenotype and to a specific genotype. The typical syndrome includes liver abscess, bacteremia, and metastatic infection. Ampicillin/amoxicillin therapy started within the previous 30 days has been associated with increased risk for this syndrome, presumably because of selection for the causative strain. Unless previous surgery has been performed, anaerobes are not generally involved in liver abscesses arising from biliary infections. In contrast, in liver abscesses arising from pelvic and other intraperitoneal sources, a mixed flora including both aerobic and anaerobic species is common; *B. fragilis* is the species most frequently isolated. With hematogenous spread of infection, usually only a single organism is encountered; this species may be *S. aureus* or a streptococcal species such as one in the *Streptococcus milleri* group. Liver abscesses may also be caused by *Candida* species; such abscesses usually follow fungemia in patients receiving chemotherapy for cancer and often present when PMNs return after a period of neutropenia. Amebic liver abscesses are not an uncommon problem (**Chap. 223**). Amebic serologic testing gives positive results in >95% of cases. In addition, polymerase chain reaction (PCR) testing has been used in recent years. Negative results from these studies help to exclude this diagnosis.

TREATMENT
Liver Abscesses

(Fig. 132-3) Drainage is the mainstay of therapy for intraabdominal abscesses, including liver abscesses; the approach can be either percutaneous (with a pigtail catheter kept in place or possibly with a device that can perform pulse lavage to fragment and evacuate the semisolid contents of a liver abscess), transluminal (with endoscopic ultrasound guidance), or surgical. However, there is growing interest in medical management alone for pyogenic liver abscesses. The drugs used for empirical therapy include the same ones used in intraabdominal sepsis and secondary bacterial peritonitis. Usually, blood cultures and a diagnostic aspirate of abscess contents should be obtained before the initiation of empirical therapy, with antibiotic choices adjusted when the results of Gram's staining and culture become available. Cases treated without definitive drainage generally require longer courses of antibiotic therapy. When percutaneous drainage was compared with open surgical drainage, the average length of hospital stay for the former was almost twice that for the latter, although both the time required for fever to resolve and the mortality rate were the same for the two procedures. The mortality rate was appreciable despite treatment, averaging 15%. Several factors predict the failure of percutaneous drainage and therefore may favor primary surgical intervention. These factors include the presence of multiple, sizable abscesses; viscous abscess contents that tend to plug the catheter; associated disease (e.g., disease of the biliary tract) requiring surgery; the presence of yeast; communication with an untreated obstructed biliary tree; or the lack of a clinical response to percutaneous drainage in 4–7 days.

Treatment of candidal liver abscesses often entails initial administration of liposomal amphotericin B (3–5 mg/kg IV daily) or an echinocandin, with subsequent fluconazole therapy (**Chap. 216**). In some cases, therapy with fluconazole alone (6 mg/kg daily) may be used—e.g., in clinically stable patients whose infecting isolate is susceptible to this drug.

Splenic Abscesses Splenic abscesses are much less common than liver abscesses. The incidence of splenic abscesses has ranged from 0.14 to 0.7% in various autopsy series. The clinical setting and the organisms isolated usually differ from those for liver abscesses. The degree of clinical suspicion for splenic abscess needs to be high because this condition is frequently fatal if left untreated. Even in the most recently published series, diagnosis was made only at autopsy in 37% of cases. Although splenic abscesses may arise occasionally from contiguous spread of infection or from direct trauma to the spleen, hematogenous spread of infection is more common. Bacterial endocarditis is the most common associated infection (**Chap. 128**). Splenic abscesses can develop in patients who have received extensive immunosuppressive therapy (particularly those with malignancy involving the spleen) and in patients with hemoglobinopathies or other hematologic disorders (especially sickle cell anemia).

Although ~50% of patients with splenic abscesses have abdominal pain, the pain is localized to the left upper quadrant in only one-half of these cases. Splenomegaly is found in ~50% of cases. Fever and leukocytosis are generally present; the development of fever preceded diagnosis by an average of 20 days in one series. Left-sided chest findings may include abnormalities to auscultation, and chest radiographic findings may include an infiltrate or a left-sided pleural effusion. CT scan of the abdomen has been the most sensitive diagnostic tool. Ultrasonography can yield the diagnosis but is less sensitive. Liver–spleen scan or gallium scan also may be useful. Streptococcal species are the most common bacterial isolates from splenic abscesses, followed by *S. aureus*—presumably reflecting the associated endocarditis. An increase in the prevalence of gram-negative aerobic isolates from splenic abscesses has been reported; these organisms often derive from a urinary tract focus, with associated bacteremia, or from another intraabdominal source. *Salmonella* species are seen fairly commonly, especially in patients with sickle cell hemoglobinopathy. Anaerobic species accounted for only 5% of isolates in the largest collected series, but the reporting of a number of "sterile abscesses" may indicate that optimal techniques for the isolation of anaerobes were not used.

TREATMENT

Splenic Abscesses

Because of the high mortality figures reported for splenic abscesses, splenectomy with adjunctive antibiotics has traditionally been considered standard treatment and remains the best approach for complex, multilocular abscesses or multiple abscesses. However, percutaneous drainage has worked well for single, small (<3-cm) abscesses in some studies and may also be useful for patients with high surgical risk. Patients undergoing splenectomy should be vaccinated against encapsulated organisms (*Streptococcus pneumoniae, Haemophilus influenzae, Neisseria meningitidis*). The most important factor in successful treatment of splenic abscesses is early diagnosis.

Perinephric and Renal Abscesses Perinephric and renal abscesses are not common. The former accounted for only ~0.02% of hospital admissions and the latter for ~0.2% in Altemeier's series of 540 intraabdominal abscesses. Before antibiotics became available, most renal and perinephric abscesses were hematogenous in origin, usually complicating prolonged bacteremia, with *S. aureus* most commonly recovered. Now, in contrast, >75% of perinephric and renal abscesses arise from a urinary tract infection. Infection ascends from the bladder to the kidney, with pyelonephritis preceding abscess development. Bacteria may directly invade the renal parenchyma from medulla to cortex. Local vascular channels within the kidney may facilitate the transport of organisms. Areas of abscess developing within the parenchyma may rupture into the perinephric space. The kidneys and adrenal glands are surrounded by a layer of perirenal fat that, in turn, is surrounded by Gerota's fascia, which extends superiorly to the diaphragm and inferiorly to the pelvic fat. Abscesses extending into the perinephric space may track through Gerota's fascia into the psoas or transversalis muscles, into the anterior peritoneal cavity, superiorly to the subdiaphragmatic space, or inferiorly to the pelvis. Of the risk factors that have been associated with the development of perinephric abscesses, the most important is concomitant nephrolithiasis obstructing urinary flow. Of patients with perinephric abscess, 20–60% have renal stones. Other structural abnormalities of the urinary tract, prior urologic surgery, trauma, and diabetes mellitus also have been identified as risk factors.

The organisms most frequently encountered in perinephric and renal abscesses are *E. coli*, *Proteus* species, and *Klebsiella* species. *E. coli*, the aerobic species most commonly found in the colonic flora, seems to have unique virulence properties in the urinary tract, including factors promoting adherence to uroepithelial cells. The urease of *Proteus* species splits urea, thereby creating a more alkaline and more hospitable environment for bacterial proliferation. *Proteus* species are frequently found in association with large struvite stones caused by the precipitation of magnesium ammonium sulfate in an alkaline environment. These stones serve as a nidus for recurrent urinary tract infection. Although a single bacterial species is usually recovered from a perinephric or renal abscess, multiple species may be found. If a urine culture is not contaminated with periurethral flora and is found to contain more than one organism, a perinephric or renal abscess should be considered in the differential diagnosis. Urine cultures may also be polymicrobial in cases of bladder diverticulum.

Candida species can cause renal abscesses. Fungi of this genus may spread to the kidney hematogenously or by ascension from the bladder. The hallmark of the latter route of infection is ureteral obstruction with large fungal balls.

The presentation of perinephric and renal abscesses is quite nonspecific. Flank pain and abdominal pain are common. At least 50% of patients are febrile. Pain may be referred to the groin or leg, particularly with extension of infection. The diagnosis of perinephric abscess, like that of splenic abscess, is frequently delayed, and the mortality rate in some series is appreciable, although lower than in the past. Perinephric or renal abscess should be most seriously considered when a patient presents with symptoms and signs of pyelonephritis and remains febrile after 4 or 5 days of treatment. Moreover, when a urine culture yields a polymicrobial flora, when a patient is known to have renal stones, or when fever and pyuria coexist with a sterile urine culture, these diagnoses should be entertained.

Renal ultrasonography and abdominal CT are the most useful diagnostic modalities. If a renal or perinephric abscess is diagnosed, nephrolithiasis should be excluded, especially when a high urinary pH suggests the presence of a urea-splitting organism.

TREATMENT

Perinephric and Renal Abscesses

Treatment for perinephric and renal abscesses, like that for other intraabdominal abscesses, includes drainage of pus and antibiotic therapy directed at the organism(s) recovered. For perinephric abscesses, percutaneous drainage is usually successful.

Psoas Abscesses The psoas muscle is another location in which abscesses are encountered. Psoas abscesses may arise from a hematogenous source, by contiguous spread from an intraabdominal or pelvic process, or by contiguous spread from nearby bony structures (e.g., vertebral bodies). Associated osteomyelitis due to spread from bone to muscle or from muscle to bone is common in psoas abscesses. When Pott's disease was common, *Mycobacterium tuberculosis* was a frequent cause of psoas abscess. Currently, either *S. aureus* or a mixture of enteric organisms including aerobic and anaerobic gram-negative bacilli is usually isolated from psoas abscesses in the United States. *S. aureus* is most likely to be isolated when a psoas abscess arises from hematogenous spread or a contiguous focus of osteomyelitis; a mixed enteric flora is the most likely etiology when the abscess has an intraabdominal or pelvic source. Patients with psoas abscesses frequently present with fever, lower abdominal or back pain, or pain referred to the hip or knee. CT is the most useful diagnostic technique.

TREATMENT

Psoas Abscesses

Treatment includes surgical drainage and the administration of an antibiotic regimen directed at the inciting organism(s).

Pancreatic Abscesses See Chap. 348.

FURTHER READING

Fazili T et al: *Klebsiella pneumoniae* liver abscess: An emerging disease. Am J Med Sci 351:297, 2016.

Hahn AW et al: New approaches to antibiotic use and review of recently approved antimicrobial agents. Med Clin North Am 100:911, 2016.

Khan R et al: Model for end-stage liver disease score predicts development of first episode of spontaneous bacterial peritonitis in patients with cirrhosis. Mayo Clin Proc 94:1799, 2019.

Li PK et al: ISPD peritonitis recommendations: 2016 update on prevention and treatment. Perit Dial Int 36:481, 2016.

Oliver A et al: Role of rifaximin in spontaneous bacterial peritonitis prevention. South Med J 111:660 2018.

Ross JT et al: Secondary peritonitis: Principles of diagnosis and intervention. BMJ 361:k1407, 2018.

Sunjaya DB et al: Prevalence and predictors of third-generation cephalosporin resistance in the empirical treatment of spontaneous bacterial peritonitis. Mayo Clin Proc 94:1499, 2019.

133 Acute Infectious Diarrheal Diseases and Bacterial Food Poisoning

Richelle C. Charles, Regina C. LaRocque

Diarrheal disease mortality has decreased substantially in the past three decades. Nevertheless, acute diarrheal disease is still a leading cause of illness globally and is associated with an estimated 1.7 million deaths per year. Among children <5 years of age, diarrheal disease is the fifth leading cause of death, with countries in South Asia and sub-Saharan Africa bearing the highest burden of disease. The morbidity from diarrhea also is significant. Recurrent intestinal infections are associated with physical and mental stunting, wasting, micronutrient deficiencies, and malnutrition. In short, diarrheal disease is a driving factor in global morbidity and mortality.

The wide range of clinical manifestations of acute gastrointestinal illnesses is matched by the wide variety of infectious agents involved, including viruses, bacteria, and parasites (**Table 133-1**). This chapter discusses factors that enable gastrointestinal pathogens to cause disease, reviews host defense mechanisms, and delineates an approach to the evaluation and treatment of patients presenting with acute diarrhea. Individual organisms causing acute gastrointestinal illnesses are discussed in detail in subsequent chapters.

PATHOGENIC MECHANISMS

Enteric pathogens have developed a variety of tactics to overcome host defenses. Understanding the virulence factors employed by these organisms is important in the diagnosis and treatment of clinical disease.

INOCULUM SIZE

The number of microorganisms that must be ingested to cause disease varies considerably from species to species. For *Shigella*, enterohemorrhagic *Escherichia coli*, *Giardia lamblia*, or *Entamoeba*, as few as 10–100 bacteria or cysts can produce infection, while 10^5–10^8 *Vibrio cholerae* organisms must be ingested to cause disease. The infective dose of *Salmonella* varies widely, depending on the species, host, and food vehicle. The ability of organisms to overcome host defenses has important implications for transmission; *Shigella*, enterohemorrhagic *E. coli*, *Entamoeba*, and *Giardia* can spread by person-to-person contact, whereas under some circumstances, *Salmonella* may need to grow in food for several hours before reaching an effective infectious dose.

ADHERENCE

Many organisms must adhere to the gastrointestinal mucosa as an initial step in the pathogenic process; thus, organisms that can compete with the normal bowel flora and colonize the mucosa have an important advantage in causing disease. Specific cell-surface proteins involved in attachment of bacteria to intestinal cells are important virulence determinants. *V. cholerae*, for example, adheres to the brush border of small-intestinal enterocytes via specific surface adhesins, including the toxin-coregulated pilus and other accessory colonization factors. Enterotoxigenic *E. coli*, which causes watery diarrhea, produces an adherence protein called *colonization factor antigen* that is necessary for colonization of the upper small intestine by the organism prior to the production of enterotoxin. Enteropathogenic *E. coli*, an agent of diarrhea in young children, and enterohemorrhagic *E. coli*, which causes hemorrhagic colitis and the hemolytic-uremic syndrome, produce virulence determinants that allow these organisms to attach to and efface the brush border of the intestinal epithelium.

TOXIN PRODUCTION

The production of one or more exotoxins is important in the pathogenesis of numerous enteric organisms. Such toxins include *enterotoxins*, which cause watery diarrhea by acting directly on secretory mechanisms in the intestinal mucosa; *cytotoxins*, which cause destruction of mucosal cells and associated inflammatory diarrhea; and *neurotoxins*, which act directly on the central or peripheral nervous system.

The prototypical enterotoxin is cholera toxin, a heterodimeric protein composed of one A and five B subunits. The A subunit contains the enzymatic activity of the toxin, while the B subunit pentamer binds holotoxin to the enterocyte surface receptor, the ganglioside G_{M1}. After the binding of holotoxin, a fragment of the A subunit is translocated across the eukaryotic cell membrane into the cytoplasm, where it catalyzes the adenosine diphosphate ribosylation of a guanosine triphosphate–binding protein and causes persistent activation of adenylate cyclase. The end result is an increase of cyclic adenosine monophosphate in the intestinal cell, which increases Cl^- secretion and decreases Na^+ absorption, leading to a loss of fluid and the production of diarrhea.

Enterotoxigenic strains of *E. coli* may produce a protein called *heat-labile enterotoxin* (LT) that is similar to cholera toxin and causes secretory diarrhea by the same mechanism. Alternatively, enterotoxigenic strains of *E. coli* may produce *heat-stable enterotoxin* (ST), one form of which causes diarrhea by activation of guanylate cyclase and elevation of intracellular cyclic guanosine monophosphate. Some enterotoxigenic strains of *E. coli* produce both LT and ST.

Bacterial cytotoxins, in contrast, destroy intestinal mucosal cells and produce the syndrome of dysentery, with bloody stools containing inflammatory cells. Enteric pathogens that produce such cytotoxins include *Shigella dysenteriae* type 1, *Vibrio parahaemolyticus*, and *Clostridium difficile*. *S. dysenteriae* type 1 and Shiga toxin–producing strains of *E. coli* produce potent cytotoxins and have been associated with outbreaks of hemorrhagic colitis and hemolytic-uremic syndrome.

Neurotoxins are usually produced by bacteria outside the host and therefore cause symptoms soon after ingestion. Included are the staphylococcal and *Bacillus cereus* toxins, which act on the central nervous system to produce vomiting.

INVASION

Dysentery may result not only from the production of cytotoxins but also from bacterial invasion and destruction of intestinal mucosal cells. Infections due to *Shigella* and enteroinvasive *E. coli* are characterized by

TABLE 133-1 Gastrointestinal Pathogens Causing Acute Diarrhea

MECHANISM	LOCATION	ILLNESS	STOOL FINDINGS	EXAMPLES OF PATHOGENS INVOLVED
Noninflammatory (enterotoxin)	Proximal small bowel	Watery diarrhea	No fecal leukocytes; mild or no increase in fecal lactoferrin	*Vibrio cholerae*, enterotoxigenic *Escherichia coli* (LT and/or ST), enteroaggregative *E. coli*, *Clostridium perfringens*, *Bacillus cereus*, *Staphylococcus aureus*, *Aeromonas hydrophila*, *Plesiomonas shigelloides*, rotavirus, norovirus, enteric adenoviruses, *Giardia lamblia*, *Cryptosporidium* spp., *Cyclospora* spp., microsporidia
Inflammatory (invasion or cytotoxin)	Colon or distal small bowel	Dysentery or inflammatory diarrhea	Fecal polymorphonuclear leukocytes; substantial increase in fecal lactoferrin	*Shigella* spp., *Salmonella* spp., *Campylobacter jejuni*, enterohemorrhagic *E. coli*, enteroinvasive *E. coli*, *Yersinia enterocolitica*, *Listeria monocytogenes*, *Vibrio parahaemolyticus*, *Clostridium difficile*, *A. hydrophila*, *P. shigelloides*, *Entamoeba histolytica*, *Klebsiella oxytoca*
Penetrating	Distal small bowel	Enteric fever	Fecal mononuclear leukocytes	*Salmonella* Typhi, *Y. enterocolitica*

Abbreviations: LT, heat-labile enterotoxin; ST, heat-stable enterotoxin.

the organisms' invasion of mucosal epithelial cells, intraepithelial multiplication, and subsequent spread to adjacent cells. *Salmonella* causes inflammatory diarrhea by invasion of the bowel mucosa but generally is not associated with the destruction of enterocytes or the full clinical syndrome of dysentery. *Salmonella* Typhi and *Yersinia enterocolitica* can penetrate intact intestinal mucosa, multiply intracellularly in Peyer's patches and intestinal lymph nodes, and then disseminate through the bloodstream to cause enteric fever—a syndrome characterized by fever, headache, relative bradycardia, abdominal pain, splenomegaly, and leukopenia.

HOST DEFENSES

Given the enormous number of microorganisms ingested with every meal, the normal host must combat a constant influx of potential enteric pathogens. Studies of infections in patients with alterations in defense mechanisms have led to a greater understanding of the variety of ways in which the normal host can protect itself against disease.

INTESTINAL MICROBIOTA

The large numbers of bacteria that normally inhabit the intestine (*the intestinal microbiota*) act as an important host defense mechanism, preventing colonization by potential enteric pathogens. Persons with fewer intestinal bacteria, such as infants who have not yet developed normal enteric colonization or patients receiving antibiotics, are at greater risk of developing infections with enteric pathogens. The composition of the intestinal microbiota is as important as the number of organisms present. More than 99% of the normal colonic microbiota is made up of anaerobic bacteria, and the acidic pH and volatile fatty acids produced by these organisms appear to be critical elements in resistance to colonization.

GASTRIC ACID

The acidic pH of the stomach is an important barrier to enteric pathogens, and an increased frequency of infections due to *Salmonella*, *G. lamblia*, and a variety of helminths has been reported among patients who have undergone gastric surgery or are achlorhydric for some other reason. Neutralization of gastric acid with antacids, proton pump inhibitors, or H_2 blockers—a common practice in the management of hospitalized patients—similarly increases the risk of enteric colonization. In addition, some microorganisms can survive the extreme acidity of the gastric environment; rotavirus and *Shigella*, for example, are highly stable to acidity.

INTESTINAL MOTILITY

Normal peristalsis is the major mechanism for clearance of bacteria from the proximal small intestine. When intestinal motility is impaired (e.g., by treatment with opiates or other antimotility drugs, anatomic abnormalities, or hypomotility states), the frequency of bacterial overgrowth and infection of the small bowel with enteric pathogens is increased. Some patients whose treatment for *Shigella* infection consists of diphenoxylate hydrochloride with atropine (Lomotil) experience prolonged fever and shedding of organisms, while patients treated with opiates for mild *Salmonella* gastroenteritis have a higher frequency of bacteremia than those not treated with opiates.

INTESTINAL MUCIN

A complex layer of mucus, produced by specialized secretory cells, covers the stomach, small intestine, and large intestine and separates the commensal microbiota from the epithelium. The thickness and constituents of this mucus barrier vary throughout the gastrointestinal tract. The mucus barrier turns over rapidly and comprises glycoproteins and a range of antimicrobial molecules and secreted immunoglobulins directed against specific microbial antigens. Enteric pathogens have evolved a wide range of strategies to overcome this barrier and thus to reach the underlying epithelium and cause disease. For example, pathogens can penetrate the mucus layer by secreting enzymes to degrade the mucus or through flagella-mediated motility. Some organisms, such as *Shigella*, secrete toxins that can diffuse through the mucus layer and disrupt the underlying epithelium. The resulting reduction of mucus production allows the pathogen to reach the cell surface.

IMMUNITY

Both cellular immune responses and antibody production play important roles in protection from enteric infections. Humoral immunity to enteric pathogens consists of systemic IgG and IgM as well as secretory IgA. The mucosal immune system may be the first line of defense against many gastrointestinal pathogens. The binding of bacterial antigens to the luminal surface of M cells in the distal small bowel and the subsequent presentation of antigens to subepithelial lymphoid tissue lead to the proliferation of sensitized lymphocytes. These lymphocytes circulate and populate all of the mucosal tissues of the body as IgA-secreting plasma cells.

GENETIC DETERMINANTS

Host genetic variation influences susceptibility to diarrheal diseases. People with blood group O show increased susceptibility to disease due to *V. cholerae*, *Shigella*, *E. coli* O157, and norovirus. Polymorphisms in genes encoding inflammatory mediators have been associated with the outcome of infection with enteroaggregative *E. coli*, enterotoxin-producing *E. coli*, *Salmonella*, *C. difficile*, and *V. cholerae*.

APPROACH TO THE PATIENT
Infectious Diarrhea or Bacterial Food Poisoning

The approach to the patient with possible infectious diarrhea or bacterial food poisoning is shown in Fig. 133-1.

HISTORY

The answers to questions with high discriminating value can quickly narrow the range of potential causes of diarrhea and help determine whether treatment is needed. Important elements of the narrative history are detailed in Fig. 133-1.

PHYSICAL EXAMINATION

The examination of patients for signs of dehydration provides essential information about the severity of the diarrheal illness and the need for rapid therapy. Mild dehydration is indicated by thirst, dry mouth, decreased axillary sweat, decreased urine output, and slight weight loss. Signs of moderate dehydration include an orthostatic fall in blood pressure, skin tenting, and sunken eyes (or, in infants, a sunken fontanelle). Signs of severe dehydration include lethargy, obtundation, feeble pulse, hypotension, and frank shock.

DIAGNOSTIC APPROACH

After the severity of illness is assessed, the clinician must distinguish between *inflammatory* and *noninflammatory* disease. Using the history and epidemiologic features of the case as guides, the clinician can then rapidly evaluate the need for further efforts to define a specific etiology and for therapeutic intervention. Examination of a stool sample may supplement the narrative history. Grossly bloody or mucoid stool suggests an inflammatory process. A test for fecal leukocytes (preparation of a thin smear of stool on a glass slide, addition of a drop of methylene blue, and examination of the wet mount) can suggest inflammatory disease in patients with diarrhea, although the predictive value of this test is still debated. A test for fecal lactoferrin, which is a marker of fecal leukocytes, is more sensitive and is available in latex agglutination and enzyme-linked immunosorbent assay formats. Causes of acute infectious diarrhea, categorized as inflammatory and noninflammatory, are listed in Table 133-1.

POSTDIARRHEA COMPLICATIONS

Chronic complications may follow the resolution of an acute diarrheal episode. The clinician should inquire about prior diarrheal illness if the conditions listed in **Table 133-2** are observed.

EPIDEMIOLOGY

TRAVEL HISTORY

Of the several million people who travel from temperate industrialized countries to tropical regions of Asia, Africa, and Central and South America each year, 20–50% experience a sudden onset of abdominal

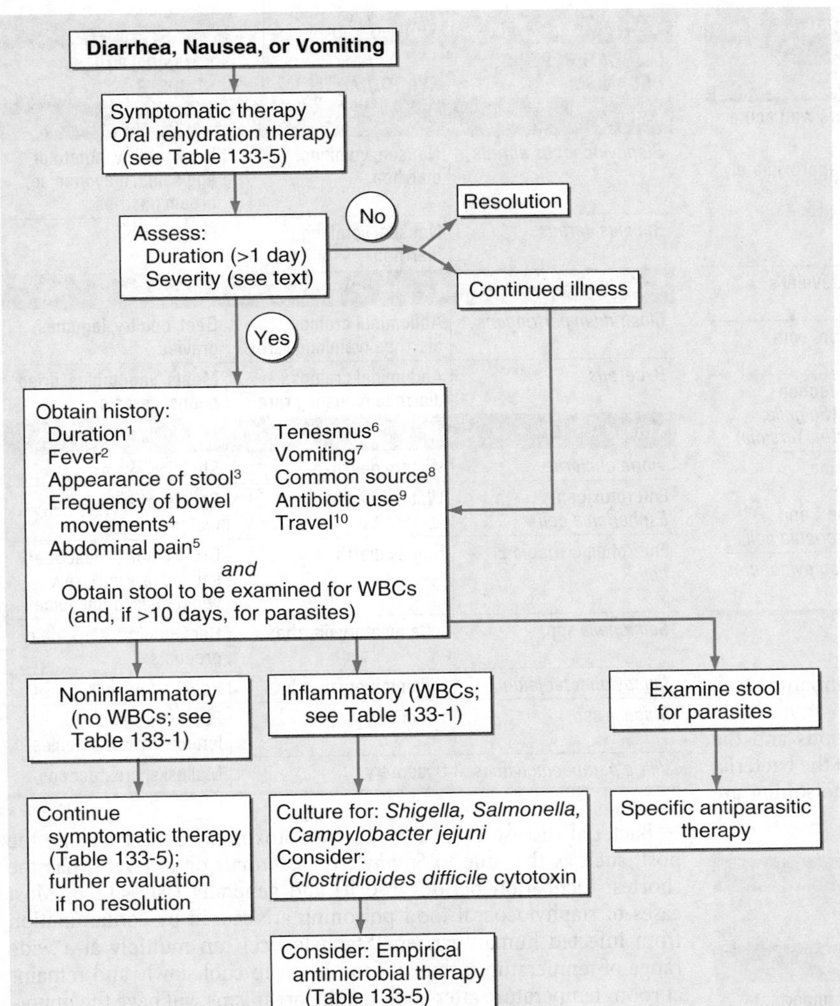

FIGURE 133-1 Clinical algorithm for the approach to patients with community-acquired infectious diarrhea or bacterial food poisoning. Key to superscripts: 1. Diarrhea lasting >2 weeks is generally defined as chronic; in such cases, many of the causes of acute diarrhea are much less likely, and a new spectrum of causes needs to be considered. 2. Fever often implies invasive disease, although fever and diarrhea may also result from infection outside the gastrointestinal tract, as in malaria. 3. Stools that contain blood or mucus indicate ulceration of the large bowel. Bloody stools without fecal leukocytes should alert the laboratory to the possibility of infection with Shiga toxin–producing enterohemorrhagic *Escherichia coli.* Bulky white stools suggest a small-intestinal process that is causing malabsorption. Profuse "rice-water" stools suggest cholera or a similar toxigenic process. 4. Frequent stools over a given period can provide the first warning of impending dehydration. 5. Abdominal pain may be most severe in inflammatory processes like those due to *Shigella, Campylobacter,* and necrotizing toxins. Painful abdominal muscle cramps, caused by electrolyte loss, can develop in severe cases of cholera. Bloating is common in giardiasis. An appendicitis-like syndrome should prompt a culture for *Yersinia enterocolitica* with cold enrichment. 6. Tenesmus (painful rectal spasms with a strong urge to defecate but little passage of stool) may be a feature of cases with proctitis, as in shigellosis or amebiasis. 7. Vomiting implies an acute infection (e.g., a toxin-mediated illness or food poisoning) but can also be prominent in a variety of systemic illnesses (e.g., malaria) and in intestinal obstruction. 8. Asking patients whether anyone else they know is sick is a more efficient means of identifying a common source than is constructing a list of recently eaten foods. If a common source seems likely, specific foods can be investigated. See text for a discussion of bacterial food poisoning. 9. Current antibiotic therapy or a recent history of treatment suggests *Clostridium difficile* diarrhea **(Chap. 134)**. Stop antibiotic treatment if possible and consider tests for *C. difficile* toxins. Antibiotic use may increase the risk of chronic intestinal carriage following salmonellosis. 10. See text (and **Chap. 124**) for a discussion of traveler's diarrhea. *(From RL Guerrant, DA Bobak: Bacterial and protozoal gastroenteritis. N Engl J Med 325:327, 1991. Copyright © 1991 Massachusetts Medical Society. Reprinted with permission from Massachusetts Medical Society.)*

cramps, anorexia, and watery diarrhea; thus, *traveler's diarrhea* is the most common travel-related infectious illness (**Chap. 124**). The time of onset is usually 3 days to 2 weeks after the traveler's arrival in a resource-poor area; most cases begin within the first 3–5 days. The illness is generally self-limited, lasting 1–5 days. The high rate of diarrhea among travelers to underdeveloped areas is related to the ingestion of contaminated food or water.

The organisms that cause traveler's diarrhea vary considerably with location (**Table 133-3**), as does the pattern of antimicrobial resistance. In all areas, enterotoxigenic and enteroaggregative strains of *E. coli* are the most common isolates from persons with the classic secretory traveler's diarrhea syndrome. Infection with *Campylobacter jejuni* is especially common in areas of Asia.

LOCATION

Closed and semi-closed communities, including day-care centers, schools, residential facilities, and cruise ships, are important settings for outbreaks of enteric infections. Norovirus, which is highly contagious and robust in surviving on surfaces, is the most common etiologic agent associated with outbreaks of acute gastroenteritis. Other common organisms, often spread by fecal–oral contact in such communities, are *Shigella, C. jejuni,* and *Cryptosporidium.* Rotavirus is rarely a cause of pediatric diarrheal outbreaks in the United States since rotavirus vaccination was broadly recommended in 2006. Similarly, hospitals are sites in which enteric infections are concentrated. Diarrhea is one of the most common manifestations of nosocomial infections. *C. difficile* is the predominant cause of nosocomial diarrhea among adults in the United States, and outbreaks of norovirus infection are common in health care settings. *Klebsiella oxytoca* has been identified as a cause of antibiotic-associated hemorrhagic colitis. Enteropathogenic *E. coli* has been associated with outbreaks of diarrhea in nurseries for newborns. One-third of elderly patients in chronic-care institutions develop a significant diarrheal illness each year; more than one-half of these cases are caused by cytotoxin-producing *C. difficile.* Antimicrobial therapy can predispose to pseudomembranous colitis by altering the normal colonic flora and allowing the multiplication of *C. difficile* (**Chap. 134**).

AGE

Globally, most morbidity and mortality from enteric pathogens involve children <5 years of age. Breast-fed infants are protected from pathogens in contaminated food and water and derive some protection from maternal antibodies, but their risk of infection rises dramatically when they begin to eat solid foods. Exposure to rotavirus is universal, with most children experiencing their first infection in the first or second year of life if not vaccinated. Older children and adults are more commonly infected with norovirus. Other organisms with higher attack rates among children than among adults include enterotoxigenic, enteropathogenic, and enterohemorrhagic *E. coli*; *Shigella*; *C. jejuni*; and *G. lamblia.*

HOST IMMUNE STATUS

Immunocompromised hosts are at elevated risk of acute and chronic infectious diarrhea. Individuals with defects in cell-mediated immunity (including those with AIDS) are at particularly high risk of invasive enteropathies, including salmonellosis, listeriosis, and cryptosporidiosis. Individuals with hypogammaglobulinemia are at particular risk of *C. difficile* colitis and giardiasis. Patients with cancer are more likely to develop *C. difficile* infection as a result of chemotherapy and frequent hospitalizations. Infectious diarrhea can be life-threatening in immunocompromised hosts, with complications including bacteremia and metastatic seeding of infection. Furthermore, dehydration may compromise renal function and increase the toxicity of immunosuppressive drugs.

TABLE 133-2 Postdiarrhea Complications of Acute Infectious Diarrheal Illness

COMPLICATION	COMMENTS
Chronic diarrhea (diarrhea lasting >4 weeks) • Lactase deficiency • Small-bowel bacterial overgrowth • Malabsorption syndromes (tropical and celiac sprue)	Occurs in ~1% of travelers with acute diarrhea • Protozoa account for approximately one-third of cases
Initial presentation or exacerbation of inflammatory bowel disease	May be precipitated by traveler's diarrhea
Irritable bowel syndrome	Occurs in ~10% of travelers with traveler's diarrhea
Reactive arthritis	Particularly likely after infection with invasive organisms (*Shigella, Salmonella, Campylobacter, Yersinia*)
Hemolytic-uremic syndrome (hemolytic anemia, thrombocytopenia, and renal failure)	Follows infection with Shiga toxin–producing bacteria (*Shigella dysenteriae* type 1 and enterohemorrhagic *Escherichia coli*)
Guillain-Barré syndrome	Particularly likely after *Campylobacter* infection

BACTERIAL FOOD POISONING

If the history and the stool examination indicate a noninflammatory etiology of diarrhea and there is evidence of a common-source outbreak, questions concerning the ingestion of specific foods and the time of onset of diarrhea after a meal can provide clues to the bacterial cause of the illness. Potential causes of bacterial food poisoning are shown in **Table 133-4**.

TABLE 133-3 Causes of Traveler's Diarrhea

ETIOLOGIC AGENT	APPROXIMATE PERCENTAGE OF CASES	COMMENTS
Bacteria	**50–75**	
Enterotoxigenic *Escherichia coli*	10–45	Single most important agent
Enteroaggregative *E. coli*	5–35	Emerging enteric pathogen with worldwide distribution
Campylobacter jejuni	5–25	More common in Asia
Shigella	0–15	Major cause of dysentery
Salmonella	0–15	—
Others	0–5	Including *Aeromonas, Plesiomonas,* and *Vibrio cholerae*
Viruses	**0–20**	
Norovirus	0–10	Associated with cruise ships
Rotavirus	0–5	Particularly common among children
Parasites	**0–10**	
Giardia lamblia	0–5	Affects hikers and campers who drink from freshwater streams
Cryptosporidium	0–5	Resistant to chlorine treatment of water sources
Entamoeba histolytica	<1	—
Cyclospora	<1	—
Other	**0–10**	
Acute food poisoning[a]	0–5	—
No pathogen identified	10–50	—

[a]For etiologic agents, see Table 133-4.

Source: After DR Hill et al: The practice of travel medicine: Guidelines by the Infectious Diseases Society of America. Clin Infect Dis 43:1499, 2006.

TABLE 133-4 Bacterial Food Poisoning

INCUBATION PERIOD, ORGANISM	SYMPTOMS	COMMON FOOD SOURCES
1–6 h		
Staphylococcus aureus	Nausea, vomiting, diarrhea	Ham, poultry, potato or egg salad, mayonnaise, cream pastries
Bacillus cereus	Nausea, vomiting, diarrhea	Fried rice
8–16 h		
Clostridium perfringens	Abdominal cramps, diarrhea (vomiting rare)	Beef, poultry, legumes, gravies
B. cereus	Abdominal cramps, diarrhea (vomiting rare)	Meats, vegetables, dried beans, cereals
>16 h		
Vibrio cholerae	Watery diarrhea	Shellfish, water
Enterotoxigenic *Escherichia coli*	Watery diarrhea	Salads, cheese, meats, water
Enterohemorrhagic *E. coli*	Bloody diarrhea	Ground beef, roast beef, salami, raw milk, raw vegetables, apple juice
Salmonella spp.	Inflammatory diarrhea	Beef, poultry, eggs, dairy products
Campylobacter jejuni	Inflammatory diarrhea	Poultry, raw milk
Shigella spp.	Dysentery	Potato or egg salad, lettuce, raw vegetables
Vibrio parahaemolyticus	Dysentery	Mollusks, crustaceans

Bacterial disease caused by an enterotoxin elaborated outside the host, such as that due to *Staphylococcus aureus* or *B. cereus*, has the shortest incubation period (1–6 h) and generally lasts <12 h. Most cases of staphylococcal food poisoning are caused by contamination from infected human carriers. Staphylococci can multiply at a wide range of temperatures; thus, if food is left to cool slowly and remains at room temperature after cooking, the organisms will have the opportunity to form enterotoxin. Outbreaks following picnics where potato salad, mayonnaise, and cream pastries have been served offer classic examples of staphylococcal food poisoning. Diarrhea, nausea, vomiting, and abdominal cramping are common, while fever is less so.

B. cereus can produce either a syndrome with a short incubation period—the *emetic* form, mediated by a staphylococcal type of enterotoxin—or one with a longer incubation period (8–16 h)—the *diarrheal* form, caused by an enterotoxin resembling *E. coli* LT, in which diarrhea and abdominal cramps are characteristic but vomiting is uncommon. The emetic form of *B. cereus* food poisoning is associated with contaminated fried rice; the organism is common in uncooked rice, and its heat-resistant spores survive boiling. If cooked rice is not refrigerated, the spores can germinate and produce toxin. Frying before serving may not destroy the preformed, heat-stable toxin.

Food poisoning due to *Clostridium perfringens* also has a slightly longer incubation period (8–14 h) and results from the survival of heat-resistant spores in inadequately cooked meat, poultry, or legumes. After ingestion, toxin is produced in the intestinal tract, causing moderately severe abdominal cramps and diarrhea; vomiting is rare, as is fever. The illness is self-limited, rarely lasting >24 h.

Not all food poisoning has a bacterial cause. Nonbacterial agents of short-incubation food poisoning include capsaicin, which is found in hot peppers, and a variety of toxins found in fish and shellfish (**Chap. 460**).

LABORATORY EVALUATION

Many cases of noninflammatory diarrhea are self-limited or can be treated empirically, and in these instances, the clinician may not need to determine a specific etiology. Potentially pathogenic *E. coli* cannot be distinguished from normal fecal flora by routine culture, and tests to detect enterotoxins are not available in most clinical laboratories. In situations in which cholera is a concern, stool should be cultured on selective media such as thiosulfate–citrate–bile salts–sucrose (TCBS) or tellurite–taurocholate–gelatin (TTG) agar; rapid diagnostic tests are also available. A latex agglutination test has made the rapid detection of rotavirus in stool practical for many laboratories, while reverse-transcriptase polymerase chain reaction (PCR) and specific antigen enzyme immunoassays have been developed for the identification of norovirus. Stool specimens should be examined by immunofluorescence-based rapid assays, or PCR or (less sensitive) standard microscopy for *Giardia* cysts or *Cryptosporidium* if the level of clinical suspicion regarding the involvement of these organisms is high.

All patients with fever and evidence of inflammatory disease acquired outside the hospital should have stool evaluated for *Salmonella*, *Shigella*, and *Campylobacter*. *Salmonella* and *Shigella* can be selected on MacConkey agar as non-lactose-fermenting (colorless) colonies or can be grown on *Salmonella–Shigella* agar or in selenite enrichment broth, both of which inhibit most organisms except these pathogens. Evaluation of nosocomial diarrhea should initially focus on *C. difficile*; stool culture for other pathogens in this setting has an extremely low yield and is not cost-effective. Toxins A and B produced by pathogenic strains of *C. difficile* can be detected by rapid enzyme immunoassays, latex agglutination tests, or PCR (**Chap. 134**). Isolation of *C. jejuni* requires inoculation of fresh stool onto selective growth medium and incubation at 42°C in a microaerophilic atmosphere. In many laboratories in the United States, *E. coli* O157:H7 is among the most common pathogens isolated from visibly bloody stools. Strains of this enterohemorrhagic serotype can be identified in specialized laboratories by serotyping but also can be identified presumptively in hospital laboratories as lactose-fermenting, indole-positive colonies of sorbitol nonfermenters (white colonies) on sorbitol MacConkey plates. If the clinical presentation suggests the possibility of intestinal amebiasis, stool should be examined by a rapid antigen detection assay or by (less sensitive and less specific) microscopy. Multiplex nucleic acid amplification methods for detection of many stool pathogens (viral, bacterial, and parasitic) are increasingly being used in clinical microbiology laboratories to decrease the time to detection of a pathogen. Although these tests may be more sensitive and rapid than standard culture methods, the lack of a microbial isolate prevents determination of antimicrobial susceptibility and typing of strains by public health authorities in order to detect and respond to common-source outbreaks. For this reason, the Centers for Disease Control and Prevention suggests that diagnosis of an enteric bacterial infection by a nucleic acid amplification method should be followed by attempted isolation of the pathogen by culture.

TABLE 133-5 Treatment of Traveler's Diarrhea on the Basis of Clinical Features[a]

CLINICAL SYNDROME	SUGGESTED THERAPY
Watery diarrhea (no blood in stool, no fever), 1 or 2 unformed stools per day without distressing enteric symptoms	Oral fluids (oral rehydration solution, Pedialyte, Lytren, or flavored mineral water) and saltine crackers
Watery diarrhea (no blood in stool, no fever), 1 or 2 unformed stools per day with distressing enteric symptoms	Bismuth subsalicylate (for adults): 30 mL or 2 tablets (262 mg/tablet) every 30 min for 8 doses; or loperamide[b]: 4 mg initially followed by 2 mg after passage of each unformed stool, not to exceed 8 tablets (16 mg) per day (prescription dose) or 4 caplets (8 mg) per day (over-the-counter dose); drugs can be taken for 2 days. Antibacterial drug[c] can be considered in selected circumstances.
Dysentery (passage of bloody stools) or fever (>37.8°C)	Antibacterial drug[c]
Vomiting, minimal diarrhea	Bismuth subsalicylate (for adults; see dose above)
Diarrhea in infants (<2 years old)	Fluids and electrolytes (oral rehydration solution, Pedialyte, Lytren); continue feeding, especially with breast milk; seek medical attention for moderate dehydration, fever lasting >24 h, bloody stools, or diarrhea lasting more than several days

[a]All patients should take oral fluids (Pedialyte, Lytren, or flavored mineral water) plus saltine crackers. If diarrhea becomes moderate or severe, if fever persists, or if bloody stools or dehydration develops, the patient should seek medical attention. [b]Loperamide should not be used by patients with fever or dysentery; its use may prolong diarrhea in patients with infection due to *Shigella* or other invasive organisms. [c]The recommended antibacterial drugs are as follows:

If the level of suspicion is low for fluoroquinolone-resistant *Campylobacter*:
Adults: (1) A fluoroquinolone such as ciprofloxacin, 750 mg as a single dose or 500 mg bid for 3 days; levofloxacin, 500 mg as a single dose or 500 mg qd for 3 days; or norfloxacin, 800 mg as a single dose or 400 mg bid for 3 days. (2) Azithromycin, 1000 mg as a single dose or 500 mg qd for 3 days. (3) Rifaximin, 200 mg tid or 400 mg bid for 3 days (not recommended for use in dysentery).
Children: Azithromycin, 10 mg/kg on day 1, 5 mg/kg on days 2 and 3 if diarrhea persists.

If fluoroquinolone-resistant *Campylobacter* is suspected (for example, following travel to Southeast Asia):
Adults: Azithromycin (at above dose for adults). *Children:* Same as for children traveling to other areas (see above).

Source: After DR Hill et al: The practice of travel medicine: Guidelines by the Infectious Diseases Society of America. Clin Infect Dis 43:1499, 2006.

TREATMENT

Infectious Diarrhea or Bacterial Food Poisoning

In many cases, a specific diagnosis is not necessary or not available to guide treatment. The clinician can proceed with the information obtained from the history, stool examination, and evaluation of dehydration severity. Empirical regimens for the treatment of traveler's diarrhea are listed in **Table 133-5**.

The mainstay of treatment is adequate rehydration. The treatment of cholera and other dehydrating diarrheal diseases was revolutionized by the promotion of oral rehydration solution (ORS), the efficacy of which depends on the fact that glucose-facilitated absorption of sodium and water in the small intestine remains intact in the presence of cholera toxin. The use of ORS has reduced cholera mortality rates from >50% (in untreated cases) to <1%. A number of ORS formulas have been used. Initial preparations were based on the treatment of patients with cholera and included a solution containing 3.5 g of sodium chloride, 2.5 g of sodium bicarbonate (or 2.9 g of sodium citrate), 1.5 g of potassium chloride, and 20 g of glucose (or 40 g of sucrose) per liter of water. Such a preparation can still be used for the treatment of severe cholera. Many causes of secretory diarrhea, however, are associated with less electrolyte loss than occurs in cholera. Beginning in 2002, the World Health Organization recommended a reduced-osmolarity/reduced-salt ORS that is better tolerated and more effective than classic ORS. This preparation contains 2.6 g of sodium chloride, 2.9 g of trisodium citrate, 1.5 g of potassium chloride, and 13.5 g of glucose (or 27 g of sucrose) per liter of water. ORS formulations containing rice or cereal as the carbohydrate source may be even more effective than glucose-based solutions. Patients who are severely dehydrated or in whom vomiting precludes oral therapy should receive IV solutions such as Ringer's lactate.

Most secretory forms of traveler's diarrhea (usually due to enterotoxigenic or enteroaggregative *E. coli* or to *Campylobacter*) can be treated effectively with rehydration, bismuth subsalicylate, or antiperistaltic agents. Antimicrobial agents can shorten the duration of illness from 3–4 days to 24–36 h but may be associated with the acquisition of multidrug-resistant organisms; their use should therefore be reserved for severe cases. Changes in diet have not been shown to have an impact on the duration of illness, while the efficacy of probiotics continues to be debated. Most individuals who present with dysentery (bloody diarrhea and fever) should be treated empirically with an antimicrobial agent (e.g., a fluoroquinolone or a macrolide) pending microbiologic analysis of stool. Individuals with shigellosis should receive a 3- to 7-day course. Individuals with more severe or prolonged *Campylobacter* infection often benefit from antimicrobial treatment as well. Because of widespread resistance of *Campylobacter* to fluoroquinolones, especially in parts of Asia, a macrolide antibiotic such as erythromycin or azithromycin may be preferred for this infection.

Treatment of salmonellosis must be tailored to the individual patient. Since administration of antimicrobial agents often prolongs intestinal colonization with *Salmonella*, these drugs are usually reserved for individuals at high risk of complications from disseminated salmonellosis, such as infants, patients with prosthetic devices, patients over age 50, and immunocompromised persons. Antimicrobial agents should not be administered to individuals (especially children) in whom enterohemorrhagic *E. coli* infection is suspected. Laboratory studies of enterohemorrhagic *E. coli* strains have demonstrated that a number of antibiotics induce replication of Shiga toxin–producing lambdoid bacteriophages, thereby significantly increasing toxin production by these strains. Clinical studies have supported these laboratory results, and antibiotics may increase by twentyfold the risk of hemolytic-uremic syndrome and renal failure during enterohemorrhagic *E. coli* infection. A clinical clue in the diagnosis of the latter infection is bloody diarrhea with low fever or none at all.

PROPHYLAXIS

Improvements in hygiene to limit fecal–oral spread of enteric pathogens will be necessary if the prevalence of diarrheal diseases is to be significantly reduced in developing countries. Travelers can reduce their risk of diarrhea by eating only hot, freshly cooked food; by avoiding raw vegetables, salads, and unpeeled fruit; and by drinking only boiled or treated water and avoiding ice. Historically, few travelers to tourist destinations adhere to these dietary restrictions. Bismuth subsalicylate is an inexpensive agent for the prophylaxis of traveler's diarrhea; it is taken at a dosage of 2 tablets (525 mg) four times a day. Treatment appears to be effective and safe for up to 3 weeks, but adverse events such as temporary darkening of the tongue, constipation, and tinnitus can occur. A meta-analysis suggests that probiotics may lessen the likelihood of traveler's diarrhea by ~15%. Prophylactic antimicrobial agents, although effective, are not generally recommended for the prevention of traveler's diarrhea except when travelers are immunosuppressed or have other underlying illnesses that place them at high risk for morbidity from gastrointestinal infection. If prophylaxis is indicated, the nonabsorbed antibiotic rifaximin can be considered.

The possibility of exerting a major impact on the worldwide morbidity and mortality associated with diarrheal diseases has led to intensive efforts to develop effective vaccines against the common bacterial and viral enteric pathogens. An effective rotavirus vaccine is available. Vaccines against *V. cholerae* are available and recommended in areas where active transmission is ongoing, although the protection they offer is incomplete and/or short lived. A new typhoid conjugate vaccine was recently prequalified and recommended by the World Health Organization for use in countries where typhoid is endemic. Large-scale effectiveness studies are underway to determine the duration of protection. At present, there are no effective commercially available vaccines against pathogenic *E. coli*, *Shigella*, *Campylobacter*, nontyphoidal *Salmonella*, norovirus, or intestinal parasites.

Acknowledgment

The authors thank Stephen B. Calderwood, MD, and Edward T. Ryan, MD, for their significant contributions to this chapter in the previous editions.

FURTHER READING

Baumler AJ, Sperandio C: Interactions between the microbiota and pathogenic bacteria in the gut. Nature 535:85, 2016.

GBD 2016 Diarrheal Disease Collaborators. Estimates of the global, regional, and national morbidity, mortality, and etiologies of diarrhea in 195 countries: A systematic analysis for the Global Burden of Disease Study 2016. Lancet Infect Dis 18:1211, 2018.

Goldenberg JZ et al: Probiotics for the prevention of pediatric antibiotic-associated diarrhea. Cochrane Database Syst Rev 12:CD004827, 2015.

Guttman JA, Finlay BB: Subcellular alterations that lead to diarrhea during bacterial pathogenesis. Trends Microbiol 16:535, 2008.

Levine MM et al: Diarrhoeal disease and subsequent risk of death in infants and children residing in low-income and middle-income countries: Analysis of the GEMS case-controlled study and 12-month GEMS-1A follow-on study. Lancet Glob Health 8:e202, 2020.

Riddle MS et al: Update on vaccines for enteric pathogens. Clin Microbiol Infect 24:1039, 2008.

Shane AL et al: 2017 Infectious Diseases Society of America clinical practice guidelines for the diagnosis and management of infectious diarrhea. Clin Infect Dis 65:e45, 2017.

Viswanathan VK et al: Enteric infection meets intestinal function: How bacterial pathogens cause diarrhoea. Nat Rev Microbiol 7:110, 2009.

134 *Clostridioides difficile* Infection, Including Pseudomembranous Colitis

Dale N. Gerding, Stuart Johnson

DEFINITION

Clostridioides difficile infection (CDI) is a unique colonic disease that is acquired most commonly in association with antimicrobial use and the consequent disruption of the normal colonic microbiota. The most commonly diagnosed diarrheal illness acquired in the hospital, CDI results from the ingestion of spores of *C. difficile* that vegetate, multiply, and secrete toxins, causing diarrhea and, in the most severe cases, pseudomembranous colitis (PMC).

ETIOLOGY AND EPIDEMIOLOGY

C. difficile is an obligately anaerobic, gram-positive, spore-forming bacillus whose spores are found widely in nature, particularly in the environment of hospitals and chronic-care facilities. CDI occurs frequently in hospitals and nursing homes (or shortly after discharge from these facilities) where the level of antimicrobial use is high and the environment is contaminated by *C. difficile* spores.

Clindamycin, ampicillin, and cephalosporins were the first antibiotics associated with CDI. The second- and third-generation cephalosporins, particularly cefotaxime, ceftriaxone, cefuroxime, and ceftazidime, are agents frequently responsible for this condition, and the fluoroquinolones (ciprofloxacin, levofloxacin, and moxifloxacin) are the most recent drug class to be implicated in hospital outbreaks. Penicillin/β-lactamase-inhibitor combinations such as ticarcillin/clavulanate and piperacillin/tazobactam pose significantly less risk. However, all antibiotics, including vancomycin (the agent most commonly used to treat CDI) and metronidazole, have been found to carry a risk of subsequent CDI. A minority of cases, especially in the community, are reported in patients without documentation of prior antibiotic exposure.

C. difficile is acquired exogenously—most often in the hospital or nursing home, but also in the outpatient setting—and is carried in the stool of both symptomatic and asymptomatic patients. The rate of fecal colonization increases in proportion to length of hospital stay and is often ≥20% among adult patients hospitalized for >2 weeks; in contrast, the rate is 1–3% among community residents. CDI is the most common health care–associated infection in the United States, with an estimated 462,100 cases in 2017. Between 2011 and 2017, the total burden of CDI in the United States decreased by 24%, which was primarily due to decreases in health care–associated CDI. The estimated burden of community-associated CDI was unchanged.

Asymptomatic fecal carriage of *C. difficile* in healthy neonates is very common, with repeated colonization by multiple strains in infants

<1–2 years of age, but associated disease in these infants is extremely rare if it occurs at all. Spores of *C. difficile* are found on environmental surfaces (where the organism can persist for months) and on the hands of hospital personnel who fail to practice good hand hygiene. Hospital epidemics of CDI have been attributed to a single *C. difficile* strain and to multiple strains present simultaneously. Other identified risk factors for CDI include older age, greater severity of underlying illness, gastrointestinal surgery, use of electronic rectal thermometers, enteral tube feeding, and antacid treatment. Use of proton pump inhibitors may be a risk factor, but this risk is probably modest, and no firm data have implicated these agents in patients who are not already receiving antibiotics.

PATHOLOGY AND PATHOGENESIS

Spores of toxigenic *C. difficile* are ingested, survive gastric acidity, germinate in the small bowel, and colonize the lower intestinal tract, where they elaborate two large toxins: toxin A (an enterotoxin) and toxin B (a cytotoxin). These toxins initiate processes resulting in the disruption of epithelial-cell barrier function, diarrhea, and pseudomembrane formation. Toxin A is a potent neutrophil chemoattractant, and both toxins glucosylate the GTP-binding proteins of the Rho subfamily that regulate the actin cell cytoskeleton. Data from studies using molecular disruption of toxin genes in isogenic mutants suggest that toxin B may be the more important virulence factor, which is consistent with the well-documented occurrence of clinical disease caused by toxin A–negative strains but not by toxin B–negative strains. Disruption of the cytoskeleton results in loss of cell shape, adherence, and tight junctions, with consequent fluid leakage. A third toxin, binary toxin CDT, was previously found in only ~6% of strains but is present in all isolates of the widely recognized epidemic NAP1/BI/027 strain (see "Global Considerations," below); this toxin is related to *C. perfringens* iota toxin. Its role in the pathogenesis of CDI has not yet been defined.

The pseudomembranes of PMC are confined to the colonic mucosa and initially appear as 1- to 2-mm whitish-yellow plaques. The intervening mucosa appears unremarkable, but, as the disease progresses, the pseudomembranes coalesce to form larger plaques and become confluent over the entire colon wall (**Fig. 134-1**). The whole colon is usually involved, but 10% of patients have rectal sparing. Viewed microscopically, the pseudomembranes have a mucosal attachment point and contain necrotic leukocytes, fibrin, mucus, and cellular debris. The epithelium is eroded and necrotic in focal areas, with neutrophil infiltration of the mucosa.

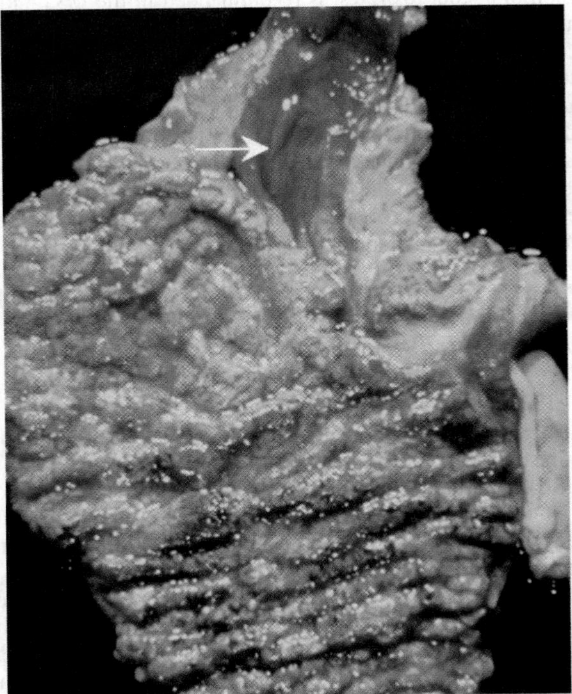

FIGURE 134-1 Autopsy specimen showing confluent pseudomembranes covering the cecum of a patient with pseudomembranous colitis. Note the sparing of the terminal ileum (*arrow*).

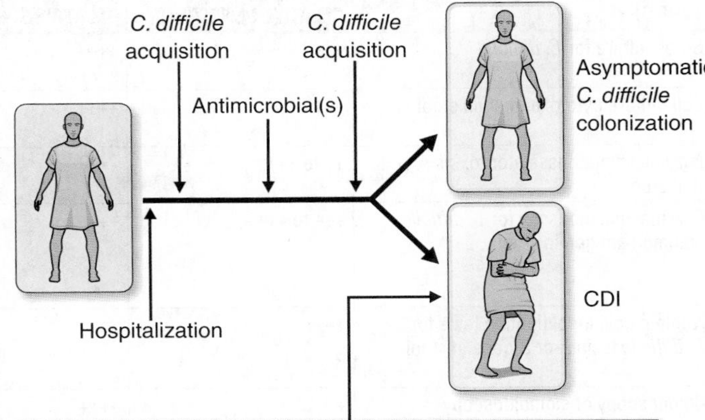

FIGURE 134-2 Pathogenesis model for hospital-acquired *Clostridioides difficile* infection (CDI). At least three events are integral to *C. difficile* pathogenesis. Exposure to antibiotics establishes susceptibility to infection. Once susceptible, the patient may acquire nontoxigenic (nonpathogenic) or toxigenic strains of *C. difficile* as a second event. Acquisition of toxigenic *C. difficile* may be followed by asymptomatic colonization or CDI, depending on one or more additional events, including an inadequate host anamnestic IgG response to *C. difficile* toxin A.

Patients colonized with *C. difficile* were initially thought to be at high risk for CDI. However, four prospective studies have shown that colonized patients who have not previously had CDI actually have a decreased risk of CDI, possibly because many of these patients are colonized by nontoxigenic strains. At least three events are proposed as essential for the development of CDI (**Fig. 134-2**). Exposure to antimicrobial agents is the first event and establishes susceptibility to CDI, most likely through disruption of the normal gastrointestinal microbiota. The second event is exposure to toxigenic *C. difficile*. Given that the majority of patients do not develop CDI after the first two events, a third event is clearly essential for its occurrence. Candidate third events include exposure to a *C. difficile* strain of particular virulence, exposure to antimicrobial agents especially likely to cause CDI, and an inadequate host immune response. The host anamnestic serum IgG antibody response to toxin A of *C. difficile* is the most likely third event that determines which patients develop diarrhea and which patients remain asymptomatic. The majority of humans probably first develop antibody to *C. difficile* toxins when colonized asymptomatically during the first year of life or after CDI in childhood. Infants are thought not to develop symptomatic CDI because they lack suitable mucosal toxin receptors that develop later in life. In adulthood, serum levels of IgG antibody to toxin A increase more in response to infection in individuals who become asymptomatic carriers than in those who develop CDI. For persons who develop CDI, increasing levels of antitoxin A during treatment correlate with a lower risk of recurrence. Two large clinical trials in which intravenous monoclonal antibodies to toxin A and toxin B were used together and as single agents in addition to standard antibiotic therapy showed that rates of recurrent CDI were significantly lower with the combination of antibodies and with the toxin B antibody alone than with placebo plus standard therapy. Antibody to toxin A alone was ineffective.

GLOBAL CONSIDERATIONS

Rates and severity of CDI in the United States, Canada, and Europe increased markedly in the early 2000s. Rates in U.S. hospitals tripled between 2000 and 2005. Hospitals in Montreal, Quebec, reported rates in 2005 that were four times higher than the 1997 baseline, with directly attributable mortality of 6.9% (increased from 1.5%). An epidemic strain, variously known as toxinotype III, REA type BI, PCR

TABLE 134-1 Relative Sensitivity and Specificity of Diagnostic Tests for *Clostridioides difficile* Infection (CDI)

TYPE OF TEST	RELATIVE SENSITIVITY[a]	RELATIVE SPECIFICITY[a]	COMMENT
Stool culture for *C. difficile*	++++	+++	Most sensitive test; specificity of ++++ if the *C. difficile* isolate tests positive for toxin; turnaround time too slow for practical use
Cell culture cytotoxin test on stool	+++	++++	With clinical data, is diagnostic of CDI; highly specific but not as sensitive as stool culture; slow turnaround time
Enzyme immunoassay for toxins A and B in stool	++ to +++	+++	With clinical data, is diagnostic of CDI; rapid results, but not as sensitive as stool culture or cell culture cytotoxin test
Enzyme immunoassay for *C. difficile* common antigen in stool	+++ to ++++	+++	Detects glutamate dehydrogenase found in toxigenic and nontoxigenic strains of *C. difficile* and other stool organisms; more sensitive and less specific than enzyme immunoassay for toxins; requires confirmation with a toxin test; rapid results
Nucleic acid amplification tests for *C. difficile* toxin A or B gene in stool	++++	+++	Detects toxigenic *C. difficile* in stool; widely used in United States for clinical testing; more sensitive than enzyme immunoassay toxin testing; marked increase in CDI diagnoses when implemented
Colonoscopy or sigmoidoscopy	+	++++	Highly specific if pseudomembranes are seen; insensitive compared with other tests

[a]According to both clinical and test-based criteria.

Note: ++++, >90%; +++, 71–90%; ++, 51–70%; +, ~50%.

ribotype 027, and pulsed-field type NAP1 (collectively designated NAP1/BI/027), likely accounted for much of the increase in incidence. Two clones of NAP1/BI/027 originated in the United States and Canada and spread to the United Kingdom, Europe, and Asia. This epidemic strain was characterized by (1) an ability to produce 16–23 times as much toxin A and toxin B as control strains in vitro, (2) the presence of binary toxin CDT, and (3) high-level resistance to all fluoroquinolones. National control policies instituted in England in 2006 resulted in a marked decline in CDI cases, and restriction of fluoroquinolones, in particular, was correlated with near elimination of fluoroquinolone-resistant strains of *C. difficile* (i.e., NAP1/BI/027) there by 2013. This epidemic strain has likewise decreased in the United States with data from the Centers for Disease Control and Prevention showing a decrease among health care–associated isolates from 31% to 15% (and from 19% to 6% in community-associated isolates) between 2011 and 2017. New strains have been and will probably continue to be implicated in outbreaks, including a strain commonly found in food animals that also carries binary toxin and has been associated with high mortality rates in human infections (toxinotype V, ribotype 078). Currently, the most frequently isolated community-associated strain in the United States is ribotype 106 (REA group DH), which was previously found to be epidemic in the United Kingdom.

■ CLINICAL MANIFESTATIONS

Diarrhea is the most common manifestation caused by *C. difficile*. Stools are almost never grossly bloody and range from soft and unformed to watery or mucoid in consistency, with a characteristic odor. Clinical and laboratory findings include fever in 28% of cases, abdominal pain in 22%, and leukocytosis in 50%. When adynamic ileus (which is seen on x-ray in ~20% of cases) results in cessation of stool passage, the diagnosis of CDI is frequently overlooked. A clue to the presence of unsuspected CDI in these patients is unexplained leukocytosis, with ≥15,000 white blood cells (WBCs)/μL. Such patients are at high risk for complications of CDI, particularly toxic megacolon and sepsis.

C. difficile diarrhea recurs after treatment in ~15–30% of cases and remains one of the most challenging treatment dilemmas. Recurrences may represent either relapses due to the same strain or reinfections with a new strain. Susceptibility to recurrence of clinical CDI is likely a result of continued disruption of the normal fecal microbiota caused by the antibiotic used to treat CDI.

■ DIAGNOSIS

The diagnosis of CDI is based on a combination of clinical criteria: (1) diarrhea (≥3 unformed stools per 24 h for ≥2 days) with no other recognized cause plus (2) detection of toxin A or B in the stool, detection of toxin-producing *C. difficile* in the stool by nucleic acid amplification testing (NAAT; e.g., polymerase chain reaction [PCR]) or by culture, or visualization of pseudomembranes in the colon. PMC is a more advanced form of CDI and is visualized at endoscopy in only ~50% of patients with diarrhea who have a positive stool culture and toxin assay for *C. difficile* (**Table 134-1**). Endoscopy is a rapid diagnostic tool in seriously ill patients with suspected PMC and an acute abdomen, but a negative result in this examination does not rule out CDI.

Despite the array of tests available for *C. difficile* and its toxins (Table 134-1), no single test has high sensitivity, high specificity, and rapid turnaround. Most laboratory tests for toxins, including enzyme immunoassays (EIAs), lack sensitivity. However, testing of multiple additional stool specimens is not recommended. NAATs (including PCR) are widely used diagnostically and are both rapid and sensitive; however, concern has been raised that PCR may detect colonization with toxigenic *C. difficile* in patients who have diarrhea for a reason other than CDI. Confirmation of the presence of toxin in the stool in addition to PCR or glutamate dehydrogenase (GDH) positivity is recommended in the European CDI guidelines for diagnosis of CDI, and inclusion of a stool toxin test is recommended in the U.S. guidelines when there are no prior criteria for stool submission. Empirical treatment is appropriate if CDI is strongly suspected on clinical grounds and stool testing is delayed. Testing of asymptomatic patients is not recommended except for epidemiologic study purposes. In particular, so-called tests of cure following treatment are not recommended because >50% of patients continue to harbor the organism and its toxin after diarrhea has ceased and test results do not always predict the recurrence of CDI. The results of such tests should not be used to restrict placement of patients in long-term care or nursing home facilities.

TREATMENT

Clostridioides difficile Infection

PRIMARY CDI

When possible, discontinuation of any ongoing antimicrobial administration is recommended as the first step in treatment of CDI. Earlier studies indicated that 15–23% of patients respond to this simple measure. However, with the advent of the NAP1/BI/027 epidemic strain and the associated rapid clinical deterioration of some patients, prompt initiation of specific CDI treatment has become the standard. General treatment guidelines include hydration and the avoidance of antiperistaltic agents and opiates, which may mask symptoms and possibly worsen disease. Nevertheless, antiperistaltic agents have been used safely with vancomycin or metronidazole treatment for mild to moderate CDI.

Oral administration of fidaxomicin or vancomycin was recommended as first-line treatment for CDI in the 2017 Infectious

TABLE 134-2 Recommendations for the Treatment of *Clostridioides difficile* Infection (CDI)

CLINICAL SETTING	TREATMENT(S)	COMMENTS
Initial episode, mild to moderate	Fidaxomicin (200 mg bid × 10 d) ***or*** Oral vancomycin (125 mg qid × 10 d)	Oral metronidazole is less effective than the other options and may necessitate a longer treatment course for response. Metronidazole (500 mg tid × 10–14 d) is recommended only if vancomycin or fidaxomicin is not readily accessible and for mild-to-moderate disease only.
Initial episode, severe	Oral vancomycin (125 mg qid × 10 d) ***or*** Fidaxomicin (200 mg bid × 10 d)	Indicators of severe disease may include leukocytosis (≥15,000 white blood cells/μL) and a creatinine level ≥1.5 mg/dL.
Initial episode, fulminant	Vancomycin (500 mg PO or via nasogastric tube) plus metronidazole (500 mg IV q8h) ***plus consider*** Rectal instillation of vancomycin (500 mg in 100 mL of normal saline as a retention enema q6–8h)	Fulminant CDI is defined as severe CDI with the addition of hypotension, shock, ileus, or toxic megacolon. The duration of treatment may need to be >2 weeks and is dictated by response.
First recurrence	Fidaxomicin (200 mg bid × 10 d) ***or*** Oral vancomycin (125 mg qid × 10 d) ***or*** Oral vancomycin followed by a taper-and-pulse regimen[a]	Treatment for the initial episode should be considered when choosing treatment for the first recurrence.
Multiple recurrences	Oral vancomycin treatment followed by a taper-and-pulse regimen ***or*** Fidaxomicin (200 mg bid × 10 d or 200 mg bid × 5 d followed by every other day × 20 d) ***or*** Vancomycin (125 mg qid × 10 d), then stop vancomycin and start rifaximin (400 mg bid × 2 weeks) ***or*** Fecal microbiota transplantation (FMT)	It is recommended that FMT given by enema be considered only after appropriate antibiotic treatment for ≥2 recurrent CDI episodes and the donor and donor specimen is screened per U.S. Food and Drug Administration recommendations.
Patients at high risk of recurrent CDI who are receiving vancomycin, fidaxomicin, or metronidazole	Bezlotoxumab 10 mg/kg given IV	Bezlotoxumab is adjuvant therapy (in addition to and during antibiotic treatment) for patients at high risk for recurrent CDI. Risk factors include age >65 years, immunocompromised host, severe CDI on presentation, and prior episode of CDI in the past 6 months.

[a]A typical taper-and-pulse vancomycin regimen following a 10-day treatment course includes: 125 mg bid × 1 week, then daily × 1 week, then q2–3d for 2–8 weeks.

Diseases Society of America (IDSA) and Society for Healthcare Epidemiology of America (SHEA) CDI guidelines. Oral metronidazole is only recommended for mild or moderate CDI when fidaxomicin or vancomycin is not available. IV vancomycin is ineffective for CDI. Fidaxomicin is available only for oral administration. Two large clinical trials comparing vancomycin and fidaxomicin indicated comparable clinical resolution of diarrhea in ~90% of patients, and the rate of recurrent CDI was significantly lower with fidaxomicin. The largest randomized controlled trial of vancomycin versus metronidazole showed that the vancomycin cure rate was superior to the metronidazole cure rate (81% vs 73%; $p = .034$) for all patients with CDI, regardless of severity. Although the mean time to resolution of diarrhea is 2–4 days, the response to metronidazole may be much slower. Treatment should not be deemed a failure until a drug has been given for at least 6 days. On the basis of data for shorter courses of vancomycin and the results of four large clinical trials, it is recommended that vancomycin or fidaxomicin be given for at least 10 days. Metronidazole was never approved for CDI by the U.S. Food and Drug Administration (FDA), and its use for CDI treatment has declined markedly after publication of the 2017 IDSA/SHEA CDI guidelines. It is important to initiate treatment with oral vancomycin for patients who appear seriously ill, particularly if they have a high WBC count (>15,000/μL) or creatinine level (≥1.5 mg/dL) **(Table 134-2)**. Small randomized trials of nitazoxanide, bacitracin, rifaximin, and fusidic acid for treatment of CDI have been conducted. These drugs have not been extensively studied, shown to be superior, or approved by the FDA for CDI, but they provide potential alternatives to vancomycin and fidaxomicin.

RECURRENT CDI

Overall, ~15–30% of successfully treated patients experience recurrences of CDI following treatment. CDI recurrence is significantly lower in patients treated with fidaxomicin than in those treated with vancomycin. Vancomycin and metronidazole have comparable recurrence rates, and metronidazole is not recommended for treatment of recurrent CDI. Patients who have a first recurrence of CDI have an even higher rate of second recurrence. Fidaxomicin is superior to vancomycin in reducing further recurrences in patients who have had one CDI recurrence (Table 134-2). Recurrent disease, once thought to be relatively mild, has now been documented to pose a significant (11%) risk of serious complications (shock, megacolon, perforation, colectomy, or death within 30 days). There is no standard treatment for multiple recurrences, but the use of vancomycin in a tapering and pulsed dosing regimen every other day for 2–8 weeks has been used for years as a practical approach to treating these patients, and recent data suggest it is still effective. Other recommended treatment options for patients with multiple CDI recurrences include fidaxomicin in standard or extended/pulsed dosing regimens, vancomycin followed by rifaximin, or fecal microbiota transplantation (FMT) via nasoduodenal tube, colonoscope, enema, or oral capsules (Table 134-2). FMT has been widely used over the past decade, and the availability of stool banks and oral capsule formulations has made this approach even more practical. The results of randomized controlled trials of FMT continue to be reported, and as would be expected, the results are not as impressive as in observational trials. However, FMT is not approved by the FDA for use in the United States, and recent FDA safety alerts regarding transmission of multidrug-resistant organisms, pathogenic *Escherichia coli*, and potential transmission of SARS-CoV-2 are a reminder that this approach should only be considered for patients who have failed appropriate antibacterial therapy and when the donor and FMT product have been rigorously screened.

In addition to antibacterial therapies, an adjunctive treatment is now available for patients who are receiving standard-of-care antibacterial agents and who are at high risk for recurrent CDI (rCDI). Bezlotoxumab, a monoclonal antibody directed against *C. difficile* toxin B, has been shown to reduce the risk of rCDI by an absolute rate of ~10% when administered to patients currently receiving vancomycin, fidaxomicin, or metronidazole. Risk factors for rCDI in the clinical trials included age >65 years, immunocompromised host, severe CDI on presentation, and prior episode of CDI in the past 6 months.

SEVERE COMPLICATED OR FULMINANT CDI

Fulminant (rapidly progressive and severe) CDI presents the most difficult treatment challenge. Patients with fulminant disease often do not have diarrhea, and their illness mimics an acute surgical abdomen. Sepsis (hypotension, fever, tachycardia, leukocytosis) may result from fulminant CDI. An acute abdomen (with or without toxic megacolon) may include signs of obstruction, ileus, colon-wall thickening and ascites on abdominal CT, and peripheral-blood leukocytosis (≥20,000 WBCs/μL). With or without diarrhea, the differential diagnosis of an acute abdomen, sepsis, or toxic megacolon should include CDI if the patient has received antibiotics in the past 2 months. Cautious sigmoidoscopy or colonoscopy to visualize PMC and an abdominal CT examination are the best diagnostic tests in patients without diarrhea.

Medical management of fulminant CDI is suboptimal because of the difficulty of delivering oral fidaxomicin, metronidazole, or vancomycin to the colon in the presence of ileus (Table 134-2). The combination of vancomycin (given orally or via nasogastric tube and by retention enema) plus IV metronidazole has been used with some success in uncontrolled studies, as has IV tigecycline in small-scale uncontrolled studies. Surgical colectomy may be life-saving if there is no response to medical management. If possible, colectomy should be performed before the serum lactate level reaches 5 mmol/L. However, mortality and morbidity associated with colectomy may be reduced by performing instead a laparoscopic ileostomy followed by colon lavage with polyethylene glycol and vancomycin infusion into the colon via the ileostomy.

PROGNOSIS

The mortality rate attributed to CDI, previously found to be 0.6–3.5%, has reached 6.9% in recent outbreaks and is progressively higher with increasing age. Most patients recover, but recurrences are common.

PREVENTION AND CONTROL

Strategies for the prevention of CDI are of two types: those aimed at preventing transmission of the organism to the patient and those aimed at reducing the risk of CDI if the organism is transmitted. Transmission of *C. difficile* in clinical practice has been prevented by gloving of personnel, elimination of the use of contaminated electronic thermometers, and use of hypochlorite (bleach) solution for environmental decontamination of patients' rooms. Hand hygiene is critical; hand washing is recommended in CDI outbreaks because alcohol hand gels are not sporicidal. CDI outbreaks have been best controlled by restricting the use of specific antibiotics, such as clindamycin, second- and third-generation cephalosporins, and fluoroquinolones. Outbreaks of CDI due to clindamycin-resistant strains have resolved promptly when clindamycin use is restricted. Future prevention strategies include use of monoclonal antibodies, vaccines, and biotherapeutics with live organisms that restore protection from colonization.

FURTHER READING

Dingle KE et al: Effects of control interventions on *Clostridium difficile* infection in England: An observational study. Lancet Infect Dis 17:411, 2017.

Guh AY et al: Trends in U.S. burden of *Clostridioides difficile* infection and outcomes. N Engl J Med 382:1320, 2020.

He M et al: Emergence and global spread of epidemic healthcare-associated *Clostridium difficile*. Nat Genet 45:109, 2013.

Hota SS et al: Oral vancomycin followed by fecal transplantation versus tapering oral vancomycin treatment for recurrent *Clostridium difficile* infection: An open-label, randomized controlled trial. Clin Infect Dis 64:265, 2016.

Johnson S et al: Vancomycin, metronidazole, or tolevamer for *Clostridium difficile* infection: Results from two multinational, randomized, controlled trials. Clin Infect Dis 59:345, 2014.

Kociolek LK et al: Natural *Clostridioides difficile* toxin immunization in colonized infants. Clin Infect Dis 70:2095, 2020.

Louie TJ et al: Fidaxomicin versus vancomycin for *Clostridium difficile* infection. N Engl J Med 364:422, 2011.

Magill SS et al: Multistate point–prevalence survey of healthcare-associated infections. N Engl J Med 370:1198, 2014.

McDonald LC et al: Clinical practice guidelines for *Clostridium difficile* infection in adults and children: 2017 update by the Infectious Diseases Society of America (IDSA) and the Society for Healthcare Epidemiology of America (SHEA). Clin Infect Dis 66:987, 2018.

Polage CR et al: Overdiagnosis of *Clostridium difficile* infection in the molecular test era. JAMA Intern Med 175:1792, 2015.

See I et al: NAP1 strain type predicts outcomes from *Clostridium difficile* infection. Clin Infect Dis 58:1394, 2014.

Wilcox MH et al: Bezlotoxumab for prevention of *Clostridium difficile* infection recurrence. N Engl J Med 376:305, 2017.

135 Urinary Tract Infections, Pyelonephritis, and Prostatitis

Kalpana Gupta, Barbara W. Trautner

Urinary tract infection (UTI) is a common and painful human illness that is rapidly responsive to modern antibiotic therapy, if the correct antibiotic is chosen for the particular urinary pathogen. In the preantibiotic era, UTI caused significant morbidity. Hippocrates, writing about a disease that appears to have been acute cystitis, said that the illness could last for a year before either resolving or worsening to involve the kidneys. When chemotherapeutic agents used to treat UTI were introduced in the early twentieth century, they were relatively ineffective, and persistence of infection after 3 weeks of therapy was common. Nitrofurantoin, which became available in the 1950s, was the first tolerable and effective agent for the treatment of UTI.

Since the most common manifestation of UTI is acute cystitis and since acute cystitis is far more prevalent among women than among men, most clinical research on UTI has involved women. Many studies have enrolled women from college campuses or large health maintenance organizations in the United States. Therefore, when reviewing the literature and recommendations concerning UTI, clinicians must consider whether the findings are applicable to their patient populations.

DEFINITIONS

UTI may be asymptomatic (subclinical infection) or symptomatic (disease). Thus, the term *urinary tract infection* encompasses a variety of clinical entities, including asymptomatic bacteriuria (ASB), cystitis, prostatitis, and pyelonephritis. The distinction between symptomatic UTI and ASB has major clinical implications. Both UTI and ASB connote the presence of bacteria in the urinary tract, usually accompanied by white blood cells and inflammatory cytokines in the urine. However, ASB occurs in the absence of symptoms attributable to the bacteria in the urinary tract and usually does not require treatment, while UTI has more typically been assumed to imply symptomatic disease that warrants antimicrobial therapy. Much of the literature concerning UTI, particularly catheter-associated infection, does not differentiate between UTI and ASB. In this chapter, the term *urinary tract infection* denotes symptomatic disease; *cystitis*, symptomatic infection of the bladder; and *pyelonephritis*, symptomatic infection of the kidneys. *Uncomplicated urinary tract infection* refers to an infection confined to the bladder, or acute cystitis. *Pyelonephritis* occurs when the infection involves the renal parenchyma. *Complicated urinary tract infection* is accompanied by symptoms that suggest the infection extends beyond the bladder, such as a fever or signs or symptoms of systemic illness. *Recurrent urinary tract infection* is not necessarily complicated; individual episodes can be uncomplicated and treated as such. *Catheter-associated bacteriuria* can be either symptomatic (CAUTI) or asymptomatic. This new approach to UTI categorization differs from the classical approach, in which men with UTI are automatically considered complicated. This updated categorization more closely reflects actual clinical practice. The key considerations in diagnostic workup and therapy for UTI are whether the patient is stable for outpatient management and whether the antimicrobial agents need to achieve adequate levels in blood and tissue.

EPIDEMIOLOGY AND RISK FACTORS

Except among infants and older adults, UTI occurs far more commonly in females than in males. During the neonatal period, the incidence of UTI is slightly higher among males than among females because male infants more commonly have congenital urinary tract anomalies. After 50 years of age, obstruction from prostatic hypertrophy becomes common in men, and the incidence of UTI is almost as high among men as among women. Between 1 year and ~50 years of age, UTI and recurrent UTI are predominantly diseases of females. The prevalence of ASB is ~5% among women between ages 20 and 40 and may be as high as 40–50% among elderly women and men.

As many as 50–80% of women in the general population acquire at least one UTI during their lifetime—uncomplicated cystitis in most cases. Recent use of a diaphragm with spermicide, frequent sexual intercourse, and a history of UTI are independent risk factors for acute cystitis. Cystitis is temporally related to recent sexual intercourse in a dose–response manner, with an increased relative risk ranging from 1.4 with one episode of intercourse in the preceding week to 4.8 with five episodes. In healthy postmenopausal women, sexual activity, diabetes mellitus, and incontinence are risk factors for UTI.

Many factors predisposing women to cystitis also increase the risk of pyelonephritis. Factors independently associated with pyelonephritis in young healthy women include frequent sexual intercourse, a new sexual partner, a UTI in the previous 12 months, a maternal history of UTI, diabetes, and incontinence. The shared risk factors for cystitis and pyelonephritis are not surprising given that pyelonephritis typically arises through the ascent of bacteria from the bladder to the upper urinary tract. However, pyelonephritis can occur without symptomatic antecedent cystitis.

About 20–30% of women who have had one episode of UTI will have recurrent episodes. Early recurrence (within 2 weeks) is usually regarded as relapse rather than reinfection and may indicate the need to evaluate the patient for a sequestered focus. Intracellular bacterial communities of infecting organisms within the bladder epithelium have been demonstrated in animal models of UTI and in exfoliated human urothelial cells, but the clinical impact of this phenomenon in humans is not yet clear. The rate of recurrence ranges from 0.3 to 7.6 infections per patient per year, with an average of 2.6 infections per year. It is not uncommon for multiple recurrences to follow an initial infection, resulting in clustering of episodes. Clustering may be related temporally to the presence of a new risk factor, to the sloughing of the protective outer bladder epithelial layer in response to bacterial attachment during acute cystitis, or possibly to antibiotic-related alteration of the normal flora. The likelihood of a recurrence decreases with increasing time since the last infection. A case–control study of predominantly white premenopausal women with recurrent UTI identified frequent sexual intercourse, use of spermicide, a new sexual partner, a first UTI before 15 years of age, and a maternal history of UTI as independent risk factors for recurrent UTI. The only consistently documented behavioral risk factors for recurrent UTI include frequent sexual intercourse and spermicide use. In postmenopausal women, major risk factors for recurrent UTI include a history of premenopausal UTI and anatomic factors affecting bladder emptying, such as cystoceles, urinary incontinence, and residual urine.

In pregnant women, ASB has clinical consequences, and both screening for and treatment of this condition are indicated. Specifically, ASB during pregnancy is associated with maternal pyelonephritis, which in turn is associated with preterm delivery. Antibiotic treatment of ASB in pregnant women can reduce the risk of pyelonephritis, preterm delivery, and low-birth-weight babies.

The majority of men with UTI have a functional or anatomic abnormality of the urinary tract, most commonly urinary obstruction secondary to prostatic hypertrophy. That said, not all men with UTI have detectable urinary abnormalities; this point is particularly relevant for men ≤45 years of age. Lack of circumcision is associated with an increased risk of UTI because *Escherichia coli* is more likely to colonize the glans and prepuce and subsequently migrate into the urinary tract of uncircumcised men.

Women with diabetes have a two- to threefold higher rate of ASB and UTI than women without diabetes; there is insufficient evidence on which to base a corresponding statement about men. Increased duration of diabetes and the use of insulin rather than oral medication are associated with an elevated risk of UTI among women with diabetes. Poor bladder function, obstruction in urinary flow, and incomplete voiding are additional factors commonly found in patients with diabetes that increase the risk of UTI. Impaired cytokine secretion may contribute to ASB in diabetic women. The sodium–glucose cotransporter 2 (SGLT2) inhibitors used for treatment of diabetes result in glycosuria. Initial concerns that these drugs as a class increased the risk of UTI are not supported by data.

ETIOLOGY

The uropathogens causing UTI vary by clinical syndrome but are usually enteric gram-negative rods that have migrated to the urinary tract. The susceptibility patterns of these organisms vary by clinical syndrome and by geography. In acute uncomplicated cystitis in the United States, the etiologic agents are highly predictable: *E. coli* accounts for 75–90% of isolates; *Staphylococcus saprophyticus* for 5–15% (with particularly frequent isolation from younger women); and *Klebsiella*, *Proteus*, *Enterococcus*, and *Citrobacter* species, along with other organisms, for 5–10%. Similar etiologic agents are found in Canada, South America, and Europe. The spectrum of agents causing uncomplicated pyelonephritis is similar, with *E. coli* predominating. In complicated UTI (e.g., CAUTI), *E. coli* remains the predominant organism, but other aerobic gram-negative rods, such as *Pseudomonas aeruginosa* and *Klebsiella*, *Proteus*, *Citrobacter*, *Acinetobacter*, and *Morganella* species, also are frequently isolated. Gram-positive bacteria (e.g., enterococci and *Staphylococcus aureus*) and yeasts also are important pathogens in complicated UTI. Data on etiology and resistance are generally obtained from laboratory surveys and should be understood in the context that organisms are identified only in cases in which urine is sent for culture—typically, when complicated UTI or pyelonephritis is suspected. Genetic sequencing of the bladder microbiome or of all the bacteria that can be identified in the bladder has consistently demonstrated that more bacterial species are present than can be identified by routine culture methods, in both symptomatic and asymptomatic states. The clinical significance of these non-cultivatable organisms is unknown but has challenged the assumption that the bladder is normally a sterile site.

The available data demonstrate a worldwide increase in the resistance of *E. coli* to specific antibiotics commonly used to treat UTI. North American, South American, and European surveys from women with acute cystitis have documented resistance rates of >20% to trimethoprim-sulfamethoxazole (TMP-SMX) in many regions and >10% to ciprofloxacin in some regions. In community-acquired infections, the increased prevalence of multidrug-resistant uropathogens has left few oral options for therapy in some cases. Since resistance rates vary by local geographic region, with individual patient characteristics, and over time, it is important to use current and local data when choosing a treatment regimen.

PATHOGENESIS

The urinary tract can be viewed as an anatomic unit linked by a continuous column of urine extending from the urethra to the kidneys. In the majority of UTIs, bacteria establish infection by ascending from the urethra to the bladder. Continuing ascent up the ureter to the kidney is the pathway for most renal parenchymal infections. However, introduction of bacteria into the bladder does not inevitably lead to sustained and symptomatic infection. The interplay of host, pathogen, and environmental factors determines whether tissue invasion and symptomatic infection will ensue (**Fig. 135-1**). For example, bacteria

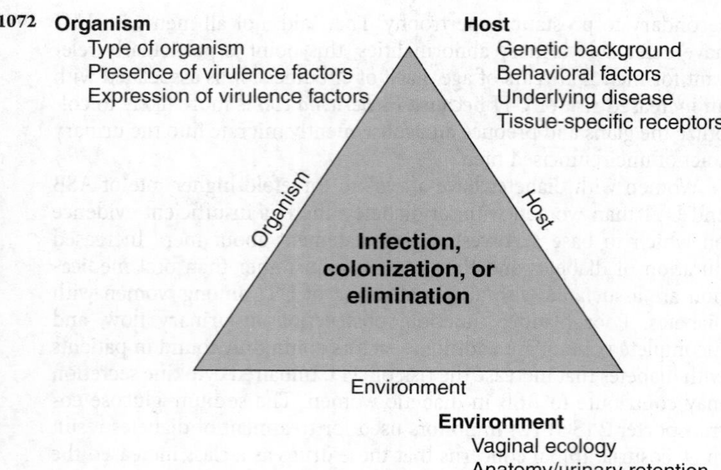

FIGURE 135-1 Pathogenesis of urinary tract infection. The relationship among specific host, pathogen, and environmental factors determines the clinical outcome.

often enter the bladder after sexual intercourse, but normal voiding and innate host defense mechanisms in the bladder eliminate these organisms. Any foreign body in the urinary tract, such as a urinary catheter or stone, provides an inert surface for bacterial colonization. Abnormal micturition and/or significant residual urine volume promotes infection. In the simplest of terms, anything that increases the likelihood of bacteria entering the bladder and staying there increases the risk of UTI.

Bacteria can gain access to the urinary tract through the bloodstream. However, hematogenous spread accounts for <2% of documented UTIs and usually results from bacteremia caused by relatively virulent organisms, such as *Salmonella* and *S. aureus*. Indeed, the isolation of either of these pathogens from a patient without a catheter or other instrumentation warrants a search for a bloodstream source. Hematogenous infections may produce focal abscesses or areas of pyelonephritis within a kidney and result in positive urine cultures. The pathogenesis of candiduria is distinct in that the hematogenous route is common. The presence of *Candida* in the urine of a non-instrumented immunocompetent patient implies either genital contamination or potentially widespread visceral dissemination.

Environmental Factors • VAGINAL ECOLOGY Vaginal ecology is an important environmental factor affecting the risk of UTI in women. Colonization of the vaginal introitus and periurethral area with organisms from the intestinal flora (usually *E. coli*) is the critical initial step in the pathogenesis of UTI. Sexual intercourse is associated with an increased risk of vaginal colonization with *E. coli* and thereby increases the risk of UTI. Nonoxynol-9 in spermicide is toxic to the normal vaginal lactobacilli and thus is likewise associated with an increased risk of *E. coli* vaginal colonization and bacteriuria. In postmenopausal women, the previously predominant vaginal lactobacilli are replaced with colonizing gram-negative bacteria. The use of topical estrogens to prevent UTI in postmenopausal women is controversial; given the side effects of systemic hormone replacement, oral estrogens should not be used to prevent UTI.

ANATOMIC AND FUNCTIONAL ABNORMALITIES Any condition that permits urinary stasis or obstruction predisposes the individual to UTI. Foreign bodies such as stones or urinary catheters provide an inert surface for bacterial colonization and formation of a persistent biofilm. Thus, vesicoureteral reflux, ureteral obstruction secondary to prostatic hypertrophy, neurogenic bladder, and urinary diversion surgery create an environment favorable to UTI. In persons with such conditions, *E. coli* strains lacking typical urinary virulence factors are often the cause of infection. Inhibition of ureteral peristalsis and decreased ureteral tone leading to vesicoureteral reflux are important in the pathogenesis of pyelonephritis in pregnant women. Anatomic factors—specifically, the distance of the urethra from the anus—are

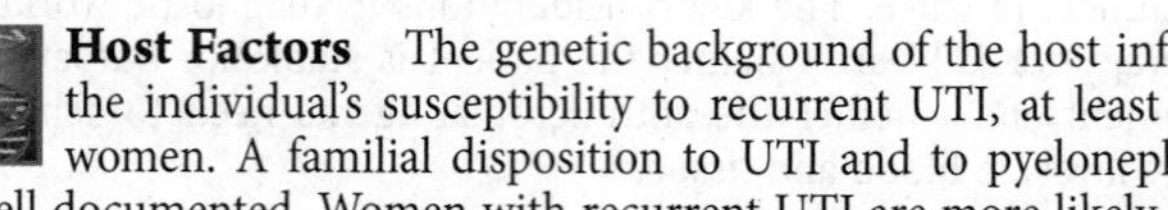

considered to be the primary reason why UTI is predominantly an illness of young women rather than of young men.

Host Factors The genetic background of the host influences the individual's susceptibility to recurrent UTI, at least among women. A familial disposition to UTI and to pyelonephritis is well documented. Women with recurrent UTI are more likely to have had their first UTI before the age of 15 years and to have a maternal history of UTI. A component of the underlying pathogenesis of this familial predisposition to recurrent UTI may be persistent vaginal colonization with *E. coli*, even during asymptomatic periods. Vaginal and periurethral mucosal cells from women with recurrent UTI bind threefold more uropathogenic bacteria than do mucosal cells from women without recurrent infection. Epithelial cells from women who are nonsecretors of certain blood group antigens may possess specific types of receptors to which *E. coli* can bind, thereby facilitating colonization and invasion. Mutations in host innate immune response genes (e.g., those coding for Toll-like receptors and the interleukin 8 receptor) also have been linked to recurrent UTI and pyelonephritis. The genetic patterns that predispose to cystitis and pyelonephritis appear to be distinct.

Microbial Factors An anatomically normal urinary tract presents a stronger barrier to infection than a compromised urinary tract. Thus, strains of *E. coli* that cause invasive symptomatic infection of the urinary tract in otherwise normal hosts often possess and express genetic virulence factors, including surface adhesins that mediate binding to specific receptors on the surface of uroepithelial cells. The best-studied adhesins are the P fimbriae, hair-like protein structures that interact with a specific receptor on renal epithelial cells. (The letter *P* denotes the ability of these fimbriae to bind to blood group antigen P, which contains a D-galactose-D-galactose residue.) P fimbriae are important in the pathogenesis of pyelonephritis and subsequent bloodstream invasion from the kidney.

Another adhesin is the type 1 pilus (fimbria), which all *E. coli* strains possess but not all *E. coli* strains express. Type 1 pili are thought to play a key role in initiating *E. coli* bladder infection; they mediate binding to mannose on the luminal surface of bladder uroepithelial cells. Toxins, metal (iron) acquisition systems, biofilm formation, and capsules also can contribute to the ability of pathogenic *E. coli* to thrive in the bladder.

APPROACH TO THE PATIENT

Clinical Syndromes

The most important issue to be addressed when a UTI is suspected is the characterization of the clinical syndrome as ASB, uncomplicated cystitis, pyelonephritis, prostatitis, or complicated UTI. This information will shape the diagnostic and therapeutic approach.

ASYMPTOMATIC BACTERIURIA

A diagnosis of ASB can be considered only when the patient does not have local or systemic symptoms referable to the urinary tract. The clinical presentation is usually bacteriuria detected incidentally when a patient undergoes a screening urine culture for a reason unrelated to the genitourinary tract. Systemic signs or symptoms such as fever, altered mental status, and leukocytosis in the setting of a positive urine culture are nonspecific and do not merit a diagnosis of symptomatic UTI unless other potential etiologies have been considered.

CYSTITIS

The typical symptoms of cystitis are dysuria, urinary frequency, and urgency. Nocturia, hesitancy, suprapubic discomfort, and gross hematuria are often noted as well. Unilateral back or flank pain suggest that the upper urinary tract is involved, and are thus inconsistent with uncomplicated cystitis. Fever likewise suggests invasive infection beyond the bladder, involving kidney, prostate, or bloodstream.

PYELONEPHRITIS

Mild pyelonephritis can present as low-grade fever with or without lower-back or costovertebral-angle pain, whereas severe pyelonephritis can manifest as high fever, rigors, nausea, vomiting, and flank and/or loin pain. Symptoms are generally acute in onset, and symptoms of cystitis may not be present. Fever is the main feature distinguishing cystitis from pyelonephritis. The fever of pyelonephritis typically exhibits a high spiking "picket-fence" pattern and resolves over 72 h of therapy. Bacteremia develops in 20–30% of cases of pyelonephritis. Patients with diabetes may present with obstructive uropathy associated with acute papillary necrosis when the sloughed papillae obstruct the ureter. Papillary necrosis may also be evident in some cases of pyelonephritis complicated by obstruction, sickle cell disease, analgesic nephropathy, or combinations of these conditions. In the rare cases of bilateral papillary necrosis, a rapid rise in the serum creatinine level may be the first indication of the condition. *Emphysematous* pyelonephritis is a particularly severe form of the disease that is associated with the production of gas in renal and perinephric tissues and occurs almost exclusively in diabetic patients **(Fig. 135-2)**. *Xanthogranulomatous* pyelonephritis occurs when chronic urinary obstruction (often by staghorn calculi), together with chronic infection, leads to suppurative destruction of renal tissue **(Fig. 135-3)**. On pathologic examination, the residual renal tissue frequently has a yellow coloration, with infiltration by lipid-laden macrophages. Pyelonephritis can also be complicated by intraparenchymal abscess formation; this development should be suspected when a patient has continued fever and/or bacteremia despite antibacterial therapy.

PROSTATITIS

Prostatitis includes both infectious and noninfectious abnormalities of the prostate gland. Infections can be acute or chronic, are almost always bacterial in nature, and are far less common than the noninfectious entity *chronic pelvic pain syndrome* (formerly known as chronic prostatitis). Acute bacterial prostatitis presents as dysuria, frequency, and pain in the prostatic pelvic or perineal area. Fever and chills are usually present, and symptoms of bladder outlet obstruction are common. Chronic bacterial prostatitis presents more insidiously as recurrent episodes of cystitis, sometimes with associated pelvic and perineal pain. Men who present with recurrent cystitis should be evaluated for a prostatic focus as well as urinary retention.

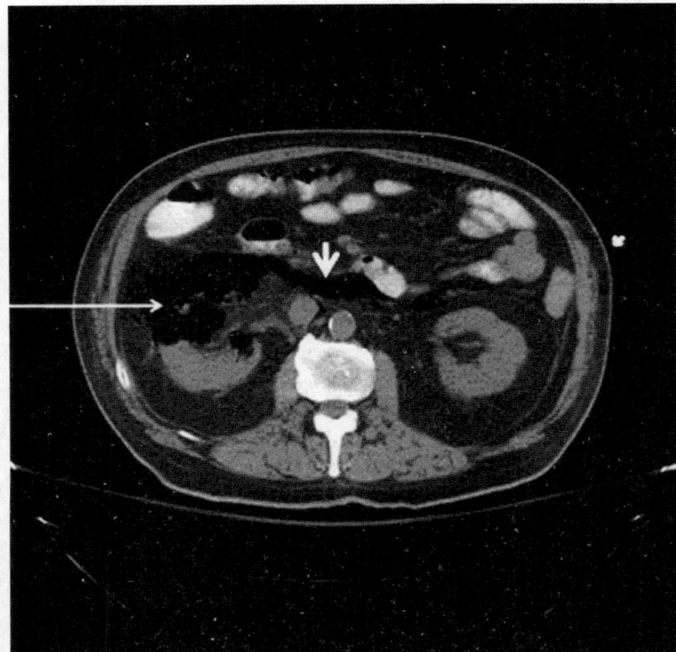

FIGURE 135-2 Emphysematous pyelonephritis. Infection of the right kidney of a diabetic man by *Escherichia coli*, a gas-forming, facultative anaerobic uropathogen, has led to destruction of the renal parenchyma (*arrow*) and tracking of gas through the retroperitoneal space (*arrowhead*).

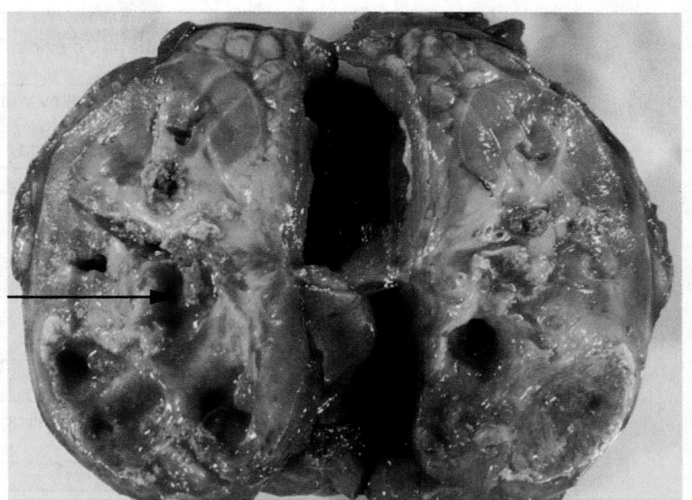

A

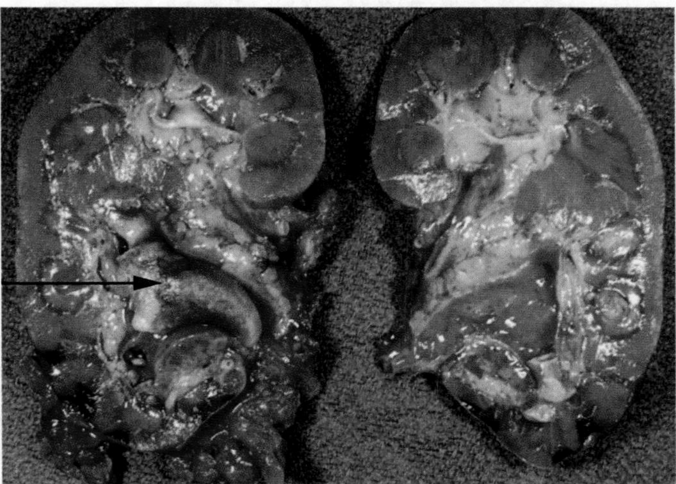

B

FIGURE 135-3 Xanthogranulomatous pyelonephritis. ***A.*** This photograph shows extensive destruction of renal parenchyma due to long-standing suppurative inflammation. The precipitating factor was obstruction by a staghorn calculus, which has been removed, leaving a depression (*arrow*). The mass effect of xanthogranulomatous pyelonephritis can mimic renal malignancy. ***B.*** A large staghorn calculus (*arrow*) is seen obstructing the renal pelvis and calyceal system. The lower pole of the kidney shows areas of hemorrhage and necrosis with collapse of cortical areas. *(Images courtesy of Dharam M. Ramnani, MD, Virginia Urology Pathology Laboratory, Richmond, VA.)*

COMPLICATED UTI

Complicated UTI presents as a systematic illness with an infectious focus in the urinary tract and frequently occurs in patients with an anatomic predisposition to infection, such as a foreign body in the urinary tract, or with factors predisposing to a delayed response to therapy.

DIAGNOSTIC TOOLS

History The diagnosis of any of the UTI syndromes or ASB begins with a detailed history **(Fig. 135-4)**. The history given by the patient has a high predictive value in uncomplicated cystitis. A meta-analysis evaluating the probability of acute UTI on the basis of history and

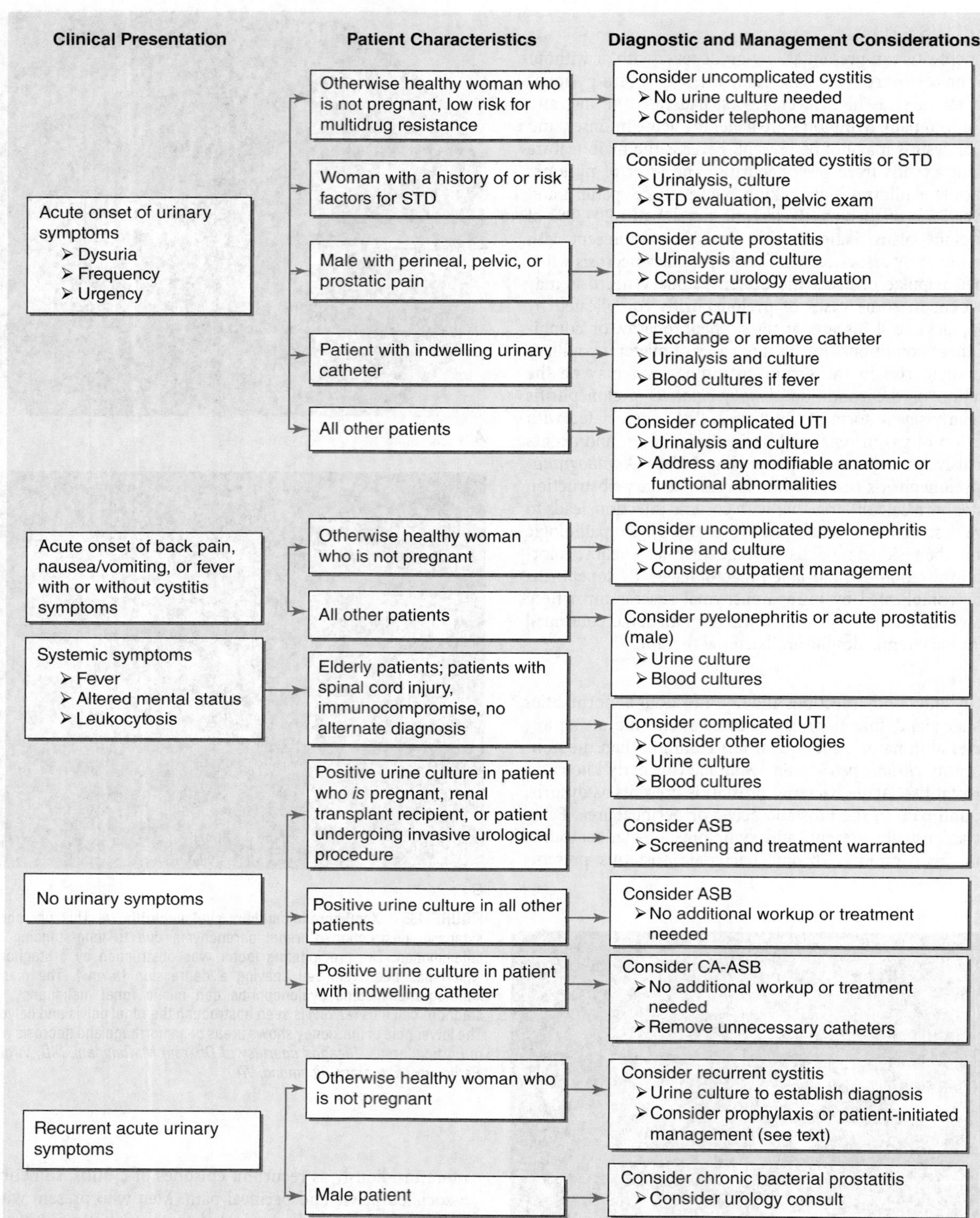

FIGURE 135-4 Diagnostic approach to urinary tract infection (UTI). ASB, asymptomatic bacteriuria; CA-ASB, catheter-associated ASB; CAUTI, catheter-associated UTI; STD, sexually transmitted disease.

physical findings concluded that, in women presenting with at least one symptom of UTI (dysuria, frequency, hematuria, or back pain) and without complicating factors, the probability of acute cystitis or pyelonephritis is 50%. The even higher rates of accuracy of self-diagnosis among women with recurrent UTI probably account for the success of patient-initiated treatment of recurrent cystitis. If vaginal discharge and complicating factors are absent and risk factors for UTI are present, then the probability of UTI is close to 90%, and no laboratory evaluation is needed. A combination of dysuria and urinary frequency in the absence of vaginal discharge increases the probability of UTI to 96%. Further laboratory evaluation with dipstick testing or urine culture is not necessary in such patients before the initiation of definitive therapy, unless concern for resistant pathogens suggests a need for urine culture.

In applying the patient's history as a diagnostic tool, the physician must remember that the studies included in the meta-analysis cited above did not enroll children, adolescents, pregnant women, men, or patients with complicated UTI. One significant concern is that sexually transmitted disease—that caused by *Chlamydia trachomatis* in particular—may be inappropriately treated as UTI. This concern is particularly relevant for female patients under the age of 25. The differential diagnosis to be considered when women present with dysuria includes cervicitis

(*C. trachomatis, Neisseria gonorrhoeae*), vaginitis (*Candida albicans, Trichomonas vaginalis*), herpetic urethritis, interstitial cystitis, and noninfectious vaginal or vulvar irritation. Women with more than one sexual partner and inconsistent use of condoms are at high risk for both UTI and sexually transmitted disease, and symptoms alone do not always distinguish between these conditions.

Urine Dipstick Test, Urinalysis, and Urine Culture Useful diagnostic tools include the urine dipstick test and urinalysis, both of which provide point-of-care information, and the urine culture, which can retrospectively confirm a prior diagnosis and provide organism susceptibility data for the patient's next UTI. Understanding the parameters of the dipstick test is important in interpreting its results. Only members of the family Enterobacteriaceae convert nitrate to nitrite, and enough nitrite must accumulate in the urine to reach the threshold of detection. If a woman with acute cystitis is forcing fluids and voiding frequently, the dipstick test for nitrite is less likely to be positive, even when *E. coli* is present. The leukocyte esterase test detects this enzyme in polymorphonuclear leukocytes in the host's urine, whether the cells are intact or lysed. Many reviews have attempted to describe the diagnostic accuracy of dipstick testing. The bottom line for clinicians is that a urine dipstick test can confirm the diagnosis of uncomplicated cystitis in a patient with a reasonably high pretest probability of this disease; either nitrite or leukocyte esterase positivity can be interpreted as a positive result. Blood in the urine also may suggest a diagnosis of UTI. A dipstick test negative for both nitrite and leukocyte esterase in this type of patient should prompt consideration of other explanations for the patient's symptoms and collection of urine for culture. A negative dipstick test is not sufficiently sensitive to rule out bacteriuria in pregnant women, in whom it is important to detect all episodes of bacteriuria.

Urine microscopy reveals pyuria in nearly all cases of cystitis and hematuria in ~30% of cases. In current practice, most hospital laboratories use an automated system rather than manual examination for urine microscopy. A machine aspirates a sample of the urine and then classifies the particles in the urine by size, shape, contrast, light scatter, volume, and other properties. These automated systems can be overwhelmed by high numbers of dysmorphic red blood cells, white blood cells, or crystals; in general, counts of bacteria are less accurate than are counts of red and white blood cells. The authors' clinical recommendation is that the patient's symptoms and presentation should outweigh an incongruent result on automated urinalysis.

The detection of bacteria in a urine culture from a patient with symptoms of cystitis can confirm the diagnosis of UTI; unfortunately, however, culture results do not become available until 24 h after the patient's presentation. Furthermore, the presence of bacteriuria does not mean the patient has urinary symptoms, so a positive urine culture is consistent with both cystitis and ASB. Identifying specific organism(s) can require an additional 24 h. Studies of women with symptoms of cystitis have found that a colony count threshold of $\geq 10^2$ bacteria/mL is more sensitive (95%) and specific (85%) than a threshold of 10^5/mL for the diagnosis of acute cystitis in women. In men, the minimal level indicating infection appears to be 10^3/mL. Urine specimens frequently become contaminated with the normal microbial flora of the distal urethra, vagina, or skin. These contaminants can grow to high numbers if the collected urine is allowed to stand at room temperature. In most instances, a culture that yields mixed bacterial species is contaminated except in settings of long-term catheterization, chronic urinary retention, or the presence of a fistula between the urinary tract and the gastrointestinal or genital tract.

DIAGNOSTIC APPROACH

The approach to diagnosis is influenced by which of the clinical UTI syndromes is suspected and presence of risk factors for resistance (Fig. 135-4).

Uncomplicated Cystitis in Women Uncomplicated cystitis in women can be treated on the basis of history alone. However, if the symptoms are not specific or if a reliable history cannot be obtained, then a urine dipstick test should be performed. A positive nitrite or leukocyte esterase result in a woman with one symptom of UTI increases the probability of UTI from 50% to ~80%, and empirical treatment can be considered without further testing. In this setting, a negative dipstick result does not rule out UTI, and a urine culture, close clinical follow-up, and possibly a pelvic examination are recommended. In women with pregnancy, suspected bacterial resistance, or recurrent UTI, a urine culture is warranted to guide appropriate therapy.

Cystitis in Men The signs and symptoms of cystitis in men are similar to those in women, but this disease differs in several important ways in the male population. Collection of urine for culture is strongly recommended when a man has symptoms of UTI, as the documentation of bacteriuria can differentiate the less common syndromes of acute and chronic bacterial prostatitis from the very common entity of chronic pelvic pain syndrome, which is not associated with bacteriuria and thus is not usually responsive to antibacterial therapy. Men with febrile UTI often have an elevated serum level of prostate-specific antigen as well as an enlarged prostate and enlarged seminal vesicles on ultrasound—findings indicative of prostate involvement. In a study of 85 men with febrile UTI, symptoms of urinary retention, early recurrence of UTI, hematuria at follow-up, and voiding difficulties were predictive of surgically correctable disorders. Men with none of these symptoms had normal upper and lower urinary tracts on urologic workup. In general, men with a first febrile UTI should have imaging performed (CT or ultrasound); if the diagnosis is unclear or if UTI is recurrent, referral for urologic consultation is appropriate.

Asymptomatic Bacteriuria The diagnosis of ASB involves both microbiologic and clinical criteria. The microbiologic criterion (including in urinary catheter–associated asymptomatic bacteriuria) is $\geq 10^5$ bacterial CFU/mL of urine. The clinical criterion is an absence of signs or symptoms referable to UTI.

TREATMENT

Urinary Tract Infections

Treatment of UTI accounts for a major proportion of antimicrobial use in ambulatory care, inpatient care, and long-term-care settings. Responsible use of antibiotics for this common infection has broad implications for preserving antibiotic effectiveness into the future. Nevertheless, antimicrobial therapy is warranted for any UTI that is truly symptomatic. The choice of antimicrobial agent, the dose, and the duration of therapy depend on the site of infection and the presence or absence of complicating conditions. Each category of UTI warrants a different approach based on the particular clinical syndrome.

Antimicrobial resistance among uropathogens varies from region to region and impacts the approach to empirical treatment of UTI. *E. coli* ST131 is the predominant multilocus sequence type found worldwide as the cause of multidrug-resistant UTI. Recommendations for treatment must be considered in the context of local resistance patterns and national differences in some agents' availability. For example, fosfomycin and pivmecillinam are not available in all countries but are considered first-line options where they are available because they retain activity against a majority of uropathogens that produce extended-spectrum β-lactamases. Thus, therapeutic choices should depend on local resistance, drug availability, and individual patient factors such as recent travel and antimicrobial use.

UNCOMPLICATED CYSTITIS IN WOMEN

Since the species and antimicrobial susceptibilities of the bacteria that cause acute uncomplicated cystitis are highly predictable, many episodes of uncomplicated cystitis can be managed over the telephone (Fig. 135-4). Most patients with other UTI syndromes require further diagnostic evaluation. Although the risk of serious complications with telephone management appears to be low, studies of telephone management algorithms generally have involved otherwise healthy women who are at low risk of complications of UTI.

In 1999, TMP-SMX was recommended as the first-line agent for treatment of uncomplicated UTI in the published guidelines of the Infectious Diseases Society of America. Since then, antibiotic resistance among uropathogens causing uncomplicated cystitis has increased, appreciation of the importance of collateral damage (as defined below) has increased, and newer agents have been studied. Unfortunately, there is no longer a single best agent for acute uncomplicated cystitis.

Collateral damage refers to the adverse ecologic effects of antimicrobial therapy, including killing of the normal flora and selection of drug-resistant organisms. The implication of collateral damage for UTI management is that a drug that is highly efficacious for the treatment of UTI is not necessarily the optimal first-line agent if it also has pronounced secondary effects on the normal flora or is likely to adversely affect resistance patterns. Drugs used for UTI that have a minimal effect on fecal flora include pivmecillinam, fosfomycin, and nitrofurantoin. In contrast, trimethoprim, TMP-SMX, quinolones, and ampicillin affect the fecal flora more significantly; these drugs are notably the agents for which rising resistance levels have been documented.

Choosing judiciously whether to initiate antibiotic therapy and then selecting the most urinary-focused agent for the shortest appropriate duration are important factors in global efforts to stem the rise of antimicrobial-resistant organisms. Several effective therapeutic regimens are available for acute uncomplicated cystitis in women (**Table 135-1**). Well-studied first-line agents include TMP-SMX and nitrofurantoin. Second-line agents include β-lactams. There is increasing experience with the use of fosfomycin for UTIs (including complicated infections), particularly for infections caused by multidrug-resistant *E. coli*. According to an advisory from the U.S. Food and Drug Administration (FDA), fluoroquinolones should not be used for uncomplicated cystitis unless no alternatives are available. Pivmecillinam is not currently available in the United States or Canada but is a popular agent in some European countries. The pros and cons of specific agents are discussed briefly below.

Traditionally, TMP-SMX has been recommended as first-line treatment for acute cystitis, and it remains appropriate to consider the use of this drug in regions with resistance rates not exceeding 20%. In women with recurrent UTI, prior cultures can be used as a guide to TMP-SMX susceptibility, although interim acquisition of resistant bacteria can occur. TMP-SMX resistance has clinical significance: in TMP-SMX-treated patients with resistant isolates, the time to symptom resolution is longer and rates of both clinical and microbiologic failure are higher. Individual host factors associated with an elevated risk of UTI caused by a strain of *E. coli* resistant to TMP-SMX include recent use of TMP-SMX or another antimicrobial agent and recent travel to an area with high rates of TMP-SMX resistance. Prior urine cultures with an organism resistant to TMP-SMX also are a strong indication of risk of resistance in the current infection. The optimal setting for empirical use of TMP-SMX is uncomplicated UTI in a female patient who has an established relationship with the practitioner and who can thus seek further care if her symptoms do not respond promptly.

Resistance to nitrofurantoin remains low despite >60 years of use, as several mutational steps are required for the development of bacterial resistance to this drug. Nitrofurantoin remains highly active against *E. coli* and most non–*E. coli* isolates. *Proteus, Pseudomonas, Serratia, Enterobacter*, and yeasts are all intrinsically resistant to this drug. Although nitrofurantoin has traditionally been prescribed as a 7-day regimen, guidelines now recommend a 5-day course, which is as effective as a 3-day course of TMP-SMX for treatment of acute cystitis; 3-day courses of nitrofurantoin are not recommended for acute cystitis. Nitrofurantoin does not reach significant levels in tissue and cannot be used to treat pyelonephritis.

Guidelines also recommend fosfomycin as a first-line agent to treat acute, uncomplicated cystitis in women. Oral fosfomycin is given as a single 3-g dose sachet (powder) that is dissolved in a glass of water and swallowed. Fosfomycin interferes with cell wall formation and is bactericidal. While fosfomycin susceptibility remains very high among *E. coli, Pseudomonas* is intrinsically resistant to fosfomycin, and its activity against *Klebsiella* species is unreliable. Fosfomycin susceptibility does not appear on standard, automated microbiological susceptibility reports.

Most fluoroquinolones are highly effective as short-course therapy for cystitis when the causative organism is susceptible to them; the exception is moxifloxacin, which may not reach adequate urinary levels. The fluoroquinolones commonly used for UTI include ciprofloxacin and levofloxacin. The two main concerns about fluoroquinolone use for acute cystitis are the propagation of fluoroquinolone resistance, not only among uropathogens but also among other organisms causing more serious and difficult-to-treat infections at other sites, and their rare but potentially serious adverse effects. For example, quinolone use in certain populations, including adults >60 years of age, has been associated with an increased risk of Achilles tendon rupture. Other potential side effects include irreversible neuropathy. An association with aortic dissection has been noted by both the FDA and the European Medicines Agency. In light of these detrimental effects, the FDA issued an advisory against using fluoroquinolones to treat acute cystitis in patients who have other therapeutic options.

β-Lactam agents generally have not performed as well as TMP-SMX or fluoroquinolones in acute cystitis. Rates of pathogen eradication are lower and relapse rates are higher with β-lactam drugs. The generally accepted explanation is that β-lactams fail to eradicate uropathogens from the vaginal reservoir. Many strains of *E. coli* that are resistant to TMP-SMX are also resistant to amoxicillin and cephalexin; thus, these drugs should be used only for patients

TABLE 135-1 Treatment Strategies for Acute Uncomplicated Cystitis

DRUG AND DOSE	ESTIMATED CLINICAL EFFICACY, %	ESTIMATED BACTERIAL EFFICACY,[a] %	COMMON SIDE EFFECTS
Nitrofurantoin, 100 mg bid × 5–7 d	87–95	82–92	Nausea, headache
TMP-SMX, 1 DS tablet bid × 3 d	86–100	85–100	Rash, urticaria, nausea, vomiting, hematologic abnormalities
Fosfomycin, 3-g single-dose sachet	83–95	78–98	Diarrhea, nausea, headache
Pivmecillinam, 400 mg bid × 3–7 d	55–82	74–84	Nausea, vomiting, diarrhea
Fluoroquinolones, dose varies by agent; 3-d regimen	81–98	78–96	Nausea, vomiting, diarrhea, headache, drowsiness, insomnia
β-Lactams, dose varies by agent; 5- to 7-d regimen[b]	79–98	74–98	Diarrhea, nausea, vomiting, rash, urticaria

[a]Microbial response as measured by reduction of bacterial counts in the urine. [b]Two trials tested cefpodoxime and one tested amoxicillin-clavulanate.

Note: Efficacy rates are averages or ranges calculated from the data and studies included in the 2010 Infectious Diseases Society of America/European Society of Clinical Microbiology and Infectious Diseases guideline for treatment of uncomplicated UTI and the 2014 *JAMA* systematic review on UTI in the outpatient setting. Ranges are estimates from published studies and may vary by specific agent and by rate of resistance.

Abbreviations: DS, double-strength; TMP-SMX, trimethoprim-sulfamethoxazole.

infected with susceptible strains. However, given rising resistance to TMP-SMX and the goal of avoiding fluoroquinolones, oral cephalosporins (such as cefpodoxime and cefixime) are increasingly appearing in UTI treatment algorithms.

Urinary analgesics are appropriate in certain situations to speed resolution of bladder discomfort. The urinary tract analgesic phenazopyridine is widely used but can cause significant nausea. Combination analgesics containing urinary antiseptics (methenamine, methylene blue), a urine-acidifying agent (sodium phosphate), and an antispasmodic agent (hyoscyamine) also are available.

Interest in the responsible use of antibiotics has led to exploration of antibiotic-sparing approaches to the treatment of acute uncomplicated cystitis. Both placebo and analgesics alone have proved inferior to antibiotics for resolution of symptoms and prevention of pyelonephritis. Delayed therapy, in which a woman receives a prescription for antibiotics but fills it only if symptoms fail to resolve in a day or two, has the potential advantage of avoiding antibiotic use in those who either do not have cystitis to begin with or have a mild case that resolves spontaneously. The downside is that women who really do have cystitis endure discomfort for a longer period and may meanwhile progress to pyelonephritis. However, one certain measure for more responsible use of antibiotics in cystitis is to treat for the correct duration; in practice, many episodes of acute cystitis are treated longer than is recommended by evidence-based guidelines.

PYELONEPHRITIS

Since patients with pyelonephritis have tissue-invasive disease, the treatment regimen chosen should have a very high likelihood of eradicating the causative organism and should reach therapeutic blood levels quickly. High rates of TMP-SMX-resistant *E. coli* in patients with pyelonephritis have made fluoroquinolones the first-line therapy for acute uncomplicated pyelonephritis. Whether the fluoroquinolones are given orally or parenterally depends on the patient's tolerance for oral intake. A randomized clinical trial demonstrated that a 7-day course of therapy with oral ciprofloxacin (500 mg twice daily, with or without an initial IV 400-mg dose) was highly effective for the initial management of pyelonephritis in the outpatient setting. Oral TMP-SMX (one double-strength tablet twice daily for 14 days) also is effective for treatment of acute uncomplicated pyelonephritis if the uropathogen is known to be susceptible. If the pathogen's susceptibility is not known and TMP-SMX is used, an initial IV 1-g dose of ceftriaxone is recommended. Oral β-lactam agents are less effective than the fluoroquinolones and should be used with caution and close follow-up. Options for parenteral therapy for uncomplicated pyelonephritis include fluoroquinolones, an extended-spectrum cephalosporin with or without an aminoglycoside, or a carbapenem. Combinations of a β-lactam and a β-lactamase inhibitor (e.g., ampicillin-sulbactam, piperacillin-tazobactam) or a carbapenem (imipenem-cilastatin, ertapenem, meropenem) can be used in patients with more complicated histories, previous episodes of pyelonephritis, anticipated antimicrobial resistance, or recent urinary tract manipulations; in general, the treatment of such patients should be guided by urine culture results. The treatment of very resistant organisms may require the use of newer, very broad-spectrum agents, in consultation with infectious disease specialists. Once the patient has responded clinically, oral therapy should be substituted for parenteral therapy.

UTI IN PREGNANT WOMEN

Nitrofurantoin, ampicillin, and the cephalosporins are considered relatively safe in early pregnancy. One retrospective case-control study suggesting an association between nitrofurantoin and birth defects has not been confirmed. Sulfonamides should clearly be avoided both in the first trimester (because of possible teratogenic effects) and near term (because of a possible role in the development of kernicterus). Fluoroquinolones are avoided because of possible adverse effects on fetal cartilage development. Ampicillin and the cephalosporins have been used extensively in pregnancy and are the drugs of choice for the treatment of asymptomatic or symptomatic UTI in this group of patients. Generally, pregnant women with ASB are treated for 4–7 days in the absence of evidence to support single-dose therapy. For pregnant women with overt pyelonephritis, parenteral β-lactam therapy with or without aminoglycosides is the standard of care.

UTI IN MEN

Since the prostate is involved in the majority of cases of febrile UTI in men, the goal in these patients is to eradicate the prostatic infection as well as the bladder infection. A 7- to 14-day course of a fluoroquinolone or TMP-SMX is recommended if the uropathogen is susceptible; clinical practice is tending toward the shorter, 7-day duration to reduce antibiotic exposure. If acute bacterial prostatitis is suspected, antimicrobial therapy should be initiated after urine and blood are obtained for cultures. Therapy can be tailored to urine culture results and should be continued for 2–4 weeks. For documented chronic bacterial prostatitis, a 4- to 6-week course of antibiotics is often necessary. Recurrences, which are not uncommon in chronic prostatitis, often warrant a 12-week course of treatment.

COMPLICATED UTI

Complicated UTI occurs in a heterogeneous group of patients, many with structural and functional abnormalities of the urinary tract and kidneys. The range of species and their susceptibility to antimicrobial agents are likewise heterogeneous. As a consequence, therapy for complicated UTI must be individualized and guided by urine culture results. Frequently, a patient with complicated UTI will have prior urine-culture data that can be used to guide empirical therapy while current culture results are pending. Xanthogranulomatous pyelonephritis is treated with nephrectomy. Percutaneous drainage can be used as the initial therapy in emphysematous pyelonephritis and can be followed by elective nephrectomy as needed. Papillary necrosis with obstruction requires intervention to relieve the obstruction and to preserve renal function.

ASYMPTOMATIC BACTERIURIA

Treatment of ASB does not decrease the frequency of symptomatic infections or complications except in pregnant women, persons undergoing urologic surgery, and perhaps neutropenic patients and renal transplant recipients. Treatment of ASB in pregnant women and patients undergoing urologic procedures should be directed by urine culture results. In all other populations, screening for and treatment of ASB are discouraged. The majority of cases of catheter-associated bacteriuria are asymptomatic and do not warrant antimicrobial therapy.

CATHETER-ASSOCIATED UTI

Multiple institutions have released guidelines for the treatment of CAUTI, which is defined by bacteriuria and symptoms in a catheterized patient. The signs and symptoms either are localized to the urinary tract or can include otherwise unexplained systemic manifestations, such as fever. The accepted threshold for bacteriuria to meet the definition of CAUTI is $\geq 10^3$ CFU/mL of urine, while the threshold for bacteriuria to meet the definition of ASB is $\geq 10^5$ CFU/mL.

As catheters provide a conduit for bacteria to enter the bladder, bacteriuria is inevitable with long-term catheter use. The typical signs and symptoms of UTI, including pain, urgency, dysuria, fever, peripheral leukocytosis, and pyuria, have less predictive value for the diagnosis of infection in catheterized patients. Furthermore, the presence of bacteria in the urine of a patient who is febrile and catheterized does not necessarily mean that the patient has CAUTI, and other explanations for the fever should be considered.

The etiology of CAUTI is diverse, and urine culture results are essential to guide treatment. Fairly good evidence supports the practice of catheter change during treatment for CAUTI. The goal is to remove biofilm-associated organisms that could serve as a nidus for reinfection. Pathology studies reveal that many patients with long-term catheters have occult pyelonephritis. A randomized trial in persons with spinal cord injury who were undergoing intermittent catheterization found that relapse was more common after 3 days of therapy than after 14 days. In general, a 7- to 14-day course of antibiotics is recommended, but further studies on the optimal duration of therapy are needed.

The best strategy for prevention of CAUTI is to avoid insertion of unnecessary catheters and to remove catheters once they are no longer necessary. Quality-improvement collaboratives that have addressed technical aspects of CAUTI prevention (such as avoidance of inappropriate catheterization) as well as team communication strategies have shown the benefit of this approach in decreasing CAUTI in both acute- and long-term-care settings. Antimicrobial catheters impregnated with silver or nitrofurazone have not been shown to provide significant clinical benefit in terms of reducing rates of symptomatic UTI. Evidence is insufficient to recommend suprapubic catheters and condom catheters as alternatives to indwelling urinary catheters as a means to prevent bacteriuria. However, intermittent catheterization may be preferable to long-term indwelling urethral catheterization in certain populations (e.g., spinal cord–injured persons) to prevent both infectious and anatomic complications.

CANDIDURIA

The appearance of *Candida* in the urine is an increasingly common complication of indwelling catheterization, particularly for patients in the intensive care unit, those taking broad-spectrum antimicrobial drugs, and those with underlying diabetes mellitus. In many studies, >50% of urinary *Candida* isolates have been found to be non-*albicans* species. The clinical presentation varies from a laboratory finding without symptoms to pyelonephritis and even sepsis. Removal of the urethral catheter results in resolution of candiduria in more than one-third of asymptomatic cases. Treatment of asymptomatic patients does not appear to decrease the frequency of recurrence of candiduria. Therapy is recommended for patients who have symptomatic cystitis or pyelonephritis and for those who are at high risk for disseminated disease. High-risk patients include those with neutropenia, those who are undergoing urologic manipulation, those who are clinically unstable, and low-birth-weight infants. Fluconazole (200–400 mg/d for 7–14 days) reaches high levels in urine and is the first-line regimen for *Candida* infections of the urinary tract. Although instances of successful eradication of candiduria by some of the newer azoles and echinocandins have been reported, these agents are characterized by only low-level urinary excretion and thus are not recommended. For *Candida* isolates with high levels of resistance to fluconazole, oral flucytosine and/or parenteral amphotericin B are options. Bladder irrigation with amphotericin B generally is not recommended.

PREVENTION OF RECURRENT UTI IN WOMEN

Recurrence of uncomplicated cystitis in reproductive-age women is common, and a preventive strategy is indicated if recurrent UTIs are interfering with a patient's lifestyle. The threshold of two or more symptomatic episodes per year is not absolute; decisions about interventions should take the patient's preferences into account.

Three prophylactic strategies are available: continuous, postcoital, and patient-initiated therapy. Continuous prophylaxis and postcoital prophylaxis usually entail low doses of TMP-SMX or nitrofurantoin. These regimens are all highly effective during the period of active antibiotic intake. Typically, a prophylactic regimen is prescribed for 6 months and then discontinued, at which point the rate of recurrent UTI often returns to baseline. If bothersome infections recur, the prophylactic program can be reinstituted for a longer period. Selection of resistant strains in the fecal flora has been documented in studies of women taking prophylactic antibiotics for 12 months.

Patient-initiated therapy involves supplying the patient with materials for urine culture and with a course of antibiotics for self-medication at the first symptoms of infection. The urine culture is refrigerated and delivered to the physician's office for confirmation of the diagnosis. When an established and reliable patient–provider relationship exists, the urine culture can be omitted as long as the symptomatic episodes respond completely to short-course therapy and are not followed by relapse.

Non-antimicrobial prevention is increasingly being studied. Lactobacillus probiotics are one appealing approach to UTI prevention, but there is a paucity of data to support this strategy. Similarly, studies of cranberry products for UTI prevention have produced mixed results. Varied dosing and product composition between studies remain an issue for providing clinical guidance.

PROGNOSIS

Cystitis is a risk factor for recurrent cystitis and pyelonephritis. ASB is common among elderly and catheterized patients but does not in itself increase the risk of death. The relationships among recurrent UTI, chronic pyelonephritis, and renal insufficiency have been widely studied. In the absence of anatomic abnormalities such as reflux, recurrent infection in children and adults does not lead to chronic pyelonephritis or to renal failure. Moreover, infection does not play a primary role in chronic interstitial nephritis; the primary etiologic factors in this condition are analgesic abuse, obstruction, reflux, and toxin exposure. In the presence of underlying renal abnormalities (particularly obstructing stones), infection as a secondary factor can accelerate renal parenchymal damage.

FURTHER READING

Grigoryan L et al: Urinary tract infections in young adults. JAMA 312:1677, 2014.

Gupta K et al: International clinical practice guidelines for the treatment of acute uncomplicated cystitis and pyelonephritis in women: A 2010 update by the Infectious Diseases Society of America and the European Society for Microbiology and Infectious Diseases. Clin Infect Dis 52:e103, 2011.

Gupta K et al: Urinary tract infection. Ann Intern Med 167:ITC49, 2017.

Hooton TM et al: Diagnosis, prevention, and treatment of catheter-associated urinary tract infection in adults: 2009 international clinical practice guidelines from the Infectious Diseases Society of America. Clin Infect Dis 50:625, 2010.

Hooton TM et al: Voided midstream urine culture and acute cystitis in premenopausal women. N Engl J Med 369;1883, 2013.

Hooton TM et al: Asymptomatic bacteriuria and pyuria in premenopausal women. Clin Infect Dis 72:1332, 2021.

Nicolle LE et al: Clinical Practice Guideline for the Management of Asymptomatic Bacteriuria: 2019 Update by the Infectious Diseases Society of America. Clin Infect Dis 68:1611, 2019.

136 Sexually Transmitted Infections: Overview and Clinical Approach

Jeanne M. Marrazzo, King K. Holmes

CLASSIFICATION AND EPIDEMIOLOGY

Worldwide, most adults acquire at least one sexually transmitted infection (STI), and many remain at risk for complications. Each day, for example, more than 1 million STIs are acquired worldwide, placing many affected persons at risk for adverse reproductive health outcomes and neoplasia. Certain STIs, such as syphilis, gonorrhea, HIV infection, hepatitis B, and chancroid, often occur in highly interconnected sexual networks characterized by high rates of partner change or multiple concurrent partners. Such networks, for example, often include persons who engage in transactional sex, men who have sex with men (MSM), and persons involved in the use of illicit drugs, particularly methamphetamine. Other STIs are distributed more evenly throughout populations. For example, chlamydial infections, genital human papillomavirus (HPV) infections, and genital herpes can spread efficiently even in relatively low-risk populations. Finally, modern technologies based on detection of nucleic acid have accelerated elucidation of the role of sexual transmission in the spread of some viruses, including Ebola virus and Zika virus, and have provided new evidence of apparent sexual transmission of several bacteria, including group C *Neisseria meningitidis* and anaerobes associated with bacterial vaginosis (BV).

In general, the product of three factors determines the initial rate of spread of any STI within a population: rate of sexual exposure of susceptible to infectious people, efficiency of transmission per exposure, and duration of infectivity of those infected. Accordingly, efforts to prevent and control STIs aim to decrease the rate of sexual exposure of susceptible to infected persons (e.g., through education and efforts to change sexual behavior norms and through control efforts aimed at reducing the proportion of the population infected); to decrease the duration of infectivity (through early diagnosis and curative or suppressive treatment); and to decrease the efficiency of transmission (through promotion of condom use and safer sexual practices, use of effective vaccines, and male medical circumcision).

In all societies, STIs rank among the most common of all infectious diseases, with at least 40 microorganisms now classified as predominantly sexually transmitted or as frequently sexually transmissible (**Table 136-1**). In developing countries, with three-quarters of the world's population and 90% of the world's STIs, factors such as population growth (especially in adolescent and young-adult age groups), rural-to-urban migration, wars, limited or no provision of reproductive health services for women, and poverty create exceptional vulnerability to disease resulting from unprotected sex. During the 1990s in China, Russia, the other states of the former Soviet Union, and South Africa, internal social structures changed rapidly as borders opened to the West, unleashing enormous new epidemics of HIV infection and other STIs. Despite advances in the provision of highly effective antiretroviral therapy worldwide, HIV remains the leading cause of death in some developing countries, and HPV and hepatitis B virus (HBV) remain important causes of cervical and hepatocellular carcinoma, respectively—two of the most common (and preventable) malignancies in the developing world. Sexually transmitted herpes simplex virus (HSV) infection causes most genital ulcer disease throughout the world, and an increasing proportion of cases of genital herpes occur in developing countries with generalized HIV epidemics, where the positive-feedback loop between HSV and HIV transmission remains intractable. Despite this consistent link, randomized trials evaluating the efficacy of antiviral therapy in suppressing HSV in both HIV-uninfected and HIV-infected persons have demonstrated no protective effect against acquisition or transmission of HIV. The World Health Organization estimated that 357 million new cases of four curable STIs—gonorrhea, chlamydial infection, syphilis, and trichomoniasis—occurred annually in recent years. Up to 50% of women of reproductive age in developing countries have BV (arguably acquired sexually). All of these curable STIs have been associated with increased risk of HIV transmission or acquisition.

In the United States, the prevalence of antibody to HSV-2 began to fall in the late 1990s, especially among adolescents and young adults; the decline was presumably due to delayed sexual debut, increased condom use, and lower rates of multiple (four or more) sex partners—all well documented by the U.S. Youth Risk Behavior Surveillance System. The estimated annual incidence of HBV infection has also declined dramatically since the mid-1980s; this decrease is probably attributable to now-widespread administration of hepatitis B vaccine in infancy. Genital HPV remains the most common sexually transmitted pathogen in the United States, infecting 60% of a cohort of initially HPV-negative, sexually active Washington state college women within 5 years in a study conducted from 1990 to 2000—i.e., during the pre-HPV immunization era. Global expansion of HPV vaccine coverage among young women has already shown promise in reducing the incidence of infection with the HPV types included in the vaccines and of conditions associated with these viruses, including invasive cervical cancer.

In industrialized countries, fear of HIV infection in the mid-1980s and through the mid-2000s, coupled with widespread behavioral interventions and better-organized systems of care for the curable STIs, initially helped curb the transmission of several STDs. However, with current antiretroviral therapy, HIV has become for many a chronic disease associated with a normal life span and high quality of life. Rates of gonorrhea and syphilis remain higher in the United States than in any other Western industrialized country.

In the United States, the Centers for Disease Control and Prevention (CDC) has compiled reported rates of STIs since 1941. The incidence of reported gonorrhea peaked at 468 cases per 100,000 population in the mid-1970s and fell to a low of 98 cases per 100,000 in 2012; in 2018, the case rate was 179.1 per 100,000 persons, which is more than an 80% increase since 2009 when the number of new cases reached an all-time low. With increased testing and more sensitive tests, the incidence of reported *Chlamydia trachomatis* infection has been increasing steadily since reporting began in 1984, reaching an all-time peak of 457.6 cases per 100,000 in 2011. The incidence of primary and secondary syphilis per 100,000 peaked at 71 cases in 1946, fell rapidly to 3.9 cases in 1956, ranged from ~10 to 15 cases through 1987 (with markedly increased rates among MSM and African Americans), and then fell to a nadir of 2.1 cases in 2000–2001 (with rates falling most rapidly among heterosexual African Americans). However, since 1996, with the introduction of highly active antiretroviral therapy, gonorrhea, syphilis, and chlamydial infection have had a remarkable resurgence among MSM in North America and Europe, where outbreaks of a rare type of chlamydial infection (lymphogranuloma venereum [LGV])

TABLE 136-1 Sexually Transmitted and Sexually Transmissible Microorganisms

BACTERIA	VIRUSES	OTHER[a]
Transmitted in Adults Predominantly by Sexual Intercourse		
Neisseria gonorrhoeae	HIV (types 1 and 2)	*Trichomonas vaginalis*
Chlamydia trachomatis	Human T-cell lymphotropic virus type 1	*Pthirus pubis*
Treponema pallidum	Herpes simplex virus type 2	
Haemophilus ducreyi	Human papillomavirus (multiple genital genotypes)	
Klebsiella (Calymmatobacterium) granulomatis	Hepatitis B virus[b]	
Ureaplasma urealyticum	Molluscum contagiosum virus	
Mycoplasma genitalium		
Sexual Transmission Repeatedly Described but Not Well Defined or Not the Predominant Mode		
Mycoplasma hominis	Cytomegalovirus	*Candida albicans*
Gardnerella vaginalis and other vaginal bacteria	Human T-cell lymphotropic virus type 2	*Sarcoptes scabiei*
Group B *Streptococcus*	Hepatitis C virus	
Mobiluncus spp.	(?) Hepatitis D virus	
Helicobacter cinaedi	Herpes simplex virus type 1	
Helicobacter fennelliae	Zika virus	
Anaerobes associated with bacterial vaginosis	Ebola virus	
Leptotrichia/Sneathia	(?) Epstein-Barr virus	
Group C *Neisseria meningitidis*	Human herpesvirus type 8	
Transmitted by Sexual Contact Involving Oral–Fecal Exposure; of Declining Importance in Men Who Have Sex with Men		
Shigella spp.	Hepatitis A virus	*Giardia lamblia*
Campylobacter spp.		*Entamoeba histolytica*

[a]Includes protozoa, ectoparasites, and fungi. [b]Among U.S. patients for whom a risk factor can be ascertained, most hepatitis B virus infections are transmitted sexually.

that had virtually disappeared during the AIDS era have occurred. In 2018, ~75% of primary and secondary syphilis cases reported to the CDC were in MSM, but incidence has also increased in women with a concomitant increase in congenital syphilis. Moreover, the uptake of oral pre-exposure prophylaxis for HIV-1 acquisition has increased among MSM since its initial approval for this purpose in 2012 and has been associated with reports of reduced condom-use frequency and concomitantly increased STI acquisition. These developments have resulted in a soaring incidence of STIs, with increasing co-infection with HIV and other sexually transmitted pathogens (particularly *Treponema pallidum*, the cause of syphilis; and *Neisseria gonorrhoeae*, the cause of gonorrhea), primarily among MSM.

MANAGEMENT OF COMMON SEXUALLY TRANSMITTED DISEASE (STD) SYNDROMES

Although other chapters discuss management of specific STIs, most patients are managed (at least initially) on the basis of presenting symptoms and signs and associated risk factors, even in industrialized countries. **Table 136-2** lists some of the most common clinical STD syndromes and their microbial etiologies. Strategies for their management are outlined below. **Chapters 201 and 202 address the management of infections with human retroviruses.**

STD care and management begin with risk assessment and proceed to clinical assessment, diagnostic testing or screening, treatment, and prevention. Risk assessment guides detection and interpretation of symptoms that could denote an STD; decisions on screening or prophylactic/preventive treatment; risk reduction counseling and intervention (e.g., hepatitis B vaccination); treatment of partners of patients with known infections; and behavioral risk reduction by the patient. Consideration of routine demographic data (e.g., gender, age, area of residence) is a simple first step in this risk assessment. For example, national guidelines strongly recommend routine screening of sexually active females ≤25 years of age for *C. trachomatis* infection. **Table 136-3** provides a set of 11 STD/HIV risk-assessment questions that clinicians can pose verbally or that health care systems can adapt (with yes/no responses) into a routine self-administered questionnaire. The initial framing statement gives permission to discuss topics that may be difficult for the patient to disclose.

Risk assessment is followed by clinical assessment (elicitation of information on specific current symptoms and signs of STDs). Confirmatory diagnostic tests (for persons with symptoms or signs) or screening tests (for those without symptoms or signs) may involve microscopic examination, culture, nucleic acid amplification tests (NAATs), or serology. Initial syndrome-based treatment should cover the most likely causes. For certain syndromes, results of rapid tests can narrow the spectrum of this initial therapy (e.g., pH of vaginal fluid for women with vaginal discharge, Gram's stain of urethral discharge for men with urethral discharge, rapid plasma reagin test for genital ulcer to assess the probability of syphilis). After the institution of treatment, STD management proceeds to the "4 Cs" of prevention and control: *c*ontact tracing (see "Prevention and Control of STIs," below), ensuring *c*ompliance with therapy, and *c*ounseling on risk reduction, including *c*ondom promotion and provision as well as motivational interviewing for risk reduction.

Consistent with current guidelines, all adults should be screened for infection with HIV-1 at least once, and more frequently if they are at elevated risk for acquisition of this infection.

TABLE 136-2 Major Sexually Transmitted Disease Syndromes and Sexually Transmitted Microbial Etiologies

SYNDROME	SEXUALLY TRANSMITTED MICROBIAL ETIOLOGIES
AIDS	HIV types 1 and 2
Urethritis: males	*Neisseria gonorrhoeae, Chlamydia trachomatis, Mycoplasma genitalium, Ureaplasma urealyticum* (subspecies *urealyticum*), *Trichomonas vaginalis*, HSV, some anaerobic bacteria, *Leptotrichia/Sneathia*
Epididymitis	*C. trachomatis, N. gonorrhoeae*, and (in older men or men who have sex with men) coliform bacteria
Lower genital tract infections: females	
Cystitis/urethritis	*C. trachomatis, N. gonorrhoeae*, HSV
Mucopurulent cervicitis	*C. trachomatis, N. gonorrhoeae, M. genitalium*
Vulvitis	*Candida albicans*, HSV
Bartholinitis	*C. albicans, T. vaginalis*
Vulvovaginitis	*C. albicans, T. vaginalis*
BV	BV-associated bacteria (see text)
Acute pelvic inflammatory disease	*N. gonorrhoeae, C. trachomatis*, BV-associated bacteria, *M. genitalium*, group B streptococci
Infertility	*N. gonorrhoeae, C. trachomatis*, BV-associated bacteria
Ulcerative lesions of the genitalia	HSV-1, HSV-2, *Treponema pallidum, Haemophilus ducreyi, C. trachomatis* (LGV strains), *Klebsiella (Calymmatobacterium) granulomatis*
Complications of pregnancy/puerperium	Several pathogens implicated
Intestinal infections	
Proctitis	*C. trachomatis, N. gonorrhoeae*, HSV, *T. pallidum*
Proctocolitis or enterocolitis	*Campylobacter* spp., *Shigella* spp., *Entamoeba histolytica, Helicobacter* spp., other enteric pathogens
Enteritis	*Giardia lamblia*
Acute arthritis with urogenital infection or viremia	*N. gonorrhoeae* (e.g., DGI), *C. trachomatis* (e.g., reactive arthritis), HBV
Genital and anal warts	HPV (30 genital types)
Mononucleosis syndrome	CMV, HIV, EBV
Hepatitis	Hepatitis viruses, *T. pallidum*, CMV, EBV
Neoplasias	
Squamous cell dysplasias and cancers of the cervix, anus, vulva, vagina, or penis	HPV (especially types 16, 18, 31, 45)
Kaposi's sarcoma, body-cavity lymphomas	HHV-8
T-cell leukemia	HTLV-1
Hepatocellular carcinoma	HBV
Tropical spastic paraparesis	HTLV-1
Scabies	*Sarcoptes scabiei*
Pubic lice	*Pthirus pubis*

Abbreviations: BV, bacterial vaginosis; CMV, cytomegalovirus; DGI, disseminated gonococcal infection; EBV, Epstein-Barr virus; HBV, hepatitis B virus; HHV-8, human herpesvirus type 8; HPV, human papillomavirus; HSV, herpes simplex virus; HTLV, human T-cell lymphotropic virus; LGV, lymphogranuloma venereum.

■ URETHRITIS IN MEN

Urethritis in men produces urethral discharge, dysuria, or both, usually without frequency of urination. Causes include *N. gonorrhoeae, C. trachomatis, Mycoplasma genitalium, Ureaplasma urealyticum, Trichomonas vaginalis*, HSV, and (rarely) adenovirus.

Until recently, *C. trachomatis* caused ~30–40% of cases of nongonococcal urethritis (NGU), particularly in heterosexual men; however, the proportion of cases due to this organism has probably declined in some populations served by effective chlamydial control programs, and older men with urethritis appear less likely to have chlamydial infection. HSV and *T. vaginalis* each cause a small proportion of NGU cases in the United States. Recently, multiple studies have consistently implicated *M. genitalium* as a probable cause of many *Chlamydia*-negative cases. Fewer studies than in the past have implicated *Ureaplasma*; the ureaplasmas have been differentiated into *U. urealyticum* and *Ureaplasma parvum*, and a few studies suggest that *U. urealyticum*—but not *U. parvum*—is associated with NGU; for this reason, neither testing nor presumptive treatment for ureaplasmas in the setting of urethritis is recommended. Coliform bacteria can cause urethritis in men who

TABLE 136-3 Eleven-Question Sexually Transmitted Disease (STD)/HIV Risk Assessment

Framing Statement	
In order to provide the best care for you today and to understand your risk for certain infections, it is necessary for us to talk about your sexual behavior.	
Screening Questions	
(1) Do you have any reason to think you might have a sexually transmitted infection? If so, what reason?	
(2) For all adolescents <18 years old: Have you begun having any kind of sex yet?	
STD History	
(3) Have you ever had any sexually transmitted infections or any genital infections? If so, which ones?	
Sexual Preference	
(4) Have you had sex with men, women, or both?	
Injection Drug Use	
(5) Have you ever injected yourself ("shot up") with drugs? (If yes, have you ever shared needles or injection equipment?)	
(6) Have you ever had sex with a gay or bisexual man or with anyone who had ever injected drugs?	
Characteristics of Partner(s)	
(7) Has your sex partner had any sexually transmitted infections? If so, which ones?	
(8) Has your sex partner had other sex partners during the time you've been together?	
STD Symptoms Checklist	
(9) Have you recently developed any of these symptoms?	
For Men	**For Women**
(a) Discharge of pus (drip) from the penis	(a) Abnormal vaginal discharge (increased amount, abnormal odor, abnormal yellow color)
(b) Genital sores (ulcers) or rash	(b) Genital sores (ulcers), rash, or itching
Sexual Practices, Past 2 Months (for patients answering yes to any of the above questions, to guide examination and testing)	
(10) Now I'd like to ask what parts of your body may have been sexually exposed to an STD (e.g., your penis, mouth, vagina, anus).	
Query About Interest in STD Screening Tests (for patients answering no to all of the above questions)	
(11) Would you like to be tested for HIV or any other STDs today? (If yes, clinician can explore which STD and why.)	

Source: Adapted from JR Curtis, KK Holmes, in KK Holmes et al (eds): *Sexually Transmitted Diseases,* 4th ed. New York, McGraw-Hill, 2008.

practice insertive anal intercourse. More recently, anaerobic bacteria that are characteristically involved in BV, especially *Leptotrichia/Sneathia* species, have occasionally been associated with urethritis in heterosexual men. Recommendations for the initial diagnosis of urethritis in men currently include specific tests only for *N. gonorrhoeae* and *C. trachomatis*; they do not yet include testing for *M. genitalium*, although a NAAT is now commercially available for the latter.

APPROACH TO THE PATIENT

Urethritis in Men

The following summarizes the approach to the male patient with suspected urethritis:

1. *Establish the presence of urethritis.* If proximal-to-distal "milking" of the urethra does not express a purulent or mucopurulent discharge, even after the patient has not voided for several hours (or preferably overnight), a Gram's-stained smear of an anterior urethral specimen obtained by passage of a small urethrogenital swab 2–3 cm into the urethra usually reveals ≥2 neutrophils per 1000× field when urethritis is present; in gonococcal infection, such a smear usually reveals gram-negative intracellular diplococci as well. Alternatively, the centrifuged sediment of the first 20–30 mL of voided urine—ideally collected as the first morning specimen—can be examined for inflammatory cells, either by microscopy showing ≥10 leukocytes per high-power field or by the leukocyte esterase test. Patients with symptoms who lack objective evidence of urethritis generally do not benefit from repeated courses of antibiotics, and other etiologies of such symptoms may be considered.
2. *Evaluate for complications or alternative diagnoses.* A brief history and examination can exclude epididymitis and systemic complications, such as disseminated gonococcal infection (DGI) and reactive arthritis. Although digital examination of the prostate gland seldom contributes to the evaluation of sexually active young men with urethritis, men with dysuria who lack evidence of urethritis as well as sexually inactive men with urethritis should undergo prostate palpation, urinalysis, and urine culture to exclude bacterial prostatitis and cystitis.
3. *Evaluate for gonococcal and chlamydial infection.* An absence of typical gram-negative diplococci on Gram's-stained smear of urethral exudate containing inflammatory cells warrants a preliminary diagnosis of NGU, as this test is 98% sensitive for the diagnosis of gonococcal urethral infection. However, most men with symptoms and/or signs of urethritis are simultaneously assessed for infection with *N. gonorrhoeae* and *C. trachomatis* by NAATs of first-catch urine. The urine specimen tested should consist of the first 10–15 mL of the stream, and if possible, patients should not have voided for the prior 2 h. Culture or NAAT for *N. gonorrhoeae* may yield positive results even when Gram's staining is negative; certain strains of *N. gonorrhoeae* can result in negative urethral Gram's stains in up to 30% of cases of urethral infection. Results of tests for gonococcal and chlamydial infection predict the patient's prognosis (with greater risk for recurrent NGU if neither chlamydiae nor gonococci are found than if either is detected) and can guide both the counseling given to the patient and the management of the patient's sexual partner(s).
4. *Treat urethritis promptly while test results are pending.*

TREATMENT

Urethritis in Men

Table 136-4 summarizes the steps in management of urethral discharge and/or dysuria in sexually active men.

In practice, if Gram's stain does not reveal gonococci, urethritis is treated with a regimen effective for NGU, such as azithromycin or doxycycline. Both are effective. Although azithromycin has been more effective than doxycycline for *M. genitalium* infection, the efficacy of azithromycin for treatment of *M. genitalium* is rapidly declining. Alternatives include moxifloxacin and pristinamycin, a streptogramin antibiotic available in some countries. If gonococci are demonstrated by Gram's stain or if no diagnostic tests are performed to exclude gonorrhea definitively, treatment should include parenteral cephalosporin therapy for gonorrhea (**Chap. 156**). Azithromycin is effective for treating *C. trachomatis* infection, which can cause urethral co-infection in men with gonococcal urethritis. Sexual partners with contact to the index patient in the past 60 days should also be tested for gonorrhea and chlamydial infection. Regardless of whether they are tested for these infections, however, they should receive the same regimen given to the male index case. Patients with confirmed persistence or recurrence of urethritis after treatment should be re-treated with the initial regimen if they did not comply with the original treatment or were reexposed to an untreated partner. Most persistent urethritis is due to *M. genitalium*, and prompt diagnostic testing and/or treatment for *M. genitalium* is recommended.

National and international guidelines do exist for treatment of gonococcal urethritis, typically with ceftriaxone. However,

TABLE 136-4 Management of Urethral Discharge in Men

USUAL CAUSES	USUAL INITIAL EVALUATION
Chlamydia trachomatis *Neisseria gonorrhoeae* *Mycoplasma genitalium* *Ureaplasma urealyticum* *Trichomonas vaginalis* Herpes simplex virus	Demonstration of urethral discharge or pyuria Exclusion of local or systemic complications Urethral Gram's stain to confirm urethritis, detect gram-negative diplococci Test for *N. gonorrhoeae, C. trachomatis*
Initial Treatment for Patient and Partners	
Treat gonorrhea (unless excluded): Ceftriaxone (500 mg IM[a])	
Management of Recurrence	
Confirm objective evidence of urethritis. If patient was reexposed to untreated or new partner, repeat treatment of patient and partner. If patient was not reexposed, consider infection with *T. vaginalis*[b] or antibiotic-resistant *M. genitalium*[c], and treat accordingly (metronidazole for trichomoniasis; azithromycin for *M. genitalium* followed by moxifloxacin if needed.	

[a]Neither oral cephalosporins nor fluoroquinolones are recommended for treatment of gonorrhea in the United States because of the emergence of increasing fluoroquinolone resistance in *N. gonorrhoeae,* especially (but not only) among men who have sex with men, and the decreasing susceptibility of a still-small proportion of gonococci to ceftriaxone (Fig. 136-1). Updates on the emergence of antimicrobial resistance in *N. gonorrhoeae* can be obtained from the Centers for Disease Control and Prevention at *http://www.cdc.gov/std.* [b]In men, the diagnosis of *T. vaginalis* infection requires nucleic acid amplification testing of a urethral swab specimen obtained before voiding. [c]*M. genitalium* is often resistant to doxycycline and azithromycin but is usually susceptible to the fluoroquinolone moxifloxacin. Moxifloxacin can be considered for treatment of refractory nongonococcal, nonchlamydial urethritis.

consensus is still lacking on treatment of urethritis that persists after treatment and cure of gonorrhea. Ideally, the approach would involve testing for potential causes of persistent urethritis (e.g., *M. genitalium*) and antimicrobial susceptibility testing in settings and populations where antimicrobial resistance is emerging. Currently, assays are available that can detect *M. genitalium*, and some experts believe it is time to integrate such testing into STD care. If *M. genitalium* is detected, the persistent urethritis can be treated with azithromycin or moxifloxacin in light of local patterns of antimicrobial susceptibility.

In heterosexual men with a high likelihood of exposure to trichomoniasis, an intraurethral swab specimen and a first-voided urine sample should be tested for *T. vaginalis* using NAAT. Presumptive treatment with metronidazole or tinidazole (2 g by mouth in a single dose) should be given. For MSM, trichomoniasis is unlikely, and consideration of a course of moxifloxacin is warranted. Because MSM also have the highest prevalence rates of antimicrobial-resistant *N. gonorrhoeae*, this possibility, even if apparently ruled out at the initial presentation, should be kept in mind.

EPIDIDYMITIS

Acute epididymitis, almost always unilateral, produces pain, swelling, and tenderness of the epididymis, with or without symptoms or signs of urethritis. This condition must be differentiated from testicular torsion, tumor, and trauma. Torsion, a surgical emergency, usually occurs in the second or third decade of life and produces a sudden onset of pain, elevation of the testicle within the scrotal sac, rotation of the epididymis from a posterior to an anterior position, and absence of blood flow on Doppler ultrasound. Persistence of symptoms after a course of therapy for epididymitis suggests the possibility of testicular tumor or of a chronic granulomatous disease, such as tuberculosis. In sexually active men under age 35, acute epididymitis is caused most frequently by *C. trachomatis* and less commonly by *N. gonorrhoeae* and is usually associated with overt or subclinical urethritis. Acute epididymitis occurring in older men or following urinary tract instrumentation is usually caused by urinary pathogens. These older men usually have no urethritis but do have bacteriuria. Similarly, epididymitis in MSM who have practiced insertive rectal intercourse is often caused by Enterobacteriaceae.

TREATMENT

Epididymitis

Ceftriaxone (500 mg as a single dose IM) followed by doxycycline (100 mg by mouth twice daily for 10 days) constitutes effective treatment for epididymitis caused by *N. gonorrhoeae* or *C. trachomatis*. Neither oral cephalosporins nor fluoroquinolones are recommended for treatment of gonorrhea in the United States because of resistance in *N. gonorrhoeae,* especially (but not only) among MSM **(Fig. 136-1)**. Given rapidly escalating rates of resistance in *N. gonorrhoeae* to azithromycin, this antibiotic is no longer recommended as co-therapy with a parenteral ceftriaxone for gonorrhea. When infection with Enterobacteriaceae is suspected, oral levofloxacin (500 mg once daily for 10 days) or ofloxacin (300 mg twice daily for 10 days) is effective for syndrome-based initial treatment of epididymitis; however, because this regimen is not effective against gonococcal or chlamydial infection, it should be combined with effective therapy for possible gonococcal or chlamydial infection of the epididymis unless bacteriuria with Enterobacteriaceae is confirmed.

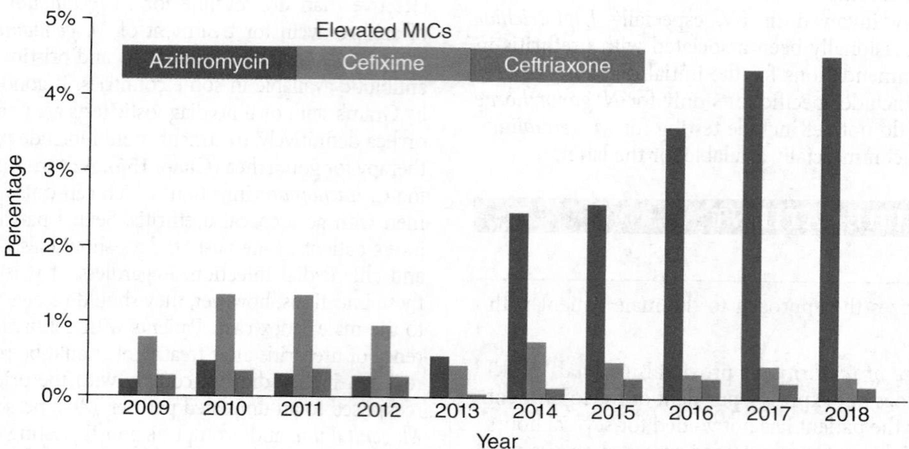

FIGURE 136-1 Percentage of *Neisseria gonorrhoeae* isolates with elevated minimal inhibitory concentrations (MICs) to azithromycin, ceftriaxone, and cefixime, United States, 2009–2018. *(From the Centers for Disease Control and Prevention: Gonococcal Isolate Surveillance Project [GISP], 2018.)*

PART 5 Infectious Diseases

URETHRITIS AND THE URETHRAL SYNDROME IN WOMEN

C. trachomatis, N. gonorrhoeae, and occasionally HSV cause symptomatic urethritis—known as *the urethral syndrome* in women—that is characterized by "internal" dysuria (usually without urinary urgency or frequency), pyuria, and an absence of *Escherichia coli* and other uropathogens at counts of $\geq 10^2$/mL in urine. In contrast, the dysuria associated with vulvar herpes or vulvovaginal candidiasis (and perhaps with trichomoniasis) is often described as "external," being caused by painful contact of urine with the inflamed or ulcerated labia or introitus. Acute onset, association with urinary urgency or frequency, hematuria, or suprapubic bladder tenderness suggests bacterial cystitis. Among women with symptoms of acute bacterial cystitis, costovertebral pain and tenderness or fever suggest acute pyelonephritis. **The management of bacterial urinary tract infection (UTI) is discussed in Chap. 135.**

Signs of vulvovaginitis, coupled with symptoms of external dysuria, suggest vulvar infection (e.g., with HSV or *Candida albicans*). Among dysuric women without signs of vulvovaginitis, bacterial UTI must be differentiated from the urethral syndrome by assessment of risk, evaluation of the pattern of symptoms and signs, and specific microbiologic testing. An STI etiology of the urethral syndrome is suggested by young age, more than one current sexual partner, a new partner within the past month, a partner with urethritis, or coexisting mucopurulent cervicitis (see below). The finding of a single urinary pathogen, such as *E. coli* or *Staphylococcus saprophyticus*, at a concentration of $\geq 10^2$/mL in a properly collected specimen of midstream urine from a dysuric woman with pyuria indicates probable bacterial UTI, whereas pyuria with $<10^2$ conventional uropathogens per milliliter of urine ("sterile" pyuria) suggests acute urethral syndrome due to *C. trachomatis* or *N. gonorrhoeae*. Gonorrhea and chlamydial infection should be sought by specific tests (e.g., NAATs of vaginal secretions collected with a swab). Among dysuric women with sterile pyuria caused by infection with *N. gonorrhoeae* or *C. trachomatis*, appropriate treatment alleviates dysuria. The role of *M. genitalium* in the urethral syndrome in women remains undefined.

VULVOVAGINAL INFECTIONS

Abnormal Vaginal Discharge If directly questioned about vaginal discharge during routine health checkups, many women acknowledge having nonspecific symptoms of vaginal discharge that do not correlate with objective signs of inflammation or with actual infection. However, unsolicited reporting of abnormal vaginal discharge often denotes BV or trichomoniasis. Specifically, an abnormally increased amount or an abnormal odor of the discharge is associated with one or both of these conditions. Cervical infection with *N. gonorrhoeae* or *C. trachomatis* does not often cause an increased amount or abnormal odor of discharge; however, when these pathogens cause cervicitis, they—like *T. vaginalis*—often result in an increased number of neutrophils in vaginal fluid, which thus takes on a yellow color. Vulvar conditions such as genital herpes or vulvovaginal candidiasis can cause vulvar pruritus, burning, irritation, or lesions as well as external dysuria (as urine passes over the inflamed vulva or areas of epithelial disruption) or vulvar dyspareunia.

Certain vulvovaginal infections may have serious sequelae. Trichomoniasis, BV, and vulvovaginal candidiasis have all been associated with increased risk of acquisition of HIV infection; BV promotes HIV transmission from HIV-infected women to their male sex partners. Vaginal trichomoniasis and BV early in pregnancy independently predict premature onset of labor. BV can also lead to anaerobic bacterial infection of the endometrium and salpinges. Vaginitis may be an early and prominent feature of toxic shock syndrome, and recurrent or chronic vulvovaginal candidiasis develops with increased frequency among women who have systemic illnesses, such as diabetes mellitus or HIV-related immunosuppression (although only a very small proportion of women with recurrent vulvovaginal candidiasis in industrialized countries actually have a serious predisposing illness).

Thus, vulvovaginal symptoms or signs warrant careful evaluation, including speculum and pelvic examination, diagnostic testing, and appropriate therapy specific for the infection identified. Unfortunately, clinicians do not always perform the tests required to establish the cause of such symptoms. Further, self-diagnosis of a specific type of infection—including vulvovaginal candidiasis—is often incorrect. The diagnosis and treatment of the three most common types of vaginal infection are summarized in **Table 136-5**.

Inspection of the vulva and perineum may reveal tender genital ulcerations or fissures (typically due to HSV infection or vulvovaginal candidiasis) or discharge visible at the introitus before insertion of a speculum (suggestive of BV or trichomoniasis). Speculum examination permits the clinician to discern whether the discharge appears abnormal and whether it emanates from the cervical os (mucoid and, if abnormal, yellow) or from the vagina (not mucoid, since the vaginal epithelium does not produce mucus). Symptoms or signs of abnormal vaginal discharge should prompt testing of vaginal fluid for pH, for a fishy odor when mixed with 10% KOH, and for certain microscopic features when mixed with saline (motile trichomonads and/or "clue cells") and with 10% KOH (pseudohyphae or hyphae indicative of vulvovaginal candidiasis). Additional objective laboratory tests, described below, are useful for establishing the cause of abnormal vaginal discharge. Gram's staining of vaginal fluid can be used to characterize the vaginal bacteria using the Nugent score but is used primarily for research purposes and requires familiarity with the morphotypes and scale involved. Of note, NAATs that characterize relative concentrations of BV-associated bacteria and certain *Lactobacillus* species are now available and offer comparable performance to clinical diagnostic criteria.

TREATMENT
Vaginal Discharge

Patterns of treatment for abnormal vaginal discharge vary widely. In developing countries, where clinics or pharmacies often dispense treatment based on symptoms alone without examination or testing, oral treatment with metronidazole—particularly with a 7-day regimen—provides reasonable coverage against both trichomoniasis and BV, the usual causes of symptoms of vaginal discharge. Metronidazole treatment of sex partners prevents reinfection of women with *T. vaginalis*, although it does not help prevent the recurrence of BV. Guidelines for syndromic management promulgated by the World Health Organization suggest consideration of treatment for cervical infection and for trichomoniasis, BV, and vulvovaginal candidiasis in women with symptoms of abnormal vaginal discharge. However, it is important to note that the majority of chlamydial and gonococcal cervical infections produce no symptoms.

In industrialized countries, clinicians treating symptoms and signs of abnormal vaginal discharge should, at a minimum, differentiate between BV and trichomoniasis because optimal management of patients and partners differs for these two conditions.

Vaginal Trichomoniasis (See also Chap. 229) Symptomatic trichomoniasis characteristically produces a profuse, yellow, purulent, homogeneous vaginal discharge and vulvar irritation, sometimes with visible inflammation of the vaginal and vulvar epithelium and petechial lesions on the cervix (the so-called strawberry cervix, best visualized by colposcopy). The pH of vaginal fluid—normally <4.7—usually rises to ≥5. Microscopic examination of vaginal discharge mixed with saline reveals motile trichomonads in most culture-positive cases. However, saline microscopy probably detects only one-half of all cases, and, especially in the absence of symptoms or signs, culture or NAAT is usually required for detection of the organism. NAAT for *T. vaginalis* is more sensitive than culture. Treatment of asymptomatic as well as symptomatic cases reduces rates of transmission and prevents later development of symptoms.

TREATMENT
Vaginal Trichomoniasis

Only nitroimidazoles (e.g., metronidazole and tinidazole) consistently cure trichomoniasis. A single 2-g oral dose of metronidazole has been the standard treatment for decades, but it is less effective

TABLE 136-5 Diagnostic Features and Management of Vaginal Infection

FEATURE	NORMAL VAGINAL EXAMINATION	VULVOVAGINAL CANDIDIASIS	TRICHOMONAL VAGINITIS	BACTERIAL VAGINOSIS (BV)
Etiology	Uninfected; lactobacilli predominant	*Candida albicans*	*Trichomonas vaginalis*	Associated with *Gardnerella vaginalis*, various anaerobic bacteria, and mycoplasmas
Typical symptoms	None	Vulvar itching and/or irritation	Profuse discharge; vulvar itching	Malodorous, slightly increased discharge
Discharge				
Amount	Variable; usually scant	Scant	Often profuse	Moderate
Color[a]	Clear or translucent	White	White or yellow	White or gray
Consistency	Nonhomogeneous, flocculent	Clumped; adherent plaques	Homogeneous	Homogeneous, low viscosity; uniformly coats vaginal walls
Inflammation of vulvar or vaginal epithelium	None	Erythema of vaginal epithelium, introitus; vulvar dermatitis, fissures common	Erythema of vaginal and vulvar epithelium; colpitis macularis	None
pH of vaginal fluid[b]	Usually ≤4.5	Usually ≤4.5	Usually ≥5	Usually >4.5
Amine ("fishy") odor with 10% KOH	None	None	May be present	Present
Microscopy[c]	Normal epithelial cells; lactobacilli predominant	Leukocytes, epithelial cells; mycelia or pseudomycelia in up to 80% of *C. albicans* culture–positive persons with typical symptoms	Leukocytes; motile trichomonads seen in 80–90% of symptomatic patients, less often in the absence of symptoms	Clue cells; few leukocytes; no lactobacilli or only a few outnumbered by profuse mixed microbiota, nearly always including *G. vaginalis* plus anaerobic species on Gram's stain (Nugent's score ≥7)
Other laboratory findings		Isolation of *Candida* spp.	Isolation of *T. vaginalis* or positive NAAT[d]	Diagnosis of BV by NAAT[d]
Usual treatment	None	Azole cream, tablet, or suppository—e.g., miconazole (100-mg vaginal suppository) or clotrimazole (100-mg vaginal tablet) once daily for 7 days Fluconazole, 150 mg orally (single dose)	Metronidazole or tinidazole, 2 g orally (single dose) Metronidazole, 500 mg PO bid for 7 days	Metronidazole, 500 mg PO bid for 7 days Metronidazole gel, 0.75%, one applicator (5 g) intravaginally once daily for 5 days Clindamycin, 2% cream, one full applicator vaginally each night for 7 days
Usual management of sexual partner	None	None; topical treatment if candidal dermatitis of penis is detected	Examination for sexually transmitted infection; treatment with metronidazole, 2 g PO (single dose)	None

[a]Color of discharge is best determined by examination against the white background of a swab. [b]A pH determination is not useful if blood is present or if the test is performed on endocervical secretions. [c]To detect fungal elements, vaginal fluid is digested with 10% KOH prior to microscopic examination; to examine for other features, fluid is mixed (1:1) with physiologic saline. Gram's stain is also excellent for detecting yeasts (less predictive of vulvovaginitis) and pseudomycelia or mycelia (strongly predictive of vulvovaginitis) and for distinguishing normal flora from the mixed flora seen in bacterial vaginosis, but it is less sensitive than the saline preparation for detection of *T. vaginalis*. [d]NAAT, nucleic acid amplification test (where available). NAAT for diagnosis of BV typically tests for combinations of BV-associated bacteria and absence of *Lactobacillus* species.

than a weeklong course; the latter is preferred. Tinidazole has a longer half-life than metronidazole, causes fewer gastrointestinal symptoms, and may be useful in treating trichomoniasis that fails to respond to metronidazole. Treatment of sexual partners, facilitated by dispensing metronidazole to the female patient to give to her partner(s), significantly reduces both the risk of reinfection and the reservoir of infection; treating partners is the standard of care. Intravaginal treatment with 0.75% metronidazole gel is not reliable for vaginal trichomoniasis. Thus, systemic use of metronidazole is still recommended throughout pregnancy for treatment of trichomoniasis. In a large randomized trial, metronidazole treatment of trichomoniasis during pregnancy was associated with an increased frequency of perinatal morbidity. However, most studies, including randomized controlled trials, have shown no adverse effects of metronidazole use during pregnancy on preterm birth or birth defects.

Bacterial Vaginosis BV is a syndrome characterized by symptoms of vaginal malodor and increased white-gray discharge, which appears homogeneous, is low in viscosity, and uniformly covers the vaginal mucosa. BV has been associated with an increased risk of acquiring several other genital infections, including those caused by HIV, *C. trachomatis*, and *N. gonorrhoeae*. Other possible risk factors include recent unprotected vaginal intercourse, having a female sex partner, and vaginal douching. Although bacteria associated with BV have been detected under the foreskin of uncircumcised men and have been associated with urethritis, metronidazole treatment of male partners has not reduced the rate of recurrence of BV among affected women.

Among women with BV, culture of vaginal fluid has shown markedly increased prevalences and concentrations of *Gardnerella vaginalis*, *Mycoplasma hominis*, and several anaerobic bacteria (e.g., *Mobiluncus*, *Prevotella* [formerly *Bacteroides*], and some *Peptostreptococcus* species) as well as an absence of hydrogen peroxide–producing *Lactobacillus* species that constitute most of the normal vaginal microbiota and help protect against cervical and vaginal infections. Broad-range polymerase chain reaction (PCR) amplification of 16S rDNA in vaginal fluid, with subsequent identification of specific bacterial species by various methods, has documented even greater bacterial diversity, including several unique species not previously identified in culture (**Fig. 136-2**) and *Atopobium vaginae*, an organism that is strongly associated with BV and is resistant to metronidazole. Other genera newly implicated in BV include *Megasphaera*, *Leptotrichia*, *Eggerthella*, and *Dialister*.

BV is conventionally diagnosed clinically with the Amsel criteria, which include any three of the following four clinical abnormalities: (1) objective signs of increased white homogeneous vaginal discharge; (2) a vaginal discharge pH of >4.5; (3) liberation of a distinct fishy odor (attributable to volatile amines such as trimethylamine) immediately after vaginal secretions are mixed with a 10% solution of KOH; and (4) microscopic demonstration of "clue cells" (vaginal epithelial cells

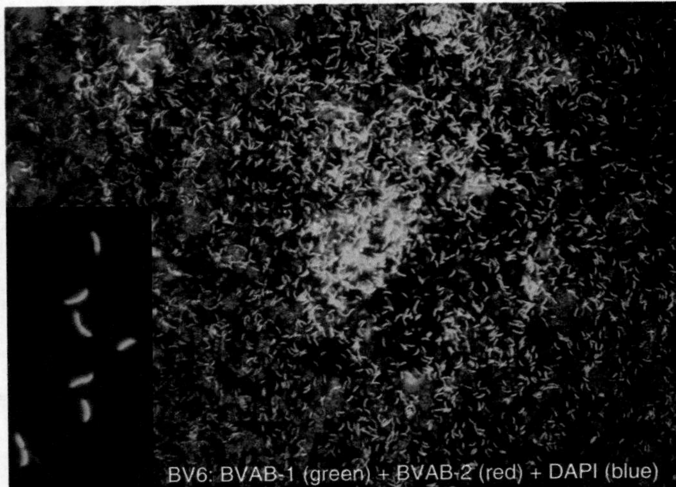

FIGURE 136-2 Broad-range polymerase chain reaction amplification of 16S rDNA in vaginal fluid from a woman with bacterial vaginosis (BV) shows a field of bacteria hybridizing with probes for BV-associated bacterium 1 (BVAB-1, visible as a thin, curved green rod) and for BVAB-2 (red). The *inset* shows that BVAB-1 has a morphology similar to that of *Mobiluncus* (curved rod). *(Adapted from DN Fredricks et al: Molecular identification of bacteria associated with bacterial vaginosis. N Engl J Med 353:1899, 2005.)*

coated with coccobacillary organisms, which have a granular appearance and indistinct borders; **Fig. 136-3**) on a wet mount prepared by mixing vaginal secretions with normal saline in a ratio of ~1:1.

TREATMENT
Bacterial Vaginosis

The standard dosage of oral metronidazole for the treatment of BV is 500 mg twice daily for 7 days. Intravaginal treatment with 2% clindamycin cream (one full applicator [5 g containing 100 mg of clindamycin phosphate] each night for 7 nights) or with 0.75% metronidazole gel (one full applicator [5 g containing 37.5 mg of metronidazole] twice daily for 5 days) is also approved for use in the United States and does not elicit systemic adverse reactions; the response to both of these treatments is similar to the response to oral metronidazole. Another nitroimidazole given orally, secnidazole, is also effective (single 2-g dose). Other alternatives include oral clindamycin (300 mg twice daily for 7 days), clindamycin ovules (100 g intravaginally once at bedtime for 3 days), and oral tinidazole (1 g daily for 5 days or 2 g daily for 3 days). Unfortunately, recurrence over the long term (i.e., several months later) is distressingly common after either oral or intravaginal treatment. A randomized trial comparing intravaginal gel containing 37.5 mg of metronidazole with a suppository containing 500 mg of metronidazole plus nystatin (the latter not marketed in the United States) showed significantly higher rates of recurrence with the 37.5-mg regimen; this result suggests that higher metronidazole dosages may be important in topical intravaginal therapy. Recurrences can be significantly lessened with the twice-weekly use of suppressive intravaginal metronidazole gel. The goal of replenishing the vaginal lactobacilli that sustain vaginal health has recently been bolstered by a randomized trial that demonstrated that weekly vaginal administration of *Lactobacillus crispatus* CTV-05 (LACTIN-V) reduced rates of recurrent BV by approximately one-third.

A meta-analysis of 18 studies concluded that BV during pregnancy substantially increased the risk of preterm delivery and of spontaneous abortion. However, in most studies, topical intravaginal treatment of BV with clindamycin during pregnancy has not reduced adverse pregnancy outcomes. Numerous trials of oral metronidazole treatment during pregnancy have given inconsistent results, and recent reviews have concluded that antenatal treatment of women with BV—including those with previous preterm delivery—did not reduce the risk of preterm delivery. The U.S. Preventive Services Task Force thus recommends against routine screening of pregnant women for BV.

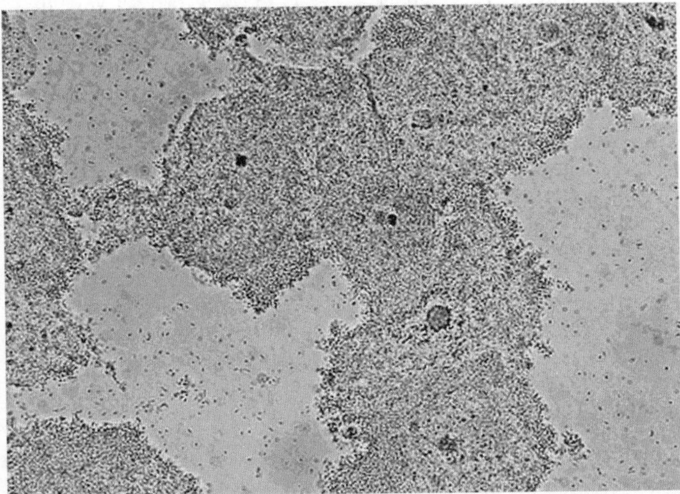

FIGURE 136-3 Wet mount of vaginal fluid showing typical clue cells from a woman with bacterial vaginosis. Note the obscured epithelial cell margins and the granular appearance attributable to many adherent bacteria (×400). *(Photograph provided by Lorna K. Rabe, reprinted with permission from S Hillier et al, in KK Holmes et al [eds]: Sexually Transmitted Diseases, 4th ed. New York, McGraw-Hill, 2008.)*

Vulvovaginal Pruritus, Burning, or Irritation Vulvovaginal candidiasis produces vulvar pruritus, burning, or irritation, generally without symptoms of increased vaginal discharge or malodor. Genital herpes can produce similar symptoms, with lesions sometimes difficult to distinguish from the fissures and inflammation caused by candidiasis. Signs of vulvovaginal candidiasis include vulvar erythema, edema, fissures, and tenderness. With candidiasis, a white scanty vaginal discharge sometimes takes the form of white thrush-like plaques or cottage cheese–like curds adhering loosely to the vaginal epithelium. *C. albicans* accounts for nearly all cases of symptomatic vulvovaginal candidiasis, which probably arise from endogenous strains of *C. albicans* that have colonized the vagina or the intestinal tract. Complicated vulvovaginal candidiasis includes cases that recur four or more times per year; are unusually severe; are caused by non-*albicans Candida* species; or occur in women with uncontrolled diabetes, debilitation, immunosuppression, or pregnancy.

In addition to compatible clinical symptoms, the diagnosis of vulvovaginal candidiasis involves the demonstration of pseudohyphae or hyphae by microscopic examination of vaginal fluid mixed with saline or 10% KOH or subjected to Gram's staining. Microscopic examination is less sensitive than culture but correlates better with symptoms. Culture is typically reserved for cases that do not respond to standard first-line antimycotic agents and is undertaken to rule out imidazole or azole resistance (often associated with *Candida glabrata*) or before the initiation of suppressive antifungal therapy for recurrent disease.

TREATMENT
Vulvovaginal Pruritus, Burning, or Irritation

Symptoms and signs of vulvovaginal candidiasis warrant treatment, usually intravaginal administration of any of several imidazole antibiotics (e.g., miconazole or clotrimazole) for 3–7 days or of a single dose of oral fluconazole (Table 136-5). Over-the-counter marketing of such preparations has reduced the cost of care and made treatment more convenient for many women with recurrent yeast vulvovaginitis. However, most women who purchase these preparations do not have vulvovaginal candidiasis, whereas many have other vaginal infections that require different treatment. Therefore, only women with classic symptoms of vulvar pruritus and a history of previous episodes of yeast vulvovaginitis documented by an experienced clinician should self-treat. Short-course topical intravaginal azole drugs are effective for the treatment of uncomplicated vulvovaginal candidiasis (e.g., clotrimazole, two 100-mg vaginal tablets daily for 3 days; or miconazole, a 1200-mg vaginal suppository as a single dose). Single-dose oral treatment with fluconazole (150 mg) is also effective and is preferred by many patients. Management of complicated cases (see above) and those that do not respond to the usual intravaginal or single-dose oral therapy often involves prolonged or periodic oral therapy; this situation is discussed extensively in the 2015 CDC STD treatment guidelines (*http://www.cdc.gov/std/treatment*). Treatment of sexual partners is not routinely indicated.

Other Causes of Vaginal Discharge or Vaginitis In the ulcerative vaginitis associated with staphylococcal toxic shock syndrome, *Staphylococcus aureus* should be promptly identified in vaginal fluid by Gram's stain and by culture. In desquamative inflammatory vaginitis, smears of vaginal fluid reveal neutrophils, massive vaginal epithelial cell exfoliation with increased numbers of parabasal cells, and gram-positive cocci; this syndrome may respond to treatment with 2% clindamycin cream, often given in combination with topical steroid preparations for several weeks. Additional causes of vaginitis and vulvovaginal symptoms include retained foreign bodies (e.g., tampons), cervical caps, vaginal spermicides, vaginal antiseptic preparations or douches, vaginal epithelial atrophy (in postmenopausal women or during prolonged breast-feeding in the postpartum period), allergic reactions to latex condoms, vaginal aphthae associated with HIV infection or Behçet's syndrome, and vestibulitis.

MUCOPURULENT CERVICITIS

Mucopurulent cervicitis (MPC) refers to inflammation of the columnar epithelium and subepithelium of the endocervix and of any contiguous columnar epithelium that lies exposed in an ectopic position on the ectocervix. MPC in women represents the "silent partner" of urethritis in men, being equally common and often caused by the same agents (*N. gonorrhoeae, C. trachomatis, M. genitalium*); however, MPC is more difficult than urethritis to recognize, given the nonspecific nature of symptoms (e.g., abnormal vaginal discharge) and the need for visualization by pelvic examination. As the most common manifestation of these serious bacterial infections in women, MPC can be a harbinger or sign of upper genital tract infection, also known as *pelvic inflammatory disease* (PID; see below). In pregnant women, MPC can lead to obstetric complications. In the pre-NAAT era, more than one-third of cervicovaginal specimens tested for *C. trachomatis, N. gonorrhoeae, M. genitalium*, HSV, and *T. vaginalis* revealed no identifiable etiology for MPC **(Fig. 136-4)**. More recent studies employing NAATs for these pathogens have still failed to identify a microbiologic etiology in nearly one-half of women with MPC. Individual bacteria associated with BV may also elicit an inflammatory reaction at the cervix; thus, BV may be a cause of MPC.

The diagnosis of MPC rests on the detection of cardinal signs at the cervix, including yellow mucopurulent discharge from the cervical os, endocervical bleeding upon gentle swabbing, and edematous cervical ectopy (see below); the latter two findings are somewhat more common with MPC due to chlamydial infection, but signs alone do not allow a distinction among the causative pathogens. Unlike the endocervicitis produced by gonococcal or chlamydial infection, cervicitis caused by HSV produces ulcerative lesions on the stratified squamous epithelium of the ectocervix as well as on the columnar epithelium. Yellow cervical mucus on a white swab removed from the endocervix indicates the presence of polymorphonuclear leukocytes (PMNs). Gram's staining may confirm their presence, although it adds relatively little to the diagnostic value of assessment for cervical signs. The presence of ≥20 PMNs per 1000× microscopic field within strands of cervical mucus not contaminated by vaginal squamous epithelial cells or vaginal bacteria indicates endocervicitis. Detection of intracellular gram-negative diplococci in carefully collected endocervical mucus is quite specific but ≤50% sensitive for gonorrhea. Therefore, NAATs for *N. gonorrhoeae* and *C. trachomatis* are always indicated in the evaluation of MPC, as is a careful evaluation of vaginal discharge for the causes of vaginitis discussed above.

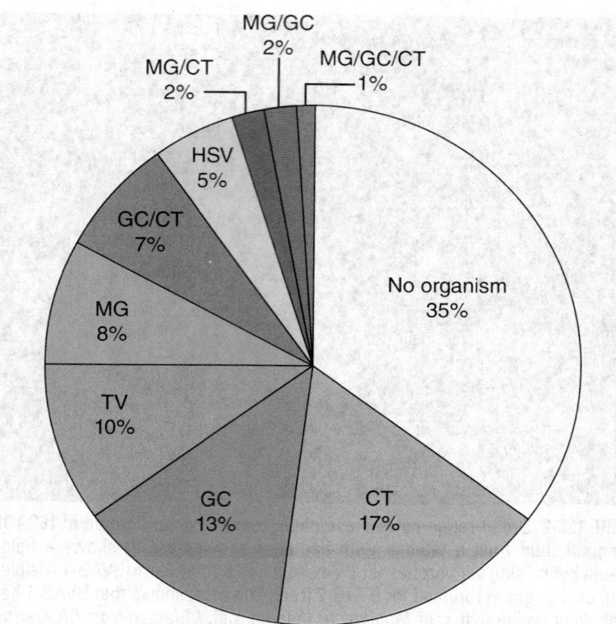

FIGURE 136-4 Organisms detected among female sexually transmitted disease clinic patients with mucopurulent cervicitis (n = 167). CT, *Chlamydia trachomatis*; GC, gonococcus; HSV, herpes simplex virus; MG, *Mycoplasma genitalium*; TV, *Trichomonas vaginalis*. *(Courtesy of Dr. Lisa Manhart; with permission.)*

TREATMENT
Mucopurulent Cervicitis

Although the above criteria for MPC are neither highly specific nor highly predictive of gonococcal or chlamydial infection in some settings, the 2015 CDC STD guidelines call for consideration of empirical treatment for MPC, pending test results, in most cases. Presumptive treatment with antibiotics active against *C. trachomatis* should be provided for women at increased risk for this common STI (risk factors: age <25 years, new or multiple sex partners, and unprotected sex), especially if follow-up cannot be ensured. Concurrent therapy for gonorrhea is indicated if the prevalence of this infection is substantial in the relevant patient population (e.g., young adults, a clinic with documented high prevalence). In this situation, therapy should include a single-dose regimen effective for gonorrhea plus treatment for chlamydial infection, as outlined in Table 136-4 for the treatment of urethritis. In settings where gonorrhea is much less common than chlamydial infection, initial therapy for chlamydial infection alone suffices, pending test results for gonorrhea. The etiology and potential benefit of treatment for endocervicitis not associated with gonorrhea or chlamydial infection have not been established. Although the antimicrobial susceptibility of *M. genitalium* is not yet well defined, the organism frequently persists after doxycycline therapy, and it currently seems reasonable to use azithromycin to treat possible *M. genitalium* infection in such cases. With resistance of *M. genitalium* to azithromycin now recognized, moxifloxacin may be a reasonable alternative. The sexual partner(s) of a woman with MPC should be examined and given a regimen similar to that chosen for the woman unless results of tests for gonorrhea or chlamydial infection in either partner warrant different therapy or no therapy.

CERVICAL ECTOPY

Cervical ectopy, often mislabeled "cervical erosion," is easily confused with infectious endocervicitis. Ectopy represents the presence of the one-cell-thick columnar epithelium extending from the endocervix out onto the visible ectocervix. In ectopy, the cervical os may contain clear or slightly cloudy mucus but usually not yellow mucopus. Colposcopy shows intact epithelium. Normally found during adolescence and early adulthood, ectopy gradually recedes through the second and third decades of life, as squamous metaplasia replaces the ectopic columnar epithelium. Oral contraceptive use favors the persistence or reappearance of ectopy, while smoking apparently accelerates squamous metaplasia. Cauterization of ectopy is not warranted. Ectopy may render the cervix more susceptible to infection with *N. gonorrhoeae, C. trachomatis*, or HIV.

PELVIC INFLAMMATORY DISEASE

The term *pelvic inflammatory disease* (PID) usually refers to infection that ascends from the cervix or vagina to involve the endometrium and/or fallopian tubes. Infection can extend beyond the reproductive tract to cause pelvic peritonitis, generalized peritonitis, perihepatitis, perisplenitis, or pelvic abscess. Rarely, infection not related to specific sexually transmitted pathogens extends secondarily to the pelvic organs (1) from adjacent foci of inflammation (e.g., appendicitis, regional ileitis, or diverticulitis) or BV, (2) as a result of hematogenous dissemination (e.g., of tuberculosis or staphylococcal bacteremia), or (3) as a complication of certain tropical diseases (e.g., schistosomiasis). Intrauterine infection can be primary (spontaneously occurring and usually sexually transmitted) or secondary to invasive intrauterine surgical procedures (e.g., dilation and curettage, termination of pregnancy, insertion of an intrauterine device [IUD], or hysterosalpingography) or to parturition.

Etiology The agents most often implicated in acute PID include the primary causes of endocervicitis (*N. gonorrhoeae, C. trachomatis*, and *M. genitalium*) and anaerobes associated with BV. In general, PID is most often caused by *N. gonorrhoeae* in settings where there is a high incidence of gonorrhea. *M. genitalium* has also been significantly associated with histopathologic diagnoses of endometritis and with salpingitis.

Anaerobic and facultative organisms (especially *Prevotella* species, peptostreptococci, *E. coli, Haemophilus influenzae*, and group B streptococci) as well as genital mycoplasmas have been isolated from the peritoneal fluid or fallopian tubes in a varying proportion (typically one-fourth to one-third) of women with PID studied in the United States. The difficulty of determining the exact microbial etiology of an individual case of PID—short of using invasive procedures for specimen collection—has implications for the approach to empirical antimicrobial treatment of this infection.

Epidemiology In the United States, the estimated annual number of initial visits to physicians' offices for PID by women 15–44 years of age fell from an average of 400,000 during the 1980s to 250,000 in 1999 and then to 51,000 in 2014. Hospitalizations for acute PID in the United States also declined steadily throughout the 1980s and early 1990s but have remained fairly constant at 70,000–100,000 per year since 1995. Important risk factors for acute PID include the presence of endocervical infection or BV, a history of salpingitis or of recent vaginal douching, and recent insertion of an IUD. Certain other iatrogenic factors, such as dilation and curettage or cesarean section, can increase the risk of PID, especially among women with endocervical gonococcal or chlamydial infection or BV. Symptoms of *N. gonorrhoeae*–associated and *C. trachomatis*–associated PID often begin during or soon after the menstrual period; this timing suggests that menstruation is a risk factor for ascending infection from the cervix and vagina. Experimental inoculation of the fallopian tubes of nonhuman primates has shown that repeated exposure to *C. trachomatis* leads to the greatest degree of tissue inflammation and damage; thus, immunopathology probably contributes to the pathogenesis of chlamydial salpingitis. Women using oral contraceptives appear to be at decreased risk of symptomatic PID, and tubal sterilization reduces the risk of salpingitis by preventing intraluminal spread of infection into the tubes.

Clinical Manifestations • **ENDOMETRITIS: A CLINICAL PATHOLOGIC SYNDROME** A study of women with clinically suspected PID who were undergoing both endometrial biopsy and laparoscopy showed that those with endometritis alone differed from those who also had salpingitis in significantly less often having lower quadrant, adnexal, or cervical motion or abdominal rebound tenderness; fever; or elevated C-reactive protein levels. In addition, women with endometritis alone differed from those with neither endometritis nor salpingitis in more often having gonorrhea, chlamydial infection, and risk factors such as douching or IUD use. Thus, women with endometritis alone were intermediate between those with neither endometritis nor salpingitis and those with salpingitis with respect to risk factors, clinical manifestations, cervical infection prevalence, and elevated C-reactive protein level. Women with endometritis alone are at lower risk of subsequent tubal occlusion and resulting infertility than are those with salpingitis.

SALPINGITIS Symptoms of nontuberculous salpingitis classically evolve from a yellow or malodorous vaginal discharge caused by MPC and/or BV to midline abdominal pain and abnormal vaginal bleeding caused by endometritis and then to bilateral lower abdominal and pelvic pain caused by salpingitis, with nausea, vomiting, and increased abdominal tenderness if peritonitis develops.

The abdominal pain in nontuberculous salpingitis is usually described as dull or aching. In some cases, pain is lacking or atypical, but active inflammatory changes are found in the course of an unrelated evaluation or procedure, such as a laparoscopic evaluation for infertility. Abnormal uterine bleeding precedes or coincides with the onset of pain in ~40% of women with PID, symptoms of urethritis (dysuria) occur in 20%, and symptoms of proctitis (anorectal pain, tenesmus, and rectal discharge or bleeding) are occasionally seen in women with gonococcal or chlamydial infection.

Speculum examination shows evidence of MPC (yellow endocervical discharge, easily induced endocervical bleeding) in the majority of women with gonococcal or chlamydial PID. Cervical motion tenderness is produced by stretching of the adnexal attachments on the side toward which the cervix is pushed. Bimanual examination reveals uterine fundal tenderness due to endometritis and abnormal adnexal tenderness due to salpingitis that is usually, but not necessarily, bilateral. Adnexal swelling is palpable in about one-half of women with acute salpingitis, but evaluation of the adnexae in a patient with marked tenderness is not reliable. The initial temperature is >38°C in only about one-third of patients with acute salpingitis. Laboratory findings include elevation of the erythrocyte sedimentation rate (ESR) in 75% of patients with acute salpingitis and elevation of the peripheral white blood cell count in up to 60%.

Unlike nontuberculous salpingitis, genital tuberculosis often occurs in older women, many of whom are postmenopausal. Presenting symptoms include abnormal vaginal bleeding, pain (including dysmenorrhea), and infertility. About one-quarter of these women have had adnexal masses. Endometrial biopsy shows tuberculous granulomas and provides optimal specimens for culture.

PERIHEPATITIS AND PERIAPPENDICITIS Pleuritic upper abdominal pain and tenderness, usually localized to the right upper quadrant (RUQ), develop in 3–10% of women with acute PID. Symptoms of perihepatitis arise during or after the onset of symptoms of PID and may overshadow lower abdominal symptoms, thereby leading to a mistaken diagnosis of cholecystitis. In perhaps 5% of cases of acute salpingitis, early laparoscopy reveals perihepatic inflammation ranging from edema and erythema of the liver capsule to exudate with fibrinous adhesions between the visceral and parietal peritoneum. When treatment is delayed and laparoscopy is performed late, dense "violin-string" adhesions can be seen over the liver; chronic exertional or positional RUQ pain ensues when traction is placed on the adhesions. Although perihepatitis, also known as the *Fitz-Hugh–Curtis syndrome*, was for many years specifically attributed to gonococcal salpingitis, most cases are now attributed to chlamydial salpingitis. In patients with chlamydial salpingitis, serum titers of microimmunofluorescent antibody to *C. trachomatis* are typically much higher when perihepatitis is present than when it is absent.

Physical findings include RUQ tenderness and usually include adnexal tenderness and cervicitis, even in patients whose symptoms do not suggest salpingitis. Results of liver function tests and RUQ ultrasonography are nearly always normal. The presence of MPC and pelvic tenderness in a young woman with subacute pleuritic RUQ pain and normal ultrasonography of the gallbladder points to a diagnosis of perihepatitis.

Periappendicitis (appendiceal serositis without involvement of the intestinal mucosa) has been found in ~5% of patients undergoing appendectomy for suspected appendicitis and can occur as a complication of gonococcal or chlamydial salpingitis.

Among women with salpingitis, HIV infection is associated with increased severity of salpingitis and with tuboovarian abscess requiring hospitalization and surgical drainage. Nonetheless, among women with HIV infection and salpingitis, the clinical response to conventional antimicrobial therapy (coupled with drainage of tuboovarian abscess, when found) has usually been satisfactory.

Diagnosis Treatment appropriate for PID must not be withheld from patients who have an equivocal diagnosis; it is better to err on the side of overdiagnosis and overtreatment. On the other hand, it is essential to differentiate between salpingitis and other pelvic pathology, particularly surgical emergencies such as appendicitis and ectopic pregnancy or the chronic syndrome of endometriosis.

Nothing short of laparoscopy definitively identifies salpingitis, but routine laparoscopy to confirm suspected salpingitis is generally impractical. Most patients with acute PID have lower abdominal pain of <3 weeks' duration, pelvic tenderness on bimanual pelvic examination, and evidence of lower genital tract infection (e.g., MPC). Approximately 60% of such patients have salpingitis at laparoscopy, and perhaps 10–20% have endometritis alone. Among the patients with these findings, a rectal temperature >38°C, a palpable adnexal mass, and elevation of the ESR to >15 mm/h also raise the probability of salpingitis, which has been found at laparoscopy in 68% of patients with one of these additional findings, 90% of patients with two, and 96% of patients with three. However, only 17% of all patients with laparoscopy-confirmed salpingitis have had all three additional findings.

In a woman with pelvic pain and tenderness, increased numbers of PMNs (30 per 1000× microscopic field in strands of cervical mucus) or leukocytes outnumbering epithelial cells in vaginal fluid (in the absence of trichomonal vaginitis, which also produces PMNs in vaginal discharge) increase the predictive value of a clinical diagnosis of acute PID, as do onset with menses, history of recent abnormal menstrual bleeding, presence of an IUD, history of salpingitis, and sexual exposure to a male with urethritis. Appendicitis or another disorder of the gut is favored by the early onset of anorexia, nausea, or vomiting; the onset of pain later than day 14 of the menstrual cycle; or unilateral pain limited to the right or left lower quadrant. Whenever the diagnosis of PID is being considered, serum assays for human β-chorionic gonadotropin should be performed; these tests are usually positive with ectopic pregnancy. Ultrasonography and MRI can be useful for the identification of tuboovarian or pelvic abscess. MRI of the tubes can also show increased tubal diameter, intratubal fluid, or tubal wall thickening in cases of salpingitis.

The primary value of laparoscopy in women with lower abdominal pain is for the exclusion of other surgical problems that cannot be resolved with noninvasive imaging. Some of the most common or serious problems that may be confused with salpingitis (e.g., acute appendicitis, ectopic pregnancy, corpus luteum bleeding, ovarian tumor) are unilateral. Unilateral pain or pelvic mass, although not incompatible with PID, is a strong indication for laparoscopy unless the clinical picture warrants laparotomy instead. Atypical clinical findings such as the absence of lower genital tract infection, a missed menstrual period, a positive pregnancy test, or failure to respond to appropriate therapy are other common indications for laparoscopy. Endometrial biopsy is relatively sensitive and specific for the diagnosis of endometritis, which correlates well with the presence of salpingitis.

Vaginal or endocervical swab specimens should be obtained for NAATs for *N. gonorrhoeae* and *C. trachomatis*. At a minimum, vaginal fluid should be evaluated for the presence of PMNs, and endocervical secretions ideally should be assessed by Gram's staining for PMNs and gram-negative diplococci, which indicate gonococcal infection. The clinical diagnosis of PID made by expert gynecologists is confirmed by laparoscopy or endometrial biopsy in ~90% of women who also have cultures positive for *N. gonorrhoeae* or *C. trachomatis*. Even among women with no symptoms suggestive of acute PID who were attending an STD clinic or a gynecology clinic in Pittsburgh, endometritis was significantly associated with endocervical gonorrhea or chlamydial infection or with BV, being detected in 26%, 27%, and 15% of women with these conditions, respectively.

TREATMENT

Pelvic Inflammatory Disease

Recommended combination regimens for ambulatory or parenteral management of PID are presented in **Table 136-6**. Women managed as outpatients should receive a combined regimen with broad activity, such as ceftriaxone (to cover possible gonococcal infection) followed by doxycycline (to cover possible chlamydial infection). Metronidazole should be strongly considered to enhance activity against anaerobes, especially if BV or trichomoniasis are present or there is a recent (3-week) history of gynecologic instrumentation; in a recent randomized trial, the addition of metronidazole to ceftriaxone and doxycycline effected reduction in endometrial anaerobes, *M. genitalium*, and pelvic tenderness.

The CDC STD treatment guidelines recommend initiation of empirical treatment for PID in sexually active young women and other women at risk for PID if they are experiencing pelvic or lower abdominal pain, if no other cause for the pain can be identified, and if pelvic examination reveals one or more of the following criteria for PID: cervical motion tenderness, uterine tenderness, or adnexal tenderness. Women with suspected PID can be treated as either outpatients or inpatients. In the multicenter Pelvic Inflammatory Disease Evaluation and Clinical Health (PEACH) trial, 831 women with mild to moderately severe symptoms and signs of PID were randomized to receive either inpatient treatment with IV cefoxitin and doxycycline or outpatient treatment with a single IM dose of cefoxitin plus oral doxycycline. Short-term clinical and microbiologic outcomes and long-term outcomes were equivalent in the two groups. Nonetheless, hospitalization should be considered when (1) the diagnosis is uncertain and surgical emergencies such as appendicitis and ectopic pregnancy cannot be excluded, (2) the patient is pregnant, (3) pelvic abscess is suspected, (4) severe illness or nausea and vomiting preclude outpatient management, (5) the patient has HIV infection, (6) the patient is assessed as unable to follow or tolerate an outpatient regimen, or (7) the patient has failed to respond

TABLE 136-6 Combination Antimicrobial Regimens Recommended for Outpatient Treatment or for Parenteral Treatment of Pelvic Inflammatory Disease

OUTPATIENT REGIMENS[a]	PARENTERAL REGIMENS
Ceftriaxone (500 mg IM once) ***plus*** Doxycycline (100 mg PO bid for 14 days) ***plus***[b] Metronidazole (500 mg PO bid for 14 days)	Initiate parenteral therapy with either of the following regimens; continue parenteral therapy until 48 h after clinical improvement; then change to outpatient therapy, as described in the text **Regimen A** Cefotetan (2 g IV q12h) *or* cefoxitin (2 g IV q6h) ***plus*** Doxycycline (100 mg IV or PO q12h) **Regimen B** Clindamycin (900 mg IV q8h) ***plus*** Gentamicin (loading dose of 2 mg/kg IV or IM, then maintenance dose of 1.5 mg/kg q8h)

[a]See text for discussion of options in the patient who is intolerant of cephalosporins.
[b]The addition of metronidazole is recommended particularly if bacterial vaginosis or trichomoniasis is present.

Source: Adapted from Centers for Disease Control and Prevention: MMWR Recomm Rep 64(RR-03):1, 2015.

to outpatient therapy. Some experts also prefer to hospitalize adolescents with PID for initial therapy, although younger women do as well as older women on outpatient therapy.

Currently, no agents other than parenteral cephalosporins provide reliable coverage for gonococcal infection. Thus, adequate oral treatment of women with serious intolerance to cephalosporins is a challenge. If penicillins are an option, amoxicillin/clavulanic acid combined with doxycycline has elicited a short-term clinical response in one trial. Clinical trials performed outside the United States support the effectiveness of oral moxifloxacin. In this case, it is imperative to perform a sensitive diagnostic test for gonorrhea (ideally, a culture to test for antimicrobial susceptibility) before initiation of therapy. For women whose PID involves quinolone-resistant *N. gonorrhoeae*, treatment is uncertain but could include parenteral gentamicin or oral azithromycin, although the latter agent has not been studied for this purpose.

For hospitalized patients, the following two parenteral regimens (Table 136-6) have given nearly identical results in a multicenter randomized trial:

1. Doxycycline plus either cefotetan or cefoxitin: Administration of these drugs should be continued by the IV route for at least 48 h after the patient's condition improves and then followed with oral doxycycline (100 mg twice daily) to complete 14 days of therapy.
2. Clindamycin plus gentamicin in patients with normal renal function: Once-daily administration of gentamicin (with combination of the total daily dose into a single daily dose) has not been evaluated in PID but has been efficacious in other serious infections and could be substituted. Treatment with these drugs should be continued for at least 48 h after the patient's condition improves and then followed with oral doxycycline (100 mg twice daily) or clindamycin (450 mg four times daily) to complete 14 days of therapy. In cases with tuboovarian abscess, clindamycin rather than doxycycline for continued therapy provides better coverage for anaerobic infection.

FOLLOW-UP

Hospitalized patients should show substantial clinical improvement within 3–5 days. Women treated as outpatients should be clinically reevaluated within 72 h. A follow-up telephone survey of women seen in an emergency department and given a prescription for 10 days of oral doxycycline for PID found that 28% never filled the prescription and 41% stopped taking the medication early (after an average of 4.1 days), often because of persistent symptoms, lack of symptoms, or side effects. Women not responding favorably to ambulatory therapy should be hospitalized for parenteral therapy and further diagnostic evaluations, including a consideration of laparoscopy. Male sex partners should be evaluated and treated empirically for gonorrhea and chlamydial infection. After completion of treatment, tests for persistent or recurrent infection with *N. gonorrhoeae* or *C. trachomatis* should be performed if symptoms persist or recur or if the patient has not complied with therapy or has been reexposed to an untreated sex partner.

SURGERY

Surgery is necessary for the treatment of salpingitis only in the face of life-threatening infection (such as rupture or threatened rupture of a tuboovarian abscess) or for drainage of an abscess. Conservative surgical procedures are usually sufficient. Pelvic abscesses can often be drained by posterior colpotomy, and peritoneal lavage can be used for generalized peritonitis.

Prognosis Late sequelae include infertility due to bilateral tubal occlusion, ectopic pregnancy due to tubal scarring without occlusion, chronic pelvic pain, and recurrent salpingitis. The overall post-salpingitis risk of infertility due to tubal occlusion in a large study in Sweden was 11% after one episode of salpingitis, 23% after two episodes, and 54% after three or more episodes. A University of Washington study found a sevenfold increase in the risk of ectopic pregnancy and an eightfold increase in the rate of hysterectomy after PID.

Prevention A randomized controlled trial designed to determine whether selective screening for chlamydial infection reduces the risk of subsequent PID showed that women randomized to undergo screening had a 56% lower rate of PID over the following year than did women receiving the usual care without screening. This report helped prompt U.S. national guidelines for risk-based chlamydial screening of young women to reduce the incidence of PID and the prevalence of post-PID sequelae, while also reducing sexual transmission of *C. trachomatis*. The CDC and the U.S. Preventive Services Task Force recommend that sexually active women ≤25 years of age be screened annually for genital chlamydial infection. Despite this recommendation, screening coverage in many primary care settings remains low.

ULCERATIVE GENITAL OR PERIANAL LESIONS

Genital ulceration reflects a set of important STIs, most of which sharply increase the risk of sexual acquisition and shedding of HIV. In a 1996 study of genital ulcers in 10 of the U.S. cities with the highest rates of primary syphilis, PCR testing of ulcer specimens demonstrated HSV in 62% of patients, *T. pallidum* in 13%, and *Haemophilus ducreyi* (the cause of chancroid) in 12–20%. Today, genital herpes represents an even higher proportion of genital ulcers in the United States and other industrialized countries.

In Asia and Africa, chancroid (**Fig. 136-5**) was once considered the most common type of genital ulcer, followed in frequency by primary syphilis and then genital herpes (**Fig. 136-6**). With increased efforts to control chancroid and syphilis and widespread use of broad-spectrum antibiotics to treat STI-related syndromes, together with more frequent recurrences or persistence of genital herpes attributable to HIV infection, PCR testing of genital ulcers now clearly implicates genital herpes as by far the most common cause of genital ulceration in most developing countries. LGV due to *C. trachomatis* (**Fig. 136-7**) and donovanosis (granuloma inguinale, due to *Klebsiella granulomatis*; **see Fig. 173-1**) continue to cause genital ulceration in some developing countries. LGV virtually disappeared in industrialized countries during the first 20 years of the HIV pandemic, but outbreaks are again occurring in Europe (including the United Kingdom), in North America, and in Australia. In these outbreaks, LGV typically presents as proctitis, with or without anal lesions, in men who report unprotected receptive anal intercourse, very often in association with HIV and/or hepatitis C virus infection; the latter may be an acute infection acquired through the same exposure. Other causes of genital ulcers include (1) candidiasis and traumatized genital warts—both readily recognized; (2) lesions due to genital involvement by more widespread dermatoses;

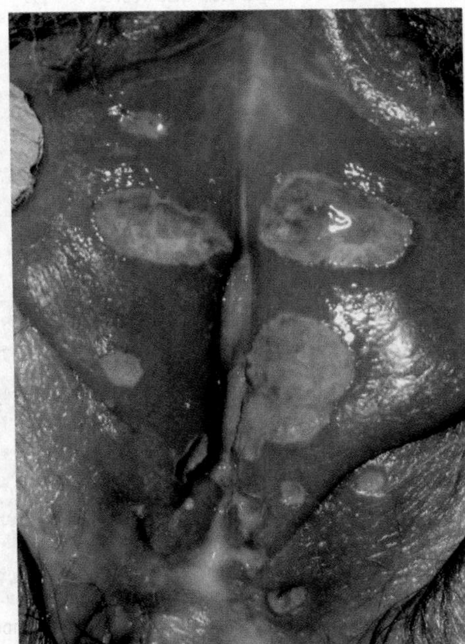

FIGURE 136-5 Chancroid: multiple, painful, punched-out ulcers with undermined borders on the labia occurring after autoinoculation.

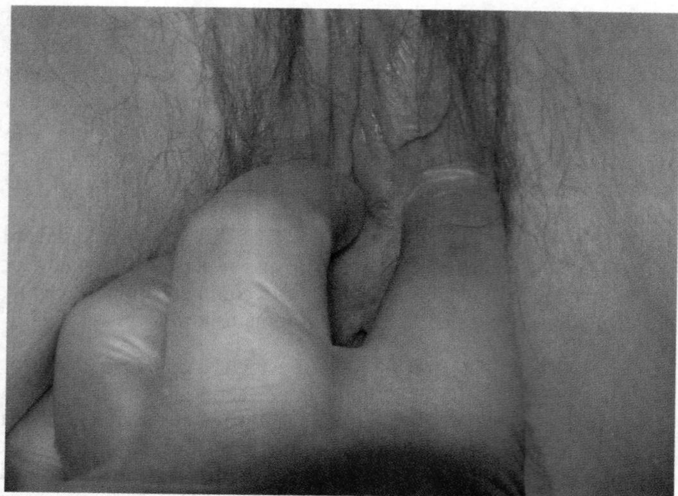

FIGURE 136-6 Genital herpes. A relatively mild, superficial ulcer is typically seen in episodic outbreaks. *(Courtesy of Michael Remington, University of Washington Virology Research Clinic.)*

(3) cutaneous manifestations of systemic diseases such as genital mucosal ulceration in Stevens-Johnson syndrome or Behçet's disease; (4) superinfections of lesions that may originally have been sexually acquired (for example, methicillin-resistant *S. aureus* complicating a genital ulcer due to HSV-2); and (5) localized drug reactions, such as the ulcers occasionally seen with topical paromomycin cream or boric acid preparations.

Diagnosis Although most genital ulcerations cannot be diagnosed confidently on clinical grounds alone, clinical findings **(Table 136-7)** and epidemiologic considerations can usually guide initial management **(Table 136-8)** pending results of specific tests. Clinicians should order a rapid serologic test for syphilis in all cases of genital ulcer and treat presumptively while awaiting serology in a patient at high risk (especially MSM). To evaluate lesions except those highly characteristic of infection with HSV (i.e., those with herpetic vesicles), dark-field microscopy, direct immunofluorescence, and a NAAT for *T. pallidum* can be useful but are rarely available. It is important to note that 30% of syphilitic chancres—the primary ulcer of syphilis—are associated with an initially nonreactive syphilis serology. All patients presenting with genital ulceration should be counseled and tested for HIV infection.

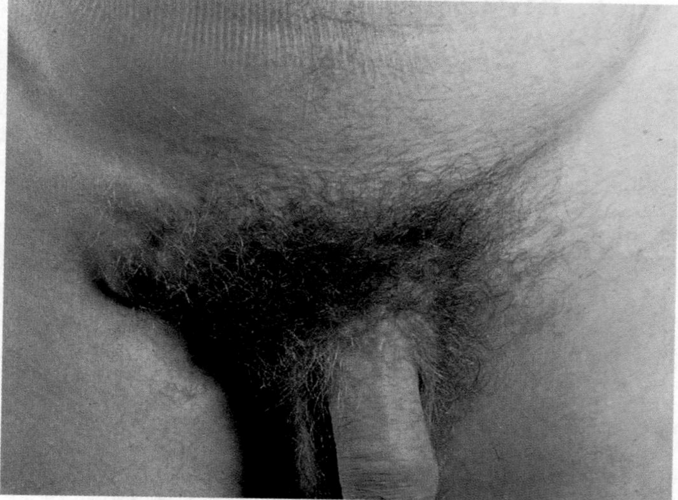

FIGURE 136-7 Lymphogranuloma venereum (LGV): striking tender lymphadenopathy occurring at the femoral and inguinal lymph nodes, separated by a groove made by Poupart's ligament. This "sign-of-the-groove" is not considered specific for LGV; for example, lymphomas may present with this sign.

Typical vesicles or pustules or a cluster of painful ulcers preceded by vesiculopustular lesions suggest genital herpes. These typical clinical manifestations make detection of the virus optional; however, many patients want confirmation of the diagnosis, and differentiation of HSV-1 from HSV-2 has prognostic implications, because the latter causes more frequent genital recurrences and is more infectious to vulnerable sex partners.

Painless, nontender, indurated ulcers with firm, nontender inguinal adenopathy suggest primary syphilis. If results of dark-field examination and a rapid serologic test for syphilis are initially negative, or if these tests are not available, presumptive therapy should be provided on the basis of the individual's risk. With historically high rates of syphilis among MSM in the United States, therapy for this infection should not be withheld pending watchful waiting and/or subsequent detection of seroconversion. Repeated serologic testing for syphilis 1 or 2 weeks after treatment of seronegative primary syphilis usually demonstrates seroconversion.

"Atypical" or clinically trivial ulcers may be more common manifestations of genital herpes than classic vesiculopustular lesions. Specific tests for HSV in such lesions are therefore indicated **(Chap. 192)**. Commercially available type-specific serologic tests for serum antibody to HSV-2 may give negative results, especially when patients present early with the initial episode of genital herpes or when HSV-1 is the cause of genital herpes (as is often the case today). Furthermore, a positive test for antibody to HSV-2 does not prove that the current lesions are herpetic because nearly one-fifth of the general population of the United States (and no doubt a higher proportion of those at risk for other STIs) becomes seropositive for HSV-2 during early adulthood. Although even "type-specific" tests for HSV-2 that are commercially available in the United States are not 100% specific, a positive HSV-2 serology does enable the clinician to tell the patient that he or she has probably had genital herpes, should learn to recognize symptoms, and should avoid sex during recurrences. In addition, because genital shedding and sexual transmission of HSV-2 often occur in the absence of symptoms and signs of recurrent herpetic lesions, persons who have a history of genital herpes or who are seropositive for HSV-2 should consider the use of condoms or suppressive antiviral therapy, both of which can reduce the risk of HSV-2 transmission to a sexual partner.

Demonstration of *H. ducreyi* by culture (or by PCR, where available) is most useful when ulcers are painful and purulent, especially if inguinal lymphadenopathy with fluctuance or overlying erythema is noted; if chancroid is prevalent in the community; or if the patient has recently had a sexual exposure elsewhere in a chancroid-endemic area (e.g., a developing country). Enlarged, fluctuant lymph nodes should be aspirated for culture or PCR to detect *H. ducreyi* as well as for Gram's staining and culture to rule out the presence of other pyogenic bacteria.

When genital ulcers persist beyond the natural history of initial episodes of herpes (2–3 weeks) or of chancroid or syphilis (up to 6 weeks) and do not resolve with syndrome-based antimicrobial therapy, then—in addition to the usual tests for herpes, syphilis, and chancroid—biopsy is indicated to exclude donovanosis as well as carcinoma and other nonvenereal dermatoses.

TREATMENT

Ulcerative Genital or Perianal Lesions

Immediate syndrome-based treatment for acute genital ulcer (after collection of all necessary diagnostic specimens at the first visit) is often appropriate before all test results become available because patients with typical initial or recurrent episodes of genital or anorectal herpes can benefit from prompt oral antiviral therapy **(Chap. 192)**; because early treatment of sexually transmitted causes of genital ulcers decreases further transmission; and because some patients do not return for test results and treatment. A thorough assessment of the patient's sexual-risk profile and medical history is critical in determining the course of initial management. The patient who has risk factors consistent with exposure to syphilis (e.g., a male patient who reports sex with other men or who has

TABLE 136-7 Clinical Features of Genital Ulcers

FEATURE	SYPHILIS	HERPES	CHANCROID	LYMPHOGRANULOMA VENEREUM	DONOVANOSIS
Incubation period	9–90 days	2–7 days	1–14 days	3 days–6 weeks	1–4 weeks (up to 6 months)
Early primary lesions	Papule	Vesicle	Pustule	Papule, pustule, or vesicle	Papule
Number of lesions	Usually one	Multiple	Usually multiple, may coalesce	Usually one; often not detected, despite lymphadenopathy	Variable
Diameter	5–15 mm	1–2 mm	Variable	2–10 mm	Variable
Edges	Sharply demarcated, elevated, round, or oval	Erythematous	Undermined, ragged, irregular	Elevated, round, or oval	Elevated, irregular
Depth	Superficial or deep	Superficial	Excavated	Superficial or deep	Elevated
Base	Smooth, nonpurulent, relatively nonvascular	Serous, erythematous, nonvascular	Purulent, bleeds easily	Variable, nonvascular	Red and velvety, bleeds readily
Induration	Firm	None	Soft	Occasionally firm	Firm
Pain	Uncommon	Frequently tender	Usually very tender	Variable	Uncommon
Lymphadenopathy	Firm, nontender, bilateral	Firm, tender, often bilateral with initial episode	Tender, may suppurate, loculated, usually unilateral	Tender, may suppurate, loculated, usually unilateral	None; pseudobuboes

Source: Reproduced with permission from RM Ballard, in KK Holmes et al (eds): *Sexually Transmitted Diseases,* 4th ed. New York, McGraw-Hill, 2008.

HIV infection) should generally receive initial treatment for syphilis. Empirical therapy for chancroid should be considered if there has been an exposure in an area of the world where chancroid occurs or if regional lymph node suppuration is evident. Finally, empirical antimicrobial therapy may be indicated if ulcers persist and the diagnosis remains unclear after a week of observation despite attempts to diagnose herpes, syphilis, and chancroid.

PROCTITIS, PROCTOCOLITIS, ENTEROCOLITIS, AND ENTERITIS

Sexually acquired *proctitis*, with inflammation limited to the rectal mucosa (the distal 10–12 cm), results from direct rectal inoculation of typical STD pathogens. In contrast, inflammation extending from the rectum to the colon (*proctocolitis*), involving both the small and the large bowel (*enterocolitis*), or involving the small bowel alone (*enteritis*) can result from ingestion of typical intestinal pathogens through oral-anal exposure during sexual contact. Anorectal pain and mucopurulent, bloody rectal discharge suggest proctitis or proctocolitis. Proctitis commonly produces tenesmus (causing frequent attempts to defecate, but not true diarrhea) and constipation, whereas proctocolitis and enterocolitis more often cause true diarrhea. In all three conditions, anoscopy usually shows mucosal exudate and easily induced mucosal bleeding (i.e., a positive "wipe test"), sometimes with petechiae or mucosal ulcers. Exudate should be sampled for Gram's staining and other microbiologic studies. Sigmoidoscopy or colonoscopy shows inflammation limited to the rectum in proctitis or disease extending at least up into the sigmoid colon in proctocolitis.

TABLE 136-8 Initial Management of Genital or Perianal Ulcer

Causative Pathogens

HSV
Treponema pallidum (primary syphilis)
Haemophilus ducreyi (chancroid)

Usual Initial Laboratory Evaluation

Dark-field examination (if available), direct FA, or PCR for *T. pallidum*
RPR, VDRL, or EIA serologic test for syphilis[a]
Culture, direct FA, ELISA, or PCR for HSV
HSV-2-specific serology (consider)
In chancroid-endemic area: PCR or culture for *H. ducreyi*

Initial Treatment

Herpes confirmed or suspected (history or sign of vesicles):
Treat for genital herpes with acyclovir, valacyclovir, or famciclovir.

Syphilis confirmed (dark-field, FA, or PCR showing *T. pallidum*, or RPR reactive):
Benzathine penicillin (2.4 million units IM once to patient, to recent [e.g., within 3 months] seronegative partner[s], and to all seropositive partners)[b]

Chancroid confirmed or suspected (diagnostic test positive, or HSV and syphilis excluded, and persistent lesion):
- Ciprofloxacin (500 mg PO as single dose) *or*
- Ceftriaxone (250 mg IM as single dose) *or*
- Azithromycin (1 g PO as single dose)

[a]If results are negative but primary syphilis is suspected, treat presumptively when indicated by epidemiologic and sexual risk assessment; repeat in 1 week. [b]The same treatment regimen is also effective in HIV-infected persons with early syphilis.

Abbreviations: EIA, enzyme immunoassay; ELISA, enzyme-linked immunosorbent assay; FA, fluorescent antibody; HSV, herpes simplex virus; PCR, polymerase chain reaction; RPR, rapid plasma reagin; VDRL, Venereal Disease Research Laboratory.

The AIDS era brought an extraordinary shift in the clinical and etiologic spectrum of intestinal infections among MSM. The number of cases of the acute intestinal STIs described above fell as high-risk sexual behaviors became less common in this group. At the same time, the number of AIDS-related opportunistic intestinal infections increased rapidly, many associated with chronic or recurrent symptoms. The incidence of these opportunistic infections has since fallen with increasingly widespread coverage of HIV-infected persons with effective antiretroviral therapy. Two species initially isolated in association with intestinal symptoms in MSM—now known as *Helicobacter cinaedi* and *Helicobacter fennelliae*—have both been isolated from the blood of HIV-infected men and other immunosuppressed persons, often in association with a syndrome of multifocal dermatitis and arthritis.

Acquisition of HSV, *N. gonorrhoeae*, or *C. trachomatis* (including LGV strains of *C. trachomatis*) during receptive anorectal intercourse causes most cases of infectious proctitis in women and MSM. Primary and secondary syphilis can also produce anal or anorectal lesions, with or without symptoms. Gonococcal or chlamydial proctitis typically involves the most distal rectal mucosa and the anal crypts and is clinically mild, without systemic manifestations. In contrast, primary proctitis due to HSV and proctocolitis due to the strains of *C. trachomatis* that cause LGV usually produce severe anorectal pain and often cause fever. Perianal ulcers and inguinal lymphadenopathy, most commonly due to HSV, can also occur with LGV or syphilis. Sacral nerve root radiculopathies, usually presenting as urinary retention, laxity of the anal sphincter, or constipation, may complicate primary herpetic proctitis. In LGV, rectal biopsy typically shows crypt abscesses, granulomas, and giant cells—findings resembling those in Crohn's disease; such findings should always prompt rectal culture and serology for LGV, which is a curable infection. Syphilis can also produce rectal granulomas, usually in association with infiltration by plasma cells or other mononuclear cells. Syphilis, LGV, and HSV infection involving the rectum can produce perirectal adenopathy that is sometimes mistaken for malignancy; syphilis, LGV, HSV infection, and chancroid involving the anus can produce inguinal adenopathy because anal lymphatics drain to inguinal lymph nodes.

Diarrhea and abdominal bloating or cramping pain without anorectal symptoms and with normal findings on anoscopy and sigmoidoscopy occur with inflammation of the small intestine (enteritis) or with proximal colitis. In MSM without HIV infection, enteritis is often attributable to *Giardia lamblia*. Sexually acquired proctocolitis is most often due to *Campylobacter* or *Shigella* species.

TREATMENT

Proctitis, Proctocolitis, Enterocolitis, and Enteritis

Acute proctitis in persons who have practiced receptive anorectal intercourse is usually sexually acquired. Such patients should undergo anoscopy to detect rectal ulcers or vesicles and petechiae after swabbing of the rectal mucosa; to examine rectal exudates for PMNs and gram-negative diplococci; and to obtain rectal swab specimens for testing for rectal gonorrhea, chlamydial infection, herpes, and syphilis. Pending test results, patients with proctitis should receive empirical syndromic treatment—e.g., with ceftriaxone (a single IM dose of 500 mg for gonorrhea) plus doxycycline (100 mg by mouth twice daily for 7 days for possible chlamydial infection) plus treatment for herpes or syphilis if indicated. If LGV proctitis is proven or suspected, the recommended treatment is doxycycline (100 mg by mouth twice daily for 21 days); alternatively, 1 g of azithromycin once a week for 3 weeks is likely to be effective but is little studied.

PREVENTION AND CONTROL OF STIs

Prevention and control of STIs require the following:

1. Reduction of the average rate of sexual exposure to STIs through alteration of sexual risk behaviors and behavioral norms among both susceptible and infected persons in all population groups. The necessary changes include reduction in the total number of sexual partners and the number of concurrent sexual partners. The U.S. Preventive Services Task Force recommends intensive behavioral counseling for all sexually active adolescents and adults who are at increased risk for STIs (grade B recommendation). Motivational interviewing is one approach that has elicited behavioral changes, including safer sex practices and more consistent contraception, that contribute to these goals.
2. Reduction of the efficiency of transmission through the promotion of safer sexual practices, the use of condoms during casual or commercial sex, vaccination against HBV and HPV infection, male circumcision (which reduces risk of acquisition of HIV infection, chancroid, and perhaps other STIs), and a growing number of other approaches (e.g., early detection and treatment of other STIs to reduce the efficiency of sexual transmission of HIV). Longitudinal studies have shown that consistent condom use is associated with significant protection of both males and females against all STIs that have been examined, including HIV, HPV, and HSV infections as well as gonorrhea and chlamydial infection. The only exceptions are probably sexually transmitted *Pthirus pubis* and *Sarcoptes scabiei* infestations.
3. Shortening of the duration of infectivity of STIs through early detection and curative or suppressive treatment of patients and their sexual partners. The availability of curative therapy for hepatitis C virus infection and suppressive therapy for HBV infection exemplifies new opportunities for shortening infectivity in major STIs.

Financial and time constraints imposed by many clinical practices, along with the reluctance of some clinicians to ask questions about stigmatized sexual behaviors, often curtail screening and prevention services. As outlined in **Fig. 136-8**, the success of clinicians' efforts to detect and treat STIs depends in part on societal efforts to teach young people how to recognize symptoms of STIs; to motivate individuals

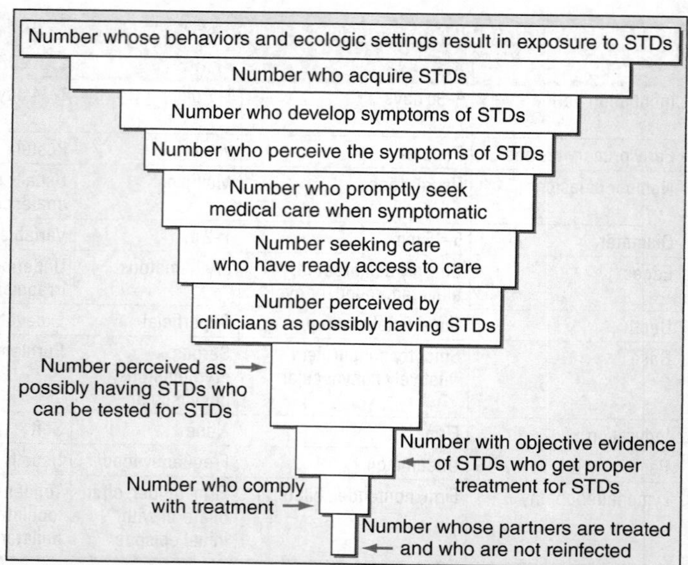

FIGURE 136-8 Critical control points for preventive and clinical interventions against sexually transmitted diseases (STDs). *(Adapted from HT Waller and MA Piot: Bull World Health Organ 41:75, 1969 and 43:1, 1970; and from "Resource allocation model for public health planning—a case study of tuberculosis control," Bull World Health Organ 48[Suppl], 1973.)*

with symptoms to seek care promptly; to educate persons who are at risk but have no symptoms about what tests they should undergo routinely; and to make high-quality, appropriate care accessible, affordable, and acceptable, especially to the young indigent patients most likely to acquire an STI.

STI RISK ASSESSMENT

Because many infected individuals develop no symptoms or fail to recognize and report symptoms, clinicians should routinely perform an STI risk assessment for teenagers and young adults as a guide to selective screening. As stated earlier, the U.S. Preventive Services Task Force recommends screening sexually active female patients ≤25 years of age for *C. trachomatis* whenever they present for health care (at least once a year); older women should be tested if they have more than one sexual partner, have begun a new sexual relationship since the previous test, or have another STI diagnosed. In women 25–29 years of age, chlamydial infection is uncommon but still may reach a prevalence of 3–5% in some settings; information provided by women in this age group on a sex partner's concurrency (whether a male partner has had another sex partner during the time they have been together) is helpful in identifying women at increased risk. In some regions of the United States, widespread selective screening and treatment of young women for cervical *C. trachomatis* infection have been associated with a 50–60% drop in prevalence. Such screening and treatment also protect the individual woman from PID. Sensitive urine-based genetic amplification tests permit expansion of screening to men, teenage boys, and girls in settings where examination is not planned or is impractical (e.g., during preparticipation sports examinations or during initial medical evaluation of adolescent girls). Vaginal swabs—collected either by the health care provider at a pelvic examination or by the woman herself—are highly sensitive and specific for the diagnosis of chlamydial and gonococcal infection; they are now the preferred type of specimen for screening and diagnosis of these infections.

Although gonorrhea is now substantially less common than chlamydial infection in women in industrialized countries, screening tests for *N. gonorrhoeae* are still appropriate for women and teenage girls attending STD clinics and for sexually active teens and young women from areas of high gonorrhea prevalence. Multiplex NAATs that combine screening for *N. gonorrhoeae* and *C. trachomatis*—and, more recently, for *T. vaginalis*—in a single low-cost assay now facilitate the prevention and control of these infections for populations at high risk.

All patients who have newly detected STIs or are at high risk for STIs according to routine risk assessment as well as all pregnant women should be encouraged to undergo serologic testing for syphilis and HIV infection, with appropriate HIV counseling before and after testing. Randomized trials have shown that risk-reduction counseling of patients with STIs significantly lowers subsequent risk of acquiring an STI; such counseling should now be considered a standard component of STI management. Preimmunization serologic testing for antibody to HBV is indicated for unvaccinated persons who are known to be at high risk, such as MSM and people who use injection drugs. In most young persons, however, it is more cost-effective to vaccinate against HBV without serologic screening. It is important to recognize that, while immunization against HBV has contributed to marked reductions in the incidence of infection with this virus, the majority of new cases that do occur are acquired through sex. In 2006, the CDC's Advisory Committee on Immunization Practices (ACIP) recommended the following: (1) Universal hepatitis B vaccination should be implemented for all unvaccinated adults in settings in which a high proportion of adults have risk factors for HBV infection (e.g., STD clinics, HIV testing and treatment facilities, drug-abuse treatment and prevention settings, health care settings targeting services to injection drug users or MSM, and correctional facilities). (2) In other primary care and specialty medical settings that provide care to adults at risk for HBV infection, health care providers should inform all patients about the health benefits of vaccination, the risk factors for HBV infection, and the persons for whom vaccination is recommended; they should vaccinate adults who report risk factors for HBV infection as well as any adult who requests protection from HBV infection. To promote vaccination in all settings, health care providers should implement standing orders to identify adults recommended for hepatitis B vaccination, should administer hepatitis B vaccine as part of routine clinical services, should not require acknowledgment of an HBV infection risk factor for adult vaccination, and should use available reimbursement mechanisms to remove financial barriers to hepatitis B vaccination.

In 2007, the ACIP made its first recommendation for routine immunization of 9- to 26-year-old girls and women with the quadrivalent HPV vaccine (against HPV types 6, 11, 16, and 18). In 2011, the ACIP recommended routine administration of quadrivalent HPV vaccine to boys at 11 or 12 years of age and to males 13–21 years of age who have not yet been vaccinated or who have not completed the three-dose vaccine series; HBV vaccination of men 22–26 years of age has also been recommended. Since that time, a nonavalent HPV vaccine has become available and has largely replaced the earlier vaccines. The optimal age for recommended vaccination is 11–12 years because of the very high risk of HPV infection after sexual debut.

Partner notification is the process of identifying and informing partners of infected patients about possible exposure to an STI and of examining, testing, vaccinating, and treating partners as appropriate. In a series of 22 reports concerning partner notification during the 1990s, index patients with gonorrhea or chlamydial infection named a mean of 0.75–1.6 partners, of whom one-fourth to one-third were infected; those with syphilis named 1.8–6.3 partners, with one-third to one-half infected; and those with HIV infection named 0.76–5.31 partners, with up to one-fourth infected. Persons who transmit infection or who have recently been infected and are still in the incubation period usually have no symptoms or only mild symptoms and seek medical attention only when notified of their exposure. Therefore, the clinician must encourage patients to participate in partner notification, must ensure that exposed persons are notified and treated, and must guarantee confidentiality to all involved. In the United States, local health departments often offer assistance in partner notification, treatment, and/or counseling. It seems both feasible and most useful to notify those partners exposed within the patient's likely period of infectiousness, which is often considered the preceding 1 month for gonorrhea, 1–2 months for chlamydial infection, and up to 3 months for early syphilis.

Persons with a new-onset STI always have a *source* contact who gave them the infection; in addition, they may have a *secondary* (*spread* or *exposed*) contact with whom they had sex after becoming infected. The identification and treatment of these two types of contacts have different objectives. Treatment of the source contact (often a casual contact) benefits the community by preventing further transmission and benefits the source contact; treatment of the recently exposed secondary contact (typically a spouse or another steady sexual partner) prevents the development of serious complications (such as PID) in the partner, reinfection of the index patient, and further spread of infection. A survey of a random sample of U.S. physicians found that most instructed patients to abstain from sex during treatment, to use condoms, and to inform their sex partners after being diagnosed with gonorrhea, chlamydial infection, or syphilis; physicians sometimes gave the patients drugs for their partners. However, follow-up of the partners by physicians was infrequent. A randomized trial compared patients' delivery of therapy to partners exposed to gonorrhea or chlamydial infection with conventional notification and advice to partners to seek evaluation for STD; patients' delivery of partners' therapy, also known as *expedited partner therapy* (EPT), significantly reduced combined rates of reinfection of the index patient with *N. gonorrhoeae* or *C. trachomatis*. State-by-state variations in regulations governing this approach have not been well defined, but the 2015 CDC STD treatment guidelines describe its potential use. EPT, which is now commonly used by many practicing physicians, is currently permissible in 39 states and potentially allowable in another 8. (Updated information on the legal status of EPT is available at *http://www.cdc.gov/std/ept*.)

In summary, clinicians and public health agencies share responsibility for the prevention and control of STIs. In the current health care environment, the role of primary care clinicians has become increasingly important in STI prevention as well as in diagnosis and treatment, and the resurgence of bacterial STIs like syphilis and LGV among MSM—particularly those co-infected with HIV—emphasizes the need for risk assessment and routine screening.

FURTHER READING

Clement ME et al: Treatment of syphilis: A systematic review. JAMA 312:1905, 2014.

Gottlieb SL et al: The global roadmap for advancing development of vaccines against sexually transmitted infections: Update and next steps. Vaccine 34:2939, 2016.

Johnston C, Corey L: Current concepts for genital herpes simplex virus infection: Diagnostics and pathogenesis of genital tract shedding. Clin Microbiol Rev 29:149, 2016.

Kirkcaldy RD et al: *Neisseria gonorrhoeae* antimicrobial resistance among men who have sex with men and men who have sex exclusively with women: The Gonococcal Isolate Surveillance Project, 2005–2010. Ann Intern Med 158:321, 2013.

Mlisana K et al: Symptomatic vaginal discharge is a poor predictor of sexually transmitted infections and genital tract inflammation in high-risk women in South Africa. J Infect Dis 206:6, 2012.

Newman L et al: Global estimates of the prevalence and incidence of four curable sexually transmitted infections in 2012 based on systematic review and global reporting. PLoS One 10:e0143304, 2015.

Price MJ et al: Risk of pelvic inflammatory disease following *Chlamydia trachomatis* infection: Analysis of prospective studies with a multistate model. Am J Epidemiol 178:484, 2013.

Unemo M et al: Sexually transmitted infections: Challenges ahead. Lancet Infect Dis 17:e235-279, 2017.

US Preventive Services Task Force: Behavioral counseling interventions to prevent sexually transmitted infections. JAMA 324:674, 2020.

Wiesenfeld HC et al: A randomized controlled trial of ceftriaxone and doxycycline, with or without metronidazole, for the treatment of acute pelvic inflammatory disease. Clin Infect Dis 13:ciaa101, 2020.

Workowski KA, Bolan GA: Sexually transmitted disease treatment guidelines, 2015. MMWR Recomm Rep 64(RR-03):1, 2015.

Zakher B et al: Screening for gonorrhea and *Chlamydia*: A systematic review for the US Preventive Services Task Force. Ann Intern Med 161:884, 2014.

137 Encephalitis

Karen L. Roos, Michael R. Wilson,
Kenneth L. Tyler

■ DEFINITION

Encephalitis is defined as an inflammation of the brain caused either by infection, usually with a virus, or from a primary autoimmune process. This chapter will focus on infectious causes of encephalitis. Many patients with encephalitis also have evidence of associated meningitis (meningoencephalitis) and, in some cases, involvement of the spinal cord or nerve roots (encephalomyelitis, encephalomyeloradiculitis).

■ CLINICAL MANIFESTATIONS

Similar to meningitis, encephalitis is typically an acute febrile illness. The patient with encephalitis commonly has an altered level of consciousness (confusion, behavioral abnormalities), or a depressed level of consciousness ranging from mild lethargy to coma, and evidence of either focal or diffuse neurologic signs and symptoms. Patients with encephalitis may have hallucinations, agitation, personality change, behavioral disorders, and, at times, a frankly psychotic state. Focal or generalized seizures occur in many patients with encephalitis. Virtually every possible type of focal neurologic disturbance has been reported in viral encephalitis; the signs and symptoms reflect the sites of infection and inflammation. The most commonly encountered focal findings are aphasia, ataxia, upper or lower motor neuron patterns of weakness, involuntary movements (e.g., myoclonic jerks, tremor), and cranial nerve deficits (e.g., ocular palsies, facial weakness). Involvement of the hypothalamic-pituitary axis may result in temperature dysregulation, diabetes insipidus, or the development of the syndrome of inappropriate secretion of antidiuretic hormone (SIADH). Even though neurotropic viruses typically cause injury in distinct regions of the central nervous system (CNS), variations in clinical presentations make it impossible to reliably establish the etiology of a specific case of encephalitis on clinical grounds alone (see "Differential Diagnosis," below).

■ ETIOLOGY

In the United States, there are an estimated ~20,000 cases of encephalitis per year, although the actual number of cases is likely to be significantly higher. Despite comprehensive diagnostic efforts, most cases of acute encephalitis with a suspected viral etiology remain of unknown cause. Hundreds of viruses are capable of causing encephalitis, although only a limited subset is responsible for most cases in which a specific cause is identified **(Table 137-1)**. The most commonly identified viruses causing sporadic cases of acute encephalitis in immunocompetent adults are herpesviruses (herpes simplex virus [HSV] **[Chap. 192]**, varicella-zoster virus [VZV] **[Chap. 193]**, Epstein-Barr virus [EBV] **[Chap. 194]**). Epidemics of encephalitis are caused by arboviruses **(Chap. 209)**, which belong to several different viral taxonomic groups including *Alphaviruses* (e.g., eastern equine encephalitis [EEE] virus and chikungunya virus), *Flaviviruses* (e.g., West Nile virus [WNV], St. Louis encephalitis virus, Japanese encephalitis virus, Powassan virus, Zika virus), and *Bunyaviruses* (e.g., California encephalitis virus serogroup, La Crosse virus, Jamestown Canyon virus). Historically, the largest number of cases of arbovirus encephalitis in the United States has been due to St. Louis encephalitis virus and the California encephalitis virus serogroup. However, since 2002, WNV has been responsible for the majority of arbovirus meningitis and encephalitis cases in the United States. WNV caused 24,657 confirmed cases of neuroinvasive disease (encephalitis, meningitis, or myelitis) in the years 1999–2018 with 2033 deaths. In 2018, there were 1658 reported cases of neuroinvasive disease (encephalitis, meningitis, acute flaccid paralysis), 908 of which were encephalitis. Preliminary data for 2019 indicate there were only 626 neuroinvasive cases with 54 deaths. It is important to recognize that WNV epidemics are unpredictable and that cases have occurred in every state in the continental United States. Since 2006, there have been increasing numbers of cases of the tick-borne Powassan virus primarily in the northeastern United States and Minnesota and Wisconsin. New causes of viral CNS infections are constantly appearing, as evidenced by the outbreak of cases of encephalitis in Southeast Asia caused by Nipah virus, a member of the Paramyxoviridae family; meningitis in Europe caused by Toscana virus, an arbovirus belonging to the Bunyavirus family; neurologic disorders associated with Zika virus, a flavivirus, in South America; and neurologic disorders associated with major epidemics of chikungunya virus, a togavirus, in Africa, India, and Southeast Asia. Dengue virus is common in >100 countries worldwide with cases on the rise in the Caribbean and Puerto Rico and rare cases reported in the United States in Florida and in southern Texas. Parechoviruses including human parechovirus 3 (HPeV3), members of the Picornavirus family, have been reported as causes of fever, sepsis, and meningitis in infants (age <3 months) in the United States and abroad.

TABLE 137-1 Viruses Causing Acute Encephalitis in North America

COMMON	LESS COMMON
Herpesviruses	Rabies
Cytomegalovirus[a]	Eastern equine encephalitis virus
Herpes simplex virus 1[b]	Powassan virus
Herpes simplex virus 2	Cytomegalovirus[a]
Human herpesvirus 6	Colorado tick fever virus
Varicella-zoster virus	Mumps
Epstein-Barr virus	Jamestown Canyon virus
Arthropod-borne viruses	
La Crosse virus	
West Nile virus[c]	
St. Louis encephalitis virus	
Zika	
Enteroviruses	

[a]Immunocompromised host. [b]The most common cause of sporadic encephalitis.
[c]The most common cause of epidemic encephalitis.

■ LABORATORY DIAGNOSIS

CSF Examination Cerebrospinal fluid (CSF) examination should be performed in all patients with suspected viral encephalitis unless contraindicated by the presence of severely increased intracranial pressure (ICP). Ideally, at least 20 mL of the initial CSF sample should be collected, with 5–10 mL stored frozen for later studies, including additional direct detection tests like virus-specific polymerase chain reaction (PCR) or metagenomic next-generation sequencing, since many neuroinvasive viruses are only transiently present in the CSF. The characteristic CSF profile is indistinguishable from that of viral meningitis and typically consists of a lymphocytic pleocytosis, a mildly elevated protein concentration, and a normal glucose concentration. A CSF pleocytosis (>5 cells/μL) occurs in >95% of immunocompetent patients with documented viral encephalitis. In rare cases, a pleocytosis may be absent on the initial lumbar puncture (LP) but present on subsequent LPs. Patients who are severely immunocompromised by HIV infection, glucocorticoid or other immunosuppressant drugs, chemotherapy, or lymphoreticular malignancies may fail to mount a CSF inflammatory response. CSF cell counts exceed 500/μL in only about 10% of patients with encephalitis. Infections with certain arboviruses (e.g., EEE virus or California encephalitis virus), mumps, and lymphocytic choriomeningitis virus (LCMV) may occasionally result in cell counts >1000/μL, but this degree of pleocytosis should suggest the possibility of nonviral infections or other inflammatory processes. Atypical lymphocytes in the CSF may be seen in EBV infection and less commonly with other viruses, including cytomegalovirus (CMV), HSV, and enteroviruses. Increased numbers of plasmacytoid or Mollaret-like large mononuclear cells have been reported in WNV encephalitis. Polymorphonuclear pleocytosis occurs in ~45% of patients with WNV encephalitis and is also a common feature in CMV myeloradiculitis in immunocompromised patients. Large numbers of CSF polymorphonuclear leukocytes may be present in patients with encephalitis due to EEE virus, echovirus 9, and, more rarely, other enteroviruses. However, persisting CSF neutrophilia should prompt consideration of bacterial infection, leptospirosis, amebic infection, and noninfectious processes such as acute hemorrhagic leukoencephalitis. About 20% of patients with encephalitis will have a significant number of red blood cells (>500/μL) in the CSF in a nontraumatic tap. The pathologic correlate of this finding may be punctate microhemorrhages of the type seen with HSV; however, CSF red blood cells occur with similar frequency and in similar numbers in patients with nonherpetic focal encephalitides. A decreased CSF glucose concentration is distinctly unusual in viral encephalitis and should suggest the possibility of bacterial, fungal, tuberculous, parasitic, leptospiral, syphilitic, sarcoid, or neoplastic meningitis. Rare patients with mumps, LCMV, or advanced HSV encephalitis and many patients with CMV myeloradiculitis have low CSF glucose concentrations.

■ CSF POLYMERASE CHAIN REACTION

CSF PCR has become the primary diagnostic test for CNS infections caused by HSV, CMV, EBV, HHV-6, and enteroviruses. In the case of VZV CNS infection, CSF PCR and detection of virus-specific IgM or intrathecal antibody synthesis both provide important aids to diagnosis. The sensitivity and specificity of CSF PCRs vary with the virus being tested. The sensitivity (~96%) and specificity (~99%) of HSV CSF PCR are equivalent to or exceed those of brain biopsy. It is important to recognize that HSV CSF PCR results need to be interpreted after considering the likelihood of disease in the patient being tested, the timing of the test in relationship to onset of symptoms, and the prior use of antiviral therapy. A negative HSV CSF PCR test performed by a qualified laboratory at the appropriate time during illness in a patient with a high likelihood of HSV encephalitis based on clinical and laboratory abnormalities significantly reduces the likelihood of HSV encephalitis but does not exclude it. For example, in a patient with a pretest probability of 35% of having HSV encephalitis, a negative HSV CSF PCR reduces the posttest probability to ~2%, and for a patient with a pretest probability of 60%, a negative test reduces the posttest probability to ~6%. In both situations, a positive test makes the diagnosis almost certain (98–99%). There have been reports of initially negative HSV CSF PCR tests that were obtained early (≤72 h) following symptom onset and that became positive when repeated 1–3 days later. The frequency of positive HSV CSF PCRs in patients with herpes encephalitis also decreases as a function of the duration of illness, with only ~20% of cases remaining positive after ≥14 days. PCR results are generally not affected by ≤1 week of antiviral therapy. In one study, 98% of CSF specimens remained PCR positive during the first week of antiviral therapy, but the numbers fell to ~50% by 8–14 days and to ~21% by >15 days after initiation of antiviral therapy.

The sensitivity and specificity of CSF PCR tests for viruses other than HSV have not been definitively characterized. Enteroviral (EV) CSF PCR appears to have a sensitivity and specificity of >95%. EV PCR sensitivity for EV-A71 may be considerably lower (~30% in some reports). Patients with EV-D68-associated acute flaccid myelitis (AFM) only rarely have a positive CSF RT-PCR (<3%) but may have a positive test on nasopharyngeal swab specimens. Parechoviruses are also not detected by standard EV RT-PCRs. The specificity of EBV CSF PCR has not been established. Positive EBV CSF PCRs associated with positive tests for other pathogens have been reported and may reflect reactivation of EBV latent in lymphocytes that enter the CNS as a result of an unrelated infectious or inflammatory process. In patients with CNS infection due to VZV, CSF antibody and PCR studies should be considered complementary because patients may have evidence of intrathecal synthesis of VZV-specific antibodies and negative CSF PCRs. In the case of WNV infection, CSF PCR appears to be less sensitive than detection of WNV-specific CSF IgM, although PCR testing remains useful in immunocompromised patients who may not mount an effective anti-WNV antibody response. The recent pandemic of disease due to SARS-CoV-2 (COVID-19) has been associated with cases of encephalopathy due to the indirect effects on the nervous system of multiorgan system failure and/or to a hyperinflammatory syndrome and disseminated intravascular coagulation, but also with rare cases of true encephalitis caused by viral CNS invasion. In both sets of patients, nasopharyngeal reverse transcriptase (RT)-PCR tests for SARS-CoV-2 are positive, but only cases with encephalitis have a positive CSF RT-PCR for SARS-CoV-2. Neuroinvasion by SARS-CoV-2 has also been detected by RT-PCR of brain tissue, and there has been demonstration of virion particles by electron microscopy in neurons and endothelial cells.

Unbiased metagenomic sequencing technologies capable of identifying infectious genomes in CSF, brain, and other tissues have recently shown great promise for rapid diagnosis of obscure cases of encephalitis and other brain infections.

CSF Culture CSF culture is generally of limited utility in the diagnosis of acute viral encephalitis. Culture may be insensitive (e.g., >95% of patients with HSV encephalitis have negative CSF cultures, as do virtually all patients with EBV-associated CNS disease) and often takes too long to significantly affect immediate therapy.

Serologic Studies and Antigen Detection For many arboviruses including WNV, serologic studies remain important diagnostic tools. Serum antibody determination is less useful for viruses with high seroprevalence rates in the general population such as HSV, VZV, CMV, and EBV. For viruses with low seroprevalence rates, diagnosis of acute viral infection can be made by documenting seroconversion between acute-phase and convalescent sera (typically obtained after 2–4 weeks) or by demonstrating the presence of virus-specific IgM antibodies. For viruses with high seroprevalence such as VZV and HSV, demonstration of synthesis of virus-specific antibodies in CSF, as shown by an increased IgG index or the presence of CSF IgM antibodies, may be useful and can provide presumptive evidence of CNS infection. Unfortunately, the delay between onset of infection and the host's generation of a virus-specific antibody response often means that serologic data are useful mainly for the retrospective establishment of a specific diagnosis, rather than in aiding acute diagnosis or management.

In patients with HSV encephalitis, antibodies to HSV-1 glycoproteins and HSV glycoprotein antigens have been detected in the CSF. Optimal detection of both HSV antibodies and antigen typically occurs after the first week of illness, limiting the utility of these tests in acute diagnosis. Nonetheless, HSV CSF antibody testing is of value in selected patients whose illness is >1 week in duration and who are CSF PCR negative for HSV. In the case of VZV infection, CSF IgM antibody tests may be positive when PCR fails to detect viral DNA, and both tests should be considered complementary rather than mutually exclusive.

Demonstration of WNV IgM antibodies is diagnostic of WNV encephalitis because IgM antibodies do not cross the blood-brain barrier, and their presence in CSF is therefore indicative of intrathecal synthesis. Timing of antibody collection may be important because the rate of CSF WNV IgM seropositivity increases during the first week after illness onset, reaching 80% or higher on day 7 after symptom onset. Although serum and CSF IgM antibodies generally persist for only a few months after acute infection, there are exceptions to this rule, and WNV serum IgM has been shown to persist in some patients for >1 year following acute infection.

MRI, CT, and EEG Patients with suspected encephalitis almost invariably undergo neuroimaging studies and often electroencephalogram (EEG). These tests help identify or exclude alternative diagnoses and assist in the differentiation between a focal and a diffuse encephalitic process. Focal findings in a patient with encephalitis should always raise the possibility of HSV encephalitis. Examples of focal findings include: (1) areas of increased signal intensity in the frontotemporal, cingulate, or insular regions of the brain on T2-weighted, fluid-attenuated inversion recovery (FLAIR), or diffusion-weighted MRI (**Fig. 137-1**); (2) focal areas of low absorption, mass effect, and contrast enhancement on CT; or (3) periodic focal temporal lobe spikes on a background of slow or low-amplitude ("flattened") activity on EEG.

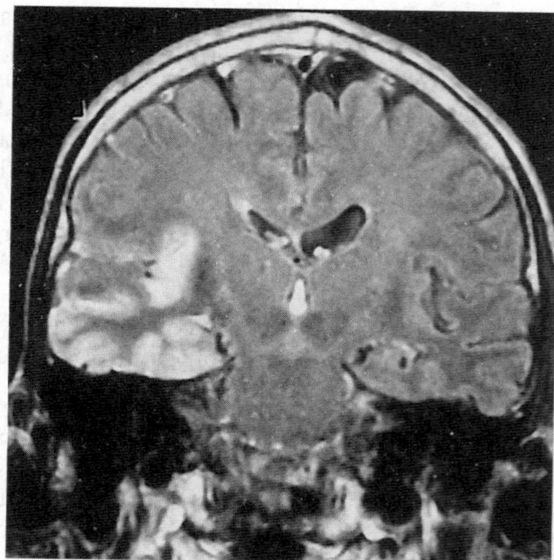

FIGURE 137-1 Coronal fluid-attenuated inversion recovery (FLAIR) magnetic resonance image from a patient with herpes simplex encephalitis. Note the area of increased signal in the right temporal lobe (*left side of image*) confined predominantly to the gray matter. This patient had predominantly unilateral disease; bilateral lesions are more common but may be quite asymmetric in their intensity.

Approximately 10% of patients with PCR-documented HSV encephalitis will have a normal MRI, although nearly 80% will have abnormalities in the temporal lobe, and an additional 10% in extratemporal regions. The lesions are typically hyperintense on T2-weighted images. The addition of FLAIR and diffusion-weighted images to the standard MRI sequences enhances sensitivity. Children with HSV encephalitis may have atypical patterns of MRI lesions and often show involvement of brain regions outside the frontotemporal areas. CT is less sensitive than MRI and is normal in up to 20–35% of patients. EEG abnormalities occur in >75% of PCR-documented cases of HSV encephalitis; they typically involve the temporal lobes but are often nonspecific. Some patients with HSV encephalitis have a distinctive EEG pattern consisting of periodic, stereotyped, sharp-and-slow complexes originating in one or both temporal lobes and repeating at regular intervals of 2–3 s. The periodic complexes are typically noted between days 2 and 15 of the illness and are present in two-thirds of pathologically proven cases of HSV encephalitis.

Significant MRI abnormalities are found in only approximately two-thirds of patients with WNV encephalitis, a frequency less than that with HSV encephalitis. When present, abnormalities often involve deep brain structures, including the thalamus, basal ganglia, and brainstem, rather than the cortex, and may only be apparent on FLAIR images. Similar MRI patterns can be observed in patients infected with other arboviruses, including other flaviviruses such as Japanese encephalitis virus and St. Louis encephalitis virus, as well the *Alphavirus* EEE virus. EEGs in patients with WNV encephalitis typically show generalized slowing that may be more anteriorly prominent rather than the temporally predominant pattern of sharp or periodic discharges more characteristic of HSV encephalitis. Patients with VZV encephalitis may show multifocal areas of hemorrhagic and ischemic infarction, reflecting the tendency of this virus to produce a CNS vasculopathy rather than a true encephalitis. Immunocompromised adult patients with CMV often have enlarged ventricles with areas of increased T2 signal on MRI outlining the ventricles and subependymal enhancement on T1-weighted postcontrast images. Prominent cerebellar T2/FLAIR abnormalities have been observed with Powassan virus encephalitis and in children with herpesviruses like EBV and VZV. **Table 137-2** highlights specific diagnostic test results in encephalitis that can be useful in clinical decision-making.

Brain Biopsy Brain biopsy is now generally reserved for patients in whom CSF PCR studies fail to lead to a specific diagnosis, who have focal abnormalities on MRI, who have no serologic evidence of autoimmune disease, and who continue to show progressive clinical deterioration despite treatment with acyclovir and supportive therapy.

TABLE 137-2 Use of Diagnostic Tests in Encephalitis

The best test for WNV encephalitis is the *CSF IgM antibody test*. The prevalence of positive CSF IgM tests increases by about 10% per day after illness onset and reaches 70–80% by the end of the first week. Serum WNV IgM can provide evidence for recent WNV infection, but in the absence of other findings does not establish the diagnosis of neuroinvasive disease (meningitis, encephalitis, acute flaccid paralysis).
Approximately 80% of patients with proven HSV encephalitis have *MRI* abnormalities involving the temporal lobes. This percentage likely increases to >90% when FLAIR and diffusion-weighted MRI sequences are also used. The absence of temporal lobe lesions on MRI reduces the likelihood of HSV encephalitis and should prompt consideration of other diagnostic possibilities.
The *CSF HSV PCR* test may be negative in the first 72 h of symptoms of HSV encephalitis. A repeat study should be considered in patients with an initial early negative PCR in whom diagnostic suspicion of HSV encephalitis remains high and no alternative diagnosis has yet been established.
Detection of *intrathecal synthesis* (increased CSF/serum HSV antibody ratio corrected for breakdown of the blood-brain barrier) of *HSV-specific antibody* may be useful in diagnosis of HSV encephalitis in patients in whom only late (>1 week after onset) CSF specimens are available and PCR studies are negative. Serum serology alone is of no value in diagnosis of HSV encephalitis due to the high seroprevalence rate in the general population.
Negative *CSF viral cultures* are of no value in excluding the diagnosis of HSV or EBV encephalitis.
VZV CSF IgM antibodies may be present in patients with a negative VZV CSF PCR. Both tests should be performed in patients with suspected VZV CNS disease.
The specificity of *EBV CSF PCR* for diagnosis of CNS infection is unknown. Positive tests may occur in patients with a CSF pleocytosis due to other causes. Detection of EBV CSF IgM or intrathecal synthesis of antibody to VCA supports the diagnosis of EBV encephalitis. Serologic studies consistent with acute EBV infection (e.g., IgM VCA, presence of antibodies against EA but not against EBNA) can help support the diagnosis.
In addition to broad-based PCR assays for bacterial and fungal infections, metagenomic next-generation sequencing (mNGS) allows for unbiased detection of nucleic acids from the whole range of infectious agents (except prions), which can then be confirmed by independent pathogen-specific techniques. Due to the sensitivity of this technology, there is a risk of false-positive results. As this technology becomes refined and the turnaround time faster, mNGS is likely to become a routine test on CSF for the diagnosis of encephalitis.

Abbreviations: CNS, central nervous system; CSF, cerebrospinal fluid; DWI, diffusion-weighted imaging; EA, early antigen; EBNA, EBV-associated nuclear antigen; EBV, Epstein-Barr virus; FLAIR, fluid-attenuated inversion recovery; HSV, herpes simplex virus; IgM, immunoglobulin M; MRI, magnetic resonance imaging; PCR, polymerase chain reaction; VCA, viral capsid antibody; VZV, varicella-zoster virus; WNV, West Nile virus.

DIFFERENTIAL DIAGNOSIS

Infection by a variety of other organisms can mimic viral encephalitis. In studies of biopsy-proven HSV encephalitis, common infectious mimics of focal viral encephalitis included mycobacteria, fungi, rickettsiae, *Listeria*, *Mycoplasma*, and other bacteria (including *Bartonella* sp.) as well as neurosyphilis. There are an increasing number of antibodies reported that cause autoimmune encephalitis, including those associated with antibodies against *N*-methyl-D-aspartate (NMDA) receptor, voltage-gated potassium channels/leucine-rich glioma inactivated protein-1 (VGKC/LGI-I), α-amino-3-hydroxy-5-methyl-4-isoxazolepropionic acid (AMPA), γ-aminobutyric acid (GABA) receptors, and glutamic acid decarboxylase (GAD 65), that can mimic that caused by viral infection. In most cases, diagnosis is made by detection of the specific autoantibodies in serum and/or CSF. NMDA receptor antibodies have been reported in up to 25% of patients with HSV encephalitis, and their presence should not exclude appropriate testing and treatment for HSV encephalitis. It has been suggested that development of NMDA receptor antibodies in patients with HSV encephalitis may contribute to delayed recovery or clinical relapse. Autoimmune encephalitis may also be associated with specific cancers (paraneoplastic) and onconeuronal antibodies (e.g., anti-Hu, Yo, Ma2, amphiphysin, CRMP5, CV2) (**Chap. 94**). Subacute or chronic forms of encephalitis may occur in association with autoantibodies against thyroglobulin and thyroperoxidase (Hashimoto's encephalopathy) and with prion diseases.

Infection caused by the ameba *Naegleria fowleri* can also cause acute meningoencephalitis (primary amebic meningoencephalitis), whereas that caused by *Acanthamoeba* and *Balamuthia* more typically produces subacute or chronic granulomatous amebic meningoencephalitis. *Naegleria* thrive in warm, iron-rich pools of water, including those found in drains, canals, and both natural and human-made outdoor pools. Infection has typically occurred in immunocompetent children with a history of swimming in potentially infected water. The CSF, in contrast to the typical profile seen in viral encephalitis, often resembles that of bacterial meningitis with a neutrophilic pleocytosis and hypoglycorrhachia. Motile trophozoites can be seen in a wet mount of warm, fresh CSF. There have been an increasing number of cases of *Balamuthia mandrillaris* amebic encephalitis mimicking acute viral encephalitis in children and immunocompetent adults. This organism has also been associated with encephalitis in recipients of transplanted organs from a donor with unrecognized infection. No effective treatment has been identified, and mortality approaches 100%.

Encephalitis can be caused by the raccoon pinworm *Baylisascaris procyonis*. Clues to the diagnosis include a history of raccoon exposure, especially of playing in or eating dirt potentially contaminated with raccoon feces. Most patients are children, and many have an associated eosinophilia.

Once nonviral causes of encephalitis have been excluded, the major diagnostic challenge is to distinguish HSV from other viruses that cause encephalitis. This distinction is particularly important because in virtually every other instance the therapy is supportive, whereas specific and effective antiviral therapy is available for HSV, and its efficacy is enhanced when it is instituted early in the course of infection. HSV encephalitis should be considered when clinical features suggest involvement of the inferomedial frontotemporal regions of the brain, including prominent olfactory or gustatory hallucinations, anosmia, unusual or bizarre behavior or personality alterations, or memory disturbance. HSV encephalitis should always be suspected in patients with signs and symptoms consistent with acute encephalitis with focal findings on clinical examination, neuroimaging studies, or EEG. The diagnostic procedure of choice in these patients is CSF PCR analysis for HSV. A positive CSF PCR establishes the diagnosis, and a negative test dramatically reduces the likelihood of HSV encephalitis (see above).

The anatomic distribution of lesions may provide an additional clue to diagnosis. Patients with rapidly progressive encephalitis and prominent brainstem signs, symptoms, or neuroimaging abnormalities may be infected by flaviviruses (WNV, St. Louis encephalitis virus, Japanese encephalitis virus), HSV, enterovirus A71 (EV-A71), rabies, or *Listeria monocytogenes*. Significant involvement of deep gray matter structures, including the basal ganglia and thalamus, should also suggest possible flavivirus infection. These patients may present clinically with prominent movement disorders (tremor, myoclonus) or parkinsonian features. Patients with WNV infection can also present with a poliomyelitis-like AFM, as can patients infected with EV-A71, EV-D68, and less commonly, other enteroviruses. Acute flaccid paralysis is characterized by the acute onset of a lower motor neuron type of weakness with flaccid tone, reduced or absent reflexes, and relatively preserved sensation. Patients often have multisegmental increased FLAIR and T2 signal in the anterior horns of the spinal cord and a CSF lymphocytic pleocytosis.

Epidemiologic factors may provide important clues to the diagnosis of viral encephalitis. Particular attention should be paid to the season of the year; the geographic location and travel history; and possible exposure to animal bites or scratches, rodents, and ticks. Although transmission from the bite of an infected dog remains the most common cause of rabies worldwide, in the United States, very few cases of dog rabies occur, and the most common risk factor is exposure to bats—although a clear history of a bite or scratch is often lacking. The classic clinical presentation of encephalitic (furious) rabies is fever, fluctuating consciousness, and autonomic hyperactivity. Phobic spasms of the larynx, pharynx, neck muscles, and diaphragm can be triggered by attempts to swallow water (*hydrophobia*) or by inspiration (*aerophobia*). Patients may also present with paralytic (dumb) rabies characterized by acute ascending paralysis. Rabies due to the bite of a bat has a different clinical presentation than classic rabies due to a dog or wolf bite. Patients present with focal neurologic deficits, myoclonus, seizures, and hallucinations; phobic spasms are not a typical feature. Patients with rabies have a CSF lymphocytic pleocytosis and may show areas of increased T2 signal abnormality in the brainstem, hippocampus, and hypothalamus. Diagnosis can be made by finding rabies virus antigen in brain tissue or in the neural innervation of hair follicles at the nape of the neck. PCR amplification of viral nucleic acid from CSF and saliva or tears may also enable diagnosis. Serology is frequently negative in both serum and CSF in the first week after onset of infection, which limits its acute diagnostic utility. No specific therapy is available, and cases are almost invariably fatal, with isolated survivors having devastating neurologic sequelae.

State public health authorities provide a valuable resource concerning isolation of particular agents in individual regions. Regular updates concerning the number, type, and distribution of cases of arboviral encephalitis can be found on the Centers for Disease Control and Prevention and U.S. Geological Survey (USGS) websites (*http://www.cdc.gov* and *http://diseasemaps.usgs.gov*).

TREATMENT

Viral Encephalitis

Specific antiviral therapy should be initiated when appropriate. Vital functions, including respiration and blood pressure, should be monitored continuously and supported as required. In the initial stages of encephalitis, many patients will require care in an intensive care unit. Basic management and supportive therapy should include careful monitoring of ICP, fluid restriction, avoidance of hypotonic intravenous solutions, and suppression of fever. Seizures should be treated with standard anticonvulsant regimens, and prophylactic therapy should be considered in view of the high frequency of seizures in severe cases of encephalitis. As with all seriously ill, immobilized patients with altered levels of consciousness, encephalitis patients are at risk for aspiration pneumonia, stasis ulcers and decubiti, contractures, deep venous thrombosis and its complications, and infections of indwelling lines and catheters.

Acyclovir is of benefit in the treatment of HSV and should be started empirically in patients with suspected viral encephalitis, especially if focal features are present, while awaiting viral diagnostic studies. Treatment should be discontinued in patients found not to have HSV encephalitis, with the possible exception of patients with severe encephalitis due to VZV or EBV. HSV, VZV, and EBV all encode an enzyme deoxypyrimidine (thymidine) kinase that phosphorylates acyclovir to produce acyclovir-5′-monophosphate. Host cell enzymes then phosphorylate this compound to form a triphosphate derivative. It is the triphosphate that acts as an antiviral agent by inhibiting viral DNA polymerase and by causing premature termination of nascent viral DNA chains. The specificity of action depends on the fact that uninfected cells do not phosphorylate significant amounts of acyclovir to acyclovir-5′-monophosphate. A second level of specificity is provided by the fact that the acyclovir triphosphate is a more potent inhibitor of viral DNA polymerase than of the analogous host cell enzymes.

Adults should receive a dose of 10 mg/kg of acyclovir intravenously every 8 h (30 mg/kg per day total dose) for 21 days. Neonatal HSV CNS infection is less responsive to acyclovir therapy than HSV encephalitis in adults; it is recommended that neonates with HSV encephalitis receive 20 mg/kg of acyclovir every 8 h (60 mg/kg per day total dose) for a minimum of 21 days.

Prior to intravenous administration, acyclovir should be diluted to a concentration ≤7 mg/mL. (A 70-kg person would receive a dose of 700 mg, which would be diluted in a volume of 100 mL.) Each dose should be infused slowly over 1 h, rather than by rapid or bolus infusion, to minimize the risk of renal dysfunction. Care should be taken to avoid extravasation or intramuscular or subcutaneous administration. The alkaline pH of acyclovir can cause local inflammation and phlebitis (9%). Dose adjustment is required in patients with impaired renal glomerular filtration. Penetration into CSF is excellent, with average drug levels ~50% of serum levels.

Complications of therapy include elevations in blood urea nitrogen and creatinine levels (5%), thrombocytopenia (6%), gastrointestinal toxicity (nausea, vomiting, diarrhea) (7%), and neurotoxicity (lethargy or obtundation, disorientation, confusion, agitation, hallucinations, tremors, seizures) (1%). Acyclovir resistance may be mediated by changes in either the viral deoxypyrimidine kinase or DNA polymerase. To date, acyclovir-resistant isolates have not been a significant clinical problem in immunocompetent individuals. However, there have been reports of clinically virulent acyclovir-resistant HSV isolates from sites outside the CNS in immunocompromised individuals, including those with AIDS.

Oral antiviral drugs with efficacy against HSV, VZV, and EBV, including acyclovir, famciclovir, and valacyclovir, have not been evaluated in the treatment of encephalitis as primary therapy. Additional oral valaciclovir following a 14- to 21-day course of intravenous acyclovir does not improve outcomes in adult patients with HSV encephalitis. The role of adjunctive intravenous glucocorticoids in treatment of HSV and VZV infection remains unclear. Experimental models and case reports of HSV encephalitis suggest that glucocorticoids may be efficacious, although no data from randomized controlled human trials are available. Ganciclovir and foscarnet, either alone or in combination, are often used in the treatment of CMV-related CNS infections, although their efficacy remains unproven. Cidofovir (see below) may provide an alternative in patients who fail to respond to ganciclovir and foscarnet, although data concerning its use in CMV CNS infections are extremely limited.

Ganciclovir is a synthetic nucleoside analogue of 2′-deoxyguanosine. The drug is preferentially phosphorylated by virus-induced cellular kinases. Ganciclovir triphosphate acts as a competitive inhibitor of the CMV DNA polymerase, and its incorporation into nascent viral DNA results in premature chain termination. Following intravenous administration, CSF concentrations of ganciclovir are 25–70% of coincident plasma levels. The usual dose for treatment of severe neurologic illnesses is 5 mg/kg every 12 h given intravenously at a constant rate over 1 h. Induction therapy is followed by maintenance therapy of 5 mg/kg every day for an indefinite period. Induction therapy should be continued until patients show a decline in CSF pleocytosis and a reduction in CSF CMV DNA copy number on quantitative PCR testing (where available). Doses should be adjusted in patients with renal insufficiency. Treatment is often limited by the development of granulocytopenia and thrombocytopenia (20–25%), which may require reduction in or discontinuation of therapy. Gastrointestinal side effects, including nausea, vomiting, diarrhea, and abdominal pain, occur in ~20% of patients. Some patients treated with ganciclovir for CMV retinitis have developed retinal detachment, but the causal relationship to ganciclovir treatment is unclear. Valganciclovir is an orally bioavailable prodrug that can generate high serum levels of ganciclovir, although studies of its efficacy in treating CMV CNS infections are limited.

Foscarnet is a pyrophosphate analogue that inhibits viral DNA polymerases by binding to the pyrophosphate-binding site. Following intravenous infusion, CSF concentrations range from 15 to 100% of coincident plasma levels. The usual dose for serious CMV-related neurologic illness is 60 mg/kg every 8 h administered by constant infusion over 1 h. Induction therapy for 14–21 days is followed by maintenance therapy (60–120 mg/kg per day). Induction therapy may need to be extended in patients who fail to show a decline in CSF pleocytosis and a reduction in CSF CMV DNA copy number on quantitative PCR tests (where available). Approximately one-third of patients develop renal impairment during treatment, which is reversible following discontinuation of therapy in most, but not all, cases. This is often associated with elevations in serum creatinine and proteinuria and is less frequent in patients who are adequately hydrated. Many patients experience fatigue and nausea. Reductions in serum calcium, magnesium, and potassium occur in ~15% of patients and may be associated with tetany, cardiac rhythm disturbances, or seizures.

Cidofovir is a nucleotide analogue that is effective in treating CMV retinitis and equivalent to or better than ganciclovir in some experimental models of murine CMV encephalitis, although data concerning its efficacy in human CMV CNS disease are limited. The usual dose is 5 mg/kg intravenously once weekly for 2 weeks, then biweekly for two or more additional doses, depending on clinical response. Patients must be prehydrated with normal saline (e.g., 1 L over 1–2 h) prior to each dose and treated with probenecid (e.g., 1 g 3 h before cidofovir and 1 g 2 and 8 h after cidofovir). Nephrotoxicity is common; the dose should be reduced if renal function deteriorates.

Intravenous ribavirin (15–25 mg/kg per day in divided doses given every 8 h) has been reported to be of benefit in isolated cases of severe encephalitis due to California encephalitis (La Crosse) virus. Ribavirin might be of benefit for the rare patients, typically infants or young children, with severe adenovirus or rotavirus encephalitis and in patients with encephalitis due to LCMV or other arenaviruses. However, clinical trials are lacking. Hemolysis, with resulting anemia, has been the major side effect limiting therapy.

No specific antiviral therapy of proven efficacy is currently available for treatment of WNV encephalitis. Patients have been treated with interferon-α, ribavirin, an Israeli IVIg preparation that contains high-titer anti-WNV antibody (Omr-IgG-am), and humanized monoclonal antibodies directed against the viral envelope glycoprotein (*www.clinicaltrials.gov*, identifiers NCT00927953 and 00515385). Omr-IgG-am did not improve outcomes in patients with WNV neuroinvasive disease, but the study design was potentially flawed as some patients received drug up to a week after symptom onset, when expected benefit may have been minimal. WNV chimeric vaccines (in which WNV envelope and premembrane proteins are inserted into the background of another flavivirus), DNA plasmid vaccines, and inactivated virus vaccines have all been tested in phase 1 clinical trials and have been found to be both safe and immunogenic in healthy adults but have not yet been tested for disease prevention in humans (see *www.clinicaltrials.gov*). Both chimeric and killed inactivated WNV vaccines have been found to be safe and effective in preventing equine WNV infection, and effective vaccines are already in human use for prevention of other flavivirus infections including Japanese encephalitis and yellow fever, suggesting that efficacy testing and commercial considerations rather than scientific issues will be the major impediment to creating a WNV vaccine.

High-quality, randomized, placebo-controlled clinical trials in patients with severe COVID-19 have identified modest beneficial effects of the experimental antiviral drug remdesivir, which acts as a false nucleoside analogue to inhibit SARS-CoV-2 replication, as well as glucocorticoids. Studies currently available have not shown significant benefit for ritonavir/lopinavir or chloroquine/hydroxychloroquine despite anecdotal reports of benefit in isolated cases. Trials of convalescent plasma derived from patients who have recovered from confirmed COVID-19 infection and of inhibitors of proinflammatory cytokines including interleukin 6, which may contribute to the hyperinflammatory state in severe COVID-19 infection, are underway.

SEQUELAE

There is considerable variation in the incidence and severity of sequelae in patients surviving viral encephalitis. In the case of EEE virus infection, nearly 80% of survivors have severe neurologic sequelae. At the other extreme are infections due to EBV, California encephalitis virus, and Venezuelan equine encephalitis virus, where severe sequelae are unusual. For example, ~5–15% of children infected with La Crosse virus have a residual seizure disorder, and 1% have persistent hemiparesis. Detailed information about sequelae in patients with HSV encephalitis treated with acyclovir is available from the NIAID-Collaborative Antiviral Study Group (CASG) trials. Of 32 acyclovir-treated patients, 26 survived (81%). Of the 26 survivors, 12 (46%) had no or only minor sequelae, 3 (12%) were moderately impaired (gainfully employed but not functioning at their previous level), and 11 (42%) were severely impaired (requiring continuous supportive care). The incidence and severity of sequelae were directly related to the age of the patient and the level of consciousness at the time of initiation of therapy. Patients with severe neurologic impairment (Glasgow Coma Scale score 6) at initiation of therapy either died or survived with severe sequelae. Young patients (<30 years) with good neurologic function at initiation of therapy did substantially better (100% survival, 62% with no or mild sequelae) compared with their older counterparts (>30 years; 64% survival, 57% no or mild sequelae). Many patients with WNV infection have sequelae, including cognitive impairment; weakness; and hyper- or hypokinetic movement disorders, including tremor, myoclonus, and parkinsonism. In a large longitudinal study of prognosis in 156 patients with WNV infection, the mean time to achieve recovery (defined as 95% of maximal predicted score on specific validated tests) was 112–148 days for fatigue, 121–175 days for physical function, 131–139 days for mood, and 302–455 days for mental function (the longer interval in each case representing patients with invasive CNS disease).

CHRONIC ENCEPHALITIS

PROGRESSIVE MULTIFOCAL LEUKOENCEPHALOPATHY

Clinical Features and Pathology Progressive multifocal leukoencephalopathy (PML) is characterized pathologically by multifocal areas of demyelination of varying size distributed throughout the brain but sparing the spinal cord and optic nerves. In addition to demyelination, there are characteristic cytologic alterations in both astrocytes and oligodendrocytes. Astrocytes are enlarged and contain hyperchromatic, deformed, and bizarre nuclei and frequent mitotic figures. Oligodendrocytes have enlarged, densely staining nuclei that contain viral inclusions formed by crystalline arrays of JC virus (JCV) particles. Patients often present with visual deficits (45%), typically a homonymous hemianopia; mental impairment (38%) (dementia, confusion, personality change); weakness, including hemi- or monoparesis; and ataxia. Seizures occur in ~20% of patients, predominantly in those with lesions abutting the cortex.

Almost all patients have an underlying immunosuppressive disorder or are receiving immunomodulatory therapy. In a recent series, the most common associated conditions were AIDS (80%), hematologic malignancies (13%), transplant recipients (5%), and chronic inflammatory diseases (2%). It has been estimated that up to 5% of AIDS patients will develop PML. Approximately 1000 cases of PML have been reported in patients being treated for multiple sclerosis and inflammatory bowel disease with natalizumab, a humanized monoclonal antibody that inhibits lymphocyte trafficking into CNS and bowel mucosa by binding to α_4 integrins. Overall risk in these patients has been estimated at ~4 PML cases per 1000 treated patients, but the risk depends on a variety of factors including anti-JCV antibody serostatus and the magnitude of the JCV antibody response, prior immunosuppressive therapy use, and duration of natalizumab therapy. Patients who lack detectable JCV antibody have a risk of developing PML of <0.1 case/1000 patients, whereas those who are JCV seropositive and have been exposed to prior immunosuppressive therapy and have received >24 months of natalizumab therapy have a risk of >1.3 cases/100 treated patients. Some recent studies suggest that extended dosing interval regimens of natalizumab (at 5- to 6-week intervals rather than the conventional 4-week interval) may significantly reduce the risk of PML. Among JCV-seropositive individuals, those with higher JCV antibody index values, presumably due to the "immunizing" effects of more frequent JCV reactivations, appear to be at higher risk than those with low antibody indices. PML cases have also been reported in patients receiving other immunomodulatory agents including rituximab, ocrelizumab, fingolimod, and dimethyl fumarate, although the relative risks have not been clearly established, and many individual cases are complicated by previous exposure to other therapies including natalizumab. The basic clinical and diagnostic features appear to be similar in HIV-associated PML and PML associated with immunomodulatory drugs with the exception of an increased likelihood of MRI enhancement of PML lesions in immunomodulatory cases. In natalizumab-associated PML, patients will also almost invariably develop clinical and radiographic worsening of lesions with discontinuation of therapy, attributed to development of immune reconstitution inflammatory syndrome (IRIS).

Diagnostic Studies The diagnosis of PML is frequently suggested by MRI. MRI reveals multifocal asymmetric, coalescing white matter lesions located periventricularly, in the centrum semiovale, in the parietal-occipital region, and in the cerebellum. These lesions have increased signal on T2 and FLAIR images and decreased signal on T1-weighted images. HIV-PML lesions are classically nonenhancing (90%), but patients with immunomodulatory drug-associated PML may have peripheral ring enhancement. PML lesions are not typically associated with edema or mass effect. CT scans, which are less sensitive than MRI for the diagnosis of PML, often show hypodense nonenhancing white matter lesions. JCV infection may also induce rare cases of encephalitis and cerebellitis in immunocompromised patients that are distinct from PML and have differing neuroimaging features.

The CSF is typically normal, although mild elevation in protein and/or IgG may be found. Pleocytosis occurs in <25% of cases, is predominantly mononuclear, and rarely exceeds 25 cells/μL. PCR amplification of JCV DNA from CSF has become an important diagnostic tool. The presence of a positive CSF PCR for JCV DNA in association with typical MRI lesions in the appropriate clinical setting is diagnostic of PML, reflecting the assay's relatively high specificity (92–100%); however, sensitivity is variable, and a negative CSF PCR does not exclude the diagnosis. In HIV-negative patients and HIV-positive patients not receiving highly active antiviral therapy (HAART), sensitivity is likely 70–90%. In HAART-treated patients, sensitivity may be closer to 60%, reflecting the lower JCV CSF viral load in this relatively more immunocompetent group. Patients with natalizumab-associated PML have highly variable amounts of JCV DNA in CSF. Some patients may have negative CSF PCRs performed in commercial laboratories, where assay detection thresholds are typically >100 JCV DNA copies/μL, but positive results in reference laboratories using supersensitive techniques (detection of 10 JCV copies/μL or less). CSF studies with quantitative JCV PCR indicate that patients with low JCV loads (<100 copies/μL) have a generally better prognosis than those with higher viral loads. Patients with negative CSF PCR studies may require brain biopsy for definitive diagnosis. In biopsy or necropsy specimens of brain, JCV antigen and nucleic acid can be detected by immunocytochemistry, in situ hybridization, or PCR amplification.

Serologic studies of JCV antibody are of modest value in diagnosis of PML due to the high basal seroprevalence level, although the absence of detectable JCV antibody may be useful in reducing the likelihood of PML in the differential diagnosis as PML results from viral reactivation in previously infected individuals and virtually all confirmed cases have been JCV seropositive at diagnosis. Antibody testing may also be useful in risk stratification of patients receiving immunomodulatory therapies.

TREATMENT

Progressive Multifocal Leukoencephalopathy

No consistently effective therapy for PML is available. There are case reports of potential beneficial effects of the 5-HT_{2a} receptor antagonist mirtazapine, which may inhibit binding of JCV to its receptor on oligodendrocytes. Retrospective noncontrolled studies have also suggested a possible beneficial effect of treatment with interferon-α. Neither of these agents has been tested in randomized controlled clinical trials. A prospective multicenter clinical trial to evaluate the efficacy of the antimalarial drug mefloquine failed to show benefit. Intravenous and/or intrathecal cytarabine were not shown to be of benefit in a randomized controlled trial in

HIV-associated PML, although some experts suggest that cytarabine may have therapeutic efficacy in situations where breakdown of the blood-brain barrier allows sufficient CSF penetration. A randomized controlled trial of cidofovir in HIV-associated PML also failed to show significant benefit. Because PML almost invariably occurs in immunocompromised individuals, any therapeutic interventions designed to enhance or restore immunocompetence should be considered; a small series of patients treated with the PD-1 inhibitor pembrolizumab demonstrated clinical improvement and stabilization. Positive results in small case series have also been reported in patients receiving infusions of BK or JC virus–specific cytotoxic T lymphocytes. Perhaps the most dramatic demonstration of the benefit of restoring immune competence is disease stabilization and, in rare cases, improvement associated with an improved immune status of HIV-positive patients with AIDS following institution of HAART. In HIV-positive PML patients treated with HAART, 1-year survival is ~50%, although up to 80% of survivors may have significant neurologic sequelae. HIV-positive PML patients with higher CD4 counts (>300/μL) and low or nondetectable HIV viral loads have a better prognosis than those with lower CD4 counts and higher viral loads. Although institution of HAART enhances survival in HIV-positive PML patients, the associated immune reconstitution in patients with an underlying opportunistic infection such as PML may also result in a severe CNS inflammatory syndrome (IRIS) associated with clinical worsening, CSF pleocytosis, and the appearance of new enhancing MRI lesions. Patients receiving natalizumab or other immunomodulatory antibodies who are suspected of having PML should have therapy immediately halted. Removal of drugs with long pharmacokinetic or biological half-lives, such as natalizumab, with plasma exchange or immunoadsorption is frequently utilized, although whether this improves outcomes has not been definitively established. Patients should be closely monitored for development of IRIS, which is generally treated with intravenous glucocorticoids, although controlled clinical trials of efficacy remain lacking.

SUBACUTE SCLEROSING PANENCEPHALITIS

Subacute sclerosing panencephalitis (SSPE) is a rare, chronic, progressive demyelinating disease of the CNS associated with a chronic nonpermissive infection of brain tissue with measles virus. The frequency has been estimated at 1 in 100,000–500,000 measles cases. An average of five cases per year is reported in the United States. The incidence has declined dramatically since the introduction of a measles vaccine. Most patients give a history of primary measles infection at an early age (2 years), which is followed after a latent interval of 6–8 years by the development of a progressive neurologic disorder. Some 85% of patients are between 5 and 15 years old at diagnosis. Initial manifestations include poor school performance and mood and personality changes. Typical signs of a CNS viral infection, including fever and headache, do not occur. As the disease progresses, patients develop progressive intellectual deterioration, focal and/or generalized seizures, myoclonus, ataxia, and visual disturbances. In the late stage of the illness, patients are unresponsive, quadriparetic, and spastic, with hyperactive tendon reflexes and extensor plantar responses.

Diagnostic Studies MRI is often normal early, although areas of increased T2 signal develop in the white matter of the brain and brainstem as disease progresses. The EEG may initially show only nonspecific slowing, but with disease progression, patients develop a characteristic periodic pattern with bursts of high-voltage, sharp, slow waves every 3–8 s, followed by periods of attenuated ("flat") background. The CSF is acellular with a normal or mildly elevated protein concentration and a markedly elevated gamma globulin level (>20% of total CSF protein). CSF antimeasles antibody levels are invariably elevated, and oligoclonal antimeasles antibodies are often present. Measles virus can be cultured from brain tissue using special cocultivation techniques. Viral antigen can be identified immunocytochemically, and viral genome can be detected by in situ hybridization or PCR amplification.

TREATMENT
Subacute Sclerosing Panencephalitis

No definitive therapy for SSPE is available. Treatment with isoprinosine (Inosiplex, 100 mg/kg per day), alone or in combination with intrathecal or intraventricular interferon-α, has been reported to prolong survival and produce clinical improvement in some patients but has never been subjected to a controlled clinical trial.

PROGRESSIVE RUBELLA PANENCEPHALITIS

This is an extremely rare disorder that primarily affects males with congenital rubella syndrome, although isolated cases have been reported following childhood rubella. After a latent period of 8–19 years, patients develop progressive neurologic deterioration. The manifestations are similar to those seen in SSPE. CSF shows a mild lymphocytic pleocytosis, slightly elevated protein concentration, markedly increased gamma globulin, and rubella virus–specific oligoclonal bands. No therapy is available. Universal prevention of both congenital and childhood rubella through the use of the available live attenuated rubella vaccine would be expected to eliminate the disease.

FURTHER READING

Cortese I et al: Pembrolizumab treatment for progressive multifocal leukoencephalopathy. N Engl J Med 380:1597, 2019.

Ramachandran PS, Wilson MR: Metagenomics for neurological infections: Expanding our imagination. Nat Rev Neurol 16:547, 2020.

Ramos-Estebanez et al: A systematic review on the role of adjunctive corticosteroids in herpes simplex virus encephalitis: Is timing critical for safety and efficacy? Antivir Ther 19:133, 2014.

Tunkel AR et al: The management of encephalitis: Clinical practice guidelines by the Infectious Diseases Society of America. Clin Infect Dis 47:303, 2008.

Tyler KL: Acute viral encephalitis. N Engl J Med 379:557, 2018.

Venkatesan A et al: International Encephalitis Consortium. Case definitions, diagnostic algorithms, and priorities in encephalitis: Consensus statement of the International Encephalitis Consortium. Clin Infect Dis 57:1114, 2013.

138 Acute Meningitis

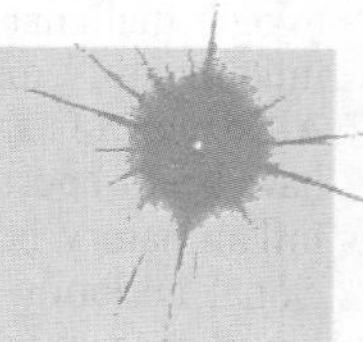

Karen L. Roos, Kenneth L. Tyler

BACTERIAL MENINGITIS

DEFINITION

Bacterial meningitis is an acute purulent infection within the subarachnoid space (SAS). It is associated with a CNS inflammatory reaction that may result in decreased consciousness, seizures, raised intracranial pressure (ICP), and stroke. The meninges, SAS, and brain parenchyma are all frequently involved in the inflammatory reaction (*meningoencephalitis*).

EPIDEMIOLOGY

Bacterial meningitis is the most common form of suppurative CNS infection, with an annual incidence in the United States of >2.5 cases/100,000 population. The organisms most often responsible for community-acquired bacterial meningitis are *Streptococcus pneumoniae* (~50%), *Neisseria meningitidis* (~25%), group B streptococci (~15%), and *Listeria monocytogenes* (~10%). *Haemophilus influenzae* type b accounts for <10% of cases of bacterial meningitis in most series. *N. meningitidis* is the causative organism of recurring epidemics of meningitis every 8–12 years.

■ ETIOLOGY

S. pneumoniae (Chap. 148) is the most common cause of meningitis in adults >20 years of age, accounting for nearly half the reported cases (1.1 per 100,000 persons per year). There are a number of predisposing conditions that increase the risk of pneumococcal meningitis, the most important of which is pneumococcal pneumonia. Additional risk factors include coexisting acute or chronic pneumococcal sinusitis or otitis media, alcoholism, diabetes, splenectomy, hypogammaglobulinemia, complement deficiency, and head trauma with basilar skull fracture and cerebrospinal fluid (CSF) rhinorrhea. The mortality rate remains ~20% despite antibiotic therapy.

The incidence of meningitis due to *N. meningitidis* (Chap. 155) has decreased with the routine immunization of 11- to 18-year-olds with the quadrivalent (serogroups A, C, W-135, and Y) meningococcal glycoconjugate vaccine. The vaccine does not contain serogroup B, which is responsible for one-third of cases of meningococcal disease. The Advisory Committee on Immunization Practices (ACIP) recommends that adolescents and young adults aged 16–23 years be vaccinated with a serogroup B meningococcal vaccine. This vaccine has become part of the required vaccination schedule for students matriculating at most American universities. There are two meningococcal group B vaccines, 4MCMenB and MenB-FHbp, both of which use outer membrane proteins as the vaccine antigens. The serogroup B polysaccharide capsule is poorly immunogenic. Neither group B vaccine reduces the risk of bacterial spread of group B meningococcus from vaccinated persons to *unimmunized* persons as the vaccines do not significantly reduce nasopharyngeal carriage of meningococci, and this remains the major source of person-to-person bacterial transmission. In contrast, nasopharyngeal carriage is reduced in vaccinated individuals who have received the conjugate vaccines that cover groups A, C, W, and Y. The presence of petechial or purpuric skin lesions can provide an important clue to the diagnosis of meningococcal infection. In some patients, the disease is fulminant, progressing to death within hours of symptom onset. Infection may be initiated by nasopharyngeal colonization, which can result in either an asymptomatic carrier state or invasive meningococcal disease. The risk of invasive disease following nasopharyngeal colonization depends on both bacterial virulence factors and host immune defense mechanisms, including the host's capacity to produce antimeningococcal antibodies and to lyse meningococci by both classic and alternative complement pathways. Individuals with deficiencies of any of the complement components, including properdin, are highly susceptible to meningococcal infections.

Gram-negative bacilli cause meningitis in individuals with chronic and debilitating diseases such as diabetes, cirrhosis, or alcoholism and in those with urinary tract infections. Gram-negative meningitis can also complicate neurosurgical procedures, particularly craniotomy, and head trauma associated with CSF rhinorrhea or otorrhea.

Otitis, mastoiditis, and sinusitis are predisposing and associated conditions for meningitis due to *Streptococcus* spp., gram-negative anaerobes, *Staphylococcus aureus, Haemophilus* spp., and Enterobacteriaceae. Meningitis complicating endocarditis may be due to viridans streptococci, *S. aureus, Streptococcus bovis*, the HACEK group (*Haemophilus* spp., *Actinobacillus actinomycetemcomitans, Cardiobacterium hominis, Eikenella corrodens, Kingella kingae*), or enterococci.

Group B *Streptococcus*, or *Streptococcus agalactiae* (Chap. 148), was previously responsible for meningitis predominantly in neonates, but it has been reported with increasing frequency in individuals aged >50 years, particularly those with underlying diseases.

L. monocytogenes (Chap. 151) is an increasingly important cause of meningitis in neonates (<1 month of age), pregnant women, individuals >60 years, and immunocompromised individuals of all ages. Infection is acquired by ingesting foods contaminated by *Listeria*. Foodborne human listerial infection has been reported from contaminated coleslaw, milk, soft cheeses, and several types of "ready-to-eat" foods, including delicatessen meat and uncooked hotdogs.

The frequency of *H. influenzae* type b (Hib) meningitis in children has declined dramatically since the introduction of the Hib conjugate vaccine, although rare cases of Hib meningitis in vaccinated children have been reported. More frequently, *H. influenzae* causes meningitis in unvaccinated children and older adults, and non-b *H. influenzae* is an emerging pathogen (Chap. 157).

S. aureus and coagulase-negative staphylococci (Chap. 142) are important causes of meningitis that occurs following invasive neurosurgical procedures, particularly shunting procedures for hydrocephalus, or as a complication of the use of subcutaneous Ommaya reservoirs for administration of intrathecal chemotherapy.

■ PATHOPHYSIOLOGY

The most common bacteria that cause meningitis, *S. pneumoniae* and *N. meningitidis*, initially colonize the nasopharynx by attaching to nasopharyngeal epithelial cells. Bacteria are transported across epithelial cells in membrane-bound vacuoles to the intravascular space or invade the intravascular space by creating separations in the apical tight junctions of columnar epithelial cells. Once in the bloodstream, bacteria are able to avoid phagocytosis by neutrophils and classic complement-mediated bactericidal activity because of the presence of a polysaccharide capsule. Bloodborne bacteria can reach the intraventricular choroid plexus, directly infect choroid plexus epithelial cells, and gain access to the CSF. Some bacteria, such as *S. pneumoniae*, can adhere to cerebral capillary endothelial cells and subsequently migrate through or between these cells to reach the CSF. Bacteria are able to multiply rapidly within CSF because of the absence of effective host immune defenses. Normal CSF contains few white blood cells (WBCs) and relatively small amounts of complement proteins and immunoglobulins. The paucity of the latter two prevents effective opsonization of bacteria, an essential prerequisite for bacterial phagocytosis by neutrophils. Phagocytosis of bacteria is further impaired by the fluid nature of CSF, which is less conducive to phagocytosis than a solid tissue substrate.

A critical event in the pathogenesis of bacterial meningitis is the inflammatory reaction induced by the invading bacteria. Many of the neurologic manifestations and complications of bacterial meningitis result from the immune response to the invading pathogen rather than from direct bacteria-induced tissue injury. As a result, neurologic injury can progress even after the CSF has been sterilized by antibiotic therapy.

The lysis of bacteria with the subsequent release of cell-wall components into the SAS is the initial step in the induction of the inflammatory response and the formation of a purulent exudate in the SAS (Fig. 138-1). Bacterial cell-wall components, such as the lipopolysaccharide (LPS) molecules of gram-negative bacteria and teichoic acid and peptidoglycans of *S. pneumoniae*, induce meningeal inflammation by stimulating the production of inflammatory cytokines and chemokines by microglia, astrocytes, monocytes, microvascular endothelial cells, and CSF leukocytes. In experimental models of meningitis, cytokines including tumor necrosis factor alpha (TNF-α) and interleukin 1β (IL-1β) are present in CSF within 1–2 h of intracisternal inoculation of LPS. This cytokine response is quickly followed by an increase in CSF protein concentration and leukocytosis. Chemokines (cytokines that induce chemotactic migration in leukocytes) and a variety of other proinflammatory cytokines are also produced and secreted by leukocytes and tissue cells that are stimulated by IL-1β and TNF-α. In addition, bacteremia and the inflammatory cytokines induce the production of excitatory amino acids, reactive oxygen and nitrogen species (free oxygen radicals, nitric oxide, and peroxynitrite), and other mediators that can induce death of brain cells, especially in the dentate gyrus of the hippocampus.

Much of the pathophysiology of bacterial meningitis is a direct consequence of elevated levels of CSF cytokines and chemokines. TNF-α and IL-1β act synergistically to increase the permeability of the blood-brain barrier, resulting in induction of vasogenic edema and the leakage of serum proteins into the SAS (Fig. 138-1). The subarachnoid exudate of proteinaceous material and leukocytes obstructs the flow of CSF through the ventricular system and diminishes the resorptive capacity of the arachnoid granulations in the dural sinuses, leading to obstructive and communicating hydrocephalus and concomitant interstitial edema.

Inflammatory cytokines upregulate the expression of selectins on cerebral capillary endothelial cells and leukocytes, promoting leukocyte

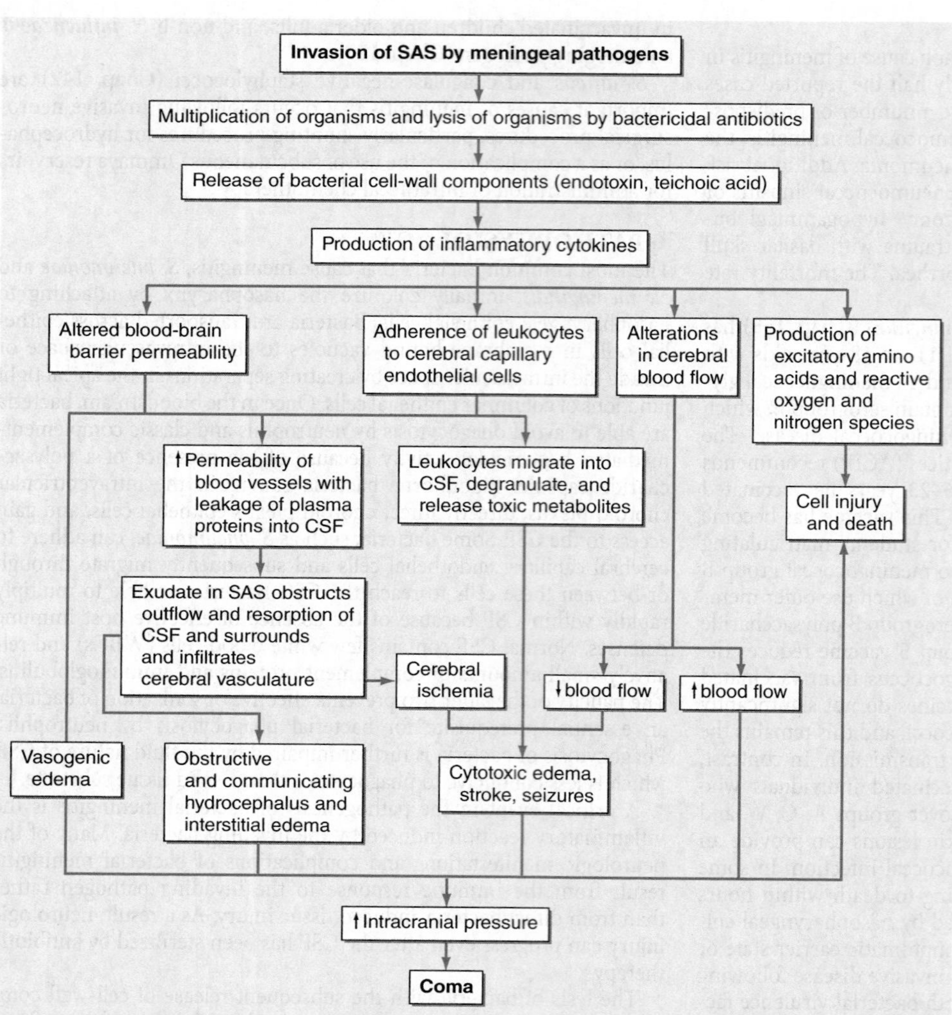

FIGURE 138-1 The pathophysiology of the neurologic complications of bacterial meningitis. CSF, cerebrospinal fluid; SAS, subarachnoid space.

adherence to vascular endothelial cells and subsequent migration into the CSF. The adherence of leukocytes to capillary endothelial cells increases the permeability of blood vessels, allowing for the leakage of plasma proteins into the CSF, which adds to the inflammatory exudate. Neutrophil degranulation results in the release of toxic metabolites that contribute to cytotoxic edema, cell injury, and death. Contrary to previous beliefs, CSF leukocytes probably do little to contribute to the clearance of CSF bacterial infection.

During the very early stages of meningitis, there is an increase in cerebral blood flow, soon followed by a decrease in cerebral blood flow and a loss of cerebrovascular autoregulation **(Chap. 307)**. Narrowing of the large arteries at the base of the brain due to encroachment by the purulent exudate in the SAS and infiltration of the arterial wall by inflammatory cells with intimal thickening (*vasculitis*) also occur and may result in ischemia and infarction, obstruction of branches of the middle cerebral artery by thrombosis, thrombosis of the major cerebral venous sinuses, and thrombophlebitis of the cerebral cortical veins. The combination of interstitial, vasogenic, and cytotoxic edema leads to raised ICP and coma. Cerebral herniation usually results from the effects of cerebral edema, either focal or generalized; hydrocephalus and dural sinus or cortical vein thrombosis may also play a role.

CLINICAL PRESENTATION

Meningitis can present as either an acute fulminant illness that progresses rapidly in a few hours or as a subacute infection that progressively worsens over several days. The classic clinical triad of meningitis is fever, headache, and nuchal rigidity, and these features each occur in >80% of adult cases of acute bacterial meningitis, although the complete classic triad is not always present. A decreased level of consciousness occurs in >75% of patients and can vary from lethargy to coma. Nausea, vomiting, and photophobia are also common complaints.

Nuchal rigidity ("stiff neck") is the pathognomonic sign of meningeal irritation and is present when the neck resists passive flexion. Kernig's and Brudzinski's signs are also classic signs of meningeal irritation. *Kernig's sign* is elicited with the patient in the supine position. The thigh is flexed on the abdomen, with the knee flexed; attempts to passively extend the knee elicit pain when meningeal irritation is present. *Brudzinski's sign* is elicited with the patient in the supine position and is positive when passive flexion of the neck results in spontaneous flexion of the hips and knees. Although commonly tested on physical examinations, the sensitivity and specificity of Kernig's and Brudzinski's signs are uncertain. Both may be absent or reduced in very young or elderly patients, immunocompromised individuals, or patients with a severely depressed mental status. The high prevalence of cervical spine disease in older individuals may result in false-positive tests for nuchal rigidity.

Seizures occur as part of the initial presentation of bacterial meningitis or during the course of the illness in 15–40% of patients. Focal seizures are usually due to focal arterial ischemia or infarction, cortical venous thrombosis with hemorrhage, or focal edema. Generalized seizure activity and status epilepticus may be due to hyponatremia, cerebral anoxia, or, less commonly, the toxic effects of antimicrobial agents.

Raised ICP is an expected complication of bacterial meningitis and the major cause of obtundation and coma in this disease. More than 90% of patients will have a CSF opening pressure >180 mmH_2O, and 20% have opening pressures >400 mmH_2O. Signs of increased ICP include a deteriorating or reduced level of consciousness, papilledema, dilated poorly reactive pupils, sixth nerve palsies, decerebrate posturing, and the Cushing reflex (bradycardia, hypertension, and irregular respirations). The most disastrous complication of increased ICP is cerebral herniation. The incidence of herniation in patients with bacterial meningitis has been reported to occur in as few as 1% to as many as 8% of cases.

Specific clinical features may provide clues to the diagnosis of individual organisms and are discussed in more detail in specific chapters devoted to individual pathogens. The most important of these clues is the rash of meningococcemia, which begins as a diffuse erythematous maculopapular rash resembling a viral exanthem; however, the skin lesions of meningococcemia rapidly become petechial. Petechiae are found on the trunk and lower extremities, in the mucous membranes and conjunctiva, and occasionally on the palms and soles.

DIAGNOSIS

When bacterial meningitis is suspected, blood cultures should be immediately obtained and empirical antimicrobial and adjunctive dexamethasone therapy initiated without delay **(Table 138-1)**. The diagnosis of bacterial meningitis is made by examination of the CSF **(Table 138-2)**. The need to obtain neuroimaging studies (CT or MRI) prior to lumbar puncture (LP) requires clinical judgment. In an immunocompetent patient with no known history of recent head trauma, a

TABLE 138-1 Antibiotics Used in Empirical Therapy of Bacterial Meningitis and Focal Central Nervous System Infections[a]

INDICATION	ANTIBIOTIC	
Preterm infants to infants <1 month	Ampicillin + cefotaxime	
Infants 1–3 months	Ampicillin + cefotaxime or ceftriaxone	
Immunocompetent children >3 months and adults <55	Cefotaxime, ceftriaxone, or cefepime + vancomycin	
Adults >55 and adults of any age with alcoholism or other debilitating illnesses	Ampicillin + cefotaxime, ceftriaxone, or cefepime + vancomycin	
Hospital-acquired meningitis, posttraumatic or postneurosurgery meningitis, neutropenic patients, or patients with impaired cell-mediated immunity	Ampicillin + ceftazidime or meropenem + vancomycin	
	TOTAL DAILY DOSE AND DOSING INTERVAL	
ANTIMICROBIAL AGENT	CHILD (>1 MONTH)	ADULT
Ampicillin	300 (mg/kg)/d, q6h	12 g/d, q4h
Cefepime	150 (mg/kg)/d, q8h	6 g/d, q8h
Cefotaxime	225–300 (mg/kg)/d, q6h	12 g/d, q4h
Ceftriaxone	100 (mg/kg)/d, q12h	4 g/d, q12h
Ceftazidime	150 (mg/kg)/d, q8h	6 g/d, q8h
Gentamicin	7.5 (mg/kg)/d, q8h[b]	7.5 (mg/kg)/d, q8h
Meropenem	120 (mg/kg)/d, q8h	6 g/d, q8h
Metronidazole	30 (mg/kg)/d, q6h	1500–2000 mg/d, q6h
Nafcillin	200 (mg/kg)/d, q6h	12 g/d, q4h
Penicillin G	400,000 (U/kg)/d, q4h	20–24 million U/d, q4h
Vancomycin	45–60 (mg/kg)/d, q6h	45–60 (mg/kg)d, q6–12h[b]

[a]All antibiotics are administered intravenously; doses indicated assume normal renal and hepatic function. [b]Doses should be adjusted based on serum peak and trough levels: gentamicin therapeutic level: peak: 5–8 μg/mL; trough: <2 μg/mL; vancomycin therapeutic level: peak: 25–40 μg/mL; trough: 5–15 μg/mL.

normal level of consciousness, and no evidence of papilledema or focal neurologic deficits, it is considered safe to perform LP without prior neuroimaging studies. If LP is delayed in order to obtain neuroimaging studies, empirical antibiotic therapy should be initiated after blood cultures are obtained. Antibiotic therapy initiated a few hours prior to LP will not significantly alter the CSF WBC count or glucose concentration, nor is it likely to prevent visualization of organisms by Gram's stain or detection of bacterial nucleic acid by polymerase chain reaction (PCR) assay.

The classic CSF abnormalities in bacterial meningitis (Table 138-2) are (1) polymorphonuclear (PMN) leukocytosis (>100 cells/μL in 90%), (2) decreased glucose concentration (<2.2 mmol/L [<40 mg/dL] and/or CSF/serum glucose ratio of <0.4 in ~60%), (3) increased protein

TABLE 138-2 Cerebrospinal Fluid (CSF) Abnormalities in Bacterial Meningitis

Opening pressure	>180 mmH_2O
White blood cells	10/μL to 10,000/μL; neutrophils predominate
Red blood cells	Absent in nontraumatic tap
Glucose	<2.2 mmol/L (<40 mg/dL)
CSF/serum glucose	<0.4
Protein	>0.45 g/L (>45 mg/dL)
Gram's stain	Positive in >60%
Culture	Positive in >80%
PCR	Detects bacterial DNA

Abbreviation: PCR, polymerase chain reaction.

concentration (>0.45 g/L [>45 mg/dL] in 90%), and (4) increased opening pressure (>180 mmH_2O in 90%). CSF bacterial cultures are positive in >70% of patients, and CSF Gram's stain demonstrates organisms in >60%.

CSF glucose concentrations <2.2 mmol/L (<40 mg/dL) are abnormal, and a CSF glucose concentration of zero can be seen in bacterial meningitis. Use of the CSF/serum glucose ratio corrects for hyperglycemia that may mask a relative decrease in the CSF glucose concentration. The CSF glucose concentration is low when the CSF/serum glucose ratio is <0.6. A CSF/serum glucose ratio <0.4 is highly suggestive of bacterial meningitis but may also be seen in other conditions, including fungal, tuberculous, and carcinomatous meningitis. It takes from 30 min to several hours for the concentration of CSF glucose to reach equilibrium with blood glucose levels; therefore, administration of 50 mL of 50% glucose (D50) prior to LP, as commonly occurs in emergency room settings, is unlikely to alter CSF glucose concentration significantly unless more than a few hours have elapsed between glucose administration and LP.

There are a number of CSF multiplex PCR pathogen assays that detect the nucleic acid of *S. pneumoniae, N. meningitidis, Escherichia coli, L. monocytogenes, H. influenzae*, and *S. agalactiae* (group B streptococci). Although these PCR assays have a rapid turnaround time, the sensitivity and specificity for bacterial meningeal pathogens is not known. Almost all patients with bacterial meningitis will have neuroimaging studies performed during the course of their illness. MRI is preferred over CT because of its superiority in demonstrating areas of cerebral edema and ischemia. In patients with bacterial meningitis, diffuse meningeal enhancement is often seen after the administration of gadolinium. Meningeal enhancement is not diagnostic of meningitis but occurs in any CNS disease associated with increased blood-brain barrier permeability.

Petechial skin lesions, if present, should be biopsied. The rash of meningococcemia results from the dermal seeding of organisms with vascular endothelial damage, and biopsy may reveal the organism on Gram's stain.

DIFFERENTIAL DIAGNOSIS

Viral meningoencephalitis, and particularly herpes simplex virus (HSV) encephalitis **(Chap. 137)**, can mimic the clinical presentation of bacterial meningitis (encephalitis). HSV encephalitis typically presents with headache, fever, altered consciousness, focal neurologic deficits (e.g., dysphasia, hemiparesis), and focal or generalized seizures. The findings on CSF studies, neuroimaging, and electroencephalogram (EEG) distinguish HSV encephalitis from bacterial meningitis. The typical CSF profile with viral CNS infections is a lymphocytic pleocytosis with a normal glucose concentration, in contrast to the PMN pleocytosis and hypoglycorrhachia characteristic of bacterial meningitis. The CSF HSV PCR has a 96% sensitivity and a 99% specificity when CSF is examined 72 h following symptom onset and in the first week of antiviral therapy. MRI abnormalities (other than meningeal enhancement) are not seen in uncomplicated bacterial meningitis. By contrast, in HSV encephalitis, on T2-weighted, fluid-attenuated inversion recovery (FLAIR) and diffusion-weighted MRI images, high-signal-intensity lesions are seen in the orbitofrontal, anterior, and medial temporal lobes in the majority of patients within 48 h of symptom onset. Some patients with HSV encephalitis have a distinctive periodic pattern on EEG.

Rickettsial disease can resemble bacterial meningitis **(Chap. 187)**. Rocky Mountain spotted fever (RMSF) is transmitted by a tick bite and caused by the bacteria *Rickettsia rickettsii*. The disease may present acutely with high fever, prostration, myalgia, headache, nausea, and vomiting. Most patients develop a characteristic rash within 96 h of the onset of symptoms. The rash is initially a diffuse erythematous maculopapular rash that may be difficult to distinguish from that of meningococcemia. It progresses to a petechial rash, then to a purpuric rash, and if untreated, to skin necrosis or gangrene. The color of the lesions changes from bright red to very dark red, then yellowish-green to black. The rash typically begins in the wrist and ankles and then spreads distally and proximally within a matter of a few hours, involving the palms and soles. Diagnosis is made by immunofluorescent staining of skin biopsy specimens. Ehrlichioses are also transmitted by a tick bite. These are small gram-negative coccobacilli of which two species cause human disease. *Anaplasma phagocytophilum* causes human granulocytic ehrlichiosis (anaplasmosis), and *Ehrlichia chaffeensis* causes human monocytic ehrlichiosis. The clinical and laboratory manifestations of the infections are similar. Patients present with fever, headache, confusion, nausea, and vomiting. Twenty percent of patients have a maculopapular or petechial rash. There is laboratory evidence of leukopenia, thrombocytopenia, and anemia, and mild to moderate elevations in alanine aminotransferases, alkaline phosphatase, and lactate dehydrogenase. Patients with RMSF and those with ehrlichial infections may have an altered level of consciousness ranging from mild lethargy to coma, confusion, focal neurologic signs, cranial nerve palsies, hyperreflexia, and seizures.

Focal suppurative CNS infections, including subdural and epidural empyema and brain abscess, should also be considered, especially when focal neurologic findings are present. MRI should be performed promptly in all patients with suspected meningitis who have focal features, both to detect the intracranial infection and to search for associated areas of infection in the sinuses or mastoid bones.

A number of noninfectious CNS disorders can mimic bacterial meningitis. Subarachnoid hemorrhage (SAH; **Chap. 429**) is generally the major consideration. Other possibilities include medication-induced hypersensitivity meningitis; chemical meningitis due to rupture of tumor contents into the CSF (e.g., from a cystic glioma or craniopharyngioma epidermoid or dermoid cyst); carcinomatous or lymphomatous meningitis; meningitis associated with inflammatory disorders such as sarcoid, systemic lupus erythematosus (SLE), and Behçet's syndrome; pituitary apoplexy; and uveomeningitic syndromes (Vogt-Koyanagi-Harada syndrome).

On occasion, subacutely evolving meningitis (**Chap. 139**) may be considered in the differential diagnosis of acute meningitis. The principal causes include *Mycobacterium tuberculosis* (**Chap. 178**), *Cryptococcus neoformans* (**Chap. 215**), *Histoplasma capsulatum* (**Chap. 212**), *Coccidioides immitis* (**Chap. 213**), and *Treponema pallidum* (**Chap. 182**).

TREATMENT

Acute Bacterial Meningitis

EMPIRICAL ANTIMICROBIAL THERAPY

(Table 138-1) Bacterial meningitis is a medical emergency. The goal is to begin antibiotic therapy within 60 min of a patient's arrival in the emergency room. Empirical antimicrobial therapy is initiated in patients with suspected bacterial meningitis before the results of CSF Gram's stain and culture are known. *S. pneumoniae* (**Chap. 146**) and *N. meningitidis* (**Chap. 155**) are the most common etiologic organisms of community-acquired bacterial meningitis. Due to the emergence of penicillin- and cephalosporin-resistant *S. pneumoniae*, empirical therapy of community-acquired suspected bacterial meningitis in children and adults should include a combination of dexamethasone, a third- or fourth-generation cephalosporin (e.g., ceftriaxone, cefotaxime, or cefepime), and vancomycin, plus acyclovir, as HSV encephalitis is the leading disease in the differential diagnosis, and doxycycline during tick season to treat tick-borne bacterial infections. Ceftriaxone or cefotaxime provides good coverage for susceptible *S. pneumoniae*, group B streptococci, and *H. influenzae* and adequate coverage for *N. meningitidis*. Cefepime is a broad-spectrum fourth-generation cephalosporin with in vitro activity similar to that of cefotaxime or ceftriaxone against *S. pneumoniae* and *N. meningitidis* and greater activity against *Enterobacter* species and *Pseudomonas aeruginosa*. In clinical trials, cefepime has been demonstrated to be equivalent to cefotaxime in the treatment of penicillin-sensitive pneumococcal and meningococcal meningitis, and it has been used successfully in some patients with meningitis due to *Enterobacter* species and *P. aeruginosa*. Cefepime has been associated with seizures, myoclonus, and encephalopathy, any of which may limit its use in critically ill patients. Ampicillin should be added to the empirical regimen for coverage of *L. monocytogenes* in individuals <3 months of age, those >55, or those with suspected impaired cell-mediated immunity because of chronic illness, organ transplantation, pregnancy, malignancy, or immunosuppressive therapy. Metronidazole is added to the empirical regimen to cover gram-negative anaerobes in patients with otitis, sinusitis, or mastoiditis. In hospital-acquired meningitis, and particularly meningitis following neurosurgical procedures, staphylococci and gram-negative organisms including *P. aeruginosa* are the most common etiologic organisms. In these patients, empirical therapy should include a combination of vancomycin and ceftazidime or meropenem. Ceftazidime or meropenem should be substituted for ceftriaxone or cefotaxime in neurosurgical patients and in neutropenic patients, because ceftriaxone and cefotaxime do not provide adequate activity against CNS infection with *P. aeruginosa*. Meropenem is a carbapenem antibiotic that is highly active in vitro against *L. monocytogenes*, has been demonstrated to be effective in cases of meningitis caused by *P. aeruginosa*, and shows good activity against penicillin-resistant pneumococci. In experimental pneumococcal meningitis, meropenem was comparable to ceftriaxone and inferior to vancomycin in sterilizing CSF cultures. When *S. pneumoniae, H. influenzae, L. monocytogenes*, or aerobic gram-negative bacilli (including *P. aeruginosa* and *E. coli*) are possible meningeal pathogens, based on predisposing and associated conditions, the combination of vancomycin plus meropenem can be recommended as empiric therapy for bacterial meningitis in children and adults. Meropenem should not be used as monotherapy.

SPECIFIC ANTIMICROBIAL THERAPY

Meningococcal Meningitis (Table 138-3) Although ceftriaxone and cefotaxime provide adequate empirical coverage for *N. meningitidis*, penicillin G remains the antibiotic of choice for meningococcal meningitis caused by susceptible strains. Isolates of *N. meningitidis* with moderate resistance to penicillin have been identified and are increasing in incidence worldwide. CSF isolates of *N. meningitidis* should be tested for penicillin and ampicillin susceptibility, and if resistance is found, cefotaxime or ceftriaxone should be substituted for penicillin. A 7-day course of intravenous antibiotic therapy is adequate for

TABLE 138-3 Antimicrobial Therapy of Central Nervous System Bacterial Infections Based on Pathogen[a]

ORGANISM	ANTIBIOTIC
Neisseria meningitides	
Penicillin-sensitive	Penicillin G or ampicillin
Penicillin-resistant	Ceftriaxone or cefotaxime
Streptococcus pneumoniae	
Penicillin-sensitive	Penicillin G
Penicillin-intermediate	Ceftriaxone or cefotaxime or cefepime
Penicillin-resistant	Ceftriaxone (or cefotaxime or cefepime) + vancomycin
Gram-negative bacilli (except *Pseudomonas* spp.)	Ceftriaxone or cefotaxime
Pseudomonas aeruginosa	Ceftazidime or cefepime or meropenem
Staphylococci spp.	
Methicillin-sensitive	Nafcillin
Methicillin-resistant	Vancomycin
Listeria monocytogenes	Ampicillin + gentamicin
Haemophilus influenzae	Ceftriaxone or cefotaxime if beta-lactamase positive; ampicillin if beta-lactamase negative
Streptococcus agalactiae	Penicillin G or ampicillin
Bacteroides fragilis	Metronidazole
Fusobacterium spp.	Metronidazole

[a]Doses are as indicated in Table 138-1.

uncomplicated meningococcal meningitis. The index case and all close contacts should receive chemoprophylaxis with a 2-day regimen of rifampin (600 mg every 12 h for 2 days in adults and 10 mg/kg every 12 h for 2 days in children >1 year). Rifampin is not recommended in pregnant women. Alternatively, adults can be treated with one dose of azithromycin (500 mg) or one intramuscular dose of ceftriaxone (250 mg). Close contacts are defined as those individuals who have had contact with oropharyngeal secretions, either through kissing or by sharing toys, beverages, or cigarettes.

Pneumococcal Meningitis Antimicrobial therapy of pneumococcal meningitis is initiated with a cephalosporin (ceftriaxone, cefotaxime, or cefepime) and vancomycin. All CSF isolates of *S. pneumoniae* should be tested for sensitivity to penicillin and the cephalosporins. Once the results of antimicrobial susceptibility tests are known, therapy can be modified accordingly (Table 138-3). For *S. pneumoniae* meningitis, an isolate of *S. pneumoniae* is considered to be susceptible to penicillin with a minimal inhibitory concentration (MIC) <0.06 μg/mL and to be resistant when the MIC is >0.12 μg/mL. Isolates of *S. pneumoniae* that have cephalosporin MICs ≤0.5 μg/mL are considered sensitive to the cephalosporins (cefotaxime, ceftriaxone, cefepime). Those with MICs of 1 μg/mL are considered to have intermediate resistance, and those with MICs ≥2 μg/mL are considered resistant. For meningitis due to pneumococci, with cefotaxime or ceftriaxone MICs ≤0.5 μg/mL, treatment with cefotaxime or ceftriaxone is usually adequate. For MIC >1 μg/mL, vancomycin is the antibiotic of choice. Rifampin can be added to vancomycin for its synergistic effect but is inadequate as monotherapy because resistance develops rapidly when it is used alone.

A 2-week course of intravenous antimicrobial therapy is recommended for pneumococcal meningitis.

Patients with *S. pneumoniae* meningitis should have a repeat LP performed 24–36 h after the initiation of antimicrobial therapy to document sterilization of the CSF. Failure to sterilize the CSF after 24–36 h of antibiotic therapy should be considered presumptive evidence of antibiotic resistance. Patients with penicillin- and cephalosporin-resistant strains of *S. pneumoniae* who do not respond to intravenous vancomycin alone may benefit from the addition of intraventricular vancomycin. The intraventricular route of administration is preferred over the intrathecal route because adequate concentrations of vancomycin in the cerebral ventricles are not always achieved with intrathecal administration.

***Listeria* Meningitis** Meningitis due to *L. monocytogenes* is treated with ampicillin for at least 3 weeks (Table 138-3). Gentamicin is added in critically ill patients (2 mg/kg loading dose, then 7.5 mg/kg per day given every 8 h and adjusted for serum levels and renal function). The combination of trimethoprim (10–20 mg/kg per day) and sulfamethoxazole (50–100 mg/kg per day) given every 6 h may provide an alternative in penicillin-allergic patients.

Staphylococcal Meningitis Meningitis due to susceptible strains of *S. aureus* or coagulase-negative staphylococci is treated with nafcillin (Table 138-3). Vancomycin is the drug of choice for methicillin-resistant staphylococci and for patients allergic to penicillin. In these patients, the CSF should be monitored during therapy. If the CSF is not sterilized after 48 h of intravenous vancomycin therapy, then either intraventricular or intrathecal vancomycin, 20 mg once daily, can be added.

Gram-Negative Bacillary Meningitis The third-generation cephalosporins—cefotaxime, ceftriaxone, and ceftazidime—are equally efficacious for the treatment of gram-negative bacillary meningitis, with the exception of meningitis due to *P. aeruginosa*, which should be treated with ceftazidime or meropenem (Table 138-3). A 3-week course of intravenous antibiotic therapy is recommended for meningitis due to gram-negative bacilli.

■ ADJUNCTIVE THERAPY

The release of bacterial cell-wall components by bactericidal antibiotics leads to the production of the inflammatory cytokines IL-1β and TNF-α in the SAS. Dexamethasone exerts its beneficial effect by inhibiting the synthesis of IL-1β and TNF-α at the level of mRNA, decreasing CSF outflow resistance, and stabilizing the blood-brain barrier. The rationale for giving dexamethasone 20 min before antibiotic therapy is that dexamethasone inhibits the production of TNF-α by macrophages and microglia only if it is administered before these cells are activated by endotoxin. Dexamethasone does not alter TNF-α production once it has been induced. The results of clinical trials of dexamethasone therapy in meningitis due to *H. influenzae*, *S. pneumoniae*, and *N. meningitidis* have demonstrated its efficacy in decreasing meningeal inflammation and neurologic sequelae such as the incidence of sensorineural hearing loss.

A prospective European trial of adjunctive therapy for acute bacterial meningitis in 301 adults found that dexamethasone reduced the number of unfavorable outcomes (15 vs 25%, $p = .03$) including death (7 vs 15%, $p = .04$). The benefits were most striking in patients with pneumococcal meningitis. Dexamethasone (10 mg intravenously) was administered 15–20 min before the first dose of an antimicrobial agent, and the same dose was repeated every 6 h for 4 days. These results were confirmed in a second trial of dexamethasone in adults with pneumococcal meningitis. Therapy with dexamethasone should ideally be started 20 min before, or not later than concurrent with, the first dose of antibiotics. It is unlikely to be of significant benefit if started >6 h after antimicrobial therapy has been initiated. Dexamethasone may decrease the penetration of vancomycin into CSF, and it delays the sterilization of CSF in experimental models of *S. pneumoniae* meningitis. As a result, to assure reliable penetration of vancomycin into the CSF, children and adults are treated with vancomycin in a dose of 45–60 mg/kg per day. Alternatively, vancomycin can be administered by the intraventricular route. In clinical trials, dexamethasone has also been shown to reduce rates of death and hearing loss with no adverse effects in patients with meningococcal meningitis.

One of the concerns for using dexamethasone in adults with bacterial meningitis is that in experimental models of meningitis, dexamethasone therapy increased hippocampal cell injury and reduced learning capacity. This has not been the case in clinical series. The efficacy of dexamethasone therapy in preventing neurologic sequelae is different between high- and low-income countries. Three large randomized trials in low-income countries (sub-Saharan Africa, Southeast Asia) failed to show benefit in subgroups of patients. The lack of efficacy of dexamethasone in these trials has been attributed to late presentation to the hospital with more advanced disease, antibiotic pretreatment, malnutrition, infection with HIV, and treatment of patients with probable, but not microbiologically proven, bacterial meningitis. The results of these clinical trials suggest that patients in sub-Saharan Africa and those in low-income countries with negative CSF Gram's stain and culture should not be treated with dexamethasone.

■ INCREASED INTRACRANIAL PRESSURE

Emergency treatment of increased ICP includes elevation of the patient's head to 30–45°, intubation, and hyperventilation (Pa_{CO_2} 25–30 mmHg), and mannitol. Patients with increased ICP should be managed in an intensive care unit; accurate ICP measurements are best obtained with an ICP monitoring device.

Treatment of increased ICP is discussed in detail in Chap. 307.

■ PROGNOSIS

Mortality rate is 3–7% for meningitis caused by *H. influenzae*, *N. meningitidis*, or group B streptococci; 15% for that due to *L. monocytogenes*; and 20% for *S. pneumoniae*. In general, the risk of death from bacterial meningitis increases with (1) decreased level of consciousness on admission, (2) onset of seizures within 24 h of admission, (3) signs of increased ICP, (4) young age (infancy) and age >50, (5) the presence of comorbid conditions including shock and/or the need for mechanical ventilation, and (6) delay in the initiation of treatment. Decreased CSF glucose concentration (<2.2 mmol/L [<40 mg/dL]) and markedly increased CSF protein concentration (>3 g/L [> 300 mg/dL]) have been predictive of increased mortality and poorer outcomes in some series. Moderate or severe sequelae occur in ~25% of survivors, although the exact incidence varies with the infecting organism. Common sequelae include decreased intellectual function, memory impairment, seizures, hearing loss and dizziness, and gait disturbances.

VIRAL MENINGITIS

■ CLINICAL MANIFESTATIONS

Immunocompetent adult patients with viral meningitis usually present with headache, fever, and signs of meningeal irritation coupled with an inflammatory CSF profile (see below). Headache is almost invariably present and often characterized as frontal or retroorbital and frequently associated with photophobia and pain on moving the eyes. Nuchal rigidity is present in most cases but may be mild and present only near the limit of neck anteflexion. Constitutional signs can include malaise, myalgia, anorexia, nausea and vomiting, abdominal pain, and/or diarrhea. Patients often have mild lethargy or drowsiness; however, profound alterations in consciousness, such as stupor, coma, or marked confusion, do not occur in viral meningitis and suggest the presence of encephalitis or other alternative diagnoses. Similarly, seizures or focal neurologic signs or symptoms or neuroimaging abnormalities indicative of brain parenchymal involvement are not typical of viral meningitis and suggest the presence of encephalitis or another CNS infectious or inflammatory process.

■ ETIOLOGY

Using a variety of diagnostic techniques, including CSF PCR, culture, and serology, a specific viral cause can be found in 60–90% of cases of viral meningitis. The most important agents are enteroviruses (including echoviruses and coxsackieviruses in addition to numbered enteroviruses), varicella-zoster virus (VZV), HSV (HSV-2 > HSV-1), HIV, and arboviruses (**Table 138-4**). CSF cultures are positive in 30–70% of patients, with the frequency of isolation depending on the specific viral agent. Approximately two-thirds of culture-negative cases of "aseptic" meningitis have a specific viral etiology identified by CSF PCR testing (see below).

■ EPIDEMIOLOGY

Viral meningitis is not a nationally reportable disease; however, it has been estimated that the incidence is ~60,000–75,000 cases per year. In temperate climates, there is a substantial increase in cases during the nonwinter months, reflecting the seasonal predominance of enterovirus and arthropod-borne virus (arbovirus) infections in the summer and fall, with a peak monthly incidence of about 1 reported case per 100,000 population.

■ LABORATORY DIAGNOSIS

CSF Examination The most important laboratory test in the diagnosis of viral meningitis is examination of the CSF. The typical profile is a pleocytosis, a normal or slightly elevated protein concentration (0.2–0.8 g/L [20–80 mg/dL]), a normal glucose concentration, and a normal or mildly elevated opening pressure (100–350 mmH_2O). Organisms are *not* seen on Gram's stain of CSF. The total CSF cell count in viral meningitis is typically 25–500/μL, although cell counts of several thousand/μL are occasionally seen, especially with infections due to lymphocytic choriomeningitis virus (LCMV) and mumps virus. Lymphocytes are typically the predominant cell. Rarely, PMNs may predominate in the first 48 h of illness, especially with infections due to echovirus 9, West Nile virus (WNV), eastern equine encephalitis (EEE) virus, or mumps. A PMN pleocytosis occurs in 45% of patients with WNV meningitis and can persist for a week or longer before shifting to a lymphocytic pleocytosis. PMN pleocytosis with low glucose may also be a feature of cytomegalovirus (CMV) infections in immunocompromised hosts. Despite these exceptions, the presence of a CSF PMN pleocytosis in a patient with suspected viral meningitis in whom a specific diagnosis has not been established should prompt consideration of alternative diagnoses, including bacterial meningitis or parameningeal infections. The CSF glucose concentration is typically normal in viral infections, although it may be decreased in 10–30% of cases due to mumps or LCMV. Rare instances of decreased CSF glucose concentration occur in cases of meningitis due to echoviruses and other enteroviruses, HSV-2, and VZV. As a rule, a lymphocytic pleocytosis with a low glucose concentration should suggest fungal or tuberculous meningitis, *Listeria* meningoencephalitis, or noninfectious disorders (e.g., sarcoid, neoplastic meningitis).

A number of tests measuring levels of various CSF proteins, enzymes, and mediators—including C-reactive protein, lactic acid, lactate dehydrogenase, neopterin, quinolinate, IL-1β, IL-6, soluble IL-2 receptor, β_2-microglobulin, and TNF—have been proposed as potential discriminators between viral and bacterial meningitis or as markers of specific types of viral infection (e.g., infection with HIV), but they remain of uncertain sensitivity and specificity and are not widely used for diagnostic purposes.

Polymerase Chain Reaction Amplification of Viral Nucleic Acid Amplification of viral-specific DNA or RNA from CSF using PCR amplification has become the single most important method for diagnosing CNS viral infections. In both enteroviral and HSV infections of the CNS, CSF PCR has become the diagnostic procedure of choice and is substantially more sensitive than viral cultures. HSV CSF PCR is also an important diagnostic test in patients with recurrent episodes of "aseptic" meningitis, many of whom have amplifiable HSV DNA in CSF despite negative viral cultures. CSF PCR is also used routinely to diagnose CNS viral infections caused by CMV, Epstein-Barr virus (EBV), VZV, and human herpesvirus 6 (HHV-6). CSF PCR tests are available for WNV but are not as sensitive as detection of WNV-specific CSF IgM. PCR is also useful in the diagnosis of CNS infection caused by *Mycoplasma pneumoniae*, which can mimic viral meningitis and encephalitis. PCR of throat washings may assist in diagnosis of enteroviral and mycoplasmal CNS infections. PCR of stool specimens may also assist in diagnosis of enteroviral infections (see below).

Viral Culture The sensitivity of CSF cultures for the diagnosis of viral meningitis and encephalitis, in contrast to its utility in bacterial infections, is generally poor. In addition to CSF, specific viruses may also be isolated from throat swabs, stool, blood, and urine. Enteroviruses and adenoviruses may be found in feces; arboviruses, some enteroviruses, and LCMV in blood; mumps and CMV in urine; and enteroviruses, mumps, and adenoviruses in throat washings. During enteroviral infections, viral shedding in stool may persist for several weeks. The presence of enterovirus in stool is not diagnostic and may result from residual shedding from a previous enteroviral infection; it also occurs in some asymptomatic individuals during enteroviral epidemics.

Serologic Studies The basic approach to the serodiagnosis of viral meningitis is identical to that discussed earlier for viral encephalitis (**see Chap. 137**). Serologic studies are important for the diagnosis of arboviruses such as WNV; however, these tests are less useful for viruses such as HSV, VZV, CMV, and EBV that have a high seroprevalence in the general population.

CSF oligoclonal gamma globulin bands occur in association with a number of viral infections. The associated antibodies are often directed against viral proteins. Oligoclonal bands also occur commonly in certain noninfectious neurologic diseases (e.g., multiple sclerosis) and may be found in nonviral infections (e.g., neurosyphilis, Lyme neuroborreliosis).

TABLE 138-4 Viruses Causing Acute Meningitis in North America

COMMON	LESS COMMON
Enteroviruses (coxsackieviruses, echoviruses, and the numbered enteroviruses) Varicella-zoster virus Herpes simplex virus 2 Epstein-Barr virus Arthropod-borne viruses (notably WNV) HIV	Herpes simplex virus 1 Human herpesvirus 6 Cytomegalovirus Lymphocytic choriomeningitis virus Mumps Zika and other non-WNV arboviruses

Abbreviation: WNV, West Nile virus.

Other Laboratory Studies All patients with suspected viral meningitis should have a complete blood count and differential, liver and renal function tests, erythrocyte sedimentation rate (ESR), and C-reactive protein, electrolytes, glucose, creatine kinase, aldolase, amylase, and lipase. Neuroimaging studies (MRI preferable to CT) are not absolutely necessary in patients with uncomplicated viral meningitis but should be performed in patients with altered consciousness, seizures, focal neurologic signs or symptoms (see "Differential Diagnosis" below), atypical CSF profiles, or underlying immunocompromising treatments or conditions.

DIFFERENTIAL DIAGNOSIS

The most important issue in the differential diagnosis of viral meningitis is to consider diseases that can mimic viral meningitis, including (1) untreated or partially treated bacterial meningitis; (2) early stages of meningitis caused by fungi, mycobacteria, or *Treponema pallidum* (neurosyphilis), in which a lymphocytic pleocytosis is common, cultures may be slow growing or negative, and hypoglycorrhachia may not be present early; (3) meningitis caused by agents such as *Mycoplasma, Listeria* spp., *Brucella* spp., *Coxiella* spp., *Leptospira* spp., and *Rickettsia* spp.; (4) parameningeal infections; (5) neoplastic meningitis; and (6) meningitis secondary to noninfectious inflammatory diseases, including medication-induced hypersensitivity meningitis, SLE and other rheumatologic diseases, sarcoidosis, Behçet's syndrome, and the uveomeningitic syndromes. Studies in children >28 days of age suggest that the presence of CSF protein >0.5 g/L (sensitivity 89%, specificity 78%) and elevated serum procalcitonin levels >0.5 ng/mL (sensitivity 89%, specificity 89%) were clues to the presence of bacterial as opposed to "aseptic" meningitis. A variety of clinical algorithms for differentiating bacterial from aseptic meningitis have been developed. One such prospectively validated system, the *bacterial meningitis score*, suggests that the probability of bacterial meningitis is 0.3% or less (negative predictive value 99.7%, 95% confidence interval 99.6–100%) in children with CSF pleocytosis who have (1) a negative CSF Gram's stain, (2) CSF neutrophil count <1000 cells/μL, (3) CSF protein <80 mg/dL, (4) peripheral absolute neutrophil count of <10,000 cells/μL, and (5) no prior history or current presence of seizures.

SPECIFIC VIRAL ETIOLOGIES

Enteroviruses (EV) **(Chap. 204)** are the most common cause of viral meningitis, accounting for >85% of cases in which a specific etiology can be identified. Cases may either be sporadic or occur in clusters. EV71 has produced large epidemics of neurologic disease outside the United States, especially in Southeast Asia, but most recently reported cases in the United States have been sporadic. Enteroviruses are the most likely cause of viral meningitis in the summer and fall months, especially in children (<15 years), although cases occur at reduced frequency year round. Although the incidence of enteroviral meningitis declines with increasing age, some outbreaks have preferentially affected older children and adults. Meningitis outside the neonatal period is usually benign. Patients present with sudden onset of fever; headache; nuchal rigidity; and often constitutional signs, including vomiting, anorexia, diarrhea, cough, pharyngitis, and myalgias. The physical examination should include a careful search for stigmata of enterovirus infection, including exanthems, hand-foot-mouth disease, herpangina, pleurodynia, myopericarditis, and hemorrhagic conjunctivitis. The CSF profile is typically a lymphocytic pleocytosis (100–1000 cells/μL) with normal glucose and normal or mildly elevated protein concentration. However, up to 15% of patients, most commonly young infants rather than older children or adults, have a normal CSF leukocyte count. In rare cases, PMNs may predominate during the first 48 h of illness. CSF reverse transcriptase PCR (RT-PCR) is the diagnostic procedure of choice and is both sensitive (>95%) and specific (>100%). CSF RT-PCR has the highest sensitivity if performed within 48 h of symptom onset, with sensitivity declining rapidly after day 5 of symptoms. RT-PCR of throat washings or stool specimens may be positive for several weeks, and positive results can help support the diagnosis of an acute enteroviral infection. The sensitivity of routine enteroviral RT-PCRs for detecting EV71 is low, and specific testing may be required. Treatment is supportive, and patients usually recover without sequelae. Chronic and severe infections can occur in neonates and in individuals with hypo- or agammaglobulinemia.

Arbovirus infections **(Chap. 209)** occur predominantly in the summer and early fall. Arboviral meningitis should be considered when clusters of meningitis and encephalitis cases occur in a restricted geographic region during the summer or early fall. In the United States, the most important causes of arboviral meningitis and encephalitis are WNV, St. Louis encephalitis virus, and the California encephalitis group of viruses. In WNV epidemics, avian deaths may serve as sentinel infections for subsequent human disease. A history of tick exposure or travel or residence in the appropriate geographic area should suggest the possibility of Colorado tick fever virus or Powassan virus infection, although nonviral tick-borne diseases, including RMSF and Lyme neuroborreliosis, may present similarly. Arbovirus meningitis is typically associated with a CSF lymphocytic pleocytosis, normal glucose concentration, and normal or mildly elevated protein concentration. However, ~45% of patients with WNV meningitis have CSF neutrophilia, which can persist for a week or more. The rarity of hypoglycorrhachia in WNV infection, the absence of positive Gram's stains, and the negative cultures help distinguish these patients from those with bacterial meningitis. Definitive diagnosis of arboviral meningitis is based on demonstration of viral-specific IgM in CSF or seroconversion. The prevalence of CSF IgM increases progressively during the first week after infection, peaking at >80% in patients with neuroinvasive disease; as a result, repeat studies may be needed when disease suspicion is high and an early study is negative. CSF RT-PCR tests are available for some viruses in selected diagnostic laboratories and at the Centers for Disease Control and Prevention (CDC), but in the case of WNV, sensitivity (~70%) of CSF RT-PCR is less than that of CSF serology. WNV CSF RT-PCR may be useful in immunocompromised patients who may have absent or reduced antibody responses.

HSV meningitis **(Chap. 192)** has been increasingly recognized as a major cause of viral meningitis in adults, and overall, it is probably second in importance to enteroviruses as a cause of viral meningitis, accounting for 5% of total cases overall and undoubtedly a higher frequency of those cases occurring in adults and/or outside of the summer-fall period when enterovirus infections are increasingly common. In adults, the majority of cases of uncomplicated meningitis are due to HSV-2, whereas HSV-1 is responsible for 90% of cases of HSV encephalitis. HSV meningitis occurs in ~25–35% of women and ~10–15% of men at the time of an initial (primary) episode of genital herpes. Of these patients, 20% go on to have recurrent attacks of meningitis. Diagnosis of HSV meningitis is usually by HSV CSF PCR because cultures may be negative, especially in patients with recurrent meningitis. Demonstration of intrathecal synthesis of HSV-specific antibody may also be useful in diagnosis, although antibody tests are less sensitive and less specific than PCR and may not become positive until after the first week of infection. Although a history of or the presence of HSV genital lesions is an important diagnostic clue, many patients with HSV meningitis give no history and have no evidence of active genital herpes at the time of presentation. Most cases of recurrent viral or "aseptic" meningitis, including cases previously diagnosed as Mollaret's meningitis, are due to HSV.

VZV meningitis **(Chap. 193)** should be suspected in the presence of concurrent chickenpox or shingles. However, it is important to recognize that VZV is being increasingly identified as an important cause of both meningitis and encephalitis in patients without rash. The frequency of VZV as a cause of meningitis is extremely variable, ranging from as low as 3% to as high as 20% in different series. Diagnosis is usually based on CSF PCR, although the sensitivity of this test is not as high as for the other herpesviruses. VZV serologic studies complement PCR testing, and the diagnosis of VZV CNS infection can be made by the demonstration of VZV-specific intrathecal antibody synthesis and/or the presence of VZV CSF IgM antibodies, or by positive CSF cultures.

EBV infections **(Chap. 194)** may also produce aseptic meningitis, with or without associated infectious mononucleosis. The presence of atypical lymphocytes in the CSF or peripheral blood is suggestive of EBV infection but may occasionally be seen with other viral infections.

EBV is almost never cultured from CSF. Serum and CSF serology help establish the presence of acute infection, which is characterized by IgM viral capsid antibodies (VCAs), antibodies to early antigens (EAs), and the absence of antibodies to EBV-associated nuclear antigen (EBNA). CSF PCR is another important diagnostic test, although false-positive results may reflect viral reactivation associated with other infectious or inflammatory processes or the presence of latent viral DNA in lymphocytes recruited due to other inflammatory conditions.

HIV meningitis should be suspected in any patient presenting with a viral meningitis with known or suspected risk factors for HIV infection. Meningitis may occur following primary infection with HIV in 5–10% of cases and less commonly at later stages of illness. Cranial nerve palsies, most commonly involving cranial nerves V, VII, or VIII, are more common in HIV meningitis than in other viral infections. Diagnosis can be confirmed by detection of HIV genome in blood or CSF. Seroconversion may be delayed, and patients with negative HIV serologies who are suspected of having HIV meningitis should be monitored for delayed seroconversion. **For further discussion of HIV infection, see Chap. 202.**

Mumps **(Chap. 207)** should be considered when meningitis occurs in the late winter or early spring, especially in males (male-to-female ratio 3:1). With the widespread use of the live attenuated mumps vaccine in the United States since 1967, the incidence of mumps meningitis has fallen by >95%; however, mumps remains a potential source of infection in nonimmunized individuals and populations. Rare cases (10–100/100,000 vaccinated individuals) of vaccine-associated mumps meningitis have been described, with onset typically 2–4 weeks after vaccination. The presence of parotitis, orchitis, oophoritis, pancreatitis, or elevations in serum lipase and amylase is suggestive of mumps meningitis; however, their absence does not exclude the diagnosis. Clinical meningitis was previously estimated to occur in 10–30% of patients with mumps parotitis; however, in a recent U.S. outbreak of nearly 2600 cases of mumps, only 11 cases of meningitis were identified, suggesting the incidence may be lower than previously suspected. Mumps infection confers lifelong immunity, so a documented history of previous infection excludes this diagnosis. Patients with meningitis have a CSF pleocytosis that can exceed 1000 cells/μL in 25%. Lymphocytes predominate in 75%, although CSF neutrophilia occurs in 25%. Hypoglycorrhachia occurs in 10–30% of patients and may be a clue to the diagnosis when present. Diagnosis is typically made by culture of virus from CSF or by detecting IgM antibodies or seroconversion. CSF PCR is available in some diagnostic and research laboratories.

LCMV infection **(Chap. 209)** should be considered when aseptic meningitis occurs in the late fall or winter and in individuals with a history of exposure to house mice (*Mus musculus*), pet or laboratory rodents (e.g., hamsters, rats, mice), or their excreta. Some patients have an associated rash, pulmonary infiltrates, alopecia, parotitis, orchitis, or myopericarditis. Laboratory clues to the diagnosis of LCMV, in addition to the clinical findings noted above, may include the presence of leukopenia, thrombocytopenia, or abnormal liver function tests. Some cases present with a marked CSF pleocytosis (>1000 cells/μL) and hypoglycorrhachia (<30%). Diagnosis is based on serology and/or culture of virus from CSF.

TREATMENT
Acute Viral Meningitis

Treatment of almost all cases of viral meningitis is primarily symptomatic and includes use of analgesics, antipyretics, and antiemetics. Fluid and electrolyte status should be monitored. Patients with suspected bacterial meningitis should receive appropriate empirical therapy pending culture results (see above). Hospitalization may not be required in immunocompetent patients with presumed viral meningitis and no focal signs or symptoms, no significant alteration in consciousness, and a classic CSF profile (lymphocytic pleocytosis, normal glucose, negative Gram's stain) if adequate provision for monitoring at home and medical follow-up can be ensured. Immunocompromised patients; patients with significant alteration in consciousness, seizures, or the presence of focal signs and symptoms suggesting the possibility of encephalitis or parenchymal brain involvement; and patients who have an atypical CSF profile should be hospitalized. Oral or intravenous acyclovir may be of benefit in patients with meningitis caused by HSV-1 or -2 and in cases of severe EBV or VZV infection. Data concerning treatment of HSV, EBV, and VZV meningitis are extremely limited. Seriously ill patients should probably receive intravenous acyclovir (15–30 mg/kg per day in three divided doses), which can be followed by an oral drug such as acyclovir (800 mg five times daily), famciclovir (500 mg tid), or valacyclovir (1000 mg tid) for a total course of 7–14 days. Patients who are less ill can be treated with oral drugs alone. Patients with HIV meningitis should receive highly active antiretroviral therapy **(Chap. 202)**. There is no specific therapy of proven benefit for patients with arboviral encephalitis, including that caused by WNV.

Patients with viral meningitis who are known to have deficient humoral immunity (e.g., X-linked agammaglobulinemia) and who are not already receiving either intramuscular gamma globulin or intravenous immunoglobulin (IVIg) should be treated with these agents. Intraventricular administration of immunoglobulin through an Ommaya reservoir has been tried in some patients with chronic enteroviral meningitis who have not responded to intramuscular or intravenous immunoglobulin.

Vaccination is an effective method of preventing the development of meningitis and other neurologic complications associated with poliovirus, mumps, measles, rubella, and varicella infection. A live attenuated VZV vaccine (Varivax) is available in the United States. Clinical studies indicate an effectiveness rate of 70–90% for this vaccine, but a booster may be required after ~10 years to maintain immunity. The recombinant zoster vaccine (RSV, Shingrix) contains recombinant VZV glycoprotein E in combination with an adjuvant ($ASO1_B$) and has greater efficacy in preventing zoster in adults aged ≥70 years than the live attenuated vaccine (Zostrax). ACIP recommends the use of the recombinant zoster vaccine in immunocompetent adults aged ≥50 years. An inactivated varicella vaccine is available for transplant recipients and others for whom live viral vaccines are contraindicated.

PROGNOSIS

In adults, the prognosis for full recovery from viral meningitis is excellent. Rare patients complain of persisting headache, mild mental impairment, incoordination, or generalized asthenia for weeks to months. The outcome in infants and neonates (<1 year) is less certain; intellectual impairment, learning disabilities, hearing loss, and other lasting sequelae have been reported in some studies.

SUBACUTE MENINGITIS

CLINICAL MANIFESTATIONS

Patients with subacute meningitis typically have an unrelenting headache, stiff neck, low-grade fever, and lethargy for days to several weeks before they present for evaluation. Cranial nerve abnormalities and night sweats may be present. **This syndrome overlaps that of chronic meningitis, discussed in detail in Chap. 139, but is included here as the meningeal pathogens of subacute meningitis can also present as an acute meningitis.**

ETIOLOGY

Common causative organisms include *M. tuberculosis, C. neoformans, H. capsulatum, C. immitis,* and *T. pallidum*. Initial infection with *M. tuberculosis* is acquired by inhalation of aerosolized droplet nuclei. Tuberculous meningitis in adults does not develop acutely from hematogenous spread of tubercle bacilli to the meninges. Rather, millet seed–sized (miliary) tubercles form in the parenchyma of the brain during hematogenous dissemination of tubercle bacilli in the course of primary infection. These tubercles enlarge and are usually caseating. The propensity for a caseous lesion to produce meningitis is determined by its proximity to the SAS and the rate at which fibrous encapsulation develops. Subependymal caseous foci cause meningitis via discharge of bacilli and tuberculous antigens into the SAS. Mycobacterial antigens produce an intense inflammatory reaction that leads to the production of a thick exudate that fills the basilar cisterns and surrounds the cranial nerves and major blood vessels at the base of the brain.

Fungal infections are typically acquired by the inhalation of airborne fungal spores. The initial pulmonary infection may be asymptomatic or present with fever, cough, sputum production, and chest pain. The pulmonary infection is often self-limited. A localized pulmonary fungal infection can then remain dormant in the lungs until there is an abnormality in cell-mediated immunity that allows the fungus to reactivate and disseminate to the CNS. The most common pathogen causing fungal meningitis is *C. neoformans*. This fungus is found worldwide in soil and bird excreta. *H. capsulatum* is endemic to the Ohio and Mississippi River valleys of the central United States and to parts of Central and South America. *C. immitis* is endemic to the desert areas of the southwest United States, northern Mexico, and Argentina.

Syphilis is a sexually transmitted disease that is manifest by the appearance of a painless chancre at the site of inoculation. *T. pallidum* invades the CNS early in the course of syphilis. Cranial nerves VII and VIII are most frequently involved.

■ LABORATORY DIAGNOSIS

The classic CSF abnormalities in tuberculous meningitis are as follows: (1) elevated opening pressure, (2) lymphocytic pleocytosis (10–500 cells/μL), (3) elevated protein concentration in the range of 1–5 g/L, and (4) decreased glucose concentration in the range of 1.1–2.2 mmol/L (20–40 mg/dL). *The combination of unrelenting headache, stiff neck, fatigue, night sweats, and fever with a CSF lymphocytic pleocytosis and a mildly decreased glucose concentration is highly suspicious for tuberculous meningitis.* The last tube of fluid collected at LP is the best tube to send for a smear for acid-fast bacilli (AFB). If there is a pellicle in the CSF or a cobweb-like clot on the surface of the fluid, AFB can best be demonstrated in a smear of the clot or pellicle. Positive smears are typically reported in only 10–40% of cases of tuberculous meningitis in adults. Cultures of CSF take 4–8 weeks to identify the organism and are positive in ~50% of adults. Culture remains the gold standard to make the diagnosis of tuberculous meningitis. PCR for the detection of *M. tuberculosis* DNA should be sent on CSF if available, but the sensitivity and specificity on CSF have not been defined. The CDC recommends the use of nucleic acid amplification tests for the diagnosis of pulmonary tuberculosis.

The characteristic CSF abnormalities in fungal meningitis are a mononuclear or lymphocytic pleocytosis, an increased protein concentration, and a decreased glucose concentration. There may be eosinophils in the CSF in *C. immitis* meningitis. Large volumes of CSF are often required to demonstrate the organism on India ink smear or grow the organism in culture. If spinal fluid examined by LP on two separate occasions fails to yield an organism, CSF should be obtained by high-cervical or cisternal puncture.

The cryptococcal polysaccharide antigen test is a highly sensitive and specific test for cryptococcal meningitis. A reactive CSF cryptococcal antigen test establishes the diagnosis. The detection of the *Histoplasma* polysaccharide antigen in CSF establishes the diagnosis of a fungal meningitis but is not specific for meningitis due to *H. capsulatum*. It may be falsely positive in coccidioidal meningitis. The CSF complement fixation antibody test is reported to have a specificity of 100% and a sensitivity of 75% for coccidioidal meningitis.

The diagnosis of syphilitic meningitis is made when a reactive serum treponemal test (fluorescent treponemal antibody absorption test [FTA-ABS] or microhemagglutination assay–*T. pallidum* [MHA-TP]) is associated with a CSF lymphocytic or mononuclear pleocytosis and an elevated protein concentration, or when the CSF Venereal Disease Research Laboratory (VDRL) test is positive. A reactive CSF FTA-ABS is not definitive evidence of neurosyphilis. The CSF FTA-ABS can be falsely positive from blood contamination. A negative CSF VDRL does not rule out neurosyphilis. A negative CSF FTA-ABS or MHA-TP rules out neurosyphilis.

TREATMENT
Subacute Meningitis

Empirical therapy of tuberculous meningitis is often initiated on the basis of a high index of suspicion without adequate laboratory support. Initial therapy is a combination of isoniazid (300 mg/d), rifampin (10 mg/kg per day), pyrazinamide (30 mg/kg per day in divided doses), ethambutol (15–25 mg/kg per day in divided doses), and pyridoxine (50 mg/d). When the antimicrobial sensitivity of the *M. tuberculosis* isolate is known, ethambutol can be discontinued. If the clinical response is good, pyrazinamide can be discontinued after 8 weeks and isoniazid and rifampin continued alone for the next 6–12 months. A 6-month course of therapy is acceptable, but therapy should be prolonged for 9–12 months in patients who have an inadequate resolution of symptoms of meningitis or who have positive mycobacterial cultures of CSF during the course of therapy. Dexamethasone therapy is recommended for HIV-negative patients with tuberculous meningitis. The dose is 12–16 mg/d for 3 weeks, and then tapered over 3 weeks.

Meningitis due to *C. neoformans* in non-HIV, nontransplant patients is treated with induction therapy with amphotericin B (AmB) (0.7 mg/kg IV per day) plus flucytosine (100 mg/kg per day in four divided doses) for at least 4 weeks if CSF culture results are negative after 2 weeks of treatment. Therapy should be extended for a total of 6 weeks in the patient with neurologic complications. Induction therapy is followed by consolidation therapy with fluconazole 400 mg/d for 8 weeks. Organ transplant recipients are treated with liposomal AmB (3–4 mg/kg per day) or AmB lipid complex (ABLC; 5 mg/kg per day) plus flucytosine (100 mg/kg per day in four divided doses) for at least 2 weeks or until CSF culture is sterile. Follow CSF yeast cultures for sterilization rather than the cryptococcal antigen titer. This treatment is followed by an 8- to 10-week course of fluconazole (400–800 mg/d [6–12 mg/kg] PO). If the CSF culture is sterile after 10 weeks of acute therapy, the dose of fluconazole is decreased to 200 mg/d for 6 months to a year. Patients with HIV infection are treated with AmB or a lipid formulation plus flucytosine for at least 2 weeks, followed by fluconazole for a minimum of 8 weeks. HIV-infected patients may require indefinite maintenance therapy with fluconazole 200 mg/d. Meningitis due to *H. capsulatum* is treated with AmB (0.7–1.0 mg/kg per day) for 4–12 weeks. A total dose of 30 mg/kg is recommended. Therapy with AmB is not discontinued until fungal cultures are sterile. After completing a course of AmB, maintenance therapy with itraconazole 200 mg two or three times daily is initiated and continued for at least 9 months to a year. *C. immitis* meningitis is treated with either high-dose fluconazole (1000 mg daily) as monotherapy or intravenous AmB (0.5–0.7 mg/kg per day) for >4 weeks. Intrathecal AmB (0.25–0.75 mg/d three times weekly) may be required to eradicate the infection. Lifelong therapy with fluconazole (200–400 mg daily) is recommended to prevent relapse. AmBisome (5 mg/kg per day) or ABLC (5 mg/kg per day) can be substituted for AmB in patients who have or who develop significant renal dysfunction. The most common complication of fungal meningitis is hydrocephalus. Patients who develop hydrocephalus should receive a CSF diversion device. A ventriculostomy can be used until CSF fungal cultures are sterile, at which time the ventriculostomy is replaced by a ventriculoperitoneal shunt.

Syphilitic meningitis is treated with aqueous penicillin G in a dose of 3–4 million units intravenously every 4 h for 10–14 days. An alternative regimen is 2.4 million units of procaine penicillin G intramuscularly daily with 500 mg of oral probenecid four times daily for 10–14 days. Either regimen is followed with 2.4 million units of benzathine penicillin G intramuscularly once a week for 3 weeks. The standard criterion for treatment success is reexamination of the CSF. The CSF should be reexamined at 6-month intervals for 2 years. The cell count is expected to normalize within 12 months, and the VDRL titer to decrease by two dilutions or revert to nonreactive within 2 years of completion of therapy.

Failure of the CSF pleocytosis to resolve or an increase in the CSF VDRL titer by two or more dilutions requires retreatment.

FURTHER READING

Centers for Disease Control and Prevention: Recommendations of the Advisory Committee on Immunization Practices for use of herpes zoster vaccines. MMWR 67:103, 2018.

Harrison LE et al: Good news and bad news-4CMenB vaccine for group B *Neisseria meningitidis*. N Engl J Med 382:376, 2020.

Heckenberg SG et al: Adjunctive dexamethasone in adults with meningococcal meningitis. Neurology 79:1563, 2012.

Roos KL et al: Acute bacterial meningitis, in *Infections of the Central Nervous System*, 4th ed. Scheld WM, Whitley RJ, Marra (eds). Philadelphia, Wolters Kluwer Health, 2014, pp 365–419.

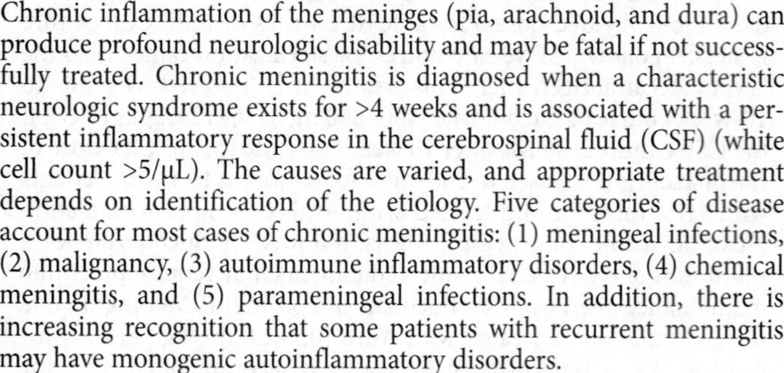

139 Chronic and Recurrent Meningitis

Avindra Nath, Walter J. Koroshetz, Michael R. Wilson

Chronic inflammation of the meninges (pia, arachnoid, and dura) can produce profound neurologic disability and may be fatal if not successfully treated. Chronic meningitis is diagnosed when a characteristic neurologic syndrome exists for >4 weeks and is associated with a persistent inflammatory response in the cerebrospinal fluid (CSF) (white cell count >5/μL). The causes are varied, and appropriate treatment depends on identification of the etiology. Five categories of disease account for most cases of chronic meningitis: (1) meningeal infections, (2) malignancy, (3) autoimmune inflammatory disorders, (4) chemical meningitis, and (5) parameningeal infections. In addition, there is increasing recognition that some patients with recurrent meningitis may have monogenic autoinflammatory disorders.

CLINICAL PATHOPHYSIOLOGY

Neurologic manifestations of chronic meningitis (**Table 139-1**) are determined by the anatomic location of the inflammation and its consequences. Persistent headache, clinical signs of hydrocephalus, meningeal signs, cranial neuropathies, radiculopathies, and cognitive or personality changes are the cardinal features. These can occur alone or in combination. When they appear in combination, it may be indicative of widespread dissemination of the inflammatory process along CSF pathways. In some cases, the presence of an underlying systemic illness points to the probable cause of the meningitis (**Fig. 139-1**). The diagnosis of chronic meningitis is usually made when the clinical presentation prompts the physician to examine the CSF for signs of inflammation. CSF is produced by the choroid plexus of the cerebral ventricles, exits through narrow foramina in the fourth ventricle into the subarachnoid space surrounding the brain and spinal cord, circulates around the base of the brain and over the cerebral hemispheres, and is resorbed by arachnoid villi projecting into the superior sagittal sinus where it mixes with blood in the venous sinuses. Recently, a cerebral lymphatic system has been identified that drains the dura mater (**Chap. 424**); however, its role in chronic meningitis has not been studied. CSF flow provides a pathway for rapid spread of infectious and other infiltrative processes over the brain, spinal cord, cranial, and spinal nerve roots. Spread from the subarachnoid space into brain parenchyma may occur via the arachnoid cuffs that surround blood vessels that penetrate brain tissue (Virchow-Robin spaces).

TABLE 139-1 Symptoms and Signs of Chronic Meningitis

SYMPTOM	SIGN
Chronic headache	± Papilledema
Neck or back pain/stiffness	Brudzinski's or Kernig's sign of meningeal irritation
Change in personality	Altered mental status—drowsiness, inattention, disorientation, memory loss, frontal release signs (grasp, suck, snout), perseveration
Facial weakness	Peripheral seventh CN paresis
Double vision	Paresis of CNs III, IV, and/or VI
Diminished vision	Papilledema, CN II (optic atrophy/inflammation)
Hearing loss	Eighth CN paresis
Arm or leg weakness	Myelopathy or radiculopathy
Numbness in arms or legs	Myelopathy or radiculopathy
Urinary retention/ incontinence	Myelopathy or radiculopathy Frontal lobe dysfunction (hydrocephalus)
Clumsiness	Ataxia

Abbreviation: CN, cranial nerve.

Intracranial Meningitis In intracranial meningitis, nociceptive nerve fibers of the meninges are stimulated by the inflammatory process, resulting in headache, neck pain, or back pain. Obstruction of CSF pathways at the cerebral aqueduct or arachnoid villi may produce hydrocephalus and signs and symptoms of raised intracranial pressure (ICP), including headache, vomiting, apathy or drowsiness, gait instability, papilledema, visual loss, impaired upgaze, or palsy of the sixth cranial nerve (CN VI). Cognitive and behavioral changes during the course of chronic meningitis may also result from vascular damage due to inflammation around the blood vessels in the subarachnoid space, causing infarction. Inflammatory deposits seeded via the CSF circulation are often prominent around the brainstem and cranial nerves and along the undersurface of the frontal and temporal lobes. Such cases, termed *basal meningitis*, often present as multiple cranial neuropathies (**Chap. 441**), with some combination of decreased vision (CN II), facial weakness (CN VII), decreased hearing (CN VIII), diplopia (CNs III, IV, and VI), sensory or motor abnormalities of the oropharynx (CNs IX, X, and XII), decreased olfaction (CN I), or decreased facial sensation and masseter weakness (CN V). Involvement of the lower CNs is more common because the inflammatory exudate tends to collect at the base of the brain.

Spinal Meningitis In spinal meningitis, injury may occur to motor and sensory nerve roots as they traverse the subarachnoid space and penetrate the meninges. These cases present as multiple radiculopathies with combinations of radicular pain, sensory loss, motor weakness, and urinary or fecal incontinence. In some cases, chronic inflammation causes arachnoiditis with clumping of the lower nerve roots and thickening of the meninges. Preferential involvement of the lower nerve roots results from inflammatory cells that gravitate to the bottom of the intrathecal space. Meningeal inflammation can encircle and damage the spinal cord, resulting in a myelopathy. Slow progressive involvement of multiple CNs and/or spinal nerve roots is likely due to chronic meningitis. Electrophysiologic testing (electromyography, nerve conduction studies, and evoked response testing) may be helpful in determining whether there is involvement of cranial and spinal nerve roots.

Systemic Manifestations In some patients, evidence of systemic disease provides clues to the underlying cause of chronic meningitis. A complete history of travel, sexual exposure, insect bites, and other modes of exposure to infectious agents should be sought. Infectious causes are often associated with fever, malaise, anorexia, and signs of localized or disseminated infection outside the nervous system. Infectious causes are of major concern in immunosuppressed patients and especially in patients with untreated HIV infection, in whom chronic meningitis is most often caused by *Mycobacterium tuberculosis* or *Cryptococcus neoformans* and may present without headache, fever, or meningeal signs. In this population, a high index of clinical suspicion

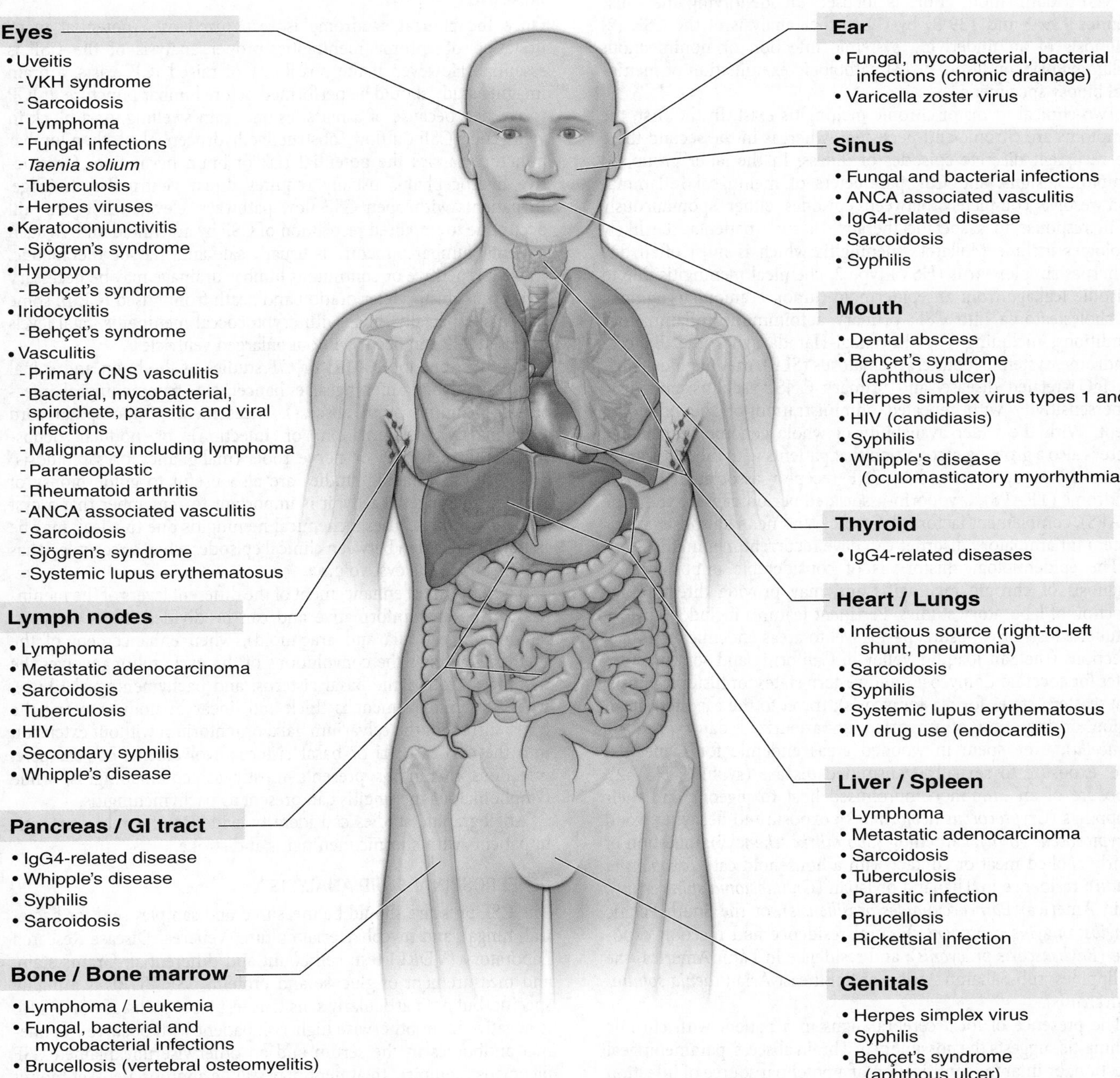

FIGURE 139-1 Systemic manifestations that may provide clues to the etiology of chronic meningitis.

needs to be maintained even when there is only mild confusion or a nonspecific headache syndrome. Noninfectious inflammatory disorders most often produce systemic manifestations first, but meningitis may be the initial manifestation. Carcinomatous meningitis, caused by CSF seeding with metastatic cancer cells, may or may not be accompanied by clinical evidence of the primary neoplasm.

APPROACH TO THE PATIENT

Chronic Meningitis

The occurrence of chronic headache, clinical signs of hydrocephalus, cranial neuropathy, radiculopathy, and/or cognitive decline in a patient should prompt consideration of a lumbar puncture for evidence of meningeal inflammation. On occasion, the diagnosis is made when a contrast-enhanced imaging study (MRI or CT) shows leakage of contrast agent into the meninges. Meningeal enhancement is always concerning with the exception of dural enhancement after lumbar puncture, neurosurgical procedures, concussion, or spontaneous CSF leakage. Once chronic meningitis is confirmed by CSF examination, effort is focused on identifying the cause (**Tables 139-2** and **139-3**) by (1) further analysis of the CSF, (2) diagnosis of an underlying systemic infection or noninfectious inflammatory condition, or (3) pathologic examination of meningeal biopsy specimens.

Two clinical forms of chronic meningitis exist. In the first, the symptoms are chronic and persistent, whereas in the second there are recurrent discrete episodes of illness. In the latter group, all symptoms, signs, and CSF parameters of meningeal inflammation resolve completely between episodes either spontaneously or in response to a specific therapy. In such patients, the likely etiologies include Mollaret's meningitis which is most often due to herpes simplex virus (HSV) type 2; chemical meningitis due to episodic leakage from an epidermoid tumor, craniopharyngioma, or cholesteatoma into CSF; primary autoimmune inflammatory conditions, including Vogt-Koyanagi-Harada syndrome, Behçet's syndrome, systemic lupus erythematosus (SLE), rheumatoid arthritis, IgG4-related disease, and primary CNS vasculitis; and drug hypersensitivity with repeated administration of the offending agent. With the wider availability of whole genome sequencing, there is also a growing recognition that patients with inherited autoinflammatory syndromes like TNF receptor–associated periodic syndrome (TRAPS), cryoporin-associated periodic fever syndrome (CAPS), complement factor I deficiency, and neonatal-onset multisystem inflammatory disorder can have recurrent meningitis.

The epidemiologic history is of considerable importance in diagnosis of chronic meningitis and may provide direction for selection of laboratory studies. Pertinent features include a history of tuberculosis or exposure; past travel to areas endemic for fungal infections (the San Joaquin Valley in California and southwestern states for coccidioidomycosis, midwestern states for histoplasmosis, southeastern states for blastomycosis); travel to the Mediterranean region or ingestion of imported unpasteurized dairy products (*Brucella*); time spent in wooded areas endemic for Lyme disease; exposure to sexually transmitted disease (syphilis; HSV-2); exposure of an immunocompromised host to pigeons and their droppings (*Cryptococcus neoformans*); exposure to decaying wood (*Cryptococcus gattii*); gardening (*Sporothrix schenckii*); ingestion of poorly cooked meat or contact with a household cat (*Toxoplasma gondii*); residence in Thailand or Japan (*Gnathostoma spinigerum*), Latin America (*Paracoccidioides brasiliensis*), or the South Pacific (*Angiostrongylus cantonensis*); rural residence and raccoon exposure (*Baylisascaris procyonis*); and residence in Latin America, the Philippines, sub-Saharan Africa, or Southeast Asia (*Taenia solium/cysticercosis*).

The presence of focal cerebral signs in a patient with chronic meningitis suggests the possibility of a brain abscess, parameningeal infection, or infarct; identification of a potential source of infection (chronic draining ear, sinusitis, dental abscess, right-to-left cardiac or pulmonary shunt, chronic pleuropulmonary infection) supports this diagnosis. In some cases, diagnosis may be established by recognition and biopsy of unusual skin lesions (Behçet's syndrome, SLE, cryptococcosis, blastomycosis, Lyme disease, sporotrichosis, trypanosomiasis, IV drug use) or enlarged lymph nodes (lymphoma, sarcoid, tuberculosis, HIV, secondary syphilis, or Whipple's disease). A careful ophthalmologic examination may reveal uveitis (Vogt-Koyanagi-Harada syndrome, sarcoid, or central nervous system [CNS] lymphoma), keratoconjunctivitis sicca (Sjögren's syndrome), or iridocyclitis (Behçet's syndrome) and is essential to assess visual loss from papilledema. Aphthous oral lesions, genital ulcers, and hypopyon (inflammatory cells in the anterior chamber of the eye) suggest Behçet's syndrome. Hepatosplenomegaly suggests lymphoma, sarcoid, tuberculosis, or brucellosis. Herpetic lesions in the genital area or on the thighs suggest HSV-2 infection. A breast nodule; a suspicious hyperpigmented skin lesion; focal bone pain; hard, fixed lymph nodes; or an abdominal mass suggests possible carcinomatous meningitis.

IMAGING

Once the clinical syndrome is recognized as a potential manifestation of chronic meningitis, proper analysis of the CSF is essential. However, if the possibility of raised ICP exists, a brain imaging study should be performed before lumbar puncture. If ICP is elevated because of a mass lesion, brain swelling, or a block in ventricular CSF outflow (obstructive hydrocephalus), then lumbar puncture carries the potential risk of brain herniation. Obstructive hydrocephalus usually requires direct ventricular drainage. In patients with open CSF flow pathways, elevated ICP can still occur due to impaired resorption of CSF by arachnoid villi. In such patients, lumbar puncture is usually safe and may be therapeutic. Indeed, repetitive or continuous lumbar drainage may be necessary to prevent abrupt deterioration and death from raised ICP. In some patients, especially those with cryptococcal meningitis, fatal levels of raised ICP can occur without enlarged ventricles.

Contrast-enhanced MRI or CT studies of the brain and spinal cord can identify meningeal enhancement, parameningeal infections (including brain abscess), encasement of the spinal cord (malignancy, inflammation, or infection), or nodular deposits on the meninges or nerve roots (malignancy or sarcoidosis) (**Fig. 139-2**). Imaging studies are also useful to guide biopsy of affected meninges. Lastly, it is important to remember that a cyst that recurrently causes a chemical meningitis due to a leak may be better visualized in between clinical episodes when a recent leak has not shrunken the cyst volume.

The patterns of enhancement of the different layers of the meninges can be very informative and can be divided into two types: leptomeningeal (pia and arachnoid), when enhancement of the meninges follows the convolutions of the gyri and/or involves the meninges around the basal cisterns; and pachymeningeal (dura), when the enhancement is thick and linear or nodular along the inner surface of the calvarium, falx, or tentorium without extension into the cortical gyri or basal cistern involvement. For example, infectious meningitis presents mostly as leptomeningitis, while lymphomatous meningitis can present as pachymeningitis.

Angiographic studies can identify evidence of cerebral arteritis in patients with chronic meningitis and stroke.

CEREBROSPINAL FLUID ANALYSIS

The CSF pressure should be measured and samples sent for bacterial, fungal, and mycobacterial culture; Venereal Disease Research Laboratory (VDRL) test; cell count and differential; Gram's stain; and measurement of glucose and protein. CSF VDRL is a highly specific, but not particularly sensitive, test for syphilis. If CSF VDRL is negative in an otherwise high-risk patient with positive treponemal antibodies in the serum and an otherwise unexplained CSF pleocytosis, empiric treatment may still be appropriate. Wet mount for fungus and parasites, India ink preparation, culture for fastidious bacteria and fungi, assays for cryptococcal antigen and oligoclonal immunoglobulin bands, and cytology should be performed. Other specific CSF tests (Tables 139-2 and 139-3) or blood tests and cultures should be ordered as indicated on the basis of the history, physical examination, or preliminary CSF results (i.e., eosinophilic, mononuclear, or polymorphonuclear meningitis). Rapid diagnosis may be facilitated by serologic tests and polymerase chain reaction (PCR) testing to identify DNA sequences in the CSF that are specific for the suspected pathogen. 16s ribosomal RNA (rRNA) PCR can be used to detect a broad range of bacterial causes of meningitis and can be particularly useful in partially treated meningitis when the yield of culture is low. 18s and 28s rRNA PCR can similarly

TABLE 139-2 Infectious Causes of Chronic Meningitis

CAUSATIVE AGENT	CSF FORMULA	HELPFUL DIAGNOSTIC TESTS	RISK FACTORS AND SYSTEMIC MANIFESTATIONS
Common Bacterial Causes			
Partially treated suppurative meningitis	Mononuclear or mixed mononuclear-polymorphonuclear cells	CSF culture and Gram's stain; CSF 16s rRNA PCR	History consistent with acute bacterial meningitis and incomplete treatment
Parameningeal infection	Mononuclear or mixed mononuclear-polymorphonuclear cells	Contrast-enhanced CT or MRI to detect parenchymal, subdural, epidural, or sinus infection	Otitis media, pleuropulmonary infection, right-to-left cardiopulmonary shunt for brain abscess; focal neurologic signs; neck, back, ear, or sinus tenderness
Mycobacterium tuberculosis	Mononuclear cells except polymorphonuclear cells in early infection (commonly <500 WBC/μL); low CSF glucose; high protein	Tuberculin skin test may be negative; interferon gamma release assay; PCR and AFB culture of CSF (sputum, urine, gastric contents if indicated); identify tubercle bacillus on acid-fast stain of CSF or protein pellicle	Exposure history; previous tuberculous illness; immunosuppressed, anti-TNF therapy or AIDS; young children; fever, meningismus, night sweats, miliary TB on x-ray or liver biopsy; stroke due to arteritis
Lyme disease (Bannwarth's syndrome) *Borrelia burgdorferi*	Mononuclear cells; elevated protein	Serum Lyme antibody titer; western blot confirmation; (patients with syphilis may have false-positive Lyme titer)	History of tick bite or appropriate exposure history; erythema chronicum migrans skin rash; arthritis, radiculopathy, Bell's palsy, meningoencephalitis–multiple sclerosis-like syndrome
Syphilis (secondary, tertiary) *Treponema pallidum*	Mononuclear cells; elevated protein	CSF VDRL; serum VDRL (or RPR); fluorescent treponemal antibody-absorbed (FTA) or MHA-TP; serum VDRL and RPR may be negative in tertiary syphilis due to waning antibody levels or earlier in the disease course due to very elevated antibody levels (prozone effect)	Appropriate exposure history; HIV-seropositive individuals at increased risk of aggressive infection; fever; lymphadenopathy; generalized, nonpruritic, mucocutaneous rash; "dementia"; cerebral infarction due to endarteritis; myelopathy
Uncommon Bacterial Causes			
Actinomyces	Polymorphonuclear cells	Anaerobic culture	Parameningeal abscess or sinus tract (oral or dental focus); pneumonitis
Nocardia	Polymorphonuclear; occasionally mononuclear cells; often low glucose	Isolation may require weeks; weakly acid fast	Associated brain abscess may be present
Brucella	Mononuclear cells (rarely polymorphonuclear); elevated protein; often low glucose	CSF antibody detection; serum antibody detection	Intake of unpasteurized dairy products; exposure to goats, sheep, cows; fever, arthralgia, myalgia, vertebral osteomyelitis
Whipple's disease *Tropheryma whipplei*	Mononuclear cells	Biopsy of small bowel or lymph node; CSF PCR for *T. whipplei;* brain and meningeal biopsy (with PAS stain and EM examination)	Diarrhea, weight loss, arthralgias, fever; dementia, ataxia, paresis, ophthalmoplegia, oculomasticatory myoclonus
Rare Bacterial Causes			
Leptospirosis (occasionally if left untreated may last 3–4 weeks)			
Fungal Causes			
Cryptococcus neoformans and *var. gattii*	Mononuclear cells; count not elevated in some patients with AIDS	India ink or fungal wet mount of CSF (budding yeast); blood and urine cultures; antigen detection in CSF	AIDS and immune suppression; pigeon exposure for *C. neoformans*, decaying wood exposure for *C. var. gattii*; skin and other organ involvement due to disseminated infection
Coccidioides immitis	Mononuclear cells (sometimes 10%–20% eosinophils); often low glucose	Antibody detection in CSF and serum, antigen detection in CSF	Exposure history—southwestern United States; increased virulence in dark-skinned races
Candida sp.	Polymorphonuclear or mononuclear	Fungal stain and culture of CSF	IV drug abuse; postsurgery; prolonged IV therapy; disseminated candidiasis, recent epidural injection
Histoplasma capsulatum	Mononuclear cells; low glucose	Fungal stain and culture of large volumes of CSF; antigen detection in CSF, serum, and urine; antibody detection in serum, CSF	Exposure history—Ohio and central Mississippi River Valley; AIDS; mucosal lesions
Blastomyces dermatitidis	Mononuclear or polymorphonuclear	Fungal stain and culture of CSF; biopsy and culture of skin, lung lesions; antibody detection in serum	Midwestern and southeastern United States; usually systemic infection; abscesses, draining sinus, ulcers
Aspergillus sp.	Mononuclear or polymorphonuclear	CSF culture	Sinusitis; granulocytopenia or immunosuppression
Sporothrix schenckii	Mononuclear cells	Antibody detection in CSF and serum; CSF culture	Traumatic inoculation; IV drug use; ulcerated skin lesion
Rare Fungal Causes			
Xylohypha (formerly *Cladosporium*) *trichoides* and other dark-walled (dematiaceous) fungi such as *Curvularia; Drechslera; Mucor*, and, after water aspiration, *Pseudallescheria boydii;* iatrogenic *Exserohilum rostratum* infection following spinal blocks			

(*Continued*)

TABLE 139-2 Infectious Causes of Chronic Meningitis (Continued)

CAUSATIVE AGENT	CSF FORMULA	HELPFUL DIAGNOSTIC TESTS	RISK FACTORS AND SYSTEMIC MANIFESTATIONS
Protozoal Causes			
Toxoplasma gondii	Mononuclear cells	Biopsy or response to empirical therapy in clinically appropriate context (including presence of antibody in serum)	Usually with intracerebral abscesses; common in HIV-seropositive patients; fever
Trypanosomiasis *Trypanosoma gambiense*, *T. rhodesiense*	Mononuclear cells; elevated protein	Elevated CSF IgM; identification of trypanosomes in CSF and blood smear	Endemic in Africa; chancre, lymphadenopathy; prominent sleep disorder
Rare Protozoal Causes			
Acanthamoeba sp. causing granulomatous amebic encephalitis and meningoencephalitis in immunocompromised and debilitated individuals; *Balamuthia mandrillaris* causing chronic meningoencephalitis in immunocompetent hosts			
Helminthic Causes			
Cysticercosis (infection with cysts of *Taenia solium*)	Mononuclear cells; may have eosinophils; glucose level may be low	Indirect hemagglutination assay in CSF; ELISA immunoblotting in serum; antigen or PCR testing in CSF	Usually with multiple cysts in basal meninges and hydrocephalus; cerebral cysts, ocular involvement; muscle calcification
Gnathostoma spinigerum	Eosinophils, mononuclear cells	Peripheral eosinophilia	History of eating raw fish; common in Thailand and Japan; ocular involvement; subarachnoid hemorrhage; painful radiculopathy
Angiostrongylus cantonensis	Eosinophils, mononuclear cells	Recovery of worms from CSF	History of eating raw shellfish; common in tropical Pacific regions; often benign; ocular involvement (rare)
Baylisascaris procyonis (raccoon ascarid)	Eosinophils, mononuclear cells	Immunoblot in CSF (Centers for Disease Control and Prevention)	Infection follows accidental ingestion of *B. procyonis* eggs from raccoon feces; ocular involvement; fatal meningoencephalitis
Rare Helminthic Causes			
Trichinella spiralis (trichinosis); *Fasciola hepatica* (liver fluke), *Echinococcus* cysts; *Schistosoma* sp. The former may produce a lymphocytic pleocytosis whereas the latter two may produce an eosinophilic response in CSF associated with cerebral cysts (*Echinococcus*) or granulomatous lesions of brain or spinal cord.			
Viral Causes			
Mumps	Mononuclear cells	Antibody in serum	No prior mumps or immunization; orchitis; may produce meningoencephalitis; may persist for 3–4 weeks
Lymphocytic choriomeningitis	Mononuclear cells; may have low glucose	Antibody in serum; PCR for LCMV in CSF	Contact with rodents or their excreta; may persist for 3–4 weeks
Echovirus	Mononuclear cells; may have low glucose	Virus isolation from CSF	Congenital hypogammaglobulinemia; history of recurrent meningitis
HIV (acute retroviral syndrome)	Mononuclear cells	PCR for HIV in blood and CSF	HIV risk factors; rash, fever, lymphadenopathy; lymphopenia in peripheral blood; syndrome may persist long enough to be considered as "chronic meningitis"; or chronic meningitis may develop in later stages (AIDS) due to HIV
Human herpes viruses	Mononuclear cells	PCR for HSV, EBV, CMV DNA; CSF antibody for HSV, EBV	Recurrent meningitis due to HSV-2 (rarely HSV-1) often associated with genital recurrences; EBV associated with myeloradiculopathy, CMV with polyradiculopathy

Abbreviations: AFB, acid-fast bacillus; CMV, cytomegalovirus; CSF, cerebrospinal fluid; CT, computed tomography; EBV, Epstein-Barr virus; ELISA, enzyme-linked immunosorbent assay; EM, electron microscopy; FTA, fluorescent treponemal antibody absorption test; HSV, herpes simplex virus; LCMV, lymphocytic choriomeningitis virus; MHA-TP, microhemagglutination assay–*T. pallidum*; MRI, magnetic resonance imaging; PAS, periodic acid–Schiff; PCR, polymerase chain reaction; RPR, rapid plasma reagin test; TB, tuberculosis; VDRL, Venereal Disease Research Laboratory test.

be useful for detecting a broad range of fungal species. In patients with suspected fungal infections, when other tests are negative, CSF assays for beta-glucans may be a useful adjunct in establishing the diagnosis. Building on progress in parallel deep sequencing and informatics, unbiased metagenomic next-generation sequencing is becoming generally available, representing an efficient and powerful method for diagnosis of challenging infectious cases.

In most categories of chronic (not recurrent) meningitis, mononuclear cells predominate in the CSF. When neutrophils predominate after 3 weeks of illness, the principal etiologic considerations are *Nocardia asteroides*, *Actinomyces israelii*, *Brucella*, *Mycobacterium tuberculosis* (5%–10% of early cases only), various fungi (*Blastomyces dermatitidis*, *Candida* spp., *Histoplasma capsulatum*, *Aspergillus* spp., *Pseudallescheria boydii*, *Cladophialophora bantiana*), and noninfectious causes (SLE, exogenous chemical meningitis). When eosinophils predominate or are present in limited numbers in a primarily mononuclear cell response in the CSF, the differential diagnosis includes parasitic diseases (*A. cantonensis*, *G. spinigerum*, *B. procyonis*, or *Toxocara canis* infection, cysticercosis, schistosomiasis, echinococcal disease, *T. gondii* infection), fungal infections (6–20% eosinophils along with a predominantly lymphocyte pleocytosis, particularly with coccidioidal meningitis), neoplastic disease (lymphoma, leukemia, metastatic carcinoma), or other inflammatory processes (sarcoidosis, hypereosinophilic syndrome).

It is often necessary to broaden the number of diagnostic tests if the initial workup does not reveal the cause. In addition, repeated samples (three or more) of large volumes of lumbar CSF may be required to diagnose certain infectious and malignant causes of chronic meningitis. Lymphomatous or carcinomatous meningitis may be diagnosed by examination of sections cut from a cell block formed by spinning down the sediment from a large volume of CSF. Flow cytometry for malignant cells may also be useful in patients

TABLE 139-3 Noninfectious Causes of Chronic Meningitis

CAUSATIVE AGENTS	CSF FORMULA	HELPFUL DIAGNOSTIC TESTS	RISK FACTORS AND SYSTEMIC MANIFESTATIONS
Malignancy	Mononuclear cells; elevated protein; low glucose	Repeated cytologic examination of large volumes of CSF; CSF exam by polarizing microscopy; clonal lymphocyte markers; deposits on nerve roots or meninges seen on myelogram or contrast-enhanced MRI; meningeal biopsy	Metastatic cancer of breast, lung, stomach, or pancreas; melanoma, lymphoma, leukemia; meningeal gliomatosis; sarcoma; cerebral dysgerminoma
Chemical compounds (may cause recurrent meningitis)	Mononuclear or PMNs; low glucose, elevated protein; xanthochromia from subarachnoid hemorrhage in week prior to presentation with "meningitis"	Contrast-enhanced CT scan or MRI; cerebral angiogram to detect aneurysm. Enhancement and clumping of nerve roots of the cauda equina in arachnoiditis/pachymeningitis	History of recent injection into the subarachnoid space; history of sudden onset of headache; recent resection of acoustic neuroma or craniopharyngioma; epidermoid tumor of brain or spine, sometimes with dermoid sinus tract; pituitary apoplexy
Primary Inflammation			
CNS sarcoidosis	Mononuclear cells; elevated protein; often low glucose	Serum and CSF angiotensin-converting enzyme levels (insensitive); biopsy of extraneural affected tissues or brain lesion/meningeal biopsy	CN palsy, especially CN VII and CN II, including optic chiasm; hypothalamic dysfunction, especially diabetes insipidus; abnormal chest radiograph; peripheral neuropathy or myopathy; longitudinally extensive transverse myelitis
Vogt-Koyanagi-Harada syndrome (recurrent meningitis)	Mononuclear cells		Recurrent meningoencephalitis with uveitis, retinal detachment, alopecia, lightening of eyebrows and lashes, dysacousia, cataracts, glaucoma
Isolated granulomatous angiitis of the nervous system	Mononuclear cells; elevated protein	Angiography; meningeal biopsy may be necessary if confined to small vessels. VZV PCR in blood, CSF and biopsy tissue	Subacute dementia; multiple cerebral infarctions; recent zoster ophthalmicus
Systemic lupus erythematosus	Mononuclear or PMNs	Anti-DNA antibody, antinuclear antibodies	Encephalopathy; seizures; stroke; transverse myelopathy; rash; arthritis
Behçet's syndrome (recurrent meningitis)	Mononuclear or PMNs; elevated protein		Oral and genital aphthous ulcers; iridocyclitis; retinal hemorrhages; pathergic lesions at site of skin puncture
Chronic benign lymphocytic meningitis	Mononuclear cells		Recovery in 2–6 months, diagnosis by exclusion
Mollaret's meningitis (recurrent meningitis)	Large endothelial cells and PMNs in first hours, followed by mononuclear cells	PCR for HSV; MRI/CT to rule out epidermoid tumor or dural cyst	Recurrent meningitis; exclude HSV-2; rare cases due to HSV-1; occasional case associated with dural cyst
Drug hypersensitivity	PMNs; occasionally mononuclear cells or eosinophils	Complete blood count (eosinophilia)	Exposure to nonsteroidal anti-inflammatory agents, sulfonamides, isoniazid, tolmetin, ciprofloxacin, penicillin, carbamazepine, lamotrigine, IV immunoglobulin, OKT3 antibodies, phenazopyridine; improvement after discontinuation of drug; recurrence with repeat exposure
Granulomatosis with polyangiitis (Wegener's)	Mononuclear cells	Chest and sinus radiographs; urinalysis; ANCA antibodies in serum; Pachymeningitis on contrast-enhanced MRI	Associated sinus, pulmonary, or renal lesions; CN palsies; skin lesions; peripheral neuropathy
Neonatal-Onset Multisystem Inflammatory Disorder	Mononuclear and PMNs	Gain of function mutation in NLRP3 gene leading to elevated IL-1β	Recurrent fever, urticaria, arthralgia, sensorineural hearing loss, papilledema, increased ICP
IgG4-Related Hypertrophic Pachymeningitis	Mild lymphocytic pleocytosis in some cases; normal to mildly increased protein; normal glucose	Serum IgG4 levels frequently elevated; ESR and C-reactive protein; Pachymeningitis on contrast-enhanced MRI; meningeal biopsy shows swirling "storiform" fibrosis with lymphocytic infiltrates, obliterative phlebitis and IgG4+ plasma cells	Headache; seizures; focal symptoms from dural involvement in spinal cord/nerve roots, clivus, periorbital, vestibular and brainstem structures. Systemic IgG4-related disease can involve many tissues including pancreas, thyroid, lungs, retroperitoneum, lacrimal, parotid and submandibular glands, orbits, kidney, aorta, liver.
TNF receptor-associated periodic fever syndrome (TRAPS)	Mononuclear cells	Mutation in TNFRSF1A gene leading to elevated TNF	Headache, seizures, tinnitus, skin rash, abdominal pain, lymphadenopathy, periorbital edema, joint pain, myalgia
Complement factor I deficiency	PMNs	Mutation in complement factor I gene leading to low serum levels of factor I (or dysfunctional factor I) and C3	Recurrent, steroid-responsive, aseptic, neutrophilic meningitis with or without encephalitis; increased risk for systemic infections with encapsulated bacteria, glomerulonephritis, systemic lupus erythematosus and leukocytoclastic vasculitis
Cryoporin-associated periodic fever syndrome (CAPS)	Mononuclear cells	heterozygous gain-of-function mutations within the *NLRP3* gene	Fever, urticaria, amyloidosis, arthralgia, sensorineural hearing loss, myalgias, papilledema, vision changes
Other: multiple sclerosis, Sjögren's syndrome, and rarer forms of vasculitis (e.g., Cogan's syndrome)			

Abbreviations: ANCA, antineutrophil cytoplasmic antibodies; CN, cranial nerve; CSF, cerebrospinal fluid; CT, computed tomography; HSV, herpes simplex virus; MRI, magnetic resonance imaging; PCR, polymerase chain reaction; PMNs, polymorphonuclear cells; TNF, tumor necrosis factor.

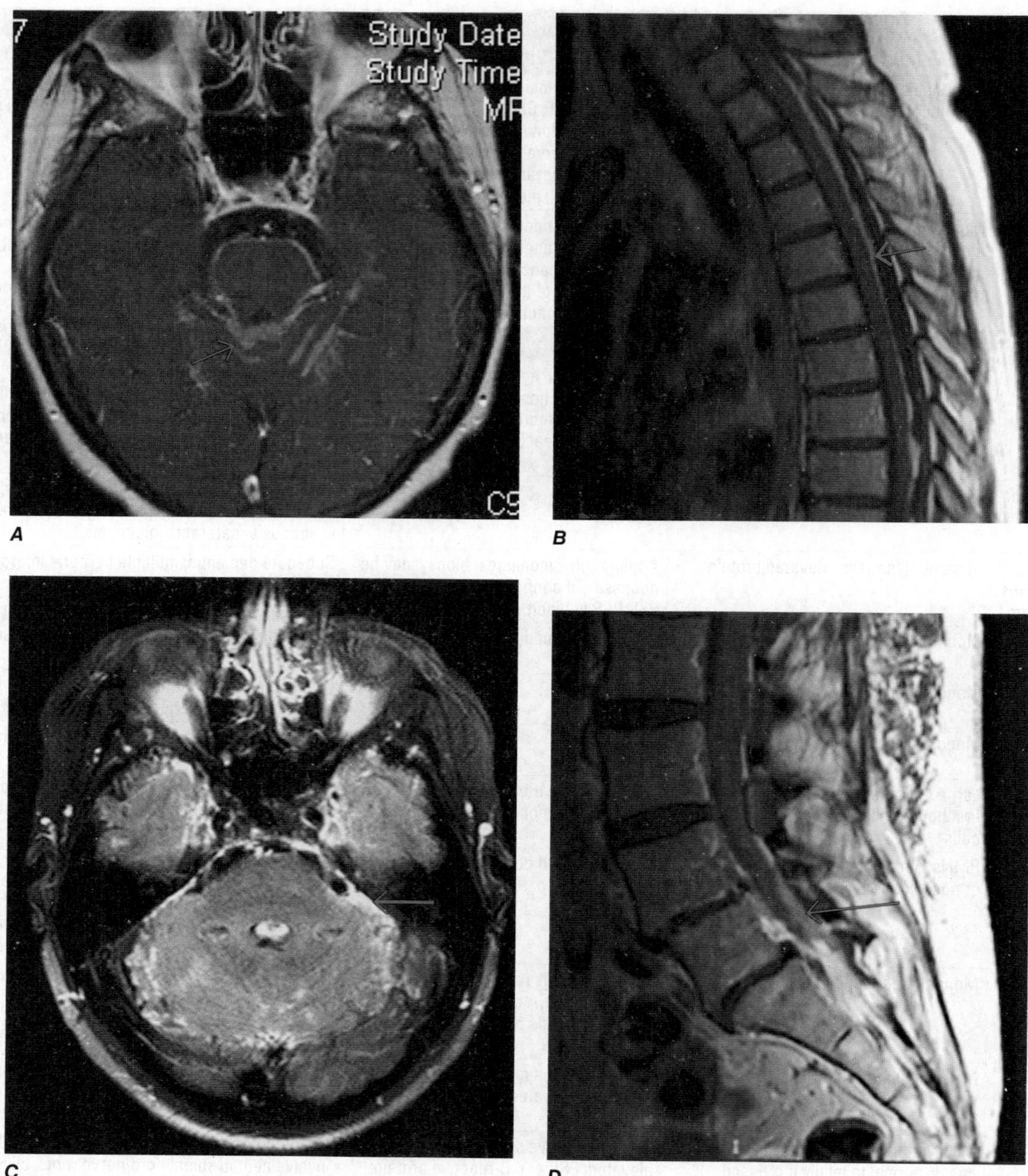

FIGURE 139-2 Chronic meningitis illustrating meningeal enhancement on contrast MRI scan. ***A*** and ***B*** are images from a patient with chronic meningitis due to carcinoma. ***C*** and ***D*** are from a patient with chronic meningitis due to Cryptococcus infection. *Arrows* point to the most prominent areas of meningeal inflammation around the brainstem and cerebellar folia (***A***), cerebellum (***C***), along the dorsal spinal cord (***B***), and clumping of roots in the cauda equina (***D***).

with suspected carcinomatous meningitis. The diagnosis of fungal meningitis may also require large volumes of CSF for culture of sediment. If standard lumbar puncture is unrewarding, a cervical cisternal tap to sample CSF near to the basal meninges may be fruitful. Ventricular fluid may appear sterile in cases with active infection in the lower lumbar space.

LABORATORY INVESTIGATION

In addition to the CSF examination, an attempt should be made to uncover pertinent underlying illnesses. Tuberculin skin test, chest radiograph, urine analysis and culture, blood count and differential, renal and liver function tests, alkaline phosphatase, sedimentation rate, antinuclear antibody, anti-Ro antibody, anti-La antibody, rheumatoid factor, and IgG4 level are often indicated. In some cases, a thorough search for a systemic site of infection is indicated. Pulmonary foci of infection may be present, particularly with fungal or tuberculous disease. Hence a CT or MRI of the chest and a sputum examination may be helpful. Abnormalities can be pursued by bronchoscopy or transthoracic needle biopsy. A tuberculin skin test is often placed, although the test has limited specificity and sensitivity for diagnosis of active disease. Where available, gamma interferon release assays may be used to diagnose latent tuberculosis. Liver, bone marrow, or lymph node biopsy may be diagnostic in some cases of miliary tuberculosis, disseminated fungal infection, sarcoidosis, or metastatic malignancy. Positron emission tomography with fluorodeoxyglucose may be useful in identifying a systemic site for biopsy in patients with suspected carcinomatous meningitis or sarcoidosis when other tests are unrevealing. Genetic testing can identify mutations that cause rare monogenic autoinflammatory disorders.

MENINGEAL BIOPSY

If CSF is not diagnostic then a meningeal biopsy should be strongly considered in patients who are severely disabled, who need chronic ventricular decompression, or whose illness is progressing rapidly. The activities of the surgeon, pathologist, microbiologist, and cytologist should be coordinated so that a large enough sample is obtained and the appropriate cultures and histologic and molecular studies, including electron-microscopic and PCR studies, are performed. The diagnostic yield of meningeal biopsy can be increased by targeting regions that enhance with contrast on MRI or CT. With current microsurgical techniques, most areas of the basal meninges can be accessed for biopsy via a limited craniotomy. In one series, MRI demonstrated meningeal enhancement in 47% of patients undergoing meningeal biopsy; biopsy of an enhancing region was diagnostic in 80% of cases, biopsy of nonenhancing regions was diagnostic in only 9%, and sarcoid (31%), and metastatic adenocarcinoma (25%) were the most common conditions identified. Tuberculosis is the most common condition identified in many reports from outside the United States.

APPROACH TO THE ENIGMATIC CASE

In approximately one-third of cases, the diagnosis is not known despite careful evaluation of CSF and potential extraneural sites of disease. A number of the organisms that cause chronic meningitis may take weeks to be identified by cultures. In enigmatic cases, several options are available, determined by the extent of the clinical deficits and rate of progression. It is prudent to wait until cultures are finalized if the patient is asymptomatic or symptoms are mild and not progressive. Unfortunately, in many cases progressive neurologic deterioration occurs, and rapid treatment is required. Ventricular-peritoneal shunts may be placed to relieve hydrocephalus, but the risk of disseminating the undiagnosed inflammatory process into the abdomen must be considered.

Empirical Treatment Diagnosis of the causative agent is essential because effective therapies exist for many etiologies of chronic meningitis, but if the condition is left untreated, progressive damage to the CNS and cranial nerves and roots is likely to occur. Occasionally, empirical therapy must be initiated when all attempts at diagnosis fail. In general, empirical therapy in the United States consists of antimycobacterial agents, amphotericin B (often combined with flucytosine) for fungal infection, and/or glucocorticoids for noninfectious inflammatory causes. It is important to direct empirical therapy of lymphocytic meningitis at tuberculosis, particularly if the condition is associated with low CSF glucose, since untreated disease can be devastating within weeks. Prolonged anti-tumor necrosis factor therapy and antiprogrammed death-1 (PD-1) inhibitors can cause reactivation of TB, and such patients who develop chronic meningitis should be treated empirically with antituberculous therapy if the etiology is uncertain. In the Mayo Clinic series, the most useful empirical therapy was administration of glucocorticoids rather than antituberculous therapy. When proceeding with empiric glucocorticoids, caution should be maintained whenever a transient response to treatment is noted, as some infectious (e.g., tuberculosis and cysticercosis) and noninfectious (e.g., lymphoma) etiologies may temporarily respond to glucocorticoid monotherapy. Carcinomatous or lymphomatous meningitis may be difficult to diagnose initially, but the diagnosis becomes evident with time.

THE IMMUNOSUPPRESSED PATIENT

Chronic meningitis is not uncommon in the course of HIV infection. Pleocytosis and mild meningeal signs often occur at the onset of HIV infection, and occasionally low-grade meningitis persists. In worldwide populations, *Mycobacterium tuberculosis* is the most common cause of chronic meningitis, followed by *Cryptococcus neoformans*. Toxoplasmosis commonly presents as intracranial abscesses and also may be associated with meningitis. Other important causes of chronic meningitis in AIDS include infection with *Nocardia*, *Candida*, or other fungi; syphilis; and lymphoma (Fig. 139-2). With HIV infection, primary CNS lymphomas may arise, which are typically positive for EBV infection. Toxoplasmosis, nocardiosis, cryptococcosis and other fungal infections are important etiologic considerations in individuals with immunodeficiency states other than AIDS, including those due to immunosuppressive medications. Because of the increased risk of chronic meningitis and the attenuation of clinical signs of meningeal irritation in immunosuppressed individuals, CSF examination should be performed for any persistent headache or unexplained change in mental state.

FURTHER READING

Baldwin K, Whiting C: Chronic meningitis: simplifying a diagnostic challenge. Curr Neurol Neurosci Rep 16:30, 2016.

Cheng TM et al: Chronic meningitis: the role of meningeal or cortical biopsy. Neurosurgery 34:590, 1994.

Kacar M et al: Hereditary systemic autoinflammatory diseases and Schnitzler's syndrome. Rheumatology 58:vi31, 2019.

Le LT, Spudich SS: HIV-associated neurologic disorders and central nervous system opportunistic infections in HIV. Semin Neurol 36:373, 2016.

Lu LX et al: IgG4-related hypertrophic pachymeningitis: Clinical features, diagnostic criteria and treatment. JAMA Neurol 71:785, 2014.

Torok ME: Tuberculous meningitis: advances in diagnosis and treatment. Br Med Bull 113:117, 2015.

Wilson MR et al: Chronic meningitis investigated via metagenomic next-generation sequencing. JAMA Neurol 75:947, 2018.

140 Brain Abscess and Empyema

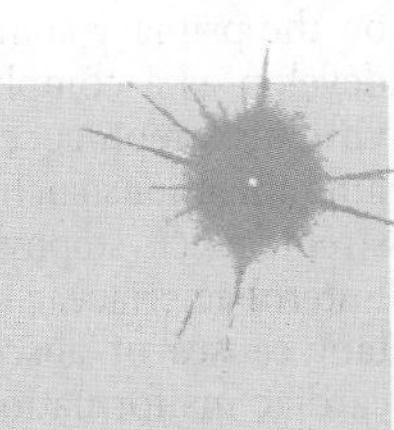

Karen L. Roos, Kenneth L. Tyler

BRAIN ABSCESS

DEFINITION

A brain abscess is a focal, suppurative infection within the brain parenchyma, typically surrounded by a vascularized capsule. The term *cerebritis* is often employed to describe a nonencapsulated brain abscess.

EPIDEMIOLOGY

A bacterial brain abscess is a relatively uncommon intracranial infection, with an incidence of ~0.3–1.3:100,000 persons per year. Predisposing conditions include otitis media and mastoiditis, paranasal sinusitis, pyogenic infections in the chest or other body sites, penetrating head trauma or neurosurgical procedures, and dental infections. In immunocompetent individuals the most important pathogens are *Streptococcus* spp. (anaerobic, aerobic, and viridans [40%]), Enterobacteriaceae (*Proteus* spp., *Escherichia coli* sp., *Klebsiella* spp. [25%]), anaerobes (e.g., *Bacteroides* spp., *Fusobacterium* spp. [30%]), and staphylococci (10%). In immunocompromised hosts with underlying HIV infection, organ transplantation, cancer, or immunosuppressive therapy, most brain abscesses are caused by *Nocardia* spp., *Toxoplasma gondii*, *Aspergillus* spp., *Candida* spp., and *C. neoformans*. In Latin America and in immigrants from Latin America, the most common cause of brain abscess is *Taenia solium* (neurocysticercosis). In India and East Asia, mycobacterial infection (tuberculoma) remains a major cause of focal CNS mass lesions.

ETIOLOGY

A brain abscess may develop (1) by direct spread from a contiguous cranial site of infection, such as paranasal sinusitis, otitis media, mastoiditis, or dental infection; (2) following head trauma or a neurosurgical procedure; or (3) as a result of hematogenous spread from a remote site of infection. In up to 25% of cases, no obvious primary source of infection is apparent (cryptogenic brain abscess).

Approximately one-third of brain abscesses are associated with otitis media and mastoiditis, often with an associated cholesteatoma. Otogenic abscesses occur predominantly in the temporal lobe (55–75%) and cerebellum (20–30%). In some series, up to 90% of cerebellar abscesses are otogenic. Common organisms include streptococci, *Bacteroides* spp., *Pseudomonas* spp., *Haemophilus* spp., and Enterobacteriaceae. Abscesses that develop as a result of direct spread of infection from the frontal, ethmoidal, or sphenoidal sinuses and those that occur due to dental infections are usually located in the frontal lobes. Approximately 10% of brain abscesses are associated with paranasal sinusitis, and this association is particularly strong in young males in their second and third decades of life. The most common pathogens in brain abscesses associated with paranasal sinusitis are streptococci (especially *Streptococcus milleri*), *Haemophilus* spp., *Bacteroides* spp., *Pseudomonas* spp., and *Staphylococcus aureus*. Dental infections are associated with ~2% of brain abscesses, although it is often suggested that many "cryptogenic" abscesses are in fact due to dental infections. The most common pathogens in this setting are streptococci, staphylococci, *Bacteroides* spp., and *Fusobacterium* spp.

Hematogenous abscesses account for ~25% of brain abscesses. Hematogenous abscesses are often multiple, and multiple abscesses often (50%) have a hematogenous origin. These abscesses show a predilection for the territory of the middle cerebral artery (i.e., posterior frontal or parietal lobes). Hematogenous abscesses are often located at the junction of the gray and white matter and are often poorly encapsulated. The microbiology of hematogenous abscesses is dependent on the primary source of infection. For example, brain abscesses that develop as a complication of infective endocarditis are often due to viridans streptococci or *S. aureus*. Abscesses associated with pyogenic lung infections such as lung abscess or bronchiectasis are often due to streptococci, staphylococci, *Bacteroides* spp., *Fusobacterium* spp., or Enterobacteriaceae. Enterobacteriaceae and *P. aeruginosa* are important causes of abscesses associated with urinary sepsis. Congenital cardiac malformations that produce a right-to-left shunt allow bloodborne bacteria to bypass the pulmonary capillary bed and reach the brain. Similar phenomena can occur with pulmonary arteriovenous malformations. The decreased arterial oxygenation and saturation from the right-to-left shunt and polycythemia may cause focal areas of cerebral ischemia, thus providing a nidus for microorganisms that bypassed the pulmonary circulation to multiply and form an abscess. Streptococci are the most common pathogens in this setting.

Abscesses that follow penetrating head trauma or neurosurgical procedures are frequently due to methicillin-resistant *S. aureus* (MRSA), *Staphylococcus epidermidis*, Enterobacteriaceae, *Pseudomonas* spp., and *Clostridium* spp.

PATHOGENESIS AND HISTOPATHOLOGY

Results of experimental models of brain abscess formation suggest that for bacterial invasion of brain parenchyma to occur, there must be preexisting or concomitant areas of ischemia, necrosis, or hypoxemia in brain tissue. The intact brain parenchyma is relatively resistant to infection. Once bacteria have established infection, brain abscess frequently evolves through a series of stages, influenced by the nature of the infecting organism and by the immunocompetence of the host. The early cerebritis stage (days 1–3) is characterized by a perivascular infiltration of inflammatory cells, which surround a central core of coagulative necrosis. Marked edema surrounds the lesion at this stage. In the late cerebritis stage (days 4–9), pus formation leads to enlargement of the necrotic center, which is surrounded at its border by an inflammatory infiltrate of macrophages and fibroblasts. A thin capsule of fibroblasts and reticular fibers gradually develops, and the surrounding area of cerebral edema becomes more distinct than in the previous stage. The third stage, early capsule formation (days 10–13), is characterized by the formation of a capsule that is better developed on the cortical than on the ventricular side of the lesion. This stage correlates with the appearance of a ring-enhancing capsule on neuroimaging studies. The final stage, late capsule formation (day 14 and beyond), is defined by a well-formed necrotic center surrounded by a dense collagenous capsule. The surrounding area of cerebral edema has regressed, but marked gliosis with large numbers of reactive astrocytes has developed outside the capsule. This gliotic process may contribute to the development of seizures as a sequela of brain abscess.

CLINICAL PRESENTATION

A brain abscess typically presents as an expanding intracranial mass lesion rather than as an infectious process. Although the evolution of signs and symptoms is extremely variable, ranging from hours to weeks or even months, most patients present to the hospital 11–12 days following onset of symptoms. The classic clinical triad of headache, fever, and a focal neurologic deficit is present in <50% of cases. The most common symptom in patients with a brain abscess is headache, occurring in >75% of patients. The headache is often characterized as a constant, dull, aching sensation, either hemicranial or generalized, and it becomes progressively more severe and refractory to therapy. Fever is present in only 50% of patients at the time of diagnosis, and its absence should not exclude the diagnosis. The new onset of focal or generalized seizure activity is a presenting sign in 15–35% of patients. Focal neurologic deficits including hemiparesis, aphasia, or visual field defects are part of the initial presentation in >60% of patients.

The clinical presentation of a brain abscess depends on its location, the nature of the primary infection if present, and the level of the intracranial pressure (ICP). Hemiparesis is the most common localizing sign of a frontal lobe abscess. A temporal lobe abscess may present with a disturbance of language (dysphasia) or an upper homonymous quadrantanopia. Nystagmus and ataxia are signs of a cerebellar abscess. Signs of raised ICP—papilledema, nausea and vomiting, and drowsiness or confusion—can be the dominant presentation of some abscesses, particularly those in the cerebellum. Meningismus is not present unless the abscess has ruptured into the ventricle or the infection has spread to the subarachnoid space.

DIAGNOSIS

Diagnosis is made by neuroimaging studies. MRI **(Fig. 140-1)** is better than CT for demonstrating abscesses in the early (cerebritis) stages and is superior to CT for identifying abscesses in the posterior fossa. Cerebritis appears on MRI as an area of low signal intensity on T1-weighted images with irregular postgadolinium enhancement and as an area of increased signal intensity on T2-weighted images. Cerebritis is often not visualized by CT scan, but when present, appears as an area of hypodensity. On a contrast-enhanced CT scan, a mature brain abscess appears as a focal area of hypodensity surrounded by ring enhancement with surrounding edema (hypodensity). On contrast-enhanced T1-weighted MRI, a mature brain abscess has a capsule that enhances surrounding a hypodense center and surrounded by a hypodense area of edema. On T2-weighted MRI, there is a hyperintense central area of pus surrounded by a well-defined hypointense capsule and a hyperintense surrounding area of edema. It is important to recognize that the CT and MRI appearance, particularly of the capsule, may be altered by treatment with corticosteroids. The distinction between a brain abscess and other focal CNS lesions such as primary or metastatic tumors may be facilitated by the use of diffusion-weighted imaging sequences on which a brain abscess typically shows increased signal due to restricted diffusion of the abscess cavity with corresponding low signal on apparent diffusion coefficient images.

Microbiologic diagnosis of the etiologic agent is most accurately determined by Gram's stain and culture of abscess material obtained by CT-guided stereotactic needle aspiration. Aerobic and anaerobic bacterial cultures and mycobacterial and fungal cultures should be obtained. Up to 10% of patients will also have positive blood cultures. Lumbar puncture (LP) should not be performed in patients with known or suspected focal intracranial infections such as abscess or empyema; cerebrospinal fluid (CSF) analysis contributes nothing to diagnosis or therapy, and LP increases the risk of herniation.

Additional laboratory studies may provide clues to the diagnosis of brain abscess in patients with a CNS mass lesion. About 50% of patients have a peripheral leukocytosis, 60% an elevated erythrocyte sedimentation rate, and 80% an elevated C-reactive protein. Blood cultures are positive in ~10% of cases overall but may be positive in >85% of patients with abscesses due to *Listeria*.

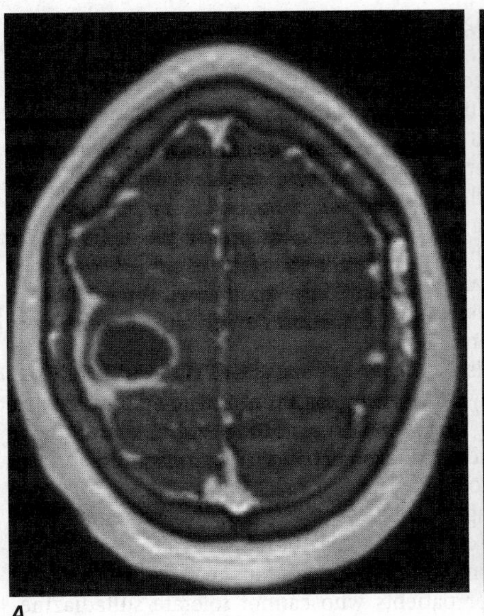
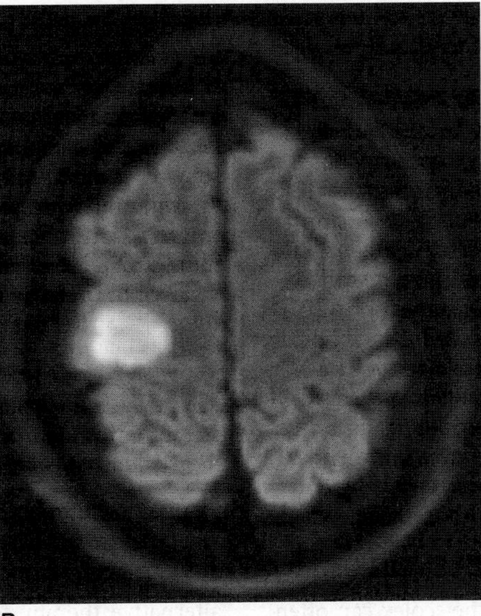
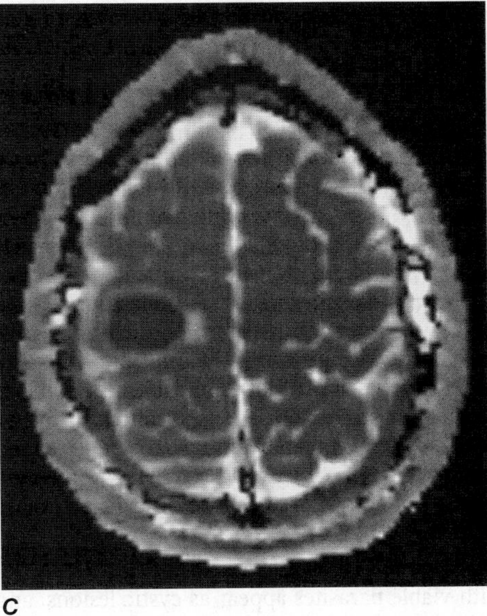

A B C

FIGURE 140-1 Pyogenic brain abscess. Note that the abscess wall enhances prominently after gadolinium administration on the magnetic resonance axial T1-weighted image (***A***). The abscess is hyperintense on the diffusion-weighted image (***B***) and dark on the apparent diffusion coefficient (ADC) image (***C***). *(Courtesy of Aaron Kamer, MD; with permission.)*

■ DIFFERENTIAL DIAGNOSIS

Conditions that can cause headache, fever, focal neurologic signs, and seizure activity include brain abscess, subdural empyema, bacterial meningitis, viral meningoencephalitis, superior sagittal sinus thrombosis, and acute disseminated encephalomyelitis. When fever is absent, primary and metastatic brain tumors become the major differential diagnosis. Less commonly, cerebral infarction or hematoma can have an MRI or CT appearance resembling brain abscess.

TREATMENT

Brain Abscess

Optimal therapy of brain abscesses involves a combination of high-dose parenteral antibiotics and neurosurgical drainage. Empirical therapy of community-acquired brain abscess in an immunocompetent patient typically includes a third- or fourth-generation cephalosporin (e.g., cefotaxime, ceftriaxone, or cefepime) and metronidazole **(see Table 138-1 for antibiotic dosages)**. In patients with penetrating head trauma or recent neurosurgical procedures, treatment should include ceftazidime as the third-generation cephalosporin to enhance coverage of *Pseudomonas* spp. and vancomycin for coverage of staphylococci. Meropenem plus vancomycin also provides good coverage in this setting.

Aspiration and drainage of the abscess under stereotactic guidance are beneficial for both diagnosis and therapy. Empirical antibiotic coverage should be modified based on the results of Gram's stain and culture of the abscess contents. Complete excision of a bacterial abscess via craniotomy or craniectomy is generally reserved for multiloculated abscesses or those in which stereotactic aspiration is unsuccessful.

Medical therapy alone is not optimal for treatment of brain abscess and should be reserved for patients whose abscesses are neurosurgically inaccessible, for patients with small (<2–3 cm) or nonencapsulated abscesses (cerebritis), and for patients whose condition is too tenuous to allow performance of a neurosurgical procedure. All patients should receive a minimum of 6–8 weeks of parenteral antibiotic therapy. The role, if any, of supplemental oral antibiotic therapy following completion of a standard course of parenteral therapy has never been adequately studied.

In addition to surgical drainage and antibiotic therapy, patients should receive prophylactic anticonvulsant therapy because of the high risk (~35%) of focal or generalized seizures. Anticonvulsant therapy is continued for at least 3 months after resolution of the abscess, and decisions regarding withdrawal are then based on the EEG. If the EEG is abnormal, anticonvulsant therapy should be continued. If the EEG is normal, anticonvulsant therapy can be slowly withdrawn, with close follow-up and repeat EEG after the medication has been discontinued.

Corticosteroids should not be given routinely to patients with brain abscesses. Intravenous dexamethasone therapy (10 mg every 6 h) is usually reserved for patients with substantial periabscess edema and associated mass effect and increased ICP. Dexamethasone should be tapered as rapidly as possible to avoid delaying the natural process of encapsulation of the abscess.

Serial MRI or CT scans should be obtained on a monthly or twice-monthly basis to document resolution of the abscess. More frequent studies (e.g., weekly) are probably warranted in the subset of patients who are receiving antibiotic therapy alone. A small amount of enhancement may remain for months after the abscess has been successfully treated.

■ PROGNOSIS

The mortality rate of brain abscess has declined in parallel with the development of enhanced neuroimaging techniques, improved neurosurgical procedures for stereotactic aspiration, and improved antibiotics. In modern series, the mortality rate is typically <15%. Significant sequelae, including seizures, persisting weakness, aphasia, or mental impairment, occur in ≥20% of survivors.

NONBACTERIAL CAUSES OF INFECTIOUS FOCAL CNS LESIONS

■ ETIOLOGY

Neurocysticercosis is the most common parasitic disease of the CNS worldwide. Humans acquire cysticercosis by the ingestion of food contaminated with the eggs of the parasite *T. solium* **(Chap. 235)**. Toxoplasmosis **(Chap. 228)** is a parasitic disease caused by *T. gondii* and acquired from the ingestion of undercooked meat and from handling cat feces.

■ CLINICAL PRESENTATION

The most common manifestation of neurocysticercosis is new-onset partial seizures with or without secondary generalization. Cysticerci may develop in the brain parenchyma and cause seizures or focal neurologic deficits. When present in the subarachnoid or ventricular spaces, cysticerci can produce increased ICP by interference with CSF flow. Spinal cysticerci can mimic the presentation of intraspinal tumors. When the cysticerci first lodge in the brain, they frequently cause little in the way of an inflammatory response. As the cysticercal cyst degenerates, it elicits an inflammatory response that may present clinically as a seizure. Eventually the cyst dies, a process that may take several years and is typically associated with resolution of the inflammatory response and, often, abatement of seizures.

Primary *Toxoplasma* infection is often asymptomatic. However, during this phase, parasites may spread to the CNS, where they become latent. Reactivation of CNS infection is almost exclusively associated with immunocompromised hosts, particularly those with HIV infection. During this phase, patients present with headache, fever, seizures, and focal neurologic deficits.

DIAGNOSIS

The lesions of neurocysticercosis are readily visualized by MRI or CT scans depending on the stage of the lesion. There are four stages of neurocysticercosis: (1) the vesicular stage, (2) the colloidal stage, (3) the granulonodular stage, and (4) the nodular-calcified stage. Lesions with viable parasites appear as cystic lesions, and the scolex can often be visualized on MRI. Cystic lesions with small nodules (scolex) within the cyst are in the vesicular stage of neurocysticercosis (**Fig. 140-2*A* and *B***). There is no significant edema surrounding a lesion in the vesicular stage. Lesions in the colloidal stage demonstrate peripheral enhancement on postcontrast imaging (**Fig. 140-2*C***) with substantial surrounding edema on T2 images (**Fig. 140-2*D***). In the granulonodular stage, on postcontrast imaging, the lesion enhances in a homogenous fashion (**Fig. 140-2*E***). On fluid-attenuated inversion recovery (FLAIR) images, there is no surrounding edema (**Fig. 140-2*F***). Parenchymal brain calcifications are the most common finding and evidence that the parasite is no longer viable. These chronic lesions are best seen on CT (**Fig. 140-2*G***) and can be difficult to detect on MRI. The most sensitive technique for the detection of these small calcific foci on MRI is susceptibility-weighted imaging (SWI). If a confirmatory test for neurocysticercosis is needed, the enzyme-linked immunotransfer blot is recommended. A funduscopic exam is also recommended for all patients with suspected neurocysticercosis.

MRI findings of toxoplasmosis consist of multiple lesions in the deep white matter, the thalamus, and basal ganglia and at the gray-white junction in the cerebral hemispheres. With contrast administration, the majority of the lesions enhance in a ringed, nodular, or homogeneous pattern and are surrounded by edema. In the presence of the characteristic neuroimaging abnormalities of *T. gondii* infection, serum IgG antibody to *T. gondii* should be obtained and, when positive, the patient should be treated.

TREATMENT

Infectious Focal CNS Lesions

Anticonvulsant therapy is initiated when the patient with neurocysticercosis presents with a seizure. There is controversy about whether or not anthelmintic therapy should be given to all patients, and recommendations are based on the stage of the lesion. Cysticerci appearing as cystic lesions in the brain parenchyma with or without pericystic edema or in the subarachnoid space at the convexity of the cerebral hemispheres should be treated with anticysticidal therapy. Cysticidal drugs accelerate the destruction of the parasites, resulting in a faster resolution of the infection. Albendazole monotherapy is recommended for patients with one to two parenchymal cysts. The dose of albendazole is 15 mg/kg per day in two daily doses for 10–14 days. A combination of albendazole plus praziquantel is recommended for patients with more than two viable cysts. Viable cysts are defined as those in the vesicular or colloidal stages (see above). The recommended dose of praziquantel is 50 mg/kg per day for 10–14 days. Prednisone or dexamethasone is begun prior to anticysticidal therapy to reduce the host inflammatory response to degenerating parasites. Only cysts in the vesicular stage, where the cyst contains living larva (scolex seen on CT or MRI), and cysts in the colloidal stage, as the larva degenerates (edema surrounds the lesion), are treated with anticysticidal therapy. Some, but not all, experts recommend anticysticidal therapy for lesions that are in the granulonodular stage (surrounded by a contrast-enhancing ring). There is universal agreement that calcified lesions do not need to be treated with anticysticidal therapy. Antiepileptic therapy can be stopped once a follow-up CT or MRI scan shows resolution of the lesion and the patient has had no seizures for 24 consecutive months. Long-term antiepileptic therapy is recommended when seizures occur after resolution of edema and resorption or calcification of the degenerating cyst.

CNS toxoplasmosis is treated with a combination of sulfadiazine, 1.5–2.0 g orally qid, plus pyrimethamine, 100 mg orally to load, then 75–100 mg orally qd, plus folinic acid, 10–15 mg orally qd. Folinic acid is added to the regimen to prevent megaloblastic anemia. Therapy is continued until there is no evidence of active disease on neuroimaging studies, which typically takes at least 6 weeks, and then the dose of sulfadiazine is reduced to 2–4 g/d and pyrimethamine to 50 mg/d. Clindamycin plus pyrimethamine is an alternative therapy for patients who cannot tolerate sulfadiazine, but the combination of pyrimethamine and sulfadiazine is more effective.

SUBDURAL EMPYEMA

A subdural empyema (SDE) is a collection of pus between the dura and arachnoid membranes (**Fig. 140-3**).

EPIDEMIOLOGY

SDE is a rare disorder that accounts for 15–25% of focal suppurative CNS infections. Sinusitis is the most common predisposing condition and typically involves the frontal sinuses, either alone or in combination with the ethmoid and maxillary sinuses. Sinusitis-associated empyema has a striking predilection for young males, possibly reflecting sex-related differences in sinus anatomy and development. It has been suggested that SDE may complicate 1–2% of cases of frontal sinusitis severe enough to require hospitalization. As a consequence of this epidemiology, SDE shows an ~3:1 male/female predominance, with 70% of cases occurring in the second and third decades of life. SDE may also develop as a complication of head trauma or neurosurgery. Secondary infection of a subdural effusion may also result in empyema, although secondary infection of hematomas, in the absence of a prior neurosurgical procedure, is rare.

ETIOLOGY

Aerobic and anaerobic streptococci, staphylococci, Enterobacteriaceae, and anaerobic bacteria are the most common causative organisms of sinusitis-associated SDE. Staphylococci and gram-negative bacilli are often the etiologic organisms when SDE follows neurosurgical procedures or head trauma. Up to one-third of cases are culture-negative, possibly reflecting difficulty in obtaining adequate anaerobic cultures.

PATHOPHYSIOLOGY

Sinusitis-associated SDE develops as a result of either retrograde spread of infection from septic thrombophlebitis of the mucosal veins draining the sinuses or contiguous spread of infection to the brain from osteomyelitis in the posterior wall of the frontal or other sinuses. SDE may also develop from direct introduction of bacteria into the subdural space as a complication of a neurosurgical procedure. The evolution of SDE can be extremely rapid because the subdural space is a large compartment that offers few mechanical barriers to the spread of infection. In patients with sinusitis-associated SDE, suppuration typically begins in the upper and anterior portions of one cerebral hemisphere and then extends posteriorly. SDE is often associated with other intracranial infections, including epidural empyema (40%), cortical thrombophlebitis (35%), and intracranial abscess or cerebritis (>25%). Cortical venous infarction produces necrosis of underlying cerebral cortex and subcortical white matter, with focal neurologic deficits and seizures (see below).

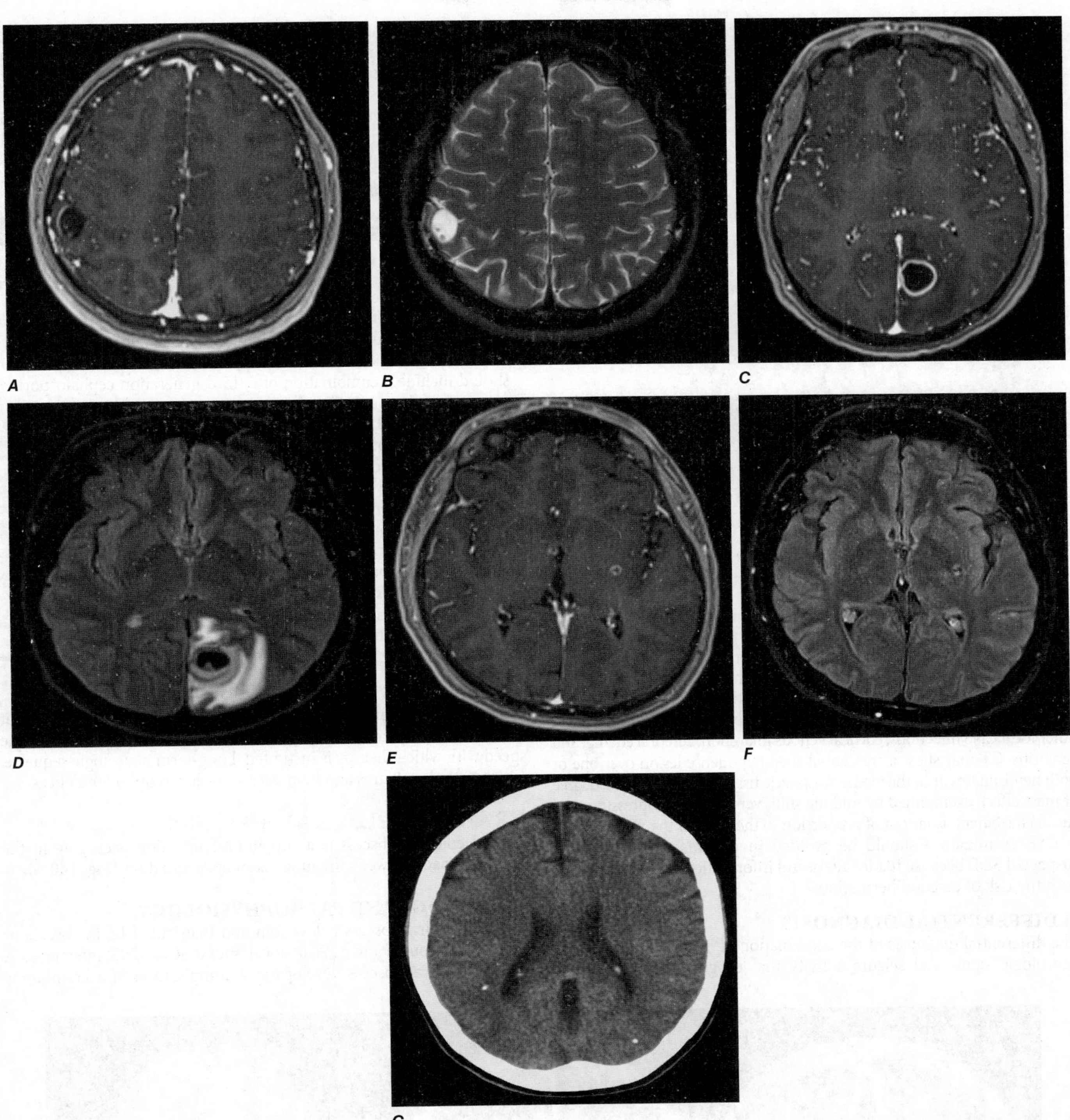

FIGURE 140-2 The four stages of neurocysticercosis. *A, B.* The vesicular stage. ***A.*** Postcontrast T1 magnetic resonance image (MRI). Note lesion in right parietal area. Small hypointense nodules within the cyst likely represent scolex. ***B.*** T2 MRI. The cyst is now visualized as a uniform hyperintense lesion with the small hypointense nodules likely representing scolex. No significant edema is present around the lesion on T2, typical for this stage of the disease. ***C, D.*** The colloidal stage. ***C.*** A medial left occipital lesion demonstrates peripheral enhancement on postcontrast imaging. ***D.*** On fluid-attenuated inversion recovery (FLAIR) MRI, the lesion has substantial surrounding hyperintense edema. ***E, F.*** The granulonodular stage. ***E.*** Postcontrast T1-weighted imaging demonstrates enhancing lesions in the left putamen and in the genu of the internal capsule near the foramen of Monro. ***F.*** These lesions demonstrate no surrounding edema on FLAIR imaging, typical for this stage of the disease. ***G.*** The nodular-calcified stage. Computed tomography scan demonstrates typical parenchymal brain calcifications. *(Courtesy of Aaron Kamer, MD; with permission.)*

CLINICAL PRESENTATION

A patient with SDE typically presents with fever and a progressively worsening headache. The diagnosis of SDE should always be suspected in a patient with known sinusitis who presents with new CNS signs or symptoms. Patients with underlying sinusitis frequently have symptoms related to this infection. As the infection progresses, focal neurologic deficits, seizures, nuchal rigidity, and signs of increased ICP commonly occur. Headache is the most common complaint at the time of presentation; initially it is localized to the side of the subdural infection, but then it becomes more severe and generalized. Contralateral hemiparesis or hemiplegia is the most common focal neurologic deficit and can occur from the direct effects of the SDE on the cortex or as a consequence of venous infarction. Seizures begin as partial motor seizures that then become secondarily generalized. Seizures may be due to the direct irritative effect of the SDE on the underlying cortex or result from cortical venous infarction (see above). In untreated SDE,

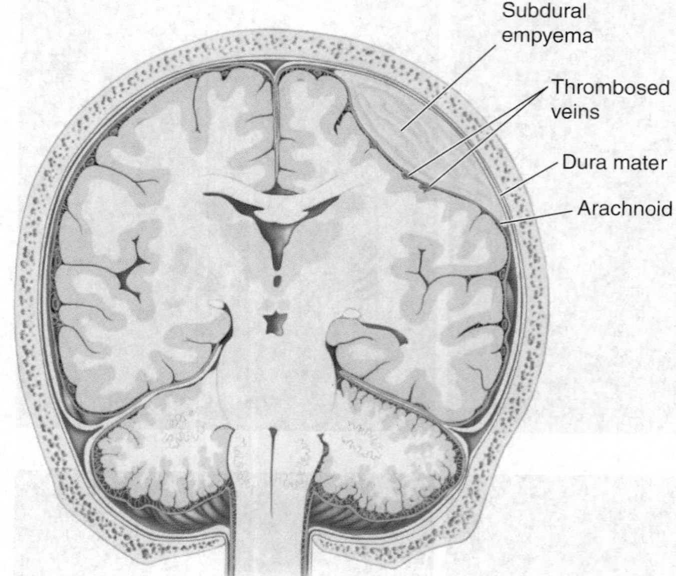

FIGURE 140-3 Subdural empyema.

the increasing mass effect and increase in ICP cause progressive deterioration in consciousness, leading ultimately to coma.

■ DIAGNOSIS

MRI **(Fig. 140-4)** is superior to CT in identifying SDE and any associated intracranial infections. The administration of gadolinium greatly improves diagnosis by enhancing the rim of the empyema and allowing the empyema to be clearly delineated from the underlying brain parenchyma. Cranial MRI is also extremely valuable in identifying sinusitis, other focal CNS infections, cortical venous infarction, cerebral edema, and cerebritis. CT may show a crescent-shaped hypodense lesion over one or both hemispheres or in the interhemispheric fissure. Frequently the degree of mass effect, exemplified by midline shift, ventricular compression, and sulcal effacement, is far out of proportion to the mass of the SDE.

CSF examination should be avoided in patients with known or suspected SDE because it adds no useful information and is associated with the risk of cerebral herniation.

■ DIFFERENTIAL DIAGNOSIS

The differential diagnosis of the combination of headache, fever, focal neurologic signs, and seizure activity that progresses rapidly to an altered level of consciousness includes subdural hematoma, bacterial meningitis, viral encephalitis, brain abscess, superior sagittal sinus thrombosis, and acute disseminated encephalomyelitis. The presence of nuchal rigidity is unusual with brain abscess or epidural empyema and should suggest the possibility of SDE when associated with significant focal neurologic signs and fever. Patients with bacterial meningitis also have nuchal rigidity but do not typically have focal deficits of the severity seen with SDE.

TREATMENT

Subdural Empyema

SDE is a medical emergency. Emergent neurosurgical evacuation of the empyema, either through craniotomy, craniectomy, or burr-hole drainage, is the definitive step in the management of this infection. Empirical antimicrobial therapy for community-acquired SDE should include a combination of a third-generation cephalosporin (e.g., cefotaxime or ceftriaxone), vancomycin, and metronidazole **(see Table 138-1 for dosages)**. Patients with hospital-acquired SDE may have infections due to *Pseudomonas* spp. or MRSA and should receive coverage with a carbapenem (e.g., meropenem) and vancomycin. Metronidazole is not necessary for antianaerobic therapy when meropenem is being used. Parenteral antibiotic therapy should be continued for a minimum of 3–4 weeks after SDE drainage. Patients with associated cranial osteomyelitis may require longer therapy. Specific diagnosis of the etiologic organisms is made based on Gram's stain and culture of fluid obtained via either burr holes or craniotomy; the initial empirical antibiotic coverage can be modified accordingly.

■ PROGNOSIS

Prognosis is influenced by the level of consciousness of the patient at the time of hospital presentation, the size of the empyema, and the speed with which therapy is instituted. Long-term neurologic sequelae, which include seizures and hemiparesis, occur in up to 50% of cases.

CRANIAL EPIDURAL ABSCESS

Cranial epidural abscess is a suppurative infection occurring in the potential space between the inner skull table and dura **(Fig. 140-5)**.

■ ETIOLOGY AND PATHOPHYSIOLOGY

Cranial epidural abscess is less common than either brain abscess or SDE and accounts for <2% of focal suppurative CNS infections. A cranial epidural abscess develops as a complication of a craniotomy

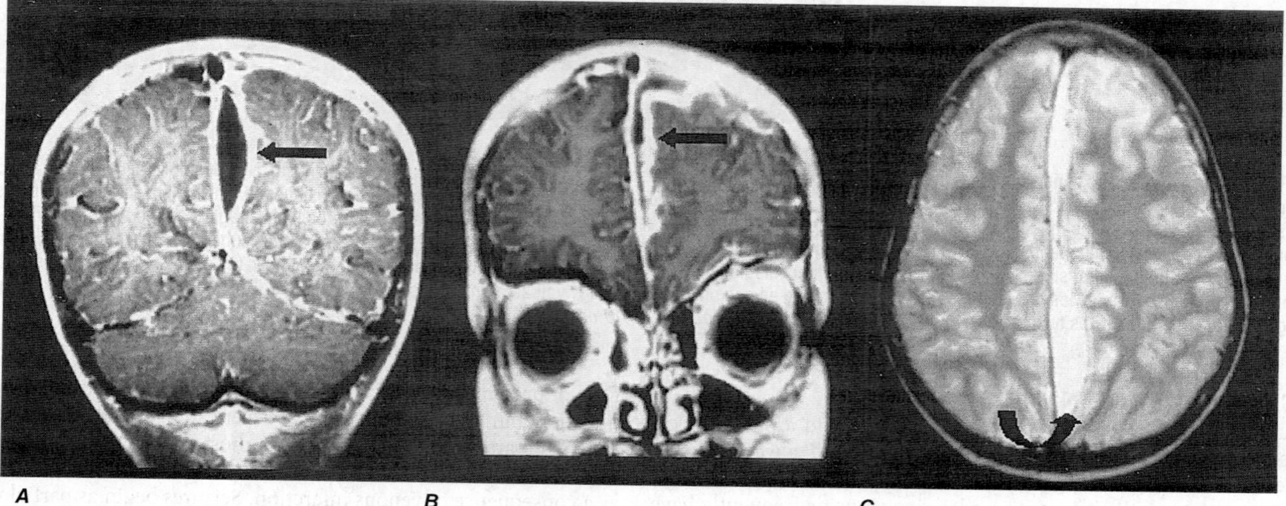

FIGURE 140-4 Subdural empyema. There is marked enhancement of the dura and leptomeninges (***A, B***, *straight arrows*) along the left medial hemisphere. The pus is hypointense on T1-weighted images (***A, B***) but markedly hyperintense on the proton density–weighted (***C***, *curved arrow*) image. *(Courtesy of Joseph Lurito, MD; with permission.)*

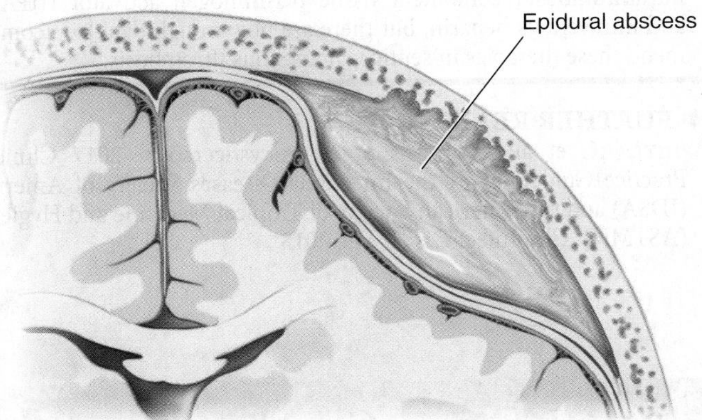

FIGURE 140-5 Cranial epidural abscess is a collection of pus between the dura and the inner table of the skull.

or compound skull fracture or as a result of spread of infection from the frontal sinuses, middle ear, mastoid, or orbit. An epidural abscess may develop contiguous to an area of osteomyelitis, when craniotomy is complicated by infection of the wound or bone flap, or as a result of direct infection of the epidural space. Infection in the frontal sinus, middle ear, mastoid, or orbit can reach the epidural space through retrograde spread of infection from septic thrombophlebitis in the emissary veins that drain these areas or by way of direct spread of infection through areas of osteomyelitis. Unlike the subdural space, the epidural space is really a potential rather than an actual compartment. The dura is normally tightly adherent to the inner skull table, and infection must dissect the dura away from the skull table as it spreads. As a result, epidural abscesses are often smaller than SDEs. Cranial epidural abscesses, unlike brain abscesses, only rarely result from hematogenous spread of infection from extracranial primary sites. The bacteriology of a cranial epidural abscess is similar to that of SDE (see above). The etiologic organisms of an epidural abscess that arises from frontal sinusitis, middle-ear infections, or mastoiditis are usually streptococci or anaerobic organisms. Staphylococci or gram-negative organisms are the usual cause of an epidural abscess that develops as a complication of craniotomy or compound skull fracture.

CLINICAL PRESENTATION

Patients present with fever (60%), headache (40%), nuchal rigidity (35%), seizures (10%), and focal deficits (5%). Development of symptoms may be insidious, as the empyema usually enlarges slowly in the confined anatomic space between the dura and the inner table of the skull. Periorbital edema and Pott's puffy tumor, reflecting underlying associated frontal bone osteomyelitis, are present in ~40%. In patients with a recent neurosurgical procedure, wound infection is invariably present, but other symptoms may be subtle and can include altered mental status (45%), fever (35%), and headache (20%). The diagnosis should be considered when fever and headache follow recent head trauma or occur in the setting of frontal sinusitis, mastoiditis, or otitis media.

DIAGNOSIS

Cranial MRI with gadolinium enhancement is the procedure of choice to demonstrate a cranial epidural abscess. The sensitivity of CT is limited by the presence of signal artifacts arising from the bone of the inner skull table. The CT appearance of an epidural empyema is that of a lens or crescent-shaped hypodense extraaxial lesion. On MRI, an epidural empyema appears as a lentiform or crescent-shaped fluid collection that is hyperintense compared to CSF on T2-weighted images. On T1-weighted images, the fluid collection may be either isointense or hypointense compared to brain. Following the administration of gadolinium, there is linear enhancement of the dura on T1-weighted images. In distinction to subdural empyema, signs of mass effect or other parenchymal abnormalities are uncommon.

TREATMENT
Epidural Abscess

Immediate neurosurgical drainage is indicated. Empirical antimicrobial therapy, pending the results of Gram's stain and culture of the purulent material obtained at surgery, should include a combination of a third-generation cephalosporin, vancomycin, and metronidazole **(see Table 138-1)**. Ceftazidime or meropenem should be substituted for ceftriaxone or cefotaxime in neurosurgical patients. Metronidazole is not necessary for antianaerobic coverage in patients receiving meropenem. When the organism has been identified, antimicrobial therapy can be modified accordingly. Antibiotics should be continued for 3–6 weeks after surgical drainage. Patients with associated osteomyelitis may require additional therapy.

PROGNOSIS

The mortality rate is <5% in modern series, and full recovery is the rule in most survivors.

SUPPURATIVE THROMBOPHLEBITIS

DEFINITION

Suppurative intracranial thrombophlebitis is septic venous thrombosis of cortical veins and sinuses. This may occur as a complication of bacterial meningitis; SDE; epidural abscess; or infection in the skin of the face, paranasal sinuses, middle ear, or mastoid.

ANATOMY AND PATHOPHYSIOLOGY

The cerebral veins and venous sinuses have no valves; therefore, blood within them can flow in either direction. The superior sagittal sinus is the largest of the venous sinuses **(Fig. 140-6)**. It receives blood from the frontal, parietal, and occipital superior cerebral veins and the diploic veins, which communicate with the meningeal veins. Bacterial meningitis is a common predisposing condition for septic thrombosis of the superior sagittal sinus. The diploic veins, which drain into the superior sagittal sinus, provide a route for the spread of infection from the meninges, especially in cases where there is purulent exudate near areas of the superior sagittal sinus. Infection can also spread to the superior sagittal sinus from nearby SDE or epidural abscess. Dehydration from vomiting, hypercoagulable states, and immunologic abnormalities, including the presence of circulating antiphospholipid antibodies, also contribute to cerebral venous sinus thrombosis. Thrombosis may extend from one sinus to another, and at autopsy, thrombi of different histologic ages can often be detected in several sinuses. Thrombosis of the superior sagittal sinus is often associated with thrombosis of superior cortical veins and small parenchymal hemorrhages.

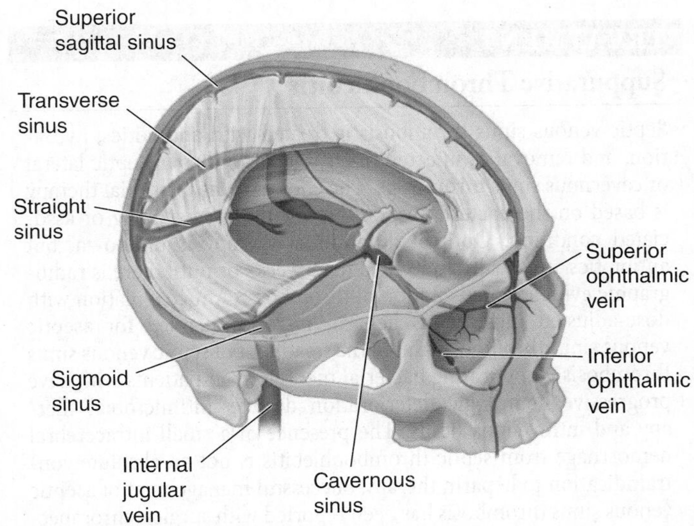

FIGURE 140-6 Anatomy of the cerebral venous sinuses.

The superior sagittal sinus drains into the transverse sinuses (Fig. 140-6). The transverse sinuses also receive venous drainage from small veins from both the middle ear and mastoid cells. The transverse sinus becomes the sigmoid sinus before draining into the internal jugular vein. Septic transverse/sigmoid sinus thrombosis can be a complication of acute and chronic otitis media or mastoiditis. Infection spreads from the mastoid air cells to the transverse sinus via the emissary veins or by direct invasion. The cavernous sinuses are inferior to the superior sagittal sinus at the base of the skull. The cavernous sinuses receive blood from the facial veins via the superior and inferior ophthalmic veins. Bacteria in the facial veins enter the cavernous sinus via these veins. Bacteria in the sphenoid and ethmoid sinuses can spread to the cavernous sinuses via the small emissary veins. The sphenoid and ethmoid sinuses are the most common sites of primary infection resulting in septic cavernous sinus thrombosis.

CLINICAL MANIFESTATIONS

Septic thrombosis of the superior sagittal sinus presents with headache, fever, nausea and vomiting, confusion, and focal or generalized seizures. There may be a rapid development of stupor and coma. Weakness of the lower extremities with bilateral Babinski's signs or hemiparesis is often present. When superior sagittal sinus thrombosis occurs as a complication of bacterial meningitis, nuchal rigidity and Kernig's and Brudzinski's signs may be present.

The oculomotor nerve, the trochlear nerve, the abducens nerve, the ophthalmic and maxillary branches of the trigeminal nerve, and the internal carotid artery all pass through the cavernous sinus (see Fig. 441-7). The symptoms of *septic cavernous sinus thrombosis* are fever, headache, frontal and retroorbital pain, and diplopia. The classic signs are ptosis, proptosis, chemosis, and extraocular dysmotility due to deficits of cranial nerves III, IV, and VI; hyperesthesia of the ophthalmic and maxillary divisions of the fifth cranial nerve and a decreased corneal reflex may be detected. There may be evidence of dilated, tortuous retinal veins and papilledema.

Headache and earache are the most frequent symptoms of *transverse sinus thrombosis*. A transverse sinus thrombosis may also present with otitis media, sixth nerve palsy, and retroorbital or facial pain (*Gradenigo's syndrome*). Sigmoid sinus and internal jugular vein thrombosis may present with neck pain.

DIAGNOSIS

The diagnosis of septic venous sinus thrombosis is suggested by an absent flow void within the affected venous sinus on MRI and confirmed by magnetic resonance venography, CT angiogram, or the venous phase of cerebral angiography. The diagnosis of thrombophlebitis of intracerebral and meningeal veins is suggested by the presence of intracerebral hemorrhage but requires cerebral angiography for definitive diagnosis.

TREATMENT

Suppurative Thrombophlebitis

Septic venous sinus thrombosis is treated with antibiotics, hydration, and removal of infected tissue and thrombus in septic lateral or cavernous sinus thrombosis. The choice of antimicrobial therapy is based on the bacteria responsible for the predisposing or associated condition. Optimal duration of therapy is unknown, but antibiotics are usually continued for 6 weeks or until there is radiographic evidence of resolution of thrombosis. Anticoagulation with dose-adjusted intravenous heparin is recommended for aseptic venous sinus thrombosis and in the treatment of septic venous sinus thrombosis complicating bacterial meningitis in patients who have progressive neurologic deterioration despite antimicrobial therapy and intravenous fluids. The presence of a small intracerebral hemorrhage from septic thrombophlebitis is not an absolute contraindication to heparin therapy. Successful management of aseptic venous sinus thrombosis has been reported with surgical thrombectomy, catheter-directed urokinase therapy, and a combination of intrathrombus recombinant tissue plasminogen activator (rtPA) and intravenous heparin, but there are not enough data to recommend these therapies in septic venous sinus thrombosis.

FURTHER READING

White AC et al: Diagnosis of Neurocysticercosis: 2017 Clinical Practice Guidelines by the Infectious Diseases Society of America (IDSA) and the American Society of Tropical Medicine and Hygiene (ASTMH). Clin Infect Dis 66:e49, 2018.

141 Infectious Complications of Bites

Sandeep S. Jubbal, Florencia Pereyra Segal, Lawrence C. Madoff

The skin is an essential component of nonspecific immunity, protecting the host from potential pathogens in the environment. Breaches in this protective barrier thus represent a form of immunocompromise that predisposes the patient to infection. Bites and scratches from animals and humans allow the inoculation of microorganisms past the skin's protective barrier into deeper, susceptible host tissues.

Each year in the United States, millions of animal-bite wounds are sustained. The vast majority are inflicted by pet dogs and cats, which number >100 million; the annual incidence of dog and cat bites has been reported as 300 bites per 100,000 population. Other bite wounds are a consequence of encounters with animals in the wild or in occupational settings. While many of these wounds require minimal or no therapy, a significant number result in infection, which may be life-threatening. The microbiology of bite-wound infections in general reflects the oropharyngeal flora of the biting animal, although organisms from the soil, the skin of the animal and the victim, and the animal's feces may also be involved.

DOG BITES

In the United States, dogs bite >4.7 million people each year and are responsible for 80% of all animal-bite wounds, an estimated 15–20% of which become infected. Each year, 800,000 Americans seek medical attention for dog bites; of those injured, 386,000 require treatment in an emergency department, with >1000 emergency department visits each day and ~30 deaths per year. Most dog bites are provoked and are inflicted by the victim's pet or by a dog known to the victim. These bites are frequently sustained during efforts to break up a dogfight. Children are more likely than adults to sustain canine bites, with the highest incidence of 6 bites per 1000 population among boys 5–9 years old. Victims are more often male than female, and bites most often involve an upper extremity. Among children <4 years old, two-thirds of all these injuries involve the head or neck. Infection typically manifests 8–24 h after the bite as pain at the site of injury with cellulitis accompanied by purulent, sometimes foul-smelling discharge. Septic arthritis and osteomyelitis may develop if a canine tooth penetrates synovium or bone. Systemic manifestations (e.g., fever, lymphadenopathy, and lymphangitis) also may occur. The microbiology of dog-bite wound infections is usually mixed and includes *Pasteurella* species, β-hemolytic streptococci, *Staphylococcus* species (including methicillin-resistant *Staphylococcus aureus* [MRSA] and *Staphylococcus intermedius*), *Neisseria* species (commonly *Neisseria weaveri*, formerly known as CDC group M-5), *Eikenella corrodens*, and *Capnocytophaga canimorsus*. Many wounds also include anaerobic bacteria such as *Actinomyces*, *Fusobacterium*, *Prevotella*, and *Porphyromonas* species.

While most infections resulting from dog-bite injuries are localized to the area of injury, many of the microorganisms involved are capable of causing systemic infection, including bacteremia, meningitis, brain abscess, endocarditis, and chorioamnionitis. These infections are particularly likely in hosts with edema or compromised lymphatic drainage in the involved extremity (e.g., after a bite on the arm in a woman who has undergone mastectomy) and in patients who are immunocompromised by medication or disease (e.g., glucocorticoid use, systemic lupus erythematosus, acute leukemia, or hepatic cirrhosis). In addition, dog bites and scratches may result in systemic illnesses such as rabies **(Chap. 208)** and tetanus **(Chap. 152)**.

Infection with *C. canimorsus* following dog-bite wounds (or licking of preexisting wounds) may result in fulminant sepsis, disseminated intravascular coagulation, and renal failure, particularly in hosts who have impaired hepatic function, who have undergone splenectomy, or who are immunosuppressed. This thin gram-negative rod is difficult to culture on most solid media but grows in a variety of liquid media. It may require up to 14 days of incubation to grow on blood cultures. The bacteria are occasionally seen within polymorphonuclear leukocytes on Wright-stained smears of peripheral blood from septic patients. Tularemia **(Chap. 170)** also has been reported to follow dog bites.

CAT BITES

Although less common than dog bites, cat bites and scratches result in infection in more than half of all cases. Because the cat's narrow, sharp canine teeth penetrate deeply into tissue, cat bites are more likely than dog bites to cause septic arthritis and osteomyelitis; the development of these conditions is particularly likely when punctures are located over or near a joint, especially in the hand. Women sustain cat bites more frequently than do men. These bites most often involve the hands and arms. Both bites and scratches from cats are prone to infection from organisms in the cat's oropharynx. *Pasteurella multocida*, a normal component of the feline oral flora, is a small gram-negative coccobacillus implicated in the majority of cat-bite wound infections. Like that of dog-bite wound infections, however, the microflora of cat-bite wound infections is usually mixed. However, the median time from bite to the appearance of signs and symptoms of wound infection is much shorter when compared to dog bites. Other microorganisms causing infection after cat bites are similar to those causing dog-bite wound infections.

The same risk factors for systemic infection following dog-bite wounds apply to cat-bite wounds. *Pasteurella* infections tend to advance rapidly, often within hours, causing severe inflammation accompanied by purulent drainage with adenitis; *Pasteurella* may also be spread by respiratory droplets from animals, resulting in pneumonia or bacteremia. Like dog-bite wounds, cat-bite wounds may result in the transmission of rabies or in the development of tetanus. Infection with *Bartonella henselae* causes cat-scratch disease **(Chap. 172)** and is an important late consequence of cat bites and scratches. Tularemia **(Chap. 170)** also has been reported to follow cat bites. Occasionally, sporotrichosis **(Chap. 219)** has been associated with scratches or bites by animals, especially domestic cats.

OTHER ANIMAL BITES

Infections have been attributed to bites from many animal species. Often these bites are sustained as a consequence of occupational exposure (farmers, laboratory workers, veterinarians) or recreational exposure (hunters and trappers, wilderness campers, owners of exotic pets). Generally, the microflora of bite wounds reflects the oral flora of the biting animal. Most members of the cat family, including feral cats, harbor *P. multocida*. Bite wounds from aquatic animals such as alligators or piranhas may contain *Aeromonas hydrophila*. Shark, moray eel, and barracuda bites, like other injuries sustained in saltwater, are often associated with infections with marine *Vibrio* species. Venomous snakebites **(Chap. 460)** result in severe inflammatory responses and tissue necrosis—conditions that render these injuries prone to infection. The snake's oral flora includes many species of aerobes and anaerobes, such as *Pseudomonas aeruginosa, Serratia marcescens, Proteus* species, *Staphylococcus epidermidis, Bacteroides fragilis*, and *Clostridium* species. Bites from nonhuman primates are highly susceptible to infection with pathogens similar to those isolated from human bites (see below). Bites from Old World monkeys (*Macaca*) may also result in the transmission of B virus (*Macacine herpesvirus 1, Herpesvirus simiae, Cercopithecine herpesvirus*), a cause of serious infection of the human central nervous system. *Actinobacillus lignieresii* has often been reported in infected wounds of humans bitten by horses, pigs, and sheep. Bites of seals, walruses, and polar bears may cause a chronic suppurative infection known as *seal finger*, which is probably due to one or more species of *Mycoplasma* colonizing these animals.

Small rodents, including rats, mice, and gerbils, as well as animals that prey on rodents may transmit *Streptobacillus moniliformis* (a microaerophilic, pleomorphic gram-negative rod) or *Spirillum minor* (a spirochete); these organisms cause a clinical illness known as *rat-bite fever*. The vast majority of cases in the United States are streptobacillary, whereas *Spirillum* infection occurs mainly in Asia.

In the United States, the risk of rodent bites is usually greatest among laboratory workers or inhabitants of rodent-infested dwellings (particularly children). Rat-bite fever is distinguished from acute bite-wound infection by its typical manifestation after the initial wound has healed. Streptobacillary disease follows an incubation period of 3–10 days. Fever, chills, myalgias, headache, and severe migratory arthralgias are usually followed by a maculopapular rash, which characteristically involves the palms and soles and may become confluent or purpuric. Complications include endocarditis, myocarditis, meningitis, pneumonia, and abscesses in many organs. *Haverhill fever* is an *S. moniliformis* infection acquired from contaminated milk or drinking water and has similar manifestations. Streptobacillary rat-bite fever was frequently fatal in the preantibiotic era. The differential diagnosis includes Rocky Mountain spotted fever, Lyme disease, leptospirosis, and secondary syphilis. The diagnosis is made by direct observation of the causative organisms in tissue or blood, by culture of the organisms on enriched media, or by serologic testing with specific agglutinins.

Spirillum infection (referred to in Japan as *sodoku*) causes pain and purple swelling at the site of the initial bite, with associated lymphangitis and regional lymphadenopathy, after an incubation period of 1–4 weeks. The systemic illness includes fever, chills, and headache. The original lesion may eventually progress to an eschar. The infection is diagnosed by direct visualization of the spirochetes in blood or tissue or by animal inoculation.

Finally, NO-1 (CDC nonoxidizer group 1) is a bacterium associated with dog- and cat-bite wounds. Infections in which NO-1 has been isolated have tended to manifest locally (i.e., as abscess and cellulitis). These infections have occurred in healthy persons with no underlying illness and in some instances have progressed from localized to systemic illnesses. The phenotypic characteristics of NO-1 are similar to those of asaccharolytic *Acinetobacter* species; i.e., NO-1 is oxidase-, indole-, and urease-negative. To date, all strains identified have been shown to be susceptible to aminoglycosides, β-lactam antibiotics, tetracyclines, quinolones, and sulfonamides.

HUMAN BITES

Human bites may be self-inflicted; may be sustained by medical personnel caring for patients; or may take place during fights, domestic abuse, or sexual activity. Human-bite wounds become infected more frequently (~10–15% of the time) than do bites inflicted by other animals. These infections reflect the diverse oral microflora of humans, which includes multiple species of aerobic and anaerobic bacteria. Common aerobic isolates include viridans streptococci, *S. aureus, E. corrodens* (which is particularly common in clenched-fist injury; see below), and *Haemophilus influenzae*. Anaerobic species, including *Fusobacterium nucleatum* and *Prevotella, Porphyromonas*, and *Peptostreptococcus* species, are isolated from 50% of wound infections due to human bites; many of these isolates produce β-lactamases. The oral flora of hospitalized and debilitated patients often includes Enterobacteriaceae in addition to the usual organisms. Hepatitis B, hepatitis C, herpes simplex virus infection, syphilis, tuberculosis, actinomycosis, and tetanus have been reported to be transmitted by human bites; it is biologically possible to transmit HIV through human bites, although this event is quite unlikely. In general, postexposure prophylaxis should be considered for bites involving severe trauma with extensive tissue damage and the presence of blood in saliva. There is essentially no risk of transmission if the skin is intact.

Human bites are categorized as either *occlusional* injuries, which are inflicted by actual biting, or *clenched-fist* injuries, which are sustained when the fist of one individual strikes the teeth of another, causing traumatic laceration of the hand. For several reasons, clenched-fist injuries, which are sometimes referred to as "fight bite" and which are more common than occlusional injuries, result in particularly serious infections. The deep spaces of the hand, including the bones, joints, and tendons, are frequently inoculated with organisms in the course of such injuries. The clenched position of the fist during injury, followed by extension of the hand, may further promote the introduction of bacteria as contaminated tendons retract beneath the skin's surface. Moreover, medical attention is often sought only after frank infection develops.

APPROACH TO THE PATIENT

Animal or Human Bites

A careful history should be elicited, including the type of biting animal, the type of attack (provoked or unprovoked), and the amount of time elapsed since injury. Local and regional public-health authorities should be contacted to determine whether an individual species could be rabid and/or to locate and observe the biting animal when rabies prophylaxis may be indicated **(Chap. 208)**. Suspicious human-bite wounds should provoke careful questioning regarding domestic or child abuse. Details on antibiotic allergies, immunosuppression, splenectomy, liver disease, mastectomy, and immunization history should be obtained. The wound should be inspected carefully for evidence of infection, including redness, exudate, and foul odor. The type of wound (puncture, laceration, or scratch); the depth of penetration; and the possible involvement of joints, tendons, nerves, and bones should be assessed. It is often useful to include a diagram or photograph of the wound in the medical record. In addition, a general physical examination should be conducted and should include an assessment of vital signs as well as an evaluation for evidence of lymphangitis, lymphadenopathy, dermatologic lesions, and functional limitations. Injuries to the hand warrant consultation with a hand surgeon for the assessment of tendon, nerve, and muscular damage. Radiographs should be obtained when bone may have been penetrated or a tooth fragment may be present. Culture and Gram's staining of all infected wounds are essential; anaerobic cultures should be undertaken if abscesses, devitalized tissue, or foul-smelling exudate is present. A small-tipped swab may be used to culture deep punctures or small lacerations. It is also reasonable to culture samples from apparently uninfected wounds due to bites inflicted by animals other than dogs and cats, since the microorganisms causing disease are less predictable in these cases. The white blood cell count should be determined and the blood cultured if systemic infection is suspected.

TREATMENT

Bite-Wound Infections

WOUND MANAGEMENT

Wound closure is controversial in bite injuries. Many authorities prefer not to attempt primary closure of wounds that are or may become infected, choosing instead to irrigate these wounds copiously, debride devitalized tissue, remove foreign bodies, and approximate the wound edges. Delayed primary closure may be undertaken after the risk of infection is over. Small uninfected wounds may be allowed to close by secondary intention. Puncture wounds due to cat bites should be left unsutured because of the high rate at which they become infected. Facial wounds are usually sutured after thorough cleaning and irrigation because of the importance of a good cosmetic result in this area and because anatomic factors such as an excellent blood supply and the absence of dependent edema lessen the risk of infection. In general, wounds >12 h old (for bites to the arm or leg) or >24 h old (for bites to the face) should not be closed primarily and may require prophylactic antibiotics (see below).

ANTIBIOTIC THERAPY

Established Infection Antibiotics should be administered for all established bite-wound infections and should be chosen in light of the most likely potential pathogens, as indicated by the biting species and by Gram's stain and culture results **(Table 141-1)**. For dog and cat bites, antibiotics should be effective against *S. aureus, Pasteurella* species, *C. canimorsus*, streptococci, and oral anaerobes. For human bites, agents with activity against *S. aureus, H. influenzae*, and β-lactamase-positive oral anaerobes should be used. The combination of an extended-spectrum penicillin with a β-lactamase inhibitor (amoxicillin/clavulanic acid, ticarcillin/clavulanic acid, ampicillin/sulbactam) appears to offer the most reliable coverage for these pathogens. Second- and third-generation cephalosporins (ceftriaxone, cefuroxime, cefoxitin, cefpodoxime) also offer substantial coverage when given in conjunction with a drug that provides anaerobic coverage (clindamycin or metronidazole). The choice of antibiotics for penicillin-allergic patients (particularly those in whom immediate-type hypersensitivity makes the use of cephalosporins hazardous) is more difficult and is based primarily on in vitro sensitivity since data on clinical efficacy are inadequate. The combination of an antibiotic active against gram-positive cocci and anaerobes (such as clindamycin) with trimethoprim-sulfamethoxazole or a fluoroquinolone, which is active against many of the other potential pathogens, would appear reasonable. Moxifloxacin, a fluoroquinolone with anaerobic coverage, can also be considered as a single agent. In vitro data suggest that azithromycin alone provides coverage against most commonly isolated bite-wound pathogens; however, this agent has variable activity against *P. multocida, E. corrodens,* and fusobacteria and thus should be avoided unless no alternative agent is available. As MRSA becomes more common in the community and evidence of its transmission between humans and their animal contacts increases, empirical use of agents active against MRSA should be considered in high-risk situations while culture results are awaited.

Antibiotics are generally given for 10–14 days, but the response to therapy must be carefully monitored. Failure to respond should prompt a consideration of diagnostic alternatives and surgical evaluation for possible drainage or debridement. Complications such as osteomyelitis or septic arthritis mandate a longer duration of therapy.

Management of *C. canimorsus* sepsis requires a 2-week course of IV penicillin G (2 million units IV every 4 h) or IV ampicillin/sulbactam (1.5–3.0 g every 6 h) along with supportive measures. Alternative agents for the treatment of *C. canimorsus* infection include cephalosporins, carbapenems, and clindamycin. Serious infection with *P. multocida* (e.g., pneumonia, sepsis, or meningitis) also should be treated with IV penicillin G. Alternative agents include a second- or third-generation cephalosporin or ciprofloxacin. Penicillin resistance is uncommon.

Bites by venomous snakes **(Chap. 460)** may not require antibiotic treatment. Because it is often difficult to distinguish signs of infection from tissue damage caused by the envenomation, many authorities continue to recommend treatment directed against the snake's oral flora—i.e., the administration of broadly active agents such as ceftriaxone (1–2 g IV every 12–24 h) or ampicillin/sulbactam (1.5–3.0 g IV every 6 h).

Seal finger appears to respond to doxycycline (100 mg twice daily for a duration guided by the response to therapy).

Presumptive or Prophylactic Therapy The use of antibiotics for patients presenting early (within 8 h) after bite injury is controversial. Although symptomatic infection frequently will not yet have manifested at this point, many early wounds will harbor pathogens, and many will become infected. Studies of antibiotic prophylaxis for wound infections are limited and have often included only

TABLE 141-1 Management of Wound Infections Following Animal and Human Bites

BITING SPECIES	COMMONLY ISOLATED PATHOGENS	PREFERRED ANTIBIOTIC(S)[a]	ALTERNATIVE IN PENICILLIN-ALLERGIC PATIENT	PROPHYLAXIS ADVISED FOR EARLY UNINFECTED WOUNDS	OTHER CONSIDERATIONS
Dog	*Staphylococcus aureus, Pasteurella multocida*, anaerobes, *Capnocytophaga canimorsus*	Amoxicillin/clavulanate (250–500 mg PO tid) or ampicillin/sulbactam (1.5–3.0 g IV q6h)	Clindamycin (150–300 mg PO qid) plus either TMP-SMX (1 DS tablet PO bid) or ciprofloxacin (500 mg PO bid)	Sometimes[b]	Consider rabies prophylaxis.
Cat	*P. multocida, S. aureus*, anaerobes	Amoxicillin/clavulanate or ampicillin/sulbactam as above	Clindamycin plus TMP-SMX as above or a fluoroquinolone	Usually	Consider rabies prophylaxis. Carefully evaluate for joint/bone penetration.
Human, occlusional	Viridans streptococci, *S. aureus, Haemophilus influenzae*, anaerobes	Amoxicillin/clavulanate or ampicillin/sulbactam as above	Erythromycin (500 mg PO qid) or a fluoroquinolone	Always	
Human, clenched-fist	As for occlusional, plus *Eikenella corrodens*	Ampicillin/sulbactam as above or imipenem (500 mg q6h)	Cefoxitin[c]	Always	Examine for tendon, nerve, or joint involvement.
Monkey	As for human bite	As for human bite	As for human bite	Always	For macaque monkeys, consider B virus prophylaxis with acyclovir.
Snake	*Pseudomonas aeruginosa, Proteus* spp., *Bacteroides fragilis, Clostridium* spp.	Piperacillin/tazobactam 3.375 g IV q6–8h	Clindamycin plus a fluoroquinolone	Sometimes, especially with venomous snakes	Administer antivenin for venomous snakebite.
Rodent	*Streptobacillus moniliformis, Leptospira* spp., *P. multocida*	Penicillin VK (500 mg PO qid)	Doxycycline (100 mg PO bid)	Sometimes	
Aquatic animal (alligator, piranha, shark, moray eel, barracuda)	*Aeromonas hydrophila*, marine *Vibrio* spp. (*Vibrio vulnificus*)	Third-generation cephalosporin (e.g., ceftriaxone, 1 g IV q24h) plus doxycycline (100 mg PO bid)	Clindamycin plus levofloxacin (750 mg PO qd) plus doxycycline	Always	Obtain prompt surgical consultation, as risk for necrotizing infection is high with *Aeromonas* and *Vibrio* spp.

[a]Antibiotic choices should be based on culture data when available. These suggestions for empirical therapy need to be tailored to individual circumstances and local conditions. IV regimens should be used for hospitalized patients. A single IV dose of antibiotics may be given to patients who will be discharged after initial management. [b]Prophylactic antibiotics are suggested for severe or extensive wounds, facial wounds, and crush injuries; when bone or joint may be involved; and when comorbidity is present (see text). [c]May be hazardous in patients with immediate-type hypersensitivity to penicillin.

Abbreviations: DS, double-strength; TMP-SMX, trimethoprim-sulfamethoxazole.

small numbers of cases in which various types of wounds have been managed according to various protocols. A meta-analysis of eight randomized trials of prophylactic antibiotics in patients with dog-bite wounds demonstrated a reduction in the rate of infection by 50% with prophylaxis. However, in the absence of sound clinical trials, many clinicians base the decision to treat bite wounds with empirical antibiotics on the species of the biting animal; the location, severity, and extent of the bite wound; and the existence of comorbid conditions in the host. All human- and monkey-bite wounds should be treated presumptively because of the high rate of infection. Most cat-bite wounds, particularly those involving the hand, should be treated. Other factors favoring treatment for bite wounds include severe injury, as in crush wounds; potential bone or joint involvement; involvement of the hands or genital region; host immunocompromise, including that due to diabetes mellitus, liver disease, or splenectomy; involvement of extremities with underlying venous and/or lymphatic compromise; and prior mastectomy on the side of an involved upper extremity. When prophylactic antibiotics are administered, they are usually given for 3–5 days.

Rabies and Tetanus Prophylaxis Rabies prophylaxis, consisting of both passive administration of rabies immune globulin (with as much of the dose as possible infiltrated into and around the wound) and active immunization with rabies vaccine, should be given in consultation with local and regional public-health authorities for some animal bites and scratches as well as for certain nonbite exposures **(Chap. 208)**. Rabies is endemic in a variety of animals, including dogs and cats, in many areas of the world. In the United States, although the majority (90%) of rabid animals reported each year are wild (including raccoons, skunks, foxes, and bats), most people receive rabies prophylaxis because of close contact with domestic animals. Furthermore, more cats than dogs are reported rabid each year. Many local health authorities require the reporting of all animal bites.

A tetanus booster immunization should be given if the patient has undergone primary immunization but has not received a booster dose in the past 5 years. Patients who have not previously completed primary immunization should be immunized and should also receive tetanus immune globulin. Elevation of the site of injury is an important adjunct to antimicrobial therapy. Immobilization of the infected area, especially the hand, also is beneficial.

Hepatitis B Prophylaxis Hepatitis B virus can be transmitted, albeit rarely, by exposure of nonintact skin to blood-free saliva. The mainstay of postexposure prophylaxis is active immunization with hepatitis B vaccine, but, in certain circumstances, hepatitis B immune globulin is recommended in addition to vaccine for added protection **(Chap. 339)**.

FURTHER READING

Abrahamian FM, Goldstein EJC: Microbiology of animal bite wound infections. Clin Microbiol Rev 24:231, 2011.

Brook I: Management of human and animal bite wounds: An overview. Adv Skin Wound Care 18:197, 2005.

Bystritsky R, Chambers H: Cellulitis and soft tissue infections. Ann Intern Med 168:ITC17, 2018.

Ellis R, Ellis C: Dog and cat bites. Am Fam Phys 90:239, 2014.

FALLOUJI MA: Traumatic love bites. Br J Surg 77:100, 1990.

FLEISHER GR: The management of bite wounds. N Engl J Med 340:138, 1999.

KAISER RM et al: Clinical significance and epidemiology of NO-1, an unusual bacterium associated with dog and cat bites. Emerg Infect Dis 8:171, 2002.

KULLBERG BJ et al: Purpura fulminans and symmetrical peripheral gangrene caused by *Capnocytophaga canimorsus* (formerly DF-2) septicemia—a complication of dog bite. Medicine (Baltimore) 70:287, 1991.

LOHIYA GS et al: Human bites: Bloodborne pathogen risk and postexposure follow-up algorithm. J Natl Med Assoc 105:92, 2013.

MARTINO R et al: Bacteremia caused by *Capnocytophaga* species in patients with neutropenia and cancer: Results of a multicenter study. Clin Infect Dis 33:e20, 2001.

MORGAN M, PALMER J: Dog bites. BMJ 334:413, 2007.

OEHLER RL et al: Bite-related and septic syndromes caused by cats and dogs. Lancet Infect Dis 9:439, 2009.

STEVENS DL et al: Practice guidelines for the diagnosis and management of skin and soft tissue infections. 2014 update by the Infectious Diseases Society of America. Clin Infect Dis 59:e10, 2014.

WEBER DJ et al: Infections resulting from animal bites. Infect Dis Clin North Am 5:663, 1991.

Section 3 Clinical Syndromes: Health Care–Associated Infections

142 Infections Acquired in Health Care Facilities

Robert A. Weinstein

Health care–associated infections affect at least 2 million patients at a cost of billions of dollars and 100,000 or more lives in U.S. hospitals annually. Guidelines from the Centers for Disease Control and Prevention (CDC) (*www.cdc.gov/hicpac/*), the Agency for Healthcare Research and Quality (*www.ahrq.gov*), and professional societies (e.g., *www.shea-online.org*; *www.idsociety.org*; *www.apic.org*; *www.his.org.uk*) have led to marked reductions in occurrence of most device-related infections (*https://www.cdc.gov/hai/data/portal/progress-report.html*)—historically, the largest drivers of nosocomial infection risk. Despite these successes, there is the seemingly unending threat of antimicrobial-resistant infections and novel pathogens. This chapter reviews the epidemiology, prevention, and control of health care–associated infections and newer challenges.

ORGANIZATION, RESPONSIBILITIES, AND SCRUTINY OF HEALTH CARE–ASSOCIATED INFECTION PROGRAMS

Over the past several decades, hospitals have refined programs for surveillance, prevention, and control of health care–associated infections. The successful deployment of these activities has been driven by accrediting agencies, primarily The Joint Commission (*www.jointcommission.org*); by payers and regulators, primarily the U.S. Centers for Medicare and Medicaid Services (CMS) (*www.cms.hhs.gov*); by quality assurance groups that grade hospitals and health care performance (e.g., *www.leapfroggroup.org*; *www.ihi.org*); and by federal agencies such as the CDC that provide landmark guidelines and recommendations. Although neither the carrot (pay-for-performance) nor the stick (nonpayment for preventable infections) appears to have had a major impact on infection rates in U.S. hospitals, the specter of public attention to infection rates has been more powerful.

SURVEILLANCE

Traditionally, infection preventionists surveyed inpatients for infections acquired in hospitals (some of which only appear after hospital discharge, i.e., community-onset, health care–associated infections). Many infection-control programs leverage electronic surveillance (e.g., for vascular catheter, surgical wound, or even clustered infections inferred from clinical microbiology data) to complement "shoe-leather" epidemiology on nursing wards. Such approaches show the increasing value of newer computer techniques, such as machine learning and artificial intelligence, and can facilitate "house-wide" surveillance, remove observer bias, and free personnel time for health care worker education and adherence monitoring. Infection control programs and surveillance activities in many nursing homes and some long-term acute-care hospitals (LTACHs) are still in formative stages, highlighting a key opportunity for intervention by regulators, advisory agencies, and payers, given the role of long-term care facilities in the transmission of antimicrobial-resistant pathogens (**Fig. 142-1**).

In the spirit of "what is measured improves," most states require public reporting of health care–associated infection. Thirty-six states require health care facilities in their jurisdictions to report to CDC's National Healthcare Safety Network (NHSN) (*https://www.cdc.gov/nhsn/index.html*) reporting system, which provides uniform definitions and facilitates transmission of data. Beginning in 2011, CMS required hospitals to report health care–associated infection data to NHSN to qualify for their full annual payment update. In subsequent years, CMS included health care–associated infection reporting requirements to NHSN as part of the Hospital Value Based Purchasing Program and Hospital Acquired Conditions Reduction Program. Increasing reliance on NHSN led to participation by >24,000 facilities (~5500 of the ~5700 acute-care hospitals in the United States, ~620 LTACHs, ~432 inpatient rehabilitation facilities, ~8150 outpatient dialysis facilities, ~5600 ambulatory surgery centers, and ~3800 skilled nursing facilities). This level of participation provides a nationwide view of health care–associated infections and antimicrobial resistance and potential access to national rates of antimicrobial use.

Results of surveillance are expressed as rates, qualified when possible by duration of risk, site of infection, patient population, and exposure to risk factors. To account for some of these variables, the CDC now uses a standardized infection ratio (SIR; *https://www.cdc.gov/nhsn/pdfs/ps-analysis-resources/nhsn-sir-guide.pdf*) as part of NHSN rate reporting. Denominators often include the number of patients exposed to a specific risk or the number of intervention days (e.g., 1000 patient-days on a ventilator). As use of invasive devices such as indwelling bladder catheters has purposely been decreased, the denominators have become smaller, but patients who still require such devices (potential numerators) often are at intrinsically higher risk—a situation that may paradoxically increase rates when device-days account for the denominator.

Temporal trends in rates should be reviewed, and rates should be compared with regional and national benchmarks that incorporate the SIR. Interhospital comparisons still may be misleading because of the wide range in risk factors and severity of underlying illnesses. Process measures usually do not require risk adjustment but some, such as adherence to hand hygiene, can be difficult to measure, leading to development of a number of innovative electronic monitoring systems that track hand-hygiene adherence. Although this approach is exciting, sustained improvements in rates remain to be seen. Major morbidity and costly outcomes (e.g., cardiac surgery wound infection rates) can identify outlier hospitals (e.g., in the highest deciles of risk) for further evaluation. Most importantly, temporal analysis of a hospital's infection rates—comparison to self over time—can help to determine if control measures are succeeding and where increased efforts should be focused.

EPIDEMIOLOGIC BASIS AND GENERAL MEASURES FOR PREVENTION AND CONTROL

Nosocomial infections follow basic epidemiologic patterns that direct prevention and control measures. Nosocomial pathogens have reservoirs, are transmitted by largely predictable routes, and require

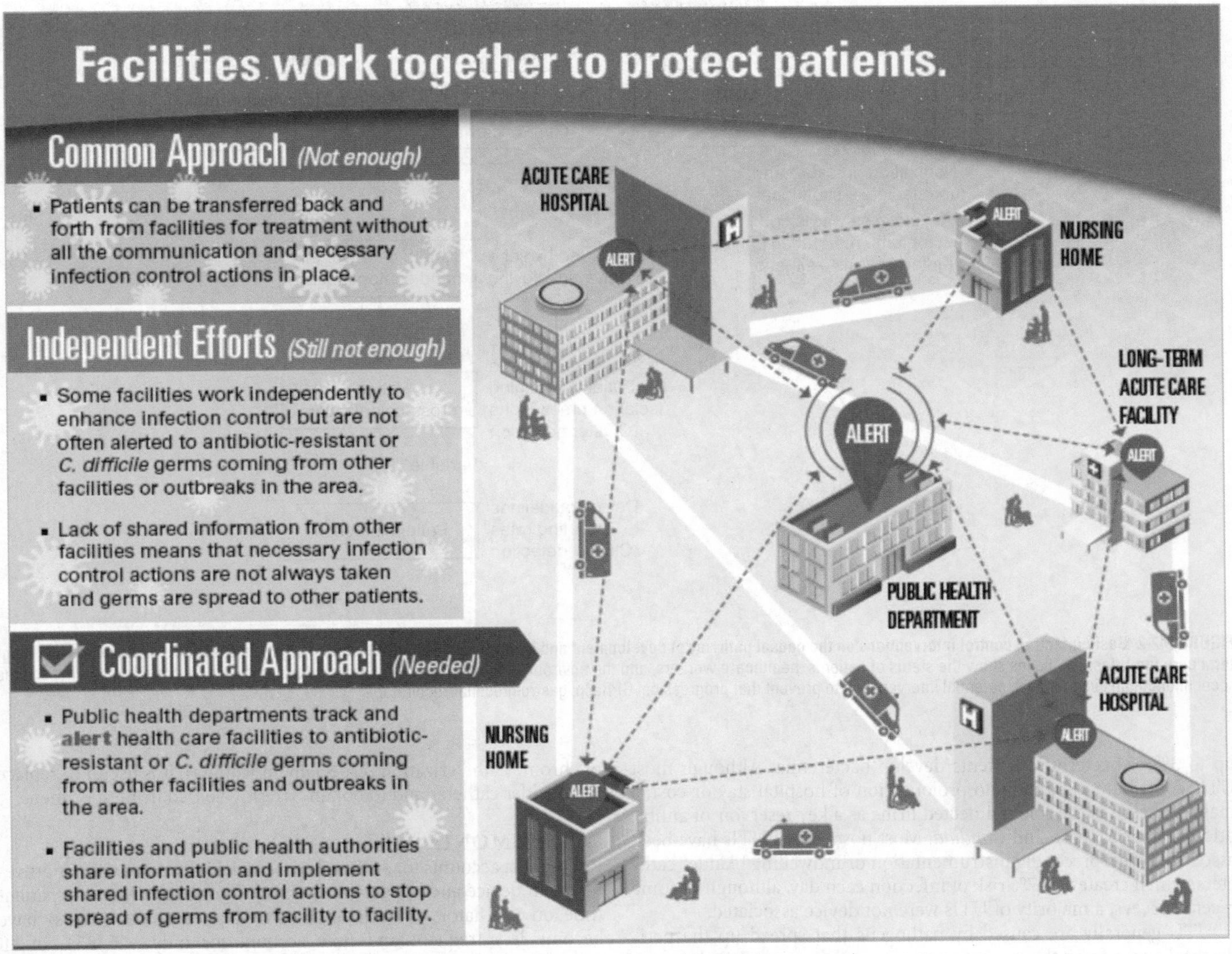

FIGURE 142-1 Regional spread and control of antimicrobial-resistance. *(From www.cdc.gov/vitalsigns/stop-spread.)*

susceptible hosts. Reservoirs and sources exist in the inanimate environment (e.g., antibiotic-resistant bacteria or *Clostridioides difficile* spores on frequently touched surfaces) and in the animate environment (e.g., infected or colonized patients and hospital visitors). The mode of transmission usually is either cross-infection (e.g., indirect spread from one patient to another on the inadequately cleaned hands of hospital personnel) or autoinoculation (e.g., aspiration of oropharyngeal flora); patient hand colonization with problem microbes also may contribute to self, environmental, and health care worker contamination. Occasionally, pathogens (e.g., group A streptococci and many respiratory viruses) are spread from person to person via large infectious droplets released by coughing or sneezing. Much less common—but often devastating in terms of epidemic risk—is true airborne spread of small or droplet nuclei (as in nosocomial chickenpox or measles) or common-source spread (e.g., by contaminated IV fluids). Factors that increase patient susceptibility include diabetes, renal insufficiency, and other comorbidities; extremes of age; abnormalities of innate defense (e.g., due to genetic polymorphisms; see **Chap. 466**); medical–surgical interventions that compromise host defenses; and epidemiologic issues, such as "colonization pressure" created by neighboring patients.

Hospital infection-control programs determine general and specific control measures based on the "causal pathway" of spread (**Fig. 142-2**). Given the prominence of cross-infection, hand hygiene is cited as the most important preventive measure. Health care worker adherence to hand hygiene is historically low. Reasons cited include inconvenience, time pressures, and skin damage from frequent washing. Sinkless alcohol rubs are quick and highly effective, and their emollients may improve hand condition. Use of alcohol hand rubs between patient contacts is recommended for all health care workers except when hands are visibly soiled or after care of a patient who is part of an outbreak of infection with *C. difficile*, whose spores resist killing by alcohol. In these cases, washing with soap and running water is recommended.

Adequate staffing is essential in acute and long-term settings to allow for attention to hand hygiene and asepsis during patient care and to provide thorough environmental cleaning.

NOSOCOMIAL AND DEVICE-RELATED INFECTIONS

The five major nosocomial infection sites are urinary, lower respiratory, surgical wound, bloodstream, and gastrointestinal (mostly *C. difficile*). The percentage of infections due to invasive devices—25–50%—has fallen in recent years, reflecting marked improvements in the use and design of devices. Intensive education, bundling of evidence-based interventions (**Table 142-1**), and use of checklists to facilitate adherence have reduced infection rates, largely through improved asepsis in handling and earlier removal of invasive devices. This progress demonstrates both the effectiveness of infection-control programs and the need to focus surveillance and interventions on control of the other 50–75% of health care–associated infections.

URINARY TRACT INFECTIONS

Urinary tract infections (UTIs) due to indwelling bladder catheters affect ~160,000 patients annually, which represents a deceased risk over the past several years, and account for ~10% of nosocomial infections;

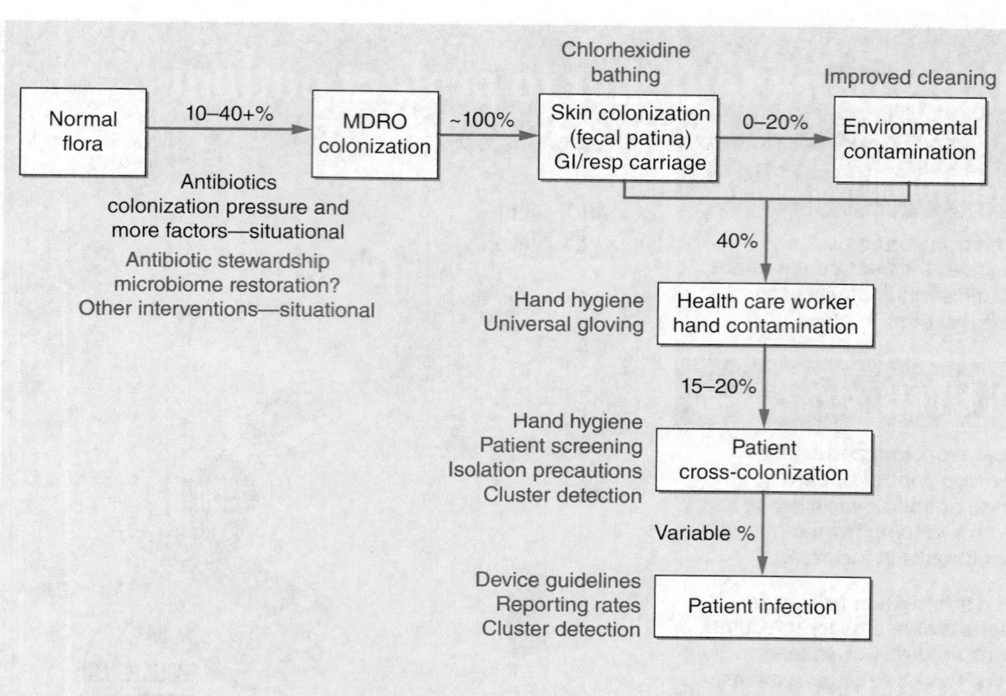

FIGURE 142-2 Basic infection control interventions on the causal pathway of development and spread of multidrug-resistance organisms (MDROs) in hospitals and long-term care facilities. The boxes show the status of patients, healthcare workers, and the environment; the %s are the likelihood of progressing along the pathway; and the recommendations in green are potential interventions to prevent that progression. GI/Resp, gastrointestinal/respiratory.

up to 3% of bacteriuric patients develop bacteremia. Although most UTIs contribute marginally to prolongation of hospital stay or cost, a major concern is the role of infected urine as a key reservoir of antibiotic-resistant bacteria and *Candida*. Most nosocomial UTIs have been associated with preceding instrumentation or indwelling bladder catheters, which create a 3–7% risk of infection each day, although in some recent surveys, a majority of UTIs were not device associated.

UTIs generally are caused by pathogens that spread up the periurethral space from the patient's perineum or gastrointestinal tract—the most common pathogenesis in women—or via intraluminal contamination of urinary catheters, usually due to cross-infection by caregivers who are emptying drainage bags. Pathogens come occasionally from inadequately disinfected equipment and rarely from contaminated supplies. The frequency with which asymptomatic UTIs occur, especially in older women, may inflate infection rates due to erroneous assumptions that the urinary tract is the source of infection in a febrile hospitalized patient.

With organized control programs to monitor key performance measures (Table 142-1), hospitals can reduce rates of catheter use and UTI. In addition, in a multicenter trial, daily chlorhexidine bathing lessened UTI risk in catheterized men. A condom catheter for men without bladder obstruction may be more acceptable than an indwelling catheter and may lessen the risk of UTI if maintained carefully. A new prevention strategy for women is use of flexible external catheters that are positioned between the labia and buttocks to wick away urine via low-pressure suction. Older strategies have included the use of topical meatal antimicrobial agents, drainage bag disinfectants, and anti-infective catheters, none of which is considered routine. The role of suprapubic catheters in preventing infection is not well defined.

Treatment of UTIs is based on the results of quantitative urine cultures **(Chap. 135)**. The most common pathogens are *Escherichia coli*, nosocomial gram-negative bacilli, enterococci, and *Candida*. Recovery of *Staphylococcus aureus* from urine cultures may result from hematogenous seeding and indicate an occult systemic infection. In patients with chronic indwelling bladder catheters, especially those in long-term-care facilities, the catheter microbiome—microorganisms living on encrustations within the catheter lumen—may differ from actual urinary tract pathogens. Thus, for suspected UTI in the setting of chronic catheterization (especially in women), it is useful to replace the bladder catheter and to obtain a freshly voided urine specimen.

PNEUMONIA

Pneumonia accounts for ~28% of nosocomial infections; with improvements in device and patient care—most importantly, lessening patient time on ventilators—ventilator-associated pneumonias (VAPs) have become less frequent and now account for only ~25–35% of all nosocomial lower respiratory tract infections. Most cases of bacterial nosocomial pneumonia are caused by aspiration of endogenous or hospital-acquired oropharyngeal or gastric flora. Nosocomial pneumonias have been associated with more deaths than have infections at any other body site. However, attributable mortality rates suggest that the risk of dying from nosocomial pneumonia is affected greatly by other factors, including comorbidities, inadequate antibiotic treatment, and the involvement of specific pathogens (particularly *Pseudomonas aeruginosa* or *Acinetobacter*). Surveillance and accurate diagnosis of pneumonia have been problematic in hospitals because many patients, especially those in the intensive care unit (ICU), have abnormal chest roentgenographs, fever, and leukocytosis potentially attributable to multiple causes. This diagnostic uncertainty has led to a refocus from VAP to ventilator-associated events (VAEs), conditions, and complications, for which worsening physiologic parameters, such as oxygenation, are key metrics. VAEs occur in as many as 5–10% of patients using mechanical ventilators.

There is increasing interest in health care–associated pneumonia in patients who are on general wards or not receiving mechanical ventilation. Viral pneumonias, which are particularly important in pediatric and immunocompromised patients, are discussed in the virology section and in **Chap. 126**.

Risk factors for nosocomial pneumonia include those events that increase colonization by potential pathogens (e.g., prior antimicrobial therapy, contaminated ventilator equipment, or decreased gastric acidity, which also may increase risk of colonization by antibiotic-resistant bacteria); those that facilitate aspiration of oropharyngeal contents into the lower respiratory tract (e.g., intubation, decreased levels of consciousness, or presence of a nasogastric tube); and those that reduce pulmonary defense mechanisms and permit overgrowth of aspirated

TABLE 142-1 Examples of Selected Components of Evidence-Based Bundled Interventions to Prevent Common Health Care–Associated Infections and Other Adverse Events[a]

Prevention of Central Venous Catheter Infections

Catheter insertion bundle

- Educate personnel about catheter insertion and care.
- Use chlorhexidine to prepare the insertion site.
- Use maximal barrier precautions and asepsis during catheter insertion.
- Consolidate insertion supplies (e.g., in an insertion kit or cart).
- Use a checklist to enhance adherence to the insertion bundle.
- Empower nurses to halt insertion if asepsis is breached.

Catheter maintenance bundle

- Cleanse patients daily with chlorhexidine.
- Maintain clean, dry dressings.
- Enforce hand hygiene among health care workers.
- Use aseptic technique when accessing transducers or vascular ports.

Ask daily: Is the catheter needed? Remove catheter if not needed or used.

Prevention of Ventilator-Associated Events

- Avoid mechanical ventilation whenever possible.
- Elevate head of bed to 30–45° to lessen aspiration risk.
- Decontaminate oropharynx regularly with chlorhexidine (controversial).
- Use aseptic care of all respiratory equipment.
- Consider using endotracheal tubes with channels for subglottic drainage of secretions.
- Give "sedation vacation" and assess readiness to extubate daily, which can shorten duration of intubation and of intensive care unit stays.
- Use deep-vein thrombosis prophylaxis (unless contraindicated).

Prevention of Surgical-Site Infections

- Choose a surgeon wisely.
- Treat *active* infections preoperatively.
- Administer prophylactic antibiotics within 1 h before surgery; discontinue within 24 h.
- Limit any hair removal to the time of surgery; use clippers or do not remove hair at all.
- Prepare surgical site with chlorhexidine-alcohol.
- Enforce operating room asepsis, e.g., minimize movement in-and-out of the room.
- Assess attention to technical surgical issues (e.g., avoiding open or prophylactic wound drains).
- Provide surveillance results to surgeons.

Prevention of Urinary Tract Infections

- Place bladder catheters only when absolutely needed (e.g., to relieve obstruction), not solely for the provider's convenience.
- Use aseptic equipment and technique for catheter insertion and urinary tract instrumentation.
- Minimize manipulation or opening of drainage systems; avoid catheter irrigation.
- Ask daily: Is the bladder catheter needed? Remove catheter if not needed.
- Use bladder scanners to avoid catheterization, e.g., for assessing urinary retention.

Prevention of Pathogen Cross-Transmission

- Cleanse hands with alcohol hand rub before and after all contacts with patients or their environments.

[a]See text for additional interventions to prevent device- and procedure-associated infections; checklists and personnel education have been recommended as management tools for each of the prevention bundles.

Source: Adapted from information presented at the following websites: *www.cdc.gov/hicpac/pubs.html; www.cdc.gov/HAI/index.html; www.ihi.org.*

pathogens (e.g., chronic obstructive pulmonary disease or upper abdominal surgery).

Several control measures can lessen risk for pneumonia (Table 142-1). Although the benefits of selective decontamination of the oropharynx and gut with nonabsorbable antimicrobial agents—a practice usually avoided in the United States because of concerns about antibiotic resistance—have been controversial, a randomized multicenter Dutch trial demonstrated lowered ICU mortality rates among patients on mechanical ventilation who underwent oropharyngeal decontamination. Nevertheless, reducing VAP rates often has not lessened overall ICU mortality, suggesting inadequacies of surveillance and that VAP often may be a marker for patients with an otherwise-heightened risk of death.

The most likely pathogens for nosocomial pneumonia and treatment options are discussed in **Chap. 126**. Of note, early-onset nosocomial pneumonia, which manifests within the first 4 days of hospitalization, is often caused by community-acquired pathogens such as *Streptococcus pneumoniae* and *Haemophilus* species, although some studies have challenged this view. Late-onset pneumonias commonly are due to *S. aureus*, *P. aeruginosa*, *Enterobacter* species, *Klebsiella pneumoniae*, or *Acinetobacter*. Shorter durations of treatment for nosocomial pneumonia can lessen emergence of resistant pathogens, and a negative nasal swab for methicillin-resistant *S. aureus* precludes the need to treat for this pathogen. In febrile patients (particularly those who have tubes inserted through the nares), occult bacterial sinusitis and otitis media should be considered.

SURGICAL-SITE (WOUND) INFECTIONS

Wound infections account for ~17% of nosocomial infections. The average wound infection has an incubation period of 5–7 days—longer than many postoperative stays. For this reason and because many procedures are now performed on an outpatient basis, the incidence of wound infections has become difficult to assess. These infections usually are caused by the patient's endogenous or hospital-acquired skin and mucosal flora and occasionally are due to airborne spread of skin squames that may be shed into the wound from members of the operating-room team or environmental sources. True airborne spread of infection is rare in operating rooms unless there is a disseminator (e.g., of group A streptococci or staphylococci) among the staff or air supply contamination (e.g., with mold). In general, the common risks for postoperative wound infection are related to the surgeon's technical skill, the patient's underlying conditions (e.g., diabetes mellitus, obesity) or advanced age, and inappropriate timing of antibiotic prophylaxis. Additional risks include the presence of drains, prolonged preoperative hospital stays, shaving of operative sites by razor the day before surgery, and prolonged duration of surgery.

The substantial global morbidity and costs associated with these infections have led to international guidelines (*http://www.who.int/gpsc/ssi-guidelines/en/*) in addition to existing national prevention programs and recommendations for bundling of preventive measures (Table 142-1). Preoperative administration of intranasal mupirocin to patients colonized with *S. aureus*, preoperative antiseptic bathing, intra- and postoperative oxygen supplementation, and attention to patients' blood glucose levels and body temperature have been controversial because of conflicting study results, but evidence seems mostly to favor these interventions. Recently debated issues include appropriate garb in operating rooms—less may be more—and the value of negative-pressure wound dressings.

The most common pathogens in postoperative wound infections are *S. aureus*, coagulase-negative staphylococci, and enteric and anaerobic bacteria. In rapidly progressing postoperative infections manifesting within 24–48 h of a surgical procedure, the level of suspicion regarding group A streptococcal or clostridial infection (**Chaps. 148 and 154**) should be high. Diagnosis of infections of prosthetic devices, such as orthopedic implants, may be complicated when pathogens are cloistered in prosthesis-adherent biofilms; cultures of sonicates from explanted prosthetic joints have been more sensitive. Treatment of postoperative wound infections requires adequate source control, i.e., drainage or surgical excision of infected or necrotic material, and antibiotic therapy aimed at the most likely or laboratory-confirmed pathogens.

INFECTIONS RELATED TO VASCULAR ACCESS AND MONITORING

Intravascular device–related bacteremias cause ~10–15% of nosocomial infections; central vascular catheters (CVCs) account for most of these bloodstream infections, although peripheral catheters are underappreciated as a source of nosocomial bacteremia. National estimates have indicated that ~72,000 primary bloodstream infections occur in the United States each year. CVC infections have had estimated attributable mortality rates of 12–25%, an excess length of hospital stay of 7–15 days, and an estimated cost of $31,000–65,000 per episode; one-third to one-half of these episodes occurred in ICUs. However, infection rates have dropped steadily since the publication of guidelines by the Healthcare Infection Control Practices Advisory Committee (HICPAC) (*www.cdc.gov/hicpac/*). With increasing care of seriously ill patients in the community, vascular catheter–associated bloodstream infections acquired in outpatient settings are becoming more frequent. Broader surveillance for infections—outside ICUs and even outside hospitals—is more routine.

Catheter-related bloodstream infections derive largely from the cutaneous microbiome at the insertion site, with pathogens migrating extraluminally to the catheter tip, usually during the first week after insertion—a risk that has been lessened greatly by use of bundled catheter-insertion guidelines. In addition, contamination of the hubs of CVCs or of the ports of needle-less systems may lead to intraluminal infection over longer periods, particularly with surgically implanted or cuffed catheters. Intrinsic (during the manufacturing process) or extrinsic (on-site in a health care facility) contamination of infusate, although rare, is the most common cause of epidemic device-related bloodstream infection. The most common pathogens isolated from vascular device–associated bacteremias include coagulase-negative staphylococci, *S. aureus* (often resistant to methicillin), enterococci, nosocomial gram-negative bacilli, and *Candida*. Many pathogens, especially staphylococci, produce extracellular polysaccharide biofilms that facilitate attachment to catheters and provide sanctuary from antimicrobial agents.

Evidence-based bundles of control measures (Table 142-1) have been strikingly effective, eliminating almost all CVC-associated infections in some ICUs, and can be effective in low-income and middle-income, as well as in high-income, countries. Additional control measures include use of a chlorhexidine-impregnated patch at the skin-catheter junction; application of semitransparent access-site dressings (for ease of bathing and site inspection and protection of the site from secretions); daily bathing of ICU patients with chlorhexidine; avoidance of the femoral site for catheterization; and rotation of peripheral catheters—an underrecognized cause of staphylococcal bacteremia—to a new site at specified intervals (e.g., every 72–96 h) rather than as clinically indicated (a debatable recommendation that may be facilitated by use of an IV therapy team).

Controversial issues have included the role of gut translocation rather than vascular-access sites as a cause of primary bacteremia in immunocompromised patients and the implications for surveillance definitions; the best frequency for rotation of CVC sites (given that guidewire-assisted catheter changes at the same site do not lessen and can even increase infection risk); the relative risk posed by peripherally inserted central catheters (PICC lines); and the risk–benefit of prophylactic use of vancomycin, alcohol, or other solutions as catheter "locks"—concentrated anti-infective solutions instilled into the catheter lumen—for high-risk patients.

Vascular device–related infection is suspected on the basis of the appearance of the catheter site or the presence of fever or bacteremia without another source in patients with vascular catheters. The diagnosis is confirmed by the recovery of the same species of microorganism from peripheral-blood cultures and from semiquantitative or quantitative cultures of the vascular catheter tip. Cultures drawn from the CVC for diagnostic purposes are convenient but risk false-positive results (e.g., due to catheter hub contamination). When infusion-related sepsis is considered (e.g., because of the abrupt onset of fever or shock temporally related to infusion therapy), a sample of the infusate or blood product should be retained for culture.

Therapy for vascular access–related infection is directed at the pathogen recovered from the blood and/or infected site. Important considerations are the need for an echocardiogram (to evaluate the patient for endocarditis), the duration of therapy, and the need to remove potentially infected catheters. In one report, approximately one-fourth of patients with intravascular catheter–associated *S. aureus* bacteremia who were studied by transesophageal echocardiography had evidence of endocarditis; this test may be useful in determining the appropriate duration of treatment.

Detailed consensus guidelines for the management of intravascular catheter–related infections have been published and recommend catheter removal in most cases of bacteremia or fungemia due to nontunneled CVCs. When attempting to salvage a potentially infected catheter, some clinicians use the "antibiotic lock" technique, which may facilitate penetration of infected biofilms, in addition to systemic antimicrobial therapy (see *www.idsociety.org/Other_Guidelines/*).

ISOLATION TECHNIQUES

Written policies for isolation of infectious patients are a staple for infection-control programs. The CDC has guidelines for all components of health care, including acute-care hospitals and long-term, ambulatory, and home-care settings (see *www.cdc.gov/hicpac/pdf/isolation/Isolation2007.pdf*), as well as recommendations for the control of multidrug-resistant organisms.

Standard precautions are designed for the care of all patients in hospitals and aim to reduce the risk of transmission of microorganisms from both recognized and unrecognized sources. These precautions include gloving and hand cleansing for potential contact with (1) blood; (2) all other body fluids, secretions, and excretions, whether or not they contain visible blood; (3) nonintact skin; and (4) mucous membranes. Depending on exposure risks, standard precautions also include use of masks, eye protection, and gowns.

Precautions for the care of patients with potentially contagious clinical syndromes (e.g., acute diarrhea) or with suspected or diagnosed colonization or infection by transmissible pathogens are based on probable routes of transmission: *airborne*, *droplet*, or *contact*, for which personnel don, at a minimum, N95 respirators, surgical face masks, or glove and gown, respectively. Sets of precautions may be combined for diseases that have more than one route of transmission (e.g., contact and airborne isolation for varicella).

Some prevalent antibiotic-resistant pathogens, particularly those that colonize the gastrointestinal tract (e.g., vancomycin-resistant enterococci [VRE] and even multidrug-resistant gram-negative bacilli such as strains of *K. pneumoniae* and other Enterobacteriaceae that produce carbapenemases [carbapenem-resistant Enterobacteriaceae, or CRE]), may be present on *intact* skin of patients in hospitals (the "fecal patina"). This issue has led some experts to recommend gloving for all contact with patients who are acutely ill and/or in high-risk units, such as ICUs or LTACHs, and daily bathing of all ICU and LTACH patients with chlorhexidine to remove this veneer of antibiotic-resistant bacteria. Wearing gloves does not replace the need for hand hygiene because hands sometimes (in up to 20% of interactions) become contaminated during wearing or removal of gloves.

Further, in response to the frequent spread of resistant pathogens in long-term care facilities, CDC recommends *enhanced barrier precautions*—use of gown and gloves for high-contact resident care activities that have been demonstrated to result in transfer of resistant strains to health care personnel (*https://www.cdc.gov/hai/containment/faqs.html*).

EPIDEMIC AND EMERGING PROBLEMS

Full-blown epidemics probably account for <5% of nosocomial infections, but mini-clusters of a few infections that result from time-limited gaps in asepsis may be more common. The investigation and control of nosocomial epidemics require that infection control personnel (1) develop a case definition, (2) confirm that an outbreak really exists (since apparent epidemics may actually be pseudo-outbreaks due to surveillance or laboratory artifacts), (3) review aseptic practices and disinfectant use, (4) determine the extent of the outbreak, (5) perform an epidemiologic investigation, which may require a case–control study to determine sources and modes of transmission, (6) work closely with microbiology personnel to culture for common sources or personnel carriers as appropriate and to provide molecular typing—by pulsed-field gel electrophoresis (PFGE) or whole genome sequencing (WGS)—of epidemiologically important isolates, and (7) heighten surveillance to judge the effect of control measures. Control measures generally include reinforcing routine aseptic practices, hand hygiene, and environmental cleaning; surveillance for additional cases and ensuring appropriate isolation (and instituting cohort isolation and nursing if needed); and implementing further controls on the basis of the investigation's findings. Examples of some emerging and potential epidemic problems and control measures follow.

VIRAL RESPIRATORY INFECTIONS: CORONAVIRUS EPIDEMICS AND PANDEMIC INFLUENZA

The world has been plagued with three coronavirus respiratory illness epidemics since 2003. Common features include initial spread as a zoonosis, e.g., from "wet" (live food) markets; suspicion that bats are a key viral reservoir; risk of person-to-person and of nosocomial spread; excess mortality compared to common viral community-acquired infections; extensive use of isolation and quarantine in some affected communities; public fear; and often marked economic impact, e.g., due to temporary stoppages of commerce.

Infections caused by the severe acute respiratory syndrome (SARS)–associated coronavirus challenged health care systems globally in 2003 (**Chap. 199**). In 2012, Middle East respiratory syndrome coronavirus (MERS-CoV) emerged as a more geographically localized problem (**Chap. 199**), related initially to exposure to camels. For SARS, basic infection-control measures helped to keep the worldwide case and death counts at ~8000 and ~800, respectively. The epidemiology of SARS—spread largely in households once patients were ill or in hospitals—contrasts markedly with that of influenza (**Chap. 200**), which is often contagious a day before symptom onset and therefore can spread rapidly in the community among nonimmune persons.

The most recent coronavirus to emerge is SARS-CoV-2 (**Chap. 199**). The resultant COVID-19 infections are less lethal than SARS was (<2% vs ~10%, respectively) but much more of a global risk because infected patients may be contagious 1–2 days before symptoms appear. COVID-19 was first recognized in Wuhan City, Hubei Province, China in late 2019 and spread rapidly within China, despite aggressive isolation and quarantine programs, and to several continents via plane and cruise ship passengers. Each infected patient appears to lead to two to three secondary cases, mostly via dispersal of large respiratory droplets, but the potential for environmental and opportunistic airborne spread (e.g., during aerosol-generating procedures), as was seen with SARS, is a concern. A larger problem is spread by minimally symptomatic patients, which has created an influenza-like risk of extensive spread in the community. While efforts are underway to develop a vaccine and effective antiviral agents, control of SARS-CoV-2 must rely on prompt case recognition (based on epidemiologic or clinical clues and widened use of polymerase chain reaction [PCR] diagnostic tests), aggressive contact tracing, isolation, quarantine of exposed individuals, and aggressive use of personal protective equipment by health care workers.

Although the three coronavirus outbreaks are dramatic, seasonal influenza, with as many as 30 million cases and 30,000 deaths, remains a daunting *annual* challenge. Control of seasonal influenza has depended on (1) use of annually updated vaccines by children, the general public, and health care workers; (2) prescription of antiviral medications for early treatment and for prophylaxis as part of outbreak control, especially for high-risk patients and in high-risk settings like nursing homes or hospitals; (3) infection control (surveillance and droplet precautions) for symptomatic patients; and (4) general use of universal respiratory hygiene and cough etiquette (basically, "cover your cough") and source containment (e.g., use of face masks and spatial separation) for outpatients with potentially infectious respiratory illnesses. In an outpatient study, health care worker use of high-efficiency N95 respirators (recommended for airborne isolation) versus procedure masks (used for droplet precautions) resulted in no significant difference in the acquisition of laboratory-confirmed influenza.

In the spring of 2009, a novel strain of influenza virus—H1N1 (swine flu) virus—caused the first influenza pandemic in four decades. This pandemic led to reexaminations of the value of nonpharmacologic interventions, such as social distancing (e.g., closing of schools and community venues), that were used in the 1918–1919 influenza pandemic. These interventions became necessary again due to the extensive community spread of COVID-19. Recombinant events that create new strains (e.g., H7N9) to which there is population-wide susceptibility continue to challenge global efforts at infection control and vaccine development (**Chap. 200**).

OTHER EMERGING VIRAL PATHOGENS

The reemergence of Ebola virus in West Africa has had a global impact on infection-control preparedness and isolation techniques, on guidelines for donning and doffing of—and design refinements for—personal protective equipment, on situational awareness, and on successful development of vaccines and antivirals (**Chap. 210**). The emergence of epidemic Zika virus disease in Brazil and its spread throughout Latin America to the United States created a major concern for pregnant women and has added to the list yet another potential blood-borne pathogen that requires blood-bank screening (**Chap. 209**).

NOSOCOMIAL DIARRHEA

Overall rates of *C. difficile*–associated diarrhea (**Chap. 134**) have increased during the past few years, especially among older patients in U.S. hospitals. This increase has been related in part to a new, more virulent strain, NAP1/BI/027, and to use of PCR testing. In 2017, 223,900 cases of *C. difficile* infection occurred and at least 12,800 people died. In a CDC multistate survey, *C. difficile* was the most common nosocomial pathogen, causing 12% of health care–associated infections. Use of WGS is improving our understanding of *C. difficile* epidemiology. For now, control measures include judicious use of all antibiotics, especially fluoroquinolone antibiotics that have been implicated in driving outbreaks; heightened suspicion for atypical presentations (e.g., toxic megacolon or leukemoid reaction without diarrhea); enhanced disinfection of isolation rooms with sporicidal agents, such as bleach; and early diagnosis, treatment, and contact precautions. Preliminary data suggest a role for probiotics in the prevention of diarrhea in patients in whom systemic antibiotic therapy is being initiated. Fecal transplantation has had dramatic results in the treatment of relapsing cases of *C. difficile*–associated diarrhea (**Chap. 134**).

Outbreaks of norovirus infection (**Chap. 203**) in health care facilities can be challenging. The virus often is introduced by ill visitors or staff. Norovirus should be suspected when nausea and vomiting are prominent aspects of bacterial culture–negative diarrheal syndromes. Contact precautions may need to be augmented by aggressive environmental cleaning (given the persistence of norovirus on inanimate objects), prevention of secondary cases in members of the cleaning staff through an emphasis on the use of personal protective equipment and hand hygiene, and active exclusion of ill staff and visitors.

CHICKENPOX

Infection-control practitioners institute a varicella exposure investigation and control plan whenever health care workers have been exposed to chickenpox (**Chap. 193**) or have worked while having or during the 24 h before developing chickenpox. Fortunately, routine varicella vaccination of children and susceptible health care employees has made nosocomial spread less common.

MYCOBACTERIA

Important measures for the control of pulmonary tuberculosis (**Chap. 178**) include prompt recognition, isolation, and treatment of cases; recognition of atypical presentations (e.g., lower-lobe infiltrates without cavitation); use of negative-pressure, 100% exhaust, private isolation rooms with closed doors, and at least 6–12 air changes per hour; use of N95 respirators by caregivers entering isolation rooms; possible use of high-efficiency particulate air-filter units and/or ultraviolet lights for disinfecting air when other engineering controls are not feasible or reliable; and follow-up testing of susceptible personnel who have been exposed to infectious patients before isolation. The use of serologic tests, rather than skin tests, in the diagnosis of latent tuberculosis has become common, and health care worker testing is now largely event-directed rather than annual.

An unprecedented multicountry outbreak of postoperative invasive *Mycobacterium chimaera* infections has been traced to contaminated heater–cooler devices used commonly during cardiac surgery.

■ GROUP A STREPTOCOCCAL INFECTIONS

The potential for an outbreak of group A streptococcal infection **(Chap. 148)** should be considered when even one or two nosocomial cases occur. Most outbreaks involve surgical wounds and are due to the presence of an asymptomatic carrier in the operating room. Investigation can be confounded by carriage at extrapharyngeal sites such as the rectum and vagina.

■ FUNGAL INFECTIONS

When dusty areas—common sources of fungal spores—are disturbed during hospital repairs or renovation, the spores become airborne. Inhalation of spores by immunosuppressed (especially neutropenic) patients creates a risk of pulmonary and/or paranasal sinus infection and disseminated aspergillosis **(Chap. 217)**. Routine surveillance among neutropenic patients for infections with filamentous fungi, such as *Aspergillus* and *Fusarium*, helps hospitals to assess environmental risks. As a matter of routine, hospitals should inspect and clean air-handling equipment; review all planned renovations with infection-control personnel and construct appropriate barriers; remove immunosuppressed patients from renovation sites; and consider the use of high-efficiency particulate air-intake filters for rooms housing immunosuppressed patients.

A major multistate iatrogenic outbreak of meningitis, localized spinal or paraspinal infection, and arthritis due to *Exserohilum rostratum* was recognized in 2012 and traced to contamination of an injectable preservative-free steroid product produced by a single compounding pharmacy **(Chap. 217)**.

Candida auris **(Chap. 216)**, a pathogen first identified in Japan in 2009, has emerged globally as a cause of invasive health care–associated infections, with several distinct aspects. The appearance on multiple continents occurred over a period of only months, markedly faster than spread of most problem pathogens. Although *C. auris* strains (clades) are similar within a region, they differ genetically between continents; some strains are resistant to multiple antifungals.

Epidemiologic and clinical features of *C. auris* include prolonged colonization of multiple body sites, especially skin and nares; high organism burdens that have facilitated nosocomial spread in acute and, particularly, long-term care hospitals; and high mortality in fungemic patients. Control currently relies on aggressive surveillance and contact precautions for colonized patients, point prevalence surveys in facilities with emerging *C. auris* problems, and cleaning of the often-extensive environmental contamination (including reusable patient care equipment) in rooms of colonized patients. Efforts to decolonize patients have been variably successful. Collaboration of infection control, public health, and laboratory personnel has been essential.

■ LEGIONELLOSIS

Nosocomial *Legionella* pneumonia **(Chap. 159)** is most often due to contamination of potable water or of water used in decorative fountains. This disease predominantly affects immunosuppressed patients, particularly those receiving glucocorticoid medications. The risk varies greatly geographically, depending on the extent of hospital water contamination and on hospital practices (e.g., the presence of decorative fountains in hospital lobbies or inappropriate use of nonsterile water in respiratory therapy equipment). If nosocomial cases are detected, environmental samples (e.g., tap water) should be cultured. If cultures yield *Legionella* and if typing of clinical and environmental isolates reveals a correlation, eradication measures should be pursued. An alternative approach is to periodically culture tap water in wards housing high-risk patients. If *Legionella* is found, a concerted effort should be made to introduce engineering controls to reduce or eliminate water-borne *Legionella* within the facility.

ANTIBIOTIC-RESISTANT BACTERIA: SURVEILLANCE, CONTROL, AND ANTIBIOTIC AND DIAGNOSTIC STEWARDSHIP

Emerging multidrug-resistant bacteria like CRE are harbingers of a potential postantibiotic era. The CDC's comprehensive 2019 Antibiotic Resistance Threat Report (*https://www.cdc.gov/drugresistance/pdf/threats-report/2019-ar-threats-report-508.pdf*) provides the updated estimate that >2.8 million antibiotic-resistant infections occur in the United States each year, and >35,000 people die as a result. The report ranks and reviews the 18 microbes currently viewed as our biggest threats and also provides a watch list of potential problems **(Table 142-2)**.

Control of resistance depends on early detection of problem pathogens that now can be facilitated by collaboration with the nationwide CDC-supported, state-based Antibiotic Resistance Laboratory Network (*https://www.cdc.gov/drugresistance/solutions-initiative/ar-lab-network.html*); on aggressive reinforcement of routine asepsis; on implementation of barrier precautions for all colonized and/or infected patients; on use of patient surveillance cultures to more fully ascertain the extent of patient colonization; on diagnostic stewardship to avoid overtreatment, e.g., of colonizing germs; on antimicrobial stewardship to lessen ecologic pressures; and on timely initiation of an epidemiologic investigation when rates increase. There is increasing interest in use of "implementation science" to close the gap between discussions of control measures and practice.

Advanced molecular diagnostics (e.g., PFGE and, more recently, WGS) can help differentiate an outbreak due to a single strain (which necessitates an emphasis on hand hygiene and an evaluation of potential common-source exposures) from a polyclonal outbreak (which requires an emphasis on antibiotic prudence and device bundles; Table 142-1), providing a form of "precision infection control." Continuing emergence of multidrug-resistant organisms suggests that control efforts have been insufficient and that heightened interventions and global strategies are needed urgently

TABLE 142-2 Bacteria and Fungi Listed in the CDC 2019 AR Threats Report

Urgent threats
Carbapenem-resistant *Acinetobacter*
Candida auris
Clostridioides difficile
Carbapenem-resistant Enterobacteriaceae
Drug-resistant *Neisseria gonorrhoeae*
Serious Threats
Drug-resistant *Campylobacter*
Drug-resistant *Candida*
ESBL-producing Enterobacteriaceae
Vancomycin-resistant *Enterococci* (VRE)
Multidrug-resistant *Pseudomonas aeruginosa*
Drug-resistant nontyphoidal *Salmonella*
Drug-resistant *Salmonella* serotype Typhi
Drug-resistant *Shigella*
Methicillin-resistant *Staphylococcus aureus* (MRSA)
Drug-resistant *Streptococcus pneumoniae*
Drug-resistant Tuberculosis
Concerning threats
Erythromycin-resistant group A *Streptococcus*
Clindamycin-resistant group B *Streptococcus*
Watch list
Azole-resistant *Aspergillus fumigatus*
Drug-resistant *Mycoplasma genitalium*
Drug-resistant *Bordetella pertussis*

Abbreviations: AR, antibiotic resistance; CDC, Centers for Disease Control and Prevention; ESBL, extended-spectrum beta-lactamase.

Source: Centers for Disease Control and Prevention. *https://www.cdc.gov/drugresistance/pdf/threats-report/2019-ar-threats-report-508.pdf.*

(see *https://www.cdc.gov/drugresistance/biggest-threats.html* and *https://www.cdc.gov/vitalsigns/stop-spread/index.html*); this need is highlighted by the creation of the U.S. Presidential Advisory Council on Combating Antibiotic-Resistant Bacteria and by the U.N. General Assembly's 2016 Declaration (see *https://www.hhs.gov/ash/advisory-committees/paccarb, http://www.un.org/pga/71/2016/09/21/press-release-hl-meeting-on-antimicrobial-resistance/*, and *https://www.gov.uk/government/publications/uk-5-year-antimicrobial-resistance-strategy-2013-to-2018*).

To facilitate tracking of resistance problems, the CDC's innovative, interactive online Antibiotic Resistance Patient Safety Atlas allows users to search state-level resistance data (*https://arpsp.cdc.gov/*). The European Centre for Disease Prevention and Control also has online resistance reporting (*http://ecdc.europa.eu/en/healthtopics/antimicrobial-resistance-and-consumption/antimicrobial_resistance/EARS-Net/Pages/EARS-Net.aspx*).

Several antibiotic resistance problems are pressing global threats. First, *S. aureus* continues to cause significant morbidity and mortality. The emergence of community-associated methicillin-resistant *S. aureus* (CA-MRSA) has been dramatic in many countries, with as many as 50% of community-acquired "staph infections" in some U.S. cities now caused by strains resistant to β-lactam antibiotics **(Chap. 147)**. The incursion of CA-MRSA into hospitals is well documented and has impacted surveillance and control of nosocomial MRSA infections. After an encouraging 17% annual reduction in incidence of hospital-onset MRSA bloodstream infections during 2005–2012, the decline slowed in 2013–2016. CA-MRSA declined less (~7% annually), whereas hospital-onset methicillin-sensitive *S. aureus* (MSSA) has not changed and CA-MSSA infections have increased (~4% per year) from 2012 to 2017.

Second, in the global emergence of multidrug-resistant gram-negative bacilli, problems include plasmid-mediated resistance to fluoroquinolones, metallo-β-lactamase–mediated resistance to carbapenems, CRE, and pan-resistant strains of *Acinetobacter*. Many multidrug-resistant gram-negative bacilli are susceptible only to colistin, to newer combination β-lactamase inhibitor drugs, or to no available agents. The increased use of colistin, which often has been futile, has led to recognition of plasmid-mediated colistin resistance in *E. coli*—first in swine-associated strains from China and now in strains from many countries, including the United States.

Transmission of CRE has been traced in a number of outbreaks to exposure to duodenoscopes used for endoscopic retrograde cholangiopancreatography. The duodenoscope is more intricate than other endoscopes and has an "elevator mechanism" that can be difficult to clean and disinfect; this problem has led to development of disposable portions of these devices.

A number of "water bug" (e.g., *Pseudomonas* spp.) outbreaks have been traced to environmental sources, such as sinks, sink drains, and bedpan hoppers. These outbreaks have called attention to the sources and reservoirs of waterborne and often antibiotic-resistant bacteria and the need for environmental interventions to control these organisms. This is reminiscent of infection control experiences in the 1970s, when waterborne bacteria were blamed for ICU respiratory infection outbreaks.

Third, there has been renewed recognition of the role of nursing homes, and now LTACHs, in the spread of resistant gram-negative bacilli such as CRE. In some LTACHs, as many as 30–50% of patients may be colonized with CREs. The frequent transfer of patients who are colonized or infected with antibiotic-resistant bacteria between long-term and acute-care facilities (Fig. 142-1) has led to studies of the regional spread of antibiotic resistance and the push to develop regional infection-control interventions (see *https://www.cdc.gov/vitalsigns/stop-spread/index.html*) aimed at the highest-risk facilities, which often drive regional resistance rates.

Fourth, there has been increasing community-based spread of *E. coli* strains harboring an enzyme, CTX-M, that renders them broadly resistant to β-lactam antibiotics. Understanding the epidemiology of these strains will be essential for development of control measures. In the meantime, community-based antibiotic stewardship has been associated in at least one trial with reduction in resistance rates.

Fifth, as a consequence of going abroad, international travelers, especially to Latin America, Asia, and Africa, may become gastrointestinal carriers of multidrug-resistant Enterobacteriaceae that express extended-spectrum β-lactamases (ESBLs). As many as 30–40% of returning travelers can have newly acquired resistant strains that can persist for as long as 6–12 months. The frequency of clinical consequences—e.g., antibiotic-resistant UTIs or familial or local spread of resistant strains—is not yet known.

Controversial control issues include the need for continuing use of contact isolation for patients colonized with more common, often community-acquired strains, such as ESBL *E. coli*, MRSA, or VRE, and duration of contact precautions. The role of single-patient rooms for contact isolation has been questioned but seems a clear choice for anyone who ever has been hospitalized. Manipulation of patients' intestinal microbiomes has been considered as a control strategy for individual patients or for outbreaks of multidrug-resistant pathogens that have a gastrointestinal reservoir, but a report of drug-resistant *E. coli* bacteremia transmitted by fecal microbiota transplant has highlighted the need for carefully controlled trials of this approach.

In several cluster-randomized controlled trials over the past ~15 years, source control—i.e., removal of patients' fecal patinas—by daily bathing with chlorhexidine has reduced the risk of bacteremia in ICU patients. "Search-and-destroy" methods—i.e., active surveillance cultures to detect and isolate the "resistance iceberg" of patients colonized with MRSA—are credited with elimination of nosocomial MRSA in the Netherlands and Denmark. In a multicenter trial in the United States, universal source control with chlorhexidine and nasal mupirocin was significantly more effective in controlling MRSA than was a search-and-destroy approach and led to control of other pathogens as well, providing a broad (horizontal) rather than a narrower (vertical) intervention (see *https://www.ahrq.gov/hai/universal-icu-decolonization/index.html*). For some pathogens, such as VRE and *C. difficile*, enforcement of environmental cleaning can markedly reduce cross-transmission risk. Newer environmental disinfection modalities, such as ultraviolet (UV) light and hydrogen peroxide mists, are appealing but sometimes limited in application by practicality and inconsistent results.

Because the excessive use of broad-spectrum antibiotics underlies many resistance problems and adverse patient events, antibiotic stewardship programs are mandatory in acute care hospitals (see *https://www.cdc.gov/getsmart/healthcare/implementation/core-elements.html*) and are being promulgated actively for long-term care and outpatient facilities (see *https://www.cdc.gov/longtermcare/prevention/antibiotic-stewardship.html* and *https://www.cdc.gov/mmwr/volumes/65/rr/rr6506a1.htm*), where implementing such programs is challenging but of great importance. In some studies, 30–50% of antibiotic courses are inappropriate—a large target for improvement efforts. The main interventions that will save the "antimicrobial commons," limit selective pressures on nosocomial flora, and protect patients are restricting use of particular agents to narrowly defined indications; treating with the shortest efficacious courses; deescalating from empiric broad-spectrum treatment as soon as possible on the basis of the results of culture and susceptibility tests; and consulting infectious disease experts for treatment of *S. aureus* bacteremia and candidemia. Reductions in total and high-risk antibiotic use have been associated with decreased risk of nosocomial *C. difficile* infections and lowered rates of antibiotic resistance in hospitals and communities.

New stewardship teams must ensure that they have a visible and effective program champion; start with interventions that are based on well-controlled trials; focus on high impact areas, such as emergency departments where therapy often is initiated; promote guidelines that are amenable to surveillance, enforcement, and sustainability; and tailor stewardship activities to comport with the motivations and identities of physicians in different specialties, recognizing that at times internists can be from Venus and surgeons from Mars.

From a One Health perspective, antimicrobial use in animal husbandry and agriculture can be an important driver of genetic resistance elements in bacteria and fungi, which then spread predominantly among humans. This concern has led to recommendations for eliminating the use of antibiotics for growth promotion and as prophylaxis for feed animals. The United States lags behind some European countries in control of veterinary and agricultural use of antimicrobial drugs.

Key to an understanding of the success of antibiotic stewardship initiatives is better surveillance of antibiotic use among humans and animals at regional and national levels.

BIOTERRORISM AND OTHER SURGE-EVENT PREPAREDNESS

The horrific attack on the World Trade Center in New York City on September 11, 2001; subsequent mailings of anthrax spores in the United States; the Boston Marathon bombing in 2013; and ongoing terrorist activities globally have made bioterrorism a prominent source of concern to hospital infection-control programs **(Chap. S3)**. The essentials for hospital preparedness entail education, internal and external communication, and situational awareness (see *https://emergency.cdc.gov/bioterrorism/*).

EMPLOYEE HEALTH SERVICE ISSUES

An institution's employee health service is critical for infection control. New employees should be processed through the service, where a contagious disease history can be taken; evidence of immunity to a variety of diseases, such as hepatitis B, chickenpox, measles, mumps, and rubella, can be sought; immunizations for hepatitis B, measles, mumps, rubella, varicella, and pertussis can be given as needed (an especially important step with the resurgence in the United States of vaccine-preventable diseases such as pertussis, mumps, and measles); baseline testing for latent tuberculosis can be performed; and education about personal responsibility for infection control can be initiated.

The employee health service must have protocols for dealing with workers exposed to contagious diseases (e.g., influenza) and those percutaneously or mucosally exposed to the blood of patients infected with HIV or hepatitis B or C virus. Protocols are also needed for dealing with caregivers who have common contagious diseases (e.g., chickenpox, group A streptococcal infection, influenza or another respiratory infection, or infectious diarrhea) and for those who have less common but high-visibility public health problems (e.g., chronic hepatitis B or C or HIV infection) for which exposure-control guidelines have been published by the CDC and by the Society for Healthcare Epidemiology of America.

■ FURTHER READING

Alp E et al: Infection control bundles in intensive care: An international cross-sectional survey in low- and middle-income countries. J Hosp Inf 101:245, 2019.

Banach DB et al: Duration of contact precautions for acute-care settings. Infect Control Hosp Epidemiol 39:127, 2018.

Carling PC: Wastewater drains: epidemiology and interventions in 23 carbapenem-resistant organism outbreaks. Infect Control Hosp Epidemiol 39:972, 2018.

Gaynes R: History of infection control in hospitals in the United States. Hygiènes 26:23, 2018.

Hsu H et al: CAUTI rates decline following change in case definition. Infect Control Hosp Epidemiol 10:1017, 2019.

Kourtis AP et al: Vital signs: Epidemiology and recent trends in methicillin-resistant and in methicillin-susceptible *Staphylococcus aureus* bloodstream infections–United States. MMWR 68:214, 2019.

Magill SS et al: Changes in prevalence of health care–associated infections in U.S. hospitals. N Engl J Med 379:1732, 2018.

Sironi M, de laTorre JC: Encouraging AWaRe-ness and discouraging inappropriate antibiotic use-the new 2019 Essential Medicines List becomes a global antibiotic stewardship tool. Lancet Infect Dis 19:1278, 2019.

Strassle PD et al: Incidence and risk factors of non-device-associated pneumonia in an acute-care hospital. Infect Control Hosp Epidemiol 41:73, 2020.

Weiner-Lastinger LM et al: Antimicrobial-resistant pathogens associated with adult healthcare-associated infections: Summary of data reported to the National Healthcare Safety Network, 2015-2017. Infect Control Hosp Epidemiol 41:1, 2020.

143 Infections in Transplant Recipients

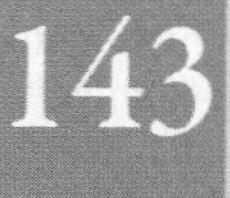

Robert W. Finberg*

The evaluation of infections in transplant recipients involves consideration of both the donor and the recipient of the transplanted cells or organ. Two central issues are of paramount importance: (1) infectious agents (particularly viruses, but also bacteria, fungi, and parasites) can be introduced into the recipient by the donor; and (2) treatment of the recipient with medicine to prevent rejection can suppress normal immune responses, greatly increasing susceptibility to infection. Thus, what might have been a latent or asymptomatic infection in an immunocompetent donor or in the recipient prior to therapy can become a life-threatening problem when the recipient becomes immunosuppressed. The pretransplantation evaluation of each patient should be guided by an analysis of both (1) what infections the recipient is currently harboring, since organisms that exist in a state of latency or dormancy before the procedure may cause fatal disease when the patient receives immunosuppressive treatment; and (2) what organisms are likely to be transmitted by the donor, particularly those to which the recipient may be naïve.

PRETRANSPLANTATION EVALUATION

■ THE DONOR

A variety of organisms have been transmitted by organ transplantation. Transmission of infections that may have been latent or not clinically apparent in the donor has resulted in the development of specific donor-screening protocols. Results from routine blood-bank studies, including those for antibodies to *Treponema pallidum* (syphilis), *Trypanosoma cruzi*, hepatitis B and C viruses, HIV-1 and -2, and human T-lymphotropic virus types 1 and 2 (HTLV-1 and -2), should be documented. Serologic studies should be ordered to identify latent infection with viruses, such as herpes simplex virus types 1 and 2 (HSV-1, HSV-2), varicella-zoster virus (VZV), cytomegalovirus (CMV), Epstein-Barr virus (EBV), and Kaposi's sarcoma–associated herpesvirus (KSHV; also known as human herpesvirus type 8); acute infection with hepatitis A virus; and infection with the common parasite *Toxoplasma gondii*. Donors should be screened for parasites, such as *Strongyloides stercoralis*, *T. cruzi*, and *Schistosoma* species, if they have lived in endemic areas. Clinicians caring for prospective organ donors should examine chest radiographs for evidence of granulomatous disease (e.g., caused by mycobacteria or fungi) and should perform skin testing or obtain blood for immune cell-based assays that detect active or latent *Mycobacterium tuberculosis* infection. An investigation of the donor's dietary habits (e.g., consumption of raw meat or fish or of unpasteurized dairy products), occupations or avocations (e.g., gardening or spelunking), and travel history (e.g., travel to areas with endemic fungi causing infections such as blastomycosis, coccidioidomycosis, and histoplasmosis) also is indicated and may mandate additional testing. A number of unusual parasites (including *Balamuthia mandrillaris*) have been identified in transplanted kidneys. Uncommonly diagnosed viruses, including lymphocytic choriomeningitis virus (LCMV), West Nile virus, Zika virus, dengue virus, and rabies virus, can be transplanted in organs and are likely to be difficult to diagnose in recipients. If an unusual parasite or uncommon virus is identified in a transplant recipient, the organ-donor organization and caregivers for recipients of other organs isolated from the same donor should be notified immediately.

Creutzfeldt-Jakob disease has been transmitted through corneal transplants; however, to what degree it can be transmitted by transfused blood is unknown. Variant Creutzfeldt-Jakob disease can be transmitted with transfused non-leukodepleted blood, posing a theoretical risk to transplant recipients.

*Deceased.

PART 5 Infectious Diseases

THE RECIPIENT

It is expected that the recipient will have been even more comprehensively assessed than the donor. Additional studies recommended for the recipient include evaluation for acute respiratory viruses and gastrointestinal pathogens in the immediate pretransplantation period. An important caveat is that, because of immune dysfunction resulting from chemotherapy or underlying chronic disease, serologic testing of the recipient may prove less reliable than usual.

THE DONOR CELLS/ORGAN

Careful attention to the sterility of the medium used to process the donor organ, combined with meticulous microbiologic evaluation, reduces rates of transmission of bacteria (or, rarely, yeasts) that may be present or grow in the organ culture medium. From 2 to >20% of donor kidneys are estimated to be contaminated with bacteria—in most cases, with the organisms that colonize the skin or grow in the tissue culture medium used to bathe the donor organ while it awaits implantation. The reported rate of bacterial contamination of transplanted stem cells (bone marrow, peripheral blood, cord blood) is as high as 17% but most commonly is ~1%. The use of enrichment columns and monoclonal antibody depletion procedures results in a higher incidence of contamination. In some cases, because of the clinical situation, contaminated cells have been infused, usually with concomitant administration of antimicrobial agents. In one series of patients receiving contaminated stem cells, 14% had fever or bacteremia, but none died. Results of cultures performed at the time of cryopreservation and at the time of thawing were helpful in guiding therapy for the recipient.

INFECTIONS IN HEMATOPOIETIC STEM CELL TRANSPLANT RECIPIENTS

Transplantation of hematopoietic stem cells (HSCs) from bone marrow or from peripheral or cord blood for cancer, immunodeficiency, or autoimmune disease is marked by a transient state of complete immunologic incompetence. Immediately after myeloablative chemotherapy and transplantation, both innate immune cells (phagocytes, dendritic cells, natural killer cells) and adaptive immune cells (T and B cells) are absent, and the host is extremely susceptible to infection. The reconstitution that follows transplantation has been likened to maturation of the immune system in neonates. The analogy does not entirely predict infections seen in HSC transplant recipients, however, because the stem cells mature in an old host who has several latent infections already. The choice among the current variety of methods for obtaining stem cells is determined by availability and by the need to optimize the chances of a cure for an individual recipient. One strategy is autologous HSC transplantation, in which the recipient's own stem cells are used. After chemotherapy, stem cells are collected and are purged (ex vivo) of residual neoplastic populations. Allogeneic HSC transplantation has the advantage of providing a graft-versus-tumor effect. In this case, the recipient is matched to varying degrees for human leukocyte antigens (HLAs) with a donor who may be related or unrelated. In some individuals, nonmyeloablative therapy (mini-allotransplantation) is used and permits recipient cells to persist for some time after transplantation while preserving the graft-versus-tumor effect and sparing the recipient intense myeloablative therapy. Cord-blood transplantation is increasingly used in adults; two independent cord-blood units are typically required for suitable neutrophil engraftment early after transplantation, even though only one of the units is likely to provide long-term engraftment. In each circumstance, a different balance is struck among the toxicity of conditioning therapy, the need for a maximal graft-versus-target effect, short-term and long-term infectious complications, and the risk of graft-versus-host disease (GVHD; acute versus chronic). The various approaches differ in terms of reconstitution speed, cell lineages introduced, and likelihood of GVHD—all factors that can produce distinct effects on the risk of infection after transplantation (**Table 143-1**). Despite these caveats, most infections occur in a predictable time frame after transplantation (**Table 143-2**).

BACTERIAL INFECTIONS

In the first month after HSC transplantation, infectious complications are similar to those in granulocytopenic patients receiving chemotherapy for acute leukemia (**Chap. 74**). Because of the anticipated 1- to 4-week duration of neutropenia and the high rate of bacterial infection in this population, many centers give prophylactic antibiotics to patients upon initiation of myeloablative therapy. Quinolones decrease the incidence of gram-negative bacteremia among these patients. Bacterial infections are common in the first few days after HSC transplantation. The organisms involved are predominantly those found on skin, mucosa, or IV catheters (*Staphylococcus aureus*, coagulase-negative staphylococci, streptococci) or aerobic bacteria that colonize the bowel (*Escherichia coli*, *Klebsiella*, *Pseudomonas*). *Bacillus cereus*, although rare, has emerged as a pathogen early after transplantation and can cause meningitis, which is unusual in these patients.

TABLE 143-1 Risk of Infection, by Type of Hematopoietic Stem Cell Transplant

TYPE OF HEMATOPOIETIC STEM CELL TRANSPLANT	SOURCE OF STEM CELLS	RISK OF EARLY INFECTION: NEUTROPHIL DEPLETION	RISK OF LATE INFECTION: IMPAIRED T- AND B-CELL FUNCTION	RISK OF ONGOING INFECTION: GVHD AND IATROGENIC IMMUNOSUPPRESSION	GRAFT-VS-TUMOR EFFECT
Autologous	Recipient (self)	High risk; neutrophil recovery sometimes prolonged	~1 year	Minimal to no risk of GVHD and late-onset severe infection	None (–)
Syngeneic (genetic twin)	Identical twin	Low risk; 1–2 weeks for neutrophil recovery	~1 year	Minimal risk of GVHD and late-onset severe infection	+/–
Allogeneic related	Sibling	Low risk; 1–2 weeks for neutrophil recovery	~1 year	Minimal to moderate risk of GVHD and late-onset severe infection	++
Allogeneic related	Child/parent (haploidentical)	Intermediate risk; 2–3 weeks for neutrophil recovery	1–2 years	Moderate risk of GVHD and late-onset severe infection	++++
Allogeneic unrelated adult	Unrelated donor	Intermediate risk; 2–3 weeks for neutrophil recovery	1–2 years	High risk of GVHD and late-onset severe infection	++++
Allogeneic unrelated cord blood	Unrelated cord-blood units (×2)	Intermediate to high risk; neutrophil recovery sometimes prolonged	Prolonged	Minimal to moderate risk of GVHD and late-onset severe infection	++++
Allogeneic mini (nonmyeloablative)	Donor (transiently coexisting with recipient cells)	Low risk; neutrophil counts close to normal	1–2+ years	Variable risk of GVHD and late-onset severe infection[a]	++++ (but develops slowly)

[a]Depending on the disparity of the match (major and minor histocompatibility antigens), GVHD may be severe or mild, the requirement for immunosuppression intense or minimal, and the risk of severe late infections coordinate with the degree of immunosuppression.

Abbreviation: GVHD, graft-versus-host disease.

TABLE 143-2 Common Sources of Infection after Hematopoietic Stem Cell Transplantation

	PERIOD AFTER TRANSPLANTATION		
INFECTION SITE	EARLY (<1 MONTH)	MIDDLE (1–4 MONTHS)	LATE (>6 MONTHS)
Disseminated	Aerobic bacteria (gram-negative, gram-positive)	*Candida, Aspergillus,* EBV	Encapsulated bacteria (*Streptococcus pneumoniae, Haemophilus influenzae, Neisseria meningitidis*)
Skin and mucous membranes	HSV	HHV-6	VZV, HPV (warts)
Lungs	Aerobic bacteria (gram-negative, gram-positive), *Candida, Aspergillus,* other molds, HSV	CMV, seasonal respiratory viruses, *Pneumocystis, Toxoplasma*	*Pneumocystis, Nocardia, S. pneumoniae*
Gastrointestinal tract	*Clostridioides difficile*	CMV, adenovirus	EBV, CMV
Kidney		BK virus, adenovirus	
Brain		HHV-6, *Toxoplasma*	*Toxoplasma,* JC virus (rare)
Bone marrow		CMV, HHV-6	CMV, HHV-6

Abbreviations: CMV, cytomegalovirus; EBV, Epstein-Barr virus; HHV-6, human herpesvirus type 6; HPV, human papillomavirus; HSV, herpes simplex virus; VZV, varicella-zoster virus.

Chemotherapy, use of broad-spectrum antibiotics, and delayed reconstitution of humoral immunity place HSC transplant patients at risk for diarrhea and colitis caused by *Clostridioides difficile* overgrowth and toxin production. Reconstitution of the bowel with microbial flora from donors ("fecal transplantation") has been successful in drug-resistant cases **(Chap. 134)**.

Beyond the first few days of neutropenia, infections with nosocomial pathogens (e.g., vancomycin-resistant enterococci, *Stenotrophomonas maltophilia, Acinetobacter* species, and extended-spectrum β-lactamase-producing gram-negative bacteria) as well as with filamentous bacteria (e.g., *Nocardia* species) become more common. Vigilance is indicated, particularly for patients with a history of active or known latent tuberculosis, even when they have been appropriately pretreated. Episodes of bacteremia due to encapsulated organisms mark the late posttransplantation period (>6 months after HSC reconstitution); patients who have undergone splenectomy and those with persistent hypogammaglobulinemia are at particular risk.

■ FUNGAL INFECTIONS

Beyond the first week after HSC transplantation, fungal infections become increasingly common, particularly among patients who have received broad-spectrum antibiotics. As in most granulocytopenic patients, *Candida* infections are most commonly seen in this setting. However, with increased use of prophylactic fluconazole, infections with *Candida albicans* resistant to fluconazole and naturally fluconazole-resistant fungi—in particular, *Aspergillus* and other non-*Aspergillus* molds (*Rhizopus, Fusarium, Scedosporium, Penicillium*)—have become more common, prompting some centers to replace fluconazole with agents such as micafungin, voriconazole, isavuconazole, or posaconazole. Identification of *Candida auris* as a pathogen has made prophylaxis and treatment of fungal infections more difficult as these organisms are often resistant to most antifungal agents. Echinocandins are recommended for initial therapy of patients with serious *Candida* infections. Treatment should be adjusted based on sensitivities. The role of antifungal prophylaxis with these different agents, in contrast to empirical treatment for suspected infection that is based on a positive β-D-glucan assay or galactomannan antigen test, remains controversial **(Chap. 74)**. Documented infection should be aggressively treated, ideally with agents of proven activity. In patients with GVHD who require prolonged or indefinite courses of glucocorticoids and other immunosuppressive agents (e.g., cyclosporine, tacrolimus [FK506, Prograf], mycophenolate mofetil [CellCept], rapamycin [sirolimus, Rapamune], antithymocyte globulin, or anti-CD52 antibody [alemtuzumab, Campath—an antilymphocyte and antimonocyte monoclonal antibody]), there is a high risk of fungal infection (usually with *Candida* or *Aspergillus*) even after engraftment and resolution of neutropenia. These patients are also at high risk for reactivation of latent fungal infection (histoplasmosis, coccidioidomycosis, or blastomycosis) in areas where endemic fungi reside and after involvement in activities such as gardening or caving. Prolonged use of central venous catheters for parenteral nutrition (lipids) increases the risk of fungemia with *Malassezia*. Some centers administer prophylactic antifungal agents to these patients. Because of the high and prolonged risk of *Pneumocystis jirovecii* pneumonia (especially among patients being treated for hematologic malignancies), most patients receive maintenance prophylaxis with trimethoprim-sulfamethoxazole (TMP-SMX) starting after engraftment and continuing for at least 1 year.

■ PARASITIC INFECTIONS

The regimen described above for the fungal pathogen *Pneumocystis* may also protect patients seropositive for the parasite *T. gondii*, which can cause pneumonia, visceral disease (occasionally), and central nervous system (CNS) lesions (more commonly). The advantages of maintaining HSC transplant recipients on daily TMP-SMX for 1 year after transplantation include some protection against *Listeria monocytogenes* and nocardiosis as well as late infections with *Streptococcus pneumoniae* and *Haemophilus influenzae* that stem from the inability of the immature immune system to respond to polysaccharide antigens.

With increasing international travel, parasitic diseases typically restricted to particular environmental niches may pose a risk of reactivation in certain patients after HSC transplantation. Thus, in recipients with an appropriate history who were not screened and/or treated before transplantation or in patients with recent exposures, evaluation for infection with *Strongyloides, Leishmania*, schistosomes, trypanosomes, or various parasitic causes of diarrheal illness (*Giardia, Entamoeba, Cryptosporidium*, microsporidia) may be warranted.

■ VIRAL INFECTIONS

HSC transplant recipients are susceptible to infection with a variety of viruses, including primary and reactivation syndromes caused by most human herpesviruses **(Table 143-3)** and acute infections caused by viruses that circulate in the community.

Herpes Simplex Virus Within the first 2 weeks after transplantation, most patients who are seropositive for HSV-1 excrete the virus from the oropharynx. The ability to isolate HSV declines with time. Administration of prophylactic acyclovir (or valacyclovir) to seropositive HSC transplant recipients has been shown to reduce mucositis and prevent HSV pneumonia (a rare condition reported almost exclusively in allogeneic HSC transplant recipients). Both esophagitis (usually due to HSV-1) and anogenital disease (commonly caused by HSV-2) may be prevented with acyclovir prophylaxis. **For further discussion, see Chap. 192.**

Varicella-Zoster Virus Reactivation of VZV manifests as herpes zoster and may occur within the first month but more commonly occurs several months after transplantation. Reactivation rates are ~40% for allogeneic HSC transplant recipients and 25% for autologous recipients. Localized zoster can spread rapidly in an immunosuppressed patient. Fortunately, disseminated disease can usually be controlled with high doses of acyclovir. Because of frequent VZV

TABLE 143-3 Herpesvirus Syndromes in Transplant Recipients

VIRUS	REACTIVATION DISEASE
Herpes simplex virus type 1	Oral lesions Esophageal lesions Pneumonia (primarily HSC transplant recipients) Hepatitis (rare)
Herpes simplex virus type 2	Anogenital lesions Hepatitis (rare)
Varicella-zoster virus	Zoster (can disseminate)
Cytomegalovirus	Associated with graft rejection Fever and malaise Bone marrow failure Pneumonitis Gastrointestinal disease
Epstein-Barr virus	B-cell lymphoproliferative disease/lymphoma Oral hairy leukoplakia (rare)
Human herpesvirus type 6	Fever Delayed monocyte/platelet engraftment Encephalitis (rare)
Human herpesvirus type 7	Undefined
Kaposi's sarcoma–associated virus (human herpesvirus type 8)	Kaposi's sarcoma Primary effusion lymphoma (rare) Multicentric Castleman's disease (rare) Marrow aplasia (rare)

Abbreviation: HSC, hematopoietic stem cell.

dissemination among patients with skin lesions, acyclovir is given prophylactically in many centers to prevent severe disease. Low doses of acyclovir appear to be effective in preventing reactivation of VZV. While the live-attenuated zoster vaccine is contraindicated in this patient population, the recombinant subunit vaccine may be given before or after transplantation. **For further discussion, see Chap. 193.**

Cytomegalovirus The onset of CMV disease (interstitial pneumonia, bone marrow suppression, graft failure, hepatitis/colitis) usually begins 30–90 days after HSC transplantation, when the granulocyte count is adequate but immunologic reconstitution has not occurred. CMV disease rarely develops earlier than 14 days after transplantation and may become evident as late as 4 months or more after the procedure. It is of greatest concern in the second month after transplantation, particularly in allogeneic HSC transplant recipients. In cases in which the donor marrow is depleted of T cells (to prevent GVHD or eliminate a T-cell tumor) and in cord-blood recipients, the disease may manifest earlier. The use of alemtuzumab to prevent GVHD in nonmyeloablative transplantation has been associated with an increase in CMV disease. Patients who receive ganciclovir for prophylaxis, preemptive treatment, or treatment (see below) may develop recurrent CMV infection even later than 4 months after transplantation, as treatment appears to delay the development of an effective immune response to CMV infection. Although CMV disease may present as isolated fever, granulocytopenia, thrombocytopenia, or gastrointestinal disease, the foremost cause of death from CMV infection in the setting of HSC transplantation is pneumonia.

With the standard use of CMV-negative or filtered blood products, CMV infection should be a major risk in allogeneic transplantation only when the recipient is CMV seropositive and the donor is CMV seronegative. This situation is the reverse of that in solid organ transplant recipients. CMV reactivates from latent reservoirs present in the recipient at a time when donor T cells (especially cord-blood T cells) are too immature to control CMV replication. If the T cells from the donor have never encountered CMV and the recipient carries the virus, the patient is at maximal risk of severe disease. Reactivation disease or superinfection with another strain from the donor also can occur in CMV-positive recipients, but clinical manifestations are typically less severe, presumably because of CMV-specific memory in transplanted donor T cells. Most patients infected with CMV who undergo HSC transplantation excrete virus, with or without clinical findings. Serious CMV disease is much more common among allogeneic than autologous recipients and is often associated with GVHD. In addition to pneumonia and marrow suppression (and, less often, graft failure), manifestations of CMV disease in HSC transplant recipients include fever with or without arthralgias, myalgias, hepatitis, and esophagitis. CMV ulcerations occur in both the lower and the upper gastrointestinal tract, and it may be difficult to distinguish diarrhea due to GVHD from that due to CMV infection. The finding of CMV in the liver of a patient with GVHD does not necessarily mean that CMV is responsible for hepatic enzyme abnormalities. It is interesting that ocular and neurologic manifestations of CMV infections are common in patients with AIDS but uncommon in patients who develop CMV disease after transplantation.

Management of CMV disease in HSC transplant recipients includes strategies directed at prophylaxis, preemptive therapy (suppression of silent replication), and treatment of disease. Prophylaxis results in a lower incidence of disease at the cost of treating many patients who otherwise would not require therapy. Because of the high fatality rate associated with CMV pneumonia in these patients and the difficulty of early diagnosis of CMV infection, prophylactic IV ganciclovir or oral valganciclovir has been used in some centers and has been shown to prevent CMV disease during the period of maximal vulnerability (from engraftment to day 120 after transplantation). Ganciclovir also prevents HSV reactivation and reduces the risk of VZV reactivation; thus, acyclovir prophylaxis should be discontinued when ganciclovir is administered. The foremost problem with the administration of ganciclovir relates to adverse effects, which include dose-related bone marrow suppression (thrombocytopenia, leukopenia, anemia, and pancytopenia). Because the frequency of CMV pneumonia is lower among autologous HSC transplant recipients (2–7%) than among allogeneic HSC transplant recipients (10–40%), prophylaxis in the former group is not routine. Letermovir, an oral agent that does not commonly cause bone marrow suppression, is effective in suppressing CMV reactivation in allogeneic HSC transplant recipients.

Preemptive treatment of CMV—that is, initiation of therapy with drugs only after CMV is detected in blood by a nucleic acid amplification test (NAAT)—is used at most centers. To limit variability between tests, the World Health Organization (WHO) has developed an international reference standard for measurement of CMV load by NAAT-based assays. A positive test (or increasing viral load) prompts the initiation of preemptive therapy with ganciclovir. Preemptive approaches that target patients who have quantitative NAAT evidence of CMV infection can still lead to unnecessary treatment of many individuals with drugs that have adverse effects on the basis of a laboratory test that is not highly predictive of disease; however, invasive disease, particularly in the form of pulmonary infection, is difficult to treat and is associated with high mortality rates. When prophylaxis or preemptive therapy is stopped, late manifestations of CMV replication may occur, although by then the HSC transplant patient is often equipped with improved graft function and is better able to combat disease. Cord-blood transplant recipients are especially vulnerable to disease caused by members of the human herpesvirus family, including CMV. Implementation of the WHO standard for CMV load measurement will facilitate large-scale comparative studies and thus the establishment of optimal guidelines for distinct patient subsets.

CMV pneumonia in HSC transplant recipients (unlike that in other clinical settings) is often treated with both IV immunoglobulin (IVIg) and ganciclovir. In patients who cannot tolerate ganciclovir, foscarnet is a useful alternative, although it may produce nephrotoxicity and electrolyte imbalance. When neither ganciclovir nor foscarnet is clinically tolerated, cidofovir can be used; however, its efficacy is less well established, and its side effects include nephrotoxicity. A lipid-conjugate form of cidofovir, brincidofovir, appears to have more activity and less toxicity than cidofovir and is in clinical trials. Transfusion of CMV-specific T cells from the donor has decreased viral load in a small series of patients; this result suggests that immunotherapy (e.g., banked T cells) may play a role in the management of this disease in the future. **For further discussion, see Chap. 195.**

Human Herpesviruses 6 and 7 Human herpesvirus type 6 (HHV-6), the cause of roseola in children, is a ubiquitous herpesvirus that is reactivated (as determined by quantitative plasma polymerase chain reaction [PCR]) in ~50% of HSC transplant recipients 2–4 weeks after transplantation. Reactivation is more common among patients requiring glucocorticoids for GVHD and among those receiving second transplants. Reactivation of HHV-6, primarily type B, may be associated with delayed monocyte and platelet engraftment. Limbic encephalitis developing after transplantation has been associated with HHV-6 in cerebrospinal fluid (CSF). The causality of the association is not well defined; in several cases, plasma viremia was detected long before the onset of encephalitis. Nevertheless, most patients with encephalitis had very high viral loads in plasma at the time of CNS illness, and viral antigen has been detected in hippocampal astrocytes. HHV-6 DNA is sometimes found in lung samples after transplantation. However, its role in pneumonitis is unclear, as co-pathogens are frequently present. While HHV-6 is susceptible to foscarnet or cidofovir (and possibly to ganciclovir) in vitro, the efficacy of antiviral treatment has not been well studied. Although treatment of HHV-6 encephalitis is recommended, there are no randomized, controlled trials demonstrating efficacy of any antiviral agent, and treatment of DNAemia (the detection of DNA in samples of plasma, whole blood, and isolated peripheral-blood leukocytes) is not recommended. Little is known about the related herpesvirus HHV-7 or its role in posttransplantation infection. **For further discussion, see Chap. 195.**

Epstein-Barr Virus Primary EBV infection can be fatal to HSC transplant recipients; EBV reactivation can cause EBV B-cell lymphoproliferative disease (EBV-LPD), which may also be fatal to patients taking immunosuppressive drugs. Latent EBV infection of B cells leads to several interesting phenomena in HSC transplant recipients. The marrow ablation that occurs as part of the HSC transplantation procedure may sometimes eliminate latent EBV from the host. Infection can then be reacquired immediately after transplantation by transfer of infected donor B cells. Rarely, transplantation from a seronegative donor may result in a cure. The recipient is then at risk for a second primary infection.

EBV-LPD can develop in the recipient's B cells (if any survive marrow ablation) but is more likely to be a consequence of outgrowth of infected donor cells. Both lytic replication and latent replication of EBV are more likely during immunosuppression (e.g., they are associated with GVHD and the use of antibodies to T cells). Although less likely in autologous transplantation, reactivation can occur in T cell–depleted autologous recipients (e.g., patients being given antibodies to T cells for the treatment of T-cell lymphoma with marrow depletion). EBV-LPD, which can become apparent as early as 1–3 months after engraftment, can cause high fevers and cervical adenopathy resembling the symptoms of infectious mononucleosis but more commonly presents as an extranodal mass. The incidence of EBV-LPD among allogeneic HSC transplant recipients is 0.6–1%, which contrasts with figures of ~5% for renal transplant recipients and up to 20% for cardiac transplant patients. In all cases, EBV-LPD is more likely to occur with high-dose, prolonged immunosuppression, especially that caused by the use of antibodies to T cells, glucocorticoids, and calcineurin inhibitors (e.g., cyclosporine, tacrolimus). Cord-blood recipients constitute another high-risk group because of delayed T-cell function. Ganciclovir, administered to preempt CMV disease, may reduce EBV lytic replication and thereby diminish the pool of B cells that can become newly infected and give rise to LPD. Increasing evidence indicates that replacement of calcineurin inhibitors with mTOR inhibitors (e.g., rapamycin) exerts an antiproliferative effect on EBV-infected B cells that decreases the likelihood of development of LPD or unrelated proliferative disorders associated with transplant-related immunosuppression.

PCR can be used to monitor EBV production after HSC transplantation. High or increasing viral loads predict an enhanced likelihood of EBV-LPD development and should prompt rapid reduction of immunosuppression and a search for nodal or extranodal disease. If reduction of immunosuppression does not have the desired effect, administration of a monoclonal antibody to CD20 (e.g., rituximab) for the treatment of B-cell lymphomas that express this surface protein has elicited dramatic responses and currently constitutes first-line therapy for CD20-positive EBV-LPD. However, long-term suppression of new antibody responses accompanies therapy, and recurrences are common. Additional B cell–directed antibodies, including anti-CD22, are under study. The role of antiviral drugs is uncertain because no available agents have been documented to have activity against the different forms of latent EBV infection. Diminishing lytic replication and virion production in these patients would theoretically produce a statistical decrease in the frequency of latent disease by decreasing the number of virions available to cause additional infection. In case reports and animal studies, ganciclovir and/or high-dose zidovudine, together with other agents, have been used to eradicate EBV-LPD and CNS lymphomas, another EBV-associated complication of transplantation. Both interferon and retinoic acid have been employed in the treatment of EBV-LPD, as has IVIg, but no large-scale prospective studies have assessed the efficacy of any of these agents. Several additional drugs are undergoing preclinical evaluation. Standard chemotherapeutic regimens are used if the disease persists after reduction of immunosuppressive agents and administration of antibodies. EBV-specific T cells generated from the donor have been used experimentally to prevent and treat EBV-LPD in allogeneic recipients, and efforts are underway to increase the activity and specificity of ex vivo–generated T cells. **For further discussion, see Chap. 194.**

Human Herpesvirus 8 (KSHV) The gammaherpesvirus KSHV, which is causally associated with Kaposi's sarcoma, primary effusion lymphoma, and multicentric Castleman's disease, has rarely resulted in disease in HSC transplant recipients, although some cases of virus-associated marrow aplasia have been reported in the peritransplantation period. The relatively low seroprevalence of KSHV in the population and the limited duration of profound T-cell suppression after HSC transplantation provide a plausible explanation for the currently low incidence of KSHV disease compared with that in recipients of solid organ transplants and patients with HIV infection. **For further discussion, see Chap. 195.**

Other (Non-Herpes) Viruses and Pneumonia The diagnosis of pneumonia in HSC transplant recipients poses special problems. Because patients have undergone treatment with multiple chemotherapeutic agents and sometimes irradiation, their differential diagnosis should include—in addition to bacterial and fungal pneumonia—CMV pneumonitis, pneumonia of other viral etiologies, parasitic pneumonia, diffuse alveolar hemorrhage, and chemical- or radiation-associated pneumonitis. Since fungi and viruses (e.g., influenza A and B viruses, respiratory syncytial virus [RSV], parainfluenza virus types 1–4, adenovirus, enterovirus, bocavirus, human metapneumovirus, coronavirus, and rhinovirus [increasingly detected by multiplex PCR]) also can cause pneumonia in this setting, it is important to obtain a specific diagnosis. Diagnostic modalities include Gram's stain, microbiologic culture, antigen testing, and—increasingly—multipathogen PCR and mass spectrometry assays. HSC transplant recipients are likely to have difficulty responding to SARS-CoV-2 infections and may have long courses of disease and/or secondary infections.

■ GLOBAL CONSIDERATIONS

M. tuberculosis has been an uncommon cause of pneumonia among HSC transplant recipients in Western countries (accounting for <0.1–0.2% of cases) but is common in Hong Kong (5.5%) and in countries where the prevalence of tuberculosis is high. The recipient's exposure history is clearly critical in an assessment of posttransplantation infections.

Both RSV and parainfluenza viruses, particularly type 3, can cause severe or even fatal pneumonia in HSC transplant recipients. Infections with both of these agents sometimes occur as disastrous nosocomial epidemics. Therapy with palivizumab or ribavirin for RSV infection remains controversial. New agents, some host-directed, are under study. Influenza also occurs in HSC transplant recipients and generally mirrors the presence of infection in the community. Progression to pneumonia is more common when infection occurs early after transplantation and when the recipient is lymphopenic. The neuraminidase inhibitors oseltamivir (oral) and zanamivir (aerosolized) are active against both influenza A virus and influenza B virus and are a reasonable treatment option. Parenteral forms of neuraminidase inhibitors, such as peramivir (intravenous), are available in some countries, and several new oral agents are still being assessed in trials. Baloxavir, a single-dose oral agent, has excellent activity, but resistance may occur. An important preventive measure is immunization of household members, hospital staff members, and other frequent contacts. Adenoviruses can be isolated from HSC transplant recipients at rates varying from 5 to ≥18%. Like CMV infection, adenovirus infection usually occurs in the first to third month after transplantation and is often asymptomatic, although pneumonia, hemorrhagic cystitis/nephritis, severe gastroenteritis with hemorrhage, and fatal disseminated infection have been reported and may be strain-specific. Banked virus-specific T-cell therapy is under study for adenovirus infection (as well as for CMV and EBV infections).

Although diverse respiratory viruses can sometimes cause severe pneumonia and respiratory failure in HSC transplant recipients, mild or even asymptomatic infection may be more common. For example, rhinoviruses and coronaviruses are frequent co-pathogens in HSC transplant recipients; however, whether they independently contribute to significant pulmonary infection is unknown. At present, the overall contribution of these viral respiratory pathogens to the burden of lower respiratory tract disease in HSC transplant recipients requires further study. Infections with parvovirus B19 (presenting as anemia or occasionally as pancytopenia) and disseminated enteroviruses (sometimes fatal) can occur. Parvovirus B19 infection can be treated with IVIg (**Chap. 197**).

Rotaviruses, a cause of gastroenteritis in HSC transplant recipients, cause disease more frequently in children. Norovirus is a common cause of vomiting and diarrhea, and symptoms can be prolonged in HSC recipients. The BK virus (a polyomavirus) is found at high titers in the urine of patients who are profoundly immunosuppressed. BK viruria may be associated with hemorrhagic cystitis in these patients. In contrast to its incidence among patients with impaired T-cell function due to AIDS (4–5%), progressive multifocal leukoencephalopathy caused by the related JC virus is relatively rare among HSC transplant recipients (**Chap. 138**). When transmitted by mosquitoes or by blood transfusion, West Nile virus (WNV) can cause encephalitis and death after HSC transplantation.

INFECTIONS IN SOLID ORGAN TRANSPLANT RECIPIENTS

Rates of morbidity and mortality among recipients of solid organ transplants (SOTs) are reduced by the use of effective antibiotics. The organisms that cause acute infections in recipients of SOTs are different from those that infect HSC transplant recipients because SOT recipients do not go through a period of neutropenia. As the transplantation procedure involves major surgery, however, SOT recipients are subject to infections at anastomotic sites and to wound infections. Compared with HSC transplant recipients, SOT patients are immunosuppressed for longer periods (often permanently). Thus, they are susceptible to many of the same organisms as patients with chronically impaired T-cell immunity (**Chap. 74**, especially **Table 74-1**). Moreover, the persistent HLA mismatch between recipient immune cells (e.g., effector T cells) and the donor organ (allograft) places the organ at permanently increased risk of infection.

During the early period (<1 month after transplantation; **Table 143-4**), infections are most commonly caused by extracellular bacteria (staphylococci, streptococci, enterococci, and *E. coli* and other gram-negative organisms, including nosocomial organisms with broad antibiotic resistance), which often originate in surgical-wound or anastomotic sites. The type of transplant largely determines the spectrum of infection. The incidence and type of surgical site infection vary dramatically with the organ transplanted, with renal transplants having the lowest incidence and intestinal and multivisceral transplants having the highest incidence and the most varied types of organisms. *S. aureus* and coagulase-negative *Staphylococcus* are among the most common causes of infection following renal transplantation, while lung transplant recipients, in addition to being infected with *Staphylococcus*, are subject to infections with *Burkholderia*, *Pseudomonas*, and *Stenotrophomonas* as well. In subsequent weeks, the consequences of the administration of agents that suppress cell-mediated immunity become apparent, and acquisition—or, more commonly, reactivation—of viruses, mycobacteria, endemic fungi, and parasites (from the recipient or from the transplanted organ) can occur. CMV infection is often a problem, particularly in the first 6 months after transplantation, and may present as severe systemic disease or as infection of the transplanted organ. HHV-6 reactivation (assessed by plasma PCR) occurs within the first 2–4 weeks after transplantation and may be associated with fever, leukopenia, and very rare cases of encephalitis. Data suggest that replication of HHV-6 and HHV-7 may exacerbate CMV-induced

TABLE 143-4 Common Infections after Solid Organ Transplantation, by Site of Infection

	PERIOD AFTER TRANSPLANTATION		
INFECTED SITE	**EARLY (<1 MONTH)**	**MIDDLE (1–4 MONTHS)**	**LATE (>6 MONTHS)**
Donor organ	Bacterial and fungal infections of the graft, anastomotic site, and surgical wound	CMV infection	EBV infection (may present in allograft organ)
Systemic	Bacteremia and candidemia (often resulting from central venous catheter colonization)	CMV infection (fever, bone marrow suppression)	CMV infection, especially in patients given early posttransplantation prophylaxis; EBV proliferative syndromes (may occur in donor organs)
Lung	Bacterial aspiration pneumonia with prevalent nosocomial organisms associated with intubation and sedation	*Pneumocystis* infection; CMV pneumonia; *Aspergillus* infection	*Pneumocystis* infection; granulomatous lung diseases (nocardial and reactivated fungal and mycobacterial diseases)
Kidney	Bacterial and fungal (*Candida*) infections (cystitis, pyelonephritis) associated with urinary tract catheters (highest risk in kidney transplantation)	BK virus infection (associated with nephropathy); JC virus infection	Bacterial infections (late urinary tract infections, usually not associated with bacteremia); BK virus infection (nephropathy, graft failure, generalized vasculopathy)
Liver and biliary tract	Cholangitis	CMV hepatitis	CMV hepatitis
Heart		*Toxoplasma gondii* infection (highest risk in heart transplantation); endocarditis (*Aspergillus* and gram-negative organisms more common than in the general population)	*T. gondii* (highest risk in heart transplantation)
Gastrointestinal tract	Peritonitis, especially after liver transplantation	Colitis secondary to *Clostridioides difficile* infection (risk can persist)	Colitis secondary to *C. difficile* infection (risk can persist)
Central nervous system		*Listeria* infection (meningitis); *T. gondii* infection; CMV infection	Listerial meningitis; cryptococcal meningitis; nocardial abscess; JC virus-associated PML

Abbreviations: CMV, cytomegalovirus; EBV, Epstein-Barr virus; PML, progressive multifocal leukoencephalopathy.

disease. CMV is associated not only with generalized immunosuppression but also with organ-specific, rejection-related syndromes: glomerulopathy in kidney transplant recipients, bronchiolitis obliterans in lung transplant recipients, vasculopathy in heart transplant recipients, and the vanishing bile duct syndrome in liver transplant recipients. A complex interplay between increased CMV replication and enhanced graft rejection is well established: elevated immunosuppression leads to increased CMV replication, which is associated with graft rejection. For this reason, considerable attention has been focused on the diagnosis, prophylaxis, and treatment of CMV infection in SOT recipients. Early transmission of WNV to transplant recipients from a donated organ or transfused blood has been reported; however, the risk of WNV acquisition has been reduced by implementation of screening procedures. In rare instances, rabies virus and lymphocytic choriomeningitis virus also have been acutely transmitted in this setting; although accompanied by distinct clinical syndromes, both viral infections have resulted in fatal encephalitis. As screening for unusual viruses is not routine, only vigilant assessment of the prospective donor is likely to prevent the use of an infected organ.

Beyond 6 months after transplantation, infections characteristic of patients with defects in cell-mediated immunity—e.g., infections with *Listeria, Nocardia, Rhodococcus*, mycobacteria, various fungi, and other intracellular pathogens—may be a problem. International patients and global travelers may experience reactivation of dormant infections with trypanosomes, *Leishmania, Plasmodium, Strongyloides*, and other parasites. Reactivation of latent *M. tuberculosis* infection, while rare in Western nations, is far more common among persons from developing countries. The recipient is typically the source, although reactivation and spread from the donor organ can occur. While pulmonary disease remains most common, atypical sites can be involved and mortality rates can be high (up to 30%). Vigilance, prophylaxis/preemptive therapy (when indicated), and rapid diagnosis and treatment of infections can be lifesaving in SOT recipients, who, unlike most HSC transplant recipients, continue to be immunosuppressed.

SOT recipients are susceptible to EBV-LPD from as early as 2 months to many years after transplantation. The prevalence of this complication is increased by potent and prolonged use of T cell–suppressive drugs. Decreasing the degree of immunosuppression may in some cases reverse the condition. Among SOT patients, those with heart and lung transplants—who receive the most intensive immunosuppressive regimens—are most likely to develop EBV-LPD, particularly in the lungs. Although the disease usually originates in recipient B cells, several cases of donor origin, particularly in the transplanted organ, have been noted. High organ-specific content of B lymphoid tissues (e.g., bronchus-associated lymphoid tissue in the lung), anatomic factors (e.g., lack of access of host T cells to the transplanted organ because of disturbed lymphatics), and differences in major histocompatibility loci between the host T cells and the organ (e.g., lack of cell migration or lack of effective T-cell/macrophage/dendritic cell cooperation) may result in defective elimination of EBV-infected B cells. SOT recipients are also highly susceptible to developing Kaposi's sarcoma and, less frequently, to the B cell–proliferative disorders associated with KSHV, such as primary effusion lymphoma and multicentric Castleman's disease. Kaposi's sarcoma is 550–1000 times more common among SOT recipients than in the general population; it can develop very rapidly after transplantation and can also occur in the allograft. However, because the seroprevalence of KSHV is very low in Western countries, Kaposi's sarcoma is not common. Recipients (or donors) from Iceland, the Middle East, Mediterranean countries, and Africa are at highest risk of disease. Data suggest that a switch of immunosuppressive agents—from calcineurin inhibitors (cyclosporine, tacrolimus) to mTOR pathway–active agents (sirolimus, everolimus)—after adequate wound healing may significantly reduce the likelihood of developing Kaposi's sarcoma and perhaps of EBV-LPD and certain other posttransplantation malignancies.

■ KIDNEY TRANSPLANTATION

See Table 143-4.

Early Infections Bacteria often cause infections that develop in the period immediately after kidney transplantation. There is a role for perioperative antibiotic prophylaxis, and each center should consider local resistance patterns. Administration within 60–120 minutes of the surgical incision is recommended. Dosing should be adjusted for weight and duration of surgery. Urinary tract infections developing soon after transplantation are usually related to anatomic alterations resulting from surgery. Such early infections may require prolonged treatment (e.g., 6 weeks of antibiotic administration for pyelonephritis). Urinary tract infections that occur >6 months after transplantation may be treated for shorter periods because they do not seem to be associated with the high rate of pyelonephritis or relapse seen with infections that occur during the first 3 months.

Prophylaxis with TMP-SMX for the first 4–6 months after transplantation decreases the incidence of early and middle-period infections (see below, Table 143-4, and **Table 143-5**).

Middle-Period Infections Because of continuing immuno-suppression, kidney transplant recipients are predisposed to lung infections characteristic of those in patients with T-cell deficiency (i.e., infections with intracellular bacteria, mycobacteria, nocardiae, fungi, viruses, and parasites). A high mortality rate associated with *Legionella pneumophila* infection (**Chap. 159**) led to the closing of renal transplant units in hospitals with endemic legionellosis.

About 50% of all renal transplant recipients presenting with fever 1–4 months after transplantation have evidence of CMV disease; CMV itself accounts for the fever in more than two-thirds of cases and thus is the predominant pathogen during this period. CMV infection (**Chap. 195**) may also present as arthralgias, myalgias, or organ-specific symptoms. During this period, this infection may represent primary disease (in the case of a seronegative recipient of a kidney from a seropositive donor) or may represent reactivation disease or superinfection.

TABLE 143-5 Prophylactic Regimens Commonly Used to Decrease Risk of Infection in Transplant Recipients[a]

RISK FACTOR	ORGANISM	PROPHYLACTIC DRUG	EXAMINATION(S)[b]
Travel to or residence in an area with known risk of endemic fungal infection	*Histoplasma, Blastomyces, Coccidioides*	Triazoles considered in context of clinical and laboratory assessment	Chest radiography, antigen testing, serology
Latent herpesviruses	HSV, VZV, CMV, EBV	Acyclovir after HSC transplantation to prevent HSV and VZV infection or reactivation; letermovir or ganciclovir to prevent CMV infection, with possible effect on EBV/KSHV (HHV-8)/HHV-6 infections in some settings	Serologic tests for HSV, VZV, CMV, HHV-6, EBV, KSHV (HHV-8); PCR
Latent fungi and parasites	*Pneumocystis jirovecii, Toxoplasma gondii*	Trimethoprim-sulfamethoxazole (or alternatives)	Serologic test for *Toxoplasma*
History of exposure to active or latent tuberculosis	*Mycobacterium tuberculosis*	Isoniazid or rifampin in patients with recent seroconversion or positive chest imaging and/or no previous treatment	Chest imaging; TST and/or cell-based assay

[a]For information on latent infection with hepatitis B or C virus, see **Chap. 341**. [b]Serologic examination, tuberculin skin test, and interferon assays may be less reliable after transplantation.

Abbreviations: CMV, cytomegalovirus; EBV, Epstein-Barr virus; HHV, human herpesvirus; HSC, hematopoietic stem cell; HSV, herpes simplex virus; KSHV, Kaposi's sarcoma–associated herpesvirus; PCR, polymerase chain reaction; TST, tuberculin skin test; VZV, varicella-zoster virus.

Patients may have atypical lymphocytosis. Unlike immunocompetent patients, however, they rarely have lymphadenopathy or splenomegaly. Therefore, clinical suspicion and laboratory confirmation are necessary for diagnosis. The clinical syndrome may be accompanied by bone marrow suppression (particularly leukopenia). CMV also causes glomerulopathy and is associated with an increased incidence of other opportunistic infections. Because of the frequency and severity of disease, a considerable effort has been made to prevent and treat CMV infection in renal transplant recipients. Ganciclovir (or valganciclovir) is beneficial for prophylaxis (when indicated) and for the treatment of serious CMV disease. The availability of valganciclovir has allowed most centers to move to oral prophylaxis for transplant recipients. Infection with the other herpesviruses may become evident within 6 months after transplantation or later. Early after transplantation, HSV may cause either oral or anogenital lesions that are usually responsive to acyclovir. Large ulcerating lesions in the anogenital area may lead to bladder and rectal dysfunction and may predispose the patient to bacterial infection. VZV may cause fatal disseminated infection in nonimmune kidney transplant recipients, but in immune patients, reactivation zoster usually does not disseminate outside the dermatome; thus, disseminated VZV infection is a less fearsome complication in kidney transplantation than in HSC transplantation. HHV-6 reactivation may occur and (although usually asymptomatic) may be associated with fever, rash, marrow suppression, or rare instances of renal impairment, hepatitis, colitis, or encephalitis.

EBV disease is more serious; it may present as an extranodal proliferation of B cells that invade the CNS, nasopharynx, liver, small bowel, heart, and other organs, including the transplanted kidney. The disease is diagnosed by identifying a mass of proliferating EBV-positive B cells. The incidence of EBV-LPD is elevated among patients who acquire EBV infection from the donor and among patients given high doses of cyclosporine, tacrolimus, glucocorticoids, and anti–T-cell antibodies. Disease may regress once immunocompetence is restored. KSHV infection can be transmitted with the donor kidney and result in the development of Kaposi's sarcoma, although it more often represents reactivation of latent infection in the recipient. Kaposi's sarcoma often appears within 1 year after transplantation, although the time of onset ranges widely (1 month to ~20 years). Avoidance of immunosuppressive agents that inhibit calcineurin has been associated with less Kaposi's sarcoma, less EBV disease, and even less CMV replication. The use of rapamycin (sirolimus) has independently led to regression of Kaposi's sarcoma.

The polyomaviruses BK virus and JC virus (polyomavirus hominis types 1 and 2) have been cultured from the urine of kidney transplant recipients (as they have from that of HSC transplant recipients) in the setting of profound immunosuppression. High levels of BK virus replication detected by PCR in urine and blood are predictive of pathology, especially in the setting of renal transplantation. JC virus may rarely cause similar disease in kidney transplantation. Urinary excretion of BK virus and BK viremia are associated with the development of ureteral strictures, polyomavirus-associated nephropathy (1–10% of renal transplant recipients), and (less commonly) generalized vasculopathy. Timely detection and early reduction of immunosuppression are critical and can reduce rates of graft loss related to polyomavirus-associated nephropathy from 90 to 10–30%. Therapeutic responses to IVIg, quinolones, leflunomide, and cidofovir have been reported, but the efficacy of these agents has not been substantiated through adequate clinical study. Most centers approach the problem by reducing immunosuppression in an effort to enhance host immunity and decrease viral titers. JC virus is associated with rare cases of progressive multifocal leukoencephalopathy. Adenoviruses may persist and cause hemorrhagic nephritis/cystitis with continued immunosuppression in these patients, but disseminated disease, like that seen in HSC transplant recipients, is much less common.

Kidney transplant recipients are also subject to infections with other intracellular organisms. These patients may develop pulmonary infections with *Mycobacterium, Aspergillus*, and *Mucor* species as well as infections with other pathogens in which the T-cell/macrophage axis plays an important role. *L. monocytogenes* is a common cause of bacteremia ≥1 month after renal transplantation and should be seriously considered in renal transplant recipients presenting with fever and headache. Kidney transplant recipients may develop *Salmonella* bacteremia, which can lead to endovascular infections and require prolonged therapy. Pulmonary infections with *Pneumocystis* are common unless the patient is maintained on TMP-SMX prophylaxis. Acute interstitial nephritis caused by TMP-SMX is rare. However, because transient increases in creatinine (artifactual) and hyperkalemia (manageable) can occur, early discontinuation of prophylaxis, especially after kidney transplantation, is recommended by some groups. Although additional monitoring is indicated, the benefits of TMP-SMX in kidney transplant recipients may outweigh the risks; otherwise, second-line prophylactic agents should be used. *Nocardia* infection **(Chap. 174)** may present in the skin, bones, and lungs or in the CNS, where it usually takes the form of single or multiple brain abscesses. Nocardiosis generally occurs ≥1 month after transplantation and may follow immunosuppressive treatment for an episode of rejection. Pulmonary manifestations most commonly consist of localized disease with or without cavities, but the disease may be disseminated. The diagnosis is made by culture of the organism from sputum or from the involved nodule. As it is for *P. jirovecii* infection, prophylaxis with TMP-SMX is often efficacious in the prevention of nocardiosis.

Toxoplasmosis can occur in seropositive patients but is less common than in other transplantation settings, usually developing in the first few months after kidney transplantation. Again, TMP-SMX is helpful in prevention. In endemic areas, histoplasmosis, coccidioidomycosis, and blastomycosis may cause pulmonary infiltrates or disseminated disease.

Late Infections Late infections (>6 months after kidney transplantation) may involve the CNS and include CMV retinitis as well as other CNS manifestations of CMV disease. Patients (particularly those whose immunosuppression has been increased) are at risk for subacute meningitis due to *Cryptococcus neoformans*. Cryptococcal disease may present in an insidious manner (sometimes as a skin infection before the development of clear CNS findings). *Listeria* meningitis may have an acute presentation and requires prompt therapy to avoid a fatal outcome. TMP-SMX prophylaxis may reduce the frequency of *Listeria* infections.

Patients who continue to take glucocorticoids are predisposed to ongoing infection. "Transplant elbow," a recurrent bacterial infection in and around the elbow that is thought to result from a combination of poor tensile strength of the skin of steroid-treated patients and steroid-induced proximal myopathy, requires patients to push themselves up with their elbows to get out of chairs. Bouts of cellulitis (usually caused by *S. aureus*) recur until patients are provided with elbow protection.

Kidney transplant recipients are susceptible to invasive fungal infections, including those due to *Aspergillus* and *Rhizopus*, which may present as superficial lesions before dissemination. Mycobacterial infection (particularly that with *Mycobacterium marinum*) can be diagnosed by skin examination. Infection with *Prototheca wickerhamii* (an achlorophyllic alga) has been diagnosed by skin biopsy. Warts caused by human papillomaviruses (HPVs) are a late consequence of persistent immunosuppression; imiquimod or other forms of local therapy are usually satisfactory. Merkel cell carcinoma, a rare and aggressive neuroendocrine skin tumor whose frequency is increased five-fold in elderly SOT (especially kidney) recipients, is causally linked to a novel polyomavirus, Merkel cell polyomavirus.

Notably, although BK virus replication and virus-associated disease can be detected far earlier, polyomavirus-associated nephropathy is clinically diagnosed at a median of ~300 days and thus qualifies as a late-onset disease. With the establishment of better screening procedures (e.g., urine cytology, urine nucleic acid load, plasma PCR), disease onset is being detected earlier (see "Middle-Period Infections," above), and preemptive strategies (decrease or modification of immunosuppression) are being instituted more promptly, as the efficacy of antiviral therapy is not well established.

HEART TRANSPLANTATION

Early Infections Sternal wound infection and mediastinitis are early complications of heart transplantation. An indolent course is common, with fever or a mildly elevated white blood cell count preceding the development of site tenderness or drainage. Clinical suspicion based on evidence of sternal instability and failure to heal may lead to the diagnosis. Common microbial residents of the skin (e.g., *S. aureus*, including methicillin-resistant strains, and *Staphylococcus epidermidis*) as well as gram-negative organisms (e.g., *Pseudomonas aeruginosa*) and fungi (e.g., *Candida*) are often involved. In rare cases, mediastinitis in heart transplant recipients can also be due to *Mycoplasma hominis* (**Chap. 188**); since this organism requires an anaerobic environment for growth and may be difficult to see on conventional medium, the laboratory should be alerted that its involvement is suspected. *M. hominis* mediastinitis has been cured with a combination of surgical debridement (sometimes requiring muscle-flap placement) and the administration of clindamycin and tetracycline. Organisms associated with mediastinitis may sometimes be cultured from pericardial fluid.

Middle-Period Infections *T. gondii* (**Chap. 228**) residing in the heart of a seropositive donor may be transmitted to a seronegative recipient. Thus, serologic screening for *T. gondii* infection is important before and in the months after cardiac transplantation. Rarely, active disease can be introduced at the time of transplantation. The overall incidence of toxoplasmosis is so high in the setting of heart transplantation that some prophylaxis is always warranted. Although alternatives are available, the most frequently used agent is TMP-SMX, which prevents infection with *Pneumocystis* as well as with *Nocardia* and several other bacterial pathogens. CMV also has been transmitted by heart transplantation. *Toxoplasma*, *Nocardia*, and *Aspergillus* can cause CNS infections. *L. monocytogenes* meningitis should be considered in heart transplant recipients with fever and headache.

CMV infection is associated with poor outcomes after heart transplantation. The virus is usually detected 1–2 months after transplantation, causes early signs and laboratory abnormalities (usually fever and atypical lymphocytosis or leukopenia and thrombocytopenia) at 2–3 months, and can produce severe disease (e.g., pneumonia) at 3–4 months. An interesting observation is that seropositive recipients usually develop viremia faster than patients whose primary CMV infection is a consequence of transplantation. Between 40 and 70% of patients develop symptomatic CMV disease in the form of (1) CMV pneumonia, the form most likely to be fatal; (2) CMV esophagitis and gastritis, sometimes accompanied by abdominal pain with or without ulcerations and bleeding; and (3) CMV syndrome, consisting of CMV in the bloodstream along with fever, leukopenia, thrombocytopenia, and hepatic enzyme abnormalities. Ganciclovir is efficacious in the treatment of CMV infection; prophylaxis with ganciclovir or possibly with other antiviral agents may reduce the overall incidence of CMV-related disease.

Late Infections EBV infection usually presents as a lymphoma-like proliferation of B cells late after heart transplantation, particularly in patients maintained on intense immunosuppressive therapy. A subset of heart and heart–lung transplant recipients may develop early fulminant EBV-LPD (within 2 months). Treatment includes the reduction of immunosuppression (if possible), the use of glucocorticoid and calcineurin inhibitor–sparing regimens, and the consideration of therapy with anti–B-cell antibodies (rituximab and possibly others). Immunomodulatory and antiviral agents continue to be studied. Ganciclovir prophylaxis for CMV disease may indirectly reduce the risk of EBV-LPD through reduced spread of replicating EBV to naïve B cells. Aggressive chemotherapy is a last resort, as discussed earlier for HSC transplant recipients. KSHV-associated disease, including Kaposi's sarcoma and primary effusion lymphoma, has been reported in heart transplant recipients. GVHD prophylaxis with sirolimus may decrease the risk of both rejection and outgrowth of KSHV-infected cells. Antitumor therapy is discussed in **Chap. 73**. Prophylaxis for *Pneumocystis* infection is required for these patients (see "Lung Transplantation, Late Infections," below).

Left Ventricular Assist Devices Increasingly, left ventricular assist devices (LVADs) have been used as a "bridge to transplant." These devices are implantable pumps that assist failing left ventricles. The internal pump is connected to an external power source through a subcutaneously tunneled cable termed a *driveline*, and they can be used for long periods (>80% lasting at least a year). However, infections are common, largely in the driveline, and affect 12–35% of patients. *S. aureus* and coagulase-negative staphylococci are the most common causes of infection, followed by enterococci, *Corynebacterium*, *P. aeruginosa*, *Klebsiella* species, and *E. coli*. A variety of prophylactic antibiotic regimens have been used by various centers. The most common cause of infection following surgery is thought to relate to trauma to the driveline, and local care of the entry site is important.

LUNG TRANSPLANTATION

Early Infections It is not surprising that lung transplant recipients are predisposed to the development of pneumonia. The combination of ischemia and the resulting mucosal damage, together with accompanying denervation and lack of lymphatic drainage, probably contributes to the high rate of pneumonia (66% in one series). The prophylactic use of high doses of broad-spectrum antibiotics for the first 3–4 days after surgery may decrease the incidence of pneumonia. Gram-negative pathogens (Enterobacteriaceae and *Pseudomonas* species) are troublesome in the first 2 weeks after surgery (the period of maximal vulnerability). Pneumonia can also be caused by *Candida* (including drug-resistant strains of *C. auris*), possibly as a result of colonization of the donor lung, and by *Aspergillus* and *Cryptococcus*. Many centers use antifungal prophylaxis (typically fluconazole or liposomal amphotericin B) for the first 1–2 weeks.

Mediastinitis may occur at an even higher rate among lung transplant recipients than among heart transplant recipients and most commonly develops within 2 weeks of surgery. In the absence of prophylaxis, pneumonitis due to CMV (which may be transmitted as a consequence of transplantation) usually presents between 2 weeks and 3 months after surgery, with primary disease occurring later than reactivation disease.

Middle-Period Infections The incidence of CMV infection, either reactivated or primary, is 75–100% if either the donor or the recipient is seropositive for CMV. CMV-induced disease after SOT appears to be most severe in recipients of lung and heart–lung transplants. Whether this severity relates to the mismatch in lung antigen presentation and host immune cells or is attributable to nonimmunologic factors is unknown. More than half of lung transplant recipients with symptomatic CMV disease have pneumonia. Difficulty in distinguishing the radiographic picture of CMV infection from that of other infections or from organ rejection further complicates therapy. CMV can also cause bronchiolitis obliterans in lung transplants. The development of pneumonitis related to HSV has led to the prophylactic use of acyclovir. Such prophylaxis may also decrease rates of CMV disease, but ganciclovir is more active against CMV and is also active against HSV. The prophylaxis of CMV infection with IV ganciclovir—or increasingly with valganciclovir, the oral alternative—is recommended for lung transplant recipients. Antiviral alternatives are discussed in the earlier section on HSC transplantation. Although the overall incidence of serious disease is decreased during prophylaxis, late disease may occur when prophylaxis is stopped—a pattern observed increasingly in recent years. With recovery from peritransplantation complications and, in many cases, a decrease in immunosuppression, the recipient is often better equipped to combat late infection.

Late Infections The incidence of *Pneumocystis* infection (which may present with a paucity of findings) is high among lung and heart–lung transplant recipients. Some form of prophylaxis for *Pneumocystis* pneumonia are indicated in all organ transplant situations (Table 143-5). Prophylaxis with TMP-SMX for 12 months after transplantation may be sufficient to prevent *Pneumocystis* disease in patients whose immunosuppression is not increased.

As in other transplant recipients, EBV infection in lung and heart–lung recipients may cause either a mononucleosis-like syndrome or EBV-LPD. The tendency of the B-cell blasts to present in the lung appears to be greater after lung transplantation than after the transplantation of other organs, possibly because of a rich source of B cells in bronchus-associated lymphoid tissue. Reduction of immunosuppression and switching of regimens, as discussed in earlier sections, cause remission in some cases, but mTOR inhibitors such as rapamycin may contribute to lung toxicity. Airway compression can be fatal, and rapid intervention may, therefore, become necessary. The approach to EBV-LPD is similar to that described in other sections.

LIVER TRANSPLANTATION

Early Infections As in other transplantation settings, early bacterial infections are a major problem after liver transplantation. Many centers administer systemic broad-spectrum antibiotics for the first 24 h or sometimes longer after surgery, even in the absence of documented infection. However, despite prophylaxis, infectious complications are common and correlate with the duration of the surgical procedure and the type of biliary drainage. An operation lasting >12 h is associated with an increased likelihood of infection. Patients who have a choledochojejunostomy with drainage of the biliary duct to a Roux-en-Y jejunal bowel loop have more fungal infections than those whose bile is drained via anastomosis of the donor common bile duct to the recipient common bile duct. Overall, liver transplant patients have a high incidence of fungal infections, and the occurrence of fungal (often candidal) infection in the setting of choledochojejunostomy correlates with re-transplantation, elevated creatinine levels, long procedures, transfusion of >40 units of blood, reoperation, preoperative use of glucocorticoids, prolonged treatment with antibacterial agents, and fungal colonization 2 days before and 3 days after surgery. Many centers give antifungal agents prophylactically in this setting.

Peritonitis and intraabdominal abscesses are common complications of liver transplantation. Bacterial peritonitis or localized abscesses may result from biliary leaks. Early leaks are especially common with live-donor liver transplants. Peritonitis in liver transplant recipients is often polymicrobial, frequently involving enterococci, aerobic gram-negative bacteria, staphylococci, anaerobes, or *Candida* and sometimes involving other invasive fungi. Only one-third of patients with intraabdominal abscesses have bacteremia. Abscesses within the first month after surgery may occur not only in and around the liver but also in the spleen, pericolic area, and pelvis. Treatment includes antibiotic administration and drainage as necessary. Not surprisingly, *C. difficile* colitis is also a problem in this setting (**Chap. 134**).

Middle-Period Infections The development of postsurgical biliary stricture predisposes patients to cholangitis. The incidence of strictures is increased in live-donor liver transplantation. Transplant recipients who develop cholangitis may have high spiking fevers and rigors but often lack the characteristic signs and symptoms of classic cholangitis, including abdominal pain and jaundice. Although these findings may suggest graft rejection, rejection is typically accompanied by marked elevation of liver function enzymes. In contrast, in cholangitis in transplant recipients, results of liver function tests (with the possible exception of alkaline phosphatase levels) are often within the normal range. Definitive diagnosis of cholangitis in liver transplant recipients requires demonstration of aggregated neutrophils in bile duct biopsy specimens. Unfortunately, invasive studies of the biliary tract (either T-tube cholangiography or endoscopic retrograde cholangiopancreatography) may themselves lead to cholangitis. For this reason, many clinicians recommend an empirical trial of therapy with antibiotics covering gram-negative organisms and anaerobes before these procedures are undertaken as well as antibiotic coverage if procedures are eventually performed.

Reactivation of viral hepatitis is a common complication of liver transplantation (**Chap. 339**). Recurrent hepatitis B and C infections, for which transplantation may be performed, are problematic. To prevent hepatitis B virus reinfection, prophylaxis with an optimal antiviral agent or combination of agents (lamivudine, adefovir, entecavir) and hepatitis B immune globulin is currently recommended, although the optimal dose, route, and duration of therapy remain controversial. Success in preventing reinfection with hepatitis B virus has increased in recent years. Complications related to hepatitis C infection are the most common reason for liver transplantation in the United States. Without treatment, reinfection of the graft with hepatitis C virus occurs in all patients, with a variable time frame. Recent studies employing direct-acting antivirals have provided impressive results in both the treatment of existing infections before transplantation and the prevention of infections after transplantation in patients with hepatitis C (**Chap. 339**).

As in other transplantation settings, reactivation disease with herpesviruses is common (Table 143-3). Herpesviruses can be transmitted in donor organs. Although CMV hepatitis occurs in ~4% of liver transplant recipients, it is usually not so severe as to require re-transplantation. Without prophylaxis, CMV disease develops in the majority of seronegative recipients of organs from CMV-positive donors, but fatality rates are lower among liver transplant recipients than among lung or heart–lung transplant recipients. Disease due to CMV has also been associated with the vanishing bile duct syndrome after liver transplantation. Liver transplant recipients with high levels of CMV respond to treatment with ganciclovir; prophylaxis with oral forms of ganciclovir or valganciclovir decreases the frequency of disease. A role for HHV-6 reactivation in early posttransplantation fever and leukopenia has been proposed, although the more severe sequelae described in HSC transplantation are unusual. HHV-6 and HHV-7 appear to exacerbate CMV disease in this setting. EBV-LPD after liver transplantation shows a propensity for involvement of the liver, and such disease may be of donor origin. See previous sections for discussion of EBV infections in SOT.

PANCREAS TRANSPLANTATION

Pancreas transplantation is most frequently performed together with or after kidney transplantation, although it may be performed alone. Transplantation of the pancreas can be complicated by early bacterial and yeast infections. Most pancreatic transplants are drained into the bowel, and the rest are drained into the bladder. A cuff of duodenum is used in the anastomosis between the pancreatic graft and either the gut or the bladder. Bowel drainage poses a risk of early intraabdominal and allograft infections with enteric bacteria and yeasts. These infections can result in loss of the graft. Bladder drainage causes a high rate of urinary tract infection and sterile cystitis; however, such infection can usually be cured with appropriate antimicrobial agents. In both procedures, prophylactic antimicrobial agents are commonly used at the time of surgery. Aggressive immunosuppression, especially when the patient receives a kidney and a pancreas from different donors, is associated with late-onset systemic fungal and viral infections; thus, many centers administer an antifungal drug and an antiviral agent (ganciclovir or a congener) for extended prophylaxis.

Issues related to the development of CMV infection, EBV-LPD, and infections with opportunistic pathogens in patients receiving a pancreatic transplant are similar to those in other SOT recipients.

COMPOSITE-TISSUE TRANSPLANTATION

Composite-tissue allotransplantation (CTA) is a new field in which, rather than a single organ, multiple tissue types composing a major body part are transplanted. The sites involved have included hands, feet, arms, legs, face, trachea, and abdominal wall. The numbers of recipients are limited. The different procedures and the associated infectious complications vary. Nevertheless, some early trends related to infectious complications have become apparent, as very intense and prolonged immunosuppression is typically required to prevent rejection. For example, in the early postoperative period, bacterial infections are especially frequent in facial transplant recipients. Perioperative prophylaxis is tailored to the organisms likely to complicate the different procedures. As in SOT recipients, complicated CMV infections have been observed in several CTA settings, particularly when the recipient is seronegative and the donor is seropositive. In some patients, anti-CMV immune globulin in addition to ganciclovir (as used in HSC transplant recipients with CMV pneumonia) was needed to control disease, and ganciclovir resistance requiring alternative therapies developed in several patients. Infectious complications from reactivation of other members of the human herpesvirus family and other latent viruses also caused significant morbidity, as discussed for SOT recipients. Prophylaxis for CMV infection, *P. jirovecii* infection, toxoplasmosis, and fungal infection is administered for several months on the basis of the limited studies available.

MISCELLANEOUS INFECTIONS IN SOLID ORGAN TRANSPLANTATION

Indwelling IV Catheter Infections The prolonged use of indwelling IV catheters for administration of medications, blood products, and nutrition is common in diverse transplantation settings and poses a risk of local and bloodstream infections. Exit-site infection is most commonly caused by staphylococcal species. Bloodstream infection most frequently develops within 1 week of catheter placement or in patients who become neutropenic. Coagulase-negative staphylococci are the most common isolates from blood. Although infective endocarditis in HSC transplant recipients is uncommon, the incidence of endocarditis among SOT recipients has been estimated to be as high as 1%, and this infection is associated with excessive high mortality in this population. Although staphylococci predominate, the involvement of fungal and gram-negative organisms may be more common than in the general population. **For further discussion of differential diagnosis and therapeutic options, see Chap. 74.**

Tuberculosis The incidence of tuberculosis within the first 12 months after SOT is greater than that observed after HSC transplantation (0.23–0.79%) and ranges broadly worldwide (1.2–15%), reflecting the prevalence of tuberculosis in local populations. Lesions suggesting prior tuberculosis on chest radiography, older age, diabetes, chronic liver disease, GVHD, and intense immunosuppression are predictive of tuberculosis reactivation and development of disseminated disease in a host with latent disease. Tuberculosis has rarely been transmitted from the donor organ. In contrast to the low mortality rate among HSC transplant recipients, mortality rates among SOT recipients are reported to be as high as 30%. Vigilance is indicated, as the presentation of disease is often extrapulmonary (gastrointestinal, genitourinary, central nervous, endocrine, musculoskeletal, laryngeal) and atypical; tuberculosis in this setting sometimes manifests as fever of unknown origin. Careful elicitation of a history and direct evaluation of both the recipient and the donor prior to transplantation are optimal. Skin testing of the recipient with purified protein derivative may be unreliable because of chronic disease and/or immunosuppression. Cell-based assays that measure interferon-γ and/or cytokine production may prove more sensitive in the future. Isoniazid toxicity has not been a significant problem except in the setting of liver transplantation. Therefore, appropriate prophylaxis should be used (see recommendations from the Centers for Disease Control and Prevention [CDC] at *www.cdc.gov/tb/topic/treatment/ltbi.htm*). An assessment of the need to treat latent disease should include careful consideration of the possibility of a false-negative test result. Pending final confirmation of suspected tuberculosis, aggressive multidrug treatment in accordance with the guidelines of the CDC, the Infectious Diseases Society of America, and the American Thoracic Society is indicated because of the high mortality rates among these patients. Altered drug metabolism (e.g., upon coadministration of antituberculous medications and certain immunosuppressive agents) can be managed with careful monitoring of drug levels and appropriate dose adjustment. Close follow-up of hepatic enzymes is warranted. Drug-resistant tuberculosis is especially problematic in these individuals **(Chap. 178)**.

SARS-CoV-2 SARS-CoV-2 infections in SOT recipients are associated with high mortality, long courses of disease, and infections with new strains of this virus after resolution of initial infections. Unfortunately, early vaccine studies indicate that SOT recipients do not respond as well as healthy controls. Further studies are needed to define optimal approaches to treatment and prevention of disease in this group. In the meantime, as with influenza, vaccination of family members and other close contacts is recommended.

Virus-Associated Malignancies In addition to malignancy associated with gammaherpesvirus infection (EBV, KSHV) and simple warts (HPV), other tumors that are virus-associated or suspected of being virus-associated are more likely to develop in transplant recipients, particularly those who require long-term immunosuppression, than in the general population. The interval to tumor development is usually >1 year. Transplant recipients develop nonmelanoma skin or lip cancers that, in contrast to de novo skin cancers, have a high ratio of squamous cells to basal cells. HPV may play a major role in these lesions. Cervical and vulvar carcinomas, which are quite clearly associated with HPV, develop with increased frequency in female transplant recipients. The frequency of Merkel cell carcinoma associated with Merkel cell polyomavirus is also increased among transplant recipients; however, it is unclear whether recipients infected with HTLV-1 are at increased risk of leukemia. Among renal transplant recipients, rates of melanoma are modestly increased and rates of cancers of the kidney and bladder are increased. Recommendations for dealing with these problems include vaccination against HPV, a switch from calcineurin inhibitors to mTOR inhibitors (see above), and reduction of immunosuppression to the lowest level possible without graft rejection.

VACCINATION OF TRANSPLANT RECIPIENTS

(See also Chap. 123) In addition to receiving antibiotic prophylaxis, transplant recipients should be vaccinated against likely pathogens **(Table 143-6)**. In the case of HSC transplant recipients, optimal responses cannot be achieved until after immune reconstitution, despite previous immunization of both donor and recipient. Recipients of an allogeneic HSC transplant must be reimmunized if they are to be protected against pathogens. The situation is less clear-cut in the case of autologous transplantation. T and B cells in the peripheral blood may reconstitute the immune response if they are transferred in adequate numbers. However, cancer patients (particularly those with Hodgkin's disease, in whom vaccination has been extensively studied) who are undergoing chemotherapy do not respond normally to immunization, and titers of antibodies to infectious agents fall more rapidly than in healthy individuals. Therefore, even immunosuppressed patients who have not undergone HSC transplantation may need booster vaccine injections. If memory cells are specifically eliminated as part of a stem cell "cleanup" procedure, it will be necessary to reimmunize the recipient with a new primary series. Optimal times for immunizations of different transplant populations are being evaluated. Yearly immunization of household and other contacts (including health care personnel) against influenza benefits the patient by preventing local spread.

In the absence of compelling data as to optimal timing, it is reasonable to administer the pneumococcal and *H. influenzae* type b conjugate vaccines to both autologous and allogeneic HSC transplant recipients beginning 12 months after transplantation. A series that includes both the 13-valent pneumococcal conjugate vaccine (Prevnar®) and the 23-valent pneumococcal polysaccharide vaccine (Pneumovax®) is now recommended (according to CDC guidelines). The pneumococcal and *H. influenzae* type b vaccines are particularly important for patients who have undergone splenectomy. The *Neisseria meningitidis* polysaccharide conjugate vaccine (Menactra® or Menveo®) also is recommended. In addition, diphtheria, tetanus, acellular pertussis, and inactivated polio vaccines can all be given at these same intervals (12 months and, as required, 24 months after transplantation). Some authorities recommend a new primary series for tetanus/diphtheria/pertussis and inactivated poliovirus vaccines beginning 12 months after transplantation. Vaccination to prevent hepatitis B and hepatitis A (both killed vaccines) also seems advisable. HPV vaccination, which can prevent genital warts as well as specific cancers, is recommended through age 26 for healthy young adults who previously have not been vaccinated or have not received the full series. Live-virus measles/mumps/rubella (MMR) vaccine can be given to autologous HSC transplant recipients 24 months after transplantation and to most allogeneic HSC transplant recipients at 24 months if they are not receiving maintenance therapy with immunosuppressive drugs and do not have ongoing GVHD. The risk of spread from a household contact is low for MMR vaccine. In parts of the world where live poliovirus vaccine is used, patients as well as contacts should be advised to receive only the killed vaccine. In the rare setting where both donor and recipient are VZV naïve and the recipient is no longer receiving acyclovir or ganciclovir prophylaxis, the patient should be counseled to receive varicella-zoster immune globulin (VariZIG®) up to 10 days after exposure to a person with chickenpox or uncovered zoster; such patients should avoid close contact with persons recently vaccinated with Varivax®. Neither patients nor their household contacts should receive vaccinia vaccine unless they have been exposed to smallpox virus. Among patients who have active GVHD and/or are taking high maintenance doses of glucocorticoids, it may be prudent to avoid all live-virus vaccines.

TABLE 143-6 Vaccination of Hematopoietic Stem Cell Transplant (HSCT) and Solid Organ Transplant (SOT) Recipients

VACCINE	TYPE OF TRANSPLANTATION: HSCT	SOT[a]
Streptococcus pneumoniae, Haemophilus influenzae, Neisseria meningitidis	Immunize after transplantation with *H. influenzae* conjugate vaccine and *N. meningitidis* conjugate vaccine. *S. pneumoniae* vaccine is given in two steps.[b]	Immunize before transplantation with *H. influenzae* conjugate and *N. meningitidis* conjugate vaccines. *S. pneumoniae* vaccine is given in two steps.[b]
Influenza	Vaccinate in the fall. Vaccinate close contacts.	Vaccinate in the fall. Vaccinate close contacts.
Polio	Administer inactivated vaccine.	Administer inactivated vaccine.
Measles/mumps/rubella	Immunize 24 months after transplantation if GVHD is absent.	Immunize before transplantation.
Diphtheria, pertussis, tetanus	Reimmunize after transplantation with primary series, DTaP. See *www.cdc.gov/vaccines/hcp/acip-recs/general-recs/immunocompetence.html*.	Immunize or boost before transplantation with Tdap; give Td boosters at 10-year intervals or as required.
Hepatitis B and A	Reimmunize after transplantation. See recommendations.	Immunize before transplantation.
Human papillomavirus	3 doses for persons 9–45 years of age[c]	3 doses for persons 9–45 years of age[c]

[a]Immunizations should be given before transplantation whenever possible. [b]Step 1: Administer one dose of the pneumococcal conjugate vaccine Prevnar® (13-valent pneumococcal vaccine, PCV13) to all transplant candidates. If a candidate has previously been vaccinated with Pneumovax® (23-valent pneumococcal vaccine, PPSV23), at least 6 months should have elapsed before Prevnar is administered. Step 2: Administer one dose of Pneumovax at least 8 weeks after vaccination with PCV13; follow with a booster dose of Pneumovax 5 years later. If the patient has previously been vaccinated with Pneumovax (i.e., before receiving Prevnar), at least 3 years should have elapsed before the second dose of Pneumovax is administered. [c]The second and third doses should follow the first dose after 1–2 months and 6 months, respectively. Centers for Disease Control and Prevention (CDC) current recommendations: *https://www.cdc.gov/vaccines/hcp/acip-recs/general-recs/immunocompetence.html*. Some authorities recommend vaccination of all transplant recipients because of the risk of new sexual contacts later in life and the potential for human papillomavirus replication in immunocompromised patients.

Note: Recommendations from the CDC should be checked regularly as they frequently change upon receipt of new clinical information and new formulations of specific vaccines. See *www.cdc.gov/vaccines/hcp/acip-recs/general-recs/immunocompetence.html*.

Abbreviations: DTaP, full-level diphtheria and tetanus toxoids and acellular pertussis, adsorbed; GVHD, graft-versus-host disease; IDSA, Infectious Diseases Society of America; Tdap, tetanus toxoid, reduced diphtheria toxoid, and acellular pertussis.

In the case of SOT recipients, administration of all the usual vaccines and of the indicated booster doses should be completed before immunosuppression, if possible, to maximize responses. If vaccinations have not been completed prior to transplantation, many centers will wait 3–6 months before vaccinating. An exception is the seasonal influenza vaccine, which can be given 1 month after transplant with good results and should be given if a delay would result in the loss of protection during the season. For patients taking immunosuppressive agents, the administration of pneumococcal vaccine should be repeated every 5 years. No data are available for the meningococcal vaccine, but it is probably reasonable to administer it along with the pneumococcal vaccine. *H. influenzae* conjugate vaccine is safe and should be efficacious in this population; therefore, its administration before transplantation is recommended. Booster doses of this vaccine are not recommended for adults. SOT recipients who continue to receive immunosuppressive drugs should not receive live-virus vaccines. A person in this group who is exposed to measles should be given measles immune globulin. Similarly, an immunocompromised patient who is seronegative for varicella and who comes into contact with a person who has chickenpox should be given varicella-zoster immune globulin as soon as possible (optimally within 96 h; up to 10 days after contact); if this is not possible, a 10- to 14-day course of acyclovir therapy should be started immediately. Upon the discontinuation of treatment, clinical disease may still occur in a small number of patients; thus, vigilance is indicated. Rapid re-treatment with acyclovir should limit the symptoms of disease. Household contacts of transplant recipients can receive live attenuated VZV vaccine, but vaccinees should avoid direct contact with the patient if a rash develops. Virus-like particle vaccines have been licensed for the prevention of infection with several HPV serotypes most commonly implicated in cervical and anal carcinomas and in anogenital and laryngeal warts. These vaccines are not live; current CDC recommendations are for three doses in immunocompromised hosts.

Immunocompromised patients who travel may benefit from some but not all vaccines **(Chaps. 123 and 124)**. In general, these patients should receive any killed or inactivated vaccine preparation appropriate to the area they are visiting; this recommendation includes the vaccines for Japanese encephalitis, hepatitis A and B, poliomyelitis, meningococcal infection, and typhoid. Live typhoid vaccines are not recommended for use in most immunocompromised patients, but an inactivated or purified polysaccharide typhoid vaccine can be used. Live yellow fever vaccine should not be administered, nor should live cholera vaccine. On the other hand, primary immunization or boosting with the purified-protein hepatitis B vaccine is indicated. Inactivated hepatitis A vaccine should also be used in the appropriate setting **(Chap. 123)**. A vaccine is now available that provides dual protection against hepatitis A and hepatitis B. If hepatitis A vaccine is not administered, travelers should consider receiving passive protection with immune globulin (the dose depending on the duration of travel in the high-risk area).

IN MEMORIAM

Dr. Robert W. Finberg, Richard M. Haidack Distinguished Professor and Chair of Medicine, University of Massachusetts Chan Medical School (2000-2020), Professor of Medicine and Chair of Infectious Diseases, Dana Farber Cancer Institute (1996-1999), passed away on August 30, 2021. In addition to this chapter, he authored Chapter 74, "Infections in Patients with Cancer." Dr. Finberg was an internationally renowned physician-scientist and an academic leader whose career spanned four decades. A brilliant talented researcher focused on viral pathogenesis he was also a consummate clinician who attended at the bedside throughout his career. Dr. Finberg played an important role in the COVID-19 pandemic by leading clinical trials for SARS-CoV-2 vaccines and therapeutics. Warm and generous with a keen wit, he was a beloved family man, colleague and friend. As an educator and mentor he truly cared about training the next generation, as evidenced by the legacy of a very large number of trainees he leaves behind. We are indebted to Dr. Finberg for his outstanding contributions to nine editions of Harrison's Principles of Internal Medicine and to his considerable and significant contributions to the field of human health.

FURTHER READING

Abbo LM et al: Surgical site infections: Guidelines from the American Society of Transplantation Infectious Diseases Community of Practice. Clin Transplant 33:e13489, 2019.

Danziger-Isakov L et al: Vaccination of solid organ transplant candidates and recipients: Guidelines from the American Society of Transplantation Infectious Diseases Community of Practice. Clin Transplant 33:e13563, 2019.

Kumar R, Ison MG: Opportunistic infections in transplant patients. Infect Dis Clin North Am 33:1143, 2019.

Pereira MR et al: COVID-19 in solid organ transplant recipients: Initial report from the US epicenter. Am J Transplant 20:1800, 2020.

White SL et al: Infectious diseases transmission in solid organ transplantation: Donor evaluation, recipient risk, and outcomes of transmission. Transplant Direct 5:e416, 2018.

Zinoviev R et al: In full flow: Left ventricular assist device infections in the modern era. Open Forum Infect Dis 7:ofaa124, 2020.

144 Treatment and Prophylaxis of Bacterial Infections

David C. Hooper, Erica S. Shenoy, Ramy H. Elshaboury

Antimicrobial agents have had a major impact on human health. Together with vaccines, they have contributed to reduced mortality, extended lifespan, and enhanced quality of life. Among drugs used in human medicine, however, they are distinctive in that their use promotes the occurrence of drug resistance in the pathogens they are designed to treat as well as in other "bystander" organisms. Indeed, the history of antimicrobial development has been driven in large part by the medical need engendered by the emergence of resistance to each generation of agents. Thus, the careful and appropriate use of antimicrobial drugs is particularly important not only for optimizing efficacy and minimizing adverse effects but also for minimizing the risk of resistance and preserving the value of existing agents. Although this chapter focuses on antibacterial agents, the optimal use of all antimicrobials depends on an understanding of each drug's mechanism of action, spectrum of activity, mechanisms of resistance, pharmacology, and adverse effect profile. This information is applied in the context of the patient's clinical presentation, underlying conditions, and epidemiology to define the site and likely nature of the infection or other condition and thus to choose the best therapy. Gathering of microbiologic information is especially important for refining therapeutic choices on the basis of documented pathogen and susceptibility data whenever possible; this information also makes it possible to choose more targeted therapy, thereby reducing the risk of selection of resistant bacteria. Durations of therapy are chosen according to the nature of the infection and the patient's response to treatment and are informed by clinical studies when they are available, with the understanding that shorter courses are less likely than longer courses to promote the emergence of resistance. This chapter and the one that follows provide specific information that is necessary for making informed choices among antibacterial agents. The mechanisms of action of antibacterial agents are discussed in detail in the text of this chapter, and mechanisms of resistance are discussed in detail in **Chap. 145**. Both types of mechanisms, which are related to each other, are summarized for the most commonly used groups of agents in **Table 145-1**. A schematic of antibacterial targets is provided in **Fig. 145-1**.

MECHANISMS OF ACTION (SEE TABLE 145-1)

Multiple essential components of bacterial cell structures and metabolism have been the targets of antibacterial agents used in clinical medicine, and the interaction of an agent with its target results in either inhibition of bacterial growth and replication (*bacteriostatic effect*) or bacterial killing (*bactericidal effect*). In general, targets have been chosen because they either do not exist in mammalian cells and physiology or are sufficiently different from their bacterial counterparts to allow selective bacterial targeting. Treatment with bacteriostatic agents is effective when the patient's host defenses are sufficient to contribute to eradication of the infecting pathogen. In patients with impaired host defenses (e.g., neutropenia) or infections at body sites with impaired or limited host defenses (e.g., meningitis and endocarditis), bactericidal agents are generally preferred.

INHIBITION OF CELL WALL SYNTHESIS

The bacterial cell wall, which is external to the cytoplasmic membrane and has no counterpart in mammalian cells, protects bacterial cells from lysis under low osmotic conditions. The cell wall is a cross-linked peptidoglycan composed of a polymer of alternating units of *N*-acetylglucosamine (NAG) and *N*-acetylmuramic acid (NAM), four-amino-acid stem peptides linked to each NAM, and a peptide cross-bridge that links adjacent stem peptides to form a netlike structure. Several steps in peptidoglycan synthesis are targets of antibacterial agents. Inhibition of cell wall synthesis generally results in a bactericidal effect that is linked to cell lysis. This effect results not only from the blocking of new cell-wall formation but from the uninhibited action of cell wall–remodeling enzymes called *autolysins*, which cleave peptidoglycan as part of normal cell-wall growth.

In gram-positive bacteria the peptidoglycan is the most external cell structure, but in gram-negative bacteria, an asymmetric lipid outer membrane is external to the peptidoglycan and contains diffusion channels called *porins*. The space between the outer membrane and the peptidoglycan and cytoplasmic membrane is referred to as the *periplasmic space*. Most antibacterial drugs enter the gram-negative bacterial cell through a porin channel, since the outer membrane is a major diffusion barrier. Although the peptidoglycan layer is thicker in gram-positive (20–80 nm) than in gram-negative (1 nm) bacteria, peptidoglycan itself constitutes only a limited diffusion barrier for antibacterial agents.

β-Lactams The β-lactam drugs, including penicillins, cephalosporins, monobactams, and carbapenems, target transpeptidase enzymes (also called *penicillin-binding proteins* or PBPs) involved in the stem-peptide cross-linking step. Inhibitors of β-lactamases—bacterial enzymes that can degrade β-lactams—are used in combination with some β-lactams to expand their spectrum of activity.

Glycopeptides and Lipoglycopeptides The glycopeptides, including vancomycin and teicoplanin, and the lipoglycopeptides, including telavancin, dalbavancin, and oritavancin, bind the two terminal D-alanine residues of the stem peptide, hindering the glycosyltransferase involved in polymerizing NAG–NAM units as well as transpeptidases. Vancomycin also binds to the lipid II intermediate that delivers cell wall precursor subunits. The additional binding of teicoplanin, telavancin, dalbavancin, and oritavancin to the bacterial cytoplasmic membrane contributes to their increased potency. Both β-lactams and glycopeptides interact with their targets external to the cytoplasmic membrane.

Bacitracin (Topical) and Fosfomycin These agents interrupt enzymatic steps in the production of peptidoglycan precursors in the cytoplasm.

INHIBITION OF PROTEIN SYNTHESIS

Most inhibitors of bacterial protein synthesis target bacterial ribosomes, whose difference from eukaryotic ribosomes allows selective antibacterial action. Some inhibitors bind to the 30S ribosomal subunit and others to the 50S subunit. Most protein synthesis–inhibiting agents are bacteriostatic; aminoglycosides are an exception and are bactericidal.

Aminoglycosides Aminoglycosides (amikacin, gentamicin, kanamycin, netilmicin, streptomycin, tobramycin, and plazomicin) bind irreversibly to 16S ribosomal RNA (rRNA) of the 30S ribosomal subunit, blocking the translocation of peptidyl transfer RNA (tRNA) from the A (aminoacyl) to the P (peptidyl) site and, at low concentrations, causing misreading of messenger RNA (mRNA) codons and thus causing the introduction of incorrect amino acids into the peptide chain; at higher concentrations, translocation of the peptide chain is blocked. Cellular uptake of aminoglycosides is dependent on the electrochemical gradient across the bacterial membrane. Under anaerobic conditions, this gradient is reduced, with a consequent reduction in the uptake and activity of the aminoglycosides. Spectinomycin is a related aminocyclitol antibiotic that also binds to 16S rRNA of the 30S ribosomal subunit but at a different site. This drug inhibits translocation of the growing peptide chain but does not trigger codon misreading and produces only a bacteriostatic effect.

PART 5 Infectious Diseases

Tetracyclines Tetracyclines (doxycycline, minocycline, tetracycline) bind reversibly to the 16S rRNA of the 30S ribosomal subunit and block the binding of aminoacyl tRNA to the ribosomal A site, thereby inhibiting peptide elongation. Active transport of tetracyclines into bacterial but not mammalian cells contributes to the selectivity of these agents. Tigecycline, a derivative of minocycline and the only available glycylcycline, acts similarly to the tetracyclines but is distinctive for its ability to circumvent the most common mechanisms of resistance to the tetracyclines. Other new tetracycline derivatives—eravacycline, a fluorocycline, and omadacycline, an aminomethylcycline—like tigecycline are notable for being little affected by prior common tetracycline resistance mechanisms.

Macrolides and Ketolides In contrast to the aminoglycosides and tetracyclines, the macrolides (azithromycin, clarithromycin, and erythromycin) and ketolides (telithromycin) bind to the 23S rRNA of the 50S ribosomal subunit. These agents block translocation of the growing peptide chain by binding to the tunnel from which the chain exits the ribosome.

Lincosamides Clindamycin is the only lincosamide in clinical use. It binds to the 23S rRNA of the 50S ribosomal subunit, interacting with both the ribosomal A and P sites and blocking peptide bond formation.

Streptogramins The only streptogramin in clinical use is a combination of quinupristin, a group B streptogramin, and dalfopristin, a group A streptogramin. Both components bind to 23S rRNA of the 50S ribosome: dalfopristin binds to both the A and P sites of the peptidyl transferase center, and quinupristin binds to a site that overlaps the macrolide-binding site, blocking the emergence of nascent peptide from the ribosome. The combination is bactericidal, but macrolide-resistant bacteria exhibit cross-resistance to quinupristin, and the remaining activity of dalfopristin alone is only bacteriostatic.

Chloramphenicol Chloramphenicol binds reversibly to the 23S rRNA of the 50S subunit in a manner that interferes with the proper positioning of the aminoacyl component of tRNA in the A site. This site of binding is near those of the macrolides and lincosamides.

Oxazolidinones Linezolid and tedizolid are the only oxazolidinones in clinical use. They bind directly to the A site in the 23S rRNA of the 50S ribosomal subunit and block binding of aminoacyl tRNA, inhibiting the initiation of protein synthesis.

Pleuromutilins Lefamulin is the only systemic pleuromutilin in clinical use. It binds to the peptidyl transferase center of the 50S ribosomal subunit and prevents the correct positioning of tRNAs, thereby inhibiting peptide bond formation and protein synthesis.

Mupirocin Mupirocin (pseudomonic acid) is used topically. It competes with isoleucine for binding to isoleucyl tRNA synthetase, depleting stores of isoleucyl tRNA and thereby inhibiting protein synthesis.

INHIBITION OF BACTERIAL METABOLISM

Available inhibitors (antimetabolites) target the pathway for synthesis of folate, which is a cofactor in a number of one-carbon transfer reactions involved in the synthesis of some nucleic acids, including the pyrimidine thymidine and all purines (adenine and guanine), as well as some amino acids (methionine and serine) and acetyl coenzyme A. Two sequential steps in folate synthesis are targeted. The selective antibacterial effect stems from the inability of mammalian cells to synthesize folate; they depend instead on exogenous sources. Antibacterial activity, however, may be reduced in the presence of high exogenous concentrations of the end products of the folate pathway (e.g., thymidine and purines) that may occur in some infections, resulting from local breakdown of leukocytes and host tissues.

Sulfonamides Sulfonamides, including sulfadiazine, sulfisoxazole, and sulfamethoxazole, inhibit dihydropteroate synthetase (DHPS), which adds *p*-aminobenzoic acid (PABA) to pteridine, producing dihydropteroate. Sulfonamides are structural analogues of PABA and act as competing enzyme substrates.

Trimethoprim Subsequent steps in folate synthesis are catalyzed by dihydrofolate synthase, which adds glutamate to dihydropteroate, and dihydrofolate reductase (DHFR), which then generates the final product, tetrahydrofolate. Trimethoprim is a structural analogue of pteridine and inhibits DHFR. Trimethoprim is available alone but is most often used in combination products that also contain sulfamethoxazole and thus block two sequential steps in folate synthesis.

INHIBITION OF DNA AND RNA SYNTHESIS OR ACTIVITY

A variety of antibacterial agents act on these processes.

Quinolones The quinolones include nalidixic acid, the first agent in the class, and newer, more widely used fluorinated derivatives (fluoroquinolones), including norfloxacin, ciprofloxacin, levofloxacin, moxifloxacin, gemifloxacin, and delafloxacin. The quinolones are synthetic compounds that inhibit bacterial DNA synthesis by interacting with the DNA complexes of two essential enzymes, DNA gyrase and DNA topoisomerase IV, which alter DNA topology. Quinolones trap enzyme–DNA complexes in such a way that they block movement of the DNA replication apparatus and can generate lethal double-strand breaks in DNA, resulting in bactericidal activity. Although mammalian cells also have type II DNA topoisomerases related to gyrase and topoisomerase IV, the structures of the mammalian enzymes are sufficiently different from those of the bacterial enzymes that quinolones have substantially selective antibacterial activity.

Rifamycins Rifampin, rifabutin, and rifapentine are semisynthetic derivatives of rifamycin B and bind the β subunit of bacterial RNA polymerase, thereby blocking elongation of mRNA. Their action is highly selective for the bacterial enzyme over mammalian RNA polymerases.

Nitrofurantoin The reduction of nitrofurantoin, a nitrofuran compound, by bacterial enzymes produces highly reactive derivatives that are thought to cause DNA strand breakage. Nitrofurantoin is used only for the treatment of lower urinary tract infections.

Metronidazole Metronidazole is a synthetic nitroimidazole with activity limited to anaerobic bacteria and certain anaerobic protozoa. Reduction of its nitro group by the electron-transport system in anaerobic bacteria produces reactive intermediates that damage DNA and result in bactericidal activity. Both nitrofurantoin and metronidazole have selective antibacterial activity because the reducing activity needed to produce active derivatives is generated only by bacterial and not mammalian enzymes.

DISRUPTION OF MEMBRANE INTEGRITY

The integrity of the bacterial cytoplasmic membrane—and, in gram-negative bacteria, the outer membrane—is important for bacterial viability. Two bactericidal drugs have membrane targets.

Polymyxins The polymyxins, including polymyxin B and polymyxin E (colistin), are cationic cyclic polypeptides that disrupt the cytoplasmic membrane and the outer membrane (the latter by binding lipopolysaccharide, which is negatively charged).

Daptomycin Daptomycin is a lipopeptide that binds the cytoplasmic membrane of gram-positive bacteria in the presence of calcium, generating a channel that leads to leakage of cytoplasmic potassium ions and membrane depolarization.

PHARMACOKINETICS AND PHARMACODYNAMICS

The term *pharmacokinetics* describes the disposition of a drug in the body, whereas *pharmacodynamics* describes the drug action on the pathogen in relation to pharmacokinetic factors. An understanding of the principles governing these two areas is required for effective drug selection, dosing, and prevention of toxicities.

PHARMACOKINETICS

The process of drug disposition consists of four principal phases: absorption, distribution, metabolism, and excretion. These phases determine the time course of drug concentrations in serum and other tissues and body fluids.

Absorption When a drug is administered, *absorption* is defined as the percentage of the dose that reaches the vasculature. The fraction of a drug, however, that reaches the systemic circulation or the pharmacologic site of action is termed *bioavailability*. The bioavailability is more relevant when non-IV routes are used—e.g., the oral, IM, SC, and topical routes. For example, since IV administration provides direct access to the systemic circulation, the bioavailability is 100%. IV and oral dosing for highly bioavailable agents result in equivalent systemic concentrations; examples of such agents include metronidazole, fluoroquinolones, tetracyclines, and linezolid. Additionally, many factors can influence a drug's oral bioavailability, including the timing of food consumption relative to drug administration, drug-metabolizing enzymes, efflux transporters, concentration-dependent solubility, and acid degradation. Underlying conditions such as diarrhea or ileus can also affect the site of drug absorption and thereby alter its bioavailability. Certain orally administered drugs may have lower bioavailability because of the *first-pass effect*—the process by which drugs are absorbed in the small intestine through the portal circulation and directly transported to the liver for metabolism before reaching their intended site of action.

Distribution *Distribution* describes the process of drug transfer reversibly between the general circulation and body tissues. After absorption into the general circulation and the central compartment (the extensively perfused organs), the drug also distributes into the peripheral compartment (less well-perfused tissues). The volume of distribution (Vd) is a pharmacokinetic parameter that describes the amount of drug in the body at a given time relative to the measured serum concentration. Properties such as the drug's lipophilicity, partition coefficient within different body tissues, protein binding, blood flow, penetration of the blood-brain barrier, and pH can affect the Vd and subsequently the concentration in various tissues. Drugs with a small Vd are limited to certain areas within the body (typically extracellular fluid), whereas those with a higher Vd penetrate extensively into tissues. Some antibacterial drugs can bind to serum proteins, resulting in typically lower Vd as only the unbound (free) fraction of the drug distributes into body tissues and fluids. Furthermore, only the unbound fraction of the drug is considered therapeutically active and available to exert antibacterial effects.

Metabolism *Metabolism* is the chemical transformation of a drug by the body. This modification can occur within several areas; the liver is the organ most commonly involved. Drugs are metabolized by enzymes, but enzyme systems have a finite capacity to metabolize a substrate. If a drug is given in a dose at which the concentration does not exceed the rate of metabolism, the metabolic process is generally linear. If the dose exceeds the amount that can be metabolized, drug accumulation and potential toxicity may occur. Drugs are metabolized through phase I or phase II reactions. In phase I reactions, the drug is made more polar through dealkylation, hydroxylation, oxidation, and deamination. Polarity increases water solubility and facilitates removal from the body (e.g., renal elimination). Phase II reactions, which include glucuronidation, sulfation, and acetylation, result in compounds larger and more polar than the parent drug. Both phases usually inactivate the parent drug, although some drugs are rendered more active. The hepatic cytochrome P450 (CYP) enzyme system is mostly responsible for phase I reactions. CYP3A4 is a common subfamily within this system that is responsible for the majority of phase I metabolism. Antibacterial drugs can be substrates, inhibitors, or inducers of a particular CYP enzyme. Inducers, e.g., rifampin, can increase the production of CYP enzymes and consequently increase the metabolism of other drugs. Inhibitors, such as macrolides, cause a decrease in enzyme activity and therefore an increase in the concentration of the interacting drug by decreasing the rate of its metabolism.

Excretion *Excretion* describes the body's mechanisms of drug elimination. Drugs can be eliminated through more than one mechanism. Renal clearance is the most common route and includes elimination through glomerular filtration, tubular secretion, and/or passive diffusion. Some agents undergo nonrenal clearance and rely on the biliary tract or the intestine for excretion. Rate of excretion affects the half-life of a drug—i.e., defined as the time it takes for the blood concentration of a drug to decrease by one-half. This value can range from minutes to days. Half-life and overall drug clearance can be extended if the organ responsible for clearance is impaired. For example, patients with renal or hepatic impairment may require dose adjustments that take delayed clearance into account and prevent drug accumulation and toxicity. For example, the majority of beta-lactam agents are cleared predominantly through glomerular filtration, and in the presence of renal impairment, the dosing interval is typically increased to account for the increased half-life.

PHARMACODYNAMICS

The term *pharmacodynamics* describes the relationship between the serum concentrations that determine the efficacy of the drug and those that may produce toxic effects. For an antibacterial agent, the pharmacodynamic focus is the type of drug exposure needed for optimal antibacterial effect in relation to the minimal inhibitory concentration (MIC)—the lowest drug concentration that inhibits the growth of a microorganism under standardized laboratory conditions. Antibacterial effect usually correlates with one or more of the following parameters: (1) concentration-dependent killing (defined as the ratio of peak serum concentration to the MIC), (2) time-dependent killing (defined as duration of drug concentrations above the MIC), or (3) the area under the concentration–time curve to the MIC (AUC/MIC) (**Fig. 144-1**).

For *concentration-dependent* killing agents, as the designation implies, the higher the drug peak concentration (C_{max}), the higher the rate and extent of bacterial killing. Aminoglycosides fit into the C_{max}/MIC model of pharmacodynamics activity, and a particular peak serum concentration is often targeted to achieve optimal killing. In contrast, *time-dependent* killing agents reach a ceiling at which higher concentrations do not result in increased effect. Rather, these agents are active against bacteria only when the drug concentration exceeds the MIC. The T > MIC predicts clinical efficacy for all β-lactams. The longer the concentration of the β-lactam remains above the MIC for an infecting pathogen during the dosing interval, the greater is the killing effect. Fluoroquinolones and vancomycin exemplify agents for which the AUC/MIC is a predictor of efficacy. For example, studies have found that an AUC/MIC ratio of >30 will maximize killing of *S. pneumoniae* by fluoroquinolones, while AUC/MIC ratios >125 are required to exert their effects against gram-negative pathogens. Finally, for some antibacterial drugs such as aminoglycosides, a *postantibiotic*

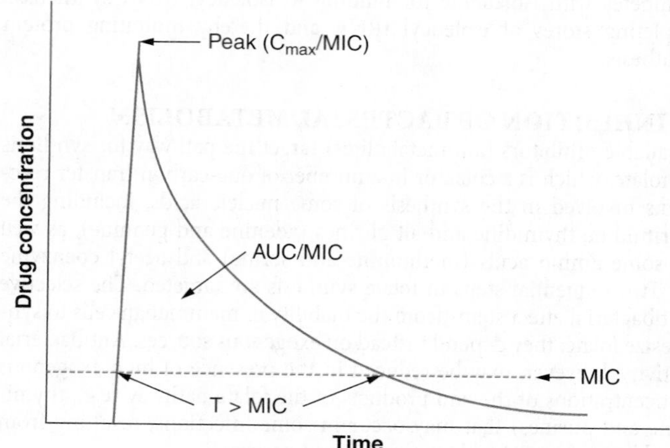

FIGURE 144-1 Pharmacokinetic and pharmacodynamic model predicting efficacy of antibacterial drugs. AUC, area under the time–concentration curve; C_{max}, peak serum concentration of drug; MIC, minimal inhibitory concentration; T > MIC, duration of drug concentrations above the MIC.

effect—the delayed regrowth of surviving bacteria after exposure to an antibiotic—supports less frequent dosing.

APPROACH TO THERAPY

The approach to antibiotic therapy is driven by host factors, site of infection, and local resistance profiles of suspected or known pathogens. Further, national and local drug shortages and formulary restrictions can affect available therapies. Regular monitoring of the patient and collection of laboratory data should be undertaken to streamline antibacterial therapy as appropriate and to investigate the possibility of treatment failure if the patient fails to respond appropriately.

EMPIRICAL AND DIRECTED THERAPY

Therapy is considered *empirical* when the causative agent has yet to be determined and therapeutic decisions are based on the severity of illness, the clinician's assessment of likely pathogens in light of the clinical syndrome, the patient's medical conditions and prior therapy, and relevant epidemiologic factors. For patients with severe illness, empirical therapy often takes the form of an antibacterial combination that provides broad coverage of diverse agents and thus ensures adequate treatment of possible pathogens while additional data are being collected. *Directed* therapy is predicated on identification of the pathogen, determination of its susceptibility profile, and establishment of the extent of the infection. Directed therapy generally allows the use of more targeted and narrower-spectrum antibacterial agents than does empirical therapy.

Information on epidemiology, exposures, and local antibacterial susceptibility patterns can help guide empirical therapy. When empirical treatment is clinically appropriate, care should be taken to obtain clinical specimens for microbiologic analysis before the initiation of therapy and to adjust therapy as new information is obtained about the patient's clinical condition and the causal pathogens. Change to directed therapy can limit unnecessary risks of drug side effects as well as selection for antibacterial resistance.

SITE OF INFECTION

The site of infection is a consideration in antibacterial therapy, largely because of the differing abilities of drugs to penetrate and achieve adequate concentrations at particular body sites. For example, to be effective in the treatment of meningitis, an agent must (1) be able to cross the blood-brain barrier and reach adequate concentrations in the cerebrospinal fluid (CSF) and (2) be active against the relevant pathogen(s). Dexamethasone, administered with or 15–20 min before the first dose of an antibacterial drug, has been shown to improve outcomes in patients with some types of acute bacterial meningitis, but its use may reduce penetration of some antibacterial agents, such as vancomycin, into the CSF. In this case, rifampin is added because its penetration is not reduced by dexamethasone. Infections at sites where pathogens are protected from normal host defenses, penetration of an antibacterial drug is limited, or local conditions (e.g., low pH) limit activity of some agents include, in addition to meningitis, osteomyelitis, prostatitis, intraocular infections, and abscesses. In such cases, consideration must be given to the route of drug delivery (e.g., intravitreal injections) as well as to interventions to drain, debride, or otherwise reduce bacterial load and necrotic material that can reduce antibacterial activity.

HOST FACTORS

Host factors, including immune function, pregnancy, allergies, age, renal and hepatic function, drug–drug interactions, comorbid conditions, and occupational or social exposures, should be considered.

Immune Dysfunction Patients with deficits in immune function that blunt the response to bacterial infection, including neutropenia, deficient humoral immunity, and asplenia (either surgical or functional), are all at increased risk of severe bacterial infection. Such patients should be treated aggressively and often broadly in the early stages of suspected infection pending results of microbiologic tests. For asplenic patients, treatment should include coverage of encapsulated organisms, particularly *Streptococcus pneumoniae*, that may cause rapidly life-threatening infection. For neutropenic patients, initial treatment typically includes antibacterial agents with broad activity against gram-negative bacteria.

Pregnancy Pregnancy affects decisions regarding antibacterial therapy in two respects. First, pregnancy is associated with an increased risk of particular infections (e.g., those caused by *Listeria*). Second, the potential risks to the fetus that are posed by specific drugs must be considered. As for other drugs, the safety of the vast majority of antibacterial agents in pregnancy has not been established, and such agents are grouped in categories B and C by the U.S. Food and Drug Administration (FDA). Drugs in categories D and X are contraindicated in pregnancy or lactation due to established risks. Note that in accordance with the Pregnancy and Lactation Labeling Final Rule (PLLR), drugs submitted to the FDA for approval after 2015 do not use the pregnancy risk categories. The risks associated with antibacterial use in pregnancy and during lactation are summarized in **Table 144-1**.

Allergies Allergies to antibiotics are among the most common allergies reported, and an allergy history should be obtained whenever possible before therapy is chosen. A detailed allergy history can shed light on the type of reaction experienced previously and on whether rechallenge with the same or a related medication is advisable (and, if so, under what circumstances). Allergies to the penicillins are most common. Although as many as 10% of patients may report an allergy to penicillin, studies suggest that more than 90% of these patients could tolerate a penicillin or cephalosporin. Adverse effects **(Table 144-2)** should be distinguished from true allergies to ensure appropriate selection of antibacterial therapy.

Drug–Drug Interactions Patients commonly receive other drugs that may interact with antibacterial agents. A summary of the most common drug–drug interactions, by antibacterial class, is provided in **Table 144-3**.

Exposures Exposures, both occupational and social, may provide clues to likely pathogens. When relevant, inquiries about exposure to ill contacts, animals, insects, and water should be included in the history, along with sites of residence and travel.

Other Host Factors Age, renal and hepatic function, and comorbid conditions are all considerations in the choice of and schedule for therapy. Dose adjustments should be made accordingly. In patients with decreased or unreliable oral absorption, IV therapy may be preferred to ensure adequate blood levels of drug and delivery of the antibacterial agent to the site of infection. In general, initial treatment for severe and life-threatening infections is given by intravenous injection to assure prompt and adequate drug delivery.

DURATION OF THERAPY

Whether empirical or directed, the duration of therapy should be determined in most clinical situations. Guidelines that synthesize available literature and expert opinion provide recommendations on therapy duration that are based on infecting organism, organ system, and patient factors. For example, the American Heart Association has published guidelines endorsed by the Infectious Diseases Society of America (IDSA) on diagnosis, antibacterial therapy, and management of complications of infective endocarditis. Similar guidelines from the IDSA exist for bacterial meningitis, urinary tract infections (including those that are catheter-associated), intraabdominal infections, community- and hospital-acquired pneumonia, skin and soft tissue infections, and other infections. In general, where data on adequate durations of therapy exist, shorter courses are preferred to reduce the likelihood of drug adverse effects and selection of resistant bacteria.

FAILURE OF THERAPY

If a patient does not respond to therapy, investigations often should include imaging and the collection of additional specimens for microbiologic testing as indicated. Failure to respond can be the result of an antibacterial regimen that does not address the underlying causative organism, the development of resistance during therapy, or the existence of a focus of infection at a site poorly penetrated by systemic

TABLE 144-1 Risks Associated with Use of Antibacterial Drugs in Pregnancy and Lactation

PREGNANCY CATEGORY[a]	ANTIBACTERIAL DRUG	FETAL RISK RECOMMENDATION[b]	BREAST-FEEDING RISK RECOMMENDATION[b]
B	Azithromycin	Limited human data. Animal data suggest low risk.	Limited human data; probably compatible
	Cephalosporins (including cephalexin, cefuroxime, cefixime, cefpodoxime, cefotaxime, ceftriaxone)	Compatible	Compatible
	Ceftazidime-avibactam	No human data; no fetal harm in animal studies	Ceftazidime is excreted into human milk in low concentrations. Avibactam is excreted into the milk of lactating rats; no human studies have been conducted.
	Ceftolozane-tazobactam	Compatible	Unknown
	Clindamycin	Compatible	Compatible
	Ertapenem	No human data; probably compatible	Limited human data; probably compatible
	Erythromycin	Compatible (except for estolate salt)	Compatible
	Meropenem and meropenem-vaborbactam	No human data. Animal data suggest low risk.	No human data; probably compatible
	Metronidazole	Human data suggest low risk.	Interrupt breast-feeding for 12–24 h after single 2-g dose. Limited human data; potential toxicity in divided doses
	Nitrofurantoin	Human data suggest risk in third trimester.	Limited human data; probably compatible. Higher risk associated with younger infants and those with G6PD deficiency
	Penicillins (including amoxicillin, ampicillin, cloxacillin)	Compatible	Compatible
	Quinupristin-dalfopristin	Compatible. Maternal benefit must far outweigh risk to embryo/fetus.	No human data; potential toxicity
	Vancomycin	Compatible	Limited human data; probably compatible
C	Chloramphenicol	Compatible	Limited human data; potential toxicity
	Fluoroquinolones	Human data suggest low risk.	Limited human data; probably compatible
	Clarithromycin	Limited human data. Animal data suggest high risk.	No human data; probably compatible
	Imipenem-cilastatin	Limited human data. Animal data suggest low risk.	Limited human data; probably compatible
	Linezolid	Compatible. Maternal benefit must far outweigh risk to embryo/fetus.	No human data; potential toxicity
	Telavancin	No human data. Animal studies have revealed evidence of teratogenicity.[c]	No human data. Animal studies have revealed evidence of teratogenicity.[c]
	Tedizolid	Limited data. Embryofetal studies in mice, rats, and rabbits have demonstrated fetal developmental toxicities. Use only if benefit outweighs risk.	Excreted in the breast milk of rats; unknown in humans; caution use
	Dalbavancin	Limited human data. At high doses in animal studies, delayed fetal maturation, increased embryo and offspring death. Use only if benefit outweighs risk.	Excreted in the breast milk of animals; unknown in humans; caution use
	Oritavancin	Limited human data. Studies in rats and rabbits demonstrated no harm at 25% of recommended human dose. Use only if benefit outweighs risk.	Excreted in the breast milk of rats; unknown in humans; caution use
C/D	Amikacin	Human data suggest low risk.	Compatible
	Gentamicin	Human data suggest low risk.	Compatible
D	Kanamycin	Human data suggest risk.	Limited human data; probably compatible
	Streptomycin	Human data suggest risk.	Compatible
	Sulfonamides	Human data suggest risk in third trimester.	Limited human data; potential toxicity. Avoid in ill, stressed, premature infants and in infants with hyperbilirubinemia or G6PD deficiency.
	Tetracyclines	Contraindicated in second and third trimesters.	Compatible
	Tigecycline	Human data suggest risk in second and third trimesters.	No human data; potential toxicity
Not assigned[d]	Cefiderocol	No controlled data in human pregnancy; animal studies have not provided evidence of fetal harm.	Unknown if excreted in human milk; excreted in animal milk.
	Eravacycline	No controlled data in human pregnancy; animal data indicate drug crosses placenta and is associated with risk at higher doses,	Unknown if excreted in human milk; excreted in animal milk. Not recommended during and for a period after treatment.
	Imipenem-cilastatin-relebactam	No controlled data in human pregnancy; animal studies have not revealed teratogenicity but have shown evidence of increased fetal loss.	Imipenem and cilastatin are excreted into human milk; no data on relebactam in human milk. Relebactam is excreted in animal milk. No human data regarding potential effect on infant.
	Lefamulin[e]	No controlled data in human pregnancy; animal studies have revealed evidence of fetal harm.	Unknown if excreted in human milk; excreted in animal milk. Breastfeeding is not recommended during use and for 2 days afterward.

(Continued)

TABLE 144-1 Risks Associated with Use of Antibacterial Drugs in Pregnancy and Lactation (Continued)

PREGNANCY CATEGORY[a]	ANTIBACTERIAL DRUG	FETAL RISK RECOMMENDATION[b]	BREAST-FEEDING RISK RECOMMENDATION[b]
	Meropenem-vaborbactam	No controlled data in human pregnancy; animal studies have revealed evidence of fetal harm (related to vaborbactam component).	Meropenem is excreted in human milk; it is unknown if vaborbactam is excreted in human milk. Data on excretion of vaborbactam in animal milk is unknown.
	Omadacycline	No controlled data in human pregnancy; however, as this is a tetracycline class antibiotic, may cause deciduous tooth discoloration and bone growth inhibition in second and third trimesters of pregnancy; animal data have demonstrated embryofetal lethality, teratogenicity, and embryofetal toxicity.	Unknown if excreted in human milk; data not available regarding excretion in animal milk. Not recommended during and for a period after treatment.
	Plazomicin	No controlled data in human pregnancy; however, aminoglycoside antibiotics are known to cause fetal harm in pregnancy.	Unknown if excreted in human milk; excreted in animal milk.

[a]*Category B: Either* animal reproduction studies have failed to demonstrate a risk to the fetus, and there are no adequate and well-controlled studies in pregnant women; *or* animal studies have shown an adverse effect, but adequate and well-controlled studies in pregnant women have failed to demonstrate a risk to the fetus in any trimester. *Category C:* Animal reproduction studies have shown an adverse effect on the fetus, and there are no adequate and well-controlled studies in humans, but potential benefits may warrant use of the drug in pregnant women despite potential risks. *Category D:* There is positive evidence of human fetal risk based on adverse reaction data from investigational or marketing experience or studies in humans, but potential benefits may warrant use of the drug in pregnant women despite potential risks. [b]Fetal risk recommendation and breast-feeding risk recommendation adapted from GG Briggs et al (eds): *Drugs in Pregnancy and Lactation*, 9th ed. Philadelphia, Lippincott Williams and Wilkins, 2011; and the U.S. Food and Drug Administration (Drugs@FDA). [c]A registry has been established to monitor pregnancy outcomes of pregnant women exposed to telavancin. Physicians are encouraged to register pregnant patients or pregnant women may enroll themselves by calling 1-855-633-8479. [d]The U.S. Food and Drug Administration is phasing out use of pregnancy categories A, B, C, D, and X. [e]A pregnancy pharmacovigilance program is available: If this drug is inadvertently administered during pregnancy or if a patient becomes pregnant while receiving this drug, healthcare providers or patients should report drug exposure by calling 1-855-5NABRIVA (1-855-56227482) to enroll.

Abbreviation: G6PD, glucose-6-phosphate dehydrogenase.

therapy. Some infections may also require surgical interventions (e.g., large abscesses, myonecrosis). Fever due to allergic drug reactions can sometimes complicate assessment of the patient's response to antibacterial treatment.

EXPERT GUIDANCE

Selected websites with the most up-to-date information and guidance for the clinician include the following:

- Johns Hopkins ABX Guide (*www.hopkins-abxguide.org*)
- IDSA Practice Guidelines (*https://www.idsociety.org/practice-guideline/practice-guidelines/#/date_na_dt/DESC/0/+/*)
- Center for Disease Dynamics, Economics and Policy Antibiotic Resistance Map (*https://resistancemap.cddep.org/AntibioticResistance.php*)
- Centers for Disease Control and Prevention Antibiotic/Antimicrobial Resistance (*www.cdc.gov/drugresistance/*)

CLINICAL USE OF ANTIBACTERIAL AGENTS

The clinical application of antibacterial therapy is guided by the spectrum of the agent and the suspected or known target pathogen. Infections for which specific antibacterial agents are among the drugs of choice are listed, along with associated pathogens and susceptibility data, in **Table 144-4**. Resistance rates of specific organisms are dynamic and should be taken into account in the approach to antibacterial therapy. While national resistance rates can serve as a reference, the most useful reference for the clinician is the most recent local laboratory antibiogram, which provides details on local resistance patterns, often on an annual or semiannual basis.

β-LACTAMS

The β-lactam class of antibiotics consists of penicillins, cephalosporins, carbapenems, and monobactams. The term *β-lactam* reflects the drugs' four-membered lactam ring, which is their core structure. The differing side chains among the agents of this family determine the spectrum of activity. All β-lactams exert a bactericidal effect by inhibiting bacterial cell-wall synthesis. The β-lactams are classified as time-dependent killing agents; therefore, their clinical efficacy is best correlated with the proportion of the dosing interval during which drug levels remain above the MIC for the targeted pathogen.

Penicillins and β-Lactamase Inhibitors Penicillin, the first β-lactam, was discovered in 1928 by Alexander Fleming. Natural penicillins, such as penicillin G, are active against non-β-lactamase-producing gram-positive and gram-negative bacteria, anaerobes, and some gram-negative cocci. Penicillin G is used for penicillin-susceptible streptococcal infections, pneumococcal and meningococcal meningitis, enterococcal endocarditis, and syphilis. The antistaphylococcal penicillins, which have potent activity against methicillin-susceptible *Staphylococcus aureus* (MSSA), include nafcillin, oxacillin, dicloxacillin, and flucloxacillin. Aminopenicillins, such as ampicillin and amoxicillin, provide added coverage beyond penicillin against gram-negative cocci, such as *Haemophilus influenzae*, and some Enterobacterales, including *Escherichia coli*, *Proteus mirabilis*, *Salmonella*, and *Shigella*. The aminopenicillins are hydrolyzed by many common β-lactamases. These drugs are commonly used for infections caused by susceptible enterococcal and streptococcal species. IV ampicillin is commonly used in meningitis and endocarditis. Oral amoxicillin may be an option for otitis media, respiratory tract infections, and urinary tract infections. The antipseudomonal penicillins include ticarcillin and piperacillin. These penicillin groups generally offer adequate anaerobic coverage; the exceptions are *Bacteroides* species (such as *Bacteroides fragilis*), which produce β-lactamases and are generally resistant. The rising prevalence of β-lactamase-producing bacteria has led to the increased use of β-lactam–β-lactamase inhibitor combinations, such as ampicillin-sulbactam, amoxicillin-clavulanate, ticarcillin-clavulanate, piperacillin-tazobactam, ceftolozane-tazobactam, ceftazidime-avibactam, meropenem-vaborbactam, and imipenem-relebactam. The β-lactamase inhibitors themselves do not have antibacterial activity (with the exception of sulbactam, which has activity against *Acinetobacter baumannii*) but typically inhibit the *S. aureus* class A β-lactamase, β-lactamases of *H. influenzae* and *Bacteroides* species, and a number of plasmid-encoded β-lactamases. These combination agents are typically used when broader-spectrum coverage is needed—e.g., in pneumonia and intraabdominal infections. Piperacillin-tazobactam is a useful agent for broad coverage in febrile neutropenic patients. Avibactam, vaborbactam, and relebactam inhibit a broader spectrum of β-lactamases than the other inhibitors, including extended-spectrum β-lactamases (ESBLs), AmpC β-lactamases, and some carbapenemases (**see Chap. 145**).

Cephalosporins The cephalosporin drug class encompasses several generations distinguished by a spectrum of antibacterial activity. The first generation (cefazolin, cefadroxil, and cephalexin) largely has activity against gram-positive bacteria, with some additional activity against *E. coli*, *P. mirabilis*, and *Klebsiella pneumoniae*. First-generation cephalosporins are commonly used for infections caused by MSSA and

TABLE 144-2 Common Adverse Reactions to Antibacterial Agents

ANTIBACTERIAL(S)	POTENTIAL ADVERSE EFFECTS	COMMENTS
β-Lactams	Hypersensitivity reactions	Range from rash to anaphylaxis. Cross-reactivity among β-lactams is related to chemical structure and side chain similarity.
	Neurotoxicity	More commonly described with cefepime and imipenem, but likely a class effect. Risk is increased in patients with history of seizures, renal impairment, and advanced age.
	Neutropenia/hematologic reactions	May be related to high doses and prolonged duration.
Vancomycin	Nephrotoxicity	Risk increases with vancomycin trough levels >20 μg/mL or concomitant administration with other potentially nephrotoxic agents. The effect is usually reversible.
	Infusion reaction formerly known as "red man syndrome"	Can be managed with a slower vancomycin infusion and pretreatment with antihistamine.
Telavancin	QT prolongation	
	Interference with coagulation tests	May falsely affect INR, PT, aPTT. Perform these tests before the next dose of telavancin (when serum drug levels are at their nadir).
	Taste disturbances	
	Nephrotoxicity	
Oritavancin	Interference with coagulation tests	May falsely affect INR, PT, aPTT. Perform these tests at least 24 h after the dose is administered.
	Gastrointestinal distress	
Dalbavancin	Gastrointestinal distress	
Daptomycin	Myopathy	Monitor CPK levels during therapy. Rhabdomyolysis has been reported but appears to be rare.
	Eosinophilic pneumonia	
Aminoglycosides	Nephrotoxicity	Associated with prolonged use; usually reversible
	Ototoxicity	Can cause both vestibular and cochlear toxicity. Ototoxicity may be irreversible.
Fluoroquinolones	QT_c prolongation	Moxifloxacin appears more likely than other quinolones to exert this effect. Risk of arrhythmia increases when these drugs are given concomitantly with other QT_c-prolonging agents.
	Tendinitis	Risk is greater among the elderly and patients receiving steroids.
	Dysglycemia	
	Exacerbation of myasthenia gravis	
Rifampin	Hepatotoxicity	Risk is greater when drug is given with other antituberculosis agents. When rifampin is given alone, LFT values may be transiently elevated without symptoms.
	Orange discoloration of body fluids	
Tetracyclines, including tigecycline, eravacycline, and omadacycline	Photosensitivity	
	Gastrointestinal distress	High incidence of diarrhea, nausea, vomiting
Macrolides	Gastrointestinal distress	Erythromycin is occasionally used as a therapeutic agent for some gastric motility disorders.
	QT_c prolongation	Azithromycin use is associated with an increased risk of death from cardiovascular causes among patients at high baseline risk.
Metronidazole	Peripheral neuropathy	Associated with prolonged use
Clindamycin	Diarrhea and pseudomembranous colitis	
Linezolid, tedizolid	Myelosuppression	Associated with prolonged use
	Optic and peripheral neuropathy	Associated with prolonged use
	Lactic acidosis	
TMP-SMX	Hypersensitivity reactions	Allergy usually associated with sulfonamide moiety
	Nephrotoxicity	Associated with high doses
	Hematologic effects	Associated with prolonged use
Nitrofurantoin	Pneumonitis and other pulmonary reactions	Associated with prolonged use
	Peripheral neuropathy	Associated with accumulation of nitrofurantoin in renal failure. Avoid use in renal impairment.
Fosfomycin	Gastrointestinal effects	
Polymyxins	Nephrotoxicity	Associated with high dose
	Neurotoxicity	Neuromuscular blockade and muscle weakness are well described and usually reversible.
Quinupristin-dalfopristin	Arthralgias and myalgias	
Chloramphenicol	Bone marrow suppression	Aplastic anemia or hematopoietic toxicity
Pleuromutilin	Gastrointestinal	Diarrhea
	QT_c prolongation	When used in conjunction with CYP3A4 substrates

Note: All systemic antibiotics have the potential to alter abdominal flora and induce *Clostridioides difficile* infection.

Abbreviations: aPTT, activated partial thromboplastin time; CPK, creatine phosphokinase; INR, international normalized ratio; LFT, liver function test; PT, prothrombin time; TMP-SMX, trimethoprim-sulfamethoxazole.

TABLE 144-3 Important Antibacterial Drug Interactions

ANTIBACTERIAL(S)	INTERACTING AGENT(S)	POTENTIAL EFFECT AND MANAGEMENT
Nafcillin	Warfarin, cyclosporine, tacrolimus	Decreased effects of interacting drug via CYP3A4 induction. Monitor levels of affected drug closely if drugs are given concomitantly.
Ceftriaxone	Calcium-containing IV solutions	Concomitant use is contraindicated in neonates (<28 days); the combination can lead to precipitation of ceftriaxone-calcium particulate. Ceftriaxone and calcium-containing solutions can be given to infants >28 days of age provided they are given sequentially and the lines are thoroughly flushed between infusions, or infused via separate lines.
Carbapenems	Valproic acid	Diminished levels of valproic acid. Monitor valproic acid levels closely if drugs are given concomitantly and consider alternative therapies.
Linezolid, tedizolid	Serotonergic and adrenergic agents (e.g., SSRIs, vasopressors)	Increased levels of serotonergic and adrenergic agents. Monitor for serotonin syndrome. Tedizolid may have less potential than linezolid to cause this drug interaction.
Quinupristin-dalfopristin	Substrates of CYP3A4 (e.g., warfarin, ritonavir, cyclosporine, diazepam, verapamil)	Can result in increased levels of interacting drug
Fluoroquinolones	Theophylline[a]	Can result in theophylline toxicity
	Sucralfate; antacids containing aluminum, calcium, or magnesium; ferrous sulfate– and zinc-containing multivitamins	Can result in decreased oral absorption of fluoroquinolones. Administer fluoroquinolone 2 h before or 6 h after interacting drug.
	Tizanidine[a]	Can result in increased levels of tizanidine and hypotensive, sedative effects. Monitor for side effects if drugs are given concomitantly.
	QT_c-prolonging drugs (e.g., azoles, sotalol, amiodarone, dofetilide, fluoxetine)	Increased risk of cardiotoxicity and arrhythmias. Monitor QT_c.
Rifampin	Substrates of CYP3A4 (e.g., warfarin, ritonavir, cyclosporine, diazepam, verapamil, protease inhibitors, voriconazole)	Can result in decreased levels of interacting drug. Avoid concomitant use if possible. If giving drugs concomitantly, monitor drug levels if possible.
	Substrates of CYP2C19 (e.g., omeprazole, lansoprazole)	
	Substrates of CYP2C9 (e.g., warfarin, tolbutamide)	
	Substrates of CYP2C8 (e.g., repaglinide, rosiglitazone)	
	Substrates of CYP2B6 (e.g., efavirenz)	
	Hormone therapy (e.g., norethindrone)	Can result in decreased levels of hormone. If oral contraceptive and rifampin are given concomitantly, use alternative or additional forms of birth control.
Tetracyclines	Antacids or drugs containing calcium, magnesium, iron, or aluminum	Can result in decreased oral absorption of tetracyclines. Administer tetracycline 2 h before or 6 h after interacting drug.
	Warfarin	Increased effect of warfarin. Monitor levels closely if drugs are given concomitantly.
	Eravacycline: Strong CYP3A4 inducers (e.g., rifampin)	Reduced eravacycline efficacy
Macrolides[b]	Substrates of CYP3A4 (e.g., warfarin, ritonavir, cyclosporine, diazepam, verapamil, amiodarone)	Avoid concomitant administration if possible.
	QT_c-prolonging agents (e.g., fluoroquinolones, sotalol)	Increased risk of cardiotoxicity and arrhythmias. Monitor QT_c.
	Protease inhibitors (e.g., ritonavir)	Can result in increased levels of both macrolides and protease inhibitors. Avoid concomitant use if possible.
	Cimetidine	Cimetidine can increase levels of macrolides.
Metronidazole	Ethanol	Can result in disulfiram-like reaction. Ethanol may be present in some formulations of oral drug suspensions (e.g., ritonavir).
	Warfarin	Can increase warfarin effects. Monitor INR closely if drugs are given concomitantly.
TMP-SMX	Warfarin	Increased effect of warfarin. Monitor levels closely if drugs are given concomitantly.
	Phenytoin	Increased levels of phenytoin. Monitor levels closely if drugs are given concomitantly.
	Methotrexate	Increased levels of methotrexate and prolonged exposure. Monitor levels closely if drugs are given concomitantly.
Oritavancin	Substrates of CYP3A4 (e.g., cyclosporine, warfarin) and CYP2D6 (e.g., aripiprazole)	Can result in decreased levels of interacting drug. Avoid concomitant use if possible. If giving drugs concomitantly, monitor drug levels if possible.
	Substrates of CYP2C19 (e.g., omeprazole) and CYP2C9 (e.g., warfarin)	
Lefamulin	QT_c-prolonging drugs (e.g., azoles, sotalol, amiodarone, dofetilide, fluoxetine)	Increased risk of cardiotoxicity and arrhythmias. Monitor QT_c.
	Strong CYP3A4 inducers (e.g., rifampin)	Reduced lefamulin efficacy
	Strong CYP3A4 strong inhibitors (e.g., ritonavir)	Increased lefamulin exposure

[a]Drug reaction described with ciprofloxacin only. [b]Clarithromycin and erythromycin are potent CYP3A4 inhibitors; the probability of a drug interaction with azithromycin is lower.

Abbreviations: INR, international normalized ratio; SSRI, selective serotonin-reuptake inhibitor; TMP-SMX, trimethoprim-sulfamethoxazole.

TABLE 144-4 Drug Indications for Specific Infections, Associated Pathogens, and Sample Susceptibility Rates

ANTIMICROBIAL(S)	INFECTIONS	COMMON PATHOGENS (% SUSCEPTIBLE); RESISTANCE AS NOTED[a]
Penicillin G	Syphilis; yaws; leptospirosis; streptococcal infections; pneumococcal infections; actinomycosis; oral and periodontal infections; meningococcal meningitis and meningococcemia; viridans streptococcal endocarditis; clostridial myonecrosis; tetanus; rat-bite fever; *Pasteurella multocida* infections; erysipeloid (*Erysipelothrix rhusiopathiae*)	*Neisseria meningitidis*; viridans streptococci (69%); *Streptococcus pneumoniae* (97% nonmeningitis; 75% meningitis)
Ampicillin, amoxicillin	Salmonellosis; acute otitis media; *Haemophilus influenzae* meningitis and epiglottitis; *Listeria monocytogenes* meningitis; *Enterococcus faecalis* UTI	*Escherichia coli* (51%); *H. influenzae* (70%); *Salmonella* spp. (85%)
Nafcillin, oxacillin	MSSA bacteremia and endocarditis	*Staphylococcus aureus* (70%); coagulase-negative staphylococci (50%)
Piperacillin-tazobactam	Intraabdominal infections (facultative enteric gram-negative bacilli and obligate anaerobes); infections caused by mixed flora (aspiration pneumonia, diabetic foot ulcers); infections caused by *Pseudomonas aeruginosa*	*P. aeruginosa* (82%)
Cefazolin	*E. coli* UTI; surgical prophylaxis; MSSA bacteremia and endocarditis	*E. coli* (82%)
Cefoxitin, cefotetan	Intraabdominal infections and pelvic inflammatory disease	*Bacteroides fragilis* (60%)[b]
Ceftriaxone	Gonococcal infections; pneumococcal meningitis; viridans streptococcal endocarditis; salmonellosis and typhoid fever; hospital-acquired infections caused by nonpseudomonal facultative gram-negative enteric bacilli	*S. pneumoniae* (91% meningitis; 99% nonmeningitis); *E. coli* (90%); *Klebsiella pneumoniae* (88%)
Ceftazidime, cefepime	Hospital-acquired infections caused by facultative gram-negative bacilli and *Pseudomonas* spp.	*P. aeruginosa* (86%)
Ceftaroline	CAP caused by *S. pneumoniae*, MSSA, *H. influenzae*, *K. pneumoniae*, *Klebsiella oxytoca*, and *E. coli*; acute bacterial skin and skin-structure infections caused by MSSA, MRSA, *Streptococcus pyogenes*, *Streptococcus agalactiae*, *E. coli*, *K. pneumoniae*, and *K. oxytoca*	Mostly susceptible; four strains of MRSA with ceftaroline MICs >4 μg/mL reported in isolates from a single Greek hospital[c]; additional case reports, including in patients without prior exposure to ceftaroline[d,e]
Ceftazidime-avibactam, meropenem-vaborbactam	Complicated UTIs (ceftazidime-avibactam and meropenem-vaborbactam) and complicated intraabdominal infections (ceftazidime-avibactam in combination with metronidazole) caused by resistant gram-negative organisms, including *Pseudomonas*, and some anaerobes	*P. aeruginosa* (84–97%)[f] MDR Enterobacterales, including carbapenem-resistant Enterobacterales that produce KPCs No activity against metallo-β-lactamases (e.g., NDM)
Ceftolozane-tazobactam	Complicated UTIs and complicated intraabdominal infections (in combination with metronidazole) caused by resistant gram-negative organisms, including *Pseudomonas*, and some anaerobes	*P. aeruginosa* (>86% overall; 60–80% of ceftazidime- and meropenem-resistant strains)[f] MDR Enterobacterales No activity against KPC-producing organisms
Imipenem, meropenem	Intraabdominal infections, infections caused by *Enterobacter* spp. and ESBL-producing gram-negative bacilli	*P. aeruginosa* (84%); *Acinetobacter calcoaceticus-baumannii* complex (85%) (meropenem susceptibilities reported)
Ertapenem	CAP; complicated UTIs, including pyelonephritis; acute pelvic infections; complicated intraabdominal infections; complicated skin and skin-structure infections, excluding diabetic foot infections accompanied by osteomyelitis or caused by *P. aeruginosa*	*Enterobacter cloacae* (90%); *K. pneumoniae* (98%)
Aztreonam	Infections caused by facultative gram-negative bacilli and *Pseudomonas* in penicillin-allergic patients	*P. aeruginosa* (69%)
Vancomycin	Bacteremia, endocarditis, and other invasive disease caused by MRSA; pneumococcal meningitis; oral formulation for CDAD	*S. aureus* (100%); *E. faecalis* (96%); *E. faecium* (34%)
Telavancin	Hospital- and ventilator-associated pneumonia or skin and soft tissue infections caused by MRSA	*S. aureus*: none reported
Dalbavancin, oritavancin	Complicated skin and soft tissue infections	*S. aureus*: rarely reported for dalbavancin,[g] rarely reported for oritavancin[h]
Daptomycin	VRE infections; MRSA bacteremia	*E. faecalis* (99.9%)[i]; *E. faecium* (99.7%)[i]; *S. aureus* (99.9%)[g]
Gentamicin, tobramycin, amikacin	Combined with penicillin for staphylococcal, enterococcal, or streptococcal endocarditis; combined with β-lactam for gram-negative bacteremia; pyelonephritis	*E. coli* (gentamicin, 91%); *P. aeruginosa* (amikacin, 82%; gentamicin, 84%); *A. calcoaceticus-baumannii* complex (gentamicin, 89%)
Azithromycin, clarithromycin, erythromycin	*Legionella*, *Campylobacter*, and *Mycoplasma* infections; CAP; GAS pharyngitis in penicillin-allergic patients; bacillary angiomatosis; gastric infections due to *Helicobacter pylori*; MAC infections	*S. pneumoniae* (60%); group A streptococci (82%); *H. pylori* (75%)[j]
Clindamycin	Severe, invasive GAS infections (with a β-lactam); infections caused by obligate anaerobes; infections caused by susceptible staphylococci	*S. aureus* (70%)
Doxycycline, minocycline	Acute bacterial exacerbations of chronic bronchitis; granuloma inguinale; brucellosis (with streptomycin); tularemia; glanders; melioidosis; spirochetal infections caused by *Borrelia* (Lyme disease and relapsing fever; doxycycline); infections caused by *Vibrio vulnificus*; some *Aeromonas* infections; infections due to *Stenotrophomonas* (minocycline); plague; ehrlichiosis; chlamydial infections (doxycycline); granulomatous infections due to *Mycobacterium marinum* (minocycline); rickettsial infections; mild CAP; skin and soft tissue infections caused by gram-positive cocci (e.g., CA-MRSA infections); leptospirosis; syphilis; and actinomycosis in the penicillin-allergic patient	*S. pneumoniae* (63%); *S. aureus* (97%)

(*Continued*)

TABLE 144-4 Drug Indications for Specific Infections, Associated Pathogens, and Sample Susceptibility Rates (Continued)

ANTIMICROBIAL(S)	INFECTIONS	COMMON PATHOGENS (% SUSCEPTIBLE); RESISTANCE AS NOTED[a]
Tigecycline	CAP caused by *S. pneumoniae, H. influenzae*, or *Legionella pneumophila*; complicated skin infections caused by *E. coli*, MRSA, MSSA, *S. pyogenes, Streptococcus anginosus, S. agalactiae, B. fragilis*; complicated intraabdominal infections caused by *E. coli*, vancomycin-susceptible *E. faecalis, Citrobacter freundii, E. cloacae, K. pneumoniae, K. oxytoca, Bacteroides* spp., *Clostridium perfringens*, and *Peptostreptococcus* spp.	Mostly susceptible, although case reports of resistance in *A. baumannii* and *K. pneumoniae*
TMP-SMX	Community-acquired UTI; CA-MRSA skin and soft tissue infections	*E. coli* (73%); *S. aureus* (95%)
Sulfonamides	Nocardial infections; leprosy (dapsone); toxoplasmosis (sulfadiazine)	Unknown
Ciprofloxacin, levofloxacin, moxifloxacin, delafloxacin	CAP (levofloxacin and moxifloxacin); UTI; bacterial gastroenteritis; hospital-acquired gram-negative enteric infections; *Pseudomonas* infections (ciprofloxacin and levofloxacin); skin and skin-structure infections (delafloxacin)	*S. pneumoniae* (99% levofloxacin); *E. coli* (79% for ciprofloxacin and levofloxacin); *P. aeruginosa* (ciprofloxacin, 76%; levofloxacin, 70%); *Salmonella* spp. (72% for ciprofloxacin and levofloxacin)
Rifampin	Staphylococcal foreign body infections (in combination with other antistaphylococcal agents); *Legionella* pneumonia; *Mycobacterium tuberculosis*; atypical nontuberculous mycobacterial infection; pneumococcal meningitis when organisms are susceptible or response is delayed	*S. aureus* (99%), although staphylococci rapidly develop resistance with monotherapy
Metronidazole	Obligate anaerobic gram-negative bacteria (e.g., *Bacteroides* spp.); abscess in lung, brain, or abdomen; bacterial vaginosis; CDAD	Mostly susceptible; resistance very rare
Linezolid, tedizolid	VRE; uncomplicated and complicated skin and soft tissue infections caused by MSSA and MRSA; CAP with concurrent bacteremia; hospital-acquired pneumonia	Mostly susceptible; resistance occasionally seen in VRE
Chloramphenicol	Infections due to gram-positive and gram-negative organisms resistant to standard alternatives (e.g., *Burkholderia*)	Unknown
Colistin	Infections due to gram-negative bacilli resistant to all other chemotherapy (e.g., *P. aeruginosa, Acinetobacter* spp., and *Stenotrophomonas maltophilia*)	*P. aeruginosa* (case reports, outbreaks)
Quinupristin-dalfopristin	VRE; complicated skin and skin-structure infections due to MSSA and *S. pyogenes*	*E. faecalis* (<20%)[k]; *E. faecium* (>90%)[k]
Mupirocin	Topical application to nares for *S. aureus* decolonization	*S. aureus* (74–100%)[l]
Nitrofurantoin	UTI caused by most gram-negative bacilli and some gram-positive organisms; prophylaxis in recurrent cystitis	*E. coli* (95%); *E. faecalis* (99%)
Fosfomycin	UTI caused by most gram-negative bacilli and some gram-positive organisms; prophylaxis in recurrent cystitis	Considered low prevalence[l]
Cefiderocol	Complicated UTIs and/or pyelonephritis caused by multidrug-resistant gram-negative bacteria, including extended-spectrum beta-lactamase- or carbapenemase-producing organisms and multidrug-resistant *P. aeruginosa, A. baumannii, Stenotrophomonas maltophilia*, and *Burkholderia cepacia* complex	Very low resistance rates in initial studies
Eravacycline	Complicated intra-abdominal infections caused by *E. coli, K. pneumoniae, C. freundii, E. cloacae, K. oxytoca, E. faecalis, E. faecium, S. aureus, S. anginosus* group, *C. perfringens, Bacteroides* spp., and *Parabacteroides distasonis*	Resistance noted in both gram-negative and gram-positive bacteria[m]
Imipenem-cilastatin-relebactam	Complicated intraabdominal infections, pneumonia, and complicated UTI including pyelonephritis caused by multidrug-resistant organisms including Enterobacterales and against some imipenem-nonsusceptible *P. aeruginosa*	Low resistance rates in initial studies
Lefamulin[e]	CAP caused by MRSA, *S. pneumoniae*, and atypical CAP pathogens	Low resistance rates in target pathogens in initial studies
Meropenem-vaborbactam	Complicated UTI caused by KPC-producing Enterobacteriaceae	Identified in KPC-producing strains of *K. pneumoniae*[n]
Omadacycline	Community-acquired bacterial pneumonia caused by *S. pneumoniae, S. aureus* (methicillin-susceptible isolates), *H. influenzae, Haemophilus parainfluenzae, K. pneumoniae, L. pneumophila, Mycoplasma pneumoniae*, and *Chlamydophila pneumoniae*	Broad spectrum overall, but resistance can occur in gram-negative isolates; not active against *Pseudomonas*
Plazomicin	Complicated UTIs caused by carbapenemase-producing Enterobacteriaceae	Resistance uncommon except in infrequent isolates with plasmid-encoded ribosome-modifying methylases

[a]Unless otherwise noted, susceptibility rates are based on isolates from the Massachusetts General Hospital Clinical Microbiology Laboratory collected between January and December 2012. Local rates will vary. [b]JA Karlowsky et al: Antimicrob Agents Chemother 56:1247, 2012. [c]RE Mendes et al: J Antimicrob Chemother 67:1321, 2012. [d]SW Long et al: Antimicrob Agents Chemother 58:6668, 2014. [e]M Nigo et al: Antimicrob Agents Chemother 61:e01235, 2017. [f]D Van Duin, RA Bonomo: Clin Infect Dis 63:234, 2016. [g]SP McCurdy et al: Antimicrob Agents Chemother 59:5007, 2015. [h]JA Karlowsky et al: Diag Microbiol Infect Dis 87:349, 2017. [i]HS Sader et al: J Chemother 23:200, 2011. [j]J Torres et al: J Clin Microbiol 39:2677, 2001. [k]WS Oh et al: Antimicrob Agents Chemother 49:5176, 2005. [l]AE Simor et al: Antimicrob Agents Chemother 51:3880, 2007; S Demirci-Duarte et al: Diagn Microbiol Infect Dis 98:115098, 2020. [m]LJ Scott: Drugs 79:315, 2019. [n]D Sun et al: Antimicrob Agents Chemother 61:e01694, 2017.

Abbreviations: CA-MRSA, community-acquired MRSA; CAP, community-acquired pneumonia; CA-UTI, community-acquired UTI; CDAD, *Clostridioides difficile*–associated diarrhea; ESBL, extended-spectrum β-lactamase; GAS, group A streptococcal; KPCs, *Klebsiella pneumoniae* carbapenemases; MAC, *M. avium* complex; MDR, multidrug-resistant; MIC, minimal inhibitory concentration; MRSA, methicillin-resistant *S. aureus*; MSSA, methicillin-susceptible *S. aureus*; NDM, New Delhi metallo-β-lactamase; TMP-SMX, trimethoprim-sulfamethoxazole; UTI, urinary tract infection; VRE, vancomycin-resistant *Enterococcus*.

streptococci (e.g., skin and soft tissue infections). Cefazolin is a popular choice for surgical prophylaxis against skin organisms. The second generation (cefamandole, cefuroxime, cefaclor, cefprozil, cefuroxime axetil, cefoxitin, and cefotetan) has additional activity against *H. influenzae* and *Moraxella catarrhalis*. Cefoxitin and cefotetan have potent activity against anaerobes as well. Second-generation cephalosporins have been used to treat community-acquired pneumonia because of their activity against *S. pneumoniae, H. influenzae*, and *M. catarrhalis*. They are also used for other mild or moderate infections, such as acute otitis media and sinusitis. The third-generation cephalosporins are characterized by greater potency against gram-negative bacilli and reduced potency against gram-positive cocci. These cephalosporins, which include cefoperazone, cefotaxime, ceftazidime, ceftriaxone, cefdinir, cefixime, and cefpodoxime, are used for infections caused by Enterobacterales, although resistance is an increasing concern. Ceftriaxone penetrates the CSF and can be used to treat meningitis caused by *H. influenzae*, *N. meningitidis*, and susceptible strains of *S. pneumoniae*. It is also used for the treatment of later-stage Lyme disease, gonococcal infections, and streptococcal endocarditis. It is noteworthy that ceftazidime is the only third-generation cephalosporin with activity against *Pseudomonas aeruginosa*, but it lacks activity against gram-positive bacteria. This drug is frequently used for pulmonary infections in cystic fibrosis, postneurosurgical meningitis, and febrile neutropenia. The fourth generation of cephalosporins includes cefepime and cefpirome, broad-coverage agents with potent activity against both gram-negative bacilli, including *P. aeruginosa*, and gram-positive cocci. The fourth generation has clinical applications similar to those of the third generation and may offer additional activity over the first, second, and third generations in the presence of certain β-lactamases. These agents can be used in bacteremia, febrile neutropenia, and intraabdominal and urinary tract infections. Ceftaroline, a fifth-generation cephalosporin, differs from the other cephalosporins in its added activity against MRSA, which is resistant to all other β-lactams. Ceftaroline's gram-negative activity is similar to that of the third-generation cephalosporins but does not include *P. aeruginosa*. Ceftaroline may be used in community-acquired pneumonia and skin infections, and emerging data support its use in more severe infections such as bacteremia. Adverse reactions to ceftaroline have included hypersensitivity reactions and neutropenia. Ceftolozane-tazobactam and ceftazidime-avibactam are novel cephalosporin–β-lactamase inhibitor combinations with activity against gram-negative bacteria, including *Pseudomonas*, and some anaerobes. Both agents have been studied in complicated intraabdominal infections and complicated urinary tract infections. Ceftolozane-tazobactam is thought to be stable against many ESBL-producing organisms because of the tazobactam component. The addition of avibactam to ceftazidime yields a combination agent with activity against AmpC-, ESBL-, and *K. pneumoniae* carbapenemase (KPC)–producing organisms. These cephalosporin–β-lactamase inhibitor combinations may be of clinical benefit in multidrug-resistant gram-negative infections.

Carbapenems Carbapenems, including doripenem, imipenem, meropenem, and ertapenem, offer the most reliable coverage for strains containing ESBLs. All carbapenems have broad activity against gram-positive cocci, gram-negative bacilli, and anaerobes. None is active against methicillin-resistant *S. aureus* (MRSA), but all are active against MSSA, *Streptococcus* species, and Enterobacterales. Ertapenem is the only carbapenem that has poor activity against *P. aeruginosa* and *Acinetobacter*. Imipenem is active against penicillin-susceptible *Enterococcus faecalis* but not *Enterococcus faecium*. Carbapenems are not active against Enterobacterales containing carbapenemases. *Stenotrophomonas maltophilia* and some *Bacillus* species are intrinsically resistant to carbapenems because of a zinc-dependent carbapenemase. Addition of vaborbactam to meropenem and relebactam to imipenem results in inhibition of AmpC β-lactamases, ESBLs, and KPCs but not metallo-carbapenemases, such as NDM (New Delhi metallo-β-lactamases).

Monobactams Aztreonam is the sole monobactam in clinical use. Its activity is limited to gram-negative bacteria and includes *P. aeruginosa* and most other Enterobacterales. This drug is inactivated by ESBLs and carbapenemases. The principal use for aztreonam is as an alternative to penicillins, cephalosporins, or carbapenems in patients with a serious β-lactam allergy. Aztreonam is structurally related to ceftazidime and should be used cautiously in individuals with a serious ceftazidime allergy. It is used in febrile neutropenia and intraabdominal infections when other β-lactams cannot be used.

Adverse Reactions to β-Lactam Drugs Agents within the β-lactam class are known for several adverse effects. Gastrointestinal side effects, mainly diarrhea, are common, but hypersensitivity reactions constitute the most common adverse effect of β-lactams. The reactions' severity can range from rash to anaphylaxis, but the rate of true anaphylactic reactions is only 0.05%. An individual with an accelerated IgE-mediated reaction to one β-lactam agent may still receive another agent within the class, but caution should be used and a β-lactam that has a dissimilar side chain and a low level of cross-reactivity would be the preferred choice. For example, the second-, third-, and fourth-generation cephalosporins and the carbapenems display very low cross-reactivity in patients with penicillin allergy. Aztreonam is the only β-lactam that has no cross-reactivity with the penicillin group. In cases of severe allergy, desensitization (a graded challenge) to the indicated β-lactam, with close monitoring, may be warranted if other antibacterial options are not suitable.

β-Lactams can rarely cause serum sickness, Stevens-Johnson syndrome, nephropathy, hematologic reactions, and neurotoxicity. Neutropenia appears to be related to high doses or prolonged use. Neutropenia and interstitial nephritis caused by β-lactams generally resolve upon discontinuation of the agent. Imipenem and cefepime are associated with an increased risk of seizure, but this risk is likely a class effect and related to high doses or doses that are not adjusted in renal impairment.

GLYCOPEPTIDES AND LIPOGLYCOPEPTIDES

Vancomycin is a glycopeptide antibiotic with activity against staphylococci (including MRSA and coagulase-negative staphylococci), streptococci (including *S. pneumoniae*), and enterococci. It is not active against gram-negative organisms. Vancomycin also displays activity against *Bacillus* species, *Corynebacterium jeikeium*, and gram-positive anaerobes such as *Peptostreptococcus*, *Actinomyces*, *Clostridium*, and *Propionibacterium* species. Vancomycin has several important clinical uses. It is used for serious infections caused by MRSA, including health care–associated pneumonia, bacteremia, osteomyelitis, and endocarditis. It is also commonly used for skin and soft tissue infections. Oral vancomycin is not absorbed systemically and is reserved for the treatment of *Clostridioides difficile* infection. Vancomycin is also an alternative for the treatment of infections caused by MSSA in patients who cannot tolerate β-lactams. Resistance to vancomycin is a rising concern. Strains of vancomycin-intermediate *S. aureus* (VISA) and vancomycin-resistant enterococci (VRE) are not uncommon. Vancomycin appears to be a concentration-dependent killer, with the AUC/MIC ratio being the best predictor of efficacy (Fig. 144-1). Guidelines recommend targeting a vancomycin trough level of 15–20 μg/mL in MRSA infections in order to maintain an AUC/MIC ratio >400. When using vancomycin, clinicians should monitor for nephrotoxicity. The risk of nephrotoxicity increases when trough levels are >20 μg/mL. Concomitant therapy with other nephrotoxic agents, such as aminoglycosides, also increases the risk. Ototoxicity was reported with early formulations of vancomycin but is currently uncommon because purer formulations are available. Both of these adverse effects are reversible upon discontinuation of vancomycin. Clinicians should be aware of the infusion reaction formerly known as "red man syndrome," a common reaction that presents as a rapid onset of erythematous rash or pruritus on the head, face, neck, and upper trunk. This reaction is caused by histamine release from basophils and mast cells and can be treated with diphenhydramine and slowing of the vancomycin infusion.

Telavancin, dalbavancin, and oritavancin are structurally similar to vancomycin and are referred to as *lipoglycopeptides*. They have antibacterial activity against *S. aureus* (including MRSA and some strains of VISA and vancomycin-resistant *S. aureus* [VRSA]), streptococci, and enterococci. Oritavancin may have activity against some strains of VRE. These lipoglycopeptide agents also provide coverage against anaerobic gram-positive organisms except for *Lactobacillus* and some *Clostridium* species. The clinical efficacy of telavancin has been demonstrated in both skin and soft tissue infections and nosocomial pneumonia, and the efficacy of dalbavancin and oritavancin has been shown in skin and soft tissue infections. The vancomycin resistance phenotype may reduce the potency of all three lipoglycopeptides, but the rate of resistance to these drugs among *S. aureus* and enterococcal isolates has been low. Adverse effects of telavancin include nephrotoxicity, metallic taste, and gastrointestinal side effects. Clinicians should be aware of the potential for electrocardiographic QT_c prolongation that can increase the risk of cardiac arrhythmias when telavancin is used concomitantly with other QT_c-prolonging agents. Telavancin may interfere with certain coagulation tests (e.g., causing false elevations in prothrombin time). Dalbavancin and oritavancin have safety profiles similar to that of vancomycin, with common effects reported as headache and gastrointestinal side effects. These glycolipopeptides should be used cautiously in patients with hypersensitivity reactions to vancomycin, as cross-allergy may be possible.

LIPOPEPTIDES

Daptomycin is a lipopeptide antibiotic with activity against a broad range of gram-positive organisms. This drug is active against staphylococci (including MRSA and coagulase-negative staphylococci), streptococci, and enterococci. Daptomycin remains active against enterococci that are resistant to vancomycin. In addition, it exhibits activity against *Bacillus*, *Corynebacterium*, *Peptostreptococcus*, and *Clostridium* species. Daptomycin's pharmacodynamic parameter for efficacy is concentration-dependent killing. Resistance to daptomycin is rare, but MICs may be higher for some VISA strains. Daptomycin can be used in skin and soft tissue infections, bacteremia, endocarditis, and osteomyelitis. It is an important alternative for MRSA and other gram-positive infections when bactericidal therapy is needed and vancomycin cannot be used. Daptomycin is generally well tolerated, and its main toxicity consists of elevation of creatine phosphokinase (CPK) levels and myopathy. CPK should be monitored during daptomycin treatment, and the drug should be discontinued if muscular toxicities occur. There have also been case reports of reversible eosinophilic pneumonia associated with daptomycin use.

AMINOGLYCOSIDES

The aminoglycosides are a class of antibacterial agents with concentration-dependent activity against most gram-negative organisms. The most commonly used aminoglycosides are gentamicin, tobramycin, and amikacin, although others, such as streptomycin, kanamycin, neomycin, and paromomycin, may be used in special circumstances. Plazomicin is a new aminoglycoside that is less affected by common resistance mechanisms and is approved for treatment of complicated urinary tract infections and acute pyelonephritis. Aminoglycosides have a significant dose-dependent postantibiotic effect; i.e., they have an antibacterial effect even after serum drug levels fall below inhibitory concentrations. The postantibiotic effect and concentration-dependent killing form the rationale behind extended-interval aminoglycoside dosing, in which a larger dose is given once daily rather than smaller doses multiple times daily. Aminoglycosides are active against gram-negative bacilli, such as Enterobacterales, *P. aeruginosa*, and *Acinetobacter*. They also enhance the activity of cell wall–active agents such as β-lactams or vancomycin against some gram-positive bacteria, including staphylococci and enterococci. This combination therapy is termed *synergistic* because the effect of both agents provides a killing effect greater than would be predicted from the effects of either agent alone. Amikacin and streptomycin have activity against *Mycobacterium tuberculosis*, and amikacin has activity against *M. avium* complex. The aminoglycosides do not have activity against anaerobes, *S. maltophilia*, or *Burkholderia cepacia* complex. Aminoglycosides are used in clinical practice in a variety of infections caused by gram-negative organisms, including bacteremia and urinary tract infections. They are frequently used either alone or in combination for the treatment of *P. aeruginosa* infection. When used in combination with a cell wall–active agent, gentamicin and streptomycin are also important for the treatment of gram-positive bacterial endocarditis. All aminoglycosides can cause nephrotoxicity and ototoxicity. The risk of nephrotoxicity is not well defined; however, some studies have indicated that the effect may be related to the duration of therapy as well as to the concomitant use of other nephrotoxic agents. Nephrotoxicity is usually reversible, but ototoxicity can be irreversible.

MACROLIDES AND KETOLIDES

The macrolides (azithromycin, clarithromycin, and erythromycin) and ketolides (telithromycin) are classes of antibiotics that inhibit protein synthesis. Compared with erythromycin (the older antibiotic), azithromycin and clarithromycin have better oral absorption and tolerability. Azithromycin, clarithromycin, and telithromycin all have broader spectra of activity than erythromycin, which is less frequently used. These agents are commonly used in the treatment of upper and lower respiratory tract infections caused by *S. pneumoniae*, *H. influenzae*, *M. catarrhalis*, and atypical organisms (e.g., *Chlamydophila pneumoniae*, *Legionella pneumophila*, and *Mycoplasma pneumoniae*); group A streptococcal pharyngitis in penicillin-allergic patients; and nontuberculous mycobacterial infections (e.g., caused by *Mycobacterium marinum* and *Mycobacterium chelonae*) as well as in the prophylaxis and treatment of *M. avium* complex infection in patients with HIV/AIDS and in combination therapy for *Helicobacter pylori* infection and bartonellosis. Enterobacterales, *Pseudomonas* species, and *Acinetobacter* species are intrinsically resistant to macrolides as a result of decreased membrane permeability, although azithromycin is active against gram-negative diarrheal pathogens. The major adverse effects of this drug class include nausea, vomiting, diarrhea and abdominal pain, prolongation of QT_c interval, exacerbation of myasthenia gravis, tinnitus and reversible deafness, especially in the elderly. Azithromycin specifically has been associated with an increased risk of death, especially among patients with underlying heart disease, because of the risk of QT_c interval prolongation and torsades de pointes arrhythmia. Erythromycin, clarithromycin, and telithromycin inhibit the CYP3A4 hepatic drug-metabolizing enzyme and can result in increased levels of coadministered drugs, including benzodiazepines, statins, warfarin, cyclosporine, and tacrolimus. Azithromycin does not inhibit CYP3A4 and therefore does not interact with these drugs.

CLINDAMYCIN

Clindamycin is a lincosamide antibiotic and is bacteriostatic against some organisms and bactericidal against others. It is used most often to treat bacterial infections caused by anaerobes (e.g., *B. fragilis*, *Clostridium perfringens*, *Fusobacterium* species, *Prevotella melaninogenicus*, and *Peptostreptococcus* species) and susceptible staphylococci and streptococci. Clindamycin is used for treatment of dental infections, anaerobic lung abscess, and skin and soft tissue infections. It is used together with bactericidal agents (penicillins or vancomycin) to inhibit new toxin synthesis in the treatment of streptococcal or staphylococcal toxic shock syndrome. Other uses include treatment of infections caused by *Capnocytophaga canimorsus*, combination therapy for babesiosis and occasionally malaria, and therapy for toxoplasmosis. Clindamycin has excellent oral bioavailability. Adverse effects include nausea, vomiting, diarrhea, *C. difficile*–associated diarrhea and pseudomembranous colitis, maculopapular rash, and rarely Stevens-Johnson syndrome.

TETRACYCLINES

The older (doxycycline, minocycline, and tetracycline) and newer (tigecycline, eravacycline, and omadacycline) tetracyclines inhibit protein synthesis and are bacteriostatic. These drugs have wide clinical uses. They are used in the treatment of skin and soft tissue infections caused by gram-positive cocci (including MRSA), spirochetal infections (e.g., Lyme disease, syphilis, leptospirosis, and relapsing fever), rickettsial infections (e.g., Rocky Mountain spotted fever, scrub typhus), atypical pneumonia, sexually transmitted infections (e.g., *Chlamydia trachomatis* infection, lymphogranuloma venereum, and granuloma inguinale), infections with *Nocardia* and *Actinomyces*, brucellosis, tularemia, Whipple's disease, and malaria. Tigecycline is a glycylcycline derived from minocycline and is available only in IV formulation. It is indicated in the treatment of complicated skin and soft tissue infections, complicated intraabdominal infections, and community-acquired bacterial pneumonia in adults. Tigecycline has activity against MRSA, vancomycin-sensitive enterococci, many Enterobacterales, and *Bacteroides* species; it has no activity against *P. aeruginosa*. This drug has been used in combination with colistin for the treatment of serious infections with multidrug-resistant gram-negative organisms. A pooled analysis of 13 clinical trials found an increased risk of death and treatment failure among patients given tigecycline alone; as a result, the FDA mandated a black box warning. Eravacycline is a fluorocycline derivative available in IV formulation with a similar spectrum but more potent than tigecycline in vitro. It has been approved for complicated intraabdominal infections. Omadacycline is an aminomethylcycline derivative available in both IV and oral formulations. It has activity similar to that of tigecycline against gram-positive pathogens but is less active against gram-negative pathogens. Omadacycline has been approved for treatment of bacterial skin and skin structure infections and community-acquired bacterial pneumonia. Tetracyclines have reduced absorption when orally coadministered with calcium- and iron-containing compounds, including milk, and doses should be spaced at least 2 h apart. The major adverse reactions to old and new tetracyclines are nausea, vomiting, diarrhea, and photosensitivity. Tetracyclines have been associated with fetal bone-growth abnormalities and should be avoided during pregnancy and in the treatment of children <8 years old.

TRIMETHOPRIM-SULFAMETHOXAZOLE

Trimethoprim-sulfamethoxazole (TMP-SMX) is an antibiotic with two components that each inhibit a separate step in folate synthesis and produce antibacterial activity. TMP-SMX is active against gram-positive bacteria such as staphylococci and streptococci; however, its use against MRSA is usually limited to community-acquired infections, and its activity against *Streptococcus pyogenes* may not be reliable. This drug is also active against many gram-negative bacteria, including *H. influenzae*, *E. coli*, *P. mirabilis*, *Neisseria gonorrhoeae*, and *S. maltophilia*. TMP-SMX is not active against anaerobes or *P. aeruginosa*. It has many uses because of its wide spectrum of activity and high oral bioavailability. Urinary tract infections, skin and soft tissue infections, and respiratory tract infections are among the common uses. Another important indication is for both prophylaxis and treatment of *Pneumocystis jirovecii* infections in immunocompromised patients. Resistance to TMP-SMX has limited its use against many Enterobacterales. Resistance rates among urinary isolates of *E. coli* are almost 25% in the United States. The most common adverse reactions associated with TMP-SMX are gastrointestinal effects such as nausea, vomiting, and diarrhea. In addition, rash is a common allergic reaction and may preclude the subsequent use of other sulfonamides. With prolonged use, leukopenia, thrombocytopenia, and granulocytopenia can develop. TMP-SMX can also cause nephrotoxicity, hyperkalemia, and hyponatremia, which are more common at high doses. TMP-SMX has several important interactions with other drugs (Table 144-3), including warfarin, phenytoin, and methotrexate.

FLUOROQUINOLONES

The fluoroquinolones include norfloxacin, ciprofloxacin, ofloxacin, levofloxacin, moxifloxacin, gemifloxacin, and delafloxacin. Ciprofloxacin and levofloxacin have the broadest spectrum of activity against gram-negative bacteria, including *P. aeruginosa* (similar to that of third-generation cephalosporins). Because of the risk of selection of resistance during fluoroquinolone treatment of serious pseudomonal infections, these agents are usually used in combination with an antipseudomonal β-lactam. Levofloxacin, moxifloxacin, gemifloxacin, and delafloxacin have additional gram-positive activity, including that against *S. pneumoniae* and some strains of MSSA, and, with the exception of delafloxacin, these agents are used for treatment of community-acquired pneumonia. Strains of MRSA are commonly resistant to all fluoroquinolones except delafloxacin. Moxifloxacin is used as one component of second-line regimens for multidrug-resistant tuberculosis. Fluoroquinolones are no longer used for treatment of gonorrhea because of common resistance in *N. gonorrhoeae*. Fluoroquinolones exhibit concentration-dependent killing, are well absorbed orally, and have elimination half-lives that usually support once- or twice-daily dosing. Oral coadministration with compounds containing high concentrations of aluminum, magnesium, or calcium can reduce fluoroquinolone absorption. The penetration of fluoroquinolones into prostate tissue supports their use for bacterial prostatitis. Fluoroquinolones are generally well tolerated but can cause central nervous system (CNS) stimulatory effects, including seizures; peripheral neuropathy; glucose dysregulation; and tendinopathy associated with Achilles tendon rupture, particularly in older patients, organ transplant recipients, and patients taking glucocorticoids. Other potential effects on connective tissues include an association with increased risk of aortic aneurysm. Worsening of myasthenia gravis also has been associated with quinolone use. Moxifloxacin causes modest prolongation of the QT_c interval and should be used with caution in patients receiving other QT_c-prolonging drugs.

RIFAMYCINS

The rifamycins include rifampin, rifabutin, and rifapentine. Rifampin is the most commonly used rifamycin. For almost all therapeutic indications, it is used in combination with other agents to reduce the likelihood of selection of high-level rifampin resistance. Rifampin is used foremost in the treatment of mycobacterial infections—specifically, as a mainstay of combination therapy for *M. tuberculosis* infection or as a single agent in the treatment of latent *M. tuberculosis* infection. In addition, it is often used in the treatment of nontuberculous mycobacterial infection. Rifampin is used in combination regimens for the treatment of staphylococcal infections, particularly prosthetic-valve endocarditis and bone infections with retained hardware. It is a component of combination therapy for brucellosis (with doxycycline) and leprosy (with dapsone for tuberculoid leprosy and with dapsone and clofazimine for lepromatous disease). Rifampin can be used alone for prophylaxis in close contacts of patients with *H. influenzae* or *N. meningitidis* meningitis. The drug has high oral bioavailability, which is further enhanced when it is taken on an empty stomach. Rifampin has several adverse effects, including elevated aminotransferase levels (14%), rash (1–5%), and gastrointestinal events such as nausea, vomiting, and diarrhea (1–2%). Its many clinically relevant interactions with other drugs (Table 144-3) mandate the clinician's careful review of the patient's medications before rifampin initiation to assess safety and the need for additional monitoring, including monitoring of drug levels.

METRONIDAZOLE

Metronidazole is used in the treatment of anaerobic bacterial infections as well as infections caused by protozoa (e.g., amebiasis, giardiasis, trichomoniasis). It is the agent of choice as a component of combination therapy for polymicrobial abscesses in the lung, brain, or abdomen, the etiology of which often includes anaerobic bacteria, and for bacterial vaginosis, pelvic inflammatory disease, and anaerobic infections, such as those due to *Bacteroides*, *Fusobacterium*, and *Prevotella* species. This drug is an alternative agent for treatment of mild to moderate *C. difficile*–associated diarrhea. Metronidazole is bactericidal against anaerobic bacteria and exhibits concentration-dependent killing. It has high oral bioavailability and tissue penetration, including penetration of the blood-brain barrier. The majority of *Actinomyces*, *Propionibacterium*, and *Lactobacillus* species are intrinsically resistant to metronidazole. The major adverse effects include nausea, diarrhea, and a metallic taste. Concomitant ingestion of alcohol may result in a disulfiram-like reaction, and patients are usually instructed to avoid alcohol during treatment. Long-term treatment carries the risk of leukopenia, neutropenia, peripheral neuropathy, and CNS toxicity manifesting as confusion, dysarthria, ataxia, nystagmus, and ophthalmoparesis. Through metronidazole's effect on the CYP2C9 drug-metabolizing enzyme, its coadministration with warfarin can result in decreased metabolism and enhanced anticoagulant effects that require close monitoring. Concomitant administration of metronidazole with lithium can result in increased serum levels of lithium and associated toxicity; coadministration with phenytoin can result in phenytoin toxicity and possibly decreased levels of metronidazole.

OXAZOLIDINONES

Linezolid is a bacteriostatic agent and is indicated for serious infections due to resistant gram-positive bacteria, such as MRSA and VRE. The intrinsic resistance of gram-negative bacteria is mediated primarily by endogenous efflux pumps. Linezolid has excellent oral bioavailability. Adverse effects include myelosuppression and ocular and peripheral neuropathy with prolonged therapy. Peripheral neuropathy may be irreversible. Linezolid is a weak, reversible monoamine oxidase inhibitor, and coadministration with sympathomimetics and foods rich in tyramine should be avoided. Linezolid has been associated with serotonin syndrome when coadministered with selective serotonin reuptake inhibitors. Tedizolid has properties similar to those of linezolid, but with lower dosing due to greater potency, it may be less likely to cause adverse hematologic and neuropathic effects.

PLEUROMUTILINS

Lefamulin is the only member of the pleuromutilin class approved for systemic use; it is available in IV and oral formulations. Lefamulin has in vitro activity against *S. aureus* (including MRSA), *S. pneumoniae*, *H. influenzae*, and atypical respiratory pathogens, including *L. pneumophila*, *M. pneumoniae*, and *C. pneumoniae*, and has been approved for treatment of community-acquired bacterial pneumonia. Adverse effects are most commonly gastrointestinal, including diarrhea (12%), nausea (5%), and vomiting (3%). Prolongation of QT_c interval and hepatic transaminase elevations occur in some patients. There can be interactions with drugs that are either inducers or inhibitors of CYP3A4 or P-glycoprotein transporter.

NITROFURANTOIN

Nitrofurantoin's antibacterial activity results from the drug's conversion to highly reactive intermediates that can damage bacterial DNA and other macromolecules. Nitrofurantoin is bactericidal, and its action is concentration dependent. It displays activity against a range of gram-positive bacteria, including *S. aureus*, *Staphylococcus epidermidis*, *Staphylococcus saprophyticus*, *E. faecalis*, *Streptococcus agalactiae*, group D streptococci, viridans streptococci, and corynebacteria, as well as gram-negative organisms, including *E. coli*, *Enterobacter*, *Salmonella*, and *Shigella* species. Nitrofurantoin is used primarily in the treatment of urinary tract infections and is preferred in the treatment of such infections in pregnancy. It may be used for the prevention of recurrent cystitis. Recently, there has been interest in the use of nitrofurantoin for treatment of urinary tract infections caused by ESBL-producing Enterobacterales such as *E. coli*, although resistance has been growing in Latin America and parts of Europe. Coadministration with magnesium should be avoided because of decreased absorption, and patients should be encouraged to take the drug with food to increase its bioavailability and decrease the risk of adverse effects, which include nausea, vomiting, and diarrhea. Nitrofurantoin may also cause pulmonary fibrosis and drug-induced hepatitis. Because the risk of adverse reactions increases with age, the use of nitrofurantoin in elderly patients is not recommended. Patients with glucose-6-phosphate dehydrogenase (G6PD) deficiency are at elevated risk for nitrofurantoin-associated hemolytic anemia.

POLYMYXINS

Colistin and polymyxin B act by disrupting bacterial cell membrane integrity and are active against the nonenteric pathogens *P. aeruginosa* and *A. baumannii* but not against *Burkholderia*. These drugs also exhibit activity against many Enterobacterales, with the exceptions of *Proteus*, *Providencia*, and *Serratia* species. They lack activity against gram-positive bacteria. Polymyxins are bactericidal and are available in IV formulations. Colistimethate is converted to the active form (colistin) in plasma. Polymyxins are most often used for infections due to pathogens resistant to multiple other antibacterial agents, including urinary tract infections, hospital-acquired pneumonia, and bloodstream infections. Nebulized formulations have been used for adjunctive treatment of refractory ventilator-associated pneumonia. The most important adverse effect is dose-dependent reversible nephrotoxicity. Neurotoxicity, including paresthesias, muscle weakness, and confusion, is reversible and less common than nephrotoxicity.

QUINUPRISTIN-DALFOPRISTIN

Quinupristin-dalfopristin contains two members of the streptogramin class of antibiotics and kills bacteria by inhibiting protein synthesis. The antibacterial spectrum of quinupristin-dalfopristin includes staphylococci (including MRSA), streptococci, and *E. faecium* (but not *E. faecalis*). This drug combination is also active against *Corynebacterium* species and *L. monocytogenes*. Quinupristin-dalfopristin is not reliably active against gram-negative organisms. It exhibits concentration-dependent killing, with an AUC/MIC ratio predicting efficacy. The clinical use of quinupristin-dalfopristin is largely for infections due to vancomycin-resistant *E. faecium* and other gram-positive bacterial infections. The drug has demonstrated efficacy in a variety of infections, including urinary tract infections, bone and joint infections, and bacteremia. Adverse effects associated with quinupristin-dalfopristin include infusion-related reactions, arthralgias, and myalgias. The arthralgias and myalgias may be severe enough to warrant drug discontinuation. Quinupristin-dalfopristin inhibits the CYP3A4 drug-metabolizing enzyme, with consequent drug interactions (Table 144-3).

FOSFOMYCIN

Fosfomycin is a phosphonic acid antibiotic that has greater activity in acidic environments and is excreted in its active form in the urine. Thus, its use is primarily for prophylaxis and treatment of uncomplicated cystitis and should be avoided if there is concern about pyelonephritis. The drug is administered as a single 3-g dose that results in high urine concentrations for up to 48 h. Fosfomycin is active against *S. aureus*, vancomycin-susceptible enterococci and VRE, and a wide range of gram-negative organisms, including *E. coli*, *Enterobacter* species, *Serratia marcescens*, *P. aeruginosa*, and *K. pneumoniae*. Notably, the vast majority of ESBL-producing Enterobacterales are susceptible to fosfomycin. *A. baumannii* and *Burkholderia* species are resistant. The emergence of resistance to fosfomycin has not been observed during treatment of cystitis but has been documented during treatment of respiratory tract infections and osteomyelitis. The few adverse effects that have been reported include nausea and diarrhea.

CHLORAMPHENICOL

The use of chloramphenicol is limited by its potentially serious toxicities. When other agents are contraindicated or ineffective, chloramphenicol represents an alternative treatment for infections, including meningitis caused by susceptible bacteria such as *N. meningitidis*, *H. influenzae*, and *S. pneumoniae*. It has also been used for the treatment of anthrax, brucellosis, *Burkholderia* infections, chlamydial infections, clostridial infections, ehrlichiosis, rickettsial infections, and typhoid fever. Adverse reactions include aplastic anemia, myelosuppression, and gray baby syndrome. Chloramphenicol inhibits the CYP2C19 and CYP3A4 drug-metabolizing enzymes and consequently increases levels of many classes of drugs.

APPROACH TO PROPHYLAXIS OF INFECTION

Antibacterial prophylaxis is indicated only in selected circumstances (**Table 144-5**) and should be supported by well-designed studies or expert panel recommendations. In all cases, the risk or severity of the infection to be prevented should be greater than the adverse consequences of antibacterial therapy, including the potential for selection of resistance. In addition, the timing and duration of antibacterial treatment should be targeted for maximal effect and minimal required exposure. Prophylaxis of surgical infections targets bacteria that may contaminate the wound during the surgical procedure, including the skin flora of the patient or operating team and the air in the operating room. Delivery of the antibacterial drug within 1 h before the surgical incision is most effective. For prolonged procedures, redosing may be necessary to maintain effective blood and tissue levels until the wound is closed. Additional dosing is not recommended after the incision is closed. In patients with nasal carriage of *S. aureus*, preoperative decolonization with nasal mupirocin reduces the rate of *S. aureus* surgical-site infections and is generally recommended for high-risk procedures such as cardiac surgery and orthopedic implantation of prosthetic devices. For dental procedures, preprocedure antibacterial drugs are given to prevent transient bacteremia during the procedure and the seeding of certain high-risk cardiac lesions. Prophylaxis is also used in nonprocedural settings in certain patients who have recurrent infections or

TABLE 144-5 Prophylaxis of Bacterial Infections in Adults

CONDITION	ANTIBACTERIAL AGENTS[a]	TIMING OR DURATION OF PROPHYLAXIS
Surgical		
Clean (cardiac, thoracic, neurologic, orthopedic, vascular, plastic)	Cefazolin (vancomycin,[b] clindamycin)	1 h before incision; re-dose with long procedures
Clean (ophthalmic)	Topical neomycin–polymyxin B–gramicidin, topical moxifloxacin	Every 5–15 min for 5 doses immediately prior to procedure
Clean-contaminated (head and neck)	Cefazolin + metronidazole, ampicillin-sulbactam[c] (clindamycin)	1 h before incision; re-dose with long procedures
Clean-contaminated (hysterectomy, gastroduodenal, biliary, unobstructed small intestine, urologic)	Cefazolin, ampicillin-sulbactam[c] (clindamycin + aminoglycoside, aztreonam, or fluoroquinolone)	1 h before incision; re-dose with long procedures
Clean-contaminated (colorectal, appendectomy)	Cefazolin + metronidazole, ampicillin-sulbactam,[c] ertapenem (clindamycin + aminoglycoside, aztreonam, or fluoroquinolone)	1 h before incision; re-dose with long procedures
Dirty (ruptured viscus)	Therapeutic regimen directed at anaerobes and gram-negative bacteria (e.g., ceftriaxone + metronidazole)	1 h before incision; re-dose with long procedures; continue for 3–5 days after procedure
Dirty (traumatic wound)	Therapeutic regimen: cefazolin (clindamycin ± aminoglycoside, aztreonam, or fluoroquinolone)	1 h before incision; re-dose with long procedures; continue for 3–5 days after procedure
Nonsurgical		
Dental, oral, or upper respiratory procedures in patients with high-risk cardiac lesions (prosthetic valves, congenital heart defects, prior endocarditis)	Amoxicillin PO, ampicillin IM (clindamycin PO, IV)	Oral agents 1 h before procedure; injection 30 min before procedure
Recurrent *S. aureus* skin infections[d]	Mupirocin[e]	Intranasal application for 5 days
Recurrent cellulitis associated with lymphatic disruption[d]	Benzathine penicillin IM monthly, oral penicillin or erythromycin twice daily	Undefined
Recurrent cystitis in women[d]	Nitrofurantoin, TMP-SMX, fluoroquinolone	After sexual intercourse *or* 3 times weekly for up to 1 year
Bite wounds	Amoxicillin-clavulanate (doxycycline, moxifloxacin)	3–5 days
Recurrent spontaneous bacterial peritonitis in cirrhotic patients[d]	Fluoroquinolone[f]	Undefined
Recurrent pneumococcal meningitis in patient with CSF leak or humoral immune defect[d]	Penicillin	Undefined
Exposure to patient with meningococcal meningitis	Rifampin, ciprofloxacin	2 days (rifampin), single dose (ciprofloxacin)
High-risk neutropenia (ANC, ≤100/μL for >7 days)[d]	Levofloxacin or ciprofloxacin[f]	Until neutropenia resolves or fever dictates use of other antibacterials

[a]Regimens in parentheses are alternatives for patients allergic to β-lactams. [b]Vancomycin may be given together with cefazolin to patients known to be colonized with methicillin-resistant *Staphylococcus aureus*. [c]Cefoxitin or cefotetan may also be considered. [d]Not considered routine for all patients, but an acceptable consideration among alternative approaches. [e]Usually coupled with bathing with chlorhexidine-containing skin antiseptic. [f]Choice of fluoroquinolone prophylaxis must be balanced against the risk of selection of resistance.

Abbreviations: ANC, absolute neutrophil count; CSF, cerebrospinal fluid; TMP-SMX, trimethoprim-sulfamethoxazole.

who are at risk of serious infection from a specific exposure (e.g., close contact with a patient with meningococcal meningitis). Extension of prophylaxis beyond the period of infection risk (24 h in the case of surgical procedures) does not add further benefit and may increase the risk of resistance selection or *C. difficile* disease.

ANTIMICROBIAL STEWARDSHIP

In an era of increasing prevalence of multidrug-resistant bacteria and with a substantial amount of inappropriate antimicrobial use, the need for rational antimicrobial prescribing has never been greater **(Chap. 145)**. *Antimicrobial stewardship* describes the practice of promoting the selection of the appropriate drug, dosage, route, and duration of antimicrobial therapy. Antimicrobial stewardship programs implement a variety of strategies to (1) improve patient care through appropriate antimicrobial use; (2) preserve a vital health care resource by curbing the development of resistance within patient populations; (3) reduce the incidence of adverse effects; and (4) control costs. The Centers for Disease Control and Prevention (CDC) guidelines, The Joint Commission (TJC) Medication Management Standards, and the Centers for Medicare and Medicaid Services (CMS) Conditions of Participation, as well as the 2015 National Action Plan for Combating Antibiotic-Resistant Bacteria, have all supported *antimicrobial stewardship* in various health care settings. Antimicrobial stewardship programs are typically multidisciplinary and often include infectious disease physicians, clinical pharmacists (usually with special training in infectious disease), clinical microbiologists, information systems specialists, infection prevention and control practitioners, and epidemiologists. These teams employ a variety of approaches to achieve the program's goals.

Established strategies of antimicrobial stewardship programs include (1) prospective audit of antimicrobial use, with intervention and feedback; (2) formulary restriction; and (3) preauthorization. *Prospective audit and feedback* are usually undertaken by an infectious disease physician or a pharmacist. In this process, orders for broad-spectrum antimicrobials (e.g., carbapenems) or agents for which more cost-effective alternatives may exist (e.g., daptomycin, ceftazidime-avibactam) are reviewed on a regular basis for appropriateness. In circumstances when antimicrobial use can be further optimized, the stewardship program team can intervene to recommend an alternative. This process has been successful in several quasi-experimental studies, resulting in declines in use of broad-spectrum drugs and decreases in adverse events, such as *C. difficile* infection. *Formulary restriction* is the inclusion of a limited set of antimicrobial agents in a hospital formulary for the purpose of limiting indiscriminate use of antimicrobials in the absence of demonstrated benefit. Such restriction coincidentally serves to avoid unnecessary drug expenditure. *Preauthorization* is the practice of requiring clinicians to obtain approval before using selected antimicrobials. Approval may be provided electronically with sophisticated Computerized Provider Order Entry (CPOE) software, after specific criteria for use are met, or after communication with an infectious disease specialist as designated by the stewardship program. These strategies have led to a decrease in *C. difficile* infections and to improvements in drug susceptibility patterns.

Additional strategies used in specific health care settings are guidelines and pathways, dose optimization, parenteral-to-oral conversion, antibiotic time-out, and de-escalation of therapy. Documentation of the indication for which each antimicrobial is prescribed is also encouraged. Finally, antimicrobial stewardship teams provide ongoing education of antimicrobial best practices. An evolving and an increasingly active area of clinical research to identify best practices, antimicrobial stewardship continues to grow as an essential service in various health care settings. The IDSA, in collaboration with several other professional organizations, has published guidelines for developing institutional antimicrobial stewardship programs (*www.idsociety.org/Antimicrobial_Agents/*).

Acknowledgment

The authors thank Christy A. Varughese for her significant contributions to this chapter in the previous editions.

FURTHER READING

Barlam TF et al: Implementing an antibiotic stewardship program: Guidelines by the Infectious Diseases Society of America and the Society for Healthcare Epidemiology of America. Clin Infect Dis 62:e51, 2016.

Bratzler DW et al: Clinical practice guidelines for antimicrobial prophylaxis in surgery. Surg Infect (Larchmt) 14:73, 2013.

Grayson ML et al (eds): *Kucers' The Use of Antibiotics. A Clinical Review of Antibacterial, Antifungal, Antiparasitic and Antiviral Drugs*, 7th ed. Boca Raton, CRC Press, 2018.

Infectious Diseases Society of America: Practice guidelines by organ system. Available at *http://www.idsociety.org/Organ_System/*. Accessed February 21, 2017.

Jeffries MN et al: Consequences of avoiding β-lactams in patients with β-lactam allergies. J Allergy Clin Immunol 137:1148, 2016.

Labreche MJ et al: Recent updates on the role of pharmacokinetics–pharmacodynamics in antimicrobial susceptibility testing as applied to clinical practice. Clin Infect Dis 61:1446, 2015.

Rotschafer J et al (eds): *Antibiotic Pharmacodynamics. Methods in Pharmacodynamics and Toxicology.* New York, Humana Press, 2016.

Shenoy ES et al: Evaluation and management of penicillin allergy: A review. JAMA 321:188, 2019.

Thomas Z et al: A multicenter evaluation of prolonged empiric antibiotic therapy in adult ICUs in the United States. Crit Care Med 43:2527, 2015.

145 Bacterial Resistance to Antimicrobial Agents

David C. Hooper

DEFINITION OF RESISTANCE

The action of antimicrobial agents on a range of targets within the bacterial cell can result in inhibition of bacterial growth or in killing of the bacterial cell **(Chap. 144)**. Reduction in or loss of an agent's antibacterial effect is referred to as *resistance*, and the properties of or alterations in the bacterium that result in reduced antimicrobial activity are termed *resistance mechanisms*. Bacteria can be resistant to single or multiple antimicrobials, as detailed in the sections that follow. The occurrence and magnitude of resistance are often assessed in clinical microbiology laboratories by measurement of the lowest drug concentration that inhibits growth of a bacterium (minimal inhibitory concentration, or MIC) with a standardized inoculum and growth conditions. MIC values are generally interpreted as representing bacterial susceptibility, intermediate susceptibility, or resistance; the interpretation is based on correlations of the MIC values with the pharmacokinetics and delivery of a drug to the site of infection in the body as well as with data from clinical trials. Thus, a clinical laboratory result of "susceptible" for a bacterium predicts a likely clinical response to an appropriately dosed antimicrobial drug by a patient infected with that organism, whereas a result of "resistant" predicts poor or no clinical response to that drug. Breakpoint MIC values for categorization of bacteria as susceptible, intermediate, or resistant are generally developed by regulatory and advisory groups and are often based on the distribution of MIC values from a large collection of recent clinical bacterial isolates. Research studies on the mechanisms and epidemiology of resistance may in some cases use different and less rigid definitions of resistance based on determination of a reproducible increase in an MIC value relative to a baseline reference MIC, independent of clinical breakpoints.

MECHANISMS OF RESISTANCE

Bacteria use a wide variety of mechanisms to block or circumvent the activity of antibacterial agents **(Table 145-1** and **Fig. 145-1)**. Although myriad, these mechanisms can generally be grouped into three categories: (1) alteration or bypassing of targets that exhibit reduced binding of the drug, (2) altered access of the drug to its target by reductions in uptake or increases in active efflux, and (3) a modification of the drug that reduces its activity. These mechanisms result from either mutations in bacterial chromosomal genes occurring spontaneously during bacterial DNA replication or the acquisition of new genes by DNA transfer from other bacteria or uptake of exogenous DNA. New genes are most often acquired on self-replicating plasmids or other DNA elements transferred from other bacteria. However, some bacteria, such as *Streptococcus pneumoniae* and *Neisseria gonorrhoeae*, can also take up fragments of environmental DNA from related bacterial species and recombine that DNA directly into their own chromosomes, a process called *transformation*. Not uncommonly, resistant bacteria have combinations of resistance mechanisms either within one category or among categories, and many plasmids contain more than one resistance gene. Thus, plasmid acquisition itself can in many cases confer resistance to multiple antibacterial agents. Resistance to multiple, structurally unrelated antibiotics can also occur by mutations that cause increased expression of certain bacterial efflux pumps, some of which have broad substrate profiles enabling transport of multiple antibacterial agents out of the cell.

Many antibacterial drugs are derived from natural products of environmental microbial species. Some genes encoding resistance to these drugs originate in the drug-producer organism to protect it from its product and have then been mobilized onto plasmids that spread into other organisms. Surviving nonproducer bacteria in the exposed natural environment may also have evolved resistance under selection pressure that adds to the reservoir of resistance mechanisms. Exposure to antibacterial agents either in nature or during human, animal, or other use then results in the selection of resistant strains within an otherwise susceptible bacterial population. In some cases, resistance mechanisms may confer disadvantages that render bacterial growth or survival fitness inferior to that of susceptible strains. In a number of examples, however, fitness defects are often mitigated over time by compensatory mutational mechanisms that make the bacteria both resistant and fit and thereby more likely to persist in a reservoir even in the absence of continued antimicrobial selection pressures. Discussed below are the major classes of antimicrobial agents currently in clinical use and the most important mechanisms of resistance encountered in clinical infections.

β-Lactams β-lactams, the largest class of antibiotics, inhibit bacterial cell-wall synthesis by binding to cell-wall transpeptidases, cross-linking enzymes that are also called penicillin-binding proteins (PBPs); PBPs are targets that are unique to bacteria and have no mammalian counterpart. The most common mechanism of resistance to β-lactams, particularly in gram-negative bacteria, is their degradation

TABLE 145-1 The Most Common Mechanisms of Resistance to Antibacterial Agents

ANTIBACTERIAL AGENT(S)	MAJOR TARGET	MECHANISM(S) OF ACTION	MECHANISM(S) OF RESISTANCE
β-Lactams (penicillins, cephalosporins, monobactams, carbapenems)	Cell-wall synthesis	Bind cell-wall cross-linking enzymes (PBPs, transpeptidases)	1. Drug inactivation by β-lactamases 2. Altered PBP targets 3. Reduced diffusion through porin channels 4. Altered iron uptake proteins (cefiderocol)
Glycopeptides and lipoglycopeptides (vancomycin, teicoplanin, telavancin, dalbavancin, oritavancin)	Cell-wall synthesis	Block cell wall glycosyltransferases by binding D-Ala-D-Ala stem-peptide terminus Teicoplanin, telavancin, dalbavancin, and oritavancin: affect membrane function	1. Altered D-Ala-D-Ala target (D-Ala-D-Lac) 2. Increased D-Ala-D-Ala target binding at sites distant from cell wall synthesis enzymes
Bacitracin	Cell-wall synthesis	Blocks lipid carrier of cell wall precursors	Active drug efflux
Fosfomycin	Cell-wall synthesis	Blocks linkage of stem peptide to NAG by enoyltransferase	1. Target enzyme overexpression 2. Drug-modifying enzymes
Aminoglycosides (gentamicin, tobramycin, amikacin, plazomicin)	Protein synthesis	Bind 30S ribosomal subunit Block translocation of peptide chain Cause misreading of mRNA	1. Drug-modifying enzymes 2. Methylation at ribosome binding site 3. Decreased permeation to target due to active efflux
Tetracyclines (tetracycline, doxycycline, minocycline)	Protein synthesis	Bind 30S ribosomal subunit Inhibit peptide elongation	1. Active drug efflux 2. Ribosomal protection proteins
Tigecycline, eravacyclin, omadacycline	Protein synthesis	Same as tetracyclines	Active drug efflux (pumps different from those affecting tetracyclines)
Macrolides (erythromycin, clarithromycin, azithromycin) and the ketolide telithromycin	Protein synthesis	Bind 50S ribosomal subunit Block peptide chain exit	1. Methylation at ribosome binding site 2. Active drug efflux
Lincosamides (clindamycin)	Protein synthesis	Bind 50S ribosomal subunit Block peptide bond formation	Methylation at ribosome binding site
Streptogramins (quinupristin, dalfopristin)	Protein synthesis	Same as macrolides	1. Same as macrolides 2. Drug-modifying enzymes
Chloramphenicol	Protein synthesis	Binds 50S ribosomal subunit Blocks aminoacyl tRNA positioning	Drug-modifying enzymes
Oxazolidinones (linezolid, tedizolid)	Protein synthesis	Bind 50S ribosomal subunit Inhibit initiation of peptide synthesis	1. Altered rRNA binding site 2. Methylation of ribosome binding site
Pleuromutilins (lefamulin)	Protein synthesis	Bind 50S ribosomal subunit Blocks peptidyl transferase center	1. Altered L3 and L4 protein binding site 2. Methylation of ribosome binding site
Mupirocin	Protein synthesis	Blocks isoleucyl tRNA synthetase	1. Acquired resistant tRNA synthetase (drug bypass) 2. Altered native tRNA synthetase target
Sulfonamides (sulfadiazine, sulfisoxazole, and sulfamethoxazole)	Folate synthesis	Inhibit dihydropteroate synthetase	Acquired resistant dihydropteroate synthetase (drug bypass)
Trimethoprim	Folate synthesis	Inhibits dihydrofolate reductase	Acquired resistant dihydrofolate reductase (drug bypass)
Quinolones (norfloxacin, ciprofloxacin, ofloxacin, levofloxacin, moxifloxacin, gemifloxacin, delafloxacin)	DNA synthesis	Inhibit DNA gyrase and DNA topoisomerase IV Enzyme–DNA–drug complex: blocks DNA replication apparatus	1. Altered target(s) 2. Active efflux 3. Protection of target from drug 4. Drug-modifying enzyme (ciprofloxacin)
Rifamycins (rifampin, rifabutin, rifapentine)	RNA synthesis	Inhibit RNA polymerase	Altered target
Nitrofurantoin	Nucleic acid synthesis	Reduces reactive drug derivatives that damage DNA	Altered drug-activating enzymes
Metronidazole	Nucleic acid synthesis	Reduces reactive drug derivatives that damage DNA	1. Altered drug-activating enzyme 2. Acquired detoxifying enzymes 3. Active efflux
Polymyxins (polymyxin B and polymyxin E [colistin])	Cell membrane	Bind LPS and disrupt both outer and cytoplasmic membranes	Altered cell-membrane charge with reduced drug binding
Daptomycin	Cell membrane	Produces membrane channel and membrane leakage	Altered cell-membrane charge with reduced drug binding

Abbreviations: LPS, lipopolysaccharide; NAG, *N*-acetylglucosamine; PBP, penicillin-binding protein.

by β-lactamases, enzymes that break down the core β-lactam ring and destroy drug activity. β-Lactamases differ in the spectrum of β-lactams they can degrade. Some β-lactamases are encoded on the bacterial chromosome, and their activity contributes to the intrinsic susceptibility profile of a particular species. Chromosomally encoded β-lactamases can be produced in varying amounts that affect the degree of resistance. In some cases, enzyme expression is physiologically induced by exposure to certain β-lactams; in other cases, enzyme expression can become constant or constitutive through mutations in genes that encode the regulators of expression of a β-lactamase gene.

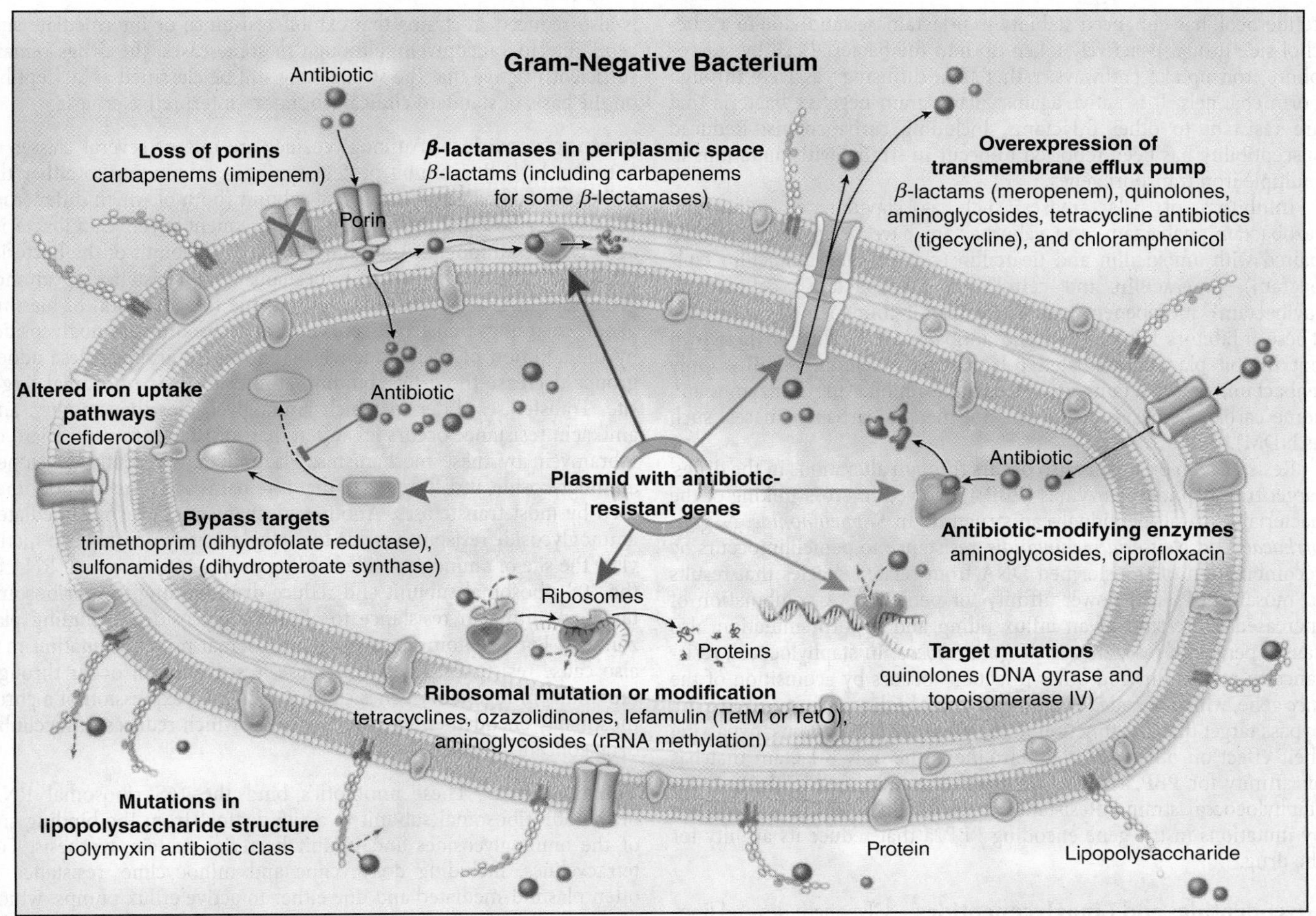

FIGURE 145-1 Antibacterial targets and mechanisms of resistance to antibacterial agents, as illustrated in a gram-negative bacterium. Similar mechanisms are found in gram-positive bacteria, but their lack of an outer membrane causes β-lactamases to be excreted outside the cell, rather than into the periplasmic space between the inner and outer membranes, and reduces the efficiency of efflux pumps because exported drugs can re-enter the cell after crossing a single membrane, rather than the two membranes in gram-negative bacteria. Red spheres indicate antibiotics. *(From AY Peleg, DC Hooper: Hospital-acquired infections due to gram-negative bacteria. N Engl J Med 362:1084, 2010. Copyright © 2010 Massachusetts Medical Society. Reprinted with permission from Massachusetts Medical Society.)*

Other β-lactamases are encoded by genes on acquired plasmids and are usually constitutively expressed. The resistance profiles due to plasmids may be present in some strains of a species but not others, depending on which plasmids the strain has acquired. In gram-positive bacteria β-lactamases are secreted into the extracellular environment, whereas in gram-negative bacteria these enzymes are secreted into the periplasmic space between the cytoplasmic and outer membranes—a limited space that permits the presence of high concentrations of β-lactamase. Thus, in gram-negative bacteria, access of β-lactams both to their target PBPs and to β-lactamases requires diffusion across the outer membrane, generally through the porin diffusion channels. Reductions in outer-membrane diffusion channels due to mutation can further augment the efficiency of β-lactamase degradation of β-lactams: slow diffusion acts together with the high enzyme concentrations in the periplasmic space to enhance drug degradation and resistance.

Most strains of *Staphylococcus aureus* produce a plasmid-encoded β-lactamase that degrades penicillin but not semisynthetic penicillins, such as oxacillin and nafcillin. The greatest diversity among β-lactamases, however, is found in gram-negative bacteria. The most common and earliest identified plasmid-encoded β-lactamases of gram-negative bacteria can inactivate all penicillins and most early-generation cephalosporins. Multiple extended-spectrum β-lactamase (ESBL) variants of these early enzymes have emerged and are now widely disseminated. These ESBLs can degrade later-generation cephalosporins (ceftriaxone, cefotaxime, ceftazidime) as well as the monobactam aztreonam, and some ESBLs also degrade the fourth-generation cephalosporin cefepime. Carbapenems (imipenem, meropenem, ertapenem, doripenem) generally are not degraded by ESBLs, but additional β-lactamases, called *carbapenemases*, which degrade carbapenems and most if not all other β-lactams, have emerged and are increasing in prevalence. In the United States, *Klebsiella pneumoniae* carbapenemases (KPCs), which are usually found in strains of *Escherichia coli* and *K. pneumoniae*, are most widespread, but New Delhi metallo-β-lactamases (NDM carbapenemases), which were found initially on the Indian subcontinent, have now appeared in several areas in the United States, as has an OXA group carbapenemase, OXA-48. In some cases, high levels of expression of an ESBL or an AmpC enzyme (see below), together with reduced porin diffusion channels, can also result in resistance to carbapenems. In *Pseudomonas aeruginosa*, resistance to carbapenems can occur by mutations that cause reductions in the OprD diffusion channel for imipenem or increased expression of efflux pumps that can remove meropenem from the bacterial cell.

The chromosomal β-lactamase of *K. pneumoniae* preferentially degrades penicillins but not cephalosporins. In contrast, the chromosomal β-lactamase of *Enterobacter* and related genera, AmpC, can degrade almost all cephalosporins but is normally expressed in only small amounts. Mutations in regulatory genes that cause increased amounts of AmpC to be produced confer full resistance to penicillins and cephalosporins; the exceptions are cefoxitin and cefepime, which are relatively stable to AmpC. Resistance to cefepime can develop, however, through the combined effects of mutations that cause increased AmpC production and decreased porin diffusion channels. Genes encoding AmpC have also been found on plasmids but are less common than plasmid-encoded ESBLs. A recent novel cephalosporin, cefiderocol, has enhanced stability to β-lactamases and, due to a catechol side group, is actively taken up into the bacterial cell by siderophore iron uptake pathways, rather than diffusing passively through porin channels. It is active against many gram-negative bacteria that are resistant to other β-lactams, including carbapenems. Reduced susceptibility has been reported to occur in strains with mutations in multiple iron transport genes.

Inhibitors of β-lactamases such as clavulanate, sulbactam, tazobactam, avibactam, and vaborbactam have been developed and paired with amoxicillin and ticarcillin (clavulanate), ampicillin (sulbactam), piperacillin and ceftolozane (tazobactam), ceftazidime (avibactam), meropenem (vaborbactam), or imipenem (relebactam). These inhibitors have little or no antibacterial activity of their own but inhibit plasmid-mediated β-lactamases, including ESBLs. Only avibactam, vaborbactam, and relebactam inhibit AmpC enzymes and some carbapenemases (KPCs but not metallo-carbapenemases, such as NDM).

Resistance to β-lactams also occurs through alterations in the drugs' target transpeptidase enzymes (PBPs) involved in cross-linking of the bacterial cell-wall peptidoglycan structure. In *S. pneumoniae*, *N. gonorrhoeae*, and *Neisseria meningitidis*, resistance to penicillin occurs by recombination of transformed DNA from related species that results in mosaic PBPs with lower affinity for penicillin. A combination of increased expression of an efflux pump and a porin mutation also causes penicillin resistance in *N. gonorrhoeae*. In staphylococci, resistance to methicillin and other β-lactams occurs by acquisition of the *mec* gene, which encodes PBP2a with reduced drug affinity. PBP2a is a bypass target that can function in the presence of β-lactams, bypassing their effect on other PBPs. Ceftaroline is the only β-lactam that has an affinity for PBP2a and is thus active against methicillin-resistant staphylococcal strains. Resistance to ceftaroline can occur, however, by mutations in the gene encoding PBP2a that reduce its affinity for the drug.

Glycopeptides and Lipoglycopeptides Glycopeptides and lipoglycopeptides inhibit bacterial cell-wall synthesis by binding to the terminal two D-alanine amino acids on the cell-wall peptidoglycan stem peptides, which are involved in peptidoglycan cross-links. In doing so, these drugs block the transpeptidase cross-linking enzymes and glycosyl transferases necessary for cell-wall synthesis. Resistance to vancomycin in enterococci is due to the acquisition of a set of *van* genes that result in (1) the production of D-alanine-D-lactate—instead of the normal D-alanine-D-alanine—at the end of the peptidoglycan stem peptide and (2) the reduction of existing D-alanine-D-alanine–terminated peptides. Vancomycin binds D-alanine-D-lactate with a 1000-fold lower affinity than D-alanine-D-alanine. The *van* genes originated in the organisms that naturally produce vancomycin and have been mobilized and reorganized in transposon mobile genetic elements and onto plasmids, which can be transferred between enterococci. In rare cases, the *van* gene cassettes have been transferred from enterococci to *S. aureus*, with the consequent generation of full vancomycin resistance. In *S. aureus*, intermediate resistance to vancomycin is more common than full vancomycin resistance and is due to a different mechanism that results from a series of several chromosomal mutations leading to a thickened and poorly cross-linked cell wall. This modified cell wall contains additional D-alanine-D-alanine–terminated stem peptides that bind vancomycin at a site distant from the cell membrane, adjacent to which new peptidoglycan is synthesized and where vancomycin binding blocks transpeptidase and transglycosylase enzymes. Thus, vancomycin's binding to these distant termini impedes its access to the proximal binding sites that result in inhibition of peptidoglycan synthesis. This intermediate-resistance phenotype was first recognized in patients receiving prolonged courses of vancomycin that created an opportunity for selection of the multiple mutations needed to produce the modified cell wall. Because of the energy costs of a thickened cell wall, this intermediate-resistance phenotype may be unstable, with strains returning to susceptibility in the absence of vancomycin selection pressure. Susceptibility to telavancin, dalbavancin, and oritavancin is also reduced in strains that exhibit resistance or intermediate susceptibility to vancomycin, although in some cases, the drugs remain sufficiently active that the strains may still be classified as susceptible on the basis of standard clinical laboratory interpretive criteria.

Aminoglycosides Aminoglycosides are one of several classes of antimicrobials that inhibit protein synthesis by binding to either the 30S or the 50S bacterial ribosomal subunit (both of which differ from eukaryotic ribosomal subunits), with consequent selective antibacterial activity. The aminoglycosides bind to the 30S subunit of the bacterial ribosome. The most common mechanism of resistance to aminoglycosides in gram-negative bacteria is due to acquisition of plasmid genes encoding transferase enzymes that modify aminoglycosides by the addition of acetyl, adenyl, or phosphate groups; these added groups decrease the drugs' binding affinity to their ribosomal target site. Transferases differ in which aminoglycosides they modify, and amikacin resistance occurs less often than resistance to gentamicin or tobramycin by these mechanisms. Plazomicin, a recently developed aminoglycoside, is distinctive in that it remains active and is not modified by most transferases. Another mechanism of plasmid-mediated aminoglycoside resistance is due to methylase enzymes that can methylate the site of aminoglycoside binding on the 16S ribosomal RNA of the 30S ribosomal subunit and reduce drug binding to its ribosome target, resulting in resistance to all aminoglycosides, including plazomicin. For streptomycin, a single ribosomal protein mutation may also cause resistance. In *P. aeruginosa*, resistance can occur through mutations in regulatory genes causing increased expression of a chromosomally encoded efflux pump, MexXY, which reduces intracellular drug concentrations.

Tetracyclines These antibiotics bind the 16S ribosomal RNA of the 30S ribosomal subunit at a site distinct from the binding site of the aminoglycosides and inhibit bacterial protein synthesis. For tetracyclines, including doxycycline and minocycline, resistance is often plasmid-mediated and due either to active efflux pumps, which are generally specific for tetracyclines, or to proteins that protect the ribosome from tetracycline action. A number of broad-spectrum, chromosomally encoded efflux pumps may also include tetracyclines among their substrates, and regulatory mutations that cause pump overexpression may confer tetracycline resistance together with resistance to other agents. There have been recent derivatives of the tetracyclines, including the glycylcycline, tigecycline, the fluorocycline, eravacycline, and the aminomethylcycline, omadacycline, which have modifications on the core tetracycline ring structure rendering them less affected or unaffected by the common tetracycline resistance mechanisms. Resistance to the newer tetracyclines can occur, however, through mutations that cause overexpression of some broad-spectrum efflux pumps, particularly in *Proteus* species. An uncommon plasmid-encoded tetracycline modification mechanism can also cause resistance to the newer agents.

Macrolides, Ketolides, Lincosamides, and Streptogramins These antibiotics are also inhibitors of bacterial protein synthesis, in this case through their binding to the 23S RNA of the 50S ribosomal subunit. They are generally active against gram-positive bacteria. Resistance to macrolides, clindamycin, and quinupristin is most often due to acquired Erm methylases that modify the drug-binding site on the ribosome, reducing drug binding. Resistance to quinupristin by this mechanism renders the quinupristin-dalfopristin combination bacteriostatic rather than bactericidal. Telithromycin, a ketolide structurally related to macrolides, has an additional binding site on the ribosome and remains active in the presence of some methylases. Methylase gene expression can be induced by exposure to most macrolides but generally not ketolides (e.g., telithromycin); however, bacterial strains constitutively expressing methylase genes can display resistance to both macrolides and ketolides. Acquired genes encoding active efflux pumps also can contribute to resistance to macrolides in streptococci and to resistance to macrolides, clindamycin, and dalfopristin in staphylococci. Plasmid-acquired, drug-modifying enzymes in staphylococci can also cause resistance to quinupristin and dalfopristin. Macrolide resistance due to 23S rRNA mutations at the site of drug binding is uncommon in staphylococci and streptococci because of the multiple copies of the rRNA genes on the chromosomes of these species; such resistance may occur more frequently, however, in mycobacteria, *Helicobacter pylori*, and *Treponema* species, which have only one or two chromosomal copies of these rRNA genes. Among gram-negative bacteria, many of which are not susceptible to current macrolides because of inadequate drug permeation, some strains with acquired genes for macrolide-modifying enzymes have been described.

Chloramphenicol Chloramphenicol inhibits bacterial protein synthesis by binding to the 23S rRNA of the 50S subunit at a site that overlaps the macrolide-binding site. Chloramphenicol is uncommonly used in human medicine because of infrequent but potentially severe bone marrow toxicity. Resistance to chloramphenicol is most often due to plasmid-encoded, drug-modifying acetyltransferases that have been found in both gram-positive and gram-negative bacteria and whose expression can be induced by drug exposure. Among staphylococci, some resistant strains have been found to have a plasmid-encoded ribosomal methylase that confers resistance to chloramphenicol, clindamycin, and oxazolidinones. As is the case for macrolides, ribosomal mutations causing resistance to chloramphenicol are uncommon because of multiple copies of rRNA genes in most human pathogens. Plasmid-encoded efflux pumps affecting chloramphenicol specifically have been found in gram-negative bacteria, and other pumps affecting chloramphenicol and oxazolidinones have been found in gram-positive bacteria.

Oxazolidinones Linezolid and tedizolid are the only members of the oxazolidinone class of antimicrobials in clinical use, and both are active against gram-positive bacteria only; lack of sufficient activity in gram-negative bacteria results from the ability of native efflux pumps in these bacteria to limit drug access to their cytoplasmic ribosome targets. Oxazolidinones target the bacterial ribosome and inhibit protein synthesis by binding to 23S rRNA of the 50S subunit at a distinct site that overlaps with the chloramphenicol-binding site. Resistance has been seen in enterococci more often than in staphylococci and, in both organisms, is most often due to mutations in multiple copies of the 23S rRNA genes that reduce drug binding to the ribosome. A plasmid-acquired ribosomal methylase gene that enables ribosomal alteration at a site that confers resistance to both linezolid and chloramphenicol has also been found in some strains of both *S. aureus* and coagulase-negative staphylococci but is not yet widespread. A plasmid-encoded active efflux pump conferring resistance to oxazolidinones (both linezolid and tedizolid) and chloramphenicol has been described in animal isolates and a small number of human isolates of *Enterococcus faecalis*.

Pleuromutilins Lefamulin was recently approved and is the only systemic pleuromutilin in clinical use. Retapamulin has been available for topical use in skin infections. Pleuromutilins inhibit bacterial protein synthesis by binding to the peptidyl transferase center in the 50S ribosomal subunit, and lefamulin is generally active against gram-positive bacteria, *Haemophilus influenzae*, *Moraxella catarrhalis*, and atypical respiratory pathogens such a *Mycoplasma pneumoniae* and *Legionella* spp. Although there is partial overlap in the site of binding of lefamulin and those of other antibacterials binding the 50S ribosomal subunit, cross-resistance with macrolides, oxazolidinones, lincosamides, and streptogramins is uncommon. Resistance to lefamulin can occur by mutations in L3 and L4 proteins of the 50S subunit that alter the lefamulin binding site. In addition, the plasmid-encoded Cfr methylase, which confers resistance to chloramphenicol and oxazolidinones, can also cause resistance to lefamulin by disrupting its binding site. Vga transporters, which cause resistance to lincosamides and streptogramins, also affect pleuromutilins.

Mupirocin Mupirocin is used only in topical formulations, most often for elimination of nasal carriage of *S. aureus*. It targets bacterial leucyl-tRNA synthetase and inhibits protein synthesis. Resistance to mupirocin occurs by either mutation in the target leucyl-tRNA synthetase (low-level resistance) or the acquisition of a plasmid-encoded resistant tRNA synthetase (high-level resistance), which bypasses drug inhibition of the native, sensitive synthetase.

Sulfonamides and Trimethoprim These agents inhibit the folate biosynthesis pathway at different steps. Sulfonamides are structurally similar to *para*-aminobenzoic acid (PABA) and competitively inhibit dihydropteroate synthetase, which, in an early step in the pathway, uses PABA to synthesize dihydropteroate, a precursor of dihydrofolate. Trimethoprim inhibits dihydrofolate reductase at a later step in the pathway that generates tetrahydrofolate. Clinical use of folate pathway inhibitors most often consists of the combination of sulfamethoxazole and trimethoprim; on occasion, however, trimethoprim or various sulfonamides are used individually. Resistance to both of these antimetabolites can result from mutation in their target enzymes or can be due to plasmid-acquired genes encoding resistant enzymes that bypass the inhibition of the native sensitive enzymes—a resistant dihydropteroate synthetase in the case of sulfonamides and a resistant dihydrofolate reductase in the case of trimethoprim. Resistance to the combination of sulfamethoxazole and trimethoprim requires that the bacterial strain have resistance mechanisms for both agents and yet is not uncommon. Resistance due to drug efflux or drug modification has been limited for both sulfonamides and trimethoprim.

Quinolones Quinolones are synthetic inhibitors of bacterial DNA synthesis. They bind to two enzymes required for DNA synthesis: DNA gyrase and DNA topoisomerase IV, which alter DNA conformation and the interlinking of replicated molecules. In addition to inhibiting the enzymes' catalytic functions of altering DNA topology, they stabilize enzyme–DNA complexes that form a barrier to the DNA replication machinery and are a precursor to lethal double-strand DNA breaks. Although related topoisomerase enzymes are involved in mammalian DNA synthesis, the mammalian and bacterial enzymes are sufficiently different from each other for quinolones to have selective activity against bacteria. Resistance to quinolones is most often due either to chromosomal mutations altering the target enzymes DNA gyrase and DNA topoisomerase IV, with consequent reduction in drug binding, or to mutations that increase the expression of native broad-spectrum efflux pumps for which quinolones (among other compounds) are substrates. In addition, three types of acquired genes can confer reduced susceptibility or low-level resistance by protecting the target enzymes, modifying some quinolones (particularly ciprofloxacin and norfloxacin) to reduce their activity, or generating an efflux of quinolones. These genes are usually located on multidrug-resistance plasmids that have spread worldwide. Their presence can promote higher levels of quinolone resistance by enhancing selection of the mutations in chromosomal target genes with exposure to quinolones and can then link quinolone resistance to resistance to other antibacterial drugs that are encoded by the same plasmid.

Rifampin and Rifabutin Antimicrobials of the rifamycin class target bacterial RNA polymerase and thereby inhibit transcription of messenger RNA and gene expression. Their activity is generally limited to gram-positive bacteria because native efflux pumps in most gram-negative bacteria reduce drug access to the cytoplasmic enzyme target. Single mutations in the β subunit of RNA polymerase constitute the principal mechanism of acquired rifampin resistance, which is high level. Thus, rifampin and other rifamycins are used for treatment of infections only in combination with other antibacterial drugs in order to reduce the likelihood of selection of high-level resistance.

Metronidazole Metronidazole is actively taken up by most anaerobic bacteria and then converted to reactive drug derivatives that nonspecifically damage cytoplasmic proteins and nucleic acids. Thus, metronidazole lacks a specific cellular target. Acquired resistance to metronidazole in *Bacteroides* species is rare. Such resistance has been reported in strains that lack the endogenous activating nitroreductase or that have acquired *nim* genes responsible for further reduction of

DNA-damaging nitroso intermediates to an inactive derivative. Active efflux and enhanced DNA repair mechanisms also have been associated with resistance.

Nitrofurantoin Nitrofurantoin is used only for treatment of lower urinary tract infections because adequate drug concentrations are found only in urine. Its mechanism of action is not fully understood but is thought to involve generation of reactive derivative molecules (as occurs with metronidazole) that damage DNA and ribosomes. Resistance to nitrofurantoin in *E. coli* can emerge through a series of mutations that progressively decrease the nitroreductase activity required for generating active nitrofuran metabolites. These mutants are also impaired in growth; this impairment possibly explains the infrequent occurrence of resistance with clinical use of nitrofurantoin.

Polymyxins Because of emerging multidrug resistance in gram-negative bacteria, colistin and polymyxin B are being used increasingly for infections due to resistant Enterobacterales, *P. aeruginosa*, and *Acinetobacter* species. Polymyxins are cationic cyclic peptide molecules that bind negatively charged lipopolysaccharides on the gram-negative bacterial outer membrane, with subsequent disruption and permeabilization of both outer-membrane and cytoplasmic-membrane structure. Thus, the polymyxins are bactericidal. Resistance is so far uncommon but can emerge during therapy through mutations that cause reductions in the negative charge of the gram-negative bacterial cell surface, thereby reducing binding of the positively charged colistin. Recently transferable plasmid-mediated colistin resistance has also been found to be due to *mcr-1*, a gene encoding a phosphoethanolamine transferase that also reduces the negative charge on the cell surface. *mcr-1*-containing enteric bacteria have now been identified in Asia, Europe, and the United States.

Daptomycin Daptomycin is active against gram-positive bacteria and interacts with and disrupts the cytoplasmic membrane in a calcium-dependent manner, resulting in bactericidal activity. The mechanisms of resistance to daptomycin are complex and involve mutations in several genes that can alter cell membrane charge and structure and reduce daptomycin binding. Resistance to daptomycin is relatively infrequent but has emerged in some *S. aureus* strains with intermediate vancomycin susceptibility from patients treated with vancomycin and not exposed to daptomycin. In some strains of methicillin-resistant *S. aureus*, daptomycin resistance has been linked to acquired susceptibility to β-lactams; combinations of daptomycin with nafcillin or ceftaroline have been successful for treatment of patients infected with resistant strains when daptomycin alone or in combination with other agents has failed. The mechanism of this effect is not yet clear but may involve alteration in surface charge and increased daptomycin binding in the presence of β-lactams. Daptomycin resistance has also been reported in enterococci.

EPIDEMIOLOGY OF RESISTANCE AND REDUCTION OF ITS OCCURRENCE

Multidrug resistance in human bacterial infections has been increasing overall in recent years, substantially limiting the number of antibiotics that can be used to treat some infections. The prevalence of resistance to various antimicrobials among human pathogens can, however, vary greatly in different geographic areas and even at different institutions in the same area. Thus, specific local data on the occurrence of various types of resistance are an important component of the choice of antimicrobials for empirical treatment of infection until the responsible pathogen is identified and its specific susceptibilities are determined by the clinical microbiology laboratory. Prompt adjustment of the initially chosen antimicrobial on the basis of species and susceptibility data to best target therapy is equally important. These principles emphasize the importance of obtaining appropriate samples for culture or other diagnostic modalities and susceptibility testing—whenever possible, prior to administration of antimicrobials. They also highlight the importance of rapid and sensitive diagnostic methods and the prompt communication of their results to clinicians to inform best choices of antimicrobials.

The overall prevalence of resistance can be affected by a number of factors, including (1) the extent of resistance reservoirs in the patient population; (2) the selection pressures from use of antimicrobials that favor resistant strains over susceptible ones; and (3) the extent by which resistance is amplified by transmission of resistant strains to patients from their environment or other persons, either directly or indirectly via the contaminated hands of health care workers when hand hygiene and other infection control practices are inadequately followed. The likelihood that an individual patient will be infected with a resistant pathogen is likewise affected by his or her history. Studies have shown that prior antibiotic treatment, prior infection with resistant pathogens, and prior hospitalizations all increase this likelihood.

These factors emphasize the importance of the appropriate use of antimicrobials (particularly, the avoidance of their use in clinical conditions in which they are not needed), the use of the shortest courses of therapy sufficient for a successful clinical outcome, and the implementation of antimicrobial stewardship programs **(Chap. 144)** as well as careful and consistent infection control practices in short- and long-term-care institutions. Antimicrobial agents are distinct among drug classes in human medicine in that—despite their clear clinical value when used appropriately—the extent of their use can compromise their future utility because of resistance. The remarkable ability of pathogens to acquire resistance is inherent in their biology and emphasizes the necessity for clinicians and institutions to pay careful attention to those factors that can be controlled through judicious antimicrobial use and rigorous infection control and prevention practices.

Efforts to address the problems caused by resistance are now being made worldwide. The U.S. Centers for Disease Control and Prevention (CDC) has recently estimated that >2.8 million resistant bacterial infections occur in the United States each year, with 35,900 deaths, and has identified particular resistant pathogens that are of greatest concern because of their overall effects on public health **(Table 145-2)**. Enteric bacteria (such as *E. coli*, *K. pneumoniae*, and *Enterobacter* spp.) and

TABLE 145-2 Antibiotic Resistance Threats in the United States, 2019

THREAT CATEGORY	ORGANISMS
Urgent	Carbapenem-resistant *Acinetobacter*
	Candida auris
	Clostridioides difficile
	Carbapenem-resistant Enterobacterales
	Drug-resistant *Neisseria gonorrhoeae*
Serious	Drug-resistant *Campylobacter*
	Drug-resistant *Candida*
	Extended-spectrum β-lactamase–producing Enterobacterales
	Vancomycin-resistant *Enterococcus*
	Multidrug-resistant *Pseudomonas aeruginosa*
	Drug-resistant nontyphoidal *Salmonella*
	Drug-resistant *Salmonella* serotype Typhi
	Drug-resistant *Shigella*
	Methicillin-resistant *Staphylococcus aureus*
	Drug-resistant *Streptococcus pneumoniae*
	Drug-resistant *Mycobacterium tuberculosis*
Concerning	Erythromycin-resistant group A *Streptococcus*
	Clindamycin-resistant group B *Streptococcus*
Watch List	Azole-resistant *Aspergillus fumagatis*
	Drug-resistant *Mycoplasma genitalium*
	Drug-resistant *Bordetella pertussis*

Source: U.S. Centers for Disease Control and Prevention.

Acinetobacter spp. that are resistant to carbapenems are included in the "urgent" category because of their increasing occurrence worldwide and because they are often highly resistant to multiple drugs, with few if any active antimicrobials available for treatment. Resistant *N. gonorrhoeae* is included in this category as well because of the ease with which gonorrhea can be spread from person to person and because few active agents are now available. Other resistances are common and also affect clinical care, often requiring use of alternatives to first-line agents that can be less effective and less well tolerated. Also affecting clinical care and considered urgent are infections due to *Clostridioides difficile*. Although not directly due to acquired resistance, *C. difficile* disease, like resistant bacterial infections, is linked to antibacterial use (by the disruption of the normal microbiome of the gastrointestinal tract rather than direct resistance selection) and to its ability as a spore-forming bacterium to be spread in health care environments. To address the problems posed by resistance and *C. difficile* disease, the CDC has emphasized a set of five core actions. (1) *Infection prevention and control:* These efforts focus on implementation of evidence-based activities to reduce the risks and incidence of device-related infections overall and on improvement of compliance with infection control practices that prevent transmission of resistant pathogens from one person to another, such as hand hygiene and isolation precautions in health care and long-term care settings. (2) *Tracking and data:* Efforts aim to increase the reporting and sharing of the occurrence of resistance to enhance epidemiologic data and inform targeting of preventive interventions. (3) *Antibiotic use and access:* Antimicrobial stewardship programs with specific components to track usage and educate clinicians on appropriate use have become required in hospitals, and the CDC has implemented efforts to reduce inappropriate use in outpatient settings, with particular attention to upper respiratory illnesses that often do not require antimicrobials because of their common self-limited viral causes. (4) *Vaccines, therapeutics, and diagnostics:* The U.S. Congress and the U.S. Food and Drug Administration, as well as agencies in other countries, have recently developed incentives and enhanced regulatory pathways for drug approval that pharmaceutical companies can use for development of antimicrobials that specifically address particular resistant pathogens. Both small and large companies have undertaken efforts in this area. New technologies for rapid detection of resistance and susceptibility are also being developed by multiple diagnostics companies in order to facilitate the appropriate choice of antimicrobials earlier in the course of illness, providing an important tool for antimicrobial stewardship programs. (5) *Environment and sanitation:* Reservoirs of resistant bacteria and resistance genes on mobile genetic elements can exist in agriculture and food production and domestic animals and have the potential for introduction into humans. Thus, antibiotic use in these environments can amplify resistance reservoirs and increase the chance of human exposure. Therefore, public health interventions addressing these issues in a One Health approach (*https://www.cdc.gov/onehealth/index.html*) are an important component of managing resistance risks.

FURTHER READING

Bush K, Bradford PA: Interplay between β-lactamases and new β-lactamase inhibitors. Nat Rev Microbiol 17:295, 2019.

Centers for Disease Control and Prevention: Antibiotic resistance threats in the United States, 2019. Available at *https://www.cdc.gov/drugresistance/pdf/threats-report/2019-ar-threats-report-508.pdf.* Accessed June 23, 2020.

French GL: Antimicrobial resistance and healthcare-associated infections, in *Hospital Epidemiology and Infection Control*, 4th ed. GC Mayhall (ed). Philadelphia, Lippincott Williams & Wilkins, 2012, pp 1297–1310.

Rice LB: Mechanisms of resistance and clinical relevance of resistance to β-lactams, glycopeptides, and fluoroquinolones. Mayo Clin Proc 87:198, 2012.

Silver LL, Bush K (eds): *Antibiotics and Antibiotic Resistance*. Cold Spring Harbor Perspectives in Medicine. New York, Cold Spring Harbor Laboratory Press, 2016.

Section 5 Diseases Caused by Gram-Positive Bacteria

146 Pneumococcal Infections

David Goldblatt, Katherine L. O'Brien

In the late nineteenth century, pairs of micrococci were first recognized in the blood of rabbits injected with human saliva by both Louis Pasteur, working in France, and George Sternberg, an American army physician. The important role of these micrococci in human disease was not appreciated at that time. By 1886, when the organism was designated "pneumokokkus" and *Diplococcus pneumoniae*, it had been isolated by many independent investigators, and its role in the etiology of pneumonia was well known. In the 1930s, pneumonia was the third leading cause of death in the United States (after heart disease and cancer) and was responsible for ~7% of all deaths both in the United States and in Europe. While pneumonia was caused by a host of pathogens, lobar pneumonia—a pattern more likely to be caused by the pneumococcus—accounted for approximately one-half of all pneumonia deaths in the United States in 1929. In 1974, the organism was reclassified as *Streptococcus pneumoniae*.

MICROBIOLOGY

Etiologic Agent Pneumococci are spherical gram-positive bacteria of the genus *Streptococcus*. Within this genus, cell division occurs along a single axis, and bacteria grow in chains or pairs—hence the name *Streptococcus*, from the Greek *streptos*, meaning "twisted," and *kokkos*, meaning "berry." At least 22 streptococcal species are recognized and are divided further into groups based on their hemolytic properties. *S. pneumoniae* belongs to the α-hemolytic group that characteristically produces a greenish color on blood agar because of the reduction of iron in hemoglobin (**Fig. 146-1**). The bacteria are fastidious and grow

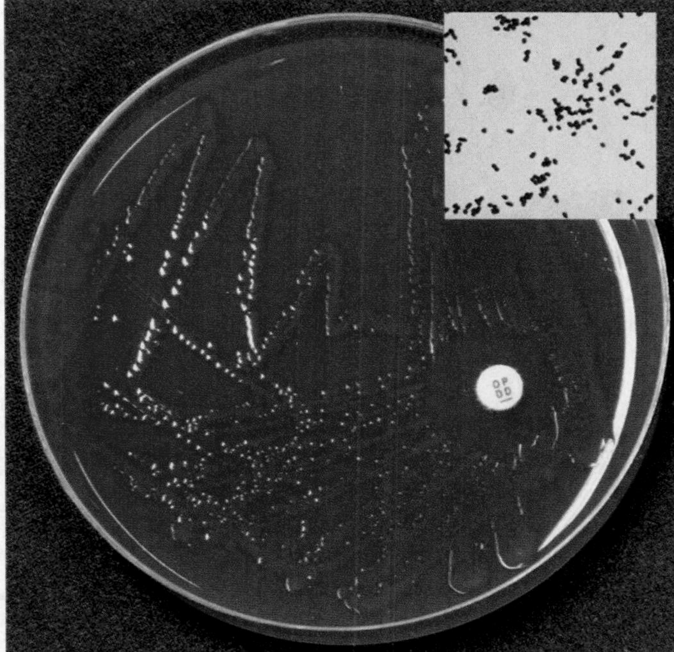

FIGURE 146-1 Pneumococci growing on blood agar, illustrating α hemolysis and optochin sensitivity (zone around optochin disk). *Inset:* Gram's stain, illustrating gram-positive diplococci. *(Photographs courtesy of Paul Turner, University of Oxford, United Kingdom.)*

best in 5% CO_2 but require a source of catalase (e.g., blood) for growth on agar plates, where they develop mucoid (smooth/shiny) colonies. Pneumococci without a capsule produce colonies with a rough surface. Unlike that of other α-hemolytic streptococci, their growth is inhibited in the presence of optochin (ethylhydrocupreine hydrochloride), and they are bile soluble.

In common with other gram-positive bacteria, pneumococci have a cell membrane beneath a cell wall, which in turn is covered by a polysaccharide capsule. Pneumococci are divided into serogroups or serotypes based on capsular polysaccharide structure, as distinguished with rabbit polyclonal antisera; capsules swell in the presence of specific antiserum (the Quellung reaction). The most recently discovered serotypes—6C, 6D, 6F, 6G, 6H, 11E, 20A, 20B and 35D—have been identified with monoclonal antibodies and by serologic, genetic, and biochemical means. The currently recognized 98 serotypes fall into 21 serogroups, and each serogroup contains two to eight serotypes with closely related capsules. Detailed genetic analysis of the locus coding for the polysaccharide capsule, the *cps* locus, continues to reveal putative novel capsular polysaccharides, variants within existing serogroups and designated with an "X." In the absence of type-specific antibody, the capsule protects the bacteria from phagocytosis by host cells and is arguably the most important determinant of pneumococcal virulence. Unencapsulated variants are occasionally identified in cases of invasive pneumococcal disease; however, when their genotype is assessed, they often contain capsular genes. Thus it is likely that they were encapsulated in vivo and have stopped producing capsule during the laboratory steps of pathogen isolation.

Virulence Factors Within the cytoplasm, cell membrane, and cell wall, many molecules that may play a role in pneumococcal pathogenesis and virulence have been identified **(Fig. 146-2)**. These proteins are often involved in direct interactions with host tissues or in concealment of the bacterial surface from host defense mechanisms. Pneumolysin (PLY) is a secreted cytotoxin thought to result in cytolysis of cells and tissues, and LytA enhances pathogenesis. A number of cell wall proteins interfere with the complement pathway, thus inhibiting complement deposition and preventing lysis and/or opsonophagocytosis. The pneumococcal H inhibitor (Hic) impedes the formation of C3 convertase, while pneumococcal surface protein C (PspC), also known as choline-binding protein A (CbpA), binds factor H and is thought to accelerate the breakdown of C3. PspA and CbpA inhibit the deposition of or degrade C3b. To avoid clearance by the mucus, pneumococci utilize the matrix metalloprotease ZmpA, which cleaves mucosal IgA to evade complement activation, preventing agglutination and thus clearance by the mucociliary flow.

The numerous pneumococcal proteins thought to be involved in adhesion include pneumococcal surface adhesin A (PsaA) and the exoglycosidases such as neuraminidase (NanA), β-galactosidase (BgaA), and β-N-Acetylglucosaminidase (StrH), which deglycosylate host glycoproteins releasing sugars as a nutrient source and exposing hidden receptors for adhesion. Once through the epithelial barrier, pneumococci utilize PLY and Mannose receptor C type lectin 1 (MRC-1/CD206) on the surface of dendritic cells and macrophages to enter cells, where they may survive intracellularly in vacuoles thus facilitating spread. To outcompete the other co-colonizing bacteria, the pneumococcus produces bacteriocins called pneumocins that mediate intraspecific competition. Some of the antigens mentioned above are potential vaccine candidates (see "Prevention," below). Biofilm production by pneumococci is now well recognized and is likely to be an important mechanism aiding survival of pneumococci in the upper respiratory tract and contributing to local disease manifestations such as otitis media.

Although the capsule surrounding the cell wall of *S. pneumoniae* is the basis for categorization by serotype, the disease potential of a

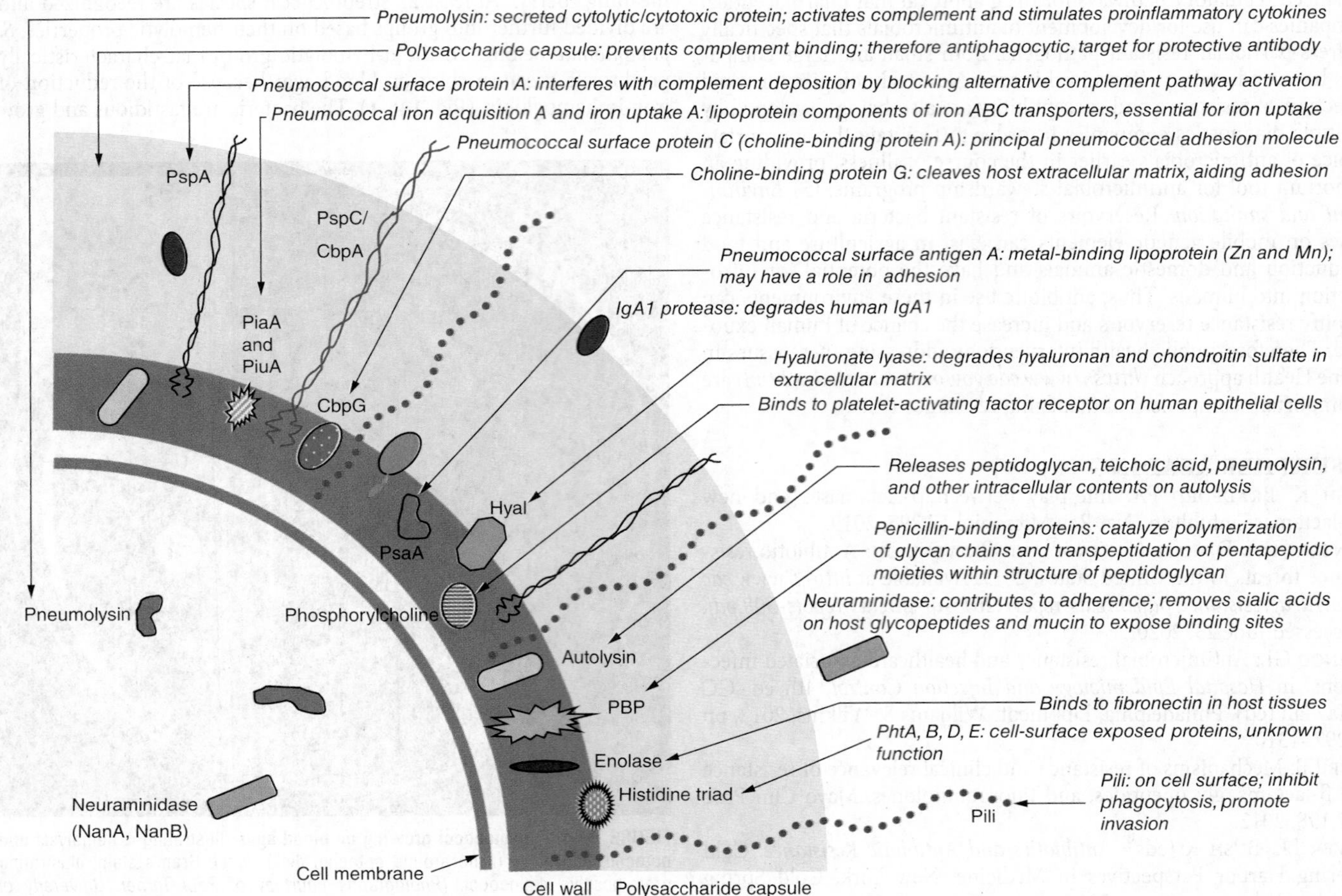

Pneumolysin: secreted cytolytic/cytotoxic protein; activates complement and stimulates proinflammatory cytokines
Polysaccharide capsule: prevents complement binding; therefore antiphagocytic, target for protective antibody
Pneumococcal surface protein A: interferes with complement deposition by blocking alternative complement pathway activation
Pneumococcal iron acquisition A and iron uptake A: lipoprotein components of iron ABC transporters, essential for iron uptake
Pneumococcal surface protein C (choline-binding protein A): principal pneumococcal adhesion molecule
Choline-binding protein G: cleaves host extracellular matrix, aiding adhesion
PspA
PspC/
CbpA
Pneumococcal surface antigen A: metal-binding lipoprotein (Zn and Mn); may have a role in adhesion
IgA1 protease: degrades human IgA1
PiaA
and
PiuA
Hyaluronate lyase: degrades hyaluronan and chondroitin sulfate in extracellular matrix
Binds to platelet-activating factor receptor on human epithelial cells
CbpG
Releases peptidoglycan, teichoic acid, pneumolysin, and other intracellular contents on autolysis
Hyal
PsaA
Penicillin-binding proteins: catalyze polymerization of glycan chains and transpeptidation of pentapeptidic moieties within structure of peptidoglycan
Neuraminidase: contributes to adherence; removes sialic acids on host glycopeptides and mucin to expose binding sites
Pneumolysin
Phosphorylcholine
Autolysin
PBP
Binds to fibronectin in host tissues
PhtA, B, D, E: cell-surface exposed proteins, unknown function
Enolase
Histidine triad
Neuraminidase
(NanA, NanB)
Pili
Pili: on cell surface; inhibit phagocytosis, promote invasion
Cell membrane
Cell wall
Polysaccharide capsule

FIGURE 146-2 Schematic diagram of the pneumococcal cell surface, with key antigens and their roles highlighted.

serotype is also related to the genetic composition of the strain. Molecular genotyping and epidemiology are therefore essential, and the gold-standard technique for epidemiologic analyses is the sequencing of housekeeping genes by multilocus sequence typing (MLST). For *S. pneumoniae*, alleles at each of seven loci (*aroE, gdh, gki, recP, spi, xpt,* and *ddl*) are sequenced and compared with all of the known alleles at that locus. The combination of seven alleles confers the unique sequence type (ST). The pneumococcal MLST website (*pubmlst.org/spneumoniae/*) facilitates the assignment of allele and ST data. Users from nearly all countries of the world and from all major public health and reference laboratories submit their data to the PubMLST site for assignment and curation. Sequence-based MLST genotyping thus provides an unambiguous nomenclature for epidemiologic investigations.

The first pneumococcal genome (a serotype 4 strain known as TIGR4) was sequenced nearly 20 years ago. With the recent advent of high-throughput and relatively inexpensive sequencing techniques, whole-genome sequencing has facilitated even more precise molecular epidemiology: seven-locus STs are simple to define, and enhanced genomic epidemiology can be performed using ribosomal MLST (rMLST; >50 ribosomal genes) and core genome MLST (cgMLST; >1300 core genes), also via the PubMLST website. The pneumococcal database currently contains nearly 50,000 isolates, more than 275,000 alleles, and nearly 15,000 genomes. This includes the PubMLST Pneumococcal Genome Library of curated, published, assembled genomes and isolate provenance data (*pubmlst.org/spneumoniae/pgl/*). All PubMLST data are publicly available and free to access. In recent years, genome sequence analyses have made major contributions to the understanding of pneumococcal molecular epidemiology, biology, diversity, pathogenicity, and vaccine impact.

■ EPIDEMIOLOGY

(See also "Global Health," below.) Pneumococcal infections remain a significant global cause of morbidity and death, particularly among children and the elderly. Rapid and dramatic changes in the epidemiology of this disease during the past 20 years in several developed countries followed the licensure and routine childhood administration of pneumococcal polysaccharide–protein conjugate vaccine (PCV). With PCV introduction in low and middle-income countries (LMIC), additional profound changes in pneumococcal ecology and disease epidemiology are occurring. The disease burden and serotype distribution in the PCV era are influenced not only by the reduction in disease caused by serotypes included in PCV but also by serotype replacement as a result of reductions in vaccine serotypes, concomitant secular trends in pneumococcal strains unrelated to vaccine use, the impact of antibiotic use on pneumococcal strain ecology, and surveillance system attributes that can themselves affect analysis of epidemiologic features of pneumococcal strains and disease.

Serotype Distribution Not all pneumococcal serotypes are equally likely to cause disease; observed serotype distributions vary by age category, disease syndrome, and geography. Geographic differences may be driven by variations in the relative prevalence of syndromes causing disease rather than by true serotype distribution differences, as certain serotypes are more common causes of some syndromes than others (e.g., pneumonia and meningitis). Most data on serotype distribution come from pediatric invasive pneumococcal disease (IPD, defined as infection of a normally sterile site); much less information on global or regional serotype distributions is available for disease in adults. In the era before PCV use, five to seven serotypes caused >60% of IPD cases among children <5 years of age in most parts of the world; seven serotypes (1, 5, 6A, 6B, 14, 19F, and 23F) accounted for ~60% of such cases in all areas of the world, but in any given region these seven serotypes may not all rank as the most common disease strains. Some serotypes (e.g., types 1 and 5) not only tend to cause disease in areas with a high disease burden but also cause waves of disease in lower-burden areas (e.g., Europe) or outbreaks (e.g., in military barracks; meningitis in sub-Saharan Africa). The widespread use of pneumococcal conjugate vaccines has significantly altered serotype-specific epidemiology, with some of the serotypes identified above now causing little invasive disease in countries with mature vaccine programs and emerging serotypes, not prominent in the pre-conjugate vaccine era, appearing as important causes of invasive disease. These include serotypes such as 15BC, 22F, 10A, 23B, 12F, 33F, 15A, 8, and 24F, while some serotypes included in PCVs such as 3 and 19A continue to cause IPD.

Nasopharyngeal Carriage Pneumococci are intermittent inhabitants of the healthy human nasopharynx and are transmitted by respiratory droplets. In children, pneumococcal nasopharyngeal ecology varies by geographic region, socioeconomic status, climate, degree of crowding, and particularly intensity of exposure to other children, with children in day-care settings having higher rates of colonization. In developed-world settings, children serve as the major vectors of pneumococcal transmission. By 1 year of age, ~50% of children have had at least one episode of pneumococcal colonization. Cross-sectional prevalence data show rates of pneumococcal carriage ranging from 20% to 50% among children <5 years of age and from 5% to 15% among young and middle-aged adults; **Fig. 146-3** shows relevant data from the United Kingdom. Data on colonization rates among healthy elderly individuals are limited. In LMICs, pneumococcal acquisition occurs much earlier, sometimes within the first few days after birth, and nearly all infants have had at least one episode of colonization by 2 months of age. Cross-sectional studies show that up to the age of 5 years, 70–90% of children carry *S. pneumoniae* in the nasopharynx, and a significant proportion of adults (sometimes >40%) also are colonized. Their high rates of colonization make adults an important source of transmission and may affect community transmission dynamics.

Invasive Disease and Pneumonia IPD develops when *S. pneumoniae* invades the bloodstream and seeds other organs or directly reaches the cerebrospinal fluid (CSF) by local extension. Pneumonia may follow aspiration of pneumococci, although only 10–30% of pneumococcal pneumonia cases are associated with a positive blood culture (and thus contribute to the measured burden of IPD). The substantial variation of IPD rates with age is illustrated by data from the United States for 1998–1999, a period prior to PCV introduction. Rates of IPD were highest among children <2 years of age and among adults ≥65 years of age (188 and 60 cases/100,000, respectively; **Fig. 146-4**). Since the introduction of PCV, IPD rates among infants and children in the United States have fallen by >75%, a decrease driven by the near elimination of vaccine-serotype IPD. A similar impact of PCV on vaccine-serotype IPD rates has been consistently observed in countries where PCV has been introduced into the routine pediatric vaccination schedule. However, the magnitudes of change in the non-vaccine-serotype IPD rate in various countries have been heterogeneous; the interpretation of this heterogeneity is a complex issue. In the United States, Canada, and Australia, rates of non-vaccine-serotype IPD have increased but the magnitude of the increase is

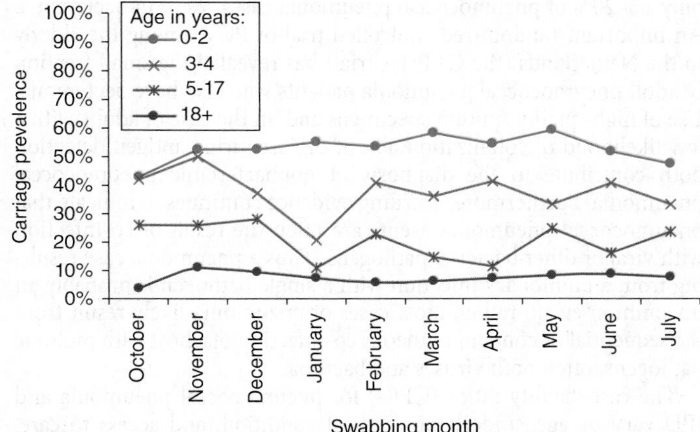

FIGURE 146-3 Prevalence of pneumococcal carriage in adults and children resident in the United Kingdom who had nasopharyngeal swabs collected monthly for 10 months (no seasonal trend; *t* test trend, >.05). *(Data adapted from D Goldblatt et al: J Infect Dis 192:387, 2005.)*

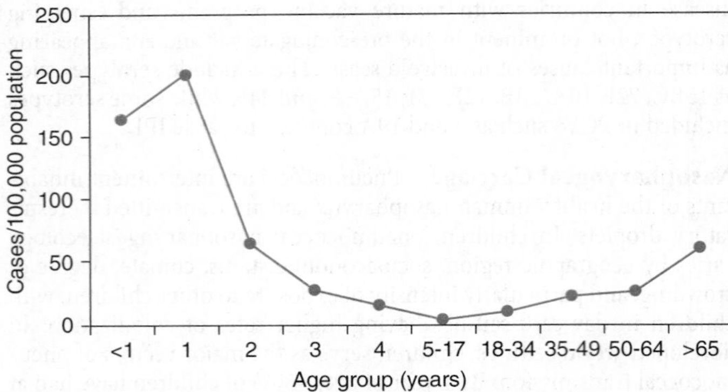

FIGURE 146-4 Rates of invasive pneumococcal disease before the introduction of pneumococcal conjugate vaccine, by age group: United States, 1998. *(Source: CDC, Active Bacterial Core Surveillance/Emerging Infectious Program Network, 2000. Data adapted from MMWR 49[RR-9], 2000.)*

generally small relative to the substantial reductions in vaccine-serotype IPD. In contrast, in other settings (e.g., Alaska Native communities and adults in the United Kingdom), the reduction in vaccine-serotype IPD has been offset by notable increases in rates of disease caused by non-vaccine serotypes. Explanations for the heterogeneity of findings include replacement disease resulting from vaccine pressure, changes in clinical case investigation, secular trends unrelated to PCV use, antibiotic pressure selecting for resistant organisms, changes in surveillance or reporting systems, rapidity of PCV introduction, and inclusion of a catch-up campaign. Serotype replacement in IPD follows the use of PCV7, PCV10, and PCV13, but the magnitude of this phenomenon is small relative to the reduction in disease from vaccine serotypes in vaccinated populations. In adults in the UK, however, where rates of IPD due to vaccine serotypes fell following PCV introduction, the increase in IPD secondary to non-vaccine serotypes is eroding the original impact of PCV. Furthermore, not all vaccine serotypes have declined and persistent disease due to serotypes 3 and 19A bas been noted in many settings.

Pneumonia is the most common of the serious pneumococcal disease syndromes and poses special challenges from a clinical and public health perspective. Most cases of pneumococcal pneumonia are not associated with bacteremia, and in these cases a definitive etiologic diagnosis is difficult or impossible. As a result, estimates of disease burden focus primarily on IPD rates and fail to include the major portion of the burden of serious pneumococcal disease. Among children, PCV trials designed to collect efficacy data on syndrome-based outcomes (e.g., radiographically confirmed pneumonia, clinically diagnosed pneumonia) have revealed the burden of culture-negative pneumococcal pneumonia. These trials have provided the means to infer that only ~5–20% of pneumococcal pneumonia cases result in bacteremia. An important randomized controlled trial of PCV among the elderly in the Netherlands (the CAPiTA trial) has revealed the small fraction of adult pneumococcal pneumonia patients who also have bacteremia. Use of high-quality sputum specimens and, in the case of adults with a low likelihood of colonization absent disease, urine antigen detection both contribute to the diagnosis of nonbacteremic pneumococcal pneumonia. Furthermore, accruing evidence continues to indicate that pneumococcal pneumonia events are often the result of co-infection with viral or other bacterial pathogens. Thus a pneumonia case resulting from a pulmonary infection with a single pathogen is probably an uncommon event; rather, most cases of pneumonia likely result from the sequential or contemporaneous co-infection of a host with multiple pathogens, often both viruses and bacteria.

The case-fatality ratios (CFRs) for pneumococcal pneumonia and IPD vary by age, underlying medical condition, and access to care. In addition, the CFR for pneumococcal pneumonia varies with the severity of disease at presentation (rather than according to whether the pneumonia episode is associated with bacteremia) and with the patient's age (from <5% among hospitalized patients 18–44 years old to >12% among those >65 years old, even when appropriate and timely management is available). Notably, the likelihood of death in the first 24 h of hospitalization did not change substantially with the introduction of antibiotics; this surprising observation highlights the fact that the pathophysiology of severe pneumococcal pneumonia among adults reflects a rapidly progressive cascade of events that often unfolds irrespective of antibiotic administration. Management in an intensive care unit can provide critical support for the patient through the acute period, with lower CFRs, while antibiotics address the underlying infection.

Rates of pneumococcal disease vary by season, with higher rates in colder than in warmer months in temperate climates; by sex, with males more often affected than females; and by risk group, with risk factors including underlying medical conditions, behavioral issues (e.g., smoking), and ethnic group. In the United States, some Native American populations (including Alaska Natives) and African Americans have higher rates of disease than the general population; the increased risk is probably attributable to socioeconomic conditions and the prevalence of underlying risk factors for pneumococcal disease. Medical conditions that increase the risk of pneumococcal infection are listed in **Table 146-1**. Outbreaks of disease are well recognized in crowded settings with susceptible individuals, such as infant day-care facilities, military barracks, and nursing homes. Furthermore, there is a clear association between preceding viral respiratory disease (especially but not exclusively influenza) and risk of secondary pneumococcal infections. The significant role of pneumococcal pneumonia in the morbidity and mortality associated with seasonal and pandemic influenza is increasingly well recognized.

Antibiotic Resistance Reduced pneumococcal susceptibility to penicillin was first noted in 1967, but not until the 1990s did reduced antibiotic susceptibility emerge as a significant clinical and public health issue, with an increasing prevalence of pneumococcal isolates resistant to single or multiple classes of antibiotics and a rising absolute

TABLE 146-1 Clinical Risk Groups for Pneumococcal Infection

CLINICAL RISK GROUP	EXAMPLES
Asplenia or splenic dysfunction	Sickle cell disease and other hemoglobinopathies, celiac disease
Chronic respiratory disease	Chronic obstructive pulmonary disease, bronchiectasis, cystic fibrosis, interstitial lung fibrosis, pneumoconiosis, bronchopulmonary dysplasia, aspiration risk, neuromuscular disease (e.g., cerebral palsy), severe asthma
Chronic heart disease	Ischemic heart disease, congenital heart disease, hypertension with cardiac complications, chronic heart failure
Chronic kidney disease	Nephrotic syndrome, chronic renal failure, renal transplantation
Chronic liver disease	Cirrhosis, biliary atresia, chronic hepatitis
Diabetes mellitus	Diabetes mellitus requiring insulin or oral hypoglycemic drugs
Immunocompromise/ immunosuppression	HIV infection, primary immunodeficiency including B-cell, T-cell, complement and some phagocytic disorders, leukemia, lymphoma, Hodgkin's disease, multiple myeloma, generalized malignancy, chemotherapy, organ or bone marrow transplantation, systemic glucocorticoid treatment for >1 month at a dose equivalent to ≥20 mg/d (children, ≥1 mg/kg per day)
Cochlear implants	...
Cerebrospinal fluid leaks	...
Miscellaneous	Infancy and old age; prior hospitalization; alcoholism; malnutrition; cigarette smoking; day-care center attendance; residence in military training camps, prisons, homeless shelters

Note: Groups for whom pneumococcal vaccines are recommended by the Advisory Committee on Immunization Practices can be found at *www.cdc.gov/vaccines/schedules/*.

magnitude of minimal inhibitory concentrations (MICs). Strains with reduced susceptibility to penicillin G, cefotaxime, ceftriaxone, macrolides, and other antibiotics are now found worldwide and account for a significant proportion of disease-causing strains in many locations, especially among children. Vancomycin resistance has not yet been observed in clinical pneumococcal strains. Lack of antimicrobial susceptibility is clearly related to a subset of serotypes, many of which disproportionately cause disease among children. Resistance phenotypes are based on a diverse array of mutational events and inter- and intraspecies gene-transfer phenomena carried out by several types of mobile genetic elements, with consequent dissemination of successful resistant clones. The vicious cycle of antibiotic exposure, selection of resistant organisms in the nasopharynx, and transmission of these organisms within the community, leading to difficult-to-treat infections and increased antibiotic exposure, has been interrupted to some extent by the introduction and routine use of PCV. The clinical implications of pneumococcal antimicrobial nonsusceptibility are addressed in "Treatment," below.

PATHOGENESIS

Pneumococci colonize the human nasopharynx from an early age; colonization acquisition events are generally described as asymptomatic, but evidence exists to associate acquisition with mild respiratory symptoms, especially in the very young. Bacteria survive in the nasopharynx protected by a variety of factors, including their bacterial capsule and the formation of a biofilm. From the nasopharynx, the bacteria spread either via the bloodstream to distant sites (e.g., brain, joint, bones, peritoneal cavity) or locally to mucosal surfaces where they can cause otitis media or pneumonia. Direct spread from the nasopharynx to the central nervous system (CNS) can occur in rare cases of skull-base fracture, although most cases of pneumococcal meningitis are secondary to hematogenous spread. The pneumococcus is not a static bacterium; rather, it modifies its expression of capsule in adaptation to the external environment. In the nasopharynx, the pneumococcus downregulates capsular expression, averting protective immunologic mechanisms that recognize capsule; rough colonies are the phenotype on culture. Upon invasion by traversal of the epithelium, the pneumococcus upregulates its capsular expression, transforming its appearance on culture to smooth colonies—a change illustrating the dynamic nature of the organism in response to the local environment. Pneumococci can cause disease in almost any organ or part of the body; however, otitis media, pneumonia, bacteremia, and meningitis are most common. Colonization is a relatively frequent event, yet disease is rare. In the nasopharynx, pneumococci survive in mucus secreted by epithelial cells and in a biofilm they create, where they can avoid local immune factors such as leukocytes and complement. The mucus itself is a component of local defense mechanisms, and the flow of mucus (driven in part by cilia in what is known as the *mucociliary escalator*) effects mechanical clearance of pneumococci. While many colonization episodes are of short duration, longitudinal studies in adults and children have revealed persistent colonization with a specific serotype over many months. Colonization eventually results in the development of capsule- and protein-specific serum IgG antibodies, which are thought to play a role in mediating clearance of bacteria from the nasopharynx. IgG antibodies to surface-exposed cell-wall or secreted proteins also appear in the circulation in an age-dependent fashion or after colonization; these antibodies are likely to have a disease-modifying and/or protective role. Recent acquisition of a new colonizing serotype is more likely to be associated with subsequent invasion, presumably as a result of the absence of type-specific immunity. Intercurrent viral infections make the host more susceptible to pneumococcal colonization, and pneumococcal disease in a colonized individual often follows perturbation of the nasopharyngeal mucosa by such infections. Local cytokine production after a viral infection is thought to upregulate adhesion factors in the respiratory epithelium, allowing pneumococci to adhere via a variety of surface adhesin molecules, including PsaA, PspA, CbpA, PspC, Hyl, pneumolysin, and the neuraminidases (Fig. 146-2). Adhesion coupled with inflammation induced by pneumococcal factors such as peptidoglycans and teichoic acids results in invasion. It is the inflammation induced by various bacterium-derived factors that is responsible for the pathology associated with pneumococcal infection. Pneumococcal cell wall–derived teichoic acids and peptidoglycans induce a variety of cytokines, including the proinflammatory cytokines interleukin (IL) 1, IL-6, and tumor necrosis factor, and activate complement via the alternative pathway. Polymorphonuclear leukocytes are thus attracted, and an intense inflammatory response is initiated. Pneumolysin also is important in local pathology, inducing proinflammatory cytokine production by local monocytes.

The pneumococcal capsule, consisting of polysaccharides with antiphagocytic properties (i.e., the capacity to resist complement deposition in the absence of type-specific antibody), plays an important role in pathogenesis. While most capsular types can cause human disease, certain capsular types are more commonly isolated from sites of infection. The reason for the dominance of some serotypes over others in IPD is unclear.

HOST DEFENSE MECHANISMS

Innate Immunity As described above, intact respiratory epithelium and a host of nonspecific or innate immune factors (e.g., mucus, splenic function, complement, neutrophils, and macrophages) constitute the first line of defense against pneumococci. Physical factors such as the cough reflex and the mucociliary escalator are important in clearing bacteria from the lungs. Immunologic factors are critical as well: C-reactive protein (CRP) binds phosphorylcholine in the pneumococcal cell wall, inducing complement activation and leading to bacterial clearance; Toll-like receptor 2 (TLR2) recognizes pneumococcal-derived lipoproteins. In animal models, the absence of host TLR2 leads to more severe infection and impaired clearance of nasopharyngeal colonization. TLR4 appears to be necessary for the proinflammatory effect of pneumolysin on macrophages. The importance of TLR recognition is underlined by descriptions of an inherited deficiency of human IL-1 receptor–associated kinase 4 (IRAK-4) that manifests as an unusual susceptibility to infection with bacteria, including *S. pneumoniae.* IRAK-4 is essential for the normal functioning of several TLRs. Other factors that interfere with these nonspecific mechanisms (e.g., viral infections, cystic fibrosis, bronchiectasis, complement deficiency, chronic obstructive pulmonary disease) all predispose to the development of pneumococcal pneumonia. Patients who lack a spleen or have abnormal splenic function (e.g., persons with sickle cell disease) are at high risk of developing overwhelming pneumococcal disease.

Acquired Immunity Acquired immunity induced following colonization or through exposure to cross-reactive antigens rests largely on the development of serum IgG antibody specific for the pneumococcal capsular polysaccharide. Nearly all polysaccharides are T-cell–independent antigens; B cells can make antibodies to such antigens without T cell help. However, in children <1–2 years old, such B-cell responses are poorly developed. This delayed ontogeny of capsule-specific IgG in young children is associated with susceptibility to pneumococcal infection (Fig. 146-5). The extremely high risk of pneumococcal infection in the absence of serum immunoglobulin (i.e., in conditions such as agammaglobulinemia) highlights the important role of capsular antibody in protection against disease. Each serotype's capsule is chemically distinct, even though for some serotypes the chemical distinction from another type may be a minor one; thus immunity tends to be serotype specific, although some cross-immunity exists. For example, conjugate vaccine–induced antibodies to serotype 6B prevent infection due to serotype 6A. However, cross-protection against serotypes within serogroups is not universal; for instance, antibodies to serotype 19F induced by some vaccines do not appear to confer protection against disease caused by serotype 19A. Antibodies to surface-exposed or secreted pneumococcal proteins (such as pneumolysin, PsaA, and PspA) also appear in the circulation with increasing age of the host and are likely to contribute to protection. Data from murine models suggest that CD4+ T cells may play a role in preventing pneumococcal colonization and disease, and experimental data derived from humans suggest that IL-17-secreting CD4+ T cells may be relevant.

APPROACH TO THE PATIENT
Pneumococcal Infections

There is no pathognomonic presentation of pneumococcal disease; patients may present with one or more clinical syndromes (e.g., pneumonia, meningitis, sepsis). *S. pneumoniae* can infect nearly any body tissue, manifesting as disease ranging in severity from mild and self-limited to life-threatening. The differential diagnosis of common clinical syndromes such as pneumonia, otitis media, fever of unknown origin, and meningitis should always include pneumococcal infection. A microbiologically confirmed diagnosis is made in only a minority of pneumococcal cases since, in most circumstances (and especially in pneumonia and otitis media), fluid from the site of infection is not available for etiologic determination, and infection of body fluids distant from the site of infection (e.g., blood in the case of pneumonia) occurs in only a minority of true pneumococcal cases. Empirical therapy that includes appropriate treatment for *S. pneumoniae* is often indicated.

Algorithms for assessment and management of ill children (Integrated Management of Childhood Illness; IMCI) have been developed for use in the developing world or in other settings where evaluation by a trained physician may not be feasible. No such algorithms for the management of adults with suspected disease exist. Children who present with signs associated with increased risk of serious disease, such as an inability to drink, convulsions, lethargy, and severe malnutrition, are categorized as having very severe disease without further evaluation by the community health care worker; are given antibiotics; and are immediately referred to a hospital for diagnosis and management. Children who present with cough and tachypnea (the latter defined according to specific age strata) are further stratified into severity categories based on the presence or absence of lower chest wall indrawing and are managed accordingly either with antibiotics alone or with antibiotics and referral to a hospital facility. Children with cough but no tachypnea are categorized as having a nonpneumonia respiratory illness.

CLINICAL MANIFESTATIONS

The clinical manifestations of pneumococcal disease depend on the site of infection and the duration of illness. Clinical syndromes are classified as noninvasive (e.g., otitis media) or invasive (e.g., bacteremic pneumonia, meningitis) according to whether a normally sterile site is infected. The pathogenesis of noninvasive illness involves contiguous spread from the nasopharynx or skin; invasive disease involves infection of a normally sterile body fluid or follows bacteremia. Regardless of the mechanism, all pneumococcal infections result from nasopharyngeal acquisition of the organism.

Pneumonia Pneumonia is the most common serious pneumococcal syndrome and is considered invasive when associated with a positive blood culture. Whether to categorize nonbacteremic pneumococcal pneumonia as invasive or noninvasive remains debatable.

Pneumococcal pneumonia can present as a mild community-acquired infection at one extreme and as a life-threatening disease requiring intubation and intensive support at the other.

PRESENTING MANIFESTATIONS The presentation of pneumococcal pneumonia does not reliably distinguish it from pneumonia of other etiologies. In a subset of cases, pneumococcal pneumonia is recognized at the outset as associated with a viral upper respiratory infection and is characterized by the abrupt onset of cough and dyspnea accompanied by fever, shaking chills, and myalgias. The cough evolves from nonpurulent to productive of sputum that is purulent and sometimes tinged with blood. Patients may describe stabbing pleuritic chest pain and significant dyspnea indicating involvement of the parietal pleura. Among the elderly, the presenting clinical symptoms may be less specific, with confusion or malaise but without fever or cough. In such cases, a high index of suspicion is required because failure to treat pneumococcal pneumonia promptly in an elderly patient is likely to result in rapid evolution of the infection, with increased severity, morbidity, and risk of death.

FINDINGS ON PHYSICAL EXAMINATION The clinical signs associated with pneumococcal pneumonia among adults include tachypnea (defined as >20 breaths/min) and tachycardia, hypotension in severe cases, and fever in most cases (although not in all elderly patients). Respiratory signs are varied, including dullness to percussion in areas of the chest with significant consolidation, crackles on auscultation, reduced expansion of the chest in some cases as a result of splinting to reduce pain, bronchial breathing in a minority of cases, pleural rub in occasional cases, and cyanosis in cases with significant hypoxemia. Among infants with severe pneumonia, chest wall indrawing and nasal flaring are common. Nonrespiratory findings can include upper abdominal pain if the diaphragmatic pleura is involved as well as mental status changes, particularly confusion in elderly patients.

DIFFERENTIAL DIAGNOSIS The differential diagnosis of pneumococcal pneumonia includes cardiac conditions such as myocardial infarction and heart failure with atypical pulmonary edema; pulmonary conditions such as atelectasis; and pneumonia caused by viral pathogens, mycoplasmas, *Haemophilus influenzae*, *Klebsiella pneumoniae*, *Staphylococcus aureus*, *Legionella*, or (in HIV-infected and otherwise immunocompromised hosts) *Pneumocystis jirovecii*. In cases with abdominal symptoms, the differential diagnosis includes cholecystitis, appendicitis, perforated peptic ulcer disease, and subphrenic abscesses. The challenge in cases with abdominal symptoms is to remember to include pneumococcal pneumonia—a nonabdominal process—in the differential diagnosis.

DIAGNOSIS Some authorities advocate treating uncomplicated, nonsevere, community-acquired pneumonia without determining the microbiologic etiology, given that this information is unlikely to alter clinical management. However, efforts to identify the cause of pneumonia are important when the disease is more severe and when the diagnosis of pneumonia is not clearly established. The gold standard for etiologic diagnosis of pneumococcal pneumonia is pathologic examination of lung tissue. In lieu of that procedure, evidence of an infiltrate on chest radiography warrants a diagnosis of pneumonia. However, cases of pneumonia without radiographic evidence do occur. An infiltrate can be absent either early in the course of the illness or with dehydration; upon rehydration, an infiltrate usually appears. The radiographic appearance of pneumococcal pneumonia is varied; it classically consists of lobar or segmental consolidation (**Fig. 146-5**) but in some cases is patchy. More than one lobe is involved in ~30% of cases. Consolidation may be associated with a small pleural effusion or empyema in complicated cases. In children, "round pneumonia," a distinctly spherical consolidation on chest radiography, is associated with a pneumococcal etiology. Round pneumonia is uncommon in adults. *S. pneumoniae* is not the only cause of such lesions; other causes, especially cancer, should be considered.

Blood drawn from patients with suspected pneumococcal pneumonia can be used for supportive or definitive diagnostic tests. Blood cultures are positive for pneumococci in a minority (<30%) of cases of pneumococcal pneumonia, as evidenced especially by vaccine clinical trials, which provide an independent method to reveal the contribution of the pneumococcus to pneumonia cases. Nonspecific findings include an elevated polymorphonuclear leukocyte count (>15,000/μL in most cases and upward of 40,000/μL in some), leukopenia in <10% of cases (a poor prognostic sign associated with a fatal outcome), and elevated values in liver function tests (e.g., both conjugated and unconjugated hyperbilirubinemia). Anemia, low serum albumin levels, hyponatremia, and elevated serum creatinine levels are all found in ~20–30% of patients.

Urinary pneumococcal antigen assays, based on identifying a ubiquitous common cell wall polysaccharide, have facilitated etiologic diagnosis, but the application of the results is confounded by the fact that nasopharyngeal colonization with the pneumococcus, in the absence of disease, also results in a positive test. In adults, therefore, a positive pneumococcal urinary antigen test has a predictive value for etiologic attribution of pneumonia because the prevalence of pneumococcal nasopharyngeal colonization is relatively low. In communities, particularly those in low-income countries, where colonization rates

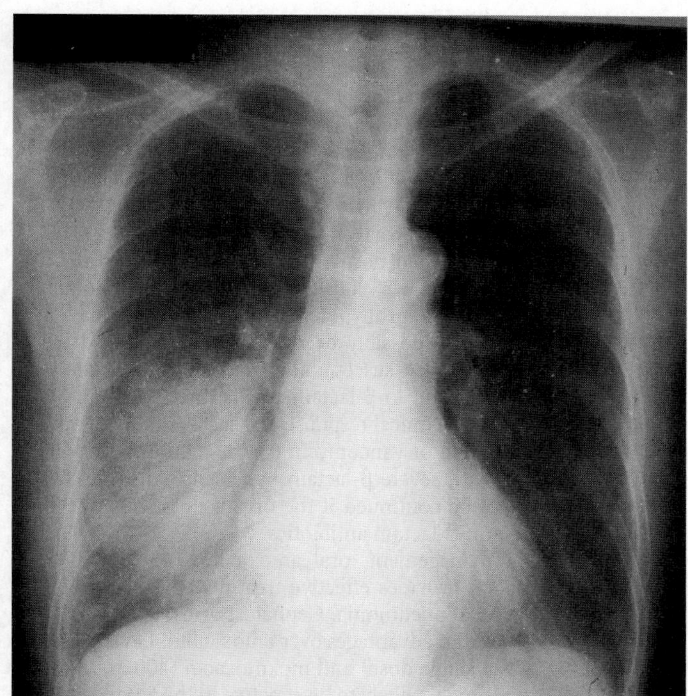

FIGURE 146-5 Chest radiograph depicting classic lobar pneumococcal pneumonia in the right lower lobe of an elderly patient's lung.

among adults are high, urine antigen assays may be less useful. The same issue holds for children, in whom a positive urinary antigen test is usually uninformative for etiologic attribution of their pneumonia illness because colonization rates are generally high. A recent advance is the development of quantitative serotype-specific urinary antigen detection assays; their application for adults and children holds promise, especially in detecting serotypes that are rarely identified in asymptomatic carriage (e.g., serotype 1), even among children.

Most cases of pneumococcal pneumonia in adults are diagnosed by Gram's staining and culture of sputum. The utility of a sputum specimen is directly related to its quality and the patient's antibiotic treatment status.

COMPLICATIONS Empyema is the most common focal complication of pneumococcal pneumonia, occurring in <5% of cases. When fluid in the pleural space is accompanied by fever and leukocytosis (even low-grade) after 4–5 days of appropriate antibiotic treatment for pneumococcal pneumonia, empyema should be considered. Parapneumonic effusions are more common than empyema, representing a self-limited inflammatory response to pneumonia. Pleural fluid with frank pus, bacteria (detected by microscopic examination), or a pH of ≤7.1 indicates empyema and demands aggressive and complete drainage, usually through chest tube insertion.

Meningitis Pneumococcal meningitis usually presents as a pyogenic condition that is clinically indistinguishable from meningitis of other bacterial etiologies. Meningitis can be the primary presenting pneumococcal syndrome or a complication of other conditions such as skull fracture, otitis media, bacteremia, or mastoiditis. Now that *H. influenzae* type b vaccine is routinely used in children, *S. pneumoniae* and *Neisseria meningitidis* are the most common bacterial causes of meningitis in both adults and children. Pyogenic meningitis, including that due to *S. pneumoniae,* is associated clinically with findings that include severe, generalized, gradual-onset headache, fever, and nausea as well as specific CNS manifestations such as stiff neck, photophobia, seizures, and confusion. Clinical signs include a toxic appearance, altered consciousness, bradycardia, and hypertension indicative of increased intracranial pressure. A small proportion of adult patients have Kernig's or Brudzinski's sign or cranial nerve palsies (particularly of the third and sixth cranial nerves).

A definitive diagnosis of pneumococcal meningitis rests on the examination of CSF for (1) evidence of turbidity (visual inspection); (2) elevated protein level, elevated white blood cell count, and reduced glucose concentration (quantitative measurement); and (3) specific identification of the etiologic agent (culture, Gram's staining, antigen testing, or polymerase chain reaction [PCR]). A blood culture positive for *S. pneumoniae* in conjunction with clinical manifestations of meningitis also is considered confirmatory. As discussed in "Pneumonia," above, detection of pneumococcal antigen in urine is considered highly specific among adults because of the low prevalence of nasopharyngeal colonization in this age group.

The mortality rate for pneumococcal meningitis is ~20%. In addition, up to 50% of survivors experience acute or chronic complications, including deafness, hydrocephalus, and mental retardation in children and diffuse brain swelling, subarachnoid bleeding, hydrocephalus, cerebrovascular complications, and hearing loss in adults.

Other Invasive Syndromes *S. pneumoniae* can cause other invasive syndromes involving virtually any body site. These syndromes include primary bacteremia without other sites of infection (bacteremia without a source; occult bacteremia), osteomyelitis, septic arthritis, endocarditis, pericarditis, and peritonitis. The essential diagnostic approach is collection of fluid from the site of infection by sterile technique and examination by Gram's staining, culture, and—when relevant—capsular antigen assay or PCR. Hemolytic-uremic syndrome can complicate invasive pneumococcal disease.

Noninvasive Syndromes The major noninvasive syndromes caused by *S. pneumoniae* are sinusitis, bacterial bronchitis, and otitis media; the latter is the most common pneumococcal syndrome and most often affects young children. The manifestations of otitis media include the acute onset of severe pain, fever, deafness, and tinnitus, most frequently in the setting of a recent upper respiratory tract infection. Clinical signs include a red, swollen, often bulging tympanic membrane with reduced movement on insufflation or tympanography. Redness of the tympanic membrane is not sufficient for the diagnosis of otitis media.

Pneumococcal sinusitis is also a complication of upper respiratory tract infections and presents with facial pain, congestion, fever, and—in many cases—persistent nighttime cough. A definitive diagnosis is made by aspiration and culture of sinus material; however, presumptive treatment is most commonly initiated after application of a strict set of clinical diagnostic criteria. Pneumococcal bronchitis is usually seen in the context of pre-existing lung conditions such as bronchiectasis or chronic obstructive pulmonary disease (COPD) and may be caused by non-typeable strains.

TREATMENT

Pneumococcal Infections

Historically, the activity of penicillin against pneumococci made parenteral penicillin G the drug of choice for disease caused by susceptible organisms, including community-acquired pneumonia. Today, parenteral β-lactam drugs such as ampicillin, cefotaxime, ceftriaxone, and cefuroxime are often used as first-line agents for community-acquired infections. Macrolides and cephalosporins are alternatives for penicillin-allergic patients. While agents such as clindamycin, tetracycline, and trimethoprim-sulfamethoxazole exhibit some activity against pneumococci, resistance to these agents is frequently encountered in different parts of the world.

Penicillin-resistant pneumococci were first described in the mid-1960s, at which point tetracycline- and macrolide-resistant strains had already been reported. Multidrug-resistant strains were first described in the 1970s, but it was during the 1990s that pneumococcal drug resistance reached pandemic proportions. The use of antibiotics selects for resistant pneumococci, and strains resistant to β-lactam agents and to multiple drugs are now found all over the world. The emergence of high rates of macrolide and fluoroquinolone resistance also has been described. Drug-resistant pneumococci are considered a serious threat by the Centers for Disease Control and Prevention.

The molecular basis of penicillin resistance in *S. pneumoniae* is the alteration of penicillin-binding protein (PBP) genes by transformation and horizontal transfer of DNA from related streptococcal species. Such alteration of PBPs results in lower affinity for penicillins. Depending on the specific PBP(s) and the number of PBPs altered, the level of resistance ranges from intermediate to high. For many years, penicillin susceptibility breakpoints have been defined by MICs as follows: susceptible, ≤0.06 μg/mL and resistant, ≥2.0 μg/mL. However, in vitro results often were not predictive of the response of a patient to treatment for pneumococcal diseases other than meningitis. Revised recommendations have been based on the penicillin G breakpoints established in 2008 by the Clinical and Laboratory Standards Institute. For IV treatment of meningitis with at least 24 million units per day in 8 divided doses, the susceptibility breakpoint remains ≤0.06 μg/mL, and MICs of ≥0.12 μg/mL indicate resistance. For IV treatment of nonmeningeal infections with 12 million units per day in 6 divided doses, the breakpoints are ≤2 μg/mL for susceptible organisms and ≥8 μg/mL for resistant organisms; a dosage of 18–24 million units per day is recommended for strains with MICs in the intermediate category.

Although guidelines for antibiotic therapy should be driven in part by local patterns of resistance, guidelines from national organizations in many countries (e.g., the Infectious Diseases Society of America/American Thoracic Society, the British Thoracic Society, the European Respiratory Society) lay out evidence-based approaches. The following guidelines for the treatment of individual sepsis syndromes are based on those advocated by the American Academy of Pediatrics and published in the 2018 *Red Book*.

MENINGITIS LIKELY OR PROVEN TO BE DUE TO *S. PNEUMONIAE*

In areas of the world with an increased prevalence of resistant pneumococci, first-line therapy for persons ≥1 month of age is a combination of vancomycin (adults, 30–60 mg/kg per day; infants and children, 60 mg/kg per day) and cefotaxime (adults, 8–12 g/d in 4–6 divided doses; children, 225–300 mg/kg per day in 1 dose or 2 divided doses) or ceftriaxone (adults, 4 g/d in 1 dose or 2 divided doses; children, 100 mg/kg per day in 1 dose or 2 divided doses). In low-prevalence areas and where the patient has not recently traveled, vancomycin is not included in first-line therapy. If children are hypersensitive to β-lactam agents (penicillins and cephalosporins), rifampin (adults, 600 mg/d; children, 20 mg/d in 1 dose or 2 divided doses) can be substituted for cefotaxime or ceftriaxone and added as a second agent. A repeat lumbar puncture should be considered after 48 h if the organism is not susceptible to penicillin and information on cephalosporin sensitivity is not yet available, if the patient's clinical condition does not improve or deteriorates, or if dexamethasone has been administered interfering with the ability to interpret clinical responses in the deteriorating patient. When antibiotic sensitivity data become available, treatment should be modified accordingly. If the isolate is sensitive to penicillin, vancomycin can be discontinued and penicillin can replace the cephalosporin, or cefotaxime or ceftriaxone can be continued alone. If the isolate displays any resistance to penicillin but is susceptible to the cephalosporins, vancomycin can be discontinued and cefotaxime or ceftriaxone continued. If the isolate exhibits any resistance to penicillin and is not susceptible to cefotaxime and ceftriaxone, vancomycin and high-dose cefotaxime or ceftriaxone can be continued and rifampin may be added. Data support the use of corticosteroids in high-income countries but do not appear to have a beneficial effect in low-income countries. This discrepancy in the efficacy of corticosteroids may be related to differences in availability of appropriate and timely medical care. Glucocorticoids significantly reduce rates of mortality, severe hearing loss, and neurologic sequelae in adults and should be administered to those with community-acquired bacterial meningitis. If dexamethasone is given to either adults or children, it should be administered before or in conjunction with the first antibiotic dose.

SEPSIS (EXCLUDING MENINGITIS)

In previously well children with noncritical illness, therapy with a recommended antibiotic should be instigated at the usually recommended dosages: ampicillin 200 mg/kg/day (doses 6h apart), cefotaxime, 75–225 mg/kg/day (doses 8 h apart), ceftriaxone, 50–75 mg/kg/day (doses 12–24 h apart) or penicillin G, 250,000–400,000 units/kg per day (in divided doses 4–6 h apart). For critically ill children, including those who have myocarditis or multilobular pneumonia with hypoxia or hypotension, vancomycin may be added if the isolate may possibly be resistant to β-lactam drugs, with its use reviewed once susceptibility data become available. If the organism is resistant to β-lactam agents, therapy should be modified on the basis of clinical response and susceptibility to other antibiotics. Clindamycin or vancomycin can be used as a first-line agent for children with severe β-lactam hypersensitivity, but vancomycin should not be continued if the organism is shown to be sensitive to other non-β-lactam antibiotics.

For outpatient management, oral amoxicillin (45–90 mg/kg/day, doses 8 h apart) provides effective treatment for virtually all cases of pneumococcal pneumonia. Cephalosporins, which are far more expensive, offer no advantages over amoxicillin. Levofloxacin (500–750 mg/d as a single dose) and moxifloxacin (400 mg/d as a single dose) also are highly likely to be effective in the United States except in patients who come from closed populations where these drugs are used widely or who have themselves been treated recently with a quinolone. Clindamycin (600–1200 mg/d every 6 h) is effective in 90% of cases and azithromycin (500 mg on day 1 followed by 250–500 mg/d) or clarithromycin (500–750 mg/d as a single dose) in 80% of cases. Treatment failure resulting in bacteremic disease due to macrolide-resistant isolates has been amply documented in patients given azithromycin empirically. As noted above, rates of resistance to all these antibiotics are relatively low in some countries and much higher in others; high-dose amoxicillin remains the best option worldwide.

The optimal duration of treatment for pneumococcal pneumonia is uncertain, but its continuation for at least 5 days once the patient becomes afebrile appears to be a prudent approach—although in adults, 5 days in total will usually suffice. Cases with a second focus of infection (e.g., empyema or septic arthritis) require longer therapy.

ACUTE OTITIS MEDIA

Amoxicillin (80–90 mg/kg per day) is recommended for infants <6 months of age and those 6–23 months of age with bilateral disease. Observation and symptom-based treatment without antibiotics are advocated for nonsevere illness and an uncertain diagnosis in children 6 months to 2 years of age and nonsevere illness (even if the diagnosis seems certain) in children >2 years of age. Although the optimal duration of therapy has not been conclusively established, a 10-day course is recommended for younger children and for children with severe disease at any age. For children >6 years old who have mild or moderate disease, a course of 5–7 days is considered adequate. Patients whose illness fails to respond should be reassessed at 48–72 h. If acute otitis media is confirmed and antibiotic treatment has not been started, administration of amoxicillin should be commenced. If antibiotic therapy fails, a change is indicated. Failure to respond to second-line antibiotics (such as high-dose amoxicillin-clavulanate) as well indicates that myringotomy or tympanocentesis may need to be undertaken in order to obtain samples for culture.

The above recommendations can also be followed for the treatment of sinusitis. Detailed information on the further management of these conditions in children has been published by the American Academy of Pediatrics, the American Academy of Family Physicians, the Pediatric Infectious Diseases Society, and the Infectious Diseases Society of America.

PREVENTION

Measures to prevent pneumococcal disease include vaccination against *S. pneumoniae* and influenza viruses, reduction of comorbidities that increase the risk of pneumococcal disease, and prevention of antibiotic overuse, which fuels pneumococcal resistance.

Capsular Polysaccharide Vaccines The 23-valent pneumococcal polysaccharide vaccine (PPSV23), containing 25 μg of each capsular polysaccharide, has been licensed for use since 1983. Recommendations for its use vary by country. The U.S. Advisory Committee on Immunization Practices (ACIP) recommends PPSV23 for all persons ≥65 years of age and for those 2–64 years of age who have underlying medical conditions that put them at increased risk for pneumococcal disease or, if infected, disease of increased severity (Table 146-1; see also *www.cdc.gov/vaccines/schedules*). The committee updated their recommendations to include the combined use of pneumococcal conjugate vaccine followed by PPSV23 in at-risk individuals (see "Polysaccharide–Protein Conjugate Vaccines," below). Revaccination 5 years after the first dose is recommended for persons >2 years of age who have underlying medical conditions but not routinely for those whose only indication is an age of ≥65 years. PPSV23 does not induce an anamnestic response, and antibody concentrations wane over time; thus revaccination is particularly important for individuals with conditions resulting in loss of antibody. Concerns about repeated revaccination have focused on safety (i.e., local reactions) and the induction of immune hyporesponsiveness. Neither the clinical relevance nor the biologic basis of hyporesponsiveness is clear, but, given the possibility of its occurrence, more than one revaccination has not been recommended.

The effectiveness of PPSV23 against IPD, pneumococcal pneumonia, all-cause pneumonia, and death is controversial, with wide variation in observations. The many published meta-analyses of PPSV efficacy have often reached opposing conclusions with regard to a given clinical entity. Generally, observational studies cite greater effectiveness than do controlled clinical trials. The consensus is that PPSV is effective against IPD but is less effective against nonbacteremic pneumococcal pneumonia. However, the results of some published trials, observational studies, and meta-analyses contradict this view. Effectiveness is often lower in the elderly and in immunodeficient patients whose condition is associated with reduced antibody responses to vaccines than in younger, healthier populations. When PPSV is effective, the duration of protection following a single dose of vaccine is estimated to be ~5 years.

What is not disputed is that improved pneumococcal vaccines are needed for adults. Even in the setting of routine pneumococcal conjugate vaccination of infants (which indirectly protects adults from vaccine-serotype strains), disease caused by serotypes not represented in the conjugate vaccine continues to be a significant burden among adults.

Polysaccharide–Protein Conjugate Vaccines Infants and young children respond poorly to PPSV, which contains T cell–independent antigens. Consequently, another class of pneumococcal vaccines, the PCVs, were developed specifically for infants and young children. The first product, a 7-valent PCV, was licensed in 2000 in the United States. Two PCV products—containing 10 and 13 serotypes, respectively—are commercially available as of 2020. The serotypes included in these PCV formulations are important causes of IPD and antibiotic resistance among young children. Randomized controlled trials have demonstrated a high degree of efficacy of PCVs against vaccine-serotype IPD as well as efficacy against pneumonia, otitis media, nasopharyngeal colonization, and all-cause mortality. PCVs are recommended by the World Health Organization for inclusion in routine childhood immunization schedules worldwide, especially in countries with high infant mortality rates. To date 144 countries have PCV in their National Immunization program, 16 are planning introduction, and 34 have no national decision.

The introduction of PCV in high-income settings has resulted in a >90% reduction in vaccine-serotype IPD among the whole population. This decline has been noted not only in those age groups immunized but also in adults and is attributable to the near elimination of vaccine-serotype nasopharyngeal colonization in immunized infants, which reduces spread to adults. This protection of unimmunized community members through vaccination of a subset of the community is termed *the indirect effect*. Increases in colonization with—and concomitantly in disease due to—non-vaccine-serotype strains (i.e., replacement colonization and disease) have been seen. The scale of replacement disease has varied geographically with the impact eroding vaccine impact significantly in the elderly in the UK while having relatively little impact in the USA (see "Epidemiology," above). Since vaccine-serotype strains are more commonly resistant to antibiotics than are non-vaccine serotypes, use of PCV has also resulted in substantial declines in the proportion and absolute rates of drug-resistant pneumococcal disease. The ACIP recommendations for the use of conjugate vaccines can be found at *www.cdc.gov/vaccines/hcp/acip-recs/vacc-specific/pneumo.html*. PCV has been shown to prevent pneumococcal infection in HIV-infected adults. In the United States, PCV13 followed by a dose of PPSV23 is now recommended for all immunocompromised children and adults. Until 2019 this was also the U.S. recommendation for those ≥65 years of age, but that recommendation has been modified. Shared decision-making with a physician should determine whether PCV13 in addition to PPSV23 is used in otherwise healthy adults ≥65 years of age. Two new extended-valency vaccines containing upwards of 15 serotypes—VAXNEUVANCE (Merck) and PREVNAR 20 (Pfizer)—were licensed in 2021.

Other Prevention Strategies Pneumococcal disease can be averted through the prevention of illnesses that predispose individuals to pneumococcal infections. Relevant measures include smoking cessation and influenza vaccination, as well as improved management and control of diabetes, HIV infection, heart disease, and lung disease. Finally, the reduction of antibiotic misuse is a strategy for the prevention of pneumococcal disease in that antimicrobial resistance directly and indirectly perpetuates organism transmission and disease in the community.

GLOBAL HEALTH

Pneumococcal infections are estimated to cause ~317,000 annual deaths worldwide among children 1–59 months of age, accounting for 9.7 % of the 3.2 million all-cause deaths and 38% of all pneumonia deaths in this age group in 2015. Reliable estimates of adult cases and deaths globally are more difficult to establish because of limited data from parts of the world where most disease occurs. Rates of pneumococcal disease and mortality vary substantially across geographic settings, with the highest rates in selected countries of sub-Saharan Africa and southern Asia, where risk factors for pneumococcal disease—including HIV infection, lack of breast feeding of infants and children, malnutrition, sickle cell disease, and limited access to medical care—are prevalent. Serotypes causing disease exhibit some heterogeneity across geographic settings, but a small number of serotypes universally account for the preponderance of disease in the absence of vaccination; accordingly, vaccine development and vaccination programs are globally relevant. Reductions in disease from pneumococcal infections are anchored in prevention through the inclusion of pneumococcal vaccines in infant immunization programs, timely assessment and appropriate treatment of persons with pneumococcal infections, and reduction of risk factors for pneumococcal disease. The availability of vaccines for the prevention of adult pneumococcal disease, particularly among the elderly, is currently restricted to high-income countries, with virtually no availability in low-income countries where most cases of disease exist.

FURTHER READING

Krone CL et al: Immunosenescence and pneumococcal disease: An imbalance in host–pathogen interactions. Lancet Respir Med 2:141, 2014.

Mackenzie GA et al: Effect of the introduction of pneumococcal conjugate vaccination on invasive pneumococcal disease in The Gambia: A population-based surveillance study. Lancet Infect Dis 16:703, 2016.

Matanock A et al: Use of 13-valent pneumococcal conjugate vaccine and 23-valent pneumococcal polysaccharide vaccine among adults aged ≥65 years. MMWR Morb Mortal Wkly Rep 68:1069, 2019.

Subramanian K et al: Pneumolysin binds to the mannose receptor C type 1 (MRC-1) leading to anti-inflammatory responses and enhanced pneumococcal survival. Nat Microbiol 4:62, 2019.

Van Der Poll T, Opal SM: Pathogenesis, treatment, and prevention of pneumococcal pneumonia. Lancet 374:1543, 2009.

■ WEBSITES

American Academy of Pediatrics: Red Book: The report of the Committee on Infectious Diseases. Available at: *aapredbook.aappublications.org.*

Cochrane: Corticosteroids for Bacterial Meningitis. Available at: *www.cochrane.org/CD004405/ARI_corticosteroids-bacterial-meningitis.*

U.S. Department of Health and Human Services: Antibiotic Resistance Threats in the United States 2019. Available at: *www.cdc.gov/drugresistance/pdf/threats-report/2019-ar-threats-report-508.pdf.*

World Health Organization: Summary of WHO Position Paper on Pneumococcal conjugate vaccines in infants and children under 5 years of age, February 2019. Available at: *www.who.int/immunization/policy/position_papers/who_pp_pcv_2019_summary.pdf.*

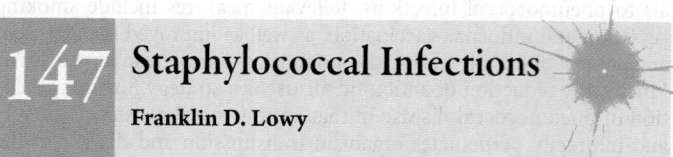

147 Staphylococcal Infections

Franklin D. Lowy

Staphylococcus aureus, the most virulent of the many (≥40) staphylococcal species, has demonstrated its versatility by remaining a major cause of morbidity and mortality worldwide despite the availability of numerous effective antistaphylococcal antibiotics. *S. aureus* is a pluripotent pathogen, causing disease through both toxin- and non-toxin-mediated mechanisms. It is responsible for numerous nosocomial and community-based infections that range from relatively minor skin and soft tissue infections (SSTIs) to life-threatening systemic infections.

The "other" staphylococci, coagulase-negative staphylococci, are less virulent than *S. aureus* but remain important pathogens in select settings, such as infections that involve prosthetic devices.

MICROBIOLOGY AND TAXONOMY

Staphylococci, gram-positive cocci in the family Micrococcaceae, form grapelike clusters on Gram's stain **(Fig. 147-1)**. These organisms (~1 μm in diameter) are catalase-positive (unlike streptococcal species), nonmotile, aerobic, and facultatively anaerobic. They are capable of prolonged survival on environmental surfaces under varying conditions. Some species have a relatively broad host range, including mammals and birds, whereas the host range for others is quite narrow—i.e., limited to one or two closely related animals.

S. aureus is generally distinguished from other staphylococcal species by coagulase production, a surface enzyme that converts fibrinogen to fibrin. However, several of the "coagulase-negative staphylococci," including *S. pseudintermedius* and *S. argenteus*, are coagulase positive. As a result, description of these other staphylococci as non–*S. aureus* staphylococci (NSaS) is more accurate.

S. aureus ferments mannitol, is positive for protein A, and produces DNAse. On blood agar plates, *S. aureus* forms golden β-hemolytic colonies; in contrast, most NSaS form small white nonhemolytic colonies. Latex kits that detect both protein A and clumping factor can distinguish *S. aureus* from most other staphylococcal species. Point of care tests also are used for the rapid detection of staphylococcal colonization.

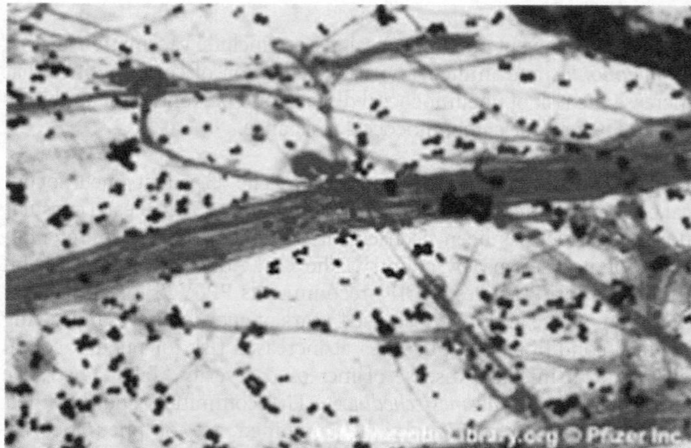

FIGURE 147-1 Gram's stain of *S. aureus* in a sputum sample, illustrating staphylococcal clusters. *(From ASM MicrobeLibrary.org. © Pfizer, Inc.)*

Newer methods such as matrix-assisted laser desorption/ionization time-of-flight mass spectrometry (MALDI-TOF) are increasingly being used for staphylococcal speciation.

Determining whether multiple staphylococcal isolates from different patients are the same or different is often relevant when there is concern that a nosocomial outbreak of staphylococcal infections is due to a common point source (e.g., a contaminated medical instrument). Molecular typing methods, such as pulsed-field gel electrophoresis and sequence-based techniques (e.g., staphylococcal protein A [SpA] typing), have been used for this purpose. More recently, whole-genome sequencing has emerged as the gold standard for discrimination among different isolates.

S. AUREUS INFECTIONS

■ EPIDEMIOLOGY

S. aureus is both a commensal and an opportunistic pathogen. Approximately 20–40% of healthy persons are colonized with *S. aureus*, with a smaller percentage (~10%) persistently colonized with the same strain. The rate of colonization is elevated among type 1 diabetics, HIV-infected patients, patients undergoing hemodialysis, injection drug users, and individuals with skin damage. The anterior nares and oropharynx are frequent sites of human colonization, although the skin (especially when damaged), vagina, axilla, and perineum also are often colonized. These colonization sites serve as potential reservoirs for future infections.

Most individuals who develop *S. aureus* infections become infected with a strain that is already a part of their own commensal flora. Breaches of the skin or mucosal membrane allow *S. aureus* to initiate infection. Person-to-person transmission of *S. aureus* also occurs, most frequently from direct personal contact with an infected body site. Spread of staphylococci in aerosols of respiratory or nasal secretions from heavily colonized individuals, although rare, has been reported.

Some diseases increase the risk of *S. aureus* infection; diabetes, for example, combines an increased rate of *S. aureus* colonization and the use of injectable insulin with the possibility of impaired leukocyte function. Individuals with congenital or acquired qualitative or quantitative defects of polymorphonuclear leukocytes (PMNs) are at increased risk of *S. aureus* infections; this group includes neutropenic patients (e.g., those receiving chemotherapeutic agents), those with chronic granulomatous disease, and those with autosomal dominant hyperimmunoglobulin E (Job syndrome) or Chédiak-Higashi syndrome. Other groups at risk include individuals with end-stage renal disease, HIV infection, skin abnormalities, or prosthetic devices.

S. aureus is a leading cause of health care–associated infections **(Chap. 142)**. It is the most common cause of surgical wound infections and is second only to NSaS as a cause of primary bacteremia. These isolates are often resistant to multiple antibiotics; thus, available therapeutic options may be limited. In the community, *S. aureus* remains an important cause of SSTIs, respiratory infections, and, especially among injection drug users, infective endocarditis. The increasing use of home infusion therapy also poses a risk of community-acquired staphylococcal infections.

In the past three decades, there has been a dramatic change in the epidemiology of infections due to methicillin-resistant *S. aureus* (MRSA). In addition to its major role as a nosocomial pathogen, MRSA has become an established community-based pathogen. Numerous outbreaks of community-associated MRSA (CA-MRSA) infections have been reported in both rural and urban settings in widely separated regions throughout the world.

This trend appears to be due in part to the dramatic increase in MRSA colonization found in the community in different parts of the world. Outbreaks of CA-MRSA infections have occurred among such diverse groups as children, prisoners, athletes, Native Americans, and drug users. Risk factors common to these outbreaks include poor hygienic conditions, close contact, contaminated material, and damaged skin. In some geographic regions of the world, the infections have been caused by a single CA-MRSA strain, while in others a variety of CA-MRSA strains have been responsible. In the United States, strain sequence type 8 (PFGE type USA300) has been the predominant clone **(Fig. 147-2)**. Although the majority of infections caused by these strains have involved the skin and soft tissue, 5–10% have been invasive and potentially life-threatening. CA-MRSA strains have also been responsible for an increasing number of nosocomial infections. Of concern has been the enhanced capacity of CA-MRSA to cause disease in immunocompetent individuals.

■ PATHOGENESIS

General Concepts *S. aureus* is a pyogenic pathogen known for its capacity to induce abscess formation at both local and distant sites (i.e., metastatic infections). This classic pathologic response to *S. aureus* defines the framework within which the infection will progress. The bacteria elicit an inflammatory response characterized by an initial intense infiltration of PMNs and a subsequent infiltration of macrophages and fibroblasts. Either the host cellular response (including the deposition of fibrin and collagen) contains the infection with the formation of a fibrinous capsule, or infection spreads to the adjoining tissue or into the bloodstream.

In toxin-mediated staphylococcal disease, infection is not invariably present. For example, in staphylococcal food poisoning, once the heat-stable enterotoxin has been released into food, symptoms can develop in the absence of viable bacteria. In staphylococcal toxic shock syndrome (TSS), conditions allowing toxin elaboration at colonization sites (e.g., the presence of a superabsorbent tampon) suffice for initiation of clinical illness.

The *S. aureus* Genome The complete genomes of *S. aureus* strains are now readily available. Among the interesting revelations are (1) the high degree of nucleotide sequence similarity of the core genomes of different strains; (2) the acquisition of a relatively large amount of genetic information by horizontal transfer from other bacterial species; and (3) the presence of unique "pathogenicity" or "genomic" islands—mobile genetic elements that contain clusters of enterotoxin and exotoxin genes and/or antimicrobial resistance determinants. Among the genes in these islands is *mecA*, the gene responsible for methicillin resistance. Methicillin resistance–containing islands have been designated staphylococcal cassette chromosome *mec* (SCC*mec*). There are different *SCCmec* types that range in size from ~20 to 60 kb. Among the more common SCC*mec* types, types 1–3 are traditionally associated with nosocomial MRSA isolates, whereas types 4–6 have been associated with epidemic CA-MRSA strains.

A relatively limited number of MRSA clones have been responsible for most community- and hospital-associated infections worldwide. A comparison of these strains with those from earlier outbreaks (e.g., the phage 80/81 strains from the 1950s) has revealed preservation of the nucleotide sequence over time. This observation suggests that these strains possess determinants that facilitate survival and spread.

Regulation of Virulence Gene Expression In both toxin-mediated and non-toxin-mediated diseases due to *S. aureus*, the expression of virulence determinants associated with infection depends on a series of regulatory genes (e.g., accessory gene regulator [*agr*] and staphylococcal accessory regulator [*sar*]) that coordinately control the expression of many virulence genes. The

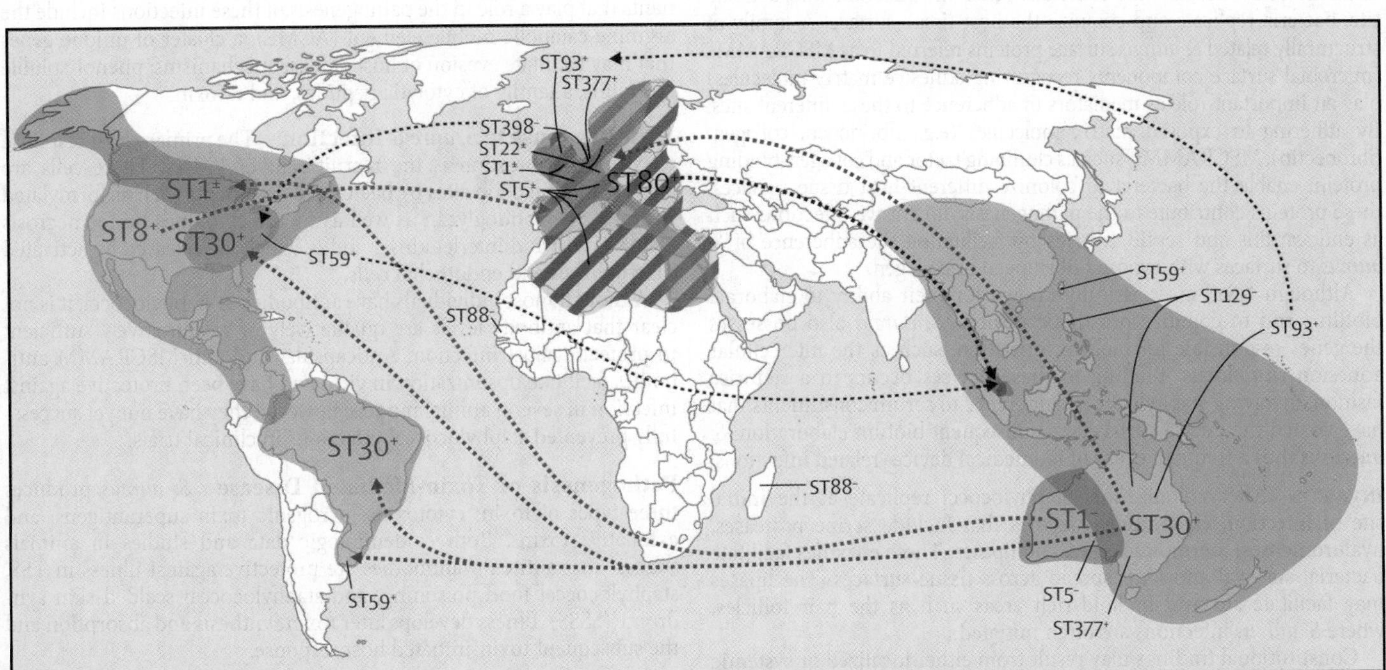

FIGURE 147-2 Global distribution of community-associated MRSA. Dotted lines indicate possible route of dissemination. Estimates of the areas are shown where infection with the main strains—i.e., ST1 *(green)*, ST8 *(red)*, ST30 *(blue)*, and ST80 *(grey hatched)*—have been reported. +, Panton Valentine Leukocidin (PVL)-positive strains; –, PVL-negative strains; ±, PVL-positive and -negative strains. *(Reproduced with permission from FR DeLeo, M Otto, BN Kreiswirth, HF Chambers: Community-associated meticillin-resistant Staphylococcus aureus. Lancet 375:1557, 2010.)*

regulatory gene *agr* is part of a quorum-sensing signal transduction pathway that senses and responds to bacterial density. Staphylococcal surface proteins are synthesized during the bacterial exponential growth phase in vitro. In contrast, many secreted proteins, such as α toxin, the enterotoxins, and assorted enzymes, are released during the post–exponential growth phase in response to transcription of the effector molecule of *agr*, RNAIII.

These regulatory genes appear to serve a similar function in vivo. Successful invasion requires the sequential expression of these different bacterial elements. Bacterial adhesins are needed to initiate colonization of host tissue surfaces. The subsequent release of various enzymes enables the colony to obtain nutritional support and permits bacteria to spread to adjacent tissues. Studies with strains in which these regulatory genes are inactivated show reduced virulence in several animal models of *S. aureus* infection.

Pathogenesis of Invasive *S. aureus* Infection Staphylococci are opportunists. For these organisms to invade the host and cause infection, some or all of the following steps are necessary: contamination and colonization of host tissue surfaces, breach of cutaneous or mucosal barriers, establishment of a localized infection, invasion, evasion of the host response, and metastatic spread. Colonizing strains or strains transferred from other exposures are introduced into damaged skin, a wound, or the bloodstream. Recurrences of *S. aureus* infections are common, apparently because of the capacity of these pathogens to persist in a quiescent state in various tissues, and then to cause recrudescent infections when suitable conditions arise.

***S. AUREUS* COLONIZATION OF BODY SURFACES** The anterior nares and oropharynx are primary sites of staphylococcal colonization. In the nares, colonization appears to involve the attachment of *S. aureus* to keratinized epithelial cells. Other factors that contribute to colonization include the influence of other resident nasal flora and their bacterial density, host factors, and nasal mucosal damage (e.g., that resulting from inhalational drug use). Other colonized body sites, such as damaged skin, the groin, and the oropharynx, may be particularly important reservoirs for CA-MRSA strains.

INOCULATION AND COLONIZATION OF TISSUE SURFACES Staphylococci may be introduced into tissue as a result of minor abrasions (e.g., mosquito bites), administration of medications such as insulin, or establishment of IV access with catheters. After introduction into a tissue site, bacteria replicate and colonize the host tissue surface. A family of structurally related *S. aureus* surface proteins referred to as MSCRAMMs (microbial surface components recognizing adhesive matrix molecules) play an important role as mediators of adherence to these different sites. By adhering to exposed matrix molecules (e.g., fibrinogen, collagen, fibronectin), MSCRAMMs, such as clumping factor and collagen-binding protein, enable the bacteria to colonize different host tissue surfaces; these proteins contribute to the pathogenesis of invasive infections such as endocarditis and septic arthritis by facilitating the adherence of *S. aureus* to surfaces with exposed fibrinogen or collagen.

Although NSaS are classically known for their ability to elaborate biofilms and to colonize prosthetic devices, *S. aureus* also possesses the genes responsible for biofilm formation, such as the intercellular adhesion (*ica*) locus. Binding to these devices occurs in a stepwise fashion, involving staphylococcal adherence to serum constituents that have coated the device surface and subsequent biofilm elaboration. *S. aureus* is thus a frequent cause of biomedical device–related infections.

INVASION After colonization, staphylococci replicate at the initial site of infection, elaborating enzymes that include serine proteases, hyaluronidases, thermonucleases, and lipases. These enzymes facilitate bacterial survival and local spread across tissue surfaces. The lipases may facilitate survival in lipid-rich areas such as the hair follicles, where *S. aureus* infections are often initiated.

Constitutional findings may result from either localized or systemic infections. The staphylococcal cell wall—consisting of alternating *N*-acetyl muramic acid and *N*-acetyl glucosamine units in combination with an additional cell wall component, lipoteichoic acid—can initiate an inflammatory response that includes the sepsis syndrome. Staphylococcal alpha (α) toxin is a critical staphylococcal toxin. It causes pore formation in various eukaryotic cells and can also initiate an inflammatory response with findings suggestive of sepsis. The *S. aureus* toxin Panton-Valentine leukocidin is cytolytic to PMNs, macrophages, and monocytes. Strains elaborating this toxin have been epidemiologically linked with cutaneous and more serious infections (i.e., pneumonia) caused by strains of CA-MRSA.

EVASION OF HOST DEFENSE MECHANISMS Staphylococci have many host immune evasion strategies that are crucial to their survival. They possess an antiphagocytic polysaccharide microcapsule. Most human *S. aureus* infections are due to strains with capsular types 5 and 8. The zwitterionic (both negatively and positively charged) *S. aureus* capsule also plays a critical role in the induction of abscess formation. Protein A, an MSCRAMM unique to *S. aureus*, acts as an Fc receptor, binding the Fc portion of IgG subclasses 1, 2, and 4 and preventing opsonophagocytosis by PMNs. Both chemotaxis inhibitory protein of staphylococci (CHIPS, a secreted protein) and extracellular adherence protein (EAP, a surface protein) interfere with PMN migration to sites of infection. There are a number of cytolytic toxins, including α toxin and Panton Valentine toxin, that are secreted by staphylococci that cause lysis of different host cells and contribute to host tissue damage.

An additional potential mechanism of *S. aureus* evasion is its capacity for intracellular survival. Both professional and nonprofessional phagocytes internalize staphylococci. Internalization by these cells may provide a sanctuary that protects bacteria against the host's defenses. This phenomenon appears to be especially relevant for hepatic Kupffer cells during staphylococcal bacteremias. The intracellular environment favors the phenotypic expression of *S. aureus* small-colony variants, which are found in patients receiving antimicrobial therapy (e.g., with aminoglycosides) and in those with cystic fibrosis or osteomyelitis. These variants, whether intra- or extracellular, may facilitate prolonged staphylococcal survival in different tissue sites and enhance the likelihood of recurrences. Finally, *S. aureus* can survive within PMNs and may use these cells to spread and seed other tissue sites.

PATHOGENESIS OF COMMUNITY-ACQUIRED MRSA INFECTIONS A number of specific virulence determinants contribute to the pathogenesis of CA-MRSA infections. A strong epidemiologic association links the presence of the gene for the Panton-Valentine leukocidin with SSTIs and with necrotizing post-influenza pneumonia. Other determinants that play a role in the pathogenesis of these infections include the arginine catabolic mobile element (ACME), a cluster of unique genes that may facilitate evasion of host defense mechanisms; phenol-soluble modulins, a family of cytolytic peptides; and α toxin.

Host Response to *S. aureus* Infection The primary host response to *S. aureus* infection is the recruitment of PMNs. These cells are attracted to infection sites by bacterial components such as formylated peptides or peptidoglycan as well as by the cytokines tumor necrosis factor (TNF) and interleukins 1 and 6, which are released by activated macrophages and endothelial cells.

Although most individuals have antibodies to staphylococci, it is not clear that antibody levels are qualitatively or quantitatively sufficient to protect against infection. Anticapsular and anti-MSCRAMM antibodies facilitate opsonization in vitro and have been protective against infection in several animal models; however, they have not yet successfully prevented staphylococcal infections in clinical trials.

Pathogenesis of Toxin-Mediated Disease *S. aureus* produces three types of toxin: cytotoxins, pyrogenic toxin superantigens, and exfoliative toxins. Both epidemiologic data and studies in animals suggest that antitoxin antibodies are protective against illness in TSS, staphylococcal food poisoning, and staphylococcal scalded-skin syndrome (SSSS). Illness develops after toxin synthesis and absorption and the subsequent toxin-initiated host response.

ENTEROTOXIN AND TOXIC SHOCK SYNDROME TOXIN 1 (TSST-1) The pyrogenic toxin superantigens are a family of small-molecular-size, structurally similar proteins that are responsible for two diseases: TSS and food poisoning. TSS results from the ability of TSST-1 and enterotoxins to function as T-cell mitogens. In the normal process of antigen presentation, the antigen is first processed within the cell, and peptides are then presented in the major histocompatibility complex (MHC) class II groove, initiating a measured T-cell response. In contrast, TSST-1 and enterotoxins bind directly to the invariant region of MHC—outside the MHC class II groove. TSST-1 and the enterotoxins can then bind T-cell receptors via the vβ chain; this binding results in a dramatic overexpansion of T-cell clones (up to 20% of the total T-cell population). The consequence of this T-cell expansion is a cytokine storm, with the release of inflammatory mediators that include interferon γ, IL-1, IL-6, TNF-α, and TNF-β. The resulting multisystem disease produces a constellation of findings that mimic those found in endotoxin shock; however, the pathogenic mechanisms differ.

A different region of the enterotoxin molecule is responsible for the symptoms of food poisoning. The enterotoxins are heat stable and can survive conditions that kill the bacteria. Illness results from the ingestion of preformed toxin; as a result, the incubation period is short (1–6 h). The toxin stimulates the vagus nerve and the vomiting center of the brain. It also appears to stimulate intestinal peristaltic activity.

EXFOLIATIVE TOXINS AND SSSS The exfoliative toxins are responsible for SSSS, most commonly seen in newborns. The toxins that produce disease in humans are of two serotypes: ETA and ETB. These toxins are serine proteases that cleave desmosomal cadherins in the superficial layer of the skin, triggering exfoliation. The result is a split in the epidermis at the granular level, which is responsible for the superficial desquamation of the skin that typifies this illness.

DIAGNOSIS

Staphylococcal infections are readily diagnosed by Gram's stain (Fig. 147-1) and microscopic examination of abscess contents or of infected tissue. Routine cultures of infected material usually are positive; blood cultures are sometimes positive even when infections are localized to extravascular sites. *S. aureus* is rarely a blood culture contaminant. Polymerase chain reaction (PCR)–based assays are now often used for the rapid diagnosis of *S. aureus* infection. A number of point-of-care tests are available to screen patients for colonization with MRSA. Determining whether patients with documented *S. aureus* bacteremia also have infective endocarditis or a metastatic focus of infection remains a diagnostic challenge. Uniformly positive cultures of blood collected over time suggest an endovascular infection such as endocarditis (see "Bacteremia, Sepsis, and Infective Endocarditis," below).

CLINICAL SYNDROMES (Table 147-1)

Skin and Soft Tissue Infections *S. aureus* causes a variety of cutaneous infections. Common factors predisposing to *S. aureus* cutaneous infection include chronic skin conditions (e.g., eczema), skin damage (e.g., insect bites, minor trauma), injections (e.g., in diabetes, injection drug use), and poor personal hygiene. These infections are characterized by the formation of pus-containing blisters, which often begin in hair follicles and spread to adjoining tissues. *Folliculitis* is a superficial infection that involves the hair follicle, with a central area of purulence (pus) surrounded by induration and erythema. *Furuncles* (boils) are more extensive, painful lesions that tend to occur in hairy, moist regions of the body and extend from the hair follicle to become a true abscess with an area of central purulence. *Carbuncles* are most often located in the lower neck and are even more severe and painful, resulting from the coalescence of other lesions that extend to a deeper layer of the subcutaneous tissue. In general, furuncles and carbuncles are readily apparent, with pus often expressible or discharging from the abscess. Other cutaneous *S. aureus* infections include impetigo and cellulitis. *S. aureus* is one of the most common causes of surgical wound infections.

Mastitis develops in 1–3% of nursing mothers. This infection of the breast, which generally presents within 2–3 weeks after delivery, is characterized by findings that range from cellulitis to abscess formation. Systemic signs, such as fever and chills, are often present in more severe cases.

TABLE 147-1 Common Illnesses Caused by *Staphylococcus aureus*

Skin and Soft Tissue Infections
Folliculitis
Abscess, furuncle, carbuncle
Cellulitis
Impetigo
Mastitis
Surgical wound infections
Musculoskeletal Infections
Septic arthritis
Osteomyelitis (hematogenous or contiguous spread)
Pyomyositis
Psoas abscess
Respiratory Tract Infections
Ventilator-associated or nosocomial pneumonia
Septic pulmonary emboli
Postviral pneumonia (e.g., influenza)
Empyema
Bacteremia and Its Complications
Sepsis, septic shock
Metastatic foci of infection (kidney, joints, bone, lung)
Infective endocarditis
Infective Endocarditis
Injection drug use–associated
Native-valve
Prosthetic-valve
Nosocomial
Device-Related Infections (e.g., intravascular catheters, prosthetic joints)
Toxin-Mediated Illnesses
Toxic shock syndrome
Food poisoning
Staphylococcal scalded-skin syndrome
Invasive Infections Associated with Community-Acquired Methicillin-Resistant *S. aureus*
Necrotizing fasciitis
Waterhouse-Friderichsen syndrome
Necrotizing pneumonia
Purpura fulminans

Musculoskeletal Infections *S. aureus* is a common cause of bone infections—both those resulting from hematogenous dissemination and those arising from contiguous spread from a soft tissue site. *Hematogenous osteomyelitis* in children most often involves the long bones. Infections present with fever and bone pain or with a child's reluctance to bear weight. The white blood cell count and erythrocyte sedimentation rate are often elevated. Blood cultures are positive in ~50% of cases. When necessary, bone biopsies for culture and histopathologic examination are usually diagnostic.

In adults, hematogenous osteomyelitis involving the long bones is less common. However, *vertebral osteomyelitis* is among the more common clinical presentations. Vertebral bone infections are most often seen in patients with endocarditis, those undergoing hemodialysis, diabetics, and injection drug users. These infections may present with intense back pain and fever but may also be clinically occult, presenting as chronic back pain with low-grade fever. *S. aureus* is the most common cause of epidural abscess, a complication that can result in neurologic compromise. Patients report difficulty voiding or walking

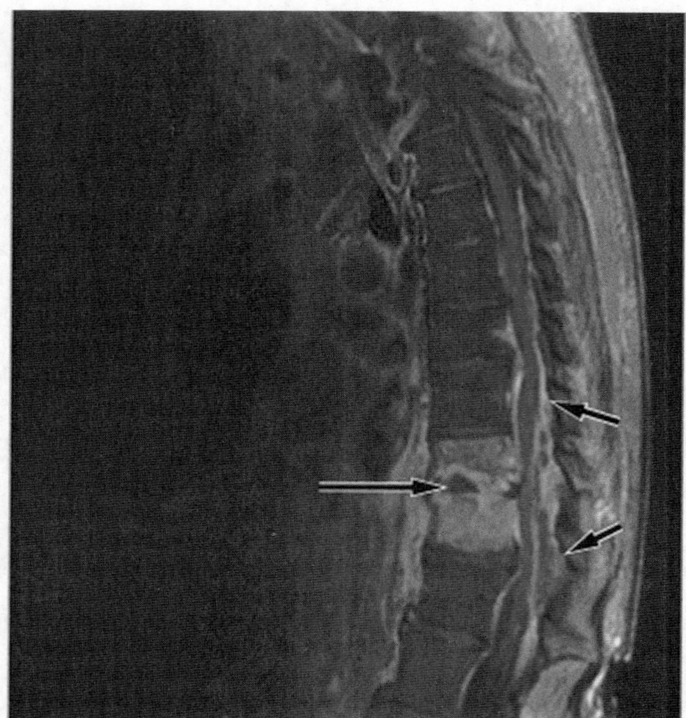

FIGURE 147-3 ***S. aureus* vertebral osteomyelitis and epidural abscess involving the thoracic disk between T9 and T10.** Sagittal postcontrast MRI of the spine illustrates destruction of the T9–T10 intervertebral space with enhancement (*long arrow*). There is impingement on the thoracic cord and an epidural collection extending from T9 through T11 (*short arrows*).

and radicular pain in addition to the symptoms associated with their osteomyelitis. Surgical intervention in this setting often constitutes a medical emergency.

MRI is the most reliable imaging modality to help establish the diagnosis of osteomyelitis **(Fig. 147-3)**. Routine x-rays are an appropriate first step, but findings may be normal for up to 14 days after the onset of symptoms. If an MRI is not possible, CT is an acceptable alternative.

Bone infections that result from contiguous spread tend to develop from soft tissue infections, such as those associated with diabetic or vascular ulcers, surgery, or trauma. Exposure of bone, a draining fistulous tract, failure to heal, or continued drainage suggests involvement of underlying bone. Bone involvement is established by bone culture and histopathologic examination (revealing evidence of PMN infiltration). Contamination of culture material from adjacent tissue can make the diagnosis of osteomyelitis difficult in the absence of pathologic confirmation. Samples obtained during surgery are the most reliable. An MRI is the most reliable radiologic test to distinguish between osteomyelitis and overlying soft tissue infection with underlying osteitis.

In both children and adults, *S. aureus* is the most common cause of *septic arthritis* in native joints. If left untreated, this infection is rapidly progressive and may be associated with extensive joint destruction. It presents with intense pain on motion of the affected joint, swelling, and fever. Aspiration of the joint reveals turbid fluid, with >50,000 PMNs/μL and gram-positive cocci in clusters seen on Gram's stain (Fig. 147-1). In adults, septic arthritis may result from trauma, surgery, or hematogenous dissemination. The most commonly involved joints include the knees, shoulders, hips, and phalanges. Infection frequently develops in joints previously damaged by osteoarthritis or rheumatoid arthritis. Iatrogenic infections resulting from aspiration or injection of agents into the joint also occur. In these settings, the patient experiences increased pain and swelling in the involved joint in association with fever.

Pyomyositis is an unusual infection of skeletal muscles that is seen primarily in tropical climates but also occurs in immunocompromised (e.g., HIV-infected) patients. It is believed to arise from occult bacteremia. Pyomyositis presents as fever, swelling, and pain overlying the involved muscle. Aspiration of fluid from the involved tissue yields pus. Although a history of trauma may be associated with the infection, its pathogenesis is poorly understood.

Respiratory Tract Infections Respiratory tract infections caused by *S. aureus* occur in selected clinical settings. *S. aureus* is a cause of serious respiratory tract infections in newborns and infants; these infections present with shortness of breath, fever, and respiratory failure. Chest x-ray may reveal pneumatoceles (shaggy, thin-walled cavities). Pneumothorax and empyema are recognized complications.

In adults, nosocomial *S. aureus* pulmonary infections are common among intubated patients in intensive care units. Nasally colonized patients are at increased risk of these infections. The clinical presentation is no different from pulmonary infections caused by other bacterial pathogens. Patients produce increased volumes of purulent sputum and develop respiratory distress, fever, and new pulmonary infiltrates. Distinguishing bacterial pneumonia from respiratory failure or other causes of new pulmonary infiltrates in critically ill patients is difficult and relies on a constellation of clinical, radiologic, and laboratory findings.

Community-acquired respiratory tract infections due to *S. aureus* often follow viral infections—most commonly influenza. Patients may present with fever, bloody sputum production, and midlung-field pneumatoceles or multiple, patchy pulmonary infiltrates. Diagnosis is made by sputum Gram's stain and culture. Blood cultures, although useful, are usually negative.

Bacteremia, Sepsis, and Infective Endocarditis *S. aureus* bacteremia may be complicated by sepsis, endocarditis, vasculitis, or metastatic seeding (establishment of suppurative collections at other tissue sites). Among the more commonly seeded tissue sites are bones, joints, kidneys, and lungs. The frequency of metastatic seeding during bacteremia has been estimated to be as high as 31%. The incidence of these complications increases with the duration of the bacteremia.

Recognition of these complications by clinical criteria alone is challenging. Comorbid conditions that are frequently seen in association with *S. aureus* bacteremia and that increase the risk of complications include diabetes, HIV infection, and renal insufficiency. Other host factors that increase the risk of complications include presentation with community-acquired *S. aureus* bacteremia, lack of an identifiable primary focus of infection, and the presence of prosthetic devices or material.

Clinically, *S. aureus* sepsis presents in a manner similar to that documented for sepsis due to other bacteria. The well-described progression of hemodynamic changes—beginning with respiratory alkalosis and clinical findings of hypotension and fever—is commonly seen. The microbiologic diagnosis is established by positive blood cultures.

The overall incidence of *S. aureus* endocarditis has increased over the past 20 years. *S. aureus* is now the leading cause of endocarditis worldwide, accounting for 25–35% of cases. This increase is due, at least in part, to the increased use of intravascular devices and, more recently, the upsurge in injection drug use. Studies using transesophageal echocardiography found an endocarditis incidence of ~25% among patients with intravascular catheter–associated *S. aureus* bacteremia. Other factors associated with an increased risk of endocarditis are hemodialysis, the presence of intravascular prosthetic devices at the time of bacteremia, and immunosuppression. Patients with implantable cardiac devices (e.g., permanent pacemakers) are at increased risk of endocarditis or device-related infections. Despite the availability of effective antibiotics, mortality rates from these infections continue to range from 20 to 40%, depending on both the host and the nature of the infection. Complications of *S. aureus* endocarditis include cardiac valvular insufficiency, peripheral emboli, metastatic seeding, vasculitis, and central nervous system (CNS) involvement (e.g., mycotic aneurysms, embolic strokes).

S. aureus endocarditis is encountered in four clinical settings: (1) right-sided endocarditis in association with injection drug use; (2) left-sided native-valve endocarditis; (3) prosthetic-valve endocarditis; and

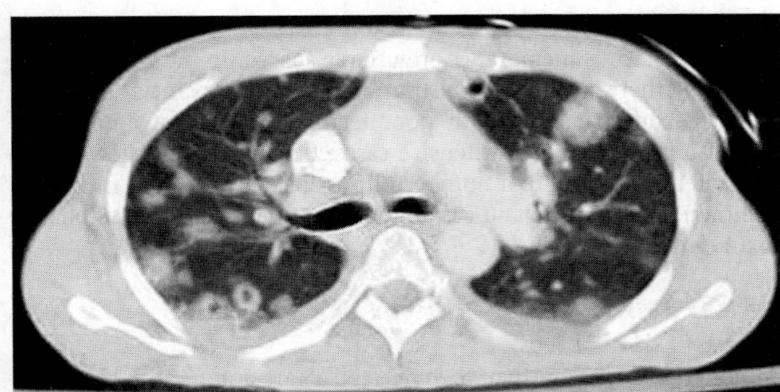

FIGURE 147-4 CT scan illustrating septic pulmonary emboli in a patient with methicillin-resistant *Staphylococcus aureus* bacteremia.

(4) nosocomial endocarditis. In each of these settings, the diagnosis is suspected from the patient's history and the recognition of physical signs suggestive of endocarditis. These findings include cardiac manifestations, such as new or changing cardiac valvular murmurs; cutaneous evidence, such as vasculitic lesions, Osler's nodes, or Janeway lesions; evidence of right- or left-sided embolic disease; and a history suggesting a risk for *S. aureus* bacteremia. In the absence of antecedent antibiotic therapy, blood cultures are almost uniformly positive. Transthoracic echocardiography, while less sensitive than transesophageal echocardiography, is less invasive and often identifies valvular vegetations. The Duke criteria **(Chap. 128)** are commonly used to help establish this diagnosis.

Acute right-sided tricuspid valvular *S. aureus* endocarditis is most often seen in patients who inject drugs. The classic presentation includes a high fever, a toxic clinical appearance, pleuritic chest pain, and the production of purulent, sometimes bloody, sputum. Chest x-rays or CT scans reveal evidence of septic pulmonary emboli (small, peripheral, circular lesions that may cavitate with time) **(Fig. 147-4)**. A high percentage of affected patients have no history of antecedent valvular damage. At the outset of their illness, patients may present with fever alone, without cardiac or other localizing findings. As a result, a high index of clinical suspicion is essential for diagnosis.

Individuals with antecedent cardiac valvular damage more commonly present with left-sided native-valve endocarditis involving the damaged valve. These patients tend to be older than those with right-sided endocarditis, their prognosis is worse, and their incidence of complications (including peripheral emboli, cardiac decompensation, cerebrovascular events and metastatic seeding) is increased.

S. aureus is one of the more common causes of prosthetic-valve endocarditis. This infection is especially fulminant in the early postoperative period and is associated with increased morbidity and mortality. In most instances, medical therapy alone is not sufficient and urgent valve replacement is necessary. Patients are prone to develop valvular insufficiency or myocardial abscesses originating from the region of valve implantation.

The increased frequency of nosocomial endocarditis (15–30% of cases, depending on the series) reflects in part the increased use of intravascular devices. This form of endocarditis is most commonly caused by *S. aureus*. These patients are often critically ill, are receiving antibiotics for various other indications, and have comorbid conditions. As a result, blood cultures may be negative and the diagnosis missed.

Prosthetic Device–Related Infections *S. aureus* accounts for a large proportion of prosthetic device–related infections. These infections include intravascular and peritoneal catheters, prosthetic valves, orthopedic devices, pacemakers, left-ventricular-assist devices, or vascular grafts. In contrast with the more indolent presentation of NSaS infections, *S. aureus* device-related infections are often acute, have both local and systemic manifestations, and tend to progress more rapidly. It is relatively common for a pyogenic collection to be present at the device site. Aspiration of these collections and performance of blood cultures are important components in establishing a diagnosis. *S. aureus* infections tend to occur more commonly soon after implantation unless the device is used for access (e.g., intravascular or hemodialysis catheters). In the latter instance, infections can occur at any time. As in most prosthetic-device infections, successful therapy usually involves removal of the device. Left in place, the device serves as a potential nidus for either persistent or recurrent infections.

Urinary Tract Infections Urinary tract infections (UTIs) are infrequently caused by *S. aureus*. The presence of *S. aureus* in the urine often suggests hematogenous dissemination. Ascending *S. aureus* infections occasionally result from instrumentation of the genitourinary tract.

Infections Associated with Community-Acquired MRSA Although skin and soft tissues are by far the most common sites of infection associated with CA-MRSA, 5–10% of these infections are invasive and can be life-threatening. The latter unique infections, including necrotizing fasciitis, necrotizing pneumonia, and sepsis with Waterhouse-Friderichsen syndrome or purpura fulminans, were rarely associated with *S. aureus* prior to the emergence of CA-MRSA. These life-threatening infections reflect the increased virulence of CA-MRSA strains.

Toxin-Mediated Diseases • FOOD POISONING *S. aureus* is among the most common causes of foodborne outbreaks in the United States. Staphylococcal food poisoning results from the inoculation of toxin-producing *S. aureus* into food by colonized food handlers. Toxin is then elaborated in such growth-promoting food as custards, potato salad, or processed meats. Even if the bacteria are killed by warming, the heat-stable toxin is not destroyed. The onset of illness is rapid, occurring within 1–6 h of ingestion; it is characterized by nausea and vomiting, although diarrhea, hypotension, and dehydration may occur. The differential diagnosis includes diarrhea of other etiologies, especially that caused by similar toxins (e.g., the toxins elaborated by *Bacillus cereus*). The rapidity of onset, the absence of fever, and the epidemic nature of the presentation (without secondary spread) should arouse suspicion of staphylococcal food poisoning. Symptoms generally resolve within 8–10 h. The diagnosis can be established by the demonstration of bacteria or the documentation of enterotoxin in the implicated food. Treatment is entirely supportive.

TOXIC SHOCK SYNDROME TSS gained attention in the early 1980s, when a nationwide outbreak occurred among young, otherwise healthy, menstruating women. Epidemiologic investigation demonstrated that these cases were associated with the use of a highly absorbent tampon recently introduced to the market. Subsequent studies established the role of TSST-1 in these illnesses. Withdrawal of the tampon from the market resulted in a rapid decline in the incidence of this disease. However, menstrual and nonmenstrual cases continue to be reported. Nonmenstrual cases are seen in patients with surgical or postpartum wound infections, especially when packing of the wound occurs.

The clinical presentation is similar in menstrual and nonmenstrual TSS. Evidence of clinical *S. aureus* infection is not a prerequisite. TSS results from the elaboration of an enterotoxin or the structurally related enterotoxin-like TSST-1. More than 90% of menstrual cases are caused by TSST-1, whereas a high percentage of nonmenstrual cases are caused by enterotoxins (e.g., enterotoxin B). TSS begins with relatively nonspecific flulike symptoms. In menstrual cases, the onset usually comes 2 or 3 days after the start of menstruation. Patients present with fever, hypotension, and erythroderma of variable intensity. Mucosal involvement is common (e.g., conjunctival hyperemia). The illness can rapidly progress to symptoms that include vomiting, diarrhea, confusion, myalgias, and abdominal pain. These symptoms reflect the multisystemic nature of the disease, with involvement of the liver, kidneys, gastrointestinal tract, and/or CNS. Desquamation of the skin occurs during convalescence, usually 1–2 weeks after the onset of illness. Laboratory findings may include azotemia, leukocytosis, hypoalbuminemia, thrombocytopenia, and liver function abnormalities.

Diagnosis of TSS still depends on a constellation of findings rather than one specific finding and on a lack of evidence of other possible infections **(Table 147-2)**. These other diagnoses include drug toxicities,

TABLE 147-2 Case Definition of *Staphylococcus aureus* Toxic Shock Syndrome

Clinical Criteria

An illness with the following clinical manifestations:

- Fever: temperature ≥102.0°F (≥38.9°C)
- Rash: diffuse macular erythroderma
- Desquamation: 1–2 weeks after rash onset
- Hypotension: systolic blood pressure ≤90 mmHg for adults or less than the fifth percentile, by age, for children <16 years old
- Multisystem involvement (≥3 of the following organ systems)
  - Gastrointestinal: vomiting or diarrhea at illness onset
  - Muscular: severe myalgia or creatine phosphokinase level at least twice ULN
  - Mucous membrane: vaginal, oropharyngeal, or conjunctival hyperemia
  - Renal: blood urea nitrogen or creatinine level at least twice ULN for laboratory or urinary sediment with pyuria (≥5 leukocytes per high-power field) in the absence of urinary tract infection
  - Hepatic: total bilirubin or aminotransferase level at least twice ULN for laboratory
  - Hematologic: platelet count $<10^5/\mu L$
  - Central nervous system: disorientation or alterations in consciousness without focal neurologic signs in the absence of fever and hypotension

Laboratory Criteria

Negative results in the following tests, if obtained:

- Blood or cerebrospinal fluid cultures for another pathogen[a]
- Serologic tests for Rocky Mountain spotted fever, leptospirosis, or measles

Case Classification

Probable: a case that meets the laboratory criteria and in which four of the five clinical criteria are fulfilled

Confirmed: a case that meets the laboratory criteria and in which all five of the clinical criteria are fulfilled, including desquamation (unless the patient dies before desquamation occurs)

[a]Blood cultures may be positive for *S. aureus*.

Abbreviation: ULN, upper limit of normal.

Source: Centers for Disease Control and Prevention (*www.cdc.gov/nndss/conditions/toxic-shock-syndrome-other-than-streptococcal/case-definition/2011/*).

viral exanthems, Rocky Mountain spotted fever, sepsis, and Kawasaki disease. Illness occurs only in persons who lack antibody to TSST-1. Recurrences are possible if antibody fails to develop after the illness.

STAPHYLOCOCCAL SCALDED-SKIN SYNDROME SSSS primarily affects newborns and children. The illness may vary from a localized blister to exfoliation of much of the skin surface. The skin is usually fragile and often tender, with thin-walled, fluid-filled bullae (**Fig. 147-5**). Gentle pressure results in rupture of the lesions, leaving denuded underlying skin. The mucous membranes are usually spared. In more generalized infection, there are often constitutional symptoms, including fever, lethargy, and irritability with poor feeding. Significant amounts of fluid can be lost in more extensive cases. Illness usually follows localized infection at one of a number of possible sites. SSSS is much less common among adults but can follow infections caused by exfoliative toxin–producing strains.

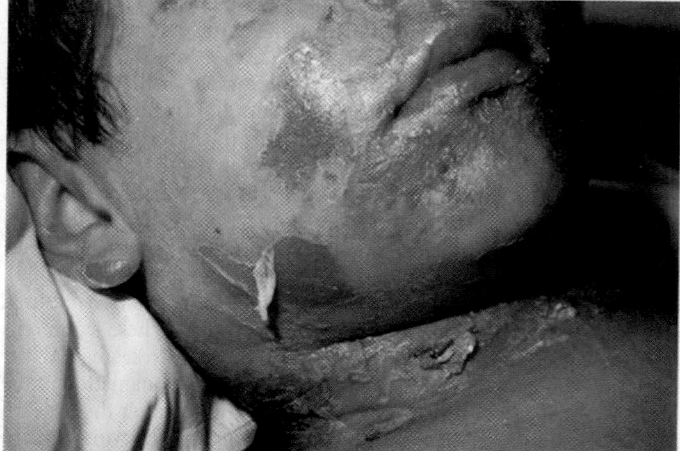

FIGURE 147-5 Staphylococcal scalded skin syndrome in a 6-year-old boy. Nikolsky's sign, with separation of the superficial layer of the outer epidermal layer, is visible. *(Adapted from LA Schenfeld: Staphylococcal scalded skin syndrome: N Engl J Med 342:1178, 2000.)*

NON-*S. AUREUS* STAPHYLOCOCCAL INFECTIONS

Although less virulent than *S. aureus*, NSaS are among the most common causes of prosthetic-device infections, including endocarditis. They also are increasingly a cause of native-valve endocarditis and life-threatening bloodstream infections in neonates and in neutropenic patients. Approximately half of the identified NSaS species have been associated with human infections. Of these species, *Staphylococcus epidermidis* is the most common human pathogen. It is part of the normal human flora and is found on the skin (where it is the most abundant bacterial species) as well as in the oropharynx and vagina. *Staphylococcus saprophyticus*, a novobiocin-resistant species, is a common pathogen in UTIs.

PATHOGENESIS

S. epidermidis is the NSaS species most often associated with prosthetic-device infections. Infection is a two-step process, with initial adhesion to the device followed by colonization. *S. epidermidis* is uniquely adapted to colonize these devices because of its capacity to elaborate the extracellular polysaccharide (glycocalyx or slime) that facilitates formation of a protective biofilm on the device surface.

Implanted prosthetic material is rapidly coated with host matrix molecules such as fibrinogen or fibronectin. These molecules serve as potential bridging ligands, facilitating initial bacterial attachment to the device surface. A number of staphylococcal surface-associated proteins, such as autolysin (AtlE), fibrinogen-binding protein, and accumulation-associated protein (AAP), appear to play a role in attachment to either modified or unmodified prosthetic surfaces. The polysaccharide intercellular adhesin facilitates subsequent staphylococcal colonization, aggregation, and accumulation on the device surface. Intercellular adhesin (*ica*) genes are more commonly found in strains of *S. epidermidis* that are associated with device infections than in strains associated with colonization of mucosal surfaces. Biofilm acts as a barrier, protecting bacteria from host defense mechanisms as well as from antibiotics while providing a suitable environment for bacterial maturation, survival, and potential spread to other tissue sites.

Two additional NSaS species, *Staphylococcus lugdunensis* and *Staphylococcus schleiferi*, produce more serious infections (native-valve endocarditis and osteomyelitis) than do other NSaS. The basis for this enhanced virulence is not known, although both species appear to share more virulence determinants with *S. aureus* (e.g., clumping factor and lipase) than do other NSaS.

The capacity of *S. saprophyticus* to cause UTIs in young women appears related to the presence of adhesins that facilitate adherence to uroepithelial cells. A 160-kDa hemagglutinin/adhesin may contribute to this affinity.

DIAGNOSIS

Although the detection of NSaS at sites of infection or in the bloodstream by standard microbiologic culture methods is not difficult, interpretation of these results is frequently problematic. Because these organisms are present in large numbers on the skin, they often contaminate cultures. It has been estimated that only 10–20% of blood cultures positive for NSaS reflect true bacteremia. Similar problems arise with cultures obtained from other sites. Among the clinical findings suggestive of true bacteremia are fever, evidence of local infection (e.g., erythema or purulent drainage at the IV catheter site), leukocytosis, and systemic signs of sepsis. Laboratory findings suggestive of true bacteremia include repeated isolation of the same strain (i.e., the same species with the same antibiogram or with a closely related DNA fingerprint) from separate cultures, growth of the strain within 48 h, and bacterial growth in both aerobic and anaerobic bottles.

CLINICAL SYNDROMES

NSaS cause a variety of prosthetic device–related infections, including those that involve prosthetic cardiac valves and joints, vascular grafts, intravascular devices, and CNS shunts. In all of these settings, the clinical presentation is similar. The signs of localized infection are often subtle, the rate of disease progression is slow, and the systemic findings are often limited. Signs of infection, such as purulent drainage, pain at the site, or loosening of prosthetic implants, are sometimes evident. Fever is frequently but not always present, and there may be mild leukocytosis. Acute-phase reactant levels, erythrocyte sedimentation rate, and C-reactive protein concentration may be elevated.

Infections that are not associated with prosthetic devices include, as noted, native-valve endocarditis due to NSaS, which accounts for ~5% of cases. Infections in preterm infants and neutropenic patients are often associated with the need for intravascular devices. *S. lugdunensis* appears to be a more aggressive pathogen in this setting, causing greater mortality and rapid valvular destruction with abscess formation than other NSaS.

TREATMENT

Staphylococcal Infections

GENERAL PRINCIPLES OF THERAPY

Source control (e.g., incision and drainage of suppurative collections or removal of infected prosthetic devices), coupled with rapid institution of appropriate antimicrobial therapy, is essential for the management of all staphylococcal infections. The emergence of MRSA as a community-based pathogen has increased the importance of culturing all sites of infection in order to determine antimicrobial susceptibility.

DURATION OF ANTIMICROBIAL THERAPY

Therapy for *S. aureus* bacteremia is generally prolonged (4–6 weeks) because of the high risk of complications (e.g., endocarditis, metastatic foci of infection). Among the findings associated with complicated bacteremias are (1) persistently positive blood cultures 96 h after institution of therapy, (2) acquisition of the infection in the community, (3) failure to promptly remove or drain an identified focus of infection (i.e., an intravascular catheter), and (4) the presence of deep-seated infections. Patients with uncomplicated bacteremias are defined by a removable focus of infection, prompt response to antimicrobial therapy (i.e., no fever or positive blood cultures after 3–4 days), no evidence of metastatic foci of infection, and no implanted prostheses. In these latter infections, short-course therapy (2 weeks) can be given; however, these findings are not always predictive of uncomplicated bacteremias. Transesophageal echocardiography to rule out endocarditis is generally necessary because neither clinical nor laboratory findings can reliably detect cardiac involvement. A thorough radiologic investigation to identify potential metastatic collections is also indicated. All symptomatic body sites must be carefully evaluated.

Recent studies have demonstrated that parenteral therapy is not always necessary to complete a course of treatment for invasive staphylococcal infections such as endocarditis or osteomyelitis.

NSaS treatment is complicated by the possibility that a single isolate may be a contaminant. Therapy for 7–14 days is recommended for documented infections (i.e., blood cultures of the same strain ≥24 hours apart) in the absence of endocarditis or additional sites of infection.

CHOICE OF ANTIMICROBIAL AGENTS

The choice of antimicrobial agents to treat both coagulase-positive and coagulase-negative staphylococcal infections is often difficult because of the prevalence of multidrug-resistant strains and the limited number of clinical trials that have compared the available agents. Staphylococcal resistance to most antibiotic families, including β-lactams, aminoglycosides, fluoroquinolones, and (to a lesser extent) glycopeptides, has increased. This trend is even more apparent with NSaS; >80% of nosocomial isolates are resistant to methicillin, and these methicillin-resistant strains are often resistant to many other antibiotics. Because the selection of antimicrobial agents for *S. aureus* infections is similar to that for NSaS infections, treatment options for these pathogens are discussed together and are summarized in **Table 147-3**.

Few strains of staphylococci (≤5%) remain susceptible to penicillin. This is a result of the widespread dissemination of plasmids containing the enzyme penicillinase. Penicillin-resistant isolates are treated with semisynthetic penicillinase-resistant penicillins (SPRPs), such as oxacillin or nafcillin. Methicillin, the first of the SPRPs, is no longer used. Cephalosporins are alternative therapeutic agents for these infections. Second- and third-generation cephalosporins offer no therapeutic advantage over first-generation cephalosporins for the treatment of staphylococcal infections, and some third-generation cephalosporins (e.g., ceftazidime) have considerably less activity. The carbapenems have excellent activity against methicillin-sensitive *S. aureus* but not against MRSA.

The isolation of MRSA was reported within 1 year of the introduction of methicillin. Since then, the prevalence of MRSA has steadily increased. In many U.S. hospitals, 40–50% of *S. aureus* isolates are resistant to methicillin. Resistance to methicillin indicates resistance to all SPRPs as well as to all cephalosporins (except ceftaroline). Production of a novel penicillin-binding protein (PBP2a) is responsible for methicillin resistance. This protein is synthesized by the *mecA* gene, which (as stated above) is part of a large mobile genetic element—a pathogenicity or genomic island—called SCC*mec*. It is hypothesized that *mecA* was acquired via horizontal transfer from related staphylococcal species. Phenotypic expression of methicillin resistance may be constitutive (i.e., expressed in all cells in a population) or heterogeneous (i.e., displayed by only a proportion of the total cell population). Detection of methicillin resistance is enhanced by growth of cultures at reduced temperatures (≤35°C for 24 h) and with increased concentrations of salt in the medium. Culture techniques are increasingly being replaced by PCR-based or other methods (e.g., latex agglutination) that allow for the rapid detection of methicillin resistance.

Either vancomycin or daptomycin are recommended as the drugs of choice for the treatment of invasive MRSA infections. MRSA susceptibility to vancomycin has decreased in many areas of the world. It is important to note that vancomycin is less effective than SPRPs for the treatment of infections due to methicillin-susceptible strains. In patients with a history of serious β-lactam allergies, alternatives to SPRPs for the treatment of invasive infections should be used only after careful consideration. Desensitization to β-lactams remains an option for life-threatening infections.

Three types of staphylococcal resistance to vancomycin have emerged. (1) Minimal inhibitory concentration (MIC; an in vitro measure of susceptibility) "creep" refers to the incremental increase in vancomycin MICs that has been detected in various geographic areas. Studies suggest that morbidity and mortality may be increased in infections due to *S. aureus* strains with vancomycin MICs of ≥1.5 μg/mL. (2) In 1997, an *S. aureus* strain with reduced susceptibility to vancomycin (vancomycin-intermediate *S. aureus* [VISA]) was reported from Japan. Subsequently, additional VISA clinical isolates were reported. These strains were resistant to methicillin and many other antimicrobial agents. The VISA strains appear to evolve (under vancomycin selective pressure) from strains that are susceptible to vancomycin but are heterogeneous, with a small proportion of the bacterial population expressing the resistance phenotype. The mechanism of VISA resistance is in part due to an abnormally thick cell wall. Vancomycin is trapped by the abnormal peptidoglycan cross-linking and is unable to gain access to its target site. Regulatory genes involved in cell wall metabolism appear to play an important role in this type of resistance. (3) In 2002, the first clinical isolate of fully vancomycin-resistant *S. aureus* (VRSA) was reported. Resistance in this and several additional clinical isolates

TABLE 147-3 Antimicrobial Therapy for Staphylococcal Infections[a]

SENSITIVITY/RESISTANCE OF ISOLATE	DRUG OF CHOICE	ALTERNATIVE(S)	COMMENTS
Parenteral Therapy for Serious Infections			
Sensitive to penicillin	Penicillin G (4 mU q4h)	Nafcillin or oxacillin (2 g q4h), cefazolin (2 g q8h), vancomycin (15–20 mg/kg q8h[b])	Fewer than 5% of isolates are sensitive to penicillin. The clinical microbiology laboratory must verify that the strain is not a β-lactamase producer.
Sensitive to methicillin; Resistant to penicillin	Nafcillin or oxacillin (2 g q4h)	Cefazolin (2 g q8h), daptomycin (6–10 mg/kg IV q24h[b,d]), vancomycin (15–20 mg/kg q8h[b])	Patients with a penicillin allergy can be treated with a cephalosporin if the allergy does not involve an anaphylactic or accelerated reaction; desensitization to β-lactams may be indicated in selected cases of serious infection when maximal bactericidal activity is needed (e.g., prosthetic-valve endocarditis[c]). Vancomycin is a less effective option than a β-lactam.
Resistant to methicillin	Vancomycin (15–20 mg/kg q8–12h[b]), daptomycin (6–10 mg/kg IV q24h[b,d]) for bacteremia, endocarditis, osteomyelitis, and complicated skin infections	Linezolid (600 mg q12h PO or IV), ceftaroline (600 mg IV q8–12h), telavancin (7.5–10 mg/kg IV q24h)[b], TMP-SMX (5 mg [based on TMP]/kg IV q8–12h)[f] Additional agents include tedizolid (200 mg once daily IV), oritavancin (single dose of 1200 mg), dalbavancin (single dose of 1500 mg), delafloxacin (300 mg q 12 h IV), omadacycline 100 mg OD). These drugs are primarily approved for the treatment of skin and soft tissue infections.[g]	Sensitivity testing is necessary before an alternative drug is selected. The efficacy of adjunctive therapy is not well established in many settings. Linezolid, ceftaroline, and telavancin have in vitro activity against most VISA and VRSA strains. See footnote for treatment of prosthetic-valve endocarditis.[c]
Resistant to methicillin with intermediate or complete resistance to vancomycin[e]	Daptomycin (6–10 mg/kg q24h[b,d]) for bacteremia, endocarditis, osteomyelitis, and complicated skin infections	Same as for methicillin-resistant strains (check antibiotic susceptibilities) *or* Ceftaroline (600 mg IV q8–12h) Newer agents include tedizolid (200 mg once daily IV or PO), oritavancin (single dose of 1200 mg), and dalbavancin (single dose of 1500 mg). These drugs are approved only for the treatment of skin and soft tissue infections.	Same as for methicillin-resistant strains; check antibiotic susceptibilities. Ceftaroline is used either alone or in combination with daptomycin.
Not yet known (i.e., empirical therapy)	Vancomycin (15–20 mg/kg q8–12h[b]), daptomycin (6–10 mg/kg q24h[b,d]) for bacteremia, endocarditis, osteomyelitis, and complicated skin infections	—	Empirical therapy is given when the susceptibility of the isolate is not known. Vancomycin with or without a β-lactam is recommended for suspected community- or hospital-acquired *Staphylococcus aureus* infections because of the increased frequency of methicillin-resistant strains in the community. If isolates with an elevated MIC to vancomycin (≥1.5 μg/mL) are common in the community, daptomycin may be preferable.
Oral Therapy for Skin and Soft Tissue Infections			
Sensitive to methicillin	Dicloxacillin (500 mg qid), cephalexin (500 mg qid), or cefadroxil (1 g q12h)	Minocycline or doxycycline (100 mg q12h[b]), TMP-SMX (1 or 2 DS tablets bid), clindamycin (300–450 mg tid), linezolid (600 mg PO q12h), tedizolid (200 mg PO q24h)	It is important to know the antibiotic susceptibility of isolates in the specific geographic region. All collections should be drained, and drainage should be cultured.
Resistant to methicillin	Clindamycin (300–450 mg tid), TMP-SMX (1 or 2 DS tablets bid), minocycline or doxycycline (100 mg q12h[b]), linezolid (600 mg bid), or tedizolid (200 mg once daily)	Delafloxacin 450 mg q 12 h, omadacycline 300 mg OD	It is important to know the antibiotic susceptibility of isolates in the specific geographic region. All collections should be drained, and drainage should be cultured.

[a]Recommended dosages are for adults with normal renal and hepatic function. [b]The dosage must be adjusted for patients with reduced creatinine clearance. [c]For the treatment of prosthetic-valve endocarditis, the addition of gentamicin (1 mg/kg q8h) and rifampin (300 mg PO q8h) is recommended, with adjustment of the gentamicin dosage if the creatinine clearance rate is reduced. [d]Daptomycin cannot be used for the treatment of pneumonia. [e]Vancomycin-resistant *S. aureus* isolates from clinical infections have been reported. [f]TMP-SMX may be less effective than vancomycin. [g]Limited data are available on the efficacy of these drugs for the treatment of invasive infections.

Abbreviations: DS, double-strength; TMP-SMX, trimethoprim-sulfamethoxazole; VISA, vancomycin-intermediate *S. aureus;* VRSA, vancomycin-resistant *S. aureus.*

Source: Modified from C Liu et al: Clin Infect Dis 52:285, 2011; DL Stevens et al: Clin Infect Dis 59:148, 2014; DL Stevens et al: Med Lett Drugs Ther 56:39, 2014; and LM Baddour et al: Circulation 132:1435, 2015.

was due to the presence of *vanA*, the gene responsible for expression of vancomycin resistance in enterococci. This observation suggested that resistance was acquired as a result of horizontal conjugal transfer from a vancomycin-resistant strain of *Enterococcus faecalis*. Several of the patients infected with the VRSA strain had both MRSA and vancomycin-resistant enterococci cultured from infection sites. The *vanA* gene is responsible for the synthesis of the dipeptide D-Ala-D-Lac in place of D-Ala-D-Ala. Vancomycin cannot bind to the altered peptide. While isolates with MICs of ≥1.5 μg/mL have been relatively common in some areas, VISA and VRSA isolates are uncommon.

Daptomycin, a parenteral bactericidal agent with antistaphylococcal activity, is approved for the treatment of bacteremia (including right-sided endocarditis) and complicated skin infections. It is not effective in respiratory infections. This drug has a unique mechanism of action: it disrupts the cytoplasmic membrane. Staphylococcal resistance to daptomycin has been reported. Resistance can emerge during therapy; patients previously treated with vancomycin may have elevated daptomycin MICs. Patients need to be monitored for rhabdomyolysis with creatine phosphokinase measurement and for eosinophilic pneumonia.

Linezolid—the first oxazolidinone—is bacteriostatic against staphylococci; it offers the advantage of comparable bioavailability after oral or parenteral administration. Cross-resistance with other inhibitors of protein synthesis has not been detected. Resistance to linezolid has been increasingly reported. Serious adverse reactions to linezolid include thrombocytopenia, occasional cases of neutropenia, and rare instances of lactic acidosis or peripheral and optic neuropathy. These reactions tend to occur after relatively prolonged courses of therapy.

Tedizolid, a second oxazolidinone, is available as both oral and parenteral preparations. It exhibits enhanced in vitro activity against antibiotic-resistant gram-positive bacteria, including staphylococci. Tedizolid is administered once a day. Data on its efficacy for the treatment of deep-seated infections are limited.

Ceftaroline is a fifth-generation cephalosporin with bactericidal activity against MRSA (including strains with reduced susceptibility to vancomycin and daptomycin). It is generally well tolerated. Ceftaroline is approved for use in nosocomial pneumonias and for SSTIs. It has increasingly been used to treat invasive MRSA infections.

Telavancin is a parenteral lipoglycopeptide derivative of vancomycin that is approved for the treatment of complicated SSTIs and for nosocomial pneumonias. The drug has two targets: the cell wall and the cell membrane. It remains active against VISA strains. Because of its potential nephrotoxicity, telavancin should be avoided in patients with renal disease.

Dalbavancin and oritavancin are long-acting, parenterally administered lipoglycopeptides that have been used to treat complicated SSTIs. Because of their long half-lives, they can be administered on a weekly basis. Both have been used as single-dose regimens for the treatment of SSTIs. Anecdotal data support their use for the treatment of invasive staphylococcal infections.

Although the quinolones are active against staphylococci in vitro, the frequency of staphylococcal resistance to these agents has increased, especially among methicillin-resistant isolates. Of particular concern in MRSA is the possibility of quinolone resistance emerging during therapy. Therefore, quinolones are not recommended for the treatment of MRSA infections. Resistance to the quinolones is most commonly chromosomal and results from mutations of the topoisomerase IV or DNA gyrase genes, although multidrug efflux pumps also may contribute. Although the newer quinolones exhibit increased in vitro activity against staphylococci, it is uncertain whether this increase translates into enhanced in vivo activity. Delafloxacin, a fluoroquinolone with broad-spectrum activity, has excellent activity against MRSA, retaining activity against some isolates resistant to other fluoroquinolones.

Tigecycline, a broad-spectrum minocycline analogue, has bacteriostatic activity against MRSA and is approved for use in SSTIs as well as intraabdominal infections caused by *S. aureus*. It is not recommended for the treatment of invasive infections.

Other older antibiotics, such as minocycline, doxycycline, clindamycin, and trimethoprim-sulfamethoxazole, continue to be successfully used to treat MRSA infections.

The benefit of antistaphylococcal combinations to enhance bactericidal activity in the treatment of deep-seated infections remains controversial. Clinical studies have not documented a therapeutic benefit from the addition of gentamicin or rifampin to single-drug regimens; recent reports have raised concern about the potential nephrotoxicity of gentamicin and adverse reactions from, or drug interactions with, rifampin. As a result, the use of gentamicin in combination with β-lactams or other antimicrobial agents is no longer routinely recommended for the treatment of invasive infections such as native-valve endocarditis. Rifampin continues to be used for the treatment of prosthetic device–related infections and for osteomyelitis.

Omadacycline and eravacycline are broad-spectrum semisynthetic tetracycline derivatives with activity against MRSA. They are currently approved for the treatment of SSTIs.

The use of bacteriophages with activity against staphylococci is now being investigated as adjunctive therapy in invasive infections.

ANTIMICROBIAL THERAPY FOR SELECTED SETTINGS

Empirical Therapy Empirical coverage for MRSA is indicated when antibiotic susceptibility is not known. Vancomycin or daptomycin are generally recommended. It remains uncertain whether daptomycin is preferable when elevated vancomycin MICs (>1.5 μg/mL) are common in a specific locale.

Salvage Therapy Salvage therapy for complicated *S. aureus* infections is sometimes needed when the bacteremia persists (i.e., for more than 3 or 4 days) despite appropriate treatment. The risk of a poor outcome (i.e., increased mortality, metastatic infections) is increased with the duration of bacteremia. There is little high-quality evidence to serve as a guide to salvage therapy. The combination of daptomycin or vancomycin with a β-lactam antibiotic (e.g., ceftaroline) has been successfully used to treat patients with persistent MRSA bacteremia, even those patients with isolates displaying reduced susceptibility to these antimicrobial agents. This combination appears to enhance the bactericidal activity of daptomycin by reducing the bacterial cell-surface charge and thus allowing enhanced daptomycin binding. For vancomycin, the combination may allow more strategic binding to the target site with reduced cell-wall thickness. Other combinations have included trimethoprim-sulfamethoxazole or rifampin combined with daptomycin. Linezolid or ceftaroline have also been used as single alternative agents.

Endocarditis *S. aureus* endocarditis is usually an acute, life-threatening infection. Thus, prompt collection of blood for cultures should be followed by immediate institution of empirical antimicrobial therapy. For native-valve endocarditis, therapy with a β-lactam is recommended. If a MRSA strain is isolated, vancomycin (15–20 mg/kg every 8–12 h, given in equal doses up to a total of 2 g, with the dose adjusted in the case of renal disease) or daptomycin (6–10 mg/kg every 24 h) is recommended. The vancomycin dose should be adjusted on the basis of trough drug levels. Patients are generally treated for 6 weeks. For prosthetic-valve endocarditis, surgery in addition to antibiotic therapy is often necessary. The combination of a β-lactam agent—or, if the isolate is β-lactam-resistant, vancomycin or daptomycin—with an aminoglycoside (gentamicin, 1 mg/kg IV every 8 h) for 2 weeks and rifampin (300 mg orally or IV every 8 h) for ≥6 weeks is recommended.

Bone and Joint Infections For hematogenous osteomyelitis or septic arthritis in children, a 4-week course of therapy is usually adequate. In adults, treatment is often more prolonged. For chronic forms of osteomyelitis, surgical debridement is necessary in combination with antimicrobial therapy. For joint infections, a critical component of therapy is the repeated aspiration or arthroscopy of the affected joint to prevent damage from leukocytes. The combination of rifampin with ciprofloxacin has been used successfully to treat or suppress prosthetic-joint infections, especially when the device cannot be removed. The efficacy of this combination may reflect enhanced activity against staphylococci in biofilms as well as the attainment of effective intracellular concentrations.

Skin and Soft Tissue Infections The increase in SSTIs caused by CA-MRSA has drawn attention to the need for initiation of appropriate empirical therapy. Even small abscesses appear to benefit from antibiotic therapy in addition to incision and drainage. Antibiotics are selected depending on local antibiotic susceptibility data; a number of oral agents have been used to treat these infections, including clindamycin, trimethoprim-sulfamethoxazole, doxycycline, linezolid, and tedizolid. Parenteral therapy is reserved for more complicated infections.

Toxic Shock Syndrome Treatment of shock is the mainstay of therapy for TSS. Both fluids and pressors may be necessary. Tampons or other packing material should be promptly removed. Some investigators recommend therapy with a combination of clindamycin and a semisynthetic penicillin or (if the isolate is resistant to methicillin) vancomycin. Clindamycin is advocated because, as a protein synthesis inhibitor, it reduces toxin production. Linezolid also appears to be effective. A semisynthetic penicillin or a glycopeptide is recommended to eliminate any potential focus of infection as well as to eradicate persistent carriage that might increase the possibility of recurrence. Intravenous immunoglobulin to treat TSS is of uncertain benefit. Glucocorticoids are not recommended for the treatment of this disease.

Other Toxin-Mediated Diseases Therapy for staphylococcal food poisoning is entirely supportive. For SSSS, antistaphylococcal therapy targets the primary site of infection.

NONTRADITIONAL APPROACHES TO ANTI-STAPHYLOCOCCAL THERAPY

In addition to the development of new antibiotics, new and nontraditional approaches to therapy are currently being investigated. These include the use of phages or phage-derived peptides, as well as probiotics and anti-virulence strategies that target selected virulence determinants.

■ PREVENTION

Primary prevention of *S. aureus* infections in the hospital setting involves hand washing and careful attention to appropriate isolation procedures. Through careful screening for MRSA carriage and strict isolation practices, several Scandinavian countries have been remarkably successful at preventing the introduction and dissemination of MRSA in hospitals.

Decolonization strategies, using both universal and targeted approaches with topical agents (e.g., mupirocin) to eliminate nasal colonization and/or chlorhexidine to eliminate colonization of additional body sites with *S. aureus*, have been successful in some clinical settings where the risk of infection is high (e.g., intensive care units). An analysis of clinical trials suggests that decolonization can reduce the incidence of postsurgical infections among people nasally colonized with *S. aureus*. The risk of recurrent admissions among patients with *S. aureus* bacteremia following discharge is high (approximately 22% within 30 days). Decolonization following discharge with mupirocin and chlorhexidine can lower the incidence of recurrent infections.

"Bundling" (the application of selected medical interventions in a sequence of prescribed steps) has reduced rates of nosocomial infections related to procedures such as the insertion of intravenous catheters, in which staphylococci are among the most common pathogens **(see Table 142-1)**. A number of immunization strategies to prevent *S. aureus* infections—both active (e.g., capsular polysaccharide–protein conjugate vaccine) and passive (e.g., clumping factor antibody)—have been investigated. However, to date, none has been successful for either prophylaxis or therapy in clinical trials.

Strategies to prevent recurrent *S. aureus* infections in the community have had limited success. Decolonization with intranasal mupirocin and chlorhexidine washes of the infected individual and the additional decolonization of household members combined with environmental cleaning of surfaces and personal items have all been studied. For individuals with extensive skin disease and recurrent infections, the use of bleach baths (e.g., one-half cup of household bleach in a half-filled bathtub) 15 minutes three times weekly may be useful.

■ FURTHER READING

Becker K et al: Coagulase-negative staphylococci. Clin Microbiol Rev 27:870, 2014.

DeLeo FR et al: Community-associated methicillin-resistant *Staphylococcus aureus*. Lancet 375:1557, 2010.

Huang SS et al: Decolonization to reduce post discharge infection risk among MRSA carriers. N Engl J Med 380:638, 2019.

Kullar R et al: When sepsis persists: A review of MRSA bacteraemia salvage therapy. J Antimicrob Chemother 71:576, 2016.

Lee AS et al: Methicillin-resistant *Staphylococcus aureus*. Nat Rev Dis Primers 4:18033:1, 2018.

Thwaites GE et al: Adjunctive rifampicin for *Staphylococcus aureus* bacteraemia (ARREST): A multicentre, randomised, double-blind, placebo-controlled trial. Lancet 391:668, 2018.

Tong SY et al: *Staphylococcus aureus* infections: Epidemiology, pathophysiology, clinical manifestations, and management. Clin Microbiol Rev 28:603, 2015.

148 Streptococcal Infections

Michael R. Wessels

Many varieties of streptococci are found as part of the normal flora colonizing the human respiratory, gastrointestinal, and genitourinary tracts. Several species are important causes of human disease. Group A *Streptococcus* (GAS, *Streptococcus pyogenes*) is responsible for streptococcal pharyngitis, one of the most common bacterial infections of school-age children, and for the postinfectious syndromes of acute rheumatic fever (ARF) and poststreptococcal glomerulonephritis (PSGN). Group B *Streptococcus* (GBS, *Streptococcus agalactiae*) is the leading cause of bacterial sepsis and meningitis in newborns and a major cause of endometritis and fever in parturient women. Viridans streptococci are the most common cause of bacterial endocarditis. Enterococci, which are morphologically similar to streptococci, are now considered a separate genus on the basis of DNA homology studies. Thus, the species previously designated as *Streptococcus faecalis* and *Streptococcus faecium* have been renamed *Enterococcus faecalis* and *Enterococcus faecium*, respectively. **The enterococci are discussed in Chap. 149.**

Streptococci are gram-positive, spherical to ovoid bacteria that characteristically form chains when grown in liquid media. Most streptococci that cause human infections are facultative anaerobes, although some are strict anaerobes. Streptococci are relatively fastidious organisms, requiring enriched media for growth in the laboratory. Clinicians and clinical microbiologists identify streptococci by several classification systems, including hemolytic pattern, Lancefield group, species name, and common or trivial name. Many streptococci associated with human infection produce a zone of complete (β) hemolysis around the bacterial colony when cultured on blood agar. The β-hemolytic streptococci that form large (≥0.5-mm) colonies on blood agar can be classified by the Lancefield system, a serologic grouping based on the reaction of specific antisera with bacterial cell-wall carbohydrate antigens. With rare exceptions, organisms belonging to Lancefield groups A, B, C, and G are all β-hemolytic, and each

TABLE 148-1 Classification of Streptococci

LANCEFIELD GROUP	REPRESENTATIVE SPECIES	HEMOLYTIC PATTERN	TYPICAL INFECTIONS
A	*S. pyogenes*	β	Pharyngitis, impetigo, cellulitis, scarlet fever
B	*S. agalactiae*	β	Neonatal sepsis and meningitis, puerperal infection, urinary tract infection, diabetic ulcer infection, endocarditis
C, G	*S. dysgalactiae* subsp. *equisimilis*	β	Cellulitis, bacteremia, endocarditis
D	Enterococci[a]: *E. faecalis, E. faecium*	Usually nonhemolytic	Urinary tract infection, nosocomial bacteremia, endocarditis
	Nonenterococci: *S. gallolyticus* (formerly *S. bovis*)	Usually nonhemolytic	Bacteremia, endocarditis
Variable or nongroupable	Viridans streptococci: *S. sanguis, S. mitis*	α	Endocarditis, dental abscess, brain abscess
	Intermedius or *milleri* group: *S. intermedius, S. anginosus, S. constellatus*	Variable	Brain abscess, visceral abscess
	Anaerobic streptococci[b]: *Peptostreptococcus magnus*	Usually nonhemolytic	Sinusitis, pneumonia, empyema, brain abscess, liver abscess

[a]See Chap. 149. [b]See Chap. 177.

is associated with characteristic patterns of human infection. Other streptococci produce a zone of partial (α) hemolysis, often imparting a greenish appearance to the agar. These α-hemolytic streptococci are further identified by biochemical testing and include *Streptococcus pneumoniae* (**Chap. 146**), an important cause of pneumonia, meningitis, and other infections, and the several species referred to collectively as the *viridans streptococci,* which are part of the normal oral flora and are important agents of subacute bacterial endocarditis. Finally, some streptococci are nonhemolytic, a pattern sometimes called γ *hemolysis.* Among the organisms classified serologically as group D streptococci, the enterococci are assigned to a distinct genus (**Chap. 149**). The classification of the major streptococcal groups causing human infections is outlined in **Table 148-1**.

GROUP A STREPTOCOCCI

Lancefield group A consists of a single species, *S. pyogenes.* As its species name implies, this organism is associated with a variety of suppurative infections. In addition, GAS can trigger the postinfectious syndromes of ARF (which is uniquely associated with *S. pyogenes* infection; **Chap. 359**) and PSGN (**Chap. 314**).

Worldwide, GAS infections and their postinfectious sequelae (primarily ARF and rheumatic heart disease) account for an estimated 500,000 deaths per year. Although data are incomplete, the incidence of all forms of GAS infection and that of rheumatic heart disease are thought to be tenfold higher in resource-limited countries than in developed countries (**Fig. 148-1**).

PATHOGENESIS

GAS elaborates a number of cell-surface components and extracellular products important in both the pathogenesis of infection and the human immune response. The cell wall contains a carbohydrate antigen that may be released by acid treatment. The reaction of such acid extracts with group A–specific antiserum is the basis for definitive identification of a streptococcal strain as *S. pyogenes.* Rarely, the group A antigen may be present on isolates of *S. dysgalactiae ssp. equisimilis,* which usually express the group C or G antigen (see "Streptococci of Groups C and G," below). The major surface protein of GAS is M protein, which is the basis for the serotyping of strains with specific antisera. The M protein molecules are fibrillar structures anchored in the cell wall of the organism that extend as hairlike projections away from the cell surface. The amino acid sequence of the distal or amino-terminal portion of the M protein molecule is variable, accounting for the antigenic variation of the different M types, while more proximal regions of the protein are relatively conserved. Traditional M-typing by serologic methods has been largely supplanted by a newer technique for assignment of M type to GAS isolates by use of the polymerase chain reaction to amplify the variable region of the *emm* gene, which encodes M protein. DNA sequence analysis of the amplified gene segment can be compared with an extensive database (developed at the Centers for Disease Control and Prevention [CDC]) for assignment of *emm* type. Use of *emm* typing has increased the number of identified *emm* types to more than 200. This method eliminates the need for typing sera, which are available in only a few reference laboratories.

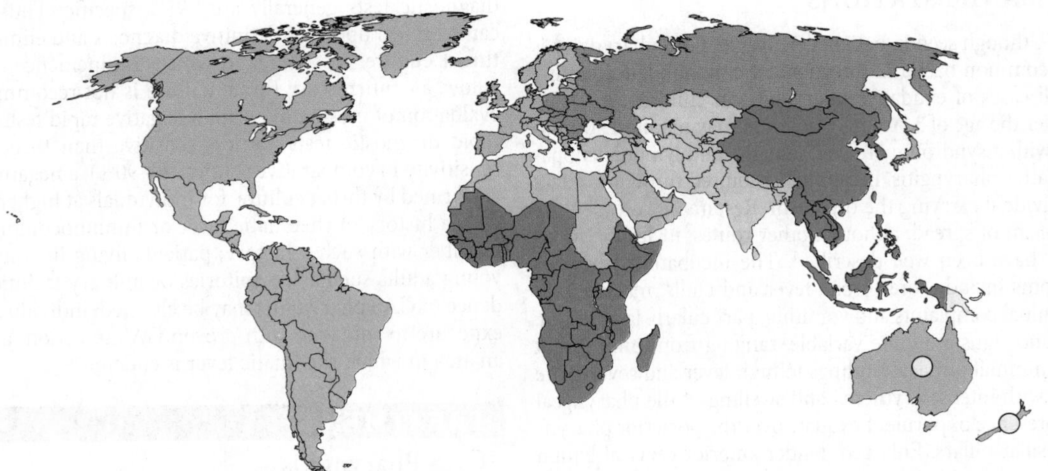

Presence of rheumatic heart disease (cases per 1000)

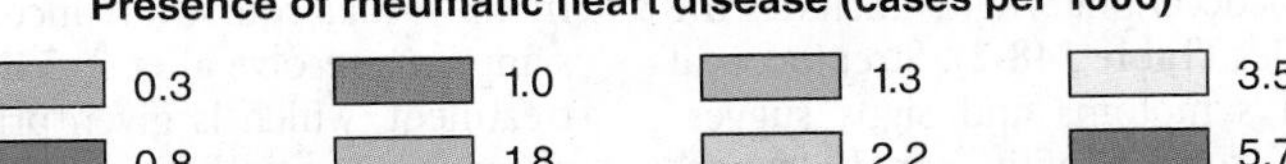

FIGURE 148-1 Prevalence of rheumatic heart disease in children 5–14 years old. The *circles* within Australia and New Zealand represent indigenous populations (and also Pacific Islanders in New Zealand). *(Reproduced with permission from JR Carapetis et al: The global burden of group A streptococcal diseases. Lancet Infect Dis 5:685, 2005.)*

The presence of M protein on a GAS isolate correlates with its capacity to resist phagocytic killing in fresh human blood. This phenomenon appears to be due, at least in part, to the binding of plasma fibrinogen to M protein molecules on the streptococcal surface, which interferes with complement activation and deposition of opsonic complement fragments on the bacterial cell. This resistance to phagocytosis may be overcome by M protein–specific antibodies; thus, individuals with antibodies to a given M type acquired as a result of prior infection are protected against subsequent infection with organisms of the same M type but not against that with different M types.

GAS also elaborates, to varying degrees, a polysaccharide capsule composed of hyaluronic acid. While most clinical isolates of GAS produce a hyaluronic acid capsule, strains of M type 4 or 22 lack a capsule, as do some isolates of M type 89. The fact that acapsular strains have been associated with pharyngitis and invasive infection implies that the capsule is not essential for virulence. The production of large amounts of capsule by certain strains imparts a characteristic mucoid appearance to the colonies. The capsular polysaccharide plays an important role in protecting GAS from ingestion and killing by phagocytes. In contrast to M protein, the hyaluronic acid capsule is a weak immunogen, and antibodies to hyaluronate have not been shown to be important in protective immunity. The presumed explanation is the apparent structural identity between streptococcal hyaluronic acid and the hyaluronic acid of mammalian connective tissues. The capsular polysaccharide may also play a role in GAS colonization of the pharynx by binding to CD44, a hyaluronic acid–binding protein expressed on human pharyngeal epithelial cells.

GAS produces a large number of extracellular products that may be important in local and systemic toxicity and in the spread of infection through tissues. These products include streptolysins S and O, toxins that damage cell membranes and account for the hemolysis produced by the organisms; streptokinase; DNAses; SpyCEP, a serine protease that cleaves and inactivates the chemoattractant cytokine interleukin 8, thereby inhibiting neutrophil recruitment to the site of infection; and several pyrogenic exotoxins. Previously known as erythrogenic toxins, the pyrogenic exotoxins cause the rash of scarlet fever. Since the mid-1980s, pyrogenic exotoxin–producing strains of GAS have been linked to unusually severe invasive infections, including necrotizing fasciitis and the streptococcal toxic shock syndrome (TSS). Several extracellular products stimulate specific antibody responses useful for serodiagnosis of recent streptococcal infection. Tests for antibodies to streptolysin O and DNase B are used most commonly for detection of preceding streptococcal infection in cases of suspected ARF or PSGN.

CLINICAL MANIFESTATIONS

Pharyngitis Although seen in patients of all ages, GAS pharyngitis is one of the most common bacterial infections of childhood, accounting for 20–40% of all cases of exudative pharyngitis in children; it is rare among those under the age of 3. Younger children may manifest streptococcal infection with a syndrome of fever, malaise, and lymphadenopathy without exudative pharyngitis. Infection is acquired through contact with another individual carrying the organism. Respiratory droplets are the usual mechanism of spread, although other routes, including foodborne outbreaks, have been well described. The incubation period is 1–4 days. Symptoms include sore throat, fever and chills, malaise, and sometimes abdominal complaints and vomiting, particularly in children. Both symptoms and signs are quite variable, ranging from mild throat discomfort with minimal physical findings to high fever and severe sore throat associated with intense erythema and swelling of the pharyngeal mucosa and the presence of purulent exudate over the posterior pharyngeal wall and tonsillar pillars. Enlarged, tender anterior cervical lymph nodes commonly accompany exudative pharyngitis.

The differential diagnosis of streptococcal pharyngitis includes the many other bacterial and viral etiologies (**Table 148-2**). Streptococcal infection is an unlikely cause when symptoms and signs suggestive of viral infection are prominent (conjunctivitis, coryza, cough, hoarseness, or discrete ulcerative lesions of the buccal or pharyngeal mucosa). Because of the range of clinical presentations of streptococcal pharyngitis and the large number of other agents that can produce the same clinical picture, diagnosis of streptococcal pharyngitis on clinical grounds alone is not reliable. The throat culture remains the diagnostic gold standard. Culture of a throat specimen that is properly collected (i.e., by vigorous rubbing of a sterile swab over both tonsillar pillars) and properly processed is the most sensitive and specific means of definitive diagnosis. A rapid diagnostic test for latex agglutination or enzyme immunoassay of swab specimens is a useful adjunct to throat culture. While precise figures on sensitivity and specificity vary, rapid diagnostic tests generally are >95% specific. Thus, a positive result can be relied upon for definitive diagnosis and eliminates the need for throat culture. In settings in which the incidence of rheumatic fever is low, a confirmatory throat culture is not recommended for routine evaluation of most adults with a negative rapid test. However, because rapid diagnostic tests are less sensitive than throat culture (relative sensitivity in comparative studies, 70–90%), a negative result should be confirmed by throat culture for individuals at higher risk such as those with a history of rheumatic fever or immunocompromise or a family member with such a history; patients living in congregate settings of young adults such as dormitories or military facilities where the incidence of GAS pharyngitis may be elevated; individuals with household exposure to someone with proven GAS infection; and those living in an area in which rheumatic fever is endemic.

TABLE 148-2 Infectious Etiologies of Acute Pharyngitis

ORGANISM	ASSOCIATED CLINICAL SYNDROME(S)
Viruses	
Rhinovirus	Common cold
Coronavirus	Common cold, COVID-19
Adenovirus	Pharyngoconjunctival fever
Influenza virus	Influenza
Parainfluenza virus	Cold, croup
Coxsackievirus	Herpangina, hand-foot-and-mouth disease
Herpes simplex virus	Gingivostomatitis (primary infection)
Epstein-Barr virus	Infectious mononucleosis
Cytomegalovirus	Mononucleosis-like syndrome
HIV	Acute (primary) infection syndrome
Bacteria	
Group A streptococci	Pharyngitis, scarlet fever
Group C or G streptococci	Pharyngitis
Mixed anaerobes	Vincent's angina
Arcanobacterium haemolyticum	Pharyngitis, scarlatiniform rash
Neisseria gonorrhoeae	Pharyngitis
Treponema pallidum	Secondary syphilis
Francisella tularensis	Pharyngeal tularemia
Corynebacterium diphtheriae	Diphtheria
Yersinia enterocolitica	Pharyngitis, enterocolitis
Yersinia pestis	Plague
Chlamydiae	
Chlamydia pneumoniae	Bronchitis, pneumonia
Chlamydia psittaci	Psittacosis
Mycoplasmas	
Mycoplasma pneumoniae	Bronchitis, pneumonia

TREATMENT

GAS Pharyngitis

In the usual course of uncomplicated streptococcal pharyngitis, symptoms resolve after 3–5 days. The course is shortened little by treatment, which is given primarily to prevent suppurative complications and ARF. Prevention of ARF depends on eradication of the organism from the pharynx, not simply on resolution of symptoms, and requires 10 days of penicillin treatment (**Table 148-3**). A first-generation cephalosporin, such as cephalexin or cefadroxil,

TABLE 148-3 Treatment of Group A Streptococcal Infections

INFECTION	TREATMENT[a]
Pharyngitis	Benzathine penicillin G (1.2 mU IM) *or* penicillin V (250 mg PO tid or 500 mg PO bid) × 10 days
	(Children <27 kg: Benzathine penicillin G [600,000 units IM] *or* penicillin V [250 mg PO bid or tid] × 10 days)
Impetigo	Same as pharyngitis
Erysipelas/cellulitis	Severe: Penicillin G (1–2 mU IV q4h)
	Mild to moderate: Procaine penicillin (1.2 mU IM bid)
Necrotizing fasciitis/ myositis	Surgical debridement *plus* penicillin G (2–4 mU IV q4h) *plus* clindamycin[b] (600–900 mg IV q8h)
Pneumonia/empyema	Penicillin G (2–4 mU IV q4h) *plus* drainage of empyema
Streptococcal toxic shock syndrome	Penicillin G (2–4 mU IV q4h) *plus* clindamycin[b] (600–900 mg IV q8h) *plus* IV immunoglobulin[b] (2 g/kg as a single dose)

[a]Penicillin allergy: A first-generation cephalosporin, such as cephalexin or cefadroxil, may be substituted for penicillin in cases of penicillin allergy if the nature of the allergy is not an immediate hypersensitivity reaction (anaphylaxis or urticaria) or another potentially life-threatening manifestation (e.g., severe rash and fever). Alternative agents for oral therapy are erythromycin (10 mg/kg PO qid, up to a maximum of 250 mg per dose) and azithromycin (a 5-day course at a dose of 12 mg/kg once daily, up to a maximum of 500 mg/d). Vancomycin is an alternative for parenteral therapy. [b]Efficacy unproven, but recommended by several experts. See text for discussion.

may be substituted for penicillin in cases of penicillin allergy if the nature of the allergy is not an immediate hypersensitivity reaction (anaphylaxis or urticaria) or another potentially life-threatening manifestation (e.g., severe rash and fever).

Alternative agents are erythromycin and azithromycin. Azithromycin offers the advantages of better gastrointestinal tolerability, once-daily dosing, and a 5-day treatment course. Resistance to erythromycin and other macrolides is common among isolates from several countries, including Spain, Italy, Finland, Japan, and Korea. Macrolide resistance may be becoming more prevalent elsewhere with the increasing use of this class of antibiotics. In areas with resistance rates exceeding 5–10%, macrolides should be avoided unless results of susceptibility testing are known.

Follow-up culture after treatment is no longer routinely recommended but may be warranted in selected cases, such as those involving patients or families with frequent streptococcal infections or those occurring in situations in which the risk of ARF is thought to be high (e.g., when cases of ARF have recently been reported in the community).

Complications Suppurative complications of streptococcal pharyngitis have become uncommon with the widespread use of antibiotics for most symptomatic cases. These complications result from the spread of infection from the pharyngeal mucosa to deeper tissues by direct extension or by the hematogenous or lymphatic route and may include cervical lymphadenitis, peritonsillar or retropharyngeal abscess, sinusitis, otitis media, meningitis, bacteremia, endocarditis, and pneumonia. Local complications, such as peritonsillar or parapharyngeal abscess formation, should be considered in a patient with unusually severe or prolonged symptoms or localized pain associated with high fever and a toxic appearance. Nonsuppurative complications include ARF (**Chap. 358**) and PSGN (**Chap. 314**), both of which are thought to result from immune responses to streptococcal infection. Penicillin treatment of streptococcal pharyngitis reduces the likelihood of ARF but not that of PSGN.

BACTERIOLOGIC TREATMENT FAILURE AND THE ASYMPTOMATIC CARRIER STATE

Surveillance cultures have shown that up to 20% of individuals in certain populations may have asymptomatic pharyngeal colonization with GAS. There are no definitive guidelines for management of these asymptomatic carriers or of asymptomatic patients who still have a positive throat culture after a full course of treatment for symptomatic pharyngitis. A reasonable course of action is to give a single 10-day course of penicillin for symptomatic pharyngitis and, if positive cultures persist, not to re-treat unless symptoms recur. Studies of the natural history of streptococcal carriage and infection have shown that the risk both of developing ARF and of transmitting infection to others is substantially lower among asymptomatic carriers than among individuals with symptomatic pharyngitis. Therefore, aggressive attempts to eradicate carriage probably are not justified under most circumstances. An exception is the situation in which an asymptomatic carrier is a potential source of infection to others. Outbreaks of food-borne infection and nosocomial puerperal infection have been traced to asymptomatic carriers who may harbor the organisms in the throat, vagina, or anus or on the skin.

TREATMENT

Asymptomatic Pharyngeal Colonization with GAS

When a carrier is transmitting infection to others, attempts to eradicate carriage are warranted. Data are limited on the best regimen to clear GAS after penicillin alone has failed. Regimens reported to have efficacy superior to that of penicillin alone for eradication of carriage include (1) a first-generation cephalosporin such as cephalexin (30 mg/kg; 500 mg maximum) twice daily for 10 days or (2) oral clindamycin (7 mg/kg; 300 mg maximum) three times daily for 10 days. A 10-day course of oral vancomycin (250 mg four times daily) and rifampin (600 mg twice daily) has eradicated rectal colonization. Single-dose azithromycin (20 mg/kg; 1000 mg maximum) has been used for mass prophylaxis/eradication of colonization in outbreak situations.

Scarlet Fever Scarlet fever consists of streptococcal infection, usually pharyngitis, accompanied by a characteristic rash (**Fig. 148-2**). The rash arises from the effects of one of several toxins, currently designated *streptococcal pyrogenic exotoxins* and previously known as *erythrogenic* or *scarlet fever toxins*. In the past, scarlet fever was thought to reflect infection of an individual lacking toxin-specific immunity with a toxin-producing strain of GAS. Susceptibility to scarlet fever was correlated with results of the Dick test, in which a small amount of erythrogenic toxin injected intradermally produced local erythema in susceptible individuals but elicited no reaction in those with specific immunity. Subsequent studies have suggested that development of the scarlet fever rash may reflect a hypersensitivity reaction requiring prior exposure to the toxin. For reasons that are not clear, scarlet fever has become less common in recent years, although large outbreaks have

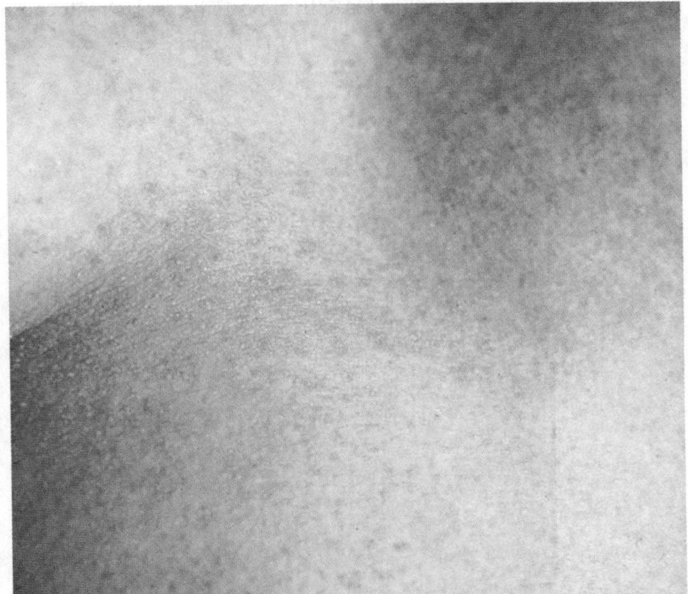

FIGURE 148-2 Scarlet fever exanthem. Finely punctate erythema has become confluent (scarlatiniform); petechiae can occur and have a linear configuration within the exanthem in body folds (Pastia's lines). *(From TB Fitzpatrick, RA Johnson, K Wolff: Color Atlas and Synopsis of Clinical Dermatology, 4th ed, New York, McGraw-Hill, 2001, with permission.)*

occurred recently in China and the United Kingdom. The symptoms of scarlet fever are the same as those of pharyngitis alone. The rash typically begins on the first or second day of illness over the upper trunk, spreading to involve the extremities but sparing the palms and soles. The rash is made up of minute papules, giving a characteristic "sandpaper" feel to the skin. Associated findings include circumoral pallor, "strawberry tongue" (enlarged papillae on a coated tongue, which later may become denuded), and accentuation of the rash in skinfolds (*Pastia's lines*). Subsidence of the rash in 6–9 days is followed after several days by desquamation of the palms and soles. The differential diagnosis of scarlet fever includes other causes of fever and generalized rash, such as measles and other viral exanthems, Kawasaki disease, TSS, and systemic allergic reactions (e.g., drug eruptions).

Skin and Soft Tissue Infections GAS—and occasionally other streptococcal species—can cause a variety of infections involving the skin, subcutaneous tissues, muscles, and fascia. While several clinical syndromes offer a useful means for classification of these infections, not all cases fit exactly into one category. The classic syndromes are general guides to predicting the level of tissue involvement in a particular patient, the probable clinical course, and the likelihood that surgical intervention or aggressive life support will be required.

IMPETIGO (PYODERMA)

Impetigo, a superficial infection of the skin, is caused primarily by GAS and occasionally by other streptococci or *Staphylococcus aureus*. Impetigo is seen most often in young children, tends to occur during warmer months, and is more common in semitropical or tropical climates than in cooler regions. Infection is more common among children living under conditions of poor hygiene. Prospective studies have shown that colonization of unbroken skin with GAS precedes clinical infection. Minor trauma, such as a scratch or an insect bite, may then serve to inoculate organisms into the skin. Impetigo is best prevented, therefore, by attention to adequate hygiene. The usual sites of involvement are the face (particularly around the nose and mouth) and the legs, although lesions may occur at other locations. Individual lesions begin as red papules, which evolve quickly into vesicular and then pustular lesions that break down and coalesce to form characteristic honeycomb-like crusts (**Fig. 148-3**). Lesions generally are not painful, and patients do not appear ill. Fever is not a feature of impetigo and, if present, suggests either infection extending to deeper tissues or another diagnosis. The classic presentation of impetigo usually poses little diagnostic difficulty. Cultures of impetiginous lesions often yield *S. aureus* as well as GAS. In almost all cases, streptococci are isolated initially, and staphylococci appear later, presumably as secondary colonizing flora. In the past, penicillin was nearly always effective against these infections. However, an increasing frequency of penicillin treatment failure suggests that *S. aureus* may have become more prominent as a cause of impetigo. *Bullous impetigo* due to *S. aureus* is distinguished from typical streptococcal infection by more extensive, bullous lesions that break down and leave thin paper-like crusts instead of the thick amber crusts of streptococcal impetigo. Other skin lesions that may be confused with impetigo include herpetic lesions—either those of orolabial herpes simplex or those of chickenpox or zoster. Herpetic lesions can generally be distinguished by their appearance as more discrete, grouped vesicles and by a positive Tzanck test or by herpes simplex virus- or varicella-zoster virus-specific PCR. In difficult cases, cultures of vesicular fluid should yield GAS (or *Staphylococcus aureus*) in impetigo and the responsible virus in herpesvirus infections.

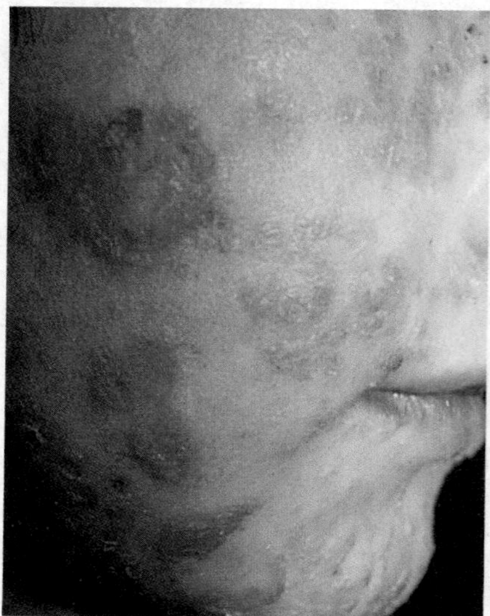

FIGURE 148-3 Impetigo is a superficial streptococcal or *Staphylococcus aureus* infection consisting of honey-colored crusts and erythematous weeping erosions. Occasionally, bullous lesions may be seen. *(Courtesy of Mary Spraker, MD; with permission.)*

TREATMENT

Streptococcal Impetigo

Treatment of streptococcal impetigo is the same as that for streptococcal pharyngitis. In view of evidence that *S. aureus* has become a relatively frequent cause of impetigo, empirical regimens should cover both streptococci and *S. aureus*. For example, either dicloxacillin or cephalexin can be given at a dose of 250 mg four times daily for 10 days. Topical mupirocin ointment also is effective. Culture may be indicated to rule out methicillin-resistant *S. aureus*, especially if the response to empirical treatment is unsatisfactory. In most areas of the world, ARF is not a sequela to streptococcal skin infections, although PSGN may follow either skin or throat infection. The reason for this difference is not known. One hypothesis is that the immune response necessary for development of ARF occurs only after infection of the pharyngeal mucosa. In addition, the strains of GAS that cause pharyngitis are generally of different M protein types than those associated with skin infections; thus the strains that cause pharyngitis may have rheumatogenic potential, while the skin-infecting strains may not. An exception to this general rule may occur among indigenous people in northern Australia and in certain Pacific island groups. Acute rheumatic fever and rheumatic heart disease are prevalent in these populations as is streptococcal impetigo/pyoderma, but not pharyngitis. This epidemiologic pattern has led investigators to suggest that skin infection may trigger acute rheumatic fever in this setting.

CELLULITIS

Inoculation of organisms into the skin may lead to *cellulitis*: infection involving the skin and subcutaneous tissues. The portal of entry may be a traumatic or surgical wound, an insect bite, or any other break in skin integrity. Often, no entry site is apparent. One form of streptococcal cellulitis, *erysipelas*, is characterized by a bright red appearance of the involved skin, which forms a plateau sharply demarcated from surrounding normal skin (**Fig. 148-4**). The lesion is warm to the touch, may be tender, and appears shiny and swollen. The skin often has a *peau d'orange* texture, which is thought to reflect involvement of superficial lymphatics; superficial blebs or bullae may form, usually 2–3 days after onset. The lesion typically develops over a few hours and is associated with fever and chills. Erysipelas tends to occur on the malar area of the face (often with extension over the bridge of the nose to the contralateral malar region) or on the lower extremities. After one episode, recurrence at the same site—sometimes years later—is not uncommon. Classic cases of erysipelas, with typical features, are almost always due to β-hemolytic streptococci, usually GAS and occasionally group C or G. Often, however, the appearance of streptococcal cellulitis is not sufficiently distinctive to permit a specific diagnosis on clinical grounds. The anatomic area involved may not be typical for erysipelas, the lesion may be less intensely red than usual and may fade into surrounding skin, and/or the patient

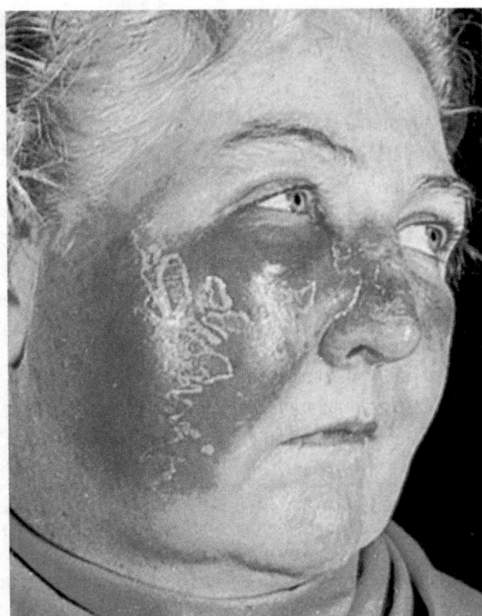

FIGURE 148-4 Erysipelas is a streptococcal infection of the superficial dermis and consists of well-demarcated, erythematous, edematous, warm plaques.

may appear only mildly ill. In such cases, it is prudent to broaden the spectrum of empirical antimicrobial therapy to include other pathogens, particularly *S. aureus*, that can produce cellulitis with the same appearance. Staphylococcal infection should be suspected if cellulitis develops around a wound or an ulcer.

Streptococcal cellulitis tends to develop at anatomic sites in which normal lymphatic drainage has been disrupted, such as sites of prior cellulitis, the arm ipsilateral to a mastectomy and axillary lymph node dissection, a lower extremity previously involved in deep venous thrombosis or chronic lymphedema, or the leg from which a saphenous vein has been harvested for coronary artery bypass grafting. The organism may enter via a dermal breach some distance from the eventual site of clinical cellulitis. For example, some patients with recurrent leg cellulitis following saphenous vein removal stop having recurrent episodes only after treatment of tinea pedis on the affected extremity. Fissures in the skin presumably serve as a portal of entry for streptococci, which then produce infection more proximally in the leg at the site of previous injury. Streptococcal cellulitis may also involve recent surgical wounds. GAS is among the few bacterial pathogens that typically produce signs of wound infection and surrounding cellulitis within the first 24 h after surgery. These wound infections are usually associated with a thin exudate and may spread rapidly, either as cellulitis in the skin and subcutaneous tissue or as a deeper tissue infection (see below). Streptococcal wound infection or localized cellulitis may also be associated with *lymphangitis*, manifested by red streaks extending proximally along superficial lymphatics from the infection site.

TREATMENT
Streptococcal Cellulitis

See Table 148-3 and **Chap. 129.**

DEEP SOFT-TISSUE INFECTIONS

Necrotizing fasciitis (*hemolytic streptococcal gangrene*) involves the superficial and/or deep fascia investing the muscles of an extremity or the trunk. The source of the infection is either the skin, with organisms introduced into tissue through trauma (sometimes trivial), or the bowel flora, with organisms released during abdominal surgery or from an occult enteric source, such as a diverticular or appendiceal abscess. The inoculation site may be inapparent and is often some distance from the site of clinical involvement; e.g., the introduction of organisms via minor trauma to the hand may be associated with clinical infection of the tissues overlying the shoulder or chest. Cases associated with the bowel flora are usually polymicrobial, involving a mixture of anaerobic bacteria (such as *Bacteroides fragilis* or anaerobic streptococci) and facultative organisms (usually gram-negative bacilli). Cases unrelated to contamination from bowel organisms are most commonly caused by GAS alone or in combination with other organisms (most often *S. aureus*). Overall, GAS is implicated in ~60% of cases of necrotizing fasciitis. The onset of symptoms is usually quite acute and is marked by severe pain at the site of involvement, malaise, fever, chills, and a toxic appearance. The physical findings, particularly early on, may not be striking, with only minimal erythema of the overlying skin. Pain and tenderness are usually severe. In contrast, in more superficial cellulitis, the skin appearance is more abnormal, but pain and tenderness are only mild or moderate. As the infection progresses (often over several hours), the severity and extent of symptoms worsen, and skin changes become more evident, with the appearance of dusky or mottled erythema and edema. The marked tenderness of the involved area may evolve into anesthesia as the spreading inflammatory process produces infarction of cutaneous nerves.

Although myositis is more commonly due to *S. aureus* infection, GAS occasionally produces abscesses in skeletal muscles (*streptococcal myositis*), with little or no involvement of the surrounding fascia or overlying skin. The presentation is usually subacute, but a fulminant form has been described in association with severe systemic toxicity, bacteremia, and a high mortality rate. The fulminant form may reflect the same basic disease process seen in necrotizing fasciitis, but with the necrotizing inflammatory process extending into the muscles themselves rather than remaining limited to the fascial layers.

TREATMENT
Deep Soft-Tissue Streptococcal Infections

Once necrotizing fasciitis is suspected, early surgical exploration is both diagnostically and therapeutically indicated. Surgery reveals necrosis and inflammatory fluid tracking along the fascial planes above and between muscle groups, without involvement of the muscles themselves. The process usually extends beyond the area of clinical involvement, and extensive debridement is required. Drainage and debridement are central to the management of necrotizing fasciitis; antibiotic treatment is a useful adjunct (Table 148-3), but surgery is life-saving. Treatment for streptococcal myositis consists of surgical drainage—usually by an open procedure that permits evaluation of the extent of infection and ensures adequate debridement of involved tissues—and high-dose penicillin (Table 148-3).

Pneumonia and Empyema GAS is an occasional cause of pneumonia, generally in previously healthy individuals. The onset of symptoms may be abrupt or gradual. Pleuritic chest pain, fever, chills, and dyspnea are the characteristic manifestations. Cough is usually present but may not be prominent. Approximately one-half of patients with GAS pneumonia have an accompanying pleural effusion. In contrast to the sterile parapneumonic effusions typical of pneumococcal pneumonia, those complicating streptococcal pneumonia are almost always infected. The empyema fluid is usually visible by chest radiography on initial presentation, and its volume may increase rapidly. These pleural collections should be drained early, as they tend to become loculated rapidly, resulting in a chronic fibrotic reaction that may require thoracotomy for removal.

Bacteremia, Puerperal Sepsis, and Streptococcal Toxic Shock Syndrome In adults, GAS bacteremia is usually associated with an identifiable local infection, whereas children may have bacteremia without an associated focal infection. Bacteremia occurs rarely with otherwise uncomplicated pharyngitis, occasionally with cellulitis or pneumonia, and relatively frequently with necrotizing fasciitis. Bacteremia without an identified source raises the possibility of endocarditis, an occult abscess, or osteomyelitis. A variety of focal infections may arise secondarily from streptococcal bacteremia, including endocarditis, meningitis, septic arthritis, osteomyelitis, peritonitis, and visceral abscesses. GAS is occasionally implicated in infectious complications of childbirth, usually endometritis and associated bacteremia. In the preantibiotic era, puerperal sepsis was commonly caused by GAS; currently, it is more often caused by GBS. Several nosocomial outbreaks of puerperal GAS infection have been traced to an asymptomatic carrier, usually someone present at delivery. The site of carriage may be the skin, throat, anus, or vagina.

Beginning in the late 1980s, several reports described patients with GAS infections associated with shock and multisystem organ failure. This syndrome was called *streptococcal toxic shock syndrome* (*TSS*) because it shares certain features with staphylococcal TSS. In 1993, a case definition for streptococcal TSS was formulated **(Table 148-4)**. The general features of the illness include fever, hypotension, renal impairment, and respiratory distress syndrome. Various types of rash have been described, but rash usually does not develop. Laboratory abnormalities include a marked shift to the left in the white blood cell differential, with many immature granulocytes; hypocalcemia; hypoalbuminemia; and thrombocytopenia, which usually becomes more pronounced on the second or third day of illness. In contrast to patients with staphylococcal TSS, the majority with streptococcal TSS are bacteremic. The most common associated infection is a soft tissue infection—necrotizing fasciitis, myositis, or cellulitis—although a variety of other associated local infections have been described, including pneumonia, peritonitis, osteomyelitis, and myometritis. Streptococcal TSS is associated with a mortality rate of ≥30%, with most deaths secondary to shock and respiratory failure. Because of its rapidly progressive and lethal course, early recognition of the syndrome is essential. Patients should receive aggressive supportive care (fluid resuscitation, pressors, and mechanical ventilation) in addition to antimicrobial therapy and, in cases associated with necrotizing fasciitis, should undergo surgical debridement. Exactly why certain patients develop this fulminant syndrome is not known. Early studies of the streptococcal strains isolated from these patients demonstrated a strong association with the production of pyrogenic exotoxin A. This association has been inconsistent in subsequent case series. Pyrogenic exotoxin A and several other streptococcal exotoxins act as superantigens to trigger release of inflammatory cytokines from T lymphocytes. Fever, shock, and organ dysfunction in streptococcal TSS may reflect, in part, the systemic effects of superantigen-mediated cytokine release.

TREATMENT

Streptococcal Toxic Shock Syndrome

In light of the possible role of pyrogenic exotoxins or other streptococcal toxins in streptococcal TSS, treatment with clindamycin has been advocated by some authorities (Table 148-3), who argue that, through its direct action on protein synthesis, clindamycin is more effective in rapidly terminating toxin production than is penicillin—a cell-wall agent. Support for this view comes from studies of an experimental model of streptococcal myositis, in which mice given clindamycin had a higher rate of survival than those given penicillin. Comparable data on the treatment of human infections are not available, although retrospective analysis has suggested a better outcome when patients with invasive soft-tissue infection are treated with clindamycin rather than with cell wall–active antibiotics. Although clindamycin resistance in GAS is uncommon among U.S. isolates (<2%), resistance rates as high as 23% have been documented in Finland. Thus, if clindamycin is used for initial treatment of a critically ill patient, penicillin should be given as well until the antibiotic susceptibility of the streptococcal isolate is known. IV immunoglobulin has been used as adjunctive therapy for streptococcal TSS (Table 148-3). Pooled immunoglobulin preparations contain antibodies capable of neutralizing the effects of streptococcal toxins. Anecdotal reports and case series have suggested favorable clinical responses to IV immunoglobulin, but no adequately powered, prospective, controlled trials have been reported. A meta-analysis of five studies of streptococcal TSS patients treated with clindamycin found that IVIG use was associated with a reduction in mortality rate from 33.7% to 15.7%.

TABLE 148-4 Proposed Case Definition for Streptococcal Toxic Shock Syndrome[a]

I. Isolation of group A streptococci (*Streptococcus pyogenes*)
   A. From a normally sterile site
   B. From a nonsterile site
II. Clinical signs of severity
   A. Hypotension *and*
   B. ≥2 of the following signs
      1. Renal impairment
      2. Coagulopathy
      3. Liver function impairment
      4. Adult respiratory distress syndrome
      5. A generalized erythematous macular rash that may desquamate
      6. Soft tissue necrosis, including necrotizing fasciitis or myositis; *or* gangrene

[a]An illness fulfilling criteria IA, IIA, and IIB is defined as a *definite* case. An illness fulfilling criteria IB, IIA, and IIB is defined as a *probable* case if no other etiology for the illness is identified.

Source: Modified from Working Group on Severe Streptococcal Infections: JAMA 269:390, 1993.

PREVENTION

No vaccine against GAS is commercially available. A formulation that consists of recombinant peptides containing epitopes of 26 M-protein types has undergone phase 1 and 2 testing in volunteers. Early results indicate that the vaccine is well tolerated and elicits type-specific antibody responses. Vaccines based on a conserved region of M protein or on a mixture of other conserved GAS protein antigens are in earlier stages of development.

Household contacts of individuals with invasive GAS infection (e.g., bacteremia, necrotizing fasciitis, or streptococcal TSS) are at greater risk of invasive infection than the general population. Asymptomatic pharyngeal colonization with GAS has been detected in up to 25% of persons with >4 h/d of same-room exposure to an index case. However, the CDC does not recommend antibiotic prophylaxis routinely for contacts of patients with invasive disease because such an approach (if effective) would require treatment of hundreds of contacts to prevent a single case. Prophylaxis may be considered for contacts of unusually severe cases or for individuals at increased risk for invasive infection.

STREPTOCOCCI OF GROUPS C AND G

Group C and group G streptococci are β-hemolytic bacteria that occasionally cause human infections similar to those caused by GAS. Strains that form small colonies on blood agar (<0.5 mm) are generally members of the *Streptococcus milleri* group (*Streptococcus intermedius, Streptococcus anginosus*; see "Viridans Streptococci," below). Large-colony group C and G streptococci of human origin are now considered a single species, *Streptococcus dysgalactiae* subspecies *equisimilis*. These organisms have been associated with pharyngitis, cellulitis and soft tissue infections, pneumonia, bacteremia, endocarditis, and septic arthritis. Puerperal sepsis, meningitis, epidural abscess, intraabdominal abscess, urinary tract infection, and neonatal sepsis also have been reported. Group C or G streptococcal bacteremia most often affects elderly or chronically ill patients and, in the absence of obvious local infection, is likely to reflect endocarditis. Septic arthritis, sometimes involving multiple joints, may complicate endocarditis or develop in its absence. Distinct streptococcal species of Lancefield group C cause infections in domesticated animals, especially horses and cattle; some human infections are acquired through contact with animals or consumption of unpasteurized milk. These zoonotic organisms include *Streptococcus equi* subspecies *zooepidemicus* and *S. equi* subspecies *equi*.

TREATMENT

Group C or G Streptococcal Infection

Penicillin is the drug of choice for treatment of group C or G streptococcal infections. Antibiotic treatment is the same as for similar syndromes due to GAS (Table 148-3). Patients with bacteremia or septic arthritis should receive IV penicillin (2–4 mU every 4 h). All group C and G streptococci are sensitive to penicillin; nearly all are inhibited in vitro by concentrations of ≤0.03 μg/mL. Occasional isolates exhibit tolerance: although inhibited by low concentrations of penicillin, they are killed only by significantly higher concentrations. The clinical significance of tolerance is unknown. Because of the poor clinical response of some patients to penicillin alone, the addition of gentamicin (1 mg/kg every 8 h for patients with normal renal function) is recommended by some authorities for treatment of endocarditis or septic arthritis due to group C or G streptococci; however, combination therapy has not been shown to be superior to penicillin treatment alone. Patients with joint infections often require repeated aspiration or open drainage and debridement for cure; the response to treatment may be slow, particularly in debilitated patients and those with involvement of multiple joints. Infection of prosthetic joints almost always requires prosthesis removal in addition to antibiotic therapy.

GROUP B STREPTOCOCCI

Identified first as a cause of mastitis in cows, streptococci belonging to Lancefield group B have since been recognized as a major cause of sepsis and meningitis in human neonates. GBS is also a frequent cause of peripartum fever in women and an occasional cause of serious infection in nonpregnant adults. Since the widespread institution of prenatal screening for GBS in the 1990s, the incidence of neonatal infection per 1000 live births has fallen from ~2–3 cases to ~0.6 case. During the same period, GBS infection in adults with underlying chronic illnesses has become more common; adults now account for a larger proportion of invasive GBS infections than do newborns. Lancefield group B consists of a single species, *S. agalactiae*, which is definitively identified with specific antiserum to the group B cell wall–associated carbohydrate antigen. A streptococcal isolate can be classified presumptively as GBS on the basis of biochemical tests, including hydrolysis of sodium hippurate (in which 99% of isolates are positive), hydrolysis of bile esculin (in which 99–100% are negative), bacitracin susceptibility (in which 92% are resistant), and production of CAMP factor (in which 98–100% are positive). CAMP factor is a phospholipase produced by GBS that causes synergistic hemolysis with β lysin produced by certain strains of *S. aureus*. Its presence can be demonstrated by cross-streaking of the test isolate and an appropriate staphylococcal strain on a blood agar plate. GBS organisms causing human infections are encapsulated by one of ten antigenically distinct polysaccharides. The capsular polysaccharide is an important virulence factor. Antibodies to the capsular polysaccharide afford protection against GBS of the same (but not of a different) capsular type.

INFECTION IN NEONATES

Two general types of GBS infection in infants are defined by the age of the patient at presentation. *Early-onset infections* occur within the first week of life, with a median age of 20 h at onset. Approximately half of these infants have signs of GBS disease at birth. The infection is acquired during or shortly before birth from the colonized maternal genital tract. Surveillance studies have shown that 5–40% of women are vaginal or rectal carriers of GBS. Approximately 50% of infants delivered vaginally by carrier mothers become colonized, although only 1–2% develop clinically evident infection. Prematurity, prolonged labor, obstetric complications, and maternal fever are risk factors for early-onset infection. The presentation of early-onset infection is the same as that of other forms of neonatal sepsis. Typical findings include respiratory distress, lethargy, and hypotension. Essentially all infants with early-onset disease are bacteremic, one-third to one-half have pneumonia and/or respiratory distress syndrome, and one-third have meningitis.

Late-onset infections occur in infants 1 week to 3 months old and, in rare instances, in older infants (mean age at onset, 3–4 weeks). The infecting organism may be acquired during delivery (as in early-onset cases) or during later contact with a colonized mother, nursery personnel, or another source. Meningitis is the most common manifestation of late-onset infection and in most cases is associated with a strain of capsular type III. Infants present with fever, lethargy or irritability, poor feeding, and seizures. The various other types of late-onset infection include bacteremia without an identified source, osteomyelitis, septic arthritis, and facial cellulitis associated with submandibular or preauricular adenitis.

TREATMENT

Group B Streptococcal Infection in Neonates

Penicillin is the agent of choice for all GBS infections. Empirical broad-spectrum therapy for suspected bacterial sepsis, consisting of ampicillin and gentamicin, is generally administered until culture results become available. If cultures yield GBS, many pediatricians continue to administer gentamicin, along with ampicillin or penicillin, for a few days until clinical improvement becomes evident. Infants with bacteremia or soft tissue infection should receive penicillin at a dosage of 200,000 units/kg per day in divided doses. For meningitis, infants ≤7 days of age should receive 250,000–450,000 units/kg per day in three divided doses; infants >7 days of age should receive 450,000–500,000 units/kg per day in four divided doses. Meningitis should be treated for at least 14 days because of the risk of relapse with shorter courses.

Prevention The incidence of GBS infection is unusually high among infants of women with risk factors: preterm delivery, early rupture of membranes (>24 h before delivery), prolonged labor, fever, or chorioamnionitis. Because the usual source of the organisms infecting a neonate is the mother's birth canal, efforts have been made to prevent GBS infections by the identification of high-risk carrier mothers and their treatment with various forms of antibiotic prophylaxis or immunoprophylaxis. Prophylactic administration of ampicillin or penicillin to such patients during delivery reduces the risk of infection in the newborn. This approach has been hampered by logistical difficulties in identifying colonized women before delivery; the results of vaginal cultures early in pregnancy are poor predictors of carrier status at delivery. The CDC recommends screening for anogenital colonization at 35–37 weeks of pregnancy by a swab culture of the lower vagina and anorectum; intrapartum chemoprophylaxis is recommended for culture-positive women and for women who, regardless of culture status, have previously given birth to an infant with GBS infection or have a history of GBS bacteriuria during pregnancy. Women whose culture status is unknown and who develop premature labor (<37 weeks), prolonged rupture of membranes (>18 h), or intrapartum fever or who have a positive intrapartum nucleic acid amplification test for GBS also should receive intrapartum chemoprophylaxis. The recommended regimen for chemoprophylaxis is a loading dose of 5 million units of penicillin G followed by 2.5 million units every 4 h until delivery. Cefazolin is an alternative for women with a history of penicillin allergy who are thought not to be at high risk for anaphylaxis. For women with a history of immediate hypersensitivity, clindamycin may be substituted, but only if the colonizing isolate has been demonstrated to be susceptible. If susceptibility testing results are not available or indicate resistance, vancomycin should be used in this situation.

Treatment of all pregnant women who are colonized or have risk factors for neonatal infection will result in exposure of up to one-third of pregnant women and newborns to antibiotics, with the attendant risks of allergic reactions and selection for resistant organisms. Although still in the developmental stages, a GBS vaccine may ultimately offer a better solution to prevention. Because transplacental passage of maternal antibodies produces protective antibody levels in newborns, efforts are underway to develop a vaccine against GBS that can be given to childbearing-age women before or during pregnancy. Results of phase 1 clinical trials of GBS capsular polysaccharide–protein conjugate vaccines suggest that a multivalent conjugate vaccine would be safe and highly immunogenic.

INFECTION IN ADULTS

The majority of GBS infections in otherwise healthy adults are related to pregnancy and parturition. Peripartum fever, the most common manifestation, is sometimes accompanied by symptoms and signs of endometritis or chorioamnionitis (abdominal distention and uterine or adnexal tenderness). Blood and vaginal swab cultures are often positive. Bacteremia is usually transitory but occasionally results in meningitis or endocarditis. Infections in adults that are not associated with the peripartum period generally involve individuals who are elderly or have an underlying chronic illness, such as diabetes mellitus or a malignancy. Among the infections that develop with some frequency in adults are cellulitis and soft tissue infection (including infected diabetic skin ulcers), urinary tract infection, pneumonia, endocarditis, and septic arthritis. Other reported infections include meningitis, osteomyelitis, and intraabdominal or pelvic abscesses. Relapse or recurrence of invasive infection weeks to months after a first episode is documented in ~4% of cases.

TREATMENT
Group B Streptococcal Infection in Adults

GBS is less sensitive to penicillin than GAS, requiring somewhat higher doses. Adults with serious localized infections (pneumonia, pyelonephritis, abscess) should receive doses of ~12 million units of penicillin G daily; patients with endocarditis or meningitis should receive 18–24 million units per day in divided doses. Vancomycin is an acceptable alternative for penicillin-allergic patients.

NONENTEROCOCCAL GROUP D STREPTOCOCCI

The main nonenterococcal group D streptococci that cause human infections were previously considered a single species, *Streptococcus bovis*. The organisms encompassed by *S. bovis* have been reclassified into two species, each of which has two subspecies: *Streptococcus gallolyticus* subspecies *gallolyticus*, *S. gallolyticus* subspecies *pasteurianus*, *Streptococcus infantarius* subspecies *infantarius*, and *S. infantarius* subspecies *coli*. Endocarditis caused by these organisms is often associated with neoplasms of the gastrointestinal tract—most frequently, a colon carcinoma or polyp—but is also reported in association with other bowel lesions. When occult gastrointestinal lesions are carefully sought, abnormalities are found in >60% of patients with endocarditis due to *S. gallolyticus* or *S. infantarius*. In contrast to the enterococci, nonenterococcal group D streptococci like these organisms are reliably killed by penicillin as a single agent, and penicillin is the agent of choice for the infections they cause.

VIRIDANS AND OTHER STREPTOCOCCI

VIRIDANS STREPTOCOCCI

Consisting of multiple species of α-hemolytic streptococci, the viridans streptococci are a heterogeneous group of organisms that are important agents of bacterial endocarditis (**Chap. 128**). Several species of viridans streptococci, including *Streptococcus salivarius*, *Streptococcus mitis*, *Streptococcus sanguis*, and *Streptococcus mutans*, are part of the normal flora of the mouth, where they live in close association with the teeth and gingiva. Some species contribute to the development of dental caries.

Previously known as *Streptococcus morbillorum*, *Gemella morbillorum* has been placed in a separate genus, along with *Gemella haemolysans*, on the basis of genetic-relatedness studies. These species resemble viridans streptococci with respect to habitat in the human host and associated infections.

The transient viridans streptococcal bacteremia induced by eating, toothbrushing, flossing, and other sources of minor trauma, together with adherence to biologic surfaces, is thought to account for the predilection of these organisms to cause endocarditis (**see Fig. 128-1**). Viridans streptococci are also isolated, often as part of a mixed flora, from sites of sinusitis, brain abscess, and liver abscess.

Viridans streptococcal bacteremia occurs relatively frequently in neutropenic patients, particularly after bone marrow transplantation or high-dose chemotherapy for cancer. Some of these patients develop a sepsis syndrome with high fever and shock. Risk factors for viridans streptococcal bacteremia include chemotherapy with high-dose cytosine arabinoside, prior treatment with trimethoprim-sulfamethoxazole or a fluoroquinolone, treatment with antacids or histamine antagonists, mucositis, and profound neutropenia.

The *S. milleri* group (also referred to as the *S. intermedius* or *S. anginosus* group) includes three species that cause human disease: *S. intermedius*, *S. anginosus*, and *Streptococcus constellatus*. These organisms are often considered viridans streptococci, although they differ somewhat from other viridans streptococci in both their hemolytic pattern (they may be α-, β-, or nonhemolytic) and the disease syndromes they cause. This group commonly produces suppurative infections, particularly abscesses of brain and abdominal viscera, and infections related to the oral cavity or respiratory tract, such as peritonsillar abscess, lung abscess, and empyema.

TREATMENT
Infection with Viridans Streptococci

Isolates from neutropenic patients with bacteremia are often resistant to penicillin; thus these patients should be treated presumptively with vancomycin until the results of susceptibility testing become available. Viridans streptococci isolated in other clinical settings usually are sensitive to penicillin. Susceptibility testing should be performed to guide treatment of serious infections.

ABIOTROPHIA AND *GRANULICATELLA* SPECIES (NUTRITIONALLY VARIANT STREPTOCOCCI)

Occasional isolates cultured from the blood of patients with endocarditis fail to grow when subcultured on solid media. These *nutritionally variant streptococci* require supplemental thiol compounds or active forms of vitamin B_6 (pyridoxal or pyridoxamine) for growth in the laboratory. The nutritionally variant streptococci are generally grouped with the viridans streptococci because they cause similar types of infections. However, they have been reclassified on the basis of 16S ribosomal RNA sequence comparisons into two separate genera: *Abiotrophia*, with a single species (*Abiotrophia defectiva*), and *Granulicatella*, with three species associated with human infection (*Granulicatella adiacens*, *Granulicatella para-adiacens*, and *Granulicatella elegans*).

TREATMENT
Infection with Nutritionally Variant Streptococci

Treatment failure and relapse appear to be more common in cases of endocarditis due to nutritionally variant streptococci than in those due to the usual viridans streptococci. Thus, the addition of gentamicin (1 mg/kg every 8 h for patients with normal renal function) to the penicillin regimen is recommended for endocarditis due to the nutritionally variant organisms.

OTHER STREPTOCOCCI

Streptococcus suis is an important pathogen in swine and has been reported to cause meningitis in humans, usually in individuals with occupational exposure to pigs. *S. suis* has been reported to be the most common cause of bacterial meningitis in Vietnam, and it has been responsible for outbreaks in China. Strains of *S. suis* associated with human infections have generally reacted with Lancefield group R typing serum and sometimes with group D typing serum as well. Isolates may be α- or β-hemolytic and are sensitive to penicillin. *Streptococcus iniae*, a pathogen of fish, has been associated with infections in humans who have handled live or freshly killed fish. Cellulitis of the hand is the most common form of human infection, although bacteremia and endocarditis have been reported. *Anaerobic streptococci*, or peptostreptococci, are part of the normal flora of the oral cavity, bowel, and vagina. **Infections caused by the anaerobic streptococci are discussed in Chap. 177.**

■ FURTHER READING

Bruckner L, Gigliotti F: Viridans group streptococcal infections among children with cancer and the importance of emerging antibiotic resistance. Semin Pediatr Infect Dis 17:153, 2006.

Parks T et al: Polyspecific intravenous immunoglobulin in clindamycin-treated patients with streptococcal toxic shock syndrome: A systematic review and meta-analysis. Clin Infect Dis 67:1434, 2018.

Raabe V, Shane A: Group B *Streptococcus* (*Streptococcus agalactiae*), in *Gram-Positive Pathogens*, 3rd ed, Fischetti V et al (eds). Washington, DC, ASM Press, 2019, pp 228–238.

Shulman ST et al: Clinical practice guideline for the diagnosis and management of group A streptococcal pharyngitis: 2012 update by the Infectious Diseases Society of America. Clin Infect Dis 55:1279, 2012.

Stevens DL, Bryant AE: Necrotizing soft tissue infections. N Engl J Med 377:2253, 2017.

149 Enterococcal Infections

William R. Miller, Cesar A. Arias, Barbara E. Murray

Enterococci have been recognized as potential human pathogens for well over a century, but only in recent years have these organisms acquired prominence as important causes of nosocomial infections. The ability of enterococci to survive and/or disseminate in the hospital environment and to acquire antibiotic resistance determinants makes the treatment of some enterococcal infections in critically ill patients a difficult challenge. Enterococci were first mentioned in the French literature in 1899; the "entérocoque" was found in the human gastrointestinal tract. The first pathologic description of an enterococcal infection dates to the same year. A clinical isolate from a patient who died as a consequence of endocarditis was initially designated *Micrococcus zymogenes*, was later named *Streptococcus faecalis* subspecies *zymogenes*, and would now be classified as *Enterococcus faecalis*. The ability of this isolate to cause severe disease in both rabbits and mice illustrated its potential lethality in the appropriate settings.

■ MICROBIOLOGY AND TAXONOMY

Enterococci are gram-positive organisms. In clinical specimens, they are usually observed as single cells, diplococci, or short chains **(Fig. 149-1)**, although long chains are noted with some strains. Enterococci were originally classified as streptococci because organisms of the two genera share many morphologic and phenotypic characteristics, including a generally negative catalase reaction. Only DNA hybridization studies and later 16S rRNA sequencing clearly demonstrated that enterococci should be grouped as a genus distinct from the streptococci. Unlike the majority of streptococci, enterococci hydrolyze esculin in the presence of 40% bile salts and grow at high salt concentrations (e.g., 6.5%) and at high temperatures (46°C). Enterococci are usually reported by the clinical laboratory to be nonhemolytic on the basis of their inability to lyse the ovine or bovine red blood cells (RBCs) commonly used in agar plates; however, some strains of *E. faecalis* do lyse RBCs from humans, horses, and rabbits due to the presence of an acquired hemolysin/cytolysin gene. The majority of clinically relevant enterococcal species hydrolyze pyrrolidonyl-β-naphthylamide (PYR); this characteristic is helpful in differentiating enterococci from organisms of the *Streptococcus gallolyticus* group (formerly known as *S. bovis*, which includes

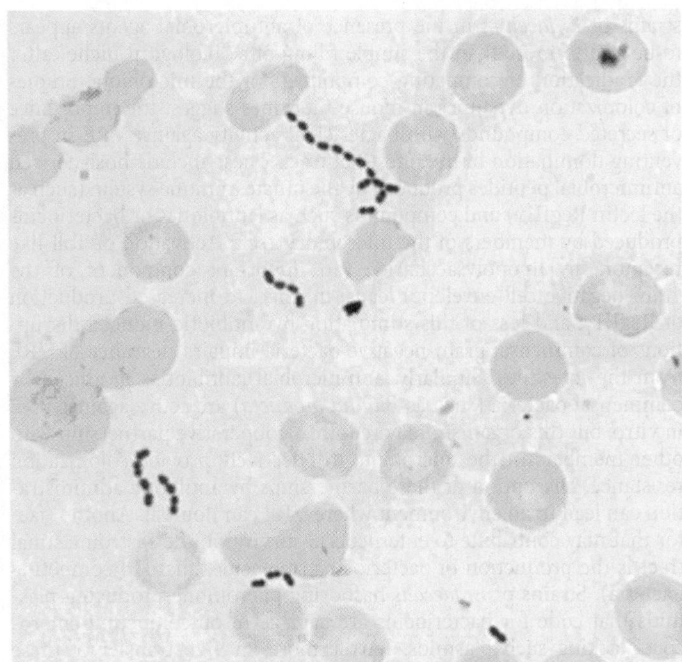

FIGURE 149-1 Gram's stain of cultured blood from a patient with enterococcal bacteremia. Oval gram-positive bacterial cells are arranged as diplococci and short chains. *(Courtesy of Audrey Wanger, PhD.)*

S. gallolyticus, *S. pasteurianus*, and *S. infantarius*) and from *Leuconostoc* species. Although many species of enterococci have been isolated from human infections, the overwhelming majority of cases are caused by two species, *E. faecalis* and *E. faecium*. Less frequently isolated species include *Enterococcus gallinarum*, *E. durans*, *E. hirae*, and *E. avium*.

■ PATHOGENESIS

Enterococci are normal inhabitants of the large bowel of human adults, although they usually make up <1% of the culturable intestinal microbiota. In the healthy human host, enterococci are typical symbionts that coexist with other gastrointestinal bacteria; in fact, the utility of certain enterococcal strains as probiotics in the treatment of diarrhea suggests their possible role in maintaining the homeostatic equilibrium of the bowel. These commensals play a role in *colonization resistance*, or the ability of a healthy gastrointestinal microbiota to impede the establishment of a population of drug-resistant bacteria such as vancomycin-resistant enterococci (VRE). Colonization resistance arises from a complex set of metabolic and immunologic interactions between the host, pathogen, and intestinal microbiota, many of which are disrupted in hospitalized or chronically ill patients.

Several studies have shown that a higher level of gastrointestinal colonization is a critical factor in the pathogenesis of enterococcal infections. However, the mechanisms by which enterococci successfully colonize the bowel and gain access to the lymphatics and/or bloodstream remain incompletely understood. Physical factors, such as stomach pH and the mucin layer on the interior of the intestinal lumen, provide a barrier and limit pathogen access to the intestinal epithelium. In the hospital setting, administration of medications that suppress stomach acid secretion, or degradation of the mucin layer by gut commensals during periods of decreased oral intake, can disrupt these protective layers.

One of the most important factors that promotes increased gastrointestinal colonization by enterococci is the administration of antimicrobial agents since enterococci are intrinsically resistant to a variety of commonly used antibacterial drugs. In particular, antibiotics that are excreted in the bile and have broad-spectrum activity (e.g., certain cephalosporins that target gram-negative bacteria or anaerobes) are usually associated with the recovery of higher numbers of enterococci from feces. However, the increased colonization by hospital-associated strains of *E. faecium* in the presence of antimicrobial agents appears to be due to more than the simple filling of a "biological niche" after the eradication of competing components of the microbiota. Studies of colonization dynamics in mouse intestines suggest the importance of secreted compounds with bactericidal activity against VRE in preventing domination of the intestinal tract. These include host-derived antimicrobial peptides produced by the innate immune system (such as the lectin RegIIIγ) and compounds such as lantibiotics or bacteriocins produced by members of the microbiota itself. Activation of Toll-like receptors by lipopolysaccharide (an important component of the gram-negative cell envelope) leads, in mice, to increased production of RegIIIγ, and loss of this stimulation by antibiotic-induced disruptions of commensal gram-negative bacteria impairs clearance of VRE from the intestines. Similarly, antimicrobial lantibiotics produced by commensal bacteria (such as *Blautia producta*) are active against VRE in vitro, but this organism may require a cooperative partnership with other members of the microbiota to effectively provide colonization resistance. Disruption of these partnerships by antibiotic administration can lead to an environment where VRE can flourish. Another factor that may contribute to enterococcal survival in the gastrointestinal tract is the production of bacteriocins (molecules that kill competing bacteria). Strains of *E. faecalis* harboring pheromone-producing plasmids that code for bacteriocins are capable of outcompeting enterococci lacking such plasmids. Furthermore, in vivo transfer of these plasmids occurs by conjugation, enhancing the survival of the recipients. In the absence of antibiotics, hospital-associated lineages of *E. faecium* seem to be less adapted for survival in the gastrointestinal tract than are commensal *E. faecium* strains. Studies examining the rate of carriage of VRE in patients after discharge from the hospital document a median time to clearance between 2 and 4 months in patients without ongoing risk factors, such as continued antibiotic use, residence in a long-term care facility, or need for hemodialysis.

Several vertebrate, worm, and insect models have been developed to study the role of possible pathogenic determinants in both *E. faecalis* and *E. faecium*. Three main groups of virulence factors may increase the ability of enterococci to colonize the gastrointestinal tract and/or cause disease. The first group, *enterococcal secreted factors*, are molecules released outside the bacterial cell that contribute to the process of infection. The best studied of these molecules include enterococcal hemolysin/cytolysin and two enterococcal proteases (gelatinase and serine protease). Enterococcal cytolysin is a heterodimeric toxin produced by some strains of *E. faecalis* that is capable of lysing human (as well as equine but not ovine) RBCs as well as polymorphonuclear leukocytes and macrophages. *E. faecalis* gelatinase and serine protease are thought to mediate virulence by several mechanisms, including the degradation of host tissues and the modification of critical components of the immune system. Mutants lacking the genes corresponding to these proteins are highly attenuated in experimental animal models of peritonitis, endocarditis, and endophthalmitis.

A second group of virulence factors, *enterococcal surface components*, includes adhesins and is thought to contribute to bacterial attachment to extracellular matrix molecules in the human host. Several molecules on the surface of enterococci have been characterized and shown to play a role in the pathogenesis of enterococcal infections. Among the characterized adhesins is *aggregation substance* of *E. faecalis*, which mediates the attachment of bacterial cells to each other, thereby facilitating conjugative plasmid exchange. Several lines of evidence indicate that aggregation substance and enterococcal cytolysin act synergistically to increase the virulence potential of *E. faecalis* strains in experimental endocarditis. The surface protein adhesin of collagen of *E. faecalis* (Ace) and its *E. faecium* homologue (Acm) are microbial surface components adhering to matrix molecules (MSCRAMMs); they recognize adhesive matrix molecules involved in bacterial attachment to host proteins such as collagen, fibronectin, and fibrinogen. Both Ace and Acm are collagen adhesins that are important in the pathogenesis of experimental endocarditis. Pili of gram-positive bacteria are important mediators of attachment to and invasion of host tissues and are considered potential targets for immunotherapy. Both *E. faecalis* and *E. faecium* have surface pili. Mutants of *E. faecalis* lacking pili are attenuated in biofilm production, experimental endocarditis, and urinary tract infections (UTIs). Other surface proteins that share structural homology with MSCRAMMs and appear to play a role in enterococcal attachment to the host and in virulence include the *E. faecalis* surface protein Esp and its *E. faecium* homologue Esp_{fm}, the second collagen adhesin of *E. faecium* (Scm), the surface proteins of *E. faecium* (Fms), SgrA (which binds to components of the basal lamina), and EcbA (which binds to collagen type V). Additional surface components apparently associated with pathogenicity include the Erl protein (a protein from the WxL family) and polysaccharides, which are thought to interfere with phagocytosis of the organism by host immune cells. Some *E. faecalis* strains appear to harbor at least three distinct classes of capsular polysaccharide; some of these polysaccharides play a role in virulence and are potential targets for immunotherapy. Teichoic acids on the enterococcal surface appear to be immunogenic, and antibodies to these molecules are protective in some animal models.

The third group of virulence factors has not been well characterized but includes the *E. faecalis* stress protein Gls24, which has been associated with enterococcal resistance to bile salts and appears to be important in the pathogenesis of endocarditis, and the hyl_{Efm}-containing plasmids of *E. faecium*, which are transferable between strains and increase gastrointestinal colonization by *E. faecium*. In mouse peritonitis, acquisition of these plasmids increased the lethality of a commensal strain of *E. faecium* and enhanced colonization of the uroepithelium. A gene encoding a regulator of oxidative stress (AsrR) has been identified as an important virulence factor of *E. faecium*.

EPIDEMIOLOGY

According to data collected from 2015 to 2017 by the National Healthcare Safety Network of the Centers for Disease Control and Prevention, enterococci are the second most common isolates (after staphylococci) from hospital-associated infections in the United States. Although *E. faecalis* remains the predominant species recovered from nosocomial infections, the isolation of *E. faecium* has increased substantially in the past 20 years and accounts for approximately one-third of all enterococcal infections identified to the species level. This point is important, since *E. faecium* is by far the most resistant and challenging enterococcal species to treat. More than 90% of *E. faecium* isolates are resistant to ampicillin (historically the most effective β-lactam agent against enterococci), while ampicillin resistance in *E. faecalis* is uncommon. Vancomycin resistance in *E. faecium* isolates ranges from 83% in acute care hospitals in the United States to up to 93% in long-term care facilities. Resistance to vancomycin in *E. faecalis* isolates is less common, with a higher incidence in device-associated infections (7.2%) than surgical-site infections (3.4%).

The dynamics of enterococcal transmission and dissemination in the hospital environment have been extensively studied, with a focus on VRE. These studies have revealed that VRE colonization of the gastrointestinal tract is a critical step in the development of enterococcal disease and that a substantial proportion of patients colonized with VRE remain colonized for prolonged periods (sometimes >1 year) and are more likely than patients without VRE colonization to develop an *Enterococcus*-related illness (e.g., bacteremia). Important factors associated with VRE colonization and persistence in the gut include prolonged hospitalization; long courses of antibiotic therapy; hospitalization in long-term care facilities, surgical units, and/or intensive care units; organ transplantation; renal failure (particularly in patients undergoing hemodialysis) and/or diabetes; high APACHE (Acute Physiology and Chronic Health Evaluation) scores; and physical proximity to patients infected or colonized with VRE or these patients' rooms. Once a patient becomes colonized with VRE, several key factors are involved in the organisms' dissemination in the hospital environment. VRE can survive exposure to heat and certain disinfectants and have been found on numerous inanimate objects in the hospital, including bed rails, medical equipment, doorknobs, gloves, telephones, and computer keyboards. Thus, health care workers and the environment play pivotal roles in enterococcal transmission from patient to patient, and infection control measures are crucial in breaking the chain of transmission. Moreover, two meta-analyses have found that, independent of the patient's clinical status, VRE infection increases the risk of death over that among individuals infected with a glycopeptide-susceptible enterococcal strain.

The epidemiology of enterococcal disease and the emergence of VRE have followed slightly different trends in other parts of the world than in the United States. In Europe, the emergence of VRE in the mid-1980s was seen primarily in isolates recovered from animals and healthy humans rather than from hospitalized patients. The presence of VRE was associated with the use of the glycopeptide avoparcin as a growth promoter in animal feeds; this association prompted the European Union to ban the use of this compound in animal husbandry in 1996. However, after an initial decrease in the isolation of VRE from animals and humans, the prevalence of hospital-associated VRE infections has slowly increased in certain European countries, with important regional differences. For example, rates of vancomycin resistance among *E. faecium* clinical isolates in Europe are highest in Greece, Ireland, Romania, Hungary, Slovakia, and Poland (25–35%), whereas rates in the Scandinavian countries and the Netherlands are <5%. These regional differences have been attributed in part to the implementation of aggressive "search-and-destroy" infection-control policies in countries such as the Netherlands; these policies have kept the frequency of nosocomial methicillin-resistant *Staphylococcus aureus* (MRSA) and VRE very low. Despite regional differences, Europe has seen a general trend of increasing rates of VRE over the past decade, though these rates continue to be much lower than in the United States. The reasons are not totally understood, although it has been postulated that this difference is related to the higher levels of human antibiotic use in the United States. Recent data have also shown increasing rates of enterococcal resistance to vancomycin in Latin American countries, with 34% of clinical *E. faecium* isolates found to be resistant in a multicenter study including hospitals from Colombia, Venezuela, Ecuador, and Peru. In Asia, rates of vancomycin resistance among enterococci appear to be similar to those in U.S. hospitals.

The ability to sequence bacterial genomes has increased our understanding of bacterial diversity, evolution, pathogenesis, and mechanisms of antibiotic resistance. The genome sequences of >8000 enterococcal strains are currently available, and some have been entirely closed and annotated. This has allowed researchers to trace the evolutionary trajectory of enterococci from their origin to the emergence of hospital-adapted clones. Sequence analysis suggests the genus appeared ~400 million years ago with the advent of terrestrial animals. Several key features aided in this transition, including the ability to recombine large portions of chromosomal DNA from the *core genome* and a malleable *accessory genome* consisting of plasmids, phages, and mobile genetic elements. This genomic plasticity contributes to the rising rates of antibiotic resistance seen within the genus and, in particular, in *E. faecium*.

A large proportion of the genomes available for analysis belong to *E. faecium*, due to its importance as a nosocomial pathogen and the epidemiologic surveillance projects to track the spread of vancomycin-resistant strains. The population can be divided into two large groups, or clades, of organisms: a hospital-associated clade A and a community-associated clade B. The hospital-associated clade appears to be evolving rapidly, and genomic comparisons suggest that this lineage emerged 75–80 years ago—a time point that coincides with the introduction of antimicrobial drugs—and evolved, perhaps continuously, from animal strains, not from human commensal isolates. Strains belonging to clade A are more frequently identified as isolates causing invasive disease and are more likely to carry drug resistance determinants, whereas clade B isolates largely retain a susceptible phenotype.

One reason for the propensity of clade A strains to acquire resistance determinants is that they more frequently lack a functional CRISPR-cas system (short for *c*lustered *r*egularly *i*nterspaced *s*hort *p*alindromic *r*epeats). These systems serve as a primitive "immune system" and provide a genome defense for bacteria to protect them from foreign DNA, such as phages, but they also serve to reduce the frequency of acquisition of resistance genes borne on mobile genetic elements. Another reason for their survival in the hospital environment is that clade A isolates tend to possess alleles of penicillin-binding protein 5 (PBP5) associated with high-level β-lactam resistance in *E. faecium* and may express higher levels of this enzyme than commensal strains.

A notable feature of the distribution of strains in clade A in some studies is that they share a relatively recent common ancestor with *E. faecium* of livestock origin. Use of antibiotics in animal husbandry as both therapeutics and growth promoters has been linked to resistance in several important contexts, including glycopeptides as mentioned above. This suggests continued surveillance, and an expanding understanding of the population structure of enterococci may help identify potential reservoirs of resistance and inform policy to limit their spread.

CLINICAL SYNDROMES

Urinary Tract Infection and Prostatitis Enterococci are well-known causes of nosocomial UTI—the most common infection caused by these organisms **(Chap. 135)**. Enterococcal UTIs are usually associated with indwelling catheterization, instrumentation, or anatomic abnormalities of the genitourinary tract, and it is often challenging to differentiate between true infection and colonization (particularly in patients with chronic indwelling catheters). Their role as pathogens in otherwise healthy premenopausal woman with acute cystitis is less clear, with data from one study suggesting that enterococci recovered from mid-stream urine cultures were not predictive of bacteriuria in a subsequent catheterized specimen. The presence of leukocytes in the urine in conjunction with systemic manifestations (e.g., fever) or local signs and symptoms of infection with no other explanation and a positive urine culture (≥10^5 CFU/mL) suggests the diagnosis. Moreover, enterococcal UTIs often occur in critically or chronically ill patients whose comorbidities may obscure the diagnosis. In many cases, removal of the indwelling catheter may suffice to eradicate the organism without specific antimicrobial therapy. In rare circumstances, UTIs caused by enterococci may run a complicated course, with the development of pyelonephritis and perinephric abscesses that may be a portal of entry for bloodstream infections (see below). Enterococci are also known causes of chronic prostatitis, particularly in men whose urinary tract has been manipulated surgically or endoscopically. These infections can be difficult to treat since the agents most potent against enterococci (i.e., aminopenicillins and glycopeptides) penetrate prostatic tissue poorly. Chronic prostatic infection can be a source of recurrent enterococcal bacteremia.

Bacteremia and Endocarditis Bacteremia without endocarditis is another frequently encountered presentation of enterococcal disease. Intravascular catheters and other devices are commonly associated with these bacteremic episodes **(Chap. 142)**. Other well-known sources of enterococcal bacteremia include the gastrointestinal and hepatobiliary tracts; pelvic and intraabdominal foci; and, less frequently, wound infections, UTIs, and bone infections. In the United States, enterococci are ranked second (after staphylococci) as etiologic agents of central line–associated bacteremia. Patients with enterococcal bacteremia usually have comorbidities and have been in the hospital for prolonged periods; they commonly have received several courses of antibiotics. Several studies indicate that the isolation of *E. faecium* from the blood may lead to worse outcomes and higher mortality rates than when other enterococcal species are isolated; this finding may be related to the higher prevalence of vancomycin and ampicillin resistance in *E. faecium* than in other enterococcal species, with the consequent reduction of therapeutic options. In some cases (usually when the gastrointestinal tract is the source), enterococcal bacteremia may be polymicrobial, with gram-negative organisms isolated at the same time. In addition, several cases have been documented in which enterococcal bacteremia was associated with *Strongyloides stercoralis* hyperinfection syndrome in immunocompromised patients.

Enterococci are important causes of community- and health care–associated endocarditis, ranking second after staphylococci in the latter infections. The presumed initial source of bacteremia leading to endocarditis is the gastrointestinal or genitourinary tract—e.g., in patients who have malignant and inflammatory conditions of the gut or have undergone procedures in which these tracts are manipulated.

The affected patients tend to be male and elderly and to have other debilitating diseases and heart conditions. Both prosthetic and native valves can be involved; mitral and aortic valves are affected most often. Community-associated endocarditis (usually caused by *E. faecalis*) also occurs in patients with no apparent risk factors or cardiac abnormalities. Endocarditis in women of childbearing age was well described in the past. The typical presentation of enterococcal endocarditis is a subacute course of fever, weight loss, malaise, and cardiac murmur; typical stigmata of endocarditis (e.g., petechiae, Osler's nodes, Roth's spots) are found in only a minority of patients. Atypical manifestations include arthralgias and manifestations of metastatic disease (splenic abscesses, hiccups, pain in the left flank, pleural effusion, and spondylodiscitis). Embolic complications are variable and can affect the brain. Heart failure is a common complication of enterococcal endocarditis, and valve replacement may be critical in curing this infection, particularly when multidrug-resistant organisms or major complications are involved. Several clinical scoring systems (designated NOVA and DENOVA) have been proposed to help differentiate enterococcal bacteremia from true endocarditis. The duration of therapy is usually 4–6 weeks, with more prolonged courses suggested for multidrug-resistant isolates in the absence of valvular replacement.

Meningitis Enterococcal meningitis is an uncommon disease (accounting for only ~4% of meningitis cases) that is usually associated with neurosurgical interventions and conditions such as shunts, central nervous system (CNS) trauma, and cerebrospinal fluid (CSF) leakage. In some instances—usually in patients with a debilitating condition, such as cardiovascular or congenital heart disease, chronic renal failure, malignancy, receipt of immunosuppressive therapy, or HIV/AIDS—presumed hematogenous seeding of the meninges is seen in infections such as endocarditis or bacteremia. Fever and changes in mental status are common, whereas overt meningeal signs are less so. CSF findings are consistent with bacterial infection—i.e., pleocytosis, with a predominance of polymorphonuclear leukocytes (average, ~500/μL), an elevated serum protein level (usually >100 mg/dL), and a decreased glucose concentration (average, 28 mg/dL). Gram's staining yields a positive result in about half of cases, with a high rate of organism recovery from CSF cultures; the most common species isolated are *E. faecalis* and *E. faecium*. Complications include hydrocephalus, brain abscesses, and stroke. As mentioned before for bacteremia, an association with *Strongyloides* hyperinfection has also been documented.

Intraabdominal, Pelvic, and Soft Tissue Infections As mentioned earlier, enterococci are part of the commensal microbiota of the gastrointestinal tract and can produce spontaneous peritonitis in cirrhotic individuals and in patients undergoing chronic ambulatory peritoneal dialysis (**Chap. 132**). These organisms are commonly found (usually along with other bacteria, including enteric gram-negative species and anaerobes) in clinical samples from intraabdominal and pelvic collections. The presence of enterococci in intraabdominal infections is sometimes considered to be of little clinical relevance. Several studies have shown that the role of enterococci in intraabdominal infections originating in the community and involving previously healthy patients is minor since surgery and broad-spectrum antimicrobial drugs that do not target enterococci are often sufficient to treat these infections successfully. In the past few decades, however, these organisms have become prominent as a cause of intraabdominal infections in hospitalized patients because of the emergence and spread of vancomycin resistance among enterococci and the increase in rates of nosocomial infections due to multidrug-resistant *E. faecium* isolates. In fact, several studies have now documented treatment failures due to enterococci, with consequently increased rates of postoperative complications and death among patients with intraabdominal infections. Thus, anti-enterococcal therapy is recommended for nosocomial peritonitis in immunocompromised and severely ill patients who have had a prolonged hospital stay, have undergone multiple procedures, have persistent abdominal sepsis and collections, or have risk factors for the development of endocarditis (e.g., prosthetic or damaged heart valves). Conversely, specific treatment for enterococci in the first episode of intraabdominal infection originating in the community and affecting previously healthy patients with no important cardiac risk factors for endocarditis does not appear to be beneficial.

Enterococci are commonly isolated from soft tissue infections (**Chap. 129**), particularly those involving surgical wounds (**Chap. 142**). In fact, these organisms rank third as agents of nosocomial surgical-site infections, with *E. faecalis* the most frequently isolated species. The clinical relevance of enterococci in some of these infections—as in intraabdominal infections—is a matter of debate; differentiating between colonization and true infection is sometimes challenging, although in some cases, enterococci have been recovered from lung, liver, and skin abscesses. Diabetic foot and decubitus ulcers are often colonized with enterococci and may be the portal of entry for bone infections.

Other Infections Enterococci are well-known causes of neonatal infections, including sepsis (mostly late-onset), bacteremia, meningitis, pneumonia, and UTI. Outbreaks of enterococcal sepsis in neonatal units have been well documented. Risk factors for enterococcal disease in newborns include prematurity, low birth weight, indwelling devices, and abdominal surgery. Enterococci have also been described as etiologic agents of bone and joint infections, including vertebral osteomyelitis, usually in patients with underlying conditions such as diabetes or endocarditis. Similarly, enterococci have been isolated from bone infections in patients who have undergone arthroplasty or reconstruction of fractures with the placement of hardware. Since enterococci can produce a biofilm that is likely to alter the efficacy of anti-enterococcal agents, treatment of infections that involve foreign material is challenging, and removal of the hardware may be necessary to eradicate the infection. Rare cases of enterococcal pneumonia, lung abscess, and spontaneous empyema have been described.

TREATMENT
Enterococcal Infections

GENERAL PRINCIPLES

Enterococci are intrinsically resistant and/or tolerant to several antimicrobial agents. (*Tolerance* is defined as lack of killing by drug concentrations 32 times higher than the minimal inhibitory concentration [MIC].) Monotherapy for endocarditis with a β-lactam antibiotic (to which many enterococci are tolerant) has produced disappointing results, with high relapse rates after the end of therapy. However, the addition of an aminoglycoside to a cell wall–active agent (a β-lactam or a glycopeptide) increases cure rates and eradicates the organisms; moreover, this combination is synergistic and bactericidal in vitro. Therefore, for many decades, combination therapy with a cell wall–active agent and an aminoglycoside was the standard of care for endovascular infections caused by enterococci. This synergistic effect can be explained, at least in part, by the increased penetration of the aminoglycoside into the bacterial cell, presumably as a result of cell-wall alterations produced by the β-lactam (or glycopeptide). Nonetheless, attaining synergistic bactericidal activity in the treatment of severe enterococcal infections—particularly those caused by *E. faecium*—has become increasingly difficult because of the development of resistance to virtually all antibiotics available for this purpose.

The treatment of *E. faecalis* differs substantially from that of *E. faecium* (**Tables 149-1 and 149-2**), mainly because of differences in resistance profiles (see below). For example, resistance to ampicillin and vancomycin is rare in *E. faecalis*, whereas these antibiotics are only infrequently useful against current isolates of *E. faecium*. Moreover, as a consequence of the challenges and therapeutic limitations posed by the emergence of drug resistance in enterococci, valve replacement may need to be considered in the treatment of endocarditis caused by multidrug-resistant enterococci. Less severe infections are often related to indwelling intravascular catheters; removal of the catheter increases the likelihood of enterococcal eradication by a subsequent short course of appropriate antimicrobial therapy.

TABLE 149-1 Suggested Regimens for the Management of Infections Caused by *Enterococcus faecalis*

CLINICAL SYNDROME	SUGGESTED THERAPEUTIC OPTIONS[a]
Endovascular infections (including endocarditis)	• Ampicillin[b] (12 g/d IV in divided doses q4h) plus ceftriaxone (2 g IV q12h) • Ampicillin[b] (12 g/d IV in divided doses q4h or by continuous infusion) or penicillin (18–30 mU/d IV in divided doses q4h or by continuous infusion) *plus* an aminoglycoside[c] • Vancomycin[d] (15 mg/kg IV per dose) plus an aminoglycoside[c] • High-dose daptomycin[e] ± another active agent[f] • Ampicillin[b] plus imipenem
Nonendovascular bacteremia[g]	• Ampicillin (12 g/d IV in divided doses q4h) or penicillin (18 mU/d IV in divided doses q4h) ± an aminoglycoside[c] or ceftriaxone • Vancomycin[d] (15 mg/kg IV per dose) • High-dose daptomycin[e] ± another active agent[f] • Linezolid (600 mg IV/PO q12h)
Meningitis	• Ampicillin (20–24 g/d IV in divided doses q4h) or penicillin (24 mU/d IV in divided doses q4h) *plus* an aminoglycoside[c,h] and consider adding ceftriaxone (2 g IV q12h) • Vancomycin (500–750 mg IV q6h)[d] *plus* an aminoglycoside[c] or rifampin • Linezolid • High-dose daptomycin[e] (plus intrathecal daptomycin) ± another active agent[f]
Urinary tract infections (uncomplicated)	• Fosfomycin (3 g PO, one dose)[i] • Ampicillin (500 mg IV or PO q6h) • Nitrofurantoin (100 mg PO q6h)

[a]Authors' preferences are underlined for each category; many of the regimens are off-label. [b]In rare cases, β-lactamase-producing isolates may be present. Because these isolates are not detected by conventional determination of the minimal inhibitory concentration, additional tests (e.g., the nitrocefin disk) are recommended for isolates from endocarditis. The use of ampicillin/sulbactam (12–24 g/d) is suggested in these cases. [c]Only if the organism does not exhibit high-level resistance (HLR) to aminoglycosides. This test is performed by the clinical microbiology laboratory only for gentamicin or streptomycin (growth of enterococci on agar containing gentamicin [500 μg/mL] or streptomycin [2000 μg/mL]). If HLR is documented, the aminoglycoside will not act synergistically with the other agent in the combination. However, HLR to one of these aminoglycosides does not indicate resistance to the other agent (as reported individually). HLR to gentamicin implies lack of synergism with tobramycin and with amikacin. Gentamicin (1–1.5 mg/kg IV q8h) and streptomycin (15 mg/kg per day IV/IM in two divided doses) are the only two recommended aminoglycosides. [d]Vancomycin is recommended only as an alternative to β-lactam agents in cases of allergy or toxicity plus the inability to desensitize. Specific pharmacologic targets for trough concentrations have not been clinically evaluated in enterococcal bacteremia; trough concentrations of 15–20 mg/L have been associated with increased rates of nephrotoxicity. Cerebrospinal fluid (CSF) concentrations in meningitis should be determined. Vancomycin-resistant strains of *E. faecalis* have been reported. [e]Consider doses of 10–12 mg/kg once daily if used in combination and 10–12 mg/kg per day if used alone. Monitoring of creatine phosphokinase levels is recommended throughout therapy because of possible rhabdomyolysis. [f]Potentially active agents may include an aminoglycoside (if HLR is not detected), ampicillin, ceftaroline, tigecycline, or a fluoroquinolone (which, if the isolate is susceptible, may be favored in meningitis). The presence of mutations in *liaFSR* seems to increase susceptibility to ampicillin and ceftaroline, and combinations of daptomycin with these compounds are bactericidal in vitro against such strains. [g]In selected cases of catheter-associated bacteremia, removal of the catheter and a short course of therapy (~5–7 days) may be sufficient. A single positive blood culture that is likely to be associated with a catheter in a patient who is otherwise doing well may not require therapy after removal of the catheter. Patients at high risk for endovascular infections or with severe disease may benefit from synergistic combination therapy. [h]The addition of intrathecal or intraventricular therapy with gentamicin (2–10 mg/d) if the organism does not exhibit HLR or with vancomycin (10–20 mg/d) when the isolate is susceptible has been suggested by some authorities. The addition of systemic rifampin (a good CSF-penetrating agent) may be considered. The combination of ampicillin and ceftriaxone may have clinical benefit (by analogy with endocarditis), but no cases treated with this combination have been reported; the authors would use this combination. [i]Approved by the U.S. Food and Drug Administration only for uncomplicated urinary tract infections caused by vancomycin-susceptible *E. faecalis*.

TABLE 149-2 Suggested Regimens for the Management of Infections Caused by Vancomycin- and Ampicillin-Resistant *Enterococcus faecium*

CLINICAL SYNDROME	SUGGESTED THERAPEUTIC OPTIONS[a]
Endovascular infections (including endocarditis)	• High-dose daptomycin[b] plus another agent[c] ± an aminoglycoside[d] • Linezolid (600 mg IV q12h) • High-dose ampicillin (if MIC is ≤64 μg/mL) ± an aminoglycoside[d] • Ampicillin plus imipenem (if the ampicillin MIC is ≤32 μg/mL) • Q/D[e] (22.5 mg/kg per day in divided doses q8h) ± another active agent[f]
Nonendovascular bacteremia[g]	• High-dose daptomycin[b] ± another agent[c] ± an aminoglycoside[d] • Linezolid (600 mg IV q12h) • Q/D (22.5 mg/kg per day in divided doses q8h) ± another active agent[f]
Meningitis	• Linezolid (600 mg IV q12h) ± another CSF-penetrating active agent[h] • High-dose daptomycin[b] (plus intraventricular daptomycin) ± another CSF-penetrating active agent[h,i] • Q/D (22.5 mg/kg per day in divided doses q8h plus intraventricular Q/D)[j] ± another active agent[h]
Urinary tract infections	• Fosfomycin (3 g PO, one dose)[k] • Nitrofurantoin (100 mg PO q6h) • Ampicillin or amoxicillin (2 g IV/PO q4–6h)[l]

[a]Authors' preferences are underlined for each category; many of these regimens are off-label. [b]Daptomycin at doses of 10–12 mg/kg once daily is suggested (off-label). Close monitoring of creatine phosphokinase levels is recommended throughout therapy because of possible rhabdomyolysis. [c]Potentially active agents may include ampicillin or ceftaroline (even if the infecting strain is resistant in vitro) or tigecycline. In vitro synergism of daptomycin with ampicillin or ceftaroline has been observed against some isolates that subsequently become nonsusceptible to daptomycin during therapy. The synergism of daptomycin and β-lactams is associated with mutations in *liaFSR*. Consider combination therapy if the minimal inhibitory concentration (MIC) of daptomycin is ≥3 μg/mL. [d]Only if the organism does not exhibit high-level resistance to aminoglycosides (see Table 149-1, footnote *c*). [e]Quinupristin/dalfopristin (Q/D) lost U.S. Food and Drug Administration (FDA) approval for infections due to vancomycin-resistant *Enterococcus*. [f]Agents that may be useful in combination with Q/D (if the isolate is susceptible to each agent) include doxycycline with rifampin (one reported case) or fluoroquinolones (one reported case). [g]In selected cases of catheter-associated bacteremia, removal of the catheter and a short course of therapy (~5–7 days) may be sufficient. A single positive blood culture that is likely to be associated with a catheter in a patient who is otherwise doing well may not require therapy after removal of the catheter. [h]Fluoroquinolones (e.g., moxifloxacin) and rifampin (if the isolate is susceptible to each agent) reach therapeutic levels in the cerebrospinal fluid. [i]Intrathecal gentamicin (2–10 mg/d) if high-level resistance is not detected. Intraventricular daptomycin has been used in two cases of meningitis [j]Intrathecal Q/D (1–5 mg/d) has been used in combination with Q/D systemic therapy in meningitis. If Q/D is chosen, simultaneous use of both systemic and intrathecal therapy is suggested. [k]Approved by the FDA only for uncomplicated urinary tract infections caused by vancomycin-susceptible *E. faecalis*. [l]Concentrations of amoxicillin and ampicillin in urine far exceed those in serum and may be potentially effective even against isolates with high MICs. Doses up to 12 g/d are suggested for isolates with MICs of ≥64 μg/mL.

CHOICE OF ANTIMICROBIAL AGENTS

Among the β-lactams, the most active are the aminopenicillins (ampicillin, amoxicillin) and ureidopenicillins (i.e., piperacillin); next most active are penicillin G and imipenem. Cephalosporins, with the possible exception of ceftaroline, are not active as monotherapy. For *E. faecium*, a combination of high-dose ampicillin (up to 30 g/d) plus an aminoglycoside has been suggested—even for ampicillin-resistant strains if the MIC is ≤64 μg/mL—since a plasma ampicillin concentration higher than this value can be achieved at high doses. The only two aminoglycosides recommended for synergistic therapy in severe enterococcal infections are gentamicin and streptomycin. This is because the most common acquired enzyme conferring high-level resistance to gentamicin also is active against tobramycin and amikacin but not streptomycin, and the resistance mechanisms causing streptomycin high-level resistance do not affect gentamicin. The use of amikacin is strongly discouraged because it is infrequently active tobramycin should never be used for the treatment of *E. faecium* infections due to the presence of a chromosomally encoded, species-specific, tobramycin-modifying enzyme and aminoglycoside monotherapy should not be employed. Vancomycin is an alternative to β-lactam drugs for the treatment of *E. faecalis* infections but is less useful against *E. faecium* because resistance is common.

As mentioned above, use of the aminoglycoside–ampicillin combination for *E. faecalis* infections has become increasingly problematic because of toxicity in critically ill patients and increased rates of high-level resistance to aminoglycosides. An observational, nonrandomized, comparative study encompassing a multicenter cohort was conducted in 17 Spanish hospitals and one Italian hospital; the results indicated that a 6-week course of ampicillin plus ceftriaxone is as effective as ampicillin plus gentamicin in the treatment of *E. faecalis* endocarditis, with less risk of toxicity. Therefore, this regimen should be considered in patients at risk for aminoglycoside toxicity or those with isolates displaying high-level resistance to aminoglycosides, and it is now recommended as first-line therapy for *E. faecalis* endocarditis. Use of dual β-lactam regimens for ampicillin-susceptible isolates of *E. faecium* has not been studied in the clinical setting. Limited in vitro data suggest that synergism between ampicillin and ceftriaxone is not reliably active against these isolates.

Linezolid is the only agent approved by the U.S. Food and Drug Administration (FDA) for the treatment of VRE infections (Table 149-2). (A prior approval for quinupristin/dalfopristin has been withdrawn.) Linezolid is not bactericidal, and its use in severe endovascular infections has produced mixed results; therefore, it is recommended only as an alternative to other agents for such infections. In addition, linezolid may cause significant toxicities (thrombocytopenia, peripheral neuropathy, optic neuritis, and lactic acidosis) when used in regimens given for >2 weeks. Nonetheless, linezolid may play a role in the treatment of enterococcal meningitis and other CNS infections, although clinical data are limited.

The lipopeptide daptomycin is a bactericidal antibiotic with potent in vitro activity against all enterococci. Although daptomycin is not approved by the FDA for the treatment of VRE or *E. faecium* infections, it has been used alone (at high dosage) or in combination with other agents (ampicillin, ceftaroline, and tigecycline) with apparent success against multidrug-resistant enterococcal infections (Tables 149-1 and 149-2). The main adverse reactions to daptomycin are elevated creatine phosphokinase levels and eosinophilic pneumonitis (rare). Daptomycin is not useful against pulmonary infections because the pulmonary surfactant inhibits its antibacterial activity.

Several meta-analyses have examined the question of which agent should be preferred for VRE bacteremia—linezolid or daptomycin. These studies concluded either no difference between the two drugs or favored linezolid due to lower all-cause and infection-related mortality, but were limited by small patient numbers and heterogenous outcomes. A subsequent large retrospective observational study from the Veterans Affairs database reported lower rates of all-cause mortality at 30 days and less microbiologic failure (i.e., positive cultures despite therapy) with daptomycin as compared to linezolid. One important observation from these investigations is that the efficacy of daptomycin is dependent on the dose, with improved outcomes seen with high-dose daptomycin therapy (≥10 mg/kg) as compared to standard-dose therapy (6 mg/kg). Genome sequencing of clinical isolates has revealed that mutations in genes associated with daptomycin resistance are not uncommon (see "Antimicrobial Resistance," below) and were associated with the emergence of resistance to daptomycin at lower simulated dosing regimens (6 mg/kg) in experimental models of infection. These data led the Clinical Laboratory and Standards Institute (CLSI) to change the daptomycin breakpoints in 2019. For *E. faecium*, all isolates with an MIC of ≤4 mg/L are placed in a "susceptible dose-dependent" category based on a dosing regimen of 8–12 mg/kg, while those with an MIC ≥8 mg/L are considered resistant. For all other enterococci, isolates are considered susceptible with an MIC of ≤2 mg/L, intermediate with an MIC of 4 mg/L, and resistant with an MIC ≥8 mg/L.

The glycylcycline drug tigecycline is active in vitro against all enterococci, regardless of the isolates' vancomycin susceptibility. However, its use as monotherapy for endovascular or severe enterococcal infections is not recommended because of low attainable blood levels. Newer generation tetracyclines, such as eravacycline and omadacycline, also display in vitro activity, but their role in the treatment of enterococcal infections remains to be evaluated.

Telavancin, a lipoglycopeptide approved by the FDA for the treatment of skin and soft tissue infections as well as hospital-associated pneumonia, is active against vancomycin-susceptible enterococci but not VRE. Likewise, dalbavancin, a lipoglycopeptide antibiotic with a long terminal half-life, has FDA approval for skin and soft tissue infections due to susceptible strains of *E. faecalis*, but no activity against VRE. Oritavancin, a novel glycopeptide with activity against VRE, has been approved for the treatment of acute bacterial skin and soft tissue infections caused by susceptible organisms, including vancomycin-susceptible *E. faecalis*. The MICs of oritavancin against VRE are low, and this compound may be a promising drug for VRE treatment in the future.

Lastly, tedizolid—a new oxazolidinone now available for clinical use—is approved only for the treatment of *E. faecalis* infections. Tedizolid is more potent than linezolid in vitro against VRE strains; however, its role in severe VRE infections remains to be determined.

ANTIMICROBIAL RESISTANCE

Resistance to β-lactam agents continues to be observed only infrequently in *E. faecalis* but is characteristic of *E. faecium*. The mechanism of ampicillin resistance in *E. faecium* is related to a penicillin-binding protein (PBP) designated PBP5, which is the critical target of β-lactam antibiotics. PBP5 exhibits low affinity for ampicillin and can synthesize cell wall in the presence of this antibiotic, even when other PBPs are inhibited. The version of this protein found in ampicillin-resistant hospital-associated strains has multiple amino-acid differences that even further decrease the affinity of PBP5 for ampicillin; these changes and/or increased production of PBP5 are the two most common mechanisms of high-level ampicillin resistance (e.g., MIC >32 μg/mL) in clinical strains.

Vancomycin is a glycopeptide antibiotic that inhibits cell-wall peptidoglycan synthesis in susceptible enterococci and has been widely used against enterococcal infections in clinical practice when the utility of β-lactams is limited by resistance, allergy, or adverse reactions. This effect is mediated by binding of the antibiotic to peptidoglycan precursors (UDP-MurNAc-pentapeptides) upon their exit from the bacterial cell cytoplasm. The interaction of vancomycin with the peptidoglycan is specific and involves the last two D-alanine residues of the precursor. The first isolates of VRE were documented in 1986, and vancomycin resistance (particularly in *E. faecium*) has since increased considerably around the world. The mechanism involves the replacement of the last D-alanine residue of peptidoglycan precursors with D-lactate (e.g., VanA and VanB) or D-serine (e.g., VanC), with consequent high- and low-level resistance, respectively. There is significant heterogeneity among isolates, but either substitution substantially decreases the affinity of vancomycin for the peptidoglycan; with the D-lactate substitution, the affinity for binding to the pentapeptide precursor is decreased by ~1000-fold. Vancomycin-resistant organisms also produce enzymes that destroy the D-alanine-D-alanine ending precursors, ensuring that additional binding sites for vancomycin are not available.

The genes encoding the machinery responsible for vancomycin resistance are located in the *van* operon and likely originated in soil bacteria. Several variants of the operon have been described, but VanA is the most common in clinical isolates in the United States, Latin America, and Europe, whereas VanB isolates are more frequent in Australia. Two enterococcal species, *E. gallinarum* and

E. casseliflavus, have intrinsic low-level resistance to vancomycin due to the presence of the VanC operon in the chromosome.

High-level resistance to aminoglycosides (of which gentamicin and streptomycin are the only two tested by clinical laboratories) abolishes the synergism observed between cell wall–active agents and the aminoglycoside. This important phenotype is routinely sought by the clinical laboratory in isolates from serious infections (Tables 149-1 and 149-2). Genes encoding aminoglycoside-modifying enzymes are usually the cause of high-level resistance to these compounds and are widely disseminated among enterococci, decreasing the options for the treatment of severe enterococcal infections. Additionally, ribosomal methyltransferases, enzymes that methylate rRNA and, as a consequence, disrupt the binding site for aminoglycosides, can also lead to high-level resistance.

Resistance to daptomycin has now been well documented in both *E. faecalis* and *E. faecium*. Daptomycin exerts its action by complexing with calcium and binding to phosphatidylglycerol in the bacterial membrane. After binding, daptomycin forms oligomers, with recent data suggesting that it displaces enzymes important for cell envelope synthesis (MurG and PlsX) and that it can form a complex with lipid II molecules critical for cell-wall synthesis, among other effects on the membrane. Resistance to this antibiotic in enterococci arises via two main pathways. The first involves mutations in genes that coordinate the cell-wall and cell-membrane stress response, most commonly a three-component system designated LiaFSR (for *l*ipid II *i*nterfering *a*ntibiotics). These mutations lead to activation of the system, with increased expression of an extracellular protein known as LiaX capable of binding daptomycin and enhancing the signaling response. In clinical isolates, mutations in LiaFSR may lead to tolerance (loss of bactericidal activity) usually in isolates with MICs near the daptomycin breakpoint (i.e., 3–4 mg/L). The second pathway involves changes in genes involved in phospholipid metabolism. It is thought that mutations priming the stress response system occur first, with the subsequent accrual of phospholipid changes leading to a fully resistant phenotype. Prior exposure to daptomycin has been identified as a risk factor for the emergence of daptomycin-resistant *E. faecium* in cancer patients. Resistance in the absence of exposure to the drug has also been well described, possibly due to the similarity of this antibiotic to antimicrobial peptides of the innate immune system. Thus, careful consideration of patient characteristics, bacterial phenotype, and daptomycin dose is warranted, and it is advisable to obtain infectious diseases consultation in complicated VRE infections.

The oxazolidonones (linezolid and tedizolid) act by binding to the ribosome and inhibiting the binding of aminoacyl-tRNAs, thus preventing protein synthesis. Resistance to this class of antibiotics is usually due to alterations of the binding site, either via mutations in the 23S rRNA genes or the presence of an rRNA methylase. Since enterococci carry multiple copies of the gene encoding the 23S rRNA, prolonged exposure to oxazolidonones can select for increasing levels of resistance by favoring propagation of the resistance allele via recombination. Changes in accessory ribosomal proteins have also been associated with linezolid resistance and may act to mitigate the fitness defects of mutations in the rRNA. More concerning is the emergence of plasmid-borne resistance genes, which can be readily transferred between enterococcal strains. Several of these genes were first recognized in bacterial isolates of animal origin, likely under the selective pressure of antibiotics such as florfenicol. The *cfr* (chloramphenicol-*f*lorfenicol *r*esistance) gene encodes an rRNA methylase that modifies the 23S rRNA, leading to increases in the MIC of linezolid. Tedizolid tends to exhibit lower MICs in the presence of *cfr*; however, animal models suggest some variants of the enzyme may compromise the activity of this drug. Two other transmissible resistance genes, *optrA* and *poxtA*, encode a ribosomal protection factor that has been implicated in linezolid resistance in enterococcal strains of human and animal origin. While still relatively rare to encounter in clinical practice, these determinants have been identified across the globe and could be an emerging source of resistance.

Tigecycline retains activity in the presence of typical tetracycline resistance determinants, including drug efflux pumps and ribosomal protection factors. However, resistance has been documented and appears to be related to changes in the S10 ribosomal protein, which is situated near the binding site for the drug.

■ FURTHER READING

Bouza E et al: The NOVA score: A proposal to reduce the need for transesophageal echocardiography in patients with enterococcal bacteremia. Clin Infect Dis 60:528, 2015.

Garcia-Solache M, Rice L: The enterococcus: A model of adaptability to its environment. Clin Microbiol Rev 32:e00058, 2019.

Khan A et al: Antimicrobial sensing coupled with cell membrane remodeling mediates antibiotic resistance and virulence in *Enterococcus faecalis*. Proc Natl Acad Sci USA 116:26925, 2019.

Lebreton F et al: Tracing the enterococci from Paleozoic origins to the hospital. Cell 169:849, 2017.

Satlin MJ et al: Development of daptomycin susceptibility breakpoints for *Enterococcus faecium* and revision of the breakpoints for other enterococcal species by the Clinical and Laboratory Standards Institute. Clin Infect Dis 70:1240, 2020.

150 Diphtheria and Other Corynebacterial Infections

William R. Bishai, John R. Murphy

DIPHTHERIA

Diphtheria is a nasopharyngeal and skin infection caused by *Corynebacterium diphtheriae*. Toxigenic strains of *C. diphtheriae* produce a protein toxin that causes systemic toxicity, myocarditis, and polyneuropathy. The toxin is associated with the formation of pseudomembranes in the pharynx during respiratory diphtheria. While toxigenic strains most frequently cause pharyngeal diphtheria, nontoxigenic strains commonly cause cutaneous disease.

■ ETIOLOGY

C. diphtheriae is a gram-positive bacillus that is unencapsulated, nonmotile, and nonsporulating. The organism was first identified microscopically in 1883 by Klebs and a year later was isolated in pure culture by Löffler in Robert Koch's laboratory. The bacteria have a characteristic club-shaped bacillary appearance and typically form clusters of parallel rays, or *palisades*, that are referred to as "Chinese characters." The specific laboratory media recommended for the cultivation of *C. diphtheriae* rely upon tellurite, colistin, or nalidixic acid for the organism's selective isolation from other autochthonous pharyngeal microbes. *C. diphtheriae* may be isolated from individuals with both nontoxigenic (*tox*$^-$) and toxigenic (*tox*$^+$) phenotypes. Uchida and Pappenheimer demonstrated that corynebacteriophage beta carries the structural gene *tox*, which encodes diphtheria toxin, and that a family of closely related corynebacteriophages are responsible for toxigenic conversion of *tox*$^-$ *C. diphtheriae* to the *tox*$^+$ phenotype. Moreover, lysogenic conversion from a nontoxigenic to a toxigenic phenotype has been shown to occur in situ. Growth of toxigenic strains of *C. diphtheriae* under iron-limiting conditions leads to the optimal expression of diphtheria toxin and is believed to be a pathogenic mechanism during human infection. Less commonly, diphtheria-like disease may be caused by *Corynebacterium ulcerans* and *Corynebacterium pseudotuberculosis*, which express the same toxin and are considered members of the *C. diphtheriae* group (discussed below).

■ EPIDEMIOLOGY

While in many regions diphtheria has been controlled in recent years with effective vaccination, there have been sporadic outbreaks in the

United States and Europe. Diphtheria is still common in the Caribbean, Latin America, and the Indian subcontinent, where mass immunization programs are not enforced. Large-scale epidemics of diphtheria have occurred in the post–Soviet Union independent states. Additional outbreaks have recently been reported in Africa and Asia. In temperate regions, respiratory diphtheria occurs year-round but is most common during winter months.

C. diphtheriae is transmitted via the aerosol route, usually during close contact with an infected person. There are no significant reservoirs other than humans. The incubation period for respiratory diphtheria is 2–5 days, but disease onset has occurred as late as 10 days after exposure. Prior to the vaccination era, most individuals over the age of 10 were immune to *C. diphtheriae*; infants were protected by maternal IgG antibodies but became susceptible after ~6 months of age. Thus, the disease primarily affected children and nonimmune young adults.

The development of diphtheria antitoxin in 1898 by von Behring and of the diphtheria toxoid vaccine in 1924 by Ramon led to the near-elimination of diphtheria in Western countries. The annual incidence rate in the United States peaked in 1921, with 206,000 cases (191 cases per 100,000) and 15,520 deaths. In contrast, since 1980, the annual figure in the United States has been fewer than 5 cases per 100,000, with only 2 cases reported from 2004 through 2017. Nevertheless, pockets of colonization persist in North America, and groups or individuals who resist vaccination remain at risk. Immunity to diphtheria induced by childhood vaccination gradually decreases in adulthood. An estimated 30% of men 60–69 years old have antitoxin titers below the protective level. In addition to older age and lack of vaccination, risk factors for diphtheria outbreaks include alcoholism, low socioeconomic status, crowded living conditions, and Native American ethnic background. An outbreak of diphtheria in Seattle, Washington, between 1972 and 1982 comprised 1100 cases, most of which were cutaneous. During the 1990s in the states of the former Soviet Union, a much larger diphtheria epidemic included more than 140,000 cases and more than 4000 deaths; at its peak in 1995, more than 50,412 cases were reported. Clonally related toxigenic *C. diphtheriae* strains of the ET8 complex were associated with this outbreak. Beginning in 1998, this epidemic was controlled by mass vaccination programs, and between 2000 and 2009 the diphtheria incidence fell by >95%, with high-burden countries such as Latvia reporting fewer than 10 cases. During the epidemic, the incidence rate was high among individuals between 16 and 50 years of age. The epidemic was attributed to multiple factors, including socioeconomic instability, migration, deteriorating public health programs, unnecessary contraindications to vaccination, low-dose vaccine formulations, frequent vaccine and antitoxin shortages, delayed implementation of vaccination and treatment in response to cases, public mistrust, and lack of awareness.

Since 2010, significant outbreaks of diphtheria and diphtheria-related mortality have continued to be reported from many developing countries, including the Dominican Republic, Nigeria, India, Laos, Thailand, Indonesia, and Brazil. Statistics collected by the World Health Organization indicated that 7321 diphtheria cases were reported in 2014, but many more cases are likely to have gone unreported. Although 86% of the global population has been adequately vaccinated, only 28% of countries have successfully vaccinated >80% of individuals in all districts.

Cutaneous diphtheria is usually a secondary infection that follows a primary skin lesion due to trauma, allergy, or autoimmunity. Most often, these isolates lack the *tox* gene and thus do not express diphtheria toxin. In tropical latitudes, cutaneous diphtheria is more common than respiratory diphtheria. In contrast to respiratory disease, cutaneous diphtheria is not reportable in the United States. Nontoxigenic strains of *C. diphtheriae* have been associated with pharyngitis in Europe, causing outbreaks among men who have sex with men and persons who use illicit IV drugs.

PATHOGENESIS AND IMMUNOLOGY

Diphtheria toxin produced by *tox*$^+$ strains of *C. diphtheriae* is the primary virulence factor in clinical disease. The toxin is synthesized in precursor form; is released as a 535-amino-acid, single-chain protein; and, in sensitive species (e.g., guinea pigs and humans, but not mice or rats), has a 50% lethal dose of ~100 ng/kg of body weight. The toxin is produced in the pseudomembranous lesion and is taken up in the bloodstream, from which it is distributed to all organ systems in the body. Once bound to its cell surface receptor (a heparin-binding epidermal growth factor–like precursor), the toxin is internalized by receptor-mediated endocytosis and enters the cytosol from an acidified early endosomal compartment. In vitro, the toxin may be separated into two chains by digestion with serine proteases: the N-terminal A fragment and the C-terminal B fragment. Delivery of the A fragment into the eukaryotic cell cytosol results in irreversible inhibition of protein synthesis by NAD$^+$-dependent ADP-ribosylation of elongation factor 2. The eventual result is the death of the cell.

In 1926, Ramon at the Institut Pasteur found that formalinization of diphtheria toxin resulted in the production of a nontoxic but highly immunogenic diphtheria toxoid. Subsequent studies showed that immunization with diphtheria toxoid elicited antibodies that neutralized the toxin and prevented most disease manifestations. In the 1930s, mass immunization of children and susceptible adults with diphtheria toxoid commenced in the United States and Europe.

Individuals with a diphtheria antitoxin titer of >0.01 U/mL are at low risk of disease. In populations where a majority of individuals have protective antitoxin titers, the carrier rate for toxigenic strains of *C. diphtheriae* decreases and the overall risk of diphtheria among susceptible individuals is reduced. Nevertheless, individuals with nonprotective titers may contract diphtheria through either travel or exposure to individuals who have recently returned from regions where the disease is endemic.

Characteristic pathologic findings of diphtheria include mucosal ulcers with a pseudomembranous coating composed of an inner band of fibrin and a luminal band of neutrophils. Initially white and firmly adherent, in advanced diphtheria the pseudomembranes turn gray or even green or black as necrosis progresses. Mucosal ulcers result from toxin-induced necrosis of the epithelium accompanied by edema, hyperemia, and vascular congestion of the submucosal base. A significant fibrinosuppurative exudate from the ulcer develops into the pseudomembrane. Ulcers and pseudomembranes in severe respiratory diphtheria may extend from the pharynx into medium-sized bronchial airways. Expanding and sloughing membranes may result in fatal airway obstruction.

APPROACH TO THE PATIENT

Diphtheria

Diphtheria, although rare in the United States and other developed countries, should be considered when a patient has severe pharyngitis, particularly when there is difficulty swallowing, respiratory compromise, or signs of systemic disease (e.g., myocarditis or generalized weakness). The leading causes of pharyngitis are respiratory viruses (rhinoviruses, influenza viruses, parainfluenza viruses, coronaviruses, adenoviruses; ~25% of cases), group A streptococci (15–30%), group C streptococci (~5%), atypical bacteria such as *Mycoplasma pneumoniae* and *Chlamydia pneumoniae* (15–20% in some series), and other viruses such as herpes simplex virus (~4%) and Epstein-Barr virus (<1% in infectious mononucleosis). Less common causes are acute HIV infection, gonorrhea, fusobacterial infection (e.g., Lemierre's syndrome), thrush due to *Candida albicans* or other *Candida* species, and diphtheria. The presence of a pharyngeal pseudomembrane or an extensive exudate should prompt consideration of diphtheria **(Fig. 150-1)**.

CLINICAL MANIFESTATIONS

Respiratory Diphtheria The clinical diagnosis of diphtheria is based on the constellation of sore throat; adherent tonsillar, pharyngeal, or nasal pseudomembranous lesions; and low-grade fever. In addition, diagnosis requires the isolation of *C. diphtheriae* or histopathologic isolation of compatible gram-positive organisms. The

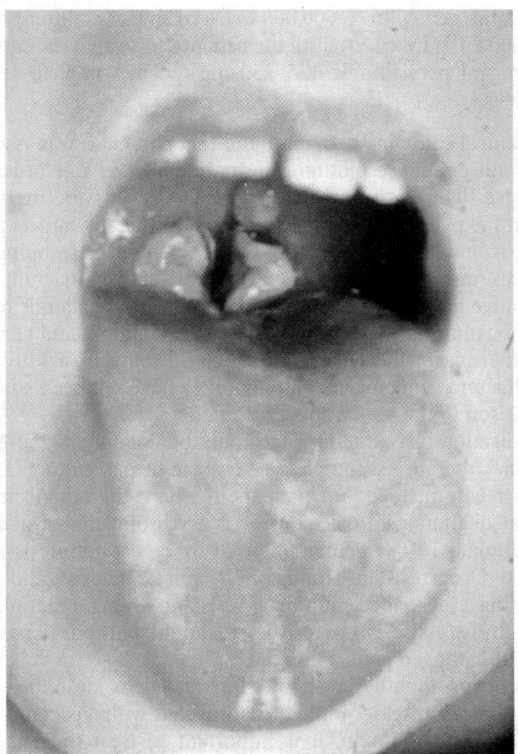

FIGURE 150-1 Respiratory diphtheria due to toxigenic *C. diphtheriae* producing exudative pharyngitis in a child displaying a pseudomembrane extending from the uvula to the pharyngeal wall. The characteristic white pseudomembrane is caused by diphtheria toxin–mediated necrosis of the respiratory epithelial layer, producing a fibrinous coagulative exudate. Submucosal edema adds to airway narrowing. The pharyngitis is acute in onset, and respiratory obstruction from the pseudomembrane may occur in severe cases. Inoculation of pseudomembrane fragments or submembranous swabs onto Löffler's or tellurite selective medium reveals *C. diphtheriae*. *(Photograph courtesy of the Centers for Disease Control and Prevention and Immunization Action Coalition, used by permission.)*

Centers for Disease Control and Prevention (CDC) recognizes *confirmed* respiratory diphtheria (laboratory proven or epidemiologically linked to a culture-confirmed case) and *probable* respiratory diphtheria (clinically compatible but not laboratory proven or epidemiologically linked). Carriers are defined as individuals who have positive cultures for *C. diphtheriae* and who either are asymptomatic or have symptoms but lack pseudomembranes. Most patients seek medical care for sore throat and fever several days into the illness. Occasionally, weakness, dysphagia, headache, and voice change are the initial manifestations. Neck edema and difficulty breathing are evident in more advanced cases and carry a poor prognosis.

The systemic manifestations of diphtheria stem from the effects of diphtheria toxin and include weakness as a result of neurotoxicity and cardiac arrhythmias or congestive heart failure due to myocarditis. Most commonly, the pseudomembranous lesion is located in the tonsillopharyngeal region. Less commonly, the lesions are located in the larynx, nares, and trachea or bronchial passages. Large pseudomembranes are associated with severe disease and a poor prognosis. A few patients develop massive swelling of the tonsils and present with "bull-neck" diphtheria, which results from edema of the submandibular and paratracheal region and is further characterized by foul breath, thick speech, and stridorous breathing. The diphtheritic pseudomembrane is gray or whitish and sharply demarcated. Unlike the exudative lesion associated with streptococcal pharyngitis, the pseudomembrane in diphtheria is tightly adherent to the underlying tissues. Attempts to dislodge the membrane may cause bleeding. Hoarseness suggests laryngeal diphtheria, in which laryngoscopy may be diagnostically helpful.

Cutaneous Diphtheria This dermatosis is characterized by punched-out ulcerative lesions with necrotic sloughing or pseudomembrane formation (**Fig. 150-2**). The diagnosis requires cultivation of *C. diphtheriae* from lesions, which most commonly occur on the lower and upper extremities, head, and trunk.

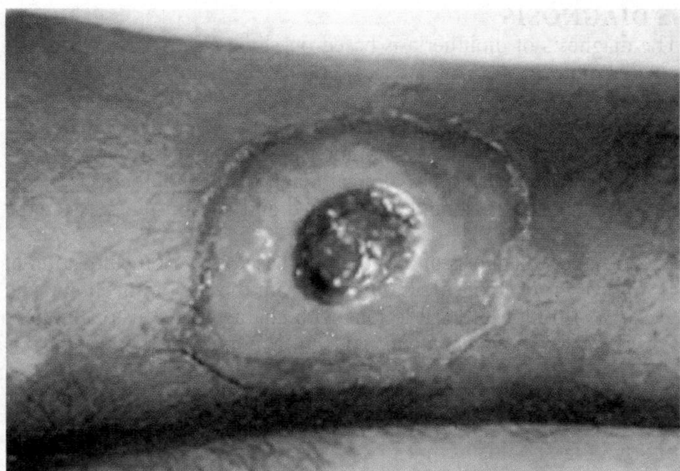

FIGURE 150-2 Cutaneous diphtheria due to nontoxigenic *C. diphtheriae* on the lower extremity. *(From the Centers for Disease Control and Prevention, Public Health Image Library [PHIL]. #1941.)*

Infections Due to Non-*diphtheriae Corynebacterium* Species and Nontoxigenic *C. diphtheriae* Non-*diphtheriae* species of *Corynebacterium* and related genera (discussed below) as well as nontoxigenic strains of *C. diphtheriae* itself have been found in bloodstream and respiratory infections, often in individuals with immunosuppression or chronic respiratory disease. These organisms can cause disease manifestations and should not necessarily be dismissed as colonizers.

Other Clinical Manifestations *C. diphtheriae* causes rare cases of endocarditis and septic arthritis, most often in patients with preexisting risk factors, such as abnormal cardiac valves, injection drug use, or cirrhosis.

COMPLICATIONS

Airway obstruction poses a significant early risk in patients presenting with advanced diphtheria. Pseudomembranes may slough and obstruct the airway or may advance to the larynx or into the tracheobronchial tree. Children are particularly prone to obstruction because of their small airways.

Polyneuropathy and myocarditis are late toxic manifestations of diphtheria. During a diphtheria outbreak in the Kyrgyz Republic in 1999, myocarditis was found in 22% and neuropathy in 5% of 676 hospitalized patients. The mortality rate was 7% among patients with myocarditis as opposed to 2% among those without myocardial manifestations. The median time to death in hospitalized patients was 4.5 days. Myocarditis is typically associated with arrhythmias and dilated cardiomyopathy.

Polyneuropathy is seen 3–5 weeks after the onset of diphtheria and has a slow indolent course. However, patients may develop severe and prolonged neurologic abnormalities. The disorders typically occur in the mouth and neck, with lingual or facial numbness as well as dysphonia, dysphagia, and cranial nerve paresthesias. More ominous signs include weakness of respiratory and abdominal muscles and paresis of the extremities. Sensory manifestations and sensory ataxia also are observed. Cranial nerve dysfunction typically precedes disturbances of the trunk and extremities because of proximity to the site of infection. Autonomic dysfunction also is associated with polyneuropathy and can lead to hypotension. Polyneuropathy is typically reversible in patients who survive the acute phase.

Other complications of diphtheria include pneumonia, renal failure, encephalitis, cerebral infarction, pulmonary embolism, and serum sickness from antitoxin therapy.

DIAGNOSIS

The diagnosis of diphtheria is based on clinical signs and symptoms plus laboratory confirmation. Respiratory diphtheria should be considered in patients with sore throat, pharyngeal exudates, and fever. Other symptoms may include hoarseness, stridor, or palatal paralysis. The presence of a pseudomembrane should prompt strong consideration of diphtheria. Once a clinical diagnosis of diphtheria is made, diphtheria antitoxin should be obtained and administered as rapidly as possible.

Laboratory diagnosis of diphtheria is based either on cultivation of *C. diphtheriae* or toxigenic *C. ulcerans* from the site of infection or on the demonstration of local lesions with characteristic histopathology. *Corynebacterium pseudodiphtheriticum*, a nontoxigenic organism, is a common component of the normal throat flora and does not pose a significant risk. Throat samples should be submitted to the laboratory for culture with the notation that diphtheria is being considered. This information should prompt cultivation on special selective medium and subsequent biochemical testing to differentiate *C. diphtheriae* from other nasopharyngeal commensal corynebacteria. All laboratory isolates of *C. diphtheriae,* including nontoxigenic strains, should be submitted to the CDC.

A diagnosis of cutaneous diphtheria requires laboratory confirmation since the lesions are not characteristic and are indistinguishable from other dermatoses. Diphtheritic ulcers occasionally—but not consistently—have a punched-out appearance (Fig. 150-2). Patients in whom cutaneous diphtheria is identified should have the nasopharynx cultured for *C. diphtheriae.* The laboratory medium for cutaneous diphtheria specimens is the same as that used for respiratory diphtheria: Löffler's or Tinsdale's selective medium in addition to nonselective medium such as blood agar. As has been mentioned, respiratory diphtheria remains a notifiable disease in the United States, whereas cutaneous diphtheria is not.

TREATMENT

Diphtheria

DIPHTHERIA ANTITOXIN

Prompt administration of diphtheria antitoxin is critical in the management of respiratory diphtheria. Diphtheria antitoxin, a horse antiserum, is effective in reducing the extent of local disease as well as the risk of complications of myocarditis and neuropathy. Rapid institution of antitoxin therapy is also associated with a significant reduction in mortality risk. Because diphtheria antitoxin cannot neutralize cell-bound toxin, prompt initiation is important. This product, which is no longer commercially available in the United States, can be obtained from the CDC Emergency Operations Center at 770-488-7100 (website: *www.cdc.gov/diphtheria/dat.html*) after first contacting the state health department. The current protocol for the use of diphtheria antitoxin involves a test dose to rule out immediate hypersensitivity. Patients who demonstrate hypersensitivity require desensitization before a full therapeutic dose of antitoxin is administered.

Given that the world supply of equine anti–diphtheria toxin is limited, a human monoclonal antibody with the potential to provide a safer alternative to equine antitoxin therapy is being developed.

ANTIMICROBIAL THERAPY

Antibiotics are used in the management of diphtheria primarily to prevent transmission to susceptible contacts. Antibiotics also prevent further toxin production and reduce the severity of local infection. Recommended treatment options for patients with respiratory diphtheria are as follows:

- Erythromycin, 500 mg IV q6h (for children: 40–50 mg/kg per day IV in two or four divided doses) until the patient can swallow comfortably; then 500 mg PO qid to complete a 14-day course
- Procaine penicillin G, 600,000 U IM q12h (for children: 12,500–25,000 U/kg IM q12h) until the patient can swallow comfortably; then oral penicillin V, 125–250 mg qid to complete a 14-day course

A clinical study in Vietnam found that penicillin was associated with a more rapid resolution of fever and a lower rate of bacterial resistance than erythromycin; however, relapses were more common in the penicillin group. Erythromycin therapy targets protein synthesis and thus offers the presumed benefit of stopping toxin synthesis more quickly than a cell wall–active β-lactam agent. Alternative therapeutic agents for patients who are allergic to penicillin or cannot take erythromycin include rifampin and clindamycin. Other reasonable antibiotics are clarithromycin, azithromycin, linezolid, and vancomycin, although they have not been studied in comparison to the agents above.

Eradication of *C. diphtheriae* should be documented after antimicrobial therapy is complete. A repeat throat culture 2 weeks later is recommended. For patients in whom the organism is not eradicated after a 14-day course of erythromycin or penicillin, an additional 10-day course followed by repeat culture is recommended. Drug-resistant strains of *C. diphtheriae* exist, and several reports have described multidrug-resistant strains, predominantly in Southeast Asia. Drug resistance should be considered when efforts at pathogen eradication fail.

Cutaneous diphtheria should be treated as described above for respiratory disease. Individuals infected with toxigenic strains should receive antitoxin. It is important to treat the underlying cause of the dermatoses in addition to the superinfection with *C. diphtheriae.*

Patients who recover from respiratory or cutaneous diphtheria should have antitoxin levels measured. If diphtheria antitoxin has been administered, this test should be performed 6 months later. Patients who recover from respiratory or cutaneous diphtheria should receive the appropriate vaccine to ensure the development of protective antibody titers.

MANAGEMENT STRATEGIES

Patients in whom diphtheria is suspected should be hospitalized in respiratory isolation rooms, with close monitoring of cardiac and respiratory function. A cardiac workup is recommended to assess the possibility of myocarditis. In patients with extensive pseudomembranes, an anesthesiology or an ear, nose, and throat consultation is recommended because of the possible need for tracheostomy or intubation. In some settings, pseudomembranes can be removed surgically. Treatment with glucocorticoids has not been shown to reduce the risk of myocarditis or polyneuropathy.

PROGNOSIS

The mortality rate for diphtheria is 5–10% but may approach 20% among children <5 years old and adults >40 years of age. Fatal pseudomembranous diphtheria typically occurs in patients with nonprotective antibody titers and in unimmunized patients. The pseudomembrane may actually increase in size from the time it is first noted. Risk factors for death include bullneck diphtheria; myocarditis with ventricular tachycardia; atrial fibrillation; complete heart block; an age of >60 years or <6 months; alcoholism; extensive pseudomembrane elongation; and laryngeal, tracheal, or bronchial involvement. Another important predictor of fatal outcome is the interval between the onset of local disease and the administration of antitoxin. Cutaneous diphtheria has a low mortality rate and is rarely associated with myocarditis or peripheral neuropathy.

PREVENTION

Vaccination Sustained campaigns for vaccination of children and adequate boosting vaccination of adults are responsible for the exceedingly low incidence of diphtheria in most developed nations. Currently, diphtheria toxoid vaccine is coadministered with tetanus vaccine (with or without acellular pertussis). DTaP (full-level diphtheria toxoid, tetanus toxoid, and acellular pertussis vaccine) is currently recommended for children up to the age of 6; DTaP replaced the earlier whole-cell pertussis vaccine DTP in 1997. Tdap is a tetanus toxoid, reduced diphtheria toxoid, and acellular pertussis vaccine formulated for adolescents and adults. Tdap was licensed for use in the United States in 2005 and is recommended for children ≥7 years old and for adults. It is recommended that all adults (i.e., persons >19 years old) receive a single dose of Tdap if they have not received it previously, regardless of the interval since the last dose of Td (tetanus and reduced-dose diphtheria toxoids, adsorbed). Tdap vaccination is a priority for health care workers, pregnant women, adults anticipating contact with infants, and adults not previously vaccinated for pertussis. Adults who have received acellular pertussis vaccine should continue to receive decennial Td booster vaccinations. **The vaccine schedule is detailed in Chap. 123.**

Prophylaxis Administration to Contacts Close contacts of diphtheria patients should undergo throat culture to determine whether they are carriers. After samples for throat culture are obtained, antimicrobial prophylaxis should be considered for all contacts, even those whose cultures are negative. The options are 7–10 days of oral erythromycin or one dose of IM benzathine penicillin G (1.2 million units for persons ≥6 years of age or 600,000 units for children <6 years of age).

Contacts of diphtheria patients whose immunization status is uncertain should receive the appropriate diphtheria toxoid–containing vaccine. The Tdap vaccine (rather than Td) is now the booster vaccine of choice for adults who have not recently received an acellular pertussis–containing vaccine. Carriers of *C. diphtheriae* in the community should be treated and vaccinated when identified.

OTHER CORYNEBACTERIAL AND *RHODOCOCCUS* INFECTIONS

Nondiphtherial corynebacteria, referred to as *diphtheroids* or *coryneforms*, are frequently considered colonizers or contaminants; however, they have been associated with invasive disease, particularly in immunocompromised patients. Importantly, even though they are termed nondiphtherial corynebacteria, *C. ulcerans* and *C. pseudotuberculosis* may produce diphtheria toxin and therefore cause severe human illness. These organisms have been isolated from the bloodstream, especially in association with catheter infection, endocarditis, prosthetic valve infection, meningitis, brain abscess, osteomyelitis, and peritonitis. Risk factors include indwelling intravenous or peritoneal catheters and neurosurgical shunts. Patients infected with these organisms are often immunosuppressed or have significant medical comorbidities. The nondiphtherial coryneforms are a collection of bacteria that are taxonomically grouped together in the genus *Corynebacterium* on the basis of their 16S rDNA signature nucleotides. Despite the shared rDNA signatures, these isolates are quite diverse. For example, their guanine-cytosine content ranges from 45 to 70%. Several nondiphtheroid corynebacteria, including *Corynebacterium jeikeium* and *Corynebacterium urealyticum*, are associated with resistance to multiple antibiotics. *Rhodococcus equi* is associated with necrotizing pneumonia and granulomatous infection, particularly in immunocompromised individuals.

MICROBIOLOGY AND LABORATORY DIAGNOSIS

These organisms are non-acid-fast, catalase-positive, aerobic or facultatively anaerobic rods. Their colonial morphologies on blood agar vary widely; some species are small and α-hemolytic (similar to lactobacilli), whereas others form large white colonies (similar to yeasts). Many nondiphtherial coryneforms require special media, such as Löffler's, Tinsdale's, or tellurite medium. These cultivation idiosyncrasies have led to a complex taxonomic categorization of the organisms.

EPIDEMIOLOGY

Humans are the natural reservoirs for several nondiphtherial coryneforms, including *C. xerosis, C. pseudodiphtheriticum, C. striatum, C. minutissimum, C. jeikeium, C. urealyticum,* and *Arcanobacterium haemolyticum.* Animal reservoirs including milk are responsible for carriage of *C. ulcerans* and *C. pseudotuberculosis.* Soil is the natural reservoir for *R. equi.*

CLINCAL MANIFESTATIONS

C. ulcerans This organism causes a diphtheria-like illness and produces both diphtheria toxin and a dermonecrotic toxin. The organism is a commensal in horses and cattle and has been isolated from cow's milk. In contrast to diphtheria, this infection is considered a zoonosis, and cases have been traced to contact with animal carriers, including dogs and pigs. *C. ulcerans* causes exudative pharyngitis, primarily during summer months, in rural areas, and among individuals exposed to animals. Treatment with antitoxin and antibiotics should be initiated when respiratory *C. ulcerans* is identified, and a contact investigation (including throat cultures to determine the need for antimicrobial prophylaxis and, in unimmunized contacts, administration of the appropriate diphtheria toxoid–containing vaccine) should be conducted. The organism grows on Löffler's, Tinsdale's, and tellurite agars as well as blood agar. In addition to exudative pharyngitis, cutaneous disease due to *C. ulcerans* has been reported. *C. ulcerans* is susceptible to a wide panel of antibiotics. Erythromycin and other macrolides appear to be the first-line agents.

C. pseudotuberculosis Infection caused by *C. pseudotuberculosis* is an important animal pathogen (most notably of sheep) that rarely causes human disease. *C. pseudotuberculosis* causes suppurative granulomatous lymphadenitis and an eosinophilic pneumonia syndrome among individuals who handle sheep; horses, cattle, goats, deer, and raw milk also have been implicated. Surgical excision of affected lymph nodes should be performed when feasible, and successful treatment with erythromycin or tetracycline has been reported. Some strains express diphtheria toxin and produce a diphtheria-like disease, which should be treated with antitoxin.

***C. jeikeium* (Group JK)** Originally described in American hospitals, *C. jeikeium* infection was subsequently reported in Europe. After a 1976 survey of diseases caused by nondiphtherial corynebacteria, CDC group JK emerged as an important opportunistic pathogen among neutropenic and HIV-infected patients. The organism has now been designated a separate species. *C. jeikeium* forms small, gray to white, glistening, nonhemolytic colonies on blood agar. It lacks urease and nitrate reductase and does not ferment most carbohydrates. The predominant syndrome associated with *C. jeikeium* is sepsis, sometimes with associated pneumonia, endocarditis, meningitis, osteomyelitis, or epidural abscess. Risk factors for *C. jeikeium* infection include hematologic malignancy, neutropenia from comorbid conditions, prolonged hospitalization, exposure to multiple antibiotics, and skin disruption. There is evidence that *C. jeikeium* is part of the inguinal, axillary, genital, and perirectal flora of hospitalized patients.

Broad-spectrum antimicrobial therapy appears to select for colonization. The organisms appear as gram-positive coccobacillary forms slightly resembling streptococci. *C. jeikeium* is resistant to the majority of antibiotic classes except oxazolidinones (e.g., linezolid) and glycopeptides (e.g., vancomycin). Effective therapy involves removal of the infectious source, whether a catheter, prosthetic joint, or prosthetic valve. Efforts have been made to prevent *C. jeikeium* infection with strict institution of infection control protocols for high-risk patients, particularly those in intensive care units.

***C. urealyticum* (Group D2)** Identified as a urease-positive nondiphtherial *Corynebacterium* in 1972, *C. urealyticum* is an opportunistic pathogen causing sepsis and urinary tract infection. *C. urealyticum* appears to be the etiologic agent of a severe urinary tract syndrome known as *alkaline-encrusted cystitis*, a chronic inflammatory bladder infection associated with deposition of ammonium magnesium phosphate on the surface and walls of ulcerating lesions in the bladder. In addition, *C. urealyticum* has been associated with pneumonia, peritonitis, endocarditis, osteomyelitis, and wound infection. It is similar to *C. jeikeium* in its resistance to most antibiotics except oxazolidinones and glycopeptides. Vancomycin therapy has been used successfully in severe infections.

C. *minutissimum* (Erythrasma) Erythrasma is a cutaneous infection producing reddish-brown, macular, scaly, pruritic intertriginous patches. The dermatologic presentation under the Wood's lamp is of coral red fluorescence. *C. minutissimum* appears to be a common cause of erythrasma, although there is evidence for a polymicrobial etiology in certain settings. This microbe has also been associated with bacteremia in patients with hematologic malignancy. Erythrasma responds to topical erythromycin, clarithromycin, clindamycin, or fusidic acid, although more severe infections may require oral macrolide therapy.

Other Nondiphtherial Corynebacteria *C. xerosis* is a human commensal found in the conjunctiva, nasopharynx, and skin. This nontoxigenic organism is occasionally identified as a source of invasive infection in immunocompromised or postoperative patients and prosthetic joint recipients. *C. amycolatum* is a closely related species but tends to demonstrate more antibiotic resistance. *C. striatum* is found in the anterior nares, skin, face, and upper torso of healthy individuals. Also nontoxigenic, this organism has been associated with invasive opportunistic infections in severely ill or immunocompromised patients. *C. glucuronolyticum* is a nonlipophilic species that causes male genitourinary tract infections such as prostatitis and urethritis. These infections may be successfully treated with a wide variety of antibacterial agents, including β-lactams, rifampin, aminoglycosides, or vancomycin; however, the organism appears to be resistant to fluoroquinolones, macrolides, and tetracyclines. *C. imitans* has been identified in eastern Europe as a nontoxigenic cause of pharyngitis. *C. auris* has been identified in children with otitis media; it is susceptible to fluoroquinolones, rifampin, tetracycline, and vancomycin but resistant to penicillin G and variably susceptible to macrolides. *C. pseudodiphtheriticum* is a nontoxigenic species that is part of the normal human flora. Human infections—particularly endocarditis of either prosthetic or natural valves and invasive pneumonia—have been reported only rarely. Although *C. pseudodiphtheriticum* may be isolated from the nasopharynx of patients with suspected diphtheria, it is part of the normal flora and does not produce diphtheria toxin. *C. propinquum*, a close relative of *C. pseudodiphtheriticum*, is part of CDC group D-1 and has been isolated from the human respiratory tract and blood. *C. afermentans* and subspecies belongs to CDC group ANF-1; it is a rare human pathogen that has been isolated from human blood and abscesses.

Rhodococcus *Rhodococcus* species are phylogenetically related to the corynebacteria. These gram-positive coccobacilli have been associated with tuberculosis-like infections in humans with granulomatous pathology. While *R. equi* is best known, other near-relative species have been identified in human infections including *R. fascians*, *R. erythropolis*, *R. rhodochrous*, *Gordonia bronchialis*, *G. sputi*, *G. terrae*, and *Tsukamurella paurometabola*.

R. equi has been recognized as a cause of pneumonia in horses since the 1920s and as a cause of related infections in cattle, sheep, and swine. It is found in soil as an environmental microbe. The organisms vary in length; appear as spherical to long, curved, clubbed rods; and produce large irregular mucoid colonies. *R. equi* cannot ferment carbohydrates or liquefy gelatin and is often acid fast. An intracellular pathogen of macrophages, *R. equi* can cause granulomatous necrosis and caseation. This organism has most commonly been identified in pulmonary infection, but infections of brain, bone, and skin also have been reported. Most commonly, *R. equi* disease manifests as nodular and/or cavitary pneumonia of the upper lobe—a picture similar to that seen in tuberculosis or nocardiosis. Most patients are immunocompromised, often by HIV infection. Subcutaneous nodular lesions also have been identified. The involvement of *R. equi* should be considered when any patient presents with a tuberculosis-like syndrome.

Infection due to *R. equi* has been treated successfully with antibiotics that penetrate intracellularly, including macrolides, clindamycin, rifampin, and trimethoprim-sulfamethoxazole. β-Lactam antibiotics have not been useful. The organism is routinely susceptible to vancomycin, which is considered the drug of choice.

Arcanobacteria *Arcanobacterium haemolyticum* was identified as an agent of wound infections in U.S. soldiers in the South Pacific during World War II. It appears to be a human commensal of the nasopharynx and skin, but it is known to cause true pharyngitis as well as chronic skin ulcers. In contrast to the much more common pharyngitis caused by *Streptococcus pyogenes*, *A. haemolyticum* pharyngitis is associated with a scarlatiniform rash on the trunk and proximal extremities in about half of cases; this illness is occasionally confused with toxic shock syndrome. Because *A. haemolyticum* pharyngitis primarily affects teenagers, it has been postulated that the rash–pharyngitis syndrome may represent co-pathogenicity, synergy, or opportunistic secondary infection with Epstein-Barr virus. *A. haemolyticum* has also been reported as a cause of bacteremia, soft tissue infections, osteomyelitis, and cavitary pneumonia, predominantly in the setting of underlying diabetes mellitus. The organism is susceptible to most β-lactams, macrolides, fluoroquinolones, clindamycin, vancomycin, and doxycycline. However, resistance to trimethoprim-sulfamethoxazole as well as tetracycline is common.

■ FURTHER READING

Kim R, Reboli AC: Other coryneform bacteria and *Rhodococcus,* in *Mandell, Douglas, and Bennett's Principles and Practice of Infectious Diseases*, 9th ed. JE Bennett et al (eds). Philadelphia, Elsevier, 2020, pp 2532–2542.

Moore LS et al: *Corynebacterium ulcerans* cutaneous diphtheria. Lancet Infect Dis 15:1100, 2015.

Saleeb PG: *Corynebacterium diphtheriae* (diphtheria), in *Mandell, Douglas, and Bennett's Principles and Practice of Infectious Diseases*, 9th ed. JE Bennett et al (eds). Philadelphia, Elsevier, 2020, pp 2526–2531.

Sharma NC et al: Diphtheria. Nat Rev Dis Primers 5:81, 2019.

Wiedermann BL: Diphtheria in the 21st century: New insights and a wake-up call. Clin Infect Dis 71:98, 2020.

151 *Listeria monocytogenes* Infections

Jennifer P. Collins, Patricia M. Griffin

Listeria monocytogenes is a ubiquitous environmental saprophyte and an intracellular pathogen in several animals. Humans develop *L. monocytogenes* infection—listeriosis—primarily through foodborne transmission. The clinical spectrum of listeriosis ranges from febrile gastroenteritis in healthy persons to invasive disease, including bacteremia and meningoencephalitis. Typical risk groups for invasive disease are pregnant women and their neonates, older adults, and immunocompromised persons.

■ MICROBIOLOGY

L. monocytogenes is a nonsporulating, facultatively anaerobic, short, gram-positive rod that grows well on blood agar, demonstrating small zones of β-hemolysis. Organisms sometimes appear gram-variable and resemble cocci, diplococci, or diphtheroids; this appearance can obscure the diagnosis. On light microscopy, *L. monocytogenes* demonstrates characteristic tumbling motility. It grows optimally at 30–37°C but can grow at refrigerator temperatures as low as 4°C. Serotypes are usually determined on the basis of somatic (O) and flagellar (H) antigens. Nearly all human illness is caused by serotypes 1/2a, 1/2b, and 4b.

■ PATHOGENESIS

L. monocytogenes lives in soil and decaying vegetable matter. Numerous bird and mammal species are reservoirs. In addition to its ability to grow at cold temperatures, *Listeria*'s tolerance to low-pH and high-salt environments facilitates its environmental survival. Human infection typically occurs through ingestion of contaminated food. The infectious dose has not been well established but is likely to be very low for persons with severely impaired cellular immunity. Increased gastric pH, such as that due to proton pump inhibitors, probably promotes the organism's survival in the gastrointestinal tract. After transcytosis across the intestinal epithelium, the bacteria travel via mesenteric lymph nodes and the bloodstream to the liver and spleen, its target organs; dissemination to other organs can occur. *L. monocytogenes* can also migrate across the blood–brain barrier and the placenta.

Virulence factors, including a pore-forming cytolysin (listeriolysin O; LLO) and phospholipases, facilitate evasion of intracellular killing by mediating escape from the internalization vacuole; the organism can then enter the host cell cytosol. The surface protein ActA facilitates direct cell-to-cell movement within the cytosol, allowing *L. monocytogenes* to avoid encountering components of the host immune system, such as antibodies and complement, during dissemination. Iron promotes listerial growth of the organism in vitro, an effect that explains why listeriosis has been associated with iron-overload conditions, including hemochromatosis.

IMMUNE RESPONSE

Although *L. monocytogenes* is ubiquitous in the environment, infection is rare because of both innate and adaptive host immune responses. Studies of mice have contributed to a detailed understanding of the immune response to infection. Activation of innate immunity is important for host survival. Interferon γ and tumor necrosis factor α (TNF-α) are among the key cytokines involved in this response. T cells are the primary drivers of the adaptive immune response, furthering the clearance of infected cells. Cytotoxic (CD8+) T cells are the main contributors to long-term immunity.

These immune mechanisms explain the association between invasive listeriosis and immunocompromising conditions, particularly impaired cellular immunity. In light of numerous reports of invasive listeriosis in patients treated with TNF-α inhibitors, the U.S. Food and Drug Administration added listeriosis to the boxed warning for this drug class. Because *L. monocytogenes* induces a vigorous cell-mediated immune response, attenuated strains that express foreign antigens are undergoing clinical trials as a cancer immunotherapy.

EPIDEMIOLOGY

More than 50 years after *L. monocytogenes* was first identified as a human pathogen, a 1983 outbreak investigation implicated coleslaw, thus establishing foodborne transmission. It is now known that *L. monocytogenes* transmission is almost always foodborne. Listeriosis is a nationally notifiable disease in the United States. According to the Centers for Disease Control and Prevention's (CDC's) Foodborne Diseases Active Surveillance Network (FoodNet), the incidence of invasive listeriosis was 2.4–3.7 cases per million persons during 2008–2019 (**Fig. 151-1**). Listeriosis is a substantial contributor to deaths from foodborne illness despite being a relatively uncommon cause of illness.

Only about 3% of cases of listeriosis are part of a recognized outbreak—i.e., have a source determined; however, outbreak investigations provide data on major food sources. Hot dogs and deli meats were the major sources of U.S. outbreaks until 2002, when an outbreak linked to turkey deli meat resulted in eight deaths and the recall of >30 million pounds of meat. After that outbreak, the U.S. Department of Agriculture's Food Safety and Inspection Service issued new regulations and intensified testing for *L. monocytogenes* in ready-to-eat meat and poultry plants, and producers added growth inhibitors. Since then, these products have rarely been implicated in outbreaks, yet the incidence of listeriosis has not declined significantly in about two decades (Fig. 151-1). Evidence that other sources are now more important is supported by the marked decline in isolations of *L. monocytogenes* from ready-to-eat meats (Fig. 151-1). Dairy products are an important source, especially soft cheese made with raw (unpasteurized) milk or produced from pasteurized milk in unsanitary facilities; ice cream and raw milk also have caused outbreaks. Raw produce is another important source; outbreaks have been traced to packaged salad, sprouts, cantaloupe and other fruit, caramel apples, and frozen vegetables. A single strain of *L. monocytogenes* can survive in a production facility for years. A small amount of contamination during production can lead to much higher levels when food is ingested because of the organism's ability to grow at refrigerator temperatures.

Most people with invasive listeriosis are older adults, whose risk increases with each decade over 59 years of age. Most other patients have impaired cellular immunity associated with hematologic malignancy, solid organ or bone marrow transplantation, HIV infection, or receipt of glucocorticoid or other immunosuppressive drugs. The group at highest risk is pregnant women, who almost always have only mild flulike symptoms but who transmit the infection to the fetus through the placenta. Some neonates may acquire infection in the hospital, as illustrated by an outbreak associated with contaminated mineral oil. Rarely, children and adults with no risk factors develop invasive listeriosis, probably through heavy contamination of food. The

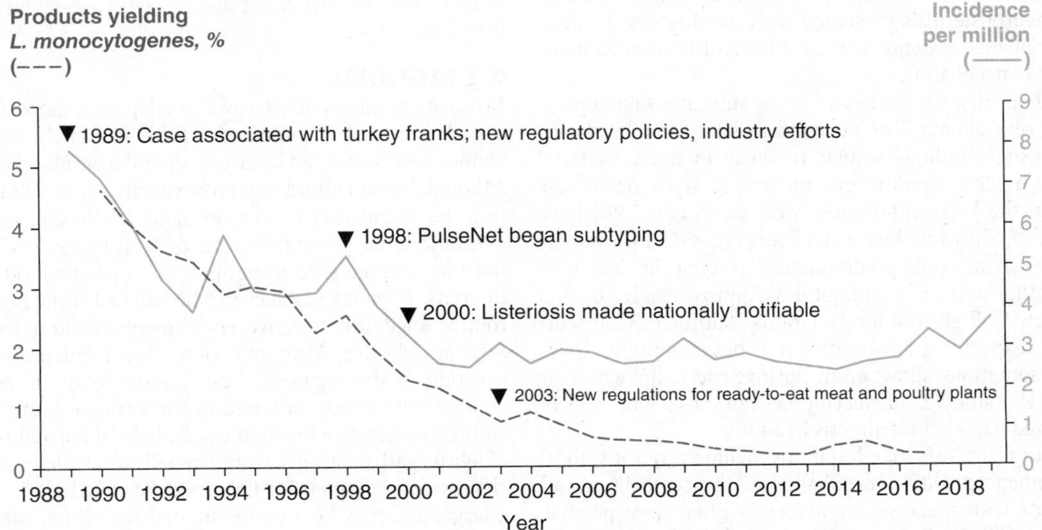

FIGURE 151-1 Incidence of listeriosis and percentage of ready-to-eat meat and poultry products with cultures that yielded *L. monocytogenes*, United States, 1989–2019. Incidence data are from the Center for Disease Control and Prevention's active sentinel site surveillance and include data from an early surveillance system (1986–1995) and from the Foodborne Diseases Active Surveillance Network (FoodNet) database (1996–2019). The incidence was 7.3 cases per million in 1986. Product data for 1990–2017 are publicly available through the U. S. Department of Agriculture Food Safety and Inspection Service Microbiological Testing Program for Ready-to-Eat Meat and Poultry Products.

diagnosis of listeriosis in a hospitalized patient with new symptoms should prompt investigation into the food provided during hospitalization as a source. In fact, outbreaks have been traced to food served to hospitalized patients, especially those with immunocompromising conditions; implicated foods include sandwiches, butter, precut celery, Camembert cheese, sausage, tuna salad, and ice cream. A large 2017–2018 outbreak of listeriosis in South Africa, linked to a ready-to-eat processed meat product, disproportionately affected people living with HIV and pregnant women. No outbreak-associated cases were detected in the 15 other countries that imported the product; this discrepancy suggests that listeriosis is underrecognized in low- to middle-income countries, particularly those with a high prevalence of HIV infection.

CLINICAL MANIFESTATIONS

L. monocytogenes infection can manifest in several ways. The incubation period differs according to host factors and dose consumed: on average, this interval is <24 h for gastroenteritis and ~11 days for invasive disease, although it can be much longer. Data from outbreak investigations suggest that the incubation period is longer in pregnant women than in nonpregnant adults.

Febrile Gastroenteritis *Listeria* organisms typically pass through healthy people without causing symptoms, but acute febrile gastroenteritis can occur. Outbreak investigations of *L. monocytogenes* febrile gastroenteritis have identified high organism density in implicated foods, suggesting that a large inoculum must be ingested to cause illness. Major manifestations are fever, diarrhea, headache, and constitutional symptoms. Illness is usually self-limited, with symptoms lasting an average of 1–3 days.

Bacteremia Bacteremia without a focus is the most common manifestation of invasive listeriosis. Major features are fever, chills, myalgias, and arthralgias, sometimes preceded by nausea or diarrhea—markers of the initial gut infection. Bacteremia can cause neurolisteriosis or localized infection at other sites, in which case the diagnosis may be suggested by neurologic or other focal findings. In a large French cohort study, the 3-month mortality rate for *L. monocytogenes* bacteremia was 46%; death was associated with older age, female sex, neoplasia, multiorgan failure, worsening of preexisting organ dysfunction, and monocytopenia (<200 cells/μL).

Neurolisteriosis *L. monocytogenes* has an affinity for the central nervous system. Neurolisteriosis is the second most common manifestation of invasive listeriosis. Signs of meningitis along with altered mental status, seizures, or focal neurologic findings suggest meningoencephalitis. A recent French cohort study found that 84% of patients with neurolisteriosis presented with meningoencephalitis. Isolate-based surveillance systems may not distinguish between meningitis and meningoencephalitis.

Onset of neurologic disease can be sudden or subacute, taking place over the course of several days. Patients typically have fever, headache, nausea, and vomiting—findings similar to those in other bacterial meningitides—but nuchal rigidity and meningeal signs occur less commonly than in the latter conditions. Most patients (~75%) have cerebrospinal fluid (CSF) white blood cell counts of <1000/μL (range, 100–5000/μL). CSF neutrophil predominance is typically less pronounced than in other bacterial meningitides. Approximately 30–40% of patients have low CSF glucose levels. Gram's staining of CSF sediment can show the expected gram-positive rods but commonly shows no organisms and sometimes shows gram-positive cocci, diplococci, or diphtheroids. In a U.S. study, *L. monocytogenes* caused <5% of cases of community-acquired bacterial meningitis in adults.

Uncommon neurolisteriosis manifestations include cerebritis, focal abscess, and rhombencephalitis (encephalitis of the cerebellum and brainstem). Patients with macroscopic abscesses often have positive blood cultures, but CSF findings may be normal in the absence of concurrent meningitis. Abscesses may be misdiagnosed as a primary or metastatic malignancy; they rarely occur in the cerebellum or spinal cord. Rhombencephalitis disproportionately affects otherwise healthy older adults. The classic presentation is biphasic, beginning with fever and headache and continuing after several days with signs of brainstem or cerebellar involvement, such as asymmetric cranial nerve palsies, ataxia, tremor, hemiparesis, or hemisensory deficits. Nearly half of patients with rhombencephalitis experience respiratory failure. The diagnosis may be delayed by the subacute course and by CSF findings, which are often only minimally abnormal. MRI is superior to CT for the diagnosis of neurolisteriosis, including rhombencephalitis.

Overall, the 3-month mortality rate for neurolisteriosis was 30% in a recent French cohort study; death was associated with the same risk factors as those documented for bacteremia. Neurolisteriosis-associated mortality was also higher among patients with a positive blood culture and among those treated with dexamethasone. Nearly half of survivors had long-term neurologic impairment.

Focal infections Hematogenous dissemination of *L. monocytogenes* infrequently causes endocarditis, pneumonia, localized abscesses in the liver or other internal organs, peritonitis, septic arthritis, osteomyelitis, urinary tract infection, or skin lesions. Direct inoculation has been reported as a rare cause of ocular infection, skin infection, and lymphadenitis.

Infection in Pregnant Women and Neonates Pregnancy-associated listeriosis is most common in the third trimester, presumably because of impaired maternal cell-mediated immunity. Typically, pregnant women either are asymptomatic or have a mild, flulike illness with fever, headache, myalgias, or arthralgias. Neurolisteriosis and death are rare in pregnant women without other risk factors. Although nearly all infected women fully recover, only a minority (~5%) have a normal delivery and postpartum course. In a study of 107 pregnancies in which *L. monocytogenes* was isolated from the mother, fetus, or neonate, 24% ended with fetal loss, 45% with premature birth, and 21% with abnormal delivery at term (i.e., fever, meconium release into amniotic fluid, abnormal fetal heart rate). Moreover, 88% of the 82 live-born neonates were ill, including 49% who required intensive care. Fetal loss is uncommon after 29 weeks of gestation. Granulomatosis infantiseptica is a severe in utero infection caused by *L. monocytogenes* and characterized by disseminated microabscesses and granulomas in the skin, liver, and spleen; most infants with this condition are stillborn or die soon after birth. Neonatal infection usually manifests in one of two ways: early-onset sepsis is hypothesized to result from in utero infection because it is typically diagnosed within 48 h after birth and is often associated with prematurity, whereas late-onset meningitis is thought to result from infection acquired at or soon after birth because it is typically diagnosed at ~2 weeks of age in full-term infants. A study of 128 pregnancy-associated listeriosis cases found that 47 (62%) of 76 ill neonates had early-onset disease. The case–fatality rate for neonatal listeriosis is 10–50%.

DIAGNOSIS

Because symptoms of listeriosis overlap with those of other infections, a high index of suspicion can facilitate timely diagnosis. Pregnant women with suspected listeriosis should have blood drawn for cultures, although blood cultures are positive only about half the time. Isolation of *L. monocytogenes* from a normally sterile site, such as blood, CSF, amniotic fluid, placental tissue, or fetal tissue, is diagnostic. *Listeria* must be distinguished from other gram-positive rods, especially diphtheroids. *L. monocytogenes* can be isolated from sterile specimens on routine medium; selective enrichment medium (such as PALCAM *Listeria* Selective Agar or Oxford Agar) enhances the capacity for isolation of the organism from nonsterile specimens, such as stool. Stool culture is not indicated in the evaluation of invasive listeriosis; culture on selective medium can be helpful for outbreak investigations of febrile gastroenteritis. Commercially available multiplex polymerase chain reaction panels for CSF specimens include *L. monocytogenes* as a target and may be a useful adjunct to culture. Matrix-assisted laser desorption/ionization time-of-flight (MALDI-TOF) mass spectrometry can rapidly identify an isolate as *L. monocytogenes.* Whole-genome sequencing has been a valuable tool for solving outbreaks of listeriosis, including a nosocomial outbreak associated with ice cream served in hospital milkshakes.

TREATMENT

Infections Caused by *Listeria monocytogenes*

L. monocytogenes treatment has not been evaluated in clinical trials. Recommendations are based on in vitro animal studies and observational clinical data. High-dose ampicillin (adult dose, 2 g IV every 4 h) or penicillin G (adult dose, 4 million units IV every 4 h) constitutes first-line therapy. Because penicillins are only weakly bactericidal against *L. monocytogenes*, many experts recommend adding gentamicin for synergy (1.0–1.7 mg/kg every 8 h if renal function is normal), particularly if the infection is severe. Small studies have had varying results with regard to the benefits of gentamicin. A large study provided evidence favoring amoxicillin–gentamicin as first-line therapy. Patients who are allergic to penicillin should undergo desensitization or be treated with trimethoprim-sulfamethoxazole (TMP-SMX; 5 mg/kg per dose of the trimethoprim component, given IV every 6–12 h). TMP-SMX should be avoided during the first trimester because it has been associated with neural tube and cardiovascular defects and in the perinatal period because it may increase the risk of kernicterus. Resistance to TMP-SMX has been reported; thus antibiotic susceptibility testing should be performed if this drug is considered. Treatment failures have been reported with meropenem despite in vitro susceptibility of the organism. *L. monocytogenes* is susceptible in vitro to several other drugs, including vancomycin, linezolid, tetracycline, macrolides, and fourth-generation fluoroquinolones (e.g., moxifloxacin), but relevant clinical reports are limited. Cephalosporins are not effective. A retrospective study of 31 patients found significantly reduced survival rates among patients treated with dexamethasone; the authors suggest avoiding this drug in neurolisteriosis. Prepartum antibiotic treatment of pregnant women with listeriosis enhances the chance of delivering a healthy infant.

The optimal duration of antibiotic therapy has not been established. Treatment duration usually depends on the clinical syndrome, disease severity, patient attributes, and response to treatment. The typical minimal treatment duration is 2 weeks for bacteremia, 2 weeks for early-onset neonatal disease, 3 weeks for meningitis, 4–6 weeks for endocarditis, and 6–8 weeks for brain abscess or encephalitis. Longer courses may be needed when patients are immunocompromised or are not improving as expected. Patients with neurolisteriosis do not routinely require a follow-up lumbar puncture if they are improving clinically during antibiotic therapy.

PREVENTION

Care of patients with listeriosis should be undertaken with standard precautions because person-to-person transmission is rare. Implementation of general precautions to prevent foodborne illness can help prevent listeriosis. These measures include fully cooking meats; washing fresh produce; cleaning hands, utensils, and kitchen surfaces after handling uncooked foods; and avoiding unpasteurized dairy products. Persons at increased risk for listeriosis should take additional precautions, including avoiding soft cheeses (particularly those made with unpasteurized milk) and either avoiding ready-to-eat and delicatessen foods (including meats, hot dogs, and smoked seafood) or heating these foods until the internal temperature is 165°F or until they are steaming hot. Additional CDC recommendations can be found at *www.cdc.gov/listeria/prevention.html*. Hospital dietary services should implement safe food-preparation procedures for immunocompromised patients and should not serve these patients higher-risk foods. Testing and treatment are not indicated for an asymptomatic person who has eaten a product recalled because of *L. monocytogenes* contamination, even if the person has risk factors for invasive listeriosis. TMP-SMX given as prophylaxis for *Pneumocystis jirovecii* infection (e.g., to persons infected with HIV or organ transplant recipients) helps prevent listeriosis.

FURTHER READING

Charlier C et al: Clinical features and prognostic factors of listeriosis: The MONALISA National Prospective Cohort Study. Lancet Infect Dis 17:510, 2017.

Farley MM: *Listeria monocytogenes*, in *Principles and Practice of Pediatric Infectious Diseases*, 5th ed, Long SS et al (eds). Philadelphia, Elselvier, 2018, pp 781–785.

Gottlieb SL et al: Multistate outbreak of listeriosis linked to turkey deli meat and subsequent changes in US regulatory policy. Clin Infect Dis 42:29, 2006.

Hof H: An update on the medical management of listeriosis. Expert Opin Pharmacother 5:1727, 2004.

McCollum JT et al: Multistate outbreak of listeriosis associated with cantaloupe. N Engl J Med 369:944, 2013.

Radoshevich L, Cossart P: *Listeria monocytogenes*: Towards a complete picture of its physiology and pathogenesis. Nat Rev Microbiol 16:32, 2018.

Silk BJ et al: Foodborne listeriosis acquired in hospitals. Clin Infect Dis 59:532, 2014.

Thomas J et al: Outbreak of listeriosis in South Africa associated with processed meat. N Engl J Med 382:632, 2020.

152 Tetanus

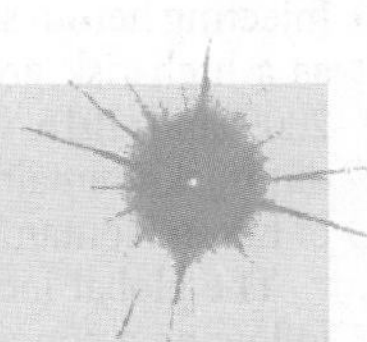

C. Louise Thwaites, Lam Minh Yen

Tetanus is an acute disease manifested by skeletal muscle spasm and autonomic nervous system disturbance. It is caused by a powerful neurotoxin produced by the bacterium *Clostridium tetani* and is completely preventable by vaccination. *C. tetani* is found throughout the world, and tetanus commonly occurs where the vaccination coverage rate is low. In developed countries, the disease is seen occasionally in individuals who are incompletely vaccinated. In any setting, established tetanus is a severe disease with a high mortality rate.

DEFINITION

Tetanus is diagnosed on clinical grounds (sometimes with supportive laboratory confirmation of the presence of *C. tetani*; see "Diagnosis," below), and case definitions are often used to facilitate clinical and epidemiologic assessments. The Centers for Disease Control and Prevention (CDC) defines probable tetanus as "an acute illness with muscle spasms or hypertonia in the absence of a more likely diagnosis." *Neonatal* tetanus is defined by the World Health Organization (WHO) as "an illness occurring in a child who has the normal ability to suck and cry in the first 2 days of life but who loses this ability between days 3 and 28 of life and becomes rigid and has spasms." Given the unique presentation of neonatal tetanus, the history generally permits accurate classification of the illness with a high degree of probability. *Maternal* tetanus is defined by the WHO as tetanus occurring during pregnancy or within 6 weeks after the conclusion of pregnancy (whether with birth, miscarriage, or abortion).

ETIOLOGY

C. tetani is an anaerobic, gram-positive, spore-forming rod whose spores are highly resilient and can survive readily in the environment throughout the world. Spores resist boiling and many disinfectants. In addition, *C. tetani* spores and bacilli survive in the intestinal systems of many animals, and fecal carriage is common. The spores or bacteria enter the body through abrasions, wounds, or (in the case of neonates) the umbilical stump. Once in a suitable anaerobic environment, the organisms grow, multiply, and release tetanus toxin, an exotoxin that enters the nervous system and causes disease. Very low concentrations of this highly potent toxin can result in tetanus (minimal lethal human dose, 2.5 ng/kg).

In 20–30% of cases of tetanus, no puncture entry wound is found. Superficial abrasions to the limbs are the most common infection sites in adults. Deeper infections (e.g., attributable to open fracture, abortion, or drug injection) are associated with more severe disease and worse outcomes. In neonates, infection of the umbilical stump can result from inadequate umbilical-cord care; in some cultures, for example, the cord is cut with grass or animal dung is applied to the stump. Circumcision or ear-piercing also can result in neonatal tetanus.

■ EPIDEMIOLOGY

Tetanus is a rare disease in the developed world. Two cases of neonatal tetanus have occurred in the United States since 2009. In 2018, 23 cases of tetanus were reported to the U.S. national surveillance system, almost all of which were in adults. Most cases occur in incompletely vaccinated or unvaccinated individuals. Vaccination status is known in 25% of cases reported in the United States between 2009 and 2015; among these cases, only 20% of patients had received three or more doses of tetanus toxoid–containing vaccine.

Persons >60 years of age are at greater risk of tetanus because antibody levels decrease over time. Approximately one-quarter of recent cases in the United States were in persons >65 years old. Diabetes is associated with increased tetanus risk, representing 13% of all cases and 25% of deaths in 2009–2015. People who inject drugs—particularly those injecting heroin subcutaneously ("skin-popping")—also are recognized as a high-risk group. Approximately 6% of all tetanus cases between 2009 and 2015 were in injection-drug users. The reasons for these outbreaks remain unclear but are thought to involve a combination of heroin contamination, skin-popping, and incomplete vaccination.

The global incidence of neonatal tetanus has reduced significantly following a concerted elimination program by WHO partnering with the United Nations Children's Fund (UNICEF) and the United Nations Population Fund (UNFPA). The incidence of tetanus among older children and adults is unknown, as few countries have good surveillance systems, although in 2015 there were estimated to be between 30,000 and 62,000 deaths from tetanus in this age group.

■ PATHOGENESIS

Genome sequencing of *C. tetani* has allowed identification of several exotoxins and virulence factors. Only those bacteria producing tetanus toxin (tetanospasmin) can cause tetanus. Although closely related to the botulinum toxins in structure and mode of action, tetanus toxin undergoes retrograde transport into the central nervous system (CNS) and thus produces clinical effects different from those caused by the botulinum toxins, which remain at the neuromuscular junction.

Tetanus toxin is intra-axonally transported to motor nuclei of the cranial nerves or ventral horns of the spinal cord. This toxin is produced as a single 150-kDa protein that is cleaved to produce heavy (100-kDa) and light (50-kDa) chains linked by a disulfide bond and noncovalent forces. The carboxy terminal of the heavy chain binds to specific membrane components in presynaptic α-motor nerve terminals; evidence suggests binding to both polysialogangliosides and membrane proteins. This binding results in toxin internalization and uptake into the nerves. Once inside the neuron, the toxin enters a retrograde transport pathway, whereby it is carried proximally to the motor neuron body. It is known that tetanus toxin exhibits several different pH-dependent conformations and therefore can interact with a variety of different receptors. During its passage from the periphery to the central nervous system, tetanus toxin can access neuronal trafficking systems and evade degradation.

Following retrograde transport in the motor neuron, the tetanus toxin undergoes translocation across the synapse to the GABA-ergic presynaptic inhibitory interneuron terminals. Here the light chain, which is a zinc-dependent endopeptidase, cleaves vesicle-associated membrane protein 2 (VAMP2, also known as *synaptobrevin*). This molecule is necessary for presynaptic binding and release of neurotransmitter; thus tetanus toxin prevents transmitter release and effectively blocks inhibitory interneuron discharge. The result is unregulated activity in the motor nervous system. Similar activity in the autonomic system accounts for the characteristic features of skeletal muscle spasm and autonomic system disturbance. The increased circulating catecholamine levels in severe tetanus are associated with cardiovascular complications.

Relatively little is known about the processes of recovery from tetanus. Recovery can take several weeks. Peripheral nerve sprouting is involved in recovery from botulism, and similar CNS sprouting may occur in tetanus. Other evidence suggests toxin degradation as a mechanism of recovery.

APPROACH TO THE PATIENT

Tetanus

The clinical manifestations of tetanus occur only after tetanus toxin has reached presynaptic inhibitory nerves. Once these effects become apparent, there may be little that can be done to affect disease progression. Treatment should not be delayed while the results of laboratory tests are awaited. Management strategies aim to neutralize remaining unbound toxin and support vital functions until the effects of the toxin have worn off. Recent interest has focused on intrathecal methods of antitoxin administration to neutralize toxin within the CNS and limit disease progression (see "Treatment," below).

■ CLINICAL MANIFESTATIONS

Tetanus produces a wide spectrum of clinical features that are broadly divided into generalized (including neonatal) and local. In the usually mild form of local tetanus, only isolated areas of the body are affected and only small areas of local muscle spasm may be apparent. If the cranial nerves are involved in localized cephalic tetanus, the pharyngeal or laryngeal muscles may spasm, with consequent aspiration or airway obstruction, and the prognosis may be poor. In the typical progression of generalized tetanus (**Fig. 152-1**), muscles of the face and jaw often are affected first, presumably because of the shorter distances toxin must travel up motor nerves to reach presynaptic terminals. Neonates typically present with an inability to suck.

In assessing prognosis, the speed at which tetanus develops is important. The incubation period (time from wound to first symptom) and the period of onset (time from first symptom to first generalized spasm) are of particular significance; shorter times are associated with worse outcome. In neonatal tetanus, the younger the infant is when symptoms occur, the worse the prognosis.

The most common initial symptoms are trismus (lockjaw), muscle pain and stiffness, back pain, and difficulty swallowing. In neonates, difficulty in feeding is the usual presentation. As the disease progresses, muscle spasm develops. Generalized muscle spasm can be very painful. Commonly, the laryngeal muscles are involved early or even in isolation. This is a life-threatening event as complete airway obstruction may ensue. Spasm of the respiratory muscles results in respiratory failure. Without ventilatory support, respiratory failure is the most common cause of death in tetanus. Spasms strong enough to produce tendon avulsions and crush fractures have been reported, but this outcome is extremely rare.

Autonomic disturbance is maximal during the second week of severe tetanus, and death due to cardiovascular events becomes the major risk. Blood pressure is usually labile, with rapid fluctuations from high to low accompanied by tachycardia. Episodes of bradycardia and heart block also can occur. Autonomic involvement is evidenced by gastrointestinal stasis, sweating, increased tracheal secretions, and acute (often high-output) renal failure.

■ DIAGNOSIS

The diagnosis of tetanus is based on clinical findings. As stated above, treatment should not be delayed while laboratory tests are conducted. Culture of *C. tetani* from a wound provides supportive evidence. Serum anti-tetanus immunoglobulin G also may be measured in a sample taken before the administration of antitoxin or immunoglobulin; levels >0.1 IU/mL (measured by standard enzyme-linked immunosorbent assay) are deemed protective and do not support the diagnosis of tetanus. If levels are below this threshold, a bioassay for serum tetanus toxin may be helpful, but a negative result does not exclude the diagnosis, and these levels are not generally performed. Polymerase chain

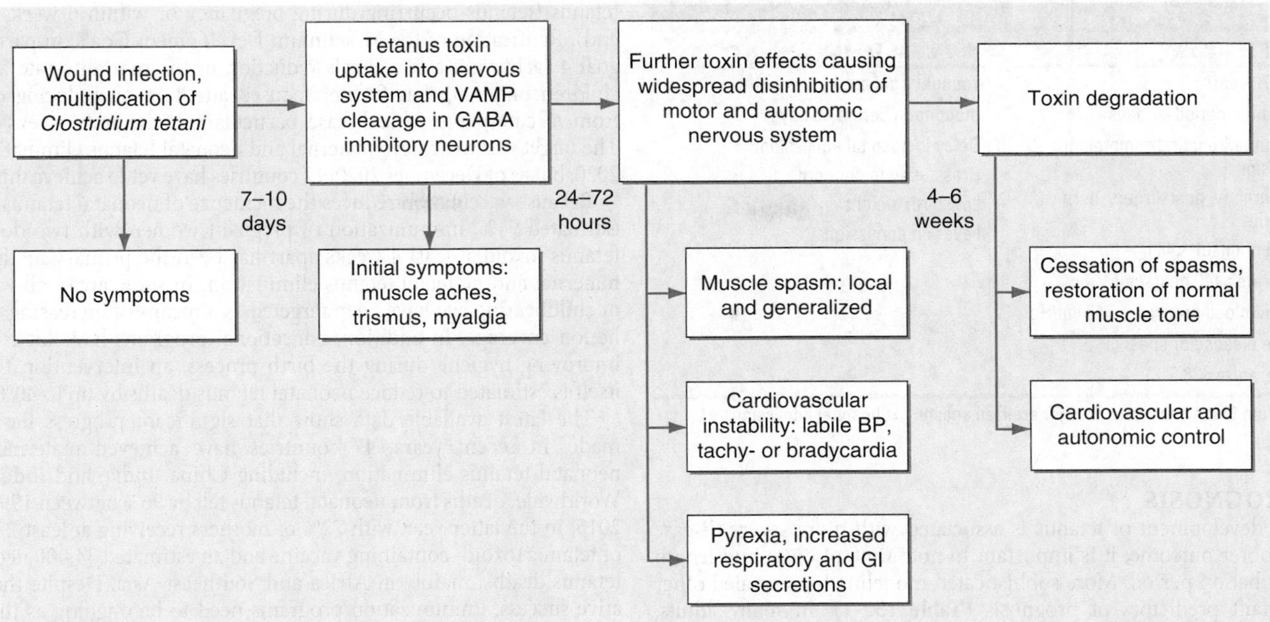

FIGURE 152-1 Clinical and pathologic progression of tetanus. BP, blood pressure; GABA, γ-aminobutyric acid; GI, gastrointestinal; VAMP, vesicle-associated membrane protein (synaptobrevin).

reaction also has been used for detection of tetanus toxin, but its sensitivity is unknown, and, similarly, a negative result does not exclude the diagnosis.

The few conditions that mimic generalized tetanus include strychnine poisoning and dystonic reactions to antidopaminergic drugs. Abdominal muscle rigidity is characteristically continuous in tetanus but is episodic in the latter two conditions. Cephalic tetanus can be confused with trismus of other etiologies, such as oropharyngeal infection. Hypocalcemia and meningoencephalitis are included in the differential diagnosis of neonatal tetanus.

TREATMENT
Tetanus

If possible, the entry wound should be identified, cleaned, and debrided of necrotic material in order to remove anaerobic foci of infection and prevent further toxin production. Metronidazole (400 mg rectally or 500 mg IV every 6 h for 7 days) is preferred for antibiotic therapy. An alternative is penicillin (100,000–200,000 IU/kg per day), although this drug theoretically may exacerbate spasms and in one study was associated with increased mortality. Failure to remove pockets of ongoing infection may result in recurrent or prolonged tetanus.

Antitoxin should be given early in an attempt to deactivate any circulating tetanus toxin and prevent its uptake into the nervous system. Two preparations are available: human tetanus immune globulin (TIG) and equine antitoxin. TIG is the preparation of choice, as it is less likely to be associated with anaphylactoid reactions. A single IM dose (500–5000 IU) is given, with a portion injected around the wound. Equine-derived antitoxin is available widely and is used in low-income countries; after hypersensitivity testing, 10,000–20,000 U is administered IM as a single dose or as divided doses. Some evidence indicates that intrathecal administration of TIG inhibits disease progression and leads to a better outcome. The results of relevant studies have been supported by a meta-analysis of trials involving both adults and neonates, with TIG doses of 50–1500 IU administered intrathecally. However, most preparations are not licensed for intrathecal use.

Spasms are controlled by heavy sedation with benzodiazepines. Chlorpromazine and phenobarbital are commonly used worldwide, and IV magnesium sulfate has been used as a muscle relaxant. A significant problem with all these treatments is that the doses necessary to control spasms also cause respiratory depression; thus, in resource-limited settings without mechanical ventilators, controlling spasms while maintaining adequate ventilation is problematic, and respiratory failure is a common cause of death. In locations with ventilation equipment, severe spasms are best controlled with a combination of sedatives or magnesium and relatively short-acting, cardiovascularly inert, nondepolarizing neuromuscular blocking agents that allow titration against spasm intensity. Infusions of propofol also have been used successfully to control spasms and provide sedation.

It is important to establish a secure airway early in severe tetanus. Ideally, patients should be nursed in calm, quiet environments because light and noise can trigger spasms. Tracheal secretions are increased in tetanus, and dysphagia due to pharyngeal involvement combined with hyperactivity of laryngeal muscles makes endotracheal intubation difficult. Patients may need ventilator support for several weeks. Thus tracheostomy is the usual method of securing the airway in severe tetanus.

Cardiovascular instability in severe tetanus is notoriously difficult to treat. Rapid fluctuations in blood pressure and heart rate can occur. Cardiovascular stability is improved by increasing sedation with IV magnesium sulfate (plasma concentration, 2–4 mmol/L or titrated against disappearance of the patella reflex), morphine, fentanyl, or other sedatives. In addition, drugs acting specifically on the cardiovascular system (e.g., esmolol, calcium antagonists, and inotropes) may be required. Short-acting drugs that allow rapid titration are preferred; particular care should be taken when longer-acting β antagonists are administered, as their use has been associated with hypotensive cardiac arrest.

Complications arising from treatment are common and include thrombophlebitis associated with diazepam injection, ventilator-associated pneumonia, central-line infections, and septicemia. In some centers, prophylaxis against deep-vein thrombosis and thromboembolism is routine.

Recovery from tetanus may take 4–6 weeks. Patients must be given a full primary course of immunization as tetanus toxin is poorly immunogenic and the immune response following natural infection is inadequate.

TABLE 152-1 Factors Associated with a Poor Prognosis in Tetanus

ADULT TETANUS	NEONATAL TETANUS
Age >70 years	Younger age, premature birth
Incubation period <7 days	Incubation period <6 days
Short time from first symptom to admission	Delay in hospital admission
Puerperal, IV, postsurgery, burn entry site	Grass used to cut cord
Period of onset[a] <48 h	Low birth weight
Heart rate >140 beats/min[b]	Fever on admission
Systolic blood pressure >140 mmHg[b]	
Severe disease or spasms[b]	
Temperature >38.5°C[b]	

[a]Time from first symptom to first generalized spasm. [b]At hospital admission.

PROGNOSIS

Rapid development of tetanus is associated with more severe disease and poorer outcome; it is important to note time of onset and length of incubation period. More sophisticated modeling has revealed other important predictors of prognosis **(Table 152-1)**. In many adults, particularly in the elderly, surviving tetanus is associated with reduced long-term functional outcome measures. Studies of children and neonates have suggested a higher incidence of neurologic sequelae. Neonates may be at increased risk of learning disabilities, behavioral problems, cerebral palsy, and deafness.

PREVENTION

Tetanus is prevented by good wound care and immunization **(Chap. 123)**. In neonates, use of safe, clean delivery and cord-care practices as well as maternal vaccination are essential. The WHO guidelines for tetanus vaccination consist of a primary course of three doses in infancy, boosters at 4–7 and 12–15 years of age, and one booster in adulthood. In the United States, the CDC suggests an additional dose at 15–18 months with booster at 11–12 years of age and every 10 years thereafter. For those with incomplete primary vaccination series in infancy, specific "catch-up" schedules are published. For those age 7 years or older, the recommendation is a three-dose primary course with 4 weeks between the first two doses, followed by a booster 6–12 months later. Catch-up schedules for those under 7 years involve a primary series of four doses of tetanus toxoid–containing vaccine if the child is under 12 months when the first dose is given, or three doses for those over 12 months at first dose.

Standard WHO recommendations for prevention of maternal and neonatal tetanus call for administration of two doses of tetanus toxoid at least 4 weeks apart to previously unimmunized pregnant women. A third dose should be given at least 6 months later, followed by one dose in subsequent pregnancies (or intervals of at least 1 year), to a total of five doses to provide long-term immunity. However, in high-risk areas, a more intensive approach has been successful, with all women of childbearing age receiving a primary course along with education on safe delivery and postnatal practices.

Individuals sustaining tetanus-prone wounds should be immunized if their vaccination status is incomplete or unknown or if their last booster was given >10 years earlier. Patients with an inadequate vaccine status who sustain wounds not classified as clean or minor should also undergo passive immunization with TIG. It is recommended that tetanus toxoid be given in conjunction with diphtheria toxoid in a preparation with or without acellular pertussis: DTaP for children <7 years old, Td for 7- to 9-year-olds, and Tdap for children >9 years old and adults.

In the early 1980s, tetanus caused more than 1 million deaths a year, accounting for an estimated 5% of maternal deaths and 14% of all neonatal deaths. In 1989, the World Health Assembly adopted a resolution to eliminate neonatal tetanus by the year 2000; elimination was defined as <1 case/1000 live births in every district in every country. By 1999, elimination was still to be achieved in 57 countries and the deadline was extended until 2005, with the additional target of eliminating maternal tetanus (tetanus occurring during pregnancy or within 6 weeks of its end). Ratification of the Millennium Development Goals, in particular goal 4 (achieving a two-thirds reduction in the mortality rate among children under 5), has further focused attention on reducing deaths from vaccine-preventable disease, particularly in the first 4 weeks of life. The target was to achieve maternal and neonatal tetanus elimination by 2020, but as of December 2020, 12 countries have yet to achieve this goal.

Because vaccination reduces the incidence of neonatal tetanus by an estimated 94%, immunization of pregnant women with two doses of tetanus toxoid at least 4 weeks apart has been the primary method of maternal and neonatal tetanus elimination. In some areas, all women of childbearing age have been targeted as a means of increasing vaccination coverage. In addition, educational programs have focused on improving hygiene during the birth process, an intervention that in itself is estimated to reduce neonatal tetanus deaths by up to 40%.

The latest available data show that significant progress has been made: in recent years, 47 countries have achieved maternal and neonatal tetanus elimination, including China, India, and Indonesia. Worldwide, deaths from neonatal tetanus fell by 96% between 1990 and 2015; in the latter year, with 72% of mothers receiving at least 2 doses of tetanus toxoid–containing vaccine and an estimated 34,000 neonatal tetanus deaths, mainly in Africa and Southeast Asia. Despite this relative success, immunization programs need to be ongoing as there is no herd immunity effect for tetanus and *C. tetani* contamination of soil and feces is widespread.

The rate of primary vaccination coverage in infancy (three doses of DTP) is 86%, but rates for the subsequent boosters necessary for long-term protection are unknown. Dedicated public health initiatives are lacking, and the continuing reports of sizable case series in the medical literature suggest that tetanus continues to pose a significant global health burden.

FURTHER READING

Borrow R et al: The immunological basis for immunization series. Module 3: Tetanus update 2018. Edited by Vaccines and Biologicals Immunization. World Health Organization, 2018.

Kyu HH et al: Mortality from tetanus between 1990 and 2015: Findings from the global burden of disease study 2015. BMC Public Health 17:179, 2017.

Rodrigo C et al: Pharmacological management of tetanus: An evidence-based review. Crit Care 18:217, 2014.

Yen LM, Thwaites CL: Tetanus. Lancet 393:1657, 2019.

WEBSITES

Centers for Disease Control and Prevention: Pink Book. Tetanus. 1997. *www.cdc.gov/vaccines/pubs/pinkbook/downloads/tetanus.pdf*.

Health Protection Agency: Tetanus: Information for health professionals. 2013. *www.gov.uk/government/publications/tetanus-advice-for-health-professionals*.

World Health Organization: Maternal and neonatal tetanus (MNT) elimination. *www.who.int/immunization/diseases/MNTE_initiative/en/*.

153 Botulism

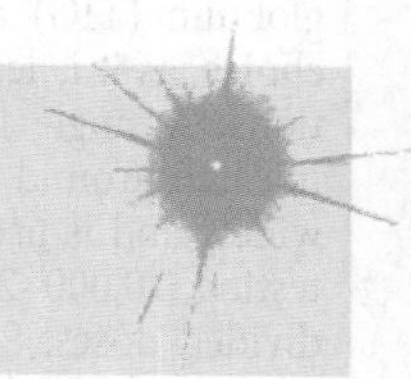

Carolina Lúquez, Jeremy Sobel

Botulism is a rare, life-threatening disease characterized by cranial nerve palsies and symmetric descending flaccid paralysis. Four forms of naturally occurring botulism have been described: foodborne botulism, infant botulism, wound botulism, and adult intestinal colonization. Other forms of botulism include iatrogenic botulism and inhalational botulism. Effective treatment depends on early clinical diagnosis.

ETIOLOGY AND PATHOGENESIS

Botulism is caused by botulinum neurotoxins (BoNTs), which are produced by *Clostridium botulinum*. Rare strains of *Clostridium butyricum* and *Clostridium baratii* can also produce BoNTs. Seven distinct serotypes of BoNT (A through G) are well characterized; serotypes A, B, E, and F reportedly cause disease in humans. Novel serotypes—BoNT/FA (or H or HA), BoNT/En, and BoNT/X—have been proposed, but the scientific community has not yet reached a consensus as to whether each represents a new serotype or a combination of known serotypes, as in the case of BoNT/FA (or H or HA), or whether they represent true toxins or botulinum-like proteins, as in the case of BoNT/En and BoNT/X. BoNTs are encoded by the *bont* gene, which is also diverse in its DNA sequence. At least 40 unique subtypes of BoNT have been identified within serotypes A, B, E, and F. By definition, a variant of BoNT represents a new subtype when its amino acid sequence differs by at least 2.6% from those of all known subtypes within that particular serotype. Although 2.6% is an arbitrary threshold, this figure has provided the basis for genetic subtype designations for the past decade, aiding in the classification of BoNTs as new DNA or amino acid sequences become publicly available. In addition, *bont* genes typically reside within two types of gene clusters. One type includes *ha* genes encoding hemagglutinin proteins, which facilitate the absorption of toxins across the epithelial barrier. The other type of cluster includes *orfX* genes that encode proteins with unknown functions. Both cluster types include an *ntnh* gene, which encodes for a nontoxic nonhemagglutinin protein. It has been proposed that these accessory proteins form a complex with BoNTs and protect them from external proteolytic activity.

Despite their structural variability, BoNTs all have a similar mechanism of action: they target neurons and block neurotransmission by cleaving SNARE-family proteins in the host, with consequent inhibition of acetylcholine release. BoNTs are metalloproteases composed of a light chain and a heavy chain. The light chain has catalytic activity, and the heavy chain contains a translocation domain and a receptor-binding domain. The receptor-binding domain of the heavy chain mediates the neurospecific binding of BoNTs, which leads to its internalization within endocytic compartments. Interaction of the translocation domain of the heavy chain with the membrane of endocytic vesicles leads to the translocation of the light chain into the cytosol. Once in the cytosol, the light chain cleaves specific SNARE-family proteins. Serotypes A and E cleave SNAP-25; serotypes B, D, F, and G cleave VAMP; and serotype C cleaves SNAP-25 and syntaxin. Cleavage of any of these proteins disrupts the assembly of synaptic fusion complexes, and this disruption inhibits the fusion of the membrane of the synaptic vesicle containing acetylcholine with the neuronal cell membrane. Clinically, the result is flaccid paralysis of voluntary muscles. The irreversible binding of BoNTs to their targets has a clinical consequence: once toxin binding has occurred, the resulting paralysis persists for weeks or months, until nerve endings have been regenerated.

BoNTs are produced by *C. botulinum* and some strains of *C. butyricum* and *C. baratii*, which are gram-positive, rod-shaped, spore-forming, anaerobic bacteria. Under most environmental conditions, *C. botulinum* exists as spores that are heat-resistant and ubiquitous in soil. In general, *C. botulinum* spores require temperatures above boiling to ensure destruction; their thermal resistance increases with higher pH and lower salt content. Spores present in foods can survive most preservation methods and, if the conditions allow it, can germinate and produce BoNTs in significant amounts to cause disease.

BoNTs are among the most toxic substances known. Extremely small amounts of BoNT can cause severe disease and death. Severity of disease varies with dose, serotype, and route of exposure. The lethal dose of BoNT in humans is not known but can be estimated by extrapolation of toxicity data from animal studies. The estimated human lethal dose of BoNT acquired via the IV or IM route is 0.1–1 ng/kg of body weight. The human lethal dose of BoNT acquired by inhalation of aerosolized toxin is estimated at 1–75 ng/kg. The degree of toxicity of BoNT acquired by the oral route is estimated to be much lower: 0.1–1 μg/kg.

As stated above, four naturally occurring and two non–naturally occurring forms of botulism are known. Foodborne botulism is caused by the ingestion of foods contaminated with BoNT. Wound botulism occurs when spores of BoNT-producing species of *Clostridium* contaminate a wound and then germinate, multiply, and produce toxin. Infant botulism is caused by BoNT-producing species of *Clostridium* colonizing the intestinal tract of infants ≤1 year of age. Adult intestinal colonization is similar to infant botulism but affects persons >1 year of age. Iatrogenic botulism occurs when a patient given injections of BoNT experiences signs of systemic botulism. BoNTs can also be aerosolized and used as a bioweapon, entering the human body by inhalation.

Foodborne Botulism Foodborne botulism is the most common form reported in many countries. Every case of foodborne botulism represents a public health emergency because of the potential for causing outbreaks. Foodborne botulism is an intoxication in which food containing preformed toxin is ingested. Spores of BoNT-producing species of *Clostridium* are ubiquitous in soil and can be found on vegetables and other foodstuffs. *C. botulinum* type E is commonly found in aquatic environments and in aquatic animals. Because the spores are found in many foods, improper preparation or storage may produce the confluence of conditions that allow germination and growth of BoNT-producing species of *Clostridium*, which in turn result in production of BoNT. Both historically and at the present time, canned foods are of concern because they create anaerobic environments. To render these foods safe, proper processing procedures in conditions of enough heat and pressure to inactivate *Clostridium* spores, along with sufficient acidity, salinity, or other preservative methods to limit the organism's growth and its production of BoNT, are required. Low-acidity foods, such as corn, peppers, potatoes, and beets, represent a higher risk. A series of botulism outbreaks from commercially canned foods in the early twentieth century resulted in standardization of retort canning methods and promulgation and enforcement of production safety codes. Consumption of fish or other foods of marine origin can cause botulism if prepared or conserved improperly. Most foodborne botulism cases in the United States are caused by home-canned vegetables such as green beans; however, commercially prepared foods, including chicken broth, carrot juice, hot dog chili sauce, and nacho cheese, have also been implicated in recent outbreaks. Marine mammal and fish products traditionally prepared by Alaskan Natives and First Peoples are the main source of botulism in Alaska and Canada.

Wound Botulism Wound botulism is caused by germination and growth of *C. botulinum* spores in a wound or necrotic tissue where they produce BoNT, which then enters circulation and produces systemic disease. Few cases of wound botulism were described in the United States until 1981, when the first case associated with injection drug use was reported. Since then, botulism cases due to injection drug use, especially in association with subcutaneous or tissue injection (skin popping) of black tar heroin, have substantially increased in the United States. Black tar heroin was introduced into the United States in the 1970s and, since the late 1980s, has become the predominant form of heroin west of the Mississippi River. Black tar heroin is contaminated with by-products of the manufacturing process, adulterants, and diluents and therefore is considered the most probable source of *C. botulinum* spores. In recent decades, the few cases of wound botulism not associated with injection drug use have been associated with vehicle crashes, gunshot wounds, open-fracture wounds, and penetrating wounds caused by contaminated objects.

Infant Botulism Infant botulism is the most common form of botulism in the United States. It affects infants ≤1 year old, with a mean age at onset of 14 weeks. It has been suggested that the intestinal microbiota in infants may induce susceptibility to botulism; animal models seem to support this claim. Spores of BoNT-producing species of *Clostridium* can enter the body by ingestion. The highly resistant spores survive passage through the stomach and colonize the intestine, where they germinate, grow, and produce BoNT in situ. Infants can continue excreting *C. botulinum* for weeks after clinical recovery. Spores of BoNT-producing species of *Clostridium* have been found in honey. Consumption of honey has been epidemiologically implicated in infant botulism; therefore, honey should not be fed to babies ≤1 year of age. Honey exposure, however, explains only a small proportion of cases. As spores are found in dust and soil, most infant botulism patients probably acquire BoNT-producing species of *Clostridium* by swallowing dust particles. Why only a few dozen infants are affected each year when presumably most infants regularly ingest clostridial spores remains unknown.

Adult Intestinal Botulism Similar to infant botulism, adult intestinal colonization is caused by spores of BoNT-producing species of *Clostridium* colonizing the large intestine, growing, and producing BoNT in situ. Although spores are routinely ingested and excreted by humans, the adult intestinal tract does not support spore germination and toxin production under normal circumstances. Adult intestinal colonization is usually associated with inborn anatomic abnormalities, gastrointestinal surgery, or prolonged use of antibiotics, which may alter the normal intestinal microbiota and facilitate colonization by BoNT-producing species of *Clostridium.* Although these associated conditions are relatively common, fewer than 30 cases of adult intestinal colonization have been reported worldwide.

Iatrogenic Botulism Iatrogenic botulism occurs in patients injected with large doses of BoNT for treatment of muscle complications related to such conditions as cerebral palsy and spastic dystonia. The small doses of botulinum toxin used for wrinkle elimination in dermatologic practice are usually insufficient to cause systemic disease. In 2004, an outbreak of four cases caused by the injection of an unlicensed, highly concentrated BoNT product for cosmetic purposes occurred in the United States. Similarly, in 2017, an outbreak of nine cases occurred in Egypt in association with an unlicensed, highly concentrated BoNT preparation.

Weaponized Inhalational Botulism BoNTs were weaponized by the biological weapons programs of several countries in the twentieth century. Aerosolized BoNTs can be used as a bioweapon, exerting their effect by entering the body through inhalation. In the United States, BoNTs are designated as Tier 1 select agents—i.e., agents that present the greatest risk of deliberate misuse with significant potential for mass casualties or devastating effects on the economy, critical infrastructure, or public confidence. Tier 1 agents pose a severe threat to public health and safety. Terrorists have attempted to use BoNT as a bioweapon: Aum Shinrikyo, a Japanese cult, tried unsuccessfully to aerosolize BoNT in terrorism attacks at multiple sites in Japan between 1990 and 1995.

■ EPIDEMIOLOGY

Foodborne Botulism In the United States, foodborne botulism is the third most common form of botulism. From 2001 to 2017, 326 foodborne botulism cases were reported, with a mean of 19 cases per year. Most cases (65%) were caused by serotype A BoNT, which was followed in frequency by serotype E (25%). Serotypes B and F caused 7% and 1% of foodborne botulism cases, respectively. Outbreaks caused by serotype E usually had a shorter incubation period, those caused by type A had higher numbers of patients who required mechanical ventilation, and those caused by type B had lower numbers of deaths.

Foodborne botulism cases are usually sporadic (i.e., cases occur singly), but small and large outbreaks can also occur. From 2001 to 2017, five foodborne botulism outbreaks affecting 10 or more people were reported in the United States (**Table 153-1**). Every case of foodborne botulism is considered a public health emergency because it may be the first in an outbreak involving additional patients.

Most foodborne botulism cases in the United States are due to a wide variety of home-canned vegetables and pickled vegetables (e.g., beets, green beans, carrots, mushrooms, asparagus, peppers, beans, mustard greens, corn, tomato sauce, olives, and pumpkin butter), vegetables baked in aluminum foil (e.g., potatoes and beets), home-canned meat-based foods (e.g., tuna, pickled pigs' feet, stew, and pasta in meat sauce), oil-based foods (e.g., pasta and jarred pesto or homemade garlic-infused oil), herbal deer antler tea, home-prepared fermented tofu, commercial clam chowder, or commercial grain and vegetable products. In Alaska, traditional Alaskan Native foods linked to foodborne botulism cases have included seal oil, seal blubber, dried herring in seal oil, fermented seal flipper, stinkheads and other fermented fish heads, stinkfish, salmon eggs, beaver tail, whitefish, fish eggs, fermented beluga, and whale blubber.

TABLE 153-1 Total Foodborne Botulism Outbreaks of 10 or More Cases Reported in the United States Between 2001 and 2017

YEAR	STATE	FOOD SOURCE	NO. OF CONFIRMED CASES
2001	Texas	Chili	16
2007	Multistate	Commercially canned hot dog chili sauce	10
2015	Ohio	Home-canned potatoes used to prepare a potato salad, served at a church potluck	27
2016	Mississippi	Pruno, illegal alcoholic beverage consumed by inmates at a federal facility	19
2017	California	Commercially produced nacho cheese, sold at a convenience store	10

Commercial food manufacturing processes include retort canning, in which high temperature and pressure destroy the highly resistant clostridial spores, and manipulations that inhibit bacterial growth, such as acidification or addition of growth inhibitors that prevent germination and growth of BoNT-producing species of *Clostridium* and the production of BoNT. However, commercial foods occasionally still cause botulism if safe manufacturing processes are not followed or fail or if foods are stored or used inappropriately by the retailer or consumer. For instance, an outbreak of 10 cases associated with commercially canned hot dog chili sauce occurred in 2007 as a result of deficiencies in the canning process. Other commercial food–associated outbreaks that occurred in the United States between 2001 and 2017 include a 2001 outbreak of 16 cases linked to chili that was stored at inappropriate temperatures and later served at a church event in Texas and a 2006 outbreak linked to commercial carrot juice, which included four cases in the United States and two cases in Canada. The investigation of the latter outbreak led to an international product recall. The juice, which had no added sugar, salt, or preservatives, was stored at inappropriate temperatures.

Pruno, an illicit prison-brewed alcoholic beverage, first caused a botulism outbreak in a California prison in 2004, affecting four prisoners. In 2011, a second outbreak due to pruno was reported and involved eight patients at a prison in Utah. In 2012, two outbreaks associated with pruno occurred in a single prison in Arizona, with four and eight cases, respectively. The largest outbreak from pruno occurred in 2016 in a Mississippi prison; 31 cases were identified, including 19 confirmed and 12 suspected.

Wound Botulism Wound botulism was once rare in the United States, but its frequency has been increasing for decades, and it is now the second most common form of botulism. Between 2001 and 2017, 372 cases of wound botulism were reported, with an average of 22 cases per year. Most cases (92%) were caused by BoNT serotype A and 5% by serotype B (5%). Most cases (95%) were among persons who injected drugs (mainly black tar heroin), and the remaining 5% of cases were due to traumatic injuries.

Infant Botulism Infant botulism is the most common form of botulism in the United States. Between 2001 and 2017, 1858 infant botulism cases were reported. BoNT serotypes A and B caused most cases (40% and 58%, respectively). Only two cases were due to serotype E. One of these two cases was due to *C. botulinum* type E and the other to *C. butyricum* type E; both cases represented the first report anywhere in this country of infant botulism due to those respective organisms. A small fraction (<1%) of cases were caused by serotype F. Of note, 13 infant botulism cases were due to strains of *C. botulinum* that can produce two BoNT serotypes (A and B or B and F).

Botulism of Other Etiologies Between 2001 and 2017, 49 cases were reported as being of "unknown or other etiology." This category includes laboratory-confirmed botulism cases that do not meet the definition of foodborne, infant, or wound botulism. Most of these cases were caused by serotype A (65%) and serotype F (25%). Many were thought to be cases of adult intestinal colonization, although confirmation of this form of botulism is not always possible.

CLINICAL MANIFESTATIONS

Botulism produces a syndrome characterized by bilateral cranial nerve palsies that may be followed by symmetric, descending flaccid paralysis that may cause respiratory arrest. There are no sensory deficits; patients are fully conscious, with normal intellectual function, although cranial nerve palsies may give a mistaken impression of altered consciousness. The incubation period (based on data for foodborne botulism cases, where exposure can be identified) is 1 or 2 days, but a range of 6 h to >7 days has been reported. Several recent systematic reviews substantiate long-known observations that the syndrome is essentially identical for all types of botulism in patients of all ages, although elicitation of the typical signs and symptoms may be challenging in infants and young children. A recent systematic review of 16 cases of botulism in pregnant women reported the same clinical syndrome as in nonpregnant individuals. In all botulism syndromes, the first neurologic manifestation usually is ptosis, which can be striking. Ocular findings of fuzzy vision or frank diplopia are caused by extraocular muscle paralysis due to palsies of cranial nerves III, IV, and VI. Flat, youthfully unlined, expressionless facies are produced by cranial nerve VII (facial nerve) palsy. Dysarthria is also a prominent manifestation. Oral and nasal regurgitation of foods or beverages is caused by cranial nerve IX (glossopharyngeal nerve) palsy. The autonomic system may be affected, producing anhidrosis manifesting as severe pharyngeal pain and erythema that has been mistaken for pharyngitis; paradoxically, other patients experience an inability to manage copious oral secretions. Autonomic dysfunction may produce hemodynamic instability requiring monitoring. Cranial nerve palsy may produce pharyngeal muscle flaccidity, causing airway collapse and respiratory arrest early in the course of illness, while reduction in diaphragmatic and accessory muscle function may cause respiratory compromise hours or days later. Cranial nerve palsies may be followed by descending symmetric flaccid paralysis of the muscles of the neck, shoulders, upper limbs, and lower limbs; proximal muscle groups of each limb are affected before distal muscle groups.

A recent analysis of 332 U.S. botulism cases found the following frequencies for patient-reported symptoms: difficulty swallowing, 86%; fatigue, 85%; blurred vision, 80%; slurred speech, 78%; double vision, 76%; shortness of breath, 65%; and dry mouth, 62%. The analysis also reported the following frequencies of observed signs: afebrile body temperature, 99%; descending paralysis, 93%; alert and oriented status, 93%; ptosis, 81%; limb weakness, 78%; decreased palatal reflex, 54%; facial palsy, 47%; and dilated pupils. Sixty-six percent of patients were intubated and received mechanical ventilation. These findings are similar to those reported in many smaller series. Rarely, asymmetry of cranial nerve palsies or distal muscle paralysis is reported and, at least in some cases (especially those described in reports based on chart abstractions), may reflect an incomplete or incompletely recorded neurologic examination. Despite intact sensorium, symptoms such as ptosis, dysarthria, and gait instability may be mistaken for diminished consciousness and lack of coordination and may be erroneously attributed to intoxication from alcohol or other substances. Paresthesias have been reported in some patients; these sensations are not explained by the known activity of botulinum toxin. Paralysis of the diaphragm and accessory muscles of respiration may occur, producing respiratory compromise. Distal tendon reflexes diminish symmetrically. Constipation due to intestinal paralysis develops in almost all patients. Nausea and vomiting may occur in foodborne botulism, preceding neurologic symptoms. Whether these manifestations are due to BoNT, other products of BoNT-producing species of *Clostridium*, or other contaminants of spoiled food is unknown. These gastrointestinal symptoms have not been reported in wound botulism.

Death in untreated patients during the first hours to days of illness is caused by airway obstruction resulting from pharyngeal muscle paralysis and inadequate tidal volume resulting from paralysis of diaphragmatic and accessory respiratory muscles. The combination of expressionless facies from cranial nerve paralysis and immobility from voluntary muscle paralysis may give patients with botulism a placid appearance that masks the agitation expected with respiratory distress. Respiratory compromise occurs early in the course of disease in a substantial proportion of patients: the largest systematic literature review to date of foodborne and wound botulism cases (402 patients) reported that the average time from symptom onset to hospitalization was 2 days and that, at hospital admission, 42% of patients had respiratory symptoms; of these patients, 42% presented with no extremity weakness. In the same review, 87% of patients who required mechanical ventilation were intubated during the first 2 days of hospitalization. The severity of disease varies greatly between patients and is probably governed by the dose of toxin to which they have been exposed. Without treatment, some patients do not progress beyond ptosis and mild palsy in one or two cranial nerves; others experience fulminant cranial nerve palsies and rapidly progressive descending flaccid paralysis eventually affecting most or all voluntary muscles as well as respiratory failure requiring intubation and mechanical ventilation within hours.

The different BoNT serotypes are associated with variations in the botulism syndrome. BoNT type A is associated with more rapid disease progression, more frequent respiratory compromise and mechanical ventilation, and longer duration of paralysis. Type B is associated with a milder syndrome, with less severe and shorter-duration paralysis. Intoxication with the rarely occurring type F produces a syndrome of rapidly progressing paralysis that often leads to respiratory failure, with more rapid recovery than occurs with other toxin types. However, all toxin types causing human illness can cause severe disease; the clinical approach is the same for all.

The paralysis of botulism can last for weeks or months—the time required for regeneration of affected nerve endings and recovery of voluntary muscle function. For severely affected patients with extensive paralysis, management consists of protracted intensive care, with detection and treatment of attendant risks not specific to botulism, such as ventilator-associated pneumonia, decubitus ulcers, and psychological trauma. More than 95% of noninfant botulism patients in the United States recover; hospital discharge is often followed by protracted rehabilitative care. The survival rate for infant botulism is near 100%.

CLINICAL DIAGNOSIS AND LABORATORY CONFIRMATION

Rapid clinical diagnosis is essential. A diagnostic aid for botulism, "Clinical Criteria to Trigger Suspicion of Botulism," has been published by botulism consultants at the Centers for Disease Control and Prevention (CDC; accessible at *https://academic.oup.com/cid/article/66/suppl_1/S38/4780423*). The paralysis of botulism lasts for weeks or months, and administration of equine-source botulinum antitoxin (BAT)—the specific therapy to arrest the progression of paralysis—depends on the correct diagnosis. At this time, laboratory confirmation of botulism, which may require ≥24 h, must take place at a specialized public health laboratory. Therefore, effective, timely treatment relies on rapid clinical diagnosis of botulism in a patient with clinically compatible findings. A clinician suspecting noninfant botulism in a patient should immediately contact the state health department's emergency 24-h line. The state will connect the clinician with a botulism clinical consultant at the CDC (or, in Alaska and California, at the state health department), who will review the case with the clinician, assist in the shipping of appropriate specimens to a public health laboratory for definitive diagnosis, and, when indicated, arrange for immediate shipping of BAT from the federal stockpile at no charge. A clinician suspecting infant botulism in a patient should immediately contact the Infant Botulism Treatment and Prevention Program's on-call physician at (510) 231-7600, who will provide consultation, assist with specimen collection, and, when indicated, assist with the provision of human-derived botulinum antitoxin (BabyBIG), a specific treatment licensed for treatment of infant botulism.

The neurologic examination is the key to clinical diagnosis of botulism, as it readily uncovers the cranial nerve deficits that are invariably present in botulism and focuses the differential diagnosis. In principle, the distinct syndrome of bilateral cranial palsies and descending flaccid paralysis in a fully conscious patient should render the diagnosis and prompt treatment of botulism straightforward. The presentation of two or more patients with this syndrome is almost pathognomonic, since other illnesses considered during the differential diagnosis of botulism do not produce outbreaks. In practice, however, sporadic (lone) cases of botulism are misdiagnosed, and sometimes the diagnosis is missed even in the setting of an outbreak. In part, these failures may be due to the rarity of botulism and the clinician's unfamiliarity with its presentation. A possible cause of misdiagnosis is failure to perform a complete neurologic examination; indeed, review of some botulism patients' charts reveals documentation of the first neurologic examination, which suggested the correct diagnosis, days after hospital admission. As stated earlier, the combination of ptosis, dysarthria, and perceived gate instability from muscle paralysis in some cases may be misinterpreted as intoxication from alcohol or other substances. In other cases, rapidly progressing botulism may result in pharyngeal collapse and respiratory distress relatively early in the course, leading the clinical team to focus on airway management and primary respiratory diagnoses and thus delaying the neurologic evaluation.

Standard clinical studies, including bloodwork and radiology, are not useful in diagnosing botulism. In contrast to the findings in Guillain-Barré syndrome (GBS; see below), lumbar-puncture cerebrospinal fluid (CSF) values—and specifically the protein level—are usually normal in botulism. The CSF protein level may be very slightly elevated in a minority of botulism cases. The fact that botulism produces no abnormal findings on brain imaging may help rule out rare basilar strokes that produce nonlateralizing symptoms. The Tensilon test helps rule out myasthenia gravis. Electromyography, when performed by an experienced practitioner, can provide support for the diagnosis. Botulism is indicated by findings consistent with neuromuscular junction blockage, normal axonal conduction, and potentiation with rapid repetitive stimulation in affected muscles.

Once a neurologic examination reveals the cranial nerve palsies of botulism and any additional bilateral flaccid paralysis, the differential diagnosis may include GBS, myasthenia gravis, Lambert-Eaton syndrome, and tick paralysis. Less likely conditions include tetrodotoxin or shellfish poisoning, antimicrobial-associated paralysis, and rarer poisonings. A careful history and physical examination can further narrow the range of diagnoses. GBS is a rare (~1 case per 100,000 population per year in the United States) autoimmune demyelinating polyneuropathy that follows acute infection by *Campylobacter jejuni*, certain viruses, and other bacteria. In 95% of cases, GBS presents as an ascending paralysis. Recent reports from Peru indicate massive outbreaks of GBS of unknown cause, challenging the previously held notion that conditions causing flaccid paralysis other than botulism occur only as sporadic cases. The 5% of GBS cases presenting as the Miller Fisher variant are characterized by the triad of ophthalmoplegia, ataxia, and areflexia, which may resemble early descending paralysis. The CSF protein level is elevated in GBS, but the increase may take place days after symptom onset; thus, normal CSF levels should be taken into account along with the duration of symptoms, and lumbar puncture may need to be repeated. Electromyography performed by an experienced operator may yield findings indicative of GBS and not botulism. A strongly positive Tensilon test, with or without the presence of autoantibodies, confirms myasthenia gravis; borderline positive Tensilon tests have been reported in botulism patients. In most stroke patients, the physical examination should reveal asymmetric paralysis and upper motor neuron signs; brain imaging can help reveal rare basilar strokes that can produce symmetric bulbar palsies. The history and physical examination should rule out Lambert-Eaton syndrome, which is characterized by proximal limb weakness in patients with advanced cancer.

Laboratory testing confirms clinically diagnosed botulism cases and determines the BoNT serotype causing the disease. In addition, laboratory testing can confirm epidemiologic data by demonstrating presence of BoNT in the suspected food. Botulism cases are confirmed by the laboratory when BoNT is identified in serum or stool specimens or when a BoNT-producing species of *Clostridium* is isolated from stool specimens or wound cultures. Identification of preformed BoNT in food consumed by patients also confirms foodborne botulism.

The gold standard for identification and serotyping of BoNT in clinical or food specimens is the mouse bioassay. The drawback is that this highly sensitive and specific method requires the use of animals. Specimens are injected IP into the mice with and without antitoxin; the mice are then observed for up to 96 h for signs of botulism. If the specimen contains BoNT at levels sufficient to affect the mice quickly, results may be available within 24 h of injection. Low levels of toxin may produce signs later, so that mice should be monitored for 4 days after injection. Many in vitro methods have been developed for detection of BoNT and BoNT-producing species of *Clostridium* in clinical and food specimens. For instance, public health laboratories in the United States can use a real-time polymerase chain reaction test that detects *bont* genes encoding serotypes A through G. This test is a useful screening method to determine whether BoNT-producing species of *Clostridium* are present in cultures of clinical specimens, but positive results must be confirmed. Another in vitro method, the Endopep mass spectrometry (Endopep-MS) assay, is highly sensitive and specific and can detect BoNT in clinical specimens and foods. The advantage of Endopep-MS is that it detects active BoNT and therefore represents an ideal alternative to the mouse bioassay. Immune-based assays can provide rapid and sensitive results; their main limitation is that they detect antigens, which may not necessarily represent active BoNT. Cell-based in vitro assays are also a possible alternative to the mouse bioassay as they detect biological activity of BoNT.

TREATMENT
Botulism

Treatment for botulism consists of two components: meticulous monitoring and supportive care, including admittance to the intensive care unit when indicated, and administration of botulinum antitoxin, the only specific therapy for botulism, as quickly as possible. Paralysis from botulism can be rapidly progressive. Vital capacity, and often hemodynamic parameters, should be frequently monitored and mechanical ventilation instituted immediately if needed. Paralysis induced by BoNT lasts weeks or months, and patients with extensive paralysis require painstaking care to avoid complications associated with protracted immobilization, including respirator-dependent pneumonia, decubitus ulcers, and psychological trauma. Patients who have recovered from severe botulism report that their appearance and immobility often led caregivers to assume they were unconscious; as a consequence, patients were sometimes subjected to painful procedures without warning and to insensitive comments. Signage should remind all caregivers that botulism patients are conscious but "locked in." Psychological support should be instituted for intubated botulism patients from the outset. With proper supportive care, >95% of botulism patients in the United States recover, even without antitoxin therapy; however, antitoxin, if promptly administered, can substantially reduce the extent and duration of illness (see below).

Botulinum antitoxin is the only specific treatment for botulism. The antitoxin prevents the progression of paralysis but does not reverse existing paralysis. If given early enough in the course of disease, it may avert respiratory compromise, obviate mechanical intubation, and forestall protracted paralysis and hospitalization along with associated complications. Accordingly, it is essential to administer antitoxin as soon as possible. A recent systematic literature review and meta-analysis covering nearly a century of the published literature in noninfant botulism patients confirmed long-known findings from smaller studies by showing significantly reduced mortality rates among patients treated with equine antitoxin, especially when treatment was administered within 48 h of symptom onset. Another large systematic literature review of pediatric noninfant botulism recently showed significantly reduced mortality risk among children treated with equine antitoxin. Published studies have demonstrated a substantial reduction in the duration and severity of illness among patients with infant botulism who are treated with human-derived botulinum antitoxin.

The equine botulinum antitoxin used to treat noninfant botulism consists of antibodies produced in horses immunized with botulinum toxoids (inactivated toxins) and toxins. The antibodies are type-specific (anti-A neutralizes BoNT type A and so forth). The currently licensed antitoxin product in the United States, heptavalent botulinum antitoxin (BAT), contains antibodies to BoNT types A, B, C, D, E, F, and G. These equine antibodies have undergone despeciation to reduce antigenicity and the risk of anaphylaxis to foreign protein. A recent systematic literature review, along with studies of BAT use, indicated that <2% of recipients experience serious adverse reactions. Administration of one vial of BAT elicits circulating antitoxin concentrations sufficient to neutralize toxin levels one to two orders of magnitude higher than those found in the serum of most botulism patients. As noted earlier, clinicians suspecting botulism in a patient should immediately call their state health department's emergency contact to be put in touch with a botulism clinical consultant who will review the case and assist in its management, including shipment of BAT from the federal stockpile at no charge. The botulinum antitoxin used to treat infants, BabyBIG, consists of human antibodies obtained from hyperimmunized volunteers. The product is licensed for treatment of infant botulism due to BoNT types A and B and, as noted earlier, can be obtained through the Infant Botulism Treatment and Prevention Program.

There is no prophylactic treatment for botulism. Persons who may have been exposed to botulinum toxin should be evaluated by a physician and carefully observed for the development of symptoms of botulism. If symptoms appear, the patient should be treated immediately with botulinum antitoxin.

PREVENTION

No vaccine is licensed for the prevention of botulism. In the United States, a botulinum toxoid vaccine was available through the CDC until 2011, but it was discontinued because of a decline in immunogenicity of some serotypes and an increase in occurrence of moderate local reactions. Several vaccine candidates are currently in clinical trials.

Because most foodborne botulism cases are caused by home-canned or home-preserved foods, the prevention of foodborne botulism depends mainly on proper preparation and preservation that ensures the destruction of spores of BoNT-producing species of *Clostridium* that may be present in the food or on the creation of an environment that will not allow the germination and growth of these spores, such as low pH or low water activity. Water activity is a measure of how much water is free, unbound, and thus available to microorganisms to use for growth. If foods have low water activity, it means they do not have much free water, and growth of *C. botulinum* will be limited or inhibited. Using pressure canners and properly cleaning items employed in the canning process can reduce the risk of foodborne botulism. Among other resources, the *USDA Complete Guide to Home Canning* provides a detailed description of safe home-canning practices. Other ways of preventing foodborne botulism include refrigerating homemade oils infused with garlic or herbs and discarding any of these oils that have not been used after 4 days; maintaining baked potatoes or similar foods wrapped in aluminum foil at temperatures above 140°F until served and then refrigerating leftovers; refrigerating canned or pickled foods after opening; and boiling home-canned foods before eating, especially those foods that are low in acid.

Wound botulism largely affects people who inject drugs, especially black tar heroin. Using safe injection practices may help prevent wound botulism and many other infections, such as HIV and hepatitis C virus infections. Thus, educating injection drug users on the prevention of wound botulism and other infections is vital in protecting their health. As wound botulism can also follow traumatic injuries, keeping wounds clean is key.

The risk factors for infant botulism are not fully understood, but possible sources of spores of BoNT-producing species of *Clostridium* include foods and dust. In most cases of infant botulism, no source of spores is identified. Honey is the only food that has been identified as an epidemiologically associated reservoir of spores of BoNT-producing species of *Clostridium*. Honey should not be fed to infants ≤1 year of age.

GLOBAL CONSIDERATIONS

Botulism has been reported from all parts of the world. The European Centre for Disease Prevention and Control has reported an average of 110 botulism cases each year from 2007 to 2018. During that period, 1315 botulism cases were reported from 25 countries, with the most cases in Italy (311 cases), Romania (239 cases), and Poland (202 cases). Foodborne botulism is the most common form of botulism in Europe. Most laboratory-confirmed cases reported from Italy, Romania, and Poland were due to BoNT serotype B. The country of Georgia has a high incidence of botulism (0.9 case per 100,000 persons) relative to rates in the European Union (<0.1/100,000) and the United States (0.01/100,000). From 1980 to 2002, a total of 879 cases of botulism were reported in Georgia; all of them were foodborne, most were associated with home-preserved vegetables, and the majority were due to serotype B. From 1958 to 1983, 986 foodborne botulism outbreaks affecting 4377 individuals were reported from China. Most cases were due to serotype A and were associated with bean products. Botulism in Thailand has been associated with fermented bamboo shoots and fermented soybeans. In 2006, a large foodborne botulism outbreak associated with bamboo shoots occurred in Thailand and affected 209 people who attended a local festival. In South America, Brazil and Argentina have reported several outbreaks of foodborne botulism. For instance, between 2001 and 2008, Brazil reported 18 outbreaks, most of which were associated with meat-based foods such as home-canned meat, homemade pork liver pâté, and commercially canned liver pâté. From 1994 to 2007, Argentina reported 36 outbreaks, most frequently involving home-canned vegetables. Although reports of foodborne botulism in Africa are rare, five outbreaks were reported in South Africa between 1959 and 2002, with the majority due to serotype B and associated with noncommercial foods. In addition, one outbreak of 91 cases was reported in Egypt in 1991 and was due to serotype E associated with a traditional salted fish.

Wound botulism cases have been reported most frequently from the United States, next most frequently from the United Kingdom, and occasionally from Italy, France, and Australia. Clusters of wound botulism are rare, but, according to a report from the European Centre for Disease Prevention and Control, 23 cases of wound botulism among people who had injected heroin were reported in Norway and Scotland between December 2014 and February 2015. Other countries that have reported wound botulism cases include Argentina, China, and Ecuador.

Although rarely reported, infant botulism cases have been noted on all continents except Africa. Outside the United States (where there were 2419 cases), Argentina reported the largest number of cases (366) and Australia the next largest number (32) between 1976 and 2006. Canada, Italy, and Japan also reported a relatively large number of cases (27, 26, and 22, respectively).

FURTHER READING

CENTERS FOR DISEASE CONTROL AND PREVENTION: Botulism in the United States, 1899–1996, *Handbook for Epidemiologists, Clinicians, and Laboratory Workers*. Atlanta, Centers for Disease Control and Prevention, 1998.

CENTERS FOR DISEASE CONTROL AND PREVENTION: National Botulism Surveillance. Available at *https://www.cdc.gov/botulism/surveillance.html*. Accessed September 27, 2020.

CHATHAM-STEPHENS K et al: Clinical features of foodborne and wound botulism: A systematic review of the literature, 1932–2015. Clin Infect Dis 66:S11, 2017.

EUROPEAN CENTRE FOR DISEASE PREVENTION AND CONTROL: *Botulism*. Available at *https://www.ecdc.europa.eu/en/botulism*. Accessed September 27, 2020.

Fleck-Derderian S et al: The epidemiology of foodborne botulism outbreaks: A systematic review. Clin Infect Dis 66:S73, 2017.

Griese SE et al: Pediatric botulism and use of equine botulinum antitoxin in children: A systematic review. Clin Infect Dis 66:S17, 2017.

Koepke R et al: Global occurrence of infant botulism, 1976–2006. Pediatrics 122:e73, 2008.

National Center for Home Food Preservation: *USDA Complete Guide to Home Canning, 2015 Revision*. Available at *https://nchfp.uga.edu/publications/publications_usda.html*. Accessed September 27, 2020.

O'Horo JC et al: Efficacy of antitoxin therapy in treating patients with foodborne botulism: A systematic review and meta-analysis of cases, 1923–2016. Clin Infect Dis 66:S43, 2017.

Peck M et al: Historical perspectives and guidelines for botulinum neurotoxin subtype nomenclature. Toxins (Basel) 9:38, 2017.

Pirazzini M et al: Botulinum neurotoxins: Biology, pharmacology, and toxicology. Pharmacol Rev 69:200, 2017.

Rao AK et al: Clinical criteria to trigger suspicion for botulism: An evidence-based tool to facilitate timely recognition of suspected cases during sporadic events and outbreaks. Clin Infect Dis 66:S38, 2017. (Also available at *https://academic.oup.com/cid/article/66/suppl_1/S38/4780423*. Accessed September 27, 2020.)

Yu PA et al: Safety and improved clinical outcomes in patients treated with new equine-derived heptavalent botulinum antitoxin. Clin Infect Dis 66:S57, 2017.

154 Gas Gangrene and Other Clostridial Infections

Amy E. Bryant, Dennis L. Stevens

The genus *Clostridium* encompasses >60 species that may be commensals of the gut microflora or may cause a variety of infections in humans and animals through the production of a plethora of proteinaceous exotoxins. *C. tetani* and *C. botulinum*, for example, cause specific clinical disease by elaborating single but highly potent toxins. In contrast, *C. perfringens* and *C. septicum* cause aggressive necrotizing infections that are attributable to multiple toxins, including bacterial proteases, phospholipases, and cytotoxins.

ETIOLOGIC AGENT

Vegetative cells of *Clostridium* species are pleomorphic, rod-shaped, and arranged singly or in short chains **(Fig. 154-1)**; the cells have rounded or sometimes pointed ends. Although clostridia stain gram-positive in the early stages of growth, they may appear to be gram-negative or gram-variable later in the growth cycle or in infected tissue specimens. Most strains are motile by means of peritrichous flagella; *C. septicum* swarms on solid media. Nonmotile species include *C. perfringens*, *C. ramosum*, and *C. innocuum*. Most species are obligately anaerobic, although clostridial tolerance to oxygen varies widely; some species (e.g., *C. septicum*, *C. tertium*) will grow but will not sporulate in air.

Clostridia produce more protein toxins than any other bacterial genus, and >25 clostridial toxins lethal to mice have been identified. These proteins include neurotoxins, enterotoxins, cytotoxins, collagenases, permeases, necrotizing toxins, lipases, lecithinases, hemolysins, proteinases, hyaluronidases, DNases, ADP-ribosyltransferases, and neuraminidases. Botulinum and tetanus neurotoxins are the most potent toxins known, with lethal doses of 0.2–10 ng/kg for humans. Epsilon toxin, a 33-kDa protein produced by *C. perfringens* types B and D, causes edema and hemorrhage in the brain, heart, spinal cord, and kidneys of animals. It is among the most lethal of the clostridial toxins and is considered a potential agent of bioterrorism. The genomic sequences of some pathogenic clostridia are now available and are

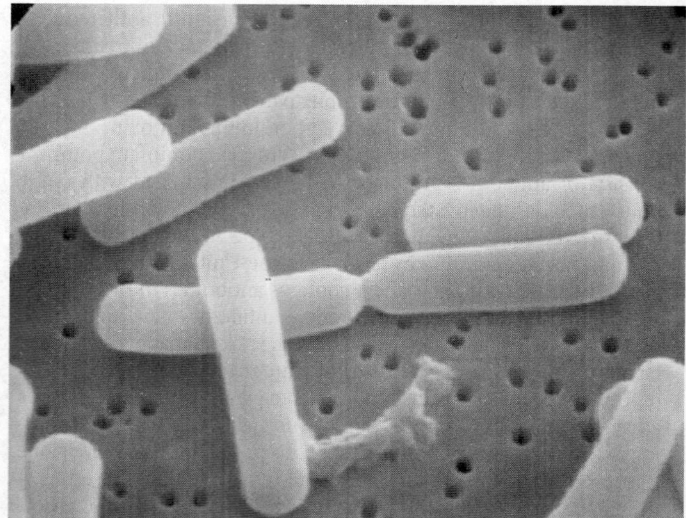

FIGURE 154-1 Scanning electron micrograph of *C. perfringens*.

likely to facilitate a comprehensive approach to understanding the virulence factors involved in clostridial pathogenesis.

EPIDEMIOLOGY AND TRANSMISSION

Clostridium species are widespread in nature, forming endospores that are commonly found in soil, feces, sewage, and marine sediments. The ecology of *C. perfringens* in soil is greatly influenced by the degree and duration of animal husbandry in a given location and is relevant to the incidence of gas gangrene caused by contamination of war wounds with soil. For example, the incidence of clostridial gas gangrene is higher in agricultural regions of Europe than in the Sahara Desert of Africa. Similarly, the incidences of tetanus and food-borne botulism are clearly related to the presence of clostridial spores in soil, water, and many foods. Clostridia are present in large numbers in the indigenous microbiota of the intestinal tract of humans and animals, in the female genital tract, and on the oral mucosa. It should be noted that not all commensal clostridia are toxigenic.

Clostridial infections remain a serious public-health concern worldwide. In developing nations, food poisoning, necrotizing enterocolitis, and gas gangrene are common because large portions of the population are poor and have little or no immediate access to health care. These infections remain prevalent in developed countries as well. Gas gangrene commonly follows knife or gunshot wounds or vehicular accidents or develops as a complication of surgery or gastrointestinal carcinoma. Severe clostridial infections have emerged as a health threat to injection drug users and to women undergoing childbirth or abortion. Historically, clostridial gas gangrene has been the scourge of the battlefield. The global political situation portends another possible scenario involving mass casualties of war or terrorism, with extensive injuries conducive to gas gangrene. Thus, there is an ongoing need to develop novel strategies to prevent or attenuate the course of clostridial infections in both civilians and military personnel. Vaccination against exotoxins important in pathogenesis would be of great benefit in developing nations and could also be used safely in at-risk populations such as the elderly, patients with diabetes who may require lower-limb surgery due to trauma or poor circulation, and those undergoing intestinal surgery. Moreover, a hyperimmune globulin would be a valuable tool for prophylaxis in victims of acute traumatic injury or for attenuation of the spread of infection in patients with established gas gangrene.

CLINICAL SYNDROMES

Life-threatening clostridial infections range from intoxications (e.g., food poisoning, tetanus) to necrotizing enteritis/colitis, bacteremia, myonecrosis, and toxic shock syndrome (TSS). **Tetanus and botulism are discussed in Chaps. 152 and 153, respectively. Colitis due to *C. difficile* is discussed in Chap. 134.**

CLOSTRIDIAL WOUND CONTAMINATION

Of open traumatic wounds, 30–80% reportedly are contaminated with clostridial species. In the absence of devitalized tissue, the presence of clostridia does not necessarily lead to infection. In traumatic injuries, clostridia are isolated with equal frequency from both suppurative and well-healing wounds. Thus, diagnosis and treatment of clostridial infection should be based on clinical signs and symptoms and not solely on bacteriologic findings.

POLYMICROBIAL INFECTIONS INVOLVING CLOSTRIDIA

Clostridial species may be found in polymicrobial infections also involving microbial components of the indigenous flora. In these infections, clostridia often appear in association with non-spore-forming anaerobes and facultative or aerobic organisms. Head and neck infections, conjunctivitis, brain abscess, sinusitis, otitis, aspiration pneumonia, lung abscess, pleural empyema, cholecystitis, septic arthritis, and bone infections all may involve clostridia. These conditions are often associated with severe local inflammation but may lack the characteristic systemic signs of toxicity and rapid progression seen in other clostridial infections. In addition, clostridia are isolated from ~66% of intraabdominal infections in which the mucosal integrity of the bowel or respiratory system has been compromised. In this setting, *C. ramosum*, *C. perfringens*, and *C. bifermentans* are the most commonly isolated species. Their presence does not invariably lead to a poor outcome. Clostridia have been isolated from suppurative infections of the female genital tract (e.g., ovarian or pelvic abscess) and from diseased gallbladders. Although the most frequently isolated species is *C. perfringens*, gangrene is not typically observed; however, gas formation in the biliary system can lead to emphysematous cholecystitis, especially in diabetic patients. *C. perfringens* in association with mixed aerobic and anaerobic microbes can cause aggressive life-threatening type I necrotizing fasciitis or Fournier's gangrene.

The treatment of mixed aerobic/anaerobic infection of the abdomen, perineum, or gynecologic organs should be based on Gram's staining, culture, and antibiotic sensitivity information. Reasonable empirical treatment consists of ampicillin or ampicillin/sulbactam combined with either clindamycin or metronidazole (**Table 154-1**). Broader gram-negative coverage may be necessary if the patient has recently been hospitalized or treated with antibiotics. Such coverage can be obtained by substituting ticarcillin/clavulanic acid, piperacillin/sulbactam, or a penem antibiotic for ampicillin or by adding a fluoroquinolone or an aminoglycoside to the regimen. Empirical treatment should be given for 10–14 days or until the patient's clinical condition improves.

ENTERIC CLOSTRIDIAL INFECTIONS

C. perfringens type A is one of the most common bacterial causes of food-borne illness in the United States and Canada. The foods typically implicated include improperly cooked meat and meat products (e.g., gravy) in which residual spores germinate and proliferate during slow cooling or insufficient reheating. Illness results from the ingestion of food containing at least ~10^8 viable vegetative cells, which sporulate in the alkaline environment of the small intestine, producing *C. perfringens* enterotoxin in the process. The diarrhea that develops within 7–30 h of ingestion of contaminated food is generally mild and self-limiting; however, in the very young, the elderly, and the immunocompromised, symptoms are more severe and occasionally fatal. Enterotoxin-producing *C. perfringens* has been implicated as an etiologic agent of persistent diarrhea in elderly patients in nursing homes and tertiary-care institutions and has been considered to play a role in antibiotic-associated diarrhea without pseudomembranous colitis.

C. perfringens strains associated with food poisoning possess the gene (*cpe*) coding for enterotoxin, which acts by forming pores in host cell membranes. *C. perfringens* strains isolated from non-food-borne diseases, such as antibiotic-associated and sporadic diarrhea, carry *cpe* on a plasmid that may be transmitted to other strains. Several methods have been described for the detection of *C. perfringens* enterotoxin in feces, including cell culture assay (Vero cells), enzyme-linked immunosorbent assay, reversed-phase latex agglutination, and polymerase chain reaction (PCR) amplification of *cpe*. Each method has its advantages and limitations.

Enteritis necroticans (gas gangrene of the bowel) is a fulminating clinical illness characterized by extensive necrosis of the intestinal mucosa and wall. Cases can occur sporadically in adults or as epidemics in people of all ages. Enteritis necroticans is caused by α toxin– and β toxin–producing strains of *C. perfringens* type C; β toxin is located on a plasmid and is mainly responsible for pathogenesis. This life-threatening infection causes ischemic necrosis of the jejunum. In Papua New Guinea during the 1960s, enteritis necroticans (known in that locale as *pigbel*) was found to be the most common cause of death in childhood; it was associated with pig feasts and occurred both sporadically and in outbreaks. Intramuscular immunization against the β toxin resulted in a decreased incidence of the disease in Papua New Guinea, although the condition remains common. Enteritis necroticans has also been recognized in the United States, the United Kingdom, Germany (where it is known as *darmbrand*), and other developed nations; especially affected are adults who are malnourished or who have diabetes, alcoholic liver disease, or neutropenia.

Necrotizing enterocolitis, a disease resembling enteritis necroticans but associated with *C. perfringens* type A, has been found in North

TABLE 154-1 Treatment of Clostridial Infections

CONDITION	ANTIBIOTIC TREATMENT	PENICILLIN ALLERGY	ADJUNCTIVE TREATMENT/NOTE
Wound contamination	None	—	Treatment should be based on clinical signs and symptoms as listed below and not solely on bacteriologic findings.
Polymicrobial anaerobic infections involving clostridia (e.g., abdominal wall, gynecologic)	Ampicillin (2 g IV q4h) *plus* Clindamycin (600–900 mg IV q6–8h) *plus* Ciprofloxacin (400 mg IV q6–8 h)	Vancomycin (1 g IV q12h) *plus* Metronidazole (500 mg IV q6h) *plus* Ciprofloxacin (400 mg IV q6–8h)	Empirical therapy should be initiated. Therapy should be based on Gram's stain and culture results and on sensitivity data when available. Add gram-negative coverage if indicated (see text).
Clostridial sepsis	Penicillin (3–4 mU IV q4–6h) *plus* Clindamycin (600–900 mg IV q6–8h)	Clindamycin alone *or* Metronidazole (as above) *or* Vancomycin (as above)	Transient bacteremia without signs of systemic toxicity may be clinically insignificant.
Gas gangrene[a]	Penicillin G (4 mU IV q4–6 h) *plus* Clindamycin (600–900 mg IV q6–8h)	Cefoxitin (2 g IV q6h) *plus* Clindamycin (600–900 mg IV q6–8h)	Emergent surgical exploration and thorough debridement are extremely important. Hyperbaric oxygen therapy may be considered after surgery and antibiotic initiation.

[a] *C. tertium* is resistant to penicillin, cephalosporins, and clindamycin. Appropriate antibiotic therapy for *C. tertium* infection is vancomycin (1 g q12h IV) or metronidazole (500 mg q8h IV).

America in previously healthy adults. It is also a serious gastrointestinal disease of low-birth-weight (premature) infants hospitalized in neonatal intensive care units. The etiology and pathogenesis of this disease have remained enigmatic for more than four decades. Pathologic similarities between necrotizing enterocolitis and enteritis necroticans include the pattern of small-bowel necrosis involving the submucosa, mucosa, and muscularis; the presence of gas dissecting the tissue planes; and the degree of inflammation. In contrast to enteritis necroticans, which most commonly involves the jejunum, necrotizing enterocolitis affects the ileum and frequently the ileocecal valve. Both diseases may manifest as intestinal gas cysts, although this feature is more common in necrotizing enterocolitis. The sources of the gas, which contains hydrogen, methane, and carbon dioxide, are probably the fermentative activities of intestinal bacteria, including clostridia. Epidemiologic data support an important role for *C. perfringens* or other gas-producing microorganisms (e.g., *C. neonatale*, certain other clostridia, or *Klebsiella* species) in the pathogenesis of necrotizing enterocolitis.

Patients with suspected clostridial enteric infection should undergo nasogastric suction and receive IV fluids. Pyrantel is given by mouth, and the bowel is rested by fasting. Benzylpenicillin (1 mU) is given IV every 4 h, and the patient is observed for complications requiring surgery. Patients with mild cases recover without surgical intervention. However, if surgical indications are present (gas in the peritoneal cavity, absent bowel sounds, rebound tenderness, abdominal rigidity), the mortality rate ranges from 35 to 100%; a fatal outcome is due in part to perforation of the intestine.

As pigbel continues to be a common disease in Papua New Guinea, consideration should be given to the use of a *C. perfringens* type C β toxoid vaccine in local areas. Two doses given 3–4 months apart are preventive.

CLOSTRIDIAL BACTEREMIA

Clostridium species are important causes of bloodstream infections. Molecular epidemiologic studies of anaerobic bacteremia have identified *C. perfringens* and *C. tertium* as the two most frequently isolated species; these organisms cause up to 79 and 5%, respectively, of clostridial bacteremias. Occasionally, *C. perfringens* bacteremia occurs in the absence of an identifiable infection at another site. When associated with myonecrosis, bacteremia has a grave prognosis.

C. septicum is also commonly associated with bacteremia. This species is isolated only rarely from the feces of healthy individuals but may be found in the normal appendix. More than 50% of patients whose blood cultures are positive for this organism have some gastrointestinal anomaly (e.g., diverticular disease) or underlying malignancy (e.g., carcinoma of the colon). In addition, a clinically important association of *C. septicum* bacteremia with neutropenia of any origin—and, more specifically, with neutropenic enterocolitis involving the terminal ileum or cecum—has been observed. Patients with diabetes mellitus, severe atherosclerotic cardiovascular disease, or anaerobic myonecrosis (gas gangrene) also may develop *C. septicum* bacteremia. *C. septicum* has been recovered from the bloodstream of cirrhotic patients, as have *C. perfringens*, *C. bifermentans*, and other clostridia. Infections of the bloodstream by *C. sordellii* and *C. perfringens* have been associated with TSS.

Bloodstream infection by *C. tertium*, either alone or in combination with *C. septicum* or *C. perfringens*, can be found in patients with serious underlying disease such as malignancy or acute pancreatitis, with or without neutropenic enterocolitis; the frequency has not been systematically studied. *C. tertium* may present special problems in terms of both identification and treatment. This organism may stain gram-negative; is aerotolerant; and is resistant to metronidazole, clindamycin, and cephalosporins.

Other clostridia from the *C. clostridioforme* group (including *C. clostridioforme*, *C. hathewayi*, and *C. bolteae*) can cause bacteremia.

The clinical importance of recognizing clostridial bacteremia—especially that due to *C. septicum*—and starting appropriate treatment immediately (Table 154-1) cannot be overemphasized. Patients with this condition usually are gravely ill, and infection may metastasize to distant anatomic sites, resulting in spontaneous myonecrosis (see next section). Alternative methods to identify bacteremia-causing clostridial species, such as PCR or other rapid diagnostic tests, are not currently available. Anaerobic blood cultures and Gram's stain interpretation remain the best diagnostic tests at this point.

CLOSTRIDIAL SKIN AND SOFT TISSUE INFECTIONS

Histotoxic clostridial species such as *C. perfringens*, *C. histolyticum*, *C. septicum*, *C. novyi*, and *C. sordellii* cause aggressive necrotizing infections of the skin and soft tissues. These infections are attributable in part to the elaboration of bacterial proteases, phospholipases, and cytotoxins. Necrotizing clostridial soft tissue infections are rapidly progressive and are characterized by marked tissue destruction, gas in the tissues, and shock; they frequently end in death. Severe pain, crepitus, brawny induration with rapid progression to skin sloughing, violaceous bullae, and marked tachycardia are characteristics found in the majority of patients.

Clostridial Myonecrosis (Gas Gangrene)

• TRAUMATIC GAS GANGRENE *C. perfringens* myonecrosis (gas gangrene) is one of the most fulminant gram-positive bacterial infections of humans. Even with appropriate antibiotic therapy and management in an intensive care unit, tissue destruction can progress rapidly. Gas gangrene is accompanied by bacteremia, hypotension, and multiorgan failure and is invariably fatal if untreated. Gas gangrene is a true emergency and requires immediate surgical debridement.

The development of gas gangrene requires an anaerobic environment and contamination of a wound with spores or vegetative organisms. Devitalized tissue, foreign bodies, and ischemia reduce locally available oxygen levels and favor outgrowth of vegetative cells and spores. Thus, conditions predisposing to traumatic gas gangrene include crush-type injury, laceration of large or medium-sized arteries, and open fractures of long bones that are contaminated with soil or bits of clothing containing the bacterial spores. Gas gangrene of the abdominal wall and flanks follows penetrating injuries such as knife or gunshot wounds that are sufficient to compromise intestinal integrity, with resultant leakage of the bowel contents into the soft tissues. Proximity to fecal sources of bacteria is a risk factor for cases following hip surgery, adrenaline injections into the buttocks, or amputation of the leg for ischemic vascular disease. In the last decade, cutaneous gas gangrene caused by *C. perfringens*, *C. novyi*, and *C. sordellii* has been described in the United States and northern Europe among persons injecting black-tar heroin subcutaneously.

The incubation period for traumatic gas gangrene can be as short as 6 h and is usually <4 days. The infection is characterized by the sudden onset of excruciating pain at the affected site and the rapid development of a foul-smelling wound containing a thin serosanguineous discharge and gas bubbles. Brawny edema and induration develop and give way to cutaneous blisters containing bluish to maroon-colored fluid. Such tissue later may become liquefied and slough. The margin between healthy and necrotic tissue often advances several inches per hour despite appropriate antibiotic therapy, and radical amputation remains the single best life-saving intervention. Shock and organ failure frequently accompany gas gangrene; when patients become bacteremic, the mortality rate exceeds 50%.

Diagnosis of traumatic gas gangrene is not difficult because the infection always begins at the site of significant trauma, is associated with gas in the tissue, and is rapidly progressive. Gram's staining of drainage or tissue biopsy is usually definitive, demonstrating large gram-positive (or gram-variable) rods, an absence of inflammatory cells, and widespread soft tissue necrosis.

SPONTANEOUS (NONTRAUMATIC) GAS GANGRENE Spontaneous gas gangrene generally occurs via hematogenous seeding of normal muscle with histotoxic clostridia—principally *C. perfringens*, *C. septicum*, and *C. novyi* and occasionally *C. tertium*—from a gastrointestinal tract portal of entry (as in colonic malignancy, inflammatory bowel disease, diverticulitis, necrotizing enterocolitis, cecitis, or distal ileitis or after gastrointestinal surgery, including colonoscopic polypectomy). These gastrointestinal pathologies permit bacterial access to the bloodstream; consequently, aerotolerant *C. septicum* can proliferate in normal tissues. Patients surviving bacteremia or spontaneous gangrene due to *C. septicum* should undergo aggressive diagnostic studies to rule out gastrointestinal pathology.

Additional predisposing host factors include leukemia, lymphoproliferative disorders, cancer chemotherapy, radiation therapy, and AIDS. Cyclic, congenital, or acquired neutropenia also is strongly associated with an increased incidence of spontaneous gas gangrene due to *C. septicum*; in such cases, necrotizing enterocolitis, cecitis, or distal ileitis is common, particularly among children.

The first symptom of spontaneous gas gangrene may be confusion followed by the abrupt onset of excruciating pain in the absence of trauma. These findings, along with fever, should heighten suspicion of spontaneous gas gangrene. However, because of the lack of an obvious portal of entry, the correct diagnosis is frequently delayed or missed. The infection is characterized by rapid progression of tissue destruction with demonstrable gas in the tissue (**Fig. 154-2**). Swelling increases, and bullae filled with clear, cloudy, hemorrhagic, or purplish fluid appear. The surrounding skin has a purple hue, which may reflect vascular compromise resulting from the diffusion of bacterial toxins into surrounding tissues. Invasion of healthy tissue rapidly ensues, with quick progression to shock and multiple-organ failure. Mortality rates in this setting range from 67 to 100% among adults; among children, the mortality rate is 59%, with the majority of deaths occurring within 24 h of onset.

PATHOGENESIS OF GAS GANGRENE In traumatic gas gangrene, organisms are introduced into devitalized tissue. It is important to recognize that, for *C. perfringens* and *C. novyi*, trauma must be sufficient to interrupt the blood supply and thereby to establish an optimal anaerobic environment for growth of these species. These conditions are not strictly required for the more aerotolerant species such as *C. septicum* and *C. tertium*, which can seed normal tissues from gastrointestinal lesions. Once introduced into an appropriate niche, the organisms proliferate locally and elaborate exotoxins.

The major *C. perfringens* extracellular toxins implicated in gas gangrene are α toxin and θ toxin. A lethal hemolysin that has both phospholipase C and sphingomyelinase activities, α toxin has been implicated as the major virulence factor of *C. perfringens*: immunization of mice with the C-terminal domain of α toxin provides protection against lethal challenge with *C. perfringens*, and isogenic α toxin–deficient mutant strains of *C. perfringens* are not lethal in a murine model of gas gangrene. Recently, a human single-chain recombinant antibody to α toxin that has significant preventive and therapeutic efficacy in mice has been developed.

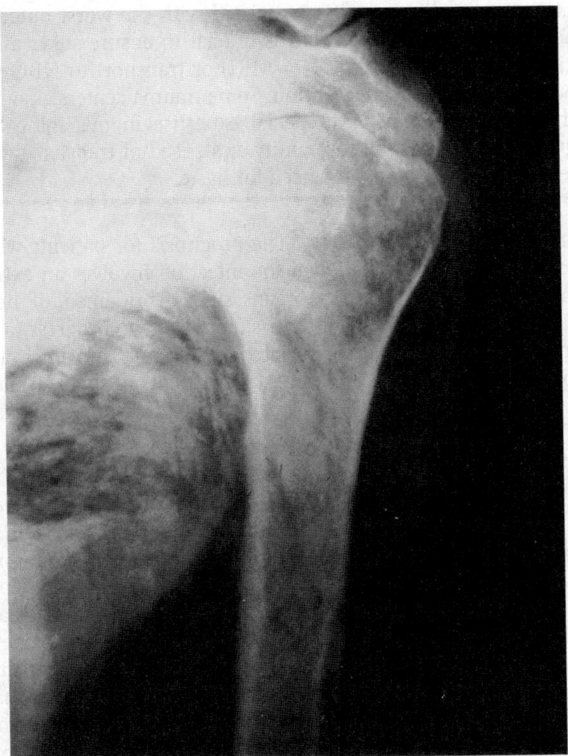

FIGURE 154-2 Radiograph of patient with spontaneous gas gangrene due to *C. septicum*, demonstrating gas in the affected arm and shoulder.

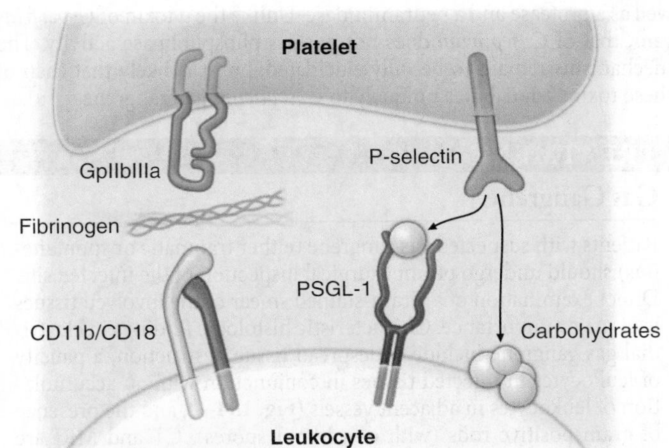

FIGURE 154-3 Schematic illustration of the molecular mechanisms of *C. perfringens* toxin–induced platelet/neutrophil aggregates. Homotypic aggregates of platelets (not shown) and heterotypic aggregates of platelets and leukocytes are due to α toxin–induced activation of the platelet fibrinogen receptor gpIIb/IIIa and upregulation of leukocyte CD11b/CD18. Binding of fibrinogen (*red*) bridges the connection between these adhesion molecules on adjacent cells. An auxiliary role for α toxin–induced upregulation of platelet P-selectin and its binding to leukocyte P-selectin glycoprotein ligand 1 (PSGL-1) or other leukocyte surface carbohydrates also has been demonstrated.

It has been shown in experimental models that the severe pain, rapid progression, marked tissue destruction, and absence of neutrophils in *C. perfringens* gas gangrene are attributable in large part to α toxin–induced occlusion of blood vessels by heterotypic aggregates of platelets and neutrophils. The formation of these aggregates, which occurs within minutes, is largely mediated by α toxin's ability to activate the platelet adhesion molecule gpIIb/IIIa (**Fig. 154-3**); the implication is that platelet glycoprotein inhibitors (e.g., eptifibatide, abciximab) may be therapeutic for maintaining tissue blood flow.

C. perfringens θ toxin (*perfringolysin O* [PFO]) is a member of the thiol-activated cytolysin family known as cholesterol-dependent cytolysins, which includes streptolysin O from group A *Streptococcus*, pneumolysin from *Streptococcus pneumoniae*, and several other toxins. Cholesterol-dependent cytolysins bind as oligomers to cholesterol in host cell membranes. At high concentrations, these toxins form ringlike pores resulting in cell lysis. At sublytic concentrations, θ toxin hyperactivates phagocytes and vascular endothelial cells. θ toxin–mediated activation of the macrophage inflammasome, with production of interleukin 1β, has also been reported.

Cardiovascular collapse and end-organ failure occur late in the course of *C. perfringens* gas gangrene and are largely attributable to both direct and indirect effects of α and θ toxins. In experimental models, θ toxin causes markedly reduced systemic vascular resistance but increased cardiac output (i.e., "warm shock"), probably via induction of endogenous mediators (e.g., prostacyclin, platelet-activating factor) that cause vasodilation. This effect is similar to that observed in gram-negative sepsis. In sharp contrast, α toxin directly suppresses myocardial contractility; the consequence is profound hypotension due to a sudden reduction in cardiac output. The roles of other endogenous mediators, such as cytokines (e.g., tumor necrosis factor, interleukin 1, interleukin 6) and vasodilators (e.g., bradykinin) have not been fully elucidated.

C. septicum produces three main toxins—α toxin (lethal, hemolytic, necrotizing activity), β toxin (DNase), and γ toxin (hyaluronidase)—as well as a protease and a neuraminidase. Unlike the α toxin of *C. perfringens*, that of *C. septicum* does not possess phospholipase activity. The mechanisms remain to be fully elucidated, but it is likely that each of these toxins contributes uniquely to *C. septicum* gas gangrene.

TREATMENT
Gas Gangrene

Patients with suspected gas gangrene (either traumatic or spontaneous) should undergo prompt surgical inspection of the infected site. Direct examination of a Gram-stained smear of the involved tissues is of major importance. Characteristic histologic findings in clostridial gas gangrene include widespread tissue destruction, a paucity of leukocytes in infected tissues in conjunction with an accumulation of leukocytes in adjacent vessels (**Fig. 154-4**), and the presence of gram-positive rods (with or without spores). CT and MRI are invaluable for determining whether the infection is localized or is spreading along fascial planes, and needle aspiration or punch biopsy may provide an etiologic diagnosis in at least 20% of cases. However, these techniques should not replace surgical exploration, Gram's staining, and histopathologic examination. When spontaneous gas gangrene is suspected, blood should be cultured since bacteremia usually precedes cutaneous manifestations by several hours.

For patients with evidence of clostridial gas gangrene, thorough emergent surgical debridement is of extreme importance. All devitalized tissue should be widely resected back to healthy viable muscle and skin so as to remove conditions that allow anaerobic organisms to continue proliferating. Closure of traumatic wounds or compound fractures should be delayed for 5–6 days until it is certain that these sites are free of infection.

Except for infection caused by *C. tertium* (see below), antibiotic treatment of traumatic or spontaneous gas gangrene (Table 154-1) consists of the administration of penicillin and clindamycin for 10–14 days. Penicillin is recommended on the basis of in vitro sensitivity data; clindamycin is recommended because of its superior efficacy over penicillin in animal models of *C. perfringens* gas gangrene and in some clinical reports. Controlled clinical trials comparing the efficacy of these agents in humans have not been performed. In the penicillin-allergic patient, clindamycin may be used alone. The superior efficacy of clindamycin is probably due to its ability to inhibit bacterial protein toxin production, its insensitivity to the size of the bacterial load or the stage of bacterial growth, and its ability to modulate the host's immune response.

Although *C. perfringens* remains largely susceptible to first-line antibiotics, antibiotic resistance has been reported. Case reports from the United Kingdom and from Spain found clindamycin-resistant *C. perfringens* in cellulitis and in a spontaneous abscess, respectively. Larger studies from Canada and Taiwan also showed increasing resistance to clindamycin among bloodstream isolates. In 2014, Marchand-Austin et al published a 2-year prospective Canadian study that examined antimicrobial susceptibility of anaerobic bacteria isolated from blood, body fluids, and abscesses. Of 1412 isolates submitted for susceptibility testing, 68 were *C. perfringens*. Of these, all were universally susceptible to penicillin but 3.8% were clindamycin-resistant. Notably, for *Clostridium* species other than *C. perfringens* (n = 289), 14.2% were penicillin-resistant and 21.6% clindamycin-resistant. A more recent study from Iran found that 21.2% of *C. perfringens* isolates were resistant to penicillin. Lastly, a 2019 study from Hungary found resistance to penicillin (2.6%) and clindamycin (3.8%) among *C. perfringens* isolates (n = 313) from tissues with gas gangrene. Among the non-perfringens gas gangrene isolates (n = 59), higher resistance to penicillin and clindamycin was observed (6.8% and 8.5%, respectively). These findings, though not universal, highlight the importance of good anaerobic microbiology susceptibility testing to provide up-to-date information to guide optimal clinical management decisions for clostridial infections.

C. tertium is resistant to penicillin, cephalosporins, and clindamycin. Appropriate antibiotic therapy for *C. tertium* infection is vancomycin (1 g every 12 h IV) or metronidazole (500 mg every 8 h IV).

The value of adjunctive treatment with hyperbaric oxygen (HBO) for gas gangrene remains controversial. Basic-science studies suggest that HBO can inhibit the growth of *C. perfringens* but not that of the more aerotolerant *C. septicum*. In vitro, blood and macerated muscle inhibit the bactericidal potential of HBO. Numerous studies in animals demonstrate little efficacy of HBO alone, whereas antibiotics alone—especially those that inhibit bacterial protein synthesis—confer marked benefits. Addition of HBO to the therapeutic regimen provides some additional benefit, but only if surgery and antibiotic administration precede HBO treatment.

In conclusion, gas gangrene is a rapidly progressive infection whose outcome depends on prompt recognition, emergent surgery, and timely administration of antibiotics that inhibit toxin production. Gas gangrene associated with bacteremia probably represents a later stage of illness and is associated with the worst outcomes. Emergent surgical debridement is crucial to ensure survival, and ancillary procedures (e.g., CT or MRI) or transport to HBO units should not delay this intervention. Some trauma centers associated with HBO units may have special expertise in managing these aggressive infections, but proximity and speed of transfer must be carefully weighed against the need for haste.

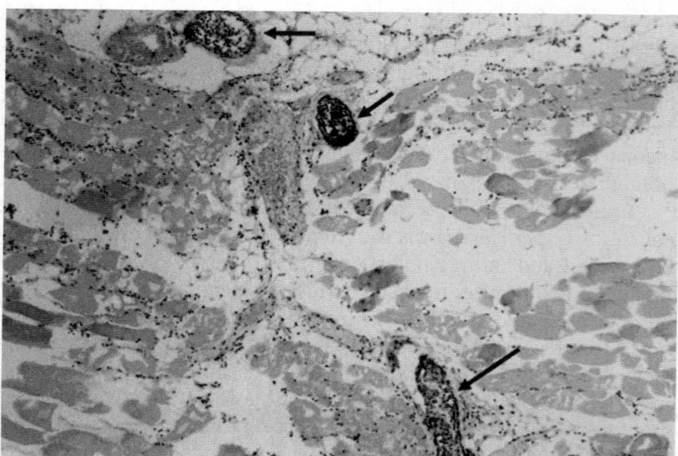

FIGURE 154-4 Histopathology of experimental gas gangrene due to *C. perfringens*, demonstrating widespread muscle necrosis, a paucity of leukocytes in infected tissues, and accumulation of leukocytes in adjacent vessels (*arrows*). These features are due to the effects of α and θ toxins on muscle cells, platelets, leukocytes, and endothelial cells.

PROGNOSIS OF GAS GANGRENE The prognosis for patients with gas gangrene is more favorable when the infection involves an extremity rather than the trunk or visceral organs, since debridement of the latter sites is more difficult. Gas gangrene is most likely to progress to shock and death in patients with associated bacteremia and intravascular hemolysis. Mortality rates are highest for patients in shock at the time of diagnosis. Mortality rates are relatively high among patients with spontaneous gas gangrene, especially that due to *C. septicum*. Survivors of gas gangrene may undergo multiple debridements and face long periods of hospitalization and rehabilitation.

PREVENTION OF GAS GANGRENE Initial aggressive debridement of devitalized tissue can reduce the risk of gas gangrene in contaminated deep wounds. Interventions to be avoided include prolonged application of tourniquets and surgical closure of traumatic wounds; patients with compound fractures are at significant risk for gas gangrene if the wound is closed surgically. Vaccination against α toxin is protective in experimental animal models of *C. perfringens* gas gangrene but has not been investigated in humans. In addition, as mentioned above, a hyperimmune globulin would represent a significant advance for prophylaxis in victims of acute traumatic injury or for attenuation of the spread of infection in patients with established gas gangrene.

Toxic Shock Syndrome Clostridial infection of the endometrium, particularly that due to *C. sordellii*, can develop after gynecologic procedures, childbirth, or abortion (spontaneous or elective, surgical or medical) and, once established, proceeds rapidly to TSS and death. Systemic manifestations, including edema, effusions, profound leukocytosis, and hemoconcentration, are followed by the rapid onset of hypotension and multiple-organ failure. Elevation of the hematocrit to 75–80% and leukocytosis of 50,000–200,000 cells/μL, with a left shift, are characteristic of *C. sordellii* infection. Pain may not be a prominent feature, and fever is typically absent. In one series, 18% of 45 cases of *C. sordellii* infection were associated with normal childbirth, 11% with medically induced abortion, and 0.4% with spontaneous abortion; the case–fatality rate was 100% in these groups. Of the infections in this series that were not related to gynecologic procedures or childbirth, 22% occurred in injection drug users, and 50% of these patients died. Other infections followed trauma or surgery (42%), mostly in healthy persons, and 53% of these patients died. Overall, the mortality rate was 69% (31 of 45 cases). Of patients who succumbed, 85% died within 2–6 days after infection onset or following procedures. Rapidly fatal, spontaneous *C. bifermentans* necrotizing endometritis with toxic shock, leukemoid reaction, and capillary leak has also been described.

Early diagnosis of *C. sordellii* infections often proves difficult for several reasons. First, the prevalence of these infections is low. Second, the initial symptoms are nonspecific and frankly misleading. Early in the course, the illness resembles any number of infectious diseases, including viral syndromes. Given these vague symptoms and an absence of fever, physicians usually do not aggressively pursue additional diagnostic tests. The absence of local evidence of infection and the lack of fever make early diagnosis of *C. sordellii* infection particularly problematic in patients who develop deep-seated infection following childbirth, therapeutic abortion, gastrointestinal surgery, or trauma. Such patients are frequently evaluated for pulmonary embolization, gastrointestinal bleeding, pyelonephritis, or cholecystitis. Unfortunately, such delays in diagnosis increase the risk of death, and, as in most necrotizing soft tissue infections, patients are hypotensive with evidence of organ dysfunction by the time local signs and symptoms become apparent. In contrast, infection is more readily suspected in injection drug users presenting with local swelling, pain, and redness at injection sites; early recognition probably contributes to the lower mortality rates in this group.

Physicians should suspect *C. sordellii* infection in patients who present within 2–7 days after injury, surgery, drug injection, childbirth, or abortion and who report pain, nausea, vomiting, and diarrhea but are afebrile. There is little information regarding appropriate treatment for *C. sordellii* infections. In fact, the interval between onset of symptoms and death is often so short that there is little time to initiate empirical antimicrobial therapy. Indeed, anaerobic cultures of blood and wound aspirates are time-consuming, and many hospital laboratories do not routinely perform antimicrobial sensitivity testing on anaerobes. Antibiotic susceptibility data from older studies suggest that *C. sordellii*, like most clostridia, is susceptible to β-lactam antibiotics, clindamycin, tetracycline, and chloramphenicol but is resistant to aminoglycosides and sulfonamides. Antibiotics that suppress toxin synthesis (e.g., clindamycin) may possibly prove useful as therapeutic adjuncts since they are effective in necrotizing infections due to other toxin-producing gram-positive organisms.

Other Clostridial Skin and Soft Tissue Infections *Crepitant cellulitis* (also called *anaerobic cellulitis*) occurs principally in diabetic patients and characteristically involves subcutaneous tissues or retroperitoneal tissues, whereas the muscle and fascia are not involved. This infection can progress to fulminant systemic disease.

Cases of *C. histolyticum* infection with cellulitis, abscess formation, or endocarditis have also been documented in injection drug users. Endophthalmitis due to *C. sordellii* or *C. perfringens* has been described. *C. ramosum* is also isolated frequently from clinical specimens, including blood and both intraabdominal and soft tissues. This species may be resistant to clindamycin and multiple cephalosporins.

FURTHER READING

Aldape MJ et al: *Clostridium sordellii* infection: Epidemiology, clinical findings, and current perspectives on diagnosis and treatment. Clin Infect Dis 43:1436, 2006.

Bodey GP et al: Clostridial bacteremia in cancer patients. A 12-year experience. Cancer 67:1928, 1991.

Bos J et al: Fatal necrotizing colitis following a foodborne outbreak of enterotoxigenic *Clostridium perfringens* type A infection. Clin Infect Dis 40:e78, 2005.

Bryant AE et al: Clostridial gas gangrene II: Phospholipase C–induced activation of platelet gpIIb/IIIa mediates vascular occlusion and myonecrosis in *C. perfringens* gas gangrene. J Infect Dis 182:808, 2000.

Leong HN et al: Management of complicated skin and soft tissue infections with a special focus on the role of newer antibiotics. Infect Drug Resist 11:1959, 2018.

Marchand-Austin A et al: Antimicrobial susceptibility of clinical isolates of anaerobic bacteria in Ontario, 2010-2011. Anaerobe 28:120-125, 2014.

Obladen M: Necrotizing enterocolitis—150 years of fruitless search for the cause. Neonatology 96:203, 2009.

Peetermans M et al: Necrotizing skin and soft-tissue infections in the intensive care unit. Clin Microbiol Infect 26:8, 2020.

Sayeed S et al: Beta toxin is essential for the intestinal virulence of *Clostridium perfringens* type C disease isolate CN3685 in a rabbit ileal loop model. Mol Microbiol 67:15, 2008.

Stevens DL, Bryant AE: Necrotizing soft tissue infections. N Engl J Med 377:2253, 2017.

Stevens DL et al: Practice guidelines for the diagnosis and management of skin and soft tissue infections: 2014 update by the Infectious Diseases Society of America. Clin Infect Dis 59:e10, 2014.

Stevens DL et al: *Clostridium*, in *Manual of Clinical Microbiology*, 11th ed, JH Jorgensen et al (eds). Washington, DC, ASM Press, 2015, pp 940–966.

Wang C et al: Hyperbaric oxygen for treating wounds: A systematic review of the literature. Arch Surg 138:272, 2003.

Section 6 Diseases Caused by Gram-Negative Bacteria

155 Meningococcal Infections

Manish Sadarangani, Andrew J. Pollard

DEFINITION

Infection with *Neisseria meningitidis* most commonly manifests as asymptomatic colonization in the nasopharynx of healthy adolescents and adults. Invasive disease occurs rarely, usually presenting as either bacterial meningitis or meningococcal septicemia. Patients may also present with occult bacteremia, pneumonia, septic arthritis, conjunctivitis, and chronic meningococcemia.

ETIOLOGY AND MICROBIOLOGY

N. meningitidis is a gram-negative aerobic diplococcus that colonizes humans only and that causes disease after transmission to a susceptible individual. Several related neisserial organisms have been recognized, including the pathogen *N. gonorrhoeae* and the commensals *N. lactamica*, *N. flavescens*, *N. mucosa*, *N. sicca*, and *N. subflava*. *N. meningitidis* is a catalase- and oxidase-positive organism that utilizes glucose and maltose to produce acid.

TABLE 155-1 Structure of the Polysaccharide Capsule of Common Disease-Causing Meningococci

MENINGOCOCCAL CAPSULAR GROUP	CHEMICAL STRUCTURE OF OLIGOSACCHARIDE	CURRENT DISEASE EPIDEMIOLOGY
A	2-Acetamido-2-deoxy-D-mannopyranosyl phosphate	Epidemic disease mainly in sub-Saharan Africa; sporadic cases worldwide
B	α-2,8-*N*-acetylneuraminic acid	Sporadic cases worldwide; propensity to cause hyperendemic disease
C	α-2,9-*O*-acetylneuraminic acid	Small outbreaks and sporadic disease
Y	4-*O*-α-D-glucopyranosyl-*N*-acetylneuraminic acid	Sporadic disease and occasional small institutional outbreaks
W	4-*O*-α-D-galactopyranosyl-*N*-acetylneuraminic acid	Sporadic disease; outbreaks of disease associated with mass gatherings; epidemics in sub-Saharan Africa
X	(α1→4) *N*-acetyl-D-glucosamine-1-phosphate	Sporadic disease and large outbreaks in the meningitis belt of Africa

Meningococci associated with invasive disease are usually encapsulated with polysaccharide, and the antigenic nature of the capsule determines an organism's capsular group (serogroup) **(Table 155-1)**. In total, 12 capsular groups have been identified (A–C, X–Z, E, W, H–J, and L), but just six of these—A, B, C, X, Y, and W (formerly W135)—account for the majority of cases of invasive disease. Group D is often listed as the thirteenth capsular group but has recently been identified as an unencapsulated variant of group C. Meningococci are commonly isolated from the nasopharynx in studies of carriage; the lack of capsule often is a result of phase variation of capsule expression, but as many as 16% of isolates lack the genes for capsule synthesis and assembly. These "capsule-null" meningococci and those that express capsules other than A, B, C, X, Y, and W are only rarely associated with invasive disease and are most commonly identified in the nasopharynx of asymptomatic carriers.

Beneath the capsule, meningococci are surrounded by an outer phospholipid membrane containing lipopolysaccharide (LPS, endotoxin) and multiple outer-membrane proteins **(Figs. 155-1 and 155-2)**. Antigenic variability in porins expressed in the outer membrane defines the serotype (PorB) and serosubtype (PorA) of the organism, and structural differences in LPS determine the immunotype. Serologic methods

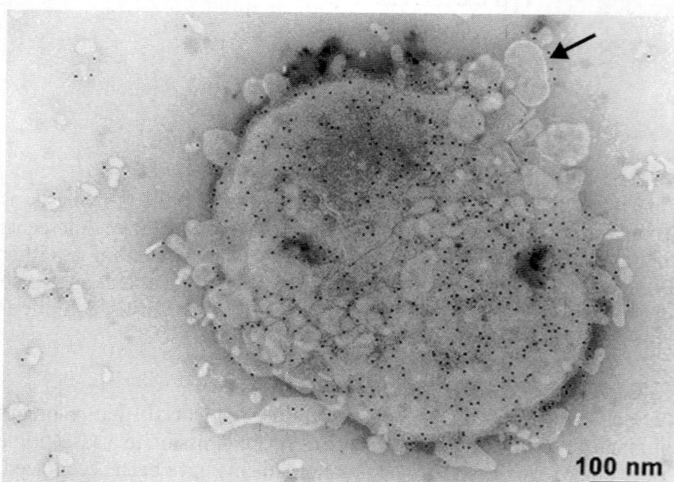

FIGURE 155-1 Electron micrograph of *Neisseria meningitidis*. Black dots are gold-labeled polyclonal antibodies binding surface opacity proteins. Blebs of outer membrane can be seen being released from the bacterial surface (*arrow*). (*Photo courtesy of D. Ferguson, Oxford University.*)

for typing of meningococci are restricted by the limited availability of serologic reagents that can distinguish among the organisms' highly variable surface proteins. Where available, high-throughput antigen gene sequencing has superseded serology for meningococcal typing. A large database of antigen gene sequences for the outer-membrane proteins PorA, PorB, FetA, Opa, NadA, Neisserial heparin binding antigen (NHBA), and factor H–binding protein (fHbp) is available online (*pubmlst.org/organisms/neisseria-spp*). The number of specialized iron-regulated proteins found in the meningococcal outer membrane (e.g., FetA and transferrin-binding proteins) highlights the organisms' dependence on iron from human sources. A thin peptidoglycan cell wall separates the outer membrane from the cytoplasmic membrane.

The structure of meningococcal populations involved in local and global spread has been studied with multilocus enzyme electrophoresis (MLEE), which characterizes isolates according to differences in the electrophoretic mobility of cytoplasmic enzymes. However, this technique was replaced by multilocus sequence typing (MLST), in which meningococci are characterized by sequence types assigned on the basis of sequences of internal fragments of 7 housekeeping genes. The online MLST database currently includes more than 15,000 unique *Neisseria* sequence types. A limited number of hyperinvasive lineages of *N. meningitidis* have been recognized and are responsible for the majority of cases of invasive meningococcal disease worldwide. Hyperinvasive lineages may be associated with more than one capsular group. The apparent genetic stability of these meningococcal clones over decades and during wide geographic spread indicates that they are well adapted to the nasopharyngeal environment of the host and to efficient transmission. While MLST has become established as the main method for meningococcal genotyping in many reference laboratories over the past 15 years, whole-genome sequencing is gradually replacing this approach, with more than 4500 genomes already available in the United Kingdom's national library.

The group B meningococcal genome is >2 megabases in length and contains 2158 coding regions. Many genes undergo phase variation that makes it possible to control their expression; this capacity is likely to be important in meningococcal adaptation to the host environment and evasion of the immune response. Meningococci can obtain DNA from their environment and can acquire new genes—including the capsular operon—such that *capsule switching* from one capsular group to another can occur.

EPIDEMIOLOGY

Patterns of Disease Up to 500,000 cases of meningococcal disease are thought to occur worldwide each year, although the numbers have been declining recently as a result of both immunization programs and secular trends. About 10% of affected individuals die. There are several patterns of disease: epidemic, outbreak (small clusters of cases), hyperendemic, and sporadic or endemic.

Epidemics have continued since the original descriptions of meningococcal disease, especially affecting the sub-Saharan meningitis belt of Africa, where tens to hundreds of thousands of cases (caused mainly by capsular group A but also by capsular groups C, W, and X) may be reported over a season and rates may be as high as 1000 cases per 100,000 population. Capsular group A epidemics took place in Europe and North America after the First and Second World Wars, and capsular group A outbreaks have been documented over the past 30 years in New Zealand, China, Nepal, Mongolia, India, Pakistan, Poland, and Russia. However, 65% of outbreaks reported in the meningitis belt between 2010 and 2017 were caused by capsular group C and 35% by capsular group W meningococci, following an immunization campaign to control capsular group A outbreaks.

Clusters of cases occur where there is an opportunity for increased transmission—i.e., in closed or semi-closed communities such as schools, colleges, universities, military training centers, and refugee camps. Recently, such clusters have been especially strongly linked with a particular clone (sequence type 11) that is mainly associated with capsular group C or W but was first described in association with capsular group B. Clusters of capsular group W disease associated with

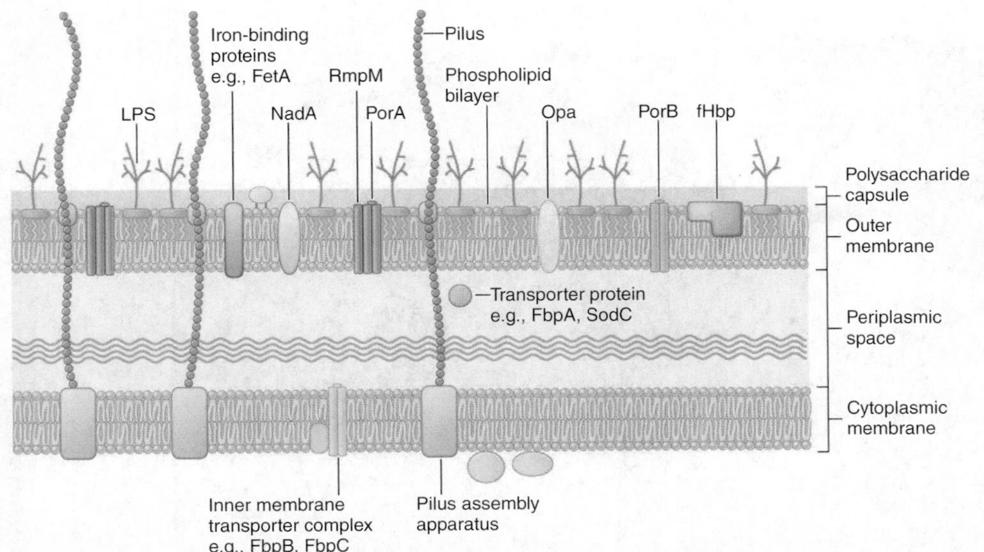

FIGURE 155-2 Cross-section through surface structures of *Neisseria meningitidis*. LPS, lipopolysaccharide. *(Reproduced with permission from M Sadarangani, AJ Pollard: Serogroup B meningococcal vaccines–an unfinished story. Lancet Infect Dis 10:112, 2010.)*

the Hajj pilgrimage in 2000/2001 led to a requirement for vaccination against meningococcal disease for travel to Saudi Arabia. Wider and more prolonged community outbreaks (hyperendemic disease) due to single clones of capsular group B meningococci account for ≥10 cases per 100,000. Regions affected in the past decade include the U.S. Pacific Northwest, New Zealand (both islands), and the province of Normandy in France.

Most countries now experience predominantly sporadic cases (0.3–5 cases per 100,000 population), with many different disease-causing clones involved and usually no clear epidemiologic link between one case and another. The disease rate and the distribution of meningococcal strains vary in different regions of the world and also in any one location over time. For example, in the United States, the rate of meningococcal disease fell from 1.2 cases per 100,000 population in 1997 to 0.10 cases per 100,000 in 2018 **(Fig. 155-3)**. Meningococcal disease in the United States was previously dominated by capsular groups B and C; however, capsular group Y emerged during the 1990s and in 2018 group B was predominant in children age <5 years, whereas adults 45 years and older were infected with groups B, C, and Y **(Fig. 155-4)**. In contrast, rates of disease in England and Wales rose to >5 cases per 100,000 during the 1990s because of an increase in cases caused by the ST11 capsular group C clone. As a result of a mass immunization program against capsular group C in 1999, capsular group B then became predominant. Introduction of a MenB vaccine since 2015 has led to a significant reduction in group B cases, with an increase in recent years of capsular group W infections (Fig. 155-4). Over the last decade, most industrialized nations have seen a general decrease in meningococcal disease; this decrease is linked to immunization against capsular group C meningococci in Europe, Canada, and Australia and to adolescent immunization programs for capsular groups A, C, Y, and W in the United States. However, other factors, including changes in population immunity and prevalent clones of meningococci (factors that, in combination, probably explain the cyclic nature of meningococcal disease rates) as well as a reduction in smoking and passive exposure to tobacco smoke (driven by bans on smoking in buildings and public spaces) across wealthy countries, are likely to have contributed to the fall in cases. Over the past decade, a hyperinvasive ST11 clone bearing a W capsule has emerged in South America and spread to the United Kingdom and has also emerged in other countries in Europe and in Australia, leading to a considerable increase in capsular group W cases. Increases in capsular group Y disease have also been noted in various countries in Europe, Canada, and South Africa.

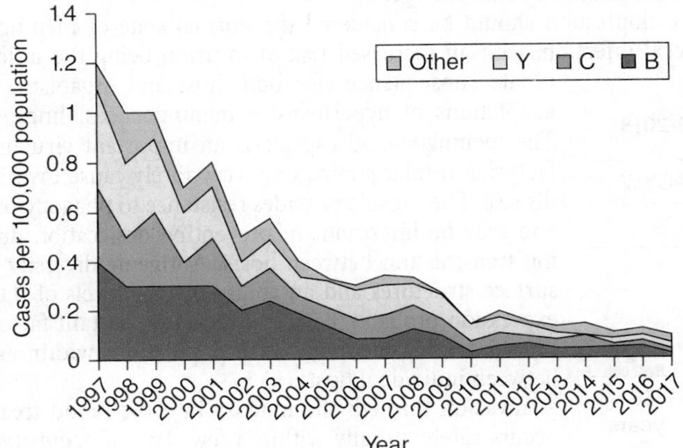

FIGURE 155-3 Meningococcal disease in the United States, 1997–2017. ABCs, active bacterial cores. *(Adapted from ABC Surveillance data, Centers for Disease Control and Prevention; www.cdc.gov.)*

Factors Associated with Disease Risk and Susceptibility The principal determinant of disease susceptibility is age, with the peak incidence in the first year of life **(Fig. 155-5)**. The susceptibility of the very young presumably results from an absence of specific adaptive immunity in combination with very close contact with colonized individuals, including parents. Compared with other age groups, infants appear to be particularly susceptible to capsular group B disease: >30% of capsular group B cases in the United States occur during the first year of life. In the early 1990s in North America, the median ages for patients with disease due to capsular groups B, C, Y, and W were 6, 17, 24, and 33 years, respectively.

After early childhood, a second peak of disease occurs among adolescents and young adults (15–25 years of age) in Europe and North America. It is thought that this peak relates to social behaviors and environmental exposures in this age group, as discussed below. Most cases of infection with *N. meningitidis* in developed countries today are sporadic, and the rarity of the disease suggests that individual susceptibility may be important. A number of factors probably contribute to individual susceptibility, including the host's genetic constitution, environment, and contact with a carrier or a case.

The best-documented genetic association with meningococcal disease is complement deficiency, chiefly of the terminal complement components (C5–9), properdin, or factor D; such a deficiency increases the risk of disease by up to 600-fold and may result in recurrent attacks. Complement components are believed to be important for the bactericidal activity of serum, which is considered the principal mechanism of immunity against invasive meningococcal disease. However, when investigated, complement deficiency is found in only a very small proportion of individuals with meningococcal disease (0.3%). Conversely, 7–20% of persons whose disease is caused by the less common capsular groups (W, X, Y, Z, E) have a complement deficiency. Complement deficiency appears to be associated with capsular group B disease only rarely. Individuals with recurrences of meningococcal disease, particularly those caused by non-B capsular groups, should be assessed for complement deficiency by measurement of total hemolytic complement activity. There is also limited evidence that hyposplenism (through reduction in phagocytic capacity) and hypogammaglobulinemia (through absence of specific antibody) increase the risk of meningococcal disease. Genetic studies have revealed various

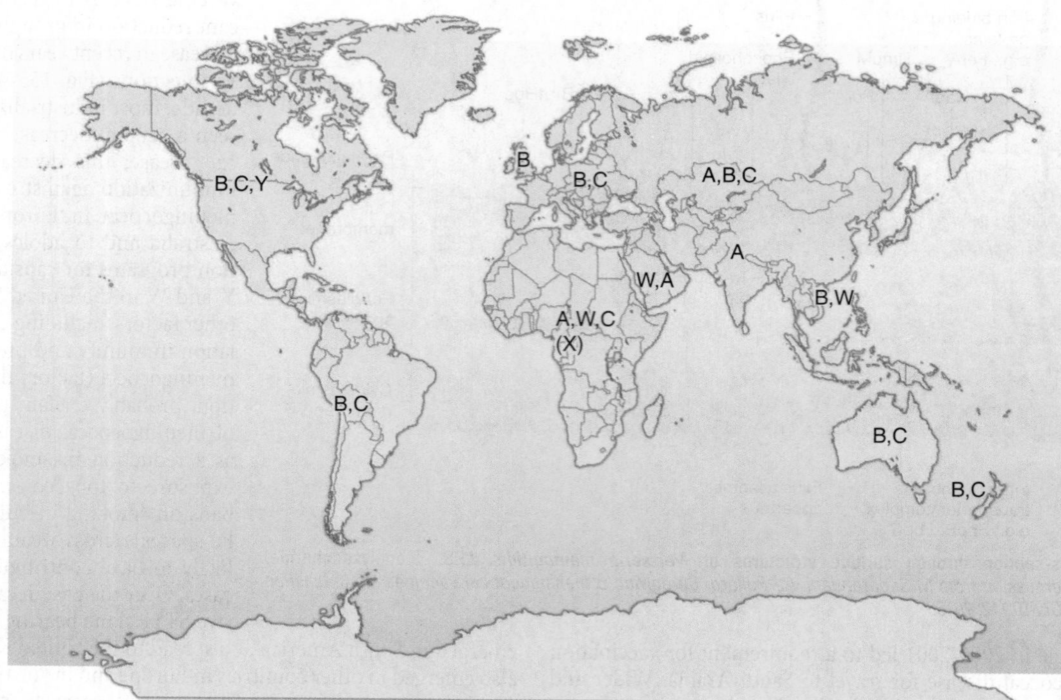

FIGURE 155-4 Global distribution of meningococcal capsular groups, 1999–2009.

associations with disease susceptibility, including complement and mannose-binding lectin deficiency, single-nucleotide polymorphisms in Toll-like receptor (TLR) 4 and complement factor H, and variants of Fc gamma receptors.

Factors that increase the chance of a susceptible individual's acquiring *N. meningitidis* via the respiratory route also increase the risk of meningococcal disease. Acquisition occurs through close contact with carriers as a result of overcrowding (e.g., in poor socioeconomic settings, in refugee camps, during the Hajj pilgrimage to Mecca, during freshman-year residence in college dormitories) and certain social behaviors (e.g., attendance at bars and nightclubs, kissing). Secondary cases may occur in close contacts of an index case (e.g., household members, persons kissing the infected individual); the risk to these contacts may be as high as 1000 times the background rate in the population. Factors that damage the nasopharyngeal epithelium also increase the risk of both colonization with *N. meningitidis* and invasive disease. The most important of these factors are tobacco smoking (odds ratio, 4.1) and passive exposure to tobacco smoke. In addition, recent viral respiratory tract infection, infection with *Mycoplasma* species, and winter or the dry season have been associated with meningococcal disease; all of these factors presumably either increase the expression of adhesion molecules in the nasopharynx, thus enhancing meningococcal adhesion, or facilitate meningococcal invasion of the bloodstream.

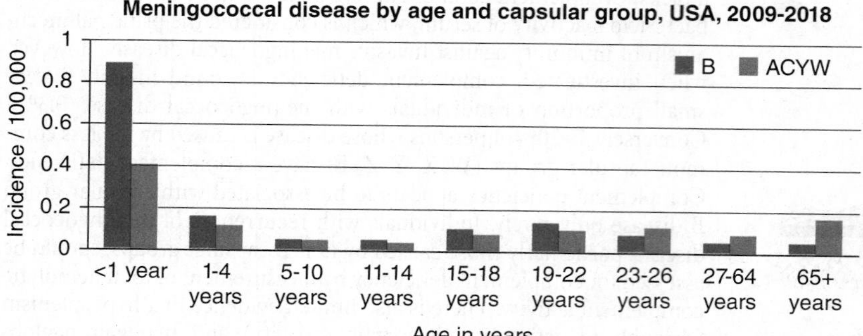

FIGURE 155-5 Age distribution of capsular groups B and ACWY meningococcal disease USA, 2009-2018. *(Adapted from www.cdc.gov/meningococcal/surveillance/surveillance-data.html#figure01.)*

PATHOGENESIS

N. meningitidis has evolved as an effective colonizer of the human nasopharynx, with asymptomatic infection rates of >25% described in some series of adolescents and young adults and among residents of crowded communities. Point-prevalence studies reveal widely divergent rates of carriage for different types of meningococci. This variation suggests that some types may be adapted to a short duration of carriage with frequent transmission to maintain the population, while others may be less efficiently transmitted but may overcome this disadvantage by colonizing for a long period. Despite the high rates of carriage among adolescents and young adults, only ~10% of adults carry meningococci, and colonization is very rare in early childhood. Many of the same factors that increase the risk of meningococcal disease also increase the risk of carriage. Colonization of the nasopharynx involves a series of interactions of meningococcal adhesins (e.g., Opa proteins and pili) with their ligands on the epithelial mucosa. *N. meningitidis* produces an IgA1 protease that is likely to reduce interruption of colonization by mucosal IgA.

Colonization should be considered the normal state of meningococcal infection, with an increased risk of invasion being the unfortunate consequence (for both host and organism) of adaptations of hyperinvasive meningococcal lineages. The meningococcal capsule is an important virulence factor: acapsular strains only very rarely cause invasive disease. The capsule provides resistance to phagocytosis and may be important in preventing desiccation during transmission between hosts. Antigenic diversity in surface structures and an ability to vary levels of their expression probably have evolved as important factors in maintaining meningococcal populations within and between individual hosts.

Invasion through the mucosa into the bloodstream occurs rarely, usually within a few days of acquisition of an invasive strain by a susceptible individual. Only occasional cases of prolonged colonization prior to invasion have been documented. Once the organism is in the bloodstream, its growth may be limited if the individual is partially immune, although bacteremia may allow seeding of another site, such as the meninges or the joints. Alternatively, unchecked proliferation may continue, resulting in high bacterial counts in the circulation. During growth, meningococci release blebs of outer membrane (Fig. 155-1) containing outer-membrane proteins and LPS. Endotoxin binds cell-bound CD14 in association with TLR4 to initiate an inflammatory cascade with the release of high levels of various mediators, including tumor necrosis factor (TNF) α, soluble TNF receptor, interleukin (IL) 1, IL-1 receptor antagonist, IL-1β, IL-6, IL-8, IL-10, plasminogen-activator inhibitor 1 (PAI-1), and leukemia inhibitory factor. Soluble CD14-bound endotoxin acts as a mediator of endothelial activation. The severity of meningococcal disease is related both to the levels of endotoxin in the blood and to the magnitude of the inflammatory response. The latter is determined to some extent by polymorphisms in the inflammatory response genes (and their inhibitors), and the release of the inflammatory cascade heralds the development of meningococcal septicemia (meningococcemia). Endothelial injury is central to many clinical features of meningococcemia, including increased vascular permeability, pathologic changes in vascular tone, loss of thromboresistance, intravascular coagulation, and myocardial dysfunction. Endothelial injury leads to increased vascular permeability (attributed to loss of glycosaminoglycans and endothelial proteins), with subsequent gross proteinuria. Leakage of fluid and electrolytes into the tissues from capillaries ("capillary leak syndrome") leads to hypovolemia, tissue edema, and pulmonary edema. Initial compensation results in vasoconstriction and tachycardia, although cardiac output eventually falls. While resuscitation fluids may restore circulating volume, tissue edema will continue to increase, and, in the lung, the consequence may be respiratory failure.

Intravascular thrombosis (caused by activation of procoagulant pathways in association with upregulation of tissue factor on the endothelium) occurs in some patients with meningococcal disease and results in purpura fulminans and infarction of areas of skin or even of whole limbs. At the same time, multiple anticoagulant pathways are downregulated through loss of endothelial thrombomodulin and protein C receptors and decreases in levels of antithrombin III, protein C, protein S, and tissue factor pathway inhibitor. Thrombolysis is also profoundly impaired in meningococcal sepsis through the release of high levels of PAI-1.

Shock in meningococcal septicemia appears to be attributable to a combination of factors, including hypovolemia, which results from the capillary leak syndrome secondary to endothelial injury, and myocardial depression, which is driven by hypovolemia, hypoxia, metabolic derangements (e.g., hypocalcemia), and cytokines (e.g., IL-6). Decreased perfusion of tissues as a result of intravascular thrombosis, vasoconstriction, tissue edema, and reduced cardiac output in meningococcal septicemia can cause widespread organ dysfunction, including renal impairment and—later in the disease—a decreased level of consciousness due to central nervous system involvement.

Bacteria that reach the meninges cause a local inflammatory response—with release of a spectrum of cytokines similar to that seen in septicemia—that presents clinically as meningitis and is thought to determine the severity of neuronal injury. Local endothelial injury may result in cerebral edema and rapid onset of raised intracranial pressure in some cases.

■ CLINICAL MANIFESTATIONS

As discussed above, the most common form of infection with *N. meningitidis* is asymptomatic carriage of the organism in the nasopharynx. Despite the location of infection in the upper airway, meningococcal pharyngitis is rarely reported; however, upper respiratory tract symptoms are common prior to presentation with invasive disease. It is not clear whether these symptoms relate to preceding viral infection (which may promote meningococcal acquisition and/or invasion) or to meningococcal acquisition itself. After acquiring the organism, susceptible individuals develop disease manifestations in 1–10 days (usually <4 days, although colonization for 11 weeks has been documented).

Along the spectrum of presentations of meningococcal disease, the most common clinical syndromes are meningitis and meningococcal septicemia. In fulminant cases, death may occur within hours of the first symptoms. Occult bacteremia is also recognized and, if untreated, progresses in two-thirds of cases to focal infection, including meningitis or septicemia. Meningococcal disease may also present as pneumonia, pyogenic arthritis or osteomyelitis, purulent pericarditis, endophthalmitis, conjunctivitis, primary peritonitis, or (rarely) urethritis. Perhaps because it is difficult to diagnose, meningococcal pneumonia is not commonly reported but is associated with capsular groups Y, W, and Z and appears most often to affect individuals >10 years of age.

Rash A nonblanching rash (petechial or purpuric) develops in >80% of cases of meningococcal disease; however, the rash is often absent early in the illness. Usually initially blanching in nature (macules, maculopapules, or urticaria) and indistinguishable from more common viral rashes, the rash of meningococcal infection becomes petechial or frankly purpuric over the hours after onset. In the most severe cases, large purpuric lesions develop (purpura fulminans; **Fig. A1-41**). Some patients (including those with overwhelming sepsis) may have no rash. While petechial rash and fever are important signs of meningococcal disease, fewer than 10% of children (and, in some clinical settings, fewer than 1% of patients) with this presentation are found to have meningococcal disease. Most patients presenting with a petechial or purpuric rash have a viral infection **(Table 155-2)**. The skin lesions exhibit widespread endothelial necrosis and occlusion of small vessels in the dermis and subcutaneous tissues, with a neutrophilic infiltrate.

Meningitis Meningococcal meningitis commonly presents as nonspecific manifestations, including fever, vomiting, and (especially in infants and young children) irritability, and is indistinguishable from other forms of bacterial meningitis unless there is an associated petechial or purpuric rash, which occurs in two-thirds of cases. Headache is rarely reported in early childhood but is more common in later childhood and adulthood. When headache is present, the following features, in association with fever or a history of fever, are suggestive of bacterial meningitis: neck stiffness, photophobia, decreased level of consciousness, seizures or status epilepticus, and focal neurologic signs. Classic signs of meningitis, such as neck stiffness and photophobia, are often absent in infants and young children with bacterial meningitis, who more usually present with fever and irritability and may have a bulging fontanelle.

While 30–50% of patients present with a meningitis syndrome alone, up to 40% of meningitis patients also present with some features of septicemia. Most deaths from meningococcal meningitis alone (i.e., without septicemia) are associated with raised intracranial pressure presenting as a reduced level of consciousness, relative bradycardia and hypertension, focal neurologic signs, abnormal posturing, and signs of brainstem involvement—e.g., unequal, dilated, or poorly reactive pupils; abnormal eye movement; and impaired corneal responses **(Chap. 28)**.

TABLE 155-2 Common Causes of Petechial or Purpuric Rashes
Enteroviruses
Influenza and other respiratory viruses
Measles virus
Epstein-Barr virus
Cytomegalovirus
Parvovirus
Deficiency of protein C or S (including postvaricella protein S deficiency)
Platelet disorders (e.g., idiopathic thrombocytopenic purpura, drug effects, bone marrow infiltration)
Henoch-Schönlein purpura, connective tissue disorders, trauma (including nonaccidental injuries in children)
Pneumococcal, streptococcal, staphylococcal, or gram-negative bacterial sepsis

Septicemia Meningococcal septicemia alone accounts for up to 20% of cases of meningococcal disease. The condition may progress from early nonspecific symptoms to death within hours. Mortality rates among children with this syndrome have been high (25–40%), but early aggressive management (as discussed below) may reduce the figure to <10%. Early symptoms are nonspecific and suggest an influenza-like illness with fever, headache, and myalgia accompanied by vomiting and abdominal pain. As discussed above, the rash, if present, may appear to be viral early in the course until petechiae or purpuric lesions develop. Purpura fulminans occurs in severe cases (Fig. A1-41), with multiple large purpuric lesions and signs of peripheral ischemia. Surveys of patients have indicated that limb pain, pallor (including a mottled appearance and cyanosis), and cold hands and feet may be prominent. Shock is manifested by tachycardia, poor peripheral perfusion, tachypnea, and oliguria. Decreased cerebral perfusion leads to confusion, agitation, or decreased level of consciousness. With progressive shock, multiorgan failure ensues; hypotension is a late sign in children, who more commonly present with compensated shock (tachycardia, poor peripheral perfusion, and normal blood pressure). Poor outcome is associated with an absence of meningism, hypotension, young age, coma, relatively low temperature (<38°C), leukopenia, and thrombocytopenia. Spontaneous hemorrhage (pulmonary, gastric, or cerebral) may result from consumption of coagulation factors and thrombocytopenia.

Chronic Meningococcemia Chronic meningococcemia, which is rarely recognized, presents as repeated episodes of petechial rash (**Fig. A1-42**) associated with fever, joint pain, features of arthritis, and splenomegaly that may progress to acute meningococcal septicemia if untreated. During the relapsing course, bacteremia characteristically clears without treatment and then recurs. The differential diagnosis includes bacterial endocarditis, acute rheumatic fever, Henoch-Schönlein purpura, infectious mononucleosis, disseminated gonococcal infection, and immune-mediated vasculitis. This condition has been associated with complement deficiencies in some cases and with inadequate sulfonamide therapy in others.

A study from the Netherlands found that half of isolates from patients with chronic meningococcemia had an underacylated lipid A (part of the surface LPS molecule) due to an *lpxL1* gene mutation, which markedly reduces the inflammatory response to endotoxin.

Postmeningococcal Reactive Disease In a small proportion of patients, an immune complex disease develops ~4–10 days after the onset of meningococcal disease, with manifestations that include a maculopapular or vasculitic rash (2% of cases), arthritis (up to 8% of cases), iritis (1%), pericarditis, and/or polyserositis associated with fever. The immune complexes involve meningococcal polysaccharide antigen and result in immunoglobulin and complement deposition with an inflammatory infiltrate. These features resolve spontaneously without sequelae. It is important to recognize this condition since a new onset of fever and rash, and/or arthritis, can lead to concerns about relapse of meningococcal disease and unnecessarily prolonged antibiotic treatment.

DIAGNOSIS

Like other invasive bacterial infections, meningococcal disease may produce elevations of the white blood cell (WBC) count and of values for inflammatory markers (e.g., C-reactive protein and procalcitonin levels or the erythrocyte sedimentation rate). Values may be normal or low in rapidly progressive disease, and a lack of rise in these laboratory test values does not exclude the diagnosis. However, in the presence of fever and a petechial rash, these elevations are suggestive of meningococcal disease. In patients with severe meningococcal septicemia, common laboratory findings include hypoglycemia, acidosis, hypokalemia, hypocalcemia, hypomagnesemia, hypophosphatemia, anemia, and coagulopathy.

Although meningococcal disease is often diagnosed on clinical grounds, in suspected meningococcal meningitis or meningococcemia, blood should routinely be sent for culture to confirm the diagnosis and to facilitate public health investigations; blood cultures are positive in up to 75% of cases. Culture media containing sodium polyanethol sulfonate, which may inhibit meningococcal growth, should be avoided. Meningococcal viability is reduced if there is a delay in transport of the specimen to the microbiology laboratory for culture or in plating of cerebrospinal fluid (CSF) samples. In countries where treatment with antibiotics before hospitalization is recommended for meningococcal disease, the majority of clinically suspected cases are culture negative. Real-time polymerase chain reaction (PCR) analysis of whole-blood samples increases the diagnostic yield by >40%, and results obtained with this method may remain positive for several days after administration of antibiotics. Indeed, in the United Kingdom, more than half of clinically suspected cases are currently identified by PCR.

Unless contraindications exist (raised intracranial pressure, uncorrected shock, disordered coagulation, thrombocytopenia, respiratory insufficiency, local infection, ongoing convulsions), lumbar puncture should be undertaken to identify and confirm the etiology of suspected meningococcal meningitis, whose presentation cannot be distinguished from that of meningitis of other bacterial causes. Some authorities have recommended a CT brain scan prior to lumbar puncture because of the risk of cerebral herniation in patients with raised intracranial pressure. However, a normal CT scan is not uncommon in the presence of raised intracranial pressure in meningococcal meningitis, and the decision to perform a lumbar puncture should be made on clinical grounds. CSF features of meningococcal meningitis (elevated protein level and WBC count, decreased glucose level) are indistinguishable from those of other types of bacterial meningitis unless a gram-negative diplococcus is identified. (Gram's staining is up to 80% sensitive for meningococcal meningitis.) CSF should be submitted for culture (sensitivity, 90%) and (where available) PCR analysis. CSF antigen testing with latex agglutination is insensitive and should be replaced by molecular diagnosis when possible.

Lumbar puncture should generally be avoided in meningococcal septicemia, as positioning for the procedure may critically compromise the patient's circulation in the context of hypovolemic shock. Delayed lumbar puncture may still be useful when the diagnosis is uncertain, particularly if molecular diagnostic technology is available.

In other types of focal infection, culture and PCR analysis of normally sterile body fluids (e.g., synovial fluid) may aid in the diagnosis. Although some authorities have recommended cultures of scrapings or aspirates from skin lesions, this procedure adds little to the diagnostic yield when compared with a combination of blood culture and PCR analysis. Urinary antigen testing also is insensitive, and serologic testing for meningococcal infection has not been adequately studied. Because *N. meningitidis* is a component of the normal human nasopharyngeal flora, identification of the organism on throat swabs has limited diagnostic value, but strains identified in the nasopharynx in the context of a probable case are likely to be those responsible for disease.

TREATMENT

Meningococcal Infections

Death from meningococcal disease is associated most commonly with hypovolemic shock (meningococcemia) and occasionally with raised intracranial pressure (meningococcal meningitis). Therefore, management should focus on the treatment of these urgent clinical issues in addition to the administration of specific antibiotic therapy. Delayed recognition of meningococcal disease or its associated physiologic derangements, together with inadequate emergency management, is associated with poor outcome. Since the disease is rare, protocols for emergency management have been developed (see *www.meningitis.org*).

Airway patency may be compromised if the level of consciousness is depressed as a result of shock (impaired cerebral perfusion) or raised intracranial pressure; this situation may require intervention. In meningococcemia, pulmonary edema and pulmonary oligemia (presenting as hypoxia) require oxygen therapy or elective endotracheal intubation. In cases with shock, aggressive fluid resuscitation (with replacement of the circulating volume several times in severe cases) and inotropic support may be necessary to maintain cardiac output. If shock persists after volume resuscitation at 40 mL/kg, the risk of pulmonary edema is high, and elective intubation is recommended to improve oxygenation and decrease the work of breathing. Metabolic derangements, including hypoglycemia, acidosis, hypokalemia, hypocalcemia, hypomagnesemia, hypophosphatemia, anemia, and coagulopathy, should be anticipated and corrected. However, aggressive fluid resuscitation with unbuffered electrolyte solutions was found to increase mortality in febrile African children. Studies of the effects of lower volumes of buffered solutions and similar studies in resource-rich settings are required. In the presence of raised intracranial pressure, management includes correction of coexistent shock and neurointensive care to maintain cerebral perfusion.

Empirical antibiotic therapy for suspected meningococcal disease consists of a third-generation cephalosporin such as ceftriaxone (75–100 mg/kg per day [maximum, 4 g/d] in one or two divided IV doses) or cefotaxime (200 mg/kg per day [maximum, 8 g/d] in four divided IV doses) to cover the various other (potentially penicillin-resistant) bacteria that may produce an indistinguishable clinical syndrome. Although unusual in most isolates, reduced meningococcal sensitivity to penicillin (a minimal inhibitory concentration of 0.12–1.0 μg/mL) has been reported.

Both meningococcal meningitis and meningococcal septicemia are conventionally treated for 7 days, although courses of 3–5 days may be equally effective. Furthermore, a single dose of ceftriaxone or an oily suspension of chloramphenicol has been used successfully in resource-poor settings. No data are available to guide the duration of treatment for meningococcal infection at other foci (e.g., pneumonia, arthritis); antimicrobial therapy is usually continued until clinical and laboratory evidence of infection has resolved. Cultures usually become sterile within 24 h of initiation of appropriate antibiotic chemotherapy.

The use of glucocorticoids for adjunctive treatment of meningococcal meningitis remains controversial since no relevant studies have had sufficient power to determine true efficacy. One large study in adults did indicate a trend toward benefit, and in clinical practice a decision to use glucocorticoids usually must precede a definite microbiologic diagnosis. Therapeutic doses of glucocorticoids are not recommended in meningococcal septicemia, but many intensivists recommend replacement glucocorticoid doses for patients who have refractory shock in association with impaired adrenal gland responsiveness, management that is supported by limited evidence.

Various other adjunctive therapies for meningococcal disease have been considered, but few have been subjected to clinical trials and none can currently be recommended. An antibody to LPS (HA1A) failed to confer a demonstrable benefit. Recombinant bactericidal/permeability-increasing protein (which is not currently available) was tested in a study that had inadequate power to show an effect on mortality rates; however, there were trends toward lower mortality rates among patients who received a complete infusion, and this group also had fewer amputations, fewer blood-product transfusions, and a significantly improved functional outcome. Given that protein C concentrations are reduced in meningococcal disease, the use of activated protein C has been considered. A survival benefit was demonstrated in adult sepsis trials; however, trials in pediatric sepsis (of particular relevance for meningococcal disease) found no benefit and indicated a potential risk of bleeding complications with use of activated protein C.

The postmeningococcal immune-complex inflammatory syndrome has been treated with nonsteroidal anti-inflammatory agents until spontaneous resolution occurs.

COMPLICATIONS

About 10% of patients with meningococcal disease die despite the availability of antimicrobial therapy and other intensive medical interventions. The most common complication of meningococcal disease (10% of cases) is scarring after necrosis of purpuric skin lesions, for which skin grafting may be necessary. The lower limbs are most often affected; next in frequency are the upper limbs, the trunk, and the face. On average, 13% of the skin surface area is involved. Amputations are necessary in 1–2% of survivors of meningococcal disease because of a loss of tissue viability after peripheral ischemia or compartment syndromes. Unless there is local infection, amputation should usually be delayed to allow the demarcation between viable and nonviable tissue to become apparent. Approximately 5% of patients with meningococcal disease suffer hearing loss, and 7% have neurologic complications. In one study, pain was reported by 21% of survivors, and in a recent analysis of capsular group B meningococcal disease (the MOSAIC study) as many as one-quarter of survivors had psychological disorders. In some investigations, the rate of complications is higher for capsular group C disease (mostly associated with the ST11 clone) than for capsular group B disease. In patients with severe hypovolemic shock, renal perfusion may be impaired and prerenal failure is common, but permanent renal replacement therapy is rarely needed.

Several studies suggest adverse psychosocial outcomes after meningococcal disease, with reduced quality of life, lowered self-esteem, and poorer neurologic development, including increased rates of attention deficit/hyperactivity disorder and special educational needs. Other studies have not found evidence of such outcomes.

PROGNOSIS

Several prognostic scoring systems have been developed to identify patients with meningococcal disease who are least likely to survive. Factors associated with a poorer prognosis are shock; young age (infancy), old age, and adolescence; coma; purpura fulminans; disseminated intravascular coagulation; thrombocytopenia; leukopenia; absence of meningitis; metabolic acidosis; low plasma concentrations of antithrombin and proteins S and C; high blood levels of PAI-1; and a low erythrocyte sedimentation rate or C-reactive protein level. The Glasgow Meningococcal Septicaemia Prognostic Score (GMSPS) performs well and may be clinically useful for severity assessment in meningococcal disease. However, scoring systems do not direct the clinician to specific interventions, and the priority in management should be recognition of compromised airways, breathing, or circulation and direct, urgent intervention. Most patients improve rapidly with appropriate antibiotics and supportive therapy. Fulminant meningococcemia is more likely to result in death or ischemic skin loss than is meningitis; optimal emergency management may reduce mortality rates among the most severely affected patients.

PREVENTION

Since mortality rates in meningococcal disease remain high despite improvements in intensive care management, immunization is the only rational approach to prevention at a population level. Secondary cases are common among household and "kissing" contacts of cases, and secondary prophylaxis with antibiotics is widely recommended for these contacts (see below).

Polysaccharide Vaccines Purified meningococcal capsular polysaccharide has been used for immunization since the 1960s. Meningococcal polysaccharide vaccines are currently formulated as either bivalent (capsular groups A and C) or quadrivalent (capsular groups A, C, Y, and W), with 50 μg of each polysaccharide per dose. Local reactions (erythema, induration, and tenderness) may occur in up to 40% of vaccinees, but serious adverse events (including febrile convulsions in young children) are very rarely reported. In adults, the vaccines are immunogenic, but immunity appears to be relatively short-lived (with antibody levels above baseline for only 2–10 years), and booster doses do not induce a further rise in antibody concentration. Indeed, a state of immunologic hyporesponsiveness has been widely reported to follow booster doses of plain polysaccharide vaccines. The repeating units of these vaccines cross-link B-cell receptors to drive specific memory B cells to become plasma cells and produce antibody. Because meningococcal polysaccharides are T cell–independent antigens, no memory B cells are produced after immunization, and the memory B-cell pool

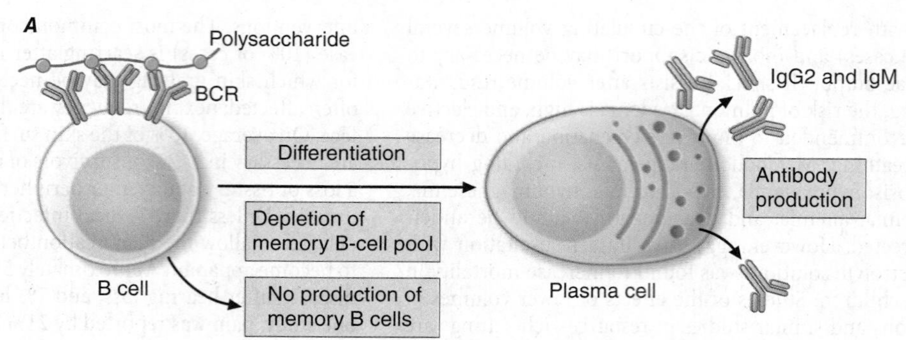

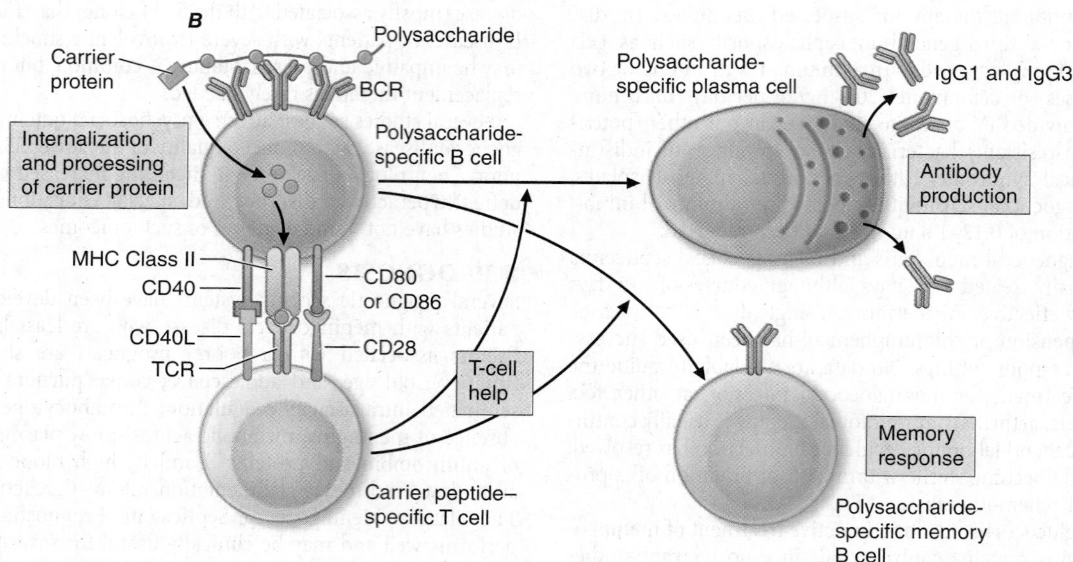

FIGURE 155-6 ***A.*** Polysaccharides from the encapsulated bacteria that cause disease in early childhood stimulate B cells by cross-linking the B-cell receptor (BCR) and driving the production of immunoglobulins. There is no production of memory B cells, and the B-cell pool may be depleted by this process such that subsequent immune responses are decreased. ***B.*** The carrier protein from protein–polysaccharide conjugate vaccines is processed by the polysaccharide-specific B cell, and peptides are presented to carrier peptide–specific T cells, with the consequent production of both plasma cells and memory B cells. MHC, major histocompatibility complex; TCR, T-cell receptor. *(Reproduced with permission from AJ Pollard: Maintaining protection against invasive bacteria with protein–polysaccharide conjugate vaccines. Nat Rev Immunol 9:213, 2009.)*

is depleted such that fewer polysaccharide-specific cells are available to respond to a subsequent dose of vaccine **(Fig. 155-6)**. The clinical relevance of hyporesponsiveness is unknown. Plain polysaccharide vaccines generally are not immunogenic in early childhood, possibly because marginal-zone B cells are involved in polysaccharide responses and maturation of the splenic marginal zone is not complete until 18 months to 2 years of age. The efficacy of the meningococcal capsular group C component is >90% in young adults; no efficacy data are available for the capsular group Y and W polysaccharides in this age group.

Group A meningococcal polysaccharides are exceptional in that they are effective in preventing disease at all ages. Two doses administered 2–3 months apart to children 3–18 months of age or a single dose administered to older children or adults has a protective efficacy rate of >95%. The vaccine was previously used widely in the control of outbreaks of meningococcal disease in the African meningitis belt. The duration of protection appears to be only 3–5 years. The plain polysaccharide vaccines have been largely superseded by protein–polysaccharide conjugate vaccines.

There is no meningococcal capsular group B plain polysaccharide vaccine because α-2,8-*N*-acetylneuraminic acid is expressed on the surface of neural cells in the fetus such that the B polysaccharide is perceived as "self" and therefore is not immunogenic in humans.

Conjugate Vaccines The poor immunogenicity of plain polysaccharide vaccines in infancy has been overcome by chemical conjugation of the polysaccharides to a carrier protein (CRM_{197}, tetanus toxoid, or diphtheria toxoid). Conjugates that contain monovalent capsular group C polysaccharide and quadrivalent vaccines with A, C, Y, and W polysaccharides have been developed, as have vaccines including various other antigen combinations (e.g., tetanus conjugates with capsular group C and/or Y polysaccharide and *Haemophilus influenzae* type b polysaccharide). After immunization, peptides from the carrier protein are conventionally thought to be presented by polysaccharide-specific B cells to peptide-specific T cells in association with major histocompatibility complex (MHC) class II molecules. (Some data suggest that carrier protein peptide may actually be presented in association with an oligosaccharide and MHCII.) The result is a T cell–dependent immune response that allows production of antibody and generation of an expanded B-cell memory pool. Unlike responses to booster doses of plain polysaccharides, responses to booster doses of conjugate vaccines have the characteristics of memory responses. Indeed, conjugate vaccines overcome the hyporesponsiveness induced by plain polysaccharides by replenishing the memory pool. The reactogenicity of conjugate vaccines is similar to that of plain polysaccharide vaccines.

The first widespread use of capsular group C meningococcal conjugate vaccine (MenC) came in 1999 in the United Kingdom after a rise in capsular group C disease. A mass vaccination campaign involving all individuals <19 years of age was undertaken, and the number of laboratory-confirmed capsular group C cases fell from 955 in 1998–1999 to just 29 in 2011–2012. The effectiveness of the immunization program was attributed both to direct protection of immunized persons and to reduced transmission of the organism in the population as a result of decreased rates of colonization among the immunized (i.e., herd immunity). Data on immunogenicity and effectiveness have shown that the duration of protection is short when the vaccine is administered in early childhood; thus booster doses are needed to maintain population immunity. In contrast, immunity after a dose of vaccine given in adolescence appears to be more prolonged.

In 2005, the first quadrivalent conjugate meningococcal vaccine containing A, C, Y, and W polysaccharides conjugated to diphtheria toxoid was initially recommended for all children >11 years of age in the United States and for persons 2–55 years of age in Canada. Such vaccines are now recommended by the Advisory Committee on Immunization Practices (ACIP) for routine administration to individuals 11–18 years of age, with a booster dose 3 years later; only a single dose is given to persons >16 years of age. These vaccines are also recommended for high-risk persons from 2 months to 55 years of age (see *www.cdc.gov/mmwr/preview/mmwrhtml/mm6324a2.htm*).

Uptake was slow initially, but current U.S. data suggest an efficacy rate of 82% in the first year after vaccination, with waning to 59% at 3–6 years after vaccination. Limited early data from the U.S. Vaccine Adverse Events Reporting System indicated that there might be a short-term increase in the risk of Guillain-Barré syndrome after immunization with the diphtheria conjugate vaccine; however, further investigation has not confirmed this finding. Quadrivalent conjugate vaccines with tetanus or CRM_{197} as carrier protein are now available in many countries and are used for high-risk groups and in routine programs for toddlers and adolescents.

A monovalent capsular group A vaccine, manufactured in India, was licensed in 2010 and rolled out to countries in the sub-Saharan African meningitis belt in a mass immunization campaign. There is strong evidence that this vaccine has been highly effective in controlling epidemic meningococcal disease in the region, with >90% reduction in disease in vaccinated populations. However, disease caused by capsular groups C, X, and W persists, and new-generation vaccines with wider coverage are being developed.

Vaccines Based on Subcapsular Antigens The lack of immunogenicity of the group B capsule has led to the development of vaccines based on subcapsular antigens. Various surface components have been studied in early-phase clinical trials. Outer-membrane vesicles (OMVs) containing outer-membrane proteins, phospholipid, and LPS can be extracted from cultures of *N. meningitidis* by detergent treatment **(Fig. 155-7)**. OMVs prepared in this way were used in efficacy trials with a Norwegian outbreak strain and reduced the incidence of group B disease among 14- to 16-year-old schoolchildren by 53%. Similarly, OMV vaccines constructed from local outbreak strains in Cuba and New Zealand have had reported efficacy rates of >70%. These OMV vaccines appear to produce strain-specific immune responses, with only limited cross-protection, and are therefore best suited to clonal outbreaks (e.g., those in Cuba and New Zealand as well as others in Norway and the province of Normandy in France).

Several purified surface proteins have been evaluated in phase 1 clinical trials but have not yet been developed further because of antigenic variability or poor immunogenicity (e.g., transferrin-binding proteins, neisserial surface protein A). Other vaccine candidates have been identified since sequencing of the meningococcal genome. The combination vaccine 4CMenB, which includes the New Zealand OMV vaccine and three recombinant proteins (neisserial adhesin A, factor H–binding protein, and neisserial heparin-binding antigen), is immunogenic from infancy and has been licensed for use in the United States, Canada, Europe, and Australia. This vaccine has been used with apparent success in the control of several university outbreaks in the United States and in a community outbreak in an area of Quebec, Canada. 4CMenB vaccine has an acceptable safety profile, with fever prominent among infants and injection-site pain frequently reported among older children and adults. The vaccine is also being used in many countries for immunization of high-risk groups. In September 2015, 4CMenB was recommended for routine use in the United Kingdom for all infants born from May 2015 onward; a recent analysis reported a 75% reduction in age groups that were fully eligible for vaccination,

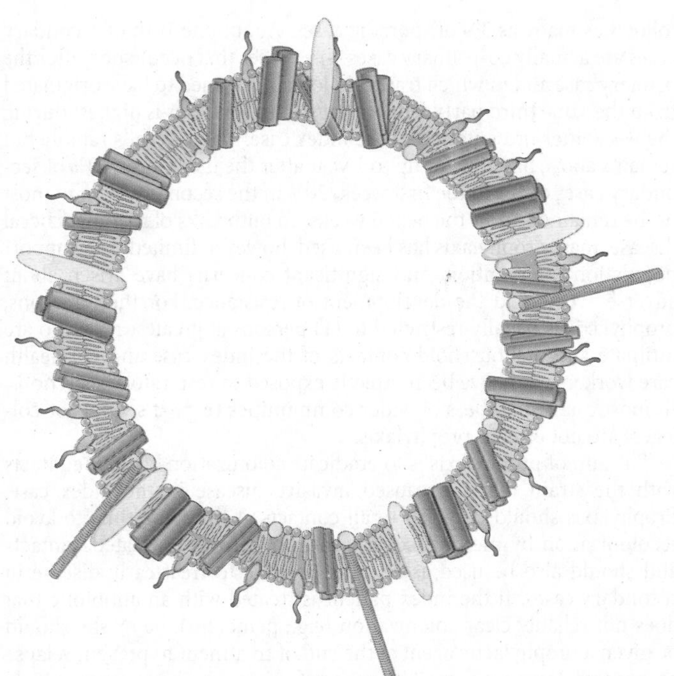

FIGURE 155-7 Illustration of meningococcal outer-membrane vesicle containing outer-membrane structures.

with a high coverage rate of 95%. The licensed schedule is 3 priming doses before 6 months of age and a booster dose at 12 months of age. A non-significant vaccine effectiveness of 53% was seen after two doses, and 59% effectiveness was found after the booster dose at 1 year of age.

Because the disease is so rare, the cost-effectiveness of capsular group B vaccine in infant immunization programs, as assessed with conventional thresholds, is borderline in the United Kingdom. Since infants are not commonly colonized with capsular group B meningococci, any impact on the total population burden of carried organisms will be small. It is therefore unlikely that an infant immunization program will provide additional value through induction of herd immunity. Rates of capsular group B carriage are higher among teenagers and young adults than at other ages (apart from infancy). A recent large cluster randomized trial in Australia found no effect of 4CMenB on carriage of disease-causing meningococci, highlighting that the benefit of this vaccine is likely to be via direct protection.

An immunogenic vaccine based on two variants of the lipoprotein factor H–binding protein (fHbp2) has been developed for use in adolescents and is licensed in the United States and Europe. The vaccine is immunogenic against representative indicator strains, inducing fourfold rises in bactericidal antibody titer in 50–92% of individuals. fHbp2 has an acceptable safety profile, with pain at the injection site, fatigue, and headache commonly reported. This vaccine can be used with a range of vaccines routinely administered in adolescence, including Tdap (tetanus–diphtheria–acellular pertussis), human papillomavirus, and MenACWY vaccines. fHbp2 has been used to control outbreaks of meningococcal disease in educational institutions in the United States, but no formal studies of its effectiveness have yet been undertaken. Studies in the UK are currently evaluating the impact of both 4CMenB and fHbp2 against meningococcal carriage amongst teenagers.

Both of the new capsular group B meningococcal vaccines are licensed for use in the United States for persons 10–25 years of age. In addition, ACIP recommends their administration to individuals at high risk of capsular group B disease, with 4CMenB administered as two doses (1–2 months apart) and fHbp2 as two doses (at 0 and 6 months) or three doses (at 0, 1–2, and 6 months).

MANAGEMENT OF CONTACTS

Close (household and kissing) contacts of individuals with meningococcal disease are at increased risk for developing secondary disease (up to 1000 times the rate for the general population); a secondary case follows as many as 3% of sporadic cases. About one-fifth of secondary cases are actually co-primary cases—i.e., cases that occur soon after the primary case and in which transmission is presumed to have originated from the same third party. The rate of secondary cases is highest during the week after presentation of the index case. The risk falls rapidly but remains above baseline for up to 1 year after the index case; 30% of secondary cases occur in the first week, 20% in the second week, and most of the remainder over the next 6 weeks. In outbreaks of meningococcal disease, mass prophylaxis has been used; however, limited data support population intervention, and significant concerns have arisen about adverse events and the development of resistance. For these reasons, prophylaxis is usually restricted to (1) persons at greatest risk who are intimate and/or household contacts of the index case and (2) health care workers who have been directly exposed to respiratory secretions. In most cases, members of wider communities (e.g., at schools or colleges) are not offered prophylaxis.

The aim of prophylaxis is to eradicate colonization of close contacts with the strain that has caused invasive disease in the index case. Prophylaxis should be given to all contacts at the same time to avoid recolonization by meningococci transmitted from untreated contacts and should also be used as soon as possible to treat early disease in secondary cases. If the index patient is treated with an antibiotic that does not reliably clear colonization (e.g., penicillin), he or she should be given a prophylactic agent at the end of treatment to prevent relapse or onward transmission. Although rifampin has been most widely used and studied, it is not the optimal agent because it fails to eradicate carriage in 15–20% of cases, rates of adverse events have been high, compliance is affected by the need for four doses, and emerging resistance has been reported. Ceftriaxone as a single IM or IV injection is highly (97%) effective in carriage eradication and can be used at all ages and in pregnancy. Reduced susceptibility of isolates to ceftriaxone has occasionally been reported. Ciprofloxacin or ofloxacin is preferred in some countries; these agents are highly effective and can be administered by mouth but are not recommended in pregnancy. Resistance to fluoroquinolones has been reported in some meningococci in North America, Europe, and Asia.

In documented capsular group A, B, C, Y, or W disease, contacts may be offered immunization (with either the MenACWY conjugate vaccine or the MenB vaccine, as appropriate) in addition to chemoprophylaxis to provide protection beyond the duration of antibiotic therapy. Mass vaccination has been used successfully to control disease during outbreaks in closed communities (educational and military establishments) as well as during epidemics in open communities.

FURTHER READING

Christensen H et al: Meningococcal carriage by age: A systematic review and meta-analysis. Lancet Infect Dis 10:853, 2010.

Cohn AC et al: Prevention and control of meningococcal disease: Recommendations of the Advisory Committee on Immunization Practices (ACIP). MMWR Recomm Rep 62(RR-2):1, 2013.

Gossger N et al: Immunogenicity and tolerability of recombinant serogroup B meningococcal vaccine administered with or without routine infant vaccinations according to different immunization schedules: A randomized controlled trial. JAMA 307:573, 2012.

Jafri RZ et al: Global epidemiology of invasive meningococcal disease. Popul Health Metr 11:17, 2013.

Ladhani SN et al: Vaccination of infants with meningococcal group B vaccine (4CMenB) in England. N Engl J Med 382:309, 2020.

Marshall HS et al: Meningococcal B vaccine and meningococcal carriage in adolescents in Australia. N Engl J Med 382:318, 2020.

Pollard AJ et al: Maintaining protection against invasive bacteria with protein–polysaccharide conjugate vaccines. Nat Rev Immunol 9:213, 2009.

Read RC et al: Effect of a quadrivalent meningococcal ACWY glycoconjugate or a serogroup B meningococcal vaccine on meningococcal carriage: An observer-blind, phase 3 randomised clinical trial. Lancet 384:2123, 2014.

Vieusseux M: Memoire sur le maladie qui a regne a Geneva au printemps de 1805. J Med Clin Pharm 11:163, 1805.

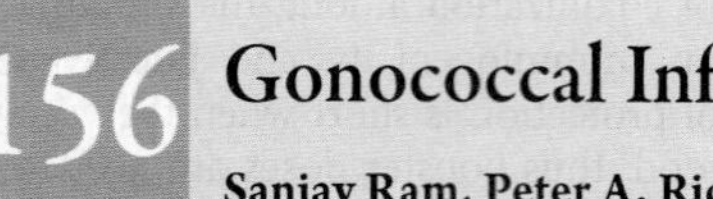

156 Gonococcal Infections

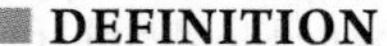

Sanjay Ram, Peter A. Rice

DEFINITION

Gonorrhea is a sexually transmitted infection (STI) of epithelium and commonly manifests as cervicitis, urethritis, proctitis, and conjunctivitis. If untreated, infections at these sites can lead to local complications such as endometritis, salpingitis, tuboovarian abscess, bartholinitis, peritonitis, and perihepatitis in female patients; periurethritis and epididymitis in male patients; and ophthalmia neonatorum in newborns. Disseminated gonococcemia is an uncommon event whose manifestations include skin lesions, tenosynovitis, arthritis, and (in rare cases) endocarditis or meningitis.

MICROBIOLOGY

Neisseria gonorrhoeae is a gram-negative, nonmotile, non-spore-forming organism that grows singly and in pairs (i.e., as monococci and diplococci, respectively). Exclusively a human pathogen, the gonococcus contains, on average, three genome copies per coccal unit; this polyploidy permits a high level of antigenic variation and the survival of the organism in its host. Gonococci, like all other *Neisseria* species, are oxidase positive. They are distinguished from other neisseriae by their ability to grow on selective media and to use glucose but not maltose, sucrose, or lactose.

EPIDEMIOLOGY

The incidence of gonorrhea had been declining steadily in the United States, but in 2018, there were ~616,000 newly reported cases—up 56% since 2015. With 87 million cases estimated by the World Health Organization to have occurred globally in 2016, gonorrhea remains a major public health problem worldwide, is a significant cause of morbidity in developing countries, and may play a role in enhancing transmission of HIV.

Gonorrhea predominantly affects young, nonwhite, unmarried, less educated members of urban populations. The number of reported cases probably represents half of the true number of cases—a discrepancy resulting from underreporting, self-treatment, nonspecific treatment without a laboratory-proven diagnosis, and asymptomatic infection. The number of reported new cases of gonorrhea in the United States rose from ~250,000 in the early 1960s to a high of 1.01 million in 1978. The recorded incidence of gonorrhea in modern times peaked in 1975, with 468 reported new cases per 100,000 population in the United States. This peak was attributable to the interaction of several variables, including improved accuracy of diagnosis, changes in patterns of contraceptive use, and changes in sexual behavior. A decline in the overall incidence of gonorrhea in the United States over the past quarter-century may have reflected increased condom use resulting from public health efforts to curtail HIV transmission. Nevertheless, in 2019, 187.8 new cases per 100,000 population were reported in this country, representing a 1-year increase of 5% and a 92% increase since the historic low in 2009; this figure is the highest among industrialized countries. Simultaneously, antibiotic resistance is increasing in the United States and other countries, prompting the U.S. Centers for Disease Control and Prevention (CDC) to name antibiotic-resistant *N. gonorrhoeae* as one of the three most urgent threats of its kind. At present, the attack rate in the United States is highest among 15- to 24-year-old women and 20- to 29-year-old men; >70% of all reported cases occur in these two groups. From the standpoint of ethnicity, rates are highest among African Americans and lowest among persons of Asian descent.

The incidence of gonorrhea is higher in developing countries than in industrialized nations. The exact incidence of any STI is difficult to ascertain in developing countries because of limited surveillance and variable diagnostic criteria. Extremely high rates of gonorrhea have been reported among aboriginal populations in Namibia and Australia. Studies in Africa have clearly demonstrated that nonulcerative STIs such as gonorrhea (in addition to ulcerative STIs) are an independent risk factor for the transmission of HIV (**Chap. 202**).

Gonorrhea is transmitted from males to females more efficiently than in the opposite direction. The rate of transmission to a woman during a single unprotected sexual encounter with an infected man is ~50–70%. Oropharyngeal gonorrhea occurs in ~20% of women who practice fellatio with infected partners. Transmission in either direction by cunnilingus is rare.

In any population, there exists a small minority of individuals who have high rates of new-partner acquisition. These "core-group members" or "high-frequency transmitters" are vital in sustaining STI transmission at the population level. Another instrumental factor in sustaining gonorrhea in the population is the large number of infected individuals who are asymptomatic or have minor symptoms that are ignored. These persons, unlike symptomatic individuals, may not cease sexual activity and therefore may continue to transmit the infection. This situation underscores the importance of contact tracing and empirical treatment of the sex partners of index cases.

PATHOGENESIS, IMMUNOLOGY, AND ANTIMICROBIAL RESISTANCE

Outer-Membrane Proteins • PILI Fresh clinical isolates of *N. gonorrhoeae* initially form piliated (fimbriated) colonies distinguishable on translucent agar. Pilus expression is rapidly switched off with unselected subculture because of rearrangements in pilus genes. This change is a basis for antigenic variation of gonococci. Piliated strains adhere better to cells derived from human mucosal surfaces and are more virulent in organ culture models and human inoculation experiments than nonpiliated variants. In a fallopian tube explant model, pili mediate gonococcal attachment to nonciliated columnar epithelial cells. This event initiates gonococcal adherence, invasion and transport through these cells to intercellular spaces near the basement membrane or directly into the subepithelial tissue. Pili are also essential for genetic competence and transformation of *N. gonorrhoeae*, which permit horizontal transfer of genetic material between different gonococcal lineages in vivo.

OPACITY-ASSOCIATED PROTEIN Another gonococcal surface protein that is important in adherence to epithelial cells is opacity-associated protein (Opa; formerly called protein II). Opa contributes to intergonococcal adhesion, which is responsible for the opaque nature of gonococcal colonies on translucent agar and the organism's adherence to a variety of eukaryotic cells, including polymorphonuclear leukocytes (PMNs). Certain Opa variants promote invasion of epithelial cells, and this effect has been linked with the ability of Opa to bind vitronectin, heparan sulfate proteoglycans, and several members of the carcinoembryonic antigen–related cell adhesion molecule (CEACAM) receptor family. Epithelial CEACAM-binding gonococci prevent exfoliation of epithelium through a mechanism that involves nitric oxide that is produced during anaerobic bacterial metabolism and upregulation of CD105 (a member of the transforming growth factor-beta receptor family), which may interfere with bacterial clearance. *N. gonorrhoeae* Opa proteins that bind CEACAM1, which is expressed by primary CD4+ T lymphocytes, suppress the activation and proliferation of these lymphocytes. Select Opa proteins can engage CEACAM3, which is expressed on neutrophils, with consequent nonopsonic phagocytosis (i.e., phagocytosis independent of antibody and complement) and killing of bacteria.

PORIN Porin (previously designated protein I) is the most abundant gonococcal surface protein. Porin molecules exist as trimers that provide anion-transporting aqueous channels through the otherwise hydrophobic outer membrane. Porin exhibits stable interstrain antigenic variation and forms the basis for gonococcal serotyping. Two main serotypes have been identified; PorB.1A strains are often associated with disseminated gonococcal infection (DGI), whereas PorB.1B strains usually cause local genital infections only. DGI strains are generally resistant to the killing action of normal human serum and do not incite a significant local inflammatory response; therefore, they may not cause symptoms at genital sites. These characteristics may be related to the ability of PorB.1A strains to bind to complement-inhibitory molecules, resulting in a diminished inflammatory response. Porin can translocate to the cytoplasmic membrane of host cells—a process that could initiate gonococcal endocytosis and invasion. PorB.1B present in outer membrane vesicles shed during bacterial growth inhibits the ability of dendritic cells to induce T-cell proliferation and may contribute to the ability of gonococci to subvert adaptive immunity.

OTHER OUTER-MEMBRANE PROTEINS Other notable outer-membrane proteins include H.8, a lipoprotein that is present in high concentration on the surface of all gonococcal strains and is an excellent target for antibody-based diagnostic testing. Transferrin-binding proteins (Tbp1 and Tbp2), lactoferrin-binding proteins (LbpA and LbpB), and hemoglobin/haptoglobin binding proteins (HpuA and HpuB) are required for scavenging iron from transferrin, lactoferrin, and heme in vivo. Transferrin and iron have been shown to enhance the attachment of iron-deprived *N. gonorrhoeae* to human endometrial cells. TdfH and TdfJ enable gonococci to scavenge host zinc from calprotectin and S100 calcium binding protein A7 (psoriasin). IgA1 protease is produced by *N. gonorrhoeae* and may protect the organism from the action of mucosal IgA.

Lipooligosaccharide Gonococcal lipooligosaccharide (LOS) consists of a lipid A and a core oligosaccharide that lacks the repeating O-carbohydrate antigenic side chain seen in many other gram-negative bacteria. Gonococcal LOS possesses marked endotoxic activity and contributes to the local cytotoxic effect in a fallopian tube model. LOS core sugars undergo a high degree of phase variation under different conditions of growth; this variation reflects genetic regulation and expression of glycotransferase genes that dictate the carbohydrate structure of LOS. These phenotypic changes may affect interactions of *N. gonorrhoeae* with elements of the humoral immune system (antibodies and complement) and may also influence direct binding of organisms to both professional phagocytes and nonprofessional phagocytes (epithelial cells). For example, gonococci that are sialylated at their LOS sites inhibit the classic pathway of complement by reducing binding of IgG and also bind complement factor H to inhibit the alternative pathway of complement. LOS sialylation may also decrease nonopsonic Opa-mediated association with neutrophils and inhibit the oxidative burst in PMNs. The binding of the unsialylated terminal lactosamine residue of LOS to an asialoglycoprotein receptor on male epithelial cells facilitates adherence and subsequent gonococcal invasion of these cells. Moreover, oligosaccharide structures in LOS can modulate host immune responses. For example, the terminal monosaccharide expressed by LOS determines the C-type lectin receptor on dendritic cells that is targeted by the bacteria. In turn, the specific C-type lectin receptor engaged influences whether a T_H1- or T_H2-type response is elicited; the latter response may be less favorable for clearance of gonococcal infection.

Host Factors In addition to gonococcal structures that interact with epithelial cells, host factors seem to be important in mediating entry of gonococci into nonphagocytic cells. Activation of phosphatidylcholine-specific phospholipase C and acidic sphingomyelinase by *N. gonorrhoeae*, which results in the release of diacylglycerol and ceramide, is a requirement for the entry of *N. gonorrhoeae* into epithelial cells. Ceramide accumulation within cells leads to apoptosis, which may disrupt epithelial integrity and facilitate entry of gonococci into subepithelial tissue. Release of chemotactic factors as a result of complement activation contributes to inflammation, as does the toxic effect of LOS in provoking the release of inflammatory cytokines.

The importance of humoral immunity in host defenses against neisserial infections is best illustrated by the predisposition of persons deficient in terminal complement components (C5 through C9) to have recurrent bacteremic gonococcal infections and recurrent meningococcal meningitis or meningococcemia. Gonococcal porin induces T cell–proliferative responses in persons with urogenital gonococcal disease. A significant increase in porin-specific interleukin (IL) 4–producing CD4+ as well as CD8+ T lymphocytes is seen in individuals with mucosal gonococcal disease. A portion of these lymphocytes that show a porin-specific T_H2-type response could traffic to mucosal surfaces and play a role in immune protection against the disease. Few data clearly indicate that protective immunity is acquired from a previous gonococcal infection, although bactericidal and opsonophagocytic antibodies to porin and LOS may offer partial protection. On the other hand, women who are infected and acquire high levels of antibody to another outer-membrane protein, Rmp (reduction modifiable protein, formerly called protein III), may be especially likely to become reinfected with *N. gonorrhoeae* because Rmp antibodies block the effect of bactericidal antibodies to porin and LOS. Rmp shows little, if any, interstrain antigenic variation; therefore, Rmp antibodies potentially may block antibody-mediated killing of all gonococci. The mechanism of blocking has not been fully characterized, but Rmp antibodies may noncompetitively inhibit binding of porin and LOS antibodies because of the proximity of these structures in the gonococcal outer membrane. In male volunteers who have no history of gonorrhea, the net effect of these events may influence the outcome of experimental challenge with *N. gonorrhoeae*. Because Rmp bears extensive homology to enterobacterial OmpA and meningococcal class 4 proteins, it is possible that these blocking antibodies result from prior exposure to cross-reacting proteins from these species and also play a role in first-time infection with *N. gonorrhoeae*.

Gonococcal Resistance to Antimicrobial Agents It is no surprise that *N. gonorrhoeae*, with its remarkable capacity to alter its antigenic structure and adapt to changes in the microenvironment, has become resistant to numerous antibiotics. The first effective agents against gonorrhea were the sulfonamides, which were introduced in the 1930s and became ineffective within a decade. Penicillin was then used as the drug of choice for the treatment of gonorrhea. By 1965, 42% of gonococcal isolates had developed low-level resistance to penicillin G. Resistance due to the production of penicillinase arose later.

Gonococci become fully resistant to antibiotics either by chromosomal mutations or by acquisition of R factors (plasmids). Two types of chromosomal mutations have been described. The first type, which is drug specific, is a single-step mutation leading to high-level resistance. The second type involves mutations at several chromosomal loci that combine to determine the level as well as the pattern of resistance. Strains with mutations in chromosomal genes were first observed in the late 1950s. As recently as 2007, chromosomal mutations accounted for resistance to penicillin, tetracycline, or both in ~16% of strains surveyed in the United States.

β-Lactamase (penicillinase)–producing strains of *N. gonorrhoeae* (PPNG) carrying β-lactamase plasmids had rapidly spread worldwide by the early 1980s. *N. gonorrhoeae* strains with plasmid-borne tetracycline resistance (TRNG) can mobilize some β-lactamase plasmids, and PPNG and TRNG occur together, sometimes along with strains exhibiting chromosomally mediated resistance (CMRNG). Penicillin, ampicillin, and tetracycline are no longer reliable for the treatment of gonorrhea and should not be used.

Quinolone-containing regimens also were recommended for treatment of gonococcal infections; the fluoroquinolones offered the advantage of antichlamydial activity when administered for 7 days. However, quinolone-resistant *N. gonorrhoeae* (QRNG) appeared soon after these agents were first used to treat gonorrhea. QRNG is particularly common in the Pacific Islands (including Hawaii) and Asia, where, in certain areas, all gonococcal strains are now resistant to quinolones. At present, QRNG is also common in parts of Europe and the Middle East. In the United States, QRNG has been identified in all areas but predominantly in states on the Pacific coast, where resistant strains were first seen. Alterations in DNA gyrase and topoisomerase IV have been implicated as mechanisms of fluoroquinolone resistance.

Resistance to spectinomycin, which has been used in the past as an alternative agent, has been reported. Because this agent usually is not associated with resistance to other antibiotics, spectinomycin can be reserved for use against multidrug-resistant strains of *N. gonorrhoeae*. Nevertheless, outbreaks caused by strains resistant to spectinomycin have been documented in Korea and England when the drug has been used for primary treatment of gonorrhea.

Third-generation cephalosporins have remained highly effective as single-dose therapy for gonorrhea, but the recent isolation of strains highly resistant to ceftriaxone (minimal inhibitory concentrations [MICs], 2 μg/mL) in Japan and some European countries is cause for concern. Even though the MICs of ceftriaxone against certain strains may reach 0.015–0.125 μg/mL (higher than the MICs of 0.0001–0.008 μg/mL for fully susceptible strains), these levels are greatly exceeded in the blood, the urethra, and the cervix when the routinely recommended parenteral dose of ceftriaxone is administered. The rising MICs of oral cefixime (the previously recommended alternative oral third-generation cephalosporin) against *N. gonorrhoeae*, combined with this drug's limited capacity to reach levels sufficiently higher than MICs in the blood, the urethra, the cervix, and especially the pharynx, have resulted in the removal of cefixime from the list of first-line agents for treatment of uncomplicated gonorrhea. *N. gonorrhoeae* strains with reduced susceptibility to ceftriaxone and cefixime (i.e., cephalosporin-intermediate/resistant strains) contain mutations in (1) the *penA* allele, which is the principal resistance determinant and encodes a penicillin-binding protein (PBP2) whose sequence can differ in up to 60–70 amino acids from that of wild-type PBP2; (2) the *m*ultiple *t*ransferable *r*esistance *r*egulator (*mtrR*) gene that results in increased drug efflux through the MtrCDE efflux pump; and (3) *penB*, which decreases drug influx through PorB.

Resistance to azithromycin can result from alterations of the ribosomal binding target by azithromycin and—as with cephalosporins—the over- and underexpression of efflux and influx systems. Combined resistance to cephalosporins and azithromycin has been reported in several instances throughout the world.

CLINICAL MANIFESTATIONS

Gonococcal Infections in Men Acute urethritis is the most common clinical manifestation of gonorrhea in male patients. The usual incubation period after exposure is 2–7 days, although the interval can be longer and most men remain asymptomatic. Strains of the PorB.1A serotype tend to cause a greater proportion of cases of mild and asymptomatic urethritis than do PorB.1B strains. When they occur, urethral discharge and dysuria, usually without urinary frequency or urgency, are the major symptoms. The discharge initially is scant and mucoid but becomes profuse and purulent within a day or two. Gram's staining of the urethral discharge may reveal PMNs and gram-negative intracellular monococci and diplococci (**Fig. 156-1**). The clinical manifestations of gonococcal urethritis are usually more severe and overt than those of nongonococcal urethritis, including urethritis caused by *Chlamydia trachomatis* (**Chap. 189**); however, exceptions are common, and it is often impossible to differentiate the causes of urethritis on clinical grounds alone. The majority of cases of urethritis seen in the United States today are not caused by *N. gonorrhoeae* and/or *C. trachomatis*. Although a number of other organisms may be responsible, many cases do not have a specific etiologic agent identified. Certain clones of *Neisseria meningitidis*, the second member of the pathogenic

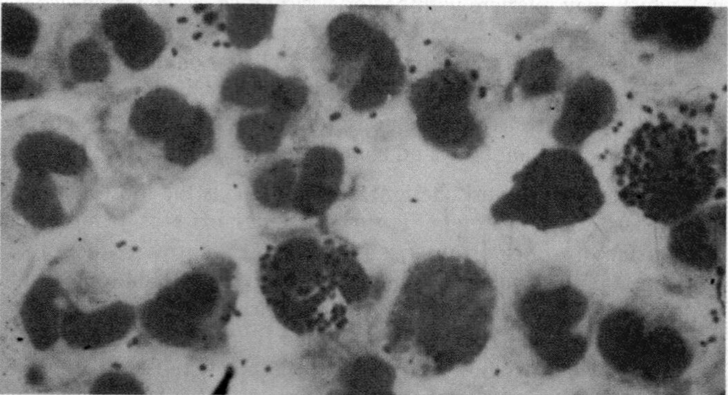

FIGURE 156-1 Gram's stain of urethral discharge from a male patient with gonorrhea shows gram-negative intracellular monococci and diplococci. *(Source: © All rights reserved. Canadian Guidelines on Sexually Transmitted Infections. Public Health Agency of Canada, modified 2020. Adapted and reproduced with permission from the Minister of Health, 2021.)*

Neisseria species, have been associated with urethritis in men who have sex with men (MSM) in Europe and in heterosexual men in the southern and midwestern United States.

Most symptomatic men with gonorrhea seek treatment and cease to be infectious. The remaining men, who are largely asymptomatic, accumulate in number over time and constitute about two-thirds of all infected men at any point in time; together with men incubating the organism who shed the organism but are asymptomatic, they serve as the source of spread of infection. Before the antibiotic era, symptoms of urethritis persisted for ~8 weeks. Epididymitis is now an uncommon complication, and gonococcal prostatitis occurs rarely, if at all. Other unusual local complications of gonococcal urethritis include edema of the penis due to dorsal lymphangitis or thrombophlebitis, submucous inflammatory "soft" infiltration of the urethral wall, periurethral abscess or fistula, inflammation or abscess of Cowper's gland, and seminal vesiculitis. Balanitis may develop in uncircumcised men.

Gonococcal Infections in Women • GONOCOCCAL CERVICITIS Mucopurulent cervicitis is a common STI diagnosis in American women and may be caused by *N. gonorrhoeae*, *C. trachomatis*, and other organisms, including *Mycoplasma genitalium* **(Chap. 188)**. Cervicitis may coexist with candidal or trichomonal vaginitis. *N. gonorrhoeae* primarily infects the columnar epithelium of the cervical os. Bartholin's glands occasionally become infected.

Women infected with *N. gonorrhoeae* usually develop symptoms. However, women who either remain asymptomatic or have only minor symptoms may delay seeking medical attention. These minor symptoms may include scant vaginal discharge issuing from the inflamed cervix (without vaginitis or vaginosis per se) and dysuria (often without urgency or frequency) that may be associated with gonococcal urethritis. Although the incubation period of gonorrhea is less well defined in women than in men, symptoms usually develop within 10 days of infection and are more acute and intense than those of chlamydial cervicitis.

The physical examination reveals a mucopurulent discharge (mucopus) issuing from the cervical os or a reddened (inflamed) cervix even in the absence of reported symptoms. Because Gram's stain is not sensitive for the diagnosis of gonorrhea in women, specimens should be submitted for culture or a nonculture assay (see "Laboratory Diagnosis," below). Edematous and friable cervical ectopy and endocervical bleeding induced by gentle swabbing are more often seen in chlamydial infection. Gonococcal infection may extend deep enough to produce dyspareunia and lower abdominal or back pain. In such cases, it is imperative to consider a diagnosis of pelvic inflammatory disease (PID) and to administer treatment for that disease **(Chaps. 136 and 189)**.

N. gonorrhoeae may also be recovered from the urethra and rectum of women with cervicitis, but these are rarely the only infected sites. Urethritis in women may produce symptoms of internal dysuria, which is often attributed to "cystitis." Pyuria in the absence of bacteriuria visible on Gram's stain of unspun urine, accompanied by urine cultures that fail to yield >10^2 colonies of bacteria usually associated with urinary tract infection, signifies the possibility of urethritis usually due to *C. trachomatis*. Urethral infection with *N. gonorrhoeae* also may occur in this context, but in this instance, urethral cultures are usually positive.

GONOCOCCAL VAGINITIS The vaginal mucosa of healthy women is lined by stratified squamous epithelium and is rarely infected by *N. gonorrhoeae*. However, gonococcal vaginitis can occur in anestrogenic women (e.g., prepubertal girls and postmenopausal women), in whom the vaginal stratified squamous epithelium is often thinned down to the basilar layer, which can be infected by *N. gonorrhoeae*. The intense inflammation of the vagina makes the physical (speculum and bimanual) examination extremely painful. The vaginal mucosa is red and edematous, and an abundant purulent discharge is often present. Infection in the urethra and in Skene's and Bartholin's glands often accompanies gonococcal vaginitis. Inflamed cervical erosion or abscesses in nabothian cysts may also occur. Coexisting cervicitis may result in pus in the cervical os.

Anorectal Gonorrhea Because the female anatomy permits the spread of cervical exudate to the rectum, *N. gonorrhoeae* is sometimes recovered from the rectum of women with uncomplicated gonococcal cervicitis. The rectum is the sole site of infection in only 5% of women with gonorrhea. Such women are usually asymptomatic but occasionally have acute proctitis manifested by anorectal pain or pruritus, tenesmus, purulent rectal discharge, and rectal bleeding. Among MSM, the frequency of gonococcal infection, including rectal infection, fell by ≥90% throughout the United States in the early 1980s, A resurgence of gonorrhea among MSM has been documented in several cities since the 1990s, the estimated rates of reported cases having more than doubled in a recent 3-year period. Gonococcal isolates from the rectum of MSM tend to be more resistant to antimicrobial agents than are gonococcal isolates from other sites. Gonococcal isolates with a mutation in *mtrR* or in the promoter region of the gene that encodes for this transcriptional regulator develop increased resistance to antimicrobial hydrophobic agents such as bile acids and fatty acids in feces and thus are found with increased frequency in MSM. This situation may have been responsible for higher rates of failure of treatment for rectal gonorrhea with older regimens consisting of penicillin or tetracyclines.

Pharyngeal Gonorrhea Pharyngeal gonorrhea is usually mild or asymptomatic, although symptomatic pharyngitis does occasionally occur with cervical lymphadenitis. The mode of acquisition is oral–genital sexual exposure, with fellatio being a more efficient means of transmission than cunnilingus. In certain female adolescent populations in the United States, pharyngeal gonorrhea has become as common as genital gonorrhea. Most cases resolve spontaneously, and transmission from the pharynx to sexual contacts is rare. Pharyngeal infection almost always coexists with genital infection. Swabs from the pharynx should be plated directly onto gonococcal selective media. Pharyngeal colonization with *N. meningitidis* needs to be differentiated from that with other *Neisseria* species. Because commensal oropharyngeal neisseriae are often resistant to antimicrobials, horizontal gene transfer between these organisms and *N. gonorrhoeae* may be important in the development of antimicrobial resistance of *N. gonorrhoeae*.

Ocular Gonorrhea in Adults Ocular gonorrhea in an adult usually results from autoinoculation of *N. gonorrhoeae* from an infected genital site. As in genital infection, the manifestations range from severe to occasionally mild or asymptomatic disease. The variability in clinical manifestations may be attributable to differences in the ability of the infecting strain to elicit an inflammatory response. Infection may result in a markedly swollen eyelid, severe hyperemia and chemosis, and a profuse purulent discharge. The massively inflamed conjunctiva may be draped over the cornea and limbus. Lytic enzymes from the infiltrating PMNs occasionally cause corneal ulceration and rarely cause perforation.

Prompt recognition and treatment of this condition are of paramount importance. Gram's stain and culture of the purulent discharge establish the diagnosis. Genital cultures also should be performed.

Gonorrhea in Pregnant Women, Neonates, and Children Gonorrhea in pregnancy can have serious consequences for both the mother and the infant. Recognition of gonorrhea early in pregnancy also identifies a population at risk for other STIs, particularly chlamydial infection, syphilis, and trichomoniasis. The risks of salpingitis and PID—conditions associated with a high rate of fetal loss—are highest during the first trimester. Pharyngeal infection, most often asymptomatic, may be more common during pregnancy because of altered sexual practices. Prolonged rupture of the membranes, premature delivery, chorioamnionitis, funisitis (infection of the umbilical cord stump), and sepsis in the infant (with *N. gonorrhoeae* detected in the newborn's gastric aspirate during delivery) are common complications of maternal gonococcal infection at term. Other conditions and microorganisms, including *Mycoplasma hominis*, *Mycoplasma genitalium*, *Ureaplasma urealyticum*, *C. trachomatis*, and bacterial vaginosis (often accompanied by infection with *Trichomonas vaginalis*), have been associated with similar complications.

The most common form of gonorrhea in neonates is ophthalmia neonatorum, which results from exposure to infected cervical secretions during parturition. Ocular neonatal instillation of a prophylactic agent (e.g., 1% silver nitrate eye drops or ophthalmic preparations containing erythromycin or tetracycline) prevents ophthalmia neonatorum but is not effective for its treatment, which requires systemic antibiotics. The clinical manifestations are acute and usually begin 2–5 days after birth. An initial nonspecific conjunctivitis with a serosanguineous discharge is followed by tense edema of the eyelids, chemosis, and a profuse, thick, purulent discharge. Corneal ulcerations that result in nebulae or perforation may lead to anterior synechiae, anterior staphyloma, panophthalmitis, and blindness. Infections described at other mucosal sites in infants, including vaginitis, rhinitis, and anorectal infection, are likely to be asymptomatic. Pharyngeal colonization has been demonstrated in 35% of infants with gonococcal ophthalmia, and coughing is the most prominent symptom in these cases. Septic arthritis (see below) is the most common manifestation of systemic infection or DGI in the newborn. The onset usually comes at 3–21 days of age, and polyarticular involvement is common. Sepsis, meningitis, and pneumonia are seen in rare instances.

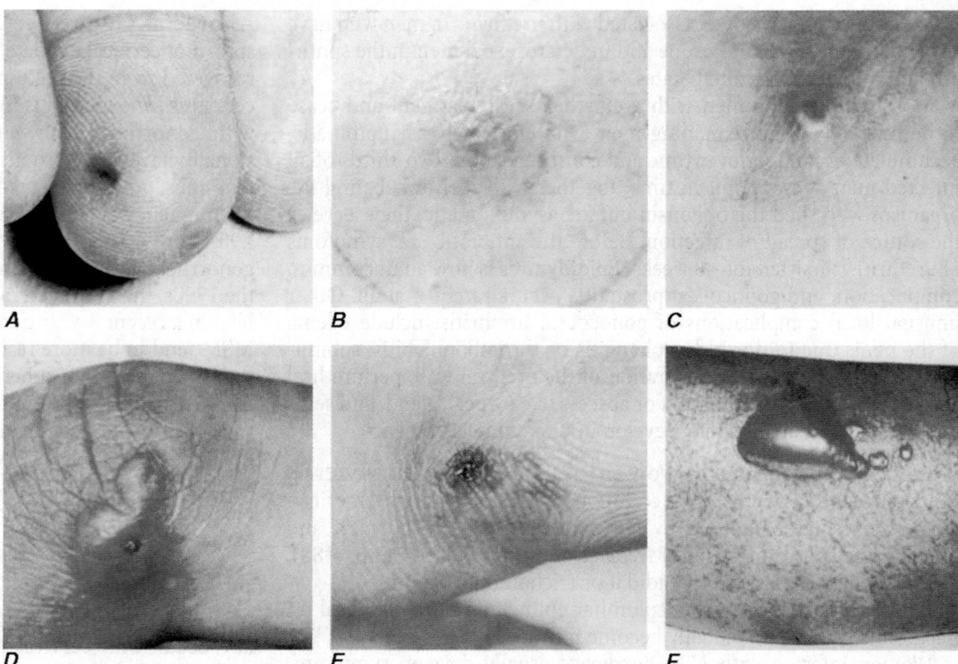

FIGURE 156-2 Characteristic skin lesions in patients with proven gonococcal bacteremia. The lesions are in various stages of evolution. ***A.*** Very early petechia on finger. ***B.*** Early papular lesion, 7 mm in diameter, on lower leg. ***C.*** Pustule with central eschar resulting from early petechial lesion. ***D.*** Pustular lesion on finger. ***E.*** Mature lesion with central necrosis (black) on hemorrhagic base. ***F.*** Bullae on anterior tibial surface. *(Reprinted with permission from TF Murphy, GI Parameswaran: Clin Infect Dis 49:124, 2009, with permission. © 2009 Infectious Diseases Society of America.)*

Any STI in children beyond the neonatal period raises the possibility of sexual abuse. Gonococcal vulvovaginitis is the most common manifestation of gonococcal infection in children beyond infancy. Anorectal and pharyngeal infections are common in these children and are frequently asymptomatic. The urethra, Bartholin's and Skene's glands, and upper genital tract are rarely involved. All children with gonococcal infection should also be evaluated for chlamydial infection, syphilis, and possibly HIV infection.

Gonococcal Arthritis Disseminated gonococcal infection (DGI; gonococcal arthritis) results from gonococcal bacteremia. In the 1970s, DGI occurred in ~0.5–3% of persons with untreated gonococcal mucosal infection. The lower incidence of DGI at present is probably attributable to a decline in the prevalence of particular strains that are likely to disseminate. Nonetheless, sporadic outbreaks of DGI still occur in North America. DGI strains resist the bactericidal action of human serum and generally do not incite inflammation at genital sites, probably because of limited generation of chemotactic factors. Strains recovered from DGI cases in the 1970s were often of the PorB.1A serotype, were highly susceptible to penicillin, and had special growth requirements—including arginine, hypoxanthine, and uracil—that made the organism more fastidious and more difficult to isolate.

Menstruation is a risk factor for dissemination, and approximately two-thirds of cases of DGI are in women. In about half of affected women, symptoms of DGI begin within 7 days of onset of menses. Complement deficiencies, especially of the components involved in the assembly of the membrane attack complex (C5 through C9), predispose to neisserial bacteremia, and persons with more than one episode of DGI should be screened with an assay for total hemolytic complement activity. DGI is also associated with the use of the complement C5-blocking monoclonal antibody eculizumab.

The clinical manifestations of DGI have sometimes been classified into two stages: a bacteremic stage, which is less common today, and a joint-localized stage with suppurative arthritis. A clear-cut progression usually is not evident. Patients in the bacteremic stage have higher temperatures, and chills more frequently accompany their fever. Painful joints are common and often occur together with tenosynovitis and skin lesions. Polyarthralgias usually include the knees, elbows, and more distal joints; the axial skeleton is generally spared. Skin lesions are seen in ~75% of patients and include papules and pustules, often with a hemorrhagic component **(Fig. 156-2; see also Fig. A1-43)**. Other manifestations of noninfectious dermatitis, such as nodular lesions, urticaria, and erythema multiforme, have been described. These lesions are usually on the extremities and number between 5 and 40. The differential diagnosis of the bacteremic stage of DGI includes reactive arthritis, acute rheumatoid arthritis, sarcoidosis, erythema nodosum, drug-induced arthritis, and viral infections (e.g., hepatitis B and acute HIV infection). The distribution of joint symptoms in reactive arthritis differs from that in DGI **(Fig. 156-3)**, as do the skin and genital manifestations **(Chap. 362)**.

Suppurative arthritis involves one or two joints, most often the knees, wrists, ankles, and elbows (in decreasing order of frequency); other joints occasionally are involved. Most patients who develop gonococcal septic arthritis do so without prior polyarthralgias or skin lesions; in the absence of symptomatic genital infection, this disease cannot be distinguished from septic arthritis caused by other pathogens. The differential diagnosis of acute arthritis in young adults is discussed in **Chap. 130**. Rarely, osteomyelitis complicates septic arthritis involving small joints of the hand.

Gonococcal endocarditis, although rare today, was a relatively common complication of DGI in the preantibiotic era, accounting for about one-quarter of reported cases of endocarditis. Another unusual complication of DGI is meningitis.

Gonococcal Infections in HIV-Infected Persons The association between gonorrhea and the acquisition of HIV has been demonstrated in several well-controlled studies, mainly in Kenya and Zaire. The nonulcerative STIs enhance the transmission of HIV three- to fivefold; transmission of HIV-infected immune cells and increased viral shedding by persons with urethritis or cervicitis may contribute **(Chap. 202)**. HIV has been detected by polymerase chain reaction (PCR) more commonly in ejaculates from HIV-positive men with gonococcal urethritis than in those from HIV-positive men with nongonococcal urethritis. PCR positivity diminishes

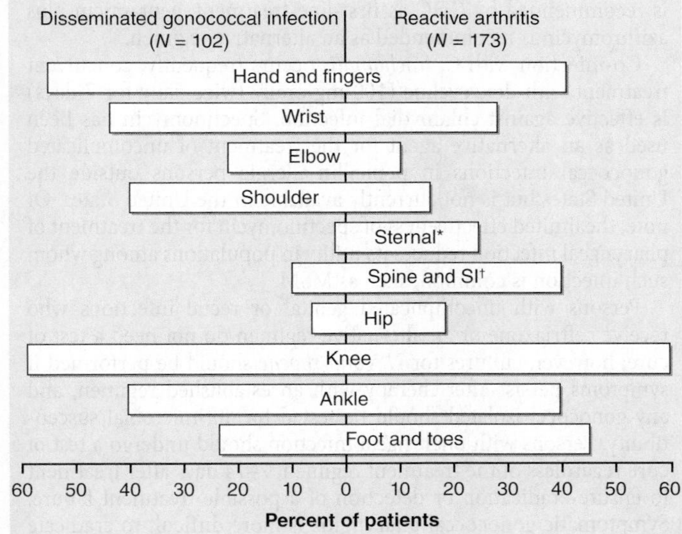

FIGURE 156-3 Distribution of joints with arthritis in 102 patients with disseminated gonococcal infection and 173 patients with reactive arthritis. *Includes the sternoclavicular joints. †SI, sacroiliac joint.

twofold after appropriate therapy for urethritis. Not only does gonorrhea enhance the transmission of HIV, but it may also increase the individual's risk for acquisition of HIV. A proposed mechanism is the significantly greater number of CD4+ T lymphocytes and dendritic cells that can be infected by HIV in endocervical secretions from women with nonulcerative STIs than in those from women with ulcerative STIs.

■ LABORATORY DIAGNOSIS

A rapid diagnosis of gonococcal infection in men may be obtained by Gram's staining of urethral exudates (Fig. 156-1). The detection of gram-negative intracellular monococci and diplococci is usually highly specific and sensitive in diagnosing gonococcal urethritis in symptomatic males but is only ~50% sensitive in diagnosing gonococcal cervicitis. Samples should be collected with Dacron or rayon swabs. Part of the sample should be inoculated onto a plate of modified Thayer-Martin or other gonococcal selective medium for culture. It is important to process all samples immediately because gonococci do not tolerate drying. If plates cannot be incubated immediately, they can be held safely for several hours at room temperature in candle extinction jars prior to incubation. If processing is to occur within 6 h, transport of specimens may be facilitated by the use of nonnutritive swab transport systems such as Stuart or Amies medium. For longer holding periods (e.g., when specimens for culture are to be mailed), culture media with self-contained CO_2-generating systems (such as the JEMBEC or Gono-Pak systems) may be used. Specimens should also be obtained for the diagnosis of chlamydial infection **(Chap. 189)**.

PMNs are often seen in the endocervix on a Gram's stain, and an abnormally increased number (≥30 PMNs per field in five 1000× oil-immersion microscopic fields) establishes the presence of an inflammatory discharge. Unfortunately, the presence or absence of gram-negative intracellular monococci or diplococci in cervical smears does not accurately predict which patients have gonorrhea, and the diagnosis in this setting should be made by culture or another suitable nonculture diagnostic method. The sensitivity of a single endocervical culture is ~80–90%. If a history of rectal sex is elicited, a rectal wall swab (uncontaminated with feces) should be cultured. A presumptive diagnosis of gonorrhea cannot be made on the basis of gram-negative diplococci in smears from the pharynx, where other *Neisseria* species are components of the normal flora.

Several nucleic acid amplification tests (NAATs), including the Roche COBAS AMPLICOR, Gen-Probe Aptima Combo 2, and BD ProbeTec ET, are now widely available on semiautomated or fully automated platforms and are commonly employed diagnostic tests for gonorrhea. These tests also detect *C. trachomatis* and are more sensitive than culture for identification of either *N. gonorrhoeae* or *C. trachomatis*. The Gen-Probe and BD tests offer the advantage that urine samples can be tested with a sensitivity similar to or greater than that obtained when urethral or cervical swab samples are assessed by other non-NAATs or culture, respectively. A point-of-care NAAT-based test (Binx *io*) for gonorrhea and chlamydia with a 30-minute turnaround time is now approved by the U.S. Food and Drug Administration (FDA). In MSM, it is important to screen the rectum and pharynx because screening urine alone will miss the majority of cases. A disadvantage of non-culture-based assays is that *N. gonorrhoeae* cannot be grown from the transport systems. Thus, a culture-confirmatory test and formal antimicrobial susceptibility testing, if needed, cannot be performed.

Because of the legal implications, the preferred method for the diagnosis of gonococcal infection in children is a standardized culture. Two positive NAATs, each targeting a different nucleic acid sequence, may be substituted for culture of the cervix or the urethra as legal evidence of infection in children. Although nonculture tests for gonococcal infection have not been approved by the FDA for use with specimens obtained from the pharynx and rectum of infected children, NAATs from these sites are preferred for diagnostic evaluation in adult victims of suspected sexual abuse, especially if the NAATs have been evaluated by the local laboratory and found to be superior. Cultures should be obtained from the pharynx and anus of both girls and boys, the urethra of boys, and the vagina of girls; cervical specimens are not recommended for prepubertal girls. For boys with a urethral discharge, a meatal specimen of the discharge is adequate for culture. Presumptive colonies of *N. gonorrhoeae* should be identified definitively by at least two independent methods.

Blood should be cultured in suspected cases of DGI. The use of Isolator blood culture tubes may enhance the yield. The probability of positive blood cultures decreases after 48 h of illness. Synovial fluid should be inoculated into blood culture broth medium and plated onto chocolate agar rather than selective medium because this fluid is not likely to be contaminated with commensal bacteria. Gonococci are infrequently recovered from early joint effusions containing <20,000 leukocytes/μL but may be recovered from effusions containing >80,000 leukocytes/μL. The organisms are seldom recovered from blood and synovial fluid of the same patient.

TREATMENT

Gonococcal Infections

Treatment failure can lead to continued transmission and the emergence of antibiotic resistance. The importance of adequate treatment with a regimen that the patient will adhere to cannot be overemphasized. Single-dose regimens have been developed for uncomplicated gonococcal infections. Treatment guidelines for gonococcal infections from the Centers for Disease Control and Prevention (CDC) were revised in 2020, and are summarized in **Table 156-1**. The third-generation cephalosporin ceftriaxone is now recommended as the first-line regimen for use at twice the previous dose (now, 500 mg IM, single dose) based on doubling of mean inhibitory concentrations (MICs) of current strains compared with MICs 20 years ago. The development of decreased sensitivity to ceftriaxone throughout the world will require the development of new effective regimens. Azithromycin, which had been recommended to provide additional treatment of gonorrhea (also to include treatment of chlamydial infection) is no longer recommended as part of a first line regimen. Resistance to azithromycin of U.S. isolates of *N. gonorrhoeae*, which had been less than 0.6% over a number of years, has increased more than sevenfold to 4.6% in the most recent year in which it was reported. If chlamydial infection cannot be excluded, concurrent treatment with doxycycline (100 mg orally twice a day for 7 days) is recommended. The recommendations for uncomplicated gonorrhea apply to HIV-infected as well as HIV-uninfected patients.

TABLE 156-1 Recommended Treatment for Gonococcal Infections: Adapted from the 2020 Guidelines for Gonococcal Infection of the Centers for Disease Control and Prevention

DIAGNOSIS	TREATMENT OF CHOICE[a]
Uncomplicated gonococcal infection of the cervix, urethra, pharynx[b], or rectum	
First-line regimen	Ceftriaxone (500 mg IM, single dose) ***plus*** Doxycycline (100 mg orally twice a day for 7 days) for treatment of chlamydial infection if chlamydial infection cannot be excluded
Alternative regimens if ceftriaxone is not available	Gentamicin (240 mg IM, single dose) plus azithromycin (2 g orally as a single dose)[c] Cefixime (800 mg PO, single dose) *or* spectinomycin (2 g IM, single dose)[d,e] ***plus*** Doxycycline (100 mg orally twice a day for 7 days) for treatment of chlamydial infection if chlamydial infection cannot be excluded
Epididymitis	**See Chap. 136**
Pelvic inflammatory disease	**See Chap. 136**
Gonococcal conjunctivitis in an adult	Ceftriaxone (1 g IM, single dose)[f]
Ophthalmia neonatorum[g]	Ceftriaxone (25–50 mg/kg IV, single dose, not to exceed 125 mg)
Disseminated gonococcal infection[h]	
Initial therapy[i]	
Patient tolerant of β-lactam drugs	Ceftriaxone (1 g IM or IV q24h; recommended) *or* cefotaxime (1 g IV q8h) *or* ceftizoxime (1 g IV q8h)
Patients allergic to β-lactam drugs	Spectinomycin (2 g IM q12h)[d]
Continuation therapy[j]	Cefixime (400 mg PO bid)
Meningitis or endocarditis	See text for specific recommendations[k]

[a]True failure of treatment with a recommended regimen is rare and should prompt an evaluation for reinfection, infection with a drug-resistant strain, or an alternative diagnosis. [b]Ceftriaxone is the most reliable agent recommended for treatment of pharyngeal infection. [c]*In vitro* synergistic killing of *N. gonorrhoeae* of gentamicin plus azithromycin is mild to moderate; azithromycin is for treatment chlamydial infection, primarily. [d]Spectinomycin is unavailable in the United States; in uncomplicated gonococcal infection it should be used at a higher dose (4 g IM, single dose) in areas of the world where increased resistance to spectinomycin exists. [e]Spectinomycin may be ineffective for the treatment of pharyngeal gonorrhea. [f]Plus lavage of the infected eye with saline solution (once). [g]Prophylactic regimens are discussed in the text. [h]Hospitalization is indicated if the diagnosis is uncertain, if the patient has the joint-localized stage with suppurative arthritis, or if the patient cannot be relied on to adhere to treatment. [i]All initial regimens should also include doxycycline (100 mg orally twice a day for 7 days) for treatment of chlamydial infection if chlamydial infection cannot be excluded; [j]gonococcal therapy should be continued for 24–48 h after clinical improvement begins, at which time the switch may be made to an oral agent (e.g., cefixime) if antimicrobial susceptibility can be documented by culture of the causative organism. If no organism is isolated and the diagnosis is secure, then treatment with ceftriaxone should be continued for at least 1 week. [k]Hospitalization is indicated to exclude suspected meningitis or endocarditis.

The currently recommended regimen for the treatment of uncomplicated gonococcal infection of the urethra, cervix, rectum, or pharynx (a single IM dose of ceftriaxone) almost always results in an effective cure. Quinolone-containing regimens are no longer recommended in the United States as first-line treatment because of widespread resistance. Rising MICs of cefixime worldwide have led the CDC to discontinue its recommendation of this agent as first-line treatment for uncomplicated gonorrhea. Multicenter trials of treatment for uncomplicated gonorrhea in the United States have shown ≥99.5% efficacy of two combination regimens and 96% efficacy in one single-agent regimen: gemifloxacin (320 mg, single oral dose) plus azithromycin (2 g, single oral dose); gentamicin (a single IM dose of 240 mg or, in individuals who weigh ≤45 kg, 5 mg/kg) plus azithromycin (2 g, single oral dose), and zoliflodacin (2 or 3 g, single oral dose). At this time, however, none of these regimens is recommended by CDC as first-line treatment; gentamicin plus azithromycin is recommended as an alternative regimen.

Co-infection with *C. trachomatis* occurs frequently; concurrent treatment with doxycycline (100 mg orally twice daily for 7 days) is effective against chlamydial infection. Spectinomycin has been used as an alternative agent for the treatment of uncomplicated gonococcal infections in penicillin-allergic persons outside the United States but is not currently available in the United States. Of note, the limited effectiveness of spectinomycin for the treatment of pharyngeal infection reduces its utility in populations among whom such infection is common, such as MSM.

Persons with uncomplicated genital or rectal infections who receive ceftriaxone or an alternative regimen do not need a test of cure; however, cultures for *N. gonorrhoeae* should be performed if symptoms persist after therapy with an established regimen, and any gonococci isolated should be tested for antimicrobial susceptibility. Persons with pharyngeal infection should undergo a test of cure regardless of the treatment regimen, 7–14 days after treatment to ensure eradication or detection of a possible treatment failure. Symptomatic gonococcal pharyngitis is more difficult to eradicate than genital infection. Persons who cannot tolerate cephalosporins may be treated with an alternative regimen. Treatment with spectinomycin results in a cure rate of ≤52%; persons given spectinomycin should have a subsequent pharyngeal sample cultured early (3–5 days) following treatment as a test of cure. A single 2-g dose of azithromycin may be used if the infecting organism is known to be sensitive or in areas where rates of resistance to azithromycin are low. Quinolones may be used if the infecting organism is known to be sensitive. If culture is not readily available and NAAT is positive, every effort should be made to perform a confirmatory culture. All isolates from test-of-cure cultures should undergo antimicrobial susceptibility testing. Because of high rates of reinfection with *N. gonorrhoeae* (and *C. trachomatis*) within 6–12 months, persons previously treated for gonorrhea should be retested 3 months after treatment.

Treatments for gonococcal epididymitis and PID are discussed in **Chap. 136**. Ocular gonococcal infections in older children and adults should be managed with a single dose of ceftriaxone combined with saline irrigation of the conjunctivae (both undertaken expeditiously), and patients should undergo a careful ophthalmologic evaluation that includes a slit-lamp examination.

DGI, particularly the joint-localized stage with suppurative arthritis, may require higher dosages and longer durations of therapy (Table 156-1). Hospitalization is indicated if the diagnosis is uncertain, if the patient has localized suppurative arthritis that requires aspiration, or if the patient cannot be relied on to comply with treatment. Open drainage is necessary only occasionally—e.g., for management of hip infections that may be difficult to drain percutaneously. Nonsteroidal anti-inflammatory agents may be indicated to alleviate pain and hasten clinical improvement of affected joints.

Gonococcal meningitis and endocarditis should be treated in the hospital with high-dose IV ceftriaxone (1–2 g IV every 12–24 h); therapy should continue for 10–14 days for meningitis and for at least 4 weeks for endocarditis. All persons who experience more than one episode of DGI should be evaluated for complement deficiency.

PREVENTION AND CONTROL

Condoms, if properly used, provide effective protection against the transmission and acquisition of gonorrhea as well as other infections that are transmitted to and from genital mucosal surfaces. Spermicidal preparations used with a diaphragm or cervical sponges impregnated with nonoxynol-9 offer some protection against gonorrhea and chlamydial infection. However, the frequent use of preparations that contain nonoxynol-9 is associated with mucosal disruption that paradoxically may enhance the risk of HIV infection in the event of exposure. All patients should be instructed to refer sex partners for evaluation and treatment. All sex partners of persons with gonorrhea should be evaluated and treated for *N. gonorrhoeae* and *C. trachomatis* infections if their last contact with the patient took place within 60 days before the onset of symptoms or the diagnosis of infection in the patient. If the patient's last potential sexual exposure to infection was >60 days before onset of symptoms or diagnosis, the patient's most recent sex partner should be treated. Partner-delivered medications or prescriptions for medications to treat gonorrhea and chlamydial infection diminish the likelihood of reinfection (or relapse) in the infected patient. In states where it is not prohibited, this approach is an option for partner management. Patients should be instructed to abstain from sexual intercourse until therapy is completed and until they and their sex partners no longer have symptoms. Greater emphasis must be placed on prevention by public health education, individual patient counseling, and behavior modification, particularly the use of condoms. Sexually active persons, especially adolescents, should be offered screening for STIs. For most male patients, NAAT of urine or a urethral swab may be used for screening. Preventing the spread of gonorrhea may help reduce the transmission of HIV. No effective vaccine for gonorrhea is yet available, but efforts to test several candidates are underway including a field trial of a licensed group B meningococcal vaccine (Bexsero), which in prototype form had been shown to reduce the incidence of gonorrhea in a population given the vaccine to control a group B meningococcal epidemic.

■ FURTHER READING

Bolan GA et al: The emerging threat of untreatable gonococcal infection. N Engl J Med 366:485, 2012.

St. Cyr S et al: Update to CDC's Treatment Guidelines for Gonococcal Infection, 2020. MMWR Morb Mortal Wkly Rep 69:1911, 2020.

Golden MR et al: Effect of expedited treatment of sex partners on recurrent or persistent gonorrhea or chlamydial infections. N Engl J Med 352:676, 2005.

Petousis-Harris EH et al: Effectiveness of a group B outer membrane vesicle meningococcal vaccine against gonorrhoea in New Zealand: A retrospective case-control study. Lancet 390:1603, 2017.

Rice PA: Gonococcal arthritis (disseminated gonococcal infection). Infect Dis Clin North Am 19:853, 2005.

Taylor SN et al: Single-dose zoliflodacin (ETX0914) for treatment of urogenital gonorrhea. N Engl J Med 379:1835, 2018.

Unemo M et al: Antimicrobial resistance expressed by *Neisseria gonorrhoeae*: A major global public health problem in the 21st century. Microbiol Spectr 4:10.1128/microbiolspec.EI10-0009-2015, 2016.

Unemo MM et al: Gonorrhoea. Nat Rev Dis Primers 5:80, 2019.

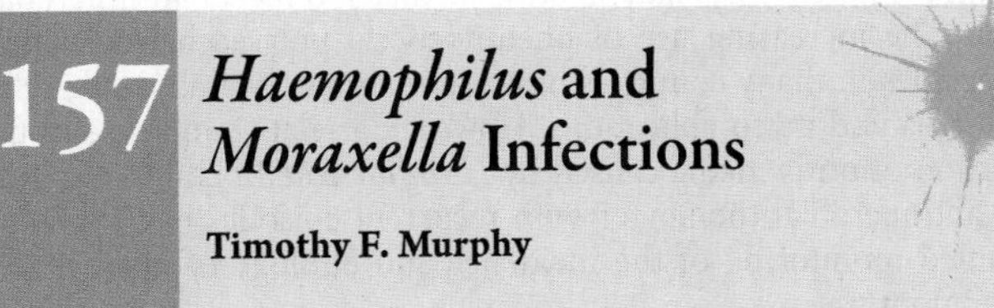

157 *Haemophilus* and *Moraxella* Infections

Timothy F. Murphy

HAEMOPHILUS INFLUENZAE

■ MICROBIOLOGY

Haemophilus influenzae was first recognized in 1892 by Pfeiffer, who erroneously concluded that the bacterium was the cause of influenza. *H. influenzae* is a small (1- × 0.3-μm) gram-negative organism of variable shape; thus, it is often described as a pleomorphic coccobacillus. In clinical specimens such as cerebrospinal fluid (CSF) and sputum, *H. influenzae* frequently stains only faintly with safranin and therefore can easily be overlooked.

H. influenzae grows both aerobically and anaerobically. Its aerobic growth requires two factors: hemin (X factor) and nicotinamide adenine dinucleotide (V factor). These requirements are used in the clinical laboratory to identify the bacterium. However, using phenotypic methods for differentiating among *Haemophilus* species has limitations, as the growing number of whole-genome sequences of *Haemophilus* isolates from the human respiratory tract is revealing complex genetic relationships among *Haemophilus* species (see "Diagnosis," below).

TABLE 157-1 Characteristics of Type b and Nontypable Strains of *Haemophilus influenzae*

FEATURE	TYPE b STRAINS	NONTYPABLE STRAINS
Capsule	Ribosyl-ribitol phosphate	Unencapsulated
Pathogenesis	Invasive infections due to hematogenous spread	Mucosal infections due to contiguous spread
Clinical manifestations	Meningitis and invasive infections in incompletely immunized infants and children	Otitis media in infants and children; lower respiratory tract infections in adults with chronic bronchitis
Evolutionary history	Basically clonal	Genetically diverse
Vaccine	Highly effective conjugate vaccines	Protein D used as carrier protein in pneumococcal vaccine approved in Europe: GSK Synflorix. Others under development

Six major serotypes of *H. influenzae* have been identified; designated *a* through *f*, they are based on antigenically distinct polysaccharide capsules. In addition, some strains lack a polysaccharide capsule and are referred to as *nontypable* strains. Type b and nontypable strains are the most relevant strains clinically (**Table 157-1**), although encapsulated strains other than type b can cause disease. *H. influenzae* was the first free-living organism to have its entire genome sequenced.

The antigenically distinct type b capsule is a linear polymer composed of ribosyl-ribitol phosphate. Strains of *H. influenzae* type b (Hib) cause disease primarily in infants and children <6 years of age. Nontypable strains are primarily mucosal pathogens but occasionally cause invasive disease.

■ EPIDEMIOLOGY AND TRANSMISSION

H. influenzae, an exclusively human pathogen, is spread by airborne droplets or by direct contact with secretions or fomites. Colonization with nontypable *H. influenzae* is a dynamic process; new strains are acquired and other strains are replaced periodically.

The widespread use of Hib conjugate vaccines in many industrialized countries has resulted in striking decreases in the rate of nasopharyngeal colonization by Hib and in the incidence of Hib infection (**Fig. 157-1**). Worldwide, invasive Hib disease occurs predominantly in unimmunized children and in those who have not completed the primary immunization series. Most World Health Organization member countries have introduced Hib conjugate vaccination, but a large number of the world's children remain unimmunized, principally in countries without national vaccine programs. Certain groups have a higher incidence of invasive Hib disease than the general population,

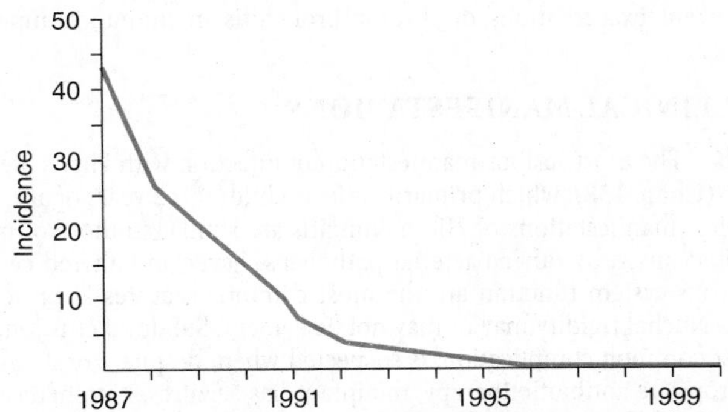

FIGURE 157-1 Estimated incidence (rate per 100,000) of invasive disease due to *Haemophilus influenzae* type b among children <5 years of age: 1987–2000. Fewer than 40 cases per year have been reported since 2000. *(Data from the Centers for Disease Control and Prevention.)*

including African-American and Australian Aboriginal children and Native American groups. Although this increased incidence has not yet been accounted for, several factors may be relevant, including age at exposure to the bacterium, socioeconomic conditions, and genetic differences.

PATHOGENESIS

Hib strains cause systemic disease by invasion and hematogenous spread from the respiratory tract to distant sites such as the meninges, bones, and joints. The type b polysaccharide capsule is an important virulence factor affecting the bacterium's ability to avoid opsonization and cause systemic disease.

Nontypable strains cause disease by local invasion of mucosal surfaces. Otitis media results when bacteria reach the middle ear by way of the eustachian tube. Adults with chronic obstructive pulmonary disease (COPD) experience recurrent lower respiratory tract infection due to nontypable strains. In addition, nontypable *H. influenzae* persist in the lower airways of adults with COPD in both extracellular and intracellular locations, contributing to the airway inflammation that is a hallmark of the disease. Nontypable strains that cause infection in adults with COPD differ in pathogenic potential and genome content from strains that cause otitis media. In the middle ear, nontypable strains form biofilms. More resistant to host clearance mechanisms and to antibiotics than are planktonic bacteria, biofilms are associated with chronic and recurrent otitis media. Nontypable *H. influenzae* persist in the human respiratory tract and cause infection by altering expression of genes through slipped-strand mispairing and through phase-variable expression of DNA methylase genes that control the expression of multiple genes that play a role in virulence.

The incidence of invasive disease caused by nontypable strains is low but appears to be increasing over the past decade. Most strains that cause invasive disease are genetically and phenotypically diverse.

IMMUNE RESPONSE

Antibody to the capsule is important in protection from infection by Hib strains. The level of (maternally acquired) serum antibody to the capsular polysaccharide, which is a polymer of polyribitol ribose phosphate (PRP), declines from birth to 6 months of age and, in the absence of vaccination, remains low until ~2 or 3 years of age. The age at the antibody nadir correlates with that of the peak incidence of type b disease. Antibody to PRP then appears partly as a result of exposure to Hib or cross-reacting antigens. Systemic Hib disease is unusual after the age of 6 years because of the presence of protective antibody. Vaccines in which PRP is conjugated to protein carrier molecules have been developed and are now used widely. These vaccines generate an antibody response to PRP in infants and effectively prevent invasive infections in infants and children.

Since nontypable strains lack a capsule, the immune response to infection is directed at noncapsular antigens. These antigens have generated considerable interest as immune targets and potential vaccine components. The human immune response to nontypable strains appears to be strain-specific, a characteristic that accounts in part for the propensity of these strains to cause recurrent otitis media and recurrent exacerbations of chronic bronchitis in immunocompetent hosts.

CLINICAL MANIFESTATIONS

Hib The most serious manifestation of infection with Hib is *meningitis* **(Chap. 138)**, which primarily affects children <2 years of age. The clinical manifestations of Hib meningitis are similar to those of meningitis caused by other bacterial pathogens. Fever and altered central nervous system function are the most common features at presentation. Nuchal rigidity may or may not be evident. Subdural effusion, the most common complication, is suspected when, despite 2 or 3 days of appropriate antibiotic therapy, the infant has seizures, hemiparesis, or continued obtundation. The overall mortality rate from Hib meningitis is ~5%, and the morbidity rate is high. Of survivors, 6% have permanent sensorineural hearing loss, and about one-fourth have a significant disability of some type. If more subtle disabilities are sought, up to half of survivors are found to have some neurologic sequelae, such as partial hearing loss and delayed language development.

Epiglottitis **(Chap. 35)** is a life-threatening Hib infection involving cellulitis of the epiglottis and supraglottic tissues. It can lead to acute upper-airway obstruction. Its unique epidemiologic features are its occurrence in an older age group (2–7 years old) than other Hib infections and its absence among Navajo Native Americans and Alaskan Eskimos. Sore throat and fever rapidly progress to dysphagia, drooling, and airway obstruction. Epiglottitis also occurs in adults.

Cellulitis **(Chap. 129)** due to Hib occurs in young children. The most common location is on the head or neck, and the involved area sometimes takes on a characteristic bluish-red color. Most patients have bacteremia, and 10% have an additional focus of infection.

Hib causes *pneumonia* in infants. The infection is clinically indistinguishable from other types of bacterial pneumonia (e.g., pneumococcal pneumonia) except that Hib is more likely to involve the pleura. Several less common invasive conditions can be important clinical manifestations of Hib infection in children. These include osteomyelitis, septic arthritis, pericarditis, orbital cellulitis, endophthalmitis, urinary tract infection, abscesses, and bacteremia without an identifiable focus.

Non–type b encapsulated strains of *H. influenzae* (types a, c, d, e, and f) are unusual causes of invasive infection manifested predominantly by bacteremia and pneumonia. *H. influenzae* type a infections are seen with increased frequency in indigenous populations of North America, and these strains are predominantly clonal. Most infections due to non–type b encapsulated strains occur in the setting of underlying conditions.

Nontypable *H. influenzae* Nontypable *H. influenzae* is the most common bacterial cause of exacerbations of COPD; these exacerbations are characterized by increased cough, sputum production, and shortness of breath. Fever is low-grade, and no infiltrates are evident on chest x-ray. Nontypable strains also cause community-acquired bacterial pneumonia in adults, especially among patients with COPD or AIDS. The clinical features of *H. influenzae* pneumonia are similar to those of other types of bacterial pneumonia, including pneumococcal pneumonia.

Nontypable *H. influenzae* is one of the three most common causes of childhood otitis media (the other two being *Streptococcus pneumoniae* and *Moraxella catarrhalis*) **(Chap. 35)**. Infants are febrile and irritable, while older children report ear pain. Symptoms of viral upper-respiratory infection often precede otitis media. The diagnosis is made by pneumatic otoscopy. An etiologic diagnosis, although not routinely sought, can be established by tympanocentesis and culture of middle-ear fluid. Clinical features associated with *H. influenzae* otitis media include a history of recurrent episodes, treatment failure, concomitant conjunctivitis, bilateral otitis media, and recent antimicrobial therapy. The increasing use of pneumococcal polysaccharide conjugate vaccines in many countries has resulted in an overall decrease in otitis media and its complications. However, a relative increase in the proportion of otitis media caused by *H. influenzae* in children failing initial antimicrobial therapy or with recurrent episodes has occurred. Continued monitoring of the incidence and etiology of otitis media will be important.

Nontypable *H. influenzae* also causes puerperal sepsis and is an important cause of neonatal bacteremia. These nontypable strains, provisionally named *Haemophilus quentini*, are closely related to but distinct from *H. haemolyticus*, tend to be of biotype IV and cause invasive disease after colonizing the female genital tract.

Nontypable *H. influenzae* causes sinusitis **(Chap. 35)** in adults and children. In addition, the bacterium is a less common cause of various invasive infections. These infections include bacteremia, empyema, adult epiglottitis, pericarditis, cellulitis, septic arthritis, osteomyelitis, endocarditis, cholecystitis, intraabdominal infections, urinary tract infections, mastoiditis, and aortic graft infection. Most *H. influenzae* invasive infections in countries where Hib vaccines are used widely are caused by nontypable strains, and a recent increased incidence of such infections has been observed. Although most strains of nontypable *H. influenzae* that cause invasive infections are genetically diverse, recent localized clusters of infections have been caused by clonally related strains. Continued monitoring will be important. Many patients with *H. influenzae* bacteremia have an underlying condition, such as HIV infection, cardiopulmonary disease, alcoholism, or cancer.

DIAGNOSIS

The most reliable method for establishing a diagnosis of invasive *H. influenzae* infection is recovery of the organism in culture in a normally sterile body site, such as blood, CSF, or joint fluid.

H. influenzae isolated from the respiratory tract must be distinguished from a complex flora and from other *Haemophilus* species. Particular caution must be used to distinguish *H. influenzae* from *Haemophilus haemolyticus*, a respiratory tract commensal that has identical growth requirements. *H. haemolyticus* has classically been distinguished from *H. influenzae* by the hemolysis of the former species on horse blood agar. However, a significant proportion of isolates of *H. haemolyticus* have now been recognized as nonhemolytic. Analysis of various genotypic markers, including 16S ribosomal sequences, superoxide dismutase, outer-membrane protein P6, protein D, and fuculose kinase, can be used to distinguish these two species. The availability of whole-genome sequences of an increasing number of *Haemophilus* isolates from the human upper respiratory tract has revealed complex genomic relationships among *Haemophilus* species, suggesting a genetic continuum between some *Haemophilus* species.

The presence of gram-negative coccobacilli in Gram-stained CSF is strong evidence for Hib meningitis. Recovery of the organism from CSF confirms the diagnosis. Cultures of other normally sterile body fluids, such as blood, joint fluid, pleural fluid, pericardial fluid, and subdural effusion, are confirmatory in other infections.

Detection of PRP is an important adjunct to culture in rapid diagnosis of Hib meningitis. Immunoelectrophoresis, latex agglutination, coagglutination, and enzyme-linked immunosorbent assay are effective in detecting PRP. These assays are particularly helpful when patients have received prior antimicrobial therapy and thus are especially likely to have negative cultures.

Because nontypable *H. influenzae* is primarily a mucosal pathogen, it is a component of a mixed flora; thus etiologic diagnosis is challenging. Nontypable *H. influenzae* infection is strongly suggested by the predominance of gram-negative coccobacilli among abundant polymorphonuclear leukocytes in a Gram-stained sputum specimen from a patient in whom pneumonia is suspected. Although bacteremia is detectable in a small proportion of patients with pneumonia due to nontypable *H. influenzae*, most such patients have negative blood cultures.

A diagnosis of otitis media is based on the detection by pneumatic otoscopy of fluid in the middle ear. An etiologic diagnosis requires tympanocentesis but is not routinely sought. An invasive procedure is also required to determine the etiology of sinusitis; thus, treatment is often empirical once the diagnosis is suspected in light of clinical symptoms and sinus radiographs.

TREATMENT

Haemophilus influenzae

Initial therapy for meningitis due to Hib should consist of a cephalosporin such as ceftriaxone or cefotaxime. For children, the dosage of ceftriaxone is 75–100 mg/kg daily given in two doses 12 h apart. The pediatric dosage of cefotaxime is 200 mg/kg daily given in four doses 6 h apart. Adult dosages are 2 g every 12 h for ceftriaxone and 2 g every 4–6 h for cefotaxime. An alternative regimen for initial therapy is ampicillin (200–300 mg/kg daily in four divided doses) plus chloramphenicol (75–100 mg/kg daily in four divided doses). Therapy should continue for a total of 1–2 weeks.

Administration of glucocorticoids to patients with Hib meningitis reduces the incidence of neurologic sequelae. The presumed mechanism is reduction of the inflammation induced by bacterial cell-wall mediators of inflammation when cells are killed by antimicrobial agents. Dexamethasone (0.6 mg/kg per day intravenously in four divided doses for 2 days) is recommended for the treatment of Hib meningitis in children >2 months of age.

Invasive infections other than meningitis are treated with the same antimicrobial agents. For epiglottitis, the dosage of ceftriaxone is 50 mg/kg daily, and the dosage of cefotaxime is 150 mg/kg daily, given in three divided doses 8 h apart. Epiglottitis constitutes a medical emergency, and maintenance of an airway is critical. The duration of therapy is determined by the clinical response. A course of 1–2 weeks is usually appropriate.

Many infections caused by nontypable strains of *H. influenzae*, such as otitis media, sinusitis, and exacerbations of COPD, can be treated with oral antimicrobial agents. Approximately 20–35% of nontypable strains produce β-lactamase (with the exact proportion depending on geographic location), and these strains are resistant to ampicillin. Several agents have excellent activity against nontypable *H. influenzae*, including amoxicillin/clavulanic acid, various extended-spectrum cephalosporins, and the macrolides azithromycin and clarithromycin. Fluoroquinolones are highly active against *H. influenzae* and are useful in adults with exacerbations of COPD. However, fluoroquinolones are not currently recommended for the treatment of children or pregnant women because of possible effects on articular cartilage.

In addition to β-lactamase production, alteration of penicillin-binding proteins—a second mechanism of ampicillin resistance—has been detected in isolates of *H. influenzae*. Although rare in the United States, these β-lactamase-negative ampicillin-resistant strains are common in Japan and are increasing in prevalence in Europe. Resistance to macrolides is also being observed with increasing frequency globally. Continued monitoring of the evolving antimicrobial susceptibility patterns of *H. influenzae* will be important.

PREVENTION

Vaccination (See also **Chap. 123**) Three conjugate vaccines that prevent invasive infections with Hib in infants and children are licensed in the United States. In addition to eliciting protective antibody, these vaccines prevent disease by reducing rates of pharyngeal colonization with Hib. The widespread use of conjugate vaccines has dramatically reduced the incidence of Hib disease in developed countries. Even though the manufacture of Hib vaccines is costly, vaccination is cost-effective. The Global Alliance for Vaccines and Immunizations has recognized the underuse of Hib conjugate vaccines.

The disease burden has been reduced in developing countries that have implemented routine vaccination (e.g., The Gambia, Chile). An important obstacle to more widespread vaccination is the lack of data on the epidemiology and burden of Hib disease in many developing countries.

All children should be immunized with an Hib conjugate vaccine, receiving the first dose at ~2 months of age, the rest of the primary series at 2–6 months of age, and a booster dose at 12–15 months of age. Specific recommendations vary for the different conjugate vaccines. The reader is referred to the recommendations of the American Academy of Pediatrics (**Chap. 123** and *www.cispimmunize.org*).

Currently, no vaccines are available specifically for the prevention of disease caused by nontypable *H. influenzae*. However, a vaccine that contains protein D—a surface protein of *H. influenzae*—conjugated to pneumococcal polysaccharides is licensed in other countries and is used widely throughout the world. The vaccine has shown partial efficacy in preventing *H. influenzae* otitis media in clinical trials. Vaccine formulations that include surface protein antigens are currently in clinical trials, and additional progress in the development of vaccines against nontypable *H. influenzae* is anticipated.

Chemoprophylaxis The risk of secondary disease is greater than normal among household contacts of patients with Hib disease. Therefore, all children and adults (except pregnant women) in households with an index case and at least one incompletely immunized contact <4 years of age should receive prophylaxis with oral rifampin. When two or more cases of invasive Hib disease have occurred within 60 days at a child-care facility attended by incompletely vaccinated children, administration of rifampin to all attendees and personnel is indicated, as it is for household contacts. Chemoprophylaxis is not indicated in nursery and child-care contacts of a single index case. The reader is referred to the recommendations of the American Academy of Pediatrics.

HAEMOPHILUS DUCREYI

Haemophilus ducreyi is the etiologic agent of chancroid (**Chap. 136**), a sexually transmitted disease characterized by genital ulceration and inguinal adenitis. In addition to being a cause of morbidity in itself, chancroid is associated with HIV infection because of the role played by genital ulceration in HIV transmission. Chancroid increases the efficiency of transmission of and the degree of susceptibility to HIV infection. *H. ducreyi* has also been recognized as an important cause of non-sexually transmitted cutaneous ulcers.

■ MICROBIOLOGY

H. ducreyi is a highly fastidious coccobacillary gram-negative bacterium whose growth requires X factor (hemin). Although, in light of this requirement, the bacterium has been classified in the genus *Haemophilus*, DNA homology and chemotaxonomic studies have established substantial differences between *H. ducreyi* and other *Haemophilus* species. Taxonomic reclassification of the organism is likely in the future but awaits further study. Ulcers contain predominantly T cells. The fact that patients who have had chancroid may have repeated infections indicates that infection does not confer protection.

■ EPIDEMIOLOGY AND PREVALENCE

The prevalence of chancroid has steadily declined in the United States and worldwide over the past decade and a half. The infection appears to be more common in developing countries. Transmission is predominantly heterosexual, and cases in males have outnumbered those in females by ratios of 3:1 to 25:1 during outbreaks. Contact with commercial sex workers and illicit drug use are strongly associated with chancroid. Most cases in developed countries are sporadic.

H. ducreyi has emerged as a major cause of cutaneous ulcers in children in developing countries, particularly in the South Pacific and Africa. Strains that cause cutaneous ulcers have genome sequences that are nearly identical to class I strains (of two related classes) of *H. ducreyi* that cause genital ulcers.

■ CLINICAL MANIFESTATIONS AND DIFFERENTIAL DIAGNOSIS

Infection is acquired as the result of a break in the epithelium during sexual contact with an infected individual. After an incubation period of 4–7 days, the initial lesion—a papule with surrounding erythema—appears. In 2 or 3 days, the papule evolves into a pustule, which spontaneously ruptures and forms a sharply circumscribed ulcer that generally is not indurated (**Fig. 157-2**). The ulcers are painful and bleed easily; little or no inflammation of the surrounding skin is evident. Approximately half of patients develop enlarged, tender inguinal lymph nodes, which frequently become fluctuant and spontaneously rupture. Patients usually seek medical care after 1–3 weeks of painful symptoms.

The presentation of chancroid does not usually include all of the typical clinical features and is sometimes atypical. Multiple ulcers can coalesce to form giant ulcers. Ulcers can appear and then resolve, with inguinal adenitis (Fig. 157-2) and suppuration following 1–3 weeks later; this clinical picture can be confused with that of lymphogranuloma venereum (**Chap. 189**). Multiple small ulcers can resemble folliculitis. Other differential diagnostic considerations include the various infections causing genital ulceration, such as primary syphilis, secondary syphilis (condyloma latum), genital herpes, and donovanosis. In rare cases, chancroid lesions become secondarily infected with bacteria; the result is extensive inflammation.

Non-sexually transmitted cutaneous ulcers caused by *H. ducreyi* resemble those of yaws caused by *Treponema pallidum* subspecies *pertenue*, which is endemic in regions where *H. ducreyi* cutaneous ulcers are seen. Ulcers caused by *H. ducreyi* are less likely than those of yaws to show central granulating tissue and less likely to have indurated edges, but substantial overlap in clinical characteristics exists.

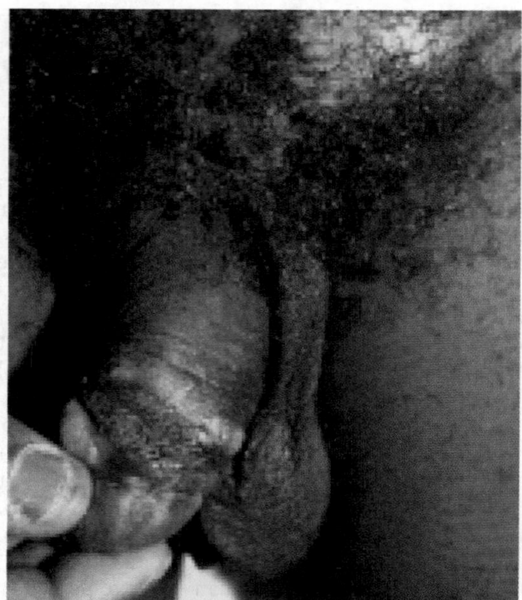

FIGURE 157-2 Chancroid with characteristic penile ulcers and associated left inguinal adenitis (bubo).

■ DIAGNOSIS

Clinical diagnosis of chancroid is often inaccurate, and laboratory confirmation should be attempted in suspected cases. An accurate diagnosis of chancroid relies on culture of *H. ducreyi* from the lesion or from an aspirate of suppurative lymph nodes. Since the organism can be difficult to grow, the use of selective and supplemented media is necessary. No polymerase chain reaction (PCR) assay for *H. ducreyi* is commercially available; such tests can be performed by Clinical Laboratory Improvement Amendment (CLIA)–certified clinical laboratories that have developed their own assays.

A probable diagnosis of sexually transmitted chancroid can be made when the following criteria are met: (1) one or more painful genital ulcers; (2) no evidence of *T. pallidum* infection by dark-field examination of ulcer exudate or by a negative serologic test for syphilis performed at least 7 days after ulcer onset; (3) a typical clinical presentation for chancroid; and (4) a negative test for herpes simplex virus in the ulcer exudate.

A serologic test for syphilis does not distinguish cutaneous ulcers due to *H. ducreyi* from those due to yaws. A PCR assay has been used in clinical studies to establish an *H. ducreyi* etiology, but, as stated above, no such assay is commercially available.

TREATMENT

Haemophilus ducreyi

Treatment regimens for both genital and cutaneous infections include (1) a single 1-g oral dose of azithromycin; (2) ceftriaxone (250 mg intramuscularly in a single dose); (3) ciprofloxacin (500 mg by mouth twice a day for 3 days); and (4) erythromycin base (500 mg by mouth three times a day for 7 days). Isolates from patients who do not respond promptly to treatment should be tested for antimicrobial resistance. In patients with HIV infection, healing may be slow and longer courses of treatment may be necessary. Clinical treatment failure in HIV-seropositive patients may reflect co-infection, especially with herpes simplex virus. Contacts of patients with chancroid should be identified and treated, whether or not symptoms are present, if they have had sexual contact with the patient during the 10 days preceding the patient's onset of symptoms.

MORAXELLA CATARRHALIS

MICROBIOLOGY

M. catarrhalis is an unencapsulated gram-negative diplococcus whose ecologic niche is the human respiratory tract. The organism was initially designated *Micrococcus catarrhalis*. Its name was changed to *Neisseria catarrhalis* in 1970 because of phenotypic similarities to commensal *Neisseria* species. On the basis of more rigorous analysis of genetic relatedness, *Moraxella catarrhalis* is now the widely accepted name for this species.

EPIDEMIOLOGY

Nasopharyngeal colonization by *M. catarrhalis* is common in infancy, with colonization rates ranging between 33% and 100% and depending on geographic location. Several factors probably account for this geographic variation, including living conditions, day-care attendance, hygiene, household smoking, and population genetics. The prevalence of colonization decreases steadily with age.

The widespread use of pneumococcal conjugate vaccines in some countries has resulted in alterations in patterns of nasopharyngeal colonization in resident populations. A relative increase in colonization by nonvaccine pneumococcal serotypes, nontypable *H. influenzae*, and *M. catarrhalis* has occurred. These changes in colonization patterns may be altering the distribution of pathogens of both otitis media and sinusitis in children.

PATHOGENESIS

M. catarrhalis causes mucosal infections of the respiratory tract by contiguous spread from its colonizing site in the upper airway. A preceding viral upper respiratory tract infection is a common inciting event for otitis media. In exacerbations of COPD, the acquisition of new strains is critical for pathogenesis. Strains exhibit substantial genetic diversity and differences in virulence properties.

The expression of several adhesin molecules with differing specificities for various host cell receptors reflects the importance of adherence to the respiratory epithelial surface in the pathogenesis of infection. *M. catarrhalis* invades multiple cell types. Its intracellular residence in lymphoid tissue provides a potential reservoir for persistence in the human respiratory tract. Like many gram-negative bacteria, *M. catarrhalis* sheds vesicles into the surrounding environment. The vesicles are internalized by host cells and mediate several virulence mechanisms, including induction of inflammation and delivery of β-lactamase, that can promote the survival of co-pathogens.

CLINICAL MANIFESTATIONS

In children, *M. catarrhalis* causes predominantly mucosal infections when the bacterium migrates from the nasopharynx to the middle ear or the sinuses **(Chap. 35)**. The inciting event for both otitis media and sinusitis is often a preceding viral infection. Overall, cultures of middle-ear fluid obtained by tympanocentesis indicate that *M. catarrhalis* causes 15–20% of cases of acute otitis media. More sensitive molecular analysis of middle ear fluid detects *M. catarrhalis* alone or with other pathogens in 30 to 50% of middle ear fluid samples from children with otitis media. Acute otitis media caused by *M. catarrhalis* or nontypable *H. influenzae* is clinically milder than otitis media caused by *S. pneumoniae*, with less fever and a lower prevalence of a red bulging tympanic membrane. However, substantial overlap makes it impossible to predict etiology in an individual child on the basis of clinical features.

A small proportion of viral upper respiratory tract infections are complicated by bacterial sinusitis. Cultures of sinus puncture aspirates show that *M. catarrhalis* accounts for ~20% of cases of acute bacterial sinusitis in children and for a smaller proportion in adults.

M. catarrhalis is a common cause of exacerbations in adults with COPD. The bacterium has been overlooked in this clinical setting because it has long been considered to be a commensal and because it is easily mistaken for commensal *Neisseria* species in cultures of respiratory secretions (see "Diagnosis," below). Several independent lines of evidence have established *M. catarrhalis* as a pathogen in COPD. These include (1) the demonstration of *M. catarrhalis* in the lower airways during exacerbations, (2) the association of exacerbation with acquisition of new strains, (3) elevations of inflammatory markers in association with *M. catarrhalis*, and (4) the development of specific immune responses following infection. *M. catarrhalis* is the second most common bacterial cause of COPD exacerbations (after *H. influenzae*), as shown in a 10-year prospective study; the distribution of exacerbations associated with new-strain acquisitions is shown in **Fig. 157-3**. Not included are culture-negative cases or cases from which a pathogen had been previously isolated. With the application of rigorous clinical criteria for defining the etiology of exacerbations (both culture-positive and culture-negative), ~10% of all exacerbations in the same study were caused by *M. catarrhalis*. The clinical features of an exacerbation due to *M. catarrhalis* are similar to those of exacerbations due to other bacterial pathogens, including *H. influenzae* and *S. pneumoniae*. The cardinal symptoms are cough with increased sputum production, sputum purulence, and dyspnea in comparison with baseline symptoms.

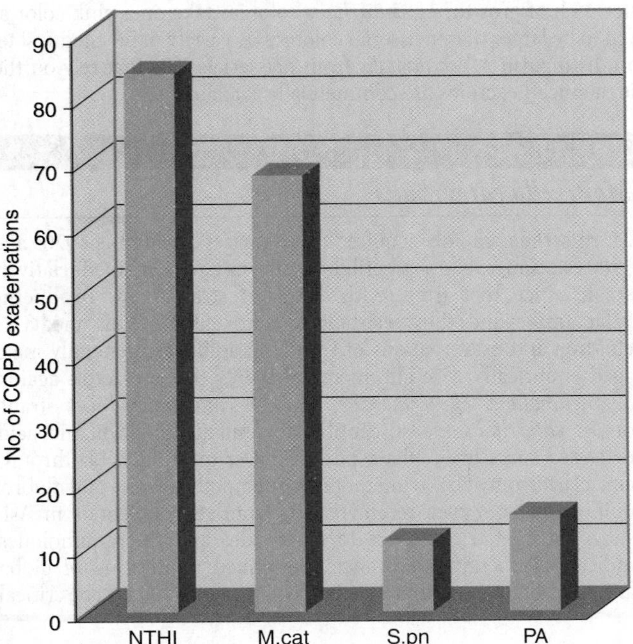

FIGURE 157-3 Cumulative results of a prospective study (1994–2004) of bacterial infection in chronic obstructive pulmonary disease (COPD) showing etiology of exacerbations. The numbers of exacerbations shown indicate the acquisition of a new strain simultaneous with clinical symptoms of an exacerbation. NTHI, nontypable *H. influenzae*; M.cat, *M. catarrhalis*; S.pn, *Streptococcus pneumoniae*; PA, *Pseudomonas aeruginosa*. *(Reproduced with permission from JC Goldstein, TF Murphy: Moraxella catarrhalis, a human respiratory tract pathogen. Clin Infect Dis 49:124, 2009.)*

Pneumonia due to *M. catarrhalis* occurs in the elderly, particularly in the setting of underlying cardiopulmonary disease, but is infrequent. Invasive infections, such as bacteremia, endocarditis, neonatal meningitis, and septic arthritis, are rare.

DIAGNOSIS

Tympanocentesis is required for etiologic diagnosis of otitis media, but this procedure is not performed routinely. Therefore, treatment of otitis media is generally empirical. Similarly, an etiologic diagnosis of sinusitis requires an invasive procedure and thus is usually not available to the clinician. Isolation of *M. catarrhalis* from an expectorated sputum sample from an adult experiencing clinical symptoms of an exacerbation is suggestive, but not diagnostic, of *M. catarrhalis* as the cause.

Upon culture, colonies of *M. catarrhalis* resemble those of commensal neisseriae that are part of the normal upper airway flora. As mentioned above, the difficulty in distinguishing colonies of *M. catarrhalis* from neisserial colonies in cultures of respiratory secretions explains in part why *M. catarrhalis* has been overlooked as a pathogen. In contrast to these *Neisseria* species, *M. catarrhalis* colonies can be slid across the agar surface without disruption (the "hockey puck sign"). In addition, after 48 h of growth, *M. catarrhalis* colonies take on a pink color and tend to be larger than neisserial colonies. A variety of biochemical tests can distinguish *M. catarrhalis* from neisseriae. Kits that rely on these biochemical reactions are commercially available.

TREATMENT
Moraxella catarrhalis

M. catarrhalis rapidly acquired β-lactamases during the 1970s and 1980s; antimicrobial susceptibility patterns have remained relatively stable since that time, with >90% of strains now producing β-lactamase and thus resistant to amoxicillin. Otitis media in children and exacerbations of COPD in adults are generally managed empirically with antimicrobial agents that are active against *S. pneumoniae*, *H. influenzae*, and *M. catarrhalis.* Most strains of *M. catarrhalis* are susceptible to amoxicillin/clavulanic acid, extended-spectrum cephalosporins, newer macrolides (azithromycin, clarithromycin), trimethoprim-sulfamethoxazole, and fluoroquinolones. However, recent reports from several centers in Asia show substantial resistance to macrolides and fluoroquinolones, indicating emerging resistance. Continued monitoring of global antimicrobial susceptibility patterns of *M. catarrhalis* will be critical.

FURTHER READING

Ahearn CP et al: Insights on persistent airway Infection by non-typeable *Haemophilus influenzae* in chronic obstructive pulmonary disease. Pathog Dis 75:ftx042, 2017.

Blakeway LV et al: Virulence determinants of *Moraxella catarrhalis*: Distribution and considerations for vaccine development. Microbiology 163:1371, 2017.

Jalalvand F, Riesbeck K: Update on non-typeable *Haemophilus influenzae*-mediated disease and vaccine development. Expert Rev Vaccines 17:503, 2018.

Lewis DA, Mitja O: *Haemophilus ducreyi*: From sexually transmitted infection to skin ulcer pathogen. Curr Opin Infect Dis 29:52, 2016.

Perez AC, Murphy TF: A *Moraxella catarrhalis* vaccine to protect against otitis media and exacerbations of COPD: An update on current progress and challenges. Hum Vacc Immunother 3:2322, 2017.

158 Infections Due to the HACEK Group and Miscellaneous Gram-Negative Bacteria

Tamar F. Barlam

THE HACEK GROUP

HACEK organisms are a group of fastidious, slow-growing, gram-negative bacteria whose growth requires an atmosphere of carbon dioxide. These organisms do not grow on media routinely used for enteric bacteria (e.g., MacConkey agar). Species belonging to this group include several *Haemophilus* species, *Aggregatibacter* (formerly *Actinobacillus*) species, *Cardiobacterium* species, *Eikenella corrodens*, and *Kingella kingae*. HACEK bacteria normally reside in the oral cavity and have been associated with local infections in the mouth. They are also known to cause severe systemic infections—such as bacteremia and bacterial endocarditis, which can develop on either native or prosthetic valves **(Chap. 128)**. In a nationwide survey in Denmark, HACEK bacteremias were most often due to *Haemophilus species*, followed by *Aggregatibacter* species. HACEK bacteremia is strongly predictive of underlying infective endocarditis (overall positive predictive value, 60%). However, this association varies significantly by organism. For example, in one study, infective endocarditis was diagnosed in 100% of patients with *Aggregatibacter actinomycetemcomitans* bacteremia, 55% with *Haemophilus parainfluenzae* bacteremia, but in no patients with *Eikenella* bacteremia.

In large series, 0.8–6% of cases of infective endocarditis are attributable to HACEK organisms, most often *Aggregatibacter* species, *Haemophilus* species, and *Cardiobacterium hominis.* Invasive infection typically occurs in patients with a history of cardiac valvular disease or prosthetic valves, often in the setting of a recent dental procedure or nasopharyngeal infection. The aortic and mitral valves are most commonly affected. The clinical course of HACEK endocarditis tends to be subacute, particularly with *Aggregatibacter* or *Cardiobacterium.* However, *K. kingae* endocarditis may have a more aggressive presentation. Compared with non-HACEK endocarditis, HACEK endocarditis occurs in younger patients and has been more frequently associated with embolic, vascular, and immunologic manifestations. Systemic embolization is common. The overall prevalence of major emboli associated with HACEK endocarditis ranges from 28% to 71% in different series. On echocardiography, valvular vegetations are seen in up to 85% of patients. *Aggregatibacter* and *Haemophilus* species cause mitral valve vegetations most often; *Cardiobacterium* is associated with aortic valve vegetations.

The microbiology laboratory should be alerted when a HACEK organism is being considered. Most cultures that ultimately yield a HACEK organism become positive within the first week, especially with improved culture systems such as BACTEC. Studies have not shown that prolonged incubation increases laboratory recovery of clinically significant HACEK isolates. Polymerase chain reaction (PCR) techniques, such as gene amplification of 16S rRNA, can facilitate the diagnosis of HACEK infection of blood or cardiac valves. Other tools, such as matrix-assisted laser desorption ionization–time of flight (MALDI-TOF) mass spectrometry performed directly on agar colonies, can increase the accuracy and speed of diagnosis of HACEK infections.

Because of HACEK organisms' slow growth, antimicrobial susceptibility testing may be difficult, and β-lactamase production may not be detected. Resistance is most commonly noted in *Haemophilus* and *Aggregatibacter* species. Etest methodology may increase the accuracy of susceptibility testing. In recent studies, ceftriaxone and levofloxacin have been active against all isolates. The overall prognosis in both native-valve and prosthetic-valve HACEK endocarditis is excellent and is significantly better than that in endocarditis caused by non-HACEK pathogens.

***Haemophilus* Species** *Haemophilus parainfluenzae* is the most common *Haemophilus* species isolated from cases of HACEK endocarditis. Of patients with HACEK endocarditis due to *Haemophilus* species, 60% have been ill for <2 months before presentation, and 19–50% develop congestive heart failure. Mortality rates as high as 30–50% were reported in older series; however, more recent studies have documented mortality rates of <5%. *H. parainfluenzae* has been isolated from other infections, such as meningitis; brain, dental, pelvic, and liver abscess; pneumonia; urinary tract infection; and septicemia.

***Aggregatibacter* Species** *Aggregatibacter* species are the most common cause of HACEK endocarditis; the species most frequently involved are *A. actinomycetemcomitans*, *A.* (formerly *Haemophilus*) *aphrophilus*, and *A. paraphrophilus*. *Aggregatibacter* is associated with prosthetic-valve endocarditis more often than are *Haemophilus* species. *A. actinomycetemcomitans* can be isolated from soft tissue infections and abscesses in association with *Actinomyces israelii*. Typically, patients who develop *Aggregatibacter* endocarditis have periodontal disease or have recently undergone dental procedures in the setting of underlying cardiac valvular damage. The disease is insidious; patients may be sick for several months before diagnosis. Frequent complications include embolic phenomena, congestive heart failure, and renal failure.

A. actinomycetemcomitans has been isolated from patients with brain abscess, meningitis, endophthalmitis, parotitis, osteomyelitis, urinary tract infection, pneumonia, and empyema, among other infections. *A. aphrophilus* is often associated with bone and joint infection and is an important cause of brain abscess. In one series, *A. aphrophilus* was isolated from brain abscesses in 10% of cases—a rate that is disproportionate to its isolation from oral flora. This species has also been described as a cause of abscess in other organ systems.

***Cardiobacterium* Species** *Cardiobacterium* species, most often *C. hominis*, cause endocarditis primarily in patients with underlying valvular heart disease or with prosthetic valves. These organisms most frequently affect the aortic valve. Many patients have signs and symptoms of long-standing infection before diagnosis, with evidence of arterial embolization, vasculitis, cerebrovascular accidents, immune complex glomerulonephritis, or arthritis at presentation. Embolization, mycotic aneurysms, and congestive heart failure are common complications. A second species, *C. valvarum*, has been described in association with endocarditis.

Eikenella corrodens *E. corrodens* is most frequently recovered from sites of infection in conjunction with other bacterial species. Clinical sources of *E. corrodens* include sites of human bite wounds (clenched-fist injuries), endocarditis, soft tissue infections, osteomyelitis, head and neck infections, respiratory infections, chorioamnionitis, gynecologic infections associated with intrauterine devices, meningitis, brain abscesses, and visceral abscesses. This organism is the least common cause of HACEK endocarditis.

Kingella kingae More than half of cases of *K. kingae* infection are bone and joint infections; the majority of the remaining infections are infective endocarditis, bacteremia, and meningitis. Invasive *K. kingae* infections with bacteremia are associated with upper respiratory tract infections and stomatitis in 80% of cases. Rates of oropharyngeal colonization with *K. kingae* are highest in the first 3 years of life (detected in ~5–10% of children) and appear higher in children regularly attending daycare; colonization coincides with an increased incidence of skeletal infections and other invasive infections due to this organism from the age of 6 months to 4 years. *K. kingae* can be transmitted from child to child and has been the cause of outbreaks among young children. *K. kingae* bacteremia can present with a petechial rash similar to that seen in *Neisseria meningitidis* sepsis.

Because of improved microbiologic methodology and molecular methods such as real-time PCR, the isolation of *K. kingae* is increasingly common. Inoculation of clinical specimens (e.g., synovial fluid) into aerobic blood culture bottles enhances recovery of this organism. PCR studies of blood or joint fluid can identify *K. kingae* in culture-negative cases. Some studies have demonstrated that *K. kingae* has surpassed *Staphylococcus aureus* as the leading cause of septic arthritis and osteomyelitis in children.

Infective endocarditis, unlike other infections with *K. kingae*, occurs in older children and adults. The majority of patients have preexisting valvular disease. There is a high incidence of complications, including arterial emboli, cerebrovascular accidents, tricuspid insufficiency, and congestive heart failure with cardiovascular collapse.

TREATMENT

HACEK Endocarditis

(**Table 158-1**) Ceftriaxone (2 g/d) is first-line therapy for HACEK endocarditis, with a favorable outcome in 80–90% of cases. Data on the use of levofloxacin (750 mg/d) for HACEK endocarditis remain limited, but this drug can be considered an alternative for treatment of patients intolerant of β-lactam therapy. Of note, *Eikenella* is resistant to clindamycin, metronidazole, and aminoglycosides.

Native-valve endocarditis should be treated for 4 weeks with antibiotics, whereas prosthetic-valve endocarditis requires 6 weeks of therapy. The cure rates for HACEK prosthetic-valve endocarditis appear to be high. Unlike prosthetic-valve endocarditis caused by other gram-negative organisms, HACEK endocarditis is often cured with antibiotic treatment alone—i.e., without surgical intervention. In a recent case-control study, 1-year mortality was significantly lower than infective endocarditis caused by viridans group *Streptococcus*.

OTHER FASTIDIOUS GRAM-NEGATIVE BACTERIA

***Capnocytophaga* Species** Like HACEK organisms, this genus of fastidious, fusiform, gram-negative coccobacilli is facultatively anaerobic and requires an atmosphere enriched in carbon dioxide for optimal growth. *Capnocytophaga* species such as *C. ochracea*, *C. gingivalis*, *C. haemolytica*, and *C. sputigena* are part of the oral flora; most infections are contiguous with the oropharynx (e.g., periodontal disease, respiratory tract infections, cervical abscesses, endophthalmitis). These organisms have also been associated with sepsis in immunocompromised hosts, particularly neutropenic patients with oral ulcerations, meningitis, endocarditis, cellulitis, osteomyelitis, and septic arthritis. *Capnocytophaga* species have been isolated from many other sites as well, usually as part of a polymicrobial infection. There is a high prevalence of resistance to β-lactams and macrolides in *Capnocytophaga*; the oral cavity serves as a reservoir for resistance genes to those agents.

C. canimorsus and *C. cynodegmi* are endogenous to the canine and feline mouth (**Chap. 141**). Patients infected with these species frequently have a history of dog or cat bites or of exposure without scratches or bites. Asplenia, glucocorticoid therapy, and alcohol abuse are predisposing conditions that can be associated with severe sepsis with shock and disseminated intravascular coagulation. Patients typically have a petechial rash that can progress from purpuric lesions to gangrene.

TABLE 158-1 Treatment of Infections Caused by HACEK-Group and Other Fastidious Gram-Negative Organisms

ORGANISMS	PREFERRED THERAPY	ALTERNATIVE AGENTS	COMMENTS
Haemophilus spp. *Aggregatibacter* spp. *Cardiobacterium* spp. *Eikenella corrodens* *Kingella kingae*	Ceftriaxone (2 g/d)	Ampicillin/sulbactam (3 g of ampicillin q6h) Levofloxacin (750 mg/d)	Ampicillin/sulbactam resistance has been described in *Haemophilus* and *Aggregatibacter* spp. Data on use of levofloxacin for endocarditis therapy are limited. Fluoroquinolones are not recommended for treatment of patients <18 years of age. Penicillin (16–18 million units q4h) or ampicillin (2 g q4h) can be used if the organism is susceptible. However, because of the slow growth of HACEK bacteria, antimicrobial testing may be difficult, and β-lactamase production may not be detected.
Capnocytophaga spp.	Ampicillin/sulbactam (1.5–3 g of ampicillin q6h)	Ceftriaxone (2 g/d q12–24h)	Penicillin (12–18 million units q4h) should be used if the isolate is known to be susceptible.
Pasteurella multocida	Ampicillin/sulbactam (1.5–3 g of ampicillin q6h)	Ceftriaxone (1–2 g/d q12–24h)	Penicillin should be used if the isolate is known to be susceptible. *P. multocida* is also susceptible to tetracyclines and fluoroquinolones.

TREATMENT
Capnocytophaga Infections

(Table 158-1) Because of increasing β-lactamase production, a penicillin derivative plus a β-lactamase inhibitor—such as ampicillin/sulbactam (1.5–3.0 g of ampicillin every 6 h)—is currently recommended for empirical treatment of infections caused by *Capnocytophaga* species. If the isolate is known to be susceptible, infections with *C. canimorsus* should be treated with penicillin (12–18 million units every 4 h). *Capnocytophaga* is also susceptible to clindamycin (600–900 mg every 6–8 h) and third-generation cephalosporins such as ceftriaxone (2 g every 12–24 h). Antibiotics should be given prophylactically to asplenic patients who have sustained dog-bite injuries.

Pasteurella multocida *P. multocida* is a fastidious, bipolar-staining, gram-negative coccobacillus that colonizes the respiratory and gastrointestinal tracts of domestic animals; oropharyngeal colonization rates are 70–90% in cats and 50–65% in dogs. *P. multocida* can be transmitted to humans through bites or scratches, via the respiratory tract from contact with contaminated dust or infectious droplets, or via deposition of the organism on injured skin or mucosal surfaces during licking. Most human infections affect skin and soft tissue; almost two-thirds of these infections are caused by cats. Patients at the extremes of age or with serious underlying disorders (e.g., cirrhosis, diabetes) are at increased risk for systemic manifestations, including meningitis, peritonitis, osteomyelitis and septic arthritis, endocarditis, septic shock, ecthyma, necrotizing fasciitis, and purpura fulminans, and are more likely not to have evidence of an animal bite. However, cases have also occurred in healthy individuals of all ages. If inhaled, *P. multocida* can cause acute respiratory tract infection, particularly in patients with underlying sinus and pulmonary disease.

TREATMENT
Pasteurella multocida Infections

(Table 158-1) *P. multocida* is susceptible to penicillin, ampicillin, ampicillin/sulbactam, second- and third-generation cephalosporins, tetracyclines, and fluoroquinolones. β-Lactamase–producing strains have been reported.

OTHER GRAM-NEGATIVE BACTERIA

Achromobacter xylosoxidans *Achromobacter* (previously *Alcaligenes*) *xylosoxidans* is an aerobic nonfermenting gram-negative organism that is probably part of the endogenous intestinal flora. It has been isolated from a variety of water sources, including well water, IV fluids, and humidifiers. Immunocompromised hosts, including patients with cancer and postchemotherapy neutropenia, cirrhosis, chronic renal failure, and cystic fibrosis, are at increased risk for infection. Nosocomial outbreaks and pseudo-outbreaks of *A. xylosoxidans* infection have been attributed to contaminated fluids, and clinical illness has been associated with isolates from many sites, including blood (often in the setting of intravascular devices). Community-acquired *A. xylosoxidans* bacteremia usually occurs in the setting of pneumonia. Metastatic skin lesions are present in one-fifth of cases. The reported mortality rate is as high as 67%—a figure similar to rates for other bacteremic gram-negative pneumonias.

TREATMENT
Achromobacter xylosoxidans Infections

(Table 158-2) Treatment is based on in vitro susceptibility testing of all clinically relevant isolates; multidrug resistance is common. Carbapenems, tigecycline, and colistin are typically the most active agents.

TABLE 158-2 Treatment Options for Other Selected Gram-Negative Bacteria[a]

ORGANISM	TREATMENT OPTIONS
Achromobacter xylosoxidans	Carbapenems, tigecycline, colistin
Aeromonas spp.	Fluoroquinolones, third- and fourth-generation cephalosporins, carbapenems, aminoglycosides
Elizabethkingia/ Chryseobacterium spp.	Fluoroquinolones, minocycline, tigecycline, piperacillin/tazobactam
Rhizobium radiobacter	Fluoroquinolones, third- and fourth-generation cephalosporins, carbapenems
Shewanella spp.	Fluoroquinolones, third- and fourth-generation cephalosporins, β-lactam/β-lactamase inhibitors, carbapenems, aminoglycosides
Chromobacterium violaceum	Carbapenems, fluoroquinolones, trimethoprim-sulfamethoxazole

[a]Treatment should be based on in vitro susceptibility testing; multidrug resistance is common among these organisms.

***Aeromonas* Species** *Aeromonas* is a facultative anaerobic gram-negative bacterium. *Aeromonas* infections are most often caused by *A. hydrophila*, *A. caviae*, *A. veronii*, and *A. dhakensis*. *Aeromonas* proliferates in potable water, freshwater, and soil. It remains controversial whether *Aeromonas* is a cause of bacterial gastroenteritis; asymptomatic colonization of the intestinal tract with *Aeromonas* occurs frequently, and no clonally related diarrheal outbreak has been documented. However, rare cases of hemolytic-uremic syndrome following bloody diarrhea have been shown to be secondary to the presence of *Aeromonas*.

Aeromonas causes health care–associated sepsis and bacteremia in infants with multiple medical problems and in immunocompromised hosts, particularly those with cancer or hepatobiliary disease, including cirrhosis. *A. caviae* is associated with health care–related bacteremia. Community-acquired infections include bacteremia, spontaneous bacterial peritonitis, biliary tract infections, and skin and soft tissue infections. Severe soft tissue infections such as necrotizing fasciitis are more common in Taiwan than in Western countries; *Aeromonas* was the most common pathogen associated with skin and soft tissue infections after the tsunami in Thailand. Along with other gram-negative organisms such as *Shewanella* and *Chromobacterium*, *Aeromonas* infections are associated with floods and other hydrologic disasters. *Aeromonas* infection and sepsis can occur in patients with trauma (including severe trauma with myonecrosis), patients with seawater-contaminated wounds, and burn patients exposed to the organism by environmental (freshwater or soil) wound contamination. Reported mortality rates range from 25% among immunocompromised adults with sepsis to >90% among patients with myonecrosis. Patients with *A. dhakensis* bacteremia have higher 14-day mortality rates than do those whose bacteremia is attributable to other species. *Aeromonas* can produce ecthyma gangrenosum (hemorrhagic vesicles surrounded by a rim of erythema with central necrosis and ulceration; **see Fig. A1-34**) resembling the lesions seen in *Pseudomonas aeruginosa* infection. This organism causes nosocomial infections related to catheters, surgical incisions, or use of leeches. Other manifestations include meningitis, peritonitis, pneumonia, and ocular infections.

TREATMENT
Aeromonas Infections

(Table 158-2) *Aeromonas* species are generally susceptible to fluoroquinolones (e.g., ciprofloxacin at a dosage of 500 mg every 12 h PO or 400 mg every 12 h IV), third- and fourth-generation cephalosporins, carbapenems, and aminoglycosides, but resistance to all those agents has been described. Because *Aeromonas* can produce various β-lactamases, including carbapenemases, susceptibility testing must be used to guide therapy. Antibiotic prophylaxis (e.g., with ciprofloxacin) is indicated when medicinal leeches are used.

***Elizabethkingia/Chryseobacterium* Species** *Elizabethkingia meningoseptica* (formerly *Chryseobacterium meningosepticum*), a nonfastidious aerobic nonfermentative gram-negative bacillus, is an important cause of nosocomial infections, including outbreaks due to contaminated fluids (e.g., contaminated sinks, disinfectants, and aerosolized antibiotics) and sporadic infections due to indwelling devices, feeding tubes, and other fluid-associated apparatuses. Most published reports have originated from Asia, particularly Taiwan. A report from South Korea described infections with a high case-fatality rate associated with mechanical ventilation. Outbreaks due to this organism have persisted until extensive cleaning of environmental surfaces and equipment has been performed. Nosocomial *E. meningoseptica* infection usually involves preterm neonates, patients with underlying immunosuppression (e.g., related to malignancy or diabetes), or patients exposed to antibiotics in intensive care. *E. meningoseptica* has been reported to cause meningitis (primarily in neonates), pneumonia, sepsis, endocarditis, bacteremia, eye infections, and soft tissue infections. Other species of *Elizabethkingia* are emerging, identified using MALDI-TOF and 16s rRNA sequencing. In a report of 86 clinical isolates, only 12 (19.8%) of the isolates were *E. meningoseptica;* the majority were *E. anophelis* (51 isolates; 59.3%). More than three-quarters of the isolates were from the lower respiratory tract, and 9.3% were from blood cultures. In a U.S. study of 11 patients with *E. anophelis* infection, all had bloodstream infections. In that series, the patients had comorbidities and recent health care exposure; there was a mortality rate of 18.2%.

Chryseobacterium indologenes has caused bacteremia, sepsis, peritonitis, meningitis, and pneumonia, typically in immunocompromised patients with indwelling devices. Mortality rates have been as high as 50% in some reports; it is unclear whether a poor prognosis is related to underlying comorbidities or to the multidrug-resistant phenotype of the organism.

TREATMENT
Elizabethkingia/Chryseobacterium Infections

(Table 158-2) These organisms are often susceptible to fluoroquinolones, minocycline, tigecycline, and rifampin. They may be susceptible to β-lactam/β-lactamase inhibitor combinations such as piperacillin/tazobactam, but multidrug-resistant isolates are increasing and can possess extended-spectrum β-lactamases and metallo-β-lactamases. In vitro susceptibility testing often indicates activity of agents used against gram-positive bacteria (e.g., vancomycin), but it is unclear that those agents are reliable clinically. Combination therapy may be needed for successful treatment. Susceptibility testing should be performed to guide the choice of optimal agents.

MISCELLANEOUS ORGANISMS

Rhizobium (formerly *Agrobacterium) radiobacter* has usually been associated with infection in the presence of medical devices, including intravascular catheter–related infections, prosthetic-joint and prosthetic-valve infections, and peritonitis caused by dialysis catheters. Cases of endophthalmitis after cataract surgery also have been described. Most *R. radiobacter* infections occur in immunocompromised hosts, especially individuals with malignancy or HIV infection. Elderly patients with septic shock, watery diarrhea, and acute renal failure also have been reported. Strains are usually susceptible to fluoroquinolones, third- and fourth-generation cephalosporins, and carbapenems (Table 158-2).

Shewanella species are ubiquitous nonfermentative gram-negative organisms found in seawater and marine environments. Human disease is caused primarily by *S. putrefaciens* and *S. algae*; *S. algae* may be the more virulent species. Most infections involve skin and soft tissue, ranging from impetigo to necrotizing fasciitis. Patients are exposed to the organism through contact of bites, open wounds, or devitalized tissue with seawater, marine animals, or fresh seafood or through ingestion of seawater or of raw or undercooked seafood, especially shellfish. *Shewanella* species also cause chronic ulcers of the lower extremities, osteomyelitis, biliary tract infections, pneumonia, bacteremia, sepsis, and potentially chronic otitis media. A fulminant course is associated with cirrhosis, hemochromatosis, diabetes mellitus, malignancy, or other severe underlying conditions. In one series of cases from Martinique, 13% of infections were fatal. These organisms are often susceptible to fluoroquinolones, third- and fourth-generation cephalosporins, β-lactam/β-lactamase inhibitors, carbapenems, and aminoglycosides (Table 158-2).

Chromobacterium violaceum is a facultative anaerobic organism found in soil and water in tropical or subtropical regions. After exposure, it can cause rare but serious—often fatal—skin and soft tissue infections of limbs although several recent reports suggest a more benign course with lower mortality. Life-threatening infections with severe sepsis and metastatic abscesses occur most often in patients with underlying illness, particularly in children with defective neutrophil function (e.g., those with chronic granulomatous disease). *C. violaceum* is frequently resistant to multiple drugs; carbapenems are most often used empirically. Fluoroquinolones and trimethoprim-sulfamethoxazole also can be active (Table 158-2).

Ochrobactrum anthropi causes infections related to central venous catheters in compromised hosts; other invasive infections such as bacteremia have been described. *Pseudomonas* (formerly *Flavimonas*) *oryzihabitans* can cause catheter-related bloodstream infections in immunocompromised patients. *Sphingobacterium* is a rare cause of human infection in immunocompromised hosts. It can colonize hospital water systems, respiratory tract equipment, and laboratory instruments. *Sphingomonas paucimobilis* is found in soil and water sources and is a rare cause of infection in both healthy and immunocompromised patients. This organism can cause bloodstream infections, respiratory distress, and sepsis. It has a predilection for bone and soft tissue infection, osteomyelitis, and septic arthritis. A different species, *Sphingomonas koreensis*, was associated with a small cluster of nosocomial cases at one hospital and was traced to a reservoir in the plumbing system. *Ralstonia* species also can contaminate water supplies, including hospital water systems. Cases of bacteremia, osteomyelitis, pneumonia, and meningitis have been described. Other organisms implicated in human infections include *Weeksella* species; *Bergeyella* species; various CDC groups; and *Oligella urethralis*. The reader is advised to consult subspecialty texts and references for further guidance on these organisms.

FURTHER READING

Chambers ST et al: HACEK infective endocarditis: Characteristics and outcomes from a large multi-national cohort. PLoS One 8:e63181, 2013.

Choi MH et al: Risk factors for *Elizabethkingia* acquisition and clinical characteristics of patients, South Korea. Emerg Infect Dis 25:42, 2019.

Kormondi S et al: Human *pasteurellosis* health risk for elderly persons living with companion animals. Emerg Infect Dis 25:229, 2019.

Lutzen L et al: Incidence of HACEK bacteremia in Denmark: A 6-year population-based study. Int J Infect Dis 68:83, 2018.

159 *Legionella* Infections

Steven A. Pergam, Thomas R. Hawn

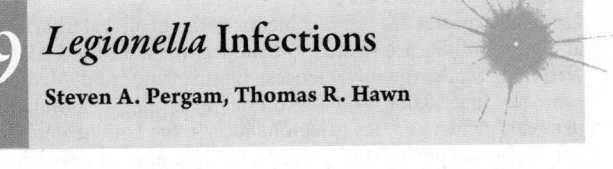

Bacteria of *Legionella* species cause two primary human diseases: *Legionella* pneumonia (often referred to as Legionnaires' disease) and Pontiac fever; collectively, these diseases are referred to as *legionellosis*. Legionnaires' disease was first described in 1976 in an outbreak among members of the American Legion participating in a conference at a hotel in Philadelphia, Pennsylvania. Since their original description,

Legionella-related infections have increased in frequency throughout the world as techniques to diagnose them have improved, clinical awareness has increased, cities have grown, and water systems have both aged and become more complex. Most cases of legionellosis are linked to waterborne exposures. These infections can be either sporadic or due to common-source community or nosocomial exposures. Outbreaks of legionellosis are well described. After exposure, legionellosis occurs primarily among persons with risk factors for disease, including older adults and those with primary organ dysfunction, immunocompromise, or other chronic illnesses. Clinical awareness is important, as the similarity of signs and symptoms of legionellosis to those of other respiratory illnesses can lead to delayed treatment. Despite appropriate therapy, *Legionella* pneumonia is associated with significant morbidity and mortality.

PATHOGEN AND PATHOGENICITY

Legionellae are aerobic gram-negative bacteria that are ubiquitous in aquatic environments, damp soil, and compost. Of the more than 60 *Legionella* species, approximately half have been documented to lead to clinical disease, but most clinical disease is driven by *Legionella pneumophila*, primarily serotype 1. The primary habitats for growth and replication of *Legionella* are amoebae and other free-living protozoa, in which these bacterial species can thrive intracellularly; humans are accidental hosts. Legionellae are reliant on host-derived amino acids and nutrients for intracellular replication. The organisms have a biphasic life cycle: a replicative phase in nutrient-rich conditions (e.g., in their protozoal hosts) and a noninfective transmissive phase under scarcity of resources. Therefore, they can persist in complex biofilms in both natural and engineered water systems (e.g., premise plumbing—a building's hot and cold water piping systems) and are phagocytized by waterborne protozoa. In premise plumbing systems, where temperature and nutrients support the protozoal hosts of legionellae, the bacteria can replicate to concentrations sufficient to cause human infection.

After exposure to *Legionella* through inhalation or aspiration of small aerosol particles, the organisms attach to immune cells and are phagocytized. After phagocytosis, they can evade intracellular defenses and replicate in human alveolar macrophages and monocytes. Pathogenic *Legionella* species have numerous virulence systems that they use to evade the human immune system, including the development of *Legionella*-containing vacuoles within immune cells, downregulation of cytokine receptors, inhibition of host protein synthesis, and avoidance of lysosomal degradation. Despite their ability to replicate and persist in the intracellular environment, innate immune components that target intracellular pathogens—specifically, pattern recognition receptors, including Toll-like receptors and nucleotide-binding oligomerization domain–like receptors—activate immune responses. Adaptive CD4 and CD8 cytotoxic T-cell involvement and these innate immune responses eventually lead to the production of interferon γ and tumor necrosis factor, the promotion of neutrophil recruitment into the lung, and other proinflammatory responses. This cascade can be beneficial and result in clearance of the pathogen. However, these inflammatory responses can also cause immunopathology and adverse outcomes. *L. pneumophila* is more cytopathogenic than most non-*pneumophila Legionella* species, a characteristic that may be partially responsible for its association with severe disease.

EPIDEMIOLOGY

Legionella species are responsible for >50% of all waterborne outbreaks and >10% of disease related to drinking water in the United States. A National Academies of Sciences, Engineering, and Medicine report estimates that 50,000–70,000 Americans develop Legionnaires' disease per year. Incidence rates of legionellosis in the United States are reportedly 2–3 cases per 100,000 persons, but higher rates have been reported in other parts of the world. Numerous global epidemiologic studies assessing legionellosis have shown an increasing prevalence over the past few decades; this increase has been hypothesized to be due to a variety of causes, including an aging population, improved diagnostics, global temperature changes, and an aging water infrastructure. Legionellosis is associated with substantial health care costs.

Legionella species are found throughout the world, but most epidemiologic data focus on legionellosis in large metropolitan areas in Australia/New Zealand, Europe, and North America. Rates of infection in other parts of the world are unknown, as surveillance systems and laboratory testing are less readily available in large portions of Africa and Asia. More than 80% of cases of Legionnaires' disease are linked to *L. pneumophila*—in particular to serotype 1, which is the most frequently isolated *Legionella* pathogen. Although *L. pneumophila* predominates as a cause of disease, species predilection varies regionally. In Australia and New Zealand, for example, the rate of disease due to *Legionella longbeachae* approaches or exceeds that for *L. pneumophila.*

As previously mentioned, most reported cases are due to *L. pneumophila* serotype 1—a reflection of its pathogenicity. However, this predominance is also due to the frequency and ease of use of urinary antigen testing that targets this pathogen and allows more effective diagnosis in the community. It is unclear how large a role non-*pneumophila* species and non–serotype 1 *L. pneumophila* play in disease. However, in studies in Europe, where respiratory cultures are more frequently collected, nearly 10% of Legionnaires' disease patients were infected with species other than *L. pneumophila.* In the United States, nearly 10% of culture-confirmed cases are due to non–serogroup 1 *L. pneumophila.* Immunosuppressed patients, such as cancer patients and transplant recipients, may be more likely to develop pneumonia caused by non-*pneumophila* species such as *Legionella micdadei, Legionella bozemanii,* and *L. longbeachae.*

Despite increases in cases in the United States (**Fig. 159-1**) and throughout the world, incident cases are still thought to be underreported. Many cohort studies of community-acquired pneumonia do not require routine testing for *Legionella* or assess only for *L. pneumophila* serotype 1 (by urinary antigen testing) and therefore may underestimate true prevalence. For example, a large administrative database of studies shows that, of patients with clinically proven community-acquired pneumonia, only 26% underwent *Legionella*-specific testing; even patients with documented risk factors for legionellosis are not always tested for *Legionella.* In studies that routinely assess for legionellosis, the prevalence of *Legionella* pneumonia ranges between 2 and 10% of all community-acquired pneumonia cases. In addition, extrapulmonary presentations and Pontiac fever are less likely to be identified or to result in presentation for health care, and this trend leads to further underestimation of the true burden of legionellosis.

Seasonality and Climate Geoclimatic changes, storms, and seasonality are thought to be important components of *Legionella*'s epidemiology. The incidence of *Legionella* disease increases in the summer and fall—specifically, in warmer weather and with increased rain and humidity. Studies that screen all respiratory samples for *Legionella* find that legionellosis is indeed diagnosed most frequently in the United States during warmer summer/fall months and periods of greater humidity. Furthermore, seasonal storms, which may disrupt water pipes or cause increased flooding, can result in contamination of water systems with soil and lead to *Legionella* exposures. There is concern that, with ongoing climate shifts and rising global temperatures, cases of legionellosis may continue to increase.

Community and Health Care–Associated Outbreaks Small and large clusters and point-source outbreaks of *Legionella* cases lead to public health investigations, but these situations account for only ~5–10% of all *Legionella* cases yearly. Outbreaks occur when two or more people become ill after shared exposures in a community. In health care systems, a single proven case should trigger a *Legionella* investigation. The Centers for Disease Control and Prevention (CDC) recommends an outbreak investigation if a singular patient with *Legionella* is identified who did not leave the facility/campus for the 10 days prior to illness onset. Additionally, an outbreak investigation within a health care system is warranted if there are at least two possible *Legionella* patients who spent any time in the hospital/long-term care facility within 12 months of each other (see "Clinical Presentations" below).

Most common outbreaks are linked to water sources dispersing aerosol droplets that increase the area of particle spread (e.g., cooling

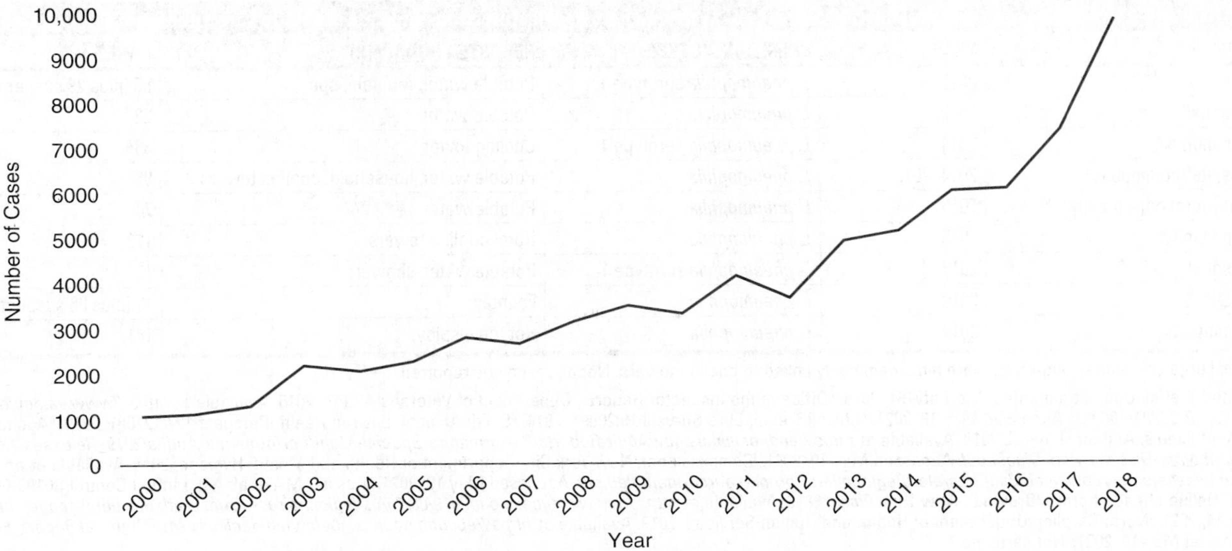

FIGURE 159-1 Increasing *Legionella* disease incidence in the United States over the past two decades (2000–2018). *(From https://www.cdc.gov/legionella/about/history.html.)*

towers or fountains) or to large building structural water systems that cause multiple prolonged exposures (e.g., those in hospitals, hotels, or apartments). The most commonly reported sources include not only cooling towers and fountains but also water misters; centralized heating, ventilation, and air-conditioning systems; hot tubs/spas; pools; ice machines; and showerheads and sinks in large premise plumbing structures (**Fig. 159-2**). When used as primary sources of water, groundwater and wells have also been associated with *Legionella* exposures. The majority of exposures are related to engineered hot-water systems, which are often maintained at temperatures that limit scalding but are ideally suited for *Legionella*'s growth. *Legionella* can also be found in cold water, particularly in warmer summer months, as a consequence of the warming water temperature; engineering issues (e.g., heating lamps in fountains); or unexpected breaks in plumbing systems (e.g., malfunctioning thermostatic mixing valves), which can lead to hot-water contamination of cold-water systems.

Buildings with inconsistent use patterns, such as hotels in seasonal travel destinations, can be linked to outbreaks of legionellosis, as water stagnation leads to low chlorine/disinfectant levels and organism proliferation can reach high enough levels to cause disease. Outbreaks have also been linked to cruise ships and boats. Because of stay-at-home orders related to the SARS-CoV-2 pandemic, there is concern that, once the affected buildings (e.g., hotels) are reopened, limited water movement and stagnation could lead to increases in cases of legionellosis. Modern buildings with water-saving devices, which aim to limit water and energy use, may increase the risk of legionellosis, as they can decrease water temperatures and limit water flow.

Outbreaks in health care and long-term care facilities are identified more frequently than outbreaks in other facilities, as they often bring together at-risk patients, prolonged water exposures, accessible testing, elevated awareness, and regulations that help ensure that cases are more easily linked to common sources. The outbreak examples listed in **Table 159-1** demonstrate the wide variety of common sources and the number of cases associated with such factors. As previously mentioned, most large outbreaks involve cooling towers, which can spread aerosol droplets over a wide area. The largest outbreak reported to date

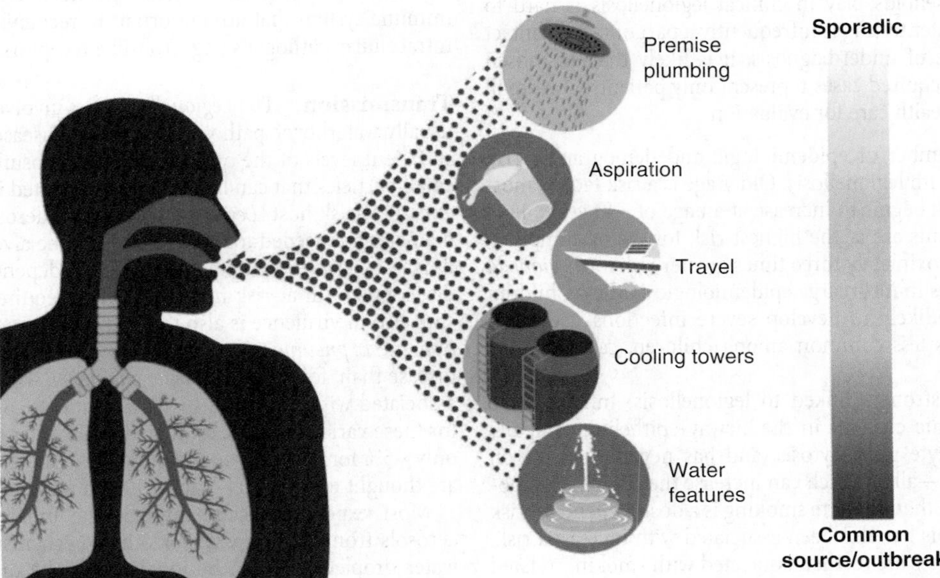

FIGURE 159-2 Sources of waterborne *Legionella* exposures and spectrum of presentation. The spectrum of sporadic to common-source outbreaks is a continuum. For example, premise plumbing in a large office building can lead to a large outbreak, and travel exposures can be related to large outbreaks. Most sporadic cases have no documented source of exposure, while outbreaks often involve mechanisms that spread water aerosol droplets over long distances (e.g., cooling towers), with a consequent ability to infect more individuals. *(Reproduced with permission from Kyoko Kurosawa.)*

TABLE 159-1 Examples of Common-Source Outbreaks of *Legionella pneumophila* Infections Indicate the Wide Variety of Sources and Cases

SITE	YEAR	SPECIES/SEROTYPE	REPORTED SOURCE(S)	CASES
Hotel[a]	2012	*L. pneumophila* serotype 1	Potable water, fountain, spa	85 (plus 29 suspected)
Hospital[b]	2012	*L. pneumophila*	Potable water	22
Community[c]	2014	*L. pneumophila* serotype 1	Cooling tower	334
Hospital/community[d]	2014–2015	*L. pneumophila*	Potable water, household, cooling towers	86
Long-term care facility[e]	2015	*L. pneumophila*	Potable water	74
Community[f]	2015	*L. pneumophila*	Hotel cooling towers	128
Hospital[g]	2018	*L. pneumophila* serotype 1	Potable water, showers	13
Hotel[h]	2019	*L. pneumophila*	Fountain	13 (plus 66 suspected)
Community[i]	2019	*L. pneumophila*	Hot tub display	141

Note: Large community outbreaks were most commonly linked to cooling towers. Not all serotypes reported.

[a]Smith SS et al: Open Forum Infect Dis 2:ofv164, 2015. [b]Office of the Inspector General, Department of Veterans Affairs, 2013. Available at *https://www.va.gov/oig/pubs/VAOIG-13-00994-180.pdf*. Accessed May 19, 2021. [c]Shivaji T et al: Euro Surveill 19:20991, 2014. [d]Smith AF et al: Environ Health Perspect 127:127001, 2019. [e]Auditor General, State of Illinois, Auditor General, 2019. Available at *https://auditor.illinois.gov/Audit-Reports/Performance-Special-Multi/Performance-Audits/2019_Releases/19-Quincy-Legionnaires-Disease-Perf-Digest.pdf*. Accessed May 19, 2021. [f]Commissioner, New York City Department of Health and Mental Hygiene, 2015. Available at *https://www1.nyc.gov/assets/doh/downloads/pdf/han/alert/legionella-in-bronx-source-identified.pdf*. Accessed May 19, 2021. [g]Kessler MA et al: Am J Infect Control S0196-6553(21)00091-2, 2021. Online ahead of print. [h]Brown E: *New York Times*, 2019. Available at *https://www.nytimes.com/2019/08/16/us/legionnaires-disease-atlanta-hotel-reopen.html*. Accessed May 14, 2021. [i]North Carolina Department of Health and Human Services, 2019. Available at *https://epi.dph.ncdhhs.gov/cd/legionellosis/MSFOutbreakReport_FINAL.pdf*. Accessed May 19, 2021. [j]Not serotype 1.

involved a cooling tower in Spain that was linked to 449 documented cases of Legionnaires' disease. Outbreaks are increasingly discussed in the media, such as outbreaks linked to cooling towers in the Bronx neighborhood of New York City, a large hotel outbreak in Atlanta, and outbreaks associated with the Flint, Michigan, water crisis. It is not uncommon for lawsuits to be initiated when deaths are linked to outbreaks.

Sporadic Cases The vast majority of cases of Legionnaires' disease occur sporadically in the community, manifesting as community-acquired pneumonia. Identification of the transmission source is more difficult in community-acquired cases than in nosocomial cases, despite reporting and review by local public health jurisdictions. In nearly 90% of all cases of legionellosis, a source of exposure is never identified. Since the spectrum of water exposures in the community is so broad and incubation periods can be long, identifying individual exposures often is not possible. Transient exposures to common sources, travel-related exposures, and exposures to less commonly linked sources (e.g., potting soil and compost) may also be hard to identify. Furthermore, studies of domestic hot water have demonstrated that 5–30% of households may have *Legionella* species detected, but the role that households play in clinical legionellosis is hard to determine, as home water testing is infrequently a part of usual contact investigations. Because of underdiagnosis, it is likely that diagnosed sporadic community-acquired cases represent only patients who are ill enough to present to health care for evaluation.

Risk Factors A number of epidemiologic and demographic risk factors are associated with legionellosis. Older age is a risk factor; most studies suggest that risk begins to increase at an age of ~40 years. Furthermore, elderly patients are at the highest risk for major complications. Males are at approximately three times greater risk for *Legionella* disease than are females in most large epidemiologic studies. Children are thought to be less likely to develop severe infections. However, since routine testing is less common among children, cases may be underreported.

Smoking has been strongly linked to legionellosis. Inhalation of smoke leads to anatomic changes in the airway epithelium, impairs neutrophil and monocyte phagocytosis, and has negative effects on airway ciliary clearance—all of which can increase the risk of pneumonia. Studies have shown that cigarette smoking is a dose-dependent risk factor. Smoking cannabis has also been associated with increased risk. Risk and severity of illness are further associated with smoking-related pulmonary diseases such as chronic obstructive pulmonary disease or emphysema, which in turn lead to increased risk for complications. Patients with other organ dysfunction/failure, such as those with renal disease (including those on dialysis), hepatic disease, nonsmoking pulmonary disease, and cardiac disease, are at increased risk for legionellosis, although it is unclear whether these factors are related to disease severity or to greater awareness and consequent recognition by health care providers.

Immunosuppressed patients are at increased risk for legionellosis and *Legionella*-related complications. Patients undergoing treatment for cancer (including recipients of hematopoietic cell transplantation) and solid organ transplant recipients are at high risk for legionellosis due to immunosuppression as well as disease- and treatment-related comorbidities. Use of prednisone and other glucocorticoids is strongly associated with legionellosis; however, in light of the heterogeneity of immunosuppressive agents and their use, it remains unclear whether most other single agents are as strongly associated with the disease. Combination immunosuppressive regimens increase risk. Patients treated with these regimens are more likely to develop non-*pneumophila* legionellosis and non–serotype 1 *L. pneumophila* infections that may be missed by routine urinary antigen testing. Patients with autoimmune diseases receiving tumor necrosis factor inhibitors, either with or without concomitant glucocorticoid use, are also at increased risk for legionellosis. Furthermore, studies suggest a possible association of legionellosis with genetic polymorphisms in components of the innate immune system that are important in recognizing and responding to intracellular pathogens (e.g., Toll-like receptors and interferon genes).

Transmission The *Legionella* species involved in human disease are usually waterborne pathogens. However, disease development requires sufficient levels of the organism at the exposure site, the formation of small particles that can be inhaled or aspirated into pulmonary alveoli, and an at-risk host. *Legionella*-containing aerosol particles <10 μm in diameter are needed for deposition into the alveoli. The infective dose during exposures is unknown but likely depends on the host: disease development in at-risk individuals may require a more limited exposure. Strain virulence is also thought to be important in disease development: *L. pneumophila* serotype 1 is more apt to lead to outbreaks and disease than, for example, *Legionella anisa*, which has only rarely been associated with disease in high-risk patients. Because of the necessity for these various factors, estimated attack rates during an exposure are only ~5% for pneumonic presentations. Attack rates for Pontiac fever are thought to be higher—up to 90% among those exposed.

Most exposures occur through the inhalation of contaminated aerosols from mists, sprays, or other mechanisms that produce small water droplets that can be inhaled into the distal alveoli. In homes, the most common sites of exposure are showerheads and sinks, which are especially apt to produce particles small enough for inhalation. The role played by aspiration or microaspiration in exposures is more controversial but is hypothesized to be a secondary route for developing pneumonia. Although human-to-human transmission is not a common pathway, a single presumptive case has been reported. After exposure, *L. pneumophila* has an incubation period of ~2–10 days; this period has been reported to be longer in immunosuppressed hosts. In contrast, symptoms of Pontiac fever occur within 24–48 h after exposure.

CLINICAL PRESENTATIONS

***Legionella* Pneumonia** *Legionella* pneumonia is the most common manifestation of legionellosis. In clinical practice, *Legionella* pneumonia is often referred to by clinicians as an "atypical pneumonia" (i.e., pneumonia that lacks the classic signs and symptoms of bronchopneumonia), and other bacterial pathogens, such as *Chlamydia pneumoniae* and *Mycoplasma pneumoniae*, are also considered as etiologic agents. Initial symptoms of *Legionella* pneumonia are nonspecific and include fever, myalgias, headache, shortness of breath, and either a dry or a productive cough (**Table 159-2**). Patients with pneumonia who present with neurologic or gastrointestinal symptoms such as anorexia, nausea, or vomiting may be more likely than others to have legionellosis. Immunosuppressed patients may present without typical symptoms such as fever. Patients who have recently traveled, who present during a known or possible *Legionella* outbreak, or who develop pneumonia while hospitalized should undergo testing for legionellosis. Patients with severe pneumonia presentations, including acute respiratory failure, and those with pneumonia and sepsis-like presentations should undergo testing for *Legionella* as per current community-acquired pneumonia guidelines.

On clinical examination, patients with *Legionella* pneumonia classically present with rales, rhonchi, and—when consolidation is present—egophony and dullness to percussion. Not all patients, particularly immunosuppressed patients, present with pulmonary findings on clinical examination. Initial laboratory findings in patients with *Legionella* pneumonia include leukocytosis or leukopenia, thrombocytopenia, and elevated liver enzyme levels; hyponatremia and/or renal dysfunction are frequent findings. Levels of nonspecific laboratory markers of inflammation, such as C-reactive protein, can also be elevated; however, procalcitonin levels may not be as useful as a diagnostic tool. Although clinical symptoms and laboratory findings tend to be nonspecific, a number of clinical prediction tools, such as the Winthrop-University Hospital Criteria and the *Legionella* Score, have been developed to assist with the diagnosis of *Legionella* pneumonia. These scoring systems may be more useful for their negative than for their positive predictive value.

An important subset of *Legionella* pneumonia cases are those that are linked to health care systems—i.e., nosocomial cases. Although cases of hospital-acquired legionellosis are rare, their identification is necessary as they may be harbingers of contamination of water systems, devices, and/or potable water sources. Because of the rarity of nosocomial cases, outbreaks have sometimes occurred over years before the source is identified within the health care system. In this regard, the CDC offers the following definitions: (1) A *presumptive* health care–associated case of Legionnaires' disease is one developing in a patient with *Legionella* pneumonia after ≥10 days of continuous stay at a health care facility during the 14 days before onset of symptoms. (2) A *possible* case is one that develops in a patient with *Legionella* pneumonia who has spent a portion of the 14 days before symptom onset in one or more health care facilities but not enough time to meet the criteria for a presumptive case. To ensure that singular cases lead to more system-wide evaluations, the CDC also recommends an investigation if a health care system detects one or more cases of presumptive health care–associated Legionnaires' disease at any time or two or more possible cases within 12 months of one another.

TABLE 159-2 Clinical and Epidemiologic Features of *Legionella* Pneumonia (Legionnaires' Disease) and Pontiac Fever

FEATURE	*LEGIONELLA* PNEUMONIA	PONTIAC FEVER
Incubation period	2–10 days[a]	24–72 h
Pathogenesis	*Legionella* infection	*Legionella* infection or exposure
Common symptoms	Abdominal or chest pain Anorexia Cough, sputum production Confusion[b] Diarrhea[b] Fatigue Fever/chills Headache Myalgias Nausea/vomiting[b] Shortness of breath	Cough Diarrhea Fatigue Fever/chills Headache Myalgias Nausea/vomiting Vertigo
Risk factors	Age >40 years Male Smoker Immunosuppressed host Neurologic disease Chronic lung disease Organ dysfunction/ chronic illness	Factors associated with increased exposure
Attack rate among exposed individuals	~5%[c]	~90%
Hospitalization rate	>90%	<1%
ICU admission rate	30–50%	Extremely low
Treatment	Antibiotics (macrolide or fluoroquinolone)	Supportive care
Case-fatality rate[d]	10%	Extremely low

[a]Incubation period in immunosuppressed hosts may be longer than 14 days. [b]This symptom is strongly associated with *Legionella* pneumonia. [c]Attack rates are highly dependent on method of exposure, level of the pathogen in source water, and host's level of risk. [d]Case-fatality rates are much higher among immunosuppressed patients and those with severe underlying lung disease, ranging from 30 to 50%.

Abbreviation: ICU, intensive care unit.

Source: Modified from *https://www.cdc.gov/legionella/clinicians/clinical-features.html*.

PONTIAC FEVER

Pontiac fever is described as an influenza-like illness whose primary symptoms are fever, headache, myalgias, chills, vertigo, nausea, vomiting, and diarrhea (Table 159-2). Compared with *Legionella* pneumonia, Pontiac fever is a milder, self-limited illness that is defined by the absence of pneumonia. Although studies have shown that Pontiac fever is associated with exposure to higher counts of colony-forming units in water sources, the role of the pathogen in the disease is not clear. Symptoms usually develop 24–48 h after exposure and can last for 2–5 days. Since many other illnesses resemble Pontiac fever, the diagnosis usually relies on the recognition of typical clinical features during an outbreak situation; therefore, cases are likely to be missed even when patients present for health care. Studies documenting specific *Legionella* species as the cause of Pontiac fever clusters find that most are due to *L. pneumophila* exposure; however, non-*pneumophila* species such as *L. anisa* have also been associated with this presentation.

Extrapulmonary Disease A number of rare presentations for legionellosis have been described. Skin and soft tissue infections that resemble cellulitis, including cases due to tap water contamination of postsurgical wounds, have been reported. Endocarditis, primarily culture-negative prosthetic valve endocarditis, and myocarditis and pericarditis have also been reported. Rarely, *Legionella* species have been associated with septic arthritis and sinusitis.

DIAGNOSIS

The diagnosis of legionellosis on the basis of clinical findings alone is difficult. Additional workup is needed to make a definitive diagnosis, even when cases are potentially linked to a possible outbreak. To make

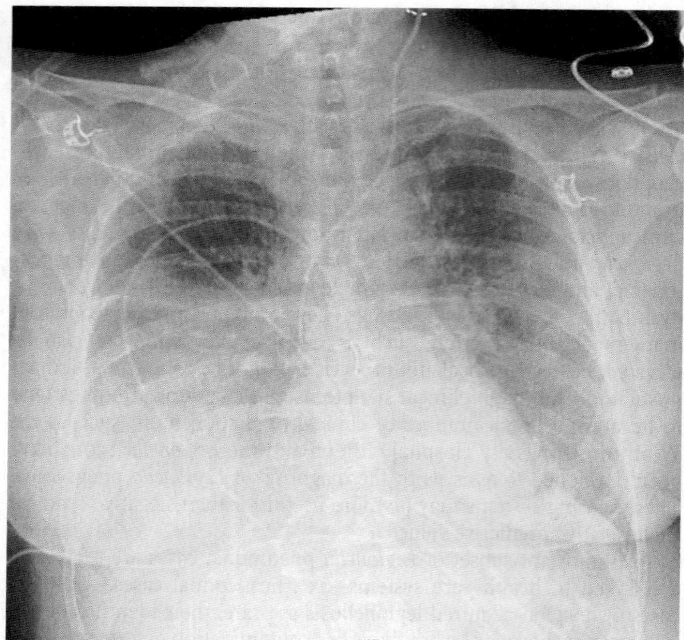

FIGURE 159-3 Chest x-ray of a patient with *Legionella* pneumonia and right-lower-lobe consolidation. A 64-year-old woman presented with fever, dry cough, and shortness of breath 7 days after returning from international travel. *Legionella* urinary antigen testing was positive for *L. pneumophila* serotype 1.

a diagnosis, laboratory confirmation is needed, and invasive procedures may be required—e.g., bronchoscopy, particularly for patients whose results on urinary antigen testing are negative and who cannot produce sufficient sputum for testing or for patients with severe disease requiring intensive care unit (ICU) admission. As current treatment guidelines for community-acquired pneumonia recommend empirical coverage that includes antibiotics active against *Legionella* species, diagnostic testing is not routine even among persons who meet the criteria for *Legionella*-specific testing. Furthermore, not all currently available diagnostic laboratory assays are accessible or rapidly available in primary care clinics, urgent care facilities, and emergency rooms where patients may present with their initial symptoms.

Radiologic Findings On chest radiography, *Legionella* pneumonia presents as focal infiltrates or consolidations, most frequently in the lower lobes, that are indistinguishable from those due to other causes of pneumonia **(Fig. 159-3)**. On CT, air-space disease in one or more lobes is often with associated ground-glass opacities **(Fig. 159-4)**; pleural effusions and lymphadenopathy are less frequently seen. In immunocompromised patients, *Legionella* can present with similar lower-lobe consolidations or atypically as pulmonary nodules—with or without cavitation—that mimic fungal infections **(Fig. 159-5)** or even as lung abscesses. Progression during early therapy is not uncommon in immunosuppressed patients.

Laboratory Diagnostics • CULTURE Cultures—of sputum, bronchoalveolar lavage fluid, lung tissue, or extrapulmonary sites—are the gold standard for diagnosis of *Legionella* pneumonia because they are critical for epidemiologic investigations. *Legionella* species require special nutrients, such as cysteine, for growth and therefore require specialized media, such as buffered charcoal yeast extract (BCYE) agar. Legionellae grow slowly, usually over 3–5 days, with non-*pneumophila* species often requiring longer incubation times. Once growth is seen, *Legionella* can be stained with standard Gram's stain, and colonies often fluoresce blue or white under ultraviolet light. *L. micdadei* is the only *Legionella* species that is also modified-acid-fast positive. Sensitivity varies with the sample but is highest among lower respiratory tract samples. At some referral centers, lower-tract samples from high-risk immunosuppressed patient populations are routinely sent for culture. Unfortunately, because of current community-acquired pneumonia guidelines, patients are often treated empirically, and many either never have samples sent for *Legionella*-specific cultures or have such samples collected only after antibiotic administration, which decreases sensitivity. Respiratory cultures from patients with legionellosis are crucial during outbreak investigations, as clinical and environmental cultures can be compared by pulsed-gel electrophoresis or molecular sequencing to help identify common-source outbreaks; cultures are also used for serotyping of *L. pneumophila*.

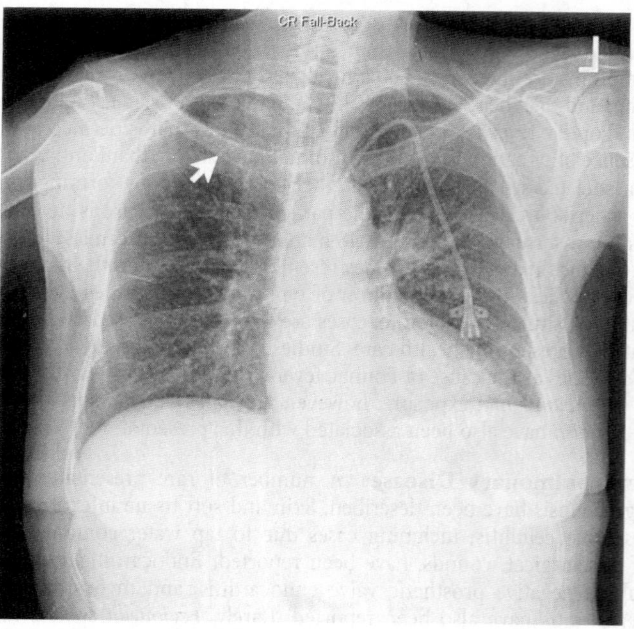

A

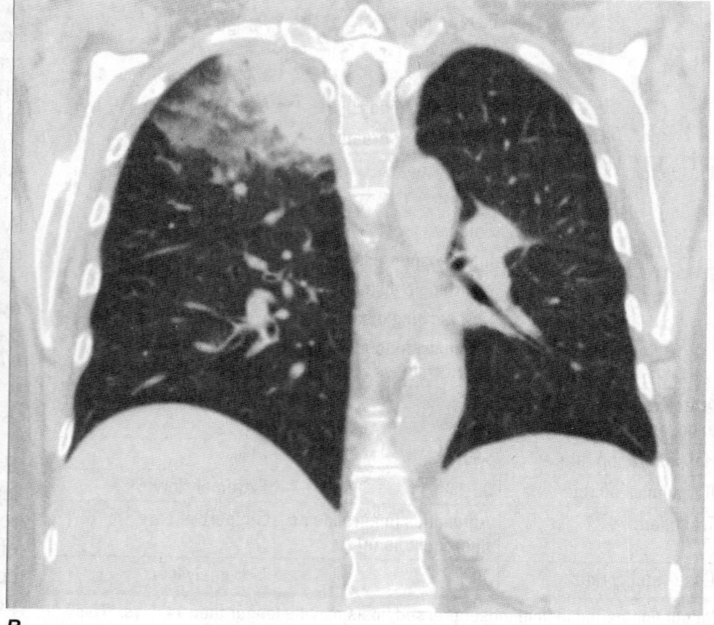

B

FIGURE 159-4 Right-upper-lobe infiltrate in a patient with *L. pneumophila* pneumonia on chest x-ray and CT. An immunosuppressed patient from a long-term care facility presented with cough, sputum production, fever, and chills. New renal insufficiency and hyponatremia were documented. A chest x-ray (***A***) was consistent with a small right-upper-lobe infiltrate (*white arrow*), which was confirmed by CT (***B***). Urinary antigen testing for *L. pneumophila* serotype 1 was negative, but polymerase chain reaction on bronchoaveolar lavage fluid was positive for *L. pneumophila*.

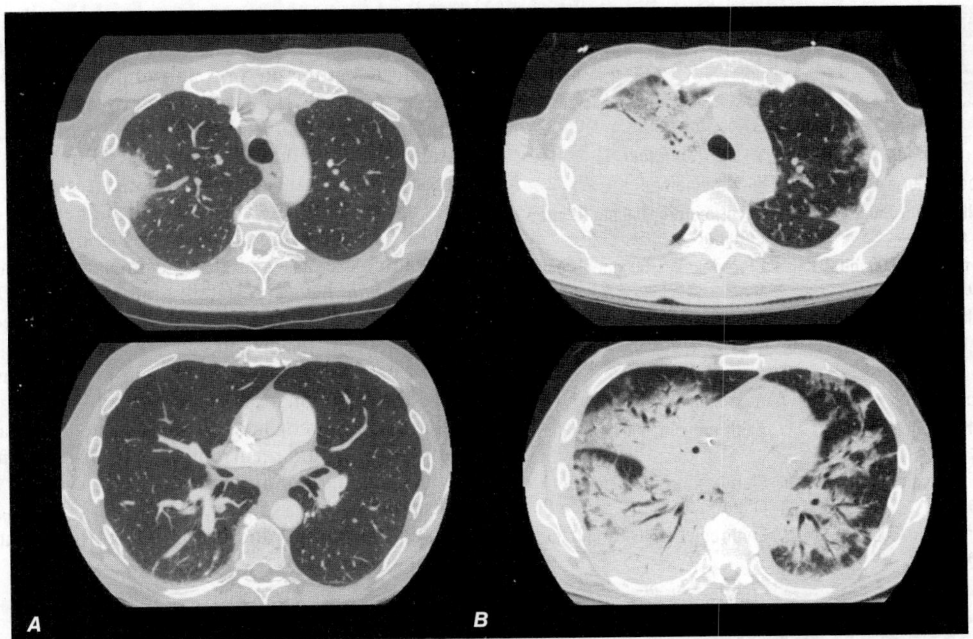

FIGURE 159-5 Nodular disease presentation on CT in an immunosuppressed patient infected with *L. micdadei*. *A.* Presenting CT scan in a hematopoietic cell transplant recipient presenting with fever and cough. A pulmonary nodule was noted in the right upper lobe. Bronchoscopy was performed; cultures were positive on day 5 for small white colonies on buffered charcoal yeast extract plates, and these colonies were eventually identified as *L. micdadei*. ***B.*** Repeat CT scan at day 12 demonstrated an enlarging nodule, diffuse infiltrates, and possible cavitation. The patient required intensive care unit admission and intubation despite appropriate targeted antibiotic therapy.

URINARY ANTIGEN TESTING *Legionella* urinary antigen tests are widely available at many hospitals and commercial laboratories and are characterized by ease of use, simple specimen collection, rapid turnaround time, high sensitivity, and the ability to detect the most prevalent *Legionella* species associated with clinical disease—*L. pneumophila* serotype 1. Urinary antigen testing has limitations, however: it detects only *L. pneumophila* serotype 1 and gives false-negative results in most cases caused by clinically important non–serotype 1 *L. pneumophila* and non-*pneumophila* species. Sensitivity for *L. pneumophila* serotype 1 is ~70% for most assays, but specificity is very high. The urinary antigen test can be negative very early in the disease and can remain positive for months after an infection, particularly in immunosuppressed patient populations; it cannot be used for patients who are anuric. Urinary antigen testing is not recommended for routine use in screening for exposures among asymptomatic patients in outbreak investigations.

SEROLOGY Acute- and convalescent-phase titers of antibody to *Legionella* have limited sensitivity in diagnosing acute Legionnaires' disease but can be useful during outbreak investigations. A case is *confirmed* by documenting a fourfold or greater rise in titer of specific serum antibody to *L. pneumophila* serogroup 1. A case is *suspected* in tests using pooled antigens by (1) a fourfold or greater rise in antibody titer to specific species (e.g., *L. longbeachae*) or non–serogroup 1 *L. pneumophila* or (2) a fourfold or greater rise in antibody titer to multiple species of *Legionella*. Some experts think that a single antibody level of ≥1:256 may be an adequate basis for diagnosing a presumptive case, but most prefer paired serology for confirmation. Serology is an imperfect tool; data suggest that as many as 20–30% of patients with proven legionellosis may not mount an antibody response that is sufficient for diagnosis, and the sensitivity and specificity of seroconversion with regard to non-*pneumophila Legionella* species are unclear among patients with altered immunity. Serology can provide important information for epidemiologic investigations, helping to identify additional cases missed by other diagnostic methods. In addition, the use of serologic testing during outbreak studies allows the investigation of patients without severe disease (e.g., those with Pontiac fever).

DIRECT FLUORESCENT ANTIBODY TESTING The sensitivity of direct fluorescent antibody (DFA) testing of sputum is lower than that of other testing modalities, ranging from 20 to 70% depending on the assay used. Most available assays target specific species (e.g., *L. pneumophila*) or serotypes. DFA testing may have a higher positive predictive value in patients with severe pneumonia or symptoms consistent with Legionnaires' disease, but it is not recommended for screening of low-risk patients because of the frequency of false-positive results.

MOLECULAR TESTING Polymerase chain reaction (PCR), loop-mediated isothermal amplification (LAMP), and other nucleic acid amplification tests are highly sensitive for lower respiratory tract specimens (e.g., sputum) and are becoming more widely available. Molecular methods can detect *Legionella* from multiple sources but are most commonly used for respiratory specimens such as sputum and bronchoalveolar lavage fluid. PCR is more sensitive than culture; in some studies, up to two to four times as many cases of lower tract disease were detected only by molecular methods. Molecular techniques also are useful in diagnosing infection in patients during antibiotic therapy. However, PCR methods are not used to determine *L. pneumophila* serotypes—information that is needed for epidemiologic investigations—and most commercially available assays target only *L. pneumophila*. Multiplex PCR tests for pneumonia and other respiratory pathogens are increasingly available and may include *L. pneumophila*.

TREATMENT

Legionella Pneumonia

Treatment of *Legionella* pneumonia involves antibiotics that target intracellular pathogens, whereas patients with Pontiac fever do not require antibiotic therapy. Macrolides and fluoroquinolones are the first-line agents for *Legionella* pneumonia according to guidelines in the United States and Europe (**Table 159-3**). Macrolides disrupt protein production critical for survival of the organism. Although erythromycin or clarithromycin is effective, azithromycin is the preferred agent, as it is easier to tolerate and is involved

TABLE 159-3 Treatment Options for *Legionella* Disease

	OPTIONS FOR INDICATED DISEASE SEVERITY[a]	
DISEASE	**MILD**	**MODERATE/SEVERE[b]**
Pontiac fever	None	N/A
Legionella pneumonia	***Either***	***Either***
	A fluoroquinolone	A fluoroquinolone
	Levofloxacin, 750 mg PO once daily; *or*	**Levofloxacin, 750 mg IV once daily;** *or*
	Ciprofloxacin, 500 mg PO bid; *or*	Ciprofloxacin, 500 mg IV bid; *or*
	Moxifloxacin, 400 mg PO once daily	Moxifloxacin, 400 mg PO bid
	or	***or***
	A macrolide	A macrolide
	Azithromycin, 500 mg PO daily; *or*	**Azithromycin, 500 mg IV daily;** *or*
	Clarithromycin, 400 mg PO daily; *or*	Clarithromycin, 400 mg IV bid; *or*
	Erythromycin, 500 mg PO daily	Erythromycin, 1000 mg IV qid
		or
		Combination therapy[c]

[a]Agents in bold type are considered first-line treatments. [b]All immunosuppressed patients should be considered to have moderate or severe disease and should be started on IV therapy if possible. All patients requiring inpatient care should receive IV therapy until their condition improves, at which point they can be switched to an oral agent. [c]Can consider combination therapy despite limited data demonstrating improved outcomes in severely ill patients. Combinations include either (1) a fluoroquinolone plus a macrolide or (2) a fluoroquinolone or a macrolide with a secondary agent. Secondary agents include doxycycline, minocycline, rifampin, and trimethoprim-sulfamethoxazole, all with varying efficacy for treatment.

Abbreviation: N/A, not applicable.

in fewer drug-drug interactions. Azithromycin and clarithromycin also reach higher intracellular concentrations than erythromycin.

Fluoroquinolones are potent agents against *Legionella* species. Data from both in vitro and in vivo models of infection suggest that fluoroquinolones may be more effective than macrolides, but no randomized clinical trials have yet compared the two drug classes for treatment of legionellosis. In nonrandomized observational studies, fluoroquinolones have been shown to be more effective than macrolides (erythromycin and clarithromycin) in terms of fever resolution and decreased duration of hospitalization; other such studies have shown no difference in outcome.

Both macrolides and fluoroquinolones are available as IV and oral formulations. Most experts prefer IV therapy during the first few days of treatment for patients with severe *Legionella* pneumonia. Secondary agents, such as rifampin, doxycycline, minocycline, and, less frequently, trimethoprim-sulfamethoxazole, have also been used, with mixed responses. Tigecycline, a third-generation glycylcycline related to tetracyclines, has been used for treatment of patients with significant antibiotic allergies. The novel aminomethylcycline antibiotic omadacycline appears to be efficacious in vitro, but its clinical efficacy has not been studied to date, and it is not currently recommended for routine use. Although data are limited, combination therapy does not appear to improve outcomes.

The duration of treatment for patients with mild disease is usually 10–14 days, but most symptoms will improve within the first 3–5 days of therapy. For immunosuppressed patients and patients with severe disease, a 3-week course of therapy is recommended. The duration of therapy for extrapulmonary manifestations of *Legionella* infection is unknown and depends on the site involved and clinical improvement. Resistance to macrolides and fluoroquinolones has been reported only rarely. Susceptibility testing is not routinely performed but is available in specialized laboratories and public health departments.

OUTCOMES

Legionella infections are associated with significant morbidity and mortality, leading to hospitalization and ICU admission of most patients who develop pneumonia. Case-fatality rates of *Legionella* pneumonia are reported to be ~10%, with death more likely among patients who are admitted to the ICU or have major comorbidities. Among patients in whom antibiotic treatment is delayed, mortality rates are approximately three times higher than among those treated earlier. Patients who develop nosocomial pneumonia attributable to health care–associated exposures, particularly those due to *L. pneumophila*, have case-fatality rates of ~25%. Death is a much more common outcome among immunocompromised hosts, whose mortality rates can reach ~30–50%. Assessment of long-term follow-up among patients who survive *Legionella* pneumonia demonstrates that more than one-quarter have ongoing complications after recovery, including recurrent hospitalizations, acute renal failure, respiratory complications, and recurrent pneumonias, among those who recover from severe disease. In contrast, recovery from Pontiac fever usually takes place within 3–5 days, as the disease is self-limiting; hospitalization, complications, and death related to Pontiac fever are extremely rare.

PREVENTION

Prevention of legionellosis starts with addressing water systems. Large municipal water systems provide water throughout the globe, but the quality of these systems varies regionally; many areas have limited access to potable water. Only limited regions have the resources to address *Legionella* water contamination; most water-monitoring agencies focus on control of enteric pathogens, such as *Escherichia coli* and other coliform bacteria, and do not have an adequate infrastructure to address *Legionella*. Even in countries and cities with more complex water systems, there is wide variation in how waterborne pathogens are addressed, and rules and regulations are often country dependent. In the Netherlands, for example, chlorination is not routine, whereas the United Kingdom and most countries in the European Union use chlorine routinely as the primary mode of disinfection for public water systems. Although regulated by the Environmental Protection Agency, management and treatment strategies in the United States vary by state and, in some instances, by city.

Prevention in the United States focuses on health care organizations and hospitals, where water-based exposures are more often linked to case fatalities. Federal requirements to reduce *Legionella* risk in the United States were first established in June 2017, when the Centers for Medicare and Medicaid Services required that all health care organizations develop and adhere to water management plans. These plans require the development of multidisciplinary teams, an understanding of the organization's water system, identification of high-risk areas (e.g., transplant units, oncology floors), identification of at-risk structures for *Legionella* growth, implementation and monitoring of control measures, methods for intervention if control measures fail, and procedures to assure documentation that policies are followed. All medical centers are required to have an awareness of water quality and to have systems in place to help prevent nosocomial *Legionella* pneumonia. Such policies leave water quality assessment, including testing for *Legionella*, up to the individual facility. In addition to hospitals, an increasing number of cities, including New York City, require similar water-management plans for cooling towers, with registration, testing, and mitigation options.

Even if detected in regional water systems, *Legionella* becomes a human pathogen only after replication in premise plumbing systems. In buildings, *Legionella* finds the ideal environment for logarithmic growth, which leads to exposures and subsequent disease. An important first step in prevention within hospitals is a review of plumbing systems to identify areas of concern and a review of impact areas such as dental clinics, ICUs, rehabilitation units, and units that house high-risk patients. Specific water features, such as therapy pools, ice machines, and decorative fountains, need policies for cleaning and disinfection. Targeted approaches to management of cooling towers, such as high-efficiency drift eliminators and routine maintenance, are important considerations. In addition, areas that have undergone recent construction or renovation should be flagged, with prevention policies in place to address the associated risks. New construction or structural updates can lead to water stagnation, while modifications to plumbing can disrupt biofilms. Units with older premise plumbing are thought to be at higher risk, but even brand new facilities can become colonized during construction, with consequent outbreaks.

Testing for *Legionella* is an important step when presumptive or possible nosocomial pneumonia cases occur and can help address a facility's potential risks. There are a number of methods for environmental testing for *Legionella*, but environmental cultures are used in most hospitals because they quantify *Legionella* levels, allow species identification/serotyping, and can link environmental sources to nosocomial outbreaks. Testing usually focuses on locations where the index patient(s) may have had potential waterborne exposures (e.g., at showers and sinks). Other adjacent areas, along with those noted to be high-risk locations within the hospital, should be considered for additional testing; positive results should widen the testing area. Proactive testing is increasingly being used to preclude nosocomial cases; however, if testing is planned, it should be coupled with a management plan that addresses how *Legionella* will be dealt with if it is found in the water system and where and how frequently testing should be done; we recommend biannual or quarterly testing of select sites within hospital systems.

If a common-source outbreak is discovered, a number of approaches can be used to address *Legionella*. Regardless of source, immediate limitation of ongoing water exposures for patients in the affected room, unit, or floor is a crucial step in avoiding additional cases. Removing or replacing water features associated with exposures, such as decorative fountains and affected equipment or plumbing devices, may be needed. Immediate interventions such as heat shock (increasing water temperatures for a limited period) and hyperchlorination may also be useful as short-term steps in addressing an outbreak.

The addition of a disinfectant to the water system is one of the most common ways to address the presence of *Legionella*. Chemical disinfection with agents such as chlorine or monochloramine and copper and silver ionization are commonly used for secondary disinfection. Use of disinfectants requires routine maintenance and monitoring of chemical or ion levels to assure that they are sufficient for prevention. Lack of monitoring and system failures have led to breakthrough nosocomial *Legionella* cases. Another option is water filtration, which either can serve as a primary method for prevention or can be used in combination with secondary disinfection. Filters—either in-line with plumbing or at point-of-use sites—can be considered for either short- or long-term prevention during an outbreak. However, filters have a limited life span, can weaken water pressure, and are costly to maintain.

FURTHER READING

Cassell K et al: Estimating the true burden of Legionnaires' disease. Am J Epidemiol 188:1686, 2019.

Centers for Disease Control and Prevention: Developing a water management program to reduce *Legionella* growth and spread in buildings: A practical guide to implementing industry standards. June 5, 2017. Available at *https://www.cdc.gov/legionella/wmp/toolkit/index.html*. Accessed May 19, 2021.

Centers for Disease Control and Prevention: Legionnaires' disease surveillance summary report, United States 2016–2017. Available at *https://www.cdc.gov/legionella/health-depts/surv-reporting/2016-17-surv-report-508.pdf*. Accessed May 19, 2021.

National Academies of Sciences, Engineering, and Medicine: *Management of Legionella in Water Systems*. Washington, DC, The National Academies Press, 2020.

Pierre DM et al: Diagnostic testing for Legionnaires' disease. Ann Clin Microbiol Antimicrob 16:1, 2017.

160 Pertussis and Other *Bordetella* Infections

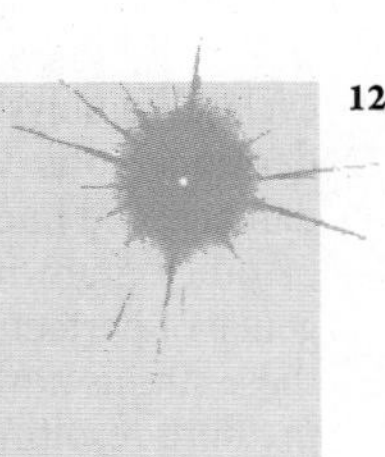

Karina A. Top, Scott A. Halperin

Pertussis is an acute infection of the respiratory tract caused by *Bordetella pertussis*. The word *pertussis* means "violent cough," which aptly describes the most consistent and prominent feature of the illness. The inspiratory sound made at the end of an episode of paroxysmal coughing gives rise to the common name for the illness, "whooping cough." However, this feature is variable: it is uncommon among infants ≤6 months of age and is frequently absent in older children and adults. The Chinese name for pertussis is "the 100-day cough," which describes the clinical course of the illness accurately. The identification of *B. pertussis* was first reported by Bordet and Gengou in 1906, and vaccines were produced over the following two decades.

MICROBIOLOGY

Of the 10 identified species in the genus *Bordetella*, only four are of major medical significance. *B. pertussis* infects only humans and is the most important *Bordetella* species causing human disease. *B. parapertussis* causes an illness in humans that is similar to pertussis but is typically milder; co-infections with *B. parapertussis* and *B. pertussis* have been documented. With improved polymerase chain reaction (PCR) diagnostic methodology, up to 20% of patients with a pertussis-like syndrome have been found to be infected with *B. holmesii*, formerly thought to be an unusual cause of bacteremia. *B. bronchiseptica* is an important pathogen of domestic animals that causes kennel cough in dogs, atrophic rhinitis and pneumonia in pigs, and pneumonia in cats. Both respiratory infection and opportunistic infection due to *B. bronchiseptica* are reported occasionally in humans. *B. petrii*, *B. hinzii*, and *B. ansorpii* have been isolated from patients who are immunocompromised.

Bordetella species are gram-negative pleomorphic aerobic bacilli that share common genotypic characteristics. *B. pertussis* and *B. parapertussis* are the most similar of the species, but *B. parapertussis* does not express the gene coding for pertussis toxin. *B. pertussis* is a slow-growing fastidious organism that requires selective medium and forms small, glistening, bifurcated colonies. Suspicious colonies are presumptively identified as *B. pertussis* by direct fluorescent antibody testing or by agglutination with species-specific antiserum. *B. pertussis* is further differentiated from other *Bordetella* species by biochemical and motility characteristics.

B. pertussis produces a wide array of toxins and biologically active products that are important in its pathogenesis and in immunity. Most of these virulence factors are under the control of a single genetic locus that regulates their production, resulting in antigenic modulation and phase variation. Although these processes occur both in vitro and in vivo, their importance in the pathobiology of the organism is unknown; they may play a role in intracellular persistence and person-to-person spread. The organism's most important virulence factor is *pertussis toxin*, which is composed of a B oligomer–binding subunit and an enzymatically active A protomer that ADP-ribosylates a guanine nucleotide–binding regulatory protein (G protein) in target cells, producing a variety of biologic effects. Pertussis toxin has important mitogenic activity, affects the circulation of lymphocytes, and serves as an adhesin for bacterial binding to respiratory ciliated cells. Other important virulence factors and adhesins are *filamentous hemagglutinin*, a component of the cell wall, and *pertactin*, an outer-membrane protein. *Fimbriae*, bacterial appendages that play a role in bacterial attachment, are the major antigens against which agglutinating antibodies are directed. These agglutinating antibodies have historically been the primary means of serotyping *B. pertussis* strains. Other virulence factors include tracheal cytotoxin, a peptidoglycan fragment, which causes inflammatory respiratory epithelial damage; adenylate cyclase-hemolysin toxin, which impairs host phagocytic cell function; dermonecrotic toxin, which may contribute to respiratory mucosal damage; and lipooligosaccharide, which has properties similar to those of other gram-negative bacterial endotoxins. Since 2010, the emergence of pertactin-negative strains has been observed worldwide, and these strains now predominate in some regions, perhaps from immune pressure resulting from the use of pertactin-containing acellular pertussis vaccines.

■ EPIDEMIOLOGY

Pertussis is a highly communicable disease, with attack rates of 80–100% among unimmunized household contacts and 20% within households in well-immunized populations. The infection has a worldwide distribution, with cyclical outbreaks every 3–5 years (a pattern that has persisted despite widespread immunization). Pertussis occurs in all months; however, in North America, its activity peaks in autumn and winter.

In developing countries, pertussis remains an important cause of infant morbidity and death. The reported incidence of pertussis worldwide has decreased as a result of improved vaccine coverage **(Fig. 160-1)**. However, coverage rates are still <60% in many developing nations; the World Health Organization (WHO) estimates that 90% of the burden of pertussis is in developing regions. In addition, over-reporting of immunization coverage and under-reporting of disease result in substantial underestimation of the global burden of pertussis. The WHO estimates that there were 161,000 deaths from pertussis among children <5 years of age in 2014.

Before the institution of widespread immunization programs in the developed world, pertussis was one of the most common infectious causes of morbidity and death. In the United States before the 1940s, between 115,000 and 270,000 cases of pertussis were reported annually, with an average yearly rate of 150 cases per 100,000 population. With universal childhood immunization, the number of reported cases fell by >90%, and mortality rates decreased even more dramatically. Only 1010 cases of pertussis were reported in 1976 **(Fig. 160-2)**. After that historic low, rates of pertussis increased slowly. In recent years, pertussis epidemics have been reported with increasing frequency in high-income countries, including Australia, the United Kingdom, and the United States. The United States experienced widespread outbreaks of pertussis in 2005, 2010, 2012, and 2014 at levels not seen in 40–50 years (48,000 reported cases in 2012).

Although thought of as a disease of childhood, pertussis can affect people of all ages and is a known cause of prolonged coughing illness in adolescents and adults. In unimmunized populations, pertussis incidence peaks during the preschool years, and well over half of children have the disease before reaching adulthood. In highly immunized populations such as those in North America, the peak incidence is among infants <1 year of age who have not completed the three-dose primary immunization series. An increase in pertussis incidence among adolescents and adults began in the late 1990s and led to the introduction of an adolescent booster dose across North America by 2006. While the disease burden among adolescents decreased initially, children 7–10 years of age emerged as a high-risk group during a major outbreak in 2010. Most of the affected children were fully immunized. Subsequent outbreaks in 2012 and 2014 showed a shift in epidemiology, with pertussis incidence increasing among adolescents while still remaining elevated among 10-year-olds. The most highly affected cohorts were those who received acellular pertussis vaccines in infancy. Although adults contribute a smaller proportion of reported cases of pertussis than do children and adolescents, this difference may be related to a greater degree of under-recognition and under-reporting. A number of studies of prolonged coughing illness suggest that *B. pertussis* may be the etiologic agent in 12–30% of adults with cough that does not improve within 2 weeks. In one study of the efficacy of an acellular pertussis vaccine in adolescents and adults, the incidence of pertussis in the placebo group was 3.7–4.5 cases per 1000 person-years. Although this prospective cohort study yielded a lower estimate than the studies of cough illness, its results still translate to ~1 million cases of pertussis annually among adults in the United States. In addition, asymptomatic pertussis infection is common and appears to contribute to disease transmission.

Severe morbidity and high mortality rates, however, are restricted almost entirely to infants. In the United States between 2008 and 2011, 83% of pertussis deaths involved infants ≤3 months and >35% of infants with pertussis required hospitalization. Although school-age children are the source of infection for most households, adults are

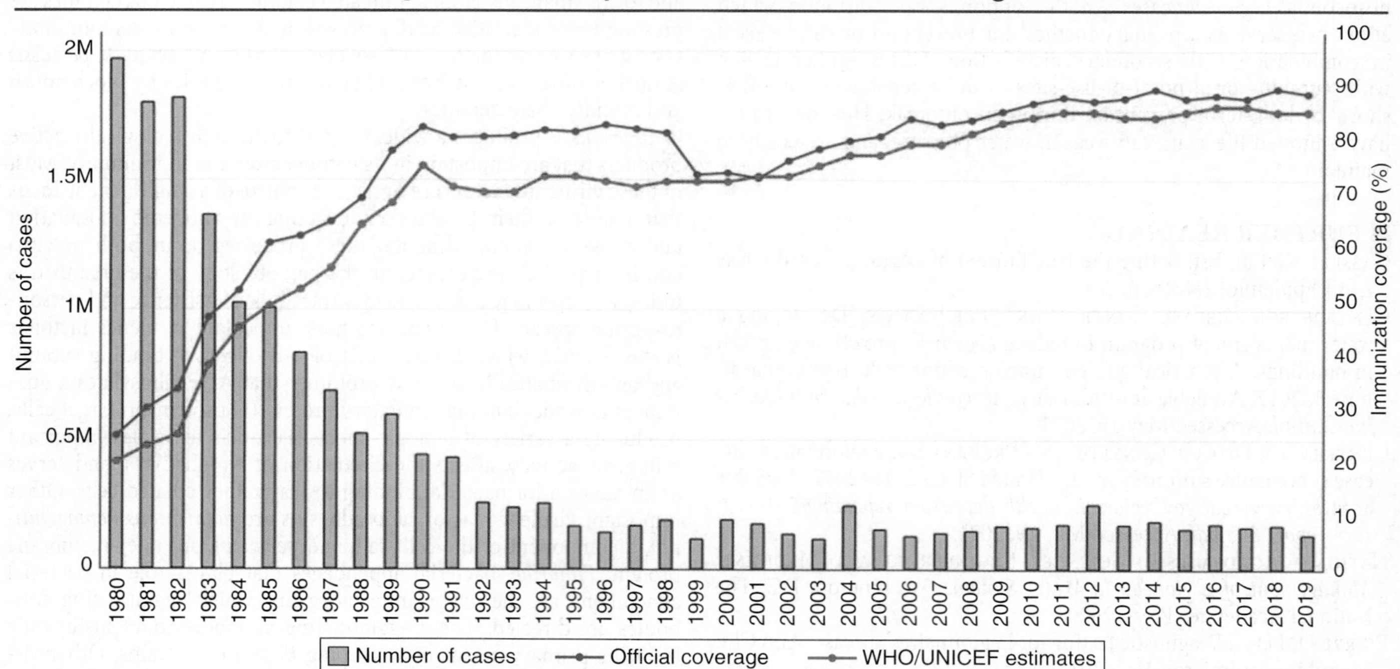

FIGURE 160-1 Global annual reported cases of pertussis and rate of coverage with DTP3 (diphtheria toxoid, tetanus toxoid, and pertussis vaccine; 3 doses), 1980–2019. *(Reproduced from www.who.int/immunization/monitoring_surveillance/burden/vpd/surveillance_type/passive/pertussis_coverage_2019.jpg. World Health Organization; 2019. License: CC BY-NC-SA 3.0 IGO. Accessed June 4, 2021.)*

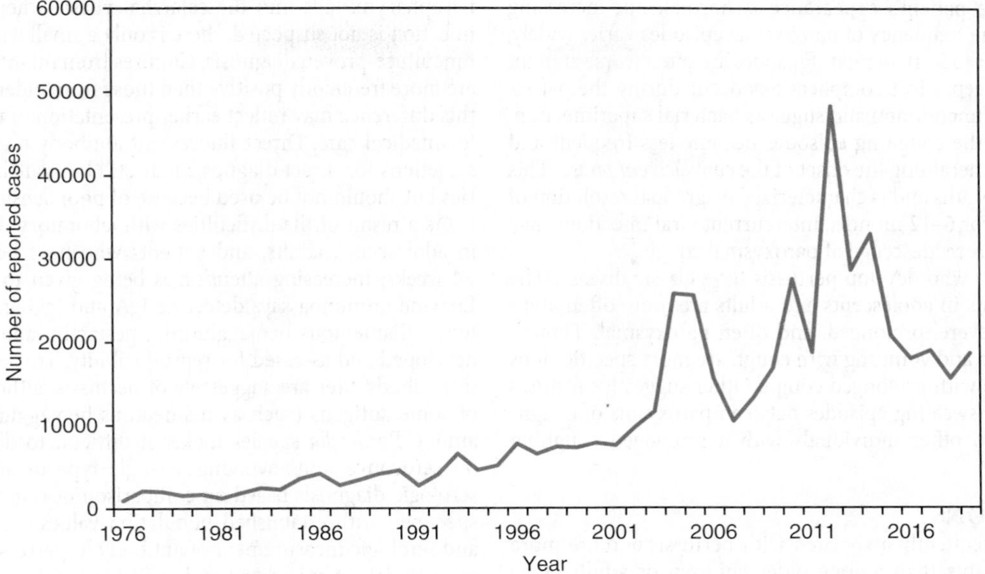

FIGURE 160-2 Reported cases of pertussis by year—United States, 1976–2019. *(From the Centers for Disease Control and Prevention, www.cdc.gov/pertussis/surv-reporting/cases-by-year.html. Accessed June 4, 2021.)*

often the source for cases in high-risk infants and may serve as the reservoir of infection between epidemic years.

PATHOGENESIS

Infection with *B. pertussis* is initiated by attachment of the organism to the ciliated epithelial cells of the nasopharynx. Attachment is mediated by surface adhesins (e.g., pertactin and filamentous hemagglutinin), which bind to the integrin family of cell-surface proteins, probably in conjunction with pertussis toxin. The role of fimbriae in adhesion and in maintenance of infection has not been fully delineated. Perhaps the result of redundancy of adhesins, no differences in virulence or clinical manifestations have been detected with the emergence of pertactin-negative strains. At the site of attachment, the organism multiplies, producing a variety of other toxins that cause local mucosal damage (tracheal cytotoxin, dermonecrotic toxin). Impairment of host defense by *B. pertussis* is mediated by pertussis toxin and adenylate cyclase-hemolysin toxin. There is local cellular invasion, with intracellular bacterial persistence; however, systemic dissemination does not occur. Systemic manifestations (lymphocytosis) result from the effects of the toxins.

The pathogenesis of the clinical manifestations of pertussis is poorly understood. It is not known what causes the hallmark paroxysmal cough. A pivotal role for pertussis toxin has been proposed but has not been confirmed. It is thought that neurologic events in pertussis, such as seizures and encephalopathy, are due to hypoxia from coughing paroxysms or apnea rather than to the effects of specific bacterial products. *B. pertussis* pneumonia, which occurs in up to 10% of infants with pertussis, is usually a diffuse bilateral primary infection. In older children and adults with pertussis, pneumonia is often due to secondary bacterial infection with streptococci or staphylococci. Deaths from pertussis among young infants are frequently associated with very high levels of leukocytosis and pulmonary hypertension.

IMMUNITY

Both humoral and cell-mediated immunity are thought to be important in pertussis. Although immunity after natural infection was thought to be lifelong, seroepidemiologic evidence demonstrates that it is not and that subsequent episodes of clinical pertussis are prevented by intermittent subclinical infection. Pertussis agglutinins were correlated with protection in early studies of whole-cell pertussis vaccines. Antibodies to pertussis toxin, filamentous hemagglutinin, pertactin, and fimbriae are all protective in animal models. Serologic correlates of protection conferred by acellular pertussis vaccines have not been established, although antibody to pertactin, fimbriae, and (to a lesser degree) pertussis toxin correlated best with protection in two efficacy trials. The duration of immunity after whole-cell pertussis vaccination is short-lived, with little protection remaining after 10–12 years. Waning of immunity is even more rapid in adolescents and children who have received all of their immunizations with acellular vaccines—i.e., within 2–4 years after the fifth or sixth dose. The type of immune response elicited may have an effect on duration of protection; natural infection and whole-cell pertussis vaccine elicit a TH1/TH17-predominant response whereas acellular pertussis vaccines stimulate a TH2-biased response.

CLINICAL MANIFESTATIONS

Pertussis is a prolonged coughing illness with clinical manifestations that vary by age **(Table 160-1)**. Although not uncommon among adolescents and adults, classic pertussis is most often seen in preschool and school-age children. After an incubation period averaging 7–10 days, an illness develops that is indistinguishable from the common cold and is characterized by coryza, lacrimation, mild cough, low-grade fever, and malaise. After 1–2 weeks, this *catarrhal phase* evolves into the *paroxysmal phase*: the cough becomes more frequent and spasmodic with repetitive bursts of 5–10 coughs, often within a single expiration. Post-tussive vomiting is frequent, with a mucous plug occasionally expelled at the end of an episode. The episode may be terminated by an audible whoop, which occurs upon rapid inspiration against a closed glottis at the end of a paroxysm. During a spasm, there may be impressive neck-vein distension, bulging eyes, tongue protrusion, and cyanosis. Paroxysms may be precipitated by noise, eating, or physical contact.

TABLE 160-1 Clinical Features of Pertussis, by Age Group and Diagnostic Status

	PERCENTAGE OF PATIENTS	
FEATURE	ADOLESCENTS AND ADULTS	INFANTS AND CHILDREN
Cough		
Paroxysmal	70–99	89–93
Worse at night	61–87	41
Whoop	8–82	69–92
Post-tussive vomiting	17–65	48–60

Source: Republished with permission of American Society for Microbiology from Pertussis: Microbiology, disease, treatment, and prevention, PE Kilgore et al: 29:449, 2016; permission conveyed through Copyright Clearance Center, Inc.

Between attacks, the patient's appearance is normal, but increasing fatigue is evident. The frequency of paroxysmal episodes varies widely, from several per hour to 5–10 per day. Episodes are often worse at night and interfere with sleep. Most complications occur during the paroxysmal stage. Fever is uncommon and suggests bacterial superinfection.

After 2–4 weeks, the coughing episodes become less frequent and less severe—changes heralding the onset of the *convalescent phase*. This phase can last 1–3 months and is characterized by gradual resolution of coughing episodes. For 6–12 months, intercurrent viral infections may be associated with a recrudescence of paroxysmal cough.

Not all individuals who develop pertussis have classic disease. The clinical manifestations in adolescents and adults are more often atypical. The cough is severe, prolonged, and often paroxysmal. Though uncommon, a whoop and vomiting with cough are more specific signs of pertussis in adults with prolonged cough. Other suggestive features are a cough at night, sweating episodes between paroxysms of coughing, and exposure to other individuals with a prolonged coughing illness.

COMPLICATIONS

Complications are frequently associated with pertussis and are more common among infants than among older children or adults. Subconjunctival hemorrhages, abdominal and inguinal hernias, pneumothoraces, and facial and truncal petechiae can result from increased intrathoracic pressure generated by severe fits of coughing. Weight loss can follow decreased caloric intake. Urinary incontinence, rib fracture, carotid artery aneurysm, and cough syncope have also been reported in adolescents and adults with pertussis. In a series of more than 1100 children <2 years of age who were hospitalized with pertussis, 27.1% had apnea, 9.4% had pneumonia, 2.6% had seizures, and 0.4% had encephalopathy; 10 children (0.9%) died. Pneumonia is reported in <5% of adolescents and adults and increases in frequency after 50 years of age. In contrast to the primary *B. pertussis* pneumonia that develops in infants, pneumonia in adolescents and adults with pertussis is usually caused by a secondary infection with encapsulated organisms such as *Streptococcus pneumoniae* or *Haemophilus influenzae*.

DIAGNOSIS

If the classic symptoms of pertussis are present, clinical diagnosis is not difficult. However, particularly in older children and adults, it is difficult to differentiate infections caused by *B. pertussis* and *B. parapertussis* from other respiratory tract infections on clinical grounds. Therefore, laboratory confirmation should be attempted in all cases. Lymphocytosis (absolute lymphocyte count $>10^8$–10^9/L) is common among young children, in whom it is unusual with other infections, but not among adolescents and adults. Culture of nasopharyngeal secretions remains the gold standard of diagnosis because of its 100% specificity, although DNA detection by PCR has replaced culture in many laboratories because of substantially increased sensitivity and quicker results. Appropriate PCR methodology must include primers to differentiate among *B. pertussis*, *B. parapertussis*, and *B. holmesii*. The best specimen is collected by nasopharyngeal aspiration, in which a fine flexible plastic catheter attached to a 10-mL syringe is passed into the nasopharynx and withdrawn while gentle suction is applied. Since *B. pertussis* is highly sensitive to drying, secretions for culture should be inoculated without delay onto appropriate medium (Bordet-Gengou or Regan-Lowe), or the catheter should be flushed with a phosphate-buffered saline solution for culture and/or PCR. An alternative to the aspirate is a Dacron or rayon nasopharyngeal swab; again, inoculation of culture plates should be immediate or an appropriate transport medium (e.g., Regan-Lowe charcoal medium) should be used. Results of PCR can be available within hours; cultures become positive by day 5 of incubation.

Nasopharyngeal cultures in untreated pertussis remain positive for a mean of 3 weeks after the onset of illness; these cultures become negative within 5 days of the institution of appropriate antimicrobial therapy. The duration of a positive PCR in untreated pertussis or after therapy is not known but exceeds that of positive cultures. Since much of the period during which the organism can be recovered from the nasopharynx falls into the catarrhal phase, when the etiology of the infection is not suspected, there is only a small window of opportunity for culture-proven diagnosis. Cultures from infants and young children are more frequently positive than those from older children and adults; this difference may reflect earlier presentation of the former age group for medical care. Direct fluorescent antibody tests of nasopharyngeal secretions for direct diagnosis may still be available in some laboratories but should not be used because of poor sensitivity and specificity.

As a result of the difficulties with laboratory diagnosis of pertussis in adolescents, adults, and patients who have been symptomatic for >4 weeks, increasing attention is being given to serologic diagnosis. Enzyme immunoassays detecting IgA and IgG antibodies to pertussis toxin, filamentous hemagglutinin, pertactin, and fimbriae have been developed and assessed for reproducibility. Two- or fourfold increases in antibody titer are suggestive of pertussis, although cross-reactivity of some antigens (such as filamentous hemagglutinin and pertactin) among *Bordetella* species makes it difficult to depend diagnostically on seroconversion involving a single type of antibody. Criteria for serologic diagnosis based on comparison of results for a single serum specimen with established population values are gaining acceptance, and serologic measurement of antibody to pertussis toxin is becoming more widely standardized and available for diagnostic purposes, particularly in outbreak settings and for surveillance.

DIFFERENTIAL DIAGNOSIS

A child presenting with paroxysmal cough, post-tussive vomiting, and whoop is likely to have an infection caused by *B. pertussis* or *B. parapertussis*; lymphocytosis increases the likelihood of a *B. pertussis* etiology. Viruses such as respiratory syncytial virus, rhinovirus, and adenovirus have been isolated from patients with clinical pertussis but probably represent co-infection, particularly in children <1 year of age.

In adolescents and adults, who often do not have paroxysmal cough or whoop, the differential diagnosis of a prolonged coughing illness is more extensive. Pertussis should be suspected when any patient has a cough that does not improve within 14 days, a paroxysmal cough of any duration, a cough followed by vomiting (adolescents and adults), or any respiratory symptoms after contact with a laboratory-confirmed case of pertussis. Other etiologies to consider include infections caused by *Mycoplasma pneumoniae*, *Chlamydia pneumoniae*, adenovirus, influenza virus, and other respiratory viruses. Use of angiotensin-converting enzyme (ACE) inhibitors, reactive airway disease, and gastroesophageal reflux disease are well-described noninfectious causes of prolonged cough in adults.

TREATMENT

Pertussis

ANTIBIOTICS

The purpose of antibiotic therapy for pertussis is to eradicate the infecting bacteria from the nasopharynx; therapy does not substantially alter the clinical course unless given early in the catarrhal phase. Macrolide antibiotics are the drugs of choice for treatment of pertussis (**Table 160-2**); macrolide-resistant *B. pertussis* strains have been reported but are rare. Trimethoprim-sulfamethoxazole is recommended as an alternative for individuals allergic to macrolides.

SUPPORTIVE CARE

Young infants have the highest rates of complication and death from pertussis; therefore, most infants (and older children with severe disease) should be hospitalized. A quiet environment may decrease the stimulation that can trigger paroxysmal episodes. Use of β-adrenergic agonists and/or glucocorticoids has been advocated by some authorities but has not been proven to be effective. Cough suppressants are not effective and play no role in the management of pertussis.

INFECTION CONTROL MEASURES

Hospitalized patients with pertussis should be placed in respiratory isolation, with the use of precautions appropriate for pathogens

TABLE 160-2 Antimicrobial Therapy for Pertussis

DRUG	ADULT DAILY DOSE	FREQUENCY	DURATION, DAYS	COMMENTS
Erythromycin estolate	500 mg	3–4 times per day	7–14	Frequent gastrointestinal side effects
Clarithromycin	500 mg	Twice a day	7	—
Azithromycin	500 mg on day 1, 250 mg subsequently	1 daily dose	5	—
Trimethoprim-sulfamethoxazole	160 mg of trimethoprim, 800 mg of sulfamethoxazole	Twice a day	14	For patients allergic to macrolides; data on effectiveness limited

Source: T Tiwari et al: Recommended antimicrobial agents for the treatment and postexposure prophylaxis of pertussis: 2005 CDC guidelines. MMWR Recomm Rep 54(RR-14):1, 2005.

spread by large respiratory droplets. Isolation should continue for 5 days after initiation of macrolide therapy or, in untreated patients, for 3 weeks (i.e., until nasopharyngeal cultures are consistently negative).

PREVENTION

Chemoprophylaxis Because the risk of transmission of *B. pertussis* within households is high, chemoprophylaxis is widely recommended for household contacts of pertussis cases regardless of their immunization status and should be initiated within 21 days of cough onset in the index case. The effectiveness of chemoprophylaxis is supported by several epidemiologic studies of institutional and community outbreaks. In the only randomized, placebo-controlled study, erythromycin estolate (50 mg/kg per day; maximum dose, 1 g/d) was effective in reducing the incidence of bacteriologically confirmed pertussis by 67%; however, there was no decrease in the incidence of clinical disease. Despite these results, authorities continue to recommend chemoprophylaxis, particularly in households with members at high risk of severe disease (children <1 year of age, pregnant women). Data on the use of the newer macrolides for chemoprophylaxis are not available, but these drugs are commonly used because of their increased tolerability and their effectiveness.

Immunization (See also Chap. 123) The mainstay of pertussis prevention is active immunization. Pertussis vaccine became widely used in North America after 1940; the reported number of pertussis cases subsequently fell by >90%. Whole-cell pertussis vaccines are prepared through the heating, chemical inactivation, and purification of whole *B. pertussis* organisms. Despite their efficacy (average estimate, 85%; range for different products, 30–100%), whole-cell pertussis vaccines are associated with adverse events—both common (fever; injection-site pain, erythema, and swelling; irritability) and uncommon (febrile seizures, hypotonic-hyporesponsive episodes). Alleged associations of whole-cell pertussis vaccine with encephalopathy, sudden infant death syndrome, and autism, although not substantiated, spawned an active anti-immunization lobby. The development of acellular pertussis vaccines, which are effective and less reactogenic, has greatly alleviated concerns about the inclusion of pertussis vaccine in the combined infant immunization series.

Although a wide variety of acellular pertussis vaccines were developed, only a few are still marketed widely; all contain pertussis toxoid and filamentous hemagglutinin. One acellular pertussis vaccine also contains pertactin, and another contains pertactin and two types of fimbriae. Adult formulations of acellular pertussis vaccines have been shown to be safe, immunogenic, and efficacious in clinical trials in adolescents and adults and are now recommended for routine immunization of these groups in several countries.

Although whole-cell vaccines are still used extensively in developing regions of the world, acellular pertussis vaccines are used exclusively for childhood immunization in much of the developed world. In light of evidence of early waning of immunity among children who received acellular pertussis vaccine in infancy, the WHO Strategic Advisory Group of Experts (SAGE) recommends that countries using whole-cell pertussis vaccine for the primary infant immunization series continue to do so. In countries using acellular pertussis vaccines in infancy, additional booster immunizations in older children, adolescents, and adults are recommended to prevent pertussis in high-risk infants. Pertussis immunization is also recommended during pregnancy to increase passive transfer of maternal antibodies to the fetus. Studies in high-income countries demonstrate that immunization of women during pregnancy is 90–93% effective at preventing pertussis in infants <2 months of age and is safe. In North America, acellular pertussis vaccines for children are given as a three-dose primary series at 2, 4, and 6 months of age, with a reinforcing dose at 15–18 months of age and a booster dose at 4–6 years of age. Adolescents (11–18 years of age) and all unvaccinated adults should receive a dose of the adult-formulation diphtheria–tetanus–acellular pertussis vaccine. Immunization is specifically recommended for health care providers, individuals in close contact with infants, and women during the third trimester of every pregnancy. Pertussis vaccine coverage among U.S. adolescents was 86.4% in 2015, and coverage among pregnant women was 48.8% in 2015–2016. However, coverage among adults remains low (23.1% in 2015). Further improvements in adult vaccine coverage may permit better control of pertussis across the age spectrum, with collateral protection of infants too young to be immunized. However, more effective vaccines with longer-lasting protection will ultimately be needed to control this disease.

FURTHER READING

De Serres G et al: Morbidity of pertussis in adolescents and adults. J Infect Dis 182:174, 2000.

Forsyth KD et al: Recommendations to control pertussis prioritized relative to economies: A Global Pertussis Initiative update. Vaccine 36:7270, 2018.

Havers FP et al: Use of tetanus toxoid, reduced diphtheria toxoid, and acellular pertussis vaccines: Updated recommendations of the Advisory Committee on Immunization Practices—United States, 2019. MMWR Morb Mortal Wkly Rep 69:77, 2020.

Kilgore PE et al: Pertussis: Microbiology, disease, treatment, and prevention. Clin Microbiol Rev 29:449, 2016.

Skoff TH: Sources of infant pertussis infection in the United States. Pediatrics 136:635, 2015.

Winter K et al: Pertussis in California: A tale of 2 epidemics. Pediatr Infect Dis J 37:324, 2018.

161 Diseases Caused by Gram-Negative Enteric Bacilli

Thomas A. Russo, James R. Johnson

GENERAL FEATURES AND PRINCIPLES

The post-antibiotic era has begun. For most people, this is the first time in their lives that an effective treatment for a bacterial infection may not exist. The Enterobacteriaceae are at the forefront of this evolving public health crisis. For example, the Centers for Disease Control and Prevention (CDC) and the World Health Organization (WHO) have designated carbapenem-resistant Enterobacteriaceae (CRE) as representing a threat level of "urgent" and "priority one, critical."

Enterobacteriaceae are responsible for a significant proportion of the deaths attributed to antimicrobial-resistant bacteria, of which an estimated 23,000 and 25,000 occur annually in the United States and the European Union, respectively, and three to five times as many (per capita) in low- and middle-income countries (e.g., Thailand). These pathogens cause a wide variety of infections involving diverse anatomic sites in both healthy and compromised hosts. Therefore, a thorough knowledge of clinical presentations and appropriate therapeutic choices is necessary for optimal outcomes. *Escherichia coli, Klebsiella, Proteus, Enterobacter, Serratia, Citrobacter, Morganella, Providencia, Cronobacter,* and *Edwardsiella* are enteric gram-negative bacilli (GNB) within the family Enterobacteriaceae that commonly cause extraintestinal infections. *Salmonella, Shigella,* and *Yersinia,* which also are in the family Enterobacteriaceae but more commonly cause gastrointestinal infections, are discussed in **Chaps. 165, 166, and 171**, respectively.

EPIDEMIOLOGY

E. coli, Klebsiella, Proteus, Enterobacter, Serratia, Citrobacter, Morganella, Providencia, Cronobacter, and *Edwardsiella* are components of the normal animal and human colonic microbiota and/or the microbiota in various environmental habitats, including long-term-care facilities (LTCFs) and hospitals. As a result, except for certain pathotypes of intestinal pathogenic *E. coli,* these genera are global pathogens. The incidence of infection due to these agents is increasing because of the combination of an aging population and increasing antimicrobial resistance. In healthy humans, *E. coli* is the predominant species of GNB in the colonic microbiota, followed by *Klebsiella* and *Proteus.* GNB (primarily *E. coli, Klebsiella,* and *Proteus*) can also colonize the oropharynx and intact skin but, in healthy individuals, tend to do so only transiently. By contrast, in LTCFs and hospital settings, a variety of GNB emerge as the dominant colonizers of both mucosal and skin epithelial surfaces, particularly in association with antimicrobial use, severe illness, and extended length of stay. LTCFs are emerging as an important reservoir for resistant GNB. Such colonization with GNB may lead to subsequent extraintestinal infection; for example, oropharyngeal colonization may lead to pneumonia, and colonic/perineal colonization may lead to urinary tract infection (UTI). The use of ampicillin or amoxicillin was associated with an increased risk of subsequent infection due to the hypervirulent pathotype of *Klebsiella pneumoniae* in Taiwan; this association suggests that changes in the quantity or prevalence of colonizing bacteria may significantly influence the risk of infection. *Serratia, Enterobacter,* and, less commonly, *Citrobacter* infection may be acquired directly through a variety of infusates (e.g., medications, blood products, non–U.S. Food and Drug Administration [FDA] approved stem cell products). *Edwardsiella* infections are acquired through freshwater and marine environment exposures and are most common in Southeast Asia.

STRUCTURE AND FUNCTION

Enteric GNB possess an extracytoplasmic outer membrane consisting of a lipid bilayer with associated proteins, lipoproteins, and polysaccharides (capsule, lipopolysaccharide). The outer membrane interfaces with the external environment, including the human host. A variety of components of the outer membrane are critical determinants in pathogenesis (e.g., capsule) and antimicrobial resistance (e.g., permeability barrier, efflux pumps). In addition, secreted products play an important role in both host infection (e.g., iron acquisition molecules) and environmental niche survival and colonization (e.g., type VI secretion systems).

PATHOGENESIS

Multiple bacterial virulence factors are required for the pathogenesis of infections caused by GNB. Possession of specialized virulence genes defines pathogens and enables them to infect the host efficiently. Hosts and their cognate pathogens have been co-adapting throughout evolutionary history. During the host–pathogen "chess match" over time, various and redundant strategies have emerged in both the pathogens and their hosts (**Table 161-1**).

TABLE 161-1 Interactions of Extraintestinal Pathogenic *Escherichia coli* with the Human Host: A Paradigm for Extracellular, Extraintestinal Gram-Negative Bacterial Pathogens

BACTERIAL GOAL	HOST OBSTACLE	BACTERIAL SOLUTION
Extraintestinal attachment	Flow of urine, mucociliary escalator	Multiple adhesins (e.g., type 1, S, and F1C fimbriae; P pili)
Nutrient acquisition for growth	Nutrient sequestration (e.g., iron via intracellular storage and extracellular scavenging via lactoferrin and transferrin)	Cellular lysis (e.g., hemolysin), multiple mechanisms for competing for iron (e.g., siderophores) and other nutrients
Initial avoidance of host bactericidal activity	Complement, phagocytic cells, antimicrobial peptides	Capsular polysaccharide, lipopolysaccharide
Dissemination (within host and between hosts)	Intact tissue barriers	Irritant tissue damage resulting in increased excretion (e.g., toxins such as hemolysin), invasion of brain endothelium
Late avoidance of host bactericidal activity	Acquired immunity (e.g., specific antibodies), treatment with antibiotics	Cell entry, acquisition of antimicrobial resistance

Intestinal pathogenic (diarrheagenic) mechanisms are discussed below. The members of the Enterobacteriaceae family that cause extraintestinal infections are primarily extracellular pathogens and therefore share certain pathogenic features. The two principal components of host defense against Enterobacteriaceae, regardless of species, are innate immunity (including intact skin and mucosal barriers; the withholding of nutrients; and the activities of complement, antimicrobial peptides, and professional phagocytes) and humoral immunity. Both susceptibility to and severity of infection are increased with dysfunction or deficiencies of these host components. By contrast, the virulence traits of intestinal pathogenic *E. coli*—i.e., the distinctive strains that can cause diarrheal disease—are for the most part different from those of extraintestinal pathogenic *E. coli* (ExPEC) and other GNB that cause extraintestinal infections. This distinction reflects site-specific differences in host environments, defense mechanisms, and physiological derangements that lead to disease.

A given enterobacterial strain usually possesses multiple adhesins for binding to a variety of host cells (e.g., in *E. coli*: type 1, S, and F1C fimbriae; P pili). Nutrient acquisition (e.g., of iron via siderophores) requires many genes that are necessary but not sufficient for pathogenesis. The ability to resist the bactericidal activity of complement and phagocytes in the absence of antibody (e.g., as conferred by capsule or the O antigen component of lipopolysaccharide) is one of the defining traits of an extracellular pathogen. Tissue damage (e.g., as mediated by *E. coli* hemolysin) may facilitate nutrient acquisition and spread within the host. Without doubt, many important virulence genes await identification.

The ability to induce septic shock is another defining feature of these genera. GNB are the most common causes of this potentially lethal syndrome. Pathogen-associated molecular pattern molecules (PAMPs; e.g., the lipid A moiety of lipopolysaccharide) stimulate a proinflammatory host response via pattern recognition receptors (e.g., Toll-like or C-type lectin receptors) that activate host defense signaling pathways; if overly exuberant, this response results in shock (**Chap. 304**). Direct bacterial damage of host tissue (e.g., by toxins) or collateral damage from the host response can result in the release of damage-associated molecular pattern molecules (DAMPs; e.g., HMGB1) that can propagate a detrimental proinflammatory host response.

Many antigenic variants (serotypes) exist in most genera of GNB. For example, *E. coli* has >150 O (somatic) antigens, 80 K (capsular) antigens, and 53 H (flagellar) antigens. This antigenic variability, which permits immune evasion and allows recurrent infection by different strains of the same species, has impeded vaccine development (**Chap. 123**).

INFECTIOUS SYNDROMES

Depending on both the host and the pathogen, GNB can infect nearly every organ or body cavity. *E. coli* can cause either intestinal or extraintestinal infection, depending on the particular pathotype, and *Edwardsiella tarda* can cause both intestinal and extraintestinal infection. *Klebsiella* causes primarily extraintestinal infection, but a toxin-producing variant of *Klebsiella oxytoca* has been associated with hemorrhagic colitis, and *Providencia alcalifaciens* and *Escherichia albertii* have been associated with gastroenteritis.

E. coli and—to a lesser degree—*Klebsiella* account for most extraintestinal infections due to GNB. These species (for *K. pneumoniae*, primarily its hypervirulent pathotype) are the most virulent pathogens within this group, as demonstrated by their ability to cause severe infections in healthy, ambulatory hosts from the community. However, the other genera of GNB are also important extraintestinal pathogens, especially among LTCF residents and hospitalized patients, in large part because of the intrinsic or acquired antimicrobial resistance of these organisms and the increasing number of individuals with compromised host defenses. The mortality rate is substantial in many GNB infections and correlates with severity of illness, underlying host status, and in some cases the antimicrobial resistance of the infecting pathogen, which can result in suboptimal therapy. Especially problematic are pneumonia, sepsis, and septic shock (arising from any site of infection), for which the associated mortality rates are 20–60%.

DIAGNOSIS

Isolation of GNB from sterile sites almost always implies infection, whereas their isolation from nonsterile sites, particularly open wounds and the respiratory tract, requires clinical correlation to differentiate colonization from infection. Clinical microbiology laboratories are increasingly incorporating newer diagnostic methodologies (e.g., matrix-assisted laser desorption–ionization–time-of-flight mass spectrometry [MALDI-TOF-MS] and polymerase chain reaction [PCR]) and immunoassays to enhance the sensitivity, accuracy, and rapidity of reporting on pathogen identification and resistance genes. This information can be used to increase the timeliness of initiation and/or the accurate selection of empirical antimicrobial therapy, thereby improving outcomes.

TREATMENT

Principles Guiding Treatment in the Era of Increasing Antimicrobial Resistance

(See also Chap. 144) Initiation of appropriate empirical antimicrobial therapy early in the course of infections due to GNB (particularly the more serious ones) leads to improved outcomes. The ever-increasing prevalence of multidrug-resistant (MDR) and extensively drug-resistant (XDR) GNB; the lag between published and current resistance rates; and variations in antimicrobial susceptibility by species, geographic location, regional antimicrobial use, and hospital site (e.g., intensive care units [ICUs] vs wards) necessitate familiarity with evolving patterns of antimicrobial resistance for the selection of appropriate empirical therapy.

Patient factors predictive of resistance in a given isolate include recent antimicrobial use, a health care association (e.g., recent or ongoing hospitalization, dialysis, residence in an LTCF, transplant, hematologic malignancy), or international travel (e.g., to Asia, Latin America, Africa, Eastern Europe). Resistance rates will almost certainly increase over time and will likely be higher than shown here by the time this chapter is published. Of concern are an increasing number of reports on resistant Enterobacteriaceae causing infections in ambulatory patients without known risk factors.

In this era of increasing antimicrobial resistance, it is critical to culture the primary site of infection before initiating antimicrobial therapy and, for systemically ill patients, to obtain blood cultures. In vitro testing may not always detect antimicrobial resistance; therefore, it is important to assess the patient's clinical response to treatment. Moreover (see discussion of AmpC β-lactamases below), resistance may emerge during therapy. In addition, drainage of abscesses, resection of necrotic tissue, and removal of infected foreign bodies, sometimes referred to collectively as "source control," are often required for cure.

For appropriately selected patients, it may be prudent initially, pending antimicrobial susceptibility results, to use two potentially active agents as a way to increase the likelihood that at least one agent will be active against the patient's organism. If broad-spectrum treatment has been initiated, it is important to switch to the most appropriate narrower-spectrum agent once antimicrobial susceptibility results become available. Such responsible antimicrobial stewardship should help disrupt the ever-escalating cycle of selection for increasingly resistant bacteria, plus decrease the likelihood of *Clostridioides difficile* infection, decrease costs, and maximize the useful longevity of available antimicrobial agents. Likewise, it is important to avoid treatment of patients who are colonized but not infected (e.g., who have a positive sputum culture without evidence of pneumonia, or a positive urine culture without clinical manifestations of UTI).

At present, the most reliably and broadly active antimicrobial agents in vitro against Enterobacteriaceae are the carbapenems (excepting imipenem, to which the Proteeae [*Proteus*, *Morganella*, *Providencia*] are intrinsically resistant); the aminoglycosides amikacin and plazomicin (excepting the Proteeae); the fourth-generation cephalosporin cefepime; the β-lactamase inhibitor combination agents piperacillin-tazobactam, ceftolozane-tazobactam, ceftazidime-avibactam, meropenem-vaborbactam; and the novel cephalosporin-siderophore cefiderocol. A limitation of imipenem/cilastatin-relebactam; the tetracycline derivatives tigecycline, omadacycline, and eravacycline; and the polymyxins B and E (colistin) (which are otherwise very active) is their poor activity against the Proteeae and *Serratia*. Furthermore, the tetracycline derivatives achieve suboptimal concentrations at several anatomic sites (including urine and blood). Clinical data are limited for cefiderocol outside of UTIs; thus, caution is in order for serious infections.

The number of antimicrobial agents effective against certain Enterobacteriaceae is shrinking, and truly pan-resistant GNB exist. Accordingly, the currently available antimicrobial drugs must be used judiciously. Extensive resistance to available agents may leave the clinician with few or no ideal therapeutic options. However, use of a regimen that takes into account the site of infection, achievable drug levels at that site (e.g., higher concentrations of many agents in urine), and pharmacodynamically guided administration strategies (e.g., prolonged infusion of β-lactam agents to maintain drug levels above the minimal inhibitory concentration [MIC]) may increase the chance for a successful outcome. In the near future, point-of-care identification of resistance mechanisms in GNB will enable a strain-specific, patient-specific precision medicine–based treatment approach that would be predicted to improve outcome.

GNB are commonly involved in polymicrobial infections, in which the role of each individual pathogen is uncertain **(Chap. 177)**. Although some GNB are more pathogenic than others, it is usually prudent, if possible, to design an antimicrobial regimen active against all of the GNB identified, because each is typically capable of pathogenicity in its own right. For patients treated initially with a broad-spectrum empirical regimen, the regimen should be de-escalated as expeditiously as possible once susceptibility results are known and the patient has responded to therapy.

Treatment duration is best individualized based on underlying host status and site of infection. However, for selected non–critically ill patients with source control and a satisfactory clinical response to therapy, 7 days of treatment may suffice.

ANTIMICROBIAL TREATMENT AND RESISTANCE MECHANISMS

The most common resistance mechanisms possessed by Enterobacteriaceae are summarized in **Table 161-2**. However, enzymatic hydrolysis (e.g., β-lactamases, of which >3000 variants have been described) and modification of antimicrobials are the major

TABLE 161-2 Common Antimicrobial Resistance Mechanisms Possessed by the Enterobacteriaceae

MECHANISM	ANTIMICROBIALS MOST SIGNIFICANTLY AFFECTED	COMMON MEDIATORS OF RESISTANCE
Efflux	Tetracyclines, fluoroquinolones (FQ)	Efflux pumps
Decreased permeability	Fosfomycin	Alterations in uptake system
Target site alteration or over-production	FQ, trimethoprim-sulfamethoxazole (TMP-SMX), and polymyxins	DNA gyrase or topoisomerase IV for FQ; enzymes for folic acid synthesis for TMP-SMX Lipid A for polymyxins
Enzymatic hydrolysis of antimicrobials	Penicillins, cephalosporins, cephamycins, carbapenems	Broad-spectrum β-lactamases (e.g., TEM, SHV) ESBLs (e.g., CTX-M, modified TEM and SHV) AmpC β-lactamases Carbapenemases (e.g., serine based KPC, SME, OXA; and metallo-based NDM, VIM, IMP)
Enzymatic modification of antimicrobials	Aminoglycosides	AAC, ANT, APH

Abbreviations: AAC, *N*-acetyltransferases; ANT, *O*-adenyltranferases; APH, *O*-phosphotransferases; CTX, cefotaxime β-lactamase; ESBL, extended-spectrum β-lactamase; IMP, active on imipenem; KPC, *Klebsiella pneumoniae* carbapenemase; NDM, New Delhi metallo-β-lactamase; OXA, oxacillinase; SHV, sulfhydryl reagent variable β-lactamase; SME, *Serratia marcescens* enzyme; TEM, temoniera β-lactamase; VIM, Verona integron-mediated metallo-β-lactamase.

mediators of resistance in GNB and will be discussed in detail below. Importantly, it is becoming increasingly recognized that MDR and XDR GNB often possess multiple plasmids and genes that encode for multiple β-lactamases.

Broad-spectrum β-lactamases mediate resistance to many penicillins and first-generation cephalosporins and are frequently expressed in enteric GNB. These enzymes are inhibited by β-lactamase inhibitors (e.g., clavulanate, sulbactam, tazobactam, avibactam). In their wild-type form, they do not hydrolyze third- and fourth-generation cephalosporins or cephamycins (e.g., cefoxitin).

Extended spectrum β-lactamases (ESBLs) are modified broad-spectrum enzymes that hydrolyze third-generation cephalosporins, aztreonam, and (in some instances) fourth-generation cephalosporins, in addition to the drugs hydrolyzed by broad-spectrum β-lactamases. GNB that express ESBLs may also exhibit porin mutations that result in decreased uptake of relevant β-lactam agents (cephalosporins, β-lactam/β-lactamase inhibitor combinations, and carbapenems), further reducing susceptibility to these agents. The prevalence of acquired ESBL production, particularly of CTX-M-type enzymes, is increasing in GNB worldwide, largely due to the presence of the corresponding genes on transferable (conjugal) plasmids, which also variably confer or are associated with resistance to fluoroquinolones, trimethoprim-sulfamethoxazole (TMP-SMX), aminoglycosides, tetracyclines, and (more recently) fosfomycin. To date, ESBLs are most prevalent in *E. coli* (especially ST131), *K. pneumoniae,* and *K. oxytoca,* but these enzymes can occur in all Enterobacteriaceae. The approximate regional prevalence of ESBL-producing GNB currently follows a descending gradient as follows: China > Eastern Europe > other parts of Asia (e.g., India) > Latin America and Africa > Western Europe, the United States, Canada, and Australia. Travel to high-prevalence regions increases the likelihood of colonization with these strains. The incidence of community-acquired infections due to ESBL-producing *Enterobacteriaceae* has increased worldwide, including in the United States.

Carbapenems are the most reliably active β-lactam agents against ESBL-expressing strains. Piperacillin-tazobactam, when active in vitro, has been used as a carbapenem-sparing alternative, but recent data from the MERINO trial do not support its use for bloodstream infections. Ceftazidime-avibactam, ceftolozane-tazobactam (less active against *Klebsiella, Enterobacter,* and *Citrobacter*), meropenem-vaborbactam, imipenem/cilastatin-relebactam, and plazomicin are active against most ESBL-producing strains and have limited clinical data that support potential utility. The roles for tigecycline, eravacycline, and omadacycline are unclear despite these agents' excellent in vitro activity against most Enterobacteriaceae; however, they are inactive against *Proteus, Morganella, Providencia,* and *Serratia.*

Oral options for the treatment of ESBL-expressing strains are limited. Fosfomycin, nitrofurantoin (for *E. coli,* 75–90% susceptible), pivmecillinam (not available in the United States), and omadacycline are the most reliably active agents. Older tetracyclines (e.g., doxycycline and minocycline) are also often active, although urine levels may be insufficient and clinical experience with gram-negative infections is limited.

AmpC β-lactamases, when induced or stably derepressed to high levels of expression, confer resistance to the same substrates as do ESBLs, plus to the cephamycins (e.g., cefoxitin and cefotetan). The genes encoding these enzymes are primarily chromosomal and therefore may not exhibit the linked resistance to TMP-SMX, aminoglycosides, and tetracyclines that is common with ESBLs. These enzymes are problematic for the clinician: resistance may develop during therapy with third-generation cephalosporins and result in clinical failure, particularly in the setting of bacteremia. Although chromosomal AmpC β-lactamases are present in nearly all members of the Enterobacteriaceae family (with the notable exceptions of *K. pneumoniae, K. oxytoca,* and *Proteus mirabilis*), the risk of clinically significant induction of high-level expression or selection of stably derepressed mutants with cephalosporin treatment is not uniform across species, being greatest with *Enterobacter cloacae, Klebsiella* (formerly *Enterobacter*) *aerogenes, Citrobacter freundii,* and *Hafnia alvei,* and less with *Serratia marcescens, Providencia,* and *Morganella morganii.* In addition, rare strains of *E. coli, K. pneumoniae,* and other Enterobacteriaceae have acquired plasmids that contain AmpC β-lactamase genes.

For AmpC-expressing strains, carbapenems are an appropriate treatment option, especially for severely ill patients. Meta-analyses support piperacillin-tazobactam as a possible option. The fourth-generation cephalosporin cefepime may be an appropriate option if the concomitant presence of an ESBL can be excluded (a task that currently exceeds the capability of most clinical microbiology laboratories) and source control is achieved. Vaborbactam and avibactam are the most potent β-lactamase inhibitors. Ceftazidime-avibactam, imipenem/cilastatin-relebactam, and cefiderocol are active in vitro, but clinical data are limited. Other carbapenem-sparing alternatives to consider if isolates are susceptible in vitro include fluoroquinolones, TMP-SMX, and aminoglycosides. Tigecycline, eravacycline, and omadacycline are active in vitro (except against *Proteus, Morganella, Providencia,* and *Serratia*).

Carbapenemases of Ambler class A (serine-based hydrolytic mechanism; *K. pneumoniae* carbapenemase [KPC], *Serratia marcescens* enzyme [SME]) and class B (metallo [zinc]-based hydrolytic mechanism; New Delhi metallo-β-lactamase [NDM], Verona integron-mediated metallo-β-lactamase [VIM], active on imipenem [IMP]) confer resistance to the same drugs as do ESBLs, plus to cephamycins and carbapenems. By contrast, Ambler class D carbapenemases (serine-based hydrolytic mechanism, e.g., oxacillinase [OXA]) hydrolyze carbapenems and penicillins, but they have minimal activity against extended-spectrum cephalosporins. As with ESBLs, carbapenemase-encoding genes may be present on transferable plasmids, which often encode linked resistance to fluoroquinolones, TMP-SMX, tetracyclines, and aminoglycosides. Transposon-mediated spread (e.g., TN4401 for KPC) is also important. Although all major carbapenemases have been described around the globe, KPC is most common in the Americas, NDM in Asia, and OXA in Europe. Asymptomatic intestinal carriage may facilitate spread.

Carbapenemase production by Enterobacteriaceae (CPE) is most prevalent in *K. pneumoniae*, followed by *Enterobacter* spp. and *E. coli*, but has been described in nearly all members of the family. *M. morganii*, *Proteus*, and *Providencia* exhibit intrinsic low-level imipenem resistance. Although for carbapenem-resistant isolates the Clinical and Laboratory Standards Institute (CLSI) no longer recommends routine identification of CPE, such data conceivably could inform epidemiologic surveillance, infection control efforts, antimicrobial stewardship, and treatment decisions, especially if susceptibility data for selected agents are not available. Genotypic and phenotypic methods can detect carbapenemase genes or activity. Each of these methodologies has pros and cons. At the time of this writing, CLSI endorses the modified carbapenem inactivation method and the Carba NP test.

For the treatment of infections due to Enterobacteriaceae that produce class A or D carbapenemases (serine-based hydrolysis; KPC, OXA, SME), ceftazidime-avibactam is emerging as a first-line agent particularly for bacteremia, but suboptimal efficacy has been observed with pneumonia and in patients on renal replacement therapy, and resistance has developed in up to 10% of cases. Polymyxins are also active. Clinical success against KPC-producing CRE has also been reported for meropenem-vaborbactam and, to a lesser extent, imipenem/cilastatin-relebactam; importantly, however, neither of these agents is active against OXA-producing CRE. For SME, based on limited in vitro data, vaborbactam is most active, followed by avibactam, whereas relebactam is significantly less active; this suggests that meropenem-vaborbactam or ceftazidime-avibactam should be viable treatment options for SME-producing CRE. Ceftazidime, cefepime, and aztreonam are active against OXA-48-like–producing CRE.

Treatment of infections due to class B metallo-β-lactamase–producing CRE is more challenging. The polymyxins B and E currently constitute one of the last lines of defense against strains that produce metallo-carbapenemases (e.g., NDM-1). However, these agents' nephrotoxicity and neurotoxicity potential, their limited clinical efficacy, and the recent emergence of the polymyxin resistance gene *mcr-1* on a stable transferable plasmid and *mcr-1*–independent resistance threaten their utility.

Aztreonam is active against metallo-carbapenemases but is hydrolyzed by ESBLs and AmpC β-lactamases, which often coexist in XDR strains. Ongoing studies are assessing aztreonam plus avibactam, a promising combination with in vitro activity against class A, B, and D enzymes, for the treatment of CRE strains that produce both NDM plus KPC or OXA. A currently available workaround involving approved drugs is co-administration of ceftazidime-avibactam and aztreonam; avibactam protects aztreonam from hydrolysis from ESBLs and AmpC β-lactamases.

Although tigecycline, eravacycline, and omadacycline are active in vitro, pharmacokinetic-pharmacodynamic limitations exist, and along with the polymyxins, they exhibit poor activity against the Proteeae and *Serratia*. Cefiderocol is active in vitro against KPC, most NDM carbapenemases, and OXA (i.e., classes A, B, and D enzymes); clinical trials for the treatment of carbapenemase-resistant GNB are in progress. Aminoglycosides, of which plazomicin is most active, may have some utility for combination therapy. Fosfomycin is often active in vitro, but clinical data in the treatment of serious infections due to CPE are limited, resistance may develop with monotherapy, and a parenteral formulation is not yet available in the United States and certain other countries. Collectively, these considerations recommend fosfomycin as a second-line agent and for use in combination therapy, except perhaps for prostatitis due to superior penetration.

Carbapenem resistance in the absence of carbapenemases can occur in the presence of ESBLs or AmpC β-lactamases in combination with porin mutations (non-CP-CRE); however, most laboratories will not be able to differentiate CPE from non-CP-CRE. The non-CP-CRE phenotype is most commonly seen in *E. coli* and *Enterobacter* spp. In general, resistance to noncarbapenem antimicrobial classes is less, but data are limited on the optimal management approach for non-CP-CRE.

β-Lactamase inhibitor resistance is an uncommon (4% of *E. coli/K. pneumoniae* blood isolates) but increasingly recognized phenotype that is characterized by resistance to β-lactamase inhibitors, but not to third-generation cephalosporins. This mechanism of resistance is distinct from production of ESBLs, AmpC β-lactamases, and carbapenemases, and is still being delineated. Limited evidence suggests that ceftriaxone is an appropriate treatment option for such strains.

Fluoroquinolone resistance is usually due to alterations in or protection of the target sites in DNA gyrase and topoisomerase IV, with or without decreased permeability and active efflux. Fluoroquinolone resistance is increasingly prevalent among GNB and is associated with resistance to other antimicrobial classes; for example, 20–80% of ESBL-producing enteric GNB are also resistant to fluoroquinolones. At present, fluoroquinolones should be considered unreliable as empirical therapy for GNB infections in critically ill patients.

Aminoglycoside resistance in Enterobacteriaceae is conferred via enzymatic modification by *N*-acetyltransferases, *O*-adenyltransferases, or *O*-phosphotransferases, which in turn affects ribosomal binding. Amikacin is less affected by these transferases than gentamicin and tobramycin and therefore is generally more active. Plazomicin is unaffected by all of these enzymes that confer resistance to amikacin, gentamicin, and tobramycin, thereby making this an important alternative agent in the treatment of selected XDR strains (excepting the Proteeae, against which plazomicin is poorly active). An as yet uncommon resistance mechanism involves 16S ribosomal RNA methylases, which prevent all aminoglycosides (including plazomicin) from binding to their target ribosomes. To date, these methylases are most common in strains that possess metallo-carbapenemases (e.g., NDM).

PREVENTION

(See also Chap. 142) Certain measures are broadly applicable for decreasing infection risk. Antimicrobial stewardship programs should be instituted to facilitate appropriate antimicrobial use, which will minimize the development of resistance. Diligent adherence to hand-hygiene protocols by health care personnel and cleaning/disinfection or single-patient use of objects that come into contact with patients (e.g., stethoscopes and blood pressure cuffs) are essential. Indwelling devices (e.g., urinary and intravascular catheters) should be used only when necessary and inserted according to an appropriate protocol; protocols for daily-use evaluation and prompt removal should be implemented. Multi-use medication vials should be avoided if possible. Oral application of chlorhexidine decreases the incidence of pneumonia among patients on ventilators. Increasing data support the implementation of universal decolonization (e.g., chlorhexidine bathing) to prevent infection in ICU patients. The public health threat from CRE has resulted in additional recommendations, especially for carbapenemase-producing CRE, which are an even greater concern. These recommendations include contact precautions for patients colonized or infected with CRE, notification to the receiving facility from facilities transferring such a patient, and daily environmental cleaning. Screening of contacts and active surveillance for these bacteria may also be appropriate.

ESCHERICHIA COLI INFECTIONS

All *E. coli* strains share a core genome of ~2000 genes. In contrast, an *E. coli* strain's ability to cause infection and the nature of such infections are defined largely by accessory (i.e., noncore, nonessential) genes that encode various virulence factors. The composition of the *E. coli* accessory genome is continuously in flux, as demonstrated by the recent evolution of Shiga toxin–producing enteroaggregative *E. coli*.

COMMENSAL STRAINS

Commensal *E. coli* variants are an important constituent of the normal intestinal microbiota that confer benefits to the host (e.g., resistance to colonization with pathogenic organisms). Such strains generally lack the specialized virulence traits that enable extraintestinal and intestinal pathogenic *E. coli* strains to cause disease outside and within the gastrointestinal tract, respectively. However, even commensal *E. coli* strains can be involved in extraintestinal infections in the presence of an aggravating factor, such as a foreign body (e.g., a urinary catheter), host compromise (e.g., local anatomic or functional abnormalities [including urinary or biliary tract obstruction] or systemic immunocompromise), or an inoculum that is large or contains a mixture of bacterial species (e.g., fecal contamination of the peritoneal cavity).

EXTRAINTESTINAL PATHOGENIC STRAINS

ExPEC strains are the most common enteric GNB to cause community-acquired and health care–associated bacterial infections. The emerging propensity of these strains to acquire new mechanisms of antimicrobial resistance (e.g., FQ resistance mutations, ESBLs, carbapenemases) poses novel challenges in managing ExPEC infection. Several ExPEC clonal groups (e.g., sequence types [STs] ST131, ST95, ST69, ST73) are recognized to have undergone global dissemination. The mechanisms underlying the epidemiologic success of such disseminated lineages remain an area of active investigation. In the case of ST131, efficient human-to-human transmission followed by colonization and long-term persistence within the intestinal microbiota appears to be a critical factor. Although acquisition of ESBL-producing *E. coli* from the food chain has been described, this appears to occur relatively uncommonly.

Like commensal *E. coli* (but unlike intestinal pathogenic *E. coli*), ExPEC strains are often found in the intestinal microbiota of healthy individuals and, except for rare chimeric ExPEC/intestinal pathogenic *E. coli* strains, do not cause gastroenteritis in humans. Entry from their site of colonization (e.g., the colon, vagina, or oropharynx) into a normally sterile extraintestinal site (e.g., the urinary tract, peritoneal cavity, or lungs) is the rate-limiting step for infection. ExPEC strains have acquired accessory genes encoding diverse virulence factors that enable the bacteria to cause infections outside the gastrointestinal tract in both normal and compromised hosts (Table 161-1). These virulence genes define ExPEC and, for the most part, are distinct from the virulence genes that enable intestinal pathogenic strains to cause diarrheal disease (**Table 161-3**). All age groups, all types of hosts, and nearly all organs and anatomic sites are susceptible to infection by ExPEC. Even previously healthy hosts can become severely ill or die when infected with ExPEC; however, adverse outcomes are more common among hosts with comorbid illnesses and host defense abnormalities. The diversity and the medical and economic impact of ExPEC infections are evident from consideration of the following specific syndromes.

Extraintestinal Infectious Syndromes • URINARY TRACT INFECTION

The urinary tract is the site most frequently infected by ExPEC. UTI is an exceedingly common infection among ambulatory patients, accounting for 1% of ambulatory care visits in the United States and second only to lower respiratory tract infection among infections responsible for hospitalization. UTIs are best considered by clinical syndrome (e.g., cystitis, pyelonephritis, catheter-associated UTI) and within the context of specific hosts (e.g., premenopausal women, compromised hosts; **Chap. 135**). *E. coli* is the single most common pathogen for all UTI syndrome/host group combinations. Each year in the United States, *E. coli* causes 80–90% of the estimated 6–8 million episodes of cystitis that occur in ambulatory, premenopausal women with an anatomically and functionally normal urinary tract (i.e., uncomplicated cystitis). Furthermore, 20% of women with an initial cystitis episode develop frequent recurrences.

Uncomplicated cystitis, the most common acute UTI syndrome, is characterized by dysuria, urinary frequency and urgency, and suprapubic pain. Progression to more severe infection is rare; the natural history is slow spontaneous symptom resolution, which antimicrobial therapy hastens. Fever and/or back pain suggest progression to pyelonephritis. Even when pyelonephritis is treated effectively, fever may take 5–7 days to resolve completely. Persistently elevated or increasing fever, flank pain, and neutrophil counts should prompt evaluation for intrarenal or perinephric abscess and/or obstruction. Pyelonephritis uncommonly causes renal parenchymal damage and loss of renal function, primarily in association with urinary obstruction, which can be preexisting or, rarely, occurs de novo in diabetic patients who develop renal papillary necrosis as a result of kidney infection. Pregnant women are at unusually high risk for developing pyelonephritis, which can adversely affect the outcome of pregnancy. As a result, prenatal screening for and treatment of asymptomatic bacteriuria during pregnancy are standard. Prostatic infection (prostatitis), a potential complication of UTI in men, can present either acutely (severe), which is rare, or in a chronic manner (recurrent cystitis), which is much more common. Acute pyelonephritis, acute prostatitis, and other systemic illnesses due to UTI can be designated collectively as *urosepsis*, *febrile UTI*, or *systemic UTI*, and may or may not be accompanied by bacteremia. The diagnosis and treatment of UTI, as detailed in **Chap. 135**, should be tailored to the individual host, the nature and site of infection, and local patterns of antimicrobial susceptibility.

ABDOMINAL AND PELVIC INFECTION The abdomen/pelvis is the second most common site of extraintestinal infection due to *E. coli*. A wide variety of clinical syndromes occur in this location, including acute peritonitis secondary to fecal contamination, spontaneous bacterial peritonitis, dialysis-associated peritonitis, diverticulitis, appendicitis, intraperitoneal or visceral abscesses (hepatic, pancreatic, splenic), infected pancreatic pseudocysts, and septic cholangitis and/or cholecystitis. In intraabdominal infections, *E. coli* can be isolated either alone or, as occurs more often, in combination with other facultative and/or anaerobic members of the intestinal microbiota (**Chap. 132**).

PNEUMONIA *E. coli* is not usually considered an important cause of pneumonia (**Chap. 126**). Indeed, enteric GNB account for only 1–3%

TABLE 161-3 Intestinal Pathogenic *Escherichia coli*

PATHOTYPE	EPIDEMIOLOGY	CLINICAL SYNDROME[a]	DEFINING MOLECULAR TRAIT	RESPONSIBLE GENETIC ELEMENT[b]
STEC/EHEC/ST-EAEC	Food, water, person-to-person; all ages, industrialized countries	Hemorrhagic colitis, hemolytic-uremic syndrome	Shiga toxin	Lambda-like Stx1- or Stx2-encoding bacteriophage
ETEC	Food, water; young children in and travelers to developing countries	Traveler's diarrhea	Heat-stable and labile enterotoxins, colonization factors	Virulence plasmid(s)
EPEC	Person-to-person; young children and neonates in developing countries	Watery diarrhea, persistent diarrhea	Localized adherence, attaching and effacing lesion on intestinal epithelium	EPEC adherence factor plasmid pathogenicity island (locus for enterocyte effacement [LEE])
EIEC	Food, water; children in and travelers to developing countries	Watery diarrhea, occasionally dysentery	Invasion of colonic epithelial cells, intracellular multiplication, cell-to-cell spread	Multiple genes contained primarily in a large virulence plasmid
EAEC	?Food, water; children in and travelers to developing countries; all ages, industrialized countries	Traveler's diarrhea, acute diarrhea, persistent diarrhea	Aggregative/diffuse adherence, virulence factors regulated by AggR	Chromosomal or plasmid-associated adherence and toxin genes

[a]Classic syndromes; see text for details on disease spectrum. [b]Pathogenesis involves multiple genes, including genes in addition to those listed.

Abbreviations: EAEC, enteroaggregative *E. coli*; EHEC, enterohemorrhagic *E. coli*; EIEC, enteroinvasive *E. coli*; EPEC, enteropathogenic *E. coli*; ETEC, enterotoxigenic *E. coli*; ST-EAEC, Shiga toxin–producing enteroaggregative *E. coli*; STEC, Shiga toxin–producing *E. coli*.

of cases of community-acquired pneumonia, in part because these organisms colonize the oropharynx only transiently in a minority of healthy individuals. However, rates of oral colonization with *E. coli* and other GNB increase with severity of illness and antibiotic use. Consequently, GNB are a more common cause of pneumonia among residents of LTCFs and are the most common cause (60–70% of cases) of hospital-acquired pneumonia (**Chap. 142**), particularly among post-operative and ICU patients (e.g., ventilator-associated pneumonia).

Pulmonary infection is usually acquired by small-volume aspiration but occasionally occurs via hematogenous spread, in which case multifocal nodular infiltrates can be seen. Tissue necrosis, probably due in part to bacterial cytotoxins, is common. Despite significant institutional variation, *E. coli* is generally the third or fourth most commonly isolated type of GNB in hospital-acquired pneumonia, accounting for 5–8% of episodes in both U.S.-based and Europe-based studies. Regardless of the host, pneumonia due to ExPEC is a serious disease, with high crude and attributable mortality rates (20–60% and 10–20%, respectively).

MENINGITIS (**See also Chap. 138**) *E. coli* is one of the leading causes of neonatal meningitis, together with group B *Streptococcus*. Most *E. coli* strains that cause neonatal meningitis possess the K1 capsular antigen and derive from a limited number of meningitis-associated clonal groups. Ventriculomegaly occurs commonly. After the first month of life, *E. coli* meningitis is uncommon, and usually accompanies surgical or traumatic disruption of the meninges or hepatic cirrhosis. In patients with cirrhosis who develop meningitis, the meninges are presumably seeded due to poor hepatic clearance of portal vein bacteremia.

CELLULITIS/MUSCULOSKELETAL INFECTION *E. coli* contributes frequently to infections of decubitus ulcers and occasionally to infections of lower-extremity ulcers and wounds in diabetic patients and other hosts with neurovascular compromise. Osteomyelitis secondary to contiguous spread can occur in these settings. *E. coli* also causes cellulitis or infections of burn sites and surgical wounds (accounting for ~10% of surgical site infections), particularly when the infection originates close to the perineum. *E. coli* causes hematogenously acquired osteomyelitis, especially of vertebral discs and bodies, accounting for up to 10% of cases in some series (**Chap. 131**). *E. coli* occasionally causes orthopedic device–associated infection or septic arthritis and rarely causes hematogenous myositis. Myositis or fasciitis of the thigh due to *E. coli* should prompt an evaluation for an abdominal source with contiguous spread.

ENDOVASCULAR INFECTION Despite being one of the most common causes of bacteremia, *E. coli* rarely seeds native heart valves. When the organism does infect native valves, it usually does so in the setting of prior valvular disease. *E. coli* infections of aneurysms, the portal vein (*pylephlebitis*), and vascular grafts are quite uncommon.

MISCELLANEOUS INFECTIONS *E. coli* can cause infection in nearly every organ and anatomic site. It occasionally causes postoperative mediastinitis or complicated sinusitis and uncommonly causes endophthalmitis, ecthyma gangrenosum, or brain abscess.

BACTEREMIA *E. coli* bacteremia can arise from infection at any extraintestinal site. In addition, *E. coli* bacteremia can arise from percutaneous intravascular devices, transrectal prostate biopsy, and the increased intestinal mucosal permeability seen in neonates and patients with advanced cirrhosis, neutropenia, chemotherapy-induced mucositis, trauma, and extensive burns. *E. coli* bacteremia due to an ESBL-producing strain also has been reported after fecal microbiota transplant in patients with increased mucosal permeability. Roughly equal proportions of *E. coli* bacteremia cases originate in the community and in health care settings. Isolation of *E. coli* from the blood is almost always clinically significant and may be accompanied by the sepsis syndrome (dysfunction of at least one organ or system) or septic shock (**Chap. 304**).

The urinary tract is the most common source for *E. coli* bacteremia, accounting for one-half to two-thirds of episodes. Bacteremia from a urinary tract source is particularly common among patients with pyelonephritis, urinary tract obstruction, or urinary instrumentation in the presence of infected urine. The abdomen is the second most common source, accounting for ~25% of episodes. Although many of these episodes result from biliary obstruction (stones, tumor) and overt bowel disruption, which typically are readily apparent, some abdominal sources (e.g., abscesses) are remarkably silent clinically and require identification via imaging studies (e.g., computed tomography). Therefore, especially given the high prevalence of asymptomatic bacteriuria among elderly and functionally compromised individuals, the physician should be cautious in attributing *E. coli* bacteremia to a urinary source in the absence of characteristic signs and symptoms of UTI. Soft tissue, bone, pulmonary infections, and intravascular catheter infections are other sources of *E. coli* bacteremia.

Diagnosis Strains of *E. coli* that cause extraintestinal infections usually grow both aerobically and anaerobically within 24 h on standard diagnostic media and are identified readily by the clinical microbiology laboratory according to routine biochemical criteria. More than 90% of ExPEC strains are rapid lactose fermenters and are indole-positive.

TREATMENT

Extraintestinal *E. coli* Infections

E. coli does not possess clinically significant intrinsic resistance to antimicrobials; however, increasing acquired resistance is making treatment problematic. Although geographic differences exist, in general, the prevalence of resistance is >20% for ampicillin, amoxicillin-clavulanate, ampicillin-sulbactam, cefazolin, TMP-SMX, and fluoroquinolones, even in community-acquired infections. This resistance precludes empirical use of these agents for serious infections. Travel outside of the United States, prior exposure to an antimicrobial agent, or exposure to a health care setting further increases the likelihood of resistance. Fortunately, >90% of isolates that cause uncomplicated cystitis remain susceptible to nitrofurantoin and fosfomycin.

From 2015 to 2017, the U.S. National Healthcare Safety Network (USNHSN) identified 24% of *E. coli* clinical isolates as ESBL-producers. Higher prevalences are reported from Asia, Eastern Europe, South America, and Africa; prevalence is also greater in isolates from health care settings, especially LTCFs. However, community-acquired UTIs caused by *E. coli* strains that produce CTX-M ESBLs are increasingly common. Oral treatment options for such strains are limited; however, in vitro and limited clinical data indicate that fosfomycin, pivmecillinam, and nitrofurantoin are highly active and can be used for cystitis, and omadacycline is predicted to be active based on in vitro data. For parenteral therapy of carbapenem-sensitive strains, the most predictably active agents (>90%) include carbapenems, amikacin, plazomicin, ceftazidime-avibactam, ceftolozane-tazobactam, meropenem-vaborbactam, imipenem/cilastatin-relebactam, piperacillin-tazobactam, polymyxins, cefiderocol, tigecycline, eravacycline, and omadacycline. Treatment of carbapenemase-producing strains is dependent of the class of enzyme produced (see "Carbapenemase" above). Uncertainty exists on the optimal treatment for non-CP-CR *E. coli*.

Empirical treatment decisions for critically ill patients should be dictated by local susceptibility patterns and patient-specific risk factors (1.2% prevalence from the USNHSN 2015–2017 data). Equally important as prompt institution of effective empirical therapy for seriously ill patients is use of appropriate narrower-spectrum agents for definitive therapy whenever possible and avoidance of treatment for patients who are colonized but not infected.

■ INTESTINAL PATHOGENIC STRAINS

Pathotypes Certain strains of *E. coli* are capable of causing diarrheal disease. (**Other important intestinal pathogens are discussed in Chaps. 133, 134, and 165–168.**) At least in the industrialized world, intestinal pathogenic *E. coli* strains are rarely encountered in the fecal flora of healthy persons, and instead appear to be essentially obligate pathogens. These strains have evolved a special ability to cause enteritis, enterocolitis, and colitis when ingested in sufficient quantities by a naive host. At least five distinct pathotypes of intestinal pathogenic *E. coli* exist: (1) Shiga toxin–producing *E. coli* (STEC), which includes the subsets enterohemorrhagic *E. coli* (EHEC) and the recently evolved Shiga toxin–producing enteroaggregative *E. coli* (ST-EAEC); (2) enterotoxigenic *E. coli* (ETEC); (3) enteropathogenic *E. coli* (EPEC); (4) enteroinvasive *E. coli* (EIEC); and (5) enteroaggregative *E. coli* (EAEC). Diffusely adherent *E. coli* (DAEC) and cytodetaching *E. coli* are additional putative pathotypes. Lastly, a variant termed adherent invasive *E. coli* (AIEC) has been associated with Crohn's disease (although a causal role remains unproven) but does not cause acute diarrheal disease.

Contaminated food and water are the primary transmission vehicles for ETEC, STEC/EHEC/ST-EAEC, EIEC, and EAEC, whereas person-to-person spread (direct or indirect) is the primary transmission route for EPEC and a secondary transmission route for STEC/EHEC/ST-EAEC. Gastric acidity confers some protection against infection; therefore, persons with decreased stomach acid levels are especially susceptible. Humans are the major reservoir for such strains (except for STEC/EHEC, for which bovines are the main carriers); host range appears to be dictated by species-specific attachment factors. Although some overlap exists, each pathotype possesses a distinctive combination of virulence traits that results in a pathotype-specific pathogenic mechanism (Table 161-3). With rare exceptions, these strains are largely incapable of causing disease outside the intestinal tract. Whereas disease due to STEC/EHEC/ST-EAEC occurs primarily in high-income countries, disease due to ETEC, EPEC, and EIEC occurs primarily in low- and middle-income countries in Asia, Africa, and Latin America, and disease due to EAEC occurs globally.

SHIGA TOXIN–PRODUCING *E. COLI* STEC/EHEC/ST-EAEC strains are pathogens that can cause hemorrhagic colitis and the hemolytic-uremic syndrome (HUS). In contrast to other intestinal pathotypes, STEC/EHEC/ST-EAEC causes infections more frequently in industrialized countries than in developing regions. Several large outbreaks resulting from the consumption of fresh produce (e.g., lettuce, spinach, sprouts) and of undercooked ground beef have received significant media attention. In addition, a dramatic 2011 outbreak—mainly in Germany—involved an EAEC strain that acquired a Shiga toxin–encoding phage, resulting in a novel genotype, ST-EAEC (O104:H4). This strain was transmitted to the primary cases by sprouted fenugreek seeds, with subsequent human-to-human transmission, and resulted in >4000 cases and 54 deaths.

STEC strains are the fourth most commonly reported cause of bacterial diarrhea in the United States (after *Campylobacter*, *Salmonella*, and *Shigella*). O157:H7 is the most prominent serotype among STEC strains, but many other serogroups have been described, including O6, O26, O45, O55, O91, O103, O111, O113, O121, and O145. Domesticated ruminant animals, particularly cattle and young calves, serve as the major reservoir for STEC/EHEC. Ground or mechanically tenderized beef—the most common food source of STEC/EHEC strains—is often contaminated with intestinal bacteria from the source animals during processing. Furthermore, manure from cattle or other animals (including in the form of fertilizer) can contaminate produce (potatoes, lettuce, spinach, sprouts, fallen fruits, nuts, strawberries), and fecal runoff from manure can contaminate water systems. Dairy products and petting zoos are additional sources of infection.

It is estimated that <10^2 colony-forming units (CFU) of STEC/EHEC/ST-EAEC can cause disease. Therefore, not only can low levels of food or environmental contamination (e.g., in water swallowed while swimming) result in disease, but person-to-person transmission (e.g., at day-care centers and in institutions) is an important route for secondary spread. Laboratory-associated infections also occur. Illness due to this group of pathogens peaks in the summer months and occurs both as outbreaks and as sporadic cases.

For STEC/EHEC/ST-EAEC, production of Shiga toxin (Stx2a-g and/or Stx1a,c,d) is a critical factor for occurrence of clinical disease, as demonstrated by the 2011 ST-EAEC outbreak. The *stx* gene is present on chromosomally integrated prophages, and various combinations of *stx* types and subtypes can occur in a given strain. *Shigella dysenteriae* strains that produce the closely related Shiga toxin Stx also can cause hemorrhagic colitis and HUS. Stx2 (especially Stx2a,c,d) appears to be more important than Stx1 in the development of HUS. All Shiga toxins studied to date are multimers; they comprise one A subunit that is enzymatically active and five identical B subunits that mediate binding to globosyl ceramides, which are membrane-associated glycolipids expressed on certain host cells. As in ricin, the Stx A subunit cleaves an adenine from the host cell's 28S rRNA, thereby irreversibly inhibiting ribosomal function (i.e., protein synthesis) and potentially leading to apoptosis.

For full pathogenicity, STEC strains require additional properties such as acid tolerance and epithelial cell adherence. Most disease-causing isolates possess the chromosomal locus for enterocyte effacement (LEE). This pathogenicity island was first described in EPEC strains; it contains genes that mediate adherence to intestinal epithelial cells and a system that subverts host cells by the translocation of bacterial proteins (type III secretion system). EHEC strains make up the subgroup of STEC strains that possess stx_1 and/or stx_2, as well as LEE. In contrast, the 2011 ST-EAEC outbreak strain lacked LEE, yet was associated with a higher proportion of patients developing HUS (22%) than the historical average for STEC/EHEC outbreaks (2–8%). Data support the essential role of the 2011 outbreak strain's EAEC-associated virulence factors (e.g., AAF/I fimbriae, serine proteases SigA, SepA) in adherence, increased inflammation, and disruption of the intestinal epithelial barrier, which in turn increased the systemic translocation of Stx2a.

After exposure to STEC/EHEC/ST-EAEC and a 3- to 4-day incubation period, colonization of the colon and perhaps the ileum results in symptoms. Colonic edema and an initial nonbloody secretory diarrhea may progress to the hallmark syndrome of grossly bloody diarrhea (identified by history or examination). Significant abdominal pain and fecal leukocytes are common (70% of cases), whereas fever is not; absence of fever can incorrectly lead to consideration of noninfectious conditions (e.g., intussusception and inflammatory or ischemic bowel disease). Occasionally, infections caused by *C. difficile*, *K. oxytoca* (see "*Klebsiella* Infections," below), *Campylobacter*, and *Salmonella* present in a similar fashion. STEC/EHEC disease is usually self-limited, lasting 5–10 days.

A feared complication of infection with STEC/EHEC strains is HUS, which occurs 2–14 days after diarrhea, most often in young children (estimated to occur in 15% of infected children <10 years of age) or elderly patients. It is estimated that in the United States >50% of all HUS cases—and 90% of HUS cases in children, which is a leading cause of acute renal failure in this latter population—are caused by STEC/EHEC. In contrast, with ST-EAEC infection, HUS occurs more commonly among nonelderly adults, especially young women. HUS is mediated by the systemic translocation of Shiga toxins. Erythrocytes may serve as carriers of Stx to endothelial cells located in the small vessels of the kidney and brain. The subsequent development of thrombotic microangiopathy (perhaps with direct toxin-mediated effects on various nonendothelial cells) commonly produces some combination of fever, hemolytic anemia, thrombocytopenia, renal failure, and encephalopathy. Stx-mediated complement activation may also play a role in the development of HUS. Although with dialysis support the mortality rate of HUS is <10%, survivors often have persisting renal and neurologic dysfunction.

ENTEROTOXIGENIC *E. COLI* ETEC is a major cause of endemic diarrhea in low- and middle-income countries and is responsible for an estimated 800 million cases annually. After weaning, children in these locales commonly experience several episodes of ETEC infection during the first 3 years of life. The incidence of disease diminishes with age, a pattern that correlates with the development of mucosal immunity to colonization factors (i.e., adhesins).

In industrialized countries, ETEC is the most common agent of traveler's diarrhea, causing 25–75% of cases. The incidence of infection may be decreased by prudent avoidance of potentially contaminated fluids and foods, particularly items that are raw, insufficiently cooked, peeled, or unrefrigerated (**Chap. 124**). ETEC infection is uncommon in the United States, but outbreaks secondary to consumption of food products imported from endemic areas have occurred. A large inoculum (10^6–10^8 CFU) is needed to produce disease, which usually develops after an incubation period of 12–72 h.

After adherence of ETEC to enterocytes via colonization factors (e.g., CFA/I, CS), disease is mediated, primarily by a heat-labile toxin (LT) and/or a heat-stable toxin (STa), leading to diarrheal disease. Disease is less severe with strains that produce only LT. Both LT and STa cause net fluid secretion via activation of adenylate cyclase and/or guanylate cyclase C (STa) in the jejunum and ileum. The result is watery diarrhea accompanied by cramps.

LT consists of an A and a pentameric B subunit and is structurally and functionally similar to cholera toxin. Strong binding of the B subunit to the GM_1 ganglioside on intestinal epithelial cells leads to the intracellular translocation of the A subunit, which functions as an ADP-ribosyltransferase. Mature STa is an 18- or 19-amino-acid secreted peptide that leads to increased intracellular concentrations of cGMP. Characteristically absent in ETEC-mediated disease are histopathologic changes within the small bowel; mucus, blood, and inflammatory cells in stool; and fever.

The disease spectrum of ETEC infection ranges from mild illness to a life-threatening, cholera-like syndrome. Although symptoms are usually self-limited (typically lasting for 3–5 days), infection may result in significant morbidity and mortality (>250,000 deaths annually, mostly from profound volume depletion) when access to health care or suitable rehydration fluids is limited and when small and/or undernourished children are affected.

ENTEROPATHOGENIC *E. COLI* EPEC causes disease primarily in young children, including neonates. The first *E. coli* pathotype recognized as an agent of diarrheal disease, EPEC was responsible for outbreaks of infantile diarrhea (including in hospital nurseries) in industrialized countries in the 1940s and 1950s. At present, EPEC infection is uncommon in high-income countries, but among infants in low- and middle-income countries, it is an important cause of diarrhea (both sporadic and epidemic), often accompanied by vomiting and fever. Breast-feeding diminishes the incidence of EPEC infection. Rapid person-to-person spread may occur.

Symptoms develop after colonization of the small bowel and a brief incubation period (1 or 2 days). Initial localized adherence to enterocytes via type IV bundle-forming pili leads to a characteristic effacement of microvilli, with the formation of cuplike, actin-rich pedestals mediated by factors in the LEE. Diarrhea production is a complex and regulated process in which host cell modulation by a type III secretion system plays an important role. Strains lacking bundle-forming pili have been categorized as atypical EPEC (aEPEC); increasing data support a role for these strains as intestinal pathogens in all age groups and among HIV-infected individuals. Diarrheal stool often contain mucus but not blood. Although EPEC diarrhea is usually self-limited (lasting 5–15 days), it may persist for weeks.

ENTEROINVASIVE *E. COLI* EIEC, a relatively uncommon (or perhaps underrecognized) cause of diarrhea, is rarely identified in the United States, although a few food-related outbreaks have been described. In low- and middle-income countries, sporadic disease is recognized infrequently in children and travelers.

EIEC shares many genetic and clinical features, as well as a common ancestor, with *Shigella*. Both are intracellular pathogens for which virulence is mediated by the presence of specific factors and by the loss or inactivation of other factors (antivirulence genes), which presumably occurred during these organisms' transition from an extracellular to an intracellular lifestyle.

Colonization and invasion of the colonic mucosa, followed by replication therein and cell-to-cell spread (in part via a type III secretion system), result in the development of inflammatory colitis. However, unlike *Shigella*, EIEC produces disease only with a large inoculum (10^8–10^{10} CFU) and is less virulent, typically causing only mild, self-limited (7–10 days), watery diarrhea. Onset generally follows an incubation period of 1–3 days. Occasionally, EIEC can cause a shigellosis-like (dysentery) syndrome characterized by fever, abdominal pain, tenesmus, and scant stool containing mucus, blood, and inflammatory cells.

ENTEROAGGREGATIVE AND DIFFUSELY ADHERENT *E. COLI* EAEC has been described primarily in low- and middle-income countries and in young children. However, recent studies indicate that it also may be a relatively common cause of diarrhea in all age groups in industrialized countries. EAEC has been recognized increasingly as an important cause of traveler's diarrhea. It is highly adapted to humans—the probable reservoir. A large inoculum is required for infection, which usually manifests as watery and sometimes persistent diarrhea in healthy but also malnourished or HIV-infected hosts.

In vitro, EAEC cells exhibit a diffuse or "stacked-brick" pattern of adherence to small-intestine epithelial cells. Virulence factors that probably are necessary for disease are regulated in large part by the transcriptional activator AggR. The pathogenesis of EAEC disease begins with intestinal adherence, which results from stimulation of epithelial mucus production and bacterial biofilm formation, the latter mediated by fimbriae and possibly the mucinase Pic and dispersin. Inflammation ensues, resulting in epithelial cell exfoliation and intestinal secretion, which is mediated by the enterotoxins Pet, EAST-1, ShET1, and HlyE.

An additional enteric pathotype, DAEC, is associated with diarrheal disease, primarily in children 2–6 years of age in some developing countries, and may cause traveler's diarrhea. The Afa/Dr adhesins may contribute to the pathogenesis of such infections.

Diagnosis Acute infectious diarrhea can be classified as noninflammatory (most commonly viral) or inflammatory (usually bacterial); the latter is suggested by grossly bloody or mucoid stools or a positive test for fecal leukocytes, lactoferrin, or calprotectin (**Chap. 133**). ETEC, EPEC, DAEC, and EAEC cause noninflammatory diarrhea. Identification of these agents can be achieved with a commercial platform (e.g., BioFire® Film Array® Gastrointestinal Panel can detect STEC, ETEC, EPEC, EAEC, and EIEC). However, organism identification is rarely needed because the associated diseases are self-limited. ETEC causes the majority and EAEC a minority of cases of noninflammatory traveler's diarrhea; here again, however, definitive diagnosis generally is not necessary for management (as discussed below). If diarrhea persists for >10 days despite treatment, *Giardia* or *Cryptosporidium* (or, in immunocompromised hosts, certain opportunistic pathogens) should be sought.

Because of the considerable public-health importance of STEC/EHEC/ST-EAEC infections, including the threat of HUS, the CDC now recommends that all patients with community-acquired diarrhea, whether inflammatory or not, be evaluated for these pathogens by simultaneous culture (to provide an isolate for strain typing and for outbreak detection and control) and detection of Shiga toxin or the corresponding genes. The rationale for testing all cases of community-acquired diarrhea, regardless of clinical features, is that bloody stool and fecal white blood cells (or lactoferrin) are not reliably present with STEC/EHEC/ST-EAEC infection. In addition, the use of both tests increases diagnostic sensitivity over that with either test alone.

O157 STEC/EHEC may be identified via culture by screening for *E. coli* strains that do not ferment sorbitol, with subsequent serotyping and testing for Shiga toxin. Selective or screening media are not available for culture-based detection of non-O157 STEC/EHEC/ST-EAEC strains. Detection of Shiga toxins or toxin genes via DNA-based, enzyme-linked immunosorbent, and cytotoxicity assays offers the advantages of rapidity and detection of non-O157 STEC/EHEC/ST-EAEC strains. Specimens positive for toxin but culture-negative for O157 should be forwarded to the local or state public-health laboratory for specialized testing.

TREATMENT

Intestinal *E. coli* Infections

The mainstay of treatment for all diarrheal syndromes is replacement of water and electrolytes. This measure is especially important for STEC/EHEC/ST-EAEC infection because appropriate volume expansion may protect against renal injury and improve outcome.

The use of prophylactic antibiotics to prevent traveler's diarrhea generally should be discouraged, especially in light of high rates of antimicrobial resistance. However, in selected patients (e.g., those who cannot afford a brief illness or are predisposed to infection), the use of rifaximin, which is nonabsorbable and is well tolerated, is reasonable.

When stools are free of mucus and blood, early patient-initiated treatment of traveler's diarrhea with a fluoroquinolone or azithromycin decreases the duration of illness, and the use of loperamide may halt symptoms within a few hours. Although dysentery caused by EIEC is self-limited, antimicrobial therapy hastens the resolution of symptoms, particularly in severe cases. In contrast, antimicrobial therapy for STEC/EHEC/ST-EAEC infection (the presence of which is suggested by grossly bloody diarrhea without fever) should be avoided because antibiotics may increase the incidence of HUS (possibly via increased production/release of Stx). In the treatment of HUS, plasmapheresis has no benefit and the value of inhibition of C5 (via eculizumab) is unresolved.

KLEBSIELLA INFECTIONS

K. pneumoniae is the most important *Klebsiella* species from a medical standpoint, causing community-acquired, LTCF-acquired, and nosocomial infections. *K. oxytoca* and *K.* (formerly *Enterobacter*) *aerogenes* are primarily pathogens in LTCFs and hospitals. *Klebsiella* species are broadly prevalent in the environment and colonize the mucosal surfaces of mammals. In healthy humans, the prevalence of *K. pneumoniae* colonization is 5–35% in the colon and 1–5% in the oropharynx; skin is usually colonized only transiently.

Most *Klebsiella* infections in Western countries are caused by "classical" *K. pneumoniae* (cKp) and occur in hospitals and LTCFs. The most common clinical syndromes due to cKp are pneumonia, UTI, abdominal infection, intravascular device infection, surgical site infection, soft tissue infection, and secondary bacteremia. cKp strains have gained notoriety because of their propensity for acquiring treatment-confounding antimicrobial resistance determinants and causing both localized and widespread outbreaks, such as with the global spread of NDM-1-producing cKp strains from India associated with medical tourism. Clonal groups STs 11, 15, 101, 307, and 258/512, many members of which produce carbapenemases, are undergoing international dissemination. Transmission within or between institutions is common. *K. pneumoniae* is nearly four-fold more transmissible than *E. coli*, and, disconcertingly, carbapenemase-producing strains are associated with increased spread compared to carbapenem-susceptible strains.

In addition, hypervirulent *K. pneumoniae* (hvKp) strains that are phenotypically and clinically distinct from cKp have emerged recently, after their initial recognition in Taiwan in 1986. Although hvKp infections have occurred globally in all ethnic groups, most cases have been reported in individuals of Asian ethnicity residing in countries from the Asian Pacific Rim, but also in Asians living in other countries. Affected individuals often have diabetes mellitus. These demographics raise the possibility of a locale-specific distribution of the organism or an increased susceptibility of Asian hosts, especially those who are diabetic. In contrast to the usual health care–associated context for cKp infections in the West, hvKp is capable of causing serious life- and organ-threatening infections in younger, healthy individuals from the community and can spread metastatically from the primary site of infection or present with multiple sites of infection. Of concern, recent reports from Asian countries have demonstrated that hvKp is responsible for an increasing number of health care–associated or hospital-acquired infections.

hvKp infection initially was characterized and distinguished from traditional infections caused by cKp strains by its (1) presentation as community-acquired monomicrobial pyogenic liver abscess (**Fig. 161-1, *top***), (2) occurrence in patients lacking a history of hepatobiliary disease, and (3) propensity for metastatic spread to distant sites. Subsequently, the hvKp pathotype has been recognized as the cause of extrahepatic abscesses and infections with or without liver involvement, including pneumonia; meningitis (in the absence of trauma or

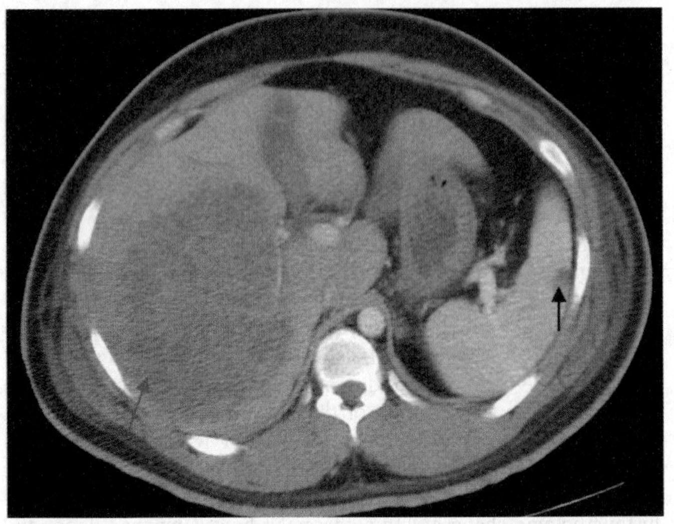

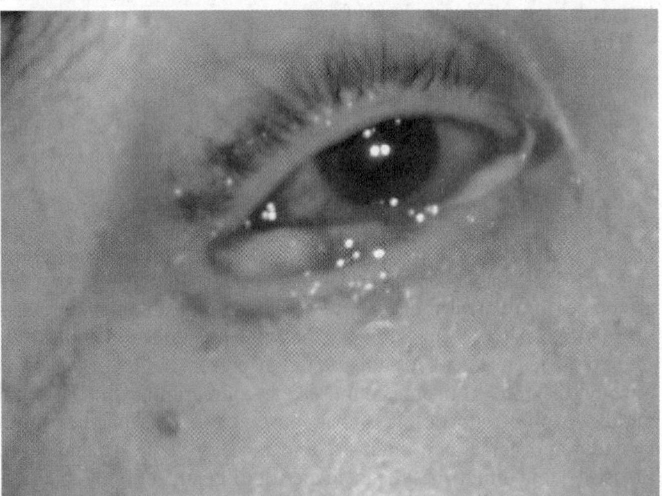

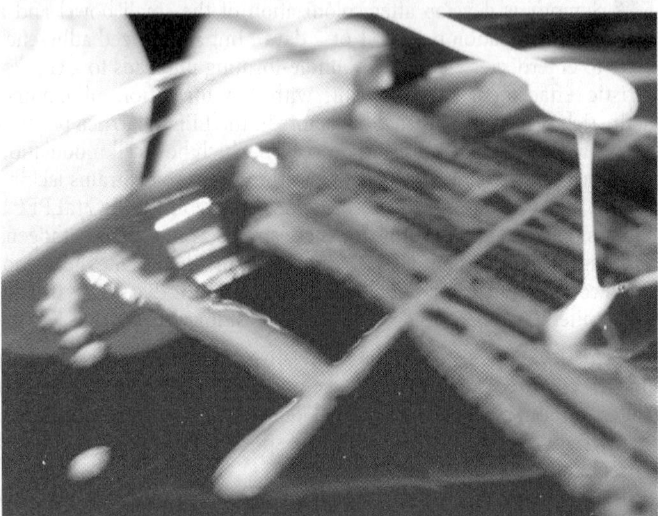

FIGURE 161-1 Hypervirulent pathotype of *K. pneumoniae* (hvKp). ***Top:*** Abdominal CT scan of a previously healthy 24-year-old Vietnamese man shows a primary liver abscess (*red arrow*) with metastatic spread to the spleen (*black arrow*). *(Courtesy of Drs. Chiu-Bin Hsaio and Diana Pomakova.)* ***Middle:*** A previously healthy 33-year-old Chinese man presented with endophthalmitis. *(AS Shon, RP Bajwa, TA Russo: Hypervirulent (hypermucoviscous) Klebsiella pneumoniae: A new and dangerous breed. Virulence 4:107, 2013.)* ***Bottom:*** A hypermucoviscous phenotype (which does not necessarily equate with a mucoid phenotype) has been associated with hvKp strains. A positive string test is shown. However, this test is not optimally sensitive or specific. Identification of the combination of the biomarkers *iucA*, *iroB*, *peg-344*, *rmpA*, and *rmpA2* is presently the most accurate means to identify hvKp.

neurosurgery); endophthalmitis (**Fig. 161-1**, ***middle***); splenic, psoas, prostatic, epidural, and brain abscesses; and necrotizing fasciitis. Survivors often suffer catastrophic morbidity, such as vision loss and major neurologic sequelae. Most recently, clinicians are faced with an even greater challenge—the confluence of antimicrobial resistance determinants possessed by cKp and the virulence factors possessed by hvKp on the same or coexisting plasmids. The result is the evolution of MDR and XDR hvKp.

K. pneumoniae subspecies *rhinoscleromatis* is the causative agent of rhinoscleroma, a granulomatous mucosal upper-respiratory infection that progresses slowly (over months or years) and causes necrosis and occasionally obstruction of the nasal passages. *K. pneumoniae* subspecies *ozaenae* has been implicated as a cause of chronic atrophic rhinitis and rarely of invasive disease in compromised hosts. *K. (Calymmatobacterium) granulomatis*, a sexually transmitted pathogen, is the causative agent of granuloma inguinale (donovanosis) that results in chronic genital ulcers (**Chap. 173**). These *Klebsiella* pathotypes are usually isolated from patients in tropical climates and are genomically distinct from both cKp and hvKp.

INFECTIOUS SYNDROMES

Pneumonia Although cKp accounts for only a small proportion of cases of community-acquired pneumonia in Western countries (**Chap. 126**), cKP and *K. oxytoca* are common causes of pneumonia among LTCF residents and hospitalized patients because of increased rates of oropharyngeal colonization with these organisms in such individuals. Mechanical ventilation is an important risk factor. In Asia and South Africa, community-acquired pneumonia due to hvKp is becoming increasingly common, rivaling *Streptococcus pneumoniae*, and may occur in younger patients with no underlying disease. *Klebsiella* is also a common cause of pneumonia in severely malnourished children in developing countries.

As in all pneumonias due to enteric GNB, typical manifestations include production of purulent sputum and evidence of airspace disease. Presentation with earlier, less extensive infection is now more common than is the classically described lobar infiltrate, bulging fissure, and currant-jelly sputum. Pulmonary infection due to hvKp that has spread metastatically (e.g., from a hepatic abscess) usually includes nodular bilateral densities, more commonly in the lower lobes. Pulmonary necrosis, pleural effusion, and empyema can occur with disease progression.

UTI cKP accounts for only 1–2% of UTI episodes among otherwise healthy adults but for 5–17% of episodes of UTI in patients with anatomic and functional abnormalities of the urinary tract, including indwelling urinary catheter use (complicated UTI). UTI due to hvKp presents more commonly as renal or prostatic abscess due to bacteremic spread than as ascending infection from the urethra and bladder.

Abdominal Infection cKp causes a spectrum of abdominal infections similar to that caused by *E. coli* but is less frequently isolated from such infections than is *E. coli*. hvKp is a common cause of monomicrobial community-acquired pyogenic liver abscess; in the Asian Pacific Rim, it has been recovered with steadily increasing frequency over the past two decades, replacing *E. coli* as the most common pathogen causing this syndrome. hvKp also is increasingly described as a cause of spontaneous bacterial peritonitis and splenic abscess.

Other Infections When cKp and *K. oxytoca* cause cellulitis or soft tissue infection, the process most frequently involves devitalized tissue (e.g., decubitus and diabetic ulcers, burn wounds) and immunocompromised hosts. cKp and *K. oxytoca* cause some cases of surgical site infection and nosocomial sinusitis as well as occasional cases of osteomyelitis contiguous to soft tissue infection, nontropical myositis, and meningitis (during the neonatal period and after neurosurgery). By contrast, hvKp has become an important cause of community-acquired monomicrobial necrotizing fasciitis, meningitis, endophthalmitis (Fig. 161-1, *middle*), and abscesses within the brain, subdural space, and epidural space, particularly in the Asian Pacific Rim but also globally. Cytotoxin-producing strains of *K. oxytoca* have been implicated as a cause of non–*C. difficile* antibiotic-associated hemorrhagic colitis.

Bacteremia *Klebsiella* infection at any site can produce bacteremia. Infections of the urinary tract, respiratory tract, and abdomen (especially hepatic abscess) each account for 15–30% of episodes of *Klebsiella* bacteremia. Intravascular device–related infections account for another 5–15% of episodes, and surgical site and miscellaneous infections account for the rest. *Klebsiella* is an occasional cause of sepsis in neonates and of bacteremia in neutropenic patients. However, like enteric GNB in general, *Klebsiella* rarely causes endocarditis or other endovascular infections, although the endocarditis can involve extensive valvular destruction.

DIAGNOSIS

Klebsiellae are readily isolated and identified in the laboratory. These organisms usually ferment lactose, although the subspecies *rhinoscleromatis* and *ozaenae* are nonfermenters and are indole-negative. hvKp usually possesses a hypermucoviscous phenotype (**Fig. 161-1**, ***bottom***), although the sensitivity and specificity of the string test are less than optimal. Identification of the combination of the biomarkers *iucA*, *iroB*, *peg-344*, *rmpA*, and *rmpA2* is presently the most accurate means to identify hvKp, although currently, this test is not routinely available.

TREATMENT

Klebsiella Infections

K. (formerly *Enterobacter*) *aerogenes* has a similar resistance profile to *E. cloacae*, the treatment of which is discussed below. *K. pneumoniae* and *K. oxytoca* have similar antibiotic resistance profiles; both are intrinsically resistant to ampicillin. The prevalence of acquired resistance in *K. pneumoniae* and *K. oxytoca* is generally >30% for amoxicillin-clavulanate, ampicillin-sulbactam, nitrofurantoin, and TMP-SMX and ~10–20% for fluoroquinolones, piperacillin-tazobactam, fosfomycin, and omadacycline.

USNHSN data from 2015–2017 identified 25% of *K. pneumoniae* as ESBL-producing strains; higher rates are reported from Asia, South America, and Africa. Although prevalent ESBL-producing strains are greatest in LTCF, isolates of cKp that produce CTX-M ESBLs are increasingly described from the community. Oral treatment for infection due to ESBL-producing strains is more challenging with *Klebsiella* than with *E. coli* because of the comparatively poor activity of nitrofurantoin, the lesser activity of fosfomycin (~80%), and limited available data regarding pivmecillinam (>80%) and omadacycline (75–100% susceptible for ESBL-producing isolates, but 60% if resistant to tetracycline).

Predictably, the ESBL-driven use of carbapenems has selected for strains of cKp and *K. oxytoca* that express carbapenemases (8–18% based on the study and locale, 8.6% prevalence from 2015–2017 USNHSN data). Treatment can be problematic for such organisms, especially those with a metallo-β-lactamase (e.g., NDM), for which the highest prevalences are in cKp and *K. oxytoca* isolates from Eastern Europe and Asia and among health care–associated isolates. Likewise, hvKp strains from Asia are also increasingly reported to produce ESBLs and carbapenemases.

Treatment options for carbapenem-resistant *Klebsiella* are similar to those described for *E. coli* and depend on the class of carbapenemase produced (see "Carbapenemase" above); consultation with relevant experts is advised. For carbapenem-sensitive strains, the most predictably active agents include carbapenems, amikacin, plazomicin, ceftazidime-avibactam, ceftolozane-tazobactam, meropenem-vaborbactam, imipenem/cilastatin-relebactam, polymyxins, cefiderocol, tigecycline, eravacycline, and omadacycline. Empirical treatment decisions for the critically ill patient should be dictated by local susceptibility patterns and patient-specific risk factors.

PROTEUS INFECTIONS

Proteus species are part of the colonic flora of a wide variety of mammals, birds, fish, and reptiles. The ability of these GNB to generate histamine from contaminated fish has implicated them in the pathogenesis of scombroid (fish) poisoning (**Chap. 460**).

P. mirabilis causes 90% of *Proteus* infections, which occur in the community, LTCFs, and hospitals. By contrast, *Proteus vulgaris* and *Proteus penneri* are associated primarily with infections acquired in LTCFs or hospitals. Correspondingly, *P. mirabilis* colonizes healthy humans (prevalence, 50%), whereas *P. vulgaris* and *P. penneri* are isolated primarily from individuals with underlying disease. By far the most common site of *Proteus* infection is the urinary tract, where the principal known urovirulence factors of *Proteus* include adhesins, flagella, IgA-IgG protease, iron acquisition systems, and urease. *Proteus* less commonly causes infection at a variety of other extraintestinal sites.

■ INFECTIOUS SYNDROMES

UTI *P. mirabilis* causes only 1–2% of UTIs in healthy women, and *Proteus* species collectively cause only 5% of hospital-acquired UTIs. However, *Proteus* is responsible for 10–15% of cases of complicated UTI, primarily those associated with catheterization; indeed, *Proteus* accounts for 20–45% of urine isolates from chronically catheterized patients. This high prevalence is due in part to bacterial production of urease, which hydrolyzes urea to ammonia and results in alkalization of the urine. In alkaline urine, organic and inorganic compounds precipitate, contributing to the formation of struvite and carbonate–apatite crystals, biofilms on catheters, and/or frank calculi. *Proteus* becomes associated with the stones and biofilms; thereafter, it usually cannot be eradicated without removal of the stones or catheter. Over time, staghorn calculi may form within the renal pelvis and lead to obstruction and renal failure. Although biologically plausible, clinical support is lacking for the concept that urine samples exhibiting unexplained alkalinity should be cultured, and that isolation of a *Proteus* species (or other urea-splitting organism) should prompt consideration of an evaluation for urolithiasis.

Other Infections *Proteus* occasionally causes pneumonia (primarily in LTCF residents or hospitalized patients), nosocomial sinusitis, intraabdominal abscesses, biliary tract infection, surgical site infection, soft tissue infection (especially decubitus and diabetic ulcers), and osteomyelitis (primarily contiguous); in rare cases, it causes non-tropical myositis. In addition, *Proteus* uncommonly causes neonatal meningitis, with the umbilicus frequently implicated as the source; this disease is often complicated by development of a cerebral abscess. Otogenic brain abscess also occurs.

Bacteremia Most episodes of *Proteus* bacteremia originate from the urinary tract, although intravascular devices and any of the less common sites of *Proteus* infection are also potential sources. Endovascular infection is rare. *Proteus* species are occasional agents of sepsis in neonates and of bacteremia in neutropenic patients.

■ DIAGNOSIS

Proteus is readily isolated and identified in the laboratory. Most strains are lactose-negative, produce H_2S, and demonstrate characteristic swarming motility on agar plates. *P. mirabilis* and *P. penneri* are indole-negative, whereas *P. vulgaris* is indole-positive. The inability to produce ornithine decarboxylase differentiates *P. penneri* from *P. mirabilis*.

TREATMENT

Proteus Infections

Intrinsic resistance occurs in all *Proteus* spp. to nitrofurantoin, polymyxins, imipenem, and the tetracycline derivatives (e.g., tigecycline, eravacycline, omadacycline) and, in *P. vulgaris* and *P. penneri*, also to ampicillin and the first- and second-generation cephalosporins. Acquired resistance (% of isolates) occurs in *P. mirabilis* to ampicillin (15–65%), and in *Proteus* spp. to fluoroquinolones (10–55%), fosfomycin (7–22%), and TMP-SMX (20–50%). In *P. mirabilis*, ampicillin-sulbactam is more active than ampicillin, with resistance prevalences of 6–18%, but the prevalence of ESBL production (which confers ampicillin-sulbactam resistance) is increasing in the United States (5–10%) and Asia (up to 60%). Isolates of *P. mirabilis* that produce CTX-M ESBLs have been recovered from ambulatory patients with no recent health care contact (see the section on the treatment of extraintestinal *E. coli* infections for treatment considerations). The use of third-generation cephalosporins can induce or select for stable de-repression of AmpC β-lactamase in *P. vulgaris*. Acquired carbapenem resistance remains relatively infrequent (<10%). However, production of a class B metallo-β-lactamase (e.g., NDM) limits treatment options due to the inherent resistance of *Proteus* spp. to polymyxins and tetracycline derivatives (see "Carbapenemase" above). For critically ill patients, agents with excellent activity overall against *Proteus* spp. (90–100% of isolates susceptible) include carbapenems (excepting imipenem), amikacin, piperacillin-tazobactam, aztreonam, cefepime, ceftazidime-avibactam, ceftolozane-tazobactam, and meropenem-vaborbactam.

ENTEROBACTER AND *CRONOBACTER* INFECTIONS

The *E. cloacae* complex is responsible for most *Enterobacter* infections, whereas *Cronobacter sakazakii* (formerly *Enterobacter sakazakii*), *Cronobacter malonaticus*, *Enterobacter cancergenus*, and *Enterobacter gergoviae* are less commonly isolated (<1% for each). *Enterobacter bugandensis* has been recently described as an agent of sepsis in neonates and was isolated from the International Space Station. *Enterobacter* spp. cause primarily health care–related infections. The organisms are widely prevalent in foods, environmental sources (including equipment at health care facilities), and a variety of animals.

Colonization with these organisms is uncommon among healthy humans, but increases significantly with LTCF residence or hospitalization. Although colonization is an important prelude to infection, direct introduction via IV lines (e.g., contaminated IV fluids or pressure monitors) or contaminated non-FDA-approved stem cell products also occurs. Extensive antibiotic resistance has developed in *Enterobacter* spp. and probably has contributed to these organisms' emergence as prominent nosocomial pathogens. Risk factors for *Enterobacter* infection include prior antibiotic treatment, comorbid disease, and ICU residency. *Enterobacter* spp. causes a spectrum of extraintestinal infections similar to those described for other GNB.

■ INFECTIOUS SYNDROMES

The most commonly encountered syndromes include pneumonia, UTI (particularly catheter-associated), intravascular device–related infection, surgical site infection, and abdominal infection (primarily postoperative or related to devices such as biliary stents). Nosocomial sinusitis, meningitis related to neurosurgical procedures (including use of intracranial pressure monitors), osteomyelitis, and endophthalmitis after eye surgery are less frequent. Neonates (particularly if low-birth-weight) are at risk for *C. sakazakii* infection, including neonatal bacteremia, necrotizing enterocolitis, and meningitis (which is often complicated by brain abscess or ventriculitis). Contaminated powdered infant formula has been implicated as a source for such neonatal infections. The WHO recommends that, to reduce the initial number of bacteria, powdered infant formula should be reconstituted with hot water (>70°C) and, to limit replication of residual bacteria, the reconstituted formula should be stored at <5°C or its storage time minimized.

Enterobacter bacteremia can result from primary infection at any anatomic site. In bacteremia of unclear origin, particularly in an outbreak setting, sources for consideration should include contaminated IV fluids or medications, blood components or plasma derivatives, catheter-flushing fluids, pressure monitors, and dialysis equipment. *Enterobacter* can also cause bacteremia in neutropenic patients. *Enterobacter* endocarditis is rare, occurring primarily in association with illicit IV drug use or prosthetic valves.

■ DIAGNOSIS

Enterobacter is readily isolated and identified in the laboratory. Most strains are lactose-positive and indole-negative.

TREATMENT
Enterobacter Infections

E. cloacae is intrinsically resistant to ampicillin, ampicillin-sulbactam, ampicillin-clavulanate, the first-generation cephalosporins, and the cephamycins. The prevalence of acquired resistance has ranged from 15 to 40% for piperacillin-tazobactam, 5 to 23% for polymyxin E, 15 to 17% for fosfomycin, 15 to 30% for TMP-SMX, and 5 to 20% for fluoroquinolones and is ~10% for omadacycline (53% if tetracycline resistant). USNHSN data from 2015–2017 identified 8.9% of *E. cloacae* isolates as presumptively ESBL-producing, based on cefepime resistance. The prevalence of ESBLs in *E. cloacae* outside of the United States is 20–50%. The use of third-generation cephalosporins can induce or select for stable de-repression of AmpC β-lactamase. Because resistance may emerge during therapy (in one study, this phenomenon was documented in 20% of clinical isolates), these agents should be avoided in the treatment of serious *Enterobacter* infection.

Cefepime is stable in the presence of AmpC β-lactamases; thus, it is a suitable option for treatment of *Enterobacter* infections so long as no coexistent ESBL is present. Overall, resistance prevalence generally ranges from 10 to 25% for cefepime and 25 to 50% for aztreonam and the third-generation cephalosporins. Carbapenem resistance remains relatively uncommon (USNHSN data from 2015–2017 identified a 5% prevalence) and is more commonly associated with increased AmpC expression and decreased permeability due to porin mutations rather than carbapenemase production, although acquisition of carbapenemase genes is increasing (see "Carbapenemase" above). Uncertainty exists on the optimal treatment for non-CP-CR-*Enterobacter* spp. Fortunately, overall, the percentage of susceptibility is high (90–99%) for carbapenems, amikacin, plazomicin, ceftazidime-avibactam, meropenem-vaborbactam, imipenem/cilastatin-relebactam, cefiderocol, tigecycline, eravacycline, and omadacycline (the latter three for tetracycline-susceptible isolates). Once susceptibility data for a patient's isolate become available, de-escalation of the antimicrobial regimen is advisable whenever possible.

SERRATIA INFECTIONS

S. marcescens causes >90%, and *Serratia liquefaciens* complex <10%, of *Serratia* infections. Serratiae are found primarily in the environment (including in health care institutions), particularly in moist settings. Serratiae have been isolated from a variety of animals, insects, and plants, but only infrequently from healthy humans. In LTCFs and hospitals, reservoirs for the organisms include the hands and fingernails of health care personnel, food, milk (on neonatal units), sinks, medical equipment or devices, IV solutions or parenteral medications (particularly those generated by compounding pharmacies), prefilled syringes and multiple-access medication vials (e.g., for heparin, propofol, saline), blood products (e.g., platelets), hand soaps and lotions, irrigation solutions, and even disinfectants such as chlorhexidine.

Infection results from either direct inoculation (e.g., via contaminated injected substances [IV fluids, medications, or recreational drugs] or snake bite) or colonization (primarily of the respiratory tract). Sporadic infection is most common, but outbreaks (often involving MDR strains in adult and neonatal ICUs) also occur. Hygiene, medication-compounding standards, sterile technique, and infection control programs are critical measures to prevent infection.

The spectrum of extraintestinal infections caused by *Serratia* is similar to that for other GNB. *Serratia* species are usually considered to cause mainly health care–associated infections; they account for 1–3% of hospital-acquired infections. However, population-based laboratory surveillance studies in Canada and Australia have demonstrated that community-acquired *Serratia* infections occur more commonly than was previously appreciated, and case reports have documented serious infection in otherwise healthy hosts. *Serratia* also is one of the pathogens associated with chronic granulomatous disease.

■ INFECTIOUS SYNDROMES

The most common primary sites of *Serratia* infection are the respiratory and genitourinary tracts, intravascular devices, the eye (contact lens–associated keratitis and other ocular infections), surgical wounds, and the bloodstream (from contaminated infusions), although most episodes of *Serratia* bacteremia arise from one of the listed focal infections rather than contaminated infusate. Less common syndromes are soft tissue infections (including myositis, fasciitis, mastitis), osteomyelitis, abdominal and biliary tract infections (usually postprocedural), and septic arthritis (primarily from intraarticular injections). Serratiae are uncommon causes of neonatal meningitis; postsurgical meningitis, endophthalmitis, or breast implant infection; and bacteremia in neutropenic patients. Endocarditis is rare, occurring most commonly in IV drug users.

■ DIAGNOSIS

Serratiae are readily cultured and identified by the laboratory and are usually lactose- and indole-negative. The red pigmentation of some *S. marcescens* strains and *Serratia rubidaea* can produce distinctive clinical findings (e.g., pink breast milk or hypopyon; pseudohemoptysis).

TREATMENT
Serratia Infections

Most *Serratia* strains (>80%) are intrinsically resistant to ampicillin, amoxicillin-clavulanate, ampicillin-sulbactam, first- and second-generation cephalosporins, cephamycins, nitrofurantoin, and polymyxins; likewise, tetracycline derivatives are poorly active. By contrast, fluoroquinolones, TMP-SMX, piperacillin-tazobactam, fosfomycin, and omadacycline are active against 85–95% of U.S. and European isolates, including those resistant to tetracycline. Both in the United States and globally, the prevalence of ESBL-producing isolates is generally low (<10%), but rates of 20–30% have been reported in Asia and Latin America. The use of third-generation cephalosporins may result in the induction or selection of variants with stable de-repression of chromosomal AmpC β-lactamases during therapy but is uncommon. Resistance prevalence generally ranges from 10 to 20% for aztreonam and the third-generation cephalosporins. Acquisition of carbapenemase-encoding genes is uncommon but increasing. Production of a class B metallo-β-lactamase (e.g., NDM) limits treatment options due to *Serratia*'s predictable resistance to polymyxins and tetracycline derivatives (see "Carbapenemase" above). For critically ill patients, the most active agents overall (>90% susceptible) are carbapenems, piperacillin-tazobactam, cefepime, amikacin, plazomicin, ceftazidime-avibactam, ceftolozane-tazobactam, and meropenem-vaborbactam.

CITROBACTER INFECTIONS

C. freundii and *Citrobacter koseri* cause most human *Citrobacter* infections, which are epidemiologically and clinically similar to *Enterobacter* infections. *Citrobacter* species are commonly present in water, food, soil, and certain animals. Colonization with these organisms is uncommon among healthy humans, but increases significantly with LTCF residence or hospitalization. *Citrobacter* species account for 1–2% of nosocomial infections. The affected hosts are usually immunocompromised and/or have comorbid disease or disruption of skin or mucosal barriers. Infection from treatment with contaminated, non-FDA-approved stem cell products has been described. *Citrobacter* causes extraintestinal infections similar to those described for other GNB.

■ INFECTIOUS SYNDROMES

The urinary tract accounts for 40–50% of *Citrobacter* infections. Less commonly involved sites include the biliary tree (particularly with stones or obstruction), the respiratory tract, surgical sites, soft tissue (e.g., decubitus ulcers), the peritoneum, and intravascular devices. Osteomyelitis (usually from a contiguous focus), central nervous system infection in adults (from neurosurgical or other types of meningeal disruption), and myositis occur rarely. *Citrobacter* (primarily *C. koseri*) also causes 1–2% of neonatal meningitis cases, of which 50–80% are complicated by brain abscess. Further, case reports in adults suggest that *C. koseri* infection has a predilection for abscess formation. *Citrobacter* bacteremia is most often due to UTI, biliary/abdominal infection, or intravascular device infection, and occurs in some neutropenic patients. Endocarditis and other endovascular infections are rare.

DIAGNOSIS

Citrobacter species are readily isolated and identified; 35–50% of isolates are lactose-positive, and 100% are oxidase-negative. *C. freundii* is indole-negative, whereas *C. koseri* is indole-positive.

TREATMENT

Citrobacter Infections

C. freundii is more extensively antibiotic-resistant than is *C. koseri*. Most *C. freundii* isolates are intrinsically resistant to ampicillin, ampicillin-sulbactam, amoxicillin-clavulanate, first-generation cephalosporins, and cephamycins. *C. koseri* exhibits intrinsic resistance to ampicillin and ampicillin-sulbactam. Overall, the prevalence of acquired resistance generally ranges from 15 to 35% for third-generation cephalosporins, piperacillin-tazobactam, fluoroquinolones, and TMP-SMX and is ~10% for nitrofurantoin and omadacycline (but 39% for omadacycline if tetracycline-resistant). The prevalence of ESBL production ranges from 5 to 30%. The use of third-generation cephalosporins may result in the induction or selection of variants with stable de-repression of chromosomal AmpC β-lactamases during therapy. Presently, <10% of isolates have acquired carbapenemases (see "Carbapenemase" above). Carbapenems, amikacin, plazomicin, fosfomycin, polymyxins, cefepime, ceftazidime-avibactam, cefiderocol, tigecycline, eravacycline, and omadacycline (the latter three if tetracycline-susceptible) are the most active agents against *Citrobacter* isolates (>90% susceptible).

MORGANELLA AND *PROVIDENCIA* INFECTIONS

M. morganii, Providencia stuartii, and (less frequently) *Providencia rettgeri* are the members of their respective genera that cause systemic human infections. *P. alcalifaciens* has been implicated as a cause of food-borne gastroenteritis. These organisms' epidemiologic associations, pathogenic properties, and clinical manifestations resemble those of *Proteus* species. *Morganella* and *Providencia* occur more commonly among LTCF residents than among hospitalized patients, largely resulting from chronic urinary catheter use. Because of these organisms' intrinsic resistance to polymyxins and tigecycline, they may become increasingly common in settings with extensive use of these agents.

INFECTIOUS SYNDROMES

These species are primarily urinary tract pathogens, causing UTIs that are most often associated with long-term (>30-day) catheterization. Such infections commonly lead to biofilm formation and catheter encrustation (sometimes causing catheter obstruction) or the development of struvite bladder or renal stones (sometimes causing renal obstruction, abscess, and extrarenal extension, and serving as foci for relapse). They can cause purple urine ("purple bag syndrome"), as can *P. mirabilis, K. pneumoniae, E. coli*, and *P. aeruginosa*. *Morganella* is also commonly isolated from snakebite infection.

Other, less common infectious syndromes due to *Morganella* and *Providencia* include surgical site infection, soft tissue infection (primarily involving decubitus and diabetic ulcers), burn site infection, pneumonia (particularly ventilator-associated), intravascular device infection, and intraabdominal infection. Rarely, the other extraintestinal infections described for GNB also occur. Bacteremia is uncommon; when it does occur, any infected site can serve as the source, but the urinary tract accounts for most cases, followed by surgical site, soft tissue, and hepatobiliary infections.

DIAGNOSIS

M. morganii and *Providencia* are readily isolated and identified. Nearly all isolates are lactose-negative and indole-positive.

TREATMENT

Morganella and *Providencia* Infections

Morganella and *Providencia* are intrinsically resistant to ampicillin, ampicillin-clavulanate, ampicillin-sulbactam, first-generation cephalosporins, nitrofurantoin, tetracyclines and derivatives (e.g., tigecycline), imipenem (but not the other carbapenems), and the polymyxins. *P. stuartii* additionally exhibits intrinsic resistance to gentamicin and tobramycin, as does *M. morganii* to second-generation cephalosporins. Fosfomycin is poorly active (>50% resistance). The prevalence of resistance generally ranges from 10 to 30% for the third-generation cephalosporins, from 10 to 40% for fluoroquinolones, and from 20 to 40% for TMP-SMX; the prevalence is more widely variable for piperacillin-tazobactam. The prevalence of ESBL production is generally <10%. The use of third-generation cephalosporins can induce or select for stable de-repression of AmpC β-lactamase for both *Morganella* and *Providencia*. The prevalence of acquired carbapenemase production is <10%. Production of a class B metallo-β-lactamase (e.g., NDM) limits treatment options due to the inherent resistance of the *Proteeae* to polymyxins and tetracycline derivatives (see "Carbapenemase" above). Overall, the most active agents (>90% of isolates susceptible) are carbapenems (excepting imipenem), amikacin, cefepime, ceftazidime-avibactam, ceftolozane-tazobactam, meropenem-vaborbactam, and cefiderocol. Removal of a colonized urinary catheter or stone is critical for eradication of UTI.

EDWARDSIELLA INFECTIONS

E. tarda is the only member of the genus *Edwardsiella* that is associated with human disease. This organism is found predominantly in freshwater and marine environments and in the associated aquatic animal species. Human acquisition occurs primarily from interaction with these reservoirs or ingestion of raw or inadequately cooked aquatic animals. *E. tarda* infection is rare in the United States, where acquisition occurs mainly along the Gulf of Mexico; recently reported cases are mostly from Asia. This pathogen shares clinical features with *Salmonella* species (as an intestinal pathogen; **Chap. 165**), *Vibrio vulnificus* (as an extraintestinal pathogen; **Chap. 168**), and *Aeromonas hydrophila* (as both an intestinal and an extraintestinal pathogen; **Chap. 158**).

INFECTIOUS SYNDROMES

Gastroenteritis is the predominant *Edwardsiella*-associated infectious syndrome (50–80% of reported cases). Self-limiting watery diarrhea is most common, but severe colitis also occurs. The most common extraintestinal infection is wound infection due to direct inoculation, which is often associated with brackish or freshwater injuries, snakebites, or fish-related trauma. A case of pneumonia occurred after a near-drowning incident. Cholecystitis, cholangitis, and hepatic abscess may be due to ascending infection via the biliary tree. Other infectious syndromes result from invasion of the gastrointestinal tract and subsequent bacteremia. A primary bacteremic syndrome, sometimes complicated by meningitis, has a 40% case–fatality rate; hematogenous seeding may result in hepatic and intra- and extraperitoneal abscesses, endocarditis, mycotic aneurysm, septic arthritis, osteomyelitis, necrotizing fasciitis, and empyema. Most hosts who develop systemic *Edwardsiella* infection have significant comorbidities (e.g., hepatobiliary disease, iron overload, cancer, or diabetes mellitus).

DIAGNOSIS

Although *E. tarda* can readily be isolated and identified, most laboratories do not routinely screen for or identify it in stool samples. Production of hydrogen sulfide is a characteristic biochemical property.

TREATMENT
Edwardsiella Infections

E. tarda is susceptible to most antimicrobial agents appropriate for use against GNB. Gastroenteritis is generally self-limiting, but treatment with a fluoroquinolone may hasten resolution. In the setting of severe sepsis, fluoroquinolones, third- and fourth-generation cephalosporins, carbapenems, and amikacin—either alone or in combination—are the safest choices pending susceptibility data.

INFECTIONS CAUSED BY MISCELLANEOUS GENERA

Other gram-negative organisms such as *Hafnia, Kluyvera, Cedecea, Pantoea, Ewingella, Leclercia, Raoultella,* and *Photorhabdus* spp. are occasionally isolated from diverse clinical specimens, including blood, sputum, urine, cerebrospinal fluid, joint fluid, bile, and wounds. Such organisms cause infection predominantly in compromised hosts or in association with an invasive procedure or foreign body. Cephalosporinases from *Kluyvera* have been implicated as the progenitors of CTX-M ESBLs. *Kluyvera* and *Raoultella* may produce carbapenemases.

FURTHER READING

Anesi JA et al: Poor clinical outcomes associated with community-onset urinary tract infections due to extended-spectrum cephalosporin-resistant Enterobacteriaceae. Infect Control Hosp Epidemiol 39:1431, 2018.

Baker TM et al: Epidemiology of bloodstream infections caused by *Escherichia coli* and *Klebsiella pneumoniae* that are piperacillin-tazobactam-nonsusceptible but ceftriaxone-susceptible. Open Forum Infect Dis 5:ofy300, 2018.

Boisen N et al: Shiga toxin 2a and enteroaggregative *Escherichia coli*—A deadly combination. Gut Microbes 6:272, 2015.

Bonten M et al: Epidemiology of *Escherichia coli* bacteremia: A systematic literature review. Clin Infect Dis 72:1211, 2021.

Cheng MP et al: Beta-lactam/beta-lactamase inhibitor therapy for potential AmpC-producing organisms: A systematic review and meta-analysis. Open Forum Infect Dis 6:ofz248, 2019.

David S et al: Epidemic of carbapenem-resistant *Klebsiella pneumoniae* in Europe is driven by nosocomial spread. Nat Microbiol 4:1919, 2019.

Gurieva T et al: The transmissibility of antibiotic-resistant Enterobacteriaceae in intensive care units. Clin Infect Dis 66:489, 2018.

Harris PNA et al: Effect of piperacillin-tazobactam vs meropenem on 30-day mortality for patients with *E coli* or *Klebsiella pneumoniae* bloodstream infection and ceftriaxone resistance: A randomized clinical trial [published correction appears in JAMA 321:2370, 2019]. JAMA 320:984, 2018.

Holy O, Forsythe S: *Cronobacter spp.* as emerging causes of healthcare-associated infection. J Hosp Infect 86:169, 2014.

Kamiyama S et al: *Edwardsiella tarda* bacteremia, Okayama, Japan, 2005-2016. Emerg Infect Dis 25:1817, 2019.

Lim C et al: Epidemiology and burden of multidrug-resistant bacterial infection in a developing country. Elife 5:E18082, 2016.

Nordmann P et al: Carbapenem resistance in Enterobacteriaceae: Here is the storm! Trends Mol Med 18:263, 2012.

Peirano G, Pitout JDD: Extended-spectrum β-lactamase-producing Enterobacteriaceae: Update on molecular epidemiology and treatment options. Drugs 79:1529, 2019.

Russo TA, Marr CM: Hypervirulent *Klebsiella pneumoniae*. Clin Microbiol Rev 32:e00001, 2019.

van Duin D et al: Molecular and clinical epidemiology of carbapenem-resistant Enterobacterales in the USA (CRACKLE-2): A prospective cohort study Lancet Infect Dis 20:731, 2020. [Erratum in Lancet Infect Dis 19:30755, 2020].

Weiner-Lastinger LM et al: Antimicrobial-resistant pathogens associated with adult healthcare-associated infections: Summary of data reported to the National Healthcare Safety Network, 2015-2017. Infect Control Hosp Epidemiol 41:1, 2020.

162 *Acinetobacter* Infections

Rossana Rosa, L. Silvia Munoz-Price

DEFINITION

Acinetobacter species were first described in 1911 and named *Micrococcus calcoaceticus*. Thereafter, the genus was renamed multiple times; since 1950, it has been known as *Acinetobacter*. *Acinetobacter* species are gram-negative, oxidase-negative, nonmotile, nonfermenting coccobacilli that are easily recovered on standard culture media. Differentiation among *Acinetobacter* species on the basis of phenotypic characteristics alone is very difficult. Molecular-based methods such as matrix-assisted laser desorption–ionization–time-of-flight mass spectrometry (MALDI-TOF-MS) and quantitative real-time polymerase chain reaction (PCR) are usually necessary to identify *Acinetobacter baumannii*, the most clinically relevant species of the genus.

ETIOLOGY AND EPIDEMIOLOGY

Acinetobacter species are naturally encountered in water and soil and have also been recovered from fruits and vegetables. In humans, *Acinetobacter* can be found on the skin and in the respiratory and gastrointestinal tracts. *A. baumannii* is capable of surviving environmental desiccation for weeks; this characteristic is important from an infection-control perspective as it allows this organism to persist in the hospital environment and on equipment.

Acinetobacter was historically considered a pathogen of hot and humid climates. In recent years, however, hospital outbreaks caused by *A. baumannii* have been reported worldwide, even in temperate climates. In the United States, the Centers for Disease Control and Prevention (CDC) estimates that 12,000 *Acinetobacter* infections occur every year, 7300 of which are caused by multidrug-resistant strains, with 500 attributable deaths. The increase in the number of infections with *A. baumannii* is suspected to be due to the rapid spread of certain genetically distinct lineages; of the three international clonal lineages (ICLs), ICL I and ICL II are multidrug resistant. The predominance of these lineages remains unexplained, although it has been proposed that this population structure is the result of two waves of expansion. The first wave followed a bottleneck (possibly linked to a restricted ecologic niche) that occurred in the distant past. The second wave is ongoing and is being driven by the rapid expansion of a limited number of multidrug-resistant clones.

Analysis of the *A. baumannii* pangenome (the sum of the core and dispensable genomes) has shown that its organization is characterized by a small core genome and a large accessory or disposable genome. This organization reflects *A. baumannii's* high plasticity, which enables it to acquire exogenous genetic material. With few exceptions, gene functions associated with virulence are found in the core genome; this observation suggests a limited role for the acquisition of new virulence traits in the recent nosocomial expansion of *A. baumannii* clones. Genes associated with resistance to antimicrobial agents are found in both the species core genome and the accessory genome. In the accessory genome, these genes have been found in alien islands, often flanked by integrases, transposases, or insertion sequences. This pattern suggests possible acquisition by horizontal gene transfer from other *Acinetobacter* strains or even from different bacterial species present in the immediate environment. Acquisition of these antimicrobial resistance genes is hypothesized to have led to the recent rapid expansion of highly homogeneous clonal lineages, whose main difference from nonclonal *A. baumannii* appears to be their antimicrobial resistance.

Health Care–Associated Infections Infections caused by *A. baumannii* occur frequently among patients admitted to intensive care units (ICUs). Risk factors for colonization and infection with this pathogen include nursing home residence, prolonged ICU stay, central venous catheterization, tracheostomy, mechanical ventilation, enteral feedings, and treatment with third-generation cephalosporins, fluoroquinolones, and carbapenems. Acquisition of carbapenem-resistant *A. baumannii* is most common among patients exposed to carbapenems. Spread of *A. baumannii* across different regions is facilitated by the movement of patients between health care systems and throughout the continuum of health care. Within the hospital, environmental spread of *A. baumannii* occurs as a result of inappropriate hand hygiene among workers providing health care for infected or colonized patients and the contamination of hospital equipment, such as respiratory therapy and ventilation equipment. The air surrounding the patient may also play a role in environmental colonization with *A. baumannii*, especially in inpatient areas without physical barriers between patients and with an inadequate number of air exchanges.

A. baumannii strains identified during hospital outbreaks are typically resistant to more antibiotic classes than strains from the community. The prevalence of colonization with *A. baumannii* at the time of admission or during a stay in a long-term acute-care hospital (LTACH) or nursing home is variable and depends on regional flora. Outbreaks of *A. baumannii* in acute-care hospitals and LTACHs that "share" patients have been described in Ohio, Michigan, Illinois, and Indiana.

Community-Acquired Infections Community-acquired infections caused by *Acinetobacter* have been described in Australia and Asia. Few cases have been reported in regions with a temperate climate, and even those few cases have taken place during warm and humid months. Risk factors for community-acquired pneumonia due to this organism include a history of alcohol abuse, diabetes mellitus, smoking, and chronic lung disease.

War Zone–Associated Infections Infections caused by *Acinetobacter* in war zones include skin and soft tissue infections associated with traumatic injuries and bloodstream infections. Outbreak investigations of *A. baumannii* infections among military personnel returning from Iraq and Afghanistan suggested the acquisition of *A. baumannii* in field hospitals rather than colonization of the skin before an injury. This view is supported by the recovery of *A. baumannii* isolates with similar genetic characteristics from inanimate surfaces in field hospitals and from patients.

Disaster Medicine *A. baumannii* is linked to infections among victims of trauma during tsunamis, earthquakes, and terrorist attacks. The types of infections most frequently observed in these settings are soft tissue injuries, but bloodstream infections and pneumonia have also been reported. In addition, outbreaks of *A. baumannii* infection in ICUs caring for disaster victims have been described.

PATHOGENESIS

Mechanisms of pathogenesis and virulence in *Acinetobacter* species have not been fully elucidated. However, *A. baumannii* seems to have greater virulence potential than other *Acinetobacter* species, as evidenced by its ability to grow at 37°C and to resist uptake by macrophages.

Initial *A. baumannii* colonization of the host and the environment is facilitated by the organism's ability to adhere to surfaces and human cells and to create biofilms. The ability to form a biofilm is phenotypically associated with exopolysaccharide production and pilus formation. A quorum-sensing molecule encoded by the *abaI* autoinducer synthase gene has been implicated in *A. baumannii* biofilm formation on abiotic surfaces. Outer-membrane porins appear to mediate cell apoptosis. *A. baumannii* can survive in harsh environments within the host and on inanimate surfaces by modifying the structure of its lipid A, with a consequent decrease in susceptibility to antibiotics and antimicrobial peptides and an increase in survival upon desiccation.

Acinetobacter species produce an extracellular capsule that protects the bacteria from external threats, including complement-mediated killing. Studies of mouse models showed that *Acinetobacter* species can increase capsule production in the presence of subinhibitory levels of antibiotic—an ability that leads to increased resistance to complement-mediated killing and a hypervirulent phenotype.

Phospholipase C and phospholipase D have been identified as virulence factors in *A. baumannii*. These enzymes exert cytotoxic effects on epithelial cells and facilitate their invasion.

Iron-acquisition systems are also important virulence mechanisms in *A. baumannii*. Through secretion of siderophores (low-molecular-mass ferric-binding compounds), *A. baumannii* is able to grow despite iron deficiencies in the surrounding environment (e.g., in the human host).

Several protein-secretion systems have been identified in *A. baumannii*. The most recently described is a type II secretion system. The substrate for this system, the LipA lipase, is required for growth on medium containing lipids as a sole carbon source. Mutants lacking the genes for the type II secretion system or its substrate exhibit defective in vivo growth in a neutropenic murine model of bacteremia. *A. baumannii* also has a type VI secretion system whose primary function seems to be to secrete antibacterial toxins that kill competing bacteria, including other strains in the same species.

The type V autotransporter system has been characterized in *A. baumannii*. In a murine systemic model of *Acinetobacter* infection, the *Acinetobacter* trimeric autotransporter mediates biofilm formation and maintenance; adherence to extracellular matrix components such as collagen I, II, and IV; and virulence.

Outer-membrane vesicles (OMVs) play a special role in protein secretion. Many *A. baumannii* strains secrete OMVs containing various virulence factors, including outer-membrane protein A (OmpA), proteases, and phospholipases. The membrane proteins in OMVs are responsible for eliciting a potent innate immune response. Several studies have shown that *A. baumannii* OMVs could be used as an acellular vaccine to effectively control *A. baumannii* infections.

Nosocomial strains of *Acinetobacter* can deploy multiple mechanisms of resistance, including alterations in porins and efflux pumps and expression of β-lactamases. More specifically, *Acinetobacter* species can reduce the expression of porins, thus hindering the passage of β-lactam antibiotics into the periplasmic space. These species can overexpress bacterial efflux pumps and decrease the concentration of β-lactam antibiotics in the periplasmic space. Efflux pumps can also actively remove quinolones, tetracyclines, chloramphenicol, disinfectants, and tigecycline. *Acinetobacter* species possess chromosomally encoded cephalosporinases and are capable of acquiring β-lactamases, including serine and metallo-β-lactamases. AmpC β-lactamases are class C β-lactamases intrinsic to all *A. baumannii* strains. Although these enzymes are expressed at low levels and are not inducible, the addition of the insertion sequence *ISAba1* next to the AmpC gene increases β-lactamase production, with resulting resistance to cephalosporins.

Carbapenem resistance in *Acinetobacter* species is mostly tied to the emergence of Ambler class D oxacillinases of group 2d, some of which are intrinsic and chromosomal (e.g., OXA-51-like) while others are acquired and are found in plasmids or are chromosomally encoded (e.g., OXA-23-like, 24 [33-like, 40-like], 58-like, 143-like, and 235-like).

CLINICAL MANIFESTATIONS

Pneumonia *A. baumannii* is a notorious cause of nosocomial pneumonia, most frequently among patients requiring prolonged mechanical ventilation. The onset of disease tends to be later than that caused by other gram-negative bacilli; however, clinical symptoms of hospital-acquired or ventilator-associated pneumonia due to *A. baumannii* are similar to those of nosocomial or ventilator-associated pneumonia due to other nosocomial pathogens. Thus, the most common indicators of infection include fever and increased sputum production. The positivity of respiratory cultures in most cases may present a challenge for the clinician, since airway colonization with *A. baumannii* is a risk factor for infection itself. Radiologic findings are nonspecific and can include lobar consolidations and pleural effusions, but cavitations are rarely seen. The crude mortality rates associated with nosocomial pneumonia due to *A. baumannii* are reported to be as high as 65%. However, since these infections occur in debilitated patients, their attributable mortality has been difficult to establish.

Community-acquired pneumonia due to *A. baumannii* is a relatively rare entity. Its clinical presentation is characterized by fever, severe respiratory symptoms, and multiple-organ dysfunction. Patients frequently have a cough productive of purulent sputum, shortness of breath, and chest pain. Imaging studies usually show lobar consolidation. Mortality rates associated with this process are >50%.

Bloodstream Infections Bloodstream infections due to *A. baumannii* are most frequent among ICU patients and usually occur in the presence of a central venous catheter or as a secondary complication of hospital-acquired or ventilator-associated pneumonia. Polymicrobial growth has been reported in 20–36% of bacteremia episodes. Fever is the most common sign of infection (developing in >95% of cases), and presentation with septic shock and disseminated intravascular coagulopathy has been described in as many as 25 to 30% of patients, respectively. *A. baumannii* bloodstream infections often result in higher hospitalization costs and longer ICU stays. Crude mortality rates from this infection are as high as 40%; however, rates can be as high as 70% from infections caused by carbapenem-resistant isolates. In patients with infections caused by extremely drug-resistant strains, poor outcomes are thought to be driven by delays in the initiation of adequate antimicrobial therapy.

Skin and Soft Tissue Infections *Acinetobacter* species have been described as part of the skin flora, yet the majority of the organisms from this genus that colonize the skin are not those associated with nosocomial infections. Discerning infection from wound colonization is challenging. Gunshot wounds and the presence of orthopedic external-fixation devices are common among patients with combat trauma–associated *A. baumannii* skin and soft tissue infections. The report on a case series of eight U.S. military patients described the clinical presentation of their infections as evolving from an edematous *peau d'orange* appearance to a sandpaper appearance with overlying vesicles and then to a necrotizing process with hemorrhagic bullae. Other case series have also included necrotizing fasciitis. *A. baumannii* is an important pathogen in burn units worldwide. Large burns provide ideal conditions for *A. baumannii* and facilitate patient-to-patient transmission. The presence of *A. baumannii* in wounds contributes to healing delays and graft loss. In addition, wound colonization is a risk factor for bloodstream infections among patients with extensive burn injuries.

A. baumannii infections resulting from trauma to soft tissues in the setting of natural disasters, such as tsunamis and earthquakes, have been reported. The implication is that *A. baumannii* should be considered in the differential diagnosis of soft tissue infections following exposure to tropical and subtropical environments.

Urinary Tract Infections *A. baumannii* is an infrequent cause of urinary tract infections. The majority of cases reported are catheter-associated infections, reflecting the ability of *A. baumannii* to form biofilms on these devices. A few reports have described community-acquired infections occurring in the setting of nephrolithiasis and after renal transplantation.

Meningitis Central nervous system infections with *A. baumannii* have been reported in the context of outbreaks, traumatic injuries, neurosurgical procedures, and external ventricular drains. One case series described a petechial rash in up to 30% of patients. *Acinetobacter* species may look similar to *Neisseria meningitidis* on a Gram's stain of cerebrospinal fluid; both appear as gram-negative paired cocci.

Other Miscellaneous Infections A few cases of *A. baumannii* keratitis associated with the use of contact lenses have been reported. Cases of native- and prosthetic-valve endocarditis have also been described.

TREATMENT

Acinetobacter Infections

Treatment of *Acinetobacter* infections is challenging because *Acinetobacter* can develop resistance to most available antibiotics. Therefore, the choice of empirical therapy should be based on local epidemiology and the patient's colonization status. Definitive therapy should be determined by antimicrobial susceptibility testing.

TABLE 162-1 Therapeutic Options for the Management of Multidrug-Resistant *Acinetobacter baumannii* Infections

ANTIBIOTIC	DOSING[a]	COMMENTS
Sulbactam	3–9 g/d (9–27 g/d if given in combination with ampicillin)	Unavailable as single drug in many countries (including the United States)
Meropenem	2 g q8h	Prolonged infusion (3–4 h) has been used; limited data
Imipenem	500 mg q6h	Prolonged infusion (3–4 h) has been used; limited data
Cefiderocol	2g q8h	Prolonged infusion (3 h) used in pharmacokinetic models
Colistin	Loading dose of 5 mg/kg followed by 2.5–5.0 mg/kg per day of colistin base given in 2–4 divided doses	Optimal dosing regimen unknown Inhaled formulation has been used as adjunct treatment in lung infections.
Polymyxin B	1.5–3 mg/kg q12h	
Tigecycline	100-mg loading dose followed by 50 mg q12h	Low serum concentrations and bacteriostatic activity limit use in bacteremia.
Minocycline	100 mg q12h	Loading dose of 200 mg IV has been used.
Eravacycline	1 mg/kg q12h	
Amikacin	15 mg/kg qd	Inhaled formulation of tobramycin has been used as adjunct treatment in lung infections.
Rifampin	600 mg qd or 600 mg q12h	Use in combination therapy
Fosfomycin	4 g q12h PO	Use in combination therapy IV formulation not available in the United States

[a]All drugs are given by the IV route unless otherwise stated.

Antimicrobial options for the management of infections caused by *A. baumannii* are displayed in **Table 162-1**.

Acinetobacter species possess intrinsic β-lactamases that inactivate first- and second-generation cephalosporins. Through acquisition of extended-spectrum β-lactamases, the organisms can also become resistant to third- and fourth-generation cephalosporins. Nevertheless, when the isolate is susceptible, β-lactam agents are the drugs of choice for the treatment of *A. baumannii*. Among β-lactamase inhibitors, sulbactam is active against *A. baumannii* and is as effective as carbapenems and polymyxins. Cefiderocol is a novel cephalosporine and is stable against many β-lactamase classes, including extended-spectrum β-lactamases, AmpC, and carbapenemases. Cefiderocol has shown in vitro activity against *A. baumannii* isolates producing OXA-23, OXA-40, OXA-58, NDM, and IMP. However, published clinical trials have not included patients with infections caused by carbapenem-resistant strains.

Carbapenems have been the preferred drugs for treatment of invasive or hospital-acquired infections. Unfortunately, surveillance data from U.S. hospitals show that up to 50% of *A. baumannii* isolates recovered from ICUs are carbapenem resistant, and rates of carbapenem resistance are even higher around the world.

Aminoglycosides are of limited utility against *A. baumannii* because of toxicity and lack of lung penetration. Inhaled formulations of tobramycin have been used with variable success.

Polymyxins are cationic detergents that fell out of use as a result of nephrotoxicity and neurotoxicity. In vitro, they are the most active agents against carbapenem-resistant *A. baumannii*. Colistin has been used in both intravenous and inhaled formulations, although the optimal dosage has not yet been determined. Combination therapy using colistin as a base has long been preferred but randomized controlled trials have failed to show improved survival compared to colistin monotherapy.

Tigecycline is a glycylcycline with clinical activity against *A. baumannii*. It reaches only low serum concentrations and therefore cannot be used for bloodstream infections. The susceptibility of isolates is variable, especially in outbreak settings, and the emergence of resistance during treatment has been reported.

Minocycline is a tetracycline that has a bacteriostatic effect on *A. baumannii*. Synergistic and bactericidal activity has been noted when minocycline is used in combination with colistin or a carbapenem.

Eravacycline is a novel tetracycline with in vitro activity against multidrug-resistant and extensively drug-resistant strains of *A. baumannii*. However, only a small number of carbapenem-resistant isolates have been included in clinical studies. Furthermore, eravacycline has been approved for the treatment of complicated intraabdominal infections but was shown to be inferior to levofloxacin and ertapenem for the management of complicated urinary tract infections.

Fosfomycin is an inhibitor of peptidoglycan synthesis that has no direct activity against *A. baumannii* but has been observed to be synergistic in vitro in combination with colistin or sulbactam. Clinical data have shown higher rates of microbiologic cure, but no differences in clinical response, with combinations of fosfomycin and colistin.

In vitro data favor combination therapy with colistin in many different regimens containing a carbapenem (imipenem, meropenem), rifampin, minocycline, ceftazidime, azithromycin, doxycycline, trimethoprim-sulfamethoxazole, or ampicillin-sulbactam. However, clinical data have not shown such combination therapy to be superior to colistin alone.

Bacteriophage therapy against multidrug-resistant *A. baumannii* has been reported with varied success rates. Furthermore, dosing and duration of therapy vary by syndrome and resistance can also arise during treatment.

COMPLICATIONS AND PROGNOSIS

Infections caused by *A. baumannii* can be associated with high mortality rates. Factors contributing to higher mortality are thought to include severity of the patient's underlying illness and drug resistance in the infecting strain.

INFECTION CONTROL AND PREVENTION

Acinetobacter species are capable of surviving on hospital surfaces for prolonged periods. In the hospital environment, *A. baumannii* has been associated with establishment of a *fecal patina*; this term refers to a coating of enteric organisms that can cover the skin of colonized patients and extend to their surrounding environment. Concentrations of enteric organisms are highest in the colonized patient's rectum, with spread in a target-like concentric pattern covering the patient's body and the surrounding environment. High-frequency touch areas in rooms occupied by patients colonized with *A. baumannii* are more likely to be contaminated. The hands, gloves, and gowns of health care workers can be contaminated after entry into the room of a patient colonized with *A. baumannii* **(Fig. 162-1)**.

Outbreaks caused by *A. baumannii* are frequently mono- or oligoclonal. A common source of infection has been identified in ~50% of outbreaks. These sources include respiratory therapy equipment, the hands of health care workers, bedside humidifiers, warm bathwater, hospital-prepared distilled water, bedpans, urine jugs, heparinized saline solution, mattresses, reusable pressure transducers in arterial lines, and fluids used for pressure lavage of wounds.

Control of multidrug-resistant *Acinetobacter* outbreaks starts with early recognition, with subsequent halting of the spread of infection throughout a facility and prevention of the establishment of an endemic strain. It is important to identify the outbreak strain and differentiate it from nonoutbreak strains so that infection control activities can be better targeted. Traditionally, the strain was identified with phenotypic typing systems (biotyping) or by determination of antimicrobial susceptibility patterns. Molecular typing systems have ushered in an era of molecular epidemiology that allows more precise identification of outbreak strains through use of techniques such as ribotyping, pulse-field gel electrophoresis, repetitive sequence-based PCR, and multilocus sequence testing.

During outbreaks, the simultaneous introduction of multiple ("bundled") measures makes it difficult to assess the impact of each individual measure. These interventions include aggressive cleaning of the general environment, active surveillance, contact isolation of colonized or infected patients, cohorting of medical staff, reinforcement of compliance with hand hygiene by health care workers, and use of aseptic care devices.

Colonization with *A. baumannii* is a strong predictor of subsequent clinical infection by this organism. Exposure to carbapenems is a risk factor for initial acquisition of this pathogen; therefore, efforts to curtail unnecessary use of antibiotics are fundamental to the prevention of

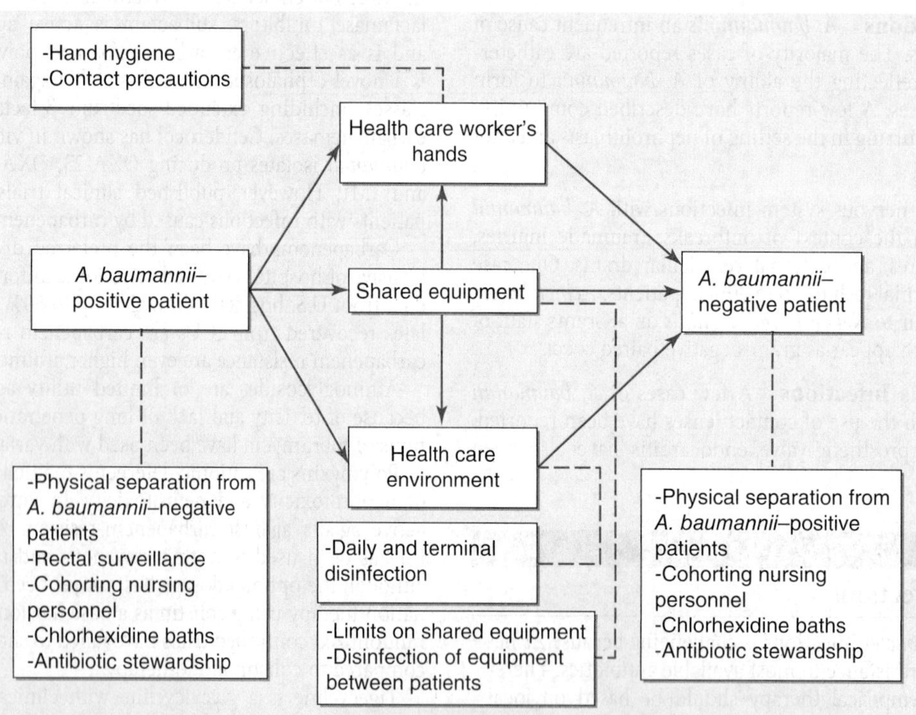

FIGURE 162-1 Strategies for the prevention of dissemination of *Acinetobacter baumannii* in health care facilities.

A. baumannii colonization of patients and the organism's establishment in health care facilities.

FURTHER READING

Adams-Haduch JM et al: Molecular epidemiology of carbapenem-nonsusceptible *Acinetobacter baumannii* in the United States. J Clin Microbiol 49:3849, 2011.

Antunes LC et al: *Acinetobacter baumannii:* Evolution of a global pathogen. Pathog Dis 71:292, 2014.

Chen W: Host innate immune responses to *Acinetobacter baumannii* infection. Front Cell Infect Microbiol 10:486, 2020.

Dexter C et al: Community-acquired *Acinetobacter baumannii*: Clinical characteristics, epidemiology and pathogenesis. Expert Rev Anti Infect Ther 13:567, 2015.

Garnacho-Montero J: Optimum treatment strategies for carbapenem-resistant *Acinetobacter baumannii:* Bacteremia. Expert Rev Anti Infect Ther 13:769, 2015.

Isler B et al: New treatment options against carbapenem-resistant *Acinetobacter baumannii* infections. Antimicrob Agents Chemother 63:e01110, 2018.

Lee CR et al: Biology of *Acinetobacter baumannii*: Pathogenesis, antibiotic resistance mechanisms, and prospective treatment options. Front Cell Infect Microbiol 7:55, 2017.

Munoz-Price LS: Controlling multi-drug resistant gram-negative bacilli in your hospital: A transformational journey. J Hosp Infect 89:254, 2015.

Munoz-Price LS, Weinstein RA: *Acinetobacter* infection. N Engl J Med 358:1271, 2008.

Peleg AY et al: *Acinetobacter baumannii*: Emergence of a successful pathogen. Clin Microbiol Rev 21:538, 2008.

Tal-Jasper R et al: Clinical and epidemiological significance of carbapenem resistance in *Acinetobacter baumannii* infections. Antimicrob Agents Chemother 60:3127, 2016.

Wong D et al: Clinical and pathophysiological overview of *Acinetobacter* infections: A century of challenges. Clin Microbiol Rev 30:409, 2017.

163 *Helicobacter pylori* Infections

John C. Atherton, Martin J. Blaser

Helicobacter pylori colonizes the stomach in ~50% of the world's human population, essentially for life unless eradicated by antibiotic treatment. Colonization with this organism is the main risk factor for peptic ulceration (**Chap. 324**) as well as for gastric adenocarcinoma and gastric mucosa-associated lymphoid tissue (MALT) lymphoma (**Chap. 80**). Treatment for *H. pylori* has revolutionized the management of peptic ulcer disease, providing a permanent cure in most cases. Such treatment also represents first-line therapy for patients with low-grade gastric MALT lymphoma. Treatment of *H. pylori* is of no benefit in the treatment of gastric adenocarcinoma, but prevention of *H. pylori* colonization or eradicative treatment could potentially prevent gastric malignancy and peptic ulceration. In contrast, increasing evidence indicates that lifelong *H. pylori* colonization may offer some protection against complications of gastroesophageal reflux disease (GERD), including esophageal adenocarcinoma. Recent research has focused on whether *H. pylori* colonization is also a risk factor for some extragastric diseases and whether it is protective against some recently emergent medical problems, such as childhood-onset asthma and other allergic and metabolic conditions.

ETIOLOGIC AGENT

Helicobacter pylori *H. pylori* is a gram-negative bacillus that has naturally colonized humans for at least 100,000 years, and probably throughout human evolution. It lives in gastric mucus, with a proportion of the bacteria adherent to the mucosa and possibly a very small number of the organisms entering cells or penetrating the mucosa; the organism's distribution is mucosal rather than systemic. Its spiral shape and flagella render *H. pylori* motile in the mucus environment. The organism has several acid-resistance mechanisms, most notably a highly expressed urease that catalyzes urea hydrolysis to produce buffering ammonia. *H. pylori* is microaerophilic (i.e., grows in low levels of oxygen), is slow-growing, and requires complex growth media in vitro.

Other *Helicobacter* Species A small proportion of gastric *Helicobacter* infections are due to species other than *H. pylori*, possibly acquired as zoonoses. These non-*pylori* gastric helicobacters are associated with low-level inflammation and occasionally with disease. In immunocompromised hosts, several nongastric (intestinal) *Helicobacter* species can cause disease with clinical features resembling those of *Campylobacter* infections; these species are covered in **Chap. 167**.

EPIDEMIOLOGY

Prevalence and Risk Factors The prevalence of *H. pylori* among adults is <30% in most parts of the United States, Europe, and Oceania as opposed to >60% in many parts of Africa, South America, and West Asia. In the United States, prevalence varies with age: up to 50% of 60-year-old persons, ~20% of 30-year-old persons, and <10% of children are colonized. *H. pylori* is usually acquired in childhood. The age association is due mostly to a birth-cohort effect whereby current 60-year-olds were more commonly colonized as children than are current children. Spontaneous acquisition or loss of *H. pylori* in adulthood is uncommon. Childhood acquisition explains why the main risk factors for infection are markers of crowding and social deprivation in childhood. Longitudinal studies have shown declining prevalences over the past half-century, concomitant with socioeconomic development and widespread antibacterial treatments.

Transmission Humans are the only important reservoir of *H. pylori*. Children may acquire the organism from their parents (most often the primary caregiver) or from other children. The former is more common in developed countries and the latter in less developed countries. Whether transmission takes place more often by the fecal–oral or the oral–oral route is unknown, but *H. pylori* is easily cultured from vomitus and gastroesophageal refluxate and is much less easily cultured from stool. Most acquisition of *H. pylori* is during the early years of childhood.

PATHOLOGY AND PATHOGENESIS

Long-term *H. pylori* colonization induces *chronic superficial gastritis*, a tissue response in the stomach that includes infiltration of the mucosa by both mononuclear and polymorphonuclear cells. (The term *gastritis* should be used specifically to describe histologic features; it has also been used to describe endoscopic appearances and even symptoms, but only magnification endoscopy correlates with microscopic findings or even with the presence of *H. pylori*, and even this is insufficient for diagnosis.) Although *H. pylori* is capable of numerous adaptations that prevent excessive stimulation of the immune system, colonization is accompanied by a considerable persistent local and systemic immune response, including the production of antibodies and cell-mediated responses. However, these responses are ineffective in clearing the bacterium. This inefficient clearing appears to be due in part to *H. pylori*'s downregulation of the immune system, which fosters its own persistence.

Most *H. pylori*–colonized persons do not develop clinical sequelae. That some persons develop overt disease whereas others do not is related to a combination of factors: bacterial strain differences, host susceptibility to disease, and environmental factors.

Bacterial Virulence Factors Several *H. pylori* virulence factors are more common among strains that are associated with disease than among those that are not. The *cag* island is a group of genes that encodes a bacterial type IV secretion system. Through this system, an effector protein, CagA, is translocated into epithelial cells, where it may be activated by phosphorylation and induces host cell signal transduction; proliferative, cytoskeletal, and inflammatory changes in the cell result. The protein at the tip of the secretory apparatus, CagL, binds to integrins on the cell surface, transducing further signaling. Finally, soluble components of the peptidoglycan cell wall enter the cell, mediated by the same secretory system. These components are recognized by the intracellular bacterial receptor Nod1, which stimulates a proinflammatory cytokine response resulting in an enhanced tissue response. Carriage of *cag*-positive strains increases the risk of both peptic ulcer and gastric adenocarcinoma. A second major host-interaction factor is the vacuolating cytotoxin VacA, which forms pores in cell membranes. VacA is polymorphic, and carriage of more active forms also increases the risk of ulcer disease and gastric cancer. Other bacterial factors that are associated with increased disease risk include adhesins, such as BabA (which binds to blood group antigens on epithelial cells).

Host Genetic and Environmental Factors The best-characterized host determinants of disease are genetic polymorphisms leading to enhanced activation of the innate immune response, including polymorphisms in cytokine genes and in genes encoding bacterial recognition proteins such as Toll-like receptors. For example, colonized people with polymorphisms in the interleukin 1 gene that increase the production of this cytokine in response to *H. pylori* infection are at increased risk of gastric adenocarcinoma. In addition, environmental cofactors are important in pathogenesis. Smoking increases the risks of duodenal ulcers and gastric cancer in *H. pylori*–positive individuals. Diets high in salt and preserved foods increase cancer risk, whereas diets high in antioxidants and vitamin C are modestly protective.

Distribution of Gastritis and Differential Disease Risk The pattern of gastric tissue response is associated with disease risk: antral-predominant gastritis is most closely linked with duodenal ulceration, whereas pan-gastritis and corpus-predominant gastritis are linked with gastric ulceration and adenocarcinoma. This difference probably explains why patients with duodenal ulceration are not at high risk of developing gastric adenocarcinoma later in life, despite being colonized by *H. pylori*.

PATHOGENESIS OF DUODENAL ULCERATION How gastric colonization causes duodenal ulceration is now becoming clearer. *H. pylori*–induced tissue responses in the gastric antrum diminish the number of somatostatin-producing D cells. Because somatostatin inhibits gastrin release, gastrin levels are higher than in *H. pylori*–negative persons, and these higher levels lead to increased meal-stimulated acid secretion from the relatively spared gastric corpus. How this situation increases duodenal ulcer risk remains controversial, but the increased acid secretion may contribute to the formation of potentially acid-protective gastric metaplasia in the duodenum. Gastric metaplasia in the duodenum may become colonized by *H. pylori* and subsequently inflamed and ulcerated.

PATHOGENESIS OF GASTRIC ULCERATION AND GASTRIC ADENOCARCINOMA The pathogenesis of these conditions is less well understood, although both arise in association with pan- or corpus-predominant gastritis. The hormonal changes described above still occur, but the tissue responses in the gastric corpus mean that it produces less acid (hypochlorhydria) despite hypergastrinemia. Gastric ulcers commonly occur at the junction of antral and corpus-type mucosa, an area that is often particularly inflamed. Gastric cancer usually arises in stomachs with extensive atrophic gastritis and hypochlorhydria, and probably stems from progressive DNA damage and the survival of abnormal epithelial cell clones. The DNA damage is thought to be due principally to reactive oxygen and nitrogen species arising from inflammatory cells, perhaps in relation to other bacteria that survive in a hypochlorhydric stomach. Longitudinal analyses of gastric biopsy specimens taken years apart from the same patient show that the common *intestinal* type of gastric adenocarcinoma follows stepwise changes from simple gastritis to gastric atrophy, metaplasia, and dysplasia. A second, *diffuse* type of gastric adenocarcinoma found more commonly in younger adults may arise directly from chronic gastritis without atrophic changes. In recent years, there has been a progressive rise in gastric cancers centered on the gastric corpus and occurring in younger adults (<50 years old) and disproportionately in females; this appears to be in the absence of *H. pylori*.

PATHOGENESIS OF GASTRIC MALT LYMPHOMA Low-grade B-cell MALT lymphomas are rare malignancies, reported at a rate of ~1 per million population per year prior to the discovery of *H. pylori*. Since then, reported rates have increased substantially, possibly reflecting overdiagnosis. These tumors arise from the substrate of chronic stimulation of lymphocyte populations by the persistent *H. pylori* colonization. Importantly, there have been numerous reports of these low-grade tumors responding dramatically to *H. pylori* eradication therapies. However, the boundary between true malignancy and benign lymphoid hypertrophy is uncertain. Among responders to *H. pylori* eradication, most do not have the characteristic t(11;18)(q21;q21) translocation of the malignancy and may not have true malignancies but rather benign polyclonal lymphoid proliferation. CagA-positive *H. pylori* strains have been significantly associated with the t(11;18)(q21;q21)–positive gastric MALT lymphoma compared with translocation-negative cases.

CLINICAL MANIFESTATIONS

Essentially all *H. pylori*–colonized persons have histologic gastritis, but only ~10–15% develop associated illnesses such as peptic ulceration, gastric adenocarcinoma, or gastric lymphoma (**Fig. 163-1**). Despite similar rates of *H. pylori* colonization, rates of these diseases among women are less than half of those among men.

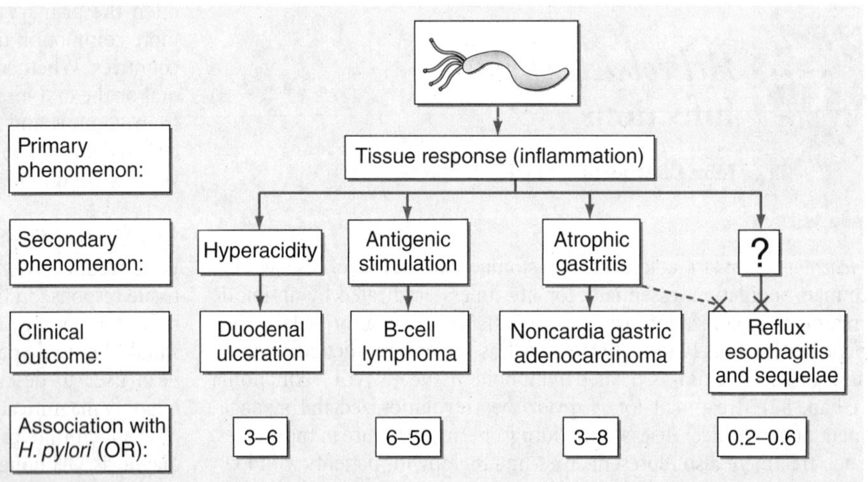

FIGURE 163-1 Schematic of the relationships between colonization with *Helicobacter pylori* and diseases of the upper gastrointestinal tract. Essentially all persons colonized with *H. pylori* develop a host response, which is generally termed *chronic gastritis*. The nature of the host's interaction with the particular bacterial population determines the clinical outcome. *H. pylori* colonization increases the lifetime risk of peptic ulcer disease, noncardia gastric cancer, and B-cell non-Hodgkin's gastric lymphoma (odds ratios [ORs] for all, >3). In contrast, a growing body of evidence indicates that *H. pylori* colonization (especially with *cagA*+ strains) protects against adenocarcinoma of the esophagus (and the sometimes related gastric cardia) and premalignant lesions such as Barrett's esophagus (ORs, <1). Although the incidences of peptic ulcer disease (cases not due to nonsteroidal anti-inflammatory drugs) and noncardia gastric cancer are declining in developed countries, the incidence of adenocarcinoma of the esophagus is increasing. *(Reproduced with permission from MJ Blaser: Hypothesis: The changing relationships of Helicobacter pylori and humans: Implications for health and disease. J Inf Dis 179:1523, 1999.)*

PEPTIC ULCER DISEASE

Worldwide, ~70% of duodenal ulcers and ~50% of gastric ulcers are related to *H. pylori* colonization (**Chap. 324**). However, in particular, the proportion of gastric ulcers caused by aspirin and nonsteroidal anti-inflammatory drugs (NSAIDs) is increasing, and in many developed countries, these drugs have overtaken *H. pylori* as a cause of gastric ulceration. The main lines of evidence supporting an ulcer-promoting role for *H. pylori* are that (1) the presence of the organism is a risk factor for the development of ulcers, (2) non-NSAID-induced ulcers rarely develop in the absence of *H. pylori*, (3) eradication of *H. pylori* virtually abolishes long-term ulcer relapse, and (4) experimental *H. pylori* infection of gerbils can cause gastric ulceration. Thus, *H. pylori* is neither necessary nor sufficient for the development of peptic ulcer disease, but it is a very strong risk factor for its occurrence, and removal of *H. pylori* changes the natural history of ulcer disease.

Gastric Adenocarcinoma and Lymphoma Prospective nested case–control studies have shown that *H. pylori* colonization is a risk factor for adenocarcinomas of the distal (noncardia) stomach (**Chap. 80**). Long-term experimental infection of gerbils also may result in gastric adenocarcinoma. Moreover, *H. pylori* may induce primary gastric lymphoma, although this condition is much less common, and the approaches to histopathologic and cytogenetic evaluations are not standardized. Many of the diagnosed low-grade gastric B-cell lymphomas are dependent on *H. pylori* for continuing growth and proliferation, and these tumors may regress either fully or partially after *H. pylori* eradication. However, they require careful short- and long-term monitoring; any that are not confined to the superficial mucosa (and, indeed, some that are) require additional treatment with chemotherapeutic agents or radiotherapy.

Functional Dyspepsia Many patients have upper gastrointestinal symptoms but have normal results on upper gastrointestinal endoscopy (so-called functional or nonulcer dyspepsia; **Chap. 324**). Because *H. pylori* is common, some of these patients will be colonized with the organism. *H. pylori* eradication leads to symptom resolution up to 15% more commonly than does placebo treatment. Whether such patients have peptic ulcers in remission at the time of endoscopy or whether a small subgroup of patients with "true" functional dyspepsia respond to *H. pylori* treatment is unclear. Either way, because functional dyspepsia is often persistent and difficult to treat, most consensus conference guidelines recommend *H. pylori* eradication in these patients. If this advice is followed, it is important to realize that only a small subgroup of patients who are treated will benefit.

Protection Against Peptic Esophageal Disease, Including Esophageal Adenocarcinoma Much interest has focused on a protective role for *H. pylori* against GERD (**Chap. 323**), Barrett's esophagus (**Chap. 323**), and adenocarcinoma of the esophagus and gastric cardia (**Chap. 80**). The main lines of evidence for this role are (1) that there is a temporal relationship between a falling prevalence of gastric *H. pylori* colonization and a rising incidence of these conditions; (2) that, in most studies, the prevalence of *H. pylori* colonization (especially with proinflammatory *cagA*$^+$ strains) is significantly lower among patients with these esophageal diseases than among control participants; and (3) that, in prospective nested studies (see above), the presence of *H. pylori* is inversely related to these cancers. The mechanism underlying this protective effect is likely *H. pylori*–induced hypochlorhydria. Because, at the individual level, GERD severity may decrease, worsen, or remain unchanged after *H. pylori* treatment, concerns about GERD should not affect decisions about whether to treat *H. pylori* in an individual patient if a clear-cut indication exists; if there is no clear indication, clinicians should carefully balance considerations of benefit and harm.

Other Pathologies *H. pylori* has an increasingly recognized role in other gastric pathologies. It may predispose some patients to iron deficiency through occult blood loss and/or hypochlorhydria and reduced iron absorption. In addition, several extragastrointestinal pathologies have been linked with *H. pylori* colonization, although evidence of causality is less strong. Studies of *H. pylori* treatment in idiopathic thrombocytopenic purpura have consistently described improvement in or even normalization of platelet counts. Potentially important but even more controversial (protective) associations are with ischemic heart disease and cerebrovascular disease. However, the strength of the latter associations is reduced if confounding factors are taken into account, and our present knowledge is incomplete. Most authorities consider the associations to be noncausal. An increasing number of studies have shown an inverse association of *cagA*$^+$ *H. pylori* with childhood-onset asthma, hay fever, and atopic disorders. These associations have been shown to be causal in animal models, but the effect size in humans has not been established.

DIAGNOSIS

Tests for *H. pylori* fall into two groups: tests that require upper gastrointestinal endoscopy and simpler tests that can be performed in the clinic (**Table 163-1**).

Endoscopy-Based Tests Endoscopy is usually unnecessary in the initial management of young patients with simple dyspepsia but is commonly used to exclude malignancy and make a positive diagnosis in older patients or those with "alarm" symptoms. If endoscopy is performed, the most convenient biopsy-based test is the biopsy urease test, in which one large or two small gastric biopsy specimens are placed into a gel containing urea and an indicator. The presence of *H. pylori* urease leads to a rise in pH and therefore to a color change, which often occurs within minutes but can require up to 24 h. Histologic examination of biopsy specimens for *H. pylori* also is accurate, provided that a special stain (e.g., a modified Giemsa, silver, or immuno-stain) permitting optimal visualization of the organism is used. If biopsy specimens are obtained from both antrum and corpus, histologic study yields additional information, including the degree and pattern of inflammation and the presence of any atrophy, metaplasia, or dysplasia. Microbiologic culture is most specific but may be insensitive because of difficulty with *H. pylori* isolation. Once the organism is cultured, its identity as *H. pylori* can be confirmed by its typical appearance on Gram's stain and its positive reactions in oxidase, catalase, and urease tests. Moreover, the organism's susceptibility to antibiotics can be determined, and this information can be clinically useful in difficult cases. The occasional biopsy specimens containing the less common non-*pylori* gastric helicobacters give weakly positive results in the

TABLE 163-1 Tests Commonly Used to Detect *Helicobacter pylori*

TEST	ADVANTAGES	DISADVANTAGES
Tests Based on Endoscopic Biopsy		
Biopsy urease test	Quick, simple	Some commercial tests not fully sensitive before 24 h
Histology	May give additional histologic information	Sensitivity dependent on experience and use of special stains
Culture	Permits determination of antibiotic susceptibility	Sensitivity dependent on experience
Noninvasive Tests		
Serology	Inexpensive and convenient; not affected by recent antibiotics or proton pump inhibitors to the same extent as breath and stool tests	Cannot be used to monitor treatment success; some commercial kits inaccurate, and most less accurate than urea breath test
^{13}C urea breath test	Inexpensive and simpler than endoscopy; useful for follow-up after treatment	Requires fasting; not as convenient as blood or stool tests
Stool antigen test	Inexpensive and convenient; useful for follow-up after treatment; may be particularly useful in children	Stool-based tests disliked by people from some cultures

biopsy urease test. Positive identification of these bacteria requires visualization of the characteristic long, tight spirals in histologic sections; they cannot easily be cultured.

Noninvasive Tests Noninvasive *H. pylori* testing is the norm if gastric cancer does not need to be excluded by endoscopy. The longest-established test (and a very accurate one) is the *urea breath test.* In this simple test, the patient drinks a solution of urea labeled with the nonradioactive isotope ^{13}C and then blows into a tube. If *H. pylori* urease is present, the urea is hydrolyzed, and labeled carbon dioxide is detected in breath samples. The *stool antigen test*, a simple and accurate test using monoclonal antibodies specific for *H. pylori* antigens, is more convenient and less expensive than the urea breath test, but some patients dislike sampling stool. The simplest tests for ascertaining *H. pylori* status are *serologic assays* measuring specific IgG levels in serum by enzyme-linked immunosorbent assay or immunoblot. The best of these tests are nearly as accurate as other diagnostic methods, but many commercial tests—especially rapid office tests—do not perform well.

Use of Tests to Assess Treatment Success The urea breath test, the stool antigen test, and biopsy-based tests can all be used to assess the success of treatment **(Fig. 163-2)**. However, because these tests are dependent on *H. pylori* load, their use <4 weeks after treatment may yield false-negative results. Early suppression of bacterial numbers may lead to false-negative results since regrowth of the organism can result in its detection weeks later. For the same reason, these tests are unreliable if performed within 4 weeks of intercurrent treatment with antibiotics or bismuth compounds or within 2 weeks of the discontinuation of proton pump inhibitor (PPI) treatment. In the assessment of treatment success, noninvasive tests are normally preferred. However, after gastric ulceration, endoscopy should be repeated to ensure healing and exclude gastric carcinoma by further histologic sampling; if PPIs have been stopped for at least 2 weeks and no antibiotics or bismuth compounds have been given for at least 6 weeks, there is an opportunity to assess treatment success with biopsy-based tests. Serologic tests are not used to monitor treatment success, as the gradual drop in titer of *H. pylori*–specific antibodies is too slow (requiring >14 weeks) to be of practical use.

TREATMENT
Helicobacter pylori Infection

INDICATIONS

The most clear-cut indications for treatment are *H. pylori*–related duodenal or gastric ulceration or low-grade gastric B-cell MALT lymphoma. Whether or not the ulcers are currently active, *H. pylori* should be eradicated in patients with documented ulcer disease to prevent relapse (Fig. 163-2). Guidelines have recommended *H. pylori* treatment for colonized patients with functional dyspepsia in case they are among the small percentage who will benefit from such therapy (beyond placebo effects). *H. pylori* eradication in the treatment of conditions not definitively known to respond has also been recommended but is not universally supported; such conditions include idiopathic thrombocytopenic purpura, vitamin B_{12} deficiency, and iron-deficiency anemia where other causes have been carefully excluded. For individuals with a strong family history of gastric cancer, treatment to eradicate *H. pylori* in the hope of reducing cancer risk is reasonable but of unproven value: it slightly reduces future cancer incidence, but there is no evidence it reduces all-cause mortality. For older dyspeptic patients in the community or those who have "alarm" symptoms (e.g., weight loss) associated with their dyspepsia, upper gastrointestinal endoscopy is indicated to seek a diagnosis and test for *H. pylori*; the decision regarding whether to eradicate the organism can then be based on indication. Endoscopy is usually considered unnecessary for young dyspeptic patients in the community who have no alarm symptoms (with the precise age cutoff dependent on local guidelines). If the community prevalence of *H. pylori* is below ~20%, such patients are treated with a short course of acid suppression using a PPI. If these patients do not respond or relapse when treatment is stopped, or if the

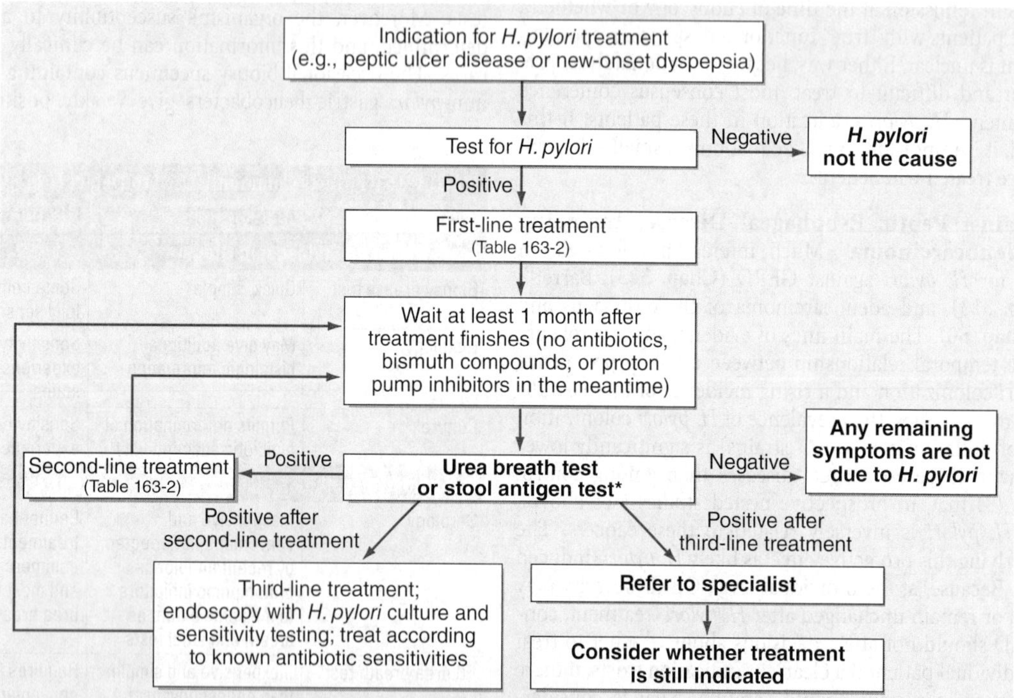

FIGURE 163-2 Algorithm for the management of *Helicobacter pylori* infection. *Note that either the urea breath test or the stool antigen test can be used in this algorithm. Occasionally, endoscopy and a biopsy-based test are used instead of either of these tests in follow-up after treatment. The main indication for these invasive tests is in follow-up after gastric ulceration; in this condition, as opposed to duodenal ulceration, it is important to check healing and exclude underlying gastric adenocarcinoma. However, even in this situation, patients undergoing endoscopy may still be receiving proton pump inhibitor therapy, which precludes *H. pylori* testing. Thus, a urea breath test or a stool antigen test is still required at a suitable interval after the end of therapy to determine whether treatment has been successful (see text). Some authorities use empirical third-line regimens, of which several have been described.

H. pylori community prevalence is >20%, many national guidelines recommend a strategy of testing for *H. pylori* noninvasively and eradicating it if it is found. This strategy will benefit patients who have peptic ulcers and the ~5–10% of patients who have functional dyspepsia responsive to *H. pylori* eradication, but most patients will be treated unnecessarily. Currently, widespread community screening for and treatment of *H. pylori* as primary prophylaxis for gastric cancer and peptic ulcers are not recommended in most countries, mainly because the extent of the consequent reduction in cancer risk is not known. Several studies have found a modestly reduced cancer risk after treatment, but the period of follow-up is still fairly short, and the magnitude of the effect in different populations remains unclear. Other reasons not to treat *H. pylori* in asymptomatic populations at present include (1) the adverse side effects (which are common and can be severe in rare cases) of the multiple-antibiotic regimens used; (2) antibiotic resistance, which may emerge in *H. pylori* or other incidentally carried bacteria; (3) the anxiety that may arise in otherwise healthy people, especially if treatment is unsuccessful; and (4) the existence of a subset of people who will develop GERD symptoms after treatment. Despite the absence of screening strategies, many doctors treat *H. pylori* if it is known to be present (particularly in children and younger adults), even when the patient is asymptomatic. The rationale is that it reduces patient concern and may reduce future gastric cancer risk and that any reduction in risk is likely to be greater in younger patients. However, such practices do not factor in any potential benefits of *H. pylori* colonization. Overall, despite widespread clinical activity in this area, most treatment of persons with asymptomatic *H. pylori* carriage is given with no firm evidence base. Because a proportion of patients (up to 70%) of those diagnosed with gastric low-grade B-cell MALT lymphomas respond to *H. pylori* eradication, it should be used in all cases, regardless of whether *H. pylori* can be detected by the diagnostic modalities used since there may be falsely negative results. However, not all of these cases represent true malignancies, so the reported success rate may reflect the eradication of benign processes. Examination of tissues for the characteristic chromosomal translocations should be done to help distinguish benign and malignant processes and to guide further therapeutic approaches. These generally are slowly progressive tumors, so the time needed for *H. pylori* eradication and subsequent evaluation will not interfere with the use of subsequent chemotherapy and/or radiotherapy, if needed.

REGIMENS

Although *H. pylori* is susceptible to a wide range of antibiotics in vitro, monotherapy is not usually successful, probably because of inadequate active antibiotic delivery to the colonization niche. Clinical failure of monotherapy prompted the development of multidrug regimens. Current regimens consist of a PPI and two or three antimicrobial agents given for 10–14 days (**Table 163-2**). The optimal regimens vary in different parts of the world, depending on the known rates of primary antibiotic resistance in most *H. pylori* strains in a particular locale. For this reason, guidelines on optimal regimens for *H. pylori* eradication in individual countries are evolving, and physicians should refer to the most up-to-date local guideline.

The two most important factors in successful *H. pylori* treatment are the patient's close compliance with the regimen and the use of drugs to which the patient's strain of *H. pylori* has not acquired resistance. Treatment failure following minor lapses in compliance is common and often leads to acquired resistance. To stress the importance of compliance, written instructions should be given to the patient, and minor side effects of the regimen should be explained. Increasing levels of primary *H. pylori* resistance to clarithromycin, levofloxacin, and—to a lesser extent—metronidazole are of growing concern. In most parts of the world (the main exception being northwestern Europe), the rate of primary clarithromycin resistance is sufficiently high that regimens containing clarithromycin plus one other antibiotic often fail; regimens with clarithromycin and two other antibiotics remain an option as the other two antibiotics are likely to eradicate *H. pylori* even if the strain is clarithromycin-resistant. When a patient is known to have been exposed—even remotely in time—to clarithromycin or a fluoroquinolone, these antibiotics usually should be avoided. Resistance to amoxicillin or tetracycline is unusual, even if these antibiotics have been given previously, and resistance to metronidazole is only partial; thus, there is no need to avoid using these antibiotics whether or not they have been previously prescribed. Whichever antibiotic regimen is used, meta-analyses show that using high rather than moderate doses of acid-suppressive PPIs with the antibiotics increases the effectiveness of the regimen. Similarly, use of vonoprazan, a highly effective potassium-competitive acid blocker, currently licensed in Japan, was associated with higher eradication rates in conjunction with amoxicillin and clarithromycin, than when a PPI was used for acid suppression.

Assessment of antibiotic susceptibilities before treatment would be optimal but is not usually undertaken because endoscopy and mucosal biopsy are necessary to obtain *H. pylori* for culture and because most microbiology laboratories are inexperienced in *H. pylori* culture. If initial *H. pylori* treatment fails, the usual approach is empirical re-treatment with another drug regimen (Table 163-2). The third-line approach ideally should be endoscopy, biopsy, and culture plus treatment based on documented antibiotic sensitivities. However, empirical third-line therapies are often used.

TABLE 163-2 Commonly Recommended Treatment Regimens for *Helicobacter pylori*

REGIMEN[a] (DURATION)	DRUG 1	DRUG 2	DRUG 3	DRUG 4
Regimen 1: OCM (14 days)[b]	Omeprazole (20 mg bid[c])	Clarithromycin (500 mg bid)	Metronidazole (500 mg bid)	—
Regimen 2: OCA (14 days)[b]	Omeprazole (20 mg bid[c])	Clarithromycin (500 mg bid)	Amoxicillin (1 g bid)	—
Regimen 3: OBTM (14 days)[d]	Omeprazole (20 mg bid[c])	Bismuth subsalicylate (2 tabs qid)	Tetracycline HCl (500 mg qid)	Metronidazole (500 mg tid)
Regimen 4: concomitant (14 days)[e]	Omeprazole (20 mg bid[c])	Amoxicillin (1 g bid)	Clarithromycin (500 mg bid)	Tinidazole (500 mg bid[f])
Regimen 5: OAL (10 days)[g]	Omeprazole (20 mg bid[c])	Amoxicillin (1 g bid)	Levofloxacin (500 mg bid)	—

[a]The recommended first-line regimens for most of the world are shown in **bold** type. [b]This regimen should be used only for populations in which the prevalence of clarithromycin-resistant strains is known to be <20%. In practice, this restriction limits the regimens' appropriate range mainly to northern Europe. [c]Many authorities and some guidelines recommend doubling this dose of omeprazole as trials show resultant increased efficacy with some antibiotic combinations. Omeprazole may be replaced with any proton pump inhibitor (PPI) at an equivalent dosage. Because extensive metabolizers of PPIs are prevalent among Caucasian populations, many authorities recommend esomeprazole (40 mg bid) or rabeprazole (20 mg bid), particularly for regimens 4 and 5. [d]Data supporting this regimen come mainly from Europe and are based on the use of bismuth subcitrate (1 tablet qid) and metronidazole (400 mg tid). This is a recommended first-line regimen in most countries and is the recommended second-line regimen in northern Europe. [e]This regimen may be used as an alternative to regimen 3. [f]Metronidazole (500 mg bid) may be used as an alternative. [g]This regimen is used as second-line treatment in many countries (particularly where quadruple or concomitant therapy is used as the first-line regimen) and as third-line treatment in others. It may be less effective where rates of fluoroquinolone use are high and is more likely to be ineffective if there is a personal history of fluoroquinolone use for previous treatment of other infections.

Non-*pylori* gastric helicobacters are treated in the same way as *H. pylori*. However, in the absence of trials, it is unclear whether a positive outcome always represents successful treatment or whether it is sometimes due to natural clearance of the bacteria.

PREVENTION

Carriage of *H. pylori* has considerable public health significance in economically richer countries, where it is associated with peptic ulcer disease and gastric adenocarcinoma, and in some, but not all, economically poorer countries, where gastric adenocarcinoma may be an even more common cause of cancer death late in life. If mass prevention were contemplated, vaccination would be the most obvious method: experimental immunization of animals has given promising results, and the first reported trial in humans has shown some efficacy. Further trials are ongoing. However, given that *H. pylori* has co-evolved with its human host over millennia, preventing colonization on a population basis may have biological and clinical costs. For example, lifelong absence of *H. pylori* is a risk factor for GERD complications, including esophageal adenocarcinoma. We have speculated that the disappearance of *H. pylori* may also be associated with an increased risk of other emergent diseases reflecting aspects of the current Western lifestyle, such as childhood-onset asthma and allergy, as supported by both epidemiologic and animal model studies.

FURTHER READING

Amieva M, Peek RM: Pathobiology of *Helicobacter pylori*–induced gastric cancer. Gastroenterology 150:64, 2016.

Anderson WF et al: The changing face of noncardia gastric cancer incidence among US non-Hispanic whites. J Natl Cancer Inst 110:608, 2018.

Arnold IC et al: *Helicobacter pylori* infection prevents allergic asthma in mouse models through the induction of regulatory T cells. J Clin Invest 121:3088, 2011.

Atherton JC, Blaser MJ: Co-adaptation of *Helicobacter pylori* and humans: Ancient history and modern implications. J Clin Invest 119:2475, 2009.

Chen Y, Blaser MJ: Inverse associations of *Helicobacter pylori* with asthma and allergies. Arch Intern Med 167:821, 2007.

Chen Y et al: Association between *Helicobacter pylori* and mortality in the NHANES II study. Gut 62:1262, 2013.

Chow WH et al: An inverse relation between *cagA*+ strains of *Helicobacter pylori* infection and risk of esophageal and gastric cardia adenocarcinoma. Cancer Res 58:588, 1998.

Deguchi H et al: Current status of *Helicobacter pylori* diagnosis and eradication therapy in Japan using a nationwide database. Digestion 101:441, 2020.

Ford AC et al: *Helicobacter pylori* eradication therapy to prevent gastric cancer in healthy asymptomatic infected individuals: Systematic review and meta-analysis of randomized controlled trials. BMJ 348:g3174, 2014.

Graham DY et al: Rifabutin-based triple therapy (RHB-105) for *Helicobacter pylori* eradication: A double-blind, randomized, controlled trial. Ann Intern Med 172:795, 2020.

Hooi JKY et al: Global prevalence of *Helicobacter pylori* infection: Systematic review and meta-analysis. Gastroenterology 153:420, 2017.

Kuo S-H et al: First-line antibiotic therapy in *Helicobacter pylori*-negative low-grade gastric mucosa-associated lymphoid tissue lymphoma. Scientific Rep 7:14333, 2017.

Linz B et al: An African origin for the intimate association between humans and *Helicobacter pylori*. Nature 445:915, 2007.

Maixner F et al: The 5300-year-old *Helicobacter pylori* genome of the Iceman. Science 351:162, 2016.

Marshall BJ, Warren JR: Unidentified curved bacilli in the stomach of patients with gastritis and peptic ulceration. Lancet 1:1311, 1984.

Plummer M et al: Global burden of gastric cancer attributable to *Helicobacter pylori*. Int J Cancer 136:487, 2015.

164 Infections Due to *Pseudomonas, Burkholderia,* and *Stenotrophomonas* Species

Reuben Ramphal

The pseudomonads are a heterogeneous group of gram-negative bacteria that have in common an inability to ferment lactose. Formerly classified in the genus *Pseudomonas*, the members of this group have been assigned to three medically important genera—*Pseudomonas, Burkholderia*, and *Stenotrophomonas*—whose biologic behaviors encompass both similarities and marked differences and whose genetic repertoires differ in many respects. The pathogenicity of most pseudomonads is based on opportunism; the exceptions are *Burkholderia pseudomallei* and *Burkholderia mallei*, which are primary pathogens.

The genus *Pseudomonas* now contains >140 species. *Pseudomonas aeruginosa*, the major pathogen of the group, is a significant cause of infections in hospitalized patients and in patients with cystic fibrosis (CF; **Chap. 291**). Cytotoxic chemotherapy, mechanical ventilation, and broad-spectrum antibiotic therapy set up conditions that predispose to colonization and infection of increasing numbers of hospitalized patients by this pathogen. Other significant members of the genus—*Pseudomonas putida, Pseudomonas fluorescens, Pseudomonas oryzihabitans*, and *Pseudomonas stutzeri*—infect humans infrequently and are generally opportunists always present in the environment.

The genus *Burkholderia* comprises >20 species, of which *Burkholderia cepacia* is most frequently encountered in Western countries. Similar to *P. aeruginosa, B. cepacia* (now referred to as the *B. cepacia* complex species) is both an opportunistic nosocomial pathogen and a cause of infection in CF. The other medically important members of this genus are *B. pseudomallei* and *B. mallei*, the etiologic agents of melioidosis and glanders, respectively.

The genus *Stenotrophomonas* contains one species of medical significance, *Stenotrophomonas maltophilia*. This organism is strictly an opportunist that "overgrows" in the setting of broad-spectrum antibiotic use.

PSEUDOMONAS AERUGINOSA

EPIDEMIOLOGY

P. aeruginosa is found in most moist environments. Soil, plants, vegetables, tap water, and countertops are all potential reservoirs for this microbe, as it has simple nutritional needs. Given the ubiquity of *P. aeruginosa*, it is clear that simple contact with the organism is not sufficient for colonization or infection. Clinical and experimental observations suggest that infection by *P. aeruginosa* occurs concomitantly with compromised host defenses, mucosal trauma, physiologic derangement, and antibiotic-mediated suppression of normal flora. Thus, it comes as no surprise that the majority of *P. aeruginosa* infections occur in intensive care units (ICUs), where these factors frequently converge. The organism is initially acquired from environmental sources, but patient-to-patient spread also occurs in CF clinics.

In the past, burned patients appeared to be unusually susceptible to *P. aeruginosa*. For example, in 1959–1963, *Pseudomonas* burn-wound sepsis was the principal cause of death in 60% of burned patients dying at the U.S. Army Institute of Surgical Research. For reasons that are unclear, *P. aeruginosa* infection in burns is no longer the major problem that it was during the 1950s and 1960s. Similarly, in the 1960s, *P. aeruginosa* appeared as a common pathogen in patients receiving cytotoxic chemotherapy at many institutions in the United States, but it has subsequently diminished in importance. Despite this subsidence, *P. aeruginosa* remains one of the most feared pathogens in this population because of its high attributable mortality.

In some parts of Asia and Latin America, *P. aeruginosa* continues to be the most common cause of gram-negative bacteremia in neutropenic patients.

In contrast to the trends for burned patients and neutropenic patients in the United States, the incidence of *P. aeruginosa* infections among patients with CF has not changed. *P. aeruginosa* remains the most common contributing factor to respiratory failure in CF and is responsible for the majority of deaths among CF patients.

LABORATORY FEATURES

P. aeruginosa is a nonfastidious, motile, gram-negative rod that grows on most common laboratory media, including blood and MacConkey agars. It is easily identified in the laboratory on primary-isolation agar plates by pigment production that confers a yellow to dark green or even bluish appearance. Colonies have a shiny "gun-metal" appearance and a characteristic fruity odor. Two of the identifying biochemical characteristics of *P. aeruginosa* are an inability to ferment lactose on MacConkey agar and a positive reaction in the oxidase test. Most strains are identified on the basis of these readily detectable laboratory features even before extensive biochemical testing is done. Some isolates from CF patients are easily identified by their mucoid appearance, which is due to the production of large amounts of the mucoid exopolysaccharide or alginate.

PATHOGENESIS

Unraveling the mechanisms that underlie disease caused by *P. aeruginosa* has proved challenging. Of the common gram-negative bacteria, no other species produces such a large number of putative virulence factors (**Table 164-1**). Yet *P. aeruginosa* rarely initiates an infectious process in the absence of host injury or compromise, and few of its putative virulence factors have been shown definitively to be involved in disease in humans. Despite its metabolic versatility and possession of multiple colonizing factors, *P. aeruginosa* exhibits no competitive advantage over enteric bacteria in the human gut; it is not a normal inhabitant of the healthy human gastrointestinal tract, despite the host's continuous environmental exposure to the organism.

Virulence Attributes Involved in Acute *P. aeruginosa* Infections

• **MOTILITY AND COLONIZATION** A general tenet of bacterial pathogenesis is that most bacteria must adhere to surfaces or colonize a host niche in order to initiate disease. Most gram-negative bacteria examined thus far possess adherence factors called *adhesins*. *P. aeruginosa* is no exception. Among its many adhesins are its pili, which demonstrate adhesive properties for a variety of cells and adhere best to injured cell surfaces. In the organism's flagellum, the flagellin molecule binds to cells, and the flagellar cap attaches to mucins through the recognition of glycan chains. Other *P. aeruginosa* adhesins include the outer core of the lipopolysaccharide (LPS) molecule, which binds to the cystic fibrosis transmembrane conductance regulator (CFTR) and aids in internalization of the organism, and the alginate coat of mucoid strains, which enhances adhesion to cells and mucins. In addition, membrane proteins and lectins have been proposed as colonization factors. The deletion of any given adhesin is not sufficient to abrogate the ability of *P. aeruginosa* to colonize surfaces. Motility is important in host invasion via mucosal surfaces in some animal models of infection; however, nonmotile strains are not uniformly avirulent. It has been well demonstrated that nonmotile strains of *P. aeruginosa* are poorly phagocytosed, possibly leading to enhancement of the virulence of this organism.

TABLE 164-1 Main Putative Virulence Factors of *Pseudomonas aeruginosa*

SUBSTANCE/ ORGANELLE	FUNCTION	VIRULENCE IN ANIMAL DISEASE
Pili	Adhesion to cells	?
Flagella	Adhesion, motility, inflammation	Yes
Lipopolysaccharide	Antiphagocytic activity, inflammation	Yes
Type III secretion system	Toxic activity (ExoU, ExoS)	Yes
Type II secretion system	Toxic activity	Yes
Proteases	Proteolytic activity	?
Phospholipases	Cytotoxicity	?
Exotoxin A	Cytotoxicity	?
Pyocyanin	Cytotoxicity	Yes

EVASION OF HOST DEFENSES The transition from bacterial colonization to disease requires the evasion of host defenses followed by invasion by the microorganism. *P. aeruginosa* appears to be well equipped for evasion. Attached bacteria inject four known toxins (ExoS or ExoU, ExoT, and ExoY) via a type III secretion system that allows the bacteria to evade phagocytic cells either by direct cytotoxicity or by inhibition of phagocytosis. Clinical studies suggest that the mortality rate is higher among patients infected by strains that secrete the ExoU toxin. Another secretion system—the type II system—secretes toxins that can kill animals, and some of its secreted toxins, such as exotoxin A, have the potential to kill phagocytic cells. Multiple proteases secreted by this system may degrade host effector molecules, such as cytokines and chemokines, that are released in response to infection.

TISSUE INJURY Among gram-negative bacteria, *P. aeruginosa* probably produces the largest number of substances that are toxic to cells and thus have the potential to injure tissues. The toxins secreted by the organism's type III secretion system are capable of injuring tissue. However, their delivery requires the adherence of the organism to cells. Thus, the effects of these toxins are likely to be local or to depend on the presence of large numbers of bacteria at the site of an infection or in the bloodstream. On the other hand, diffusible toxins, secreted by the organism's type II secretion system, can act freely wherever they come into contact with cells. Possible effectors of this system include exotoxin A, at least four different proteases, and at least two phospholipases. In addition to these secreted toxins, rhamnolipids, pyocyanins—the pigments that confer the characteristic color and odor of *P. aeruginosa* colonies—and hydrocyanic acid, are produced by *P. aeruginosa* and are all capable of causing host tissue injury and even neutrophil death.

INFLAMMATORY COMPONENTS The inflammatory responses to the lipid A component of *Pseudomonas* LPS and to its flagellin, mediated through the Toll-like receptor (TLR) system (principally TLR4 and TLR5, respectively), are thought to represent important factors in disease causation. Although these inflammatory responses are required for successful defense against *P. aeruginosa* (i.e., in their absence, animals are defenseless against *P. aeruginosa* infection), florid responses are likely to result in disease. Thus, when the sepsis syndrome and septic shock develop in *P. aeruginosa* infection, they are probably the result of the host response to one or both of these substances, but injury to the lung by *Pseudomonas* toxins may also result in sepsis syndromes, possibly by causing cell death and the release of cellular components (e.g., heat-shock proteins) that may activate the TLR or another proinflammatory system. Thus, the virulence of this bacterium in acute infections is likely to be multifactorial with a great redundancy of effector molecules being produced.

Chronic *P. aeruginosa* Infections

Chronic infection due to *P. aeruginosa* occurs mainly in the lungs in the setting of structural pulmonary diseases. The classic example is CF; others include bronchiectasis and chronic relapsing panbronchiolitis, a disease seen in Japan and some Pacific Islands. A hallmark of these illnesses is severely defective mucociliary clearance leading to mucus stasis and mucus accumulation in the lungs. There is probably a common factor that selects for *P. aeruginosa* colonization in these lung diseases—perhaps the adhesiveness of *P. aeruginosa* for mucus, a phenomenon that is not noted for most other common gram-negative bacteria, and/or the ability of *P. aeruginosa* to evade host defenses in mucus. Furthermore, *P. aeruginosa* undergoes evolutionary adaptations and diversification in ways that allow its prolonged survival in the lung without an early fatal outcome for the host. The strains found in CF patients exhibit minimal production of virulence factors. Many strains lose the ability to produce pili and flagella, and most become complement-sensitive because of the loss of the O side chain of their LPS molecules. In addition, most strains found in CF patients overproduce a mucoid exopolysaccharide. These changes probably dampen the host response, allowing the organism to survive in CF mucus. *P. aeruginosa* is also believed to lose its ability to secrete many of its injectable toxins during growth in mucus. Although the alginate coat is thought to play a role in the organism's survival, alginate is not essential as nonmucoid strains may predominate for long periods. In short, virulence in chronic infections may be mediated by the chronic but attenuated host inflammatory response, which injures the lungs over decades.

CLINICAL MANIFESTATIONS

P. aeruginosa causes infections at almost all sites in the body but shows a rather marked predilection for the lungs. The infections encountered most commonly in hospitalized patients are described below.

Bacteremia Crude mortality rates exceeding 50% have been reported among patients with *P. aeruginosa* bacteremia. Consequently, this clinical entity has been much feared, and its management has been attempted with the use of multiple antibiotics. Recent publications report attributable mortality rates of 28–44%, with the precise figure depending on the adequacy and timing of treatment and the seriousness of the underlying disease. In the past, the patient with *P. aeruginosa* bacteremia classically was neutropenic or had a burn injury. Today, however, a minority of such patients have bacteremic *P. aeruginosa* infections. Rather, *P. aeruginosa* bacteremia is seen most often in patients in ICUs with the lungs, the urinary tract, central venous lines, or wounds being the most important portals for systemic invasion.

The clinical presentation of *P. aeruginosa* bacteremia rarely differs from that of sepsis in general **(Chap. 304)**. Patients are usually febrile, but those who are most severely ill may be in shock or even hypothermic. The only point differentiating this entity from gram-negative sepsis of other causes may be the distinctive skin lesions (ecthyma gangrenosum) of *Pseudomonas* infection, which occur almost exclusively in markedly neutropenic patients and patients with AIDS. These small or large, painful, reddish, maculopapular lesions have a geographic margin; they are initially pink, then darken to purple, and finally become black and necrotic **(Fig. 164-1)**. Histopathologic studies indicate that the lesions are due to vascular invasion and are teeming with bacteria. Although similar lesions may occur in aspergillosis, mucormycosis, and occasionally *Staphylococcus aureus* bacteremia, their presence in a neutropenic patient generally suggests *P. aeruginosa* bacteremia as the most likely cause.

TREATMENT

P. aeruginosa Bacteremia

(Table 164-2) Antimicrobial treatment of *P. aeruginosa* bacteremia has been controversial. Combination therapy with an antipseudomonal β-lactam and an aminoglycoside became the standard of care because of the dismal outcome of single-drug therapy, mainly with aminoglycosides and polymixins, prior to 1971—first for *P. aeruginosa* bacteremia in febrile neutropenic patients and then extrapolated to all *P. aeruginosa* bacteremic infections in both neutropenic and nonneutropenic patients.

Following the introduction of new antipseudomonal drugs, a number of studies have revisited the choice between combination treatment and monotherapy for *Pseudomonas* bacteremia. Although some clinicians still favor combination therapy, most recent observational studies indicate that a single modern antipseudomonal β-lactam agent to which the isolate is sensitive is as efficacious as a combination. Even in patients at greatest risk of early death from *P. aeruginosa* bacteremia (i.e., those with fever and neutropenia), empirical antipseudomonal monotherapy is deemed to be as efficacious as empirical combination therapy by the practice guidelines of the Infectious Diseases Society of America (IDSA). One firm conclusion is that monotherapy with an aminoglycoside is not optimal.

There are, of course, institutions and countries where rates of susceptibility of *P. aeruginosa* to first-line antibiotics are <80%. Thus, when a septic patient with a high probability of *P. aeruginosa* infection is encountered in such settings, empirical combination therapy should be administered until the pathogen is identified and susceptibility data become available. Thereafter, whether one or two agents should be continued remains a matter of individual preference. Recent studies suggest that extended infusions of β-lactams such as cefepime, piperacillin/tazobactam, or meropenem may result in better outcomes of *Pseudomonas* bacteremia and possibly of *Pseudomonas* pneumonia. The duration of antibiotic therapy has now become an important consideration due to the increasing isolation of multiple drug-resistant (MDR) and extensively drug-resistant (XDR) *P. aeruginosa* strains. Recently published studies now strongly support the use of shorter courses of therapy (7 days) rather than the longer duration (10–14 days) that is commonly recommended for many cases of *Pseudomonas* bacteremia.

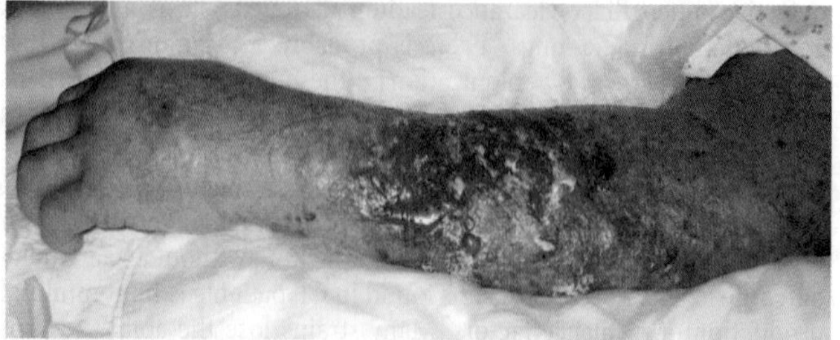

FIGURE 164-1 Ecthyma gangrenosum in a neutropenic patient 3 days after onset.

Acute Pneumonia Respiratory infections are the most common of all infections caused by *P. aeruginosa*. *P. aeruginosa* is common in both hospital-acquired pneumonia (HAP) and ventilator-associated pneumonia (VAP). This organism appears first or second among the causes of VAP. However, much debate centers on the actual role of *P. aeruginosa* in VAP. Many of the relevant data are based on cultures of sputum or endotracheal tube aspirates and may represent nonpathogenic colonization of the tracheobronchial tree, biofilms on the endotracheal tube, or simple tracheobronchitis.

Older reports of *P. aeruginosa* pneumonia described patients with an acute clinical syndrome of fever, chills, cough, and necrotizing pneumonia indistinguishable from other gram-negative bacterial pneumonias. The traditional accounts described a fulminant infection. Chest radiographs demonstrated bilateral pneumonia, often with nodular densities with or without cavities. This picture is now remarkably rare. Today, the typical patient is on a ventilator, has a slowly progressive infiltrate, and has been colonized with *P. aeruginosa* for days. While some cases may progress rapidly over 48–72 h, they are the exceptions. Nodular densities are not commonly seen. However, infiltrates may go on to necrosis. Necrotizing pneumonia has also been seen in the community (e.g., after inhalation of hot-tub water contaminated with *P. aeruginosa*). The typical patient has fever, leukocytosis, and purulent sputum, and the chest radiograph shows a new infiltrate or the expansion of a preexisting infiltrate. A sputum Gram's stain showing mainly polymorphonuclear leukocytes (PMNs) in conjunction with a culture positive for *P. aeruginosa* in this setting suggests a diagnosis of acute *P. aeruginosa* pneumonia.

There have been increasing reports of the occurrence of community-acquired *P. aeruginosa* pneumonia among patients with underlying lung diseases. While this undoubtedly occurs, it is difficult to make this diagnosis with a great degree of certainty with the use of sputum cultures in a population prone to airway colonization by multiple strains of bacteria. The patient population in whom the possibility of a community-acquired *P. aeruginosa* pneumonia should be considered is the neutropenic patient, given the pivotal role that neutrophils play in defense against this bacterium. Such a patient, whether hospitalized or admitted from the community with a pneumonia, should be treated empirically for *P. aeruginosa*.

TABLE 164-2 Antibiotic Treatment of Infections Due to *Pseudomonas aeruginosa* and Related Species

INFECTION	ANTIBIOTICS AND DOSAGES	OTHER CONSIDERATIONS
Bacteremia		
Nonneutropenic host	Ceftazidime (2 g q8h IV) *or* cefepime (2 g q8h IV) *or* piperacillin/tazobactam (3.375 g q4h IV) *or* imipenem (500 mg q6h IV) *or* meropenem (1 g q8h IV) *or* doripenem (500 mg q8h IV) ***Optional:*** Amikacin (7.5 mg/kg q12h or 15 mg/kg q24h IV)	Add an aminoglycoside for patients in shock and in regions or hospitals where rates of resistance to the primary β-lactam agents are high. Tobramycin may be used instead of amikacin (susceptibility permitting). The duration of therapy is 7 days for nonneutropenic patients. Neutropenic patients should be treated until no longer neutropenic.
Neutropenic host	Cefepime (2 g q8h IV) *or* all the other agents above (except doripenem) in the above dosages	
Endocarditis	Antibiotic regimens as for bacteremia for 6–8 weeks	Resistance during therapy is common. Surgery is required for relapse.
Pneumonia	Drugs and dosages as for bacteremia, except that the available carbapenems should not be the sole primary drugs because of high rates of resistance during therapy.	IDSA guidelines recommend the addition of an aminoglycoside or ciprofloxacin. The duration of therapy is 7 days.
Bone infection, malignant otitis externa	Cefepime or ceftazidime at the same dosages as for bacteremia; aminoglycosides not a necessary component of therapy; ciprofloxacin (500–750 mg q12h PO) may be used	Duration of therapy varies with the drug used (e.g., 6 weeks for a β-lactam agent; at least 3 months for oral therapy except in puncture-wound osteomyelitis, for which the duration should be 2–4 weeks).
Central nervous system infection	Ceftazidime or cefepime (2 g q8h IV) *or* meropenem (1 g q8h IV)	Abscesses or other closed-space infections may require drainage. The duration of therapy is ≥2 weeks.
Eye infection		
Keratitis/ulcer	Topical therapy with tobramycin/ciprofloxacin/levofloxacin eyedrops	Use maximal strengths available or compounded by pharmacy. Therapy should be administered for 2 weeks or until the resolution of eye lesions, whichever is shorter.
Endophthalmitis	Ceftazidime or cefepime as for central nervous system infection ***plus*** Topical therapy	
Urinary tract infection (UTI)	Ciprofloxacin (500 mg q12h PO) *or* levofloxacin (750 mg q24h) *or* any aminoglycoside (total daily dose given once daily). Cefepime or ceftazidime (1g q8h) *or* piperacillin/tazobactam (4.5 g q8h)	Uncomplicated cystitis may be treated for 3 days with oral agents. Relapse may occur if an obstruction or a foreign body is present. The duration of therapy for complicated UTI is 7–10 days (up to 2 weeks for pyelonephritis).
Multidrug- and extreme drug-resistant *P. aeruginosa* infection	Ceftazidime/avibactam (2.5 g q8h, infused over 2 h) *or* ceftolozane/tazobactam (1.5 g q8h) *or* meropenem/vaborbactam (2 g q8h) or imipenem/relebactam (500 mg q6h) *or* cefiderocol (2 g q8h) *or* colistin (100 mg q12h IV for the shortest possible period to obtain a clinical response)	Higher doses of ceftolozane/tazobactam may be required for pneumonias. The colistin doses used have varied. Dosage adjustment for colistin is required in renal failure. Inhaled colistin may be added for pneumonia (100 mg q12h).
Burkholderia cepacia complex infection	Meropenem (1 g q8h IV) *or* TMP-SMX (1600/320 mg q12h IV) for 14 days	Resistance to both agents is increasing. Do not use them in combination because of possible antagonism.
Melioidosis (*B. pseudomallei*), Glanders (*B. mallei*)	Ceftazidime (2 g q6h) *or* meropenem (1 g q8h) *or* imipenem (500 mg q6h) for 2 weeks ***followed by*** TMP-SMX (1600/320 mg q12h PO) for 3 months	
Stenotrophomonas maltophilia infection	TMP-SMX (1600/320 mg q12h IV) *plus* ticarcillin/clavulanate (3.1 g q4h IV) for 14 days	Resistance to all agents is increasing. Levofloxacin or tigecycline may be alternatives, but there is little published clinical experience with these agents.

Abbreviations: IDSA, Infectious Diseases Society of America; TMP-SMX, trimethoprim-sulfamethoxazole.

TREATMENT

Acute Pneumonia

(Table 164-2) Therapy for *P. aeruginosa* pneumonia remains unsatisfactory. Reports suggest mortality rates of 40–80%, but how many of these deaths are attributable to underlying disease remains unknown. The drugs of choice for *P. aeruginosa* pneumonia are similar to those given for bacteremia. A potent antipseudomonal β-lactam drug is the mainstay of therapy. Failure rates were high when aminoglycosides were used as single agents, possibly because of their poor penetration into the airways and their binding to airway secretions. Nonetheless, for the treatment of patients at high risk of death, some experts suggest the combination of a β-lactam agent and an antipseudomonal fluoroquinolone or aminoglycoside. As for the duration of therapy, recent IDSA/American Thoracic Society (ATS) guidelines recommend 7 days of treatment for HAP or VAP, even when *P. aeruginosa* is the offending organism. However, the outcome in neutropenic patients is poor, especially if accompanied by bacteremia; thus, therapy needs to be extended until neutropenia resolves.

Chronic Respiratory Tract Infections *P. aeruginosa* is responsible for chronic infections of the airways associated with a number of underlying or predisposing conditions—most commonly CF (**Chap. 291**). A state of chronic colonization beginning early in childhood is seen in some Asian populations with chronic or diffuse panbronchiolitis, a disease of unknown etiology. *P. aeruginosa* is one of the organisms that colonizes damaged bronchi in bronchiectasis, a disease secondary to multiple causes in which profound structural abnormalities of the airways result in mucus stasis.

TREATMENT

Chronic Respiratory Tract Infections

Optimal management of chronic *P. aeruginosa* lung infection has not been determined. Patients respond clinically to antipseudomonal therapy, but the organism is rarely eradicated. Because eradication is unlikely, the aim of treatment for chronic infection is to quell exacerbations of inflammation. The regimens used are similar to those used for pneumonia, but an aminoglycoside is almost always added because resistance is common in chronic disease.

However, it may be appropriate to use an inhaled aminoglycoside preparation in order to maximize airway drug levels. MDR strains are now commonly found in such patients given their increased life span and the repeated courses of antibiotics they receive.

Endovascular Infections Infective endocarditis due to *P. aeruginosa* is a disease of IV drug users whose native valves are involved. This organism has also been reported to cause prosthetic-valve endocarditis. Sites of prior native-valve injury due to the injection of foreign material such as talc or fibers probably serve as niduses for bacterial attachment to the heart valve. The manifestations of *P. aeruginosa* endocarditis resemble those of other forms of endocarditis in IV drug users except that the disease is more indolent than *S. aureus* endocarditis. While most disease involves the right side of the heart, left-sided involvement is not rare, and multivalvular disease is common. Fever is a common manifestation, as is pulmonary involvement (due to septic emboli to the lungs). Thus, patients may also experience chest pain and hemoptysis. Involvement of the left side of the heart may lead to signs of cardiac failure, systemic emboli, and local cardiac involvement with sinus of Valsalva abscesses and conduction defects. Skin manifestations are rare in this disease, and ecthyma gangrenosum is not commonly seen in these patients. Vertebral **osteomyelitis** and sternoclavicular joint septic arthritis are uncommon but pathognomic complications of this disease. The diagnosis is based on positive blood cultures along with clinical signs of endocarditis.

TREATMENT
Endovascular Infections

(Table 164-2) It has been customary to use synergistic antibiotic combinations in treating *P. aeruginosa* endocarditis because of the development of resistance during therapy with a single antipseudomonal β-lactam agent. Which combination therapy is preferable is unclear, as all combinations have failed. Treatment is likely to more often be successful in cases of right-sided endocarditis. Cases of *P. aeruginosa* endocarditis that relapse during or fail to respond to therapy are often caused by resistant organisms and may require surgical therapy. Other considerations for valve replacement are similar to those in other forms of endocarditis (**Chap. 128**).

Bone and Joint Infections *P. aeruginosa* is an infrequent cause of bone and joint infections. However, *Pseudomonas* bacteremia or infective endocarditis caused by the injection of contaminated illicit drugs has been documented to result in vertebral osteomyelitis and sternoclavicular joint arthritis. The clinical presentation of vertebral *P. aeruginosa* osteomyelitis is more indolent than that of staphylococcal osteomyelitis. The duration of symptoms in IV drug users with vertebral osteomyelitis due to *P. aeruginosa* varies from weeks to months. Fever is not uniformly present; when present, it tends to be low grade. There may be mild tenderness at the site of involvement. Blood cultures are usually negative unless there is concomitant endocarditis. The erythrocyte sedimentation rate (ESR) is generally elevated. Vertebral osteomyelitis due to *P. aeruginosa* has also been reported in the elderly, in whom it originates from urinary tract infections (UTIs). The infection generally involves the lumbosacral area because of a shared venous drainage (Batson's plexus) between the lumbosacral spine and the pelvis. Sternoclavicular septic arthritis due to *P. aeruginosa* is seen almost exclusively in IV drug users. This disease may occur with or without endocarditis, and a primary site of infection often is not found. Plain radiographs show joint or bone involvement. Treatment of these forms of disease is generally successful.

Pseudomonas osteomyelitis of the foot most often follows puncture wounds through sneakers and mostly affects children. The main manifestation is pain in the foot, sometimes with superficial cellulitis around the puncture wound and tenderness on deep palpation of the wound. Multiple joints or bones of the foot may be involved. Systemic symptoms are generally absent, and blood cultures are usually negative. Radiographs may or may not be abnormal, but the bone scan is usually positive, as are MRI studies. Needle aspiration usually yields a diagnosis. Prompt surgery, with exploration of the nail puncture tract and debridement of the involved bones and cartilage, is generally recommended in addition to antibiotic therapy.

Osteomyelitis due to *P. aeruginosa* is also seen following trauma and with decubitus ulcers. In these settings, the cause of osteomyelitis is often polymicrobial, and the role of *P. aeruginosa* can be questioned. It is therefore critical that deep bone biopsies be requested to ascertain its significance.

TREATMENT
Bone and Joint Infections

The treatment of bone and joint infections due to *P. aeruginosa* is often governed by the primary *Pseudomonas* infection. Since endocarditis is often the primary infection, the agents used for endocarditis will dictate treatment. In other situations, a 6-week course of therapy with an antipseudomonal β-lactam is recommended, and in case of puncture-wound osteomyelitis, oral ciprofloxacin may be used.

Central Nervous System (CNS) Infections CNS infections due to *P. aeruginosa* are relatively rare. Involvement of the CNS is almost always secondary to a surgical procedure, head trauma, implanted devices, and rarely bacteremia. The entity seen most often is postoperative or posttraumatic meningitis. Subdural or epidural infection occasionally results from contamination of these areas. Embolic disease arising from endocarditis in IV drug users and leading to brain abscesses has also been described. The cerebrospinal fluid (CSF) profile of *P. aeruginosa* meningitis is no different from that of pyogenic meningitis of any other etiology.

TREATMENT
Central Nervous System Infections

(Table 164-2) Treatment of *Pseudomonas* meningitis is difficult; little information has been published. However, the general principles involved in the treatment of meningitis apply, including the need for high doses of bactericidal antibiotics to attain high drug levels in the CSF. The agent with which there is the most published experience in *P. aeruginosa* meningitis is ceftazidime, but other antipseudomonal β-lactam drugs that reach reasonable CSF concentrations, such as cefepime, piperacillin/tazobactam, and meropenem, have also been used successfully. Other forms of *P. aeruginosa* CNS infection, such as brain abscesses and epidural and subdural empyema, generally require surgical drainage in addition to antibiotic therapy.

Eye Infections Eye infections due to *P. aeruginosa* occur mainly as a result of direct inoculation into the tissue during trauma or surface injury by contact lenses. Keratitis and corneal ulcers are the most common types of eye disease and are often associated with contact lenses (especially the extended-wear variety). Keratitis can be slowly or rapidly progressive, but the classic description is disease progressing over 48 h to involve the entire cornea, with opacification and sometimes perforation. *P. aeruginosa* keratitis should be considered a medical emergency because of the rapidity with which it can progress to loss of sight. *P. aeruginosa* endophthalmitis secondary to bacteremia is the most devastating of *P. aeruginosa* eye infections. The disease is fulminant, with severe pain, chemosis, decreased visual acuity, anterior uveitis, vitreous involvement, and panophthalmitis. It is also a rare complication of cataract removal with lens insertion.

TREATMENT
Eye Infections

(Table 164-2) The usual therapy for keratitis is the administration of topical antibiotics. Therapy for endophthalmitis includes the use of high-dose local and systemic antibiotics (to achieve higher drug concentrations in the eye) and vitrectomy.

Ear Infections *P. aeruginosa* infections of the ears vary from mild swimmer's ear to serious life-threatening infections with neurologic sequelae. Swimmer's ear is common among children and results from infection of moist macerated skin of the external ear canal. Most cases resolve with treatment, but some patients develop chronic drainage. Swimmer's ear is managed with topical antibiotic agents (otic solutions). The use of hearing aids may also predispose to this type of infection. The most serious form of *Pseudomonas* infection involving the ear has been given various names: two of these designations, *malignant otitis externa* and *necrotizing otitis externa*, are now used for the same entity. This disease was originally described in elderly diabetic patients, in whom the majority of cases still occur. However, it has also been described in patients with AIDS and in elderly patients without underlying diabetes or immunocompromise. The usual presenting symptoms are decreased hearing and ear pain, which may be severe and lancinating. The pinna is usually painful, and the external canal may be tender. The ear canal almost always shows signs of inflammation, with granulation tissue and exudate. Tenderness anterior to the tragus may extend as far as the temporomandibular joint and mastoid process. A small minority of patients have systemic symptoms. Patients in whom the diagnosis is made late may present with cranial nerve palsies, most commonly cranial nerve VII or even with cavernous venous sinus thrombosis. The ESR is invariably elevated (≥100 mm/h). The diagnosis is made on clinical grounds in severe cases; however, the "gold standard" is a positive technetium-99 bone scan in a patient with otitis externa due to *P. aeruginosa*. In diabetic patients, a positive bone scan constitutes presumptive evidence for this diagnosis and should prompt biopsy or empirical therapy.

TREATMENT
Ear Infections

(Table 164-2) Given the infection of the ear cartilage, sometimes with mastoid or petrous ridge involvement, patients with malignant (necrotizing) otitis externa are treated as for osteomyelitis.

Urinary Tract Infections UTIs due to *P. aeruginosa* generally occur as a complication of a catheter in the urinary tract, an obstruction or stone in the genitourinary system, urinary tract instrumentation, or surgery. A *P. aeruginosa* UTI occurring in the community often signals the presence of an abnormality in the urinary tract. It has been reported that the urinary tract is the second most important site of infection leading to *Pseudomonas* bacteremia.

TREATMENT
Urinary Tract Infections

(Table 164-2) Most *P. aeruginosa* UTIs are considered complicated infections that must be treated longer than uncomplicated cystitis. In general, a 7- to 10-day course of treatment suffices, with 10–14 days of therapy in cases of pyelonephritis. Urinary catheters, stents, or stones should be removed to prevent relapse, which is common and may not be due to antibiotic resistance but rather to factors such as a foreign body that has been left in place or an ongoing obstruction. Removal of a urinary catheter will allow shorter courses of antibiotic therapy if that is the only predisposing factor.

Skin and Soft Tissue Infections Besides pyoderma (ecthyma) gangrenosum in neutropenic patients, folliculitis and other papular or vesicular lesions due to *P. aeruginosa* have been extensively described and are collectively referred to as *dermatitis*. Multiple outbreaks have been linked to whirlpools, spas, and swimming pools. To prevent such outbreaks, the growth of *P. aeruginosa* in the home and in recreational environments must be controlled by proper chlorination of water. Most cases of hot-tub folliculitis are self-limited, requiring only the avoidance of exposure to the contaminated source of water.

Toe-web infections occur especially often in the tropics, and the "green-nail syndrome" is caused by *P. aeruginosa* paronychia, which results from frequent submersion of the hands in water. In the latter entity, the green discoloration results from diffusion of pyocyanin into the nail bed. *P. aeruginosa* remains a prominent cause of burn wound infections in some parts of the world. The management of these infections is best left to specialists in burn wound care.

Infections in Febrile Neutropenic Patients In febrile neutropenia, *P. aeruginosa* has historically been the organism against which empirical coverage is always essential. Although in Western countries these infections are now less common, their importance has not diminished because of persistently high mortality rates. In other parts of the world, *P. aeruginosa* continues to be a significant problem in febrile neutropenia, causing a larger proportion of infections in febrile neutropenic patients than any other single organism. For example, *P. aeruginosa* was responsible for 28% of documented infections in 499 febrile neutropenic patients in one study from the Indian subcontinent and for 31% of such infections in another. In a large study of infections in leukemia patients from Japan, *P. aeruginosa* was the most frequently documented cause of bacterial infection. In studies performed in North America, northern Europe, and Australia, the incidence of *P. aeruginosa* bacteremia in febrile neutropenia was quite variable. In a review of 97 reports published between 1987 and 1994, the incidence was reported to be 1–2.5% among febrile neutropenic patients given empirical therapy and 5–12% among patients with microbiologically documented infections. The most common clinical syndromes encountered were bacteremia, pneumonia, and soft tissue infections manifesting mainly as ecthyma gangrenosum.

TREATMENT
Infections in Febrile Neutropenic Patients

(Table 164-2) Compared with rates three decades ago, improved rates of response to antibiotic therapy have been reported in many studies. A study of 127 patients demonstrated a reduction in the mortality rate from 71 to 25% with the introduction of ceftazidime and imipenem. Because neutrophils—the normal host defenses against this organism—are absent in febrile neutropenic patients, maximal doses of antipseudomonal β-lactam antibiotics should be used for the management of *P. aeruginosa* bacteremia in this setting.

Infections in Patients with AIDS *P. aeruginosa* infections were well documented in patients with AIDS before the advent of antiretroviral therapy. Since the introduction of protease inhibitors, *P. aeruginosa* infections in AIDS patients have been seen less frequently but still occur, particularly in the form of sinusitis. While this entity is now uncommon in developed nations, there are still large numbers of patients with untreated HIV infection or poorly controlled disease in developing nations who are likely to suffer from *P. aeruginosa* infections. The clinical presentation of *Pseudomonas* infection (especially pneumonia and bacteremia) in AIDS patients is remarkable in that, although the illness may appear not to be severe, the infection may nonetheless be fatal. Patients with bacteremia may have only a low-grade fever and may present with ecthyma gangrenosum. Pneumonia, with or without bacteremia, is perhaps the most common type of *P. aeruginosa* infection. Patients with *P. aeruginosa* pneumonia exhibit the classic clinical signs and symptoms of pneumonia, such as fever, productive cough, and chest pain. The infection may be lobar or multilobar and shows no predisposition for any particular location. The most striking feature is the high frequency of cavitary disease.

TREATMENT
Infections in Patients with AIDS

Therapy for any of these conditions in AIDS patients is no different from that in other patients. However, relapse is the rule unless the patient's CD4+ T-cell count rises to >50/μL or suppressive antibiotic therapy is given. In attempts to achieve cures and prevent relapses, therapy tends to be more prolonged than in the case of an immunocompetent patient.

Gastrointestinal Infections A poorly understood syndrome caused by *P. aeruginosa* has been described in the Far East and has been called *Shanghai fever* and *Pseudomonas enterocolitis*. This syndrome occurs in young children; its occurrence in adults appears to be rare. Shanghai fever manifests as severe enteric disease, sepsis with invasive disease, and complications, whereas *Pseudomonas* enterocolitis is characterized by prolonged fever with bloody or mucoid diarrhea mimicking bacterial enterocolitis. The mortality rate ranges between 23 and 89%, with ecthyma gangrenosum occurring in >50% of cases. Early recognition and treatment have led to a reduction in the mortality rate. There is an above-average occurrence of the *exoU* gene among *Pseudomonas* isolates from patients with this syndrome.

Multidrug-Resistant Infections (Table 164-2) *P. aeruginosa* has a notorious propensity to develop antibiotic resistance. Over three decades, the impact of resistance was minimized by the rapid development of several potent antipseudomonal β-lactams and fluoroquinolones. However, rates of resistance to these agents that revolutionized the treatment of *P. aeruginosa* have risen to the point where some are almost unusable empirically because of the worldwide emergence of strains carrying determinants that mediate resistance. Extremely high rates of MDR strains have been reported from Eastern and Southern Europe, Latin America, India, and China, especially in ICUs. Physicians have had to resort to drugs such as colistin and polymyxin B, which were discarded decades ago. This surge in resistance is mediated by multiple mechanisms sometimes converging in individual strains. Chief among these are chromosomal or plasmid-borne penicillinases, extended-spectrum β-lactamases, cephalosporinases, and carbapenemases. Any of these may be combined with permeability mutations and efflux pump overexpression. The greatest nemesis in this regard is the worldwide presence of carbapenemases in *P. aeruginosa* leading to resistance to most β-lactams except some of the newest agents recently developed. These new agents are generally combinations of a cephalosporin or a carbapenem most often with a novel β-lactamase inhibitor. Several have been approved for clinical use, and all are active against MDR *P. aeruginosa* to varying degrees. Currently approved agents include ceftolozane/tazobactam, ceftazidime/avibactam, meropenem/vaborbactam, and imipenem/relebactam. A novel cephalosporin, cefiderocol, which uses the iron uptake pathway of *P. aeruginosa*, also demonstrates activity against MDR strains. Since MDR and XDR *P. aeruginosa* are unpredictable in regard to the underlying mechanisms of resistance, laboratory testing is absolutely required before the use of any of these agents. Most academic institutions restrict the use of these agents as there are concerns about the development of resistance, as has already been noted, as well the cost implications of misuse.

BURKHOLDERIA SPECIES

BURKHOLDERIA CEPACIA COMPLEX

The *B. cepacia* complex (BCC) gained notoriety as the cause of a rapidly fatal syndrome of respiratory distress and septicemia (the "cepacia syndrome") in CF patients. Of the more than 20 species of this complex, the three most frequently seen in CF patients are *B. cenocepacia*, *B. multivorans*, and *B. stabilis*. In addition to their occurrence in CF, members of this complex were not uncommonly encountered in ICU patients (previously designated *Pseudomonas cepacia*) and patients with chronic granulomatous disease, in whom they caused lung disease. BCC organisms are environmental organisms that inhabit moist environments and are found in the rhizosphere. They possess multiple virulence factors that may play roles in disease as well as colonizing factors that are capable of binding to lung mucus—an ability that may explain the predilection of *B. cepacia* for the lungs in CF. *B. cenocepacia* is motile, secretes elastase, and possesses components of an injectable toxin-secretion system like that of *P. aeruginosa*; its LPS is among the most potent of all LPSs in stimulating an inflammatory response in the lungs. Inflammation may be the major cause of the lung disease seen in the "cepacia" syndrome. Besides infecting the lungs in CF, the BCC organisms appear as airway colonizers during broad-spectrum antibiotic therapy and are causes of VAP, catheter-associated infections, and wound infections.

TREATMENT

B. cepacia Complex Infections

BCC organisms are intrinsically resistant to many antibiotics, rendering empiric treatment difficult. Therefore, treatment must be tailored according to sensitivities. Trimethoprim-sulfamethoxazole (TMP-SMX), meropenem, and minocycline are the most active agents in vitro and may be started as first-line agents (Table 164-2). However, recent reports indicate that there has been increasing resistance to these agents especially in CF patients. Some strains are susceptible to third-generation ureidopenicillins, advanced cephalosporins, and fluoroquinolones, and these agents may be used against isolates known to be susceptible. Newer antibiotics such as ceftolozane/tazobactam and ceftazidime/avibactam show good activity against MDR strains in vitro. However, there is very limited clinical experience with these agents.

BURKHOLDERIA PSEUDOMALLEI

B. pseudomallei is the causative agent of melioidosis, a disease of humans and animals that is geographically restricted to Southeast Asia and northern Australia, with occasional cases in countries such as India and China. This organism may be isolated from individuals returning directly from these endemic regions and from military personnel who have served in endemic regions. Symptoms of this illness may develop only at a later date because of the organism's ability to cause latent infections, which has been attributed to its ability to survive within cells. *B. pseudomallei* is found in soil and water. Humans and animals are infected by inoculation, inhalation, or ingestion; only rarely is the organism transmitted from person to person. Humans are not colonized without being infected. Among the pseudomonads, *B. pseudomallei* is perhaps the most virulent. Host compromise is not an essential prerequisite for disease, although many patients have common underlying medical diseases (e.g., diabetes renal failure or alcohol abuse). *B. pseudomallei* is a facultative intracellular organism whose replication in PMNs and macrophages may be aided by the possession of a polysaccharide capsule. The organism also possesses elements of a type III secretion system that plays a role in its intracellular survival. During infection, there is a florid inflammatory response whose role in disease is unclear.

B. pseudomallei causes a wide spectrum of conditions, ranging from asymptomatic infection to abscesses, pneumonia, and disseminated disease. It is a significant cause of fatal community-acquired pneumonia and septicemia in endemic areas, with mortality rates as high as 44% reported in Thailand. Acute pulmonary infection is the most commonly diagnosed form of melioidosis. Pneumonia may be asymptomatic (with routine chest radiographs showing mainly upper-lobe infiltrates) or may present as severe necrotizing disease. *B. pseudomallei* also causes chronic pulmonary infections with systemic manifestations that mimic those of tuberculosis, including chronic cough, fever, hemoptysis, night sweats, and cavitary lung disease. Besides pneumonia, the other principal form of *B. pseudomallei* disease is skin ulceration with associated lymphangitis and regional lymphadenopathy. Spread from the lungs or skin, which is most often documented in debilitated individuals, gives rise to septicemic forms of melioidosis that carry a high mortality rate.

TREATMENT

B. pseudomallei Infections

B. pseudomallei is susceptible to advanced penicillins, cephalosporins, and carbapenems (Table 164-2). Treatment is divided into two stages: an intensive 2-week phase of therapy with ceftazidime or a carbapenem followed by at least 12 weeks of oral TMP-SMX to eradicate the organism and prevent relapse. Australian guidelines for treating this condition recommend longer periods of intensive therapy—4–8 weeks for severe infections, osteomyelitis, and CNS infections. The recognition of this bacterium as a potential agent of biologic warfare has stimulated interest in the development of a vaccine.

BURKHOLDERIA MALLEI

B. mallei causes the equine disease glanders in Africa, Asia, and South America. The organism was eradicated from Europe and North America decades ago. The last case seen in the United States occurred in 2001 in a laboratory worker; before that, *B. mallei* had last been seen in this country in 1949. In contrast to the other organisms discussed in this chapter, *B. mallei* is not an environmental organism and does not persist outside its equine hosts. Consequently, *B. mallei* infection is an occupational risk for handlers of horses, equine butchers, and veterinarians in areas of the world where it still exists. The polysaccharide capsule is a critical virulence determinant; diabetics are thought to be especially susceptible to infection by this organism. The organism is transmitted from animals to humans by inoculation into the skin, where it causes local infection with nodules and lymphadenitis. Regional lymphadenopathy is common. Respiratory secretions from infected horses are extremely infectious. Inhalation results in clinical signs of typical pneumonia but may also cause an acute febrile illness with ulceration of the trachea. The organism may disseminate from the skin or lungs to cause septicemia with signs of sepsis. The septicemic form is frequently associated with shock and a high mortality rate. The infection may also enter a chronic phase and present as disseminated abscesses. *B. mallei* infection may present as early as 1–2 days after inhalation or (in cutaneous disease) may not become evident for months.

TREATMENT

B. mallei Infections

The antibiotic susceptibility pattern of *B. mallei* is similar to that of *B. pseudomallei*; in addition, the organism is susceptible to the macrolides azithromycin and clarithromycin. *B. mallei* infection should be treated with the same drugs and for the same duration as melioidosis.

STENOTROPHOMONAS MALTOPHILIA

S. maltophilia is the only potential human pathogen among a genus of ubiquitous organisms found in the rhizosphere (i.e., the soil that surrounds the roots of plants). The organism is an opportunist that is acquired from the environment but is even more limited than *P. aeruginosa* in its ability to colonize patients or cause infections. Immunocompromise is not sufficient to permit these events; rather, major perturbations of the human flora are usually necessary for the establishment of *S. maltophilia*. Accordingly, most cases of human infection occur in the setting of very broad-spectrum antibiotic therapy with agents such as advanced cephalosporins and carbapenems, which eradicate the normal flora and other pathogens. The remarkable ability of *S. maltophilia* to resist virtually all classes of antibiotics is attributable to the possession of antibiotic efflux pumps and of two β-lactamases (L1 and L2) that mediate β-lactam resistance, including that to carbapenems. It is fortunate that the virulence of *S. maltophilia* appears to be limited. Although a serine protease is present in some strains, virulence is probably a result of the host's inflammatory response to components of the organism such as LPS and flagellin. *S. maltophilia* is most commonly found in the respiratory tract of ventilated patients, where the distinction between its roles as a colonizer and as a pathogen is often difficult to make. However, *S. maltophilia* does cause pneumonia and bacteremia in such patients, and these infections have led to septic shock. Also common is central venous line–associated infection (with or without bacteremia), which has been reported most often in patients with cancer. *S. maltophilia* is a rare cause of ecthyma gangrenosum in neutropenic patients. It has been isolated from ~5% of CF patients but is not believed to be a significant pathogen in this setting.

TREATMENT

S. maltophilia Infections

The intrinsic resistance of *S. maltophilia* to most antibiotics renders infection difficult to treat. The antibiotics to which it is most often (although not uniformly) susceptible are TMP-SMX, ticarcillin/clavulanate, levofloxacin, and tigecycline (Table 164-2). Consequently, a combination of TMP-SMX and ticarcillin/clavulanate is recommended for initial therapy pending susceptibility testing. Catheters must be removed in the treatment of bacteremia. The treatment of VAP due to *S. maltophilia* is much more difficult than that of bacteremia, with frequent development of resistance during therapy. The newest β-lactam/β-lactamase inhibitor combinations show mixed results against this organism.

FURTHER READING

Bauer KA et al: Extended-infusion cefepime reduces mortality in patients with *Pseudomonas aeruginosa* infections. Antimicrob Agents Chemother 57:2907, 2013.

Bowers DR et al: Outcomes of appropriate empiric combination versus monotherapy for *Pseudomonas aeruginosa* bacteremia. Antimicrob Agents Chemother 157:1270, 2013.

Brooke JS: *Stenotrophomonas maltophilia*: An emerging global opportunistic pathogen. Clin Microbiol Rev 25:2, 2012.

Cattaneo C et al: *P. aeruginosa* bloodstream infections among hematological patients: An old or new question? Ann Hematol 91:1299, 2012.

Chuang C-H et al: Shanghai fever: A distinct *Pseudomonas aeruginosa* enteric disease. Gut 63:736, 2014.

Fabre V et al: Antibiotic therapy for *Pseudomonas aeruginosa* bloodstream infections: How long is long enough? Clin Infect Dis 69:2011, 2019.

Horcajada JP et al: Epidemiology and treatment of multidrug-resistant and extensively drug-resistant *Pseudomonas aeruginosa* infections. Clin Microbiol Rev 32:e00031, 2019.

Kalil AC et al: Executive summary: Management of adults with hospital-acquired and ventilator-associated pneumonia: 2016 clinical practice guidelines by the Infectious Diseases Society of America and the American Thoracic Society. Clin Infect Dis 63:575, 2016.

Peña C et al: Influence of virulence genotype and resistance profile in the mortality of *Pseudomonas aeruginosa* bloodstream infections. Clin Infect Dis 60:539, 2015.

Van Zandt KE et al: Glanders: An overview of infections in humans. Orphanet J Rare Dis 8:131, 2013.

Wunderlink RG et al: Cefiderocol versus high-dose, extended-infusion meropenem for the treatment of Gram-negative nosocomial pneumonia (APEKS-NP): A randomized, double-blind, phase 3, non-inferiority trial. Lancet Infect Dis 21:213, 2021.

165 Salmonellosis

David A. Pegues, Samuel I. Miller

Bacteria of the genus *Salmonella* are highly adapted for growth in both humans and animals and cause a wide spectrum of disease. The growth of serotypes *Salmonella* Typhi and *Salmonella* Paratyphi is restricted to human hosts, in whom these organisms cause enteric (typhoid) fever. The remaining serotypes (nontyphoidal *Salmonella*, or NTS) can colonize the gastrointestinal tracts of a broad range of animals, including mammals, reptiles, birds, and insects. More than 200 serotypes of *Salmonella* are pathogenic to humans, in whom they often cause gastroenteritis and can be associated with localized infections and/or bacteremia.

ETIOLOGY

This large genus of gram-negative bacilli within the family Enterobacteriaceae consists of two species: *Salmonella enterica*, which contains six subspecies, and *Salmonella bongori*. *S. enterica* subspecies I includes almost all the serotypes pathogenic for humans. Members of the seven

Salmonella subspecies are classified into >2500 serotypes (serovars); for simplicity, *Salmonella* serotypes (most of which are named for the city where they were identified) are often used as the species designation. For example, the full taxonomic designation *S. enterica* subspecies *enterica* serotype Typhimurium can be shortened to *Salmonella* serotype Typhimurium or simply *S.* Typhimurium. Serotyping is based on antigenically diverse surface structures: the somatic O antigen (lipopolysaccharide cell-wall components), the surface Vi antigen (restricted to *S.* Typhi and *S.* Paratyphi C), and the flagellar H antigen.

Salmonellae are gram-negative, non-spore-forming, facultatively anaerobic bacilli that measure 2–3 μm by 0.4–0.6 μm. The initial identification of salmonellae in the clinical microbiology laboratory is based on growth characteristics. Salmonellae, like other Enterobacteriaceae, produce acid on glucose fermentation, reduce nitrates, and do not produce cytochrome oxidase. In addition, all salmonellae except *Salmonella* Gallinarum-Pullorum are motile by means of peritrichous flagella, and all but *S.* Typhi produce gas (H_2S) on sugar fermentation. Notably, only 1% of clinical isolates ferment lactose; a high level of suspicion must be maintained to detect these rare clinical lactose-fermenting isolates.

Although serotyping of all surface antigens can be used for formal identification, most laboratories perform a few simple agglutination reactions that define specific O-antigen serogroups, designated A, B, C_1, C_2, D, and E. Strains in these six serogroups cause ~99% of *Salmonella* infections in humans and other warm-blooded animals. Molecular typing methods, including pulsed-field gel electrophoresis, multiple-locus variable-number tandem repeat analysis, and whole-genome sequencing, are used in epidemiologic investigations to differentiate *Salmonella* strains of a common serotype.

PATHOGENESIS

All *Salmonella* infections begin with ingestion of organisms, most commonly in contaminated food or water. The infectious dose ranges from 200 colony-forming units (CFU) to 10^6 CFU, and the ingested dose is an important determinant of incubation period and disease severity. Conditions that decrease either stomach acidity (an age of <1 year, acid suppression therapy, or achlorhydric disease) or intestinal integrity (inflammatory bowel disease, cytotoxic chemotherapy, prior gastrointestinal surgery, or alteration of the intestinal microbiome by antibiotic administration) increase susceptibility to *Salmonella* infection.

Once *S.* Typhi and *S.* Paratyphi reach the small intestine, they penetrate the mucus layer of the gut and traverse the intestinal layer through phagocytic microfold (M) cells that reside within Peyer's patches. Salmonellae can trigger the formation of membrane ruffles in normally nonphagocytic epithelial cells. These ruffles reach out and enclose adherent bacteria within large vesicles by *bacterium-mediated endocytosis*. This process is dependent on the direct delivery of *Salmonella* proteins into the cytoplasm of epithelial cells by the specialized bacterial type III secretion system. These bacterial proteins mediate alterations in the actin cytoskeleton that are required for *Salmonella* uptake.

After crossing the epithelial layer of the small intestine, *S.* Typhi and *S.* Paratyphi, which cause enteric (typhoid) fever, are phagocytosed by macrophages. These salmonellae survive the antimicrobial environment of the macrophage by sensing environmental signals that trigger alterations in regulatory systems of the phagocytosed bacteria. For example, PhoP/PhoQ (the best-characterized regulatory system) triggers the alteration of the outer membrane by increasing the synthesis and transport of different outer-membrane proteins, lipopolysaccharides, and glycerophospholipids, so that the altered bacterial surface can resist microbicidal activities and potentially alter host cell signaling. In addition, salmonellae encode a second type III secretion system that directly delivers bacterial proteins across the phagosome membrane into the macrophage cytoplasm. This secretion system functions to remodel the *Salmonella*-containing vacuole, promoting bacterial survival and replication.

Once phagocytosed, typhoidal salmonellae disseminate throughout the body in macrophages via the lymphatics and colonize reticuloendothelial tissues (liver, spleen, lymph nodes, and bone marrow). Patients have relatively few or no signs and symptoms during this initial incubation stage. Signs and symptoms, including fever and abdominal pain, probably result from secretion of cytokines by macrophages and epithelial cells in response to bacterial products that are recognized by innate immune receptors when a critical number of organisms have replicated. Over time, the development of hepatosplenomegaly is likely to be related to the recruitment of mononuclear cells and the development of a specific acquired cell-mediated immune response to *S.* Typhi colonization. The recruitment of additional mononuclear cells and lymphocytes to Peyer's patches during the several weeks after initial colonization/infection can result in marked enlargement and necrosis of the Peyer's patches, which may be mediated by bacterial products that promote cell death as well as the inflammatory response. In the case of *S.* Typhi, many strains produce a toxin, which probably contributes to systemic symptoms as well as the unusual neuropsychiatric states that can be seen in severe typhoidal illness.

In contrast to enteric fever, which is characterized by an infiltration of mononuclear cells into the small-bowel mucosa, NTS gastroenteritis is characterized by massive polymorphonuclear leukocyte infiltration into both the large- and small-bowel mucosa. This response appears to depend on the induction of interleukin 8, a strong neutrophil chemotactic factor, which is secreted by intestinal cells as a result of nontyphoidal *Salmonella* colonization and translocation of bacterial proteins into host cell cytoplasm. The degranulation and release of toxic substances by neutrophils may result in damage to the intestinal mucosa, causing the inflammatory diarrhea observed with nontyphoidal gastroenteritis. An additional important factor in the persistence of NTS in the intestinal tract and the organism's capacity to compete with endogenous flora is the ability to utilize the sulfur-containing compound tetrathionate for metabolism in a microaerophilic environment. In the presence of intestinal inflammation, tetrathionate is generated from thiosulfate produced by epithelial cells through inflammatory cell production of reactive oxygen species.

ENTERIC (TYPHOID) FEVER

Enteric (typhoid) fever is a systemic disease characterized by fever and abdominal pain and caused by dissemination of *S.* Typhi or *S.* Paratyphi. The disease was initially called *typhoid fever* because of its clinical similarity to typhus. In the early 1800s, typhoid fever was clearly defined pathologically as a unique illness on the basis of its association with enlarged Peyer's patches and mesenteric lymph nodes. In 1869, given the anatomic site of infection, the term *enteric fever* was proposed as an alternative designation to distinguish typhoid fever from typhus. However, to this day, the two designations are used interchangeably.

EPIDEMIOLOGY

In contrast to other *Salmonella* serotypes, the etiologic agents of enteric fever—*S.* Typhi and *S.* Paratyphi serotypes A, B, and C—have no known hosts other than humans. Most commonly, food-borne or waterborne transmission results from fecal contamination by ill or asymptomatic chronic carriers. Sexual transmission between male partners has been described. Health care workers occasionally acquire enteric fever after exposure to infected patients or during processing of clinical specimens and cultures.

With improvements in food handling and water/sewage treatment, enteric fever has become rare in developed nations. In 2017, worldwide there were an estimated 14.3 million cases of enteric fever with 136,000 deaths. The annual incidence is highest (>100 cases/100,000 population) in South Central and Southeast Asia; medium (10–100 cases/100,000) in the rest of Asia, Africa, Latin America, and Oceania (excluding Australia and New Zealand); and low in other parts of the world (**Fig. 165-1**). A high incidence of enteric fever correlates with mixing of drinking water with human sewage. In endemic regions, enteric fever is more common in poor neighborhoods in large cities than rural areas and among young children and adolescents than among other age groups. Risk factors include fecally contaminated drinking water or ice, flooding, food and drinks purchased from street vendors, raw fruits and vegetables grown in fields fertilized with sewage, ill household contacts, lack of hand washing and toilet access, and evidence of prior *Helicobacter pylori* infection (an association probably

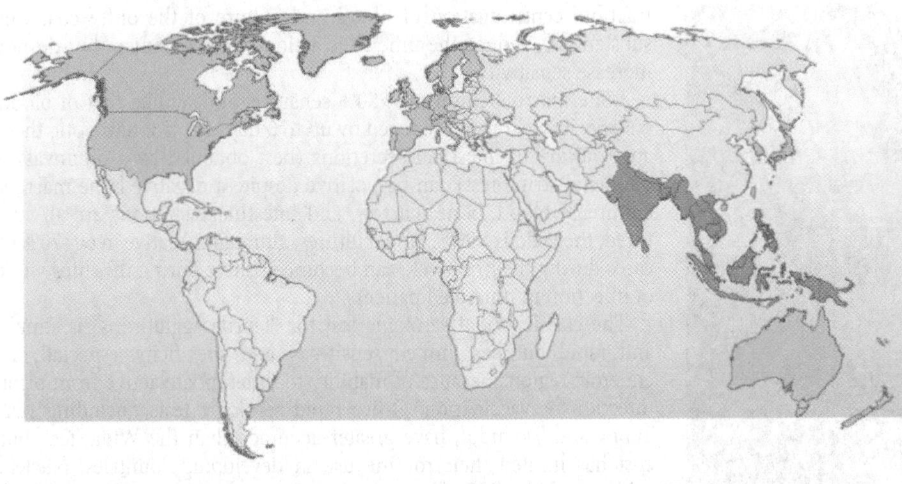

FIGURE 165-1 Annual incidence of typhoid fever per 100,000 population. *(Reproduced with permission from JA Crump: The global burden of typhoid fever. Bull World Health Organ 82:346, 2004.)*

related to chronically reduced gastric acidity). It is estimated that there is one case of paratyphoid fever for every four cases of typhoid fever, but the incidence of infection associated with S. Paratyphi A appears to be increasing, especially in India; this increase may be a result of vaccination for S. Typhi.

Multidrug-resistant (MDR) strains of S. Typhi emerged in the 1980s in China and Southeast Asia and have since disseminated widely. These strains contain plasmids encoding resistance to chloramphenicol, ampicillin, and trimethoprim—antibiotics long used to treat enteric fever. With the increased use of fluoroquinolones to treat MDR enteric fever in the 1990s, MDR strains of S. Typhi and S. Paratyphi with decreased susceptibility to ciprofloxacin (DSC; minimal inhibitory concentration [MIC], ≥0.125 μg/mL) or ciprofloxacin resistance (MIC, ≥1 μg/mL) emerged on the Indian subcontinent and have spread with human migration first to southern Asia and more recently to Eastern and Southern Africa. These strains represent clone H58, which increasingly has been associated with clinical treatment failure of fluoroquinolones. Testing of isolates for resistance to the first-generation quinolone nalidixic acid detects many but not all strains with reduced susceptibility to ciprofloxacin and is no longer recommended. Since 2017, a large outbreak of plasmid-mediated ceftriaxone-resistant S. Typhi H58 has been ongoing, centered in urban slums in Pakistan. The outbreak predominantly has affected children aged 15 and younger and is associated with fecally contaminated drinking water.

In 2015, there were 309 cases of typhoid fever and 71 cases of paratyphoid fever reported in the United States. Median age of patients with typhoid fever was 23 years and paratyphoid fever 29 years. Most cases of enteric fever were associated with international travel (78%), predominantly to Indian, Pakistan, and Bangladesh, and visiting friends and family. Only 3% of travelers diagnosed with typhoid fever had received S. Typhi vaccine within the previous 5 years. In 2015, 66% of S. Typhi in the United States were DSC, and ~10% were resistant to ampicillin, chloramphenicol, and trimethoprim-sulfamethoxazole (TMP-SMX). Infection with DSC S. Typhi was associated with travel to the Indian subcontinent. In the United States, domestically acquired cases of enteric fever are less often DSC or MDR compared to travel-associated cases and are most often sporadic, although outbreaks linked to contaminated food products and previously unrecognized chronic carriers continue to occur.

■ CLINICAL COURSE

Enteric fever is a misnomer, in that the hallmark features of this disease—fever and abdominal pain—are variable. While fever is documented at presentation in >75% of cases, abdominal pain is reported in only 30–40%. Thus, a high index of suspicion for this potentially fatal systemic illness is necessary when a person presents with fever and a history of recent travel to a developing country.

The mean incubation period for S. Typhi is 10–14 days but ranges from 5 to 21 days, depending on the inoculum size and the host's health and vaccination status. The most prominent symptom is prolonged fever (38.8°–40.5°C [101.8°–104.9°F]), which can continue for up to 4 weeks if untreated. S. Paratyphi A is thought to cause milder disease than S. Typhi, with predominantly gastrointestinal symptoms. However, a prospective study of 669 consecutive cases of enteric fever in Kathmandu, Nepal, found that the infections caused by these organisms were clinically indistinguishable. In this series, symptoms reported on initial medical evaluation included headache (80%), chills (35–45%), cough (30%), sweating (20–25%), myalgias (20%), malaise (10%), and arthralgia (2–4%). Gastrointestinal manifestations included anorexia (55%), abdominal pain (30–40%), nausea (18–24%), vomiting (18%), and diarrhea (22–28%) more commonly than constipation (13–16%). Physical findings included coated tongue (51–56%), splenomegaly (5–6%), and abdominal tenderness (4–5%).

Early physical findings of enteric fever include rash ("rose spots"; 30%), hepatosplenomegaly (3–6%), epistaxis, and relative bradycardia at the peak of high fever (<50%). Rose spots **(Fig. 165-2; see also Fig. A1-9)** make up a faint, salmon-colored, blanching, maculopapular rash located primarily on the trunk and chest. The rash is evident in ~30% of patients at the end of the first week and resolves without a trace after 2–5 days. Patients can have two or three crops of lesions, and *Salmonella* can be cultured from punch biopsies of these lesions. The faintness of the rash makes it difficult to detect in highly pigmented patients.

Complications of typhoid fever are estimated to occur in ~27% of hospitalized patients and correlate with a longer duration of symptoms before hospitalization, host factors (host genetics, immunosuppression, acid suppression therapy, previous exposure, and vaccination status), strain virulence and inoculum, and choice of antibiotic therapy. Gastrointestinal bleeding (6%) and intestinal perforation (1%) most commonly occur in the third and fourth weeks of illness and result from hyperplasia, ulceration, and necrosis of the ileocecal Peyer's patches at the initial site of *Salmonella* infiltration **(Fig. 165-3)**. Both complications are life-threatening and require immediate fluid resuscitation and surgical intervention, with broadened antibiotic coverage for polymicrobial peritonitis **(Chap. 132)** and treatment of gastrointestinal hemorrhages, including bowel resection. Neurologic manifestations

FIGURE 165-2 "Rose spots," the rash of enteric fever due to *Salmonella* Typhi or *Salmonella* Paratyphi.

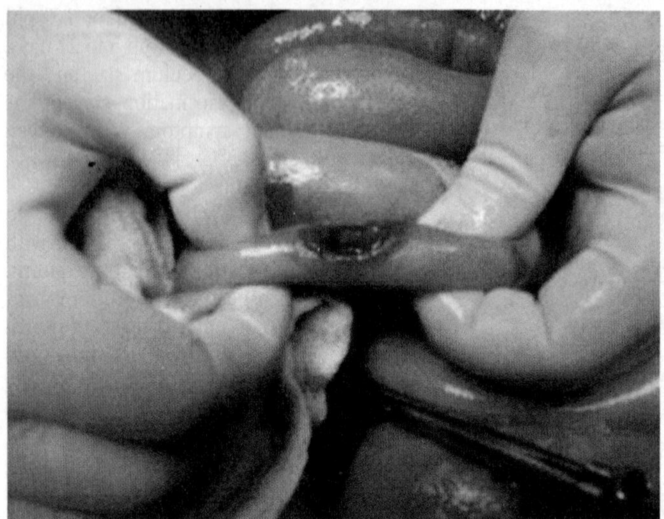

FIGURE 165-3 Typical ileal perforation associated with *Salmonella* Typhi infection. *(From JM Saxe, R Cropsey: Is operative management effective in treatment of perforated typhoid? Am J Surg 189:342, 2005.)*

occur in 2–40% of patients and include meningitis, Guillain-Barré syndrome, neuritis, and neuropsychiatric symptoms (described as "muttering delirium" or "coma vigil"), with picking at bedclothes or imaginary objects.

Uncommon complications whose incidences are reduced by prompt antibiotic treatment include disseminated intravascular coagulation, hematophagocytic syndrome, pancreatitis, hepatic and splenic abscesses and granulomas, endocarditis, pericarditis, myocarditis, orchitis, hepatitis, glomerulonephritis, pyelonephritis and hemolytic-uremic syndrome, severe pneumonia, arthritis, osteomyelitis, endophthalmitis, and parotitis. Up to 10% of patients develop mild relapse, usually within 2–3 weeks of fever resolution and in association with the same strain type and susceptibility profile.

Up to 10% of untreated patients with typhoid fever excrete *S.* Typhi in the feces for up to 3 months, and 2–5% develop chronic asymptomatic carriage, shedding *S.* Typhi in either urine or stool for >1 year. Chronic carriage is more common among women, infants, and persons who have biliary abnormalities or concurrent bladder infection with *Schistosoma haematobium*. *S.* Typhi and other salmonellae are adapted to survive in the gallbladder environment by forming biofilms on gallstones and invading gallbladder epithelial cells. Chronic carriage is associated with an increased risk of gallbladder cancer, which is much more common in locales where *S.* Typhi is common, such as the Indian subcontinent.

DIAGNOSIS

Because the clinical presentation of enteric fever is relatively nonspecific, the diagnosis needs to be considered in any febrile traveler returning from a developing region, especially the Indian subcontinent, the Philippines, or Latin America. Other diagnoses that should be considered in these travelers include malaria, hepatitis, bacterial enteritis, dengue fever, rickettsial infections, leptospirosis, amebic liver abscesses, and acute HIV infection (**Chap. 124**). Other than a positive culture, no specific laboratory test is diagnostic for enteric fever. In 15–25% of cases, leukopenia and neutropenia are detectable. Leukocytosis is more common among children, during the first 10 days of illness, and in cases complicated by intestinal perforation or secondary infection. Other nonspecific laboratory findings include moderately elevated values in liver function tests and muscle enzyme levels.

The definitive diagnosis of enteric fever requires the isolation of *S.* Typhi or *S.* Paratyphi from blood, bone marrow, other sterile sites, rose spots, stool, or intestinal secretions. The diagnostic sensitivity of blood culture is only ~60% and is lower with low blood sample volume and among patients with prior antimicrobial use or in the first week of illness, reflecting the small number of *S.* Typhi organisms (i.e., <15/mL) typically present in the blood. Because almost all *S.* Typhi organisms in blood are associated with the mononuclear cell/platelet fraction, centrifugation of blood and culture of the buffy coat can substantially reduce the time to isolation of the organism but do not increase sensitivity.

Bone marrow culture is >80% sensitive, and, unlike that of blood culture, its yield is not reduced by up to 5 days of prior antibiotic therapy. Culture of intestinal secretions (best obtained by a noninvasive duodenal string test) can be positive despite a negative bone marrow culture. If blood, bone marrow, and intestinal secretions are all cultured, the yield is >90%. Stool cultures, although negative in 60–70% of cases during the first week, can become positive during the third week of infection in untreated patients.

The classic Widal serologic test for "febrile agglutinins" is simple and rapid but has limited sensitivity and specificity, especially in endemic regions because of inability to differentiate active from prior infection or vaccination. Other rapid serologic tests, including IDL Tubex and Typhidot, have greater accuracy than the Widal test, but cost has limited their routine use in developing countries. Nucleic acid–based identification methods are not yet commercially available.

TREATMENT

Enteric (Typhoid) Fever

Enteric fever is associated with an overall case-fatality rate of 2.5%, and it rises to 4.5% among hospitalized patients. Prompt administration of appropriate antibiotic therapy prevents severe complications of enteric fever and reduces mortality to <1%. The initial choice of antibiotics depends on the susceptibility of the *S.* Typhi and *S.* Paratyphi strains in the area of residence or travel (**Table 165-1**). For treatment of drug-susceptible typhoid fever,

TABLE 165-1 Antibiotic Therapy for Enteric Fever in Adults

INDICATION	AGENT	DOSAGE (ROUTE)	DURATION, DAYS
Empirical Treatment			
	Ceftriaxone[a]	2 g/d (IV)	10–14
	Azithromycin[b]	1 g/d (PO)	5
Fully Susceptible			
Optimal treatment	Ciprofloxacin[c]	500 mg bid (PO) or 400 mg q12h (IV)	5–7
	Azithromycin	1 g/d (PO)	5
Alternative treatment	Amoxicillin	1 g tid (PO) or 2 g q6h (IV)	14
	Chloramphenicol	25 mg/kg tid (PO or IV)	14–21
	Trimethoprim-sulfamethoxazole	160/800 mg bid (PO)	7–14
Multidrug-Resistant, Fluoroquinolone-Susceptible			
Optimal treatment	Ceftriaxone[a]	2 g/d (IV)	10–14
	Azithromycin	1 g/d (PO)	5
Alternative treatment	Ciprofloxacin	500 mg bid (PO) or 400 mg q12h (IV)	5–14
Fluroquinolone-Resistant			
Optimal treatment	Ceftriaxone	2 g/d (IV)	10–14
	Azithromycin	1 g/d (PO)	5
Ceftriaxone-Resistant			
Optimal treatment	Meropenem[d]	1 g q8h (IV)	10–14
	Azithromycin	1 g/d (PO)	5
Eradication of Carriage			
Optimal treatment	Ciprofloxacin	500–750 mg bid (PO)	28
Alternative treatment	Amoxicillin[e]	2 g tid (PO)	28–42

[a]Or another third-generation cephalosporin (e.g., cefotaxime, 2 g q8h IV; or cefixime, 400 mg bid PO). [b]Or 1 g on day 1 followed by 500 mg/d PO for 6 days. [c]Or ofloxacin, 400 mg bid PO for 2–5 days. [d]Or imipenem 500 mg q6h IV. [e]If fluroquinolone resistant and ampicillin susceptible.

fluoroquinolones are the most effective class of agents, with cure rates of ~98% and relapse and fecal carriage rates of <2%. Experience is most extensive with ciprofloxacin. Short-course ofloxacin therapy is similarly successful against infection caused by quinolone-susceptible strains. However, because of the high prevalence of strains of S. Typhi and S. Paratyphi with decreased susceptibility to ciprofloxacin (MIC >0.125 μg/mL) on the Indian subcontinent, in Nepal, and in some locales in Africa, fluoroquinolones should no longer be used for empirical treatment of enteric fever in these regions. Patients infected with DSC strains of S. Typhi or S. Paratyphi should be treated with ceftriaxone or azithromycin. Patients with concern for ceftriaxone-resistant S. Typhi infection should be treated empirically with a carbapenem.

Ceftriaxone, cefotaxime, and (oral) cefixime are effective for treatment of MDR enteric fever, including that caused by DSC and fluoroquinolone-resistant strains. These agents clear fever in ~1 week, with failure rates of ~5–10%, fecal carriage rates of <3%, and relapse rates of 3–6%. Oral azithromycin results in defervescence in 4–6 days, with rates of relapse and convalescent stool carriage of <3%. Against DSC strains, azithromycin is associated with lower rates of treatment failure and shorter durations of hospitalization than are fluoroquinolones. Despite efficient in vitro killing of *Salmonella*, first- and second-generation cephalosporins as well as aminoglycosides are ineffective in the treatment of clinical infections.

Most patients with uncomplicated enteric fever can be managed at home with oral antibiotics and antipyretics. Patients with persistent vomiting, diarrhea, and/or abdominal distension should be hospitalized and given supportive therapy as well as a parenteral third-generation cephalosporin, a fluoroquinolone, or carbapenem depending on the susceptibility profile. Therapy should be administered for at least 10 days or for 5 days after fever resolution.

In a randomized, prospective, double-blind study of critically ill patients with enteric fever (i.e., those with shock and obtundation) in Indonesia in the early 1980s, the administration of dexamethasone (an initial dose of 3 mg/kg followed by eight doses of 1 mg/kg every 6 h) with chloramphenicol was associated with a substantially lower mortality rate than was treatment with chloramphenicol alone (10% vs 55%). Although this study has not been repeated in the "post-chloramphenicol era," severe enteric fever remains one of the few indications for glucocorticoid treatment of an acute bacterial infection.

The 2–5% of patients who develop chronic carriage of *Salmonella* can be treated for 4 weeks with oral ciprofloxacin or other fluoroquinolones, with an eradication rate of ~80%. Oral amoxicillin is associated with lower eradication rates than fluoroquinolones but can be considered in persons with fluoroquinolone-resistant strains that are susceptible to ampicillin. In cases of anatomic abnormality (e.g., biliary or kidney stones), eradication often requires both antibiotic therapy and surgical correction.

PREVENTION AND CONTROL

Theoretically, it is possible to eliminate the salmonellae that cause enteric fever because they survive only in human hosts and are spread by contaminated food and water. However, given the high prevalence of the disease in developing countries that lack adequate sewage disposal and water treatment, this goal is currently unrealistic. Thus, travelers to developing countries should be advised to monitor their food and water intake carefully and to strongly consider immunization against S. Typhi.

Two typhoid vaccines are commercially available in the United States: (1) Ty21a, an oral live attenuated S. Typhi vaccine (given on days 1, 3, 5, and 7, with revaccination with a full four-dose series every 5 years); in January 2021, manufacture of Ty21a was suspended due to COVID-19-related reductions in international travel; and (2) Vi CPS, a parenteral vaccine consisting of purified Vi polysaccharide from the bacterial capsule (given in a single dose, with a booster every 2 years). The minimal age for vaccination is 6 years for Ty21a and 2 years for Vi CPS. In a recent meta-analysis of 18 randomized clinical trials of vaccines for preventing typhoid fever in populations in endemic areas, the cumulative efficacy was 50% for Ty21a at 2.5 to 3 years and 55% for Vi CPS at 3 years. Although data on typhoid vaccines in travelers are limited, recent evidence suggests that typhoid vaccines are moderate effective (80%) in U.S. travelers. Currently, there is no licensed vaccine for paratyphoid fever.

Vi CPS typhoid vaccine is poorly immunogenic in children <5 years of age because of T cell–independent properties. In contrast, in a 2001 study, a prototype conjugated typhoid vaccine Vi-rEPA (Vi antigen conjugated to *Pseudomonas aeruginosa* exotoxin A) had 91% efficacy at 27 months in preventing typhoid fever in Vietnamese children 2–5 years of age. This vaccine is not commercially available. In a 2019 randomized clinical trial, a Vi polysaccharide–tetanus toxoid conjugate vaccine (Vi-TT) reduced the incidence of blood culture–confirmed typhoid fever by 82% compared to a control meningococcal vaccine among 6-month-old to 16-year-old children in Nepal. Seroconversion was 99% after Vi-TT vaccination. The World Health Organization now recommends Vi-TT administered as a single 0.5-mL dose for infants and children from 9 months to 15 years of age in high-burden settings. In typhoid-endemic areas, immunization with Vi-TT or Vi CPS is recommended for HIV-infected and other immunocompromised persons. The Vi-TT vaccine is not licensed in the United States.

Typhoid vaccine is not required for international travel, but it is recommended for travelers to areas where there is a moderate to high risk of exposure to S. Typhi, especially those who are traveling to southern Asia and other developing regions of Asia, Africa, the Caribbean, and Central and South America and who will be exposed to potentially contaminated food and drink. Typhoid vaccine should be considered even for persons planning <2 weeks of travel to high-risk areas. In addition, clinical microbiology or research laboratory staff at risk of occupational exposure to S. Typhi and household contacts of known S. Typhi carriers should be vaccinated. Because the protective efficacy of vaccine can be overcome by the high inocula that are commonly encountered in food-borne exposures, immunization is an adjunct and not a substitute for the avoidance of high-risk foods and beverages. Immunization is not recommended for the management of persons who may have been exposed in a common-source outbreak.

Enteric fever is a notifiable disease in the United States. Individual health departments have their own guidelines for allowing ill or colonized food handlers or health care workers to return to their jobs. The reporting system enables public health departments to identify potential source patients and to treat chronic carriers in order to prevent further outbreaks. In addition, because 1–4% of patients with S. Typhi infection become chronic carriers, it is important to monitor patients (especially child-care providers and food handlers) for chronic carriage and to treat this condition if indicated.

NONTYPHOIDAL SALMONELLOSIS

EPIDEMIOLOGY

Worldwide, NTS causes ~93 million enteric infections and 155,000 deaths annually. In the United States, NTS causes ~12 million illnesses annually, and the incidence has remained relatively unchanged during the past two decades. In 2017, the incidence of NTS infection in the United States was 16.0 cases per 100,000 persons—the second highest rate after *Campylobacter* (19.1 cases per 100,000 persons) among the 10 food-borne enteric pathogens under active surveillance. The four most common serotypes were Enteritidis, Typhimurium, Newport, and Javiana, which together accounted for ~40% of U.S. NTS infections.

The incidence of nontyphoidal salmonellosis is highest during the rainy season in tropical climates and during the warmer months in temperate climates—a pattern coinciding with the peak in food-borne outbreaks. Rates of morbidity and mortality associated with NTS are highest among the elderly, infants, and immunocompromised individuals, including those with hemoglobinopathies, HIV infection, or infections that cause blockade of the reticuloendothelial system (e.g., bartonellosis, malaria, schistosomiasis, histoplasmosis). NTS account for a significant majority of illnesses and hospitalizations associated with U.S. multistate food-borne outbreaks.

Invasive NTS disease is a major cause of global morbidity and mortality, especially in sub-Saharan Africa and Southeast Asia, causing an estimated annual 535,00 cases and 77,500 deaths. Invasive NTS disease is not as common as *Salmonella* enterocolitis but is associated with a much higher case–fatality rate (14.5%), especially in children; the elderly; those with poor nutrition, malaria, or HIV infection; and in areas of low sociodemographic development. In sub-Saharan Africa, specific endemic NTS strain types, including *S.* Typhimurium sequence type (ST) 131, *S.* Enteritidis sequence type 11, *S.* Dublin, and *S.* Isangi, are the predominant cause of invasive NTS disease.

Unlike *S.* Typhi and *S.* Paratyphi, whose only reservoir is humans, NTS can be acquired from multiple animal and plant reservoirs that are part of the typical food supply. Transmission is most commonly associated with food products of animal origin (especially eggs, poultry, undercooked ground meat, and dairy products), fresh produce contaminated with animal waste, and contact with animals or their environments. In the United States, NTS are the second most common cause of food-borne outbreaks after norovirus, causing 30% of outbreaks and 35% of outbreak-associated illnesses.

S. Enteritidis infection associated with chicken eggs emerged as a major cause of food-borne disease during the 1980s and 1990s. *S.* Enteritidis infection of the ovaries and upper oviduct tissue of hens results in contamination of egg contents before shell deposition. Infection is spread to egg-laying hens from breeding flocks and through contact with rodents and manure. The number of *S.* Enteritidis outbreaks and the proportion attributable to egg-containing foods have continued to decline since the mid-1990s; these declines have coincided with interventions in the egg-producing and food service industries. Despite these control efforts, outbreaks of *S.* Enteritidis infection associated with shell eggs continue to occur. In 2010, a national outbreak of *S.* Enteritidis infection resulted in >1900 reported illnesses and the recall of 500 million eggs. Transmission via contaminated eggs can be prevented by cooking eggs until the yolk is solidified and pasteurizing egg products.

Salmonella serotype 4,[5],12:i:-, an antigenic variant of *S.* Typhimurium that lacks the second stage flagellar antigen, has dramatically emerged as a foodborne pathogen associated with pigs and pork products. This serotype is now the second most common NTS in Europe and the fifth most common in the United States. These strains are multidrug resistant; in addition to resistance to ampicillin, streptomycin, sulfonamides, and tetracycline, strains from the United States also have phenotypic resistance to the veterinary antimicrobials enrofloxacin and cefdinir, which are widely used in pork production.

Centralization of food processing and widespread food distribution have contributed to the increased incidence of NTS in developed countries. NTS account for a significant majority of illnesses and hospitalizations associated with multistate foodborne outbreaks in the United States. Manufactured foods to which recent multistate *Salmonella* outbreaks have been traced include peanut butter; milk products, including infant formula; and various processed foods, including packaged breakfast cereal, salsa, frozen prepared meals, and snack foods. Large outbreaks also have been linked to fresh produce, including alfalfa sprouts, nuts/seeds, cantaloupe, mangoes, papayas, tomatoes, and raw meal replacement powder; these items become contaminated by manure or water at a single site and then are widely distributed.

An estimated 6% of sporadic *Salmonella* infections in the United States are attributed to contact with reptiles or amphibians, especially iguanas, snakes, turtles, and lizards. Other pets, including hedgehogs, birds, rodents, baby chicks, ducklings, dogs, and cats, also are potential sources of NTS. Compared to foodborne outbreaks, outbreaks of NTS linked to animal contact more commonly affect young children (<1–4 years of age), result in hospitalization, and are more sustained.

Increasing antibiotic resistance in NTS species is a global problem and has been linked to the widespread use of antimicrobial agents in food animals and especially in animal feed. In the early 1990s, *S.* Typhimurium definitive phage type 104 (DT104), characterized by resistance to at least five antibiotics (ampicillin, chloramphenicol, streptomycin, sulfonamides, and tetracyclines; R-type ACSSuT), emerged worldwide. In 2015, resistance to at least ACSSuT was reported in 2.7% of U.S. NTS isolates, including 10.8% of *S.* Typhimurium isolates. Acquisition is associated with exposure to ill farm animals and to various meat products, including uncooked or undercooked ground beef. Although probably no more virulent than susceptible *S.* Typhimurium strains, DT104 strains are associated with an increased risk of bloodstream infection and hospitalization.

Because of increased resistance to conventional antibiotics such as ampicillin and TMP-SMX, extended-spectrum cephalosporins and fluoroquinolones have emerged as the agents of choice for the treatment of MDR NTS infections. In 2015, 2.7% of NTS strains in the United States were resistant to ceftriaxone. Most ceftriaxone-resistant isolates contain plasmid-encoded AmpC β-lactamases that were probably acquired by horizontal genetic transfer from *Escherichia coli* strains in food-producing animals—an event linked to the widespread use of the veterinary cephalosporin ceftiofur.

Since the early 2000s, strains of DSC NTS (MIC, ≥0.125 μg/mL) have emerged and have been associated with delayed response and treatment failure. In 2015, 5.8% of NTS isolates in the United States were DSC. These strains have diverse resistance mechanisms, including single and multiple mutations in the DNA gyrase genes *gyr*A and *gyr*B, mutations in the chromosomally encoded quinolone resistance–determining region, and plasmid-encoded quinolone resistance genes that are not reliably detected by nalidixic acid susceptibility testing or standard ciprofloxacin disk diffusion. In 2012, the U.S. Clinical Laboratory Standards Institute proposed a lower ciprofloxacin susceptibility breakpoint (≥0.06 μg/mL) for all *Salmonella* species to address this issue. Because commercial test systems do not contain ciprofloxacin concentrations low enough to allow use of this breakpoint, laboratories need to determine the ciprofloxacin MIC by Etest or another alternative method.

While NTS strains with decreased susceptibility to azithromycin (MIC, ≥32 μg/mL) remain uncommon in the United States (0.3% in 2015), in 2018–2019, there was an outbreak of 255 cases of azithromycin-resistant *S.* Newport infection in 32 states linked to beef obtained in the United States and soft cheese obtained in Mexico. Sporadic cases of carbapenemase-resistant NTS have been reported in Europe, North Africa, and southern Asia.

CLINICAL MANIFESTATIONS

Gastroenteritis Infection with NTS most often results in gastroenteritis indistinguishable from that caused by other enteric pathogens. Nausea, vomiting, and diarrhea occur 6–48 h after the ingestion of contaminated food or water. Patients often experience abdominal cramping and fever (38–39°C [100.5–102.2°F]). Diarrheal stools are usually loose, nonbloody, and of moderate volume. However, large-volume watery stools, bloody stools, or symptoms of dysentery may occur. Rarely, NTS causes pseudoappendicitis or an illness that mimics inflammatory bowel disease.

Gastroenteritis caused by NTS is usually self-limited. Diarrhea resolves within 3–7 days and fever within 72 h. Stool cultures remain positive for 4–5 weeks after infection and—in rare cases of chronic carriage (<1%)—for >1 year. Persistent NTS infection and relapsing diarrhea have been described in a small fraction of Israeli patients and were associated with in-host single nucleotide mutations in key virulence regulators. For acute NTS gastroenteritis, antibiotic treatment usually is not recommended and may prolong fecal carriage. Neonates, the elderly, and immunosuppressed patients (e.g., transplant recipients, HIV-infected persons) with NTS gastroenteritis are especially susceptible to dehydration and invasive infection and may require hospitalization and antibiotic therapy. Acute NTS gastroenteritis was associated with a threefold increased risk of dyspepsia and irritable bowel syndrome at 1 year in a study from Spain.

Bacteremia and Endovascular Infections Up to 8% of patients with NTS gastroenteritis develop bacteremia; of these, 5–10% develop localized infections. Bacteremia and metastatic infection are most common with *Salmonella* Choleraesuis and *Salmonella* Dublin and among infants, the elderly, and immunocompromised patients, especially those with HIV infection. NTS endovascular infection should be suspected in high-grade or persistent bacteremia, especially with preexisting valvular heart disease, atherosclerotic vascular disease, prosthetic vascular graft, or aortic aneurysm. Arteritis should be suspected in elderly patients with prolonged fever and back, chest, or abdominal pain developing after an episode of gastroenteritis. Endocarditis and arteritis are rare (<1% of cases) but are associated with potentially fatal complications, including valve perforation, endomyocardial abscess, infected mural thrombus, pericarditis, mycotic aneurysms, aneurysm rupture, aortoenteric fistula, and vertebral osteomyelitis.

Invasive NTS disease is among the most common causes of bacteremia in children and in HIV-infected adults in sub-Saharan Africa and Southeast Asia, causing 39% of community-acquired bloodstream infection in one study. NTS bacteremia among these children is not associated with diarrhea and has been associated with poor nutritional status, malaria, sickle cell disease, and HIV infection. *S.* Typhimurium ST 131, the most common cause of invasive NTS disease in sub-Saharan Africa, forms a specific clade that is associated with genome reduction and loss of traits required for environmental stress resistance, likely contributing to making this strain more human adapted, perhaps as a result of carriage by immunosuppressed individuals with HIV.

Localized Infections • INTRAABDOMINAL INFECTIONS Intraabdominal infections due to NTS are rare and usually manifest as hepatic or splenic abscesses or as cholecystitis. Risk factors include hepatobiliary anatomic abnormalities (e.g., gallstones), abdominal malignancy, and sickle cell disease (especially with splenic abscesses). Eradication of the infection often requires surgical correction of abnormalities and percutaneous drainage of abscesses.

CENTRAL NERVOUS SYSTEM INFECTIONS NTS meningitis most commonly develops in infants 1–4 months of age and in adults with HIV infection. It often results in severe sequelae (including seizures, hydrocephalus, brain infarction, and mental retardation), with death in up to 60% of cases. Other rare central nervous system infections include ventriculitis, subdural empyema, and brain abscesses.

PULMONARY INFECTIONS NTS pulmonary infections usually present as lobar pneumonia, and complications include lung abscess, empyema, and bronchopleural fistula formation. The majority of cases occur in patients with lung cancer, structural lung disease, sickle cell disease, or glucocorticoid use.

URINARY AND GENITAL TRACT INFECTIONS Urinary tract infections caused by NTS present as either cystitis or pyelonephritis. Risk factors include malignancy, urolithiasis, structural abnormalities, HIV infection, and renal transplantation. NTS genital infections are rare and include ovarian and testicular abscesses, prostatitis, and epididymitis. Like other focal infections, both genital and urinary tract infections can be complicated by abscess formation.

BONE, JOINT, AND SOFT TISSUE INFECTIONS *Salmonella* osteomyelitis most commonly affects the femur, tibia, humerus, or lumbar vertebrae and is most often seen in association with sickle cell disease, hemoglobinopathies, or preexisting bone disease (e.g., fractures). Prolonged antibiotic treatment is recommended to decrease the risk of relapse and chronic osteomyelitis. Septic arthritis occurs in the same patient population as osteomyelitis and usually involves the knee, hip, or shoulder joints. Reactive arthritis can follow NTS gastroenteritis and is seen most frequently in persons with the HLA-B27 histocompatibility antigen. NTS rarely can cause soft tissue infections, usually at sites of local trauma in immunosuppressed patients.

DIAGNOSIS

The diagnosis of NTS infection is based on isolation of the organism from freshly passed stool or from blood or another ordinarily sterile body fluid. *Salmonella* is increasingly identified by culture-independent diagnostic tests due to increased sensitivity, rapid turnaround, and ability to detect multiple enteric pathogens in one test. Culture-independent positive specimens should have primary isolation performed to replicate results and recover NTS isolates. All NTS isolates should be referred to local public health departments for serotyping. Blood cultures should be obtained whenever a patient has prolonged or recurrent fever. Endovascular infection should be suspected if there is high-grade bacteremia (>50% of three or more blood cultures positive). Echocardiography, CT, and indium-labeled white cell scanning are used to identify localized infection. When another localized infection is suspected, joint fluid, abscess drainage, or cerebrospinal fluid should be cultured, as clinically indicated.

TREATMENT

Nontyphoidal Salmonellosis

Antibiotics should not be used routinely to treat uncomplicated NTS gastroenteritis. The symptoms are usually self-limited, and the duration of fever and diarrhea is not significantly decreased by antibiotic therapy. In addition, antibiotic treatment has been associated with increased rates of relapse, prolonged gastrointestinal carriage, and adverse drug reactions. Dehydration secondary to diarrhea should be treated with fluid and electrolyte replacement.

Preemptive antibiotic treatment (**Table 165-2**) should be considered for patients at increased risk for invasive NTS infection, including neonates (probably up to 3 months of age); persons >50 years of age with known or suspected atherosclerosis; and patients with immunosuppression, cardiac valvular or endovascular abnormalities, or significant joint disease. Treatment should consist of an oral or IV antibiotic administered for 48–72 h or

TABLE 165-2 Antibiotic Therapy for Nontyphoidal *Salmonella* Infection in Adults

INDICATION	AGENT	DOSAGE (ROUTE)	DURATION, DAYS
Preemptive Treatment[a]			
	Ciprofloxacin[b]	500 mg bid (PO)	2–3
Severe Gastroenteritis[c]			
	Ciprofloxacin	500 mg bid (PO) or 400 mg q12h (IV)	7
	Azithromycin	500 mg once daily	5
	Trimethoprim-sulfamethoxazole	160/800 mg bid (PO)	7
	Amoxicillin	1 g tid (PO)	7
	Ceftriaxone	1–2 g/d (IV)	7
Bacteremia			
	Ceftriaxone[d]	2 g/d (IV)	7–14
	Ciprofloxacin	400 mg q12h (IV), then 500 mg bid (PO)	
Endocarditis or Arteritis			
	Ceftriaxone	2 g/d (IV)	42
	Ciprofloxacin	400 mg q8h (IV), then 750 mg bid (PO)	
	Ampicillin	2 g q4h (IV)	
Meningitis			
	Ceftriaxone	2 g q12h (IV)	14–21
	Ampicillin	2 g q4h (IV)	
Other Localized Infection			
	Ceftriaxone	2 g/d (IV)	14–28
	Ciprofloxacin	500 mg bid (PO) or 400 mg q12h (IV)	
	Ampicillin	2 g q6h (IV)	

[a]Consider for neonates; persons >50 years of age with possible atherosclerotic vascular disease; and patients with immunosuppression, endovascular graft, or joint prosthesis. [b]Or ofloxacin, 400 mg bid (PO). [c]Consider on an individualized basis for patients with severe diarrhea and high fever who require hospitalization. [d]Or cefotaxime, 2 g q8h (IV).

until the patient becomes afebrile. Immunocompromised persons may require up to 7–14 days of therapy. The <1% of persons who develop chronic carriage of NTS should receive a prolonged antibiotic course, as described above for chronic carriage of S. Typhi.

Because of the increasing prevalence of antibiotic resistance, empirical therapy for life-threatening NTS bacteremia or focal NTS infection should include a third-generation cephalosporin or a fluoroquinolone (Table 165-2). If the bacteremia is low-grade (<50% of blood cultures positive), the patient should be treated for 7–14 days. Patients with HIV/AIDS and NTS bacteremia should receive 1–2 weeks of IV antibiotic therapy followed by 4 weeks of oral therapy with a fluoroquinolone. Patients whose infections relapse after this regimen should receive long-term suppressive therapy with a fluoroquinolone or TMP-SMX, as indicated by bacterial sensitivities.

If the patient has endocarditis or arteritis, treatment for 6 weeks with an IV β-lactam antibiotic (such as ceftriaxone or ampicillin) is indicated. IV ciprofloxacin followed by prolonged oral therapy is an option. Early surgical resection of infected aneurysms or other infected endovascular sites is recommended. Patients with infected prosthetic vascular grafts that cannot be resected have been maintained successfully on chronic suppressive oral therapy. For extraintestinal nonvascular infections, a 2- to 4-week course of antibiotic therapy (depending on the infection site) is usually recommended. In chronic osteomyelitis, abscess, or urinary or hepatobiliary infection associated with anatomic abnormalities, surgical resection or drainage may be required in addition to prolonged antibiotic therapy for eradication of infection.

PREVENTION AND CONTROL

Despite widespread efforts to prevent or reduce bacterial contamination of animal-derived food products and to improve food-safety education and training, recent declines in the incidence of NTS in the United States have been modest compared with those of other food-borne pathogens. This observation probably reflects the complex epidemiology of NTS. Identifying effective risk-reduction strategies requires monitoring of every step of the food supply chain, including farm sources, slaughter and processing of raw animal or plant products, storage and transport, and preparation of finished foods. Contaminated food can be made safe for consumption by pasteurization, irradiation, or proper cooking. All cases of NTS infection should be reported to local public health departments because tracking and monitoring of these cases can identify the source(s) of infection and help authorities anticipate large outbreaks. Prudent use of antimicrobial agents in both humans and animals is needed to limit the emergence of MDR *Salmonella*. In developing countries, immunogenic conjugated vaccines against NTS and rapid, point-of-care diagnostics are critically needed to reduce the morbidity and mortality associated with invasive NTS infection.

FURTHER READING

Cruz Espinoza LM et al: Occurrence of typhoid fever complications and their relation to duration of illness preceding hospitalization: A systematic literature review and meta-analysis. Clin Infect Dis 69(Suppl 6):S435, 2019.

GBD 2017 Non-Typhoidal Salmonella Invasive Disease Collaborators: The global burden of non-typhoidal salmonella invasive disease: A systematic analysis for the Global Burden of Disease Study 2017. Lancet Infect Dis 19:1312, 2019.

Milligan R et al: Vaccines for preventing typhoid fever. Cochrane Database Syst Rev 5:CD001261, 2018.

Onwuezobe IA et al: Antimicrobials for treating symptomatic non-typhoidal *Salmonella* infection. Cochrane Database Syst Rev CD001167, 2012.

Shakya M et al: Phase 3 efficacy analysis of a typhoid conjugate vaccine trial in Nepal. N Engl J Med 381:2209, 2019.

Singeltary LA et al: Loss of multicellular behavior in epidemic African nontyphoidal *Salmonella enterica* serovar Typhimurium ST313 strain D23580. mBio 7:e02265, 2015.

Wain J et al: Typhoid fever. Lancet 385:1136, 2015.

166 Shigellosis

Philippe J. Sansonetti, Jean Bergounioux

The discovery of *Shigella* as the etiologic agent of dysentery—a clinical syndrome of fever, intestinal cramps, and frequent passage of small, bloody, mucopurulent stools—is attributed to the Japanese microbiologist Kiyoshi Shiga, who isolated the Shiga bacillus (now known as *Shigella dysenteriae* type 1) from patients' stools in 1897 during a large and devastating dysentery epidemic. *Shigella* cannot be distinguished from *Escherichia coli* by DNA hybridization and remains a separate species only on historical and clinical grounds.

ETIOLOGIC AGENT

Shigella is a non-spore-forming, gram-negative bacterium that, unlike *E. coli*, is nonmotile and does not produce gas from sugars, decarboxylate lysine, or hydrolyze arginine. Some serovars produce indole, and occasional strains utilize sodium acetate. *Shigella dysenteriae*, *Shigella flexneri*, *Shigella boydii*, and *Shigella sonnei* (serogroups A, B, C, and D, respectively) can be differentiated on the basis of biochemical and serologic characteristics.

Genome sequencing of *E. coli* K12, *S. flexneri* 2a, *S. sonnei*, *S. dysenteriae* type 1, and *S. boydii* has revealed that these species have ~93% of genes in common. The three major genomic "signatures" of *Shigella* are (1) a 215-kb virulence plasmid that carries most of the genes required for pathogenicity (particularly invasive capacity); (2) the lack or alteration of genetic sequences encoding products (e.g., lysine decarboxylase) that, if expressed, would attenuate pathogenicity; and (3) in *S. dysenteriae* type 1, the presence of genes encoding Shiga toxin, a potent cytotoxin.

EPIDEMIOLOGY

The human intestinal tract represents the major reservoir of *Shigella*, which is also found (albeit rarely) in the higher primates. Because excretion of shigellae is greatest in the acute phase of disease, the bacteria are transmitted most efficiently by the fecal–oral route via hand carriage; however, some outbreaks reflect foodborne or waterborne transmission. In impoverished areas, *Shigella* can be transmitted by flies. The high-level infectivity of *Shigella* is reflected by the very small inoculum required for experimental infection of volunteers (100 colony-forming units [CFU]), by the very high attack rates during outbreaks in day-care centers (33–73%), and by the high rates of secondary cases among family members of sick children (26–33%). Shigellosis can also be transmitted sexually.

Throughout history, *Shigella* epidemics have often occurred in settings of human crowding under conditions of poor hygiene—e.g., among soldiers in campaigning armies, inhabitants of besieged cities, groups on pilgrimages, and refugees in camps. Epidemics follow a cyclical pattern in areas such as the Indian subcontinent and sub-Saharan Africa. These devastating epidemics, which are most often caused by *S. dysenteriae* type 1, are characterized by high attack and mortality rates. In Bangladesh, for instance, an epidemic caused by *S. dysenteriae* type 1 was associated with a 42% increase in mortality rate among children 1–4 years of age. Apart from these epidemics, shigellosis is mostly an endemic disease, with 99% of cases occurring in the developing world and the highest prevalences in the most impoverished areas, where personal and general hygiene is below standard. *S. flexneri* isolates predominate in the least developed areas, whereas *S. sonnei* is more prevalent in economically emerging countries and in the industrialized world.

Prevalence in the Developing World In a review published under the auspices of the World Health Organization (WHO), the total annual number of cases in 1966–1997 was estimated at 165 million, and 69% of these cases occurred in children <5 years of age. In this review, the annual number of deaths was calculated to range between 500,000 and 1.1 million. Data (2000–2004) from six Asian countries indicate that, even though the incidence of shigellosis remains stable, mortality rates associated with this disease may have decreased significantly, possibly as a result of improved nutritional status. However, extensive and essentially uncontrolled use of antibiotics, which may also account for declining mortality rates, has increased the rate of emergence of multidrug-resistant *Shigella* strains. A 2013 prospective matched case-control study of children <5 years of age emphasizes the importance of *Shigella* in the burden and etiology of diarrheal diseases in developing countries. *Shigella* is one of the top four pathogens associated with moderate to severe diarrhea and is now ranked first among children 12–59 months of age. These moderate to severe cases account for an 8.5-fold increase in mortality incidence over the average diarrheal disease-related mortality. The study's authors conclude that *Shigella* remains a major pathogen to be targeted by health care programs.

An often-overlooked complication of shigellosis is the short- and long-term impairment of the nutritional status of infected children in endemic areas. Combined with anorexia, the exudative enteropathy resulting from mucosal abrasions contributes to rapid deterioration of the patient's nutritional status. Shigellosis is thus a major contributor to stunted growth among children in developing countries.

Peaking in incidence in the pediatric population, endemic shigellosis is rare among young and middle-aged adults, probably because of naturally acquired immunity. Incidence then increases again in the elderly population.

Prevalence in the Industrialized World In pediatric populations, local outbreaks occur when proper and adapted hygiene policies are not implemented in group facilities such as day-care centers and institutions for the mentally retarded. In adults, as in children, sporadic cases occur among travelers returning from endemic areas, and rare outbreaks of varying size can follow waterborne or foodborne infections.

PATHOGENESIS AND PATHOLOGY

Shigella infection occurs essentially through oral contamination via direct fecal–oral transmission, the organism being poorly adapted to survive in the environment. Resistance to low-pH conditions allows *Shigella* to survive passage through the gastric barrier, an ability that may explain in part why a small inoculum (as few as 100 CFU) is sufficient to cause infection.

The watery diarrhea that usually precedes the dysenteric syndrome is attributable to active secretion and abnormal water reabsorption—a secretory effect at the jejunal level described in experimentally infected rhesus monkeys. This initial purge is probably due to the combined action of an enterotoxin (ShET-1) and mucosal inflammation. The dysenteric syndrome, manifested by bloody and mucopurulent stools, reflects invasion of the mucosa.

The pathogenesis of *Shigella* is essentially determined by a large virulence plasmid of 214 kb comprising ~100 genes, of which 25 encode a type III secretion system that inserts into the membrane of the host cell to allow effectors to transit from the bacterial cytoplasm to the host cell cytoplasm (**Fig. 166-1**). Bacteria are thereby able to invade intestinal epithelial cells by inducing their own uptake either directly at the opening of colonic crypts, or following the initial crossing of the epithelial barrier through M cells (the specialized translocating epithelial cells in the follicle-associated epithelium that covers mucosal lymphoid nodules). *Shigella* induces apoptosis of subepithelial resident macrophages. Once inside the cytoplasm of intestinal epithelial cells, *Shigella* effectors trigger the cytoskeletal rearrangements necessary to direct uptake of the organism into the epithelial cell. The *Shigella*-containing vacuole is then quickly lysed, releasing bacteria into the cytosol.

Intracellular shigellae next use cytoskeletal components to propel themselves inside the infected cell; when the moving organism and the host cell membrane come into contact, cellular protrusions form and are engulfed by neighboring cells. This series of events permits bacterial cell-to-cell spread.

Cytokines released by a growing number of infected intestinal epithelial cells attract increased numbers of immune cells (particularly polymorphonuclear leukocytes [PMNs]) to the infected site, thus further destabilizing the epithelial barrier, exacerbating inflammation, and leading to the acute colitis that characterizes shigellosis. Evidence indicates that some type III secretion system–injected effectors can control the extent of inflammation, thus facilitating bacterial survival.

Shiga toxin produced by *S. dysenteriae* type 1 increases disease severity. This toxin belongs to a group of A1-B5 protein toxins whose B subunit binds to the receptor globotriaosylceramide on the target cell surface and whose catalytic A subunit is internalized by receptor-mediated endocytosis and interacts with the subcellular machinery to inhibit protein synthesis by expressing RNA *N*-glycosidase activity on 28S ribosomal RNA. This process leads to inhibition of binding of the amino-acyl-tRNA to the 60S ribosomal subunit and thus to a general shutoff of cell protein biosynthesis. Shiga toxins are translocated from the bowel into the circulation. After binding of the toxins to target cells in the kidney, pathophysiologic alterations may result in hemolytic-uremic syndrome (HUS; see below).

CLINICAL MANIFESTATIONS

The presentation and severity of shigellosis depend to some extent on the infecting serotype but even more on the age and the immunologic and nutritional status of the host. Poverty and poor standards of hygiene are strongly related to the number and severity of diarrheal episodes, especially in children <5 years old who have been weaned.

Shigellosis typically evolves through four phases: incubation, watery diarrhea, dysentery, and the postinfectious phase. The incubation period usually lasts 1–4 days but may be as long as 8 days. Typical initial manifestations are transient fever, limited watery diarrhea, malaise, and anorexia. Signs and symptoms may range from mild abdominal discomfort to severe cramps, diarrhea, fever, vomiting, and tenesmus. The manifestations are usually exacerbated in children, with temperatures up to 40°–41°C (104.0°–105.8°F) and more severe anorexia and watery diarrhea. This initial phase may represent the only clinical manifestation of shigellosis, especially in developed countries. Otherwise, dysentery follows within hours or days and is characterized by uninterrupted excretion of small volumes of bloody mucopurulent stools with increased tenesmus and abdominal cramps. At this stage, *Shigella* produces acute colitis involving mainly the distal colon and the rectum. Unlike most diarrheal syndromes, dysenteric syndromes rarely present with dehydration as a major feature. Endoscopy shows an edematous and

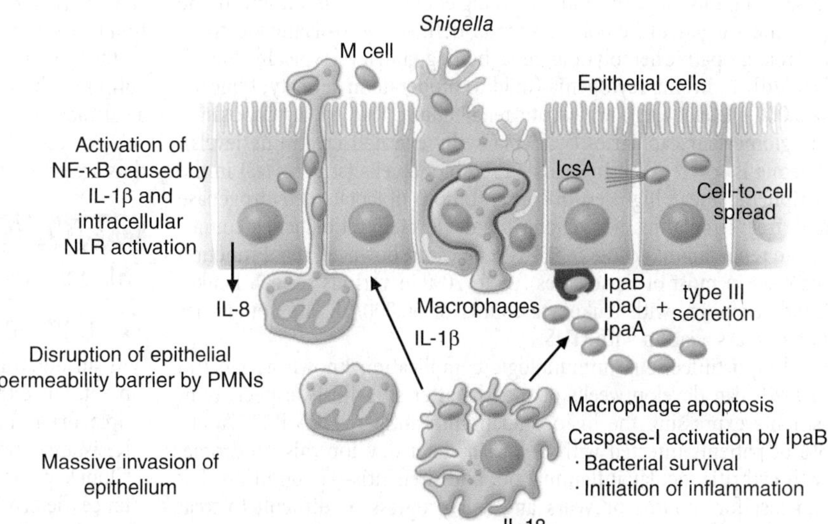

FIGURE 166-1 Invasive strategy of *Shigella flexneri*. IL, interleukin; NF-κB, nuclear factor κB; NLR, NOD-like receptor; PMN, polymorphonuclear leukocyte.

hemorrhagic mucosa, with ulcerations and possibly overlying exudates resembling pseudomembranes. The extent of the lesions correlates with the number and frequency of stools and with the degree of protein loss by exudative mechanisms. Most episodes are self-limited and resolve without treatment in 1 week. With appropriate treatment, recovery takes place within a few days to a week, with no sequelae.

Acute life-threatening complications are seen most often in children <5 years of age (particularly those who are malnourished) and in elderly patients. Risk factors for death in a clinically severe case include nonbloody diarrhea, moderate to severe dehydration, bacteremia, absence of fever, abdominal tenderness, and rectal prolapse. Major complications are predominantly intestinal (e.g., toxic megacolon, intestinal perforations, rectal prolapse) or metabolic (e.g., hypoglycemia, hyponatremia, dehydration). Bacteremia is rare and is reported most frequently in severely malnourished and HIV-infected patients. Alterations of consciousness, including seizures, delirium, and coma, may occur, especially in children <5 years old, and are associated with a poor prognosis; fever and severe metabolic alterations are more often the major causes of altered consciousness than is meningitis or the Ekiri syndrome (toxic encephalopathy associated with bizarre posturing, cerebral edema, and fatty degeneration of viscera), which has been reported mostly in Japanese children. Pneumonia, vaginitis, and keratoconjunctivitis due to *Shigella* are rarely reported. In the absence of serious malnutrition, severe and very unusual clinical manifestations, such as meningitis, may be linked to genetic defects in innate immune functions (i.e., deficiency in interleukin 1 receptor–associated kinase 4 [IRAK-4]) and may require genetic investigation.

Two complications of particular importance are toxic megacolon and HUS. Toxic megacolon is a consequence of severe inflammation extending to the colonic smooth-muscle layer and causing paralysis and dilation. The patient presents with abdominal distention and tenderness, with or without signs of localized or generalized peritonitis. The abdominal x-ray characteristically shows marked dilation of the transverse colon (with the greatest distention in the ascending and descending segments); thumbprinting caused by mucosal inflammatory edema; and loss of the normal haustral pattern associated with pseudopolyps, often extending into the lumen. Pneumatosis coli is an occasional finding. If perforation occurs, radiographic signs of pneumoperitoneum may be apparent. Predisposing factors (e.g., hypokalemia and use of opioids, anticholinergics, loperamide, psyllium seeds, and antidepressants) should be investigated.

Shiga toxin produced by *S. dysenteriae* type 1 has been linked to HUS in developing countries but rarely in industrialized countries, where enterohemorrhagic *E. coli* (EHEC) predominates as the etiologic agent of this syndrome. HUS is an early complication that most often develops after several days of diarrhea. Clinical examination shows pallor, asthenia, and irritability and, in some cases, bleeding of the nose and gums, oliguria, and increasing edema. HUS is a nonimmune (Coombs-negative) hemolytic anemia defined by a diagnostic triad: microangiopathic hemolytic anemia (hemoglobin level typically <80 g/L [<8 g/dL]), thrombocytopenia (mild to moderate in severity; typically <60,000 platelets/μL), and acute renal failure due to thrombosis of the glomerular capillaries (with markedly elevated creatinine levels). Anemia is severe, with fragmented red blood cells (*schizocytes*) in the peripheral smear, high serum concentrations of lactate dehydrogenase and free circulating hemoglobin, and elevated reticulocyte counts. Acute renal failure occurs in 55–70% of cases; however, renal function recovers in most of these cases (up to 70% in various series). Leukemoid reactions, with leukocyte counts of 50,000/μL, are sometimes noted in association with HUS.

The postinfectious immunologic complication known as *reactive arthritis* can develop weeks or months after shigellosis, especially in patients expressing the histocompatibility antigen HLA-B27. About 3% of patients infected with *S. flexneri* later develop this syndrome, with arthritis, ocular inflammation, and urethritis—a condition that can last for months or years and can progress to difficult-to-treat chronic arthritis. Postinfectious arthritis occurs only after infection with *S. flexneri* and not after infection with the other *Shigella* serotypes.

LABORATORY DIAGNOSIS

The differential diagnosis in patients with a dysenteric syndrome depends on the clinical and environmental context. In developing areas, infectious diarrhea caused by other invasive pathogenic bacteria (*Salmonella*, *Campylobacter jejuni*, *Clostridium difficile*, *Yersinia enterocolitica*) or parasites (*Entamoeba histolytica*) should be considered. Only bacteriologic and parasitologic examinations of stool can truly differentiate among these pathogens. A first flare of inflammatory bowel disease, such as Crohn's disease or ulcerative colitis **(Chap. 326)**, should be considered in patients in industrialized countries. Despite the similarity in symptoms, anamnesis discriminates between shigellosis, which usually follows recent travel in an endemic zone, and these other conditions.

Microscopic examination of stool smears shows erythrophagocytic trophozoites with very few PMNs in *E. histolytica* infection, whereas bacterial enteroinvasive infections (particularly shigellosis) are characterized by high PMN counts in each microscopic field. However, because shigellosis often manifests only as watery diarrhea, systematic attempts to isolate *Shigella* are necessary.

The "gold standard" for the diagnosis of *Shigella* infection remains the isolation and identification of the pathogen from fecal material. One major difficulty, particularly in endemic areas where laboratory facilities are not immediately available, is the fragility of *Shigella* and its common disappearance during transport, especially with rapid changes in temperature and pH. In the absence of a reliable enrichment medium, buffered glycerol saline or Cary-Blair medium can be used as a holding medium, but prompt inoculation onto isolation medium is essential. The probability of isolation is higher if the portion of stools that contains bloody and/or mucopurulent material is directly sampled. Rectal swabs can be used, as they offer the highest rate of successful isolation during the acute phase of disease. Blood cultures are positive in fewer than 5% of cases but should be done when a patient presents with a clinical picture of severe sepsis.

In addition to quick processing, the use of several media increases the likelihood of successful isolation: a nonselective medium such as bromocresol-purple agar lactose; a low-selectivity medium such as MacConkey or eosin-methylene blue; and a high-selectivity medium such as Hektoen, *Salmonella-Shigella*, or xylose-lysine-deoxycholate agar. After incubation on these media for 12–18 h at 37°C (98.6°F), shigellae appear as non-lactose-fermenting colonies that measure 0.5–1 mm in diameter and have a convex, translucent, smooth surface. Suspected colonies on nonselective or low-selectivity medium can be subcultured on a high-selectivity medium before being specifically identified or can be identified directly by standard commercial systems on the basis of four major characteristics: glucose positivity (usually without production of gas), lactose negativity, H_2S negativity, and lack of motility. The four *Shigella* serogroups (A–D) can then be differentiated by additional characteristics. This approach adds time and difficulty to the identification process; however, after presumptive diagnosis, the use of serologic methods (e.g., slide agglutination, with group- and then type-specific antisera) should be considered. Group-specific antisera are widely available; in contrast, because of the large number of serotypes and subserotypes, type-specific antisera are rare and more expensive and thus are often restricted to reference laboratories.

TREATMENT

Shigellosis

ANTIBIOTIC SUSCEPTIBILITY OF *SHIGELLA*

As an enteroinvasive disease, shigellosis requires antibiotic treatment. Since the mid-1960s, however, increasing resistance to multiple drugs has been a dominant factor in treatment decisions. Resistance rates are highly dependent on the geographic area. Clonal spread of particular strains and horizontal transfer of resistance determinants, particularly via plasmids and transposons, contribute to multidrug resistance. The current global status—i.e., high rates of resistance to classic first-line antibiotics such as amoxicillin—has led to a rapid switch to quinolones such as nalidixic acid. However, resistance to such early-generation quinolones has also emerged and spread quickly as a result of chromosomal mutations affecting DNA gyrase and topoisomerase IV; this resistance has necessitated the use of later-generation quinolones as first-line antibiotics in many areas. For instance, a review of the antibiotic resistance history of *Shigella* in India found that, after their introduction in the late 1980s, the second-generation quinolones norfloxacin, ciprofloxacin, and ofloxacin were highly effective in the treatment of shigellosis, including cases caused by multidrug-resistant strains of *S. dysenteriae* type 1. However, investigations of subsequent outbreaks in India and Bangladesh detected resistance to norfloxacin, ciprofloxacin, and ofloxacin in 5% of isolates. In the United States, the resistance rate of *Shigella* to fluoroquinolones reached 87% during 2014–2015. The incidence of multidrug resistance parallels the widespread, uncontrolled use of antibiotics and calls for the rational use of effective drugs. Despite the alarming proportion of resistant *Shigella*, there is a lack of studies assessing the resistance of community-acquired strains.

ANTIBIOTIC TREATMENT OF SHIGELLOSIS (TABLE 166-1)

With effective antibiotic therapy clinical improvement occurs within 48 h, resulting in a decreased risk of complications and death, shorter duration of symptoms, and elimination of *Shigella* from the stool. Because of the ready transmissibility of *Shigella*, current public health recommendations in the United States are that every case be treated with antibiotics. The use of fluoroquinolones (first-line, preferably ciprofloxacin), and cephalosporins and β-lactams (second-line) for 7–10 days is recommended for the treatment of shigellosis. Whereas infections caused by non-*dysenteriae Shigella* in immunocompetent individuals are routinely treated with a 3-day course of antibiotics, it is recommended that *S. dysenteriae* type 1 infections be treated for 5 days and that *Shigella* infections in immunocompromised patients be treated for 7–10 days.

Treatment for shigellosis must be adapted to the clinical context, with the recognition that the most fragile patients are children <5 years old, who represent two-thirds of all cases worldwide. There are few data on the use of quinolones in children, but *Shigella*-induced dysentery is a well-recognized indication for their use. The half-life of ciprofloxacin is longer in infants than in older individuals. The ciprofloxacin dose generally recommended for children is 30 mg/kg per day in two divided doses. Adults living in areas with high standards of hygiene are likely to develop milder, shorter-duration disease, whereas infants in endemic areas can develop severe, sometimes fatal, dysentery. In the former setting, treatment will remain minimal and bacteriologic proof of infection will often come after symptoms have resolved; in the latter setting, antibiotic treatment and more aggressive measures, possibly including resuscitation, are often required.

Vaccine studies for *S. flexneri* have been impaired by the lack of optimal animal models. New findings document the immunogenicity and preclinical efficacy effects of *S. flexneri* vaccine in mice and suggest that further work can help elucidate relevant immune responses and, ultimately, its clinical efficacy in humans.

TABLE 166-1 Recommended Antimicrobial Therapy for Shigellosis

ANTIMICROBIAL AGENT	TREATMENT SCHEDULE: CHILDREN	TREATMENT SCHEDULE: ADULTS	LIMITATIONS
First-Line			
Ciprofloxacin	15 mg/kg	500 mg	
	2 times per day for 3 days, PO		
Second-Line			
Pivmecillinam	20 mg/kg	100 mg	Cost
	4 times per day for 5 days PO		No pediatric formulation Frequent administration Emerging resistance
Ceftriaxone	50–100 mg/kg	–	Efficacy not validated Must be injected
	Once a day IM for 2–5 days		
Azithromycin	6–20 mg/kg	1–1.5 g	Cost
	Once a day for 1–5 days PO		Efficacy not validated Minimum inhibitory concentration near serum concentration Rapid emergence of resistance and spread to other bacteria

Source: Reproduced with permission from World Health Organization: Guidelines for the control of shigellosis, including epidemics due to Shigella dysenteriae type 1.

REHYDRATION AND NUTRITION

Shigella infection rarely causes significant dehydration. Cases requiring aggressive rehydration (particularly in industrialized countries) are uncommon. In developing countries, malnutrition remains the primary indicator for diarrhea-related death, highlighting the importance of nutrition in early management. Rehydration should be oral unless the patient is comatose or presents in shock. Because of the improved effectiveness of reduced-osmolarity oral rehydration solution (especially for children with acute noncholera diarrhea), the WHO and UNICEF now recommend a standard solution of 245 mOsm/L (sodium, 75 mmol/L; chloride, 65 mmol/L; glucose [anhydrous], 75 mmol/L; potassium, 20 mmol/L; citrate, 10 mmol/L). In shigellosis, the coupled transport of sodium and glucose may be variably affected, but oral rehydration therapy remains the easiest and most efficient form of rehydration, especially in severe cases.

Nutrition should be started as soon as possible after completion of initial rehydration. Early refeeding is safe, well tolerated, and clinically beneficial. Because breast-feeding reduces diarrheal losses and the need for oral rehydration in infants, it should be maintained in the absence of contraindications (e.g., maternal HIV infection).

NONSPECIFIC, SYMPTOM-BASED THERAPY

Antimotility agents have been implicated in prolonged fever in volunteers with shigellosis. These agents are suspected of increasing the risk of toxic megacolon and are thought to have been responsible for HUS in children infected by EHEC strains. For safety reasons, it is better to avoid antimotility agents in bloody diarrhea.

TREATMENT OF COMPLICATIONS

There is no consensus regarding the best treatment for toxic megacolon. The patient should be assessed frequently by both medical and surgical teams. Anemia, dehydration, and electrolyte deficits (particularly hypokalemia) may aggravate colonic atony and should be actively treated. Nasogastric aspiration helps to deflate the colon. Parenteral nutrition has not been proven to be beneficial. Fever persisting beyond 48–72 h raises the possibility of local perforation or abscess. Most studies recommend colectomy if, after 48–72 h, colonic distention persists. However, some physicians recommend continuation of medical therapy for up to 7 days if the patient seems to be improving clinically despite persistent megacolon without free perforation. Intestinal perforation, either isolated or complicating toxic megacolon, requires surgical treatment and intensive medical support.

Rectal prolapse must be treated as soon as possible. With the health care provider using surgical gloves or a soft warm wet cloth and the patient in the knee-chest position, the prolapsed rectum is gently pushed back into place. If edema of the rectal mucosa is evident (rendering reintegration difficult), it can be osmotically reduced by the application of gauze impregnated with a warm solution of saturated magnesium sulfate. Rectal prolapse often relapses but usually resolves along with the resolution of dysentery.

HUS must be treated by water restriction, including discontinuation of oral rehydration solution and potassium-rich alimentation. Hemofiltration is usually required.

PREVENTION

Hand washing after defecation or handling of children's feces and before handling of food is recommended. Stool decontamination (e.g., with sodium hypochlorite), together with a cleaning protocol for medical staff as well as for patients, has proven useful in limiting the spread of infection during *Shigella* outbreaks. Ideally, patients should have a negative stool culture before their infection is considered cured. Recurrences are rare if therapeutic and preventive measures are correctly implemented.

Although several live attenuated oral and subunit parenteral vaccine candidates have been produced and are undergoing clinical trials, no vaccine against shigellosis is currently available. Especially given the rapid progression of antibiotic resistance in *Shigella*, a vaccine is urgently needed.

FURTHER READING

Arena ET et al: Bioimage analysis of *Shigella* infection reveals targeting of colonic crypts. Proc Natl Acad Sci USA 112:E3282, 2015.

Bennish ML, Wojtyniak BJ: Mortality due to shigellosis: Community and hospital data. Rev Infect Dis 13(Suppl 4):S245, 1991.

Cossart P, Sansonetti PJ: Bacterial invasion: The paradigms of enteroinvasive pathogens. Science 304:242, 2004.

Kotloff KL et al: The incidence, aetiology, and adverse clinical consequences of less severe diarrhoeal episodes among infants and children residing in low-income and middle-income countries: A 12-month case-control study as a follow-on to the Global Enteric Multicenter Study (GEMS). Lancet Glob Health 7:E568, 2019.

Mani S et al: Status of vaccine research and development for *Shigella*. Vaccine 34:2887, 2016.

Niyogi SK: Shigellosis. J Microbiol 43:133, 2005.

Phalipon A, Sansonetti PJ: *Shigella's* ways of manipulating the host intestinal innate and adaptive immune system: A tool box for survival? Immunol Cell Biol 85:119, 2007.

Traa BS et al: Antibiotics for the treatment of dysentery in children. Int J Epidemiol 39(Suppl 1):i70, 2010.

World Health Organization: Guidelines for the control of shigellosis, including epidemics due to *Shigella dysenteriae* type 1. WHO Library Cataloguing-in-Publication Data. *www.who.int/cholera/publications/shigellosis/en/*.

167 Infections Due to *Campylobacter* and Related Organisms

Martin J. Blaser

DEFINITION

Bacteria of the genus *Campylobacter* and of the related genera *Arcobacter* and *Helicobacter* (**Chap. 163**) cause a variety of inflammatory conditions. Although acute diarrheal illnesses are most common, these organisms may cause infections in virtually all parts of the body, especially in compromised hosts, and these infections may have late nonsuppurative sequelae. The designation *Campylobacter* comes from the Greek for "curved rod" and refers to the organism's vibrio-like morphology.

ETIOLOGY

Campylobacters are motile, non-spore-forming, curved, gram-negative rods. Originally known as *Vibrio fetus*, these bacilli were reclassified as a new genus in 1973 after their dissimilarity to other vibrios was recognized. More than 20 species have since been identified. These species are currently divided into three genera: *Campylobacter*, *Arcobacter*, and *Helicobacter*. Not all of the species are pathogens of humans. The human pathogens fall into two major groups: those that primarily cause diarrheal disease and those that cause extraintestinal infection. The principal diarrheal pathogen is *Campylobacter jejuni*, which accounts for 80–90% of all cases of recognized illness due to campylobacters and related genera. Other organisms that can cause diarrheal disease include *Campylobacter coli, Campylobacter upsaliensis, Campylobacter lari, Campylobacter hyointestinalis, Campylobacter fetus, Arcobacter butzleri, Arcobacter cryaerophilus, Helicobacter cinaedi*, and *Helicobacter fennelliae*. The two *Helicobacter* species causing diarrheal disease, *H. cinaedi* and *H. fennelliae*, are intestinal rather than gastric organisms; in terms of the clinical features of the illnesses they cause, these species most closely resemble *Campylobacter* rather than *Helicobacter pylori* (**Chap. 163**) and thus are considered in this chapter. The pathogenic roles of *Campylobacter concisus, Campylobacter ureolyticus*, and *Campylobacter troglodytis* are uncertain. A new subspecies—*C. fetus* subspecies *testudinum*—has been described, chiefly in Asian patients; the very close resemblance of human isolates to strains isolated from reptiles suggests a food source.

The major species causing extraintestinal illnesses is *C. fetus*. However, any of the diarrheal agents listed above may cause systemic or localized infection as well, especially in compromised hosts. Neither aerobes nor strict anaerobes, these microaerophilic organisms are adapted for survival in the gastrointestinal mucous layer. This chapter focuses on *C. jejuni* and *C. fetus* as the major pathogens and prototypes for their groups. The key features of infection are listed by species (excluding *C. jejuni*, described in detail in the text below) in **Table 167-1**.

EPIDEMIOLOGY

Campylobacters are found in the gastrointestinal tract of many animals used for food (including poultry, cattle, sheep, and swine) and many household pets (including birds, dogs, and cats). These microorganisms often do not cause illness in their animal hosts, but occasionally this can occur (especially in puppies). In most cases, campylobacters are transmitted to humans in raw or undercooked food products or through direct contact with infected animals. In the United States and other developed countries, ingestion of contaminated poultry that has not been sufficiently cooked is the most common mode of acquisition (30–70% of cases). Other modes include ingestion of raw (unpasteurized) milk or untreated water, contact with infected household pets, ingestion of contaminated seafood, travel to developing countries (campylobacters being a leading cause of traveler's diarrhea; **Chaps. 124 and 133**), oral–anal sexual contact, cross-contamination from any of these sources, and (occasionally) contact with an index case who is incontinent of stool.

Campylobacter infections are common. Active surveillance of foodborne infections in the United States estimates the incidence of diarrheal disease due to campylobacters at ~20 cases per 100,000 persons—similar in incidence to *Salmonella* and more common than *Shigella*. Infections occur throughout the year, but the incidence peaks during summer and early autumn. Persons of all ages are affected; however, attack rates for *C. jejuni* are highest among young children and young adults, whereas those for *C. fetus* are highest at the extremes of age. Systemic infections due to *C. fetus* (and to other *Campylobacter* and related species) are most common among compromised hosts. Persons at increased risk include those with AIDS, immunoglobulin deficiencies, neoplasia, liver disease, diabetes mellitus, and generalized atherosclerosis as well as neonates and pregnant women; proton pump inhibitor use also increases risk. However, apparently healthy nonpregnant persons occasionally develop transient *Campylobacter* bacteremia as part of a gastrointestinal illness (0.1–1% of cases).

In contrast, in many developing countries where sanitation is poor, *C. jejuni* infections are hyperendemic, with the highest rates among children <2 years old. According to large prospective cohort studies in low- to middle-income countries, *Campylobacter* infections—even when asymptomatic—are associated with short stature (stunting). Rates of clinically apparent infection fall with age, as does the illness-to-infection ratio, consistent with development of immunity.

TABLE 167-1 Clinical Features Associated with Infection Due to "Atypical" *Campylobacter* and Related Species Implicated as Causes of Human Illness

SPECIES	COMMON CLINICAL FEATURES	LESS COMMON CLINICAL FEATURES	ADDITIONAL INFORMATION
Campylobacter coli	Fever, diarrhea, abdominal pain	Bacteremia[a]	Clinically indistinguishable from *C. jejuni*
Campylobacter fetus	Bacteremia,[a] sepsis, meningitis, vascular infections	Diarrhea, relapsing fevers	Not usually isolated from media containing cephalothin or incubated at 42°C
Campylobacter upsaliensis	Watery diarrhea, low-grade fever, abdominal pain	Bacteremia, abscesses	Difficult to isolate because of cephalothin susceptibility
Campylobacter lari	Abdominal pain, diarrhea	Colitis, appendicitis	Seagulls frequently colonized; organism often transmitted to humans via contaminated water
Campylobacter hyointestinalis	Watery or bloody diarrhea, vomiting, abdominal pain	Bacteremia	Causes proliferative enteritis in swine
Helicobacter fennelliae	Chronic mild diarrhea, abdominal cramps, proctitis	Bacteremia[a]	Best treated with fluoroquinolones
Helicobacter cinaedi	Chronic mild diarrhea, abdominal cramps, proctitis	Bacteremia[a]	Best treated with fluoroquinolones; identified in healthy hamsters
Campylobacter jejuni subspecies *doylei*	Diarrhea	Chronic gastritis, bacteremia[b]	Uncertain role as human pathogen
Arcobacter cryaerophilus	Diarrhea	Bacteremia	Poultry, seafood sources. Cultured under aerobic conditions
Arcobacter butzleri	Fever, diarrhea, abdominal pain, nausea; or asymptomatic	Bacteremia, appendicitis	Cultured under aerobic conditions; enzootic in nonhuman primates
Campylobacter sputorum	Pulmonary, perianal, groin, and axillary abscesses; diarrhea	Bacteremia	Three clinically relevant biovars: *sputorum, faecalis,* and *paraureolyticus*

[a]In immunocompromised hosts, especially HIV-infected persons. [b]In children.
Source: Adapted from BM Allos, MJ Blaser: Clin Infect Dis 20:1092, 1995.

PATHOLOGY AND PATHOGENESIS

C. jejuni infections may be subclinical, especially in hosts in developing countries who have had multiple prior infections and may be partially immune. Symptomatic infections mostly occur within 2–4 days (range, 1–7 days) of exposure to the organism. The sites of tissue injury include the jejunum, ileum, and colon. Biopsies show an acute nonspecific inflammatory reaction, with neutrophils, monocytes, and eosinophils in the lamina propria, as well as damage to the epithelium, including loss of mucus, glandular degeneration, and crypt abscesses. Biopsy findings may be consistent with Crohn's disease or ulcerative colitis, but these "idiopathic" chronic inflammatory diseases should not be diagnosed unless infectious colitis, *specifically including* that due to infection with *Campylobacter* species and related organisms, has been ruled out.

The components of protective immunity to *Campylobacter* in humans are poorly understood. The high frequency of *C. jejuni* infections and their severity and recurrence among immunoglobulin-deficient patients suggest that antibodies are important in protective immunity. Experience from field studies and human experimental infection models suggests that immune protection may be short-lived or incomplete in the absence of continuous exposure. Knowledge of the pathogenesis of infection is also incomplete. Both the motility of the strain and its capacity to adhere to host tissues appear to favor disease, but classic enterotoxins and cytotoxins (including cytolethal distending toxin) appear not to play substantial roles in tissue injury or disease production. The organisms have been visualized within the epithelium, albeit in low numbers. The documentation of a significant tissue response and occasionally of *C. jejuni* bacteremia further suggests that tissue invasion is clinically significant, and in vitro studies are consistent with this pathogenic feature.

The pathogenesis of *C. fetus* infections is better defined. Virtually all clinical isolates of *C. fetus* possess a proteinaceous capsule-like structure (an S-layer) that renders the organisms resistant to complement-mediated killing and opsonization. As a result, *C. fetus* can cause bacteremia and can seed sites beyond the intestinal tract. The ability of the organism to switch the S-layer proteins expressed—a phenomenon that results in antigenic variability—may contribute to the chronicity and high rate of recurrence of *C. fetus* infections in compromised hosts.

CLINICAL MANIFESTATIONS

The clinical features of infections due to *Campylobacter* and the related *Arcobacter* and intestinal *Helicobacter* species causing enteric disease appear to be highly similar. *C. jejuni* can be considered the prototype, in part because it is by far the most common enteric pathogen in the group. A prodrome of fever, headache, myalgia, and/or malaise often occurs 12–48 h before the onset of diarrheal symptoms. The most common signs and symptoms of the intestinal phase are diarrhea, abdominal pain, and fever. The degree of diarrhea varies from several loose watery stools to visibly bloody stools (~10% of cases in adults); most patients presenting for medical attention have ≥10 bowel movements on the worst day of illness. Abdominal pain usually consists of cramping and may be the most prominent symptom. Pain is usually generalized but may become localized; *C. jejuni* infection may cause pseudoappendicitis. Fever may be the only initial manifestation of *C. jejuni* infection, a situation mimicking the early stages of typhoid fever. Febrile young children may develop convulsions. *Campylobacter* enteritis is generally self-limited; however, symptoms persist for >1 week in 10–20% of patients seeking medical attention, and clinical relapses occur in 5–10% of untreated patients. Studies of common-source epidemics indicate that milder illnesses or asymptomatic infections may commonly occur.

C. fetus may cause a diarrheal illness similar to that due to *C. jejuni*, especially in immunocompetent hosts. This organism also may cause either intermittent diarrhea or nonspecific abdominal pain without localizing signs. Sequelae are uncommon, and the outcome is benign. *C. fetus* may also cause a prolonged relapsing systemic illness (with fever, chills, and myalgias) that has no obvious primary source; this manifestation is especially common among compromised hosts. Secondary seeding of an organ (e.g., meninges, brain, bone, urinary tract, or soft tissue) complicates the course, which may be fulminant. *C. fetus* infections have a tropism for vascular sites: endocarditis, mycotic aneurysm, and septic thrombophlebitis may all occur. Infection during pregnancy often leads to fetal death. A variety of *Campylobacter* species and *H. cinaedi* can cause recurrent cellulitis with fever and bacteremia in immunocompromised hosts.

COMPLICATIONS

Except in infection with *C. fetus*, bacteremia is uncommon, developing most often in immunocompromised hosts and at the extremes of age. Three patterns of extraintestinal infection have been noted: (1) transient bacteremia in a normal host with enteritis (benign course, no specific treatment needed); (2) sustained bacteremia or focal infection in a normal host (bacteremia originating from enteritis, with patients responding well to antimicrobial therapy); and (3) sustained bacteremia or focal infection in a compromised host. Enteritis may not be clinically apparent. Antimicrobial therapy, possibly prolonged, is necessary for suppression or cure of these infections.

Campylobacter, Arcobacter, and intestinal *Helicobacter* infections in patients with AIDS or immunoglobulin-deficient patients (most often common variable immunodeficiency) may be severe, persistent, and extraintestinal; relapse after cessation of therapy is common. Immunoglobulin-deficient patients also may develop osteomyelitis and an erysipelas-like rash or cellulitis.

Local suppurative complications of infection include cholecystitis, pancreatitis, and cystitis; distant complications include meningitis, endocarditis, arthritis, peritonitis, cellulitis, and septic abortion. All these complications are rare, except in immunocompromised hosts. Hepatitis, interstitial nephritis, and the hemolytic-uremic syndrome occasionally complicate acute infection. The two most common postinfectious sequelae are reactive arthritis and Guillain-Barré syndrome. Reactive arthritis has been reported in up to 2.5% of cases, although nonspecific rheumatologic symptoms are more common (~10%). Reactive arthritis may develop several weeks after infection, especially in persons with the HLA-B27 phenotype. The knees are most frequently involved, but involvement of the ankles, wrists, and small joints of the hands is common, with an average of 3.2 joints affected. Guillain-Barré syndrome or its Miller Fisher (cranial polyneuropathy) variant follow either symptomatic or asymptomatic *Campylobacter* infections uncommonly—i.e., in 1 of every 1000–2000 cases or, for certain *C. jejuni* serotypes (such as O19), in 1 of every 100–200 cases. Despite the low frequency of this complication, it is estimated that *Campylobacter* infections, because of their high incidence, may trigger 20–40% of all cases of Guillain-Barré syndrome. The presence of sialylated lipopolysaccharides on *C. jejuni* strains prompts a form of molecular mimicry that promotes autoimmune recognition of sialylated cell-surface molecules on axons. Immunoproliferative small-intestinal disease (*alpha chain disease*), a form of lymphoma that originates in small-intestinal mucosa-associated lymphoid tissue (MALToma), has been associated with *C. jejuni*; antimicrobial therapy has led to marked clinical improvement.

DIAGNOSIS

In patients with *Campylobacter* enteritis, peripheral leukocyte counts reflect the severity of the inflammatory process. In addition, stools from nearly all *Campylobacter*-infected patients presenting for medical attention in the United States contain leukocytes or erythrocytes. Gram- or Wright-stained fecal smears should be examined in all suspected cases. When the diagnosis of *Campylobacter* enteritis is suspected on the basis of findings indicating inflammatory diarrhea (fever, fecal leukocytes), clinicians can ask the microbiology laboratory to attempt the visualization of organisms with characteristic vibrioid morphology by direct microscopic examination of stools with Gram's staining or to use phase-contrast or dark-field microscopy to identify the organisms' characteristic "darting" motility. Confirmation of the diagnosis of *Campylobacter* infection is based on identification of an isolate from cultures of stool, blood, or another site; specific species can be identified by MALDI-TOF (matrix-assisted laser desorption/ionization–time of flight) mass spectrometry. *Campylobacter*-specific media should be used to culture stools from all patients with inflammatory or bloody diarrhea. Because all *Campylobacter* species are fastidious, they will not be isolated unless selective media or other selective techniques are used. Failure to isolate campylobacters from stool by culture does not entirely rule out their presence. Although culture remains the diagnostic gold standard, species-specific real-time polymerase chain reaction (PCR) techniques appear more sensitive than culture. Although PCR and other culture-independent diagnostic test (CIDTs), including antigen detection tests, may detect nonviable bacteria and may be falsely positive, they are now used frequently to diagnose infection with *Campylobacter* and other enteric bacteria in clinical microbiology laboratories. The detection of the organisms in stool in the United States by culture almost always implies active or recent infection, but CIDT positivity is more questionable.

In any event, follow-up testing after the clinical resolution of an acute infection is rarely needed. *Campylobacter sputorum* and related organisms found in the oral cavity are commensals that only rarely have pathogenic significance. Because of the low levels of metabolic activity of *Campylobacter* species in standard blood culture media, *Campylobacter* bacteremia is difficult to detect.

DIFFERENTIAL DIAGNOSIS

The symptoms of *Campylobacter* enteritis are not sufficiently unusual to distinguish this illness from that due to *Salmonella, Shigella, Yersinia,* enterohemorrhagic *Escherichia coli,* and other pathogens. The combination of fever and fecal leukocytes or erythrocytes is indicative of inflammatory diarrhea, and definitive diagnosis is based on culture, CIDTs, or demonstration of the characteristic organisms on stained fecal smears. Extraintestinal *Campylobacter* illness is diagnosed by culture. Infection due to *Campylobacter* should be suspected in the setting of septic abortion, and that due to *C. fetus* should be suspected specifically in the setting of septic thrombophlebitis. It is important to reiterate that (1) the presentation of *Campylobacter* enteritis may mimic that of ulcerative colitis or Crohn's disease, (2) *Campylobacter* enteritis is much more common than either of the latter (especially among young adults), and (3) biopsy may not distinguish among these entities. Thus, a diagnosis of inflammatory bowel disease should not be made until *Campylobacter* infection has been ruled out, especially in persons with a history of foreign travel, significant animal contact, immunodeficiency, or exposure incurring a high risk of transmission.

TREATMENT
Campylobacter Infection

Fluid and electrolyte replacement is central to the treatment of diarrheal illnesses (**Chap. 133**). Even among patients presenting for medical attention with *Campylobacter* enteritis, not all clearly benefit from specific antimicrobial therapy. Indications for therapy include high fever, bloody diarrhea, severe diarrhea, persistence for >1 week, and worsening of symptoms. A 3-day course of azithromycin (500 mg once daily) is the regimen of choice. A 1-day regimen of azithromycin (1000 mg given as two 500-mg tablets) can also be used. Alternative regimens for adults consist of fluoroquinolones—ciprofloxacin (500 mg by mouth twice daily for 3 days) or levofloxacin (750 mg daily for 3 days)—but resistance to this class of agents as well as to tetracyclines is substantial; ~27% of U.S. human isolates of *Campylobacter* in 2014 were resistant to ciprofloxacin, and rates are higher in many other countries; thus, travel-related *Campylobacter* infections should be considered a priori to be fluoroquinolone-resistant. Because macrolide resistance usually is much less common (<10%), these drugs are the empirical agents of choice. Patients infected with antibiotic-resistant strains are at increased risk of adverse outcomes. Use of antimotility agents, which may prolong the duration of symptoms and have been associated with toxic megacolon and with death, is not recommended. Of note, *C. jejuni* and *C. coli* are resistant to trimethoprim and β-lactam antibiotics, including penicillin and most cephalosporins.

For patients with immunocompromising conditions and uncomplicated enteritis caused by *C. jejuni*, therapy duration should be extended to 7–14 days. For systemic infections, treatment with a carbapenem (imipenem, 500 mg IV every 6 h; or meropenem, 1–2 g IV every 8 h) should be started empirically, and susceptibility testing should always be performed. For life-threatening illness, gentamicin (1.0–1.7 mg/kg IV every 8 h after a loading dose of 1.5–2 mg/kg) can be added. In the absence of endovascular involvement, therapy for systemic infections should be administered for 7–14 days. For immunocompromised patients with systemic infections due to *C. fetus* and for patients with endovascular infections due to any species, prolonged therapy (up to 4 weeks) is usually necessary. For recurrent infections in immunocompromised hosts, lifelong therapy/prophylaxis is sometimes necessary.

■ PROGNOSIS

Nearly all patients recover fully from *Campylobacter* enteritis, either spontaneously or after antimicrobial therapy. Volume depletion probably contributes to the few deaths that are reported. As stated above, occasional patients develop reactive arthritis or Guillain-Barré syndrome or its variants. Systemic infection with *C. fetus* is much more often fatal than that due to related species; this higher mortality rate reflects in part the population affected. Prognosis depends on the rapidity with which appropriate therapy is begun. Otherwise healthy hosts usually survive *C. fetus* infections without sequelae. Compromised hosts often have recurrent and/or life-threatening infections due to a variety of *Campylobacter* species.

■ FURTHER READING

Amour C et al: Epidemiology and impact of *Campylobacter* infection in children in 8 low-resource settings: Results from the MAL-ED Study. Clin Infect Dis 63:1171, 2016.

Costa D, Iraola G: Pathogenomics of emerging *Campylobacter* Species. Clin Microbiol Rev 32:e00072, 2019.

Dai L et al: New and alternative strategies for the prevention, control, and treatment of antibiotic-resistant *Campylobacter*. Transl Res 223:76, 2020.

Fernández-Cruz A et al: *Campylobacter* bacteremia: Clinical characteristics, incidence, and outcome over 23 years. Medicine (Baltimore) 89:319, 2010.

Man SM: The clinical importance of emerging *Campylobacter* species. Nat Rev Gastroenterol Hepatol 8:669, 2011.

Marder EP et al: Incidence and trends of infections with pathogens transmitted commonly through food and the effect of increasing use of culture-independent diagnostic tests on surveillance—Foodborne Diseases Active Surveillance Network, 10 U.S. sites, 2013–2016. Morb Mortal Wkly Rep 66:397, 2017.

Montgomery MP et al: Multidrug-resistant *Campylobacter jejuni* outbreak linked to puppy exposure–United States, 2016-2018. Morb Mortal Wkly Rep 67:1032, 2018.

Riddle MS et al: ACG clinical guideline: Diagnosis, treatment, and prevention of acute diarrheal infections in adults. Am J Gastroenterol 111:602, 2016.

Same RG, Tamma PD: *Campylobacter jejuni* infections in children. Pediatr Rev 39:533, 2018.

Ternhag A et al: A meta-analysis of the effects of antibiotic treatment on duration of symptoms caused by infection with *Campylobacter* species. Clin Infect Dis 44:696, 2007.

168 Cholera and Other Vibrioses

Matthew K. Waldor, Edward T. Ryan

Members of the genus *Vibrio* cause a number of important infectious syndromes. Classic among them is cholera, a devastating diarrheal disease caused by *Vibrio cholerae* that has been responsible for seven global pandemics and much suffering over the past two centuries. Epidemic cholera remains a significant public-health concern in the developing world today. Other vibrioses caused by other *Vibrio* species include syndromes of diarrhea, soft tissue infection, or primary sepsis. All *Vibrio* species are highly motile, facultatively anaerobic, curved gram-negative rods with one or more flagella. In nature, vibrios most commonly reside in tidal rivers and bays under conditions of moderate salinity. They proliferate in the summer months when water temperatures exceed 20°C. As might be expected, the illnesses they cause also increase in frequency during the warm months.

CHOLERA

■ DEFINITION

Cholera is an acute diarrheal disease that can, in a matter of hours, result in profound, rapidly progressive dehydration and death. Accordingly, *cholera gravis* (the severe form) is a much-feared disease, particularly in its epidemic presentation. Fortunately, prompt aggressive fluid repletion and supportive care can obviate the high mortality that is historically associated with cholera. Although the term *cholera* has occasionally been applied to any severely dehydrating secretory diarrheal illness, whether infectious in etiology or not, it now refers to disease caused by *V. cholerae* serogroup O1 or O139—i.e., the serogroups with epidemic potential.

■ MICROBIOLOGY AND EPIDEMIOLOGY

The species *V. cholerae* is classified into >200 serogroups based on the carbohydrate constituents of their lipopolysaccharide (LPS) O antigens. Although some non-O1 *V. cholerae* serogroups (strains that do not agglutinate in antisera to the O1 group antigen) have occasionally caused sporadic outbreaks of diarrhea, serogroup O1 was, until the emergence of serogroup O139 in 1992 (see below), the exclusive cause of epidemic cholera. The O1 serogroup is further subdivided into two serotypes, termed *Inaba* and *Ogawa*. Two biotypes of *V. cholerae* O1, classical and El Tor, have been described, but the former is thought to be extinct.

The natural habitat of *V. cholerae* is coastal salt water and brackish estuaries, where the organism lives in close relation to plankton. *V. cholerae* can also exist in freshwater in the presence of adequate nutrients and warmth. Humans become infected incidentally but, once infected, can act as vehicles for spread. Ingestion of water contaminated by human feces is the most common means of acquisition of *V. cholerae*. Consumption of contaminated food also can contribute to spread. There is no known animal reservoir. Although the infectious dose is relatively high, it is markedly reduced in hypochlorhydric persons, in those using antacids, and when gastric acidity is buffered by a meal. Cholera is predominantly a pediatric disease in endemic areas, but it affects adults and children equally when newly introduced into a population. In endemic areas, the burden of disease is often greatest during "cholera seasons" associated with high temperatures, heavy rainfall, and flooding, but cholera can occur year-round.

Cholera is native to the Ganges delta on the Indian subcontinent. Since 1817, seven global pandemics have occurred. The current (seventh) pandemic—the first due to the El Tor biotype—began in Indonesia in 1961 and spread in serial waves throughout Asia as *V. cholerae* El Tor displaced the endemic classical biotype, which is thought to have caused the previous six pandemics. In the early 1970s, El Tor cholera erupted in Africa, causing major epidemics before becoming a persistent endemic problem. Currently, >95% of cholera cases reported annually to the World Health Organization (WHO) are from Africa and Asia (**Fig. 168-1**), but the true burden and distribution of cholera are unknown because the diagnosis is often syndromic and many countries with endemic cholera do not report cholera to the WHO. It is possible that >1–4 million cases of cholera occur yearly (of which only ~200,000 are reported to the WHO) and that these cases result in >20,000–140,000 deaths annually (of which <2000 are reported to the WHO).

After a century without cholera in Latin America, the current cholera pandemic reached Central and South America in 1991. Following an initial explosive spread that affected millions, the burden of disease has markedly decreased in Latin America. In 2010, a severe cholera outbreak began in Haiti, a country with no recorded history of this disease. Several lines of evidence indicate that cholera was likely introduced into Haiti by United Nations security forces from Asia, raising the possibility that asymptomatic carriers of *V. cholerae* play an important role in transmitting cholera over long distances. The Haitian outbreak involved >800,000 individuals, resulting in thousands of deaths. In 2016, an outbreak of cholera occurred in Yemen in the setting of a civil war and population displacement and the breakdown of health infrastructure. The outbreak is still ongoing and has resulted

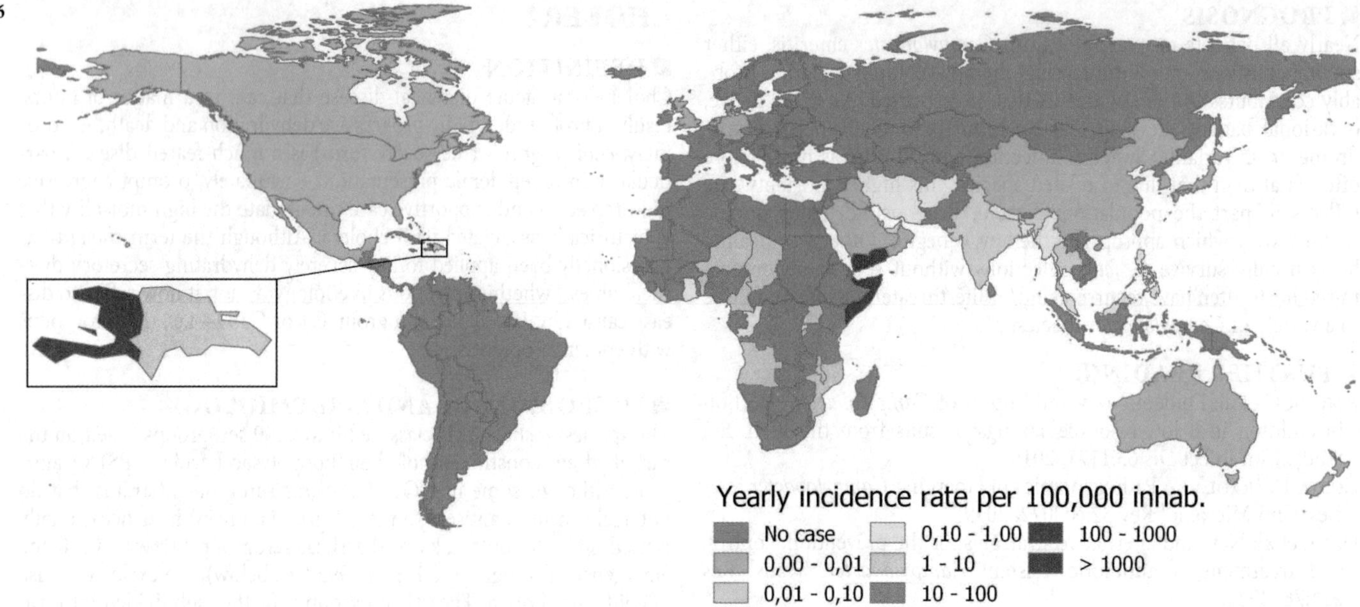

FIGURE 168-1 World distribution of cholera in 2016–2018. WHO, World Health Organization. *(Reproduced with permission from Dr. M. Piarroux, Université de la Méditerranée, France.)*

in over 1.2 million cases and thousands of deaths. The recent history of cholera has been punctuated by such severe outbreaks, especially among impoverished or displaced persons. These outbreaks are often precipitated by war or other circumstances that lead to the breakdown of public-health measures. Such was similarly the case in the camps for Rwandan refugees set up in 1994 around Goma, Zaire; in 2008–2009 in Zimbabwe; and in 2015 in South Sudan and the Democratic Republic of the Congo.

Sporadic endemic infections due to *V. cholerae* O1 strains related to the seventh-pandemic strain have been recognized along the U.S. Gulf Coast of Louisiana and Texas. These infections are typically associated with the consumption of contaminated, locally harvested shellfish. Occasionally, cases in U.S. locations remote from the Gulf Coast have been linked to shipped-in Gulf Coast seafood.

In October 1992, a large-scale outbreak of clinical cholera caused by a new serogroup, O139, occurred in southeastern India. The organism appears to be a derivative of El Tor O1 but has a distinct LPS and an immunologically related O-antigen polysaccharide capsule. (O1 organisms are not encapsulated.) After an initial spread across 11 Asian countries, *V. cholerae* O139 has once again been almost entirely replaced by O1 strains. The clinical manifestations of disease caused by *V. cholerae* O139 are indistinguishable from those of O1 cholera. Immunity to one, however, is not protective against the other.

■ PATHOGENESIS

In the final analysis, cholera is a toxin-mediated disease. The watery diarrhea characteristic of cholera is due to the action of cholera toxin, a potent protein enterotoxin elaborated by the organism in the small intestine. The toxin-coregulated pilus (TCP), so named because its synthesis is regulated in parallel with that of cholera toxin, is essential for *V. cholerae* to survive and multiply in (colonize) the small intestine. Production of cholera toxin, TCP, and several other virulence factors are coordinately regulated by ToxR. This protein modulates the expression of genes coding for virulence factors in response to environmental signals via a cascade of regulatory proteins. Additional regulatory processes, including bacterial responses to the density of the bacterial population (in a phenomenon known as *quorum sensing*), modulate the virulence of *V. cholerae*.

Once established in the human small bowel, the organism produces cholera toxin, which consists of a monomeric enzymatic moiety (the A subunit) and a pentameric binding moiety (the B subunit). The B pentamer binds to GM_1 ganglioside, a glycolipid on the surface of epithelial cells that serves as the toxin receptor and makes possible the delivery of the A subunit to its cytosolic target. The activated A subunit (A_1) irreversibly transfers ADP-ribose from nicotinamide adenine dinucleotide to its specific target protein, the GTP-binding regulatory component of adenylate cyclase. The ADP-ribosylated G protein upregulates the activity of adenylate cyclase; the result is the intracellular accumulation of high levels of cyclic adenosine monophosphate (AMP). In intestinal epithelial cells, cyclic AMP inhibits the absorptive sodium-transport system in villus cells and activates the secretory chloride-transport system in crypt cells, and these events lead to the accumulation of sodium chloride in the intestinal lumen. Because water moves passively to maintain osmolality, isotonic fluid accumulates in the lumen. When the volume of that fluid exceeds the capacity of the rest of the gut to resorb it, watery diarrhea results. Unless the wasted fluid and electrolytes are adequately replaced, shock (due to profound dehydration) and acidosis (due to loss of bicarbonate) follow. Although perturbation of the adenylate cyclase pathway is the primary mechanism by which cholera toxin causes excess fluid secretion, cholera toxin also enhances intestinal secretion via prostaglandins and/or neural histamine receptors.

The *V. cholerae* genome is composed of two circular chromosomes. Lateral gene transfer has played a key role in the evolution of epidemic *V. cholerae*. The genes encoding cholera toxin (*ctxAB*) are part of the genome of a bacteriophage, CTXΦ. The receptor for this phage on the *V. cholerae* surface is the intestinal colonization factor TCP. Because *ctxAB* is part of a mobile genetic element (CTXΦ), horizontal transfer of this bacteriophage may account for the emergence of new toxigenic *V. cholerae* serogroups. Many of the other genes important for *V. cholerae* pathogenicity, including the genes encoding the biosynthesis of TCP, those encoding accessory colonization factors, and those regulating virulence gene expression, are clustered together in the *V. cholerae* pathogenicity island. Similar clustering of virulence genes is found in other bacterial pathogens. It is believed that pathogenicity islands are acquired by horizontal gene transfer. *V. cholerae* O139 is probably derived from an El Tor O1 strain that acquired the genes for O139 O-antigen synthesis by horizontal gene transfer.

■ CLINICAL MANIFESTATIONS

Individuals infected with *V. cholerae* O1 or O139 exhibit a range of clinical manifestations. Some individuals are asymptomatic or have only mild diarrhea; others present with the sudden onset of explosive and life-threatening diarrhea (*cholera gravis*). The reasons for the range in signs and symptoms of disease are incompletely understood

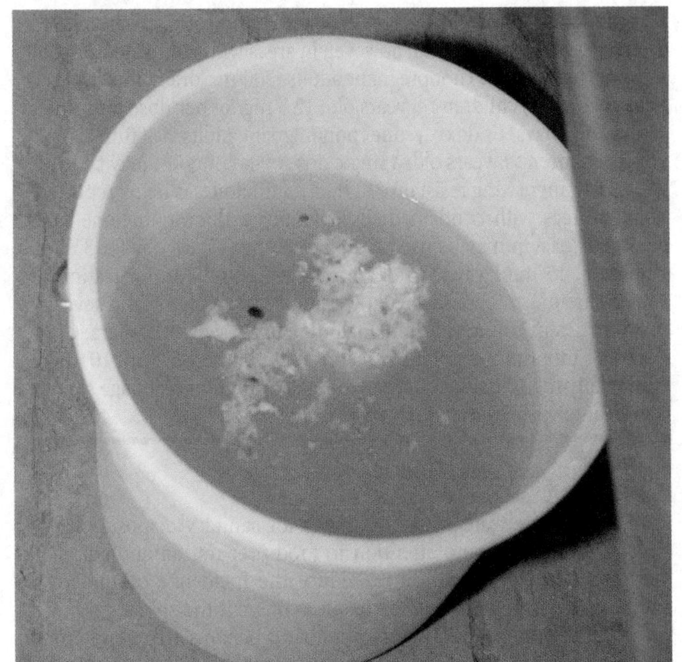

FIGURE 168-2 Rice-water cholera stool. Note floating mucus and gray watery appearance. *(Courtesy of Dr. A. S. G. Faruque, International Centre for Diarrhoeal Disease Research, Dhaka; with permission.)*

but include the level of preexisting immunity, blood type (persons with type O blood are at greatest risk of severe disease if infected, whereas those with type AB are at least risk), and nutritional status. In a nonimmune individual, after a 24- to 48-h incubation period, cholera characteristically begins with the sudden onset of painless watery diarrhea that may quickly become voluminous. Patients often vomit. In severe cases, volume loss can exceed 250 mL/kg in the first 24 h. If fluids and electrolytes are not replaced, hypovolemic shock and death may ensue. Fever is usually absent. Muscle cramps due to electrolyte disturbances are common. The stool has a characteristic appearance: a nonbilious, gray, slightly cloudy fluid with flecks of mucus, no blood, and a somewhat fishy, inoffensive odor. It has been called "rice-water" stool because of its resemblance to the water in which rice has been washed (**Fig. 168-2**). Clinical symptoms parallel volume contraction: at losses of <5% of normal body weight, thirst develops; at 5–10%, postural hypotension, weakness, tachycardia, and decreased skin turgor are documented; and at >10%, oliguria, weak or absent pulses, sunken eyes (and, in infants, sunken fontanelles), wrinkled ("washerwoman") skin, somnolence, and coma are characteristic. Complications derive exclusively from the effects of volume and electrolyte depletion and include renal failure due to acute tubular necrosis. Thus, if the patient is adequately treated with fluid and electrolytes, complications are averted and the process is self-limited, resolving in a few days.

Laboratory data usually reveal an elevated hematocrit (due to hemoconcentration) in nonanemic patients; mild neutrophilic leukocytosis; elevated levels of blood urea nitrogen and creatinine consistent with prerenal azotemia; normal sodium, potassium, and chloride levels; a markedly reduced bicarbonate level (<15 mmol/L); and an elevated anion gap (due to increases in serum lactate, protein, and phosphate). Arterial pH is usually low (~7.2).

DIAGNOSIS

Cholera should be suspected when a patient ≥5 years of age develops acute watery diarrhea in an area known to have cholera or develops severe dehydration or dies from acute watery diarrhea, even in an area where cholera is not known to be present. The clinical suspicion of cholera can be confirmed by the identification of *V. cholerae* in stool; however, the organism must be specifically sought. With experience, it can be detected directly by dark-field microscopy on a wet mount of fresh stool, and its serotype can be discerned by immobilization with specific antisera. Laboratory isolation of the organism requires the use of a selective medium such as taurocholate-tellurite-gelatin (TTG) agar or thiosulfate-citrate-bile salts-sucrose (TCBS) agar. If a delay in sample processing is expected, Carey-Blair transport medium and/or alkaline-peptone water-enrichment medium may be used as well. In endemic areas, there is little need for biochemical confirmation and characterization, although these tasks may be worthwhile in places where *V. cholerae* is an uncommon isolate. Standard microbiologic biochemical testing for Enterobacteriaceae will suffice for identification of *V. cholerae*. All vibrios are oxidase-positive. Point-of-care antigen-detection cholera dipstick assays are now commercially available for use in the field or where laboratory facilities are lacking.

TABLE 168-1 Assessing the Degree of Dehydration in Patients with Cholera

DEGREE OF DEHYDRATION	CLINICAL FINDINGS
None or mild, but diarrhea	Thirst in some cases; <5% loss of total body weight
Moderate	Thirst, postural hypotension, weakness, tachycardia, decreased skin turgor, dry mouth/tongue, no tears; 5–10% loss of total body weight
Severe	Unconsciousness, lethargy, or "floppiness"; weak or absent pulse; inability to drink; sunken eyes (and, in infants, sunken fontanelles); >10% loss of total body weight

TREATMENT

Cholera

Death from cholera is due to hypovolemic shock; thus, treatment of individuals with cholera first and foremost requires fluid resuscitation and management. In light of the level of dehydration (**Table 168-1**) and the patient's age and weight, euvolemia should first be rapidly restored, and adequate hydration should then be maintained to replace ongoing fluid losses (**Table 168-2**). Administration of oral rehydration solution (ORS) takes advantage of the

TABLE 168-2 Treatment of Cholera, Based on Degree of Dehydration[a]

DEGREE OF DEHYDRATION, PATIENT'S AGE (WEIGHT)	TREATMENT[b]
None or Mild, but Diarrhea[c]	
<2 years	1/4–1/2 cup (50–100 mL) of ORS, to a maximum of 0.5 L/d
2–9 years	1/2–1 cup (100–200 mL) of ORS, to a maximum of 1 L/d
≥10 years	As much ORS as desired, to a maximum of 2 L/d
Moderate[c,d]	
<4 months (<5 kg)	200–400 mL of ORS
4–11 months (5–<8 kg)	400–600 mL of ORS
12–23 months (8–<11 kg)	600–800 mL of ORS
2–4 years (11–<16 kg)	800–1200 mL of ORS
5–14 years (16–<30 kg)	1200–2200 mL of ORS
≥15 years (≥30 kg)	2200–4000 mL of ORS
Severe[c]	
All ages and weights	Undertake IV fluid replacement with Ringer's lactate (or, if not available, normal saline). Give 100 mL/kg in the first 3-h period (or the first 6-h period for children <12 months old); start rapidly, then slow down. Give a total of 200 mL/kg in the first 24 h. Continue until the patient is awake, can ingest ORS, and no longer has a weak pulse.

[a]Adapted from World Health Organization: First steps for managing an outbreak of acute diarrhoea. Global Task Force on Cholera Control, 2009 (updated 2010; *http://www.who.int/cholera/publications/firststeps/en/*). [b]Continue normal feeding during treatment. [c]Reassess regularly; monitor stool and vomit output. [d]Volumes of ORS listed should be given within the first 4 h.

Abbreviation: ORS, oral rehydration solution.

TABLE 168-3 Composition of World Health Organization Reduced-Osmolarity Oral Rehydration Solution (ORS)[a,b]

CONSTITUENT	CONCENTRATION, mmol/L
Na^+	75
K^+	20
Cl^-	65
Citrate[c]	10
Glucose	75
Total osmolarity	245

[a]Contains (per package, to be added to 1 L of drinking water): NaCl, 2.6 g; $Na_3C_6H_5O_7 \cdot 2H_2O$, 2.9 g; KCl, 1.5 g; and glucose (anhydrous), 13.5 g. [b]If prepackaged ORS is unavailable, a simple homemade alternative can be prepared by combining 3.5 g (~1/2 teaspoon) of NaCl with either 50 g of precooked rice cereal or 6 teaspoons of table sugar (sucrose) in 1 L of drinking water. In that case, potassium must be supplied separately (e.g., in orange juice or coconut water). [c]10 mmol of citrate per liter, which supplies 30 mmol of HCO_3/L.

hexose-Na^+ co-transport mechanism to move Na^+ across the gut mucosa together with an actively transported molecule such as glucose (or galactose); Cl^- and water follow. This transport mechanism remains intact even when cholera toxin is active. ORS may be made by adding safe water to prepackaged sachets containing salts and sugar or by adding 0.5 teaspoon (i.e., a small spoonful) of table salt and 6 level teaspoons (i.e., 6 small spoonfuls) of table sugar to 1 L of safe water. Potassium intake in bananas or green coconut water should be encouraged. A number of ORS formulations are available, and the WHO now recommends "low-osmolarity" ORS for treatment of individuals with dehydrating diarrhea of any cause (**Table 168-3**). If available, rice-based ORS is considered superior to standard ORS in the treatment of cholera. ORS can be administered via a nasogastric tube to individuals who cannot ingest fluid; however, optimal management of individuals with severe dehydration includes the administration of IV fluid and electrolytes. Because profound acidosis (pH <7.2) is common in this group, Ringer's lactate is the best choice among commercial products (**Table 168-4**); it must be used with additional potassium supplements, preferably given by mouth. The total fluid deficit in severely dehydrated patients (>10% of body weight) can be replaced safely within the first 3–4 h of therapy, half within the first hour. Transient muscle cramps and tetany are common. Thereafter, oral therapy can usually be initiated, with the goal of maintaining fluid intake equal to fluid output. However, patients with continued large-volume diarrhea may require prolonged IV treatment to match gastrointestinal fluid losses. Severe hypokalemia can develop but will respond to potassium given either IV or orally. In the absence of adequate staff to monitor the patient's progress, the oral route of rehydration and potassium replacement is safer than the IV route.

Although not necessary for cure, the use of an antibiotic to which the organism is susceptible diminishes the duration and volume of fluid loss and hastens clearance of the organism from the stool. Adjunctive antibiotics should therefore be administered to patients with moderate or severe dehydration due to cholera. In many areas, macrolides such as erythromycin (adults, 250 mg orally four times a day for 3 days; children, 12.5 mg/kg per dose four times a day for 3 days) or azithromycin (adults, a single 1-g dose; children, a single 20-mg/kg dose) are the agents of choice. Increasing resistance to tetracyclines is widespread; however, in areas with confirmed susceptibility, tetracycline (nonpregnant adults, 500 mg orally four times a day for 3 days; children >8 years old, 12.5 mg/kg per dose four times a day for 3 days) or doxycycline (nonpregnant adults, a 300-mg single dose; children >8 years old, a single dose of 4–6 mg/kg) may be used. Similarly, increasing resistance to fluoroquinolones is being reported, but in areas with confirmed susceptibility, a fluoroquinolone such as ciprofloxacin may be used (adults, 500 mg twice a day for 3 days; children, 15 mg/kg twice a day for 3 days). Oral administration of supplemental zinc is associated with decreased volume and severity of diarrhea in young children, including in those with cholera. Children <6 months of age with cholera should be treated with 10 mg of zinc daily for 10 days; children from 6 to <60 months of age should be treated with 20 mg of oral zinc daily for 10 days.

TABLE 168-4 Electrolyte Composition of Cholera Stool and of Intravenous Rehydration Solution

	CONCENTRATION, mmol/L			
SUBSTANCE	NA+	K+	CL−	BASE
Stool				
Adult	135	15	100	45
Child	100	25	90	30
Ringer's lactate	130	4[a]	109	28

[a]Potassium supplements, preferably administered by mouth, are required to replace the usual potassium losses from stool.

PREVENTION

Provision of safe water and of facilities for sanitary disposal of feces, improved nutrition, and attention to food preparation and storage in the household can significantly reduce the incidence of cholera. In addition, precautions should be taken to prevent the spread of cholera via infected and potentially asymptomatic persons from endemic to nonendemic regions of the world (as was probably the case in the outbreak in Haiti; see "Microbiology and Epidemiology," above).

Much effort has been devoted to the development of an effective cholera vaccine over the past few decades, with a particular focus on oral vaccine strains. In an attempt to maximize mucosal responses, two types of oral cholera vaccine have been developed: oral killed vaccines and live attenuated vaccines. Currently, three oral killed cholera vaccines have been prequalified by the WHO and are available internationally. BivWC (Shanchol™; Shantha Biotechnics, Hyderabad, India) contains both biotypes and serotypes of *V. cholerae* O1 and *V. cholerae* O139 without supplemental cholera toxin B subunit. A related vaccine is produced in South Korea (Euvichol™, Euvichol-Plus™; Eubiologics, Seoul). WC-rBS (Dukoral®; Valneva, Lyon, France) contains both biotypes and serotypes of *V. cholerae* O1 supplemented with 1 mg of recombinant cholera toxin B subunit per dose. The vaccines are administered as a two- or three-dose regimen, with doses usually separated by 14 days. They provide ~60–85% protection for the first few months. Booster immunizations of WC-rBS are recommended after 2 years for individuals ≥6 years of age and after 6 months for children 2–5 years of age. For BivWC, which was developed more recently, no formal recommendation regarding booster immunizations exists. However, BivWC was associated with ~60% protection over 5 years among recipients of all ages in a study in Kolkata, India; the rate of protection among children ≤5 years of age approximated 40%. In outbreak situations, even a single dose of BivWC can provide some protection: 40% and 63% adjusted protection for 6 months for all and severely dehydrating cholera, respectively; although there was no evidence of protection in children younger than 5 years of age. Models predict significant herd immunity when vaccination coverage rates exceed 50%. The killed vaccines have been safely administered among populations with high rates of HIV infection.

Oral live attenuated vaccines for *V. cholerae* O1 are also in development. These strains have in common their lack of the genes encoding cholera toxin. One such vaccine, CVD 103-HgR (Vaxchora™; PaxVax, Redwood City, CA), is approved by the U.S. Food and Drug Administration for use in travelers to cholera-endemic regions. The vaccine was 90 and 80% efficacious against severe cholera after experimental infection of North American volunteers 10 days and 90 days after vaccination, respectively. Vaxchora is approved for use in individuals 2–64 years of age; no recommendations concerning the timing or need for booster vaccinations are currently available. Other live attenuated vaccine candidate strains have been prepared from El Tor and O139 *V. cholerae* and have been tested in studies of volunteers. An advantage of live attenuated cholera vaccines is that they may induce protection after a single oral dose. Conjugate and subunit cholera vaccines are also being developed.

Recognizing that it may be decades before safe water and adequate sanitation become a reality for those most at risk of cholera, the WHO has recommended incorporation of cholera vaccination into comprehensive control strategies and has established an international stockpile of oral killed cholera vaccine to assist in outbreak responses. A global strategy on cholera control was launched in 2017. This country-by-country approach aims to reduce cholera deaths by 90% and to eliminate cholera in as many as 20 countries by 2030. Integral components of this strategy are advancing water, sanitation, and hygiene (WASH) programs, as well as use of cholera vaccine. From 2016–2020, >64 million doses of cholera vaccine have been requested from the Global Vaccine Stockpile, and >33 million doses have been shipped to requesting countries for use in control programs.

OTHER *VIBRIO* SPECIES

The genus *Vibrio* includes several human pathogens that do not cause cholera. Abundant in coastal waters throughout the world, noncholera vibrios can reach high concentrations in the tissues of filter-feeding mollusks. As a result, human infection commonly follows the ingestion of seawater or of raw or undercooked shellfish (**Table 168-5**). Most noncholera vibrios can be cultured on blood or MacConkey agar, which contains enough salt to support the growth of these halophilic species. In the microbiology laboratory, the species of noncholera vibrios are distinguished by standard biochemical tests. The most important of these organisms are *Vibrio parahaemolyticus* and *Vibrio vulnificus*. Vibriosis causes an estimated 80,000 illnesses and 100 deaths in the United States every year.

The two major types of syndromes for which these noncholera vibrios are responsible are gastrointestinal illness (due to *V. parahaemolyticus*, non-O1/O139 *V. cholerae*, *Vibrio mimicus*, *Vibrio fluvialis*, *Vibrio hollisae*, and *Vibrio furnissii*) and soft tissue infections (due to *V. vulnificus*, *Vibrio alginolyticus*, and *Vibrio damselae*). *V. vulnificus* is also a cause of primary sepsis in some compromised individuals.

■ SPECIES ASSOCIATED PRIMARILY WITH GASTROINTESTINAL ILLNESS

V. parahaemolyticus Widespread in marine environments, the halophilic *V. parahaemolyticus* is the leading seafood-borne bacterial cause of enteritis worldwide. This species was originally implicated in enteritis in Japan in 1953, accounting for 24% of reported cases in one study—a rate that presumably was due to the common practice of eating raw seafood in that country. In the United States, common-source outbreaks of diarrhea caused by this organism have been linked to the consumption of undercooked or improperly handled seafood or of other foods contaminated by seawater. Since the mid-1990s, the incidence of *V. parahaemolyticus* infections has increased in several countries, including the United States. Serotypes O3:K6, O4:K68, and O1:K-untypable, which are genetically related to one another, account in part for this increase. The enteropathogenicity of *V. parahaemolyticus* is associated with its ability to cause hemolysis via a thermostable direct hemolysin (Vp-TDH). Although the mechanisms by which the organism causes diarrhea are not fully defined, most *V. parahaemolyticus* genomes encode two type III secretion systems, which directly inject toxic bacterial proteins into host cells. The activity of one of these secretion systems is required for intestinal colonization and virulence in animal models. *V. parahaemolyticus* should be considered a possible etiologic agent in all cases of diarrhea that can be linked epidemiologically to seafood consumption or to the sea itself. The incidence of *V. parahaemolyticus* infection in the United States may be increasing, with this species accounting for almost half of all *Vibrio* isolates reported in this country in 2014.

Infections with *V. parahaemolyticus* can result in two distinct gastrointestinal presentations. The more common of the two presentations (including nearly all cases in North America) is characterized by watery diarrhea, usually occurring in conjunction with abdominal cramps, nausea, and vomiting and accompanied in ~25% of cases by fever and chills. After an incubation period of 4 h to 4 days, symptoms develop and persist for a median of 3 days. Dysentery, the less common presentation, is characterized by severe abdominal cramps, nausea, vomiting, and bloody or mucoid stools. *V. parahaemolyticus* also causes rare cases of wound infection and otitis and very rare cases of sepsis.

Most cases of *V. parahaemolyticus*–associated gastrointestinal illness, regardless of the presentation, are self-limited. Fluid replacement should be stressed. Antimicrobial agents may be of benefit in moderate or severe disease. Doxycycline, fluoroquinolones, macrolides, or third-generation cephalosporins are usually used. Deaths are extremely rare among immunocompetent individuals. Severe infections are associated with underlying diseases, including diabetes, preexisting liver disease, iron-overload states, or immunosuppression.

Non-O1/O139 (Noncholera) *V. cholerae* The heterogeneous non-O1/O139 *V. cholerae* organisms cannot be distinguished from *V. cholerae* O1 or O139 by routine biochemical tests but do not agglutinate in O1 or O139 antiserum. Non-O1/O139 strains have caused several well-studied food-borne outbreaks of gastroenteritis and have also been responsible for sporadic cases of otitis media, wound infection, and bacteremia. Generally, non-O1/O139 *V. cholerae* strains do not produce cholera toxin and do not cause large epidemics of diarrheal disease. Like other vibrios, non-O1/O139 *V. cholerae* organisms are widely distributed in marine environments. In most instances, recognized cases in the United States have been associated with the consumption of raw oysters or with recent travel. The broad clinical spectrum of diarrheal illness caused by these organisms is probably due to the group's heterogeneous virulence attributes.

In the United States, about half of all non-O1/O139 *V. cholerae* isolates are from stool samples. The typical incubation period for gastroenteritis due to these organisms is <2 days, and the illness lasts for ~2–7 days. Patients' stools may be copious and watery or may be partly formed, less voluminous, and bloody or mucoid. Diarrhea can result in severe dehydration. Many cases include abdominal cramps, nausea, vomiting, and fever. Like those with cholera, patients who are seriously dehydrated should receive oral or IV fluids; the value of antibiotics is not clear.

Extraintestinal infections due to non-O1/O139 *V. cholerae* commonly follow occupational or recreational exposure to seawater.

TABLE 168-5 Features of Selected Noncholera Vibrioses

ORGANISM	VEHICLE OR ACTIVITY	HOST AT RISK	SYNDROME
Vibrio parahaemolyticus	Shellfish, seawater	Normal	Gastroenteritis
	Seawater	Normal	Wound infection
Non-01/0139 *Vibrio cholerae*	Shellfish, travel	Normal	Gastroenteritis
	Seawater	Normal	Wound infection, otitis media
Vibrio vulnificus	Shellfish	Immunosuppressed[a]	Sepsis, secondary cellulitis
	Seawater	Normal, immunosuppressed[a]	Wound infection, cellulitis
Vibrio alginolyticus	Seawater	Normal	Wound infection, cellulitis, otitis
	Seawater	Burned, other immunosuppressed	Sepsis

[a]Especially with liver disease or hemochromatosis.

Source: Table 161-3 in *Harrison's Principles of Internal Medicine*, 14th edition.

Around 10% of non-O1/O139 *V. cholerae* isolates come from cases of wound infection, 10% from cases of otitis media, and 20% from cases of bacteremia (which is particularly likely to develop in patients with liver disease). Extraintestinal infections should be treated with antibiotics. Information to guide antibiotic selection and dosing is limited, but most strains are sensitive in vitro to tetracycline, ciprofloxacin, and third-generation cephalosporins.

SPECIES ASSOCIATED PRIMARILY WITH SOFT TISSUE INFECTION OR BACTEREMIA

(See also Chap. 129)

V. vulnificus Infection with *V. vulnificus* is rare, but this organism is the most common cause of severe *Vibrio* infections in the United States. Like most vibrios, *V. vulnificus* proliferates in the warm summer months and requires a saline environment for growth. In the United States, infections in humans typically occur in coastal states between May and October and most commonly affect men >40 years of age. *V. vulnificus* has been linked to two distinct syndromes: primary sepsis, which usually occurs in patients with underlying liver disease, and primary wound infection, which generally affects people without underlying disease. (*Vulnificus* is Latin for "wound maker.") Some authors have suggested that *V. vulnificus* also causes gastroenteritis independent of other clinical manifestations. *V. vulnificus* is endowed with a number of virulence attributes, including a capsule that confers resistance to phagocytosis and to the bactericidal activity of human serum as well as a cytolysin. Measured as the 50% lethal dose in mice, the organism's virulence is considerably increased under conditions of iron overload; this observation is consistent with the propensity of *V. vulnificus* to infect patients who have hemochromatosis.

Primary sepsis most often develops in patients who have cirrhosis or hemochromatosis. However, *V. vulnificus* bacteremia can also affect individuals who have hematopoietic disorders or chronic renal insufficiency, those who are using immunosuppressive medications or alcohol, or (in rare instances) those who have no known underlying disease. After a median incubation period of 16 h, the patient develops malaise, chills, fever, and prostration. One-third of patients develop hypotension, which is often apparent at admission. Cutaneous manifestations develop in most cases (usually within 36 h of onset) and characteristically involve the extremities (the lower more often than the upper). In a common sequence, erythematous patches are followed by ecchymoses, vesicles, and bullae. In fact, sepsis and hemorrhagic bullous skin lesions suggest the diagnosis in appropriate settings. Necrosis and sloughing may also be evident. Laboratory studies reveal leukopenia more often than leukocytosis, thrombocytopenia, or elevated levels of fibrin-split products. *V. vulnificus* can be cultured from blood or cutaneous lesions. The mortality rate approaches 50%, with most deaths due to uncontrolled sepsis **(Chap. 304)**. Accordingly, prompt treatment is critical and should include empirical antibiotic administration, aggressive debridement, and general supportive care. *V. vulnificus* is sensitive in vitro to a number of antibiotics, including tetracycline, fluoroquinolones, and third-generation cephalosporins. Data from animal models suggest that either a fluoroquinolone or the combination of a tetracycline and a third-generation cephalosporin should be used in the treatment of *V. vulnificus* septicemia.

V. vulnificus–associated soft tissue infection can complicate either a fresh or an old wound that comes into contact with seawater; the patient may or may not have underlying disease. After a short incubation period (4 h to 4 days; mean, 12 h), the disease begins with swelling, erythema, and (in many cases) intense pain around the wound. These signs and symptoms are followed by cellulitis, which spreads rapidly and is sometimes accompanied by vesicular, bullous, or necrotic lesions. Metastatic events are uncommon. Most patients have fever and leukocytosis. *V. vulnificus* can be cultured from skin lesions and occasionally from the blood. Prompt antibiotic therapy and debridement are usually curative.

V. alginolyticus First identified as a pathogen of humans in 1973, *V. alginolyticus* occasionally causes eye, ear, and wound infections. This species is the most salt-tolerant of the vibrios and can grow in salt concentrations of >10%. Most clinical isolates come from superinfected wounds that presumably become contaminated at the beach. Although its severity varies, *V. alginolyticus* infection tends not to be serious and generally responds well to antibiotic therapy and drainage. Cases of otitis externa, otitis media, and conjunctivitis due to this pathogen have been described. Tetracycline treatment usually results in cure. *V. alginolyticus* is a rare cause of bacteremia in immunocompromised hosts.

FURTHER READING

Domman D et al: Integrated view of *Vibrio cholerae* in the Americas. Science 358:789, 2017.

Islam MS et al: Environmental reservoirs of *Vibrio cholera*. Vaccine 38(Suppl 1):A52, 2020.

Qadri F et al: Emergency deployment of oral cholera vaccine for the Rohingya in Bangladesh. Lancet 391:1877, 2018.

Qadri F et al: Efficacy of a single-dose regimen of inactivated whole-cell oral cholera vaccine: Results from 2 years of follow-up of a randomised trial. Lancet Infect Dis 18:666, 2018.

Weill FX et al: Genomic history of the seventh pandemic of cholera in Africa. Science 358:785, 2017.

World Health Organization: Cholera vaccines: WHO position paper. Wkly Epidemiol Rec 92:477, 2017.

169 Brucellosis

Nicholas J. Beeching

DEFINITION

Brucellosis is a bacterial zoonosis transmitted directly or indirectly to humans from infected animals, predominantly domesticated ruminants and swine. The disease is known colloquially as *undulant fever* because of its remittent character. Although brucellosis commonly presents as an acute febrile illness, its clinical manifestations vary widely, and definitive signs indicative of the diagnosis may be lacking. Thus the clinical diagnosis usually must be supported by the results of bacteriologic and/or serologic tests.

ETIOLOGIC AGENTS

Human brucellosis is caused by strains of *Brucella*, a bacterial genus that was previously suggested, on genetic grounds, to comprise a single species, *B. melitensis*, with a number of biologic variants exhibiting particular host preferences. This view was challenged on the basis of detailed differences in chromosomal structure and host preference. The traditional classification into nomen species is now favored both because of these differences and because this classification scheme closely reflects the epidemiologic patterns of the infection. The nomen system recognizes *B. melitensis*, which is the most common cause of symptomatic disease in humans and for which the main sources are sheep, goats, and camels; *B. abortus*, which is usually acquired from cattle or buffalo; *B. suis*, which is generally acquired from swine but has one variant enzootic in reindeer and caribou and another in rodents; and *B. canis*, which is acquired most often from dogs. *B. ovis*, which causes reproductive disease in sheep, has not been clearly implicated in human disease, while rare human infections have been reported with *B. neotomae*, which is found in desert rodents. Two relatively new species, *B. ceti* and *B. pinnipedialis*, have been identified in marine mammals, including seals and dolphins. At least one case of laboratory-acquired human disease due to one of these species has been described, and several cases of natural human infection have been reported. As infections in marine mammals appear to be widespread, more cases of zoonotic infection in humans may be identified. Other newly reported species include *B. microti* (isolated from field voles),

B. papionis (from baboons), *B. vulpis* (from foxes), and *B. inopinata* (from a patient with a breast implant). Additional novel strains have been described in diverse species, including frogs, bats, and various rodents, and the genus likely will expand further in forthcoming years. Moreover, it has become apparent that *Brucella* is closely related to the genus *Ochrobactrum*, which includes environmental bacteria sometimes associated with opportunistic infections. Genomics-based studies are beginning to elucidate the pathway of evolution from free-living soil bacteria to highly successful intracellular pathogens.

All brucellae are small, gram-negative, unencapsulated, nonsporulating rods or coccobacilli. They grow aerobically on peptone-based medium incubated at 37°C; the growth of some types is improved by supplementary CO_2. In vivo, brucellae behave as facultative intracellular parasites. The organisms are sensitive to sunlight, ionizing radiation, and moderate heat; they are killed by boiling and pasteurization but are resistant to freezing and drying. Their resistance to drying renders brucellae stable in aerosol form, facilitating airborne transmission. The organisms can survive for up to 2 months in soft cheeses made from goat's or sheep's milk; for at least 6 weeks in dry soil contaminated with infected urine, vaginal discharge, or placental or fetal tissues; and for at least 6 months in damp soil or liquid manure kept in cool dark conditions. Brucellae are easily killed by a wide range of common disinfectants used under optimal conditions but are likely to be much more resistant at low temperatures or in the presence of heavy organic contamination.

EPIDEMIOLOGY

Brucellosis is a zoonosis whose occurrence and control are closely related to its prevalence in domesticated animals. Its distribution is worldwide apart from the few countries where it has been eradicated from the animal reservoir. The true global prevalence of human brucellosis is unknown because of the imprecision of diagnosis and the inadequacy of reporting and surveillance systems in many countries. Recently, there has been increased recognition of the high incidence of brucellosis in India, Pakistan, Sri Lanka and parts of China, and of importations to countries in Oceania, such as Fiji, and in Asia, such as Thailand and Vietnam. In Europe, the incidence of brucellosis in a country is inversely related to gross domestic product, and, in both developed and less well-resourced settings, human brucellosis is related to rural poverty and inadequate access to medical care. Failure of veterinary control programs due to conflicts or for economic reasons contributes further to the emergence and re-emergence of disease, as seen currently in some eastern Mediterranean countries.

Even in well-resourced settings, the true incidence of brucellosis in domesticated animals may be 10–20 times higher than the reported figures. Bovine brucellosis has been the target of control programs in many parts of the world and has been eradicated from the cattle populations of much of northern Europe, Australia, New Zealand, and Canada, among other nations. Its incidence has been reduced to a low level in the United States and most western European countries, with a varied picture in other parts of the world. Efforts to eradicate *B. melitensis* infection from sheep and goat populations have been much less successful. These efforts have relied heavily on vaccination programs, which have tended to fluctuate with changing economic and political conditions. In some countries (e.g., Israel), *B. melitensis* has caused serious outbreaks in cattle. Infections with *B. melitensis* still pose a major public health problem in Mediterranean countries; in western, central, and southern Asia; and in parts of Africa and South and Central America. Infections with *B. abortus* are common in cattle-rearing communities in African countries such as Kenya and Uganda. Canine infection with *B. canis* is present on most continents—the incidence appears to be increasing in North America and in several European countries, often associated with importation of dogs from an endemic area.

Human brucellosis is usually associated with occupational or domestic exposure to infected animals or their products. Farmers, shepherds, goatherds, veterinarians, and employees in slaughterhouses and meat-processing plants in endemic areas are occupationally exposed to infection. Feral pig hunters are at risk of infection with *B. suis* in several countries, including Australia. Family members of individuals involved in animal husbandry may be at risk, although it is often difficult to differentiate food-borne infection from environmental contamination under these circumstances. Laboratory workers who handle cultures or infected samples also are at risk. Travelers and urban residents usually acquire the infection through consumption of contaminated foods. In countries that have eradicated the disease, new cases are most commonly acquired abroad. Dairy products, especially soft cheeses, unpasteurized milk, and ice cream, are the most frequently implicated sources of infection; raw meat and bone marrow may be sources under exceptional circumstances. Infections acquired through cosmetic treatments using materials of fetal origin have been reported. Person-to-person transmission is extremely rare, as is transfer of infection by blood or tissue donation. Although brucellosis is a chronic intracellular infection, there is no evidence for increased prevalence or severity among individuals with HIV infection or with immunodeficiency or immunosuppression of other etiologies.

Brucellosis may be acquired by ingestion, inhalation, or mucosal or percutaneous exposure. Accidental injection or ingestion of the live vaccine strains of *B. abortus* (S19 and RB51) and *B. melitensis* (Rev 1) can cause disease. *B. melitensis* and *B. suis* have historically been developed as biological weapons by several countries and could be exploited for bioterrorism (**Chap. S3**). This possibility should be borne in mind in the event of sudden unexplained outbreaks.

IMMUNITY AND PATHOGENESIS

Exposure to brucellosis elicits both humoral and cell-mediated immune responses. The mechanisms of protective immunity against human brucellosis are presumed to be similar to those documented in laboratory animals, but such generalizations must be interpreted with caution. The response to infection and its outcome are influenced by the virulence, phase, and species of the infecting strain. Differences have been reported between *B. abortus* and *B. suis* in modes of cellular entry and subsequent compartmentalization and processing. Antibodies promote clearance of extracellular brucellae by bactericidal action and by facilitation of phagocytosis by polymorphonuclear and mononuclear phagocytes; however, antibodies alone cannot eradicate infection. Organisms taken up by macrophages and other cells can establish persistent intracellular infections. The key target cell is the macrophage, and bacterial mechanisms for suppressing intracellular killing and apoptosis result in very large intracellular populations. Opsonized bacteria are actively phagocytosed by neutrophilic granulocytes and by monocytes. In these and other cells, initial attachment takes place via specific receptors, including Fc, C3, fibronectin, and mannose-binding proteins. Opsonized—but not unopsonized—bacteria trigger an oxidative burst inside phagocytes. Unopsonized bacteria are internalized via similar receptors but at much lower efficiency. Smooth strains enter host cells via lipid rafts. Smooth lipopolysaccharide (LPS), β-cyclic glucan, and possibly an invasion–attachment protein (IalB) are involved in this process. Tumor necrosis factor α (TNF-α) produced early in the course of infection stimulates cytotoxic lymphocytes and activates macrophages, which can kill intracellular brucellae (probably mainly through production of reactive oxygen and nitrogen intermediates) and may clear infection. However, virulent *Brucella* cells can suppress the TNF-α response, and control of infection in this situation depends on macrophage activation and interferon γ (IFN-γ) responses. Cytokines such as interleukin 12(IL-12) promote production of IFN-γ, which drives T_H1-type responses and stimulates macrophage activation. Inflammatory cytokines, including IL-4, IL-6, and IL-10, downregulate the protective response. As in other types of intracellular infection, it is assumed that initial replication of brucellae takes place within cells of the lymph nodes draining the point of entry. Subsequent hematogenous spread may result in chronic localizing infection at almost any site, although the reticuloendothelial system, musculoskeletal tissues, and genitourinary system are most frequently targeted. Both acute and chronic inflammatory responses develop in brucellosis, and the local tissue response may include granuloma formation with or without necrosis and caseation. Abscesses may also develop, especially in chronic localized infection.

The determinants of pathogenicity of *Brucella* have not been fully characterized, and the mechanisms underlying the manifestations of brucellosis are incompletely understood. The organism is a "stealth" pathogen whose survival strategy is centered on several processes that avoid triggering innate immune responses and that permit survival within monocytic cells. These processes include evasion of intracellular destruction by restricting the fusion of type IV secretion system–dependent *Brucella*-containing vacuoles with lysosomal compartments, inhibition of apoptosis of infected mononuclear cells, and prevention of dendritic cell maturation, antigen presentation, and activation of naïve T cells. The smooth *Brucella* LPS, which has an unusual O-chain and core-lipid composition, has relatively low endotoxin activity and plays a key role in pyrogenicity and in resistance to phagocytosis and serum killing in the nonimmune host. In addition, LPS is believed to play a role in suppressing phagosome–lysosome fusion and diverting the internalized bacteria into vacuoles located in endoplasmic reticulum, where intracellular replication takes place. Specific exotoxins have not been isolated, but a type IV secretion system (VirB) that regulates intracellular survival and trafficking has been identified. In *B. abortus* this system can be activated extracellularly, but in *B. suis* it is activated (by low pH) only during intracellular growth. Brucellae then produce acid-stable proteins that facilitate the organisms' survival in phagosomes and may enhance their resistance to reactive oxygen intermediates. A type III secretion system based on modified flagellar structures also has been inferred, although not yet confirmed. Virulent brucellae are resistant to defensins and produce a Cu-Zn superoxide dismutase that increases their resistance to reactive oxygen intermediates. A hemolysin-like protein may trigger the release of brucellae from infected cells.

CLINICAL FEATURES

Brucellosis almost invariably causes fever, which may be associated with profuse sweats, especially at night. In endemic areas, brucellosis may be difficult to distinguish from the many other causes of fever. However, two features recognized in the nineteenth century distinguish brucellosis from other tropical fevers, such as typhoid and malaria: (1) Left untreated, the fever of brucellosis shows an undulating pattern that persists for weeks before the commencement of an afebrile period that may be followed by relapse. (2) The fever of brucellosis is associated with musculoskeletal symptoms and signs in about one-half of all patients.

The clinical syndromes caused by the different nomen species are similar, although *B. melitensis* tends to be associated with a more acute and aggressive presentation and *B. suis* with focal abscess induction. *B. abortus* infections may be more insidious in onset and more likely to become chronic. *B. canis* infections are generally regarded as less severe but, like other species, can cause serious disease such as endocarditis.

The incubation period varies from 1 week to several months, and the onset of fever and other symptoms may be abrupt or insidious. In addition to experiencing fever and sweats, patients become increasingly apathetic and fatigued; lose appetite and weight; and have nonspecific myalgia, headache, and chills. Overall, the presentation of brucellosis often fits one of three patterns: febrile illness that resembles typhoid but is less severe; fever and acute monoarthritis, typically of the hip or knee, in a young child; and long-lasting fever, misery, and low-back or hip pain in an older man. In an endemic area (e.g., much of the Middle East), a patient with fever and difficulty walking into the clinic would be regarded as having brucellosis until it was proven otherwise.

Diagnostic clues in the patient's history include travel to an endemic area, employment in a diagnostic microbiology laboratory, consumption of unpasteurized milk products (including soft cheeses), contact with animals, accidental inoculation with veterinary *Brucella* vaccines, and—in an endemic setting—a history of similar illness in the family (documented in almost 50% of cases). Focal features are present in the majority of patients. The most common are musculoskeletal pain and physical findings in the peripheral and axial skeleton (~40% of cases). Osteomyelitis more commonly involves the lumbar and low thoracic vertebrae than the cervical and high thoracic spine. Individual joints that are most commonly affected by septic arthritis are the knee, hip, sacroiliac, shoulder, and sternoclavicular joints; the pattern may be one of monoarthritis or polyarthritis. Osteomyelitis may also accompany septic arthritis.

TABLE 169-1 Radiology of the Spine: Differentiation of Brucellosis from Tuberculosis

	BRUCELLOSIS	TUBERCULOSIS
Site	Lumbar and others	Dorsolumbar
Vertebrae	Multiple or contiguous	Contiguous
Diskitis	Late	Early
Body	Intact until late	Morphology lost early
Canal compression	Rare	Common
Epiphysitis	Anterosuperior	General: upper and lower disk regions, central, subperiosteal
Osteophyte	Anterolateral (parrot beak)	Unusual
Deformity	Wedging uncommon	Anterior wedge, gibbus
Recovery	Sclerosis, whole-body	Variable
Paravertebral abscess	Small, well-localized	Common and discrete loss, transverse process
Psoas abscess	Rare	More likely

In addition to the usual causes of vertebral osteomyelitis or septic arthritis, the most important disease in the differential diagnosis is tuberculosis. This point influences the therapeutic approach as well as the prognosis, given that several antimicrobial agents used to treat brucellosis are also used to treat tuberculosis. Septic arthritis in brucellosis progresses slowly, starting with small pericapsular erosions. In the vertebrae, anterior erosions of the superior end plate are typically the first features to become evident, with eventual involvement and sclerosis of the whole vertebra. Anterior osteophytes eventually develop, but vertebral destruction or impingement on the spinal cord is rare and usually suggests tuberculosis (**Table 169-1**).

Other systems may be involved in a manner that resembles typhoid. About one-quarter of patients have a dry cough, usually with few changes visible on the chest x-ray, although pneumonia, empyema, intrathoracic adenopathy, or lung abscess can occur. Sputum or pleural effusion cultures are rarely positive in such cases, which respond well to standard brucellosis treatment. One-quarter of patients have hepatosplenomegaly, and 10%–20% have significant lymphadenopathy; the differential diagnosis includes glandular fever–like illness such as that caused by Epstein-Barr virus, *Toxoplasma*, cytomegalovirus, HIV, or *Mycobacterium tuberculosis*. Up to 10% of men have acute epididymo-orchitis, which must be distinguished from mumps and from surgical problems such as torsion. Prostatitis, inflammation of the seminal vesicles, salpingitis, and pyelonephritis all occur. There is an increased incidence of fetal loss among infected pregnant women, although teratogenicity has not been described and the tendency toward abortion is much less pronounced in humans than in farm animals.

Neurologic involvement is common, with depression and lethargy whose severity may not be fully appreciated by either the patient or the physician until after treatment. A small proportion of patients develop lymphocytic meningoencephalitis that mimics neurotuberculosis, atypical leptospirosis, or noninfectious conditions and that may be complicated by intracerebral abscess, a variety of cranial nerve deficits, or ruptured mycotic aneurysms.

Endocarditis occurs in ~1% of cases, most often affecting the aortic valve (natural or prosthetic). Any site in the body may be involved in metastatic abscess formation or inflammation; the female breast and the thyroid gland are affected particularly often. Nonspecific maculopapular rashes and other skin manifestations are uncommon and are rarely noticed by the patient even if they develop.

DIAGNOSIS

Because the clinical picture of brucellosis is not distinctive, the diagnosis must be based on a history of potential exposure, a presentation consistent with the disease, and supporting laboratory findings. Results of routine biochemical assays are usually within normal limits, although serum levels of hepatic enzymes and bilirubin may be elevated. Peripheral leukocyte counts are usually normal or low, with relative lymphocytosis. Mild anemia may be documented. Thrombocytopenia and disseminated intravascular coagulation with raised levels of fibrinogen degradation products can develop. The erythrocyte sedimentation rate and C-reactive protein levels are often normal but may be raised.

In body fluids such as cerebrospinal fluid (CSF) or joint fluid, lymphocytosis and low glucose levels are the norm. Elevated CSF levels of adenosine deaminase cannot be used to distinguish tubercular meningitis, as they may also be found in brucellosis. Biopsied samples of tissues such as lymph node or liver may show noncaseating granulomas without acid/alcohol-fast bacilli. The radiologic features of bony disease develop late and are much more subtle than those of tuberculosis or septic arthritis of other etiologies, with less bone and joint destruction. Isotope scanning is more sensitive than plain x-ray and continues to give positive results long after successful treatment.

Isolation of brucellae from blood, CSF, bone marrow, or joint fluid or from a tissue aspirate or biopsy sample is definitive, and attempts at isolation are usually successful in 50%–70% of cases. Blood culture using modern nonradiometric or similar signaling systems (e.g., Bactec) usually become positive within 7 days. Clinicians should alert the laboratory to the possibility of brucellosis if suspected, as all cultures should be handled under containment conditions appropriate for dangerous pathogens. *Brucella* species may be misidentified as *Agrobacterium*, *Ochrobactrum*, or *Psychrobacter (Moraxella) phenylpyruvicus* by the gallery identification strips commonly used in the diagnostic laboratory. In recent years, matrix-assisted laser desorption ionization time-of-flight mass spectrometry (MALDI-TOF MS) has emerged as a powerful tool in bacterial identification. The relative homogeneity of classical *Brucella* species makes identification beyond the genus level by routine approaches challenging, although further improvements may facilitate discrimination at the species level, particularly in reference laboratories. The place of this technique in routine diagnostic practice will depend on further refinements. Meanwhile, the author is aware of cases in which blood culture isolates have been identified incorrectly using MALDI-TOF MS.

The peripheral blood–based polymerase chain reaction (PCR) has enormous potential to detect bacteremia, to predict relapse, and to exclude "chronic brucellosis." This method is more sensitive and is certainly quicker than blood culture, and it does not carry the attendant biohazard risk posed by culture. Nucleic acid amplification techniques are now quite widely used, although no single standardized procedure has been adopted. Primers for the spacer region between the genes encoding the 16S and 23S ribosomal RNAs (*rrs-rrl*), various outer-membrane protein–encoding genes, the insertion sequence *IS711*, and the protein BCSP31 are sensitive and specific. Blood and other tissues are the most suitable samples for analysis. The clinical significance of prolonged PCR positivity, commonly seen in blood after successful treatment, remains controversial.

Serologic examination often provides the only positive laboratory findings in brucellosis. In acute infection, IgM antibodies appear early and are followed by IgG and IgA. All these antibodies are active in agglutination tests, whether performed by tube, plate, or microagglutination methods. The majority of patients have detectable agglutinins at this stage. As the disease progresses, IgM levels decline, and the avidity and subclass distribution of IgG and IgA change. The result is reduced or undetectable agglutinin titers. However, the antibodies are detectable by alternative tests, including the complement fixation test, Coomb's antiglobulin test, and enzyme-linked immunosorbent assays. There is no clear cutoff value for a diagnostic titer. Rather, serology results must be interpreted in the context of exposure history and clinical presentation. In endemic areas or in settings of potential occupational exposure, agglutinin titers of 1:320–1:640 or higher are considered diagnostic; in nonendemic areas, a titer of ≥1:160 is considered significant. Repetition of tests after 2–4 weeks may demonstrate a rising titer.

In most centers, the standard agglutination test (or a derivative such as the microagglutination test) is still the mainstay of serologic diagnosis. In an endemic setting, >90% of patients with acute bacteremia have standard agglutination titers of at least 1:320 at the time of clinical presentation. Some investigators rely on the Rose Bengal test, which has been only partially validated for human diagnostic use but can be used for screening. Dipstick assays for anti-*Brucella* IgM have been developed but are uncommonly utilized. Other near-patient or point-of-care tests are still in developmental stages.

Antibody to the *Brucella* LPS O chain—the dominant antigen—is detected by all the conventional tests that employ smooth *B. abortus* cells as antigen. Because *B. abortus* cross-reacts with *B. melitensis* and *B. suis*, there is no advantage in replicating the tests with these antigens. Cross-reactions also occur with the O chains of some other gram-negative bacteria, including *Yersinia enterocolitica* O:9, *Escherichia coli* O157, *Francisella tularensis*, *Salmonella enterica* group N, *Stenotrophomonas maltophilia*, and *Vibrio cholerae*. Cross-reactions do not occur with the cell-surface antigens of rough *Brucella* strains such as *B. canis* or *B. ovis*; serologic tests for these nomen species must employ an antigen prepared from either one. Similarly, the live *B. abortus* vaccine strain RB51 does not elicit antibody responses in serologic tests that use smooth antigens, and this fact must be taken into account if serologic tests are employed in attempts to identify or follow the course of infections in persons accidentally exposed to the vaccine.

TREATMENT

Brucellosis

The broad aims of antimicrobial therapy are to treat and relieve the symptoms of current infection and to prevent relapse. Focal disease presentations may require specific intervention in addition to more prolonged and tailored antibiotic therapy. In addition, tuberculosis must always be excluded, or—to prevent the emergence of resistance—therapy must be tailored to specifically exclude drugs active against tuberculosis (e.g., rifampin used alone) or to include a full antituberculous regimen.

Early experience with streptomycin monotherapy showed that relapse was common; thus dual therapy with tetracyclines became the norm. This is still the most effective combination, but alternatives may be used, with the options depending on local or national policy about the use of rifampin for the treatment of nonmycobacterial infection. For the several antimicrobial agents that are active in vivo, efficacy can usually be predicted by in vitro testing. However, numerous *Brucella* strains show in vitro sensitivity to a whole range of antimicrobials that are therapeutically ineffective, including assorted β-lactams. Moreover, the use of fluoroquinolones remains controversial despite the good in vitro activity and white-cell penetration of most agents of this class. Low intravacuolar pH is probably a factor in the poor performance of these drugs.

For adults with acute nonfocal brucellosis (duration, <1 month), a 6-week course of therapy incorporating at least two antimicrobial agents is required. Complex or focal disease may necessitate ≥3 months of therapy. Adherence to the therapeutic regimen is very important, and poor adherence underlies almost all cases of apparent treatment failure; such failure is rarely due to the emergence of drug resistance, although increasing resistance to trimethoprim-sulfamethoxazole (TMP-SMX) has been reported at one center. There is good retrospective evidence that a 3-week course of two agents is as effective as a 6-week course for treatment and prevention of relapse in children, but this has not yet been investigated in prospective studies.

The gold standard for the treatment of brucellosis in adults is IM streptomycin (0.75–1 g daily for 14–21 days) together with doxycycline (100 mg twice daily for 6 weeks). In both clinical trials and observational studies, relapse follows such treatment in 5%–10% of cases. The usual alternative regimen (and the current World Health Organization recommendation) is rifampin (600–900 mg/d) plus doxycycline (100 mg twice daily) for 6 weeks. The relapse/failure rate is ~10% in trial conditions but rises to >20% in many nontrial situations, possibly because doxycycline levels are reduced and clearance rates increased by concomitant rifampin administration. Patients who cannot tolerate or receive tetracyclines (children, pregnant women) can be given high-dose TMP-SMX instead (two or three standard-strength tablets twice daily for adults, depending on weight).

Increasing evidence supports the use of an aminoglycoside such as gentamicin (5–6 mg/kg per day for at least 2 weeks) instead of streptomycin. Shorter courses have been associated with high failure rates in adults. A 5- to 7-day course of therapy with gentamicin and a 3-week course of TMP-SMX may be adequate for children with uncomplicated disease, but prospective trials are still needed to support this recommendation. Early experience with fluoroquinolone monotherapy was disappointing, although it was suggested that ofloxacin or ciprofloxacin, given together with rifampin for 6 weeks, might be an acceptable alternative to the other 6-week regimens for adults. A substantial meta-analysis did not support the use of fluoroquinolones in first-line treatment regimens, and these drugs are not recommended by an expert consensus group (the Ioannina Recommendations) except in the context of well-designed clinical trials. However, a more recent meta-analysis is more supportive of the efficacy of these drugs, and an adequately powered prospective study will be needed to resolve their role in standard combination therapy. A triple-drug regimen—doxycycline and rifampin combined with an initial course of an aminoglycoside—was superior to double-drug regimens in a meta-analysis. The triple-drug regimen should be considered for all patients with complicated disease and for those for whom treatment adherence is likely to be a problem.

Focal neurologic disease due to *Brucella* species requires prolonged treatment (i.e., for 3–6 months), usually with ceftriaxone supplementation of a standard regimen. *Brucella* endocarditis is treated with at least three drugs (an aminoglycoside, a tetracycline, and rifampin), and many experts add ceftriaxone and/or a fluoroquinolone to reduce the need for valve replacement. Treatment is usually given for at least 4–6 months, and clinical endpoints for its discontinuation are often difficult to define. Surgery is still required for the majority of cases of infection of prosthetic heart valves and prosthetic joints.

There is no evidence base to guide prophylaxis after exposure to *Brucella* organisms (e.g., in the laboratory), inadvertent immunization with live vaccine intended for use in animals, or exposure to deliberately released brucellae. Most authorities have recommended the administration of rifampin plus doxycycline for 3 weeks after a low-risk exposure (e.g., an unspecified laboratory accident) and for 6 weeks after a major exposure to aerosol or injected material. However, such regimens are poorly tolerated, and doxycycline monotherapy of the same duration may be substituted. (Monotherapy is the standard recommendation in the United Kingdom but not in the United States.) Rifampin should be omitted after exposure to vaccine strain RB51, which is resistant to rifampin, and replaced by another agent such as TMP-SMX in combination with doxycycline. After significant brucellosis exposure, expert consultation is advised for women who are (or may be) pregnant.

PROGNOSIS AND FOLLOW-UP

Relapse occurs in up to 30% of poorly compliant patients. Thus patients should ideally be followed clinically for up to 2 years to detect relapse, which responds to a prolonged course of the same therapy used originally. The general well-being and the body weight of the patient are more useful guides than serology to lack of relapse. IgG antibody levels detected by the standard agglutination test and its variants can remain in the diagnostic range for >2 years after successful treatment. Complement fixation titers usually fall to normal within 1 year of cure. Immunity is not solid; patients can be reinfected after repeated exposures. Fewer than 1% of patients die of brucellosis. When the outcome is fatal, death is usually a consequence of cardiac involvement; more rarely, it results from severe neurologic disease. Despite the low mortality rate, recovery from brucellosis is slow, and the illness can cause prolonged inactivity, with domestic and economic consequences.

The existence of a prolonged chronic brucellosis state after successful treatment remains controversial. Evaluation of patients in whom this state is considered (often those with work-related exposure to brucellae) includes careful exclusion of malingering, nonspecific chronic fatigue syndromes, and other causes of excessive sweating, such as alcohol abuse and obesity. In the future, the availability of more sensitive assays to detect *Brucella* antigen or DNA may help to identify patients with ongoing infection.

PREVENTION

Vaccines based on live attenuated *Brucella* strains, such as *B. abortus* strain 19BA or 104M, have been used in some countries to protect high-risk populations but have displayed only short-term efficacy and high reactogenicity. Subunit vaccines have been developed but are of uncertain value and cannot be recommended at present. Research in this area has been stimulated by interest in biodefense (**Chap. S3**) and may eventually yield new products. The mainstay of veterinary prevention is a national commitment to testing and slaughter of infected herds/flocks (with compensation for owners), control of animal movement, and active immunization of animals. These measures are usually sufficient to control human disease as well. In their absence, pasteurization of all milk products before consumption is sufficient to prevent nonoccupational animal-to-human transmission. All cases of brucellosis in animals and humans should be reported to the appropriate public health authorities.

FURTHER READING

Ariza J et al: Perspectives for the treatment of brucellosis in the 21st century: The Ioannina recommendations. PLoS Med 4:e317, 2007.

Beeching NJ et al: Brucellosis. BMJ Best Practice, 2019. *https://bestpractice.bmj.com/topics/en-us/911.*

Centers for Disease Control and Prevention: Brucellosis. *https://www.cdc.gov/brucellosis/index.html.*

Dean AS et al: Clinical manifestations of human brucellosis: a systematic review and metaanalysis. PLoS Negl Trop Dis 6:e1929, 2012.

Norman FF et al: Imported brucellosis: a case series and literature review. Travel Med Infect Dis 14:182, 2016.

Yagupsky P et al: Laboratory diagnosis of human brucellosis. Clin Microbiol Rev 33:e00073, 2019.

170 Tularemia

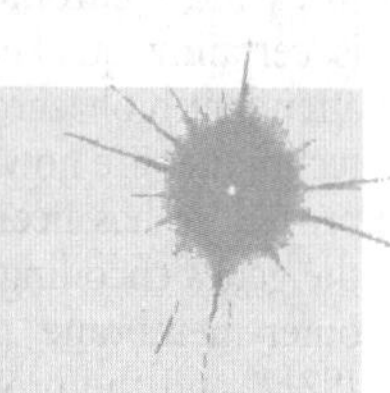

Max Maurin, Didier Raoult

DEFINITION

Tularemia is a zoonosis caused by the gram-negative, facultative intracellular bacterium *Francisella tularensis*. This microorganism was isolated first in 1911 by McCoy and Chapin from rodents in Tulare County, California, and then from humans in 1914 by Wherry and Lamb. Because of taxonomic evolution, only two subspecies of *F. tularensis* are currently associated with tularemia: *F. tularensis* subsp. *tularensis* and *F. tularensis* subsp. *holarctica* are responsible for type A and type B tularemia, respectively. These two subspecies are highly virulent human pathogens belonging to category A of potential biological threat agents, as defined by the U.S. Centers for Disease Control and Prevention.

FRANCISELLA SPECIES, SUBSPECIES, AND CLADES

The *Francisella* genus currently comprises seven species. *F. tularensis* is split into four subspecies: *F. tularensis* subsp. *tularensis* (type A); *F. tularensis* subsp. *holarctica* (type B); *F. tularensis* subsp. *mediasiatica*, restricted to central Asia and Russia, but never associated with human diseases; and *F. tularensis* subsp. *novicida*, an aquatic bacterium and rare opportunistic human pathogen. Molecular methods (especially those based on whole genome sequencing) have now allowed the characterization of a large number of *F. tularensis* genotypes, which are divided into clades and subclades. The major clades are A1 (divided into A1a and A1b) and A2 for type A strains, and B4, B6, B12, and B16 for type B strains. These clades vary in geographic distribution, virulence, and resistance to macrolides; clade B12 strains are naturally highly resistant to erythromycin.

EPIDEMIOLOGY

■ GEOGRAPHIC DISTRIBUTION

Tularemia-endemic areas are mainly distributed in the Northern Hemisphere (**Fig. 170-1**). Human tularemia cases are described in North America (the United States, Canada, and part of Central America), Asia (Japan, China, Mongolia, Russia, Pakistan, Turkey, Iran, Kazakhstan, Georgia, Armenia, and Azerbaijan), and Europe (almost all countries except Iceland, Ireland, the United Kingdom, Portugal, and the southern Balkan countries). Type A strains are classically restricted to North America, although a few strains (probably imported laboratory strains) have been detected from arthropods in Slovakia. Type B strains are classically found in the whole Northern Hemisphere but have also been detected in southern Australia. In the United States, human tularemia cases predominate in southern and central states (especially, in order of decreasing incidence, Arkansas, Oklahoma, South Dakota, Kansas, Missouri, North Dakota, and Nebraska) and, to a lesser extent, in eastern states (mainly Massachusetts and Martha's Vineyard) and western states (especially California, Oregon, and Montana).

There is a specific, complex, and overlapping geographic distribution of *F. tularensis* clades and subclades (Fig. 170-1). Clade A1 is found throughout North America, while clade A2 is restricted to the U.S. western states. Clade B4 predominates in North America but has also been detected in Scandinavia, Germany, and western China. Clade B6 is spread throughout western Europe (with a predominance of subclade B44), but also in central Europe, Scandinavia, and North America. Clade B12 has been found mainly in eastern Europe, Scandinavia, and Asia (e.g., Russia and China). Finally, clade B16 is currently restricted to Japan, Turkey, Australia, and western China.

■ RESERVOIRS AND MODES OF TRANSMISSION

F. tularensis can infect a wide range of mammals, birds, amphibians, reptiles, and fish, causing many of these vertebrate species to develop severe and often fatal infections. Because this organism can infect so many animal species, the actual animal reservoir of *F. tularensis* remains unknown. However, small terrestrial and semi-aquatic rodents (including mice, gerbils, beavers, lemmings, and voles) and lagomorphs (hares and rabbits) are the predominant animal sources for human tularemia cases.

Some arthropods are able to transmit *F. tularensis* between animal species, including from animals to humans. Ixodidae ticks are the primary vectors of tularemia and may also represent a reservoir due to transstadial transmission of *F. tularensis*. Mosquitoes (especially *Aedes* species) are vectors of this microorganism in Sweden and Finland. Other blood-sucking arthropods (especially tabanids) may also transmit tularemia in restricted areas. *F. tularensis* survives for weeks or months in contaminated soil or water environments, which possibly represent other natural reservoirs of this bacterium.

The modes of transmission of *F. tularensis* to humans are varied, reflecting the ubiquitous nature of this microbe. A common mode of infection is direct contact with infected animals or, less frequently, through animal bites. Lagomorphs and other game animals as well as small rodents are most frequently involved. Domestic animals, especially cats and dogs, are occasionally involved in transmission to humans or as recipients of the microbe from wild animals. Tularemia can also be acquired through the consumption of contaminated food products (especially those from game animals) or water (often nonpotable water from water wells or spring water). Arthropod-borne tularemia cases mainly occur through tick bites except in Sweden and Finland, where mosquitoes are the primary vectors. Human infections also occur through contact with contaminated soil or water environments or inhalation of contaminated dust.

■ AT-RISK EXPOSURES AND POPULATIONS

In endemic areas, the people most at risk for tularemia are those frequently exposed to wild animals, arthropod bites (mainly those of ticks), or contaminated hydrotelluric environments.

Occupational Risk Tularemia is recognized as an occupational disease in most endemic countries. The high-risk occupational groups include breeders, farmers, veterinarians, game wardens, forest rangers,

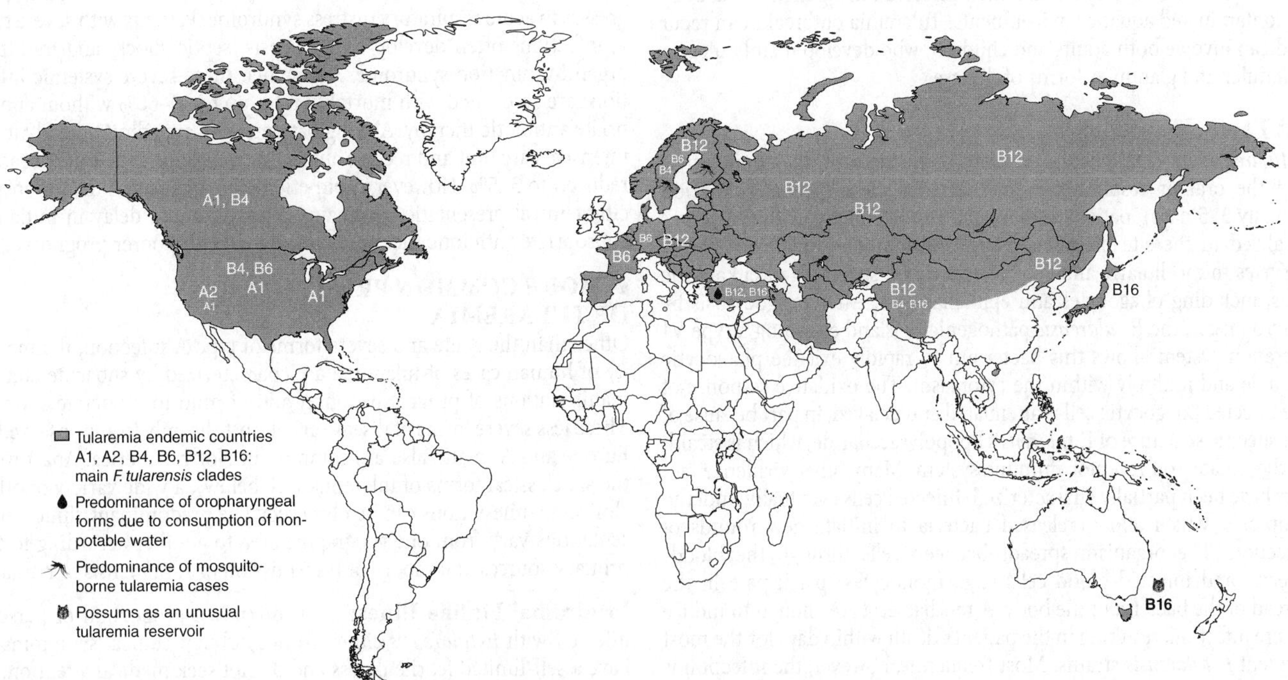

FIGURE 170-1 Global distribution of reported (or strongly suspected) autochthonous human tularemia cases. The major clades detected in specific areas—A1, A2, B4, B6, B12, and B16—are shown. In most countries, the actual endemic areas are poorly defined. The actual distribution of clades and subclades is complex and overlapping. Lagomorphs, small rodents, and ticks are the primary sources of human tularemia cases except in the indicated specific situations.

landscapers, trappers, tanners, slaughterhouse workers, renderers, zoological park employees, butchers who handle game meat, military personnel (especially during the navigation of military obstacle courses), and laboratory personnel handling *F. tularensis* cultures.

Leisure-Associated Risk The leisure activities potentially associated with exposure to *F. tularensis* include hunting, trapping, gardening, mowing the lawn, canyoneering, fishing or swimming in contaminated fresh water, and walking or biking in forests and other areas infested with ticks. Owning pets that may carry *F. tularensis* (especially unusual animals such as prairie dogs) is also a risk factor.

At-Risk Populations and Seasonal Variations The most at-risk population varies according to the geographic area and the predominant mode(s) of contamination. When infections occur through contact with wildlife fauna and tick bites, middle-aged men living in rural areas are most frequently involved. Game-related contamination usually occurs during the hunting (autumn and winter) seasons, while tick-borne tularemia cases are more frequent during the warm season. Infections caused by the consumption of contaminated water occur throughout the year and involve men, women, and children. Mosquito-borne tularemia cases predominate during the warm season in both adults and children in Scandinavia.

NATURAL CYCLES OF *F. TULARENSIS*

The highly variable epidemiologic and clinical aspects of tularemia in different geographic areas suggest several *F. tularensis* natural cycles. These cycles probably vary with the predominant animal reservoirs, arthropod vectors, climatic conditions, and *F. tularensis* species and lineages. However, two cycles have been hypothesized to explain the spatiotemporal maintenance of tularemia. In the *terrestrial* cycle, lagomorphs, terrestrial rodents, and ticks are considered primarily involved. Human infections occur mainly through contact with the terrestrial wildlife fauna and tick bites. This cycle is characterized by sporadic tularemia cases in the most exposed population (often middle-aged men), with a predominance of ulceroglandular and glandular forms. In the *aquatic* cycle, semi-aquatic rodents and the aquatic environment play a significant role. In Turkey, most patients are infected through the consumption of nonpotable water (especially spring water). Water-borne tularemia outbreaks have occurred, involving both adults and children, with a predominance of oropharyngeal forms. In Sweden and Finland, mosquito-borne tularemia cases predominate. These arthropods are likely infected during their larval cycle in contaminated aquatic environments. Tularemia outbreaks can recur and can involve both adults and children, who develop mainly ulceroglandular and glandular forms of disease.

PATHOGENESIS

F. tularensis inoculation can occur through the skin, the conjunctiva, and the oral or respiratory route. After a short incubation period (usually 3–5 days), patients experience a flulike illness with symptoms localized to the site of initial tissue invasion. The organism mainly survives intracellularly and can infect a broad spectrum of eukaryotic cells, including phagocytes and epithelial cells. After phagocytosis by macrophages, the *F. tularensis* pathogenicity island encoding a type VI secretion system allows this bacterium to rapidly exit the phagocytic vacuole and multiply within the cytoplasm. The oxidative response of the infected phagocytic cell is attenuated and delayed, in part because of the specific structure of *F. tularensis* lipopolysaccharide, which is stealth to the innate Toll receptor immune system. Many other virulence factors have been partially characterized. Infected cells eventually undergo apoptosis, which allows released bacteria to initiate new rounds of infection. The organism spreads between cells through the bloodstream, and infected blood cells (e.g., monocytes) participate in the spread of the bacteria in the body. A few bacteria are enough to induce severe infection, resulting in the patient's death within days for the most virulent *F. tularensis* strains. Most frequently, however, the infection is controlled both by the humoral and cellular immune responses.

The earliest infected organs—and thus the earliest clinical manifestations—depend on the route of infection. Infection through the skin results in a local inoculation lesion and development of regional lymphadenopathy within days. Conjunctival inoculation leads to conjunctivitis with local lymphadenopathy. The oral route of infection manifests as pharyngitis with cervical lymphadenopathy, but intestinal involvement may occasionally lead to enteritis and other intraabdominal organ involvement. The inhalation of a contaminated aerosol can result in acute, subacute, or chronic pneumonia. All these localized infections can lead to *F. tularensis* bacteremia (hence the term *tularemia*) and secondary infection of almost all organs.

CLINICAL MANIFESTATIONS

Tularemia can be considered as two separate diseases: a severe, often life-threatening disease observed in North America and caused by the most virulent type A strains; and a disease of mild to moderate severity, with protean clinical manifestations that often resemble those of other infectious diseases; in fact, these other diseases typically are initially suspected before the diagnosis of tularemia is made. The incubation period of tularemia is typically short (3–5 days on average) but can last up to 3 weeks.

SEVERE TYPE A TULAREMIA

The most virulent strains of *F. tularensis* subsp. *tularensis* (genotype A1b) can cause severe systemic disease, usually of acute onset. These infections justify the classification of *F. tularensis* as a Tier 1 select agent in the United States and most other countries. For severe type A tularemia cases, the most frequently reported mode of contamination is the inhalation of an infected aerosol. This event results in the rapid development of acute, life-threatening pneumonia or pleuropneumonia, which is the most severe presentation of the so-called pneumonic form of tularemia. Systemic infections are acquired through other modes of contamination, including ingestion of contaminated food or water and arthropod bites. A severe typhoid-like disease (referred to as the typhoidal form of tularemia) is consistent with a combination of high fever, sepsis, and neurologic symptoms (ranging from confusion to deep coma), but no localized infection (e.g., no skin inoculation lesion and no lymphadenopathy). The acute pneumonic and typhoidal forms of tularemia are usually associated with *F. tularensis* bacteremia, although bloodstream infection may not be detected at hospital admission because of its intermittent and temporary nature.

Severe type A tularemia is not restricted to persons with compromised immunity or underlying disorders and can occur in young, healthy adults. If untreated, the acute pneumonic form rapidly progresses to acute respiratory distress syndrome. Patients with severe type A infections often develop severe sepsis, septic shock, and multiple-organ dysfunction syndrome. Altogether, these severe systemic infections are associated with mortality rates up to 40–60% without appropriate antibiotic therapy. Among patients who are admitted early to an intensive care unit and receive appropriate antibiotics, the death rate is reduced to 3–5%. However, rapid etiologic diagnosis of these nonspecific clinical presentations remains difficult, and a delay in initiating appropriate antibiotic therapy is associated with poorer prognosis.

MORE COMMON PRESENTATIONS OF TULAREMIA

Other than the acute and severe forms of type A infection, the majority of human cases of tularemia are characterized by subacute clinical manifestations of progressive onset and of mild to moderate severity. These less severe forms of disease are almost the only forms observed in Europe and Asia and also are common in North America. Apart from the six classical forms of tularemia (see below), a wide variety of other clinical manifestations can be observed. The predominant clinical presentations vary from one geographic area to another according to the primary sources and modes of transmission of *F. tularensis* to humans.

Prodromal Flulike Illness An unknown proportion of persons infected with *F. tularensis* either do not develop clinical symptoms or have a self-limited febrile illness and do not seek medical attention. In symptomatic patients, early clinical manifestations usually correspond to a flulike illness and may include fever, headache, chills, fatigue, malaise, arthralgia, and myalgia.

Classical Forms of Tularemia Following the prodromal period, tularemia usually evolves into one of six classical clinical forms, which are occasionally combined.

ULCEROGLANDULAR FORM This form is the most common and typical presentation of tularemia worldwide. It occurs after *F. tularensis* inoculation through the skin (e.g., during manipulation of an infected animal or via an arthropod bite). A cutaneous inoculation lesion develops that may be papular or vesicular but that often evolves to a skin ulcer persisting for several weeks before healing. A few days after infection, regional lymphadenopathy develops at locations that vary with the inoculation site (e.g., axillary, epitrochlear, or inguinal). The differential diagnosis of the combination of a skin lesion and regional lymphadenopathy is difficult and includes cat-scratch disease caused by *Bartonella henselae* (**Chap. 172**) as well as several rickettsioses (**Chap. 187**). However, in patients with the above clinical presentation, tularemia should be considered.

GLANDULAR FORM The glandular form is similar to the ulceroglandular form, but the skin lesion either has not developed or has healed by the time the patient seeks medical attention. This form is a common but clinically less typical presentation. Because many infectious agents may cause regional lymphadenopathy, the diagnosis of tularemia is often delayed.

OCULOGLANDULAR FORM Infection through the conjunctiva usually leads to painful granulomatous unilateral conjunctivitis. Bilateral conjunctivitis due to contamination of both eyes rarely occurs. Within a few days, swollen periauricular lymphadenopathy develops. Thus, tularemia is a rare etiology of Parinaud oculoglandular syndrome. *B. henselae* (the cause of cat-scratch disease) is the most common etiology of this syndrome, but tularemia should be considered as an alternative diagnosis.

OROPHARYNGEAL FORM The oral route of contamination (usually via the hands or through consumption of contaminated water or food) corresponds to painful pharyngitis and the development within days of submandibular or cervical lymphadenopathy. The oropharyngeal form resembles a group A streptococcal infection (**Chap. 148**), but with swollen cervical lymphadenopathy in most patients and almost no efficacy of β-lactam therapy. This form may also include digestive symptoms of variable severity, including nausea and vomiting, abdominal pain, bloody diarrhea, and occasionally the involvement of other intraabdominal organs.

PNEUMONIC FORM The inhalation of an *F. tularensis*–contaminated aerosol may result in pneumonia or pleuropneumonia. However, the most common presentations of this clinical form consist of subacute lung involvement with low-grade fever and mild pulmonary symptoms (dry cough, moderate dyspnea, and mild chest pain). Some patients suffer from prolonged clinical symptoms, with intermittent fever, fatigue, progressive weight loss, and deterioration in general condition. The diagnosis is usually delayed for weeks or months until chest x-ray or CT reveals hilar or mediastinal lymphadenopathy, often with no or only minor pulmonary lesions. Tuberculosis and lymphoma are usually suspected first. The tularemia diagnosis is usually fortuitous and obtained thanks to histologic and bacteriologic analysis of surgically removed mediastinal or hilar lymph nodes.

TYPHOIDAL FORM In Europe and Asia, a diagnosis of typhoidal tularemia may be considered in patients presenting with sepsis and confusion but without a localized infection (no skin lesion, lymphadenopathy, pharyngitis, or conjunctivitis). However, the prognosis of this form of illness is much better than that of type A infections in North America. Many of these patients experience *F. tularensis* bacteremia. Fatal cases are rare and most often occur in debilitated and elderly patients.

Skin Manifestations Apart from skin inoculation lesions, tularemia patients may present with various other types of skin involvement. Reported manifestations include skin rash, Sweet syndrome, dermatitis, urticaria, acneiform eruption, vasculitis-like eruption, lymphangitis, cellulitis, subcutaneous abscesses, erythema nodosum, erythema multiforme, and livedo reticularis.

Complications Up to 20–30% of symptomatic tularemia patients with common clinical presentations require hospitalization, either in the early stage of the disease—because of severe clinical symptoms—or after several weeks or months of evolution—because of an unfavorable course.

BACTEREMIA, SEPSIS, AND SEPTIC SHOCK These complications are rare among patients with the above classical forms of tularemia and have been reported more frequently in immunocompromised persons, transplant recipients, persons with severe underlying disorders, and the elderly.

LYMPH NODE SUPPURATION, SOFT TISSUE INFECTIONS, AND DEEP ABSCESSES Because of delayed diagnosis, 30–40% of tularemia patients with regional lymphadenopathy experience a progression to lymph node suppuration, which can spontaneously drain through a skin fistula. Soft tissue infections usually occur in the area adjacent to suppurative lymphadenopathy and may consist of cellulitis or subcutaneous abscesses. Periauricular lymphadenopathy may lead to parotid infection. Myositis and rhabdomyolysis have also been reported. Deep abscesses of variable location may occur through the diffusion of a lymph node suppuration into the surrounding tissues or through hematogenous spread of bacteria.

OCULAR COMPLICATIONS Tularemia conjunctivitis rarely evolves to more severe ocular infections. Rare cases of dacryocystitis, keratitis, chorioretinitis, cyclitis, and optic neuritis have been reported.

OTITIS Otitis media is a rare complication likely occurring as a complication of oropharyngeal tularemia or direct inoculation of *F. tularensis* through a tympanic perforation.

MENINGITIS, MENINGOENCEPHALITIS, AND NEUROLOGIC DISEASE Meningitis and meningoencephalitis are hematogenous complications that, although uncommon, can occur as an inaugural and unique clinical manifestation. Their clinical presentation is not specific, and a tularemia diagnosis is usually established by isolation of *F. tularensis* from cerebrospinal fluid. Meningitis has been more commonly reported in the United States than in Europe and Asia. Other rare neurologic complications include cerebral abscesses, polyneuritis cranialis, ataxia, and Guillain-Barré syndrome.

CARDIOVASCULAR INFECTIONS Endocarditis (including prosthetic valve endocarditis), myocarditis, pericarditis, and aortitis are rare complications of tularemia. Therefore, diagnosis may be particularly challenging unless blood cultures allow rapid isolation of *F. tularensis*.

ABDOMINAL INFECTIONS Rare abdominal complications include granulomatous hepatitis, peritonitis, acute renal failure, and liver or spleen abscesses or nodules.

OSTEOARTICULAR INFECTIONS Osteoarticular infections, including osteomyelitis, arthritis, and prosthetic joint infections, are rare hematogenous complications of tularemia.

ADVERSE PREGNANCY OUTCOMES Tularemia is not considered a disease responsible for complications during pregnancy or fetal abnormalities. A single tularemia case in the first trimester of pregnancy, followed by intrauterine fetal death in the third trimester, has been reported.

DIAGNOSIS

A tularemia diagnosis is often missed or delayed. This delay may be related to inadequate knowledge of this disease by some clinicians, lack of specific clinical symptoms, and a high frequency of mild disease with spontaneous recovery. Once clinically suspected, a diagnosis of tularemia usually is readily confirmed by specific laboratory tests.

■ NONSPECIFIC BIOLOGIC FINDINGS

Routine blood tests usually are not very informative in the diagnosis of tularemia. The leukocyte count can be normal or moderately high, usually with a relative increase in mononuclear cells. Moderate thrombocytopenia is more frequently observed. The erythrocyte sedimentation rate is usually elevated, and the C-reactive protein level may also be slightly elevated. Levels of liver enzymes, including alkaline phosphatase, aspartate aminotransferase, alanine aminotransferase, and gamma-glutamyl transpeptidase, can be moderately elevated. High levels of creatine phosphokinase are found in patients with rhabdomyolysis.

RADIOLOGIC FINDINGS

Radiologic examinations (e.g., CT, MRI, ultrasonography) may be useful for detecting and specifying the extent of lymphadenopathy and lung or other organ involvement. Although usually not specific to tularemia, radiologic findings may include superficial or deep lymphadenopathies; soft tissue, lymph node, or other organ abscesses; brain tissue involvement; cardiovascular disease; lung or pleural involvement; and osteoarticular lesions. The pneumonic form of tularemia may be associated with variable radiologic findings, including unilateral or bilateral infiltrates, lung consolidation, lung abscess, cavitary lesions, pleural effusion, and hilar or mediastinal enlargement due to lymphadenopathy.

CLINICAL SAMPLES

Blood samples should be collected in blood culture bottles (aerobic and anaerobic) when patients have febrile disease. On the basis of clinical manifestations, biological samples can be obtained for culture and polymerase chain reaction (PCR) testing, including samples of cutaneous biopsies or exudates (especially from the inoculation lesion), conjunctival or pharyngeal exudates, lymph node aspirates or biopsies, various suppurations and abscesses, sputum and other lower respiratory tract secretions, pleural and other serous fluid, cerebrospinal fluid, and organ biopsies.

SEROLOGIC DIAGNOSIS

A serum sample should be collected as early as possible and analyzed for antibodies to *F. tularensis*. Ideally, a second serum sample should be collected at least 2 weeks later. The serologic diagnosis of tularemia is widely used and is sensitive. Antibodies are measured by different techniques, depending on the laboratory. Assays include the microagglutination test, immunofluorescence assays (IFAs), enzyme-linked immunosorbent assays (ELISAs), and Western blots. The IFA and ELISA methods allow separate titration of IgM- and IgG-type antibodies. Significant antibody titers (i.e., titers above the cutoff of the technique used) are usually detected 2–3 weeks after disease onset, with ELISAs allowing the earliest detection. Antibody titers peak 4–6 weeks after disease onset and then decline progressively over the following months. However, in many patients, residual IgG titers and, to a lesser extent, IgM titers persist for several years.

False-negative results may be obtained in the early stage of tularemia or in the rare patients who do not mount a significant antibody response. False-positive results classically arise as a result of antigenic cross-reactions between *F. tularensis* and other bacterial species, including *Brucella* spp. and *Yersinia enterocolitica*. The risk of false-positive results linked to antigenic cross-reactions is high in patients with antibody titers close to the cutoff thresholds. In addition, the long-term persistence of anti–*F. tularensis* antibodies in patients with past infection may also lead to false-positive results. Lack of kinetics between antibody titers in early and (when available) late serum samples may allow the differentiation of recent from past infections.

CULTURE-BASED DIAGNOSIS

F. tularensis is a highly infectious and virulent bacterium. Cultures of this pathogen should be handled in a biosafety level 3 laboratory to prevent the contamination of laboratory personnel. Blood-enriched media (especially chocolate agar supplemented with vitamins) are needed to isolate this fastidious-growth bacterium. Current blood culture systems are adequate for *F. tularensis* isolation within 5 days of incubation. *F. tularensis* may also be isolated from various other clinical samples.

F. tularensis can be presumptively identified by Gram's staining (small gram-negative coccobacilli), a few biochemical tests, agglutination, and matrix-assisted laser desorption/ionization–time of flight (MALDI-TOF) mass spectrometry. Molecular tests are the gold standard for determination of the involved species, subspecies, and genotype (see below).

MOLECULAR DIAGNOSIS

F. tularensis DNA can be detected in blood or other clinical samples. Available real-time PCR is both rapid and accurate. Whole genome sequencing of a large number of *F. tularensis* strains has allowed the development of molecular tests for the detection and identification of this pathogen at the species, subspecies, or genotype level. The fact that PCR tests usually remain positive despite 1–2 weeks of antibiotic therapy may help establish the diagnosis of tularemia, whereas specific cultures can be negative at that point.

Blood samples may be PCR-positive, especially when collected from patients with *F. tularensis* bacteremia. However, PCR results are more frequently positive for other clinical samples, especially samples of lymph nodes, skin ulcers, and conjunctival and pharyngeal exudates. It is interesting that lymph node tissue surgically removed because of suppuration several weeks after disease onset are PCR-positive in >90% of cases, whereas *F. tularensis* is rarely isolated from these samples.

OPTIMIZED DIAGNOSTIC STRATEGY

Molecular tests are the most useful diagnostic tools for rapid tularemia diagnosis. In the acute phase of the disease, *F. tularensis* DNA can be detected in various biologic samples collected in light of clinical manifestations, including blood, skin inoculation lesions, conjunctival or pharyngeal exudates, sputum or pleural fluid, and cerebrospinal fluid. Real-time PCR can provide a rapid (within 2 h) and accurate diagnosis of acute pneumonic tularemia, especially in the context of bioterrorism. Molecular tests are also useful in patients with late clinical manifestations, especially those with lymph node suppuration. The combination of several molecular tests allows a rapid search for several pathogens responsible for similar clinical manifestations. For example, in patients with a skin inoculation lesion and regional lymphadenopathy, PCR testing of a skin lesion biopsy allows rapid detection of *B. henselae*, *Rickettsia* spp., and *F. tularensis*.

F. tularensis culture remains the most specific diagnostic technique, providing definitive diagnostic confirmation whatever the site of its isolation, although this pathogen is most frequently isolated from blood samples. However, isolation of *F. tularensis* is challenging and classically has <10% sensitivity.

Serologic methods remain useful in patients with common clinical forms of tularemia when no clinical sample is available for culture or PCR. Serologic findings must be interpreted according to the clinical and epidemiologic context. Only seroconversion or a fourfold or greater rise in *F. tularensis* antibody titers between two serum samples collected at least 2 weeks apart is considered a diagnostic confirmation of tularemia. A single antibody titer higher than the cutoff should be interpreted cautiously and may represent a false-positive result.

TREATMENT

Tularemia

ANTIBIOTIC THERAPY

Three antibiotic classes are commonly used for tularemia treatment: the aminoglycosides, the tetracyclines, and the fluoroquinolones. No acquired resistance to these antibiotics has been reported in natural strains of *F. tularensis*. Chloramphenicol is now rarely used because of bone marrow toxicity. The β-lactams are considered ineffective and the macrolides only poorly effective; however, azithromycin is bacteriostatic in vitro against *F. tularensis* (except for B12 genotypes). **Table 170-1** summarizes current treatment recommendations for patients in the United States and Europe.

The aminoglycosides streptomycin and gentamicin remain the gold standard for the treatment of severe tularemia because of their significant and rapid bactericidal activity against *F. tularensis*. Doxycycline or a fluoroquinolone are usually prescribed for treating common clinical forms of mild to moderate severity.

TABLE 170-1 Guidelines for Tularemia Treatment and Postexposure Prophylaxis

REGION, PATIENT GROUP	
United States, Nonpregnant Adults[a]	
First line	Streptomycin, 1 g IM bid, 10 days; *or* Gentamicin,[b] 5 mg/kg IM or IV daily, 10 days
Second line	Doxycycline, 100 mg IV bid, 14–21 days; *or* Chloramphenicol,[b] 15 mg/kg IV qid, 14–21 days; *or* Ciprofloxacin,[b] 400 mg IV bid, 10 days
Prophylaxis	Doxycycline, 100 mg PO bid, 14 days; *or* Ciprofloxacin,[b] 500 mg PO bid, 14 days
United States, Pregnant Women[a]	
First line	Gentamicin,[b] 5 mg/kg IM or IV daily, 10 days; *or* Streptomycin, 1 g IM bid, 10 days
Second line	Doxycycline, 100 mg IV bid, 14–21 days; *or* Ciprofloxacin,[b] 400 mg IV bid, 10 days
Prophylaxis	Ciprofloxacin,[b] 500 mg PO bid, 14 days; *or* Doxycycline, 100 mg PO bid, 14 days
Europe, Nonpregnant Adults and Pregnant Women	
First line	Gentamicin, 5 mg/kg IM or IV daily or bid, 10 days; *or* Streptomycin, 1 g IM bid, 10 days
Second line[c]	Ciprofloxacin, 400 mg IV bid, then 500 mg PO bid, 14 days; *or* Ofloxacin, 400 mg IV bid, then 400 mg PO bid, 14 days; *or* Levofloxacin, 500 mg IV daily, then 500 mg PO daily, 14 days
Third line[c]	Doxycycline, 100 mg IV bid, then 100 mg PO bid, 21 days
Prophylaxis	Ciprofloxacin, 500 mg PO bid, 14 days; *or* Ofloxacin, 400 mg PO bid, 14 days; *or* Levofloxacin, 500 mg PO daily, 14 days; *or* Doxycycline, 100 mg PO bid, 14 days[d]

[a]Persons beginning with IM or IV doxycycline, ciprofloxacin, or chloramphenicol can switch to oral antibiotic administration when clinically indicated. [b]Not a use approved by the U.S. Food and Drug Administration. [c]Persons beginning with IV treatment can switch to oral antibiotic administration when clinically indicated. [d]Second line.

The fluoroquinolones are usually associated with lower rates of treatment failure and relapse than doxycycline.

However, the efficacy of antibiotic treatment varies dramatically with the type and duration of clinical manifestations and with immune status. Antibiotic efficacy is usually poor in curing suppurated lymphadenopathies or other soft tissue or organ abscesses. No standardized treatment has been defined for tularemia complications such as meningitis, endocarditis, and osteoarticular infections. The same holds for infections occurring in immunocompromised patients. The combination of an aminoglycoside with either doxycycline or a fluoroquinolone is often used in these specific situations, although the superiority of dual therapy over monotherapy has not been demonstrated.

For pregnant women in the United States, gentamicin is advocated as first-line treatment and doxycycline or a fluoroquinolone as second-line treatment. All these antibiotics have potential side effects on the mother and the fetus and thus are classically avoided before childbirth—most importantly, during the first trimester of pregnancy. Azithromycin has been used successfully in a few pregnant women with mild disease in western Europe, where tularemia cases are caused only by type B *F. tularensis* strains susceptible to this antibiotic.

SURGICAL TREATMENT

Removal of suppurated lymph nodes in tularemia patients with regional lymphadenopathy is the leading cause of surgical intervention. The combination of surgery and appropriate antibiotic therapy is the most effective treatment of this complication. Several surgeries are sometimes necessary for definite cure. Surgery may also be needed in other clinical situations, including skin or subcutaneous abscesses, cellulitis, deep abscesses, endocarditis, osteoarticular infections, and ocular complications.

PROGNOSIS

The prognosis of patients with tularemia depends on the patient's immune status, the clinical form of disease, and the involved *F. tularensis* strain. Classically, spontaneous mortality rates range from 5 to 15% for type A tularemia and are <1% for type B disease. With receipt of appropriate antibiotic therapy, <2% of type A tularemia patients die. The pneumonic and typhoidal forms have been associated with mortality rates up to 30%. A more recent evaluation of mortality rates in culture-confirmed tularemia cases in the United States highlighted significant variations depending on the involved *F. tularensis* genotype: 24% for A1b, 4% for A1a, 7% for B, and 0% for A2 strains. Therefore, an accurate prognostic evaluation of type A tularemia will require genotyping of the causative *F. tularensis* strain.

PREVENTION

LACK OF HUMAN-TO-HUMAN TRANSMISSION

Human-to-human transmission of *F. tularensis* is considered unlikely. In the literature, such transmission has been reported in only two specific situations: the autopsy of a person who died of tularemia and organ transplantation from a person who died of tularemia. Thus, no isolation measures for tularemia patients are necessary during routine medical care, even those with the pneumonic form of disease.

EXPOSURE PREVENTION

The most effective prophylactic measures against tularemia are those reducing the risk of exposure to *F. tularensis*. Persons manipulating potentially contaminated animals (especially lagomorphs and small rodents) or their carcasses should wear appropriate protective equipment (gloves, glasses, a respiratory mask, and protective clothing). Use of repellants against arthropods (especially ticks) is also essential in tularemia-endemic areas. Water-borne and food-borne tularemia cases can be prevented by consuming potable water and well-cooked food. Hydrotelluric sources of contamination are more challenging to identify and, therefore, to avoid. Finally, laboratory personnel handling *F. tularensis* cultures should work in biosafety level 3 facilities with appropriate safety equipment.

POSTEXPOSURE PROPHYLAXIS

The most at-risk situation is exposure to an *F. tularensis* aerosol. A highly suspected *F. tularensis* aerosol inhalation requires postexposure antibiotic prophylaxis. The need for such treatment is more easily identified for laboratory personnel handling *F. tularensis* cultures. Current recommendations are to treat the exposed person with either doxycycline or a fluoroquinolone for 14 days (Table 170-1). Subsequent medical and possibly serologic monitoring is usually carried out. At least 1 month of surveillance after the end of treatment seems reasonable.

VACCINATION

The live vaccine strain (LVS), a virulence-attenuated type B strain of *F. tularensis*, was widely used before and after World War II to vaccinate highly exposed persons (especially laboratory staff). This vaccine has been abandoned because of its limited efficacy against severe type A pneumonia, unstable colony phenotype, and potentially severe side effects at the inoculation site as well as fear of a potential reversion of LVS to a virulent strain. In recent years, significant efforts have been made to develop new and safer vaccines. *F. tularensis* mutants for metabolic enzymes, virulence factors, or regulatory proteins have been developed. However, no vaccine has currently been authorized by the U.S. Food and Drug Administration or by health protection agencies in other countries.

FURTHER READING

Bossi P et al: Bichat guidelines for the clinical management of tularaemia and bioterrorism-related tularaemia. Euro Surveill 9:E9, 2004.

Centers for Disease Control and Prevention: Tularemia: United States. Available at *https://www.cdc.gov/tularemia/index.html*. Accessed October 3, 2020.

Dennis DT et al: Tularemia as a biological weapon: Medical and public health management. JAMA 285:2763, 2001.

Maurin M, Gyuranecz M: Tularaemia: Clinical aspects in Europe. Lancet Infect Dis 16:113, 2016.

World Health Organization: *WHO Guidelines on Tularaemia*. Geneva, WHO Press, 2007.

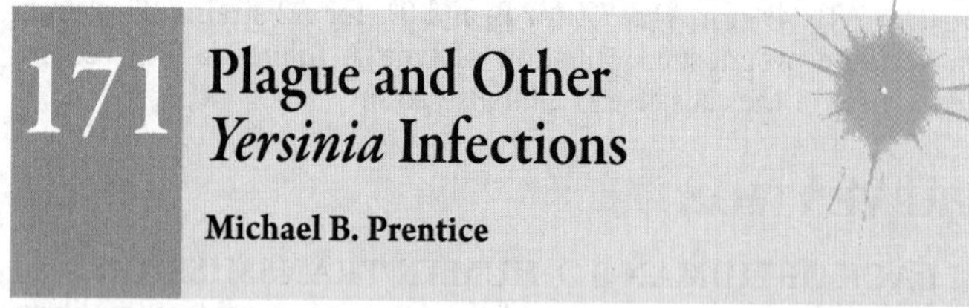

171 Plague and Other *Yersinia* Infections

Michael B. Prentice

PLAGUE

Plague is a systemic zoonosis caused by *Yersinia pestis*. It predominantly affects small rodents in rural areas of Africa, Asia, and the Americas and is usually transmitted to humans by an arthropod vector (the flea). Less often, infection follows contact with animal tissues or respiratory droplets. Plague is an acute febrile illness that is treatable with antimicrobial agents, but mortality rates among untreated patients are high. Ancient DNA studies have confirmed that both the fourteenth-century Black Death and the sixth-century Plague of Justinian in Europe were due to *Y. pestis* infection. Patients can present with the bubonic, septicemic, or pneumonic form of the disease. Although there is concern about epidemic spread of plague by the respiratory route, this is not the most common route of plague transmission, and established infection-control measures for respiratory plague exist. However, the fatalities associated with plague and the capacity for infection via the respiratory tract mean that *Y. pestis* fits the profile of a potential agent of bioterrorism (**Chap. S3**). Consequently, measures have been taken to restrict access to the organism, including legislation affecting diagnostic and research procedures in some countries (e.g., the United States).

ETIOLOGY

The genus *Yersinia* comprises gram-negative bacteria of the order *Enterobacterales* (class *Gammaproteobacteria*). Overwhelming taxonomic and paleogenomic evidence shows *Y. pestis* recently evolved from *Yersinia pseudotuberculosis*, an enteric pathogen of mammals spread by the fecal–oral route, and thus has a phenotype distinctly different from that of *Y. pestis*. When grown in vivo or at 37°C, *Y. pestis* forms an amorphous capsule made from a plasmid-specified fimbrial protein, Caf or fraction 1 (F1) antigen, which is an immunodiagnostic marker of infection.

EPIDEMIOLOGY

Human plague generally follows an outbreak in a host rodent population (epizootic). Mass deaths among the rodent primary hosts lead to a search by fleas for new hosts, with consequent incidental infection of other mammals. The precipitating cause for an epizootic may ultimately be related to climate or other environmental factors. The reservoir for *Y. pestis* causing enzootic plague in natural endemic foci between epizootics (i.e., when the organism may be difficult to detect in rodents or fleas) is a topic of ongoing research and may not be the same in all regions. The enzootic/epizootic pattern may be the result of complex dynamic interactions of host rodents that have different plague susceptibilities with different flea vectors; alternatively, an environmental reservoir may be important.

GLOBAL FEATURES

In general, the enzootic areas for plague are lightly populated regions of Africa, Asia, and the Americas (**Fig. 171-1**). Between January 2013 and December 2018, 2886 cases of plague with a global case–fatality rate of 17% were notified to the World Health Organization (WHO) under the International Health Regulations. More than 97% of these cases were in Africa. The majority of cases in each year were from the island of Madagascar, which in 2017 experienced an urban outbreak of over 2400 clinically suspected cases, with an unusually high proportion of pneumonic plague (78%). A decline in reports from the Democratic Republic of the Congo (DRC) may reflect ongoing conflict in that country affecting surveillance rather than a true decrease. In the past decade, outbreaks of pneumonic plague have been recorded in the DRC, Uganda, Algeria, Madagascar, China, and Peru.

Plague was introduced into North America via the port of San Francisco in 1900 as part of the Third Pandemic, which spread around the world from Hong Kong. The disease is presently enzootic on the western side of the continent from southwestern Canada to Mexico. Most human cases in the United States occur in two regions:

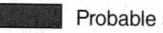

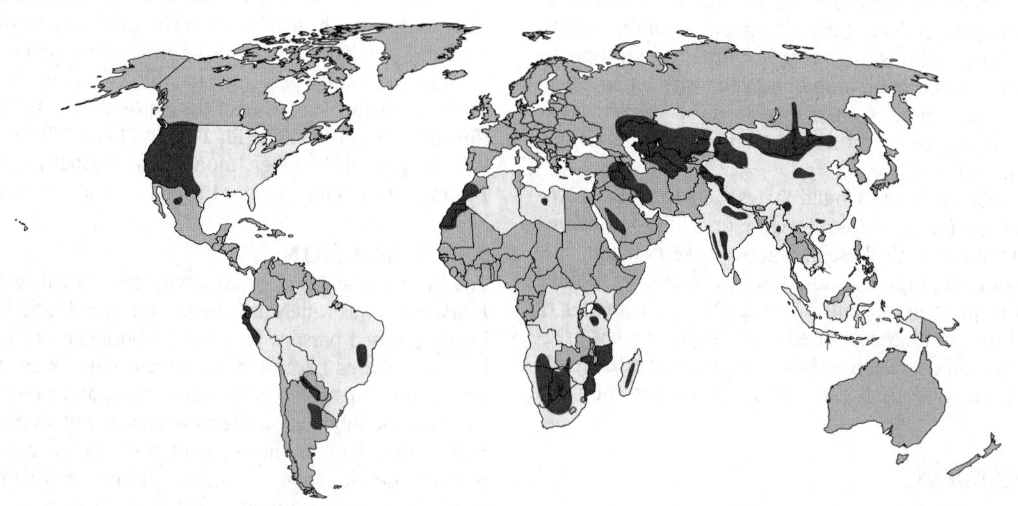

FIGURE 171-1 Approximate global distribution of *Yersinia pestis*. *(Compiled from WHO, CDC, and country sources. From DT Dennis, GL Campbell: Plague and other Yersinia infections, in Harrison's Principles of Internal Medicine, 17th ed, AS Fauci et al [eds]. New York, McGraw-Hill, Chap. 152, 2008.)*

"Four Corners" (the junction point of New Mexico, Arizona, Colorado, and Utah), especially northern New Mexico, northern Arizona, and southern Colorado; and further west in California, southern Oregon, and western Nevada *(www.cdc.gov/plague/maps/)*. From 1970 to 2017, 482 cases of plague were reported in the United States; in recent decades incidence has fallen to an average of 7 cases per year. Most cases occur from May to October—the time of year when people are outdoors and rodents and their fleas are most plentiful. Prior animal contact occurs in at least 50% of cases, and about 60% of these include domestic animals (usually dogs or cats) that brought wild animals or plague-infected fleas home. Infected cats or dogs may transmit plague directly to humans by the respiratory route. A slightly lower percentage of prior animal contacts involve direct handling of living or dead wild small mammals (e.g., rabbits, hares, prairie dogs) or wild carnivores (e.g., wildcats, coyotes, mountain lions). In 2014, an outbreak of nonfatal pneumonic plague in Colorado affected four people exposed to an infected dog, with possible interhuman transmission in one case. Prior to this report, the most recent case of person-to-person transmission in the United States occurred in the Los Angeles pneumonic plague outbreak of 1924.

Plague most often develops in areas with poor sanitary conditions and infestations of rats—in particular, the widely distributed roof rat *Rattus rattus* and the brown rat *Rattus norvegicus* (which serves as a laboratory model of plague). Rat control in warehouses and shipping facilities has been recognized as important in preventing the spread of plague since the early twentieth century and features in the current WHO International Health Regulations. Urban rodents acquire infection from wild rodents, and the proximity of the former to humans increases the risk of transmission. The oriental rat flea *Xenopsylla cheopis* is the most efficient vector for transmission of plague among rats and onward to humans in Asia, Africa, and South America.

Worldwide, bubonic plague is the predominant form reported (80–95% of suspected cases), with mortality rates of 10–20%. The mortality rate is higher (22%) in the small proportion of patients (10–20%) with primary septicemic plague (i.e., systemic *Y. pestis* sepsis with no bubo; see "Clinical Manifestations," below) and is highest with primary pulmonary plague. The latter is generally the least common of the main plague presentations, but, as in the 2017 Madagascar outbreak, it is occasionally predominant. Mortality rates of 50% or more for primary pulmonary plague are reported with delayed antimicrobial treatment in small case series from the older literature. Rare outbreaks of pharyngeal plague following consumption of raw or undercooked camel or goat meat have been reported.

A total of 744 (82%) of the 913 plague cases with clinically documented features (out of 1006 cases reported in total) in the United States from 1900 to 2012 were bubonic disease, 87 (10%) were septicemic disease, and 74 (8%) were pneumonic disease; 6 cases (1%) were pharyngeal. Sixteen percent of cases were fatal in the postantibiotic era from 1942 onward compared with 66% in the period 1900–1941.

PATHOGENESIS

As mentioned earlier, genetic evidence shows *Y. pestis* is a clone derived from the enteric pathogen *Y. pseudotuberculosis* in the recent evolutionary past (7000–50,000 years ago). The change from infection by the fecal–oral route to a two-stage life cycle, with alternate parasitization of arthropod and mammalian hosts, occurred as a result of two plasmid gene acquisitions (*pla* on pPCP1/pPst and *ymt* on pFra/pMT1), and the inactivation of a handful of *Y. pseudotuberculosis* genes, in conjunction with preexisting properties of the *Y. pseudotuberculosis* ancestor, including the presence of a virulence plasmid, pYV, and the capacity to cause septicemia. In the arthropod-parasitizing portion of its life cycle, *Y. pestis* multiplies and forms biofilm-embedded aggregates in the flea midgut after ingestion of a blood meal containing bacteria. In some fleas, biofilm-embedded bacteria eventually fill the proventriculus (a valve connecting the esophagus to the midgut) and block normal blood feeding. Both "blocked" fleas and those containing masses of biofilm-embedded *Y. pestis* without complete blockage inoculate *Y. pestis* into each bite site. The ability of *Y. pestis* to colonize and multiply in the flea requires phospholipase D encoded by the *ymt* gene on the pFra (pMT1) plasmid, and biofilm synthesis requires the chromosomal *hms* locus shared with *Y. pseudotuberculosis*. Three *Y. pseudotuberculosis* genes inhibiting biofilm formation or promoting its degradation are inactivated in *Y. pestis*, together with urease (urease activity otherwise causes acute flea gastrointestinal toxicity). Blockage takes days or weeks to come about after initial infection of the flea and is followed by the flea's death. Many flea vectors (including *X. cheopis*) are also able to transmit plague in an early-phase unblocked state for up to a week after feeding, but 10 fleas in this state are required to infect a mammalian host (mass transmission).

Y. pestis disseminates from the site of inoculation in the mammalian host in a process initially dependent on plasminogen activator Pla, which is encoded by the small pPCP1 (pPst) plasmid. This surface protease activates mammalian plasminogen, degrades complement, and adheres to the extracellular matrix component laminin. Pla is essential for the high-level virulence of *Y. pestis* in mice by subcutaneous or intradermal injection (laboratory proxies for fleabites) and for the development of primary pneumonic plague. When actual fleabite inoculation is used in mouse models, the fimbrial capsule-forming protein (Ca1 or fraction 1; F1 antigen) encoded on pFra increases the efficiency of transmission, and plasminogen activator is required for the formation of buboes.

Paleogenomics (sequencing of DNA extracts from teeth of ancient human remains) shows that *Y. pestis* was a common cause of death in Eurasia in the Bronze age. Remarkably, the *ymt* gene is absent from the pFra (pMT1) plasmid in *Y. pestis* sequences from remains more than 4000 years old, while *pla* is present. This suggests that plague was a common fatal human infection before flea-borne transmission was possible, presumably spread by the pneumonic or gastrointestinal route.

Macrophages, neutrophils, and dendritic cells are all involved in the innate immune response to flea-transmitted *Y. pestis*. The organism is taken up by macrophages but avoids being killed by autophagy and can also survive and replicate in neutrophils. Rapid transport of the bacteria to regional lymph nodes occurs. *Y. pestis* then undergoes extracellular replication with full expression of its antiphagocytic systems: the type III secretion machines and their effectors encoded by pYV as well as the F1 capsule. These factors prevent neutrophil uptake, and the type III secretion effectors also block extrusion of microbicidal DNA by neutrophils and trigger apoptotic cell death. Immune cell targeting follows binding of the N-formylpeptide receptor (FPR1) on phagocytic cells by LcrV, the needle cap protein of the type III secretion system. Overproduction of LcrV also exerts an anti-inflammatory effect, reducing host immune responses. Likewise, *Y. pestis* lipopolysaccharide is modified to minimize stimulation of host Toll-like receptor 4, thereby reducing protective host inflammatory responses during peripheral infection and prolonging host survival with high-grade bacteremia—an effect that probably enhances the pathogen's subsequent transmission by fleabite.

Replication of *Y. pestis* in a regional lymph node results in the local swelling of the lymph node and periglandular region known as a *bubo*. On histology, the node is found to be hemorrhagic or necrotic, with thrombosed blood vessels, and the lymphoid cells and normal architecture are replaced by large numbers of bacteria and fibrin. Periglandular tissues are inflamed and also contain large numbers of bacteria in a serosanguineous, gelatinous exudate.

Continued spread through the lymphatic vessels to contiguous lymph nodes produces second-order primary buboes. Infection is initially contained in the infected regional lymph nodes, although transient bacteremia can be detected. As infection progresses, spread via efferent lymphatics to the thoracic duct produces high-grade bacteremia. Hematogenous spread to the spleen, liver, and secondary buboes follows, with subsequent uncontrolled septicemia leading to death. In some patients, this septicemic phase occurs without obvious prior bubo development or lung disease (septicemic plague). Hematogenous spread to the lungs results in secondary plague pneumonia, with bacteria initially more prominent in the interstitium than in the air spaces (the reverse being the case in primary plague pneumonia). Hematogenous spread to other organs, including the meninges, can occur.

CLINICAL MANIFESTATIONS

Bubonic Plague After an incubation period of 2–6 days, the onset of bubonic plague is sudden and is characterized by fever (>38°C), malaise, myalgia, dizziness, and increasing pain due to progressive lymphadenitis in the regional lymph nodes near the fleabite or other inoculation site. Lymphadenitis manifests as a tense, tender swelling (bubo) that, when palpated, has a boggy consistency with an underlying hard core. Generally, there is one painful and erythematous bubo with surrounding periganglionic edema. The bubo is most commonly inguinal but can also be crural, axillary (**Fig. 171-2**), cervical, or submaxillary, depending on the site of the bite. Abdominal pain from intraabdominal node involvement can occur without other visible signs. Children are most likely to present with cervical or axillary buboes.

The differential diagnosis includes acute focal lymphadenopathy of other etiologies, such as streptococcal or staphylococcal infection, tularemia, cat-scratch disease, tick typhus, infectious mononucleosis, or lymphatic filariasis. These infections do not progress as rapidly, are not as painful, and are associated with visible cellulitis or ascending lymphangitis—both of which are absent in plague.

Without treatment, *Y. pestis* dissemination occurs and causes serious illness, including pneumonia (secondary pneumonic plague) and meningitis. Secondary pneumonic plague can be the source of person-to-person transmission of respiratory infection by productive cough (droplet infection), with the consequent development of primary plague pneumonia. Appropriate treatment of bubonic plague results in fever resolution within 2–5 days, but buboes may remain enlarged for >1 week after initial treatment and can become fluctuant.

Primary Septicemic Plague A minority (10–25%) of infections with *Y. pestis* present as gram-negative septicemia (hypotension, shock) without preceding lymphadenopathy. Septicemic plague occurs in all age groups, but persons >40 years of age are at elevated risk. Some chronic conditions may predispose to septicemic plague: in 2009 in the United States, a fatal laboratory-acquired infection with an attenuated *Y. pestis* strain manifested as septicemic plague in a 60-year-old researcher with diabetes mellitus and undiagnosed hemochromatosis. These conditions also carry an increased risk of septicemia with other pathogenic *Yersinia* species. The term *septicemic plague* can be confusing since most patients with buboes have detectable bacteremia

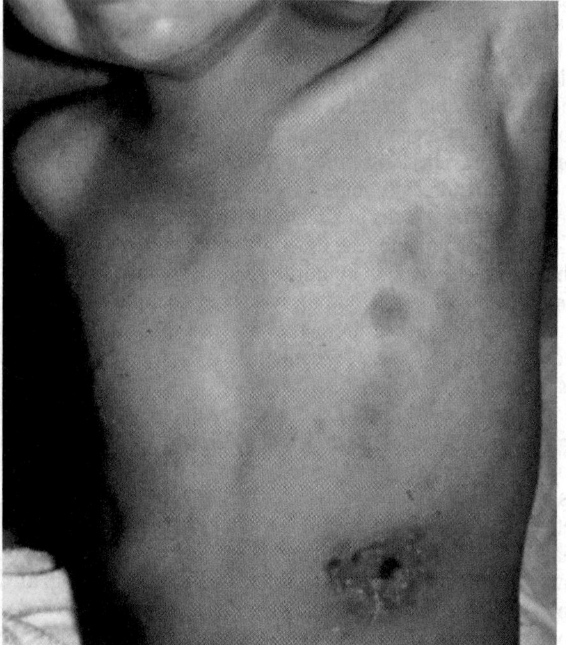

FIGURE 171-2 Plague patient in the southwestern United States with a left axillary bubo and an unusual plague ulcer and eschar at the site of the infective flea bite. *(Reproduced with permission from AS Fauci et al: Harrison's Principles of Internal Medicine, 17th ed. New York: McGraw-Hill; 2008.)*

at some stage, with or without systemic signs of sepsis. In laboratory experiments, however, septicemic disease without histologic changes in lymph nodes is seen in a minority of mice infected via fleabites.

Pneumonic Plague Primary pneumonic plague results from inhalation of infectious bacteria in droplets expelled from another person or an animal with primary or secondary plague pneumonia. This syndrome has a short incubation period, averaging from a few hours to 2–3 days (range, 1–7 days), and is characterized by a sudden onset of fever, headache, myalgia, weakness, nausea, vomiting, and dizziness. Respiratory signs—cough, dyspnea, chest pain, and sputum production with hemoptysis—typically arise after 24 h. Progression of initial segmental pneumonitis to lobar pneumonia and then to bilateral lung involvement may occur (**Fig. 171-3**). The possible release of aerosolized *Y. pestis* bacteria in a bioterrorist attack, manifesting as an outbreak of primary pneumonic plague in nonendemic regions or in an urban setting where plague is rarely seen, has been a source of public health concern. Secondary pneumonic plague is a consequence of bacteremia occurring in ~10–15% of patients with bubonic plague. Bilateral alveolar infiltrates are seen on chest x-ray, and diffuse interstitial pneumonitis with scanty sputum production is typical.

Meningitis Meningeal plague is uncommon, occurring in ≤6% of plague cases reported in the United States. Presentation with headache and fever typically occurs >1 week after the onset of bubonic or septicemic plague and may be associated with suboptimal antimicrobial therapy (delayed therapy, penicillin administration, or low-dose tetracycline treatment) and cervical or axillary buboes.

Pharyngitis Symptomatic plague pharyngitis can follow the consumption of contaminated meat from an animal dying of plague or contact with persons or animals with pneumonic plague. This condition can resemble tonsillitis, with peritonsillar abscess and cervical lymphadenopathy. Asymptomatic pharyngeal carriage of *Y. pestis* can also occur in close contacts of patients with pneumonic plague.

LABORATORY DIAGNOSIS

Because of the scarcity of laboratory facilities in regions where human *Y. pestis* infection is most common, and because of the potential significance of *Y. pestis* isolation in a nonendemic area or an area from which human plague has been absent for many years, the WHO recommends an initial presumptive diagnosis followed by reference laboratory confirmation (**Table 171-1**). In the United States, comprehensive national diagnostic facilities for plague have been in place since 1999 (Laboratory Response Network for Biological Threats; *emergency.cdc.gov/lrn/*) to detect possible use of biological terrorism agents, including *Y. pestis*. Routine diagnostic clinical microbiology laboratories that are included in this network as sentinel-level laboratories use joint protocols from the Centers for Disease Control and Prevention (CDC) and the American Society for Microbiology *(https://asm.org/Articles/Policy/Laboratory-Response-Network-LRN-Sentinel-Level-C)* to identify suspected *Y. pestis* isolates and to refer these specimens to LRN reference laboratories for confirmatory tests. *Y. pestis* is designated a "Tier 1 select agent" under the Public Health Security and Bioterrorism Preparedness and Response Act of 2002 and subsequent executive orders; the provisions of this act, the Patriot Act of 2001, and related executive orders apply to all U.S. laboratories and individuals working with *Y. pestis*. Details of the applicable regulations are available from the CDC (*www.selectagents.gov*).

Yersinia species are gram-negative coccobacilli (short rods with rounded ends) 1–3 μm in length and 0.5–0.8 μm in diameter. *Y. pestis* in particular appears bipolar (with a "closed safety pin" appearance) and pleomorphic when stained with a polychromatic stain (Wayson or Wright-Giemsa; **Fig. 171-4**). Its lack of motility distinguishes *Y. pestis* from other *Yersinia* species, which are motile at 25°C and nonmotile at 37°C. Transport medium (e.g., Cary-Blair medium) preserves the viability of *Y. pestis* if transport is delayed.

The appropriate specimens for diagnosis of bubonic, pneumonic, and septicemic plague are bubo aspirate, bronchoalveolar lavage fluid or sputum, and blood, respectively. Culture of postmortem organ biopsy samples also can be diagnostic. A bubo aspirate is obtained

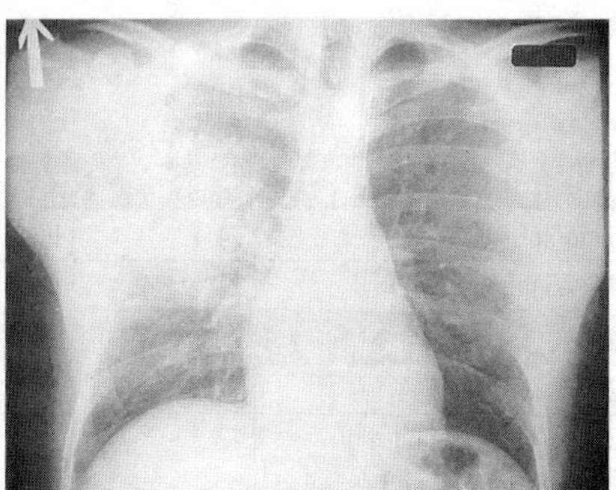

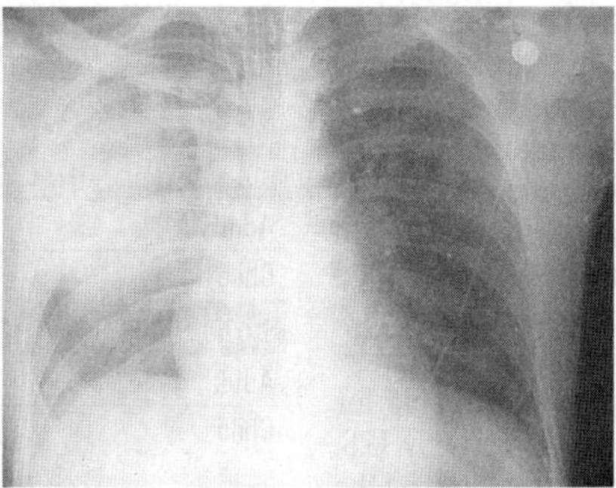

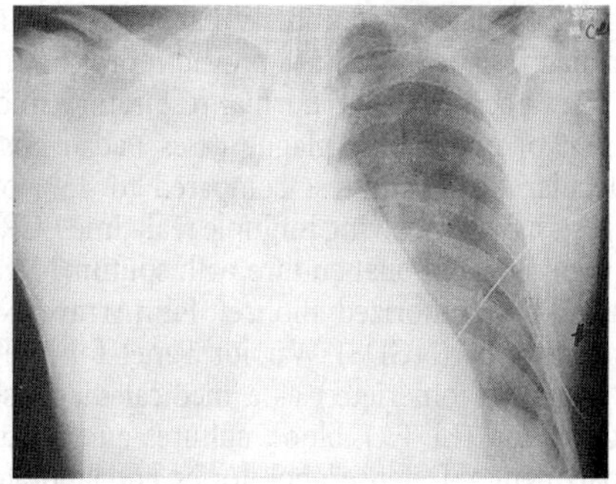

FIGURE 171-3 Sequential chest radiographs of a patient with fatal primary plague pneumonia. ***Left:*** Upright posteroanterior film taken at admission to hospital emergency department on third day of illness, showing segmental consolidation of right upper lobe. ***Center:*** Portable anteroposterior film taken 8 h after admission, showing extension of pneumonia to right middle and right lower lobes. ***Right:*** Portable anteroposterior film taken 13 h after admission (when patient had clinical acute respiratory distress syndrome), showing diffuse infiltration throughout right lung and patchy infiltration of left lower lung. A cavity later developed at the site of initial right-upper-lobe consolidation. *(Reproduced with permission from AS Fauci et al: Harrison's Principles of Internal Medicine, 17th ed. New York: McGraw-Hill; 2008.)*

by injection of 1 mL of sterile normal saline into a bubo under local anesthetic and aspiration of a small amount of (usually blood-stained) fluid. The WHO has provided interim guidance on how to aspirate buboes and collect sputum from patients with suspected pneumonic plague (*www.who.int/csr/disease/plague/collecting-sputum-samples.PDF*). Gram's staining of these specimens may reveal gram-negative rods, which are shown by Wayson or Wright-Giemsa staining to be bipolar. These bacteria may even be visible in direct blood smears in septicemic plague (Fig. 171-4); this finding indicates very high numbers of circulating bacteria and a poor prognosis.

Y. pestis grows on nutrient agar and other standard laboratory media but forms smaller colonies than do other Enterobacteriaceae.

TABLE 171-1 World Health Organization Case Definitions of Plague

Suspected Case
Compatible clinical presentation
And
Consistent epidemiologic features, such as exposure to infected animals or humans and/or evidence of fleabites and/or residence in or travel to a known endemic focus within the previous 10 days
Presumptive Case
Meeting the definition of a suspected case
Plus
Putative new or reemerging focus: ≥2 of the following tests positive
• Microscopy: gram-negative coccobacilli in material from bubo, blood, or sputum; bipolar appearance of Wayson or Wright-Giemsa staining
• F1 antigen detected in bubo aspirate, blood, or sputum
• A single anti-F1 serology without evidence of previous *Yersinia pestis* infection or immunization
• PCR detection of *Y. pestis* in bubo aspirate, blood, or sputum
Known endemic focus: ≥1 of the above tests positive
Confirmed Case
Meeting the definition of a suspected case
Plus
• Identification of an isolate from a clinical sample as *Y. pestis* (colonial morphology and 2 of the following 4 tests positive: phage lysis of cultures at 20–25°C and 37°C; F1 antigen detection; PCR; *Y. pestis* biochemical profile)
Or
• A fourfold rise in anti-F1 titer in paired serum samples
Or
• In endemic areas when no other confirmatory test can be performed, a positive rapid diagnostic test with immunochromatography to detect F1 antigen

Abbreviation: PCR, polymerase chain reaction.

Source: Reproduced with permission from Interregional meeting on prevention and control of plague, World Health Organization, 2006.

Specimens should be inoculated onto nutrient-rich media such as sheep blood agar (SBA), into nutrient-rich broth such as brain-heart infusion broth, and onto selective agar such as MacConkey or eosin methylene blue (EMB) agar. *Yersinia*-specific CIN (cefsulodin, triclosan [Irgasan], novobiocin) agar can be useful for culture of contaminated specimens, such as sputum. Blood should be cultured in a standard blood culture system. The optimal growth temperature is <37°C (25–29°C), with pinpoint colonies only on SBA at 24 h. Slower growth occurs at 37°C. *Y. pestis* is oxidase-negative, catalase-positive, urease-negative, indole-negative, and lactose-negative. Automated biochemical or mass spectrometry identification systems can misidentify *Y. pestis* as *Y. pseudotuberculosis* or other bacterial species.

Reference laboratory tests for definitive identification of isolates include direct immunofluorescence for F1 antigen; specific polymerase chain reaction (PCR) for targets such as F1 antigen, the pesticin gene, and the plasminogen activator gene; and specific bacteriophage lysis. PCR can also be applied to diagnostic specimens, as can direct immunofluorescence for F1 antigen (produced in large amounts by *Y. pestis*) by slide microscopy. An immunochromatographic test strip for F1 antigen detection by monoclonal antibodies in clinical specimens has been devised in Madagascar. This method is effective for both laboratory and near-patient use and is now widely used in endemic countries. A similar test strip for Pla antigen has been developed and could be used to detect wild-type or engineered F1-negative virulent strains. In

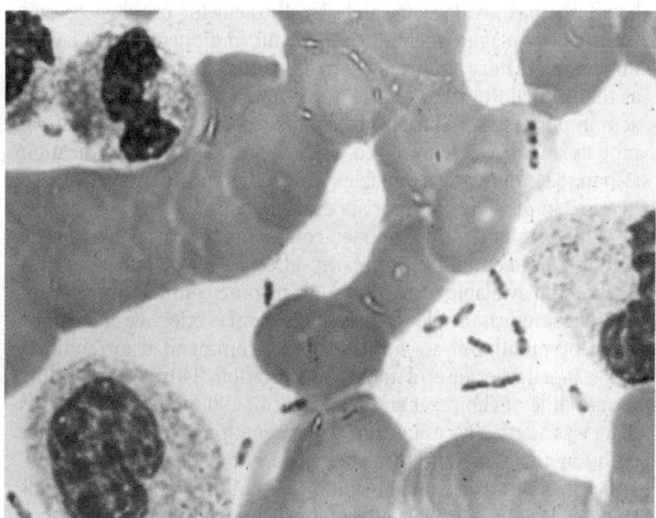

FIGURE 171-4 Peripheral-blood smear from a patient with fatal plague septicemia and shock, showing characteristic bipolar-staining *Yersinia pestis* bacilli (Wright's stain, oil immersion). *(Reproduced with permission from AS Fauci et al: Harrison's Principles of Internal Medicine, 17th ed. New York: McGraw-Hill; 2008.)*

the 2017 Madagascar outbreak, diagnosis by F1-antigen strip or molecular diagnosis from sputum proved more challenging than from bubo aspirates because of the normal respiratory microbiota. Twenty-three percent of pneumonic plague cases had a positive culture, strip, or molecular diagnostic test compared to 45% of bubonic cases. This suggests assays involving multiple real-time PCR targets are required to augment conventional culture with sputum. *Yersinia pestis* is included in the FDA-authorized Biofire® FilmArray® Next Generation Diagnostic System (NGDS) Warrior Panel for use with the FilmArray® 2.0 system (Biomérieux) as a medical diagnostic device suitable for whole blood (EDTA), blood cultures and sputum specimens by U.S. Department of Defense laboratories, and laboratories designated by the Department of Defense. Detailed phylogeographic DNA sequence data based on culture collections have been accumulated to trace plague evolution, and this approach could be adapted in the future to real-time clinical plague epidemiology.

In the absence of other positive laboratory diagnostic tests, a retrospective serologic diagnosis may be made on the basis of rising titers of hemagglutinating antibody to F1 antigen. Enzyme-linked immunosorbent assays (ELISAs) for IgG and IgM antibodies to F1 antigen are also available.

The white blood cell (WBC) count is generally raised (to 10,000–20,000/μL) in plague, with neutrophilic leukocytosis and a left shift (numerous immature neutrophils); in some cases, however, the WBC count is normal or leukopenia develops. WBC counts are occasionally very high, especially in children (>100,000/μL). Levels of fibrinogen degradation products are elevated in a majority of patients, but platelet counts are usually normal or low-normal. However, disseminated intravascular coagulation, with low platelet counts, prolonged prothrombin times, reduced fibrinogen, and elevated fibrinogen degradation product levels, occurs in a significant minority of patients.

TREATMENT

Plague

Guidelines for the treatment of plague are given in **Table 171-2**. A 10- to 14-day course of antimicrobial therapy (or a course continued until 2 days after fever subsides) is recommended. Streptomycin has historically been the parenteral treatment of choice for plague and is approved for this indication by the FDA. Although not yet approved by the FDA for plague, gentamicin has proved safe and effective in clinical trials in Tanzania and Madagascar and in retrospective reviewed cases in the United States. In view of streptomycin's adverse-reaction profile and limited availability, some experts now recommend gentamicin over streptomycin. The FDA has approved levofloxacin, moxifloxacin, and ciprofloxacin for prophylaxis and treatment of plague (including septicemic and pneumonic plague) under a regulatory approach based on animal studies alone, known as the Animal Rule. Levofloxacin has more efficacy than ciprofloxacin in postexposure prophylaxis of inhalational anthrax in animal models and has also received FDA approval for this indication (**Chap. S3**); thus it is a suitable agent for prophylaxis against two diseases in possible bioterrorism exposures.

While systemic chloramphenicol therapy is available in the resource-poor countries primarily affected by plague, it is less likely to be available or used in high-income countries because of its adverse-effect profile. Tetracyclines are also effective and can be given by mouth but are not generally recommended for children age <7 years because of tooth discoloration. Doxycycline is the tetracycline of choice; at an oral dosage of 100 mg twice daily, this drug was as effective as intramuscular gentamicin (2.5 mg/kg twice daily) in a trial in Tanzania. There is recent evidence that doxycycline does not cause dental staining in children because it binds calcium less readily than other tetracyclines. Because of reduced efficacy in some non-human primate models of pneumonic plague, CDC recommends doxycycline as a first line agent for bubonic plague and an alternative agent for septicemic and pneumonic plague.

TABLE 171-2 Guidelines for the Treatment of Plague

DRUG	DAILY DOSE	DOSING INTERVAL, h	ROUTE
Gentamicin			
Adult	5 mg/kg[a]	24	IM/IV
Child	4.5-7.5 mg/kg[a]	24	IM/IV
Streptomycin			
Adult	2 g	12	IM
Child	30 mg/kg (maximum 1 g per dose)	12	IM
Levofloxacin			
Adult (child >50 kg)	750 (500-750) mg	24	PO/IV
Child <50 kg and ≥6 months of age	16 mg/kg (maximum, 250 mg/dose)	12	PO/IV
Ciprofloxacin			
Adult	1500 mg	12	PO
	1200 mg	8	IV
Child	30-45 mg/kg (maximum, 500 mg/dose)	8-12	PO
	20-30 mg/kg (maximum, 400 mg/dose)	8-12	IV
Moxifloxacin			
Adult	400 mg (no loading dose)	24	PO/IV
Doxycycline			
Adult and child ≥45 kg	200 mg (200 mg loading dose)	12	PO/IV
Child <45 kg	4.4 mg/kg (maximum, 100 mg/dose), 4.4 mg/kg loading dose	12	PO/IV
Tetracycline			
Adult	2 g	6	PO/IV
Child >8 yr	40–50 mg/kg	6	PO/IV
Chloramphenicol			
Adult	50-100 mg/kg	6	PO/IV
Child >2 yr	50-100 mg/kg (maximum, 4 g)	6	PO/IV

[a]Aminoglycoside dose is adjusted with impaired renal function. No trial data have been published for once-daily gentamicin therapy for plague in adults or children, but this regimen is efficacious in gram-negative sepsis of other etiologies and has been successful in a recent outbreak of pneumonic plague in the Democratic Republic of the Congo. Neonates (up to 1 week of age) should receive gentamicin at 4 mg/kg IV once daily.

Source: TV Inglesby et al: Plague as a biological weapon: Medical and public health management. Working Group on Civilian Biodefense. JAMA 283:2281, 2000; and *https://www.cdc.gov/plague/healthcare/clinicians.html*. For detailed guidelines on recommended regimens for pneumonic vs bubonic plague, plague meningitis, treatment during pregnancy and lactation, and neonatal infection see CA Nelson et al: Antimicrobial treatment and prophylaxis of plague: Recommendations for naturally acquired infections and bioterrorism response. MMWR Recomm Rep 70(No. RR-3):1, 2021.

Although *Y. pestis* is sensitive to β-lactam drugs in vitro and these drugs have been efficacious against plague in some animal models, the response to penicillins has been poor in some clinical cases; thus β-lactams and macrolides are not generally recommended as first-line therapy. Chloramphenicol, alone or in combination, is recommended for some focal complications of plague (e.g., meningitis, endophthalmitis, myocarditis) because of its tissue penetration properties. Fluoroquinolones, effective in vitro and in animal models, are recommended in guidelines for possible bioterrorism-associated pneumonic plague and are increasingly used in plague therapy.

PREVENTION

In endemic areas, the control of plague in humans is based on reduction of the likelihood of being bitten by infected fleas or exposed to infected droplets from either humans or animals with plague pneumonia. In the United States, residence and outdoor activity or contact with wild or pet animals in rural areas of western states where epizootics occur are the main risk factors for infection. To assess potential risks to humans in specific areas, surveillance for *Y. pestis* infection among animal plague hosts and vectors is carried out regularly as well as in response to observed animal die-offs. Personal protective measures include avoidance of areas where a plague epizootic has been identified and publicized (e.g., by warning signs or closure of campsites). Sick or dead animals should not be handled by the general public. Hunters, zoologists and pet-owners should wear gloves if handling wild-animal carcasses in endemic areas. General measures to avoid rodent fleabite during outdoor activity are appropriate and include the use of insect repellent, insecticide, and protective clothing. General measures to reduce peridomestic and occupational human contact with rodents are advised and include rodent-proofing of buildings and food-waste stores and removal of potential rodent habitats (e.g., woodpiles and junk heaps). Flea control by insecticide treatment of wild rodents is an effective means of minimizing human contact with plague if an epizootic is identified in an area close to human habitation. Any attempt to reduce rodent numbers must be preceded by flea suppression to reduce the migration of infected fleas to human hosts. An oral F1-V subunit vaccine using raccoon poxvirus (RCN) as a vector (sylvatic plague vaccine) is partially protective against plague when administered to wild prairie dogs in field trials and may in the future provide a means of reducing the risk of human exposure to *Y. pestis*.

Patients in whom pneumonic plague is suspected should be managed in isolation (with negative pressure, if available), with droplet precautions observed until pneumonia is excluded or effective antimicrobial therapy has been given for 48 h. Review of the literature published before the advent of antimicrobial agents suggests that the main infective risk is posed by patients in the final stages of disease who are coughing up sputum with plentiful visible blood and/or pus. Cotton and gauze masks were protective in these circumstances. Current surgical masks capable of barrier protection against droplets, including large respiratory particles, are probably protective, but the differential diagnosis of fever and hemoptysis in plague-endemic areas includes aerosol-transmitted infections such as tuberculosis. In addition, WHO guidance recommends that personal protective equipment for potential aerosol-generating procedures (e.g., collection of respiratory samples from patients with suspected or confirmed plague) should include a fit-tested N95 face mask, a gown, gloves, and a face shield or goggles.

Antimicrobial Prophylaxis Postexposure antimicrobial prophylaxis lasting 7 days is recommended following household, hospital, or other close contact with persons with untreated pneumonic plague. (*Close contact* is defined as contact with a patient at <2 m.) In animal aerosol-infection studies, levofloxacin and ciprofloxacin are associated with higher survival rates than doxycycline (**Table 171-3**).

TABLE 171-3 Guidelines for Plague Prophylaxis

DRUG	DAILY DOSE	DOSING INTERVAL, h	ROUTE
Doxycycline			
Adult	200 mg	12 or 24	PO
Child ≥8 y	≥45 kg: adult dose	12	PO
	≤45 kg: 2.2 mg/kg bid (maximum, 200 mg)	12	PO
Tetracycline			
Adult	2 g	6 or 12	PO
Child ≥8 y	40 mg/kg (maximum 500 mg/dose)	6 or 12	PO
Levofloxacin			
Adult and child >50 kg	500-750 mg	24	PO
Child <50 kg and ≥6 months of age	16 mg/kg (maximum, 250 mg/dose)	12	PO
Ciprofloxacin			
Adult	1-1.5 g	12	PO
Child	30 mg/kg (maximum 750 mg dose)	12	PO

Source: TV Inglesby et al: Plague as a biological weapon: Medical and public health management. Working Group on Civilian Biodefense. JAMA 283:2281, 2000; *https://www.cdc.gov/plague/healthcare/clinicians.html*; CA Nelson et al: Antimicrobial treatment and prophylaxis of plague: Recommendations for naturally acquired infections and bioterrorism response. MMWR Recomm Rep 70(No. RR-3):1, 2021.

Immunization Studies with candidate plague vaccines in animal models show that neutralizing antibody provides protection against exposure but that cell-mediated immunity is critical for protection and clearance of *Y. pestis* from the host. A killed whole-cell vaccine used in humans required multiple doses, caused significant local and systemic reactions, and was not protective against pneumonic plague; this vaccine is not currently available. A live attenuated vaccine based on strain EV76 is still used in countries of the former Soviet Union and China but has significant side effects. Different subunit vaccines devised by governmental agencies in the United States, UK, and China all comprising recombinant F1 (rF1) and various recombinant V (rV) proteins produced in *Escherichia coli*, combined either as a fusion protein or as a mixture, purified, and adsorbed to aluminum hydroxide for injection are close to licensing. This combination protects mice and various nonhuman primates in laboratory models of bubonic and pneumonic plague and has been evaluated in phase 2 clinical trials. Prelicensing field-efficacy studies (phase 3 trials) are difficult to devise because of plague epidemiology. In the United States, the FDA will assess plague vaccines for human use under the Animal Rule, using efficacy data from animal studies and antibodies and other correlates of immunity from human vaccinees (*www.fda.gov/emergencypreparedness/counterterrorism/medicalcountermeasures/mcmregulatoryscience/ucm391604.htm*), and the rF1-V subunit vaccine has orphan drug status. The World Health Organization has produced a target product profile (TPP) for phase 3 trial design and prioritization of the 17 known vaccine candidates. These include protein subunit vaccines, live-attenuated vaccines, and bacterial, viral, and bacteriophage vectors, or outer membrane vesicles, carrying *Y. pestis* antigens. Antigens other than F1 and V are being investigated because of the recovery of F1-negative *Y. pestis* strains from natural sources and the observation that F1 antigen is not required for virulence in primate models of pneumonic plague.

YERSINIOSIS

Yersiniosis is a zoonotic infection with an enteropathogenic *Yersinia* species, usually *Y. enterocolitica* or *Y. pseudotuberculosis*. The usual hosts for these organisms are pigs and other wild and domestic animals; humans are usually infected by the oral route, and outbreaks from contaminated food occur. Yersiniosis is most common in childhood and in colder climates. Patients present with abdominal pain and sometimes with diarrhea (which may not occur in up to 50% of cases). *Y. enterocolitica* is more closely associated with terminal ileitis and *Y. pseudotuberculosis* with mesenteric adenitis, but both organisms may cause mesenteric adenitis and symptoms of abdominal pain and tenderness that result in pseudoappendicitis, with the surgical removal of a normal appendix. Diagnosis was historically based on culture of the organism or convalescent serology, but proprietary multiplex PCR systems for gastrointestinal infection diagnosis now include *Y. enterocolitica*. *Y. pseudotuberculosis* and some rarer strains of *Y. enterocolitica* (serogroup O:8) are especially likely to cause systemic infection, which is also more likely in patients with diabetes or iron overload. Systemic sepsis is treatable with antimicrobial agents, but postinfective arthropathy responds poorly to such therapy. Sixteen other *Yersinia* species lacking the virulence plasmid pYV common to *Y. pestis*, *Y. pseudotuberculosis*, and *Y. enterocolitica* are now recognized. These are, at most, opportunistic pathogens of humans (*Y. aldovae*, *Y. aleksiciae*, *Y. bercovieri*, *Y. entomophaga*, *Y. frederiksenii*, *Y. hibernica*, *Y. intermedia*, *Y. kristensenii*, *Y. massiliensis*, *Y. mollaretii*, *Y. nurmii*, *Y. pekkanenii*, *Y. rohdei*, *Y. similis*, *Y. ruckeri*, and *Y. wautersii*). Whole genome sequencing has recently detected several more probable novel *Yersinia* species. Molecular phylogeny shows that *Y. enterocolitica* is more distantly related to *Y. pseudotuberculosis* than these other

Yersinia species, and the similar virulence plasmid they share has probably been acquired independently by at least one of the two since the species diverged.

EPIDEMIOLOGY

Y. enterocolitica *Y. enterocolitica* is found worldwide and has been isolated from a wide variety of wild and domestic animals and environmental samples, including samples of food and water. In vitro, *Y. enterocolitica* is resistant to predation by the protozoon *Acanthamoeba castellani* and can survive inside it, suggesting a possible mode of environmental persistence. Strains are differentiated by combined biochemical reactions (biovar) and serogroup, and increasingly by whole genome sequence. Most clinical infections are associated with serogroups O:3, O:9, and O:5,27, with a declining number of O:8 infections in North America. Some O:8 infections, previously confined to North America, have been reported from Europe and Japan in recent years, and O:8 infections caused a high percentage of yersiniosis cases in Poland in 2008–2011, with a subsequent decline. Yersiniosis, >99% due to *Y. enterocolitica*, remains the third commonest bacterial food-borne zoonosis reported in Europe, especially prevalent in Germany and Scandinavia. The incidence is highest among children; children <4 years of age are more likely to present with diarrhea than are older children. Abdominal pain with mesenteric adenitis and terminal ileitis is more prominent among older children and adults. Septicemia is more likely in patients with preexisting conditions such as diabetes mellitus, liver disease, any condition involving iron overload (including thalassemia and hemochromatosis), advanced age, malignancy, or HIV/AIDS. As in enteritis of other bacterial etiologies, postinfective complications such as reactive arthritis occur mainly in individuals who are HLA-B27 positive. Erythema nodosum (Fig. A1-39) following *Yersinia* infection is not associated with HLA-B27 and is more common among women than among men.

Consumption or preparation of raw pork products (such as chitterlings) and some processed pork products is strongly linked with infection because a high percentage of pigs carry pathogenic *Y. enterocolitica* strains. Outbreaks of *Y. enterocolitica* infection have been associated with consumption of milk (pasteurized, unpasteurized, and chocolate-flavored) and various foods contaminated with spring water. Person-to-person transmission is suspected in a few cases (e.g., in nosocomial and familial outbreaks) but is much less likely with *Y. enterocolitica* than with other causes of gastrointestinal infection, such as *Salmonella*. A multivariate analysis indicates that contact with companion animals is a risk factor for *Y. enterocolitica* infection among children in Sweden, and low-level colonization of dogs and cats with *Y. enterocolitica* has been reported. Transfusion-associated septicemia due to *Y. enterocolitica*, while recognized as a very rare but frequently fatal event for >30 years, has been difficult to eradicate.

Y. pseudotuberculosis *Y. pseudotuberculosis* is much less frequently reported as a cause of human disease than *Y. enterocolitica*, and infection with *Y. pseudotuberculosis* is more likely to present as fever and abdominal pain due to mesenteric lymphadenitis and to be identified from a blood culture isolate. This organism is associated with wild mammals (rodents, rabbits, and deer), birds, and domestic pigs. Although outbreaks are generally rare, several have recently occurred in Finland in association with consumption of lettuce, raw carrots, or unpasteurized milk. Strains have historically been differentiated by combined biochemical reactions (biovar) and serogroup. Multilocus sequence typing shows that some strains previously assigned to *Y. pseudotuberculosis* belong to the closely related but distinct species now called *Yersinia wautersii* (opportunistic pathogenic) and *Yersinia similis* (nonpathogenic).

PATHOGENESIS

The usual route of infection is oral. Studies with both *Y. enterocolitica* and *Y. pseudotuberculosis* in animal models suggest that initial replication in the small intestine is followed by invasion of Peyer's patches of the distal ileum via M cells, with onward spread to mesenteric lymph nodes. The liver and spleen also can be involved after oral infection. The characteristic histologic appearance of enteropathogenic *Yersinia* after invasion of host tissues is as extracellular microabscesses surrounded by an epithelioid granulomatous lesion.

Experiments involving oral infection of mice with tagged *Y. enterocolitica* show that only a very small proportion of bacteria in the gut invade tissues. Individual bacterial clones from an orally inoculated pool give rise to each microabscess in a Peyer's patch, and the host restricts the invasion of previously infected Peyer's patches. A prior model positing progressive bacterial spread from Peyer's patches and mesenteric lymph nodes to the liver and spleen appears to be inaccurate: spread of *Y. pseudotuberculosis* and *Y. enterocolitica* to the liver and spleen of mice occurs independently of regional lymph node colonization and in mice lacking Peyer's patches.

Invasion requires the expression of several nonfimbrial adhesins, such as invasin (Inv) and—in *Y. pseudotuberculosis*—*Yersinia* adhesin A (YadA). Inv interacts directly with β1 integrins, which are expressed on the apical surfaces of M cells but not enterocytes. YadA of *Y. pseudotuberculosis* interacts with extracellular matrix proteins such as collagen and fibronectin to facilitate host cell integrin association and invasion. YadA of *Y. enterocolitica* lacks a crucial N-terminal region and binds collagen and laminin but not fibronectin and does not cause invasion. Inv is chromosomally encoded, whereas YadA is encoded on the virulence plasmid pYV. YadA also helps to confer serum resistance in *Y. enterocolitica* by binding host complement regulators such as factor H and C4-binding protein. Another chromosomal gene, *ail* (attachment and invasion locus), encodes the extracellular protein Ail, which is the main factor conferring serum resistance in *Y. pseudotuberculosis* by binding these complement regulators.

By binding to host cell surfaces, YadA allows targeting of immune effector cells by the pYV plasmid–encoded type III secretion system (injectisome). As a consequence, the host's innate immune response is altered; toxins (*Yersinia* outer proteins, or Yops) are injected into host macrophages, neutrophils, and dendritic cells, affecting signal transduction pathways, resulting in reduced phagocytosis and inhibited production of reactive oxygen species by neutrophils, and triggering apoptosis of macrophages. Other factors functional in invasive disease include yersiniabactin (Ybt), a siderophore produced by some strains of *Y. pseudotuberculosis* and *Y. enterocolitica* as well as other *Enterobacterales*. Ybt allows bacteria to access iron from saturated lactoferrin during infection and reduces production of reactive oxygen species by innate immune effector cells, thereby decreasing bacterial killing. *Y. pseudotuberculosis* and *Y. pestis* make other siderophores apart from Ybt.

CLINICAL MANIFESTATIONS

Self-limiting diarrhea is the most common reported presentation in infection with pathogenic *Y. enterocolitica*, especially in children <4 years of age, who form the single largest group in most case series. Blood may be detected in diarrheal stool. Older children and adults are more likely than younger children to present with abdominal pain, which can be localized to the right iliac fossa—a situation that often leads to laparotomy for presumed appendicitis (pseudoappendicitis). Appendectomy is not indicated for *Yersinia* infection causing pseudoappendicitis. Thickening of the terminal ileum and cecum is seen on endoscopy and ultrasound, with elevated round or oval lesions that may overlie Peyer's patches. Mesenteric lymph nodes are enlarged. Ulcerations of the mucosa are noted on endoscopy. Gastrointestinal complications include granulomatous appendicitis, a chronic inflammatory condition affecting the appendix that is responsible for ≤2% of cases of appendicitis; *Yersinia* is involved in a minority of cases. *Y. enterocolitica* infection can present as acute pharyngitis with or without other gastrointestinal symptoms. Fatal *Y. enterocolitica* pharyngitis has been recorded. Mycotic aneurysm can follow *Y. enterocolitica* bacteremia, as can focal infection (abscess) in many other sites and body compartments (liver, spleen, kidney, bone, meninges, endocardium).

Y. pseudotuberculosis infection is more likely to present as abdominal pain and fever than as diarrhea. A superantigenic toxin—*Y. pseudotuberculosis* mitogen (YPM)—is produced by strains seen in eastern Russia in association with Far Eastern scarlet-like fever, a childhood illness with desquamating rash, arthralgia, and toxic shock. A similar illness is recognized in Japan (Izumi fever) and Korea. Similarities have been noted with Kawasaki disease, the idiopathic acute systematic vasculitis of childhood. There is an epidemiologic link between exposure of populations to superantigen-positive *Y. pseudotuberculosis* and an elevated incidence of Kawasaki disease.

Y. enterocolitica or *Y. pseudotuberculosis* septicemia presents as a severe illness with fever and leukocytosis, often without localizing features, and is significantly associated with predisposing conditions such as diabetes mellitus, liver disease, and iron overload. Hemochromatosis combines several of these risk factors. Administration of iron chelators like deferoxamine, which provide iron accessible to *Yersinia* (and have an inhibitory effect on neutrophil function), may result in *Yersinia* septicemia in patients with iron overload who presumably have an otherwise mild gastrointestinal infection. HIV/AIDS has been associated with *Y. pseudotuberculosis* septicemia. The unusual phenomenon of transfusion-associated septicemia is linked to the ability of *Y. enterocolitica* to multiply at refrigerator temperature (psychrotrophy). Typically, the transfused unit has been stored for >20 days, and it is believed that small numbers of yersiniae from an apparently healthy donor with subclinical bacteremia are amplified to very high numbers by growth inside the bag at ≤4°C, with consequent septic shock after transfusion. Complete prevention of this very rare event (1 case in several million transfused units in countries such as the United States and France) without unacceptable restriction in the blood supply has not yet been devised.

POSTINFECTIVE PHENOMENA

As in other invasive intestinal infections (salmonellosis, shigellosis), reactive arthritis (articular arthritis of multiple joints developing within 2–4 weeks of a preceding infection) occurs as a result of autoimmune activity initiated by the deposition of bacterial components (not viable bacteria) in joints in combination with the immune response to invading bacteria. The majority of individuals affected by reactive arthritis due to *Yersinia* are HLA-B27 positive. Myocarditis with electrocardiographic ST-segment abnormalities may occur with *Yersinia*-associated reactive arthritis. Most *Yersinia*-associated cases follow *Y. enterocolitica* infection (presumably because it is more common than infection with other species), but *Y. pseudotuberculosis*–associated reactive arthritis is also well documented in Finland, where sporadic and outbreak infections with *Y. pseudotuberculosis* are more common than in other countries. Of infected individuals identified in a recent *Y. pseudotuberculosis* serotype O:3 outbreak in Finland, 12% developed reactive arthritis affecting the small joints of the hands and feet, knees, ankles, and shoulders and lasting >6 months in most cases. Erythema nodosum (**Fig. A1-39**) occurs after *Yersinia* infection (more commonly in women) with no evidence of HLA-B27 linkage.

There is a long-standing association between antithyroid and anti-*Yersinia* antibodies. Antibody evidence of prior *Y. enterocolitica* infection in Graves' disease and increased levels of antithyroid antibody in patients with *Y. enterocolitica* antibodies were first noted in the 1970s. *Y. enterocolitica* contains a thyroid-stimulating hormone (TSH)–binding site that is recognized by antibodies to TSH from Graves' disease patients. Raised titers of antibodies to *Y. enterocolitica* whole cells and Yops have been found in some series of Graves' disease patients but not in others. It remains unclear whether this cross-reactivity is significant in the etiology of Graves' disease.

LABORATORY DIAGNOSIS

Standard laboratory culture methods can be used to isolate enteropathogenic *Yersinia* species from sterile samples, including blood and cerebrospinal fluid. Culture on specific selective media (CIN agar), with or without pre-enrichment in broth or phosphate-buffered saline at either 4°C or 16°C, is the basis of most schema for isolation of yersiniae from stool or other nonsterile samples. Outside known high-incidence areas, specific culture may only be carried out by laboratories on request, or if a multiplex PCR screen detects *Y. enterocolitica*-specific DNA in feces. Several CE-marked, FDA-approved kits for enteric pathogens now offer *Y. enterocolitica* detection (the precise assay targets are not disclosed), and their use has increased detection of *Y. enterocolitica*. A standard for PCR detection of pathogenic *Y. enterocolitica* and *Y. pseudotuberculosis* in food samples is available from the International Organization for Standardization.

Matrix-assisted laser desorption ionization time of flight (MALDI-TOF) mass spectrometry systems can speciate isolates of *Y. enterocolitica* and *Y. pseudotuberculosis* (but cannot separate *Y. similis* or *Y. pestis* from *Y. pseudotuberculosis*). Virulence plasmid–negative strains of *Y. enterocolitica* can be isolated from cultures of stool from asymptomatic individuals, especially after cold enrichment. These strains usually differ in biotype (typically biovar 1a) from virulence plasmid–possessing strains; although some display apparent pathogenicity in a mouse model and all are pathogenic in an insect model, virulence plasmid–negative strains are not commonly accepted as human pathogens. Because of the frequency with which the virulence plasmid is lost on laboratory subculture, combined biochemical identification (with biotyping according to a standard schema) and serologic identification are usually required to interpret the significance of an isolate of *Y. enterocolitica* from a nonsterile site. Most pathogenic *Y. enterocolitica* strains currently isolated from humans are of serogroup O:3/biovar 4 or serogroup O:9/biovar 2; this pattern holds even in the United States, where serogroup O:8/biovar 1B strains were previously predominant. Whole genome DNA sequencing applying a *Yersinia* genus-wide seven-gene MLST scheme can speciate *Y. enterocolitica*, *Y. pestis*, and *Y. pseudotuberculosis* and differentiate *Y. enterocolitica* biotypes. A core-genome MLST scheme has recently been developed, providing an even more detailed population structure and revealing novel as yet phenotypically undefined *Yersinia* species.

Agglutinating or ELISA antibody titers to specific O-antigen types are used in the retrospective diagnosis of both *Y. enterocolitica* and *Y. pseudotuberculosis* infections. IgA and IgG antibodies persist in patients with reactive arthritis. Serologic cross-reactions between *Y. enterocolitica* serogroup O:9 and *Brucella* are due to the similarity of their lipopolysaccharide structures. Multiple assays are required to cover even the predominant serogroups (*Y. enterocolitica* O:3, O5,27, and O:9; *Y. pseudotuberculosis* O:1a, O:1b, and O:3), and these assays are generally available only in reference laboratories. ELISA and Western blot tests for antibodies to Yops, which are expressed by all pathogenic strains of *Y. enterocolitica* and *Y. pseudotuberculosis*, also are available; most of the positivity in these assays probably relates to previous infection with *Y. enterocolitica*.

TREATMENT

Yersiniosis

Most cases of diarrhea caused by enteropathogenic *Yersinia* are self-limiting. Data from clinical trials do not support antimicrobial treatment for adults or children with *Y. enterocolitica* diarrhea. Systemic infections with bacteremia or focal infections outside the gastrointestinal tract generally require antimicrobial therapy. Infants <3 months of age with documented *Y. enterocolitica* infection may require antimicrobial treatment because of the increased likelihood of bacteremia in this age group. *Y. enterocolitica* strains nearly always express β-lactamases. Because of the relative rarity of systemic *Y. enterocolitica* infection, there are no clinical trial data to guide antimicrobial choice or to suggest the optimal dose and duration of therapy. On the basis of retrospective case series and in vitro sensitivity data, fluoroquinolone therapy is effective for bacteremia in adults; for example, ciprofloxacin is given at a typical dose of 500 mg twice daily by mouth or 400 mg twice daily IV for at least 2 weeks (longer if positive blood cultures persist). A third-generation cephalosporin is an alternative—e.g., cefotaxime (typical dose, 6–8 g/d in 3 or 4 divided doses) or ceftriaxone. In children, third-generation cephalosporins are effective; for example, cefotaxime is given to children ≥1 month of age at a typical dose of 75–100 mg/kg per day in 3 or 4 divided doses, with an increase to 150–200 mg/kg per day in severe cases (maximal daily dose, 8–10 g). Amoxicillin and amoxicillin/clavulanate have shown poor efficacy in case series. Trimethoprim-sulfamethoxazole, gentamicin, and imipenem are all active in vitro. *Y. pseudotuberculosis* strains do not express β-lactamase but are intrinsically resistant to polymyxin. Because human infection with *Y. pseudotuberculosis* is less common than that with *Y. enterocolitica*, less case information is available; however, studies in mice suggest that ampicillin is ineffective. Drugs similar to those used against *Y. enterocolitica* should be used. The best results have been obtained with a quinolone.

Some trials of treatment for reactive arthritis (with a large proportion of cases due to *Yersinia*) found that 3 months of oral ciprofloxacin therapy did not affect outcome. One trial in which the same therapy was given specifically for *Y. enterocolitica*–reactive arthritis found that, while outcome indeed was not affected, there was a trend toward faster remission of symptoms in the treated group. Follow-up 4–7 years after initial antibiotic treatment of reactive arthritis (predominantly following *Salmonella* and *Yersinia* infections) demonstrated apparent efficacy in the prevention of chronic arthritis in HLA-B27-positive individuals. A trial showing that azithromycin therapy did not affect outcome in reactive arthritis included cases thought to have followed yersiniosis, although no breakdown of cases was provided.

PREVENTION AND CONTROL

Current control measures are similar to those used against other enteric pathogens like *Salmonella* and *Campylobacter*, which colonize the intestine of food animals. The focus is on safe handling and processing of food. No vaccine is effective in preventing intestinal colonization of food animals by enteropathogenic *Yersinia*. Consumption of food made from raw pork (which is popular in Germany and Belgium) should be discouraged at present because it is not possible to eliminate contamination with the enteropathogenic *Yersinia* strains found worldwide in pigs. Exposure of infants to raw pig intestine during domestic preparation of chitterlings is inadvisable. Modification of abattoir technique in Scandinavian countries from the 1990s onward included the removal of pig intestines in a closed plastic bag; levels of carcass contamination with *Y. enterocolitica* were reduced, but such contamination was not eliminated. Experimental pig herds free of pathogenic *Y. enterocolitica* O:3 (and also of *Salmonella*, *Campylobacter*, *Toxoplasma*, and *Trichinella*) have been established by selective breeding in Norway but remain rare. In the food industry, vigilance is required because of the potential for large outbreaks if small numbers of enteropathogenic yersiniae contaminate any ready-to-eat food whose safe preservation is based on refrigeration before consumption.

The rare phenomenon of contamination of blood for transfusion has proved impossible to eradicate. However, leukodepletion is now practiced in most blood transfusion centers, primarily to prevent non-hemolytic febrile transfusion reactions and alloimmunization against HLA antigens. This measure reduces but does not eliminate the risk of *Yersinia* blood contamination.

Notification of yersiniosis is now obligatory in some countries.

FURTHER READING

Plague

Bertherat E: Plague around the world in 2019. Wkly Epidemiol Rec 94:289, 2019.

Campbell SB et al: Animal exposure and human plague, United States, 1970–2017. Emerg Infect Dis 25:2270, 2019.

Demeure C et al: *Yersinia pestis* and plague: An updated view on evolution, virulence determinants, immune subversion, vaccination and diagnostics. Microbes Infect 21:202, 2019.

Hinnebusch BJ et al: Ecological opportunity, evolution, and the emergence of flea-borne plague. Infect Immun 84:1932, 2016.

Kool JL: Risk of person-to-person transmission of pneumonic plague. Clin Infect Dis 40:1166, 2005.

Nelson CA et al: Antimicrobial treatment and prophylaxis of plague: Recommendations for naturally acquired infections and bioterrorism response. MMWR Recomm Rep 70(No. RR-3):1, 2021.

Randremanana R et al: Epidemiological characteristics of an urban plague epidemic in Madagascar, August-November, 2017: An outbreak report. Lancet Infect Dis 19:537, 2019.

Sun W et al: Plague vaccine: Recent progress and prospects. NPJ Vaccines 4:11. 2019.

Yersiniosis

Francis MS et al: The pathogenic Yersiniae—advances in the understanding of physiology and virulence. Front Cell Infect Microbiol 9:119, 2019.

Savin C et al: Genus-wide *Yersinia* core-genome multilocus sequence typing for species identification and strain characterization. Microbial Genomics 5:e000301, 2019.

172 *Bartonella* Infections, Including Cat-Scratch Disease

Michael Giladi, Moshe Ephros

Bartonella species are fastidious, facultative intracellular, slow-growing, gram-negative bacteria that cause a broad spectrum of diseases in humans. This genus includes >40 distinct species or subspecies, of which at least 16 have been recognized as confirmed or potential human pathogens; *Bartonella bacilliformis*, *Bartonella quintana*, and *Bartonella henselae* are most commonly identified (**Table 172-1**). Most *Bartonella* species have successfully adapted to survival in specific domestic or wild mammals. Prolonged intraerythrocytic infection in these animals creates a niche where the bacteria are protected from both innate and adaptive immunity and which serves as a reservoir for human infections. *Bartonella* characteristically evades the host immune system by modification of its virulence factors (e.g., lipopolysaccharides or flagella) and by attenuation of the immune response. *B. bacilliformis* and *B. quintana*, which are not zoonotic, are exceptions. Arthropod vectors are often involved. Isolation and characterization of *Bartonella* species are difficult and require special techniques. Clinical presentation generally depends on both the infecting *Bartonella* species and the immune status of the infected individual. *Bartonella* species are susceptible to many antibiotics in vitro; however, clinical responses to therapy and studies in animal models suggest that the minimal inhibitory concentrations of many antimicrobial agents correlate poorly with the drugs' in vivo efficacies in patients with *Bartonella* infections.

CAT-SCRATCH DISEASE

DEFINITION AND ETIOLOGY

Usually a self-limited illness, cat-scratch disease (CSD) has two general clinical presentations. *Typical* CSD, the more common, is characterized by subacute regional lymphadenopathy; *atypical* CSD is the collective designation for numerous extranodal manifestations involving various organs. *B. henselae* is the principal etiologic agent of CSD. Rare cases have been associated with *Afipia felis* and other *Bartonella* species.

EPIDEMIOLOGY

CSD occurs worldwide, favoring warm and humid climates. In temperate climates, incidence peaks during fall and winter. Adults are affected nearly as frequently as children. Intrafamilial clustering is rare, and person-to-person transmission does not occur. Apparently healthy bacteremic cats constitute the major reservoir of *B. henselae*, and cat fleas (*Ctenocephalides felis*) may be responsible for cat-to-cat transmission. CSD usually follows contact with cats (especially kittens), but other animals (e.g., dogs) have been implicated as possible reservoirs in rare instances. In the United States, the estimated annual disease incidence is ~5 cases per 100,000 population. About 5% of patients are hospitalized.

PATHOGENESIS

Although cat fleas are likely responsible for cat-to-cat transmission, the mode of cat-to-human transmission is undetermined. *B. henselae*–infected

TABLE 172-1 *Bartonella* Species Known or Suspected to Be Human Pathogens

BARTONELLA SPECIES[a]	DISEASE(S)[b]	RESERVOIR HOST(S)[c]	ARTHROPOD VECTOR
B. henselae	Cat-scratch disease, bacillary angiomatosis, bacillary peliosis, bacteremia, endocarditis	Cats, other felines	Cat fleas (*Ctenocephalides felis*): associated with cat-to-cat, but not with cat-to-human, transmission
B. quintana	Trench fever, chronic bacteremia, bacillary angiomatosis, endocarditis	Humans	Human body lice (*Pediculus humanus corporis*)
B. bacilliformis	Carrión's disease	Humans	Sandflies (*Lutzomyia verrucarum*)
B. elizabethae	Endocarditis	Rats, dogs	Unknown
B. grahamii[d]	Lymphadenopathy	Mice, voles	Fleas
B. vinsonii subsp. *arupensis*	Endocarditis, febrile illness	Mice, dogs	Ticks
B. vinsonii subsp. *berkhoffii*	Endocarditis	Domestic dogs, coyotes, gray foxes	Ticks
B. washoensis	Endocarditis, myocarditis, meningitis	Squirrels, possibly other rodents	Fleas
B. alsatica	Endocarditis, lymphadenitis, vascular graft infection	Rabbits	Fleas
B. koehlerae	Endocarditis	Cats	Unknown
B. clarridgeiae	Possibly cat-scratch disease	Cats	Unknown
B. rochalimae	Bacteremia, fever, splenomegaly	Unknown	Possibly fleas
B. tamiae	Bacteremia, fever, myalgia, rash	Unknown	Unknown
B. melophagi	Various clinical manifestations	Sheep	Sheep keds
B. ancashensis	Verruga peruana	Unknown	Unknown
Candidatus B. mayotimonensis[e]	Endocarditis	Bats	Unknown

[a]Many other *Bartonella* species exist but are not recognized as human pathogens. [b]Animal-associated *Bartonella* species (*B. henselae, B. doshiae, B. schoenbuchensis,* and *B. tribocorum*) were isolated from blood of patients who reported tick bites and chronic symptoms such as fatigue and myalgia. DNA of *B. henselae, B. vinsonii* subsp. *berkhoffii, B. koehlerae,* or *B. melophagi* or co-infection with more than one *Bartonella* species was detected by polymerase chain reaction in blood samples from patients with extensive arthropod and animal exposure who presented with chronic neurologic or neurocognitive syndromes. The causal relationship between bacteremia with these pathogens, tick bites, and clinical manifestations needs to be established. [c]Animals are implicated when existing evidence supports their infection with *Bartonella* species. Data supporting animal-to-human transmission may be lacking. [d]Retinitis may also be associated with *B. grahamii.* [e]*Candidatus* is a taxonomic status for bacteria that cannot be described in sufficient detail to warrant establishment of a novel taxon or cannot be cultured or propagated in culture media. The phylogenetic relatedness of these bacteria has been determined by gene amplification and sequence analysis.

cats' saliva spreads to claws by self-licking, and *B. henselae*–contaminated flea feces can be inoculated by a scratch or a bite. Infection of mucous membranes or conjunctivae via droplets or licking may occur as well. With lymphatic drainage to one or more regional lymph nodes in immunocompetent hosts, a T_H1 response can result in necrotizing granulomatous lymphadenitis. Dendritic cells, along with their associated chemokines, play a role in the host inflammatory response and granuloma formation.

■ CLINICAL MANIFESTATIONS AND PROGNOSIS

Of patients with CSD, 85–90% have *typical* disease. The primary lesion, a small (0.3- to 1-cm) painless erythematous papule or pustule, develops at the inoculation site within days to 2 weeks in about one-third to two-thirds of patients (**Fig. 172-1*A, B***). Lymphadenopathy develops 1–3 weeks or longer after cat contact. The affected lymph node(s) are enlarged and usually painful, sometimes have overlying erythema, and suppurate in ~10% of cases (**Fig. 172-1*C, D,* and *E***). Axillary/epitrochlear nodes are most commonly involved, followed by head/neck nodes and inguinal/femoral nodes. Approximately 50% of patients have fever, malaise, and anorexia. A smaller proportion experience weight loss and night sweats mimicking the presentation of lymphoma. Fever is usually low-grade but infrequently rises to ≥39°C. Resolution is slow, requiring weeks (for fever, pain, and accompanying signs and symptoms) to months (for node shrinkage).

Atypical CSD occurs in 10–15% of patients in the absence or presence of lymphadenopathy. Atypical disease includes Parinaud's oculoglandular syndrome (granulomatous conjunctivitis with ipsilateral preauricular lymphadenitis; Fig. 172-1*E*), hepatosplenic disease, neuroretinitis (often presenting as unilateral deterioration of vision; **Fig. 172-1*F***) and other ophthalmologic manifestations, neurologic manifestations (encephalitis, seizures, myelitis, cerebellitis, facial and other cranial or peripheral palsies), fever of unknown origin, pneumonitis, debilitating myalgia, arthritis or arthralgia (affecting mostly women >20 years old), osteomyelitis (including multifocal disease), tendinitis, and dermatologic manifestations (including erythema nodosum [**see Fig. A1-39**], sometimes accompanying arthropathy). CSD-associated fever of unknown origin is a unique syndrome that may be severe and debilitating, often mimics malignancy, and may present with multiorgan involvement, including hepatosplenic space-occupying lesions, abdominal/mediastinal lymphadenopathy, ocular disease, and multifocal osteomyelitis. Fever may be continuous or relapsing. Other manifestations and syndromes (pleural effusion, idiopathic thrombocytopenic purpura, Henoch-Schönlein purpura, erythema multiforme [**see Fig. A1-24**], glomerulonephritis, myocarditis) have also been associated with CSD. In elderly patients (>60 years old), lymphadenopathy is more often absent but encephalitis and fever of unknown origin are more common than in younger patients. In immunocompetent individuals, CSD—whether typical or atypical—usually resolves without treatment and without sequelae, although some of the ophthalmologic manifestations may occasionally result in moderate to severe vision loss. Lifelong immunity is the rule.

■ DIAGNOSIS

Routine laboratory tests usually yield normal or nonspecific results. Histopathology initially shows lymphoid hyperplasia and later demonstrates stellate granulomata with necrosis, coalescing microabscesses, and occasional multinucleated giant cells—findings that, although nonspecific, may narrow the differential diagnosis. Serologic testing (immunofluorescence or enzyme immunoassay) is the most commonly used laboratory diagnostic approach, with variable sensitivity and specificity. CSD serodiagnosis is often based on the presence of IgG alone (i.e., in the absence of IgM), and seroconversion may take a few weeks; these two factors may pose difficulties in the interpretation of serologic results. Other tests are of low sensitivity (culture, Warthin-Starry silver staining), of low specificity (cytology, histopathology), or of limited availability in routine diagnostic laboratories (polymerase chain reaction [PCR], immunohistochemistry). PCR of pus aspirated from lymph nodes or the primary inoculation lesion is highly sensitive and specific and is particularly useful for definitive and rapid diagnosis in seronegative patients. PCR of a lymph node biopsy specimen may be less sensitive, perhaps because of sampling error.

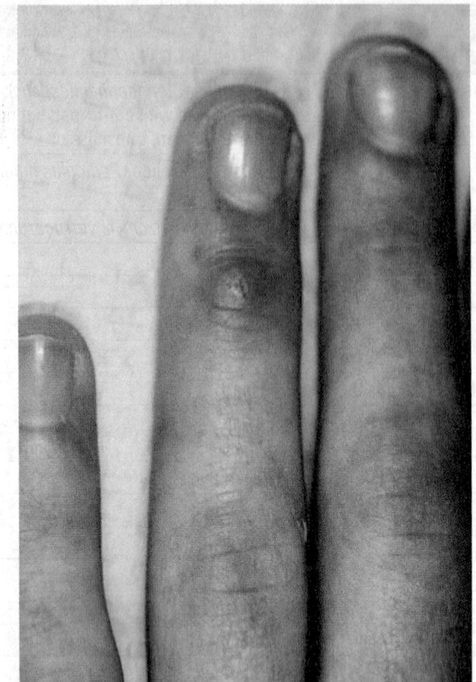

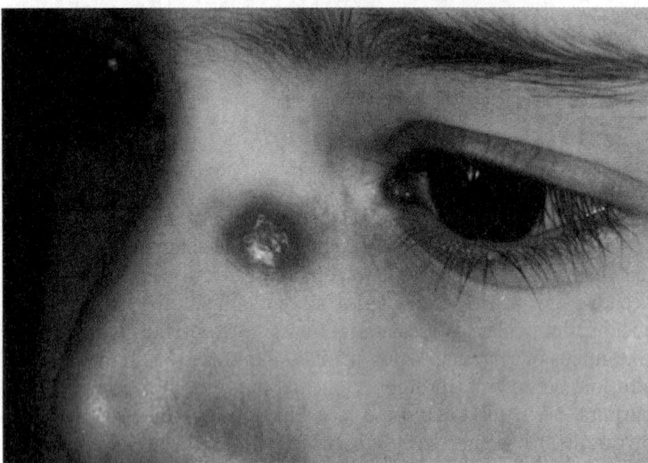

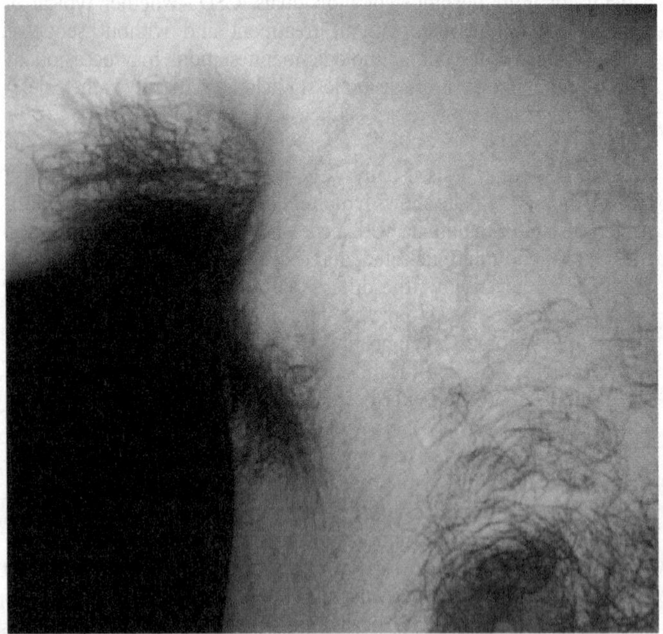

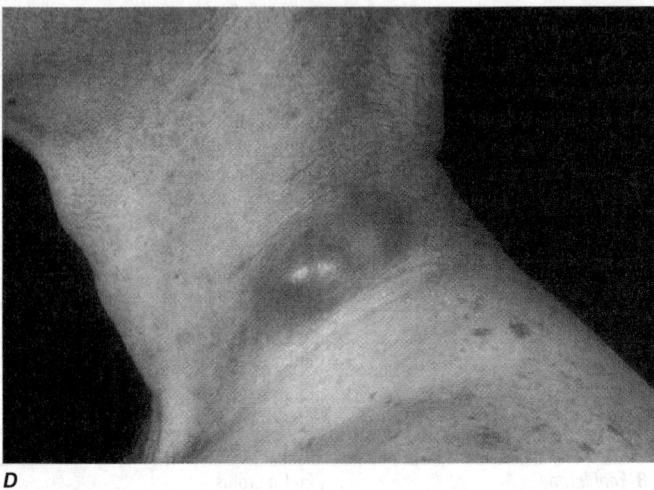

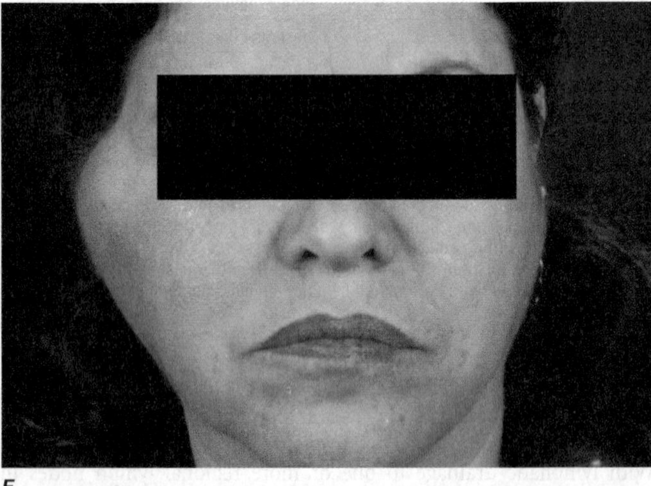

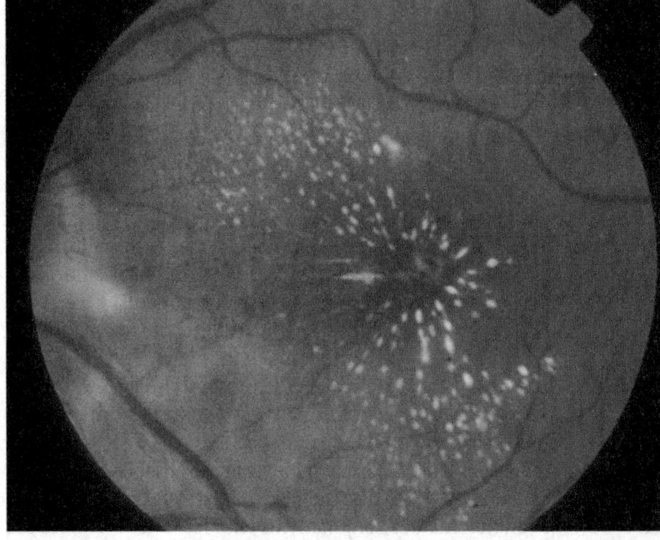

FIGURE 172-1 Manifestations of cat-scratch disease. ***A.*** Primary inoculation lesion. Axillary and epitrochlear lymphadenitis appeared 2 weeks later. ***B.*** Primary inoculation lesion. Submental lymphadenitis appeared 10 days later. ***C.*** Axillary lymphadenopathy of 2 weeks' duration. The overlying skin appears normal. ***D.*** Cervical lymphadenopathy of 6 weeks' duration. The overlying skin is red. Thick, odorless pus (12 mL) was aspirated. ***E.*** Preauricular lymphadenopathy. ***F.*** Left-eye neuroretinitis. Note papilledema and stellate macular exudates ("macular star").

APPROACH TO THE PATIENT

Cat-Scratch Disease

A history of cat contact, a primary inoculation lesion, and regional lymphadenopathy—especially axillary/epitrochlear lymphadenopathy—are highly suggestive of CSD. A characteristic clinical course and corroborative laboratory tests make the diagnosis very likely. Conversely, when acute- and convalescent-phase sera are negative (as is the case in 10–20% of CSD patients), when spontaneous regression of lymph node size does not occur, and particularly when constitutional symptoms persist, malignancy must be ruled out. Pyogenic lymphadenitis, mycobacterial infection, brucellosis, syphilis, tularemia, plague, toxoplasmosis, sporotrichosis, and histoplasmosis should also be considered. In clinically suspected CSD in a seronegative individual, fine-needle aspiration may be adequate and PCR can confirm the diagnosis. When data are less supportive of CSD, lymph node biopsy rather than fine-needle aspiration is preferred. In seronegative CSD patients with lymphadenopathy and severe complications (e.g., encephalitis or neuroretinitis), early biopsy is important to establish a specific diagnosis.

TREATMENT

Cat-Scratch Disease

(Table 172-2) Treatment regimens are based on only minimal data. Suppurative nodes should be drained by large-bore needle aspiration and not by incision and drainage to avoid chronic draining tracts. Systemic antibiotics are recommended in immunocompromised patients.

PREVENTION

Avoiding cats (especially kittens) and instituting flea control are options for immunocompromised patients and for patients with valvular heart disease.

TRENCH FEVER AND CHRONIC BACTEREMIA

DEFINITION AND ETIOLOGY

Trench fever, also known as *5-day fever* or *quintan fever*, is a febrile illness caused by *B. quintana*. It was first described as an epidemic in the trenches of World War I; however, recent paleomicrobiological studies have provided evidence that *B. quintana* has been associated with human infection for 4000 years. This infection recently reemerged as chronic bacteremia seen most often in homeless people, also referred to as *urban* or *contemporary trench fever*.

EPIDEMIOLOGY

In addition to epidemics during World Wars I and II, sporadic outbreaks of trench fever have been reported in many regions of the world. The human body louse has been identified as the vector and humans as the only known reservoir. After a hiatus of several decades during which trench fever was almost forgotten, small clusters of cases of *B. quintana* chronic bacteremia were reported sporadically, primarily from the United States and France, in HIV-uninfected homeless people. Alcoholism and louse infestation were identified as risk factors.

CLINICAL MANIFESTATIONS

The typical incubation period is 15–25 days (range, 3–38 days). "Classical" trench fever, as described in 1919, ranges from a mild febrile illness to a recurrent or protracted and debilitating disease. Fever is often periodic, lasting 4–5 days with 5-day (range, 3- to 8-day) intervals between episodes. Other symptoms and signs include headache, back and limb pain, profuse sweating, shivering, myalgia, arthralgia, splenomegaly, a maculopapular rash in occasional cases, and nuchal rigidity in some cases. Untreated, the disease usually lasts 4–6 weeks. Death is rare. The clinical spectrum of *B. quintana* bacteremia in homeless people ranges from asymptomatic infection to a febrile illness with headache, severe leg pain, and thrombocytopenia. Endocarditis sometimes develops.

TABLE 172-2 Antimicrobial Therapy for Disease Caused by *Bartonella* Species in Adults

DISEASE	ANTIMICROBIAL THERAPY
Typical cat-scratch disease	Not routinely indicated; for patients with extensive lymphadenopathy, consider azithromycin (500 mg PO on day 1, then 250 mg PO once a day for 4 days)
Cat-scratch disease neuroretinitis	Value of systemic antibiotics is controversial, particularly when visual acuity is not significantly compromised. For more severe cases, doxycycline (100 mg PO bid) *plus* rifampin (300 mg PO bid) for 4–6 weeks is given. Consider adding systemic glucocorticoids.
Other atypical cat-scratch disease manifestations[a]	As per neuroretinitis. Treatment duration should be individualized.
Trench fever or chronic bacteremia with *B. quintana*	Gentamicin (3 mg/kg IV once a day for 14 days) *plus* doxycycline (200 mg PO once a day or 100 mg PO bid for 6 weeks)
Suspected *Bartonella* endocarditis	Gentamicin[b] (1 mg/kg IV q8h for ≥14 days) *plus* doxycycline (100 mg PO/IV bid for 6 weeks[c]) *plus* ceftriaxone (2 g IV once a day for 6 weeks)
Confirmed *Bartonella* endocarditis	As for suspected *Bartonella* endocarditis *minus* ceftriaxone
Bacillary angiomatosis	Erythromycin[d] (500 mg PO qid for 3 months) *or* Doxycycline (100 mg PO bid for 3 months)
Bacillary peliosis	Erythromycin[d] (500 mg PO qid for 4 months) *or* Doxycycline (100 mg PO bid for 4 months)
Carrión's disease	
Oroya fever	Chloramphenicol (500 mg PO/IV qid for 14 days) *plus* another antibiotic (β-lactam preferred) *or* Ciprofloxacin (500 mg PO bid for 10 days) +/– ceftriaxone (1–2 g IV once a day for 10 days)
Verruga peruana	Azithromycin (500 mg PO once a day for 7 days) *or* Ciprofloxacin (500 mg PO bid for 7–10 days) *or* Rifampin (10 mg/kg PO once a day, to a maximum of 600 mg, for 14 days) *or* Streptomycin (15–20 mg/kg IM once a day for 10 days)

[a]Data on treatment efficacy for encephalitis and hepatosplenic cat-scratch disease are lacking. Therapy similar to that given for neuroretinitis is reasonable. [b]Some experts recommend gentamicin at 3 mg/kg IV once a day. If gentamicin is contraindicated, rifampin (300 mg PO bid) can be added to doxycycline for documented *Bartonella* endocarditis. [c]Some experts recommend extending oral doxycycline therapy for 3–6 months. [d]Other macrolides are probably effective and may be substituted for erythromycin or doxycycline.

Source: Recommendations are modified from JM Rolain et al: Antimicrob Agents Chemother 48:1921, 2004.

DIAGNOSIS

Definitive diagnosis requires isolation of *B. quintana* by blood culture. Some patients have positive blood cultures for several weeks. Patients with acute trench fever typically develop significant titers of antibody to *Bartonella*, whereas those with chronic *B. quintana* bacteremia may be seronegative. Patients with high titers of IgG antibodies should be evaluated for endocarditis. In epidemics, trench fever should be differentiated from epidemic louse-borne typhus and relapsing fever, which occur under similar conditions and share many features.

TREATMENT

B. quintana Bacteremia

(Table 172-2) In a small, randomized, placebo-controlled trial involving homeless people with *B. quintana* bacteremia, therapy with gentamicin and doxycycline was superior to administration of placebo in eradicating bacteremia. Treatment of bacteremia is important, even in clinically mild cases, to prevent endocarditis. Optimal therapy for trench fever without documented bacteremia is uncertain.

BARTONELLA ENDOCARDITIS

DEFINITION AND ETIOLOGY

Coxiella burnetii (**Chap. 187**) and *Bartonella* species are the most common pathogens in culture-negative endocarditis (**Chap. 128**). In France, for example, *Bartonella* species were identified as the etiologic agents in 28% of 348 cases of culture-negative endocarditis. Prevalence, however, varies by geographic location and epidemiologic setting. In addition to *B. quintana* and *B. henselae* (the most common *Bartonella* species implicated in endocarditis, the former more commonly than the latter), other *Bartonella* species have reportedly caused rare cases (Table 172-1).

EPIDEMIOLOGY

Bartonella endocarditis has been reported worldwide. Most patients are adults; more are male than female. Risk factors associated with *B. quintana* endocarditis include homelessness, alcoholism, and body louse infestation; however, individuals with no risk factors have had *Bartonella* endocarditis diagnosed as well. *B. henselae* endocarditis is associated with exposure to cats. Most cases involve native rather than prosthetic valves; the aortic valve accounts for ~60% of cases. Patients with *B. henselae* endocarditis usually have preexisting valvulopathy, whereas *B. quintana* often infects normal valves.

CLINICAL MANIFESTATIONS

Clinical manifestations are usually characteristic of subacute endocarditis of any etiology. However, a substantial number of patients have a prolonged, minimally febrile or even afebrile indolent illness, with mild nonspecific symptoms lasting weeks or months before the diagnosis is made. Initial echocardiography may not show vegetations. Acute, aggressive disease is rare.

DIAGNOSIS

Blood cultures, even with use of special techniques (lysis centrifugation or EDTA-containing tubes), are positive in only ~25% of cases—mostly those caused by *B. quintana* and only rarely those caused by *B. henselae*. Prolonged incubation of cultures (up to 6 weeks) is required. Serologic tests—either immunofluorescence or enzyme immunoassay—usually demonstrate high-titer (≥1:800) IgG antibodies to *Bartonella*. Because of cross-antigenicity, routine serology does not distinguish between *B. quintana* and *B. henselae* and may also be low-titer cross-reactive with other pathogens, such as *C. burnetii* and *Chlamydia* species. Identification of *Bartonella* to the species level is usually accomplished by application of PCR and DNA sequencing methods to valve tissue.

TREATMENT

Bartonella Endocarditis

(Table 172-2) For patients with culture-negative endocarditis suspected to be due to *Bartonella* species, empirical treatment consists of gentamicin, doxycycline, and ceftriaxone; the major role of ceftriaxone in this regimen is to adequately treat other potential causes of culture-negative endocarditis, including members of the HACEK group (**Chap. 158**). Once a diagnosis of *Bartonella* endocarditis has been established, ceftriaxone is discontinued. Aminoglycosides, the only antibiotics known to be bactericidal against *Bartonella*, should be included in the regimen for ≥2 weeks. Indications for valvular surgery are the same as in subacute endocarditis due to other pathogens; however, the proportion of patients who undergo surgery (~60%) is high, probably as a consequence of delayed diagnosis.

BACILLARY ANGIOMATOSIS AND PELIOSIS

DEFINITION AND ETIOLOGY

Bacillary angiomatosis (sometimes called *bacillary epithelioid angiomatosis* or *epithelioid angiomatosis*) is a disease of severely immunocompromised patients, is caused by *B. henselae* or *B. quintana*, and is characterized by neovascular proliferative lesions involving various organs. Both species cause cutaneous lesions; hepatosplenic lesions are caused only by *B. henselae*, whereas subcutaneous and lytic bone lesions are more frequently associated with *B. quintana*. Bacillary peliosis is a closely related angioproliferative disorder caused by *B. henselae* and involving primarily the liver (peliosis hepatis) but also the spleen and lymph nodes. Bacillary peliosis is characterized by blood-filled cystic structures whose size ranges from microscopic to several millimeters.

EPIDEMIOLOGY

Bacillary angiomatosis and bacillary peliosis occur primarily in HIV-infected persons (**Chap. 202**) with CD4+ T-cell counts of <100/μL but also affect other immunosuppressed patients and, in rare instances, immunocompetent patients. The incidence has decreased since the introduction of effective antiretroviral therapy and the routine use of rifabutin and macrolides to prevent *Mycobacterium avium* complex infection in AIDS patients. Contact with cats or cat fleas increases the risk of *B. henselae* infection. Risk factors for *B. quintana* infection are low income, homelessness, and body louse infestation.

CLINICAL MANIFESTATIONS

Bacillary angiomatosis presents most commonly as one or more cutaneous lesions that are not painful and may be tan, red, or purple in color. Subcutaneous, often tender nodules, superficial ulcerated plaques (**Fig. 172-2**), and verrucous growths are also seen. Nodular forms resemble those seen in fungal or mycobacterial infections. Painful osseous lesions, most often involving long bones, may underlie cutaneous lesions and occasionally develop in their absence. Other organs are rarely involved. Patients usually have constitutional symptoms, including fever, chills, malaise, headache, anorexia, weight loss, and night sweats. In patients with advanced immunodeficiency, *B. henselae* and *B. quintana* are important causes of fever of unknown origin. In osseous disease, lytic lesions are generally seen on radiography, and technetium scan shows focal uptake. The differential diagnosis of cutaneous bacillary angiomatosis includes Kaposi's sarcoma, pyogenic granuloma, subcutaneous tumors, and verruga peruana. In bacillary peliosis, hypodense hepatic areas are usually evident on imaging.

PATHOLOGY

Bacillary angiomatosis consists of lobular proliferations of small blood vessels lined by enlarged endothelial cells interspersed with mixed infiltrates of neutrophils and lymphocytes, with predominance of the former. Histologic examination of organs with bacillary peliosis reveals small blood-filled cystic lesions partially lined by endothelial cells that can be several millimeters in size. Peliotic lesions are surrounded by fibromyxoid stroma containing inflammatory cells, dilated capillaries, and clumps of granular material. Warthin-Starry silver staining of bacillary angiomatosis and peliosis lesions reveals clusters of bacilli. Cultures are usually negative.

DIAGNOSIS

Bacillary angiomatosis and bacillary peliosis are diagnosed by histologic examination. Blood cultures may be positive.

TREATMENT

Bacillary Angiomatosis and Peliosis

(Table 172-2) Prolonged therapy with a macrolide or doxycycline is recommended for both bacillary angiomatosis and bacillary peliosis.

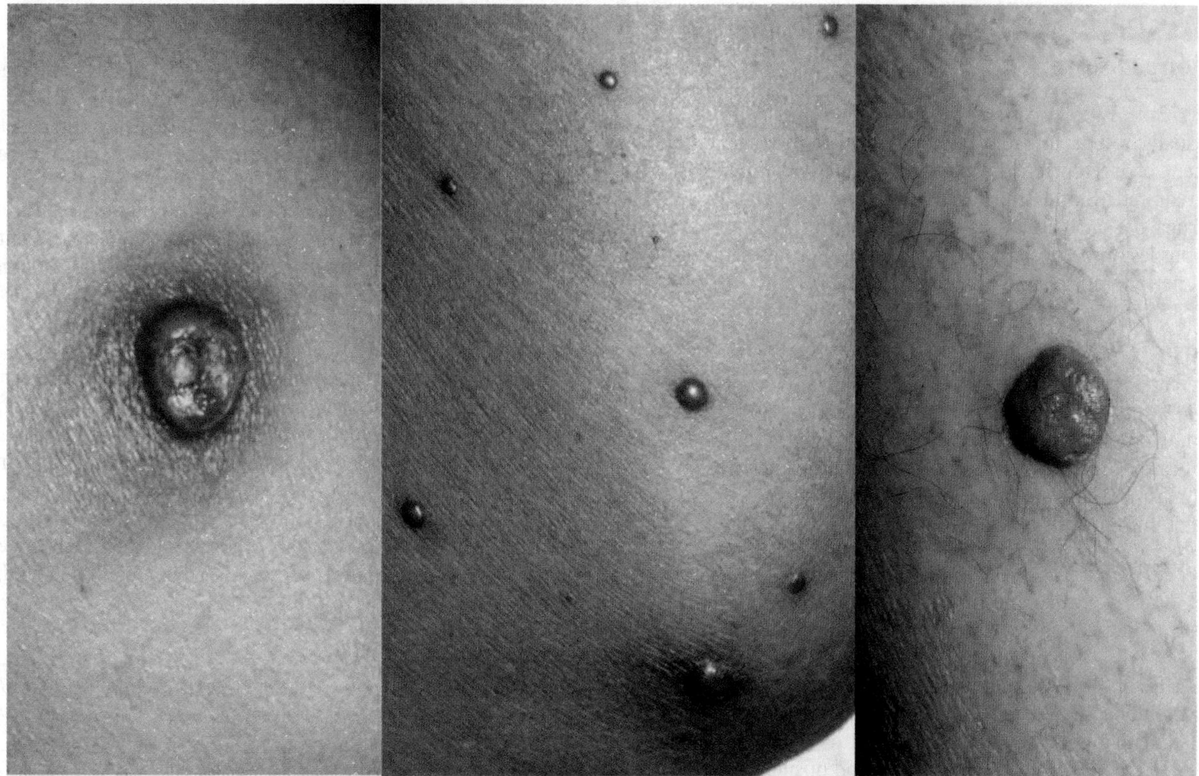

FIGURE 172-2 Lesions of cutaneous bacillary angiomatosis (BA) in three severely immunocompromised AIDS patients. Left panel shows a 1.5-cm ulcerated, bleeding BA lesion with an erythematous base; middle panel shows numerous small, 2-mm, scattered angiomatous BA lesions; right panel shows a 2.0-cm friable BA lesion on the thigh. *(Photos courtesy of Timothy Berger, MD; Jordan Tappero, MD, MPH; and Jane Koehler, MA, MD.)*

PREVENTION

Reasonable strategies for HIV-infected persons consist of control of cat-flea infestation and avoidance of cat scratches (for prevention of *B. henselae*) and avoidance and treatment of body louse infestation (for prevention of *B. quintana*). Primary prophylaxis is not recommended, but suppressive therapy with a macrolide or doxycycline is indicated in HIV-infected patients with bacillary angiomatosis or bacillary peliosis until CD4+ T-cell counts are >200/μL. Relapse may necessitate lifelong suppressive therapy in individual cases.

CARRIÓN'S DISEASE (OROYA FEVER AND VERRUGA PERUANA)

DEFINITION AND ETIOLOGY

Carrión's disease is a biphasic disease caused by *B. bacilliformis*. Oroya fever is the initial, bacteremic, systemic form, and verruga peruana is its late-onset, eruptive manifestation.

EPIDEMIOLOGY AND PREVENTION

Infection is endemic to the geographically restricted Andes valleys of Peru, Ecuador, and Colombia (~500–3200 m above sea level). Sporadic epidemics occur. The disease is transmitted by the phlebotomine sandfly *Lutzomyia verrucarum*. Maternal-fetal transmission as well as transmission by blood transfusion have been reported. Humans are the only known reservoir of *B. bacilliformis*. Sandfly control measures (e.g., insecticides) and personal protection measures (e.g., repellents, screening, bed nets) may decrease the risk of infection.

PATHOGENESIS

After inoculation by the sandfly, bacteria invade the blood vessel endothelium and proliferate; the reticuloendothelial system and various organs may also be involved. Upon reentry into blood vessels, *B. bacilliformis* invades, replicates, and ultimately destroys erythrocytes, with consequent massive hemolysis and sudden, severe anemia. Microvascular thrombosis results in end-organ ischemia. Survivors sometimes develop cutaneous hemangiomatous lesions characterized by various inflammatory cells, endothelial proliferation, and the presence of *B. bacilliformis* (verruga peruana).

CLINICAL MANIFESTATIONS

The incubation period is 3 weeks (range, 2–14 weeks). Oroya fever may present as a nonspecific bacteremic febrile illness without anemia or as an acute, severe hemolytic anemia with hepatomegaly and jaundice of rapid onset leading to vascular collapse and clouded sensorium. Myalgia, arthralgia, lymphadenopathy, and abdominal pain may develop. Temperature is elevated but not extremely so; high fever may suggest intercurrent infection. Subclinical asymptomatic infection also occurs. In verruga peruana, red, hemangioma-like, cutaneous vascular lesions of various sizes appear either weeks to months after systemic illness or with no previous suggestive history. These lesions persist for months up to 1 year. Mucosal and internal lesions may also develop.

DIAGNOSIS AND APPROACH TO THE PATIENT

Systemic illness (with or without anemia) or the development of cutaneous lesions in a person who has been to an endemic area raises the possibility of *B. bacilliformis* infection. Severe anemia with exuberant reticulocytosis—and sometimes thrombocytopenia—can occur. In systemic illness, Giemsa-stained blood films may show typical intraerythrocytic bacilli. Blood and bone marrow cultures may be positive, but growth is slow (1–6 weeks) and requires lower incubation temperature. Serologic assays may be helpful. Diagnosis of verruga peruana is largely clinical, although biopsy may be required to confirm the diagnosis. Several PCR assays have been described; however, their role in diagnosis remains to be clinically validated. Differential diagnosis includes coendemic systemic febrile illnesses (e.g., typhoid fever, malaria, brucellosis) and diseases producing cutaneous vascular lesions (e.g., hemangiomata, bacillary angiomatosis, Kaposi's sarcoma).

TREATMENT

Carrión's Disease

(Table 172-2) Antibiotic therapy for systemic *B. bacilliformis* infection usually results in rapid defervescence. Additional antibiotic treatment of intercurrent infection (particularly salmonellosis) is often required. Blood transfusion may be necessary. Treatment of verruga peruana usually is not always required. Patients with numerous lesions, especially lesions that have been present for only a short period, may respond well to antibiotic therapy.

COMPLICATIONS AND PROGNOSIS

Mortality rates associated with Oroya fever have been reported to be as high as 40% without treatment but are considerably lower (~10%) with treatment. Complications such as bacterial superinfection and neurologic and cardiac manifestations occur frequently. Generalized massive edema (anasarca) and petechiae are associated with poor outcome. Permanent immunity usually develops.

FURTHER READING

DENG H et al: Molecular mechanisms of *Bartonella* and mammalian erythrocyte interactions: A review. Front Cell Infect Microbiol 8:431, 2018.

FOURNIER PE et al: Epidemiologic and clinical characteristics of *Bartonella quintana* and *Bartonella henselae* endocarditis: A study of 48 patients. Medicine (Baltimore) 80:245, 2001.

GOMES C, RUIZ J: Carrion's disease: The sound of silence. Clin Microbiol Rev 31:e56, 2018.

KOEHLER JE et al: Molecular epidemiology of *Bartonella* infections in patients with bacillary angiomatosis-peliosis. N Engl J Med 337:1876, 1997.

LANDES M et al: Cat scratch disease presenting as fever of unknown origin is a unique clinical syndrome. Clin Infect Dis 71:2818, 2020.

ROLAIN JM et al: Recommendations for treatment of human infections caused by *Bartonella* species. Antimicrob Agents Chemother 48:1921, 2004.

ROSE SR, KOEHLER JE: *Bartonella* including cat scratch disease, in *Principles and Practice of Infectious Diseases*, 9th ed, GL Mandell et al (eds). Philadelphia, Elsevier, Inc. 2020, pp 2824-2843.

173 Donovanosis

Nigel O'Farrell

Donovanosis is a chronic, progressive bacterial infection that usually involves the genital region. The condition is generally regarded as a sexually transmitted infection of low infectivity. This infection has been known by many other names, the most common being *granuloma inguinale*.

ETIOLOGY

The causative organism has been reclassified as *Klebsiella granulomatis comb nov* on the basis of phylogenetic analysis, although there is ongoing debate about this decision. Some authorities consider the original nomenclature (*Calymmatobacterium granulomatis*) to be more appropriate in light of analysis of 16S rRNA gene sequences.

Donovanosis was first described in Calcutta in 1882, and the causative organism was recognized by Charles Donovan in Madras in 1905. He identified the characteristic Donovan bodies, measuring 1.5 × 0.7 μm, in macrophages and the stratum malpighii. The organism was not reproducibly cultured until the mid-1990s, when its isolation in peripheral-blood monocytes and human epithelial cell lines was reported.

EPIDEMIOLOGY

Donovanosis has an unusual geographic distribution that has included Papua New Guinea, parts of southern Africa, India, the Caribbean, French Guyana, Brazil, and Aboriginal communities in Australia. In Australia, donovanosis has been almost entirely eliminated through a sustained program backed by strong political commitment and resources at the primary health care level. In South Africa, donovanosis is also very close to elimination. Although few cases are now reported in the United States, donovanosis was once prevalent in this country, with 5000–10,000 cases recorded in 1947. The largest epidemic recorded was in Dutch South Guinea, where 10,000 cases were identified in a population of 15,000 (the Marind-anim) between 1922 and 1952.

Donovanosis is associated with poor hygiene and is more common in lower socioeconomic groups than in those who are better off and in men than in women. Infection in sexual partners of index cases occurs to a limited extent. Donovanosis is a risk factor for HIV infection (**Chap. 202**).

Globally, the incidence of donovanosis has decreased significantly in recent times. This decline probably reflects a greater focus on effective management of genital ulcers because of their role in facilitating HIV transmission.

CLINICAL FEATURES

A lesion starts as a papule or subcutaneous nodule that later ulcerates after trauma. The incubation period is uncertain, but experimental infections in humans indicate a duration of ~50 days. Four types of lesions have been described: (1) the classic ulcerogranulomatous lesion (**Fig. 173-1**), a beefy red ulcer that bleeds readily when touched; (2) a hypertrophic or verrucous ulcer with a raised irregular edge; (3) a necrotic, offensive-smelling ulcer causing tissue destruction; and (4) a sclerotic or cicatricial lesion with fibrous and scar tissue.

The genitals are affected in 90% of patients and the inguinal region in 10%. The most common sites of infection are the prepuce, coronal sulcus, frenum, and glans in men and the labia minora and fourchette in women. Cervical lesions may mimic cervical carcinoma. In men, lesions are associated with lack of circumcision. Lymphadenitis is uncommon. Extragenital lesions occur in 6% of cases and may involve the lip, gums, cheek, palate, pharynx, larynx, and chest. Hematogenous spread with involvement of liver and bone has been reported. During pregnancy, lesions tend to develop more quickly and respond more slowly to treatment. Polyarthritis and osteomyelitis are rare complications. In newborn infants, donovanosis may present with ear infection. Cases in children have been attributed to sitting on the laps of infected adults. As the incidence of donovanosis has decreased, the number of unusual case reports has appeared to be increasing.

Complications include neoplastic changes, pseudoelephantiasis, and stenosis of the urethra, vagina, or anus.

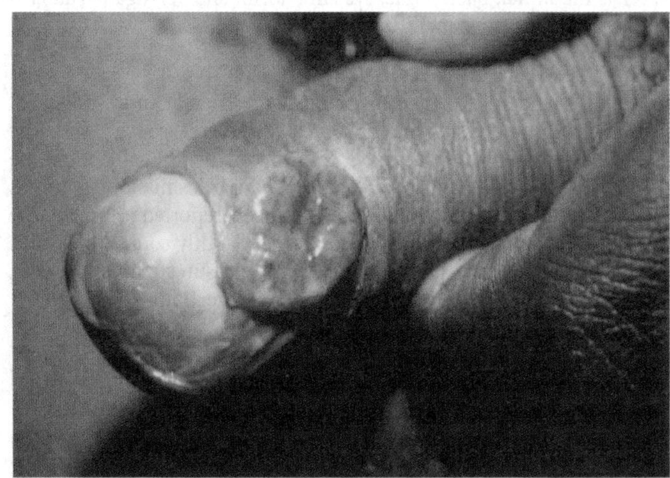

FIGURE 173-1 Ulcerogranulomatous penile lesion of donovanosis, with some hypertrophic features.

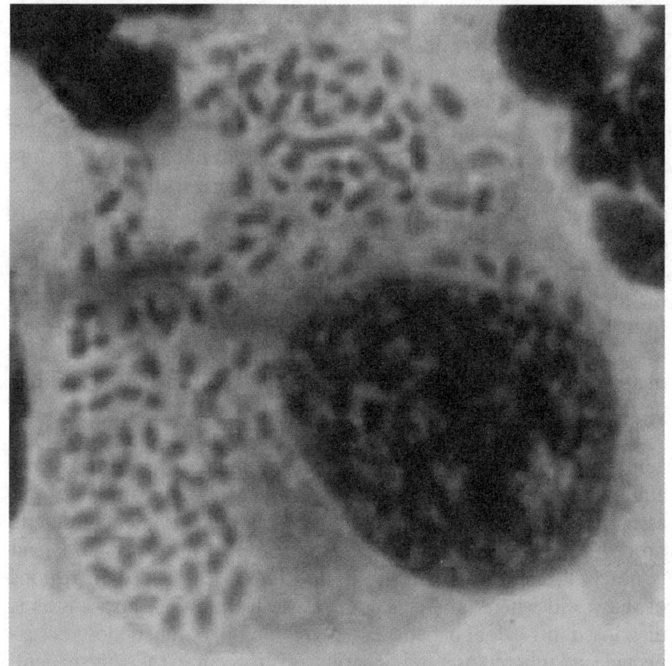

FIGURE 173-2 Pund cell stained by rapid Giemsa (RapiDiff) technique. Numerous Donovan bodies are visible.

■ DIAGNOSIS

A clinical diagnosis of donovanosis made by an experienced practitioner on the basis of the lesion's appearance usually has a high positive predictive value. The diagnosis is confirmed by microscopic identification of Donovan bodies (**Fig. 173-2**) in tissue smears. Preparation of a good-quality smear is important. If donovanosis is suspected on clinical grounds, the smear for Donovan bodies should be taken before swab samples are collected to be tested for other causes of genital ulceration so that enough material can be collected from the ulcer. A swab should be rolled firmly over an ulcer previously cleaned with a dry swab to remove debris. Smears can be examined in a clinical setting by direct microscopy with a rapid Giemsa or Wright's stain. Alternatively, a piece of granulation tissue crushed and spread between two slides can be used. Donovan bodies can be seen in large, mononuclear (Pund) cells as gram-negative intracytoplasmic cysts filled with deeply staining bodies that may have a safety-pin appearance. These cysts eventually rupture and release the infective organisms. Histologic changes include chronic inflammation with infiltration of plasma cells and neutrophils. Epithelial changes include ulceration, microabscesses, and elongation of rete ridges.

A diagnostic polymerase chain reaction (PCR) test was based on the observation that two unique base changes in the *phoE* gene eliminate Hae111 restriction sites, enabling differentiation of *K. granulomatis comb nov* from related *Klebsiella* species. PCR analysis with a colorimetric detection system can now be used in routine diagnostic laboratories. A genital ulcer multiplex PCR that includes *K. granulomatis* has been developed. Serologic tests are only poorly specific and are not currently used.

The differential diagnosis of donovanosis includes primary syphilitic chancres, secondary syphilis (condylomata lata), chancroid, lymphogranuloma venereum, genital herpes, neoplasm, and amebiasis. Mixed infections are common. Histologic appearances should be distinguished from those of rhinoscleroma, leishmaniasis, and histoplasmosis.

TREATMENT

Donovanosis

Many patients with donovanosis present quite late with extensive ulceration. They may be embarrassed and have low self-esteem related to their disease. Reassurance that they have a treatable condition is important, as are the administration of antibiotics and the monitoring of patients for an adequate interval (see below). Epidemiologic treatment of sexual partners and advice about how to improve genital hygiene are recommended.

TABLE 173-1 Effective Antibiotics for the Treatment of Donovanosis

ANTIBIOTIC	ORAL DOSE
Azithromycin	1 g on day 1, then 500 mg daily for 7 days or 1 g weekly for 4 weeks
Trimethoprim-sulfamethoxazole	960 mg bid for 14 days
Doxycycline	100 mg bid for 14 days
Erythromycin	500 mg qid for 14 days (in pregnant women)
Tetracycline	500 mg qid for 14 days

The recommended drug regimens for donovanosis are shown in **Table 173-1**. Gentamicin can be added if the response is slow. Ceftriaxone, chloramphenicol, and norfloxacin also are effective. Patients treated for 14 days should be monitored until lesions have healed completely. Those treated with azithromycin probably do not need such rigorous follow-up.

Surgery may be indicated for very advanced lesions.

■ CONTROL AND PREVENTION

Donovanosis is probably the cause of genital ulceration that is most readily recognizable clinically. Donovanosis is now limited to a few specific locations, and its global eradication is a distinct possibility.

■ FURTHER READING

MULLER EE, KULARATNE R: The changing epidemiology of genital ulcer disease in South Africa: Has donovanosis been eliminated? Sex Transm Infect 96:596, 2020.

O'FARRELL N: Donovanosis, in *Sexually Transmitted Diseases*, 4th ed. KK Holmes et al (eds). McGraw-Hill, 2008, pp 701–708.

RAJAM RV, RANGIAH PN: Donovanosis (granuloma inguinale, granuloma venereum). Monogr Ser World Health Organ 24:1, 1954.

SEHGAL VN, PRASAD AL: Donovanosis. Current concepts. Int J Dermatol 5:8, 1986.

Section 7 Miscellaneous Bacterial Infections

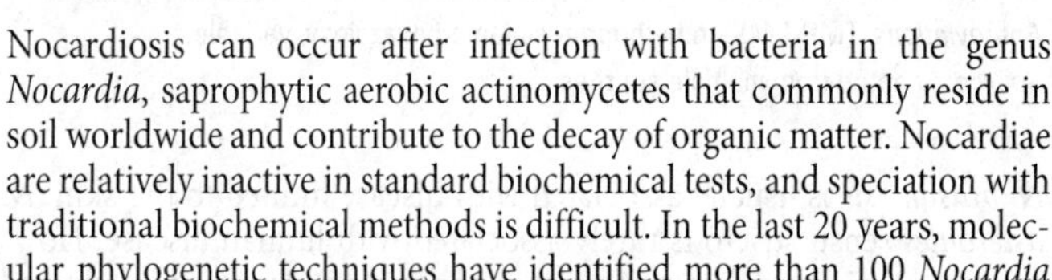

174 Nocardiosis

Gregory A. Filice

Nocardiosis can occur after infection with bacteria in the genus *Nocardia*, saprophytic aerobic actinomycetes that commonly reside in soil worldwide and contribute to the decay of organic matter. Nocardiae are relatively inactive in standard biochemical tests, and speciation with traditional biochemical methods is difficult. In the last 20 years, molecular phylogenetic techniques have identified more than 100 *Nocardia* species, more than 50 of which are implicated in human disease.

In the past, the majority of isolates associated with pneumonia and systemic disease were identified biochemically as *Nocardia asteroides*, but the lineage of the type strain was muddled, and most human isolates in fact belong to other species. Nine species or species complexes are commonly associated with human disease (**Table 174-1**). Most systemic disease involves *N. cyriacigeorgica*, *N. farcinica*, *N. pseudobrasiliensis*, and species in the *N. transvalensis* and *N. nova* complexes.

TABLE 174-1 *Nocardia* **Species Most Commonly Associated with Human Disease and Their In Vitro Susceptibility Patterns**

SPECIES	SUSCEPTIBLE TO[a]	RESISTANT TO[b]
N. abscessus	Amikacin, amoxicillin/clavulanate, ampicillin, ceftriaxone, gentamicin, linezolid, minocycline, tigecycline, tobramycin, TMP-SMX	Ciprofloxacin, clarithromycin (v), imipenem (v), moxifloxacin
N. brevicatena/paucivorans complex (*N. brevicatena, N. paucivorans, N. carnea*, others)	Amikacin, ampicillin, ceftriaxone, ciprofloxacin (v), clarithromycin (v), gentamicin, imipenem, linezolid, minocycline (v), moxifloxacin, tigecycline, tobramycin, TMP-SMX	Amoxicillin/clavulanate (v)
N. nova complex (*N. nova, N. veterana, N. africana, N. kruczakiae, N. elegans*, others)	Amikacin, ampicillin (v), ceftriaxone (v), clarithromycin, gentamicin (v), imipenem, linezolid, tigecycline (v), TMP-SMX	Amoxicillin/clavulanate, ciprofloxacin, minocycline, moxifloxacin, tobramycin
N. transvalensis complex (*N. blacklockiae, N. wallacei*, others)	Ceftriaxone (v), ciprofloxacin (v), linezolid, moxifloxacin, TMP-SMX (v)	Amikacin (v), amoxicillin/clavulanate (v), ampicillin, clarithromycin, gentamicin, imipenem, minocycline (v), tobramycin
N. farcinica	Amikacin, amoxicillin/clavulanate (v), linezolid, moxifloxacin (v), TMP-SMX	Ampicillin, ceftriaxone, ciprofloxacin (v), clarithromycin, gentamicin, imipenem (v), minocycline, tigecycline (v), tobramycin
N. cyriacigeorgica	Amikacin, ceftriaxone, gentamicin, linezolid, tigecycline, tobramycin, TMP-SMX	Amoxicillin/clavulanate, ampicillin, ciprofloxacin, clarithromycin, imipenem (v), minocycline, moxifloxacin
N. brasiliensis	Amikacin, amoxicillin/clavulanate, linezolid, tigecycline, tobramycin, TMP-SMX	Ampicillin, ceftriaxone (v), ciprofloxacin, clarithromycin, imipenem, minocycline (v), moxifloxacin
N. pseudobrasiliensis	Amikacin (v), ciprofloxacin, clarithromycin, linezolid, tobramycin, TMP-SMX (v)	Amoxicillin/clavulanate, ampicillin, ceftriaxone, imipenem, minocycline
N. otitidiscaviarum complex	Amikacin, gentamicin (v), linezolid, tobramycin (v), TMP-SMX	Amoxicillin/clavulanate, ampicillin, ceftriaxone, ciprofloxacin, clarithromycin, imipenem, minocycline (v), moxifloxacin (v)

[a]From 85 to 100% of isolates are susceptible unless the drug name is followed by (v), in which case 50–84% are susceptible. [b]From 0 to 15% of isolates are susceptible unless the drug name is followed by (v), in which case 16–49% are susceptible.

Abbreviations: TMP-SMX, trimethoprim-sulfamethoxazole; v, variable.

Source: Adapted from multiple sources.

N. brasiliensis is usually associated with disease limited to the skin. *N. asteroides* sensu stricto is rarely associated with human disease. However, most clinical laboratories cannot speciate isolates accurately and may identify them simply as *N. asteroides* or *Nocardia* species.

EPIDEMIOLOGY

Pulmonary and/or systemic nocardiosis occurs worldwide. The annual incidence, estimated on three continents (North America, Europe, and Australia), is ~0.375 case per 100,000 persons and may be increasing. There is some geographic variation in species frequencies; for example, *N. asiatica, N. beijingensis, and N. terpenica* infections appear to be more commonly involved in cases from eastern Asia. However, exact species prevalences are difficult to determine precisely since nocardial infections are not reportable and most publications consist of case reports or case series.

Mycetoma is an indolent, slowly progressive disease of skin and underlying tissues with nodular swellings and draining sinuses. Actinomycetoma refers to cases of mycetoma associated with actinomycetes as opposed to fungi or other bacterial orders, and nocardia strains commonly associated with actinomycetoma include *N. brasiliensis, N. otitidiscaviarum*, and *N. transvalensis* complex. Mycetoma occurs mainly in tropical and subtropical regions. Most cases are reported from Sudan, Mexico, and India. The most important risk factors are lower socioeconomic status and frequent contact with soil or vegetable matter; accordingly, many patients are laborers or women who perform outdoor chores like gathering wood.

Pulmonary and/or systemic nocardiosis is more common among adults than among children and more common among males than among females. Nearly all cases are sporadic, but outbreaks have been associated with contamination of the hospital environment, cosmetic procedures, and parenteral illicit drug use. Person-to-person spread is not well documented. There is no known seasonality. In regions of the world where tuberculosis is relatively common, nocardiosis is diagnosed in 1–5% of patients in whom pulmonary tuberculosis is suspected, and tuberculosis and nocardiosis can occur in the same patient.

The majority of cases of pulmonary or disseminated disease occur in people with a host defense defect. Most have deficient cell-mediated immunity, especially that associated with lymphoma, transplantation, glucocorticoid therapy, or AIDS. In transplant recipients, nocardiosis has been associated with high-dose prednisone, elevated calcineurin inhibitor concentrations, and cytomegalovirus disease. The incidence is ~140-fold greater among patients with AIDS and ~340-fold greater among bone marrow transplant recipients than in general populations. In AIDS, nocardiosis usually affects persons with <250 CD4+ T lymphocytes/μL. Nocardiosis has also been associated with pulmonary alveolar proteinosis, tuberculosis and other mycobacterial diseases, chronic granulomatous disease, interleukin 12 deficiency, and autoantibodies to granulocyte-macrophage colony-stimulating factor (GM-CSF). Any child with nocardiosis and no known cause of immunosuppression should undergo tests to determine the adequacy of the phagocytic respiratory burst. Cases have been associated with newer immunomodulating drugs, especially with tumor necrosis factor and calcineurin inhibitors. *Nocardia* is frequently isolated from and may persist in respiratory secretions of patients with cystic fibrosis and may be associated with deterioration of lung function, but this association has not been convincingly established.

PATHOLOGY AND PATHOGENESIS

Pneumonia and disseminated disease are both thought to follow inhalation of fragmented bacterial mycelia. The characteristic histologic feature of nocardiosis is an abscess with extensive neutrophil infiltration and prominent necrosis. Granulation tissue usually surrounds the lesions, but extensive fibrosis or encapsulation is uncommon.

Actinomycetoma is characterized by suppurative inflammation with sinus tract formation. Granules—microcolonies composed of dense masses of bacterial filaments extending radially from a central core—are occasionally observed in histologic preparations. The granules are frequently found in discharges from lesions of actinomycetoma but almost never in discharges from lesions in other forms of nocardiosis.

Nocardiae have evolved a number of properties that enable them to survive within phagocytes, including neutralization of oxidants, prevention of phagosome–lysosome fusion, and prevention of phagosome acidification. Neutrophils phagocytose the organisms and limit their growth but do not kill them efficiently. Cell-mediated immunity is important for definitive control and elimination of nocardiae. Antibodies to GM-CSF have been found in the majority of patients with alveolar proteinosis and appear to be central to the pathogenesis of this disease. Nocardiae stimulate the production of GM-CSF in phagocytes in vitro, and nocardial infection has been observed in several patients with autoantibodies to GM-CSF, most of whom had not had

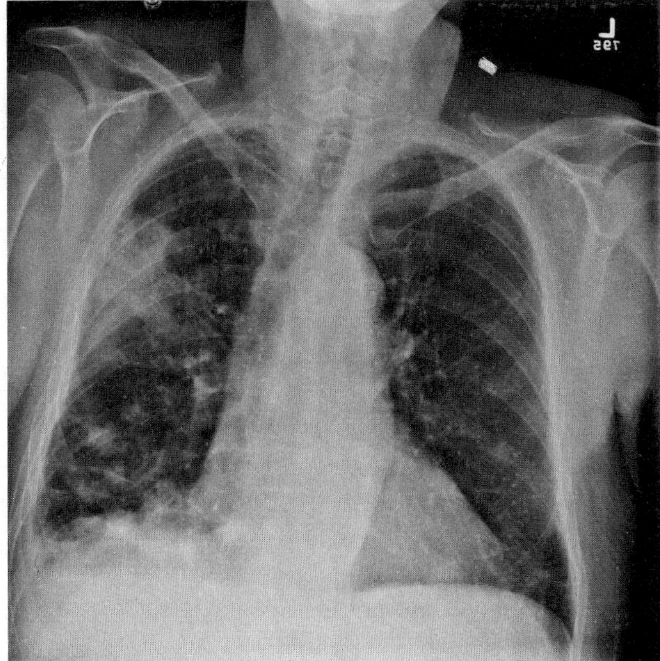

FIGURE 174-1 **Nocardial pneumonia.** A dense infiltrate with a possible cavity and several nodules are apparent in the right lung.

pulmonary alveolar proteinosis. The relationships between pulmonary alveolar proteinosis, nocardiosis, and antibodies to GM-CSF remain incompletely defined.

■ CLINICAL MANIFESTATIONS

Respiratory Tract Disease Pneumonia, the most common form of nocardial disease in the respiratory tract, is typically subacute; symptoms have usually been present for days or weeks at presentation. The onset is occasionally more acute in immunosuppressed patients. Cough is prominent and produces small amounts of thick, purulent sputum that is not malodorous. Fever, anorexia, weight loss, and malaise are common; dyspnea, pleuritic pain, and hemoptysis are less common. Remissions and exacerbations over several weeks are frequent. Roentgenographic patterns vary, but some are highly suggestive of nocardial pneumonia. Infiltrates vary in size and are typically dense. Single or multiple nodules are common (**Figs. 174-1 and 174-2**), sometimes suggesting tumors or metastases. Infiltrates and nodules tend to cavitate (Fig. 174-2). Empyema is present in one-quarter of cases.

Nocardiosis may spread directly from the lungs to adjacent tissues. Pericarditis, mediastinitis, and superior vena cava syndrome have all been reported. Nocardial laryngitis, tracheitis, bronchitis, and sinusitis are much less common than pneumonia. In the major airways, disease often presents as a nodular or granulomatous mass. Nocardiae are sometimes isolated from respiratory secretions of persons without apparent nocardial disease, usually individuals who have underlying lung or airway abnormalities.

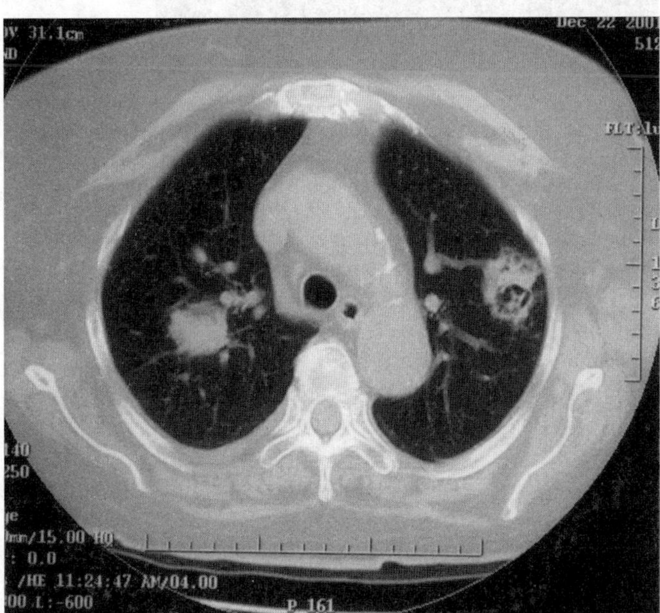

FIGURE 174-2 **Nocardial pneumonia.** A computed tomography scan shows bilateral nodules, with cavitation in the nodule in the left lung.

Extrapulmonary Disease In half of all cases of pulmonary nocardiosis, disease appears outside the lungs. In one-fifth of cases of disseminated disease, lung disease is not apparent. The most common site of dissemination is the brain. Other common sites include the skin and supporting structures, kidneys, bones, muscles, and eyes, but almost any organ can be involved. Peritonitis has been reported in patients undergoing peritoneal dialysis. Nocardiae have been recovered from blood in a few cases of pneumonia, disseminated disease, or central venous catheter infection. Nocardial endocarditis occurs rarely and can affect either native or prosthetic valves.

The typical manifestation of extrapulmonary dissemination is a subacute abscess. A minority of abscesses outside the lungs or central nervous system (CNS) form fistulas and discharge small amounts of pus. In CNS infections, brain abscesses are usually supratentorial, are often multiloculated, and may be single or multiple (**Fig. 174-3**). Cases in the posterior fossa and spinal cord have been reported, but they are less common. Brain abscesses tend to burrow into the ventricles or extend out into the subarachnoid space. The symptoms and signs are somewhat more indolent than those of other types of bacterial brain abscess. Meningitis is uncommon and is usually due to spread from a nearby brain abscess. Nocardiae are not easily recovered from cerebrospinal fluid (CSF).

Disease following Transcutaneous Inoculation Disease that follows transcutaneous nocardial inoculation usually takes one of three forms: cellulitis, lymphocutaneous syndrome, or actinomycetoma.

Cellulitis generally begins 1–3 weeks after a recognized breach of the skin, often with soil contamination. Subacute cellulitis, with pain, swelling, erythema, and warmth, develops over days to weeks. The lesions are usually firm and not fluctuant. Disease may progress to involve underlying muscles, tendons, bones, or joints. Dissemination is

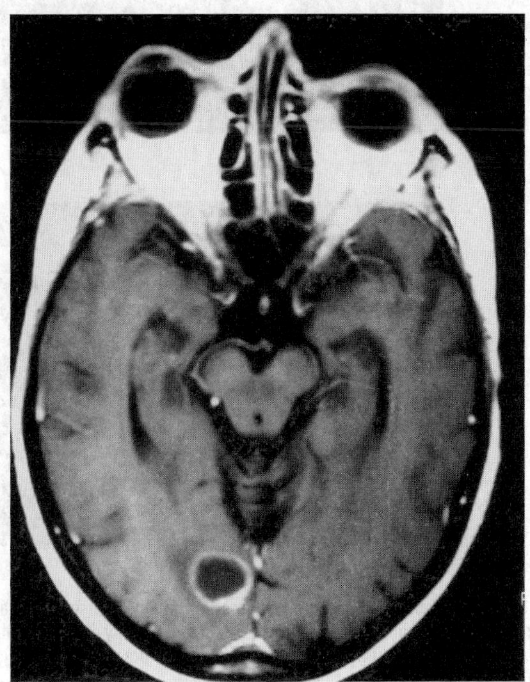

FIGURE 174-3 **Nocardial abscesses** in the right occipital lobe.

rare. *N. brasiliensis* and species in the *N. otitidiscaviarum* complex are most common in cellulitis cases.

Lymphocutaneous disease usually begins as a pyodermatous nodule at the site of inoculation, with central ulceration and purulent or honey-colored drainage. Subcutaneous nodules often appear along lymphatics that drain the primary lesion. Most cases of nocardial lymphocutaneous syndrome are associated with *N. brasiliensis*. Similar disease occurs with other pathogens, most notably *Sporothrix schenckii* (**Chap. 219**) and *Mycobacterium marinum* (**Chap. 180**).

Actinomycetoma usually begins with a nodular swelling, sometimes at a site of local trauma. Lesions (**Fig. 174-4*A***) typically develop on the feet or hands but may involve the posterior part of the neck, the upper back, the head, and other sites. The nodule eventually breaks down, and a fistula appears, typically followed by others. The fistulas tend to come and go, with new ones forming as old ones disappear. The discharge is serous or purulent, may be bloody, and often contains 0.1- to 2-mm white granules consisting of masses of mycelia (**Figs. 174-4*C* and 174-4*D***). The lesions spread slowly along fascial planes to involve adjacent areas of skin, subcutaneous tissue, and bone. Over months or years, there may be extensive deformation of the affected part. Lesions involving soft tissues are only mildly painful; those affecting bones or joints are more so (**Fig. 174-4*B***). Systemic symptoms are absent or minimal, but mycetoma cases are often associated with prolonged, severe disability. Infection rarely disseminates from actinomycetoma, but lesions on the head, neck, and trunk can invade locally to involve deep organs.

Eye Infections Nocardia species are uncommon causes of subacute keratitis, usually following eye trauma. Nocardial endophthalmitis can develop after eye surgery. In one series, nocardiae accounted for more than half of culture-proved cases of endophthalmitis after cataract surgery. Endophthalmitis can also occur during disseminated disease. Nocardial infection of lachrymal glands has been reported.

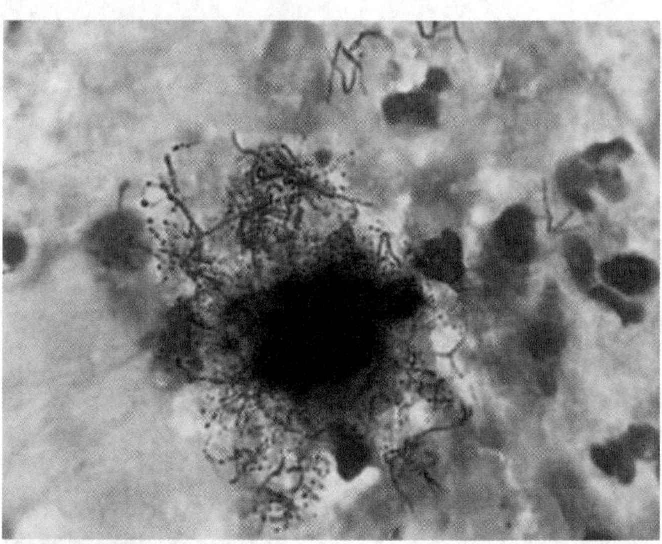

FIGURE 174-5 Gram-stained sputum from a patient with nocardial pneumonia. *(Image provided by Charles Cartwright and Susan Nelson, Hennepin County Medical Center, Minneapolis, MN.)*

DIAGNOSIS

The first step in diagnosis is examination of sputum or pus for crooked, branching, beaded, gram-positive filaments 1 μm wide and up to 50 μm long (**Fig. 174-5**). Most nocardiae are acid-fast in direct smears if a weak acid is used for decolorization (e.g., in the modified Kinyoun, Ziehl-Neelsen, and Fite-Faraco methods). The organisms often take up silver stains. Recovery from specimens containing a mixed flora can be improved with selective media (colistin–nalidixic acid agar, modified Thayer-Martin agar, or buffered charcoal–yeast extract agar).

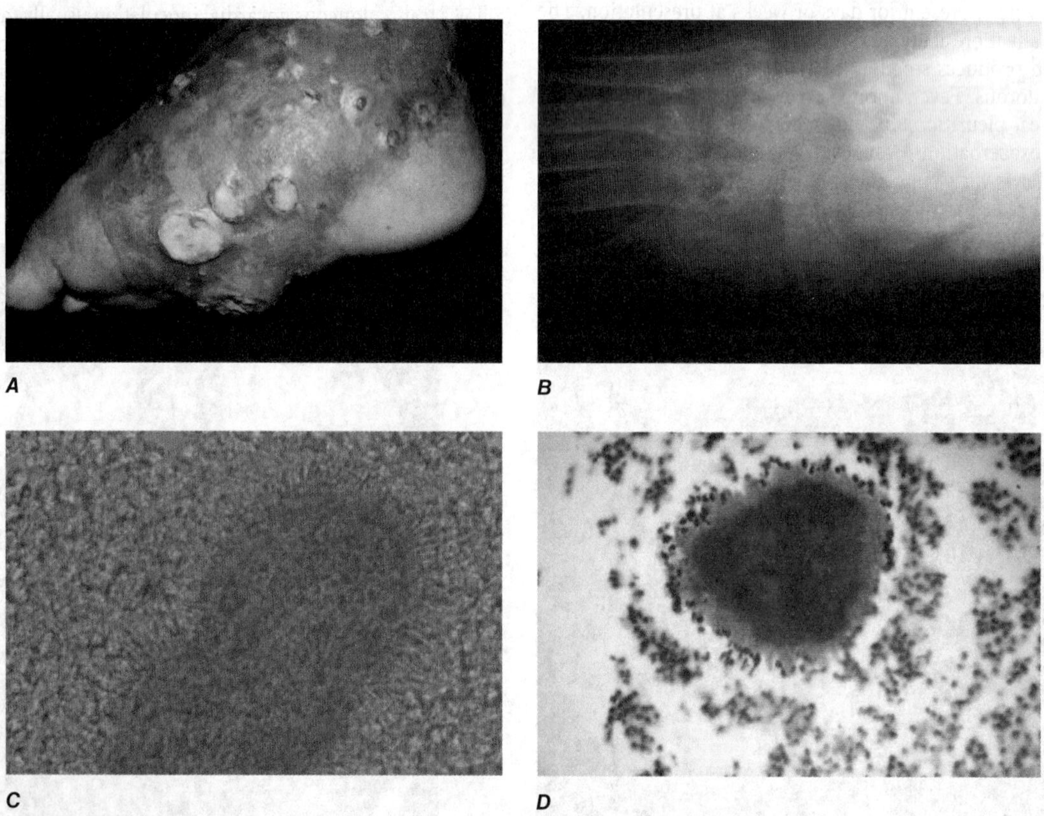

FIGURE 174-4 *Nocardia brasiliensis* mycetoma. *A.* Draining sinuses and giant white grains with a seropurulent discharge. ***B.*** Radiography of the foot showing marked soft tissue enlargement and bony lytic lesions. ***C.*** Direct microscopy of grains stained with Lugol's iodine (×40). ***D.*** Periodic acid–Schiff stain of skin biopsy (×40). *(Images provided by Roberto Arenas and Mahreen Ameen, St. John's Institute of Dermatology, Guy's & St Thomas' NHS Trust, London, UK. Reprinted from R Arenas, M Ameen: Lancet Infect Dis 10:66, 2010, with permission from Elsevier.)*

Nocardiae grow well on most fungal and mycobacterial media, but procedures used for decontamination of specimens for mycobacterial culture can kill nocardiae and should not be used when nocardiae are suspected.

Nocardiae grow relatively slowly; colonies may take up to 2 weeks to appear and may not develop their characteristic appearance—white, yellow, or orange, with aerial mycelia and delicate, dichotomously branched substrate mycelia—for up to 4 weeks. Several blood culture systems support nocardial growth, although nocardiae may not be detected for up to 2 weeks. The growth of nocardiae is so different from that of more common pathogens that the laboratory should be alerted when nocardiosis is suspected in order to maximize the likelihood of isolation.

In nocardial pneumonia, sputum smears are often negative. Unless the diagnosis can be made in smear-negative cases by sampling lesions in more accessible sites, bronchoscopy or lung aspiration is usually necessary. To evaluate the possibility of dissemination in patients with nocardial pneumonia, a careful history should be obtained and a thorough physical examination performed. Suggestive symptoms or signs should be pursued with further diagnostic tests. MRI or CT with contrast of the brain should be done when feasible in cases of pulmonary or disseminated disease. When clinically indicated, CSF or urine should be concentrated and then cultured. Actinomycetoma, eumycetoma (cases involving fungi; **Chap. 219**), and botryomycosis (cases involving cocci or bacilli, often *Staphylococcus aureus*) are difficult to distinguish clinically but are readily distinguished with microbiologic testing or biopsy. Granules should be sought in any discharge. Suspect particles should be washed in saline, examined microscopically, and cultured. Granules in actinomycetoma cases are usually white, pale yellow, pink, or red. Viewed microscopically, they consist of tight masses of fine filaments (0.5–1 μm wide) radiating outward from a central core (Fig. 174-5). Granules from eumycetoma cases are white, yellow, brown, black, or green; under the microscope, they appear as masses of broader filaments (2–5 μm wide) encased in a matrix. Granules of botryomycosis consist of loose masses of cocci or bacilli. Organisms can also be seen in wound discharge or histologic specimens. The most reliable way to differentiate among the various organisms associated with mycetoma is by culture.

Isolation of nocardiae from sputum or blood occasionally represents colonization, transient infection, or contamination. In typical cases of respiratory tract colonization, Gram-stained specimens are negative and cultures are only intermittently positive. A positive sputum culture in an immunosuppressed patient usually reflects disease. When nocardiae are isolated from sputum of an immunocompetent patient without apparent nocardial disease, the patient should be observed carefully without treatment. A patient with a host-defense defect that increases the risk of nocardiosis should usually receive antimicrobial treatment.

Nocardia DNA has been detected in respiratory tract samples from patients with proven or suspected pulmonary nocardiosis, other chronic lung diseases, and healthy controls. The sensitivity and specificity of DNA testing has not been well defined.

Species are definitively determined by molecular techniques. Matrix-assisted laser desorption/ionization/time-of-flight (MALDI-TOF) mass spectrometry is accurate in 75% or more cases when compared with genetic testing. MALDI-TOF is much more practical for clinical laboratories and is becoming common in laboratories in high-resource countries.

Because nocardiosis is uncommon, data on the relation between susceptibility test results for specific drugs and clinical outcomes in patients treated with these drugs are meager. Careful clinical monitoring is essential, and consultation with clinicians who have experience with nocardiosis is often needed. Susceptibility to antimicrobial agents in vitro is best determined with a Clinical Laboratory Standards Institute (CLSI)-approved broth dilution test. Susceptibility testing with E-test or BACTEC radiometric methods is less definitive. Nocardial growth is slower than the growth of most clinically important bacteria, and nocardiae tend to clump in suspension so that susceptibility-test end points are difficult to read; thus experience is necessary for reliable reading of results. If an isolate can be accurately speciated, its susceptibility to antimicrobial drugs can be predicted with reasonable accuracy.

Speciation by molecular methods or MALDI-TOF is not practical in many resource-poor countries. As a result, therapy for nocardiosis is often initiated without definitive speciation or knowledge of susceptibility results. For mild or moderate cases, therapy with drugs known to be effective against most isolates is usually adequate. For severe cases or cases that do not respond promptly to antimicrobial therapy, isolates should be sent to a laboratory experienced with *Nocardia* for identification and susceptibility testing whenever possible.

TREATMENT
Nocardiosis

Trimethoprim-sulfamethoxazole (TMZ-SMX) is the drug of choice for most cases (**Tables 174-1** and **174-2**). Reported rates of TMP-SMX susceptibility have varied widely, and controversy has ensued about the reliability of sulfonamides for therapy. However, clinical responses to appropriate sulfonamide treatment around the world are usually satisfactory. At the outset, 10–20 mg/kg of TMP and 50–100 mg/kg of SMX are given each day in two divided doses. Later, daily doses can be decreased to as little as 5 mg/kg and 25 mg/kg, respectively. In persons with sulfonamide allergies, desensitization usually allows continuation of therapy with these effective and inexpensive drugs.

Clinical experience with other oral drugs is limited. Minocycline (100–200 mg twice a day) is often effective; other tetracyclines are usually less effective. Linezolid is the most consistently active antimicrobial agent, but adverse effects become common and limiting in many patients after 2–3 weeks. Amoxicillin (875 mg) combined with clavulanate (125 mg), given twice a day, has been effective in *N. brasiliensis* cases and some *N. farcinica* cases. Among the quinolones, moxifloxacin and gemifloxacin appear to be most active.

Amikacin, the best-established parenteral drug except in cases involving the *N. transvalensis* complex, is given in doses of 5–7.5 mg/kg every 12 h or 15 mg/kg every 24 h. Serum drug levels should be monitored during prolonged therapy in patients with diminished renal function and in the elderly. Ceftriaxone and imipenem are usually effective except as indicated in Table 174-1. Tigecycline appears to be active in vitro against some species, but little clinical experience has been reported.

Patients with severe disease are initially treated with a combination including TMP-SMX, amikacin, and ceftriaxone or imipenem. Clinical improvement is usually noticeable after 1–2 weeks of therapy but may take longer, especially with CNS disease. After definite

TABLE 174-2 Treatment Duration for Nocardiosis

DISEASE	DURATION
Pulmonary or systemic	
Intact host defenses	6–12 months
Deficient host defenses	12 months[a]
CNS disease	12 months[b]
Cellulitis, lymphocutaneous syndrome	2 months
Osteomyelitis, arthritis, laryngitis, sinusitis	4 months
Actinomycetoma	6–12 months after clinical cure
Keratitis	Topical: until apparent cure
	Systemic: until 2–4 months after apparent cure

[a]In some patients with AIDS and CD4+ T lymphocyte counts of <200/μL or with chronic granulomatous disease, therapy for pulmonary or systemic disease must be continued indefinitely. [b]If all apparent central nervous system (CNS) disease has been excised, the duration of therapy may be reduced to 6 months.

clinical improvement, therapy can be continued with a single oral drug, usually TMP-SMX. Some experts use two or more drugs for the entire course of therapy, but whether multiple drugs are better than a single agent is not known, and additional drugs increase the risk of toxicity. In patients with nocardiosis who need immunosuppressive therapy for an underlying disease or prevention of transplant rejection, immunosuppressive therapy should be continued.

Use of SMX and TMP in high-risk populations to prevent *Pneumocystis* disease or urinary tract infections appears to reduce but not eliminate the risk of nocardiosis. The incidence of nocardiosis is low enough that prophylaxis solely to prevent this disease is not recommended.

Surgical management of nocardial disease is similar to that of other bacterial diseases. Brain abscesses should be aspirated, drained, or excised if the diagnosis is unclear, if an abscess is large and accessible, or if an abscess fails to respond to chemotherapy. Small or inaccessible brain abscesses should be treated medically; clinical improvement should be noticeable within 1–2 weeks. Brain imaging should be repeated to document the resolution of lesions, although abatement on images often lags behind clinical improvement.

Antimicrobial therapy usually suffices for nocardial actinomycetoma. In deep or extensive cases, drainage or excision of heavily involved tissue may facilitate healing, but structure and function should be preserved whenever possible. Keratitis is treated with a topical sulfonamide or amikacin drops plus a sulfonamide or an alternative drug given by mouth.

Nocardial infections tend to relapse (particularly in patients with chronic granulomatous disease), and long courses of antimicrobial therapy are necessary (Table 174-2). If disease is unusually extensive or if the response to therapy is slow, the recommendations in Table 174-2 should be exceeded.

With appropriate treatment, the mortality rate for pulmonary or disseminated nocardiosis outside the CNS should be <5%. CNS disease carries a higher mortality rate. Patients should be followed carefully for at least 6 months after therapy has ended. Actinomycetoma often responds better to therapy than mycetoma associated with fungi, but relapses occur in a minority of patients, and disability often persists.

■ FURTHER READING

Abbas M et al: The disabling consequences of mycetoma. PLoS Negl Trop Dis 12:e0007019, 2018.

Body B et al: Evaluation of the Vitek MS v3.0 Matrix-Assisted Laser Desorption Ionization–Time of Flight Mass Spectrometry System for identification of mycobacterium and nocardia. J Clin Microbiol 56:e00237, 2018.

Coussement J et al: *Nocardia* infection in solid organ transplant recipients: A multicenter European case-control study. Clin Infect Dis 63:338, 2016.

Haussaire D et al: Nocardiosis in the south of France over a 10-years period, 2004–2014. Int J Infect Dis 57:13, 2017.

Huang L et al: Clinical features, identification, antimicrobial resistance patterns of *Nocardia* species in China: 2009–2017. Diagn Microbiol Infect Dis 94:165, 2019.

Mei-Zahav M et al: The spectrum of nocardia lung disease in cystic fibrosis. Pediatr Infect Dis J 34:909, 2015.

Paige EK, Spelman D: Nocardiosis: 7-year experience at an Australian tertiary hospital. Intern Med J 49:373, 2019.

Rosen LB et al: Nocardia-induced granulocyte macrophage colony-stimulating factor is neutralized by autoantibodies in disseminated/extrapulmonary nocardiosis. Clin Infect Dis 60:1017, 2015.

Schlaberg R et al: Susceptibility profiles of nocardia isolates based on current taxonomy. Antimicrob Agents Chemother 58:795, 2014.

Viscuse PV, Mohabbat AB: 69-year-old woman with fatigue, dyspnea, and lower extremity pain. Mayo Clin Proc. 94:149, 2019.

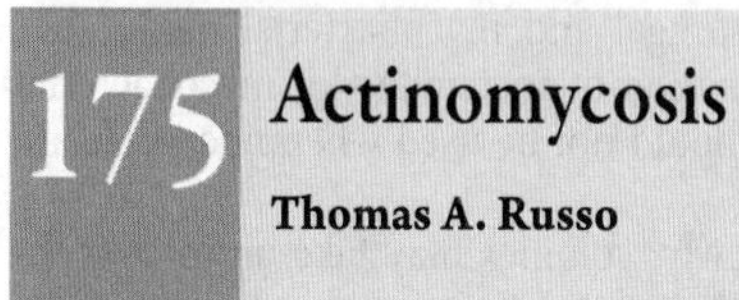
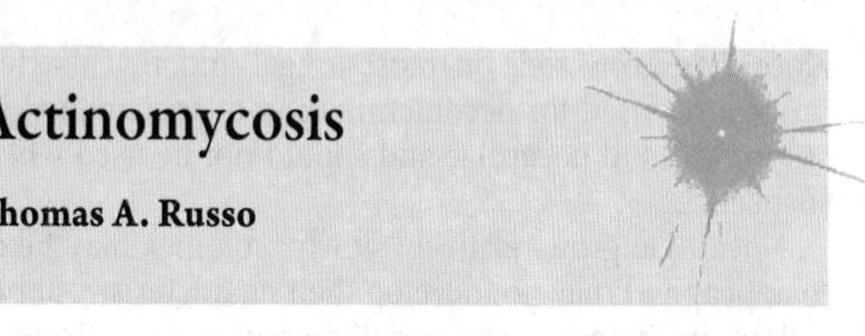

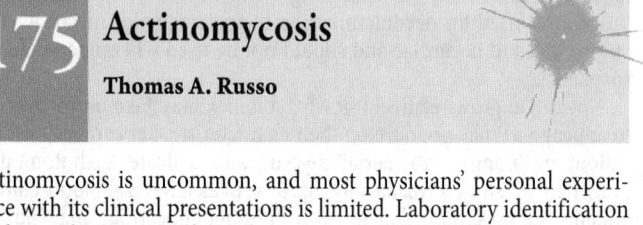

175 Actinomycosis

Thomas A. Russo

Actinomycosis is uncommon, and most physicians' personal experience with its clinical presentations is limited. Laboratory identification of the etiologic agents from the order Actinomycetales is not routine. Thus, actinomycosis remains a diagnostic challenge, even for a skilled clinician. However, this infection is usually curable with medical therapy alone. Therefore, an awareness of the full spectrum of clinical syndromes can expedite diagnosis and treatment and minimize unnecessary surgical interventions, morbidity, and mortality.

Classical actinomycosis is an indolent, slowly progressive infection caused by anaerobic or microaerophilic bacteria, primarily of the genus *Actinomyces*, that colonize the mouth, colon, and vagina. Mucosal disruption may lead to infection at virtually any site in the body. In vivo growth of actinomycetes usually results in the formation of characteristic clumps called *grains* or *sulfur granules*. The clinical presentations of actinomycosis are myriad. Common in the preantibiotic era, actinomycosis has diminished in incidence, as has its timely recognition. Actinomycosis has been called the most misdiagnosed disease, and it has been said that no disease is so often missed by experienced diagnosticians.

Three "classic" clinical presentations that should prompt consideration of this unique infection are (1) the combination of chronicity, progression across tissue boundaries, and mass-like features (mimicking malignancy, with which it is often confused); (2) the development of a sinus tract, which may spontaneously resolve and recur; and (3) a refractory or relapsing infection after a short course of therapy, since cure of established actinomycosis requires prolonged treatment.

■ ETIOLOGIC AGENTS

Actinomycosis is most commonly caused by *A. israelii, A. naeslundii, A. odontolyticus, A. viscosus, A. meyeri, A. graevenitzii*, and *A. gerencseriae*. Infections due to *A. neuii* have been increasingly recognized. Most if not all actinomycotic infections are polymicrobial. *Aggregatibacter (Actinobacillus) actinomycetemcomitans, Eikenella corrodens*, Enterobacteriaceae, and species of *Fusobacterium, Bacteroides, Capnocytophaga, Staphylococcus*, and *Streptococcus* are commonly isolated with actinomycetes in various combinations, depending on the site of infection. Their contribution to the pathogenesis of actinomycosis is uncertain.

Comparative 16S rRNA gene sequencing has led to the identification of an ever-expanding list of *Actinomyces* species and a reclassification of some species to other genera. At present, 53 species and 2 subspecies have been recognized (*https://www.bacterio.net/genus/actinomyces*), with at least 25 species implicated as causes of human disease. *A. europaeus, A. neuii, A. radingae, A. turicensis, A. cardiffensis, A. urogenitalis, A. hongkongensis, A. georgiae, A. massiliensis, A. timonensis*, and *A. funkei* as well as two former *Actinomyces* species—*Trueperella* (*Arcanobacterium*) *pyogenes* and *Trueperella* (*Arcanobacterium*) *bernardiae*—and *Propionibacterium propionicum* are additional causes of human actinomycosis, albeit not always with a "classic" presentation.

■ EPIDEMIOLOGY

Actinomycosis has no geographic boundaries and occurs throughout life, with a peak incidence in the middle decades. Males have a threefold higher incidence than females, possibly because of poorer dental hygiene and/or more frequent trauma. Improved dental hygiene and the initiation of antimicrobial treatment before actinomycosis fully develops have probably contributed to a decrease in incidence since the advent of antibiotics. Individuals who do not seek or have access to health care, those who have an intrauterine contraceptive device (IUCD) in place for a prolonged period (see "Pelvic Disease," below), and those who receive bisphosphonate treatment (see "Oral–Cervicofacial Disease," below) are probably at higher risk.

PATHOGENESIS AND PATHOLOGY

The etiologic agents of actinomycosis are members of the normal oral flora and are often cultured from the bronchi, the gastrointestinal tract, and the female genital tract. The critical step in the development of actinomycosis is disruption of the mucosal barrier. Local infection may ensue. Once established, actinomycosis spreads contiguously in a slow, progressive manner, ignoring tissue planes. Although acute inflammation may initially develop at the infection site, the hallmark of actinomycosis is the characteristic chronic, indolent phase manifested by lesions that usually appear as single or multiple indurations. Central necrosis consisting of neutrophils and sulfur granules develops and is virtually diagnostic. The fibrotic walls of the mass are typically described as "wooden." The responsible bacterial and/or host factors have not been identified. Over time, sinus tracts to the skin, adjacent organs, or bone may develop. In rare instances, distant hematogenous seeding may occur; lymphatic spread and associated lymphadenopathy are uncommon. As mentioned above, these unique features of actinomycosis mimic malignancy, with which it is often confused.

Foreign bodies appear to facilitate infection. This association most frequently involves IUCDs. Reports have described an association of actinomycosis with HIV infection; transplantation; common variable immunodeficiency; chronic granulomatous disease; treatment with anti–tumor necrosis factor α agents, glucocorticoids, or bisphosphonates; and radio- or chemotherapy. Ulcerative mucosal infections (e.g., by herpes simplex virus or cytomegalovirus) may facilitate disease development.

CLINICAL MANIFESTATIONS

Oral–Cervicofacial Disease Actinomycosis occurs most frequently at an oral, cervical, or facial site, usually as a soft tissue swelling, abscess, mass, or ulcerative lesion that is often mistaken for a neoplasm. Dental diseases or procedures are common precipitating factors. The angle of the jaw is generally involved, but a diagnosis of actinomycosis should be considered with any mass lesion or relapsing infection in the head and neck. Radiation therapy and especially bisphosphonate treatment have been recognized as contributing to an increasing incidence of actinomycotic infection of the mandible and maxilla (**Fig. 175-1**). Canaliculitis (commonly due to *P. propionicum*), otitis, sinusitis, and laryngeal disease also can develop. Pain, fever, and leukocytosis are variably reported. Contiguous extension to the cranium, cervical spine, or thorax is a potential sequela.

Thoracic Disease Thoracic actinomycosis, which may be facilitated by aspirated foreign material, usually follows an indolent progressive course, with involvement of the pulmonary parenchyma and/or the pleural space. Chest pain, fever, and weight loss are common. A cough, when present, is variably productive. The usual radiographic finding is either a mass lesion or pneumonia. On CT, central areas of low attenuation and ring-like rim enhancement may be seen; cavitary disease may develop. More than 50% of cases include pleural thickening, effusion, or empyema (**Fig. 175-2**). Rarely, pulmonary nodules or endobronchial lesions occur. Lesions suggestive of actinomycosis include those that cross fissures or pleura; extend into the mediastinum, contiguous bone, or chest wall (*empyema necessitatis*); or are associated with a sinus tract. In the absence of these findings, thoracic actinomycosis is usually mistaken for a neoplasm or pneumonia due to more usual causes.

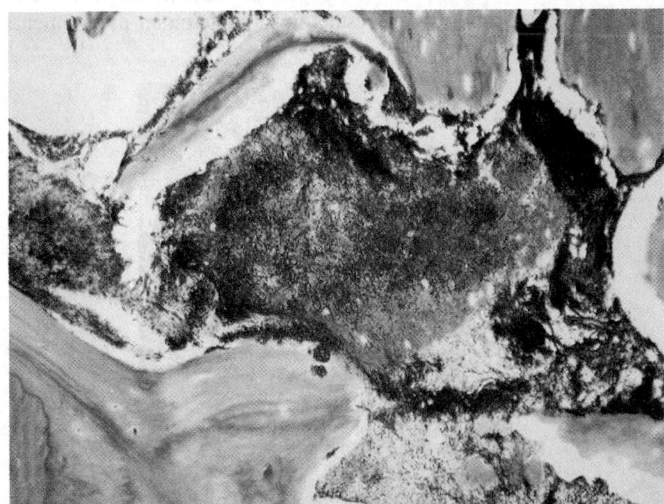

FIGURE 175-1 Bisphosphonate-associated maxillary osteomyelitis due to *Actinomyces viscosus*. A sulfur granule is seen within the bone. *(Reprinted with permission from NH Naik, TA Russo: Bisphosphonate related osteonecrosis of the jaw: The role of Actinomyces. Clin Infect Dis 49:1729, 2009. © 2009 Oxford University Press.)*

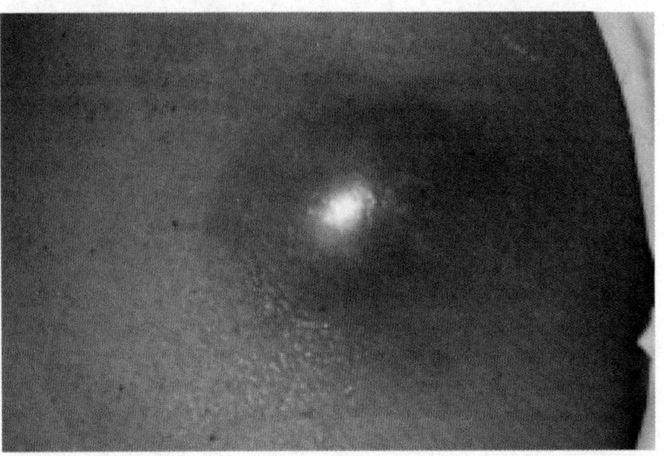

A

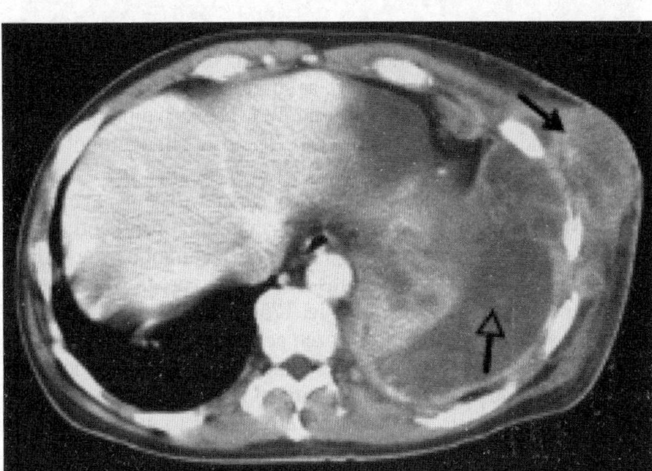

B

FIGURE 175-2 Thoracic actinomycosis. *A.* A chest wall mass from extension of pulmonary infection. ***B.*** Pulmonary infection is complicated by empyema (*open arrow*) and extension to the chest wall (*closed arrow*). *(Courtesy of Dr. C. B. Hsiao, Division of Infectious Diseases, Department of Medicine, State University of New York at Buffalo.)*

Mediastinal infection is uncommon, usually arising from thoracic extension but rarely from perforation of the esophagus, trauma, or extension of head and neck or abdominal disease. The structures within the mediastinum and the heart can be involved in various combinations; consequently, the possible presentations are diverse. Primary endocarditis (in which *A. neuii* has been increasingly described), esophageal infection, and isolated disease of the breast occur.

Abdominal Disease Abdominal actinomycosis poses a great diagnostic challenge. Months or years usually pass from the inciting event (e.g., appendicitis, diverticulitis, peptic ulcer disease, spillage of gallstones or bile during cholecystectomy, foreign-body perforation, bowel surgery, or ascension from IUCD-associated pelvic disease) to clinical recognition. Because of the flow of peritoneal fluid and/or the direct extension of primary disease, virtually any abdominal organ, region, or space can be involved. The disease usually presents as an abscess, a mass, or a mixed lesion that is often fixed to underlying tissue and mistaken for a tumor. On CT, enhancement is most often heterogeneous and adjacent bowel is thickened. Sinus tracts to the abdominal wall, to the perianal region, or between the bowel and other organs may develop and mimic inflammatory bowel disease (**Chap. 326**). Recurrent disease or a wound or fistula that fails to heal suggests actinomycosis.

Hepatic infection usually presents as one or more abscesses or masses (**Fig. 175-3**). Isolated disease presumably develops via hematogenous seeding from cryptic foci. Imaging and percutaneous techniques have resulted in improved diagnosis and treatment.

All levels of the urogenital tract can be infected. Renal disease usually presents as pyelonephritis and/or renal and perinephric abscess. Bladder involvement, usually due to extension of pelvic disease, may result in ureteral obstruction or fistulas to bowel, skin, or uterus. *Actinomyces* can be detected in urine with appropriate stains and cultures.

Pelvic Disease Actinomycotic involvement of the pelvis occurs most commonly in association with an IUCD but can also be associated with other foreign bodies, such as surgical mesh. When an IUCD is in place or has been used but removed, pelvic symptoms should prompt consideration of actinomycosis. The risk, although not quantified, appears small. The disease rarely develops when the IUCD has been in place for <1 year, but the risk increases with time. Symptoms are typically indolent; fever, weight loss, abdominal pain, and abnormal vaginal bleeding or discharge are the most common. The earliest stage of disease—often endometritis—commonly progresses to pelvic masses or a tuboovarian abscess (**Fig. 175-4**). Unfortunately, because the diagnosis is often delayed, a "frozen pelvis" mimicking malignancy or endometriosis can develop by the time of recognition, which may lead to unnecessary surgery. Cancer antigen 125 levels may be elevated, further contributing to misdiagnosis. In contrast to malignancy and tuberculosis, pelvic actinomycosis only uncommonly includes ascites and lymphadenopathy. An endometrial biopsy may enable diagnosis in a minimally invasive fashion.

Actinomyces-like organisms (ALOs), which are identified in Papanicolaou-stained specimens in (on average) 7% of women using an IUCD, have a low positive predictive value for diagnosis. The detection of ALOs in an asymptomatic patient warrants education and close follow-up but not removal of the IUCD unless a suitable contraceptive alternative is agreed on. In the presence of symptoms that cannot be accounted for, it seems prudent to remove the IUCD and—if advanced disease is excluded—to initiate a 14-day course of empirical treatment for possible early endometritis.

Central Nervous System Disease Actinomycosis of the central nervous system (CNS) is rare. Single or multiple brain abscesses are most common. Individuals with hereditary hemorrhagic telangiectasia are at increased risk for brain abscess with *Actinomyces* as the potential etiologic agent. An abscess usually appears on CT as a ring-enhancing lesion with a thick wall that may be irregular or nodular. Magnetic resonance perfusion and spectroscopy findings have also been described, as have primary meningitis, epidural or subdural space infection, and cavernous sinus syndrome.

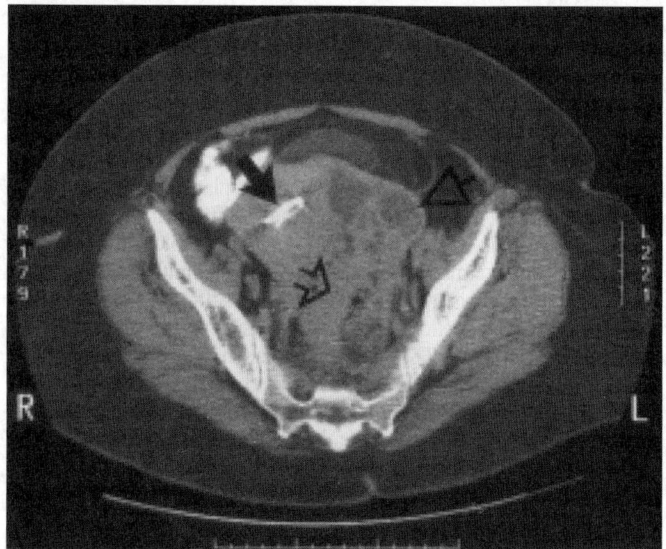

FIGURE 175-4 Computed tomogram showing pelvic actinomycosis associated with an intrauterine contraceptive device. The device is encased by endometrial fibrosis (*solid arrow*); also visible are paraendometrial fibrosis (*open triangular arrowhead*) and an area of suppuration (*open arrow*).

Musculoskeletal and Soft Tissue Infection Actinomycotic infection of bones and joints is usually due to adjacent soft tissue infection but may be associated with trauma, injections, surgery (e.g., prostheses), osteoradionecrosis and bisphosphonate osteonecrosis (limited to mandibular and maxillary bones), or hematogenous spread. Because of slow disease progression, new bone formation and bone destruction can be seen concomitantly. Infection of soft tissue is uncommon and is usually a result of trauma. Actinomycetoma is a slowly progressive infection of the skin and subcutaneous tissue that is usually seen in warm climates. Despite the name being suggestive of *Actinomyces* as a causative agent, it is most commonly caused by *Nocardia* or *Actinomadura* species (**Chap. 174**).

Disseminated Disease Hematogenous dissemination of disease from any location rarely results in multiple-organ involvement.

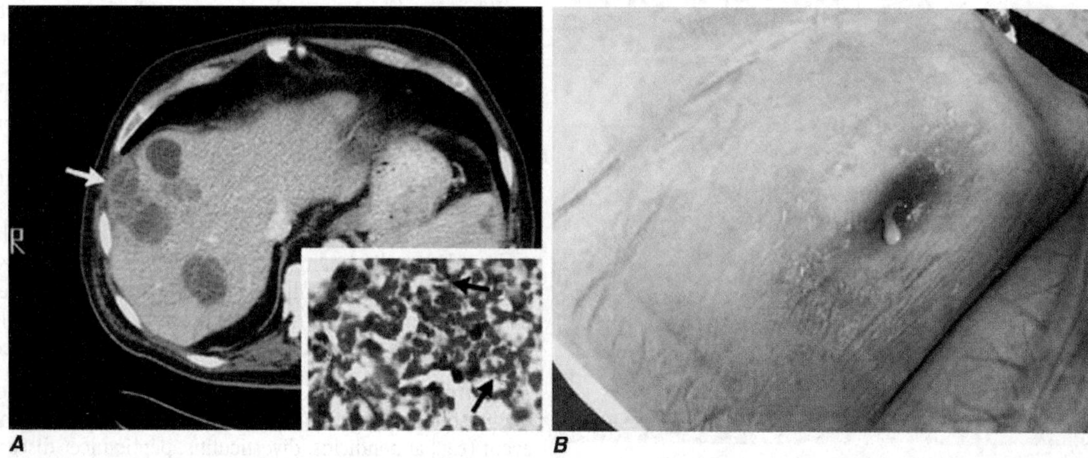

FIGURE 175-3 Hepatic–splenic actinomycosis. *A.* Computed tomogram showing multiple hepatic abscesses and a small splenic lesion due to *Actinomyces israelii*. Arrow indicates extension outside the liver. *Inset:* Gram's stain of abscess fluid demonstrating beaded filamentous gram-positive rods. ***B.*** Subsequent formation of a sinus tract. *(Reprinted with permission from Saad M: Actinomyces hepatic abscess with cutaneous fistula. N Engl J Med 353:e16, 2005. © 2005 Massachusetts Medical Society. All rights reserved.)*

A. meyeri is most commonly involved. The lungs and liver are most often affected, with the presentation of multiple nodules mimicking disseminated malignancy. The clinical presentation may be surprisingly indolent given the extent of disease.

DIAGNOSIS

The diagnosis of actinomycosis is rarely considered. All too often, actinomycosis is first mentioned by the pathologist after extensive surgery. Since medical therapy alone is frequently sufficient for cure, the challenge for the clinician is to consider the possibility of actinomycosis, to diagnose it in the least invasive fashion, and to avoid unnecessary surgery. The clinical and radiographic presentations that suggest actinomycosis are discussed above. Of note, hypermetabolism has been demonstrated by ^{18}F-fluorodeoxyglucose positron emission tomography (FDG-PET) in actinomycotic disease. Aspirations and biopsies (with or without CT or ultrasound guidance) are being used successfully to obtain clinical material for diagnosis, although surgery may be required. The microscopic identification of sulfur granules (an in vivo matrix of bacteria, calcium phosphate, and host material) in pus or tissues, which increases with the examination of additional histopathologic sections and the use of positively charged slides to optimize adhesion, is the most common means of diagnosis. Occasionally, these granules are identified grossly from draining sinus tracts or pus. Although sulfur granules are a defining characteristic of actinomycosis, granules also are found in mycetoma **(Chaps. 174 and 219)** and botryomycosis (a chronic suppurative bacterial infection of soft tissue or, in rare cases, visceral tissue that produces clumps of bacteria resembling granules). These entities can easily be differentiated from actinomycosis with appropriate histopathologic and microbiologic studies. Microbiologic identification of actinomycetes is often precluded by prior antimicrobial therapy or failure to perform appropriate microbiologic cultures. For optimal yield, the avoidance of even a single dose of antibiotics is mandatory. Although some species can grow aerobically, isolation is maximized under anaerobic conditions, usually requiring 5–7 days but potentially up to 2–4 weeks. The use of 16S rRNA gene amplification and sequencing by clinical microbiology laboratories is increasing and is enhancing diagnostic sensitivity and specificity. Matrix-assisted laser desorption/ionization time-of-flight mass spectrometry (MALDI-TOF MS) holds similar promise, but databases are still being optimized. Because actinomycetes are components of the normal oral and genital-tract flora, their identification in the absence of sulfur granules in sputum, bronchial washings, and cervicovaginal secretions is of little significance.

TREATMENT

Actinomycosis

Decisions about treatment are based on the collective clinical experience of the past 70 years. Actinomycosis requires prolonged treatment with high doses of antimicrobial agents; suitable antimicrobial agents and those deemed unreliable are listed in **Table 175-1**. The need for intensive treatment is presumably due to the drugs' poor penetration of the thick-walled masses common in this infection and/or the sulfur granules themselves, which may represent a biofilm. Although therapy must be individualized, the IV administration of 18–24 million units of penicillin daily for 2–6 weeks, followed by oral therapy with penicillin or amoxicillin (total duration, 6–12 months), is a reasonable guideline for serious infections and bulky disease. For penicillin-allergic patients, tetracyclines, ceftriaxone, or carbapenems are reasonable alternatives. Less extensive disease, particularly that involving the oral–cervicofacial region or the isolation of *Actinomyces* in the absence of tissue changes associated with actinomycosis, may be cured with a shorter course. For home IV therapy, the ease of once-a-day dosing makes ceftriaxone appealing in certain circumstances; however, a greater body of literature supporting its efficacy would be desirable. The availability of portable infusion pumps for home therapy allows for both the appropriate dosing and practical administration of IV

TABLE 175-1 Appropriate and Inappropriate Antibiotic Therapy for Actinomycosis[a]

CATEGORY	AGENT
Extensive successful clinical experience[b]	Penicillin: 3–4 million units IV q4h[c,d]
	Amoxicillin: 500 mg PO q6h
	Erythromycin: 500–1000 mg IV q6h or 500 mg PO q6h[c]
	Tetracycline: 500 mg PO q6h
	Doxycycline: 100 mg IV or PO q12h
	Minocycline: 100 mg IV or PO q12h
	Clindamycin: 900 mg IV q8h or 300–450 mg PO q6h[c]
Anecdotal successful clinical experience	Ceftriaxone[d]
	Ceftizoxime
	Imipenem-cilastatin
	Piperacillin-tazobactam
Agents predicted to be efficacious on the basis of in vitro activity	Vancomycin
	Linezolid
	Quinupristin-dalfopristin
	Rifampin
	Ertapenem[d]
	Tigecycline[d]
	Azithromycin[d]
Agents that should be avoided	Metronidazole
	Aminoglycosides
	Oxacillin, dicloxacillin
	Cephalexin
	Fluoroquinolones

[a]Additional coverage for concomitant "companion" bacteria may be required. [b]Controlled evaluations have not been performed. Dose and duration require individualization depending on the host, site, and extent of infection. As a general rule, a maximal parenteral antimicrobial dose for 2–6 weeks followed by oral therapy, for a total duration of 6–12 months, is required for serious infections and bulky disease, whereas a shorter course may suffice for less extensive disease, particularly in the oral–cervicofacial region. Monitoring the impact of therapy with CT or MRI is advisable when appropriate. [c]Recent in vitro data have demonstrated resistance in up to 33% of isolates. [d]This agent can be considered for at-home parenteral therapy; penicillin requires a continuous infusion pump.

penicillin. For infections in critical sites (e.g., CNS), this approach remains the safest until more information is available on other agents. The pharmacokinetic properties, availability of oral and parenteral formulations, and potential efficacy of azithromycin also make this agent appealing. Unfortunately, few in vitro and no clinical data exist on its use to treat actinomycosis. If therapy is extended beyond the resolution of measurable disease, the risk of relapse—a clinical hallmark of this infection—will be minimized; CT and MRI are generally the most sensitive and objective techniques by which to accomplish this goal. A similar approach is reasonable for immunocompromised patients, although refractory disease has been described in HIV-infected individuals. While the role played by "companion" microbes in actinomycosis is unclear, many isolates are pathogens in their own right, and a regimen covering these organisms during the initial treatment course is reasonable. Isolation of *Actinomyces* from blood cultures in the absence of defined infection may represent contamination or transient bacteremia from a mucosal site of colonization, in which case treatment may not be necessary.

Combined medical–surgical therapy is still advocated in some reports. However, an increasing body of literature now supports an initial attempt at cure with medical therapy alone, even in extensive disease. CT and MRI should be used to monitor the response to therapy. In most cases, either surgery can be avoided or a less extensive procedure can be used. This approach is particularly valuable in sparing critical organs, such as the bladder or the reproductive organs in women of childbearing age. For a well-defined abscess, percutaneous drainage in combination with medical therapy is a reasonable approach. When a critical location is involved (e.g., the epidural space, the CNS), when there is significant hemoptysis, or when suitable medical therapy fails, surgical intervention may be appropriate. In the absence of optimal data, the combination of a prolonged course of antimicrobial therapy and resection—at least of necrotic bone for bisphosphonate-related osteonecrosis of the jaw (BRONJ)—is a reasonable approach.

FURTHER READING

Barberis C et al: Antimicrobial susceptibility of clinical isolates of *Actinomyces* and related genera reveals an unusual clindamycin resistance among *Actinomyces urogenitalis* strains. J Glob Antimicrob Resist 8:115, 2017.

Bonnefond S et al: Clinical features of actinomycosis: A retrospective, multicenter study of 28 cases of miscellaneous presentations. Medicine 95:e3923, 2016.

Fong P et al: Identification and diversity of *Actinomyces* species in a clinical microbiology laboratory in the MALDI-TOF MS era. Anaerobe 54:151, 2018.

Heo SH et al: Imaging of actinomycosis in various organs: A comprehensive review. Radiographics 34:19, 2014.

Jeffery-Smith A et al: Is the presence of *Actinomyces* spp. in blood culture always significant? J Clin Microbiol 54:1137, 2016.

Karanfilian KM et al: Cervicofacial actinomycosis. Int J Dermatol 59:1185, 2020.

Kononen E, Wade WG: *Actinomyces* and related organisms in human infections. Clin Microbiol Rev 28:419, 2015.

Lo Muzio L et al: The contribution of histopathological examination to the diagnosis of cervico-facial actinomycosis: A retrospective analysis of 68 cases. Eur J Clin Microbiol Infect Dis 33:1915, 2014.

Lynch T et al: Species-level identification of *Actinomyces* isolates causing invasive infections: Multiyear comparison of Vitek MS (matrix-assisted laser desorption ionization-time of flight mass spectrometry) to partial sequencing of the 16S rRNA gene. J Clin Microbiol 54:712, 2016.

Qiu L et al: Pulmonary actinomycosis imitating lung cancer on (18) F-FDG PET/CT: A case report and literature review. Korean J Radiol 16:1262, 2015.

Yang WT, Grant M: *Actinomyces neuii*: A case report of a rare cause of acute infective endocarditis and literature review. BMC Infect Dis 19:511, 2019.

176 Whipple's Disease

Thomas A. Russo, Seth R. Glassman

Whipple's disease (WD), described by George Whipple in 1907, is a chronic infection caused by *Tropheryma whipplei*. Most commonly, years pass from the onset of symptoms to the recognition of the disease because of its rarity, its various manifestations mimicking other conditions, and the need to perform nonroutine diagnostic tests. The long-held belief that WD is an infection was supported by observations on its responsiveness to antimicrobial therapy in the 1950s and the identification of bacilli via electron microscopy in small-bowel biopsy specimens in the 1960s. This hypothesis was finally confirmed by amplification and sequencing of a partial 16S rRNA polymerase chain reaction (PCR)–generated amplicon from duodenal tissue in 1991. The subsequent successful cultivation of *T. whipplei* enabled whole-genome sequencing and the development of additional diagnostic tests. The development of PCR-based diagnostics has broadened our understanding of both the epidemiology of and the clinical syndromes attributable to *T. whipplei*. Exposure to *T. whipplei*, which appears to be much more common than has been appreciated, can be followed by asymptomatic carriage, acute disease, or chronic infection. Chronic infection—WD—is a rare development after exposure. "Classic" WD is manifested by some combination of arthralgias/arthritis, weight loss, chronic diarrhea, abdominal pain, and fever. Variable involvement at other sites also occurs; neurologic and cardiac disease are most common. Acute infection and chronic organ disease in the absence of intestinal involvement (see "Isolated Infection," below) are described with increasing frequency. Since untreated WD is often fatal and delayed diagnosis may lead to irreparable organ damage (e.g., in the central nervous system [CNS]), knowledge of the clinical scenarios in which Whipple's should be considered and of an appropriate diagnostic strategy is mandatory.

ETIOLOGIC AGENT

T. whipplei is a weakly staining gram-positive bacillus. Genomic sequence data have revealed that the organism has a small (<1-megabase) chromosome, with many biosynthetic pathways absent or incomplete. This finding is consistent with a host-dependent intracellular pathogen or a pathogen that requires a nutritionally rich extracellular environment. It is one of the slowest growing human pathogens, with a doubling time of 18 days. A genotyping scheme based on a variable region has disclosed >100 genotypes to date. All genotypes appear to be capable of causing similar clinical syndromes.

EPIDEMIOLOGY

WD is rare but has been increasingly recognized since the advent of PCR-based diagnostic tools. Prevalence had been previously estimated at 1–3 cases per 1 million population, although a recent U.S. epidemiologic survey places the number closer to 10 cases per million. Seroprevalence studies indicate that ~50% of Western Europeans and ~75% of Africans from rural Senegal have been exposed to *T. whipplei*. Higher prevalence may be attributable to differences in sanitation. Humans are the only known host. In most studies, males more commonly develop WD; WD is more common in Caucasians and increases with age. To date, no clear animal or environmental reservoir has been demonstrated. However, the organism has been identified by PCR in sewage water and human feces. Workers with direct exposure to sewage are more likely to be asymptomatically colonized than controls, a pattern suggesting fecal–oral spread. Fecal PCR detection rates of 38% among family members of carriers or patients with infection support oral–oral or fecal–oral spread, although a common environmental exposure cannot be excluded. Further, the development of acute *T. whipplei* pneumonia in children raises the possibility of droplet or airborne transmission.

PATHOGENESIS AND PATHOLOGY

Rates of asymptomatic carriage of *T. whipplei* are far higher than rates of chronic infection (<0.01% of those exposed). Both decreased host pathogen-specific inflammatory response and pathogen-driven modulation of host inflammatory response likely play a role in establishing chronic infection. The human leukocyte antigen (HLA) alleles DRB1*13 and DQB1*06, which stimulate humoral rather than cell-mediated immune responses, are associated with an increased risk of infection. However, only a minority of infected patients possess these haplotypes, suggesting a role for other host factors. IRF4, a transcription factor involved with the immune response, could be such a factor as evidenced by four related family members with WD who possessed IFR4 haploinsufficiency due to a loss-of-function mutation; the distribution of WD in this extended family was consistent with an autosomal dominant trait with incomplete penetrance.

Flow cytometry performed in WD patients demonstrates B-cell subset abnormalities when compared to matched controls. Chronic infection is associated with an impaired T_H1 response, enhanced production of anti-inflammatory cytokines, increased activity of regulatory T cells, M2 polarization of macrophages with diminished antimicrobial activity and impaired phagosome–lysosome fusion and ensuing apoptosis, and blunted development of *T. whipplei*–specific T cells. Therapies that blunt cell-mediated host immune responses (e.g. systemic glucocorticoids or anti–tumor necrosis factor α [TNF-α] agents) may accelerate progression of chronic disease. Impaired cell-mediated immunity may play a role in establishing chronic carriage of *T. whipplei* as is evidenced by higher rates of detection in the secretions of HIV-infected persons.

T. whipplei has a tropism for myeloid cells, which it invades and in which it can avoid being killed. Infiltration of infected tissue by large numbers of foamy macrophages containing periodic acid–Schiff (PAS)–staining inclusions (representing ingested bacteria) is a characteristic and most common finding. With gastrointestinal disease progression, villus atrophy, lymphangiectasia, crypt hyperplasia, and apoptosis of surface epithelial cells are observed in the small intestine, with resultant diarrhea due to decreased absorption and increased leak of water and solutes. Occasionally, involvement of lymphatic or hepatic tissue may manifest as noncaseating granulomas that can mimic sarcoid or granulomatous vasculitis.

■ CLINICAL MANIFESTATIONS

Asymptomatic Colonization/Carriage Studies using primarily PCR have detected *T. whipplei* sequence in stool, saliva, duodenal tissue, and (rarely) blood in the absence of symptoms. Although prevalence rates are still being defined, in Western European countries, detection in saliva (0.2%) is less common than that in stool (1–11%) and appears to occur only with concomitant fecal carriage. The prevalence of fecal carriage is elevated among individuals with exposure to waste water or sewage (12–26%) and among children living in tropical Africa and Asia (20–48%). A duration of carriage of 7 years for the same strain has been described in a sewer worker. Evolution of the carrier state into chronic disease is uncommon. Bacterial loads are lighter in asymptomatic carriage than in active disease.

Acute Infection *T. whipplei* has been implicated as a cause of acute gastroenteritis in children. It was also detected via PCR in the blood of 4.6% of febrile patients (75% of whom were <15 years of age) from two rural villages in Senegal as opposed to 0.25% of healthy controls. Further, *T. whipplei* has been implicated as a cause of acute pneumonia. These data suggest that primary acquisition may result in symptomatic pulmonary or intestinal infection or a febrile syndrome, which perhaps are more common than is generally appreciated.

Chronic Infection • **"CLASSIC" WD** So-called classic WD was the initial clinical syndrome recognized, with consequent identification of *T. whipplei*. This chronic infection is defined by involvement of the duodenum and/or jejunum that develops over years. In most individuals, the initial phase of disease manifests primarily as intermittent, often symmetrical, occasionally chronic, and rarely destructive migratory oligo- or polyarthralgias/seronegative arthritis involving the knees, wrists, ankles, and metacarpal-interphalangeal joints most commonly. Less frequently, spondylitis, sacroiliitis, discitis, tenosynovitis, bursitis, and prosthetic hip infection also have been described. Intermittent fever, myalgias, and skin nodules may accompany joint symptoms. Tests for rheumatoid factor and antinuclear antibody are usually negative. This initial stage is often confused with a variety of rheumatologic disorders and, on average, lasts 6–8 years before gastrointestinal symptoms commence. Treatment of presumed inflammatory arthritis with immunosuppressive agents (e.g., glucocorticoids, anti-TNF-α, anakinra) can accelerate progression of the disease process; thus, screening for WD prior to initiation of immunosuppressant therapy may be appropriate, depending on the clinical scenario. Alternatively, antimicrobial therapy for another indication may reduce symptoms, and this situation should also prompt consideration of WD. The intestinal symptoms that develop in the majority of cases are characterized by diarrhea with accompanying weight loss and may be associated with fever and abdominal pain. Occult gastrointestinal blood loss, vitamin deficiencies, hepatosplenomegaly (10–15%), and ascites (10%) are less common. Anemia and hypereosinophilia may be detected. The most common finding on abdominal CT is mesenteric and/or retroperitoneal lymphadenopathy (usually raising concern about lymphoma). The endoscopic or video-capsule observation of pale, yellow, or shaggy mucosa with erythema or ulceration past the first portion of the duodenum suggests WD (**Fig. 176-1**). When endoscopy with duodenal biopsy is nondiagnostic, a video-capsule study may assist in identifying more distal lesions for subsequent biopsy. ^{18}F-Fluorodeoxyglucose positron emission tomography (FDG-PET) studies in patients with WD suggest the entire small bowel can be involved. Diagnostic misdirection can be caused by co-infection with *Giardia lamblia*, which is occasionally identified. The intestinal phase can also be confused with Crohn's or celiac disease. In addition to rheumatologic and intestinal disease, neurologic (6–63%), cardiac (17–55%), pulmonary (10–50%), lymphatic (10–55%), ocular (5–10%), dermal (5–30%), and less commonly other sites are variably involved in classic WD.

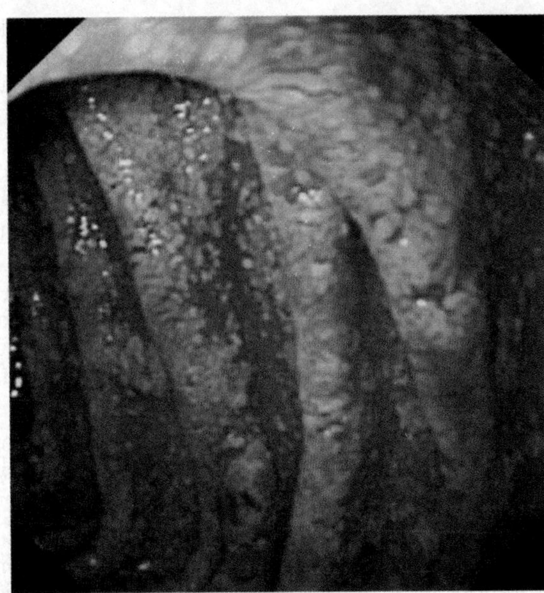

FIGURE 176-1 Endoscopic view of the jejunal mucosa demonstrating a thickened, granular mucosa and "white spots" due to dilated lacteals. *(Reprinted with permission from J Bureš et al: Whipple's disease: Our own experience and review of the literature. Gastroenterol Res Pract, 2013.)*

Neurologic Disease CNS disease, defined by PCR-based detection of *T. whipplei* in cerebrospinal fluid (CSF), develops in ~50% of patients, many of whom are asymptomatic. A variety of neurologic manifestations have been reported and portend a poor prognosis. The most common are cognitive changes including memory impairment progressing to dementia, personality and mood alterations, hypothalamic involvement (e.g., polyuria/polydipsia, sleep-cycle disorders), and supranuclear ophthalmoplegia. In addition, neuro-ophthalmologic manifestations of WD include supranuclear gaze palsy (usually vertical), oculomasticatory and oculofacial myorhythmia (highly suggestive of Whipple's), nystagmus, and retrobulbar neuritis. Focal neurologic presentations (dependent on lesion location), seizures, ataxia, meningitis, encephalitis, rhombo- or limbic encephalitis, hydrocephalus, myelopathy, myoclonus, choreiform movements, and distal polyneuropathy also have been described. Neurologic sequelae occur with CNS disease, and the mortality risk is significant.

MRI results may be normal. Identified lesions (solitary or multifocal) are usually T2 and fluid-attenuated inversion recovery (FLAIR) hyperintense and may enhance with gadolinium. All sites can be involved, and the nature of lesions is variable (e.g., nodular, infiltrative, tumor-like). Although imaging findings are myriad and are not diagnostic, the median temporal lobe, midbrain, hypothalamus, and thalamus are commonly affected. FDG-PET may reveal increased uptake. CSF analysis may be normal; when abnormal, leukocytosis (generally lymphocyte-predominant) and an elevated protein concentration are common. A low CSF glucose level has been reported.

Cardiac Disease Endocarditis is increasingly recognized in WD (85% of cases in males), causes 2.6–6.3% of culture-negative endocarditis cases, and may be complicated by congestive heart failure (40% of cases), embolic events, arrhythmias, mycotic aneurysm, or rarely hypotension. Fever is often absent, and the Duke clinical criteria are rarely met. Vegetations are identified by echocardiography in 50–75% of cases. All valves, alone or in combination, can be affected; most commonly involved are the aortic and mitral valves. Preexisting valvular disease is found in only a minority of cases, although infection of bioprosthetic valves has been described. Mural, myocardial, or pericardial disease also occurs alone or in combination with valvular involvement. Constrictive pericarditis develops infrequently. Diagnosis of cardiac disease is rarely made prior to surgical intervention.

Pulmonary Disease Some combination of interstitial disease, nodules, parenchymal infiltrate, and pleural effusion is observed. An association with pulmonary hypertension has also been reported. The clinical significance of *T. whipplei* sequence identified in bronchoalveolar lavage fluid (BALF) from asymptomatic HIV-infected individuals or in a case of interstitial lung disease is unresolved but suggests caution in diagnosing "isolated" pneumonia on the basis of sequence alone. Notably, while the bacterium seems to exist in the airways of HIV-infected persons at higher rates, its presence is not clearly associated with increased inflammation or a discernible decrease in lung function.

Lymphatic Disease Mesenteric and retroperitoneal lymphadenopathy are common with intestinal disease, and mediastinal adenopathy may be associated with pulmonary infection. Peripheral adenopathy is less common.

Ocular Disease (Non–Neuro-Ophthalmologic) Uveitis is the most common form of ocular disease, usually presenting as a change in vision or "floaters." Anterior (anterior chamber), intermediate (vitreous), and posterior (retina/choroid) uveitis can occur alone or in combination. Treatment with glucocorticoids alone can worsen uveitis and unmask extraocular disease. Likewise, use of local or systemic glucocorticoids after ocular surgery can precipitate ocular infection, likely as a result of asymptomatic or subclinical disease. Keratitis, crystalline keratopathy, and optic neuritis also have been reported. Patients may be misdiagnosed with sarcoid or Behçet's disease prior to the recognition of Whipple's.

Dermatologic Disease Skin hyperpigmentation (melanoderma), particularly in light-exposed areas in the absence of adrenal dysfunction, is suggestive of WD. A variety of other cutaneous manifestations have been described, including erythematous macular lesions, nonthrombocytopenic purpura, subcutaneous nodules, and hyperkeratosis.

Miscellaneous Sites Thyroid, renal, testicular, epididymal, gallbladder, skeletal muscle, and bone marrow involvement have all been described. In fact, almost any organ can be involved in classic WD, with varying frequency, variable combinations, and myriad signs and symptoms. As a result, WD should be considered in the setting of a chronic multisystemic process. Despite its rarity, the combination of rheumatologic and intestinal disease with weight loss, with or without neurologic and cardiac involvement, warrants heightened suspicion.

ISOLATED INFECTION This entity has been defined as infection in the absence of intestinal symptoms, although an occasional small-bowel biopsy may be PAS-positive or more commonly PCR-positive in this setting. "Isolated infection" is something of a misnomer since multiple nonintestinal sites of *T. whipplei* infection are not uncommon. Infection at the same nonintestinal sites (single or multiple) that are variably involved in classic WD may also present as "isolated infection." Further, intestinal disease can subsequently develop. Endocarditis, neurologic disease, uveitis, rheumatologic manifestations, and pulmonary involvement are most commonly described. Signs and symptoms are similar to those described for *T. whipplei* infection of these sites in classic WD. With enhanced PCR-based diagnostic capabilities, *T. whipplei* infection without concomitant intestinal involvement (of which endocarditis is the best example) will probably be diagnosed increasingly often.

REINFECTION/RELAPSING DISEASE/IMMUNE RECONSTITUTION INFLAMMATORY SYNDROME (IRIS) It has been suggested that, if an underlying host immune defect places an individual at risk for chronic infection, then that person may be at risk for reinfection due to occupational exposure or contact with family members who are asymptomatically colonized. One case of apparent reinfection that was due to a different genotype supports this contention.

Optimal treatment regimens and durations are still being defined. However, it is clear, especially in the setting of occult or overt CNS disease, that treatment with oral tetracycline or trimethoprim-sulfamethoxazole (TMP-SMX) alone may result in disease relapse. Relapses or perhaps reinfections occurring years to decades after initial therapy have been described.

As in patients treated for HIV or mycobacterial disease, IRIS has been described in up to 17% of patients treated for *T. whipplei* infection. Prior immunosuppressive therapy increases the likelihood of IRIS, in which inflammation recurs after an initial clinical response to treatment and loss of PCR detection of *T. whipplei*. Manifestations include the development of fever, arthritis, skin lesions, subcutaneous nodules, pleuritis, uveitis, and orbital and periorbital inflammation; some cases have been fatal.

DIAGNOSIS

Considering *T. whipplei* infection and ensuring that the appropriate tests are performed are the critical steps in making the diagnosis, which otherwise will likely be missed. Serology is of little value since patients with active infection usually mount a poor IgM/IgG response to *T. whipplei* and a positive result most likely reflects prior exposure and clearance. The clinical presentation will in part dictate which clinical specimens are most likely to enable the diagnosis. In the presence (and perhaps the absence) of gastrointestinal symptoms, postbulbar duodenal biopsies should be performed, although a normal macroscopic appearance is common. As a general rule, diagnostic yield is greater for tissue specimens than for body fluids. Biopsy of normal-appearing skin may detect *T. whipplei* in the setting of classic WD and serve as a minimally invasive means to establish the diagnosis. It is prudent to collect CSF even in the absence of CNS symptoms; asymptomatic disease is common, the CNS is the most common site for relapse, and thus the information gained by CSF examination could influence the design and duration of the treatment regimen.

The diagnosis of classic WD was originally based on histologic findings in intestinal biopsy specimens. Although this diagnostic procedure remains important, it is not optimally sensitive. Infiltration of the lamina propria with macrophages containing PAS-positive inclusions that are resistant to diastase is observed. However, PAS is nonspecific, also yielding positive results with mycobacteria (which can be differentiated with Ziehl-Neelsen stain and culture), *Rhodococcus equi*, *Bacillus cereus*, *Corynebacterium* species, and *Histoplasma* species. *T. whipplei* can be detected by silver stain, Brown-Brenn (weakly positive), or acridine orange and is not stained by calcofluor. Staining of other tissues or fluids (e.g., ocular aspirations) for PAS-positive inclusions in macrophages can be performed to support the diagnosis. The sensitivity of identification of PAS-positive inclusions in WD may be decreased by anti-TNF-α therapy. Electron microscopy can be used to identify the trilaminar cell wall of *T. whipplei*. When available, immunohistochemistry has greater specificity and sensitivity than PAS staining and can be performed on archived fixed tissue. Alternatively, the use of fluorescence in situ hybridization (FISH) has been reported as a complementary diagnostic tool with various tissue samples.

The development and implementation of specific PCR-based diagnostics have significantly increased the sensitivity and specificity of *T. whipplei* identification. PCR can be applied to affected tissues (with greater sensitivity for non-formalin-fixed than for formalin-fixed tissue) in support of histologic findings and to various body fluids (e.g., CSF; aqueous or vitreous humor; joint, pericardial, or pleural fluid; BALF; blood; urine). It is important to note that the interpretation of a PCR-based diagnostic approach must take into account limitations such as false-positive results due to sample contamination, false-negative results due to low organism load, poor sample quality, inadequate DNA extraction, and variability in performance of various PCR assays. As with all diagnostic tests, consideration of pretest probability is critical for interpretation and a negative result does not exclude WD. Urine PCR for T. *whipplei* infection may hold promise for the noninvasive diagnosis of classic and isolated WD. In a recent study of 12 cases, urine PCR was positive in 9 (75%) of 12 cases prior to treatment compared to 0 (0%) of 110 controls, including 11 controls that were presumed carriers in which feces PCR was positive, although there was no evidence of disease. In addition, urine PCR is a potential tool to evaluate success of WD therapy. Saliva and fecal PCR is inappropriate as the sole diagnostic tool for WD due to a low positive predictive value, which more commonly identifies colonization, not disease; a positive result requires confirmation from appropriate end-organ tissue or body fluid.

T. whipplei has been successfully cultured from blood, CSF, synovial fluid, BALF, valve tissue, duodenal tissue, skeletal muscle, and lymph nodes, but culture is not practical since it takes months to obtain a positive result.

Affected anatomic sites in WD patients may demonstrate uptake on FDG-PET, which in turn could guide tissue sampling for use in specific tests.

TREATMENT

Whipple's Disease

Data on treatment are emerging, but the optimal regimen and duration for chronic infection, which may depend on the sites involved (e.g., CNS and heart valve), are unclear. Appropriate treatment usually results in a rapid—and at times remarkable—clinical response (e.g., in CNS disease), but eradication requires prolonged treatment. Maintenance of a durable response has been more challenging because of both relapse and host predisposition to reinfection.

Rates of relapse, particularly of CNS disease, were unacceptable with oral tetracycline or TMP-SMX monotherapy. Sequence data now indicate that TMP is not active against *T. whipplei* (given the absence of dihydrofolate reductase in *T. whipplei*) and that resistance to SMX and sulfadiazine can occur. However, a randomized controlled trial in 40 patients, who received either ceftriaxone (2 g IV q24h) or meropenem (1 g IV q8h) for 2 weeks followed by oral TMP-SMX (160/800 mg) twice a day for 1 year, demonstrated outstanding efficacy. The only case in which therapy failed—an asymptomatic CNS infection that was not eradicated by either regimen—was subsequently cured with oral minocycline and chloroquine (250 mg/d after a loading dose). A follow-up trial reported similar efficacy with a regimen of ceftriaxone (2 g IV q24h) for 2 weeks followed by oral TMP-SMX for 3 months. One issue in these trials was that the doses—and perhaps the duration of ceftriaxone and meropenem treatment as well—were not optimal for CNS infection. By contrast, in a small retrospective series, outcome was better in patients treated with oral doxycycline (100 mg twice a day) plus hydroxychloroquine (200 mg three times a day; to raise phagosome pH and increase drug activity in vitro) than in patients initially treated with TMP-SMX.

Until more data become available, it seems prudent—at least in asymptomatic/symptomatic CNS disease (which is present in many cases of WD)—first to administer CNS-optimized doses of IV ceftriaxone (2 g q12h) or meropenem (2 g q8h) for 2–4 weeks and then to treat with oral doxycycline, or minocycline plus hydroxychloroquine for at least 1 year, if tolerated. Although TMP-SMX has been frequently used as the oral alternative with reported success, a number of relapses or reinfections with TMP-SMX treatment have been reported, thereby suggesting caution for its use in patients with infection in critical locations such as the CNS and the heart. Although data on the use of PCR to guide therapy do not exist, it seems reasonable that continued *T. whipplei* detection by PCR, especially in the CSF and perhaps urine, should dictate at least continuation of therapy or perhaps consideration of an alternative regimen when in conjunction with a poor clinical response.

As molecular diagnostics become more available, *T. whipplei* may be increasingly recognized as a cause of endocarditis, and thus, timely recognition may result in cure with medical management alone. Surgery may be needed in the setting of endocarditis with significant valve dysfunction or myocardial abscess. Current European guidelines for the treatment of endocarditis caused by *T. whipplei* recommend oral doxycycline plus hydroxychloroquine for ≥18 months or, alternatively, ceftriaxone (2 g q24h IV) or penicillin (2 million units q4h IV) plus streptomycin (1 g q24h IV) for 2–4 weeks followed by oral TMP-SMX (800 mg q12h); a small study from Spain reported that treatment durations of 12–13 months with these regimens or variations were efficacious.

Data on isolated infection and certain site-specific treatment issues are even more limited. Anecdotal reports describe successful treatment of uveitis with oral TMP-SMX with or without rifampin, whereas treatment with tetracycline alone has resulted in relapse. Although a role for adjunctive intraocular therapy has been reported, the data are unclear on this point. There is a single case report of clearance of infection in a chronically relapsing patient by the addition of interferon gamma to antimicrobials. The supplementation to antimicrobials may be a consideration to address refractory disease or potential issues with antibiotic resistance.

Although data on the treatment of foreign body–associated infection are virtually nonexistent, medical treatment for a prosthetic hip infection was apparently successful; however, follow-up was limited.

The occurrence of a Jarisch-Herxheimer reaction within 24 h of treatment initiation has been described, with rapid resolution. The addition of glucocorticoids may be beneficial in the management of IRIS, and thalidomide has been used in steroid-refractory cases.

Importantly, although data are lacking, due to the inherent risk of relapse or reinfection, lifelong suppressive therapy with doxycycline after completion of the initial treatment regimen has been advocated. Regardless of the therapeutic approach chosen, an effort to ensure compliance and close follow-up for potential relapse or reinfection, which can occur many years after an apparent cure, will maximize the chances for a good outcome.

FURTHER READING

Bally JF et al: Systematic review of movement disorders and oculomotor abnormalities in Whipple's disease. Mov Disord 33:1700, 2018.

Crews NR et al: Diagnostic approach for classic compared with localized Whipple disease. Open Forum Infect Dis 5:ofy136, 2018.

Damaraju D et al: Clinical problem-solving: A surprising cause of chronic cough. N Engl J Med 373:561, 2015.

Guérin A et al: IRF4 haploinsufficiency in a family with Whipple's disease. Elife 7:e32340, 2018.

Gunther U et al: Gastrointestinal diagnosis of classical Whipple disease: Clinical, endoscopic, and histopathologic features in 191 patients. Medicine 94:e714, 2015.

Lagier JC, Raoult D: Whipple's disease and *Tropheryma whipplei* infections: When to suspect them and how to diagnose and treat them. Curr Opin Infect Dis 31:463, 2018.

McGee M et al: *Tropheryma whipplei* endocarditis: Case presentation and review of the literature. Open Forum Infect Dis 6:ofy330, 2018.

Meunier M et al: Rheumatic and musculoskeletal features of Whipple disease: A report of 29 cases. J Rheumatol 40:2061, 2013.

Moter A et al: Potential role for urine polymerase chain reaction in the diagnosis of Whipple's Disease. Clin Infect Dis 68:1089, 2019.

Watanuki S et al: Sutton's Law: Keep going where the money is. J Gen Intern Med 30:1711, 2015.

177 Infections Due to Mixed Anaerobic Organisms

Neeraj K. Surana, Dennis L. Kasper

Anaerobes comprise the predominant class of bacteria of the normal human microbiota that reside on mucous membranes and predominate in many infectious processes, particularly those arising from mucosal surfaces. These organisms generally cause disease subsequent to the breakdown of mucosal barriers and the leakage of the microbiota into normally sterile sites. Infections resulting from contamination by the microbiota are usually polymicrobial and involve both aerobic and anaerobic bacteria. However, the difficulties encountered in handling specimens in which anaerobes may be important and the technical challenges entailed in cultivating and identifying these organisms in clinical microbiology laboratories continue to leave the anaerobic etiology of an infectious process unproven in many cases. Therefore, an understanding of the types of infections in which anaerobes can play a role is crucial in selecting appropriate microbiologic tools to identify the organisms in clinical specimens and in choosing the most appropriate treatment, including antibiotics and surgical drainage or debridement of the infected site. This chapter focuses on infections caused by anaerobic bacteria other than *Clostridium* species, which are covered elsewhere (**Chaps. 134 and 154**).

HISTORICAL PERSPECTIVE

Anaerobic organisms were first identified by Antonie van Leeuwenhoek in 1680—nearly a century before oxygen itself was discovered. Leeuwenhoek set up culture medium (crushed pepper powder and clean rainwater) in two glass tubes—one open to ambient air and the other sealed closed—that he incubated for several days. Although he did not expect to observe anything in the sealed tube, he was surprised to find "animalcules" in both tubes. He noted that these bacteria in the sealed tube were "bigger than the biggest sort" in the tube left open to air. It was not until the mid- to late nineteenth century that Leeuwenhoek's findings were confirmed by Pasteur and others. However, these principles described by Leeuwenhoek underlie the basic pathogenesis of anaerobic infections: development of an anaerobic environment in a closed space is due to consumption of oxygen by aerobic organisms and results in the outgrowth of anaerobic organisms.

DIFFERENCES BETWEEN ANAEROBIC AND AEROBIC ORGANISMS

Anaerobic bacteria can be categorized as *obligate anaerobes* (killed in the presence of ≥0.5% oxygen), *aerotolerant organisms* (can tolerate the presence of oxygen but cannot use it for growth), and *facultative anaerobes* (can grow in the presence or absence of oxygen). Most clinically relevant anaerobes, such as *Bacteroides fragilis, Prevotella melaninogenica,* and *Fusobacterium nucleatum*, are relatively aerotolerant. These organisms contrast with *obligate aerobes*, which require high concentrations of oxygen for growth, and *microaerophilic organisms*, which are damaged by atmospheric concentrations of oxygen (~21%) but require low concentrations of oxygen (typically 2–10%) for growth. Given that molecular oxygen can reduce to superoxide (O_2^-) and hydrogen peroxide (H_2O_2), which are damaging to cells, the ability to tolerate the presence of oxygen is due, in part, to the expression of superoxide dismutase and catalase. The variation in anaerobic organisms tolerating anywhere from <0.5 to 8% O_2 may reflect the amount of these enzymes that is produced.

Furthermore, aerobic and anaerobic organisms differ in their energy metabolism. Cellular respiration requires establishment of an electrochemical gradient across the membrane, resulting in an electric potential (often related to a proton gradient) across the membrane. In aerobic respiration, electrons are shuttled through an electron transport chain, with oxygen as the final electron acceptor. Anaerobic organisms can metabolize energy by either anaerobic respiration or fermentation. Given that the final electron acceptor in anaerobic respiration (e.g., sulfate, nitrate, carbon dioxide, or fumarate) is not as highly oxidizing as oxygen, this pathway is less efficient than aerobic respiration and produces less ATP per glucose molecule. In contrast, fermentation does not use an electrochemical gradient. Rather, it releases energy from an organic molecule (e.g., pyruvate and its derivatives) via substrate-level phosphorylation and is therefore a less efficient process than either aerobic or anaerobic respiration; for comparison, fermentation results in ~5% of the energy released by aerobic respiration. For these reasons, facultative anaerobes will preferentially utilize oxygen if it is available; in oxygen-limiting situations, organisms will use anaerobic respiration rather than fermentative processes, if possible.

ANAEROBES OF THE HUMAN MICROBIOTA

Most human mucocutaneous surfaces harbor a rich indigenous normal microbiota composed of aerobic and anaerobic bacteria. These surfaces are dominated by anaerobic bacteria, which often account for 99.0–99.9% of the cultivable microbiota and range in concentration from 10^3/mL in the nose to 10^{12}/mL in gingival scrapings and the colon (**Table 177-1**). It is interesting that anaerobes inhabit many areas of the body that are exposed to air: skin, nose, mouth, and throat. Anaerobes are thought to reside in the portions of these sites that either are relatively well protected from oxygen (e.g., gingival crevices) or have a local anaerobic environment conferred by neighboring aerobic organisms (e.g., tooth surfaces). The ability to cultivate these organisms is improving, and—with strict attention to anaerobic conditions—more than 80% of the microscopic counts in fecal samples can be cultured. However, culture-independent approaches (e.g., sequencing of the 16S rDNA gene) show that the overwhelmingly diverse low-abundance bacterial species present in the microbiota remain uncultivated. Several projects, including the Human Microbiome Project (funded by the U.S. National Institutes of Health) and MetaHIT (financed by the European Commission), have characterized the normal microbiota of healthy individuals and have demonstrated the presence of >10,000 different bacterial species in the collective human microbiota. The human gut alone harbors >1000 bacterial species, with 100–200 species present in any given individual.

The major reservoir of anaerobic bacteria is the lower gastrointestinal tract, but these organisms are also present in considerable numbers in the oral cavity, skin, and female genital tract (Table 177-1). In the oral cavity, the ratio of anaerobic to aerobic bacteria ranges from 1:1 on the surface of a tooth to 1000:1 in the gingival crevices. *Prevotella* and *Porphyromonas* species make up much of the indigenous oral anaerobic microbiota. *Fusobacterium* and *Bacteroides* (non–*B. fragilis* group) species are present in lower numbers. Anaerobic bacteria are not found in appreciable numbers in the normal stomach and proximal small intestine. In the distal ileum, the microbiota begins to resemble that of the

TABLE 177-1 The Anaerobic Human Microbiota: An Overview

ANATOMIC SITE	TOTAL BACTERIA[a]	ANAEROBIC/AEROBIC RATIO	POTENTIAL PATHOGEN(S)
Nose	10^3–10^4	2:1	*Peptostreptococcus* spp., *Prevotella* spp.
Oral cavity			
Saliva	10^8–10^9	10:1	*Fusobacterium nucleatum, Prevotella melaninogenica, Prevotella oralis* group, *Bacteroides ureolyticus* group, *Peptostreptococcus* spp.
Tooth surface	10^{10}–10^{11}	1:1	
Gingival crevices	10^{11}–10^{12}	10^3:1	
Gastrointestinal tract			
Stomach	10^0–10^3	1:10	*Lactobacillus* spp.
Duodenum	10^1–10^5	1:1	*Lactobacillus* spp., *Streptococcus* spp.
Jejunum	10^3–10^6	1:1	*Streptococcus* spp., *Lactobacillus* spp., *Peptostreptococcus* spp.
Ileum	10^4–10^9	10:1	*Bacteroides* spp., *Streptococcus* spp., *Enterococcus* spp.
Cecum and colon	10^{11}–10^{12}	10^3:1	*Bacteroides* spp. (principally members of the *B. fragilis* group), *Prevotella* spp., *Clostridium* spp.
Female genital tract	10^7–10^9	10:1	*Peptostreptococcus* spp., *Bacteroides* spp., *Prevotella bivia*
Skin	10^4–10^6	100:1	*Cutibacterium acnes*

[a]Per gram or milliliter.

colon, where the ratio of anaerobes to aerobic species is high (~1000:1). The predominant anaerobes in the human intestine belong to the phyla Bacteroidetes and Firmicutes and include a number of *Prevotella* and *Bacteroides* species (e.g., members of the *B. fragilis* group, such as *B. fragilis, B. thetaiotaomicron, B. ovatus, B. vulgatus, B. uniformis*, and *Parabacteroides distasonis*) as well as various *Clostridium, Peptostreptococcus, Blautia*, and *Fusobacterium* species. In the female genital tract, there are ~10^9 organisms/mL of secretions, with an anaerobe-to-aerobe ratio of ~10:1. The predominant anaerobes in the female genital tract are *Prevotella, Bacteroides, Fusobacterium, Clostridium*, and the anaerobic *Lactobacillus* species. The skin microbiota contains anaerobes as well; *Cutibacterium acnes* (which was previously *Propionibacterium acnes* and will be considered as one of the *Propionibacterium* species for the remainder of this chapter) is the predominant species, and other species of propionibacteria and peptostreptococci are present in lower numbers.

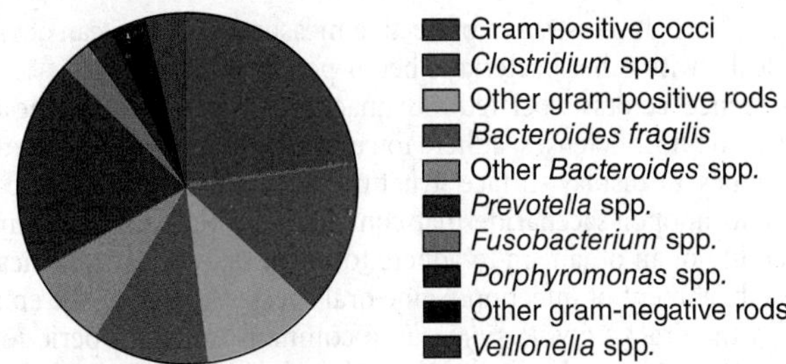

FIGURE 177-1 Distribution of anaerobic organisms isolated from clinical materials. *(Data combined from Y Park et al: Clinical features and prognostic factors of anaerobic infections: A 7-year retrospective study. Korean J Intern Med 24:13, 2009; and Japanese Association for Anaerobic Infections Research: Anaerobic infections (general): Epidemiology of anaerobic infections. J Infect Chemother 17[Suppl 1]:4, 2011.)*

ANAEROBES AND HUMAN HEALTH

Commensal anaerobes have been implicated as crucial mediators of physiologic, metabolic, and immunologic functions in the mammalian host. The intestinal microbiota is essential for fermenting dietary carbohydrates into forms that are more usable by the host, among which polysaccharides are the most abundant biological source of energy. Of the organisms found within the intestines, *Bacteroides* species express the widest array of polysaccharide-degrading enzymes, providing important nutrients for both the host and other commensal organisms. For example, *B. thetaiotaomicron* expresses 172 glycosyl hydrolases. The anaerobic intestinal microbiota is also responsible for the production of secreted products that promote human health (e.g., vitamin K and bile acids useful in fat absorption and cholesterol regulation).

One of the most important roles that anaerobes serve as components of the normal colonic microbiota is the promotion of resistance to colonization. The presence of commensal bacteria effectively interferes with colonization by potentially pathogenic bacterial species through the depletion of oxygen and nutrients, the production of enzymes and toxic end products, and the modulation of the host's intestinal innate immune response. For example, the normal intestinal microbiota plays an important role in protection against enteric infections, including those due to *Salmonella enterica* serotype Typhimurium and *Clostridium difficile*.

The anaerobic intestinal microbiota also has immunomodulatory properties that help regulate the immune system. The first example of this role was demonstrated with *B. fragilis*, which can balance the effector functions of T cells in the peripheral immune system and induce colonic regulatory T cells via expression of polysaccharide A (PSA). Moreover, *B. fragilis* expresses a glycosphingolipid that regulates the number of colonic invariant natural killer T cells. There are now numerous examples of commensal anaerobes that can modulate different aspects of the intestinal and extraintestinal immune system—everything from specific effector T cells to dendritic cells to antimicrobial peptides.

Clearly, the gut microbiota confers many benefits, and its dysregulation may play a role in the pathogenesis of diseases characterized by inflammation and aberrant immune responses, such as inflammatory bowel disease, rheumatoid arthritis, multiple sclerosis, asthma, and type 1 diabetes. Furthermore, the gut microbiota has been associated with obesity and metabolic syndrome. A more complete discussion of the intersection between the microbiota and human health is covered elsewhere (**Chap. 471**).

ETIOLOGY

There are >10,000 species of bacteria—the overwhelming majority of which are anaerobes—in the human microbiota, with each individual colonized by hundreds of species. Anaerobic infections occur when the harmonious relationship between the host and the host's microbiota is disrupted. Any site in the body is susceptible to infection with these indigenous organisms if they are introduced into otherwise sterile tissue, either through disruption of mucosal surfaces (e.g., intestinal perforation, ischemia, surgery) or via direct inoculation of organisms into tissue (e.g., bite wounds, trauma). Because the sites that are colonized by anaerobes contain many species of bacteria, the resulting infections are often polymicrobial, involving multiple species of anaerobes in combination with synergistically acting facultative and/or microaerophilic organisms.

Despite the complex array of bacteria in the normal microbiota, relatively few genera are isolated commonly from human infections (**Fig. 177-1**). While the specific organisms identified vary with the site and source of infection, the etiologic agents typically reflect the neighboring microbiota. For example, organisms normally found in the oro- and nasopharyngeal microbiota (e.g., *P. melaninogenica, Fusobacterium necrophorum, F. nucleatum, Peptostreptococcus* species, *Porphyromonas gingivalis, Porphyromonas asaccharolytica*, and *Actinomyces* species) can cause disease in contiguous areas, including odontogenic infections, peripharyngeal space infections, chronic sinusitis, and pleuropulmonary infections. In female genital tract infections, organisms normally colonizing the vagina (e.g., *Prevotella bivia* and *Prevotella disiens*) are the most common isolates. *Escherichia coli* and *B. fragilis*, both of which are components of the intestinal microbiota, are the most commonly identified isolates from intraabdominal abscesses. Indeed, the *B. fragilis* group, which encompasses 25 species and includes *B. thetaiotaomicron, B. vulgatus, B. uniformis*, and *B. ovatus*, contains the anaerobic organisms among the most frequently isolated from clinical infections.

It is useful to think about anaerobic infectious etiologies with regard not only to their anatomic location but also to their microbiologic features. While many anaerobic gram-negative bacilli cause disease (e.g., *Prevotella, Bacteroides, Fusobacterium*, and *Porphyromonas* species), *Veillonella* species, which are part of the oral and intestinal microbiota, are among the few anaerobic gram-negative cocci that have been implicated in human disease. Similarly, the peptostreptococci (e.g., *P. micros, P. asaccharolyticus*, and *P. anaerobius*) and *Finegoldia magnus* (which was previously *Peptostreptococcus magnus* and will be considered as part of the peptostreptococci for the remainder of this chapter) are the chief anaerobic gram-positive cocci that have pathogenic potential. *Clostridium* species are the primary anaerobic spore-forming gram-positive rods that produce human disease (**Chap. 154**). Uncommonly, anaerobic gram-positive non-spore-forming bacilli cause infection; *C. acnes*, a component of the skin microbiota and a cause of foreign-body infections, and *Actinomyces* species are relevant examples.

PATHOGENESIS

First and foremost, anaerobic infections require an anaerobic environment with a lowered oxidation-reduction potential. In some circumstances, this environment can occur directly—e.g., in tissue ischemia, trauma, surgery, or a perforated viscus. In many other situations, the infection is polymicrobial, and the facultative organisms maintain a lowered oxidation-reduction potential in the local microenvironment that allows for the propagation of obligate anaerobes. Once the proper anaerobic environment is established, the organisms must still contend with the host's immune defenses. Similar to aerobic organisms, anaerobes express an array of virulence factors that help evade host defenses, they can form abscesses as a protective measure, and they can act synergistically with other bacteria to better persist in the host.

Virulence factors associated with anaerobes typically confer the ability to evade host defenses, adhere to cell surfaces, produce toxins and/or enzymes, or display surface structures such as capsular polysaccharides and lipopolysaccharide that contribute to pathogenic potential. The ability of an organism to adhere to host tissues is often critical to the establishment of infection. Some oral species adhere to the epithelium in the oral cavity. *P. gingivalis*, a common isolate in periodontal disease, has fimbriae that facilitate attachment. In supragingival plaque, many oral anaerobes are able to attach directly to aerobic bacteria (e.g., *Streptococcus* species) that are adherent to the tooth's surface. *F. nucleatum* is a notable example of these secondary colonizers: it expresses receptors to which almost all oral bacteria can bind and serves as an important bridge between the primary colonizers and subsequent layers of bacteria. *B. fragilis* synthesizes pili, fimbriae, and hemagglutinins that aid in attachment to host cell surfaces in the intestine.

Anaerobic bacteria produce a number of exoproteins that can enhance the organisms' virulence. *P. gingivalis* produces a collagenase that enhances tissue destruction. Exotoxins produced by clostridial species, including botulinum toxins, tetanus toxin, *C. difficile* toxins A and B, and five toxins produced by *Clostridium perfringens*, are among the most virulent bacterial toxins in mouse lethality assays. Anaerobic gram-negative bacteria, such as *B. fragilis, P. gingivalis*, and *Prevotella intermedia*, possess lipid A molecules (endotoxins) that are 100–1000 times less biologically potent than endotoxins associated with aerobic gram-negative bacteria; these differences may relate to variations in acylation status, length of fatty acids, and number of phosphate groups. This relative biologic inactivity may account for the lower frequency of disseminated intravascular coagulation and purpura in anaerobic gram-negative bacteremia than in facultative and aerobic gram-negative bacillary bacteremia. An exception is the lipopolysaccharide from *Fusobacterium*, which may account for the severity of Lemierre syndrome (see "Complications of Anaerobic Head and Neck Infections," below).

The most extensively studied virulence factor of the nonsporulating anaerobes is the capsular polysaccharide complex of *B. fragilis*. This organism is unique among anaerobes in its potential for virulence during growth at normally sterile sites. Although it constitutes only 0.5–1% of the normal colonic microbiota, *B. fragilis* is the anaerobe most commonly isolated from intraabdominal infections and bacteremia. In an animal model of intraabdominal sepsis, the capsular polysaccharide was identified as the major virulence factor of *B. fragilis*; this polymer plays a specific, central role in the induction of abscesses. A series of detailed biologic and molecular studies of this virulence factor showed that *B. fragilis* produces at least eight distinct capsular polysaccharides, far more than the number reported for any other encapsulated bacterium. *B. fragilis* can exhibit distinct surface polysaccharides either alone or in combination by regulating the expression of these different capsules in an on–off manner through a reversible inversion of DNA segments within the promoters for operons containing the genes required for polysaccharide synthesis. Structural analysis of two of these polysaccharides, PSA and polysaccharide B (PSB), revealed that each polymer consists of repeating units with positively charged free amino groups and negatively charged groups. This structural feature is rare among bacterial polysaccharides, and the ability of PSA—and, to a lesser extent, PSB—to induce abscesses in animals depends on this zwitterionic charge motif. Intraabdominal abscess induction is related to the capacity of PSA to stimulate macrophages to release cytokines and chemokines—in particular, interleukin (IL) 8, IL-17, and tumor necrosis factor α (TNF-α)—from resident peritoneal cells through a Toll-like receptor 2–dependent mechanism. The release of cytokines and chemokines results in the chemotaxis of polymorphonuclear neutrophils (PMNs) into the peritoneum, where they adhere to mesothelial cells induced by TNF-α to upregulate their expression of intercellular adhesion molecule 1 (ICAM-1). PMNs adherent to ICAM-1-expressing cells probably represent the nidus for an abscess. PSA also activates T cells to produce certain cytokines, including IL-17 and interferon γ, that are necessary for abscess formation.

These virulence factors not only promote persistence of the anaerobe that produces them but also aid in the survival of bystander organisms and result in bacterial synergies. Clinically, these synergies are evidenced by the fact that anaerobic infections typically involve three to six different organisms. Examples of this synergistic pathogenesis include creation of a favorable environment for growth (e.g., establishment and maintenance of an anaerobic environment by facultative organisms), inhibition of host defenses (e.g., production of short-chain fatty acids and succinic acid that inhibit the ability of phagocytes to clear facultative organisms), provision of necessary growth factors for other organisms (e.g., oral diphtheroids that produce vitamin K, which is needed by *P. melaninogenica*), and creation of tissue damage that promotes spread of the infection. In these ways, facultative and obligate anaerobes synergistically potentiate abscess formation.

APPROACH TO THE PATIENT

Infections Due to Anaerobic Bacteria

The physician must consider several points when approaching the patient with a possible infection due to anaerobic bacteria.

1. The organisms colonizing mucosal sites are commensals, very few of which typically cause disease. When these organisms do cause disease, it often occurs in proximity to the mucosal site they colonize.
2. For anaerobes to cause tissue infection, they must spread beyond the normal mucosal barriers.
3. Conditions favoring the propagation of anaerobic bacteria, particularly a lowered oxidation-reduction potential, are necessary. These conditions exist at sites of trauma, tissue destruction, compromised vascular supply, and necrosis.
4. Frequently, a complex array of infecting microbes can be found, occasionally with >10 different species isolated from a suppurative site.
5. Anaerobic organisms tend to be found in abscess cavities or in necrotic tissue. The failure of an abscess to yield organisms on routine culture is a clue that the abscess is likely to contain anaerobic bacteria. Often smears of this "sterile pus" are found to be teeming with bacteria when Gram's stain is applied. Although some facultative organisms (e.g., *Staphylococcus aureus*) are also capable of causing abscesses, abscesses in organs or deeper body tissues should call anaerobic infection to mind.
6. Gas is found in many anaerobic infections of deep tissues but is not diagnostic because it can be produced by aerobic bacteria as well.
7. Although a putrid-smelling infection site or discharge is considered diagnostic for anaerobic infection, this manifestation usually develops late in the course and is present in only 30–50% of cases.
8. Some species (the best example being the *B. fragilis* group) require specific therapy. However, many synergistic infections can be cured with antibiotics directed at some but not all of the organisms involved. Antibiotic therapy, combined with debridement and drainage, disrupts the interdependent relationship among the bacteria, and some species that are resistant to the antibiotic do not survive without the co-infecting organisms.
9. Manifestations of severe sepsis and disseminated intravascular coagulation are unusual in patients with purely anaerobic infection.

EPIDEMIOLOGY

Difficulties in the performance of appropriate cultures, contamination of cultures by components of the normal microbiota, and the lack of readily available, reliable culture techniques have made it challenging to obtain accurate data on the incidence or prevalence of anaerobic infections. However, anaerobic infections are encountered frequently, with anaerobes comprising 7–8% and 13–15% of bacteria isolated from inpatients and outpatients, respectively. Bacteremia and soft

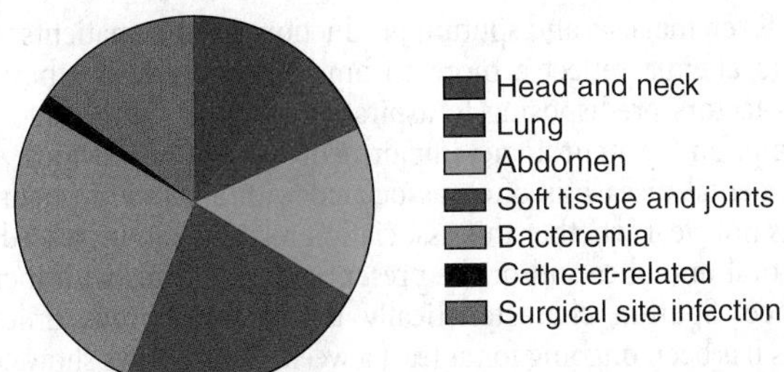

FIGURE 177-2 Distribution of types of infection from which anaerobic organisms were cultured at a single hospital over a 7-year period. Head and neck infections included sinusitis, otitis media, and retropharyngeal abscess; abdominal infections included liver abscess, biliary tract infection, bowel obstruction, and intraabdominal abscess; catheter-related infections included those related to peritoneal dialysis catheters and ventriculoperitoneal shunts. *(Data from Y Park et al: Clinical features and prognostic factors of anaerobic infections: A 7-year retrospective study. Korean J Intern Med 24:13, 2009.)*

tissue infections are the most common types of anaerobic infection (**Fig. 177-2**). Typically, anaerobic bacteria account for <1% of all cases of bacteremia.

CLINICAL MANIFESTATIONS

Although anaerobes can cause infection anywhere in the body, certain clinical findings and characteristics are commonly found. These include abscess formation, putrid purulence (due to volatile fatty acid by-products), septic thrombophlebitis, tissue necrosis, and failure to respond clinically to broad-spectrum antibiotics that lack activity against anaerobes.

Anaerobic Infections of the Mouth, Head, and Neck

Anaerobic bacteria are commonly involved in infections of the mouth, head, and neck (**Chap. 35**). The predominant isolates are components of the normal microbiota of the upper airways—mainly *Prevotella* species, *P. asaccharolytica*, *Fusobacterium* species, peptostreptococci, and microaerophilic streptococci.

OROFACIAL INFECTIONS The most common oral infections are odontogenic and include dental caries and periodontal disease (gingivitis and periodontitis). While dental caries usually manifest with pain, sensitivity, and discoloration of the tooth, periodontal disease involves inflammation of the gums and underlying tissue. In its more severe forms, periodontitis can result in difficulty chewing, loose teeth, and occasionally tooth loss. Severe orofacial infections typically develop as a consequence of dental infection, and the infection can spread from the tooth to different anatomic areas that provide the least resistance, resulting in periapical, periodontal, or pericoronal infections. If the dental surface is completely breached, an endodontic infection (pulpitis) can occur. In late stages of pulpitis, the tooth is generally very sensitive to heat, but cold stimuli may provide relief. Left untreated, pulpitis can progress to invade the alveolar bone and develop into a periapical abscess. The abscesses, particularly those involving the second and third molars, can occasionally extend into the submandibular, sublingual, and submental spaces (*Ludwig's angina*). This infection results in marked local swelling of tissues, with pain, trismus, and superior and posterior displacement of the tongue. Submandibular swelling of the neck and obstruction by the tongue can impair swallowing and cause respiratory obstruction. In some cases, tracheotomy is lifesaving.

Microbiologically, dental caries begin with the binding of *Streptococcus mutans* and *Streptococcus sanguis* to the tooth surface, with subsequent further colonization by anaerobes. In contrast, periodontitis is typically associated with *P. gingivalis*, *Tannerella forsythensis*, *Aggregatibacter actinomycetemcomitans*, and *Treponema denticola*. *Fusobacterium*, *Actinomyces*, *Peptostreptococcus*, and *Bacteroides* species (other than *B. fragilis*) are the organisms most commonly isolated from periapical abscesses.

ACUTE NECROTIZING ULCERATIVE GINGIVITIS Gingivitis may become a necrotizing infection (*trench mouth*, *Vincent's stomatitis*). The onset of disease is usually sudden and is associated with painful bleeding gums, foul breath, and a bad taste. The gingival mucosa, especially the papillae between the teeth, becomes ulcerated and may be covered by a yellowish-white or gray "pseudomembrane," which is removable with gentle pressure. Patients may become systemically ill, developing fever, malaise, cervical lymphadenopathy, and leukocytosis. The infection can sometimes extend into the pharynx, resulting in an extremely sore throat, foul breath, and tonsillar pillars that are swollen, red, ulcerated, and covered by a pseudomembrane. *Prevotella*, *Treponema*, and *Fusobacterium* species have been implicated.

In some cases, acute necrotizing gingivitis can rapidly progress to noma (*cancrum oris*), a gangrenous infection that destroys the soft and hard tissues related to the oral cavity. Noma occurs most frequently in young children (1–4 years of age) who have immune dysfunction related to malnutrition and endemic infections (particularly measles). This infection occurs worldwide but is most common in sub-Saharan Africa, where the incidence is 1–7 cases per 1000 children. Although the pathogenesis is not fully understood, infections with *F. necrophorum* and *P. intermedia* are thought to be key drivers of this disease. Without treatment, the mortality rate is 70–90%.

PERIPHARYNGEAL SPACE INFECTIONS These infections arise from the spread of organisms from the upper airways to potential spaces formed by the fascial planes of the head and neck. The etiology is typically polymicrobial and represents the normal microbiota of the mucosa of the originating site.

Peritonsillar abscess (*quinsy*) is the most common peripharyngeal infection and occurs as a complication of acute tonsillitis. Consistent with its association with tonsillitis, adolescents are most commonly affected. Patients present with a sore throat, dysphagia, peritonsillar swelling, muffled voice, and uvular deviation to the contralateral side. The abscess material typically grows group A *Streptococcus* in conjunction with obligate anaerobes (e.g., *Bacteroides*, *Prevotella*, and *Peptostreptococcus* species) (**Chap. 35**). Retropharyngeal abscesses typically occur in children 2–4 years of age, although they can occur at any age. Although a suppurative infection of the retropharyngeal lymph nodes is the usual precursor to these abscesses in children, foreign-body ingestion and/or local trauma is more commonly the inciting factor in adults. The clinical presentation shares many features with peritonsillar abscesses, but difficulty extending the neck and torticollis are more common with retropharyngeal abscesses. The etiologic agents are the same as in peritonsillar abscesses, with additional aerobic organisms (e.g., *S. aureus*, viridans streptococci) also playing a role.

SINUSITIS AND OTITIS Anaerobic bacteria have been implicated in chronic sinusitis but play little role in acute sinusitis. Numerous studies related to the microbiology of chronic sinusitis have been conducted; on average, anaerobic bacteria have been found in two-thirds of patients, with many studies demonstrating their presence in >90% of patients. Anaerobic bacteria represent ~40% of all bacteria cultured, with *Peptostreptococcus*, *Prevotella*, and *Porphyromonas* species the most commonly isolated anaerobes. *S. aureus* and Enterobacteriaceae are the aerobes most commonly recovered in chronic sinusitis. Anaerobic bacteria have been isolated in ~60% of cases of chronic suppurative otitis media in children, but they are not involved in acute otitis media.

COMPLICATIONS OF ANAEROBIC HEAD AND NECK INFECTIONS Direct extension of these infections into contiguous areas can result in additional disease manifestations. Cranial spread of these infections can result in osteomyelitis of the skull or mandible or in intracranial infections, such as brain abscess and subdural empyema. Caudal spread can produce mediastinitis or pleuropulmonary infection. Hematogenous complications can also result from anaerobic infections of the head and neck. Bacteremia, which occasionally is polymicrobial, can lead to endocarditis or other distant infections. Lemierre's syndrome (**Chap. 35**), which is usually due to *F. necrophorum*, is an acute oropharyngeal infection with secondary septic thrombophlebitis of the internal jugular vein and frequent septic emboli, most commonly to the lung. This infection typically begins with pharyngitis, which is followed by local invasion in the lateral pharyngeal space, with resultant internal jugular vein thrombophlebitis.

Central Nervous System (CNS) Infections CNS infections associated with anaerobic bacteria are brain abscess, epidural abscess, and subdural empyema, in which anaerobes are recovered in up to 30, 20, and 10% of cases, respectively. The frequency with which anaerobes are recovered depends in large part on the underlying reason for the infection. For example, brain abscesses are typically due to hematogenous seeding, contiguous spread, penetrating head trauma, or recent surgical intervention. Anaerobic bacteria are most commonly associated with brain abscesses resulting from contiguous spread (related to otogenic, odontogenic, and sinus infections), and the pathogens recovered are the same as in these antecedent infections. Facultative or microaerophilic streptococci and coliforms are often part of a mixed infecting flora in brain abscesses. The location of the abscess may also provide insight into the pathogens. Abscesses in the frontal lobe (often associated with sinusitis) are due to anaerobes, streptococci, and staphylococci; temporal lobe and cerebellar abscesses are often related to the oral microbiota and middle-ear pathogens.

Obligate anaerobes rarely cause meningitis. Only one obligate anaerobe was identified in a seminal study of 188 bacterial meningitis isolates, and a U.S. national surveillance study of 18,642 such isolates collected between 1977 and 1981 found only five obligate anaerobes. This low incidence may be due, in part, to the fact that many clinical microbiology laboratories do not routinely culture cerebrospinal fluid (CSF) for anaerobes.

Pleuropulmonary Infections The lungs are constantly seeded with organisms from the oral microbiota via subclinical microaspiration that normally occurs in all people. Even though the lung is the site of oxygen exchange and is therefore an overwhelmingly aerobic environment, the organisms most abundant in the lower respiratory tract (as assessed by culture-independent methods) include anaerobes such as *Prevotella* and *Veillonella* species, with oral microaerophilic streptococcal species (e.g., the *Streptococcus milleri* group) also present in significant abundances. In patients who have impaired bacterial clearance (due to decreased cough, dysfunctional mucociliary transport, or alcohol intoxication) and/or increased rates of aspiration (due to neurologic disorders, impaired consciousness, or swallowing dysfunction), these anaerobic bacteria can establish an infection and result in aspiration pneumonia, lung abscess, or empyema. These anaerobic infections have an indolent course that may serve as a clinical clue differentiating them from conditions with other etiologies (e.g., chemical pneumonitis, pneumococcal pneumonia) that often present more acutely.

ASPIRATION PNEUMONIA Bacterial aspiration pneumonia must be distinguished from two other clinical syndromes associated with aspiration that are not of bacterial etiology. One syndrome results from aspiration of food or, rarely, other foreign bodies. Obstruction of major airways typically results in difficulty breathing, atelectasis, and moderate nonspecific inflammation. Therapy consists of removal of the foreign body. The second aspiration syndrome relates to chemical pneumonitis caused by inhalation or aspiration of alveolar irritants. Perhaps the most common cause of chemical pneumonitis is *Mendelson syndrome*, which results from regurgitation and aspiration of acidic gastric juices. Pulmonary inflammation—including the destruction of the alveolar lining, with transudation of fluid into the alveolar space—occurs with remarkable rapidity. This syndrome typically develops within 4–6 h, often following anesthesia when the gag reflex is depressed. The patient becomes tachypneic, tachycardic, and hypoxic, often in the absence of fever. The leukocyte count may rise, and the chest x-ray may evolve from normal to a complete bilateral "whiteout" within 8–24 h. Sputum production is minimal. The pulmonary signs and symptoms often resolve quickly with symptom-based therapy, but this condition can culminate in respiratory failure due, in part, to pulmonary edema. Antibiotic therapy is not indicated unless bacterial superinfection occurs.

In contrast to these syndromes, bacterial aspiration pneumonia develops over a period of several days or weeks rather than hours. The pathogenesis includes some combination of an increased bacterial burden, increased virulence of the organisms aspirated, and potential airway damage related to aspiration of gastric fluid. Patients generally report fever, malaise, and sputum production. In some patients, weight loss and anemia reflect a more chronic process. Usually the history reveals factors predisposing to aspiration, such as significant alcohol consumption or neurologic impairment due to a previous stroke. Severe dental disease is often associated with aspiration pneumonia, but it is not clear whether this association relates to an increased number of oral microbes and/or the presence of organisms with increased virulence. Sputum characteristically is not malodorous unless the process has been ongoing for at least a week. Chest x-rays show consolidation in dependent pulmonary segments: in the basilar segments of the lower lobes if the patient has aspirated while upright and in either the posterior segment of the upper lobe (usually on the right side, given that the right mainstem bronchus has a more vertical orientation) or the superior segment of the lower lobe if the patient has aspirated while supine.

A mixed bacterial population with many PMNs is evident on Gram's staining of sputum. Expectorated sputum is unreliable for anaerobic cultures because of inevitable contamination by the normal oral microbiota. Reliable specimens for culture can be obtained by transtracheal or transthoracic aspiration—techniques that are rarely used at present. Although the culture of protected-brush specimens or bronchoalveolar lavage fluid obtained by bronchoscopy is controversial, more recent data suggest that these approaches can be used without oropharyngeal contamination and can recover anaerobic organisms from the lower respiratory tract in a site-directed manner. Further research is needed to determine how these approaches compare with the previous gold standards.

ANAEROBIC LUNG ABSCESSES (See also Chap. 127) These abscesses result from subacute anaerobic pulmonary infection. The clinical presentation typically involves a history of constitutional signs and symptoms (including malaise, weight loss, fever, night sweats, and foul-smelling sputum) that have typically persisted for 1–3 weeks prior to hospitalization. Patients who develop lung abscesses often, but not always, have an antecedent dental infection. Abscess cavities may be single or multiple and generally occur in dependent pulmonary segments (**Fig. 177-3**). The differential diagnosis for lung abscesses includes pneumonia (including necrotizing pneumonia), a purulent pleural effusion with a bronchopleural fistula, and a pneumatocele. Of note, infection with some aerobic organisms, particularly *S. aureus*, can develop into a lung abscess without an anaerobic component. Approximately 90% of cases have an anaerobe identified—usually three to six isolates per sample—if careful attention is paid to handling and processing of the abscess sample. The most common isolates include peptostreptococci, *Prevotella* and *Porphyromonas* species, and *F. nucleatum*. An important finding is that ~90% of cultures also demonstrate the presence of aerobic organisms, such as *S. aureus*, *Streptococcus pneumoniae*, and *Klebsiella pneumoniae*. Consistent with the notion that anaerobes are contributing to disease, patients often do not improve clinically until they receive an antibiotic regimen that includes anaerobic coverage.

EMPYEMA Empyema is a manifestation of long-standing anaerobic pulmonary infection and manifests with thick, purulent material in the pleural space, often in association with a bronchopleural fistula. Alternatively, a subdiaphragmatic infection may extend into the pleural space and similarly result in an empyema. The clinical presentation resembles that of other anaerobic pulmonary infections and may include foul-smelling sputum, pleuritic chest pain, and marked chest-wall tenderness. This disease process must be differentiated from a parapneumonic effusion resulting from more routine causes of pneumonia (e.g., *S. pneumoniae*). In the latter instance, the fluid is a thin exudate that has a mean white blood cell (WBC) count of ~5000 cells/mL, a lactate dehydrogenase level of >200 IU/L, and a pH of ~7.4. In contrast, empyema is characterized by foul-smelling thick pus with a mean WBC count of ~55,000 cells/mL, a lactate dehydrogenase level of >1000 IU/L, and a pH of <7.2 as well as loculations and a thick pleural peel on imaging. Drainage and occasionally decortication of the visceral and parietal pleura are required. Defervescence, a return to a feeling of well-being, and resolution of the process may require several months, particularly in the absence of surgical intervention.

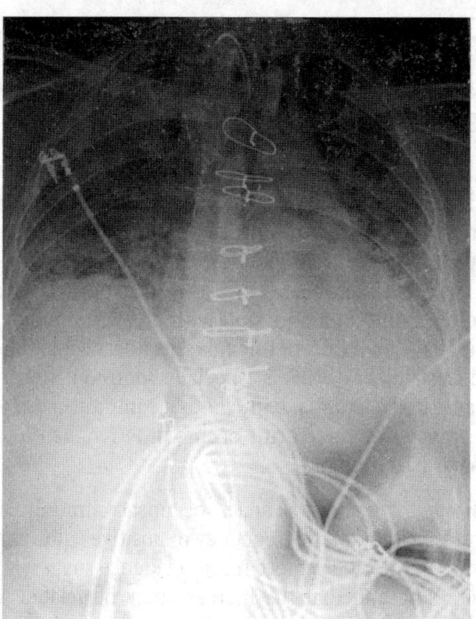
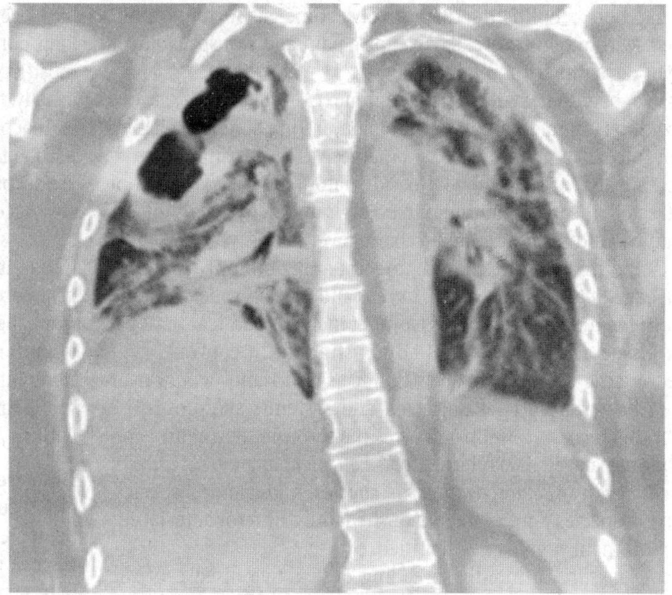

FIGURE 177-3 Chest radiograph (*left*) and CT image (*right*) of a lung abscess. The patient aspirated while supine and developed an abscess in the posterior segment of the right upper lobe. Cultures were pretreated and grew only *Klebsiella pneumoniae*. *(Images provided by Gita N. Mody, MD, MPH, Division of Cardiothoracic Surgery, Department of Surgery, The University of North Carolina at Chapel Hill.)*

Intraabdominal Infections Breach of the gut mucosal surface (e.g., due to trauma, intestinal perforation, or malignancy) allows members of the microbiota to enter the normally sterile peritoneum. Accordingly, the offending organisms reflect the microbiota in the affected intestinal region. For example, recovery of *Candida* species from intraabdominal infections should prompt evaluation of the stomach and proximal small bowel for potential perforation. Furthermore, a study of patients with perforated and gangrenous appendicitis demonstrated that virtually all samples yielded *E. coli* and members of the *B. fragilis* group; peptostreptococci and *Bilophila wadsworthia*—additional components of the appendiceal and colonic microbiota—were also recovered from >50% of samples. Notably, some studies have identified an average of 10 different bacterial species, with an anaerobe-to-aerobe ratio of ~3:1. Given that >1000 bacterial species are present in the colonic microbiota, the dominance of such a limited repertoire of bacterial genera and species recovered in intraabdominal infections reflects a combination of two factors: the increased propensity of these organisms to result in intraabdominal abscesses and the difficulty faced by clinical microbiology laboratories in culturing the diverse organisms present in these samples. **See Chap. 132 for a complete discussion of intraabdominal infections.**

Neutropenic enterocolitis (typhlitis) involves marked thickening of the bowel wall (typically >4 mm) in the setting of neutropenia, abdominal pain, and fever. This condition most commonly affects the cecum and may extend to the neighboring terminal ileum and/or proximal colon, but any intestinal region may be involved. Typhlitis generally occurs after 1–2 weeks of chemotherapy-induced neutropenia associated with treatment of hematologic or, less commonly, solid tumor malignancies, but it can occur regardless of the cause of neutropenia. At least 5% of adults hospitalized for malignancy are thought to develop typhlitis, but this is likely an underestimate. Although the right lower quadrant is the most common location of abdominal pain and tenderness, these symptoms are absent in nearly half of cases; moreover, some patients, particularly those taking glucocorticoids, may not experience abdominal pain at all. Given the weakened integrity of the bowel wall and the associated neutropenia, patients often develop bacteremia due to one or more organisms related to the microbiota of the affected intestinal segment. Patients who develop bacteremia due to *Clostridium septicum* often have relatively severe disease, and identification of this organism is highly associated with the presence of malignancy—notably, colon cancer. Medical management including bowel rest, intestinal decompression, and broad-spectrum antibiotic administration is generally successful, although surgical intervention may be required in cases of persistent intestinal bleeding, necrotic bowel, or clinical deterioration suggestive of an ongoing intestinal process.

Pelvic Infections Anaerobes are frequently encountered in pelvic inflammatory disease, pelvic abscess, endometritis, tubo-ovarian abscess, septic abortion, and postoperative or postpartum infections. These infections are often of mixed etiology, involving both anaerobes and coliforms; pure anaerobic infections without coliform or other facultative bacterial species occur more often in pelvic than in intraabdominal sites. The major anaerobic pathogens in pelvic abscesses are *P. bivia*, *P. disiens*, and the *B. fragilis* group, but many other anaerobes have also been implicated. **See Chap. 136 for a complete discussion of pelvic inflammatory disease.**

Anaerobic bacteria have been thought to be contributing factors in bacterial vaginosis. This syndrome of unknown etiology is characterized by a profuse malodorous discharge and a change in bacterial ecology that results in replacement of the *Lactobacillus*-dominated normal microbiota with an overgrowth of anaerobic bacterial species. Culture-based and culture-independent approaches have identified numerous organisms, including *Gardnerella vaginalis*, peptostreptococci, genital mycoplasmas, and species within the genera *Prevotella*, *Mobiluncus*, *Atopobium*, *Leptotrichia*, *Megasphaera*, and *Eggerthella*. This wide array of implicated bacteria may reflect differences in the overall disease spectrum of bacterial vaginosis and/or a shared physiologic response to these different organisms.

Skin and Soft Tissue Infections Similar to other anatomic sites, skin or soft tissue injured by trauma, ischemia, or surgery creates a suitable environment for anaerobic infections. The infecting bacteria either are introduced directly (e.g., wounds associated with intestinal surgery, decubitus ulcers, or human bites) or originate in contiguous areas (e.g., cutaneous abscesses, rectal abscesses, and axillary sweat gland infections [*hidradenitis suppurativa*]). Anaerobes also are often cultured from foot ulcers of diabetic patients. The most common locations for anaerobic cellulitis include the neck, trunk, groin (including the genitalia), and legs. The deep soft tissue infections associated with anaerobic bacteria are gas gangrene, synergistic cellulitis (both progressive and necrotizing), necrotizing fasciitis, and myositis **(Chaps. 129 and 154)**.

Gas gangrene (crepitus cellulitis) is most often due to *C. perfringens*, although other clostridial species have been implicated as well. This infection involves extensive gas formation in the tissue leading to crepitus and a thin, dark, occasionally malodorous discharge. True gas gangrene typically presents with fever and tenderness around the lesion and can rapidly spread; in contrast, there are somewhat more indolent forms of anaerobic cellulitis that may involve some gas formation but often present without fever or extensive local pain and can spread over the course of days rather than minutes.

Progressive bacterial synergistic gangrene (*Meleney gangrene*) is characterized by an area of exquisite pain, redness, and swelling followed by ulceration. As the ulcer enlarges, it is surrounded by a violaceous ring that fades into a pink edematous border. If it is not promptly treated, the ulcer continues to enlarge, and new, distant ulcers may emerge. Symptoms are limited to pain; fever is not typical. Peptostreptococci and microaerophilic streptococci are commonly found in the leading edge of the lesions, and *S. aureus* and *Proteus* species can be isolated from the ulcerated lesion. Treatment includes surgical removal of necrotic tissue and antimicrobial administration. In contrast, synergistic necrotizing cellulitis involves the deep fascia and occurs near the point of bacterial entry. Pain, fever, and systemic symptoms are common. If this form of cellulitis involves the scrotum, perineum, and anterior abdominal wall, it is referred to as *Fournier gangrene*. *S. aureus*, the *B. fragilis* group, *Peptostreptococcus* species, *Clostridium* species, *Fusobacterium* species, and members of the family Enterobacteriaceae are the predominant organisms identified.

Necrotizing fasciitis, a rapidly spreading destructive disease of the fascia, is usually attributed to group A streptococci (**Chap. 148**) but can also be a mixed infection involving anaerobes and aerobes. Polymicrobial necrotizing fasciitis differs from stereotypical group A streptococcal necrotizing fasciitis in that the initial erythematous, swollen, tender lesions progress over 3–5 days (as opposed to 1–3 days), with consequent skin breakdown and cutaneous gangrene. Fever, subcutaneous gas, development of anesthesia (often before skin necrosis), and a foul-smelling discharge are common. The particular clinical findings sometimes suggest the causative agent: regional lymphadenopathy suggests the *B. fragilis* group; necrosis and gangrene suggest *Clostridium* species, peptostreptococci, the *B. fragilis* group, and Enterobacteriaceae; bullous lesions suggest Enterobacteriaceae; a foul-smelling odor suggests *Bacteroides* and *Clostridium* species; and subcutaneous gas suggests peptostreptococci, *Clostridium* species, and the *B. fragilis* group. Moreover, diabetic infections are often associated with *Bacteroides* species, Enterobacteriaceae, and *S. aureus*, and infections related to trauma are associated with *Clostridium* species.

Although *S. aureus* is the typical cause of myositis, anaerobes—particularly *C. perfringens*—are often recovered from patients with pyogenic myositis. In anaerobic streptococcal myonecrosis, peptostreptococci are often identified along with group A streptococci or *S. aureus*. Patients typically present with fever, muscle pain, fatigue, and an elevated creatinine kinase level suggestive of muscle inflammation.

Bone and Joint Infections A comprehensive review of the world literature on anaerobic bone infections included >650 cases. Of these, ~400 cases were caused by *Actinomyces* species; anaerobic cocci and *Bacteroides*, *Fusobacterium*, and *Clostridium* species were most commonly identified in the remaining cases. Actinomycotic involvement of the jaw was the most common bone infection, with the mandible involved four times as frequently as the maxilla. Patients with cervicofacial actinomycosis (**Chap. 175**) are often described as having a "lumpy jaw" because of the prominent soft tissue swelling that is sometimes mistaken for malignancy or granulomatous disease. These infections can be chronic in nature, can include the development of sinus tracts, can progress across normal tissue boundaries, and can require prolonged antibiotic treatment to prevent relapse. The vertebrae are the second most common location for *Actinomyces* infection; involvement of the thorax, abdomen, or pelvis is much less frequent.

Osteomyelitis involving anaerobes other than *Actinomyces* species most commonly develops by extension of an adjacent infection (e.g., soft tissue, paranasal sinus, or middle-ear infection). For example, diabetic foot ulcers and decubitus ulcers may be complicated by mixed aerobic–anaerobic osteomyelitis (**Chap. 131**). Hematogenous seeding of bone by anaerobes is uncommon and is thought to occur in fewer than 10% of cases. The most common sites of anaerobic osteomyelitis are the head (skull and jaw) and the extremities. Fusobacteria have been isolated in pure culture from infections of the mastoid, mandible, and maxilla. *Clostridium* species have been reported as anaerobic pathogens in cases of osteomyelitis of the long bones following trauma. Anaerobic and microaerophilic cocci are most frequently isolated from infections involving the skull or mastoid; usually, these organisms are present in mixed cultures.

In contrast to anaerobic osteomyelitis, anaerobic arthritis (**Chap. 130**) is uncommon, typically involving a single isolate, and most cases are secondary to hematogenous spread. Although *Fusobacterium* species accounted for nearly one-third of cases in the preantibiotic era, *C. acnes*, peptostreptococci, and *B. fragilis* are now among the more frequent causes of anaerobic septic arthritis. Peptostreptococci and *C. acnes* are often found in association with prosthetic joints, *Fusobacterium* species have a predilection for the sternoclavicular and sacroiliac joints, and clostridial arthritis is especially common after trauma. As a frequent cause of bacteremia, *B. fragilis* is a common cause of anaerobic septic arthritis; however, arthritis occurs in fewer than 5% of patients with *B. fragilis* bacteremia.

Bacteremia *B. fragilis* is the anaerobe most commonly isolated from blood cultures. Although the frequency of positive cultures appeared to be decreasing in the 1980s, more recent evidence suggests that the rate is now increasing and that the increase may be related to changing demographics, with more patients who are elderly, immunocompromised, and/or receiving medications that may disrupt the mucosal barrier (e.g., chemotherapy). The source of bacteremia is most often an abscess in the abdomen, female genital tract, or soft tissue. At a large tertiary-care U.S. hospital, 0.8% of all positive blood cultures yielded an anaerobic gram-negative bacillus, with 0.5% yielding *B. fragilis*. A similar study in France revealed that 0.6% of all positive blood cultures yielded an anaerobic organism; 60% of these isolates were *Bacteroides* species, and 22% were *Clostridium* species. *Peptostreptococcus* and *Fusobacterium* species are also recovered with significant frequency.

Once the organism in the blood has been identified, both the portal of bloodstream entry and the underlying problem that probably led to seeding of the bloodstream can often be deduced from an understanding of the organism's normal site of residence. For example, mixed anaerobic bacteremia including *B. fragilis* usually implies a colonic pathology, with mucosal disruption from neoplasia, diverticulitis, or some other inflammatory lesion. The initial manifestations are determined by the portal of entry and reflect the localized condition. Although the clinical manifestations of *B. fragilis* bacteremia (e.g., rigors, hectic fevers) are similar to those of aerobic gram-negative bacillary bacteremia, the incidence of septic shock is lower with *B. fragilis*. This difference may be due to differences in the immunostimulatory effects of the different endotoxin structures.

In virtually all cases, isolation of a member of the *B. fragilis* group from blood indicates underlying infection that is associated with a mortality rate of 60% if untreated. It has been suggested that the mortality rate depends in part on the species recovered (*B. thetaiotaomicron* > *P. distasonis* > *B. fragilis*), but it is unclear whether differences in mortality rates relate to intrinsic differences in the virulence of these organisms, in their antimicrobial susceptibility profiles, and/or in the host's immune response. Case–fatality rates appear to increase with the increasing age of the patient (with reported rates of >66% among patients >60 years old), with the isolation of multiple species from the bloodstream, and with the failure to surgically remove a focus of infection.

Endocarditis (**See also Chap. 128**) Although gram-negative anaerobic bacteria only rarely cause endocarditis, their involvement is associated with significant mortality rates (21–43%). Members of the *B. fragilis* group are the most commonly identified gram-negative anaerobes in endocarditis. Anaerobic streptococci, which are often classified incorrectly, are likely responsible for this disease more frequently than is generally appreciated. Compared to aerobic bacterial endocarditis, endocarditis due to *Bacteroides* species is less likely to be associated with a history of cardiovascular disease and more likely to involve thromboembolic complications.

DIAGNOSIS

There are three critical steps in the diagnosis of anaerobic infection: (1) proper collection of specimens; (2) rapid transport of the specimens to the microbiology laboratory, preferably in anaerobic transport media; and (3) proper handling of the specimens by the laboratory. Specimens must be collected by meticulous sampling of infected sites, with avoidance of contamination by the normal microbiota. Samples from sites known to harbor numerous anaerobes (e.g., the mouth, nose, vagina, feces) are not acceptable for anaerobic culture as the presence of the normal microbiota will complicate interpretation of the results in a clinically meaningful manner. In contrast, samples from normally sterile locations (e.g., blood, pleural fluid, peritoneal fluid, CSF, and aspirates or biopsy samples from normally sterile sites) are appropriate for anaerobic culture in clinical microbiology laboratories. As a general rule, liquid or tissue specimens are preferred; if swab specimens must be used, special anaerobic swab systems should be used to help maintain persistence of anaerobes. Liquid samples should be collected in an air-free syringe that is then capped, injected into anaerobic transport bottles, or quickly transported to the clinical microbiology laboratory for immediate culture.

Because of the time and difficulty involved in the isolation of anaerobic bacteria, the diagnosis of anaerobic infections must frequently be based on presumptive evidence. As mentioned previously, anaerobic infections are sometimes suggested by specific clinical factors, such as origins from a site with an anaerobic-rich microbiota (e.g., the intestinal tract, oropharynx), the presence of an abscess, involvement of sites with lowered oxidation-reduction potential (e.g., avascular necrotic tissues), a foul odor, and the presence of gas in tissues. None of these features is necessarily pathognomonic or required for the diagnosis of an anaerobic infection, but these are helpful clues to keep in mind when constructing a differential diagnosis.

When cultures of obviously infected sites or purulent material yield no growth, streptococci only, or a single aerobic species (such as *E. coli*) and Gram's staining reveals a mixed bacterial population, the involvement of anaerobes should be suspected; the implication is that the anaerobic microorganisms have failed to grow because of inadequate transport and/or culture techniques. It is also important to remember that prior antibiotic therapy reduces the cultivability of these bacteria. Failure of an infection to respond to antibiotics that are not active against anaerobes (e.g., aminoglycosides and—in some circumstances—penicillin, cephalosporins, or tetracyclines) suggests an anaerobic etiology.

TREATMENT

Anaerobic Infections

Similar to successful therapy for other types of infection, treatment for anaerobic infections requires the administration of appropriate antibiotics, surgical debridement of devitalized tissues, and drainage of any large abscess. Any mucosal breach must be closed promptly to prevent ongoing infection.

ANTIBIOTIC THERAPY AND RESISTANCE

The antibiotics used to treat anaerobic infections should be active against both aerobic and anaerobic organisms because many of these infections are of mixed etiology. Antibiotic regimens can usually be selected empirically on the basis of the location of infection (which provides insight into the likely species involved), the severity of infection, and knowledge of local antimicrobial resistance patterns. Other factors influencing the selection of antibiotics include need for penetration into certain organs (such as the brain) and associated toxicity (**Chap. 144**). As with all infections, the general maxim is to use the least broad-spectrum agent(s) possible so as to minimize the impact on the normal microbiota and the development of resistance.

Because of the slow growth rate of many anaerobes, the lack of standardized testing methods and of clinically relevant standards for resistance, and the generally good results obtained with empirical therapy, the role of antibiotic susceptibility testing of these organisms has been limited in most clinical microbiology laboratories. Instead, isolates are sent to reference laboratories for susceptibility testing when an infection is serious (e.g., brain abscess, meningitis, joint infection), is refractory, or requires prolonged therapy (e.g., osteomyelitis, prosthetic joint infection, endocarditis). Such testing should also be considered when a patient is not responding to antimicrobial therapy as expected; multidrug-resistant anaerobes have been reported. Antimicrobial susceptibility testing is also helpful in monitoring the activity of new drugs and recording current resistance patterns among anaerobic pathogens.

The need for susceptibility testing of anaerobic organisms is highlighted by increasing rates of antimicrobial resistance, geographic and institutional differences in susceptibility profiles, species-specific antibiograms, and the potential for worse clinical outcomes when ineffective antibiotics are used. These differences preclude making any sweeping generalizations regarding antibiotic therapy for anaerobic infections. For example, rates of resistance to piperacillin-tazobactam have remained low (≤1%) for all *Bacteroides* species in the United States, but *B. thetaiotaomicron* isolates in Korea have a notably higher resistance rate (17%). Clindamycin was historically effective against members of the *B. fragilis* group, but rates of resistance have increased to 30–43% in the United States and are >80% in some parts of the world. Furthermore, metronidazole is effective against many different anaerobic organisms and is considered a first-line agent for many anaerobic infections worldwide, but, in a population of Colombian patients with refractory periodontitis, 45% of *Fusobacterium* isolates and 25% of *Prevotella* and *Porphyromonas* strains were resistant to metronidazole; this finding underscores the importance of understanding the local antibiogram and of assessing susceptibility profiles in refractory disease.

Empirical Therapy Not every anaerobe isolated must be specifically targeted by the antibiotic regimen. Given that infections involving anaerobes are typically polymicrobial, that the cultivation and identification of anaerobes are challenging (i.e., not all organisms may be recovered), and that organisms often depend on one another for persistence, clinical resolution of the infection is often achieved with empirical antibiotics targeting the bulk of the organisms recovered. Antibiotics that demonstrate no useful activity against anaerobes include aminoglycosides, monobactams, and trimethoprim-sulfamethoxazole. With the caveat that susceptibility profiles may change with time and geography, the antibiotics that are commonly used as empirical therapy against anaerobic bacteria include metronidazole, β-lactam/β-lactamase inhibitor combinations, clindamycin, carbapenems, and chloramphenicol (**Table 177-2**).

Metronidazole is active against gram-negative anaerobes, including nearly all isolates of *Bacteroides* species, and gram-positive spore-forming organisms, such as *C. difficile* (**Chap. 134**) and other *Clostridium* species. Given intrinsically reduced susceptibility, metronidazole is clinically unreliable against gram-positive non-spore-forming organisms, such as *Actinomyces*, *Propionibacterium*, *Lactobacillus*, *Bifidobacterium*, *Eubacterium*, and *Peptostreptococcus*.

TABLE 177-2 Antimicrobial Therapy That Is Typically Active Against Commonly Encountered Anaerobes

ANTIBIOTIC(S)	CAVEATS
Metronidazole	This drug is clinically unreliable against gram-positive non-spore-forming anaerobes (e.g., *Actinomyces* spp., *Propionibacterium* spp., *Peptostreptococcus* spp.).
β-Lactam/β-lactamase inhibitor combinations (ampicillin-sulbactam, ticarcillin–clavulanic acid, piperacillin-tazobactam)	Rates of resistance are increasing in some gram-negative anaerobes. The newer cephalosporin/β-lactamase combinations have limited anaerobic activity.
Clindamycin	Rates of resistance are increasing in *Bacteroides* spp.
Carbapenems (meropenem, imipenem, ertapenem, doripenem)	Rates of resistance are currently very low (<5%), although some carbapenemase-producing strains have been identified.
Chloramphenicol	Some clinical failures have been noted, even when the isolate is found to be susceptible by in vitro testing.

Of note, a few metronidazole-resistant *Bacteroides* isolates have been identified in the United States, and rates of such resistance have been increasing in Europe. Moreover, the rate of resistance to metronidazole has probably been greatly underestimated in some countries (e.g., the United Kingdom) that use metronidazole susceptibility to discriminate between obligate and facultative anaerobes (with obligate anaerobes defined by their susceptibility). Although the majority of metronidazole-resistant isolates have been identified in patients who have been exposed to the drug, resistant organisms have also been found in metronidazole-naïve patients.

More than 90% of clinical isolates from the *B. fragilis* group produce β-lactamases that are predominantly active against cephalosporins and that are highly active, cell associated, and produced constitutively. Thus, members of the *B. fragilis* group are presumed to be resistant to penicillin and ampicillin but may remain susceptible to extended-spectrum penicillins, particularly in combination with a β-lactamase inhibitor (e.g., ampicillin-sulbactam, piperacillin-tazobactam). Rates of resistance to ampicillin-sulbactam are increasing, particularly in *P. distasonis*, which has a reported resistance rate of 21% in the United States. Because β-lactamase production is not common in *Clostridium* species, these combination agents are usually effective. Of note, the newer cephalosporin/β-lactamase inhibitors (e.g., ceftolozane-tazobactam, ceftazidime-avibactam) have limited anaerobic activity.

Clindamycin is active against many anaerobes. However, rates of resistance to clindamycin among *Bacteroides* species increased in the United States from 7% in 1981 to 33% in 2010–2012. Resistance to clindamycin among non-*Bacteroides* gram-negative anaerobes is much less common (<10%). Some *Clostridium* species are resistant to clindamycin, although *C. perfringens* typically is not.

Carbapenems (ertapenem, doripenem, meropenem, and imipenem) are active against anaerobes, with fewer than 3% of *Bacteroides* isolates resistant. There is little difference among resistance rates for specific species, and, of the carbapenems, imipenem typically has the lowest resistance rate. Although the β-lactamase produced by most *Bacteroides* species is unable to inactivate carbapenems, rare *B. fragilis* strains have been reported to produce a carbapenemase.

Resistance to chloramphenicol is rare in *Bacteroides* species. Nationwide surveys in the United States have identified no resistant organisms, but some isolates with elevated minimal inhibitory concentrations (MICs)—i.e., 16 μg/mL—have been noted. Although chloramphenicol has excellent in vitro activity against all clinically relevant anaerobes, some clinical failures have been documented. Therefore, this drug may be less preferable if other active agents are available.

Other antibiotics with more variable activity against anaerobes include the fluoroquinolones and tigecycline. Although many fluoroquinolones (e.g., ciprofloxacin, levofloxacin, ofloxacin) display reasonable activity against anaerobic organisms other than *Bacteroides* species, these agents exhibit poor activity against the *B. fragilis* group. Rates of resistance to moxifloxacin are relatively high (39–83%) among *Bacteroides* isolates obtained in the United States but are much lower among *B. fragilis* and *B. thetaiotaomicron* isolates collected in Korea (8 and 2%, respectively) or Taiwan (8 and 15%, respectively). Tigecycline is active against most anaerobic bacteria, although MICs are somewhat higher for *Clostridium* species. Tigecycline's efficacy for treatment of complicated intraabdominal infections is comparable to that of imipenem, and it is therefore recommended as single-agent therapy for these infections.

Infections at Specific Sites In clinical situations, specific antibiotic regimens and durations must be tailored to the initial site of infection; the reader is referred to specific chapters on infections at specific sites for recommendations. In general, anaerobic infections are often broadly categorized as originating above or below the diaphragm. This distinction is clinically useful in that the predominant pathogens—and therefore the empirical antibiotic regimens—differ between these two categories of infection.

Infections above the diaphragm usually reflect the orodental microbiota, which includes *Prevotella*, *Porphyromonas*, *Fusobacterium*, and *Bacteroides* species other than the *B. fragilis* group along with streptococci (both aerobic and microaerophilic). Accordingly, antibiotic regimens should cover both aerobic and anaerobic bacteria. Given that >70% of these infections include a β-lactamase-producing organism, β-lactam drugs (penicillins and cephalosporins) are poor options as monotherapy. The recommended regimens include clindamycin, a β-lactam/β-lactamase inhibitor combination, or metronidazole in combination with a drug active against microaerophilic and aerobic streptococci (e.g., penicillin).

Anaerobic infections arising below the diaphragm (e.g., colonic and intraabdominal infections) must be treated specifically with agents active against *Bacteroides* species, including *B. fragilis*. Single agents suitable for this purpose include cefoxitin, moxifloxacin, a β-lactam/β-lactamase inhibitor combination, or a carbapenem. A two-drug regimen is an alternative, with one drug active against anaerobes and the other against coliforms (e.g., metronidazole with either a cephalosporin or a fluoroquinolone). In addition, if the clinician suspects that gram-positive facultative organisms such as enterococci are involved, therapeutic regimens should include ampicillin or vancomycin. Although clindamycin and cefotetan were previously considered acceptable options for intraabdominal infections involving anaerobes, these drugs are no longer recommended because of escalating rates of resistance in the *B. fragilis* group. Ampicillin-sulbactam is not recommended because of high rates of resistance among community-acquired strains of *E. coli* rather than because of resistance in anaerobic bacteria.

CNS infections involving anaerobic organisms may be treated with metronidazole, a carbapenem, chloramphenicol, or—if only gram-positive anaerobes are involved—penicillin. Clindamycin and cefoxitin have poor penetration into the CSF and should not be used. Cases of osteomyelitis in which a polymicrobial infection is identified from a bone biopsy specimen should be treated with a regimen that covers both aerobes and anaerobes, as some organisms that are often regarded as a contaminant (e.g., *C. acnes*) may have a pathogenic role. When an anaerobic organism is recognized as a major or sole pathogen infecting a joint, the duration of treatment should be similar to that used for arthritis caused by aerobic bacteria (**Chap. 130**).

Although not every anaerobe needs to be covered with pathogen-directed therapy in most polymicrobial infections, several studies of *Bacteroides* bacteremia have clearly demonstrated that patients receiving effective therapy have lower mortality rates and more rapid sterilization of blood cultures than patients receiving ineffective therapy.

FAILURE OF THERAPY

Anaerobic infections that fail to respond to treatment or that relapse should be reassessed. Potential causes include an uncontrolled source of infection (e.g., ongoing intestinal leak into the peritoneum), superinfection with a new organism, and/or antibiotic failure. Additional imaging may be useful to discern whether surgical drainage or debridement is warranted. Obtaining additional culture specimens will help identify whether an organism resistant to the antibiotics being used is present. Strong consideration should be given to obtaining susceptibility profiles for the isolates.

FURTHER READING

Brook I: Antimicrobial therapy of anaerobic infections. J Chemother 28:143, 2016.

Cooley L, Teng J: Anaerobic resistance: Should we be worried? Curr Opin Infect Dis 32:523, 2019.

Finegold SM: Anaerobes: Problems and controversies in bacteriology, infections, and susceptibility testing. Rev Infect Dis 12(Suppl 2):S223, 1990.

Kierzkowska M et al: Trends and impact in antimicrobial resistance among *Bacteroides* and *Parabacteroides* species in 2007-2012 compared to 2013-2017. Microb Drug Resist 26:1452, 2020.

Styrt B, Gorbach SL: Recent developments in the understanding of the pathogenesis and treatment of anaerobic infections (2). N Engl J Med 321:240, 1989.

Wexler HM: *Bacteroides*: The good, the bad, and the nitty-gritty. Clin Microbiol Rev 20:593, 2007.

Section 8 **Mycobacterial Diseases**

178 Tuberculosis

Mario C. Raviglione, Andrea Gori

Tuberculosis (TB), which is caused by bacteria of the *Mycobacterium tuberculosis* complex, is one of the oldest diseases known to affect humans and the top cause of infectious death worldwide excluding COVID-19. Population genomic studies suggest that *M. tuberculosis* may have emerged ~70,000 years ago in Africa and subsequently disseminated along with anatomically modern humans, expanding globally during the Neolithic Age as human density started to increase. Progenitors of *M. tuberculosis* are likely to have affected prehominids. This disease most often affects the lungs, although other organs are involved in up to one-third of cases. If properly treated, TB caused by drug-susceptible strains is curable in the vast majority of cases. If untreated, the disease may be eventually fatal in over 70% of people. Transmission usually takes place through the airborne spread of droplet nuclei produced by patients with infectious pulmonary TB. Through pharmacological prophylaxis the development of the disease can be prevented in those who have contracted TB infection.

ETIOLOGIC AGENT

Mycobacteria belong to the family Mycobacteriaceae and the order Actinomycetales. Of the pathogenic species belonging to the *M. tuberculosis* complex, which comprises eight distinct subgroups, the most common and important agent of human disease by far is *M. tuberculosis* (*sensu stricto*). A closely related organism isolated from cases in West, Central, and East Africa is *M. africanum*. The complex includes some zoonotic members, such as *M. bovis* (the bovine tubercle bacillus—characteristically resistant to pyrazinamide, once an important cause of TB transmitted by unpasteurized milk, and currently responsible for 140,000 human cases worldwide in 2019, half of them in Africa) and *M. caprae* (related to *M. bovis*). In addition, other organisms that have been reported rarely as causing TB include *M. pinnipedii* (a bacillus infecting seals and sea lions in the southern hemisphere and recently isolated from humans), *M. mungi* (isolated from banded mongooses in southern Africa), *M. orygis* (described in oryxes and other Bovidae in Africa and Asia and a potential cause of infection in humans), and *M. microti* (the "vole" bacillus, a less virulent organism). Finally, *M. canetti* is a rare isolate from East African cases that produces unusual smooth colonies on solid media and is considered closely related to a supposed progenitor type. There is no known environmental reservoir for any of these organisms.

M. tuberculosis is a rod-shaped, non-spore-forming, thin aerobic bacterium measuring 0.5 μm by 3 μm. Mycobacteria, including *M. tuberculosis*, are often neutral on Gram's staining. However, once stained, the bacilli cannot be decolorized by acid alcohol; this characteristic justifies their classification as acid-fast bacilli (AFB; **Fig. 178-1**). Acid fastness is due mainly to the organisms' high content of mycolic acids, long-chain cross-linked fatty acids, and other cell-wall lipids. Microorganisms other than mycobacteria that display some acid fastness include species of *Nocardia* and *Rhodococcus*, *Legionella micdadei*, and the protozoa *Isospora* and *Cryptosporidium*. In the mycobacterial cell wall, lipids (e.g., mycolic acids) are linked to underlying arabinogalactan and peptidoglycan. This structure results in very low permeability of the cell wall, thus reducing the effectiveness of most antibiotics. Another molecule in the mycobacterial cell wall, lipoarabinomannan, is involved in the pathogen–host interaction and facilitates the survival of *M. tuberculosis* within macrophages.

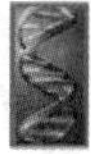

The complete genome sequence of *M. tuberculosis* comprises 4.4 million base pairs, 4043 genes encoding 3993 proteins, and 50 genes encoding stable RNAs; its high guanine-plus-cytosine content (65.6%) is indicative of an aerobic "lifestyle." A large proportion of genes are devoted to the production of enzymes involved in cell wall metabolism. Substantial genetic variability exists among the innumerable *M. tuberculosis* strains from different parts of the world. Based on such genetic variability it is possible to distinguish and compare different strains. Their distinction is important to study transmission dynamics and identify outbreaks. Starting in the 1990s, reproducible genotyping methods were developed to type the bacterium. Initially, they included insertion sequence 6110 (IS6110), restriction fragment length polymorphism (RFLP) typing, and spoligotyping. Lately, most studies utilize mycobacterial interspersed repetitive unit variable number tandem repeats (MIRU-VTNRs) and whole genome sequencing analysis.

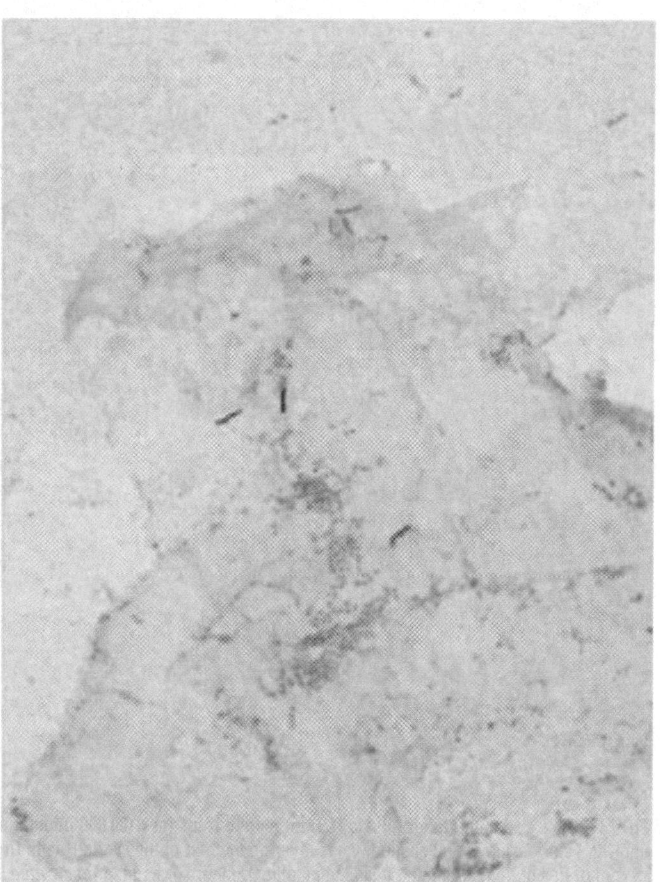

FIGURE 178-1 Acid-fast bacillus smear showing *M. tuberculosis* bacilli. *(Courtesy of the Centers for Disease Control and Prevention, Atlanta.)*

EPIDEMIOLOGY

In 2019, 7.1 million new cases of TB (all forms, both pulmonary and extrapulmonary) were reported to the World Health Organization (WHO) by its member states; 97% of cases were reported from low- and middle-income countries. However, because of insufficient case detection and incomplete notification, reported cases represent only about two-thirds of the total estimated cases. The WHO estimated that 10 million (range 9-11 million; rate 130 per 100,000 people) new (incident) cases of TB occurred worldwide in 2019, 97% of them in low- and middle-income countries of Asia (6.1 million), Africa (2.4 million), the Middle East (0.8 million), and Latin America (0.28 million). Eight countries accounted for two-thirds of all new cases: India, Indonesia, China, the Philippines, Pakistan, Nigeria, Bangladesh, and South Africa. Of all cases, 57% occurred in male patients, 32% in female patients, and 11% in children. It is further estimated that 1.4 million (range, 1.3–1.6 million) deaths from TB, including 0.21 million among people with HIV co-infection, occurred in 2019; 98% of these deaths were in low- and middle-income countries. Estimates of TB incidence rates (per 100,000 population) and numbers of TB-related deaths in 2018 are depicted in **Figs. 178-2 and 178-3**, respectively. During the

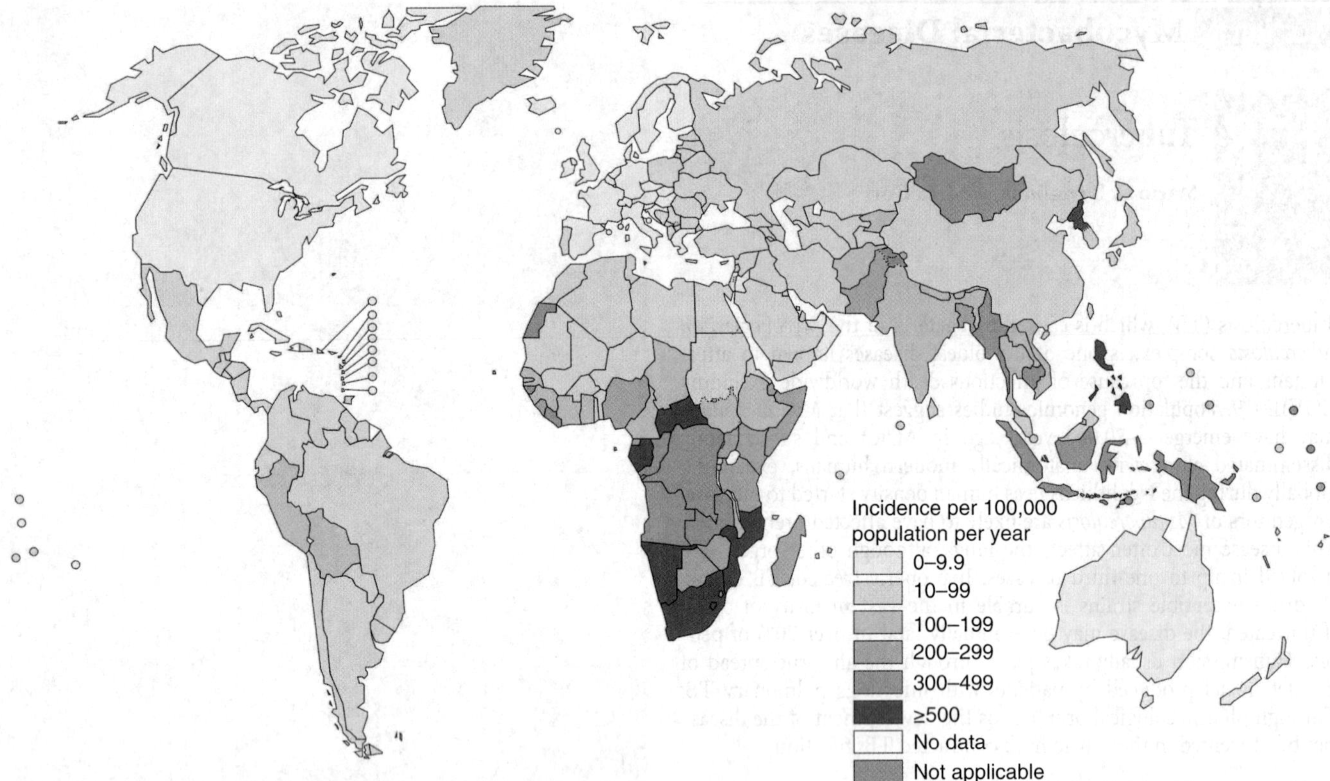

FIGURE 178-2 Estimated tuberculosis (TB) incidence rates (per 100,000 population) in 2018. The designations used and the presentation of material on this map do not imply the expression of any opinion whatsoever on the part of the World Health Organization (WHO) concerning the legal status of any country, territory, city, or area or of its authorities or concerning the delimitation of its frontiers or boundaries. *Dotted, dashed,* and *white lines* represent approximate border lines for which there may not yet be full agreement. *(Reproduced with permission from Global Tuberculosis Report 2019. Geneva, World Health Organization; 2019.)*

late 1980s and early 1990s, numbers of reported cases of TB increased in high-income countries after years of decline. These increases were related largely to immigration from countries with a high incidence of TB; the worldwide spread of the HIV epidemic; social problems, such as increase in urbanization and the related increased urban poverty, homelessness, and drug abuse; and dismantling of TB services. During the past few years, numbers of reported cases have begun to decline again or have stabilized in most industrialized nations. In the United States, with the re-establishment of stronger control programs, the decline resumed in 1993, and during the period 2007–2012, the decline rate was 6.5% annually on average. Later, between 2012 and 2019 this annual rate slowed down to 2.1%. In 2019, 8920 cases of TB

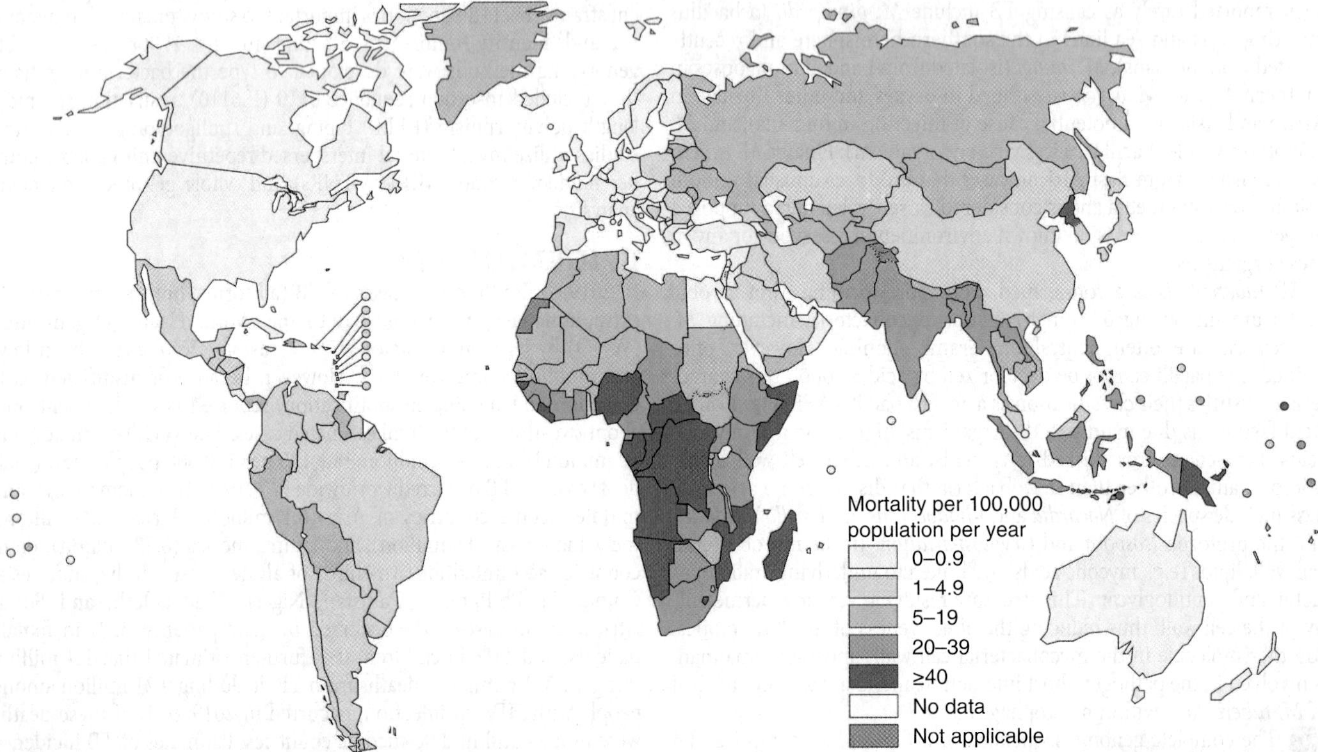

FIGURE 178-3 Estimated tuberculosis (TB) mortality rates in HIV-negative people in 2018. *(See disclaimer in Fig. 178-2. Reproduced with permission from Global Tuberculosis Report 2019. Geneva, World Health Organization; 2019.)*

(2.7 cases/100,000 population) were preliminarily reported to the U.S. Centers for Disease Control and Prevention (CDC).

In the United States, TB is uncommon among young white adults of European descent, who have only rarely been exposed to *M. tuberculosis* infection during recent decades. In contrast, because of a high risk of transmission in the past, the prevalence of *M. tuberculosis* infection is relatively high among elderly whites. In general, adults ≥65 years of age have the highest incidence rate per capita and children <14 years of age the lowest. Among U.S.-born persons, African Americans accounted for the highest proportion of cases (35%; 905 in 2019), followed by white persons (756 cases), and Hispanic/Latinos (628). TB in the United States is also a disease of adult members of the HIV-infected population (4.9% of all cases), the foreign-born population (71% of all cases in 2019), and disadvantaged/marginalized populations. Of the 6322 cases reported among non-U.S.-born persons in the United States in 2019, 33% occurred in Hispanic/Latinos and 47% in persons born in Asia. Overall, the highest rates per capita were among non-U.S.-born Asians (26 cases/100,000 population) and native Hawaiian/Pacific Islanders (25 cases/100,000 population). A total of 515 deaths was caused by TB in the United States in 2017. In Canada, TB cases and rates per 100,000 population have been increasing between 2014 and 2017 (from 1615/4.5 to 1796/4.9). In 2017, 1796 TB cases were reported (4.9 cases/100,000 population); 72% (1290) of these cases occurred in foreign-born persons, and 17.4% (313 cases) occurred in Canadian-born Indigenous Peoples, whose per capita rate is disproportionately high (21.5 cases/100,000 population). The highest rate was found in the territory of Nunavut, at 265 cases/100,000 population—a rate similar to that in many highly endemic countries. Similarly, in Europe, TB has reemerged as an important public health problem, mainly as a result of cases among immigrants from high-incidence countries and among marginalized populations, often in large urban settings such as London. In 2018, 36% of all cases reported from England occurred in London, 82% of them among people born abroad; although decreasing, the rate per capita (19 cases/100,000 population) is twice as high as that of England with a borough (Newham) reaching 47 cases per 100,000 population. Likewise, in most Western European countries, there are more cases annually among foreign-born than native populations.

Recent data on global trends indicate that in 2019 the TB incidence was stable or falling in most regions; this trend began in the early 2000s and appears to have continued, with an average annual decline of 1.7% globally and 2.3% between 2018 and 2019. This global decrease is explained largely by the reduction in TB incidence in sub-Saharan Africa, where rates had risen steeply since the 1980s as a result of the HIV epidemic and the lack of capacity of health systems and services to deal with the problem effectively, and, less so, in Eastern Europe, where incidence increased rapidly during the 1990s because of a deterioration in socioeconomic conditions and the health care infrastructure (although, after peaking in 2001, incidence in Eastern Europe has since declined slowly).

Of the estimated 10 million new cases of TB in 2019, 8.2% (0.82 million) were associated with HIV co-infection, and 73% of these HIV-associated cases occurred in Africa. An estimated 0.21 million persons with HIV-associated TB died in 2019. Furthermore, an estimated 465,000 (range 400,000-535,000) cases of rifampin- (also called rifampicin) resistant TB (RR-TB) and multidrug-resistant TB (MDR-TB)—a form of the disease caused by bacilli resistant at least to isoniazid and rifampin—occurred in 2019, representing 3.3% and 18%, respectively, of all new and previously treated cases. Only 44% of these cases were diagnosed because of a lack of culture and drug susceptibility testing (DST) capacity in many settings worldwide. As a consequence, an estimated 200,000 people with MDR/RR-TB died in 2019. The countries of the former Soviet Union reported the highest proportions of MDR/RR disease among new TB cases (37% in Belarus, 35% in Russia, 29% in Kyrgyzstan, Moldova, and Ukraine). Overall, half of all MDR/RR-TB cases occur in India (27%), China (14%), and the Russian Federation (9%). Since 2006, 131 countries, including the United States, have reported cases of extensively drug-resistant TB (XDR-TB), in which MDR-TB is compounded by additional resistance to any fluoroquinolones and at least one of the injectable drugs amikacin, kanamycin, and capreomycin. (N.B: In January 2021, the WHO published the following new definitions: (i) Pre-XDR-TB, as TB caused by *Mycobacterium tuberculosis* strains that fulfill the definition of MDR/RR-TB and that are also resistant to any fluoroquinolone. (ii) XDR-TB, as TB caused by *Mycobacterium tuberculosis* strains that fulfill the definition of MDR/RR-TB and that are also resistant to any fluoroquinolone and at least one additional Group A drug including levofloxacin or moxifloxacin, bedaquiline and linezolid.) About 6.2% of the MDR-TB cases worldwide may be XDR-TB, but the vast majority of XDR-TB cases remain undiagnosed because reliable methods for DST are lacking and laboratory capacity is limited mainly in low-income countries. Lately, a few cases deemed resistant to all anti-TB drugs have been reported; however, this information must be interpreted with caution because susceptibility testing for several second-line drugs is neither accurate nor reproducible.

FROM EXPOSURE TO INFECTION

M. tuberculosis is most commonly transmitted from a person with infectious pulmonary TB by droplet nuclei containing *M. tuberculosis* bacteria, which are aerosolized by coughing, sneezing, or speaking. The tiny droplets dry rapidly; the smallest (<5–10 μm in diameter) may remain suspended in the air for several hours and may reach the terminal air passages when inhaled. There may be as many as 3000 infectious nuclei per cough. Other routes of transmission of tubercle bacilli (e.g., through the skin or the placenta) are uncommon and of no epidemiologic significance. The risk of transmission and of subsequent acquisition of *M. tuberculosis* infection is determined mainly by exogenous factors, although endogenous factors may also play a role. The probability of contact with a person who has an infectious form of TB, the intimacy and duration of that contact, the degree of infectiousness of the case, and the shared environment in which the contact takes place are all important determinants of the likelihood of transmission. Several studies of close-contact situations have clearly demonstrated that TB patients whose sputum contains AFB visible by microscopy (sputum smear–positive cases) are the most likely to transmit the infection. The most infectious patients have cavitary pulmonary disease or, much less commonly, laryngeal TB and produce sputum containing as many as 10^5–10^7 AFB/mL. Patients with sputum smear–negative/culture-positive TB are less infectious, although they have been responsible for up to 20% of transmission in some studies in the United States. Those with culture-negative pulmonary TB and extrapulmonary TB are essentially noninfectious. Because persons with both HIV infection and TB are less likely to have cavitations, they may be less infectious than persons without HIV co-infection. Crowding in poorly ventilated rooms is one of the most important factors in the transmission of tubercle bacilli because it increases the intensity of contact with a case. The virulence of the transmitted organism is also an important factor in establishing infection. Endogenous factors such as the degree of immune competence are also important. In particular, HIV-infected patients, persons undergoing cancer treatment, or those administered immunosuppressive drugs may be at higher risk of TB infection acquisition.

Because of delays in seeking care and in making a diagnosis, it has been estimated that, in high-prevalence settings, up to 20 contacts (or 3–10 people per year) may be infected by each AFB-positive case before the index case is diagnosed. Attempts to estimate the basic reproductive number R_0 for TB have resulted in a wide range of values depending on environmental conditions and social behaviors of populations: from 0.24 in the Netherlands during the period 1933–2007 to 4.3 in China in 2012 reflecting the status of disease control.

FROM INFECTION TO DISEASE

Unlike the risk of acquiring infection with *M. tuberculosis*, the risk of developing disease after being infected depends largely on endogenous factors, such as the individual's innate immunologic and nonimmunologic defenses and the level at which the individual's cell-mediated immunity is functioning. Clinical illness directly following infection is classified as *primary TB* and is common among children in the first few years of life and among immunocompromised persons. Although primary TB may be severe and disseminated, it generally is not associated

TABLE 178-1 Risk Factors for Active Tuberculosis in Persons Who Have Been Infected with Tubercle Bacilli

FACTOR	RELATIVE RISK/ODDS[a]
Recent infection (<1 year)	12.9
Fibrotic lesions (spontaneously healed)	2–20
Comorbidities and iatrogenic causes	
HIV infection	21–>30
Silicosis	30
Chronic renal failure/hemodialysis	10–25
Diabetes	2–4
IV drug use	10–30
Excessive alcohol use	3
Immunosuppressive treatment	10
Tumor necrosis factor α inhibitors	4–5
Gastrectomy	2–5
Jejunoileal bypass	30–60
Posttransplantation period (renal, cardiac)	20–70
Tobacco smoking	2–3
Malnutrition and severe underweight	2

[a]Old infection = 1.

with high-level transmissibility. When infection is acquired later in life, the chance is greater that the mature immune system will contain it at least temporarily. Bacilli, however, may persist for years before reactivating to produce *secondary* (or *postprimary*) *TB*, which, because of frequent cavitation, is more often infectious than is primary disease. Overall, it is estimated that up to 10% of infected persons will eventually develop active TB in their lifetime—half of them during the first 18 months after infection. The risk is much higher among immunocompromised individuals and, particularly, HIV-infected persons. Reinfection of a previously infected individual, which is common in areas with high rates of TB transmission, may also favor the development of disease. At the height of the TB resurgence in the United States in the early 1990s, molecular typing and comparison of strains of *M. tuberculosis* suggested that up to one-third of cases of active TB in some inner-city communities were due to recent transmission rather than to reactivation of old infection. Age is an important determinant of the risk of disease after infection. Among infected persons, the incidence of TB is highest during late adolescence and early adulthood; the reasons are unclear. The incidence among women peaks at 25–34 years of age. In this age group, rates among women may be higher than those among men, whereas at older ages the opposite is true. The risk increases in the elderly, possibly because of waning immunity and comorbidity.

A variety of diseases and conditions favor the development of active TB (**Table 178-1**). In absolute terms, the most potent risk factor for TB among infected individuals is clearly HIV co-infection, which suppresses cellular immunity. The risk that infection will proceed to active disease is directly related to the patient's degree of immunosuppression. In a study of HIV-co-infected, tuberculin skin test (TST)–positive persons, this risk varied from 2.6 to 13.3 cases/100 person-years and increased as the CD4+ T-cell count decreased.

NATURAL HISTORY OF DISEASE

Studies conducted in various countries before the advent of antimicrobial TB therapy showed that untreated TB is often fatal. About one-third of patients died within 1 year after diagnosis. Historical data also show that 55% of sputum smear-positive cases were dead within 5 years and up to 86% (weighted mean 70%) within 10 years. A lower case fatality rate, around 20%, was estimated for untreated paucibacillary smear-negative cases at 5 years. Of the survivors at 5 years, ~60% had undergone spontaneous remission, while the remainder were still excreting tubercle bacilli. With effective, timely, and proper antimicrobial TB treatment, patients have a very high chance of being cured. However, improper use of anti-TB drugs, while reducing mortality rates, may also result in large numbers of chronic infectious cases, often with drug-resistant bacilli.

PATHOGENESIS AND IMMUNITY

INFECTION AND MACROPHAGE INVASION

The interaction of *M. tuberculosis* with the human host begins when droplet nuclei containing viable microorganisms, propelled into the air by infectious patients, are inhaled by a close bystander. Although the majority of inhaled bacilli are trapped in the upper airways and expelled by ciliated mucosal cells, a fraction (usually <10%) reach the alveoli, a unique immunoregulatory environment. There, in the very early phases of infection, the predominant cells infected by *M. tuberculosis* are myeloid dendritic cells. Subsequently, alveolar macrophages that have not yet been activated (prototypic alternatively activated macrophages) phagocytose the bacilli. Adhesion of mycobacteria to macrophages results largely from binding of the bacterial cell wall to a variety of macrophage cell-surface receptor molecules, including complement receptors, the mannose receptor, the immunoglobulin G Fcγ receptor, and type A scavenger receptors. Surfactants may also play a role in the early phase of interaction between the host and the pathogen, and surfactant protein D can prevent phagocytosis. Phagocytosis is enhanced by complement activation leading to opsonization of bacilli with C3 activation products such as C3b and C3bi. Concomitantly, binding of certain receptors, such as the mannose receptor, regulates postphagocytic events like phagosome–lysosome fusion and inflammatory cytokine production. After a phagosome forms, the survival of *M. tuberculosis* in the cell seems to depend in part on reduced acidification due to lack of assembly of a complete vesicular proton-adenosine triphosphatase. A complex series of events is generated by the bacterial cell-wall lipoglycan lipoarabinomannan, which inhibits the intracellular increase of Ca^{2+}. Thus, the Ca^{2+}/calmodulin pathway (leading to phagosome–lysosome fusion) is impaired, and the bacilli survive within the phagosomes by blocking fusion. The *M. tuberculosis* phagosome inhibits the production of phosphatidylinositol 3-phosphate, which normally earmarks phagosomes for membrane sorting and maturation (including phagolysosome formation), which would destroy the bacteria. Bacterial factors block the host defense of autophagy, in which the cell sequesters the phagosome in a double-membrane vesicle (*autophagosome*) that is destined to fuse with lysosomes. If the bacilli are successful in arresting phagosome maturation, then replication begins and the macrophage eventually ruptures and releases its bacillary contents. This process is mediated by the ESX-1 secretion system that is encoded by genes contained in the region of difference 1 (RD1). Other uninfected phagocytic cells are then recruited to continue the infection cycle by ingesting dying macrophages and their bacillary content, thus, in turn, becoming infected themselves and expanding the infection.

VIRULENCE OF TUBERCLE BACILLI

M. tuberculosis must be viewed as a complex formed by a multitude of strains that differ in virulence and are capable of producing a variety of manifestations of disease. Since the elucidation of the *M. tuberculosis* genome in 1998, large mutant collections have been generated, and many bacterial genes that contribute to *M. tuberculosis* virulence have been found. Moreover, different patterns of virulence defects have been defined in various animal models—predominantly mice but also guinea pigs, rabbits, and nonhuman primates. The *katG* gene encodes for a catalase/peroxidase enzyme that protects against oxidative stress and is required for isoniazid activation and subsequent bactericidal activity. RD1 is a 9.5-kb locus that encodes two key small protein antigens—6-kDa early secretory antigen (ESAT-6) and culture filtrate protein-10 (CFP-10)—as well as a putative secretion apparatus that may facilitate their egress; the absence of this locus in the vaccine strain *M. bovis* bacille Calmette-Guérin (BCG) is a key attenuating mutation. In *M. marinum*, a mutation in the RD1 virulence locus encoding the ESX-1 secretion system impairs the capacity of apoptotic macrophages to recruit uninfected cells for further rounds of infection. The results are less replication and fewer new granulomas. These observations in *M. marinum* are similar in part to events related to the virulence of *M. tuberculosis*; however, ESX-1, although necessary, is probably insufficient to explain virulence, and other mechanisms may be in play. Mutants lacking key enzymes of bacterial biosynthesis become auxotrophic for the missing substrate and often are totally unable to proliferate in animals; these include the *leuCD* and *panCD* mutants, which require leucine and pantothenic acid, respectively. The isocitrate lyase gene (*icl1*) encodes a key step in the glyoxylate shunt that facilitates bacterial growth on fatty acid substrates; this gene is required for long-term persistence of *M. tuberculosis* infection in mice with chronic TB. *M. tuberculosis* mutants in regulatory genes such as sigma factor C and sigma factor H (*sigC* and *sigH*) are associated with normal bacterial growth in mice, but they fail to elicit full tissue pathology. Finally, the mycobacterial protein CarD (expressed by the *carD* gene) seems essential for the control of rRNA transcription that is required for mycobacterial replication and persistence in the host cell. Its loss exposes mycobacteria to oxidative stress, starvation, DNA damage, and ultimately sensitivity to killing by a variety of host mutagens and defense mechanisms.

INNATE RESISTANCE TO INFECTION

Several observations suggest that genetic factors play a key role in innate resistance to infection with *M. tuberculosis* and the development of disease. The existence of this resistance, which is polygenic in nature, is suggested by the differing degrees of susceptibility to TB in different populations. This mechanism of elimination of the pathogen may be accompanied by negative results in the TST and interferon-γ (IFN-γ) release assays (IGRAs). In mice, a gene called *Nramp1* (natural resistance–associated macrophage protein 1) plays a regulatory role in resistance/susceptibility to mycobacteria. The human homologue NRAMP1, which maps to chromosome 2q, may play a role in determining susceptibility to TB, as is suggested by a study among West Africans. Studies of mice identified a novel host resistance gene, *ipr1*, that is encoded within the *sst1* locus; *ipr1* encodes an IFN-inducible nuclear protein that interacts with other nuclear proteins in macrophages primed with IFNs or infected by *M. tuberculosis.* In addition, polymorphisms in multiple genes, such as those encoding for various major histocompatibility complex alleles, IFN-γ, T-cell growth factor β, interleukin (IL) 10, mannose-binding protein, IFN-γ receptor, Toll-like receptor 2, vitamin D receptor, and IL-1, have been associated with susceptibility to TB.

THE HOST RESPONSE, GRANULOMA FORMATION, AND "LATENCY"

In the initial stage of host–bacterium interaction, prior to the onset of an acquired cell-mediated immune (CMI) response, *M. tuberculosis* disseminates widely through the lymph vessels, spreading to other sites in the lungs and other organs, and undergoes a period of extensive growth within naïve inactivated macrophages; additional naïve macrophages are recruited to the early granuloma. How the bacillus accesses the parenchymal tissue still needs to be elucidated: it may directly infect epithelial cells or transmigrate through infected macrophages across the epithelium. Infected dendritic cells or monocytes then begin to transport bacilli to the lymphatic system. Studies suggest that *M. tuberculosis* uses specific virulence mechanisms to subvert host cellular signaling and to elicit an early regulated proinflammatory response that promotes granuloma expansion and bacterial growth during this key early phase. A study of *M. marinum* infection in zebrafish has delineated one molecular mechanism by which mycobacteria induce granuloma formation. The mycobacterial protein ESAT-6 induces secretion of matrix metalloproteinase 9 (MMP9) by nearby epithelial cells that are in contact with infected macrophages. MMP9 in turn stimulates recruitment of naïve macrophages, thus inducing granuloma maturation and bacterial growth. Disruption of MMP9 function results in reduced bacterial growth. Another study has shown that *M. tuberculosis*–derived cyclic AMP is secreted from the phagosome into host macrophages, subverting the cell's signal transduction pathways and stimulating an elevation in the secretion of tumor necrosis factor α (TNF-α) as well as further proinflammatory cell recruitment. Ultimately, the chemoattractants and bacterial products released during the repeated rounds of cell lysis and infection of newly arriving macrophages enable dendritic cells to access bacilli; these cells migrate to the draining lymph nodes and present mycobacterial antigens to T lymphocytes. At this point, the development of cell-mediated and humoral immunity begins. These initial stages of infection are usually asymptomatic.

About 2–4 weeks after infection, two host responses to *M. tuberculosis* develop: a macrophage-activating CMI response and a tissue-damaging response. The *macrophage-activating response* is a T-cell mediated phenomenon resulting in the activation of macrophages that are capable of killing and digesting tubercle bacilli. The *tissue-damaging response* is the result of a delayed-type hypersensitivity reaction to various bacillary antigens; it destroys inactivated macrophages that contain multiplying bacilli but also causes caseous necrosis of the involved tissues (see below). Although both of these responses can inhibit mycobacterial growth, it is the balance between the two that determines the forms of TB that will develop subsequently. With the development of specific immunity and the accumulation of large numbers of activated macrophages at the site of the primary lesion, granulomatous lesions (*tubercles*) are formed. These lesions consist of accumulations of lymphocytes and activated macrophages that evolve toward epithelioid and giant cell morphologies. Initially, the tissue-damaging response can limit mycobacterial growth within macrophages. As stated above, this response, mediated by various bacterial products, not only destroys macrophages but also produces early solid necrosis in the center of the tubercle. Although *M. tuberculosis* can survive, its growth is inhibited within this necrotic environment by low oxygen tension and low pH. At this point, some lesions may heal by fibrosis, with subsequent calcification, whereas inflammation and necrosis occur in other lesions. Some observations have challenged the traditional view that any encounter between mycobacteria and macrophages results in chronic infection. It is possible that an immune response capable of eradicating early infection may sometimes develop as a consequence, for instance, of disabling mutations in mycobacterial genomes rendering their replication ineffective. Individual granulomas that are formed during this phase of infection can vary in size and cell composition; some can contain the spread of mycobacteria, while others cannot. TB infection ensues as a result of this dynamic balance between the microorganism and the host. For many years, TB infection has been called "latent TB infection (LTBI)." This terminology was used to define a state of persistent immune response to stimulation by *M. tuberculosis* antigens with no evidence of clinically manifest, active TB. The qualification "latent" may offer some convenience of distinguishing infection from disease, albeit an inaccurate description of a process that encompasses bacterial generations that are not dormant. It has been speculated that *latency* may therefore be an inaccurate term because bacilli may remain active during this "latent" stage, forming biofilms in necrotic areas within which they temporarily hide. Thus some have proposed the term *persister* as more accurate to indicate the behavior of the bacilli in this phase. It is important to recognize that infection and disease represent not a binary state but rather a continuum along which infection will eventually move in the direction of full containment or disease. The ability to predict, through systemic biomarkers, which affected individuals will progress toward disease would be of immense value in devising prophylactic interventions at scale.

MACROPHAGE-ACTIVATING RESPONSE

Cell-mediated immunity is critical at this early stage. In the majority of infected individuals, local macrophages are activated when bacillary antigens processed by macrophages stimulate T lymphocytes to release a variety of lymphokines. These activated macrophages aggregate around the lesion's center and effectively neutralize tubercle bacilli without causing further tissue destruction. In the central part of the lesion, the necrotic material resembles soft cheese (*caseous necrosis*)—a phenomenon that may also be observed in other conditions, such as neoplasms. Even when healing takes place, viable bacilli may remain dormant within macrophages or in the necrotic material for many years. These "healed" lesions in the lung parenchyma and hilar lymph nodes may later undergo calcification.

DELAYED-TYPE HYPERSENSITIVITY

In a minority of cases, the macrophage-activating response is weak, and mycobacterial growth can be inhibited only by intensified delayed hypersensitivity reactions, which lead to lung tissue destruction. The lesion tends to enlarge further, and the surrounding tissue is progressively damaged. At the center of the lesion, the caseous material liquefies. Bronchial walls and blood vessels are invaded and destroyed, and cavities are formed. The liquefied caseous material, containing large amount of bacilli, is drained through bronchi. Within the cavity, tubercle bacilli multiply, spill into the airways, and are discharged into the environment through expiratory maneuvers such as coughing and talking. In the early stages of infection, bacilli are usually transported by macrophages to regional lymph nodes, from which they gain access to the central venous return; from there they reseed the lungs and may also disseminate beyond the pulmonary vasculature throughout the body via the systemic circulation. The resulting extrapulmonary lesions may undergo the same evolution as those in the lungs, although most tend to heal. In young children with poor natural immunity, hematogenous dissemination may result in fatal miliary TB or tuberculous meningitis.

ROLE OF MACROPHAGES AND MONOCYTES

While cell-mediated immunity confers partial protection against *M. tuberculosis*, humoral immunity plays a less well-defined role in protection (although evidence is accumulating on the existence of antibodies to lipoarabinomannan, which may prevent dissemination of infection in children). In cell-mediated immunity, two types of cells are essential: macrophages, which directly phagocytose tubercle bacilli, and T cells (mainly CD4+ T lymphocytes, although the role of CD8+ T cells has recently been the subject of much research), which induce protection through the production of cytokines, especially IFN-γ. After infection with *M. tuberculosis*, alveolar macrophages secrete various cytokines responsible for a number of events (e.g., the formation of granulomas) as well as systemic effects (e.g., fever and weight loss). However, alternatively activated alveolar macrophages may be particularly susceptible to *M. tuberculosis* growth early on, given their more limited proinflammatory and bactericidal activity, which is related in part to being bathed in surfactant. New monocytes and macrophages attracted to the site are key components of the immune response. Their primary mechanism is probably related to production of oxidants (such as reactive oxygen intermediates or nitric oxide) that have antimycobacterial activity and increase the synthesis of cytokines such as TNF-α and IL-1, which in turn regulate the release of reactive oxygen intermediates and reactive nitrogen intermediates. In addition, macrophages can undergo apoptosis—a defensive mechanism to prevent the release of cytokines and bacilli via their sequestration in the apoptotic cell. Recent work also describes the involvement of neutrophils in the host response, although the timing of their appearance and their effectiveness remain uncertain.

ROLE OF T LYMPHOCYTES

Alveolar macrophages, monocytes, and dendritic cells are also critical in processing and presenting antigens to T lymphocytes, primarily CD4+ and CD8+ T cells; the result is the activation and proliferation of CD4+ T lymphocytes, which are crucial to the host's defense against *M. tuberculosis*. Qualitative and quantitative defects of CD4+ T cells explain the inability of HIV-infected individuals to contain mycobacterial proliferation. Activated CD4+ T lymphocytes can differentiate into cytokine-producing T_H1 or T_H2 cells. T_H1 cells produce IFN-γ—an activator of macrophages and monocytes—and IL-2. T_H2 cells produce IL-4, IL-5, IL-10, and IL-13 and may also promote humoral immunity. The interplay of these various cytokines and their cross-regulation determine the host's response. The role of cytokines in promoting intracellular killing of mycobacteria, however, has not been entirely elucidated. IFN-γ may induce the generation of reactive nitrogen intermediates and regulate genes involved in bactericidal effects. TNF-α is also important. Although its precise mechanisms are complex and not yet fully clarified, a model has been suggested that foresees an ideal setting for TNF-α between excessive activation—with consequent worsening of immunopathological reactions—and insufficient activation—with resulting lack of containment—in the control of TB infection. Observations made originally in transgenic knockout mice and more recently in humans suggest that other T-cell subsets, especially CD8+ T cells, may play an important role. CD8+ T cells have been associated with protective activities via cytotoxic responses and lysis of infected cells as well as with production of IFN-γ and TNF-α. Finally, natural killer cells act as co-regulators of CD8+ T-cell lytic activities, and γδ T cells are increasingly thought to be involved in protective responses in humans.

MYCOBACTERIAL LIPIDS AND PROTEINS

Lipids are involved in mycobacterial recognition by the innate immune system, and lipoproteins (such as 19-kDa lipoprotein) trigger potent signals through Toll-like receptors present in blood dendritic cells. *M. tuberculosis* possesses various protein antigens. Some are present in the cytoplasm and cell wall; others are secreted. That the latter are more important in eliciting a T lymphocyte response is suggested by experiments documenting the appearance of protective immunity in animals after immunization with live, protein-secreting mycobacteria. Among the antigens that may play a protective role are the 30-kDa (or 85B) and ESAT-6 antigens. Protective immunity is probably the result of reactivity to many different mycobacterial antigens. These antigens are being incorporated into newly designed vaccines on various platforms.

SKIN-TEST REACTIVITY

Coincident with the appearance of immunity, delayed-type hypersensitivity to *M. tuberculosis* develops. This reactivity is the basis of the TST, which is used primarily for the diagnosis of *M. tuberculosis* infection in persons without symptoms. The cellular mechanisms responsible for TST reactivity are related mainly to previously sensitized CD4+ T lymphocytes, which are attracted to the skin-test site. There, they proliferate and produce cytokines. Although delayed hypersensitivity is associated with protective immunity (TST-positive persons are less susceptible to a new *M. tuberculosis* infection than TST-negative persons), it by no means guarantees protection against reactivation. In fact, cases of active TB are often accompanied by strongly positive skin-test reactions. There is also evidence of reinfection with a new strain of *M. tuberculosis* in patients previously treated for active disease. This evidence underscores the fact that previous infection or active TB may not confer fully protective immunity.

CLINICAL MANIFESTATIONS

TB is classified as pulmonary, extrapulmonary, or both. Depending on several factors linked to host immunological status and bacterial strains, extrapulmonary TB may occur in 10–40% of patients. Furthermore, up to two-thirds of HIV-infected patients with TB may have both pulmonary and extrapulmonary TB or extrapulmonary TB alone.

PULMONARY TB

Pulmonary TB is conventionally categorized as primary or postprimary (adult-type, secondary). This distinction has been challenged by molecular evidence from TB-endemic areas indicating that a large percentage of cases of adult pulmonary TB result from recent infection (either primary infection or reinfection) and not from reactivation.

Primary Disease Primary pulmonary TB occurs soon after the initial infection. It may be asymptomatic or may present with fever and occasionally pleuritic chest pain. In areas of high TB transmission, this form of disease is often seen in children. Because most inspired air is distributed to the middle and lower lung zones, these areas are most commonly involved in primary TB. The lesion forming after initial infection (*Ghon focus*) is usually peripheral and accompanied by transient hilar or paratracheal lymphadenopathy, which may or may not be visible on standard chest radiography (CXR) (**Fig. 178-4**). Some patients develop erythema nodosum on the legs (**see Fig. A1-39**) or phlyctenular conjunctivitis. In the majority of cases, the lesion heals spontaneously and becomes evident only as a small calcified nodule. Pleural reaction overlying a subpleural focus is also common. The Ghon focus, with or without overlying pleural reaction, thickening, and regional lymphadenopathy, is referred to as the *Ghon complex*.

In young children with immature cell-mediated immunity and in persons with impaired immunity (e.g., those with malnutrition or HIV infection), primary pulmonary TB may progress rapidly to clinical illness. The initial lesion increases in size and can evolve in different ways. Pleural effusion, which is found in up to two-thirds of cases,

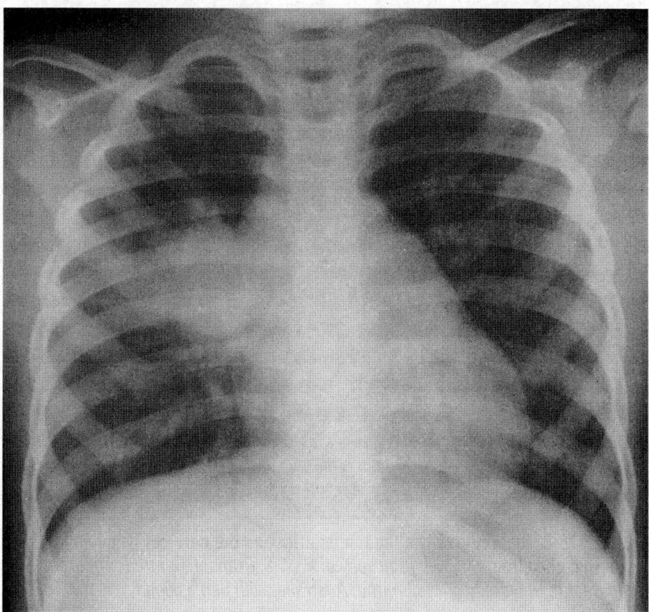

FIGURE 178-4 Chest radiograph showing right hilar lymph node enlargement with infiltration into the surrounding lung tissue in a child with primary tuberculosis. *(Courtesy of Prof. Robert Gie, Department of Paediatrics and Child Health, Stellenbosch University, South Africa; with permission.)*

results from the penetration of bacilli into the pleural space from an adjacent subpleural focus. In severe cases, the primary site rapidly enlarges, its central portion undergoes necrosis, and cavitation develops (*progressive primary TB*). TB in young children is almost invariably accompanied by hilar or paratracheal lymphadenopathy due to the spread of bacilli from the lung parenchyma through lymphatic vessels. Enlarged lymph nodes may compress bronchi, causing total obstruction with distal collapse, partial obstruction with large-airway wheezing, or a ball-valve effect with segmental/lobar hyperinflation. Lymph nodes may also rupture into the airway with development of pneumonia, often including areas of necrosis and cavitation, distal to the obstruction. Bronchiectasis (**Chap. 290**) may develop in any segment/lobe damaged by progressive caseating pneumonia. Occult hematogenous dissemination commonly follows primary infection. However, in the absence of a sufficient acquired immune response, which usually contains the infection, disseminated or miliary disease may result (**Fig. 178-5**). Small granulomatous lesions develop in multiple organs

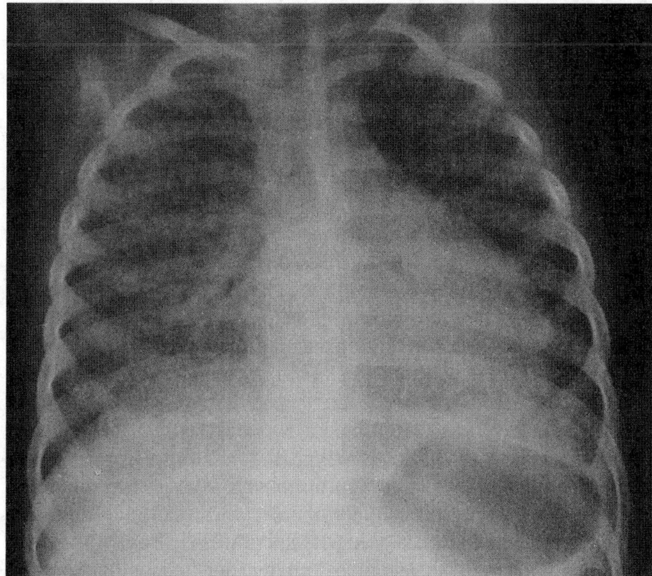

FIGURE 178-5 Chest radiograph showing bilateral miliary (millet-sized) infiltrates in a child. *(Courtesy of Prof. Robert Gie, Department of Paediatrics and Child Health, Stellenbosch University, South Africa; with permission.)*

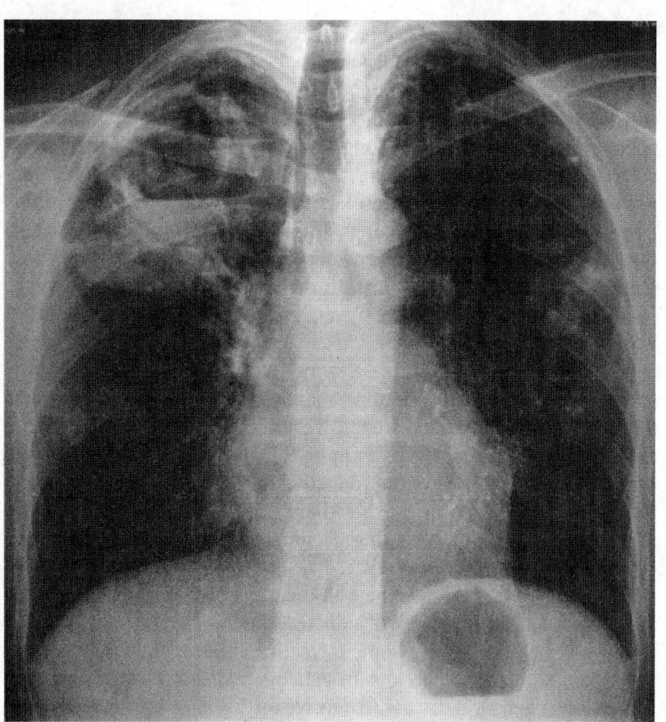

FIGURE 178-6 Chest radiograph showing a right-upper-lobe infiltrate and a cavity with an air-fluid level in a patient with active tuberculosis. *(Courtesy of Dr. Andrea Gori, Infectious Diseases Unit, Fondazione IRCCS Ca' Granda Ospediale Maggiore Policlinico, University of Milan, Milan, Italy; with permission.)*

and may cause locally progressive disease or result in tuberculous meningitis; this is a particular concern in very young children and immunocompromised persons (e.g., patients with HIV infection).

Postprimary (Adult-Type) Disease Also referred to as *reactivation* or *secondary TB*, postprimary TB is probably most accurately termed *adult-type TB* because it may result from endogenous reactivation of distant or recent infection (primary infection or reinfection). It is usually localized to the apical and posterior segments of the upper lobes, where the substantially higher mean oxygen tension (compared with that in the lower zones) favors mycobacterial growth. The superior segments of the lower lobes are also frequently involved. The extent of lung parenchymal involvement varies greatly, from small infiltrates to extensive cavitary disease. With cavity formation, liquefied necrotic contents are ultimately discharged into the airways and may undergo bronchogenic spread, resulting in satellite lesions within the lungs that may in turn undergo cavitation (**Figs. 178-6 and 178-7**). Massive involvement of pulmonary segments or lobes,

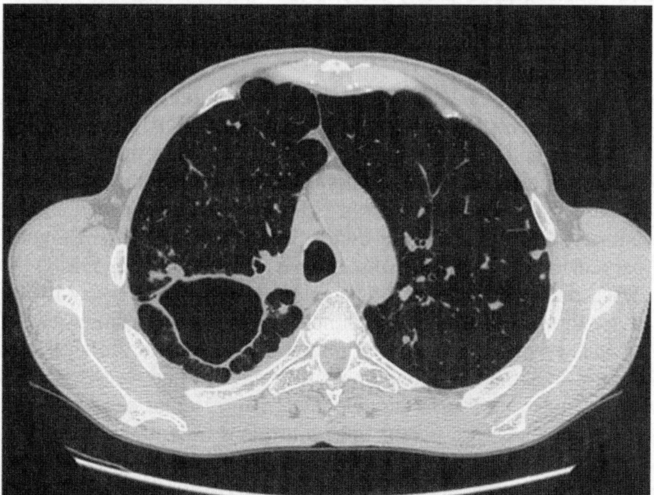

FIGURE 178-7 CT scan showing a large cavity in the right lung of a patient with active tuberculosis. *(Courtesy of Dr. Elisa Busi Rizzi, National Institute for Infectious Diseases, Spallanzani Hospital, Rome, Italy; with permission.)*

with coalescence of lesions, produces caseating pneumonia. While up to one-third of untreated patients reportedly succumb to severe pulmonary TB within a few months after onset (the classic "galloping consumption" of the past), others may undergo a process of spontaneous remission or proceed along a chronic, progressively debilitating course ("consumption" or *phthisis*). Under these circumstances, some pulmonary lesions become fibrotic and may later calcify, but cavities persist in other parts of the lungs. Individuals with such chronic disease continue to discharge tubercle bacilli into the environment. Most patients respond to treatment, with defervescence, decreasing cough, weight gain, and a general improvement in well-being within several weeks.

Early in the course of disease, symptoms and signs are often nonspecific and insidious, consisting mainly of fever, often diurnal and night sweats due to defervescence, weight loss, anorexia, general malaise, and weakness. However, in up to 90% of cases, cough eventually develops—often initially nonproductive and limited to the morning and subsequently accompanied by the production of purulent sputum, sometimes with blood streaking. Hemoptysis develops in 20–30% of cases, and massive hemoptysis may ensue as a consequence of the erosion of a blood vessel in the wall of a cavity. Hemoptysis, however, may also result from rupture of a dilated vessel in a cavity (*Rasmussen's aneurysm*) or from aspergilloma formation in an old cavity. Pleuritic chest pain sometimes develops in patients with subpleural parenchymal lesions or pleural disease. Extensive disease may produce dyspnea and, in rare instances, adult respiratory distress syndrome. Physical findings are of limited use in pulmonary TB. Many patients have no abnormalities detectable by chest examination, whereas others have detectable rales in the involved areas during inspiration, especially after coughing. Occasionally, rhonchi due to partial bronchial obstruction and classic amphoric breath sounds in areas with large cavities may be heard. Systemic features include fever (often low-grade and intermittent) in up to 80% of cases and wasting. Absence of fever, however, does not exclude TB. In some recurrent cases and among people with low Karnofsky score, finger clubbing has been reported. The most common hematologic findings are mild anemia, leukocytosis, and thrombocytosis with a slightly elevated erythrocyte sedimentation rate and/or C-reactive protein level. None of these findings is consistent or sufficiently accurate for diagnostic purposes. Hyponatremia due to the syndrome of inappropriate secretion of antidiuretic hormone has also been reported.

■ EXTRAPULMONARY TB

In descending order of frequency, the extrapulmonary sites most commonly involved in TB are the lymph nodes, pleura, genitourinary tract, bones and joints, meninges, peritoneum, and pericardium. However, virtually any organ system may be affected. As a result of hematogenous dissemination in HIV-infected individuals, extrapulmonary TB is seen more commonly today than in the past in settings of high HIV prevalence.

Lymph Node TB (Tuberculous Lymphadenitis) The most common presentation of extrapulmonary TB in both HIV-seronegative individuals and HIV-infected patients (35% of cases worldwide and >40% of cases in the United States in recent series), lymph node disease is particularly frequent among HIV-infected patients and among children (Fig. 178-8). In the United States, besides children, women (particularly non-Caucasians) seem to be especially susceptible. Once caused mainly by *M. bovis*, tuberculous lymphadenitis today is due largely to *M. tuberculosis*. Lymph node TB presents as painless swelling of the lymph nodes, most commonly at posterior cervical and supraclavicular sites (a condition historically referred to as *scrofula*). Lymph nodes are usually discrete in early disease but develop into a matted nontender mass over time; a fistulous tract draining caseous material may result. Associated pulmonary disease is present in fewer than 50% of cases, and systemic symptoms are uncommon except in HIV-infected patients. The diagnosis is established by fine-needle aspiration biopsy (with a yield of up to 80%) or surgical excision biopsy. Bacteriologic confirmation is achieved in the vast majority of cases, granulomatous lesions with or without visible AFBs are typically seen, and cultures are positive in 70–80% of cases. Among HIV-infected patients, granulomas are less well organized and are frequently absent entirely, but bacterial loads are heavier than in HIV-seronegative patients, with higher yields from microscopy and culture. Differential diagnosis includes a variety of infectious conditions, neoplastic diseases such as lymphomas or metastatic carcinomas, and rare disorders like Kikuchi's disease (necrotizing histiocytic lymphadenitis), Kimura's disease, and Castleman's disease.

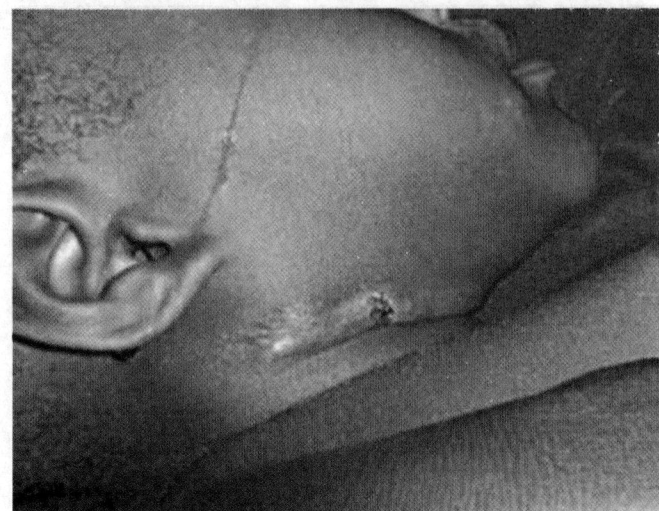

FIGURE 178-8 Tuberculous lymphadenitis affecting the cervical lymph nodes in a 2-year-old child from Malawi. *(Courtesy of Prof. S. Graham, Centre for International Child Health, University of Melbourne, Australia; with permission.)*

Pleural TB Involvement of the pleura accounts for ~20% of extrapulmonary cases in the United States and elsewhere. Isolated pleural effusion usually reflects recent primary infection, and the collection of fluid in the pleural space represents a hypersensitivity response to mycobacterial antigens. Pleural disease may also result from contiguous parenchymal spread, as in many cases of pleurisy accompanying postprimary disease. Depending on the extent of reactivity, the effusion may be small, remain unnoticed, and resolve spontaneously or may be sufficiently large to cause symptoms such as fever, pleuritic chest pain, and dyspnea. Physical findings are those of pleural effusion: dullness to percussion and absence of breath sounds. CXR reveals the effusion and, in up to one-third of cases, also shows a parenchymal lesion. Thoracentesis is required to ascertain the nature of the effusion and to differentiate it from manifestations of other etiologies. The fluid is straw-colored and at times hemorrhagic; it is an exudate with a protein concentration >50% of that in serum (usually ~4–6 g/dL), a normal to low glucose concentration, a pH of ~7.3 (occasionally <7.2), and detectable white blood cells (usually 500–6000/μL). Neutrophils may predominate in the early stage, but lymphocyte predominance is the typical finding later. Mesothelial cells are generally rare or absent. AFBs are rarely seen on direct smear, and cultures often may be falsely negative for *M. tuberculosis*; positive cultures are more common among postprimary cases. Determination of the pleural concentration of adenosine deaminase may be a useful screening test, and TB may be excluded if the value is very low. Lysozyme is also present in the pleural effusion. Measurement of IFN-γ, either directly or through stimulation of sensitized T cells with mycobacterial antigens, can be diagnostically helpful. Needle biopsy of the pleura is often required for diagnosis and is recommended over pleural fluid analysis; it reveals granulomas and/or yields a positive culture in up to 80% of cases. Pleural biopsy can yield a positive result in ~75% of cases when real-time automated nucleic acid amplification is used (the Xpert MTB/RIF assay [Cepheid; Sunnyvale, CA]; see "Nucleic Acid Amplification Technology," below); testing of pleural fluid with this assay is not recommended because of low sensitivity. This form of pleural TB responds rapidly to chemotherapy and may resolve spontaneously. Concurrent glucocorticoid administration may reduce the duration of fever and/or chest pain but is not of proven benefit.

Tuberculous empyema is a less common complication of pulmonary TB. It is usually the result of the rupture of a cavity, with spillage of a large number of organisms into the pleural space. This process may create a bronchopleural fistula with evident air in the pleural space. CXR shows hydropneumothorax with an air-fluid level. The pleural fluid is purulent and thick and contains large numbers of lymphocytes. Acid-fast smears and mycobacterial cultures are often positive. Surgical drainage is usually required as an adjunct to chemotherapy. Tuberculous empyema may result in severe pleural fibrosis and restrictive lung disease. Removal of the thickened visceral pleura (*decortication*) is occasionally necessary to improve lung function.

TB of the Upper Airways Nearly always a complication of advanced cavitary pulmonary TB, TB of the upper airways may involve the larynx, pharynx, and epiglottis. Symptoms include hoarseness, dysphonia, and dysphagia in addition to chronic productive cough. Findings depend on the site of involvement, and ulcerations may be seen on laryngoscopy. Acid-fast smear of the sputum is often positive, but biopsy may be necessary in some cases to establish the diagnosis. Carcinoma of the larynx may have similar features but is usually painless.

Genitourinary TB Genitourinary TB, which accounts for ~10–15% of all extrapulmonary cases in the United States and elsewhere, may involve any portion of the genitourinary tract. Clinical manifestations are cryptic and protean. Patients may be asymptomatic and their disease discovered only after destructive lesions of the kidneys have developed. Symptoms are often nonspecific, and include those of urinary tract infection with frequency, dysuria, nocturia and hematuria, and abdominal or flank pain. Without a high index of suspicion, this form of TB may result in delayed diagnosis with irreversible organ damage. Up to 75% of patients have abnormalities on CXR suggesting previous or concomitant pulmonary disease. Urinalysis gives abnormal results in 90% of cases, revealing pyuria and hematuria. The documentation of culture-negative pyuria in acidic urine should raise the suspicion of TB. IV pyelography, abdominal CT, or MRI (Fig. 178-9) may show deformities and obstructions; calcifications and ureteral strictures are suggestive findings. Culture of three morning urine specimens yields a definitive diagnosis in nearly 90% of cases. Severe ureteral strictures may lead to hydronephrosis, serious renal damage, and, ultimately, renal failure. Genital TB is diagnosed more commonly in female than in male patients. In female patients, it affects the fallopian tubes and the endometrium and may cause infertility, pelvic pain, and menstrual abnormalities. Diagnosis requires biopsy or culture of specimens obtained by dilation and curettage. In male patients, genital TB preferentially affects the epididymis, producing a slightly tender mass that may drain externally through a fistulous tract; orchitis and prostatitis may also develop. In almost half of cases of genitourinary TB, urinary tract disease is also present. Genitourinary TB responds well to chemotherapy.

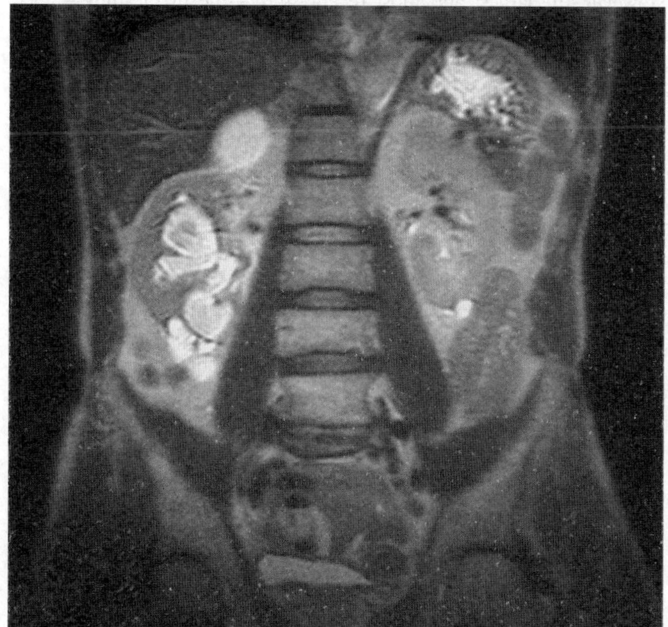

FIGURE 178-9 MRI of culture-confirmed renal tuberculosis. T2-weighted coronary plane: coronal sections showing several renal lesions in both the cortical and the medullary tissues of the right kidney. *(Courtesy of Dr. Alberto Matteelli, Department of Infectious Diseases, University of Brescia, Italy; with permission.)*

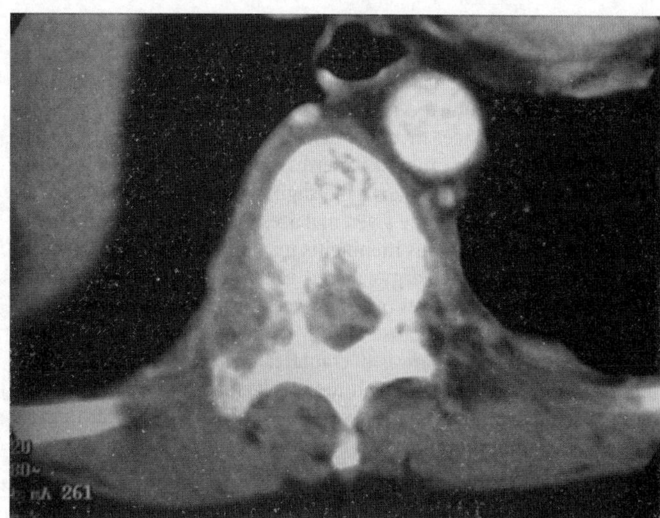

FIGURE 178-10 CT scan demonstrating destruction of the right pedicle of T10 due to Pott's disease. The patient, a 70-year-old Asian woman, presented with back pain and weight loss and had biopsy-proven tuberculosis. *(Courtesy of Charles L. Daley, MD, University of California, San Francisco; with permission.)*

Skeletal TB In the United States, TB of the bones and joints is responsible for ~10% of extrapulmonary cases. In bone and joint disease, pathogenesis is related to reactivation of hematogenous foci or to spread from adjacent paravertebral lymph nodes. Weight-bearing joints (the spine in 40% of cases, the hips in 13%, and the knees in 10%) are most commonly affected. Spinal TB (Pott's disease or tuberculous spondylitis; Fig. 178-10) often involves two or more adjacent vertebral bodies. Whereas the upper thoracic spine is the most common site of spinal TB in children, the lower thoracic and upper lumbar vertebrae are usually affected in adults. From the anterior superior or inferior angle of the vertebral body, the lesion slowly reaches the adjacent body, later affecting the intervertebral disk. With advanced disease, collapse of vertebral bodies results in kyphosis (*gibbus*). A paravertebral "cold" abscess may also form. In the upper spine, this abscess may track to and penetrate the chest wall, presenting as a soft tissue mass; in the lower spine, it may reach the inguinal ligaments or present as a psoas abscess. CT or MRI reveals the characteristic lesion and suggests its etiology. The differential diagnosis includes tumors and other infections. Pyogenic bacterial osteomyelitis, in particular, involves the disk very early and produces rapid sclerosis. Aspiration of the abscess or bone biopsy confirms the tuberculous etiology, as cultures are usually positive and histologic findings highly typical. A catastrophic complication of Pott's disease is paraplegia, which is usually due to an abscess or a lesion compressing the spinal cord. Paraparesis due to a large abscess is a medical emergency and requires rapid drainage. TB of the hip joints, usually involving the head of the femur, causes pain; TB of the knee produces pain and swelling. If the disease goes unrecognized, the joints may be destroyed. Diagnosis requires examination of the synovial fluid, which is thick in appearance, with a high protein concentration and a variable cell count. Although synovial fluid culture is positive in a high percentage of cases, synovial biopsy and tissue culture may be necessary to establish the diagnosis. Skeletal TB responds to chemotherapy, but severe cases may require surgery.

Tuberculous Meningitis and Tuberculoma TB of the central nervous system (CNS) accounts for ~5% of extrapulmonary cases in the United States. It is seen most often in young children but also develops in adults, especially those infected with HIV. Tuberculous meningitis results from the hematogenous spread of primary or postprimary pulmonary TB or from the rupture of a subependymal tubercle into the subarachnoid space. In more than half of cases, evidence of old pulmonary lesions or a miliary pattern is found on CXR. The disease often presents subtly as headache and slight mental changes after a prodrome of weeks of low-grade fever, malaise, anorexia, and irritability. If not recognized, tuberculous meningitis may evolve acutely with severe headache, confusion, lethargy, altered sensorium, and neck rigidity. Typically, the disease evolves over 1–2 weeks, a course longer than that of bacterial meningitis. Because meningeal involvement is pronounced at the base of the brain, paresis of cranial nerves (ocular nerves in particular) is a frequent finding, and the involvement of cerebral arteries may produce focal ischemia. The ultimate evolution is toward coma, with hydrocephalus and intracranial hypertension.

Lumbar puncture is the cornerstone of diagnosis. In general, examination of cerebrospinal fluid (CSF) reveals a high leukocyte count (up to 1000/μL), usually with a predominance of lymphocytes but sometimes with a predominance of neutrophils in the early stage; a protein content of 1–8 g/L (100–800 mg/dL); and a low glucose concentration. However, any of these three parameters can be within the normal range. AFBs are infrequently seen on direct smear of CSF sediment, and repeated lumbar punctures increase the yield. Culture of CSF is diagnostic in up to 80% of cases and remains the gold standard. Real-time automated nucleic acid amplification (the Xpert MTB/RIF assay) has a sensitivity of up to 80% and is the preferred initial diagnostic option. Treatment should be initiated immediately upon a positive Xpert MTB/RIF result. A negative result does not exclude a diagnosis of TB and requires further diagnostic workup. Imaging studies (CT and MRI) may show hydrocephalus and abnormal enhancement of basal cisterns or ependyma. If unrecognized, tuberculous meningitis is uniformly fatal. This disease responds to chemotherapy; however, neurologic sequelae are documented in 25% of treated cases, in most of which the diagnosis has been delayed. Clinical trials have demonstrated that patients given adjunctive glucocorticoids may experience faster resolution of CSF abnormalities and elevated CSF pressure, resulting in lower rates of death or severe disability and relapse. In one study, adjunctive dexamethasone significantly enhanced the chances of survival among persons >14 years of age but did not reduce the frequency of neurologic sequelae. The dexamethasone schedule was (1) 0.4 mg/kg per day given IV with tapering by 0.1 mg/kg per week until the fourth week, when 0.1 mg/kg per day was administered; followed by (2) 4 mg/d given by mouth with tapering by 1 mg per week until the fourth week, when 1 mg/d was administered. The WHO now recommends that adjuvant glucocorticoid therapy with either dexamethasone or prednisolone, tapered over 6–8 weeks, should be used in CNS TB.

Tuberculoma, an uncommon manifestation of TB of the CNS, presents as one or more space-occupying lesions and usually causes seizures and focal signs. CT or MRI reveals contrast-enhanced ring lesions, but biopsy is necessary to establish the diagnosis.

Gastrointestinal TB Gastrointestinal TB is uncommon, making up only 3.5% of extrapulmonary cases in the United States. Various pathogenetic mechanisms are involved: swallowing of sputum with direct seeding, hematogenous spread, or (largely in developing areas) ingestion of milk from cows affected by bovine TB. Although any portion of the gastrointestinal tract may be affected, the terminal ileum and the cecum are the sites most commonly involved. Abdominal pain (at times similar to that associated with appendicitis) and swelling, obstruction, hematochezia, and a palpable mass in the abdomen are common findings at presentation. Fever, weight loss, anorexia, and night sweats are also common. With intestinal wall involvement, ulcerations and fistulae may simulate Crohn's disease; the differential diagnosis of this entity is always difficult. Anal fistulae should prompt an evaluation for rectal TB. Because surgery is required in most cases, the diagnosis can be established by histologic examination and culture of specimens obtained intraoperatively.

Tuberculous peritonitis follows either the direct spread of tubercle bacilli from ruptured lymph nodes and intraabdominal organs (e.g., genital TB in women) or hematogenous seeding. Nonspecific abdominal pain, fever, and ascites should raise the suspicion of tuberculous peritonitis. The coexistence of cirrhosis (**Chap. 342**) in patients with tuberculous peritonitis complicates the diagnosis. In tuberculous peritonitis, paracentesis reveals an exudative fluid with a high protein content and leukocytosis that is usually lymphocytic (although neutrophils occasionally predominate). The yield of direct smear and culture is relatively low; culture of a large volume of ascitic fluid can increase the yield, but peritoneal biopsy (with a specimen best obtained by laparoscopy) is often needed to establish the diagnosis.

Pericardial TB (Tuberculous Pericarditis) Due either to direct extension from adjacent mediastinal or hilar lymph nodes or to hematogenous spread, pericardial TB has often been a disease of the elderly in countries with low TB prevalence. However, it also develops frequently in HIV-infected patients. Case-fatality rates are as high as 40% in some series. The onset may be subacute, although an acute presentation, with dyspnea, fever, dull retrosternal pain, and a pericardial friction rub, is possible. An effusion eventually develops in many cases; cardiovascular symptoms and signs of cardiac tamponade may ultimately appear (**Chap. 270**). In the presence of effusion, TB must be suspected if the patient belongs to a high-risk population (HIV-infected, originating in a high-prevalence country); if there is evidence of previous TB in other organs; or if echocardiography, CT, or MRI shows effusion and thickness across the pericardial space. A definitive diagnosis can be obtained by pericardiocentesis under echocardiographic guidance. The pericardial fluid must be submitted for biochemical, cytologic, and microbiologic evaluation. The effusion is exudative in nature, with a high count of lymphocytes and monocytes. Hemorrhagic effusion is common. Direct smear examination is very rarely positive. Culture of pericardial fluid reveals *M. tuberculosis* in up to two-thirds of cases, whereas pericardial biopsy has a higher yield. High levels of adenosine deaminase, lysozyme, and IFN-γ may suggest a tuberculous etiology.

Without treatment, pericardial TB is usually fatal. Even with treatment, complications may develop, including chronic constrictive pericarditis with thickening of the pericardium, fibrosis, and sometimes calcification, which may be visible on a chest radiograph. Systematic reviews and meta-analyses show a trend toward benefit from glucocorticoid treatment with regard to death and constrictive pericarditis. However, the largest and most recent study—the IMPI study—failed to show such a benefit. Of the patients enrolled in this trial, 67% were infected with HIV, and only a fraction were receiving antiretroviral treatment (ART). A supplemental analysis among HIV-negative people showed a small mortality benefit, as did another small study among HIV-infected people. The WHO currently recommends that, in patients with tuberculous pericarditis, initial adjuvant glucocorticoid therapy may be used. The 2016 guidelines of the American Thoracic Society (ATS), the CDC, and the Infectious Diseases Society of America (IDSA), on the other hand, suggest that glucocorticoid therapy should not be routinely administered.

Caused by direct extension from the pericardium or by retrograde lymphatic extension from affected mediastinal lymph nodes, tuberculous myocarditis is an extremely rare disease. Usually, it is fatal and is diagnosed postmortem.

Miliary or Disseminated TB Miliary TB is due to hematogenous spread of tubercle bacilli. Although in children it is often the consequence of primary infection, in adults it may be due to either recent infection or reactivation of old disseminated foci. The lesions are usually yellowish granulomas 1–2 mm in diameter that resemble millet seeds (thus the term *miliary*, coined by nineteenth-century pathologists). Clinical manifestations are nonspecific and protean, depending on the predominant site of involvement. Fever, night sweats, anorexia, weakness, and weight loss are presenting symptoms in the majority of cases. At times, patients have a cough and other respiratory symptoms due to pulmonary involvement as well as abdominal symptoms.

Physical findings include hepatomegaly, splenomegaly, and lymphadenopathy. Eye examination may reveal choroidal tubercles, which are pathognomonic of miliary TB, in up to 30% of cases. Meningismus occurs in fewer than 10% of cases.

A high index of suspicion is required for the diagnosis of miliary TB. Frequently, CXR (Fig. 178-5) reveals a miliary reticulonodular pattern (more easily seen on underpenetrated film), although no radiographic abnormality may be evident early in the course and among HIV-infected patients. Other radiologic findings include large infiltrates, interstitial infiltrates (especially in HIV-infected patients), and pleural effusion. Sputum-smear microscopy is negative in most cases. Various hematologic abnormalities may be seen, including anemia with leukopenia, lymphopenia, neutrophilic leukocytosis and leukemoid reactions, and polycythemia. Disseminated intravascular coagulation has been reported. Elevation of alkaline phosphatase levels and other abnormal values in liver function tests are detected in patients with severe hepatic involvement. TST results may be negative in up to half of cases, but reactivity may be restored during chemotherapy. Bronchoalveolar lavage and transbronchial biopsy are more likely to provide bacteriologic confirmation, and granulomas are evident in liver or bone-marrow biopsy specimens from many patients. If it goes unrecognized, miliary TB is lethal; with proper early treatment, however, it is amenable to cure. Glucocorticoid therapy has not proved beneficial.

A rare presentation seen in the elderly, *cryptic miliary TB* has a chronic course characterized by mild intermittent fever, anemia, and—ultimately—meningeal involvement preceding death. An acute septicemic form, *nonreactive miliary TB*, occurs very rarely and is due to massive hematogenous dissemination of tubercle bacilli. Pancytopenia is common in this form of disease, which is rapidly fatal. At postmortem examination, multiple necrotic but nongranulomatous ("nonreactive") lesions are detected.

Less Common Extrapulmonary Forms TB may cause chorioretinitis, uveitis, panophthalmitis, and painful hypersensitivity-related phlyctenular conjunctivitis. Tuberculous otitis is rare and presents as hearing loss, otorrhea, and tympanic membrane perforation. In the nasopharynx, TB may simulate granulomatosis with polyangiitis. Cutaneous manifestations of TB include primary infection due to direct inoculation, abscesses and chronic ulcers, scrofuloderma, lupus vulgaris (a smoldering disease with nodules, plaques, and fissures), miliary lesions, and erythema nodosum. Tuberculous mastitis results from retrograde lymphatic spread, often from the axillary lymph nodes. Adrenal TB is a manifestation of disseminated disease presenting rarely as adrenal insufficiency. Finally, congenital TB results from transplacental spread of tubercle bacilli to the fetus or from ingestion of contaminated amniotic fluid. This rare disease affects the liver, spleen, lymph nodes, and various other organs.

Post-TB Complications TB may cause persisting pulmonary damage in patients whose infection has been considered cured on clinical grounds. Chronic impairment of lung functions, bronchiectasis, aspergillomas, and chronic pulmonary aspergillosis **(Chap. 217)** have been associated with TB. Chronic pulmonary aspergillosis may manifest as simple aspergilloma (fungal ball) or chronic cavitary aspergillosis. Early studies revealed that, especially in the presence of large residual cavities, *Aspergillus fumigatus* may colonize the lesion and produce symptoms such as respiratory impairment, hemoptysis, persistent fatigue, and weight loss, often resulting in the erroneous diagnosis of TB recurrence. The detection of *Aspergillus* precipitins (IgG) in the blood suggests chronic pulmonary aspergillosis, as do radiographic abnormalities such as thickening of the pleura and cavitary walls or the presence of a fungal ball inside the cavity. Treatment is difficult. Recent preliminary studies on the use of itraconazole for ≥6 months indicate improvement or stabilization of 60–75% of the radiologic and clinical manifestations. Surgical removal of lesions is risky except in simple aspergilloma.

HIV-Associated TB (See also Chap. 202) TB is one of the most common diseases among HIV-infected persons worldwide. Responsible for up to 30% of all HIV-related mortality (208,000 deaths per year), TB is likely the main cause of death in this population. In certain urban settings in some African countries, the prevalence of HIV infection among TB patients reaches 70–80% **(Fig. 178-11)**.

A person with a positive TST who acquires HIV infection has a 3–13% annual risk of developing active TB, with the exact risk depending on the degree of immunosuppression when observation begins. Furthermore, a new TB infection acquired by an HIV-infected individual may evolve into active disease in a matter of weeks rather

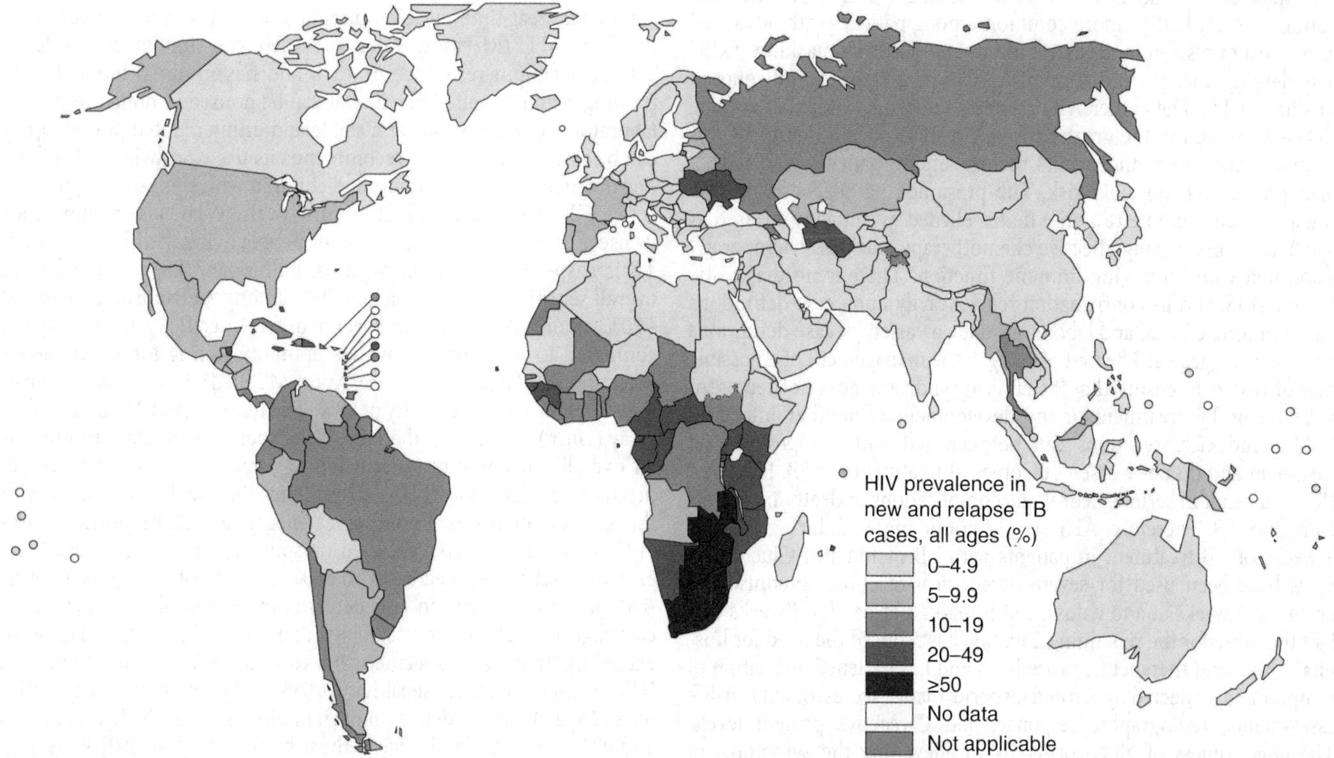

FIGURE 178-11 Estimated HIV prevalence in new and relapse tuberculosis (TB) cases in 2018. *(See disclaimer in Fig. 178-2. Reproduced with permission from Global Tuberculosis Report 2019. Geneva, World Health Organization; 2019.)*

than months or years. TB can appear at any stage of HIV infection, and its presentation varies with the stage. When cell-mediated immunity is only partially compromised, pulmonary TB presents in a typical manner (Figs. 178-6 and 178-7), with upper-lobe infiltrates and cavitation and without significant lymphadenopathy or pleural effusion. In late stages of HIV infection, when the CD4+ T-cell count is <200/μL, a primary TB–like pattern, with diffuse interstitial and subtle infiltrates, little or no cavitation, pleural effusion, and intrathoracic lymphadenopathy, is more common. However, these forms are becoming less common because of the expanded use of ART. Overall, sputum smears are less frequently positive among TB patients with HIV infection than among those without; thus the diagnosis of TB with traditional technology may be difficult, especially in view of the variety of HIV-related pulmonary conditions mimicking TB. Extrapulmonary TB is common among HIV-infected patients. In various series, extrapulmonary TB—alone or in association with pulmonary disease—has been documented in 40–60% of all cases in individuals co-infected with HIV. The most common forms are lymphatic, disseminated, pleural, and pericardial. Mycobacteremia and meningitis are also common, particularly in advanced HIV disease. The diagnosis of TB in HIV-infected patients may be complicated not only by the increased frequency of sputum-smear negativity (up to 40% in culture-proven pulmonary cases) but also by atypical radiographic findings, a lack of classic granuloma formation in the late stages, and a negative TST. The Xpert MTB/RIF assay is the preferred initial diagnostic option for pulmonary TB ensuring a sensitivity of 81% and a specificity of 98%, and therapy should be started on the basis of a positive result because treatment delays may be fatal. A negative Xpert MTB/RIF result, however, does not exclude a diagnosis of TB. Culture remains the gold standard. Recent assessment of a test based on the detection of mycobacterial lipoarabinomannan antigen in urine has shown favorable results in assisting with the detection of TB in HIV-positive people (see "Additional Diagnostic Procedures," below).

The *immune reconstitution inflammatory syndrome* (*IRIS*) or *TB immune reconstitution disease* consists of exacerbations in systemic manifestations (lymphadenopathy, fever) or respiratory signs (worsening of pulmonary infiltrations, pleural effusion) as well as laboratory or radiographic manifestations of TB. This syndrome has been associated with the administration of ART and occurs in ~10% of HIV-infected TB patients. Usually developing 1–3 months after initiation of ART, IRIS is more common among patients with advanced immunosuppression and extrapulmonary TB. "Unmasking IRIS" may develop after the initiation of ART in patients with undiagnosed subclinical TB. The earlier ART is started and the lower the baseline CD4+ T-cell count, the greater the risk of IRIS. Death due to IRIS is relatively infrequent and occurs mainly among patients who have a high preexisting mortality risk. The presumed pathogenesis of IRIS consists of an immune response that is elicited by antigens released as bacilli are killed during effective chemotherapy and that is temporally associated with improving immune function. There is no diagnostic test for IRIS, and its confirmation relies heavily upon case definitions incorporating clinical and laboratory data; a variety of case definitions have been suggested. The first priority in the management of a possible case of IRIS is to ensure that the clinical syndrome does not represent a failure of TB treatment or the development of another infection. Mild paradoxical reactions can be managed with symptom-based treatment and do not worsen outcomes of treatment for TB. However, IRIS can result in serious neurologic complications or death in patients with CNS TB. Therefore, ART should not be initiated during the first 8 weeks of TB treatment in patients with TB meningitis. Glucocorticoids have been used for severe paradoxical reactions; prednisolone given for 4 weeks at a low dosage (1.5 mg/kg per day for 2 weeks and half that dose for the remaining 2 weeks) has reduced the need for hospitalization and therapeutic procedures and has hastened alleviation of symptoms, as reflected by Karnofsky performance scores, quality-of-life assessments, radiographic response, and C-reactive protein levels. The effectiveness of glucocorticoids in alleviating the symptoms of IRIS is probably linked to suppression of proinflammatory cytokine concentrations as these medications reduce serum concentrations of IL-6, IL-10, IL-12p40, TNF-α, IFN-γ, and IFN-γ-inducible protein 10. Recommendations for the prevention and treatment of TB in HIV-infected individuals are provided below.

DIAGNOSIS

The key to the early diagnosis of TB is a high index of suspicion. Diagnosis is not difficult in persons belonging to high-risk populations who present with typical symptoms and a classic chest radiograph showing upper-lobe infiltrates with cavities (Fig. 178-6). On the other hand, the diagnosis can easily be missed in an elderly nursing-home resident or a teenager with a focal infiltrate. Often, the diagnosis is first entertained when the chest radiograph of a patient being evaluated for respiratory symptoms is abnormal. If the patient has no complicating medical conditions that cause immunosuppression, the chest radiograph may show typical upper-lobe infiltrates with cavitation (Fig. 178-6). The longer the delay between the onset of symptoms and the diagnosis, the more likely is the finding of cavitary disease. In contrast, immunosuppressed patients, including those with HIV co-infection, may have "atypical" findings on CXR—e.g., lower-zone infiltrates without cavity formation—or interstitial disease only.

The several approaches to the diagnosis of TB require, above all, a well-organized microbiology laboratory network with an appropriate distribution of tasks at different levels of the health care system. Besides clinical assessment and radiography, screening and referral are the principal tasks at the peripheral and community levels. Diagnosis at a secondary level (e.g., a traditional district hospital in a high-incidence setting) can be accomplished nowadays through real-time automated nucleic acid amplification technology (e.g., the Xpert MTB/RIF assay, which also allows detection of drug resistance) or through traditional AFB microscopy, where new tools have not yet been introduced. At a tertiary level, additional technology is necessary, including molecular tests, rapid culture, and DST.

■ NUCLEIC ACID AMPLIFICATION TECHNOLOGY

Several test systems based on amplification of mycobacterial nucleic acid have become available in the past few years and are now the preferred first-line diagnostic tests. These tests are progressively replacing smear microscopy, as they ensure rapid confirmation of all types of TB. One system that permits rapid diagnosis of TB with high specificity and sensitivity (approaching that of liquid culture) is the fully automated, real-time nucleic acid amplification technology known as the Xpert MTB/RIF assay. Xpert MTB/RIF can simultaneously detect TB and rifampin resistance in <2 h and has minimal biosafety and training requirements. Therefore, it can be housed in nonconventional laboratory settings as long as a stable and uninterrupted power supply can be assured. The WHO recommends its use worldwide as the first-line diagnostic test in all adults and children with signs or symptoms of active TB. Given the test's high sensitivity, the WHO also recommends its use as the initial diagnostic test for people living with HIV in whom TB is suspected. In the diagnosis of pulmonary TB, this test has an overall sensitivity of 85% reaching 98% among AFB-positive cases and ~70% among AFB-negative specimens; its specificity is 98%. When compared to phenotypic drug susceptibility testing for simultaneous detection of rifampin resistance, Xpert MTB/RIF has an overall sensitivity of 96% and a specificity of 98%. The newer Xpert MTB/RIF Ultra assay (Ultra), which uses the same GeneXpert diagnostic platform, has an overall sensitivity of 90% including "trace calls" (i.e., the "noise" produced by detection of DNA from nonviable bacilli) as positive with the greatest increases among smear-negative, culture-positive cases (+17%) and among HIV-infected persons (+12%). If "trace calls" are excluded, sensitivity decreases to 86%. Because of this greater sensitivity and the capacity to also detect nonviable bacilli, the new Ultra cartridge has 2% lower specificity than the original test. However, excluding "trace calls," specificity increases to 98%. Among people with HIV co-infection, Ultra sensitivity is 88% and specificity 95%. Sensitivity and specificity for detection of rifampin resistance by Ultra are 94% and 99%, respectively, similar to those by the Xpert MTB/RIF assay.

In the diagnosis of extrapulmonary TB, Xpert MTB/RIF and Ultra should be the initial test applied to CSF from patients in whom TB meningitis is suspected as well as a replacement test (preferable to conventional microscopy, culture, and histopathology) for selected nonrespiratory specimens—those obtained by gastric lavage, fine-needle aspiration, or pleural or other biopsies. Sensitivity varies according to specimen type being the lowest in pleural fluid (50% with Xpert MTB/RIF and 71% with Ultra) and the highest in synovial fluid (97%) and lymph node biopsy (100% with Ultra). "Trace calls" in specimens from persons with extrapulmonary TB, as well as for HIV-infected patients and children, should be considered true positives, given the high risk of severe morbidity and premature death, while among other cases they warrant additional tests to confirm the diagnosis of TB and prevent overtreatment. Among patients with a recent history of TB, "trace calls" may represent false positivity due to DNA from dead bacilli under degradation.

Truenat MTB and MTC Plus are two newly introduced rapid molecular tests with a sensitivity of 83% and 89%, respectively, if compared to bacteriological culture, and with specificity of 98% and 99%, respectively. Truenat MTB-Rif Dx detects rifampin resistance with a sensitivity of 93% and a specificity of 95%. These rapid tests, developed in India by MolBio Diagnostics Pvt Ltd Goa, have accuracy comparable to that of Xpert MTB/RIF and Ultra. Being portable and battery-operated, they can be used in the most peripheral care settings. New high-throughput automated platforms for TB diagnosis and drug-resistant variants are becoming available (Abbott RealTime MTB and RIF/INH, FluoroType MTBDR, BD Max MDR-TB). These platforms are suitable for centralized laboratories and have the advantage of processing a large number of samples in a reasonable time. Sensitivity is higher than 91% and specificity ranges from 97 to 100%. Head-to-head studies with Xpert MTB/RIF have shown comparable performance. Another available molecular test for detection of *M. tuberculosis* is based on the loop-mediated isothermal amplification (LAMP) temperature-independent technology that amplifies DNA, is relatively simple to use, and is interpreted through a visual display. The TB-LAMP assay (LoopampTM *M. tuberculosis* complex detection kit; Eiken Chemical Company, Japan) requires minimal laboratory infrastructure and has few biosafety requirements. It may be used as a replacement for sputum-smear microscopy for the diagnosis of adult pulmonary TB and as a follow-up test to smear microscopy for the further investigation of smear-negative specimens from adults with suspected pulmonary TB. The TB-LAMP assay should not replace rapid molecular tests that detect both TB and rifampin resistance, and its usefulness in HIV-infected people in whom TB is suspected remains unclear.

AFB MICROSCOPY

In many low- and middle-income settings, a presumptive diagnosis is still commonly based on the finding of AFB on microscopic examination of a diagnostic specimen, such as a smear of expectorated sputum or of tissue (e.g., a lymph node biopsy). Although inexpensive, AFB microscopy has relatively low sensitivity (40–60%) in culture-confirmed cases of pulmonary TB. The traditional method—light microscopy of specimens stained with Ziehl-Neelsen basic fuchsin dyes—is satisfactory, although time consuming and operator dependent. Most modern laboratories processing large numbers of diagnostic specimens use auramine–rhodamine staining and fluorescence microscopy; this approach is more sensitive than the Ziehl-Neelsen method. However, it is expensive because it requires high-cost mercury vapor light sources and a darkroom. Less expensive light-emitting diode (LED) fluorescence microscopes are now recommended by the WHO as the microscopy tool of choice. They are as sensitive as—or more sensitive than—traditional fluorescence microscopes. As a result, conventional light and fluorescence microscopes are being replaced with this more recent technology, especially in developing countries. For patients with signs or symptoms of pulmonary TB, it has been recommended that one or two sputum specimens, preferably collected early in the morning, should be submitted to the laboratory for AFB smear and mycobacterial culture. If tissue is obtained, it is critical that the portion of the specimen intended for culture not be put in preservation fluid such as formaldehyde. The use of AFB microscopy in examining urine or gastric lavage fluid is limited by the low numbers of organisms, which can cause false-negative results, or the presence of commensal mycobacteria, which can cause false-positive results.

MYCOBACTERIAL CULTURE

Definitive diagnosis depends on the isolation and identification of *M. tuberculosis* from a clinical specimen. Commercial liquid-culture systems such as the Mycobacterial Growth Indicator Tube (MGIT) system (Becton Dickinson; Franklin Lakes, NJ) are recommended by the WHO as the reference standard for culture. The MGIT system uses a fluorescent compound sensitive to the presence of oxygen dissolved in the liquid medium. The appearance of fluorescence, detected by fluorometric technology, indicates active growth of mycobacteria. MGIT cultures usually become positive after a period ranging from 10 days to 2–3 weeks; the tubes are read weekly until the eighth week of incubation before the result is declared to be negative. Specimens may also be inoculated onto egg- or agar-based medium (e.g., Löwenstein-Jensen or Middlebrook 7H10 or 7H11) and incubated at 37°C (under 5% CO_2 for Middlebrook medium). Because most species of mycobacteria, including *M. tuberculosis*, grow slowly, 4–8 weeks may be required before growth is detected on these conventional culture media. Although *M. tuberculosis* may be identified presumptively on the basis of growth time and colony pigmentation and morphology, a variety of biochemical tests have traditionally been used to speciate mycobacterial isolates. In modern, well-equipped laboratories, commercial liquid culture for isolation and species identification by molecular methods or high-pressure liquid chromatography of mycolic acids has replaced isolation on solid media and identification by biochemical tests. A low-cost, rapid immunochromatographic lateral-flow assay based on detection of MTP64 antigen may also be used for species identification of the *M. tuberculosis* complex in culture isolates. These new methods, which are increasingly used in limited-resource settings, have decreased the time required for bacteriologic confirmation of TB to 2–3 weeks.

DRUG SUSCEPTIBILITY TESTING

Universal DST is considered by the WHO as the current standard of care for all TB patients and should consist of DST to at least rifampin for all initial isolates of *M. tuberculosis*, as rifampin resistance is an excellent proxy for MDR-TB diagnosis. Susceptibility testing is particularly important if one or more risk factors for drug resistance are identified or if the patient either fails to respond to initial therapy or has a relapse after the completion of treatment (see "Treatment Failure and Relapse," below). In addition, expanded and rapid susceptibility testing for isoniazid and key second-line anti-TB drugs (especially the fluoroquinolones and the injectable drugs) is mandatory when RR-TB is found in order to guide selection of the appropriate treatment regimens. Susceptibility testing may be conducted directly by molecular techniques (with the clinical specimen) or indirectly (with mycobacterial cultures) on solid or liquid medium. Results are obtained rapidly by direct susceptibility testing on liquid medium, with an average reporting time of 3 weeks. With indirect testing on solid medium, results may not be available for ≥8 weeks. Highly reliable genotypic methods for the rapid identification of genetic mutations in gene regions known to be associated with resistance to rifampin (such as those in *rpo*B) and isoniazid (such as those in *kat*G and *inh*A) have been developed and are being widely implemented for screening of patients at increased risk of drug-resistant TB. Apart from the Xpert MTB/RIF, Xpert MTB/RIF Ultra, and Truenat MTB-Rif Dx assays, which, as mentioned above, effectively detect rifampin resistance, the most widely used tests are molecular line probe assays (LPAs). LPAs are a family of DNA strip-based tests capable of detecting bacterial DNA and identifying drug resistance-associated mutations. After extraction of DNA from *M. tuberculosis* isolates or from clinical specimens, the resistance gene regions are amplified by polymerase chain reaction (PCR), and labeled and probe-hybridized PCR products are detected by colorimetric development. This assay reveals the presence of *M. tuberculosis* as well as mutations in target resistance-gene regions. Given the rapidity and accuracy of commercially available LPAs, the WHO recommends that they (rather than phenotypic culture-based tests) may be used to detect resistance to isoniazid and rifampin when patients have sputum smear–positive specimens or a cultured isolate of *M. tuberculosis*. These recommendations do not eliminate the need for conventional culture-based testing to identify resistance to other drugs and to monitor emergence of additional drug resistance. A similar approach has been developed for second-line anti-TB drugs, such as the fluoroquinolones and the injectable drugs kanamycin, amikacin, and capreomycin. Therefore, second-line LPAs (instead of phenotypic culture-based DST) are now recommended by the WHO as the initial test for rapid detection of resistance to the fluoroquinolones or the second-line injectable drugs in isolates from patients with confirmed RR-TB or MDR-TB. As with first-line LPAs, these recommendations do not eliminate the need for conventional phenotypic, culture-based testing to identify resistance to other drugs and to monitor for the emergence of additional resistance. Detection of pyrazinamide resistance is important among persons with MDR/RR-TB. The WHO has recently recommended the use of a LPA with reverse hybridization-based technology in culture isolates rather than phenotypic culture-based DST. Finally, a few noncommercial, inexpensive culture and susceptibility testing methods (e.g., microscopically observed drug susceptibility, nitrate reductase, and colorimetric redox indicator assays) have been used in resource-limited settings. Their use is restricted to national reference laboratories with proven proficiency and adequate external quality control as an interim solution while genotypic or automated liquid-culture technology is introduced.

Whole genome sequencing (WGS) of *M. tuberculosis* provides comprehensive information on mutations conferring resistance and is a promising alternative to existing phenotypic and molecular DST methods. Recent studies have confirmed the potential for WGS to identify genetic polymorphisms that reliably predict drug susceptibility phenotype within a clinically relevant timeframe and a comparable cost range. The clinical use of WGS, however, has been hampered by the requirement for a culture sample before DNA processing. Recently, amplification and sequencing of relevant genomic targets directly from sputum samples have been successfully tested and targeted new-generation sequencing (tNGS) is now a possible option. Evidence is accumulating supporting the clinical application of NGS-based diagnostic systems for TB to replace traditional diagnostic tests in the future.

RADIOGRAPHIC PROCEDURES

CXR is a rapid imaging technique that has historically been used as a primary tool to detect pulmonary TB. CXR has high sensitivity but poor specificity. Although TB may often present with typical patterns strongly suggesting the disease, some abnormalities seen in TB are also present in several other lung conditions. The initial suspicion of pulmonary TB is often based on abnormal CXR findings in a patient undergoing triage for respiratory symptoms. The presence of lesions suggestive of TB should prompt bacteriologic investigations in all cases, without exception. Although the "classic" picture is that of upper-lobe disease with infiltrates and cavities (Fig. 178-6), virtually any radiographic pattern—from a normal film or a solitary pulmonary nodule to diffuse alveolar infiltrates in a patient with adult respiratory distress syndrome—may be seen. In the era of HIV/AIDS, no radiographic pattern can be considered pathognomonic, but CXR can assist in diagnosing TB or ruling it out before initiation of any preventive treatment. CXR is also helpful as a screening test used preceding rapid molecular assays to improve their predictive value. Digital CXR technology, which allows display of images in a digital format on a computer screen instead of on x-ray film, offers several advantages: the procedure time is reduced, the running costs are lower, the imaging is of superior quality, and telemedicine assistance is available, including computer-aided detection (CAD) and interpretation of findings using software programs that analyze digital imaging for abnormalities compatible with TB. However, the limited evidence available suggests that while sensitivity may be high, specificity is variable. A recent systematic review of CAD studies concluded that the diagnostic accuracy of this technology is still limited and that generalizability to low-prevalence settings is still uncertain.

CT (Fig. 178-7) may be useful in interpreting questionable findings on plain CXR and in diagnosing some forms of extrapulmonary TB (e.g., intrabdominal disease, Pott's disease; Fig. 178-10). A recent study has shown the potential of positron emission tomography combined with CT for detection of subclinical disease that may be progressing toward full-blown TB in HIV-infected people. MRI is useful in the diagnosis of bone lesions and intracranial TB.

ADDITIONAL DIAGNOSTIC PROCEDURES

Other diagnostic tests may be used when pulmonary TB is suspected. Sputum induction by ultrasonic nebulization of hypertonic saline may be useful for patients who cannot produce a sputum specimen spontaneously. Frequently, patients with radiographic abnormalities that are consistent with other diagnoses (e.g., bronchogenic carcinoma) undergo fiberoptic bronchoscopy with bronchial brushings and endobronchial or transbronchial biopsy of the lesion. Bronchoalveolar lavage of a lung segment containing an abnormality may also be performed. In all cases, it is essential that specimens be submitted for molecular testing with the Xpert MTB/RIF assay, mycobacterial culture, and AFB smear. For the diagnosis of primary pulmonary TB in children, who often do not expectorate sputum, induced sputum specimens and specimens from early-morning gastric lavage may yield positive results in the Xpert MTB/RIF assay or on culture.

Invasive diagnostic procedures are indicated for patients with suspected extrapulmonary TB. In addition to testing of specimens from involved sites (e.g., CSF for tuberculous meningitis, pleural fluid and biopsy samples for pleural disease), biopsy and culture of bone marrow and liver tissue have a good diagnostic yield in disseminated (miliary) TB, particularly in HIV-infected patients, who also have a high frequency of positive blood cultures. Xpert MTB/RIF should always be the initial diagnostic test in patients where TB meningitis is suspected; any positive results should prompt immediate treatment initiation, while negative results should be followed up by additional testing. In some cases, the results of culture or Xpert MTB/RIF are negative but a clinical diagnosis of TB is supported by consistent epidemiologic evidence (e.g., a history of close contact with an infectious patient) and a compatible clinical and radiographic response to treatment. In the United States and other industrialized countries with low rates of TB, some patients with limited abnormalities on CXR and sputum positive for AFB are infected with nontuberculous mycobacteria, most commonly organisms of the *M. avium* complex or *M. kansasii* (**Chap. 180**). Factors favoring the diagnosis of nontuberculous mycobacterial disease over TB include an absence of risk factors for TB and the presence of underlying chronic pulmonary disease.

Patients with HIV-associated TB pose several diagnostic problems (see "HIV-Associated TB," above). HIV-infected patients with sputum culture–positive, AFB-positive TB may present with a normal chest radiograph. The Xpert MTB/RIF assay is the preferred rapid diagnostic test in this population of patients because of its simplicity and increased sensitivity (~60–70% among AFB-negative, culture-positive cases and 97–98% among AFB-positive cases). With the advent of ART, the occurrence of disseminated *M. avium* complex disease that can be confused with TB has become much less common. A test based on the detection of mycobacterial lipoarabinomannan antigen in urine has emerged as a potentially useful point-of-care test for TB in HIV-infected persons with low CD4+ T-cell counts. The lateral-flow urine lipoarabinomannan assay can be performed manually and read by eye. After a systematic review of the evidence, the WHO recommends that this assay be used to assist in the diagnosis of TB in HIV-positive adults who have signs and symptoms of TB and a CD4+ T-cell count of ≤100 cells/μL or in HIV-positive patients who are seriously ill regardless of CD4+ T-cell count or with an unknown CD4+ count. The WHO recommends that this test not be used, pending information on recent promising technological test advances, for TB diagnosis or as a screening test for TB in any other patient categories. One limitation of the available lipoarabinomannan point-of-care test, AlereLAM (Alere Determine TB LAM Ag), is the low sensitivity (45%). A novel assay, FujiLAM (SILVAMP TB LAM) has recently shown a sensitivity of 70%.

SEROLOGIC AND OTHER DIAGNOSTIC TESTS FOR ACTIVE TB

Several serologic tests based on detection of antibodies to a variety of mycobacterial antigens have been carefully assessed by the WHO and found not to be useful as diagnostic aids because of their low sensitivity and specificity and their poor reproducibility. In 2011, after a rigorous evaluation of these tests, the WHO issued a "negative" recommendation in order to prevent their abuse in the private sector of many resource-limited countries. Various methods aimed at detection of mycobacterial antigens in diagnostic specimens are being investigated but are limited at present by low sensitivity. Determinations of adenosine deaminase and IFN-γ levels in pleural fluid may be useful adjunctive tests in the diagnosis of pleural TB; their utility in the diagnosis of other forms of extrapulmonary TB (e.g., pericardial, peritoneal, and meningeal) is less clear.

BIOMARKERS

In view of the limitations of current diagnostics, research on TB biomarkers and multiple marker biosignatures that could be used as a point-of-care test for disease or triage is a high priority and has been crystallized in well-defined target product profiles by the WHO. Recent systematic reviews revealed that promising host biomarkers under study, such as antibodies, cytokines, chemokines, and RNA signatures, by far exceed pathogen biomarkers that can be obtained from urine or blood. However, currently, candidate biomarkers require additional studies to fully assess their performance.

DIAGNOSIS OF *M. TUBERCULOSIS* INFECTION

Two tests currently exist for identification of individuals with TB infection: the TST and IGRA, both of which measure host immunological response to TB antigens. These tests have limitations, especially in settings or populations with high TB and/or HIV prevalence.

Tuberculin Skin Testing In 1891, Robert Koch discovered that components of *M. tuberculosis* in a concentrated liquid-culture medium, subsequently named "old tuberculin," were capable of eliciting a skin reaction when injected subcutaneously into patients with TB. In 1932, Seibert and Munday purified this product by ammonium sulfate precipitation to produce an active protein fraction known as *tuberculin purified protein derivative* (*PPD*). In 1941, PPD-S, developed by Seibert and Glenn, was chosen as the international standard. Later, the WHO and UNICEF sponsored large-scale production of a master batch of PPD (RT23) and made it available for general use. The greatest limitation of PPD is its lack of mycobacterial species specificity, a property due to the large number of proteins in this product that are highly conserved in the various species. In addition, subjectivity of the skin-reaction interpretation that is dependent on the operator, deterioration of the product, and batch-to-batch variations limit the usefulness of PPD.

The skin test with tuberculin PPD (TST) is most widely used in screening for TB infection. It probably measures the response to antigenic stimulation by T cells that reside in the skin rather than the response of recirculating memory T cells. The test is of limited value in the diagnosis of active TB because of its relatively low sensitivity and specificity and its inability to discriminate between TB infection and active disease. False-negative reactions are common in immunosuppressed patients and in those with overwhelming TB. False-positive reactions may be caused by infections with nontuberculous mycobacteria (**Chap. 180**) and by BCG vaccination. A repeated TST can produce larger reaction sizes due to either boosting or true conversion. The "boosting phenomenon" is a spurious TST conversion resulting from boosting of reactivity on a subsequent TST 1–5 weeks after the initial test. Distinguishing boosting from true conversion is difficult yet important and can be based on clinical and epidemiologic considerations. For instance, true conversions are likely after BCG vaccination in a previously TST-negative person or in a close contact of an infectious patient.

IFN-γ Release Assays Two in vitro assays that measure T-cell release of IFN-γ in response to stimulation with the highly TB-specific RD1-encoded antigens ESAT-6 and CFP-10 were introduced in the early 2000s and are commercially available. The T-SPOT.TB test (Oxford Immunotec; Oxford, United Kingdom) is an enzyme-linked immunospot assay, and the QuantiFERON-TB Gold test (Qiagen GmbH; Hilden, Germany) is a whole-blood enzyme-linked immunosorbent assay for measurement of IFN-γ. The QuantiFERON-TB Gold In-Tube (QFT-GIT) assay, which facilitates blood collection and initial incubation, also contains another specific antigen, TB7.7. These tests mainly measure the response of recirculating memory CD4+ T cells—normally part of a reservoir in the spleen, bone marrow, and lymph nodes—to persisting bacilli-producing antigenic signals. However, CD8+ cells can also release IFN-γ in vitro in response to stimulation with TB antigens, and they seem to do so especially in the early phase of infection and in the phase of reactivation. Therefore, a new version of the QFT-GIT assay, called QuantiFERON-TB Gold Plus (QFT-Plus), has been developed that operates through two antigen tubes: TB1, containing long peptides from ESAT-6 and CFP-10 and inducing a CD4+ T-cell response, and TB2 that also contains shorter peptides stimulating CD8+ cells. The QFT-Plus may have an increased sensitivity, compared to QFT-GID, but this conclusion needs confirmation.

In settings or population groups with low TB and HIV burdens, IGRAs have previously been reported to be more specific than the TST as a result of less cross-reactivity with BCG vaccination and sensitization by nontuberculous mycobacteria; i.e., RD1 antigens are not encoded in the genome of either BCG strains or most nontuberculous mycobacteria. Recent studies suggest that IGRAs may not perform well in serial testing (e.g., among health care workers) and that interpretation of results depends on cutoff values used to define positivity. Potential advantages of IGRAs include logistical convenience, the need for fewer patient visits to complete testing, and the avoidance of somewhat subjective measurements (e.g., skin induration). However, IGRAs require that blood be drawn and then delivered to the laboratory in a timely fashion. IGRAs also require that testing be performed by specially trained technicians in a laboratory setting. These requirements pose challenges similar to those faced with the TST, including cold-chain requirements and batch-to-batch variations. Because of higher specificity and greater availability of resources, IGRAs have usually replaced the TST for TB infection diagnosis in low-incidence, high-income settings. However, in high-incidence TB and HIV settings and population groups, evidence about the performance and usefulness of IGRAs is still limited, and cost considerations may currently limit wider use.

A number of national guidelines on the use of IGRAs for TB infection testing have been issued. In the United States, an IGRA is preferred to the TST for most persons over the age of 5 years who are being screened for TB infection. However, for individuals at high risk of progression to active TB (e.g., HIV-infected persons), either test—or, to optimize sensitivity, both tests—may be used. Because of the paucity of data on the use of IGRAs in children, the TST is preferred for TB infection testing of children aged <5 years. In Canada and some European countries, a two-step approach for those with positive TSTs—i.e., an initial TST followed by an IGRA—is often recommended. However, a TST may boost an IGRA response if the interval between the two tests exceeds 3 days.

In conclusion, both the TST and IGRA, although useful as diagnostic aids, are imperfect tests for TB infection: while they can identify infected persons, they have low predictive value in identifying individuals with the highest risk of progression toward disease, cannot differentiate between active TB and TB infection, cannot distinguish new infections from reinfections, and display reduced sensitivity in immunocompromised patients.

TREATMENT

Tuberculosis

The two main aims of TB treatment are (1) to prevent morbidity and death by curing TB while preventing recurrences and emergence of drug resistance, and (2) to interrupt transmission by rendering patients noninfectious to others. Chemotherapy for TB became possible with the discovery of streptomycin in 1943. Randomized clinical trials clearly indicated that the administration of streptomycin to patients with chronic TB reduced mortality rates and led to cure in the majority of cases. However, monotherapy with streptomycin was soon associated with the development of resistance to this drug and the resulting failure of treatment. With the introduction into clinical practice of para-aminosalicylic acid (PAS) and isoniazid, it became axiomatic in the early 1950s that cure of TB required the concomitant administration of at least two agents to which the organism was susceptible. Furthermore, early clinical trials demonstrated that a long period of treatment—i.e., 12–24 months—was required to prevent recurrence. The introduction of rifampin in the early 1970s heralded the era of effective short-course chemotherapy, with a treatment duration of <12 months. The discovery that pyrazinamide, which was first used in the 1950s, augmented the potency of isoniazid/rifampin regimens led to the use of a 6-month course of this triple-drug regimen as standard therapy. Streptomycin was added as the fourth drug mainly to prevent the emergence of drug resistance. These four drugs (with streptomycin replaced by ethambutol) still form the basis of the optimal treatment regimen for rifampin-susceptible TB. The emergence of drug-resistant TB in the 1990s prompted attempts to standardize the approach to treatment of this condition mainly on the basis of expert opinion. This event has also stimulated research on and development of new anti-TB agents in the past 15 years. In 2013 and 2014, respectively, bedaquiline and delamanid—the first two drugs specifically developed for TB during nearly half a century—received conditional approval by the US Food and Drug Administration (FDA) and other drug-regulatory authorities; approval was based on the results of phase 2b clinical trials in which the drugs were added to the 18- to 24-month WHO-recommended regimen for MDR-TB. Bedaquiline and delamanid are now being used increasingly for treatment of MDR-TB under specific conditions. In 2019, another new drug, pretomanid, was approved by the FDA as part of a new combination regimen with bedaquiline and linezolid for patients with MDR-TB caused by a strain with additional resistance to a fluoroquinolone or a second-line injectable drug, or were intolerant of therapy, or in whom treatment had failed.

DRUGS

Four major drugs are considered first-line agents for the treatment of TB: isoniazid, rifampin, pyrazinamide, and ethambutol. **Table 178-2** presents currently recommended dosages in adults and children. Some studies have suggested increased effectiveness when isoniazid, rifampin, and pyrazinamide are given at higher dosage; thus if these findings are confirmed, dosages may be revised in the future. These drugs are well absorbed after oral administration, with peak serum levels at 2–4 h and nearly complete elimination within 24 h. Isoniazid and rifampin, two key anti-TB drugs, are recommended on the basis of their bactericidal activity (i.e., their ability to rapidly reduce the number of viable organisms and render patients noninfectious). All four agents are recommended in light of their sterilizing activity (i.e., their ability to sterilize the affected tissues, measured in terms of the ability to prevent relapses) and the lowered risk that drug-resistant mutant bacilli will be selected when the drugs are used in combination. Two additional rifamycins, rifapentine and rifabutin, are also available; however, their level of cross-resistance with rifampin is high. For a detailed discussion of the drugs used for the treatment of TB, see **Chap. 181.**

Because of a lower degree of effectiveness and tolerability, several classes of second-line drugs are generally used only for the treatment of patients with drug-resistant TB. These agents have previously been classified in various manners to facilitate a standardized approach to their use. In the latest WHO guidance on the treatment of MDR-TB, they are now grouped in three ranked categories for the purpose of designing more individualized regimens of 18–20 months' duration. Group A drugs include three classes of oral agents: the fluoroquinolones levofloxacin and moxifloxacin; the oxazolidinone linezolid; and the recently introduced diarylquinoline bedaquiline, which was granted accelerated approval by the FDA in late 2012. Group B drugs include two other oral agents: clofazimine and cycloserine (or its analogue terizidone). Group C drugs include the nitroimidazole delamanid; imipenem-cilastatin or meropenem; the injectable aminoglycosides amikacin and streptomycin (the latter formerly a first-line agent, now rarely used for drug-resistant TB because resistance levels worldwide are high and it is more toxic than the other drugs in the same class); ethionamide or prothionamide; and PAS. In addition, the first-line anti-TB drugs ethambutol and pyrazinamide (both included in Group C) as well as high-dose isoniazid (only for the shorter regimen; see below) are used for MDR-TB treatment. Information about drugs used in the treatment of drug-resistant TB (including dosages) can be found in the following WHO Handbook: *http://apps.who.int/iris/bitstream/10665/130918/1/9789241548809_eng.pdf.* Recent information from the phase 3 clinical trial of delamanid (a drug granted accelerated approval by the European Medicines Agency [EMA] in late 2013) added to an optimized longer WHO background regimen shows that treatment success is not different from that obtained with the addition of placebo. The future role of delamanid as a replacement drug in MDR-TB treatment remains to be assessed. The new classification scheme excludes the second-line injectable aminoglycoside kanamycin and the polypeptide capreomycin. Amithiozone, which has been associated with severe and at times fatal skin reactions—including Stevens-Johnson syndrome—among HIV-infected patients, is no longer recommended. Finally, amoxicillin–clavulanic acid is recommended only as an adjunct to carbapenems.

TABLE 178-2 Recommended Dosage[a] for Initial Treatment of Tuberculosis in Adults and Children

	DAILY DOSE	
DRUG	ADULT	PEDIATRIC
Isoniazid	5 mg/kg, max 300 mg	10 (7–15) mg/kg, max 300 mg
Rifampin	10 mg/kg, max 600 mg	15 (10–20) mg/kg, max 600 mg
Pyrazinamide	25 mg/kg, max 2 g	35 (30–40) mg/kg
Ethambutol[b]	15 mg/kg	20 (15–25) mg/kg

[a]The duration of treatment with individual drugs varies by regimen, as detailed in Table 178-3. [b]In certain settings, streptomycin (15 mg/kg daily, with a maximal dose of 1 g; or 25–30 mg/kg thrice weekly, with a maximal dose of 1.5 g) can replace ethambutol in the initial phase of treatment. However, streptomycin generally is no longer considered a first-line drug.

Source: Based on recommendations of the American Thoracic Society/Infectious Diseases Society of America/Centers for Disease Control and Prevention and the World Health Organization.

REGIMENS

Standard regimens are divided into an intensive (bactericidal) phase and a continuation (sterilizing) phase. During the intensive phase, the majority of tubercle bacilli are killed, symptoms resolve, and usually the patient becomes noninfectious. The continuation phase is required to eliminate persisting mycobacteria and prevent relapse.

The treatment regimen of choice for virtually all forms of drug-susceptible TB in adults consists of a 2-month initial (intensive) phase of isoniazid, rifampin, pyrazinamide, and ethambutol followed by a 4-month continuation phase of isoniazid and rifampin (**Table 178-3**). This regimen can cure TB in >90% of patients. In children, most forms of TB in the absence of HIV infection or suspected isoniazid resistance can be safely treated without ethambutol in the intensive phase. Treatment should be given daily throughout the course. Systematic reviews have demonstrated that the use of an intermittent thrice-weekly regimen in the intensive phase is associated with increased risk of treatment failure, relapse, and acquisition of drug resistance. Furthermore, a thrice-weekly regimen in the continuation phase only has also been associated with increased rates of failure and relapse, while a twice-weekly regimen in the continuation phase increased the risk of acquisition of drug resistance as well as rates of failure and relapse. Therefore, the WHO now recommends that TB treatment in all cases be administered daily. The 2016 guidelines by the ATS, the CDC, and the IDSA, while recommending daily administration of drugs, include a provision for use of intermittent thrice-weekly supervised regimens among patients who are not infected with HIV and are at low risk of relapse (i.e., have pulmonary TB caused by drug-susceptible

TABLE 178-3 Recommended Antituberculosis Treatment Regimens

	INITIAL PHASE		CONTINUATION PHASE	
INDICATION	DURATION, MONTHS	DRUGS	DURATION, MONTHS	DRUGS
New smear- or culture-positive cases	2	HRZE[a,b]	4	HR[a,c]
New culture-negative cases	2	HRZE[a]	4	HR[a,d]
Pregnancy	2	HRE[e]	7	HR
Relapses and treatment default[f]	← Tailored according to rapid drug susceptibility testing →			
Failures[f]	← Tailored according to rapid drug susceptibility testing →			
Resistance (or intolerance) to H	Throughout (6)	RZEQ		
Resistance (or intolerance) to R	← Same as for MDR-TB; see below →			
MDR-TB (resistance to at least H + R)	← See Tables 178-4 and 178-5 →			
XDR-TB	← See Table 178-4 →			
Intolerance to Z	2	HRE	7	HR

[a]All drugs should be given daily. [b]A 4-month regimen of 8 weeks of once-daily rifapentine, isoniazid, pyrazinamide and moxifloxacin followed by 9 weeks of once-daily rifapentine, isoniazid, and moxifloxacin is a possible alternative. [c]A clinical trial showed that HIV-negative patients with noncavitary pulmonary tuberculosis who have negative sputum AFB smears after the initial phase of treatment can be given once-weekly rifapentine/isoniazid in the continuation phase. However, this regimen is rarely used. [d]The American Thoracic Society, the Centers for Disease Control and Prevention, and the Infectious Diseases Society of America suggest that a 2-month continuation phase could be used in HIV-seronegative patients with sputum smear–negative and culture-negative TB. [e]The 6-month regimen with pyrazinamide can probably be used safely during pregnancy and is recommended by the WHO and the International Union Against Tuberculosis and Lung Disease. If pyrazinamide is not included in the initial treatment regimen, the minimal duration of therapy is 9 months. [f]The availability of rapid molecular methods to identify drug resistance allows initiation of a proper regimen at the start of treatment.

Abbreviations: E, ethambutol; H, isoniazid; MDR-TB, multidrug-resistant tuberculosis; Q, a quinolone antibiotic; R, rifampin; WHO, World Health Organization; XDR-TB, extensively drug-resistant tuberculosis; Z, pyrazinamide.

organisms that, at the start of treatment, is noncavitary and/or sputum smear–negative). The same guidelines suggest that a 4-month regimen consisting of isoniazid, rifampin, pyrazinamide, and ethambutol may be adequate for treatment of HIV-negative adults with sputum smear–negative and culture-negative pulmonary TB (i.e., paucibacillary TB).

A continuation phase of once-weekly rifapentine and isoniazid is effective in HIV-seronegative patients without cavitation on CXR. In general, however, this regimen should be used with great caution. Patients with cavitary pulmonary TB and delayed sputum-culture conversion (i.e., those who remain culture-positive at 2 months) should be retested immediately for drug-resistant TB, and a change of regimen should be considered. A full course of 6 months with four-drug therapy should be performed not including interruptions of >4 weeks. In some developing countries where the ability to ensure adherence to treatment is limited, a continuation-phase regimen of daily isoniazid and ethambutol for 6 months has been used in the past. This regimen is clearly associated with a higher rate of relapse, treatment failure, and death, especially among HIV-infected patients, and is no longer recommended by the WHO. Several studies attempting to reduce treatment duration to 4 months by using fluoroquinolones (with moxifloxacin replacing ethambutol or isoniazid, or gatifloxacin replacing ethambutol) were conducted over the last decade. The main finding was that shorter (4-month) fluoroquinolone-containing regimens are associated with significantly higher rates of relapse at 18 months than the standard 6-month rifampin-containing regimen. In addition, the studies showed no reduction in adverse events with the fluoroquinolone-containing regimen and no difference in all-cause and TB-related mortality rates. Therefore, shortening of the treatment duration to 4 months through the use of fluoroquinolones has not been recommended. However, the recent Tuberculosis Trials Consortium Study 31/AIDS Clinical Trials Group A5349 (Study 31/A5349) showed that a 4-month daily regimen that included isoniazid, pyrazinamide, rifapentine at a daily dose of 1200 mg and moxifloxacin at a daily dose of 400 mg was noninferior to the standard 6-month regimen and had a similar adverse event profile. In early 2021, this option was therefore considered by the WHO as a possible alternative to the old standard provided that rigorous antibacterial stewardship is ensured especially to prevent fluoroquinolone resistance and that rifapentine becomes more widely available. Alternative regimens for patients who exhibit drug intolerance or adverse reactions are listed in Table 178-3. However, severe side effects prompting discontinuation of any of the first-line drugs and use of these alternative regimens are uncommon. To prevent isoniazid-related neuropathy, pyridoxine (10–25 mg/d) should be added to the regimen given to persons at high risk of vitamin B_6 deficiency (e.g., alcoholics; malnourished persons; pregnant and lactating women; and patients with conditions such as chronic renal failure, diabetes, and HIV infection, which are also associated with neuropathy). Finally, to facilitate absorption of rifampin, the drug should be taken on an empty stomach and without meals.

PATIENT CARE AND SUPPORT

Poor adherence to treatment is one of the most important impediments to cure. Moreover, the tubercle bacilli harbored by patients who do not fully adhere to the prescribed regimen are likely to become resistant to the drugs to which they are irregularly exposed. Both patient- and provider-related factors may affect adherence. Patient-related factors include a lack of belief that the illness is worth the cost of adherence; the existence of concomitant medical conditions (notably alcohol or substance abuse); lack of social support; fear of the stigma and discrimination associated with TB; and poverty, with attendant joblessness and homelessness. Provider-related factors that may prevent adherence include lack of support, education, and encouragement of patients and inconvenient clinical services.

A variety of interventions to increase the chances of completion of the months-long treatment course are available. First, a package of social support interventions that are complementary and not mutually exclusive, consisting of educational, psychological, and material goods and services, may enable people with TB to address hurdles to treatment adherence. Health education and counseling on the disease's seriousness and solutions and on the importance of treatment adherence until cure should be provided to all patients at the start of and throughout the course of TB therapy. Psychological support (i.e., counseling sessions or peer-group support) can be particularly relevant in the context of the stigma and discrimination often affecting people with TB and their families. Material support (e.g., food or financial support in forms such as meals, food baskets, food supplements, food vouchers, transport subsidies, living allowances, housing incentives, or financial bonuses) reduces indirect costs incurred by patients or their attendants in accessing health services and mitigates the consequences of income loss related to the disease.

Second, it is paramount that health services be arranged to meet the needs and reasonable expectations of patients. Components of optimal health services include a suitable geographic location, a schedule responsive to patients' needs, functional channels of communication between patients and their health care providers (e.g., a telephone short-messaging system, audio/video call capability, home or workplace visits), and a staff willing and competent to care for people with TB, to address their concerns, and to base the care they provide on sound ethical standards.

Third, it is crucial to offer the patient a suitable option for treatment administration that minimizes the chance of nonadherence. Such options traditionally include unsupervised, self-administered therapy; in-person directly observed therapy (DOT); and nondaily DOT (e.g., supervision not for every dose but weekly or a few times per week) at a location mutually agreed on by patient and health care provider, with supervisory responsibility delegated to a qualified person. Direct supervision of adherence is crucial in view of the lack of tools to accurately predict adherence to self-administered treatment and of the public health importance of TB. The WHO, along with the ATS, the CDC, and the IDSA, states that ideally all patients should have their therapy directly supervised, especially during the initial phase, with proper social support based on a patient-centered approach as described above. In several countries, personnel to supervise therapy are usually available through TB control programs of local public health departments, often involving members of the community who are accepted by the patient and who have been properly trained and educated by health workers to undertake the supervisory role. Direct supervision with social support has been shown to significantly increase the proportion of patients completing treatment in all settings and to lessen the chances of treatment failure, relapse, and default. In general, community- or home-based DOT is recommended over health facility–based DOT or unsupervised treatment; DOT administered by trained lay providers or health care workers is recommended over DOT administered by family members. Recently, comparison of video-observed therapy (VOT) with in-person DOT has shown similar outcomes. In a multicenter, analyst-blinded, randomized controlled superiority trial of VOT through daily remote observation using a smartphone app versus DOT done 3–5 times weekly at home, community, or clinic settings, VOT was superior to DOT in ensuring scheduled observation of drug intake. Therefore, VOT can replace DOT when Internet access is good and video communication technology (e.g., smartphones, tablets, computers) is available. The system can be appropriately organized and operated by health care providers and patients. Other digital health tools can facilitate the monitoring of adherence, including digital medication monitors; these monitors can register when the pillbox is opened, with options to emit audio signals or a short message to remind patients to take medicines. These tools are customized to the needs and preferences of the individual patient and the provider.

In addition to the above measures promoting adherence, provision of fixed-dose combination products that reduce the number of tablets the patient needs to swallow is recommended over separate drug formulations. Various fixed-dose combination products are available (e.g., isoniazid/rifampin, isoniazid/rifampin/pyrazinamide, and isoniazid/rifampin/pyrazinamide/ethambutol). Fixed-dose combinations increase patient satisfaction and minimize the likelihood of prescription error or of development of drug resistance resulting from monotherapy if a drug is out of stock or the patient prefers one drug over others. In addition, these combinations facilitate programmatic management of procurement and supply. In the past, the bioavailability of rifampin was found to be substandard in some formulations of fixed-dose combinations. Medical regulatory authorities should ensure that combination products are of good quality; however, top standards for drug quality assurance are not always operative, especially in limited-resource countries. Prescribers should be aware of this potential problem.

MONITORING TREATMENT RESPONSE AND DRUG TOXICITY

Bacteriologic evaluation through commercial liquid-culture systems (or—when liquid-culture capacity is not yet available—through smear microscopy) is essential in monitoring the response to TB treatment. In addition, the patient's weight should be monitored regularly and the drug dosage adjusted with any significant weight change. Patients with pulmonary disease should have their sputum examined monthly until cultures become negative to allow early detection of treatment failure. With the recommended 6-month standard first-line regimen, >80% of drug-susceptible TB patients will have negative sputum cultures at the end of the second month of treatment. By the end of the third month, the sputum of virtually all patients should be culture negative. In some patients, especially those with extensive cavitary disease and large numbers of organisms, AFB smear conversion may lag behind culture conversion as a result of the expectoration and microscopic visualization of dead bacilli. Therefore, as capacity is built, smear microscopy should be progressively abandoned as a monitoring tool in favor of liquid culture. As noted above, patients with cavitary disease in whom sputum culture conversion does not occur by 2 months require immediate testing or retesting for drug resistance. When a patient's sputum cultures or smears remain positive at ≥3 months despite good adherence, treatment failure caused by drug resistance is likely. The pattern of drug resistance should guide the choice of the best treatment option (see below). A sputum specimen should be collected at the end of treatment to document cure. In settings where mycobacterial cultures are not yet available, monitoring by AFB smear examination should be undertaken at 2, 5, and 6 months. Bacteriologic monitoring of patients with extrapulmonary TB is more difficult and often is not feasible. In these cases, the response to treatment must be assessed clinically with the help of medical imaging.

Monitoring of the response to chemotherapy by nucleic acid amplification technology, such as the Xpert MTB/RIF assay, is not suitable because these tests can produce positive results due to nonviable bacilli. Likewise, serial chest radiographs are not recommended because radiographic changes may lag behind bacteriologic response and are not highly sensitive. After the completion of treatment, neither sputum examination nor CXR is recommended for routine follow-up purposes. However, a chest radiograph obtained at the end of treatment may be useful for comparative purposes should the patient develop symptoms of recurrent TB months or years later. Patients should be instructed to report promptly for medical assessment if they develop any such symptoms.

During treatment, patients should also be monitored for drug toxicity. The most common adverse reaction of significance among people treated for drug-susceptible TB is hepatitis. Patients should be carefully educated about the signs and symptoms of drug-induced hepatitis (e.g., dark urine, loss of appetite, nausea) and should be instructed to discontinue treatment promptly and see their health care provider if these manifestations occur. Although biochemical monitoring is not routinely recommended, all adult patients should undergo baseline assessment of liver function (e.g., measurement of serum levels of hepatic aminotransferases and bilirubin). Older patients, those with concomitant diseases, those with a history of hepatic disease (especially hepatitis C), and those using alcohol daily should be monitored especially closely (i.e., monthly), with repeated measurements of aminotransferases, during the initial phase of treatment. Up to 20% of patients have small increases (up to three times the upper limit of normal) in serum levels of aspartate aminotransferase that are not accompanied by symptoms and are of no consequence. Suspension of treatment should be considered for patients with symptomatic hepatitis, especially when accompanied by at least a three-fold increase in serum levels of AST and/or ALT, and for patients without symptoms of hepatic injury who have marked (at least five-fold) elevations in serum levels of AST and/or ALT. Drugs should be reintroduced one at a time after liver function has returned to normal. Hypersensitivity reactions usually require the discontinuation of all drugs and rechallenge to determine which agent is the culprit. Because of the variety of regimens available, it usually is not necessary—although it is possible—to desensitize patients. Hyperuricemia and arthralgia caused by pyrazinamide can usually be managed by the administration of acetylsalicylic acid; however, pyrazinamide treatment should be stopped if the patient develops gouty arthritis. Individuals who develop autoimmune thrombocytopenia secondary to rifampin therapy should not receive the drug thereafter. Similarly, the occurrence of optic neuritis with ethambutol is an indication for permanent discontinuation of this drug. Other common manifestations of drug intolerance, such as pruritus and gastrointestinal upset, can generally be managed without the interruption of therapy. Treatment with second-line agents for drug-resistant TB is associated with a variety of adverse drug reactions that are more frequent and severe than in patients receiving first-line TB regimens (see below). The likelihood of drug–drug interactions is also higher when second-line regimens are used.

TREATMENT FAILURE AND RELAPSE

As stated above, treatment failure should be suspected when a patient's cultures (or sputum smears, when cultures are not available) remain positive after 3 months of treatment. In the management of such patients, it is imperative that the current isolate be urgently retested (or tested for the first time if, for some reason, rapid molecular susceptibility testing was not performed at the start of treatment) for susceptibility to first-line agents and, if resistance to rifampin is detected, to second-line agents as well. The treatment approach should start with molecular testing for—at the least—resistance to rifampin and isoniazid. Because results are expected to become available within a few days, changes in the regimen can be postponed until that time. However, if the patient's clinical condition is deteriorating rapidly, an earlier change in regimen may be indicated. A cardinal rule in the latter situation is always to add more than one drug, preferably two or three, at a time to a failing regimen; in practice, starting an empirical regimen for MDR-TB (see "Drug-Resistant TB," below) is warranted. The patient may continue to take isoniazid and rifampin along with these new agents pending the results of susceptibility tests.

Patients who experience a recurrence after apparently successful treatment (i.e., a relapse) are less likely to harbor drug-resistant strains than are patients in whom treatment has failed. Acquired resistance is uncommon among strains from patients in whom relapse follows the proper completion of a standard 6-month regimen. The treatment decision depends on a general assessment of the risk of drug resistance, the severity of the case, and the results of rapid susceptibility testing. Patients whose treatment has been interrupted and who have a high likelihood of MDR-TB should receive an empirical MDR-TB regimen that includes second-line agents (Table 178-3). Once drug susceptibility results are available, the regimen can be adjusted accordingly.

DRUG-RESISTANT TB

Strains of *M. tuberculosis* resistant to individual drugs arise by spontaneous point mutations in the mycobacterial genome that occur at low but predictable rates (10^{-7}–10^{-10} for the key drugs). Resistance to rifampin is associated with mutations in the *rpoB* gene in 95% of cases, that to isoniazid with mutations mainly in the *katG* gene (50–95% of cases) and the *inhA* gene promoter region (up to 45%), that to pyrazinamide in the *pncA* gene (up to 98%), that to ethambutol in the *embB* gene (50–65%), that to the fluoroquinolones in the *gyrA–gyrB* genes (75–95%), and that to the aminoglycosides mainly in the *rrs* gene (up to 80%); the C-12T mutation is the most common mutation in the *eis* promoter region associated with aminoglycoside resistance, especially in Eastern European countries. Because there is no cross-resistance among the commonly used classes of drugs, the probability that a strain will be resistant to two drug classes is the product of the probabilities of resistance to each drug class and thus is low. The development of drug-resistant TB almost invariably follows monotherapy—i.e., the failure of the health care provider to prescribe at least two drugs to which tubercle bacilli are susceptible; of the patient to absorb or take properly prescribed therapy; or of the bioavailability of poor-quality drugs or preparations (e.g., due to crushing of tablets). Drug-resistant TB may be either primary or acquired. In primary drug resistance, the patient is infected from the start by a drug-resistant strain. Acquired resistance develops in the infecting strain during treatment. In North America, Western Europe, most of Latin America, and the Persian Gulf states, rates of primary resistance are generally low and isoniazid resistance is most common. In the United States, although rates of primary isoniazid resistance have been stable at ~7–8%, the rate of primary MDR-TB has declined from 2.5% in 1993 to <1% since 2000. As described above, MDR-TB is an increasingly serious problem in some regions, especially in the countries of the former Soviet Union and some countries of Asia (**Fig. 178-12**). Even more serious is the occurrence of MDR strains that are also resistant to additional second-line agents used in treatment, such as the fluoroquinolones. Creation of

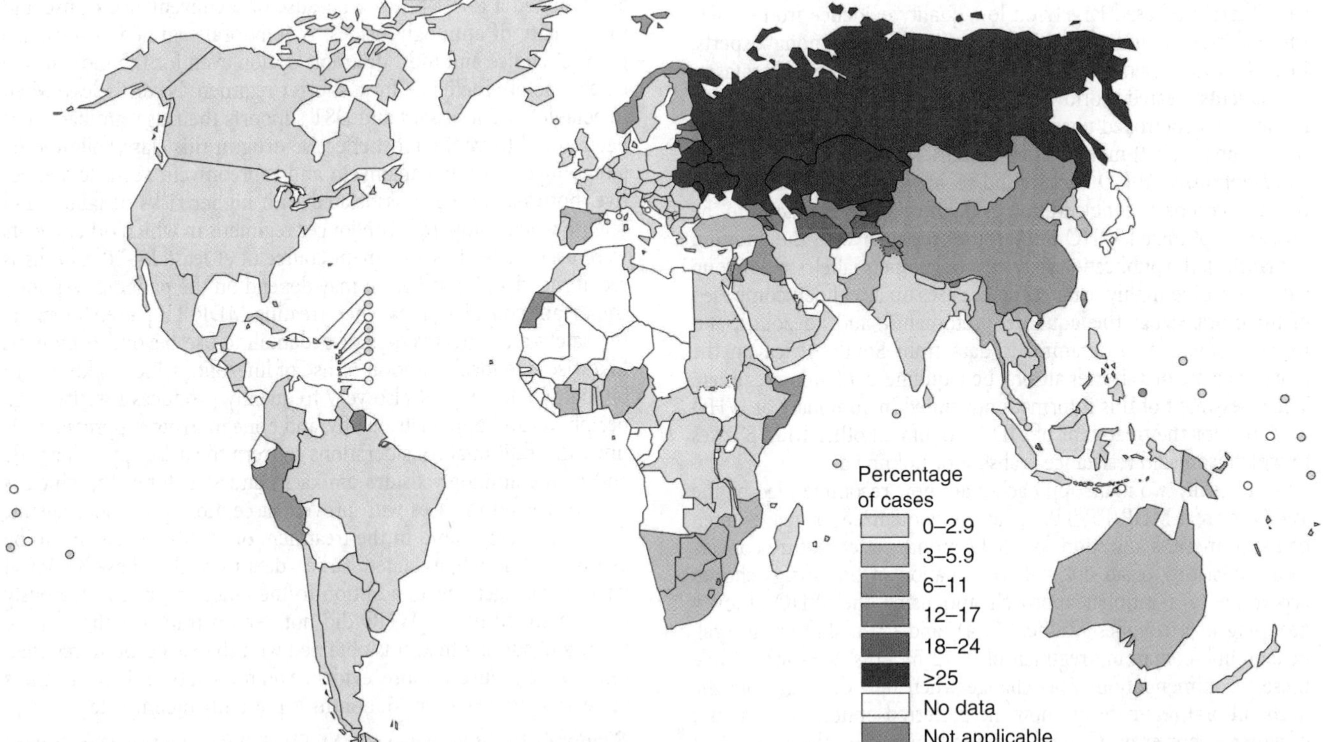

FIGURE 178-12 Percentage of new cases of multidrug-resistant/rifampin-resistant tuberculosis (TB) in all countries surveyed by the World Health Organization (WHO) Global Drug Resistance Surveillance Project during 1994–2018. Figures are based on the most recent year for which data have been reported, which varies among countries. Data reported before the year 2002 are not shown. *(See disclaimer in Fig. 178-2. Reproduced with permission from Global Tuberculosis Report 2019. Geneva, World Health Organization; 2019.)*

drug-resistant TB can be prevented by adherence to the principles of sound treatment: inclusion of at least two quality-assured, bactericidal drugs to which the organism is susceptible; use of effective combination regimens; supervision of treatment with patient support; and verification that patients complete the prescribed course. The use of fixed-dose combination products may prevent selective drug intake and therefore possibly protect against the creation of drug resistance. Transmission of drug-resistant strains can be prevented by the implementation of respiratory infection-control measures (see below) and by early detection of people with active TB followed by immediate initiation of treatment with an effective regimen.

Isoniazid-Resistant TB For the treatment of patients with isoniazid-resistant disease, a combination of rifampin, ethambutol, pyrazinamide, and levofloxacin for 6 months is recommended. This fluoroquinolone-containing regimen should not be used until rifampin resistance has been excluded by a reliable diagnostic test to avoid inadvertent treatment of MDR-TB with an inadequate regimen. Ideally, a laboratory test for susceptibility should also be done for the fluoroquinolones and pyrazinamide. If the fluoroquinolone is contraindicated because of intolerance or resistance, the patient can be given a 6-month regimen of rifampin, ethambutol, and pyrazinamide. Isoniazid probably does not contribute to a successful outcome in these regimens but may be retained (also to facilitate treatment with the four-drug fixed-dose formulation). Other drugs, such as the injectable aminoglycosides, are unlikely to play a role in the treatment of most isoniazid-resistant TB cases. However, they may be considered in the presence of additional resistance (e.g., to pyrazinamide or ethambutol) or of drug intolerance.

RR-, MDR-TB MDR-TB, in which bacilli are resistant to (at least) isoniazid and rifampin, is more difficult to manage than is disease caused by drug-susceptible organisms because these two bactericidal drugs are the most potent first-line agents available and because associated resistance to other first-line drugs as well (e.g., ethambutol) is not uncommon. Treatment for RR-TB and MDR-TB has traditionally been a topic of much debate, given its complexity, long duration, toxicity, and limited efficacy; the cost of most second-line drugs; and the lack of randomized controlled clinical trials to support combinations. Until recently, recommendations were therefore based largely on low-quality evidence from observational studies and on best-practice consensus among experts. Recent developments include the accrual of individual datasets for patients treated worldwide, the release of findings from two randomized controlled phase 3 clinical trials (the STREAM Stage 1 trial comparing a 9-month, shorter MDR-TB regimen with the previous optimized WHO background regimen; and Otsuka's phase 3 trial 213 comparing the addition of the new drug delamanid to the previous optimized WHO background regimen with the addition of placebo), the publication of results of an open-label, single group study enrolling highly drug-resistant cases on a regimen composed of three oral drugs (bedaquiline, pretomanid, and linezolid), and the assessment of programmatic data from South Africa on the large-scale use of a shorter all-oral bedaquiline-containing regimen. The assessment of this information resulted in an update of WHO guidance for the treatment of MDR-TB and all other RR-TB cases in which isoniazid resistance is absent or unknown.

As a result, two main approaches are now recommended by the WHO to treat MDR/RR-TB: (1) an individualized longer regimen of 18–20 months' duration (or 15-17 months after culture conversion) consisting of an optimal combination of oral drugs chosen according to a rational approach and using the WHO priority grouping of medicines (**Table 178-4**); and (2) a shorter, all-oral, bedaquiline-containing regimen of 9–12 months' duration. While these recommendations may change when new data indicate the need, all-oral regimens are now the preferred options and the use of either a shorter or a longer regimen depends on the assessment of the severity of disease, knowledge of drug resistance pattern, and history of previous treatment.

TABLE 178-4 Groups of Drugs Recommended for Use in Longer MDR-TB Regimens and Approach to the Design of a Longer Regimen for Adults and Children

GROUP	DRUG
Group A: Drugs to be prioritized and included in all regimens, unless they cannot be used	Levofloxacin *or* moxifloxacin Bedaquiline Linezolid
Group B: Drugs to be added in all regimens, unless they cannot be used	Clofazimine Cycloserine *or* terizidone
Group C: Drugs to be used to complete the regimen and when drugs from groups A and B cannot be used	Ethambutol Delamanid Pyrazinamide Imipenem-cilastatin *or* meropenem Amikacin *or* streptomycin Ethionamide *or* prothionamide *p*-Aminosalicylic acid

Source: Adapted from the World Health Organization, 2018.

Longer MDR-TB Regimen In MDR/RR-TB patients where infecting strains have or are presumed to have additional resistance (e.g., resistance to the fluoroquinolones), in those who have severe pulmonary or extrapulmonary disease, or those who have been treated previously with second-line drugs, a longer regimen is recommended. Table 178-4 shows the priority grouping of drugs recommended by the WHO and the approach to the design of a longer regimen for both adults and children. As much as possible, the regimen is composed of all group A agents and at least one group B agent. The use of bedaquiline and linezolid is promoted, together with a fluoroquinolone (levofloxacin or moxifloxacin), whenever possible, in all patients. Clofazimine and cycloserine (group B) are the two preferred options to be added to group A drugs. Group C drugs can replace group A and B agents that cannot be used, and the choice should be based on drug susceptibility testing, drug resistance levels in the population, the patient's history of previous use of these drugs, and potential intolerance or toxicity. The injectable agents (e.g., amikacin, streptomycin, and the carbapenems) are assigned a lower priority because of inconvenience of use and the toxicity of aminoglycosides. A fully oral regimen is thus also the first choice and most desirable option even for the most severe cases who are ineligible for a shorter regimen. Nevertheless, when injectables are necessary and DST supports their use, amikacin has been found to be the most effective drug in this class, followed by streptomycin, while kanamycin and capreomycin seem less effective, both having been associated with higher risks of failure and relapse when compared with longer regimens in which other agents were used instead. A treatment course of at least 18–20 months is recommended, but duration may depend on the patient's response. Important considerations when treating MDR-TB patients include the safety and effectiveness of bedaquiline use beyond 6 months. Likewise, the ideal duration of use of linezolid, which is known to be highly effective but also very frequently produces toxicity (e.g., peripheral and optic neuropathy, and bone marrow suppression), is unclear. Additional considerations concern the use of pyrazinamide and of the aminoglycosides amikacin and streptomycin, which is now restricted to cases with proven susceptibility to those agents. The role of delamanid in the treatment of MDR-TB remains to be assessed, although, as stated earlier, data from the phase 3 clinical trial of this agent as an addition to the longer regimen previously recommended by the WHO did not demonstrate a higher rate of treatment success than was obtained with the background regimen plus placebo. Furthermore, evidence on the safety and effectiveness of delamanid given for >6 months is presently incomplete.

Shorter MDR-TB Regimen In MDR/RR-TB patients with no extensive pulmonary disease or severe extrapulmonary disease, without history of previous treatment with second-line drugs, and whose infecting strains are not resistant to the fluoroquinolones, a shorter, all-oral, bedaquiline-containing regimen is recommended. Recent observational programmatic data from South Africa, assessed by WHO in 2019, showed that a fully oral regimen starting with 6 months of bedaquiline accompanied by 4–6 months of levofloxacin or moxifloxacin, ethionamide, ethambutol, pyrazinamide, high-dose isoniazid (10–15 mg/kg per day), and clofazimine, and followed by 5 months of levofloxacin (or moxifloxacin), clofazimine, pyrazinamide and ethambutol, was associated with low toxicity and better outcomes than the older, standardized, injectable-containing regimen when used in patients, including the HIV-infected, with no extensive pulmonary disease or severe extrapulmonary disease, fluoroquinolone resistance, or previous history of second-line drug use. The WHO therefore now recommends the adoption of this regimen and the progressive phasing-out of the previously recommended injectable-containing shorter regimen. The WHO also recommends that any modifications of a shorter regimen, where injectables are replaced by drugs other than bedaquiline, should be tested under operational research conditions and not adopted on a large programmatic scale until evidence shows their safety, tolerability, and efficacy.

The criteria used to define eligible patients are listed in **Table 178-5**. Adults and children eligible for the shorter regimen may still be offered the option of a new longer regimen if their completion of the full duration is adequately supported; with the longer regimen, the likelihood of relapse-free cure could be increased, and its administration is fully oral. As with any anti-TB regimen, the risk of creating additional resistance is high if the regimen is used incorrectly (e.g., in someone with preexisting fluoroquinolone resistance).

As in past recommendations, informed consent should be sought from patients treated with all MDR-TB regimens, and active TB drug safety monitoring is recommended. Patients taking QT interval–prolonging drugs (bedaquiline, delamanid, clofazimine, and fluoroquinolones) should be closely monitored, with electrocardiography performed at the start of treatment and repeated during treatment; patients with a QTc interval >500 ms or a history of ventricular arrhythmias should not be given these drugs. Patients taking amikacin should undergo serial audiometry to detect any hearing loss early on. Incentives and other forms of support can encourage patients not to interrupt treatment.

MDR-TB patients with additional resistance to fluoroquinolones and other second-line medicines have fewer treatment options and a poorer prognosis. However, the new longer regimen offers more options for a reasonably effective and tolerable regimen. The design of regimens for complex patterns of MDR-TB follows the same principles outlined in Table 178-4 through the selection of agents likely to be effective and tolerated. Observational studies have shown that aggressive management in such patients, with early drug susceptibility testing, use of a rational combination of at least five effective drugs, strict adherence to directly observed therapy, monthly bacteriologic monitoring, and intensive patient support, may—besides interrupting transmission—increase the chances of cure and avert death. For patients with localized disease and sufficient pulmonary reserve, lobectomy or wedge resection may be considered as part of treatment. A novel regimen composed of bedaquiline, the new nitroimidazole compound pretomanid, and linezolid (BPaL) administered orally for 6 months has been tested by the Global Alliance for TB Drug Development in South Africa in an open-label, single-group study enrolling 109 patients with MDR-TB caused by a strain with additional resistance to a fluoroquinolone or a second-line injectable drug, or were intolerant of therapy, or in whom treatment had failed. The cure rate was 90% after a 6-month course of treatment; the main toxicity, due to linezolid, consisted of peripheral neuropathy (81%) and myelosuppression (48%), which were manageable with dose reduction or interruption of the drug. Based on these findings, in August 2019 the FDA approved the new drug pretomanid under the Limited Population Pathway for Antibacterial and Antifungal Drugs (LPAD pathway) as part of a three-drug, 6-month, all-oral regimen for the treatment of a population of patients with MDR-TB caused by a strain with additional resistance to a fluoroquinolone or a second-line injectable drug, or who were intolerant of therapy, or in whom treatment had failed. Although approved by the FDA and proven as highly efficacious in the only trial available, in late 2019 the WHO suggested that this new 6–9 month regimen be used either under operational research conditions until more information is available on safety and efficacy or as a last resort in difficult-to-treat individual patients. A new, dose-blinded study reported in 2021 suggested that BPaL regimens where linezolid was used at reduced daily dose (from 1200 mg to 600 mg) and/or for a shorter period of time (from 6 to 2 months) were safer. Another regimen being tested by the Global Alliance is composed of bedaquiline, pretomanid, moxifloxacin, and pyrazinamide (BPaMZ). In a phase 2B trial, MDR-TB patients became culture-negative within 8 weeks of treatment three times faster than drug-sensitive TB patients treated with the standard regimen. The BPaMZ regimen is now being tested for both MDR-TB and drug-susceptible TB, with the aim of reducing treatment duration to 6 months and 4 months, respectively. Results are expected in late 2021.

Because the management of MDR-TB is complicated by both social and medical factors, care of seriously ill patients is ideally provided in specialized centers or, in their absence, in the context of programs with adequate resources and capacity, including community support. When patients are in stable condition, treatment and care on an ambulatory basis at a decentralized health care facility should be prioritized as this approach may increase treatment success and reduce loss to follow-up. This approach should not, however, preclude hospitalization when it is necessary. Respiratory infection-control measures should be observed throughout. As part of a patient-centered approach, palliative and end-of-life care should be provided as a priority when all recommended treatment options have been exhausted.

TABLE 178-5 Criteria for Offering a Shorter All-Oral Regimen (9–11 Months) to Patients with Confirmed Multidrug- or Rifampin-Resistant (MDR/RR) Tuberculosis (TB)

- Confirmed absence of resistance to or lack of suspicion of the ineffectiveness of a drug in the shorter MDR-TB regimen (except for isoniazid resistance)
- No history of exposure to one or more second-line drugs used in the shorter MDR-TB regimen (including bedaquiline) for >1 month
- Confirmed fluoroquinolone-susceptible disease
- No intolerance to drugs used in the shorter MDR-TB regimen or risk of toxicity (e.g., drug–drug interactions)
- No pregnancy
- No extensive pulmonary disease
- No disseminated, meningeal, or central nervous system TB
- Availability of all drugs in the shorter MDR-TB regimen

Source: Adapted from the World Health Organization, 2019.

HIV-ASSOCIATED TB

Several observational studies and randomized controlled trials have shown that treatment of HIV-associated TB with anti-TB drugs and simultaneous use of ART is associated with significant reductions in mortality risk and AIDS-related events. Evidence from randomized controlled trials shows that early initiation of ART during anti-TB treatment is associated with a 34–68% reduction in mortality rates, with especially good results in patients with CD4+ T-cell counts of <50/μL. Therefore, the main aim in the management of HIV-associated TB is to initiate anti-TB treatment and to immediately consider initiating or continuing ART. All HIV-infected TB patients, regardless of CD4+ T-cell count, are candidates for ART, which optimally is initiated as soon as possible after the diagnosis of TB and with the strong recommendation to start within the first 8 weeks of anti-TB therapy; ART should be started within the first 2 weeks of TB treatment for profoundly immunosuppressed patients with CD4+ T-cell counts of <50/μL. In general, the standard 6-month daily regimen is equally efficacious in HIV-negative and HIV-positive patients with drug-susceptible TB. However, in the uncommon situation where an HIV-infected patient cannot receive ART, prolongation of the continuation phase of TB treatment by 3 months can be considered. As in any other TB patient, intermittent regimens should not be used in HIV-infected people. As for any other adult living with HIV (**Chap. 202**), first-line ART for TB patients consists of two nucleoside reverse transcriptase inhibitors plus a nonnucleoside reverse transcriptase inhibitor or an integrase or protease inhibitor. Recent guidelines have also considered a two-drug treatment consisting of one nucleoside reverse transcriptase inhibitor plus an integrase inhibitor. Although TB treatment modalities are similar to those in HIV-negative patients, adverse drug reactions may be more pronounced in HIV-infected patients. In this regard, three important considerations are relevant: an increased frequency of paradoxical reactions, interactions between ART components and rifamycins, and development of rifampin monoresistance with intermittent treatment. IRIS—i.e., the exacerbation of symptoms and signs of TB—has been described above. Rifampin, a potent inducer of enzymes of the cytochrome P450 system, lowers serum levels of many HIV protease inhibitors and some nonnucleoside reverse transcriptase inhibitors—essential drugs used in ART. In such cases, rifabutin, which has much less enzyme-inducing activity, has been used in place of rifampin. However, dosage adjustments for rifabutin and protease or integrase inhibitors are still being assessed. Several clinical trials have found that patients with HIV/TB co-infection whose degree of immunosuppression is advanced (e.g., CD4+ T-cell counts of <100/μL) are prone to treatment failure and relapse with rifampin-resistant organisms when treated with "highly intermittent" (i.e., once- or twice-weekly) rifamycin-containing regimens. Consequently, it is now recommended that all TB patients who are infected with HIV, like all other TB patients with rifampin-susceptible disease, receive a rifampin-containing regimen on a daily basis. Because recommendations are frequently updated, consultation of the following websites is advised: *www.who.int/hiv*, *www.who.int/tb*, *www.cdc.gov/hiv*, and *www.cdc.gov/tb*.

SPECIAL CLINICAL SITUATIONS

Although comparative clinical trials of treatment for extrapulmonary TB are limited, the available evidence indicates that most forms of disease should be treated with a 6-month regimen recommended for patients with pulmonary disease. For TB meningitis, the ATS, the CDC, and the IDSA recommend extension of the continuation phase for 7–10 months. The WHO and the American Academy of Pediatrics recommend that children with bone and joint TB, tuberculous meningitis, or miliary TB receive up to 12 months of treatment (2-month induction treatment followed by 10-month consolidation treatment). Treatment for TB may be complicated by underlying medical problems that require special consideration. As a rule, patients with chronic renal failure should not receive aminoglycosides and should receive ethambutol only if serum drug levels can be monitored. Isoniazid, rifampin, and pyrazinamide may be given in the usual doses in cases of mild to moderate renal failure, but the dosages of isoniazid and pyrazinamide should be reduced for all patients with severe renal failure except those undergoing hemodialysis. Patients with hepatic disease pose a special problem because of the hepatotoxicity of isoniazid, rifampin, and pyrazinamide. Patients with severe hepatic disease may be treated with ethambutol, streptomycin, and possibly another drug (e.g., a fluoroquinolone); if required, isoniazid and rifampin may be administered under close supervision. The use of pyrazinamide by patients with liver failure should be avoided. Silicotuberculosis necessitates the extension of therapy by at least 2 months.

The regimen of choice for pregnant women (Table 178-3) is 9 months of treatment with isoniazid and rifampin supplemented by ethambutol for the first 2 months. Although the WHO has recommended routine use of pyrazinamide for pregnant women in combination with isoniazid and rifampin, this drug has not been recommended for pregnant women in the United States because of insufficient data documenting its safety in pregnancy. Streptomycin is contraindicated because it is known to cause eighth-cranial-nerve damage in the fetus. The thioamides, bedaquiline, and delamanid should also be avoided in the treatment of pregnant women with MDR-TB. Treatment for TB is not a contraindication to breastfeeding; most of the drugs administered will be present in small quantities in breast milk, albeit at concentrations far too low to provide any therapeutic or prophylactic benefit to the child.

Medical consultation on difficult-to-manage cases is provided by the US CDC Regional Training and Medical Consultation Centers (*www.cdc.gov/tb/education/rtmc/*).

PREVENTION

The primary way to prevent TB is to diagnose and isolate infectious cases rapidly and to administer appropriate treatment until patients are rendered noninfectious (usually 2–4 weeks after the start of proper treatment) and the disease is cured. Additional strategies include BCG vaccination and preventive treatment of persons with TB infection who are at high risk of developing active disease.

BCG VACCINATION

Historically one of the most used vaccines in the history of medicine, BCG was derived from an attenuated strain of *M. bovis* and was first administered to humans in 1921. Many BCG vaccines are available worldwide; all are derived from the original strain, but the vaccines vary in efficacy, ranging from 80% to nil in randomized, placebo-controlled trials. A similar range of efficacy was found in observational studies (case-control, historic cohort, and cross-sectional) in areas where infants are vaccinated at birth. These studies and a meta-analysis also found higher rates of efficacy in the protection of infants and young children from serious disseminated forms of childhood TB, such as tuberculous meningitis and miliary TB. BCG vaccine is safe and rarely causes serious complications. The local tissue response begins 2–3 weeks after vaccination, with scar formation and healing within 3 months. Side effects—most commonly, ulceration at the vaccination site and regional lymphadenitis—occur in 1–10% of vaccinated persons. Some vaccine strains have caused osteomyelitis in ~1 case per million doses administered. Disseminated BCG infection ("BCGitis") and death have occurred in 1–10 cases per 10 million doses administered, although this problem is restricted almost exclusively to persons with impaired immunity, such as children with severe combined immunodeficiency syndrome or adults with HIV infection. BCG vaccination induces TST reactivity, which tends to wane with time. The presence or size of TST reactions after vaccination does not predict the degree of protection afforded.

BCG vaccine is recommended for routine use at birth in countries or among populations with high TB prevalence (**Fig. 178-13**). However, because of the low risk of transmission of TB in the United States and other high-income countries, the variability in protection afforded by BCG, and its impact on the TST, the vaccine is not recommended for general use. HIV-infected adults and children should not receive BCG vaccine. Moreover, infants whose HIV status is unknown but who have signs and symptoms consistent with HIV infection or who are born to HIV-infected mothers should not receive BCG.

Over the past decade, renewed research and development efforts have been made toward a new TB vaccine, and several candidates have been developed and tested. The MVA-85A was the first new TB vaccine to be tested in a phase 2B proof-of-concept trial in infants in South Africa. Results published in 2013 showed that MVA-85A was well tolerated and modestly immunogenic but did not confer significant protection against clinical TB or *M. tuberculosis* infection. A second, more promising candidate vaccine, M72/AS01$_E$, a subunit vaccine pairing two *M. tuberculosis* antigens (32A and 39A) with the adjuvant M72/AS01$_E$, was recently tested in a randomized trial among 3575 patients with *M. tuberculosis* infection to prevent development of active disease. TB developed in 13 participants among those receiving the vaccine and in 26 among those receiving placebo with an estimated efficacy of 49.7% at 36 months. Adverse events were not different in the two groups. This vaccine is now being considered for further development.

As of the end of 2020, 14 candidate vaccines were in various stages of clinical trials. They included whole-cell or mycobacterial whole-cell

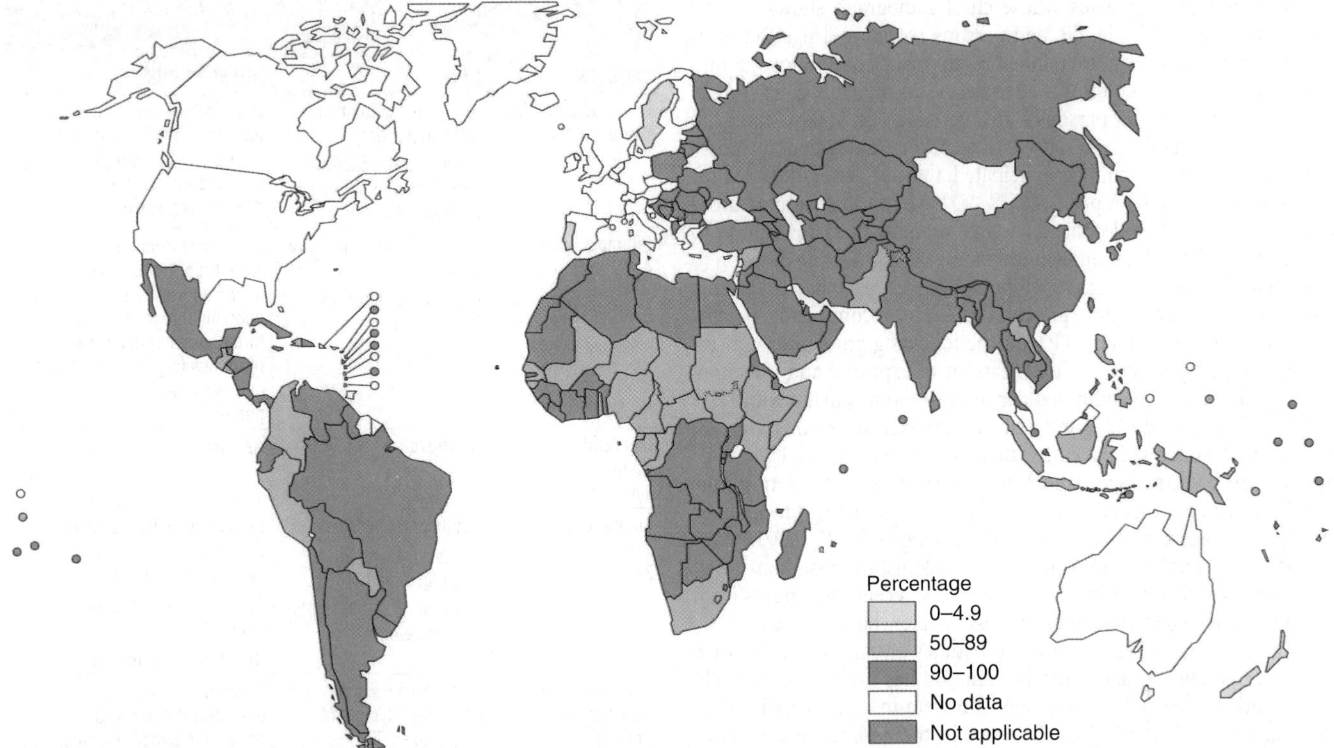

FIGURE 178-13 Coverage of BCG vaccination in 2018. The target population of BCG coverage varies depending on national policies but is typically for the number of live births in the year of reporting. *(See disclaimer in Fig. 178-2. Reproduced with permission from Global Tuberculosis Report 2019. Geneva, World Health Organization; 2019.)*

or lysates, viral vector vaccines, and adjuvant recombinant protein vaccines. Several challenges must be faced in the development of a TB vaccine. For instance, the lack of predictive animal models and protection correlates renders trials long and expensive. Furthermore, the decision about whether a candidate vaccine should be developed for prevention of infection (preexposure) or prevention of reactivation (postexposure) without an exact understanding of its precise mechanism of action is complex. Therefore, introduction of a new vaccine on a large scale is not likely in the near future. This step will require an intensified and much larger investment in research and development.

TB PREVENTIVE TREATMENT (TPT)

It is estimated that 1.7 billion people—more than one-quarter of the human population—have been infected with *M. tuberculosis.* Although only a small fraction of these infections will progress toward active disease in a lifetime, new active cases will continue to emerge from this pool of infected individuals. Therefore, TPT (also called *chemoprophylaxis* or *preventive chemotherapy*, and previously referred to as *treatment of latent TB infection*) is a fundamental intervention in TB control and elimination strategies.

Infection can be tested using TST or IGRA, although these tests just measure host immune response to TB antigens. Unfortunately, at present, there is no gold-standard diagnostic test that can confirm true infection (as opposed to immunologic memory of previous exposure) or predict which infected individuals will develop active TB. As a result, decisions to treat infection should include consideration of the risk of progression in an individual. For skin testing, five tuberculin units of polysorbate-stabilized PPD should be injected intradermally into the volar surface of the forearm (i.e., the Mantoux method). Multipuncture tests are not recommended. Reactions are read at 48–72 h as the transverse diameter (in millimeters) of induration; the diameter of erythema is not considered. In some persons, TST reactivity wanes with time but can be recalled by a second skin test administered ≥1 week after the first (i.e., two-step testing). For persons periodically undergoing the TST, such as health care workers and individuals admitted to long-term-care institutions, initial two-step testing may preclude subsequent misclassification of those who have boosted reactions as TST converters. The cutoff for a positive TST (and thus for TPT) is related both to the probability that the reaction represents true infection and to the likelihood that the individual, if truly infected, will develop TB. **Table 178-6** suggests possible conventional cutoff by risk group. Thus, positive reactions for persons with HIV infection, recent close contacts of infectious cases, organ transplant recipients,

TABLE 178-6 Tuberculin Reaction Size and Cutoff for Tuberculosis (TB) Preventive Treatment

RISK GROUP	TUBERCULIN REACTION SIZE, mm
HIV-infected persons	≥5
Recent contacts of a patient with TB	≥5[a]
Organ transplant recipients	≥5
Persons with fibrotic lesions consistent with old TB on chest radiography	≥5
Persons who are immunosuppressed—e.g., due to the use of glucocorticoids or tumor necrosis factor α inhibitors	≥5
Persons with high-risk medical conditions[b]	≥5
Recent immigrants (≤5 years) from high-prevalence countries	≥10
Injection drug users	≥10
Mycobacteriology laboratory personnel; residents and employees of high-risk congregate settings[c]	≥10
Children <5 years of age; children and adolescents exposed to adults in high-risk categories	≥10
Low-risk persons[d]	≥15

[a]Tuberculin-negative contacts, especially children, should receive prophylaxis for 2–3 months after contact ends and should then undergo repeat tuberculin skin testing (TST). Those whose results remain negative should discontinue prophylaxis. HIV-infected contacts should receive a full course of treatment regardless of TST results. [b]These conditions include silicosis and end-stage renal disease managed by hemodialysis. [c]These settings include correctional facilities, nursing homes, homeless shelters, and hospitals and other health care facilities. [d]Except for employment purposes where longitudinal TST screening is anticipated, TST is not indicated for these low-risk persons. A decision to treat should be based on individual risk/benefit considerations.

Source: Adapted from Centers for Disease Control and Prevention: TB elimination—treatment options for latent tuberculosis infection (2011). Available at *http://www.cdc.gov/tb/publications/factsheets/testing/skintestresults.pdf.*

previously untreated persons whose chest radiograph shows fibrotic lesions consistent with old TB, and persons receiving drugs that suppress the immune system are defined as an area of induration ≥5 mm in diameter. A 10-mm cutoff is used to define positive reactions in most other at-risk persons. For persons with a very low risk of developing TB if infected, a cutoff of 15 mm is used. (Except for employment purposes where longitudinal screening is anticipated, the TST is not indicated for these low-risk persons.) A positive IGRA is based on the manufacturer's recommendations. Good clinical practice requires that, in addition to test results, epidemiologic and clinical factors also guide the decision to implement TPT and that active TB be definitively excluded before the initiation of a prophylactic regimen. The WHO recommends systematic testing for infection and TPT for the following groups at high risk of progression from infection to disease or of exposure and infection: adults, adolescents and children older than 12 months living with HIV; infants with HIV aged <12 months who are contacts of persons with TB; all household contacts of patients with infectious pulmonary TB including children <5 years of age; patients with silicosis, patients starting anti-TNF treatment, patients on dialysis, and patients preparing for organ or hematologic transplantation. In addition, testing and TPT may be considered for persons living or working in at-risk institutional or crowded settings, such as prisoners, health care workers, recent immigrants from high-TB-burden countries, and homeless people who use drugs.

Some TST- and IGRA-negative individuals are also candidates for TPT. Once an appropriate clinical evaluation has excluded active TB, infants and children <5 years of age who were in contact with infectious cases should be offered TPT even in the absence of a positive test for TB infection. HIV-infected persons >1 year of age who have been exposed to an infectious TB patient should receive TPT regardless of the TST result. Any HIV-infected candidate for TPT must be screened carefully to exclude active TB, which would necessitate full disease treatment. The use of a clinical algorithm based on four signs/symptoms (current cough, fever, weight loss, and night sweats) helps to decide which HIV-infected person can start TPT. The absence of all four symptoms tends to exclude active TB in people living with HIV. The presence of one of these four manifestations, on the other hand, warrants further investigation for active TB before TPT is started. Although a test of TB infection is prudent before starting TPT, this test is not an absolute requirement—given the logistical challenges—among contacts aged <5 years and people living with HIV in high-TB-incidence and low-resource settings.

Among people living with HIV and receiving ART, conversion of the TST from negative to positive can occur during the first few months of TPT. Conversions (from negative to positive) and reversions (from positive to negative) are more common with IGRAs than with TSTs among serially tested health care workers in the United States.

TPT in selected persons at risk aims at preventing active disease and, in the absence of an immunizing vaccine, is a critical component of TB elimination strategies. Potential candidates for TPT are listed in Table 178-6. This intervention is based on the results of a large number of randomized, placebo-controlled clinical trials demonstrating that a 6- to 9-month course of isoniazid reduces the risk of active TB in infected people by up to 90%. Analysis of available data indicated that the optimal duration of treatment with this drug was ~9 months. In the absence of reinfection, the protective effect is believed to be lifelong. Clinical trials have shown that isoniazid reduces rates of TB among TST-positive persons with HIV infection. Studies in HIV-infected patients have also demonstrated the effectiveness of shorter TPT regimens containing a rifamycin. Several TPT regimens (**Table 178-7**) can be used. The most widely used has been that based on isoniazid alone at a daily dose of 5 mg/kg (up to 300 mg/d) for 9 months. On the basis of cost–benefit analyses and concerns about feasibility, a 6-month period of treatment at the same dose is considered adequate by the WHO. An alternative regimen for adults is 4 months of daily rifampin, which should also be effective against isoniazid-resistant strains. A 3-month regimen of daily isoniazid and rifampin is used in some countries (e.g., the United Kingdom) for both adults and children who are known not to have HIV infection. A previously recommended 2-month regimen of rifampin and pyrazinamide has been associated with serious or even fatal hepatotoxicity and is not recommended. The rifampin-containing regimens should be considered for persons who are likely to have been infected with an isoniazid-resistant strain. A clinical trial showed that a regimen of isoniazid (900 mg) and rifapentine (900 mg), given once weekly for 12 weeks, is as effective as the standard 9-month isoniazid regimen. This regimen was associated with higher rates of treatment completion (82% vs 69%) and less hepatotoxicity (0.4% vs 2.7%) than isoniazid alone, although the rate of permanent discontinuation due to an adverse event was higher (4.9% vs 3.7%).

TABLE 178-7 Recommended Regimens and Drug Dosages for Tuberculosis Preventive Treatment[a]

REGIMEN	DOSE	ADVERSE EVENTS
Isoniazid alone for 6 or 9 months	Adults: 5 mg/kg (max, 300 mg) per day Children <10 years of age: 10 mg/kg per day (range, 7–15 mg)	Drug-induced liver injury, nausea, vomiting, abdominal pain, skin rash, peripheral neuropathy, dizziness, drowsiness, seizure
Rifampin alone for 4 months	Adults: 10 mg/kg per day Children <10 years of age: 15 mg/kg (range, 10–20 mg) per day	Flulike syndrome, skin rash, drug-induced liver injury, anorexia, nausea, abdominal pain, neutropenia, thrombocytopenia, renal reactions (e.g., acute tubular necrosis and interstitial nephritis)
Isoniazid plus rifampin for 3 months	As above	As above
Rifapentine plus isoniazid for 3 months	Adults and children: Isoniazid: 15 mg/kg (900 mg) weekly Rifapentine: 15–30 mg/kg (900 mg) weekly	Hypersensitivity reactions, petechial skin rash, drug-induced liver injury Anorexia, nausea, abdominal pain Hypotensive reactions
Rifapentine plus isoniazid for 1 month	Age >13 years only: Isoniazid 300 mg and rifapentine 600 mg daily (28 doses)	Essentially like those of isoniazid alone with neutropenia more common and elevation in liver enzyme levels and neuropathy less common

[a]See text for full description of evidence on and limitations of these regimens.
Source: Reproduced with permission from World Health Organization.

Currently, the isoniazid–rifapentine regimen is not recommended for children <2 years of age or pregnant women. Recently, an open-label, randomized, phase 3 noninferiority trial has shown that among HIV-infected persons, a 1-month regimen of daily rifapentine plus isoniazid was noninferior to the 9-month daily isoniazid regimen and ensured a higher treatment completion. As a result, the WHO has included a 1-month regimen composed of daily isoniazid (300 mg) and rifapentine (600 mg) among the available options for people aged 13 years or more. Rifampin and rifapentine are contraindicated in HIV-infected individuals receiving protease inhibitors, most nonnucleoside reverse transcriptase inhibitors (e.g., nevirapine), and, for those with chronic hepatitis B, tenofovir alafenamide. However, efavirenz and tenofovir disoproxil can be used for simultaneous administration with a rifamycin without dose adjustment. However, the dose of the integrase inhibitor dolutegravir needs to be increased to 50 mg twice daily when given together with rifampin, a dose that is usually well tolerated and gives equivalent efficacy in viral suppression and recovery of CD4+ cell count compared with efavirenz. Administration of rifapentine with raltegravir was found to be safe and well tolerated. A recent phase 1/2 trial of the 3-month regimen isoniazid plus rifapentine and dolutegravir in adults with HIV reported good tolerance and viral load suppression, no adverse events of grade >3, and did not indicate that rifapentine reduced dolutegravir levels sufficiently to require dose adjustment. Clinical trials to assess the efficacy of long-term isoniazid administration (i.e., for at least 3 years) among people living with HIV in high-TB-transmission settings have shown that this regimen can be more effective than 9 months of isoniazid and is therefore recommended under those circumstances. Studies looking at whether briefer treatment with rifapentine-based regimens could achieve similar efficacies have been undertaken. Isoniazid should not be given to persons with active liver disease. All isoniazid recipients at increased risk of hepatotoxicity (e.g., those abusing alcohol daily and those with a history of liver disease) should undergo baseline and then monthly assessment of liver function; they should be carefully educated about hepatitis and instructed to discontinue use of the drug immediately should any symptoms develop. Moreover, these patients should be seen and questioned monthly during therapy about adverse reactions and should be given no more than a 1-month supply of drug at each visit. Persons receiving high-dose isoniazid and who are at risk of vitamin B6 (pyridoxine) deficiency, as listed above, should receive pyridoxine to prevent peripheral neuropathy.

TPT among persons likely to have been infected by a multidrug-resistant strain is a challenge because no clinical trial results are available to guide treatment. Close observation for early signs of disease is one option. However, in selected high-risk household contacts of patients with MDR-TB (e.g., children, recipients of immunosuppressive therapy), TPT may be considered on the basis of individualized risk assessment and clinical criteria. In the absence of evidence of efficacy of any regimen, important factors in the decision to treat include intensity of exposure, certainty about a source case, information on the drug resistance pattern of the index case, and potential adverse events. Confirmation of infection with available testing is generally required. Drug selection should be based on the drug susceptibility profile of the index case. One regimen recommended by the WHO is daily levofloxacin (750–1000 mg daily among adults) for 6 months.

It may be more difficult to ensure adherence to TPT than when treating those with active TB. If family members of patients with active TB are being treated, adherence and monitoring may be easier. When feasible, supervised therapy may increase the likelihood of completion. As in active cases, the provision of incentives may also be helpful. Currently, no evidence shows that large-scale use of TPT leads to significant development of drug resistance. However, before TPT begins, it is mandatory to carefully exclude active TB in order to prevent undertreatment and promote development of drug resistance.

PRINCIPLES OF TB CONTROL

The highest priority in any TB control program is the prompt detection of cases and the provision of treatment to all TB patients under proper case-management conditions, including DOT and social support. In addition, screening of high-risk groups, including immigrants from high-prevalence countries, migrant workers, prisoners, homeless individuals, substance abusers, and HIV-seropositive persons, is recommended. TST- or IGRA-positive high-risk persons should receive TPT as described above. Contact investigation is an important component of efficient TB control. In the United States and other countries worldwide, a great deal of attention has been given to the transmission of TB (particularly in association with HIV co-infection) in institutional settings such as hospitals, homeless shelters, and prisons. Measures to limit such transmission include respiratory isolation of persons with suspected TB until they are proven to be noninfectious (at least by sputum AFB smear negativity), proper ventilation in rooms of patients with infectious TB, use of ultraviolet irradiation in areas of increased risk of TB transmission, correct use of personal protective equipment, and periodic screening of personnel who may come into contact with known or unsuspected cases of TB. In the past, radiographic surveys, especially those conducted with portable equipment and miniature films, were advocated for case finding. Today, however, the prevalence of TB in industrialized countries is sufficiently low that "mass miniature radiography" is not cost effective.

In high-prevalence countries, most TB control programs have made remarkable progress in reducing morbidity and mortality since the mid-1990s by adopting and implementing the standards and strategies internationally promoted by the WHO. Between 2000 and 2018, more than 60 million lives are estimated to have been saved. The essential elements of good TB care and control were established in the mid-1990s and consist of well-defined interventions that were the basis of the "DOTS strategy": early detection of cases and bacteriologic confirmation of the diagnosis; administration of standardized short-course chemotherapy, with direct supervision to ensure adherence to treatment and the provision of social support to patients; availability of drugs of proven quality, with an effective supply and management system; and a monitoring and evaluation system, including assessment of treatment outcomes—e.g., cure, completion of treatment without bacteriologic proof of cure, death, treatment failure, and default—in all cases registered and notified as well as measurement of the impact of control methods on classical TB indicators such as mortality, incidence, prevalence, and drug resistance. In 2006, the WHO indicated that, besides pursuing these essential elements that remain the fundamental components of any control strategy, additional steps had to be undertaken in order to reach international TB control targets. These steps included addressing HIV-associated TB and MDR-TB with additional measures; operating in harmony with general health services; engaging all care providers beyond the public providers; empowering people with TB and their communities; and enabling and promoting research. Evidence-based International Standards for Tuberculosis Care—focused on diagnosis, treatment, and public health responsibilities—were introduced for wide adoption by medical and professional societies, academic institutions, and all practitioners worldwide.

Care and control of HIV-associated TB are particularly challenging in poor countries because existing interventions require collaboration between HIV/AIDS and TB programs as well as standard services. TB programs must test every patient for HIV in order to provide access to trimethoprim-sulfamethoxazole prophylaxis against common infections and ART. HIV/AIDS programs must regularly screen persons living with HIV/AIDS for active TB, provide TPT, and ensure infection control in settings where people living with HIV congregate.

Early and active case detection is considered an important intervention not only among persons living with HIV/AIDS but also among other vulnerable populations, as it reduces transmission in a community and provides early effective care. Additional measures are indicated for the management of MDR-TB, RR-TB, and other forms of drug-resistant TB; they include upgrades of laboratory capacity to perform rapid DST and ensure surveillance of drug resistance; availability of drug regimens that are recommended for RR/MDR-TB, with assured quality of drugs; and infection control measures in all settings where patients with drug-resistant forms of TB may congregate. In the new era of the United Nations Sustainable Development Goals (2016–2030), the approach to TB control and care needs to evolve further and become multisectoral and more holistic. Engagement beyond dedicated programs and even the health sector is now essential. Therefore, the new "End TB" strategy promoted by the WHO since 2016 builds on three pillars and relies on increased investments and efforts by all governments, their national programs, and a multitude of partners within and beyond the health sector: (1) integrated, patient-centered care and prevention; (2) bold policies and supportive systems; and (3) intensified research and innovation. The first pillar incorporates all technological innovations, such as early diagnostic approaches (including universal DST and systematic screening of identified, setting-specific, high-risk groups); well-designed treatment regimens for all forms of TB; proper management of HIV-associated TB and other comorbidities; and preventive treatment of persons at high risk. The second pillar is fundamental and is normally beyond the scope of dedicated programs, relying on policies forged by the highest-level health and governmental authorities: availability of adequate human and financial resources; engagement of civil organizations and all relevant public and private providers to pursue proper care for all patients and prevention for all people at risk; a policy of universal health coverage (which, together with social protection, implies avoidance of catastrophic expenditures caused by TB among the poorest); regulatory frameworks for case notifications, vital registration, quality and rational use of medicines, and infection control; social protection mechanisms as part of poverty alleviation strategies; and promotion of interventions against the broader determinants of TB. Finally, the third pillar of the new strategy emphasizes intensification of research and development on new tools and interventions as well as optimal implementation and rapid adoption of new tools in endemic countries. Besides specific clinical care and control interventions as described in this chapter, elimination of TB in a society ultimately will require control and mitigation of the multitude of direct risk factors (e.g., HIV infection, smoking, alcohol abuse, diabetes) and socioeconomic determinants (e.g., extreme poverty, inadequate living conditions and poor housing, malnutrition, indoor air pollution) with clearly implemented policies within the health sector and other sectors linked to human development and welfare.

FURTHER READING

Conradie F et al: Treatment of highly drug-resistant pulmonary tuberculosis. N Engl J Med 382:893, 2020.

Dorman SE et al: Four-month rifapentine regimens with or without moxifloxacin for tuberculosis. N Engl J Med 384:1705, 2021.

Getahun H et al: Latent *Mycobacterium tuberculosis* infection. N Engl J Med 372:2127, 2015.

Nahid P et al: An Official American Thoracic Society/Centers for Disease Control and Prevention/European Respiratory Society/Infectious Diseases Society of America clinical practice guideline: Treatment of drug-resistant tuberculosis. Am J Respir Crit Care Med 200:e93, 2019.

Nahid P et al: An Official American Thoracic Society/Centers for Disease Control and Prevention/Infectious Diseases Society of America clinical practice guidelines: Treatment of drug-susceptible tuberculosis. Clin Infect Dis 63:853, 2016.

Pai M et al: Tuberculosis. Nat Rev Dis Primers 2:16076, 2016.

Swindells S et al: One month of rifapentine plus isoniazid to prevent HIV-related tuberculosis. N Engl J Med 380:1001, 2019.

Tait DR et al: Final analysis of a trial of M72/AS01 vaccine to prevent tuberculosis. N Engl J Med 381:2429, 2019.

Uplekar M et al: WHO's new End TB strategy. Lancet 385:1799, 2015.

WEBSITES

World Health Organization: Global tuberculosis report 2020, Geneva, WHO, 2020. *https://www.who.int/publications/i/item/9789240013131*

World Health Organization: Treatment of tuberculosis. Guidelines for treatment of drug-susceptible tuberculosis and patient care. 2017 update. Geneva, WHO, 2017. *https://apps.who.int/iris/bitstream/handle/10665/255052/9789241550000-eng.pdf?sequence=1*

World Health Organization: WHO Consolidated Guidelines on Tuberculosis, Module 4: Treatment. Drug-Resistant Tuberculosis Treatment. Geneva, WHO, 2020. *https://www.who.int/publications/i/item/9789240007048*

World Health Organization: WHO consolidated guidelines on tuberculosis. Module 3: Diagnosis. Rapid diagnostics for tuberculosis detection. 2021 update. Geneva, WHO, 2021. *https://www.who.int/publications/i/item/9789240029415*

179 Leprosy

Jan H. Richardus, Hemanta K. Kar, Zoica Bakirtzief, Wim H. van Brakel

Leprosy, also referred to as Hansen's disease, is a chronic infectious disease caused by *Mycobacterium leprae*. The clinical manifestations are largely confined to the skin, peripheral nervous system, eyes, and upper respiratory tract. The differing immune responses to *M. leprae* result in a spectrum of disease ranging from tuberculoid to lepromatous leprosy. *M. leprae* has a predilection for peripheral nerves, and immunologically mediated reactional states can cause nerve damage to the face, arms, and legs; this damage often results in disability, which in turn can lead to stigma and social exclusion. The physical disfigurement that accompanies leprosy has left marks on society that have endured long after the disease's disappearance in many countries. In everyday language, leprosy has become a metaphor for a horrible condition that warrants social exclusion. Leprosy is a neglected disease and is often thought no longer to exist. However, 202,185 new cases from 150 countries were reported in 2019. A general lack of awareness among both the public and medical practitioners often delays diagnosis and treatment and thus results in irreversible impairments. Early diagnosis and treatment of leprosy and leprosy reactions can cure the disease and prevent most chronic complications.

ETIOLOGY

M. leprae is an obligate, intracellular, acid-fast staining, rod-shaped bacterium, measuring 1–8 µm in length and 0.3 µm in diameter. *M. leprae* mostly appears irregularly stained and fragmented or granular, in which case the organism is usually considered to be dead. The few bacteria that are brightly and uniformly stained are thought to be solid, viable bacilli. The morphologic index is a measure of uniformly stained solid bacilli on slit-skin smear examination and is calculated as the percentage of viable bacilli among the total number of bacilli counted under oil-immersion microscopy. On slit-skin smear examination at the lepromatous end of the disease spectrum, *M. leprae* is predominantly found in clumps or globi within macrophages (*lepra cells*). Inside these cells, *M. leprae* multiplies in unrestricted fashion, and hundreds of bacilli may be present; the organisms are arranged in parallel arrays placed side by side as a result of the presence of surface lipids (*glial substances*). The bacteriologic index is a logarithmic-scaled measure of the density of bacilli of all forms found in the dermis upon slit-skin smear examination, varying from 0 to 6+ (with or without globi) from the tuberculoid to the lepromatous end of the disease spectrum. The bacteriological index falls an average of 1 log unit per year with multidrug therapy. *M. leprae* infects mainly macrophages and Schwann cells. It has never been grown in artificial media. Reproduction occurs by binary fission, and the organism grows slowly (over 12–14 days) in the footpads of mice. The temperature required for survival and proliferation—between 27°C and 30°C—explains the greater impact of the disease on surface areas such as the skin, peripheral nerves, testicles, and upper airways, with less inner visceral involvement. *M. leprae* remains viable for 9 days in the environment.

Ultrastructural Characteristics of *M. leprae* Electron microscopy reveals that *M. leprae* has a cytoplasm, plasma membrane, cell wall, and capsule. The cytoplasm contains structures common in gram-positive microorganisms. The plasma membrane has a permeable lipid bilayer containing interacting proteins—the protein surface antigens. Similar to that of other mycobacteria, *M. leprae*'s cell wall, which is attached to the plasma membrane, is composed of peptidoglycans bound to branched-chain polysaccharides; these peptidoglycans are arabinogalactans, which support mycolic acids, and lipoarabinomannan (LAM). The capsule—the outermost structure—contains lipids, particularly phthiocerol dimycocerosate and phenolic glycolipid (PGL-1), which has a trisaccharide bound to lipid by a molecule of phenol. Because this trisaccharide is antigenically specific for *M. leprae*, its detection is helpful in serologic diagnosis of leprosy.

Genome of *M. leprae* Comparative analysis of the genomics of single-nucleotide polymorphisms indicates that four distinct strains of *M. leprae* originated in East Africa or Central Asia. A mutation spread to Europe and subsequently underwent two separate mutations that were then followed by spread to West Africa and the Americas. The genome of *M. leprae* is circular. Its estimated molecular mass is 2.2×10^9 Da, with 3,268,203 base pairs and a guanine-plus-cytosine content of 57.8%.

Culture Difficulties Compared to the genome of *Mycobacterium tuberculosis*, that of *M. leprae* underwent reductive evolution, resulting in a smaller genome rich in inactive or entirely deleted genes. This reductive evolution, gene decay, and genome downsizing all may explain the unusually long generation time and may account for the inability to culture the leprosy bacillus in artificial media. As a result, propagation of *M. leprae* has been restricted to animal models, including the armadillo and normal, athymic, and gene-knockout mice. These systems have provided the basic resources for genetic, metabolic, and antigenic studies of the bacillus. Growth of *M. leprae* in mouse footpads also provides a tool for assessing the viability of the bacteria and testing the drug susceptibility of clinical isolates.

Immunologic Properties of *M. leprae* *M. leprae* induces both humoral and cell-mediated immune responses. The immunogenic components of *M. leprae* include polysaccharides and proteins. Polysaccharide components induce mainly a humoral immune response, whereas protein components induce both humoral and cell-mediated immune responses. The immunogens in *M. leprae* form two distinct groups: cytoplasmic antigens and antigens from the mycobacterial cell. As mentioned above, a species-specific phenolic glycolipid, PGL-1, has been identified in *M. leprae*. Other varieties of *M. leprae* antigens identified with monoclonal antibodies include antigens of 18, 28, 7, 14, 36, 65, and 70 kDa that may possibly induce an immune response.

Mycobacterium lepromatosis In 2008, a new mycobacterial species, *M. lepromatosis*, was isolated from patients with a special type of diffuse lepromatous leprosy known as *diffuse leprosy of Lucio and Latapí*. This clinical variety of leprosy is found mainly in Mexico and Central America. *M. lepromatosis* is very similar to *M. leprae* microbiologically and clinically. Microbiologically, both species are acid-fast and noncultivable and preferably infect skin and peripheral nerves. Clinically, differentiation of *M. lepromatosis* from *M. leprae* in individual patients is not diagnostically necessary since both organisms respond well to the same antimycobacterial regimens.

EPIDEMIOLOGY

Incidence, Prevalence, and Disability The true incidence of leprosy is difficult to establish because the figure is very low and because the initial signs and symptoms are often insidious, and thus not all cases are detected as they occur. In 2019, as stated earlier, 202,185 new cases were reported to the World Health Organization (WHO) from 150 countries. New case detection per year is commonly used as a proxy for incidence, but operational factors, such as the intensity of case detection, the use of surveys, the use of contact tracing, the level of community awareness, and the quality and availability of health care, have a profound effect on case detection rates. In nonendemic countries around the world, leprosy is often misdiagnosed simply because it is not considered.

The registered prevalence of leprosy is defined as the number of patients receiving treatment at a point in time (usually at the end of a calendar year). The registered prevalence is a proxy measure for true prevalence, which would include existing cases that have not yet been detected. The two factors that determine the registered prevalence are the new case detection rate and the duration of treatment; changes in either factor will affect the registered prevalence.

The WHO leprosy disability grading system scores patients according to the presence of disabilities of the eyes, hands, and feet. For the hands and feet, grade 0 means no anesthesia and no visible impairment; grade 1 signifies anesthesia but no visible impairment; and grade 2 indicates visible impairment. For the eyes, grade 0 signifies no eye problems due to leprosy and no evidence of visual loss; grade 1 signifies eye problems due to leprosy without severe effects on vision; and grade 2 indicates severe visual impairment (vision score worse than 6/60; inability to count fingers at 6 meters) and also includes lagophthalmos, iridocyclitis, and corneal opacities. The sum score for these six body sites is called the Eye-Hand-Foot (EHF) score and is used as an overall indicator of the impairment status of a person with leprosy. Leprosy-related grade 2 disability is usually reported as the proportion of people with such disability at any site among patients newly diagnosed with leprosy in a specific year.

The global trend in new case detection since 1985 is presented in **Fig. 179-1**. The trend was remarkably static up to the year 2001, with a peak around the year 2000; fell dramatically between 2001 and 2005; and has leveled off since 2006. The most important factor contributing to the fast downward trend was the decline in leprosy control activities following the declaration by the WHO in 2000 that leprosy was eliminated as a "public health problem." *Elimination* was defined as a prevalence of <1 case per 10,000 population at the global level. The attainment of this target was a great achievement but led many to believe that the problem of leprosy was solved altogether. This misunderstanding in turn led to reduced political commitment to leprosy control programs and facilities, with consequent downsizing and decreased funding. The stabilization of the new case detection rate at just over 200,000 cases annually since 2006 indicates that transmission of *M. leprae* is continuing unabated, posing an enormous challenge in leprosy control.

Sex, Age, and Geographic Distribution Approximately 40% of all reported leprosy patients are women, but the low proportion in some countries raises concerns about underdiagnosis in women due to poor access to health services, illiteracy, low status, and other cultural factors. The age-specific incidence often shows a bimodal pattern, with peaks in the teenage years and in adulthood. Around 8% of all newly detected cases are found in children (<15 years of age), a measure that is often taken as an indicator of continued (recent) transmission. Leprosy is rare among children <5 years of age. Around 5% of all patients have a grade 2 disability.

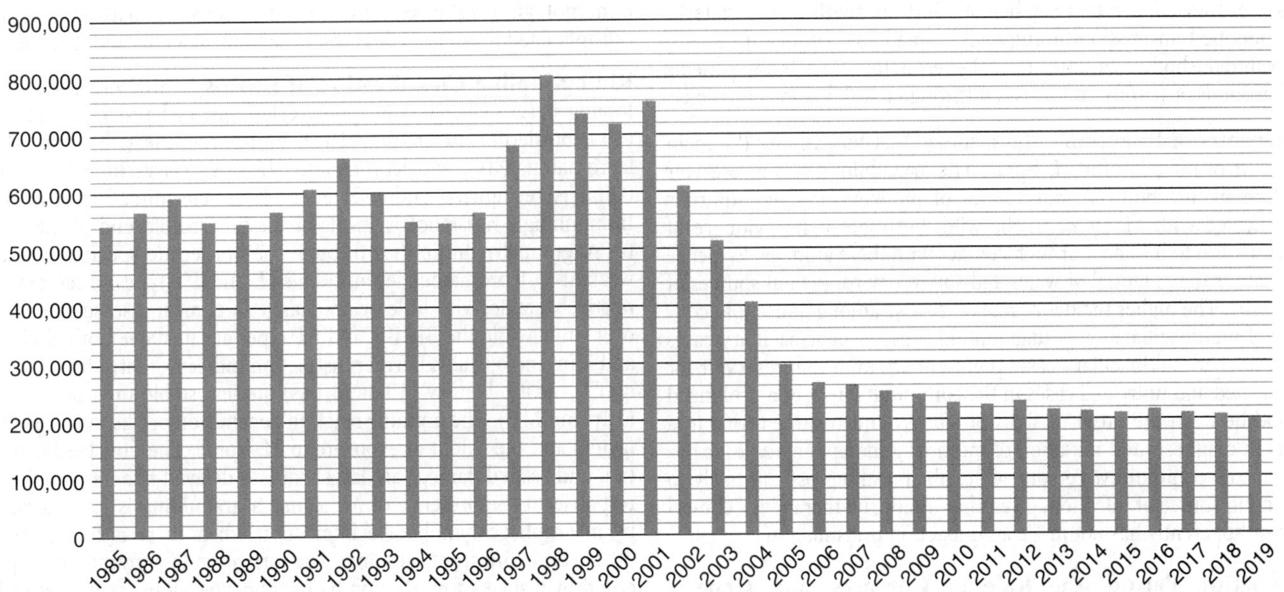

FIGURE 179-1 Global trend in leprosy new-case detection, 1985–2019.

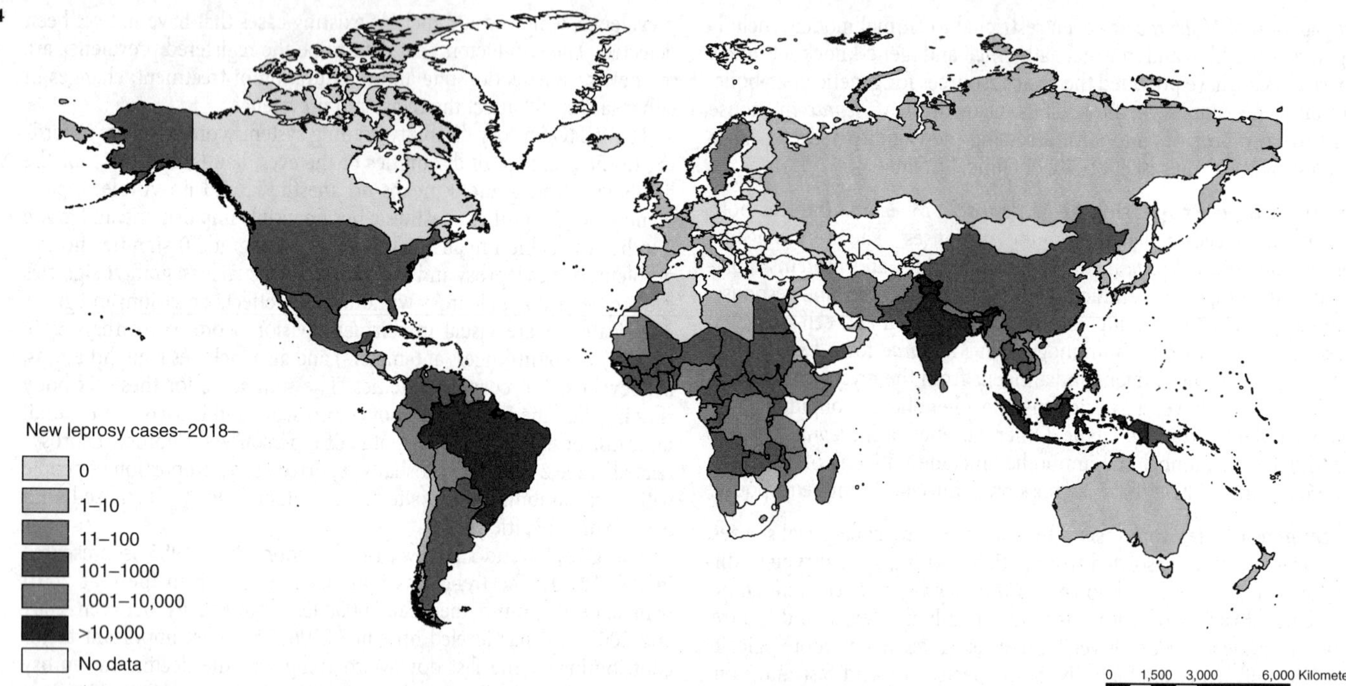

FIGURE 179-2 Geographic distribution of new leprosy cases, 2018. *(Reproduced with permission from Global leprosy update, 2018: moving towards a leprosy-free world. Wkly Epidemiol Rec 35/36:389, 2019.)*

There are large variations among world regions and countries in new case detection rates. Approximately 80% of global new case detection is reported from India, Brazil, and Indonesia. There are also distinct geographic variations within countries, with differences between urban and rural communities and clustering of cases at the village or neighborhood level. Geographic variations can be due to differences in health service provision, socioeconomic development, isolation, and poverty. **Figure 179-2** depicts the geographic distribution of new leprosy cases in 2018.

Transmission Understanding of the transmission of *M. leprae* is limited. The existing evidence is largely circumstantial because of the long incubation period from exposure to disease, the inability to culture *M. leprae*, and the difficulty of diagnosing both infection and early disease. *M. leprae* organisms can be shed in large numbers from the mouth and nose of patients with untreated multibacillary leprosy (droplet infection) and sometimes from damaged skin, but it is unclear whether patients with paucibacillary leprosy can spread the bacillus. There is evidence for transmission between humans and—in southern U.S. states—for zoonotic transmission through wild armadillos. The main route of entry into the body is assumed to be the respiratory tract, but in patients with wounds or tattoos, transmission through the skin also is possible.

Reservoirs of Infection It is assumed that humans are the main reservoir of infection for *M. leprae*. The armadillo is also a reservoir for human infection. Certain species of monkeys and red squirrels are infected with *M. leprae* in the wild, but there is no evidence of transmission to humans through contact with these animals. Evidence is weak for the potential of water and soil as environmental sources of *M. leprae*. The higher incidence rate of leprosy among household contacts of multibacillary cases than among those of paucibacillary cases suggests that multibacillary cases represent an important reservoir for undetected and untreated cases in the community; that is, a prolonged period between the onset of signs of leprosy and treatment due to a delay in diagnosis and initiation of multidrug therapy increases exposure in the community. Persons with subclinical leprosy are likely to be a main source of infection, given that multidrug therapy for clinical leprosy apparently has not made an impact on transmission.

Incubation Period, the Role of Contacts, and Genetic Susceptibility The incubation period of leprosy is estimated to range from 2 to ≥10 years. The incubation period for multibacillary leprosy appears to be longer (5 to ≥10 years) than that for paucibacillary leprosy (~2–5 years). Poverty-associated factors such as low level of education, poor hygiene, and food shortages have been identified as risk factors for leprosy, but the most important risk factors are associated with intimacy and duration of contact with a leprosy patient, in particular with an index case with multibacillary leprosy, and the intensity of contact with and physical distance from the index patient. Increasing evidence from studies in twins and from observational studies supports host genetic susceptibility to leprosy. Ongoing studies are exploring the mechanism underlying genetic susceptibility to leprosy and its clinical manifestations.

PATHOGENESIS

Whatever the route of *M. leprae*'s entry into the human body, the pathogenic process usually starts in the peripheral nerves. Once bacilli are engulfed by Schwann cells, the histopathologic changes in nerve and skin—and thus the type of leprosy that develops—depend on the immunologic resistance of the person infected, in particular on the cell-mediated immune (CMI) response to the bacillus and its antigens.

Ridley-Jopling Classification of Leprosy In 1962, Ridley and Jopling described five overlapping categories of leprosy: tuberculoid (TT), borderline tuberculoid (BT), mid-borderline (BB), borderline lepromatous (BL), and lepromatous (LL). An early clinical manifestation is recognized and referred to as indeterminate leprosy (IL). Immunologic resistance is strong at the tuberculoid end of the spectrum, gradually diminishes through the borderline spectrum, and is weakest in lepromatous leprosy. The LL and TT types of leprosy are relatively stable, with little or no change in clinical disease expression over time, while the BL, BB, and BT types are unstable both clinically and immunologically. Further distinction indicates that subpolar types of TT and LL leprosy (TTs and LLs) are less stable than polar types (TTp and LLp). The immune reaction depends on predisposing genetic factors and the extent of exposure to *M. leprae*. The host tissue's reaction and related damage are largely due to delayed hypersensitivity. In response to the presence of *M. leprae*, a granuloma is formed either by macrophage-lymphocyte interaction when there is immunity or otherwise by macrophages only. The formation of a granuloma is preceded by a stage of infiltration by lymphocytes alone, as is seen in IL. Because of the strong immune response toward the tuberculoid end of the spectrum, macrophages, along with many lymphocytes, become fixed epithelioid cells, and groups of these cells become giant cells. The tuberculoid granuloma leads to nerve destruction resulting in anesthesia and muscle weakness. The cellular response is less focal and less destructive in the borderline portion of the spectrum; consequently, there is less damage to nerves and few bacilli are present. In BL leprosy, there are macrophage granulomas along with lymphocytes, but little nerve damage and more bacilli. In LL leprosy, bacilli multiply within Schwann cells and perineural cells. Liberated bacilli from these cells are engulfed by histiocytes, becoming wandering macrophages and traveling throughout the body to other nerves and tissues via blood, lymph, and tissue fluids. In addition, there are diffuse lepromas in LL leprosy that consist of histiocytes and/or macrophages, with very few lymphocytes and plasma cells. The bacilli are packed within macrophages called *globi* and outside macrophages either singly or in small groups.

WHO Simplified Clinical Classification of Leprosy Ridley-Jopling classification requires clinical and pathologic expertise that does not exist in many settings. The WHO has therefore introduced a simplified classification system based on slit-skin smear: patients with negative slit-skin smear results at all body sites are classified as having paucibacillary leprosy, whereas patients with positive smears at any body site are classified as having multibacillary leprosy. However, because slit-skin smear facilities are not available or dependable in many countries, most leprosy control programs use clinical criteria only for classifying leprosy and deciding on the appropriate treatment regimen for individual patients. In this circumstance, paucibacillary leprosy is defined as one to five skin lesions and no or only one involved peripheral nerve, while multibacillary leprosy is defined as six or more skin lesions and/or more than one involved peripheral nerve.

CLINICAL MANIFESTATIONS

Leprosy is a disease affecting mainly the skin, cutaneous and peripheral nerves, mucous membranes, and, less commonly, other sites such as joints, lymph nodes, eyes, and testes. Other systemic manifestations may occur, particularly in BL and LL disease, with or without leprosy reactions. Most dermal and cutaneous nerves feeding skin lesions are affected—e.g., the supraorbital, great auricular, radial cutaneous, infrapatellar, superficial fibular, and sural nerves and the cutaneous nerves of the thigh. The peripheral nerves involved include the ulnar, median, radial (in upper limbs), lateral popliteal, and posterior tibial (in lower limbs). The cranial nerves commonly involved are the trigeminal and facial.

Indeterminate Leprosy (IL) This early clinical type manifests as one or a few hypopigmented or faintly erythematous, ill-defined to well-defined macular lesions measuring 1–5 cm in diameter. These lesions invariably occur on the external aspects of the limbs, buttocks, and face, with mild to moderate impairment of touch and/or thermal sensations. There is no thickening of the corresponding cutaneous and peripheral nerves. IL is often, but not always, the first clinical sign of leprosy. This type either heals spontaneously or progresses to a determinate form of the disease (TT, BT, BB, BL, or LL), depending on CMI status.

Tuberculoid (TT) Leprosy TT leprosy (Fig. 179-3) presents either as a well-defined, hypopigmented macule or as a raised, erythematous/brown/copper-colored plaque with a well-defined edge. The lesions may be found on any part of the skin and are characterized by complete loss of fine touch and temperature sensations over their surface. Skin lesions are single or few (up to three) in number and can be of any size, but they seldom measure >10 cm in diameter. In plaque-type lesions, the raised clear-cut edge often slopes inward to a flattened and sometimes hypopigmented central area, acquiring an annular configuration. The skin surface of both macular and plaque lesions is dry, hairless, and anesthetic because of destruction of underlying superficial cutaneous nerves. Larger corresponding cutaneous nerves are thickened in a limited number of cases. On the face, sensory impairment may be difficult to demonstrate because of the generous and bilateral supply of sensory nerve endings. Autonomic nerve damage within the lesion is responsible for surface dryness and loss of sweating over the lesion. A solitary peripheral-nerve trunk in the vicinity of a lesion may be thickened, with sensory loss of the area supplied and with or without motor disfigurement. On slit-skin smear examination, no acid-fast bacilli (AFB) are normally found. The lepromin skin test is strongly positive, signifying good host CMI status.

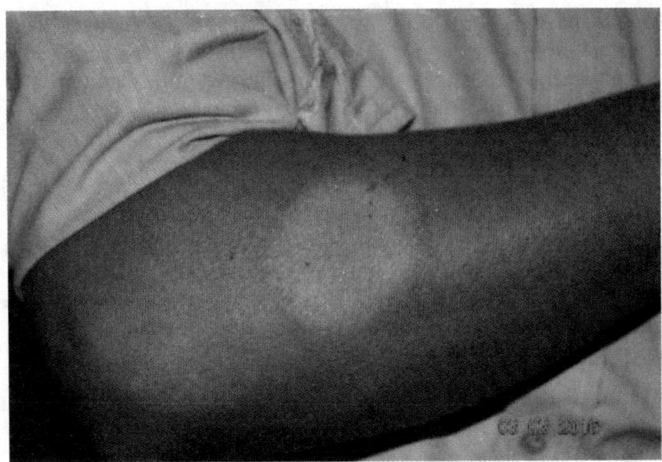

FIGURE 179-3 Tuberculoid (TT) leprosy. Hypopigmented macular lesion with a well-defined edge and loss of fine-touch sensation. *(From Dr. H. K. Kar, with permission.)*

Borderline Tuberculoid (BT) Leprosy BT leprosy (Fig. 179-4) is characterized by either macular or plaque-type lesions numbering three to nine or more and asymmetrically located on any part of the body, with variable sizes and contours. The margins of the lesions range from poorly defined to well defined; sometimes both forms of margin are seen in one lesion. There may be smaller satellite lesions around a larger one, especially on sides where the margin is less defined; this characteristic indicates downgrading of the lesion from TT to BT leprosy. The edges of plaque lesions may slope outward in contrast to TT lesions, which slope inward; plaques may gradually fade outward and eventually blend into normal-looking skin. Loss of sensation is less intense than it is in TT lesions and dryness on the surface less conspicuous. Several peripheral nerves are likely to be enlarged in an asymmetrical pattern, with sensory and motor deficits. One of the most striking features of BT leprosy is susceptibility to a type 1 leprosy reaction (T1R; see below) that exacerbates skin lesions and/or peripheral nerves. If not diagnosed and treated early, disease in these patients tends to downgrade across the spectrum to BB, BL, or LLs leprosy, with an increasing bacteriologic index and a regressed CMI response causing nerve damage along the way. Slit-skin smears show bacteriologic indices varying from negative to 1+.

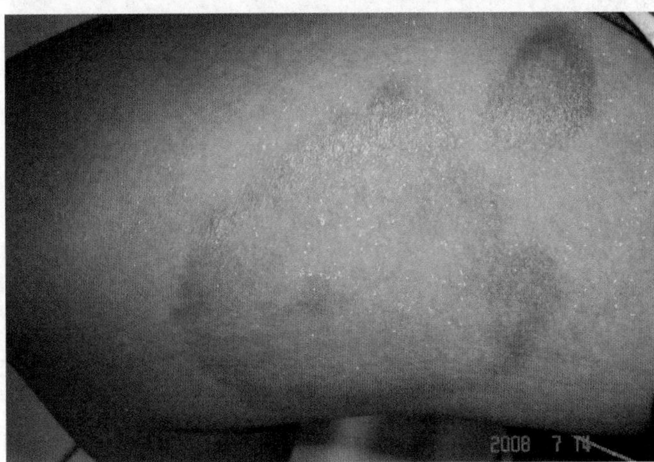

FIGURE 179-4 Borderline tuberculoid (BT) leprosy. Macular lesion with irregular, moderately defined edge and satellite lesion, with loss of sensation. *(From Dr. W. H. van Brakel, with permission from NLR.)*

Mid-Borderline (BB) Leprosy This form of leprosy is unstable. Many cases downgrade toward BL and LLs disease, especially if not treated. There are multiple plaque lesions and, not infrequently, macular lesions; the lesions are of various shapes and sizes, are bilateral, and usually occur in a more or less symmetrical distribution. In annular lesions, the inner edge is well demarcated and "punched out," and the outer edge is ill defined and merges with normal-looking skin. The surface of the lesions is moderately shiny and the central area looks pale. There is minimal loss of sensation over the lesions. Nerve damage is variable in BB leprosy. Many nerves may be thickened, and this effect may be asymmetrical. BB leprosy is not commonly observed and rapidly changes its spectrum—rarely to BT leprosy but more often to BL disease. The lepromin test is negative. Slit-skin smears of lesions show a moderate number of AFB (2+ to 3+).

Borderline Lepromatous (BL) Leprosy In BL leprosy (Fig. 179-5) there are numerous bilateral, round or oval, macular, diffusely infiltrated, erythematous or hypopigmented lesions with moderately defined borders. The lesions are usually 2–3 cm in diameter, may have a coppery hue, and tend to become symmetrical. Some loss of sensation may be detected, particularly over older lesions; however, no loss of sensation is observed over fresh lesions. With disease progression, papules, nodules, and plaques develop over the macular lesions. In untreated patients, new ill-defined skin lesions continue to develop. Widespread but asymmetrical thickening of peripheral nerves, with or without tenderness, leads to sensory and motor deficits. The lepromin test gives negative results, as it does in all degrees of lepromatous leprosy. Slit-skin smear examination of lesions shows a bacteriologic index varying from 3+ to 4+.

Lepromatous (LL) Leprosy LL leprosy (Fig. 179-6) presents with innumerable bilateral, symmetrically distributed, diffusely indurated, erythematous, copper-colored or skin-colored patches or plaques. There is no loss of sensation over these lesions, which have a smooth, shiny surface. The lesions spread over the face, earlobes, ears, extensor aspects of the upper and lower extremities, back, and buttocks. Induration can readily be recognized when lesions are viewed tangentially under natural sunlight. The induration initially is of a finer type but gradually becomes coarse, and lesions then progress to papules, plaques, and nodules. Bilateral earlobe thickening and eyebrow loss occur. Coarse induration on the face sometimes results in gross skin folds that lead to an appearance referred to as "lion face," particularly when associated with loss of eyebrows and thickening of earlobes. Of all cases of LL leprosy, 10–15% are of the polar type (LLp) from the time of lesion onset; the remaining cases downgrade from the untreated borderline spectrum to subpolar LLs leprosy. Patients with LLs disease develop nerve damage during the borderline stages. In LLp disease, involvement of peripheral nerves occurs late and is bilateral and symmetrical, with sensory loss in a "glove-and-stocking" distribution. Slit-skin smear examination shows a bacteriologic index of 4+ to 6+ with globi.

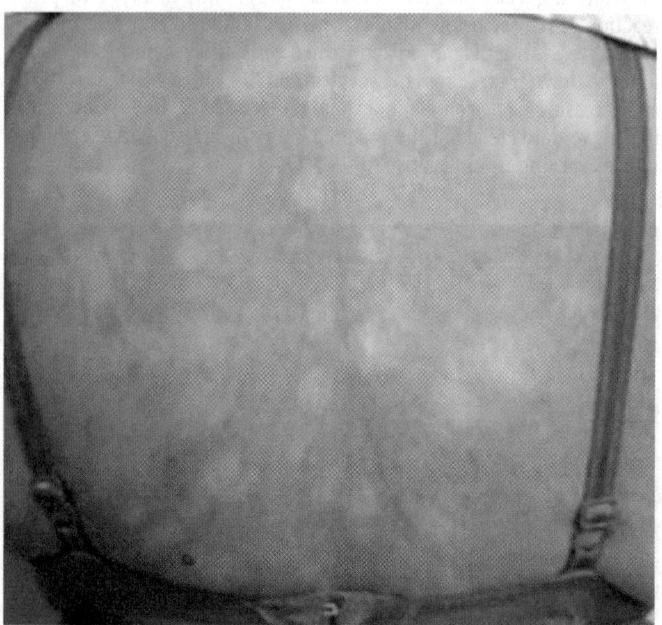

FIGURE 179-5 Borderline lepromatous (BL) leprosy. Numerous diffusely infiltrated erythematous and hypopigmented macules, downgrading from borderline tuberculoid to lepromatous leprosy. *(From Dr. C. L. M. van Hees, Department of Dermatology, Erasmus MC, University Medical Center, Rotterdam, the Netherlands, with permission.)*

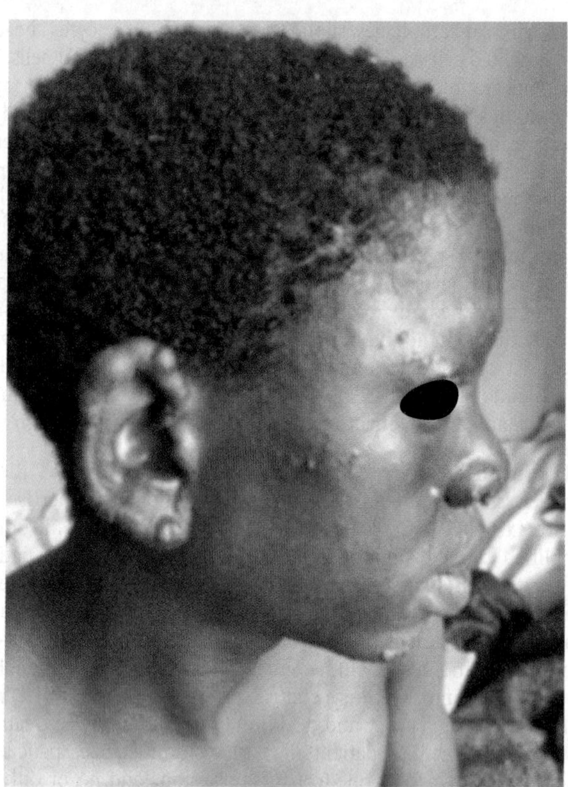

FIGURE 179-6 Lepromatous (LL) leprosy. Multiple nodules on ears and face and loss of eyebrows. *(From Dr. K. Mponda, Department of Dermatology, Queen Elisabeth Central Hospital, Blantyre, Malawi, with permission.)*

SYSTEMIC INVOLVEMENT In LL leprosy, AFB are found in the lymph nodes, spleen, liver, bone marrow, adrenal glands, smooth and striated muscles, tooth pulp, testes, oral cavity, nose, larynx, and eyes. Involvement of the testes leads first to sterility and then to gynecomastia and impotence. Eye involvement includes corneal anesthesia; early on, this manifestation is due to bacillary infiltration of corneal nerves, while later it arises from damage to the ophthalmic division of the trigeminal nerve. In addition, eye involvement includes episcleritis, iridocyclitis, iris atrophy, cataract and glaucoma, lagophthalmos, corneal ulceration and perforation, and blindness. The nose is the portal of entry for *M. leprae* and is the earliest site of involvement in LL leprosy. Edema and mucosal thickening occur in the inferior turbinate and nasal septum, with crusting and epistaxis. Later, patients develop chronic rhinitis with loss of smell sensation. Septal perforation due to bony destruction, with typical saddle-nose disfigurement, is common in advanced LL disease. In late-stage LL leprosy, ulceration of the tongue, pharynx, hard and soft palates (leading to palate perforation), tonsillar pillars, and uvula occurs. In the hands, slow resorption sets in, starting from the distal end of the terminal phalanx and proceeding proximally to involve the middle and proximal phalanges.

HISTOID LEPROSY Histoid leprosy is a rare form of LL leprosy in which waxy, shiny, firm, symmetrical or asymmetrical nodules and plaques are observed over normal-looking skin. Histologic examination of these lesions shows specific spindle-cell granulomas. Slit-skin smear examination reveals high bacteriologic and microbiologic indices without globi in most cases.

DIFFUSE LEPROSY OF LUCIO AND LATAPÍ This rare form of non-nodular LL leprosy occurring in Mexico and Central America is characterized by diffuse shiny infiltration of the skin and widespread sensory loss. The skin looks waxy and has a shiny appearance ("lepra bonita," or beautiful leprosy), with obvious diffuse induration of the earlobes and forehead as well as loss of eyebrows, sometimes eyelashes, and not infrequently all body hair. This form of leprosy can be complicated by an unusual reaction known as Lucio's phenomenon (see below).

Primary Neuritic Leprosy In some countries, such as India and Nepal, primary neuritic disease is observed in 2–10% of all leprosy cases, with only peripheral nerve involvement and no skin lesions. Nerve thickening and sensory loss occur in the affected area, with or without a motor deficit. Primary neuritic leprosy, even though not described by Ridley and Jopling, can manifest at different points along the disease spectrum. For practical purposes, primary neuritic leprosy is classified as paucibacillary or multibacillary on the basis of the absence or presence of AFB in nerve biopsy sections or the number of thickened nerves (single or multiple).

LEPROSY REACTIONS

Leprosy reactions are immunologic phenomena that occur before, during, or after treatment. They are severe complications that need to be diagnosed and treated early to prevent nerve function impairment and subsequent disfigurement as well as blindness.

Type 1 Leprosy Reaction (T1R) T1R is a delayed hypersensitivity reaction associated with sudden alteration of CMI status and leading to a shift in the patient's position on the leprosy spectrum. This reaction is marked by infiltration of lesions by activated CD4+ T lymphocytes, especially T helper cells. T1R is also called a *reversal reaction* because of the upgrading of CMI status. T1R is usually observed in the borderline portion of the spectrum. Skin lesions are characterized by acute swelling and redness (**Fig. 179-7**). Nerves may be painful and tender because of neuritis, with consequent nerve damage and disfigurement. In the severe form of T1R, nerve abscesses may be formed. Loss of nerve function can be much less obvious than usual when it occurs without other signs of inflammation. This "silent neuritis" may lead to sensory and motor impairment in the hands, feet, and face. Arthralgia or arthritis sometimes occurs. Rarely, the patient may develop fever and malaise, tenosynovitis, and edema of the feet and hands.

Type 2 Leprosy Reaction (T2R) T2R, also known as ENL (erythema nodosum leprosum), is an immune complex–mediated syndrome (i.e., an antigen–antibody reaction involving complement) that causes inflammation of the skin, nerves, and other organs as well as general malaise. ENL is an example of a type III hypersensitivity reaction (Coombs and Gell classification) or Arthus phenomenon. This reaction occurs mostly during multidrug therapy but can also develop in untreated patients. Evanescent, pink-to-red maculopapular, papular, nodular, or plaque lesions suddenly appear and are usually accompanied by constitutional symptoms like malaise and fever, with or without painful swelling in the joints (**Fig. 179-8**). These crops of skin lesions present on the outer aspects of the thighs, legs, and face. They are painful or tender and warm, blanch with light finger pressure, and last for a few days. The lesions change in color from pink/red to bluish and brownish after 24–48 h and turn dark in a week. Rarely, ENL lesions become vesicular, pustular, bullous, and necrotic and break down to produce ulceration (erythema nodosum necroticans). The patient may have other associated signs such as lymph node enlargement, myositis, arthritis, synovitis, rhinitis, epistaxis, laryngitis, iridocyclitis, glaucoma, painful dactylitis, acute epididymoorchitis, nephritis and renal failure, hepatosplenomegaly, anemia, and—at a later stage—amyloidosis. Severe T2R may include swollen, painful, and tender nerve trunks with sensory and motor deficits.

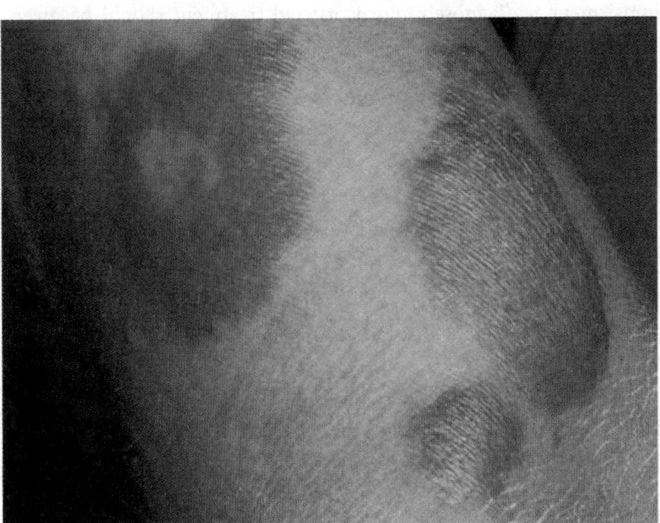

FIGURE 179-7 Type 1 leprosy reaction. Increased inflammation of existing lesions. *(From Dr. W. H. van Brakel, with permission from NLR.)*

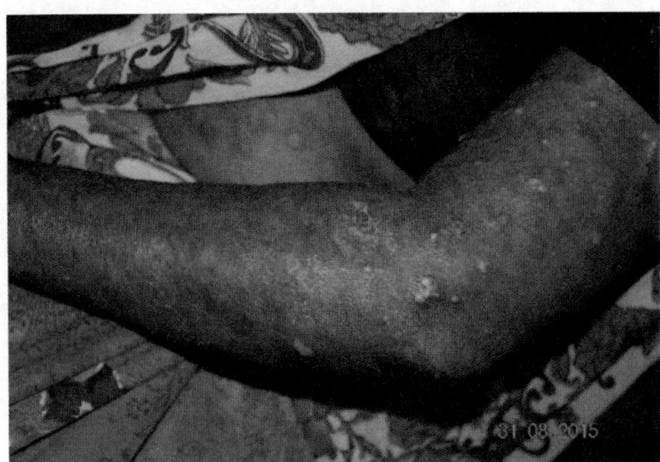

FIGURE 179-8 Type 2 leprosy reaction. Erythema nodosum leprosum, with pustular lesions. *(From Dr. H. K. Kar, with permission.)*

Lucio's Phenomenon Lucio's phenomenon is observed in diffuse leprosy of Lucio and Latapí and may be a variant of erythema nodosum necroticans. Marked vasculitis and thrombosis of the superficial and deep vessels result in hemorrhage and infarction of the skin. Clinically, the skin reaction begins as slightly indurated, bluish-red, ill-defined, painful, and rarely palpable plaques with an erythematous halo, usually developing on one limb but sometimes on other areas of the body. The lesions are irregular or triangular. After a few days, they become purplish at the center; a central hemorrhagic infarct may develop with or without blister formation, and a necrotic eschar that detaches easily and leaves an ulcer of irregular shape may follow later. The ulcer heals, leaving a superficial scar. Patients remain afebrile throughout.

Nerve Function Impairment, Neuritis, and Disfigurement The terms *nerve function impairment, nerve damage, neuropathy*, and *neuritis* are often used interchangeably for the sensory, motor, and/or autonomic nerve deficits that occur because of the pathologic processes resulting from *M. leprae* infection of the nerve. Neuritis (nerve inflammation) in leprosy is usually a subacute, demyelinating, and unremitting event involving cutaneous nerves and larger peripheral nerves. "Silent neuritis" or "quiet nerve paralysis" is defined as progressive sensory or motor impairment in the absence of symptoms such as pain, paresthesia, or tenderness of the nerve and with no obvious signs of leprosy reactions. Neuritis can occur at any time during leprosy but is more common and severe during leprosy reactions, mainly in T1R. Sensory and motor neuropathy can lead to secondary impairments in the upper and lower extremities, such as muscle atrophy, mobile- and fixed-joint contractures, bone absorption of digits, and cracks and wounds.

DIAGNOSIS

Clinical Diagnosis Three cardinal signs indicate a diagnosis of leprosy. The diagnosis can be established when two of these three signs are present:

1. Hypopigmented or erythematous skin lesion(s) with definite loss or impairment of sensation: The clinical presentation of skin patches or plaques is diagnostic when it is associated with a definite loss or impairment of sensation (light touch, pain, and/or temperature). Diagnostic dilemmas arise in the indeterminate stage of leprosy because of variable loss of sensation and the presence of facial lesions (i.e., because the density of innervation in the face can compensate for damage to certain nerve branches).
2. Involvement of the peripheral nerves, as demonstrated by definite thickening with sensory impairment: Thickening of a peripheral nerve should be assessed by palpation of the affected nerve and comparison with the corresponding contralateral nerve. In multibacillary leprosy, thickening of nerves is often bilateral. Nerve tenderness is established by the application of mild pressure on the nerve during palpation with the fingertips. The peripheral nerves commonly palpated in a leprosy patient are the greater auricular, ulnar, radial, radial cutaneous, median, lateral popliteal, posterior tibial, sural, and superficial peroneal nerves.
3. A positive result for AFB in slit-skin smears, establishment of the presence of AFB in a skin smear or biopsy sample, or a positive result in a biopsy PCR.

Diagnostic Tools • TESTING OF SKIN SENSATION Light-touch sensation is tested with cotton wool or a feather. Pain is assessed as the patient's ability to distinguish between the sharp and blunt ends of a wooden or bamboo toothpick. Thermal sensation thresholds are assessed with computer-assisted sensory testing equipment.

SLIT-SKIN SMEAR Normally a slit-skin smear is taken from four sites: the right earlobe, the forehead above the eyebrows, the chin, and the left buttock in men or the left upper thigh in women. The material is stained with Ziehl-Neelsen reagent and examined with a light microscope. The bacteriologic index is determined with a standard logarithmic scale and graded from 0 to 6. The microbiologic index is determined as the percentage of solid, stained AFB.

SKIN BIOPSY A skin biopsy is done to confirm the diagnosis of leprosy, to classify the disease, to support the diagnosis of reactions, and to determine cure after the completion of multidrug therapy. When macular lesions are suspected of reflecting IL, a biopsy sample should be taken from the middle of a lesion; with plaques, a sample should be obtained from the active indurated edge. When there are numerous skin lesions with different morphologies, more than one biopsy sample is required for proper evaluation of the disease spectrum. Identification of early lesions of leprosy by histopathologic techniques is enhanced by immunochemical staining, which reveals the presence of *M. leprae* antigens.

PGL-1 ANTIBODY TEST PGL-1 is a specific lipid on the *M. leprae* cell wall. A PGL-1 ELISA has been used for serologic diagnosis of leprosy, yielding positive results in 90–95% of multibacillary cases and in 25–60% of paucibacillary cases. Using PGL-1 antigen and adopting an immunochromatographic technique, a rapid lateral-flow assay—the ML flow test—has been developed for detection of antibody to PGL-1. This assay gives positive results in 92–97% of patients with multibacillary leprosy and in 32–40% of patients with paucibacillary disease.

LEPROMIN TEST The lepromin (or Mitsuda) skin test measures cellular immunity against lepromin. A bacillary suspension standardized by the number of inactivated *M. leprae* it contains is injected just under the skin. The reaction to lepromin is measured as induration in millimeters 3–4 weeks after intradermal inoculation. The result provides information about the ability of an individual's T cells to respond to *M. leprae* and the likelihood of granuloma formation in that individual. A negative lepromin test is generally seen in patients with LL or BL leprosy, indicating the lack of a protective cellular response.

GENE AMPLIFICATION (PCR) TECHNIQUE Gene amplification significantly enhances the detection of *M. leprae*, especially in bacteriologic index–negative leprosy and cases that do not fulfill the criteria for the cardinal signs of leprosy. The several PCR methods developed to amplify different gene stretches in *M. leprae* include conventional DNA-based PCR, reverse-transcription PCR, and multiplex PCR. As major genes for detection of disease targets, PCR uses *M. leprae*–specific genes encoding 36-kDa antigen, 18-kDa antigen, 65-kDa antigen complex 85, 16S ribosomal RNA (rRNA), and repetitive sequences. These assays are sensitive to as few as 1–10 bacilli and yield positive results in 60–75% of smear-negative cases. Multiplex PCR employing the genes encoding the repetitive element RLEP, SodA, and 16S rRNA can be used for early diagnosis and for the diagnosis of subclinical infection among household contacts.

Differential Diagnosis Leprosy is often diagnosed late, with a consequent increase in the risk of nerve damage and its ensuing disabilities. The hypopigmented macules of leprosy must be differentiated from a variety of conditions, including pityriasis alba, vitiligo, progressive macular hypomelanosis, pityriasis versicolor, pityriasis rosea, postinflammatory hypopigmentation, sarcoidosis, post–kala-azar dermal leishmaniasis, and morphea. In the analysis of plaques and nodular lesions, conditions such as granuloma annulare, cutaneous sarcoidosis, cutaneous leishmaniasis, lupus miliaris disseminatus faciei, nodular histiocytosis, lupus erythematosus, cutaneous T-cell lymphomas (especially mycosis fungoides), and secondary syphilis should be kept in mind. ENL lesions must be differentiated from erythema nodosum of other etiologies, nodular vasculitis, and cutaneous polyarteritis nodosa. In the case of mononeuropathy lesions, diabetes, amyloidosis, and myxedema must be considered. With polyneuropathy lesions of acute onset, Guillain-Barré syndrome and toxic polyneuropathy must be given consideration.

Diagnostic Tools for Nerve Function Impairment All sensory modalities, autonomic function, and motor function of motor nerves may be affected in leprosy to varying degrees. The modalities mediated by small unmyelinated fibers, such as pain and warm temperature sensation and autonomic function, are often affected first. Clinically detectable impairment of touch sensation and motor function frequently follows after several months. Unfortunately, tools that allow reliable and safe testing of pain and temperature sensation and autonomic function often are not available at peripheral health facilities, but simple and reliable tests of touch sensation and motor function do provide a reflection of the underlying neuropathy.

TOUCH SENSATION TESTING The ulnar and median nerves and the posterior tibial nerve are usually tested for touch sensation. The most reliable test is the Semmes-Weinstein monofilament (SWM) test. If the impairment is of <6 months' duration and/or new nerve function impairment is diagnosed, glucocorticoid treatment should be given. Because filaments are not available in most peripheral health centers, the WHO recommends that a ballpoint pen be used instead. The testing protocol is the same as in the SWM test: the stimulus is delivered by touching the test sites with the tip of a ballpoint pen held at an angle of ~45° relative to the skin.

VOLUNTARY MUSCLE TESTING Motor function of the hands and feet should be evaluated by voluntary muscle testing. The muscle functions most affected in leprosy are eye closure (facial nerve), finger abduction (ulnar nerve), thumb opposition (median nerve), wrist extension (radial nerve), and ankle extension (common peroneal nerve). Strength is assessed with a WHO-recommended system as strong, weak, or paralyzed.

NERVE CONDUCTION TESTS Testing of nerve conduction parameters is sensitive in detecting early signs of peripheral neuropathy in leprosy. Sensory nerve conduction parameters are often affected several months ahead of clinical tests (e.g., the SWM test). However, a trial of glucocorticoid treatment of such early changes did not show improved long-term outcomes, perhaps suggesting that the glucocorticoids are unable to switch off or reverse the pathologic process.

ULTRASOUND TESTING OF NERVES Palpable enlargement of certain peripheral nerves is one of the cardinal signs of leprosy. Definite enlargement is easy to establish, but milder degrees are much harder to diagnose by palpation. Ultrasound imaging and measurement of nerve diameters—even with portable equipment—can detect nerve enlargement accurately. This technique may be used to support the diagnosis of leprosy and may indicate the onset of neuropathy that warrants anti-inflammatory treatment.

OTHER TESTS OF PERIPHERAL NERVE FUNCTION Pain and temperature sensation are commonly affected in leprosy neuropathy. However, these sensations are difficult to test safely and reliably under field conditions. Studies have shown that heat detection thresholds are often affected several months before touch sensation is impaired. Laser Doppler measurement of autonomic vasomotor reflexes is a sensitive method for detection of peripheral autonomic nerve damage in leprosy patients.

TREATMENT
Leprosy, Leprosy Reactions, And Other Major Manifestations

TREATMENT OF LEPROSY

Multidrug Therapy Only one multidrug regimen is recommended by the WHO for the treatment of leprosy. This regimen consists of a combination of two or three of the following drugs: rifampin, dapsone, and clofazimine (**Table 179-1**). The keystone of WHO-recommended multidrug therapy for multibacillary leprosy is a monthly dose of rifampin together with daily doses of dapsone and daily and monthly doses of clofazimine. Patients with paucibacillary leprosy are treated with two drugs, receiving monthly doses of rifampin and daily doses of dapsone. The treatment duration is 12 months for multibacillary disease and 6 months for paucibacillary disease. Provided that patients complete therapy, treatment failure rates are very low.

Some studies have investigated a uniform regimen of three drugs for 6 months. In a recent systematic review of evidence on the potential benefits and risks of this shorter regimen, the WHO concluded that relevant evidence is limited and inconclusive, with a potential increase in the risk of relapse. Therefore, the WHO does not recommend a shortened treatment duration for multibacillary leprosy.

The WHO further recommends supervised intake, but actual practice varies among countries. Through the WHO, multidrug therapy is provided free of charge as blister packs for adults to all countries reporting leprosy. Blister packs are also provided for 10- to 14-year-olds, while younger children are given doses adjusted according to body weight (Table 179-1).

TABLE 179-1 WHO-Recommended Multidrug Treatment for Leprosy

DRUG, AGE GROUP	PAUCIBACILLARY LEPROSY[a]	MULTIBACILLARY LEPROSY[b]
Dapsone		
Adult	100 mg/d	100 mg/d
Child age 10–14 years	50 mg/d	50 mg/d
Child <10 years	Dose adjusted to body weight	Dose adjusted to body weight
Rifampin		
Adult	600 mg monthly	600 mg monthly
Child 10–14 years	450 mg monthly	450 mg monthly
Child <10 years	Dose adjusted to body weight	Dose adjusted to body weight
Clofazimine[c]		
Adult	—	50 mg/d plus 300 mg monthly
Child 10–14 years	—	50 mg/d plus 150 mg monthly
Child <10 years	—	Dose adjusted to body weight

[a]Duration: 6 doses (6 blister packs). [b]Duration: 12 doses (12 blister packs). [c]In 2018, the World Health Organization (WHO) suggested including clofazimine in the multidrug therapy regimen for paucibacillary leprosy as well, but it is questionable whether this suggestion will be implemented because of the possibility that skin discoloration might compromise compliance. In addition, this alteration would involve a major change in the production of blister packs, which currently do not include clofazimine for paucibacillary leprosy patients (in line with the original WHO recommendation).

Adverse Events • **Rifampin** Rifampin acts by inhibiting DNA-dependent RNA polymerase, thereby interfering with bacterial RNA synthesis. Rifampin is well absorbed orally. Hepatotoxicity may occur with a mild transient elevation of hepatic aminotransferases, but this reaction is rare at the dosages and intervals recommended for leprosy and is not an indication for discontinuation of treatment. Because rifampin is given only monthly in WHO-recommended multidrug therapy regimens, the adverse effects recognized from its use in tuberculosis probably do not occur. A monthly dose of rifampin probably does not cause induction of hepatic cytochrome p450, but this outcome has not been formally assessed. Urine discoloration occurs but is harmless.

Dapsone Dapsone (4,4-diaminodiphenyl sulfone [DDS]) acts by blocking folic acid synthesis and is only weakly bactericidal. Oral absorption is good, and the drug has a long half-life averaging 28 h. Dapsone has a poor safety profile, and its use should be monitored carefully. In the doses recommended for leprosy, it can cause mild hemolysis and may cause anemia or, rarely, psychosis. Glucose-6-phosphate dehydrogenase deficiency seldom causes a problem, and enzyme levels are not routinely tested before the start of multidrug treatment. On the other hand, the "DDS syndrome" (also called the *dapsone hypersensitivity syndrome*) is a severe adverse event that is not uncommon in some countries. It usually develops 6 weeks after the commencement of dapsone administration and manifests as fever, skin rash, eosinophilia, lymphadenopathy, hepatitis, and encephalopathy. Other rare but severe cutaneous adverse reactions are erythema multiforme, Stevens-Johnson syndrome, toxic epidermal necrolysis, and exfoliative dermatitis. The fatality rate for DDS syndrome is 10%, with death occurring from liver failure, sepsis, and bone marrow failure. Most patients require treatment with systemic glucocorticoids. In all cases, dapsone treatment must be stopped. Agranulocytosis, hepatitis, and cholestatic jaundice occur rarely with dapsone therapy.

Clofazimine Clofazimine is a brick-red, fat-soluble crystalline dye. The mechanism of its weakly bactericidal action against *M. leprae* is not known. High drug concentrations are found in the intestinal mucosa, mesenteric lymph nodes, and body fat. The most noticeable adverse event is skin discoloration ranging from red to purple or black, with the degree of discoloration depending on the dosage. Clofazimine can accumulate in active leprosy skin lesions, thus making them more prominent. The abnormal pigmentation usually fades within 6–12 months of clofazimine discontinuation, although traces of discoloration may remain for up to 4 years. The skin discoloration associated with clofazimine is psychologically distressing for many people. Patients often stop taking the drug because the discoloration is socially disabling for them, alerting their social environment to the fact that they are taking anti-leprosy medication and thus breaking confidentiality about treatment. Urine, sputum, and sweat may become pink during clofazimine administration. Clofazimine also produces a characteristic ichthyosis on the shins and forearms. Adverse gastrointestinal events ranging from mild cramps to diarrhea and weight loss may result from clofazimine crystal deposition in the wall of the small bowel.

Relapse The cure rate for leprosy with multidrug therapy is 99%, but relapse is possible. In multibacillary leprosy, relapse is defined as the multiplication of *M. leprae*, with an increase of at least 2+ over the previous value in the bacteriologic index at any single site;

this change usually occurs in conjunction with evidence of clinical deterioration (e.g., new skin patches or nodules and/or new nerve damage). Relapse rates are well below 1% except among a small proportion of patients who have a very high bacillary load at the start of treatment (bacteriologic index ≥4). In different studies, four to seven relapses were recorded per 100 person-years. These relapses usually occurred <5 years after the end of multidrug therapy. Since antimicrobial resistance to the combination of drugs used in multidrug treatment is rare, patients with relapse can be re-treated with the same multibacillary regimen.

Recognizing a relapse in paucibacillary leprosy can be difficult, as symptoms may resemble T1R. However, relapse of paucibacillary disease is very rare. Administration of a therapeutic trial with glucocorticoids to patients with new lesions may help distinguish between these two phenomena: a definite improvement within 4 weeks of initiation of glucocorticoid therapy indicates T1R, whereas a lack of response favors the diagnosis of a clinical relapse. Patients with multibacillary disease who present with a relapse are re-treated with the multidrug regimen regardless of any change in classification. Patients with paucibacillary disease require 2 years of monitoring after treatment and patients with multibacillary disease at least 5 years. Re-infection by different strains of *M. leprae* is possible and can be confused with relapse.

Rifampin Resistance and Second-Line Drugs Resistance to rifampin has been reported from several countries, although the number of patients involved is small. Evidence on the potential benefits and risks of using alternative regimens for drug-resistant leprosy is not available. Therefore, recommendations provided by the WHO for second-line regimens are based on expert opinion and the known activity of alternative drugs, including the likelihood of cross-resistance. For rifampin-resistant leprosy, the WHO guidelines recommend daily treatment with at least two second-line drugs—clarithromycin, minocycline, or a quinolone (ofloxacin, levofloxacin, or moxifloxacin)—plus clofazimine for 6 months, followed by clofazimine plus one of the second-line drugs daily for an additional 18 months. Leprosy patients infected with *M. leprae* resistant to both rifampin and ofloxacin may be treated daily with the following regimen: clarithromycin, minocycline, and clofazimine for 6 months, followed by clarithromycin or minocycline plus clofazimine for an additional 18 months.

TREATMENT OF LEPROSY REACTIONS

Type 1 Reactions Oral, short-acting glucocorticoids are the treatment of choice for T1R. Prednisolone is used most often in an initial dose of 1 mg/kg of body weight once a day, usually with a maximum of 60–80 mg. If standard treatment protocols are followed, as they are in most leprosy programs in endemic countries, an initial dose of 40 mg of prednisolone is recommended by the WHO. The dose is tapered slowly, usually by 5 mg every 2 weeks over a period of 20 weeks—a schedule that results in better outcomes and lower reaction relapse rates than the previously recommended 12-week glucocorticoid regimen. However, the clinical response should guide treatment. Patients should be examined every 2 weeks, and the examination should include a quick nerve function assessment. Not infrequently, the reaction flares up again once the daily glucocorticoid dose is tapered to <10–20 mg. The potential benefits of longer treatment should be balanced against the risks of prolonged glucocorticoid use, especially at higher doses.

Type 2 Reactions Mild first-time T2R (or ENL) reactions with localized skin nodules may be treated with aspirin and pentoxifylline. If a rapid effect is needed, the most effective drug to date is thalidomide, which rapidly suppresses clinical signs, including nerve impairment and iritis. However, the drug is blacklisted in many countries because of its teratogenicity. If available, it should be given with great caution to women of childbearing age—only after careful counseling and a negative pregnancy test and with strict adherence to contraception. A dose of 100–200 mg is given either once or twice daily. In acute first episodes, thalidomide treatment should be tapered down and stopped after 1–2 weeks. If tissues other than the skin are affected—e.g., the eyes (iritis/uveitis), testes (orchitis), kidneys (nephritis), or joints (arthritis)—longer treatment may be needed until signs and symptoms have resolved. In patients with severe recurrent ENL, a daily thalidomide maintenance dose of 50 mg may be effective in suppressing new episodes. Because of the restricted availability and use of thalidomide, patients with acute ENL are usually treated with glucocorticoids. T2R tends to be transient, often resolving in ~2 weeks. The treatment strategy is therefore to suppress the acute signs and symptoms with high-dose oral prednisolone, quickly tapering treatment in 2–3 weeks either to zero or to a low maintenance dose if the patient has had previous attacks. High-dose clofazimine also is effective in preventing recurrent ENL, but attainment of a maximal effect takes several weeks. The usual regimen is 300 mg daily for 1 month, followed by 200 mg daily for 1 month and, subsequently, 100 mg daily as a maintenance dose for as long as necessary. Prolonged use of high-dose clofazimine may cause significant adverse gastrointestinal effects. An important side effect of clofazimine is a dark discoloration of the skin. While discoloration resolves gradually after the drug is discontinued, it is one main reason that patients dislike or even refuse to take clofazimine.

TREATMENT AND PROGNOSIS OF NERVE FUNCTION IMPAIRMENT

Episodes of sensory or motor nerve function impairment without skin signs are common. Neuropathy may occur without obvious neuritis. Still, the treatment of such "silent neuropathy" is the same as that for T1R. High-dose prednisolone is the drug of choice. Some experts think that patients will benefit from nerve decompression surgery, but evidence from randomized controlled trials is lacking.

If glucocorticoid treatment is started shortly after the development of nerve function impairment, the prognosis for full recovery is good. Generally, some recovery can still be expected up to 6 months after onset, but the likelihood of recovery diminishes with every new episode. Generally, nerve function impairment that has persisted for >6 months does not benefit from glucocorticoid treatment.

TREATMENT OF (NEUROPATHIC) PAIN

Pain is common in people affected by leprosy and is often of neuropathic origin. Little evidence-based information is currently available on the origin and treatment of pain in leprosy. Generally, for the treatment of neuropathic pain, three classes of medication are available: tricyclic antidepressants, phenothiazines, and anticonvulsants (carbamazepine, oxcarbazepine, gabapentin, and pregabalin). These agents can be combined with analgesics and anti-inflammatory drugs according to the patient's needs.

DISEASE MANAGEMENT DURING TREATMENT

Leprosy can be cured effectively, but the long duration of multidrug therapy means that careful management is needed to help the patient complete treatment. Regular visits to a health center may invoke questions from community members that may threaten the patient's privacy, thus causing the patient mental distress and jeopardizing treatment adherence. Counseling is essential, as are patient-friendly arrangements for collecting treatment drugs. The disease, its treatment, and its possible complications should be discussed, including a consideration of disease prognosis, the resolution of skin patches, skin discoloration by clofazimine, the lack of contagiousness during multidrug therapy, and the capacity for unrestricted family relations, including marital life and sexual activity. Possible stigmatization, including self-stigmatization, also should be discussed.

Because of the diverse complications that are possible, especially in patients with multibacillary leprosy, a multidisciplinary approach to patient management is required. In low-income countries, the responsibility for treatment usually lies with a leprosy control officer or a general medical practitioner. In middle- and high-income countries, the main treatment responsibility usually falls to a dermatologist. Additional support should come from a neurologist or neurophysiologist for the diagnosis of nerve function impairment, and a rehabilitation physician, physiotherapist, infectious disease specialist, and/or psychologist may be needed. Occasionally, specialist support with regard to orthotics as well as in ophthalmology, occupational therapy, reconstructive surgery, and/or community-based rehabilitation is indicated.

Supervised Multidrug Therapy Regular treatment is important, especially the supervised 4-weekly dose of rifampin and clofazimine. However, treatment adherence can be facilitated by flexible arrangements; for example, patients can be allowed to take home more than one 4-week blister pack if they will be away for travel or seasonal labor. In such cases, a family member or another responsible person can be asked to supervise the monthly dose.

Monthly Nerve Function Assessment Since nerve damage can be insidious and silent, it is important to conduct a brief nerve function assessment at each clinic visit during multidrug therapy. This regular assessment is especially important in patients with known risk factors for nerve function impairment. At highest risk are patients with multibacillary disease, who already have nerve damage at the start of treatment. Their risk of additional nerve damage is as high as 65%. Multibacillary leprosy patients without nerve function impairment at diagnosis and paucibacillary leprosy patients *with* such impairment at diagnosis have a 16% chance of developing damage and additional damage, respectively. Patients with paucibacillary disease who do not have nerve function impairment at diagnosis are at lowest risk (3%); for them, an assessment at the start and completion of multidrug therapy can be sufficient. Leprosy reactions and new nerve damage may also occur after completion of multidrug treatment. While the risk diminishes with time, these manifestations can occur up to 3 years after the conclusion of therapy.

Health Education During treatment, patients will have questions that need to be addressed in order to ensure their treatment adherence. Sensitive questions may arise regarding everyday life within the family and at work that, if not addressed properly, could lead to social withdrawal and mental health issues. Crucial points for health education are at diagnosis and at completion of treatment. When communicating the diagnosis, the physician must explain that the disease is caused by a curable microbial infection and must cover the possible discomforts of drug intake, the interruption of disease transmission through drug intake, and the importance of adhering to treatment to achieve a cure. At the completion of multidrug therapy, the emphasis should be on separating the concept of cure (bacterial activity) from the sequelae of the disease (nerve function impairment, leprosy reactions, and disabilities) and explaining that the patient may need to continue receiving health care, including reconstructive surgery, for the sequelae. Patients often associate cure with the absence of symptoms, which is not accurate in leprosy. Some patients will experience discomfort during bacterial activity but will have no sequelae after treatment. In others, nerve function impairment or leprosy reactions may cause disfigurement with physical discomfort after cure; these sequelae will need further management. Disabilities such as claw hand or neuropathic foot require chronic care.

Guidelines after the Completion of Multidrug Therapy Patients should receive counseling at release from treatment. The topics covered should include reassurance that the person is no longer contagious, that in some patients hypopigmentation in skin lesions may not resolve for a long time, and that skin discoloration due to clofazimine will gradually disappear in the following months. Nerve impairment may continue to improve after release from treatment, but this is by no means certain. Most important, patients should be instructed to return to the clinic if any new skin signs or fresh nerve damage occurs. This situation is not uncommon, is usually due to a leprosy reaction, and should be managed carefully from both a medical and a social perspective, since patients and persons in their environment will interpret this development as "leprosy coming back." Patients at risk of further episodes of reaction and/or additional nerve function impairment (e.g., patients with preexisting nerve function impairment and multibacillary infection or patients who have experienced a reactional episode during therapy) should be asked to return for a check-up every 6 months for at least 3 years after being released from treatment.

REHABILITATION AND SOCIAL ASPECTS

Physical Rehabilitation Peripheral neuropathy and its secondary disabling consequences often require physical rehabilitation. This effort may include reconstructive surgery in the case of facial, ulnar, median, or posterior tibial paralysis. In this case, pre- and postoperative physical therapy is of crucial importance. Physical therapy is also indicated when muscles are not completely paralyzed or when contractures are too stiff to allow surgery. Since paralysis is usually accompanied by sensory and autonomic neuropathy, occupational therapy also is helpful; therapists teach patients how to minimize the risk of further injury and other techniques for prevention of disabilities. The key principle is teaching patients and former patients to self-manage their disabilities. In many programs, this teaching occurs in the setting of self-care groups. A well-tested and evidence-based self-care routine for hands and feet consists of inspection, soaking, scraping, and oiling (ISSO). Specifically, in ISSO, the person inspects the affected limbs for hotspots (evidence of too much stress on an area of skin): wounds, cracks, and calluses. Next the affected limb(s) are soaked in plain water for 15 minutes. While the skin is wet, areas with excess calluses are scraped with a rough stone or another rough object. The skin is then rubbed with petroleum jelly or another nonfragrant oil in order to trap moisture in the skin. If this routine is performed daily, the skin can be kept supple and in good condition, despite sensory and autonomic damage. If sensation on the soles of the feet is impaired, the person must wear protective footwear. Simple footwear (e.g., sandals or sneakers) available at the local market is adequate as long as it has a strong sole and a soft insole of ethylene-vinyl acetate or microcellular rubber that distributes pressure—an especially important feature when foot muscles are weak or paralyzed or the architecture of the foot is damaged, as is often the case with neuropathy. In high-resource settings, tailor-made orthopedic shoes can be provided.

Mental and Social Support Like other chronic health conditions, leprosy requires patients to cope with the burden of new routines in everyday life. In addition to coping with stigma, they must organize themselves for prolonged treatment, prevention of disabilities, and rehabilitation activities. Moreover, like other neglected tropical diseases (see "Neglected Tropical Diseases," below), leprosy may lead to poor mental health. Such diseases are accompanied by social exclusion in the form of poor access to services such as health care, education, employment, and housing. This exclusion accounts for common mental health comorbidities in leprosy patients and their family members, including depression, anxiety, and suicidal thoughts. Leprosy is probably the most notorious of all stigmatized health conditions, and social stigmatization is the most common issue that triggers mental suffering. Other infectious diseases that raise this issue include HIV infection, tuberculosis, and neglected tropical diseases like lymphatic filariasis, Buruli ulcer, and dermal leishmaniasis. Although the reasons for stigmatization vary, the manifestations and interventions that effectively reduce stigma are similar across conditions and countries. Therefore, joint interventions addressing health-related stigmas for multiple conditions would be strategically and financially attractive. The need to introduce mental health care in leprosy services is pressing. Therapeutic group meetings among institutionalized patients and self-care groups at the community level, with a focus on prevention of disabilities and mental well-being, are known to ameliorate depression, encourage self-acceptance, and promote confidence.

NEGLECTED TROPICAL DISEASES Leprosy is one of a medically diverse group of 20 neglected tropical diseases (NTDs). This group includes infectious diseases caused by bacteria, viruses, fungi, and parasites as well as some noninfectious conditions, such as podoconiosis and snakebite. NTDs have been grouped together because they affect

1.5 billion of the poorest people on Earth and have been widely neglected in domains such as public policy, funding, and the development of diagnostics and treatments. Leprosy is the archetypical NTD, featuring all of the common characteristics: a treatable infectious disease, a known population at risk, available preventive chemotherapy, disease complications that may lead to severe disabilities, and a pervasive social stigma that leads to discrimination, social exclusion, and severe mental health consequences. Nevertheless, the priority accorded to leprosy on the public health agenda of most endemic countries is very low. By joining hands in advocacy, fundraising, and development of joint control strategies, health care organizations can substantially raise the priority profile of NTDs, benefiting each of the individual disease control programs. Such a joint approach serves the goal of universal health coverage and helps to strengthen health services more effectively than vertical programs are ever able to do on their own.

PREVENTION AND CONTROL

Interruption of Transmission and Novel Preventive Strategies Leprosy control was traditionally based on early case detection and multidrug treatment. Apart from health education and leprosy awareness campaigns, no preventive measures were available. In the 1990s, authorities hoped that the transmission of *M. leprae* in the community could be interrupted through timely detection of cases and provision of multidrug therapy, leading to a decline in leprosy incidence. Unfortunately, this has not been the case (Fig. 179-1). The inability to reduce leprosy incidence in many countries and the heightened interest in neglected tropical diseases have invigorated research into new techniques for the diagnosis of disease and infection, leprosy vaccines, enhanced postexposure chemoprophylaxis regimens, epidemiologic tools (e.g., geographic information systems for identifying leprosy hotspots), surveillance of antimicrobial resistance, and alternative drugs and drug treatment regimens.

Vaccines against Leprosy The bacille Calmette-Guérin (BCG) vaccine used against tuberculosis provides varying degrees of protection against leprosy and is used routinely as postexposure immunoprophylaxis for contacts of leprosy patients in Brazil. Two promising vaccine candidates are in the pipeline: the MIP vaccine from India, which is based on killed *Mycobacterium indicus pranii,* and the synthetic LepVax vaccine developed by the University of Washington's Infectious Disease Research Institute in the United States. If proven effective, these vaccines, like the BCG vaccine, will be used as postexposure prophylaxis for contacts of leprosy patients. Trials are in early stages, and sufficient proof of efficacy will take years.

Postexposure Chemoprophylaxis The introduction of postexposure chemoprophylaxis (PEP) for household and other close contacts of leprosy patients is an important innovation. A large randomized controlled trial has shown that single-dose rifampin, given once to household contacts, neighbors, and social contacts, reduces the recipients' risk of leprosy by ~60%. Implementation studies have shown that PEP with single-dose rifampin is feasible and well accepted by patients, contacts, and health workers in a variety of health care settings. Furthermore, modeling studies have indicated the potential impact of PEP on transmission of *M. leprae* in endemic populations. This intervention was included in the 2018 WHO Guidelines for the Diagnosis, Treatment, and Prevention of Leprosy and is currently being introduced in many countries. Research is ongoing into enhanced PEP regimens for those close contacts who are at increased risk of leprosy (e.g., blood-related household contacts and close contacts of multibacillary leprosy patients).

"Zero Leprosy" The WHO has formulated its new Global Leprosy Strategy 2021–2030. As in the organization's previous strategy, a holistic approach to leprosy control is advocated, focusing on zero infection and disease, zero disability, and zero stigma and discrimination. For 2030, the WHO is setting ambitious targets of achieving 120 countries with zero new autochthonous leprosy cases, reducing the annual number of new cases detected by 70%, reducing the rate of new cases with grade 2 disability per million population (as a proxy for detection delay) by 90%, and reducing the rate of new child cases with leprosy per million children (as a proxy for recent transmission) by 90%. Widespread implementation of PEP with single-dose rifampin is one of the key strategies to achieve these goals. The "Triple Zero Strategy" (*zeroleprosy.org*) has also been embraced by the partners united in the Global Partnership for Zero Leprosy, the International Federation of Anti-Leprosy Associations, the Novartis Foundation, the Sasakawa Health Foundation, and the International Association for Integration, Dignity, and Economic Advancement.

The outlook for achieving "zero leprosy" in the coming decades is better than ever before, but this goal is admittedly very ambitious. It can be reached only when all leprosy-endemic countries enhance their leprosy control activities to include (1) active case-finding strategies, including improved diagnosis; (2) contact screening; (3) implementation of PEP; (4) improved prevention of disability services; and (5) activities to reduce stigma and discrimination and to promote the social inclusion and mental well-being of affected patients and their families. Coincident with these efforts, an important threat must be confronted. With the waning of interest in leprosy and the integration of management of the disease into nonspecialized health systems, the number of medical doctors and health workers at the primary care level who have experience in diagnosing and treating leprosy has decreased substantially all over the world. Once lost, expertise is difficult to regain. Therefore, new energy and resources need to be invested in bolstering technical capacity for all aspects of leprosy services, with a view to strengthening the health system in an integrated way and leaving no one behind.

Acknowledgement

We thank Dr. Colette L.M. van Hees, dermatologist at Erasmus MC, University Medical Center Rotterdam, for critical review of this chapter.

FURTHER READING

Bratschi MW et al: Current knowledge on *Mycobacterium leprae* transmission: A systematic literature review. Lepr Rev 86:142, 2015.

Kumar B, Kar HK (eds.): *IAL Textbook of Leprosy*, 2nd ed. New Delhi, Jaypee Brothers Medical Publishers (P) Ltd, 2017.

Scollard DM, Gillis TP (eds): *International Textbook of Leprosy*. Available at *https://internationaltextbookofleprosy.org*. Accessed February 7, 2021.

Smith WC et al: The missing millions: A threat to the elimination of leprosy. PLoS Negl Trop Dis 9 e0003658, 2015.

World Health Organization: Guidelines for the diagnosis, treatment and prevention of leprosy. New Delhi, WHO Regional Office for South-East Asia, 2018. Available at *https://apps.who.int/iris/handle/10665/274127*. Accessed February 7, 2021.

180 Nontuberculous Mycobacterial Infections

Steven M. Holland

Several terms—nontuberculous mycobacteria (NTM), atypical mycobacteria, mycobacteria other than tuberculosis, and environmental mycobacteria—all refer to mycobacteria other than *Mycobacterium tuberculosis*, its close relatives (*M. bovis, M. caprae, M. africanum, M. pinnipedii, M. canetti*), and *M. leprae*. The number of identified species of NTM is growing and will continue to do so because of the use of DNA sequence typing for speciation. The number of known species currently exceeds 199. NTM are highly adaptable and can inhabit hostile environments, including industrial solvents.

EPIDEMIOLOGY

NTM are ubiquitous in soil and water. Specific organisms have recurring niches, such as *M. simiae* in certain aquifers, *M. fortuitum* in pedicure baths, and *M. immunogenum* in metalworking fluids. Most NTM cause disease in humans only rarely unless some aspect of host defense is impaired, as in bronchiectasis, or breached, as by inoculation (e.g., liposuction, trauma, cardiac surgery). There are few instances of human-to-human transmission of NTM, which occurs almost exclusively in cystic fibrosis. Because infections due to NTM are rarely reported to health agencies and because their identification is sometimes problematic, reliable data on incidence and prevalence are lacking. Disseminated disease denotes significant immune dysfunction (e.g., advanced HIV infection), whereas pulmonary disease, which is much more common, is highly associated with pulmonary epithelial defects but not with systemic immunodeficiency.

In the United States, the incidence and prevalence of pulmonary infection with NTM, mostly in association with bronchiectasis (**Chap. 290**), have for many years been several-fold higher than the corresponding figures for tuberculosis, and rates of the former are increasing among the elderly as rates of tuberculosis continue to fall. Among patients with cystic fibrosis, who often have bronchiectasis, rates of clinical infection with NTM range from 3% to 15%, with even higher rates among older patients. Although NTM may be recovered from the sputa of many individuals, it is critical to differentiate active disease from commensal harboring of the organisms. A scheme to help with the proper diagnosis of pulmonary infection caused by NTM has been developed by the American Thoracic Society and is widely used. The bulk of nontuberculous mycobacterial disease in North America is due to *M. kansasii*, organisms of the *M. avium* complex (MAC), and *M. abscessus*.

In Europe, Asia, and Australia, the distribution of NTM in clinical specimens is roughly similar to that in North America, with MAC species and rapidly growing organisms such as *M. abscessus* encountered frequently. *M. xenopi* and *M. malmoense* are especially prominent in northern Europe. *M. ulcerans* causes the distinct clinical entity Buruli ulcer, which occurs throughout tropical zones, especially in western Africa. *M. marinum* is a common cause of cutaneous and tendon infections in coastal regions and among individuals exposed to fish tanks or swimming pools.

The true international epidemiology of infections due to NTM is hard to determine because the isolation of these organisms often is not reported and speciation often is not performed for *M. tuberculosis* or NTM. The latter issue poses an especially important problem during therapy for tuberculosis when smears positive for acid-fast bacilli are considered evidence of treatment failure. The increasing ease of identification and speciation of these organisms is already having a major impact on the description of the dynamic international epidemiology of tuberculosis and NTM infections.

PATHOBIOLOGY

Because exposure to NTM is essentially universal and disease is rare, it can be assumed that normal host defenses against these organisms must be strong and that otherwise healthy individuals in whom significant disease develops are highly likely to have specific susceptibility factors that permit NTM to become established, multiply, and cause disease. At the advent of HIV infection, CD4+ T lymphocytes were recognized as key effector cells against NTM; the development of disseminated MAC disease was highly correlated with a decline in CD4+ T lymphocyte numbers. Such a decrease has also been implicated in disseminated MAC infection in patients with idiopathic CD4+ T lymphocytopenia. Potent inhibitors of tumor necrosis factor α (TNF-α), such as infliximab, adalimumab, certolizumab, golimumab, and etanercept, neutralize this critical cytokine, with consequent inhibition of granuloma formation. The occasional result is severe mycobacterial or fungal infection; these associations indicate that TNF-α is a crucial element in mycobacterial control. However, in cases without the above risk factors, much of the genetic basis of susceptibility to disseminated infection with NTM is accounted for by specific mutations in the interferon γ (IFN-γ)/interleukin 12 (IL-12) synthesis and response pathways.

Mycobacteria are typically phagocytosed by macrophages, which respond with the production of IL-12, a heterodimer composed of IL-12p35 and IL-12p40 moieties that together make up IL-12p70. IL-12 activates T lymphocytes and natural killer cells through binding to its receptor (composed of IL-12Rβ1 and IL-12Rβ2/IL-23R), with consequent phosphorylation of STAT4. IL-12 stimulation of STAT4 leads to secretion of IFN-γ, which activates neutrophils and macrophages to produce reactive oxidants, to increase expression of the major histocompatibility complex and Fc receptors, and to concentrate certain antibiotics intracellularly. Signaling by IFN-γ through its receptor (composed of IFN-γR1 and IFN-γR2) leads to phosphorylation of STAT1, which in turn regulates IFN-γ-responsive genes, such as those coding for IL-12 and TNF-α. TNF-α signals through its own receptor via a downstream complex containing the nuclear factor κB (NF-κB) essential modulator (NEMO). Therefore, the positive feedback loop between IFN-γ and IL-12/IL-23 drives the immune response to mycobacteria and other intracellular infections. These genes are known to be the critical ones in the pathway of mycobacterial control: specific Mendelian mutations have been identified in *IFNGR1, IFNGR2, STAT1, GATA2, ISG15, IRF8, IL-12A, IL-12RB1, IL-12RB2, CYBB* (which encodes the gp91*phox* protein of the NADPH oxidase), *SPP2A*, and *IKBKG* (which encodes NEMO) (**Fig. 180-1**). Despite the identification of genes associated with disseminated disease, only ~70% of cases of disseminated nontuberculous mycobacterial infections that are not associated with HIV infection have a genetic diagnosis; the implication is that more mycobacterial susceptibility genes and pathways remain to be identified.

In contrast to the recognized genes and mechanisms associated with disseminated nontuberculous mycobacterial infection, the best-recognized underlying condition for pulmonary infection with NTM is bronchiectasis (**Chap. 290**). Most of the well-characterized forms of bronchiectasis, including cystic fibrosis, primary ciliary dyskinesia, STAT3-deficient hyper-IgE syndrome, and idiopathic bronchiectasis, have high rates of association with nontuberculous mycobacterial infection. The precise mechanism by which bronchiectasis predisposes to locally destructive but not systemic involvement is unknown.

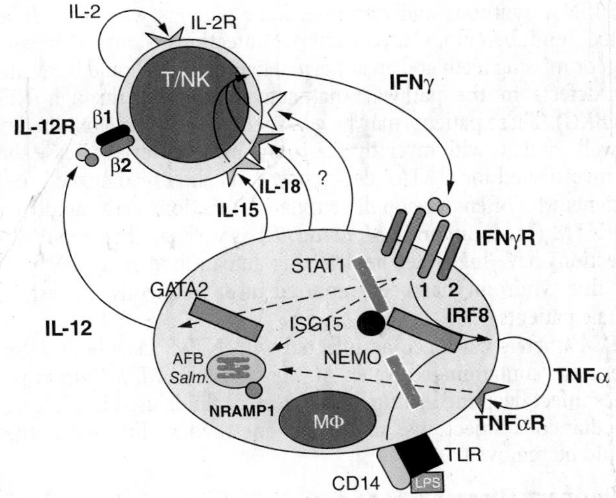

FIGURE 180-1 Cytokine interactions of infected macrophages (MΦ) with T and natural killer (NK) lymphocytes. Infection of macrophages by mycobacteria (AFB) leads to the release of heterodimeric interleukin 12 (IL-12). IL-12 acts on its receptor complex (IL-12R), with consequent STAT4 activation and production of homodimeric interferon γ (IFNγ). Through its receptor (IFNγR), IFNγ activates STAT1, stimulating the production of tumor necrosis factor α (TNFα) and leading to the killing of intracellular organisms such as mycobacteria, salmonellae (*Salm.*), and some fungi. Homotrimeric TNFα acts through its receptor (TNFαR) and requires nuclear factor κB essential modulator (NEMO) to activate nuclear factor κB, which also contributes to the killing of intracellular bacteria. Both IFNγ and TNFα lead to upregulation of IL-12. TNFα-blocking antibodies work either by blocking the ligand (infliximab, adalimumab, certolizumab, golimumab) or by providing soluble receptor (etanercept). Mutations in *IFNGR1, IFNGR2, IL12B, IL12RB1, IL12RB2, STAT1, GATA2, ISG15, IRF8, CYBB*, and *IKBKG* (NEMO) have been associated with predisposition to mycobacterial infections. Other cytokines, such as IL-15 and IL-18, also contribute to IFNγ production. Signaling through the Toll-like receptor (TLR) complex and CD14 also upregulates TNFα production. IRF8, interferon regulatory factor 8; ISG15, interferon-stimulated gene 15; LPS, lipopolysaccharide; NRAMP1, natural resistance-associated macrophage protein 1.

Unlike disseminated or pulmonary infection, "hot-tub lung" represents pulmonary hypersensitivity to NTM—most commonly MAC organisms—growing in underchlorinated water, often in indoor hot tubs.

CLINICAL MANIFESTATIONS

Disseminated Disease Disseminated MAC or *M. kansasii* infections in patients with advanced HIV infection are now uncommon in North America because of effective antimycobacterial prophylaxis and improved treatment of HIV infection. When such mycobacterial disease was common, the portal of entry was the bowel, with spread to bone marrow and the bloodstream. Surprisingly, disseminated infections with rapidly growing NTM (e.g., *M. abscessus*, *M. fortuitum*) are very rare in HIV-infected patients, even in those with advanced HIV infection. Because these organisms are of low intrinsic virulence and disseminate only in conjunction with impaired immunity, disseminated disease can be indolent and progressive over weeks to months. Typical manifestations of malaise, fever, and weight loss are often accompanied by organomegaly, lymphadenopathy, and anemia. Because special cultures or stains are required to identify the organisms, the most critical step in diagnosis is to suspect infection with NTM. Blood cultures may be negative, but involved organs typically have significant organism burdens, sometimes with a grossly impaired granulomatous response.

In a child, disseminated involvement (i.e., involvement of two or more organs) without an underlying iatrogenic cause should prompt an investigation of the IFN-γ/IL-12 pathway. Recessive mutations in *IFNGR1* and *IFNGR2* typically lead to severe infection with NTM. In contrast, dominant negative mutations in *IFNGR1*, which lead to over-accumulation of a defective interfering mutant receptor on the cell surface, inhibit normal IFN-γ signaling and thus lead to nontuberculous mycobacterial osteomyelitis. Dominant negative mutations in *STAT1* and recessive mutations in *IL-12RB1* can produce variable phenotypes consistent with their residual capacities for IFN-γ synthesis and response. Male patients who have disseminated nontuberculous mycobacterial infections along with conical, peg, or missing teeth and an abnormal hair pattern should be evaluated for defects in the pathway that activates NF-κB through NEMO (*IKBKG*). These patients may have associated immune globulin defects as well. Patients with myelodysplasia and mycobacterial disease should be investigated for GATA2 deficiency. A recently recognized group of patients who often develop disseminated infections with rapidly growing NTM (predominantly *M. abscessus*) as well as other opportunistic infections have high-titer neutralizing autoantibodies to IFN-γ. Thus far, this syndrome has been reported most frequently in East Asian female patients.

IV catheters can become infected with NTM, usually as a consequence of contaminated water. *M. abscessus* and *M. fortuitum* sometimes infect deep indwelling lines as well as fluids used in eye surgery, subcutaneous injections, and local anesthetics. Infected catheters should be removed.

Pulmonary Disease Lung disease is by far the most common form of nontuberculous mycobacterial infection in North America and the rest of the industrialized world. In North America, rates of NTM lung disease far exceed rates of tuberculosis. The clinical presentation typically consists of months or years of throat clearing, nagging cough, and slowly progressive fatigue. Patients will often have seen physicians multiple times and received symptom-based or transient therapy before the diagnosis is entertained and samples are sent for mycobacterial stains and cultures. Because not all patients can produce sputum, bronchoscopy may be required for diagnosis. The typical lag between onset of symptoms and diagnosis is ~5 years in older women. Predisposing factors include underlying lung diseases such as bronchiectasis (**Chap. 290**), pneumoconiosis (**Chap. 289**), chronic obstructive pulmonary disease (**Chap. 292**), primary ciliary dyskinesia (**Chap. 290**), α_1 antitrypsin deficiency (**Chap. 292**), and cystic fibrosis (**Chap. 291**). Bronchiectasis and nontuberculous mycobacterial infection often coexist and progress in tandem. This situation makes causality difficult to determine in a given index case, but bronchiectasis is certainly among the most critical predisposing factors that are exacerbated by infection.

MAC organisms are the most common causes of pulmonary nontuberculous mycobacterial infection in North America, but rates vary somewhat by region. MAC infection most commonly develops during the sixth or seventh decade of life in women who have had months or years of nagging intermittent cough and fatigue, with or without sputum production or chest pain. The constellation of pulmonary disease due to NTM in a tall and thin woman who may have chest wall abnormalities is often referred to as Lady Windermere syndrome, after an Oscar Wilde character of the same name. In fact, pulmonary MAC infection does afflict older nonsmoking white women more than men, with onset at ~60 years. Patients tend to be taller and thinner than the general population, with high rates of scoliosis, mitral valve prolapse, and pectus anomalies. Whereas male smokers with upper-lobe cavitary disease tend to carry the same single strain of MAC indefinitely, nonsmoking females with nodular bronchiectasis tend to carry several strains of MAC simultaneously, with changes over the course of their disease.

M. kansasii can cause a clinical syndrome that strongly resembles tuberculosis, consisting of hemoptysis, chest pain, and cavitary lung disease. The rapidly growing NTM, such as *M. abscessus*, have been associated with esophageal motility disorders such as achalasia. Patients with pulmonary alveolar proteinosis are prone to pulmonary nontuberculous mycobacterial and *Nocardia* infections; the underlying mechanism may be inhibition of alveolar macrophage function due to the autoantibodies to granulocyte-macrophage colony-stimulating factor found in many of these patients.

Cervical Lymph Nodes The most common form of nontuberculous mycobacterial infection among young children in North America is isolated cervical lymphadenopathy, caused most frequently by MAC organisms but also by other NTM. The cervical swelling is typically firm and relatively painless, with a paucity of systemic signs. Because the differential diagnosis of painless adenopathy includes malignancy, many children have infection with NTM diagnosed inadvertently at biopsy; cultures and special stains may not have been requested because mycobacterial disease was not ranked high in the differential. Local fistulae usually resolve completely with resection and/or antibiotic therapy. Likewise, the entity of isolated pediatric intrathoracic nontuberculous mycobacterial infection, which is probably related to cervical lymph node infection, is usually mistaken for cancer. In neither isolated cervical nor isolated intrathoracic infections with NTM have children with underlying immune defects been commonly identified, nor do the affected children usually go on to develop other opportunistic infections.

Skin and Soft Tissue Disease Cutaneous involvement with NTM usually requires a break in the skin for introduction of the bacteria. Pedicure bath–associated infection with *M. fortuitum* is more likely if skin abrasion (e.g., during leg shaving) has occurred just before the pedicure. Outbreaks of skin infection are often caused by rapidly growing NTM (especially *M. abscessus*, *M. fortuitum*, and *M. chelonae*) acquired via skin contamination from surgical instruments (especially in cosmetic surgery), injections, and other procedures. These infections are typically accompanied by painful, erythematous, draining subcutaneous nodules, usually without associated fever or systemic symptoms.

M. marinum lives in many water sources and can be acquired from fish tanks, swimming pools, barnacles, and fish scales. This organism typically causes papules or ulcers ("fish-tank granuloma"), but the infection can progress to tendinitis with significant impairment of manual dexterity. Lesions appear days to weeks after inoculation of organisms by a typically minor trauma (e.g., incurred during the cleaning of boats or the handling of fish). Tender nodules due to *M. marinum* can advance up the arm in a pattern also seen with *Sporothrix schenckii* (*sporotricoid spread*). The typical carpal-tendon involvement may be the first presenting manifestation and may lead to surgical exploration or steroid injection. The index of suspicion for

M. marinum infections must be high to ensure that proper specimens obtained during procedures are sent for culture.

M. ulcerans, another waterborne skin pathogen, is found mainly in the tropics, especially in tropical areas of Africa. Infection follows skin trauma or insect bites that allow admission to contaminated water. The skin lesions are typically painless, clean ulcers that slough and can cause osteomyelitis. The toxin mycolactone accounts for the modest host inflammatory response and the painless ulcerations.

DIAGNOSIS

NTM can be detected on acid-fast or fluorochrome smears of sputum or other body fluids. When the organism burden is high, the organisms may appear as gram-positive beaded rods, but this finding is unreliable. (In contrast, nocardiae may appear as gram-positive and beaded but filamentous bacteria.) Again, the requisite and most sensitive step in the diagnosis of any mycobacterial disease is to think of including it in the differential. In almost all laboratories, mycobacterial sample processing, staining, and culture are conducted separately from routine bacteriologic tests; thus many infections go undiagnosed because of the physician's failure to request the appropriate test. In addition, mycobacteria usually require separate blood culture media. NTM are broadly differentiated into rapidly growing (<7 days) and slowly growing (≥7 days) forms. Because *M. tuberculosis* typically takes ≥2 weeks to grow, many laboratories refuse to consider culture results final until 6 weeks have elapsed. Newer techniques using liquid culture media permit more rapid isolation of mycobacteria from specimens than is possible with traditional media. Species more readily detected with incubation at 30°C include *M. marinum*, *M. haemophilum*, and *M. ulcerans*. *M. haemophilum* prefers iron supplementation or blood, whereas *M. genavense* requires supplemented medium with the additive mycobactin J. Bacterial formation of pigment in light conditions (*photochromogenicity*) or dark conditions (*scotochromogenicity*) or a lack of bacterial pigment formation (*nonchromogenicity*) was historically used to help categorize NTM. In contrast to NTM colonies, *M. tuberculosis* colonies are beige, rough, dry, and flat. Current identification schemes reliably use biochemical, nucleic acid, or cell wall composition, as assessed by high-performance liquid chromatography or mass spectrometry, for speciation. With the remarkable decline in U.S. cases of tuberculosis over recent decades, NTM have become the mycobacteria most commonly isolated from humans in North America. However, not all isolations of NTM, especially from the lung, reflect pathology and require treatment. Whereas identification of an organism in a blood or organ biopsy specimen in a compatible clinical setting is diagnostic, the American Thoracic Society recommends that pulmonary infection due to NTM be diagnosed only when disease is clearly demonstrable—i.e., in an appropriate clinical and radiographic setting (nodules, bronchiectasis, cavities) and with repeated isolation of NTM from expectorated sputum or recovery of NTM from bronchoscopy or biopsy specimens. Given the large number of species of NTM and the importance of accurate diagnosis for the implementation of proper therapy, identification of these organisms is ideally taken to the species level.

The purified protein derivative (PPD) of tuberculin is delivered intradermally to evoke a memory T cell response to mycobacterial antigens. This test is variously referred to as the PPD test, the tuberculin skin test, and the Mantoux test, among other designations. Unfortunately, the cutaneous immune response to these tuberculosis-derived filtrate proteins does not differentiate well between infection with some NTM and that with *M. tuberculosis*. Because intermediate reactions (~10 mm) to PPD in latent tuberculosis and nontuberculous mycobacterial infections can overlap significantly, the progressive decline in active tuberculosis in the United States means that NTM probably account for increasing proportions of PPD reactivity. In addition, *bacille Calmette-Guérin* (BCG) can cause some degree of cross-reactivity, posing problems of interpretation for patients who have received BCG vaccine. Assays to measure the elaboration of IFN-γ in response to the relatively tuberculosis-specific proteins ESAT6 and CFP10 form the basis for IFN-γ-release assays (IGRAs). These assays can be performed with whole blood or on membranes. It is important to note that *M. marinum*, *M. kansasii*, and *M. szulgai* also have ESAT6 and CFP10 and may cause false-positive reactions in IGRAs. Despite cross-reactivity with NTM, large PPD reactions (>15 mm) most commonly signify tuberculosis. Conversely, in the setting of anti-IFNg autoantibodies the IGRA test is indeterminate (failure of IFNg detection in response to specific antigens and mitogens, due to neutralizing anti-IFNg autoantibodies).

Isolation of NTM from blood specimens is clear evidence of disease. Whereas rapidly growing mycobacteria may proliferate in routine blood culture media, slow-growing NTM typically do not; thus it is imperative to suspect the diagnosis and to use the correct bottles for cultures. Isolation of NTM from a biopsy specimen constitutes strong evidence for infection, but cases of laboratory contamination do occur. Identification of organisms on stained sections of biopsy material confirms the authenticity of the culture. Certain NTM require lower incubation temperatures (*M. genavense*) or special additives (*M. haemophilum*) for growth. Some NTM (e.g., *M. tilburgii*) remain noncultivable but can be identified molecularly in clinical samples.

The radiographic appearance of nontuberculous mycobacterial disease in the lung depends on the underlying disease, the severity of the infection, and the imaging modality used. The advent and increase in the use of CT has allowed the identification of characteristic changes that are highly consistent with nontuberculous mycobacterial infection, such as the "tree-in-bud" pattern of bronchiolar inflammation (**Fig. 180-2**). Involvement of the lingual and right-middle lobes is commonly seen on chest CT but is difficult to appreciate on plain film. Severe bronchiectasis and cavity formation are common in more advanced disease. Isolation of NTM from respiratory samples can be confusing. *M. gordonae* is often recovered from respiratory samples but is not usually seen on smear and is almost never a pathogen. Patients with bronchiectasis occasionally have NTM recovered from sputum culture with a negative smear. The American Thoracic Society has developed guidelines for the diagnosis of infection with MAC, *M. abscessus*, and *M. kansasii*. A positive diagnosis requires the growth of NTM from two of three sputum samples, regardless of smear findings; a positive bronchoscopic alveolar sample, regardless of smear findings; or a pulmonary parenchyma biopsy sample with granulomatous inflammation or mycobacteria found on section and NTM found on culture. These guidelines probably apply to other NTM as well.

Although many laboratories use DNA probes to identify *M. tuberculosis*, MAC, *M. gordonae*, and *M. kansasii*, speciation of NTM helps determine the antimycobacterial therapy to be used. Only testing of MAC organisms for susceptibility to clarithromycin and of *M. kansasii* for susceptibility to rifampin is indicated; few data support other in vitro susceptibility tests, attractive though they appear. MAC isolates that have not been exposed to macrolides are almost always susceptible. NTM that have persisted beyond a course of antimicrobial therapy

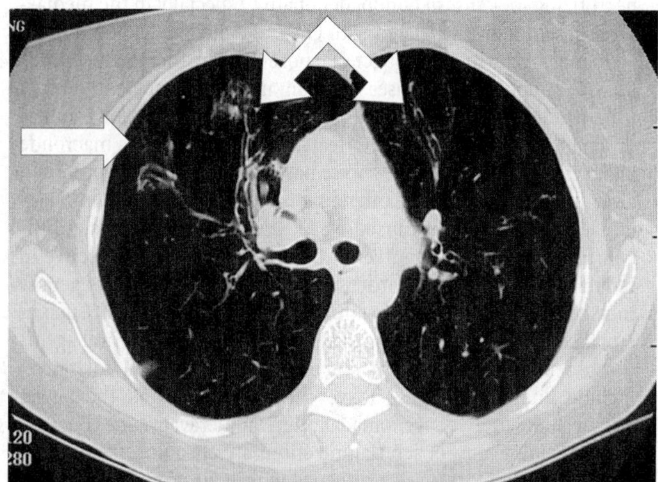

FIGURE 180-2 Chest CT of a patient with pulmonary *Mycobacterium avium* complex infection. *Arrows* indicate the "tree-in-bud" pattern of bronchiolar inflammation (peripheral right lung) and bronchiectasis (central right and left lungs).

 are often tested for antibiotic susceptibility, but the value and meaning of these tests are undetermined.

PREVENTION

Prophylaxis of MAC disease in patients infected with HIV is started when the CD4+ T lymphocyte count falls to <50/μL. Azithromycin (1200 mg weekly), clarithromycin (1000 mg daily), or rifabutin (300 mg daily) is effective. Macrolide prophylaxis in immunodeficient patients who are susceptible to NTM (e.g., those with defects in the IFN-γ/IL-12 axis) has not been prospectively validated but seems prudent.

TREATMENT

Nontuberculous Mycobacteria

NTM cause chronic infections that evolve relatively slowly over a period of weeks to years. Therefore, it is rarely necessary to initiate treatment on an emergent basis before the diagnosis is clear and the infecting species is known. Treatment of NTM is complex, often poorly tolerated, and potentially toxic. Just as in tuberculosis, inadequate single-drug therapy is almost always associated with the emergence of antimicrobial resistance and relapse.

MAC infection often requires multidrug therapy, the foundation of which is a macrolide (clarithromycin or azithromycin), ethambutol, and a rifamycin (rifampin or rifabutin). For disseminated nontuberculous mycobacterial disease in HIV-infected patients, the use of rifamycins poses special problems—i.e., rifamycin interactions with protease inhibitors. For pulmonary MAC disease, thrice-weekly administration of a macrolide, a rifamycin, and ethambutol has been successful. Therapy is prolonged, generally continuing for 12 months after culture conversion; typically, a course lasts for at least 18 months. Other drugs with activity against MAC organisms include IV and aerosolized aminoglycosides, fluoroquinolones, and clofazimine. In elderly patients, rifabutin can exert significant toxicity. However, with only modest efforts, most antimycobacterial regimens are well tolerated by most patients. Resection of cavitary lesions or severely bronchiectatic segments has been advocated for some patients, especially those with macrolide-resistant infections. The success of therapy for pulmonary MAC infections depends on whether disease is nodular or cavitary and on whether it is early or advanced, ranging from 20 to 80%.

M. kansasii lung disease is similar to tuberculosis in many ways and is also effectively treated with isoniazid (300 mg/d), rifampin (600 mg/d), and ethambutol (15 mg/kg per day). Other drugs with very high-level activity against *M. kansasii* include clarithromycin, fluoroquinolones, and aminoglycosides. Treatment should continue until cultures have been negative for at least 1 year. In most instances, *M. kansasii* infection is easily cured. Bulky, severe, necrotizing *M. kansasii* lymphadenopathy, especially in the mediastinum, is strongly associated with GATA2 deficiency.

Rapidly growing mycobacteria pose special therapeutic problems. Extrapulmonary disease in an immunocompetent host is usually due to inoculation (e.g., via surgery, injections, or trauma) or to line infection and is often treated successfully with a macrolide and another drug (with the choice based on in vitro susceptibility), along with removal of the offending focus. In contrast, pulmonary disease, especially that caused by *M. abscessus*, is extremely difficult to cure. Repeated courses of treatment are usually effective in reducing the infectious burden and symptoms. Therapy generally includes a macrolide along with an IV-administered agent such as amikacin, a carbapenem, cefoxitin, or tigecycline. Other oral agents (used according to in vitro susceptibility testing and tolerance) include fluoroquinolones, doxycycline, linezolid, and the newer tetracycline family drugs, omadacycline and eravacycline. Because nontuberculous mycobacterial infections are chronic, care must be taken in the long-term use of drugs with neurotoxicities, such as linezolid and ethambutol. Prophylactic pyridoxine has been suggested in these cases. Durations of therapy for *M. abscessus* lung disease are difficult to predict because so many cases are chronic and require intermittent therapy. Expert consultation and management are strongly recommended.

Once recognized, *M. marinum* infection is highly responsive to antimicrobial therapy and is cured relatively easily with any combination of a macrolide, ethambutol, and a rifamycin. Therapy should be continued for 1–2 months after clinical resolution of isolated soft-tissue disease; tendon and bone involvement may require longer courses in light of clinical evolution. Other drugs with activity against *M. marinum* include sulfonamides, trimethoprim-sulfamethoxazole, doxycycline, and minocycline.

Treatment of the other NTM is less well defined, but macrolides and aminoglycosides are usually effective, with other agents added as indicated. Expert consultation is strongly encouraged for difficult or unusual infections due to NTM.

PROGNOSIS

The outcomes of nontuberculous mycobacterial infections are closely tied to the underlying condition (e.g., IFN-γ/IL-12 pathway defect, cystic fibrosis) and can range from recovery to death. With no or inadequate treatment, symptoms and signs can be debilitating, including persistent cough, fever, anorexia, and severe lung destruction. With treatment, patients typically regain strength and energy. The optimal duration of therapy when NTM persist in sputum is unknown, but treatment in this situation can be prolonged. In general, for severe underlying immunodeficiencies, hematopoietic stem cell transplantation is recommended and may be helpful in the resolution of severe mycobacterial disease.

GLOBAL CONSIDERATIONS

In many countries, pulmonary tuberculosis is diagnosed by smear alone, which is also the method used for monitoring of response and relapse. However, examination of mycobacteria from the affected "relapsed" patients shows that a significant proportion of isolates are actually NTM. Overall, as rates of tuberculosis decline, the proportion of positive smears caused by NTM will increase. Advances in speciation will distinguish tuberculosis from nontuberculous mycobacterial infections and thereby affect rates of assumed relapse and resistance, leading to more targeted and appropriate therapy.

FURTHER READING

Flume PA et al: Advances in bronchiectasis: Endotyping, genetics, microbiome, and disease heterogeneity. Lancet 392:880, 2018.

Holland SM et al: Case 28-2017. A 13-month-old girl with pneumonia and a 33-year-old woman with hip pain. N Engl J Med 377:1077, 2017.

Hong GH et al: Natural history and evolution of anti-interferon-γ autoantibody-associated immunodeficiency syndrome in Thailand and the United States. Clin Infect 71:53, 2020.

Kim RD et al: Pulmonary nontuberculous mycobacterial disease: Prospective study of a distinct preexisting syndrome. Am J Respir Crit Care Med 178:1066, 2008.

Lovell JP et al: Mediastinal and disseminated *Mycobacterium kansasii* disease in GATA2 deficiency. Ann Am Thorac Soc 13:2169, 2016.

Marras TK et al: Relative risk of all-cause mortality in patients with nontuberculous mycobacterial lung disease in a US managed care population. Respir Med 145:80, 2018.

Olivier KN et al: Inhaled amikacin for treatment of refractory pulmonary nontuberculous mycobacterial disease. Ann Am Thorac Soc 11:30, 2014.

Spinner MA et al: GATA2 deficiency: A protean disorder of hematopoiesis, lymphatics, and immunity. Blood 123:809, 2014.

Szymanski EP et al: Pulmonary nontuberculous mycobacterial infection. A multisystem, multigenic disease. Am J Respir Crit Care Med 192:618, 2015.

Wu UI et al: Patients with idiopathic pulmonary nontuberculous mycobacterial disease have normal Th1/Th2 cytokine responses but diminished Th17 cytokine and enhanced granulocyte-macrophage colony-stimulating factor production. Open Forum Infect Dis 6:ofz484, 2019.

181 Antimycobacterial Agents

Divya Reddy, Sebastian G. Kurz, Max R. O'Donnell

Agents used for the treatment of mycobacterial infections, including tuberculosis (TB), leprosy, and infections due to nontuberculous mycobacteria (NTM), are administered in multiple-drug regimens for prolonged courses. Currently, >160 species of mycobacteria have been identified, the majority of which do not cause disease in humans. While the incidence of disease caused by *Mycobacterium tuberculosis* has been declining in the United States, TB remains a leading cause of morbidity and mortality in low- and middle-income countries—for example, in sub-Saharan Africa and Asia, where the HIV epidemic rages. Well-organized infrastructure for early diagnosis, treatment of TB infection and disease, and development of effective drug regimens and vaccines remain vital to the global strategies for TB control (**Chaps. 472 and 474**). Infections with NTM have gained in clinical prominence in the United States and other developed countries. These largely environmental organisms often establish infection in immunocompromised patients or in persons with structural lung disease.

TUBERCULOSIS

GENERAL PRINCIPLES

The earliest recorded human case of TB dates back 9000 years. Early treatment modalities, such as bloodletting, were replaced by the sanatorium movement in the late nineteenth century, which focused on fresh air, nutrition, and bed rest to treat consumptive patients and came with the benefit of isolating infected individuals. The discovery of streptomycin in 1943 launched the era of antibiotic treatment for TB. Over subsequent decades, the discovery of additional agents and the use of multiple-drug regimens allowed progressive shortening of the treatment course from years to as little as 6 months for drug-susceptible TB. Latent TB infection (LTBI) and active TB disease are diagnosed by history, physical examination, radiographic imaging, tuberculin skin test, interferon-γ release assays, acid-fast staining, mycobacterial cultures, and/or new molecular diagnostics. LTBI is treated with isoniazid plus rifapentine (weekly for 3 months), rifampin (daily for 4 months), isoniazid plus rifampin (daily for 3 months), or isoniazid (optimally daily or twice weekly for 6–9 months) (**Table 181-1**). The 3-month, weekly regimen of isoniazid with rifapentine is currently the regimen of choice in children >2 years of age and in all adults including HIV-positive individuals. The regimen is not recommended for pregnant women and for persons with hypersensitivity reactions to isoniazid or rifampin. Shorter duration rifamycin-based regimens (rifampin alone for 4 months or for 3 months in combination with isoniazid) are currently preferred for the treatment of LTBI over isoniazid for 6–9 months in adults and children due to their effectiveness, safety, and tolerability. Caution is advised in HIV-positive individuals due to potential for drug interactions, lack of definitive data on effectiveness, and the possibility of subclinical TB disease that could facilitate the development of rifampin resistance.

Completions rates of a self-administered, once-weekly regimen of isoniazid plus rifapentine for 3 months with monthly monitoring were found to be noninferior to those seen with directly observed therapy (DOT) in the United States, and thus, this regimen is considered an acceptable strategy for treating LTBI in countries with a focus on secondary prevention of TB disease. Recently, a 1-month daily regimen of rifapentine and isoniazid in HIV-positive individuals was found to be noninferior to 9 months of isoniazid; this regimen will be included in the new World Health Organization (WHO) LTBI treatment guidelines.

For active or suspected TB disease, clinical factors, including HIV co-infection, symptom duration, radiographic appearance, and public health concerns about TB transmission, drive diagnostic testing and treatment initiation. Confirmation of active TB relies on detection of *M. tuberculosis* via culture or molecular testing. A combination of drugs is used for the treatment of TB disease (**Table 181-2**). For drug-susceptible disease, a standardized regimen is used with an intensive phase consisting of four drugs—isoniazid, rifampin, pyrazinamide, and ethambutol—given for 2 months, which is followed by a continuation phase of isoniazid and rifampin for 4 months, for a total treatment duration of 6 months. U.S. guidelines recommend extension of the continuation phase to 7 months (for a total treatment duration of 9 months) for patients with cavitary disease; if the 2-month course of pyrazinamide is not completed; or if sputum cultures remain positive beyond 2 months of treatment (delayed culture conversion), which also warrants evaluation for development of drug resistance.

Treatment of TB in patients co-infected with HIV poses significant challenges, but some progress is being made. To improve survival, current recommendations include initiation of antiretroviral therapy (ART) in HIV patients co-infected with *M. tuberculosis* within 2 weeks of the initiation of treatment for TB (except TB meningitis) if the CD4+ T-cell count is ≤50/μL and by 8–12 weeks of TB treatment initiation if the CD4+ T-cell count is ≥50/μL. Interactions of rifampin with protease inhibitors or nonnucleoside reverse transcriptase inhibitors can be significant and require close monitoring and dose adjustments. Reassuringly, a recent study comparing the safety and efficacy of rifampin for 4 months in patients with LTBI showed that it was as effective as isoniazid for 9 months and was also well tolerated and safe for treatment in persons living with HIV. Rifabutin is an alternative drug of choice in HIV patients co-infected with *M. tuberculosis,* as it is a less potent cytochrome P3A inhibitor than rifampin. The TB immune reconstitution inflammatory syndrome (IRIS) may appear as early as 1 week after initiation of ART and manifests as paradoxical worsening or unmasking of existing TB infection. Conservative management consists of continued administration of ART and TB medications. However, severe or debilitating IRIS has been treated in reported case series with varying doses of glucocorticoids. A randomized, double-blind, placebo-controlled trial showed that a 4-week course of prednisone significantly reduced need for hospitalization and hastened symptom improvement and quality of life in TB IRIS. Intermittent antimycobacterial therapy

TABLE 181-1 Regimens for the Treatment of Latent Tuberculosis Infection in Adults

REGIMEN	SCHEDULE	DURATION	COMMENTS
Isoniazid plus rifapentine	900 mg (15 mg/kg) weekly plus 900 mg (for weight >50 kg) weekly	3 months	Directly observed therapy is recommended for once-weekly treatment in HIV-positive and -negative individuals. This regimen may be supplemented with pyridoxine (25–50 mg/d).
Rifampin	600 mg/d (10 mg/kg)	4 months	Recommended in HIV-negative individuals and in children. Data on effectiveness in HIV-positive patients are unavailable.
Isoniazid plus rifampin	300 mg/d (5 mg/kg) plus 600 mg/d (10 mg/kg)	3 months	Risk of hepatotoxicity may be higher with the combination regimen compared to that of the individual drugs.
Isoniazid	300 mg/d (5 mg/kg) Alternative: 900 mg twice weekly (15 mg/kg)	6–9 months (6 months acceptable)	Supplement with pyridoxine (25–50 mg daily) 6 months' duration strongly recommended for HIV-negative patients and conditional for HIV-positive patients. 9 months may be more effective but with higher risk of hepatic toxicity. Twice-weekly regimens require directly observed therapy.

Source: Sterling TR et al. Guidelines for the treatment of latent tuberculosis infection: Recommendations from the National Tuberculosis Controllers Association and CDC, 2020. MMWR Recomm Rep 69(No. RR-1):1, 2020.

TABLE 181-2 Simplified Approach to Treatment of Active Tuberculosis (TB) in Adults

CULTURE RESULTS	INTENSIVE PHASE	CONTINUATION PHASE	EXTENSION OF TOTAL TREATMENT
Culture-positive, drug-susceptible	HRZE for 2 months, daily[a] or 3 times per week (with dose adjustment)	HR for 4 months, daily or 5 days per week *or* HR for 4 months, 3 times per week[b] (with dose adjustment)	Continuation phase extended to 7 months if 2 months of Z is not completed, if the patient is infected with HIV and is not receiving antiretroviral therapy, or if culture conversion is prolonged and/or cavitation is evident on chest radiography (U.S. guidelines)[c]
Culture-negative	HRZE for 2 months	HR for 2 months, daily or 2 or 3 times per week[d]	Continuation phase extended to 4 months if the patient is infected with HIV
Extrapulmonary, drug-susceptible	HRZE for 2 months	HR for 4–7 months, daily or 5 days per week[e]	Continuation phase extended to 10 months in TB meningitis; 7 months recommended by some authorities for bone/joint TB

[a]Daily treatment is preferred; however, thrice-weekly therapy in the intensive phase (with or without an initial 2 weeks of daily therapy) may be considered in patients who are not infected with HIV and are at low risk of relapse (i.e., in pulmonary tuberculosis caused by drug-susceptible organisms that, at the start of treatment, is noncavitary and/or smear negative). [b]Use regimen with caution in HIV patients and/or those with cavitary disease, as missed doses can lead to treatment failure, relapse, and acquired drug resistance. [c]Culture conversion is prolonged if it occurs beyond 2 months. [d]Twice-weekly treatment regimens are not recommended in patients infected with HIV and those with cavitary pulmonary disease suspected to be TB. [e]Standard daily 6-month TB treatment regimen is considered to be adequate for most forms of extrapulmonary TB, including miliary TB. For TB meningitis, the addition of glucocorticoids is recommended.

Abbreviations: E, ethambutol; H, isoniazid; R, rifampin; Z, pyrazinamide.

Sources: Official American Thoracic Society/Centers for Disease Control and Prevention/Infectious Diseases Society of America: Clinical practice guidelines: Treatment of drug-susceptible tuberculosis. Clin Infect Dis 63:e147, 2016.

in patients infected with HIV and *M. tuberculosis* has been associated with low plasma levels of several key TB drugs and with higher rates of treatment failure or relapse; therefore, intermittent twice-weekly therapy for TB in HIV-co-infected individuals is not recommended.

Adherence to medications is critical in achieving a cure with antimycobacterial therapy. In addition to DOT by trained staff, either in the clinic or at home, case management interventions such as patient education/counseling, field/home visits, and patient reminders are also recommended to improve treatment adherence. Use of mobile health technologies, including video DOT, text messaging, and next-generation electronic pillboxes, shows promise in promoting TB adherence. In drug-susceptible TB, monthly dispensing of TB medications is also advised for all patients to allow essential clinical monitoring for hepatotoxicity due to these medications. Clinical monitoring includes at least monthly assessment for symptoms (nausea, vomiting, abdominal discomfort, and unexplained fatigue) and signs (jaundice, dark urine, light stools, diffuse pruritus) of hepatotoxicity, although the latter represent comparatively late manifestations (**Table 181-3**). The presence

TABLE 181-3 Monitoring and Clinical Management of Tuberculosis (TB) Treatment in Adults[a]

DRUG	ASSESSMENT	MANAGEMENT
LTBI Treatment		
With hepatic risk factors[b], check ALT and bilirubin at baseline. If ALT is ≥3 × ULN or total bilirubin is >2 × ULN, defer treatment and reevaluate.		
Isoniazid	Determine whether hepatic risk factors are present. If so, obtain baseline and periodic ALT and bilirubin values	If ALT is 5 × ULN (or 3 × ULN with symptoms)[c] or if bilirubin reaches jaundice levels (usually >2 × ULN), interrupt treatment. With normalization, consider an alternative agent.
Rifampin	Same as above	Same as above
TB Treatment		
Check ALT, bilirubin, platelets, creatinine, and hepatitis panel for all patients at baseline. If hepatic risk factors are present, check ALT and bilirubin monthly.		
Isoniazid	If ALT is >5 × ULN (or >3 × ULN with hepatitis symptoms)[c]	Obtain history of alcohol consumption and concomitant drug use. In most instances, discontinue H, Z, R, and other hepatotoxic drugs. Consider alternative agents. Obtain viral hepatitis serologies. Rechallenge: With normalization of liver enzymes, R and H may be sequentially reintroduced. With no recurrence of hepatotoxicity, Z is not resumed in many cases. Alternative rechallenge protocols have been used.
Rifampin	If primary elevation is in bilirubin and alkaline phosphatase, most likely due to rifampin	Discontinue R if total bilirubin reaches jaundice levels (usually >2 × ULN). May try to reintroduce; if not tolerated, may substitute Q.
Ethambutol	Decrease in visual acuity or color vision on monthly screening	Discontinue ethambutol and repeat ocular examination. Peripheral neuropathy may be a precursor of ocular toxicity; if it occurs, consider repeat ocular examination.
Pyrazinamide	If ALT is >5 × ULN (or >3 × ULN with symptoms)[c]	Same as for H.
Fluoroquinolone, bedaquiline, delamanid	QTc prolongation is a concern and should be monitored, especially if drugs are used in combination	Asymptomatic QTc prolongation should prompt consideration of stopping known QT-prolonging drugs and/or close monitoring, depending on the clinical situation and degree of prolongation. Symptomatic QTc prolongation (e.g., palpitations or arrhythmias) should prompt discontinuation of drugs.
Linezolid	Visual impairment; monitor for peripheral neuropathy and bone marrow suppression including anemia, thrombocytopenia, and leukopenia	Discontinue linezolid if visual toxicity develops. Rechallenge after complete resolution, especially with a lower dose, is an option. Stop if peripheral neuropathy or bone marrow suppression develops.

[a]All regimens require monthly clinical monitoring. [b]Hepatic risk factors: chronic alcohol use, viral hepatitis, preexisting liver disease, pregnancy or ≤3 months postpartum, hepatotoxic medications. [c]Relevant manifestations include nausea, vomiting, abdominal pain, jaundice, or unexplained fatigue.

Abbreviations: ALT, alanine aminotransferase; H, isoniazid; LTBI, latent tuberculosis infection; Q, fluoroquinolone; QTc, corrected QT interval; R, rifampin; ULN, upper limit of normal; Z, pyrazinamide.

Sources: JJ Saukkonen et al: An official ATS statement: Hepatotoxicity of antituberculosis therapy. Am J Respir Crit Care Med 174:935, 2006; American Thoracic Society/Centers for Disease Control and Prevention/Infectious Diseases Society of America: Treatment of tuberculosis. Am J Respir Crit Care Med 167:603, 2003; WHO consolidated guidelines on drug-resistant tuberculosis treatment. Geneva: World Health Organization; 2019. License: CC BY-NC-SA 3.0 IGO.

of such symptoms and signs mandates provisional discontinuation of potentially hepatotoxic agents; discontinuation at the onset of hepatitis symptoms reduces the risk of progression to fatal hepatitis. Although biochemical monitoring is not routinely recommended, baseline assessment of liver function is recommended in adults including testing of at least serum alanine aminotransferase (ALT) and total bilirubin levels (Table 181-3). **(See Chap. 178 for further details.)** For patients with active TB, monthly mycobacterial cultures of sputum are recommended until it is certain that the organisms have been cleared and the patient has responded to therapy or until no sputum is available for culture.

If significant clinical improvement does not occur or the patient's condition deteriorates over the course of therapy, possibilities include treatment failure due to nonadherence, poor medication absorption, or the development of resistance. For patients co-infected with HIV and *M. tuberculosis*, IRIS, which is a diagnosis of exclusion, should also be a consideration. Drug susceptibility testing should be repeated at this point. If resistance is documented or strongly suspected, at least two efficacious drugs to which the isolate is susceptible or which the patient has not already taken should be added to the therapeutic regimen.

Multidrug-resistant tuberculosis (MDR-TB) is defined as disease caused by a strain of *M. tuberculosis* that is resistant to both isoniazid and rifampin—the most efficacious of the first-line TB drugs. The risk of MDR-TB is elevated in patients presenting from geographic areas in which ≥5% of incident cases are MDR-TB and in patients previously treated for TB. Treatment regimens for MDR-TB are rapidly evolving, and in 2019, the WHO issued a new classification of second-line agents to treat drug-resistant disease **(See Table 178-4)**. Current WHO recommendations are emphasizing an all-oral bedaquiline-containing regimen with the goal to limit treatment duration to 9–11 months compared to conventional durations of 18–20 months **(Table 181-4)**.

Results from several recent large clinical trials have formed the basis of these recommendations. The "Bangladesh regimen" was the first short-course MDR-TB regimen systematically studied in the STREAM-1 trial and was able to reduce treatment duration to 9–12 months with favorable outcomes in up to 90% of patients. It consists of a seven-drug intensive phase (kanamycin, prothionamide, isoniazid, fluoroquinolone, ethambutol, pyrazinamide, and clofazimine) and a four-drug continuation phase (fluoroquinolone, ethambutol, pyrazinamide, and clofazimine). In 2018, a large meta-analysis, which pooled individual data from >12,000 patients enrolled in 50 trials, assessed the role of individual drugs to treat MDR-TB. This analysis showed an association of significantly better treatment outcomes with the use of linezolid, bedaquiline, clofazimine, carbapenems, and later generation fluoroquinolones and worse outcomes with kanamycin and capreomycin in these patients. As a result of this analysis, oral drug combinations are now prioritized, while several traditional second-line drugs, including kanamycin and capreomycin, are no longer recommended. A further step toward a shortened all-oral regimen was the Nix-TB study, which showed that a 6-month regimen of bedaquiline, pretomanid, and linezolid (BPaL regimen) for treatment of highly drug-resistant TB was associated with favorable outcomes (absence of clinical or bacteriologic treatment failure or relapse within 6 months of treatment completion) in 89% of patients. While a major breakthrough, caution has been raised regarding higher rate of side effects mostly due to linezolid and lack of a control arm. The BPaL regimen is currently recommended under operational research conditions only.

The shift toward all-oral regimens of shortened duration has been made possible by the introduction of novel drugs, most prominently bedaquiline and pretomanid, as well as the repurposing of existing agents for MDR-TB treatment (e.g., linezolid, clofazimine). High cost and limited access to these new drugs are barriers that need to be addressed to facilitate global adaptation of these new regimens.

FIRST-LINE ANTITUBERCULOSIS DRUGS

The following discussion of individual anti-TB agents focuses on treatment of TB in adults, unless otherwise noted. Several agents are being actively investigated during the current remarkable period of drug development for TB treatment.

Isoniazid Isoniazid is a critical drug for treatment of both TB disease and LTBI. Isoniazid has excellent bactericidal activity against both intracellular and extracellular, actively dividing *M. tuberculosis*. This drug is bacteriostatic against slowly dividing organisms. In treatment of LTBI, isoniazid is generally well tolerated, has well-established efficacy, and is inexpensive. In this setting, the drug is taken daily, which is the preferred dosing schedule, or intermittently (i.e., twice weekly) using DOT for 6 months, which has been found to be equivalent to the traditional 9 months in most settings. A weekly isoniazid and rifapentine regimen, administered over 3 months under DOT, has been shown to be noninferior to daily isoniazid given for 9 months and had a higher treatment completion rate than the single-drug regimen. More recent evidence also suggests that completion rates of a self-administered 3-month regimen of weekly isoniazid and rifapentine are noninferior to those seen with DOT in the United States. It is expected that a 1-month daily regimen in combination with rifapentine will be added to new WHO guidelines.

TABLE 181-4 Simplified Approach to Treatment of Drug-Resistant Tuberculosis (TB) in Adults[a]

CULTURE RESULTS	INTENSIVE PHASE	CONTINUATION PHASE	EXTENSION OF TOTAL TREATMENT
Resistant to H	Lfx RZE[b] for 6 months	…	Prolonged culture conversion and/or evidence of cavitation on chest radiography
Resistant to HR (MDR)[c]			
WHO short course regimen[d]	Bdq, Lfx or Mfx, Eto, E, Z, Hh, Cfz for 4–6 months	Lfx or Mfx, Cfz, Z, E for 5 months	Prolonged culture conversion, delayed response, and/or evidence of cavitation on chest radiography
WHO extended regimen[e]	At least five effective second-line agents, including all group A and at least one group B, add group C if intolerant to A or B drugs for 5–7 months	4 drugs for a total of 18–20 months or for 15–17 months after culture conversion	Prolonged culture conversion, delayed response, and/or evidence of cavitation on chest radiography

[a]Drug-resistant TB treatment regimens should be constructed and care provided in close consultation with experienced drug-resistant TB clinicians. Surgical management should also be considered in appropriate cases. [b]Prolonged pyrazinamide duration may be associated with increased risk of liver toxicity. [c]Monoresistance to R is rare and should be treated as MDR. [d]The WHO short-course regimen is for patients with no prior exposure to second-line drugs and documented fluoroquinolone susceptibility only. Patients with treatment intolerance to antimycobacterial agents, disseminated TB, or pregnancy should be excluded from short-course regimens. It is currently not endorsed by U.S. societies. [e]Patients who do not qualify for WHO short-course regimens should be treated using extended MDR-TB treatment regimens. The construction of extended regimens is guided by the requirement for selection of effective antimycobacterial agents, the need to combine sufficient medicines to maximize relapse-free survival, and the need to minimize toxicity.

Abbreviations: Bdq, bedaquiline; Cfz, clofazimine; E, ethambutol; Eto, ethionamide; H, isoniazid; Hh, high-dose isoniazid; Lfx, levofloxacin; MDR, multidrug resistant; Mfx, moxifloxacin; Pa, pretomanid; Q, fluoroquinolone; R, rifampin; WHO, World Health Organization; Z, pyrazinamide.

Sources: Official American Thoracic Society/Centers for Disease Control and Prevention/Infectious Diseases Society of America: Clinical practice guidelines: Treatment of drug-resistant tuberculosis. Am J Respir Crit Care Med 200:e93, 2019; World Health Organization consolidated guidelines on drug-resistant tuberculosis treatment. WHO 2019; Rapid Communication: Key changes to the treatment of drug-resistant tuberculosis, WHO December 2019.

For treatment of TB disease, isoniazid is used in combination with other agents to ensure killing of both actively dividing *M. tuberculosis* and slowly growing "persister" mycobacteria. Unless the organism is resistant, the standard regimen includes isoniazid, rifampin, ethambutol, and pyrazinamide (Table 181-2). Isoniazid is often given together with 25–50 mg of pyridoxine daily to prevent drug-related peripheral neuropathy.

MECHANISM OF ACTION Isoniazid is a prodrug activated by the mycobacterial KatG catalase-peroxidase; isoniazid is coupled with reduced nicotinamide adenine dinucleotide (NADH). The resulting isonicotinic acyl–NADH complex blocks the mycobacterial ketoenoylreductase known as InhA through binding to its substrate and inhibiting fatty acid synthase and ultimately mycolic acid synthesis. Mycolic acids are essential components of the mycobacterial cell wall. KatG activation of isoniazid also results in the release of free radicals that have antimycobacterial activity, including nitric oxide.

The minimal inhibitory concentrations (MICs) of isoniazid for wild-type (untreated) susceptible strains are <0.1 μg/mL for *M. tuberculosis* and 0.5–2 μg/mL for *M. kansasii.*

PHARMACOLOGY Isoniazid is the hydrazide of isonicotinic acid, a small, water-soluble molecule. The usual adult oral daily dose of 300 mg results in peak serum levels of 3–5 μg/mL within 30 min to 2 h after ingestion—well in excess of the MICs for most susceptible strains of *M. tuberculosis*. Both oral and IM preparations of isoniazid reach effective levels in the body, although antacids and high-carbohydrate meals may interfere with oral absorption. Isoniazid diffuses well throughout the body, reaching therapeutic concentrations in body cavities and fluids, with concentrations in cerebrospinal fluid (CSF) comparable to those in serum.

Isoniazid is metabolized in the liver via acetylation by *N*-acetyltransferase 2 (NAT2) and hydrolysis. Both fast- and slow-acetylation phenotypes occur; patients who are "fast acetylators" may have lower serum levels of isoniazid, whereas "slow acetylators" may have higher levels and experience more toxicity. Satisfactory isoniazid levels are attained in the majority of homozygous fast NAT2 acetylators given a dose of 6 mg/kg and in the majority of homozygous slow acetylators given only 3 mg/kg. Genotyping is increasingly being used to characterize isoniazid-related pharmacogenomic responses.

Isoniazid's interactions with other drugs are due primarily to its inhibition of the cytochrome P450 system. Among the drugs with significant isoniazid interactions are warfarin, carbamazepine, benzodiazepines, acetaminophen, clopidogrel, maraviroc, dronedarone, salmeterol, tamoxifen, eplerenone, and phenytoin.

DOSING The recommended daily dose of isoniazid for the treatment of TB is 5 mg/kg for adults and 10 mg/kg for children (U.S. guidelines recommend 10–15 mg), with a maximal daily dose of 300 mg for both. For intermittent therapy in adults (usually twice per week), the dose is 15 mg/kg, with a maximal daily dose of 900 mg. Isoniazid does not require dosage adjustment in patients with renal disease. When the 12-dose, 3-month weekly LTBI regimen is used, the dose of isoniazid is 15 mg/kg, with a maximal dose of 900 mg, and the drug is co-administered with rifapentine. The novel 1-month regimen uses isoniazid 300 mg in conjunction with rifapentine for people aged >13 years without weight adjustment.

RESISTANCE Although isoniazid, along with rifampin, is the mainstay of TB treatment regimens, ~7% of clinical *M. tuberculosis* isolates in the United States are resistant. Rates of primary isoniazid resistance among untreated patients are significantly higher in many populations born outside the United States. Five separate pathways for isoniazid resistance have been elucidated. Most strains have amino acid changes in either the catalase-peroxidase gene (*katG*) or the mycobacterial ketoenoylreductase gene (*inhA*). Less frequently, alterations in *kasA*, the gene for an enzyme involved in mycolic acid elongation, and loss of NADH dehydrogenase 2 activity confer isoniazid resistance. In 20–30% of isoniazid-resistant *M. tuberculosis* isolates, increased expression of efflux pump genes, such as *efpA*, *mmpL7*, *mmr*, *p55*, and the Tap-like gene *Rv1258c*, has been implicated as the underlying mechanism of resistance.

ADVERSE EFFECTS Although isoniazid is generally well tolerated, drug-induced liver injury and peripheral neuropathy are significant adverse effects associated with this agent. Isoniazid may cause asymptomatic transient elevation of aminotransferase levels (often termed *hepatic adaptation*) in up to 20% of recipients. Other adverse reactions include rash (2%), fever (1.2%), anemia, acne, arthritic symptoms, a systemic lupus erythematosus–like syndrome, optic atrophy, seizures, and psychiatric symptoms. Symptomatic hepatitis occurs in <0.1% of persons treated with isoniazid alone for LTBI, and fulminant hepatitis with hepatic failure occurs in <0.01%. Isoniazid-associated hepatitis is idiosyncratic, but its incidence increases with age, with daily alcohol consumption, and in women who are within 3 months postpartum.

In patients who have liver disorders or HIV infection, who are pregnant or in the 3-month postpartum period, who have a history of liver disease (e.g., hepatitis B or C, alcoholic hepatitis, or cirrhosis), who use alcohol regularly, who have multiple medical problems, or who have other risk factors for chronic liver disease, the risks and benefits of isoniazid treatment for LTBI should be weighed. If treatment is undertaken, these patients should have serum concentrations of ALT determined at baseline. Routine baseline hepatic ALT testing based solely on an age of >35 years is optional and depends on individual concerns. Monthly biochemical monitoring during isoniazid treatment is indicated for patients whose baseline liver function tests yield abnormal results and for persons at risk for hepatic disease, including the groups just mentioned. Guidelines recommend that isoniazid be discontinued in the presence of hepatitis symptoms or jaundice and an ALT or AST level three times the upper limit of normal or in the absence of symptoms with an ALT or AST level five times the upper limit of normal (Table 181-3).

Peripheral neuropathy associated with isoniazid occurs in up to 2% of patients given 5 mg/kg. Isoniazid appears to interfere with pyridoxine (vitamin B_6) metabolism. The risk of isoniazid-related neurotoxicity is greatest for patients with preexisting disorders that also pose a risk of neuropathy, such as HIV infection; for those with diabetes mellitus, alcohol abuse, or malnutrition; and for those simultaneously receiving other potentially neuropathic medications, such as stavudine. These patients should be given prophylactic pyridoxine (25–50 mg/d).

Rifampin

Rifampin is a semisynthetic derivative of *Amycolatopsis rifamycinica* (formerly known as *Streptomyces mediterranei*). The most active antimycobacterial agent available, rifampin is the keystone of first-line treatment for TB. Introduced in 1968, this drug eventually permitted dramatic shortening of the TB treatment course. Rifampin has both sterilizing and bactericidal activity against dividing and nondividing *M. tuberculosis*. The drug is also active against an array of other organisms, including some gram-positive and gram-negative bacteria, *Legionella*, *M. kansasii*, and *Mycobacterium marinum*.

MECHANISM OF ACTION Rifampin exerts both intracellular and extracellular bactericidal activities. Like other rifamycins, rifampin specifically binds to and inhibits mycobacterial DNA-dependent RNA polymerase, blocking RNA synthesis. Susceptible strains of *M. tuberculosis* as well as *M. kansasii* and *M. marinum* are inhibited by rifampin concentrations of 1 μg/mL.

PHARMACOLOGY Rifampin is a fat-soluble, complex macrocyclic molecule readily absorbed after oral administration. Serum levels of 10–20 μg/mL are achieved 2.5 h after the usual adult oral dose of 10 mg/kg (given without food). Rifampin has a half-life of 1.5–5 h. The drug distributes well throughout most body tissues, including CSF. Rifampin turns body fluids such as urine, saliva, sputum, and tears a reddish-orange color—an effect that offers a simple means of assessing patients' adherence to this medication. Rifampin is excreted primarily through the bile and enters the enterohepatic circulation; <30% of a dose is renally excreted.

As a potent inducer of the hepatic cytochrome P450 system, rifampin can decrease the half-life of some drugs, such as digoxin, warfarin, phenytoin, prednisone, cyclosporine, methadone, oral contraceptives, clarithromycin, azole antifungal agents, quinidine, antiretroviral protease inhibitors, and nonnucleoside reverse transcriptase inhibitors. The Centers for Disease Control and Prevention (CDC) has issued guidelines for the management of drug interactions during treatment of HIV and *M. tuberculosis* co-infection (*www.cdc.gov/tb/*).

DOSING The daily dosage of rifampin is 10 mg/kg for adults and 10–20 mg/kg for children, with a maximum of 600 mg/d for both. The drug is given once daily, twice weekly, or three times weekly. No adjustments of dose or frequency are necessary in patients with renal insufficiency.

RESISTANCE Resistance to rifampin in *M. tuberculosis*, *M. leprae*, and other organisms is the consequence of spontaneous, mostly missense point mutations in a core region of the bacterial gene coding for the β subunit of RNA polymerase (*rpoB*). RNA polymerase altered in this manner is no longer subject to inhibition by rifampin. Most rapidly and slowly growing NTM harbor intrinsic resistance to rifampin, for which the mechanism has yet to be determined.

ADVERSE EFFECTS Adverse events associated with rifampin are infrequent and generally mild. Hepatotoxicity due to rifampin alone is uncommon in the absence of preexisting liver disease and often consists of isolated hyperbilirubinemia rather than aminotransferase elevation. Other adverse reactions include rash, pruritus, gastrointestinal symptoms, and pancytopenia. Rarely, a hypersensitivity reaction may occur with intermittent therapy, manifesting as fever, chills, malaise, rash, and—in some instances—renal and hepatic failure.

Pyrazinamide A nicotinamide analog, pyrazinamide is an important bactericidal drug used in the initial phase of TB treatment. Its administration for the first 2 months of therapy with rifampin and isoniazid allows treatment duration to be shortened from 9 to 6 months and decreases rates of relapse.

MECHANISM OF ACTION Pyrazinamide's antimycobacterial activity is essentially limited to *M. tuberculosis*. The drug is more active against slowly replicating organisms than against actively replicating organisms. Pyrazinamide is a prodrug that is converted by the mycobacterial pyrimidase to the active form, pyrazinoic acid (POA). This agent is active only in acidic environments (pH <6.0), as are found within phagocytes or granulomas. The exact mechanism of action of POA is unclear, but fatty acid synthetase I may be the primary target in *M. tuberculosis*. Susceptible strains of *M. tuberculosis* are inhibited by pyrazinamide concentrations of 16–50 μg/mL at pH 5.5.

PHARMACOLOGY AND DOSING Pyrazinamide is well absorbed after oral administration, with peak serum concentrations of 20–60 μg/mL at 1–2 h after ingestion of the recommended adult daily dose of 15–30 mg/kg (maximum, 2 g/d). It distributes well to various body compartments, including CSF, and is an important component of treatment for tuberculous meningitis. The serum half-life of the drug is 9–11 h with normal renal and hepatic function. Pyrazinamide is metabolized in the liver to POA, 5-hydroxypyrazinamide, and 5-hydroxy-POA. A high proportion of pyrazinamide and its metabolites (~70%) is excreted in the urine. The dosage must be adjusted according to the level of renal function in patients with reduced creatinine clearance.

ADVERSE EFFECTS At the higher dosages used previously, hepatotoxicity was seen in as many as 15% of patients treated with pyrazinamide. However, at the currently recommended dosages, hepatotoxicity now occurs less commonly when this drug is administered with isoniazid and rifampin during the treatment of TB. Older age, active liver disease, HIV infection, and low albumin levels may increase the risk of hepatotoxicity. The use of pyrazinamide with rifampin for the treatment of LTBI is no longer recommended because of unacceptable rates of hepatotoxicity and death in this setting. Hyperuricemia is a common adverse effect of pyrazinamide therapy that usually can be managed conservatively. Clinical gout is rare.

Although pyrazinamide is recommended by international TB organizations for routine use in pregnancy, it is not recommended in the United States because of inadequate teratogenicity data.

RESISTANCE The basis of pyrazinamide resistance in *M. tuberculosis* is a mutation in the *pncA* gene coding for pyrazinamidase, the enzyme that converts the prodrug to active POA. Resistance to pyrazinamide is associated with loss of pyrazinamidase activity, which prevents conversion of pyrazinamide to POA. Of pyrazinamide-resistant *M. tuberculosis* isolates, 72–98% have mutations in *pncA*. Conventional methods of testing for susceptibility to pyrazinamide may produce both false-negative and false-positive results because the high-acidity environment required for the drug's activation also inhibits the growth of *M. tuberculosis*. There is some controversy as to the clinical significance of in vitro pyrazinamide resistance.

Ethambutol Ethambutol is a bacteriostatic antimycobacterial agent first synthesized in 1961. A component of the standard first-line regimen, ethambutol provides synergy with the other drugs in the regimen and is generally well tolerated. Susceptible species include *M. tuberculosis*, *M. marinum*, *M. kansasii*, and organisms of the *Mycobacterium avium* complex (MAC); however, among first-line drugs, ethambutol is the least potent against *M. tuberculosis*. This agent is also used in combination with other agents in the continuation phase of treatment when patients cannot tolerate isoniazid or rifampin or are infected with organisms resistant to either of the latter drugs.

MECHANISM OF ACTION Ethambutol is bacteriostatic against *M. tuberculosis*. Its primary mechanism of action is the inhibition of the arabinosyltransferases involved in cell wall synthesis, which probably inhibits the formation of arabinogalactan and lipoarabinomannan. The MIC of ethambutol for susceptible strains of *M. tuberculosis* is 0.5–2 μg/mL.

PHARMACOLOGY AND DOSING From a single dose of ethambutol, 75–80% is absorbed within 2–4 h of administration. Serum levels peak at 2–4 μg/mL after the standard adult daily dose of 15 mg/kg. Ethambutol is well distributed throughout the body except in the CSF; a dosage of 25 mg/kg is necessary for attainment of a CSF level half of that in serum. For intermittent therapy, the dosage is 25–35 mg/kg thrice weekly. To prevent toxicity, the dosage must be lowered and the frequency of administration reduced for patients with renal insufficiency.

ADVERSE EFFECTS Ethambutol is usually well tolerated and has no significant interactions with other drugs. Optic neuritis, the most serious adverse effect reported, typically presents as reduced visual acuity, central scotoma, and loss of the ability to see green (or, less commonly, red). The cause of this neuritis is unknown, but it may be due to an effect of ethambutol on the amacrine and bipolar cells of the retina. Symptoms typically develop several months after initiation of therapy, but ocular toxicity soon after initiation of ethambutol has been described. The risk of ocular toxicity is dose dependent, with occurrence in 1–5% of patients, and can be increased by renal insufficiency. The routine use of ethambutol in younger children is not recommended because monitoring for visual complications can be difficult. If drug-resistant TB is suspected, ethambutol can be used for treatment of children.

All patients starting therapy with ethambutol should have a baseline test for visual acuity, visual fields, and color vision and should undergo an examination of the optic fundus. Visual acuity and color vision should be monitored monthly or less often as needed. Cessation of ethambutol in response to early symptoms of ocular toxicity usually results in reversal of the deficit within several months. Recovery of all visual function may take up to 1 year. In the elderly and in patients whose symptoms are not recognized early, deficits may be permanent. Some experts think that supplementation with hydroxycobalamin (vitamin B_{12}) is beneficial for patients with ethambutol-related ocular toxicity. Other adverse effects of ethambutol are rare. Peripheral sensory neuropathy occurs in rare instances.

RESISTANCE Ethambutol resistance in *M. tuberculosis* and NTM is associated primarily with missense mutations in the *embB* gene that encodes for arabinosyltransferase. Mutations have been found in resistant strains at codon 306 in 50–70% of cases. Mutations at *embB*306 can cause significantly increased MICs of ethambutol, resulting in clinical resistance.

OTHER RIFAMYCIN DRUGS

Rifabutin Rifabutin, a semisynthetic derivative of rifamycin S, inhibits mycobacterial DNA-dependent RNA polymerase. Rifabutin is recommended in place of rifampin for the treatment of TB in HIV-co-infected individuals who are taking protease inhibitors or nonnucleoside reverse transcriptase inhibitors, particularly nevirapine. A study in India showed better TB treatment outcomes in HIV-co-infected patients given daily rifabutin plus atazanavir/ritonavir than in those given thrice-weekly rifabutin plus atazanavir/ritonavir. Rifabutin's effect on hepatic enzyme induction is less pronounced than that of rifampin. Protease inhibitors may cause significant increases in rifabutin levels through inhibition of hepatic metabolism. Rifabutin is more active in vitro than rifampin against MAC organisms and other NTM, but its clinical superiority has not been established.

PHARMACOLOGY Like rifampin, rifabutin is lipophilic and is absorbed rapidly after oral administration, reaching peak serum levels 2–4 h after ingestion. Rifabutin distributes best to tissues, reaching levels 5–10 times higher than those in plasma. Unlike rifampin, rifabutin and its metabolites are partially cleared by the hepatic microsomal system. Rifabutin's slow clearance results in a mean serum half-life of 45 h—much longer than the 3- to 5-h half-life of rifampin. Clarithromycin (but not azithromycin) and fluconazole appear to increase rifabutin levels by inhibiting hepatic metabolism.

ADVERSE EFFECTS The most common adverse effects of rifabutin treatment are gastrointestinal; other reactions include rash, headache, asthenia, chest pain, myalgia, and insomnia. Less common adverse reactions include fever, chills, a flulike syndrome, anterior uveitis, hepatitis, *Clostridium difficile*–associated diarrhea, a diffuse polymyalgia syndrome, and yellow skin discoloration ("pseudo-jaundice"). Laboratory abnormalities include neutropenia, leukopenia, thrombocytopenia, and increased levels of liver enzymes. Rifabutin appears to be better tolerated by the majority (72%) of adult TB patients who have developed rifampin-related adverse effects. Female patients, those co-infected with hepatitis B or hepatitis C, and those with rifampin-related arthralgias, dermatologic reactions, and cholestasis are more likely to develop mild to severe rifabutin-related adverse effects.

RESISTANCE Similar to rifampin resistance, rifabutin resistance is mediated by mutations in *rpoB*.

Rifapentine Rifapentine is a semisynthetic cyclopentyl rifamycin, sharing a mechanism of action with rifampin. Rifapentine is lipophilic and has a prolonged half-life that permits weekly or twice-weekly dosing. Therefore, rifapentine is the subject of intensive clinical investigation aimed at determining optimal dosing and frequency of administration. Currently, it is an alternative to rifampin in the continuation phase of treatment for noncavitary drug-susceptible pulmonary TB in HIV-seronegative patients who have negative sputum smears at completion of the initial phase of treatment. When administered in these specific circumstances, rifapentine (10 mg/kg, up to 600 mg) is given once weekly with isoniazid. Because of higher rates of relapse, this regimen is not recommended for patients with TB disease and HIV co-infection; moreover, it has not been approved for children <12 years of age. In a phase 2 study, substituting daily rifapentine for rifampin yielded higher rates of sputum sterilization after 2 months of intensive treatment. Higher doses of rifapentine (20 mg/kg vs 10 mg/kg) had better results and were safe and well tolerated. Regimens containing high doses of rifapentine are being evaluated to see whether they can shorten the TB treatment course to <6 months.

PHARMACOLOGY Rifapentine's absorption is improved when the drug is taken with food. After oral administration, rifapentine reaches peak serum concentrations in 5–6 h and achieves a steady state in 10 days. The half-life of rifapentine and its active metabolite, 25-desacetyl rifapentine, is ~13 h. The administered dose is excreted via the liver (70%).

ADVERSE EFFECTS The adverse effects profile of rifapentine is similar to that of other rifamycins. Rifapentine is teratogenic in animal models and is relatively contraindicated in pregnancy.

RESISTANCE Rifapentine resistance is mediated by mutations in *rpoB*. Mutations that cause resistance to rifampin also cause resistance to rifapentine.

SECOND-LINE ANTITUBERCULOSIS DRUGS

Second-line anti-TB agents are indicated for treatment of drug-resistant TB, for patients who are intolerant or allergic to first-line agents, and when first-line supplemental agents are unavailable. According to their usability, they are divided into three WHO groups.

Group A • **FLUOROQUINOLONES** Fluoroquinolones inhibit mycobacterial DNA gyrase and topoisomerase IV, preventing cell replication and protein synthesis, and are bactericidal. Given their excellent activity, they have been investigated for their potential to shorten the course of treatment for drug-susceptible TB from 6 to 4 months. In contrast to prior trials, a recent large, open-label randomized controlled trial (TBTC Study 31) yielded promising results for shortening of TB treatment. Patients with drug susceptible TB disease were randomized to receive either standard six-month TB regimen or 4-month regimen containing rifapentine (8 weeks of once-daily rifapentine, isoniazid, pyrazinamide, and ethambutol followed by 9 weeks of once-daily rifapentine and isoniazid) or 4-month regimen containing rifapentine and moxifloxacin (8 weeks of once-daily rifapentine, isoniazid, pyrazinamide, and moxifloxacin followed by 9 weeks of once-daily rifapentine, isoniazid, and moxifloxacin). The trial demonstrated that a four-month regimen using daily rifapentine and moxifloxacin (but not the rifapentine only regimen) was non-inferior to the standard six-month TB treatment regimen using an end point of TB-free survival 12 months after randomization. Combining once daily rifapentine with moxifloxacin allows for synergistic action on sputum conversion in a compliance-friendly once-daily option. Current recommendations continue to be for a standard six-month regimen though it is anticipated that these results will inform future guidelines. Gatifloxacin has fallen out of favor because of significant dysglycemia. Ciprofloxacin and ofloxacin are no longer recommended for the treatment of TB because of poor efficacy. Despite documented resistance to early-generation fluoroquinolones (e.g., ofloxacin and ciprofloxacin), use of a later-generation fluoroquinolone in patients with drug-resistant TB has been associated with favorable outcomes. Fluoroquinolones are also considered safe alternatives for patients who develop treatment-limiting adverse effects from first-line agents. Levofloxacin and moxifloxacin have both been used effectively in the treatment of MDR-TB. The optimal dose of levofloxacin for this indication is being actively studied, but doses of at least 750 mg are commonly used. High-dose moxifloxacin (800 mg) is recommended for standardized shorter MDR-TB regimens.

The fluoroquinolones are well absorbed orally, reach high serum levels, and distribute well into body tissues and fluids. Their absorption is decreased by co-ingestion with products containing multivalent cations, such as antacids. Adverse effects are relatively infrequent (0.5–10% of patients) and include gastrointestinal intolerance, rashes, dizziness, and headache. Most studies of fluoroquinolone side effects have been based on relatively short-term administration for bacterial infections, but trials have now shown the relative safety and tolerability of fluoroquinolones administered for months during TB treatment in adults. Although the potential to prolong the QTc interval, leading to cardiac arrhythmias, has been a source of concern with fluoroquinolones, cessation of treatment due to this adverse effect is rare. Because the benefits may outweigh the risks in treatment of drug-resistant TB, there is increasing interest in the use of fluoroquinolones in children, which has traditionally been avoided because of the risks of tendon rupture and cartilage damage.

Multiple courses of empirical fluoroquinolone therapy for presumed community-acquired pneumonia are associated with delayed diagnosis of active pulmonary TB and increased fluoroquinolone resistance in *M. tuberculosis*. Mutations in the genes encoding for DNA gyrase (*gyrA* and *gyrB*) are implicated in the majority of cases—but not all cases—of clinical resistance to fluoroquinolones.

DIARYLQUINOLINES Bedaquiline (TMC207 or R207910) is a diarylquinoline with a novel mechanism of action: inhibition of the mycobacterial ATP synthetase proton pump. Bedaquiline is bactericidal for *M. tuberculosis*. Resistance has been reported due to point mutations in the *atpE* gene encoding for subunit c of ATP synthetase. Clinical bedaquiline resistance has also been reported due to nontarget mutations in Rv0678 (a negative repressor of the MmpL5 efflux pump) and PepQ (a cytoplasmic peptidase), both of which may cause cross-resistance to clofazimine. Bedaquiline is metabolized by the hepatic cytochrome CYP3A4. Rifampin lowers bedaquiline levels by 50%, and protease inhibitors also interact significantly with this drug. Because efavirenz induces CYP3A4, there is concern about lower bedaquiline levels with co-administration. In a study of co-treatment with bedaquiline and efavirenz in healthy volunteers, bedaquiline levels were reduced by only 20%; however, in a study modeling chronic co-administration of these two drugs, the reduction in bedaquiline levels was estimated to be 50%, leading many national TB programs to avoid efavirenz co-administration with bedaquiline.

The oral bioavailability of bedaquiline appears to be excellent. The dosage is 400 mg/d for the first 2 weeks and then 200 mg thrice weekly typically for 6 months total. The elimination half-life is long (>14 days). A single dose of this drug can inhibit the growth of *M. tuberculosis* for up to 1 week through a combination of long plasma half-life, high-level tissue penetration, and long tissue half-life. Bedaquiline added to a background regimen improved the 2-month sputum culture–conversion rate in multicenter, randomized placebo-controlled trials, and these results led to approval by the U.S. Food and Drug Administration (FDA). However, the death rate in one trial was higher in the bedaquiline arm than in the control arm (11.4% vs 2.5%); the result was a "black box" warning from the FDA, which also included QT prolongation. Subsequent studies have not found an association with significant mortality. The CDC has made a provisional recommendation for the use of bedaquiline for 24 weeks in adults with laboratory-confirmed pulmonary MDR-TB when no other effective treatment regimen can be provided. Bedaquiline is an integral part of all shorter course, oral MDR treatment regimens endorsed by the WHO.

OXAZOLIDINONES Linezolid is an oxazolidinone used primarily for the treatment of drug-resistant gram-positive bacterial infections. However, this drug is active in vitro against *M. tuberculosis* and NTM. Several case series have suggested that linezolid may help clear mycobacteria relatively rapidly when included in a regimen for the treatment of complex cases of drug-resistant TB. Linezolid's mechanism of action is disruption of protein synthesis by binding to the 50S bacterial ribosome. Linezolid has nearly 100% oral bioavailability, with good penetration into tissues and fluids, including CSF. Clinical resistance to linezolid has been reported and is typically associated with mutations in the 23S rRNA and in two ribosomal proteins, L3 (*rplC*) and L4 (*rplD*). Adverse effects may include optic and peripheral neuropathy, pancytopenia, and lactic acidosis and are usually associated with higher doses. Linezolid is a weak monoamine oxidase inhibitor and can be associated with the serotonin syndrome when given concomitantly with serotonergic drugs (primarily antidepressants such as selective serotonin reuptake inhibitors). It has been shown that ~80% of patients with MDR-TB can be successfully treated with linezolid-containing, individualized anti-TB regimens based on drug sensitivity testing. Replacement of ethambutol with linezolid for 2–4 weeks during the intensive phase of treatment of drug-susceptible TB is currently being evaluated for possible faster sputum conversion and a shorter treatment regimen. For MDR-TB treatment, linezolid is usually administered at a dose of 600 mg (or less in some cases) once daily, which appears to be effective. A single daily dose is associated with fewer adverse events than twice-a-day dosing.

Sutezolid, a modified version of oxazolidinones and protein synthesis inhibitor, is found to have higher early bactericidal activity compared to linezolid and is currently undergoing phase 2A trials. It is currently FDA approved for complex skin infections and appears to have less frequent side effects compared to linezolid; the adverse effects profile of long-term exposure compared with that of linezolid needs further investigation.

Group B • **CLOFAZIMINE** Clofazimine is a fat-soluble riminophenazine dye used primarily in the treatment of leprosy worldwide. It is currently gaining popularity in the management of drug-resistant TB because of its low cost and its intracellular and extracellular activity. By increasing reactive oxidant species and causing membrane destabilization, clofazimine may promote killing of antibiotic-tolerant *M. tuberculosis* "persister" organisms. In addition to antimicrobial activity, the drug has other pharmacologic activities, such as anti-inflammatory, pro-oxidative, and immunopharmacologic properties. Clofazimine has a half-life of ~70 days in humans, and average steady-state concentrations are achieved at ~1 month. Intake with fatty meals can improve its low and variable rates of absorption (45–62%). Common side effects include gastrointestinal intolerance, and reversible orange to brownish discoloration of skin, bodily fluids, and secretions. Dose adjustment may be necessary in patients with severe hepatic impairment. Clofazimine was studied as part of a regimen developed in Bangladesh for potential shortening of the MDR-TB treatment course. A meta-analysis suggested that inclusion of clofazimine in a multidrug regimen for treatment of MDR-TB was associated with a favorable outcome. Newer analogues with improved pharmacokinetics and alternative formulations of clofazimine (liposomal, nanosuspension, inhalational) are being studied.

CYCLOSERINE Cycloserine is an analog of the amino acid D-alanine and prevents bacterial cell-wall synthesis. It inhibits the action of enzymes, including alanine racemase, that are involved in the production of peptidoglycans. Cycloserine is active against a range of bacteria, including *M. tuberculosis*. Mechanisms of mycobacterial resistance are not well understood, but overexpression of alanine racemase can confer resistance in *Mycobacterium smegmatis*. Cycloserine is well absorbed after oral administration and is widely distributed throughout body fluids, including CSF. The usual adult dosage is 250 mg two or three times per day. Serious potential side effects include seizures and psychosis (with suicide in some cases), peripheral neuropathy, headache, somnolence, and allergic reactions. Drug levels are monitored to achieve optimal dosing and to reduce the risk of adverse effects, especially in patients with renal failure. Cycloserine should be administered as DOT only with caution and with support from experienced TB physicians to patients with epilepsy, active alcohol abuse, severe renal insufficiency, or a history of depression or psychosis.

Group C • **NITROIMIDAZOLES** The prodrugs delamanid (OPC-67683) and pretomanid (PA 824) are novel nitro-dihydroimidazooxazole derivatives that are activated by *M. tuberculosis*–specific flavin-dependent nitroreductases and whose antimycobacterial activity is attributable to inhibition of mycolic acid biosynthesis. Delamanid was shown in a randomized, placebo-controlled, multinational clinical trial to significantly improve the culture conversion rate at 2 months. QT prolongation occurred significantly more often in delamanid-treated patients, but no clinically relevant events were reported. In a subsequent randomized phase 3 trial, there was no significant difference in 6 months sputum conversion between delamanid and placebo among patients with an optimized background regimen. Currently, it is part of several ongoing clinical trials including combination with bedaquiline. It is recommended for the use in children younger than 6 years with rifampicin-resistant TB. Usual adult dose is 100 mg twice daily.

Pretomanid, the second novel agent from this class, has shown promising results in the treatment of drug-resistant TB in combination with bedaquiline. A combination of pretomanid with moxifloxacin and pyrazinamide for treatment of drug-susceptible TB was found to have higher culture conversation rates at 8 weeks compared to HRZE; however, a subsequent phase 3 study raised concern for higher frequency of potentially fatal hepatotoxicity. It is currently being evaluated in several phase 3 clinical trials in various combinations, including with fluoroquinolones and pyrazinamide. Based on the previously mentioned results with the BPaL regimen (Nix-TB study), the FDA has granted approval for specific highly resistant TB cases. Adult treatment dose is 200 mg administered daily.

AMOXICILLIN-CLAVULANATE AND CARBAPENEMS β-Lactam agents are largely ineffective for the treatment of *M. tuberculosis* because of resistance conferred by a hydrolyzing class A β-lactamase, BlaC. Carbapenems are poor substrates of BlaC, and clavulanic acid leads to irreversible inhibition. While the use of either amoxicillin-clavulanic acid or carbapenems alone for highly resistant forms of TB has been anecdotally reported with unclear results, the combination of meropenem and clavulanic acid turned out to be highly active in vitro. Recently, the combination was found to have effective early bactericidal activity, and in a large individual patient data meta-analysis, the combination was associated with positive outcomes. Nevertheless, the need to administer these carbapenems intravenously and the lack of information on the drugs' long-term side effects have restricted their use to certain severe cases only. Recommended daily doses are either imipenem-cilastatin 1 g (each component) IV twice daily or meropenem 1 g IV three times daily, each in combination with clavulanic acid 125 mg oral twice daily, which is only available in combination with amoxicillin.

AMINOGLYCOSIDES Aminoglycosides have played a time-honed role in the treatment of mycobacterial infections. Amikacin and streptomycin are aminoglycosides that exert mycobactericidal activity by binding to the 16S ribosomal subunit. The spectrum of antibiotic activity for amikacin and streptomycin includes *M. tuberculosis*, several NTM species, and aerobic gram-negative and gram-positive bacteria. Due to the need of intravenous or painful intramuscular injections and their serious side effect profile, the WHO recommends limiting their use with the increased availability of novel oral agents. Kanamycin and capreomycin, a cyclic polypeptide similar to aminoglycosides, are no longer recommended due to worse treatment outcomes and increased mortality. This recommendation is based on a large individual patient-level meta-analysis of observational cohort studies and is likely due to increased toxicity seen with these agents. Streptomycin was the first antimycobacterial agent used for the treatment of TB. Derived from *Streptomyces griseus*, streptomycin is bactericidal against dividing *M. tuberculosis* organisms but has only low-level early bactericidal activity. In developing countries, it continues to be widely used due to its low cost. The usual daily dose of streptomycin (given IM either daily or 5 days per week) is 15 mg/kg for adults and 20–40 mg/kg for children, with a maximum of 1 g/d for both with dose reduction recommended for patients ≥60 years of age or with renal impairment. Central nervous system penetration is poor.

Amikacin resistance is less widespread, and streptomycin-resistant strains may still be susceptible. The usual daily adult dosage is 15–30 mg/kg given IM or IV (maximal daily dose, 1 g). It is frequently used to treat severe nontuberculous mycobacterial infections.

Mycobacterial resistance to aminoglycosides is due to mutations in the genes encoding the 16S ribosomal RNA gene (*rrs*). Adverse effects of both amikacin and streptomycin include ototoxicity (in up to 10% of recipients, with auditory dysfunction occurring more commonly than vestibulotoxicity), nephrotoxicity, and neurotoxicity.

ETHIONAMIDE Ethionamide is a derivative of isonicotinic acid. Its mechanism of action is through inhibition of the *inhA* gene product enoyl–acyl carrier protein (acp) reductase, which is involved in mycolic acid synthesis. Ethionamide is bacteriostatic against metabolically active *M. tuberculosis* and some NTM. It is used in the treatment of drug-resistant TB, but its use is limited by severe gastrointestinal reactions (including abdominal pain, nausea, and vomiting) as well as significant central and peripheral neurologic side effects, reversible hepatitis (in ~5% of recipients), hypersensitivity reactions, and hypothyroidism. Ethionamide should be taken with food to reduce gastrointestinal effects and with pyridoxine (50–100 mg/d) to limit neuropathic side effects.

PARA-AMINOSALICYLIC ACID Para-aminosalicylic acid (PAS; 4-aminosalicylic acid) is an oral agent used in the treatment of drug-resistant TB. Its bacteriostatic activity is due to inhibition of folate synthesis and of iron uptake. PAS has relatively little activity as an anti-TB agent. Adverse effects may include high-level nausea, vomiting, and diarrhea. PAS may cause hemolysis in patients with glucose-6-phosphate dehydrogenase deficiency. The drug should be taken with acidic foods to improve absorption. Enteric-coated PAS granules (4 g orally every 8 h) appear to be better tolerated than other formulations and produce higher therapeutic blood levels. PAS has a short half-life (1 h), and 80% of the dose is excreted in the urine.

DRUGS IN DEVELOPMENT

The pipeline of novel TB drugs is rapidly changing. We direct the reader to the Working Group on New TB Drugs for the most up-to-date information (*https://www.newtbdrugs.org/pipeline/clinical*).

NONTUBERCULOUS MYCOBACTERIA

More than 150 species of NTM have been identified. Only a minority of these environmental organisms, which are extensively found in soil and water, are important human pathogens. NTM cause extensive disease primarily in persons with preexisting pulmonary disease or immunocompromise but can also cause nodular/bronchiectatic disease in otherwise seemingly healthy hosts. Disseminated infections with NTM are common in immunocompromised individuals. NTM are also important causes of skin and soft tissue infections in surgical settings. The two major classes of NTM are the slow-growing and rapidly growing species; subcultures of the latter grow within 1 week. The growth characteristics of NTM have diagnostic, therapeutic, and prognostic implications. The rate of growth can provide useful preliminary information within a specific clinical context, in that growth within 2–3 weeks is much more likely to indicate an NTM than *M. tuberculosis*. When NTM do grow from cultures, colonization should be distinguished from active disease in order to optimize the risk and benefit of prolonged treatment with multiple medications. According to the recommendations of the American Thoracic Society and the Infectious Diseases Society of America, significant clinical manifestations and/or radiographic evidence of progressive disease consistent with NTM infection as well as either reproducible sputum culture results or a single positive culture from bronchoscopy are required for the diagnosis of NTM pulmonary disease. Isolation of NTM from blood or from an infected extrapulmonary site, such as soft tissue or bone, is usually indicative of disseminated or local NTM infection (**Chap. 180**). Treatment of NTM disease is prolonged and requires multiple medications. Side effects of the regimens employed are common, and intermittent therapy is often used to mitigate these adverse events. Treatment regimens depend on the NTM species, the extent or type of disease, and—to some degree—drug susceptibility test results.

THERAPEUTIC CONSIDERATIONS FOR SPECIFIC NTM

Slowly Growing Mycobacteria Slowly growing mycobacteria can be divided into three categories based on their pigment-producing capabilities and—if they do produce pigment—their requirement for light to do so. *Photochromogens*, including *M. marinum* and *M. kansasii*, can produce yellowish-orange pigment only when exposed to light. *Scotochromogens*, including *Mycobacterium gordonae* and *Mycobacterium scrofulaceum*, can make pigment regardless of light exposure. MAC organisms and *Mycobacterium ulcerans* are *nonchromogens*—i.e., are incapable of making pigment irrespective of light exposure.

***MYCOBACTERIUM AVIUM* COMPLEX** Among the NTM, MAC organisms most commonly cause human disease. In immunocompetent hosts, MAC species are most often found in conjunction with underlying significant lung disease, such as chronic obstructive pulmonary disease or bronchiectasis. For patients with nodular or bronchiectatic MAC lung disease, an initial regimen consisting of clarithromycin or azithromycin, rifampin or rifabutin (the latter is preferred for HIV patients receiving ART), and ethambutol is given three times per week for at least 12 months after culture conversion. A daily regimen of these three drugs, with consideration of amikacin or streptomycin in the initial treatment phase, is recommended for patients with fibrocavitary MAC lung disease or severe nodular/bronchiectatic disease. Routine initial testing for macrolide resistance is recommended, as is testing at 6 months with a failing regimen (i.e., with cultures persistently positive for NTM). Interpretation of susceptibility tests to drugs other than macrolides and aminoglycosides is hampered by poor correlation with clinical outcomes. Amikacin has been reformulated as a liposomal suspension with increased penetration into airway biofilms. The

CONVERT trial showed that addition of inhaled liposomal amikacin to standard three-drug regimen of azithromycin or clarithromycin, rifampin, and ethambutol in treatment-refractory (persistent sputum positivity after at least 6 months) MAC lung disease significantly increases culture conversion rates from 9 to 26% at 6 months. Respiratory adverse events (primarily dysphonia, cough, and dyspnea) were reported in 87.4% of patients receiving inhaled liposomal amikacin compared to 50% in the standard therapy group; however, rates of serious adverse events were not different between the regimens. Inhaled liposomal amikacin is now approved for use in refractory pulmonary MAC infections (persistent positive cultures after at least 6 months of treatment). It is currently being evaluated as a first-line agent and as a replacement for rifampin in the treatment of MAC lung disease.

Surgical resection should be considered for individuals whose infection is localized to one lung, who have adequate lung function to tolerate lung resection, who have had a poor response to medical therapy, and/or who have developed macrolide-resistant MAC disease.

Treatment of MAC in persons living with HIV should be initiated in consultation with an infectious diseases specialist. For HIV-infected patients with well-controlled HIV disease and CD4 T-cell counts in the normal range, MAC treatment is identical to patients without HIV disease except that drug-drug interactions between antimycobacterial agents and ART should be carefully considered. HIV-infected patients with low CD4 count (CD4+ T-cell count >100/μL) are at risk for disseminated MAC infection. MAC disease in these patients is generally treated with clarithromycin, ethambutol, and rifabutin. Azithromycin may be preferred to clarithromycin depending on adverse effects and patient tolerance. Amikacin and fluoroquinolones are often used in salvage regimens. Treatment for disseminated MAC infection in AIDS patients may be lifelong in the absence of immune reconstitution. Therapy is recommended for at least 12 months after culture conversion and at least 6 months of effective immune reconstitution with ART (CD4+ T-cell count >100/μL).

MYCOBACTERIUM KANSASII *M. kansasii* is the second most common NTM causing human disease in the United States. It is also the second most common cause of NTM pulmonary disease in the United States, where it is most commonly reported in the southeastern region. *M. kansasii* infection can be treated with rifampin, ethambutol, and either isoniazid or macrolide; therapy continues for at least 18 months or for 12 months after culture conversion. The American Thoracic Society and the Infectious Diseases Society of America recommend routine susceptibility testing to rifampin only. Resistance to isoniazid and ethambutol can be acquired during therapy but is usually associated with rifampin resistance as well. Rifampin-resistant *M. kansasii* is treated with a three-drug regimen including agents such as ciprofloxacin, azithromycin, ethambutol, rifabutin, amikacin, trimethoprim-sulfamethoxazole, and streptomycin after drug susceptibility testing.

MYCOBACTERIUM MARINUM *M. marinum* is an NTM found in salt water and freshwater, including swimming pools and fish tanks. It is a cause of localized soft tissue infections, which may require surgical management. Combination regimens include clarithromycin and either ethambutol or rifampin. Other agents with activity against *M. marinum* include doxycycline, minocycline, and trimethoprim-sulfamethoxazole. Drug susceptibility testing is recommended only if the swab remains culture positive after 3 months of appropriate therapy.

Rapidly Growing Mycobacteria Rapidly growing mycobacteria causing human disease include *Mycobacterium abscessus, Mycobacterium fortuitum*, and *Mycobacterium chelonae*. Treatment of these mycobacteria is complex and should be undertaken with input from experienced clinicians. It is important to note that testing rapidly growing mycobacteria for macrolide resistance is tricky, as an inducible *erm* gene may confer in vivo macrolide resistance to isolates that are susceptible in vitro.

M. abscessus is the third most common NTM pathogen in the United States. It is endemic in the southeastern states between Texas and Florida. Skin, soft tissue, and bone infections occur, usually after accidental trauma or surgery. This organism appears to have a predilection to cause lung infections in white nonsmoking women aged >60 who have no preexisting lung disease. *M. abscessus* isolates are usually resistant to standard anti-TB regimens. Skin and soft tissue infections are usually treated for a minimum of 4 months with a macrolide (clarithromycin or azithromycin) and a parenteral agent such as amikacin, cefoxitin, or imipenem. Bone infections are treated for at least 6 months. This regimen can be used for the treatment of lung infections but is often unsuccessful because of drug adverse effects and toxicities. A regimen comprising a combination of at least three active drugs (amikacin, linezolid, tigecycline, imipenem, azithromycin, provided the organism is macrolide susceptible) is recommended on the basis of in vitro drug susceptibility testing. A recent meta-analysis has shown that overall therapeutic efficiency rates in *M. abscessus* lung infection are low at ~35%; however, incorporation of amikacin, imipenem, linezolid, and/or tigecycline was associated with improved outcomes. Conversely, macrolide resistance has been associated with worse outcomes. Surgical resection should be considered in all patients with good lung reserve and a localized infection.

DRUGS FOR THE TREATMENT OF NTM

Clarithromycin Clarithromycin is a macrolide antibiotic with broad activity against many gram-positive and gram-negative bacteria as well as NTM. This drug is active against MAC organisms and many other NTM species, inhibiting protein synthesis by binding to the 50S mycobacterial ribosomal subunit. NTM resistance to macrolides is probably caused by overexpression of the gene *ermB*, with consequent methylation of the binding site. Strains of *M. abscessus* subsp. *abscessus* harbor an inducible macrolide resistance mechanism coded by *erm41*, which leads to ribosomal methylation and becomes apparent after macrolide incubation of 3–5 days, significantly hampering treatment success. Twenty percent of strains have a nonfunctional *erm41* gene. Clarithromycin is well absorbed orally and distributes well to tissues. It is cleared both hepatically and renally; the dosage should be reduced in renal insufficiency. Clarithromycin is a substrate for and inhibits cytochrome 3A4 and should not be administered with cisapride, pimozide, or terfenadine because cardiac arrhythmias may occur. Numerous drugs interact with clarithromycin through the CYP3A4 metabolic pathway. Rifampin lowers clarithromycin levels; conversely, rifampin levels are increased by clarithromycin. However, the clinical relevance of this interaction does not appear to be great.

For patients with nodular/bronchiectatic MAC infection, the dosage of clarithromycin is 500 mg, given morning and evening three times a week. For the treatment of fibrocavitary or severe nodular/bronchiectatic MAC infection, a dose of 500–1000 mg is given daily. Disseminated MAC infection is treated with 1000 mg daily. Clarithromycin is used in combination regimens that typically include ethambutol and a rifamycin in order to avoid the development of macrolide resistance. Adverse effects include frequent gastrointestinal intolerance, hepatotoxicity, headache, rash, and rare instances of hypoglycemia. Clarithromycin is contraindicated during pregnancy because of its teratogenicity in animal models.

Azithromycin Azithromycin is a derivative of erythromycin. Although technically an azalide and not a macrolide, it works similarly to macrolides, inhibiting protein synthesis through binding to the 50S ribosomal subunit. Azithromycin is preferred over clarithromycin due to once-daily dosing, better tolerability, fewer drug interactions, and equal efficacy. Resistance to azithromycin is almost always associated with complete cross-resistance to clarithromycin. Azithromycin is well absorbed orally, with good tissue penetration and a prolonged half-life (~48 h). The usual dosage for treatment of MAC infection is 250 mg daily or 500 mg three times per week. Azithromycin is used in combination with other agents to avoid the development of resistance. For prophylaxis against disseminated MAC infection in immunocompromised individuals, a dose of 1200 mg once per week is given. Because azithromycin is not metabolized by cytochrome P450, it interacts with few drugs. Adjustment of the dosage on the basis of renal function is not necessary.

Amikacin Liposome Inhalation Suspension (ALIS) ALIS is a new formulation of the aminoglycoside amikacin, which allows for improved penetration in the lung with reduced toxicity. It is now approved for treatment of refractory MAC lung infection with persistent sputum positivity at 6 months while on appropriate background regimen. Typical dose is 590 mg (one vial once a day) for 6 months along with the standard three-drug regimen of macrolide, rifampin, and ethambutol. Dosage adjustments in patients with hepatic and renal dysfunction are not required. Half-life elimination typically occurs in ~5.9–9.5 h. Respiratory side effects such as bronchospasm, cough, dysphonia, and dyspnea are common. Monitoring for systemic aminoglycoside toxicity should be considered.

Imipenem Imipenem primarily inhibits cell-wall biosynthesis by binding to the penicillin-binding proteins. It is rapidly gaining importance for the treatment of *M. abscessus* with a meta-analysis showing improved outcomes with its inclusion in a multidrug regimen. It is dosed at 500 mg to 1 g twice to three times a day as part of a combination regimen for the treatment of *M. abscessus.* Half-life of imipenem is ~1 h, and because it is metabolized in the kidneys, dosing adjustment is needed with renal dysfunction. Adverse effects include anemia, thrombocythemia, and liver dysfunction.

Cefoxitin Cefoxitin is a second-generation parenteral cephalosporin with activity against rapidly growing NTM, particularly *M. abscessus* and *M. chelonae*. Its mechanism of action against NTM is unknown but may involve inactivation of cell-wall synthesis enzymes. High doses are used for treatment of NTM: 200 mg/kg IV three or four times per day, with a maximal daily dose of 12 g. The half-life of cefoxitin is ~1 h, with primary renal clearance that requires adjustment in renal insufficiency. Adverse effects are uncommon but include gastrointestinal manifestations, rash, eosinophilia, fever, and neutropenia.

Newer Drugs Three newer classes of drugs—the oxazolidinones, the glycylcyclines, and the ketolides—are currently being evaluated for possible use in the treatment of NTM infections, especially those caused by *M. abscessus*. Approximately 50% of *M. abscessus* isolates have shown some degree of susceptibility in vitro to linezolid, an oxazolidinone. Tigecycline, which is a glycylcycline and a tetracycline derivative, and telithromycin, a ketolide, also appear to have in vitro activity against *M. abscessus*. These drugs, however, have not yet been clinically tested in patients.

In addition, some anti-TB drugs, including clofazimine and bedaquiline, are being evaluated as alternative agents for the treatment of refractory NTM infections. In particular, clofazimine appears to act synergistically in combination with amikacin, bedaquiline, or tigecycline. The exact role of these agents in the treatment of refractory NTM infections remains unclear. Suppressive therapy with periodic parenteral/oral drugs to limit disease progression and control symptoms may be an appropriate alternative to curative treatment.

CONCLUSION

Treatment of mycobacterial infections requires multiple-drug regimens that often exert significant side effects with the potential to limit tolerability. The prolonged duration of treatment has vastly improved results over those obtained in past decades, but drugs and regimens that will shorten treatment duration and limit adverse drug effects and interactions are needed.

FURTHER READING

Collaborative Group for the Meta-Analysis of Individual Patient Data in MDR-TB Treatment–2017: Treatment correlates of successful outcomes in pulmonary multidrug-resistant tuberculosis: An individual patient data meta-analysis. Lancet 392:821, 2018.

Daley CL et al: Treatment of nontuberculous mycobacterial pulmonary disease: An official ATS/ERS/ESCMID/IDSA clinical practice guideline. Clin Infect Dis 71:e1, 2020.

Nahid P et al: Official American Thoracic Society/Centers for Disease Control and Prevention/Infectious Diseases Society of America clinical practice guidelines: Treatment of drug-susceptible tuberculosis. Clin Infect Dis 63:e147, 2016.

Sterling TR et al: Guidelines for the treatment of latent tuberculosis infection: Recommendations from the National Tuberculosis Controllers Association and CDC, 2020. MMWR Recomm Rep 69 (No. RR-1):1, 2020.

World Health Organization: Consolidated guidelines on drug-resistant tuberculosis treatment. Geneva: World Health Organization, 2019. License: CC BY-NC-SA 3.0 IGO.

Section 9 Spirochetal Diseases

182 Syphilis

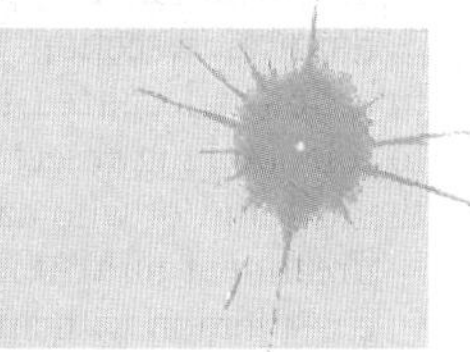

Sheila A. Lukehart

DEFINITION

Syphilis, a chronic systemic infection caused by *Treponema pallidum* subspecies *pallidum*, is usually sexually transmitted and is characterized by episodes of active disease interrupted by asymptomatic periods (latency). After an incubation period averaging 2–6 weeks, a primary lesion appears—often associated with regional lymphadenopathy—and then resolves without treatment. The secondary stage, with generalized mucosal and cutaneous lesions and generalized lymphadenopathy, also resolves spontaneously and is followed by a latent period of subclinical infection lasting years or decades. Central nervous system (CNS) invasion may occur early in infection, and CNS involvement may be symptomatic or asymptomatic. In the preantibiotic era, one-third of untreated patients developed tertiary syphilis, characterized by destructive mucocutaneous, skeletal, or parenchymal lesions; aortitis; or late CNS manifestations.

ETIOLOGY

The Spirochaetales include five genera that are pathogenic for humans and for a variety of other animals: *Leptospira* species (leptospirosis, Chap. 184); *Borrelia* and *Borreliella* species (relapsing fever and Lyme disease, respectively; Chaps. 185 and 186); *Brachyspira* species (gastrointestinal infections); and *Treponema* species (syphilis and the endemic treponematoses; see also Chap. 183). The *Treponema* subspecies include *T. pallidum* subsp. *pallidum* (venereal syphilis); *T. pallidum* subsp. *pertenue* (yaws); *T. pallidum* subsp. *endemicum* (endemic syphilis or bejel); and *T. carateum* (pinta). Historically, the subspecies were distinguished by the clinical syndromes they produce, but phylogenetic analyses of whole genome sequences from a relatively small number of strains (excluding *T. carateum*) yield the three named subspecies groupings. Whether these groupings represent geographical variation or true biological differences is unclear. The crossing of subspecies boundaries by some "molecular signatures" and the recent recognition of treponemes of the *endemicum* genotype in sexually acquired genital ulcers (chancres) and secondary rashes (Chap. 183) support the concept of a genetic and clinical "continuum" among strains and subspecies of the pathogenic treponemes.

T. pallidum subspecies are thin spiral organisms, with a cell body surrounded by a trilaminar cytoplasmic membrane, a delicate peptidoglycan layer, and a lipid-rich outer membrane. Endoflagella wind around the cell body in the periplasmic space and are responsible for motility.

Historically, *T. pallidum* could not be cultured in vitro, but long-term propagation of the Nichols strain of *T. pallidum* in complex medium with eukaryotic cells was recently reported. To date, the *pertenue* and *endemicum* subspecies have not been cultured. All *T. pallidum* subspecies have severely limited metabolic capabilities and are highly dependent on host-derived amino acids, carbohydrates, and lipids. Genetic analyses have revealed the existence of a 12-member gene family (*tpr*) encoding outer-membrane antigens. One member, TprK, has discrete variable regions that undergo antigenic variation during infection, providing a mechanism for immune evasion.

The only known natural host for *T. pallidum* subsp. *pallidum* (referred to hereafter as *T. pallidum*) is the human. *T. pallidum* can infect many mammals, but only humans, higher apes, and a few laboratory animals develop syphilitic lesions. Rabbits are used to propagate *T. pallidum* and serve as the animal model that best reflects human disease and immunopathology.

TRANSMISSION AND EPIDEMIOLOGY

Nearly all cases of syphilis are acquired by sexual contact with infectious lesions (i.e., the chancre, mucous patch, skin rash, or condylomata lata; **see Fig. A1-20**). Less common modes of transmission include nonsexual skin contact, infection in utero, blood transfusion, and organ transplantation.

SYPHILIS IN THE UNITED STATES

Following the introduction of penicillin therapy in the 1940s, the number of cases of syphilis of all stages reported in the United States declined 95% to a low of 31,575 cases in 2000, with 5979 reported cases of primary and secondary (P&S) syphilis. (P&S cases are infectious and are a better indicator of disease activity than total syphilis cases.) Since 2000, total cases have increased 3.6-fold to 115,045, and the number of P&S cases has increased nearly sixfold, with 35,063 cases reported in 2018 (**Fig. 182-1**). Nationally, ~54% of these cases were in men who have sex with men (MSM), ~41.6% of whom are co-infected with HIV. From 2017 to 2018, P&S cases rose 11.7% among all men and 34.2% among women, with increases in all racial and ethnic groups and in all geographic regions of the United States. Because the incidence of congenital syphilis parallels that of infectious syphilis in women, the striking increase in early syphilis in women has resulted in a dramatic increase in congenital syphilis. In 2018, 1306 cases of congenital syphilis were reported, resulting in 78 stillbirths and 16 infant deaths. Since 2014, the number of reported cases in infants <1 year of age has increased nearly threefold. Data from 2018 show that nearly 12% of women with syphilis reported injecting drugs in the past 12 months and nearly 8% reported heroin use.

The populations at highest risk for acquiring syphilis have changed over time, with outbreaks among MSM in the pre-HIV era of the late 1970s and early 1980s, as well as at present. The dramatic recent increases in syphilis and other sexually transmitted infections in MSM may be due to unprotected sex between persons who are HIV concordant and to disinhibition facilitated by highly effective antiretroviral therapy (ART). Many MSM diagnosed with syphilis have had syphilis previously, and more frequent (every 3 months) screening for syphilis and other sexually transmitted infections is warranted in such high-risk populations. Cases of P&S syphilis among African Americans increased 2.7-fold between 2000 and 2018, and the rate (28.1 per 100,000 population) remains higher than rates for other racial/ethnic groups.

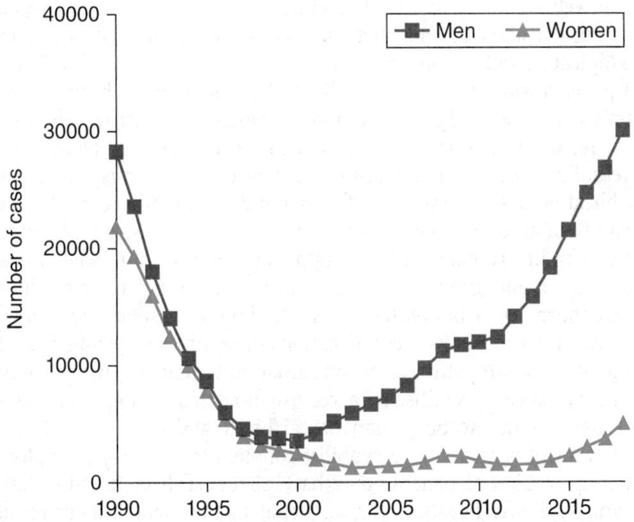

FIGURE 182-1 Primary and secondary syphilis in the United States, 1990–2018, by sex. *(Data from the Centers for Disease Control and Prevention.)*

Of individuals named as sexual contacts of persons with infectious syphilis, many will have developed manifestations of syphilis when they are first seen, and ~30% of asymptomatic contacts examined within 30 days of exposure actually have incubating infection and will later develop infectious syphilis if not treated. Thus, identification and treatment of all recently exposed sexual contacts continue to be important aspects of syphilis control.

GLOBAL SYPHILIS

Syphilis remains a significant health problem globally; the number of new infections is estimated at 6–8 million per year. The regions most affected include sub-Saharan Africa, South America, China, and Southeast Asia. The incidence rate for total syphilis in China continues to rise, and rates of P&S syphilis have increased dramatically among MSM in many European, Asian, and South American countries. Globally, through efforts by World Health Organization (WHO), progress has been made in the prevention of congenital syphilis, although there are still ~988,000 pregnant women with syphilis per year, with 661,000 cases of congenital syphilis including 200,000 stillbirths and infant deaths.

NATURAL COURSE AND PATHOGENESIS OF UNTREATED SYPHILIS

T. pallidum rapidly penetrates intact mucous membranes or microscopic abrasions in skin and, within a few hours, enters the lymphatics and blood to produce systemic infection and metastatic foci long before the appearance of a primary lesion. Blood from a patient with incubating or early syphilis is infectious. The generation time of *T. pallidum* during early disease is estimated to be ~30 h, and the incubation period of syphilis is inversely proportional to the number of organisms transmitted. The 50% infectious dose for intradermal inoculation in humans has been calculated to be 57 organisms, and the treponeme concentration generally reaches 10^7/g of tissue before a clinical lesion appears. The median incubation period in humans (~21 days) suggests an average inoculum of 500–1000 infectious organisms for naturally acquired disease; the incubation period rarely exceeds 6 weeks.

The primary lesion appears at the site of inoculation, usually persists for 4–6 weeks, and then heals spontaneously. Histopathologic examination shows perivascular infiltration, chiefly by CD4+ and CD8+ T lymphocytes, plasma cells, and macrophages, with capillary endothelial proliferation and subsequent obliteration of small blood vessels. The cellular infiltration produces a T_H1-type cytokine profile, consistent with the activation of macrophages. Phagocytosis of opsonized organisms by activated macrophages ultimately causes their destruction, resulting in spontaneous resolution of the chancre.

The generalized parenchymal, constitutional, mucosal, and cutaneous manifestations of secondary syphilis usually appear ~6–12 weeks after infection, although primary and secondary manifestations may occasionally overlap. In contrast, some patients may enter the latent stage without ever recognizing secondary lesions. The histopathologic features of secondary maculopapular skin lesions include hyperkeratosis of the epidermis, capillary proliferation with endothelial swelling in the superficial dermis, and—in the deeper dermis—perivascular infiltration by CD8+ T lymphocytes, CD4+ T lymphocytes, macrophages, and variable numbers of plasma cells. *T. pallidum* disseminates during the first days to weeks of infection, invading many tissues, including the CNS; cerebrospinal fluid (CSF) abnormalities can be detected in as many as 40% of patients during the secondary stage. Clinical hepatitis and immune complex–induced glomerulonephritis are rare, but recognized, manifestations of secondary syphilis. Generalized nontender lymphadenopathy is noted in 85% of patients with secondary syphilis. The paradoxical appearance of secondary manifestations, even after the development of an immune response that clears primary lesions, likely results from immune evasion due to antigenic variation of TprK surface antigens. Secondary lesions generally subside within

2–6 weeks, and the infection enters the latent stage, which is detectable only by serologic testing. In the preantibiotic era, up to 25% of untreated patients experienced at least one cutaneous relapse of secondary lesions, usually during the first year. Therefore, identification and examination of sexual contacts are most important for patients with syphilis of <1 year's duration.

In the preantibiotic era, about one-third of patients with untreated latent syphilis developed clinically apparent tertiary disease, the most common types being the gumma (a usually benign granulomatous lesion); cardiovascular syphilis (usually involving the vasa vasorum of the ascending aorta and resulting in aneurysm); and late symptomatic neurosyphilis (tabes dorsalis and paresis). In Western countries today, specific treatment for early and latent syphilis and coincidental therapy (i.e., therapy with antibiotics active against treponemes, but given for other conditions) have nearly eliminated tertiary syphilis. Asymptomatic CNS involvement, however, is still demonstrable in up to 40% of persons with early syphilis and 25% of patients with late latent syphilis, and modern cases of general paresis and tabes dorsalis are being reported from China. The factors that contribute to the development and progression of tertiary disease are unknown.

CLINICAL MANIFESTATIONS

PRIMARY SYPHILIS

The typical primary chancre usually begins as a single painless papule that rapidly erodes and becomes indurated, with a characteristic cartilaginous consistency on palpation of the edge and base of the ulcer. Multiple primary lesions are seen in a minority of patients. In heterosexual men, the chancre is usually located on the penis, where it is readily seen (**Fig. 182-2; see also Fig. A1-17**), but in MSM, it may also be found in the anal canal, rectum, or mouth. Oral sex has been identified as the source of infection in some MSM. In women, common primary sites are the cervix, vaginal wall, and labia, as well as anal canal and mouth. Consequently, primary syphilis goes unrecognized in women and MSM more often than in heterosexual men.

Atypical primary lesions are common, and may be multiple, small, or partially resolved. Therefore, syphilis should be considered in the evaluation of trivial or atypical dark-field-negative genital lesions. The lesions that most commonly must be differentiated from those of primary syphilis include those caused by herpes simplex virus infection (**Chap. 192**), chancroid (**Chap. 157**), traumatic injury, and donovanosis (**Chap. 173**). Regional (usually inguinal) lymphadenopathy accompanies the primary syphilitic lesion, appearing within 1 week of lesion onset. The nodes are firm, nonsuppurative, and painless. Inguinal lymphadenopathy is bilateral and may occur with anal as well as with genital chancres. The chancre generally heals within 4–6 weeks (range, 2–12 weeks), but lymphadenopathy may persist for months.

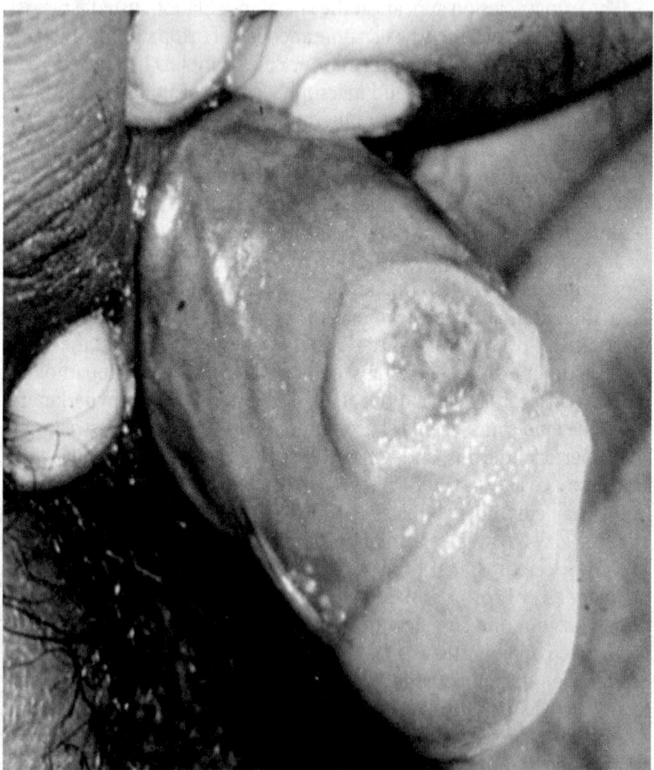

FIGURE 182-2 Primary syphilis with a firm, nontender chancre.

SECONDARY SYPHILIS

The classical manifestations of the secondary stage include mucocutaneous or cutaneous lesions and generalized nontender lymphadenopathy. The healing primary chancre may still be present in ~15% of cases—more frequently in persons with concurrent HIV infection. The skin rash consists of macular, papular, papulosquamous, and occasionally pustular syphilides; often more than one form is present simultaneously. The eruption may be very subtle, and 25% of patients with a discernible rash may be unaware that they have dermatologic manifestations. Initial lesions are pale red or pink, nonpruritic, discrete macules distributed on the trunk and extremities; these macules progress to papular lesions that are distributed widely and that frequently involve the palms and soles (**Fig. 182-3; see also Figs. A1-18 and A1-19**). Rarely, severe necrotic lesions (*lues maligna*) may appear and are more commonly reported in HIV-infected individuals. Involvement of the hair follicles may result in patchy alopecia of the scalp hair, eyebrows, or beard in up to 5% of cases.

In warm, moist, intertriginous areas (commonly the perianal region, vulva, and scrotum), papules can enlarge to produce broad, moist, pink or gray-white, highly infectious lesions (*condylomata lata*; **see Fig. A1-20**) in 10% of patients with secondary syphilis. Superficial mucosal erosions (*mucous patches*) occur in 10–15% of patients and commonly involve the oral or genital mucosa (**see Fig. A1-21**). The typical mucous patch is a painless silver-gray erosion surrounded by a red periphery. *T. pallidum* DNA has been detected in oral mucosal swabs from persons with early syphilis, but who have no visible oral lesions. The implications of this finding for transmission are unclear but warrant further research.

Constitutional signs and symptoms that may accompany or precede secondary syphilis include sore throat (15–30%), fever (5–8%), weight loss (2–20%), malaise (25%), anorexia (2–10%), headache (10%), and meningismus (5%). *Acute meningitis* occurs in only 1–2% of cases, but CSF cell and protein concentrations are increased in up to 40% of early syphilis cases, and viable *T. pallidum* organisms have been recovered from CSF during primary and secondary syphilis in 30% of cases, sometimes without other CSF abnormalities. Persons with current or recent secondary syphilis may present with ocular or otic manifestations. Ocular findings include pupillary abnormalities and optic neuritis as well as the classic iritis or uveitis. The diagnosis of ocular syphilis is often considered in affected patients only after they fail to respond to topical steroid therapy. Anterior uveitis has been reported in 5–10% of patients with secondary syphilis, and *T. pallidum* has been demonstrated in aqueous humor from such patients. Permanent blindness may result without prompt diagnosis and treatment. Otic syphilis may present as sensorineural hearing loss, vertigo, or tinnitus. The recent publication of several reports of ocular and otic syphilis reminds clinicians to inquire about neurologic manifestations in all stages of syphilis infection. In a recent study, 7.9% of patients with syphilis, when asked, reported recent vision or hearing changes, and more than half of those had abnormal CSF or ophthalmologic findings consistent with syphilis.

Less often recognized complications of secondary syphilis include hepatitis, nephropathy, gastrointestinal involvement (hypertrophic gastritis, patchy proctitis, or a rectosigmoid mass—sometimes mistakenly assumed to be malignant), arthritis, and periostitis. Hepatic involvement is common in syphilis; although it is usually asymptomatic, up to 25% of patients may have abnormal liver function tests. Frank syphilitic hepatitis is rare. Renal involvement usually results from immune complex deposition and produces proteinuria associated with an acute nephrotic syndrome. Like those of primary syphilis, most

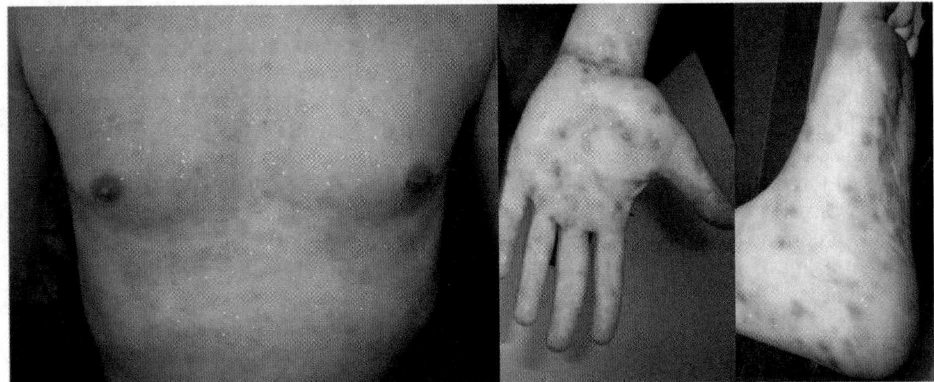

FIGURE 182-3 Secondary syphilis. ***Left:*** Maculopapular truncal eruption. ***Middle:*** Papules on the palms. ***Right:*** Papules on the soles. *(Photos courtesy of Jill McKenzie and Christina Marra.)*

manifestations of the secondary stage resolve spontaneously, usually within 1–6 months.

LATENT SYPHILIS

Positive serologic tests for syphilis, together with a normal CSF examination and the absence of clinical manifestations of syphilis, indicate a diagnosis of latent syphilis in an untreated person. The diagnosis may be made following routine serologic screening or may be suspected due to a history of primary or secondary lesions, a history of exposure to syphilis, or the delivery of an infant with congenital syphilis. A previous nonreactive serologic test or clear history of lesions or exposure may help to establish the duration of infection, which is an important factor in the selection of appropriate therapy. *Early latent* syphilis is limited to the first year after infection, whereas *late latent* syphilis is defined as that of ≥1 year's (or unknown) duration. The classical definition of early latent syphilis would include a person whose secondary rash has resolved, as well as a person whose chancre has healed but who has not yet developed secondary manifestations. The Centers for Disease Control and Prevention (CDC) have recently revised the case definitions for surveillance and reporting purposes to better reflect the recognition that some clinical manifestations may appear at several stages of infection. These definitions include the traditional primary and secondary stages, as well as "syphilis, early nonprimary nonsecondary," describing infections of <12 months' duration, and "syphilis, unknown duration or late," encompassing the previous late latent and late (tertiary) classifications. In this new scheme, neurologic, ocular, otic, and late clinical manifestations are reported separately in the context of their separate primary, secondary, early nonprimary nonsecondary, and unknown duration or late categories.

It was previously thought that untreated late latent syphilis had three possible outcomes: (1) persistent lifelong infection; (2) development of tertiary syphilis; or (3) spontaneous cure, with reversion of serologic tests to negative. Although progression to clinically evident late syphilis is very rare today, the occurrence of spontaneous microbiologic cure is in doubt.

Because *T. pallidum* continues to be present throughout untreated infection, it may seed the bloodstream intermittently during the latent stage, and a pregnant woman with latent syphilis may infect her fetus in utero. Moreover, syphilis has been transmitted through blood transfusion or organ donation from patients with latent syphilis.

REINFECTION SYPHILIS

A growing number of individuals, particularly MSM, are acquiring multiple episodes of syphilis, with important implications for clinical presentation and serologic testing. Although no national data are available, 32% of enrollees (mostly MSM) in a recent 18-year longitudinal study of CNS involvement were known to have had multiple episodes of syphilis. It is well recognized that, after treatment, persons with past syphilis are less likely to revert to nonreactive in the Venereal Disease Research Laboratory (VDRL)/rapid plasma reagin (RPR) than persons with first episode syphilis, and treponemal tests will remain reactive. However, several recent studies also indicate that subsequent episodes of syphilis are more likely to be asymptomatic than initial episodes, less likely to have *T. pallidum* identified in blood or CSF, and less likely to have laboratory-defined neurosyphilis. These cases would be detectable only by serologic screening, reinforcing the utility of frequent screening in high-risk populations.

INVOLVEMENT OF THE CNS

Traditionally, neurosyphilis has been considered a late manifestation of syphilis, but this view is inaccurate. CNS syphilis represents a continuum encompassing early invasion (usually within the first weeks of infection), months to years of asymptomatic involvement, and, in some cases, development of early or late neurologic manifestations. Early neurosyphilis includes asymptomatic or symptomatic meningitis and meningovascular syphilis; late neurosyphilis includes tabes dorsalis and general paresis.

Asymptomatic Neurosyphilis The diagnosis of asymptomatic neurosyphilis is made in patients who lack neurologic symptoms and signs but who have CSF abnormalities, including mononuclear pleocytosis, increased protein concentration, or reactivity in the CSF VDRL test. CSF abnormalities are demonstrated in up to 40% of cases of untreated primary or secondary syphilis and in 25% of cases of untreated latent syphilis. *T. pallidum* has been recovered by inoculation into rabbits of CSF from up to 30% of patients with primary or secondary syphilis but less frequently from patients with syphilis of >1 year's duration. The presence of *T. pallidum* in CSF is often associated with other CSF abnormalities, but organisms can be recovered from patients with otherwise normal CSF. Although the prognostic implications of these findings in early syphilis are uncertain, it may be appropriate to conclude that even patients with early syphilis who have CSF abnormalities do indeed have asymptomatic neurosyphilis and should be treated for neurosyphilis; such treatment is particularly important in patients with concurrent untreated HIV infection. Before the advent of penicillin, the risk of development of clinical neurosyphilis in untreated asymptomatic persons was roughly proportional to the intensity of CSF changes, with the overall cumulative probability of progression to clinical neurosyphilis ~20% in the first 10 years of infection but increasing with time. In several large studies, neurosyphilis was associated with an RPR titer of ≥1:32, regardless of clinical stage or HIV infection status. While most experts agree that neurosyphilis is more common among persons with untreated HIV infection, the immune reconstitution seen with effective ART may have a protective effect against development of clinical neurosyphilis in HIV-infected persons with syphilis. Nonetheless, RPR titer ≥1:32 is still associated with reactive CSF VDRL, even in persons taking effective ART. HIV-uninfected persons with untreated latent syphilis and normal CSF probably run a very low risk of subsequent neurosyphilis.

Symptomatic Neurosyphilis The major clinical categories of symptomatic neurosyphilis include early meningeal and meningovascular and late parenchymatous syphilis. The last category includes general paresis and tabes dorsalis. The onset of symptoms usually occurs <1 year after infection for meningeal syphilis, up to 10 years after infection for meningovascular syphilis, at ~20 years for general paresis, and at 25–30 years for tabes dorsalis. Neurosyphilis is more frequently symptomatic in patients co-infected with untreated HIV, particularly those with low CD4+ T lymphocyte counts. In addition, evidence suggests that syphilis infection worsens the cognitive impairment seen in HIV-infected persons and that this effect persists after treatment for syphilis.

Meningeal syphilis may present as headache, nausea, vomiting, neck stiffness, cranial nerve involvement, seizures, and changes in mental status. This condition may be concurrent with or may follow the secondary stage. Patients presenting with uveitis, iritis, or hearing loss often have meningeal syphilis, but these clinical findings can also be seen in patients with normal CSF.

Meningovascular syphilis reflects meningitis together with inflammatory vasculitis of small, medium, or large vessels. The most common presentation is a stroke syndrome involving the middle cerebral artery of a relatively young adult. However, unlike the usual thrombotic or embolic stroke syndrome of sudden onset, meningovascular syphilis often becomes manifest after a subacute encephalitic prodrome (with headaches, vertigo, insomnia, and psychological abnormalities), which is followed by a gradually progressive vascular syndrome.

The manifestations of *general paresis* reflect widespread late parenchymal damage and include abnormalities corresponding to the mnemonic *paresis: p*ersonality, *a*ffect, *r*eflexes (hyperactive), *e*ye (e.g., Argyll Robertson pupils), *s*ensorium (illusions, delusions, hallucinations), *i*ntellect (a decrease in recent memory and in the capacity for orientation, calculations, judgment, and insight), and *s*peech. *Tabes dorsalis* is a late manifestation of syphilis that presents as symptoms and signs of demyelination of the posterior columns, dorsal roots, and dorsal root ganglia, including ataxia, foot drop, paresthesia, bladder disturbances, impotence, areflexia, and loss of positional, deep-pain, and temperature sensations. The small, irregular Argyll Robertson pupil, a feature of both tabes dorsalis and paresis, reacts to accommodation but not to light. *Optic atrophy* also occurs frequently in association with tabes.

■ OTHER MANIFESTATIONS OF LATE SYPHILIS

The slowly progressive inflammatory process leading to tertiary disease begins early during infection, although these manifestations may not become clinically apparent for years or decades. Early syphilitic aortitis first becomes evident soon after secondary lesions subside, and treponemes that trigger the development of gummas may have seeded the tissue years earlier.

Cardiovascular Syphilis Cardiovascular manifestations, usually appearing 10–40 years after infection, are attributable to endarteritis obliterans of the vasa vasorum, which provide the blood supply to large vessels; *T. pallidum* DNA has been detected by polymerase chain reaction (PCR) in aortic tissue. Cardiovascular involvement results in uncomplicated aortitis, aortic regurgitation, saccular aneurysm (usually of the ascending aorta), or coronary ostial stenosis. In the preantibiotic era, symptomatic cardiovascular complications developed in ~10% of persons with untreated late syphilis. Today, cardiovascular syphilis is rarely seen in the developed world.

Late Benign Syphilis (Gumma) Gummas are usually solitary lesions ranging from microscopic to several centimeters in diameter. Histologic examination shows a granulomatous inflammation, with a central area of necrosis due to endarteritis obliterans. *T. pallidum* has been detected by PCR in these lesions, and penicillin treatment results in rapid resolution, confirming the treponemal stimulus for the inflammation. Common sites include the skin and skeletal system; however, any organ (including the brain) may be involved. Gummas of the skin produce indolent, painless, indurated nodular or ulcerative lesions that may resemble other chronic granulomatous conditions. Skeletal gummas may affect any bone or cartilage. Upper respiratory gummas can lead to perforation of the nasal septum or palate.

■ CONGENITAL SYPHILIS

Transmission of *T. pallidum* across the placenta from a syphilitic woman to her fetus may occur at any stage of pregnancy, but fetal damage generally does not occur until after the fourth month of gestation when fetal immunologic competence begins to develop. This timing suggests that the pathogenesis of congenital syphilis, like that of adult syphilis, depends on the host immune response rather than on a direct toxic effect of *T. pallidum*. The risk of fetal infection during untreated early maternal syphilis is ~75–95%, decreasing to ~35% for maternal syphilis of >2 years' duration. Adequate treatment of the woman before the 16th week of pregnancy should prevent fetal damage, and treatment before the third trimester should adequately treat the infected fetus. Untreated maternal infection may result in a rate of fetal loss of up to 40% with second-trimester spontaneous abortion, stillbirth, prematurity, and neonatal death. Among infants born alive, only fulminant congenital syphilis is clinically apparent at birth, and these babies have a very poor prognosis. The most common clinical problem is the healthy-appearing baby born to a mother with a positive serologic test.

Routine serologic testing for syphilis in early pregnancy is cost-effective in virtually all populations, even in areas with a low prenatal prevalence of syphilis. Low-tech point-of-care tests have been developed and widely implemented to facilitate antenatal testing in resource-poor settings. Globally, the past 10 years have seen a dramatic reduction in congenital syphilis in the face of relatively steady rates of maternal syphilis, showing the effectiveness of increased antenatal screening and treatment. Progress has been uneven, however, with major advances in Thailand, Cuba, several Baltic States, and India, but continuing high levels in Africa and China. Periodic lack of penicillin availability in low- and middle-income countries prevents treatment of seropositive women. Integration of programs to prevent congenital syphilis with programs to prevent maternal transmission of HIV would be highly cost-effective but is hampered by the restrictions placed on HIV-focused funds.

All pregnant women should be screened at their first antenatal visit. Where the prevalence of syphilis in women is high or when the patient is at high risk of reinfection, serologic testing should be repeated in the third trimester and at delivery. Neonatal congenital syphilis must be differentiated from other generalized congenital infections, including rubella, cytomegalovirus or herpes simplex virus infection, and toxoplasmosis, as well as from erythroblastosis fetalis.

Manifestations of congenital syphilis may appear early (within the first 2 years of life, often at 2–10 weeks of age) or late (after 2 years). The earliest manifestations of congenital syphilis include rhinitis, or "snuffles" (23%); mucocutaneous lesions (35–41%); bone changes (61%), including periostitis detectable by x-ray examination of long bones; hepatosplenomegaly (50%); lymphadenopathy (32%); anemia (34%); jaundice (30%); thrombocytopenia; and leukocytosis. CNS invasion by *T. pallidum* is detectable in 22% of infected neonates. Neonatal death is usually due to pulmonary hemorrhage, secondary bacterial infection, or severe hepatitis. Late congenital syphilis (untreated after 2 years of age) is subclinical in 60% of cases; the clinical spectrum in the remainder of cases may include interstitial keratitis (which occurs at 5–25 years of age), eighth-nerve deafness, and recurrent arthropathy. Neurosyphilis was documented in about one-quarter of untreated patients with late congenital syphilis in the preantibiotic era. Gummatous periostitis occurs at 5–20 years of age and, as in nonvenereal endemic syphilis, tends to cause destructive lesions of the palate and nasal septum. Classic stigmata include *Hutchinson's teeth* (centrally notched, widely spaced, peg-shaped upper central incisors), "mulberry" molars (sixth-year molars with multiple, poorly developed cusps), saddle nose, and saber shins.

LABORATORY EXAMINATIONS

■ DEMONSTRATION OF THE ORGANISM

Historically, dark-field microscopy and immunofluorescence antibody staining have been used to identify *T. pallidum* in moist lesions such as chancres or condylomata lata, but these tests are rarely available outside of research laboratories. Sensitive and specific PCR tests have been developed but are not commercially available, although a number of laboratories perform in-house validated PCR testing. The recent advances in cultivation of *T. pallidum* in a tissue culture system have not yet been implemented in clinical laboratories.

T. pallidum can be found in tissue by immunofluorescence or immunohistochemical methods using specific monoclonal or polyclonal antibodies to *T. pallidum*. Silver stains should be interpreted with caution because artifacts resembling *T. pallidum* are often seen. *T. pallidum* DNA has been detected by PCR in lesion swabs, tissue samples, blood, CSF, ocular fluid, urine, and oropharyngeal swabs.

■ SEROLOGIC TESTS FOR SYPHILIS

Treponemal and Lipoidal Tests There are two types of serologic tests for syphilis: lipoidal (so-called nontreponemal) and treponemal.

Both are reactive in persons with any treponemal infection, including syphilis, yaws, pinta, and endemic syphilis.

The most widely used lipoidal antibody tests are the RPR and VDRL tests, which measure IgG and IgM directed against a cardiolipin-lecithin-cholesterol antigen complex. The RPR test is easier to perform and uses unheated serum or plasma; it is the test of choice for rapid serologic diagnosis in a clinical setting. The VDRL test remains the standard for examining CSF and is superior to the RPR for this purpose. Either test is recommended for screening and for quantitation of serum antibody. The titer reflects disease activity, rising during early syphilis, often exceeding 1:32 in secondary syphilis, and declining slowly thereafter without therapy. After treatment for early syphilis, a persistent fall by fourfold or more (e.g., a decline from 1:32 to 1:8) is considered an adequate response. VDRL titers do not correspond directly to RPR titers, and sequential quantitative testing (as for response to therapy) must employ a single test. A reactive VDRL/RPR screening test must be confirmed by a treponemal test to rule out a biological false-positive reaction.

Treponemal tests measure antibodies to native or recombinant *T. pallidum* antigens and include the fluorescent treponemal antibody–absorbed (FTA-ABS) test and the *T. pallidum* particle agglutination (TPPA) test, both of which are more sensitive for primary syphilis than the lipoidal tests. When used to confirm reactive lipoidal test results, treponemal tests have a very high positive predictive value for diagnosis of syphilis.

Treponemal enzyme or chemiluminescence immunoassays (EIAs/CIAs), based largely on reactivity to recombinant antigens, are now widely used as screening tests by large laboratories. When these tests are used for screening, a high proportion of sera reactive by EIA/CIA are nonreactive by lipoidal tests. Such sera should be examined in the TPPA test, which includes different antigens and a different platform. If the TPPA test is nonreactive, the patient is unlikely to have syphilis; if it is reactive, the patient is likely to have current or past syphilis. Both lipoidal and treponemal tests may be nonreactive in early primary syphilis, although treponemal tests are slightly more sensitive (85–90%) during this stage than lipoidal tests (~80%). All tests are reactive during secondary syphilis. (Fewer than 1% of patients with high titers have a lipoidal test that is nonreactive or weakly reactive with undiluted serum but is reactive with diluted serum—the *prozone phenomenon.*) VDRL and RPR sensitivity and titers may decline in untreated persons with late latent syphilis, but treponemal tests remain reactive in late syphilis. After treatment for early syphilis, lipoidal test titers will generally decline or the tests will become nonreactive, whereas treponemal tests often remain reactive after therapy and are not helpful in determining the infection status of persons with past syphilis. There is some concern in the literature about persons in whom the lipoidal test titer fails to become nonreactive or remains reactive in low titer after treatment. The implications in such cases are unclear, but re-treatment rarely achieves the desired goal and is not recommended in the absence of clinical findings.

False-Positive Serologic Tests for Syphilis The lipid antigens of nontreponemal tests are similar to those found in human tissues, and these tests may be reactive (usually with titers ≤1:8) in persons without treponemal infection, largely limited to persons with autoimmune conditions or injection drug use. Among patients being screened for syphilis because of risk factors, clinical suspicion, or history of exposure, ~1% of reactive tests are falsely positive. In a patient with a false-positive nontreponemal test, syphilis is excluded by a nonreactive treponemal test.

False-positive reactions may also occur with treponemal tests, particularly the EIA/CIA tests. Screening a low-prevalence population for syphilis with a treponemal test may result in true-positive reactions being outnumbered by false-positive reactions, leading to unnecessary treatment. Thus, screening with lipoidal tests is highly recommended.

EVALUATION FOR NEUROSYPHILIS

Involvement of the CNS is detected by examination of CSF for mononuclear pleocytosis (>5 white blood cells/μL), increased protein concentration (>45 mg/dL), or CSF VDRL reactivity. Elevated CSF cell counts and protein concentrations are not specific for neurosyphilis and may be confounded by HIV co-infection. Because CSF pleocytosis may also be due to HIV, some studies have suggested using a CSF white cell cutoff of 20 cells/μL as diagnostic of neurosyphilis in HIV-infected patients with syphilis. The CSF VDRL test is highly specific and, when reactive, is considered diagnostic of neurosyphilis; however, this test is insensitive and may be nonreactive even in cases of symptomatic neurosyphilis. The RPR test should not be substituted for the VDRL test for CSF examination. The FTA-ABS test on CSF is reactive far more often than the CSF VDRL test in all stages of syphilis, but reactivity may reflect passive transfer of serum antibody into the CSF. A nonreactive FTA-ABS test on CSF, however, may be used to rule out asymptomatic neurosyphilis. Measuring CXCL13 in CSF has been demonstrated to distinguish between neurosyphilis and HIV-related CSF abnormalities.

All *T. pallidum*–infected patients with signs or symptoms consistent with neurologic disease (e.g., meningitis, hearing loss) or ophthalmic disease (e.g., uveitis, iritis) should have a CSF examination, regardless of disease stage. The appropriate management of asymptomatic persons is less clear. Lumbar puncture on all asymptomatic patients with untreated syphilis is impractical and unnecessary. Even at high doses, penicillin G benzathine fails to result in treponemicidal drug levels in CSF, and viable *T. pallidum* have been isolated from the CSF of patients (with and without HIV infection) after penicillin G benzathine treatment for early syphilis. Therefore, it is important to identify those persons at higher risk for having or developing neurosyphilis so that appropriate treatment may be given. Large-scale prospective studies have provided evidence-based guidelines for determining which syphilis patients may benefit most from CSF examination. Specifically, patients with RPR titers of ≥1:32 are at higher risk of having neurosyphilis (11-fold and 6-fold higher in HIV-infected and HIV-uninfected persons, respectively), as are HIV-infected patients with CD4+ T-cell counts of ≤350/μL. Persons with active tertiary syphilis and those in whom treatment failure is suspected should also have their CSF examined to determine appropriate therapy.

EVALUATION OF HIV-INFECTED PATIENTS FOR SYPHILIS

Because persons at highest risk for syphilis are also at increased risk for HIV infection, these two infections frequently coexist. There is evidence that syphilis and other genital ulcer diseases are important risk factors for acquisition and transmission of HIV infection. Some manifestations of syphilis may be altered in patients with concurrent untreated HIV infection, and multiple cases of neurologic relapse after standard therapy have been reported in these patients.

Persons with newly diagnosed HIV infection should be tested for syphilis; conversely, all patients with newly diagnosed syphilis should be tested for HIV infection. Some authorities, persuaded by reports of persistent *T. pallidum* in CSF of HIV-infected persons after standard therapy for early syphilis, recommend CSF examination for evidence of neurosyphilis for all co-infected patients, regardless of the stage of syphilis, with treatment for neurosyphilis if CSF abnormalities are found. Others, on the basis of their own clinical experience, think that standard therapy—without CSF examination—is sufficient for all cases of early syphilis in HIV-infected patients without neurologic signs or symptoms. As described above, RPR titer and CD4+ T-cell count can be used to identify patients at higher risk of neurosyphilis for lumbar puncture, although some cases of neurosyphilis will be missed even when these criteria are used. Serologic testing after treatment is important for all patients with syphilis, particularly for those also infected with HIV.

TREATMENT

Syphilis

TREATMENT OF ACQUIRED SYPHILIS

The CDC's 2015 guidelines for the treatment of syphilis are summarized in **Table 182-1** and are discussed below. Penicillin G is the drug of choice for all stages of syphilis. *T. pallidum* is killed by very low concentrations of penicillin G, although a long period of

TABLE 182-1 Recommendations for the Treatment of Syphilis[a]

STAGE OF SYPHILIS	PATIENTS WITHOUT PENICILLIN ALLERGY	PATIENTS WITH CONFIRMED PENICILLIN ALLERGY
Primary, secondary, or early latent	*CSF normal or not examined:* Penicillin G benzathine (single dose of 2.4 mU IM) *CSF abnormal:* Treat as neurosyphilis.	*CSF normal or not examined:* Doxycycline (100 mg PO bid) or tetracycline HCl (500 mg PO qid) for 2 weeks *CSF abnormal:* Treat as neurosyphilis.
Late latent (or latent of unknown duration), cardiovascular, or benign tertiary	*CSF normal or not examined:* Penicillin G benzathine (2.4 mU IM weekly for 3 weeks) *CSF abnormal:* Treat as neurosyphilis.	*CSF normal and patient not infected with HIV:* Doxycycline (100 mg PO bid) or tetracycline HCl (500 mg PO qid) for 4 weeks *CSF normal and patient infected with HIV:* Desensitize and treat with penicillin if compliance cannot be assured. *CSF abnormal:* Treat as neurosyphilis.
Neurosyphilis (asymptomatic or symptomatic)	Aqueous crystalline penicillin G (18–24 mU/d IV, given as 3–4 mU q4h or continuous infusion) for 10–14 days *or* Aqueous procaine penicillin G (2.4 mU/d IM) plus oral probenecid (500 mg qid), both for 10–14 days	Desensitize and treat with penicillin.
Syphilis in pregnancy	According to stage	Desensitize and treat with penicillin.

[a]See text for indications for CSF examination.

Abbreviations: CSF, cerebrospinal fluid; mU, million units.

Source: Adapted from the 2015 Sexually Transmitted Diseases Treatment Guidelines from the Centers for Disease Control and Prevention. Available from *https://www.cdc.gov/std/tg2015/default.htm.*

exposure to penicillin is required because of the unusually slow rate of multiplication of the organism. The efficacy of penicillin against syphilis remains undiminished after 75 years of use, and there is no evidence of penicillin resistance in *T. pallidum*. Other antibiotics effective in syphilis include the tetracyclines and the cephalosporins. Aminoglycosides and spectinomycin inhibit *T. pallidum* only in very large doses, and the sulfonamides and most quinolones are inactive. Azithromycin showed significant promise as an effective oral agent against *T. pallidum*; however, strains harboring 23S rDNA mutations that confer macrolide resistance are widespread. Such strains represent >80–90% of recent isolates from large U.S., European, and Chinese cities, although the prevalence of resistant strains varies by geographic location. Routine treatment of syphilis with azithromycin is not recommended. Careful follow-up of any patient treated for syphilis with azithromycin must be assured.

Early Syphilis Patients and Their Contacts Penicillin G benzathine is the most widely used agent for the treatment of early syphilis (2.4 million units; Table 182-1), and for preventive treatment of individuals exposed to infectious syphilis within the previous 3 months. *The regimens recommended for prevention are the same as those recommended for early syphilis.* Penicillin G benzathine cures >95% of cases of early syphilis, although clinical relapse can follow treatment, particularly in patients with untreated HIV infection. Because the risk of neurologic relapse may be higher in HIV-infected patients, CSF examination is recommended for HIV-seropositive individuals with syphilis of any stage, particularly those with a serum RPR titer of ≥1:32 or a CD4+ T-cell count of ≤350/μL. Therapy appropriate for neurosyphilis should be given if there is any evidence of CNS infection.

Late Latent Syphilis or Syphilis of Unknown Duration If the CSF is normal or is not examined, the recommended treatment is penicillin G benzathine (7.2 million units total; Table 182-1). If CSF abnormalities are found, the patient should be treated for neurosyphilis.

Tertiary Syphilis CSF examination should be performed. If the CSF is normal, the recommended treatment is penicillin G benzathine (7.2 million units total; Table 182-1). If CSF is abnormal, the patient should be treated for neurosyphilis. The clinical response to treatment for benign tertiary syphilis is usually impressive, but responses in cardiovascular syphilis are not dramatic because aortic aneurysm and aortic regurgitation cannot be reversed by antibiotics.

Syphilis in Penicillin-Allergic Patients For penicillin-allergic patients with syphilis, a 2-week (early syphilis) or 4-week (late or late latent syphilis) course of therapy with doxycycline or tetracycline is recommended (Table 182-1). These regimens appear to be quite effective in early syphilis but have not been tested for late or late latent syphilis, and compliance may be problematic. Limited studies suggest that ceftriaxone (1 g/d, given IM or IV for 8–10 days) is effective for early syphilis. These nonpenicillin regimens have not been carefully evaluated in HIV-infected individuals and should be used with caution. If compliance and follow-up are not assured, penicillin-allergic HIV-infected persons with late latent or late syphilis should be desensitized and treated with penicillin.

Neurosyphilis Penicillin G benzathine, even at high doses, does not produce treponemicidal concentrations of penicillin G in CSF and should not be used for treatment of neurosyphilis. Asymptomatic neurosyphilis may relapse as symptomatic disease after treatment with benzathine penicillin, and the risk of relapse may be higher in HIV-infected patients. Both symptomatic and asymptomatic neurosyphilis should be treated with aqueous penicillin (Table 182-1). Administration of either IV aqueous crystalline penicillin G or of IM aqueous procaine penicillin G plus oral probenecid in recommended doses is thought to ensure treponemicidal concentrations of penicillin G in CSF. The clinical response to penicillin therapy for meningeal syphilis is dramatic, but treatment of neurosyphilis with existing parenchymal damage may only arrest disease progression. No data suggest that additional therapy (e.g., penicillin G benzathine for 3 weeks) would be beneficial after treatment for neurosyphilis.

The use of antibiotics other than penicillin G for the treatment of neurosyphilis has not been studied, although limited data suggest that 1–2 g/d of IV ceftriaxone for 10–14 days may be used. In patients with confirmed penicillin allergy, desensitization and treatment with penicillin are recommended.

Management of Syphilis in Pregnancy Every pregnant woman should undergo a lipoidal screening test at her first prenatal visit and, if at high risk of re-exposure, again in the third trimester and at delivery. In the untreated pregnant patient with presumed syphilis, expeditious treatment appropriate to the stage of the disease is essential. Patients should be warned of the risk of a Jarisch-Herxheimer reaction, which may be associated with mild premature contractions but rarely results in premature delivery.

Penicillin is the only recommended agent for the treatment of syphilis in pregnancy. If the patient has a documented penicillin allergy, desensitization and penicillin therapy should be undertaken according to the CDC's 2015 guidelines. After treatment, a quantitative nontreponemal test should be repeated monthly throughout pregnancy to assess therapeutic efficacy. Treated women whose antibody titers rise by fourfold or whose titers do not decrease by fourfold over a 3-month period should be re-treated.

EVALUATION AND MANAGEMENT OF CONGENITAL SYPHILIS

Whether or not they are infected, newborn infants of women with reactive serologic tests may themselves have reactive tests because of transplacental transfer of maternal IgG antibodies.

For asymptomatic infants born to women treated adequately with penicillin during the first or second trimester of pregnancy, monthly quantitative nontreponemal tests may be performed to monitor for appropriate reduction in antibody titers. Rising or persistent titers indicate infection, and the infant should be treated. Detection of neonatal IgM antibody is insensitive, and no commercially available test is currently recommended.

An infant should be treated at birth if (1) the treatment status of the seropositive mother is unknown; (2) the mother received inadequate or nonpenicillin therapy; (3) the mother received penicillin therapy in the third trimester; or (4) the infant may be difficult to follow. The CSF should be examined to obtain baseline values before treatment. Penicillin is the only recommended drug for the treatment of syphilis in infants. Specific recommendations for the treatment of infants and older children are included in the CDC's 2015 treatment guidelines.

JARISCH-HERXHEIMER REACTION

A dramatic although self-limited reaction consisting of fever, chills, myalgia, headache, tachycardia, increased respiratory rate, increased circulating neutrophil count, and vasodilation with mild hypotension may follow the initiation of treatment for syphilis. This reaction is thought to be a response to lipoproteins released by dying *T. pallidum* organisms. The Jarisch-Herxheimer reaction occurs in ~50% of patients with primary syphilis, 90% of those with secondary syphilis, and a lower proportion of persons with later-stage disease. Defervescence takes place within 12–24 h. In secondary syphilis, erythema and edema of cutaneous lesions may increase. Patients should be warned to expect such developments, which can be managed with symptom-based treatment. Steroid therapy is not required for this mild transient reaction.

FOLLOW-UP EVALUATION OF RESPONSES TO THERAPY

Efficacy of treatment should be assessed by clinical evaluation and monitoring of the quantitative VDRL or RPR titer for a fourfold decline (e.g., from 1:32 to 1:8). Patients with primary or secondary syphilis should be examined 6 and 12 months after treatment, and persons with latent or late syphilis at 6, 12, and 24 months. More frequent clinical and serologic examination (3, 6, 9, 12, and 24 months) is recommended for patients concurrently infected with HIV, regardless of the stage of syphilis.

After successful treatment of seropositive first-episode primary or secondary syphilis, the VDRL or RPR titer progressively declines; the test becomes nonreactive by 12 months in 40–75% of seropositive primary cases and in 20–40% of secondary cases. In patients with HIV infection or a history of prior syphilis, VDRL and RPR tests are less likely to become nonreactive. Rates of decline of serologic titers appear to be slower, and serologically defined treatment failures more common, among HIV-infected patients than among those without HIV co-infection; however, effective ART may reduce these differences. Re-treatment should be considered if serologic responses are not adequate or if clinical signs persist or recur. Because it is difficult to differentiate treatment failure from reinfection, the CSF should be examined, with treatment for neurosyphilis if CSF is abnormal and treatment for late latent syphilis if CSF is normal. A minority of patients treated for early syphilis may experience a one-dilution titer increase within 14 days after treatment; however, this early elevation does not significantly affect the serologic outcome at 6 months after treatment. Patients treated for late latent syphilis frequently have low initial VDRL or RPR titers and may not have a fourfold decline after therapy with penicillin. In such patients, re-treatment is not warranted unless the titer rises or signs and symptoms of syphilis appear. Because treponemal tests may remain reactive despite treatment for seropositive syphilis, these tests are not useful in following the response to therapy.

The activity of neurosyphilis (symptomatic or asymptomatic) correlates best with CSF pleocytosis, and this measure provides the most sensitive index of response to treatment. Repeat CSF examinations should be performed every 6 months until the cell count is normal. An elevated CSF cell count falls to normal in 3–12 months in adequately treated HIV-uninfected patients. The persistence of mild pleocytosis in HIV-infected patients may be due to the presence of HIV in CSF; this scenario may be difficult to distinguish from treatment failure. Elevated levels of CSF protein fall more slowly, and the CSF VDRL titer declines gradually over several years. In patients treated for neurosyphilis, a fourfold reduction in serum RPR titer has been positively correlated with normalization of CSF abnormalities; this correlation is stronger in HIV-uninfected patients and in HIV-infected patients receiving effective ART.

IMMUNITY TO SYPHILIS

The rate of development of acquired resistance to *T. pallidum* after natural or experimental infection depends on both the size of the infecting inoculum and the duration of infection before treatment. Both humoral and cellular responses are important in the healing of early lesions. Cellular infiltration, predominantly by T lymphocytes and macrophages, produces an interferon γ–dominated cytokine milieu and results in the clearance of organisms by activated macrophages. Specific antibodies to surface antigens enhance phagocytosis. Antigenic variation of the TprK protein contributes to development of subsequent stages of syphilis, persistence of infection, and susceptibility to reinfection with another strain. Comparative genomic studies have revealed genes with sequence variations among *T. pallidum* strains, leading to development of molecular typing methods used to examine syphilis outbreaks. Recent work has demonstrated that immunization with the outer-membrane protein Tp0751 significantly reduces dissemination of *T. pallidum* during syphilis infection in an animal model. Vaccine studies with this and other antigens are underway.

■ FURTHER READING

Beale MA et al: Genomic epidemiology of syphilis reveals independent emergence of macrolide resistance across multiple circulating lineages. Nat Commun 10:3255, 2019.

Dombrowski JC et al: Prevalence estimates of complicated syphilis. Sex Transm Dis 42:702, 2015.

Edmondson DG et al: Long-term in vitro culture of the syphilis spirochete *Treponema pallidum* subsp. *pallidum*. mBio 9:e01153, 2018.

Kenyon C et al: Repeat syphilis is more likely to be asymptomatic in HIV-infected individuals: A retrospective cohort analysis with important implications for screening. Open Forum Infect Dis 5:ofy096, 2018.

Marra CM et al: Previous syphilis alters the course of subsequent episodes of syphilis. Clin Infect Dis 71:1243, 2020.

183 Endemic Treponematoses

Sheila A. Lukehart, Lorenzo Giacani

The endemic treponematoses are chronic diseases that are transmitted by direct contact, usually during childhood and, like syphilis, can cause severe late manifestations years after initial infection. These diseases are caused by very close relatives of *Treponema pallidum* subspecies *pallidum*, the etiologic agent of venereal syphilis **(Chap. 182)**. Yaws, pinta, and endemic syphilis (bejel) have traditionally been distinguished from venereal syphilis by mode of transmission, age of acquisition, geographic distribution, and clinical features; however, there is overlap for each of these factors. Our "knowledge" about these infections is based on observations by health care workers who have visited endemic areas during the past 70 years. Except for the ongoing programs of mass drug administration (MDA) for yaws eradication promoted by the World Health Organization (WHO), virtually no well-designed studies of the natural history, diagnosis, or treatment of

TABLE 183-1 Comparison of the Treponemes and Associated Diseases

FEATURE	VENEREAL SYPHILIS	YAWS	ENDEMIC SYPHILIS (BEJEL)	PINTA
Organism	*T. pallidum* subsp. *pallidum*	*T. pallidum* subsp. *pertenue*	*T. pallidum* subsp. *endemicum*	*T. carateum*
Common modes of transmission	Sexual, transplacental	Skin-to-skin	Mouth-to-mouth or via shared drinking/eating utensils[a]	Skin-to-skin
Usual age of acquisition	Sexual maturity or in utero	Early childhood	Early childhood, recently adulthood	Late childhood
Primary lesion	Cutaneous ulcer (chancre)	Papilloma, often ulcerative	Mucosal papule, rarely seen	Nonulcerating papule with satellites, pruritic
Common location	Genital, oral, anal	Extremities	Oral	Extremities, face
Secondary lesions	Cutaneous rash and mucocutaneous lesions; condylomata lata	Cutaneous papillomatous or ulcerative lesions; condylomata lata, osteoperiostitis	Mucocutaneous lesions (mucous patch, split papule, condylomata lata); osteoperiostitis	Pintides, pigmented, pruritic
Infectious relapses	~25%	Common	Unknown	Unknown
Late complications	Gummas, cardiovascular and central nervous system involvement[b]	Destructive gummas of skin, bone, cartilage	Destructive gummas of skin, bone, cartilage	Nondestructive, dyschromic, achromic macules

[a]Sexual transmission has been recently postulated for endemic syphilis (see text). [b]Central nervous system involvement and congenital infection in the endemic treponematoses have been postulated by some investigators (see text).

these infections have been conducted. The classically defined treponemal infections are compared and contrasted in **Table 183-1**.

■ EPIDEMIOLOGY

Generally, yaws flourishes in moist tropical areas (**Fig. 183-1**); endemic syphilis has been found primarily in arid climates of West Africa and the Middle East; and pinta has been found in temperate foci in the Americas. Because no recent epidemiologic data are available for bejel and pinta, the current extent of these infections as classically described is unknown. The endemic treponematoses have traditionally been limited to rural areas of developing nations and have been seen in developed countries primarily among recent immigrants from endemic regions.

In a WHO-sponsored mass eradication campaign from 1952 to 1969, >160 million people in Africa, Asia, and South America were examined for treponemal infections, and >50 million cases, contacts, and persons with latent infections were treated. This campaign reduced the prevalence of active yaws from >20% to <1% in many areas. In subsequent decades, lack of focused surveillance and diversion of resources resulted in documented resurgence of these infections in some regions. Of nearly 100 countries previously endemic for yaws, there are 15 countries with current yaws cases, and three others with suspected cases; there are no data for the remaining countries. In 2018, a total of 80,472 suspected cases were reported, primarily from countries in which focused yaws detection and treatment trials are ongoing. Areas of resurgent yaws morbidity in Africa include Ivory Coast, Ghana, Togo, Benin, Central African Republic, Nigeria, and Democratic Republic of the Congo. The prevalence of endemic syphilis is estimated to be >10% in some regions of northern Ghana, Mali, Niger, Burkina Faso, and Senegal, although data are scarce. In Asia and the Pacific Islands, reports document active outbreaks of yaws in

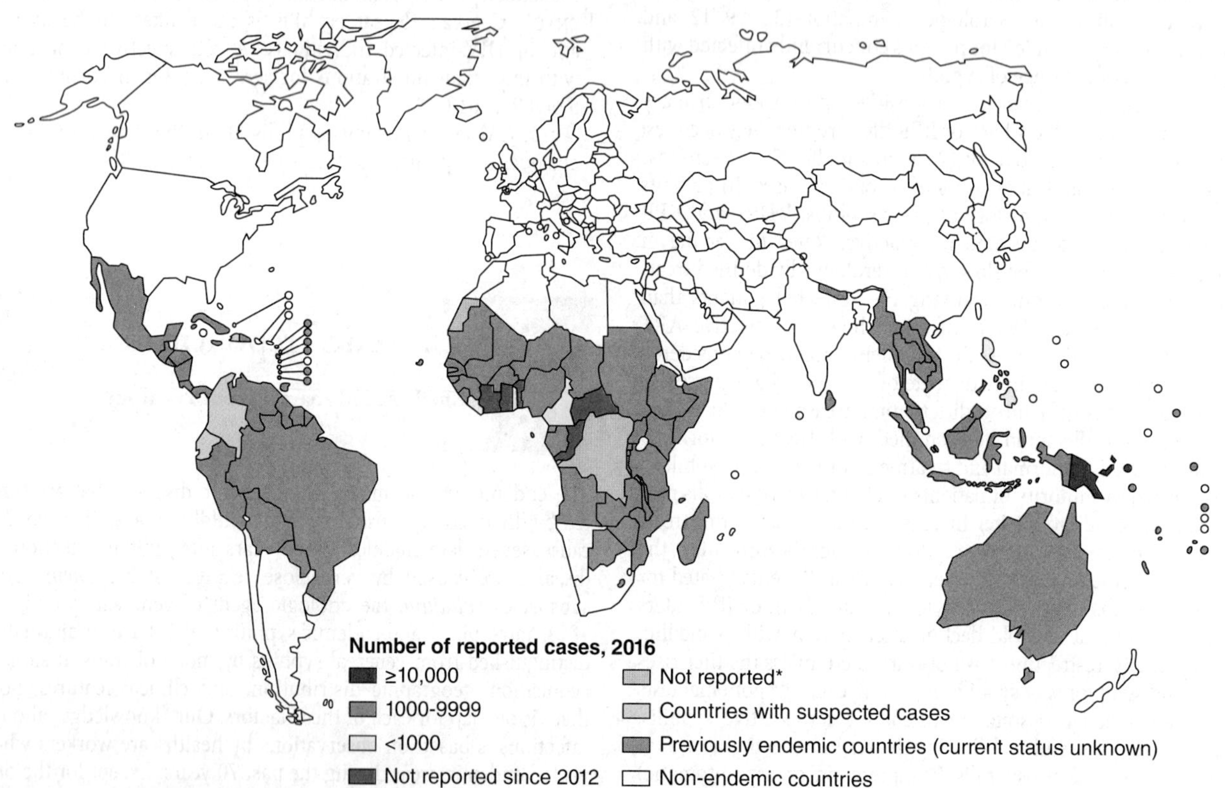

FIGURE 183-1 Geographic distribution of yaws in 2016. *No data reported since 2008 (Timor Leste) or 2009 (Democratic Republic of Congo). *(Adapted from http://www.who.int/yaws/epidemiology/Yaws_map_2012.png?ua=1. 2016 data available at http://apps.who.int/gho/data/node.main.NTDYAWSNUM?lang=en and http://apps.who.int/gho/data/node.main.NTDYAWSEND?lang=en. Reprinted with permission from World Health Organization.)*

Indonesia, Papua New Guinea, the Solomon Islands, East Timor, and Vanuatu. India actively renewed its focus on yaws control in 1996, achieved zero-case status in 2003, declared elimination in 2006, and was declared yaws-free in 2016. In the Americas, suspected yaws cases have been reported in Haiti, Colombia, and Ecuador, with insufficient recent data for Peru, Brazil, Guyana, Surinam, and many Caribbean islands. Pinta is thought to be limited to Central America and northern South America, where it is found rarely and only in very remote villages. Evidence of yaws-like and genital lesions, with treponemal seroreactivity, has been found in several species of wild nonhuman primates (NHPs) in sub-Saharan Africa and has led to speculation that there may be an animal reservoir for yaws. Organisms very closely related at the genomic level to known *T. pallidum* subspecies *pertenue* isolates have been identified in lesions from affected NHPs, although direct NHP-human transmission has not been confirmed.

MICROBIOLOGY

The etiologic agents of the endemic treponematoses are listed in Table 183-1. These little-studied organisms are morphologically identical to *T. pallidum* subspecies *pallidum* (the agent of venereal syphilis), and no definitive antigenic differences among them have been identified to date. A controversy has existed about whether the pathogenic treponemes are truly separate organisms, as genome sequencing indicates that yaws, bejel, and syphilis treponemes are 99.8% identical, and several studies support the ability of these pathogens to exchange DNA between subspecies. Three of the four etiologic agents are classified as subspecies of *T. pallidum*; the fourth (*T. carateum*) remains a separate species simply because no organisms have been available for genetic studies. Based on analysis of a limited number of strains and clinical samples available for genomic studies, molecular signatures—assessed using approaches ranging from restriction fragment length polymorphism to whole genome sequencing—have been identified that can differentiate the *T. pallidum* subspecies. Whether these minor genetic differences are related to distinct clinical characteristics of these diseases has not been determined. Full genome sequencing of a previously unclassified *Treponema* strain (Fribourg-Blanc), which was isolated from a baboon in 1966 and can cause experimental infection in humans, shows a very high degree of homology with available strains of *T. pallidum* subspecies *pertenue*. Recent genomic analyses of additional samples from nonhuman primates indicate a very close genetic relationship with known yaws isolates, but the importance of the nonhuman primate reservoir for human infection is not yet known.

CLINICAL FEATURES

All of the treponemal infections, including syphilis, are chronic and are characterized by defined disease stages, with a localized primary lesion, disseminated secondary lesions, periods of latency, and possible late lesions. Primary and secondary stages are more frequently overlapping in yaws and endemic syphilis than in venereal syphilis, and the late manifestations of pinta are very mild relative to the destructive lesions of the other treponematoses. The current preference is to divide the clinical course of the endemic treponematoses into "early" and "late" stages.

Historically, the major clinical distinctions made between venereal syphilis and the nonvenereal infections are the apparent lack of congenital transmission and of central nervous system (CNS) involvement in the nonvenereal infections. It is not known whether these distinctions are entirely accurate. Because of the high degree of genetic relatedness among the organisms, there is little biological reason to think that *T. pallidum* subspecies *endemicum* and *T. pallidum* subspecies *pertenue* would be unable to cross the blood-brain barrier or to invade the placenta. These organisms are like *T. pallidum* subspecies *pallidum* in that they obviously disseminate from the site of initial infection and can persist for decades. The lack of recognized congenital infection may be due to the fact that childhood infections often reach the latent stage (low bacterial load) before girls reach sexual maturity, thus reducing the likelihood of fetal infection. Neurologic involvement may go unrecognized because of the lack of trained medical personnel in endemic regions, the delay of many years between infection and possible CNS manifestations, or a low rate of symptomatic CNS disease. Some published evidence supports congenital transmission as well as cardiovascular, ophthalmologic, and CNS involvement in yaws and endemic syphilis. Although the reported studies have been small, have failed to control for other causes of CNS abnormalities, and in some instances have not included serologic confirmation, it may be erroneous to accept unquestioningly the frequently repeated belief that these organisms fail to cause such manifestations.

Yaws Also known as *pian*, *framboesia*, or *bouba*, yaws is characterized by the development of one or several primary lesions ("mother yaw") followed by multiple disseminated skin lesions. All early skin lesions are infectious and may persist for many months; cutaneous relapses are common during the first 5 years. Late manifestations, affecting ~10% of untreated persons, are destructive lesions of skin, bone, and joints.

The infection is transmitted by direct contact with infectious lesions, often during play or group sleeping, and may be enhanced by disruption of the skin by insect bites or abrasions. While *T. pallidum* subspecies *pertenue* DNA has been detected on flies and fomites from endemic regions, there is not yet convincing evidence of insect or fomite transmission of infection. After an average of 3–4 weeks, the first lesion begins as a papule—usually on an extremity—and then enlarges (particularly during moist warm weather) to become ulcerated (**Fig 183-2*A***) or papillomatous ("raspberry-like"—thus the name "framboesia"). Notably, recent data indicate that a large proportion of ulcerative lesions in yaws-endemic regions contain *Haemophilus ducreyi*, either as the sole etiologic agent or in combination with *T. pallidum* subspecies *pertenue*. (*H. ducreyi* DNA has also been detected on flies and fomites, as described above for *T. pallidum* subspecies *pertenue*.) Regional lymphadenopathy develops, and the lesion usually heals within 6 months; dissemination is thought to occur during the early weeks of infection. A generalized secondary eruption, accompanied by generalized lymphadenopathy, appears either concurrent with or after the primary lesion; may take several forms—macular, papular, or papillomatous (**Fig. 183-2*B***); and may become secondarily infected with other bacteria, including *H. ducreyi*. Painful papillomatous lesions on the soles of the feet result in a crablike gait ("crab yaws"), and periostitis (**Fig. 183-2*C***) may result in nocturnal bone pain and polydactylitis

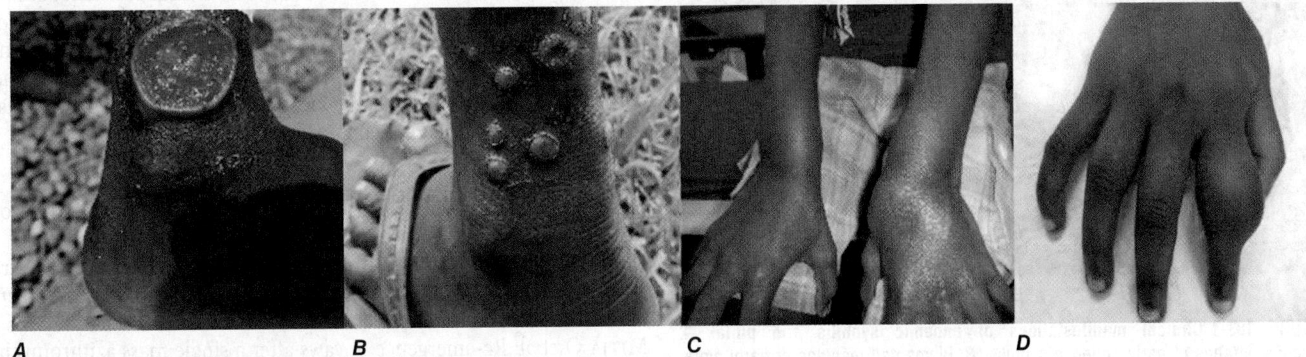

FIGURE 183-2 Clinical manifestations of early yaws. *A.* Primary ulcer. ***B.*** Secondary papillomata. ***C.*** Periostitis, ***D.*** Polydactylitis. *(Photos were taken during a yaws elimination trial in Papua New Guinea and are published with permission from Dr. Oriol Mitjà.)*

(Fig. 183-2*D*). Late yaws is manifested by gummas of the skin and long bones, hyperkeratoses of the palms and soles, osteitis and periostitis, and hydrarthrosis. The late gummatous lesions are characteristically extensive. Destruction of the nose, maxilla, palate, and pharynx is termed *gangosa* and is similar to the destructive lesions seen in leprosy and leishmaniasis.

Endemic Syphilis The early lesions of endemic syphilis (*bejel, siti, dichuchwa, njovera, skerljevo*) are localized primarily to mucocutaneous and mucosal surfaces. The infection is reportedly transmitted by direct contact, by kissing, by premastication of food, or by sharing of drinking and eating utensils. Recently, however, *T. pallidum* subspecies *endemicum* has been identified in genital lesions (assumed to be chancres) and in secondary lesions in several settings (Paris, Cuba, Japan), suggesting sexual transmission. The initial lesion, usually an intraoral papule, may go unrecognized and is followed by mucous patches on the oral mucosa (**Fig. 183-3*A***) and mucocutaneous lesions resembling the condylomata lata of secondary syphilis. This eruption may last for months or even years, and treponemes can readily be demonstrated in early lesions. Periostitis and regional lymphadenopathy are common. After a variable period of latency, late manifestations may appear, including osseous and cutaneous gummas. Destructive gummas, osteitis, and gangosa are more common in endemic syphilis than in yaws.

Pinta Pinta (*mal del pinto, carate, azul, purupuru*) is the most benign of the treponemal infections. This disease has three stages that are characterized by marked changes in skin color (**Fig. 183-3*B***), but pinta does not appear to cause destructive lesions or to involve tissues other than the skin. The initial papule is most often located on the extremities or face and is pruritic. After 1 to many months of infection, numerous disseminated secondary lesions (*pintides*) appear. These lesions are initially red but become deeply pigmented, ultimately turning a dark slate blue. The secondary lesions are infectious and highly pruritic and may persist for years. Late pigmented lesions are called *dyschromic macules* and contain treponemes. Over time, most pigmented lesions show varying degrees of depigmentation, becoming brown and eventually white and giving the skin a mottled appearance. White achromic lesions are characteristic of the late stage.

DIAGNOSIS

Diagnosis of the endemic treponematoses is based on clinical manifestations and, when available, dark-field microscopy and serologic testing. The same serologic tests that are used for venereal syphilis (**Chap. 182**) become reactive during all treponemal infections. To date there is no antibody test that can discriminate among the treponemal infections. The nonvenereal treponemal infections should be considered in the evaluation of a reactive syphilis serology in any person who has emigrated from an endemic area. Sensitive polymerase chain reaction assays can be used to confirm treponemal infection and identify the etiologic agent in research laboratories.

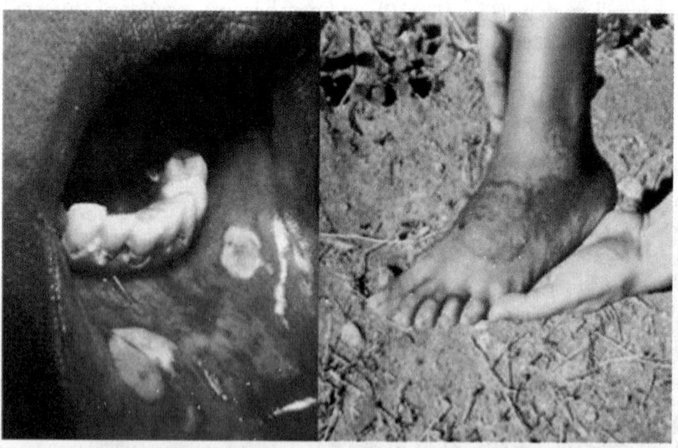

FIGURE 183-3 Clinical manifestations of endemic syphilis and pinta. *A.* Mucous patches of early endemic syphilis. ***B.*** Pigmented macules of early pinta. *(Photos reprinted with permission from PL Perine et al: Handbook of Endemic Treponematoses. Geneva, World Health Organization, Color Plates 54, 60; 1984.)*

TREATMENT

Endemic Treponematoses

The current WHO-recommended therapy for patients and their contacts includes either azithromycin (30 mg/kg, up to a maximum of 2 g) or benzathine penicillin G (1.2 million units IM for adults; 600,000 units for children <10 years old); these two drugs have been shown to be equivalent in a recent study. The recommended dose of benzathine penicillin G is half of that recommended for early venereal syphilis, yet no controlled efficacy studies have been conducted. Evidence of genetic resistance to penicillin is lacking, although relapsing lesions have been reported after penicillin treatment in Papua New Guinea.

The efficacy of single-dose azithromycin provided the WHO's revitalized yaws eradication program with a much easier regimen for use in mass treatment. Macrolide resistance has become common in circulating strains of *T. pallidum* subspecies *pallidum* in many parts of the world, and analysis of yaws samples from Papua New Guinea has yielded evidence of mutations for resistance to macrolide antibiotics, including azithromycin, in a small number of patients. Further surveillance is essential. Limited data suggest the efficacy of tetracycline for treatment of yaws, but no data exist for other endemic treponematoses. Based solely on experience with venereal syphilis, it is thought that doxycycline or tetracycline (at doses appropriate for syphilis; **Chap. 182**) are alternatives, in addition to azithromycin, for patients allergic to penicillin. A Jarisch-Herxheimer reaction (**Chap. 182**) may follow treatment of endemic treponematoses. Nontreponemal serologic titers (in the Venereal Disease Research Laboratory [VDRL] slide test or the rapid plasma reagin [RPR] test) usually decline after effective therapy, but patients may not become seronegative.

CONTROL

Buoyed by the successful elimination of yaws in India and the availability of an inexpensive, single-dose oral drug for treatment, in 2012, the WHO renewed its efforts to eradicate yaws globally by 2020. Based on the results of several pilot programs of MDA, however, the target year for eradication will likely be extended. Initial enthusiasm has been dampened by several factors: (1) Pilot studies have indicated that a very high level of MDA coverage must be achieved and that multiple rounds of MDA are needed in the affected areas. Treatment must be followed by careful case detection and targeted treatment of cases and contacts. (2) Azithromycin resistance has emerged during the pilot study in Papua New Guinea. Although subsequent treatment with benzathine penicillin G was able to contain the spread of resistant organisms, such evidence suggests that there may be only a short window of time during which countries can successfully use azithromycin for yaws eradication. Antibiotic resistance is of particular concern if multiple rounds of MDA are required. Further, given the ongoing campaigns against trachoma using low-dose azithromycin MDA, often in populations also at high risk for yaws, more widespread macrolide resistance seems inevitable. (3) Lastly, the possible animal reservoir needs be evaluated, particularly in Africa. Yaws elimination will require rapid implementation and scale-up of high-level drug coverage in endemic areas and continued careful surveillance by local health centers will be essential for success of this timely and important effort.

FURTHER READING

Giacani L, Lukehart SA: The endemic treponematoses. Clin Microbiol Rev 27:89, 2014.

Knauf S et al: Nonhuman primates across sub-Saharan Africa are infected with the yaws bacterium *Treponema pallidum* subsp. *pertenue*. Emerg Microbes Infect 7:157, 2018.

Mitjà O et al: Re-emergence of yaws after a single mass azithromycin treatment followed by targeted treatment: A longitudinal study. Lancet 391:1599, 2018.

184 Leptospirosis

Jiři F. P. Wagenaar, Marga G.A. Goris

Leptospirosis is a globally important zoonotic disease whose apparent reemergence is illustrated by recent outbreaks on virtually all continents. The disease is caused by pathogenic *Leptospira* species and is characterized by a broad spectrum of clinical manifestations, varying from asymptomatic infection to fulminant, fatal disease. In its mild form, leptospirosis may present as nonspecific symptoms such as fever, headache, and myalgia. Severe leptospirosis, characterized by jaundice, renal dysfunction, and hemorrhagic diathesis, is often referred to as *Weil's syndrome*. With or without jaundice, severe pulmonary hemorrhage is increasingly recognized as an important presentation of severe disease.

■ ETIOLOGIC AGENT

Leptospira species are spirochetes belonging to the order Spirochaetales and the family Leptospiraceae. Traditionally, the genus *Leptospira* comprised two species: the pathogenic *L. interrogans* and the free-living *L. biflexa*, now designated *L. interrogans* sensu lato and *L. biflexa* sensu lato, respectively. Sixty-four *Leptospira* species with pathogenic (17 species), intermediate (21 species), and nonpathogenic (26 species) status have now been described on the basis of phylogenetic analyses (**Fig. 184-1**). Genome sequences of all *Leptospira* species have been published, and this will undoubtedly lead to a better understanding of the pathogenesis of leptospirosis. However, classification based on serologic differences better serves clinical, diagnostic, and epidemiologic purposes. Pathogenic *Leptospira* species are divided into serovars according to their antigenic composition. There are more than 260 known pathogenic serovars, which are arranged in 26 serogroups.

Leptospires are coiled, thin, highly motile organisms that have hooked ends and two periplasmic flagella, with polar extrusions from the cytoplasmic membrane that are responsible for motility (**Fig. 184-2**). These organisms are 6–20 μm long and ~0.1 μm in diameter; they stain poorly but can be seen microscopically by dark-field examination and after silver impregnation staining of tissues. Leptospires require special media and conditions for growth; it may take weeks to months for cultures to become positive.

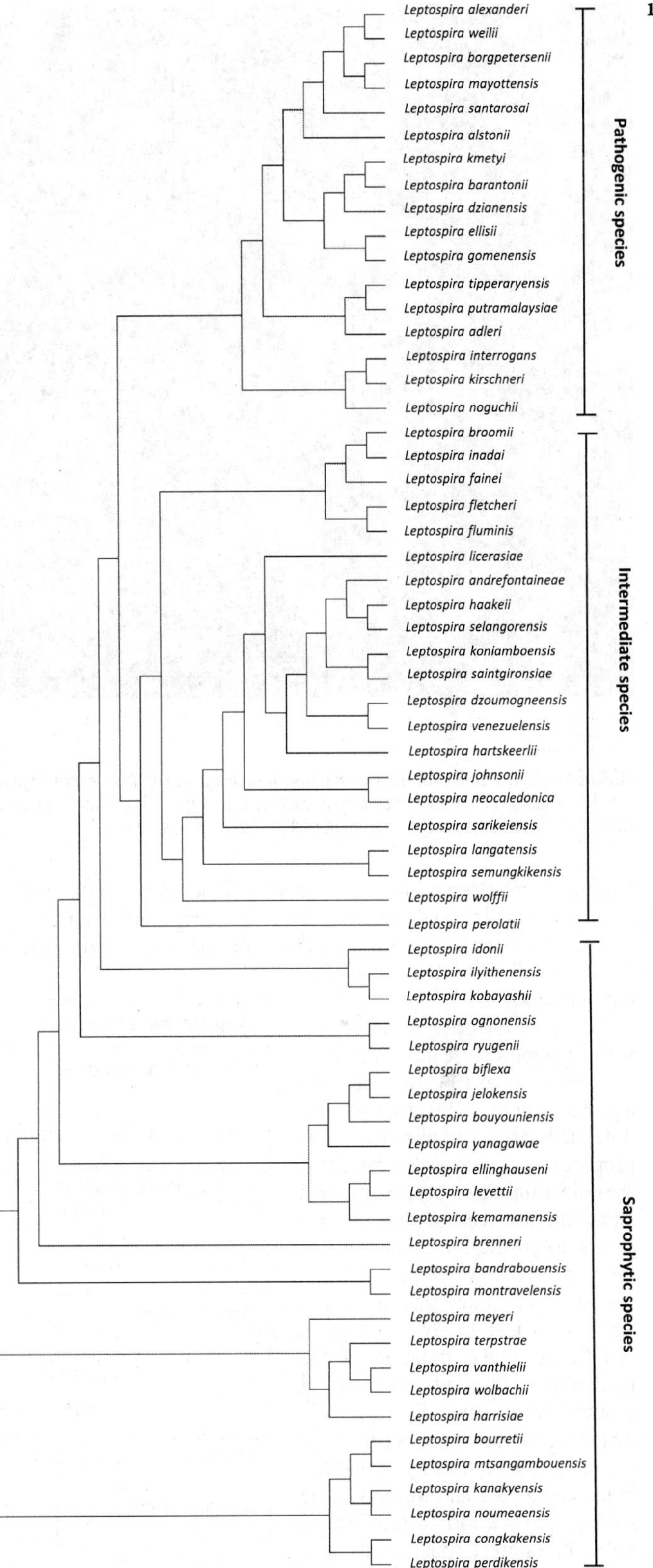

FIGURE 184-1 Differentiation of pathogenic, intermediate, and nonpathogenic (saprophytic) *Leptospira* species by molecular phylogenetic analysis using core genomes comparison (CgMLST). *(Reproduced with permission from Dr. A Ahmed, Leptospirosis Reference Center, Academic Medical Center, Medical Microbiology, Amsterdam, The Netherlands.)*

■ EPIDEMIOLOGY

Leptospirosis has a worldwide distribution but occurs most commonly in the tropics and subtropics because the climate and occasionally poor hygienic conditions favor the pathogen's survival and distribution. In most countries, leptospirosis is an underappreciated problem. Most cases occur in men, with a peak incidence during the summer and fall in both the Northern and Southern Hemispheres and during the rainy season in the tropics.

Reliable data on morbidity and mortality from leptospirosis have gradually started to appear. Current information on global human leptospirosis varies but indicates that ~1 million severe cases occur per year, with a mean case–fatality rate of nearly 10%.

As a zoonosis, leptospirosis affects almost all mammalian species and represents a significant veterinary burden. Rodents, especially rats, are the most important reservoir, although other wild mammals as well as domestic and farm animals may also harbor these microorganisms. Leptospires establish a symbiotic relationship with their host and can persist in the urogenital tract for years. Some serovars are generally associated with particular animals—e.g., Icterohaemorrhagiae and Copenhageni with rats, Grippotyphosa with voles, Hardjo with cattle, Canicola with dogs, and Pomona with pigs—but may occur in other animals as well.

Leptospirosis presents as both an endemic and an epidemic disease. Transmission of leptospires may follow direct contact with urine, blood, or tissue from an infected animal or, more commonly, exposure to environmental contamination. The dogma that human-to-human transmission is very rare is challenged by recent findings on household clustering, asymptomatic renal colonization, and prolonged excretion of leptospires. (Both of the latter features imply human infection sources that are not recognized.) Because leptospires can survive in a humid environment for many months, water is an important vehicle in their transmission. Epidemics of leptospirosis are not well understood.

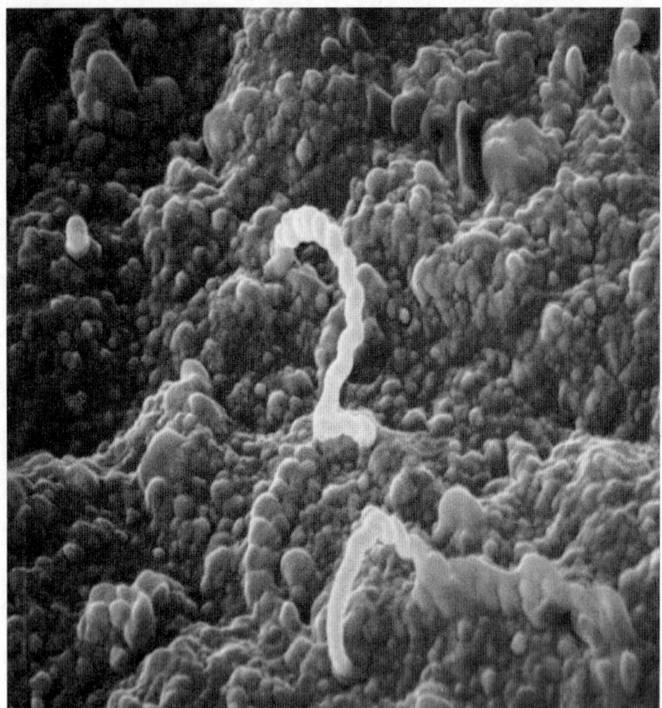

FIGURE 184-2 Transmission electron microscopic image of *Leptospira interrogans* invading equine conjunctival tissue. *(Image kindly provided by Dr. JE Nally, National Animal Disease Center, U.S. Department of Agriculture, Ames, IA.)*

Outbreaks may result from exposure to floodwaters contaminated by urine from infected animals, as has been reported from several countries. However, it is also true that outbreaks may occur without floods, and floods often occur without outbreaks.

The vast majority of infections with *Leptospira* cause no or only mild disease in humans. A small percentage of infections (~1%) lead to severe, potentially fatal complications. The proportion of leptospirosis cases that are mild is unknown because patients either do not seek or do not have access to medical care or because the nonspecific symptoms are interpreted as an influenza-like illness. Reported cases surely represent a significant underestimation of the total number. Certain occupational groups are at especially high risk, including veterinarians, agricultural workers, sewage workers, slaughterhouse employees, and workers in the fishing industry. Risk factors include direct or indirect contact with animals, including exposure to water and soil contaminated with animal urine. Leptospirosis has also been recognized in deteriorating inner cities and suburban areas where rat and mouse populations are expanding.

Recreational exposure and domestic-animal contact are prominent sources of leptospirosis. Recreational freshwater activities, such as canoeing, windsurfing, swimming, and waterskiing, place persons at risk for infection. Several outbreaks have followed sporting events. For example, an outbreak took place in 1998 among athletes after a triathlon in Springfield, Illinois. Ingestion of one or more swallows of lake water during the swimming leg of the triathlon was a prominent risk factor for illness. Heavy rains that preceded the triathlon, with consequent agricultural runoff, are likely to have increased the level of leptospiral contamination in the lake water. In another outbreak, 42% of participants contracted leptospirosis during the 2000 Eco-Challenge-Sabah multisport endurance race in Malaysian Borneo. Swimming in the Segama River was shown to be an independent risk factor. Furthermore, outbreaks among athletes participating in the recently popular mud-runs are increasingly reported.

In addition, leptospirosis is a traveler's disease. Large proportions of patients acquire the infection while traveling in tropical countries, usually during adventurous activities such as whitewater rafting, jungle trekking, and caving. Recent data from the GeoSentinel Global Surveillance Network described in detail 180 returned travelers (mostly male; 74%) with leptospirosis from January 1997 through December 2016. Infection was predominantly acquired in Southeast Asia (52% [n=93]; mainly [n=52] from Thailand); overall 110 patients (59%) were hospitalized, and one patient died. Transmission via laboratory accidents has been reported but is rare. New data indicate that leptospirosis may develop after unanticipated immersion in contaminated water (e.g., in an automobile accident) more frequently than has generally been thought and can also result from an animal bite.

PATHOGENESIS

Transmission occurs through cuts, abraded skin, or mucous membranes, especially the conjunctival and oral mucosa. After entry, the highly motile organisms proliferate, cross tissue barriers, and disseminate hematogenously to all organs (leptospiremic phase). During this initial incubation period, leptospires can be isolated from the bloodstream (**Fig. 184-3**). Clearly, *Leptospira* are able to survive in the nonimmune host by evading parts of the innate immune response such as complement-mediated killing and phagocytosis; however,

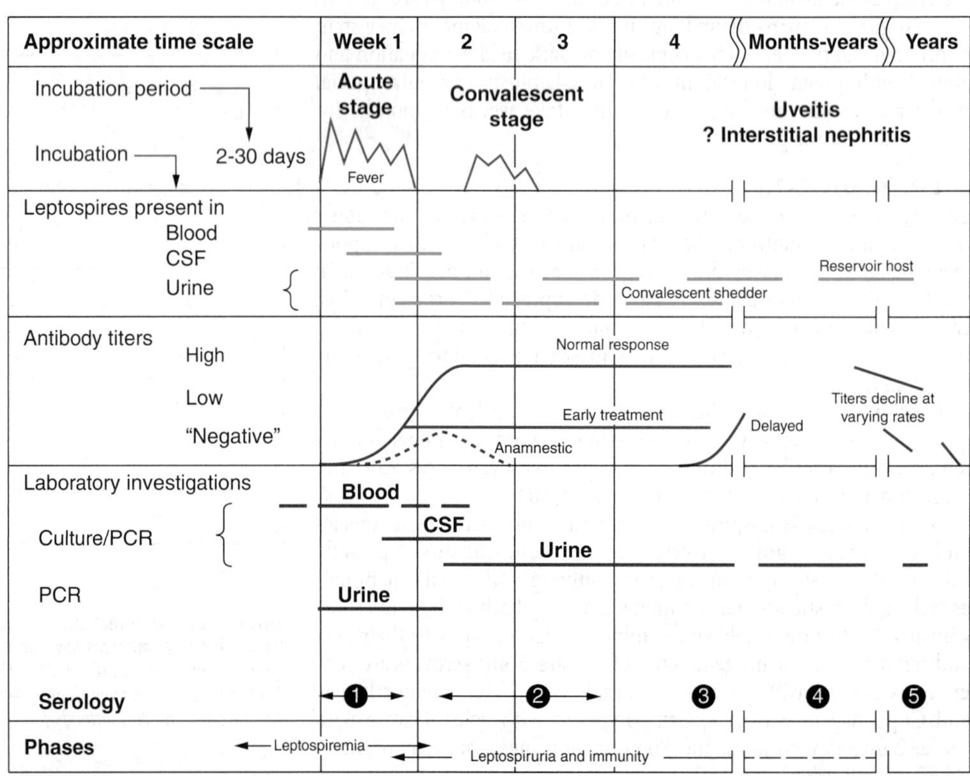

FIGURE 184-3 Biphasic nature of leptospirosis and relevant investigations at different stages of disease. Specimens 1 and 2 for serology are acute-phase serum samples; specimen 3 is a convalescent-phase serum sample that may facilitate detection of a delayed immune response; and specimens 4 and 5 are follow-up serum samples that can provide epidemiologic information, such as the presumptive infecting serogroup. CSF, cerebrospinal fluid. *(Republished with permission of American Society for Microbiology, from Leptospirosis, PN Levett, 14:296, 2001; permission conveyed through Copyright Clearance Center, Inc.)*

earlier studies have highlighted the relation between an exaggerated proinflammatory immune response and mortality. During the immune phase, the appearance of antibodies coincides with the disappearance of leptospires from the blood. However, the bacteria persist in various organs, including liver, lung, kidney, heart, and brain. Autopsy findings illustrate the involvement of multiple organ systems in severe disease. Renal pathology shows both acute tubular damage and interstitial nephritis. Acute tubular lesions progress in time to interstitial edema and acute tubular necrosis. Severe nephritis is observed in patients who survive long enough to develop it and seems to be a secondary response to acute epithelial damage. The reported deregulation of the expression of several transporters along the nephron contributes to impaired sodium absorption, tubular potassium wasting, and polyuria. Histopathology of the liver shows focal necrosis (widespread hepatocellular necrosis is usually not found), foci of inflammation, and plugging of bile canaliculi. Hepatocyte apoptosis has also been documented. Experimental work showed infiltration of *Leptospira* in Disse space (perisinusoidal space) and migration between hepatocytes with detachment of the intercellular junctions and disruption of bile canaliculi leading to bile leakage. Petechiae and hemorrhages are observed in the heart, lungs (**Fig. 184-4**), kidneys (and adrenals), pancreas, liver, gastrointestinal tract (including retroperitoneal fat, mesentery, and omentum), muscles, prostate, testes, and brain (subarachnoid bleeding). Several studies show an association between hemorrhage and thrombocytopenia. Although the underlying mechanisms of thrombocytopenia have not been elucidated, it seems likely that platelet consumption plays an important role. A consumptive coagulopathy may occur, with elevated markers of coagulation activation (thrombin–antithrombin complexes, prothrombin fragments 1 and 2, D-dimer), diminished anticoagulant markers (antithrombin, protein C), and deregulated fibrinolytic activity. Overt disseminated intravascular coagulation (DIC) has been documented in several studies. Elevated plasma levels of soluble E-selectin and von Willebrand factor in patients with leptospirosis reflect endothelial cell activation. Experimental models show that pathogenic leptospires or leptospiral proteins are able to activate endothelial cells in vitro and to disrupt endothelial-cell barrier function, promoting dissemination. Platelets have been shown to aggregate on activated endothelium in the human lung, whereas histology reveals swelling of activated endothelial cells but no evident vasculitis or necrosis. Immunoglobulin and complement deposition have been demonstrated in lung tissue involved in pulmonary hemorrhage.

Leptospira species have a typical double-membrane cell wall structure harboring a variety of membrane-associated proteins, including an unusually high number of lipoproteins. The peptidoglycan layer is located close to the cytoplasmic membrane. The lipopolysaccharide (LPS) in the outer membrane has an unusual structure with relatively low endotoxic potency. However, host immunity depends on the production of circulating antibodies to serovar-specific LPS. It is unclear whether other antigens play a significant role in protective humoral immunity.

Pathogenic *Leptospira* contain a variety of genes coding for proteins involved in motility and in cell and tissue adhesion and invasion that represent (potential) virulence factors. Many of these are surface-exposed outer-membrane proteins (OMPs). It is likely that several surface-exposed proteins mediate pathogen–host cell interactions, and these proteins may represent candidate vaccine components. Although animal-model studies have shown various degrees of vaccine efficacy for various putative virulence-associated OMPs, it is not yet clear whether such proteins elicit acceptable levels of sterilizing immunity. Ongoing breakthroughs in genetic manipulation of *Leptospira* and whole-genome sequencing will undoubtedly provide more insight into the biology and virulence of this pathogen.

CLINICAL MANIFESTATIONS

Although leptospirosis is a potentially fatal disease with bleeding and multiorgan failure as its clinical hallmarks, the majority of cases are thought to be relatively mild, presenting as the sudden onset of a febrile illness. The incubation period is usually 1–2 weeks but ranges from 2 to 30 days. Leptospirosis is classically described as biphasic. The acute *leptospiremic phase* is characterized by fever of 3–10 days' duration, during which time the organism can be cultured from blood and detected by polymerase chain reaction (PCR). During the *immune phase*, resolution of symptoms may coincide with the appearance of antibodies, and leptospires can be cultured from the urine. The distinction between the first and second phases is not always clear: milder cases do not always include the second phase, and severe disease may be monophasic and fulminant. The idea that distinct clinical syndromes are associated with specific serogroups has been refuted, although some serovars tend to cause more severe disease than others.

Mild Leptospirosis Most patients are asymptomatic or only mildly ill and do not seek medical attention. Serologic evidence of past inapparent infection is frequently found in persons who have been exposed but have not become ill. Mild symptomatic leptospirosis usually presents as a flulike illness of sudden onset, with fever, chills, headache, nausea, vomiting, abdominal pain, conjunctival suffusion (redness without exudate), and myalgia. Muscle pain is intense and especially affects the calves, back, and abdomen. The headache is intense, localized to the frontal or retroorbital region (resembling that occurring in dengue), and sometimes accompanied by photophobia. Aseptic meningitis may be present and is more common among children than among adults. Although *Leptospira* can be cultured from the cerebrospinal fluid (CSF) in the early phase, the majority of cases follow a benign course with regard to the central nervous system; symptoms disappear within a few days but may persist for weeks.

Physical examination may include any of the following findings, none of which is pathognomonic for leptospirosis: fever, conjunctival suffusion, pharyngeal injection, muscle tenderness, lymphadenopathy, rash, meningismus, hepatomegaly, and splenomegaly. If present, the rash is often transient; may be macular, maculopapular, erythematous, or hemorrhagic (petechial or ecchymotic); and may be misdiagnosed as due to scrub typhus or viral infection. Lung auscultation may reveal crackles. Mild jaundice may be present.

The natural course of mild leptospirosis usually involves spontaneous resolution within 7–10 days, but persistent symptoms have been documented. In the absence of a clinical diagnosis and antimicrobial therapy, the mortality rate in mild leptospirosis is low.

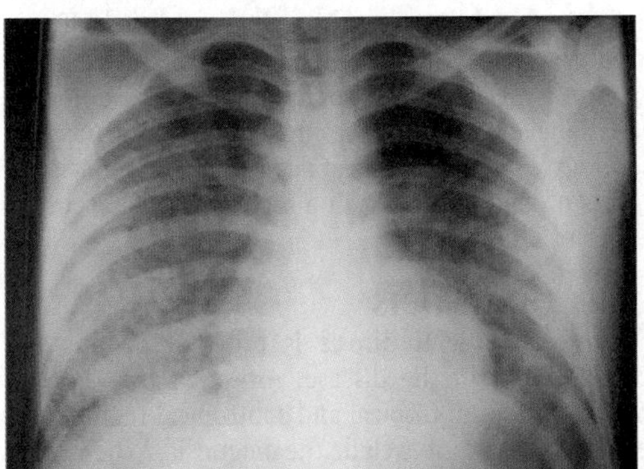
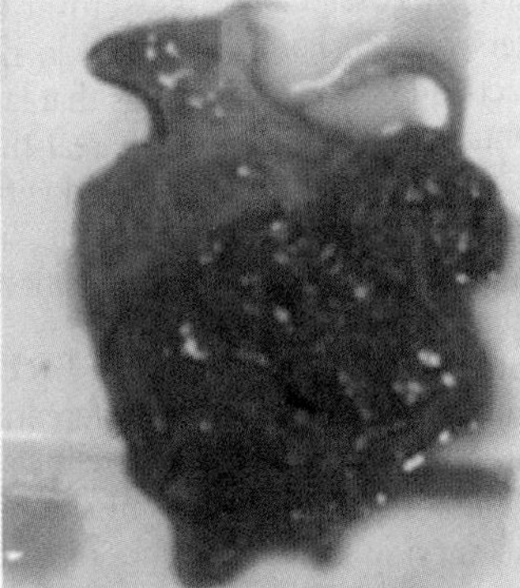

FIGURE 184-4 Severe pulmonary hemorrhage in leptospirosis. ***Left panel:*** Chest x-ray. ***Right panel:*** Gross appearance of right lower lobes of lung at autopsy. This patient, a 15-year-old from the Peruvian Amazonian city of Iquitos, died several days after presentation with acute illness, jaundice, and hemoptysis. Blood culture yielded *Leptospira interrogans* serovar Copenhageni/Icterohaemorrhagiae. *(Adapted with permission from E Segura et al: Clin Infect Dis 40:343, 2005. © 2005 by the Infectious Diseases Society of America.)*

Severe Leptospirosis Although the onset of severe leptospirosis may be no different from that of mild leptospirosis, severe disease is often rapidly progressive and is associated with a case–fatality rate ranging from 1% to 50%. Higher mortality rates are associated with an age >40 years, altered mental status, acute renal failure, respiratory insufficiency, hypotension, and arrhythmias. The classic presentation, often referred to as *Weil's syndrome*, encompasses the triad of hemorrhage, jaundice, and acute kidney injury.

Patients die of septic shock with multiorgan failure and/or severe bleeding complications that most commonly involve the lungs (pulmonary hemorrhage), gastrointestinal tract (melena, hemoptysis), urogenital tract (hematuria), and skin (petechiae, ecchymosis, and bleeding from venipuncture sites). Pulmonary hemorrhage (with or without jaundice) is now recognized as a widespread public health problem, presenting with cough, chest pain, respiratory distress, and hemoptysis that may not be apparent until patients are intubated.

Jaundice occurs in 5–10% of all patients with leptospirosis; it can be profound and give an orange cast to the skin but usually is not associated with fulminant hepatic necrosis. Physical examination may reveal an enlarged and tender liver.

Acute kidney injury is common in severe disease, presenting after several days of illness, and can be either nonoliguric or oliguric. Typical electrolyte abnormalities include hypokalemia and hyponatremia. Loss of magnesium in the urine is uniquely associated with leptospiral nephropathy. Hypotension is associated with acute tubular necrosis, oliguria, or anuria, requiring fluid resuscitation and sometimes vasopressor therapy. Hemodialysis can be lifesaving, with renal function typically returning to normal in survivors.

In severe leptospirosis, an altered mental status may reflect leptospiral meningitis. The diagnosis of leptospirosis meningitis may be challenging since patients may be anicteric, or lack other diagnostic hallmarks of severe leptospirosis. Without proper antibiotic treatment, a mortality rate of 13% has been reported; in contrast, among patients treated with antibiotics, the mortality rate is 2%. Neurologic sequelae are described until months after acute illness.

Other syndromes include (necrotizing) pancreatitis, cholecystitis, skeletal muscle involvement, and rhabdomyolysis with moderately elevated serum creatine kinase levels. Cardiac involvement is commonly reflected on the electrocardiogram as nonspecific ST- and T-wave changes. Repolarization abnormalities and arrhythmias are considered poor prognostic factors. Myocarditis has been described. Rare hematologic complications include hemolysis, thrombotic thrombocytopenic purpura, and hemolytic-uremic syndrome.

Long-term symptoms following severe leptospirosis include fatigue, myalgia, malaise, and headache and may persist for years. Autoimmune-associated uveitis, a potentially chronic condition, is a recognized sequela of leptospirosis.

DIAGNOSIS

The clinical diagnosis of leptospirosis should be based on an appropriate exposure history combined with any of the protean manifestations of the disease. Returning travelers from endemic areas usually have a history of recreational freshwater activities or other mucosal or percutaneous contact with contaminated surface waters or soil. For nontravelers, recreational or accidental water/soil contact and occupational hazards that involve direct or indirect animal contact should be explored (see "Epidemiology," above).

Although biochemical, hematologic, and urinalysis findings in acute leptospirosis are nonspecific, certain patterns may suggest the diagnosis. Laboratory results usually show signs of a bacterial infection, including leukocytosis with a left shift and elevated markers of inflammation (C-reactive protein level, procalcitonin, and erythrocyte sedimentation rate). Thrombocytopenia (platelet count $\leq 100 \times 10^9/L$) is common and is associated with bleeding and renal failure. In severe disease, signs of coagulation activation may be present, varying from borderline abnormalities to a serious derangement compatible with DIC as defined by international criteria. The kidneys are invariably involved in leptospirosis. Related findings range from urinary sediment changes (leukocytes, erythrocytes, and hyaline or granular casts) and mild proteinuria in mild disease to renal failure and azotemia in severe leptospirosis. Nonoliguric hypokalemic renal insufficiency (see "Clinical Manifestations," above) is characteristic of early leptospirosis. Serum bilirubin levels may be high, whereas rises in aminotransferase and alkaline phosphatase levels are usually moderate. Although clinical symptoms of pancreatitis are not a common finding, amylase levels are often elevated. When symptoms of meningitis develop, examination of the CSF shows pleocytosis that can range from a few cells to >1000 cells/μL, with a predominance of lymphocytes. Predominant polymorphonuclear pleocytosis has been reported. This phenomenon may be related to the timing of the lumbar puncture: polymorphonuclear cells are thought to be found in early disease and are later replaced by lymphocytes. Although protein and glucose levels in the CSF are usually normal, protein levels may be slightly elevated.

In severe leptospirosis, pulmonary radiographic abnormalities are more common than would be expected on the basis of physical examination (Fig. 184-4). The most common radiographic finding is a patchy bilateral alveolar pattern that corresponds to scattered alveolar hemorrhage. These abnormalities predominantly affect the lower lobes. Other findings include pleura-based densities (representing areas of hemorrhage) and diffuse ground-glass attenuation typical of acute respiratory distress syndrome (ARDS).

A definitive diagnosis of leptospirosis is based on isolation of the organism from the patient, on a positive result in the PCR, or on seroconversion or a rise in antibody titer. In cases with strong clinical evidence of infection, a single antibody titer of 1:200–1:800 (depending on whether the case occurs in a low- or high-endemic area) in the microscopic agglutination test (MAT) is required. Preferably, a fourfold or greater rise in titer is detected between acute- and convalescent-phase serum specimens. Antibodies generally do not reach detectable levels until the second week of illness. The antibody response can be affected by early treatment with antibiotics.

The MAT, which uses a battery of live leptospiral strains, and the enzyme-linked immunosorbent assay (ELISA), which uses a broadly reacting antigen, are the standard serologic procedures. The MAT usually is available only in specialized laboratories and is used for determination of the antibody titer and for tentative identification of the involved leptospiral serogroup—and, when epidemiologic background information is available, the putative serovar. This point underscores the importance of testing antigens representative of the serovars prevalent in the particular geographic area. However, cross-reactions occur frequently, and thus definitive identification of the infecting serovar or serogroup is not possible without isolation of the causative organism. Because serologic testing lacks sensitivity in the early acute phase of the disease (up to day 5), it cannot be used as the basis for a timely decision about whether to start treatment.

In addition to the MAT and the ELISA, various rapid tests with diagnostic value have been developed, and some of these are commercially available. These rapid tests mainly apply lateral flow, (latex) agglutination, or ELISA methodology and are reasonably sensitive and specific, although results reported in the literature vary, probably as a consequence of differences in test interpretation, (re)exposure risks, serovar distribution, and the use of biased serum panels. These methods do not require culture or MAT facilities and are useful in settings that lack a strong medical infrastructure. PCR methodologies, notably real-time PCR, have become increasingly widely implemented. Compared with serology, PCR offers a great advantage: the capacity to confirm the diagnosis of leptospirosis with a high degree of accuracy during the first 5 days of illness.

DIFFERENTIAL DIAGNOSIS

The differential diagnosis of leptospirosis is broad, reflecting the diverse clinical presentations of the disease. Although leptospirosis transmission is more common in tropical and subtropical regions, the absence of a travel history does not exclude the diagnosis. When fever, headache, and myalgia predominate, influenza and other common and less common (e.g., dengue and chikungunya) viral infections should be considered. Malaria, typhoid fever, ehrlichiosis, viral hepatitis, and acute HIV infection may mimic the early stages of leptospirosis and are important to recognize. Rickettsial diseases, dengue, and hantavirus infections (hemorrhagic fever with renal syndrome or hantavirus cardiopulmonary syndrome) share epidemiologic and clinical features with leptospirosis. Dual infections have been reported. In this light, it is advisable to conduct serologic testing for rickettsiae, dengue virus, and hantavirus when leptospirosis is suspected. When bleeding is detected, dengue hemorrhagic fever and other viral hemorrhagic fevers, including hantavirus infection, yellow fever, Rift Valley fever, filovirus infections, and Lassa fever, should be considered.

TREATMENT

Leptospirosis

Severe leptospirosis should be treated with IV penicillin (**Table 184-1**) as soon as the diagnosis is considered. *Leptospira* are highly susceptible to a broad range of antibiotics, including the β-lactam antibiotics, cephalosporins, aminoglycosides, and macrolides, but are not susceptible to vancomycin, rifampicin, metronidazole, and chloramphenicol. Early intervention may prevent the development of major organ-system failure or lessen its severity. Although studies supporting antibiotic therapy have produced conflicting results, clinical trials are difficult to perform in settings where patients frequently present for medical care with late stages of disease. Antibiotics are less likely to benefit patients in whom organ damage has already occurred. Two open-label randomized studies comparing penicillin with parenteral cefotaxime, parenteral ceftriaxone, and doxycycline showed no significant differences among the antibiotics with regard to complications and mortality risk. Thus ceftriaxone, cefotaxime, or doxycycline is a satisfactory alternative to penicillin for the treatment of severe leptospirosis. Antimicrobial susceptibility testing is not routine practice in individual cases of leptospirosis; to date, however, antibiotic resistance has not been reported in isolates from patients or the environment.

In mild cases, oral treatment with doxycycline, azithromycin, ampicillin, or amoxicillin is recommended. In regions where rickettsial diseases are coendemic, doxycycline or azithromycin is the drug of choice. In rare instances, a Jarisch-Herxheimer reaction develops within hours after the initiation of antimicrobial therapy.

Aggressive supportive care for leptospirosis is essential and can be life-saving. Patients with nonoliguric renal dysfunction require aggressive fluid and electrolyte resuscitation to prevent dehydration and precipitation of oliguric renal failure. Peritoneal dialysis or hemodialysis should be provided to patients with oliguric renal failure. Rapid initiation of hemodialysis has been shown to reduce mortality risk and typically is necessary only for short periods. Patients with pulmonary hemorrhage may have reduced pulmonary compliance (as seen in ARDS) and may benefit from mechanical ventilation with low tidal volumes to avoid high ventilation pressures. Evidence is contradictory for the use of glucocorticoids and desmopressin as adjunct therapy for pulmonary involvement associated with severe leptospirosis.

TABLE 184-1 Treatment and Chemoprophylaxis of Leptospirosis in Adults[a]

INDICATION	REGIMEN
Treatment	
Mild leptospirosis	Doxycycline[b] (100 mg PO bid) *or* Amoxicillin (500 mg PO tid) *or* Ampicillin (500 mg PO tid)
Moderate/severe leptospirosis	Penicillin (1.5 million units IV or IM q6h) *or* Ceftriaxone (2 g/d IV) *or* Cefotaxime (1 g IV q6h) *or* Doxycycline[b] (loading dose of 200 mg IV, then 100 mg IV q12h)
Chemoprophylaxis	
	Doxycycline[b] (200 mg PO once a week) *or* Azithromycin (250 mg PO once or twice a week)

[a]All regimens are given for 7 days. [b]Doxycycline should not be given to pregnant women or children. [c]The efficacy of doxycycline prophylaxis in endemic or epidemic settings remains unclear. Experiments in animal models and a cost-effectiveness model indicate that azithromycin has a number of characteristics that may make it efficacious in treatment and prophylaxis.

PROGNOSIS

Most patients with leptospirosis recover. However, post-leptospirosis symptoms, mainly of a depression-like nature, may occur and persist for years after the acute disease. Mortality rates are highest among patients who are elderly and those who have severe disease (pulmonary hemorrhage, Weil's syndrome). Leptospirosis during pregnancy is associated with high fetal mortality rates. Long-term follow-up of patients with renal failure and hepatic dysfunction has documented good recovery of renal and hepatic function.

PREVENTION

Individuals who may be exposed to *Leptospira* through their occupations or their involvement in recreational freshwater activities should be informed about the risks. Measures for controlling leptospirosis include avoidance of exposure to urine and tissues from infected animals through proper eyewear, footwear, and other protective equipment. Targeted rodent control strategies could be considered.

Vaccines for agricultural and companion animals are generally available, and their use should be encouraged. The veterinary vaccine used in a given area should contain the serovars known to be present in that area. Unfortunately, some vaccinated animals still excrete leptospires in their urine. Vaccination of humans against a specific serovar prevalent in an area has been undertaken in some European and Asian countries and has proved effective. Although a large-scale trial of vaccine in humans has been reported from Cuba, no conclusions can be drawn about efficacy and adverse reactions because of insufficient details on study design. The efficacy of chemoprophylaxis with doxycycline (200 mg once a week) or azithromycin (in pregnant women and children) is being disputed, but focused pre- and postexposure administration is indicated in instances of well-defined short-term exposure (Table 184-1).

FURTHER READING

Adler A: *Leptospira and Leptospirosis*, 1st ed. Berlin Heidelberg, Springer-Verlag, 2015.

de Vries SG et al: Leptospirosis among returned travelers: A GeoSentinel Site Survey and Multicenter Analysis–1997–2016. Am J Trop Med Hyg 99:127, 2018.

Haake DA, Levett PN: Leptospirosis in humans. Curr Top Microbiol Immunol 387:65, 2015.

van Samkar A et al: Suspected leptospiral meningitis in adults: Report of four cases and review of the literature. Neth J Med 73:464, 2015.

Vincent AT et al: Revisiting the taxonomy and evolution of pathogenicity of the genus Leptospira through the prism of genomics. PLoS Negl Trop Dis 13:e0007270, 2019.

185 Relapsing Fever and *Borrelia miyamotoi* Disease

Alan G. Barbour

Relapsing fever is caused by infection with any of several species of *Borrelia* spirochetes. Physicians in ancient Greece distinguished relapsing fever from other febrile disorders by its characteristic clinical presentation: two or more fever episodes separated by varying periods of well-being. In the nineteenth century, relapsing fever was one of the first diseases to be associated with a specific microbe by virtue of its characteristic laboratory finding: the presence of large numbers of spirochetes of the genus *Borrelia* in the blood.

The host responds with systemic inflammation that results in an illness ranging from a flulike syndrome to sepsis. Other manifestations are the consequences of central nervous system (CNS) involvement and disordered hemostasis. Antigenic variation of the spirochetes' surface proteins accounts for the infection's relapsing course. Acquired immunity follows the serial development of antibodies to each of the several variants appearing during an infection. Treatment with antibiotics results in rapid cure but at the risk of a moderate to severe Jarisch-Herxheimer reaction.

Louse-borne relapsing fever (LBRF) caused large epidemics well into the twentieth century and currently occurs in northeastern Africa and among migrants from that area. At present, however, most cases of relapsing fever are tick-borne in origin. Sporadic cases and small outbreaks are focally distributed on most continents, with Africa and Central Asia most affected. In North America, the majority of reports of relapsing fever have been from the western United States and Canada.

Another member of the genus, *Borrelia miyamotoi*, causes an acute febrile illness with nonspecific constitutional symptoms and occasionally meningoencephalitis in the same geographic distribution as Lyme disease (**Chap. 186**) in Eurasia and North America.

ETIOLOGIC AGENT

Coiled, thin microscopic filaments that swim in one direction and then coil up before heading in another were first observed in the blood of patients with relapsing fever in the 1880s. These microbes were categorized as spirochetes and assigned to the genus *Borrelia*. The breakthrough cultivation medium was rich in ingredients, ranging from simple (e.g., *N*-acetylglucosamine) to more complex (e.g., serum). The limited biosynthetic capacity of *Borrelia* cells is accounted for by a genome content one-quarter that of *Escherichia coli*.

Like other spirochetes, the helix-shaped *Borrelia* cells have two membranes, the outer of which is more loosely secured than in other double-membrane bacteria, such as *E. coli*. As a consequence, fixed organisms with damaged membranes can assume a variety of morphologies in smears and histologic preparations. The flagella of spirochetes run between the two membranes and are not on the cell surface. Although technically gram-negative, the 10- to 20-μm-long *Borrelia* cells, with a diameter of 0.2–0.3 μm, are too narrow to be seen by microscopy of Gram-stained slides.

EPIDEMIOLOGY

The several species of *Borrelia* that cause relapsing fever have restricted geographic distributions (**Table 185-1**). The exception is *Borrelia recurrentis*, which is also the only species transmitted by an insect. LBRF is acquired from a body louse (*Pediculus humanus corporis*), or possibly a head louse (*Pediculus capitis*), with humans serving as the reservoir. Acquisition occurs not from the bite itself but from either rubbing the insect's feces into the bite site with the fingers in response to irritation or inoculation into the conjunctivae or a wound. Although LBRF transmission is currently limited to Ethiopia, Eritrea, and Somalia, the disease has had a global distribution in the past, and that potential remains. Epidemics of LBRF, often in association with typhus, can occur under circumstances of famine, refugee migration, war, and pervasive homelessness. Transmission of LBRF can occur in camps of migrants at a distance from their home countries.

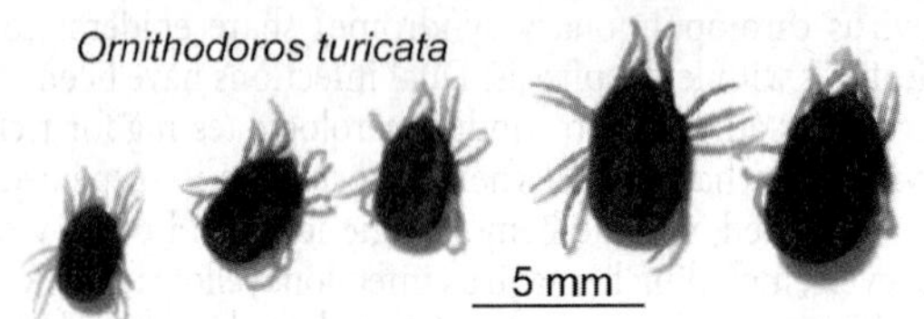

FIGURE 185-1 ***Ornithodoros turicata*** **soft ticks** of different ages.

All other known species of relapsing fever agents are tick-borne—in most cases, by soft ticks of the genus *Ornithodoros* (**Fig. 185-1**). Tick-borne relapsing fever (TBRF) is found on most continents but is absent in tropical or arctic environments. For most species, the reservoirs of infection are small to medium-sized mammals, usually rodents but sometimes pigs and other domestic animals living around human habitats. However, one species, *Borrelia duttonii* in sub-Saharan Africa, is largely maintained by tick transmission between human hosts. In North America, TBRF occurs as single cases or small case clusters through transient exposure of persons to infested buildings or caves where mammals have nests or sleep in less populated areas. The two main *Borrelia* species involved in North America are *Borrelia hermsii* in the mountainous west and *Borrelia turicatae* in arid southwestern and south-central regions. The soft tick vectors typically feed for no more than 30 min, usually while the victim is sleeping. Transovarial transmission from one generation of ticks to the next means that infection risk may persist in an area long after incriminated mammalian reservoirs have been removed.

Borrelia miyamotoi belongs to the same clade as relapsing fever species but instead is transmitted to humans from other mammals by hard ticks (e.g., *Ixodes scapularis* in the eastern United States) that also transmit Lyme disease, babesiosis, anaplasmosis, and a viral encephalitis. *B. miyamotoi* is acquired through outdoor activities and through contact with ticks in forested and shrubby areas during recreation, work, or activities around the home, similarly to Lyme disease (**Chap. 186**). Among residents of most areas where *B. miyamotoi* and *Borreliella* (also called *Borrelia*) *burgdorferi* coexist, the prevalence of antibodies to the former is about one-third of that to the latter. In contrast to *B. burgdorferi*, the transmission of *B. miyamotoi* to the host begins soon after the tick begins to feed.

PATHOGENESIS AND IMMUNITY

TBRF spirochetes enter the body in the tick's saliva with the onset of feeding. From an inoculum of a few cells, the spirochetes proliferate

TABLE 185-1 Relapsing Fever *Borrelia* Species, by Geographic Region, Vector, and Primary Reservoir

SPECIES	REGION(S)	ARTHROPOD VECTOR(S)	PRIMARY RESERVOIR
B. crocidurae	Africa	*Ornithodoros erraticus, Ornithodoros sonrai* (soft ticks)	Mammals
B. duttonii	Africa	*O. moubata*	Humans
B. hermsii	North America	*O. hermsi*	Mammals
B. hispanica	Europe, North Africa	*O. erraticus*	Mammals
B. johnsonii	North America	*Carios kellyi* (soft ticks)	Bats
B. kalaharica	Africa	*O. savignyi*	Mammals
B. mazzottii	Mexico, Central America	*O. talaje*	Mammals
B. miyamotoi	Eurasia, North America	*Ixodes* species (hard ticks)	Mammals
B. persica	Eurasia	*O. tholozani*	Mammals
B. recurrentis	Africa, global[a]	*Pediculus humanus corporis* (human body louse)	Humans
B. turicatae	North America	*O. turicata*	Mammals
B. venezuelensis	Central and South America	*O. rudis*	Mammals

[a]Although transmission is currently limited to Ethiopia and adjacent countries, *B. recurrentis* infection has had a global distribution in the past, and that potential remains.

in the blood, doubling every 6 h to numbers of 10^6–10^7/mL or more. *Borrelia* species are extracellular pathogens; their presence inside cells connotes dead bacteria after phagocytosis. Binding of the spirochetes to erythrocytes leads to aggregation of red blood cells, their sequestration in the spleen and liver, and hepatosplenomegaly and anemia. A bleeding disorder is probably the consequence of thrombocytopenia, impaired hepatic production of clotting factors, and/or blockage of small vessels by aggregates of spirochetes, erythrocytes, and platelets. Some species are neurotropic and enter the brain, where they are comparatively sheltered from host immunity. Relapsing fever spirochetes can cross the maternal-fetal barrier and cause placental damage and inflammation, leading to intrauterine growth retardation and congenital infection.

Although *Borrelia* species do not have potent exotoxins or a lipopolysaccharide endotoxin, they have abundant lipoproteins that activate Toll-like receptors on host cells, which leads to a proinflammatory process similar to that in endotoxemia, with elevations of tumor necrosis factor α, interleukin 6, and interleukin 8 concentrations.

IgM antibodies specific for the serotype-defining surface lipoprotein appear after a few days of infection and soon reach a concentration that causes lysis of bacteria in the blood through either direct bactericidal action or opsonization. The release of lipoproteins and other bacterial products from dying bacteria provokes a "crisis," during which there can be an increase in temperature, hypotension, and other signs of shock. A similar phenomenon occurring in some patients soon after the initiation of antibiotic treatment is characterized by an abrupt worsening of the patient's condition, which is called a Jarisch-Herxheimer reaction (JHR).

CLINICAL MANIFESTATIONS

Relapsing fever presents with the sudden onset of fever. Febrile periods are punctuated by intervening afebrile periods of a few days; this pattern occurs at least twice. The patient's temperature is ≥39°C and may be as high as 43°C. The first fever episode often ends in a crisis lasting ~15–30 min and consisting of rigors, a further elevation in temperature, and increases in pulse and blood pressure. The crisis phase is followed by profuse diaphoresis, falling temperature, and hypotension, which usually persist for several hours. In LBRF, the first episode of fever is unremitting for 3–6 days; it is usually followed by a single milder episode. In TBRF, multiple febrile periods last 1–3 days each. In both forms, the interval between fevers ranges from 4 to 14 days, sometimes with symptoms of malaise and fatigue.

The symptoms that accompany the fevers are usually nonspecific. Headache, neck stiffness, arthralgia, myalgia, and vomiting may accompany the first and subsequent febrile episodes. An enlarging spleen and liver cause abdominal pain. A nonproductive cough is common during LBRF and—in combination with fever and myalgias—may suggest influenza. Acute respiratory distress syndrome may occur during TBRF.

On physical examination, the patient may be delirious or apathetic. There may be body lice in the patient's clothes or signs of insect bites. In regions with *B. miyamotoi* infection, a hard tick may be embedded in the skin. Epistaxis, petechiae, and ecchymoses are common during LBRF but not in TBRF. Splenomegaly or spleen tenderness is common in both forms of relapsing fever. The majority of patients with LBRF and ~10% of patients with TBRF have discernible hepatomegaly.

Localizing neurologic findings are more common in TBRF than in LBRF. In North America, *B. turicatae* infection has neurologic manifestations more often than *B. hermsii* infection. Meningoencephalitis can result in residual hemiplegia or aphasia. Myelitis and radiculopathy may develop. Unilateral or bilateral Bell's palsy and deafness from seventh or eighth cranial nerve involvement are the most common forms of cranial neuritis and typically present in the second or third febrile episode, not the first. Visual impairment from unilateral or bilateral iridocyclitis or panophthalmitis may be permanent. In LBRF, neurologic manifestations such as altered mental state or stiff neck are thought to be secondary to systemic inflammation rather than to direct invasion of the nervous system.

Myocarditis appears to be common in both forms of relapsing fever and accounts for some deaths. Most commonly, myocarditis is evidenced by gallops on cardiac auscultation, a prolonged QT_c interval, and cardiomegaly and pulmonary edema on chest radiography.

General laboratory studies are not specific. Mild to moderate normocytic anemia is common, but frank hemolysis and hemoglobinuria do not develop. Leukocyte counts are usually in the normal range or only slightly elevated, and leukopenia can occur during the crisis. Platelet counts can fall below 50,000/μL. C-reactive protein and procalcitonin levels are elevated. Laboratory evidence of hepatitis can be found, with elevated serum concentrations of unconjugated bilirubin and aminotransferases; the prothrombin and partial thromboplastin times may be moderately prolonged.

Analysis of the cerebrospinal fluid (CSF) is indicated in cases of suspected relapsing fever with signs of meningitis or meningoencephalitis. The presence of mononuclear pleocytosis and mildly to moderately elevated protein levels justifies intravenous antibiotic therapy in TBRF.

The manifestations and course of *B. miyamotoi* disease are not as distinctive as those of relapsing fever. The most common presentation is fever without respiratory symptoms starting 1–2 weeks after a tick bite. Patients have been hospitalized with a presumptive diagnosis of undifferentiated sepsis. Meningoencephalitis with spirochetes in the CSF was documented in immunodeficient adults but may also occur in immunocompetent individuals. If the patient has coexisting early Lyme disease, there may be erythema migrans, the localized skin rash.

DIAGNOSIS

Relapsing fever should be considered in a patient with the characteristic fever pattern and a history of recent exposure—i.e., within 1–2 weeks before illness onset—to body lice or soft-bodied ticks in geographic areas with documented current or past transmission. Because of the longevity of the ticks and the transovarial transmission of the pathogen in the ticks, a case of relapsing fever may be diagnosed many years after the last case reported in that locale. The lice may be on the clothes of a migrant. While the risks for *B. miyamotoi* disease are similar to those for Lyme disease, prompt removal of an embedded tick after the exposure may not reduce the risk of infection of this pathogen.

With the exception of *B. miyamotoi* infection, the bedrock for laboratory diagnosis of LBRF and TBRF remains direct detection of the spirochetes by microscopy of the blood. Manual differential counts of white blood cells by Wright stain usually reveal spirochetes in thin blood smears if their concentration is ≥10^5/mL and several oil-immersion fields are examined (**Fig. 185-2**). But the preferred stains are Giemsa-Wright or Giemsa alone. The density of *B. miyamotoi* in the blood is not high enough for use of a blood smear alone for diagnosis. For LBRF and TBRF, the preferred time to obtain a blood specimen is between the fever's onset and its peak. Lower concentrations of spirochetes may be revealed by a thick blood smear that is treated with 0.5% acetic acid before staining. An alternative is a wet mount of anticoagulated blood mixed with saline and examined by phase-contrast or dark-field microscopy for motile spirochetes.

Polymerase chain reaction (PCR) and similar DNA amplification procedures are increasingly used for examination of blood or CSF in cases of suspected relapsing fever. PCR may reveal circulating spirochetes between febrile episodes. PCR is the preferred procedure for direct detection of *B. miyamotoi* in blood or CSF.

Culture of blood or CSF in Barbour-Stoenner-Kelly broth medium or equivalent is an option for isolation of *Borrelia* species. However, few laboratories offer this service. An alternative for tick-borne *Borrelia* species, but not *B. recurrentis*, is inoculation of blood or CSF into severe combined immunodeficient mice and examination of the animal's blood after a few days.

Options for serologic confirmation of infection are limited, and results may be misleading. Whole cell-based assays, such as enzyme-linked immunosorbent assay (ELISA) and immunoblot, and the C6-peptide ELISA for Lyme disease may be positive in relapsing fever or *B. miyamotoi* disease through antigenic cross-reactivities among these spirochetes. A commercially available assay based on GlpQ, a protein antigen of all relapsing fever *Borrelia* species (including *B. miyamotoi*) but not of any Lyme disease species, has better specificity, but commonly is negative at a time when a blood smear or PCR assay

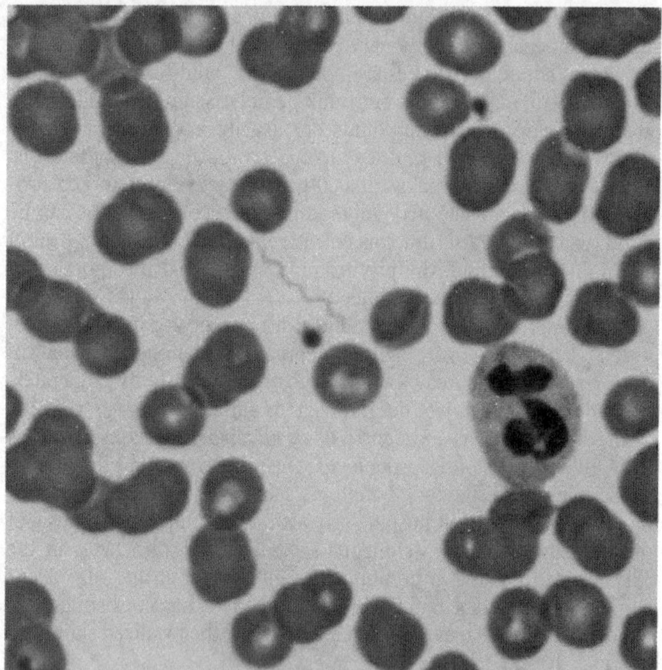

FIGURE 185-2 Photomicrograph of tick-borne relapsing fever spirochete (*Borrelia turicatae*) in a Giemsa-Wright–stained thin blood smear. Included in the figure are a polymorphonuclear leukocyte and two platelets.

would be positive. The results of current GlpQ-based assays cannot be used to differentiate between different *Borrelia* species as to etiology.

■ DIFFERENTIAL DIAGNOSIS

Depending on the patient's history of residential, occupational, travel, and recreational exposures, the differential diagnosis of relapsing fever includes one or more of the following infections that feature either periodicity in the fever pattern or an extended single febrile period with nonspecific constitutional symptoms: Colorado tick fever, Rocky Mountain spotted fever and other rickettsioses, ehrlichiosis, anaplasmosis, tick-borne viral infection, rat bite fever, and babesiosis in North America, Europe, Russia, and northeastern Asia. Elsewhere in the Americas and Asia and in most of Africa, malaria, typhoid fever, typhus and other rickettsioses, dengue, and leptospirosis may also be considered. There may be co-infections of malaria, typhus, or typhoid with TBRF or LBRF. *B. miyamotoi* infection may coexist with Lyme disease, anaplasmosis, or babesiosis in North America.

TREATMENT
Relapsing Fever

Penicillin and tetracyclines have been the antibiotics of choice for relapsing fever for several decades. Erythromycin and chloramphenicol have been long-standing alternative choices. There is no evidence of acquired resistance to these antibiotics. *Borrelia* species are also susceptible to second- and third-generation cephalosporins. These spirochetes are also relatively resistant to rifampin, sulfonamides, and aminoglycosides. Spirochetes are no longer detectable in the blood within a few hours after the first dose of an effective antibiotic.

Under conditions of limited resources or in the midst of an epidemic, a single dose of antibiotic usually suffices for successful treatment of LBRF (**Fig. 185-3**). For adults, a single dose of oral tetracycline (500 mg), oral doxycycline (200 mg), or intramuscular penicillin G procaine (800,000 units) is effective. The corresponding doses for children are oral tetracycline at 12.5 mg/kg, oral doxycycline at 5 mg/kg, and intramuscular penicillin G procaine at 200,000–400,000 units. When an adult patient is stuporous or nauseated, the intravenous dose of tetracycline is 250–500 mg. Tetracyclines are contraindicated in pregnant and nursing women and in children <9 years old; for individuals in these groups who are allergic to penicillin, oral erythromycin (500 mg for adults and 12.5 mg/kg for children) is an alternative. While there is little reported experience with other macrolides, such as azithromycin, these are likely to be as effective as erythromycin.

But there are shortcomings of single-dose therapies for LBRF. With penicillin alone, recurrence may occur in up to 20% of patients, and the frequency of JHR was higher after tetracycline than penicillin. For treatment of LBRF in adults in Ethiopia, a regimen that reduces rates of both recurrence and JHR has been a single dose of 400,000 units of intramuscular penicillin G procaine

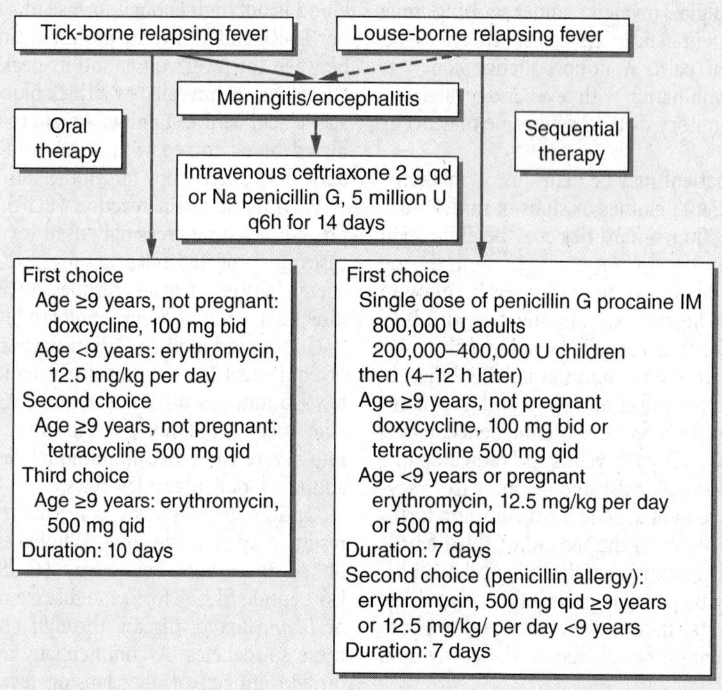

FIGURE 185-3 Algorithm for treatment of relapsing fever. If it is not known whether the patient has tick-borne or louse-borne relapsing fever, the patient should be treated for the tick-borne form. The *dashed line* indicates that central nervous system invasion in louse-borne relapsing fever is uncommon.

followed several hours later or the next day by doxycycline (100 mg orally twice daily) or tetracycline (500 mg or 12.5 mg/kg orally every 6 h) for 7 days.

The accumulated anecdotal reports on TBRF therapy indicate a recurrence rate of ≥20% after single-dose treatment, plausibly due to the propensity of some tick-borne species to invade the CNS. Accordingly, multiple antibiotic doses are recommended. The preferred treatment for adults is a 10-day course of doxycycline (100 mg twice daily) or tetracycline (500 mg or 12.5 mg/kg orally every 6 h). When tetracyclines are contraindicated, the alternative is erythromycin (500 mg or 12.5 mg/kg orally every 6 h) for 10 days. If a β-lactam antibiotic is given and CNS involvement is confirmed or suspected, it is preferably administered intravenously rather than orally. For adults, the regimen is penicillin G (5 million units IV every 6 h) or ceftriaxone (2 g IV daily) for 10–14 days. Under conditions of limited resources or when CNS involvement is not suspected, oral penicillin V potassium (500 mg or 12.5 mg/kg every 6–8 h) for 10 days is used.

The JHR during treatment of relapsing fever can be severe and may end in death if precautions are not in place for close monitoring for at least 24 h and with provision of parenteral cardiovascular and volume support as needed. Apprehension, rigors, fever, and hypotension occur within 1–3 h of initiation of antibiotic treatment and may be accompanied by a further decrease in the platelet count. The incidence of the JHR is 20–60% in LBRF after the first antibiotic dose. JHR may also be encountered when a patient with unsuspected relapsing fever is treated with other types of antibiotics, such ciprofloxacin, that have suboptimal effects.

Experience with the treatment of *B. miyamotoi* infection is limited, but this organism likely has the same antibiotic susceptibilities as other *Borrelia* species. Therapy for *B. miyamotoi* disease follows the guidelines for Lyme disease. This would include parenteral therapy for CNS involvement. In absence of contraindications, doxycycline (100 mg twice daily) is the preferred choice for uncomplicated *B. miyamotoi* infection, because of the antibiotic's efficacy for anaplasmosis and Lyme disease. If JHR occurs, it is generally milder than is observed in relapsing fever.

PROGNOSIS

The mortality rates for untreated LBRF and TBRF are in the ranges of 10–70% and 4–10%, respectively, and are largely determined by coexisting conditions, such as malnutrition, dehydration, or another infection. With prompt antibiotic treatment, the mortality rate is 2–5% for LBRF and <2% for TBRF. Features associated with a poor prognosis include concurrence with malaria, typhus, or typhoid; pregnancy; stupor or coma on admission; diffuse bleeding; poor liver function; myocarditis; and bronchopneumonia. The mortality rate from the JHR in LBRF, in the absence of adequate monitoring and resuscitation measures, is ~5%. Relapsing fever during pregnancy frequently leads to abortion or stillbirth, but congenital malformations have not been reported. Although spirochetes or their remnants may persist in the CNS or other sequestered sites after bacteremia has resolved, posttreatment sequelae and prolonged disability have not been not documented for relapsing fever or *B. miyamotoi* disease. Partial immunity against reinfection seems to develop in residents of areas with perennial elevated risk.

PREVENTION

There is no vaccine for LBRF, TBRF, or *B. miyamotoi* disease. Reduction of exposure to lice and ticks is the key strategy for prevention. LBRF can be prevented through improved personal hygiene, reduction of crowding, better access to hot water (≥60° C) for clothes washing, and selected use of pesticides. Clothing is an important factor in maintaining the human body louse. The risk of TBRF can be reduced by construction of houses with concrete or sealed plank floors and without thatched roofs or mud walls. Houses and cabins in forested areas pose a risk in western North America when rodents nest in the roof, attic, or wall spaces or under the structure. Buildings infested with *Ornithodoros* ticks can be treated with pesticides and then rodent-proofed. If residing in a high-risk environment, individuals should not sleep on the floor, and beds should be moved away from the wall. Individuals with recreational or occupational exposure to caves, where mammals, including bats, may reside, merit advice about the risk of TBRF. Following exposure at a site of TBRF risk, treatment with doxycycline (either a single dose of 100 mg or 200 mg on day 1 followed by 100 mg/d for 4 days) was efficacious in preventing infection in a placebo-controlled trial. Recommendations for preventing *B. miyamotoi* infection follow those for reducing risk of Lyme disease from exposure to the vector hard ticks (**Chap. 186**).

FURTHER READING

Barbour AG, Schwan TG: Borrelia, in *Bergey's Manual of Systematics of Archaea and Bacteria*. WB Whitman et al (eds). John Wiley & Sons, Inc., 2018, pp 1-22.

Binenbaum Y et al: Single dose of doxycycline for the prevention of tick-borne relapsing fever. Clin Infect Dis 71:1768, 2020.

Butler T: The Jarisch-Herxheimer reaction after antibiotic treatment of spirochetal infections: A review of recent cases and our understanding of pathogenesis. Am J Trop Med Hyg 96:46, 2017.

Christensen J et al: Tickborne relapsing fever, Bitterroot Valley, Montana, USA. Emerg Infect Dis 21:217, 2015.

Gugliotta JL et al: Meningoencephalitis from Borrelia miyamotoi in an immunocompromised patient. N Engl J Med 368:240, 2013.

Isenring E et al: Infectious disease profiles of Syrian and Eritrean migrants presenting in Europe: A systematic review. Travel Med Infect Dis 25:65, 2018.

Krause PJ et al: *Borrelia miyamotoi* infection in nature and in humans. Clin Microbiol Infect 21:631, 2015.

Moran-Gilad J et al: Postexposure prophylaxis of tick-borne relapsing fever: Lessons learned from recent outbreaks in Israel. Vector Borne Zoonotic Dis 13:791, 2013.

Nordmann T et al: Outbreak of louse-borne relapsing fever among urban dwellers in Arsi Zone, Central Ethiopia, from July to November 2016. Am J Trop Med Hyg 98:1599, 2018.

Salih SY, Mustafa D: Louse-borne relapsing fever: II. Combined penicillin and tetracycline therapy in 160 Sudanese patients. Trans R Soc Trop Med Hyg 71:49, 1977.

Schwan TG et al: Tick-borne relapsing fever and *Borrelia hermsii*, Los Angeles County, California, USA. Emerg Infect Dis 15:1026, 2009.

Telford SR et al: Blood smears have poor sensitivity for confirming *Borrelia miyamotoi* disease. J Clin Microbiol 57:e01468, 2019.

von Both U, Alberer M: Images in clinical medicine. *Borrelia recurrentis* infection. N Engl J Med 375:e5, 2016.

Warrell DA: Louse-borne relapsing fever (*Borrelia recurrentis* infection). Epidemiol Infect 147:e106, 2019.

Wormser GP et al: Borrelia miyamotoi: An emerging tick-borne pathogen. Am J Med 132:136, 2019.

186 Lyme Borreliosis

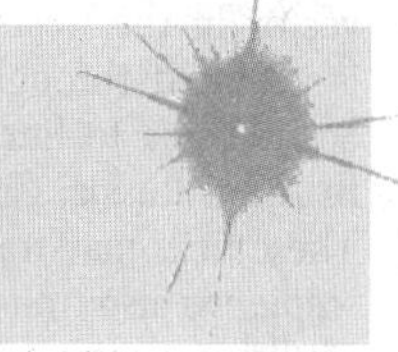

Allen C. Steere

DEFINITION

Lyme borreliosis is caused by a spirochete, *Borrelia* (also called *Borreliella*) *burgdorferi sensu lato*, that is transmitted by ticks of the *Ixodes ricinus* complex. The infection usually begins with a characteristic expanding skin lesion, erythema migrans (EM; stage 1, localized infection). After several days or weeks, the spirochete may spread to many different sites (stage 2, disseminated infection). Possible manifestations of disseminated infection include secondary annular skin lesions, meningitis, cranial neuritis, radiculoneuritis, peripheral neuritis, carditis, atrioventricular nodal block, or migratory musculoskeletal pain.

Months or years later (usually after periods of latent infection), intermittent or persistent arthritis, chronic encephalopathy or polyneuropathy, or acrodermatitis may develop (stage 3, persistent infection). Most patients experience early symptoms of the illness during the summer, but the infection may not become symptomatic until it progresses to stage 2 or 3.

Lyme disease was recognized as a separate entity in 1976 because of a geographic cluster of children in Lyme, Connecticut, who were thought to have juvenile rheumatoid arthritis. It became apparent that Lyme disease was a multisystemic illness that affected primarily the skin, nervous system, heart, and joints. Epidemiologic studies of patients with EM implicated certain *Ixodes* ticks as vectors of the disease. Early in the twentieth century, EM had been described in Europe and attributed to *I. ricinus* tick bites. In 1982, a previously unrecognized spirochete, now called *Borrelia burgdorferi*, was recovered from *Ixodes scapularis* ticks and then from patients with Lyme disease. The entity is now called Lyme disease or Lyme borreliosis.

ETIOLOGIC AGENT

B. burgdorferi, the causative agent of Lyme disease, is a fastidious microaerophilic bacterium. The spirochete's genome is quite small (~1.5 Mb) and consists of a highly unusual linear chromosome of 950 kb as well as 17–21 linear and circular plasmids. The most remarkable aspect of the *B. burgdorferi* genome is that there are sequences for more than 100 known or predicted lipoproteins—a larger number than in any other organism. The spirochete has few proteins with biosynthetic activity and depends on its host for most of its nutritional requirements. It has no sequences for recognizable toxins.

Currently, 20 closely related borrelial species are collectively referred to as *B. burgdorferi sensu lato* (i.e., "*B. burgdorferi* in the general sense"). The human infection Lyme borreliosis is caused primarily by three pathogenic genospecies: *B. burgdorferi sensu stricto* ("*B. burgdorferi* in the strict sense," hereafter referred to simply as *B. burgdorferi*), *Borrelia garinii*, and *Borrelia afzelii*. *B. burgdorferi* is the major cause of the infection in the United States; all three genospecies are found in Europe, and *B. garinii* is the major cause in Asia.

Strains of *B. burgdorferi* have been subdivided according to several typing schemes: one based on sequence variation of outer-surface protein C (OspC), a second based on differences in the 16S–23S rRNA intergenic spacer region (RST or IGS), and a third called *multilocus sequence typing*. From these typing systems, it is apparent that strains of *B. burgdorferi* differ in pathogenicity. OspC type A (RST1) strains seem to be particularly virulent and may have played a role in the emergence of Lyme disease in epidemic form in the northeastern United States in the late twentieth century.

EPIDEMIOLOGY

The 20 known genospecies of *B. burgdorferi sensu lato* live in nature in enzootic cycles involving 14 species of ticks that are part of the *I. ricinus* complex. *I. scapularis* (**Fig. 461-1**) is the principal vector in the eastern United States from Maine to Georgia and in the midwestern states of Wisconsin, Minnesota, and Michigan. *I. pacificus* is the vector in the western states of California and Oregon. The disease is acquired throughout Europe (from Ireland and Great Britain to Scandinavia to European Russia), where *I. ricinus* is the vector, and in Asian Russia, China, and Japan, where *I. persulcatus* is the vector. These ticks may transmit other agents as well. In the United States, *I. scapularis* also transmits *Babesia microti*; *Anaplasma phagocytophilum*; *Ehrlichia* species Wisconsin; *Borrelia miyamotoi*; *Borrelia mayonii*; and, in rare instances, Powassan encephalitis virus (the deer tick virus) (see "Differential Diagnosis," below). In Europe and Asia, *I. ricinus* and *I. persulcatus* also transmit tick-borne encephalitis virus.

Ticks of the *I. ricinus* complex have larval, nymphal, and adult stages. They require a blood meal at each stage. The risk of infection in a given area depends largely on the density of these ticks as well as their feeding habits and animal hosts, which have evolved differently in different locations. For *I. scapularis* in the northeastern United States, the white-footed mouse and certain other rodents are the preferred hosts of the immature larvae and nymphs. It is critical that both of the tick's immature stages feed on the same host because the life cycle of the spirochete depends on horizontal transmission: in early summer from infected nymphs to mice and in late summer from infected mice to larvae, which then molt to become the infected nymphs that will begin the cycle again the following year. It is the tiny nymphal tick that is primarily responsible for transmission of the disease to humans, which peaks during the early summer months. White-tailed deer, which are not involved in the life cycle of the spirochete, are the preferred host for the adult stage of *I. scapularis* and seem to be critical to the tick's survival.

Lyme disease is now the most common vector-borne infection in the United States and Europe. Since surveillance was begun by the Centers for Disease Control and Prevention (CDC) in 1982, the number of cases in the United States has increased dramatically. More than 30,000 new cases are now reported each summer, but the actual number of new cases is probably closer to 300,000 annually. In Europe, reported frequencies of the disease are highest in the middle of the continent and in Scandinavia.

PATHOGENESIS AND IMMUNITY

To maintain its complex enzootic cycle, *B. burgdorferi* must adapt to two markedly different environments: the tick and the mammalian host. The spirochete expresses outer-surface protein A (OspA) in the midgut of the tick, whereas OspC is upregulated as the organism travels to the tick's salivary gland. There, OspC binds a tick salivary-gland protein (Salp15), which is required for infection of the mammalian host. The tick usually must be attached for at least 24 h for transmission of *B. burgdorferi*.

After injection into the human skin, the spirochete downregulates OspC and upregulates the VlsE lipoprotein. This protein undergoes extensive antigenic variation, which is necessary for spirochetal survival. After several days to weeks, *B. burgdorferi* may migrate outward in the skin, producing EM, and may spread hematogenously or in the lymph to other organs. The only known virulence factors of *B. burgdorferi* are surface proteins that allow the spirochete to attach to mammalian proteins, integrins, glycosaminoglycans, or glycoproteins. For example, spread through the skin and other tissue matrices may be facilitated by the binding of human plasminogen and its activators to the surface of the spirochete. Some *Borrelia* strains bind complement regulator–acquiring surface proteins (FHL-1/reconectin, or factor H), which help to protect spirochetes from complement-mediated lysis. Dissemination of the organism in the blood is facilitated by binding to the fibrinogen receptor ($\alpha_{IIb}\beta_3$) on activated platelets and the vitronectin receptor ($\alpha_v\beta_3$) on endothelial cells. As the name indicates, spirochetal decorin-binding proteins A and B bind decorin, a glycosaminoglycan on collagen fibrils, and *B. burgdorferi* also binds directly to native type 1 collagen lattices. This binding may explain why the organism is commonly aligned with collagen fibrils in the extracellular matrix in the heart, nervous system, or joints.

To control and eradicate *B. burgdorferi*, the host mounts both innate and adaptive immune responses, resulting in macrophage- and antibody-mediated killing of the spirochete. As part of the innate immune response, complement may lyse the spirochete in the skin. Cells at affected sites release potent proinflammatory cytokines, including interleukin 6, tumor necrosis factor α, interleukin 1β, and interferon γ (IFN-γ). Patients who are homozygous for a Toll-like receptor 1 polymorphism (1805GG), particularly when infected with highly inflammatory *B. burgdorferi* RST1 strains, have exceptionally high levels of proinflammatory cytokines. The purpose of the adaptive immune response appears to be the production of specific antibodies, which opsonize the organism—a step necessary for optimal spirochetal killing. Studies with protein arrays expressing ~1200 *B. burgdorferi* proteins detected antibody responses to a total of 120 spirochetal proteins (particularly outer-surface lipoproteins) in a population of patients with Lyme arthritis. Histologic examination of all affected tissues reveals an infiltration of lymphocytes, macrophages, and plasma cells with some degree of vascular damage, including mild vasculitis or hypervascular occlusion. These findings suggest that the spirochete may have been present in or around blood vessels.

In enzootic infection, *B. burgdorferi* spirochetes must survive this immune assault only during the summer months before returning to larval ticks to begin the cycle again the following year. In contrast, infection of humans is a dead-end event for the spirochete. Within several weeks or months, innate and adaptive immune mechanisms—even without antibiotic treatment—control widely disseminated infection, and generalized systemic symptoms wane. However, without antibiotic therapy, spirochetes may survive in localized niches for several more years. For example, *B. burgdorferi* infection in the United States may cause persistent arthritis or, in rare cases, subtle encephalopathy or polyneuropathy. Thus, immune mechanisms seem to succeed eventually in the near or total eradication of *B. burgdorferi* from selected niches, including the joints or nervous system, and symptoms resolve in most patients.

CLINICAL MANIFESTATIONS

Early Infection: Stage 1 (Localized Infection) Because of the small size of nymphal ixodid ticks, most patients do not remember the preceding tick bite. After an incubation period of 3–32 days, EM usually begins as a red macule or papule at the site of the tick bite that expands slowly to form a large annular lesion (**Fig. 186-1**). As the lesion increases in size, it often develops a bright red outer border and partial central clearing. The center of the lesion sometimes becomes intensely erythematous and indurated, vesicular, or necrotic. In other instances, the expanding lesion remains an even, intense red; several red rings are found within an outside ring; or the central area turns blue before the lesion clears. Although EM can be located anywhere, the thigh, groin, and axilla are particularly common sites. The lesion is warm but not often painful. Approximately 20% of patients do not exhibit this characteristic skin manifestation.

Early Infection: Stage 2 (Disseminated Infection) In cases in the United States, *B. burgdorferi* often spreads hematogenously to many sites within days or weeks after the onset of EM. In these cases, patients may develop secondary annular skin lesions similar in appearance to the initial lesion. Skin involvement is commonly accompanied by severe headache, mild stiffness of the neck, fever, chills, migratory musculoskeletal pain, arthralgias, and profound malaise and fatigue. Less common manifestations include generalized lymphadenopathy or splenomegaly, hepatitis, sore throat, nonproductive cough, conjunctivitis, iritis, or testicular swelling. Except for fatigue and lethargy, which are often constant, the early signs and symptoms of Lyme disease are typically intermittent and changing. Even in untreated patients, the early symptoms usually become less severe or disappear within several weeks. In ~15% of patients, the infection presents with these nonspecific systemic symptoms.

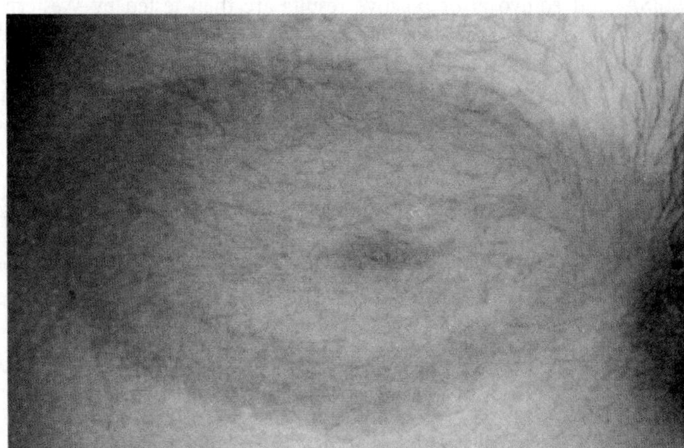

FIGURE 186-1 A classic erythema migrans lesion (9 cm in diameter) is shown near the right axilla. The lesion has partial central clearing, a bright red outer border, and a target center. *(Courtesy of Vijay K. Sikand, MD; with permission.)*

Symptoms suggestive of meningeal irritation may develop early in Lyme disease when EM is present but usually are not associated with cerebrospinal fluid (CSF) pleocytosis or an objective neurologic deficit. After several weeks or months, ~15% of untreated patients develop frank neurologic abnormalities, including meningitis, subtle encephalitic signs, cranial neuritis (including bilateral facial palsy), motor or sensory radiculoneuropathy, peripheral neuropathy, mononeuritis multiplex, cerebellar ataxia, or myelitis—alone or in various combinations. In children, the optic nerve may be affected because of inflammation or increased intracranial pressure, and these effects may lead to blindness. In the United States, the usual pattern consists of fluctuating symptoms of meningitis accompanied by facial palsy and peripheral radiculoneuropathy. Lymphocytic pleocytosis (~100 cells/μL) is found in CSF, often along with elevated protein levels and normal or slightly low glucose concentrations. In Europe and Asia, the first neurologic sign is characteristically radicular pain, which is followed by the development of CSF pleocytosis (meningopolyneuritis or *Bannwarth's syndrome*); meningeal or encephalitic signs are frequently absent. These early neurologic abnormalities usually resolve completely within months, but in rare cases, chronic neurologic disease may occur later.

Within several weeks after the onset of illness, ~8% of patients develop cardiac involvement. The most common abnormality is a fluctuating degree of atrioventricular block (first-degree, Wenckebach, or complete heart block). Some patients have more diffuse cardiac involvement, including electrocardiographic changes indicative of acute myopericarditis, left ventricular dysfunction evident on radionuclide scans, or (in rare cases) cardiomegaly or fatal pancarditis. Cardiac involvement lasts for only a few weeks in most patients but may recur in untreated patients. A few cases of mitral or aortic valve endocarditis have been reported, in one case occurring years after acute cardiac involvement of Lyme disease. Chronic cardiomyopathy caused by *B. burgdorferi* has been reported in Europe.

During this stage, musculoskeletal pain is common. The typical pattern consists of migratory pain in joints, tendons, bursae, muscles, or bones (usually without joint swelling) lasting for hours or days and affecting one or two locations at a time.

Late Infection: Stage 3 (Persistent Infection) Months after the onset of infection, ~60% of patients in the United States who have received no antibiotic treatment develop frank arthritis. The typical pattern comprises intermittent attacks of oligoarticular arthritis in large joints (especially the knees), lasting for weeks or months in a given joint. A few small joints or periarticular sites also may be affected, primarily during early attacks. The number of patients who continue to have recurrent attacks decreases each year. However, in a small percentage of cases, involvement of large joints—usually one or both knees—is persistent and may lead to erosion of cartilage and bone.

White cell counts in joint fluid range from 500 to 110,000/μL (average, 25,000/μL); most of these cells are polymorphonuclear leukocytes. Tests for rheumatoid factor or antinuclear antibodies usually give negative results. Examination of synovial biopsy samples reveals fibrin deposits, villous hypertrophy, vascular proliferation, microangiopathic lesions, and a heavy infiltration of lymphocytes and plasma cells.

Although most patients with Lyme arthritis respond well to antibiotic therapy, a small percentage in the northeastern United States have persistent postinfectious (also called postantibiotic or antibiotic-refractory) Lyme arthritis for months or even for several years after receiving oral and IV antibiotic therapy for 2 or 3 months. Although more often these patients are initially infected with OspA type A (RST1) strains of *B. burgdorferi*, this complication is not thought to result from persistent infection. Results of culture and polymerase chain reaction (PCR) for *B. burgdorferi* in synovial tissue obtained in the postantibiotic period have been uniformly negative. Rather, the basic pathogenetic feature of postinfectious Lyme arthritis is the development of an excessive, dysregulated proinflammatory immune response during the infection, characterized by exceptionally high IFN-γ levels, which persists in the postinfectious period. Risk factors for excessively high IFN-γ responses include presentation of an epitope of *B. burgdorferi* OspA (OspA$^{164-175}$) by certain class II major histocompatibility complex molecules (particularly HLA-DRBI*0401); a Toll-like receptor 1 polymorphism 1805GG in patients who were infected with OspC type A (RST1) *B. burgdorferi* strains; and an imbalance of the CD4+ T effector/regulatory cell ratio in which the majority of CD4+CD25+ T cells, which are ordinarily regulatory T cells, become IFN-γ-secreting T effector cells.

The consequences of this excessive proinflammatory response in Lyme synovia include vascular damage, autoimmune and cytotoxic processes, and tumor-like fibroblast proliferation and fibrosis. An important driver of innate immune responses may be persistence of *B. burgdorferi* peptidoglycan in synovial fluid, which may be especially difficult to clear. In addition, four autoantigens that are targets of T and B cell responses in patients with Lyme disease, particularly those with postinfectious arthritis, have now been identified: endothelial cell growth factor, matrix metalloproteinase-10, apolipoprotein B-100, and annexin A2, which may have a role in persistent inflammation.

Although rare, chronic neurologic involvement also may become apparent from months to several years after the onset of infection, sometimes after long periods of latent infection. The most common form of chronic central nervous system involvement is subtle encephalopathy affecting memory, mood, or sleep, and the most common form of peripheral neuropathy is an axonal polyneuropathy manifested as either distal paresthesia or spinal radicular pain. Patients with encephalopathy frequently have evidence of memory impairment in neuropsychological tests and abnormal results in CSF analyses. In cases of polyneuropathy, electromyography generally shows extensive abnormalities of proximal and distal nerve segments. Encephalomyelitis or leukoencephalitis, a rare manifestation of Lyme borreliosis associated primarily with *B. garinii* infection in Europe, is a severe neurologic disorder that may include spastic paraparesis, upper motor neuron bladder dysfunction, and, rarely, lesions in the periventricular white matter.

Acrodermatitis chronica atrophicans, the late skin manifestation of Lyme borreliosis, has been associated primarily with *B. afzelii* infection in Europe and Asia. It has been observed especially often in elderly women. The skin lesions, which are usually found on the acral surface of an arm or leg, begin insidiously with reddish-violaceous discoloration; they become sclerotic or atrophic over a period of years.

The basic patterns of Lyme borreliosis are similar worldwide, but there are regional variations, primarily between the illness found in North America, which is caused exclusively by *B. burgdorferi*, and that found in Europe, which is caused primarily by *B. afzelii* and *B. garinii*. With each of the *Borrelia* species, the infection usually begins with EM. However, *B. burgdorferi* strains in the eastern United States often disseminate widely; they are particularly arthritogenic, and especially OspC type A (RST1) strains may cause postinfectious arthritis. *B. garinii* typically disseminates less widely, but it is especially neurotropic and may cause borrelial encephalomyelitis. *B. afzelii* often infects only the skin but may persist in that site, where it may cause several different dermatoborrelioses, including acrodermatitis chronica atrophicans.

Post-Lyme Syndrome (Chronic Lyme Disease) Despite resolution of the objective manifestations of the infection with antibiotic therapy, ~10% of patients (although the reported percentages vary widely) continue to have subjective pain, neurocognitive manifestations, or fatigue symptoms. These symptoms usually improve and resolve within months but may last for years. At the far end of the spectrum, the symptoms may be similar to or indistinguishable from chronic fatigue syndrome (**Chap. 450**) and fibromyalgia (**Chap. 373**). Compared with symptoms of active Lyme disease, post-Lyme symptoms tend to be more generalized or disabling. They include marked fatigue, severe headache, diffuse musculoskeletal pain, multiple symmetric tender points in characteristic locations, pain and stiffness in many joints, diffuse paresthesias, difficulty with concentration, and sleep disturbances. Patients with this condition lack evidence of joint inflammation, have normal neurologic test results, and may exhibit anxiety and depression. In contrast, late manifestations of Lyme disease, including arthritis, encephalopathy, and neuropathy, are usually associated with minimal systemic symptoms. Currently, no evidence indicates that persistent subjective symptoms after recommended courses of antibiotic therapy are caused by active infection.

DIAGNOSIS

The culture of *B. burgdorferi* in Barbour-Stoenner-Kelly (BSK) medium permits definitive diagnosis, but this method has been used primarily in research studies. Moreover, with a few exceptions, positive cultures have been obtained only early in the illness—particularly from biopsy samples of EM skin lesions, less often from plasma samples, and occasionally from CSF samples. Later in the infection, PCR is greatly superior to culture for the detection of *B. burgdorferi* DNA in joint fluid; this is the major use for PCR testing in Lyme disease. However, because *B. burgdorferi* DNA may persist for at least weeks after spirochetal killing with antibiotics, detection of spirochetal DNA in joint fluid is not an accurate test of active joint infection in Lyme disease and cannot be used reliably to determine the adequacy of antibiotic therapy. The sensitivity of PCR determinations in CSF from patients with neuroborreliosis has been much lower than that in joint fluid. With current methods, there seems to be little if any role for PCR in the detection of *B. burgdorferi* DNA in blood or urine samples, although this is an area of active research. A potential drawback is that PCR must be carefully controlled to prevent contamination.

Because of the problems associated with direct detection of *B. burgdorferi*, Lyme disease is usually diagnosed by the recognition of a characteristic clinical picture accompanied by serologic confirmation. Although serologic testing may yield negative results during the first several weeks of infection, almost all patients have a positive antibody response to *B. burgdorferi* after that time when a two-test approach of enzyme-linked immunosorbent assay (ELISA) and Western blot or a protocol of two enzyme immunoassays (EIAs) is used. The limitation of serologic tests is that they do not clearly distinguish between active and inactive infection. After antibiotic therapy, the amount of antibody declines but the results of Western blot, a nonquantitative test, do not change much (or very slowly). Thus, patients with previous Lyme disease—particularly in cases progressing to late stages—often remain seropositive for years, even after adequate antibiotic therapy. In addition, ~10% of patients are seropositive because of asymptomatic infection. If individuals with past or asymptomatic *B. burgdorferi* infection subsequently develop another illness, the positive serologic test for Lyme disease may cause diagnostic confusion. According to an algorithm published by the American College of Physicians (**Table 186-1**), serologic testing for Lyme disease is recommended only for patients with at least an intermediate pretest probability of Lyme disease, such as those with oligoarticular arthritis. It should not be used as a screening procedure in patients with pain or fatigue syndromes. In such patients, the probability of a false-positive serologic result is higher than that of a true-positive result.

For serologic analysis of Lyme disease in the United States, the CDC recommends a two-step approach in which samples are first tested by ELISA, and equivocal or positive results are then tested by Western blot. This is called the conventional two-test approach. During the first weeks of infection, both IgM and IgG responses to the spirochete should be determined, preferably in both acute- and convalescent-phase serum samples. Approximately 20–30% of patients have a

TABLE 186-1 Algorithm for Testing for and Treating Lyme Disease

PRETEST PROBABILITY	EXAMPLE	RECOMMENDATION
High	Patients with erythema migrans	Empirical antibiotic treatment without serologic testing
Intermediate	Patients with oligoarticular arthritis	Serologic testing and antibiotic treatment if test results are positive
Low	Patients with nonspecific symptoms (myalgias, arthralgias, fatigue)	Neither serologic testing nor antibiotic treatment

Source: Adapted from the recommendations of the American College of Physicians (G Nichol et al: Ann Intern Med 128:37, 1998).

positive response detectable in acute-phase samples (usually only a positive IgM response), whereas ~70–80% have a positive response during convalescence (2–4 weeks later). After 4–8 weeks of infection (by which time most patients with active Lyme disease have disseminated infection), the sensitivity and specificity of the IgG response to the spirochete are both very high—in the range of 99%—as determined by the two-test approach of ELISA and Western blot. At this point and thereafter, a single test (that for IgG) is usually sufficient. In persons with illness of >2 months' duration, a positive IgM test result alone is likely to be false-positive and therefore should not be used to support the diagnosis.

According to current criteria adopted by the CDC, an IgM Western blot is considered positive if two of the following three bands are present: 23, 39, and 41 kDa. However, the combination of two such bands may still represent a false-positive result. Misuse or misinterpretation of IgM blots has been a factor in the incorrect diagnosis of Lyme disease in patients with other illnesses. An IgG blot is considered positive if 5 of the following 10 bands are present: 18, 23, 28, 30, 39, 41, 45, 58, 66, and 93 kDa. In European cases, no single set of criteria for the interpretation of immunoblots results in high levels of sensitivity and specificity in all countries.

A new methodology called the modified two-test approach, which is now approved by the U.S. Food and Drug Administration, is a two-test approach using two EIAs, thereby dispensing with the Western blot. One such method employs a whole–*B. burgdorferi* sonicate ELISA followed by a VlsE C6 peptide IgG ELISA. This approach, which gives simply a positive or a negative result, increases sensitivity during the first several weeks of infection without compromising specificity. For more complex cases or in those with late infection, it is still valuable to determine antibody specificities to multiple spirochetal proteins, as is done with Western blots. More recently, line immunoblots or other multiplexed antibody platforms have been developed as substitutes for Western blots. These assays allow more objective interpretation, and some platforms can provide quantitative data about antibody responses to many spirochetal proteins. After successful antibiotic treatment, antibody titers decline slowly, but responses (including that to the VlsE C6 peptide) may persist for years. Moreover, not only the IgG but also the IgM response may persist for years after therapy. Therefore, even a positive IgM response cannot be interpreted as confirmation of recent infection or reinfection unless the clinical picture is appropriate.

DIFFERENTIAL DIAGNOSIS

Classic EM is a slowly expanding erythema, often with partial central clearing. If the lesion expands little, it may represent the red papule of an uninfected tick bite. If the lesion expands rapidly, it may represent cellulitis (e.g., streptococcal cellulitis) or an allergic reaction, perhaps to tick saliva. Patients with secondary annular lesions may be thought to have erythema multiforme, but neither the development of blistering mucosal lesions nor the involvement of the palms or soles is a feature of *B. burgdorferi* infection. In the eastern United States, an EM-like skin lesion, sometimes with mild systemic symptoms, may be associated with *Amblyomma americanum* tick bites. However, the cause of this southern tick-associated rash illness (STARI) has not yet been identified. This tick may also transmit *Ehrlichia chaffeensis*, a rickettsial agent (**Chap. 187**).

As stated above, *I. scapularis* ticks in the United States may transmit not only *B. burgdorferi* but also *B. microti*, the red blood cell parasite causing babesiosis (**Chap. 225**); *A. phagocytophilum*, the agent of human granulocytotropic anaplasmosis (**Chap. 187**); *B. miyamotoi*, a relapsing fever spirochete (**Chap. 185**); *B. mayonii* and *Ehrlichia* species Wisconsin, newly recognized species that occur in the upper midwestern United States; or (rarely) Powassan encephalitis virus (the deer tick virus, which is closely related to European tick-borne encephalitis virus), which may cause fatal infection (**Chap. 209**). Although babesiosis and anaplasmosis are most often asymptomatic, infection with any of these agents may cause nonspecific systemic symptoms, particularly in the young or the elderly, and co-infected patients may have more severe or persistent symptoms than patients infected with a single agent. Standard blood counts may yield clues regarding the presence of co-infection with *Anaplasma* or *Babesia*. Anaplasmosis may cause leukopenia or thrombocytopenia, and babesiosis may cause thrombocytopenia or (in severe cases) hemolytic anemia. IgM serologic responses may confuse the diagnosis. For example, *A. phagocytophilum* may elicit a positive IgM response to *B. burgdorferi*. The frequency of co-infection in different studies has been variable. In one prospective study, 4% of patients with EM had evidence of co-infection.

Facial palsy caused by *B. burgdorferi*, which occurs in the early disseminated phase of the infection (often in July, August, or September), is usually recognized by its association with EM. However, in rare cases, facial palsy without EM may be the presenting manifestation of Lyme disease. In such cases, both the IgM and the IgG responses to the spirochete are usually positive. The most common infectious agents that cause facial palsy are herpes simplex virus type 1 (Bell's palsy; **Chap. 192**) and varicella-zoster virus (Ramsay Hunt syndrome; **Chap. 193**).

Later in the infection, oligoarticular Lyme arthritis most resembles peripheral spondyloarthropathy in an adult or the pauciarticular form of juvenile idiopathic arthritis in a child. Patients with Lyme arthritis usually have the strongest IgG antibody responses seen in Lyme borreliosis, with reactivity to many spirochetal proteins.

The most common problem in diagnosis is to mistake Lyme disease for chronic fatigue syndrome (**Chap. 450**) or fibromyalgia (**Chap. 373**). This difficulty is compounded by the fact that a small percentage of patients do in fact develop these chronic pain or fatigue syndromes in association with or soon after Lyme disease. Moreover, a counterculture has emerged that ascribes pain and fatigue syndromes to chronic Lyme disease when there is little or no evidence of *B. burgdorferi* infection. In such cases, the term *chronic Lyme disease*, which is equated with chronic *B. burgdorferi* infection, is a misnomer, and the use of prolonged, dangerous, and expensive antibiotic treatment is not warranted.

TREATMENT
Lyme Borreliosis

ANTIBIOTIC TREATMENT

As outlined in the algorithm in **Fig. 186-2**, the various manifestations of Lyme disease can usually be treated successfully with orally administered antibiotics; the exceptions are severe objective neurologic abnormalities and third-degree atrioventricular heart block, which are generally treated with IV antibiotics, and arthritis that does not respond to oral therapy. For early Lyme disease, doxycycline is effective and can be administered to men and nonpregnant women. An advantage of this regimen is that it is also effective against *A. phagocytophilum*, *B. miyamotoi*, and *B. mayonii*, which are transmitted by the same tick that transmits the Lyme disease agent. Amoxicillin, cefuroxime axetil, and erythromycin or its congeners are second-, third-, and fourth-choice alternatives, respectively, for the treatment of Lyme disease. In children, amoxicillin is effective (not >2 g/d); in cases of penicillin allergy, cefuroxime axetil or erythromycin may be used. In contrast to second- or third-generation cephalosporin antibiotics, first-generation cephalosporins, such as cephalexin, are not effective. For patients with infection localized to the skin, a 14-day course of therapy is generally sufficient; in contrast, for patients with early disseminated infection, a 21-day course is recommended. Approximately 15% of patients experience a Jarisch-Herxheimer-like reaction during the first 24 h of therapy. In multicenter studies, >90% of patients whose early Lyme disease was treated with these regimens had satisfactory outcomes. Although some patients reported symptoms after treatment, objective evidence of persistent infection or relapse was rare, and re-treatment was usually unnecessary.

Oral administration of doxycycline or amoxicillin for 30 days is recommended for the initial treatment of Lyme arthritis in patients who do not have concomitant neurologic involvement. Among patients with arthritis who do not respond to oral

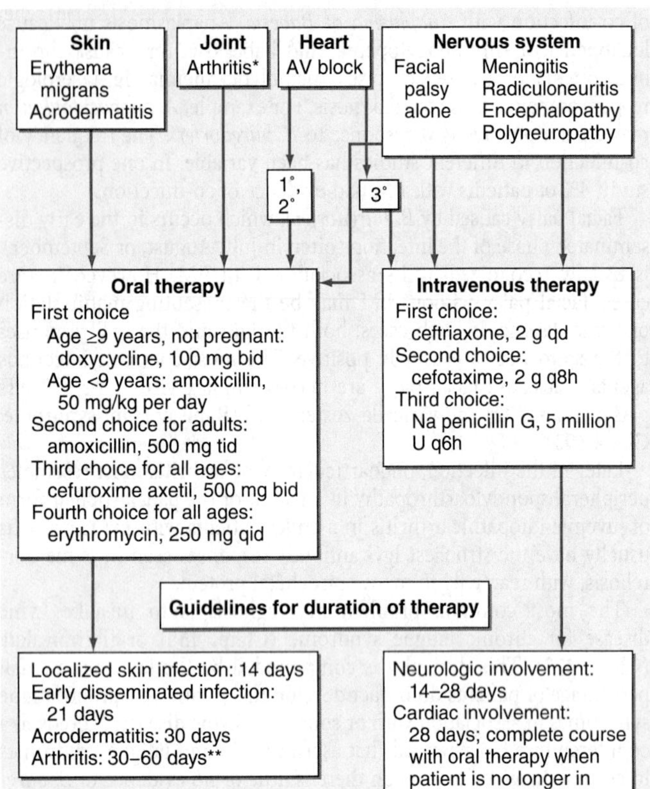

FIGURE 186-2 Algorithm for the treatment of the various early or late manifestations of Lyme borreliosis. AV, atrioventricular. *For arthritis, oral therapy should be tried first; if arthritis is unresponsive, IV therapy should be administered. **For Lyme arthritis, IV ceftriaxone (2 g given once a day for 14–28 days) also is effective and is necessary for patients who do not respond to oral therapy. However, compared with oral treatment, this regimen is less convenient to administer, has more side effects, and is more expensive.

antibiotics, re-treatment with IV ceftriaxone for 28 days is appropriate. In patients with arthritis in whom joint inflammation persists for months or even several years after both oral and IV antibiotics, treatment with nonsteroidal anti-inflammatory agents, therapy with disease-modifying antirheumatic drugs, or synovectomy may be successful.

In the United States, parenteral antibiotic therapy is usually used for severe objective neurologic abnormalities. Patients with such abnormalities are most commonly treated with IV ceftriaxone for 14–28 days, but IV cefotaxime or IV penicillin G for the same duration also may be effective. In Europe, similar results have been obtained with oral doxycycline and IV antibiotics in the treatment of acute neuroborreliosis. Although systematic trials have not been conducted in the United States, oral doxycycline is now used by some clinicians in this country for the treatment of patients with less severe neurologic abnormalities, such as facial palsy alone or uncomplicated Lyme meningitis. In patients with high-degree atrioventricular block or a PR interval of >0.3 s, IV therapy for at least part of the course and cardiac monitoring are recommended, but the insertion of a permanent pacemaker is not necessary.

It is unclear how and whether asymptomatic infection should be treated, but patients with such infection are often given a course of oral antibiotics. Because maternal–fetal transmission of *B. burgdorferi* seems to occur rarely (if at all), standard therapy for the manifestations of the illness is recommended for pregnant women. Long-term persistence of *B. burgdorferi* has not been documented in any large series of patients after treatment with currently recommended regimens. Although an occasional patient requires a second course of antibiotics, there is no indication for multiple, repeated antibiotic courses in the treatment of Lyme disease.

CHRONIC LYME DISEASE

After appropriately treated Lyme disease, a small percentage of patients continue to have subjective symptoms, primarily musculoskeletal pain, neurocognitive difficulties, or fatigue. This *chronic Lyme disease* or *post-Lyme syndrome* is sometimes a disabling condition that is similar to chronic fatigue syndrome or fibromyalgia. Five double-blind, placebo-controlled trials conducted in the United States and Europe have failed to show benefit of further antibiotic therapy in these patients. For example, in a large study, one group of patients with post-Lyme syndrome received IV ceftriaxone for 30 days followed by oral doxycycline for 60 days, while another group received IV and oral placebo preparations for the same durations. No significant differences were found between groups in the numbers of patients reporting that their symptoms had improved, become worse, or stayed the same. Such patients are best treated for the relief of symptoms rather than with prolonged courses of antibiotics.

PROPHYLAXIS AFTER A TICK BITE

The risk of infection with *B. burgdorferi* after a recognized tick bite is so low that antibiotic prophylaxis is not routinely indicated. However, if an attached, engorged *I. scapularis* nymph is found or if follow-up is anticipated to be difficult, a single 200-mg dose of doxycycline, which usually prevents Lyme disease when given within 72 h after the tick bite, may be administered.

PROGNOSIS

The response to treatment is best early in the disease. Later treatment of Lyme borreliosis is still effective, but the period of convalescence may be longer. Eventually, most patients recover with minimal or no residual deficits.

REINFECTION

Reinfection may occur after EM when patients are treated with antimicrobial agents. In such cases, the immune response is not adequate to provide protection from subsequent infection. However, patients who develop an expanded immune response to the spirochete over a period of months (e.g., those with Lyme arthritis) have protective immunity for a period of years and rarely, if ever, acquire the infection again.

PREVENTION

Protective measures for the prevention of Lyme disease may include the avoidance of tick-infested areas, the use of repellents and acaricides, tick checks, and modification of landscapes in or near residential areas. Although a vaccine for Lyme disease used to be available, the manufacturer has discontinued its production. Another company is planning testing of a similar vaccine in both the United States and Europe. However, no vaccine is currently available commercially for the prevention of this infection.

FURTHER READING

Arvikar SL, Steere AC: Diagnosis and treatment of Lyme arthritis. Infect Dis Clin North Am 29:269, 2015.

Aucott JN: Posttreatment Lyme disease syndrome. Infect Dis Clin North Am 29:309, 2015.

Branda JA, Steere AC: Laboratory diagnosis of Lyme borreliosis. Clin Micro Rev 34:e00018, 2021.

Branda JA et al: Two-tiered antibody testing for Lyme disease with use of 2 enzyme immunoassays, a whole-cell sonicate enzyme immunoassay followed by a VlsE C6 peptide enzyme immunoassay. Clin Infect Dis 53:541, 2011.

Klempner MS et al: Two controlled trials of antibiotic treatment in patients with persistent symptoms and a history of Lyme disease. N Engl J Med 345:85, 2001.

Lantos PM et al: Clinical practice guidelines by the Infectious Diseases Society of America (IDSA), American Academy of Neurology, and the American College of Rheumatology (ACR): 2020 guidelines for the prevention, diagnosis, and treatment of Lyme disease. Clin Infect Dis 72:1, 2021.

Li X et al: Burden and viability of *Borrelia burgdorferi* in skin or joints of patients with erythema migrans or Lyme arthritis. Arthritis Rheum 63:2238, 2011.
Lochhead RB et al: Robust interferon signature and suppressed tissue repair gene expression in synovial tissue from patients with postinfectious, *Borrelia burgdorferi*-induced Lyme arthritis. Cell Microbiol 21:e12954, 2019.
Oschmann P et al: Stages and syndromes of neuroborreliosis. J Neurol 245:262, 1998.
Steere AC: Lyme disease. N Engl J Med 345:115, 2001.
Steere AC: Posttreatment Lyme disease syndromes: Distinct pathogenesis caused by maladaptive host responses. J Clin Invest 130:2148, 2020.
Steere AC et al: Prospective study of serologic tests for Lyme disease. Clin Infect Dis 47:188, 2008.
Steere AC et al: Lyme borreliosis. Nat Rev Dis Primers 2:16090, 2016.

Section 10 Diseases Caused by Rickettsiae, Mycoplasmas, and Chlamydiae

187 Rickettsial Diseases

David H. Walker, J. Stephen Dumler, Lucas S. Blanton, Chantal P. Bleeker-Rovers

Rickettsiae are a heterogeneous group of small, obligately intracellular, gram-negative coccobacilli and short bacilli, most of which are transmitted by a tick, mite, flea, or louse vector. Except in the case of louse-borne typhus, humans are incidental hosts. Among rickettsiae, *Coxiella burnetii*, *Rickettsia prowazekii*, and *Rickettsia typhi* have the well-documented ability to survive for an extended period outside the reservoir or vector and to be extremely infectious: inhalation of a single *Coxiella* microorganism can cause pneumonia. High-level infectivity and severe illness after inhalation make *R. prowazekii*, *R. rickettsii*, *R. typhi*, *R. conorii*, and *C. burnetii* bioterrorism threats (**Chap. S3**).

Clinical infections with rickettsiae can be classified according to (1) the taxonomy and diverse microbial characteristics of the agents, which belong to seven genera (*Rickettsia*, *Orientia*, *Ehrlichia*, *Anaplasma*, *Neorickettsia*, "*Candidatus* Neoehrlichia," and *Coxiella*); (2) epidemiology; or (3) clinical manifestations. The clinical manifestations of all the acute presentations are similar during the first 5 days: fever, headache, and myalgias with or without nausea, vomiting, and cough. As the course progresses, clinical manifestations—including a macular, maculopapular, or vesicular rash; eschar; pneumonitis; and meningoencephalitis—vary from one disease to another. Given the many etiologic agents with varied mechanisms of transmission, geographic distributions, and associated disease manifestations, the consideration of rickettsial diseases as a single entity poses complex challenges (**Table 187-1**).

Establishing the etiologic diagnosis of rickettsioses is very difficult during the acute stage of illness, and definitive diagnosis usually requires the examination of serum samples during the acute and convalescent phases of illness. Heightened clinical suspicion is based on epidemiologic data, history of exposure to vectors or reservoir animals, travel to endemic locations, clinical manifestations (sometimes including rash or eschar), and characteristic laboratory findings (including thrombocytopenia, normal or low white blood cell [WBC] counts, elevated hepatic enzyme levels, and hyponatremia). Such suspicion should prompt empirical treatment. Doxycycline is the empirical drug of choice for most of these infections. Only one agent, *C. burnetii*, has been documented to cause chronic illness. One other species, *R. prowazekii*, causes recrudescent illness (Brill-Zinsser disease) when latent infection is reactivated years after resolution of the acute illness.

Rickettsial infections dominated by fever may resolve without further clinical evolution. However, after nonspecific early manifestations, the illnesses can also evolve along one or more of several principal clinical lines: (1) development of a macular or maculopapular rash; (2) development of an eschar at the site of tick or mite feeding, which can occur during the incubation period; (3) development of a vesicular rash (often in rickettsialpox, *R. parkeri* infection and African tick-bite fever); (4) development of pneumonitis with chest radiographic opacities and/or rales (Q fever and severe cases of Rocky Mountain spotted fever [RMSF], Mediterranean spotted fever [MSF], louse-borne typhus, human monocytotropic ehrlichiosis [HME], human granulocytotropic anaplasmosis [HGA], scrub typhus, and murine typhus); (5) development of meningoencephalitis (louse-borne typhus and severe cases of RMSF, scrub typhus, HME, murine typhus, MSF, and [rarely] Q fever); and (6) progressive hypotension and multiorgan failure as seen with sepsis or toxic shock syndromes (RMSF, MSF, louse-borne typhus, murine typhus, scrub typhus, HME, HGA, and neoehrlichiosis).

Epidemiologic clues to the transmission of a particular pathogen include (1) environmental exposure to ticks, fleas, or mites during the season of activity of the vector species for the disease in the appropriate geographic region (spotted fever and typhus rickettsioses, scrub typhus, ehrlichiosis, anaplasmosis); (2) travel to or residence in an endemic geographic region during the incubation period (Table 187-1); (3) exposure to parturient ruminants, cats, and dogs (Q fever); (4) exposure to flying squirrels (*R. prowazekii* infection); and (5) history of previous louse-borne typhus (recrudescent typhus).

Clinical laboratory findings such as thrombocytopenia (particularly in spotted fever and typhus rickettsioses, ehrlichiosis, anaplasmosis, and scrub typhus), normal or low WBC counts, mild to moderate serum elevations of hepatic aminotransferases, and hyponatremia suggest some common pathophysiologic mechanisms.

Application of these clinical, epidemiologic, and laboratory principles requires consideration of a rickettsial diagnosis and knowledge of the individual diseases.

TICK-, MITE-, LOUSE-, AND FLEA-BORNE RICKETTSIOSES

These diseases, caused by organisms of the genera *Rickettsia* and *Orientia* in the family Rickettsiaceae, result from endothelial cell infection and increased vascular permeability. Pathogenic rickettsial species are very closely related, have small genomes (as a result of reductive evolution, which eliminated many genes for biosynthesis of intracellularly available molecules), and are traditionally separated into typhus and spotted fever groups on the basis of lipopolysaccharide antigens. Some diseases and their agents (e.g., *R. africae*, *R. parkeri*, and *R. sibirica*) are too similar to require separate descriptions. Indeed, the similarities among MSF (*R. conorii* [all strains] and *R. massiliae*), North Asian tick typhus (*R. sibirica*), Japanese spotted fever (*R. japonica*), and Flinders Island spotted fever (*R. honei*) far outweigh their minor variations. The Rickettsiaceae that cause life-threatening infections are, in order of decreasing case–fatality rate, *R. rickettsii* (RMSF); *R. prowazekii* (louse-borne typhus); *Orientia tsutsugamushi* (scrub typhus); *R. conorii* (MSF); *R. typhi* (murine typhus); and, in rare cases, other spotted fever–group (SFG) organisms. Some agents (e.g., *R. parkeri*, *R. africae*, *Rickettsia* 364D, *R. akari*, *R. slovaca*, *R. honei*, *R. felis*, *R. massiliae*, *R. helvetica*, *R. heilongjiangensis*, *R. aeschlimannii*, and *R. monacensis*) have never been documented to cause a fatal illness. The most prevalent SFG rickettsia in the United States, *R. amblyommatis*, has been circumstantially associated with asymptomatic seroconversion in most persons and with self-limited illness in others.

ROCKY MOUNTAIN SPOTTED FEVER

Epidemiology RMSF occurs in 47 states (with the highest prevalence in the south-central and southeastern states) as well as in Canada, Mexico, and Central and South America. The infection is transmitted by *Dermacentor variabilis*, the American dog tick, in the

TABLE 187-1 Features of Selected Rickettsial Infections

DISEASE	ORGANISM	TRANSMISSION	GEOGRAPHIC RANGE	INCUBATION PERIOD, DAYS	DURATION, DAYS	RASH, %	ESCHAR, %	LYMPHADENOPATHY[a]
Rocky Mountain spotted fever	*Rickettsia rickettsii*	Tick bite: *Dermacentor andersoni, D. variabilis*	United States	2–14	10–20	90	<1	+
		Amblyomma cajennense sensu lato, *A. aureolatum*	Central/South America					
		Rhipicephalus sanguineus	Mexico, Brazil, United States					
Mediterranean spotted fever	*R. conorii*	Tick bite: *R. sanguineus, R. pumilio*	Southern Europe, Africa, Middle East, central Asia	5–7	7–14	97	50	+
African tick-bite fever	*R. africae*	Tick bite: *A. hebraeum, A. variegatum*	Sub-Saharan Africa, West Indies	4–10	4–19	50	90	+++
Maculatum disease	*R. parkeri*	Tick bite: *A. maculatum, A. triste, A. tigrinum, A. ovale*	United States, South America	2–10	6–16	88	94	++
Pacific Coast tick fever	*Rickettsia* 364D	Tick bite: *D. occidentalis*	United States	3–9	5–14	14	100	+++
Rickettsialpox	*R. akari*	Mite bite: *Liponyssoides sanguineus*	United States, Ukraine, Turkey, Mexico, Croatia	10–17	3–11	100	90	+++
Tick-borne lymphadenopathy	*R. slovaca*	Tick bite: *D. marginatus, D. reticularis*	Europe	7–9	17–180	5	100	++++
Flea-borne spotted fever	*R. felis*	Flea (mechanism undetermined): *Ctenocephalides felis*	Worldwide	8–16	8–16	80	15	—
Epidemic typhus	*R. prowazekii*	Louse feces: *Pediculus humanus humanus*, fleas and lice of flying squirrels, or recrudescence	Worldwide	7–14	10–18	80	None	—
Murine typhus	*R. typhi*	Flea feces: *Xenopsylla cheopis, C. felis*, others	Worldwide	8–16	9–18	80	None	—
Human monocytotropic ehrlichiosis	*Ehrlichia chaffeensis*	Tick bite: *A. americanum, D. variabilis*	United States	1–21	3–21	26	None	++
Ewingii ehrlichiosis	*E. ewingii*	Tick bite: *A. americanum*	United States	1–21	4–21	0	None	
Unnamed ehrlichiosis	*E. muris* ssp. *eauclairensis*	Tick bite: *Ixodes scapularis*	United States	Unknown	3–14	12	None	
Human granulocytotropic anaplasmosis	*Anaplasma phagocytophilum*	Tick bite: *I. scapularis, I. ricinus, I. pacificus, I. persulcatus, Haemaphysalis concinna*	United States, Europe, Asia	4–8	3–14	Rare	None	—
Unnamed disease	*A. capra*	*I. persulcatus*	Northeastern China, France	Unknown	11–21	17	9	+
Neoehrlichiosis	"*Candidatus* Neoehrlichia mikurensis"	Tick bite: *I. ricinus, I. persulcatus, Haemaphysalis concinna*	Europe, China	≥8	11–75	10	None	
Scrub typhus	*Orientia tsutsugamushi*	Mite bite: *Leptotrombidium deliense*, others	Asia, Australia, Pacific and Indian Ocean islands	9–18	6–21	50	35	+++
Q fever	*Coxiella burnetii*	Inhalation of aerosols of infected parturition material (goats, sheep, cattle, cats, others), ingestion of infected milk or milk products	Worldwide except New Zealand, Antarctica	3–30	5–57	<1	None	—

[a]++++, severe; +++, marked; ++, moderate; +, present in a small proportion of cases; —, not a noted feature.

eastern two-thirds of the United States and California; by *D. andersoni*, the Rocky Mountain wood tick, in the western United States; by *Rhipicephalus sanguineus*, the brown dog tick, in Mexico, Arizona, and probably Brazil; and by *Amblyomma sculptum, A. mixtum, A. patinoi, A. cajennense, A. tonelliae*, and *A. aureolatum* in Central and/or South America. Maintained partially by transovarian transmission from one generation of ticks to the next, *R. rickettsii* can be acquired by uninfected ticks through the ingestion of a blood meal from rickettsemic small mammals or by co-feeding adjacent to an infected tick.

Humans become infected during tick season (in the Northern Hemisphere, from April to September), although some cases occur in winter. The mortality rate was 20–25% in the preantibiotic era and has been reported at ~3–5% in the postantibiotic era, principally because of delayed diagnosis and treatment. Recent reporting of a relatively low mortality rate (0.4%) for spotted fever rickettsiosis is likely an artifact related to the abundance of less pathogenic SFG rickettsial species and to a relatively low proportion of diagnostically confirmed cases. Indeed, the reported case-fatality rates in confirmed cases in the United States and in parts of Arizona, where *R. rickettsii* is the sole infecting SFG species, are 9% and 10%, respectively. The case-fatality rate is highest among children (<10 years of age) and in the later decades of life (>70 years). For unknown reasons, the case-fatality rate of RMSF in Mexico and Brazil approaches 50%.

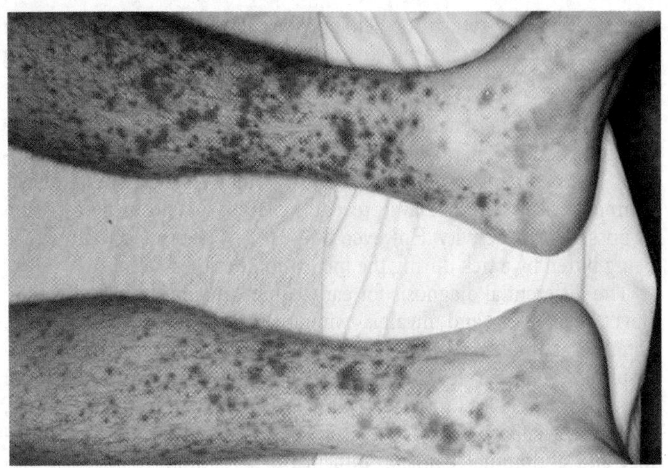

FIGURE 187-1 ***A.*** Petechial lesions of Rocky Mountain spotted fever on the lower legs and soles of a young, previously healthy patient. ***B.*** Close-up of lesions from the same patient. *(Photos courtesy of Dr. Lindsey Baden; with permission.)*

Pathogenesis *R. rickettsii* organisms are inoculated into the dermis along with secretions of the tick's salivary glands after ≥6 h of feeding. The rickettsiae spread lymphohematogenously throughout the body and infect numerous foci of contiguous endothelial cells. The dose-dependent incubation period is ~1 week (range, 2–14 days). Occlusive thrombosis and ischemic necrosis are not the fundamental pathologic bases for tissue and organ injury. Instead, increased vascular permeability, with resulting edema, hypovolemia, and ischemia, is responsible. Consumption of platelets results in thrombocytopenia in 32–52% of patients, but disseminated intravascular coagulation (DIC) with hypofibrinogenemia is rare. Activation of platelets, generation of thrombin, and activation of the fibrinolytic system all appear to be homeostatic physiologic responses to endothelial injury by nonocclusive hemostatic plugs.

Clinical Manifestations Early in the illness, when medical attention usually is first sought, RMSF is difficult to distinguish from many self-limiting viral illnesses. Fever, headache, malaise, myalgia, nausea, vomiting, and anorexia are the most common symptoms during the first 3 days. The patient becomes progressively more ill as vascular infection and injury advance. In one large series, only one-third of patients were diagnosed with presumptive RMSF early in the clinical course and treated appropriately as outpatients. In the tertiary-care setting, RMSF is all too often recognized only when late severe manifestations, developing at the end of the first week or during the second week of illness in patients without appropriate treatment, prompt return to a physician or hospital and admission to an intensive care unit.

The progressive nature of the infection is clearly manifested in the skin. Rash is evident in only 14% of patients on the first day of illness and in only 49% during the first 3 days. Macules (1–5 mm) appear first on the wrists and ankles and then on the remainder of the extremities and the trunk. Later, more severe vascular damage results in frank hemorrhage at the center of the maculopapule, producing a petechia that does not disappear upon compression (**Fig. 187-1**). This sequence of events is sometimes delayed or aborted by effective treatment. However, the rash is a variable manifestation, appearing on day 6 or later in 20% of cases and not appearing at all in 9–16% of cases. Petechiae occur in 41–59% of cases, appearing on or after day 6 in 74% of cases that manifest a rash. Involvement of the palms and soles, often considered diagnostically important, usually develops relatively late in the course (after day 5 in 43% of cases) and does not develop at all in 18–64% of cases.

Hypovolemia leads to prerenal azotemia and (in 17% of cases) hypotension. Infection of the pulmonary microcirculation leads to noncardiogenic pulmonary edema; 12% of patients have acute respiratory distress syndrome, and 8% require mechanical ventilation. Cardiac involvement manifests as dysrhythmia in 7–16% of cases.

Besides respiratory failure, central nervous system (CNS) involvement is the other important determinant of the outcome of RMSF. Encephalitis, presenting as confusion or lethargy, is apparent in 26–28% of cases. Progressively severe encephalitis manifests as stupor or delirium in 21–26% of cases, ataxia in 18%, coma in 10%, and seizures in 8%. Numerous focal neurologic deficits have been reported. Meningoencephalitis results in cerebrospinal fluid (CSF) pleocytosis in 34–38% of cases; usually there are 10–100 cells/μL and a mononuclear predominance, but occasionally there are >100 cells/μL and a polymorphonuclear predominance. The CSF protein concentration is increased in 30–35% of cases, but the CSF glucose concentration is usually normal.

Acute kidney injury, often reversible with rehydration, is caused by acute tubular necrosis in severe cases with shock. Hepatic injury with increased serum aminotransferase concentrations (38% of cases) is due to multifocal death of individual hepatocytes without hepatic failure. Jaundice is recognized in 9% of cases and an elevated serum bilirubin concentration in 18–30%.

Life-threatening bleeding is rare. Anemia develops in 30% of cases and is severe enough to require transfusions in 11%. Blood is detected in the stool or vomitus of 10% of patients, and death has followed massive upper-gastrointestinal hemorrhage.

Other characteristic clinical laboratory findings include increased plasma levels of proteins of the acute-phase response (C-reactive protein, fibrinogen, ferritin, and others), hypoalbuminemia, and hyponatremia (in 56% of cases) due to the appropriate secretion of antidiuretic hormone in response to the hypovolemic state. Myositis occurs occasionally, with marked elevations in serum creatine kinase levels and multifocal rhabdomyonecrosis. Ocular involvement includes conjunctivitis in 30% of cases and retinal vein engorgement, flame hemorrhages, arterial occlusion, and papilledema with normal CSF pressure in some instances.

Severe RMSF can present as sepsis or septic shock. In untreated fatal cases, death occurs 8–15 days after onset. A rare presentation, fulminant RMSF, is fatal within 5 days after onset. This fulminant presentation is seen most often in male black patients with glucose-6-phosphate dehydrogenase (G6PD) deficiency and may be related to an undefined effect of hemolysis on the rickettsial infection. Although survivors of RMSF usually return to their previous state of health, permanent sequelae, including neurologic deficits and gangrene necessitating amputation of extremities, may follow severe illness.

Diagnosis The diagnosis of RMSF during the acute stage is more difficult than is generally appreciated. The most important epidemiologic factor is a history of exposure to a potentially tick-infested environment within the 14 days preceding disease onset during a season of possible tick activity. However, only 60% of patients actually recall being bitten by a tick during the incubation period.

The differential diagnosis for early clinical manifestations of RMSF (fever, headache, and myalgia without a rash) includes influenza, enteroviral infection, infectious mononucleosis, viral hepatitis, leptospirosis, typhoid fever, gram-negative or gram-positive bacterial sepsis, HME, HGA, murine typhus, sylvatic flying-squirrel typhus, and rickettsialpox. Enterocolitis may be suggested by nausea, vomiting, and abdominal pain; prominence of abdominal tenderness has resulted in exploratory laparotomy. CNS involvement can masquerade as bacterial or viral meningoencephalitis. Cough, pulmonary signs, and chest radiographic opacities can lead to a diagnostic consideration of bronchitis or pneumonia.

At presentation during the first 3 days of illness, only 3% of patients exhibit the classic triad of fever, rash, and history of tick exposure. When a rash appears, a diagnosis of RMSF should be considered. However, many illnesses considered in the differential diagnosis also can be associated with a rash, including rubeola, rubella, meningococcemia, disseminated gonococcal infection, secondary syphilis, toxic shock syndrome, drug hypersensitivity, immune thrombocytopenic purpura, thrombotic thrombocytopenic purpura, Kawasaki syndrome, and immune complex vasculitis. Conversely, any person in an endemic area with a provisional diagnosis of one of the above illnesses could have RMSF. Thus, if a viral infection is suspected during RMSF season in an endemic area, it should always be kept in mind that RMSF can mimic viral infection early in the course; if the illness worsens over the next couple of days after initial presentation, the patient should return for reevaluation.

The most common serologic test for confirmation of the diagnosis is the indirect immunofluorescence assay. Not until 7–10 days after onset is a reactive titer of ≥64 first detectable. The sensitivity and specificity of the indirect immunofluorescence IgG assay are 89–100% and 99–100%, respectively. Detection of IgM is no more sensitive in early illness and is subject to nonspecific cross-reactivity. It is important to understand that serologic tests for RMSF are usually negative at the time of presentation for medical care and that treatment should not be delayed while a positive serologic result is awaited.

The only diagnostic test that has proven useful during the acute illness is immunohistologic examination of a cutaneous biopsy sample from a rash lesion for *R. rickettsii*. Examination of a 3-mm punch biopsy from such a lesion is 70% sensitive and 100% specific, and polymerase chain reaction (PCR) on a rash biopsy would likely yield even higher sensitivity. PCR amplification for detection of *R. rickettsii* DNA in peripheral blood is not adequately sensitive. Although rickettsiae are present in large quantities in heavily infected foci of endothelial cells, there are relatively low quantities in the circulation. Cultivation of rickettsiae in cell culture is feasible but is seldom undertaken because of technical difficulty and biohazard concerns. The recent dramatic increase in the reported incidence of RMSF correlates with the use of single-titer SFG cross-reactive enzyme immunoassay serology. Few cases are specifically determined to be caused by *R. rickettsii*. Currently, many febrile persons who do not have RMSF present with cross-reactive antibodies, possibly because of previous exposure to the highly prevalent SFG rickettsia *R. amblyommatis*.

TREATMENT

Rocky Mountain Spotted Fever

The drug of choice for the treatment of both children and adults with RMSF is doxycycline. Because of the severity of RMSF, immediate empirical administration of doxycycline should be strongly considered for any patient with a consistent clinical presentation in the appropriate epidemiologic setting. Doxycycline is administered orally (or, with coma or vomiting, intravenously) at 100 mg twice daily. For children with suspected RMSF, up to five courses of doxycycline may be administered with minimal risk of dental staining. In patients with allergy to doxycycline, desensitization should be considered. Once considered an alternative during pregnancy, chloramphenicol is not readily available in the United States. Although available in much of the world, it is less effective than doxycycline. Fortunately, there is little evidence to support the occurrence of tetracycline-associated adverse events in mothers (hepatotoxicity) and fetuses (staining of deciduous teeth and teratogenicity) who receive doxycycline. The antirickettsial drug should be administered until the patient is afebrile and improving clinically—usually 3–5 days after defervescence. β-Lactam antibiotics, erythromycin, and aminoglycosides have no role in the treatment of RMSF, and sulfa-containing drugs are associated with more adverse outcomes than no treatment at all. There is little clinical experience with fluoroquinolones, clarithromycin, and azithromycin, which are not recommended. The most seriously ill patients are managed in intensive care units, with careful administration of fluids to achieve optimal tissue perfusion without precipitating noncardiogenic pulmonary edema. In some severely ill patients, hypoxemia requires intubation and mechanical ventilation; oliguric or anuric acute renal failure requires renal replacement therapy; seizures necessitate the use of antiseizure medication; anemia or severe hemorrhage necessitates transfusions of packed red blood cells; or bleeding with severe thrombocytopenia requires platelet transfusions.

Prevention Avoidance of tick bites is the only available preventive approach. Use of protective clothing and tick repellents, inspection of the body once or twice a day, and removal of ticks before they inoculate rickettsiae reduce the risk of infection. Prophylactic doxycycline treatment of tick bites has no proven role in preventing RMSF.

MEDITERRANEAN SPOTTED FEVER (BOUTONNEUSE FEVER), AFRICAN TICK-BITE FEVER, AND OTHER TICK-BORNE SPOTTED FEVERS

Epidemiology and Clinical Manifestations *R. conorii* is prevalent in southern Europe, Africa, and southwestern and south-central Asia. The disease is characterized by high fever, rash, and—in most geographic locales—an inoculation eschar (*tâche noire*) that appears before the onset of fever at the site of the tick bite. A severe form of the disease (mortality rate, 50%) occurs in patients with diabetes, alcoholism, or heart failure.

African tick-bite fever, caused by *R. africae*, occurs in rural areas of sub-Saharan Africa and in the Caribbean islands and is transmitted by *Amblyomma hebraeum* and *A. variegatum* ticks. The average incubation period is 4–10 days. The mild illness consists of headache, fever, eschar, and regional lymphadenopathy. *Amblyomma* ticks, a high portion of which are infected with *R. africae*, often feed in groups, with the consequent development of multiple eschars. Rash may be vesicular, sparse, or absent altogether. Because of tourism in sub-Saharan Africa, African tick-bite fever is the rickettsiosis most frequently imported into Europe and North America. Maculatum disease, a similar disease caused by the closely related species *R. parkeri*, is transmitted by *A. maculatum* and found in a low percentage of *A. americanum* ticks in the United States. It is also transmitted by *A. triste* in South America and Arizona as well as *A. tigrinum* and *A. ovale* in South America.

R. japonica causes Japanese spotted fever, which also occurs in Korea and China. Similar diseases in northern Asia are caused by *R. sibirica* and *R. heilongjiangensis*. Queensland tick typhus due to *R. australis* is transmitted by *Ixodes holocyclus* ticks. Flinders Island spotted fever, found on the island for which it is named as well as in Tasmania, mainland Australia, and Asia, is caused by *R. honei*. In Europe, patients infected with *R. slovaca* after a wintertime *Dermacentor* tick bite usually manifest an afebrile illness with an eschar (usually on the scalp) and painful regional lymphadenopathy.

Diagnosis Diagnosis of these tick-borne spotted fevers is based on clinical and epidemiologic findings and is confirmed by serology, immunohistochemical demonstration of rickettsiae in skin biopsy specimens, cell-culture isolation of rickettsiae, or PCR of skin biopsy, eschar biopsy or swab, or blood samples. Serologic diagnosis detects antibodies to antigens shared among SFG rickettsiae, hindering identification of the etiologic species. In an endemic area, a possible diagnosis of rickettsial spotted fevers should be considered when patients present with fever, rash, and/or a skin lesion consisting of a black necrotic lesion or a crust surrounded by erythema.

TREATMENT
Tick-Borne Spotted Fevers

As with RMSF, severe cases should be treated with doxycycline (100 mg bid orally) for 3–5 days after defervescence. Alternative agents for milder disease include doxycycline (100 mg bid orally for 1–5 days), chloramphenicol (500 mg qid orally for 7–10 days), and ciprofloxacin (750 mg bid orally for 7 days). Pregnant patients may be treated with josamycin (3 g/d orally for 5 days) where available. Data on the efficacy of treatment of mildly ill children with clarithromycin or azithromycin should not be extrapolated to adults or to patients with moderate or severe illness.

■ RICKETTSIALPOX
R. akari infects mice and their mites (*Liponyssoides sanguineus*), which maintain the organisms by transovarial transmission.

Epidemiology Rickettsialpox is recognized principally in New York City, but cases have also been reported in other urban and rural locations in the United States and in Ukraine, Croatia, Mexico, and Turkey. Investigation of eschars suspected of representing bioterrorism-associated cutaneous anthrax revealed that rickettsialpox occurs more frequently than previously realized.

Clinical Manifestations A papule forms at the site of the mite's feeding, develops a central vesicle, and becomes a 1- to 2.5-cm painless black crusted eschar surrounded by an erythematous halo (**Fig. 187-2**). Enlargement of the regional lymph nodes draining the eschar suggests initial lymphogenous spread. After an incubation period of 10–17 days, during which the eschar and regional lymphadenopathy frequently go unnoticed, disease onset is marked by malaise, chills, fever, headache, and myalgia. A macular rash appears 2–6 days after onset and usually evolves sequentially into papules, vesicles, and crusts that heal without scarring (**Fig. 187-3**); in some cases, the rash remains macular or maculopapular. Some patients develop nausea, vomiting, abdominal pain, cough, conjunctivitis, or photophobia. Without treatment, fever lasts 6–10 days.

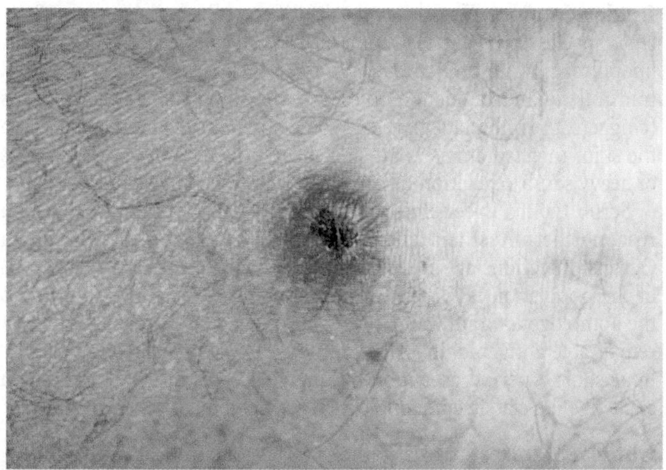

FIGURE 187-2 Eschar at the site of the mite bite in a patient with rickettsialpox. *(Reprinted from A Krusell et al: Emerg Infect Dis 8:727, 2002. Photo obtained by Dr. Kenneth Kaye.)*

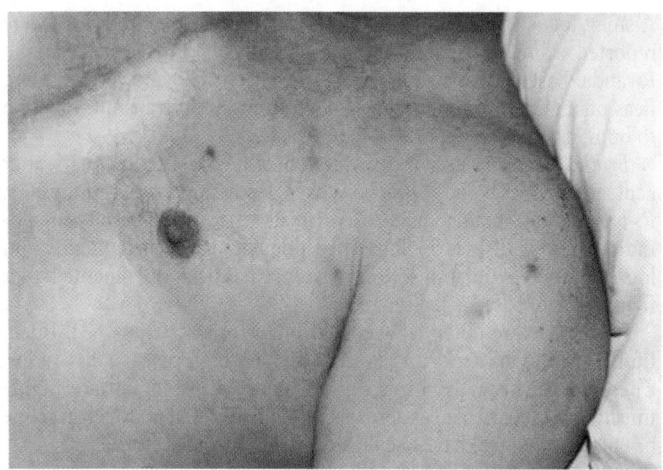

A

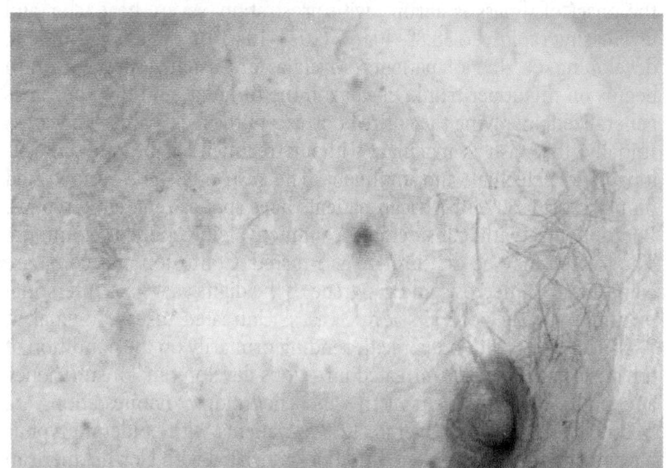

B

FIGURE 187-3 ***A.*** Papulovesicular lesions on the trunk of the patient with rickettsialpox shown in Fig. 187-2. ***B.*** Close-up of lesions from the same patient. *(Reprinted from A Krusell et al: Emerg Infect Dis 8:727, 2002. Photos obtained by Dr. Kenneth Kaye.)*

Diagnosis and Treatment Clinical, epidemiologic, and convalescent serologic data establish the diagnosis of an SFG rickettsiosis that is seldom pursued further. Doxycycline is the drug of choice for treatment.

■ FLEA-BORNE SPOTTED FEVER
Rickettsia felis is suspected to cause an emerging rickettsiosis worldwide. Maintained transovarially in the geographically widespread cat flea, *Ctenocephalides felis*, the infection has been described as moderately severe, with fever, rash, and headache as well as CNS, gastrointestinal, and pulmonary symptoms on the basis of PCR, which often detects organisms in healthy persons. Patient isolates and serologic support are lacking.

■ EPIDEMIC (LOUSE-BORNE) TYPHUS

Epidemiology The human body louse (*Pediculus humanus corporis*) lives in clothing under poor hygienic conditions and usually in impoverished cold areas. Lice acquire *R. prowazekii* when they ingest blood from a rickettsemic patient. The rickettsiae multiply in the louse's midgut epithelial cells and are shed in its feces. The infected louse leaves a febrile person and deposits infected feces on its subsequent host during its blood meal; the patient autoinoculates the organisms by scratching. The louse is killed by the rickettsiae and does not pass *R. prowazekii* to its offspring.

Epidemic typhus haunts regions afflicted by wars and disasters. An outbreak involved 100,000 people in refugee camps in Burundi in 1997.

A small focus was documented in Russia in 1998, sporadic cases were reported from Algeria, and frequent outbreaks occurred in Peru and Rwanda. Eastern flying squirrels (*Glaucomys volans*) and their lice and fleas maintain *R. prowazekii* in a zoonotic cycle and transmit infection to humans.

Brill-Zinsser disease is a recrudescent illness occurring years after acute epidemic typhus, probably as a result of waning immunity. *R. prowazekii* remains latent for years; its reactivation results in sporadic cases of disease in louse-free populations or in epidemics in louse-infested populations. Recrudescence has been documented after flying squirrel–associated typhus.

Rickettsiae are potential agents of bioterrorism (**Chap. S3**). Infections with *R. prowazekii* and *R. rickettsii* have high case–fatality ratios. These organisms cause difficult-to-diagnose diseases and are highly infectious when inhaled as aerosols. Organisms resistant to tetracycline or chloramphenicol have been developed in the laboratory.

Clinical Manifestations After an incubation period of ~1–2 weeks, the onset of illness is abrupt, with prostration, severe headache, and fever rising rapidly to 38.8°–40.0°C (102°–104°F). Cough is prominent, developing in 70% of patients. Myalgias are usually severe. A rash begins on the upper trunk, usually on the fifth day, and then becomes generalized, involving the entire body except the face, palms, and soles. Initially, this rash is macular; without treatment, it becomes maculopapular, petechial, and confluent. The rash often goes undetected on black skin; 60% of African patients have spotless epidemic typhus. Photophobia, with considerable conjunctival injection, is common. The tongue may be dry, brown, and furred. Confusion and coma are common. Skin necrosis and gangrene of the digits as well as interstitial pneumonia may occur in severe cases. Untreated disease is fatal in 7–40% of cases, with outcome depending primarily on the condition of the host. Patients with untreated infections develop renal insufficiency and multiorgan involvement in which neurologic manifestations are frequently prominent. Overall, 12% of patients with epidemic typhus have neurologic involvement. Infection associated with North American flying squirrels is a milder illness; whether this milder disease is due to host factors (e.g., better health status) or attenuated virulence is unknown.

Diagnosis and Treatment Epidemic typhus is sometimes misdiagnosed as typhoid fever in tropical countries (**Chap. 165**). The means even for serologic studies are often unavailable in settings of louse-borne typhus. Epidemics can be recognized by the serologic or immunohistochemical diagnosis of a single case or by detection of *R. prowazekii* in a louse found on a patient. Doxycycline (100 mg bid) is administered orally or—if the patient is comatose or vomiting—intravenously and continued until 3–5 days after defervescence. Under epidemic conditions, a single 200-mg oral dose can be tried but fails in some cases. Pregnant patients should be evaluated individually and treated with chloramphenicol early in pregnancy or with doxycycline late in pregnancy.

Prevention Prevention of epidemic typhus involves control of body lice. Clothes should regularly be changed and laundered in hot water, and insecticides can be used every 6 weeks to control the louse population.

■ ENDEMIC MURINE TYPHUS

Epidemiology *R. typhi* is maintained in mammalian host–flea cycles, with rats (*Rattus rattus* and *R. norvegicus*) and the Oriental rat flea (*Xenopsylla cheopis*) as the classic zoonotic niche. Fleas acquire *R. typhi* from rickettsemic rats and carry the organism throughout their life span. Nonimmune rats and humans are infected when rickettsia-laden flea feces contaminate pruritic bite lesions; less frequently, the flea bite transmits the organisms. Transmission can also occur via inhalation of aerosolized rickettsiae from flea feces. Infected rats appear healthy, although they are rickettsemic for ~2 weeks.

Murine typhus occurs mainly in Texas and southern California, where the classic rat–flea cycle is absent and an opossum–cat flea (*C. felis*) cycle is highly suspected. Globally, endemic typhus occurs mainly in warm (often coastal) areas throughout the tropics and subtropics, where it is highly prevalent though often unrecognized. The incidence peaks from April through July in Texas and during the warm months of summer and early fall in other geographic locations. Patients seldom recall exposure to fleas, although exposure to animals such as cats, opossums, and rats is reported in nearly 40% of cases.

Clinical Manifestations The incubation period of experimental murine typhus averages 11 days (range, 8–16 days). Headache, myalgia, arthralgia, nausea, and malaise develop 1–3 days before onset of chills and fever. Patients often experience nausea and vomiting.

The duration of untreated illness averages 12 days (range, 9–18 days). Rash occurs in approximately half of all patients. It is present in only 13% of patients at presentation for medical care (usually ~4 days after onset of fever), appearing an average of 2 days later in half of the remaining patients. The initial macular rash is often faint and detected by careful inspection of the axilla or the inner surface of the arm. Subsequently, the rash becomes maculopapular, involving the trunk more often than the extremities; it is seldom petechial and rarely involves the face, palms, or soles. A rash is detected in only 20% of patients with darkly pigmented skin.

Pulmonary involvement is frequently prominent; 35% of patients have a hacking, nonproductive cough, and 23% of patients who undergo chest radiography have pulmonary densities due to interstitial pneumonia, pulmonary edema, and pleural effusions. Bibasilar rales are the most common pulmonary sign. Less common clinical manifestations include abdominal pain, confusion, stupor, seizures, ataxia, coma, and jaundice. Clinical laboratory studies frequently reveal anemia and leukopenia early in the course, leukocytosis late in the course, thrombocytopenia, hyponatremia, hypoalbuminemia, increased serum levels of hepatic aminotransferases, and prerenal azotemia. Complications can include respiratory failure, hematemesis, cerebral hemorrhage, and hemolysis. Severe illness necessitates the admission of 10% of hospitalized patients to an intensive care unit. Greater severity is generally associated with old age, underlying disease, and treatment with a sulfonamide; the case–fatality rate is 1%.

Diagnosis and Treatment Serologic studies of acute- and convalescent-phase serum samples can provide a diagnosis, and an immunohistochemical method for identification of typhus group-specific antigens in biopsy samples has been developed. Cultivation is used infrequently and is not widely available. PCR of the blood is not adequately sensitive. When endemic typhus is suspected, patients should be treated empirically with doxycycline (100 mg twice daily by mouth for 7 days). Chloramphenicol, ciprofloxacin, and azithromycin are less effective alternatives.

■ SCRUB TYPHUS

Epidemiology *O. tsutsugamushi* differs substantially from *Rickettsia* species both genetically and in cell-wall composition (i.e., it lacks lipopolysaccharide). *O. tsutsugamushi* is maintained by transovarial transmission in trombiculid mites. After hatching, infected larval mites (chiggers, the only stage that feeds on a host) inoculate organisms into the skin. Infected chiggers are particularly likely to be found in areas of heavy scrub vegetation during the wet season, when mites lay eggs.

Scrub typhus is endemic and reemerging in eastern and southern Asia, northern Australia, and islands of the western Pacific and Indian Oceans. Infections are prevalent in these regions; in some areas, >3% of the population is infected or reinfected each month. Immunity to the homologous strain wanes over 1–3 years, and the organisms exhibit remarkable antigenic diversity with loss of cross-protective immunity in as short a period as 1 month. Emerging cases in Chile and Africa challenge the classic epidemiology of scrub typhus.

Clinical Manifestations Illness varies from mild and self-limiting to fatal. After an incubation period of 6–21 days, onset is characterized by fever, headache, myalgia, cough, and gastrointestinal symptoms. Some patients recover spontaneously after a few days. The classic case description includes an eschar where the chigger has fed, regional lymphadenopathy, and a maculopapular rash—signs that are seldom seen in indigenous patients. In fact, <50% of Westerners develop an eschar, and <40% develop a rash (on day 4–6 of illness). Severe cases typically manifest with encephalitis and interstitial pneumonia due to vascular injury. The case-fatality rate for untreated classic cases is 6% but would probably be lower if all mild cases were diagnosed.

Diagnosis and Treatment Serologic assays (indirect fluorescent antibody, indirect immunoperoxidase, and enzyme immunoassays) are the mainstays of laboratory diagnosis. PCR amplification of *Orientia* genes from eschars is effective, but less so for blood. Patients are treated with oral doxycycline (100 mg twice daily for 7–15 days), azithromycin (500 mg for 3 days), or chloramphenicol (500 mg four times daily for 7–15 days).

Some cases of scrub typhus in Thailand are poorly responsive to doxycycline or chloramphenicol but respond to azithromycin and rifampin.

EHRLICHIOSES AND ANAPLASMOSIS

Ehrlichioses are acute febrile infections caused by members of the family Anaplasmataceae, which is made up of obligately intracellular organisms of five genera: *Ehrlichia*, *Anaplasma*, *Wolbachia*, "*Candidatus* Neoehrlichia," and *Neorickettsia*. The bacteria reside in vertebrate reservoirs and target vacuoles of hematopoietic—and, for some species, endothelial—cells **(Fig. 187-4)**. Four *Ehrlichia* species, two *Anaplasma* species, and one *Neoehrlichia* species are transmitted by ticks to humans and cause infection that can be severe and prevalent. *E. chaffeensis*, the agent of HME, and *E. muris* subsp. *eauclairensis* infect predominantly mononuclear phagocytes; *E. ewingii* and *A. phagocytophilum* infect neutrophils. Infections with "*Candidatus* Neoehrlichia mikurensis" and *A. capra* are less well characterized but have been reported to grow in endothelium and human erythrocytes, respectively.

Ehrlichia, "*Candidatus* Neoehrlichia," and *Anaplasma* are maintained by horizontal tick-mammal-tick transmission, and humans are only inadvertently infected. Wolbachiae are associated with human filariasis, since they are important for filarial viability and pathogenicity; antibiotic treatment targeting wolbachiae is a strategy for filariasis control. Neorickettsiae parasitize flukes (trematodes) that in turn parasitize aquatic snails, fish, and insects. Only a single human neorickettsiosis has been described: sennetsu fever, an infectious mononucleosis-like illness first identified in 1953 in association with the ingestion of raw fish containing *N. sennetsu*-infected flukes.

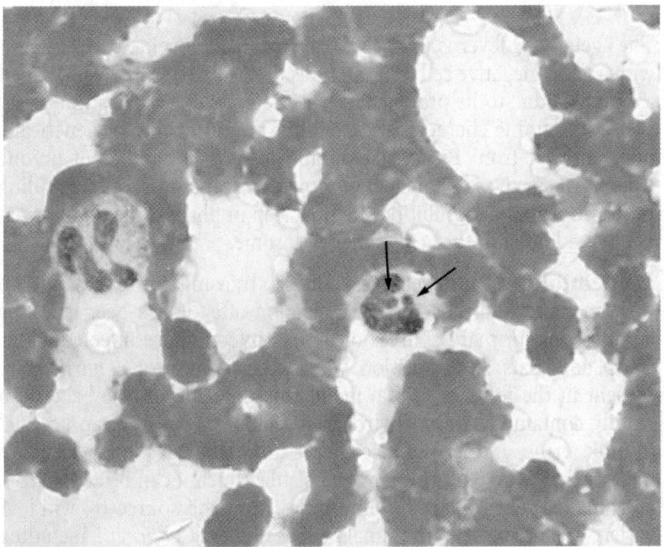

FIGURE 187-4 Peripheral-blood smear from a patient with human granulocytotropic anaplasmosis. A neutrophil contains two morulae (vacuoles filled with *A. phagocytophilum*). *(Photo courtesy of Dr. J. Stephen Dumler.)*

HUMAN MONOCYTOTROPIC EHRLICHIOSIS

Epidemiology More than 20,732 cases of *E. chaffeensis* infection had been reported to the U.S. Centers for Disease Control and Prevention (CDC) as of January 2020. However, active prospective surveillance documented an incidence as high as 414 cases per 100,000 population in some U.S. regions. Most *E. chaffeensis* infections are identified in the south-central, southeastern, and mid-Atlantic states, but cases have also been recognized in California, New York, New England, and midwestern states. All stages of the Lone Star tick (*A. americanum*), which is expanding its geographic range, feed on white-tailed deer—a major reservoir. Dogs and coyotes also serve as reservoirs and often lack clinical signs. Tick bites and exposures are frequently reported by patients in rural areas, and 64% of infections occur in May through July. The median age of HME patients is 55 years; however, 11% of infections occur in children ≤19 years of age, and these include severe and fatal infections. Of patients with HME, 59% are male.

E. chaffeensis has been detected in South and Central America, Africa, and Asia.

Clinical Manifestations *E. chaffeensis* disseminates hematogenously from the dermal blood pool created by the feeding tick. After a median incubation period of 8 days, illness develops. Clinical manifestations are undifferentiated and include fever (97% of cases), headache (70%), myalgia (68%), and malaise (77%). Less frequently observed are nausea, vomiting, and diarrhea (28–57%); cough (30%); rash (29% overall, 6% at presentation); and confusion (20%). HME can be severe: 77% of patients with confirmed cases are hospitalized, and 2% die. Life-threatening complications include renal failure, meningoencephalitis, acute respiratory distress syndrome, a DIC-like syndrome, pneumonia, septic shock, cardiac failure, hepatitis, hemorrhage, and—in immunocompromised patients—overwhelming ehrlichial infection; patients with diabetes, cancer, organ transplantation, asplenia, hepatitis C, or HIV infection have a 2.3 relative risk for death. Laboratory findings are valuable in the differential diagnosis of HME; 66% of patients have leukopenia (initially lymphopenia, later neutropenia), 86% have thrombocytopenia, and 89% have elevated serum levels of hepatic aminotransferases. Despite low blood cell counts, the bone marrow is hypercellular, and noncaseating granulomas can be present. Vasculitis is not a component of HME.

Diagnosis HME can be fatal. If not given empirical doxycycline treatment, 39% and 40% of patients with HME require admission to an intensive care unit and mechanical ventilation, respectively; these measures are necessary in no patients receiving prompt empirical treatment. In addition, hospital stay and illness duration are lengthened in untreated patients by 8 and 12 days, respectively. The diagnosis is suggested by fever, known tick exposure in the preceding 3 weeks, thrombocytopenia and/or leukopenia, and increased serum aminotransferase activities. Morulae are demonstrated in <10% of peripheral-blood smears. HME can be confirmed during active infection by PCR amplification of *E. chaffeensis* nucleic acids in blood obtained before the start of doxycycline therapy. Retrospective serodiagnosis requires a consistent clinical picture and a fourfold increase in *E. chaffeensis* antibody titer to ≥128 in paired serum samples obtained ~3 weeks apart. Separate specific diagnostic tests are necessary for HME and HGA (see below).

EWINGII EHRLICHIOSIS AND *EHRLICHIA MURIS EAUCLAIRENSIS* INFECTIONS

Ehrlichia ewingii resembles *E. chaffeensis* in its tick vector (*A. americanum*) and vertebrate reservoirs (white-tailed deer and dogs). *E. muris eauclairensis* causes human infections after *Ixodes scapularis* tick exposure in Wisconsin and Minnesota. *E. ewingii* and *E. muris* illnesses are similar to but less severe than HME. Many cases occur in immunocompromised patients. Human infections with *E. canis* have been documented as subclinical ehrlichemia. No specific serologic diagnostic tests for these other ehrlichiae are readily available, and *E. chaffeensis* serologic tests can be positive when the infecting agent is actually a different species of *Ehrlichia*.

■ "*CANDIDATUS* NEOEHRLICHIA MIKURENSIS" INFECTION

"*Candidatus* Neoehrlichia mikurensis," a bacterium in a phylogenetic clade between *Ehrlichia* and *Anaplasma*, was originally identified in *Ixodes ricinus* ticks from the Netherlands and in mice and *Ixodes ovatus* ticks from Japan. By means of broad-range 16S rRNA gene amplification and sequence analysis, this organism was identified as the cause of severe and sometimes prolonged febrile illnesses in European immunocompromised patients with tick bites or exposures and in Chinese patients developing a mild febrile illness after being bitten by *Ixodes persulcatus* and *Haemaphysalis concinna* ticks. The clinical presentation is similar to those of HME and HGA. Specific diagnostic methods have been developed but are not widely available.

TREATMENT
Ehrlichioses

Doxycycline is effective for HME as well as other ehrlichioses; the use of this drug in "*Candidatus* N. mikurensis" infection is associated with disease resolution. Therapy with doxycycline (100 mg given PO or IV twice daily) or tetracycline (250–500 mg given PO every 6 h) lowers hospitalization rates and shortens fever duration. *E. chaffeensis* is not susceptible to chloramphenicol in vitro, and the use of this drug is controversial. While a few reports document *E. chaffeensis* persistence in humans, this finding is rare; most infections are cured by short courses of doxycycline continuing for 3–5 days after defervescence. Although poorly studied for this indication, rifampin may be suitable when doxycycline is contraindicated.

Prevention HME, *E. ewingii* ehrlichiosis, *E. muris* ehrlichiosis, and "*Candidatus* N. mikurensis" infection can be prevented by the avoidance of ticks in endemic areas. The use of protective clothing and tick repellents, careful postexposure tick searches, and prompt removal of attached ticks probably diminish infection risk.

■ HUMAN GRANULOCYTOTROPIC ANAPLASMOSIS

Epidemiology As of January 2021, 45,186 cases of HGA had been reported to the CDC, most in the upper-midwestern and northeastern United States. The global geographic distribution is similar to that of Lyme disease because of the shared *Ixodes* tick vectors. Natural reservoirs for *A. phagocytophilum* are white-footed mice, squirrels, and white-tailed deer in the United States and red deer in Europe. HGA incidence peaks in May through July, but the disease can occur throughout the year with exposure to *Ixodes* ticks. HGA often affects males (59%) and older persons (median age, 51 years).

Clinical Manifestations Seroprevalence rates are high in endemic regions; thus, it seems likely that most individuals develop subclinical infections. The incubation period for HGA is 4–8 days, after which the disease manifests as fever (75–100% of cases), myalgia (73%), headache (82%), and malaise (97%). A minority of patients develop nausea, vomiting, or diarrhea (20–40%); cough (27%); or confusion (17%). A rash in HGA (5%) almost invariably reflects co-infection with *Borrelia*, resulting in erythema migrans. Most patients develop thrombocytopenia (80%) and/or leukopenia (63%) with increased serum hepatic aminotransferase levels (80%).

Life-threatening complications occur most often in the elderly and include renal failure, adult respiratory distress syndrome, a toxic shock–like syndrome, pneumonia, and a DIC- or sepsis-like syndrome. Meningoencephalitis is rare in documented cases of HGA. Other documented neurologic sequelae include brachial plexopathy, cranial nerve involvement, and demyelinating polyneuropathy. Infection of patients with a preexisting immunocompromising condition (diabetes, immunosuppressive medications, asplenia, arthritis) is associated with a 3.0 relative risk for life-threatening complications. Of patients with HGA, 31% are hospitalized, and 7% require intensive care. The case–fatality rate is 0.3%, but the relative risk for death is 16 if infection occurs with an immunosuppressive condition. Neither vasculitis nor granulomas are components of HGA. While patients can be co-infected with *Borrelia burgdorferi* and *Babesia microti* (transmitted by the same tick vector[s]), there is little evidence that these infections increase the severity or persistence of HGA. HGA transmitted by transfusion (including the transfusion of leukoreduced blood or platelets) has now been reported in at least nine cases, including a fatality.

Diagnosis HGA should be included in the differential diagnosis of influenza-like illnesses during seasons with *Ixodes* tick activity (May through December), especially in the context of a known tick bite or exposure. Concurrent thrombocytopenia, leukopenia, or elevated serum levels of alanine or aspartate aminotransferase further increase the likelihood of HGA. Many HGA patients develop Lyme disease antibodies in the absence of clinical findings consistent with that diagnosis. Thus, HGA should be considered in the differential diagnosis of atypical severe Lyme disease presentations. Peripheral-blood film examination for neutrophil morulae can yield a diagnosis in 20–75% of infections. PCR testing of blood from patients with active disease before doxycycline therapy is sensitive and specific. Serodiagnosis is retrospective, requiring a fourfold increase in *A. phagocytophilum* antibody titer (to ≥128) in paired serum samples obtained 1 month apart. Since seroprevalence is high in some regions, a single acute-phase titer should not be used for diagnosis.

***Anaplasma capra* Infection** Human infection by *A. capra*, first isolated from goat blood, was identified in 28 patients from northeastern China. Patients presented with fever, headache, malaise, dizziness, myalgias, and chills, but these manifestations were less severe than in HGA. Hospitalization was recorded for 18% of patients, and 14% had underlying disorders, including hyperglycemia, hypertension, coronary heart disease, diabetes, and cancer. Five patients had severe manifestations, including one with encephalitic signs and *A. capra* DNA present in CSF. *A. capra* is found most often in *I. persulcatus* ticks in this region. All patients responded to doxycycline treatment and survived.

TREATMENT
Human Granulocytotropic Anaplasmosis

No prospective studies of therapy for HGA have been conducted. However, doxycycline (100 mg PO twice daily) is effective. Rifampin therapy is associated with improvement of HGA in pregnant women and children. Most treated patients defervesce within 24–48 h.

Prevention HGA prevention requires tick avoidance. Transmission can be documented as few as 4 h after a tick bite.

Q FEVER

The agent of Q fever is *C. burnetii*, a small pleomorphic coccobacillus with a gram-negative cell wall, that was first isolated in 1935 and called a rickettsia due to its presence in ticks, intracellular replication, small size, and staining characteristics, but it is now known to be genetically quite distinct from Rickettsiaceae and to have a number of unique features. It survives in harsh environments, escapes intracellular killing in macrophages by inhibiting the final step in phagosome maturation, and has adapted to the acidic phagolysosome.

Epidemiology Q fever is a zoonosis: transmission of *C. burnetii* to humans typically occurs by inhalation after it has been shed by animals. The primary sources of human infection are infected cattle, sheep, and goats. At parturition, when large amounts of *C. burnetii* are present in the fetus, placenta, membranes, and fluids, the bacterium readily contaminates the environment. Smaller amounts can be shed in milk, urine, and feces. Once shed, *C. burnetii* can remain viable in manure, hay, soil, etc., for many years after which it can be aerosolized and inhaled, even after traveling miles from the source by wind. A variety of other vertebrate animals can be hosts of *C. burnetii*, including birds, cats, dogs, rabbits, skunks, raccoons, deer, bears, sloths, kangaroos, and marine animals. *C. burnetii* has also been found in several tick species, which could be important for maintenance of the agent in veterinary populations, but the majority of human Q fever cases are associated with aerosol transmission from infected livestock. Infections in animals are usually asymptomatic, but abortions and stillbirth have been observed in pregnant goats and sheep. Because it is easily dispersed as an aerosol and because of the extremely low infectious dose required for human infection (probably between 1 and 10 viable bacteria), *C. burnetii* is a potential agent of bioterrorism (**Chap. S3**), with a high infectivity rate and pneumonia as the major manifestation.

Persons at risk for Q fever include abattoir workers, veterinarians, farmers, and other individuals who have contact with infected animals (particularly newborn animals). In Canada and the Netherlands, 65% and 72%, respectively, of persons living and/or working on dairy cattle farms were seropositive, and in the United States, 22% of veterinarians were seropositive, compared to ~3% of the population overall. The organism is shed in milk for weeks to months after parturition. An outbreak of Q fever associated with ingestion of raw milk confirmed the oral route of transmission, although this route is uncommon. In rare instances, person-to-person transmission follows labor and childbirth in an infected woman, autopsy of an infected individual, or blood transfusion. Multiple outbreaks involving laboratory staff have been reported in the past. Some evidence suggests that *C. burnetii* can be sexually transmitted among humans. Some unusual modes of *C. burnetii* transmission to humans include treatment with live fetal sheep cells, which was responsible for cases in six persons in Germany, and percutaneous infection after crushing an infected tick between the fingers.

Infections due to *C. burnetii* occur in most geographic locations except New Zealand and Antarctica. Several factors influence the epidemiology: environmental conditions such as high concentrations of animals, high animal pregnancy rates, dry weather, and the strength and direction of winds. In addition to differences between strains of *C. burnetii*, the inherent variability in human susceptibility to *C. burnetii* can influence transmission and development of disease. Some people become sick after exposure, whereas others have only mild symptoms that are not sufficient to lead them to seek medical assistance, and ~60% have asymptomatic seroconversion. Q fever continues to be endemic in Australia and France. In Cayenne, French Guiana, Q fever is hyperendemic: 40% of all community-acquired pneumonias are caused by *C. burnetii*. The largest known outbreak occurred between 2007 and 2010 in the Netherlands. Over 4000 cases were reported, and over 40,000 people were infected. The outbreak was due to a combination of high-density goat farming in areas with large urban populations and environmental factors. Farms where spread did not occur had high vegetation density and lower groundwater concentrations.

Young age seems to be protective against disease caused by *C. burnetii*. In a large outbreak in Switzerland, symptomatic infection occurred five times more often among persons >15 years of age than among younger individuals. In many outbreaks, men are affected more commonly than women.

Clinical Manifestations • ACUTE Q FEVER The incubation period is 3–30 days. The primary manifestations of acute Q fever differ geographically. During the Dutch outbreak, but also in Canada and Croatia, pneumonia is the more common presentation. In some countries where Q fever is endemic, such as France and Israel, hepatitis is more common. These differences could reflect the route of infection (i.e., ingestion of contaminated milk for hepatitis and inhalation of contaminated aerosols for pneumonia) or strain differences. In the Dutch outbreak, sequelae of infection in pregnant women were rare; this was not the case among pregnant women elsewhere. Pericarditis, myocarditis, acalculous cholecystitis, pancreatitis, lymphadenitis, spontaneous rupture of the spleen, transient hypoplastic anemia, hemolytic anemia, hemophagocytic lymphohistiocytosis, optic neuritis, and erythema nodosum are less common manifestations.

The symptoms of acute Q fever are nonspecific; common among them are fever, extreme fatigue, photophobia, and severe headache that is frequently retro-orbital. Other symptoms include chills, sweats, nausea, vomiting, and diarrhea. Cough develops in about half of patients with Q fever pneumonia. A nonspecific rash may be evident in 4–18% of patients. The WBC count is usually normal. Thrombocytopenia occurs in ~25% of patients, and reactive thrombocytosis frequently develops during recovery. Biochemical markers of autoimmunity, such as anticytoplasmic antibodies (ANCA), antinuclear antibodies (ANA), anti-smooth muscle antibodies, or antiphospholipid antibodies, are often present in acute Q fever. Chest radiography can show opacities similar to those seen in pneumonia caused by other pathogens.

Acute Q fever occasionally complicates pregnancy. In one series, it resulted in premature birth in 35% of cases and in abortion or neonatal death in 43%. Neonatal death and lower infant birth weight are reported up to three times more often among women seropositive for *C. burnetii* in some areas but not others.

Q FEVER FATIGUE SYNDROME Prolonged fatigue follows Q fever in up to 20% of cases and can be accompanied by a constellation of symptoms, including headaches, sweats, arthralgia, and myalgias. Several hypotheses regarding the etiology exist, including biopsychological etiology with *C. burnetii* acting as trigger for fatigue development, host and genetic factors, and cytokine dysregulation. A randomized controlled trial including 155 patients with strictly diagnosed Q fever fatigue syndrome showed that long-term treatment with doxycycline did not reduce fatigue severity compared to placebo, so antibiotics should not be prescribed for these patients. Cognitive behavioral therapy aimed at fatigue-related cognitions and behaviors thought to perpetuate symptoms was effective in reducing fatigue severity in the short term. The beneficial effect of this treatment, however, was not maintained after 1 year.

CHRONIC Q FEVER Although it has recently been proposed that this entity be renamed *persistent Q fever*, we prefer the term *chronic Q fever*. Following primary infection, 1–5% of all patients develop chronic Q fever. Chronic Q fever endocarditis, infected aneurysms, or infected vascular prostheses are most frequently observed. The primary infection often has not been recognized or was asymptomatic, and the duration between primary infection and manifestation of chronic infection may be several years. The largest observed interval between acute infection and diagnosis of chronic Q fever was >9 years. Risk factors for the development of chronic Q fever include valvulopathy or prior valve surgery, aneurysms, vascular prostheses, renal insufficiency, older age, immunocompromised state, and malignancy. Diagnosing chronic Q fever is difficult, as patients often present with nonspecific symptoms, such as fever, night sweats, weight loss, fatigue, and malaise. Fever can be absent and is frequently low grade. C-reactive protein is often low or even normal. Chronic Q fever endocarditis differs from endocarditis caused by other bacteria, manifesting as endothelium-covered nodules on the valves, aortic root abscess, or new or rapidly increasing valve insufficiency. A high index of suspicion is necessary for timely diagnosis. Patients with chronic Q fever are often ill for >1 year before the diagnosis is made. The disease should be suspected in all patients with culture-negative endocarditis. In addition, all patients with valvular heart disease, an aneurysm or vascular prosthesis and unexplained weight loss, fever, stroke, unexpected aneurysm growth, and/or progressive heart failure should be tested for *C. burnetii* infection. Other manifestations of chronic Q fever include lymphadenitis and bone infection including vertebral osteomyelitis and prosthetic joint infection. Of 249 patients with proven chronic Q fever in the Netherlands, 61% developed complications. The most frequently observed complications were acute aneurysms, heart failure, and noncardiac abscesses. One in six patients with vascular chronic Q fever develops arterial fistula, including aortoenteric fistula, aortocaval fistula, aortobronchial fistula, and arteriocutaneous fistula. PCR positivity at any time during the disease, presence of prosthetic material, and older age were associated with complications. Q fever–related mortality was 25% in patients diagnosed with chronic Q fever after the Dutch outbreak. Chronic Q fever–related mortality was highest in patients with both endocarditis and vascular infection (33%), followed by patients with vascular infection only (25%), and was lowest in endocarditis patients (12%).

Diagnosis Culture of *C. burnetii* from buffy-coat blood samples or tissue specimens is possible but requires a biosafety level 3 laboratory and is not used in clinical practice. PCR detects *C. burnetii* DNA in blood and tissue specimens, including paraffin-embedded samples. The detection of antibodies to *C. burnetii* is the most commonly used method for the diagnosis of Q fever. Available serologic assays are indirect fluorescent antibody (IFA) assay, enzyme-linked immunosorbent assay (ELISA), and complement fixation test (CFT), with IFA being the gold standard. IFA tests are useful for the detection of and discrimination between acute and chronic infection and have excellent sensitivity and specificity. The diagnosis of acute Q fever is dependent on seroconversion, defined as a fourfold increase in IgG titer for phase II antigens between acute- and convalescent-phase samples. In the first 1–2 weeks of illness, PCR on blood or serum can also be positive. A high phase I IgG titer (e.g., >512) is suggestive of chronic Q fever, but alone, it is not enough for a definite diagnosis. A positive PCR for *C. burnetii* in blood or tissue in the absence of an acute infection confirms the diagnosis, but PCR on blood is negative in the majority of patients and tissue samples are often very difficult to obtain. The diagnosis of chronic Q fever should be based on a combination of clinical, laboratory, and imaging criteria. There has been debate on the optimal set of criteria, but the Dutch literature-based consensus guideline (**Table 187-2**) appears to be the most sensitive and is easy to use.

Valvular vegetations are detected in only 12% of patients with Q fever endocarditis by transthoracic echocardiography, but the rate of detection is higher (21–50%) with transesophageal echocardiography. Fluorodeoxyglucose positron emission tomography combined with CT (FDG-PET/CT) can detect not only prosthetic valvular infection but also intravascular infection elsewhere, osteomyelitis, and lymphadenitis. In native valve endocarditis, specificity is very high but sensitivity is low, so a normal FDG-PET/CT scan cannot exclude native valve endocarditis. A study including 273 FDG-PET/CT scans performed at diagnosis in patients suspected of chronic Q fever showed that, even after serology, PCR, and often ultrasound or CT had been performed, FDG-PET/CT led to a change in diagnosis or treatment in 20% of patients. Adding FDG uptake in a heart valve as a major criterion to the Duke criteria led to a 1.9-fold increase of definite endocarditis diagnoses. Of 218 scans performed during follow-up, 57% resulted in treatment adjustment. In case of suspected chronic Q fever, FDG-PET/CT should be considered.

TABLE 187-2 Diagnostic Criteria for Chronic Q Fever as Defined by the Dutch Q Fever Consensus Group

PROVEN CHRONIC Q FEVER	PROBABLE CHRONIC Q FEVER	POSSIBLE CHRONIC Q FEVER
1. Positive *Coxiella burnetii* PCR in blood or tissue[a] *OR* 2. IFA ≥1:800 or 1:1024 for *C. burnetii* phase I IgG *AND* Definite endocarditis according to the modified Duke criteria *OR* Proven large vessel or prosthetic infection by imaging studies ([18]FDG-PET, CT, MRI, or AUS)	IFA ≥1:800 or 1:1024 for *C. burnetii* phase I IgG *AND AT LEAST ONE OF THE FOLLOWING:* Valvulopathy not meeting the major criteria of the modified Duke criteria Known aneurysm and/or vascular or cardiac valve prosthesis without signs of infection by means of TEE/TTE, [18]FDG-PET, CT, MRI, or AUS Suspected osteomyelitis or hepatitis as manifestation of chronic Q fever Pregnancy Symptoms and signs of chronic infection, such as fever, weight loss, night sweats, hepatosplenomegaly, and persistently raised ESR and CRP Granulomatous tissue inflammation, proven by histologic examination Immunocompromised state	IFA ≥1:800 or 1:1024 for *C. burnetii* phase I IgG *without* manifestations meeting the criteria for proven or probable chronic Q fever

[a]In absence of acute infection.

Abbreviations: AUS, abdominal ultrasound; CRP, C-reactive protein; [18]FDG-PET, fluorodeoxyglucose positron emission tomography; ESR, erythrocyte sedimentation rate; IFA, indirect fluorescent antibody assay; PCR, polymerase chain reaction; TEE, transesophageal echocardiography; TTE, transthoracic echocardiography.

TREATMENT
Q Fever

ANTIBIOTICS

In vitro, *C. burnetii* is susceptible to doxycycline, quinolones, trimethoprim-sulfamethoxazole (TMP-SMX), macrolides, and rifampin. Although antimicrobial susceptibility testing is not routinely performed and resistance to doxycycline does not appear to be a common problem in clinical practice, doxycycline-resistant isolates do exist.

Treatment of acute Q fever with doxycycline (100 mg twice daily for 14 days) is usually successful. Quinolones also are effective. When Q fever is diagnosed during pregnancy, treatment with TMP-SMX is recommended for the duration of the pregnancy.

Treatment with doxycycline and hydroxychloroquine for 6–12 months following acute infection should be considered in patients with valve abnormalities, a prosthetic heart valve, an aneurysm, or vascular prosthesis. This appeared to be effective in preventing progression to chronic Q fever in patients with valvulopathy. The exact indications and duration of prophylaxis should be based on a careful consideration of possible benefits and side effects.

Decisions on treatment of chronic Q fever are challenging, so consultation with an infectious diseases expert is recommended. There is no indication for antibiotic therapy in those with possible chronic Q fever (only elevated phase I IgG without symptoms or an infectious focus). Addition of hydroxychloroquine (to alkalinize the phagolysosome) renders doxycycline bactericidal against *C. burnetii*, and the combination of doxycycline 100 mg twice daily with 200 mg hydroxychloroquine three times daily is currently the favored regimen. It is advised to determine serum levels of doxycycline aiming for concentrations between 5 and 10 mg/L. Patients treated with this regimen must be advised about photosensitivity and retinal toxicity risks; however, side effects should not lead to cessation of therapy too easily since it appears to be the most effective approach for this serious infection that has a high mortality despite treatment. Patients treated with hydroxychloroquine are at risk for developing retinopathy, so they should be evaluated by an ophthalmologist before starting treatment and every 6–12 months during the course of therapy. If doxycycline-hydroxychloroquine cannot be used, the regimen chosen should include at least two antibiotics active against *C. burnetii*. In a study including 322 patients with chronic Q fever, treatment with doxycycline combined with a quinolone appeared to be a safe alternative.

Minimum treatment duration is 18 months for native valve endocarditis and other manifestations without prosthetic material and 24 months for patients with prosthetic valve endocarditis or infected vascular prostheses. Many patients with vascular infection need prolonged treatment before the infection resolves, and surgical intervention is often necessary to remove an infected graft if the patient does not respond to antibiotic therapy. Abscesses need drainage for antibiotic therapy to be successful. A fourfold decrease in phase I IgG and the disappearance of phase II IgM was found to be a favorable prognostic indicator for patients with Q fever endocarditis, but defining cure of chronic Q fever after the minimum treatment duration should be based on a combination of imaging (if abnormal at diagnosis), decline of serologic titers, negativity of PCR on blood or serum, and improvement of symptoms.

FOLLOW-UP

After acute Q fever, patients without risk factors for developing chronic Q fever should be evaluated clinically and serologically after 6 months. When IgG phase I is <1024 and clinical symptoms do not suggest chronic infection, follow-up can be stopped. For patients with a very high risk of developing chronic Q fever who have received antibiotics for 6–12 months or patients with immunosuppression or other risk factors not treated with antibiotics for a prolonged period of time, follow-up with serology and PCR every 3–6 months for 2 years is recommended. During treatment of chronic Q fever, patients should be followed every 3 months to evaluate symptoms, side effects, serology, and PCR. When new complications are suspected, imaging should be repeated. After the end of treatment, relapse has been described up to 5 years later. It is therefore recommended to continue monitoring with serology and PCR until a minimum of 5 years after end of treatment.

Prevention A whole-cell vaccine (Q-Vax) licensed in Australia effectively prevents Q fever in abattoir workers. Vaccine is given only to people without a history of Q fever and negative results in both serologic and skin testing that is performed with intradermal diluted *C. burnetii* vaccine. Cases among abattoir workers in Australia declined dramatically as a result of a vaccination program.

Good animal-husbandry practices are important in preventing widespread contamination of the environment by *C. burnetii*. These practices include isolating aborting animals for up to 14 days, raising feed bunks to prevent contamination of feed by excreta, destroying aborted materials (by burning and burying fetal membranes and stillborn animals), and wearing masks and gloves when handling aborted materials. Vaccination of sheep and goats and a culling program were effective in the Netherlands outbreak.

During an outbreak of Q fever and for 4 weeks after it ceases, blood donations should not be accepted from individuals who live in the affected area.

Acknowledgment

The authors thank Thomas Marrie, MD, for his significant contributions to this chapter in the previous editions.

FURTHER READING

Biggs HM et al: Diagnosis and management of tickborne rickettsial diseases: Rocky Mountain spotted fever and other spotted fever group rickettsioses, ehrlichioses, and anaplasmosis—United States. MMWR 65:1, 2016.

Eldin C et al: From Q fever to *Coxiella burnetii* infection: A paradigm change. Clin Microbiol Rev 30:115, 2017.

Ismail N, McBride JW: Tick-borne emerging infections: Ehrlichiosis and anaplasmosis. Clin Lab Med 37:317, 2017.

Straily A et al: Antibody titers reactive with *Rickettsia rickettsii* in blood donors and implications for surveillance of spotted fever rickettsiosis in the United States. J Infect Dis 221:1371, 2020.

Weitzel T et al: Scrub typhus in continental Chile, 2016-2018. Emerg Infect Dis 25:1214, 2019.

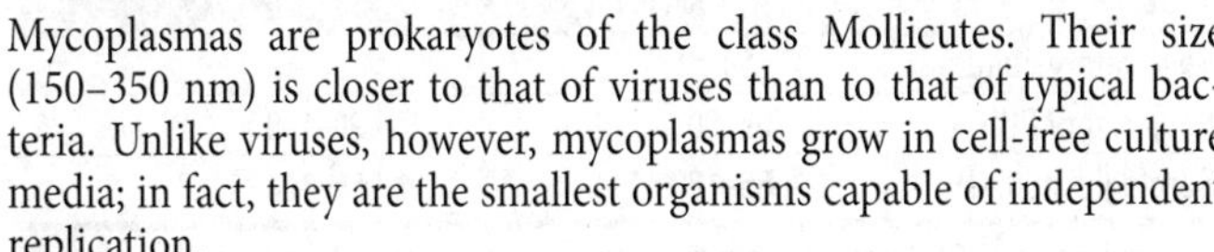

188 Infections Due to Mycoplasmas

R. Doug Hardy

Mycoplasmas are prokaryotes of the class Mollicutes. Their size (150–350 nm) is closer to that of viruses than to that of typical bacteria. Unlike viruses, however, mycoplasmas grow in cell-free culture media; in fact, they are the smallest organisms capable of independent replication.

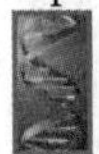

The entire genomes of many *Mycoplasma* species have been sequenced and have been found to be among the smallest of all prokaryotic genomes. Sequencing information for these genomes has helped define the minimal set of genes necessary for cellular life. The absence of genes related to the synthesis of amino acids, fatty acid metabolism, and cholesterol dictates the mycoplasmas' parasitic or saprophytic dependence on a host for exogenous nutrients and necessitates the use of complex fastidious media to culture these organisms. Mycoplasmas lack a cell wall and are bound only by a cell membrane. The absence of a cell wall explains the inactivity of β-lactam antibiotics (penicillins and cephalosporins) against infections caused by these organisms.

At least 13 *Mycoplasma* species, 2 *Acholeplasma* species, and 2 *Ureaplasma* species have been isolated from humans. Most of these species are thought to be normal inhabitants of oral and urogenital mucous membranes. *M. pneumoniae*, *M. hominis*, *M. genitalium*, *U. urealyticum*, and *U. parvum* have been shown conclusively to be pathogenic in immunocompetent humans. *M. pneumoniae* primarily infects the respiratory tract, while *M. hominis*, *M. genitalium*, *U. urealyticum*, and *U. parvum* are associated with a variety of genitourinary tract disorders and neonatal infections. Other mycoplasmas may cause disease in immunocompromised persons.

MYCOPLASMA PNEUMONIAE

PATHOGENESIS

M. pneumoniae is generally thought to act as an extracellular pathogen. Although the organism has been shown to exist and replicate within human cells, it is not known whether these intracellular events contribute to the pathogenesis of disease. *M. pneumoniae* attaches to ciliated respiratory epithelial cells by means of a complex terminal organelle at the tip of one end of the organism. Cytoadherence is mediated by interactive adhesins and accessory proteins clustered on this organelle. After extracellular attachment, *M. pneumoniae* causes injury to host respiratory tissue. The mechanism of injury is thought to be mediated by the production of hydrogen peroxide and of an ADP-ribosylating and vacuolating cytotoxin of *M. pneumoniae* that has many similarities to pertussis toxin. Because mycoplasmas lack a cell wall, they also lack cell wall–derived stimulators of the innate immune system, such as lipopolysaccharide, lipoteichoic acid, and murein (peptidoglycan) fragments. However, lipoproteins from the mycoplasmal cell membrane appear to have inflammatory properties, probably acting through Toll-like receptors (primarily TLR2) on macrophages and other cells. Lung biopsy specimens from patients with *M. pneumoniae* respiratory tract infection reveal an inflammatory process involving the trachea, bronchioles, and peribronchial tissue, with a monocytic infiltrate that coincides with a luminal exudate of polymorphonuclear leukocytes.

Experimental evidence indicates that innate immunity provides most of the host's defense against mycoplasmal infection in the lungs, whereas cellular immunity may actually play an immunopathogenic role, exacerbating mycoplasmal lung disease. Humoral immunity appears to provide protection against dissemination of *M. pneumoniae* infection; patients with humoral immunodeficiencies do not have more severe lung disease than do immunocompetent patients in the early stages of infection but more often develop disseminated infection resulting in syndromes such as arthritis, meningitis, and osteomyelitis. The immunity that follows severe *M. pneumoniae* infections is more protective and longer-lasting than that following mild infections. Genuine second attacks of *M. pneumoniae* pneumonia have been reported infrequently.

EPIDEMIOLOGY

M. pneumoniae infection occurs worldwide. It is likely that the incidence of upper respiratory illness due to *M. pneumoniae* is up to 20 times that of pneumonia caused by this organism. Infection is spread from one person to another by respiratory droplets expectorated during coughing and results in clinically apparent disease in an estimated 80% of cases. The incubation period for *M. pneumoniae* is 2–4 weeks; therefore, the time-course of infection in a specific population may be several weeks long. Intrafamilial attack rates are as high as 84% among children and 41% among adults. Outbreaks of *M. pneumoniae* illness often occur in institutional settings such as military bases, boarding schools, and summer camps. Infections tend to be endemic, with sporadic epidemics every 4–7 years.

Most significantly, *M. pneumoniae* is a major cause of community-acquired respiratory illness in both children and adults and is often grouped with *Chlamydia pneumoniae* and *Legionella* species as one of the most important bacterial causes of "atypical" community-acquired pneumonia. For community-acquired pneumonia in adults, *M. pneumoniae* is the most frequently detected "atypical" organism. Analysis of 13 studies of community-acquired pneumonia published between 1996 to 2001 (which included 6207 ambulatory and hospitalized adults) showed that the overall prevalence of *M. pneumoniae* was 22.7%; by comparison, the prevalence of *C. pneumoniae* was 11.7%, and that of *Legionella* species was 4.6%. The summation of 26 more recent investigations of "atypical" organisms in community-acquired pneumonia in adults published between 2002 to 2015 found the overall prevalence of *M. pneumoniae* was 7.2%; by comparison, the prevalence of *C. pneumoniae* was 4.3%, and that of *Legionella* species was 2.8%. *M. pneumoniae* pneumonia is also referred to as Eaton agent pneumonia (the organism having first been isolated in the early 1940s by Monroe Eaton), primary atypical pneumonia, and "walking" pneumonia.

CLINICAL MANIFESTATIONS

Upper Respiratory Tract Infections and Pneumonia Acute *M. pneumoniae* infections generally manifest as pharyngitis, tracheobronchitis, reactive airway disease/wheezing, or a nonspecific upper respiratory syndrome. Little evidence supports the commonly held belief that this organism is an important cause of otitis media, with or without bullous myringitis. Pneumonia develops in 3–13% of infected individuals; its onset is usually gradual, occurring over several days, but may be more abrupt. Although *Mycoplasma* pneumonia may begin with a sore throat, the most common presenting symptom is cough. The cough is typically nonproductive, but some patients produce sputum. Headache, malaise, chills, and fever are noted in the majority of patients.

On physical examination, wheezes or rales are detected in ~80% of patients with *M. pneumoniae* pneumonia. In many patients, however, pneumonia can be diagnosed only by chest radiography. The most common radiographic pattern is that of peribronchial pneumonia with thickened bronchial markings, streaks of interstitial infiltration, and areas of subsegmental atelectasis. Segmental or lobar consolidation is not uncommon. While clinically evident pleural effusions are infrequent, lateral decubitus views reveal that up to 20% of patients have pleural effusions.

Overall, the clinical presentation of pneumonia in an individual patient is not useful for differentiating *M. pneumoniae* pneumonia from other types of community-acquired pneumonia. The possibility of *M. pneumoniae* infection deserves particular consideration when community-acquired pneumonia fails to respond to treatment with a penicillin or a cephalosporin—antibiotics that are ineffective against mycoplasmas. Symptoms usually resolve within 2–3 weeks after the onset of illness. Although *M. pneumoniae* pneumonia is generally self-limited, appropriate antimicrobial therapy significantly shortens the duration of clinical illness. Infection uncommonly results in critical illness and only rarely in death. In some patients, long-term recurrent wheezing or reactive airway disease may follow the resolution of acute pneumonia. The significance of chronic infection, especially as it relates to asthma, is an area of active investigation.

Extrapulmonary Manifestations An array of extrapulmonary manifestations may develop during *M. pneumoniae* infection. The most significant are neurologic, dermatologic, cardiac, rheumatologic, and hematologic in nature. Extrapulmonary manifestations can be a result of disseminated infection, especially in patients with humoral immunodeficiencies (e.g., septic arthritis); postinfectious autoimmune phenomena (e.g., Guillain-Barré syndrome); or possibly ADP-ribosylating toxin. Overall, these manifestations are uncommon, given the frequency of *M. pneumoniae* infection. Notably, many patients with extrapulmonary *M. pneumoniae* disease do not have respiratory disease.

Skin eruptions described with *M. pneumoniae* infection include erythematous (macular or maculopapular), vesicular, bullous, petechial, and urticarial rashes. In some reports, 17% of patients with *M. pneumoniae* pneumonia have had an exanthem. Erythema multiforme major (Stevens-Johnson syndrome) is the most clinically significant skin eruption associated with *M. pneumoniae* infection; it appears to occur more commonly with *M. pneumoniae* than with other infectious agents.

A wide spectrum of neurologic manifestations has been reported with *M. pneumoniae* infection. The most common are meningoencephalitis, encephalitis, Guillain-Barré syndrome, and aseptic meningitis. *M. pneumoniae* has been implicated as a likely etiologic agent in 5–7% of cases of encephalitis. Other neurologic manifestations may include cranial neuropathy, acute psychosis, cerebellar ataxia, acute demyelinating encephalomyelitis, cerebrovascular thromboembolic events, and transverse myelitis.

Hematologic manifestations of *M. pneumoniae* infection include hemolytic anemia, aplastic anemia, cold agglutinins, disseminated intravascular coagulation, and hypercoagulopathy. When anemia does occur, it generally develops in the second or third week of illness.

In addition, hepatitis, glomerulonephritis, pancreatitis, myocarditis, pericarditis, rhabdomyolysis, and arthritis (septic and reactive) have been convincingly ascribed to *M. pneumoniae* infection. Septic arthritis has been described most commonly in hypogammaglobulinemic patients.

DIAGNOSIS

Clinical findings, nonmicrobiologic laboratory tests, and chest radiography are not useful for differentiating *M. pneumoniae* pneumonia from other types of community-acquired pneumonia. In addition, since *M. pneumoniae* lacks a cell wall, it is not visible on Gram's stain. Although of historical interest, the measurement of cold agglutinin titers is no longer recommended for the diagnosis of *M. pneumoniae* infection because the findings are nonspecific and assays specific for *M. pneumoniae* are now available.

Acute *M. pneumoniae* infection can be diagnosed by polymerase chain reaction (PCR) detection of the organism in respiratory tract secretions or by isolation of the organism in culture (**Table 188-1**). Oropharyngeal, nasopharyngeal, and pulmonary specimens are all acceptable for diagnosing *M. pneumoniae* pneumonia. Other bodily fluids, such as cerebrospinal fluid, are acceptable for extrapulmonary infection. *M. pneumoniae* culture (which requires special media) is not recommended for routine diagnosis because the organism may take weeks to grow and is often difficult to isolate from clinical specimens. In contrast, PCR allows rapid, specific diagnosis earlier in the course of clinical illness.

The diagnosis can also be established by serologic tests for IgM and IgG antibodies to *M. pneumoniae* in paired (acute- and convalescent-phase) serum samples; enzyme-linked immunoassay is the recommended serologic method. An acute-phase sample alone is not adequate for diagnosis, as antibodies to *M. pneumoniae* may not develop until 2 weeks into the illness; therefore, it is important to test paired samples. In addition, IgM antibody to *M. pneumoniae* can persist for up to 1 year after acute infection. Thus its presence may indicate recent rather than acute infection.

The combination of PCR of respiratory tract secretions and serologic testing constitutes the most sensitive and rapid approach to the diagnosis of *M. pneumoniae* infection.

TABLE 188-1 Diagnostic Tests for Respiratory *Mycoplasma pneumoniae* Infection[a]

TEST	SENSITIVITY, %	SPECIFICITY, %
Respiratory culture	≤60	100
Respiratory PCR	65–90	90–100
Serologic studies[b]	55–100	55–100

[a]A combination of PCR and serology is suggested for routine diagnosis. If macrolide resistance is suspected, resistance testing by culture and/or PCR is available.
[b]Acute- and convalescent-phase serum samples are recommended.

Abbreviation: PCR, polymerase chain reaction.

TREATMENT

Mycoplasma pneumoniae Infections

Although in the majority of untreated cases symptoms resolve within 2–3 weeks without significant associated morbidity, *M. pneumoniae* pneumonia can be a serious illness that responds to appropriate antimicrobial therapy (**Table 188-2**). Randomized, double-blind, placebo-controlled trials in adults have demonstrated that antimicrobial treatment significantly decreases the duration of fever, cough, malaise, hospitalization, and radiologic abnormalities in *M. pneumoniae* pneumonia. Treatment options for acute *M. pneumoniae* infection include macrolides (e.g., oral azithromycin, 500 mg on day 1, then 250 mg/d on days 2–5), tetracyclines (e.g., oral doxycycline, 100 mg twice daily for 7–14 days), and respiratory fluoroquinolones. However, ciprofloxacin and ofloxacin are *not* recommended because of their high minimal inhibitory concentrations against *M. pneumoniae* isolates and their poor performance in experimental studies. A 7- to 14-day course of quinolone therapy appears adequate. Even though appropriate antibiotic therapy significantly reduces the duration of respiratory illness, it does not appear to shorten the duration of detection of *M. pneumoniae* by culture or PCR; therefore, a test of cure or eradication is not suggested.

In Japan and China, very high levels (up to ≥90%) of *M. pneumoniae* resistance to macrolides have been reported. In Europe and to a lesser degree in the United States, macrolide-resistant *M. pneumoniae* is emerging. In the United States, national surveillance from 2018 found that 10.2% of isolates demonstrated macrolide resistance. Furthermore, national surveillance from 2015–2018 found macrolide resistance of 15.2–21.7% in the eastern United States and 1.9–2.8% in the western United States. Clinical studies have demonstrated that, when treated with macrolides, patients with community-acquired pneumonia due to macrolide-resistant *M. pneumoniae* experience a significantly longer duration of symptoms than do patients infected with macrolide-sensitive organisms; thus macrolide resistance in *M. pneumoniae* does appear to have clinical significance. If macrolide resistance is prominent in a particular geographic locale or is suspected, then a nonmacrolide antibiotic should be considered for treatment; in addition, in these instances, a respiratory sample may be sent to a mycoplasma reference laboratory for the detection of macrolide resistance by culture or PCR.

While the 2019 Infectious Diseases Society of America and American Thoracic Society guidelines do not recommend routinely using corticosteroids in community-acquired pneumonia, some clinical literature suggests that the addition of glucocorticoids to an antibiotic regimen may be of value for the treatment of severe or refractory *M. pneumoniae* pneumonia. A 2019 meta-analysis of 24 randomized controlled trials in children found that use of corticosteroids in macrolide-refractory *M. pneumoniae* pneumonia significantly reduced hospital days and duration of fever. Clinical literature in adults also shows benefit, but these data are limited and more observational in nature.

The roles of antimicrobial drugs, glucocorticoids, and IV immunoglobulin in the treatment of neurologic disease due to *M. pneumoniae* remain unknown.

TABLE 188-2 Antimicrobial Agents of Choice for *Mycoplasma* Infections[a]

ORGANISM(S)	DRUGS
Mycoplasma pneumoniae	Azithromycin, clarithromycin, erythromycin, doxycycline, levofloxacin, moxifloxacin, gemifloxacin (*not* ciprofloxacin or ofloxacin)
Ureaplasma urealyticum, *Ureaplasma parvum*	Azithromycin, clarithromycin, erythromycin, doxycycline
Mycoplasma hominis	Doxycycline, clindamycin
Mycoplasma genitalium	Azithromycin, moxifloxacin

[a]Antimicrobial resistance has been reported in mycoplasmas, as described in the text.

UROGENITAL MYCOPLASMAS

■ EPIDEMIOLOGY

M. hominis, *M. genitalium*, *U. urealyticum*, and *U. parvum* can cause urogenital tract disease. The significance of isolation of these organisms in a variety of other syndromes is unknown and in some cases is being investigated. *M. fermentans* has not been shown convincingly to cause human disease.

While urogenital mycoplasmas may be transmitted to a fetus during passage through a colonized birth canal, sexual contact is the major mode of transmission, and the risk of colonization increases dramatically with increasing numbers of sexual partners. In asymptomatic women, these mycoplasmas may be found throughout the lower urogenital tract. The vagina yields the largest number of organisms; next most densely colonized are the periurethral area and the cervix. Ureaplasmas are isolated less often from urine than from the cervix, but *M. hominis* is found with approximately the same frequency at these two sites. Ureaplasmas are isolated from the vagina of 40–80% of sexually active, asymptomatic women and *M. hominis* from 21–70%. The two microorganisms are found concurrently in 31–60% of women. In men, colonization with each organism is less prevalent. Mycoplasmas have been isolated from urine, semen, and the distal urethra of asymptomatic men.

■ CLINICAL MANIFESTATIONS

Urethritis, Pyelonephritis, and Urinary Calculi In many episodes of *Chlamydia*-negative nongonococcal urethritis, ureaplasmas may be the causative agent. These organisms may also cause chronic voiding symptoms in women. The common presence of ureaplasmas in the urethra of asymptomatic men may suggest either that only certain serovars are pathogenic or that predisposing factors, such as lack of immunity, must exist in persons who develop symptomatic infection. Alternatively, disease may develop only upon initial exposure to ureaplasmas. Ureaplasmas have been implicated in epididymitis. *M. genitalium* also appears to cause urethritis. *M. genitalium* and ureaplasmas do not have a known role in prostatitis. *M. hominis* does not appear to play a primary etiologic role in urethritis, epididymitis, or prostatitis.

Evidence suggests that *M. hominis* causes up to 5% of cases of acute pyelonephritis. Ureaplasmas have not been associated with this disease.

Ureaplasmas play a limited role in the production of urinary calculi. The frequency with which ureaplasmas reach the kidney, the predisposing factors that allow them to do so, and the relative frequency of urinary tract calculi induced by this organism (compared with other organisms) are not known.

Pelvic Inflammatory Disease *M. hominis* can cause pelvic inflammatory disease. In most episodes, *M. hominis* occurs as part of a polymicrobial infection, but the organism may play an independent role in a limited number of cases. Data also support an association of *M. genitalium* with pelvic inflammatory disease. Ureaplasmas are not thought to cause pelvic inflammatory disease.

Postpartum and Postabortal Infection Studies implicate *M. hominis* as the primary pathogen in ~5–10% of women who have postpartum or postabortal fever; ureaplasmas have been implicated to a lesser degree. These infections are generally self-limited; however, if symptoms persist, specific antimicrobial therapy should be given. Ureaplasmas also appear to play a role in occasional postcesarean wound infections.

Nonurogenital Infection In rare instances, *M. hominis* causes nonurogenital infections, such as brain abscess, wound infection, poststernotomy mediastinitis, endocarditis, and neonatal meningitis. These infections are most common among immunocompromised and hypogammaglobulinemic patients. Ureaplasmas and *M. hominis* can cause septic arthritis in immunodeficient patients. Ureaplasmas probably cause neonatal pneumonitis; their possible causal role in the development of bronchopulmonary dysplasia—the chronic lung disease of premature infants—has been extensively investigated, with most studies indicating at least a significant association. It is unclear whether ureaplasmas and *M. hominis* cause infertility, spontaneous abortion, premature labor, low birth weight, or chorioamnionitis.

DIAGNOSIS

Culture and PCR are both appropriate methods for the isolation of urogenital mycoplasmas. Culture of these organisms, however, requires special techniques and media that generally are available only at larger medical centers and reference laboratories. Serologic testing is not recommended for the clinical diagnosis of urogenital *Mycoplasma* infections.

TREATMENT

Urogenital *Mycoplasma* Infections

Because colonization with urogenital mycoplasmas is common, it appears at present that their isolation from the urogenital tract in the absence of disease generally does not warrant treatment. Macrolides and doxycycline are considered the antimicrobial agents of choice for *Ureaplasma* infections (Table 188-2). *Ureaplasma* resistance to macrolides, doxycycline, quinolones, and chloramphenicol has been reported. *M. hominis* is resistant to macrolides. Doxycycline is generally the drug of choice for *M. hominis* infections, although resistance has been reported. Clindamycin is generally active against *M. hominis*. Quinolones are active in vitro against *M. hominis*. For *M. genitalium*, the initial treatment of choice appears to be azithromycin; moxifloxacin has been successfully used to treat *M. genitalium* resistant to azithromycin.

FURTHER READING

Getman D et al: *Mycoplasma genitalium* prevalence, coinfection, and macrolide antibiotic resistance frequency in a multicenter clinical study cohort in the United States. J Clin Microbiol 54:2278, 2016.

Waites KB et al: *Mycoplasma pneumoniae* from the respiratory tract and beyond. Clin Microbiol Rev 30:747, 2017.

Waites KB et al: Macrolide-resistant *Mycoplasma pneumoniae* in the United States as determined from a national surveillance program. J Clin Microbiol 57:e00968, 2019.

Workowski KA, Bolan GA: Sexually transmitted diseases treatment guidelines, 2015. MMWR Recomm Rep 64:1, 2015.

189 Chlamydial Infections

Charlotte A. Gaydos, Thomas C. Quinn

Chlamydiae are obligate intracellular bacteria that cause a wide variety of diseases in humans and animals.

ETIOLOGIC AGENTS

The chlamydiae were originally classified as four species in the genus *Chlamydia*: *C. trachomatis, C. pneumoniae, C. psittaci*, and *C. pecorum* (the last species being found in ruminants). The *C. psittaci* group has been separated into three species: *C. psittaci, C. felis*, and *C. abortus*. The mouse pneumonitis strain (MoPn) is now classified as *C. muridarum*, and the guinea pig inclusion conjunctivitis strain (GPIC) is now designated *C. caviae*.

C. trachomatis is divided into two biovars: trachoma and LGV (lymphogranuloma venereum). The trachoma biovar causes two major types of disease in humans: ocular trachoma, the leading infectious cause of preventable blindness in the developing world; and urogenital infections, which are sexually or neonatally transmitted. The 18 serovars of *C. trachomatis* fall into three groups: the trachoma serovars A, B, Ba, and C; the oculogenital serovars D–K; and the LGV serovars L_1–L_3. Serovars can be distinguished by serologic typing with monoclonal antibodies or by molecular gene typing. However, serovar identification usually is not important clinically, since the antibiotic susceptibility pattern is the same for all three groups. The one exception applies when LGV is suspected on clinical grounds; in this situation, serovar determination is important because a longer treatment duration is required for LGV strains.

BIOLOGY, GROWTH CYCLE, AND PATHOGENESIS

BIOLOGY

During their intracellular growth, chlamydiae produce characteristic intracytoplasmic inclusions that can be visualized by direct fluorescent antibody or Giemsa staining of infected clinical material, such as conjunctival scrapings or cervical or urethral epithelial cells. Chlamydiae are nonmotile, gram-negative, obligate intracellular bacteria that replicate within the cytoplasm of host cells, forming the characteristic membrane-bound inclusions that are the basis for some diagnostic tests. Originally considered to be large viruses, chlamydiae differ from viruses in possessing RNA and DNA as well as a cell wall that is quite similar in structure to the cell wall of typical gram-negative bacteria. However, chlamydiae lack peptidoglycan; their structural integrity depends on disulfide binding of outer-membrane proteins.

GROWTH CYCLE

Among the defining characteristics of chlamydiae is a unique growth cycle that involves alternation between two highly specialized morphologic forms (**Figs. 189-1 and 189-2**): the elementary body, which is the infectious form and is specifically adapted for extracellular survival, and the metabolically active and replicating reticulate body, which is not infectious, is adapted for an intracellular environment, and does

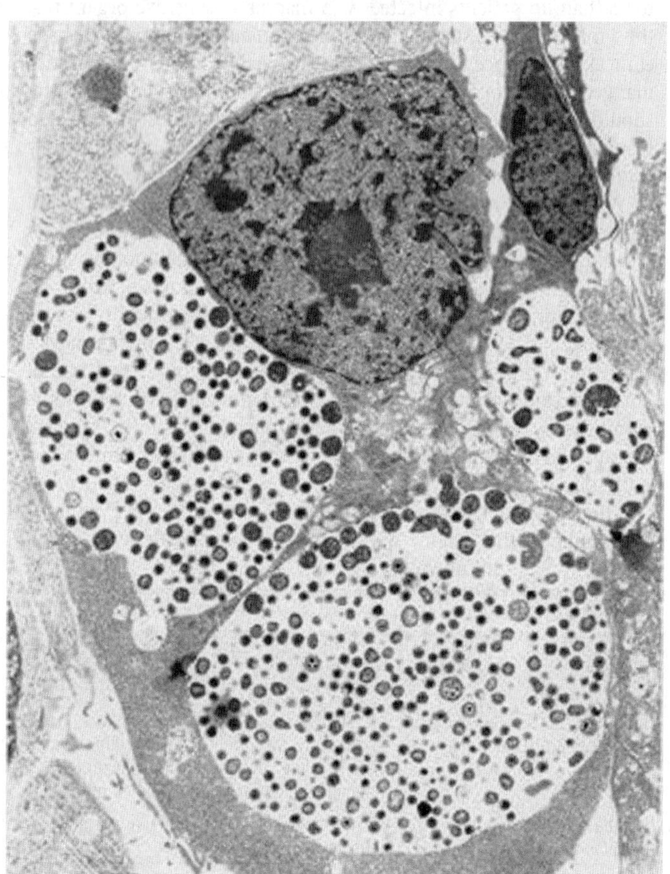

FIGURE 189-1 Chlamydial intracellular inclusions filled with smaller dense elementary bodies and larger reticulate bodies. *(Reprinted with permission from WE Stamm: Chlamydial infections, in Harrison's Principles of Internal Medicine, 17th ed, AS Fauci et al [eds]. New York, McGraw-Hill, 2008, p 1070.)*

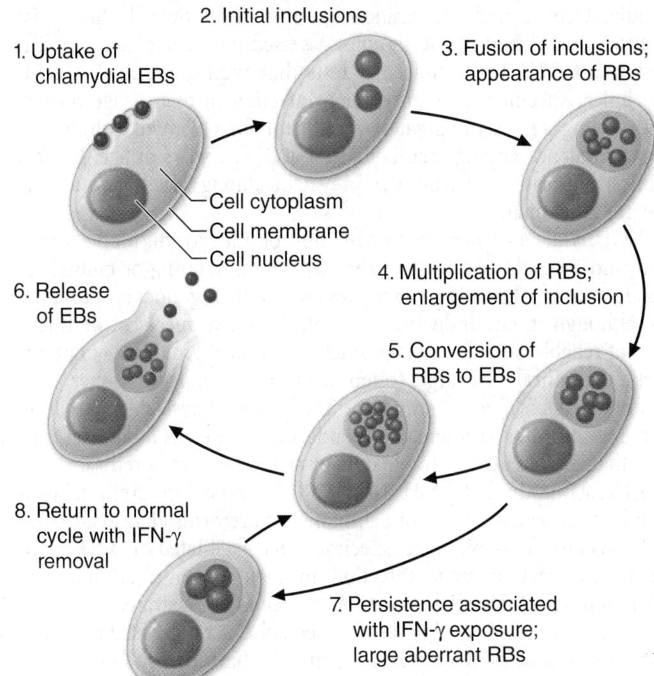

FIGURE 189-2 Chlamydial life cycle. EBs, elementary bodies; IFN-γ, interferon γ; RBs, reticulate bodies. *(Reproduced with permission from WE Stamm: Chlamydial infections, in AS Fauci et al [eds]: Harrison's Principles of Internal Medicine, 17th ed. New York, McGraw-Hill, 2008.)*

not survive well outside the host cell. The biphasic growth cycle begins with attachment of the elementary body (diameter, 0.25–0.35 μm) at specific sites on the surface of the host cell. The elementary body enters the cell through a process similar to receptor-mediated endocytosis and resides in an inclusion, where the entire growth cycle is completed. The chlamydiae prevent phagosome–lysosome fusion. The inclusion membrane is modified by insertion of chlamydial antigens. Once the elementary body has entered the cell, it reorganizes into a reticulate body, which is larger (0.5–1 μm) and contains more RNA. After ~8 h, the reticulate body starts to divide by binary fission. The intracytoplasmic, membrane-bound inclusion body containing the reticulate bodies increases in size as the reticulate bodies multiply. Approximately 18–24 h after infection of the cell, these reticulate bodies begin to become elementary bodies by a reorganization or condensation process that is poorly understood. After rupture of the inclusion body, the elementary bodies are released to initiate another cycle of infection.

Chlamydiae are susceptible to many broad-spectrum antibiotics and possess a number of enzymes, but they have a very restricted metabolic capacity. None of these metabolic reactions result in the production of energy. Chlamydiae have thus been considered to be energy parasites that use the ATP produced by the host cell for their own metabolic functions. Many aspects of chlamydial molecular biology are not well understood, but the sequencing of several chlamydial genomes and new proteomics research have provided researchers with many relevant tools for elucidating the biology of the life cycle.

■ PATHOGENESIS

Genital infections are primarily caused by *C. trachomatis* serovars D–K, with serovars D, E, and F involved most frequently. Molecular typing of the major outer-membrane protein gene (*omp1*) from which serovar differences arise has been used to demonstrate that polymorphisms can occur in isolates from patients who are exposed frequently to multiple infections, while less variation is observed in isolates from less sexually active populations. Polymorphisms in the major outer-membrane protein may provide antigenic variation, and the different forms allow persistence in the community because immunity to one is not protective against the others.

The trachoma biovar is essentially a parasite of squamocolumnar epithelial cells; the LGV biovar is more invasive and involves lymphoid cells. As is typical of chlamydiae, *C. trachomatis* strains are capable of causing chronic, clinically inapparent, asymptomatic infections. Because the duration of the chlamydial growth cycle is ~48–72 h, the incubation period of sexually transmitted chlamydial infections is relatively long—generally 1–3 weeks. *C. trachomatis* causes cell death as a result of its replicative cycle and can induce cell damage whenever it persists. However, few toxic effects are demonstrated, and cell death because of chlamydial replication is not sufficient to account for disease manifestations, the majority of which are due to immunopathologic mechanisms or nonspecific host responses to the organism or its by-products.

In recent years, the entire genomes of various chlamydial species have been sequenced, the field of proteomics has become established, host innate immunity has been more precisely delineated, and innovative host cell–chlamydial interaction studies have been conducted. As a result, many insights have been gained into how chlamydiae adapt and replicate in their intracellular environment and produce disease. These insights into pathogenesis include information on the regulation of gene expression, protein localization, the type III secretion system, the roles of CD4+ and CD8+ T lymphocytes in the host response, and T lymphocyte trafficking.

The chlamydial heat-shock protein, which shares antigenic epitopes with similar proteins of other bacteria and with human heat-shock protein, may sensitize the host, and repeated infections may cause host cell damage. Persistent or recurrent chlamydial infections are associated with fibrosis, scarring, and complications following simple squamocolumnar epithelial infections. A common endpoint of these late consequences is scarring of mucous membranes. Genital complications can lead to pelvic inflammatory disease (PID) and its late consequences of infertility, ectopic pregnancy, and chronic pelvic pain, while ocular infections may lead to blinding trachoma. High levels of antibody to human heat-shock protein have been associated with tubal factor infertility and ectopic pregnancy. Without adequate therapy, chlamydial infections may persist for several years, although symptoms—if present—usually abate.

Pathogenic mechanisms of *C. pneumoniae* have yet to be completely elucidated. The same is true for *C. psittaci*, except that this agent infects cells very efficiently and causes disease that may reflect direct cytopathic effects.

C. TRACHOMATIS INFECTIONS

■ GENITAL INFECTIONS (SEE ALSO CHAP. 136)

Spectrum Although chlamydiae cause a number of human diseases, localized lower genital tract infections caused by *C. trachomatis* and the sequelae of such infections are the most important in terms of medical and economic impact. Oculogenital infections due to *C. trachomatis* serovars D–K are transmitted during sexual contact or from mother to baby during childbirth and are associated with many syndromes, including cervicitis, salpingitis, acute urethral syndrome, endometritis, ectopic pregnancy, infertility, and PID in female patients; urethritis, proctitis, and epididymitis in male patients; and conjunctivitis and pneumonia in infants. Women bear the greatest burden of morbidity because of the serious sequelae of these infections. Untreated infections lead to PID, and multiple episodes of PID can lead to tubal factor infertility and chronic pelvic pain. Studies estimate that up to 80–90% of women and >50% of men with *C. trachomatis* genital infections lack symptoms; other patients have very mild symptoms. Thus, a large reservoir of infected persons continues to transmit infection to sexual partners.

As their designations reflect, the LGV serovars (L_1, L_2, and L_3) cause LGV, an invasive sexually transmitted disease (STD) characterized by acute lymphadenitis with bubo formation and/or acute hemorrhagic proctitis (see "LGV," below).

Epidemiology • GLOBAL EPIDEMIOLOGY *C. trachomatis* genital infections are global in distribution. The World Health Organization (WHO) estimates that in 2016, 124.3 million new cases of chlamydia occurred among adults and adolescents aged 15–49 years worldwide, with a global incidence rate for chlamydia in 2016 to be 34 cases per

1000 women (95% uncertainty interval [UI], 25–45) and 33 per 1000 men (95% UI, 21–48) This figure makes chlamydial infection the most prevalent bacterial sexually transmitted infection in the world. The associated morbidity is substantial, and the economic cost is high.

U.S. EPIDEMIOLOGY In the United States, these infections are the most commonly reported of all infectious diseases. In 2018, 1,758,668 cases were reported to the U.S. Centers for Disease Control and Prevention (CDC); however, the CDC estimates that 2–3 million new cases occur per year, with substantial underreporting due to lack of screening in some populations. Rates of infection have increased every year; higher rates among women than among men reflect the focus on expansion of screening programs for women during the past 25 years. Use of increasingly sensitive diagnostic nucleic acid amplification tests, an increased emphasis on case reporting, and improvements in the information systems used have elevated the number of cases reported every year. The CDC and other professional organizations recommend annual screening of all sexually active women <25 years of age as well as rescreening of previously infected individuals at 3 months. The 2018 case count corresponds to 539.9 cases per 100,000 population. Women have the highest infection rates (692.7 cases per 100,000) compared to the rate among men (380.6 cases per 100,000). Interestingly, with the increased availability of urine testing and extragenital testing, men—including gay, bisexual, and other men who have sex with men (MSM)—are increasingly being tested for chlamydial infection. From 2017 to 2018, rates of chlamydial infection in men increased by 5.7%, whereas rates in women rose by only 1.3% for age 15–19 years and 0.8% for age 20–24 years during this period. Chlamydial infection rates vary among different racial and ethnic minority populations.

The aforementioned statistics are based on case reporting. Studies based on screening surveys estimate that the U.S. prevalence of *C. trachomatis* cervical infection is 5% among asymptomatic female college students and prenatal patients, >10% for women seen in family planning clinics, and >20% for women seen in STD clinics. The prevalence of genital *C. trachomatis* infections varies substantially by geographic locale, with the highest rates in the southeastern United States. The prevalence of *C. trachomatis* in the cervix of pregnant women is 5–10 times higher than that of *Neisseria gonorrhoeae*. The prevalence of genital infection with either agent is highest among women who are between the ages of 20 and 24. Recurrent infections are common in these risk groups and are often acquired from untreated sexual partners. The use of oral contraception and the presence of cervical ectopy also confer an increased risk. The proportion of infections that are asymptomatic appears to be higher for *C. trachomatis* than for *N. gonorrhoeae*, and symptomatic *C. trachomatis* infections are clinically less severe. Mild or asymptomatic *C. trachomatis* infections of the fallopian tubes nonetheless cause ongoing tubal damage and infertility. The costs of *C. trachomatis* infections and their complications to the U.S. health care system have recently been estimated to be >$516.7 million annually.

Clinical Manifestations • **NONGONOCOCCAL AND POSTGONOCOCCAL URETHRITIS** *C. trachomatis* is the most common cause of nongonococcal urethritis (NGU) and postgonococcal urethritis (PGU). The designation *PGU* refers to NGU developing in men 2–3 weeks after treatment of gonococcal urethritis with single doses of agents such as penicillin or cephalosporins, which lack antimicrobial activity against chlamydiae. Current treatment regimens for gonorrhea have evolved and now include combination therapy with ceftriaxone and azithromycin; this current regimen is effective against concomitant chlamydial infection. Thus, both the incidence of PGU and the causative role of *C. trachomatis* in this syndrome have declined.

In the United States, most of the estimated 2 million cases of acute urethritis are NGU, and *C. trachomatis* is implicated in 30–50% of these cases. The cause of most of the remaining cases of NGU is uncertain, but recent evidence suggests that *Mycoplasma genitalium, Trichomonas vaginalis*, and herpes simplex virus (HSV) cause some cases. The rate of involvement of *C. trachomatis* in urethral infection ranges from 3–7% among asymptomatic men to 15–20% among symptomatic men attending STD clinics. One recent multisite study of men in Baltimore, Seattle, Denver, and San Francisco reported an overall chlamydial prevalence of 7% in urine samples assessed by nucleic acid amplification tests (NAATs)—molecular tests that amplify the nucleic acids in clinical specimens. As in women, infection in men is age related, with young age as the greatest risk factor for chlamydial urethritis. The prevalence among men is highest at 20–24 years of age. In STD clinics, urethritis is usually less prevalent among MSM than among heterosexual men.

NGU is diagnosed by documentation of a leukocyte urethral exudate and by exclusion of gonorrhea by Gram's staining or culture. *C. trachomatis* urethritis is generally less severe than gonococcal urethritis, although in any individual patient, these two forms of urethritis cannot reliably be differentiated solely on clinical grounds. Symptoms include urethral discharge (often whitish and mucoid rather than frankly purulent), dysuria, and urethral itching. Physical examination may reveal meatal erythema and tenderness as well as a urethral exudate that is often demonstrable only by stripping of the urethra.

At least one-third of male patients with *C. trachomatis* urethral infection have no evident signs or symptoms of urethritis. The availability of NAATs for first-void urine specimens has facilitated broader-based testing for asymptomatic infection in male patients. As a result, asymptomatic chlamydial urethritis has been demonstrated in 5–10% of sexually active male adolescents screened at school-based clinics or community centers. Such patients generally have pyuria (≥15 leukocytes per 400× microscopic field in the sediment of first-void urine), a positive leukocyte esterase test, or an increased number of leukocytes on a Gram-stained smear prepared from a urogenital swab inserted 1–2 cm into the anterior urethra. When specific diagnostic tests for chlamydiae are not available, the examination of an endourethral specimen for increased leukocytes is useful in differentiating between true urethritis and functional symptoms in symptomatic patients or in making a presumptive diagnosis of *C. trachomatis* infection in high-risk but asymptomatic men (e.g., male patients in STD clinics, sex partners of women with nongonococcal salpingitis or mucopurulent cervicitis, fathers of children with inclusion conjunctivitis). Alternatively, urethritis can be assayed noninvasively by examination of a first-void urine sample for pyuria, either by microscopy or by the leukocyte esterase test. Urine (or a urethral swab) can also be tested directly for chlamydiae by DNA amplification methods (NAATs), as described below (see "Detection Methods").

EPIDIDYMITIS Chlamydial urethritis may be followed by acute epididymitis, but this condition is rare, generally occurring in sexually active patients <35 years of age; in older men, epididymitis is usually associated with gram-negative bacterial infection and/or instrumentation procedures. An estimated 50–70% of cases of acute epididymitis are caused by *C. trachomatis*. The condition usually presents as unilateral scrotal pain with tenderness, swelling, and fever in a young man, often occurring in association with chlamydial urethritis. The illness may be mild enough to treat with oral antibiotics on an outpatient basis or severe enough to require hospitalization and parenteral therapy. Testicular torsion should be excluded promptly by radionuclide scan, Doppler flow study, or surgical exploration in a teenager or young adult who presents with acute unilateral testicular pain without urethritis. The possibility of testicular tumor or chronic infection (e.g., tuberculosis) should be excluded when a patient with unilateral intrascrotal pain and swelling does not respond to appropriate antimicrobial therapy.

REACTIVE ARTHRITIS Reactive arthritis consists of conjunctivitis, urethritis (or, in female patients, cervicitis), arthritis, and characteristic mucocutaneous lesions. It may develop in 1–2% of cases of NGU and is thought to be the most common type of peripheral inflammatory arthritis in young men. *C. trachomatis* has been recovered from the urethra of 16–44% of patients with reactive arthritis and 69% of men who have signs of urogenital inflammation at the time of examination. Antibodies to *C. trachomatis* have also been detected in 46–67% of patients with reactive arthritis, and *Chlamydia*-specific cell-mediated immunity has been documented in 72%. In addition, *C. trachomatis* has been isolated from synovial biopsy samples from 15 of 29 patients in a number of small series and from a smaller proportion of synovial fluid specimens. Chlamydial nucleic acids have been identified in synovial membranes and chlamydial elementary bodies in joint fluid. The pathogenesis of reactive arthritis is unclear, but this condition probably represents an abnormal host response to a number of infectious agents, including those associated with bacterial gastroenteritis (e.g., *Salmonella, Shigella, Yersinia,* or *Campylobacter*), or to infection with *C. trachomatis* or *N. gonorrhoeae.* Since >80% of affected patients have the HLA-B27 phenotype and since other mucosal infections produce an identical syndrome, chlamydial infection is thought to initiate an aberrant hyperreactive immune response that produces inflammation of the involved target organs in these genetically predisposed individuals. Evidence of exaggerated cell-mediated and humoral immune responses to chlamydial antigens in reactive arthritis supports this hypothesis. The finding of chlamydial elementary bodies and DNA in joint fluid and synovial tissue from patients with reactive arthritis suggests that chlamydiae may actually spread from genital to joint tissues in these patients—perhaps in macrophages.

NGU is the initial manifestation of reactive arthritis in 80% of patients, typically occurring within 14 days after sexual exposure. The urethritis may be mild and may even go unnoticed by the patient. Similarly, gonococcal urethritis may precede reactive arthritis, but co-infection with an agent of NGU is difficult to rule out. The urethral discharge may be purulent or mucopurulent, and patients may or may not report dysuria. Accompanying prostatitis, usually asymptomatic, has been described. Arthritis usually begins ~4 weeks after the onset of urethritis but may develop sooner or, in a small percentage of cases, may actually precede urethritis. The knees are most frequently involved; next most commonly affected are the ankles and small joints of the feet. Sacroiliitis, either symmetrical or asymmetrical, is documented in two-thirds of patients. Mild bilateral conjunctivitis, iritis, keratitis, or uveitis is sometimes present but lasts for only a few days. Finally, dermatologic manifestations occur in up to 50% of patients. The initial lesions—usually papules with a central yellow spot—most often involve the soles and palms and, in ~25% of patients, eventually epithelialize and thicken to produce keratoderma blenorrhagicum. Circinate balanitis is usually painless and occurs in fewer than half of patients. The initial episode of reactive arthritis usually lasts 2–6 months.

PROCTITIS Primary anal or rectal infections with *C. trachomatis* have been described in women and MSM who practice anal intercourse. In these infections, rectal involvement is initially characterized by severe anorectal pain, a bloody mucopurulent discharge, and tenesmus. Oculogenital serovars D–K and LGV serovars L_1, L_2, and L_3 have been found to cause proctitis. The LGV serovars are far more invasive and cause much more severely symptomatic disease, including severe ulcerative proctocolitis that can be clinically confused with HSV proctitis. Histologically, LGV proctitis may resemble Crohn's disease in that giant cell formation and granulomas are detected. In the United States and Europe, cases of LGV proctitis occur almost exclusively in MSM, many of whom have HIV infection.

The less invasive non-LGV serovars of *C. trachomatis* cause mild proctitis. Many infected individuals are asymptomatic, and in these cases, infection is diagnosed only by routine culture or NAAT of rectal swabs. The number of fecal leukocytes is usually abnormal in both asymptomatic and symptomatic cases. Sigmoidoscopy may yield normal findings or may reveal mild inflammatory changes or small erosions or follicles in the lower 10 cm of the rectum. Histologic examination of rectal biopsies generally shows anal crypts and prominent follicles as well as neutrophilic infiltration of the lamina propria. Chlamydial proctitis is best diagnosed by isolation of *C. trachomatis* from the rectum and documentation of a response to appropriate therapy. NAATs are reportedly more sensitive than culture for diagnosis and are also specific.

MUCOPURULENT CERVICITIS Although most women with chlamydial infections of the cervix have no symptoms, almost half generally have local signs of infection on examination. Cervicitis is usually characterized by the presence of a mucopurulent discharge, with >20 neutrophils per microscopic field visible in strands of cervical mucus in a thinly smeared, Gram-stained preparation of endocervical exudate. Hypertrophic ectopy of the cervix may also be evident as an edematous area near the cervical os that is congested and bleeds easily on minor trauma (e.g., when a specimen is collected with a swab). A Papanicolaou smear shows increased numbers of neutrophils as well as a characteristic pattern of mononuclear inflammatory cells, including plasma cells, transformed lymphocytes, and histiocytes. Cervical biopsy shows a predominantly mononuclear cell infiltrate of the subepithelial stroma. Clinical experience and collaborative studies indicate that a cutoff of >30 polymorphonuclear leukocytes (PMNs)/1000× field in a Gram-stained smear of cervical mucus correlates best with chlamydial or gonococcal cervicitis.

Clinical recognition of chlamydial cervicitis depends on a high index of suspicion and careful cervical examination. No genital symptoms are specifically correlated with chlamydial cervical infection. The differential diagnosis of a mucopurulent discharge from the endocervical canal in a young, sexually active woman includes gonococcal endocervicitis, salpingitis, endometritis, and intrauterine contraceptive device–induced inflammation. Diagnosis of cervicitis is based on the presence of PMNs on a cervical swab as noted above; the presence of chlamydiae is confirmed by either culture or NAAT.

PELVIC INFLAMMATORY DISEASE Inflammation of sections of the fallopian tube is often referred to as salpingitis or PID. The proportion of acute salpingitis cases caused by *C. trachomatis* varies geographically and with the population studied. It has been estimated that *C. trachomatis* causes up to 50% of PID cases in the United States. PID occurs via ascending intraluminal spread of *C. trachomatis* or *N. gonorrhoeae* from the lower genital tract. Mucopurulent cervicitis is often followed by endometritis, endosalpingitis, and finally pelvic peritonitis. Evidence of mucopurulent cervicitis is often found in women with laparoscopically verified salpingitis. Similarly, endometritis, demonstrated by an endometrial biopsy showing plasma cell infiltration of the endometrial epithelium, is documented in most women with laparoscopy-verified chlamydial (or gonococcal) salpingitis. Chlamydial endometritis can also occur in the absence of clinical evidence of salpingitis. Histologic evidence of endometritis has been correlated with a syndrome consisting of vaginal bleeding, lower abdominal pain, and uterine tenderness in the absence of adnexal tenderness. Chlamydial salpingitis produces milder symptoms than gonococcal salpingitis and may be associated with less marked adnexal tenderness. Thus, mild adnexal or uterine tenderness in a sexually active woman with cervicitis suggests chlamydial PID.

Chronic untreated endometrial and tubal inflammation can result in tubal scarring, impaired tubal function, tubal occlusion, and infertility even among women who report no prior treatment for chlamydial infection. *C. trachomatis* has been particularly implicated in "subclinical" PID on the basis of a lack of history of PID among *Chlamydia*-seropositive women with tubal damage and detection of chlamydial DNA or antigen among asymptomatic women with tubal infertility. These data suggest that the best method to prevent PID and its sequelae is surveillance and control of lower genital tract infections along with diagnosis and treatment of sex partners and prevention of reinfections. Promotion of early symptom recognition and health care presentation may reduce the frequency and severity of sequelae of PID.

PERIHEPATITIS Fitz-Hugh–Curtis syndrome was originally described as a complication of gonococcal PID. However, studies over the past several decades have suggested that chlamydial infection is more commonly associated with perihepatitis than is *N. gonorrhoeae.* Perihepatitis should be suspected in young, sexually active women who develop right-upper-quadrant pain, fever, or nausea. Evidence of salpingitis may or may not be found on examination. Frequently, perihepatitis is strongly associated with extensive tubal scarring, adhesions, and inflammation observed at laparoscopy, and high titers of antibody to the 57-kDa chlamydial heat-shock protein have been documented. Culture and/or serologic evidence of *C. trachomatis* is found in three-fourths of women with this syndrome.

URETHRAL SYNDROME IN WOMEN In the absence of infection with uropathogens such as coliforms or *Staphylococcus saprophyticus*, *C. trachomatis* is the pathogen most commonly isolated from college women with dysuria, frequency, and pyuria. Screening studies can recover *C. trachomatis* at both the cervix and the urethra; in up to 25% of infected women, the organism is isolated only from the urethra. The urethral syndrome in women consists of dysuria and frequency in conjunction with chlamydial urethritis, pyuria, and no bacteriuria or urinary pathogens. Although symptoms of the urethral syndrome may develop in some women with chlamydial infection, the majority of women attending STD clinics for urethral chlamydial infection do not have dysuria or frequency. Even in women with chlamydial urethritis causing the acute urethral syndrome, signs of urethritis such as urethral discharge, meatal redness, and swelling are uncommon. However, mucopurulent cervicitis in a woman presenting with dysuria and frequency strongly suggests *C. trachomatis* urethritis. Other correlates of chlamydial urethral syndrome include a duration of dysuria of >7–10 days, lack of hematuria, and lack of suprapubic tenderness. Abnormal urethral Gram's stains showing >10 PMNs/1000× field in women with dysuria but without coliform bacteriuria support the diagnosis of chlamydial urethritis. Other possible diagnoses include gonococcal or trichomonal infection of the urethra.

INFECTION IN PREGNANCY AND THE NEONATAL PERIOD Infections during pregnancy can be transmitted to infants during delivery. Approximately 20–30% of infants exposed to *C. trachomatis* in the birth canal develop conjunctivitis, and 10–15% subsequently develop pneumonia. Consequently, all newborn infants receive ocular prophylaxis at birth to prevent ophthalmia neonatorum. Without treatment, conjunctivitis usually develops at 5–19 days of life and often results in a profuse mucopurulent discharge. Roughly half of infected infants develop clinical evidence of inclusion conjunctivitis. However, it is impossible to differentiate chlamydial conjunctivitis from other forms of neonatal conjunctivitis (e.g., that due to *N. gonorrhoeae, Haemophilus influenzae, Streptococcus pneumoniae*, or HSV) on clinical grounds; thus, laboratory diagnosis is required. Inclusions within epithelial cells are often detected in Giemsa-stained conjunctival smears, but these smears are considerably less sensitive than cultures or NAATs for chlamydiae. Gram-stained smears may show gonococci or occasional small gram-negative coccobacilli in *Haemophilus* conjunctivitis, but smears should be accompanied by cultures or NAATs for these agents.

C. trachomatis has also been isolated frequently and persistently from the nasopharynx, rectum, and vagina of infected infants—occasionally for >1 year in the absence of treatment. In some cases, otitis media results from perinatally acquired chlamydial infection. Pneumonia may develop in infants from 2 weeks to 4 months of age. *C. trachomatis* is estimated to cause 20–30% of pneumonia cases in infants <6 months of age. Epidemiologic studies have linked chlamydial pulmonary infection in infants with increased occurrence of subacute lung disease (bronchitis, asthma, wheezing) in later childhood.

LYMPHOGRANULOMA VENEREUM *C. trachomatis* serovars L_1, L_2, and L_3 cause LGV, an invasive systemic STD. The peak incidence of LGV corresponds with the age of greatest sexual activity: the second and third decades of life. The worldwide incidence of LGV is falling, but the disease is still endemic and a major cause of morbidity in parts of Asia, Africa, South America, and the Caribbean. LGV is rare in industrialized countries; for more than a decade, the reported incidence in the United States has been only 0.1 case per 100,000 population. In the Bahamas, an apparent outbreak of LGV was described in association with a concurrent increase in heterosexual infection with HIV. Reports of outbreaks with the newly identified variant L_{2b} in Europe, Australia, and the United States indicate that LGV is becoming more prevalent among MSM. These cases have usually presented as hemorrhagic proctocolitis in HIV-positive men. More widespread use of NAATs for identification of rectal infections may have enhanced case recognition.

LGV begins as a small painless papule that tends to ulcerate at the site of inoculation, often escaping attention. This primary lesion heals in a few days without scarring and is usually recognized as LGV only in retrospect. LGV strains of *C. trachomatis* have occasionally been recovered from genital ulcers and from the urethra of men and the endocervix of women who present with inguinal adenopathy; these areas may be the primary sites of infection in some cases. Proctitis is more common among people who practice receptive anal intercourse, and an elevated white blood cell count in anorectal smears may predict LGV in these patients. Ulcer formation may facilitate transmission of HIV infection and other sexually transmitted and blood-borne diseases.

As NAATs for *C. trachomatis* are being used more often, increasing numbers of cases of LGV proctitis are being recognized in MSM, including HIV-infected MSM. Such patients present with anorectal pain and mucopurulent, bloody rectal discharge. Sigmoidoscopy reveals ulcerative proctitis or proctocolitis, with purulent exudate and mucosal bleeding. Histopathologic findings in the rectal mucosa include granulomas with giant cells, crypt abscesses, and extensive inflammation. These clinical, sigmoidoscopic, and histopathologic findings may closely resemble those of Crohn's disease of the rectum.

The most common presenting picture in heterosexual men and women is the *inguinal syndrome*, which is characterized by painful inguinal lymphadenopathy beginning 2–6 weeks after presumed exposure; in rare instances, the onset comes after a few months. The inguinal adenopathy is unilateral in two-thirds of cases, and palpable enlargement of the iliac and femoral nodes is often evident on the same side as the enlarged inguinal nodes. The nodes are initially discrete, but progressive periadenitis results in a matted mass of nodes that becomes fluctuant and suppurative. The overlying skin becomes fixed, inflamed, and thin, and multiple draining fistulas finally develop. Extensive enlargement of chains of inguinal nodes above and below the inguinal ligament ("the sign of the groove") is not specific and, although not uncommon, is documented in only a minority of cases. Spontaneous healing usually takes place after several months; inguinal scars or granulomatous masses of various sizes persist for life. Massive pelvic lymphadenopathy may lead to exploratory laparotomy.

Constitutional symptoms are common during the stage of regional lymphadenopathy and, in cases of proctitis, may include fever, chills, headache, meningismus, anorexia, myalgias, and arthralgias. Other systemic complications are infrequent but include arthritis with sterile effusion, aseptic meningitis, meningoencephalitis, conjunctivitis, hepatitis, and erythema nodosum (**Fig. A1-39**). Complications of untreated anorectal infection include perirectal abscess; anal fistulas; and rectovaginal, rectovesical, and ischiorectal fistulas. Secondary bacterial infection probably contributes to these complications. Rectal stricture is a late complication of anorectal infection and usually develops 2–6 cm from the anal orifice—i.e., at a site within reach on digital rectal examination. A small percentage of cases of LGV in men present as chronic progressive infiltrative, ulcerative, or fistular lesions of the penis, urethra, or scrotum. Associated lymphatic obstruction may produce elephantiasis. When urethral stricture occurs, it usually involves the posterior urethra and causes incontinence or difficulty with urination.

Diagnosis • DETECTION METHODS

Historically, chlamydiae were cultivated in the yolk sac of embryonated eggs. The organisms can be grown more easily in tissue culture, but cell culture—once considered the diagnostic gold standard—has been replaced by nonculture assays (**Table 189-1**). In general, culture for chlamydiae in clinical specimens is now performed only in specialized laboratories. The first nonculture assays, such as direct fluorescent antibody staining of clinical material and enzyme immunoassay (EIA), have been replaced by NAATs, which are currently recommended by the CDC as the diagnostic assays of choice. At present, six NAAT assays cleared by the U.S. Food and Drug Administration (FDA) are commercially available, some of which are available as high-throughput robotic platforms. Point-of-care rapid diagnostic assays are becoming available; they are of increasing interest since patients can potentially be treated before leaving the clinic, thus preventing forward transmission while patients wait for results from tests with longer turnaround times.

CHOICE OF SPECIMEN Cervical and urethral swabs have traditionally been used for the diagnosis of STDs in female and male patients, respectively. However, given the greatly increased sensitivity and specificity of NAATs, less invasive samples (e.g., urine for both sexes and vaginal swabs for women) can be used. For screening of asymptomatic women, the CDC now recommends that self-collected or

TABLE 189-1 Diagnostic Tests for Sexually Transmitted and Perinatal *Chlamydia trachomatis* Infection

INFECTION	SUGGESTIVE SIGNS/SYMPTOMS	PRESUMPTIVE DIAGNOSIS[a]	CONFIRMATORY TEST OF CHOICE
Men			
NGU, PGU	Discharge, dysuria	Gram's stain with >4 neutrophils per oil-immersion field; no gonococci	Urine or urethral NAAT for *C. trachomatis*
Epididymitis	Unilateral intrascrotal swelling, pain, tenderness; fever; NGU	Gram's stain with >4 neutrophils per oil-immersion field; no gonococci; urinalysis with pyuria	Urine or urethral NAAT for *C. trachomatis*
Women			
Cervicitis	Mucopurulent cervical discharge, bleeding and edema of the zone of cervical ectopy	Cervical Gram's stain with ≥20 neutrophils per oil-immersion field in cervical mucus	Urine, cervical, or vaginal NAAT for *C. trachomatis*
Salpingitis	Lower abdominal pain, cervical motion tenderness, adnexal tenderness or masses	*C. trachomatis* always potentially present in salpingitis	Urine, cervical, or vaginal NAAT for *C. trachomatis*
Urethritis	Dysuria and frequency without hematuria	MPC; sterile pyuria; negative routine urine culture	Urine or urethral NAAT for *C. trachomatis*
Adults of Either Sex			
Proctitis	Rectal pain, discharge, tenesmus, bleeding; history of receptive anorectal intercourse	Negative gonococcal culture and Gram's stain; at least 1 neutrophil per oil-immersion field in rectal Gram's stain	Rectal NAAT for *C. trachomatis* or culture
Reactive arthritis	NGU, arthritis, conjunctivitis, typical skin lesions	Gram's stain with >4 neutrophils per oil-immersion field; lack of gonococci indicative of NGU	Urine or urethral NAAT for *C. trachomatis*
LGV	Regional adenopathy, primary lesion, proctitis, systemic symptoms	None	Culture of LGV strain from node or rectum, occasionally from urethra or cervix; NAAT for *C. trachomatis* from these sites; LGV CF titer, ≥1:64; MIF titer, ≥1:512
Neonates			
Conjunctivitis	Purulent conjunctival discharge 6–18 days after delivery	Negative culture and Gram's stain for gonococci, *Haemophilus* spp., pneumococci, staphylococci	Conjunctival NAAT for *C. trachomatis*; FA-stained scraping of conjunctival material
Infant pneumonia	Afebrile, staccato cough, diffuse rales, bilateral hyperinflation, interstitial infiltrates	None	Chlamydial culture or NAAT of sputum, pharynx, eye, rectum; MIF antibody to *C. trachomatis*—fourfold change in IgG or IgM antibody titer

[a]A presumptive diagnosis of chlamydial infection is often made in the syndromes listed when gonococci are not found. A positive test for *Neisseria gonorrhoeae* does not exclude the involvement of *C. trachomatis*, which often is present in patients with gonorrhea.

Abbreviations: CF, complement-fixing; FA, fluorescent antibody; LGV, lymphogranuloma venereum; MIF, microimmunofluorescence; MPC, mucopurulent cervicitis; NAAT, nucleic acid amplification test; NGU, nongonococcal urethritis; PGU, postgonococcal urethritis.

Source: Reproduced with permission from WE Stamm: Chlamydial infections, in AS Fauci et al [eds]: *Harrison's Principles of Internal Medicine*, 17th ed. New York, McGraw-Hill, 2008.

clinician-collected vaginal swabs, which are slightly more sensitive than urine, be used. Urine screening tests are often used in outreach screening programs, however. For symptomatic women undergoing a pelvic examination, cervical swab samples are desirable because they have slightly higher chlamydial counts. For male patients, a urine specimen is the sample of choice, but self-collected penile-meatal swabs have been shown to be very effective.

ALTERNATIVE SPECIMEN TYPES Ocular samples from babies and adults can be assessed by NAATs. Samples from extragenital rectal and pharyngeal sites have been used previously to detect chlamydiae by NAATs with validation studies, but now several commercially available NAAT tests have FDA clearance for extragenital samples.

OTHER DIAGNOSTIC ISSUES Because NAATs detect nucleic acids instead of live organisms, they should be used with caution as test-of-cure assays. Residual nucleic acid from cells rendered noninfective by antibiotics may continue to yield a positive result in NAATs for as long as 3 weeks after therapy when viable organisms have actually been eradicated. Therefore, clinicians should not use NAATs for test of cure until after 3 weeks. The CDC currently does not recommend a test of cure after treatment for infection with *C. trachomatis*. However, because incidence studies have demonstrated that previous chlamydial infection increases the probability of becoming reinfected, the CDC does recommend that previously infected individuals be rescreened 3 months after treatment.

SEROLOGY Serologic testing may be helpful in the diagnosis of LGV and neonatal pneumonia caused by *C. trachomatis*. The serologic test of choice is the microimmunofluorescence (MIF) test, in which high-titer purified elementary bodies mixed with embryonated chicken yolk sac material are affixed to a glass microscope slide to which dilutions of sera are applied. After incubation and washing, fluorescein-conjugated IgG or IgM antibody is applied. The test is read with an epifluorescence microscope, with the highest dilution of serum producing visible fluorescence designated as the titer. The MIF test is not widely available except in research laboratories and is highly labor intensive. Although the complement fixation (CF) test can also be used, it employs lipopolysaccharide (LPS) as the antigen and therefore identifies the pathogen only to the genus level. Single-point titers of >1:64 support a diagnosis of LGV, for which it is difficult to demonstrate rising antibody titers—i.e., paired serum samples are difficult to obtain since the disease often results in the patient's being seen by the physician after the acute stage. Any antibody titer of >1:16 is considered significant evidence of exposure to chlamydiae. However, serologic testing is never recommended for diagnosis of uncomplicated genital infections of the cervix, urethra, and lower genital tract or for *C. trachomatis* screening of asymptomatic individuals.

TREATMENT

C. trachomatis Genital Infections

A 7-day course of oral doxycycline (100 mg twice daily) or a single 1-g oral dose of azithromycin are the primary recommended regimens of treatment for uncomplicated chlamydial infections. Alternative 7-day oral regimens include erythromycin (500 mg four times daily), or a fluoroquinolone (ofloxacin, 300 mg twice daily; or levofloxacin, 500 mg/d) can be used. The single 1-g oral dose of azithromycin is as effective as a 7-day course of doxycycline for the treatment of uncomplicated genital *C. trachomatis* infections in adults. Azithromycin causes fewer adverse gastrointestinal reactions than do older macrolides such as erythromycin. The single-dose regimen of azithromycin has great appeal for the treatment of patients with uncomplicated chlamydial infection (especially those without symptoms and those with a likelihood of poor compliance) and of the sexual partners of infected patients. These advantages must be weighed against the considerably greater cost of azithromycin. Whenever possible, the single 1-g dose should be given as directly observed therapy. Although not approved by the FDA for use in pregnancy, this regimen appears to be safe and effective for this purpose. Amoxicillin (500 mg three times daily for 7 days) or erythromycin (500 mg four times daily) can also be given as an alternative to pregnant women. The fluoroquinolones are contraindicated in pregnancy. A 2-week course of treatment is recommended for complicated chlamydial infections (e.g., PID, epididymitis) and at least a 3-week course of doxycycline (100 mg orally twice daily) or erythromycin base (500 mg orally four times daily) for LGV. Failure of treatment with a tetracycline in genital infections usually indicates poor compliance or reinfection rather than involvement of a drug-resistant strain. To date, clinically significant drug resistance has not been observed in *C. trachomatis*.

Treatment or testing for chlamydiae should be considered among *N. gonorrhoeae*–infected patients because of the frequency of co-infection. Systemic treatment with erythromycin has been recommended for ophthalmia neonatorum and for *C. trachomatis* pneumonia in infants. For the treatment of adult inclusion conjunctivitis, a single 1-g dose of azithromycin was as effective as standard 10-day treatment with doxycycline. Recommended treatment regimens for both bubonic and anogenital LGV include tetracycline, doxycycline, or erythromycin for 21 days.

SEX PARTNERS

The continued high prevalence of chlamydial infections in most parts of the United States is due primarily to the failure to diagnose—and therefore treat—patients with symptomatic or asymptomatic infection and their sex partners. Urethral or cervical infection with *C. trachomatis* has been well documented in a high proportion of the sex partners of patients with NGU, epididymitis, reactive arthritis, salpingitis, and endocervicitis. If possible, confirmatory laboratory tests for chlamydiae should be undertaken in these individuals, but even persons without positive tests or evidence of clinical disease who have recently been exposed to proven or possible chlamydial infection (e.g., NGU) should be offered therapy. A novel approach is partner-delivered therapy, in which infected patients receive treatment and are also provided with single-dose azithromycin to give to their sex partner(s).

NEONATES AND INFANTS

In neonates with conjunctivitis or infants with pneumonia, erythromycin ethylsuccinate or estolate can be given orally at a dosage of 50 mg/kg per day, preferably in four divided doses, for 2 weeks. Careful attention must be given to compliance with therapy—a frequent problem. Relapses of eye infection are common after topical treatment with erythromycin or tetracycline ophthalmic ointment and may also follow oral erythromycin therapy. Thus, follow-up cultures should be performed after treatment. Both parents should be examined for *C. trachomatis* infection and, if diagnostic testing is not readily available, should be treated with doxycycline or azithromycin.

Prevention Since many chlamydial infections are asymptomatic, effective control and prevention must involve periodic screening of individuals at risk. Selective cost-effective screening criteria have been developed. Among women, young age (generally <25 years) is a critical risk factor for chlamydial infections in nearly all studies. Other risk factors include mucopurulent cervicitis; multiple, new, or symptomatic male sex partners; and lack of barrier contraceptive use. In some settings, screening based on young age may be as sensitive as criteria that incorporate behavioral and clinical measures. Another strategy is universal testing of all patients in high-prevalence clinic populations (e.g., STD clinics, juvenile detention facilities, and family planning clinics).

The effectiveness of selective screening in reducing the prevalence of chlamydial infection among women has been demonstrated in several studies. In the Pacific Northwest, where extensive screening began in family planning clinics in 1998 and in STD clinics in 1993, the prevalence declined from 10% in the 1980s to <5% in 2000. Similar trends have occurred in association with screening programs elsewhere. In addition, screening can effect a reduction in upper genital tract disease. In Seattle, women at a large health maintenance organization who were screened for chlamydial infection on a routine basis had a lower incidence of symptomatic PID than did women who received standard care and underwent more selective screening.

In settings with low to moderate prevalence, the prevalence at which selective screening becomes more cost-effective than universal screening must be defined. Most studies have concluded that universal screening is preferable in settings with a chlamydial prevalence of >3–7%. Depending on the criteria used, selective screening is likely to be more cost-effective when prevalence falls below 3%. Nearly all regions of the United States have now initiated screening programs, particularly in family planning and STD clinics. Along with single-dose therapy, the availability of highly sensitive and specific diagnostic NAATs using urine specimens and self-obtained vaginal swabs makes it feasible to mount an effective nationwide *Chlamydia* control program, with screening of high-risk individuals in traditional health care settings and in novel outreach and community-based settings. The U.S. Preventive Services Task Force has named *Chlamydia* screening as a Grade B recommendation, which means that private insurance and Medicare will cover the cost of screening under the Affordable Care Act.

TRACHOMA

Epidemiology Trachoma—a sequela of ocular disease in developing countries—continues to be a leading cause of preventable infectious blindness worldwide. The WHO estimates that ~6 million people have been blinded by trachoma and that ~1.3 million people in developing countries still suffer from preventable blindness due to trachoma; certainly, hundreds of millions live in trachoma-endemic areas. Foci of trachoma persist in Australia, the South Pacific, and Latin America. *C. trachomatis* serovars A, B, Ba, and C are isolated from patients with clinical trachoma in areas of endemicity in developing countries in Africa, the Middle East, Asia, and South America.

The trachoma-hyperendemic areas of the world are in northern and sub-Saharan Africa, the Middle East, drier regions of the Indian subcontinent, and Southeast Asia. In hyperendemic areas, the prevalence of trachoma is essentially 100% by the second or third year of life. Active disease is most common among young children, who are the reservoir for trachoma. By adulthood, active infection is infrequent but sequelae result in blindness. In such areas, trachoma constitutes the major cause of blindness.

Trachoma is transmitted through contact with discharges from the eyes of infected patients. Transmission is most common under poor hygienic conditions and most often takes place between family members or between families with shared facilities. Flies can also transfer the mucopurulent ocular discharges, carrying the organisms on their legs from one person to another. The International Trachoma Initiative founded by the WHO in 1998 aims to eliminate blinding trachoma globally by 2020.

Clinical Manifestations Both endemic trachoma and adult inclusion conjunctivitis present initially as conjunctivitis characterized by small lymphoid follicles in the conjunctiva. In regions with hyperendemic classic blinding trachoma, the disease usually starts insidiously before the age of 2 years. Reinfection is common and probably contributes to the pathogenesis of trachoma. Studies using polymerase chain reaction (PCR) or other NAATs indicate that chlamydial DNA is often present in the ocular secretions of patients with trachoma, even in the absence of positive cultures. Thus, persistent infection may be more common than was previously thought.

The cornea becomes involved, with inflammatory leukocytic infiltrations and superficial vascularization (pannus formation). As the inflammation continues, conjunctival scarring eventually distorts the eyelids, causing them to turn inward so that the lashes constantly abrade the eyeball (trichiasis and entropion); eventually the corneal epithelium is abraded and may ulcerate, with subsequent corneal scarring and blindness. Destruction of the conjunctival goblet cells, lacrimal ducts, and lacrimal gland may produce a "dry-eye" syndrome, with resultant corneal opacity due to drying (xerosis) or secondary bacterial corneal ulcers.

Communities with blinding trachoma often experience seasonal epidemics of conjunctivitis due to *H. influenzae* that contribute to the intensity of the inflammatory process. In such areas, the active infectious process usually resolves spontaneously in affected persons at 10–15 years of age, but conjunctival scars continue to shrink, producing trichiasis and entropion with subsequent corneal scarring in adults. In areas with milder and less prevalent disease, the process may be much slower, with active disease continuing into adulthood; blindness is rare in these cases.

Eye infection with oculogenital *C. trachomatis* strains in sexually active young adults presents as an acute onset of unilateral follicular conjunctivitis and preauricular lymphadenopathy similar to that seen in acute conjunctivitis caused by adenovirus or HSV. If untreated, the disease may persist for 6 weeks to 2 years. It is frequently associated with corneal inflammation in the form of discrete opacities ("infiltrates"), punctate epithelial erosions, and minor degrees of superficial corneal vascularization. Very rarely, conjunctival scarring and eyelid distortion occur, particularly in patients treated for many months with topical glucocorticoids. Recurrent eye infections develop most often in patients whose sexual partners are not treated with antimicrobial agents.

Diagnosis The clinical diagnosis of classic trachoma can be made if two of the following signs are present: (1) lymphoid follicles on the upper tarsal conjunctiva; (2) typical conjunctival scarring; (3) vascular pannus; or (4) limbal follicles or their sequelae, Herbert pits. The clinical diagnosis of endemic trachoma should be confirmed by laboratory tests in children with relatively marked degrees of inflammation. Intracytoplasmic chlamydial inclusions are found in 10–60% of Giemsa-stained conjunctival smears in such populations, but chlamydial NAATs are more sensitive and are often positive when smears or cultures are negative. Follicular conjunctivitis in European or American adults living in trachomatous regions is rarely due to trachoma.

TREATMENT
Trachoma

Adult inclusion conjunctivitis responds well to treatment with the same regimens used in uncomplicated genital infections—namely, azithromycin (a 1-g single oral dose) or doxycycline (100 mg twice daily for 7 days). Simultaneous treatment of all sexual partners is necessary to prevent ocular reinfection and chlamydial genital disease. Topical antibiotic treatment is not required for patients who receive systemic antibiotics.

PSITTACOSIS

Psittacine birds and many other avian species act as natural reservoirs for *C. psittaci*–type organisms, common pathogens in domestic mammals and birds. The species *C. psittaci,* which now includes only avian strains, affects humans only as a zoonosis. (The other strains previously included in this species have been placed into different species that reflect the animals they infect: *C. abortus, C. muridarum, C. suis, C. felis,* and *C. caviae.*) Although all birds are susceptible, pet birds (parrots, parakeets, macaws, and cockatiels) and poultry (turkeys and ducks) are most frequently involved in transmission of *C. psittaci* to humans. Exposure is greatest in poultry-processing workers and in owners of pet birds. Infectious forms of the organisms are shed from both symptomatic and apparently healthy birds and may remain viable for several months. *C. psittaci* can be transmitted to humans by direct contact with infected birds or by inhalation of aerosols from avian nasal discharges and from infectious avian fecal or feather dust. Transmission from person to person has never been demonstrated.

The diagnosis is usually established serologically. Psittacosis in humans may present as acute primary atypical pneumonia (which can be fatal in up to 10% of untreated cases); as severe chronic pneumonia; or as a mild illness or asymptomatic infection in persons exposed to infected birds.

EPIDEMIOLOGY

Fewer than 50 confirmed cases of psittacosis are reported in the United States each year, although many more cases probably occur than are reported. Control of psittacosis depends on control of avian sources of infection. A pandemic of psittacosis was once stopped by banning shipment or importation of psittacine birds. Birds can receive prophylaxis in the form of a tetracycline-containing feed. Imported birds are currently quarantined for 30 days of treatment.

CLINICAL MANIFESTATIONS

Typical symptoms include fever, chills, muscular aches and pains, severe headache, hepato- and/or splenomegaly, and gastrointestinal symptoms. Cardiac complications may involve endocarditis and myocarditis. Fatal cases were common in the preantibiotic era. As a result of quarantine of imported birds and improved veterinary-hygienic measures, outbreaks and sporadic cases of psittacosis are now rare. Severe pneumonia requiring management in an intensive care unit may develop. Endocarditis, hepatitis, and neurologic complications may occur, and fatal cases have been reported. The incubation period is usually 5–19 days but can last as long as 28 days.

DIAGNOSIS

Previously, the most widely used serologic test for diagnosing chlamydial infections was the genus-specific CF test, in which assay of paired serum specimens often shows fourfold or greater increases in antibody titer. The CF test remains useful, but the gold standard of serologic tests is now the MIF test, which is not widely available (see section on diagnosis of *C. trachomatis* genital infection, above). Any antibody titer above 1:16 is considered significant evidence of exposure to chlamydiae, and a fourfold titer rise in paired sera in combination with a clinically compatible syndrome can be used to diagnose psittacosis. Some commercially available serologic tests based on measurement of antibodies to LPS can be useful when the clinical diagnosis is consistent with bird exposure; however, since these tests are reactive for all chlamydiae (i.e., all chlamydiae contain LPS), caution must be used in their interpretation. *C. psittaci* is now considered a biohazard category A biothreat agent and has been associated with laboratory-acquired infections. The CDC does not recommend testing for this agent when psittacosis is suspected, especially by culture.

TREATMENT
Psittacosis

The antibiotic of choice is tetracycline; the dosage for adults is 250 mg four times a day, continued for at least 3 weeks to avoid relapse. Severely ill patients may need cardiovascular and respiratory support. Erythromycin (500 mg four times a day by mouth) is an alternative therapy.

C. PNEUMONIAE INFECTIONS

C. pneumoniae is a common cause of human respiratory diseases, such as pneumonia and bronchitis. This organism reportedly accounts for as many as 10% of cases of community-acquired pneumonia, most of which are diagnosed by serology. Serologic studies have linked *C. pneumoniae* to atherosclerosis; isolation and PCR detection in cardiovascular tissues have also been reported. These findings suggest an expanded range of diseases and syndromes for *C. pneumoniae.* Large-scale case–cohort studies have demonstrated some association of *C. pneumoniae* with lung cancer, as evaluated by serology.

EPIDEMIOLOGY

Primary infection occurs mainly in school-aged children and reinfection in adults. Seroprevalence rates of 40–70% show that *C. pneumoniae* is widespread in both industrialized and developing countries. Seropositivity usually is first detected at school age, and rates generally increase by ~10% per decade. About 50% of individuals have detectable antibody at 30 years of age, and most have detectable antibody by the eighth decade of life. Although, as mentioned, serologic evidence suggests that *C. pneumoniae* may be associated with up to 10% of cases of community-acquired pneumonia, most of this evidence is based not on paired serum samples but rather on a single high IgG titer. Some doubt exists about the true prevalence and etiologic role of *C. pneumoniae* in atypical pneumonia, especially since reports of cross-reactivity have raised questions about the specificity of serology when only a single serum sample is used for diagnosis.

PATHOGENESIS

Little is known about the pathogenesis of *C. pneumoniae* infection. It begins in the upper respiratory tract and, in many persons, persists as a prolonged asymptomatic condition of the upper respiratory mucosal surfaces. However, evidence of replication within vascular endothelium and synovial membranes of joints shows that, in at least some individuals, the organism is transported to distant sites, perhaps within macrophages. A *C. pneumoniae* outer-membrane protein may induce host immune responses whose cross-reactivity with human proteins results in an autoimmune reaction.

The role of *C. pneumoniae* in the etiology of atherosclerosis has been discussed since 1988, when Finnish researchers presented serologic evidence of an association of this organism with coronary heart disease and acute myocardial infarction. Subsequently, the organism was identified in atherosclerotic lesions by culture, PCR, immunohistochemistry, and transmission electron microscopy; however, discrepant study results (including those of animal studies) and failure of large-scale treatment studies have raised doubts as to the etiologic role of *C. pneumoniae* in atherosclerosis. Epidemiologic studies have demonstrated an association between serologic evidence of *C. pneumoniae* infection and atherosclerotic disease of the coronary and other arteries. In addition, *C. pneumoniae* has been identified in atherosclerotic plaques by electron microscopy, DNA hybridization, and immunocytochemistry. The organism has been recovered in culture from atheromatous plaques—a result indicating the presence of viable replicating bacteria in vessels. Evidence from animal models supports the hypothesis that *C. pneumoniae* infection of the upper respiratory tract is followed by recovery of the organism from atheromatous lesions in the aorta and that the infection accelerates the process of atherosclerosis, especially in hypercholesterolemic animals. Antimicrobial treatment of the infected animals reverses the increased risk of atherosclerosis. In humans, two small trials in patients with unstable angina or recent myocardial infarction suggested that antibiotics reduce the likelihood of subsequent untoward cardiac events. However, larger-scale trials have not documented an effect of various antichlamydial regimens on the risk of these events.

CLINICAL MANIFESTATIONS

C. pneumoniae was first reported as the etiologic agent of mild atypical pneumonia in military recruits and college students. The clinical spectrum of *C. pneumoniae* infection includes acute pharyngitis, sinusitis, bronchitis, and pneumonitis, primarily in young adults. The clinical manifestations of primary infection appear to be more severe and prolonged than those of reinfection. The pneumonitis of *C. pneumoniae* pneumonia resembles that of *Mycoplasma* pneumonia in that leukocytosis is frequently lacking and patients often have prominent antecedent upper respiratory tract symptoms, fever, nonproductive cough, mild to moderate illness, minimal findings on chest auscultation, and small segmental infiltrates on chest x-ray. In elderly patients, pneumonia due to *C. pneumoniae* can be especially severe and may necessitate hospitalization and respiratory support.

Chronic infection with *C. pneumoniae* has been reported among patients with chronic obstructive pulmonary disease and may play a role in the natural history of asthma, including exacerbations. The clinical symptoms of respiratory infections caused by *C. pneumoniae* are nonspecific and do not differ from those caused by other agents of atypical pneumonia, such as *Mycoplasma pneumoniae.*

DIAGNOSIS

Serology, PCR amplification, and culture can be used to diagnose *C. pneumoniae* infection. Serology has been the traditional diagnostic method. The gold standard serologic test is the MIF test (see section on diagnosis of *C. trachomatis* genital infection, above). Any antibody titer >1:16 is considered significant evidence of exposure to chlamydiae. According to a CDC-sponsored expert working group, the diagnosis of acute *C. pneumoniae* infection requires demonstration of a fourfold rise in titer in paired serum samples. There are no official recommendations for diagnosis of chronic infections, although many research studies have used high titers of IgA as an indicator. The older CF tests and EIAs for LPS are not recommended, as they are not specific for *C. pneumoniae* but identify the chlamydiae only to the genus level. The organism is very difficult to grow in tissue culture but has been cultivated in HeLa cells, HEp-2 cells, and HL cells. Although NAATs are commercially available for *C. trachomatis*, only research-based PCR assays are available for *C. pneumoniae.*

TREATMENT

C. pneumoniae Infections

Although few controlled trials of treatment have been reported, *C. pneumoniae* is inhibited in vitro by erythromycin, tetracycline, azithromycin, clarithromycin, gatifloxacin, and gemifloxacin. Recommended therapy consists of 2 g/d of either tetracycline or erythromycin for 10–14 days. Other macrolides (e.g., azithromycin) and some fluoroquinolones (e.g., levofloxacin and gatifloxacin) also appear to be effective.

FURTHER READING

Centers for Disease Control and Prevention: *Sexually Transmitted Disease Surveillance, 2018.* Atlanta, GA: U.S. Department of Health and Human Services, 2019. *https://www.cdc.gov/std/chlamydia/stats.htm.*

Elwell C et al: Chlamydia cell biology and pathogenesis. Nat Rev Microbiol 14:385, 2016.

Gaydos CA, Essiq A: Chlamydiaceae, in *Manual of Clinical Microbiology,* 11th ed. JH Jorgensen et al (eds). Washington, DC, ASM Press, 2015, pp 1106–1121.

Goller JL et al: Population attributable fraction of pelvic inflammatory disease associated with chlamydia and gonorrhoea: A cross-sectional analysis of Australian sexual health clinic data. Sex Transm Infect 92:525, 2016.

Hammerschlag MR et al: *Chlamydia pneumoniae,* in *Mandell, Douglas, and Bennett's Principles and Practice of Infectious Diseases,* 9th ed. JE Bennett, R Dolin, MJ Blaser (eds). Philadelphia, Elsevier, 2020, Chapter 182.

Kuypers J et al: Principles of laboratory diagnosis of STIs, in *Sexually Transmitted Diseases,* 4th ed. KK Holmes et al (eds). New York, McGraw-Hill, 2008, pp 937–948.

Papp JR et al: Recommendations for the laboratory-based detection of *Chlamydia trachomatis* and *Neisseria gonorrhoeae*, 2014. MMWR 63(RR-02):1, 2014.

Rowley J et al: Chlamydia, gonorrhea, trichomoniasis and syphilis: Global prevalence and incidence estimates, 2016. Bull World Health Organ 97:548, 2019.

Schachter J, Stephens RS: Biology of *Chlamydia trachomatis*, in *Sexually Transmitted Diseases*, 4th ed. KK Holmes et al (eds). New York, McGraw-Hill, 2008, pp 555–574.
Taylor HR: *Trachoma: A Blinding Scourge from the Bronze Age to the Twenty-First Century*. East Melbourne, Victoria, Australia, Centre for Eye Research Australia/Haddington Press, 2008, 282 pp.
Workowski KA, Bolan GA: Sexually transmitted diseases treatment guidelines, 2015. MMWR Recomm Rep 64(Rr-03):1, 2015.

Section 11 Viral Diseases: General Considerations

190 Principles of Medical Virology

David M. Knipe

Viruses are obligate intracellular parasites that must enter cells to replicate. Infection often injures the host cell—hence the name "virus," derived from the Latin word *virus* for poison or toxin. Viruses are one of the simplest life forms and, at the minimum, have a nucleic acid genome with a protein coat. They do not divide by division, as do cells; instead, viruses are programmed to disassemble inside cells, to use their nucleic acid genome to encode viral proteins that replicate their genomic nucleic acid, and then to assemble the progeny genomes into viral particles. The progeny viruses are secreted or released from the host cell as extracellular *virions* that infect surrounding cells. Viruses depend on the host cell for many of the enzymes and organelles that synthesize carbohydrates, lipids, nucleic precursors and nucleic acids, and high-energy molecules, including the host cell's ribosomes, which are used to make viral proteins. In the process of taking over the host cell, viruses inhibit normal cell metabolic pathways and cause damage to the cell in a process that results in the *cytopathic effect* (CPE). Injury to cells and cell death can cause tissue damage and contribute to virus-induced disease.

Viruses are distinct from other intracellular parasites such as viroids, virusoids, prions, and intracellular bacteria. *Viroids* are small, circular, single-stranded RNA infectious pathogens of plants that do not have a protein coat, while *virusoids* are small, circular-RNA, infectious pathogens that depend on viruses to provide the proteins for their replication and protein coat. *Prions* are misfolded proteins that spread from one cell to another, causing the same protein molecules to misfold in the new cell. The misfolded proteins in prions cause cellular damage (**Chap. 438**).

VIRUS STRUCTURE

There are many different virus structures, but nearly all are formed from a few fundamental structural elements. The minimal virion particle is composed of a complex of nucleic acids (the *genome*) and a protein shell (the *capsid*) (**Fig. 190-1**). The combination of the genome and the capsid is called the *nucleocapsid*. The genome is protected within the capsid. The external surface of virions can consist of either the protein capsid or a lipid envelope around the capsid (Fig. 190-1).

Viral genomes can consist of single- or double-stranded RNA or DNA and can comprise one or more genome segments. Single-stranded (ss) genomes are designated as *positive strand* (+) if they contain the sequences encoding the open reading frames for viral proteins, while they are designated as *negative strand* (–) if they contain only complementary sequences. Thus, a positive-strand RNA viral genome can be translated into a viral protein upon entry into the host cell, while a negative-strand genome must be copied into complementary RNA molecules for translation. This dilemma is solved in negative-strand viruses by the loading of transcriptases onto the viral genome prior to encapsidation; these enzymes transcribe the genome into viral mRNA upon entry into and uncoating within the cell.

Viral capsids are made of repeating protein subunits because their genomes have limited coding capacity. The capsids are constructed with a few structural units or capsomers packed into a symmetrical arrangement. Capsids are usually organized in one of two ways: (1) an *icosahedral* or *spherical* symmetry based on an icosahedron with two-, three-, and fivefold axes of symmetry formed from 20 triangular faces or (2) a *helical* symmetry. However, viruses occasionally have more complex structures (e.g., the poxviruses) (Fig. 190-1).

Enveloped viruses (e.g., measles virus) are efficient in infecting cells because the viral lipid membrane fuses easily with the plasma membrane of the host cell or with internal membranes to deliver the nucleocapsid to the cytoplasm of the host cell. Thus, these viruses are highly transmissible. The lipid envelope is susceptible to disruption by detergents or organic solvents; thus, enveloped viruses such as measles virus and influenza virus can be inactivated by soap and water or alcohol-based hand sanitizers. In contrast, unenveloped viruses (e.g., norovirus or poliovirus) have a tough protein shell whose resistance to small-intestine bile salts—a surfactant that emulsifies lipids—allows them to infect the intestine. Unenveloped viruses, especially those that infect the gastrointestinal tract, are not inactivated by detergents or organic solvents and must be inactivated by peroxide or hypochlorite or removed by washing with soap and water.

CLASSIFICATION OF VIRUSES

Viruses have been classified as a free-standing group because they are not formally related to organisms within any of the major kingdoms. The highest level of viral classification was originally the family, but some families have been grouped into orders as more has been learned about them. The major viruses of clinical interest can be conveniently classified into a number of families (**Table 190-1**), each of which has characteristic virion and genome structures (**Fig. 190-2**). Classification of viruses into families, genera, and species is based on multiple criteria, including type of genomic nucleic acid (i.e., RNA or DNA; ss positive or negative strand or double strand), capsid symmetry (helical, icosahedral, or complex), presence or absence of an envelope, mode of replication, and tropism (preferred cell type for replication) or type of disease it causes. Recent sequence analysis of viral genomes has refined and revised some of the original virus classifications. The International Committee on Taxonomy of Viruses specifies both formal and common names for viruses. For example, herpes simplex virus 1 (HSV-1) is the common name for human herpesvirus 1.

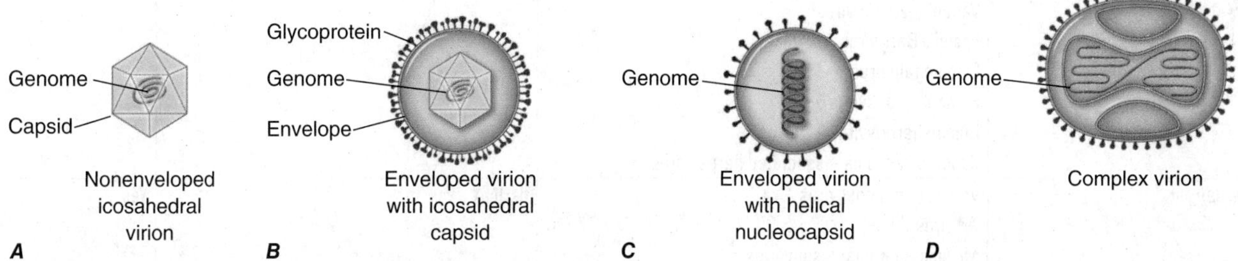

FIGURE 190-1 Schematic diagrams of the major forms of human viruses. ***A.*** Icosahedral capsid without an envelope. ***B.*** Icosahedral capsid with a lipid envelope. ***C.*** Helical capsid with a lipid envelope. ***D.*** Complex virion.

TABLE 190-1 Major Families of Human Pathogenic Viruses

FAMILY	REPRESENTATIVE VIRUSES	TYPE OF RNA/DNA	LIPID ENVELOPE
Picornaviridae	Coxsackievirus Echovirus Enteroviruses, including poliovirus Rhinoviruses Hepatitis A virus	(+) RNA	No
Caliciviridae	Norovirus	(+) RNA	No
Hepeviridae	Hepatitis E virus	(+) RNA	No
Togaviridae	Rubella virus Eastern equine encephalitis virus Western equine encephalitis virus	(+) RNA	Yes
Flaviviridae	Yellow fever virus Dengue virus St. Louis encephalitis virus West Nile virus Zika virus Hepatitis C virus Hepatitis G virus	(+) RNA	Yes
Coronaviridae	SARS-CoV-1 SARS-CoV-2 Middle East respiratory syndrome virus	(+) RNA	Yes
Rhabdoviridae	Rabies virus Vesicular stomatitis virus	(–) RNA	Yes
Filoviridae	Marburg virus Ebola virus	(–) RNA	Yes
Paramyxoviridae	Parainfluenza virus Respiratory syncytial virus Newcastle disease virus Mumps virus Rubeola (measles) virus	(–) RNA	Yes
Orthomyxoviridae	Influenza A, B, and C viruses	(–) RNA, 8 segments	Yes
Bunyaviridae	Hantavirus California encephalitis virus Sandfly fever virus	(–) RNA, 3 segments	Yes
Arenaviridae	Lymphocytic choriomeningitis virus Lassa fever virus South American hemorrhagic fever virus	(–) RNA, 2 segments	Yes
Reoviridae	Rotavirus Reovirus Colorado tick fever virus	dsRNA, 10–12 segments	No
Retroviridae	Human T lymphotropic virus 1 and 2 Human immunodeficiency virus 1 and 2	(+) RNA, 2 identical segments	Yes
Hepadnaviridae	Hepatitis B virus	dsDNA with ss portions	Yes
Parvoviridae	Parvovirus B19	ssDNA	No
Papillomaviridae	Human papillomaviruses	dsDNA	No
Polyomaviridae	JC virus BK virus Merkel cell polyoma virus	…	…
Adenoviridae	Human adenoviruses	dsDNA	No
Herpesviridae	Herpes simplex virus 1 and 2 Varicella-zoster virus Epstein-Barr virus Cytomegalovirus Human herpesvirus 6 Human herpesvirus 7 Kaposi's sarcoma–associated herpesvirus	dsDNA	Yes
Poxviridae	Variola (smallpox) virus Orf virus Molluscum contagiosum virus	dsDNA	Yes

Abbreviations: ds, double-stranded; ss, single-stranded.

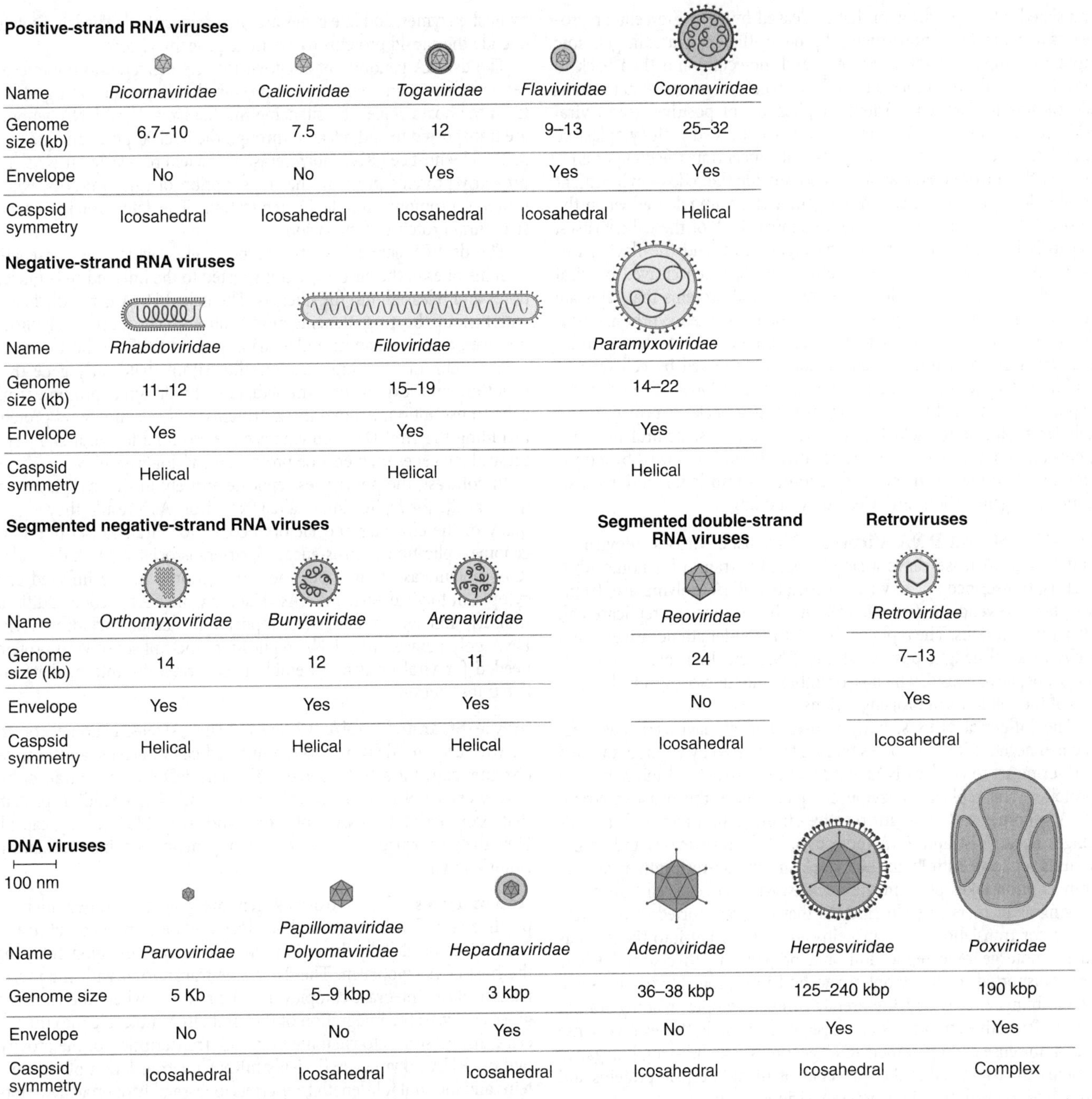

Positive-strand RNA viruses

Name	*Picornaviridae*	*Caliciviridae*	*Togaviridae*	*Flaviviridae*	*Coronaviridae*
Genome size (kb)	6.7–10	7.5	12	9–13	25–32
Envelope	No	No	Yes	Yes	Yes
Caspsid symmetry	Icosahedral	Icosahedral	Icosahedral	Icosahedral	Helical

Negative-strand RNA viruses

Name	*Rhabdoviridae*	*Filoviridae*	*Paramyxoviridae*
Genome size (kb)	11–12	15–19	14–22
Envelope	Yes	Yes	Yes
Caspsid symmetry	Helical	Helical	Helical

Segmented negative-strand RNA viruses

Name	*Orthomyxoviridae*	*Bunyaviridae*	*Arenaviridae*
Genome size (kb)	14	12	11
Envelope	Yes	Yes	Yes
Caspsid symmetry	Helical	Helical	Helical

Segmented double-strand RNA viruses

Name	*Reoviridae*
Genome size (kb)	24
Envelope	No
Caspsid symmetry	Icosahedral

Retroviruses

Name	*Retroviridae*
Genome size (kb)	7–13
Envelope	Yes
Caspsid symmetry	Icosahedral

DNA viruses

100 nm

Name	*Parvoviridae*	*Papillomaviridae* *Polyomaviridae*	*Hepadnaviridae*	*Adenoviridae*	*Herpesviridae*	*Poxviridae*
Genome size	5 Kb	5–9 kbp	3 kbp	36–38 kbp	125–240 kbp	190 kbp
Envelope	No	No	Yes	No	Yes	Yes
Caspsid symmetry	Icosahedral	Icosahedral	Icosahedral	Icosahedral	Icosahedral	Complex

FIGURE 190-2 Schematic diagrams of viruses of the major families that infect humans. The viruses are grouped by genotype, and the virions are drawn approximately to scale. Prototype viruses of each family are listed in Table 190-1. *(Source: Modified from Fig. 185-2 in Harrison's Principles of Internal Medicine, 20th ed.)*

VIRAL REPLICATION IN CELLS

Viral replication takes place in the host cell by the following steps: binding, entry, uncoating, transport to the site of replication, transcription of mRNA, translation of viral proteins, replication of the input genome, assembly of progeny viral particles, and egress from the cell. All viruses must enter cells by mechanisms that allow virus binding to the cell surface and subsequent crossing of the plasma membrane and/or other membranes to gain entry into the cytoplasm. After entry, the mechanisms of replication diverge for the different viruses, depending on the nature of the viral genome.

■ VIRAL ENTRY

Viruses bind to specific receptors on the cell surface and generally enter by one of three pathways: (1) fusion of the envelope with the surface plasma membrane; (2) endocytosis followed by fusion with the endosome membrane; or (3) lysis of the endosome or formation of pores in the endosome. Viruses often bind to a charged molecule on the surface of cells to concentrate themselves thereon. They then bind more specifically to a protein or carbohydrate molecule, and this binding triggers endocytosis or fusion of the viral envelope with the cellular plasma membrane. Endocytosis can occur by any of several mechanisms, including clathrin-mediated endocytosis, macropinocytosis, micropinocytosis, and caveolar endocytosis. After viral entry into endocytic vesicles, acidification of the vesicles leads to conformational changes in the viral glycoproteins, fusion of the viral envelope with the endocytic membrane, and release of the nucleocapsid into the cytoplasm. At the entry stage or later, the genome must be uncoated or the capsid opened sufficiently to allow transcription, translation, and/or replication.

■ VIRAL REPLICATION STRATEGIES

Positive-Strand RNA Viruses The RNA genomes of the picornaviruses, caliciviruses, hepeviruses, togaviruses, flaviviruses, and coronaviruses can be translated in the cytoplasm directly after removal of the capsid coat or uncoating. The picornaviral genomic RNA is translated into a polyprotein that is cleaved by viral and cellular proteases to generate (1) nonstructural proteins that replicate the genomic RNA to complementary negative-strand molecules and then back to positive-strand RNA molecules and (2) structural proteins that assemble capsids for progeny virions. Replication of positive-strand viral RNA takes place in replication complexes associated with cytoplasmic membranes, often in membrane sacs that concentrate the components, protect them from host responses, and provide the redox environment needed for optimal replication. Progeny virions are released when the host cell lyses. The positive-strand genome RNA of the caliciviruses, hepatitis E virus (a hepevirus), the togaviruses, and the flaviviruses is translated to generate a polyprotein, which, when cleaved by viral and cellular proteases, yields the nonstructural proteins that replicate the viral genome to a negative-strand copy and then synthesize new full-length positive strands and a subgenomic mRNA that encodes the structural proteins. Progeny virions are released by cell lysis or budding, depending on whether the virus is enveloped. The flavivirus genome is translated into one polyprotein that is cleaved by viral and cellular proteases to yield the nonstructural and structural proteins. Replication of the genome to the negative strand is followed by a transition back to the positive-strand genome for translation and encapsidation. Progeny virions are released by budding.

Negative-Strand RNA Viruses The rhabdoviruses, filoviruses, and paramyxoviruses have a single negative strand of genome RNA that is transcribed by a virion-associated RNA polymerase (transcriptase) to yield subgenomic mRNAs that encode the replicase and structural proteins. The replicase copies the full-length negative-strand RNA to a full-length positive-strand RNA and then back to a full-length negative strand, which is assembled into nucleocapsids that bud out of the cell to form progeny virions.

The influenza viruses, bunyaviruses, and arenaviruses have segmented negative RNA genomes that are transcribed by virion-associated transcriptases to yield mRNAs that encode nonstructural and structural proteins. The replicase enzyme complex copies the negative-strand RNA genomes to full-length positive-strand copies and back to full-length negative-strand RNA molecules. The bunyaviruses and arenaviruses replicate entirely in the cytoplasm. In contrast, influenza viral transcription takes place in the nucleus, with nascent cell transcripts serving as primers to yield mRNAs that are transported to the cytoplasm for translation. Viral proteins are transported into the nucleus to promote genome replication, and progeny negative-strand RNAs are transported to the cytoplasm to bud into progeny virions. Some of the bunyaviruses and the arenaviruses have open reading frames on the "negative strand." Thus, these viruses use both negative-sense and ambisense coding of their RNA genomes. The full-length negative strands are assembled in the correct assortment in capsid proteins and then bud to yield infectious progeny virions.

Double-Stranded RNA Viruses The reoviruses and rotaviruses consist of multiple double-stranded (ds) RNA molecules that are transcribed by virion-associated, RNA-dependent RNA polymerases (transcriptases) to yield mRNAs encoding nonstructural and structural proteins. Following viral protein synthesis, replication of positive-strand RNAs to form dsRNA molecules and assembly into viral capsids occur in cytoplasmic viral factories. Progeny viruses are released when infected cells lyse.

Double-Stranded DNA Viruses Most dsDNA viral genomes are transported to the infected cell's nucleus for transcription and replication. The host cell recognizes foreign DNA that is not fully loaded with histone nucleosomes with a normal pattern and tries to epigenetically silence these molecules; DNA viruses have evolved mechanisms to overcome these epigenetic silencing mechanisms. The dsDNA genomes of the papovaviruses and papillomaviruses are coated with nucleosomal chromatin in the virion and therefore are delivered to the nucleus in a form that is not recognized as foreign. Viral early gene expression is promoted by an enhancer adjacent to the early gene promoter, which is transcribed by host cell RNA polymerase II to yield the early mRNAs. The early proteins promote viral DNA replication by host enzymes, and late genes are then transcribed. The late proteins encode the capsid proteins to assemble progeny virions.

The dsDNA genomes of adenoviruses are delivered to the infected cell's nucleus coated with a viral protein that hides the viral genomes from the host's epigenetic silencing mechanisms. Viral DNA genomes are transported to and released through the nuclear pores and are transcribed by host cell RNA polymerase II to yield pre-early mRNAs. The pre-early proteins promote the transcription of early mRNAs, whose proteins promote viral DNA replication. The late proteins encode structural proteins of the virion.

The dsDNA genomes of the herpesviruses, which are not coated with histones in the virion, are transported to the infected cell's nuclear pores and released into the nucleus. The naked DNA is rapidly loaded with histones bearing silencing modifications by host cell mechanisms; however, a viral enhancer and a virion protein that uses host enzymes to drive chromatin reorganization allow immediate-early gene transcription and expression. Immediate-early proteins promote early gene transcription. Among the E proteins, eight or nine viral proteins including the viral DNA polymerase are essential for viral DNA synthesis. Late genes then encode proteins for virion assembly.

In contrast, the poxviruses replicate entirely in the cytoplasm—an unusual site for replication of a dsDNA virus. As a result, they encode many of the enzymes and factors needed for viral transcription and genome replication. A virus-encoded, virion-associated, DNA-dependent RNA polymerase transcribes the viral genome in the infected cell's cytoplasm to yield early mRNAs. The early mRNAs encode additional transcription factors and DNA replication factors, including a viral DNA polymerase. After DNA replication, the full set of viral proteins needed for viral progeny assembly is generated by intermediate and late transcription.

Single-Stranded DNA Viruses The ssDNA genomes of the parvoviruses are delivered to the infected cell's nucleus, and host cell enzymes copy the ssDNA into dsDNA. The dsDNA is then transcribed by the cell's RNA polymerase II to yield mRNAs encoding proteins that promote viral DNA replication and assemble progeny capsids. How the parvoviruses deal with host epigenetic silencing mechanisms is not known.

Retroviruses The retrovirus genome consists of two identical positive-strand ssRNA molecules, which are not translated but instead copied into dsDNA by the virion *reverse transcriptase* upon entry into the host cell's cytoplasm. The dsDNA is transported with the reverse transcriptase–integrase complex into the nucleus, where the viral integrase catalyzes the integration of the viral DNA molecule into the host cell's chromosomes to yield the provirus. Transcription of the provirus by host RNA polymerase II yields mRNA for translation of viral proteins and for viral full-length transcripts for assembly of progeny virions.

VIRAL EFFECTS ON THE HOST CELL

Many viruses inhibit cellular macromolecular processes, such as host cell transcription and protein synthesis, in an attempt to optimize their own replication by usurping the host cell's machinery and biochemical precursors. These inhibitory events can lead to cell injury and ultimately to cell death, or necrosis. The effects are often manifest by progressive changes in cell structure, detachment from the substrate and rounding up, and eventual lysis. Collectively, these changes are referred to as the CPE. Cells may detect infection as described below and initiate a pathway called *programmed cell death*, or apoptosis, in an attempt to limit viral infection.

Some viruses induce host cell growth to optimize their own replication or to amplify the host cells. Papovaviruses, papillomaviruses, and adenoviruses induce the cellular S phase to activate functions needed for viral DNA replication. These viruses also target cellular proteins that control cell growth, inactivating or degrading them to allow the cell cycle to progress to the S phase. Studies of the mechanisms of these viral effects on host cells have identified cellular tumor-suppressor genes such as the *p53* and retinoblastoma *pRB* genes. Epstein-Barr virus induces proliferation to amplify its latent-infection host cell, a B cell. However, the viral mechanisms sometimes induce immortalization of a cell that has already undergone or later undergoes the oncogenic transformation leading to a cancer cell. Some retroviruses encode altered versions of host genes that can induce transformation. Collectively, these DNA viruses and retroviruses are called *tumor viruses.*

HOST ANTIVIRAL RESPONSES AND VIRAL ANTAGONISTIC MECHANISMS

Host cells have evolved numerous mechanisms for resisting viral infection. They encode constitutively expressed proteins that inhibit viral replication in a process called *intrinsic resistance*. One well-known host resistance factor is the rhesus macaque Trim5α protein, which inhibits human immunodeficiency virus (HIV) type 1 infection soon after the viral core enters the cytoplasm.

Viruses have in turn evolved mechanisms by which to evade or neutralize resistance factors in cells of their host species. The promyelocytic leukemia (PML) protein and its associated proteins in nuclear domain 10 (ND-10) structures in the nucleus of human cells restrict HSV replication, but HSV has evolved a gene product—infected cell protein 0 (ICP0), an E3 ubiquitin ligase—that promotes the degradation of the PML protein and thwarts this antiviral mechanism. Nevertheless, PML protein expression is increased by interferon (IFN) signaling, and the elevated levels are sufficient to reduce wild-type HSV infection. Thus, during HSV infection, there is a race between IFN expression and ICP0 expression.

TYPES OF CELLULAR INFECTIONS

The balance of proviral and antiviral factors in a cell defines whether it is permissive or nonpermissive for viral replication. An infection in which progeny virus is produced is a *productive* infection. If a cell becomes infected but does not die, a virus may establish a *persistent* infection. A *chronic* infection can result if infectious virus is continually produced. An *abortive* infection occurs when infection begins but is not completed. In abortive infections, the cell may (1) die, if enough CPEs are exerted, as described above; (2) undergo oncogenic transformation; or (3) harbor a latent infection in which no infectious virus is found but the virus can reactivate at a later time. Examples of these outcomes are the abortive oncogenic infection of cells by Merkel cell polyomavirus, chronic infection of liver cells by hepatitis B virus, and latent infection of neurons by HSV.

STAGES OF INFECTION OF A HOST

The stages of viral infection are (1) entry into the host, (2) primary replication and disease at the site of entry, (3) spread through the host, (4) secondary replication and disease at new sites, (5) persistence or clearance by the host immune response, and (6) transmission or release from the host. Infection of a host can be acute, chronic, or latent.

Entry Keratinized skin cells are not viable and therefore are not good host cells for viral replication. Thus, viruses must enter the host at a mucosal surface (e.g., at oral, respiratory, and nasal sites), through a body opening (e.g., by inhalation or ingestion), or through a break in the skin (e.g., the sites of mosquito or other insect bites). For example, papillomaviruses and HSV enter at breaks in the skin, while Zika and dengue viruses can be introduced via insect bites.

Primary Replication and Disease Viruses replicate at the site of entry into the body (i.e., the primary site of infection), are shed back into the environment, and may cause entry-site disease and/or spread to cause systemic illness. For example, influenza viruses can infect the respiratory mucosa. Noroviruses and rotaviruses can infect epithelial cells in the gastrointestinal tract. Dengue and Zika viruses can infect dendritic cells in the tissues after a mosquito bite. If viral infection injures cells and tissues and causes disease at the entry site, the incubation period between exposure and disease can be as short as 1 or 2 days.

Viral Spread Some viral infections remain localized at the primary site, but others spread from the primary site to secondary sites where the viruses infect new cells and cause disease. This spread may take place through the lymph and the bloodstream (*viremia*). Measles virus, for example, replicates initially in the respiratory epithelium, and infected dendritic cells spread through the lymph to lymph nodes where T cells and monocytes are infected and transmit virus through the bloodstream to organs and lymph nodes throughout the body. Systemic disease can result from the disseminated infection, and viral spread into the skin causes the classic measles rash. The incubation period of 10–14 days from exposure to clinical symptoms reflects the time involved for multiple rounds of viral replication and spread within the body before the classic rash symptoms appear. Similarly, dendritic cells and macrophages infected with dengue virus can travel through the circulatory system and transmit virus to secondary sites where infection and disease can follow.

Alternatively, viral spread may occur via neuronal pathways by transsynaptic spread of virions. Rabies virus spreads transsynaptically from the periphery to the central nervous system to cause encephalitis. HSV-1 causes a primary infection at mucosal surfaces and then enters the axon of a sensory neuron and establishes latent infection in the neuron's cell body. Reactivation usually leads to a recurrent infection at the site of primary infection, but occasionally, the virus can move along nerve tracts to the central nervous system and cause encephalitis.

Host Immune Responses Acute viral infection is blunted by the rapid innate immune response and then controlled by the later adaptive immune response.

INNATE IMMUNITY The first arm of the host's immune response—the innate immune response—is rapid, with recognition of general patterns of viral molecules but not of specific antigens, whose recognition occurs during the later adaptive response. Using pattern recognition receptors, host cells recognize foreign molecules with patterns contained in microbes—i.e., pathogen-associated molecular patterns (PAMPs). Recognition of the foreign molecules leads to activation of innate signaling pathways that induce the expression of IFNs, cytokines, and other host gene products, including those attributable to IFN-stimulated genes, which serve as antiviral effector molecules. Viral ssRNA is recognized by Toll-like receptor 7 (TLR7) and TLR8, which induce transcription of type I IFN genes and IFN-stimulated genes. IFNs act on the producing cell in an autocrine manner and on surrounding cells in a paracrine manner to induce expression of antiviral genes and to activate antiviral mechanisms. dsRNA is recognized by TLR3, which activates expression of type I IFNs. ssRNA and dsRNA are recognized by retinoic acid–inducible gene I (RIG-I) and melanoma differentiation-associated antigen 5 (MDA5), which induce type I IFN expression. Viral glycoproteins are recognized by TLR2 and TLR4. Viral DNA is recognized by the cytoplasmic cGAS receptor, which activates type I IFN expression, and by the nuclear IFN-inducible protein 16 (IFI16) receptor, which activates IFN expression in some cell types and epigenetic silencing of the viral DNA genome in many cell types. IFI16 can therefore act as a constitutively expressed resistance factor or as an IFN-stimulated gene. Innate responses also direct the induction of the later, more specific adaptive immune responses.

ADAPTIVE IMMUNITY Viral antigens are presented as peptides to both CD4+ and CD8+ T cells by antigen-presenting cells to induce these T cells to develop into antigen-specific T cells. Viral antigens are also presented to B cells, which induce differentiation of antibody-producing B cells. Antibodies can bind to virions and neutralize their infectivity by preventing their binding to receptors, their entry, their uncoating, or other steps in infection (**Fig. 190-3**). Antibodies can also bind to viral antigens on the surface of virions and infected cells and promote phagocytosis, antibody-dependent cytotoxicity, and complement-mediated lysis. T cells recognize viral peptides bound to major histocompatibility complex molecules on the surface of infected cells and produce cytokines that exert an antiviral effect or activate cell-killing mechanisms. Thus, the host's adaptive immune responses can target either virions or infected cells and can clear infection.

VIRAL EVOLUTION

Because viral RNA-dependent RNA polymerases are error prone and do not have editing functions, sequence changes are frequently introduced into their genomes. These alterations can lead to populations

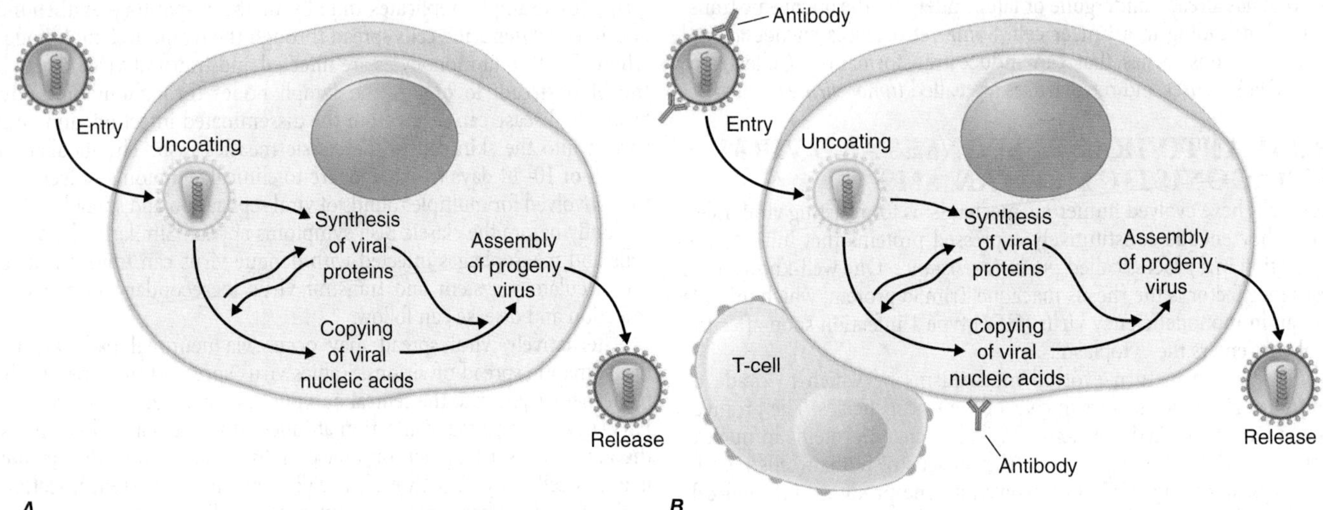

FIGURE 190-3 Steps in viral infection of a host cell and effects of immune effector mechanisms. ***A.*** Steps in viral infection of a host cell. The steps include entry into the cell, uncoating of the viral genomic nucleic acid, synthesis of viral proteins, copying of viral nucleic acids, assembly of progeny virus, egress, and release from the host cell. ***B.*** Mechanisms of immune effector mechanisms. Antibodies can bind to the extracellular virion and neutralize infectivity by preventing binding to the cellular receptor, preventing entry at other steps, preventing uncoating, or preventing other steps of infection. T cells recognize antigenic peptides presented on the surface of infected cells and produce antiviral cytokines and/or activate cell killing.

or swarms of viruses with divergent sequences among a viral population in an individual. Upon drug selection, immune pressure, or host restriction, preexisting variants can emerge as the new major form of a virus. Differences in replicative ability can lead to enrichment of more fit viruses and loss of less fit variants. This trend has been observed in the COVID-19 pandemic as more fit variants have become the dominant forms of SARS-CoV-2 in the population.

Viruses with segmented genomes can undergo genome reassortment in cells co-infected with two viral strains, the result being a new genetic composition for a given virus. For example, new segments can arise in influenza virus isolates thought to be reassortants between the extant human strains and animal or avian strains, such as those from porcine or avian species. This type of event is the cause of the major shifts in influenza viruses that occur periodically over a decade. These major changes due to reassortment and acquisition of a new genome segment are referred to as *antigenic shift*, as opposed to the small changes due to sequence variation, which are designated *antigenic drift*.

Especially in DNA viruses but—under special circumstances—also in RNA viruses such as coronaviruses, viral genomes can undergo recombination between two strains of virus and generate recombinant genomes with new combinations of genes that may be more or less fit.

Viral variants can acquire the ability to infect cells of new host species or to jump species barriers. *Zoonotic* infection occurs when a virus spreads from animals to humans, as is thought to have occurred with both SARS-CoV-1 and SARS-CoV-2. The original viral ancestor of these viruses—endemic in bats—is thought to have spread to other animals sold in the markets of China, and viral variants then arose that could efficiently infect humans. Evolution of variants that could efficiently infect and be transmitted by humans as agents of respiratory infection led to the COVID-19 pandemic.

MOLECULAR EPIDEMIOLOGY OF VIRUSES

Several molecular techniques allow easy genotyping of virus isolates. Direct sequencing, analysis of polymorphisms in restriction endonuclease cleavage sites, and polymerase chain reaction (PCR) analysis allow a search for genotypic markers in isolates, with sequencing being the most precise definition of a viral strain. When these types of tests are applied, some viruses (e.g., influenza virus and measles virus) are found to have mainly one strain prevalent in the population at a given time. Thus, only one virus strain spreads through the population. For other viruses, such as HIV or HSV, nearly every unrelated isolate can be differentiated by these tests, and many strains are latent and spreading within the population and are evolving in parallel. With these molecular techniques, genotypic markers can be used to determine whether a virus has been transmitted from one individual to another.

Genomic sequencing studies of SARS-CoV-2 have identified a number of major strains circulating at any given time. As new variants have arisen, each has become the dominant circulating strain.

DETECTION AND QUANTIFICATION OF VIRUSES

Viruses and viral infections need to be detected and quantified for both clinical and scientific purposes. Diagnostic virology employs the scientific principles described above to detect viruses and evidence of infection in clinical samples, to define the type of virus present in a sample, and in some cases to quantify the amount of virus or the viral load in a patient. Scientific studies use these principles for detection and quantification of viruses in laboratory stocks and for measurement of viral replication.

DETECTION OF INFECTIOUS VIRUS

Biologic assays must be used to detect and measure infectious virus. Infectivity can be measured as either the ability to infect animals and cause disease or the ability to infect cultured cells and cause CPE. For example, SARS-CoV-1 virus was first isolated by the introduction of an oropharyngeal swab sample into Vero cell cultures and detection of CPE.

DETECTION OF VIRAL PARTICLES, THEIR COMPONENTS, AND VIRAL GENE PRODUCTS

Viral Particles Electron microscopy (EM) must be used to visualize virions directly, because viruses (other than the poxviruses) are smaller than the resolution of the light microscope. Virions can be visualized by EM with negative staining of the virions themselves or by transmission EM of infected cells. As stated above, SARS viral particles were first visualized in sections of Vero cells infected with samples from patients. The cell culture supernatant showed coronavirus particles by negative-staining EM. The latter method has also been used to detect viral particles in stool during outbreaks of gastroenteritis. Antibodies specific for viral capsid proteins are often used in this assay to concentrate the virus and enhance its detection.

Viral Nucleic Acids Viral nucleic acids are detected by amplification methods involving PCR with specific primers, which amplifies very small numbers of viral nucleic acid molecules. These methods can use direct amplification of DNA in clinical samples to detect and quantify viral DNA genomes; alternatively, they can use reverse transcription of RNA followed by PCR to detect a DNA product in clinical samples as a means to detect viral RNA sequences. Multiple primers can be used in a multiplex reaction to detect multiple pathogens. The process of nucleic acid isolation, reverse transcription, and PCR has been automated, and high-throughput instruments measure the HIV load in serum samples. HSV-1 DNA can be measured in cerebrospinal fluid as a rapid assay for HSV encephalitis. These methods have also been transferred to rapid assays for point-of-care detection of viral genomes.

Viral Antigens Viral antigens can be detected by immunologic methods such as immunofluorescence and enzyme immunosorbent assay (EIA). Immunofluorescence involves fixation and permeabilization of cells or tissues from clinical specimens and reaction with either (1) an antiviral antibody conjugated to a fluorophore (direct immunofluorescence) or (2) an antiviral antibody followed by an anti-immunoglobulin antibody conjugated to a fluorophore (indirect immunofluorescence), with detection of the fluorophore by fluorescence microscopy in either case.

The EIA entails the immobilization of an antiviral antibody on a substrate such as a microtiter well, incubation of the patient's sample in the well, and further incubation with an antibody linked to an enzyme. The bound enzyme is then measured by production of a colored substrate that can be read spectrophotometrically.

Hemagglutination Some viruses have the ability to cross-link and agglutinate red blood cells of specific species, a process called *hemagglutination.* Viral titer is measured by the inverse of the last dilution of the sample that causes hemagglutination.

Quantitative Assays of Viruses Viruses can be quantified in terms of virion particle numbers and/or infectivity. The number of virion particles in a sample can be determined by negative staining and observation by EM. The numbers of viral DNA genomes can be determined by PCR, and RNA genomes can be determined by reverse transcriptase PCR (RT-PCR), as described above. Alternatively, purified viral particles can be quantified biochemically by spectrophotometric assays that measure viral protein.

The number of infectious particles can be quantified by an endpoint dilution assay in which the virus is diluted until only one-half of cultures are infected; this concentration is designated the tissue culture infectious dose for 50% of cultures, or $TCID_{50}$. An alternative assay can determine at what dose one-half of experimental animals die of viral disease (lethal dose for 50% of test animals, or LD_{50}). A more quantitative assay of infectivity is the plaque assay. A plaque is an area of visualized localized CPE. In the plaque assay, dilutions of the virus sample are placed on cells attached to a culture dish, and after adsorption of the virus to cells, the cells are overlaid with semisolid medium or medium containing antibody, which prevents virus diffusion through the medium. Virus then spreads only cell to cell, causing a restricted area of CPE—a plaque—on the cellular monolayer. The number of plaques formed by each dilution of virus defines the titer in plaque-forming units (PFUs) per volume of virus stock.

For viruses that infect humans, the ratio of viral particles to infectious units, or the particle-to-PFU ratio, is always much greater than 1—usually 10–1000. This result signifies a large excess of particles that are defective and/or that do not score as infectious in laboratory assays. Thus, for experimental purposes, following input virus particles, either visually or biochemically, does not guarantee that the observer is following the real infection pathway. Accordingly, clinical preparations of viruses used for vaccines, vaccine vectors, gene therapy vectors, and oncolytic viruses need to be defined precisely and specifically in terms of particles versus infectious units for accurate and safe dosing. As an example, a recent adenovirus-based COVID vaccine was quantified on the basis of spectrophotometric measurement of purified virions. After the trial was initiated, lower than expected reactogenicity led to a reexamination of the vaccine dose. An excipient discovered in the vaccine was found to cause errors in spectrophotometric measurement that led to an overestimate of the virus concentration. Parallel measurements of viral genomes with RT-PCR allowed a more accurate measurement of the vaccine vector batches, and the dose was revised to one-half of the original level. This example illustrates the importance of precise measurements of viral particles and infectious particles in clinical preparations of viruses.

DETECTION OF VIRUS-SPECIFIC ANTIBODIES

The presence of virus-specific antibodies provides evidence of prior infection with a virus or prior exposure to viral antigens through immunization; thus, antibody tests are extremely important clinically. The most common tests for antibodies are the enzyme-linked immunosorbent assay (ELISA) and the Western blot or immunoblot assay. An ELISA involves the immobilization of viral antigen on a substrate such as a microtiter well, its incubation with the patient's serum, and further incubation with an antibody to human IgG coupled to an enzyme. The amount of bound antibody is measured by detection of a colored product made by the bound enzyme. The Western blot assay involves the resolution of viral proteins in a polyacrylamide gel, their transfer to a membrane, incubation with the patient's serum, and further incubation with antibody to human IgG coupled to an enzyme. Proteins with bound antibodies are detected as a colored product made by the bound antibody. The Western blot detects antigen of a specific size and therefore is more specific than ELISA. For example, HIV serologic testing involves high-throughput ELISA screening followed by a Western blot assay to confirm the specificity of any positive ELISA result.

In a hemagglutination inhibition assay, antibodies specific for viral surface proteins are detected by their ability to block hemagglutination.

IMMUNIZATION AGAINST VIRAL DISEASES

Viral vaccines are among the most effective biomedical and public health measures that have been implemented: millions of deaths have been prevented by their use. These vaccines are safe because extensive protocols have been developed for monitoring vaccine safety both before and after licensure. Historically, viral vaccines were based on either inactivated virus or live attenuated viruses, as exemplified by the Salk polio vaccine and the Sabin live attenuated polio vaccine, respectively. Both of these vaccines were quite successful, offering individual advantages. Further vaccine types have been developed, including those based on recombinant proteins, viral vectors, and, most recently, mRNA. For each virus, the optimal antigen and immunization strategy must be developed on the basis of the virus-specific immune correlates, antibodies, or T cells needed for immunologic protection against infection and disease. These concepts are discussed in greater detail in **Chap. 123**.

ANTIVIRAL THERAPEUTICS

ANTIVIRAL DRUGS

Viruses replicate in human cells and use much of the host cell's machinery. Therefore, antiviral drugs must target virus-specific events to optimize safety. Viral targets for drugs have been identified in studies of the mechanisms of viral infection and replication (**Chap. 191**). Many of the most successful antiviral drugs target viral enzymes; examples include the anti-HSV drugs that target the virus DNA polymerases and thymidine kinase (**Chap. 191**) and the HIV drugs that target the virus reverse transcriptase, protease, and integrase (**Chap. 202**).

VIRUSES AS THERAPEUTICS

Viruses have been engineered for a number of medical purposes, including gene delivery and tumor cell killing. As described above, viruses have been developed as vaccines and vaccine vectors. For example, vesicular stomatitis virus–based vectors have been employed as Ebola vaccines. Adenovirus-based vectors have been used as AIDS vaccine vectors and are now being used as COVID-19 vaccine vectors. Viral recombinants, including those of retroviruses and adeno-associated viruses, have been approved as vectors for delivery of genes to cells for treatment of single-gene defects. Retroviruses integrate into the cell's chromosomes and are maintained with stable expression of the transgene, although some concerns have arisen about possible activation of neighboring promoters and adverse effects due to that activation. Adeno-associated viruses are not integrated but are stably maintained and capable of durable expression of the transgene. Adenoviruses and herpesviruses are also being tested as gene therapy vectors. Finally, an attenuated strain of HSV expressing granulocyte-macrophage colony-stimulating factor has been approved for treatment of melanoma because of its oncolytic and immunotherapeutic properties. Many additional studies are assessing viruses for use as vectors and for immunotherapeutic and oncolytic applications.

SUMMARY

As obligate intracellular parasites, viruses enter host cells, replicate, and spread in the form of progeny viruses. Injury to the host cell resulting from viral entry may lead to tissue and organ damage. Basic knowledge of the mechanisms underlying infection by and replication of viruses that infect humans is the foundation for medical studies of viral pathogenesis, viral vaccines, antiviral drugs, and the use of viruses as therapeutics. A broad knowledge of all viruses is essential to our preparedness for the next viral epidemic or pandemic.

FURTHER READING

Helenius A: Virus entry: Looking back and moving forward. J Mol Biol 43:1853, 2018.

Howley PM et al (eds): *Fields Virology: Vol. 1: Emerging Viruses*, 7th ed. Philadelphia, Wolters Kluwer/Lippincott Williams & Wilkins Health, 2020.

Knipe DM, Howley PM (eds): *Fields Virology*, 6th ed. Philadelphia, Wolters Kluwer/Lippincott Williams & Wilkins Health, 2013.

Knipe DM et al: Ensuring vaccine safety. Science 370:1274, 2020.

Ksiazek TG et al: A novel coronavirus associated with severe acute respiratory syndrome. N Engl J Med 348:1953, 2003.

Voysey M et al: Safety and efficacy of the ChAdOx1 nCoV-19 vaccine (AZD1222) against SARS-CoV-2: An interim analysis of four randomised controlled trials in Brazil, South Africa, and the UK. Lancet 397:99, 2021.

Zhou P et al: A pneumonia outbreak associated with a new coronavirus of probable bat origin. Nature 579:270, 2020.

191 Antiviral Chemotherapy, Excluding Antiretroviral Drugs

Jeffrey I. Cohen, Eleanor Wilson

Most antiviral drugs inhibit viral DNA or RNA replication, but other activities, such as virus entry, viral RNA transcription, cleavage of proteins by the viral protease, virus uncoating after infection, and virus release from cells, are all targeted by different licensed antiviral agents. Inhibition of viral replication does not eliminate the virus in the cell; host cell immune responses are important for viral clearance. Antiviral drugs usually do not eradicate latent viral infections, but instead usually inhibit viral replication; thus, when treatment is stopped, the virus can reactivate and replicate again. Resistance to antiviral agents due to mutations in viral proteins is not uncommon and is more common for RNA viruses with a higher mutation rate than for DNA viruses. This difference may explain the observation that drug-resistant DNA viruses are a greater problem in immunocompromised patients, whereas drug-resistant RNA viruses can be found in healthy persons as well. Patients may harbor a mixture of drug-resistant and drug-sensitive viruses that is dynamic and changes under pressure from the drug. Combination therapy with more than one antiviral agent, each with a different mechanism of action, may be more effective than monotherapy, particularly against RNA viruses, which may be present as mixtures with different resistance patterns. Antiviral testing can be performed in patients who do not respond to antiviral drugs or whose response diminishes. For some viruses, such testing involves the sequencing of selected viral genes; however, in many cases, it involves the growth of virus in the presence of different concentrations of the drug, which is a laborious, time-consuming process. Response to antiviral therapy has traditionally been assessed clinically, but quantitative PCR has been useful in monitoring the response to therapy for viruses that circulate in the blood (e.g., cytomegalovirus [CMV], hepatitis B and C viruses [HBV and HCV, respectively]). Systemic therapy with antivirals is usually more effective than topical therapy but is more commonly associated with side effects.

ANTIVIRAL DRUGS FOR HERPESVIRUS INFECTIONS

ACYCLOVIR, VALACYCLOVIR, FAMCICLOVIR, AND PENCICLOVIR

Acyclovir is an analogue of deoxyguanosine and is phosphorylated to the monophosphate form by viral thymidine kinase in cells infected with herpes simplex virus (HSV) or varicella-zoster virus (VZV). Cellular protein kinases further phosphorylate the drug to the active triphosphate form, which inhibits viral DNA polymerase; the drug is incorporated into viral DNA to terminate its replication. Valacyclovir, a valine ester of acyclovir, is absorbed much better than acyclovir; its rapid conversion to acyclovir in the liver and intestine results in plasma acyclovir levels approximately four times higher than are attained with oral acyclovir. Acyclovir and valacyclovir are approved by the U.S. Food and Drug Administration (FDA) for treatment of initial episodes of genital herpes, recurrent genital herpes, varicella, and zoster (**Table 191-1**). Valacyclovir is also approved for treatment of herpes labialis (cold sores), for suppression of recurrences of genital herpes, and for reduction of transmission of genital HSV. The doses of acyclovir and valacyclovir used for treating VZV infections are higher than those used for HSV infections since VZV is less susceptible to inhibition by these drugs. Both drugs exhibit poor activity against CMV. Intravenous acyclovir is used for severe disease requiring hospitalization; oral acyclovir or valacyclovir is used for outpatient therapy; and topical acyclovir, penciclovir, and docosanol are approved for treatment of orolabial herpes but are much less effective than the oral drugs.

Acyclovir is excreted by the kidneys. Thus the dose of acyclovir or valacyclovir needs to be reduced with renal insufficiency. Central nervous system (CNS) side effects that occur with IV acyclovir or oral valacyclovir are more common with the higher drug levels seen in persons with renal insufficiency. Reversible renal insufficiency due to crystallization of the drug in renal tubules can occur with IV acyclovir, especially in persons who are dehydrated. Headache, nausea, rash, and diarrhea have been reported with acyclovir. Mutations in the HSV or VZV thymidine kinase or, less commonly, in viral DNA polymerase can result in resistance to acyclovir or valacyclovir. Viruses lacking thymidine kinase activity are also resistant to famciclovir and ganciclovir. Acyclovir- and valacyclovir-resistant HSV and VZV are rare in immunocompetent persons. Resistant virus is treated with foscarnet or, less commonly, cidofovir. Mucosal disease due to resistant virus in immunocompromised persons is sometimes treated with topical foscarnet, trifluridine, or cidofovir.

Famciclovir is a diacetyl ester of penciclovir that is converted to penciclovir in the intestine and liver. Penciclovir is a guanosine analogue that is less potent than acyclovir, but, because of its longer intracellular half-life, its activity is similar to that of acyclovir. Penciclovir is phosphorylated by HSV and VZV thymidine and cellular kinases and has activity similar to that of acyclovir for HSV and VZV infections. Famciclovir is approved for treatment of zoster, suppression of genital herpes, and treatment of recurrent mucocutaneous herpes in patients with HIV infection. Famciclovir is excreted by the kidneys, and the dose is adjusted for renal insufficiency. Side effects are uncommon and can include headache, nausea, and diarrhea. Resistance due to mutations in viral thymidine kinase or DNA polymerase can occur.

TABLE 191-1 Antiviral Drugs for Herpesvirus Treatment and Prophylaxis in Adults

DISEASE	DRUG	ROUTE	ADULT DOSE	COMMENTS
Orolabial herpes, primary episode	Acyclovir	Oral	400 mg tid × 7–10 d	Reduces duration of fever, lesions, and virus shedding
	Valacyclovir	Oral	1 g bid × 7–10 d	
	Famciclovir	Oral	500 mg bid or 250 mg tid × 7–10 d	
Orolabial herpes, recurrence	Acyclovir	Oral	400 mg 5 times daily × 5 d	Reduces duration of lesions by 1–2 d if given during prodrome
	Valacyclovir	Oral	2 g bid × 1 d	
	Famciclovir	Oral	1500 mg × 1 d	
Orolabial herpes, suppression	Acyclovir	Oral	400 mg bid	In patients with >6 recurrences per year, reduces number of recurrences by ~50% and increases time to first recurrence
	Valacyclovir	Oral	500 mg or 1 g once daily	
	Famciclovir	Oral	500 mg bid	
Genital herpes, primary episode	Acyclovir	Oral	400 mg tid or 200 mg 5 times daily × 7–10 d	Reduces duration of symptoms, genital lesions, and virus shedding by 2, 4, and 7 d, respectively
	Valacyclovir	Oral	1 g bid × 7–10 d	
	Famciclovir	Oral	250 mg tid × 7–10 d	
Genital herpes, recurrence	Acyclovir	Oral	800 mg tid × 2 d or 400 mg tid × 5 d	Reduces duration of symptoms, genital lesions, and virus shedding by 1–2 d
	Valacyclovir	Oral	500 mg bid × 3 d or 1 g daily × 5 d	
	Famciclovir	Oral	500 mg once, then 250 mg bid × 2 d	
Genital herpes suppression	Acyclovir	Oral	400 mg bid	In patients with >6 recurrences per year, reduces recurrence rates from 80–85% to 25–30%, reduces virus shedding and transmission
	Valacyclovir	Oral	250 mg bid	
	Famciclovir	Oral	500 mg to 1 g daily	
HSV encephalitis	Acyclovir	IV	10–15 mg/kg q8h × 14–21 d	Reduces mortality and sequelae
HSV keratitis	Acyclovir	Topical	3% ophthalmic ointment, 5 times daily	Shortens duration of disease; acyclovir better tolerated, especially with prolonged treatment
	Trifluridine	Topical	1% ophthalmic solution, 1 drop q2h when awake (9 drops daily max)	
	Vidarabine	Topical	3% ointment, ½-inch ribbon 5 times daily	
Mucocutaneous herpes in immunocompromised patient	Acyclovir	IV	5 mg/kg q8h × 7–14 d	IV acyclovir reduces time to healing, duration of pain, and duration of virus shedding
	Valacyclovir	Oral	500 mg to 1 g bid × 7–10 d	
	Famciclovir	Oral	500 mg bid × 7–10 d	
Varicella	Acyclovir	Oral	20 mg/kg (800 mg max) 5 times daily × 5 d	Has modest effect on symptoms, reduces fever duration by 1 day
	Valacyclovir	Oral	20 mg/kg (1 g max) tid × 5 d	
Zoster	Acyclovir	Oral	800 mg 5 times daily × 7 d	Reduces time for last new lesion formation, virus shedding, and pain duration
	Valacyclovir	Oral	1 g tid × 7 d	
	Famciclovir	Oral	500 mg tid × 7 d	
Varicella or zoster, disseminated	Acyclovir	IV	10 mg/kg q8h × 7 d	Reduces time for last new lesion formation and virus shedding; reduces cutaneous dissemination
Cytomegalovirus disease	Ganciclovir	IV	5 mg/kg q12h × 14–21 d, then 5 mg/kg daily (maintenance dose)	Neutropenia and thrombocytopenia common after 1 week
	Valganciclovir	Oral	900 mg bid × 14–21 d, then 90 mg daily (maintenance dose)	Levels and side effects similar to ganciclovir
	Foscarnet	IV	60 mg/kg q8h × 14–21 d, then 90–120 mg daily (maintenance dose)	Nephrotoxicity, electrolyte abnormalities; give with additional saline
	Cidofovir	IV	5 mg/kg once weekly twice, then every other week	Nephrotoxicity; give with probenecid and saline

Oral acyclovir reduces the duration of pain and other symptoms, time to healing, and shedding in patients with their first episode of genital herpes when treatment is begun within 6 days of infection. Acyclovir, valacyclovir, and famciclovir are all effective for treatment of primary and recurrent genital and orolabial herpes as well as for suppressive therapy for these conditions. Topical acyclovir cream reduces shedding and time to healing by 1–2 days if given within 1 day of symptom onset in persons with recurrent genital or orolabial herpes. Oral acyclovir or valacyclovir reduces the severity of varicella when given within 1 day of onset of the rash. Oral acyclovir, famciclovir, or valacyclovir shortens the duration of pain and rash associated with zoster if given within 3 days of onset. Oral valacyclovir is more effective than oral acyclovir and is generally preferred since it has better oral bioavailability and does not need to be given as frequently. Suppressive valacyclovir therapy for genital herpes reduces transmission to uninfected partners by 50%. Intravenous acyclovir is used for herpes encephalitis and disseminated HSV or VZV disease.

GANCICLOVIR AND VALGANCICLOVIR

Ganciclovir is a deoxyguanosine analog that is phosphorylated by UL97 protein kinase in cells infected with CMV and converted to its active form, ganciclovir triphosphate, by cellular protein kinases. Ganciclovir triphosphate inhibits both viral DNA polymerase and incorporation of guanosine triphosphate into viral DNA. Valganciclovir is a valine ester of ganciclovir and is converted to ganciclovir in the liver and intestine. Valganciclovir has much better oral bioavailability than ganciclovir; plasma levels of oral valganciclovir and IV ganciclovir are similar. Ganciclovir and valganciclovir are used for treatment and prevention of CMV disease in immunocompromised patients and are approved for prevention of CMV infection in transplant recipients and for treatment of CMV retinitis. Ganciclovir is effective against HSV, VZV, human herpesvirus type 6 (HHV-6), and herpes B virus. This drug is excreted by the kidneys, and dose adjustment is required in renal insufficiency. Ganciclovir therapy often results in neutropenia and thrombocytopenia after 1 week. Less commonly, ganciclovir has been associated with CNS symptoms, particularly at high plasma drug levels. Mutations in

CMV UL97 protein kinase or, less commonly, UL54 viral DNA polymerase can result in resistance to ganciclovir or valganciclovir. CMV with mutations in protein kinase is usually sensitive to foscarnet and cidofovir, while CMV with mutations in both protein kinase and DNA polymerase is usually sensitive only to foscarnet. Mutations are more common among persons who are highly immunocompromised and who have been taking the drug for a long time. Resistant virus is treated with foscarnet or cidofovir.

Ganciclovir and valganciclovir are used for treating severe CMV infections in immunocompromised patients, including colitis, pneumonitis, retinitis, and encephalitis. Induction therapy, given two or three times daily, is usually followed by less frequently administered maintenance therapy. Oral valganciclovir has activity similar to that of intravenous ganciclovir. Ganciclovir and valganciclovir are used for prevention of CMV infection in transplant recipients when given either preemptively (on the basis of viremia) or prophylactically. Ganciclovir reduces developmental delay in infants with congenital CMV disease involving the CNS and reduces hearing loss in infants with asymptomatic congenital CMV infection. Ganciclovir and valganciclovir are used for treatment of HHV-6 encephalitis, HHV-8–associated Castleman disease in patients with poorly controlled HIV infection, and severe HSV or VZV disease when acyclovir is unavailable.

FOSCARNET

Foscarnet is a pyrophosphate analogue that directly inhibits herpesvirus DNA polymerases by blocking the pyrophosphate binding site in the enzyme. Foscarnet does not require additional phosphorylation (unlike acyclovir, cidofovir, or ganciclovir) in virus-infected cells for its activity. This drug is approved for treatment of CMV retinitis and mucocutaneous acyclovir-resistant HSV disease. It is also used to treat ganciclovir-resistant CMV and acyclovir-resistant VZV. Foscarnet is given intravenously and is excreted by the kidneys; dose adjustment is required in renal insufficiency. Up to one-third of patients receiving foscarnet develop nephrotoxicity with elevated levels of creatinine and blood urea nitrogen, and proteinuria. Renal tubular acidosis and interstitial nephritis also have been reported. Renal insufficiency is more common among persons who are dehydrated, given other nephrotoxic drugs, or given high doses or rapid infusions of foscarnet. Administering IV saline before and after each foscarnet dose and giving the drug over an adequate period can reduce nephrotoxicity. Renal insufficiency is often reversible after treatment when the drug is stopped. Other side effects include hypomagnesemia and hypocalcemia, which can be associated with arrhythmias, paresthesias, and seizures. Other metabolic abnormities include hypokalemia, hypophosphatemia, or hyperphosphatemia. Foscarnet can also cause headache, fever, rash, diarrhea, acute dystonia, tremors, hemorrhagic cystitis, genital ulcerations, anemia, and abnormal liver function values. Mutations in CMV DNA polymerase (UL54) or in HSV or VZV DNA polymerase can result in resistance to foscarnet. CMV, HSV, and VZV can become resistant to foscarnet; some strains of CMV are resistant to foscarnet, ganciclovir, and cidofovir; and HSV can become resistant to acyclovir and foscarnet. Foscarnet is typically used to treat CMV retinitis, HHV-6 encephalitis, or drug-resistant severe CMV, HSV, or VZV infections in immunocompromised patients. Topical foscarnet has been used to treat acyclovir-resistant mucosal infections due to HSV.

CIDOFOVIR

Cidofovir is an analogue of deoxycytidine monophosphate and is phosphorylated in cells to its active diphosphate form. The diphosphate form of cidofovir competes with deoxycytidine triphosphate for incorporation into herpesvirus DNA. The drug inhibits replication of all human herpesviruses as well as poxviruses, papillomaviruses, polyomaviruses, and adenoviruses. Cidofovir is approved for treatment of CMV retinitis in patients with AIDS; it is also used for treatment of infections caused by CMV exhibiting ganciclovir resistance due to mutations in UL97 protein kinase and of those caused by HSV or VZV displaying mutations in thymidine kinase. Because cidofovir is excreted by the kidneys, dose adjustment is required in renal insufficiency. About one-fifth of patients receiving cidofovir develop nephrotoxicity, and the drug is associated with metabolic acidosis and glucosuria. Cidofovir therapy is preceded by at least 1 L of saline, and probenecid is given 3 h before, 2 h after, and 8 h after each dose to reduce nephrotoxicity. An additional 1 L of saline is recommended during treatment or immediately thereafter. About one-fourth of patients receiving cidofovir develop neutropenia; additional side effects include ocular hypotony, uveitis, iritis, headache, nausea, vomiting, diarrhea, and rash. Mutations in CMV DNA polymerase (UL54) or HSV DNA polymerase can result in resistance to cidofovir. Some strains of CMV exhibiting ganciclovir resistance due to mutations in viral DNA polymerase are resistant to cidofovir, whereas many CMV and HSV strains exhibiting foscarnet resistance due to mutations in DNA polymerase may retain sensitivity to cidofovir. Cidofovir is typically used to treat ganciclovir- and/or foscarnet-resistant severe CMV disease or acyclovir- and/or foscarnet-resistant HSV disease in immunocompromised patients. Cidofovir has been used as preemptive therapy against CMV infection in transplant recipients. It has also been used to treat severe adenovirus infections, adenovirus or BK virus hemorrhagic cystitis, BK nephropathy, and severe molluscum contagiosum, although controlled studies have not been performed. Topical cidofovir has been used to treat acyclovir-resistant HSV mucosal infections and anogenital warts.

LETERMOVIR

Letermovir is a dihydroquinazolin that inhibits the CMV DNA terminase complex (UL51, UL59), which is required for cleavage and packaging of CMV into nucleocapsids. The drug has no activity against other human herpesviruses. Letermovir is approved for prophylaxis of CMV infection and disease in adult CMV-seropositive recipients of an allogeneic hematopoietic stem cell transplant. Letermovir is metabolized by the liver and excreted in the feces; dose adjustment is not required if the creatinine clearance rate (CrCl) is >10 mL/min. The dose of letermovir must be decreased in persons taking cyclosporine. Letermovir therapy results in reduced levels of voriconazole and increased levels of sirolimus, tacrolimus, cyclosporine, and other drugs metabolized by CYP2C8 or transported by OAT1B1/3. Side effects of letermovir include headache, nausea, diarrhea, and peripheral edema. Letermovir does not cause nephrotoxicity and is not myelosuppressive. Resistance to letermovir occurs more frequently in vitro than resistance to ganciclovir or foscarnet, and clinically significant letermovir resistance due to mutations in UL56 in patients with CMV disease has been reported; resistance may be less common when the drug is used for prophylaxis in patients with low or undetectable CMV levels. When given to CMV-seropositive patients, starting a median of 8 days after hematopoietic stem cell transplantation and continuing for 14 weeks, letermovir reduced the incidence of clinically significant CMV infection by 38% compared with placebo. While anecdotes describe the use of letermovir for treatment of CMV disease, resistance may develop quickly.

TRIFLURIDINE AND VIDARABINE

Trifluridine is a thymidine analogue that is incorporated into viral DNA and inhibits its synthesis. Vidarabine is approved for topical therapy of herpes keratitis and has also been used topically to treat acyclovir-resistant mucosal HSV infections. Trifluridine is active against acyclovir-resistant HSV, CMV, and vaccinia virus. Vidarabine is an adenosine analogue that is incorporated into viral DNA and inhibits viral DNA polymerase. Both trifluridine and vidarabine are used for topical therapy only.

INVESTIGATIONAL AND OTHER AGENTS

Brincidofovir is a phospholipid conjugate of cidofovir that is rapidly taken up by cells and converted into cidofovir. It is active against herpesviruses (including most strains of ganciclovir-resistant CMV), poxviruses, adenovirus, and polyomaviruses. It does not cause nephrotoxicity and is not myelosuppressive. Diarrhea is the most common side effect. The drug has been associated with intestinal toxicity and acute graft-versus-host disease of the gastrointestinal tract. The drug did not meet its primary endpoints in trials for adenovirus disease or CMV prophylaxis. Clinical trials of oral brincidofovir have been discontinued, although it is still being developed for treatment of smallpox.

It is available for patients with serious adenovirus or poxvirus infections as part of the expanded access program. An IV formulation, which, it is hoped, will cause less gastrointestinal toxicity, is being tested for adenovirus viremia.

Maribavir is a benzimidazole that inhibits the CMV UL97 protein kinase and reduces the egress of viral particles from the nucleus. The drug is active against most strains of ganciclovir- and foscarnet-resistant CMV. In phase 3 trials, maribavir was unsuccessful in preventing CMV disease in transplant recipients; it is currently being tested as therapy for CMV infections refractory to treatment with other antiviral agents.

Pritelivir inhibits the helicase–primase complex required for replication of HSV. This drug has reduced viral shedding in patients with recurrent genital herpes and is being tested for use against acyclovir-resistant HSV mucocutaneous infection. Pritelivir is available as an expanded access drug for acyclovir-resistant HSV infection.

Amenamevir is a helicase–primase inhibitor under development for HSV and VZV infections.

ANTIVIRAL DRUGS FOR RESPIRATORY VIRUS INFECTIONS

INFLUENZA

Neuraminidase Inhibitors Oseltamivir, zanamivir, and peramivir are neuraminidase inhibitors that inhibit cleavage of sialic acid, which is required for the release of influenza virus from infected cells and its spread to other cells.

Oseltamivir phosphate is an oral prodrug that is cleaved by esterases in the liver, gastrointestinal tract, and blood to oseltamivir carboxylate, the more active form. It is approved for treatment of uncomplicated influenza A or B disease when given ≤48 h after symptom onset and for prophylaxis of influenza A and B in persons ≥1 year of age (**Table 191-2**). Oseltamivir is much less active against influenza B than against influenza A. The drug is excreted by the kidneys, and the dose is adjusted in renal insufficiency. The most common side effects are nausea, abdominal pain, and vomiting. Although CNS side effects have been reported, particularly in children, it is unclear whether they are due to the drug or to influenza virus infection itself. Resistance to oseltamivir can develop as a result of mutations in the viral neuraminidase or in the hemagglutinin. Oseltamivir-resistant virus has been transmitted from person to person. Resistance has been reported in ~15% of healthy children and ~1% of adults; resistance is more common among immunocompromised persons.

Zanamivir is approved for treatment of uncomplicated influenza A and B in adults and children ≥7 years of age who have had symptoms for ≤2 days and for prophylaxis in persons ≥5 years of age. Because zanamivir has poor oral bioavailability, it is given as a powder through an inhaler. Thus, use of the drug can be difficult for young children and some elderly patients. Inhalation of zanamivir may cause bronchospasm, particularly in persons with underlying lung disease; it is not recommended for persons with asthma, chronic obstructive pulmonary disease, or other airway disease. Zanamivir is more active than oseltamivir against influenza B. It is also active against some isolates of influenza virus that are resistant to oseltamivir; resistance to zanamivir is less common than that to oseltamivir.

Peramivir is approved for treating uncomplicated influenza in patients ≥2 years of age who have had symptoms for ≤2 days. Because of its long half-life, it is given as a single IV dose. Peramivir is highly active against both influenza A and B. The drug is excreted by the kidneys, and the dose is adjusted in renal insufficiency. The most common side effect is diarrhea. While peramivir-resistant virus is rare in healthy persons, peramivir-resistant virus has been isolated from immunocompromised persons.

Oseltamivir, zanamivir, and peramivir are effective for treatment of uncomplicated influenza A and B, including disease caused by avian influenza viruses (e.g., H5N1, H7N9, and H9N2). None of the neuraminidase inhibitors is approved by the FDA for complicated influenza or for persons requiring hospitalization for the disease. While not licensed for the treatment of persons with complicated disease, inpatients, and pregnant women, oseltamivir is considered the drug of choice in these settings. The efficacy of zanamivir is similar to that of oseltamivir in hospitalized patients. Treatment is most effective when begun within 2 days of symptom onset and should be started as early as possible; such early treatment reduces symptoms by ~1 day in persons with uncomplicated disease. For persons with influenza requiring hospitalization and with pneumonia, treatment with oseltamivir or zanamivir is recommended even later. Treatment may reduce the risk of complications and death in hospitalized patients with influenza.

Oseltamivir and zanamivir (but not peramivir) are approved for prophylaxis of influenza, especially in institutions where outbreaks can be severe, and for prophylaxis in persons who have been exposed to the virus, are at high risk for disease complications, and have not recently been vaccinated. The efficacy of oseltamivir and zanamivir for prophylaxis is estimated to be ~70–90%. For persons at institutions, prophylaxis is given for at least 2 weeks and for up to 1 week after outbreaks resolve. For other high-risk persons, prophylaxis is given within 2 days of exposure and continued for 1 week after exposure. Since neuraminidase inhibitors reduce virus release from cells, they should not be given 2 days before or within 2 weeks after receipt of live, attenuated influenza vaccine. Resistance has been reported during treatment with oseltamivir or peramivir, especially in immunocompromised persons; oseltamivir-resistant viruses are usually sensitive to zanamivir.

TABLE 191-2 Antiviral Drugs for Respiratory Virus Treatment and Prophylaxis in Adults

DISEASE	DRUG	ROUTE	ADULT DOSE	COMMENTS
Influenza A, B	Oseltamivir	Oral	Treatment: 75 mg bid × 5 d Prophylaxis: 75 mg/d	Shortens duration of symptoms by 1 d when given within 2 d of onset; reduces complications; considered drug of choice for patients with complications of influenza
Influenza A, B	Zanamivir	Inhaled	Treatment: 10 mg bid × 5 d Prophylaxis: 10 mg/d	Shortens duration of symptoms by 1–2 d when given within 2 d of onset; requires patient training for use; can cause bronchospasm; not recommended for persons with asthma or chronic obstructive pulmonary disease
Influenza A, B	Peramivir	IV	600 mg once	Shortens duration of symptoms by 1–2 d when given within 2 d of onset
Influenza A, B	Baloxavir	Oral	40 mg once; if >80 kg, 80 mg once	Shortens duration of symptoms by 1 d when given within 2 d of onset; active against virus resistant to neuraminidase inhibitors
Influenza A	Amantadine	Oral	Treatment: 100 mg bid × 5 d Prophylaxis: 200 mg/d	Most influenza virus strains are resistant; use only if virus is known to be sensitive.
Influenza A	Rimantadine	Oral	Treatment: 100 mg bid × 5 d Prophylaxis: 200 mg/d	Most influenza virus strains are resistant; use only if virus is known to be sensitive.
Respiratory syncytial virus	Ribavirin	Inhaled	Aerosol from reservoir containing 20 mg/mL for 12–18 h/d × 3–6 d	Reduces severity of symptoms in hospitalized infants with lower respiratory tract disease; anecdotal reports of reduced progression to lower respiratory tract disease and mortality in stem cell transplant patients
SARS-CoV-2	Remdesivir	IV	200 mg on day 1, then 100 mg qd × 4 d	Reduces duration of hospitalization in some studies. Duration of treatment extended up to 10 days if no improvement.

Baloxavir Baloxavir inhibits the cap-dependent endonuclease that is important in initiating synthesis of influenza virus mRNA. This drug is approved by the FDA as a single oral dose for postexposure prophylaxis of influenza and for treatment of uncomplicated influenza in persons ≥12 years of age who have had symptoms for ≤48 h. Baloxavir inhibits influenza A and B viruses, including avian strains and strains that are resistant to neuraminidase inhibitors. The drug's efficacy is similar to that of the neuraminidase inhibitors in persons with uncomplicated influenza and reduces symptoms by ~1 day. In addition, baloxavir exhibits efficacy similar to that of oseltamivir for reducing symptoms in high-risk patients. However, its effectiveness in patients hospitalized with complications of influenza is unknown. Reduced sensitivity of influenza virus to baloxavir has been associated with mutations in the viral polymerase acidic protein after one dose. The incidences of nausea and vomiting are lower with baloxavir than with oseltamivir. Levels of the drug are lower if it is taken with dairy products, polyvalent cation-containing laxatives or antacids, or oral supplements containing calcium, iron, magnesium, selenium, or zinc. Since baloxavir reduces virus replication, it should not be given 2 days before or within 2 weeks after receipt of live, attenuated influenza vaccine.

Adamantanes Amantadine and rimantadine inhibit the influenza virus's M2 protein and its uncoating and membrane fusion. While these drugs are active against influenza A, resistance is widespread and can develop rapidly; thus, the adamantanes are not recommended as treatment or prophylaxis for influenza unless the virus is known to be sensitive.

■ RESPIRATORY SYNCYTIAL VIRUS

Ribavirin Ribavirin is an analogue of guanosine and inhibits replication of numerous RNA and DNA viruses. The drug inhibits viral RNA synthesis and capping of viral mRNA and in some cases increases the viral RNA mutation rate to lethal levels for some viruses. Ribavirin inhibits replication of respiratory syncytial virus (RSV), influenza virus, parainfluenza virus, and many other RNA viruses in vitro. While the drug has been used to treat numerous viral infections, including Lassa fever and hepatitis E, it is approved by the FDA only for use against RSV and as a component of combination therapy for hepatitis C. Aerosolized ribavirin is approved for treatment of hospitalized infants and young children with severe lower respiratory tract infections due to RSV; it is given for 18 h per day and is most effective when used early in the course of these severe infections. Ribavirin is given in a generator that yields an aerosol of particles small enough to reach the lower respiratory tract; the level of systemic absorption is low. The aerosolized form of the drug can induce bronchospasm, sudden deterioration of respiratory function (especially in infants), and rash and can precipitate in ventilators, interfering with their function. Ribavirin is mutagenic and teratogenic in animals; accordingly, it is not recommended for use in pregnant women, and the exposure of health care workers should be minimized with personal protective equipment. In early studies, ribavirin reduced the shedding of RSV and the severity of symptoms in hospitalized infants with lower respiratory tract disease who were not on mechanical ventilation, the duration of oxygen supplementation, and the duration of time on mechanical ventilation in infants. More recent analyses of the literature suggest that the efficacy of the drug in these settings is much less certain, and the drug is not recommended for routine use by the American Academy of Pediatrics. In retrospective studies, ribavirin has been reported to reduce the risk of progression of RSV from upper to lower respiratory tract disease in stem cell transplant recipients and to reduce mortality rates in these patients. In a retrospective study, the outcome of treatment with oral ribavirin was similar to that obtained with the aerosolized drug in hematopoietic stem cell transplant recipients with RSV disease. Ribavirin has not been shown to affect the clinical course of patients with parainfluenza and is not recommended for their treatment. Ribavirin costs more than $25,000 per day.

Palivizumab Palivizumab, a humanized monoclonal antibody to RSV F protein, is approved for prevention of lower respiratory tract disease due to RSV in pediatric patients at high risk of RSV disease, including premature infants and children with bronchopulmonary dysplasia.

■ SARS-COV-2 (SEE CHAP. 199)

Remdesivir is converted in cells to an adenosine triphosphate analogue that inhibits the RNA-dependent RNA polymerase of several viruses. The drug is approved by the FDA for treatment of persons ≥12 years of age with SARS-CoV-2 requiring hospitalization; it shortens the duration of hospitalization in persons with lower respiratory tract disease. While the results of studies with the drug vary, it is recommended by the National Institutes of Health for patients with SARS-CoV-2 who require supplemental oxygen while hospitalized. The drug is given IV and is not recommended in persons with a GFR <30 mL/min. Serum transaminase elevations have been reported in healthy persons receiving remdesivir, and liver enzymes should be monitored before and during treatment. Chloroquine inhibits the activity of remdesivir in vitro; hydroxychloroquine or chloroquine phosphate should not be given with remdesivir.

■ INVESTIGATIONAL AGENTS FOR RESPIRATORY VIRUS INFECTIONS

Favipiravir (T705) inhibits viral RNA polymerases and is active against influenza and other RNA viruses. It is approved for treatment of emerging influenza viruses in Japan. Presatovir is an RSV fusion inhibitor that was ineffective in two trials of RSV disease. DAS181 (Fludase) is a sialidase that cleaves sialic acid, a receptor for influenza A and B and parainfluenza viruses; it did not improve the clinical outcomes of patients with influenza, but in case reports transplant recipients with parainfluenza have improved clinically with the drug. Laninamivir octanoate inhibits the neuraminidase of influenza A and B viruses and is approved for treating influenza in Japan. RSV604 interacts with the RSV nucleocapsid and is undergoing phase 2 studies in transplant recipients.

Molnupiravir is an oral ribonucleoside analog that inhibits replication of SARS-CoV-2. The drug reduced the risk of hospitalization or death in patients with mild-to-moderate COVID-19 by ~50% in a phase 3 clinical trial. AT-527 is an oral nucleotide prodrug that reduced SARS-CoV-2 viral loads in patients hospitalized with COVID-19 in a phase 2 clinical trial. PF-07321332 is an oral SARS-CoV-2 protease inhibitor that is being tested in combination with low dose ritonavir in a phase 2/3 clinical trial for prevention of COVID-19 infection.

ANTIVIRAL DRUGS FOR HUMAN PAPILLOMAVIRUS AND POXVIRUS INFECTIONS

Interferon α (IFN-α) inhibits replication of many RNA and DNA viruses in vitro. IFN-α is approved by the FDA for intralesional treatment of external anogenital warts caused by human papillomavirus (HPV). It is effective in resolving lesions in ~50% of cases, with a recurrence rate of ~25%.

Imiquimod is a toll-like receptor 7 agonist that induces production of IFN-α and other cytokines. It is approved as a topical cream for treatment of external genital and perianal warts caused by HPV in persons ≥12 years of age. This drug is effective in resolving lesions in ~40% of cases.

Tecovirimat is approved by the FDA for treatment of smallpox and inhibits replication of monkeypox and vaccinia viruses. Resistance to tecovirimat developed in a person treated with the drug for progressive vaccinia.

INVESTIGATIONAL ANTIVIRAL DRUGS FOR PICORNAVIRUS

Pocapavir inhibits picornaviruses by inhibiting virus uncoating and is being developed to reduce poliovirus shedding; resistance to the drug develops rapidly.

ANTIVIRAL DRUGS FOR HEPATITIS B VIRUS INFECTION

Eight drugs of two classes are approved for the treatment of chronic HBV infection in the United States. One class, the nucleos(t)ide analogues, act as chain-terminating competitive inhibitors of HBV

TABLE 191-3 Antiviral Drugs for Chronic Hepatitis B Treatment in Adults

DRUG	ROUTE AND DOSE	DEVELOPMENT OF RESISTANCE	COMMON SIDE EFFECTS[a]	TREATMENT MONITORING	COMMENTS
Interferons					
Pegylated α2a Pegylated α2b	SC injection; 180 μg/w for 48 w SC injection; 1.5 μg/kg/w for 48 w	Not described in long term studies.	Side effects are common and include fevers, chills, myalgia, fatigue, neurotoxicity, and leukopenia. Autoantibodies can develop, particularly antithyroid antibodies.	Complete blood counts should be performed biweekly for the first month and then monthly, renal and liver function testing monthly, thyroid function testing every 3 months.	Best treatment response seen among patients with HBV genotype A infection While pegylated interferon α2b is approved for HCV, it is used for HBV.
Nucelos(t)ide Analogues					
Lamivudine	Oral; 100 mg daily	30% after 1 year; 70% after 5 years	Malaise or fatigue, GI symptoms (nausea/vomiting, abdominal pain, diarrhea), headache, upper respiratory tract infection	Renal and liver function testing every 3–6 months Assessment of lactic acid level HBV DNA and serologic testing every 3–6 months	Monotherapy recommended if duration of therapy is to be <1 year, as in prophylaxis against HBV reactivation with immunosuppression or chemotherapy
Adefovir	Oral; 10 mg daily	20–29% after 5 years Adefovir is usually active against lamivudine-resistant HBV strains.	Headache, asthenia, GI symptoms (abdominal pain, nausea)	Renal and liver function testing every 6 months Assessment of lactic acid level HBV DNA and serologic testing every 3–6 months	—
Telbivudine	Oral; 600 mg daily	11–25% after 2 years Cross-resistance is common between lamivudine- and telbivudine-resistant HBV strains.	Headache, fatigue, GI symptoms (abdominal pain)	Measurement of creatine kinase level if there is concern about myopathy Renal and liver function testing every 3–6 months Assessment of lactic acid level HBV DNA and serologic testing every 3–6 months	—
Entecavir	Oral; 0.5–1 mg daily	1–2% after 5 years in nucleos(t)ide-naïve patients; 60% in lamivudine-resistant patients	Headache, fatigue, elevated alanine aminotransferase level	Renal and liver function testing every 3–6 months Assessment of lactic acid level HBV DNA and serologic testing every 3–6 months	Recommended as first-line therapy Dose of 0.5 mg daily in treatment-naïve patients, 1 mg daily in treatment-experienced patients Dose adjusted in renal dysfunction
Tenofovir disoproxil	Oral; 300 mg daily	No resistance after up to 7 years of treatment	Headache, fatigue, nasopharyngitis, upper respiratory tract infection, nausea	Renal and liver function testing every 3–6 months Phosphorus assessment in patients with chronic kidney disease Assessment of lactic acid level HBV DNA and serologic testing every 3–6 months	Recommended as first-line therapy Dosing frequency—but not dose—reduced in chronic kidney disease May be used during pregnancy; possible risk of low birth weight
Tenofovir alafenamide	Oral; 25 mg daily	No long-term follow-up data available	Headache, fatigue, nasopharyngitis, upper respiratory tract infection	Renal and liver function testing every 3–6 months Phosphorus assessment in patients with chronic kidney disease Assessment of lactic acid level HBV DNA and serologic testing every 3–6 months	Recommended as first-line therapy May be used during pregnancy; possible risk of low birth weight
Emtricitabine	Oral; 200 mg daily	Not defined	Headache, GI symptoms (nausea, diarrhea, abdominal pain), fatigue, depression, insomnia, abnormal dreams, rash, asthenia, increased cough, rhinitis	Renal and liver function testing every 3–6 months Assessment of lactic acid level HBV DNA and serologic testing every 3–6 months	While not approved for treatment of chronic HBV infection, used interchangeably with lamivudine Dosing frequency adjusted in chronic kidney disease

[a]For emtricitabine, side effects were assessed only in combination with antiretroviral therapy.

Abbreviation: GI, gastrointestinal.

reverse transcriptase; the other class, the exogenous IFNs, mimics and augments the role of endogenous interferons (**Table 191-3**). The goal of therapy for chronic hepatitis B is to reduce the risk of hepatic inflammation, which can cause liver fibrosis progressing to cirrhosis, liver failure, and hepatocellular carcinoma. Virologic responses (defined by suppression of HBV replication), biochemical responses (improvement or normalization of liver function values), and histologic responses (the degree of hepatic fibrosis visualized on liver biopsy) are often achievable with current treatments. However, loss of hepatitis B e antigen (HBeAg), viral clearance with loss of hepatitis B surface antigen (HBsAg), and viral protection (defined by a hepatitis B surface antibody [HBsAb] titer of >10 IU/mL) are uncommon with current therapies.

Treatment with a nucleos(t)ide analogue is considered first-line therapy for chronic HBV infection because of its favorable side effect profile and ease of administration. All drugs in this class are given by mouth once daily. While all nucleos(t)ide analogues carry a warning for lactic acidosis and severe hepatomegaly, these adverse events were observed in patients taking older nucleoside analogues (such as stavudine and didanosine for the treatment of HIV) and have not occurred in clinical trials of nucleos(t)ides for chronic HBV infection. The main risk of nucleos(t)ide therapy for chronic hepatitis B consists of virus rebound and subsequent hepatitis flare following treatment cessation, which can occur in up to 20% of patients and rarely may lead to hepatic failure. Comparative studies of nucleos(t)ide analogues have demonstrated that newer drugs (entecavir and tenofovir) are associated with lower rates of viral resistance than older agents (lamivudine and adefovir), but, if viral replication is effectively suppressed, histologic and biochemical improvement will occur in ~60–75% of patients, without significant differences between antiviral agents or combinations. However, rates of HBsAg clearance remain extremely low (<1–5%).

IFN-based therapies are associated with slightly higher rates of serologic response and lower rates of viral resistance, but also with lower rates of biochemical and virologic responses (<40% for both). Response rates are somewhat higher when IFNs are combined with nucleos(t)ide therapy in naïve patients: overall rates of HBsAg loss after 48 weeks of combination therapy with pegylated IFN-α2a and tenofovir disoproxil fumarate (TDF) were low but significantly higher than when either was given alone: 9.1% versus 0 with TDF alone ($p<.001$) and 2.8% with IFN alone ($p<.005$). However, no significant difference was observed when IFN was added to the regimen administered to patients already receiving nucleos(t)ide therapy. IFN-based treatments often are not tolerated because of side effects and drug interactions and are generally reserved for patients with favorable HBV genotype A infection with HBeAg-positive active disease (characterized by viral loads of ≥20,000 IU/mL and aminotransferase levels greater than two times the upper limit of normal) and those in whom a short course of treatment is preferred (e.g., women who are planning to become pregnant).

LAMIVUDINE

Lamivudine is an oral cytidine analogue that competitively inhibits the viral reverse transcriptase activity of both HIV and HBV, preventing viral replication. Lamivudine has been used for prophylaxis against HBV reactivation during immunosuppression following liver transplantation or chemotherapy, particularly when the duration of prophylaxis is expected to be relatively short. Long-term use can be limited by a low threshold of viral resistance: rates approach 30% among patients treated for 1 year and reach 70% after 5 years of therapy. Changes in the YMDD motif of the HBV DNA polymerase are associated with reduced lamivudine efficacy.

While not approved for the treatment of chronic HBV infection, emtricitabine is a cytosine analogue similar in structure, activity, and resistance to lamivudine. It offers no advantage over lamivudine, but emtricitabine is available in combination tablets coformulated with tenofovir (both TDF and tenofovir alafenamide fumarate [TAF]). When appropriate, as in cases of established nucleoside resistance or in patients with HIV/HBV co-infection requiring lifelong antiviral therapy, these coformulations can be used with monitoring recommendations and expectations for clinical response similar to those for lamivudine and tenofovir.

ADEFOVIR

Adefovir dipivoxil is the oral prodrug of adefovir—a monophosphate nucleotide analogue of adenosine. This drug is active against HBV, HIV, some herpesviruses (HSV and CMV), and poxviruses. Treatment-limiting side effects (including rare nephrotoxicity) preclude the use of the higher doses required to inhibit HIV (60–120 mg daily), which are not FDA-approved for this indication. Studies of a 10-mg dose for HBV infection demonstrated an excellent safety and tolerability profile and led to FDA approval for the treatment of chronic HBV infection. Adefovir is effective in the treatment of naïve HBV-infected patients and those infected with lamivudine-resistant HBV. Viral resistance to adefovir is slower to emerge than resistance to lamivudine but still develops in 20–30% of patients after 5 years of treatment. Because adefovir dipivoxil is renally cleared, routine monitoring of renal function (every 6 months) is advised.

TELBIVUDINE

A β-L enantiomer of thymidine, telbivudine was approved by the FDA in 2006 for the treatment of chronic HBV infection. Telbivudine was shown to result in virologic, biochemical, and histologic improvement in patients with chronic HBV infection. Telbivudine-resistant HBV is generally cross-resistant with lamivudine-resistant virus but usually is still susceptible to adefovir or tenofovir. After 2 years of therapy, strains resistant to telbivudine were noted in 25% of HBeAg-positive patients and 11% of HBeAg-negative patients; this resistance has limited its use. Because telbivudine is rapidly absorbed and renally metabolized, the dose is reduced in patients with a CrCl of <50 mL/min. Telbivudine is generally well tolerated, but increases in creatinine kinase and fatigue and myalgias have been observed.

ENTECAVIR

Entecavir is a cyclopentyl guanosine analogue that, once triphosphorylated, blocks HBV polymerase in multiple ways, inhibiting both reverse transcription of the HBV negative strand and positive-strand synthesis. Entecavir effectively inhibits HBV replication, with resulting biochemical and histologic improvement. This drug is active against some lamivudine-resistant HBV strains, but only at concentrations 20- to 30-fold higher than those obtained with the standard 0.5-mg dose; thus a higher dose (1 mg daily) of entecavir is recommended for patients with previous lamivudine exposure. Entecavir resistance leading to viral rebound is uncommon among patients naïve to HBV treatment but may occur in up to 60% of patients with prior lamivudine resistance after 4 years of entecavir treatment. Entecavir-resistant strains retain susceptibility to tenofovir and occasionally adefovir. Entecavir is generally well tolerated and highly bioavailable but should be taken on an empty stomach because food interferes with its absorption. The drug is renally cleared, and dosing should be adjusted for a CrCl of <50 mL/min.

TENOFOVIR

Tenofovir is a nucleotide analogue of adenosine monophosphate with activity against both retroviruses and hepadnaviruses. Tenofovir potently inhibits HBV replication. Clinically significant resistance to tenofovir has not been observed with up to 7 years of therapy. It is available in two prodrug forms, TDF and TAF. Both formulations of tenofovir are approved by the FDA for the treatment of both HIV infection and HBV infection and are renally excreted. Because of structural similarities among TDF, adefovir, and cidofovir (the latter two drugs can cause proximal renal tubular toxicity), TDF carries a warning for renal toxicity, including Fanconi syndrome and diabetes insipidus, but these risks have not been found in large clinical trials of hepatitis B treatment. Rather, a small decline (by ~5 mg/dL) has been noted in the glomerular filtration rate over 2 years of TDF therapy. A mild decline in bone mineral density has been observed after 5 years of TDF treatment, but the clinical significance of this change is unknown and the risk of fracture remained low. Routine monitoring of renal function during TDF therapy is indicated, and dose frequency should be reduced in chronic kidney disease. TAF has greater stability than TDF, with higher drug concentrations within hepatocytes and less systemic exposure. A comparative study revealed that, while TAF carries the same risks, the magnitude of decline in glomerular filtration rate (GFR) and bone mineral density was 25–30% of that observed with TDF.

INTERFERONS

IFNs have a broad spectrum of antiviral activity in addition to modulating the immune system. IFNs are given IM, SC, or IV. Recombinant α, β, γ, and λ IFNs have been evaluated in a variety of viral infections.

IFNs may also be pegylated: linkage of INF-α to polyethylene glycol results in slower absorption, decreased clearance, and more sustained serum IFN concentrations, thereby permitting a more convenient, once-weekly dosing schedule. In many instances, pegylated IFN has supplanted standard IFN.

Adverse effects of IFN include fever, myalgia, fatigue, somnolence, depression, confusion, leukopenia, and development of autoantibodies, including antithyroid antibodies. Pegylated IFN-α2a is approved by the FDA for therapy in patients with chronic hepatitis B. While pegylated IFN-α2b has been reported to be useful for HBV infection, this drug is not approved for treatment of hepatitis B in the United States.

IFNs have undergone extensive study in the treatment of chronic HBV infection. The administration of standard IFN-α2b for 16–24 weeks to patients with stable chronic HBV infection resulted in the loss of markers for HBV replication (e.g., HBeAg and HBV DNA) in 33–37% of cases; 8% of patients also cleared HBsAg. In most patients who lose HBeAg and HBV DNA, serum aminotransferases return to normal levels, and both short- and long-term improvements in liver histopathology have been described. Predictors of a favorable response to standard IFN therapy include low pretherapy levels of HBV DNA, high pretherapy serum levels of alanine aminotransferase (ALT), a short duration of chronic HBV infection, and active liver inflammation on biopsy. Poor responses are seen in immunosuppressed patients, including those infected with HIV.

At high doses, IFN-α and pegylated IFN-α are active against hepatitis D virus infection. In hepatitis D, a sustained virologic response (SVR) was achieved in 25–35% of patients treated with IFN-α but in only 17–43% of patients treated with pegylated IFN-α.

Several IFN preparations have been studied and approved as therapeutic options for chronic HCV infection; often these preparations combine IFN with ribavirin, a nonspecific nucleoside analogue with the antiviral effects discussed below. The approval of directly acting antiviral agents in 2014 led to revised guidance, and IFN therapy is no longer recommended for the treatment of hepatitis C.

ANTIVIRAL DRUGS FOR HEPATITIS C INFECTION

Several targeted therapies with directly acting antiviral drugs (DAAs) are effective against HCV (**Table 191-4**). Combination DAA therapy is now the standard of care for the treatment of chronic HCV infection, regardless of genotype or fibrosis stage. HCV therapeutics have three drug targets: the NS5B RNA-dependent RNA polymerase, the NS3/4 protease, and NS5A, a zinc-binding phosphoprotein that is integral for HCV RNA replication. Treatment duration varies, usually from 8 to 24 weeks. The goal of HCV treatment is to suppress the level of viral replication; if levels of HCV RNA in the plasma remain undetectable when assessed 12 weeks after the end of treatment, an SVR has been achieved. The SVR is considered synonymous with cure, as it is associated with durable suppression of HCV replication, lower all-cause and liver-related mortality, and a reduced risk of hepatocellular carcinoma. These benefits have been confirmed in patients with and without advanced liver disease and cirrhosis who received IFN-sparing, combination DAA–based regimens.

In general, first-line DAA-based regimens for chronic HCV infection are so effective that cure rates exceed 90%. An SVR is not obtained in a small subset of patients: up to 6% for genotype 1 (the most common genotype) and >10% for genotype 3 (historically the most difficult to treat). Two pangenotypic regimens are approved specifically for re-treatment of chronic HCV infection after treatment failure: glecaprevir/pibrentasvir and sofosbuvir/velpatasvir/voxilaprevir. While some amino acid substitutions and polymorphisms can impact the efficacy of HCV treatment with combination DAA–based regimens, the clinical significance of this reduced susceptibility varies greatly between regimens and by genotype/subtype. In the setting of unfavorable viral genetics (viral subgenotypes or viral variants with resistance-associated polymorphisms) or advanced fibrosis, treatment efficacy can frequently be improved by extension of the treatment course or the addition of ribavirin. Review of the online joint American Association for the Study of Liver Diseases/Infectious Diseases Society of America's HCV Guidelines is useful. In addition, for all DAA-based treatments, checking for drug–drug interactions before the initiation of therapy is recommended.

Most regimens are well tolerated, but all DAAs carry a black-box warning about reactivation of HBV following HCV suppression. In some cases, fulminant hepatitis, hepatic flare, and death have occurred in patients with untreated HBV infection who underwent treatment for chronic HBV infection. These risks are rare and can be safely managed with routine monitoring; treatment of HCV should not be deferred because of HBV co-infection.

SOFOSBUVIR AND SOFOSBUVIR-CONTAINING REGIMENS

Sofosbuvir Sofosbuvir is the prodrug of a uridine inhibitor of the HCV NS5B RNA-dependent RNA polymerase. The active uridine nucleoside triphosphate results in termination of viral RNA replication. Sofosbuvir is approved by the FDA for the treatment of HCV genotypes 1–4 and is active against genotypes 1–6. Resistance to sofosbuvir is conferred by an S282T substitution in the NS5B protein, but clinically significant resistance to sofosbuvir treatment has rarely been encountered and virologic breakthrough during sofosbuvir treatment is exceedingly rare. Sofosbuvir is approved for use with other DAAs and is available both individually and as part of three fixed-dose combination regimens: as two-drug regimens with the NS5A protein inhibitors ledipasvir and velpatasvir, respectively, and as a three-drug regimen with velpatasvir and the protease inhibitor voxilaprevir. Both sofosbuvir and its active metabolite are renally cleared, and while the FDA has approved this drug only for patients with an estimated GFR of ≥30 mL/min, several studies have demonstrated its safety and efficacy even in end-stage renal disease and for patients undergoing dialysis. Sofosbuvir has not been associated with significant toxicity or drug interactions with one notable exception: sofosbuvir potentiates amiodarone and may cause severe bradycardia, especially if coadministered with amiodarone and a β-blocker.

Sofosbuvir/Ledipasvir Ledipasvir is an NS5A protein inhibitor that is available only in combination with sofosbuvir. The fixed-dose combination of ledipasvir and sofosbuvir is effective against genotypes 1, 4, and 6. The standard duration of treatment is 12 weeks for genotype 1 (all subgenotypes), genotype 4, and genotype 6; however, treatment duration may be reduced to 8 weeks in treatment-naïve, genotype 1–infected noncirrhotic patients with baseline HCV RNA levels below 6 million copies/mL. Treatment should be extended to 24 weeks or ribavirin should be added in patients who have decompensated cirrhosis or previous DAA exposure. Ledipasvir is excreted via the biliary route, and no adjustment is needed for mild or moderate renal impairment. Several studies have shown that sofosbuvir/ledipasvir is safe in end-stage renal disease, but it remains FDA-approved only for patients with a CrCl of >30 mL/min. No dose reduction is required for decompensated cirrhosis (Child–Turcotte–Pugh class B or C). Ledipasvir absorption is improved with food intake and is inhibited by antacids or proton-pump inhibitors. Ledipasvir is an inhibitor of P-glycoprotein and may increase levels of tenofovir; renal function should be monitored in patients receiving both medications, although clinically significant interactions are unlikely during the relatively short period of treatment. Ledipasvir is generally well tolerated, and clinical trials have shown only a small increase in side effects, including headache and fatigue, over those occurring with placebo.

Sofosbuvir/Velpatasvir While chemically similar to ledipasvir, velpatasvir has an expanded spectrum of activity and exhibits improved efficacy over ledipasvir against HCV genotypes 2 and 3. Velpatasvir is available only in combination with sofosbuvir for the treatment of naïve patients with genotype 1–6 infection and all stages of fibrosis, including decompensated cirrhosis. In contrast to sofosbuvir/ledipasvir treatment, shortening of the duration of sofosbuvir/velpatasvir therapy in these patients is not indicated. Similar to ledipasvir, velpatasvir should be taken with food, and coadministration with antacids or

TABLE 191-4 Antiviral Drugs for Hepatitis C Treatment in Adults[a]

DRUG FORMULATION	ROUTE, DOSE, DURATION	MECHANISM(S) OF ACTION	SPECTRUM OF ACTIVITY	COMMON SIDE EFFECTS	COMMENTS
Sofosbuvir	Oral; 400 mg daily; duration varies (12–24 w)	Nucleoside analogue	Genotypes 1–6	Headache, fatigue	Should be combined with at least one other DAA from a different class.
Sofosbuvir/ledipasvir	Oral; 400 mg/90 mg daily; 8, 12, or 24 w	Nucleoside analogue/ NS5A inhibitor	Genotypes 1, 4, and 6	Headache, fatigue	Avoid coadministration with antacid medications.
Sofosbuvir/velpatasvir	Oral; 400 mg/100 mg daily; 12 w	Nucleoside analogue/ NS5A inhibitor	Genotypes 1–6	Headache, fatigue	Avoid coadministration with antacid medications.
Sofosbuvir/velpatasvir/ voxilaprevir	Oral; 400 mg/100 mg/100 mg once daily; 12 w	Nucleoside analogue/ NS5A inhibitor/protease inhibitor	Genotypes 1–6	Headache, fatigue, diarrhea, nausea	Approved for re-treatment of patients with previous DAA experience. Avoid coadministration with antacid medications.
Paritaprevir/ritonavir/ ombitasvir + dasabuvir	Oral; 2 75-mg tablets/50 mg/12.5 mg once daily + 1 250-mg tablet (dasabuvir) bid; 12 or 24 w	Protease inhibitor/ boosting agent/NS5A inhibitor + nonnucleoside polymerase inhibitor	Genotypes 1a and 1b	Fatigue, nausea, pruritis, insomnia, and asthenia	Should be combined with ribavirin in patients with genotype 1a infection. Monitor hepatic function monthly during treatment.
Elbasvir/grazoprevir	Oral; 50 mg/100 mg once daily; 12 or 16 w	NS5A inhibitor/protease inhibitor	Genotypes 1 and 4	Fatigue, anemia, headache, nausea	Pretreatment testing for resistance-associated substitutions recommended in patients infected with genotype 1a. Monitor hepatic function panel at 8 w and again at 12 w if patient is receiving 16 w of treatment.
Glecaprevir/pibrentasvir	Oral; 3 100-mg tablets/ 40 mg once daily; 8, 12, or 16 w	NS5A inhibitor/protease inhibitor	Genotypes 1–6	Headache, fatigue	—
Simeprevir	Oral; 150-mg capsule once daily; 12 w	Protease inhibitor	Genotypes 1a, 1b, and 4	Rash, pruritus, nausea	Recommended only in combination with sofosbuvir; no longer considered a first- or second-line regimen. Baseline testing for resistance-associated polymorphism Q80K recommended.
Daclatasvir	Oral; 60-mg tablet once daily; 12 w Dose reduced to 30 mg once daily when taken with a strong CYP3A inhibitor Dose increased to 90 mg once daily when taken with moderate CYP3A inducers	NS5A inhibitor	Genotypes 1 and 3	Headache, fatigue	Use recommended only along with sofosbuvir—with or without ribavirin—for genotype 1 or 3 infection; no longer considered a first- or second-line regimen.
Ribavirin	Oral; 3–6 200-mg capsules once daily or in divided doses, based on weight, history of cardiovascular disease, and renal function	Nucleoside analogue, also unknown mechanisms	Unknown, used for all genotypes	Anemia, nausea, teratogenic in pregnancy	Used only as combined therapy with DAAs or interferon. Complete blood counts should be monitored after 2 w of treatment and as clinically indicated thereafter. Dose may be adjusted based on anemia and renal function.

[a]While these drugs are approved by the FDA for chronic, but not acute HCV, they have been recommended for acute HCV by both the Infectious Diseases Society of America and the American Association for the Study of Liver Diseases.

Abbreviation: DAA, directly acting antiviral agent.

proton-pump inhibitors should be avoided. Velpatasvir is in general well tolerated, and reported side effects are minimal.

Sofosbuvir/Velpatasvir/Voxilaprevir Available in a triple-drug combination with sofosbuvir and velpatasvir, voxilaprevir is a NS3/NS4A protease inhibitor that is active against HCV genotypes 1–6. The fixed-dose combination is recommended for the re-treatment of patients with genotype 1–6 infection in whom an SVR has not been attained after previous combination DAA treatment and for the treatment of naïve genotype 3–infected patients with cirrhosis. In patients with NS5A protein inhibitor–experienced genotype 3 infection, SVR rates are lower in response to sofosbuvir/velpatasvir/voxilaprevir; thus the addition of ribavirin is recommended in these patients. A 12-week course is recommended for most patients, including those with compensated cirrhosis. Voxilaprevir is not recommended for patients with decompensated cirrhosis (see "Protease Inhibitors and Protease Inhibitor–Containing Regimens," below) or those with significant renal impairment and a CrCl of <30 mL/min. Voxilaprevir, like other protease inhibitors, is metabolized by the CYP3A system, and the effect of voxilaprevir may be reduced in the presence of other CYP inducers.

Sofosbuvir/Daclatasvir The combination of sofosbuvir with daclatasvir—the only NS5A protein inhibitor available individually rather than coformulated with other DAAs—is approved for the treatment of HCV genotypes 1 and 3. Daclatasvir binds the N terminus of the NS5A protein, both inhibiting viral RNA replication and blocking virion assembly. It is given in combination with sofosbuvir for 12 weeks and is safe for the treatment of patients with decompensated cirrhosis. Daclatasvir is a substrate of CYP3A, and the dose should be adjusted when given with other CYP3A substrates; i.e., the dose should be reduced if daclatasvir is given with a strong CYP3A inhibitor and increased if it is given with moderate CYP3A4 inducers. Daclatasvir absorption is not affected by food, and daclatasvir is highly protein bound. The dose does not need to be adjusted for renal impairment, and side effects are uncommon.

PROTEASE INHIBITORS AND PROTEASE INHIBITOR–CONTAINING REGIMENS

Protease inhibitors are specifically designed to inhibit the HCV NS3/4A protease by mimicking the HCV polypeptide and, when bound by the viral protease, form a covalent bond with the catalytic NS3 serine residues, blocking further activity and preventing proteolytic cleavage of the HCV polyprotein into NS4A, NS4B, NS5A, and NS5B proteins. As a class, the protease inhibitors are hepatically metabolized and therefore should not be administered to patients with decompensated (Child–Turcotte–Pugh class B or C) cirrhosis. For patients receiving protease inhibitors, the current recommendation is that liver function tests should be monitored monthly.

Simeprevir Simeprevir inhibits the HCV NS3/4A protease and is active against HCV genotype 1 (subgenotype 1b > 1a) and genotype 4. About one-third of patients infected with HCV genotype 1b have a polymorphism (Q80K) in the NS3 protein that results in resistance of the virus to the drug; thus, if simeprevir is used, the infecting virus should be tested for this polymorphism. Simeprevir absorption is increased when it is taken with food. The drug is nearly all protein bound, and it is excreted through the biliary tract. Dose adjustment is not required for renal dysfunction. Simeprevir is metabolized by the CYP3A system and should not be given to patients with decompensated cirrhosis. In the past simeprevir was usually combined with sofosbuvir for 12 weeks, but with newer options this drug combination is no longer recommended as either a first- or second-line regimen.

Paritaprevir/Ritonavir/Ombitasvir/Dasabuvir The combination of paritaprevir (boosted with ritonavir), ombitasvir, and dasabuvir is a fixed-dose regimen for the treatment of HCV. Paritaprevir is an NS3/NS4A protease inhibitor with activity against genotypes 1a and 1b, 4, and 6. Paritaprevir is coformulated with the HIV protease inhibitor ritonavir, not for antiviral activity, but as a CYP3A inhibitor; ritonavir coformulation boosts paritaprevir levels, allowing once-daily dosing. Ombitasvir is an NS5A protein inhibitor with activity against genotypes 1a and 1b as well as genotypes 2, 3, and 5. Dasabuvir is a nonnucleoside polymerase inhibitor of the HCV NS5B polymerase; its allosteric inhibition of the polymerase effectively prevents the interaction of the polymerase with its binding site. The combination is approved for the treatment of HCV genotype 1b infection and can be used with the addition of ribavirin for the treatment of genotype 1a infection. Treatment duration is 12 weeks for patients without cirrhosis and 24 weeks for patients with compensated cirrhosis. The medications in the combination are metabolized by the CYP2C and CYP3A systems. The coadministration of paritaprevir with ritonavir results in clinically significant CYP3A4 interactions. Caution regarding drug interactions should be taken in the treatment of patients co-infected with HIV and HCV who are receiving antiretroviral therapy. No dose adjustment is required in renal insufficiency or end-stage renal disease requiring dialysis, but use of this drug combination is contraindicated in decompensated cirrhosis. Rarely, hepatic decompensation has been reported in patients receiving the combination, and patients should have liver function monitored monthly during this treatment.

Elbasvir/Grazoprevir The coformulation of elbasvir, an NS5A replication complex inhibitor, and grazoprevir, an NS3/NS4A protease inhibitor, is active against HCV genotypes 1 and 4. However, its efficacy in the treatment of HCV genotype 1a is reduced in the presence of baseline resistance–associated polymorphisms in the NS5A protein at positions M28, Q30, L31, and Y93; thus, in patients infected with genotype 1a, baseline resistance testing should be performed and, if the result is positive, ribavirin should be added and the combination therapy should be extended to improve response rates. Susceptibility to grazoprevir is reduced with NS5A protein D168 substitutions, but few resistant isolates have been noted in cases of virologic failure; thus, testing for these substitutions before therapy is not recommended. Treatment duration is 12 weeks (genotype 1b or genotype 1a without baseline resistance–associated polymorphisms) or 16 weeks (in combination with ribavirin in patients with baseline NS5A protein polymorphisms and in genotype 4–infected patients with previous IFN exposure). Absorption of grazoprevir and elbasvir is unaffected by food, and the dose does not need to be adjusted in patients with chronic kidney disease or those who are undergoing dialysis. Elbasvir, like grazoprevir, is a substrate of the CYP3A system; coadministration with moderate or strong CYP3A inducers or with strong inhibitors is not recommended. Both components are well tolerated, and few side effects have been reported. The use of this drug combination, as with all those containing protease inhibitors, is contraindicated in decompensated cirrhosis.

Glecaprevir/Pibrentasvir The newest approved DAA-combination treatment consists of glecaprevir, a pangenotypic NS3/NS4A protease inhibitor, and pibrentasvir, a pangenotypic NS5A protein inhibitor. Each medication individually has a high genetic barrier to resistance and is active against HCV genotypes 1–6. In patients infected with genotypes other than genotype 3, baseline resistance has no influence on glecaprevir treatment efficacy, and NS3/NS4A baseline polymorphisms have not been noted to correlate with virologic failure. Treatment duration varies with fibrosis and treatment experience: an 8-week course of therapy is recommended for treatment-naïve patients who are infected with any genotype and have any degree of fibrosis up to compensated cirrhosis, including patients with genotype 3 infection, while treatment-experienced cirrhotic patients should receive 12 weeks of treatment, and patients with prior NS5A protein inhibitor exposure with or without compensated cirrhosis should receive 16 weeks of therapy. The combination of glecaprevir/pibrentasvir should be taken with food. Clearance is via biliary excretion; therefore, no dose adjustment is required in end-stage renal disease. Because of the protease component, the combination of glecaprevir/pibrentasvir is not appropriate for patients with decompensated cirrhosis. Glecaprevir and pibrentasvir are only weak CYP3A inducers, but they inhibit the P glycoprotein, breast cancer resistance protein (BCRP), and organo anion transporter P1 (OATP1) drug transporters. When taken with other drugs that are substrates for these transporters, concentrations of both drugs may be increased. The combination regimen is generally well tolerated; mild headache, fatigue, diarrhea, and nausea have been reported.

RIBAVIRIN

Ribavirin, a synthetic oral triazole guanosine analogue, weakly inhibits both DNA and RNA polymerases, but its primary mechanism in HCV treatment is not well understood. It may promote infidelity of RNA viral replication, giving rise to unfit or less fit viral mutations, and also appears to stimulate IFN-response genes and modulate adaptive immune responses. The role of ribavirin in HCV therapy has changed over time. Ribavirin played an integral role in HCV treatment during the IFN era and, combined with sofosbuvir, was required as part of IFN-sparing regimens before other DAAs were available. However, adverse drug effects associated with higher doses (in heavier patients)—including hemolytic anemia, which is increased with renal failure—are frequently treatment-limiting. Other side effects include rash, myalgia, and fatigue. Ribavirin is teratogenic, and its use in women with child-bearing potential is therefore limited.

With the advent of several combination DAA-only, IFN-sparing regimens, there are often multiple ribavirin-free options for treatment. However, there are still several indications for ribavirin augmentation of combination DAA-based therapy. Most importantly, ribavirin improves the SVR rate by an average of 5% in treatment-naïve and treatment-experienced patients with genotype 1 infection, particularly that due to subgenotype 1a. The addition of ribavirin to treatment with paritaprevir/ritonavir/ombitasvir plus dasabuvir is recommended for patients with genotype 1a or 4 infection as well as for patients infected with genotype 1a who are receiving elbasvir/grazoprevir with baseline NS5A protein resistance–associated substitutions to overcome reduced susceptibility to elbasvir. Ribavirin is frequently included in regimens for re-treatment of genotype 1–infected, therapy-experienced patients with cirrhosis in order to preserve SVR rates while shortening re-treatment duration. SVR rates at 12 weeks were comparable in treatment-experienced cirrhotic patients receiving 24 weeks of ledipasvir/sofosbuvir and those receiving 12 weeks of ledipasvir/sofosbuvir plus ribavirin. Ribavirin also improves outcomes in treatment-experienced patients with genotype 3 infection—an ongoing therapeutic challenge even in the setting of current pangenotypic regimens. Ribavirin improves treatment response in other clinical settings as well, specifically in patients with decompensated cirrhosis for whose treatment protease inhibitors cannot be used and in patients with genotype 2 infection in resource-limited settings where ribavirin is more affordable than fixed-dose combination DAA regimens. Because of its broad antiviral effects, ribavirin is not known to select for any particular resistance-associated amino acid substitutions.

Absorption of ribavirin is improved by administration with food, and the drug is excreted renally. Lowering the dose of the drug may reduce toxicity. While determining red blood cell counts and hemoglobin levels after 2 weeks of therapy is recommended to monitor for hemolytic anemia, ribavirin can be administered safely to most patients for the relatively short period of DAA-based therapy. In patients with renal insufficiency and those with end-stage renal disease who are undergoing dialysis, the dose must be adjusted and the patient closely monitored for anemia.

In a recent large-scale study, ribavirin was effective in the treatment of chronic infection with hepatitis E virus, which can cause chronic inflammatory hepatitis in immunosuppressed patients, particularly solid-organ transplant recipients.

■ INTERFERON

Pegylated interferon combined with ribavirin is no longer used for the treatment of hepatitis C, as response rates are inferior and treatment is less well tolerated than with DAAs.

■ FURTHER READING

Acosta E et al: Advances in the development of therapeutics for cytomegalovirus infections. J Infect Dis 221(Suppl 1):S32, 2020.

American Association for the Study of Liver Diseases/Infectious Diseases Society of America: Recommendations for testing, managing, and treating hepatitis C. Available at *http://www.hcvguidelines.org*. Accessed October 18, 2020.

Chou R et al: Screening for hepatitis C virus infection in adolescents and adults: Updated evidence report and systematic review for the US Preventive Services Task Force. JAMA 323:976, 2020.

Gnann JW Jr, Whitley RJ: Genital herpes. N Engl J Med 375:666, 2016.

Ison MG et al: Early treatment with baloxavir marboxil in high-risk adolescent and adult outpatients with uncomplicated influenza (CAPSTONE-2): A randomised, placebo-controlled, phase 3 trial. Lancet Infect Dis 20:1204, 2020.

Koh C et al: Pathogenesis of and new therapies for hepatitis D. Gastroenterology 156:461, 2019.

Spyrou E et al: Hepatitis B: Current status of therapy and future therapies. Gastroenterol Clin North Am 2020;49:215, 2020.

Tang LE et al: Chronic hepatitis B infection: A review. JAMA 319:1802, 2018.

Uyeki T et al: Clinical practice guidelines by the Infectious Diseases Society of America: 2018 update on diagnosis, treatment, chemoprophylaxis, and institutional outbreak management of seasonal influenza. Clin Infect Dis 68:e1, 2019.

Venkatesan S et al: Neuraminidase inhibitors and hospital length of stay: A meta-analysis of individual participant data to determine treatment effectiveness among patients hospitalized with nonfatal 2009 pandemic influenza A (H1N1) virus infection. J Infect Dis 221:356, 2020.

Section 12 Infections Due to DNA Viruses

192 Herpes Simplex Virus Infections

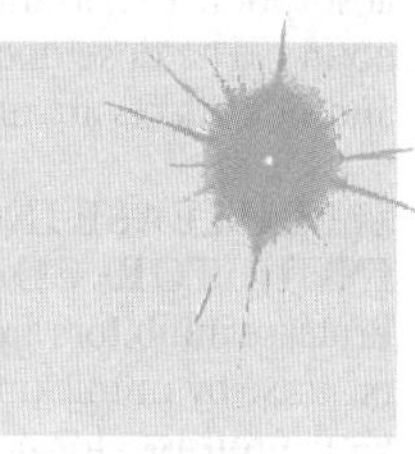

Lawrence Corey

■ DEFINITION

Herpes simplex viruses (HSV-1, HSV-2; *Herpesvirus hominis*) produce a variety of infections involving mucocutaneous surfaces, the peripheral nervous system (PNS), the central nervous system (CNS), and—on occasion—visceral organs. Prompt recognition and treatment reduce the morbidity and mortality rates associated with HSV infections.

■ ETIOLOGIC AGENT

The genome of HSV is a 152-kb linear, double-stranded DNA molecule (molecular weight, ~100 × 10^6) that encodes >90 transcription units with 84 identified proteins. The genomic structures of the two HSV subtypes are similar. The overall genomic sequence homology between HSV-1 and HSV-2 is ~50%, whereas the proteome homology is >80%. The homologous sequences are distributed over the entire genome map, and most of the polypeptides specified by one viral type are antigenically related to polypeptides of the other viral type. Many type-specific regions unique to HSV-1 and HSV-2 proteins do exist, and a number of them appear to be important in host immunity. These type-specific regions have been used to develop serologic assays that distinguish between the two viral subtypes. Either restriction endonuclease analysis or sequencing of viral DNA can be used to distinguish between the two subtypes and among strains of each subtype. Recombinant viruses (HSV-1/HSV-2) do circulate in nature. The variability of nucleotide sequences from clinical strains of HSV-1 and HSV-2 is such that HSV isolates obtained from two individuals can be differentiated by restriction enzyme patterns or genomic sequences. Moreover, epidemiologically related sources, such as sexual partners, mother–infant pairs, or persons involved in a common-source outbreak, can be inferred from such patterns. Deep sequencing of sequential isolates suggests that more than one variant of HSV-1 or HSV-2 can be found in a single individual.

The viral genome is packaged in a regular icosahedral protein shell (capsid) composed of 162 capsomeres (**Chap. 190**). The outer covering of the virus is a lipid-containing membrane (envelope) acquired as the DNA-containing capsid buds through the inner nuclear membrane of the host cell. Between the capsid and lipid bilayer of the envelope is the tegument. Viral replication has both nuclear and cytoplasmic phases. Initial attachment to the cell membrane involves interactions of viral glycoproteins C and B with several cellular heparan sulfate–like surface receptors. Subsequently, viral glycoprotein D binds to cellular co-receptors that belong to the tumor necrosis factor receptor family of proteins, the immunoglobulin superfamily (nectin family), or both. The ubiquity of these receptors contributes to the wide host range of herpesviruses. HSV replication is highly regulated. After fusion and entry, the nucleocapsid enters the cytoplasm and several viral proteins are released from the virion. Some of these viral proteins shut off host protein synthesis (by increasing cellular RNA degradation), whereas others "turn on" the transcription of immediate early genes of HSV replication. These immediate early gene products, designated *α genes*, are required for synthesis of the subsequent polypeptide group: the β polypeptides, many of which are regulatory proteins and enzymes required for DNA replication. Most current antiviral drugs interfere with β proteins, such as viral thymidine kinase (TK) and DNA polymerase. The third (γ) class of HSV genes encodes viral structural and tegument proteins and mostly requires viral DNA replication for expression. New antiviral drugs directed at viral assembly and release are under development.

After viral genome replication and structural protein synthesis, nucleocapsids are assembled in the cell's nucleus. Envelopment occurs as the nucleocapsids bud through the inner nuclear membrane into the perinuclear space. In some cells, viral replication in the nucleus forms two types of inclusion bodies: type A basophilic Feulgen-positive bodies that contain viral DNA and eosinophilic inclusion bodies that are devoid of viral nucleic acid or protein and represent a "scar" of viral infection. Enveloped virions are then transported via the endoplasmic reticulum and the Golgi apparatus to the cell surface.

Viral genomes are maintained by some neuronal cells in a repressed state called *latency*. Latency, which is associated with transcription of only a limited number of virus-encoded RNAs, accounts for the presence of viral DNA and RNA in neural tissue at times when infectious virus cannot be isolated. Maintenance and growth of neural cells from latently infected ganglia in tissue culture result in production of infectious virions (*explantation*) and in subsequent permissive infection of susceptible cells (*co-cultivation*). Activation of the viral genome may then occur, resulting in *reactivation*—the normal pattern of regulated viral gene expression and replication and HSV release. The release of virions from the neuron follows a complex process of anterograde transport down the length of neuronal axons. In experimental animals, ultraviolet light, systemic and local immunosuppression, and trauma to the skin or ganglia are associated with reactivation.

A noncoding region of the viral genome initially felt to be three noncoding regions and now felt to be a more diverse set of noncoding RNAs and micro-RNAs (miRNAs) collectively referred to as the latency-associated transcripts (LATs) is found in the nuclei of latently infected neurons, and deletion mutants of the LAT region exhibit reduced efficiency in their later reactivation. HSV DNA copy number is highly variable between neurons, with no direct correlation between HSV DNA copy numbers and LAT positivity. Substitution of HSV-1 LATs for HSV-2 LATs induces an HSV-1 reactivation pattern, suggesting this region of the genome apparently maintains—rather than establishes—latency. Viral miRNA appears to silence expression of the key neurovirulence factor infected-cell protein 34.5 (ICP34.5) and to bind in an antisense configuration to the immediate-early protein ICP0 messenger RNA to prevent expression, which is vital to HSV reactivation. While certain viral transcripts are known to be necessary for reactivation from latency, the molecular mechanisms of HSV latency are not fully understood, and strategies to interrupt or maintain latency in neurons are in developmental stages.

While latency is the predominant state of virus on a per-neuron basis, the high frequency of oral and genital tract reactivation for HSV-1 and HSV-2 suggests that the viruses are rarely quiescent within the entire biomass of ganglionic tissue. The virus appears to be in a dynamic state—"mostly suppressed"—but with continual individual cells showing various degrees of viral transcriptional activity, and only a few of these infected neurons giving rise to actual reactivation. There is increasing recognition that HSV infection of the autonomic ganglia plays an important role in both initial and reactivation infections. In fact, deaths of animals from HSV-2 infection appear to be related to autonomic dysfunction of the bowel. Both HSV-1 and HSV-2 are shed subclinically. Most persons infected with HSV-2 and HSV-1 have frequent subclinical bursts of reactivation lasting 2–6 h, and the host tissue-based immune system can contain viral reactivation in the tissue before the development of clinical reactivation.

PATHOGENESIS

Exposure to HSV at mucosal surfaces or abraded skin sites permits entry of the virus into cells of the epidermis and dermis and initiation of viral replication therein. HSV infections are usually acquired subclinically. Whether clinical or subclinical, HSV acquisition is associated with sufficient viral replication to permit infection of sensory and/or autonomic nerve endings. On entry into the neuronal cell, the virus—or, more likely, the nucleocapsid—is transported intra-axonally to the nerve cell bodies in ganglia. Viral particles tether onto cellular proteins that motor along microtubules from axon tips (neurite endings) to neuronal cell bodies. In humans, the transit interval of spread to the ganglia after virus inoculation into peripheral tissue is unknown. During the initial phase of infection, viral replication occurs in ganglia and contiguous neural tissue. Virus then spreads to other mucocutaneous surfaces through centrifugal migration of infectious virions via peripheral nerves. This mode of spread helps explain the large surface area involved, the high frequency of new lesions distant from the initial crop of vesicles that is characteristic in patients with primary genital or oral–labial HSV infection, and the ability to recover virus from neural tissue distant from neurons innervating the inoculation site. Contiguous spread of locally inoculated virus also may take place and allow further mucosal extension of disease. Recent studies have demonstrated HSV viremia—another mechanism for extension of infection throughout the body—in ~30–40% of persons with primary HSV-2 infection; latent infection with both viral subtypes in both sensory and autonomic ganglia has been demonstrated. For HSV-1 infection, trigeminal ganglia are most commonly infected, although extension to the inferior and superior cervical ganglia also occurs. With genital infection, sacral nerve root ganglia (S2–S5) are most commonly affected. Autonomic ganglia, pelvic nerves, and vaginal nerve roots are commonly infected.

After resolution of primary disease, infectious HSV can no longer be cultured from the ganglia; however, neuronal infection, as defined by the presence of viral DNA, persists in ganglionic cells in the anatomic regions of the initial infection. The mechanism of reactivation from latency is unknown, although increasingly evidence of limited viral genes or miRNAs is identified in latently infected neurons. Evidence exists for viral antigen and activated host T cells at the ganglia and periphery, and immune responses in ganglia as well as peripheral tissue appear to influence the frequency and severity of HSV reactivation. HSV-specific T cells have been recovered from peripheral nerve root ganglia. Many of these resident CD8+ T cells are juxtaposed with latently HSV-1-infected neurons in the trigeminal ganglia and can block reactivation with both interferon (IFN) γ release and granzyme B–mediated degradation of the immediate-early protein ICP4. In addition, there appears to be a latent viral load in the ganglia that correlates positively with the number of neurons infected and the rate of reactivation but inversely with the number of T cells present. It is not known whether reactivating stimuli transiently suppress these immune cells, independently upregulate transcription of lytic genes, or both. Moreover, host containment in the mucosa has been demonstrated. Once virus reaches the dermal–epidermal junction, there are three possible outcomes: (1) rapid host containment of infection near the site of reactivation; (2) spread of small amounts of virus into the epidermis, with a micro-ulceration associated with low-titer subclinical shedding; and (3) widespread replication and necrosis of epithelial cells and subsequent clinical recurrence (the latter defined clinically by a skin blister and ulceration). Histologically, herpetic lesions involve a thin-walled vesicle or ulceration in the basal region, multinucleated cells that may include intranuclear inclusions, necrosis, and an acute inflammatory response. Re-epithelialization occurs once viral replication is restricted, almost always in the absence of a scar.

Analysis of the DNA from sequential isolates of HSV or from isolates from multiple infected ganglia in any one individual has revealed similar, if not identical, restriction endonuclease or DNA sequence patterns in most persons. As more sensitive genomic technologies are developed, evidence of multiple strains of the same subtype is increasingly being reported. For example, infection of individual neurons with multiple strains of drug-susceptible and drug-resistant virus in severely immunosuppressed patients indicates that ganglia can be reseeded during chronic infection. Because exposure to mucosal shedding is relatively common during a person's lifetime, current data suggest that exogenous infection with different strains of the same subtype does occur. The role strain variation plays in the varied reactivation pattern of disease is unknown.

IMMUNITY

Host responses influence the acquisition of HSV disease, the severity of infection, resistance to the development of latency, the maintenance of latency, and the frequency of recurrences. Both antibody-mediated and cell-mediated reactions are clinically important. Immunocompromised patients with defects in cell-mediated immunity experience more severe and more extensive HSV infections than those with deficits in humoral immunity, such as agammaglobulinemia. Experimental ablation of lymphocytes indicates that T cells play a major role in preventing lethal disseminated disease, although antibodies help reduce titers of virus in neural tissue. Some clinical manifestations of HSV appear to be related to the host immune response (e.g., stromal opacities associated with recurrent herpetic keratitis). The surface viral glycoproteins have been shown to be targets of antibodies that mediate neutralization and immune-mediated cytolysis (antibody-dependent cell-mediated cytotoxicity [ADCC]). Monoclonal antibodies to HSV viral glycoproteins have, in experimental infections, conferred protection against subsequent neurologic disease or ganglionic latency, and controlled studies in humans of monoclonal antibodies on disease reactivation are not available. Multiple cell populations, including neutrophils, macrophages, and a variety of T lymphocytes, play a role in host defenses against HSV infections, as do lymphokines generated by T lymphocytes. In animals, passive transfer of primed lymphocytes confers protection from subsequent HSV challenge. Maximal protection usually requires the activation of multiple T-cell subpopulations, including cytotoxic T cells and T cells responsible for delayed hypersensitivity. The latter may confer protection by the antigen-stimulated release of lymphokines (e.g., IFNs), which in turn have a direct antiviral effect and both activate and enhance a variety of specific and nonspecific effector cells. The HSV virion contains a variety of genes that are directed at the inhibition of host responses. These include gene *ICP47*, which can bind to the cellular transporter-activating protein TAP-1 and reduce the ability of this protein to bind HSV peptides to human leukocyte antigen class I, thereby reducing recognition of viral proteins by cytotoxic T cells of the host. This effect can be overcome by the addition of IFN-γ, but this reversal requires 24–48 h; thus, the virus has time to replicate and invade other host cells. Entry of infectious HSV-1 and HSV-2 inhibits several signaling pathways of both CD4+ and CD8+ T cells, leading to their functional impairment in killing and influencing the spectrum of their cytokine secretion. Therapeutic vaccination with a replication-defective HSV lacking gD, the major neutralizing protein, produced enhanced ADCC activity and subsequent reduction in reactivation in the guinea pig model of HSV-2, suggesting that immune responses to cell-associated virus may play an important role in disease resolution.

HSV-specific CD8+ T-cell responses appear to be an important component in viral clearance from lesions. Immunosuppressed patients with frequent and prolonged HSV lesions have fewer functional CD8+ T cells directed at HSV. HSV-specific CD8+ T cells have been shown to persist in the genital skin at the dermal–epidermal junction contiguous to nerve endings for months after lesion resolution. Even during clinical quiescence, these CD8+ T cells make both antiviral and cytotoxic proteins indicative of immune surveillance. These resident memory CD8+ T cells appear to be "first responders" capable of controlling viral reactivation at the site of viral release into the dermis. This rapid "on and off" interplay between the virus and the host helps explain the variability in clinical disease severity between episodes in any single individual. Differences of 30–60 min in host responses can result in 100- to 1000-fold differences in viral levels and can determine whether an episode of disease is subclinical or clinical.

There is a strong association between the magnitude of the CD8+ T-lymphocyte response and the clearance of virus from genital lesions. The location, effectiveness, and longevity of the CD8+ T lymphocytes (and other influencers of immune effector functions such as natural killer or CD4+ T-cell responses) may be important in the expression of disease and the likelihood of transmission over time.

EPIDEMIOLOGY

Seroepidemiologic studies have documented HSV infections worldwide. The past 15 years have shown that the prevalence of HSV-2 is even higher in the developing than in the developed world. In sub-Saharan Africa, HSV-2 seroprevalence among pregnant women may approach 60%, and annual acquisition rates among teenage girls may verge on 20%. The global incidence has been estimated at ~23.6 million infections per year, with >490 million infected persons worldwide. As in the developed world, the rate of HSV-2 coital acquisition as well as the serologic prevalence are higher among women than among men. Most of this HSV-2 acquisition is preceded by acquisition of HSV-1; the frequency of genital HSV-1 in middle- and low-income countries is low at present.

Infection with HSV-1 is acquired more frequently and earlier in life than infection with HSV-2. From 70 to 90% of adults have antibodies to HSV-1 by the fifth decade of life. In populations of low socioeconomic status, most persons acquire HSV-1 infection before the third decade of life. Antibodies to HSV-2 are not detected routinely until puberty. Antibody prevalence rates correlate with past sexual activity and vary greatly among different population groups. There is evidence that the prevalence of HSV-2 has decreased slightly over the past decade or so in the United States. Serosurveys indicate that 15–20% of the U.S. population has antibodies to HSV-2. In most routine obstetric and family planning clinics, 15 to 30% of women have HSV-2 antibodies, although only 10% of those who are seropositive for HSV-2 report a history of genital lesions. As many as 50% of heterosexual adults attending sexually transmitted disease clinics have antibodies to HSV-2. A wide variety of serologic surveys has catalogued the widespread epidemic of HSV-2 in Central America, South America, and Africa. In Africa, HSV-2 seroprevalence has ranged from 40 to 70% in obstetric and other sexually experienced populations. Antibody prevalence rates average ~5–10% higher among women than among men.

Many studies continue to show that both incident and—more importantly—prevalent HSV-2 infection enhances the acquisition rate of HIV-1. More specifically, HSV-2 infection is associated on a population basis with a two- to fourfold increase in HIV-1 acquisition. This association has been amply demonstrated in heterosexual men and women in both the developed and developing worlds. Epidemiologically, regions of the world with high HSV-2 prevalence and selected populations within such regions have a higher population-based incidence of HIV-1.

An important observation is that HSV-2 facilitates the spread of HIV into low-risk populations; prevalent HSV-2 appears to increase the risk of HIV infection by seven- to ninefold on a per-coital basis. Mathematical models suggest that ~33–50% of HIV-1 infections may be attributable to HSV-2 both in men who have sex with men (MSM) and in heterosexual women in sub-Saharan Africa. In addition, HSV-2 is more frequently reactivated in and transmitted by persons co-infected with HIV-1 than in persons not co-infected. Thus, most areas of the world with a high HIV-1 prevalence also have a high HSV-2 prevalence. The shedding of HIV-1 virions from herpetic lesions in the genital region facilitates the spread of HIV through sexual contact. HSV-2 reactivation is associated with a localized persistent inflammatory response consisting of high concentrations of CCR5-enriched CD4+ T cells as well as inflammatory dendritic cells in the submucosa of the genital skin. These cells can support HIV infection and replication and thus are likely to account for the increased risk of HIV acquisition among persons with genital herpes. Unfortunately, antiviral therapy does not reduce this subclinical postreactivation inflammation, probably because of the inability of current antiviral agents to prevent the release of small amounts of HSV antigen into the genital mucosa.

Several studies suggest that many cases of "asymptomatic" genital HSV-2 infection are, in fact, simply unrecognized or confined to anatomic regions of the genital tract that are not easily visualized. Asymptomatic seropositive persons shed virus on mucosal surfaces almost as frequently as do those with symptomatic disease. This large reservoir of unidentified carriers of HSV-2 and the frequent asymptomatic reactivation of the virus from the genital tract have fostered the continued spread of genital herpes throughout the world.

HSV infections occur throughout the year. Transmission can result from contact with persons who have active ulcerative lesions or with persons who have no clinical manifestations of infection but who are shedding HSV from mucocutaneous surfaces. HSV reactivation on genital skin and mucosal surfaces is common. In fact, recent studies indicate that most HSV-1 and HSV-2 episodes last 2–6 h; thus, replication of the virus and clearance by the host are rapid. Even with once-daily sampling, HSV DNA can be detected on 20–30% of days by polymerase chain reaction (PCR). Corresponding figures for HSV-1 in oral secretions are similar. Rates of shedding are highest during the initial years after acquisition, with viral shedding occurring on as many as 30–50% of days during this period. Immunosuppressed patients shed HSV from mucosal sites at an even higher frequency (20–80% of days). These high rates of mucocutaneous reactivation suggest that exposure to HSV from sexual or other close contact (kissing, sharing of glasses or silverware) is common and help explain the continuing spread and high seroprevalence of HSV infections worldwide. Reactivation rates vary widely among individuals. Among HIV-positive patients, a low CD4+ T-cell count and a high HIV-1 load are associated with increased rates of HSV reactivation. Daily antiviral chemotherapy for HSV-2 infection can reduce shedding rates but does not eliminate shedding, as measured by PCR or culture.

CLINICAL SPECTRUM

HSV has been isolated from nearly all visceral and mucocutaneous sites. The clinical manifestations and course of HSV infection depend on the anatomic site involved, the age and immune status of the host, and the antigenic type of the virus. Primary HSV infections (i.e., first infections with either HSV-1 or HSV-2 in which the host lacks HSV antibodies in acute-phase serum) are frequently accompanied by systemic signs and symptoms. Compared with recurrent episodes, primary infections, which involve both mucosal and extramucosal sites, are characterized by a longer duration of symptoms and virus isolation from lesions. The incubation period ranges from 1 to 26 days (median, 6–8 days). Both viral subtypes can cause genital and oral–facial infections, and the infections caused by the two subtypes are clinically indistinguishable. However, the frequency of reactivation of infection is influenced by anatomic site and virus type. Genital HSV-2 infection is twice as likely to reactivate and recurs 8–10 times more frequently than genital HSV-1 infection. Conversely, oral–labial HSV-1 infection recurs more frequently than oral–labial HSV-2 infection. Asymptomatic shedding rates follow the same pattern.

Oral–Facial Infections Gingivostomatitis and pharyngitis are the most common clinical manifestations of first-episode HSV-1 infection, whereas recurrent herpes labialis is the most common clinical manifestation of reactivation HSV-1 infection. HSV pharyngitis and gingivostomatitis usually result from primary infection and are most common among children and young adults. Clinical symptoms and signs, which include fever, malaise, myalgias, inability to eat, irritability, and cervical adenopathy, may last 3–14 days. Lesions may involve the hard and soft palate, gingiva, tongue, lip, and facial area. HSV-1 or HSV-2 infection of the pharynx usually results in exudative or ulcerative lesions of the posterior pharynx and/or tonsillar pillars. Lesions of the tongue, buccal mucosa, or gingiva may occur later in the course in one-third of cases. Fever lasting 2–7 days and cervical adenopathy are common. It can be difficult to differentiate HSV pharyngitis clinically from bacterial pharyngitis, *Mycoplasma pneumoniae* infections, and pharyngeal ulcerations of noninfectious etiologies (e.g., Stevens-Johnson syndrome). No substantial evidence suggests that reactivation of oral–labial HSV infection is associated with symptomatic recurrent pharyngitis.

Reactivation of HSV from the trigeminal ganglia may be associated with asymptomatic virus excretion in the saliva, development of intraoral mucosal ulcerations, or herpetic ulcerations on the vermilion border of the lip or external facial skin. About 50–70% of seropositive patients undergoing trigeminal nerve-root decompression and 10–15% of those undergoing dental extraction develop oral–labial HSV infection a median of 3 days after these procedures. Clinical differentiation of intraoral mucosal ulcerations due to HSV from aphthous, traumatic, or drug-induced ulcerations is difficult.

In immunosuppressed patients, HSV infection may extend into mucosal and deep cutaneous layers. Friability, necrosis, bleeding, severe pain, and inability to eat or drink may result. The lesions of HSV mucositis are clinically similar to mucosal lesions caused by cytotoxic drug therapy, trauma, or fungal or bacterial infections. Persistent ulcerative HSV infections are among the most common infections in patients with AIDS. HSV and *Candida* infections often occur concurrently. Systemic antiviral therapy speeds the rate of healing and relieves the pain of mucosal HSV infections in immunosuppressed patients. The frequency of HSV reactivation during the early phases of transplantation or induction chemotherapy is high (50–90%), and prophylactic systemic antiviral agents such as intravenous (IV) acyclovir and penciclovir or the oral congeners of these drugs are used to reduce reactivation rates. Patients with atopic eczema may also develop severe oral–facial HSV infections (*eczema herpeticum*), which may rapidly involve extensive areas of skin and occasionally disseminate to visceral organs. Extensive eczema herpeticum has resolved promptly with the administration of IV acyclovir. Erythema multiforme may also be associated with HSV infections (**see Figs. 56-9 and A1-24**); some evidence suggests that HSV infection is the precipitating event in ~75% of cases of cutaneous erythema multiforme. HSV antigen has been demonstrated both in circulatory immune complexes and in skin lesion biopsy samples from these cases. Patients with severe HSV-associated erythema multiforme are candidates for chronic suppressive oral antiviral therapy.

HSV-1 and varicella-zoster virus (VZV) have been implicated in the etiology of Bell's palsy (flaccid paralysis of the mandibular portion of the facial nerve). Some but not all trials have documented quicker resolution of facial paralysis with the prompt initiation of antiviral therapy, with or without glucocorticoids. However, other trials have shown little benefit. There are advantages to the use of both antiviral drugs and glucocorticoids for moderate to severe Bell's palsy. Some experts feel glucocorticoids alone are preferred for mild disease.

Genital Infections First-episode primary genital herpes is characterized by fever, headache, malaise, and myalgias. Pain, itching, dysuria, vaginal and urethral discharge, and tender inguinal lymphadenopathy are the predominant local symptoms. Widely spaced bilateral lesions of the external genitalia are characteristic (**Fig. 192-1**). Lesions may be present in varying stages, including vesicles, pustules, or painful erythematous ulcers. The cervix and urethra are involved in >80% of women with first-episode infections. First episodes of genital herpes in patients who have had prior HSV-1 infection are occasionally associated with systemic symptoms: prior HSV-1 infection is associated with faster healing than true primary genital herpes. Detection of HSV DNA in serum has been found in ~30% of cases of true primary genital herpes.

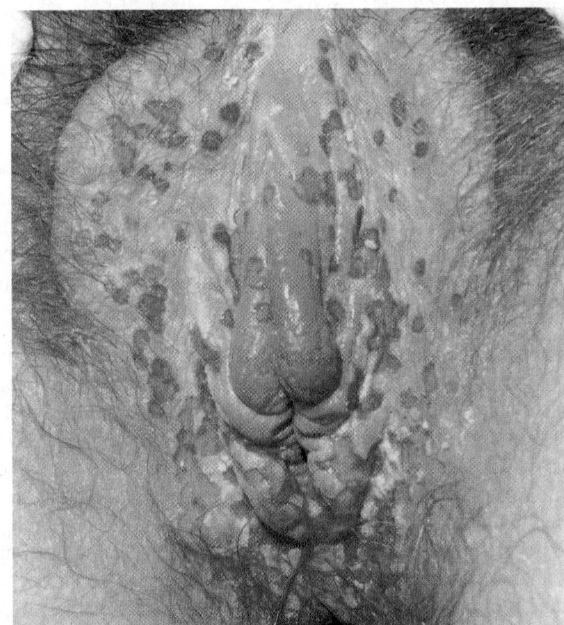

FIGURE 192-1 Genital herpes: primary vulvar infection, with multiple, extremely painful, punched-out, confluent, shallow ulcers on the edematous vulva and perineum. Micturition is often very painful. Associated inguinal lymphadenopathy is common. *(Reprinted with permission from K Wolff et al: Fitzpatrick's Color Atlas & Synopsis of Clinical Dermatology, 5th ed. New York, McGraw-Hill, 2005.)*

The clinical courses of acute first-episode genital herpes are similar for HSV-1 and HSV-2 infection. However, the recurrence rates of genital disease differ with the viral subtype: the 12-month recurrence rates among patients with first-episode HSV-2 and HSV-1 infections are ~90% and ~55%, respectively (median number of recurrences, 4 and <1, respectively). Recurrence rates for genital HSV-2 infections vary greatly among individuals and over time within the same individual. HSV has been isolated from the urethra and urine of men and women without external genital lesions. A clear mucoid discharge and dysuria are characteristics of symptomatic HSV urethritis. HSV has been isolated from the urethra of 5% of women with the dysuria–frequency syndrome. Occasionally, HSV genital tract disease is manifested by endometritis and salpingitis in women and by prostatitis in men. About 15% of cases of HSV-2 acquisition are associated with nonlesional clinical syndromes, such as aseptic meningitis, cervicitis, or urethritis. A more complete discussion of the differential diagnosis of genital herpes is presented in **Chap. 136**.

Both HSV-1 and HSV-2 can cause symptomatic or asymptomatic rectal and perianal infections. HSV proctitis is usually associated with rectal intercourse. However, subclinical perianal shedding of HSV is detected in women and men who report no rectal intercourse. This phenomenon is due to the establishment of latency in the sacral dermatome from prior genital tract infection, with subsequent reactivation in epithelial cells in the perianal region. Such reactivations are often subclinical. Symptoms of HSV proctitis include anorectal pain, anorectal discharge, tenesmus, and constipation. Sigmoidoscopy reveals ulcerative lesions of the distal 10 cm of the rectal mucosa. Rectal biopsies show mucosal ulceration, necrosis, polymorphonuclear and lymphocytic infiltration of the lamina propria, and (in occasional cases) multinucleated intranuclear inclusion-bearing cells. Perianal herpetic lesions are also found in immunosuppressed patients receiving cytotoxic therapy. Extensive perianal herpetic lesions and/or HSV proctitis is common among patients with HIV infection.

Herpetic Whitlow Herpetic whitlow—HSV infection of the finger—may occur as a complication of primary oral or genital herpes by inoculation of virus through a break in the epidermal surface or by direct introduction of virus into the hand through occupational or some other type of exposure. Clinical signs and symptoms include abrupt-onset edema, erythema, and localized tenderness of the infected finger. Vesicular or pustular lesions of the fingertip that are indistinguishable from lesions of pyogenic bacterial infection are seen. Fever, lymphadenitis, and epitrochlear and axillary lymphadenopathy are common. The infection may recur. Prompt diagnosis (to avoid unnecessary and potentially exacerbating surgical therapy and/or transmission) is essential. Antiviral therapy is usually recommended (see below).

Herpes Gladiatorum HSV may infect almost any area of skin. Mucocutaneous HSV infections of the thorax, ears, face, and hands have been described among wrestlers. Transmission of these infections is facilitated by trauma to the skin sustained during wrestling. Several recent outbreaks have illustrated the importance of prompt diagnosis and therapy to contain the spread of this infection.

Eye Infections HSV infection of the eye is the most common cause of corneal blindness in the United States. HSV keratitis presents as an acute onset of pain, blurred vision, chemosis, conjunctivitis, and characteristic dendritic lesions of the cornea. Use of topical glucocorticoids may exacerbate symptoms and lead to involvement of deep structures of the eye. Debridement, topical antiviral treatment, and/or IFN therapy hastens healing. However, recurrences are common, and the deeper structures of the eye may sustain immunopathologic injury. Stromal keratitis due to HSV appears to be related to T-cell–dependent destruction of deep corneal tissue. An HSV-1 epitope that is autoreactive with T cell–targeting corneal antigens has been postulated to be a factor in this infection. Chorioretinitis, usually a manifestation of disseminated HSV infection, may occur in neonates or in patients with HIV infection. HSV and VZV can cause acute necrotizing retinitis as an uncommon but severe manifestation. While VZV infection is the most common cause of acute retinal necropsy, both HSV-1 and HSV-2 may also be associated with this syndrome. Emergent ophthalmology consultation is recommended; both systemic and intravitical antiviral therapy is recommended.

Central and Peripheral Nervous System Infections HSV accounts for 10–20% of all cases of sporadic viral encephalitis in the United States. The estimated incidence is ~2.3 cases per 1 million persons per year. Cases are distributed throughout the year, and the age distribution appears to be biphasic, with peaks at 5–30 and >50 years of age. HSV-1 causes >95% of cases.

The pathogenesis of HSV encephalitis varies. In children and young adults, primary HSV infection may result in encephalitis; presumably, exogenously acquired virus enters the CNS by neurotropic spread from the periphery via the olfactory bulb. However, most adults with HSV encephalitis have clinical or serologic evidence of mucocutaneous HSV-1 infection before the onset of CNS symptoms. In ~25% of the cases examined, the HSV-1 strains from the oropharynx and brain tissue of the same patient differ; thus, some cases may result from reinfection with another strain of HSV-1 that reaches the CNS. Two theories have been proposed to explain the development of actively replicating HSV in localized areas of the CNS in persons whose ganglionic and CNS isolates are similar. Reactivation of latent HSV-1 infection in trigeminal or autonomic nerve roots may be associated with extension of virus into the CNS via nerves innervating the middle cranial fossa. HSV DNA has been demonstrated by DNA hybridization in brain tissue obtained at autopsy—even from healthy adults. Thus, reactivation of long-standing latent CNS infection may be another mechanism for the development of HSV encephalitis. Recent studies have identified genetic polymorphisms among families with a high frequency of HSV encephalitis. Peripheral-blood mononuclear cells, fibroblasts, and neurons from these patients (predominantly children) appear to secrete reduced levels of IFN in response to HSV. Genetic mutations in *TLR3* documented in patients with HSV encephalitis suggest that some cases of sporadic HSV encephalitis may be related to host genetic determinants.

The clinical hallmark of HSV encephalitis has been the acute onset of fever and focal neurologic symptoms and signs, especially in the temporal lobe (**Fig. 192-2**). Clinical differentiation of HSV encephalitis from other viral encephalitides, focal infections, or noninfectious processes is difficult. Elevated cerebrospinal fluid (CSF) protein levels, leukocytosis (predominantly lymphocytes), and red blood cell counts due to hemorrhagic necrosis are common. While brain biopsy has been the gold standard for defining HSV encephalitis, a highly sensitive and specific PCR for detection of HSV DNA in CSF has largely replaced biopsy for defining CNS infection. Although titers of antibody to HSV in CSF and serum increase in most cases of HSV encephalitis, they rarely do so earlier than 10 days into the illness and, therefore, although useful in retrospect, generally are not helpful in establishing an early clinical diagnosis. In rare cases, demonstration of HSV antigen, HSV DNA, or HSV replication in brain tissue obtained by biopsy is highly sensitive; examination of such tissue also provides the opportunity to identify alternative, potentially treatable causes of encephalitis. Antiviral therapy with acyclovir reduces the rate of death from HSV encephalitis. Most authorities recommend the administration of IV acyclovir to patients with presumed HSV encephalitis until the diagnosis is confirmed or an alternative diagnosis is made. All confirmed cases should be treated with IV acyclovir (30 mg/kg per day in three divided doses for 14–21 days). After the completion of therapy, the clinical recurrence of encephalitis requiring more treatment has been reported. For this reason, some authorities prefer to treat initially for 21 days, and many continue therapy until HSV DNA has been eliminated from the CSF. Even with therapy, neurologic sequelae are common, especially among persons >50 years of age.

HSV DNA has been detected in CSF from 3 to 15% of persons presenting to the hospital with aseptic meningitis. HSV meningitis, which is usually seen in association with primary genital HSV infection, is an acute, self-limited disease manifested by headache, fever, and mild photophobia and lasting 2–7 days. Lymphocytic pleocytosis in the

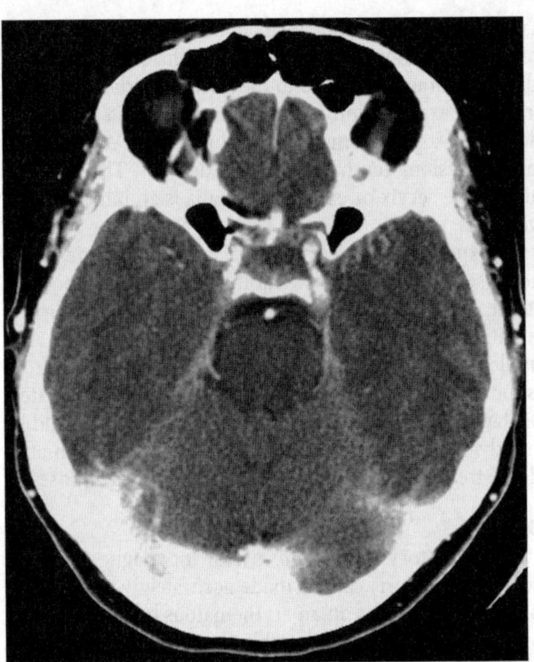

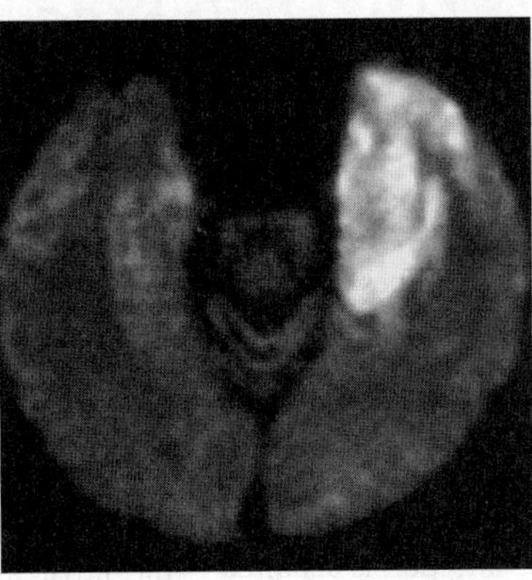

FIGURE 192-2 **Computed tomography and diffusion-weighted magnetic resonance imaging scans** of the brain of a patient with left-temporal-lobe herpes simplex virus encephalitis.

CSF is characteristic. Neurologic sequelae of HSV meningitis are rare. HSV is the most commonly identified cause of recurrent lymphocytic meningitis (*Mollaret's meningitis*). Demonstration of HSV antibodies in CSF or persistence of HSV DNA in CSF can establish the diagnosis. For persons with frequent recurrences of HSV meningitis, daily antiviral therapy has reduced the frequency of recurrent episodes of symptomatic meningitis.

Autonomic nervous system dysfunction, especially of the sacral region, has been reported in association with both HSV and VZV infections. Numbness, tingling of the buttocks or perineal areas, urinary retention, constipation, CSF pleocytosis, and (in males) impotence may occur. Symptoms appear to resolve slowly over days or weeks. Occasionally, hypoesthesia and/or weakness of the lower extremities persists for many months. Transitory hypoesthesia of the area of skin innervated by the trigeminal nerve and vestibular system dysfunction (as measured by electronystagmography) are the predominant signs of disease. Rarely, transverse myelitis, manifested by a rapidly progressive symmetric paralysis of the lower extremities or Guillain-Barré syndrome, follows HSV infection. Similarly, PNS involvement (Bell's palsy) or cranial polyneuritis may be related to reactivation of HSV-1 infection.

There is increasing experimental evidence suggesting an association between herpesvirus pathogens, specifically HSV-1, and the development of sporadic Alzheimer's disease (AD). HSV-1 DNA is detected in brain tissue of patients with AD, and epidemiologically, HSV-1 antibodies are a significant risk factor for later AD onset. A wide variety of models of AD indicate that HSV-1 infection can induce neuronal death, tau phosphorylation, and intracellular expression of isoforms of amyloid precursor protein cleavage products that produce multicellular-like plaque structures associated with AD. There are no cogent data to indicate antiviral therapy would be of benefit to anyone with AD.

Visceral Infections HSV infection of visceral organs usually results from viremia, and multiple-organ involvement is common. Occasionally, however, the clinical manifestations of HSV infection involve only the esophagus, lung, or liver. HSV esophagitis may result from direct extension of oral-pharyngeal HSV infection into the esophagus or may occur de novo by reactivation and spread of HSV to the esophageal mucosa via the vagus nerve. The predominant symptoms of HSV esophagitis are odynophagia, dysphagia, substernal pain, and weight loss. Multiple oval ulcerations appear on an erythematous base with or without a patchy white pseudomembrane. The distal esophagus is most commonly involved. With extensive disease, diffuse friability may spread to the entire esophagus. Neither endoscopic nor barium examination can reliably differentiate HSV esophagitis from *Candida* esophagitis or from esophageal ulcerations due to thermal injury, radiation, or corrosives. Endoscopically obtained secretions—for cytologic examination and culture or DNA detection by PCR—provide the most useful material for diagnosis. Systemic antiviral therapy usually reduces the severity and duration of symptoms and heals esophageal ulcerations.

HSV pneumonitis is uncommon except in severely immunosuppressed patients and may result from extension of herpetic tracheobronchitis into lung parenchyma. Focal necrotizing pneumonitis usually ensues. Hematogenous dissemination of virus from sites of oral or genital mucocutaneous disease may also occur, producing bilateral interstitial pneumonitis. Bacterial, fungal, and parasitic pathogens are commonly present in HSV pneumonitis. The mortality rate from untreated HSV pneumonia in immunosuppressed patients is high (>80%). HSV has also been isolated from the lower respiratory tract of persons with acute respiratory distress syndrome and prolonged intubation. Most authorities believe that the presence of HSV in tracheal aspirates in such settings is due to reactivation of HSV in the tracheal region and localized tracheitis in persons with long-term intubation. Such patients should be evaluated for extension of HSV infection into the lung parenchyma. While retrospective reviews of HSV tracheitis in intensive care unit patients suggest benefit from antiviral therapy, well-powered controlled trials assessing the role of antiviral agents used against HSV in ventilation-associated morbidity and mortality have not been conducted. The role of lower respiratory tract HSV infection in overall rates of morbidity and mortality associated with these conditions is unclear. HSV is an uncommon cause of hepatitis in immunocompetent patients. HSV infection of the liver is associated with fever, abrupt elevations of bilirubin and serum aminotransferase levels, and leukopenia (<4000 white blood cells/μL). Disseminated intravascular coagulation may also develop.

Other reported complications of HSV infection include monarticular arthritis, adrenal necrosis, idiopathic thrombocytopenia, and glomerulonephritis. Disseminated HSV infection in immunocompetent patients is rare. In immunocompromised patients, burn patients, or malnourished individuals, HSV occasionally disseminates to other visceral organs, such as the adrenal glands, pancreas, small and large intestines, and bone marrow. Dissemination, even recurrent dissemination, is being increasingly recognized in persons with chronic lymphocytic leukemia. Rarely, primary HSV infection in pregnancy disseminates and may be associated with the death of both mother and fetus. This uncommon event is usually related to the acquisition of primary infection in the third trimester. Disseminated HSV infection is best detected by the presence of HSV DNA in plasma or blood.

Neonatal HSV Infections Of all HSV-infected populations, neonates (infants <6 weeks) have the highest frequency of visceral and/or CNS infection. Without therapy, the overall rate of death from neonatal herpes is 65%; <10% of neonates with CNS infection develop normally. Although skin lesions are the most commonly recognized features of disease, many infants do not develop lesions at all or do so only well into the course of disease. Neonatal infection is usually acquired perinatally from contact with infected genital secretions at delivery. Congenitally infected infants have been reported. Of neonatal HSV infections, 30–50% are due to HSV-1 and 50–70% to HSV-2. The risk of developing neonatal HSV infection is 10 times higher for an infant born to a mother who has recently acquired HSV than for other infants. Neonatal HSV-1 infections may also be acquired through postnatal contact with immediate family members who have symptomatic or asymptomatic oral–labial HSV-1 infection or through nosocomial transmission within the hospital. All neonates with presumed herpes should be treated with IV acyclovir and then placed on maintenance oral antiviral therapy for the first 6–12 months of life. Antiviral chemotherapy with high-dose IV acyclovir (60 mg/kg per day) has reduced the mortality rate from neonatal herpes to ~15%. However, rates of morbidity, especially among infants with HSV-2 infection involving the CNS, are still very high.

HSV in Pregnancy In the United States, 21% of all pregnant women and 51% of non-Hispanic black pregnant women are seropositive for HSV-2. However, the risk of mother-to-child transmission of HSV in the perinatal period is highest when the infection is acquired near the time of labor—that is, in previously HSV-seronegative women. The clinical manifestations of recurrent genital herpes—including the frequency of subclinical versus clinical infection, the duration of lesions, pain, and constitutional symptoms—are similar in pregnant and nonpregnant women. Recurrences increase in frequency over the course of pregnancy. However, when women are seropositive for HSV-2 at the outset of pregnancy, no effect on neonatal outcomes (including birth weight and gestational age) is seen. First-episode infections in pregnancy have more severe consequences for mother and infant. Maternal visceral dissemination during the third trimester occasionally occurs, as does premature birth or intrauterine growth retardation. The acquisition of primary disease in pregnancy, whether related to HSV-1 or HSV-2, carries the risk of transplacental transmission of virus to the neonate and can result in spontaneous abortion, although this outcome is relatively uncommon. For newly acquired genital HSV infection during pregnancy, most authorities recommend treatment with acyclovir (400 mg three times daily) or valacyclovir (500–1000 mg twice daily) for 7–10 days. However, the impact of this intervention on transmission is unknown. The high HSV-2 prevalence rate in pregnancy and the low incidence of neonatal disease (1 case per 6000–20,000 live births) indicate that only a few infants are at risk of acquiring HSV. Therefore, cesarean section is not warranted for all women with recurrent genital disease. Because intrapartum transmission of infection accounts for the majority of cases, abdominal delivery need be considered only for women who are shedding HSV at delivery. Several studies have shown no correlation between recurrence of viral shedding before delivery and viral shedding at term. Hence, weekly virologic monitoring and amniocentesis are not recommended.

The frequency of transmission from mother to infant is markedly higher among women who acquire HSV near term (30–50%) than among those in whom HSV-2 infection is reactivated at delivery (<1%). Although maternal antibody to HSV-2 is protective, antibody to HSV-1 offers little or no protection against neonatal HSV-2 infection. Primary genital infection with HSV-1 leads to a particularly high risk of transmission during pregnancy and accounts for an increasing proportion of neonatal HSV cases. Moreover, during reactivation, HSV-1 appears more transmissible to the neonate than HSV-2. Only 2% of women who are seropositive for HSV-2 have HSV-2 isolated from cervical secretions at delivery, and only 1% of infants exposed in this manner develop infection, presumably because of the protective effects of maternally transferred antibodies and perhaps lower viral titers during reactivation. Despite the low frequency of transmission of HSV in this setting, 30–50% of infants with neonatal HSV are born to mothers with established genital herpes.

Isolation of HSV by cervicovaginal swab at the time of delivery is the greatest risk factor for intrapartum HSV transmission (relative risk = 346); however, culture-negative, PCR-positive cases of intrapartum transmission are well described. New acquisition of HSV (odds ratio [OR] = 49), isolation of HSV-1 versus HSV-2 (OR = 35), cervical versus vulvar HSV detection (OR = 15), use of fetal scalp electrodes (OR = 3.5), and young maternal age confer further risk of transmission, whereas cesarean delivery is protective (OR = 0.14). Physical examination poorly predicts the absence of shedding, and PCR far exceeds culture in terms of sensitivity and speed. Therefore, PCR detection at the onset of labor should be used to aid clinical decision-making for women with HSV-2 antibody. Because cesarean section appears to be an effective means of reducing maternal–fetal transmission, patients with recurrent genital herpes should be encouraged to come to the hospital early at the time of delivery for careful examination of the external genitalia and cervix as well as collection of a swab sample for viral isolation. Women who have no evidence of lesions can have a vaginal delivery. The presence of active lesions on the cervix or external genitalia is an indication for cesarean delivery.

If first-episode exposure has occurred (e.g., if HSV serologies show that the mother is seronegative or if the mother is HSV-1-seropositive and the isolate at delivery is found to be HSV-2), many authorities would initiate antiviral therapy for the infant with IV acyclovir. At a minimum, samples for viral cultures and PCR should be obtained from the throat, nasopharynx, eyes, and rectum of these infants immediately and at 5- to 10-day intervals. Lethargy, skin lesions, or fever should be evaluated promptly. All infants from whom HSV is isolated 24 h after delivery should be treated with IV acyclovir at recommended doses.

DIAGNOSIS

Both clinical and laboratory criteria are useful for diagnosing HSV infections. A clinical diagnosis can be made accurately when characteristic multiple vesicular lesions on an erythematous base are present. However, herpetic ulcerations may resemble skin ulcerations of other etiologies. Mucosal HSV infections may also present as urethritis or pharyngitis without cutaneous lesions. Thus, laboratory studies to confirm the diagnosis and to guide therapy are recommended. While staining of scrapings from the base of the lesions with Wright's, Giemsa's (Tzanck preparation), or Papanicolaou's stain to detect giant cells or intranuclear inclusions of *Herpesvirus* infection is a well-described procedure, few clinicians are skilled in this technique, the sensitivity of staining is low (<30% for mucosal swabs), and these cytologic methods do not differentiate between HSV and VZV infections.

HSV infection is best confirmed in the laboratory by detection of virus, viral antigen, or viral DNA in scrapings from lesions. HSV DNA detection by PCR is the most sensitive laboratory technique for detecting mucosal or visceral HSV infections and is the recommended test for laboratory confirmation of a diagnosis. HSV causes a discernible cytopathic effect in a variety of cell culture systems, and this effect can be identified within 48–96 h after inoculation. Spin-amplified culture with subsequent staining for HSV antigen has shortened the time needed to identify HSV to <24 h. Culture is indicated when antiviral sensitivity testing is required. The sensitivity of all detection methods depends on the stage of the lesions (with higher sensitivity for vesicular than for ulcerative lesions), on whether the patient has a first or a recurrent episode of the disease (with higher sensitivity in first than in recurrent episodes), and on whether the sample is from an immunosuppressed or an immunocompetent patient (with more antigen or DNA in immunosuppressed patients). Laboratory confirmation permits subtyping of the virus; information on subtype may be useful epidemiologically and may help to predict the frequency of reactivation after first-episode oral–labial or genital HSV infection.

Both type-specific and type-common antibodies to HSV develop during the first several weeks after infection and persist indefinitely. Serologic assays with whole-virus antigen preparations, such as complement fixation, neutralization, indirect immunofluorescence, passive hemagglutination, radioimmunoassay, and enzyme-linked immunosorbent assay, are useful for differentiating uninfected (seronegative) persons from those with past HSV-1 or HSV-2 infection, but they do not reliably distinguish between the two viral subtypes. Serologic assays that identify antibodies to the type-specific glycoprotein G of the two viral subtypes (G1 and G2) are available commercially and can distinguish reliably between the human antibody responses to HSV-1 and HSV-2. Point-of-care assays that provide results from capillary blood or serum during a clinic visit are available. A western blot assay that can detect several HSV type-specific proteins can also be used. The presence of type-specific HSV-2 antibody implies past HSV-2 infection—i.e., latent infection and likely subclinical reactivation.

Acute- and convalescent-phase serum samples can be useful in demonstrating seroconversion during primary HSV-1 or HSV-2 infection.

However, few available tests report titers, and increases in index values do not reflect first episodes in all patients. Serologic assays based on type-specific proteins should be used to identify asymptomatic carriers of HSV-1 or HSV-2. No reliable IgM method for defining acute HSV infection is available.

Several studies have shown that persons with previously unrecognized HSV-2 infection can be taught to identify symptomatic reactivations. Individuals seropositive for HSV-2 should be told about the high frequency of subclinical reactivation on mucosal surfaces that are not visible to the eye (e.g., cervix, urethra, perianal skin) or in microscopic ulcerations that may not be clinically symptomatic. Transmission of infection during such episodes is well established. HSV-2-seropositive persons should be educated about the high likelihood of subclinical shedding and the role that condoms (male or female) may play in reducing transmission. Antiviral therapy with valacyclovir (500 mg once daily) has been shown to reduce the transmission of HSV-2 between sexual partners.

TREATMENT

Herpes Simplex Virus Infections

Many aspects of mucocutaneous and visceral HSV infections are amenable to antiviral chemotherapy. For mucocutaneous infections, acyclovir and its congeners famciclovir and valacyclovir have been the mainstays of therapy. Several antiviral agents are available for topical use in HSV eye infections: idoxuridine, trifluorothymidine, topical vidarabine, and cidofovir. For HSV encephalitis and neonatal herpes, IV acyclovir is the treatment of choice.

All licensed antiviral agents for use against HSV inhibit the viral DNA polymerase. One class of drugs, typified by the drug acyclovir, is made up of substrates for the HSV enzyme TK. Acyclovir, ganciclovir, famciclovir, and valacyclovir are all selectively phosphorylated to the monophosphate form in virus-infected cells. Cellular enzymes convert the monophosphate form of the drug to the triphosphate, which is then incorporated into the viral DNA chain. Acyclovir is the agent most frequently used for the treatment of HSV infections and is available in IV, oral, and topical formulations. Valacyclovir, the valyl ester of acyclovir, offers greater bioavailability than acyclovir and thus can be administered less frequently. Famciclovir, the oral formulation of penciclovir, is clinically effective in the treatment of a variety of HSV-1 and HSV-2 infections. Ganciclovir is active against both HSV-1 and HSV-2; however, it is more toxic than acyclovir, valacyclovir, and famciclovir and generally is not recommended for the treatment of HSV infections. Anecdotal case reports suggest that ganciclovir may also be less effective than acyclovir for the treatment of HSV infections. All three recommended compounds—acyclovir, valacyclovir, and famciclovir—have proved effective in shortening the duration of symptoms and lesions of mucocutaneous HSV infections in both immunocompromised and immunocompetent patients (**Table 192-1**). IV and oral formulations prevent reactivation of HSV in seropositive immunocompromised patients during induction chemotherapy or in the period immediately after bone marrow or solid organ transplantation. Chronic daily suppressive therapy reduces the frequency of reactivation disease among patients with frequent genital or oral–labial herpes. Only valacyclovir has been subjected to clinical trials that demonstrated reduced transmission of HSV-2 infection between sexual partners. IV acyclovir (30 mg/kg per day, given as a 10-mg/kg infusion over 1 h at 8-h intervals) is effective in reducing rates of death and morbidity from HSV encephalitis. Early initiation of therapy is a critical factor in outcome. The major side effect associated with IV acyclovir is transient renal insufficiency, usually due to crystallization of the compound in the renal parenchyma. This adverse reaction can be avoided if the medication is given slowly over 1 h and the patient is well hydrated. Because CSF levels of acyclovir average only 30–50% of plasma levels, the dosage of acyclovir used for treatment of CNS infection (30 mg/kg per day) is double that used for treatment of mucocutaneous or visceral disease (15 mg/kg per day). Even higher doses of IV acyclovir are used for neonatal HSV infection (60 mg/kg per day in three divided doses). Antiviral drugs neither eradicate latent infection nor affect the risk, frequency, or severity of subclinical or clinical recurrence after the drug is discontinued.

Increasingly, shorter courses of therapy are being used for recurrent mucocutaneous infection with HSV-1 or HSV-2 in immunocompetent patients. One-day courses of famciclovir and valacyclovir are clinically effective, more convenient, and generally less costly than longer courses of therapy (Table 192-1). These short-course regimens should be reserved for immunocompetent hosts.

SUPPRESSION OF MUCOCUTANEOUS HERPES

Recognition of the high frequency of subclinical reactivation provides a well-accepted rationale for the use of daily antiviral therapy to suppress reactivations of HSV, especially in persons with frequent clinical reactivations (e.g., those with recently acquired genital HSV infection). Immunosuppressed persons, including those with HIV infection, may also benefit from daily antiviral therapy. Daily acyclovir and valacyclovir reduce the frequency of HSV reactivations among HIV-positive persons. Regimens used include acyclovir (400–800 mg twice daily), famciclovir (500 mg twice daily), and valacyclovir (500 mg twice daily); valacyclovir at a dose of 4 g/d was associated with thrombotic thrombocytopenic purpura in one study of HIV-infected persons. Daily acyclovir therapy is associated with a modest reduction in the titer of HIV RNA in plasma (0.5-$\log_{10}$ reduction) and in the genital mucosa (0.33-$\log_{10}$ reduction).

REDUCED HSV TRANSMISSION TO SEXUAL PARTNERS

Once-daily valacyclovir (500 mg) has been shown to reduce transmission of HSV-2 between sexual partners. Transmission rates are higher from males to females and among persons with frequent HSV-2 reactivation. Serologic screening can be used to identify at-risk couples. Daily valacyclovir appears to be more effective at reducing subclinical shedding than daily famciclovir.

ACYCLOVIR RESISTANCE

Clinically relevant acyclovir-resistant strains of HSV do occur. Most of these strains have an altered substrate specificity for phosphorylating acyclovir. Thus, cross-resistance to famciclovir and valacyclovir is usually found. Occasionally, an isolate with altered TK specificity arises and is sensitive to famciclovir but not to acyclovir. In some patients infected with TK-deficient virus, higher doses of acyclovir are associated with clearing of lesions. In others, clinical disease progresses despite high-dose therapy. The majority of clinically significant acyclovir resistance has been seen in immunocompromised patients. HSV-2 isolates appear to be more resistant than HSV-1 strains. The frequency of acyclovir resistance is not well characterized or monitored; the lack of appreciable change in the past 40 years probably reflects the reduced transmission of TK-deficient mutants. Isolation of HSV from lesions persisting despite adequate dosages and blood levels of acyclovir should raise the suspicion of acyclovir resistance. Clinical management of acyclovir resistance is challenging. Therapy with the antiviral drug foscarnet (40–80 mg/kg IV every 8 h until clinical resolution) is the only clinically demonstrated approach (**Chap. 191**). Because of its toxicity and cost, this drug is usually reserved for patients with extensive mucocutaneous infections. Cidofovir is a nucleotide analogue and exists as a phosphonate or monophosphate form. Most TK-deficient strains of HSV are sensitive to cidofovir. Cidofovir ointment speeds healing of acyclovir-resistant lesions. No well-controlled trials of systemic cidofovir have been reported. Occasional cases may respond to topical imiquimod. True TK-negative variants of HSV appear to have a reduced capacity to spread because of altered neurovirulence—a feature important in the relatively infrequent presence of such strains in immunocompetent populations, even with increasing use of antiviral drugs. A new class of drugs that inhibit HSV-specific helicase/primase activity (pritelivir) is under clinical investigation and may offer a better toxicity profile for the treatment of acyclovir-resistant strains of HSV.

TABLE 192-1 Antiviral Chemotherapy for Herpes Simplex Virus (HSV) Infection

I. **Mucocutaneous HSV infections**

A. *Infections in immunosuppressed patients*

1. *Acute symptomatic first or recurrent episodes:* IV acyclovir (5 mg/kg q8h) or oral acyclovir (400 mg qid), famciclovir (500 mg bid or tid), or valacyclovir (500 mg bid) is effective. Treatment duration may vary from 7 to 14 days. IV therapy may be given for 2–7 days until clinical improvement and followed by oral therapy.
2. *Suppression of reactivation disease (genital or oral–labial):* IV acyclovir (5 mg/kg q8h) or oral valacyclovir (500 mg bid) or acyclovir (400–800 mg 3–5 times per day) prevents recurrences during the 30-day period immediately after transplantation. Longer-term HSV suppression is often used for persons with continued immunosuppression. In bone marrow and renal transplant recipients, oral valacyclovir (2 g/d) is also effective in reducing cytomegalovirus infection. Oral valacyclovir at a dose of 4 g/d has been associated with thrombotic thrombocytopenic purpura after extended use in HIV-positive persons. In HIV-infected persons, oral acyclovir (400–800 mg bid), valacyclovir (500 mg bid), or famciclovir (500 mg bid) is effective in reducing clinical and subclinical reactivations of HSV-1 and HSV-2.

B. *Infections in immunocompetent patients*

1. *Genital herpes*
   a. *First episodes:* Oral acyclovir (200 mg 5 times per day or 400 mg tid), valacyclovir (1 g bid), or famciclovir (250 mg tid) for 7–14 days is effective. IV acyclovir (5 mg/kg q8h for 5 days) is given for severe disease or neurologic complications such as aseptic meningitis.
   b. *Symptomatic recurrent genital herpes:* Short-course (1- to 3-day) regimens are preferred because of low cost, likelihood of adherence, and convenience. Oral acyclovir (800 mg tid for 2 days), valacyclovir (500 mg bid for 3 days), valacyclovir (1 g orally once a day for 3 days), or famciclovir (750 or 1000 mg bid for 1 day, a 1500-mg single dose, or 500 mg stat followed by 250 mg q12h for 2 days) effectively shortens lesion duration. Other options include oral acyclovir (200 mg 5 times per day), valacyclovir (500 mg bid), and famciclovir (125 mg bid for 5 days).
   c. *Suppression of recurrent genital herpes:* Oral acyclovir (400–800 mg bid) or valacyclovir (500 mg daily) is given. Patients with >9 episodes per year should take oral valacyclovir (1 g daily or 500 mg bid) or famciclovir (250 mg bid or 500 mg bid).
2. *Oral–labial HSV infections*
   a. *First episode:* Oral acyclovir is given (200 mg 5 times per day or 400 mg tid); an oral acyclovir suspension can be used (600 mg/m^2 qid). Oral famciclovir (250 mg bid) or valacyclovir (1 g bid) has been used clinically. The duration of therapy is 5–10 days.
   b. *Recurrent episodes:* If initiated at the onset of the prodrome, single-dose or 1-day therapy effectively reduces pain and speeds healing. Regimens include oral famciclovir (a 1500-mg single dose or 750 mg bid for 1 day) or valacyclovir (a 2-g single dose or 2 g bid for 1 day). Self-initiated therapy with 6-times-daily topical penciclovir cream effectively speeds healing of oral–labial HSV infection. Topical acyclovir cream has also been shown to speed healing.
   c. *Suppression of reactivation of oral–labial HSV:* If started before exposure and continued for the duration of exposure (usually 5–10 days), oral acyclovir (400 mg bid) prevents reactivation of recurrent oral–labial HSV infection associated with severe sun exposure.
3. *Surgical prophylaxis of oral or genital HSV infection:* Several surgical procedures, such as laser skin resurfacing, trigeminal nerve-root decompression, and lumbar disk surgery, have been associated with HSV reactivation. IV acyclovir (3–5 mg/kg q8h) or oral acyclovir (800 mg bid), valacyclovir (500 mg bid), or famciclovir (250 mg bid) effectively reduces reactivation. Therapy should be initiated 48 h before surgery and continued for 3–7 days.
4. *Herpetic whitlow:* Oral acyclovir (200 mg) is given 5 times daily (alternative: 400 mg tid) for 7–10 days.
5. *HSV proctitis:* Oral acyclovir (400 mg 5 times per day) is useful in shortening the course of infection. In immunosuppressed patients or in patients with severe infection, IV acyclovir (5 mg/kg q8h) may be useful.
6. *Herpetic eye infections:* In acute keratitis, topical trifluorothymidine, vidarabine, idoxuridine, acyclovir, penciclovir, and interferon are all beneficial. Debridement may be required. Topical steroids may worsen disease.

II. **Central nervous system HSV infections**

A. *HSV encephalitis:* IV acyclovir (10 mg/kg q8h; 30 mg/kg per day) is given for 10 days or until HSV DNA is no longer detected in cerebrospinal fluid.

B. *HSV aseptic meningitis:* No studies of systemic antiviral chemotherapy exist. If therapy is to be given, IV acyclovir (15–30 mg/kg per day) should be used.

C. *Autonomic radiculopathy:* No studies are available. Most authorities recommend a trial of IV acyclovir.

III. **Neonatal HSV infections:** IV acyclovir (60 mg/kg per day, divided into 3 doses) is given. The recommended duration of IV treatment is 21 days. Monitoring for relapse should be undertaken. Continued suppression with oral acyclovir suspension should be given for 3–4 months.

IV. **Visceral HSV infections**

A. *HSV esophagitis:* IV acyclovir (15 mg/kg per day) is given. In some patients with milder forms of immunosuppression, oral therapy with valacyclovir or famciclovir is effective.

B. *HSV pneumonitis:* No controlled studies exist. IV acyclovir (15 mg/kg per day) should be considered.

V. **Disseminated HSV infections:** No controlled studies exist. IV acyclovir (5 mg/kg q8h) should be tried. Adjustments for renal insufficiency may be needed. No definite evidence indicates that therapy will decrease the risk of death.

VI. **Erythema multiforme associated with HSV:** Anecdotal observations suggest that oral acyclovir (400 mg bid or tid) or valacyclovir (500 mg bid) will suppress erythema multiforme.

VII. **Infections due to acyclovir-resistant HSV:** IV foscarnet (40 mg/kg IV q8h) should be given until lesions heal. The optimal duration of therapy and the usefulness of its continuation to suppress lesions are unclear. Some patients may benefit from cutaneous application of trifluorothymidine or 1% cidofovir gel, both of which must be compounded at a pharmacy. These preparations should be applied once daily for 5–7 days. Topical imiquimod can be considered. The helicase primase inhibitor pritelivir is being studied for treatment of acyclovir-resistant HSV infection. IV cidofovir (5 mg/kg weekly) may be considered.

VIII. **Acyclovir and pregnancy:** No adverse effects to the fetus or newborn have been attributable to acyclovir. Acyclovir can be used in all stages of pregnancy and among women who are breastfeeding (the drug can be found in breast milk). Suppressive acyclovir treatment in late pregnancy (acyclovir 400 mg orally tid or valacyclovir 500 mg orally bid from ~34 weeks until delivery) reduces the frequency of cesarean delivery among women with recurrent genital herpes. Such treatment may not protect against transmission to neonates.

ACYCLOVIR EFFICACY IN THE DEVELOPING WORLD

Initial studies of acyclovir-like drugs were performed solely in the developed world. While acyclovir, valacyclovir, and famciclovir are effective in the developing world, their clinical and virologic benefits, especially in reducing the frequency of genital lesions among patients in Africa, seem reduced from those in European and U.S. populations. The mechanism of this phenomenon is uncertain. Acyclovir therapy does not reduce the rate of HIV acquisition; however, HIV load among MSM in the U.S. decreased by 1.3 $\log_{10}$ in contrast to 0.9 $\log_{10}$ among Peruvian MSM and 0.5 $\log_{10}$ among African women. Curiously, the anti-HIV drug tenofovir reduces HSV-2 acquisition among women in Africa, although it has no demonstrable clinical benefit or antiviral effects among persons with established HSV-2 infection in studies in the United States. The reasons for these disparate results are unclear.

PREVENTION

Efforts to control HSV disease on a population basis through suppressive antiviral therapy and/or educational programs have been limited. Barrier forms of contraception (especially condoms) decrease the likelihood of transmission of HSV infection, particularly during periods of asymptomatic viral excretion. When lesions are present, HSV infection may be transmitted by skin-to-skin contact despite the use of a condom. Nevertheless, the available data suggest that consistent condom use is an effective means of reducing the risk of genital HSV-2 transmission. Chronic daily antiviral therapy with valacyclovir can also be partially effective in reducing acquisition of HSV-2, especially among susceptible women. There are no comparative efficacy studies of valacyclovir versus condom use. Most authorities suggest both approaches. The need for a vaccine to prevent acquisition of HSV infection is great, especially in light of the role HSV-2 plays in enhancing the acquisition and transmission of HIV-1.

A substantial portion of neonatal HSV cases could be prevented by reducing the acquisition of HSV by women in the third trimester of pregnancy. Neonatal HSV infection can result from either the acquisition of maternal infection near term or the reactivation of infection at delivery in the already-infected mother. Women without known genital herpes should be counseled to abstain from vaginal intercourse during the third trimester with partners known to have or suspected of having genital herpes. Some authorities have recommended that antiviral therapy with acyclovir or valacyclovir be given to HSV-2-infected women in late pregnancy as a means of reducing reactivation of HSV-2 at term. Data are not available to support the efficacy of this approach, and the high treatment-to-prevention ratio makes this a difficult if not dubious public health strategy, even though it can reduce the frequency of HSV-associated cesarean delivery.

FURTHER READING

Centers for Disease Control and Prevention: 2015 Sexually transmitted diseases treatment guidelines. Available at *https://www.cdc.gov/std/tg2015/herpes.htm.*

James C et al: Herpes simplex virus: Global infection prevalence and incidence estimates, 2016. Bull World Health Organ 98:315, 2020.

Looker KJ et al: Global and regional estimates of the contribution of herpes simplex virus type 2 infection to HIV incidence: A population attributable fraction analysis using published epidemiological data. Lancet Infect Dis 20:240, 2020.

Mahant S et al: Neonatal herpes simplex virus infection among Medicaid-enrolled children: 2009–2015. Pediatrics 143:e20183233, 2019.

Yousuf W et al: Herpes simplex virus type 1 in Europe: Systematic review, meta-analyses and meta-regressions. BMJ Global Health 5:e002388, 2020.

193 Varicella-Zoster Virus Infections

Richard J. Whitley

DEFINITION

Varicella-zoster virus (VZV) causes two distinct clinical syndromes: varicella (chickenpox) and herpes zoster (shingles). Chickenpox, a ubiquitous and extremely contagious infection, is usually a benign illness of childhood characterized by an exanthematous vesicular rash. With reactivation of latent VZV (which is most common after the sixth decade of life), herpes zoster presents as a dermatomal vesicular rash and is usually associated with severe pain.

ETIOLOGY

Early in the twentieth century, similarities in the histopathologic features of skin lesions resulting from varicella and herpes zoster were described. Viral isolates from patients with each of these diseases produced similar pathology in tissue culture—specifically, the appearance of eosinophilic intranuclear inclusions and multinucleated giant cells. These results suggested that the viruses were biologically similar. Restriction endonuclease analyses of viral DNA from a patient with chickenpox who subsequently developed herpes zoster verified the molecular identity of the two viruses responsible for these different clinical presentations.

VZV is a member of the family Herpesviridae, sharing with other members such structural characteristics as a lipid envelope surrounding a nucleocapsid with icosahedral symmetry, a total diameter of ~180–200 nm, and centrally located double-stranded DNA that is ~125,000 bp in length.

PATHOGENESIS AND PATHOLOGY

Primary Infection Transmission occurs readily by the respiratory route; the subsequent localized replication of the virus at an undefined site (presumably the nasopharynx) leads to seeding of the lymphatic/reticuloendothelial system and ultimately to the development of viremia. Viremia in patients with chickenpox is reflected in the diffuse and scattered nature of the skin lesions and can be confirmed by the recovery of VZV from the blood (rarely) or routinely by the detection of viral DNA in either blood or lesions by polymerase chain reaction (PCR). Vesicles involve the corium and dermis, with degenerative changes characterized by ballooning, the presence of multinucleated giant cells, and eosinophilic intranuclear inclusions. Infection may involve localized blood vessels of the skin, resulting in necrosis and epidermal hemorrhage. With the evolution of disease, the vesicular fluid becomes cloudy because of the recruitment of polymorphonuclear leukocytes and the presence of degenerated cells and fibrin. Ultimately, the vesicles either rupture and release their fluid (which includes infectious virus) or are gradually reabsorbed.

Recurrent Infection The mechanism of reactivation of VZV that results in herpes zoster is unknown. The virus infects dorsal root ganglia during chickenpox, where it remains latent until reactivated. Histopathologic examination of representative dorsal root ganglia during active herpes zoster demonstrates hemorrhage, edema, and lymphocytic infiltration. Latent virus has been detected in sensory (dorsal, cranial, and enteric) ganglia.

Active replication of VZV in other organs, such as the lung or the brain, can occur during either chickenpox or herpes zoster but is uncommon in the immunocompetent host. Pulmonary involvement is characterized by interstitial pneumonitis, multinucleated giant cell formation, intranuclear inclusions, and pulmonary hemorrhage. Central nervous system (CNS) infection leads to histopathologic evidence of perivascular cuffing similar to that encountered in measles and other viral encephalitides. Focal hemorrhagic necrosis of the brain, characteristic of herpes simplex virus (HSV) encephalitis, develops infrequently in VZV infection.

EPIDEMIOLOGY AND CLINICAL MANIFESTATIONS

Chickenpox Humans are the only known reservoir for VZV. Chickenpox is highly contagious, with an attack rate of at least 90% among susceptible (seronegative) individuals. Persons of both sexes and all races are infected equally. The virus is endemic in the population at large; however, it becomes epidemic among susceptible individuals during seasonal peaks—namely, late winter and early spring in the temperate zone. Much of our knowledge of the disease's natural history and incidence predates the licensure of the chickenpox vaccine in 1995. Historically, children 5–9 years old were most commonly affected, accounting for 50% of all cases. Most other cases involved children 1–4 and 10–14 years old. Approximately 10% of the population of the United States over the age of 15 was susceptible to infection. VZV vaccination during the second year of life has dramatically changed the

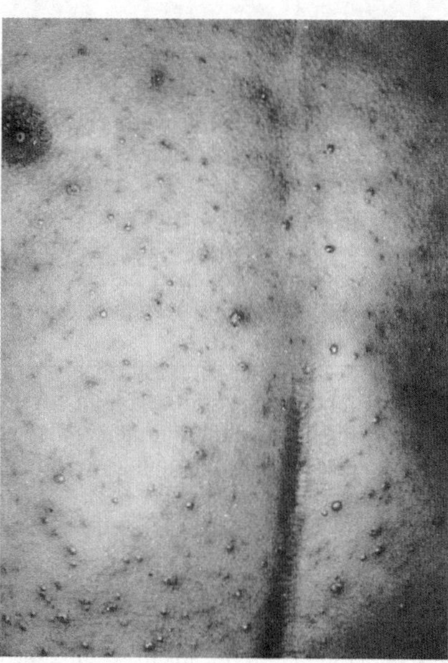

FIGURE 193-1 Varicella lesions at various stages of evolution: vesicles on an erythematous base, umbilical vesicles, and crusts.

epidemiology of infection, causing a significant decrease in the annualized incidence of chickenpox, as noted below.

The incubation period of chickenpox ranges from 10 to 21 days but is usually 14–17 days. Secondary attack rates in susceptible siblings within a household are 70–90%. Patients are infectious ~48 h before the onset of the vesicular rash, during the period of vesicle formation (which generally lasts 4–5 days), and until all vesicles are crusted.

Clinically, chickenpox presents as a rash, low-grade fever, and malaise, although a few patients develop a prodrome 1–2 days before onset of the exanthem. In the immunocompetent patient, chickenpox is usually a benign illness associated with lassitude and with body temperatures of 37.8°–39.4°C (100°–103°F) of 3–5 days' duration. The skin lesions—the hallmark of the infection—include maculopapules, vesicles, and scabs in various stages of evolution (**Fig. 193-1; see also Fig. A1-30**). These lesions, which evolve from maculopapules to vesicles over hours to days, appear on the trunk and face and rapidly spread to involve other areas of the body. Most are small and have an erythematous base with a diameter of 5–10 mm. Successive crops appear over a 2- to 4-day period. Lesions can also be found on the mucosa of the pharynx and/or the vagina. Their severity varies from one person to another. Some individuals have very few lesions, while others have as many as 2000. Younger children tend to have fewer vesicles than older individuals. Within families, secondary and tertiary cases are associated with a larger number of vesicles than the first family case. Immunocompromised patients—both children and adults, particularly those with leukemia—have lesions (often with a hemorrhagic base) that are more numerous and take longer to heal than those of immunocompetent patients. Immunocompromised individuals are also at greater risk for visceral complications, which occur in 30–50% of cases and are fatal 15% of the time in the absence of antiviral therapy.

The most common infectious complication of varicella is secondary bacterial superinfection of the skin, which is usually caused by *Streptococcus pyogenes* or *Staphylococcus aureus,* including strains that are methicillin-resistant. Skin infection results from excoriation of lesions after scratching. Gram's staining of skin lesions may help clarify the etiology of unusually erythematous and pustulated lesions.

The most common extracutaneous site of involvement in children is the CNS. The syndrome of acute cerebellar ataxia and meningeal inflammation generally appears ~21 days after onset of the rash and rarely develops in the pre-eruptive phase. The cerebrospinal fluid (CSF) contains lymphocytes and elevated levels of protein. CNS involvement is a benign complication of VZV infection in immunocompetent children and generally does not require hospitalization. Aseptic meningitis, encephalitis, transverse myelitis, and Guillain-Barré syndrome can also occur. Encephalitis is reported in 0.1–0.2% of children with chickenpox. Reye's syndrome can occur in children concomitantly treated with aspirin, and therefore, aspirin is no longer utilized. Other than supportive care, no specific therapy (e.g., acyclovir administration) has proved efficacious for patients with CNS involvement.

Varicella pneumonia, the most serious complication following chickenpox, develops more often in adults (up to 20% of cases) than in children and is particularly severe in pregnant women. Pneumonia due to VZV usually has its onset 3–5 days into the illness and is associated with tachypnea, cough, dyspnea, and fever. Cyanosis, pleuritic chest pain, and hemoptysis are frequently noted. Roentgenographic evidence of disease consists of nodular infiltrates and interstitial pneumonitis. Resolution of pneumonitis parallels improvement of the skin rash; however, patients may have persistent fever and compromised pulmonary function for weeks.

Other complications of chickenpox include myocarditis, corneal lesions, nephritis, arthritis, bleeding diatheses, acute glomerulonephritis, and hepatitis. Hepatic involvement, distinct from Reye's syndrome and usually asymptomatic, is common in chickenpox and is generally characterized by elevated levels of liver enzymes, particularly aspartate and alanine aminotransferases.

Perinatal varicella is associated with mortality rates as high as 30% when maternal disease develops within 5 days before delivery or within 48 h thereafter. Illness in this setting is unusually severe because the newborn does not receive protective transplacental antibodies and has an immature immune system. *Congenital varicella,* with clinical manifestations of limb hypoplasia, cicatricial skin lesions, and microcephaly at birth, is extremely uncommon.

Herpes Zoster Herpes zoster (shingles) is a sporadic disease that results from reactivation of latent VZV from dorsal root ganglia. Most patients with shingles have no history of recent exposure to other individuals with VZV infection. Herpes zoster occurs at all ages, but its incidence is highest (5–10 cases per 1000 persons) among individuals in the sixth decade of life and beyond. Data suggest that at least 1.2 million cases occur annually in the United States. Recurrent herpes zoster is exceedingly rare except in immunocompromised hosts, especially those with AIDS.

Herpes zoster is characterized by a unilateral vesicular dermatomal eruption, often associated with severe pain. The dermatomes from T3 to L3 are most frequently involved. If the ophthalmic branch of the trigeminal nerve is involved, *zoster ophthalmicus* results. The factors responsible for the reactivation of VZV are not known. In children, reactivation is usually benign; in adults, it can be debilitating because of pain. The onset of disease is heralded by pain within the dermatome, which may precede lesions by 48–72 h; an erythematous maculopapular rash evolves rapidly into vesicular lesions (**Fig. 193-2**). In the normal host, these lesions may remain few in number and continue to form for only 3–5 days. The total duration of disease is generally 7–10 days; however, it may take as long as 2–4 weeks for the skin to return to normal. Patients with herpes zoster can transmit infection to seronegative individuals, resulting in chickenpox. In a few patients, characteristic localization of pain to a dermatome with serologic evidence of herpes zoster has been reported in the absence of skin lesions, an entity known as *zoster sine herpetica.* When branches of the trigeminal nerve are involved, lesions may appear on the face, in the mouth, in the eye, or on the tongue. *Zoster ophthalmicus* is usually a debilitating condition that can result in blindness in the absence of antiviral therapy. In *Ramsay Hunt syndrome,* pain and vesicles appear in the external auditory canal, and patients lose their sense of taste in the anterior two-thirds of the tongue while developing ipsilateral facial palsy. The geniculate ganglion of the sensory branch of the facial nerve is involved.

In both normal and immunocompromised hosts, the most debilitating complication of herpes zoster is pain associated with acute neuritis and postherpetic neuralgia. Postherpetic neuralgia is uncommon in young individuals; however, at least 50% of patients over age 50 report some degree of pain in the involved dermatome for months after the resolution of cutaneous disease. Changes in sensation in the dermatome, resulting in either hypo- or hyperesthesia, are common.

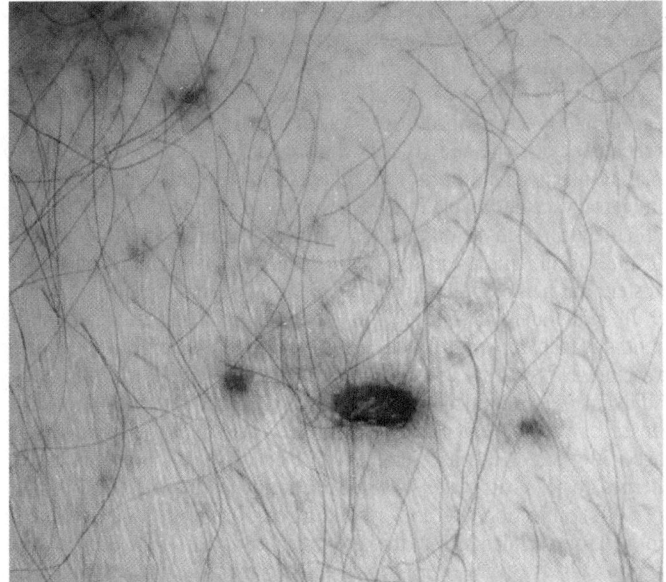

FIGURE 193-2 Close-up of lesions of disseminated zoster. Note lesions at different stages of evolution, including pustules and crusting. *(Photo courtesy of Lindsey Baden; with permission.)*

CNS involvement may follow localized herpes zoster. Many patients without signs of meningeal irritation have CSF pleocytosis and moderately elevated levels of CSF protein. Symptomatic meningoencephalitis is characterized by headache, fever, photophobia, meningitis, and vomiting. A rare manifestation of CNS involvement is granulomatous angiitis with contralateral hemiplegia, which can be diagnosed by cerebral arteriography. Other neurologic manifestations include transverse myelitis with or without motor paralysis.

Like chickenpox, herpes zoster is more severe in immunocompromised than immunocompetent individuals. Lesions continue to form for >1 week, and scabbing is not complete in most cases until 3 weeks into the illness. Patients with Hodgkin's disease and non-Hodgkin's lymphoma are at greatest risk for progressive herpes zoster. Cutaneous dissemination (**Fig. 193-3**) develops in ~40% of these patients. Among patients with cutaneous dissemination, the risk of pneumonitis, meningoencephalitis, hepatitis, and other serious complications is increased by 5–10%. However, even in immunocompromised patients, disseminated zoster is rarely fatal.

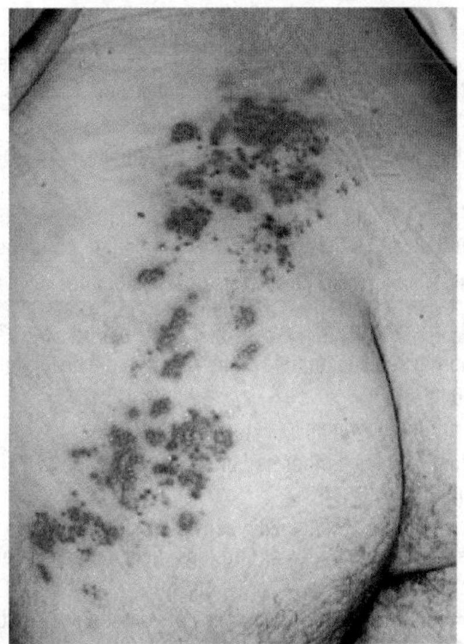

FIGURE 193-3 Herpes zoster in an HIV-infected patient is seen as hemorrhagic vesicles and pustules on an erythematous base grouped in a dermatomal distribution.

Recipients of hematopoietic stem cell transplants are at particularly high risk of VZV infection. Of all cases of post-transplantation VZV infection, 30% occur within 1 year (50% of these within 9 months); 45% of the patients involved have cutaneous or visceral dissemination. The mortality rate in this situation is 10%. Postherpetic neuralgia, scarring, and bacterial superinfection are especially common in VZV infections occurring within 9 months of transplantation. Among infected patients, concomitant graft-versus-host disease increases the chance of dissemination and/or death.

DIFFERENTIAL DIAGNOSIS

The diagnosis of chickenpox is not difficult. The characteristic rash and a history of recent exposure should lead to a prompt diagnosis. Other viral infections that can mimic chickenpox include disseminated HSV infection in patients with atopic dermatitis and the disseminated vesiculopapular lesions sometimes associated with coxsackievirus infection, echovirus infection, or atypical measles. However, these rashes are more commonly morbilliform with a hemorrhagic component rather than vesicular or vesiculopustular. Rickettsialpox (**Chap. 187**) is sometimes confused with chickenpox; however, rickettsialpox can be distinguished easily by detection of the "herald spot" at the site of the mite bite and the development of a more pronounced headache. Serologic testing is also useful in differentiating rickettsialpox from varicella and can confirm susceptibility in adults unsure of their chickenpox history. Monkeypox should be considered in travelers returning from endemic areas (**Chap. 196**). Concern about smallpox has increased because of the threat of bioterrorism (**Chap. S3**). The lesions of smallpox are larger than those of chickenpox and are all at the same stage of evolution at any given time.

Unilateral vesicular lesions in a dermatomal pattern should lead rapidly to the diagnosis of herpes zoster, although the occurrence of shingles without a rash has been reported. Both HSV and coxsackievirus infections can cause dermatomal vesicular lesions. Supportive diagnostic virology and fluorescent staining of skin scrapings with monoclonal antibodies are helpful in ensuring the proper diagnosis. In the prodromal stage of herpes zoster, the diagnosis can be exceedingly difficult and may be made only after lesions have appeared or by retrospective serologic assessment.

LABORATORY FINDINGS

Unequivocal confirmation of the diagnosis is possible only through the isolation of VZV in susceptible tissue-culture cell lines, the demonstration of either seroconversion or a fourfold or greater rise in antibody titer between acute-phase and convalescent-phase serum specimens, or the detection of VZV DNA by PCR. Specimens for detection of VZV DNA by PCR include lesions, blood, and saliva. A rapid impression can be obtained by a Tzanck smear, with scraping of the base of the lesions in an attempt to demonstrate multinucleated giant cells; however, the sensitivity of this method is low (~60%). PCR technology for the detection of viral DNA in vesicular fluid is available in many diagnostic laboratories and has become the diagnostic method of choice. Direct immunofluorescent staining of cells from the lesion base or detection of viral antigens by other assays (such as the immunoperoxidase assay) is also useful. The most frequently employed serologic tools for assessing host response are the immunofluorescent detection of antibodies to VZV membrane antigens, the fluorescent antibody to membrane antigen (FAMA) test, immune adherence hemagglutination, and enzyme-linked immunosorbent assay (ELISA). The FAMA test and the ELISA appear to be most sensitive.

TREATMENT

Varicella-Zoster Virus Infections

Medical management of chickenpox in the immunologically normal host is directed toward the prevention of avoidable complications. Obviously, good hygiene includes daily bathing and soaks. Secondary bacterial infection of the skin can be avoided by meticulous skin care, particularly with close cropping of fingernails.

Pruritus can be decreased with topical dressings or the administration of antipruritic drugs. Tepid water baths and wet compresses are better than drying lotions for the relief of itching. Administration of aspirin to children with chickenpox should be avoided because of the association of aspirin derivatives with the development of Reye's syndrome. Acyclovir (800 mg by mouth five times daily), valacyclovir (1 g three times daily), or famciclovir (250 mg three times daily) for 5–7 days is recommended for adolescents and adults with chickenpox of ≤24 h duration. (Valacyclovir is licensed for use in children and adolescents. Famciclovir is recommended but not licensed for varicella.) Likewise, acyclovir therapy may be of benefit to children <12 years of age if initiated early in the disease (<24 h) at a dose of 20 mg/kg every 6 h. The advantages (i.e., pharmacokinetics) of the second-generation agents valacyclovir and famciclovir are described in **Chap. 191.**

Aluminum acetate soaks for the management of herpes zoster can be both soothing and cleansing. Patients with herpes zoster benefit from oral antiviral therapy, as evidenced by accelerated healing of lesions and resolution of zoster-associated pain with acyclovir, valacyclovir, or famciclovir. Acyclovir is administered at a dosage of 800 mg five times daily for 7–10 days. However, valacyclovir and famciclovir have superior pharmacokinetics and pharmacodynamics and should be used preferentially. Famciclovir, the prodrug of penciclovir, is at least as effective as acyclovir and perhaps more so; the dose is 500 mg by mouth three times daily for 7 days. Valacyclovir, the prodrug of acyclovir, accelerates healing and resolution of zoster-associated pain more promptly than acyclovir. The dose is 1 g by mouth three times daily for 5–7 days. Compared with acyclovir, both famciclovir and valacyclovir offer the advantage of less frequent administration. All three of these drugs are now available as generic products.

In severely immunocompromised hosts (e.g., transplant recipients, patients with lymphoproliferative malignancies), both chickenpox and herpes zoster (including disseminated disease) should be treated, at least at the outset, with IV acyclovir, which reduces the occurrence of visceral complications but has no effect on healing of skin lesions or pain. The dose is 10 mg/kg every 8 h for 7 days. For low-risk immunocompromised hosts, oral therapy with valacyclovir or famciclovir appears beneficial. If medically feasible, it is desirable to decrease immunosuppressive treatment concomitant with the administration of IV acyclovir.

Patients with varicella pneumonia typically require ventilatory support. Persons with zoster ophthalmicus should be referred immediately to an ophthalmologist. Therapy for this condition consists of the administration of analgesics for severe pain and the use of atropine. Acyclovir, valacyclovir, and famciclovir all accelerate healing. Decisions regarding the use of corticosteroids should be made by the ophthalmologist.

The management of acute neuritis and/or postherpetic neuralgia can be particularly difficult. In addition to the judicious use of analgesics ranging from nonnarcotics to narcotic derivatives, drugs such as gabapentin, pregabalin, amitriptyline hydrochloride, lidocaine (patches), and fluphenazine hydrochloride are reportedly beneficial for pain relief. In one study, glucocorticoid therapy administered early in the course of localized herpes zoster significantly accelerated such quality-of-life improvements as a return to usual activity and termination of analgesic medications. The dose of prednisone administered orally was 60 mg/d on days 1–7, 30 mg/d on days 8–14, and 15 mg/d on days 15–21. This regimen is appropriate only for relatively healthy elderly persons with moderate or severe pain at presentation. Patients with osteoporosis, diabetes mellitus, glycosuria, or hypertension may not be appropriate candidates. Glucocorticoids should not be used without concomitant antiviral therapy.

PREVENTION

Three methods are used for the prevention of VZV infections. First, a live attenuated varicella vaccine (Oka) is recommended for all children >1 year of age (up to 12 years of age) who have not had chickenpox and for adults known to be seronegative for VZV. Two doses are recommended for all children: the first at 12–15 months of age and the second at ~4–6 years of age. VZV-seronegative persons >13 years of age should receive two doses of vaccine at least 1 month apart. The vaccine is both safe and efficacious. Breakthrough cases are mild and may result in spread of the vaccine virus to susceptible contacts. The universal vaccination of children has resulted in a decreased incidence of chickenpox in sentinel communities. Furthermore, inactivation of the vaccine virus significantly decreases the occurrence of herpes zoster after hemotopoietic stem cell transplantation.

In individuals >50 years of age, only one shingles vaccine is currently available in the United States, namely Shingrix. It is a subunit vaccine (HZ/su) that consists of VZV glycoprotein E and the $AS01_B$ adjuvant. A randomized, placebo-controlled study administered two doses of vaccine or placebo 1 month apart to 15,411 participants aged 50 years or older. Overall vaccine efficacy for the prevention of herpes zoster virus was 97.2% (95% confidence interval, 93.7-99.0%; p <.001). Injection-site and systemic reactions were more frequent in vaccine recipients, but the proportions of participants who had serious adverse events were similar in the vaccine and placebo groups. The Advisory Committee on Immunization Practices has therefore recommended that persons in this age group be offered this vaccine in order to reduce the frequency of shingles and the severity of postherpetic neuralgia. Of note, vaccine immunity wanes over time, and reassessment of current recommendations or the use of a promising inactivated vaccine in development will be required.

A second approach is to administer varicella-zoster immune globulin (VZIG) to individuals who are susceptible, are at high risk for developing complications of varicella, and have had a significant exposure. This product should be given within 96 h (preferably within 72 h) of the exposure but may be administered up to 10 days with similar efficacy. Indications for administration of VZIG appear in **Table 193-1**, which has been adapted from the American Academy of Pediatrics Redbook.

Lastly, antiviral therapy can be given as prophylaxis to individuals at high risk who are ineligible for vaccination or who are beyond the 96-h window after direct contact. While the initial studies have used acyclovir, similar benefit can be anticipated with either valacyclovir or

TABLE 193-1 Recommendations for VZIG Administration

Exposure Criteria
1. Significant exposure to a person with chickenpox or zoster
a. Household: residence in the same household
b. Playmate: face-to-face indoor play
c. Hospital
Varicella: same 2- to 4-bed room or adjacent beds in a large ward, face-to-face contact with an infectious staff member or patient, visit by a person deemed contagious
Zoster: intimate contact (e.g., touching or hugging) with a person deemed contagious
d. Newborn infant: onset of varicella in the mother ≤5 days before delivery or ≤48 h after delivery; VZIG not indicated if the mother has zoster
2. Patient should receive VZIG as soon as possible but not >96 h after exposure.
Candidates (Provided They Have Significant Exposure) Include
1. Immunocompromised susceptible children without a history of varicella or varicella immunization
2. Susceptible pregnant women
3. Newborn infants whose mother had onset of chickenpox within 5 days before or within 48 h after delivery
4. Hospitalized premature infant (≥28 weeks of gestation) whose mother lacks a reliable history of chickenpox or serologic evidence of protection against varicella
5. Hospitalized premature infant (<28 weeks of gestation or ≤1000-g birth weight), regardless of maternal history of varicella or VZV serologic status

Abbreviation: VZIG, varicella-zoster immune globulin.

Note: Table is adapted from the American Academy of Pediatrics *Red Book.*

famciclovir. Therapy is instituted 7 days after intense exposure. At this time, the host is midway into the incubation period. This approach significantly decreases disease severity, if not totally preventing disease.

FURTHER READING

Arvin A: Aging, immunity, and the varicella-zoster virus. N Engl J Med 352:2266, 2005.

Cohen JI: A new vaccine to prevent herpes zoster. N Engl J Med 372:2149, 2015.

Gershon AA et al: Varicella zoster virus infection. Nat Rev Dis Primers 1:15016, 2015.

Gnann JW, Whitley RJ: Herpes zoster. N Engl J Med 347:340, 2002.

Hata A et al: Use of an inactivated varicella vaccine in recipients of hematopoietic-cell transplants. N Engl J Med 347:26, 2002.

Kimberlin DW, Whitley RJ. Varicella-zoster vaccine for the prevention of herpes zoster. N Engl J Med 356:1338, 2007.

Lai H et al: Efficacy of an adjuvanted herpes zoster subunit vaccine in older adults. N Engl J Med 372:2087, 2015.

Levin MJ et al: Varicella zoster immune globulin (VARIZIG) administration up to 10 days after varicellas exposure in pregnant women, immunocompromised participants, and infants: Varicellas outcomes and safety results from a large, open-label, expanded access program. PLoS One 14:e0217749, 2019.

Morrison VA et al: Long-term persistence of zoster vaccine efficacy. Clin Infect Dis 60:900, 2015.

Nguyen HQ et al: Decline in mortality due to varicella after implementation of varicella vaccination in the United States. N Engl J Med 352:450, 2005.

Oxman MN et al: A vaccine to prevent herpes zoster and postherpetic neuralgia in older adults. N Engl J Med 352:2271, 2005.

Seward JF et al: Varicella disease after introduction of varicella vaccine in the United States, 1995-2000. JAMA 287:606, 2002.

Seward JF et al: Contagiousness of varicella in vaccinated cases: A household contact study. JAMA 292:704, 2004.

Shaw J, Gershon AA: Varicella virus vaccination in the United States. Viral Immunol 31:96, 2018.

Willis ED et al: Herpes zoster vaccine live: A 10 year review of post-marketing safety experience. Vaccine 35:7231, 2017.

Wutzler P et al: Varicella vaccination–the global experience. Expert Rev Vaccines 16:833, 2017.

194 Epstein-Barr Virus Infections, Including Infectious Mononucleosis

Jeffrey I. Cohen

DEFINITION

Epstein-Barr virus (EBV) is the cause of heterophile-positive infectious mononucleosis (IM), which is characterized by fever, sore throat, lymphadenopathy, and atypical lymphocytosis. EBV is also associated with several tumors, including nasopharyngeal and gastric carcinoma, Burkitt's lymphoma, Hodgkin's lymphoma, T-cell lymphoma, and (in patients with immunodeficiencies) B-cell lymphoma and smooth muscle tumors. The virus is a member of the family Herpesviridae. The two types of EBV that are widely prevalent in nature are not distinguishable by conventional serologic tests.

EPIDEMIOLOGY

EBV infections occur worldwide. These infections are most common in early childhood, with a second peak during late adolescence. By adulthood, >90% of individuals have been infected and have antibodies to the virus. IM is usually a disease of young adults. In lower socioeconomic groups and in areas of the world with deficient standards of hygiene (e.g., developing regions), EBV tends to infect children at an early age, and IM is uncommon. In areas with higher standards of hygiene, infection with EBV is often delayed until adulthood, and IM is more prevalent.

EBV is spread by contact with oral secretions. The virus is frequently transmitted from asymptomatic adults to infants and among young adults by transfer of saliva during kissing. Transmission by less intimate contact is rare. EBV has been transmitted by blood transfusion and by bone marrow transplantation. More than 90% of asymptomatic seropositive individuals shed the virus in oropharyngeal secretions. Shedding is increased in immunocompromised patients and those with IM.

PATHOGENESIS

EBV is transmitted by salivary secretions. The virus infects the epithelium of the oropharynx and the salivary glands and is shed from these cells. While B cells may become infected after contact with epithelial cells, studies suggest that lymphocytes in the tonsillar crypts can be infected directly. The virus then spreads through the bloodstream. The proliferation and expansion of EBV-infected B cells along with reactive T cells during IM result in enlargement of lymphoid tissue. Polyclonal activation of B cells leads to the production of antibodies to host-cell and viral proteins. During the acute phase of IM, up to 1 in every 100 B cells in the peripheral blood is infected by EBV; after recovery, 1–50 in every 1 million B cells is infected. During IM, there is an inverted CD4+/CD8+ T-cell ratio. The percentage of CD4+ T cells decreases, while there are large clonal expansions of CD8+ T cells; up to 40% of CD8+ T cells are directed against EBV antigens during acute infection. Memory B cells, not epithelial cells, are the reservoir for EBV in the body. When patients are treated with acyclovir, shedding of EBV from the oropharynx stops but the virus persists in B cells.

The EBV receptor (CD21) on the surface of B cells is also the receptor for the C3d component of complement. Another EBV receptor (CD35) on B cells binds to CD21. Human leukocyte antigen class II serves as a co-receptor for EBV entry into B cells. EBV infection of epithelial cells occurs by virus binding to ephrin A2 and results in viral replication and production of virions. When B cells are infected by EBV in vitro, they become transformed and can proliferate indefinitely. During latent infection of B cells, the EBV nuclear antigens (EBNAs), latent membrane proteins (LMPs), multiple microRNAs, and small EBV RNAs (EBERs) are expressed in vitro. EBV-transformed B cells secrete immunoglobulin; only a small fraction of these cells produce virus.

Cellular immunity is more important than humoral immunity in controlling EBV infection. In the initial phase of infection, suppressor T cells, natural killer (NK) cells, and nonspecific cytotoxic T cells are important in controlling the proliferation of EBV-infected B cells. Levels of markers of T-cell activation and serum interferon γ are elevated. Later in infection, human leukocyte antigen–restricted cytotoxic T cells that recognize EBNAs and LMPs and destroy EBV-infected cells are generated.

If T-cell immunity is compromised, EBV-infected B cells may begin to proliferate. When EBV is associated with lymphoma in immunocompetent persons, virus-induced proliferation is but one step in a multistep process of neoplastic transformation. In many EBV-containing tumors, LMP-1 mimics members of the tumor necrosis factor receptor family (e.g., CD40), transmitting growth-proliferating signals.

CLINICAL MANIFESTATIONS

Signs and Symptoms Most EBV infections in infants and young children either are asymptomatic or present as mild pharyngitis with or without tonsillitis. In contrast, ~75% of infections in adolescents present as IM. IM in the elderly often presents with nonspecific symptoms, including prolonged fever, fatigue, myalgia, and malaise. In contrast, pharyngitis, lymphadenopathy, splenomegaly, and atypical lymphocytes are relatively rare in elderly patients.

TABLE 194-1 Signs and Symptoms of Infectious Mononucleosis

MANIFESTATION	MEDIAN PERCENTAGE OF PATIENTS (RANGE)
Symptoms	
Sore throat	75 (50–87)
Malaise	47 (42–76)
Headache	38 (22–67)
Abdominal pain, nausea, or vomiting	17 (5–25)
Chills	10 (9–11)
Signs	
Lymphadenopathy	95 (83–100)
Fever	93 (60–100)
Pharyngitis or tonsillitis	82 (68–90)
Splenomegaly	51 (43–64)
Hepatomegaly	11 (6–15)
Rash	10 (0–25)
Periorbital edema	13 (2–34)
Palatal enanthem	7 (3–13)
Jaundice	5 (2–10)

The incubation period for IM in young adults is ~4–6 weeks. A prodrome of fatigue, malaise, and myalgia may last for 1–2 weeks before the onset of fever, sore throat, and lymphadenopathy. Fever is usually low-grade and is most common in the first 2 weeks of the illness; however, it may persist for >1 month. Common signs and symptoms are listed along with their frequencies in **Table 194-1**. Lymphadenopathy and pharyngitis are most prominent during the first 2 weeks of the illness, while splenomegaly is more prominent during the second and third weeks. Lymphadenopathy most often affects the posterior cervical nodes but may be generalized. Enlarged lymph nodes are frequently tender and symmetric but are not fixed in place. Pharyngitis, often the most prominent sign, can be accompanied by enlargement of the tonsils with an exudate resembling that of streptococcal pharyngitis. A morbilliform or papular rash, usually on the arms or trunk, develops in ~5% of cases (**Fig. 194-1**). Earlier studies reported that many patients treated with penicillin derivatives develop a macular rash; penicillin-associated rashes are not predictive of future adverse reactions to penicillins. More recent studies suggest that EBV-associated rashes may occur with similar frequency in those exposed to penicillin derivatives and those not taking these drugs. Erythema nodosum (**Fig. A1-39**) and erythema multiforme (**Fig. A1-24**) also have been described (**Chap. 58**). The severity of the disease correlates with the

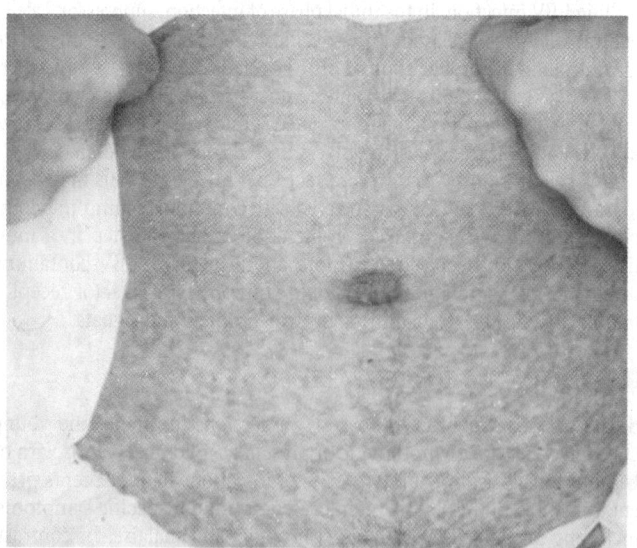

FIGURE 194-1 Rash in a patient with infectious mononucleosis due to Epstein-Barr virus. *(Courtesy of Maria Turner, MD; with permission.)*

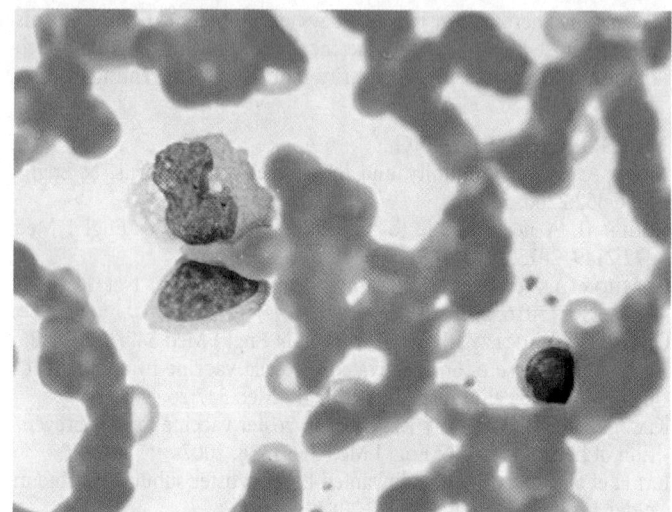

FIGURE 194-2 Atypical lymphocytes from a patient with infectious mononucleosis due to Epstein-Barr virus.

levels of CD8+ T cells and EBV DNA in the blood. Most patients have symptoms for 2–4 weeks, but nearly 10% have fatigue that persists for ≥6 months.

Laboratory Findings The white blood cell count is usually elevated and peaks at 10,000–20,000/μL during the second or third week of illness. Lymphocytosis is usually demonstrable, with >10% atypical lymphocytes. The latter cells are enlarged lymphocytes that have abundant cytoplasm, vacuoles, and indentations of the cell membrane (**Fig. 194-2**). CD8+ T cells predominate among the atypical lymphocytes. Low-grade neutropenia and thrombocytopenia are common during the first month of illness. Liver function is abnormal in >90% of cases. Serum levels of aminotransferases and alkaline phosphatase are usually mildly elevated. The serum concentration of bilirubin is elevated in ~40% of cases.

Complications Most cases of IM are self-limited. Deaths are very rare and are most often due to central nervous system (CNS) complications, splenic rupture, upper-airway obstruction, or bacterial superinfection.

When CNS complications develop, they usually do so during the first 2 weeks of EBV infection; in some patients, especially children, they are the only clinical manifestations of acute infection. Heterophile antibodies and atypical lymphocytes may be absent. Meningitis and encephalitis are the most common neurologic abnormalities, and patients may present with headache, meningismus, or cerebellar ataxia. Acute hemiplegia and psychosis also have been described. The cerebrospinal fluid contains mainly lymphocytes, with occasional atypical lymphocytes. Most cases resolve without neurologic sequelae. Acute EBV infection has also been associated with cranial nerve palsies (especially those involving cranial nerve VII), Guillain-Barré syndrome, acute transverse myelitis, and peripheral neuritis.

Autoimmune hemolytic anemia occurs in ~2% of cases during the first 2 weeks. In most cases, the anemia is Coombs-positive, with cold agglutinins directed against the red blood cell antigen. Most patients with hemolysis have mild anemia that lasts for 1–2 months, but some patients have severe disease with hemoglobinuria and jaundice. Nonspecific antibody responses may also include rheumatoid factor, antinuclear antibodies, anti–smooth muscle antibodies, antiplatelet antibodies, and cryoglobulins. IM has been associated with red-cell aplasia, severe granulocytopenia, thrombocytopenia, pancytopenia, and hemophagocytic lymphohistiocytosis. The spleen ruptures in <0.5% of cases. Splenic rupture is more common among male than female patients and may manifest as abdominal pain, referred shoulder pain, or hemodynamic compromise.

Hypertrophy of lymphoid tissue in the tonsils or adenoids can result in upper-airway obstruction, as can inflammation and edema of the epiglottis, pharynx, or uvula. About 10% of patients with IM develop streptococcal pharyngitis after their initial sore throat resolves.

Other rare complications associated with acute EBV infection include hepatitis (which can be fulminant), myocarditis or pericarditis, pneumonia with pleural effusion, interstitial nephritis, genital ulcerations, and vasculitis.

EBV-Associated Diseases Other Than IM EBV-associated lymphoproliferative disease has been described in patients with congenital or acquired immunodeficiency, including those with severe combined immunodeficiency, patients with AIDS, and recipients of bone marrow or organ transplants who are receiving immunosuppressive drugs (especially cyclosporine). Proliferating EBV-infected B cells infiltrate lymph nodes and multiple organs, and patients present with fever and lymphadenopathy or gastrointestinal symptoms. Pathologic studies show B-cell hyperplasia or poly- or monoclonal lymphoma.

X-linked lymphoproliferative disease is a recessive disorder of young boys who have a normal response to childhood infections but develop fatal lymphoproliferative disorders after infection with EBV. The protein associated with most cases of this syndrome (SAP, encoded by *SH2D1A*) binds to a protein that mediates interactions of B and T cells. Most patients with this syndrome die of acute IM. Others develop hypogammaglobulinemia, malignant B-cell lymphomas, aplastic anemia, or agranulocytosis. Disease resembling X-linked lymphoproliferative disease, but with more prominent hemophagocytosis, has also been associated with mutations in *BIRC4*. Mutations in *ITK*, *MAGT1*, *CORO1A*, *CD70*, or *CD27* are associated with inability to control EBV and lymphoma. Mutations in other genes, such as *GATA2*, *PIK3CD*, *CTPS1*, *RSGRP*1, *TNFRSF9*, and several genes associated with severe combined immunodeficiency, also can predispose to severe or fatal EBV disease as well as other infections. Moreover, IM has proved fatal to some patients with no obvious preexisting immune abnormality.

Oral hairy leukoplakia (**Fig. 194-3**) is an early manifestation of infection with HIV in adults (**Chap. 202**). Most patients present with raised, white corrugated lesions on the tongue (and occasionally on the buccal mucosa) that contain EBV DNA. Children infected with HIV can develop lymphoid interstitial pneumonitis; EBV DNA is often found in lung tissue from these patients.

Patients with chronic fatigue syndrome may have titers of antibody to EBV that are elevated but are not significantly different from those in healthy EBV-seropositive adults. These patients do not have elevated levels of EBV DNA in the blood. While some patients have malaise and fatigue that persist for weeks or months after IM, persistent EBV infection is not a cause of chronic fatigue syndrome. Chronic active EBV infection is very rare and is distinct from chronic fatigue syndrome. The affected patients have an illness lasting >6 months, with elevated levels of EBV DNA in the blood (in T cells, NK cells, or B cells); high titers of antibody to EBV; and evidence of organ involvement, including hepatosplenomegaly, lymphadenopathy, and hepatitis, pneumonitis, uveitis, or neurologic disease. Some have somatic mutations in *DD3X* and other tumor driver genes.

EBV is associated with several malignancies. About 15% of cases of Burkitt's lymphoma in the United States and ~90% of those in Africa are associated with EBV (**Chap. 108**). African patients with Burkitt's lymphoma have high levels of antibody to EBV, and their tumor tissue usually contains viral DNA. Malaria in African patients may impair cellular immunity to EBV and induce polyclonal B-cell activation with an expansion of EBV-infected B cells. In addition, malaria may target B cells and result in expansion of germinal centers, with consequently increased activity of activation-induced cytidine deaminase, which can mutate DNA. These changes may enhance the proliferation of B cells with elevated EBV DNA in the bloodstream, thereby increasing the likelihood of a *c-myc* translocation—the hallmark of Burkitt's lymphoma. EBV-containing Burkitt's lymphoma also occurs in patients with AIDS.

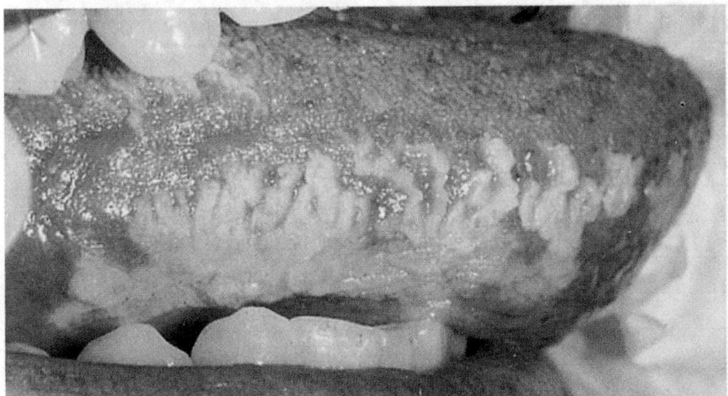

FIGURE 194-3 Oral hairy leukoplakia often presents as white plaques on the lateral surface of the tongue and is associated with Epstein-Barr virus infection.

Anaplastic nasopharyngeal carcinoma is common in southern China and is uniformly associated with EBV; the affected tissues contain viral DNA and antigens. Patients with nasopharyngeal carcinoma often have elevated titers of antibody to EBV (**Chap. 77**). Measurement of EBV DNA in plasma is useful for early detection of nasopharyngeal carcinoma. High levels of EBV plasma DNA before treatment or detectable levels of EBV DNA after radiation therapy correlate with lower rates of overall survival and relapse-free survival among patients with nasopharyngeal carcinoma.

Worldwide, the most common EBV-associated malignancy is gastric carcinoma. About 9% of these tumors are EBV-positive including >90% of gastric lymphoepithelioma-like carcinomas (**Chap. 80**).

EBV has been associated with Hodgkin's lymphoma, especially the mixed-cellularity type (**Chap. 109**). Patients with Hodgkin's lymphoma often have elevated titers of antibody to EBV. In about half of cases in the United States, viral DNA and antigens are found in Reed-Sternberg cells. The risk of EBV-positive Hodgkin's lymphoma is significantly increased in young adults for several years after EBV-seropositive IM. About 50% of non-Hodgkin's lymphomas in patients with AIDS are EBV-positive.

EBV is present in B cells of lesions from patients with lymphomatoid granulomatosis. In some cases, EBV DNA has been detected in tumors from immunocompetent patients with angiocentric nasal NK/T-cell lymphoma, aggressive NK leukemia/lymphoma, T-cell lymphoma, and CNS lymphoma. Studies have demonstrated viral DNA in leiomyosarcomas from AIDS patients and in smooth-muscle tumors from organ transplant recipients. Virtually all CNS lymphomas in AIDS patients are associated with EBV. Studies have found that a history of IM and higher levels of antibodies to EBNA before the onset of disease is more common in persons with multiple sclerosis than in the general population; additional research on a possible causal relationship is needed.

DIAGNOSIS

Serologic Testing (Fig. 194-4) The heterophile test is used for the diagnosis of IM in children and adults. In the test for this antibody, human serum is absorbed with guinea pig kidney, and the heterophile titer is defined as the greatest serum dilution that agglutinates sheep, horse, or cow erythrocytes. The heterophile antibody does not interact with EBV proteins. A titer of ≥40 is diagnostic of acute EBV infection in a patient who has symptoms compatible with IM and atypical lymphocytes. Tests for heterophile antibodies are positive in 40% of patients with IM during the first week of illness and in 80–90% during the third week. Therefore, repeated testing may be necessary, especially if the initial test is performed early. Tests usually remain positive for 3 months after the onset of illness, but heterophile antibodies can persist for up to 1 year. These antibodies usually are not detectable in children <5 years of age, in the elderly, or in patients presenting with symptoms not typical of IM. The commercially available monospot test for heterophile antibodies is somewhat more sensitive than the classic heterophile test. The monospot test is ~75% sensitive and ~90% specific compared with EBV-specific serologies (see below). False-positive monospot results are more common among persons with connective tissue disease, lymphoma, viral hepatitis, and malaria.

EBV-specific antibody testing is used for patients with suspected acute EBV infection who lack heterophile antibodies and for patients with atypical infections. Titers of IgM and IgG antibodies to viral capsid antigen (VCA) are elevated in the serum of >90% of patients

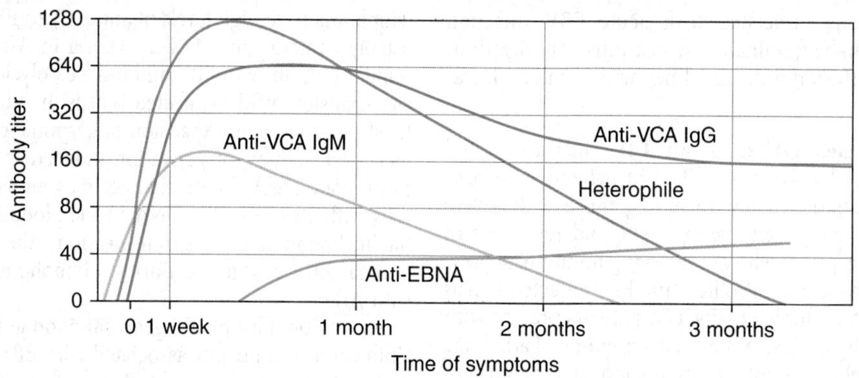

FIGURE 194-4 Pattern of Epstein-Barr virus (EBV) serology during acute infection. EBNA, Epstein-Barr nuclear antigen; VCA, viral capsid antigen. *(Reproduced with permission from JI Cohen, in NS Young et al [eds]: Clinical Hematology. Philadelphia, Mosby, 2006.)*

at the onset of disease. IgM antibody to VCA is most useful for the diagnosis of acute IM because it is present at elevated titers only during the first 2–3 months of the disease; in contrast, IgG antibody to VCA usually is not useful for diagnosis of IM but often is used to assess past exposure to EBV because it persists for life. Seroconversion to EBNA positivity also is useful for the diagnosis of acute infection with EBV. Antibodies to EBNA become detectable relatively late (3–6 weeks after the onset of symptoms) in nearly all cases of acute EBV infection and persist for the lifetime of the patient. These antibodies may be lacking in immunodeficient patients and in those with chronic active EBV disease.

Titers of other antibodies also may be elevated in IM; however, these elevations are less useful for diagnosis. Antibodies to early antigens are detectable 3–4 weeks after the onset of symptoms in patients with IM. About 70% of individuals with IM have antibodies to early antigen diffuse (EA-D) during the illness; the presence of EA-D antibodies is especially likely in patients with relatively severe disease. These antibodies usually persist for only 3–6 months. Levels of EA-D antibodies are elevated in patients with nasopharyngeal carcinoma or chronic active EBV infection. Antibodies to early antigen restricted (EA-R) are often found at elevated titers in patients with African Burkitt's lymphoma or chronic active EBV infection; however, they are not useful for diagnosis. IgA antibodies to EBV antigens have proved useful for the identification of patients with nasopharyngeal carcinoma and of persons at high risk for the disease.

Other Studies Detection of EBV DNA, RNA, or proteins has been valuable in demonstrating the association of the virus with various malignancies. The polymerase chain reaction has been used to detect EBV DNA in the cerebrospinal fluid of some AIDS patients with CNS lymphomas and to monitor the amount of EBV DNA in the blood of patients with lymphoproliferative disease. Detection of high levels of EBV DNA in blood for a few days to several weeks after the onset of IM may be useful if serologic studies yield equivocal results. Culture of EBV from throat washings or blood is not helpful in the diagnosis of acute infection, since EBV persists in the oropharynx and in B cells for the lifetime of the infected individual.

Differential Diagnosis Whereas ~90% of cases of IM are due to EBV, 5–10% of cases are due to cytomegalovirus (CMV) **(Chap. 195)**. CMV is the most common cause of heterophile-negative mononucleosis; less common causes of IM and differences from IM due to EBV are shown in **Table 194-2**.

TREATMENT

EBV-Associated Disease

Therapy for IM consists of supportive measures, with rest and analgesia. Excessive physical activity during the first month should be avoided to reduce the possibility of splenic rupture, which often necessitates splenectomy. Glucocorticoid therapy is not indicated for uncomplicated IM and in fact may predispose to bacterial superinfection. Prednisone (40–60 mg/d for 2–3 days, with subsequent tapering of the dose over 1–2 weeks) has been used for the prevention of airway obstruction in patients with severe tonsillar hypertrophy, for autoimmune hemolytic anemia, for hemophagocytic lymphohistiocytosis, and for severe thrombocytopenia. Glucocorticoids have also been administered to rare patients with severe malaise and fever and to patients with severe CNS or cardiac disease.

Acyclovir has had no significant clinical impact on IM in controlled trials. In one study, the combination of acyclovir and prednisolone had no significant effect on the duration of symptoms of IM.

Acyclovir, at a dosage of 400–800 mg five times daily, has been effective for the treatment of oral hairy leukoplakia (despite

TABLE 194-2 Differential Diagnosis of Infectious Mononucleosis

ETIOLOGY	SIGN OR SYMPTOM: FEVER	ADENOPATHY	SORE THROAT	ATYPICAL LYMPHOCYTES	DIFFERENCES FROM EBV MONONUCLEOSIS
EBV infection	+	+	+	+	—
CMV infection	+	±	±	+	Older age at presentation, longer duration of fever
HIV infection	+	+	+	±	Diffuse rash, oral/genital ulcers, aseptic meningitis
Toxoplasmosis	+	+	±	±	Less splenomegaly; exposure to cats or raw meat
HHV-6 infection	+	+	+	+	Older age at presentation
Streptococcal pharyngitis	+	+	+	–	No splenomegaly, less fatigue
Viral hepatitis	+	±	–	±	Higher aminotransferase levels
Rubella	+	+	±	±	Maculopapular rash, no splenomegaly
Lymphoma	+	+	+	+	Fixed, nontender lymph nodes
Drugs[a]	+	+	–	±	Occurs at any age

[a]Most commonly phenytoin, carbamazepine, sulfonamides, or minocycline.

Abbreviations: CMV, cytomegalovirus; EBV, Epstein-Barr virus; HHV, human herpesvirus.

common relapses). Post-transplantation EBV lymphoproliferative disease (**Chap. 143**) generally does not respond to antiviral therapy. When possible, therapy should be directed toward reduction of immunosuppression. Antibody to CD20 (rituximab) has been effective in some cases. Infusions of donor lymphocytes are often effective for stem cell transplant recipients, although graft-versus-host disease can occur. Infusions of HLA-matched EBV-specific cytotoxic T cells have been used to prevent EBV lymphoproliferative disease in high-risk settings as well as to treat the disease. Interferon α administration, cytotoxic chemotherapy, and radiation therapy (especially for CNS lesions) also have been used. Infusion of autologous EBV-specific cytotoxic T lymphocytes has shown promise in small studies of patients with nasopharyngeal carcinoma and Hodgkin's lymphoma. Treatment of several cases of X-linked lymphoproliferative disease with antibody to CD20 resulted in a successful outcome of what otherwise would probably have been fatal acute EBV infection.

PREVENTION

The isolation of patients with IM is unnecessary. A vaccine directed against the major EBV glycoprotein reduced the frequency of IM but did not affect the rate of asymptomatic infection in a phase 2 trial. Additional vaccines are under development.

FURTHER READING

Chan KCA et al: Analysis of plasma Epstein-Barr virus DNA to screen for nasopharyngeal cancer. N Engl J Med 377:513, 2017.

Chen YP et al: Nasopharyngeal carcinoma. Lancet 394:64, 2019.

Cohen JI et al: Epstein-Barr virus NK and T cell lymphoproliferative disease: Report of a 2018 international meeting. Leuk Lymphoma 61:808, 2020.

Dierickx D, Habermann TM: Post-transplantation lymphoproliferative disorders in adults. N Engl J Med 378:549, 2018.

McLaughlin LP et al: Adoptive T cell therapy for Epstein-Barr virus complications in patients with primary immunodeficiency disorders. Front Immunol 9:556, 2018.

Murray PG, Young LS: An etiological role for the Epstein-Barr virus in the pathogenesis of classical Hodgkin lymphoma. Blood 134:591, 2019.

Tangye SG, Latour S: Primary immunodeficiencies reveal the molecular requirements for effective host defense against EBV infection. Blood 135:644, 2020.

195 Cytomegalovirus and Human Herpesvirus Types 6, 7, and 8

Camille Nelson Kotton, Martin S. Hirsch

CYTOMEGALOVIRUS

DEFINITION

Cytomegalovirus (CMV), which was initially isolated from patients with congenital cytomegalic inclusion disease, is now recognized as an important pathogen in all age groups. In addition to inducing severe birth defects, CMV causes a wide spectrum of disorders in older children and adults, ranging from an asymptomatic subclinical infection to a mononucleosis syndrome in healthy individuals to disseminated disease in immunocompromised patients. Human CMV is one of several related species-specific viruses that cause similar diseases in various animals. All are associated with the production of characteristic enlarged cells—hence the name *cytomegalovirus*.

CMV, a β-herpesvirus, has double-stranded DNA, four species of mRNA, a protein capsid, and a lipoprotein envelope. Like other herpesviruses, CMV demonstrates icosahedral symmetry, replicates in the cell nucleus, and can cause either a lytic and productive or a latent infection. CMV can be distinguished from other herpesviruses by certain biologic properties, such as host range and type of cytopathology. Viral replication is associated with the production of large intranuclear inclusions and smaller cytoplasmic inclusions. CMV appears to replicate in a variety of cell types in vivo; in tissue culture it grows preferentially in fibroblasts. Although there is little evidence that CMV is oncogenic in vivo, it does transform fibroblasts in rare instances, and genomic transforming fragments have been identified.

EPIDEMIOLOGY

CMV has a worldwide distribution. In many regions of the world, nearly all adults are seropositive for CMV, whereas only half of adults in the United States and Canada are seropositive. In regions where the prevalence of CMV antibody is high, immunocompromised adults are more likely to undergo reactivation disease rather than primary infection. Data generated in specific regions should be considered in the context of local seropositivity rates, when appropriate.

Of newborns in the United States, 0.5–2.0% are infected with CMV; the percentages are higher in less developed regions. Communal living and poor personal hygiene facilitate spread. Perinatal and early childhood infections are common. CMV may be present in breast milk, saliva, feces, and urine. Transmission has occurred among young children in day-care centers and has been traced from infected toddler to pregnant mother to developing fetus. When an infected child introduces CMV into a household, 50% of susceptible family members seroconvert within 6 months.

CMV is not readily spread by casual contact but rather requires repeated or prolonged intimate exposure for transmission. In late adolescence and young adulthood, CMV is often transmitted sexually, and asymptomatic carriage in semen or cervical secretions is common. Antibody to CMV is present at detectable levels in a significant proportion of sexually active men and women, who may harbor several strains simultaneously. Transfusion of blood products containing viable leukocytes may transmit CMV, with a frequency of 0.14–10% per unit transfused. Transfusion of leukocyte-reduced or CMV-seronegative blood significantly decreases the risk of CMV transmission.

Once infected, an individual generally carries CMV for life, similar to other herpes viruses. The infection usually remains silent. CMV reactivation syndromes develop more frequently, however, when T lymphocyte–mediated immunity is compromised—for example, after organ transplantation, with lymphoid neoplasms and certain acquired immunodeficiencies (in particular, HIV infection; **Chap. 202**), or during critical illness in intensive care units. Most primary CMV infections in organ transplant recipients (**Chap. 143**) result from transmission via the graft or blood products. In CMV-seropositive transplant recipients, infection results from reactivation of latent virus in the recipients or from infection by a new strain from the donor. CMV infection may be associated with diseases as diverse as coronary artery stenosis and malignant gliomas, although these associations require further validation.

PATHOGENESIS

Congenital CMV infection can result from either primary or reactivation infection of the mother. However, clinical disease in the fetus or newborn is related largely to primary maternal infection (**Table 195-1**). The major factors determining the severity of congenital infection are unclear, although a deficient capacity to produce precipitating antibodies and to mount T-cell responses to CMV is associated with relatively severe disease.

Primary infection with CMV in late childhood or adulthood is often associated with a vigorous T-lymphocyte response that may contribute to the development of a mononucleosis syndrome similar to the sequelae of infection with Epstein-Barr virus (**Chap. 194**). The hallmark of such infection is the appearance of atypical lymphocytes in the peripheral blood; these cells are predominantly activated CD8+

TABLE 195-1 Cytomegalovirus (CMV) Disease in the Immunocompromised Host

POPULATION	RISK FACTORS	PRINCIPAL SYNDROME(S)	TREATMENT	PREVENTION
Fetus	Primary maternal infection/ early pregnancy	Cytomegalic inclusion disease	Ganciclovir followed by valganciclovir for symptomatic neonates	Avoidance of exposure; education of pregnant women about risks
Organ transplant recipient	Seropositivity of donor and/or recipient; potent immunosuppressive regimen; treatment of rejection	Febrile leukopenia (CMV syndrome); gastrointestinal disease; pneumonia	Ganciclovir or valganciclovir, ± CMV immunoglobulin	Prophylaxis with ganciclovir or valganciclovir or preemptive therapy
Hematopoietic stem cell transplant recipient	Graft-vs-host disease; older age of recipient; seropositive recipient; viremia	Pneumonia; gastrointestinal disease	Ganciclovir or valganciclovir or foscarnet, ± CMV immunoglobulin	Prophylaxis with letermovir, ganciclovir, or valganciclovir or preemptive therapy
Person with HIV	<50 CD4+ T cells/μL; CMV seropositivity	Retinitis; gastrointestinal disease; neurologic disease	Ganciclovir, valganciclovir, foscarnet, or cidofovir	Oral valganciclovir

T lymphocytes. Polyclonal activation of B cells by CMV contributes to the development of rheumatoid factors and other autoantibodies during mononucleosis.

Once acquired, CMV persists indefinitely in host tissues. The sites of persistent infection may include multiple cell types and various organs. Transmission via blood transfusion or organ transplantation is due primarily to silent infections in these tissues. If the host's T-cell responses become compromised by disease or by iatrogenic immunosuppression, latent virus can reactivate to cause a variety of syndromes. Chronic antigenic stimulation in the presence of immunosuppression (for example, after organ transplantation) appears to be an ideal setting for CMV activation and CMV disease. Certain particularly potent suppressants of T-cell immunity (e.g., antithymocyte globulin, alemtuzumab) are associated with a high rate of clinical CMV syndromes. CMV may itself contribute to further T-lymphocyte hyporesponsiveness, which often precedes superinfection with other opportunistic pathogens such as bacteria, molds, and *Pneumocystis*.

PATHOLOGY

Cytomegalic cells in vivo (presumed to be infected epithelial cells) are two to four times larger than surrounding cells and often contain an 8- to 10-μm intranuclear inclusion that is eccentrically placed and is surrounded by a clear halo, producing an "owl's eye" appearance. Smaller granular cytoplasmic inclusions are demonstrated occasionally. Cytomegalic cells are found in a wide variety of organs, including the salivary gland, lung, liver, kidney, intestine, pancreas, adrenal gland, and central nervous system.

The cellular inflammatory response to infection consists of plasma cells, lymphocytes, and monocyte-macrophages. Granulomatous reactions occasionally develop, particularly in the liver. Immunopathologic reactions may contribute to CMV disease. Immune complexes have been detected in infected infants, sometimes in association with CMV-related glomerulopathies. Immune-complex glomerulopathy has also been observed in some CMV-infected patients after renal transplantation.

CLINICAL MANIFESTATIONS

Congenital CMV Infection Fetal infections range from subclinical to severe and disseminated. CMV seroconversion rates during pregnancy range from 1% to 7%. Of infants born to mothers with primary CMV infections during pregnancy, 5–20% will develop clinical manifestations, with a mortality rate of ~5%. Petechiae, hepatosplenomegaly, and jaundice are the most common presenting features (60–80% of cases). They can have "blueberry muffin"–like hemorrhagic purpuric eruptions, which when biopsied show histopathology with dermal erythropoiesis. Infections during the first trimester are associated with up to 40–50% of infected neonates developing sensorineural complications. Microcephaly with or without cerebral calcifications, intrauterine growth retardation, and prematurity are reported in 30–50% of cases. Inguinal hernias and chorioretinitis are less common. Laboratory abnormalities include elevated alanine aminotransferase levels in serum, thrombocytopenia, conjugated hyperbilirubinemia, hemolysis, and elevated protein levels in cerebrospinal fluid. The prognosis for severely infected infants is poor, and few survivors escape intellectual or hearing difficulties later in childhood. The differential diagnosis of cytomegalic inclusion disease in infants includes syphilis, toxoplasmosis, bacterial sepsis, and infection with a variety of viruses, including rubella, Zika, or herpes simplex virus.

Most congenital CMV infections are clinically inapparent at birth. Of asymptomatically infected infants, 7–11% develop sensorineural hearing loss over a 5-year period.

Perinatal CMV Infection The newborn may acquire CMV at delivery by passage through an infected birth canal or by postnatal contact with infected breast milk or other maternal secretions. Of infants who are breast-fed for >1 month by seropositive mothers, 40–60% become infected. Iatrogenic transmission can result from blood transfusion; use of leukocyte-reduced or CMV-seronegative blood products for transfusion into low-birth-weight seronegative infants or seronegative pregnant women decreases risk.

The great majority of infants infected at or after delivery remain asymptomatic. However, protracted interstitial pneumonitis has been associated with perinatally acquired CMV infection, particularly in premature infants, and occasionally has been accompanied by infection with *Chlamydia trachomatis*, *Pneumocystis*, or *Ureaplasma urealyticum*. Poor weight gain, adenopathy, rash, hepatitis, anemia, and atypical lymphocytosis may also be found, and CMV excretion often persists for months or years.

CMV Mononucleosis The most common clinical manifestation of CMV infection in immunocompetent hosts beyond the neonatal period is a heterophile antibody–negative mononucleosis syndrome, which may develop spontaneously or follow transfusion of leukocyte-containing blood products. Although the syndrome occurs at all ages, it most often involves sexually active young adults. With incubation periods of 20–60 days, the illness generally lasts for 2–6 weeks. Prolonged high fevers, sometimes with chills, profound fatigue, and malaise, characterize this disorder. Myalgias, headache, and splenomegaly are common, but in CMV mononucleosis (as opposed to Epstein-Barr virus mononucleosis), exudative pharyngitis and cervical lymphadenopathy are rare. Occasional patients develop rubelliform rashes, often after exposure to ampicillin or certain other antibiotics. Less common are interstitial or segmental pneumonia, myocarditis, pleuritis, arthritis, splanchnic vein thrombosis, and encephalitis. In rare cases, Guillain-Barré syndrome complicates CMV mononucleosis. The characteristic laboratory abnormality of CMV mononucleosis is relative lymphocytosis in peripheral blood, with >10% atypical lymphocytes. Total leukocyte counts may be low, normal, or markedly elevated. Although significant jaundice is uncommon, serum aminotransferase and alkaline phosphatase levels are often moderately elevated. Heterophile antibodies are absent; however, transient immunologic abnormalities are common and may include the presence of cryoglobulins, rheumatoid factors, cold agglutinins, and antinuclear antibodies. Hemolytic anemia, thrombocytopenia, and granulocytopenia complicate recovery in rare instances.

Most patients recover without sequelae, although postviral asthenia may persist for months. The excretion of CMV in urine, genital secretions, and/or saliva often continues for months or years. Rarely, CMV infection is fatal in immunocompetent hosts; survivors can have recurrent episodes of fever and malaise, sometimes associated with autonomic nervous system dysfunction (e.g., attacks of sweating or flushing).

CMV Infection in the Immunocompromised Host (Table 195-1) CMV is the most common viral pathogen complicating organ transplantation (**Chap. 143**). In recipients of kidney, heart, lung, liver, pancreas, and vascularized composite (hand, face, other) transplants, CMV infection may result in a variety of clinical manifestations, including fever and leukopenia, hepatitis, colitis, pneumonitis, esophagitis, gastritis, and retinitis. CMV disease is an independent risk factor for both graft loss and death. Without prophylaxis, the period of maximal risk is between 1 and 4 months after transplantation. Disease likelihood and viral replication levels generally are greater after primary infection than after reactivation. Molecular studies indicate that seropositive organ transplant recipients are susceptible to infection with donor-derived, genotypically variant CMV. Reactivation infection, although common, is less likely than primary infection to be clinically significant. The overall risk of clinical disease is related to various factors, such as serologic mismatch (donor seropositive, recipient seronegative), degree of immunosuppression, use of antilymphocyte antibodies, lack of anti-CMV prophylaxis, and co-infection with other pathogens. The transplanted organ is particularly vulnerable as a target for CMV infection; thus, there is a tendency for CMV hepatitis to follow liver transplantation and for CMV pneumonitis to follow lung transplantation.

CMV viremia occurs in roughly one-third of hematopoietic stem cell transplant (HSCT) recipients; the risk of severe disease may be reduced by prophylaxis or preemptive therapy with antiviral drugs. The risk is greatest in the first 100 days after transplantation, and identified risk factors include certain types of immunosuppressive therapy, an allogeneic (rather than an autologous) graft, acute graft-versus-host disease, older age, and recipient seropositivity prior to transplant.

CMV is an important pathogen in patients with advanced HIV infection (**Chap. 202**), in whom it may cause retinitis or disseminated disease, particularly when peripheral-blood CD4+ T-cell counts fall below 50/μL. As treatment for underlying HIV infection has improved, the incidence of serious CMV infections (e.g., retinitis) has decreased. During the first few weeks after institution of highly active antiretroviral therapy, however, acute flare-ups of CMV retinitis may occur secondary to an immune reconstitution inflammatory syndrome.

Syndromes produced by CMV in immunocompromised hosts ("CMV syndrome") often begin with fatigue, fever, malaise, anorexia, night sweats, and arthralgias or myalgias. Liver function abnormalities, leukopenia, thrombocytopenia, and atypical lymphocytosis may be observed during these episodes. Without treatment, CMV infection may progress to more severe end-organ disease. The development of tachypnea, hypoxemia, and nonproductive cough signals respiratory involvement. Radiologic examination of the lung often shows bilateral interstitial or reticulonodular infiltrates that begin in the periphery of the lower lobes and spread centrally and superiorly; localized segmental, nodular, or alveolar patterns are less common. The differential diagnosis includes *Pneumocystis* infection; other viral, bacterial, or fungal infections; pulmonary hemorrhage; and injury secondary to irradiation or to treatment with cytotoxic drugs.

Gastrointestinal CMV involvement may be localized or extensive and almost exclusively affects immunocompromised hosts. Colitis is the most common clinical manifestation in organ transplant recipients. Ulcers of the esophagus, stomach, small intestine, or colon may result in bleeding or perforation. Clinicians should be aware that blood tests such as CMV antigenemia and viral load testing may yield negative results in the setting of intestinal disease. CMV infection may lead to exacerbations of underlying ulcerative colitis. Hepatitis occurs frequently, particularly after liver transplantation. Acalculous cholecystitis and adrenalitis also have been described.

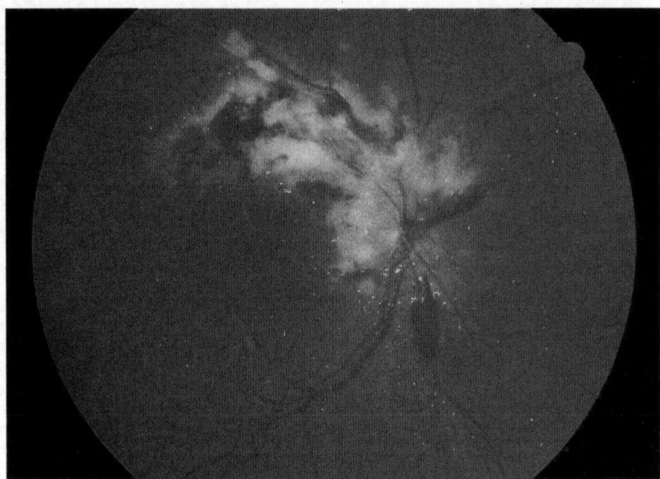

FIGURE 195-1 Cytomegalovirus infection in a patient with AIDS may appear as an arcuate zone of retinitis with hemorrhages and optic disk swelling. Often CMV is confined to the retinal periphery, beyond view of the direct ophthalmoscope.

CMV rarely causes meningoencephalitis in otherwise healthy individuals. Two forms of CMV encephalitis are seen in people with HIV. One resembles HIV encephalitis and presents as progressive dementia; the other is a ventriculoencephalitis characterized by cranial-nerve deficits, nystagmus, disorientation, lethargy, and ventriculomegaly. In immunocompromised patients, CMV can also cause subacute progressive polyradiculopathy, which is often reversible if recognized and treated promptly.

CMV retinitis is an important cause of blindness in immunocompromised patients, particularly patients with advanced AIDS (**Chap. 202**). Early lesions consist of small, opaque, white areas of granular retinal necrosis that spread in a centrifugal manner and are later accompanied by hemorrhages, vessel sheathing, and retinal edema (**Fig. 195-1**). CMV retinopathy must be distinguished from that due to other conditions, including toxoplasmosis, candidiasis, and herpes simplex virus infection.

Fatal CMV infections are often associated with persistent viremia and the involvement of multiple organ systems. Progressive pulmonary infiltrates, pancytopenia, hyperamylasemia, and hypotension are characteristic features that are frequently found in conjunction with a terminal bacterial, fungal, or protozoan superinfection. Extensive adrenal necrosis with CMV inclusions is often documented at autopsy, as is CMV involvement of many other organs.

■ DIAGNOSIS

CMV infection usually cannot be diagnosed reliably on clinical grounds alone. Isolation of CMV or detection of its antigens or DNA in appropriate clinical specimens is the preferred approach. The most common method of detection is quantitative nucleic acid testing (QNAT) for CMV by polymerase chain reaction (PCR) technology, for which blood or other specimens can be used; some centers use a CMV antigenemia test, an immunofluorescence assay that detects CMV antigens (pp65) in peripheral-blood leukocytes. Such assays may yield a positive result several days earlier than culture methods. QNAT may predict the risk for disease progression, particularly in immunocompromised hosts. CMV DNA in cerebrospinal fluid is useful in the diagnosis of CMV encephalitis or polyradiculopathy. Recent introduction of an international testing standard has helped reduce variation in viral load test results.

Virus excretion and/or viremia is readily detected by culture of appropriate specimens on human fibroblast monolayers. If CMV titers are high, as is common in congenital disseminated infection and in AIDS, characteristic cytopathic effects may be detected within a few days. However, in some situations (e.g., CMV mononucleosis), viral titers are low, and cytopathic effects may take several weeks to appear. Many laboratories expedite diagnosis with an overnight tissue-culture method (shell vial assay) involving centrifugation and an immunocytochemical detection technique employing monoclonal antibodies to an immediate-early CMV antigen. Isolation of virus from urine, stool, or saliva does not, by itself, constitute proof of acute infection, since excretion from these sites may continue for months or years after illness. Detection of viremia by QNAT or antigenemia testing is a better predictor of acute infection.

A variety of serologic assays detect antibody to CMV. An increased level of IgG antibody to CMV may not be detectable for up to 4 weeks after primary infection. Detection of CMV-specific IgM is sometimes useful in the diagnosis of recent or active infection; however, circulating rheumatoid factors may result in occasional false-positive IgM tests. Serology is more helpful when used to predict risk of CMV infection and disease in transplant recipients and is not recommended to diagnose acute disease.

PREVENTION

Prevention of CMV infection and disease in organ transplant and HSCT recipients is usually based on one of two methods: universal prophylaxis or preemptive therapy. With universal prophylaxis, antiviral drugs are used for a defined period, often 3 or 6 months. One clinical trial demonstrated that, in CMV-seronegative kidney transplant recipients with seropositive donors, prophylaxis with (val)ganciclovir was more effective at prevention when given for 200 days rather than 100 days. With preemptive therapy, patients are monitored weekly for CMV viremia, and antiviral treatment is initiated once viremia is detected. Because of the bone marrow–suppressive effects of universal prophylaxis, preemptive therapy has been more commonly employed in HSCT recipients; letermovir, which has recently been approved, allows prophylaxis in higher-risk patients. For patients with HIV infection, CMV end-organ disease is best prevented by using antiretroviral therapy sufficient to maintain CD4+ T-cell counts above 100/μL. Primary prophylaxis with ganciclovir or valganciclovir is not recommended.

Several additional measures are useful for the prevention of CMV transmission to CMV-naïve, high-risk patients. The use of CMV-seronegative or leukocyte-depleted blood significantly decreases the rate of transfusion-associated transmission. In a placebo-controlled trial, a CMV glycoprotein B vaccine reduced infection rates among 464 CMV-seronegative women; this outcome raises the possibility that this experimental vaccine will reduce rates of congenital infection, but further studies must validate this approach. A conditionally replication-defective virus, termed V160, is in a phase 2 clinical trial; the vaccine was derived from the AD169 live attenuated virus and genetically modified to restore expression of the gH/gL/pUL128-131 pentameric complex. A CMV glycoprotein B vaccine with MF59 adjuvant appeared effective in reducing the risk and duration of viremia in both seropositive and seronegative renal transplant recipients at risk for CMV infection. CMV immune globulin has been studied in a variety of clinical situations (primary CMV infection in pregnancy, HSCT, solid organ transplantation), with conflicting results, and is used much less often in the era of multiple effective antiviral agents.

Prophylactic acyclovir or valacyclovir at high doses may reduce rates of CMV infection and disease in renal transplant recipients; neither drug is effective in the treatment of active CMV disease.

TREATMENT

Cytomegalovirus Infection

Ganciclovir is a guanosine derivative that has considerably more activity against CMV than its congener acyclovir. After intracellular conversion by a viral phosphotransferase encoded by CMV gene region UL97, ganciclovir triphosphate is a selective inhibitor of CMV DNA polymerase. Several clinical studies have indicated response rates of 70–90% among people with HIV who are given ganciclovir for the treatment of CMV retinitis or colitis. In severe infections (e.g., CMV pneumonia in HSCT recipients), ganciclovir is sometimes combined with CMV immune globulin. Prophylactic or suppressive ganciclovir may be useful in high-risk HSCT or organ transplant recipients (e.g., those who are CMV-seropositive before transplantation). In many people with HIV, persistently low CD4+ T-cell counts, and CMV disease, clinical and virologic relapses occur promptly if treatment with ganciclovir is discontinued. Therefore, prolonged maintenance regimens are recommended for such patients. Resistance to ganciclovir is more common among patients treated for >3 months and is usually related to mutations in the CMV UL97 gene (or, less commonly, the UL54 gene). The advent of CMV genotyping for resistance mutations has made it possible to rapidly obtain information regarding optimal treatment approaches against clinically resistant virus.

Valganciclovir is an orally bioavailable prodrug that is rapidly metabolized to ganciclovir in intestinal tissues and the liver. Approximately 60–70% of an oral dose of valganciclovir is absorbed. An oral valganciclovir dose of 900 mg results in ganciclovir blood levels similar to those obtained with an IV ganciclovir dose of 5 mg/kg. Valganciclovir appears to be as effective as IV ganciclovir for both CMV induction (treatment) and maintenance regimens, also offering the advantage of oral dosing. Furthermore, the adverse event profiles and rates of resistance for the two drugs are similar.

Ganciclovir or valganciclovir therapy for CMV disease consists of a 14- to 21-day induction course (5 mg/kg IV twice daily for ganciclovir or 900 mg PO twice daily for valganciclovir), sometimes followed by maintenance therapy (e.g., valganciclovir, 900 mg/d). Peripheral-blood neutropenia develops in roughly one-quarter of treated patients but may be ameliorated by granulocyte colony-stimulating factor or granulocyte-macrophage colony-stimulating factor. Whether to use maintenance therapy should depend on the overall level of immunocompromise and the risk of recurrent disease. Discontinuation of maintenance therapy should be considered in people with HIV who, while receiving antiretroviral therapy, have a sustained (3- to 6-month) increase in CD4+ T-cell counts to >100/μL. Compared with shorter (6-week) courses, prolonged (6-month) courses of valganciclovir had beneficial effects on hearing and developmental outcomes in infants with congenital CMV infection.

For treatment of CMV retinitis, some clinicians prefer intravitreal injections of ganciclovir or foscarnet (see below) plus oral valganciclovir to intravenous ganciclovir, although no clinical trials have compared these approaches. *Foscarnet* (sodium phosphonoformate) inhibits CMV DNA polymerase. Because this agent does not require phosphorylation to be active, it is also effective against most ganciclovir-resistant isolates. Foscarnet is less well tolerated than ganciclovir and causes considerable toxicity, including renal dysfunction, hypomagnesemia, hypokalemia, hypocalcemia, genital ulcers, dysuria, nausea, and paresthesia. Moreover, foscarnet administration requires the use of an infusion pump and close clinical monitoring. With aggressive hydration and dose adjustments for renal dysfunction, the toxicity of foscarnet can be reduced. The use of foscarnet should be avoided when a saline load cannot be tolerated (e.g., in cardiomyopathy). The approved induction regimen is 60 mg/kg every 8 h for 2 weeks, although 90 mg/kg every 12 h is equally effective and no more toxic. Maintenance infusions should deliver 90–120 mg/kg once daily. No oral preparation is available. Foscarnet-resistant virus may emerge during extended therapy. This drug is used more frequently after HSCT than in other situations to avoid the myelosuppressive effects of ganciclovir; in general, foscarnet is also the first choice for infections with ganciclovir-resistant CMV.

Cidofovir is a nucleotide analogue with a long intracellular half-life that allows intermittent IV administration. Induction regimens of 5 mg/kg weekly for 2 weeks are followed by maintenance regimens of 3–5 mg/kg every 2 weeks. Cidofovir can cause severe nephrotoxicity through dose-dependent proximal tubular cell injury; however, this adverse effect can be tempered somewhat by saline hydration and probenecid. Cidofovir is used primarily for ganciclovir-resistant virus.

Experimental therapies such as maribavir have been reported to be effective for treatment of infection after HSCT and for resistant/refractory CMV infections, for which a phase 3 trial is underway. Letermovir has efficacy for prophylaxis after HSCT but induces rapid development of resistance when used during active infection.

HUMAN HERPESVIRUS (HHV) TYPES 6, 7, AND 8

HHV-6 AND HHV-7

HHV-6 and -7 seropositivity rates are generally high throughout the world. HHV-6 was first isolated in 1986 from peripheral-blood leukocytes of six persons with various lymphoproliferative disorders. Two genetically distinct variants (HHV-6A and HHV-6B) are now recognized. HHV-6 appears to be transmitted by saliva and possibly by genital secretions.

Infection with HHV-6 frequently occurs during infancy as maternal antibody wanes. The peak age of acquisition is 9–21 months; by 24 months, seropositivity rates approach 80%. Older siblings appear to serve as a source of transmission. In addition, congenital infection may occur, and ~1% of newborns are infected with HHV-6; placental infection with HHV-6 has been described. Congenital infection is generally asymptomatic, although subtle neurologic defects have been described. Most postnatally infected children develop symptoms (fever, fussiness, and diarrhea). A minority develop exanthem subitum (roseola infantum; **see Fig. A1-5**), a common illness characterized by fever with subsequent rash. In addition, ~10–20% of febrile seizures without rash during infancy are caused by HHV-6. After initial infection, HHV-6 persists in peripheral-blood mononuclear cells as well as in the central nervous system, salivary glands, and female genital tract.

In older age groups, HHV-6 has been associated with mononucleosis syndromes; in immunocompromised hosts, encephalitis, pneumonitis, syncytial giant-cell hepatitis, and disseminated disease are seen. In transplant recipients, HHV-6 infection may also be associated with graft dysfunction. Acute HHV-6-associated limbic encephalitis has been reported in hematopoietic stem cell transplant recipients and is characterized by memory loss, confusion, seizures, hyponatremia, and abnormal electroencephalographic and MRI results. High plasma loads of HHV-6 DNA in HSCT recipients are associated with allelic-mismatched donors, use of glucocorticoids, delayed monocyte and platelet engraftment, development of limbic encephalitis, and increased all-cause mortality rates. Mesial temporal lobe epilepsy has been associated with HHV-6 infections, and, like many other viruses, HHV-6 has been implicated in the pathogenesis of multiple sclerosis, although further study is needed to distinguish between association and etiology.

HHV-7 was isolated in 1990 from T lymphocytes from the peripheral blood of a healthy 26-year-old man. The virus is frequently acquired during childhood, albeit at a later age than HHV-6. HHV-7 is commonly present in saliva, which is presumed to be the principal source of infection; breast milk and cervical secretions may also carry the virus. Viremia can be associated with either primary or reactivation infection. The most common clinical manifestations of childhood HHV-7 infections are fever and seizures. Some children present with respiratory or gastrointestinal signs and symptoms. An association has been made between HHV-7 and pityriasis rosea, but evidence is insufficient to indicate a causal relationship.

Clustering of HHV-6, HHV-7, and CMV infections in transplant recipients can make it difficult to sort out the roles of the various agents in individual clinical syndromes. HHV-6 and HHV-7 appear to be susceptible to ganciclovir and foscarnet, although definitive evidence of clinical response is lacking.

HHV-8

Unique herpesvirus-like DNA sequences were reported during 1994 and 1995 in tissues derived from Kaposi's sarcoma (KS) and body cavity–based lymphoma occurring in people with HIV. The virus from which these sequences were derived is designated HHV-8 or Kaposi's sarcoma–associated herpesvirus (KSHV). HHV-8, which infects B lymphocytes, macrophages, and both endothelial and epithelial cells, appears to be causally related not only to KS and a subgroup of AIDS-related B cell body cavity–based lymphomas (primary effusion lymphomas) but also to multicentric Castleman disease, a lymphoproliferative disorder of B cells. The association of HHV-8 with several other diseases has been reported but not confirmed.

HHV-8 seropositivity occurs worldwide, with areas of high endemicity influencing rates of disease. Unlike other herpesvirus infections, HHV-8 infection is much more common in some geographic areas (e.g., central and southern Africa) than in others (North America, Asia, northern Europe). In high-prevalence areas, infection occurs in childhood, and seropositivity is associated with families having numerous children who share eating and drinking utensils; HHV-8 may be transmitted in saliva. In low-prevalence areas, infections typically occur in adults, probably with sexual transmission. Concurrent epidemics of HIV-1 and HHV-8 infections among certain populations (e.g., men who have sex with men) in the late 1970s and early 1980s appear to have resulted in the frequent association of AIDS and KS. Transmission of HHV-8 may also be associated with organ transplantation, injection drug use, and blood transfusion; however, transmission via organ transplantation or blood transfusion in the United States appears to be quite rare.

Primary HHV-8 infection in immunocompetent children may manifest as fever and maculopapular rash. Among individuals with intact immunity, chronic asymptomatic infection is the rule, and neoplastic disorders generally develop only after subsequent immunocompromise. Immunocompromised persons with primary infection may present with fever, splenomegaly, lymphoid hyperplasia, pancytopenia, or rapid-onset KS. Quantitative analysis of HHV-8 DNA suggests a predominance of latently infected cells in KS lesions and frequent lytic replication in multicentric Castleman disease. The KS-associated herpesvirus inflammatory cytokine syndrome (KICS)—consisting of fever, lymphadenopathy, hepatosplenomegaly, cytopenias, and high levels of HHV-8, human and viral interleukin 6, and human interleukin 10—has been described in some HIV-infected patients and is associated with a high mortality rate.

Effective antiretroviral therapy for HIV-infected individuals has led to a marked reduction in rates of KS among persons dually infected with HHV-8 and HIV in resource-rich areas. HHV-8 itself is susceptible in vitro to ganciclovir, foscarnet, and cidofovir. A small, randomized, double-blind, placebo-controlled, crossover trial suggested that oral valganciclovir administered once daily reduced HHV-8 replication. However, clinical benefits of valganciclovir or other drugs in HHV-8 infection have not yet been demonstrated. Sirolimus inhibits the progression of dermal KS in kidney transplant recipients while providing effective immunosuppression. Rituximab alone or in combination with chemotherapy can lead to a survival of >90% at 5 years in HHV-8–associated multicentric Castleman's disease.

FURTHER READING

CYTOMEGALOVIRUS

GUNKEL J et al: Outcome of preterm infants with postnatal cytomegalovirus infection. Pediatrics 141:e20170635, 2018.

KIMBERLIN DW et al: Valganciclovir for symptomatic congenital cytomegalovirus disease. N Engl J Med 372:933, 2015.

KOTTON CN et al: The third international consensus guidelines on the management of cytomegalovirus in solid-organ transplantation. Transplantation 102:900, 2018.

LERUEZ-VILLE M et al: Cytomegalovirus infection during pregnancy: State of the science. Am J Obstet Gynecol 223:330, 2020.

PLOTKIN SA et al: The status of vaccine development against the human cytomegalovirus. J Infect Dis 5:S113, 2020.

RAWLINSON WD et al: Congenital cytomegalovirus infection in pregnancy and the neonate: Consensus recommendations for prevention, diagnosis, and therapy. Lancet Infect Dis 17:e177, 2017.

WHITLEY R (ed): Cytomegalovirus infection: Advancing strategies for prevention and treatment. J Infect Dis 221:S1, 2020.

HUMAN HERPESVIRUS (HHV) TYPES 6, 7, AND 8

CESARO S et al: Incidence and outcome of Kaposi sarcoma after hematopoietic stem cell transplantation: A retrospective analysis and a review of the literature, on behalf of infectious diseases working party of EBMT. Bone Marrow Transplant 55:110, 2019.

CRABTREE KL et al: Association of household food- and drink-sharing practices with human herpesvirus 8 seroconversion in a cohort of Zambian children. J Infect Dis 216:842, 2017.

El-Mallawany NK et al: Kaposi sarcoma herpesvirus inflammatory cytokine syndrome-like clinical presentation in human immunodeficiency virus-infected children in Malawi. Clin Infect Dis 69:2022, 2019.

Lurain K et al: Treatment of Kaposi sarcoma herpesvirus-associated multicentric Castleman disease. Hematol Oncol Clin North Am 32:75, 2018.

Madan RP et al: Human herpesvirus 6, 7, and 8 in solid organ transplantation: Guidelines from the American Society of Transplantation Infectious Diseases Community of Practice. Clinical Transplantation 33:e13518, 2019.

196 Molluscum Contagiosum, Monkeypox, and Other Poxvirus Infections

Inger K. Damon

POXVIRUSES

DEFINITION AND ETIOLOGY

Poxviruses are a family of double-stranded DNA viruses whose genomic structure is generally conserved across subfamilies, genera, and species. The central portion of the genome, which can range up to 200 kb, encodes the open reading frames (ORFs) required for replication or packaging of virions. The left and right ends of the genome encode immune evasion genes or host interaction ORFs. The complement of ORFs across different genera is largely responsible for differences in disease manifestations and/or virus host range. Four genera of poxviruses include species that can infect humans; in addition, an incompletely classified poxvirus has been reported to cause human illness. **Table 196-1** identifies these viruses, the majority of which are zoonotic, and lists some of their epidemiologic characteristics.

TABLE 196-1 Poxviruses Causing Infection in Humans

GENUS, SPECIES	GEOGRAPHY	ZOONOTIC CHARACTERISTICS
Orthopoxvirus		
Variola	Eradicated, formerly worldwide	Solely a human pathogen
Monkeypox	Africa	Squirrel species, Gambian rats, and dormice implicated as potential reservoir species; other species effective in transmitting disease to humans (pet North American prairie dogs); can be acquired during hunting/preparation of African wildlife for nutritional protein source
Cowpox	Europe	Rodents as reservoir; outbreaks associated with rodent pet trade; cats also effective transmitters of illness; previously, dairy cow teat lesions linked to human cutaneous lesions
Vaccinia and vaccinia-like viruses (e.g., buffalopox, Cantagalo, Araçatuba)	India and South America	Rodents suspected as a potential reservoir; localized lesions on cattle or other ruminants (e.g., water buffalo for buffalopox) responsible for most human infections
AK2015	United States (Alaska)	Under investigation
Akhmeta	Georgia (country)	Woodmice (*Apodemus* spp.)
Molluscipoxvirus		
Molluscum contagiosum	Worldwide	Thought to be solely a human pathogen; closely related viruses described in other mammals
Parapoxvirus		
Orf	Worldwide	Handling of infected sheep and goats primarily responsible for transmission to humans; fomites?
Pseudocowpox	Worldwide	Handling of infected dairy cattle; fomites?
Bovine papular stomatitis	Worldwide	Handling of infected beef cattle
Deerpox	U.S. deer herds	Handling of infected deer
Sealpox	Seal/pinniped colonies worldwide	Handling of infected pinnipeds
Yatapoxvirus		
Tanapox	Africa	Possible nonhuman primate reservoir
Unclassified poxvirus		
NY-014[a]	United States (New York State)	Unknown

[a]Possibly an orthopoxvirus.

EPIDEMIOLOGY

Most poxviruses that infect humans are spread through contact, not by the respiratory route, and thus are less prone to cause epidemics. The notable exceptions are species of *Orthopoxvirus* (variola and monkeypox viruses), which can be transmitted by both respiratory droplets and direct contact. In what seems to have been a rare circumstance near the end of global efforts to eradicate smallpox, it was reported that the variola virus appeared to transmit via aerosol in a German hospital in Meschede. Monkeypox virus is thought to be transmitted through handling of or other direct contact with infected animals leading to percutaneous or permucosal exposure; it then may spread between humans by either the respiratory or the contact route.

Of concern, increasing numbers of monkeypox cases are reported from countries where the disease is considered endemic, and more numerous outbreaks have been reported in the past few years. Numerous cases have been reported in Nigeria, Cameroon, the Central African Republic, and the Democratic Republic of the Congo over the past 5 years. In some instances, these are the first national reports of the disease since it was identified in humans in the late 1970s and 1980s; thus, the increases may possibly be attributable to greater surveillance efforts. A recent modeling study sponsored by the World Health Organization (WHO) looked at the effective reproductive rate (R0) and suggested that monkeypox may now be a disease capable of spreading as an epidemic through human interactions and that such spread does not require repeated exposures to infected wildlife. This observation is in contradistinction to the findings of WHO-sponsored studies completed in the 1980s as part of the certification of smallpox eradication. This spreading of disease may be, in part, due to waning immunity provided by smallpox (vaccinia virus) vaccine.

Other orthopoxviruses (Table 196-1) are thought to spread only via contact or percutaneous/permucosal exposures to infected animals (or humans). Molluscum contagiosum virus (MCV) likely spreads through direct contact with and percutaneous exposure to another infected human; like variola virus, MCV is considered to be a pathogen of humans only. The epidemiology of tanapox is poorly understood. Simian reservoirs are postulated, and the potential for vector-borne infection is hypothesized. Human infections with parapoxviruses occur through direct contact with and percutaneous exposure to lesions developing at the site of contact. Other epidemiologic factors are outlined in Table 196-1.

PATHOGENESIS

The pathogenesis of *Orthopoxvirus* infections is thought to involve systemic spread of disease from the site of virus inoculation to local lymph nodes, a subsequent phase in which additional lymphoreticular tissues are seeded, and finally the development of symptomatic (febrile) viremia that seeds the skin. The severity of disease is affected by the degree to which the innate immune and interferon responses control the initial stages of infection. In immunocompromised persons, more severe systemic manifestations are seen. A case in point involves the adverse events associated with smallpox (vaccinia virus) vaccination. Individuals with intact immune systems develop a lesion at the inoculation site 3–4 days after vaccination; this lesion becomes vesicular and pustular 7–10 days after inoculation. In some instances, lymphangitis, lymphadenopathy, and/or fever are noted. After 14 days, the lesion begins to scab over. In contrast, persons with atopic dermatitis or eczema can develop eczema vaccinatum, and those with immunosuppression or immunocompromise can develop progressive vaccinia. In these instances, the spread or growth of the vaccinia virus goes unchecked, and systemic spread of disease or progressive growth of the virus-induced lesion (the latter without an inflammatory response) is noted. Generalized vaccinia, with dissemination of the rash, has been documented in HIV/AIDS patients. Inflammatory rash responses are often misclassified as generalized vaccinia. Other poxvirus infections—with the possible exception of *Yatapoxvirus* infection, in which disease pathogenesis is poorly understood—likely involve only local growth of the virus at the site of inoculation or reinoculation. In some immunocompromised hosts, the lesions caused by *Parapoxvirus* infections can become quite large; such lesions are referred to as "giant orf."

APPROACH TO THE PATIENT

Poxviruses

Usually the patient presents to the clinician with nodular or vesiculopustular lesions. Important elements of the history are travel, occupation (with greater risk in laboratory workers, farmers, hunters, and health care workers), how the lesions have progressed, and the history of fever with respect to rash onset. During the patient's assessment, contact precautions should be used, and if monkeypox or smallpox is being considered, respiratory precautions, including use of a negative-pressure isolation room, should be implemented.

CLINICAL MANIFESTATIONS

The first clinical sign of systemic poxvirus infection is fever, which is followed by rash onset days later. With systemic *Orthopoxvirus* infections (specifically, smallpox and monkeypox), the rash evolves through classic macular, papular, vesicular, and pustular phases (the last with umbilication). A centrifugal distribution, with lesions more prominent on the extremities than on the trunk (**Fig. 196-1**), is classic. Lesions are often prominent on the palms of the hands, the soles of the feet, and the face. Secondary or tertiary fever can develop; tertiary fever is sometimes a hallmark of bacterial superinfection. Once the lesions scab over and the scabs separate from the skin, the patient is no longer infectious. Patients infected with tanapox virus initially present with a very high fever, are often thought to have malaria, and later develop 1–10 nodular lesions. Other *Orthopoxvirus* infections are more localized in their presentation, with lesions likely developing directly at the site of contact with the virus. Akhmeta, AK2015, vaccinia, and cowpox virus infections are typically associated with a localized rash or lesion. In immunocompromised patients, presentation of these *Orthopoxvirus* infections can be protracted or disseminated.

Individuals infected with other poxviruses that cause localized disease (parapoxviruses and MCV) seldom report a febrile phase and instead notice the slow and gradual development of a nodular-papular lesion or lesions. The lesion of molluscum contagiosum has a classic pearly appearance. "Giant" *Parapoxvirus* infections have been reported in immunocompromised individuals. MCV infections are painless, without an obvious accompanying inflammatory response; they persist but then gradually regress after 6–12 months. The differential diagnosis in poxvirus infections includes varicella, yaws, papillomavirus infection, and (particularly in *Parapoxvirus* infections) cutaneous anthrax.

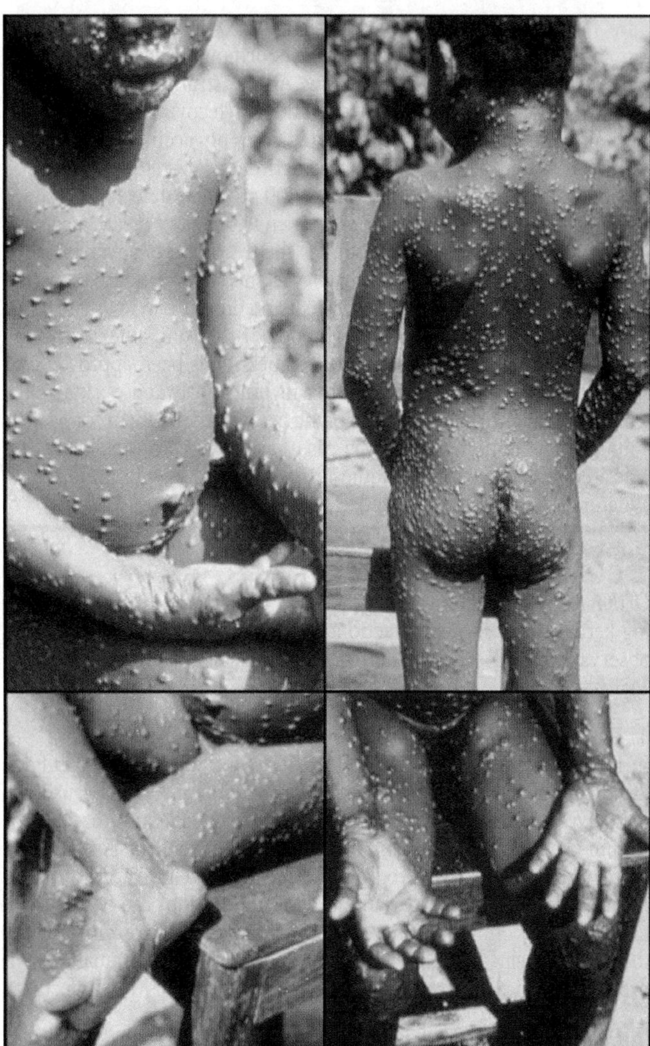

FIGURE 196-1 These images from 1997 were obtained during an investigation into an outbreak of monkeypox that took place in the Democratic Republic of the Congo (formerly Zaire). These photographs from the World Health Organization show the face, back, feet, and hands of a young boy with the characteristic maculopapular cutaneous rash of monkeypox, which is similar in appearance to the rash caused by smallpox virus. *(Source: Centers for Disease Control and Prevention.)*

DIAGNOSIS

Currently, the most common laboratory tool for diagnosis of poxvirus infection involves nucleic acid testing. Nucleic acid–based diagnostics include polymerase chain reaction and sequencing to fully characterize the isolate in some cases. This technology has led to the identification of a number of new poxviruses that can cause human infection, including Akhmeta, AK2015, and NY-014. The orthopoxviruses grow well in most standard clinical laboratory tissue cultures. The parapoxviruses are difficult to isolate via culture (primary cells are best), and MCV cannot be cultured. Electron microscopy identifies the characteristic large, brick-shaped virus particles on negative stain if *Orthopoxvirus*, *Yatapoxvirus*, or MCV is present. Parapoxviruses have an ovoid structure with crisscross spicules on negative-stain electron microscopy. MCV has a classic appearance, with Henderson-Patterson bodies, on pathologic analysis of a biopsy sample. Serologic assays can demonstrate orthopoxvirus reactivity, but most are unable to distinguish between *Orthopoxvirus* species because of their broad antigenic similarity.

TREATMENT

Poxvirus

Treatment of poxvirus infections is largely supportive and aims to avoid secondary bacterial infection if substantial areas of the skin are involved. Recently, as part of smallpox preparedness efforts, an antiviral agent active against the orthopoxviruses has been approved by the U.S. Food and Drug Administration (FDA) for the treatment of smallpox. This drug, TPOXX (tecovirimat), has been used investigationally to treat isolated cases of vaccinia virus infection associated with smallpox vaccination or laboratory exposure. The recommended dose for adults is 600 mg twice daily for 14 days. Bioavailability is best if the drug is taken with a fatty meal. Vaccinia immune globulin is also licensed for the treatment of adverse reactions to smallpox (vaccinia virus) vaccine. The standard dose is 6000 U/kg IV; dosing can be repeated, and doses of up to 9000 U/kg can be used. For treatment of orthopoxviruses, one other antiviral drug—brincidofovir (trade name Tembexa) has been approved by the FDA for treatment of smallpox in June 2021, and cocktails of monoclonal antibodies are also being assessed. Treatment for MCV infection is done on a case-by-case basis if quicker resolution is desired; curettage, topical liquid nitrogen, and some immunomodulators have been investigated.

COMPLICATIONS

Orthopoxvirus infections can often seed tissues around the eye, causing keratitis and corneal infections that can lead to blindness. Careful observation of the eye should be undertaken. Trifluridine is active against ocular infections.

PROGNOSIS

In immunocompetent hosts, most poxvirus infections are self-limited; the exceptions are the generalized *Orthopoxvirus* infections caused by monkeypox virus and variola virus, whose case–fatality rates are 2–30%. Immunocompromised hosts may have more severe *Orthopoxvirus* and *Parapoxvirus* infections (progressive vaccinia, eczema vaccinatum) or atypical presentations (e.g., giant orf). MCV infections can be diffuse in immunocompromised persons. In AIDS patients, effective antiretroviral therapy will help clear MCV. Immune reconstitution inflammatory syndrome (IRIS) has been associated with recrudescence of MCV infections.

PREVENTION

Awareness of occupational risks and institution of appropriate barrier precautions effectively prevent most poxvirus infections. For prevention of *Orthopoxvirus* infections, vaccination with vaccinia virus (smallpox vaccine) is at least 85% effective. During the smallpox eradication era, administration of a qualified vaccine 3–5 years earlier was viewed as 100% protective. During monkeypox surveillance efforts in Zaire (now the Democratic Republic of the Congo) in the 1980s, vaccination 3–19 years earlier was 85% protective against disease among household contacts of monkeypox patients. The duration of efficacy is unclear. These estimates of protection were developed for the replicative forms of vaccinia virus–based smallpox vaccines. A new replication-deficient *Orthopoxvirus* vaccine, JYNNEOS, has been licensed in the United States for the prevention of smallpox and monkeypox disease. This vaccine, which undergoes no more than one round of replication in mammalian cells, is less reactogenic than the historic, replication-competent vaccinia virus–based smallpox vaccines.

SELECT POXVIRUS INFECTIONS

MOLLUSCUM CONTAGIOSUM

Molluscum contagiosum virus is likely the most common poxvirus infection that will be seen by practitioners in the United States. Disease is transmitted through contact, usually through nonintact skin. Children are affected, likely transmitting disease through play activities. In HIV or AIDS patients, disease can be severe. Genital involvement can be seen in adults. Clinical disease is usually recognized by the development of flesh-colored papules, sometimes umbilicated as they mature. Little inflammation surrounds the painless lesions. Diagnosis is usually made by the classic presentation (umbilication can be used to differentiate from papilloma virus infections). However, skin biopsies of lesions will demonstrate a characteristic pathology, and PCR tests are also available for diagnostic verification. Clinical management varies; there is no specific systemic treatment. Various localized measures have been attempted—whether physical methods to remove the lesions or use of topical immunomodulatory agents (imiquimod). With HIV/AIDS, a successful antiretroviral regimen that reconstitutes the immune response is usually sufficient to clear the virus. Clearance in immunocompetent hosts can take months. Simple barrier precautions can prevent transmission of the virus infection.

MONKEYPOX VIRUS

Monkeypox disease is endemic in regions of western and central Africa and has been exported outside of Africa a number of times in the past 20 years. Both exported disease and endemic disease have occurred in those who have had contact with infected animals and contact with or respiratory exposure to other humans with disease. The infected individual will likely seek medical attention when classic vesiculopustular lesions develop. These lesions—which manifest at least a week after a fever and that may be attributed to a flulike illness—develop at least 2 weeks after the initial exposure to infection. Lesions can be sparse or profuse in number. As discussed previously, a centrifugal distribution is usually seen, and palms and soles can also be affected. Lesions on the face should be carefully evaluated, especially if near the eye; conjunctival involvement can result in corneal involvement with blindness as a sequela. Death was reported in up to 10% of unvaccinated (with a prior smallpox vaccination) individuals in an African study performed in the 1980s; all deaths were in children under the age of 6. Diagnosis at the rash stage of illness is easily achieved through evaluation of scrapings from a rash lesion or the scab from a healing rash lesion. High levels of virus can be found and can be detected through PCR analysis of the primary material or cultures derived from the scrapings or scab. Although there is no licensed treatment in the United States, TPOXX—licensed for the treatment of smallpox—has activity against monkeypox virus and other orthopoxviruses and has shown treatment benefit in animals challenged with monkeypox. The Centers for Disease Control and Prevention holds an Investigational New Drug license for the use of the product to treat human laboratory-confirmed monkeypox disease. JYNNEOS is an U.S. Food and Drug Administration-licensed vaccine for the prevention of monkeypox disease.

OTHER POXVIRUS INFECTIONS OF HUMANS

With respect to other poxvirus infections (and with the exception of tanapox disease, which may have an arthropod vector), most other poxvirus infections are initially acquired through exposure and contact with an animal's infection. Tanapox has rarely been seen in the United States and is seen mostly in travelers returning from West or Central Africa. The *Orthopoxvirus* infections caused by cowpox and the vaccinia-like viruses are typically acquired initially through contact with an infected animal. Human-to-human transmission can also occur via contact with the lesion(s) of the infected human. In Europe, human cowpox infections have recently been associated with the pet rat trade, and vaccinia-like viruses (e.g., Belo Horizonte, Cantagalo, Aracatuba) are reported in handlers of dairy cattle in South America. Similarly buffalopox has been reported in those inhabitants of the Indian subcontinent exposed to infectious lesions on water buffalo. In the United States, vaccinia, the virus known as the substrate for smallpox vaccine, has caused infections in laboratory workers studying the virus in the laboratory. Parapoxviruses are only spread to humans through contact with an infected animal's lesions.

Characterization of the rash can help to identify the source of the poxvirus infection. The rash lesions of tanapox are nodular, develop days after a high fever, and are initially often thought to be symptomatic of malaria. The rash lesions of *Parapoxvirus* infections begin as erythematous papules, develop into a "target" lesion, and then become nodular and papilloma-like. *Orthopoxvirus* lesions develop through classical popular, vesicular and pustular phases before scabbing. Laboratory diagnoses can be achieved through scrapings of the rash or the scab and nucleic acid analyses of the material; common approaches are to use PCR or sequencing methods.

Treatment of the lesions is usually supportive; the aim is preventing secondary bacterial infections. Orthopoxvirus infections may be amenable to investigational treatment with TPOXX or brincidofovir. As mentioned above, vaccinia immune globulin is licensed for the treatment of vaccinia infections.

FURTHER READING

Beer EM, Rao VB: A systematic review of the epidemiology of human monkeypox outbreaks and implications for outbreak strategy. PLoS Negl Trop Dis 13:e0007791, 2019.

Meza-Romero R et al: Molluscum contagiosum: An update and review of new perspectives in etiology, diagnosis, and treatment. Clin Cosmet Investig Dermatol 12:373, 2019.

197 Parvovirus Infections

Kevin E. Brown

Parvoviruses, members of the family Parvoviridae, are small (diameter, ~22 nm), nonenveloped, icosahedral viruses with a linear single-strand DNA genome of ~5000 nucleotides. These viruses are dependent on either rapidly dividing host cells or helper viruses for replication. At least five groups of parvoviruses infect humans: parvovirus B19 (B19V), dependoparvoviruses (adeno-associated viruses; AAVs), human tetraparvoviruses (PARV4 and PARV5), human bocaparvoviruses (HBoVs), and human protoparvoviruses (bufavirus, tusavirus, and cutavirus). Human dependoparvoviruses are nonpathogenic and will not be considered further in this chapter.

PARVOVIRUS B19

DEFINITION

B19V is the type member of the genus *Erythroparvovirus*. On the basis of viral sequence, B19V is divided into three genotypes (designated 1, 2, and 3), but only a single B19V antigenic type has been described. Genotype 1 is predominant in most parts of the world; genotype 2 is rarely associated with active infection; and genotype 3 appears to predominate in parts of western Africa.

EPIDEMIOLOGY

B19V exclusively infects humans, and infection is endemic in virtually all parts of the world. Transmission occurs predominantly via the respiratory route and is followed by the onset of rash and arthralgia. By the age of 15 years, ~50% of children have detectable IgG antibody to B19V; this figure rises to >90% among the elderly. In pregnant women, the estimated annual seroconversion rate is ~1%. Within households, secondary infection rates approach 50%.

Detection of high-titer B19V in blood is not unusual (see "Pathogenesis," below). Transmission can occur as a result of transfusion, most commonly of pooled components. To reduce the risk of transmission, plasma pools are screened by nucleic acid amplification technology, and high-titer pools are discarded. B19V is resistant to both heat and solvent-detergent inactivation.

PATHOGENESIS

B19V replicates primarily in erythroid progenitors. This specificity is due in part to the limited tissue distribution of the primary B19V receptor, blood group P antigen (globoside). Infection leads to high-titer viremia, with $>10^{12}$ virus particles (or IU)/mL detectable in the blood at the apex (**Fig. 197-1**), and virus-induced cytotoxicity results

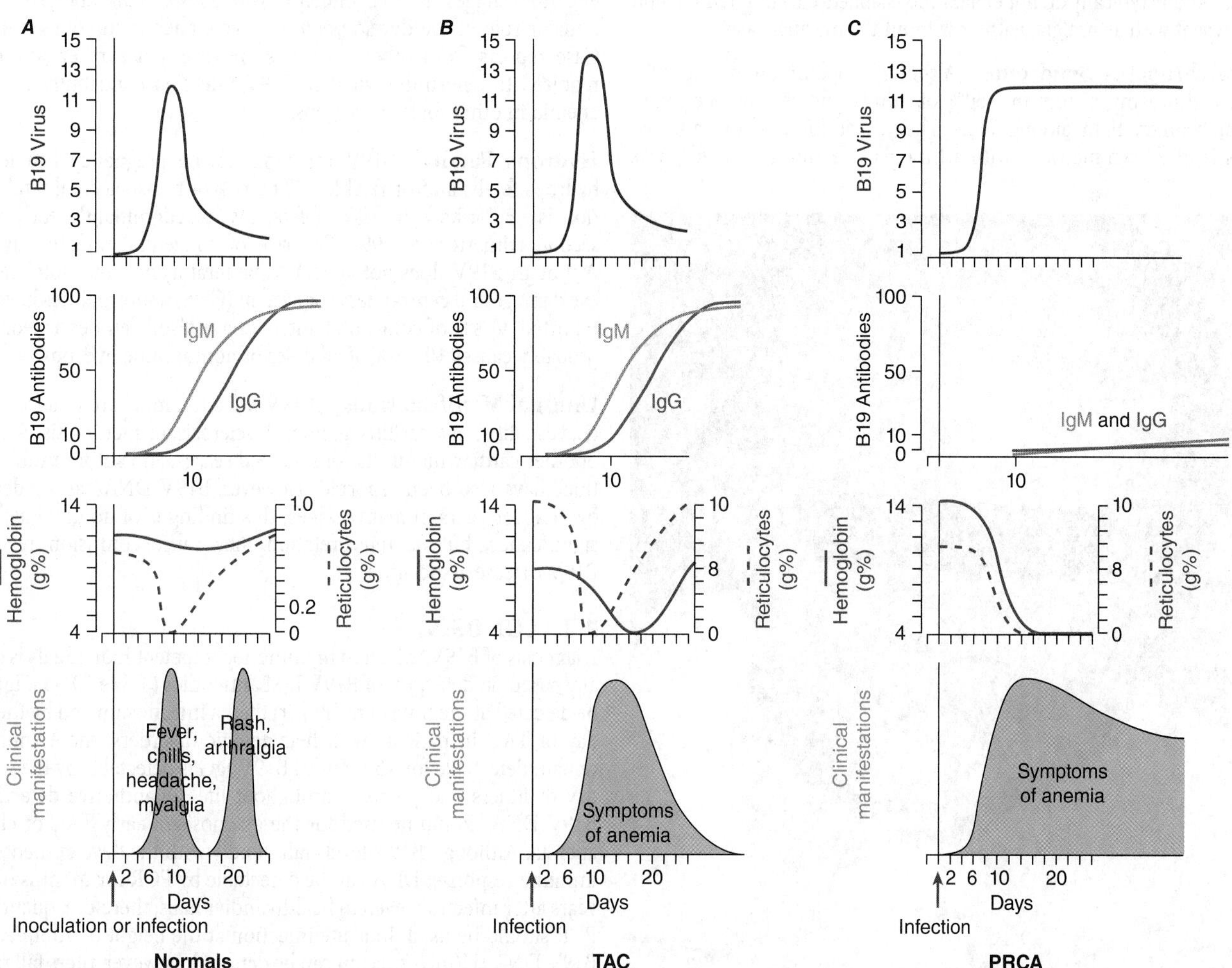

FIGURE 197-1 Schematic of the time course of parvovirus B19 infection in (***A***) normals (erythema infectiosum), (***B***) transient aplastic crisis (TAC), and (***C***) chronic anemia/pure red cell aplasia (PRCA). *(From NS Young, KE Brown: Parvovirus B19. N Engl J Med 350:586, 2004. Copyright © 2004 Massachusetts Medical Society. Reprinted with permission from Massachusetts Medical Society.)*

in cessation of red cell production. In immunocompetent individuals, viremia and arrest of erythropoiesis are transient and resolve as the IgM and IgG antibody response is mounted. In individuals with normal erythropoiesis, there is only a minimal drop in hemoglobin levels; however, in those with increased erythropoiesis (especially with hemolytic anemia), this cessation of red cell production can induce a transient crisis with severe anemia (Fig. 197-1). Similarly, if an individual (or, after maternal infection, a fetus) does not mount a neutralizing antibody response and halt the lytic infection, erythroid production is compromised and chronic anemia develops (Fig. 197-1).

The immune-mediated phase of illness, which begins 2–3 weeks after infection as the IgM response peaks, manifests as the rash of fifth disease together with arthralgia and/or frank arthritis. Low-level B19V DNA can be detected by polymerase chain reaction (PCR) in blood and tissues for months to years after acute infection. The B19V receptor is found in a variety of other cells and tissues, including megakaryocytes, endothelial cells, placenta, myocardium, and liver. Infection of these tissues by B19V may be responsible for some of the more unusual presentations of the infection. Rare individuals who lack P antigen are naturally resistant to B19V infection.

CLINICAL MANIFESTATIONS

Erythema Infectiosum Most B19V infections are asymptomatic or are associated with only a mild nonspecific illness. The main manifestation of symptomatic B19V infection is erythema infectiosum, also known as *fifth disease* or *slapped-cheek disease* (**Figs. 197-2 and A1-1A**). Infection begins with a minor febrile prodrome ~7–10 days after exposure, and the classic facial rash develops several days later; after 2–3 days, the erythematous macular rash may spread to the extremities in a lacy reticular pattern. However, its intensity and distribution vary, and B19V-induced rash is difficult to distinguish from other viral exanthems. Adults typically do not exhibit the "slapped-cheek" phenomenon but present with arthralgia, with or without the macular rash.

Polyarthropathy Syndrome Although uncommon among children, arthropathy occurs in ~50% of adults and is more common among women than among men. The distribution of the affected joints is often symmetrical, with arthralgia affecting the small joints of the hands and occasionally the ankles, knees, and wrists. Resolution usually occurs within a few weeks, but recurring symptoms can continue for months. The illness may mimic rheumatoid arthritis, and rheumatoid factor can often be detected in serum. B19V infection may trigger rheumatoid disease in some patients and has been associated with juvenile idiopathic arthritis.

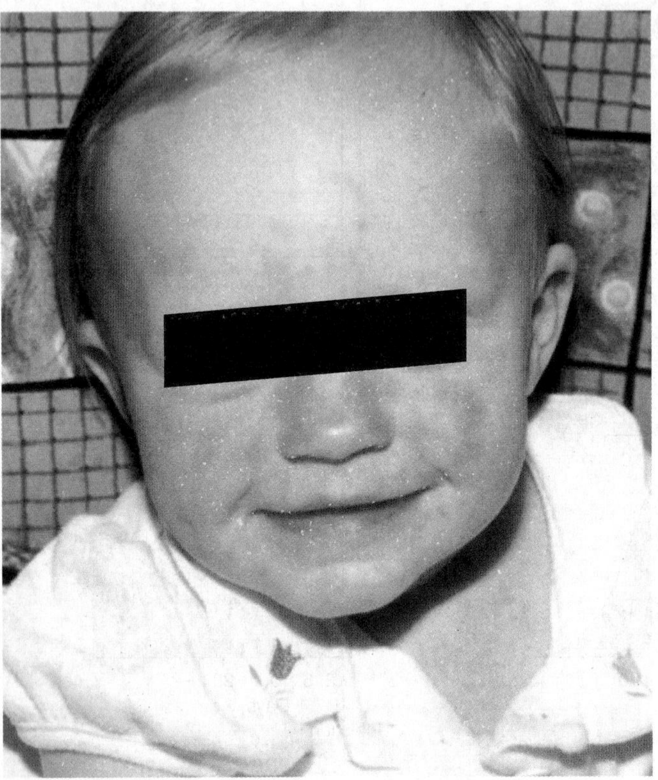

FIGURE 197-2 Young child with erythema infectiosum, or fifth disease, showing typical "slapped-cheek" appearance.

Transient Aplastic Crisis Asymptomatic transient reticulocytopenia occurs in most individuals with B19V infection. However, in patients who depend on continual rapid production of red cells, infection can cause transient aplastic crisis (TAC). Affected individuals include those with hemolytic disorders, hemoglobinopathies, red cell enzymopathies, and autoimmune hemolytic anemias. Patients present with symptoms of severe anemia (sometimes life-threatening) and a low reticulocyte count, and bone marrow examination reveals an absence of erythroid precursors and characteristic giant pronormoblasts. As its name indicates, the illness is transient, and anemia resolves with the cessation of cytopathic infection in the erythroid progenitors.

Pure Red Cell Aplasia/Chronic Anemia Chronic B19V infection has been reported in a wide range of immunosuppressed patients, including those with congenital immunodeficiency, AIDS (**Chap. 202**), lymphoproliferative disorders (especially acute lymphocytic leukemia), and transplantation (**Chap. 143**). Patients have persistent anemia with reticulocytopenia, absent or low levels of B19V IgG, high titers of B19V DNA in serum, and—in many cases—scattered giant pronormoblasts in bone marrow. Rarely, nonerythroid hematologic lineages also are affected. Transient neutropenia, lymphopenia, and thrombocytopenia (including idiopathic thrombocytopenic purpura) have been observed. B19V occasionally causes a hemophagocytic syndrome.

Studies in Papua New Guinea, Gabon, and Ghana, where malaria is endemic, suggest that co-infection with *Plasmodium* and B19V plays a major role in the development of severe anemia in young children. Case reports from other countries are rare, but further studies are required to determine whether B19V infection contributes to severe anemia in other malarial regions.

Hydrops Fetalis B19V infection during pregnancy can lead to hydrops fetalis and/or fetal loss. The risk of transplacental fetal infection is ~30%, and the risk of fetal loss (predominantly early in the second trimester) is ~9%. The risk of congenital infection is <1%. Although B19V does not appear to be teratogenic, anecdotal cases of eye damage and central nervous system (CNS) abnormalities have been reported. Cases of congenital anemia have also been described. B19V probably causes 10–20% of all cases of nonimmune hydrops.

Unusual Manifestations B19V infection may rarely cause hepatitis, vasculitis, myocarditis, glomerulosclerosis, or meningitis. A variety of other cardiac manifestations, CNS diseases, and autoimmune infections have also been reported. However, B19V DNA can be detected by PCR for years in many tissues; this finding is of no known clinical significance, but its interpretation may cause confusion regarding B19V disease association.

DIAGNOSIS

Diagnosis of B19V infection in immunocompetent individuals is generally based on detection of B19V IgM antibodies (**Table 197-1**). IgM can be detected at the time of rash in erythema infectiosum and by the third day of TAC in patients with hematologic disorders; these antibodies remain detectable for ~3 months. B19V IgG is detectable by the seventh day of illness and persists throughout life. Quantitative detection of B19V DNA should be used for the diagnosis of early TAC or chronic anemia. Although B19V levels fall rapidly with the development of the immune response, DNA can be detectable by PCR for months or even years after infection, even in healthy individuals; therefore, quantitative PCR should be used. In acute infection at the height of viremia, $>10^{12}$ B19V DNA IU/mL of serum can be detected; however, titers fall rapidly within 2 days. Patients with aplastic crisis or B19V-induced chronic anemia generally have $>10^5$ B19V DNA IU/mL.

TABLE 197-1 Diseases Associated with Human Parvovirus B19 Infection and Methods of Diagnosis

DISEASE	HOSTS	IgM	IgG	PCR	QUANTITATIVE PCR
Fifth disease	Healthy children	Positive	Positive	Positive	>10^4 IU/mL
Polyarthropathy syndrome	Healthy adults (more often women)	Positive within 3 months of onset	Positive	Positive	>10^4 IU/mL
Transient aplastic crisis	Patients with increased erythropoiesis	Negative/positive	Negative/positive	Positive	Often >10^{12} IU/mL, but rapidly decreases
Persistent anemia/pure red cell aplasia	Immunodeficient or immunocompetent patients	Negative/weakly positive	Negative/weakly positive	Positive	Often >10^{12} IU/mL, but should be >10^6 in the absence of treatment
Hydrops fetalis/congenital anemia	Fetuses (<20 weeks)	Negative/positive	Positive	Positive amniotic fluid or tissue	n/a

Abbreviations: IU, international units (1 IU equals ~1 genome); n/a, not applicable; PCR, polymerase chain reaction.

TREATMENT

Parvovirus B19 Infection

No antiviral drug effective against B19V is available, and treatment of B19V infection often targets symptoms only. TAC precipitated by B19V infection frequently necessitates symptom-based treatment with blood transfusions. In patients receiving chemotherapy, temporary cessation of treatment may result in an immune response and resolution. If this approach is unsuccessful or not applicable, commercial immune globulin (IVIg; Gammagard, Sandoglobulin) from healthy blood donors can cure or ameliorate persistent B19V infection in immunosuppressed patients. Generally, the dose used is 400 mg/kg daily for 5–10 days. Like patients with TAC, immunosuppressed patients with persistent B19V infection should be considered infectious. Administration of IVIg is not beneficial for erythema infectiosum or B19V-associated polyarthropathy. Intrauterine blood transfusion can prevent fetal loss in some cases of fetal hydrops.

PREVENTION

No vaccine has been approved for the prevention of B19V infection, although vaccines based on B19V virus-like particles expressed in insect cells are known to be highly immunogenic. Phase 1 trials of a putative vaccine were discontinued because of adverse side effects.

HUMAN TETRAPARVOVIRUSES (PARV4/5)

DEFINITION

The PARV4 viral sequence was initially detected in a patient with an acute viral syndrome. Similar sequences, including the related PARV5 sequence, have been detected in pooled plasma collections. The DNA sequence of PARV4/5 is distinctly different from that of all other parvoviruses, and this virus is now classified as a member of the newly described genus *Tetraparvovirus.*

EPIDEMIOLOGY

PARV4 DNA is commonly found in plasma pools but at lower concentrations than the levels of B19V DNA found before in plasma pools prior to screening. The higher levels of PARV4 DNA and IgG antibody in tissues (bone marrow and lymphoid tissue) and sera from IV drug users than in the corresponding specimens from control patients suggest that the virus is transmitted predominantly by parenteral means in the United States and Europe. Evidence for nonparenteral transmission in other parts of the world is limited.

CLINICAL MANIFESTATIONS

To date, PARV4/5 infection has been associated only with mild clinical disease (rash and/or transient aminotransferase elevation).

HUMAN BOCAPARVOVIRUSES

DEFINITION

Animal bocaparvoviruses are associated with mild respiratory symptoms and enteritis in young animals. Human bocavirus 1 (HBoV1) was originally identified in the respiratory tract of young children with lower respiratory tract infections. More recently, HBoV1 and the related viruses HBoV2, HBoV3, and HBoV4 have all been identified in human fecal samples.

EPIDEMIOLOGY

Seroepidemiologic studies with HBoV virus-like particles suggest that HBoV infection is common. Worldwide, most individuals are infected before the age of 5 years.

CLINICAL MANIFESTATIONS

HBoV1 DNA is found in respiratory secretions from 2–20% of children with acute respiratory infection, often in the presence of other pathogens; in these circumstances, the role of HBoV1 in disease pathogenesis is unknown. Clinical disease due to HBoV1 is associated with evidence of primary infection (IgG seroconversion or the presence of IgM), HBoV1 DNA in serum, or high-titer HBoV1 DNA (>10^4 genome copies/mL) in respiratory secretions. Symptoms are not dissimilar from those of other viral respiratory infections, and cough and wheezing are commonly reported. There is no specific treatment for HBoV infection. The role of HBoVs in childhood gastroenteritis remains to be established.

HUMAN PROTOPARVOVIRUSES

DEFINITION

Bufavirus, tusavirus, and cutavirus were all identified in clinical samples by a metagenomics approach used for identifying new pathogens. These viruses are classified as members of the *Protoparvovirus* group along with the original prototype member of the Parvoviridae, minute virus of mice.

EPIDEMIOLOGY

Little is known about the epidemiology of these viruses. Antibodies against bufavirus were very low in Finland and the United States (<4%) but >50% in countries like Iraq, Iran, and Kenya. In contrast, antibodies against cutavirus were only found in <6% of all populations and tusavirus antibodies in none. To date, tusavirus has been identified in only a single patient with diarrhea in Tunisia, and it is not clear if it is a human pathogen.

CLINICAL MANIFESTATIONS

Although bufavirus DNA is found in 0.2–4% of stools from children and adults with diarrhea in many countries, often it is detected in conjunction with other viruses. The role of bufavirus in childhood gastroenteritis remains to be confirmed. Similarly, although cutavirus has been found in biopsies of individuals with cutaneous T-cell lymphoma and melanoma, it has also been found in skin swabs from healthy individuals.

FURTHER READING

Crabol Y et al: Intravenous immunoglobulin therapy for pure red cell aplasia related to human parvovirus B19 infection: A retrospective study of 10 patients and review of the literature. Clin Infect Dis 56:968, 2013.

GUIDO M et al: Human bocavirus: Current knowledge and future challenges. World J Gastroenterol 22:8684, 2016.
MAPLE PA et al: Identification of past and recent parvovirus B19 infection in immunocompetent individuals by quantitative PCR and enzyme immunoassays: A dual-laboratory study. J Clin Microbiol 52:947, 2014.
MATTHEWS PC et al: Human parvovirus 4 'PARV4' remains elusive despite a decade of study F1000 Res 6:82, 2017.
SÖDERLUND-VENERMO M: Emerging human parvoviruses: The rocky road to fame. Ann Rev Virol 6:71, 2019.
SÖDERLUND-VENERMO M et al: Human parvoviruses, in *Clinical Virology*, 4th ed. DD Richman et al (eds). Washington, DC, ASM Press, 2016, pp 679–700.
SU C-C et al: Effects of antibodies against human parvovirus B19 on angiogenic signaling. Mol Med Rep 21:1320, 2020.

198 Human Papillomavirus Infections

Darron R. Brown, Aaron C. Ermel

Interest in human papillomavirus (HPV) infection began in earnest in the 1980s after Harold zur Hausen postulated that infection with these viruses was associated with cervical cancer. It is now recognized that HPV infection of the human genital tract is extremely common and causes clinical conditions ranging from asymptomatic infection to genital warts (condylomata acuminata); dysplastic lesions and invasive cancers of the anus, penis, vulva, vagina, and cervix; and a subset of oropharyngeal cancers. This chapter describes the epidemiology of HPV as a virus and a pathogen, the natural history of HPV infections and associated cancers, strategies to prevent infection and HPV-associated disease, and treatment modalities for some conditions caused by HPV.

PATHOGENESIS

Overview HPV is an icosahedral, nonenveloped, 8000-base-pair, double-stranded DNA virus with a diameter of 55 nm. Like the genomes of other papillomaviruses, HPV's genome consists of an early (E) gene region, a late (L) gene region, and a noncoding region, which contains regulatory elements. The E1, E2, E5, E6, and E7 proteins are expressed early in the growth cycle and are necessary for viral replication and cellular transformation. The E6 and E7 proteins are responsible for malignant transformation, targeting the human cell-cycle regulatory molecules p53 and Rb (retinoblastoma protein) for degradation, respectively. Translation of the L1 and L2 transcripts and splicing of an E1^E4 transcript occur later. The L1 gene encodes the 54-kDa major capsid protein that makes up the majority of the virus shell; the 77-kDa L2 minor protein contributes a smaller percentage of the capsid mass.

More than 125 HPV types have been identified and are numerically designated on the basis of a unique L1 gene sequence. Approximately 40 HPV types are regularly identified in the anogenital tract; these types are subdivided into high-risk and low-risk categories depending on the associated risk of cervical cancer. For example, HPV types 6 and 11 cause genital warts and ~10% of low-grade cervical lesions and are thus designated low risk. HPV types 16 and 18 cause dysplastic lesions and a high percentage of invasive cancers of the cervix and are therefore considered high risk.

HPV targets basal keratinocytes after microtrauma allows exposure of these cells to the virus. The HPV replication cycle is completed as keratinocytes undergo differentiation. Virions are assembled in the nuclei of differentiated keratinocytes and can be detected by electron microscopy. Infection is transmitted by contact with virus contained in these desquamated keratinocytes (or with free virus) from an infected individual.

The Immune Response to HPV Infection Unlike many viral infections, HPV infection has no viremic phase. This lack of viremia may account for the incomplete antibody response to HPV infection. Natural HPV infection of the genital tract gives rise to a serum antibody response in 60–70% of individuals. Significant, although incomplete, protection against type-specific reinfection is associated with the presence of neutralizing antibodies. Serum antibodies likely reach the cervical epithelium and secretions by transudation and exudation. Therefore, protection against infection relates to the amount of neutralizing antibody at the site of infection and lasts as long as sufficient levels of neutralizing antibodies are present.

A cell-mediated immune response plays an important role in controlling progression of HPV infection. Histologic examination of lesions in individuals who experience regression of genital warts demonstrates infiltration by T cells and macrophages. CD4+ T-cell regulation is particularly important in controlling HPV infections, as evidenced by the higher rates of infection and disease in immunosuppressed individuals, particularly those who are infected with HIV. Specific T-cell responses may be measured against HPV proteins, the most important of which appear to be the E2 and E6 proteins. In women with HPV type 16 cervical infection, a strong T-cell response to type 16–derived E2 protein is associated with a lack of progression of cervical disease. However, measurable changes occur in the innate and adaptive immune systems of patients with HPV-associated cancers. There is suppression of the antigen-presentation process as well as suppression of antitumor activity. The end result is a reduction of HPV-specific antitumor immune responses and an increase in immunosuppressive cellular responses.

THE NATURAL HISTORY OF HPV-ASSOCIATED MALIGNANCY

HPV is transmitted by vaginal or anal intercourse, oral sex, and probably by touching a partner's genitalia. In cross-sectional and longitudinal studies, ~40% of young women demonstrate evidence of HPV infection, with peaks during the teens and early twenties, soon after first coital experience. The number of lifetime sexual partners correlates with the likelihood of HPV infection and the subsequent risk of HPV-associated malignancy. HPV infection may occur in a monogamous person if that person's partner is infected.

Most HPV infections become undetectable after 6–9 months, a phenomenon known as "clearance." However, with prolonged follow-up and frequent sampling, the same HPV types may again be detected months or even years later. It is still debated whether such episodic detection indicates viral latency followed by reactivation or represents reinfection with an identical HPV type.

While HPV is the causative agent of several cancers, most attention has focused on cervical cancer, which is the second most common cancer in women worldwide. More than 500,000 women are diagnosed and 275,000 die from invasive cervical cancer annually. More than 85% of all cervical cancer cases, as well as deaths, occur in women living in low-income countries, especially countries in sub-Saharan Africa, Asia, and South and Central America.

Evidence collected over 25 years shows that HPV causes nearly 100% of cervical cancers. Persistent HPV infection is the most significant risk factor for cervical cancer; relative risks range from 10 to 20 and exceed 100 in prospective and case–control studies, respectively. The time from HPV infection to cervical cancer may exceed 20 years. Cervical cancer peaks in the fifth and sixth decades of life for women living in developed countries and as much as a decade earlier for women living in resource-poor countries. Persistent carriers of oncogenic HPV types are at greatest risk for high-grade cervical dysplasia and cancer.

Why HPV infections in some women but not others eventually lead to malignancy is not clear. Although oncogenic HPV infection is necessary for the development of cervical malignancy, only ~3–5%

of infected women will ever develop this cancer, even in the absence of cytologic screening. Biomarkers that can predict which women will develop cervical cancer are not available. Immunosuppression in general plays a significant role in redetection/reactivation of HPV infections, while other factors, such as smoking, hormonal changes, chlamydial infection, and nutritional deficits, have an impact on viral persistence and cancer.

The International Agency for Research on Cancer has concluded that HPV types 16, 18, 31, 33, 35, 39, 45, 51, 52, 56, 58, and 59 are carcinogenic in the uterine cervix. HPV type 16 is particularly virulent and causes 50% of cervical cancers. Worldwide, HPV types 16 and 18 cause at least 70% of cervical squamous cell carcinomas and 85% of cervical adenocarcinomas. Oncogenic types other than 16 or 18 cause the remaining 30% of cervical cancers. HPV types 16 and 18 also cause nearly 90% of anal cancers worldwide.

In addition to cervical and anal cancer, other HPV-associated cancers include vulvar and vaginal cancer (caused by HPV in 50–70% of cases), penile cancer (caused by HPV in 50% of cases), and at least 65% of oropharyngeal squamous cell carcinomas (OPSCCs). Over the past two decades, an epidemic of OPSCC related to oncogenic HPV infection, primarily HPV type 16, has developed. Rates of OPSCC in the United States have been increasing in men from a low of 0.27 case per 100,000 in 1973 to 0.57 case per 100,000 per year in 2004; rates in women have remained relatively stable at ~0.17 per 100,000 per year. The greatest increase in the incidence of OPSCC is among white men 40–50 years of age. Nearly 14,000 new cases were diagnosed in the United States in 2013. OPSCCs of the base of the tongue and tonsil cancer have increased annually by rates of 1.3 and 0.6%, respectively. Few data are available from developing countries about OPSCC.

THE EFFECTS OF HIV ON HPV-ASSOCIATED DISEASE

HIV infection accelerates the natural history of HPV infections. HIV-infected individuals are more likely than other individuals to develop genital warts, and their lesions are more recalcitrant to treatment. HIV infection has been consistently associated with precancerous cervical lesions, including low-grade cervical intraepithelial lesions (CIN) and CIN 3, the immediate precursor to cervical cancer. Women with HIV/AIDS have significantly higher rates of cervical cancer as well as subsets of some vulvar, vaginal, and oropharyngeal tumors (**Chap. 70**) than women in the general population. Studies indicate a direct relationship between low CD4+ T lymphocyte count and the risk of cervical cancer. Some studies show a reduced likelihood of HPV infection and precancerous lesions of the cervix in HIV-infected women given antiretroviral therapy (ART). However, the incidence of cervical cancer in HIV-infected women has not changed significantly since ART was introduced, possibly because of preexisting oncogenic HPV infections that occurred before ART was initiated.

The burden of HPV-associated cancers is expected to increase in HIV-infected patients, given the prolonged life expectancies provided with ART. For women living in developing countries where cervical cancer screening is not widely available, this trend will have significant consequences. Thus, elucidating the interactions of HIV infection and cervical cancer with cofactors such as diet, other sexually transmitted infections, and environmental exposures is an important focus of research that impacts women living in low- and middle-income countries.

Similar to that of cervical cancer, the incidence of anal cancer is strongly influenced by HIV infection. HIV-infected men who have sex with men (MSM) and HIV-infected women have much higher rates of anal cancer than HIV-uninfected populations. Specifically, the incidence among HIV-infected MSM has been found to be as high as 130 cases per 100,000, as opposed to 5 cases per 100,000 among HIV-negative MSM. The advent of ART has not impacted the incidence of anal cancer and high-grade anal intraepithelial neoplasia in the HIV-infected patient population.

More information regarding screening, prevention, and treatment in the HIV-infected population can be found at the Department of Health and Human Services website (*aidsinfo.nih.gov/guidelines*).

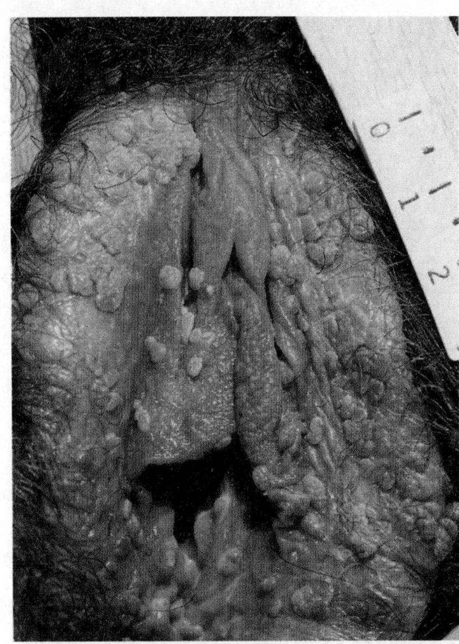

FIGURE 198-1 Warts of the vulva and vagina caused by human papillomavirus. *(Reproduced with permission from K Wolff et al: Fitzpatrick's Color Atlas and Synopsis of Clinical Dermatology, 8th ed. New York: McGraw-Hill, 2013.)*

CLINICAL MANIFESTATIONS OF HPV INFECTION

HPV infects the male urethra, penis, and scrotum and the female vulva, vagina, and cervix. Perianal, anal, and oropharyngeal infections occur in both genders. Genital warts are caused primarily by HPV type 6 or 11 and appear as soft sessile growths with a surface that is either smooth or rough with multiple finger-like projections. Penile genital warts are usually 2–5 mm in diameter and often occur in groups. A second type of penile lesion, the keratotic plaque, is slightly raised above normal epithelium and has a rough, often pigmented surface. **Figs. 198-1–198-3** show vulvar and vaginal, penile, and perianal warts, respectively.

Vulvar warts are soft, whitish papules that are either sessile or have multiple fine, finger-like projections. These lesions are most often located in the introitus and labia. In nonmucosal areas, vulvar lesions are similar in appearance to those in men: dry and keratotic. Vulvar lesions can appear as smooth, sometimes pigmented papules that may coalesce. Vaginal lesions appear as multiple areas of elongated papillae. Biopsy of vulvar or vaginal lesions may reveal malignancy; differentiation based on clinical exam is not always reliable.

Subclinical cervical HPV infections are common, and the cervix may appear normal on examination. Cervical lesions often appear as

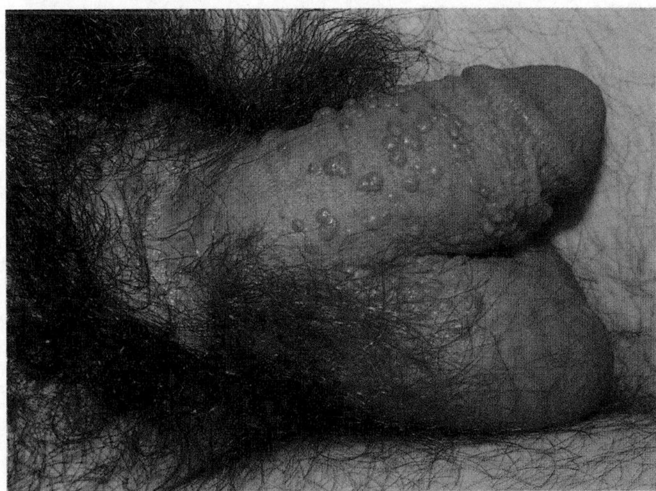

FIGURE 198-2 Penile genital warts caused by human papillomavirus. *(Reproduced with permission from K Wolff et al: Fitzpatrick's Color Atlas and Synopsis of Clinical Dermatology, 8th ed. New York: McGraw-Hill, 2013.)*

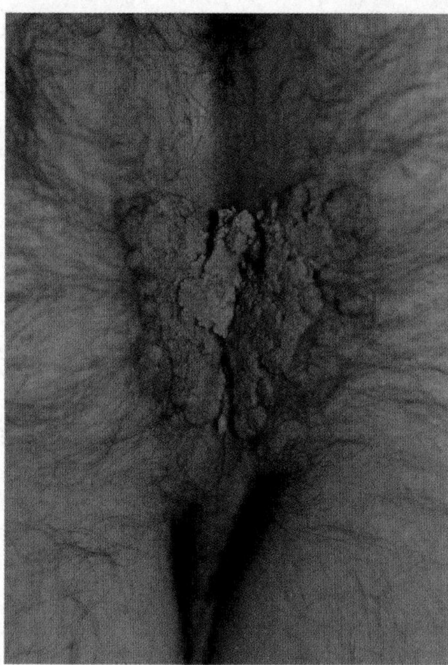

FIGURE 198-3 Perianal warts caused by human papillomavirus. *(Reproduced with permission from K Wolff et al: Fitzpatrick's Color Atlas and Synopsis of Clinical Dermatology, 8th ed. New York: McGraw-Hill, 2013.)*

papillary proliferations near the transformation zone. Irregular vascular loops are present beneath the surface epithelium. Patients who develop cervical cancer from HPV infection may present with a variety of symptoms. Early carcinomas appear eroded and bleed easily. More advanced carcinomas present as ulcerated lesions or as an exophytic cervical mass. Some cervical carcinomas are located in the cervical canal and may be difficult to see. Bleeding, symptoms of a mass lesion in late stages, and metastatic disease that may manifest as bowel or bladder obstruction due to direct extension of the tumor have also been described.

Patients with squamous cell cancer of the anus (**Chap. 81**) have more variable presentations. The most common presentations include rectal bleeding and pain or a mass sensation. Twenty percent of patients who are diagnosed with anal cancer may not present with any specific symptoms at the time of diagnosis, and the lesion is found fortuitously.

PREVENTION OF HPV INFECTION AND DISEASE

Behaviors That Can Reduce Exposure to HPV HPV infections are transmitted through direct contact with infected genital skin or mucosal surfaces and secretions. Does abstinence reduce HPV infections? For both men and women, numerous studies indicate that HPV infection and HPV-associated diseases correlate with the number of lifetime sexual partners, and people with no history of sexual intercourse have a lower detection rate of HPV. Fewer studies look at nonpenetrative sex and the risk of HPV infection and disease, but several studies indicate that HPV can be spread by *any* sexual intimacy, including touching, oral sex, or use of sex toys. It is therefore possible that individuals who have not partaken in penetrative sex can become infected.

Use of latex condoms reduces the risk of HPV infection and HPV-associated disease, such as genital warts and cervical precancers. Correct and consistent condom use has also been associated with regression of CIN in women and regression of HPV-associated penile lesions in men. As a preventive measure, condom use should be considered partially effective at best and not a substitute for cervical cancer screening or vaccination against HPV.

HPV Vaccines The development of HPV vaccines effective in preventing infection and HPV-associated disease represents a major development in the past decade. The vaccines use virus-like particles (VLPs) that consist of the HPV L1 major capsid protein. The L1 protein self-assembles into VLPs when expressed in eukaryotic cells (i.e., yeast or insect cells). These VLPs contain the same epitopes as actual HPV virions. However, they do not contain genetic material and therefore cannot transmit infection. The immunogenicity of the HPV vaccines relies on development of conformational neutralizing antibodies directed toward epitopes displayed on viral capsids.

Several large vaccine trials have been completed and demonstrate the high degree of safety and efficacy of HPV vaccines. There have been three HPV vaccines developed, tested, and U.S. Food and Drug Administration (FDA) approved, as described below.

BIVALENT VACCINE (CERVARIX) The bivalent HPV vaccine contains L1 VLPs of HPV types 16 and 18 and is marketed under the name of Cervarix (GlaxoSmithKline). This vaccine was tested in 18,644 women 15–25 years of age residing in the United States, South America, Europe, and Asia. It is administered by intramuscular injection three times (months 0, 1, and 6). The primary endpoints of the study included vaccine efficacy against persistent infections with HPV types 16 and 18. Investigators also assessed vaccine efficacy against CIN grade 2 or higher due to HPV 16 and 18 in women who had no evidence of HPV 16 or 18 infection at baseline. Vaccine efficacy related to HPV 16 or HPV 18 was 94.9% (95% confidence interval [CI], 87.7–98.4%) against CIN 2 or worse; 91.7% (95% CI, 66.6–99.1%) against CIN 3 or worse; and 100% (95% CI, –8.6–100%) against adenocarcinoma in situ (AIS). Adverse events associated with the bivalent vaccine were evaluated in phase 3 trials in a subset of 3077 women who received vaccine and 3080 women who received hepatitis A vaccine. Injection-site adverse events (pain, redness, and swelling) and systemic adverse events (fatigue, headache, and myalgia) were reported more frequently in the HPV vaccine group than in the control group. Serious adverse events, new-onset chronic disease, or medically significant conditions occurred in the same proportion (3.5%) of HPV vaccine recipients and control vaccine recipients. The bivalent HPV vaccine is approved in the United States for prevention of cervical cancer, CIN2 or worse, AIS, and CIN 1 caused by HPV types 16 and 18. This vaccine is approved for females 9–25 years of age. Cervarix is not currently marketed in the United States.

QUADRIVALENT VACCINE (GARDASIL) The quadrivalent L1 VLP vaccine (HPV types 6, 11, 16, and 18) is marketed under the name Gardasil (Merck). It is administered intramuscularly three times (months 0, 2, and 6). A combined efficacy analysis based on data from four randomized double-blind clinical studies including >20,000 participants was performed; results demonstrated that vaccine efficacy against external genital warts was 98.9% (95% CI, 93.7–100%). Vaccine efficacy was 95.2% (95% CI, 87.2–98.7%) against CIN; 100% (95% CI, 92.9–100%) against type 16- or 18-related CIN 2/3 or AIS; and 100% (95% CI, 55.5–100.0%) against type 16- or 18-related vulvar intraepithelial neoplasia grades 2 and 3 (VIN 2/3) and against vaginal intraepithelial neoplasia grades 2 and 3 (VaIN 2/3).

Safety data on the quadrivalent HPV vaccine are available from seven clinical trials, including nearly 12,000 women 9–26 years of age who received the vaccine and ~10,000 women who received aluminum-containing or saline placebo. A larger proportion of young women reported injection-site adverse events in the vaccine groups than in the placebo groups. Systemic adverse events were reported by similar proportions of vaccine and placebo recipients and were described as mild or moderate for most participants. The types of serious adverse events reported were similar for the two groups. Ten persons who received the quadrivalent vaccine and seven persons who received placebo died during the course of the trials; no deaths were considered to be vaccine related.

During the course of studies on the quadrivalent HPV vaccine, surveillance data for development of new medical conditions were collected for up to 4 years after vaccination. No statistically significant differences in the incidence of any medical conditions between vaccine and placebo recipients were demonstrated; this result indicated a very high safety profile for the vaccine. A recent safety review by the FDA and the Centers for Disease Control and Prevention (CDC) examined events related to Gardasil that had been reported to the Vaccine Adverse Events Reporting System (VAERS). The adverse events were consistent with what was seen in previous safety studies of the vaccine. Of note, rates of syncope and venous thrombotic events were higher with Gardasil than those usually observed with other vaccines.

The quadrivalent HPV vaccine is approved for (1) vaccination of females ages 9–26 years of age to prevent genital warts and cervical cancer caused by HPV types 6, 11, 16, and 18; (2) vaccination of the same population to prevent precancerous or dysplastic lesions, including cervical AIS, CIN 2/3, VIN 2/3, VaIN 2/3, and CIN 1; (3) vaccination of males 9–26 years of age to prevent genital warts caused by HPV types 6 and 11; and (4) vaccination of people ages 9–26 years to prevent anal cancer and associated precancerous lesions due to HPV types 6, 11, 16, and 18. While the duration of protection has not been established, no evidence of waning protection has been found after a three-dose series of the quadrivalent HPV vaccine, even after 10 years of follow-up from clinical trials. The quadrivalent HPV vaccine is no longer available in the United States but is still available in many other countries, although production is not likely to continue in the future.

NINE-VALENT VACCINE (GARDASIL-9) In 2014, the FDA approved a new nine-valent L1 VLP vaccine. The nine-valent vaccine is marketed under the name Gardasil-9 (Merck). It is administered intramuscularly three times (months 0, 2, and 6). The nine-valent vaccine targets HPV types 6, 11, 16, and 18 (the types also targeted by the quadrivalent HPV vaccine) as well as five additional oncogenic HPV types (31, 33, 45, 52, and 58). HPV types 16 and 18 together cause up to 80% of all cervical cancers worldwide, and worldwide data show that HPV types 31, 33, 35, 45, 52, and 58 are the next most frequently detected types in invasive cervical cancers. Mathematical models estimate that the level of protection conferred by the nine-valent HPV vaccine against all HPV-associated squamous cell cancers worldwide could be raised to 90%.

In clinical studies of females 16–26 years of age, the nine-valent HPV vaccine generated a noninferior antibody response to HPV types 6, 11, 16, and 18 compared to the quadrivalent HPV vaccine. Bridging immunologic studies in male and female vaccine recipients 9–15 years of age and in males 16–26 years of age indicated that the lower bound of the 95% CIs of the geometric mean titer ratio and seroconversion rates met criteria for noninferiority for all HPV types represented in the vaccine. In female recipients 16–26 years of age, vaccine efficacy against the combined endpoint of high-grade cervical, vulvar, or vaginal disease caused by any of the five additional oncogenic HPV types was 96.7% (95% CI, 80.9–99.8%). Like the other available HPV vaccines, the nine-valent HPV vaccine is safe and extremely well tolerated. The nine-valent HPV vaccine has an FDA indication for prevention of cervical, vaginal, vulvar, and anal cancer and genital warts due to vaccine types.

CROSS-PROTECTION OF HPV VACCINES Women who receive any of the available HPV vaccines produce neutralizing antibodies to virus types that are closely related to type 16 or 18. Analyses of data from clinical trials suggest that the HPV vaccines may offer limited cross-protection against nonvaccine virus types. Over short periods, the bivalent vaccine appears more efficacious against HPV types 31, 33, and 45 than the quadrivalent vaccine, but differences in study design make direct comparisons difficult, if not impossible. In addition, in the bivalent vaccine trials, vaccine efficacy against persistent infections with HPV types 31 and 45 waned over time, whereas efficacy against persistent infection with HPV type 16 or 18 remained stable. These results suggest that cross-protection is likely to be shorter lived than efficacy against infection and disease caused by vaccine types.

TWO-DOSE VERSUS THREE-DOSE SCHEDULE FOR HPV VACCINATION In an effort to simplify the dosing schedule and potentially reduce costs and improve vaccine uptake, a two-dose schedule has been considered. In several randomized vaccine trials among adolescent girls, geometric mean concentrations (GMCs) of antibodies to HPV type 16 were shown to be noninferior up to 24 months after a two-dose schedule to GMCs after a three-dose schedule. Numerous countries have adopted a two-dose HPV vaccination schedule. In the United States, the CDC now recommends two doses of HPV vaccine (at 0 and 6–12 months) for persons starting the vaccination series before the fifteenth birthday, as the immunologic response is rigorous in this age group. Three doses of HPV vaccine (at 0, 1–2, and 6 months) are recommended for persons starting the vaccination series on or after the fifteenth birthday and for persons with certain immunocompromising conditions, including HIV/AIDS.

RECOMMENDATIONS FOR HPV VACCINATION The most recent guidelines for HPV vaccination from the Advisory Committee on Immunization Practices (ACIP) are summarized below and provided in detail at *https://www.cdc.gov/mmwr/volumes/68/wr/mm6832a3.htm.*

No prevaccination testing of any kind is recommended to establish whether or not the HPV vaccine should be administered to an individual to determine if the vaccine will or will not be effective. The HPV vaccine should be administered, if possible, before exposure to HPV through sexual activity because the vaccines are preventative against specific HPV types and have no effect on preexisting, type-specific HPV infections. Either the bivalent (where available) or nine-valent HPV vaccines may be used. An individual can begin a vaccine series with one HPV vaccine and then complete the series with another. For those who have completed a vaccination series with the bivalent or quadrivalent vaccine, an additional full series (three doses) of vaccination with the nine-valent vaccine may be given, but there are no data to determine the effectiveness of this approach.

For children, adolescents, and adults (male and female) 9–26 years of age, the ACIP recommends HPV vaccination at age 11 or 12 years, although vaccination can be initiated at 9 years of age. "Catch-up" HPV vaccination is recommended for men and women through 26 years of age who are not adequately vaccinated.

For adults (male and female) 27–45 years of age, catch-up HPV vaccination is not routinely recommended. Instead, the ACIP now recommends shared clinical decision-making regarding HPV vaccination for certain adults 27–45 years of age who are not adequately vaccinated (see below). HPV vaccines are not licensed for use in adults older than 45 years of age. For women, cervical cancer screening should continue according to age-specific guidelines regardless of having received an HPV vaccine (see cervical cancer screening section below).

SHARED CLINICAL DECISION-MAKING FOR ADULTS 27–45 YEARS OF AGE A discussion with adults 27–45 years of age should occur prior to routine recommendation of the HPV vaccine. HPV infection occurs soon after first sexual activity in most people, and vaccine effectiveness is therefore lower in older individuals due to prior infections. HPV exposure usually decreases among older age groups. Although HPV vaccination is safe for adults 27–45 years of age, the benefit to the population is likely to be minimal. However, some men and women who are not vaccinated may be at risk for acquisition of new HPV infections and could therefore benefit from HPV vaccination.

In considering HPV vaccination of adults 27–45 years of age, some key points emphasized by the ACIP that should be discussed include the following:

- HPV is a common sexually transmitted infection, and most HPV infections are asymptomatic and do not lead to clinical disease.
- Most sexually active adults have been exposed to HPV, although not necessarily all of the HPV types targeted by vaccines.
- Some adults are at risk for acquiring new HPV infections through sexual activity. For example, having a new sex partner is a risk factor for acquiring a new HPV infection.
- Persons in a long-term, mutually monogamous sexual partnership are unlikely to acquire a new HPV infection.
- Antibody testing cannot determine whether a person is immune or susceptible to a specific HPV type.
- HPV vaccines are very effective in persons who have not been exposed to vaccine-type HPV before vaccination.
- Vaccine effectiveness is likely to be lower among persons with multiple lifetime sex partners because these individuals have probably had previous infections with vaccine-type HPV.
- HPV vaccines are prophylactic (i.e., they prevent new HPV infections). They have no utility in preventing established HPV infection from progressing to clinical disease, and they do not have a role in treatment of HPV-associated disease.

RECOMMENDATIONS FOR HPV VACCINATION IN PEOPLE LIVING WITH HIV (PLWH) Guidelines for HPV vaccination of PLWH are summarized below and can be found in detail at *https://aidsinfo.nih.gov/guidelines/html/4/adult-and-adolescent-opportunistic-infection/343/human-papillomavirus*.

HPV vaccines are safe in PLWH. Administration of HPV vaccines generates high levels of antibody against HPV types represented in vaccine, although antibody levels are generally lower than in those who are HIV-uninfected. In addition, immune responses appear stronger among PLWH who have the highest CD4 counts and the lowest HIV viral loads. Studies also indicate that HPV vaccination induces an anamnestic response in PLWH. Regarding efficacy in protecting against HPV-associated disease, one randomized, double-blind, clinical trial evaluated the efficacy of the quadrivalent HPV vaccine in adults with HIV infection older than 27 years in prevention of new anal HPV infections or improvement in high-grade dysplastic anal lesions. The trial did not show efficacy, but study participants had high levels of HPV infection at baseline.

HPV vaccination is recommended for girls and boys with HIV infection 11–26 years of age. Because some individuals with HIV infection (similar to HIV-uninfected individuals) have had many sex partners prior to vaccination, HPV vaccination may be less beneficial in these patients than in those with few or no lifetime sex partners. Current data do not support vaccination for those PLWH older than 26 years. The public health benefit for HPV vaccination of PLWH in this age range is likely to be minimal. However, although most PLWH ages 27–45 years will not benefit from the vaccine, there may be situations that suggest the possibility of vaccine benefit, and the same shared clinical decision-making (described above) between the provider and patient is recommended.

SCREENING FOR HPV-ASSOCIATED CANCER

Once HPV infection occurs, prevention of HPV-associated disease relies on screening. At present, screening for cervical cancer is widely accepted as cost-effective in preventing cervical cancer. Anal screening is accepted for screening in high-risk groups, though no national guidelines exist for screening intervals or ages for initiation and cessation of screening. In resource-rich countries, the primary method of cervical cancer screening is cytology via Pap smear. The American Society of Colposcopy and Cervical Pathology (ASCCP) guidelines recommend initiation of cervical cancer screening at age 21, no matter the age of sexual debut. Women 21–29 years old should have a Pap smear every 3 years if their initial and subsequent Pap smears are normal. Although adolescent and young women often test HPV DNA-positive, they are at very low risk of cervical cancer. Because the presence of HPV DNA does not correlate with the presence of high-grade squamous intraepithelial neoplasia, co-testing (testing for HPV DNA at the time of Pap smear) is not recommended for women in this age group.

As a method of determining the need for colposcopy, HPV DNA co-testing is recommended for women 25–29 years of age in whom cytology detects abnormal squamous cells of undetermined significance (ASCUS). Women 30–65 should have a Pap smear every 3 years if testing for HPV DNA is not performed. The screening interval for women in this age group can be extended to every 5 years if HPV DNA co-testing is performed and results are negative. HPV testing is not recommended for partners of women with HPV or for screening of conditions other than cervical cancer.

The role of HPV DNA testing as a primary screen for cervical cancer is changing. In the United States, there are two commercially available assays (cobas HPV Test [Roche Diagnostics] and the BD Onclarity HPV Assay [Becton, Dickinson and Company]) that are FDA approved for primary screening using HPV DNA testing. However, more assays may gain approval for usage as the feasibility and evidence for their use in various populations globally come to light. These tests can be used to detect HPV DNA in specimens obtained from the cervix without cervical cytology for women ≥25 years of age. A positive result for HPV type 16 or 18 has a high enough positive predictive value in the general population that these women should have colposcopy performed. If high-risk HPV types are detected other than HPV 16 or HPV 18, then cytology can be obtained. The complete set of algorithms for appropriate age-specific screening guidelines, HPV DNA testing, and the management of abnormal Pap smears are available through the ASCCP at *http://asccp.org/guidelines*.

For women ≤30 years of age who are infected with HIV, cervical cytology is the preferred method of cervical cancer screening and HPV DNA co-testing is not recommended. Cervical cancer screening should begin within 1 year of diagnosis of HIV infection, regardless of the mode of HIV transmission. If the first Pap smear is normal, then subsequent Pap smears should be performed annually until three negative tests are obtained. Cytology can then be obtained every 3 years. For women ≥30 years old, Pap testing is performed in the same manner as for younger women. However, HPV DNA co-testing can be used in women of this age group. If cytology and HPV DNA co-testing are negative, the next exam can be performed in 3 years. Positive HPV DNA co-test results are treated in the same manner as in HIV-uninfected women.

Women residing in developing countries with a lack of access to cervical screening programs have a higher rate of cervical cancer and a poorer cancer-specific survival. Approximately 75% of women living in developed countries have been screened in the past 5 years, as opposed to ~5% of women living in developing countries. Economic and logistic obstacles likely impede routine cervical cancer screening for these populations. Many poor countries rely on an alternative method—visual inspection with acetic acid (VIA)—for cervical cancer screening. While some studies show a reduction in cervical cancer mortality in communities where VIA is widely utilized, other studies do not. In addition, the low specificity of VIA is problematic. As newer methods that use detection of oncogenic HPV DNA become available, even resource-limited countries may be able to replace VIA with such methods and achieve a reduction in cervical cancers as a result.

Currently, there is no broad consensus regarding the screening for anal cancer and its precursors, including high-grade anal intraepithelial lesions. The reason is a lack of understanding of optimal treatment for low- or high-grade anal dysplasia found during cytologic screening. Current HIV treatment guidelines suggest that there may be a benefit to screening, but an effect on the associated morbidity and mortality of anal squamous cell cancer has not been consistently demonstrated. The incidence of HPV-associated head and neck cancers in the United States has overtaken the incidence of cervical cancer as of 2020, but there are no established guidelines for screening for HPV-associated head and neck cancers. However, HPV vaccination is likely to be effective for both anal and head and neck cancers associated with HPV.

TREATMENT

HPV-Associated Disease

A variety of treatment modalities are available for various HPV infections, but none has been proven to eliminate HPV from tissue adjacent to the destroyed and infected tissue. Treatment efficacies are limited by frequent recurrences, presumably due to reinfection from an infected partner, reactivation of latent virus, or autoinoculation from nearby infected cells. The goals of treatment include prevention of viral transmission, eradication of premalignant lesions, and reduction of symptoms.

Therapies are generally successful in eliminating visible lesions and grossly diseased tissue. Different therapies are indicated for genital warts, vaginal and cervical disease, and perianal and anal disease.

THERAPEUTIC OPTIONS

Imiquimod Imiquimod (5 or 3.75% cream) is a patient-applied topical immunomodulatory agent thought to activate immune cells by binding to a Toll-like receptor that leads to an inflammatory response. Imiquimod 5% cream is applied to genital warts at bedtime three times per week for up to 16 weeks. Warts are cleared in ~56% of patients, more often in women than in men; recurrence rates approach 13%. Local inflammatory side effects are

TABLE 198-1 Recommended Treatments for Genital Warts Caused by Human Papillomavirus[a]

TREATMENT	IMIQUIMOD	CRYOTHERAPY	INTERFERON	SURGICAL REMOVAL	LASER
Effectiveness	Good	Good	Good	Excellent	Excellent
Recurrence	Frequent	Frequent	Frequent	Frequent	Frequent
Adverse effects	Frequent, mild to moderate	Mild, well tolerated	Frequent, moderately severe	Mild, well tolerated	Mild to moderate, well tolerated
Availability	Fair	Good	Fair	Good	Fair
Cost	Expensive	Inexpensive	Very expensive	Moderately expensive	Very expensive

[a]Imiquimod can be self-administered. All other treatments must be administered by a clinician.

common. Rates of clearance of genital warts are not as high with the 3.75% formulation as with the 5% preparation, but the duration of treatment is shorter (daily application required for a maximum of 8 weeks) and fewer local and systemic adverse reactions occur. Imiquimod should not be used to treat vaginal, cervical, or anal lesions. The safety of imiquimod during pregnancy has not been established.

Interferon Recombinant interferon α is used for intralesional treatment of genital warts, including perianal lesions. The recommended dosage is 1.0×10^6 IU of interferon into each lesion three times weekly for 3 weeks. Interferon therapy causes clearance of infected cells by immune-boosting effects. Adverse events include headache, nausea, vomiting, fatigue, and myalgia. Interferon therapy is costly and should be reserved for severe cases that do not respond to less expensive treatments. Interferon should not be used to treat vaginal, cervical, or anal lesions.

Cryotherapy Cryotherapy (liquid nitrogen treatment) for HPV-associated lesions causes cellular death. Genital warts usually disappear after two or three weekly sessions but often recur. Cryotherapy, which is nontoxic and is not associated with significant adverse reactions, can also be used for diseased cervical tissue. Local pain occurs frequently.

Surgical Methods Exophytic lesions can be surgically removed after intradermal injection of 1% lidocaine. This treatment is well tolerated but can cause scarring and requires hemostasis. Genital warts can also be destroyed by electrocautery, in which no additional hemostasis is required.

Laser Therapy Laser treatment affords destruction of exophytic lesions and other HPV-infected tissue while preserving normal tissue. Local anesthetics are generally adequate. Efficacy for genital lesions is at least equal to that of other therapies (60–90%), with low recurrence rates (5–10%). Complications include local pain, vaginal discharge, periurethral swelling, and penile or vulvar swelling. Laser therapy has also been used successfully for cervical dysplasia and anal disease caused by HPV.

Therapeutic Vaccines The innate and adaptive immune systems are altered in patients with HPV-associated cancers. Antitumor immune responses are blunted by specific viral mechanisms. Numerous therapeutic vaccines that are being developed are designed to enhance the cell-mediated response to the HPV E6 and E7 oncoproteins, which are expressed in HPV-associated cancers. Such vaccines would enhance the ability to treat HPV-associated cancers, conditions that are very difficult to treat with current modalities. However, while progress has been made, no HPV vaccine is currently available for treatment of HPV infection or HPV-associated disease.

Other Therapies Both trichloroacetic acid and bichloroacetic acid are caustic agents that destroy warts by coagulation of proteins. Neither of these agents is recommended for treatment. Sinecatechins (15% ointment) and podophyllotoxin (0.05% solution or gel and 0.15% cream) are occasionally used for external genital warts, but other modalities listed above are as or more effective and are better tolerated.

RECOMMENDATIONS FOR TREATMENT

Table 198-1 lists available treatments for genital warts. An optimal therapy for HPV-related genital tract disease that combines high efficacy, low toxicity, low cost, and low recurrence is not available. For genital warts of the penis or vulva, cryotherapy is the safest, least expensive, and most effective modality. However, all available modalities for treatment of genital warts carry high rates of recurrence. Guidelines for the treatment of genital warts can be found on the CDC website (*https://www.cdc.gov/std/tg2015/warts.htm*).

Women with vaginal lesions should be referred to a gynecologist experienced in colposcopy and treatment of these lesions. Treatment of cervical disease involves careful inspection, biopsy, and histopathologic grading to determine the severity and extent of disease. Women with evidence of HPV-associated cervical disease should be referred to a gynecologist familiar with HPV and experienced in colposcopy. Optimal follow-up of these patients includes colposcopic examination of the cervix and vagina on a yearly basis. Guidelines from the American College of Obstetricians and Gynecologists are available for the treatment of cervical dysplasia and cancer.

For anal or perianal lesions, cryotherapy or surgical removal is safest and most effective. Anoscopy and/or sigmoidoscopy should be performed in patients with perianal lesions, and suspicious lesions should be biopsied to rule out malignancy.

COUNSELING PATIENTS REGARDING HPV DISEASE

Most sexually active adults will be infected with HPV during their lives. The only way to avoid acquiring an HPV infection is to abstain from sexual activity, including intimate touching and oral sex. Practicing safe sex (partner reduction, use of condoms) may help reduce HPV transmission. Most HPV infections will be controlled by the immune system and cause no symptoms or disease. Some infections lead to genital warts and cervical precancers. Genital warts can be treated for cosmetic reasons and to prevent spread of infection to others. Even after resolution of genital warts, latent HPV may persist in normal-appearing skin or mucosa and thus theoretically may be transmitted to uninfected partners. Precancerous cervical lesions should be treated to prevent progression to cancer.

FURTHER READING

Clifford GM et al: Carcinogenicity of human papillomavirus (HPV) types in HIV-positive women: A meta-analysis from HPV infection to cervical cancer. Clin Infect Dis 64:1228, 2017.

Curry SJ et al: Screening for cervical cancer: US Preventive Services Task Force Recommendation Statement. JAMA 320:674, 2018.

De Sanjosé S et al: The natural history of human papillomavirus infection. Best Pract Res Clin Obstet Gynaecol 47:2, 2018.

Garland SM et al: Impact and effectiveness of the quadrivalent human papillomavirus vaccine: A systematic review of 10 years of real-world experience. Clin Infect Dis 63:519, 2016.

Giuliano AR et al: Efficacy of quadrivalent HPV vaccine against HPV infection and disease in males. N Engl J Med 364:401, 2011.

Gravitt PE, Winer RL: Natural history of HPV infection across the lifespan: Role of viral latency. Viruses 9:265, 2017.

LOPALCO PL: Spotlight on the 9-valent HPV vaccine. Drug Des Devel Ther 11:35, 2016.

ROSENBLUM HG et al: Declines in prevalence of human papillomavirus vaccine-type infection among females after introduction of vaccine—United States, 2003-2018. MMWR Morb Mortal Wkly Rep 70:415, 2021.

SCHIFFMAN M et al: Carcinogenic human papillomavirus infection. Nat Rev Dis Primers 2:16086, 2016.

SERRANO B et al: Epidemiology and burden of HPV-related disease. Best Pract Res Clin Obstet Gynaecol 47:14, 2018.

SMALL W JR et al: Cervical cancer: A global health crisis. Cancer 123:2404, 2017.

WENTZENSEN N et al: Eurogin 2016 roadmap: How HPV knowledge is changing screening practice. Int J Cancer 140:2192, 2017.

Section 13 Infections Due to DNA and RNA Respiratory Viruses

199 Common Viral Respiratory Infections, Including COVID-19

James E. Crowe, Jr.

The most common and frequent infections in humans are respiratory virus infections. Influenza viruses and coronaviruses have been the agents responsible for the largest infectious disease pandemics. These viruses are easily transmitted by contact, droplets, and fomites. Furthermore, transmission can occur before the appearance of symptoms. These viruses are also associated with a large reproductive number (the number of secondary infections generated from one infected individual to others). Some classical respiratory viruses (e.g., rhinoviruses) enter the body through the respiratory tract, replicating and causing disease only in cells of the respiratory epithelium. Other, more systemic viruses (e.g., measles virus and severe acute respiratory syndrome [SARS] coronavirus) spread via the bloodstream and cause systemic disease; however, they also may enter through and cause disease in the respiratory tract. Although infections with systemic viruses often induce lifelong immunity against disease, respiratory viruses that do not cause high-grade viremia usually can reinfect the same host many times throughout life. Reinfection with the same virus is common because of incomplete or waning immunity after natural infection. Hundreds of different viruses cause infection of the respiratory tract, and within each virus type, there can be a nearly unlimited diversity of field strains that vary antigenically, geographically, and over time (e.g., antigenically drifting influenza viruses or coronaviruses). Specific antiviral treatment options are limited, and only a few licensed vaccines are available. **For further discussion of common respiratory virus infections, see Chap. 35 and syndrome-specific chapters.**

Common viral respiratory infections can be categorized in several ways, including by site of anatomic involvement, disease syndrome, or etiologic agent.

ANATOMIC SITES IN THE HUMAN RESPIRATORY TRACT

The type of respiratory disease that develops during virus infection is dictated to a large degree by the cell types and tissue organization in the respiratory tract. The vocal cords mark the transition between the upper and lower respiratory tracts. The upper respiratory tract is a complex anatomic system with interconnected structures, including the sinuses, middle-ear spaces, Eustachian tubes, conjunctiva, nasopharynx, oropharynx, and larynx. The tonsils and the adenoids are large collections of lymphoid tissue in the pharynx that participate in immunity but also are susceptible to infections. The lower respiratory tract structures include the trachea, bronchi, bronchioles, alveolar spaces, and lung tissue, including epithelial cells and blood vessels. The epithelial cell types that line the respiratory tract are varied in morphology and function, and their susceptibility to different virus infections varies. The principal types of cells in the major airways are ciliated or nonciliated epithelial cells, goblet cells, and Clara cells. Smooth-muscle cells form major tissue structures around the epithelial structures of the large airways of the lower respiratory tract down to the level of the bronchioles, and these cells are reactive to intrinsic and extrinsic signals, including viral infection or exposure to allergens or pollutants. The pathologic process of wheezing is driven by smooth-muscle contraction and obstruction of airways caused by mucus accumulation and epithelial sloughing in the lumen. Reactive airways causing wheezing are most often due to constriction of lumen size at the level of the bronchioles (which have the narrowest lumen diameter of the airways). The lung does not have smooth-muscle or ciliated cells but instead possesses pneumocytes of types I and II. Pneumonia (**Chap. 126**) is an infection of the pneumocytes in the lung tissue and the alveolar spaces. The alveolar spaces also contain cells of the monocyte lineage, such as macrophages, which patrol the air spaces.

DISEASE SYNDROMES

Since different respiratory viruses tend to have a predilection for replication in differing cells or regions of the respiratory tract, it is possible for the well-trained clinician with epidemiologic information to understand the most likely associations of viruses with clinical syndromes. The clinical diagnoses for virus infections in the upper respiratory tract are rhinitis or the common cold, sinusitis, otitis media, conjunctivitis, pharyngitis, tonsillitis, and laryngitis. In reality, some upper respiratory tract infections affect more than one upper respiratory tract anatomic site during a single infection, such as the classical pattern of pharyngoconjunctival fever during adenovirus infection. Lower respiratory tract syndromes also can be associated easily with anatomic region, including tracheitis, bronchitis, bronchiolitis, pneumonia, and exacerbations of reactive airway disease or asthma. Bronchiolitis is a disease condition characterized by trapping of air in the lungs with difficulty in expiration (i.e., wheezing); it is caused by inflammation or infection of the bronchioles, the smallest and most highly resistant airways. Again, mixed syndromes occur, such as laryngotracheitis, usually termed croup. Croup, a disease condition characterized by difficulty in inspiration associated with a barky cough, is caused by inflammation or infection of the larynx, trachea, and bronchi. When respiratory symptoms occur in the context of a respiratory viral illness with significant systemic signs, infection with particular agents can be suspected (e.g., influenza, measles, SARS, SARS-CoV-2, or hantavirus pulmonary syndrome [HPS]), with exposure history taken into account.

ETIOLOGIC AGENTS

■ RESPIRATORY VIRUSES CAUSING DISEASE IN IMMUNOCOMPETENT HOSTS

Children have more frequent respiratory virus infections than adults; thus, it was natural that many early discoveries about the viral causes of respiratory infections came from pediatric studies. The principal causes of acute viral respiratory infections were determined in large epidemiologic studies in the 1960s and 1970s, when cell culture of infectious agents became available. More recently, studies of viral epidemiology have been conducted in adults, especially in special populations such as the elderly, nursing home residents, and immunocompromised individuals. Rapid antigen detection tests (based on immunoassays for detection of viral proteins) became available for respiratory syncytial virus (RSV) and influenza virus in the 1980s. With the availability of sensitive and specific molecular tests, such as reverse transcription combined with the polymerase chain reaction (RT-PCR), studies in the past several decades have greatly increased the extent to which we understand the causes of viral respiratory infections. Multiplex panels of RT-PCR tests capable of detecting a dozen or more viruses are commonly available for clinical testing of respiratory secretions. Nested multiplex PCR assays performed in two stages provide sensitive tests that have been especially helpful in studies of infection in adults, who often shed much lower concentrations of virus in secretions than do children. Typically, influenza viruses, RSV, and human metapneumovirus (hMPV) are the most common causes of serious lower respiratory tract disease in otherwise healthy subjects; parainfluenza viruses (PIVs) and adenoviruses also cause substantial disease. Rhinoviruses (the most common cause of the common cold syndrome) have been increasingly associated with lower respiratory tract syndromes. Rhinovirus infection is so common, even in asymptomatic individuals, that it has been hard to establish clear figures for the role of rhinovirus in lower respiratory disease. COVID-19 and the associated public health measures deployed in 2020–2021 altered the epidemiology of respiratory viruses such that conventional viruses were greatly reduced in incidence. Generally, about two-thirds of cases of respiratory illness in a research setting can be associated with a specific viral agent. Besides the viruses mentioned above (and discussed below), several additional viruses identified with molecular tools have been associated with respiratory illness. Still, it is fair to say that our diagnostic tools remain suboptimal since a specific infectious agent is not identified in approximately one-third of clinical respiratory illnesses in large surveillance studies. It is likely that in most of these cases pathogens are not detected because of the very low titers of virus in patient samples at the time of clinical presentation, which may occur after the period of peak virus shedding. It is also possible that novel agents are yet to be identified. As emerging tools for microbiome and "virome" studies (with sequencing of all nucleic acids in a sample) are applied in these settings in coming years, new agents and new associations with disease will probably be discovered.

■ RESPIRATORY VIRUSES CAUSING DISEASE IN IMMUNOCOMPROMISED HOSTS

Special populations of patients are susceptible not only to the conventional respiratory viruses discussed above but also to agents causing symptoms during reactivation of latent viruses or new infections with opportunistic agents. Most prominently, reactivating latent viruses, such as herpes simplex virus (HSV) and cytomegalovirus (CMV) and adenoviruses, cause disease in immunocompromised humans. Patients at most risk are those with hematopoietic stem cell or solid organ transplantation, leukopenia caused by chemotherapy, or advanced HIV-AIDS. In immunosuppressed patients with pneumonia, CMV is the virus recovered most frequently during deep respiratory tract diagnostic procedures such as bronchoalveolar lavage. These patients also are highly susceptible to more frequent and more severe disease caused by common respiratory viruses, including RSV, hMPV, PIVs, influenza viruses, rhinoviruses, and adenoviruses. Conventional acute respiratory viruses can cause chronic and sometimes fatal infections in these populations. Nosocomial transmission of respiratory viruses occurs in hematopoietic stem cell transplantation units, and the frequency of transmission can be high, with entire units affected.

■ SPECIFIC VIRAL CAUSES OF RESPIRATORY DISEASE

Orthomyxoviridae: Influenza Viruses (See also Chap. 200)

Influenza virus infection and influenza syndrome usually are associated with fever, myalgias, fatigue, sore throat, headache, and cough. Influenza causes severe and even fatal pneumonia, particularly in elderly patients, nursing home residents, immunocompromised persons, and very young children. Influenza pneumonia has an unusually high rate of complication by bacterial superinfection, with staphylococcal and streptococcal bacterial pneumonia occurring in as many as 10% of cases in some clinical series.

Influenza is a single-stranded, segmented, negative-sense, RNA genome virus of the family *Orthomyxoviridae*. There are three (sero) types of influenza viruses: A, B, and C. Influenza A and C viruses infect multiple species, whereas influenza B virus infects humans almost exclusively. Type A viruses appear to be the most virulent for humans and most commonly cause severe disease manifestations, although type B viruses cause substantial morbidity. On the basis of antibody response, influenza A viruses can be subdivided into 18 different hemagglutinin (H) surface protein subtypes and 11 neuraminidase (N) surface protein subtypes. The subtypes that have caused major pandemics in humans are H1N1, which caused the 1918 pandemic; H2N2, which caused the 1957 pandemic; H3N2, which caused the 1968 pandemic; and H1N1pdm2009, which caused the 2009 pandemic. Currently, two type A subtypes (H1N1 and H3N2) and two type B lineages (Yamagata and Victoria) cause annual seasonal epidemics.

Major pandemics caused by new influenza viruses are always possible. Many highly pathogenic influenza viruses circulate in aquatic birds. Occasionally, avian viruses infect humans directly after close contact with infected wild birds or poultry. Co-housing of pigs (which have both avian and human influenza virus receptors) with poultry may increase the risk of reassortment of human and animal or bird viruses; reassortment can make the zoonotic viruses more fit for replication in humans. Several outbreaks of avian influenza have occurred in limited numbers of humans to date, and there is the risk of a worldwide pandemic with avian influenza viruses if a strain acquires the potential to spread efficiently from human to human. H5N1 influenza virus infection of humans, predominantly by direct chicken-to-human transmission, occurred during an epizootic in Hong Kong's poultry population in 1997. The disease affected many types of wild and domestic birds and caused a high rate of systemic disease and death in infected humans. This virus, carried in the gastrointestinal tract of wild birds, has spread throughout Asia and beyond and continues to evolve antigenically. Avian H7N7 and H7N9 viruses also have caused zoonotic outbreaks. A significant outbreak of H7N9 virus infection began in China in March 2013, with high mortality, and there have been six outbreaks to date, the largest in 2016–2017 with 766 human infections. H7N9 is considered to have high potential to cause a future pandemic. H1N2 virus is endemic in pigs and affects humans with close contact. An H3N2 variant virus that differs antigenically from seasonal human viruses is endemic in pigs and occasionally infects children who have close contact with pigs in the United States. Rare human cases caused by H6, H9, and H10 subtype viruses have been reported. Type B influenza viruses co-circulate in humans during seasonal epidemics. Type B viruses mutate less frequently than type A viruses. The slower evolution of type B viruses is probably linked to the fact that they are almost exclusively human pathogens. There is only one B type of influenza, but these viruses began to diverge into two antigenically distinguishable lineages in the 1970s. The two virus lineages were named after the initial designated representative strains—B/Victoria/2/87 and B/Yamagata/16/88—and can be distinguished by serologic or genotyping laboratory tests. The evolution of B viruses over time spurred the inclusion of two type B virus antigens in seasonal influenza vaccines, expanding some multivalent vaccines from trivalent (H1N1, H3N2, B) to a quadrivalent format. During the COVID-19 pandemic, the diversity of influenza in humans has been reduced, as strains in lineage B/Yamagata and one clade of H3N2 known as 3c3.A were not detected.

Pneumoviridae (the formal species names of family *Pneumoviridae* were updated in 2019; Table 199-1)

• **RESPIRATORY SYNCYTIAL VIRUS** Human RSV (hRSV) is a single-stranded, negative-sense, nonsegmented, RNA genome virus of the genus *Pneumovirus* in the family *Paramyxoviridae*. Infection is ubiquitous, affecting most humans in the first several years of life and causing reinfections throughout life. RSV is among the most transmissible viruses of humans. Disease epidemics occur yearly, typically between October or November and March in temperate regions. RSV is one of the most common viral causes of severe lower respiratory tract illness in the elderly and in children; it is among the most important causes of hospitalization of elderly and infant patients throughout the world. There is only one serotype of RSV, but antigenic variability does occur in circulating field strains. In immune serum reciprocal cross-neutralization studies, the two antigenic subgroups, A and B, appear to be ~25% antigenically related; this relatedness may partially explain

TABLE 199-1 Family *Pneumoviridae*, Human Pathogens with Current Species Names, the International Committee on Taxonomy of Viruses: 2019 Release

GENUS	CURRENT SPECIES NAME	FORMER SPECIES NAME
Metapneumovirus	*Human metapneumovirus (hMPV)*	Same
Orthopneumovirus	*Human orthopneumovirus*	Human respiratory syncytial virus (hRSV)

TABLE 199-2 Family *Paramyxoviridae* Human Pathogens with Current Species Names, the International Committee on Taxonomy of Viruses: 2019 Release

GENUS	CURRENT SPECIES NAME	FORMER SPECIES NAME
Respirovirus	*Human respirovirus 1*	Human parainfluenza virus type 1 (hPIV1)
	Human respirovirus 3	Human parainfluenza virus type 3 (hPIV3)
Orthorubulavirus	*Mumps orthorubulavirus*	Mumps virus
	Human orthorubulavirus 2	Human parainfluenza type 2 (hPIV2)
	Human orthorubulavirus 4	Human parainfluenza type 4a (hPIV4a)
	Human orthorubulavirus 4	Human parainfluenza type 4b (hPIV4b)
	Mammalian orthorubulavirus 5	Parainfluenza type 5 (PIV5)

the susceptibility of humans to reinfection, which is very common and can be caused by viruses of the same subgroup or even the same strain. However, reinfection in otherwise healthy adults usually is associated with mild disease confined to the upper respiratory tract. Severe lower respiratory tract disease is common in the elderly, especially in frail institutionalized elderly populations. Immunocompromised patients of any age also are at risk of severe or prolonged disease, especially recipients of hematopoietic stem cell transplants. Wheezing is common with primary infection in children (bronchiolitis), and there is a strong association of RSV infection early in life and subsequent asthma, although it is unclear whether severe childhood RSV causes asthma or is the first manifestation of reactive airway disease. RSV causes exacerbations of asthma and is associated with acute exacerbations of chronic obstructive pulmonary disease (COPD), also referred to as acute exacerbations of chronic bronchitis (AECB).

HUMAN METAPNEUMOVIRUS hMPV was discovered only in 2001 but probably has always been present in human populations. Infection occurs first in early childhood, and reinfections are common throughout life. This virus is similar in many respects to RSV. It belongs to the family *Paramyxoviridae* and is a member of the genus *Pneumovirus*. It causes both upper and lower respiratory disease. It appears to be somewhat less virulent than RSV, causing about half as much severe lower respiratory tract disease, probably because it does not possess the nonstructural genes that RSV expresses in infected cells to abrogate the effect of host innate immune effectors like interferons. The clinical features of lower respiratory tract infections caused by hMPV are like those of such infections caused by other paramyxoviruses, most often including cough, coryza, and wheezing. Like RSV, hMPV plays an important role in exacerbations of asthma or COPD and causes pneumonia or wheezing in frail and institutionalized elderly individuals and immunocompromised patients.

Paramyxoviridae (the formal species names of family *Paramyxoviridae* were updated in 2019; Table 199-2)

• **HUMAN PARAINFLUENZA VIRUSES** The human PIVs (hPIV) are a group of four distinct serotypes (designated 1–4) of single-stranded, negative-sense RNA viruses belonging to the family *Paramyxoviridae*. hPIV3 most commonly causes severe disease, and repeated infection is common throughout life, although secondary infections often are mild or asymptomatic. Primary infections in children manifest as laryngotracheitis (croup), while subsequent infections typically are limited to the upper respiratory tract. hPIVs are detected with sensitive RT-PCR tests or, more classically, by cell culture with immunofluorescent microscopy or hemadsorption in reference laboratories.

MEASLES VIRUS (See also Chap. 205) Measles virus is also a paramyxovirus but of the genus *Morbillivirus*. This virus causes a systemic infection known as rubeola but also can manifest with respiratory symptoms. Measles virus probably is the most contagious respiratory virus infection of humans: it is transmitted efficiently not only by direct contact with infected persons or fomites (like other respiratory viruses) but also by small-particle aerosols. Measles virus infection is preventable by vaccination but is so infectious that cases are inevitable—even in the United States—whenever vaccination rates fall below 90–95% in a population. The virus causes systemic illness, sometimes including severe pneumonia, when primary infection occurs in an unvaccinated adult or an immunocompromised person of any age. Therefore, vigilance in maintaining high vaccination rates is critical. With primary infection, the illness in children is typically milder; however, mortality rates in lower-resource countries are high, especially among persons with underlying risk factors, including malnutrition.

Symptoms of measles include ≥3 days of high fever and a classical set of upper and lower respiratory tract symptoms sometimes termed "the 3 Cs": cough, coryza, and conjunctivitis. Unlike most respiratory viruses, measles virus circulates in the bloodstream and thus causes disseminated infection with systemic manifestations. Usually, a characteristic diffuse maculopapular rash appears within days of fever onset. Koplik's spots (see Fig. A1-2)—typical mucosal lesions in the mouth that appear briefly—are considered diagnostic of measles infection in the setting of the typical rash and fever.

Picornaviridae

A wide variety of picornaviruses cause respiratory disease, including nonpolio enteroviruses, rhinoviruses, and parechoviruses (Chap. 204). The designations of these viruses can be confusing: the *Enterovirus*, rhinovirus, and *Parechovirus* species names were changed (with the approval of the International Committee on Taxonomy of Viruses) to remove references to host species names (such as the formerly used terms human, simian, etc.). These changes are summarized in **Table 199-3**. The genus *Enterovirus* consists of 15 species, including enteroviruses A through L and rhinoviruses A through C. The genus *Parechovirus* contains six species, one of which—Parechovirus A—encompasses 19 types: human parechovirus (HPeV) 1 through 19. These viruses exhibit seasonal patterns that differ from those of most other acute respiratory viruses. Rhinovirus infections occur year-round. *Enterovirus* infections occur most commonly in the summer months in temperate areas.

RHINOVIRUSES Rhinoviruses have single-stranded, positive-sense RNA genomes. Rhinoviruses A through C represent species in the *Enterovirus* genus of the family *Picornaviridae*. Rhinoviruses are the most common viral infective agents in humans and the most frequent cause of the common cold. Field isolates of rhinovirus are exceptionally diverse; they can be classified by serotyping into >100 serotypes or, alternatively, by genotyping into a large number of genotypes that cause cold symptoms. At the time of writing in 2021, the species Rhinovirus A contained 80 types, Rhinovirus B had 32 types, and Rhinovirus C had 57 types. The viral particles are icosahedral in structure and are nonenveloped. Rhinoviruses are responsible for at least half of all cases of the common cold. Rhinovirus-induced common colds may be complicated in children by otitis media and in adults by sinusitis. Most adults, in fact, have radiographic evidence of sinusitis during the common cold, which resolves without therapy. Therefore, the primary disease is probably best termed *rhinosinusitis*. Rhinovirus infection is associated with exacerbations of reactive airway disease in children and asthma in adults. It is not clear whether rhinovirus is restricted to the upper respiratory tract and only indirectly induces inflammatory responses that affect the lower respiratory tract or whether the viruses spread to the lower respiratory tract. In the past, it was thought that these viruses did

TABLE 199-3 Enterovirus, Rhinovirus, and Parechovirus Species Names, the International Committee on Taxonomy of Viruses: 2019 Release

GENUS	CURRENT SPECIES NAME	FORMER SPECIES NAME
Enterovirus (now 15 species)	Enterovirus A: consists of 25 serotypes, including coxsackieviruses and some nonpolio enteroviruses that cause respiratory disease	Human enterovirus A
	Enterovirus B: consists of 63 serotypes, including some coxsackieviruses, echoviruses, and nonpolio enteroviruses	Human enterovirus B
	Enterovirus C: consists of 23 serotypes, including the polioviruses	Human enterovirus C
	Enterovirus D: consists of 5 serotypes and includes enterovirus D68	Human enterovirus D
	Rhinoviruses A–C	Human rhinoviruses A–C
Parechovirus (now 6 species)	Parechovirus A: consists of 19 types (1–19). Human parechoviruses (HPeVs) 1 and 2 are common human pathogens.	HPeV-1 and HPeV-2 were formerly classified in the genus *Enterovirus* as echoviruses 22 and 23, respectively.

not often replicate or cause disease in the lower respiratory tract. However, recent studies have discerned strong epidemiologic associations of rhinoviruses with wheezing and asthma exacerbations, including episodes severe enough to require hospitalization. Rhinovirus C has been associated with more severe disease syndromes, such as pneumonia or exacerbation of COPD. Rhinoviruses likely can infect the lower airways to some degree, inducing a local inflammatory response. Another possibility is that significant local infection of the upper respiratory tract may induce regional elaboration of mediators that causes lower airway disease. The association of rhinovirus infection with lower respiratory tract illness is difficult to study because diagnosis by cell culture is not sensitive. RT-PCR diagnostic tests are difficult to interpret because they are often positive for prolonged periods and even asymptomatic individuals may have a positive test. Comprehensive serologic studies to confirm infection are difficult because of the large number of serotypes. Nevertheless, most experts believe rhinoviruses are a common cause of serious lower respiratory tract illness.

ENTEROVIRUSES Nonpolio enteroviruses are common and distributed worldwide. Although infection often is asymptomatic, these viruses cause outbreaks of clinical respiratory disease, sometimes with fatal consequences. The species Enterovirus A consists of 25 serotypes, including coxsackieviruses and some nonpolio enteroviruses that cause respiratory disease. Coxsackieviruses cause oral lesions and often are associated in children with hand-foot-and-mouth disease. The pharyngitis associated with this infection characteristically manifests with herpangina, a clinical syndrome of ulcers or small vesicles on the palate that often involves the tonsillar fossa and is associated with fever, difficulty swallowing, and throat pain. Outbreaks commonly occur in young children during the summer. Enterovirus A71 also causes large outbreaks of hand-foot-and-mouth disease, especially in Asia, sometimes leading to neurologic complications and even death. The species Enterovirus B consists of >90 serotypes, including the echoviruses (*echo* being an acronym for *e*nteric *c*ytopathic *h*uman *o*rphan, which may be an archaic notion since most echoviruses are associated with human diseases, most commonly in children). Echoviruses can be isolated from many children with upper respiratory tract infections during the summer months. Echovirus 11 has been associated with laryngotracheitis or croup. Epidemiologic studies also have associated echoviruses with epidemic pleurodynia, an acute illness characterized by sharp chest pain and fever. The species Enterovirus C consists of 23 serotypes, including the polioviruses. The species Enterovirus D consists of five serotypes, including enterovirus D68, which has been associated with wheezing and a polio-like syndrome in children.

PARECHOVIRUSES The genus *Parechovirus* comprises six species, one of which is Parechovirus A, which can affect humans. The most common member of the genus *Parechovirus*, HPeV-1, is a frequent human pathogen. The genus also includes the closely related HPeV-2. HPeVs usually cause mild respiratory or gastrointestinal illness. Most infections occur in young children. The seroprevalence of HPeV-1 and HPeV-2 is high among adults.

Adenoviridae Viruses of the family *Adenoviridae* infect both humans and animals. As their designation indicates, adenoviruses were first isolated in human lymphoid tissues from surgically removed adenoids. In fact, some serotypes establish persistent asymptomatic infections in tonsil and adenoid tissues, and virus shedding can occur for months or years. These double-stranded DNA viruses are <100 nm in diameter and have nonenveloped icosahedral morphology. The large double-stranded DNA genome is linear and nonsegmented. The seven major human adenovirus species (designated A through G) fall into 57 immunologically distinct serotypes. Human respiratory tract infections are caused mainly by the B and C species. Adenovirus infections can occur throughout the year. Many serotypes cause sporadic outbreaks, while others appear to be endemic in particular locations. Respiratory illnesses include mild disease such as the common cold and lower respiratory tract illnesses including croup, bronchiolitis, and pneumonia. Conjunctivitis is associated with infection by the B and D species. A particular constellation of symptoms referred to as pharyngoconjunctival fever is frequently associated with acute adenovirus infection. In contrast, gastroenteritis has been associated most frequently with virus serotypes 40 and 41 of species F. Immunocompromised patients are highly susceptible to severe disease during infection with respiratory adenoviruses. The syndrome of acute respiratory disease (ARD), especially common in stressful or crowded living conditions, was first recognized among military recruits during World War II and has continued to be a problem when vaccination has been suspended temporarily because of lapses in vaccine supply. ARD is most often associated with adenovirus types 4 and 7. Adenovirus vaccine containing live adenovirus types 4 and 7 taken orally as two tablets, which prevents most illness caused by these two virus types, is only available for U.S. military personnel 17–50 years of age. It is recommended by the Department of Defense for military recruits entering basic training or other military personnel at high risk for adenovirus infection.

Coronaviridae Members of the genus *Coronavirus* also contribute to respiratory illness, including severe disease. Dozens of coronaviruses affect animals. In the twentieth century, only two representative strains of human coronaviruses were known to cause disease: 229E (HCoV-229E) and OC43 (HCoV-OC43). An outbreak of infection with SARS-associated coronavirus (SARS-CoV) first showed that animal coronaviruses have the potential to cross from other species to humans, with devastating effects. The one major SARS-CoV epidemic to date (2002–2003) encompassed >8000 cases, with mortality rates approaching 10%. SARS-CoV causes a systemic illness with a respiratory route of entry. In contrast to most other viral pneumonias, SARS lacks upper respiratory symptoms, although cough and dyspnea occur in most patients. Typically, patients present with a nonspecific illness manifesting as fever, myalgia, malaise, and chills or rigors; watery diarrhea may occur as well. Investigators have reported the identification of a fourth human coronavirus, HCoV-NL63. Evidence is emerging that this new group 1 coronavirus is a common respiratory pathogen of humans, causing both upper and lower respiratory tract illness. HCoV-HKU1 was first described in January 2005 after its detection in a patient with pneumonia. Several cases of respiratory illness have been associated with this virus, but its infrequent identification suggests that this group 2 coronavirus has caused a low incidence of illness to date. The Middle

East respiratory syndrome coronavirus (MERS-CoV), first isolated in 2012, causes severe disease in humans, with ~35% mortality and >2500 cases reported to date. MERS-CoV is a zoonotic virus (transmitted between animals and people). The virus likely emerged from bats in the Middle East, although studies have shown that humans are infected through direct or indirect contact with an intermediate host—infected dromedary camels.

COVID-19 SARS-CoV-2 emerged in an outbreak in Wuhan, China, that spread worldwide causing a severe pandemic. SARS-CoV-2 is the cause of a respiratory disease called COVID-19. The virus is a member of lineage B of the *Betacoronavirus* genus that not only includes the highly pathogenic viruses SARS-CoV-1 (which caused a smaller epidemic in 2002–2003) and MERS-CoV (a lineage C virus that caused small epidemics in 2012, 2015, and 2018), but also contains the lineage A common cold viruses CoV-OC43 and CoV-HKU1 and MERS-CoV. These are enveloped, positive-sense RNA viruses encoded by a viral RNA genome that is quite large, a single linear RNA segment of nearly 30,000 nucleotides that encodes four structural proteins, designated the S (spike), E (envelope), M (membrane), and N (nucleocapsid) proteins, and a large polyprotein that is cleaved into 16 nonstructural proteins in infected cells. The trimeric S protein is primed by the transmembrane protease serine 2 (TMPRSS2) to facilitate entry of SARS-CoV-2. SARS-CoV-2 S protein is a type 1 fusion machine that also mediates attachment using a receptor binding domain (RBD) that binds to the human angiotensin-converting enzyme 2 (hACE2) protein receptor.

EPIDEMIOLOGY OF COVID-19 The virus may have spilled over from a bat reservoir and was first detected in humans in late 2019 in Wuhan, China; it rapidly spread by human-to-human transmission through all provinces of China and then worldwide. The World Health Organization (WHO) designated SARS-CoV-2 a Public Health Emergency of International Concern on January 30, 2020, and declared the outbreak a pandemic on March 11, 2020. By August 2021, the virus had caused >200 million confirmed cases and >4.3 million deaths worldwide. The basic reproduction number (R_0) (the expected number of cases generated directly by one case in a population in which all individuals are susceptible to infection) of SARS-CoV-2 has been estimated to be between 5 and 6, which is substantially higher than that of seasonal influenza (typically 1–2). Densely populated settings such as prisons, cruise ships, nursing homes, airplanes, and large indoor gatherings facilitate even higher transmission efficiency. Transmission in outdoor settings is thought to be much less common. Health care workers and those working in dentistry have high potential for exposure. Certain individuals may have contributed to extraordinarily high transmission events (so-called "superspreaders"). Transmission does occur in school settings, although schools have not been considered a primary driver of population transmission. Spread of SARS-CoV-2 is believed to be primarily via respiratory droplets transmitted between persons in proximity when the droplets make direct contact with mucous membranes. Airborne transmission by small particle from person-to-person may occur, but airborne transmission over long distances is unlikely. Fomite transmission by contact with contaminated surfaces is considered a possible but not dominant mode of transmission; therefore, handwashing in environments of exposure makes sense. Large-scale frequent surface decontamination efforts have been deployed in public spaces, but the effect of these cleanings on reducing transmission is uncertain.

In July 2020, a more infectious variant virus with S protein amino acid variant G614 replaced the original D614 strain as the dominant form in the pandemic. Thousands of virus variants have been reported with sequences organized in an ever-evolving clade structure, including strains designated "Variants of Concern" with evidence of impact of S protein polymorphisms on the sensitivity of diagnostic tests, the effectiveness of antiviral drug or antibody treatments, or the preventive efficacy of vaccines. Such variants have independently arisen in diverse geographic areas and then spread widely. Some variants may exhibit a higher capacity to transmit from one person to another or to cause severe disease or death in infected individuals. The probability of dying for a person who is infected (the infection fatality rate) varies substantially across locations, depending on local factors including the population age and structure, number of nursing homes, and case mix of infected and deceased individuals. The infection rate, determined with seroprevalence studies, is difficult to ascertain reliably. Most locations appear to have an infection fatality rate of ~0.20%.

Advanced age is the principal risk factor for severe illness from COVID-19 (marked by need for hospitalization, intensive care, and mechanical ventilation). Over 95% of COVID-19 deaths occur in people over age 45, and >80% of deaths occur in people over age 65. Preexisting social and health disparities put some groups of people at increased risk of illness or death from COVID-19, including people with disabilities and many racial/ethnic minority groups. Male sex is associated with higher risk of severe disease (odds ratio, ~1.8). Most individuals who die have preexisting comorbidities. The risk of severe COVID-19 illness increases markedly with elevated body mass index (BMI). Overweight condition (BMI >25 kg/m^2 but <30 kg/m^2), obesity (BMI ≥30 kg/m^2 but <40 kg/m^2), and severe obesity (BMI of ≥40 kg/m^2) are risk factors for progressively increased severe COVID-19. Substance use, such as alcohol, opioid, or cocaine use disorder, and current or former smoking both increase risk. Pregnant women are more likely to suffer more severe illness. Most other medical conditions increase the risk of severe illness, but conditions that especially increase risk are as follows: (1) chronic lung diseases, including COPD, moderate-to-severe asthma, cystic fibrosis, and pulmonary hypertension interstitial lung disease; (2) cancer or cancer treatments, including hematologic malignancies, solid organ transplant, and stem cell transplant; (3) immunodeficiency, including primary immunodeficiency caused by inherited genetic defects or secondary or acquired immunodeficiency caused by prolonged use of corticosteroids, other immunosuppressive drugs, or HIV type 1 (HIV-1) infection; (4) hemoglobin blood disorders, including thalassemia or sickle cell disease; (5) cerebrovascular disease, such as stroke; (6) cognitive impairment or other neurologic conditions; (7) heart conditions, including arterial hypertension, heart failure, coronary artery disease, and cardiomyopathies; (8) obstructive sleep apnea; (9) chronic inflammatory, autoimmune diseases and rheumatic diseases; (10) type 1 or type 2 diabetes mellitus; (11) chronic liver disease, especially cirrhosis; and (12) genetic conditions, especially Down syndrome. A multisystem inflammatory syndrome in children (MIS-C) has been associated with COVID-19, comprising a persistent fever, involvement of multiple organ systems (including gastrointestinal, dermatologic, cardiac, renal, hematologic, and neurologic), and elevated circulating inflammatory markers. The highest risk individuals for MIS-C in the United States are Black and Latino children aged 3 to 12 years. A similar syndrome in adults (MIS-A) may occur rarely.

PREVENTATIVE MEASURES FOR COVID-19 Early in the epidemic, public health methods for prevention were mostly limited to nonpharmaceutical interventions, including social distancing (staying at least 6 feet from other people in public to avoid infection), social isolation (staying away from other people when infected), quarantine (staying at home for 14 days after potential exposure), limiting travel, and working from home. When a local epidemic persists, prior to entering health care settings, patients should be screened for clinical signs or symptoms common in COVID-19, especially fever, respiratory symptoms (cough, dyspnea, sore throat), myalgias, and anosmia/hyposmia. Universal masking should be required in health care settings during epidemic conditions. A medical (surgical) mask should be universally used by health care workers, patients, and visitors. A respirator (N95 or higher protection) without an exhalation valve is an alternative and should be used by health care workers in place of a medical mask during procedures that generate aerosols. When patients cannot wear masks, goggles or a face shield may provide some additional protection for health care workers. In general, in public settings during epidemic conditions, well-fitting cloth masks are indicated.

CLINICAL MANIFESTATIONS OF COVID-19 The disease course varies widely, including asymptomatic infection, mild disease, moderate disease, or severe disease requiring hospitalization, oxygen therapy, intensive care, and mechanical ventilation. A substantial proportion of patients (possibly a third of those infected) are asymptomatic, but those individuals can transmit the virus to others. Most individuals with symptomatic infection have mild disease (no pneumonia). Severe disease, typically requiring hospitalization and involving pneumonia and associated manifestations (dyspnea, radiographic involvement of more than half of the lung, and/or hypoxia with oxygen saturation ≤94%), is common. Critical disease with manifestations of respiratory failure requiring mechanical ventilation, multiorgan failure, or shock occurs and requires intensive care.

DIAGNOSIS OF COVID-19 The specific diagnosis of infection typically is made using nucleic acid amplification testing of respiratory tract secretions. Nasopharyngeal swabs are used mostly commonly, while saliva testing also has been implemented, especially in large-scale population screening efforts. Other more general laboratory testing during severe or critical illness reveals widespread abnormalities consistent with systemic disease including lymphopenia and thrombocytopenia; elevated inflammatory markers, such as interleukin 6 (IL-6), tumor necrosis factor α, ferritin, and C-reactive protein; elevated liver enzymes and lactate dehydrogenase; elevated markers of acute kidney injury; elevated D-dimer and prothrombin time; and elevated troponin and creatine phosphokinase. Research-grade tests show that beneficial components of the adaptive immune response, including antibodies and T cells, also arise during the first 1–2 weeks after exposure. Chest radiographs may exhibit abnormal findings such as consolidation and ground-glass opacities that are distributed bilaterally, especially in the lower lung regions, but also may be normal despite respiratory compromise. Chest computed tomography (CT) has features (ground-glass opacifications with or without mixed consolidation, pleural thickening, interlobular septal thickening, and air bronchograms) that can be systematically interpreted as typical, indeterminate, or atypical for COVID-19. Chest CT may be more sensitive than radiographs, but CT should be used principally for medical management of respiratory disease, not as a primary diagnostic tool for COVID-19. Lung ultrasound also has been used to image the lungs to detect some COVID-19 abnormalities.

CLINICAL COURSE OF COVID-19 The onset of disease is manifest typically within 4–5 days after exposure and nearly always within 14 days. Symptoms include cough, fever, myalgia, headache, dyspnea, sore throat, and gastrointestinal symptoms of nausea, vomiting, or diarrhea. Sudden onset of dysgeusia and anosmia (loss of taste and smell) occurs in a substantial number of cases, which typically resolves in weeks to months. Diverse dermatologic findings occur in patients with COVID-19 **(see Fig. A1-57 (A-C))**. General decline of health status, including onset or worsening of dementia, can occur in older individuals, especially those with cognitive impairment. Mental health consequences of the acute disease, isolation measures, and medical management regimens are common, including depression and social anxiety.

COMPLICATIONS OF COVID-19 Severe complications of infection can occur. The major complication in patients with severe disease is acute respiratory distress syndrome requiring oxygen therapy and mechanical ventilation. Thromboembolic complications are common in severe disease mostly occurring as venous thromboembolism, including pulmonary embolism or deep vein thrombosis. Events stemming from arterial thrombosis, including acute stroke or ischemia of the limbs, are reported. Cardiac complications manifest as heart failure, myocardial injury, or arrhythmias and cardiovascular syndromes, especially shock. Encephalopathy occurs commonly in critically ill patients, and delirium in the intensive care unit setting reduces overall survival. Other neurologic complications including seizures, ataxia, or motor or sensory deficits have been reported. Those with COVID-19 disease and laboratory markers of excessive inflammatory response can exhibit a pattern of persistent fever and multiorgan disease with high risk of fatal outcome. An excessive proinflammatory host response to SARS-CoV-2 infection likely contributes directly to pulmonary pathology and severity of COVID-19. Manifestations typically mediated by autoantibodies have been reported. Disease is usually caused by direct viral pathogenesis in tissues or the associated immune response, but secondary bacterial or fungal infections do occur, usually as bacteremia or respiratory infections.

MANAGEMENT OF COVID-19 General medical management of COVID-19 is focused on severe respiratory illness and systemic disease manifestations. As bacterial infection is an uncommon complication of COVID-19, antibiotics are not generally indicated, but when the diagnosis is uncertain, empiric antibiotic regimens for community-acquired or health care–associated pneumonia should be considered. Nonpharmacologic social measures to reduce transmission of SARS-CoV-2 have greatly reduced the incidence of influenza virus infection, but in communities in which influenza is circulating, empiric influenza antiviral treatment is recommended for patients hospitalized with suspected or documented COVID-19. Since there is such a substantial risk of thromboembolic complications, many experts recommend pharmacologic prophylaxis of venous thromboembolism for all hospitalized patients with COVID-19. Nonsteroidal anti-inflammatory drugs (NSAIDs) are often used as antipyretic agents, but questions have been raised about a possible association between NSAID use and worse outcomes with COVID-19; when possible, the preferred antipyretic agent is acetaminophen. Immunosuppressed individuals are at higher risk of severe illness or death; therefore, on a case-by-case basis, providers should decide whether to continue immunomodulatory agents such as steroids or other immunosuppressive drugs that were indicated for preexisting conditions prior to onset of COVID-19. Generally, experts agree that the best course usually is to continue common preexisting medications of aspirin, statins, and angiotensin-converting enzyme inhibitors or angiotensin receptor blockers.

The time to recovery from COVID-19 is affected by the severity of disease, the individual's preexisting comorbidities, and age. Generally, symptomatic infection is an acute syndrome that resolves in 2 weeks in ~80% of persons, especially following mild or moderate disease. Individuals with severe disease often require longer for recovery, on the order of several months. However, a subset of individuals with infection progress to a recurring or persisting pattern of symptoms, most commonly including fatigue, cognitive deficits, cough, dyspnea, or chest pain. Those with severe acute pulmonary or cardiac injury may have persisting respiratory or cardiac impairment. Diverse long-term adverse mental health consequences of infection are common, and the public health measures used to manage the pandemic also have led to social isolation with adverse mental health consequences.

OVERVIEW OF APPROACH TO SPECIFIC TREATMENTS FOR COVID-19 The approach to specific treatment of COVID-19 of varying levels of severity is under study in 2021 in thousands of clinical studies; summaries of registered international clinical trials are available at the *clinicaltrials.gov* and WHO websites. Availability of trial enrollment varies by locale, and local availability of medications or other interventions may affect what treatments are possible. Standardized medical regimens that are optimal for individuals with varied severity of disease are not fully established. At this time, only general principles of treatment can be asserted with confidence. The groups of medicines most explored to date based on mechanisms of action are antivirals and immunomodulators. Antivirals (including small-molecule inhibitors and polyclonal or monoclonal antibodies) have the most potential to alter the clinical course early in infection, since they may reduce the peak titer of virus, a parameter that is likely correlated with severity of disease. Later in the clinical course, anti-inflammatory medications may be of more benefit since the pathogenesis of disease is driven increasingly more over time by tissue inflammation and systemic inflammatory responses than by direct viral cytopathic effect.

We recommend consulting up-to-date recommendations from groups authorized to provide expert or governmental guidelines, including the National Institutes of Health COVID-19 Treatment Guidelines Panel in the United States (*https://www.covid19treatmentguidelines.nih.gov*), the National Health Service in the United Kingdom (*https://www.england.nhs.uk/coronavirus/*), and the Infectious Diseases Society of America (*https://www.idsociety.org/practice-guideline/covid-19-guideline-treatment-and-management/*). Many but not all the guidelines from such groups are harmonized. The strongest evidence for mortality or clinical benefit from clinical trials to date supports the use of the anti-inflammatory glucocorticoid dexamethasone, the antiviral small-molecule drug remdesivir (with or without the Janus kinase 1 and 2 inhibitor baricitinib), tocilizumab (a monoclonal antibody against the IL-6 receptor), and SARS-CoV-2–specific human monoclonal antibodies. In a phase 3 clinical trial, molnupiravir, an oral ribonucleoside analog that inhibits replication of SARS-CoV-2, reduced the risk of hospitalization or death in patients with mild-to-moderate COVID-19 by ~50%. AT-527–an oral nucleotide prodrug--reduced SARS-CoV-2 viral loads in a phase 2 clinical trial in hospitalized patients with COVID-19. The Emergency Use Authorization (EUA) authority allows the U.S. Food and Drug Administration (FDA) to facilitate availability and use of medical countermeasures prior to full licensure when the secretary of the Department of Health and Human Services declares that an EUA is appropriate for a public health emergency (*https://www.fda.gov/emergency-preparedness-and-response/mcm-legal-regulatory-and-policy-framework/emergency-use-authorization#infoMedDev*). As of May 2021, only the following drugs and biologic therapeutic products had obtained persisting EUA for treatment of COVID-19: (1) remdesivir for certain hospitalized COVID-19 patients; (2) a remdesivir plus baricitinib combination; (3) two different SARS-CoV-2 spike protein–specific monoclonal antibody cocktails bamlanivimab plus etesevimab or REGEN-COV (casirivimab plus imdevimab); and (4) COVID-19 convalescent plasma (containing SARS-CoV-2 polyclonal antibodies). Three vaccines had obtained EUA for prevention of COVID-19: (1) the two-dose Pfizer-BioNTech mRNA vaccine; (2) the two-dose Moderna mRNA vaccine; and (3) the single-dose adenovirus-based Janssen vaccine.

Individuals who are infected but have mild disease can be treated with supportive care only. Outpatients with certain high-risk factors may be eligible for therapy with monoclonal antibodies or convalescent plasma following exposure (postexposure prophylaxis) or during early mild infection (treatment). Individuals with severe respiratory disease (marked by hypoxia [oxygen saturation ≤94% on room air]) are administered oxygen therapy and tracheal intubation and mechanical ventilation if respiratory failure occurs.

SMALL-MOLECULE ANTIVIRAL DRUGS Remdesivir (GS-5734, a novel nucleotide analogue) is an enzyme inhibitor that was known prior to the pandemic to exhibit in vitro inhibitory activity against the coronavirus RNA–dependent, RNA polymerases of SARS-CoV-1 and MERS-CoV. Thus, remdesivir was identified soon after the outbreak as a promising therapeutic candidate antiviral drug because of its in vitro activity against SARS-CoV-2. The intravenous drug is now approved for hospitalized children ≥12 years and adults with COVID-19 with any level of severity. The efficacy is difficult to assess because of the many covariates in trials including differences in disease severity, concomitant therapies, comorbidities, and other factors. Its efficacy may be highest in those with mild to moderate disease, such as cases requiring low-flow oxygen. A cohort study of 2344 U.S. veterans hospitalized with COVID-19, however, showed remdesivir therapy was not associated with improved 30-day survival but was associated with a significant increase in median time to hospital discharge. The FDA issued an EUA for the Janus kinase inhibitor baricitinib to be used only in combination with remdesivir in COVID-19 patients requiring oxygen or mechanical ventilation. Janus kinase inhibitors such as baricitinib typically are used for treatment of rheumatoid arthritis because of their known immunomodulatory effects, which probably also improve inflammation during COVID-19, but baricitinib also may mediate some direct antiviral effects by interfering with viral entry into cells.

GLUCOCORTICOIDS Systemic treatment with glucocorticoids including dexamethasone, prednisone, methylprednisolone, and hydrocortisone reduces inflammation during severe COVID-19 and may be of clinical benefit, especially in reducing mortality or the need for mechanical ventilation; dexamethasone has the most data supporting benefit in COVID-19. Patients treated with high-dose glucocorticoids should be monitored for common adverse effects, especially hyperglycemia and increased risk of co-infection.

OTHER IMMUNOMODULATORS Beyond systemic glucocorticoids, additional immunomodulators have been studied and may be of benefit in certain circumstances. Careful studies of laboratory markers of inflammation showed that elevated blood levels of D-dimer, ferritin, C-reactive protein, and IL-6 are associated with severe COVID-19. The prior approval of two classes of FDA-approved IL-6 inhibitors (monoclonal antibodies binding to either the IL-6 cytokine itself [siltuximab] or to the IL-6 receptor [sarilumab or tocilizumab]) allowed rapid testing of the hypothesis that reducing the effects of elevated IL-6 could benefit subjects with severe COVID-19. The most robust data for efficacy exists for tocilizumab, and many experts suggest adding tocilizumab to dexamethasone therapy in patients with severe or progressive COVID-19. The use of many additional types of immunomodulators including bradykinin pathway inhibitors, hematopoietic colony-stimulating factors, complement inhibitors, and other cytokine or kinase inhibitors has been reported in case reports or case series, but there is insufficient evidence to support their use outside of clinical trial settings. Interferons are a family of cytokine mediators that alert or activate the immune system to viral infection, and interferon β has in vitro antiviral effects against many viruses including SARS-CoV-2. Intravenous, subcutaneous, or inhaled interferon β is being tested, but to date, there is insufficient evidence to support its use.

ANTIBODY-BASED THERAPIES Passive immunization with SARS-CoV-2 antibodies to achieve antiviral immunity or therapeutic effect has been tested using human monoclonal antibodies (mAbs) or convalescent plasma. Human mAbs are recombinant proteins made in the laboratory based on the genes encoding an antibody obtained typically from a single SARS-CoV-2–specific B cell isolated from the peripheral blood of a convalescent individual. Three mAb products have obtained EUA for use in outpatients with laboratory-confirmed mild-to-moderate SARS-CoV-2 infection who are at high risk for progressing to severe disease and/or hospitalization. The cocktail bamlanivimab plus etesevimab (EUA now revoked) and the cocktail casirivimab plus imdevimab each contain two antibodies binding to different epitopes on the RBD of the SARS-CoV-2 spike protein that mediates attachment and fusion of the virus into cells. Sotrovimab is a single mAb with a similar action. Ongoing surveillance studies of circulating SARS-CoV-2 variants have identified variants that exhibit reduced susceptibility to individual mAbs. Therefore, a cocktail approach is preferred for preventing or treating COVID-19, and ongoing surveillance is needed to determine if any variants will arise that escape both antibodies in this type of cocktail. Convalescent plasma (blood plasma taken from people who have recovered from COVID-19) contains polyclonal SARS-CoV-2 antibodies, and theoretically, this feature could prevent escape of variant antibodies from the limited specificities in the two-antibody mAb cocktails. However, the typical overall composite titer of SARS-CoV-2–neutralizing antibodies in convalescent plasma following a single primary infection is moderately low, limiting its effectiveness and reproducibility. In August 2020, the FDA issued an EUA for convalescent plasma for the treatment of hospitalized patients with COVID-19, regardless of titer of antibodies to SARS-CoV-2. In February 2021, the FDA revised the convalescent plasma EUA to limit the authorization to selected high-titer units of COVID-19 convalescent plasma and only for the treatment of hospitalized COVID-19 patients early in the disease course or hospitalized patients with impaired humoral immunity.

TREATMENT OF COMPLICATIONS Bacterial superinfection of COVID-19 probably occurs, but the incidence is uncertain. There are insufficient data to recommend empiric broad-spectrum antimicrobial therapy in the absence of another indication, although some experts routinely administer broad-spectrum antibiotics as empiric therapy for bacterial pneumonia to all patients with COVID-19 and moderate or severe hypoxemia. Ideally, providers initiating empiric therapy should attempt to deescalate or stop antibiotics if there is no ongoing evidence of bacterial infection. Many other complications of COVID-19 occur, including acute respiratory distress syndrome, acute cardiac injury, arrhythmias, thromboembolic events, acute kidney injury, and shock. Management of these more generalized complications is discussed elsewhere. Several EUAs have been issued for medical management of complications during COVID-19, including replacement solutions for continuous renal replacement therapy and drugs for sedation via continuous infusion in intensive care. Anticoagulation in the face of COVID-19–associated thromboembolic events is an especially complex situation and requires expert consultation.

Herpesviridae Several herpesviruses cause upper respiratory infections, especially infection of the oral cavity. Herpes simplex pharyngitis is associated with characteristic clinical findings, such as acute ulcerative stomatitis and ulcerative pharyngitis. HSV types 1 and 2—also called human herpesvirus (HHV) 1 and 2, respectively—both cause oral lesions (**Chap. 192**), although >90% of oral infections are caused by HSV-1. Primary oral disease can be severe, especially in young children, who sometimes are admitted for rehydration therapy as a result of poor oral intake. A significant proportion of individuals suffer recurrences of symptomatic disease consisting of vesicles on the lips. Epstein-Barr virus (EBV) mononucleosis syndrome (**Chap. 194**) is often marked by acute or subacute exudative pharyngitis; in some cases, tonsillar swelling in EBV pharyngitis is so severe that airway occlusion appears imminent. Most of the viruses in the family *Herpesviridae*—including CMV (**Chap. 195**); EBV; varicella-zoster virus (VZV; **Chap. 193**); and HHV-6, -7, and -8 (**Chap. 195**)—can cause severe disease in immunocompromised patients, especially hematopoietic stem cell transplant recipients.

***Parvoviridae:* Human Bocavirus** Human bocavirus (HBoV) was identified in 2005 in respiratory samples from children with lower respiratory tract disease. Sequence analysis of the genome revealed that the virus is a member of the genus *Bocavirus* (subfamily *Parvovirinae*, family *Parvoviridae*). This virus has been identified as the sole agent in a limited number of respiratory samples from individuals with respiratory tract disease, especially hospitalized young children, but the virus is also commonly found by RT-PCR tests in respiratory samples from healthy subjects.

***Retroviridae:* HIV** Pharyngitis occurs with primary HIV infection and may be associated with mucosal erosions and lymphadenopathy (**Chap. 202**).

***Papovaviridae:* Polyomaviruses** Polyomaviruses are small, double-stranded, DNA-genome, nonenveloped icosahedral viruses that may be oncogenic. Two major polyomaviruses, JC and BK viruses, are known to infect humans. Of adults in the United States, ≥80% are seropositive for these viruses. JC virus can infect the respiratory system, kidneys, or brain. BK virus infection causes a mild respiratory infection or pneumonia and can involve the kidneys of immunosuppressed transplant recipients.

EPIDEMIOLOGY

AGE

Age (along with the associated factor of prior exposure history) is a major determinant of risk for symptomatic disease during respiratory virus infection. Primary infection with most of the acute respiratory viruses often is more severe than secondary infection. Indeed, reinfection with most of these viruses occurs throughout life, but primary infection is much more likely to be associated with severe lower respiratory tract disease, while secondary infection typically is asymptomatic or associated with upper respiratory tract symptoms only. As these infections are ubiquitous, most primary infections (and thus many of the severe cases) occur during the first few years of life. Later, exposure to young children (in populations such as parents of young children and daycare workers) is a risk factor for frequent reinfection. Despite a lifetime of previous exposures, the risk of severe disease increases with age in the elderly, probably because of immune senescence and general medical decline.

SEASON

Infections with most of the conventional respiratory viruses (e.g., influenza virus, RSV, and hMPV) occur in winter. Typically, there is one dominant virus sweeping through a local community at any one time, a pattern that suggests some population-level interference with transmission. However, outbreaks can be closely spaced, and co-circulation of different viruses or antigenically diverse strains of one virus does occur. In the United States, some regional differences in seasonality have been noted; for example, RSV often appears in Florida and other southeastern states first. Seasons are, of course, reversed in the Northern and Southern hemispheres, so that winter epidemics occur roughly from November to March in the United States but from April to August in Australia; therefore, "winter" epidemics are almost always occurring somewhere in the world. Seasonal variances differ in the tropics, where acute respiratory viral infections are more common in the rainy season.

RISK FACTORS FOR DISEASE

Infection with these viruses is nearly universal, but disease expression varies among individuals infected with identical viruses. Therefore, investigators have sought to identify risk factors for severe disease. Most single risk factors identified have a moderate effect on the incidence of severe disease, but an accumulation of factors is associated with high risk. Underlying lung disease is a major factor, especially diseases associated with the need for chronic oxygen supplementation. COPD is one of the most profound risk factors. Other severe underlying medical conditions, especially cardiovascular disease, also enhance risk. Smoking (or exposure to wood smoke), low socioeconomic status, and male gender all contribute to a minor increase in the risk of lower respiratory tract illness. Obesity causes a chronic state with features of inflammation that are associated with impaired immunity, reduced response to vaccination, and higher susceptibility to severe disease. Close exposure to infected people is a major factor. For instance, living in close quarters (e.g., housing for military trainees, college dormitories, or nursing homes) puts groups of individuals at risk for rapid outbreaks. A breakdown in isolation and hand-washing compliance procedures can lead to cycles of nosocomial transmission of infection in hospital inpatient wards and intensive care units. In assessments of severe lower respiratory tract illness, a history of travel to an area with unusual agents should be considered carefully (e.g., exposure to avian influenza outbreaks in Asia, exposure to MERS-CoV in the Middle East). In 2020–2021, the dominance of the SARS-CoV-2 outbreak and the associated health measures deployed reduced the incidence of conventional respiratory viruses.

TRANSMISSION

Most respiratory viruses are transmitted by two principal modes: fomites or large-particle aerosols of respiratory droplets spread directly from person to person by coughing or sneezing. Fomite transmission occurs indirectly when infected respiratory droplets are deposited on the hands or on inanimate objects and surfaces, with subsequent transfer of secretions to a susceptible person's nose or conjunctiva. Most respiratory viruses do not spread by small-particle aerosols across rooms or down halls, although measles virus and VZV do spread in this manner. Therefore, contact and droplet precautions are sufficient to prevent transmission in most settings; hand washing is especially critical in health care settings during the winter. Intensive studies of the SARS-CoV-2 pandemic are ongoing (see previous sections on COVID-19), but many experts agree that exposure to large-particle droplets likely is one of the major ways that SARS-CoV-2 spreads.

APPROACH TO THE PATIENT
Common Viral Respiratory Infections

The principal interventions that make a difference in the care of patients with acute respiratory virus infections are supportive, and these factors should be managed meticulously. Hypoxia is managed with supplemental oxygen and respiratory failure with mechanical ventilation. Because the tachypnea and fever that often accompany pneumonia and wheezing frequently result in dehydration, fluid management is important. The astute clinician can narrow the etiologic possibilities on the basis of epidemiologic knowledge; information about viruses circulating in the community (widely available from local reference laboratories, county and state health departments, and the U.S. Centers for Disease Control and Prevention [CDC]); and the patient's exposure history, age, and immunologic status, including vaccination status. Proper use of rapid diagnostic tests is important. When diagnostic tests are applied only to samples from individuals at high risk of exposure to an infectious agent in the appropriate season, the positive predictive value of the test is increased. A central medical decision is whether to use a specific antibacterial or antiviral agent to treat a respiratory infection. Antibiotics do not improve the outcome of uncomplicated respiratory virus infections in otherwise healthy subjects. Some viral infections, especially influenza, can be complicated by secondary bacterial infection. There are only a limited number of licensed antiviral drugs, which should be used when a specific viral etiology is determined. Antiviral treatment generally is effective only when administered early in the course of illness.

CLINICAL MANIFESTATIONS

The common cold is characterized by nasal congestion, sneezing, rhinorrhea, cough, and sore throat. Laryngitis is accompanied by hoarseness or dysphonia. Acute bronchitis is characterized by a dry or productive cough of <3 weeks' duration (most prevalent in winter) in the absence of signs and symptoms of pneumonia and of evidence of pneumonia on chest radiography and is primarily caused by viruses. Bacteria play a more prominent role in chronic bronchitis. Bronchiolitis is an acute illness with wheezing and evidence of upper respiratory infection, primarily seen in the winter in infants and young children. The typical clinical manifestations of acute pneumonia include cough, sputum production, dyspnea, and chest pain. More systemic signs and symptoms also occur in pneumonia, including fever, fatigue, sweats, headache, myalgia, and occasionally nausea, abdominal pain, and diarrhea.

DIAGNOSIS

The clinical diagnosis of a respiratory syndrome and the anatomic location of infection are based on history, physical examination, and radiography. A specific viral etiology can be determined by specific diagnostic tests. The gold standard for diagnosing a respiratory viral infection is virus isolation, performed by inoculation of cell cultures with fresh secretions and use of multiple cell types in a reference laboratory staffed by experienced technologists. Direct or indirect fluorescent antibody detection can be used to visualize virus-infected cells in nasal secretions. Rapid antigen-based diagnostic tests are used to detect influenza virus or RSV proteins in nasopharyngeal secretions. The most sensitive tests typically are RT-PCR molecular diagnostic tests that amplify and detect the presence of viral genomic RNA or DNA in respiratory secretions. Multiplex panels assaying a sample for a dozen or more common respiratory viruses are available. These tests must be used and interpreted carefully because of their extreme sensitivity. If care is not taken, it is relatively easy to contaminate a PCR test in the laboratory with small amounts of DNA from a previous reaction. In addition, because a viral genome can sometimes persist in nasal secretions for weeks after an infection resolves, a positive test may indicate a recently resolved rather than a currently acute infection. Despite these limitations, PCR tests generally are considered the most sensitive and specific tests available. Chest radiographs should be obtained for all patients with suspected pneumonia.

TREATMENT
Common Viral Respiratory Infections

INFLUENZA (SEE ALSO CHAP. 200)

Several drugs are licensed in the United States for the treatment or prophylaxis of influenza. Neuraminidase inhibitors act on both influenza A and B viruses by serving as transition-state analogs of the viral neuraminidase that is needed to release newly budded virion progeny from the surface of infected cells. The cell surface normally is coated heavily with the viral receptor sialic acid. Oseltamivir is administered orally and is effective for the prevention or treatment of uncomplicated influenza in otherwise healthy adults. Observational studies indicate that oseltamivir also may be beneficial during serious illness. The drug is generally well tolerated, with primarily gastrointestinal toxicity. Zanamivir, a powder that is administered through oral inhalation, exhibits effectiveness like that of oseltamivir. Moreover, zanamivir is active against some influenza virus strains that are resistant to oseltamivir. Inhalation of zanamivir powder may cause bronchospasm in patients with COPD or asthma. Peramivir is a neuraminidase inhibitor that acts as a transition-state analog inhibitor of the influenza neuraminidase enzyme that is administered intravenously as a single 600-mg dose. It is efficacious in acute, uncomplicated influenza and was approved by the FDA in 2014 for treatment of individuals who cannot take oral or inhaled medications. Laninamivir was approved in Japan for prophylaxis (2013) or treatment (2010) of influenza; it is under investigation in the United States. It is a polymeric zanamivir conjugate that is delivered by oral inhalation, and it exhibits greater potency and longer retention times than conventional zanamivir. Baloxavir marboxil is a new class of drug for influenza. It is a prodrug whose metabolism releases the active agent baloxavir acid that inhibits influenza virus cap-dependent endonuclease activity in infected cells. This activity is used by the virus for a process in which the first 10–20 residues of a host cell RNA are removed and used as the 5′ cap and primer to initiate the synthesis of the influenza mRNA (a process sometimes termed "cap snatching"). Baloxavir marboxil was approved by the FDA in 2018 for treatment of acute uncomplicated flu within 2 days of illness onset in otherwise healthy people 12 years and older or those at high risk of developing flu-related complications. In 2020, the FDA approved an updated indication to include postexposure prevention of influenza for people ≥12 years old after contact with an infected person. The adamantanes amantadine and rimantadine were used in the past for the treatment of influenza A infection. These drugs interfere with the ion channel activity caused by the M2 protein of influenza A viruses, which is needed for viral particle uncoating after endocytosis. Widespread resistance occurs in many currently circulating influenza A viruses; therefore, the adamantanes should not be used unless isolate sensitivity is demonstrated, and in most influenza seasons, the CDC does not advise their use. When they are used, they are administered orally and display efficacy against uncomplicated influenza A caused by susceptible strains. The effectiveness of these drugs in serious illness has not been established. Toxicity with rimantadine generally manifests as gastrointestinal intolerance. Toxicity with amantadine is primarily associated with central nervous system symptoms.

RSV INFECTION

Ribavirin is a nucleoside antimetabolite prodrug whose activation by kinases in the cell results in a 5′-triphosphate nucleotide form that inhibits RNA replication. The drug was licensed in an aerosol formula in the United States in 1986 for treatment of children with severe RSV-induced lower respiratory tract infection. The efficacy of aerosolized ribavirin therapy remains uncertain despite several clinical trials. Most centers use it infrequently, if ever, in otherwise healthy infants with severe RSV disease. Intravenous ribavirin has been used for adenovirus, hantavirus, measles virus, PIV, and influenza virus infections, although a good risk/benefit profile has not been clearly established for any of these uses.

OTHER VIRAL TARGETS

Pleconaril, an oral drug with good bioavailability for treatment of infections caused by picornaviruses, has been tested for treatment of rhinovirus infection. This drug acts by binding to a hydrophobic pocket in the VP1 protein and stabilizing the protein capsid, preventing release of viral RNA into the cell. Pleconaril reduces mucus secretions and other symptoms and is being further examined for this indication. Acyclovir and related compounds are guanine-analogue antiviral drugs used in the treatment of herpesvirus infections. HSV stomatitis in immunocompromised patients is treated with famciclovir or valacyclovir, and immunocompetent patients with severe oral disease compromising oral intake are sometimes treated with these agents. These compounds have also been used prophylactically to prevent the recurrence of outbreaks, with mixed results. Intravenous acyclovir is effective against HSV or VZV pneumonia in immunocompromised patients. Ganciclovir, given together with human immunoglobulin, may reduce the mortality rates associated with CMV pneumonia in hematopoietic stem cell transplant recipients and has been used as monotherapy in other patient groups. Cidofovir is a nucleotide analog with activity against many viruses, including adenoviruses. Intravenous cidofovir has been effective in the management of severe adenoviral infection in immunocompromised patients but may cause serious nephrotoxicity.

COMPLICATIONS: CO-INFECTIONS

Co-infections with two or more viruses can occur because of the overlap in the winter season of these viruses in temperate areas. In general, in careful studies using cell culture techniques for virus isolation, two or more viruses were isolated from respiratory secretions of otherwise healthy adults with acute respiratory illness in ~5–10% of cases. There is little evidence that more severe disease occurs during co-infections. The incidence of positive results in two molecular diagnostic tests (generally RT-PCR for these RNA viruses) is expected to be higher than that of culture because, as discussed above, molecular tests can remain positive for an extended period after shedding of infectious virus has ended.

PREVENTION

VACCINES

Numerous vaccines against influenza viruses have been licensed. In the United States, trivalent and quadrivalent inactivated intramuscular vaccines (covering H3N2, H1N1, and one or two B antigens) and a live attenuated trivalent vaccine for intranasal administration are available (although components of the live attenuated vaccine were only ~3% effective during the 2013–2016 seasons and that vaccine was not available during the 2016–2018 seasons). Vaccines are effective when the vaccine strains chosen for inclusion are highly related antigenically to the epidemic strain, but occasional antigenic mismatches cause negligible efficacy of a vaccine component. Antigenic drift caused by point mutations in the hemagglutinin (HA) and neuraminidase (NA) molecules leads to antigenic divergence, requiring the production of new vaccines each year. The segmented influenza genome allows reassortment of two viruses during co-infection of one individual or animal; sometimes the consequence is a major antigenic shift resulting in a pandemic. On average, pandemics occur every 20–30 years. There is current concern about the potential for an H5N1 or H7N9 pandemic, and experimental vaccines are being tested for these viruses.

Vaccines were developed for adenovirus serotypes 4 and 7 and were approved for prevention of epidemic respiratory illness among military recruits. Essentially, these vaccines consisted of unmodified viruses given by the enteric route in capsules instead of by the respiratory route—the natural route of infection leading to disease. Inoculation by the altered route resulted in an immunizing asymptomatic infection. Most U.S. military recruits are vaccinated against adenovirus, and epidemic disease recurs in the absence of vaccination.

Live attenuated and subunit vaccine candidates against RSV are under development and are being tested in clinical trials. Subunit RSV vaccines are being tested for maternal immunization and in the elderly. There are no licensed vaccines against rhinoviruses; as there is little or no cross-protection between serotypes, it will be challenging to develop a vaccine covering >100 serotypes. Efforts to develop seasonal coronavirus vaccines are in the preclinical stage.

PASSIVE PROTECTION WITH IMMUNOTHERAPY

Palivizumab, a humanized mouse monoclonal antibody to the F protein of RSV, is licensed for prevention of RSV hospitalization in high-risk infants, in half or more of whom it is effective. Experimental treatment of both immunocompetent and immunocompromised RSV-infected individuals has been reported, but the efficacy of this approach has not been established. Next-generation antibodies with higher potency and an extended half-life of ~90 days are being tested. In 2019, the FDA granted Breakthrough Therapy designation for a potential next-generation RSV monoclonal antibody—MEDI8897. This designation was based on a favorable primary analysis of the phase 2B trial that demonstrated the safety and efficacy of this RSV-neutralizing human monoclonal antibody.

ISOLATION PROCEDURES, PERSONAL PROTECTIVE EQUIPMENT, AND HAND WASHING

Most respiratory viruses are spread by direct contact—i.e., body-surface to body-surface contact and physical transfer of microorganisms between a susceptible person and an infected person. Poor hand hygiene is probably the most common cause of contact transmission of viruses, which occurs often in family, school, and workplace settings. Transmission between health care workers and patients also takes place when hand-washing compliance is low. Fomites (objects or substances capable of carrying infectious organisms), including instruments, stethoscopes, and other objects in medical environments, can contribute to transmission. Small-particle-mediated airborne transmission can occur but is probably not the dominant mode of transmission for most respiratory viruses. Particle size affects the epidemiology of airborne pathogens. The composition and size distribution of the generated particles affect the duration of suspension of the infectious agents in the air, the distance across which they can be transported, the interval during which the virus remains infectious, and the site of deposition in the airway of a susceptible host. Direct exposure to large-particle aerosols (e.g., exposure at close range—up to 3 ft—to a cough or sneeze) causes some transmission. Particles of small size can remain suspended in the air for long periods; for instance, particles of ~1 μm can remain suspended for hours. However, in general, only a few respiratory viruses are thought to be transmitted by small-particle aerosols. Protection from transmission in health care environments can be achieved by proper implementation of and adherence to established procedures for the appropriate level of precaution.

Standard and Contact Precautions Standard precautions, the basic level of infection control that is always used in the care of all patients, reduces the risk of transmission of viruses from respiratory tract secretions and mucous membranes. Contact precautions, the second level, require a single room for the patient when possible and the use of additional personal protective equipment, including the wearing of clean, nonsterile gloves when touching a patient or coming into contact with secretions. Fluid-resistant nonsterile gowns are used to protect skin and clothing during activities where contact with secretions is anticipated, and providers should wear each gown for the care of only one patient. A face mask is used when there is potential for direct contact with respiratory secretions. Eye protection (goggles or face shields) is worn in anticipation of potential splashing of respiratory secretions. Good hand hygiene should always follow any patient contact, including washing for 20 s with soap and warm water or cleaning with an alcohol-based hand rub. Providers should attempt to avoid the contamination of clothing and the transfer of microorganisms to other patients, surfaces, or environments.

Droplet Precautions Large-particle droplets are generated during sneezing and coughing and during the performance of some medical procedures, such as airway suctioning in critical care units or bronchoscopy. Such droplets may contain viruses, but their range is usually limited to about 3 ft. Transmission of large-particle droplets occurs when they are deposited on the nasal mucosa or conjunctivae. To prevent transmission in these settings, providers should implement droplet precautions. They should wear a face mask, such as a surgical mask, for close contact (within 3 ft of the patient). Patients also should wear a face mask when exiting the examination room and should avoid coming into close contact with other patients.

Airborne Precautions Airborne transmission occurs through the dissemination of airborne droplet nuclei (particles of ≤5 μm) or evaporated droplets containing viruses that can remain suspended in the air for long periods. Certain viruses that are carried by the airborne route can be inhaled by a susceptible host in the same room or over a long distance from the source patient, depending on environmental factors such as temperature and ventilation. Viruses transmitted by this route are SARS-CoV, measles virus, and VZV. Patients with these infections should be managed with personal respiratory protection and special ventilation and air handling. Providers should wear an N95 respirator selected with fit-testing, which must be repeated annually. Powered air-purifying respirators (PAPRs) are used in some cases. The patient should be housed in an airborne-infection isolation room—a negative-pressure room that has a minimum of six air exchanges per hour and exhausts through high-efficiency particulate air (HEPA) filtration or directly to the outside.

GLOBAL CONSIDERATIONS

HENDRA AND NIPAH VIRUSES

These emerging paramyxoviruses, which are grouped in their own new genus (*Henipavirus*), may not be respiratory pathogens in a conventional sense, but they probably infect humans by the respiratory route. Nipah virus is a newly recognized zoonotic virus, named after the location in Malaysia where it was first identified in 1999. It has caused disease in humans who have had contact with infectious animals. Hendra virus (formerly called equine morbillivirus) is another closely related zoonotic paramyxovirus and was first isolated in Australia in 1994. The viruses have caused only a few localized outbreaks, but their wide host range and ability to cause high mortality raise concerns for the future. The natural host of these viruses is thought to be a certain species of fruit bat present in Australia and the Pacific. Pigs may be an intermediate host for transmission to humans in Nipah infection and horses in Hendra infection. Although the mode of transmission from animals to humans is not defined, inoculation of infected materials onto the respiratory tract probably plays a role. The clinical presentation usually appears to be an influenza-like syndrome that progresses to encephalitis, includes respiratory illness, and causes death in about half of identified cases.

BUNYAVIRIDAE: HANTAVIRUS

Intermittent outbreaks of hantavirus infection occur in South America and cause a severe lung infection: HPS. In addition, >400 cases of HPS have been reported in the United States. The disease was first recognized during an outbreak in 1993. About one-third of recognized cases end in death. The Four Corners outbreak (at the intersection of the northwestern corner of New Mexico, the northeastern corner of Arizona, the southeastern corner of Utah, and the southwestern corner of Colorado) is well known; however, cases now have been reported in a total of 32 states. Patients with HPS usually present with an influenza-like illness, including fever. Findings on physical examination are nonspecific, often consisting only of fever and elevated respiratory and heart rates. In addition to respiratory symptoms, abdominal pain is common. Diagnosis is often delayed until illness becomes severe, at which point intubation and mechanical ventilation may be required for respiratory support.

SUMMARY

Viruses are the leading causes of acute lower respiratory tract infection in most populations. Influenza virus and RSV are the most common pathogens; hMPV, PIV3, and rhinoviruses account for most other acute viral respiratory infections. Infection in otherwise healthy adults generally leads to partial immunity to these pathogens, with protection against severe lower respiratory disease. However, reinfection, with upper respiratory tract illness, is common throughout life. Special populations such as immunocompromised patients, institutionalized frail elderly patients, and patients with COPD are at highest risk for severe disease.

FURTHER READING

Arons MM et al: Presymptomatic SARS-CoV-2 infections and transmission in a skilled nursing facility. N Engl J Med 382:2081, 2020.

Beard KR et al: Treatment of influenza with neuraminidase inhibitors. Curr Opin Infect Dis 31:51, 2018.

Centers for Disease Control and Prevention: Infection control guidance. Available at *https://www.cdc.gov/coronavirus/2019-ncov/hcp/infection-control-recommendations.html*. Updated February 23, 2021. Accessed May 9, 2021.

Centers for Disease Control and Prevention: Updated healthcare infection prevention and control recommendations in response to COVID-19 vaccination. Available at *https://www.cdc.gov/coronavirus/2019-ncov/hcp/infection-control-after-vaccination.html*. Updated April 27, 2021. Accessed May 9, 2021.

Centers for Disease Control and Prevention: Interim clinical considerations for use of mRNA COVID-19 vaccines currently authorized in the United States. Available at *https://www.cdc.gov/vaccines/covid-19/info-by-product/clinical-considerations.html*. Accessed January 7, 2021.

Diaz-Decaro JD et al: Critical evaluation of FDA-approved respiratory multiplex assays for public health surveillance. Expert Rev Mol Diagn 18:631, 2018.

Falsey AR et al: Bacterial complications of respiratory tract viral illness: A comprehensive evaluation. J Infect Dis 208:432, 2013.

Fendrick AM et al: The economic burden of non-influenza-related viral respiratory tract infection in the United States. Arch Intern Med 163:487, 2013.

Fry AM et al: Seasonal trends of human parainfluenza viral infections: United States, 1990–2004. Clin Infect Dis 43:1016, 2006.

Infectious Diseases Society of America: Guidelines on the treatment and management of patients with COVID-19. Available at *https://www.idsociety.org/practice-guideline/covid-19-guideline-treatment-and-management/*. Published April 11, 2020. Updated April 14, 2021. Accessed May 9, 2021.

Iuliano AD et al: Estimates of global seasonal influenza-associated respiratory mortality: A modelling study. Lancet 391:1285, 2018.

Johnston SL et al: The relationship between upper respiratory infections and hospital admissions for asthma: A time-trend analysis. Am J Respir Crit Care Med 154:654, 1996.

McMichael TM et al: COVID-19 in a long-term care facility - King County, Washington, February 27-March 9, 2020. MMWR Morb Mortal Wkly Rep 69:339, 2020.

Monto AS, Cavallaro JJ: The Tecumseh study of respiratory illness. II. Patterns of occurrence of infection with respiratory pathogens, 1965–1969. Am J Epidemiol 94:280, 1971.

National Health Service England: Coronavirus guidance for clinicians and NHS managers. Available at *https://www.england.nhs.uk/coronavirus/*. Accessed May 9, 2021.

National Institutes of Health: COVID-19 Treatment Guidelines Panel. Coronavirus Disease 2019 (COVID-19) treatment guidelines. Available at *https://www.covid19treatmentguidelines.nih.gov/*. Updated April 23, 2021. Accessed May 9, 2021.

Segaloff HE et al: The impact of obesity and timely antiviral administration on severe influenza outcomes among hospitalized adults. J Med Virol 90:212, 2018.

U.S. Food and Drug Administration: Emergency use authorization. Available at *https://www.fda.gov/emergency-preparedness-and-response/mcm-legal-regulatory-and-policy-framework/emergency-use-authorization#infoMedDev*. Accessed May 9, 2021.

Wang D et al: Clinical characteristics of 138 hospitalized patients with 2019 novel coronavirus-infected pneumonia in Wuhan, China. JAMA 323:1061, 2020.

Williams JV et al: Human metapneumovirus infection plays an etiologic role in acute asthma exacerbations requiring hospitalization in adults. J Infect Dis 192:1149, 2005.

200 Influenza

Kathleen M. Neuzil, Peter F. Wright

DEFINITION

The term *influenza* represents both a clinically defined respiratory illness accompanied by systemic symptoms of fever, malaise, and myalgia and the name of the orthomyxoviruses that cause this syndrome. Although this term is sometimes used more generally to denote any viral respiratory illness, many features distinguish influenza from these other illnesses, most particularly its systemic symptoms, its propensity to cause sharply peaked winter epidemics in temperate climates, and its capacity to spread rapidly among close contacts. The morbidity and mortality associated with influenza epidemics are documented closely in the United States by the Centers for Disease Control and Prevention (CDC), which records clinical cases of influenza-like illness, cases of virologically documented influenza, and excess deaths due to pneumonia and influenza combined.

ETIOLOGIC AGENTS

Three influenza viruses occur in humans: A, B, and C. These viruses are irregularly circular in shape, measure 80–120 nm in diameter, and have a lipid envelope and prominent spikes that are formed by the two surface glycoproteins, hemagglutinin (H) and neuraminidase (N) (**Fig. 200-1**). The hemagglutinin functions as the viral attachment protein, binding to sialic acid receptors on the cells that line the superficial epithelium of the respiratory tract. The neuraminidase cleaves the virus from the cell membrane to facilitate its release from the cell and prevents self-aggregation of viruses. Influenza A viruses have eight single-strand negative-sense RNA segments in their genomes that encode hemagglutinin and neuraminidase as well as internal genes, including polymerase, matrix, nucleoprotein, and nonstructural genes. The segmented nature of the genome allows gene *reassortment*; an analogy for reassortment is the shuffling of a deck of cards. Reassortment takes place when a single cell is infected with two different strains.

Among the influenza viruses, the A viruses are of paramount importance for several reasons: (1) the plasticity of their genomes, which enables them to react to the prevailing immunity in the community by modifying their immunogenic epitopes, particularly on the hemagglutinin surface protein (*antigenic drift*); (2) the segmentation of their genomes, which allows genes coding both surface and internal proteins to be reassorted between influenza A variants (*antigenic shift*); and (3) their extensive mammalian and avian reservoirs, in which multiple variants with distinct hemagglutinin and neuraminidase genes lie in wait. As a result of all of these factors, influenza A virus has the ability, particularly after an antigenic shift, to cause a worldwide epidemic (*pandemic*). The most severe influenza A pandemic in modern history took place in 1918; ~50 million deaths were attributed to the culpable influenza A H1N1 virus in the years surrounding 1918.

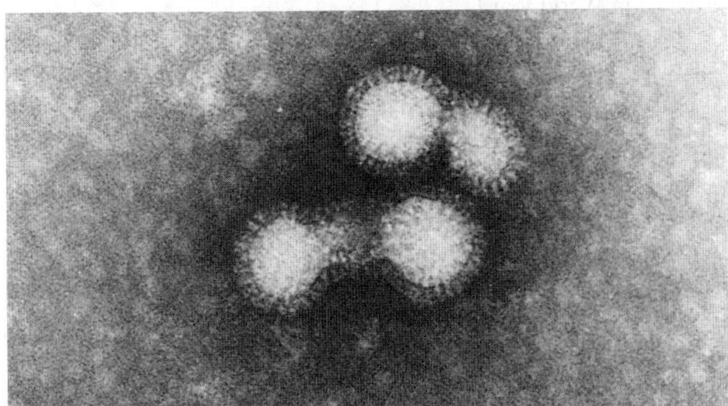

FIGURE 200-1 An electron micrograph of influenza A virus (×40,000). *(YZ Cohen, R Dolin: Influenza, in Harrison's Principles of Internal Medicine, 19th ed. DL Kasper et al [eds]. New York: McGraw-Hill, 2015, p 1209.)*

The influenza A viruses are further classified by their surface glycoproteins (H and N), the geographic location of their isolation, their sequential number among isolated viruses, and their year of isolation. Thus, for the 2021–22 season, U.S.-licensed influenza vaccines will contain an influenza A/Victoria/2570/2019 (H1N1)pdm09-like virus (for egg-based vaccines) or an influenza A/Wisconsin/588/2019 (H1N1)pdm09-like virus (for cell-based and recombinant vaccines); an influenza A/Cambodia/e0826360/2020 (H3N2)-like virus; influenza B/Washington/02/2019 (Victoria lineage)-like virus; and an influenza B/Phuket/3073/2013 (Yamagata lineage)-like virus.

EPIDEMIOLOGY

Influenza virus causes outbreaks during the cooler months of the year and thus has a mirror-image season in the antipodes compared with that in the Northern Hemisphere. The circulation of strains in the Southern Hemisphere has some predictive value for vaccine composition in the Northern Hemisphere, and vice versa. This information is important as the degree of antigenic drift is one determinate of vaccine efficacy. Vaccine composition typically must change in at least one component yearly in anticipation of the predicted circulating strains.

A typical outbreak begins in early winter and lasts 4–5 weeks in a given community, although its impact on the country as a whole will be of considerably longer duration. When excess mortality occurs, an influenza outbreak is classified as an *epidemic*. Influenza's impact is reflected in increased school and work absenteeism, increased visits to emergency departments and primary care physicians, and increased hospitalizations, particularly of elderly patients and individuals with underlying cardiopulmonary disease. The impact often is most easily recognized in the pediatric population, whose school absenteeism quickly peaks.

Influenza's global spread and causative strain(s) in a given year are well documented by the surveillance networks of the World Health Organization (WHO) and the CDC. The severity of an epidemic depends on the transmissibility and virulence of the viral strain, the susceptibility of the population, the adaptation of the virus to its human host, and the degree of antigenic match to the recommended vaccine. None of these parameters is totally predictable for influenza A.

Influenza is largely spread by small- and large-particle droplets; spread is undoubtedly facilitated by the coughing and sneezing that accompany the illness. Within families, the illness is often introduced by a preschool or school-aged child. In the United States, influenza virus circulation in first-quarter 2020 declined sharply within 2 weeks of the COVID-19 emergency declaration and widespread implementation of community mitigation measures and travel restrictions. The decline occurred in other Northern Hemisphere countries and the tropics. In 2020, Southern Hemisphere temperate climates had virtually no influenza circulation. Influenza activity remained at low levels at the start of the 2020–2021 Northern Hemisphere season. While changes in health care–seeking behavior and testing priorities during the pandemic may have contributed, such declines in influenza detection were noted even in areas with continued or increased testing, implicating community mitigation measures as the most likely reason.

Influenza A Viruses When a major shift in the hemagglutinin and/or the neuraminidase occurs, with introduction of a new serotype from an animal or avian reservoir, an influenza A strain has the potential to cause a pandemic. In modern influenza history, such shifts

TABLE 200-1 Emergence of Antigenic Subtypes of Influenza A Virus Associated with Pandemic or Epidemic Disease

YEARS	SUBTYPE	EXTENT OF OUTBREAK
1889–1890	H2N8[a]	Severe pandemic
1900–1903	H3N8[a]	Moderate epidemic
1918–1919	H1N1[b] (formerly HswN1)	Severe pandemic
1933–1935	H1N1[b] (formerly H0N1)	Mild epidemic
1946–1947	H1N1	Mild epidemic
1957–1958	H2N2	Severe pandemic
1968–1969	H3N2	Moderate pandemic
1977–1978[c]	H1N1	Mild pandemic
2009–2010[d]	H1N1	Pandemic

[a]As determined by retrospective serologic survey of individuals alive during those years ("seroarchaeology"). [b]Hemagglutinins formerly designated as Hsw and H0 are now classified as variants of H1. [c]From this time until 2016–2017, viruses of the H1N1 and H3N2 subtypes circulated in alternating years or concurrently. [d]A novel influenza A/H1N1 virus emerged to cause this pandemic.

Source: Adapted from YZ Cohen, R Dolin. Influenza. In: Kasper DL, et al, eds. *Harrison's Principles of Internal Medicine.* 19th ed. New York, McGraw-Hill; 2015:1209.

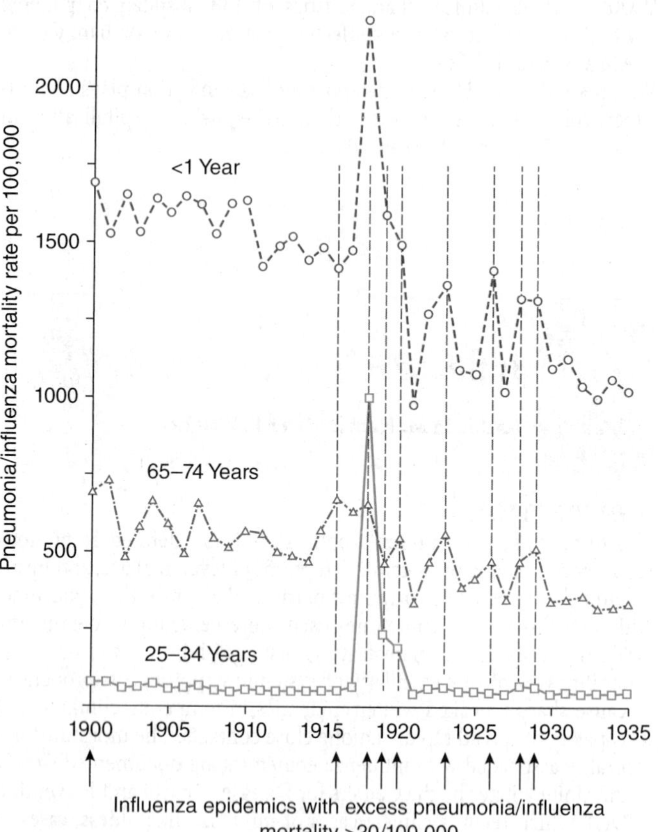

FIGURE 200-2 Excess pneumonia/influenza deaths in 1900–1953, demonstrating the dramatic peaks of deaths among young infants and young adults (25–34 years of age) in 1918. *(Data are from public health records collated by the PF Wright.)*

occurred in 1918 (H1N1), 1957 (H2N2), 1968 (H3N2), 1977 (H1N1), and 2009 (H1N1pdm) (**Table 200-1**). On the basis of seroarchaeology (the analysis of serum antibody profiles in the elderly), epidemics that took place in the 1890s have been attributed to H3N2 and H2N2 viruses. Epidemics typical of influenza have been documented throughout recorded history.

In some epidemics, a younger age group proves especially susceptible. This is the case with current H1N1 epidemics, where individuals born before 1968 had likely been exposed to related viral strains and thus were relatively protected against the current strain. The 1918 epidemic was striking in this regard: the most severely infected individuals were infants and previously healthy young adults—the latter being a group not typically found to have high influenza mortality (**Fig. 200-2**). The 1918 epidemic increased all-cause mortality and led to more deaths than all military losses in World War I. In spite of the attention paid to the risk and impact of pandemic disease, it is generally appreciated that—with the exception of 1918—cumulatively more illness occurs during yearly epidemics combined than in pandemics.

All of the annual influenza A epidemics in the past 50 years have been caused by H1N1 and/or H3N2 strains. H2N2 strains circulated between 1957 and 1968, and H1N1 strains circulated prior to that, including in 1918. However, potentially pandemic viruses continue to emerge, mostly in Asia, with higher-numbered hemagglutinins (e.g., H5, H6, H7, H8, H9) reflecting some of the 18 distinct H and 11 distinct N subtypes in avian reservoirs. Most cases of these potentially pandemic illnesses have occurred in individuals who have had direct contact with domesticated birds or who have visited live-bird markets, which are common in Asia. In addition to the global aeronautic movement of infected people, bird migration is one mechanism for rapid global spread. It is not clear why higher-numbered avian hemagglutinin strains have not acquired the degree of transmissibility necessary to cause pandemic disease.

Avian and Swine Influenza Viruses The full panoply of influenza viruses is found in domestic and migratory wild birds. It is postulated that epithelial cells in the swine respiratory tract may play a specific role as a "mixing vessel," allowing the reassortment of genes from avian and human sources and thereby permitting the transmission of avian viruses to humans. The nature of the sialic acid receptors for influenza virus hemagglutinin partially accounts for host preference. Humans have largely α-2,6-galactose receptors, while birds have α-2,3-galactose receptors. Swine have both types of receptors on their respiratory epithelial cells—hence their postulated role in facilitating reassortment and host adaptation of avian strains to growth in humans. Strains such as 2009 H1N1pdm (pandemic) had genes of avian, swine, and human origin. Some avian strains—notably H5 strains—are highly pathogenic in humans, as was the 1918 strain. The reasons for the high pathogenicity of certain strains are not entirely clear. Virulence and transmissibility often appear to be separate genetic traits.

After the sequencing of the 1918 virus recovered from the lungs of bodies buried in the Arctic permafrost, the virus was genetically reconstructed under carefully controlled isolation conditions. In animal studies of this viable 1918 virus, both the hemagglutinin and the ribonucleoprotein contributed to high levels of replication accompanied by an abnormally enhanced innate immune response characterized by proinflammatory cytokines. Perhaps this "cytokine storm" is the best explanation for the enhanced illness occurring in young, immunologically vigorous individuals in the 1918 pandemic. Sequencing demonstrated that the 1918 virus was of avian origin. Although the 1918 virus was first identified in military camps in the United States, its impact cannot be attributed to the disruption of war: the illness was well documented in countries such as Iceland that were not directly involved in World War I.

The same concerns about a "cytokine storm" have been raised with regard to the H5N1 viruses that first emerged in Hong Kong in 1996. These viruses exhibited high pathogenicity in individuals who had direct contact with domestic fowl, with mortality rates close to 50%, but also displayed poor human-to-human transmissibility. Pathogenicity appears to be a function not just of the viruses' surface proteins, but also of an optimal gene constellation including all eight segmented influenza genes. However, unlike the 1918 strain, the H5N1 viruses have, to date, caused only sporadic disease, as have other limited clusters of a highly pathogenic H7N9 virus.

Influenza B and C Viruses The influenza B viruses are more genetically stable than the influenza A viruses and are mainly associated with human infection. Two lineages of influenza B have circulated for the past 40 years (B/Yamagata-like and B/Victoria-like viruses), and it has proven very difficult to predict which strain will be dominant in

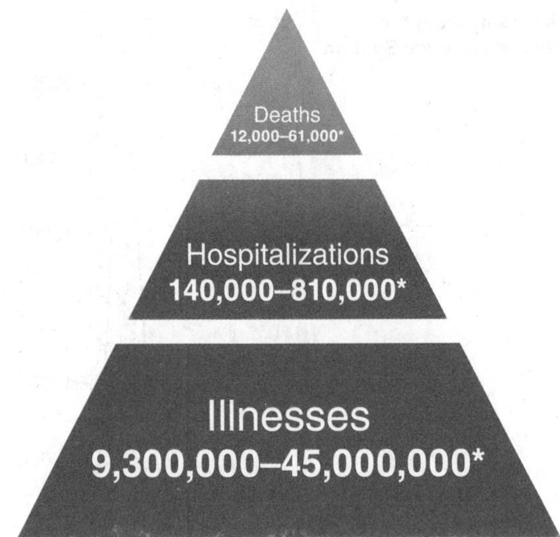

FIGURE 200-3 Pyramid of impact of influenza illness. *The top range of these burden estimates is from the 2017–2018 flu season. These are preliminary and may change as data are finalized. *(From https://www.cdc.gov/flu/about/burden/index.html.)*

a given year. This issue has led to the incorporation of representatives of both influenza B lineages plus influenza A/H1N1 and H3N2 viruses into a quadrivalent vaccine.

Influenza C viruses cause intermittent mild disease and have attracted little attention. These viruses have been the subject of fewer than 10 publications annually since the year 2000.

Influenza-Associated Morbidity and Mortality Influenza virus infects people of all ages and causes mild to severe illness, and even death in some cases. The impact of influenza is highly variable from year to year and can be depicted as a pyramid of illnesses, medical visits, hospitalizations, and deaths (**Fig. 200-3**). Infection rates are highest among children, with complications and hospitalizations from seasonal influenza being greatest among certain high-risk groups during most epidemics. These groups are assigned the highest priority for vaccination and other preventive and therapeutic measures. Their caregivers and close contacts are also prioritized targets of interventions (**Table 200-2**).

Mortality attributable to influenza, reported as excess over the anticipated sine-wave curve of pneumonia and influenza deaths during the year, has been between 12,000 to 61,000 deaths annually over the past decade. The dramatic effect of the COVID-19 pandemic on excess pneumonia and influenza mortality data is evident from the comparison of 2020 data with data from the prior three seasons (**Fig. 200-4**). Influenza-associated pediatric mortality is based on laboratory confirmation rather than modeling estimates. During the 2015–2020 influenza seasons, an estimated 95 to 195 children have died annually from influenza disease.

TABLE 200-2 High-Risk Groups Who Should Be Assigned a High Priority for Influenza Immunization and Treatment[a]

High-Risk Group
Children 6–59 months of age
Adults ≥50 years of age
Persons with chronic pulmonary (including asthma), cardiovascular (except isolated hypertension), renal, hepatic, neurologic, hematologic, or metabolic disorders (including diabetes mellitus)
Persons who are immunocompromised (any cause, including medications or HIV infection)
Women who are or plan to be pregnant during the influenza season
Children and adolescents (6 months through 18 years of age) who are receiving aspirin- or salicylate-containing medications and who might be at risk for Reye syndrome
Residents of nursing homes and other long-term-care facilities
American Indians/Alaska Natives
Persons who are extremely obese (BMI ≥40)
Contacts and Caregivers
Caregivers and contacts of those at risk: health care personnel in inpatient and outpatient care settings who have the potential for exposure to patients or to infectious materials, medical emergency-response workers, autopsy personnel, employees of nursing home and long-term-care facilities who have contact with patients or residents, and students and trainees in these professions who have contact with patients
Household contacts and caregivers of children ≤59 months (i.e., <5 years) of age (particularly contacts of infants <6 months old) and adults ≥50 years of age
Household contacts (including children) and caregivers of persons who are in a high-risk group

[a]No hierarchy is implied by order of listing.

Source: Centers for Disease Control and Prevention 2020–2021 summary of recommendations for influenza vaccine (*https://www.cdc.gov/mmwr/volumes/69/rr/rr6908a1.htm#T2_up*).

PATHOGENESIS AND IMMUNITY

At a cellular level, influenza virus binds to sialic acid receptors and enters the epithelial cell through receptor-mediated endocytosis. The virus then enters an endosome, where acidification promotes proteolytic cleavage of the hemagglutinin, exposing a fusion domain. The influenza hemagglutinin undergoes a marked structural reorganization in this cleavage step. Hemagglutinin cleavage may be one of the factors that restrict viral growth to epithelial cells, as a unique protease in the respiratory milieu is required for this cleavage to occur. The fusion domain allows the viral RNA to enter the cytoplasm. The nucleoprotein is transported into the nucleus of the cell, where transcription to a positive-sense RNA and replication take place. Viral proteins then assemble on the apical surface of the infected cell and, after incorporation of cellular membrane, bud from the membrane back into the mucosal milieu.

Influenza infection is initiated in the upper respiratory tract via aerosolized virus. The cells infected with influenza virus are primarily the ciliated cells of the respiratory tract. Denudation of the superficial epithelium probably accounts for much of the symptomatology and may predispose to secondary bacterial infections. The onset of symptoms follows an incubation period that, for a viral illness, is very short: 48–72 h. The infection spreads to the lungs but, even there, remains confined to the epithelial layer.

Influenza virus is associated with systemic symptoms of fever, malaise, and myalgia. These manifestations are presumed to be mediated by cytokines, and excess cytokine production has been implicated in the acute toxicity of H5N1 and other highly pathogenic influenza viruses.

The immune response to influenza virus occurs at the systemic and mucosal levels and involves both T and B cells. The B-cell responses are directed primarily toward antigenic epitopes on the two surface glycoproteins—i.e., hemagglutinin and neuraminidase. At a structural level, the four recognized epitopes on the hemagglutinin, largely confined to the globular head of the protein, collectively constitute the targets for hemagglutination inhibition (HAI) antibodies. HAI and neutralizing antibodies are highly correlated; HAI antibody levels are used as a measure of susceptibility to clinical infection and thus as a measure of vaccine-induced protection. In a child or an adult without prior vaccination or with the emergence of a distinctly new strain, serum HAI antibody is a surrogate for protection. However, in individuals with both vaccine-induced and natural immunity, the protective efficacy of a vaccine based on serum HAI antibody is more difficult to predict.

There is now considerable research interest in the induction and protective role of broadly neutralizing antibodies that recognize less antigenically variable regions on the stalk of the hemagglutinin. The results of these studies have led to investments toward research and development of a universal influenza vaccine, although no such vaccines are yet available in clinical practice.

The role of T-cell immunity, which primarily recognizes internal protein epitopes, remains unclear in humans. However, T-cell immunity is thought to play a role in clearance of an influenza infection that

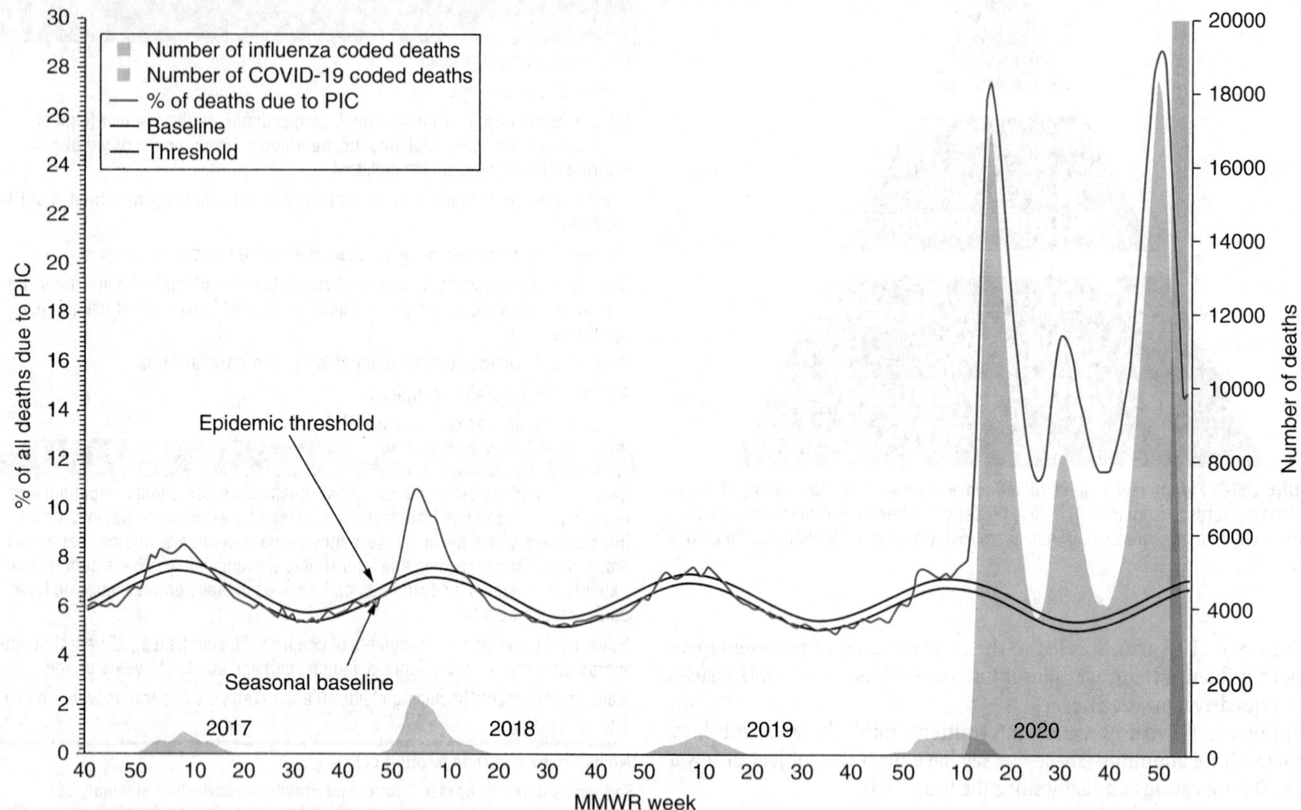

FIGURE 200-4 Pneumonia, Influenza, and COVID-19 Mortality; MMWR, *Morbidity and Mortality Weekly Report*; PIC, pneumonia, influenza, COVID-19. Data through the week ending January 23, 2021, as of January 28, 2021. *(From https://www.cdc.gov/flu/weekly/index.htm.)*

quite reproducibly develops 8–10 days after exposure. A role for T cells in protection against acquisition of infection has also been proposed.

CLINICAL MANIFESTATIONS

Influenza is primarily a respiratory illness causing cough, sore throat and rhinorrhea, or nasal congestion. The illness has a sudden onset and is epidemiologically linked to close contact with persons who have similar symptoms and often to community-wide respiratory illness. What distinguishes influenza from most other respiratory viral illnesses is the degree of accompanying fever, chills, fatigue, myalgia, and malaise. SARS-CoV-2 is the exceptional respiratory virus that also has a remarkable systemic component (**Chap. 199**). Symptoms of influenza typically begin within 48–72 h of exposure. The constellation of symptoms caused by an H3N2 viral strain, A/Port Chalmers 1/73, was followed prospectively in young seronegative children. Although these data involve children and a viral strain circulating 45 years ago, they present a representative picture of influenza today except that irritability in a young child is more specifically recognized as malaise, myalgia, and headache in an adult (**Table 200-3**).

Respiratory symptoms, particularly recurrent cough, persist well beyond the 2–5 days of systemic symptoms. There is a postinfectious delay in return to normal levels of activity. Pulmonary function is persistently decreased after acute influenza. Persons with a regular exercise routine (e.g., runners) note a decrease from their prior level of performance that typically lasts for a month or more. In the elderly, the respiratory presentation may be less prominent, but there is often a decline in baseline activity and a loss of appetite.

On physical examination, the patient with influenza appears ill and rheumy, with sweating, coughing, nonpurulent conjunctivitis, and diffuse pharyngeal erythema. With lower respiratory involvement, pulmonary examination typically reveals nonlocalizing scattered rales, rhonchi, and wheezes. When present, localized pulmonary findings suggest relatively complicated pneumonia with a bacterial component. Muscle pain may be elicited by pressure, particularly in the calves and thighs. There are rare gastrointestinal findings. No rash is associated with influenza.

COMPLICATIONS

Most persons who become ill with influenza virus infection recover without serious complications or sequelae. Complications of influenza occur most commonly in persons ≥65 years of age, young children, persons of all ages with underlying cardiopulmonary disease and immunosuppression, and women who are in the second or third trimester of pregnancy.

Respiratory Complications Pneumonia characterized by progressive air hunger, localized pulmonary findings on physical examination, and radiographic findings of diffuse infiltrates or consolidation is the most common complication of influenza. Pneumonia in influenza can be primary influenza viral pneumonia, secondary bacterial pneumonia, or mixed viral and bacterial pneumonia. Primary viral

TABLE 200-3 Clinical Observations in 24 Seronegative Children Examined during Influenza A/Port Chalmers Infection

CONDITION/EVENT	NO. OF PATIENTS
Coryza	22
Fever (temperature >38.4°C [>101°F])	21
Cough	21
Pharyngitis	20
Irritability	20
Fever (temperature >39.5°C [>103°F])	13
Anorexia	12
Tonsillitis	8
Vomiting	7
Otitis	6
Pneumonia	6
Diarrhea	6
Hoarseness	4
Croup	1

pneumonia is characterized by increasing dyspnea, persistent fever, and—in more severe cases—cyanosis. Primary influenza pneumonia was typical in the 1918 pandemic and occurs with H5N1 virus, as initially described in Hong Kong in 1997. Pathologically, a marked inflammatory reaction in the alveolar septa is characterized by infiltration of monocytes, lymphocytes, and macrophages, with variable numbers of neutrophils. Destruction and hemorrhage are seen in the respiratory epithelium. Large amounts of virus can be recovered from the lungs.

In secondary bacterial pneumonia or mixed viral and bacterial pneumonia, illness may be biphasic, with evidence of recovery from the primary influenza illness followed by recrudescence of fever and pulmonary symptoms. Localizing findings may be detected on pulmonary examination and/or x-ray. The development of secondary bacterial infection is not surprising, as influenza de-epithelializes the airways and destroys ciliary function, allowing bacterial contamination. Another proposed mechanism for bacterial/viral enhancement is the production by *Staphylococcus* and *Pseudomonas* of proteases that enhance cleavage of the influenza hemagglutinin and thereby facilitate viral replication. The risk of secondary bacterial disease is greatest in elderly patients and those with chronic obstructive pulmonary disease (COPD).

Some influenza strains cause laryngotracheobronchitis, bronchiolitis, or croup in children. Otitis media—a common accompaniment to influenza in children—may also be due to a combination of influenza virus and bacteria.

Extrapulmonary Complications Although influenza is believed to spread only rarely beyond the respiratory epithelial cells, where unique endogenous proteases facilitate hemagglutinin cleavage and productive infection, this disease causes not only prominent systemic complaints but also a variety of extrapulmonary manifestations. The most common extrapulmonary manifestation of influenza is myositis, which is seen more often in influenza B and is characterized by severe muscle pain, elevated creatinine phosphokinase levels, and myoglobinuria that can lead to renal failure. The muscles are extremely tender to touch. Myo/pericarditis is seen less frequently. However, a consistent epidemiologic link exists between influenza epidemics and excess cardiovascular hospitalizations.

Neurologic involvement, while rare, does occur following influenza infection. Influenza-associated encephalopathy or encephalitis is characterized by rapid progression within a few days of influenza infection. Transverse myelitis and Parkinsonian symptoms have been reported. Postinfectious acute demyelinating encephalomyelitis can follow influenza as well as other viral infections. The literature is mixed on the benefit and reliability of efforts to establish a polymerase chain reaction (PCR)–based diagnosis in this condition. MRI shows distinctive multifocal, symmetric brain lesions affecting the thalamus, brainstem tegmentum, cerebral periventricular white matter, and cerebellar medulla. Neurologic manifestations are more frequent in children as compared to adults. Children most commonly present with febrile seizures, increased seizure frequency among those with seizure disorders, or self-limited encephalopathy. More serious manifestations of meningitis, encephalitis, and focal brain lesions may occur, particularly in children with preexisting neurologic conditions.

Guillain-Barré syndrome can develop after influenza and was reported after a widespread influenza vaccination effort in the fall of 1976 that was undertaken in anticipation of a swine influenza epidemic (which never materialized). Until aspirin was recognized as a cofactor in its precipitation, Reye syndrome, an acute hepatic decompensation, was seen commonly in children and adolescents with influenza, particularly those infected with influenza B virus. Subsequently, the use of aspirin for fever control and symptom relief in children with viral infections was strongly discouraged, and Reye syndrome has virtually disappeared from clinical practice.

LABORATORY FINDINGS AND DIAGNOSIS

There is a strong argument for establishing a microbiologic diagnosis from both an individual-patient and a public-health perspective. This information is particularly valuable early in the season, when the extent of influenza and the precise circulating strain(s) are uncertain; in the management of high-risk or hospitalized patients; in settings such as long-term-care facilities and hospitals, where the institution of specific infection-control measures is appropriate; and in any patient with influenza-like illness if the test results will influence clinical management.

Influenza virus is most easily recovered from nasopharygeal specimens. If nasopharyngeal specimens are not available, nasal and throat swab specimens should be collected and combined together for influenza testing over single specimens from either site. These samples are most effectively collected with a flocked swab.

When available, rapid molecular assays (i.e., nucleic acid amplification test [NAAT]) are preferred over rapid influenza diagnostic tests and immunofluorescence assays in inpatients and outpatients to improve detection of influenza virus infection. Not only is this the most sensitive and specific method, it also provides opportunities to identify the strain with some specificity. Many such NAATs are multiplex, and target a panel of common respiratory pathogens—influenza, respiratory syncytial virus, parainfluenzavirus, and coronaviruses including SARS-CoV-2—an advantage in the ill hospitalized patient and during outbreaks of other respiratory pathogens. Clinicians should not use viral culture for initial or primary diagnosis of influenza because results will not be available in a timely manner to inform clinical management, but viral culture can be considered to confirm negative test results from rapid influenza diagnostic tests and immunofluorescence assays, such as during an institutional outbreak, and to provide isolates for further characterization.

Serologic confirmation of infection is also possible but requires paired serum samples, with the convalescent-phase sample obtained 2 weeks after infection. Mucosal antibody assays that are now being developed can detect strain-specific antibodies in paired mucosal specimens and yield insights into the importance of mucosal immunity in protection against influenza.

Other laboratory tests are of limited value. Mild leukopenia is seen in influenza, and a white blood cell count above 15,000/μL suggests a secondary bacterial component in influenzal pneumonia.

DIFFERENTIAL DIAGNOSIS

Influenza may be diagnosed clinically based on an acute presentation of a febrile respiratory illness during high periods of influenza circulation. However, less common presentations of influenza, and cases occurring outside of peak influenza season, are frequently misdiagnosed on the basis of symptoms alone. Influenza symptoms and signs may overlap with symptoms of other respiratory viruses. Respiratory syncytial virus often co-circulates with influenza virus; it particularly affects the youngest children, causing bronchiolitis, but it can also infect the elderly, leading to an influenza-like nonspecific respiratory illness and a decline in mobility, nutrition, and pulmonary function, with resultant hospitalization.

Patients with COVID-19 have a wide range of symptoms reported, ranging from mild to severe illness. Many of these symptoms—fever, chills, cough, shortness of breath, fatigue, muscle aches, headaches, congestion, or runny nose—overlap with the symptoms of influenza. While new loss of taste (ageusia) or smell (anosmia) may distinguish COVID-19 from influenza, they are reported in the minority of infected persons. When SARS-CoV-2 and influenza viruses are co-circulating, clinicians should consider both viruses, as well as co-infection, in patients with acute respiratory illness symptoms. The similar clinical presentations reiterate the importance of testing in order to inform treatment decisions.

IMMUNIZATION

Vaccination is the best approach to prevent influenza. The vaccines currently available in the United States are increasing in number and diversity (**Table 200-4**). These vaccines fall into two broad categories: parenterally administered inactivated influenza vaccines and intranasally administered live-attenuated influenza vaccines. Current vaccines are further classified based on production substrate (eggs, cell),

TABLE 200-4 Categories of Vaccines Licensed for Prevention of Seasonal Influenza, United States

		NONREPLICATING VACCINES			
	LIVE ATTENUATED	STANDARD INACTIVATED	HIGH-DOSE INACTIVATED	RECOMBINANT	ADJUVANTED INACTIVATED
ROUTE	Intranasal	Intramuscular	Intramuscular	Intramuscular	Intramuscular
APPROVED AGES	2–49 years	≥6 months	≥65 years	≥18 years	≥65 years
HA[a]	15	15	60	45	15
SUBSTRATE	Eggs	Eggs/cell culture	Eggs	Cell culture	Eggs
NUMBER OF STRAINS	4	4	4	4	3/4

[a]Hemagglutinin content in micrograms per strain.

antigen dose and valence (trivalent or quadrivalent), and the presence or absence of adjuvants. Current inactivated influenza vaccines are designed with the common goal to induce immunity to the hemagglutinin surface glycoprotein of the influenza virus. No effort is made to standardize the neuraminidase content.

As the viral surface hemagglutinin undergoes frequent antigenic drift, the seasonal influenza vaccine is reformulated as often as twice annually to match the strains projected to circulate in the following influenza season. The decision about vaccine composition must be made approximately 10 months before the seasonal peak in influenza virus circulation; this decision is made by committees at the World Health Organization (WHO). Subsequently, the US Food and Drug Administration (FDA), which has regulatory authority over vaccines in the United States, convenes an advisory committee that considers the recommendations of WHO, reviews and discusses similar data, and makes a final decision regarding vaccine virus composition of influenza vaccines licensed and marketed in the United States. This timing can result in a mismatch of vaccine composition with the viral strains that are actually prevalent in the upcoming season. Influenza vaccine is unique in being given seasonally in the months immediately preceding an outbreak in temperate climates. In the United States, vaccine is typically available starting in August or September.

The performance of current influenza vaccines varies by year, vaccine formulation, and the underlying age, health condition, and prior virus and vaccine exposure of the recipient. Unfortunately, the relative contribution of each of these factors has not been well elucidated, given the many variables involved and the complex interplay of infection and host response. Depending upon the degree to which vaccine strains match circulating strains, seasonal influenza vaccines will confer more or less protection, as antibody against influenza is for the most part strain-specific. A meta-analysis of randomized controlled trials of influenza vaccine efficacy over 12 influenza seasons showed inactivated influenza vaccines had a pooled efficacy of 59% (95% CI, 51%–67%) among those aged 18–65 years. Since 2004–2005, the CDC has estimated the effectiveness of seasonal influenza vaccine to prevent laboratory-confirmed influenza associated with medically attended respiratory illness. During that period, effectiveness ranged from approximately 40%–60% across all age groups during seasons when most circulating influenza vaccines are antigenically similar to the recommended influenza vaccine components; effectiveness was lower in years with strain mismatch. Importantly, studies support that influenza vaccine mitigates disease severity. For example, observational studies in children support that influenza vaccination reduces intensive care unit hospitalizations and deaths by an estimated 74% and 65%, respectively.

Newer technologies have been developed to overcome some of the limitations of current vaccines. The first fully recombinant vaccine was approved by the FDA in 2017. Both recombinant and cell-based vaccines may overcome the egg-adaptation of vaccine strains that may contribute to diminished vaccine effectiveness. Oil-in-water adjuvanted vaccines and high-dose vaccines elicit greater immune responses than traditional inactivated influenza vaccines and are approved in the United States for persons ≥65 years of age. In most head-to-head comparisons, high-dose vaccines have shown superior effectiveness to standard dose. While evidence is more limited, select comparisons of recombinant and adjuvanted vaccines with standard vaccines likewise show improved effectiveness.

In head-to-head comparisons in pediatric populations in the 1990s, a live, attenuated, intranasally administered vaccine (LAIV) exhibited an efficacy exceeding that of injected inactivated vaccines. LAIV is a desirable option in children given the ease of intranasal administration and theoretical advantage of stimulating mucosal immunity by the topical route. However, in the 2014–2016 influenza seasons, LAIV had lower replicative fitness and no demonstrable efficacy assignable to the vaccine's H1N1 component. Consequently, advisory committees in the United States and elsewhere suspended the recommendations for use of LAIV until manufacturing improvements allowed reinstatement of recommendations for its use in 2018. Since that time, LAIV has performed comparably to inactivated influenza vaccines in annual effectiveness assessments.

Inactivated influenza vaccines have been licensed for more than 60 years and have a robust safety and tolerability profile. While local reactions are most common following inactivated influenza vaccines, rare adverse events may occur. These include Guillain-Barré syndrome, identified in 1976 and less frequently during other years; oculorespiratory syndrome, first recognized in 2000; and febrile seizures first reported in young children in Australia in 2010. Adjuvanted vaccines in general cause more local pain and erythema than unadjuvanted vaccines. LAIVs have been associated with excess wheezing and hospitalizations in children younger than 2 years, and thus are not licensed for use in this age group.

Vaccine-specific recommendations for use, the approved age range of each product, the route of administration, and the anticipated side effects are updated annually by the CDC (*https://www.cdc.gov/vaccines/hcp/acip-recs/vacc-specific/flu.html*). In the United States, routine annual influenza vaccination is recommended for all persons 6 months of age and older. No preferential recommendation is made for one influenza vaccine product over another for persons for whom more than one licensed, recommended, and appropriate product is available. Two doses of vaccine should be given to children <9 years of age who are getting their first or second yearly vaccination. Groups at special risk of experiencing or transmitting influenza and for whom influenza immunization is a particularly high priority are listed in Table 200-2.

In general, influenza vaccine is not recommended for persons with a history of severe allergic reaction to the vaccine or to components other than egg. Manufacturer package inserts and updated CDC guidance should be consulted for information on contraindications and precautions for individual influenza vaccines, including specific guidance for persons with a history of egg allergy. A history of Guillain-Barré syndrome within 6 weeks of a previous dose of influenza vaccine is considered a precaution for the use of all influenza vaccines.

TREATMENT

Influenza

Antiviral therapy for influenza has been limited by the paucity of available drugs, the short duration of symptoms in uncomplicated influenza, and the changing patterns of drug resistance in influenza viral strains. In the past, influenza A infection could be treated with the M-2 channel blockers amantadine and rimantadine. Widespread resistance has currently relegated these compounds to historical interest only.

Neuraminidase inhibitors have been the mainstay for treatment of influenza A and B viruses for many years. As their name implies, these drugs inhibit the influenza neuraminidase and thus limit the egress of influenza virus from an infected cell. They are most effective in patients whose influenza illness is recognized early and confirmed by rapid diagnostic testing or on the basis of clinical and epidemiologic evidence. In experimental trials, these drugs hasten the resolution of symptoms if given within 48 h of infection. There are indications for their use both prophylactically—either throughout the season or, when a case is recognized in a close contact, in the short term—and therapeutically. The anticipated effect of early administration is the resolution of symptoms 1–2 days sooner than without treatment. The use of neuraminidase inhibitors is recommended for complicated influenza infections in hospitalized patients in the absence of formal proof of efficacy and when diagnosis may have been delayed. All the available neuraminidase inhibitors carry a risk of development of resistance, particularly with prolonged administration (e.g., to an immunodeficient individual with persistent recovery of influenza virus). Resistance to neuraminidase inhibitors is not widespread among currently circulating influenza A or B strains, but its development has been demonstrated in the laboratory, and clinical resistance could influence the utility of these drugs.

The defined risk groups who can benefit from neuraminidase inhibitors include children <2 years of age, adults >65 years of age, patients with chronic conditions, immunosuppressed individuals, pregnant women, women who have delivered infants ≤2 weeks previously, patients <19 years old who are receiving long-term aspirin treatment, Native Americans (including Alaska Natives), morbidly obese individuals, and residents of nursing homes or chronic-care facilities. This list resembles that of candidates whose vaccination is a high priority (Table 200-2). Use of neuraminidase inhibitors should be considered in selected high-risk cases despite a history of vaccination.

The available neuraminidase inhibitors are oral oseltamivir, nasal-spray zanamivir, and intravenous peramivir. Oseltamivir, which is most widely used, is an orally absorbed drug that is converted to its active component, oseltamivir carboxylate, in the liver. Gastrointestinal symptoms, especially nausea, may accompany the administration of oseltamivir. Because zanamivir is not orally bioavailable, it is given as an inhaled dry powder dispersed through a Diskhaler device.

The usual duration of therapy with either oral oseltamivir or intranasal zanamivir is 5 days, with twice-a-day dosing. Oseltamivir is preferred for treatment of pregnant women and is approved for treatment at any age, beginning at 14 days of life in infants. Poor oral intake or absorption is a contraindication to the use of oseltamivir, although this drug can also be given by oro/nasal tube. Asthma and COPD are relative contraindications to the use of intranasal zanamivir; this agent is approved for treatment in persons 7 years and older. For hospitalized patients with suspected or confirmed influenza, initiation of antiviral treatment with oral or enterically administered oseltamivir is recommended as soon as possible. For patients who cannot tolerate or absorb oral or enterically administered oseltamivir, the use of a single infusion of intravenous peramivir should be considered. Peramivir is licensed for individuals ≥2 years of age. The most current recommendations and details on influenza antiviral drug use and release are available through the CDC (*https://www.cdc.gov/flu/professionals/antivirals/summary-clinicians.htm#summary*).

In 2018, a first-in-class compound, baloxavir marboxil (XOFLUZA), was approved by the FDA for persons 12 years and older for prophylaxis or treatment of uncomplicated influenza within 2 days of onset of illness. Baloxavir inhibits cap-dependent endonuclease, has activity against influenza A and B, and is a single-dose formulation. In clinical studies, if given within 48 hours of symptoms, baloxavir decreased symptom duration, viral shedding, and antibiotic use in healthy individuals with uncomplicated influenza. However, development of resistance is a concern with 2–10% of the trial participants who received baloxavir showing viral escape with reduced drug susceptibility. CDC does not recommend use of baloxavir in pregnant women, breastfeeding mothers, outpatients with complicated or progressive illness, severely immunosuppressed patients, or hospitalized patients because of lack of information on use of baloxavir for these groups.

Other critical aspects of treatment include maintenance of fluid and electrolyte balance, oxygen supplementation, fever control with nonsteroidal anti-inflammatory drugs, and treatment of suspected secondary bacterial complications with antibiotics. Appropriate respiratory isolation of patients should be practiced in accordance with local hospital guidelines.

FURTHER READING

Barry JM: *The Great Influenza: The Story of the Deadliest Pandemic in History*. New York, Penguin Books, 2005.

Chung JR: Effects of influenza vaccination in the United States during the 2018–2019 influenza season. Clin Infect Dis 71:e368, 2020.

Erbelding EJ: A universal influenza vaccine: The strategic plan for the National Institute of Allergy and Infectious Diseases. J Infect Dis 218:347, 2018.

Fineberg HV: Pandemic preparedness and response—lessons from the H1N1 influenza of 2009. N Engl J Med 370:1335, 2014.

Kash JC, Taubenberger JK: The role of viral, host, and secondary bacterial factors in influenza pathogenesis. Am J Pathol 185:1528, 2015.

Osterholm MT et al: Efficacy and effectiveness of influenza vaccines: A systemic review and meta-analysis. Lancet Infect Dis 12:36, 2012.

Treanor JJ: Influenza vaccination. N Engl J Med 375:1261, 2016.

Uyeki TM et al: Novel influenza A viruses and pandemic threats. Lancet 398:2172, 2017.

Watanabe T et al: 1918 influenza virus hemagglutinin (HA) and the viral RNA polymerase complex enhance viral pathogenicity, but only HA induces aberrant host responses in mice. J Virol 87:5239, 2013.

Wright PF et al: Correlates of immunity to influenza as determined by challenge of children with live, attenuated influenza vaccine. Open Forum Infect Dis 3:108, 2016.

Section 14 Infections Due to Human Immunodeficiency Virus and Other Human Retroviruses

201 The Human Retroviruses

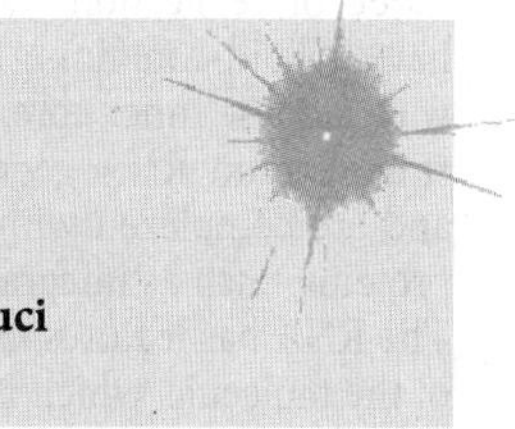

Dan L. Longo, Anthony S. Fauci

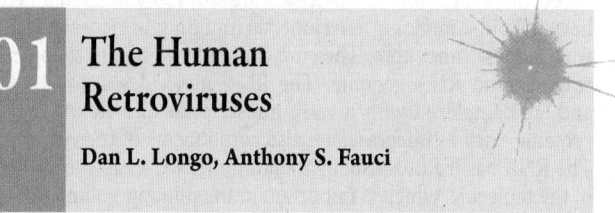

The retroviruses, which make up a large family (Retroviridae), infect mainly vertebrates. These viruses have a unique replication cycle whereby their genetic information is encoded by RNA rather than DNA. Retroviruses contain an RNA-dependent DNA polymerase (a reverse transcriptase) that directs the synthesis of a DNA form of the viral genome after infection of a host cell. The designation *retrovirus* denotes that information in the form of RNA is transcribed into DNA in the host cell—a sequence that overturned a central dogma of molecular biology: that information passes unidirectionally from DNA to RNA to protein. The observation that RNA was the source of genetic information in the causative agents of certain animal tumors led to a number of paradigm-shifting biologic insights regarding not only the direction of genetic information passage but also the viral etiology of certain cancers and the concept of oncogenes as normal host genes scavenged and altered by a viral vector.

TABLE 201-1 Classification of Retroviruses: The Family Retroviridae

GENUS	EXAMPLE(S)	FEATURE
Alpharetrovirus	Rous sarcoma virus	Contains *src* oncogene
Betaretrovirus	Mouse mammary tumor virus	Exogenous or endogenous
Gammaretrovirus	Abelson murine leukemia virus	Contains *abl* oncogene
Deltaretrovirus	HTLV-1	Causes T-cell lymphoma and neurologic disease
Epsilonretrovirus	Walleye dermal sarcoma virus	Not known to be pathogenic in humans
Lentivirus	HIV-1, HIV-2	Causes AIDS
Spumavirus	Simian foamy virus	Not known to be pathogenic in humans

The family Retroviridae includes seven subfamilies (**Table 201-1**). Members of two of the families infect humans with pathologic consequences: the deltaretroviruses, of which human T-cell lymphotropic virus (HTLV) type 1 is the most important in humans; and the lentiviruses, of which HIV is the most important in humans.

The wide variety of interactions of a retrovirus with its host range from completely benign events (e.g., silent carriage of endogenous retroviral sequences in the germline genome of many animal species) to rapidly fatal infections (e.g., exogenous infection with an oncogenic virus such as Rous sarcoma virus in chickens). The ability of retroviruses to acquire and alter the structure and function of host cell genetic sequences has revolutionized our understanding of molecular carcinogenesis. The viruses can insert into the germline genome of the host cell and behave as a transposable or movable genetic element. They can activate or inactivate genes near the site of integration into the genome. They can rapidly alter their own genome by recombination and mutation under selective environmental stimuli.

Most human viral diseases occur as a consequence of tissue destruction either directly by the virus itself or indirectly by the host's response to the virus. Although these mechanisms are operative in retroviral infections, retroviruses have additional mechanisms of inducing disease, including the malignant transformation of an infected cell and the induction of an immunodeficiency state through selective destruction or dysfunction of immune-competent cells that renders the host susceptible to opportunistic diseases (infections and neoplasms; **Chap. 202**).

STRUCTURE AND LIFE CYCLE

All retroviruses are similar in structure, genome organization, and mode of replication. Retroviruses are 70–130 nm in diameter and have a lipid-containing envelope surrounding an icosahedral capsid with a dense inner core. The core contains two identical copies of the single-strand RNA genome. The RNA molecules are 8–10 kb long and are complexed with reverse transcriptase and tRNA. Other viral proteins, such as integrase, are also components of the virion particle. The RNA has features usually found in mRNA: a cap site at the 5′ end of the molecule, which is important in the initiation of mRNA translation, and a polyadenylation site at the 3′ end, which influences mRNA turnover (i.e., messages with shorter polyA tails turn over faster than messages with longer polyA tails). However, the retroviral RNA is not translated; instead, it is transcribed into DNA. The DNA form of the retroviral genome is called a *provirus*.

The replication cycle of retroviruses proceeds in two phases (**Fig. 201-1**). In the first phase, the virus enters the cytoplasm after binding to one or more specific cell-surface receptors; the viral RNA and reverse transcriptase synthesize a double-strand DNA version of the RNA template; and the provirus moves into the nucleus and integrates into the host cell genome. This proviral integration is permanent. Although some animal retroviruses integrate into a single specific site of the host genome in every infected cell, the human retroviruses integrate randomly. This first phase of replication depends entirely on gene products in the virus. The second phase includes the synthesis and processing of viral genomes, mRNAs, and proteins using

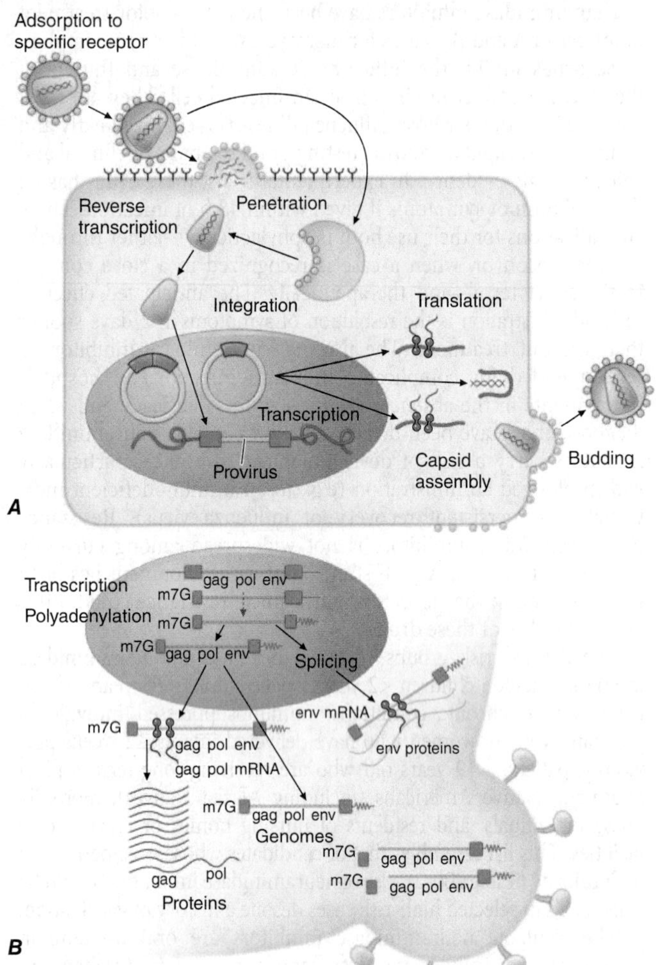

FIGURE 201-1 The life cycle of retroviruses. ***A.*** Overview of virus replication. The retrovirus enters a target cell by binding to a specific cell-surface receptor; once the virus is internalized, its RNA is released from the nucleocapsid and is reverse-transcribed into proviral DNA. The provirus is inserted into the genome and then transcribed into RNA; the RNA is translated; and virions assemble and are extruded from the cell membrane by budding. ***B.*** Overview of retroviral gene expression. The provirus is transcribed, capped, and polyadenylated. Viral RNA molecules then have one of three fates: they are exported to the cytoplasm, where they are packaged as the viral RNA in infectious viral particles; they are spliced to form the message for the envelope polyprotein; or they are translated into Gag and Pol proteins. Most of the messages for the Pol protein fail to initiate Pol translation because of a stop codon before its initiation; however, in a fraction of the messages, the stop codon is missed, and the Pol proteins are translated. *(Reproduced with permission from JM Coffin, in BN Fields, DM Knipe [eds]: Fields Virology. New York, Raven, 1990.)*

host cell machinery, often under the influence of viral gene products. Virions are assembled and released from the cell by budding from the membrane; host cell membrane proteins are frequently incorporated into the envelope of the virus. Proviral integration occurs during the S-phase of the cell cycle; thus, in general, nondividing cells are resistant to retroviral infection. Only the lentiviruses are able to infect nondividing cells. Once a host cell is infected, it is infected for the life of the cell.

Retroviral genomes include both coding and noncoding sequences (**Fig. 201-2**). In general, noncoding sequences are important recognition signals for DNA or RNA synthesis or processing events and are located in the 5′ and 3′ terminal regions of the genome. All retroviral genomes are terminally redundant, containing identical sequences called *long terminal repeats* (LTRs). The ends of the retroviral RNA genome differ slightly in sequence from the integrated retroviral DNA. In the latter, the LTR sequences are repeated in both the 5′ and the 3′ terminus of the virus. The LTRs contain sequences involved in initiating the expression of the viral proteins, the integration of the provirus, and the polyadenylation of viral RNAs. The primer binding site, which is critical for the initiation of reverse transcription, and the

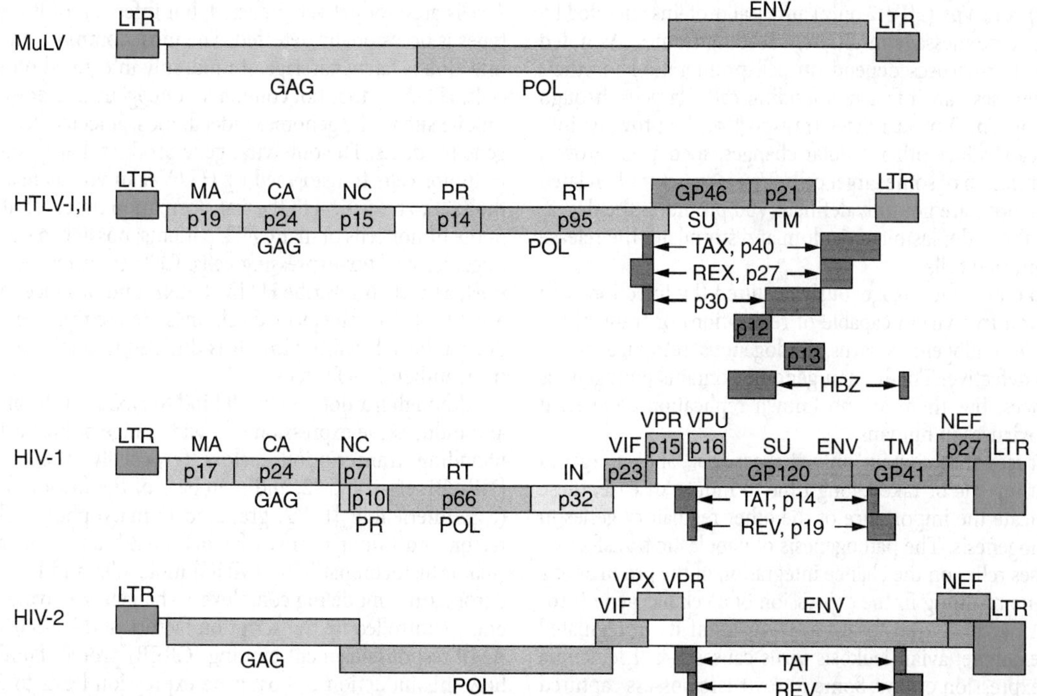

FIGURE 201-2 Genomic structure of retroviruses. The murine leukemia virus MuLV has the typical three structural genes: *gag, pol,* and *env*. The *gag* region gives rise to three proteins: matrix (MA), capsid (CA), and nucleic acid–binding (NC) proteins. The *pol* region encodes both a protease (PR) responsible for cleaving the viral polyproteins and a reverse transcriptase (RT). In addition, HIV *pol* encodes an integrase (IN). The *env* region encodes a surface protein (SU) and a small transmembrane protein (TM). The human retroviruses have additional gene products translated in each of the three possible reading frames. HTLV-1 and HTLV-2 have *tax* and *rex* genes with exons on either side of the *env* gene. HIV-1 and HIV-2 have six accessory gene products: *tat, rev, vif, nef, vpr,* and either *vpu* (in HIV-1) or *vpx* (in HIV-2). The genes for these proteins are located mainly between the *pol* and *env* genes. GP, glycoprotein; HBZ, HTLV-1 basic leucine zipper domain–containing protein; LTR, long terminal repeat.

viral packaging sequences are located outside the LTR sequences. The coding regions include the *gag* (group-specific antigen, core protein), *pol* (RNA-dependent DNA polymerase), and *env* (envelope) genes. The *gag* gene encodes a precursor polyprotein that is cleaved to form three to five capsid proteins; a fraction of the Gag precursor proteins also contain a protease responsible for cleaving the Gag and Pol polyproteins. A Gag-Pol polyprotein gives rise to the protease that is responsible for cleaving the Gag-Pol polyprotein. The *pol* gene encodes three proteins: the reverse transcriptase, the integrase, and the protease. The reverse transcriptase copies the viral RNA into the double-strand DNA provirus, which inserts itself into the host cell DNA via the action of integrase. The protease cleaves the Gag-Pol polyprotein into smaller protein products. The *env* gene encodes the envelope glycoproteins: one protein that binds to specific surface receptors and determines what cell types can be infected and a smaller transmembrane protein that anchors the complex to the envelope. Fig. 201-3 shows how the retroviral gene products make up the virus structure.

HTLVs have a region between *env* and the 3′ LTR that encodes several proteins and transcripts in overlapping reading frames (Fig. 201-2). Tax is a 40-kDa protein that does not bind to DNA but induces the expression of host cell transcription factors that alter host cell gene expression and is capable of inducing cell transformation under certain circumstances. Rex is a 27-kDa protein that regulates the expression of viral mRNAs. Other transcripts from this region (p12, p13, and p30) tend to restrict expression of viral genes and diminish the immunogenicity of infected cells. The protein of *HBZ*, a product of the complementary proviral DNA strand, interacts with many cellular transcription factors and signaling proteins. It stimulates proliferation of infected cells and is the only viral product universally expressed in HTLV-1-infected tumor cells. These proteins are produced from messages that are similar but that are spliced differently from overlapping but distinct exons.

The lentiviruses in general, and HIV-1 and -2 in particular, contain a larger genome than other pathogenic retroviruses. They contain an untranslated region between *pol* and *env* that encodes portions of several proteins, varying with the reading frame into which the mRNA is spliced. Tat is a 14-kDa protein that augments the expression of virus from the LTR. The Rev protein of HIV-1, similar to the Rex protein of HTLV, regulates RNA splicing and/or RNA transport. The Nef protein downregulates CD4, the cellular receptor for HIV; alters host T cell–activation pathways; and enhances viral infectivity. The Vif protein is necessary for the proper assembly of the HIV nucleoprotein core in many types of cells; without Vif, proviral DNA is not efficiently produced in these infected cells. In addition, the Vif protein targets APOBEC (apolipoprotein B mRNA-editing enzyme catalytic polypeptide, a cytidine deaminase that mutates the viral sequence) for proteasomal degradation, thus blocking its virus-suppressing effect. Vpr,

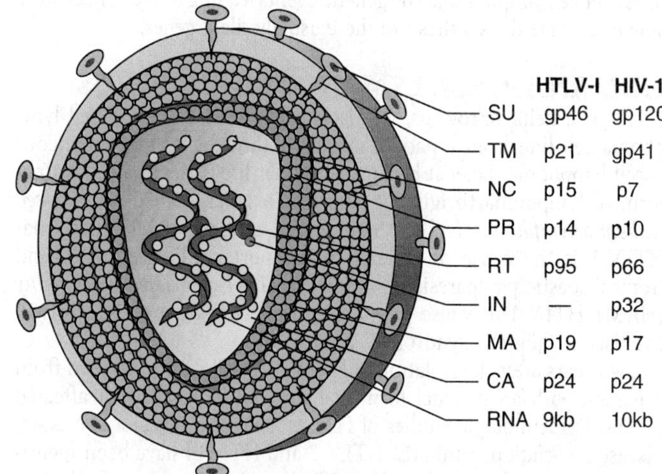

FIGURE 201-3 Schematic structure of human retroviruses. The surface glycoprotein (SU) is responsible for binding to receptors of host cells. The transmembrane protein (TM) anchors SU to the virus. NC is a nucleic acid–binding protein found in association with the viral RNA. A protease (PR) cleaves the polyproteins encoded by the *gag, pol,* and *env* genes into their functional components. RT is reverse transcriptase, and IN is an integrase present in some retroviruses (e.g., HIV-1) that facilitates insertion of the provirus into the host genome. The matrix protein (MA) is a Gag protein closely associated with the lipid of the envelope. The capsid protein (CA) forms the major internal structure of the virus, the core shell.

Vpu (HIV-1 only), and Vpx (HIV-2 only) are viral proteins encoded by translation of the same message in different reading frames. As noted above, oncogenic retroviruses depend on cell proliferation for their replication; lentiviruses can infect nondividing cells, largely through effects mediated by Vpr. Vpr facilitates transport of the provirus into the nucleus and can induce other cellular changes, such as G_2 growth arrest and differentiation of some target cells. Vpx is structurally related to Vpr, but its functions are not fully defined. Vpu promotes the degradation of CD4 in the endoplasmic reticulum and stimulates the release of virions from infected cells.

Retroviruses can be either exogenously acquired (by infection with an infected cell or a free virion capable of replication) or transmitted in the germline as endogenous virus. Endogenous retroviruses are often replication defective. The human genome contains endogenous retroviral sequences, but there are no known replication-competent endogenous retroviruses in humans.

In general, viruses that contain only the *gag, pol*, and *env* genes either are not pathogenic or take a long time to induce disease; these observations indicate the importance of the other regulatory genes in viral disease pathogenesis. The pathogenesis of neoplastic transformation by retroviruses relies on the chance integration of the provirus at a spot in the genome resulting in the expression of a cellular gene (protooncogene) that becomes transforming by virtue of its unregulated expression. For example, avian leukosis virus causes B-cell leukemia by inducing the expression of *myc*. Some retroviruses possess captured and altered cellular genes near their integration site, and these viral oncogenes can transform the infected host cell. Viruses that have oncogenes often have lost a portion of their genome that is required for replication. Such viruses need helper viruses to reproduce, a feature that may explain why these acute transforming retroviruses are rare in nature. All human retroviruses identified to date are exogenous and are not acutely transforming (i.e., they lack a transforming oncogene).

These remarkable properties of retroviruses have led to experimental efforts to use them as vectors to insert specific genes into particular cell types, a process known as *gene therapy* or *gene transfer*. The process could be used to repair a genetic defect or to introduce a new property that could be used therapeutically; for example, a gene (e.g., thymidine kinase) that would make a tumor cell susceptible to killing by a drug (e.g., ganciclovir) could be inserted. One source of concern about the use of retroviral vectors in humans is that replication-competent viruses might rescue endogenous retroviral replication, with unpredictable results. This concern is not merely hypothetical: the detection of proteins encoded by endogenous retroviral sequences on the surface of cancer cells implies that the genetic events leading to the cancer were able to activate the synthesis of these usually silent genes.

HUMAN T-CELL LYMPHOTROPIC VIRUS

HTLV-1, a delta retrovirus, was isolated in 1980 from a T-cell lymphoma cell line from a patient originally thought to have cutaneous T-cell lymphoma. Later it became clear that the patient had a distinct form of lymphoma (originally reported in Japan) called *adult T-cell leukemia/lymphoma* (ATL). Serologic data have determined that HTLV-1 is the cause of at least two important diseases: ATL and tropical spastic paraparesis, also called *HTLV-1-associated myelopathy* (HAM). HTLV-1 may also play a role in infective dermatitis, arthritis, uveitis, and Sjögren's syndrome.

Two years after the isolation of HTLV-1, HTLV-2 was isolated from a patient with an unusual form of hairy cell leukemia that affected T cells. Epidemiologic studies of HTLV-2 failed to reveal a consistent disease association. Similarly, HTLV-3 and HTLV-4 have been identified but have no known disease association.

BIOLOGY AND MOLECULAR BIOLOGY

Because the biology of HTLV-1 and that of HTLV-2 are similar, the following discussion will focus on HTLV-1.

Human glucose transporter protein 1 (GLUT-1) functions as a receptor for HTLV-1, probably acting together with neuropilin-1 (NRP1) and heparan sulfate proteoglycans. The heparan sulfate proteoglycans do not appear to be involved with HTLV-2 cell entry. Generally, only T cells are productively infected, but infection of B cells and other cell types is occasionally detected. The most common outcome of HTLV-1 infection is latent carriage of randomly integrated provirus in CD4+ T cells. HTLV-1 does not contain an oncogene and does not insert into a unique site in the genome. Indeed, most infected cells express no viral gene products. The only viral gene product that is routinely expressed in tumor cells transformed by HTLV-1 in vivo is *hbz*. The *tax* gene is thought to be critical to the transformation process but is not expressed in the tumor cells of many ATL patients, possibly because of the immunogenicity of *tax*-expressing cells. Cells transformed in vitro, by contrast, actively transcribe HTLV-1 RNA and produce infectious virions. Most HTLV-1-transformed cell lines are the result of the infection of a normal host T cell in vitro. It is difficult to establish cell lines derived from authentic ATL cells.

Although *tax* does not itself bind to DNA, it is located in the nucleus and induces the expression of a wide range of host cell gene products, including transcription factors (especially c-rel/nuclear factor κB [NF-κB], ets-1 and -2, and members of the fos/jun family), cytokines (e.g., interleukin [IL] 2, granulocyte-macrophage colony-stimulating factor, and tumor necrosis factor), membrane proteins and receptors (major histocompatibility [MHC] molecules and IL-2 receptor α), and chromatin remodeling complexes. The genes activated by *tax* are generally controlled by transcription factors of the c-rel/NF-κB and cyclic AMP response element binding (CREB) protein families. It is unclear how this induction of host gene expression leads to neoplastic transformation; *tax* can interfere with G_1 and mitotic cell-cycle checkpoints, block apoptosis, inhibit DNA repair, and promote antigen-independent T cell proliferation. Induction of a cytokine-autocrine loop has been proposed; however, IL-2 is not the crucial cytokine. The involvement of IL-4, IL-7, and IL-15 has been proposed.

In light of the irregular expression of *tax* in ATL cells, it has been suggested that *tax* is important in the early phases of transformation but is not essential for the maintenance of the transformed state. The maintenance role is thought to be due to *hbz* expression. As is clear from the epidemiology of HTLV-1 infection, transformation of an infected cell is a rare event and may depend on heterogeneous second, third, or fourth genetic hits. No consistent chromosomal abnormalities have been described in ATL; however, aneuploidy is common, and individual cases with p53 mutations and translocations involving the T cell receptor genes on chromosome 14 have been reported. *Tax* may repress certain DNA repair enzymes, permitting the accumulation of genetic damage that would normally be repaired. However, the molecular pathogenesis of HTLV-1-induced neoplasia is not fully understood.

FEATURES OF HTLV-1 INFECTION

Epidemiology HTLV-1 infection is transmitted in at least three ways: from mother to child, especially via breast milk; through sexual activity, more commonly from men to women; and through the blood—via contaminated transfusions or contaminated needles. The virus is most commonly transmitted perinatally. Compared with HIV, which can be transmitted in cell-free form, HTLV-1 is less infectious, and its transmission usually requires cell-to-cell contact.

HTLV-1 is endemic in southwestern Japan and Okinawa, where >1 million persons are infected. Antibodies to HTLV-1 are present in the serum of up to 35% of Okinawans, 10% of residents of the Japanese island of Kyushu, and <1% of persons in nonendemic regions of Japan. Despite this high prevalence of infection, only ~500 cases of ATL are diagnosed in this area each year. Clusters of infection have been noted in other areas of eastern Asia, such as Taiwan; in the Caribbean basin, including northeastern South America; in northwestern South America; in central and southern Africa; in Italy, Israel, Iran, and Papua New Guinea; in the Arctic; and in the southeastern part of the United States (**Fig. 201-4**). An estimated 5–10 million persons have HTLV-1 infection worldwide.

Progressive spastic or ataxic myelopathy developing in an individual who is HTLV-1 positive (i.e., who has serum antibodies to HTLV-1) may be due to direct infection of the nervous system with the virus, but

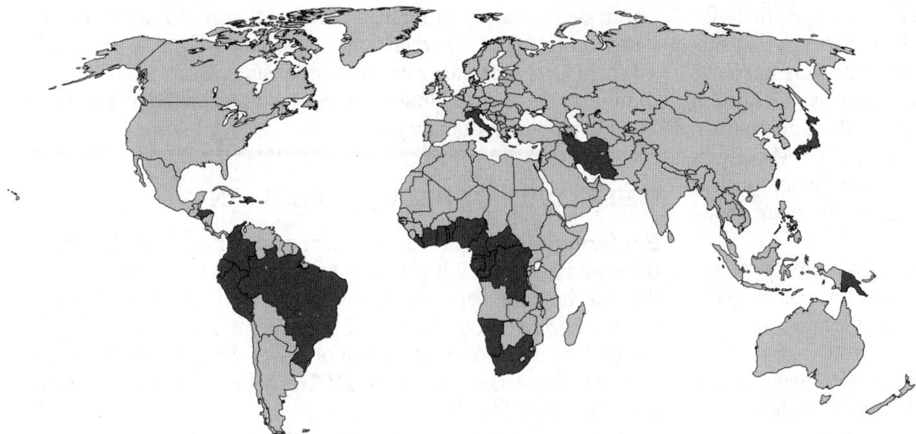

FIGURE 201-4 **Global distribution of HTLV-1 infection.** Countries with a prevalence of HTLV-1 infection of 1–5% are shaded darkly. Note that the distribution of infected patients is not uniform in endemic countries. For example, the people of southwestern Japan and northeastern Brazil are more commonly affected than those in other regions of those countries.

destruction of the pyramidal tracts appears to involve HTLV-1-infected CD4+ T cells; a similar disorder may result from infection with HIV or HTLV-2. In rare instances, patients with HAM are seronegative but have detectable antibody to HTLV-1 in cerebrospinal fluid (CSF).

The cumulative lifetime risk of developing ATL is 3% among HTLV-1-infected patients, with a threefold greater risk among men than among women; a similar cumulative risk is projected for HAM (4%), but with women more commonly affected than men. The distribution of these two diseases overlaps the distribution of HTLV-1, with >95% of affected patients showing serologic evidence of HTLV-1 infection. The latency period between infection and the emergence of disease is 20–30 years for ATL. For HAM, the median latency period is ~3.3 years (range, 4 months to 30 years). The development of ATL is rare among persons infected by blood products; however, ~20% of patients with HAM acquire HTLV-1 from contaminated blood. ATL is more common among perinatally infected individuals, whereas HAM is more common among persons infected via sexual transmission.

Associated Diseases • ATL Four clinical types of HTLV-1-induced neoplasia have been described: acute, lymphomatous, chronic, and smoldering. All of these tumors are monoclonal proliferations of CD4+ postthymic T cells with clonal proviral integrations and clonal T cell receptor gene rearrangements.

ACUTE ATL About 60% of patients who develop malignancy have classic acute ATL, which is characterized by a short clinical prodrome (~2 weeks between the first symptoms and the diagnosis) and an aggressive natural history (median survival period, 6 months). The clinical picture is dominated by rapidly progressive skin lesions, pulmonary involvement, hypercalcemia, and lymphocytosis with cells containing lobulated or "flower-shaped" nuclei (**see Fig. 108-7**). The malignant cells have monoclonal proviral integrations and express CD4, CD3, and CD25 (low-affinity IL-2 receptors) on their surface. Serum levels of CD25 can be used as a tumor marker. Anemia and thrombocytopenia are rare. The skin lesions may be difficult to distinguish from those in mycosis fungoides. Lytic bone lesions, which are common, do not contain tumor cells but rather are composed of osteolytic cells, usually without osteoblastic activity. Despite the leukemic picture, bone marrow involvement is patchy in most cases.

The hypercalcemia of ATL is multifactorial; the tumor cells produce osteoclast-activating factors (tumor necrosis factor α, IL-1, lymphotoxin) and can also produce a parathyroid hormone–like molecule. Affected patients have an underlying immunodeficiency that makes them susceptible to opportunistic infections similar to those seen in patients with AIDS (**Chap. 202**). The pathogenesis of the immunodeficiency is unclear. Pulmonary infiltrates in ATL patients reflect leukemic infiltration half the time and opportunistic infections with organisms such as *Pneumocystis* and other fungi the other half. Gastrointestinal symptoms are nearly always related to opportunistic infection. *Strongyloides stercoralis* is a gastrointestinal parasite that has a pattern of endemic distribution similar to that of HTLV-1. HTLV-1-infected persons also infected with this parasite may develop ATL more often or more rapidly than those without *Strongyloides* infections. Serum concentrations of lactate dehydrogenase and alkaline phosphatase are often elevated in ATL. About 10% of patients have leptomeningeal involvement leading to weakness, altered mental status, paresthesia, and/or headache. Unlike other forms of central nervous system (CNS) lymphoma, ATL may be accompanied by normal CSF protein levels. The diagnosis depends on finding ATL cells in the CSF (**Chap. 108**).

LYMPHOMATOUS ATL The lymphomatous type of ATL occurs in ~20% of patients and is similar to the acute form in its natural history and clinical course, except that circulating abnormal cells are rare and lymphadenopathy is evident. The histology of the lymphoma is variable but does not influence the natural history. In general, the diagnosis is suspected on the basis of the patient's birthplace (see "Epidemiology," above) and the presence of skin lesions and hypercalcemia. The diagnosis is confirmed by the detection of antibodies to HTLV-1 in serum.

CHRONIC ATL Patients with the chronic form of ATL generally have normal serum levels of calcium and lactate dehydrogenase and no involvement of the CNS, bone, or gastrointestinal tract. The median duration of survival for these patients is 2 years. In some cases, chronic ATL progresses to the acute form of the disease.

SMOLDERING ATL Fewer than 5% of patients have the smoldering form of ATL. In this form, the malignant cells have monoclonal proviral integration; <5% of peripheral-blood cells exhibit typical morphologic abnormalities; hypercalcemia, adenopathy, and hepatosplenomegaly do not develop; the CNS, the bones, and the gastrointestinal tract are not involved; and skin lesions and pulmonary lesions may be present. The median survival period for this small subset of patients appears to be ≥5 years.

HAM (TROPICAL SPASTIC PARAPARESIS) In contrast to ATL, in which there is a slight predominance of male patients, HAM affects female patients disproportionately. HAM resembles multiple sclerosis in certain ways (**Chap. 444**). The onset is insidious. Symptoms include weakness or stiffness in one or both legs, back pain, and urinary incontinence. Sensory changes are usually mild, but peripheral neuropathy may develop. The disease generally takes the form of slowly progressive and unremitting thoracic myelopathy; one-third of patients are bedridden within 10 years of diagnosis, and one-half are unable to walk unassisted by this point. Patients display spastic paraparesis or paraplegia with hyperreflexia, ankle clonus, and extensor plantar responses. Cognitive function is usually spared; cranial nerve abnormalities are unusual.

MRI reveals lesions in both the white matter and the paraventricular regions of the brain as well as in the spinal cord. Pathologic examination of the spinal cord shows symmetric degeneration of the lateral columns, including the corticospinal tracts; some cases involve the posterior columns as well. The spinal meninges and cord parenchyma contain an inflammatory infiltrate that includes CD8+ T cells with myelin destruction.

HTLV-1 is not usually found in cells of the CNS but may be detected in a small population of lymphocytes present in the CSF. In general, HTLV-1 replication is greater in HAM than in ATL, and patients with HAM have a stronger immune response to the virus. Antibodies to HTLV-1 are present in the serum and appear to be produced in the CSF of HAM patients, where titers are often higher than in the serum. The pathophysiology of HAM may involve the induction of autoimmune destruction of neural cells by T cells with specificity for viral components such as Tax or Env proteins. One theory is that susceptibility to HAM may be related to the presence of human leukocyte antigen (HLA) alleles capable of presenting viral antigens in a fashion that leads to autoimmunity. Insufficient data are available to confirm an HLA association. However, antibodies in the sera of HAM patients have been shown to bind a neuron-specific antigen (heteronuclear ribonuclear protein A1 [hnRNP A1]) and to interfere with neurotransmission in vitro.

It is unclear what factors influence whether HTLV-1 infection will cause disease and, if it does, whether it will induce a neoplasm (ATL) or an autoimmune disorder (HAM). Differences in viral strains, the susceptibility of particular MHC haplotypes, the route of HTLV-1 infection, the viral load, and the nature of the HTLV-1-related immune response are putative factors, but few definitive data are available.

OTHER PUTATIVE HTLV-1-RELATED DISEASES Even in the absence of the full clinical picture of HAM, bladder dysfunction is common in HTLV-1-infected women. In areas where HTLV-1 is endemic, diverse inflammatory and autoimmune diseases have been attributed to the virus, including uveitis, dermatitis, pneumonitis, rheumatoid arthritis, and polymyositis. However, a causal relationship between HTLV-1 and these illnesses has not been established.

Prevention Women in endemic areas should not breast-feed their children, and blood donors should be screened for serum antibodies to HTLV-1. As in the prevention of HIV infection, the practice of safe sex and the avoidance of needle sharing are important.

TREATMENT

HTLV-1 Infection

For the small number of patients who develop HTLV-1–related disease, therapies are not curative. In patients with the acute and lymphomatous types of ATL, the disease progresses rapidly. Hypercalcemia is generally controlled by glucocorticoid administration and cytotoxic therapy directed against the neoplasm. The tumor is highly responsive to combination chemotherapy that is used against other forms of lymphoma; however, patients are susceptible to overwhelming bacterial and opportunistic infections, and ATL relapses within 4–10 months after remission in most cases. The combination of interferon α and zidovudine may extend survival. Because viral replication is not clearly associated with ATL progression, zidovudine is probably effective through its cytotoxic effects (as a chain-terminating thymidine analogue) rather than its antiviral effects. Selected series have reported high rates of response and a 40% rate of 5-year survival; however, this level of response has not been universal. LSG15, a multidrug chemotherapy program developed in Japan, induces complete responses in about one-third of patients, about half of whom survive for >2 years; however, the median survival time is about 13 months. High-dose therapy with bone marrow transplantation has been widely tested in Japan. Median survival has not been influenced by this treatment; however, up to 25% of patients survive free of disease for 4 years. Lenalidomide has been reported to have a 42% response rate in patients with relapsed ATL, extending median survival to 20 months despite a short 4-month progression-free survival period. Mogamulizumab, an antibody to CCR4 (a receptor for a number of chemokines, including RANTES and TARC), improved response rates when added to chemotherapy. An experimental approach using an yttrium-90-labeled or toxin-conjugated antibody to the IL-2 receptor appears promising but is not widely available. Patients with the chronic or smoldering form of ATL may be managed with an expectant approach: treat any infections, and watch and wait for signs of progression to acute disease.

Patients with HAM may obtain some benefit from the use of glucocorticoids to reduce inflammation. Antiretroviral regimens have not been effective. In one study, danazol (200 mg three times daily) produced significant neurologic improvement in five of six treated patients, with resolution of urinary incontinence in two cases, decreased spasticity in three, and restoration of the ability to walk after confinement to a wheelchair in two. Antibody to IL-15 receptor β chain has been tested with some promising clinical effects in small numbers of patients. Physical therapy and rehabilitation are important components of management.

FEATURES OF HTLV-2 INFECTION

Epidemiology HTLV-2 is endemic in certain Native American tribes and in Africa. It is generally considered to be a New World virus that was brought from Asia to the Americas 10,000–40,000 years ago during the migration of infected populations across the Bering land bridge. The mode of transmission of HTLV-2 is probably the same as that of HTLV-1 (see above). HTLV-2 may be less readily transmitted sexually than HTLV-1.

Studies of large cohorts of injection drug users with serologic assays that reliably distinguish HTLV-1 from HTLV-2 indicated that the vast majority of HTLV-positive cohort members were infected with HTLV-2. The seroprevalence of HTLV in a cohort of 7841 injection drug users from drug treatment centers in Baltimore, Chicago, Los Angeles, New Jersey (Asbury Park and Trenton), New York City (Brooklyn and Harlem), Philadelphia, and San Antonio was 20.9%, with >97% of cases due to HTLV-2. The seroprevalence of HTLV-2 was higher in the Southwest and the Midwest than in the Northeast. In contrast, the seroprevalence of HIV-1 was higher in the Northeast than in the Southwest or the Midwest. Approximately 3% of the cohort members were infected with both HTLV-2 and HIV-1. The seroprevalence of HTLV-2 increased linearly with age. Women were significantly more likely than men to be infected with HTLV-2; the virus is thought to be more efficiently transmitted from male to female than from female to male.

Associated Diseases Although HTLV-2 was isolated from a patient with a T cell variant of hairy cell leukemia, this virus has not been consistently associated with a particular disease and in fact has been thought of as "a virus searching for a disease." However, evidence is accumulating that HTLV-2 may play a role in certain neurologic, hematologic, and dermatologic diseases. These data require confirmation, particularly in light of the previous confusion regarding the relative prevalences of HTLV-1 and HTLV-2 among injection drug users.

Prevention Avoidance of needle sharing, adherence to safe-sex practices, screening of blood (by assays for HTLV-1, which also detect HTLV-2), and avoidance of breast-feeding by infected women are important principles in the prevention of spread of HTLV-2.

HUMAN IMMUNODEFICIENCY VIRUS

HIV-1 and HIV-2 are members of the lentivirus subfamily of Retroviridae and are the only lentiviruses known to infect humans. The lentiviruses are slower-acting than viruses that cause acute infection (e.g., influenza virus) but not than other retroviruses. The features of acute primary infection with HIV resemble those of more classic acute infections. The characteristic chronicity of HIV disease is consistent with the designation *lentivirus*. **For a detailed discussion of HIV, see Chap. 202.**

FURTHER READING

El Hajj H et al: Novel treatments of adult T cell leukemia lymphoma. Front Microbiol 11:1062, 2020.

Katsuya H et al: Treatment and survival among 1594 patients with ATL. Blood 126:2570, 2015.

Ma G et al: Multifaceted functions and roles of HBA in HTLV-1 pathogenesis. Retrovirology 13:16, 2016.

Moir S et al: Pathogenic mechanisms of HIV disease. Annu Rev Pathol 6:223, 2011.

Tsukasaki K et al: Diagnostic approaches and established treatments for adult T-cell leukemia lymphoma. Front Microbiol 11:1207, 2020.

Yamauchi J et al: An update on human T-cell leukemia virus type I (HTLV-1)-associated myelopathy/tropical spastic paraparesis (HAM/TSP) focusing on clinical and laboratory biomarkers. Pharmacol Ther 218:107669, 2021.

202 Human Immunodeficiency Virus Disease: AIDS and Related Disorders

Anthony S. Fauci, Gregory K. Folkers, H. Clifford Lane

The Acquired Immune Deficiency Syndrome (AIDS) was first recognized in the United States in the summer of 1981, when the U.S. Centers for Disease Control and Prevention (CDC) reported the unexplained occurrence of *Pneumocystis jirovecii* (formerly *P. carinii*) pneumonia in five previously healthy homosexual men in Los Angeles and of Kaposi's sarcoma (KS) with or without *P. jirovecii* pneumonia and other opportunistic infections in 26 previously healthy homosexual men in New York, San Francisco, and Los Angeles. The disease was soon recognized in male and female injection drug users; in hemophiliacs and blood transfusion recipients; among female sexual partners of men with AIDS; and among infants born to mothers with AIDS. In 1983, human immunodeficiency virus (HIV) was isolated from a patient with lymphadenopathy, and by 1984 it was demonstrated clearly to be the causative agent of AIDS. In 1985, a sensitive enzyme-linked immunosorbent assay (ELISA) was developed; this led to an appreciation of the scope and evolution of the HIV epidemic at first in the United States and other developed nations and ultimately among developing nations throughout the world (see "HIV Infection and AIDS Worldwide," below). The staggering worldwide evolution of the HIV pandemic has been matched by an explosion of information in the areas of HIV virology, pathogenesis (both immunologic and virologic), treatment of HIV disease, treatment and prophylaxis of the opportunistic diseases associated with HIV infection, and prevention of HIV infection. The information flow related to HIV disease is enormous and continues to expand, and it has become almost impossible for the health care generalist to stay abreast of the literature. The purpose of this chapter is to present the most current information available on the scope of the pandemic; on its pathogenesis, treatment, and prevention; and on prospects for vaccine development. Above all, the aim is to provide a solid scientific basis and practical clinical guidelines for a state-of-the-art approach to the care of persons with HIV.

DEFINITION

The current CDC classification system for HIV infection and AIDS categorizes patients based on clinical conditions associated with HIV infection together with the level of the CD4+ T lymphocyte count. A confirmed HIV case can be classified in one of five HIV infection stages (0, 1, 2, 3, or unknown). If there was a negative HIV test within 6 months of the first HIV infection diagnosis, the stage is 0 and remains 0 until 6 months after diagnosis. Advanced HIV disease (AIDS) is classified as stage 3 if one or more specific opportunistic illness has been diagnosed (**Table 202-1**). Otherwise, the stage is determined by CD4+ T lymphocyte test results and immunologic criteria (**Table 202-2**). If none of these criteria apply (e.g., because of missing information on CD4+ T lymphocyte test results), the stage is U (unknown).

The definition and staging criteria of AIDS are complex and comprehensive and were established for surveillance purposes rather than for the practical care of patients. Thus, the clinician should not focus on whether the patient fulfills the strict definition of AIDS, but should view HIV disease as a spectrum ranging from primary infection, with or without the acute syndrome, to the relatively asymptomatic stage, to advanced stages associated with opportunistic diseases (see "Pathophysiology and Pathogenesis," below).

TABLE 202-1 CDC Stage 3 (AIDS)-Defining Opportunistic Illnesses in HIV Infection

Bacterial infections, multiple or recurrent[a]
Candidiasis of bronchi, trachea, or lungs
Candidiasis of esophagus
Cervical cancer, invasive[b]
Coccidioidomycosis, disseminated or extrapulmonary
Cryptococcosis, extrapulmonary
Cryptosporidiosis, chronic intestinal (>1 month's duration)
Cytomegalovirus disease (other than liver, spleen, or nodes), onset at age >1 month
Cytomegalovirus retinitis (with loss of vision)
Encephalopathy attributed to HIV
Herpes simplex: chronic ulcers (>1 month's duration) or bronchitis, pneumonitis, or esophagitis (onset at age >1 month)
Histoplasmosis, disseminated or extrapulmonary
Isosporiasis, chronic intestinal (>1 month's duration)
Kaposi's sarcoma
Lymphoma, Burkitt's (or equivalent term)
Lymphoma, immunoblastic (or equivalent term)
Lymphoma, primary, of brain
Mycobacterium avium complex or *Mycobacterium kansasii*, disseminated or extrapulmonary
Mycobacterium tuberculosis of any site, pulmonary,[b] disseminated, or extrapulmonary
Mycobacterium, other species or unidentified species, disseminated or extrapulmonary
Pneumocystis jirovecii (previously known as *Pneumocystis carinii*) pneumonia
Pneumonia, recurrent[b]
Progressive multifocal leukoencephalopathy
Salmonella septicemia, recurrent
Toxoplasmosis of brain, onset at age >1 month
Wasting syndrome attributed to HIV

[a]Only among children age <6 years. [b]Only among adults, adolescents, and children age ≥6 years.

Source: MMWR 63(RR-03), April 11, 2014.

ETIOLOGIC AGENT

HIV is the etiologic agent of AIDS; it belongs to the family of human retroviruses (Retroviridae) and the subfamily of lentiviruses (**Chap. 201**). Nononcogenic lentiviruses cause disease in other animal species, including sheep, horses, goats, cattle, cats, and monkeys. The four retroviruses known to cause human disease belong to two distinct groups: the human T lymphotropic viruses (HTLV)-1 and HTLV-2, which are transforming retroviruses; and the human immunodeficiency viruses, HIV-1 and HIV-2, which cause cytopathic effects either directly or indirectly (**Chap. 201**). The most common cause of HIV disease throughout the world, and certainly in the United States, is HIV-1, which comprises several subtypes with different geographic distributions (see "Molecular Heterogeneity of HIV-1," below). HIV-2 was first identified in 1986 in West African patients and was originally confined to West Africa. However, cases traced to West Africa or to sexual contacts with West Africans have been identified throughout the world. The currently defined groups of HIV-1 (M, N, O, P) and the HIV-2 groups A through H each are likely derived from a separate transfer to humans from a nonhuman primate reservoir. HIV-1 viruses likely came from chimpanzees and/or gorillas, and HIV-2 from sooty mangabeys. The AIDS pandemic is primarily caused by the HIV-1 M group viruses. Although HIV-1 group O and HIV-2 viruses have been found in numerous countries, including those in the developed world, they have caused much more localized epidemics. Reported infections with group N and group P viruses are rare and confined almost entirely to residents of Cameroon or travelers from Cameroon. The taxonomic relationship between primate lentiviruses is shown in **Fig. 202-1**.

MORPHOLOGY OF HIV

Electron microscopy shows that the HIV virion is an icosahedral structure (**Fig. 202-2**) containing numerous external spikes formed

TABLE 202-2 CDC HIV Infection Stages 1–3 Based on Age-Specific CD4+ T Lymphocyte Count or CD4+ T Lymphocyte Percentage of Total Lymphocytes[a]

	AGE ON DCATE OF CD4 T+ LYMPHOCYTE TEST					
	<1 YEAR		1–5 YEARS		6 YEARS THROUGH ADULT	
STAGE[a]	CELLS/µL	%	CELLS/µL	%	CELLS/µL	%
1	≥1500	≥34	≥1000	≥30	≥500	≥26
2	750–1499	26–33	500–999	22–29	200–499	14–25
3	<750	<26	<500	<22	<200	<14

[a]The stage is based primarily on the CD4+ T lymphocyte count; the CD4+ T lymphocyte count takes precedence over the CD4+ T lymphocyte percentage, and the percentage is considered only if the count is missing.

Source: MMWR 63(RR-03), April 11, 2014.

by the two major envelope proteins, the external gp120 and the transmembrane gp41. The HIV envelope exists as a trimeric heterodimer. The virion buds from the surface of the infected cell (Fig. 202-2***A***) and incorporates a variety of host cellular proteins into its lipid bilayer. The structure of HIV-1 is schematically diagrammed in Fig. 202-2***B***.

REPLICATION CYCLE OF HIV

HIV is an RNA virus whose hallmark is the reverse transcription of its genomic RNA to DNA by the enzyme *reverse transcriptase*. The replication cycle of HIV begins with the high-affinity binding via surface-exposed residues within the gp120 protein to its receptor on the host cell surface, the CD4 molecule (**Fig. 202-3**). The CD4 molecule is a 55-kDa protein found predominantly on a subset of T lymphocytes that are responsible for helper function in the immune system (**Chap. 349**). Once it binds to CD4, the gp120 protein undergoes a conformational change that facilitates binding to one of two major co-receptors. The two major co-receptors for HIV-1 are CCR5 and CXCR4. Both receptors belong to the family of seven-transmembrane-domain G protein–coupled cellular receptors, and the use of one or the other or both receptors by the virus for entry into the cell is an important determinant of the cellular tropism of the virus. Cell-to-cell spread is also facilitated by accessory molecules such as the C-type lectin receptor *DC-SIGN* expressed on certain dendritic cells (DCs) that bind to the HIV gp120 envelope protein, allowing virus captured on DCs to spread to CD4+ T cells. Following binding of the envelope protein to the CD4 molecule associated with the above-mentioned conformational change in the viral envelope gp120, fusion with the host cell membrane occurs via the newly exposed gp41 molecule penetrating the plasma membrane of the target cell and then coiling upon itself to bring the virion and target cell together (**Fig. 202-4**). Following fusion, uncoating of the capsid protein shell is initiated—a step that facilitates reverse transcription and leads to formation of the preintegration complex, composed of viral RNA, enzymes, and accessory proteins and surrounded by capsid and matrix proteins (Fig. 202-3). All these post-fusion viral components constitute the HIV replication complex, including the outer capsid shell, which plays an integral role in supporting reverse transcription of viral RNA. As the preintegration complex traverses the cytoplasm to reach the nucleus, the viral reverse transcriptase enzyme catalyzes the reverse transcription of the genomic RNA into DNA, resulting in the formation of double-stranded HIV proviral DNA. At several steps of the replication cycle, the virus is vulnerable to various cellular factors that can block the progression of infection. The cytoplasmic tripartite motif-containing protein 5-α (TRIM5-α) is a host restriction factor that interacts with retroviral capsids, causing their premature disassembly and induction of innate immune responses. The apolipoprotein B mRNA editing enzyme (catalytic polypeptide-like 3 [APOBEC3]) family of cellular proteins also inhibits progression of virus infection after virus has entered the cell and prior to entering the nucleus. APOBEC3 proteins, which are incorporated into virions and released into the cytoplasm of a newly infected cell, bind to the single minus-strand DNA intermediate and deaminate viral cytidine, causing hypermutation of retroviral genomes. HIV has evolved a powerful strategy to protect itself from APOBEC. The viral protein Vif targets APOBEC3 for proteasomal degradation. SAMHD1 is another post-entry host factor that prevents reverse transcription by depleting pools of deoxynucleotides (dNTPs). The type I interferon (IFN)-induced myxovirus resistance protein 2 (MX2) is another restriction factor associated with innate immunity that inhibits HIV-1 nuclear entry.

With activation of the cell, the viral DNA accesses the nuclear pore and is transferred from the cytoplasm to the nucleus, where it is integrated into the host cell chromosomes through the action of another virally encoded enzyme, *integrase* (Fig. 202-3). HIV proviral DNA integrates into the host genomic DNA preferentially in regions of active transcription and regional hotspots. This provirus may remain transcriptionally inactive (latent) or it may manifest varying levels of gene expression, up to active transcription and production of virus depending on the metabolic state of the infected cell.

Cellular activation plays an important role in the replication cycle of HIV and is critical to the pathogenesis of HIV disease (see "Pathogenesis and Pathophysiology," below). Following initial binding, fusion, and

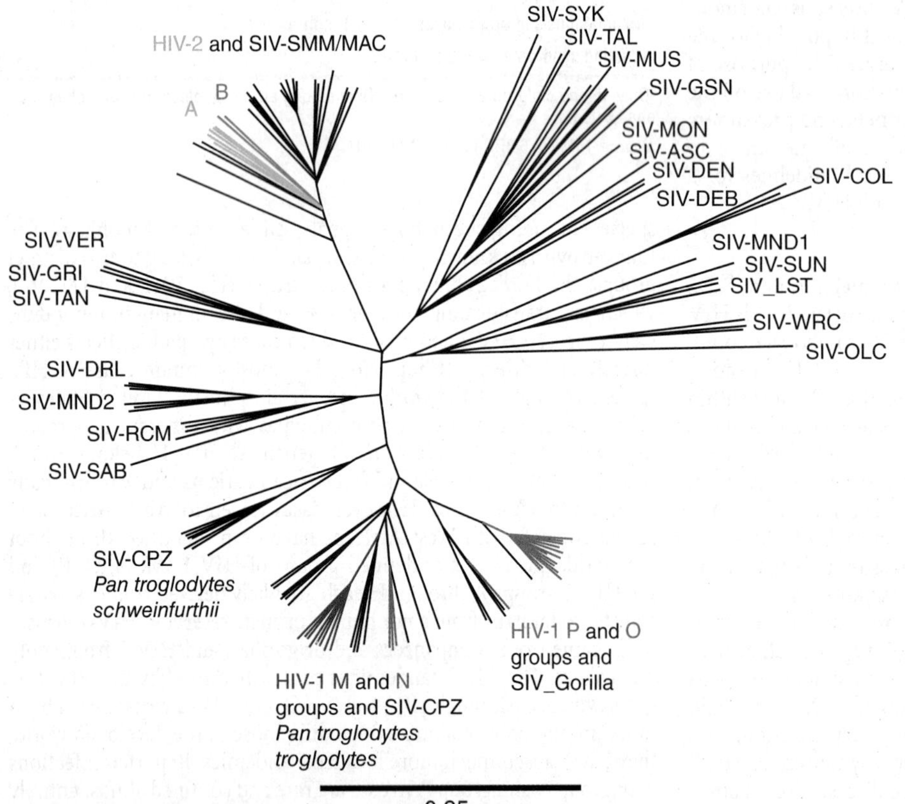

FIGURE 202-1 A phylogenetic tree based on the nearly complete genomes (*gag* through *nef* genes) of primate immunodeficiency viruses. The scale (0.25) indicates a 25% phylogenetically corrected genetic distance at the nucleotide level. Clades in color represent viruses (HIV-1, HIV-2) identified in humans after relatively recent transfers from chimpanzee, gorilla, and sooty mangabey reservoirs. *(Prepared by Brian Foley, PhD, of the HIV Sequence Database, Theoretical Biology and Biophysics Group, Los Alamos National Laboratory; additional information at www.hiv.lanl.gov/content/sequence/HelpDocs/subtypes.html.)*

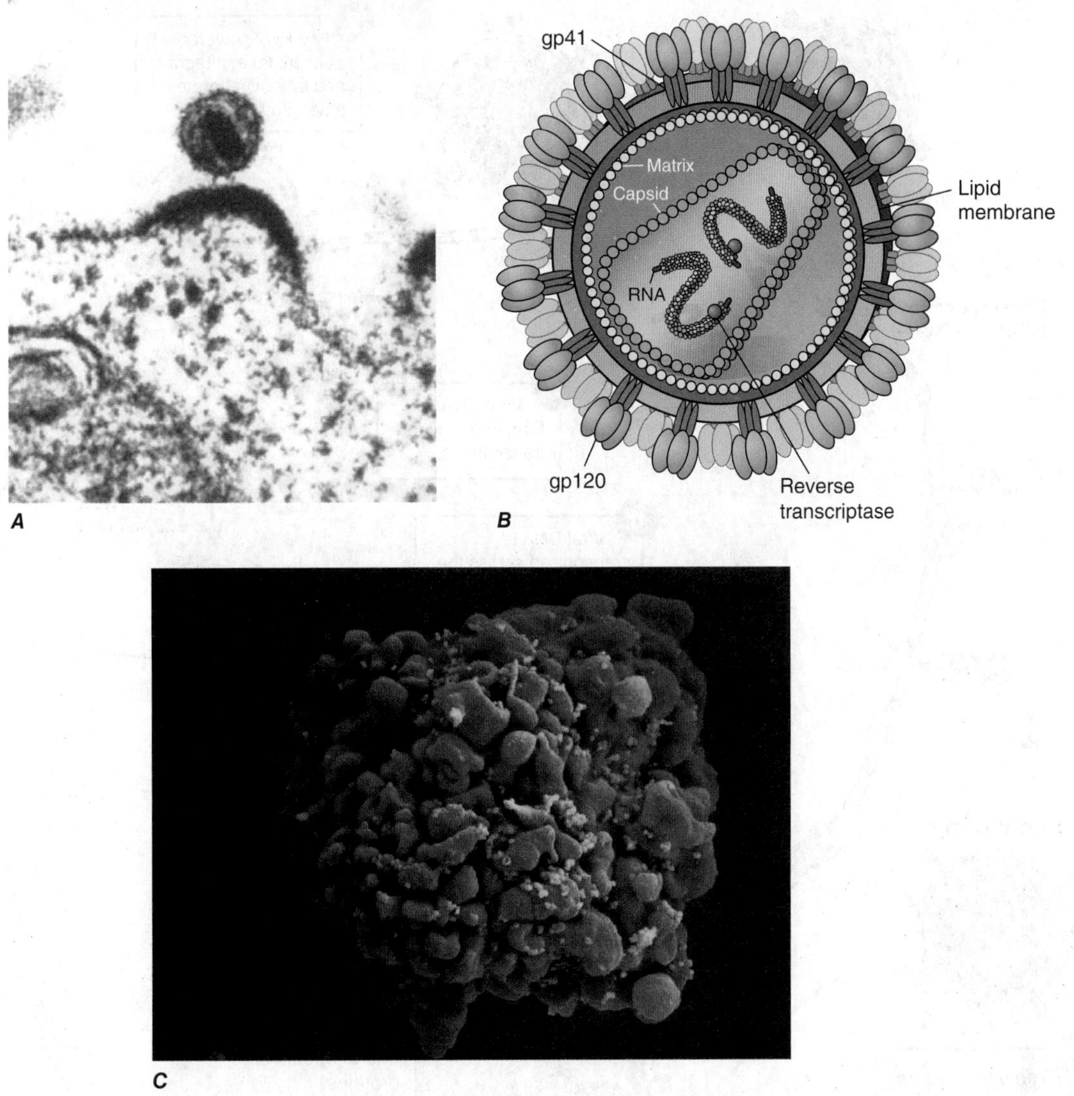

FIGURE 202-2 ***A.*** Electron micrograph of HIV. Figure illustrates a typical virion following budding from the surface of a CD4+ T lymphocyte, together with two additional incomplete virions in the process of budding from the cell membrane. ***B.*** Structure of HIV-1, including the gp120 envelope, gp41 transmembrane components of the envelope, genomic RNA, enzyme reverse transcriptase, p18(17) inner membrane (matrix), and p24 core protein (capsid). *(Courtesy by George V. Kelvin.) (Adapted from RC Gallo: Sci Am 256:46, 1987.)* ***C.*** Scanning electron micrograph of HIV-1 virions infecting a human CD4+ T lymphocyte. The original photograph was imaged at 20,000× magnification. Cell is approximately 10 microns in diameter, and the HIV particles are approximately 120 nanometers. *(Courtesy of Elizabeth R. Fischer, Rocky Mountain Laboratories, National Institute of Allergy and Infectious Diseases.)*

internalization of the nucleic acid contents of virions into the target cell, incompletely reverse-transcribed DNA intermediates are labile in quiescent cells and do not integrate efficiently into the host cell genome unless cellular activation occurs shortly after infection. Furthermore, some degree of activation of the host cell is required for the initiation of transcription of the integrated proviral DNA into either genomic RNA or mRNA. This latter process may not necessarily be associated with the detectable expression of the classic cell-surface markers of activation, especially given that cell-associated HIV RNA transcribed from competent or defective proviruses can be detected in infected resting CD4+ T cells. In this regard, activation of HIV expression from the latent state depends on the interaction of various cellular and viral factors. Following transcription, HIV mRNA is translated into proteins that undergo modification through glycosylation, myristoylation, phosphorylation, and cleavage. The viral particle is formed by the assembly of HIV proteins, enzymes, and genomic RNA at the plasma membrane of the cells. Budding of the progeny virion through the lipid bilayer of the host cell membrane is the point at which the core acquires its external envelope and where the host restriction factor tetherin can inhibit the release of budding particles. Tetherin is an IFN-induced type II transmembrane protein that interferes with virion detachment, although the HIV accessory protein Vpu counteracts this effect through direct interactions with tetherin. During or soon after budding, the virally encoded protease catalyzes the cleavage of the gag-pol precursor to yield the mature virion. Progression through the virus replication cycle is profoundly influenced by a variety of viral regulatory gene products. Likewise, each point in the replication cycle of HIV is a real or potential target for therapeutic intervention. Thus far, the reverse transcriptase, protease, and integrase enzymes as well as the process of virus–target cell binding and fusion have proved to be susceptible to pharmacologic disruption.

HIV GENOME

Figure 202-5 illustrates schematically the arrangement of the HIV genome. Like other retroviruses, HIV-1 has genes that encode the structural proteins of the virus: *gag* encodes the proteins that form the core of the virion (including p24 antigen); *pol* encodes the enzymes responsible for protease processing of viral proteins, reverse transcription, and integration; and *env* encodes the envelope glycoproteins. However, HIV-1 is more complex than other retroviruses, particularly those of the nonprimate group, in that it also contains at least six other regulatory genes (*tat, rev, nef, vif, vpr,* and *vpu*), which code for proteins involved in the modification of the host cell to enhance virus growth and the regulation of viral gene expression. Several of these

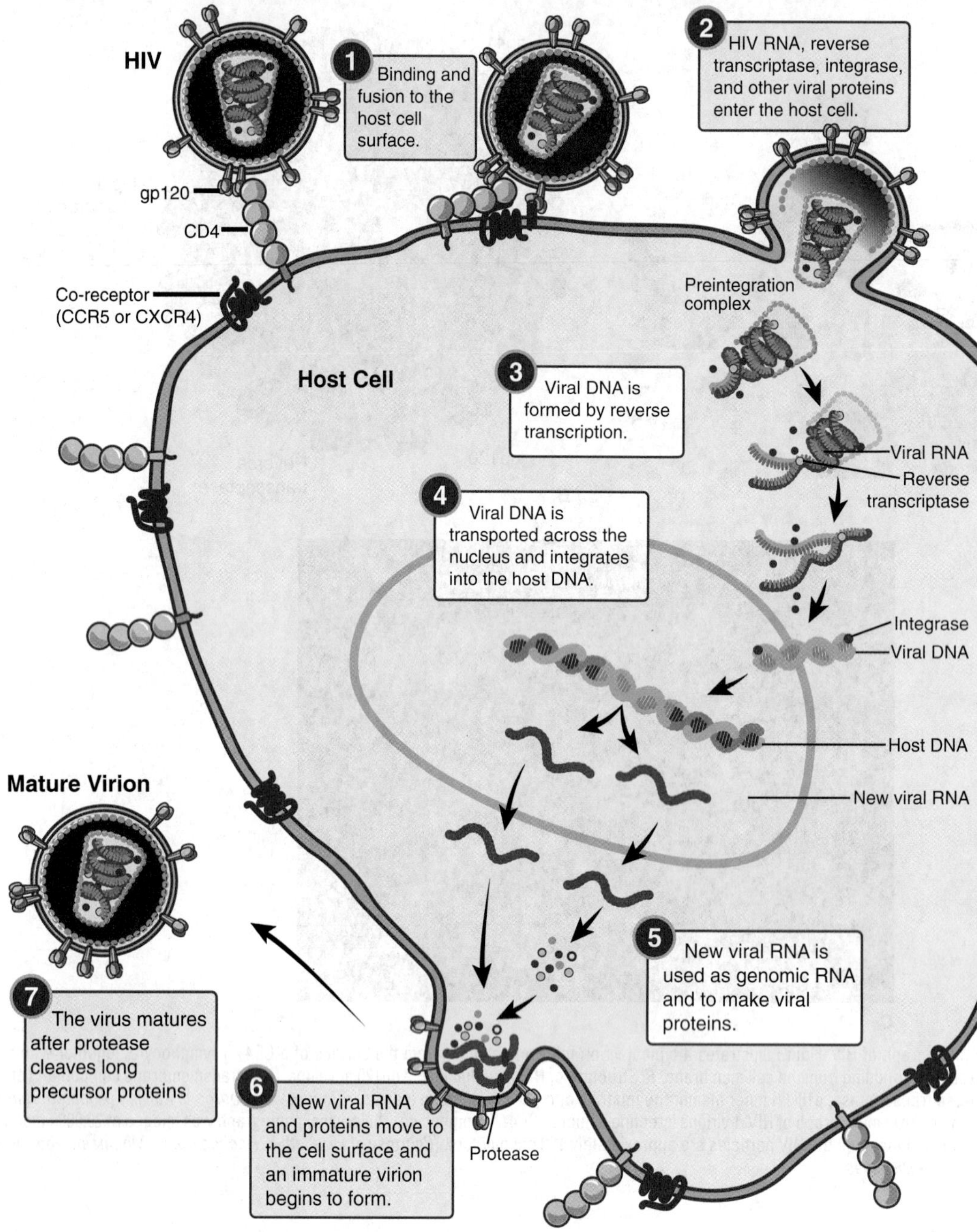

HIV

1 Binding and fusion to the host cell surface.

2 HIV RNA, reverse transcriptase, integrase, and other viral proteins enter the host cell.

gp120

CD4

Co-receptor (CCR5 or CXCR4)

Preintegration complex

Host Cell

3 Viral DNA is formed by reverse transcription.

Viral RNA

Reverse transcriptase

4 Viral DNA is transported across the nucleus and integrates into the host DNA.

Integrase

Viral DNA

Host DNA

New viral RNA

Mature Virion

5 New viral RNA is used as genomic RNA and to make viral proteins.

7 The virus matures after protease cleaves long precursor proteins

6 New viral RNA and proteins move to the cell surface and an immature virion begins to form.

Protease

FIGURE 202-3 The replication cycle of HIV. See text for description. *(From the National Institute of Allergy and Infectious Diseases.)*

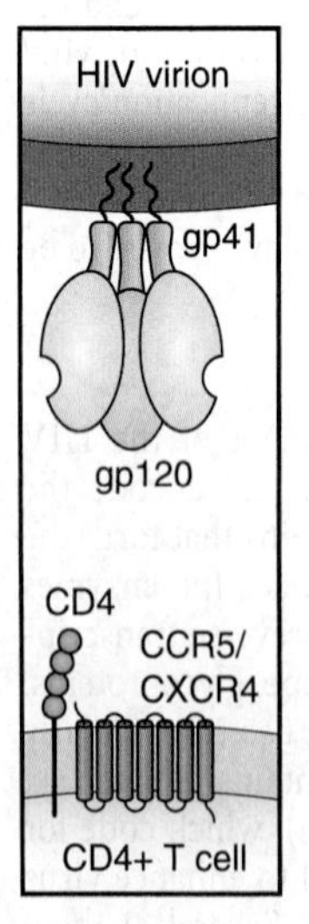

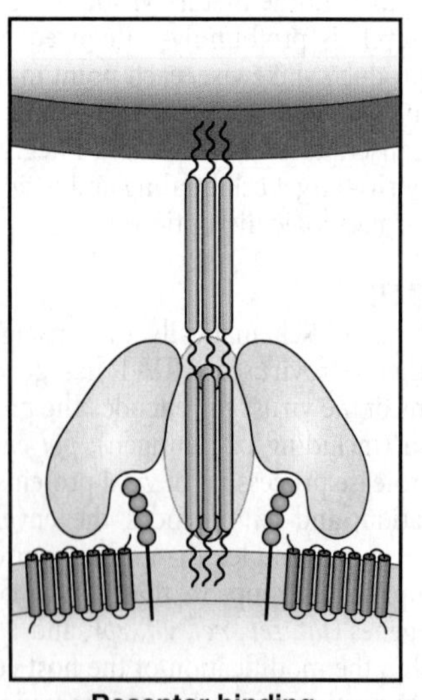

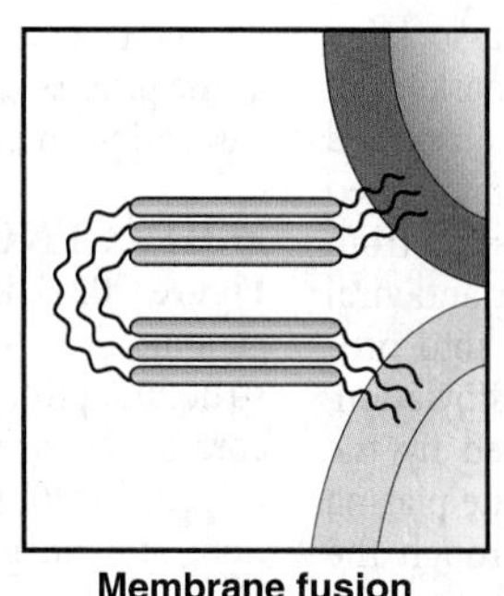

FIGURE 202-4 Binding and fusion of HIV-1 with its target cell. HIV-1 binds to its target cell via the CD4 molecule, leading to a conformational change in the gp120 molecule that allows it to bind to the co-receptor CCR5 (for R5-using viruses). The virus then firmly attaches to the host cell membrane in a coiled-spring fashion via the newly exposed gp41 molecule. Virus-cell fusion occurs as the transitional intermediate of gp41 undergoes further changes to form a hairpin structure that draws the two membranes into close proximity (see text for details). *(Adapted from Montefiori D, Moore JP: HIV vaccines. Magic of the occult? Science 283:336, 1999.)*

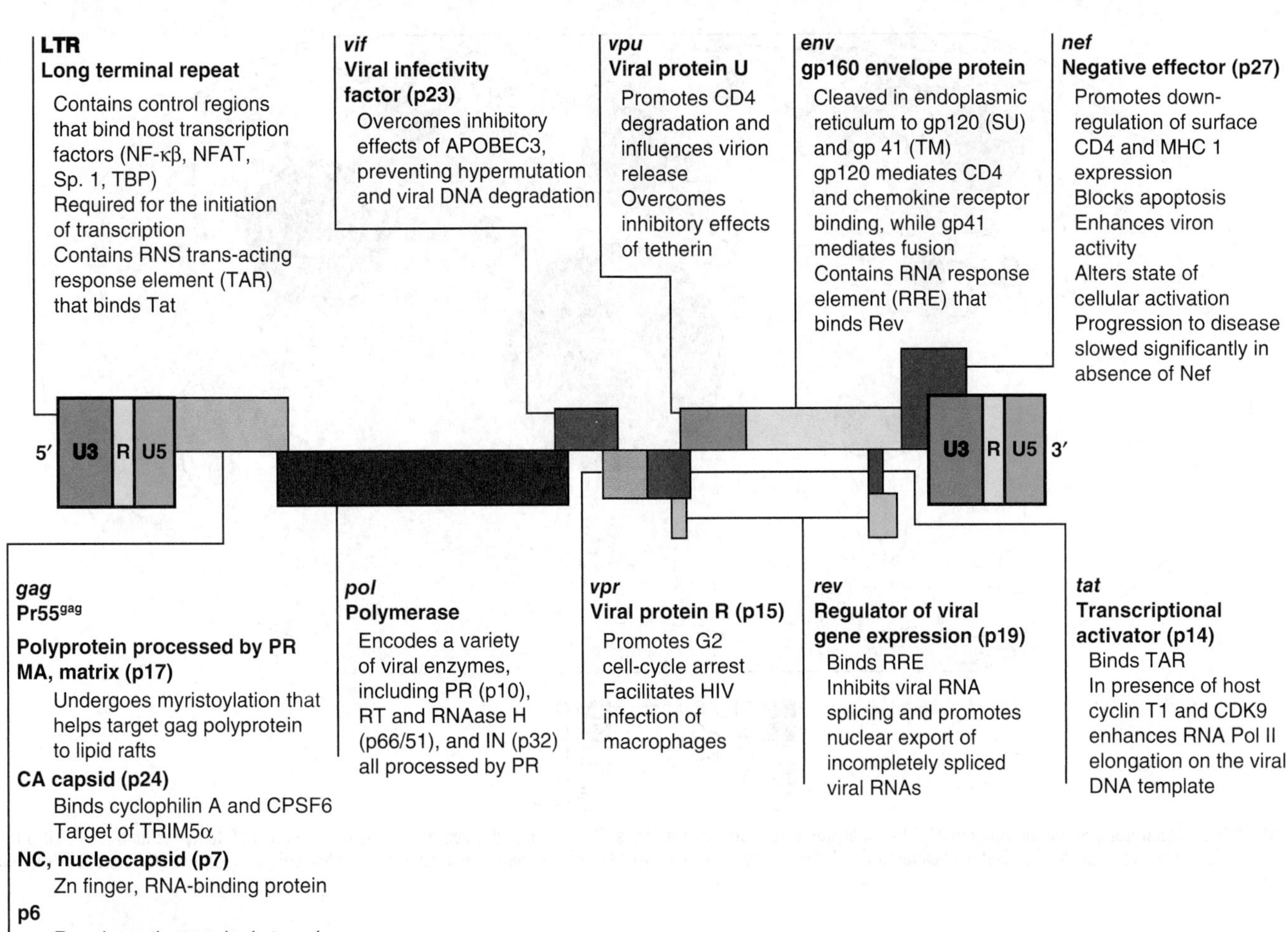
LTR
Long terminal repeat
Contains control regions that bind host transcription factors (NF-κβ, NFAT, Sp. 1, TBP)
Required for the initiation of transcription
Contains RNS trans-acting response element (TAR) that binds Tat
vif
Viral infectivity factor (p23)
Overcomes inhibitory effects of APOBEC3, preventing hypermutation and viral DNA degradation
vpu
Viral protein U
Promotes CD4 degradation and influences virion release
Overcomes inhibitory effects of tetherin
env
gp160 envelope protein
Cleaved in endoplasmic reticulum to gp120 (SU) and gp 41 (TM)
gp120 mediates CD4 and chemokine receptor binding, while gp41 mediates fusion
Contains RNA response element (RRE) that binds Rev
nef
Negative effector (p27)
Promotes down-regulation of surface CD4 and MHC 1 expression
Blocks apoptosis
Enhances viron activity
Alters state of cellular activation
Progression to disease slowed significantly in absence of Nef
5′
U3
R
U5
U3
R
U5
3′
gag
Pr55gag
Polyprotein processed by PR
MA, matrix (p17)
Undergoes myristoylation that helps target gag polyprotein to lipid rafts
CA capsid (p24)
Binds cyclophilin A and CPSF6
Target of TRIM5α
NC, nucleocapsid (p7)
Zn finger, RNA-binding protein
p6
Regulates the terminal steps in virion budding through interactions with TSG101 and ALIX 1
Incorporates Vpr into viral particles
pol
Polymerase
Encodes a variety of viral enzymes, including PR (p10), RT and RNAase H (p66/51), and IN (p32) all processed by PR
vpr
Viral protein R (p15)
Promotes G2 cell-cycle arrest
Facilitates HIV infection of macrophages
rev
Regulator of viral gene expression (p19)
Binds RRE
Inhibits viral RNA splicing and promotes nuclear export of incompletely spliced viral RNAs
tat
Transcriptional activator (p14)
Binds TAR
In presence of host cyclin T1 and CDK9 enhances RNA Pol II elongation on the viral DNA template

FIGURE 202-5 Organization of the genome of the HIV provirus together with a summary description of its 9 genes encoding 15 proteins. *(Reproduced with permission from WC Greene et al: Charting HIV's remarkable voyage through the cell: Basic science as a passport to future therapy. Nat Med 8:673, 2002.)*

proteins are thought to play a role in the pathogenesis of HIV disease; their various functions are listed in Fig. 202-5. Flanking these genes are the long terminal repeats (LTRs), which contain regulatory elements involved in gene expression (Fig. 202-5). The major difference between the genomes of HIV-1 and HIV-2 is the fact that HIV-2 lacks the *vpu* gene and has a *vpx* gene not contained in HIV-1.

MOLECULAR HETEROGENEITY OF HIV-1

Molecular analyses of HIV isolates reveal varying levels of sequence diversity over all regions of the viral genome. For example, the degree of difference in the coding sequences of the viral envelope protein ranges from a few percent (very close, among isolates from the same infected individual) to more than 50% (extreme diversity, between isolates from the different groups of HIV-1: M, N, O, and P). The changes tend to cluster in hypervariable regions. HIV can evolve by several means, including simple base substitution, insertions and deletions, recombination, and gain and loss of glycosylation sites. HIV sequence diversity arises directly from the limited fidelity of the reverse transcriptase, i.e., a tendency toward copying errors. The balance of immune pressure and functional constraints on proteins influences the regional level of variation within proteins. For example, Envelope, which is exposed on the surface of the virion and is under immune selective pressure from both antibodies and cytolytic T lymphocytes, is extremely variable, with clusters of mutations in hypervariable domains. In contrast, reverse transcriptase, with important enzymatic functions, is relatively conserved, particularly around the active site. The extraordinary variability of HIV-1 contrasts markedly with the relative stability of HTLV-1 and 2.

The four groups (M, N, O and P) of HIV-1 are the result of four separate chimpanzee-to-human (or possibly gorilla-to-human for groups O and P) transfers. Group M (major), which is responsible for most of the infections in the world, has diversified into subtypes and intersubtype recombinant forms, due to "sub-epidemics" within humans after one of those transfers.

Among primate lentiviruses, HIV-1 is most closely related to viruses isolated from chimpanzees and gorillas (Fig. 202-1). The chimpanzee subspecies *Pan troglodytes troglodytes* has been established to be the natural reservoir of the HIV-1 M and N groups. The rare viruses of the HIV-1 O and P groups are most closely related to viruses found in Cameroonian gorillas. The M group comprises ten subtypes, or *clades*, designated A, B, C, D, F, G, H, J, K and L, as well as more than 100 known circulating recombinant forms (CRFs) and numerous unique recombinant forms. Intersubtype recombinants are generated by infection of an individual with two subtypes that then recombine and create a virus with a selective advantage. These CRFs range from highly prevalent forms such as CRF01_AE, common in southeast Asia, and CRF02_AG from west and central Africa, to a large number of CRFs that are relatively rare, either because they are of a more recent origin (newly recombined) or because they have not broken out into a major population. The subtypes and CRFs create the major lineages of the M group of HIV-1. HIV-1 M group subtype C dominates the global pandemic, and although there is much speculation that it is

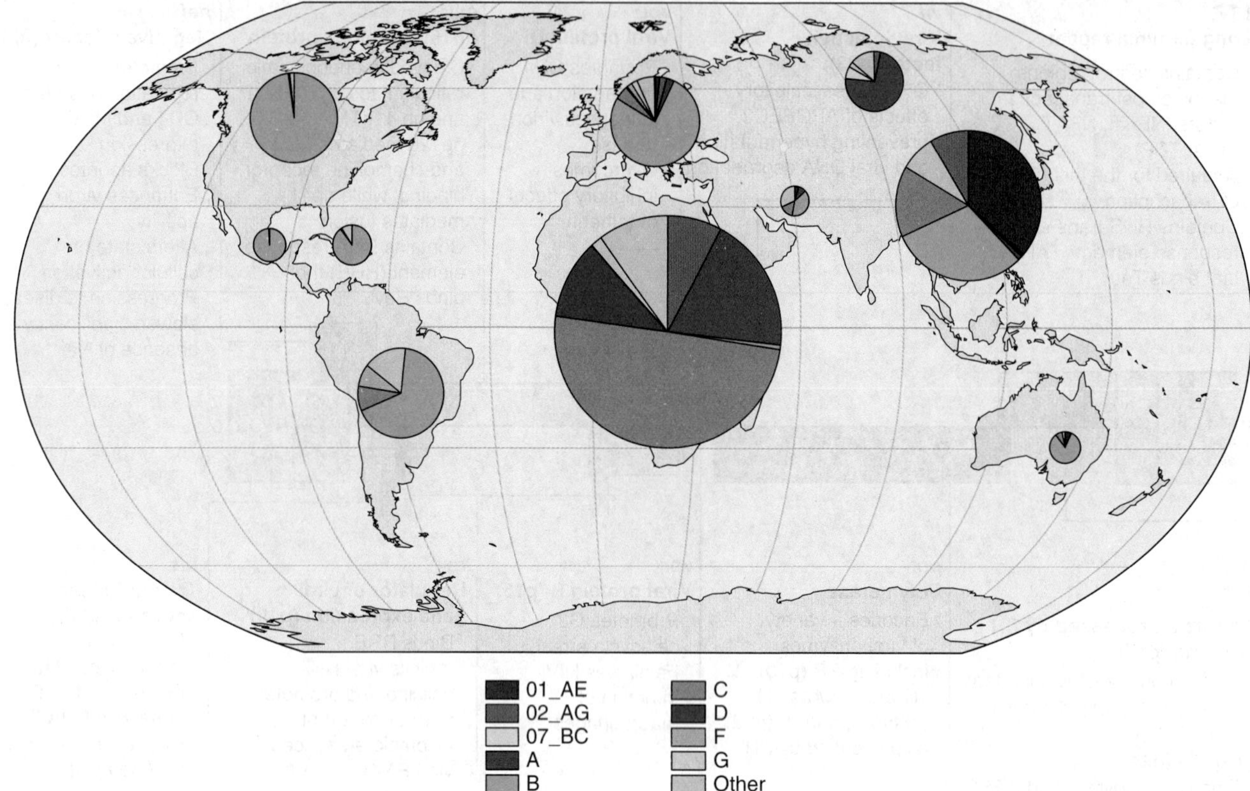

FIGURE 202-6 Global geographic distribution of HIV-1 subtypes and recombinant forms. Distributions derived from relative frequency of subtypes among >860,000 HIV genomic sequences in the Los Alamos National Laboratory HIV Sequence Database. (Additional information available at *www.hiv.lanl.gov/components/sequence/HIV/geo/geo.comp.*)

more transmissible than other subtypes, solid data on variations in transmissibility between subtypes are lacking. Human population densities, access to prevention and treatment, prevalence of genital ulcers, iatrogenic transmissions, and other confounding host factors are all possible reasons why one subtype has spread more than another.

Figure 202-6 schematically diagrams the worldwide distribution of HIV-1 subtypes by region. Nine strains account for the vast majority of HIV infections globally: HIV-1 subtypes A, B, C, D, F, G and three of the CRFs, CRF01_AE, CRF02_AG, and CRF07_BC. Subtype C viruses (of the M group) are by far the most common form worldwide, likely accounting for ~50% of prevalent infections worldwide. In sub-Saharan Africa, home to approximately two-thirds of all individuals living with HIV/AIDS, most infections are caused by subtype C, with smaller proportions of infections caused by subtype A, subtype D, CRF02_AG, and other subtypes and recombinants. In South Africa, the country with the largest number of prevalent infections (7.8 million in 2020), 98% of the HIV-1 isolates sequenced are of subtype C. In Asia, HIV-1 isolates of the CRF01_AE lineage and subtypes B and C predominate. CRF01_AE accounts for most infections in south and southeast Asia, while >95% of infections in India, home to an estimated 2.3 million HIV-infected individuals, are of subtype C (see "HIV Infection and AIDS Worldwide," below). Subtype B viruses are overwhelmingly predominant in the United States, Canada, certain countries in South America, western Europe, and Australia. It is thought that, purely by chance, subtype B was seeded into the United States and Europe in the late 1970s, thereby establishing an overwhelming founder effect. Many countries have co-circulating viral subtypes that are giving rise to new CRFs. Sequence analyses of HIV-1 isolates from infected individuals indicate that recombination among viruses of different clades likely occurs when an individual is infected with viruses of more than one subtype, particularly in geographic areas where subtypes overlap, and more often in sub-epidemics driven by injection drug use than in those driven by sexual transmission.

The extraordinary diversity of HIV, reflected by the presence of multiple subtypes, circulating recombinant forms, and continuous viral evolution, has implications for possible differential rates of transmission, rates of disease progression, and the development of resistance to antiretroviral drugs. This diversity may also prove to be a formidable obstacle to HIV vaccine development, as a broadly useful vaccine would need to induce protective responses against a wide range of viral strains.

TRANSMISSION

HIV is transmitted primarily by sexual contact (both heterosexual and male to male); by blood and blood products; and by infected mothers to infants intrapartum, perinatally, or via breast milk. After four decades of experience and observations, there is no evidence that HIV is transmitted by any other modality. **Table 202-3** lists the estimated risk of HIV transmission for various types of exposures.

■ SEXUAL TRANSMISSION

HIV infection is predominantly a sexually transmitted infection (STI) worldwide. By far the most common mode of infection, particularly in developing countries, is heterosexual transmission, although in many western countries male-to-male sexual transmission dominates. Although a wide variety of factors including viral load and the presence of ulcerative genital diseases influence the efficiency of heterosexual transmission of HIV, such transmission is generally inefficient. A recent systemic review found a low per-act risk of heterosexual transmission in the absence of antiretrovirals: 0.04% for female-to-male transmission and 0.08% for male-to-female transmission during vaginal intercourse in the absence of antiretroviral therapy or condom use (Table 202-3).

HIV has been demonstrated in seminal fluid both within infected mononuclear cells and in cell-free material. The virus appears to concentrate in the seminal fluid, particularly in situations where there are increased numbers of lymphocytes and monocytes in the fluid, as seen in genital inflammatory states such as urethritis and epididymitis, conditions closely associated with other STIs. The virus has also been demonstrated in cervical smears and vaginal fluid. There is an elevated risk of HIV transmission associated with unprotected receptive anal intercourse (URAI) among both men and women compared to the risk

TABLE 202-3 Estimated Per-Act Probability of Acquiring HIV from an Infected Source, By Exposure Act

TYPE OF EXPOSURE	RISK PER 10,000 EXPOSURES
Parenteral	
Blood transfusion	9250
Needle-sharing during injection drug use	63
Percutaneous (needle-stick)	23
Sexual	
Receptive anal intercourse	138
Insertive anal intercourse	11
Receptive penile-vaginal intercourse	8
Insertive penile-vaginal intercourse	4
Receptive oral intercourse	Low
Insertive oral intercourse	Low
Other[a]	
Biting	Negligible
Spitting	Negligible
Throwing body fluids (including semen or saliva)	Negligible
Sharing sex toys	Negligible

[a]HIV transmission through these exposure routes is technically possible but unlikely and not well documented.

Source: CDC, *www.cdc.gov/hiv/risk/estimates/riskbehaviors.html.*

associated with unprotected receptive vaginal intercourse. Although data are limited, the per-act risk for HIV transmission via URAI has been estimated to be ~1.4% (Table 202-3). The risk of HIV acquisition associated with URAI is higher than that seen in penile-vaginal intercourse probably because only a thin, fragile rectal mucosal membrane separates the deposited semen from potentially susceptible cells in and beneath the mucosa, and micro-trauma of the mucosal membrane has been associated with anal intercourse. Anal douching and sexual practices that traumatize the rectal mucosa also increase the likelihood of infection. It is likely that anal intercourse provides at least two modalities of infection: (1) direct inoculation into blood in cases of traumatic tears in the mucosa; and (2) infection of susceptible target cells, such as Langerhans cells, in the mucosal layer in the absence of trauma. Insertive anal intercourse also confers an increased risk of HIV acquisition compared to insertive vaginal intercourse in the receptive partner since the vaginal mucosa is several layers thicker than the rectal mucosa and less likely to be traumatized during intercourse. Nonetheless, the virus can be transmitted to either partner through vaginal intercourse. As noted in Table 202-3, male-to-female HIV transmission is more efficient than female-to-male transmission. The differences in reported transmission rates between men and women may be due in part to the prolonged exposure of the vaginal and cervical mucosa to infected seminal fluid; the endometrium also can be exposed to virus when semen enters through the cervical os. By comparison, the penis and urethral orifice of the uninfected male partner are exposed relatively briefly to infected vaginal fluid.

Among various cofactors examined in studies of heterosexual HIV transmission, the presence of other STIs has been strongly associated with HIV transmission. In this regard, there is a close association between genital ulcerations and transmission, owing to both susceptibility to infection and infectivity. Infections with microorganisms such as *Treponema pallidum* **(Chap. 182)**, *Haemophilus ducreyi* **(Chap. 157)**, and herpes simplex virus (HSV; **Chap. 192**) are important causes of genital ulcerations linked to transmission of HIV. In addition, pathogens responsible for non-ulcerative inflammatory STIs such as those caused by *Chlamydia trachomatis* **(Chap. 189)**, *Neisseria gonorrhoeae* **(Chap. 156)**, and *Trichomonas vaginalis* **(Chap. 229)** also are associated with an increased risk of transmission of HIV infection. Bacterial vaginosis, an infection related to sexual behavior, but not strictly an STI, also may be linked to an increased risk of transmission of HIV infection. Several studies have suggested that treating STIs and genital tract syndromes may help prevent transmission of HIV. This effect is most prominent in populations in which the prevalence of HIV infection is relatively low. It is noteworthy that this principle may not apply to the treatment of HSV infections since it has been shown that even following anti-HSV therapy with resulting healing of HSV-related genital ulcers, HIV acquisition is not reduced. Biopsy studies revealed that the likely explanation is that HIV receptor–positive inflammatory cells persisted in the genital tissue despite the healing of ulcers, and so HIV-susceptible targets remained at the site.

The quantity of HIV-1 in plasma (viral load) is a primary determinant of the risk of HIV-1 transmission. In a cohort of heterosexual couples in Uganda discordant for HIV infection and not receiving antiretroviral therapy, the mean serum HIV RNA level was significantly higher among HIV-infected subjects whose partners seroconverted than among those whose partners did not seroconvert. In fact, transmission was rare when the infected partner had a plasma level of <1700 copies of HIV RNA per milliliter, even when genital ulcer disease was present **(Fig. 202-7)**. The rate of HIV transmission per coital act was highest during the early stage of HIV infection when plasma HIV RNA levels were high and in advanced disease with high viral set points.

Antiretroviral therapy dramatically reduces plasma viremia in most HIV-infected individuals (see "Antiretroviral Therapy" and "HIV Prevention," below) and is associated with a dramatic reduction in risk of transmission, an approach widely referred to as *treatment as prevention* or TasP. Multiple studies have demonstrated that if the viral load of a person with HIV is reduced by antiretroviral therapy to below detectable levels as measured by conventional commercial assays, there is essentially no chance of sexual transmission to the person's sexual partner. This is true for heterosexuals as well as men who have sex with men, leading to the commonly used description of this phenomenon as "undetectable equals untransmittable" or "U=U."

Multiple studies including large, randomized, controlled trials clearly have indicated that male *circumcision* is associated with a lower risk of acquisition of HIV infection for heterosexual men. Studies also suggest that circumcision is protective against HIV acquisition for men who have sex with men reporting mainly or only insertive sex. The benefit of circumcision may be due to increased susceptibility of uncircumcised men to ulcerative STIs, as well as to other factors such as microtrauma to the foreskin and glans penis. In addition, the highly vascularized inner layer of foreskin tissue contains a high density of Langerhans cells as well as increased numbers of CD4+ T cells, macrophages, and other cellular targets for HIV. Finally, the moist environment under the foreskin may promote the presence or persistence of microbial flora that, via inflammatory changes, may lead to even higher concentrations of target cells for HIV in the foreskin. In addition, randomized clinical trials have demonstrated that male circumcision also reduces herpes simplex virus (HSV) type 2, human papillomavirus virus (HPV), and genital ulcer disease in men as well as HPV, genital ulcer disease, bacterial vaginosis, and *Trichomonas vaginalis* infections among female partners of circumcised men. Thus, there may be an

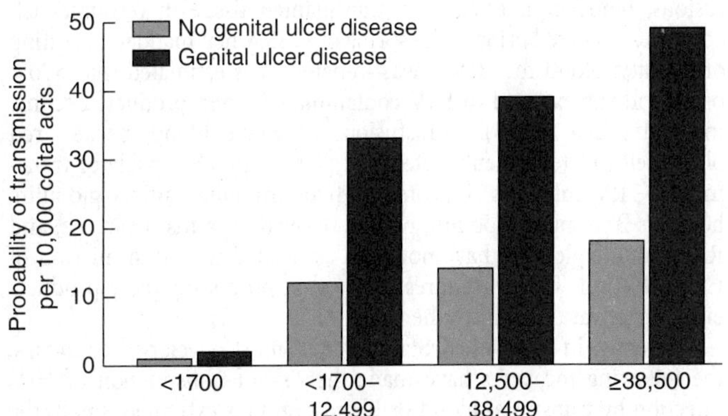

FIGURE 202-7 Probability of HIV transmission per coital act among monogamous, heterosexual, HIV-serodiscordant couples in Uganda. *(From RH Gray et al: Lancet 357:1149, 2001.)*

added indirect benefit of diminution of risk for HIV acquisition to the female sexual partners of circumcised men.

In some studies, the use of oral contraceptives was associated with an increase in incidence of HIV infection over and above that which might be expected by not using a condom for birth control. This phenomenon may be due to drug-induced changes in the cervical mucosa, rendering it more vulnerable to penetration by the virus. Adolescent girls might also be more susceptible to infection upon exposure due to the properties of an immature genital tract with increased cervical ectopy or exposed columnar epithelium.

Oral sex is a much less efficient mode of transmission of HIV than is anal intercourse or vaginal intercourse (Table 202-3). Multiple studies have reported that the incidence of transmission of infection by oral sex among couples discordant for HIV is extremely low. However, there have been well-documented reports of HIV transmission that likely resulted from fellatio or cunnilingus. Therefore, the assumption that oral sex is completely safe is not warranted.

The association of alcohol consumption and illicit drug use with unsafe sexual behavior, both homosexual and heterosexual, leads to an increased risk of sexual transmission of HIV. Methamphetamine and other so-called club drugs such as 3,4-methylenedioxymethamphetamine (MDMA; also known as "ecstasy"), ketamine, gamma-hydroxybutyrate (GHB), and inhaled nitrites (known as "poppers"), sometimes taken in conjunction with PDE-5 inhibitors such as sildenafil (Viagra), tadalafil (Cialis), or vardenafil (Levitra), have been associated with risky sexual practices and increased risk of HIV infection, particularly among men who have sex with men.

TRANSMISSION THROUGH INJECTION DRUG USE

HIV can be transmitted to injection drug users (IDUs) who are exposed to HIV while sharing injection paraphernalia such as needles, syringes, the water in which drugs are mixed, or the cotton through which drugs are filtered. Parenteral transmission of HIV during injection drug use does not require IV puncture; subcutaneous ("skin popping") or intramuscular ("muscling") injections can transmit HIV as well, even though these behaviors are sometimes erroneously perceived as low risk. Among IDUs, the risk of HIV infection increases with the duration of injection drug use; the frequency of needle sharing; the number of partners with whom paraphernalia are shared, comorbid psychiatric conditions such as antisocial personality disorder; the use of cocaine in injectable form or smoked as "crack"; and the use of injection drugs in a geographic location with a high prevalence of HIV infection. As noted in Table 202-3, the per-act risk of transmission from injection drug use with a contaminated needle has been estimated to be approximately 0.6%.

TRANSMISSION BY TRANSFUSED BLOOD AND BLOOD PRODUCTS

HIV can be transmitted to individuals who receive HIV-contaminated blood transfusions, blood products, or transplanted tissue. The vast majority of HIV infections acquired via contaminated blood transfusions, blood components, or transplanted tissue in resource-rich countries occurred prior to the spring of 1985, when mandatory testing of donated blood for HIV-1 was initiated. It is estimated that >90% of individuals exposed to HIV-contaminated blood products become infected (Table 202-3). Transfusions of whole blood, packed red blood cells, platelets, leukocytes, and plasma are all capable of transmitting HIV infection. In contrast, hyperimmune gamma globulin, hepatitis B immune globulin, plasma-derived hepatitis B vaccine, and Rh_0 immune globulin have not been associated with transmission of HIV infection. The procedures involved in processing these products either inactivate or remove the virus.

Currently, in the United States and in most developed countries, the following measures have made the risk of transmission of HIV infection by transfused blood or blood products extremely small: the screening of blood donations for antibodies to HIV-1 and HIV-2 and determination of the presence of HIV nucleic acid usually in minipools of several specimens; the careful selection of potential blood donors with health history questionnaires to exclude individuals with risk behavior; and opportunities for self-deferral and the screening out of HIV-negative individuals with serologic testing for infections that have shared risk factors with HIV, such as hepatitis B and C and syphilis. The chance of infection of a hemophiliac via clotting factor concentrates has essentially been eliminated because of standard screening of blood together with the added layer of safety resulting from heat treatment of the concentrates. It is currently estimated that the risk of infection with HIV in the United States via transfused screened blood is approximately 1 in 2 million units. Since nearly 21 million blood components are transfused in the United States each year, completely eliminating the risk of transfusion-related HIV transmission likely will not be possible. Transmission of HIV (both HIV-1 and HIV-2) by blood or blood products is still an ongoing threat in certain developing countries where routine screening of blood is not universally practiced. Furthermore, there have been reports in certain countries of sporadic breakdowns in routinely available screening procedures in which contaminated blood was transfused, resulting in small clusters of patients becoming infected.

OCCUPATIONAL TRANSMISSION OF HIV: HEALTH CARE WORKERS, LABORATORY WORKERS, AND THE HEALTH CARE SETTING

There is a small but definite occupational risk of HIV transmission to health care workers and laboratory personnel and potentially others who work with HIV-containing materials, particularly when sharp objects are used. More than 300,000 health care workers are stuck with needles or other sharp medical instruments in the United States each year. The global number of HIV infections among health care workers attributable to sharps injuries has been estimated to be 1000 cases (range, 200–5000) per year. In the United States, a total of 58 documented cases of occupational HIV transmission to health care workers, and 150 possible transmissions have been reported by the CDC. Since 1999, only one confirmed case (a laboratory technician sustaining a needle puncture while working with a live HIV culture in 2008) has been reported.

Exposures that place a health care worker at potential risk of HIV infection are percutaneous injuries (e.g., a needle stick or cut with a sharp object) or contact of mucous membrane or nonintact skin (e.g., exposed skin that is chapped, abraded, or afflicted with dermatitis) with blood, tissue, or other potentially infectious body fluids. Large, multi-institutional studies have indicated that the risk of HIV transmission following skin puncture from a needle or a sharp object that was contaminated with blood from a person with documented HIV infection is ~0.23% and after a mucous membrane exposure it is ~0.09% (see "HIV and the Health Care Worker," below) if the injured and/or exposed person is not treated within 24 hours with antiretroviral drugs. The risk of hepatitis B virus (HBV) infection following a similar type of exposure is ~6–30% in nonimmune individuals; if a susceptible worker is exposed to HBV, postexposure prophylaxis with hepatitis B immune globulin and initiation of HBV vaccine is >90% effective in preventing HBV infection. The risk of HCV infection following percutaneous injury is ~1.8% **(Chap. 339)**.

Rare HIV transmission after nonintact skin exposure has been documented, but the average risk for transmission by this route has not been precisely determined; however, it is estimated to be less than the risk for mucous membrane exposure. Transmission of HIV through intact skin has not been documented. All health care workers experiencing a puncture wound or mucous membrane exposures involving blood from a patient with documented HIV infection should be treated prophylactically with combination antiretroviral therapy (ART). This practice, referred to as *postexposure prophylaxis* or PEP, has dramatically reduced the occurrence of puncture-related transmissions of HIV to health care workers.

In addition to blood and visibly bloody body fluids, semen and vaginal secretions also are considered potentially infectious; however, they have not been implicated in occupational transmission from patients to health care workers. The following fluids also are considered potentially infectious: cerebrospinal fluid, synovial fluid, pleural fluid, peritoneal fluid, pericardial fluid, and amniotic fluid. The risk for transmission after exposure to fluids or tissues other than HIV-infected blood has not been quantified, but it is probably considerably lower than the risk after blood exposures. Feces, nasal secretions, saliva, sputum, sweat, tears, urine, and vomitus are not considered potentially infectious for HIV unless they are visibly bloody. Rare cases of HIV transmission via human bites have been reported, but not in the setting of occupational exposure.

An increased risk for HIV infection following percutaneous exposures to HIV-infected blood is associated with exposures involving a relatively large quantity of blood, as in the case of a device visibly contaminated with the patient's blood, a procedure that involves a hollow-bore needle placed directly in a vein or artery, or a deep injury. Factors that might be associated with mucocutaneous transmission of HIV include exposure to an unusually large volume of blood and prolonged contact. In addition, the risk increases for exposures to blood from untreated patients with high levels of HIV in the blood. Since the beginning of the HIV epidemic, there have been rare instances where transmission of infection from a health care worker to patients seemed highly probable. Despite this small number of documented cases, the risk of HIV transmission involving infected health care workers to patients is extremely low in developed countries—in fact, too low to be measured accurately. In this regard, several retrospective epidemiologic studies have been performed tracing thousands of patients of HIV-infected dentists, physicians, surgeons, obstetricians, and gynecologists, and no cases of HIV transmission that could be linked to the health care providers were identified other than the already identified documented cases.

Breaches in infection control and the reuse of contaminated syringes, failure to properly sterilize surgical instruments, and/or hemodialysis equipment also have resulted rarely in the transmission of HIV from patient to patient in hospitals, nursing homes, and outpatient settings. Finally, these very rare occurrences of transmission of HIV as well as HBV and HCV to and from health care workers in the workplace underscore the importance of the use of universal precautions when caring for all patients (see below and **Chap. 142**).

■ MOTHER-TO-CHILD TRANSMISSION OF HIV

HIV infection can be transmitted from an infected mother to her fetus during pregnancy, during delivery, or by breast-feeding. This remains a persistent form of transmission of HIV infection in certain developing countries. Virologic analyses of aborted fetuses indicate that HIV can be transmitted to the fetus during the first or second trimesters of pregnancy. However, maternal transmission to the fetus occurs most commonly in the perinatal period. Two studies performed in Rwanda and the Democratic Republic of Congo (then called Zaire) indicated that among all mother-to-child transmissions of HIV, the relative proportions were 23–30% before birth, 50–65% during birth, and 12–20% via breast-feeding.

In the absence of antiretroviral therapy for the mother during pregnancy, labor, and delivery, and for the fetus prophylactically following birth, the probability of transmission of HIV from mother to infant/fetus ranges from 15 to 25% in industrialized countries and from 25% to 35% in developing countries. These differences may relate to the adequacy of prenatal care as well as to the stage of HIV disease and the general health of the mother during pregnancy. Higher rates of transmission have been reported to be associated with many factors—the best documented of which is the presence of high maternal levels of plasma viremia, with the risk increasing linearly with the level of maternal plasma viremia. It is very unlikely that mother-to-child transmission will occur if the mother's level of plasma viremia is <1000 copies of HIV RNA/mL of blood and extremely unlikely if the level is <50 copies/mL. Increased mother-to-child transmission is also correlated with closer human leukocyte antigen (HLA) match between mother and child. A prolonged interval between membrane rupture and delivery is another well-documented risk factor for transmission. Other conditions that are potential risk factors, but that have not been consistently demonstrated, are the presence of chorioamnionitis at delivery; STIs during pregnancy; illicit drug use during pregnancy; cigarette smoking; preterm delivery; and obstetrical procedures such as amniocentesis, amnioscopy, fetal scalp electrodes, and episiotomy. Today, the rate of mother-to-child transmission has fallen to less than 1% in pregnant women who are receiving ART for their HIV infection. Such treatment, combined with cesarean section delivery, has rendered mother-to-child transmission of HIV an extremely unusual event in the United States and other developed nations. In this regard, both the United States Public Health Service and the World Health Organization guidelines recommend that all HIV-infected pregnant women receive life-long ART for the health of the mother (regardless of plasma HIV RNA copy number or CD4+ T-cell counts) as well as to prevent perinatal transmission.

Breast-feeding is an important modality of transmission of HIV infection in certain developing countries, particularly where mothers continue to breast-feed for prolonged periods. The risk factors for mother-to-child transmission of HIV via breast-feeding include detectable levels of HIV in breast milk, the presence of mastitis, low maternal CD4+ T-cell counts, and maternal vitamin A deficiency. The risk of HIV infection via breast-feeding is highest in the early months of breast-feeding. In addition, exclusive breast-feeding has been reported to carry a lower risk of HIV transmission than mixed feeding. In developed countries, breast feeding of babies by an HIV-infected mother is contraindicated since alternative forms of adequate nutrition, i.e., formulas, are readily available. In developing countries, where breast-feeding may be essential for the overall health of the infant, the continuation of ART in the infected mother during the period of breastfeeding markedly diminishes the risk of transmission of HIV to the infant. In fact, treatment of a pregnant woman with ART should be provided for the benefit of the woman as much as for the prevention of mother-to-child transmission and should be continued beyond the pregnancy, for life.

■ TRANSMISSION OF HIV BY OTHER BODY FLUIDS

Although HIV can be isolated typically in low titers from saliva of a small proportion of infected individuals, there is no convincing evidence that saliva can transmit HIV infection, either through kissing or through other exposures, such as occupationally to health care workers. Saliva contains endogenous antiviral factors; among these factors, HIV-specific immunoglobulins of IgA, IgG, and IgM isotypes are detected readily in salivary secretions of infected individuals. It has been suggested that large glycoproteins such as mucins and thrombospondin 1 sequester HIV into aggregates for clearance by the host. In addition, multiple soluble salivary factors inhibit HIV to various degrees in vitro, probably by targeting host cell receptors rather than the virus itself. Perhaps the best studied of these, secretory leukocyte protease inhibitor (SLPI), blocks HIV infection in several cell culture systems, and it is found in saliva at levels that approximate those required for inhibition of HIV in vitro. In this regard, higher salivary levels of SLPI in breast-fed infants were associated with a decreased risk of HIV transmission through breast milk. It has also been suggested that submandibular saliva reduces HIV infectivity by stripping gp120 from the surface of virions, and that saliva-mediated disruption and lysis of HIV-infected cells occurs because of the hypotonicity of oral secretions. Transmission of HIV by a human bite can occur but is a rare event. Although virus can be identified, if not isolated, from virtually any body fluid, there is no evidence that HIV transmission can occur as a result of exposure to tears, sweat, or urine. However, there have been isolated cases of transmission of HIV infection by body fluids that may or may not have been contaminated with blood. Most of these situations occurred in the setting of a close relative providing intensive nursing care for a person with HIV without observing universal precautions, underscoring the importance of adhering to such precautions in the handling of body fluids and wastes from HIV-infected individuals.

EPIDEMIOLOGY

■ HIV INFECTION AND AIDS WORLDWIDE

HIV infection/AIDS is a global pandemic, with cases reported from virtually every country. At the end of 2020, an estimated 37.7 million

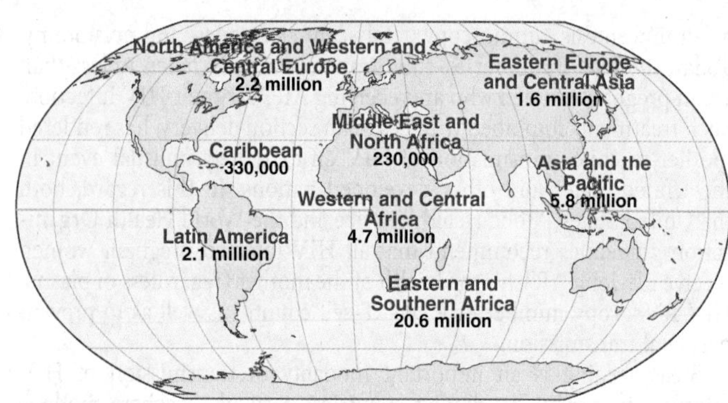

FIGURE 202-8 Estimated number of adults and children living with HIV infection as of December, 2020. Total: 37.7 million (30.2 million–45.1 million). *(From Joint United Nations Programme on HIV/AIDS [UNAIDS].)*

individuals were living with HIV infection, according to the Joint United Nations Programme on HIV/AIDS (UNAIDS). An estimated 95% of people living with HIV/AIDS reside in low- and middle-income countries; ~50% are female, and 1.7 million are children <15 years. The regional distribution of these cases is illustrated in **Fig. 202-8**. The estimated number of people living with HIV—i.e., the global prevalence—has increased nearly fivefold since 1990, reflecting the combined effects of continued high rates of new HIV infections and the life-prolonging impact of antiretroviral therapy (**Fig. 202-9**). In 2020, the global prevalence of HIV infection among persons 15–49 years of age was 0.7%, with rates varying widely by country and region as illustrated in **Fig. 202-10**.

In 2020, an estimated 1.5 million new cases of HIV infection occurred worldwide, including 150,000 among children <15 years; about one-third of new infections were among people age 15–24 years. Globally, members of certain high-risk populations are disproportionately affected by HIV infection. Sex workers; people who inject drugs; transgender people; prisoners; gay men and other men who have sex with men; the clients of sex workers; and the sexual partners of these key populations accounted for 65% of all new HIV infections in 2020 (**Fig. 202-11**).

New HIV infections globally have fallen by 52% since their peak in 1997 (Fig. 202-9). Reductions in global HIV incidence likely reflect progress with HIV prevention efforts and the increased provision to HIV-infected people of antiretroviral therapy, which makes them much less likely to transmit the virus to sexual partners. Among adults, the estimated number of new infections declined by about 50% from 1997 to 2020. During the same period a ~70% reduction in HIV infections among children <15 years was observed, progress due largely to the increasing availability of antiretroviral medications to prevent the transmission of HIV from mother to infant. An estimated 27.5 million people globally were on antiretroviral therapy as of December 2020.

In 2020, global AIDS deaths totaled 680,000 (including 99,000 children <15 years), a 64% decrease since the peak in 2004 that coincides with a rapid expansion of access to antiretroviral therapy (**Fig. 202-12**). Since the beginning of the HIV pandemic, an estimated 36.3 million persons globally have died of an AIDS-related illness.

The HIV epidemic has occurred in "waves" in different regions of the world, each wave having somewhat different characteristics depending on the demographics of the country and region in question and the timing of the introduction of HIV into the population. Although the AIDS epidemic was first recognized in the United States and shortly thereafter in Western Europe, it very likely began in sub-Saharan Africa (see above), a region particularly devastated by the epidemic.

The 20 countries of **Eastern and Southern Africa** are home to about 6% of the world's population but had 20.6 million people living with HIV in 2020, >50% of the global total (Fig. 202-8). Almost all countries in the region have generalized epidemics, that is, their national prevalence is >1%. In eight countries in the region, >10% of the adult population age 15–49 has HIV infection (Fig. 202-10). South Africa has the highest number of people living with HIV in the world (7.8 million); Eswatini (formerly known as Swaziland) has the highest adult HIV prevalence globally (26.8%). Recent data indicate declining HIV incidence and prevalence in many countries in the region, although generally at levels that remain high. Heterosexual exposure is the primary mode of HIV transmission in most countries in the region, as is the case throughout sub-Saharan Africa. Women and girls account for ~60 percent of all HIV infections in the region.

The 25 countries of **Western and Central Africa** are home to 4.7 million people living with HIV, of whom 410,000 are children. HIV prevalence in most of the countries is relatively low compared with East and Southern Africa. HIV prevalence among adults across the region overall stands at 1.3% However, there is wide variation between countries, ranging from 0.2% in Niger to 7.3% in Equatorial Guinea. An estimated 43% of new infections in the region in 2020 occurred in Nigeria, a large country with an HIV seroprevalence rate of 1.3%. As in East and Southern Africa, heterosexual transmission accounts for most HIV transmission in West and Central Africa.

The **Middle East and North Africa** region has one of the lowest HIV prevalence rates in the world (<0.1%), although new infections increased by 7% from 2010 to 2020. In 2020, an estimated 230,000 people were living with HIV in the region. Cases are largely concentrated among IDUs, men who have sex with men, and sex workers and their clients.

In **Asia and the Pacific**, an estimated 5.8 million people were living with HIV at the end of 2020. HIV infections in Asia and the Pacific declined by 21% between 2010 and 2020, with reductions in Thailand and Vietnam offset by increases in Pakistan and the Philippines. In this region, HIV prevalence is highest in southeast Asian countries, with wide variation in trends between different countries. Among countries in Asia, only Thailand has an adult seroprevalence rate that reaches 1%.

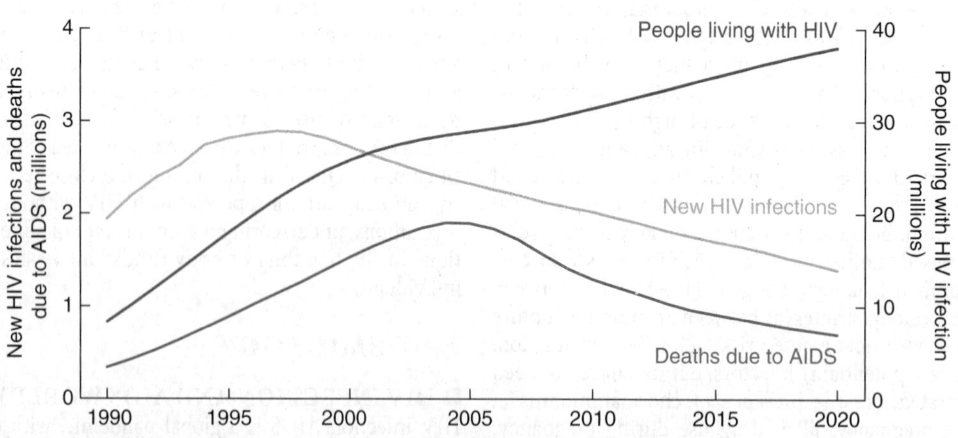

FIGURE 202-9 Global estimates of HIV incidence, AIDS deaths, and HIV prevalence 1990–2020. *(From UNAIDS.)*

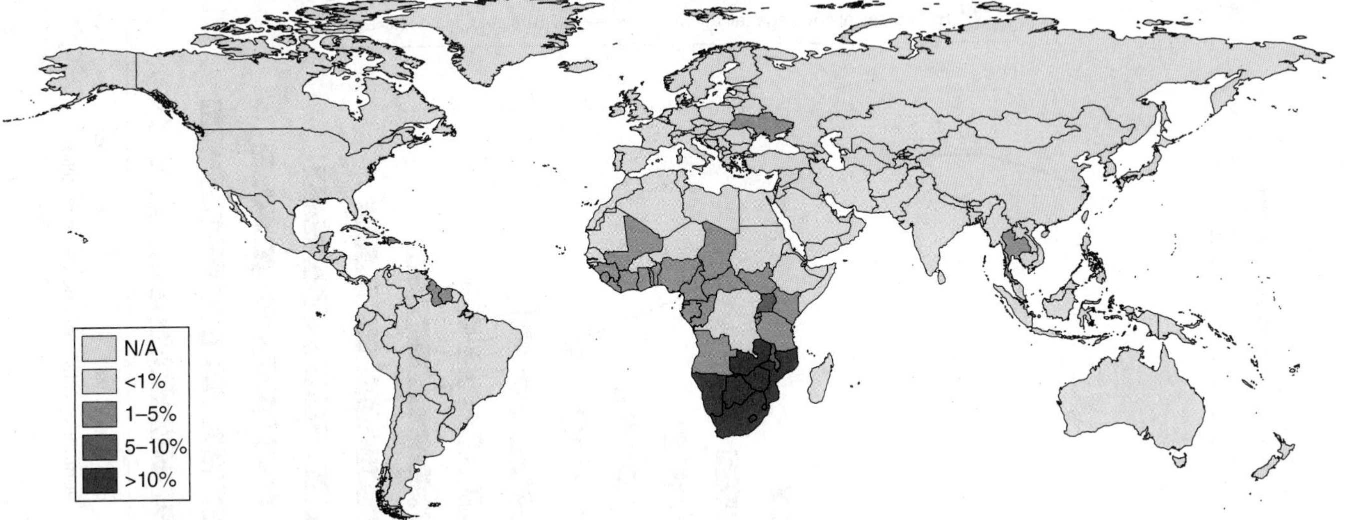

FIGURE 202-10 Adult HIV prevalence rates by country, 2020. Data are estimates for adults age 15–49 years. *(From UNAIDS.)*

However, the populations of many Asian nations are so large that even low infection and seroprevalence rates result in large numbers of people living with HIV. In this regard, three populous countries—China, India, and Indonesia—account for around three-quarters of all people living with HIV in the region. Key populations (Fig. 202-11) and their partners accounted for an estimated 94% of new HIV infections in the region in 2020, and ~30% of new HIV infections were among young people (age 15–24 years). Rising numbers of new infections among gay men and other men who have sex with men are a major concern.

The HIV epidemic continues to expand in **Eastern Europe and Central Asia**, with a 43% increase in annual new HIV infections and 32% increase in AIDS deaths between 2010 and 2020. The Russian Federation and Ukraine account for the majority of the 1.6 million people living with HIV in the region, where the epidemic has been driven by injection drug use. Key populations and their sexual partners account for the vast majority of new infections in the region.

Approximately 2.1 million people were living with HIV/AIDS in **Latin America** at the end of 2020. The rate of new HIV infections remained steady from 2010 to 2020. Brazil is home to the largest number of HIV-infected persons (930,000) in the region. In the **Caribbean**, an estimated 330,000 people are living with HIV.

Approximately 2.2 million people were living with HIV/AIDS in **North America and Western and Central Europe** at the end of 2020. While modes of transmission vary greatly by country, HIV disproportionately affects men who have sex with men. In Western and Central Europe, 11 countries saw HIV infections decline by more than 20% from 2010 to 2020, while 16 countries, mostly in Central Europe, experienced increases or had limited declines in new HIV infections. North America saw decreases in HIV diagnoses among gay and bisexual men and heterosexuals and a small increase among people who inject drugs.

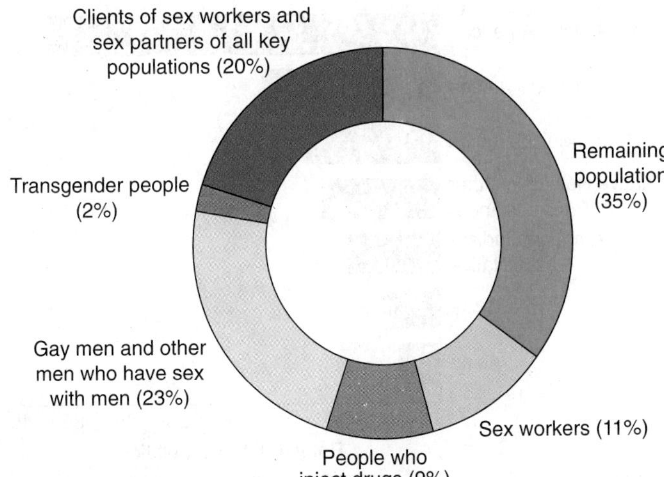

FIGURE 202-11 Global distribution of new HIV infections by population. Data for 2020. *(Reproduced with permission from UNAIDS.)*

HIV INFECTION IN THE UNITED STATES

At the end of 2019, an estimated 1.2 million individuals in the United States were living with HIV infection, ~13% of whom were unaware of their infection. As illustrated in **Fig. 202-13**, only about 57% of HIV-infected people in the United States have been able to negotiate the steps in the HIV "care continuum," from diagnosis, to entering into care and receiving antiretroviral therapy, and ultimately to achieving a suppressed viral load (see "Treatment," below).

Nearly two-thirds of people living with HIV in the United States are Black/African American or Hispanic/Latino, and ~60% are men who have sex with men, according to CDC estimates. The HIV prevalence rate among all individuals age 13 years or older in the United States is ~0.4%. Approximately 1.4% of Black/African-American adults are living with HIV in the United States, more than any other racial/ethnic group.

The estimated annual number of new HIV infections in the United States has fallen by more than two-thirds since its height in late 1980s of about 130,000 per year. CDC data indicate that progress has stalled in recent years, at about 34,000 to 38,000 new HIV infections each year. The estimated distribution of incident HIV cases in 2019 is shown in **Fig. 202-14**.

In the United States, the burden of HIV infection is not evenly distributed across states and regions. In most areas of the country, HIV is concentrated in urban areas. In the southern United States, larger percentages of diagnoses are in smaller metropolitan and nonmetropolitan areas. HIV has disproportionately affected minority populations in the United States in both urban and rural areas. Among those diagnosed with HIV (regardless of stage of infection) in 2019, 42% percent were Blacks/African Americans, a group that constitutes only 13% of the U.S. population. Hispanics/Latinos, 18% of the U.S. population, accounted for 29% of new HIV diagnoses. The estimated rate of new HIV diagnoses in 2019 by race/ethnicity per 100,000 population in the United States is shown in **Fig. 202-15**.

Perinatal HIV transmission, from an HIV-infected mother to her baby, has declined significantly in the United States, largely due to the implementation of guidelines for the universal counseling and voluntary HIV testing of pregnant women and the use of antiretroviral therapy for pregnant women and newborn infants to prevent infection. In 2019, 61 children were newly diagnosed with HIV infection in the United States, down from a peak of ~1750 in 1991.

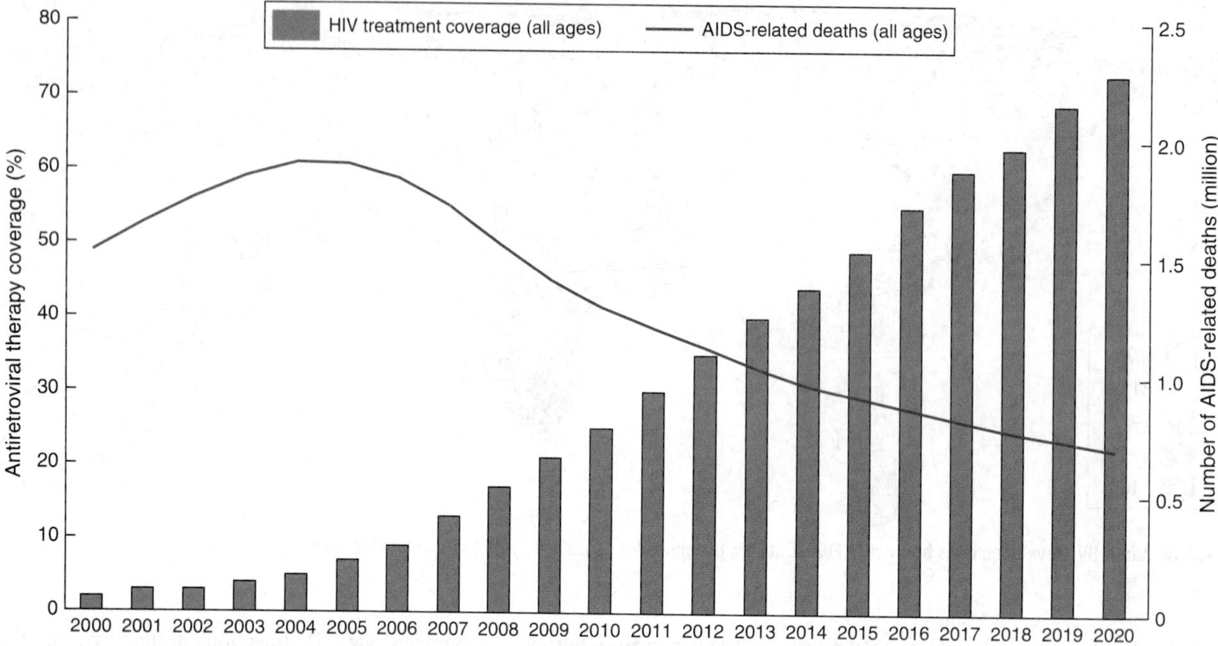

FIGURE 202-12 Global antiretroviral therapy coverage and number of AIDS-related deaths, 2000–2020. *(From UNAIDS).*

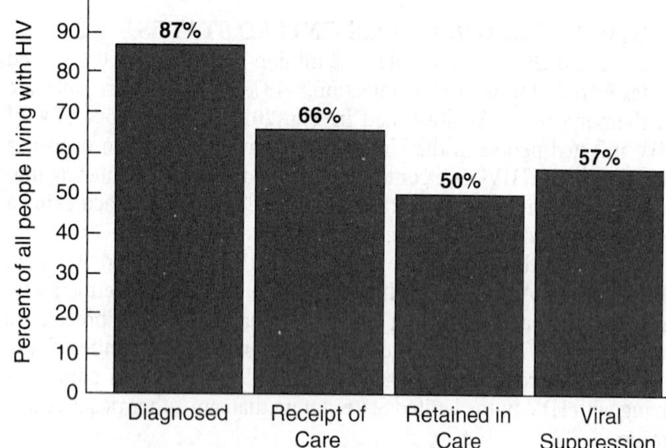

FIGURE 202-13 Estimated percentage of HIV-infected people engaged at selected stages of the continuum of HIV care in the United States. Data for 2019. Receipt of medical care defined as ≥1 test (CD4 count or viral load); retained in care, ≥2 tests (CD4 or VL) ≥3 months apart in 2019; viral suppression, <200 copies/mL on the most recent VL test. *(From Centers for Disease Control and Prevention [CDC]: HIV Surveillance Supplemental Report 26[No. 2], 2021.)*

The rate of HIV-related deaths in the United States rose steadily through the 1980s and peaked in 1995. Since then, the HIV death rate has fallen fourfold (**Fig. 202-16**). This trend is likely due to several factors, including improved prophylaxis and treatment of opportunistic infections, growing experience among the health professions in caring for HIV-infected individuals, improved access to health care, and a decrease in new infections. However, the most influential factor clearly has been the increased use of combination antiretroviral therapy (ART), generally administered in a combination of three or four agents.

PATHOPHYSIOLOGY AND PATHOGENESIS

The hallmark of HIV disease is a profound immunodeficiency resulting primarily from a progressive quantitative and qualitative deficiency of the subset of T lymphocytes referred to as *helper T cells* occurring in a setting of aberrant immune activation. The *helper* subset of T cells is defined phenotypically by the presence on its surface of the CD4 molecule (**Chap. 349**), which serves as the primary cellular receptor for HIV. A co-receptor also must be present together with CD4 for efficient binding, fusion, and entry of HIV-1 into its target cells (Figs. 202-3 and 202-4). HIV-1 uses two major co-receptors, CCR5 and CXCR4, for fusion and entry; these co-receptors are also the primary receptors for

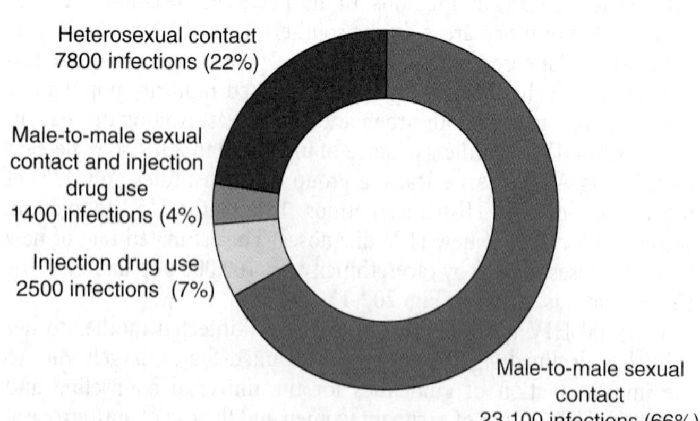

FIGURE 202-14 Estimated distribution of new HIV infections in the United States by transmission category. Total: 34,800. Incidence estimate for 2019. *(From CDC: HIV Surveillance Supplemental Report 26 [No. 1], 2021.)*

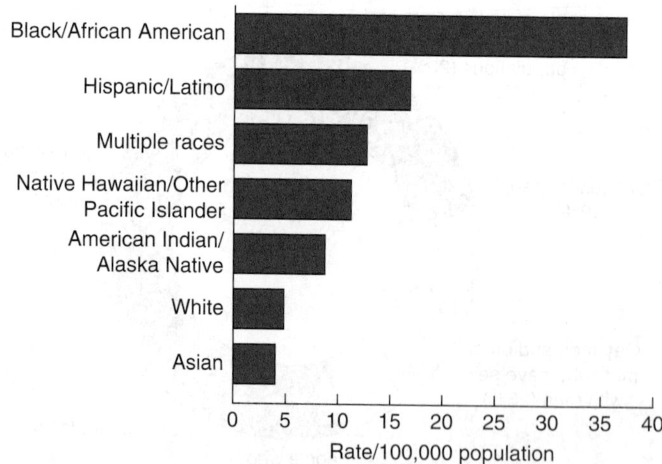

FIGURE 202-15 Estimated rate of HIV infections (including children) diagnosed during 2019 in the United States, by race/ethnicity (per 100,000 population). *(From CDC.)*

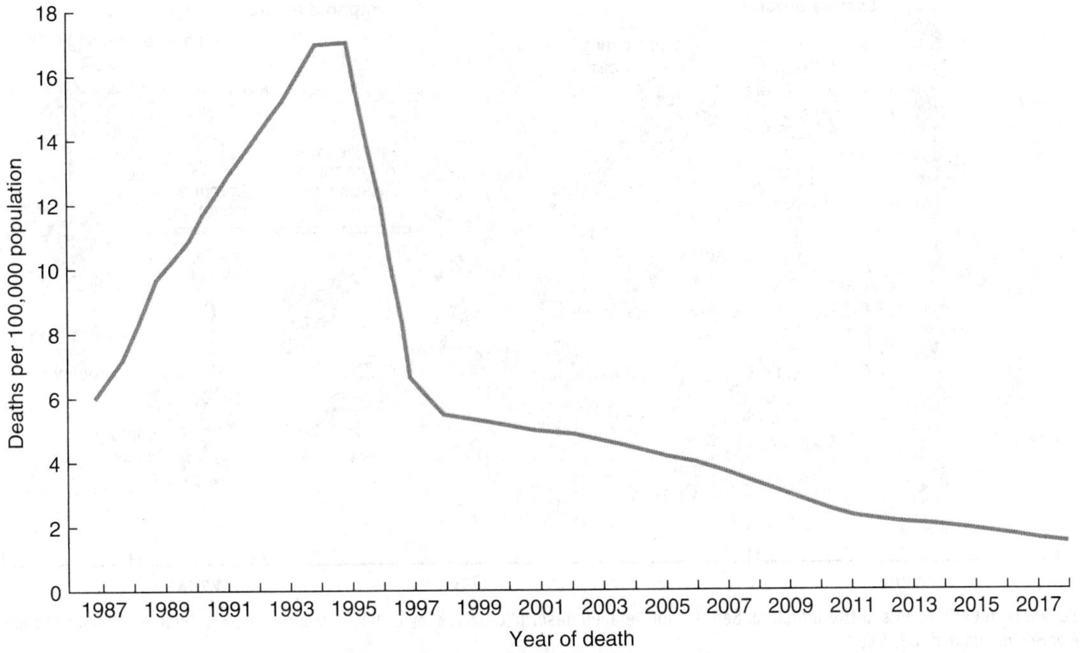

FIGURE 202-16 Trends in annual age-adjusted rates of death due to HIV infection, United States, 1987–2018. Age distribution based on 2000 population. *(From CDC.)*

certain chemoattractant cytokines termed *chemokines* and belong to the seven-transmembrane-domain G protein–coupled family of receptors. Multiple mechanisms responsible for cellular depletion and/or immune dysfunction of CD4+ T cells have been demonstrated in vitro. These include direct infection and destruction of these cells by HIV, as well as indirect effects such as immune clearance of infected cells; cell death associated with aberrant immune activation and inflammation, including caspase 1–mediated pyroptosis prompted by tissue CD4+ T cells undergoing abortive/nonproductive HIV infection; and immune exhaustion due to persistent cellular activation with resulting cellular dysfunction. Patients with CD4+ T-cell levels below certain thresholds are at high risk of developing a variety of opportunistic diseases, particularly the infections and neoplasms that are AIDS-defining illnesses. Some features of AIDS, such as Kaposi's sarcoma and certain neurologic abnormalities, cannot be explained completely by the immunodeficiency caused by HIV infection, since these complications may occur prior to the development of severe immunologic impairment.

The combination of viral pathogenic and immunopathogenic events that occur during the course of HIV disease from the moment of initial (primary) infection through the development of advanced-stage disease is complex and varied. It is important to appreciate that the pathogenic mechanisms of HIV disease are multifactorial and multiphasic and are different at different stages of the disease. Therefore, it is essential to consider the typical clinical course of an untreated individual with HIV to better appreciate these pathogenic events (**Fig. 202-17**).

EARLY EVENTS IN HIV INFECTION: PRIMARY INFECTION AND INITIAL DISSEMINATION OF VIRUS

Using rectal or vaginal mucosal transmission in nonhuman primates as a model, the earliest events (within hours) that occur following exposure of HIV to the mucosal surface determine whether an infection will be established or aborted as well as the subsequent course of events following infection. Although the mucosal barrier is relatively effective in limiting access of HIV to susceptible targets in the submucosal tissue, the virus can cross the barrier by transport on Langerhans cells, an epidermal type of DC, just beneath the surface or through microscopic rents in the mucosa. Significant disruptions in the mucosal barrier as seen in ulcerative genital disease facilitate viral entry and increase the efficiency of infection. Virus then seek susceptible targets, which are primarily CD4+ T cells that are spatially dispersed in the mucosa. This spatial dispersion of targets provides a significant obstacle to the establishment of infection. Such obstacles account for the low efficiency of sexual transmission of HIV (see "Sexual Transmission," above). Both "partially" resting CD4+ T cells and activated CD4+ T cells serve as early amplifiers of infection. Resting CD4+ T cells are more abundant; however, activated CD4+ T cells support productive

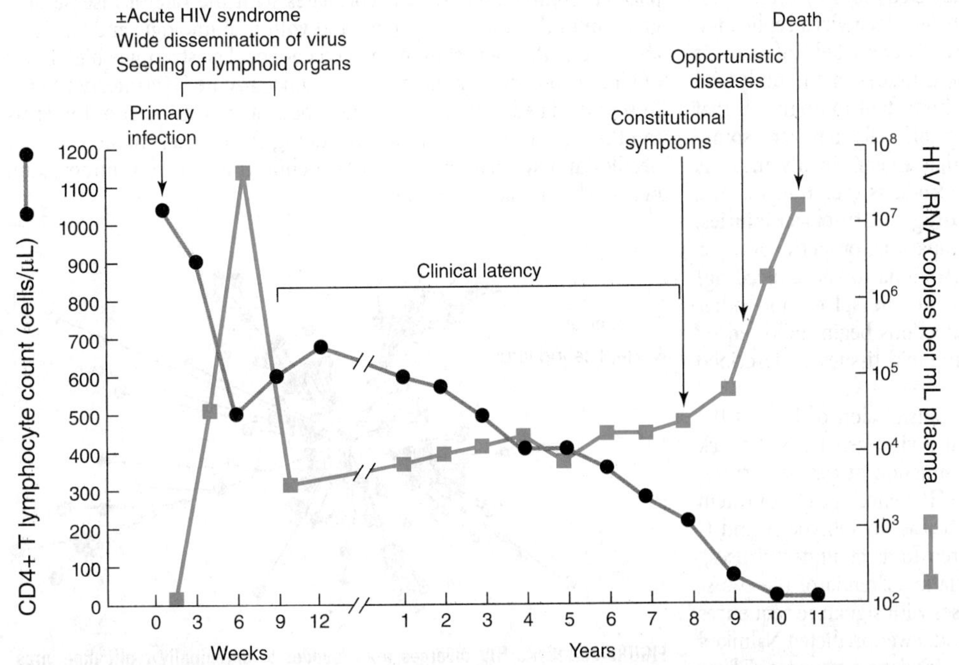

FIGURE 202-17 Typical course of an untreated HIV-infected individual. See text for detailed description. *(From G Pantaleo, C Graziosi, AS Fauci: The Immunopathogenesis of Human Immunodeficiency Virus Infection. N Engl J Med 328:327, 1993. Copyright © 1993 Massachusetts Medical Society. Reprinted with permission from Massachusetts Medical Society.)*

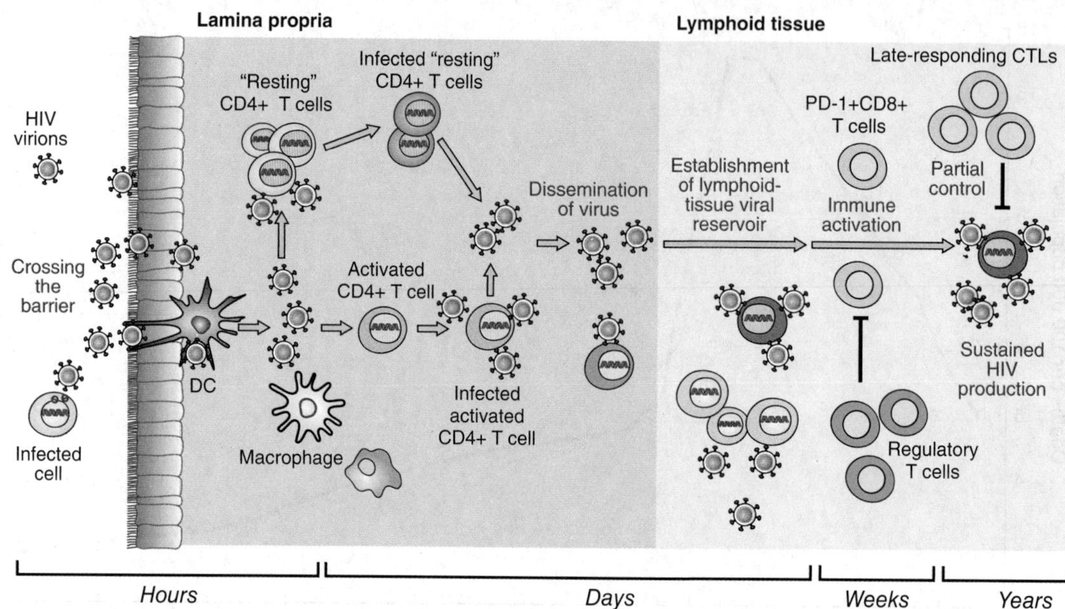

FIGURE 202-18 Summary of early events in HIV infection. See text for detailed description. CTLs, cytolytic T lymphocytes; HIV, human immunodeficiency virus. *(Adapted from AT Haase: Nat Rev Immunol 5:783, 2005.)*

infection and thus generate larger amounts of virus. For infection to become established, the basic reproductive rate (R_0) must become equal to or greater than 1, i.e., each infected cell would infect at least one other cell. Once infection is established, the virus replicates in lymphoid cells in the mucosa, the submucosa, and to some extent the lymphoreticular tissues that drain the gut or genital tissues. For a variable period ranging from a few to several days, the virus is typically not detected in the plasma. This period is referred to as the "eclipse" phase of infection. As more virus is produced within several days to weeks, it is disseminated, first to the draining lymph nodes and then to other lymphoid compartments where it has easy access to dense concentrations of CD4+ T-cell targets, allowing for a burst of high-level plasma viremia that is readily detectable by currently available assays **(Fig. 202-18)**. The gut-associated lymphoid tissue (GALT) is a target of HIV infection and the location where large numbers of CD4+ T cells (usually memory cells) are infected and depleted, both by direct viral effects and by activation-associated apoptosis. Once virus replication reaches this threshold and virus is widely disseminated, infection is firmly established throughout the lymphoid tissues of the body and persists for the life of the individual. It is important to point out that the efficiency of initial infection of susceptible cells may vary somewhat with the route of infection. Virus that enters directly into the bloodstream via infected blood or blood products (i.e., transfusions, use of contaminated needles for injection drugs, sharp-object injuries, maternal-to-fetal transmission either intrapartum or perinatally, or sexual intercourse where there is enough trauma to cause bleeding) is likely first cleared from the circulation to the spleen and other lymphoid organs, where primary focal infections begin, followed by wider dissemination throughout other lymphoid tissues as described above.

It has been demonstrated that sexual transmission of HIV is the result of a single infectious event and that a viral genetic bottleneck exists for transmission with selective transmission of certain viruses. In this regard, certain characteristics of the HIV envelope glycoprotein have a major influence on transmission, at least in subtype A and C viruses. Transmitting viruses, often referred to as "founder viruses," are usually underrepresented in the circulating viremia of the transmitting partner and are less-diverged viruses with signature sequences including shorter V1–V2 loop sequences and fewer predicted N-linked glycosylation sites relative to the major circulating variants. These viruses are almost exclusively R5 strains and are usually sensitive to neutralizing antibody. Once replication proceeds in the newly infected partner, the founder virus diverges and accumulates glycosylation sites, becoming progressively more resistant to neutralization **(Fig. 202-19)**.

The acute burst of viremia and wide dissemination of virus in primary HIV infection may be associated with an *acute HIV syndrome*, which occurs to varying degrees in ~50% of individuals within 2 to 4 weeks of initial infection (see below). This syndrome is usually associated with millions of copies of HIV RNA per milliliter of plasma that last for several weeks. Acute mononucleosis-like symptoms are well correlated with the presence of high levels of plasma viremia. Virtually all patients develop some degree of plasma viremia during primary infection, which contributes to virus dissemination throughout the lymphoid tissue, even though they may remain asymptomatic or not recall experiencing symptoms. The initial level of plasma viremia in primary HIV infection does not necessarily determine the rate of disease progression; however, the set point of the level of steady-state plasma viremia after ~1 year correlates with the rate of disease progression in the untreated patient and with immunologic and virologic aberrancies that persist in the treated patient. The strikingly high levels of viremia observed in many patients during acute HIV infection is felt to be associated with a higher likelihood of transmission of the virus to others by a variety of routes including sexual transmission, shared needles and syringes, and mother-to-child transmission intrapartum, perinatally, or via breast milk.

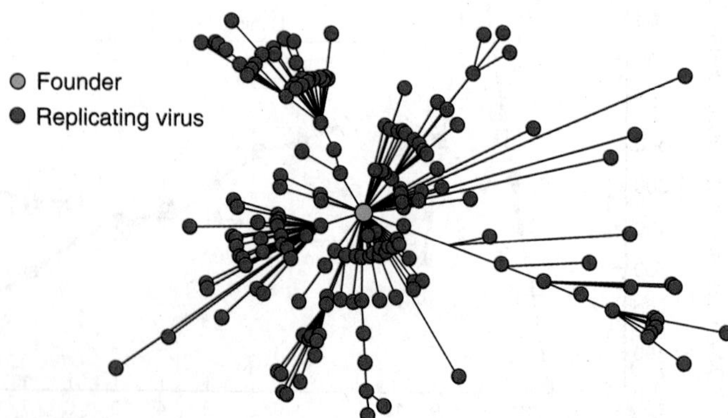

FIGURE 202-19 As HIV diverges from founder to chronically replicating virus, it accumulates N-linked glycosylation sites. See text for detailed description. *(Adapted from CA Derdeyn et al: Science 303:2019, 2004; B Chohan et al: J Virol 79:6528, 2005; and BF Keele et al: Proc Natl Acad Sci USA 105:7552, 2008.)*

ESTABLISHMENT OF CHRONIC INFECTION

Persistence of Virus Replication HIV infection is unique among human viral infections. Despite the robust cellular and humoral immune responses that are mounted following primary infection (see "Immune Response to HIV," below), once infection has been established the virus succeeds in escaping complete immune-mediated clearance, paradoxically seems to thrive on immune activation, and is never eliminated completely from the body. Rather, a chronic infection develops and persists with varying degrees of continual virus replication in the untreated patient for a median of ~10 years before the patient becomes clinically ill (see "Advanced HIV Disease," below). It is this establishment of a chronic, persistent infection that is the hallmark of HIV disease. Throughout the often-protracted course of chronic infection, virus replication can invariably be detected in untreated patients by widely available molecular assays that measure copies of virion-associated HIV RNA in plasma (copies per milliliter). Levels of virus vary greatly in most untreated patients, usually ranging from fewer than 50 to greater than a million copies of HIV RNA per milliliter of plasma. Studies using highly sensitive molecular techniques have demonstrated that even in treated patients in whom plasma viremia is suppressed to below detection (lower limit, 20–50 copies of HIV RNA per milliliter depending on assay kit manufacturer) by ART, there is a continual low level of virion production in the majority of infected patients. In other human viral infections, with some exceptions, if the host survives, the virus is completely cleared from the body and a state of immunity against subsequent infection develops. HIV infection very rarely kills the host during primary infection. Certain viruses, such as HSV (**Chap. 192**), are not completely cleared from the body after infection, but instead enter a latent state; in these cases, clinical latency is accompanied by microbiologic latency. This is not the case with HIV infection as described above. Chronicity associated with persistent virus replication can also be seen in certain cases of HBV and HCV infections (**Chap. 341**); however, in these infections the immune system is not a target of the virus.

Escape of HIV from Effective Immune System Control Inherent to the establishment of chronicity of HIV infection is the ability of the virus to evade adequate control and elimination by both the cellular and humoral immune responses. There are several mechanisms whereby the virus accomplishes this evasion. Paramount among these is the establishment of a sustained level of replication associated with the generation of viral diversity via mutation and recombination. The selection of mutants that escape control by CD8+ cytolytic T lymphocytes (CTLs) is critical to the propagation and progression of HIV infection. The high rate of virus replication associated with inevitable mutations also contributes to the inability of antibody to neutralize and/or clear the autologous virus. Furthermore, for reasons that remain unclear, the humoral immune system does not readily produce classic neutralizing antibodies against the HIV envelope and does so only after years of persistent virus replication and after the infection is firmly established (see below). Extensive analyses of sequential HIV isolates and host responses have demonstrated that viral escape from B-cell and CD8+ T-cell responses occurs early after infection and allows the virus to stay one step ahead of effective immune responses. Virus-specific CD8+ CTLs expand greatly during primary HIV infection, and they likely represent the high-affinity responses that would be expected to be most efficient in eliminating virus-infected cells; however, viral control is generally incomplete as viral replication persists at relatively high levels in the majority of individuals. In addition to viral escape from CTLs through high rates of mutation, it is thought that the initially strong immune response becomes qualitatively dysfunctional owing to the overwhelming immune activation associated with persistent viral replication, leading to immune "exhaustion" that affects both arms of adaptive immunity. Several studies have indicated that exhaustion of HIV-specific CD8+ T cells during prolonged immune activation is associated with upregulation of several inhibitory receptors, such as the programmed death (PD) 1 molecule (of the B7-CD28 family of molecules), T-cell immunoreceptor with Ig and ITIM domains (TIGIT), T-cell immunoglobulin and mucin domain–containing molecule 3 (Tim-3), and lymphocyte activating gene 3 (Lag-3), collectively referred to as *immune-checkpoint receptors*. Upregulation of these surface proteins restricts polyreactivity and proliferative capacity, functional attributes of CD8+ T cells that are essential for effective killing of pathogens. Another mechanism contributing to the evasion by HIV of immune system control is the downregulation of HLA class I molecules on the surface of HIV-infected cells by the viral proteins Nef, Tat, and Vpu, resulting in the lack of ability of CD8+ CTLs to recognize and kill infected target cells. Although this downregulation of HLA class I molecules would seem to favor elimination of HIV-infected cells by natural killer (NK) cells, this latter mechanism does not remove HIV-infected cells effectively (see below). Another potential means of escape of HIV-infected cells from elimination by CD8+ CTLs is the sequestration of infected cells in immunologically privileged sites such as the central nervous system (CNS), as well as the low frequency of virus-specific CD8+ CTLs in areas of lymphoid tissues, namely germinal centers, where HIV actively replicates.

The principal targets of neutralizing antibodies against HIV are the envelope proteins gp120 and gp41. HIV employs at least three mechanisms to evade neutralizing antibody responses: hypervariability in the primary sequence of the envelope, extensive glycosylation of the envelope, and conformational masking of neutralizing epitopes. Several studies that have followed the evolution of the humoral immune response to HIV from the earliest points after primary infection indicate that the virus continually mutates to escape the emerging antibody response such that the sequential antibodies that are induced do not neutralize the currently autologous virus. *Broadly neutralizing antibodies* capable of neutralizing a wide range of primary HIV isolates in vitro occur in only about 20% of HIV-infected individuals, and, when they do occur, 2 to 3 years of infection with continual virus replication are generally required to drive the affinity maturation of the antibodies. Unfortunately, by the time these broadly neutralizing antibodies are formed, they are ineffective in containing the virus currently replicating in the patient. Persistent viremia also results in exhaustion of B cells like the exhaustion reported for CD8+ T cells, adding to the defects in the humoral response to HIV.

CD4+ T-cell help is essential for the integrity of both humoral and cell-mediated antigen-specific immune responses. HIV preferentially infects activated CD4+ T cells including HIV-specific CD4+ T cells, and so this loss of viral-specific helper T-cell responses has profoundly negative consequences for the immunologic control of HIV replication. Furthermore, this loss occurs early in the course of infection, and animal studies indicate that 40–70% of all memory CD4+ T cells in the GALT are eliminated during acute infection. During chronic HIV viremia, CD4+ T cells also exhibit evidence of exhaustion, including by upregulation of the cytotoxic T lymphocyte–associated antigen 4 (CTLA-4), also a member of the B7-CD28 family.

Finally, the escape of HIV from immune-mediated elimination during primary infection allows the formation of a pool of latently infected CD4+ T cells, referred to as the *viral reservoir*, that may not be recognized or completely eliminated by virus-specific CTLs or by ART (see below). Thus, despite a potent immune response and the marked downregulation of virus replication following primary HIV infection, HIV succeeds in establishing a state of chronic infection with a variable degree of persistent virus replication. During this period most patients make the clinical transition from acute primary infection to variable periods of clinical latency or smoldering disease activity (see below).

The HIV Reservoir: Obstacles to the Eradication of Virus A pool of latently infected, resting CD4+ T cells that serves as at least one component of the persistent reservoir of virus exists in virtually all HIV-infected individuals, including those who are receiving ART. Such cells carry an integrated form of HIV DNA in the genome of the host and can remain in this state until an activation signal drives the expression of HIV transcripts. Only a small fraction of the latently infected cells in the viral reservoir contain replication-competent virus, with the overwhelming majority of cells containing defective proviruses incapable of a full replication cycle. However, upon activation of the reservoir variable degrees of sustained virus replication invariably

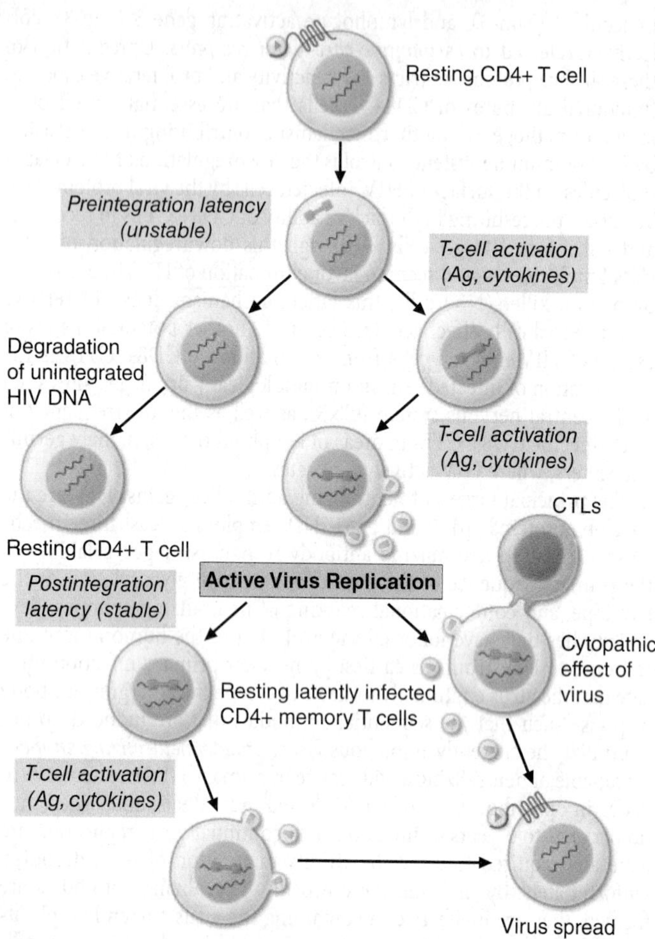

FIGURE 202-20 Generation of latently infected, resting CD4+ T cells in HIV-infected individuals. See text for details. Ag, antigen; CTLs, cytolytic T lymphocytes. *(Courtesy of TW Chun.)*

occur. This form of latency is to be distinguished from preintegration latency, in which HIV enters a resting CD4+ T cell and, in the absence of an activation signal, reverse transcription of the HIV genome occurs to a certain extent but the resulting proviral DNA fails to integrate into the host genome. This period of preintegration latency may last hours to days, and if no activation signal is delivered to the cell, the proviral DNA loses its capacity to initiate a productive infection. If these cells do become activated prior to decay of the preintegration complex, reverse transcription proceeds to completion and the virus continues along its replication cycle (see above and **Fig. 202-20**). The pool of cells that are in the postintegration state of latency is established early during primary HIV infection. Despite the suppression of plasma viremia to <50 copies per milliliter by potent regimens of ART administered over several years, this pool of latently infected cells persists and can give rise to replication-competent virus upon cellular activation ex vivo. Modeling studies built on projections of decay curves have estimated that in such a setting of prolonged viral suppression, it would require many years to the entire life of the host for the pool of latently infected cells to be eliminated. This has not been documented to occur spontaneously in any patients very likely because the latent viral reservoir is long-lived and is continually replenished by the low levels of persistent virus replication that may remain below the limits of detection of current assays (see below) as well as by the expansion by proliferation of the pool of latently infected cells (Fig. 202-20), even in patients who for the most part are treated successfully. Reservoirs of HIV-infected cells, latent or otherwise, can exist in a number of compartments including the lymphoid tissue, peripheral blood, and the CNS (likely in cells of the monocyte/macrophage lineage) as well as in other unidentified locations. Over the past several years attempts have been made to eliminate HIV in the latent viral reservoir using agents that activate resting CD4+ T cells and/or reinitiate viral expression without systemic activation during the course of ART; however, such attempts, referred to as "shock and kill," have been unsuccessful. Thus, this persistent reservoir of infected cells remains a major obstacle to the goal of eradication of virus from infected individuals and hence a classic "cure," despite the favorable clinical outcomes that have resulted from ART. Consequently, intense efforts are being directed toward investigating the feasibility of achieving ART-free HIV remission through passive transfer of long-acting broadly neutralizing antibodies and therapeutic agents that could enhance the host immune responses against the virus.

Viral Dynamics The dynamics of viral production and turnover have been quantified using mathematical modeling in the setting of the administration of reverse transcriptase and protease inhibitors to HIV-infected individuals in clinical studies. Treatment with these drugs resulted in a precipitous decline in the level of plasma viremia, which typically fell by well over 90% within 2 weeks. It was determined on the basis of modeling the kinetics of viral decline and the emergence of resistant mutants during therapy that 93–99% of the circulating virus originated from recently infected, rapidly turning over CD4+ T cells and that ~1–7% of circulating virus originated from longer-lived cells, likely monocytes/macrophages. A negligible amount of circulating virus originated from the pool of latently infected cells (**Fig. 202-21**). It was also determined that the half-life of a circulating virion was ~30–60 min and that of productively infected cells was 1 day. Given the relatively steady level of plasma viremia and of infected cells, it appears that extremely large amounts of virus (~10^{10}–10^{11} virions) are produced and cleared from the circulation each day. In addition, data suggest that the minimal duration of the HIV-1 replication cycle in vivo is ~2 days. Other studies have demonstrated that the decrease in plasma viremia that results from treatment with ART correlates closely with a decrease in virus replication in lymph nodes, further confirming that lymphoid tissue is the main site of HIV replication and the main source of plasma viremia.

The level of steady-state viremia, called the viral *set point*, at ~1 year following acquisition of HIV infection has important prognostic implications for the progression of HIV disease in the untreated patient. It has been demonstrated that, as a group, untreated HIV-infected individuals who have a low set point at 6 months to 1 year following infection progress to AIDS much more slowly than do individuals whose set point is very high at that time (**Fig. 202-22**).

Clinical Latency versus Microbiologic Latency With the exception of certain long-term nonprogressors and "elite controllers" of HIV replication, the level of CD4+ T cells in the blood inevitably decreases

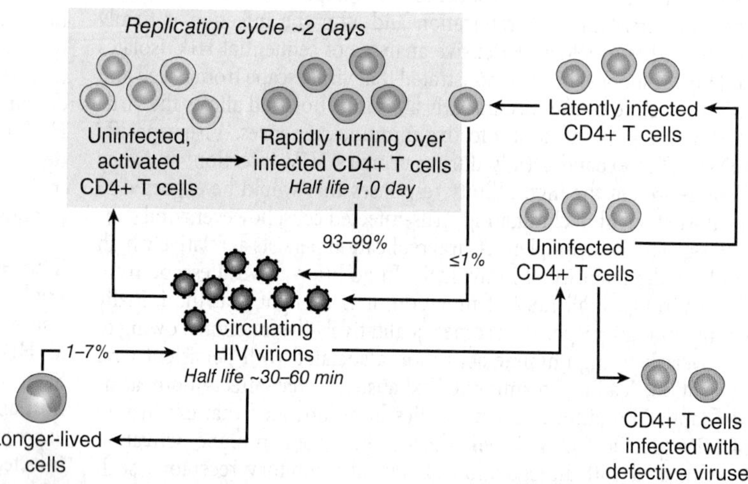

FIGURE 202-21 Dynamics of HIV infection in vivo. See text for detailed description. *(Adapted from Perelson AS, Neumann AU, Markowitz M, Leonard JM, Ho DD: HIV-1 dynamics in vivo: virion clearance rate, infected cell life-span, and viral generation time. Science 271:1582, 1996.)*

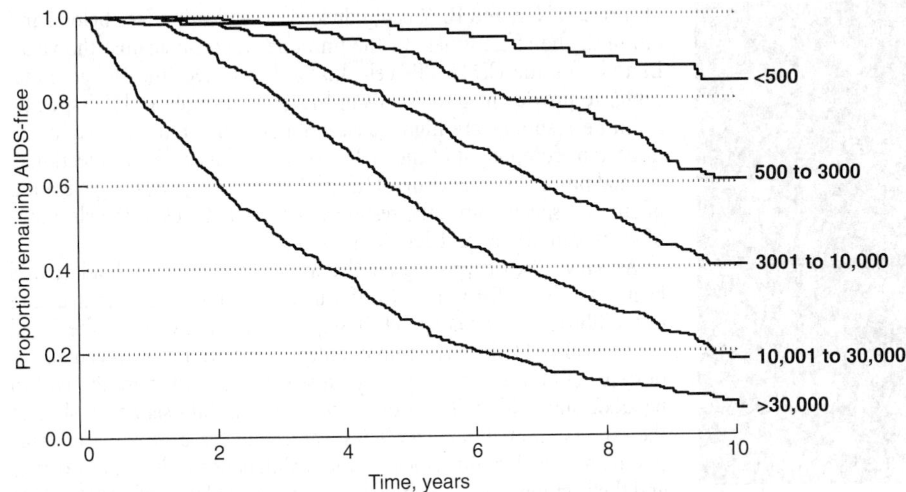

FIGURE 202-22 Relationship between levels of virus and rates of disease progression. Kaplan-Meier curves showing proportion of 1604 patients remaining AIDS-free over 10 years, stratified by baseline HIV-1 RNA categories (copies per milliliter). *(From Multicenter AIDS Cohort Study; JW Mellors, A Muñoz, JV Giorgi, JB Margolick, CJ Tassoni, P Gupta, LA Kingsley, JA Todd, AJ Saah, R Detels, JP Phair, CR Rinaldo Jr.)*

progressively in viremic HIV-infected individuals in the absence of ART. The decline in CD4+ T cells may be gradual or abrupt, the latter usually reflecting a significant spike in the level of plasma viremia. Most patients are relatively asymptomatic while this progressive decline is taking place (see below) and are often described as being in a state of *clinical latency*. However, this term is misleading; it does not mean disease latency, since progression, although slow in many cases and often without symptoms, is generally relentless as evidenced by readily detectable plasma viremia, during this period. Furthermore, clinical latency should not be confused with microbiologic latency since varying levels of virus replication inevitably occur during this period of clinical latency. Even in those rare patients, such as elite controllers, who have <50 copies of HIV RNA per milliliter in the absence of therapy, there is virtually always some degree of low-level ongoing virus replication.

ADVANCED HIV DISEASE

In untreated patients or in patients in whom therapy has not adequately controlled virus replication, after a variable period, usually measured in years, the CD4+ T-cell count falls below a critical level (<200/μL) and the patient becomes highly susceptible to opportunistic disease (Fig. 202-17). For this reason, the CDC case definition of stage 3 (AIDS) includes all HIV-infected individuals >5 years of age with CD4+ T-cell counts below this level (Table 202-2). Patients may experience constitutional signs and symptoms or may develop an opportunistic disease abruptly without any prior symptoms. The depletion of CD4+ T cells continues to be progressive and unrelenting in this phase. It is not uncommon for CD4+ T-cell counts in the untreated patient to drop to as low as 10/μL or even to zero. In countries where ART as well as prophylaxis and treatment for opportunistic infections are readily accessible, survival is increased dramatically even in those patients with advanced HIV disease. In contrast, untreated patients who progress to this severest form of immunodeficiency usually succumb to opportunistic infections or neoplasms (see below).

LONG-TERM SURVIVORS, LONG-TERM NONPROGRESSORS, AND ELITE CONTROLLERS

It is important to distinguish between the terms *long-term survivor* and *long-term nonprogressor*. Long-term nonprogressors are by definition long-term survivors; however, the reverse is not always true. Predictions from one study that antedated the availability of effective ART estimated that ~13% of homosexual/bisexual men who were infected at an early age may remain free of clinical AIDS for >20 years. Many of these individuals may have gradually progressed in their degree of immune deficiency; however, they certainly survived for a considerable period. With the advent of effective ART, the survival of HIV-infected individuals has dramatically increased. Early in the AIDS pandemic, prior to the availability of antiretroviral therapy, if a patient presented with a life-threatening opportunistic infection, the median survival was 26 weeks from the time of presentation. Currently, an HIV-infected 20-year-old individual who is appropriately treated with ART can expect to live at least 50 years according to mathematical model projections. In the face of ART, long-term survival is now commonplace. Definitions of long-term nonprogressors have varied considerably over the years, and so such individuals constitute a heterogeneous group. Long-term nonprogressors were first described in the 1990s. Originally, individuals were considered to be long-term nonprogressors if they had been infected with HIV for a long period (≥10 years), their CD4+ T-cell counts were in the normal range, their plasma viremia remained relatively low (undetectable to several thousand copies of HIV RNA/ml plasma), and they remained clinically stable over years without receiving ART. Approximately 5–15% of HIV-infected individuals fell into this broader nonprogressor category. However, this group was rather heterogeneous and over time a significant proportion of these individuals progressed and ultimately required antiretroviral therapy. From this broader group, a much smaller subgroup of "elite" controllers was identified, and they constituted a fraction of 1% of HIV-infected individuals. These elite controllers, by definition, have extremely low levels of plasma viremia that is often undetectable by standard assays and normal CD4+ T-cell counts. It is noteworthy that their HIV-specific immune response, especially HIV-specific CD8+ CTLs that can clear infected CD4+ T cells, is robust and clearly superior to those of HIV-infected progressors. In this group of elite controllers certain HLA class I haplotypes are overrepresented, particularly HLA-B57-01 and HLA-B27-05. Outside of the subgroup of elite controllers, a number of other genetic factors have been shown to be involved to a greater or lesser degree in the control of virus replication and thus in the rate of HIV disease progression (see "Genetic Factors in HIV-1 and AIDS Pathogenesis," below).

LYMPHOID ORGANS AND HIV PATHOGENESIS

Regardless of the portal of entry of HIV, lymphoid tissues are the major anatomic sites for the establishment and propagation of HIV infection. Despite the use of measurements of plasma viremia to determine the level of disease activity, virus replication occurs mainly in lymphoid tissue and not in blood; indeed, the level of plasma viremia directly reflects virus production in lymphoid tissue.

Some patients experience progressive generalized lymphadenopathy early in the course of the infection; others experience varying degrees of transient lymphadenopathy. Lymphadenopathy reflects the cellular activation and immune response to the virus in the lymphoid tissue, which is generally characterized by follicular or germinal center hyperplasia. Lymphoid tissue involvement is a common denominator of virtually all patients with HIV infection, even those without easily detectable lymphadenopathy.

Examinations of lymph tissue and peripheral blood in patients and monkeys during various stages of HIV and SIV infection, respectively, have led to substantial insight into the pathogenesis of HIV disease. In most of the original human studies, peripheral lymph nodes were the predominant sources for analyses into changes in lymphoid tissues associated with HIV and SIV infection, whereas more recent studies have expanded to include the GALT, where the earliest burst of virus replication occurs associated with marked depletion of CD4+ T cells. A variety of techniques, including sensitive molecular approaches to measure the level of HIV DNA or RNA and imaging approaches to visualize virus and cells in location or suspension, have been employed to describe events associated with HIV disease. During acute HIV infection resulting from mucosal transmission, virus replication

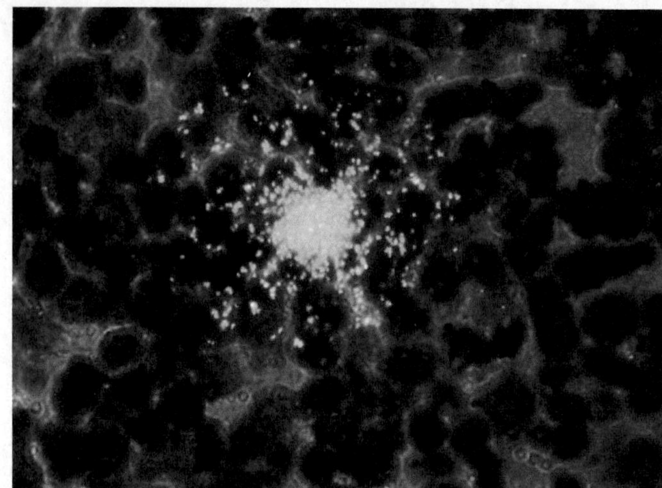

FIGURE 202-23 HIV in the lymph node of an HIV-infected individual. An individual cell infected with HIV shown expressing HIV RNA by in situ hybridization using a radiolabeled molecular probe. Original ×500. *(Reproduced with permission from G Pantaleo et al: HIV infection is active and progressive in lymphoid tissue during the clinically latent stage of disease. Nature 362:355, 1993.)*

progressively amplifies from scattered lymphoid cells in the lamina propria of the gut to draining lymph nodes, leading to high levels of plasma viremia. The GALT plays a major role in the amplification of virus replication, and virus is disseminated from replication in the GALT to peripheral lymphoid tissues. A profound degree of cellular activation occurs within lymphoid tissues (see below) and is reflected in follicular or germinal center hyperplasia. At this time copious amounts of extracellular virions (both infectious and defective) are trapped on the processes of the follicular dendritic cells (FDCs) that form the stromal cell network in the light zones of lymph node germinal centers. Virions that have bound complement components on their surfaces attach to the surface of FDCs via interactions with complement receptors and likely via Fc receptors that bind to antibodies that are attached to the virions. The use of in situ hybridization techniques, including those that allow detection of viral RNA in the context of tissue architecture, has revealed that HIV is primarily expressed in CD4+ T cells of the paracortical area and, to a lesser extent, in specialized CD4+ T cells (see below) in light zones of germinal centers (Fig. 202-23). The persistence of trapped virus on the surface of FDC likely reflects both a long-lived viral reservoir and virus that is replaced by continual expression in nearby CD4+ T cells. The trapped virus, either as whole virion or shed envelope, also serves as a continual activator of CD4+ T cells, thus driving further virus replication.

During the early stages of HIV disease, the architecture of lymphoid tissues is generally preserved and may even be hyperplastic owing to an increased presence of B cells and specialized CD4+ T cells called follicular helper CD4+ T cells (TF_H) in prominent germinal centers. Extracellular virions can be seen by electron microscopy attached to FDC processes. The trapping of antigen is a physiologically normal function for the FDCs, which present antigen to B cells and secrete factors such as CXCL13 that retain B and TF_H cells in the light zones of germinal centers. These FDC functions, along with stimulatory factors produced by TF_H cells, contribute to the generation of B-cell memory. However, in the case of HIV, persistent cellular activation, resulting in a shift to secretion of proinflammatory cytokines such as interleukin (IL) 1β, tumor necrosis factor (TNF) α, IFN-γ, and IL-6, can induce viral replication (see below) and diminish the effectiveness of the immune response against the virus. In addition, the CD4+ TF_H cells that are recruited into the germinal center to provide help to B cells in the generation of an HIV-specific immune response are highly susceptible to infection and may be an important component of the HIV reservoir. Thus, in HIV infection, a normal physiologic function of the immune system, i.e., the generation of an HIV-specific immune response that contributes to the clearance of virus, can also have deleterious consequences.

As HIV disease progresses, the architecture of lymphoid tissues begins to show disruption. Confocal microscopy reveals destruction of the fibroblastic reticular cell (FRC) and FDC networks in the T-cell zone and B-cell follicles/germinal centers, respectively. The mechanisms of destruction are not completely understood, but they are thought to be associated with collagen deposition causing fibrosis and a shift in the expression of certain cytokines, namely decreases in IL-7 and lymphotoxin-α, which are critical to the maintenance of lymphoid tissues and their lymphocyte constituents, and increased levels of transforming growth factor (TGF)-β. As the disease progresses to an advanced stage, there is complete disruption of the architecture of the lymphoid tissues, accompanied by dissolution of the FRC and FDC networks. At this point, the lymph nodes are "burnt out." This destruction of lymphoid tissue compounds the immunodeficiency of HIV disease and contributes both to the inability to control HIV replication and to the inability to mount adequate immune responses against opportunistic pathogens and vaccination. The events from primary infection to the ultimate destruction of the immune system are illustrated in **Fig. 202-24**. In nonhuman primate studies and some human studies that have examined GALT following SIV or HIV infection, the basal level of cellular activation combined with virus-mediated activation leads to the rapid infection and elimination of an estimated 50–90% of CD4+ T cells in the gut.

THE ROLE OF IMMUNE ACTIVATION AND INFLAMMATION IN HIV PATHOGENESIS

Activation of the immune system and variable degrees of inflammation are essential components of any appropriate immune response to a foreign antigen. However, immune activation and inflammation, which are aberrant in certain individuals with HIV, play a critical role in the pathogenesis of HIV disease as well as other chronic conditions associated with HIV infection. Immune activation and inflammation in individuals with HIV contribute substantially to (1) the replication of HIV, (2) the induction of immune dysfunction, and (3) the increased incidence of chronic conditions such as premature cardiovascular disease (**Table 202-4**).

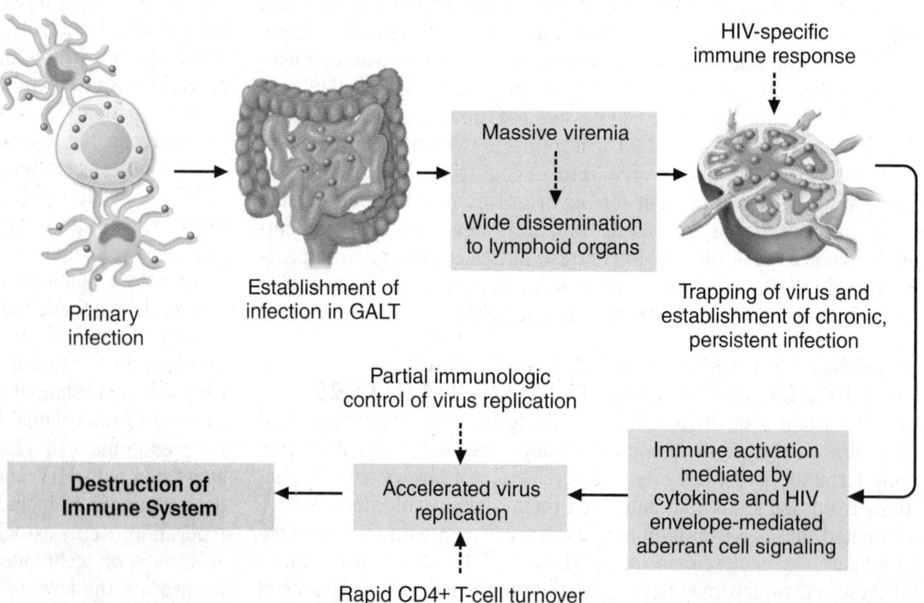

FIGURE 202-24 Events that transpire from primary HIV infection through the establishment of chronic persistent infection to the ultimate destruction of the immune system. See text for details. CTLs, cytolytic T lymphocytes; GALT, gut-associated lymphoid tissue.

TABLE 202-4 Conditions Associated with Persistent Immune Activation and Inflammation in Patients with HIV Infection

Accelerated aging syndrome
Bone fragility
Cancers
Cardiovascular disease
Diabetes
Kidney disease
Liver disease
Neurocognitive dysfunction

INDUCTION OF HIV REPLICATION BY ABERRANT IMMUNE ACTIVATION The immune system is normally in a state of homeostasis, awaiting perturbation by foreign antigenic stimuli. Once the immune response deals with and clears the antigen, the system returns to relative quiescence (**Chap. 349**). This is generally not the case in HIV infection where, in the untreated patient, virus replication is invariably persistent with very few exceptions and as a result immune activation is persistent. HIV replicates most efficiently in activated CD4+ T cells; in HIV infection, chronic activation provides the cell substrates necessary for persistent virus replication throughout the course of HIV disease, particularly in the untreated patient. Even in certain patients receiving ART whose levels of plasma viremia are suppressed to <50 copies per milliliter, there are low but detectable degrees of virus replication that drives low-level persistent immune activation. In addition, immune activation may result from RNA transcription of the integrated DNA of defective proviruses. From a virologic standpoint, although quiescent CD4+ T cells can be infected with HIV, albeit inefficiently, reverse transcription, integration, and virus spread are much more efficient in activated cells. Furthermore, cellular activation induces expression of virus in cells latently infected with HIV. In essence, immune activation and inflammation provide the engine that drives HIV replication. In addition to endogenous factors such as cytokines, a number of exogenous factors such as other microbes that are associated with heightened cellular activation can enhance HIV replication and thus may play a role in HIV pathogenesis.

Co-infection with a range of viruses, such as HSV types 1 and 2, cytomegalovirus (CMV), human herpesvirus (HHV) 6, Epstein-Barr virus (EBV), HBV, HCV, adenovirus, and HTLV-1 have been shown to upregulate HIV expression. In addition, infestation with nematodes has been shown to be associated with a heightened state of immune activation that facilitates HIV replication; in certain studies, deworming of the infected host has resulted in a decrease in plasma viremia. Two diseases of extraordinary global health significance, malaria and tuberculosis (TB), have been shown to increase HIV viral load in dually infected individuals. Globally, *Mycobacterium tuberculosis* is the most common opportunistic infection in HIV-infected individuals (**Chap. 178**). In addition to the fact that individuals with HIV are more likely to develop active TB after exposure and to reactivate latent TB, it has been demonstrated that active TB can accelerate the course of HIV infection. It has also been shown that levels of plasma viremia are greatly elevated in individuals with HIV who have active TB and who are not receiving ART, compared with pre-TB levels and levels of viremia after successful treatment of the active TB. The situation is similar in the interaction between HIV and malaria parasites (**Chap. 224**). Acute infection with *Plasmodium falciparum* of individuals with HIV increases viral load, and the increased viral load is reversed by effective treatment of malaria.

MICROBIAL TRANSLOCATION AND PERSISTENT IMMUNE ACTIVATION One proposed mechanism of persistent immune activation involves the disruption of the mucosal barrier in the gut due to HIV replication in submucosal lymphoid tissue. As a result of this disruption, there is an increase in the products of bacteria, particularly lipopolysaccharide (LPS), that translocate from the bowel lumen through the damaged mucosa to the circulation, leading to persistent systemic immune activation and inflammation. This effect can persist even after the HIV viral load is brought to <50 copies/mL by ART. Other related factors that are thought to contribute to the pathogenesis of HIV include depletion in the GALT of IL-17–producing T cells, which are responsible for defense against extracellular bacteria and fungi, as well as alterations in gut microbiota and the metabolic pathways involved.

PERSISTENT IMMUNE ACTIVATION AND INFLAMMATION INDUCE IMMUNE DYSFUNCTION The immune activated state in HIV infection is reflected by hyperactivation of B cells leading to hypergammaglobulinemia; increased lymphocyte turnover; activation of monocytes; expression of activation markers and immune checkpoint receptors on CD4+ and CD8+ T cells; increased activation-associated cellular apoptosis and pyroptosis; lymph node hyperplasia, particularly during the chronic phase prior to disease progression; increased secretion of proinflammatory cytokines, particularly IL-6 and type I interferons; elevated levels of high-sensitivity C-reactive protein, CXC chemokine ligand 10 (CXCL10), D-dimer, neopterin, β_2-microglobulin, soluble (s) CD14, sTNFR, sCD27, sCD163, and sCD40L; and autoimmune phenomena (see "Autoimmune Phenomena," below). Even in the absence of direct infection of a target cell, HIV envelope proteins can interact with cellular receptors (CD4 molecules and chemokine receptors) to deliver potent activation signals resulting in calcium flux, the phosphorylation of certain proteins involved in signal transduction, co-localization of cytoplasmic proteins including those involved in cell trafficking, immune dysfunction, and, under certain circumstances, apoptosis and pyroptosis. From an immunologic standpoint, chronic exposure of the immune system to a particular antigen over an extended period may ultimately lead to an inability to sustain an adequate immune response to the antigen in question. In many chronic viral infections, including HIV infection, persistent viremia is associated with "functional exhaustion" of virus-specific T cells, decreasing their capacity to proliferate and perform effector functions. It has been demonstrated that this phenomenon of immune exhaustion may be mediated, at least in part, by the upregulation of inhibitory receptors on HIV-specific T cells, such as PD-1, LAG-3 and Tim-3 that are shared by both CD4+ and CD8+ T cells, as well as CTLA-4 on CD4+ and 2B4 and CD160 on CD8+ T cells. Furthermore, the ability of the immune system to respond to a broad spectrum of non-HIV antigens may be compromised if immunocompetent bystander cells are maintained in a state of chronic activation.

The deleterious effects of chronic immune activation on the progression of HIV disease are well established. As in most conditions of persistent antigen exposure, the host must maintain sufficient activation of antigen (HIV)-specific responses but must also prevent excessive activation and potential immune-mediated damage to tissues. Certain studies suggest that normal immunoregulatory mechanisms that act to keep hyperimmune activation in check, particularly CD4+, FoxP3+, and CD25+ regulatory T cells (T-regs), may be dysfunctional or depleted in the context of advanced HIV disease. One possibility is a role for the inhibitory receptor LAG-3 (see below), overexpressed on exhausted T cells and shown to inhibit the proliferation of T-regs.

Apoptosis Apoptosis is a form of programmed cell death that is a normal mechanism for the elimination of effete cells in organogenesis as well as in the cellular proliferation that occurs during a normal immune response (**Chap. 349**). Apoptosis can occur by intrinsic or extrinsic pathways, the latter of which is largely dependent on cellular activation, and in this regard the aberrant cellular activation associated with HIV disease is correlated with a heightened state of apoptosis. HIV can trigger activation-induced cell death through the upregulation of the death receptors, such as Fas/CD95, TNFR1, or TNF-related apoptosis-inducing ligand (TRAIL) receptors 1 and 2. Their corresponding ligands FasL, TNF, and TRAIL also are upregulated in HIV disease. HIV-induced stress and alterations in homeostasis also can trigger intrinsic apoptosis due to the downregulation of antiapoptotic proteins such as Bcl-2. Other mechanisms of HIV-induced cell death have been described, including autophagy, necrosis, necroptosis, and pyroptosis. The phenomenon of pyroptosis, an inflammatory form of cell death involving the upregulation of the proinflammatory enzyme caspase 1 and release of the proinflammatory cytokines IL-1β and IL-18, has been linked to a bystander effect of HIV replication on depletion of CD4+ T cells (see "Pathophysiology and Pathogenesis," above). The process of pyroptosis generates multimeric complexes called inflammasomes, which can also be activated by LPS. Certain viral gene products have been associated with enhanced susceptibility to apoptosis; these include Env, Tat, and Vpr. In contrast, Nef has been shown to possess antiapoptotic properties. The intensity of apoptosis correlates with the general state of activation of the immune system and not with the stage of disease or with viral burden. A number of studies, including those examining lymphoid tissue, have demonstrated that the rate of apoptosis is elevated in HIV infection and that apoptosis is seen in "bystander" cells such as CD8+ T cells and B cells as well as in uninfected CD4+ T cells. It is likely that this bystander apoptosis of immunocompetent cells related to immune activation contributes to the general immunologic abnormalities in HIV disease.

MEDICAL CONDITIONS ASSOCIATED WITH PERSISTENT IMMUNE ACTIVATION AND INFLAMMATION IN HIV DISEASE It has become clear, as the survival of HIV-infected individuals has increased, that a number of previously unrecognized medical complications are associated with HIV disease—and that these complications relate to chronic immune activation and inflammation (Table 202-4). These complications can appear even after patients have experienced years of ART-induced adequate control of viral replication (plasma viremia < 50 copies per milliliter of plasma) for several years. Other chronic conditions that have been reported include bone fragility, certain cancers, diabetes, kidney and liver disease, and neurocognitive dysfunction, thus presenting an overall picture of accelerated aging.

Autoimmune Phenomena Autoimmune phenomena are commonly observed in HIV-infected individuals and they reflect, at least in part, chronic immune activation and the dysregulation of B and T cells. Although these phenomena usually occur in the absence of autoimmune disease, a wide spectrum of clinical manifestations that may be associated with autoimmunity have been described (see "Immunologic and Rheumatologic Diseases," below). Autoimmune phenomena include antibodies against autoantigens expressed on intact lymphocytes and other cells, or against proteins released from dying cells. Antiplatelet and anti-erythrocyte antibodies have some clinical relevance in that they may contribute to thrombocytopenia and autoimmune hemolytic anemia, respectively, in HIV disease (see below). Antibodies to nuclear and cytoplasmic components of cells have been reported, as have antibodies to cardiolipin and phospholipids, as well as surface receptors, including CD4, and serum proteins. However, these manifestations are relatively low in the era of ART. Molecular mimicry, either from opportunistic pathogens or from HIV itself, also is a trigger or cofactor in autoimmunity. Antibodies against the HIV envelope proteins, especially gp41, often cross-react with host proteins; the best-known examples are antibodies directed against the membrane-proximal external region (MPER) of gp41 that also react with phospholipids and cardiolipin. The phenomenon of polyreactive HIV-specific antibodies may be beneficial to the host (see "Immune Response to HIV," below).

The increased occurrence and/or exacerbation of certain autoimmune diseases have been reported in HIV infection; these diseases include psoriasis, idiopathic thrombocytopenic purpura, autoimmune hemolytic anemia, Graves' disease, antiphospholipid syndrome, and primary biliary cirrhosis. Most of these manifestations were described prior to the advent of ART and have decreased in frequency since its widespread use. However, with increasing availability of ART, an *immune reconstitution inflammatory syndrome* (IRIS) has been increasingly observed in infected individuals, particularly those with low CD4+ T-cell counts (see below). IRIS is an autoimmune-like phenomenon characterized by a paradoxical deterioration of clinical condition, which is usually compartmentalized to a particular organ system, in individuals in whom ART has recently been initiated. It is associated with a decrease in viral load and at least partial recovery of immune competence, which is usually associated with increases in CD4+ T-cell counts. The immunopathogenesis of this syndrome is felt to be related to an increase in immune response against the presence of residual antigens that are usually microbial and is most commonly seen with underlying mycobacterial (*Mycobacterium tuberculosis* [TB] or *avium* complex [MAC]), fungal (cryptococcal) and viral (CMV, HHV) infections. This syndrome is discussed in more detail below.

CYTOKINES AND OTHER SOLUBLE FACTORS IN HIV PATHOGENESIS

The immune system is homeostatically regulated by a complex network of immunoregulatory cytokines, which are pleiotropic and redundant and operate in an autocrine and paracrine manner. They are expressed continuously, even during periods of apparent quiescence of the immune system. On perturbation of the immune system by antigenic challenge, the expression of cytokines increases to varying degrees (**Chap. 349**). Cytokines that are important components of this immunoregulatory network are thought to play major roles in HIV disease, during both the early and chronic phases of infection. A potent proinflammatory "cytokine storm" is induced during the acute phase of HIV infection, likely a response by inflammatory cells to virus replicating at very high levels. Cytokines and chemokines that are induced during this early phase include the type I interferon IFN-α, IL-15, and CXCL10, followed by IL-6, IL-12, and TNF-α, and a delayed peak of the anti-inflammatory cytokine IL-10. Soluble factors of innate immunity also are induced shortly after infection, including neopterin and β-microglobulin. Several of these early-expressed cytokines and factors are not downregulated following the early phase of HIV infection, as seen in other self-resolving viral infections, and persist during the chronic phase of infection and contribute to maintaining high levels of immune activation. Among the cytokines and factors associated with early innate immune responses, they are intended to contain viral replication, although paradoxically most are potent inducers of HIV expression/replication because of their ability to induce immune activation that leads to enhanced viral production and an increase in readily available target cells for HIV (activated CD4+ T cells). The induction of IFN-α, one of the first cytokines induced during primary HIV infection and an important element of innate immune sensing, is thought to play a particularly important role in HIV pathogenesis by inducing a large number of IFN-associated genes that activate the immune system, alter the homeostasis of CD4+ T cells, and influence the virus variants that are selected during the HIV transmission bottleneck. Other cytokines that are elevated during the chronic phase of HIV infection and linked to immune activation include IFN-γ, the *CC-chemokine* RANTES (CCL5), macrophage inflammatory protein (MIP)-1β (CCL4), and IL-18.

Several specific cytokines and soluble factors have been associated with HIV pathogenesis at various stages of disease, in various tissues or organs, and in the regulation of HIV replication. Plasma levels of IP-10 are predictive of disease progression, whereas the proinflammatory cytokine IL-6, marker of monocyte/macrophage activation soluble CD14 (sCD14), and coagulation marker D-dimer are associated with increased risk of all-cause mortality in HIV-infected individuals. In particular, IL-6, sCD14, and D-dimer are associated with increased risk of cardiovascular disease and other causes of death, even in individuals receiving ART. IL-18 has also been shown to play a role in the development of the HIV-associated lipodystrophy syndrome. Elevated levels of TNF-α and IL-6 have been demonstrated in plasma and cerebrospinal fluid (CSF), and increased expression of TNF-α, IL-1β, IFN-γ, and IL-6 has been demonstrated in the lymph nodes of HIV-infected individuals prior to disease progression and a shift to TGF-β in advanced disease (see "Lymphoid Organs and HIV Pathogenesis, above). RANTES (CCL5), MIP-1α (CCL3), and MIP-1β (CCL4) (**Chap. 349**) inhibit infection by and spread of R5 HIV-1 strains, while *stromal cell–derived factor* (SDF) 1 inhibits infection by and spread of X4 strains. The mechanisms whereby the CC-chemokines RANTES (CCL5), MIP-1α (CCL3), and MIP-1β (CCL4) inhibit infection of R5 strains of HIV, or SDF-1 blocks X4 strains of HIV, involve blocking of the binding of the virus to its co-receptors, the CC-chemokine receptor CCR5 and the CXC-chemokine receptor CXCR4, respectively. Other soluble factors that have not yet been fully characterized, such as soluble CD8 antiviral factor (CAF), also have been shown to suppress HIV replication, independent of co-receptor usage.

TABLE 202-5 Proposed Mechanisms of CD4+ T-Cell Dysfunction and Depletion	
DIRECT MECHANISMS	**INDIRECT MECHANISMS**
Loss of plasma membrane integrity due to viral budding	Aberrant intracellular signaling events
Accumulation of unintegrated viral DNA Activation of DNA-dependent protein kinase during viral integration into host genome	Autoimmunity
Interference with cellular RNA processing	Innocent bystander killing of viral antigen–coated cells
Intracellular gp120-CD4 autofusion events	Apoptosis, pyroptosis (caspase 1–associated inflammation), autophagy
Syncytia formation	Inhibition of lymphopoiesis from reduced survival cytokines and lymphoid tissue integrity Activation-induced cell death Elimination of HIV-infected cells by virus-specific immune responses

■ LYMPHOCYTE TURNOVER IN HIV INFECTION

The immune systems of patients with HIV infection are characterized by a profound increase in lymphocyte turnover that is immediately reduced with effective ART. Studies utilizing in vivo or in vitro labeling of lymphocytes in the S-phase of the cell cycle have demonstrated a tight correlation between the degree of lymphocyte turnover and plasma viremia. This increase in turnover is seen in CD4+ and CD8+ T lymphocytes as well as B lymphocytes and can be observed in peripheral blood and lymphoid tissue. Mathematical models derived from these data suggest that one can view the lymphoid pool as consisting of dynamically distinct subpopulations of cells that are differentially affected by HIV infection. A major consequence of HIV infection appears to be a shift in cells from a more quiescent pool to a pool with a higher turnover rate. It is likely that a consequence of a higher rate of turnover is a higher rate of cell death. It has been suggested that the more rapid decline in CD4+ compared with CD8+ T cells may be linked to alterations in inflammatory and homeostatic cytokines that cause increased activation-induced death without replenishment of CD4+ T cells. (See **Table 202-5** for additional mechanisms of depletion.)

■ THE ROLE OF VIRAL RECEPTORS AND CO-RECEPTORS IN HIV PATHOGENESIS

CCR5 AND CXCR4 As mentioned above, HIV-1 utilizes two major co-receptors along with CD4 to bind to, fuse with, and enter target cells; these co-receptors are CCR5 and CXCR4, which are also receptors for certain endogenous chemokines. Strains of HIV that utilize CCR5 as a co-receptor are referred to as *R5 viruses*. Strains of HIV that utilize CXCR4 are referred to as *X4 viruses*. Many virus strains are *dual tropic* in that they utilize both CCR5 and CXCR4; these are referred to as *R5X4 viruses*.

The natural chemokine ligands for the major HIV co-receptors can readily block entry of HIV. For example, the CC-chemokines RANTES (CCL5), MIP-1α (CCL3), and MIP-1β (CCL4), which are the natural ligands for CCR5, block entry of R5 viruses, whereas SDF-1, the natural ligand for CXCR4, blocks entry of X4 viruses. The mechanism of inhibition of viral entry is a steric inhibition of binding that is not dependent on signal transduction (**Fig. 202-25**).

The transmitting virus is almost invariably an R5 virus that predominates during the early stages of HIV disease, although in the era of deep sequencing, more X4 variants have been detected in early disease than previously reported. In the absence of ART or in therapeutic failures, there is a transition to a predominantly X4 virus in approximately half of individuals infected with subtype B virus. The transition is often preceded by dual R5X4 strains, and detection of X4 variants is associated with a relatively rapid decline in CD4+ T-cell counts,

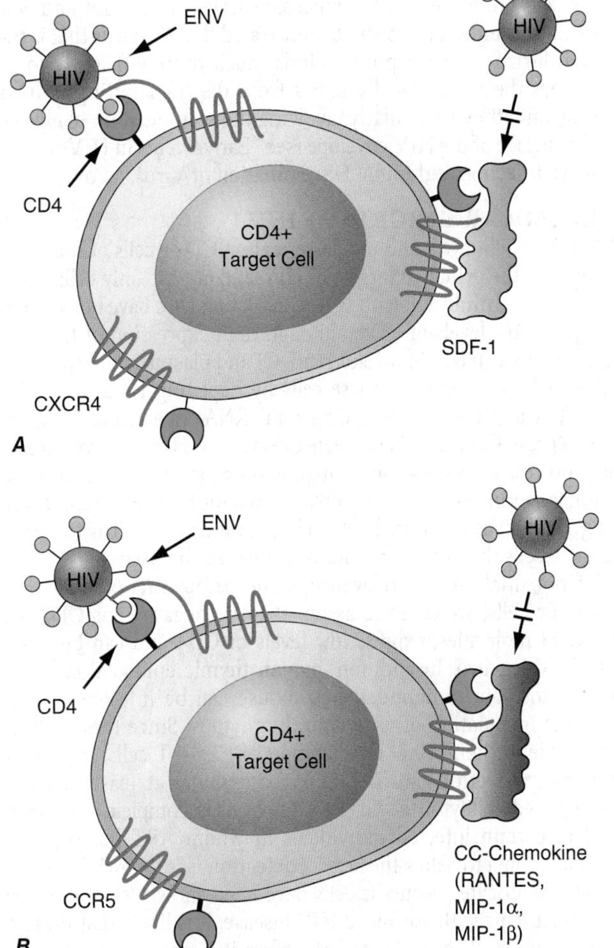

FIGURE 202-25 Model for the role of co-receptors CXCR4 and CCR5 in the efficient binding and entry of X4 (***A***) and R5 (***B***) strains of HIV-1, respectively, into CD4+ target cells. Blocking of this initial event in the virus life cycle can be accomplished by inhibition of binding to the co-receptor by the normal ligand for the receptor in question. The ligand for CXCR4 is stromal cell–derived factor (SDF-1); the ligands for CCR5 are RANTES, MIP-1α, and MIP-1β.

increased HIV plasma viremia, and progression of disease. However, the other half of infected individuals progress in their disease while maintaining predominance of an R5 virus, and individuals infected with non-subtype B clades more rarely switch from CCR5 tropism to CXCR4 tropism than those infected with subtype B. The reason for this difference is unclear.

The basis for the tropism of different envelope glycoproteins for either CCR5 or CXCR4 relates to the ability of the HIV envelope, including the third variable region (V3 loop) of gp120, to interact with these co-receptors. In this regard, binding of gp120 to CD4 induces a conformational change in gp120 that increases its affinity for the relevant co-receptor. Finally, R5 viruses are more efficient in infecting monocytes/macrophages and microglial cells of the brain (see "Neuropathogenesis in HIV Disease," below).

THE INTEGRIN α4β7 The integrin *α4β7* is an accessory receptor for HIV. It is not essential for the binding and infection of a CD4+ T cell by HIV; however, it likely plays an important role in the transmission of HIV at mucosal surfaces such as the genital tract and gut and contributes somewhat to the pathogenesis of HIV disease. The integrin α4β7, which is the gut homing receptor for peripheral T cells, binds in its activated form to a specific tripeptide in the V2 loop of gp120, resulting in rapid activation of leukocyte function–associated antigen 1 (LFA-1), the central integrin in the establishment of virologic synapses, which facilitate efficient cell-to-cell spread of HIV. It has been demonstrated that $\alpha4\beta7^{high}$ CD4+ T cells are more susceptible to productive infection than are $\alpha4\beta7^{low\text{–}neg}$ CD4+ T cells because this cellular subset is enriched with metabolically active CD4+ T cells that are CCR5^{high}. These cells are present in the mucosal surfaces of the gut and genital tract. Importantly, it has been demonstrated that the virus that is transmitted during sexual exposure binds much more efficiently to α4β7 than does the virus that diversifies from the transmitting virus over time by mutation, particularly involving the accumulation of glycogens on the surface of the HIV envelope (see "Early Events in HIV Infection: Primary Infection and Initial Dissemination of Virus," above).

CELLULAR TARGETS OF HIV

CD4+ T lymphocytes and to a lesser extent CD4+ cells of the myeloid lineage are the principal targets of HIV and are the only cells that can be productively infected with HIV. Circulating DCs have been reported to express low levels of CD4, although high expression of the restriction factor SAMHD1 in myeloid (mDC) and plasmacytoid (pDC) DCs limits HIV replication in these cells by depleting intracellular pools of dNTPs and directly degrading viral RNA. Epidermal Langerhans cells express CD4 and have been infected by HIV in vivo, although they too restrict replication by high expression of the host restriction factor, langerin. As has been shown in vivo for DCs, FDCs, and B cells, Langerhans cells are more likely to bind and transfer virus to activated CD4+ T cells than to be productively infected themselves.

Of potential clinical relevance is the demonstration that thymic precursor cells, which were assumed to be negative for CD3, CD4, and CD8 molecules, express low levels of CD4 and can be infected with HIV in vitro. In addition, human thymic epithelial cells transplanted into an immunodeficient mouse can be infected with HIV by direct inoculation of virus into the thymus. Since these cells may play a role in the normal regeneration of CD4+ T cells, it is possible that their infection and depletion contribute, at least in part, to the impaired ability of the CD4+ T-cell pool to completely reconstitute itself in certain infected individuals in whom ART has suppressed plasma viremia to below the level of detection (see below). In addition, CD34+ monocyte precursor cells have been shown to be infected in vivo in patients with advanced HIV disease. It is likely that these cells express low levels of CD4, and therefore it is not essential to invoke CD4-independent mechanisms to explain the infection. The clinical relevance of this finding is unclear.

QUALITATIVE AND QUANTITATIVE ABNORMALITIES OF MONONUCLEAR CELLS

CD4+ T Cells The primary immunopathogenic lesion in HIV infection involves CD4+ T cells, and the range of CD4+ T-cell abnormalities in advanced HIV infection is broad. The defects are both quantitative and qualitative and ultimately impact virtually every limb of the immune system, indicating the critical dependence of the integrity of the immune system on the inducer/helper function of CD4+ T cells. In advanced HIV disease, most of the observed immune defects can ultimately be explained by the quantitative depletion of CD4+ T cells. However, T-cell dysfunction can be demonstrated in patients early in the course of infection, even when the CD4+ T-cell count is in the low-normal range. The degree and spectrum of dysfunctions increase as the disease progresses, reflecting the range of CD4+ T-cell functional heterogeneity, especially in lymphoid tissues. One of the first sites of intense HIV replication is in the GALT where CD4+ T_H17 cells reside; they are important for host defense against extracellular pathogens in the intestinal mucosa and help maintain the integrity of the gut epithelium. In HIV infection, they are depleted by direct and indirect effects of viral replication and cause loss of gut homeostasis and integrity, as well as a shift toward a T_H1 phenotype. Studies have shown that even after many years of ART, normalization of the CD4+ T cells in the GALT remains incomplete. In lymph nodes, HIV perturbs another important subset of the CD4+ helper T lineage, namely TF_H cells (see "Lymphoid Organs and HIV Pathogenesis," above). TF_H cells, which are derived either directly from naïve CD4+ T cells or from other T_H precursors, migrate into B-cell follicles during germinal center reactions and provide help to antigen-specific B cells through cell–cell interactions and secretion of cytokines to which B cells respond, the most important of which is IL-21. In addition, it has been shown that HIV-infected individuals with broadly neutralizing antibodies have higher frequencies of memory TF_H CD4+ T cells. As with T_H17 cells, TF_H cells are highly susceptible to HIV infection. However, in contrast to T_H17 and most other CD4+ T-cell subsets, the number of TF_H cells is increased in lymph nodes of HIV-infected individuals, especially those who are viremic. It is unclear whether this increase is helpful to responding B cells, although the likely outcome is that the increase in numbers is detrimental to the quality of the humoral immune response against HIV (see "Immune Response to HIV," below). In addition, defects of central memory cells are a critical component of HIV immunopathogenesis. The progressive loss of antigen-specific CD4+ T cells has important implications for the control of HIV infection. In this regard, there is a correlation between the maintenance of HIV-specific CD4+ T-cell proliferative responses and improved control of infection. Essentially every T-cell function has been reported to be abnormal at some stage of HIV infection. Loss of polyfunctional HIV-specific CD4+ T cells, especially those that produce IL-2, occurs early in disease, whereas IFN-producing CD4+ T cells are maintained longer and do not correlate with control of HIV viremia. Other abnormalities include impaired expression of IL-2 receptors, defective IL-2 production, reduced expression of the IL-7 receptor (CD127), and a decreased proportion of CD4+ T cells that express CD28, a major co-stimulatory molecule necessary for the normal activation of T cells, which is also depleted as a result of aging. Cells lacking expression of CD28 do not respond normally to activation signals and may express markers of terminal activation including HLA-DR, CD38, and CD45RO. As mentioned above ("The Role of Immune Activation and Inflammation in HIV Pathogenesis"), a subset of CD4+ T cells referred to as *T regulatory cells*, or T-regs, may be involved in damping aberrant immune activation that propagates HIV replication. The presence of these T-reg cells correlates with lower viral loads and higher CD4+/CD8+ T-cell ratios. A loss of this T-reg capability with advanced disease may be detrimental to the control of virus replication.

It is difficult to explain completely the profound immunodeficiency noted in HIV-infected individuals solely based on direct infection and quantitative depletion of CD4+ T cells. This is particularly apparent during the early stages of HIV disease, when CD4+ T-cell numbers may be only marginally decreased. In this regard, it is likely that CD4+ T-cell dysfunction results from a combination of depletion of cells due to direct infection of the cell and a number of virus-related but indirect effects on the cell such as elimination of "innocent bystander cells" (Table 202-5). Several of these effects have been demonstrated ex vivo and/or by the analysis of cells isolated from the peripheral blood. Soluble viral proteins, particularly gp120, can bind with high affinity to the CD4 molecules on uninfected T cells and monocytes; in addition, virus and/or viral proteins can bind to DCs or FDCs. HIV-specific antibody can recognize these bound molecules and potentially collaborate in the elimination of the cells by ADCC. HIV envelope glycoproteins gp120 and gp160 manifest high-affinity binding to the CD4 molecule as well as to various chemokine receptors. Intracellular signals transduced by gp120 through both CD4 and CCR5/CXCR4 have been associated with a number of immunopathogenic processes including anergy, apoptosis, and abnormalities of cell trafficking. The molecular mechanisms responsible for these abnormalities include dysregulation of the T-cell receptor–phosphoinositide pathway, p56lck activation, phosphorylation of focal adhesion kinase, activation of the MAP kinase and ras signaling pathways, and downregulation of the co-stimulatory molecules CD40 ligand and CD80.

The inexorable decline in CD4+ T-cell counts that occurs in most untreated HIV-infected individuals may result in part from the inability of the immune system to regenerate over an extended period of time the rapidly turning over CD4+ T-cell pool efficiently enough to compensate for both HIV-mediated and naturally occurring attrition of cells. In this regard, the degree and duration of decline of CD4+ T cells at the time of initiation of therapy is an important predictor of the restoration of these cells. A person who maintains a very low CD4+ T-cell count for a considerable period before the initiation of ART almost invariably has an incomplete reconstitution of such cells. At least two major mechanisms may contribute to the failure of the CD4+ T-cell pool to reconstitute itself adequately over the course of HIV infection. The first is the destruction of lymphoid precursor cells, including thymic and bone marrow progenitor cells; the other is the gradual disruption of the lymphoid tissue architecture and microenvironment, which is essential for efficient regeneration of immunocompetent cells. Finally, during the advanced stages of CD4+ T lymphopenia, there are increased serum levels of the homeostatic cytokine IL-7. It was initially felt that this elevation was a homeostatic response to the lymphopenia; however, recent findings suggest that the increase in serum IL-7 was a result of reduced utilization of the cytokine related to the loss of cells expressing the IL-7 receptor, CD127, which serves as a normal physiologic regulator of IL-7 production.

CD8+ T Cells A relative CD8+ T lymphocytosis is generally associated with high levels of HIV plasma viremia and likely reflects an immune response to the virus as well as dysregulated homeostasis associated with generalized immune activation. During the late stages of HIV infection, there may be a significant reduction in the numbers of CD8+ T cells despite the presence of high levels of viremia. HIV-specific CD8+ CTLs have been demonstrated in HIV-infected individuals early in the course of disease, and their emergence often coincides with a decrease in plasma viremia—an observation that is a factor in the proposal that virus-specific CTLs can control HIV disease for a finite period of time in a certain percentage of infected individuals. However, emergence of HIV escape mutants that ultimately evade these HIV-specific CD8+ T cells has been described in most HIV-infected individuals who are not receiving ART. In addition, as the disease progresses, the functional capability of these cells gradually decreases, at least in part due to the persistent nature of HIV infection that causes functional exhaustion via the upregulation of inhibitory receptors such as PD-1, TIGIT, LAG-3, and TIM-3 on HIV-specific CD8+ T cells (see "The Role of Immune Activation and Inflammation in HIV Pathogenesis," above). As chronic immune activation persists, there are also systemic effects on CD8+ T cells, such that as a population they assume an abnormal phenotype characterized by expression of activation markers such as co-expression of HLA-DR and CD38 with an absence of expression of the IL-2 receptor (CD25) and a reduced expression of the IL-7 receptor (CD127). In addition, CD8+ T cells lacking CD28 expression are increased in HIV disease, reflecting a skewed expansion of a less differentiated CD8+ T-cell subset. This skewing of subsets is also associated with diminished polyfunctionality, a qualitative difference that distinguishes elite controllers from progressors. Elite controllers can also be distinguished from progressors by the maintenance in the former of a high proliferative capacity of their HIV-specific CD8+ T cells coupled to increases in perforin expression and elimination of infected targets, characteristics that are markedly diminished in advanced HIV disease. It has been reported that the phenotype of CD8+ T cells in HIV-infected individuals may be of prognostic significance. Those individuals whose CD8+ T cells developed a phenotype of HLA-DR+/CD38– following seroconversion had stabilization of their CD4+ T-cell counts, whereas those whose CD8+ T cells developed a phenotype of HLA-DR+/CD38+ had a more aggressive course and a poorer prognosis. In addition to the defects in HIV-specific CD8+ CTLs, functional defects in other MHC-restricted CTLs, such as those directed against influenza and CMV, have been demonstrated. CD8+ T cells secrete a variety of soluble factors that inhibit HIV replication, including the CC-chemokines RANTES (CCL5), MIP-1α (CCL3), and MIP-1β (CCL4) and potentially several yet-unidentified factors. The presence of high levels of HIV viremia in vivo as well as exposure of CD8+ T cells in vitro to HIV envelope, both of which are associated with aberrant immune activation, have been shown to be associated with a variety of cellular functional abnormalities. Furthermore, since the integrity of CD8+ T-cell function depends in part on adequate inductive signals from CD4+ T cells, the defect in CD8+ CTLs is likely compounded by the quantitative loss and qualitative dysfunction of CD4+ T cells.

B Cells The predominant defect in B cells from HIV-infected individuals is one of aberrant cellular activation, which is reflected by increased propensity to terminal differentiation and immunoglobulin secretion, as well as increased expression of markers of activation and exhaustion. As a result of activation and differentiation in vivo and induction of inhibitory pathways of regulation, B cells from HIV viremic patients manifest a decreased capacity to undergo cell signaling and mount a proliferative response ex vivo. B cells from HIV-infected individuals manifest enhanced spontaneous secretion of immunoglobulins in vitro, a process that reflects their highly differentiated state in vivo. There is also an increased incidence of EBV-related B-cell lymphomas in HIV-infected individuals that are likely due to combined effects of defective T-cell immune surveillance and increased B-cell turnover that increases the risk of oncogenesis. Untransformed B cells cannot be infected with HIV, although HIV or its products can activate B cells directly. B cells from patients with high levels of viremia bind virions to their surface via the CD21 complement receptor. It is likely that in vivo activation of B cells by replication-competent or defective virus as well as viral products during the viremic state accounts at least in part for their activated phenotype. B-cell subpopulations from HIV-infected individuals undergo a number of changes over the course of HIV disease, including the attrition of resting memory B cells and replacement with several aberrant memory and differentiated B-cell subpopulations that collectively express reduced levels of CD21 and either increased expression of activation markers or inhibitory receptors associated with functional exhaustion. The more activated and differentiated B cells are also responsible for increased secretion of immunoglobulins and increased susceptibility to Fas-mediated apoptosis. In more advanced disease, there is also the appearance of immature B cells associated with CD4+ T-cell lymphopenia. Despite increased frequencies of germinal center B cells and CD4+ TF_H cells, both of which are required for effective humoral immunity, cognate B-cell–CD4+ T-cell interactions in lymphoid tissues are perturbed in HIV-infected individuals, especially those with persistent viremia. In vivo, the aberrant activated state of B cells manifests itself by hypergammaglobulinemia and by the presence of circulating immune complexes that bind the B cells and restrict their capacity to respond to further stimulation. HIV-infected individuals respond poorly to primary and secondary immunizations with protein and polysaccharide antigens. Using immunization with influenza vaccine, it has been demonstrated that there is a memory B-cell defect in HIV-infected individuals, particularly those with high levels of HIV viremia. There is also evidence that responses to HIV and non-HIV antigens in infected individuals, especially those who remain viremic, are enriched in abnormal subsets of B cells that either are highly prone to apoptosis or show signs of functional exhaustion. Taken together, these B-cell defects are likely responsible at least in part for the inadequate humoral response to HIV as well as to decreased response to vaccinations and the increase in certain bacterial infections seen in advanced HIV disease in adults. In addition, they likely contribute to the inadequacy of host defenses against bacterial infections that play a role in the increased morbidity and mortality of HIV-infected children. The absolute number of circulating B cells also may be depressed in HIV infection; this phenomenon likely reflects increased activation-induced apoptosis as well as a redistribution of cells out of the circulation and into the lymphoid tissue—phenomena that are associated with ongoing viral replication.

Monocytes/Macrophages Circulating monocytes are generally normal in number in HIV-infected individuals; however, there is evidence of increased activation within this lineage. The increased level of sCD14 and other biomarkers (see above) reported in HIV-infected individuals is an indirect marker of monocyte activation in vivo. Levels of sCD14 can remain elevated in individuals whose plasma viremia has been suppressed by ART for several years, an indicator of the residual immune activation and inflammation observed in HIV infection and effects on the monocyte/macrophage lineage. A number of other abnormalities of circulating monocytes have been reported in HIV-infected individuals, many of which may be related directly or indirectly to aberrant in vivo immune activation. In this regard, increased levels of lipopolysaccharide (LPS) are found in the sera of HIV-infected individuals due, at least in part, to translocation across the gut mucosal barrier (see above). LPS is a highly inflammatory bacterial product that preferentially binds to macrophages through CD14 and Toll-like receptors, resulting in cellular activation. In the peripheral blood, expansion of monocytes that express the intermediate and non-classical marker CD16 and markers of activation (HLA-DR) and stimulation (CD40 and CD86) has been described, especially in viremic individuals. Activated monocytes are also responsible for secretion of inflammatory cytokines and chemokines observed in HIV infection, including CXCL10, IL-1β, and IL-6. Monocytes express the CD4 molecule and several co-receptors for HIV on their surface, and thus are potential targets of HIV infection. However, in vivo infection of circulating monocytes is difficult to demonstrate, although infection of tissue macrophages and macrophage-lineage cells in the brain (infiltrating macrophages or resident microglial cells) and lung (pulmonary alveolar macrophages) can be demonstrated easily. Tissue macrophages are an important source of HIV during the inflammatory response associated with opportunistic infections and can serve as persistent reservoirs of HIV infection, thus representing an obstacle to the eradication of HIV by antiretroviral drugs.

Dendritic and Langerhans Cells DCs and Langerhans cells are not productively infected with HIV, likely in part due to their expression of host restriction factors, including APOBEC3G and SAMHD1 (see above). However, they are thought to play an important role in the initiation of HIV infection by virtue of the ability of HIV to bind to cell-surface C-type lectin receptors, particularly DC-SIGN (see above) and langerin. However, while langerin provides a host barrier for replication by trafficking HIV to acidic compartments for degradation, DC-SIGN retains HIV in early endosomal compartments. This allows efficient presentation of intact virus to CD4+ T-cell targets that become infected; complexes of infected CD4+ T cells and DCs provide an optimal microenvironment for virus replication. Furthermore, pDCs secrete large amounts of IFN-α in response to viral infections and as such play an important role in innate sensing of HIV during early phase of infection. The numbers of circulating pDCs and mDCs are decreased in HIV infection through mechanisms that remain unclear, although several studies have shown increased lymphoid tissue recruitment of DCs associated with lymphoid hyperplasia and inflammation. The mDCs are also involved in the initiation of adaptive immunity in draining lymph nodes by presenting antigen to T cells and B cells, as well as by secreting cytokines such as IL-12, IL-15, and IL-18 that activate other immune cells, although these functions are perturbed in HIV infection.

Natural Killer Cells and Innate Lymphoid Cells NK cells represent the prototypical member of innate lymphoid cells (ILCs) that collectively provide tissue homeostasis and immunosurveillance against virus-infected cells, certain tumor cells, and allogeneic cells (Chap. 349). There are no convincing data that HIV productively infects NK cells in vivo; however, functional abnormalities in NK cells have been observed throughout the course of HIV disease, and the severity of these abnormalities increases as disease progresses. NK cells are part of the innate immune system and act by direct killing of infected cells and secretion of antiviral cytokines and chemokines. In early HIV infection there is an increase in the activation of NK cells, and the capacity to secrete IFN-γ is maintained, although they manifest reduced cytotoxic function as a result of altered maturation. During chronic HIV infection, both NK cell cytotoxicity and cytokine secretion become impaired. Given that HIV infection of target cells down-regulates HLA-A and B, but not HLA-C and D molecules, this may explain in part the relative inability of NK cells to kill HIV-infected target cells. However, the NK cell impairments, especially in patients with high levels of virus replication, are associated with an expansion of an "anergic" CD56–/CD16+ NK cell subset. This abnormal subset of NK cells manifests an increased expression of inhibitory NK cell receptors (iNKRs) and a substantial decrease in expression of natural cytotoxicity receptors (NCRs) and shows a markedly impaired lytic activity. The overrepresentation of this abnormal subset of NK cells may explain in part the observed defects in NK cell function in HIV-infected individuals and likely begins to occur during primary infection. The relative expression of iNKRs and NCRs—as well as their ligands, which include HLA class I molecules—has an impact on the antiviral functions associated with NK cells, including direct killing and ADCC. Polymorphisms in iNKR and NCR alleles have been linked to HIV-1 disease outcomes, and there are indications that the early control of HIV may be mediated by cytotoxic NK cell-mediated responses. NK cells may also serve as sources of HIV-inhibitory soluble factors, including CC-chemokines such as MIP-1α (CCL3), MIP-1β (CCL4), and RANTES (CCL5). Finally, both inflammatory cytokines and alterations in the GALT of HIV infected individuals disrupt NK cells and other ILCs.

GENETIC FACTORS IN HIV-1 AND AIDS PATHOGENESIS

Candidate gene approaches and genome-wide association studies (GWAS) have identified polymorphisms in host genes that contribute to inter-individual variation in (1) the risk of acquiring HIV, (2) the steady-state levels of HIV that are established soon after infection (virologic set point), (3) the rate at which untreated HIV infection progresses to AIDS defined by a CD4+ T-cell count that is lower than 200 cells/mm^3 and/or development of AIDS-defining illnesses, (4) the level of immune reconstitution (e.g., CD4+ cell counts) achieved and risk of non-AIDS-associated diseases after initiation of virally suppressive antiretroviral therapy (ART), and (5) adverse reactions to antiretroviral agents. The key polymorphisms that influence these five outcomes are summarized in **Table 202-6**, and their identification has greatly advanced our understanding of the genes that influence HIV-AIDS pathogenesis and ART-associated immune reconstitution. Of particular interest are polymorphisms in two chromosomal regions, as they are associated with consistent effects on HIV acquisition, virologic set point, and/or rates of HIV disease progression: the region in chromosome 3 that includes the gene that encodes the HIV co-receptor *CC chemokine receptor 5* (*CCR5*) and the *major histocompatibility locus* (*MHC*) in chromosome 6 (**Fig. 202-26**).

GENETICS OF CCR5: FROM BENCH TO BEDSIDE While the discovery of CCR5 as a major co-receptor for cell entry of HIV-1 was established by in vitro studies, genetic association studies established its seminal role in HIV pathogenesis. Initial in vitro studies revealed that a 32-bp deletion (*Δ32*) in the coding region of *CCR5* contributes to resistance to CCR5 using R5 strains of HIV. The *CCR5 Δ32* allele encodes a truncated protein that is not expressed on the cell surface. Congruently, genotype-phenotype association studies in large cohorts demonstrated that individuals homozygous for the *CCR5 Δ32* allele (*Δ32/Δ32*) lack CCR5 surface expression and are highly resistant to acquiring HIV infection; heterozygosity for the *CCR5 Δ32* allele is associated with a lower risk of acquiring HIV.

The distribution of the *CCR5 Δ32* allele is population specific. Approximately 1% of individuals of European ancestry are homozygous for the *CCR5 Δ32* allele. Depending on the geographic region in Europe, up to 18% of individuals are heterozygous for the *CCR5 Δ32* allele. The *CCR5 Δ32* allele is rare in other populations. The evolutionary pressure that resulted in the emergence of the *CCR5 Δ32* allele in the European population remains unknown and has been speculated to be secondary to an ancestral pandemic, such as the plague.

Subsequent studies identified single nucleotide variants (SNVs) in the promoter (regulatory) region of *CCR5* that influence gene expression levels. Alleles bearing specific cassettes of linked polymorphisms (haplotypes) were identified and designated as human haplogroups A to G*2 (*HHA* to *HHG*2*) (Fig. 202-26). The *CCR5 Δ32* polymorphism is found on the *HHG*2* haplotype. *CCR5* haplotypes *A–D* versus *E–G*2* differ by bearing GT versus AC at polymorphic sites rs1799987 and rs1799988 (Fig. 202-26). *CCR5-HHA* haplotype represents the ancestral haplotype (found in chimpanzees) and is associated with lower *CCR5* gene expression, whereas the *CCR5-HHE* haplotype is associated with higher CCR5 expression. Methylation of DNA is a common epigenetic signaling mechanism that cells use to lock genes in the "off" position, and polymorphisms in *CCR5* haplotypes may mediate their effects by influencing DNA methylation levels in the *CCR5* locus. The *CCR5-HHE* and *CCR5-HHA* haplotypes are more sensitive and

TABLE 202-6 Host Genetic Factors Influencing HIV/AIDS Pathogenesis and Therapy Responses

GENE[a]	GENETIC VARIATION	MECHANISMS[b]	GENETIC ASSOCIATIONS[c]
Genes in MHC Locus			
HLA-B	*B*27* and *B*57*	Altered presentation of specific HIV antigens	Slower progression to AIDS; lower viral load
	*B*35*	Restriction of specific HIV peptide presentation	Faster progression to AIDS; higher viral load
	HLA-Bw4	Providing ligands for activating KIR	Slower progression to AIDS
	*B*57:01*	Altered presentation of specific HIV antigens (as above). Possible abacavir-specific activation of cytokine-producing CD8+ T cells in carriers of this allele	Slower progression to AIDS. Higher risk of abacavir-associated hypersensitivity
	HLA-B –21M allele	–21M allele enhances HLA-E expression levels, which correlates with higher HLA-A expression and inhibition of NKG2A-expressing cells	The –21M allele associates with higher viral load, reduced CD4+ counts, and accelerated disease progression
	*B*57:03* bearing the rs2523608-A allele	Altered presentation of specific HIV antigens	Variant overexpressed in HIV-1 controllers of African descent
HLA class I allele	Homozygosity of *HLA*-class I alleles	Reduced repertoire for epitope recognition	Faster progression to AIDS; increased risk of mother-to-child transmission
	Shared donor-recipient *HLA* alleles	Preadaptation of HIV strains	Faster disease progression to AIDS
	Rare *HLA* alleles	Limited adaptation of HIV strains; less frequent escape mutants	Protection against HIV infection
HLA class II allele	*HLA-DRB1* alleles	Influence protein specificity of CD4+ T-cell responses to HIV Gag and Nef proteins	*HLA-DRB1*15:02*—lower viral load *HLA-DRB1*03:01*—higher viral load
HLA extended haplotype	A1-B8-DR3-DQ2 (AH 8.1)	Increased proinflammatory responses; higher TNF-α production	Faster progression to AIDS
HLA-C	rs9264942-C allele (35 kb upstream of *HLA-C*) in linkage with rs67384697-Del	Increased expression of HLA-C by reducing binding of miRNA-148a	Decreased viral load set point
	rs5010528-G (1 kb upstream of HLA-C)	Unknown	Higher risk of developing nevirapine-associated hypersensitivity
HCP5	rs2395029-G	Linkage disequilibrium with *HLA-B*57:01*	Lower viral load and slower progression to AIDS
MICA	Noncoding SNV near *MICA*, rs4418214-T	May affect HLA class I peptide presentation—linkage with protective *HLA-B* alleles	Enriched in HIV-1 controllers
PSORS1C3	rs3131018-A	May affect HLA class I peptide presentation	Enriched in HIV-1 controllers
ZNRD1	rs9261174-C	Possible interference in processing of HIV transcripts; influence *ZNRD1* expression	Slower disease progression to AIDS
Chemokine Receptors			
CCR5	rs333: 32-bp deletion in the ORF (Δ32) found in persons of European descent	Truncated CCR5 protein; reduced co-receptor activity of R5 HIV strain	*Δ32/Δ32*: CCR5-null state associated with resistance to acquiring HIV infection
			Δ32/wild type: slower progression to AIDS; better CD4+ T-cell recovery during ART
	Promoter SNVs, haplotypes (*HHA* to *HHG*2*)	Altered CCR5 expression, e.g., HHE haplotype correlates with high CCR5 expression	HHE/HHE: increased HIV susceptibility and faster progression to AIDS
	rs1015164 G→ A (34kb downstream from *CCR5* and close to *CCRL2*)	Increases expression of the lncRNA *RP11-24-11.2*, which corresponds to an antisense transcript that overlaps CCR5 (*CCR5AS*); results in increased CCR5 expression	rs1015164A allele associated with higher viral load
CCR2	rs1799864: SNV in ORF (64 V→I)	Linkage with polymorphisms in *CCR5* promoter	64I-bearing haplotype associated with delayed progression to AIDS
CCRL2	rs3204849: SNV in ORF (167 Y→F)	SNV in linkage with *CCR5* haplotype	167F associated with accelerated progression to AIDS and PCP
CXCR6	rs2234358 G→T in the 3′UTR	Trafficking of effector T cells and activation of NK T cells; minor HIV co-receptor	Prevalence of rs2234358-T lower in long-term nonprogressors and viremic controllers of African descent
CX3CR1	SNVs in ORF: rs3732379 (249 V→I) and rs3732378 (280 T→M)	Alleles bearing 249I and 280M reduce receptor expression and binding of fractalkine, the CX3CR1 ligand	249I and 280M associated with faster AIDS progression in persons of European descent
DARC	rs2814778: promoter SNV (–46T→C) found in persons of African descent	–46C/C associated with absent *DARC* expression (Duffy null), low neutrophil counts, and altered circulating chemokine levels as well as HIV binding to RBCs and trans-infection of HIV-1	–46C/C: increased risk of acquiring HIV but slower HIV disease progression; Duffy null–associated low neutrophil trait associated with increased HIV risk
Chemokines			
CCL3L, CCL4L	Gene copy number of *CCL3L* and *CCL4L*	High numbers of *CCL3L* and *CCL4L* gene-containing segmental duplications correlate with high *CCL3L* and *CCL4L* levels	Gene copy number lower than population median associated with increased HIV-AIDS susceptibility and lower CD4+ T-cell recovery during ART
CCL5	Promoter SNVs	Altered gene expression	Influence HIV-AIDS susceptibility
CCL2	rs1024611: Promoter SNV (–2578 T→G)	–2578G allele: increased *CCL2* expression and monocyte recruitment	–2578G/G associated with increased risk of developing HIV-1–associated dementia and faster AIDS onset

(*Continued*)

TABLE 202-6 Host Genetic Factors Influencing HIV/AIDS Pathogenesis and Therapy Responses (Continued)

GENE[a]	GENETIC VARIATION	MECHANISMS[b]	GENETIC ASSOCIATIONS[c]
CXCL12	rs7919208: promoter SNV (G→A)	rs7919208A creates a new transcription factor binding site associated with increased *CXCL12* expression	rs7919208A associated with higher susceptibility to HIV-related non-Hodgkin lymphoma
Cytokines			
IL-6	rs1800795: Promoter SNV (–174 G→C)	–174G/G associated with increased IL-6 and CRP levels	–174G/G associated with high risk of KS development and variable recovery of CD4+ T cells during ART
IL-7RA	rs6897932: Coding SNV (244 T→I)	244 I/I associated with increased signal transduction and proliferation in response to IL-7	244 I/I associated with faster CD4+ T-cell recovery during ART
IL-10	rs1800872: Promoter SNV (–592 C→A),	–592A associated with decreased IL-10 levels	–592A associated with increased HIV infection risk and AIDS progression rate
Drug-Metabolizing Enzyme Gene			
CYP2B6	Multiple variants (e.g., rs3745274 [516 G→ T], i.e., *CYP2B6*6*)	*CYP2B6* variants influence enzyme activity	516T/T associated with higher risk of adverse reactions to efavirenz
Innate Immunity Genes			
MBL	Alleles defined by 3 coding SNVs	Low plasma concentration and structural variation of MBL protein	Slow progression to AIDS with heterozygosity for coding SNVs
	X allele (promoter SNV –221)	Decreased levels of MBL protein	Faster progression to AIDS with X/X genotype
APOBEC3G	rs8177832: ORF SNV (186 H→R)	Reduced anti–HIV-1 activity	186R associated with rapid AIDS progression in persons of African descent
APOBEC3F	Haplotype tagged by rs2076101 in ORF (231 I→V)	231V variant may influence Vif-mediated *APOBEC3F* degradation	231V associated with lower viral load, slower progression to AIDS and PCP
TLR7	rs179008: ORF SNV (32A→T) on Chr. X	Lower TLR7 mRNA translation efficiency and impaired TLR7-dependent IFN-α production	rs179008-T associated with lower viral load and cell-associated HIV-1 DNA in women
PARD3B	rs11884476 near exon 20 (C→G)	Direct interaction with HIV signaling through SMAD family of proteins	rs11884476-G associated with slower progression to AIDS
IFNL4	rs368234815: Frameshift mutation (TT→ΔG)	Polymorphism in *IFNL4* gene in linkage with a *IFNL3* variant; this haplotype influences *IFNL3* levels	rs368234815-ΔG associated with higher prevalence of AIDS-defining illnesses and potentially increased HIV-1 infection risk
	rs8099917 T→G	Unknown	rs8099917-G associated with higher susceptibility to KS
Others			
ApoE	E4 allele defined by two coding SNVs	ApoE is an HIV-1–inducible inhibitor of HIV-1 replication and infectivity in macrophages	E4/E4 associated with rapid AIDS progression and HIV-associated dementia
ApoL1/MYH9	Several risk haplotypes, including G1	Overexpression of the *ApoL1* kidney risk variants may increase kidney cell death	Increased risk for HIV-associated nephropathy
RYR3	rs2229116: ORF SNV (A →G)	Unknown; potential impact on calcium signaling and homeostasis	rs2229116-G associated with subclinical atherosclerosis during ART
PROX1	rs17762192-G; 36kb upstream of *PROX1*	Unknown; presumably due to its impact on *PROX1* expression, which is a negative regulator of IFN-γ	rs17762192-G associated with reduced rate of HIV disease progression
Gene–Gene Interaction			
KIR+HLA	*KIR3DS1* interaction with *HLA-Bw4-80Ile*	Altered NK cell activity required to eliminate HIV-infected cells	*KIR3DS1/HLA-Bw4-80Ile* associated with delayed AIDS onset
	KIR2DL3 interaction with *HLA-C1*	Reduction of inhibitory KIR likely results in increased immune activation, impaired killing of latently infected cells, and a higher proviral burden	*HLA-C1*[+] *KIR2DL*[+] associated with better immune recovery during ART
	KIR3DL1 I47V interaction with *HLA-B*57:01*	Variation in an immune NK cell receptor that binds *B*57:01*, modifying the protective effect of *B*57:01*	Increasing copy numbers of 47V associated with lower viral load in persons carrying *HLA-B*57*
LILRB2+HLA	*LILRB2* interaction with HLA class I	Regulation of dendritic cells by *LILRB2-HLA* engagement	Control of HIV-1
CCL3L1+ CCR5	Low *CCL3L1* gene copies + detrimental *CCR5* genotypes	Low *CCL3L1* and high *CCR5* expression	Increased HIV/AIDS susceptibility and reduced immune reconstitution during ART

[a]Representative genes and polymorphisms and [b]possible mechanisms are listed. [c]Some of the associations are population specific and may display cohort-specific effects. Most of the associations were derived from persons of European descent.

Note: APOBEC, apolipoprotein B mRNA editing enzyme, catalytic polypeptide-like; ApoE, apolipoprotein E; ApoL1, apolipoprotein L1; ART, antiretroviral therapy; CCL, CC ligand; CCL3L, CCL3-like; CCR5, CC chemokine receptor 5; CCR5AS, CCR5 antisense RNA; CCRL2, CC chemokine receptor like 2; CRP, C-reactive protein; CYP2B6, cytochrome P450 family 2 subfamily B member 6; CXCL12, chemokine (C-X-C motif) ligand 12; CXCR6, chemokine (C-X-C motif) receptor 6; CX3CR1, chemokine (C-X3-C motif) receptor 1; DARC, Duffy antigen receptor for chemokines; Del, deletion; HCP5, HLA class I histocompatibility antigen protein P5; HHE, human haplogroup E; HLA, human leukocyte antigen; IFN, interferon; IFNL4, interferon λ4 gene; IFNL3, interferon λ3 gene; IL, interleukin; IL-7RA, interleukin 7 receptor-α; KIR, killer cell immunoglobulin-like receptors; KS, Kaposi sarcoma; LILRB2, leukocyte immunoglobulin-like receptor B2; MBL, mannose-binding lectin; MHC, major histocompatibility complex; MICA, MHC class I polypeptide-related sequence A; MYH9, myosin heavy chain 9; NK, natural killer; ORF, open reading frame; PARD3B, par-3 family cell polarity regulator beta; PCP, *Pneumocystis jirovecii* pneumonia; PROX1, prospero homeobox 1; PSORS1C3, psoriasis susceptibility 1 candidate 3; RYR3, ryanodine receptor 3; SMAD, mothers against decapentaplegic homolog; SNV, single nucleotide variant; rs#, SNV identification number; TLR7, toll-like receptor 7; TNF-α, tumor necrosis factor α; UTR, untranslated region; VL, viral load; ZNRD1, zinc ribbon domain containing 1; +, present; –, absent.

Sources: Sunil K. Ahuja, MD, Weijing He, MD, Reviews for additional information: P An et al: Trends Genet 26:119, 2010; J Fellay: Antivir Ther 14:731, 2009; RA Kaslow et al: J Infect Dis 191:S68, 2005; D van Manen et al: Retrovirology 9:70, 2012; MP Martin et al: Immunol Rev 254:245, 2013; S Limou et al: Front Immunol 4:118, 2013; PJ McLaren et al: Curr Opin HIV AIDS 10:110, 2015; PJ McLaren et al: Proc Natl Acad Sci USA 112:14658, 2015; PJ McLaren, M Carrington: Nat Immunol 16:577, 2015; P An et al: PLoS Genet 12:e1005921, 2016; F Pereyra et al: Science 330:1551, 2010; I Bartha et al: PLoS Comput Biol 13:e1005339, 2017; S Kulkarni et al: Nat Immunol 20:824, 2019; S Le Clerc et al: Front Genet 10:799 2019; V Kalidasan et al: Front Microbiol 11:46 2020; SN Gingras et al: Hum Genet 139:865 2020.

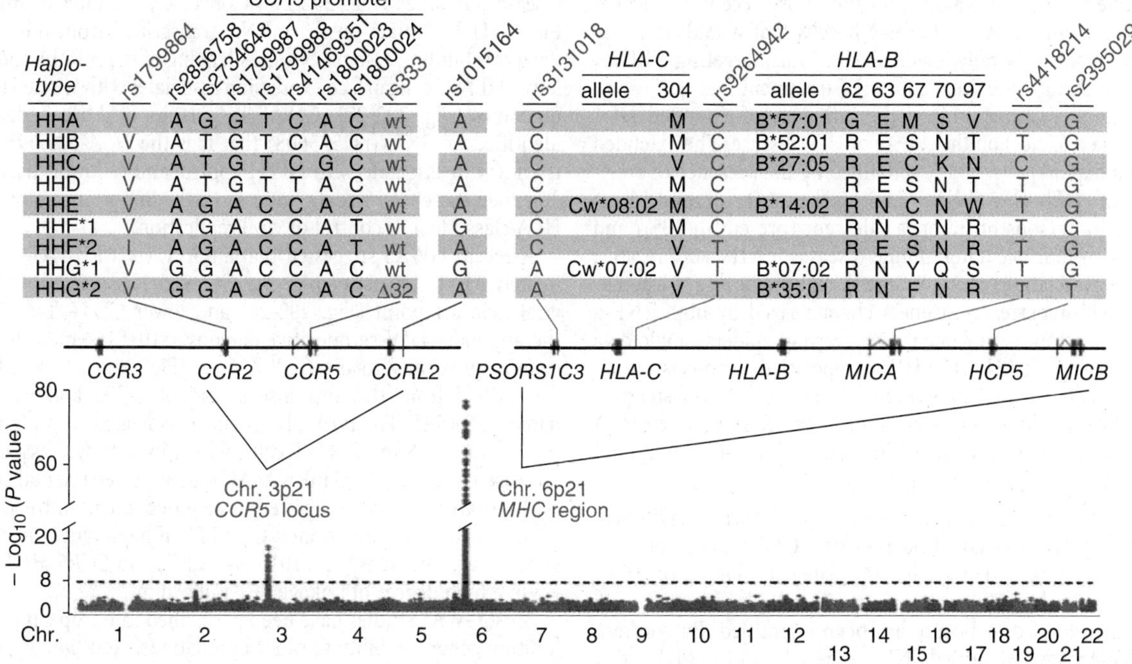

FIGURE 202-26 Schema depicting haplotypes within two regions that contribute significantly to HIV-AIDS susceptibility. *Top:* Haplotypes (Left, *CCR5*; Right, HLA alleles). *Bottom:* GWAS Manhattan plots schematized. Chr: chromosome. *Horizontal dotted line:* genome level significance threshold.

resistant, respectively, to T-cell activation–induced demethylation of the *CCR5* locus.

In worldwide populations, *HHE* and *HHC* are prevalent haplotypes, whereas the ancestral *HHA* haplotype is more common in persons of African ancestry. The associations of *CCR5* haplotypes with HIV acquisition and/or HIV disease course are largely consistent with their effects on *CCR5* gene expression. For example, homozygosity for the *CCR5-HHE* haplotype is associated with an increased risk of acquiring HIV, progressing rapidly to AIDS, and reduced immune recovery during ART. The *HHA* haplotype is associated with slower disease progression in African populations and has been speculated to be a basis for why chimpanzees (who all carry the ancestral *CCR5-HHA* haplotype) naturally infected with simian immunodeficiency virus resist disease progression. The pairing of the *HHC* and *CCR5 Δ32*-bearing *HHG*2* haplotypes (*HHC/HHG*2* genotype) is associated with a lower risk of acquiring HIV infection and slower rate of HIV disease progression, whereas the pairing of the *HHE* haplotype with the *HHG*2* haplotype is associated with the opposite effects. The *CCR2*-64I–bearing *HHF*2* haplotype is associated with a slower HIV disease course.

Consistent with these genetic associations, polymorphisms in genes encoding ligands for CCR5 have also been associated with variable HIV susceptibility and disease progression rates. Examples include copy number variations of *CCL3L1* and SNVs in *CCL5*. The sum of these studies established a pivotal role of CCR5 and its ligands in HIV-AIDS pathogenesis and, potentially, immune recovery.

The discovery that the *CCR5 Δ32/Δ32* genotype is associated with strong resistance to HIV infection, and that uninfected persons bearing this genotype did not appear to have impaired immunity, led to the development of two kinds of novel therapies. First, it spurred the development of a new class of therapies approved by the U.S. Food and Drug Administration: entry inhibitors (e.g., maraviroc) that block the interaction of CCR5 with the HIV envelope. Second, it led to the evaluation of novel experimental cellular therapies. An HIV-infected patient with acute myelogenous leukemia was given an allogeneic stem cell transplantation from an HLA-compatible person whose cells lacked expression of CCR5 due to the *Δ32/Δ32* genotype. There was no evidence of HIV-1 infection for 13 years in the patient who underwent the transplant; the patient eventually died due to recurrence of leukemia. This observation provided a proof of concept for an HIV cure and led to the development of additional novel cellular therapies involving autologous transplantation of CD4+ T cells in which the *CCR5* gene is inactivated ex vivo using new gene editing procedures. Similar cellular strategies have had mixed success, mainly due to the latent viral reservoir in various tissues.

DISCOVERY OF HLA CLASS I ALLELES THAT ASSOCIATE WITH VIROLOGIC CONTROL OF HIV INFECTION There is a strong association between variations within the *HLA-B* gene with protective (e.g., *HLA-B*57* and *HLA-B*27* alleles) or detrimental (e.g., *HLA-B*35* allele) outcomes during HIV infection. Carriage of the *HLA-B*57* and/or *HLA-B*27* alleles is associated with slower disease progression. The beneficial effects of these alleles may relate in part to their associations with a lower virologic set point as well as to higher cell-mediated immunity in HIV-infected persons. The protective effect of the *HLA-B*57* and *HLA-B*27* alleles on the HIV disease course is underscored by the finding that the prevalence of these alleles is higher among persons with long-term nonprogression and persons who control HIV replication spontaneously (elite controllers). In contrast, the *HLA-B*35* allele has been associated with faster progression to AIDS and higher viral load. The prevalence of the *HLA-B* alleles differs between populations. *HLA-B*57:01* in Europeans and *HLA-B*57:03* in persons of African descent are the protective alleles. In some populations (e.g., Japanese) where the *HLA-B*57/HLA-B*27* alleles are absent, *HLA-B*51* is associated with a protective phenotype.

Possession of the protective *HLA-B* alleles is associated with broader and stronger CD8+ T-cell responses to HIV epitopes. The mechanisms underlying the differential effects of the *HLA-B* alleles on the course of HIV disease may relate to differences in the ability of antigen-presenting cells to present immunodominant HIV epitopes to T helper or cytotoxic T lymphocytes in the context of MHC-encoded molecules. This may result in differential immune responses that influence viral replication. In this regard, the *HLA-B* alleles that impact the course of HIV disease differ in their amino acid residues in the HLA-B peptide-binding groove; this difference may play a critical role in virologic control.

The *HLA-B –21M* allele does not influence *HLA-B* gene expression; however, it is in linkage with *HLA-B* haplotypes that are associated with higher *HLA-A* and *HLA-E* expression. Higher *HLA-A* levels associate with poorer control of HIV as well as higher viral load, reduced CD4+ T-cell counts, and accelerated progression to AIDS. HLA-E is the ligand for natural killer (NK) cell NKG2A, an inhibitory receptor. Engagement of NKG2A with HLA-E inhibits NK cells that would normally be potent eliminators of virally infected cells. Thus, targeting NKG2A might provide a therapeutic avenue for HIV treatment.

Investigators have also examined the influence of extended *HLA* haplotypes (linked alleles) on the course of HIV disease. The extended *HLA* ancestral haplotype (AH) 8.1 is defined by the presence of *HLA-A1*, *HLA-B8*, and *HLA-DR3* alleles. AH 8.1 is the most common ancestral haplotype in persons of European descent (present in 10%) and is associated with multiple autoimmune diseases in HIV-seronegative persons. These associations of AH 8.1 are thought to be due to a genetically determined hyperresponsiveness characterized by high TNF-α production and lack of complement C4A. Strong epidemiologic data indicate that carriage of AH 8.1 in HIV-seropositive persons is associated with a rapid decline in the number of CD4+ T cells and faster progression to AIDS development. Gene–gene interactions between HLA alleles and other genes (e.g., killer cell immunoglobulin-like receptors) also may influence HIV disease progression rates.

POLYMORPHISMS IDENTIFIED BY GWAS THAT ASSOCIATE WITH VIROLOGIC CONTROL AND DISEASE PROGRESSION GWAS have not identified additional genetic variations that associate with the risk of HIV-1 acquisition, presumably due to a paucity of well-characterized risk cohorts in which level of exposure has been quantified. By contrast, large-scale GWAS have identified SNVs, especially in the MHC, that influence HIV viral load, including in a large group of individuals termed "HIV controllers (including elite controllers)" who spontaneously (without ART) control viral replication. GWAS in HIV-infected persons of European ancestry identified four SNVs in genes in the HLA class I loci that associated with virologic control. These SNVs are within or in the vicinity of *PSORS1C3*, *HLA-C*, *MICA*, and *HCP5* genes (Fig. 202-26). As noted in this figure, the individual effects of these alleles are difficult to discern because of linkage disequilibrium. The protective effects of the SNVs in *HCP5* and *MICA* may relate to their linkage with known protective *HLA-B* alleles. The protective *HCP5* allele is in linkage disequilibrium with the *HLA-B*57:01* allele, and the protective *MICA* allele tags with the *HLA-B*57:01* and *HLA-B*27:05* alleles. The protective *HLA-C* SNV is associated with higher HLA-C expression, which has been associated with viral control and better HIV outcomes. This protective SNV (rs9264942; T→C) resides 35 kb upstream of the *HLA-C* gene and is in strong linkage disequilibrium with a 3′-UTR indel263 SNV (rs67384697; G→deletion), generating the T-G or C-deletion haplotypes (**Fig. 202-27**). miR-148a binds to the 3′-UTR region encompassing the rs67384697 SNV and silences *HLA-C* expression. Binding of miR-148a to the 3′-UTR is disrupted on the mRNA transcribed from the C-deletion haplotype; this disruption associates with less silencing of the mRNA and therefore higher HLA-C cell surface expression, which associates with better HIV disease outcomes (Fig. 202-27). Conversely, binding of miR-148a to the 3′-UTR is intact on the mRNA transcribed from the T-G haplotype; this binding associates with silencing of the mRNA and therefore lower HLA-C cell surface expression associates with worse HIV disease outcomes (Fig. 202-27). GWAS in persons of African descent have identified an SNV (rs2523608) that tags the *HLA-B*57:03* allele that is known to associate with HIV-1 control and a slower disease course. Together, these GWAS data underscore the importance of variations in HLA class I loci in control of viral replication.

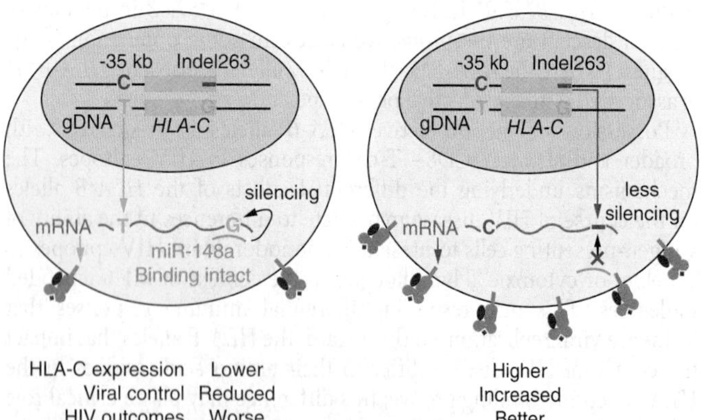

FIGURE 202-27 Linkage disequilibrium between two variants in the HLA-C locus and their influence on binding of miR-148a to the 3′-untranslated region (UTR). Altered binding of miR-148a associates with HLA-C protein expression levels and, in turn, viral control and HIV disease outcomes. Effects associated with T-G (left) and C-del (right) haplotypes are depicted. C-del: C-deletion. The C-deletion haplotype prevents binding of miR-148a to 3′-UTR of HLA-C (less silencing). Kb, kilobase.

A recent GWAS suggested that an SNV (rs1015164G→A) approximately 34 kb downstream of the *CCR5* loci associated with a higher viral load set point (Fig. 202-26) and lower CD4+ T-cell counts in therapy-naïve HIV-seropositive persons. rs1015164 maps to a lncRNA gene in proximity to the *CCRL2* gene (Fig. 202-26). The lncRNA is transcribed from the antisense strand of *CCR5* and was therefore named *CCR5AS*. The rs1015164A allele associated with higher expression of *CCR5AS* in CD4+ T cells, which in turn was associated with increased levels of *CCR5* mRNA. Although the detrimental effect of the rs1015164A allele was suggested to be independent of the detrimental effects of the abovementioned *CCR5-HHE* haplotype, further investigation is warranted as the rs1015164A allele and *CCR5-HHE* haplotype are in a high degree of linkage disequilibrium.

Most GWAS studies have been performed in European populations, limiting generalizability to other populations. Additionally, GWAS are generally not suitable for identifying rare variants (<1% prevalence). Therefore, next-generation sequencing (NGS) approaches were suggested to identify these rare variants. However, a recent NGS study suggests that exonic variants with large effect sizes are unlikely to have a major contribution to host control of HIV infection. Mathematical modeling revealed that variations in host genes may explain about 10% of the observed variability in HIV viral load, whereas viral genetic diversity may explain 29% of the variability.

GENETIC ASSOCIATIONS WITH SPECIFIC AIDS AND NON-AIDS CONDITIONS

Carotid artery disease Many of the non-AIDS events in HIV-seropositive individuals resemble those attributable to immune senescence and those found in the HIV-seronegative aging population. A functional SNV in the ryanodine receptor 3 (*RYR3*) gene was found to be associated with an increased risk of common carotid intima–media thickness (cIMT), which is a surrogate for subclinical atherosclerosis. Functional studies on *RYR3* and its isoforms demonstrate a major role of these receptors in modulating endothelial function and atherogenesis via calcium-signaling pathways, providing a biologically plausible mechanism by which the SNV in *RYR3* may associate with increased cIMT risk.

Kidney disease HIV-1–associated nephropathy (HIVAN) is a form of focal sclerosing glomerulonephritis caused by direct infection of kidney epithelial cells with HIV. HIVAN is more common in persons of African descent. There is evidence that polymorphisms in the *MYH9* gene and in the neighboring *APOL1* gene are a strong determinant of susceptibility to HIVAN in persons of African descent. The effect of carrying two *APOL1* risk alleles explains nearly 35% of HIVAN. Overexpression of the *APOL1* kidney risk variants may associate with increased kidney cell death.

HIV-associated neurocognitive disorder HIV-associated neurocognitive disorder (HAND) comprises a spectrum of neurocognitive deficits due to HIV infection. Variations in the apolipoprotein E (*ApoE*) gene have strong associations with Alzheimer's disease in the HIV-seronegative population. In HIV-seropositive persons, possession of the *E4/E4* genotype has been associated with dementia, peripheral neuropathy, and impairment in cognition as well as immediate and delayed verbal memory. Macrophage recruitment and activation play a central role in the development of many of the HAND syndromes. Variations in chemokines that play an influential role in macrophage activation and recruitment, namely *CCL2* (*MCP-1*) and *CCL3* (*MIP-1α*), have been shown to influence the risk of developing HAND. Variations in mitochondrial genes also have been associated with a risk of AIDS and

HAND. A GWAS identified a polymorphism in chromosome 14 in the T-cell receptor α locus that may influence neurocognitive outcomes.

HIV-1-associated *Pneumocystis* pneumonia Human Apobec3 cytidine deaminases are intrinsic resistance factors to HIV-1. However, HIV-1 encodes a viral infectivity factor (Vif) that degrades *APOBEC3* proteins. Association studies suggest a role of genetic variations in the APOBEC3 family in HIV disease. A common haplotype derived from 6 SNVs in the *APOBEC3F* gene and tagged by a codon-changing variant is associated with a significantly lower viral load set point, slower rate of progression to AIDS, and delayed development of *Pneumocystis jirovecii* pneumonia (PCP). In addition, a coding SNV in the *CCRL2* gene is associated with accelerated progression to AIDS and rapid development of PCP.

HIV-related non-Hodgkin lymphoma (NHL) The relative risk of developing NHL in HIV-seropositive persons is highly elevated compared with the general population. NHL represents approximately 34% of all identified cancers in HIV-seropositive persons. A recent GWAS identified a promoter SNV in the *CXCL12* gene that was associated with higher susceptibility to develop HIV-related NHL. The effect of this SNV is likely causal as it creates new transcription factor binding sites, impacting *CXCL12* expression.

ASSOCIATIONS WITH ART-RELATED ADVERSE EVENTS Abacavir, an effective antiretroviral agent, is associated with significant risk of hypersensitivity reactions (2–9% of cases). Interestingly, while the *HLA-B*57:01* allele is associated with a slower HIV disease course, possession of this allele is associated with a higher risk of abacavir-associated hypersensitivity, possibly due to the abacavir-specific activation of cytokine-producing CD8+ T cells only in *HLA-B*57:01* carriers. Pharmacogenetic screening for the *HLA-B*57:01* allele is recommended before initiation of abacavir treatment.

The antiretroviral agent nevirapine is associated with hypersensitivity reactions in 6–10% of patients, including Stevens–Johnson syndrome (SJS) and toxic epidermal necrolysis (TEN). rs5010528G, a strong proxy for *HLA-C*04:01* carriage, was associated with high risk of SJS and TEN during nevirapine treatment. In addition, efavirenz was among the first antiretroviral agents to be co-formulated into single-pill regimens for mass rollout globally. Several genetic variants in the drug-metabolizing enzyme CYP2B6 have been associated with high efavirenz plasma concentrations and increased risk of adverse neuropsychiatric effects. For example, homozygosity for one such variant, rs3745274 T/T, increases the risk of adverse reactions to efavirenz up to five folds, and this risk genotype is much more common in Africans (13.7%) than Europeans (5.6%).

NEUROPATHOGENESIS IN HIV DISEASE

While there has been a remarkable decrease in the incidence of the severe forms of HIV encephalopathy among those with access to treatment in the era of effective ART, HIV-infected individuals can still experience milder forms of neurocognitive impairment despite adequate ART. Factors that contribute to the neurocognitive decline include lack of complete control of HIV replication in the brain; production of HIV proteins that may be neurotoxic; low CD4+ T-cell nadir; chronic immune activation; comorbidities such as drug abuse, microvascular disease, older age, and diabetes; and the potential for neurotoxicity of certain antiretroviral drugs. HIV has been demonstrated in the brain and CSF of infected individuals with and without neuropsychiatric abnormalities. As opposed to lymphoid tissues, there are no resident lymphocytes in the brain. The main cell types that are infected in the brain in vivo are the perivascular macrophages and the microglial cells, which can sometimes form syncytia resulting in multinucleated giant cells; low-level viral replication is also seen in perivascular astrocytes. It has been proposed that monocytes that have already been infected in the blood can migrate into the brain, where they then reside as macrophages, or macrophages can be directly infected while residing within the brain. The precise mechanisms whereby HIV enters the brain are unclear; however, they are thought to relate, at least in part, to the ability of virus-infected and immune-activated macrophages to induce adhesion molecules such as E-selectin and vascular cell adhesion molecule 1 (VCAM-1) on brain endothelium. Other studies have demonstrated that HIV gp120 enhances the expression of intercellular adhesion molecule 1 (ICAM-1) in glial cells and HIV Tat protein can disrupt the tight junctions of the brain endothelial cells to facilitate entry of HIV-infected cells into the CNS. Virus isolates from the brain are preferentially R5 strains as opposed to X4 strains; in this regard, HIV-infected individuals who are heterozygous for *CCR5-Δ32* appear to be relatively protected against the development of HIV encephalopathy. Once HIV enters the brain due to pressures of the local environment, it evolves to develop distinct sequences in the env, tat, and LTR genes. These unique sequences have been associated with neurocognitive dysfunction; however, it is unclear if they are causal (see below).

HIV-infected individuals may manifest white matter lesions as well as neuronal loss. The white matter lesions are due to axonal injury and a disruption of the blood-brain barrier and not due to demyelination. Given the absence of evidence of HIV infection of neurons, HIV-mediated effects on neurons are thought to involve indirect pathways whereby viral proteins, particularly gp120 and Tat, trigger the release of endogenous neurotoxins from macrophages and to a lesser extent from astrocytes. In addition, it has been demonstrated that both HIV-1 Nef and Tat can induce chemotaxis of leukocytes, including monocytes, into the CNS. Neurotoxins can be released from monocytes as a consequence of infection and/or immune activation. Monocyte-derived neurotoxic factors have been reported to kill neurons via a variety of mechanisms including activation of the *N*-methyl-D-aspartate (NMDA) receptors and induction of oxidative stress. In addition, HIV gp120 shed by virus-infected monocytes could cause neurotoxicity by antagonizing the function of vasoactive intestinal peptide (VIP), by elevating intracellular calcium levels, and by decreasing neurotrophic factor levels in the cerebral cortex. A variety of monocyte-derived cytokines can contribute directly or indirectly to the neurotoxic effects in HIV infection; these include TNF-α, IL-1, IL-6, TGF-β, IFN-γ, platelet-activating factor, and endothelin. Furthermore, among the CC-chemokines, elevated levels of monocyte chemotactic protein-1 (MCP-1 or CCL-2) in the brain and CSF have been shown to correlate best with the presence and degree of HIV encephalopathy in ART-naïve patients. In addition, infection and/or activation of monocyte-lineage cells can result in increased production of eicosanoids, quinolinic acid, nitric oxide, excitatory amino acids such as L-cysteine and glutamate, arachidonic acid, platelet-activating factor, free radicals, TNF-α, and TGF-β, which may contribute to neurotoxicity. Astrocytes may play diverse roles in HIV neuropathogenesis. Reactive gliosis or astrocytosis has been demonstrated in the brains of HIV-infected individuals, and TNF-α and IL-6 have been shown to induce astrocyte proliferation. In addition, astrocyte-derived IL-6 can induce HIV expression in infected cells in vitro. Furthermore, it has been suggested that astrocytes may downregulate macrophage-produced neurotoxins. Evidence of neuronal injury can be demonstrated by measuring neurofilament levels in CSF. Treatment with ART leads to improvement in neuropsychiatric manifestations and a decrease in these cytokine levels in CSF, suggesting that they are driven by the virus or by its products. However, even in patients on long-term ART, there may be evidence of persistently activated lymphocytes in the CSF. It is unclear if these lymphocytes may contribute to neuronal injury in the brain or are critical for controlling the CNS viral reservoir. However, some individuals may develop a subacute encephalitis due to an IRIS reaction (see below). This often occurs weeks or a few months after initiation of ART in individuals with low CD4+ T-cell counts. It is thought that the recovery of CD4+ T cells causes a lymphocyte response to the CNS HIV reservoir. The contribution of host genetic factors to development of neuropsychiatric manifestations of HIV infection has not been well studied. However, evidence supports the role of several genetic factors including the E4 allele for apoE in an increased risk of HIV-associated neurocognitive disorders and peripheral neuropathy.

It has also been suggested that the CNS may serve as a relatively sequestered site for a reservoir of latently infected cells that might be a barrier for the eradication of virus by ART (see "The HIV Reservoir: Obstacles to the Eradication of Virus," above).

■ PATHOGENESIS OF KAPOSI'S SARCOMA

There are at least four distinct epidemiologic forms of KS: (1) the classic form that occurs in older men of predominantly Mediterranean or eastern European Jewish backgrounds with no recognized contributing factors; (2) the equatorial African form that occurs in all ages, also without any recognized precipitating factors; (3) the form associated with organ transplantation and its attendant iatrogenic immunosuppressed state; and (4) the form associated with HIV-1 infection. In the latter two forms, KS is an opportunistic disease; in HIV-infected individuals, unlike typical opportunistic infections, its occurrence is not strictly related to the level of depression of CD4+ T-cell counts. The pathogenesis of KS is complex; fundamentally, it is an angioproliferative disease that is not a true neoplastic sarcoma, at least not in its early stages. It is a manifestation of excessive proliferation of spindle cells that are believed to be of vascular origin and have features in common with endothelial and smooth-muscle cells. In HIV disease the development of KS is dependent on the interplay of a variety of factors including HIV-1 itself, human herpes virus 8 (HHV-8), immune activation, and cytokine secretion. Numerous epidemiologic and virologic studies have clearly linked HHV-8, which is also referred to as *Kaposi's sarcoma–associated herpesvirus* (KSHV), to KS not only in HIV-infected individuals but also in individuals with the other forms of KS. HHV-8 is a γ-herpesvirus related to EBV and *herpesvirus saimiri*. It encodes a homologue to human IL-6 and, in addition to KS, has been implicated in the pathogenesis of body cavity lymphoma, multiple myeloma, and monoclonal gammopathy of undetermined significance. Sequences of HHV-8 are found universally in the lesions of KS, and patients with KS are virtually all seropositive for HHV-8. HHV-8 DNA sequences can be found in the B cells of 30–50% of patients with KS and 7% of patients with AIDS without clinically apparent KS.

Between 1 and 2% of eligible blood donors are positive for antibodies to HHV-8, while the prevalence of HHV-8 seropositivity in HIV-infected men is 30–35%. The prevalence of HHV-8 seropositivity in HIV-infected women is ~4%. This finding is reflective of the lower incidence of KS in women. It has been debated whether HHV-8 is the transforming agent in KS; the bulk of the cells in the tumor lesions of KS are not neoplastic cells. However, it has been demonstrated that endothelial cells can be transformed in vitro by HHV-8. In this regard, HHV-8 possesses genes, including homologues of the IL-8 receptor, Bcl-2, and cyclin D, that can potentially transform the host cell. Despite the complexity of the pathogenic events associated with the development of KS in HIV-infected individuals, HHV-8 is the etiologic agent of this disease. The initiation and/or propagation of KS requires an activated state and is mediated, at least in part, by cytokines. A number of factors, including TNF-α, IL-1β, IL-6, granulocyte-macrophage colony-stimulating factor (GM-CSF), basic fibroblast growth factor, and oncostatin M, function in an autocrine and paracrine manner to sustain the growth and chemotaxis of the KS spindle cells. In this regard, KSHV-derived IL-6 has been demonstrated to induce proliferation of lymphoma cells and to inhibit the cytostatic effects of IFN-α on KSHV-infected lymphoma cells.

IMMUNE RESPONSE TO HIV

As detailed above and below, following the initial burst of viremia during primary infection, HIV-infected individuals mount robust immune responses that in most cases substantially curtail the levels of plasma viremia and likely contribute to delaying the ultimate development of clinically apparent disease for a median of 10 years in untreated individuals. This immune response contains elements of both humoral and cell-mediated immunity involving both adaptive and innate immune responses (Table 202-7; Fig. 202-28). It is directed against multiple antigenic determinants of the HIV virion as well as against viral proteins expressed on the surface of infected cells. Ironically, those CD4+ T cells with T-cell receptors specific for HIV are theoretically those CD4+ T cells most likely to be activated—and thus to serve as early targets for productive HIV infection and the cell death or dysfunction associated with infection. Thus, an early consequence of HIV infection is interference with and decrease of the helper T-cell population needed to generate an effective immune response.

TABLE 202-7 Elements of the Immune Response to HIV

Humoral immunity
Binding antibodies
Neutralizing antibodies
Type specific
Group specific
Broadly neutralizing
Antibodies participating in antibody-dependent cellular cytotoxicity (ADCC)
Protective
Pathogenic (bystander killing)
Enhancing antibodies
Complement
Cell-mediated immunity
Helper CD4+ T lymphocytes
Class I MHC–restricted cytotoxic CD8+ T lymphocytes
CD8+ T-cell–mediated inhibition (noncytolytic)
ADCC
Natural killer cells

Abbreviation: MHC, major histocompatibility complex.

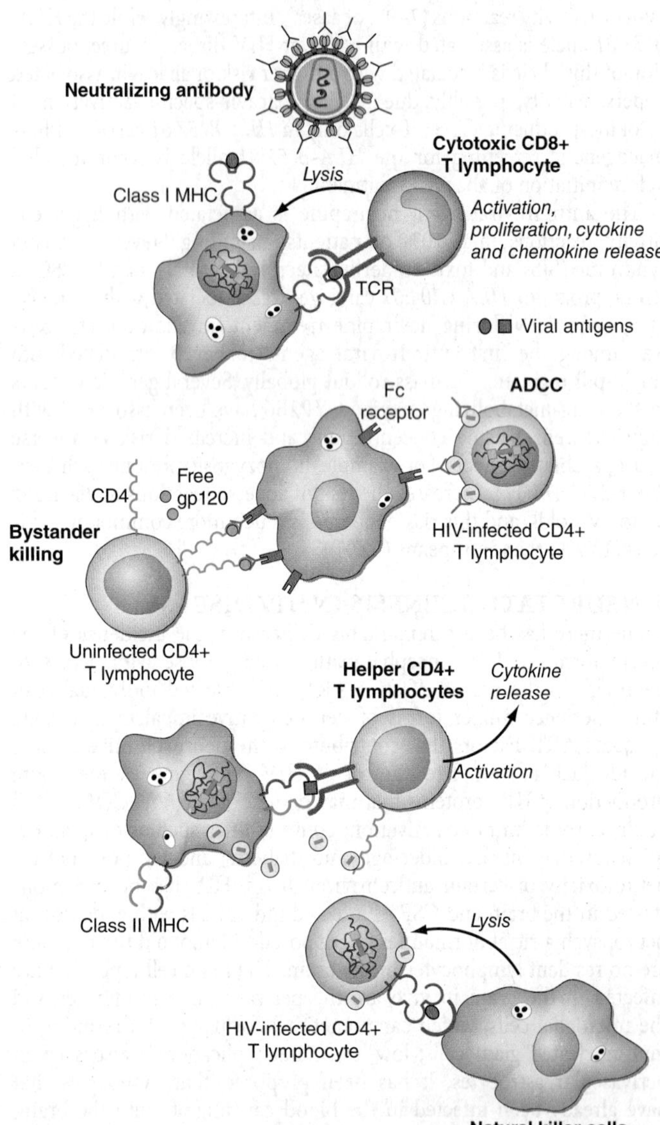

FIGURE 202-28 Schematic representation of the different immunologic effector mechanisms thought to be active in the setting of HIV infection. Detailed descriptions are given in the text. ADCC, antibody-dependent cellular cytotoxicity; MHC, major histocompatibility complex; TCR, T-cell receptor.

Although a great deal of investigation has been directed toward delineating and better understanding the components of this immune response, it remains unclear which immunologic effector mechanisms are most important in delaying progression of infection and which, if any, play a role in the pathogenesis of HIV disease. This lack of knowledge has also hampered the ability to develop an effective vaccine for HIV disease.

HUMORAL IMMUNE RESPONSE

Antibodies to HIV usually appear within 3–6 weeks and almost invariably within 12 weeks of primary infection (**Fig. 202-29**); rare exceptions are in individuals who have defects in the ability to produce HIV-specific antibodies. Detection of these antibodies forms the basis of many diagnostic screening tests for HIV infection. The appearance of HIV-binding antibodies detected by ELISA and Western blot assays occurs prior to the appearance of neutralizing antibodies; the latter generally appear following the initial decreases in plasma viremia and are more closely related to the appearance of HIV-specific CD8+ T lymphocytes. The first antibodies detected are those directed against the immunodominant region of the envelope gp41, followed by the appearance of antibodies to the structural or gag protein p24 and the gag precursor p55. Antibodies to p24 gag are followed by the appearance of antibodies to the outer envelope glycoprotein (gp120), the gag protein p17, and the products of the *pol* gene (p31 and p66). In addition, one may see antibodies to the low-molecular-weight regulatory proteins encoded by the HIV genes *vpr*, *vpu*, *vif*, *rev*, *tat*, and *nef*. On rare occasions, levels of HIV-specific antibodies may decline during treatment of acute HIV infection.

While antibodies to multiple antigens of HIV are produced, the precise functional significance of these different antibodies is unclear. The only viral proteins that elicit neutralizing antibodies are the envelope proteins gp120 and gp41. Antibodies directed toward the envelope proteins of HIV have been characterized both as being protective and as possibly contributing to the pathogenesis of HIV disease. Among the protective antibodies are those that function to neutralize HIV directly and prevent the spread of infection to additional cells, as well as those that participate in ADCC. The first neutralizing antibodies are directed against the autologous infecting virus and appear after approximately 12 to 24 weeks of infection. Due to its high rate of mutation the virus is usually able to quickly escape these (and subsequent) neutralizing antibodies. One important mechanism of immune escape is the addition of N-linked glycosylation sites, forming a glycan shield that interferes with envelope recognition by these initial antibodies.

A number of broad and potent HIV-neutralizing envelope-specific antibodies have been isolated from HIV-infected individuals in studies

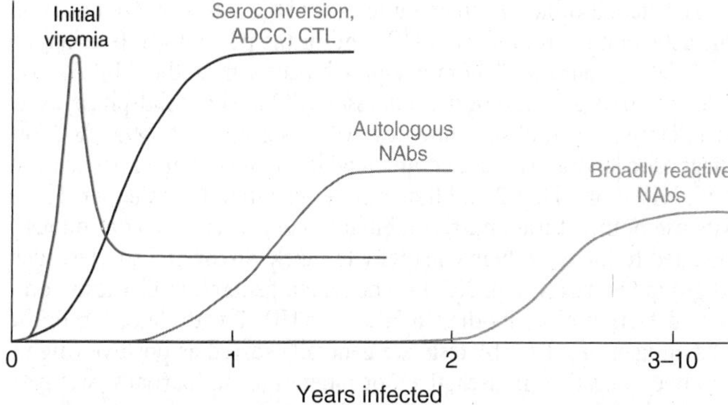

FIGURE 202-29 Relationship between initial HIV viremia and the development of antibodies to HIV. Within 3 to 6 weeks of initial HIV infection, nonneutralizing antibodies to HIV appear. These antibodies are capable of mediating antibody-dependent cellular cytotoxicity (ADCC). The decline in plasma viremia generally correlates with the appearance of cytotoxic T lymphocytes (CTL). After approximately 3 months, autologous neutralizing antibodies (NAbs) capable of neutralizing prior circulating strains of HIV appear. After 2 or more years, broadly reactive NAbs appear. *(Republished with permission of Annual Reviews, Inc. from The Role of Antibodies in HIV Vaccines, JR Mascola and DC Monteori, 28:413, 2010; permission conveyed through Copyright Clearance Center, Inc.)*

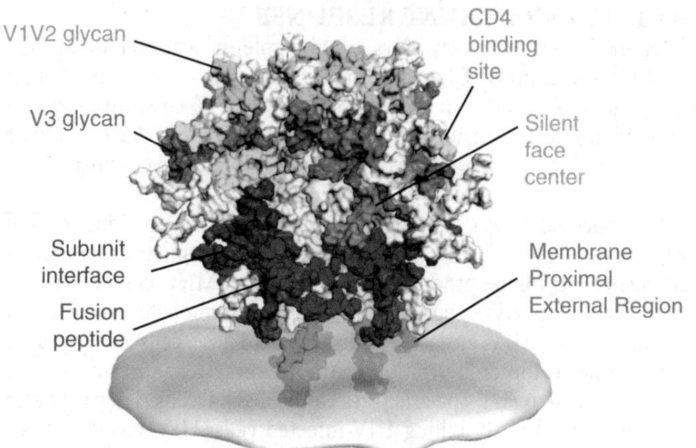

FIGURE 202-30 Known targets of broadly neutralizing antibodies against HIV-1. *(Courtesy of J Stuckey, GY Chuang.)*

designed to better understand the host response to HIV infection. Approximately 20% of patients develop antibodies capable of neutralizing highly diverse strains. These usually appear 2 or more years following infection in the face of continual viremia. These studies have revealed at least five major sites within the HIV envelope trimer that are able to elicit broadly neutralizing antibodies. These sites include antibodies directed toward the CD4 binding site (CD4bs) of gp120, those binding glycan-dependent epitopes in the V1/V2 region of gp120, those near the base of the V3 region of gp120, those binding to the gp120/gp41 bridge, and those binding to the membrane-proximal region of gp41 (**Fig. 202-30**). Several of these antibodies contain unique features including high levels of somatic hypermutation, selective germline gene usage (especially for CD4bs antibodies), and long heavy chain complementary determining regions (especially CDRH3). Of note, while these antibodies are broadly neutralizing in vitro, their precise in vivo significance is unclear and the patients from whom they were derived demonstrate evidence of ongoing viral replication unless treated with ART.

The other major class of protective antibodies are those that participate in ADCC, a form of cell-mediated immunity (**Chap. 342**) in which NK cells that bear Fc receptors are armed with specific anti-HIV antibodies that bind to the NK cells via their Fc portion. These armed NK cells then bind to and destroy cells expressing HIV antigens. The levels of anti-envelope antibodies capable of mediating ADCC are highest in the earlier stages of HIV infection. Antibodies to both gp120 and gp41 have been shown to participate in ADCC-mediated killing of HIV-infected cells. In vitro, IL-2 can augment ADCC-mediated killing.

In addition to playing a role in host defense, HIV-specific antibodies have also been implicated in disease pathogenesis. Antibodies directed to gp41, when present in low titer, have been shown in vitro to be capable of facilitating infection of cells through an Fc receptor–mediated mechanism known as *antibody enhancement*. Thus, the same regions of the envelope protein of HIV that give rise to antibodies capable of mediating ADCC can also elicit the production of antibodies that can facilitate infection of cells in vitro. In addition, it has been postulated that anti-gp120 antibodies that participate in the ADCC killing of HIV-infected cells might also kill uninfected CD4+ T cells if the uninfected cells had bound free gp120, a phenomenon referred to as *bystander killing*.

One of the most primitive components of the humoral immune system is the complement system (**Chap. 342**). This element of innate immunity consists of ~30 proteins that are found circulating in blood or associated with cell membranes. While HIV alone is capable of directly activating the complement cascade, the resulting lysis is weak due to the presence of host cell regulatory proteins captured in the virion envelope during budding. It is possible that complement-opsonized HIV virions have increased infectivity in a manner analogous to antibody-mediated enhancement.

■ CELLULAR IMMUNE RESPONSE

T-cell–mediated immunity plays a major role in host defense against most viral infections (Chap. 342) and is thought to be an important component of the host immune response to HIV. T-cell immunity can be divided into two major categories: that mediated by *helper/inducer CD4+ T cells* and that mediated by *cytotoxic/immunoregulatory CD8+ T cells*.

HIV-specific CD4+ T cells can be detected in the majority of HIV-infected patients through the use of flow cytometry to measure intracellular cytokine production in response to MHC class II tetramers pulsed with HIV peptides or through lymphocyte proliferation assays utilizing HIV antigens such as p24. These cells likely play a critical role in the orchestration of the immune response to HIV by providing help to HIV-specific B cells and CD8+ T cells. They may also be capable of directly killing HIV-infected cells. HIV-specific CD4+ T cells may be preferential targets of HIV infection by HIV-infected antigen-presenting cells during the generation of an immune response to HIV (Fig. 202-28). However, they also are likely to undergo clonal expansions in response to HIV antigens and thus survive as a population of cells despite the virus. No clear correlations exist between levels of HIV-specific CD4+ T lymphocytes and plasma HIV RNA levels; however, in the setting of high viral loads, CD4+ T-cell responses to HIV antigens appear to shift from one of proliferation and IL-2 production to one of IFN-γ production. Thus, while a reverse correlation exists between the level of p24-specific proliferation and levels of plasma HIV viremia, the nature of the causal relationship between these parameters is unclear.

MHC class I–restricted, HIV-specific CD8+ T cells have been identified in the peripheral blood of patients with HIV-1 infection. These cells include CTLs that produce perforins and granzyme, and T cells that can be induced by HIV antigens to express an array of cytokines such as IFN-γ, IL-2, MIP-1β, and TNF-α. Multiple HIV antigens, including Gag, Env, Pol, Tat, Rev, and Nef, can elicit CD8+ T-cell responses. CTLs have been identified in the peripheral blood of patients within weeks of HIV infection and prior to the appearance of plasma virus. The selective pressure they exert on the evolution of the population of circulating viruses reflects their potential role in control of HIV infection. These CD8+ T lymphocytes, through their HIV-specific antigen receptors, bind to and cause the lytic destruction of target cells bearing autologous MHC class I molecules presenting HIV antigens. Two types of CTL activity can be demonstrated in the peripheral blood or lymph node mononuclear cells of HIV-infected individuals. The first type directly lyses appropriate target cells in culture without prior in vitro stimulation (*spontaneous CTL activity*). The other type of CTL activity reflects the *precursor frequency of CTLs* (CTLp); this type of CTL activity can be demonstrated by stimulation of CD8+ T cells in vitro with a mitogen such as phytohemagglutinin or anti-CD3 antibody.

In addition to CTLs, CD8+ T cells capable of being induced by HIV antigens to express cytokines such as IFN-γ also appear in the setting of HIV-1 infection. It is not clear whether these are the same or different effector pools compared with those cells mediating cytotoxicity; in addition, the relative roles of each in host defense against HIV are not fully understood. It does appear that these CD8+ T cells are driven to in vivo expansion by HIV antigen. There is a direct correlation between levels of CD8+ T cells capable of producing IFN-γ in response to HIV antigens and plasma levels of HIV-1 RNA. Thus, while these cells are clearly induced by HIV-1 infection, in most instances they are not able to effectively control infection. One exception may be a subset of patients who control viral replication in the absence of antiretroviral drugs and are referred to as *elite nonprogressors* (see "Long-Term Survivors, Long-Term Nonprogressors, and Elite Controllers," above). The peripheral blood of these patients contains a population of CD8+ T cells that undergo substantial in vitro proliferation in response to HIV antigens and express perforin and granzyme.

At least three other forms of cell-mediated immunity to HIV have been described: non-cytolytic CD8+ T-cell–mediated suppression of HIV replication, ADCC, and NK cell activity. *Non-cytolytic CD8+ T-cell–mediated suppression of HIV replication* refers to the ability of CD8+ T cells from an HIV-infected patient to inhibit the replication of HIV in tissue culture without killing infected targets. There is no requirement for HLA compatibility between the CD8+ T cells and the HIV-infected cells. This effector mechanism is thus nonspecific and appears to be mediated by soluble factor(s) including the CC-chemokines RANTES (CCL5), MIP-1α (CCL3), and MIP-1β (CCL4). These CC-chemokines are potent suppressors of HIV replication and operate at least in part via blockade of the HIV co-receptor (*CCR5*) for R5 (macrophage-tropic) strains of HIV-1 (see above). *ADCC*, as described above in relation to humoral immunity, involves the killing of HIV-expressing cells by NK cells armed with specific antibodies directed against HIV antigens. Finally, *NK cells* alone have been shown to be capable of killing HIV-infected target cells in tissue culture. This primitive cytotoxic mechanism of host defense is directed toward nonspecific surveillance for neoplastic transformation and viral infection through recognition of altered class I MHC molecules.

DIAGNOSIS AND LABORATORY MONITORING OF HIV INFECTION

The establishment of HIV as the causative agent of AIDS and related syndromes early in 1984 was followed by the rapid development of sensitive screening tests for HIV infection. By March 1985, blood donors in the United States were routinely screened for antibodies to HIV. In 1996, blood banks in the United States added the p24 antigen capture assay to the screening process to help identify the rare infected individuals who were donating blood in the time (up to 3 months) between infection and the development of antibodies. In 2002, the ability to detect early infection with HIV was further enhanced by the licensure of nucleic acid testing (NAT) as a routine part of blood donor screening. These refinements decreased the interval between infection and detection (window period) from 22 days for antibody testing to 16 days with p24 antigen testing and subsequently to 12 days with NAT. The development of sensitive assays for monitoring levels of plasma viremia ushered in a new era of being able to monitor the progression of HIV disease more closely. Utilization of these tests, coupled with the measurement of levels of CD4+ T lymphocytes in peripheral blood, is essential in the management of patients with HIV infection.

■ DIAGNOSIS OF HIV INFECTION

The CDC has recommended that screening for HIV infection be performed as a matter of routine health care. The diagnosis of HIV infection depends on the demonstration of antibodies to HIV and/or the direct detection of HIV or one of its components. As noted above, antibodies to HIV generally appear in the circulation 3–12 weeks following infection. In addition to laboratory-based screening tests, several home tests are available.

The standard blood screening tests for HIV infection are based on the detection of antibodies to HIV and/or the p24 antigen (see below) of HIV. A common laboratory-based platform is the ELISA, also referred to as an *enzyme immunoassay* (EIA). This solid-phase assay is an extremely good screening test with a sensitivity of >99.5%. Most diagnostic laboratories use commercial kits that contain antigens from both HIV-1 and HIV-2 and thus can detect antibodies to either. These kits use both natural and recombinant antigens and are continuously updated to increase their sensitivity to newly discovered species, such as group O viruses (Fig. 202-1). The fourth-generation EIA tests combine detection of antibodies to HIV-1 or HIV-2 with detection of the p24 antigen of HIV. EIA tests are generally scored as positive (highly reactive), negative (nonreactive), or indeterminate (partially reactive). While the EIA is an extremely sensitive test, it is not optimal with regard to specificity. This is particularly true in studies of low-risk individuals, such as volunteer blood donors. In this latter population, as few as 10% of EIA-positive individuals are subsequently confirmed to have HIV infection. Among the factors associated with false-positive EIA tests are antibodies to class II antigens (such as may be seen following pregnancy, blood transfusion, or transplantation), autoantibodies, hepatic disease, recent influenza vaccination, acute viral infections, and administration of an HIV vaccine. For these reasons, anyone suspected of having HIV infection based on a positive or inconclusive fourth-generation EIA result should have the result confirmed with a more specific assay such as an HIV-1– or HIV-2–specific antibody immunoassay, a Western blot, or a plasma HIV RNA level. One can estimate whether an individual has a recent infection with HIV-1 by comparing the results on a standard EIA test that will score positive for all infected individuals with the results on an assay modified to be less sensitive ("detuned assay") that will score positive for individuals with established HIV infection and negative for individuals with recent infection. In rare instances, an HIV-infected individual treated early in the course of infection may revert to a negative EIA. This does *not* indicate clearing of infection; rather, it signifies levels of ongoing exposure to virus or viral proteins insufficient to maintain a measurable antibody response. When these individuals have discontinued therapy, viruses and antibodies have reappeared.

CDC recommendations indicate that a positive fourth-generation assay confirmed by a second HIV-1– or HIV-2–specific immunoassay or a plasma HIV RNA level is adequate for diagnosis. The Western blot, which had previously been used for a confirmatory test, is no longer used for this purpose.

A guideline for the use of these serologic tests in attempting to make a diagnosis of HIV infection is depicted in **Fig. 202-31**. In patients in whom HIV infection is suspected, the appropriate initial test is a fourth-generation HIV-1/2 antigen antibody immunoassay. If the result is negative, unless there is strong reason to suspect early HIV infection (as in a patient exposed within the previous 3 months), the diagnosis is ruled out and retesting should be performed only as clinically indicated. If the immunoassay is indeterminate or positive, the test should be repeated. If the repeat is negative on two occasions, one can assume that the initial positive reading was due to a technical error in the performance of the assay and that the patient is negative. If the repeat is indeterminate or positive, one should proceed to an HIV-1/HIV-2 antibody differentiation immunoassay such as the Bio-Rad Genius. If testing is positive for HIV-1 and/or HIV-2 one may make a diagnosis of HIV-1 and/or HIV-2 infection. If the HIV-1/HIV-2 antibody testing is negative or indeterminate one should proceed to HIV-1 RNA testing with a nucleic acid test (NAT; see below). If the NAT is positive, in the presence of a negative antibody test, one can make a diagnosis of acute HIV-1 infection. If the NAT test is negative for HIV-1 one should consider additional testing for HIV-2 RNA. One can conclude a false-positive fourth-generation test in the setting of repeated negative or indeterminate HIV-2/HIV-2 antibody tests in the setting of negative NAT tests.

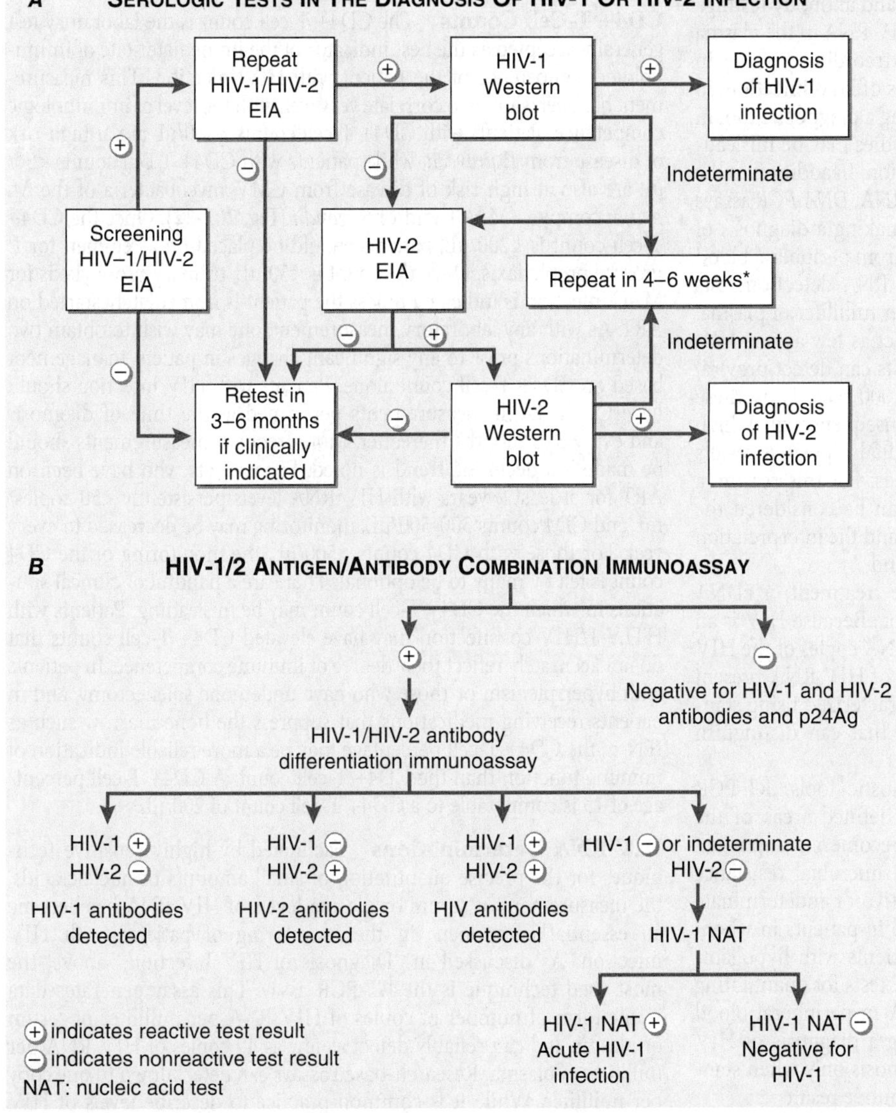

FIGURE 202-31 Serologic tests for the diagnosis of HIV-1 or HIV-2 infection. ***A.*** Algorithm including the use of a Western blot. *Stable indeterminate Western blot 4–6 weeks later makes HIV infection unlikely. However, it should be repeated twice at 3-month intervals to rule out HIV infection. Alternatively, one may test for HIV-1 p24 antigen or HIV RNA. EIA, enzyme immunoassay. ***B.*** CDC algorithm not including the use of a Western blot. *(Adapted from stacks.cdc.gov/view/cdc/23446.)*

In addition to these standard laboratory-based assays for detecting antibodies to HIV, a series of point-of-care tests can provide results in 1 to 60 minutes. While the sensitivity and specificity of these tests are generally quite high, it is generally recommended that any positive results be confirmed with standard laboratory testing. Currently one rapid test kit is available for use at home (OraQuick) as well as several tests for which the sample is obtained at home and mailed to the lab. A positive result with any of these tests should be followed with confirmatory laboratory testing by a healthcare professional.

A variety of laboratory tests are available for the direct detection of HIV or its components (**Table 202-8**). These tests may be of considerable help in making a diagnosis of HIV infection when the antibody determination assays are indeterminate. In addition, the tests detecting levels of HIV RNA can be used to determine prognosis and to assess the response to antiretroviral therapies. The simplest, least expensive, and most rarely used of the direct detection tests is the *p24 antigen capture assay.* This is an EIA-type assay in which the solid phase consists of antibodies to the p24 antigen of HIV. It detects the viral protein p24 in the blood of HIV-infected individuals where it exists either as free antigen or complexed to anti-p24 antibodies. It is currently part of the fourth-generation HIV-1/2 antigen antibody immunoassay test recommend for initial screening. Overall, ~30% of individuals with untreated HIV infection have detectable levels of free p24 antigen. This increases to ~50% when samples are treated with a weak acid to dissociate antigen-antibody complexes. Throughout the course of HIV infection, an equilibrium exists between p24 antigen and anti-p24 antibodies. During the first few weeks of infection, before an immune response develops, there is a brisk rise in p24 antigen levels. After the development of anti-p24 antibodies, these levels decline.

TABLE 202-8 Characteristics of Tests for Direct Detection of HIV

TEST	TECHNIQUE	SENSITIVITY[a]	COST/TEST[b]
Immune complex–dissociated p24 antigen capture assay	Measurement of levels of HIV-1 core protein in an EIA-based format following dissociation of antigen-antibody complexes by weak acid treatment	Positive in 50% of patients; detects down to 15 pg/mL of p24 protein	$1–2
HIV RNA by PCR	Target amplification of HIV-1 RNA via reverse transcription followed by PCR	Reliable to 40 copies/mL of HIV RNA	$75–150
HIV RNA by bDNA	Measurement of levels of particle-associated HIV RNA in a nucleic acid capture assay employing signal amplification	Reliable to 50 copies/mL of HIV RNA	$75–150
HIV RNA by TMA	Target amplification of HIV-1 RNA via reverse transcription followed by T7 RNA polymerase	Reliable to 100 copies/mL of HIV RNA	$225
HIV RNA by NASBA	Isothermal nucleic acid amplification with internal controls	Reliable to 80 copies/mL of HIV RNA	$75–150

[a]Sensitivity figures refer to those approved by the U.S. Food and Drug Administration. [b]Prices may be lower in large-volume settings.

Abbreviations: bDNA, branched DNA; cDNA, complementary DNA; EIA, enzyme immunoassay; NASBA, nucleic acid sequence–based amplification; PCR, polymerase chain reaction; TMA, transcription-mediated amplification.

Late in the course of infection, when circulating levels of virus are high, p24 antigen levels also increase, particularly when detected by techniques involving dissociation of antigen-antibody complexes. The p24 antigen capture assay has its greatest use as a screening test for HIV infection in patients suspected of having the acute HIV syndrome (see below), as high levels of p24 antigen are present prior to the development of antibodies. Its use as a stand-alone test for routine blood donor screening for HIV infection has been replaced by use of NAT or "fourth-generation" assays that combine antigen and antibody testing.

The ability to measure and monitor levels of HIV RNA in the plasma of patients with HIV infection has been of extraordinary value in furthering our understanding of the pathogenesis of HIV infection, in monitoring the response to ART, and in providing a diagnostic tool in settings where measurements of anti-HIV antibodies may be misleading, such as in acute infection and neonatal infection. In addition to the commercially available tests for measuring HIV RNA, *DNA PCR* assays also are employed by research laboratories for making a diagnosis of HIV infection by amplifying HIV proviral DNA from peripheral blood mononuclear cells. The commercially available RNA detection tests have a sensitivity of 40–80 copies of HIV RNA per milliliter of plasma. Research laboratory–based RNA assays can detect as few as one HIV RNA copy per milliliter, while the DNA PCR tests can detect proviral DNA at a frequency of one copy per 10,000–100,000 cells. Thus, these tests are extremely sensitive. One frequent consequence of a high degree of sensitivity is some loss of specificity, and false-positive results have been reported with each of these techniques. For this reason, a positive EIA with a positive HIV RNA assay can be considered the "gold standard" for a diagnosis of HIV infection, and the interpretation of other test results must be done with this in mind.

In the RT-PCR technique, following DNAse treatment, a cDNA copy is made of all RNA species present in plasma. Because HIV is an RNA virus, this will result in the production of DNA copies of the HIV genome in amounts proportional to the amount of HIV RNA present in plasma. This cDNA is then amplified and characterized using standard PCR techniques, employing primer pairs that can distinguish genomic cDNA from messenger cDNA.

In addition to being diagnostic and prognostic tools, RT-PCR and DNA-PCR also are useful for amplifying defined areas of the HIV genome for sequence analysis and have become an important technique for studies of sequence diversity and microbial resistance to antiretroviral agents. In patients with a positive or indeterminate EIA test and an indeterminate Western blot, and in patients in whom serologic testing may be unreliable (such as patients with hypogammaglobulinemia or advanced HIV disease), these tests for quantitating HIV RNA in plasma or detecting proviral DNA in peripheral blood mononuclear cells are valuable tools for making a diagnosis of HIV infection; however, they should be used for diagnosis only when standard serologic testing has failed to provide a definitive result.

LABORATORY MONITORING OF PATIENTS WITH HIV INFECTION

The integration of clinical and laboratory data is essential to optimal management of patients with HIV infection. The close relationship between clinical manifestations of HIV infection and CD4+ T-cell count has made measurement of CD4+ T-cell numbers a routine part of the evaluation of HIV-infected individuals. The discovery of HIV as the cause of AIDS led to the development of sensitive tests that allow one to monitor the levels of HIV in the blood. Determinations of peripheral blood CD4+ T-cell counts and measurements of the plasma levels of HIV RNA provide a powerful set of tools for determining prognosis and monitoring response to therapy.

CD4+ T-Cell Counts The CD4+ T-cell count is the laboratory test generally accepted as the best indicator of the immediate state of immunologic competence of the patient with HIV infection. This measurement has been shown to correlate very well with the level of immunologic competence. Patients with CD4+ T-cell counts <200/μL are at high risk of disease from *P. jirovecii*, while patients with CD4+ T-cell counts <50/μL are also at high risk of disease from CMV, mycobacteria of the *M. avium* complex (MAC), and/or *T. gondii* (**Fig. 202-32**). Once the CD4+ T-cell count is <200/μL, patients should be placed on a regimen for *P. jirovecii* prophylaxis. Once the count is <50/μL, primary prophylaxis for MAC infection is indicated unless the patient is immediately started on ART. As with any laboratory measurement, one may wish to obtain two determinations prior to any significant changes in patient management based on CD4+ T-cell count alone. Patients with HIV infection should have CD4+ T-cell measurements performed at the time of diagnosis and every 3–6 months thereafter. More frequent measurements should be made if a declining trend is noted. For patients who have been on ART for at least 2 years with HIV RNA levels persistently <50 copies/mL and CD4 counts 300-500/μL, monitoring may be decreased to every year. For those with CD4 counts >500/μL, the monitoring of the CD4 count is felt by many to be optional. There are a handful of clinical situations in which the CD4+ T-cell count may be misleading. Patients with HTLV-1/HIV co-infection may have elevated CD4+ T-cell counts that do not accurately reflect their degree of immune competence. In patients with hypersplenism or those who have undergone splenectomy, and in patients receiving medications that suppress the bone marrow such as IFN-α, the CD4+ T-cell percentage may be a more reliable indication of immune function than the CD4+ T-cell count. A CD4+ T-cell percentage of 15 is comparable to a CD4+ T-cell count of 200/μL.

HIV RNA Determinations Facilitated by highly sensitive techniques for the precise quantitation of small amounts of nucleic acids, the measurement of serum or plasma levels of HIV RNA has become an essential component in the monitoring of patients with HIV infection. As discussed in "Diagnosis of HIV Infection," above, the most used technique is the RT-PCR assay. This assay generates data in the form of number of copies of HIV RNA per milliliter of serum or plasma and can reliably detect as few as 40 copies of HIV RNA per milliliter of plasma. Research-based assays can detect down to one copy per milliliter. While it is common practice to describe levels of HIV RNA below these cut-offs as "undetectable," this is a term that should be avoided as it is imprecise and leaves the false impression that the level of virus is 0. By utilizing more sensitive, nested PCR techniques and by studying tissue levels of virus as well as plasma levels, HIV RNA can be detected in virtually every patient with HIV infection.

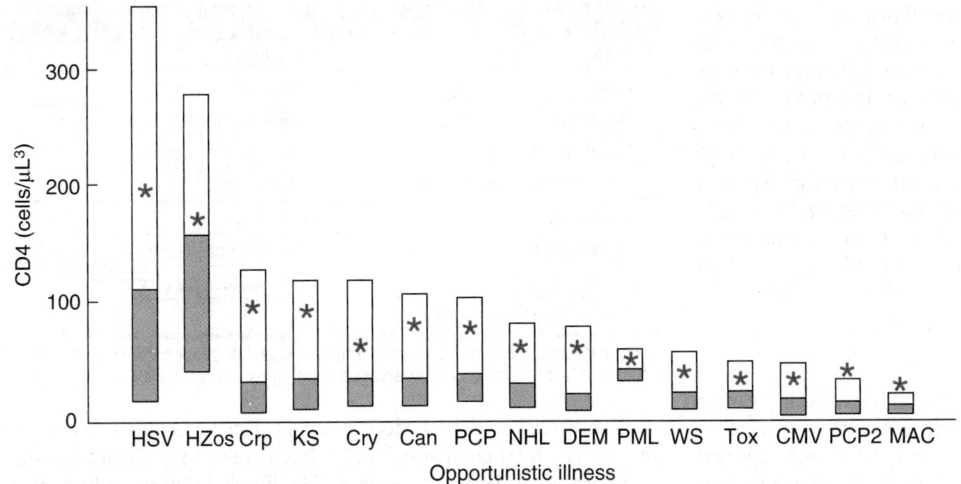

FIGURE 202-32 Relationship between CD4+ T-cell counts and the development of opportunistic diseases. Boxplot of the median (line inside the box), first quartile (bottom of the box), third quartile (top of the box), and mean (asterisk) CD4+ lymphocyte count at the time of the development of opportunistic disease. Can, candidal esophagitis; CMV, cytomegalovirus infection; Crp, cryptosporidiosis; Cry, cryptococcal meningitis; DEM, AIDS dementia complex; HSV, herpes simplex virus infection; HZos, herpes zoster; KS, Kaposi's sarcoma; MAC, *Mycobacterium avium* complex bacteremia; NHL, non-Hodgkin's lymphoma; PCP, primary *Pneumocystis jirovecii* pneumonia; PCP2, secondary *P. jirovecii* pneumonia; PML, progressive multifocal leukoencephalopathy; Tox, *Toxoplasma gondii* encephalitis; WS, wasting syndrome. *(From Annals of Internal Medicine, RD Moore, RE Chaisson: Natural History of Opportunistic Disease in an HIV-Infected Urban Clinical Cohort. 124(7):633-642, 1996. Copyright © 1996 American College of Physicians. All Rights Reserved. Reprinted with the permission of American College of Physicians, Inc.)*

There are a few notable exceptions to this that involve patients who underwent cytoreductive therapy followed by bone marrow transplant from *CCR5Δ32* homozygous donors.

Measurements of changes in HIV RNA levels over time have been of great value in delineating the relationship between levels of virus and rates of disease progression (Fig. 202-22), the rates of viral turnover, the relationship between immune system activation and viral replication, and the time to development of drug resistance. HIV RNA measurements are greatly influenced by the state of activation of the immune system and may fluctuate greatly in the setting of secondary infections or immunization. For these reasons, decisions based on HIV RNA levels should never be made on a single determination. Measurements of plasma HIV RNA levels should be made at the time of HIV diagnosis and every 3–6 months thereafter in the untreated patient. Following the initiation of therapy or any change in therapy, plasma HIV RNA levels should be monitored approximately every 4 weeks until the effectiveness of the therapeutic regimen is determined by the development of a new steady-state level of HIV RNA. In most instances of effective antiretroviral therapy, the plasma level of HIV RNA will drop to <50 copies/mL within 6 months of the initiation of treatment. During therapy, levels of HIV RNA should be monitored every 3–6 months to evaluate the continuing effectiveness of therapy.

HIV Resistance Testing The availability of multiple antiretroviral drugs as treatment options has generated a great deal of interest in the potential for measuring the sensitivity of an individual's HIV viral quasispecies to different antiretroviral agents. HIV resistance testing can be done through either genotypic or phenotypic measurements. In the genotypic assays, sequence analyses of the HIV genomes obtained from patients are compared with sequences of viruses with known antiretroviral resistance profiles. In the phenotypic assays, the in vivo growth of patient-derived viral isolates or genetically constructed pseudoviruses is compared with the growth of reference strains of the virus in the presence or absence of different antiretroviral drugs. These tests are quite good at identifying those antiretroviral agents that have been utilized in the past and suggesting agents that may be of future value in a given patient. Resistance testing is recommended at the time of initial diagnosis and, if therapy is not initiated at that time, at the time of initiation of ART. Drug resistance testing is also indicated in the setting of virologic failure and should be performed while the patient is still on the failing regimen because of the propensity for the pool of HIV quasispecies to rapidly revert to wild-type in the absence of the selective pressures of ART. In the hands of experts, resistance testing enhances the short-term ability to decrease viral load by ~0.5 log compared with changing drugs merely based on drug history. In addition to the use of resistance testing to help in the selection of new drugs in patients with virologic failure, it may also be of value in selecting an initial regimen for treatment of therapy-naïve individuals. This is particularly true in geographic areas with a high level of background resistance. The patient needs to have an HIV-1 RNA level above 500–1000 copies/mL for an accurate resistance determination. Resistance assays lose their consistency at lower levels of plasma viremia.

Co-Receptor Tropism Assays Following the licensure of maraviroc as the first CCR5 antagonist for the treatment of HIV infection (see below), it became necessary to be able to determine whether a patient's virus was likely to respond to this treatment. Patients tend to have CCR5-tropic virus early in the course of infection, with a trend toward CXCR4 viruses later in disease. The antiretroviral agent maraviroc is effective only against CCR5-tropic viruses. Because the genotypic determinants of cellular tropism are poorly defined, a phenotypic assay is necessary to determine this property of HIV. The Trofile assay (Monogram Biosciences) is available to make this determination. This assay clones the envelope regions of the patient's virus into an indicator virus that is then used to infect target cells expressing either CCR5 or CXCR4 as their co-receptor. The assay takes weeks to perform and is expensive. Another, less costly option is to obtain a genotypic assay of the V3 region of HIV-1 and then employ a computer algorithm to predict viral tropism from the sequence. While this approach is less expensive than the classic phenotypic assay, there are fewer data to validate its predictive value.

Other Tests A variety of other laboratory tests have been studied as potential markers of HIV disease activity. Among these are quantitative culture of replication-competent HIV from plasma, peripheral blood mononuclear cells, or resting memory CD4+ T cells; circulating levels of β_2-microglobulin, soluble IL-2 receptor, IgA, acid-labile endogenous IFN, or TNF-α; and the presence or absence of activation markers such as CD38, HLA-DR, and PD-1 on CD4+ or CD8+ T cells. Nonspecific serologic markers of inflammation and/or coagulation such as IL-6, D-dimer, and sCD14 have been shown to have a high correlation with all-cause mortality (**Table 202-9**). While these measurements have value as markers of disease activity and help to increase our understanding of the pathogenesis of HIV disease, they do not currently play a major role in the monitoring of patients with HIV infection.

CLINICAL MANIFESTATIONS

The clinical consequences of HIV infection encompass a spectrum ranging from an acute syndrome associated with primary infection to a prolonged asymptomatic state to advanced disease. It is best to

TABLE 202-9 Association between High-Sensitivity CRP, Il-6, and D-Dimer with All-Cause Mortality in Patients with HIV Infection

	UNADJUSTED		ADJUSTED	
MARKER	ODDS RATIO (FOURTH/FIRST)	*P*	ODDS RATIO (FOURTH/FIRST)	*P*
Hs-CRP	2.0	.05	2.8	.03
IL-6	8.3	<.0001	11.8	<.0001
D-dimer	12.4	<.0001	26.5	<.0001

Abbreviations: Hs-CRP, high-sensitivity C-reactive protein; IL-6, interleukin 6.

Source: From LH Kuller et al: PLoS Med 5:e203, 2008.

regard HIV disease as beginning at the time of primary infection and progressing through various stages. As mentioned above, active virus replication and progressive immunologic impairment occur throughout the course of HIV infection in most patients. Except for the rare, true, "elite" virus controllers or long-term nonprogressors (see "Long-Term Survivors, Long-Term Nonprogressors, and Elite Controllers," above), HIV disease in untreated patients inexorably progresses even during the clinically latent stage. Since the mid-1990s, ART has had a major impact on preventing and reversing the progression of disease over extended periods of time in a substantial proportion of adequately treated patients. Today, a person diagnosed with HIV infection and treated with ART has a close to normal life expectancy.

ACUTE HIV INFECTION

It is estimated that 50–70% of individuals with HIV infection experience an acute clinical syndrome ~3–6 weeks after primary infection (**Fig. 202-33**). Varying degrees of clinical severity have been reported, and although it has been suggested that symptomatic seroconversion leading to the seeking of medical attention indicates an increased risk for an accelerated course of disease, there does not appear to be a correlation between the level of the initial burst of viremia in acute HIV infection and the subsequent course of disease. The typical clinical findings in the acute HIV syndrome are listed in **Table 202-10**; they occur along with a burst of plasma viremia. It has been reported that several symptoms of the acute HIV syndrome (fever, skin rash, pharyngitis, and myalgia) occur less frequently in those infected by injection drug use compared with those infected by sexual contact. The syndrome is typical of an acute viral syndrome and has been likened to acute infectious mononucleosis. Symptoms usually persist for one to several weeks and gradually subside as an immune response to HIV develops and the levels of plasma viremia decrease. Opportunistic infections have been reported during this stage of infection, reflecting the immunodeficiency that results from reduced numbers of CD4+ T cells and likely also from the dysfunction of CD4+ T cells owing to viral protein and endogenous cytokine-induced perturbations of cells (Table 202-5) associated with the extremely high levels of plasma viremia. The Fiebig staging system has been used to describe the different stages of acute HIV infection, ranging from stage 1 (HIV RNA positive alone) to stage VI (HIV RNA and full Western blot positive). A number of immunologic abnormalities accompany the acute HIV syndrome, including multiphasic perturbations of the numbers of circulating lymphocyte subsets. The numbers of total lymphocytes and T-cell subsets (CD4+ and CD8+) are initially reduced. An inversion of the CD4+/CD8+ T-cell ratio occurs later because of a rise in the number of CD8+ T cells. In fact, there may be a selective and transient expansion

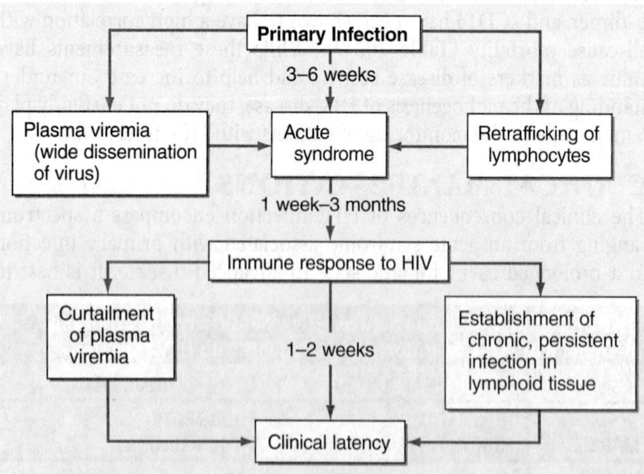

FIGURE 202-33 The acute HIV syndrome. See text for detailed description. *(From G Pantaleo, C Graziosi, AS Fauci: The Immunopathogenesis of Human Immunodeficiency Virus Infection. N Engl J Med 328:327, 1993. Copyright © 1993 Massachusetts Medical Society. Reprinted with permission from Massachusetts Medical Society.)*

TABLE 202-10 Clinical Findings in the Acute HIV Syndrome

General	Neurologic
Fever	Meningitis
Pharyngitis	Encephalitis
Lymphadenopathy	Peripheral neuropathy
Headache/retroorbital pain	Myelopathy
Arthralgias/myalgias	Dermatologic
Lethargy/malaise	Erythematous maculopapular rash
Anorexia/weight loss	Mucocutaneous ulceration
Nausea/vomiting/diarrhea	

Source: Reproduced with permission from B Tindall, DA Cooper: Primary HIV infection: Host responses and intervention strategies. AIDS 5:1, 1991.

of CD8+ T-cell subsets, as determined by T-cell receptor analysis (see above). The total circulating CD8+ T-cell count may remain elevated or return to normal; however, CD4+ T-cell levels usually remain somewhat depressed, although there may be a slight rebound toward normal. Lymphadenopathy occurs in ~70% of individuals with primary HIV infection. Most patients recover spontaneously from this syndrome and many are left with only a mildly depressed CD4+ T-cell count that remains stable for a variable period before beginning its progressive decline; in some individuals, the CD4+ T-cell count returns to the normal range. Approximately 10% of patients manifest a fulminant course of immunologic and clinical deterioration after primary infection, even after the disappearance of initial symptoms. In most patients, primary infection with or without the acute syndrome is followed by a prolonged period of clinical latency or smoldering low disease activity.

THE ASYMPTOMATIC STAGE—CLINICAL LATENCY

Although the length of time from initial infection to the development of clinical disease varies greatly, the median time for untreated patients is ~10 years. As emphasized above, HIV disease with active virus replication is ongoing and progressive during this asymptomatic period. The rate of disease progression is directly correlated with HIV RNA levels. Patients with high levels of HIV RNA in plasma progress to symptomatic disease faster than do patients with low levels of HIV RNA (Fig. 202-22). Some patients referred to as *long-term nonprogressors* show little if any decline in CD4+ T-cell counts over extended periods of time. These patients generally have extremely low levels of HIV RNA; a subset, referred to as *elite nonprogressors*, exhibits HIV RNA levels <50 copies/mL. Certain other patients remain entirely asymptomatic even though their CD4+ T-cell counts show a steady progressive decline to extremely low levels. In these patients, the appearance of an opportunistic disease may be the first manifestation of HIV infection. During the asymptomatic period of HIV infection, the average rate of CD4+ T-cell decline is ~50/μL per year in an untreated patient. When the CD4+ T-cell count falls to <200/μL, the resulting state of immunodeficiency is severe enough to place the patient at high risk for opportunistic infections and neoplasms and, hence, for clinically apparent disease.

SYMPTOMATIC DISEASE

Symptoms of HIV disease can appear at any time during the course of HIV infection. Generally, the spectrum of illnesses that one observes changes as the CD4+ T-cell count declines. The more severe and life-threatening complications of HIV infection occur in patients with CD4+ T-cell counts <200/μL. A diagnosis of AIDS is made in any individual age 6 years and older with HIV infection and a CD4+ T-cell count <200/μL (stage 3, Table 202-2) and in anyone with HIV infection who develops one of the HIV-associated diseases considered to be indicative of a severe defect in cell-mediated immunity (Table 202-1). While the causative agents of the secondary infections are characteristically opportunistic organisms such as *P. jirovecii*, atypical mycobacteria, CMV, and other organisms that do not ordinarily cause disease in the absence of a compromised immune system, they also include several common bacterial and mycobacterial pathogens. Following the widespread use of ART and implementation of guidelines for the prevention of opportunistic infections (**Table 202-11**),

TABLE 202-11 NIH/CDC/IDSA 2013 Guidelines for the Prevention of Opportunistic Infections in Persons Infected with HIV

PATHOGEN	INDICATIONS	FIRST CHOICE(S)	ALTERNATIVES
Recommended as Standard of Care for Primary and Secondary Prophylaxis			
Pneumocystis jirovecii	CD4+ T-cell count <200/μL *or* Oropharyngeal candidiasis *or* Prior bout of PCP	Trimethoprim-sulfamethoxazole (TMP-SMX), 1 DS tablet qd PO *or* TMP-SMX, 1 SS tablet qd PO	Dapsone 50 mg bid PO or 100 mg/d PO *or* Dapsone 50 mg/d PO + Pyrimethamine 50 mg/week PO + Leucovorin 25 mg/week PO *or* (Dapsone 200 mg PO + Pyrimethamine 75 mg PO + Leucovorin 25 mg weekly PO) *or* Aerosolized pentamidine, 300 mg via Respirgard II nebulizer every month *or* Atovaquone 1500 mg/d PO *or* TMP-SMX 1 DS tablet 3×/week PO
	May stop prophylaxis if CD4+ T-cell count >200/μL for ≥3 months		
Mycobacterium tuberculosis			
Isoniazid sensitive	Skin test >5 mm *or* Positive IFN-γ release assay *or* Prior positive test without treatment *or* Close contact with case of active pulmonary TB Same with high probability of exposure to drug-resistant TB	(Isoniazid 300 mg PO + Pyridoxine 25 mg PO) qd × 9 months *or* Isoniazid 900 mg PO twice weekly + Pyridoxine 25 mg PO daily × 9 months	Rifabutin (dose adjusted based on cART regimen) or rifampin 600 mg PO qd × 4 months
Drug resistant	Consult local public health authorities		
Mycobacterium-avium complex	CD4+ T-cell count <50/μL unless ART immediately initiated	Azithromycin 1200 mg weekly PO or 600 mg twice weekly PO *or* Clarithromycin 500 mg bid PO	Rifabutin (dose adjusted based on cART regimen)
	Prior documented disseminated disease	Clarithromycin 500 mg bid PO + Ethambutol 15 (mg/kg)/d PO	Azithromycin 500–600 mg/d PO + Ethambutol 15 (mg/kg)/d PO
	May stop prophylaxis once ART initiated		
Toxoplasma gondii	TOXO IgG antibody positive and CD4+ T-cell count <100/μL	TMP-SMX 1 DS tablet PO qd	TMP-SMX 1 DS 3× weekly PO *or* TMP-SMX, 1 SS PO daily *or* Dapsone 50 mg/d PO + Pyrimethamine 50 mg weekly PO + Leucovorin 25 mg weekly PO *or* (Dapsone 200 mg PO + Pyrimethamine 75 mg PO + Leucovorin 25 mg PO) weekly *or* Atovaquone 1500 mg PO daily ± (Pyrimethamine 25 mg PO + Leucovorin 10 mg PO) daily
	Prior toxoplasmic encephalitis and CD4+ T-cell count <200/μL	Sulfadiazine 2000–4000 mg in 2–4 divided doses daily PO + Pyrimethamine 25–50 mg/d PO + Leucovorin 10–25 mg/d PO	Clindamycin 600 mg q8h PO + Pyrimethamine 25–50 mg/d PO + Leucovorin 10–25 mg/d PO *or* TMP-SMX 1 DS tablet bid *or*

(*Continued*)

TABLE 202-11 NIH/CDC/IDSA 2013 Guidelines for the Prevention of Opportunistic Infections in Persons Infected with HIV (Continued)

PATHOGEN	INDICATIONS	FIRST CHOICE(S)	ALTERNATIVES
			Atovaquone 750–1500 mg PO bid ± (Pyrimethamine 25 mg/d PO + Leucovorin 10 mg/d PO) or Sulfadiazine 2000–4000 mg/d (in 2–4 divided doses) PO
Toxoplasma gondii	May stop prophylaxis if CD4+ T-cell count >200/μL for ≥3 months		
Varicella zoster virus	Significant exposure to chickenpox or shingles in a patient with no history of immunization or prior exposure to either	Varicella zoster immune globulin, IM, within 10 d of exposure (800-843-7477)	Acyclovir 800 mg PO 5 × day for 5–7 days *or* Valacyclovir 1 g PO tid for 5–7 days
Cryptococcus neoformans	Prior documented disease	Fluconazole 200 mg/d PO	Itraconazole 200 mg/d PO
	May stop prophylaxis if CD4+ T-cell count >100/μL, no evidence of active fungal infection, and HIV RNA levels <500 copies/mL for >3 months		
Histoplasma capsulatum	Prior documented disease or CD4+ T-cell count <150 μL and high risk (endemic area or occupational exposure)	Itraconazole 200 mg bid PO	Fluconazole 400 mg/d PO
	May stop prophylaxis after 1 year if CD4+ T-cell count >150/μL and patient on cART for ≥6 months		
Coccidioides immitis	Prior documented disease *or* positive serology and CD4+ T-cell count <250/μL if from a disease endemic area. (For this indication prophylaxis can be stopped if CD4+ T-cell count ≥250 for 6 months.)	Fluconazole 400 mg/d PO	
Penicillium marneffei	Prior documented disease Patients with CD4+ T-cell counts <100 who live or stay in northern Thailand, Southern China, or Vietnam	Itraconazole 200 mg/d PO	Fluconazole 400 mg PO once weekly
	May stop secondary prophylaxis in patients on ARV therapy with CD4+ T-cell count >100/μL for ≥6 months		
Salmonella species	Prior recurrent bacteremia	Ciprofloxacin 500 mg bid PO for ≥6 months	
Bartonella	Prior infection	Doxycycline 200 mg/d PO *or* Azithromycin 1200 mg weekly PO *or* Clarithromycin 500 mg bid PO	
	May stop if CD4+ T-cell count >200/μL for >3 months		
Cytomegalovirus	Prior end-organ disease	Valganciclovir 900 mg bid PO	Cidofovir 5 mg/kg every other week IV + Probenecid *or* Foscarnet 90–120 (mg/kg)/d IV
	May stop prophylaxis if CD4+ T-cell count >100/μL for 6 months and no evidence of active CMV disease Restart if prior retinitis and CD4+ T cells <100/μL		
Immunizations Generally Recommended			
Hepatitis B virus	All susceptible (anti-HBc- and anti-HBs-negative) patients	Hepatitis B vaccine: 3 doses	
Hepatitis A virus	All susceptible (anti-HAV-negative) patients	Hepatitis A vaccine: 2 doses	
Influenza virus	All patients annually	Inactivated trivalent influenza virus vaccine 1 dose yearly	Oseltamivir 75 mg PO qd *or* Rimantadine or amantadine 100 mg PO bid (influenza A only)
Streptococcus pneumoniae	All patients, preferably before CD4+ T-cell count ≤200/μL	Pneumococcal conjugated vaccine (13) 0.5 mL IM × 1 followed in 8 weeks or more by pneumococcal polysaccharide vaccine (23) if CD4+ T-cell count >200/μL	
	Patients initially immunized at a CD4+ T-cell count <100/μL whose CD4+ T-cell count then increases to>200/μL	Reimmunize	
Human papillomavirus	All patients 13–26 years of age	HPV vaccine; 3 doses	

(*Continued*)

TABLE 202-11 NIH/CDC/IDSA 2013 Guidelines for the Prevention of Opportunistic Infections in Persons Infected with HIV (Continued)

PATHOGEN	INDICATIONS	FIRST CHOICE(S)	ALTERNATIVES
Recommended for Prevention of Severe or Frequent Recurrences			
Herpes simplex	Frequent/severe recurrences	Valacyclovir 500 mg bid PO *or* Acyclovir 400 mg bid PO *or* Famciclovir 500 mg bid PO	
Candida	Frequent/severe recurrences	Fluconazole 100–200 mg/d PO	Posaconazole 400 mg bid PO

Abbreviations: ARV, antiretroviral; bid, twice daily; cART, combination antiretroviral therapy; DS, double-strength; IM, intramuscular; PCP, *Pneumocystis jirovecii* pneumonia; PO, by mouth; qd, daily; SS, single-strength; TB, tuberculosis; tid, three times a day.

the incidence of these secondary infections has decreased dramatically (Fig. 202-34). Overall, the clinical spectrum of HIV disease is constantly changing as patients live longer and new and better approaches to treatment and prophylaxis are developed. In addition to the classic, original AIDS-defining illnesses, patients with HIV infection also have an increase in several serious non-AIDS illnesses, including non-AIDS-related cancers and cardiovascular, renal, and hepatic disease. Non-AIDS events now dominate the disease burden for patients with HIV infection successfully treated with ART (Table 202-4). In developed countries, AIDS-related illnesses are responsible for only ~25% of deaths in patients with HIV infection. A similar percentage of deaths are due to non-AIDS-defining malignancies, and cardiovascular disease and liver disease each account for approximately 15% of deaths. The physician providing care to a patient with HIV infection must be well versed in general internal medicine as well as HIV-related opportunistic diseases. In general, it should be stressed that a key element of treatment of symptomatic complications of HIV disease, whether they are primary or secondary, is achieving good control of HIV replication through the use of ART and instituting primary and secondary prophylaxis for opportunistic infections as indicated.

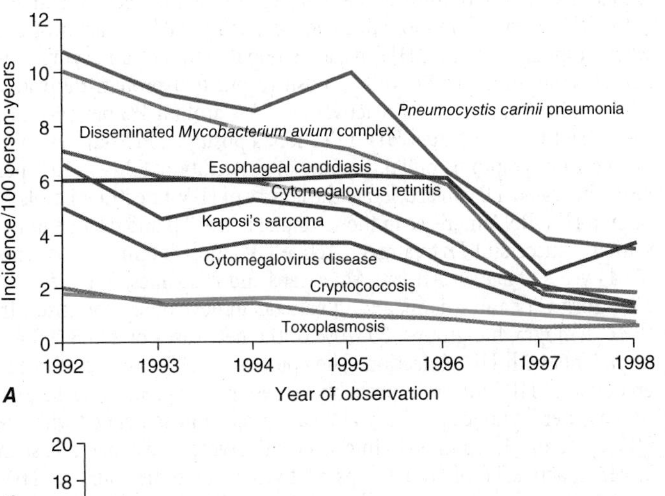

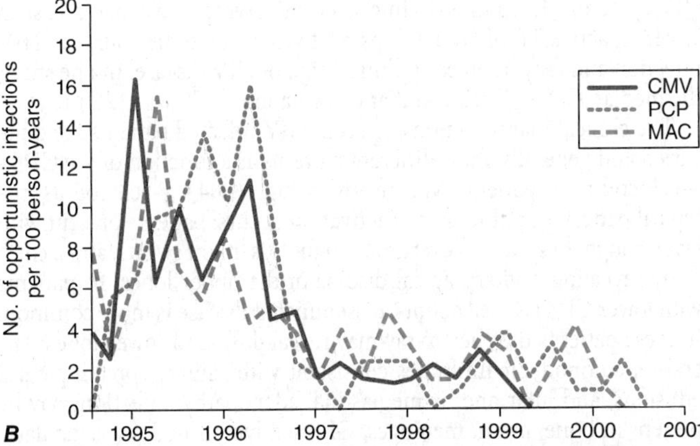

FIGURE 202-34 ***A.*** Decrease in the incidence of opportunistic infections and Kaposi's sarcoma in HIV-infected individuals with CD4+ T-cell counts <100/μL from 1992 through 1998. *(JE Kaplan et al: Epidemiology of human immunodeficiency virus-associated opportunistic infections in the United States in the era of highly active antiretroviral therapy. Clin Infect Dis 30Suppl1(s1):S5, 2000, with permission.)* ***B.*** Quarterly incidence rates of cytomegalovirus (CMV), *Pneumocystis jirovecii* pneumonia (PCP), and *Mycobacterium avium* complex (MAC) from 1995 to 2001. *(Reproduced with permission from Palella FJ Jr et al; HIV Outpatient Study Investigators. Durability and predictors of success of highly active antiretroviral therapy for ambulatory HIV-infected patients. AIDS 16:1617, 2002.)*

Diseases of the Respiratory System Acute bronchitis and sinusitis are prevalent during all stages of HIV infection. The most severe cases tend to occur in patients with lower CD4+ T-cell counts. Sinusitis presents as fever, nasal congestion, and headache. The diagnosis is made by CT or MRI. The maxillary sinuses are most commonly involved; however, disease is also frequently seen in the ethmoid, sphenoid, and frontal sinuses. While some patients may improve without antibiotic therapy, radiographic improvement is quicker and more pronounced in patients who have received antimicrobial therapy. It is postulated that this high incidence of sinusitis results from an increased frequency of infection with encapsulated organisms such as *H. influenzae* and *Streptococcus pneumoniae*. In patients with low CD4+ T-cell counts one may see mucormycosis infections of the sinuses. In contrast to the course of this infection in other patient populations, mucormycosis of the sinuses in patients with HIV infection may progress more slowly. In this setting aggressive, frequent local debridement in addition to local and systemic amphotericin B may result in effective treatment.

Pulmonary disease is one of the most frequent complications of HIV infection. The most common manifestation of pulmonary disease is pneumonia. Three of the 10 most common AIDS-defining illnesses are recurrent bacterial pneumonia, tuberculosis, and pneumonia due to the unicellular fungus *P. jirovecii*. Other major causes of pulmonary infiltrates include other mycobacterial infections, other fungal infections, nonspecific interstitial pneumonitis, KS, and lymphoma.

Bacterial pneumonia is seen with an increased frequency in patients with HIV infection, with 0.8–2.0 cases per 100 person-years. Patients with HIV infection are particularly prone to infections with encapsulated organisms. *S. pneumoniae* (**Chap. 141**) and *H. influenzae* (**Chap. 152**) are responsible for most cases of bacterial pneumonia in patients with AIDS. This may be a consequence of altered B-cell function and/or defects in neutrophil function that may be secondary to HIV disease (see above). Pneumonias due to *S. aureus* (**Chap. 142**) and *P. aeruginosa* (**Chap. 159**) also are reported to occur with an increased frequency in patients with HIV infection. *S. pneumoniae* (pneumococcal) infection may be the earliest serious infection to occur in patients with HIV disease. This can present as pneumonia, sinusitis, and/or bacteremia. Patients with untreated HIV infection have a six-fold increase in the incidence of pneumococcal pneumonia and a 100-fold increase in the incidence of pneumococcal bacteremia. Pneumococcal disease may be seen in patients with relatively intact immune systems. In one study, the baseline CD4+ T-cell count at the time of a first episode of pneumococcal pneumonia was ~300/μL. Of interest is the fact that the inflammatory response to pneumococcal infection appears proportional to the CD4+ T-cell count. Due to this high risk of pneumococcal disease, immunization with the conjugated pneumococcal vaccine followed by booster immunization with the 23-valent pneumococcal polysaccharide vaccine is one of the generally recommended prophylactic measures for patients with HIV infection.

This is likely most effective if given while the CD4+ T-cell count is >200/μL and, if given to patients with lower CD4+ T-cell counts, should be repeated once the count has been above 200 for 6 months. Although clear guidelines do not exist, it also makes sense to repeat immunization every 5 years. The incidence of bacterial pneumonia is cut in half when patients quit smoking.

Pneumocystis pneumonia (PCP) is caused by the fungus *P. jirovecii* and was once the hallmark of AIDS. It has dramatically declined in incidence following the development of effective prophylactic regimens and the widespread use of ART. It is, however, still the single most common cause of pneumonia in patients with HIV infection in the United States and can be identified as a likely etiologic agent in 25% of cases of pneumonia in patients with HIV infection, with an incidence of about 1 case per 100 person-years. Approximately 30% of cases of HIV-associated PCP occur in patients who are unaware of their HIV status. The risk of PCP is greatest among those who have experienced a previous bout of PCP and those who have CD4+ T-cell counts of <200/μL. Overall, 79% of patients with PCP have CD4+ T-cell counts <100/μL and 95% of patients have CD4+ T-cell counts <200/μL. Recurrent fever, night sweats, thrush, and unexplained weight loss also are associated with an increased incidence of PCP. For these reasons, it is strongly recommended that all patients with CD4+ T-cell counts <200/μL (or a CD4 percentage <15) receive some form of PCP prophylaxis. The incidence of PCP is approaching zero in patients with known HIV infection receiving appropriate ART and prophylaxis. In the United States, primary PCP is now occurring at a median CD4+ T-cell count of 36/μL, while secondary PCP is occurring at a median CD4+ T-cell count of 10/μL.

Patients with PCP generally present with fever and a cough that is usually nonproductive or productive of only scant amounts of white sputum. They may complain of a characteristic retrosternal chest pain that is worse on inspiration and is described as sharp or burning. HIV-associated PCP may have an indolent course characterized by weeks of vague symptoms and should be included in the differential diagnosis of fever, pulmonary complaints, or unexplained weight loss in any patient with HIV infection and <200 CD4+ T cells/μL. The most common finding on chest x-ray is either a normal film, if the disease is suspected early, or a faint bilateral interstitial infiltrate. The classic finding of a dense perihilar infiltrate is unusual in patients with AIDS. In patients with PCP who have been receiving aerosolized pentamidine for prophylaxis, one may see an x-ray picture of upper lobe cavitary disease, reminiscent of TB. Other less common findings on chest x-ray include lobar infiltrates and pleural effusions. Thin-section CT may demonstrate a patchy ground-glass appearance. Routine laboratory evaluation is usually of little help in the differential diagnosis of PCP. A mild leukocytosis is common, although this may not be obvious in patients with prior neutropenia. Elevation of lactate dehydrogenase is common. Arterial blood-gases may indicate hypoxemia with a decline in Pa_{O_2} and an increase in the arterial-alveolar (a–A) gradient. Arterial blood-gas measurements not only aid in making the diagnosis of PCP but also provide important information for staging the severity of the disease and directing treatment (see below). A definitive diagnosis of PCP requires demonstration of the organism in samples obtained from induced sputum, bronchoalveolar lavage, transbronchial biopsy, or open-lung biopsy. PCR has been used to detect specific DNA sequences for *P. jirovecii* in clinical specimens where histologic examinations have failed to make a diagnosis.

In addition to pneumonia, other clinical problems have been reported in HIV-infected patients as a result of infection with *P. jirovecii*. Otic involvement may be seen as a primary infection, presenting as a polypoid mass involving the external auditory canal. In patients receiving aerosolized pentamidine for prophylaxis against PCP, one may see a variety of extrapulmonary manifestations of *P. jirovecii*. These include ophthalmic lesions of the choroid, a necrotizing vasculitis that resembles Buerger disease, bone marrow hypoplasia, and intestinal obstruction. Other organs that have been involved include lymph nodes, spleen, liver, kidney, pancreas, pericardium, heart, thyroid, and adrenals. Organ infection may be associated with cystic lesions that may appear calcified on CT or ultrasound.

The standard treatment for PCP or disseminated pneumocystosis is trimethoprim-sulfamethoxazole (TMP-SMX). A high (20–85%) incidence of side effects, particularly skin rash and bone marrow suppression, is seen with TMP-SMX in patients with HIV infection. Alternative treatments for mild to moderate PCP include dapsone/trimethoprim, clindamycin/primaquine, and atovaquone. IV pentamidine is the treatment of choice for severe disease in the patient unable to tolerate TMP-SMX. For patients with a Pa_{O_2} <70 mmHg or with an a–A gradient >35 mmHg, adjunct glucocorticoid therapy should be used in addition to specific antimicrobials. Overall, treatment should be continued for 21 days and followed by secondary prophylaxis. Prophylaxis for PCP is indicated for any HIV-infected individual who has experienced a prior bout of PCP, any patient with a CD4+ T-cell count of <200/μL or a CD4 percentage <15, any patient with unexplained fever for >2 weeks, and any patient with a recent history of oropharyngeal candidiasis. The preferred regimen for prophylaxis is TMP-SMX, one double-strength tablet daily. This regimen also provides protection against toxoplasmosis and some bacterial respiratory pathogens. For patients who cannot tolerate TMP-SMX, alternatives for prophylaxis include dapsone plus pyrimethamine plus leucovorin, aerosolized pentamidine administered by the Respirgard II nebulizer, and atovaquone. Primary or secondary prophylaxis for PCP can be discontinued in those patients treated with ART who maintain good suppression of HIV (<50 copies/mL) and CD4+ T-cell counts >200/μL for at least 3 months.

M. tuberculosis, once thought to be on its way to extinction in the United States, experienced a resurgence associated with the HIV epidemic **(Chap. 173)**. Worldwide, approximately one-third of all AIDS-related deaths are associated with TB, and TB is the primary cause of death for 10–15% of patients with HIV infection. In the United States ~5% of untreated AIDS patients have active TB. Patients with HIV infection are more likely to have active TB by a factor of 100 when compared with an HIV-negative population. For an asymptomatic HIV-negative person with a positive purified protein derivative (PPD) skin test, the risk of reactivation TB is around 1% per year. For the patient with untreated HIV infection, a positive PPD skin test, and no signs or symptoms of TB, the rate of reactivation TB is 7–10% per year. Untreated TB can accelerate the course of HIV infection. Levels of plasma HIV RNA increase in the setting of active TB and decline in the setting of successful TB treatment. Active TB is most common in patients 25–44 years of age, in African Americans and Hispanics, in patients in New York City and Miami, and in patients in developing countries. In these demographic groups, 20–70% of the new cases of active TB are in patients with HIV infection. The epidemic of TB embedded in the epidemic of HIV infection probably represents the greatest health risk to the general public and the health care profession associated with the HIV epidemic. In contrast to infection with atypical mycobacteria such as MAC, active TB often develops relatively early in the course of HIV infection and may be an early clinical sign of HIV disease. In one study, the median CD4+ T-cell count at presentation of TB was 326/μL.

The clinical manifestations of TB in HIV-infected patients are quite varied and generally show different patterns as a function of the CD4+ T-cell count. In patients with relatively high CD4+ T-cell counts, the typical pattern of pulmonary reactivation occurs: patients present with fever, cough, dyspnea on exertion, weight loss, night sweats, and a chest x-ray revealing cavitary apical disease of the upper lobes. In patients with lower CD4+ T-cell counts, disseminated disease is more common. In these patients the chest x-ray may reveal diffuse or lower-lobe bilateral reticulonodular infiltrates consistent with miliary spread, pleural effusions, and hilar and/or mediastinal adenopathy. Infection may be present in bone, brain, meninges, GI tract, lymph nodes (particularly cervical lymph nodes), and viscera. Some patients with advanced HIV infection and active TB may have no symptoms of illness, and thus screening for TB should be part of the initial evaluation of every patient with HIV infection. Approximately 60–80% of HIV-infected patients with TB have pulmonary disease, and 30–40% have extrapulmonary disease. Respiratory isolation and a negative-pressure room should be used for patients in whom a diagnosis of pulmonary TB is being considered. This approach is critical to limit nosocomial and community spread of infection. Culture of the organism from an involved site provides a definitive diagnosis. Blood cultures are positive in 15% of patients. This figure is higher in patients with lower CD4+ T-cell counts. In the setting of fulminant disease, one cannot rely on the accuracy of a negative PPD skin test to rule out a diagnosis of TB. In addition, IFN-γ release assays may be difficult to interpret due to high backgrounds as a consequence of HIV-associated immune activation. TB is one of the conditions associated with HIV infection for which cure is possible with appropriate therapy. Therapy for TB is generally the same in the HIV-infected patient as in the HIV-negative patient (**Chap. 173**). Due to the possibility of multidrug-resistant or extensively drug-resistant TB, drug susceptibility testing should be performed to guide therapy. Due to pharmacokinetic interactions, adjusted doses of rifabutin and/or changes in ART are required when treating TB in the setting of HIV infection. Treatment is most effective in programs that involve directly observed therapy. Initiation of ART and/or anti-TB therapy may be associated with clinical deterioration due to immune reconstitution inflammatory syndrome (IRIS) reactions. These are most common in patients initiating both treatments at the same time, may occur as early as 1 week after initiation of ART therapy, and are seen more frequently in patients with advanced HIV disease. For these reasons it is recommended that initiation of ART be delayed in antiretroviral-naïve patients with CD4 counts >50 cells/μL until 2–4 weeks following the initiation of treatment for TB. For patients with lower CD4 counts the benefits of more immediate ART outweigh the risks of IRIS, and ART should be started as soon as possible in those patients. Effective prevention of active TB can be a reality if the health care professional is aggressive in looking for evidence of latent or active TB by making sure that all patients with HIV infection receive a PPD skin test or evaluation with an IFN-γ release assay. Anergy testing is not of value in this setting. Since these tests rely on the host mounting an immune response to *M. tuberculosis*, patients with CD4+ T-cell counts <200 cells/μL should be retested if their CD4+ T-cell counts rise to persistently above 200. Patients at risk of continued exposure to TB should be tested annually. HIV-infected individuals with a skin-test reaction of >5 mm, those with a positive IFN-γ release assay, or those who are close household contacts of persons with active TB should receive treatment with 9 months of isoniazid and pyridoxine.

Atypical mycobacterial infections are also seen with an increased frequency in patients with HIV infection. Infections with at least 12 different mycobacteria have been reported, including *M. bovis* and representatives of all four Runyon groups. The most common atypical mycobacterial infection is with *M. avium* or *M. intracellulare* species—the *Mycobacterium avium* complex (MAC). Infections with MAC are seen mainly in patients in the United States and are rare in Africa. It has been suggested that prior infection with *M. tuberculosis* decreases the risk of MAC infection. MAC infections probably arise from organisms that are ubiquitous in the environment, including both soil and water. There is little evidence for person-to-person transmission of MAC infection. The presumed portals of entry are the respiratory and GI tracts. MAC infection is a late complication of HIV infection, occurring predominantly in patients with CD4+ T-cell counts of <50/μL. The average CD4+ T-cell count at the time of diagnosis is 10/μL. The most common presentation is disseminated disease with fever, weight loss, and night sweats. At least 85% of patients with MAC infection are mycobacteremic, and large numbers of organisms can often be demonstrated on bone marrow biopsy. The chest x-ray is abnormal in ~25% of patients, with the most common pattern being that of a bilateral, lower-lobe infiltrate suggestive of miliary spread. Alveolar or nodular infiltrates and hilar and/or mediastinal adenopathy also can occur. Other clinical findings include endobronchial lesions, abdominal pain, diarrhea, and lymphadenopathy. Anemia and elevated liver alkaline phosphatase are common. The diagnosis is made by the culture of blood or involved tissue. The finding of two consecutive sputum samples positive for MAC is highly suggestive of pulmonary infection. Cultures may take 2 weeks to turn positive. Therapy consists of a macrolide, usually clarithromycin, with ethambutol. Some physicians elect to add a third drug from among rifabutin, ciprofloxacin, or amikacin in patients with extensive disease. Therapy is continued until resolution of clinical signs and symptoms, negative cultures, and CD4+ T-cell counts >100/μL for 3–6 months in the setting of ART. Primary prophylaxis for MAC is indicated in patients with HIV infection and CD4+ T-cell counts <50/μL not immediately starting ART. (Table 202-11). This may be discontinued in patients in whom ART induces a sustained suppression of viral replication regardless of the change in CD4+ T-cell count.

Rhodococcus equi is a gram-positive, pleomorphic, acid-fast, non-spore-forming bacillus that can cause pulmonary and/or disseminated infection in patients with advanced HIV infection. Fever and cough are the most common presenting signs. Radiographically one may see cavitary lesions and consolidation. Blood cultures are often positive. Treatment is based on antimicrobial sensitivity testing.

Fungal infections of the lung, in addition to PCP, can be seen in patients with AIDS. Patients with pulmonary cryptococcal disease present with fever, cough, dyspnea, and, in some cases, hemoptysis. A focal or diffuse interstitial infiltrate is seen on chest x-ray in >90% of patients. In addition, one may see lobar disease, cavitary disease, pleural effusions, and hilar or mediastinal adenopathy. More than half of patients are fungemic, and 90% of patients have concomitant CNS infection. *Coccidioides immitis* is a mold that is endemic in the southwest United States. It can cause a reactivation pulmonary syndrome in patients with HIV infection. Most patients with this condition will have CD4+ T-cell counts <250/μL. Patients present with fever, weight loss, cough, and extensive, diffuse reticulonodular infiltrates on chest x-ray. One may also see nodules, cavities, pleural effusions, and hilar adenopathy. While serologic testing is of value in the immunocompetent host, serologies are negative in 25% of HIV-infected patients with coccidioidal infection. Invasive aspergillosis is not an AIDS-defining illness and is generally not seen in patients with AIDS in the absence of neutropenia or administration of glucocorticoids. When it does occur, *Aspergillus* infection may have an unusual presentation in the respiratory tract of patients with AIDS, where it gives the appearance of a pseudomembranous tracheobronchitis. Primary pulmonary infection of the lung may be seen with *histoplasmosis*. The most common pulmonary manifestation of histoplasmosis, however, is in the setting of disseminated disease, presumably due to reactivation. In this setting respiratory symptoms are usually minimal, with cough and dyspnea occurring in 10–30% of patients. The chest x-ray is abnormal in ~50% of patients, showing either a diffuse interstitial infiltrate or diffuse small nodules, and the urine will often be positive for *Histoplasma* antigen.

Two forms of *idiopathic interstitial pneumonia* have been identified in patients with HIV infection: lymphoid interstitial pneumonitis (LIP) and nonspecific interstitial pneumonitis (NIP). LIP, a common finding in children, is seen in about 1% of adult patients with untreated HIV infection. This disorder is characterized by a benign infiltrate of the lung and is thought to be part of the polyclonal activation of lymphocytes seen in the context of HIV and EBV infections. Transbronchial biopsy is diagnostic in 50% of the cases, with an open-lung biopsy required for diagnosis in the remainder of cases. This condition is generally self-limited, and no specific treatment is necessary. Severe cases have been managed with brief courses of glucocorticoids. Although rarely a clinical problem since the use of ART, evidence of NIP may be seen in up to half of all patients with untreated HIV infection. Histologically, interstitial infiltrates of lymphocytes and plasma cells in a perivascular and peribronchial distribution are present. When symptomatic, patients present with fever and nonproductive cough occasionally accompanied by mild chest discomfort. Chest x-ray is usually normal or may reveal a faint interstitial pattern. Like LIP, NIP is a self-limited process for which no therapy is indicated other than appropriate management of the underlying HIV infection. HIV-related pulmonary arterial hypertension (HIV-PAH) is seen in ~0.5% of HIV-infected individuals. Patients may present with an array of symptoms including shortness of breath, fatigue, syncope, chest pain, and signs of right-sided heart failure. Chest x-ray reveals dilated pulmonary vessels and right-sided cardiomegaly with right ventricular hypertrophy seen on electrocardiogram. ART does not appear to be of clear benefit, and the prognosis is quite poor with a median survival in the range of 2 years.

Neoplastic diseases of the lung including KS and lymphoma are discussed below in the section on neoplastic diseases.

Diseases of the Cardiovascular System Heart disease is a relatively common postmortem finding in HIV-infected patients (25–75% in autopsy series). The most common form of heart disease is coronary heart disease. In one large series the overall rate of myocardial infarction (MI) was 3.5/1000 patient-years, 28% of these events were fatal, and MI was responsible for 7% of all deaths in the cohort. In patients with HIV infection, cardiovascular disease may be associated with classic risk factors such as smoking, a direct consequence of HIV infection, or a complication of ART. Patients with HIV infection have higher levels of triglycerides, lower levels of high-density lipoprotein cholesterol, and a higher prevalence of smoking than cohorts of individuals without HIV infection. The finding that the rate of cardiovascular disease events was lower in patients on antiretroviral therapy than in those randomized to undergo a treatment interruption identified a clear association between HIV replication and risk of cardiovascular disease. In one study, a baseline CD4+ T-cell count of <500/μL was found to be an independent risk factor for cardiovascular disease comparable in magnitude to that attributable to smoking. While the precise pathogenesis of this association remains unclear, it is likely related to the immune activation and increased propensity for coagulation seen because of HIV replication. Exposure to HIV protease inhibitors and certain reverse transcriptase inhibitors has been associated with increases in total cholesterol and/or risk of MI. Any increases in the risk of death from MI resulting from the use of certain antiretrovirals must be balanced against the marked increases in overall survival brought about by these drugs.

Another form of heart disease associated with HIV infection is a dilated cardiomyopathy associated with congestive heart failure (CHF) referred to as *HIV-associated cardiomyopathy*. This generally occurs as a late complication of HIV infection and, histologically, displays elements of myocarditis. For this reason, some have advocated it be treated with IV immunoglobulin (IVIg). HIV can be directly demonstrated in cardiac tissue in this setting, and there is debate over whether HIV plays a direct role in this condition. Patients present with typical findings of CHF including edema and shortness of breath. Patients with HIV infection may also develop cardiomyopathy as side effects of IFN-α or nucleoside analogue therapy. These are reversible once therapy is stopped. KS, cryptococcosis, Chagas' disease, and toxoplasmosis can involve the myocardium, leading to cardiomyopathy. In one series, most patients with HIV infection and a treatable myocarditis were found to have myocarditis associated with toxoplasmosis. Most of these patients also had evidence of CNS toxoplasmosis. Thus, MRI or double-dose contrast CT scan of the brain should be included in the workup of any patient with advanced HIV infection and cardiomyopathy.

A variety of other cardiovascular problems are found in patients with HIV infection. Pericardial effusions may be seen in the setting of advanced HIV infection. Predisposing factors include TB, CHF, mycobacterial infection, cryptococcal infection, pulmonary infection, lymphoma, and KS. While pericarditis is quite rare, in one series 5% of patients with HIV disease had pericardial effusions that were considered to be moderate or severe. Tamponade and death have occurred in association with pericardial KS, presumably owing to acute hemorrhage. Nonbacterial thrombotic endocarditis has been reported and should be considered in patients with unexplained embolic phenomena. IV pentamidine, when given rapidly, can result in hypotension as a consequence of cardiovascular collapse.

Diseases of the Oropharynx and Gastrointestinal System Oropharyngeal and GI diseases are common features of HIV infection. They are most frequently due to secondary infections. In addition, oral and GI lesions may occur with KS and lymphoma.

Oral lesions, including *thrush*, *hairy leukoplakia*, and *aphthous ulcers* (**Fig. 202-35**), are particularly common in patients with untreated HIV infection. Thrush, due to *Candida* infection, and oral hairy leukoplakia, presumed due to EBV, are usually indicative of fairly advanced immunologic decline; they generally occur in patients with CD4+ T-cell counts of <300/μL. In one study, 59% of patients with oral candidiasis went on to develop AIDS in the next year. Thrush appears as a white, cheesy exudate, often on an erythematous mucosa in the posterior oropharynx. While most commonly seen on the soft palate, early lesions are often found along the gingival vestibule. The diagnosis is made by direct examination of a scraping for pseudohyphal elements. Culturing is of no diagnostic value, as patients with HIV infection may have a positive throat culture for *Candida* in the absence of thrush. Oral hairy leukoplakia presents as white, frondlike lesions, generally along the lateral borders of the tongue and sometimes on the adjacent buccal mucosa (Fig. 202-35). Despite its name, oral hairy leukoplakia is not considered a premalignant condition. Lesions are associated with florid replication of EBV. While usually more disconcerting as a sign of HIV-associated immunodeficiency than a clinical problem in need of treatment, severe cases of oral hairy leukoplakia have been reported to respond to topical podophyllin or systemic therapy with anti-herpesvirus agents. Aphthous ulcers of the posterior oropharynx also are seen with regularity in patients with untreated HIV infection (Fig. 202-35). These lesions are of unknown etiology and can be quite painful and interfere with swallowing. Topical anesthetics provide immediate symptomatic relief of short duration. The fact that thalidomide is an effective treatment for this condition suggests that the pathogenesis may involve the action of tissue-destructive cytokines. Palatal, glossal, or gingival ulcers may also result from cryptococcal disease or histoplasmosis.

Esophagitis (**Fig. 202-36**) may present with odynophagia and retrosternal pain. Upper endoscopy is generally required to make an accurate diagnosis. Esophagitis may be due to *Candida*, CMV, or HSV. While CMV tends to be associated with a single large ulcer, HSV infection is more often associated with multiple small ulcers. The esophagus may also be the site of KS and lymphoma. Like the oral mucosa, the esophageal mucosa may have large, painful ulcers of unclear etiology that may respond to thalidomide. While achlorhydria is a common problem in patients with HIV infection, other gastric problems are generally rare. Among the neoplastic conditions involving the stomach are KS and lymphoma.

Infections of the small and large intestine leading to diarrhea, abdominal pain, and occasionally fever are among the most significant GI problems in HIV-infected patients. They include infections with bacteria, protozoa, and viruses.

Bacteria may be responsible for infections of the GI tract in patients with HIV infection. Infections with enteric pathogens such as *Salmonella*, *Shigella*, and *Campylobacter* are more common in men who have sex with men and are often more severe and more apt to relapse in patients with HIV infection. Patients with untreated HIV have approximately a 20-fold increased risk of infection with *S. typhimurium*. They may present with a variety of nonspecific symptoms including fever, anorexia, fatigue, and malaise of several weeks' duration. Diarrhea is common but may be absent. Diagnosis is made by culture of blood and stool. Long-term therapy with ciprofloxacin is the recommended treatment. HIV-infected patients also have an increased incidence of *S. typhi* infection in areas of the world where typhoid is a problem. *Shigella* spp., particularly *S. flexneri*, can cause severe intestinal disease in HIV-infected individuals. Up to 50% of patients with GI disease will develop bacteremia. *Campylobacter* infections occur with an increased frequency in patients with HIV infection. While *C. jejuni* is the strain most frequently isolated, infections with many other strains have been reported. Patients usually present with crampy abdominal pain, fever, and bloody diarrhea. Infection may also present as proctitis. Stool examination reveals the presence of fecal leukocytes. Systemic infection can occur, with up to 10% of infected patients exhibiting bacteremia. Most strains are sensitive to erythromycin. Abdominal pain and diarrhea may be seen with MAC infection, and patients with HIV infection may have persistent diarrhea due to enteroaggregative *E. coli*.

Fungal infections may also be a cause of diarrhea in patients with HIV infection. Histoplasmosis, coccidioidomycosis, and penicilliosis have all been identified as a cause of fever and diarrhea in patients with HIV infection. Peritonitis has been seen with *C. immitis*.

Cryptosporidia, microsporidia, and *Isospora belli* (**Chap. 224**) are the most common opportunistic protozoa that infect the GI tract and cause diarrhea in HIV-infected patients. Cryptosporidial infection may

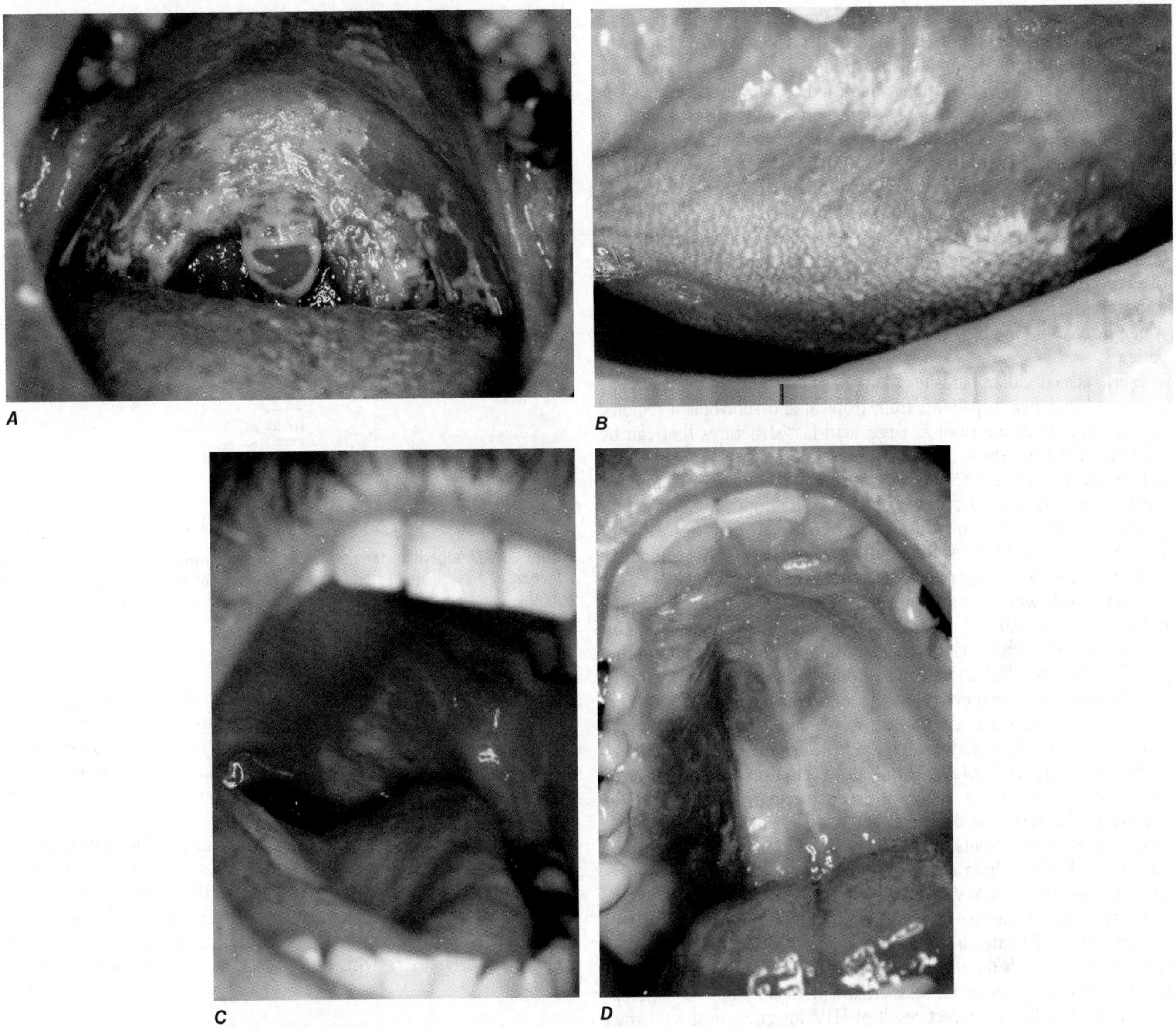

A

B

C

D

FIGURE 202-35 Various oral lesions in HIV-infected individuals. ***A.*** Thrush. ***B.*** Hairy leukoplakia. ***C.*** Aphthous ulcer. ***D.*** Kaposi's sarcoma.

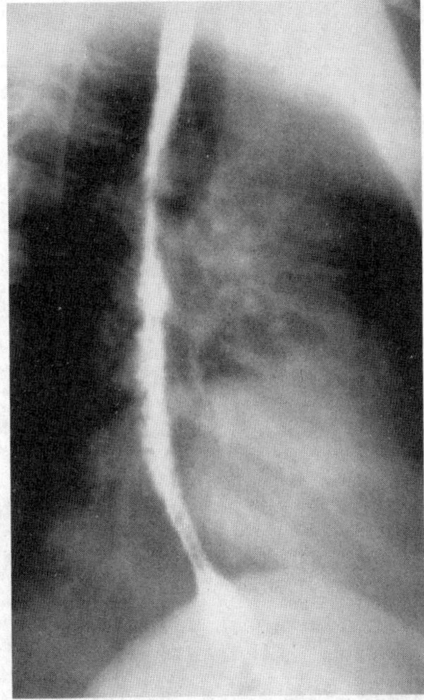

FIGURE 202-36 Barium swallow of a patient with *Candida* esophagitis. The flow of barium along the mucosal surface is grossly irregular.

present in a variety of ways, ranging from a self-limited or intermittent diarrheal illness in patients in the early stages of HIV infection to a severe, life-threatening diarrhea in severely immunodeficient individuals. In patients with untreated HIV infection and CD4+ T-cell counts of <300/μL, the incidence of cryptosporidiosis is ~1% per year. In 75% of cases the diarrhea is accompanied by crampy abdominal pain, and 25% of patients have nausea and/or vomiting. Cryptosporidia may also cause biliary tract disease in the HIV-infected patient, leading to cholecystitis with or without accompanying cholangitis and pancreatitis secondary to papillary stenosis. The diagnosis of cryptosporidial diarrhea is made by stool examination or biopsy of the small intestine. The diarrhea is noninflammatory, and the characteristic finding is the presence of oocysts that stain with acid-fast dyes. Therapy is predominantly supportive and marked improvements have been reported in the setting of effective ART. Treatment with up to 2000 mg/d of nitazoxanide (NTZ) is associated with improvement in symptoms or a decrease in shedding of organisms in about half of patients. Its overall role in the management of this condition remains unclear. Patients can minimize their risk of developing cryptosporidiosis by avoiding contact with human and animal feces, by not drinking untreated water from lakes or rivers, and by not eating raw shellfish.

Microsporidia are small, unicellular, obligate intracellular parasites that reside in the cytoplasm of enteric cells (**Chap. 224**). The main species causing disease in humans is *Enterocytozoon bieneusi*. The clinical manifestations are similar to those described for cryptosporidia and include abdominal pain, malabsorption, diarrhea, and cholangitis. The small size of the organism may make it difficult to detect; however, with the use of chromotrope-based stains, organisms can be identified in stool samples by light microscopy. Definitive diagnosis generally depends on electron-microscopic examination of a stool specimen, intestinal aspirate, or intestinal biopsy specimen. In contrast to cryptosporidia, microsporidia have been noted in a variety of extraintestinal locations, including the eye, brain, sinuses, muscle, and liver, and they have been associated with conjunctivitis and hepatitis. The most effective way to deal with microsporidia in a patient with HIV infection is to restore the immune system by treating the HIV infection with ART. Albendazole, 400 mg bid, has been reported to be of benefit in some patients.

I. belli is a coccidian parasite (Chap. 224) most commonly found as a cause of diarrhea in patients from tropical and subtropical regions. Its cysts appear in the stool as large, acid-fast structures that can be differentiated from those of cryptosporidia based on size, shape, and number of sporocysts. The clinical syndromes of *Isospora* infection are identical to those caused by cryptosporidia. The important distinction is that infection with *Isospora* is generally relatively easy to treat with TMP-SMX. While relapses are common, a thrice-weekly regimen of TMP-SMX appears adequate to prevent recurrence.

CMV colitis was once seen as a consequence of advanced immunodeficiency in 5–10% of patients with AIDS. It is much less common with the advent of ART. CMV colitis presents as diarrhea, abdominal pain, weight loss, and anorexia. The diarrhea is usually nonbloody, and the diagnosis is achieved through endoscopy and biopsy. Multiple mucosal ulcerations are seen at endoscopy, and biopsies reveal characteristic intranuclear and cytoplasmic inclusion bodies. Secondary bacteremias may result as a consequence of thinning of the bowel wall. Treatment is with either valganciclovir/ganciclovir or foscarnet for 3–6 weeks. Relapses are common, and maintenance therapy is typically necessary in patients whose HIV infection is poorly controlled. Patients with CMV disease of the GI tract should be carefully monitored for evidence of CMV retinitis.

In addition to disease caused by specific secondary infections, patients with HIV infection may also experience a chronic diarrheal syndrome for which no etiologic agent other than HIV can be identified. This entity is referred to as *AIDS enteropathy* or *HIV enteropathy*. It is most likely a direct result of HIV infection in the GI tract and improves with ART. Histologic examination of the small bowel in these patients reveals low-grade mucosal atrophy with a decrease in mitotic figures, suggesting a hyporegenerative state. Patients often have decreased or absent small-bowel lactase and malabsorption with accompanying weight loss.

The initial evaluation of a patient with HIV infection and diarrhea should include a set of stool examinations, including culture, examination for ova and parasites, and examination for *Clostridium difficile* toxin. Approximately 50% of the time this workup will demonstrate infection with pathogenic bacteria, mycobacteria, or protozoa. If the initial stool examinations are negative, additional evaluation, including upper and/or lower endoscopy with biopsy, will yield a diagnosis of microsporidial or mycobacterial infection of the small intestine ~30% of the time. In patients for whom this diagnostic evaluation is nonrevealing, a presumptive diagnosis of HIV enteropathy can be made if the diarrhea has persisted for >1 month. An algorithm for the evaluation of diarrhea in patients with HIV infection is given in Fig. 202-37.

Rectal lesions are common in HIV-infected patients, particularly the perirectal ulcers and erosions due to the reactivation of HSV (Fig. 202-38). These lesions may appear quite atypical, as denuded skin without vesicles. They typically respond well to treatment with valacyclovir, famciclovir, or foscarnet. Other rectal lesions encountered in patients with HIV infection include condylomata acuminata, KS, and intraepithelial neoplasia (see below).

Hepatobiliary Diseases Diseases of the hepatobiliary system are a major problem in patients with HIV infection. It has been estimated that approximately 15% of the deaths of patients with HIV infection are related to liver disease. While this is predominantly a reflection of the problems encountered in the setting of co-infection with hepatitis B or C, it is also a reflection of the hepatic injury, ranging from hepatic steatosis to hypersensitivity reactions to immune reconstitution, that can be seen in the context of ART.

The prevalence of co-infection with HIV and hepatitis viruses varies by geographic region. In the United States, ~90% of HIV-infected individuals have evidence of infection with HBV; 6–14% have chronic HBV infection; 5–50% of patients are co-infected with HCV; and co-infections with hepatitis D, E, and/or G viruses are common. Among IV drug users with HIV infection, rates of HCV infection

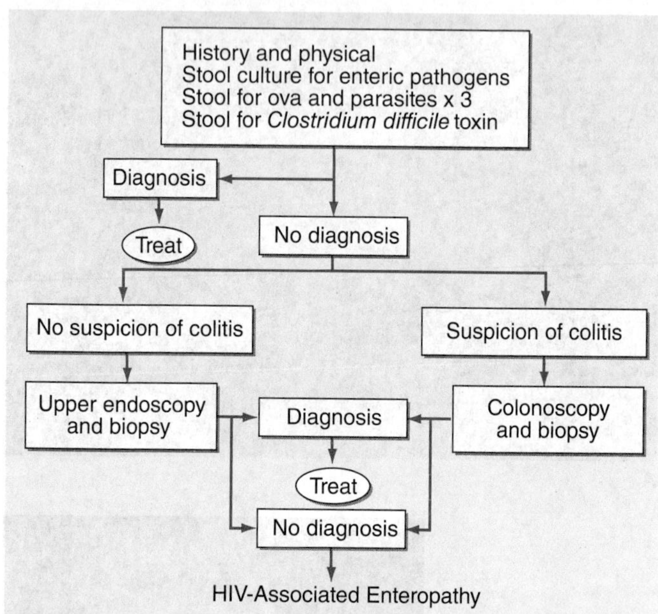

FIGURE 202-37 Algorithm for the evaluation of diarrhea in a patient with HIV infection. HIV-associated enteropathy is a diagnosis of exclusion and can be made only after other, generally treatable, forms of diarrheal illness have been ruled out.

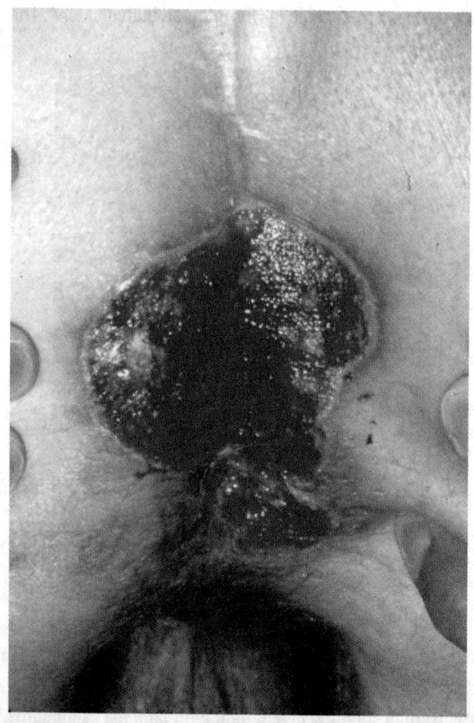

FIGURE 202-38 Severe, erosive perirectal herpes simplex in a patient with AIDS.

range from 70 to 95%. HIV infection has a significant impact on the course of hepatitis virus infection. It is associated with approximately a threefold increase in the development of persistent hepatitis B surface antigenemia. Patients infected with both HBV and HIV have decreased evidence of inflammatory liver disease. The presumption that this is due to the immunosuppressive effects of HIV infection is supported by the observations that this situation can be reversed, and one may see the development of more severe hepatitis following the initiation of effective ART. In studies of the impact of HIV on HBV infection, four- to tenfold increases in liver-related mortality rates have been noted in patients with HIV and active HBV infection compared to rates in patients with either infection alone. There is, however, only a slight increase in overall mortality rate in HIV-infected individuals who are also hepatitis B surface antigen (HBsAg)–positive. IFN-α is less successful as treatment for HBV in patients with HIV co-infection. Lamivudine, emtricitabine, adefovir/tenofovir/entecavir, and telbivudine alone or in combination are useful in the treatment of hepatitis B in patients with HIV infection. It is important to remember that all the above-mentioned drugs also have activity against HIV and should not be used alone in patients with HIV infection, to avoid the emergence of quasispecies of HIV resistant to these drugs. For this reason, the treatment of hepatitis B infection in a patient with HIV infection should always be done in the setting of ART, and alterations in ART need to take into account that the current regimen is also treating HBV. HCV infection is more severe in the patient with HIV infection; it does not appear to affect overall mortality rates in HIV-infected individuals when other variables such as age, baseline CD4+ T-cell count, and use of ART are taken into account. In the setting of HIV and HCV co-infection, levels of HCV are approximately tenfold higher than in the HIV-negative patient with HCV infection. There is a 50% higher overall mortality rate with a five-fold increased risk of death due to liver disease in patients chronically infected with both HCV and HIV. Use of directly acting agents for the treatment of HCV leads to cure rates approaching 100%, even in patients with HIV co-infection. Successful treatment of HCV in HIV-infected patients decreases mortality. Hepatitis A virus infection is not seen with an increased frequency in patients with HIV infection. It is recommended that all patients with HIV infection who have not experienced natural infection be immunized with hepatitis A and/or hepatitis B vaccines. Infection with hepatitis G virus, also known as GB virus C, is seen in ~50% of patients with HIV infection. For reasons that are currently unclear, there are data to suggest that patients with HIV infection co-infected with this virus have a decreased rate of progression to AIDS.

A variety of other infections also may involve the liver. Granulomatous hepatitis may be seen as a consequence of mycobacterial or fungal infections, particularly MAC infection. Hepatic masses may be seen in the context of TB, peliosis hepatis, or fungal infection. Among the fungal opportunistic infections, *C. immitis* and *Histoplasma capsulatum* are those most likely to involve the liver. Biliary tract disease in the form of papillary stenosis or sclerosing cholangitis has been reported in the context of cryptosporidiosis, CMV infection, and KS. When no diagnosis can be made, the term *AIDS cholangiopathy* is used. Hemophagocytic lymphohistiocytosis of the liver has been seen in the setting of Hodgkin's disease and may occur prior to diagnosis of the underlying neoplasm.

Many of the drugs used to treat HIV infection are metabolized by the liver and can cause liver injury. Fatal hepatic reactions have been reported with a wide array of antiretrovirals including nucleoside analogues, nonnucleoside analogues, and protease inhibitors. Nucleoside analogues work by inhibiting DNA synthesis. This can result in toxicity to mitochondria, which can lead to disturbances in oxidative metabolism. This may manifest as hepatic steatosis and, in severe cases, lactic acidosis and fulminant liver failure. It is important to be aware of this condition and to watch for it in patients with HIV infection receiving nucleoside analogues. It is reversible if diagnosed early and the offending agent(s) discontinued. Nevirapine has been associated with at times fatal fulminant and cholestatic hepatitis, hepatic necrosis, and hepatic failure. Indinavir may cause mild to moderate elevations in serum bilirubin in 10–15% of patients in a syndrome similar to Gilbert's syndrome. A similar pattern of hepatic injury may be seen with atazanavir. In the patient receiving ART with an unexplained increase in hepatic transaminases, strong consideration should be given to drug toxicity.

Pancreatic injury is most commonly a consequence of drug toxicity, notably that secondary to pentamidine or dideoxynucleosides. While up to half of patients in some series have biochemical evidence of pancreatic injury, <5% of patients show any clinical evidence of pancreatitis that is not linked to a drug toxicity.

Diseases of the Kidney and Genitourinary Tract Diseases of the kidney or genitourinary tract may be a direct consequence of HIV infection, due to an opportunistic infection or neoplasm, or related to drug toxicity. Overall, microalbuminuria is seen in ~20% of untreated HIV-infected patients; significant proteinuria is seen in closer to 2%. The presence of microalbuminuria has been associated with an increase in all-cause mortality. *HIV-associated nephropathy* (HIVAN) was first described in IDUs and was initially thought to be IDU nephropathy in patients with HIV infection; it is now recognized as a true direct complication of HIV infection. Although most patients with this condition have CD4+ T-cell counts <200/μL, HIV-associated nephropathy can be an early manifestation of HIV infection and is also seen in children. Over 90% of reported cases have been in African-American or Hispanic individuals; the disease is not only more prevalent in these populations but also more severe and is the third leading cause of end-stage renal failure among African Americans age 20–64 in the United States. Proteinuria is the hallmark of this disorder. Edema and hypertension are rare. Ultrasound examination reveals enlarged, hyperechogenic kidneys. A definitive diagnosis is obtained through renal biopsy. Histologically, focal segmental glomerulosclerosis is present in 80%, and mesangial proliferation in 10–15% of cases. Prior to effective antiretroviral therapy, this disease was characterized by relatively rapid progression to end-stage renal disease. Patients with HIV-associated nephropathy should be treated for their HIV infection. Treatment with angiotensin-converting enzyme (ACE) inhibitors and/or prednisone, 60 mg/d, also has been reported to be of benefit in some cases. The incidence of this disease in patients receiving adequate ART has not been well defined; however, the impression is that it has decreased in frequency and severity. It is the leading cause of end-stage renal disease in patients with HIV infection.

Among the drugs commonly associated with renal damage in patients with HIV disease are pentamidine, amphotericin, adefovir, cidofovir, tenofovir, and foscarnet. Switching from TDF to TAF may lead to a decrease in renal injury from tenofovir. TMP-SMX may compete for tubular secretion with creatinine and cause an increase in the serum creatinine level. The pharmacokinetic booster cobicistat, a component of several fixed-drug ART formulations, inhibits renal tubular secretion of creatinine leading to increased serum creatinine levels without a true decline in glomerular filtration rate. Sulfadiazine may crystallize in the kidney and result in an easily reversible form of renal shutdown, while indinavir or atazanavir may form renal calculi. Adequate hydration is the mainstay of treatment and prevention for these latter two conditions.

Genitourinary tract infections are seen with a high frequency in patients with HIV infection; they present with skin lesions, dysuria, hematuria, and/or pyuria and are managed in the same fashion as in patients without HIV infection. Infections with HSV are covered below ("Dermatologic Diseases"). Infections with *T. pallidum*, the etiologic agent of *syphilis*, play an important role in the HIV epidemic. In HIV-negative individuals, genital syphilitic ulcers as well as the ulcers of chancroid are major predisposing factors for heterosexual transmission of HIV infection. While most HIV-infected individuals with syphilis have a typical presentation, a variety of formerly rare clinical problems may be encountered in the setting of dual infection. Among them are *lues maligna*, an ulcerating lesion of the skin due to a necrotizing vasculitis; unexplained fever; nephrotic syndrome; and neurosyphilis. The most common presentation of syphilis in the HIV-infected patient is that of *condylomata lata*, a form of secondary syphilis. Neurosyphilis may be asymptomatic or may present as acute meningitis, neuroretinitis, deafness, or stroke. The rate of neurosyphilis may be as high as 1% in patients with HIV infection, and one should consider a lumbar puncture to look for neurosyphilis in all patients with HIV infection and secondary syphilis. As a consequence of the immunologic abnormalities seen in the setting of HIV infection, diagnosis of syphilis through standard serologic testing may be challenging. On the one hand, a significant number of patients have false-positive Venereal Disease Research Laboratory (VDRL) tests due to polyclonal B-cell activation. On the other hand, the development of a new positive VDRL may be delayed in patients with new infections, and the anti–fluorescent treponemal antibody (anti-FTA) test may be negative due to immunodeficiency. Thus, dark-field examination of appropriate specimens should be performed in any patient in whom syphilis is suspected, even if the patient has a negative VDRL. Similarly, any patient with a positive serum VDRL test, neurologic findings, and an abnormal spinal fluid examination should be considered to have neurosyphilis and treated accordingly, regardless of the CSF VDRL result. In any setting, patients treated for syphilis need to be carefully monitored to ensure adequate therapy. Approximately one-third of patients with HIV infection will experience a Jarisch-Herxheimer reaction upon initiation of therapy for syphilis.

Vulvovaginal candidiasis is a common problem in women with HIV infection. Symptoms include pruritus, discomfort, dyspareunia, and dysuria. Vulvar infection may present as a morbilliform rash that may extend to the thighs. Vaginal infection is usually associated with a white discharge, and plaques may be seen along an erythematous vaginal wall. Diagnosis is made by microscopic examination of the discharge for pseudohyphal elements in a 10% potassium hydroxide solution. Mild disease can be treated with topical therapy. More serious disease can be treated with fluconazole. Other causes of vaginitis include *Trichomonas* and mixed bacteria.

Diseases of the Endocrine System and Metabolic Disorders

A variety of endocrine and metabolic disorders are seen in the context of HIV infection. These may be a direct consequence of HIV infection, secondary to opportunistic infections or neoplasms, or related to medication side effects. Between 33 and 75% of patients with HIV infection receiving thymidine analogues or protease inhibitors as a component of ART develop a syndrome often referred to as *lipodystrophy*, consisting of elevations in plasma triglycerides, total cholesterol, and apolipoprotein B, as well as hyperinsulinemia and hyperglycemia. Many of the patients have been noted to have a characteristic set of body habitus changes associated with fat redistribution, consisting of truncal obesity coupled with peripheral wasting (**Fig. 202-39**). Truncal obesity is apparent as an increase in abdominal girth related to increases in mesenteric fat, a dorsocervical fat pad ("buffalo hump") reminiscent of patients with Cushing's syndrome, and enlargement of the breasts. The peripheral wasting, or lipoatrophy, is particularly noticeable in the face and buttocks and by the prominence of the veins in the legs. These changes may develop at any time ranging from ~6 weeks to several years following the initiation of ART. Approximately 20% of the patients with HIV-associated lipodystrophy meet the criteria for the *metabolic syndrome* as defined by The International Diabetes Federation or The U.S. National Cholesterol Education Program Adult Treatment Panel III. The lipodystrophy syndrome has been reported in association with regimens containing a variety of different drugs, and while initially reported in the setting of protease inhibitor therapy, it appears that similar changes can also be induced by protease-sparing regimens. It has been suggested that the lipoatrophy changes are particularly severe in patients receiving the thymidine analogues stavudine and zidovudine. Current treatment guidelines avoid these drugs and recommend drugs with fewer of these side effects. National Cholesterol Education Program (NCEP) guidelines should be followed in the management of these lipid abnormalities (**Chap. 400**), and consideration should be given to changing the components of ART with avoidance of thymidine analogues (azidothymidine and stavudine) and offending protease inhibitors. Due to concerns regarding drug interactions, the most utilized lipid-lowering agents in this setting are gemfibrozil and atorvastatin. In addition, lactic acidosis is associated with ART. This is most often seen with nucleoside analogue reverse transcriptase inhibitors and can be fatal.

Patients with advanced HIV disease may develop hyponatremia due to the syndrome of inappropriate antidiuretic hormone (vasopressin) secretion (SIADH) because of increased free-water intake and decreased free-water excretion. SIADH is usually seen in conjunction with pulmonary or CNS disease. Low serum sodium may also be due to adrenal insufficiency; a concomitant high serum potassium should alert one to this possibility. Hyperkalemia may be secondary to adrenal insufficiency; HIV nephropathy; or medications, particularly trimethoprim and pentamidine. Hypokalemia may be seen in the setting of tenofovir or amphotericin therapy. Adrenal gland disease may be due to mycobacterial infections, CMV

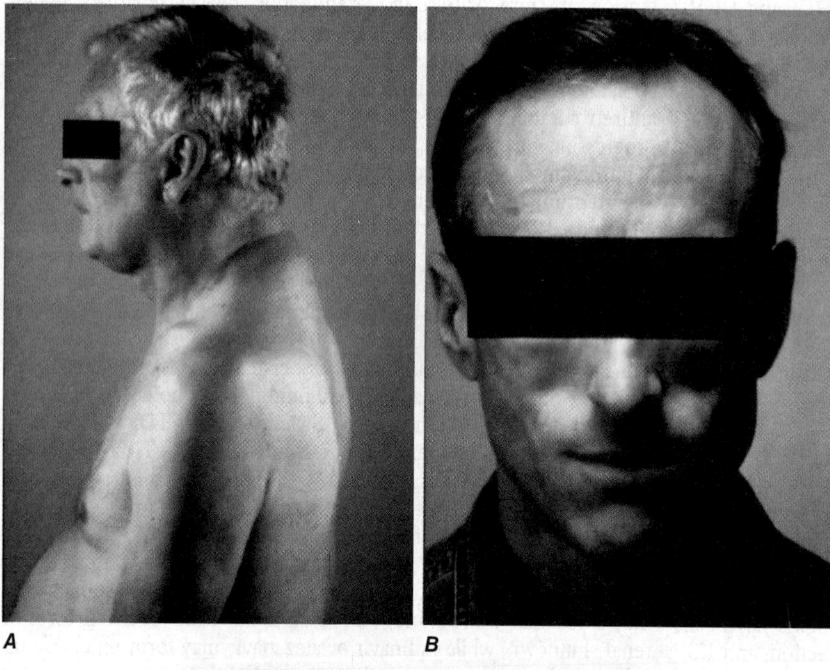

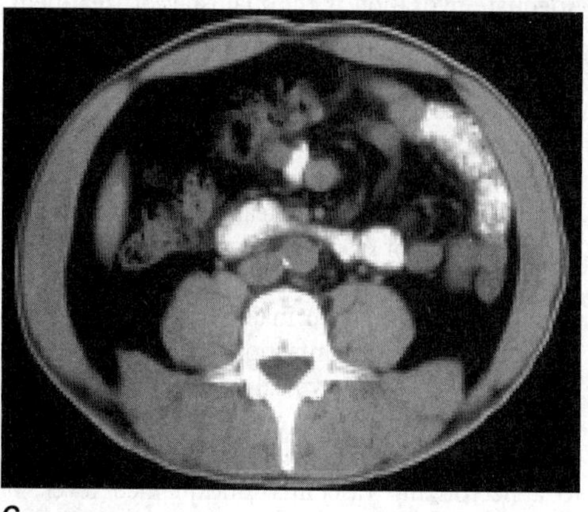

FIGURE 202-39 Characteristics of lipodystrophy. ***A.*** Truncal obesity and buffalo hump. ***B.*** Facial wasting. ***C.*** Accumulation of intraabdominal fat on CT scan.

disease, cryptococcal disease, histoplasmosis, or ketoconazole toxicity. Iatrogenic Cushing's syndrome with suppression of the hypothalamic-pituitary-adrenal axis may be seen with the use of local glucocorticoids (injected or inhaled) in patients receiving ritonavir or cobicistat. This is due to inhibition of the hepatic enzyme CYP3A4 by ritonavir leading to prolongation of the glucocorticoid half-life.

Thyroid function may be altered in 10–15% of patients with HIV infection. Both hypo- and hyperthyroidism may be seen. The predominant abnormality is subclinical hypothyroidism. In the setting of ART, up to 10% of patients have been noted to have elevated thyroid-stimulating hormone levels, suggesting that this may be a manifestation of immune reconstitution. Immune-reconstitution Graves' disease may occur as a late (9–48 months) complication of ART. In advanced HIV disease, infection of the thyroid gland may occur with opportunistic pathogens, including *P. jirovecii*, CMV, mycobacteria, *Toxoplasma gondii*, and *Cryptococcus neoformans*. These infections are generally associated with a nontender, diffuse enlargement of the thyroid gland. Thyroid function is usually normal. Diagnosis is made by fine-needle aspirate or open biopsy.

Depending on the severity of disease, HIV infection is associated with *hypogonadism* in 20–50% of men and is lowest in the setting of ART. While this is generally a complication of underlying illness, testicular dysfunction may also be a side effect of ganciclovir therapy. In some surveys, up to two-thirds of patients report decreased libido and one-third complain of erectile dysfunction. Androgen-replacement therapy should be considered in patients with symptomatic hypogonadism. HIV infection does not seem to have a significant effect on the menstrual cycle outside the setting of advanced disease.

Immunologic and Rheumatologic Diseases Immunologic and rheumatologic disorders are common in patients with HIV infection and range from excessive immediate-type hypersensitivity reactions (**Chap. 347**) to an increase in the incidence of reactive arthritis (**Chap. 355**) to conditions characterized by a diffuse infiltrative lymphocytosis. The occurrence of these phenomena is an apparent paradox in the setting of the profound immunodeficiency and immunosuppression that characterizes HIV infection and reflects the complex nature of the immune system and its regulatory mechanisms.

Drug allergies are the most significant allergic reactions occurring in HIV-infected patients and appear to become more common as the disease progresses. They occur in up to 65% of patients who receive therapy with TMP-SMX for PCP. In general, these drug reactions are characterized by erythematous, morbilliform eruptions that are pruritic, tend to coalesce, and are often associated with fever. Nonetheless, ~33% of patients can be maintained on the offending therapy, and thus these reactions are not an immediate indication to stop the drug. Anaphylaxis is extremely rare in patients with HIV infection, and patients who have a cutaneous reaction during a single course of therapy can still be considered candidates for future treatment or prophylaxis with the same agent. The one exception to this is the nucleoside analogue abacavir, where fatal hypersensitivity reactions have been reported with rechallenge. This hypersensitivity is strongly associated with the HLA-B5701 haplotype, and a hypersensitivity reaction to abacavir is an absolute contraindication to future therapy. For other agents, including TMP-SMX, desensitization regimens are moderately successful. While the mechanisms underlying these allergic-type reactions remain unknown, patients with HIV infection have been noted to have elevated IgE levels that increase as the CD4+ T-cell count declines. The numerous examples of patients with multiple drug reactions suggest that a common pathway is involved.

HIV infection shares many similarities with a variety of autoimmune diseases, including a substantial polyclonal B-cell activation that is associated with a high incidence of antiphospholipid antibodies, such as anticardiolipin antibodies, VDRL antibodies, and lupus-like anticoagulants. In addition, HIV-infected individuals have an increased incidence of antinuclear antibodies. Despite these serologic findings, there is no evidence that HIV-infected individuals have an increase in two of the more common autoimmune diseases, i.e., systemic lupus erythematosus and rheumatoid arthritis. In fact, it has been observed that these diseases may be somewhat ameliorated by the concomitant presence of HIV infection, suggesting that an intact CD4+ T-cell limb of the immune response plays an integral role in the pathogenesis of these conditions. Similarly, there are anecdotal reports of patients with common variable immunodeficiency (**Chap. 344**), characterized by hypogammaglobulinemia, who have had a normalization of Ig levels following the development of HIV infection, suggesting a possible role for overactive CD4+ T-cell immunity in certain forms of that syndrome. The one autoimmune disease that may occur with an increased frequency in patients with HIV infection is a variant of primary Sjögren's syndrome (**Chap. 354**) in which patients with HIV infection develop a syndrome consisting of parotid gland enlargement, dry eyes, and dry mouth. This condition is associated with lymphocytic infiltrates of the salivary gland and lung. One also can see peripheral neuropathy, polymyositis, renal tubular acidosis, and hepatitis. In contrast to Sjögren's syndrome, in which the lymphocytic infiltrates are composed predominantly of CD4+ T cells, in patients with HIV infection the infiltrates are composed predominantly of CD8+ T cells. In addition, while patients with Sjögren's syndrome are mainly women who have autoantibodies to Ro and La and who frequently have HLA-DR3 or B8 MHC haplotypes, HIV-infected individuals with this syndrome are usually African-American men who do not have anti-Ro or anti-La and who most often are HLA-DR5. This syndrome appears to be less common with the increased use of effective ART. The term *diffuse infiltrative lymphocytosis syndrome* (DILS) is used to describe this entity and to distinguish it from Sjögren's syndrome.

Approximately one-third of HIV-infected individuals experience arthralgias; furthermore, 5–10% are diagnosed as having some form of reactive arthritis, such as Reiter's syndrome or psoriatic arthritis as well as undifferentiated spondyloarthropathy (**Chap. 355**). These syndromes occur with increasing frequency as the competency of the immune system declines. This association may be related to an increase in the number of infections with organisms that may trigger a reactive arthritis with progressive immunodeficiency or to a loss of important regulatory T cells. Reactive arthritides in HIV-infected individuals generally respond well to standard treatment; however, therapy with methotrexate has been associated with an increase in the incidence of opportunistic infections and should be used with caution and only in severe cases.

HIV-infected individuals also experience a variety of joint problems without obvious cause that are referred to generically as *HIV-* or *AIDS-associated arthropathy*. This syndrome is characterized by subacute oligoarticular arthritis developing over a period of 1–6 weeks and lasting 6 weeks to 6 months. It generally involves the large joints, predominantly the knees and ankles, and is nonerosive with only a mild inflammatory response. X-rays are nonrevealing. Nonsteroidal anti-inflammatory drugs are only marginally helpful; however, relief has been noted with the use of intraarticular glucocorticoids. A second form of arthritis also thought to be secondary to HIV infection is called *painful articular syndrome*. This condition, reported as occurring in as many as 10% of AIDS patients, presents as an acute, severe, sharp pain in the affected joint. It affects primarily the knees, elbows, and shoulders; lasts 2–24 h; and may be severe enough to require narcotic analgesics. The cause of this arthropathy is unclear; however, it is thought to result from a direct effect of HIV on the joint. This condition is reminiscent of the fact that other lentiviruses, in particular the caprine arthritis-encephalitis virus, are capable of directly causing arthritis.

A variety of other immunologic or rheumatologic diseases have been reported in HIV-infected individuals, either de novo or in association with opportunistic infections or drugs. Using the criteria of widespread musculoskeletal pain of at least 3 months' duration and the presence of at least 11 of 18 possible tender points by digital palpation, 11% of an HIV-infected cohort containing 55% IDUs were diagnosed as having *fibromyalgia* (**Chap. 366**). While the incidence of frank arthritis was less in this population than in other studied populations that consisted predominantly of men who have sex with men, these data support the concept that there are musculoskeletal problems that occur as a direct result of HIV infection. CNS angiitis and polymyositis also have been reported in HIV-infected individuals. Septic arthritis is surprisingly rare, especially given the increased incidence of staphylococcal bacteremias seen in this population. When septic arthritis has been reported, it has usually been due to *Staphylococcus aureus*, systemic fungal infection with *C. neoformans*, *Sporothrix schenckii*, or *H. capsulatum* or to systemic mycobacterial infection with *M. tuberculosis*, *M. haemophilum*, *M. avium*, or *M. kansasii*.

Patients with HIV infection treated with ART have been found to have an increased incidence of osteonecrosis or avascular necrosis of the hip and shoulders. In a study of asymptomatic patients, 4.4% were found to have evidence of osteonecrosis on MRI. While precise cause-and-effect relationships have been difficult to establish, this complication has been associated with the use of lipid-lowering agents, systemic glucocorticoids, and testosterone; bodybuilding exercise; alcohol consumption; and the presence of anticardiolipin antibodies. Osteoporosis has been reported in 7% of women with HIV infection, with 41% of women demonstrating some degree of osteopenia. Several studies have documented decreases in bone mineral density of 2–6% in the first 2 years following the initiation of ART. This may be particularly apparent with tenofovir-containing regimens.

Immune Reconstitution Inflammatory Syndrome (IRIS) Following the initiation of effective ART, a paradoxical worsening of preexisting, untreated, or partially treated opportunistic infections may be noted. One may also see exacerbations of pre-existing autoimmune conditions or the development of new autoimmune conditions following the initiation of antiretrovirals (**Table 202-12**). IRIS related to a known pre-existing infection or neoplasm is referred to as *paradoxical IRIS*, while IRIS associated with a previously undiagnosed condition is referred to as *unmasking IRIS*. The term *immune reconstitution disease (IRD)* is sometimes used to distinguish IRIS manifestations related to opportunistic diseases from IRIS manifestations related to autoimmune diseases. IRD is particularly common in patients with underlying untreated mycobacterial or fungal infections. Some form of IRIS is seen in 10–30% of patients following the initiation of ART, depending on the clinical setting, and is most common in patients starting therapy with CD4+ T-cell counts <50 cells/μL who have a precipitous drop in HIV RNA levels following the initiation of ART. Signs and symptoms may appear anywhere from 2 weeks to 2 years after the initiation of ART and can include localized lymphadenitis, prolonged fever, pulmonary infiltrates, hepatitis, increased intracranial pressure, uveitis, sarcoidosis, and Graves' disease. The clinical course can be protracted, and severe cases can be fatal. The underlying mechanism appears to be related to a phenomenon similar to type IV hypersensitivity reactions and reflects the immediate improvements in immune function that occur as levels of HIV RNA drop and the immunosuppressive effects of HIV infection are controlled. In severe cases, the use of immunosuppressive drugs such as glucocorticoids may be required to blunt the inflammatory component of these reactions while specific antimicrobial therapy takes effect.

Diseases of the Hematopoietic System Disorders of the hematopoietic system including lymphadenopathy, anemia, leukopenia, and/or thrombocytopenia are common throughout the course of HIV infection and may be the direct result of HIV, manifestations of secondary infections and neoplasms, or side effects of therapy (**Table 202-13**). Direct histologic examination and culture of lymph node or bone marrow tissue are often diagnostic. A significant percentage of bone marrow aspirates from patients with HIV infection have been reported to contain lymphoid aggregates, the precise significance of which is unknown. Initiation of ART will lead to reversal of most hematologic complications that are the direct result of HIV infection.

TABLE 202-12 Characteristics of Immune Reconstitution Inflammatory Syndrome (IRIS)

Paradoxical worsening of an existing clinical condition or abrupt appearance of a new clinical finding (unmasking) is seen following the initiation of antiretroviral therapy
Occurs weeks to months following the initiation of antiretroviral therapy
Is most common in patients starting therapy with a CD4+ T-cell count <50/μL who experience a precipitous drop in viral load
Is frequently seen in the setting of tuberculosis; particularly when cART is starting soon after initiation of anti-TB therapy
Can be fatal

TABLE 202-13 Causes of Bone Marrow Suppression in Patients with HIV Infection

HIV infection	Medications
Mycobacterial infections	Zidovudine
Fungal infections	Dapsone
B19 parvovirus infection	Trimethoprim/sulfamethoxazole
Lymphoma	Pyrimethamine
	5-Flucytosine
	Ganciclovir
	Interferon α
	Trimetrexate
	Foscarnet

Some patients, otherwise asymptomatic, may develop *persistent generalized lymphadenopathy* as an early clinical manifestation of HIV infection. This condition is defined as the presence of enlarged lymph nodes (>1 cm) in two or more extrainguinal sites for >3 months without an obvious cause. The lymphadenopathy is due to marked follicular hyperplasia in the node in response to HIV infection. The nodes are generally discrete and freely movable. This feature of HIV disease may be seen at any point in the spectrum of immune dysfunction and is not associated with an increased likelihood of developing AIDS. Paradoxically, a loss in lymphadenopathy or a decrease in lymph node size outside the setting of ART may be a prognostic marker of disease progression. In patients with CD4+ T-cell counts >200/μL, the differential diagnosis of lymphadenopathy includes TB, KS, Castleman's disease, and lymphoma. In patients with more advanced disease, lymphadenopathy may also be due to atypical mycobacterial infection, toxoplasmosis, systemic fungal infection, or bacillary angiomatosis. While indicated in patients with CD4+ T-cell counts <200/μL, lymph node biopsy is not indicated in patients with early-stage disease unless there are signs and symptoms of systemic illness, such as fever and weight loss, or unless the nodes begin to enlarge, become fixed, or coalesce. Monoclonal gammopathy of unknown significance (MGUS) (**Chap. 107**), defined as the presence of a serum monoclonal IgG, IgA, or IgM in the absence of a clear cause, has been reported in 3% of patients with HIV infection. The overall clinical significance of this finding in patients with HIV infection is unclear, although it has been associated with other viral infections, non-Hodgkin's lymphoma, and plasma cell malignancy.

Anemia is the most common hematologic abnormality in HIV-infected patients and, in the absence of a specific treatable cause, is independently associated with a poor prognosis. While generally mild, anemia can be quite severe and require chronic blood transfusions. Among the specific reversible causes of anemia in the setting of HIV infection are drug toxicity, systemic fungal and mycobacterial infections, nutritional deficiencies, and parvovirus B19 infections. The antiretroviral zidovudine may block erythroid maturation prior to its effects on other marrow elements. A characteristic feature of zidovudine therapy is an elevated mean corpuscular volume (MCV). Another drug used in patients with HIV infection that has a selective effect on the erythroid series is dapsone. This drug can cause a serious hemolytic anemia in patients who are deficient in glucose-6-phosphate dehydrogenase and can create a functional anemia in others through induction of methemoglobinemia. Folate levels are usually normal in HIV-infected individuals; however, vitamin B_{12} levels may be depressed as a consequence of achlorhydria or malabsorption. True autoimmune hemolytic anemia is rare, although ~20% of patients with HIV infection may have a positive direct antiglobulin test as a consequence of polyclonal B-cell activation. Infection with parvovirus B19 may also cause anemia. It is important to recognize this possibility given the fact that it responds well to treatment with IVIg. Erythropoietin levels in patients with HIV infection and anemia are generally lower than expected given the degree of anemia. Treatment with erythropoietin may result in an increase in hemoglobin levels. An exception to this is a subset of patients with zidovudine-associated anemia in whom erythropoietin levels may be quite high.

During the course of HIV infection, neutropenia may be seen in approximately half of patients. In most instances it is mild; however, it can be severe and can put patients at risk of spontaneous bacterial infections. This is most frequently seen in patients with severely advanced HIV disease and in patients receiving any of a number of potentially myelosuppressive therapies. In the setting of neutropenia, diseases that are not commonly seen in HIV-infected patients, such as aspergillosis or mucormycosis, may occur. Both granulocyte colony-stimulating factor (G-CSF) and GM-CSF increase neutrophil counts in patients with HIV infection regardless of the cause of the neutropenia. Earlier concerns about the potential of these agents to also increase levels of HIV were not confirmed in controlled clinical trials.

Thrombocytopenia may be an early consequence of HIV infection. Approximately 3% of patients with untreated HIV infection and CD4+ T-cell counts ≥400/μL have platelet counts <150,000/μL. For untreated patients with CD4+ T-cell counts <400/μL, this incidence increases to 10%. Thrombocytopenia is more common in patients with hepatitis C co-infection, cirrhosis, and/or ongoing high-level HIV replication. Thrombocytopenia is rarely a serious clinical problem in patients with HIV infection and generally responds well to successful ART. Clinically, it resembles the thrombocytopenia seen in patients with idiopathic thrombocytopenic purpura (**Chap. 111**). Immune complexes containing anti-gp120 antibodies and anti-anti-gp120 antibodies have been noted in the circulation and on the surface of platelets in patients with HIV infection. Patients with HIV infection have also been noted to have a platelet-specific antibody directed toward a 25-kDa component of the surface of the platelet. Other data suggest that the thrombocytopenia in patients with HIV infection may be due to a direct effect of HIV on megakaryocytes. Whatever the cause, it is very clear that the most effective medical approach to this problem has been the use of ART. For patients with platelet counts <20,000/μL, a more aggressive approach combining IVIg or anti-Rh Ig for an immediate response and ART for a more lasting response is appropriate. Rituximab has been used with some success in otherwise refractory cases. Splenectomy is a rarely needed option and is reserved for patients refractory to medical management. Because of the risk of serious infection with encapsulated organisms, all patients with HIV infection about to undergo splenectomy should be immunized with vaccines to prevent disease from *S. pneumoniae*, *N. meningitidis*, and *H. influenzae* type b. It should be noted that, in addition to causing an increase in the platelet count, removal of the spleen will result in an increase in the peripheral blood lymphocyte count, making CD4+ T-cell counts unreliable markers of immunocompetence. In this setting, the clinician should rely on the CD4+ T-cell percentage for making diagnostic decisions with respect to the likelihood of opportunistic infections. A CD4+ T-cell percentage of 15 is approximately equivalent to a CD4+ T-cell count of 200/μL. In patients with early HIV infection, thrombocytopenia has also been reported as a consequence of classic thrombotic thrombocytopenic purpura (**Chap. 111**). This clinical syndrome, consisting of fever, thrombocytopenia, hemolytic anemia, and neurologic and renal dysfunction, is a rare complication of early HIV infection. As in other settings, the appropriate management is the use of salicylates and plasma exchange. Other causes of thrombocytopenia include lymphoma, mycobacterial infections, and fungal infections.

The incidence of venous thromboembolic disease such as deep-vein thrombosis or pulmonary embolus is approximately 1% per year in patients with HIV infection. This is approximately 10 times higher than that seen in an age-matched population. Factors associated with an increased risk of clinical thrombosis include age >45, history of an opportunistic infection, lower CD4 count, and estrogen use. Abnormalities of the coagulation cascade, including decreased protein S activity, increases in factor VIII, anticardiolipin antibodies, PAR-1 expression on T cells, or lupus-like anticoagulant, have been reported in more than 50% of patients with HIV infection. The clinical significance of this increased propensity toward thromboembolic disease is likely reflected in the observation that elevations in D-dimer are strongly associated with all-cause mortality in patients with HIV infection (Table 202-9).

Dermatologic Diseases Dermatologic problems occur in >90% of patients with HIV infection. From the macular, roseola-like rash seen with the acute seroconversion syndrome to extensive end-stage KS, cutaneous manifestations of HIV disease can be seen throughout the course of HIV infection. Among the more common nonneoplastic problems are seborrheic dermatitis, folliculitis, and opportunistic infections. Extrapulmonary pneumocystosis may cause a necrotizing vasculitis. Neoplastic conditions are covered in a separate section below.

Seborrheic dermatitis occurs in 3% of the general population and in up to 50% of patients with HIV infection. Seborrheic dermatitis increases in prevalence and severity as the CD4+ T-cell count declines. In HIV-infected patients, seborrheic dermatitis may be aggravated by concomitant infection with *Pityrosporum*, a yeastlike fungus; use of topical antifungal agents has been recommended in cases refractory to standard topical treatment.

Folliculitis is among the most prevalent dermatologic disorders in patients with HIV infection and is seen in ~20% of patients. It is more common in patients with CD4+ T-cell counts <200 cells/μL. *Pruritic papular eruption* is one of the most common pruritic rashes in patients with HIV infection. It appears as multiple papules on the face, trunk, and extensor surfaces and may improve with ART. *Eosinophilic pustular folliculitis* is a rare form of folliculitis that is seen with increased frequency in patients with HIV infection. It presents as multiple, urticarial perifollicular papules that may coalesce into plaque-like lesions. Skin biopsy reveals an eosinophilic infiltrate of the hair follicle, which in certain cases has been associated with the presence of a mite. Patients typically have an elevated serum IgE level and may respond to treatment with topical anthelmintics. Pruritus is a common symptom in patients with HIV infection and can lead to *prurigo nodularis*. Patients with HIV infection have also been reported to develop a severe form of *Norwegian scabies* with hyperkeratotic psoriasiform lesions.

Both *psoriasis* and *ichthyosis*, although they are not reported to be increased in frequency, may be particularly severe when they occur in patients with HIV infection. Preexisting psoriasis may become guttate in appearance and more refractory to treatment in the setting of HIV infection.

Reactivation herpes zoster (*shingles*) is seen in 10–20% of patients with HIV infection. This reactivation syndrome of varicella-zoster virus indicates a modest decline in immune function and may be the first indication of clinical immunodeficiency. In one series, patients who developed shingles did so an average of 5 years after HIV infection. In a cohort of patients with HIV infection and localized zoster, the subsequent rate of the development of AIDS was 1% per month. In that study, AIDS was more likely to develop if the outbreak of zoster was associated with severe pain, extensive skin involvement, or involvement of cranial or cervical dermatomes. The clinical manifestations of reactivation zoster in HIV-infected patients, although indicative of immunologic compromise, are not as severe as those seen in other immunodeficient conditions. Thus, while lesions may extend over several dermatomes, involve the spinal cord, and/or be associated with frank cutaneous dissemination, visceral involvement has not been reported. In contrast to patients without a known underlying immunodeficiency state, patients with HIV infection tend to have recurrences of shingles with a relapse rate of ~20%. Valacyclovir, acyclovir, or famciclovir is the treatment of choice. Foscarnet may be of value in patients with acyclovir-resistant virus.

Infection with *herpes simplex virus* in HIV-infected individuals is associated with recurrent orolabial, genital, and perianal lesions as part of recurrent reactivation syndromes (**Chap. 187**). As HIV disease progresses and the CD4+ T-cell count declines, these infections become more frequent and severe. Lesions often appear as beefy red, are exquisitely painful, and tend to occur high in the gluteal cleft (Fig. 202-37).

Perirectal HSV may be associated with proctitis and anal fissures. HSV should be high in the differential diagnosis of any HIV-infected patient with a poorly healing, painful perirectal lesion. In addition to recurrent mucosal ulcers, recurrent HSV infection in the form of *herpetic whitlow* can be a problem in patients with HIV infection, presenting with painful vesicles or extensive cutaneous erosion. Valacyclovir, acyclovir, or famciclovir is the treatment of choice in these settings. It is noteworthy that even subclinical reactivation of herpes simplex may be associated with increases in plasma HIV RNA levels.

Diffuse skin eruptions due to *Molluscum contagiosum* may be seen in patients with advanced HIV infection. These flesh-colored, umbilicated lesions resemble those of *Penicillium marnefei* or *Cryptococcosis.* They tend to regress with effective ART and can also be treated with local therapy. Similarly, *condyloma acuminatum* lesions may be more severe and more widely distributed in patients with low CD4+ T-cell counts. Imiquimod cream may be helpful in some cases. Atypical mycobacterial infections may present as erythematous cutaneous nodules, as may fungal infections, *Bartonella*, *Acanthamoeba*, and KS. Cutaneous infections with *Aspergillus* have been noted at the site of IV catheter placement.

The skin of patients with HIV infection is often a target organ for drug reactions (**Chap. 56**). Although most skin reactions are mild and not necessarily an indication to discontinue therapy, patients may have particularly severe cutaneous reactions, including erythroderma, *Stevens-Johnson syndrome*, and toxic epidermal necrolysis, as a reaction to drugs—particularly sulfa drugs, nonnucleoside reverse transcriptase inhibitors, abacavir, amprenavir, darunavir, fosamprenavir, and tipranavir. Similarly, patients with HIV infection are often quite photosensitive and burn easily following exposure to sunlight or as a side effect of radiation therapy (**Chap. 57**).

HIV infection and its treatment may be accompanied by cosmetic changes of the skin that are not of great clinical importance but may be troubling to patients. Yellowing of the nails and straightening of the hair, particularly in African-American patients, have been reported as a consequence of HIV infection. Zidovudine therapy has been associated with elongation of the eyelashes and the development of a bluish discoloration to the nails, again more common in African-American patients. Therapy with clofazimine may cause a yellow-orange discoloration of the skin and urine.

Neurologic Diseases Clinical disease of the nervous system accounts for a significant degree of morbidity in a high percentage of patients with HIV infection (**Table 202-14**). The neurologic problems that occur in HIV-infected individuals may be either primary to the pathogenic processes of HIV infection or secondary to opportunistic infections or neoplasms. Among the more frequent opportunistic diseases that involve the CNS are toxoplasmosis, cryptococcosis, progressive multifocal leukoencephalopathy, and primary CNS lymphoma. Other less common problems include mycobacterial infections; syphilis; and infection with CMV, herpes zoster, HTLV-1, *Trypanosoma cruzi*, or *Acanthamoeba*. Overall, secondary diseases of the CNS have been reported to occur in approximately one-third of patients with AIDS. These data antedate the widespread use of ART, and this frequency is considerably lower in patients with suppressed viral replication. Primary processes related to HIV infection of the nervous system are reminiscent of those seen with other lentiviruses, such as the maedi-visna virus of sheep.

TABLE 202-14 Neurologic Diseases in Patients with HIV Infection

Opportunistic infections	HIV-1 infection
Toxoplasmosis	Aseptic meningitis
Cryptococcosis	HIV-associated neurocognitive disorders (HAND), including HIV encephalopathy/AIDS dementia complex
Progressive multifocal leukoencephalopathy	Myelopathy
Cytomegalovirus	Vacuolar myelopathy
Syphilis	Pure sensory ataxia
Mycobacterium tuberculosis	Paresthesia/dysesthesia
HTLV-1 infection	Peripheral neuropathy
Amebiasis	Acute inflammatory demyelinating polyneuropathy (Guillain-Barré syndrome)
Neoplasms	Chronic inflammatory demyelinating polyneuropathy (CIDP)
Primary CNS lymphoma	Mononeuritis multiplex
Kaposi's sarcoma	Distal symmetric polyneuropathy
	Myopathy

Neurologic problems directly attributable to HIV occur throughout the course of infection and may be inflammatory, demyelinating, or degenerative in nature. The term *HIV-associated neurocognitive disorders* (HAND) is used to describe a spectrum of disorders that range from asymptomatic neurocognitive impairment (ANI) to minor neurocognitive disorder (MND) to clinically severe dementia. The most severe form, *HIV-associated dementia* (HAD), also referred to as the *AIDS dementia complex*, or *HIV encephalopathy*, is considered an AIDS-defining illness. Many HIV-infected patients have some neurologic problem during the course of their disease. Even in the setting of suppressive ART, approximately 50% of HIV-infected individuals can be shown to have mild to moderate neurocognitive impairment using sensitive neuropsychiatric testing. As noted in the section on pathogenesis, damage to the CNS may be a direct result of viral infection of the CNS macrophages or glial cells or may be secondary to the release of neurotoxins and potentially toxic cytokines such as IL-1β, TNF-α, IL-6, and TGF-β. It has been reported that HIV-infected individuals with the E4 allele for apoE are at increased risk for AIDS encephalopathy and peripheral neuropathy. Virtually all patients with HIV infection have some degree of nervous system involvement with the virus. This is evidenced by the fact that CSF findings are abnormal in ~90% of untreated patients, even during the asymptomatic phase of HIV infection. CSF abnormalities include pleocytosis (50–65% of patients), detection of viral RNA (~75%), elevated CSF protein (35%), and evidence of intrathecal synthesis of anti-HIV antibodies (90%). It is important to point out that evidence of infection of the CNS with HIV does not imply impairment of cognitive function. The neurologic function of an HIV-infected individual should be considered normal unless clinical signs and symptoms suggest otherwise.

Aseptic meningitis may occur at any time in the course of HIV infection; however, it is rare following the development of AIDS. This suggests that clinical aseptic meningitis in the context of HIV infection is an immune-mediated disease. In the setting of acute primary infection, patients may experience a syndrome of headache, photophobia, and meningismus. Rarely, an acute encephalopathy due to encephalitis may occur. Cranial nerve involvement may be seen, predominantly cranial nerve VII but occasionally V and/or VIII. CSF findings include a lymphocytic pleocytosis, elevated protein level, and normal glucose level. This syndrome, which cannot be clinically differentiated from other viral meningitides (**Chap. 134**), usually resolves spontaneously within 2–4 weeks; however, in some patients, signs and symptoms may become chronic.

Fungal meningitis is the leading infectious cause of meningitis in patients with AIDS (**Chap. 210**). While the vast majority of these are due to *C. neoformans*, up to 12% may be due to *C. gattii*. Cryptococcal meningitis is the initial AIDS-defining illness in ~2% of patients and generally occurs in patients with CD4+ T-cell counts <100/μL. Cryptococcal meningitis is particularly common in untreated patients with AIDS in Africa, occurring in ~5% of patients. Most patients present with a picture of subacute meningoencephalitis with fever, nausea, vomiting, altered mental status, headache, and meningeal signs. The incidence of seizures and focal neurologic deficits is low. The CSF profile may be normal or may show only modest elevations in WBC or protein levels and decreases in glucose. The opening pressure in the CSF is usually elevated. In addition to meningitis, patients may develop cryptococcomas and cranial nerve involvement. Approximately one-third of patients also have pulmonary disease. Uncommon manifestations of cryptococcal infection include skin lesions that resemble *molluscum contagiosum*, lymphadenopathy, palatal and glossal ulcers, arthritis, gastroenteritis, myocarditis, and prostatitis. The prostate gland may serve as a reservoir for smoldering cryptococcal infection. The diagnosis of cryptococcal meningitis is made by identification of organisms in spinal fluid with india ink examination or by the detection of cryptococcal antigen. Blood cultures for fungus are often positive. A biopsy may be needed to make a diagnosis of CNS cryptococcoma and to distinguish inadequately treated infection from immune reconstitution syndrome. Initial treatment is with IV amphotericin B 0.7 mg/kg daily, or liposomal amphotericin 4–6 mg/kg daily, with flucytosine 25 mg/kg qid for at least 2 weeks if possible. Decreases in renal function in association with amphotericin can lead to increases in flucytosine levels and subsequent bone marrow suppression. Therapy continues with amphotericin alone until the CSF culture turns negative followed by fluconazole 400 mg/d PO for 8 weeks, and then fluconazole 200 mg/d until the CD4+ T-cell count has increased to >200 cells/μL for 6 months in response to ART. Repeated lumbar puncture may be required to manage increased intracranial pressure. Symptoms may recur with initiation of ART as an immune reconstitution syndrome (see above). Other fungi that may cause meningitis in patients with HIV infection are *C. immitis* and *H. capsulatum*. Meningoencephalitis has also been reported due to *Acanthamoeba* or *Naegleria*.

HIV-associated dementia consists of a constellation of signs and symptoms of CNS disease. While this is generally a late complication of HIV infection that progresses slowly over months, it can be seen in patients with CD4+ T-cell counts >350 cells/μL. A major feature of this entity is the development of dementia, defined as a decline in cognitive ability from a previous level. It may present as impaired ability to concentrate, increased forgetfulness, difficulty reading, or increased difficulty performing complex tasks. Initially these symptoms may be indistinguishable from findings of situational depression or fatigue. In contrast to "cortical" dementia (such as Alzheimer's disease), aphasia, apraxia, and agnosia are uncommon, leading some investigators to classify HIV encephalopathy as a "subcortical dementia" characterized by defects in short-term memory and executive function (see below). In addition to dementia, patients with HIV encephalopathy may also have motor and behavioral abnormalities. Among the motor problems are unsteady gait, poor balance, tremor, and difficulty with rapid alternating movements. Increased tone and deep tendon reflexes may be found in patients with spinal cord involvement. Late stages may be complicated by bowel and/or bladder incontinence. Behavioral problems include apathy, irritability, and lack of initiative, with progression to a vegetative state in some instances. Some patients develop a state of agitation or mild mania. These changes usually occur without significant changes in level of alertness. This contrasts with the finding of somnolence in patients with dementia due to toxic/metabolic encephalopathies.

HIV-associated dementia is the initial AIDS-defining illness in ~3% of patients with HIV infection and thus only rarely precedes clinical evidence of immunodeficiency. Clinically significant encephalopathy eventually develops in ~25% of untreated patients with AIDS. As immunologic function declines, the risk and severity of HIV-associated dementia increases. Autopsy series suggest that 80–90% of patients with HIV infection have histologic evidence of CNS involvement. Several classification schemes have been developed for grading HIV encephalopathy; a commonly used clinical staging system is outlined in **Table 202-15**.

The precise cause of HIV-associated dementia remains unclear, although the condition is thought to be a result of a combination of direct effects of HIV on the CNS and associated immune activation. HIV has been found in the brains of patients with HIV encephalopathy by Southern blot, in situ hybridization, PCR, and electron microscopy. Multinucleated giant cells, macrophages, and microglial cells appear to be the main cell types harboring virus in the CNS. Histologically, the major changes are seen in the subcortical areas of the brain and include pallor and gliosis, multinucleated giant cell encephalitis, and vacuolar myelopathy. Less commonly, diffuse or focal spongiform changes occur in the white matter. Areas of the brain involved in motor function, language, and judgment are most severely affected.

There are no specific criteria for a diagnosis of HIV-associated dementia, and this syndrome must be differentiated from other diseases that affect the CNS of HIV-infected patients (Table 202-14). The diagnosis of dementia depends on demonstrating a decline in cognitive function. This can be accomplished objectively with the use of a Mini-Mental Status Examination (MMSE) in patients for whom prior scores are available. For this reason, it is advisable for all patients with a diagnosis of HIV infection to have a baseline MMSE. However, changes in MMSE scores may be absent in patients with mild HIV encephalopathy. Imaging studies of the CNS, by either MRI or CT, often demonstrate evidence of cerebral atrophy (**Fig. 202-40**). MRI may also reveal small areas of increased density on T2-weighted images. Lumbar puncture is an important element of the evaluation of patients with HIV infection and neurologic abnormalities. It is generally most helpful in ruling out or making a diagnosis of opportunistic infections. In HIV encephalopathy, patients may have the nonspecific findings of an increase in CSF cells and protein level. While HIV RNA can often be detected in the spinal fluid and HIV can be cultured from the CSF, this finding is not specific for HIV encephalopathy. There appears to be no correlation between the presence of HIV in the CSF and the presence of HIV encephalopathy. Elevated levels of macrophage chemoattractant protein (MCP-1), β_2-microglobulin, neopterin, and quinolinic acid (a metabolite of tryptophan reported to cause CNS injury) have been noted in the CSF of patients with HIV encephalopathy. These findings

TABLE 202-15 Clinical Staging of HAND According to Frascati Criteria

STAGE	NEUROCOGNITIVE STATUS[a]	FUNCTIONAL STATUS[b]
Asymptomatic	1 SD below mean in 2 cognitive domains	No impairments in activities of daily living
Mild neurocognitive disorder	1 SD below mean in 2 cognitive domains	Impairments in activities of daily living
HIV-associated dementia	2 SD below mean in 2 cognitive domains	Notable impairments in activities of daily living

[a]Neurocognitive testing should include assessment of at least 5 domains, including attention-information processing, language, abstraction-executive, complex perceptual motor skills, memory (including learning and recall), simple motor skills, or sensory perceptual skills. Appropriate norms must be available to establish the number of domains in which performance is below 1 SD. [b]Functional status is typically assessed by self-reporting but might be corroborated by a collateral source. No agreed measures exist for HIV-associated neurocognitive disorder criteria. Note that, for diagnosis of HIV-associated neurocognitive disorder, other causes of dementia must be ruled out and potential confounding effects of substance use or psychiatric illness should be considered.

Source: Adapted from A Antinori et al: Neurology 69:1789, 2007.

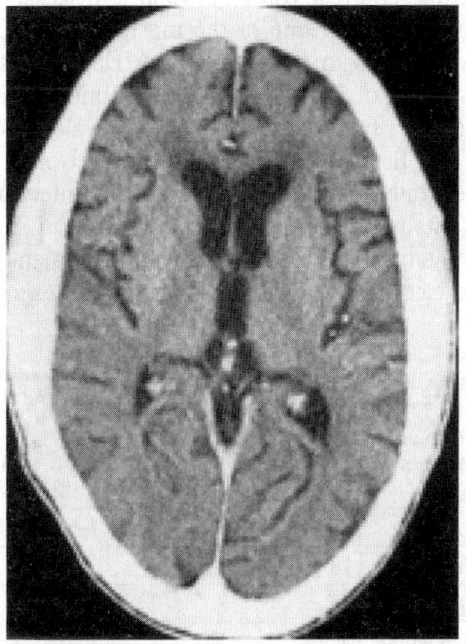

FIGURE 202-40 AIDS dementia complex. Postcontrast CT scan through the lateral ventricles of a 47-year-old man with AIDS, altered mental status, and dementia. The lateral and third ventricles and the cerebral sulci are abnormally prominent. Mild white matter hypodensity is seen adjacent to the frontal horns of the lateral ventricles.

suggest that these factors as well as inflammatory cytokines may be involved in the pathogenesis of this syndrome.

Combination antiretroviral therapy is of benefit in patients with HIV-associated dementia. Improvement in neuropsychiatric test scores has been noted for both adult and pediatric patients treated with antiretrovirals. The rapid improvement in cognitive function noted with the initiation of ART suggests that at least some component of this problem is quickly reversible, again supporting at least a partial role of soluble mediators in the pathogenesis. It should also be noted that these patients have an increased sensitivity to the side effects of neuroleptic drugs. The use of these drugs for symptomatic treatment is associated with an increased risk of extrapyramidal side effects; therefore, patients with HIV encephalopathy who receive these agents must be monitored carefully. It is felt by many physicians that the decrease in the prevalence of severe cases of HAND brought about by ART has resulted in an increase in the prevalence of milder forms of this disorder.

Seizures may be a consequence of opportunistic infections, neoplasms, or HIV encephalopathy (**Table 202-16**). The seizure threshold is often lower than normal in patients with advanced HIV infection due in part to the frequent presence of electrolyte abnormalities. Seizures are seen in 15–40% of patients with cerebral toxoplasmosis, 15–35% of patients with primary CNS lymphoma, 8% of patients with cryptococcal meningitis, and 7–50% of patients with HIV encephalopathy. Seizures may also be seen in patients with CNS tuberculosis, aseptic meningitis, and progressive multifocal leukoencephalopathy. Seizures may be the presenting clinical symptom of HIV disease. In one study of 100 patients with HIV infection presenting with a first seizure, cerebral mass lesions were the most common cause, responsible for 32 of the 100 new-onset seizures. Of these 32 cases, 28 were due to toxoplasmosis and 4 to lymphoma. HIV encephalopathy accounted for an additional 24 new-onset seizures. Cryptococcal meningitis was the third most common diagnosis, responsible for 13 of the 100 seizures. In 23 cases, no cause could be found, and it is possible that these cases represent a subcategory of HIV encephalopathy. Of these 23 cases, 16 (70%) had 2 or more seizures, suggesting that anticonvulsant therapy is indicated in all patients with HIV infection and seizures unless a rapidly correctable cause is found. Due to a variety of drug–drug interactions between antiseizure medications and antiretrovirals, drug levels need to be monitored carefully.

Patients with HIV infection may present with *focal neurologic deficits* from a variety of causes. The most common causes are toxoplasmosis, progressive multifocal leukoencephalopathy, and CNS lymphoma. Other causes include cryptococcal infections (discussed above; also **Chap. 210**), stroke, and reactivation of Chagas' disease.

Toxoplasmosis has been one of the most common causes of secondary CNS infections in patients with AIDS, but its incidence is decreasing in the era of ART. It is most common in patients from the Caribbean and from France, where the seroprevalence of *T. gondii* is around 50%. This figure is closer to 15% in the United States. Toxoplasmosis is generally a late complication of HIV infection and usually occurs in patients with CD4+ T-cell counts <200/μL. Cerebral toxoplasmosis is thought to represent a reactivation of latent tissue cysts. It is 10 times more common in patients with antibodies to the organism than in patients who are seronegative. Patients diagnosed with HIV infection should be screened for IgG antibodies to *T. gondii* during the time of their initial workup. Those who are seronegative should be counseled about ways to minimize the risk of primary infection including avoiding the consumption of undercooked meat and careful hand washing after contact with soil or changing the cat litter box. The most common clinical presentation of cerebral toxoplasmosis in patients with HIV infection is fever, headache, and focal neurologic deficits. Patients may present with seizure, hemiparesis, or aphasia as a manifestation of these focal deficits or with a picture more influenced by the accompanying cerebral edema and characterized by confusion, dementia, and lethargy, which can progress to coma. The diagnosis is usually suspected on the basis of MRI findings of multiple lesions in multiple locations, although in some cases only a single lesion is seen. Pathologically, these lesions generally exhibit inflammation and central necrosis and, as a result, demonstrate ring enhancement on contrast MRI (**Fig. 202-41**) or, if MRI is unavailable or contraindicated, on double-dose contrast CT. There is usually evidence of surrounding edema. In addition to toxoplasmosis, the differential diagnosis of single or multiple enhancing mass lesions in the HIV-infected patient includes primary CNS lymphoma and, less commonly, TB or fungal or bacterial abscesses. The definitive diagnostic procedure is brain biopsy. However, given the morbidity rate that can accompany this procedure, it is usually reserved for the patient who has failed 2–4 weeks of empiric therapy for toxoplasmosis. If the patient is seronegative for *T. gondii*, the likelihood that a mass lesion is due to toxoplasmosis is <10%. In that setting, one may choose to be more aggressive and perform a brain biopsy sooner. Standard treatment is sulfadiazine and pyrimethamine with leucovorin as needed for a minimum of 4–6 weeks. Alternative therapeutic regimens include clindamycin in combination with pyrimethamine; atovaquone plus pyrimethamine; and azithromycin plus pyrimethamine plus rifabutin. Relapses are common, and it is recommended that patients with a history of prior toxoplasmic encephalitis receive maintenance therapy with sulfadiazine, pyrimethamine, and leucovorin as long as their CD4+ T-cell counts remain <200 cells/μL. Patients with CD4+ T-cell counts <100/μL and IgG antibody to *Toxoplasma* should receive primary prophylaxis for toxoplasmosis. Fortunately, the same daily regimen of a single double-strength tablet of TMP-SMX used for *P. jirovecii* prophylaxis provides adequate primary protection against toxoplasmosis. Secondary prophylaxis/maintenance therapy for toxoplasmosis may be discontinued in the setting of effective ART and increases in CD4+ T-cell counts to >200/μL for 6 months.

JC virus, a human polyomavirus that is the etiologic agent of *progressive multifocal leukoencephalopathy* (PML), is an important opportunistic pathogen in patients with AIDS (**Chap. 133**). While ~80% of

TABLE 202-16 Causes of Seizures in Patients with HIV Infection

DISEASE	OVERALL CONTRIBUTION TO FIRST SEIZURE, %	FRACTION OF PATIENTS WHO HAVE SEIZURES, %
HIV encephalopathy	24–47	7–50
Cerebral toxoplasmosis	28	15–40
Cryptococcal meningitis	13	8
Primary central nervous system lymphoma	4	15–30
Progressive multifocal leukoencephalopathy	1	20

Source: From DM Holtzman et al: Am J Med 87:173, 1989.

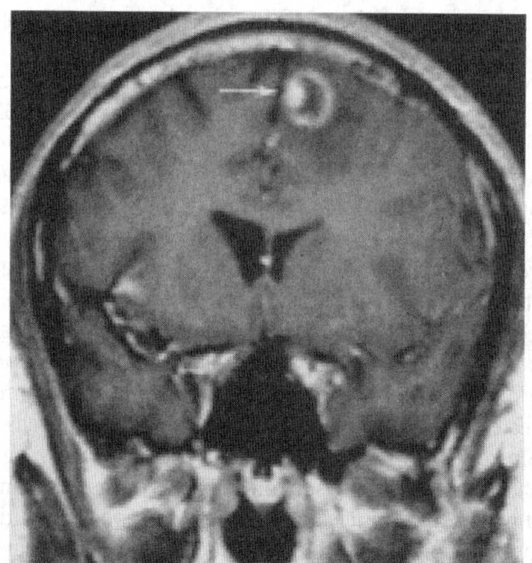

FIGURE 202-41 Central nervous system toxoplasmosis. A coronal postcontrast T1-weighted MRI scan demonstrates a peripheral enhancing lesion in the left frontal lobe, associated with an eccentric nodular area of enhancement (*arrow*); this so-called eccentric target sign is typical of toxoplasmosis.

the general adult population has antibodies to JC virus, indicative of prior infection, <10% of healthy adults show any evidence of ongoing viral replication. PML is the only known clinical manifestation of JC virus infection. It is a late manifestation of AIDS and is seen in ~1–4% of patients with AIDS. The lesions of PML begin as small foci of demyelination in subcortical white matter that eventually coalesce. The cerebral hemispheres, cerebellum, and brainstem may all be involved. Patients typically have a protracted course with multifocal neurologic deficits, with or without changes in mental status. Approximately 20% of patients experience seizures. Ataxia, hemiparesis, visual field defects, aphasia, and sensory defects may occur. Headache, fever, nausea, and vomiting are rarely seen. Their presence should suggest another diagnosis. MRI typically reveals multiple, nonenhancing white matter lesions that may coalesce and have a predilection for the occipital and parietal lobes. The lesions show signal hyperintensity on T2-weighted images and diminished signal on T1-weighted images. The measurement of JC virus DNA levels in CSF has a diagnostic sensitivity of 76% and a specificity of close to 100%. Prior to the availability of ART, most patients with PML died within 3–6 months of the onset of symptoms. Paradoxical worsening of PML has been seen with initiation of ART as an immune reconstitution syndrome. There is no specific treatment for PML; however, a median survival of 2 years and survival of >15 years have been reported in patients with PML treated with ART for their HIV disease. Despite having a significant impact on survival, only ~50% of patients with HIV infection and PML show neurologic improvement with ART. Studies with other antiviral agents such as cidofovir have failed to show clear benefit. Factors influencing a favorable prognosis for PML in the setting of HIV infection include a CD4+ T-cell count >100/μL at baseline and the ability to maintain an HIV viral load of <500 copies/mL. Baseline HIV-1 viral load does not have independent predictive value of survival. PML is one of the few opportunistic infections that continues to occur with some frequency despite the widespread use of ART.

Reactivation American trypanosomiasis may present as acute meningoencephalitis with focal neurologic signs, fever, headache, vomiting, and seizures. Accompanying cardiac disease in the form of arrhythmias or heart failure should increase the index of suspicion. The presence of antibodies to *T. cruzi* supports the diagnosis. In South America, reactivation of *Chagas' disease* is considered to be an AIDS-defining condition and may be the initial AIDS-defining condition. Most cases occur in patients with CD4+ T-cell counts <200 cells/μL. Lesions appear radiographically as single or multiple hypodense areas, typically with ring enhancement and edema. They are found predominantly in the subcortical areas, a feature that differentiates them from the deeper lesions of toxoplasmosis. *T. cruzi* amastigotes, or trypanosomes, can be identified from biopsy specimens or CSF. Other CSF findings include elevated protein and a mild (<100 cells/μL) lymphocytic pleocytosis. Organisms can also be identified by direct examination of the blood. Treatment consists of benzimidazole (2.5 mg/kg bid) or nifurtimox (2 mg/kg qid) for at least 60 days, followed by maintenance therapy for the duration of immunodeficiency with either drug at a dose of 5 mg/kg three times a week. As is the case with cerebral toxoplasmosis, successful therapy with antiretrovirals may allow discontinuation of therapy for Chagas' disease.

Stroke may occur in patients with HIV infection. In contrast to the other causes of focal neurologic deficits in patients with HIV infection, the symptoms of a stroke are sudden in onset. Patients with HIV infection have an increased prevalence of many classic risk factors associated with stroke, including smoking and diabetes. It has been reported that HIV infection itself can lead to an increase in carotid artery stiffness. The relative increase in risk for stroke as a consequence of HIV infection is more pronounced in women and in individuals between the ages of 18 and 29. Among the secondary infectious diseases in patients with HIV infection that may be associated with stroke are vasculitis due to cerebral varicella zoster or neurosyphilis and septic embolism in association with fungal infection. Other elements of the differential diagnosis of stroke in the patient with HIV infection include atherosclerotic cerebral vascular disease, thrombotic thrombocytopenic purpura, and cocaine or amphetamine use.

Primary CNS lymphoma is discussed below in the section on neoplastic diseases.

Spinal cord disease, or myelopathy, is present in ~20% of patients with AIDS, often as part of HIV-associated neurocognitive disorder. In fact, 90% of the patients with HIV-associated myelopathy have some evidence of dementia, suggesting that similar pathologic processes may be responsible for both conditions. Three main types of spinal cord disease are seen in patients with AIDS. The first of these is a vacuolar myelopathy, as mentioned above. This condition is pathologically similar to subacute combined degeneration of the cord, such as that occurring with pernicious anemia. Although vitamin B_{12} deficiency can be seen in patients with AIDS as a primary complication of HIV infection, it does not appear to be responsible for most cases of myelopathy seen in patients with HIV infection. However, it should be included in the differential diagnosis. Vacuolar myelopathy is characterized by a subacute onset and often presents with gait disturbances, predominantly ataxia and spasticity; it may progress to include bladder and bowel dysfunction. Physical findings include evidence of increased deep tendon reflexes and extensor plantar responses. The second form of spinal cord disease involves the dorsal columns and presents as a pure sensory ataxia. The third form is also sensory in nature and presents with paresthesias and dysesthesias of the lower extremities. In contrast to the cognitive problems seen in patients with HIV encephalopathy, these spinal cord syndromes do not respond well to antiretroviral drugs, and therapy is mainly supportive.

One important disease of the spinal cord that also involves the peripheral nerves is a *myelopathy* and *polyradiculopathy* seen in association with CMV infection. This entity is generally seen late in the course of HIV infection and is fulminant in onset, with lower extremity and sacral paresthesias, difficulty in walking, areflexia, ascending sensory loss, and urinary retention. The clinical course is rapidly progressive over a period of weeks. CSF examination reveals a predominantly neutrophilic pleocytosis, and CMV DNA can be detected by CSF PCR. Therapy with ganciclovir or foscarnet can lead to rapid improvement, and prompt initiation of therapy is important in minimizing the degree of permanent neurologic damage. Combination therapy with both drugs should be considered in patients who have been previously treated for CMV disease. Other diseases involving the spinal cord in patients with HIV infection include HTLV-1-associated myelopathy (HAM) (**Chap. 196**), neurosyphilis (**Chap. 177**), infection with herpes simplex (**Chap. 187**) or varicella-zoster (**Chap. 188**), TB (**Chap. 173**), and lymphoma (**Chap. 104**).

Peripheral neuropathies are common in patients with HIV infection. They occur at all stages of illness and take a variety of forms. Early in the course of HIV infection, an acute inflammatory demyelinating polyneuropathy resembling Guillain-Barré syndrome may occur (**Chap. 439**). In other patients, a progressive or relapsing-remitting inflammatory neuropathy resembling chronic inflammatory demyelinating polyneuropathy (CIDP) has been noted. Patients commonly present with progressive weakness, areflexia, and minimal sensory changes. CSF examination often reveals a mononuclear pleocytosis, and peripheral nerve biopsy demonstrates a perivascular infiltrate suggesting an autoimmune etiology. Plasma exchange or IVIg has been tried with variable success. Because of the immunosuppressive effects of glucocorticoids, they should be reserved for severe cases of CIDP refractory to other measures. Another autoimmune peripheral neuropathy seen in patients with AIDS is mononeuritis multiplex (**Chaps. 439 and 356**) due to a necrotizing arteritis of peripheral nerves. The most common peripheral neuropathy in patients with HIV infection is a *distal sensory polyneuropathy* (DSPN) also referred to as painful sensory neuropathy (HIV-SN), predominantly sensory neuropathy, or distal symmetric peripheral neuropathy. This condition may be a direct consequence of HIV infection or a side effect of ART with dideoxynucleosides. It is more common in taller individuals, older individuals, and those with lower CD4 counts. Two-thirds of patients with AIDS may be shown by electrophysiologic studies to have some evidence of peripheral nerve disease. Presenting symptoms are usually painful burning sensations in the feet and lower extremities. Findings on examination include a stocking-type sensory loss to pinprick, temperature, and touch sensation and a loss of ankle reflexes. Motor changes are mild and are usually limited to weakness of the intrinsic foot muscles. Response of this condition to antiretrovirals has been variable, perhaps because antiretrovirals are responsible for the problem in some instances. When due to dideoxynucleoside therapy, patients with lower extremity peripheral neuropathy may complain of a sensation that they are walking on ice. Other entities in the differential diagnosis of peripheral neuropathy include diabetes mellitus, vitamin B_{12} deficiency, and side effects from metronidazole or dapsone. For distal symmetric polyneuropathy that fails to resolve following the discontinuation of dideoxynucleosides, therapy is symptomatic; gabapentin, carbamazepine, tricyclics, or analgesics may be effective for dysesthesias. Treatment-naïve patients may respond to ART.

Myopathy may complicate the course of HIV infection; causes include HIV infection itself, zidovudine, and the generalized wasting syndrome (discussed below). HIV-associated myopathy may range in severity from an asymptomatic elevation in creatine kinase levels to a subacute syndrome characterized by proximal muscle weakness and myalgias. Quite pronounced elevations in creatine kinase may occur in asymptomatic patients, particularly after exercise. The clinical significance of this as an isolated laboratory finding is unclear. A variety of both inflammatory and noninflammatory pathologic processes have been noted in patients with more severe myopathy, including myofiber necrosis with inflammatory cells, nemaline rod bodies, cytoplasmic bodies, and mitochondrial abnormalities. Profound muscle wasting, often with muscle pain, may be seen after prolonged zidovudine therapy. This toxic side effect of the drug is dose-dependent and is related to its ability to interfere with the function of mitochondrial polymerases. It is reversible following discontinuation of the drug. Red ragged fibers are a histologic hallmark of zidovudine-induced myopathy.

Ophthalmologic Diseases Ophthalmologic problems occur in ~50% of patients with advanced HIV infection. The most common abnormal findings on funduscopic examination are cotton-wool spots. These are hard white spots that appear on the surface of the retina and often have an irregular edge. They represent areas of retinal ischemia secondary to microvascular disease. At times they are associated with small areas of hemorrhage and thus can be difficult to distinguish from CMV retinitis. In contrast to CMV retinitis, however, these lesions are not associated with visual loss and tend to remain stable or improve over time.

One of the most devastating consequences of HIV infection is CMV retinitis. Patients at high risk of CMV retinitis (CD4+ T-cell count <100/μL) should undergo an ophthalmologic examination every 3–6 months. The majority of cases of CMV retinitis occur in patients with a CD4+ T-cell count <50/μL. Prior to the availability of ART, this CMV reactivation syndrome was seen in 25–30% of patients with AIDS. In the ART era this has dropped to close to 2%. CMV retinitis usually presents as a painless, progressive loss of vision. Patients may also complain of blurred vision, "floaters," and scintillations. The disease is usually bilateral, although typically it affects one eye more than the other. The diagnosis is made on clinical grounds by an experienced ophthalmologist. The characteristic retinal appearance is that of perivascular hemorrhage and exudate. In situations where the diagnosis is in doubt due to an atypical presentation or an unexpected lack of response to therapy, vitreous or aqueous humor sampling with molecular diagnostic techniques may be of value. CMV infection of the retina results in a necrotic inflammatory process, and the visual loss that develops is irreversible. CMV retinitis may be complicated by rhegmatogenous retinal detachment as a consequence of retinal atrophy in areas of prior inflammation. Therapy for CMV retinitis consists of oral valganciclovir, IV ganciclovir, or IV foscarnet, with cidofovir as an alternative. Combination therapy with ganciclovir and foscarnet has been shown to be slightly more effective than either ganciclovir or foscarnet alone in the patient with relapsed CMV retinitis. A 3-week induction course is followed by maintenance therapy with oral valganciclovir. If CMV disease is limited to the eye, intravitreal injections of ganciclovir or foscarnet may be considered. Intravitreal injections of cidofovir are generally avoided due to the increased risk of uveitis and hypotony. Maintenance therapy is continued until the CD4+ T-cell count remains >100 μL for >6 months. The majority of patients with HIV infection and CMV disease develop some degree of uveitis with the initiation of ART. The etiology of this is unknown; however, it has been suggested that this may be due to the generation of an enhanced immune response to CMV as an IRIS (see above). In some instances, this has required the use of topical glucocorticoids.

Both HSV and varicella zoster virus can cause a rapidly progressing, bilateral, necrotizing retinitis referred to as the *acute retinal necrosis syndrome*, or *progressive outer retinal necrosis* (PORN). This syndrome, in contrast to CMV retinitis, is associated with pain, keratitis, and iritis. It is often associated with orolabial HSV or trigeminal zoster. Ophthalmologic examination reveals widespread pale gray peripheral lesions. This condition is often complicated by retinal detachment. It is important to recognize and treat this condition with IV acyclovir as quickly as possible to minimize the loss of vision.

Several other secondary infections may cause ocular problems in HIV-infected patients. *P. jirovecii* can cause a lesion of the choroid that may be detected as an incidental finding on ophthalmologic examination. These lesions are typically bilateral, are from half to twice the disc diameter in size, and appear as slightly elevated yellow-white plaques. They are usually asymptomatic and may be confused with cotton-wool spots. Chorioretinitis due to toxoplasmosis can be seen alone or, more commonly, in association with CNS toxoplasmosis. KS may involve the eyelid or conjunctiva, while lymphoma may involve the retina. Syphilis may lead to a uveitis that is highly associated with the presence of neurosyphilis.

Additional Disseminated Infections and Wasting Syndrome Infections with species of the small, gram-negative, *Rickettsia*-like organism *Bartonella* (**Chap. 167**) are seen with increased frequency in patients with HIV infection. While it is not considered an AIDS-defining illness by the CDC, many experts view infection with *Bartonella* as indicative of a severe defect in cell-mediated immunity. It is usually seen in patients with CD4+ T-cell counts <100/μL and is a significant cause of unexplained fever in patients with advanced HIV infection. Among the clinical manifestations of *Bartonella* infection are bacillary angiomatosis, cat-scratch disease, and trench fever. *Bacillary angiomatosis* is usually due to infection with *B. henselae* and is linked to exposure to flea-infested cats. It is characterized by a vascular proliferation that leads to a variety of skin lesions that have been confused with the skin lesions of KS. In contrast to the lesions of KS, the lesions of bacillary angiomatosis generally blanch, are painful, and typically occur in the setting of systemic symptoms. Infection can extend to the lymph nodes, liver (peliosis hepatis), spleen, bone, heart, CNS, respiratory tract, and GI tract. *Cat-scratch disease* is also due to infection with *B. henselae* and generally begins with a papule at the site of inoculation. This is followed several weeks later by the development of regional adenopathy and malaise. Infection with *B. quintana* is transmitted by lice and has been associated with case reports of trench fever, endocarditis, adenopathy, and bacillary angiomatosis. The organism is quite difficult to culture, and diagnosis often relies on identifying the organism in biopsy specimens using the Warthin-Starry or similar stains, PCR, and/or seroconversion. Treatment is with either doxycycline or erythromycin for at least 3 months.

Histoplasmosis is an opportunistic infection that is seen most frequently in patients in the Mississippi and Ohio River valleys, Puerto Rico, the Dominican Republic, and South America. These are all areas in which infection with *H. capsulatum* is endemic (**Chap. 207**). Because of this limited geographic distribution, histoplasmosis is only seen in approximately 0.5% of AIDS cases in the United States. Histoplasmosis is generally a late manifestation of HIV infection; however, it may be the initial AIDS-defining condition. In one study, the median CD4+ T-cell count for patients with histoplasmosis and AIDS was 33/μL. While disease due to *H. capsulatum* may present as a primary infection of the lung, disseminated disease, presumably due to reactivation, is the most common presentation in HIV-infected patients. Patients usually present with a 4- to 8-week history of fever and weight loss. Hepatosplenomegaly and lymphadenopathy are each seen in about 25% of patients. CNS disease, either meningitis or a mass lesion, is seen in 15% of patients. Bone marrow involvement is common, with thrombocytopenia, neutropenia, and anemia occurring in 33% of patients. Approximately 7% of patients have mucocutaneous lesions consisting of a maculopapular rash and skin or oral ulcers. Respiratory symptoms are usually mild, with chest x-ray showing a diffuse infiltrate or diffuse small nodules in ~50% of cases. The gastrointestinal tract may be involved. Diagnosis is made by silver staining of tissue, by culturing the organisms from blood, bone marrow, or tissue, or by detecting antigen in blood or urine. Treatment is typically with liposomal amphotericin B followed by maintenance therapy with oral itraconazole until the serum *Histoplasma* antigen is <2 units, the patient has been on antiretrovirals for at least 6 months, and the CD4 count is >150 cells/μL. In the setting of mild infection, it may be appropriate to initiate therapy with itraconazole alone.

Following the spread of HIV infection to southeast Asia, disseminated infection with the fungus *Penicillium marneffei* was recognized as a complication of HIV infection and is considered an AIDS-defining condition in those parts of the world where it occurs. *P. marneffei* is the third most common AIDS-defining illness in Thailand, following TB and cryptococcosis. It is more frequently diagnosed in the rainy than the dry season. Clinical features include fever, generalized lymphadenopathy, hepatosplenomegaly, anemia, thrombocytopenia, and papular skin lesions with central umbilication resembling the lesions of *Molluscum contagiosum*. Treatment is with amphotericin B followed by itraconazole until the CD4+ T-cell count is >100 cells/μL for at least 6 months.

Visceral leishmaniasis (**Chap. 221**) is recognized with increasing frequency in patients with HIV infection who live in or travel to areas endemic for this protozoal infection transmitted by sandflies. The clinical presentation is one of hepatosplenomegaly, fever, and hematologic abnormalities. Lymphadenopathy and other constitutional symptoms may be present. A chronic, relapsing course is seen in two-thirds of co-infected patients. Organisms can be detected by PCR and, with special techniques, isolated from cultures of bone marrow aspirates. Histologic stains are often diagnostic but may be negative. Antibody titers are of little help. Patients with HIV infection usually respond well initially to standard therapy with amphotericin B or pentavalent antimony compounds. Eradication of the organism is difficult, however, and relapses are common.

Patients with HIV infection are at a slightly increased risk of infection with malaria and of clinical malaria. This is particularly true for patients from nonendemic areas who are at risk for primary infection and in patients with lower CD4+ T-cell counts. HIV-positive individuals with CD4+ T-cell counts <300 cells/μL have a poorer response to malaria treatment than others. Co-infection with malaria is associated with a modest increase in HIV viral load. The risk of malaria may be decreased with TMP-SMX prophylaxis.

Generalized wasting is an AIDS-defining condition; it is defined as involuntary weight loss of >10% associated with intermittent or constant fever and chronic diarrhea or fatigue lasting >30 days in the absence of a defined cause other than HIV infection. Prior to the widespread use of ART it was the initial AIDS-defining condition in ~10% of patients with AIDS in the United States. Generalized wasting is rarely seen today with the earlier initiation of antiretrovirals. A constant feature of this syndrome is severe muscle wasting with scattered myofiber degeneration and occasional evidence of myositis. Glucocorticoids may be of some benefit; however, this approach must be carefully weighed against the risk of compounding the immunodeficiency of HIV infection. Androgenic steroids, growth hormone, and total parenteral nutrition have been used as therapeutic interventions with variable success.

Neoplastic Diseases The neoplastic diseases considered to be AIDS-defining conditions are Kaposi's sarcoma, non-Hodgkin's lymphoma, and invasive cervical carcinoma. In addition, there is also an increase in the incidence of a variety of non-AIDS-defining malignancies including Hodgkin's disease; multiple myeloma; leukemia; melanoma; and cervical, brain, testicular, oral, lung, gastric, liver, renal, and anal cancers. Since the introduction of potent ART, there has been a marked reduction in the incidence of KS (Fig. 202-34). The non-AIDS-defining malignancies now account for more morbidity and mortality in patients with HIV infection than the AIDS-defining malignancies and are responsible for approximately 10% of the deaths in patients with HIV infection. Rates of non-Hodgkin's lymphoma have declined; however, this decline has not been as dramatic as the decline in rates of KS. In contrast, ART has had little effect on human papillomavirus (HPV)-associated malignancies. As patients with HIV infection live longer, a wider array of cancers is seen in this population. While some may only reflect known risk factors (e.g., smoking, alcohol consumption, co-infection with other viruses such as hepatitis B) that are increased in patients with HIV infection, some may be a direct consequence of HIV and are clearly increased in patients with lower CD4+ T-cell counts.

Kaposi's sarcoma is a multicentric neoplasm consisting of multiple vascular nodules appearing in the skin, mucous membranes, and viscera. The clinical course of KS ranges from indolent, with only minor skin or lymph node involvement, to fulminant, with extensive cutaneous and visceral involvement. In the initial period of the AIDS epidemic, KS was a prominent clinical feature of the first cases of AIDS, occurring in 79% of the patients diagnosed in 1981. By 1989 it was seen in only 25% of cases, by 1992 the number had decreased to 9%, and by 1997 the number was <1%. HHV-8 (KSHV) has been strongly implicated as a viral cofactor in the pathogenesis of KS.

Clinically, KS has varied presentations and may be seen at any stage of HIV infection, even in the presence of a normal CD4+ T-cell count. The initial lesion may be a small, raised, reddish-purple nodule on the skin (**Fig. 202-42**), a discoloration on the oral mucosa (Fig. 202-34*D*), or a swollen lymph node. Lesions often appear in sun-exposed areas, particularly the tip of the nose, and have a propensity to occur in areas of trauma (Koebner phenomenon). Because of the vascular nature of the tumors and the presence of extravasated red blood cells in the lesions, their colors range from reddish to purple to brown and often take the appearance of a bruise, with yellowish discoloration and tattooing. Lesions range in size from a few millimeters to several centimeters in diameter and may be either discrete or confluent. KS lesions

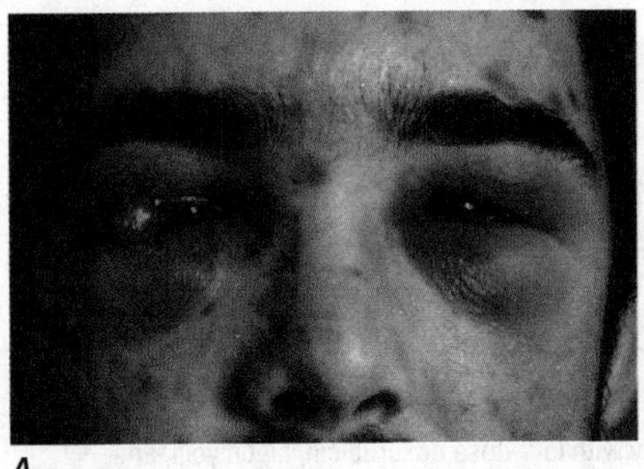
A

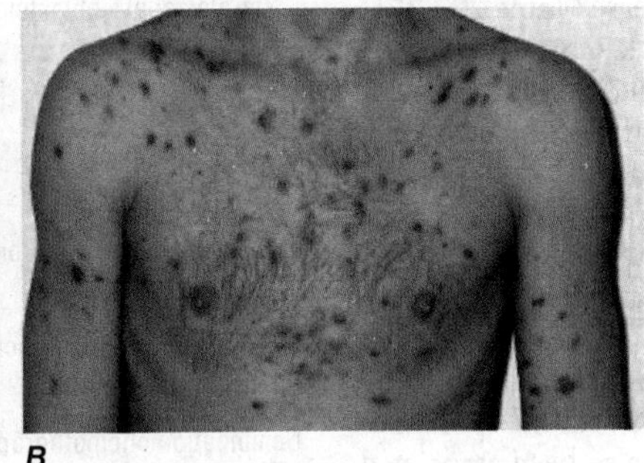
B

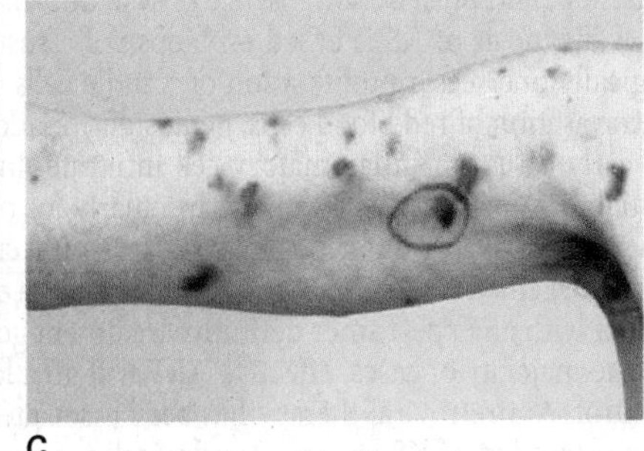
C

FIGURE 202-42 Kaposi's sarcoma in three patients with AIDS demonstrating ***(A)*** periorbital edema and bruising; ***(B)*** classic truncal distribution of lesions; and ***(C)*** upper extremity lesions.

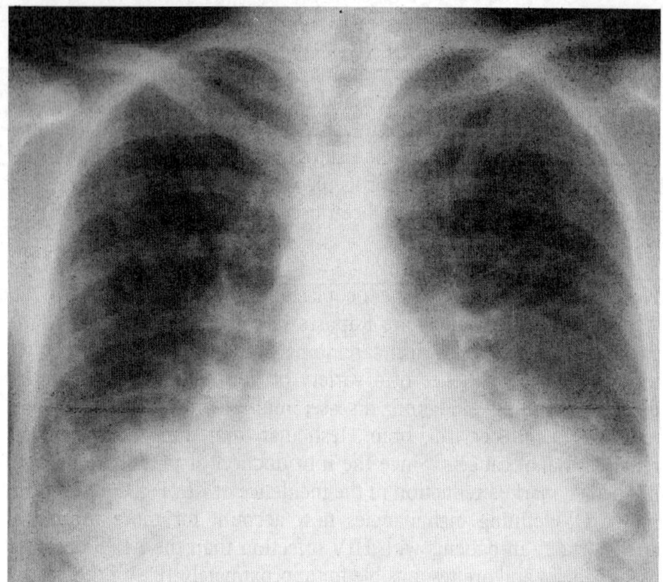

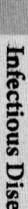

FIGURE 202-43 Chest x-ray of a patient with AIDS and pulmonary Kaposi's sarcoma. The characteristic findings include dense bilateral lower lobe infiltrates obscuring the heart borders and pleural effusions.

TABLE 202-17 National Institute of Allergy and Infectious Diseases AIDS Clinical Trials Group TIS Staging System for Kaposi's Sarcoma

PARAMETER	GOOD RISK (STAGE 0): ALL OF THE FOLLOWING	POOR RISK (STAGE 1): ANY OF THE FOLLOWING
Tumor (T)	Confined to skin and/or lymph nodes and/or minimal oral disease	Tumor-associated edema or ulceration Extensive oral lesions GI lesions Nonnodal visceral lesions
Immune system (I)	CD4+ T-cell count ≥200/μL	CD4+ T-cell count <200/μL
Systemic illness (S)	No B symptoms[a]	B symptoms[a] present
	Karnofsky performance status ≥70	Karnofsky performance status <70
	No history of opportunistic infection, neurologic disease, lymphoma, or thrush	History of opportunistic infection, neurologic disease, lymphoma, or thrush

[a]Defined as unexplained fever, night sweats, >10% involuntary weight loss, or diarrhea persisting for more than 2 weeks.

most commonly appear as raised macules; however, they can also be papular, particularly in patients with higher CD4+ T-cell counts. Confluent lesions may give rise to surrounding lymphedema and may be disfiguring when they involve the face and disabling when they involve the lower extremities or the surfaces of joints. Apart from skin, the lymph nodes, GI tract, and lung are the organ systems most commonly affected by KS. Lesions have been reported in virtually every organ, including the heart and the CNS. In contrast to most malignancies, in which lymph node involvement implies metastatic spread and a poor prognosis, lymph node involvement may be seen very early in KS and is of no special clinical significance. In fact, some patients may present with disease limited to the lymph nodes. These are generally patients with relatively intact immune function and thus the patients with the best prognosis. Pulmonary involvement with KS generally presents with shortness of breath. Some 80% of patients with pulmonary KS also have cutaneous lesions. The chest x-ray characteristically shows bilateral lower lobe infiltrates that obscure the margins of the mediastinum and diaphragm (Fig. 202-43). Pleural effusions are seen in 70% of cases of pulmonary KS, a fact that is often helpful in the differential diagnosis. GI involvement is seen in 50% of patients with KS and usually takes one of two forms: (1) mucosal involvement, which may lead to bleeding that can be severe; these patients sometimes also develop symptoms of GI obstruction if lesions become large; and (2) biliary tract involvement. KS lesions may infiltrate the gallbladder and biliary tree, leading to a clinical picture of obstructive jaundice similar to that seen with sclerosing cholangitis. Several staging systems have been proposed for KS. One in common use was developed by the National Institute of Allergy and Infectious Diseases AIDS Clinical Trials Group; it distinguishes patients on the basis of tumor extent, immunologic function, and presence or absence of systemic disease (Table 202-17).

A diagnosis of KS is based on biopsy of a suspicious lesion. Histologically one sees a proliferation of spindle cells and endothelial cells, extravasation of red blood cells, hemosiderin-laden macrophages, and, in early cases, an inflammatory cell infiltrate. Included in the differential diagnosis are lymphoma (particularly for oral lesions), bacillary angiomatosis, and cutaneous mycobacterial infections.

Management of KS (Table 202-18) should be carried out in consultation with an expert since definitive treatment guidelines do not exist. In the majority of cases, effective ART will go a long way in achieving control. Antiretroviral therapy has been associated with the spontaneous regression of KS lesions. Paradoxically, it has also been associated with the initial appearance of KS as a form of IRIS. For patients in whom tumor persists or is compromising vital functions or in whom control of HIV replication is not possible, a variety of options exist. In some cases, lesions remain quite indolent, and many of these patients can be managed with no specific treatment. Fewer than 10% of AIDS patients with KS die as a consequence of their malignancy, and death from secondary infections is considerably more common. Thus, whenever possible one should avoid treatment regimens that may further suppress the immune system and increase susceptibility to opportunistic infections. Treatment is indicated under two main circumstances. The first is when a single lesion or a limited number of easily accessible lesions are causing significant discomfort or cosmetic problems, such as with prominent facial lesions, lesions overlying a joint, or lesions in the oropharynx that interfere with swallowing or breathing. Under these circumstances, treatment with localized radiation, intralesional vinblastine, topical 9-*cis*-retinoic acid, or cryotherapy may be helpful. It should be noted that patients with HIV infection are particularly sensitive to the side effects of radiation therapy. This is especially true with respect to the development of radiation-induced mucositis; doses of radiation directed at mucosal surfaces, particularly in the head and neck region, should be adjusted accordingly. The second indication for KS-directed treatment is for patients with a large number of lesions or in patients with visceral involvement. In these patients, systemic therapy, either IFN-α or chemotherapy, should be considered. The single most important determinant of response appears to be the CD4+ T-cell count. This relationship between response rate and baseline CD4+ T-cell count is particularly true for IFN-α. The response rate to IFN-α for patients with CD4+ T-cell counts >600/μL is ~80%, while

TABLE 202-18 Management of AIDS-Associated Kaposi's Sarcoma

Observation and optimization of antiretroviral therapy

Single or limited number of lesions

- Radiation
- Intralesional vinblastine
- Cryotherapy

Extensive disease

- Initial therapy
  - Interferon α (if CD4+ T cells >150/μL)
  - Liposomal daunorubicin
- Subsequent therapy
  - Liposomal doxorubicin
  - Paclitaxel

Combination chemotherapy with low-dose doxorubicin, bleomycin, and vinblastine (ABV)

Targeted radiation

the response rate for patients with counts <150/μL is <10%. In contrast to the other systemic therapies, IFN-α provides an added advantage of having antiretroviral activity; thus, it may be the appropriate first choice for single-agent systemic therapy for early patients with disseminated disease. A variety of chemotherapeutic agents also have been shown to have activity against KS. Five of them—liposomal daunorubicin, liposomal doxorubicin, vinblastine, paclitaxel, and the thalidomide analogue pomalidomide—have been approved by the FDA for this indication. Liposomal daunorubicin and pomalidomide are approved as first-line therapy for patients with advanced KS despite ART. They have fewer side effects than conventional chemotherapy. In contrast, liposomal doxorubicin and paclitaxel are approved only for KS patients who have failed standard chemotherapy. Response rates vary from 23 to 88%, appear to be comparable to what had been achieved earlier with combination chemotherapy regimens, and are greatly influenced by CD4+ T-cell count. Vinblastine is most commonly used as an intralesional injection or as part of a combination regimen.

Lymphomas occur with an increased frequency in patients with congenital or acquired T-cell immunodeficiencies (**Chap. 344**). AIDS is no exception; at least 6% of all patients with AIDS develop lymphoma at some time during the course of their illness. This is a 10- to 20-fold increase in incidence compared with the general population. In contrast to the situation with KS, primary CNS lymphoma, and most opportunistic infections, the incidence of AIDS-associated systemic lymphomas has not experienced a dramatic decrease as a consequence of the widespread use of effective ART. Lymphoma occurs in all risk groups, with the highest incidence in patients with hemophilia and the lowest incidence in patients from the Caribbean or Africa with heterosexually acquired infection. Lymphoma is a late manifestation of HIV infection, generally occurring in patients with CD4+ T-cell counts <200/μL. As HIV disease progresses, the risk of lymphoma increases. The attack rate for lymphoma increases exponentially with increasing duration of HIV infection and decreasing level of immunologic function. At 3 years following a diagnosis of HIV infection, the risk of lymphoma is 0.8% per year; by 8 years after infection, it is 2.6% per year. As individuals with HIV infection live longer as a consequence of improved ART and better treatment and prophylaxis of opportunistic infections, it is anticipated that the incidence of lymphomas may increase.

Three main categories of lymphoma are seen in patients with HIV infection: grade III or IV immunoblastic lymphoma, Burkitt's lymphoma, and primary CNS lymphoma. Approximately 90% of these lymphomas are B cell in phenotype; more than half contain EBV DNA. Some are associated with KSHV. These tumors may be either monoclonal or oligoclonal in nature and are probably in some way related to the pronounced polyclonal B-cell activation seen in patients with AIDS.

Immunoblastic lymphomas account for ~60% of the cases of lymphoma in patients with AIDS. The majority of these are diffuse large B-cell lymphomas (DLBCL). They are generally high grade and would have been classified as diffuse histiocytic lymphomas in earlier classification schemes. This tumor is more common in older patients, increasing in incidence from 0% in HIV-infected individuals <1 year old to >3% in those >50 years of age. Two variants of immunoblastic lymphoma that are seen primarily in HIV-infected patients are primary effusion lymphoma (PEL) and its solid variant, plasmacytic lymphoma of the oral cavity. PEL, also referred to as body cavity lymphoma, presents with lymphomatous pleural, pericardial, and/or peritoneal effusions in the absence of discrete nodal or extranodal masses. The tumor cells do not express surface markers for B cells or T cells and are felt to represent a preplasmacytic stage of differentiation. While both KSHV and EBV DNA sequences have been found in the genomes of the malignant cells from patients with body cavity lymphoma, KSHV is felt to be the driving force behind the oncogenesis (see above).

Small noncleaved cell lymphoma (*Burkitt's lymphoma*) accounts for ~20% of the cases of lymphoma in patients with AIDS. It is most frequent in patients 10–19 years old and usually demonstrates characteristic c-*myc* translocations from chromosome 8 to chromosome 14 or 22. Burkitt's lymphoma is not commonly seen in the setting of immunodeficiency other than HIV-associated immunodeficiency, and

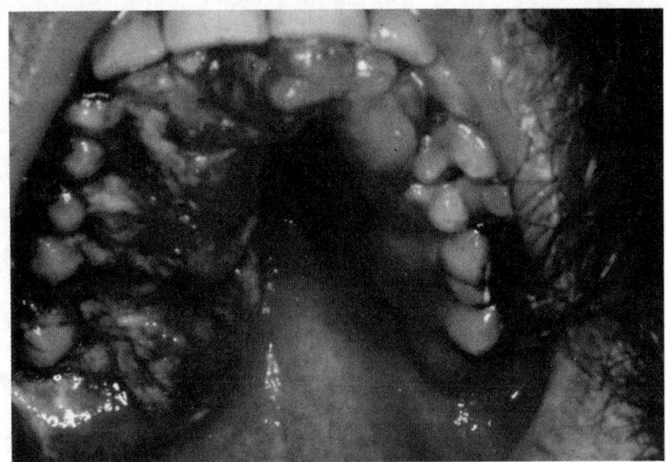

FIGURE 202-44 Immunoblastic lymphoma involving the hard palate of a patient with AIDS.

the incidence of this particular tumor is more than 1000-fold higher in the setting of HIV infection than in the general population. In contrast to African Burkitt's lymphoma, where 97% of the cases contain EBV genome, only 50% of HIV-associated Burkitt's lymphomas are EBV-positive.

Primary CNS lymphoma accounts for ~20% of the cases of lymphoma in patients with HIV infection. In contrast to HIV-associated Burkitt's lymphoma, primary CNS lymphomas are usually positive for EBV. In one study, the incidence of Epstein-Barr positivity was 100%. This malignancy does not have a predilection for any particular age group. The median CD4+ T-cell count at the time of diagnosis is ~50/μL. Thus, CNS lymphoma generally presents at a later stage of HIV infection than does systemic lymphoma. This may explain, at least in part, the poorer prognosis for this subset of patients.

The clinical presentation of lymphoma in patients with HIV infection is quite varied, ranging from focal seizures to rapidly growing mass lesions in the oral mucosa (**Fig. 202-44**) to persistent unexplained fever. At least 80% of patients present with extranodal disease, and a similar percentage have B-type symptoms of fever, night sweats, and/or weight loss. Virtually any site in the body may be involved. The most common extranodal site is the CNS, which is involved in approximately one-third of all patients with lymphoma. Approximately 60% of these cases are primary CNS lymphoma. Primary CNS lymphoma generally presents with focal neurologic deficits, including cranial nerve findings, headaches, and/or seizures. MRI or CT generally reveals a limited number (one to three) of 3- to 5-cm lesions (**Fig. 202-45**). The lesions often show ring enhancement on contrast administration and may occur in any location. Contrast enhancement is usually less pronounced than that seen with toxoplasmosis. Lesions of CNS lymphoma are most commonly seen deep in the white matter. The main diseases in the differential diagnosis are cerebral toxoplasmosis and cerebral Chagas' disease. In addition to the 20% of lymphomas in HIV-infected individuals that are primary CNS lymphomas, CNS disease is also seen in HIV-infected patients with systemic lymphoma. Approximately 20% of patients with systemic lymphoma have CNS disease in the form of leptomeningeal involvement. This fact underscores the importance of lumbar puncture in the staging evaluation of patients with systemic lymphoma.

Systemic lymphoma is seen at earlier stages of HIV infection than primary CNS lymphoma. In one series the mean CD4+ T-cell count was 226/μL. In addition to lymph node involvement, systemic lymphoma may commonly involve the GI tract, bone marrow, liver, and lung. GI tract involvement is seen in ~25% of patients. Any site in the GI tract may be involved, and patients may complain of difficulty swallowing or abdominal pain. The diagnosis is usually suspected on the basis of CT or MRI of the abdomen. Bone marrow involvement is seen in ~20% of patients and may lead to pancytopenia. Liver and lung involvement are each seen in ~10% of patients. Pulmonary disease may present as a mass lesion, multiple nodules, or an interstitial infiltrate.

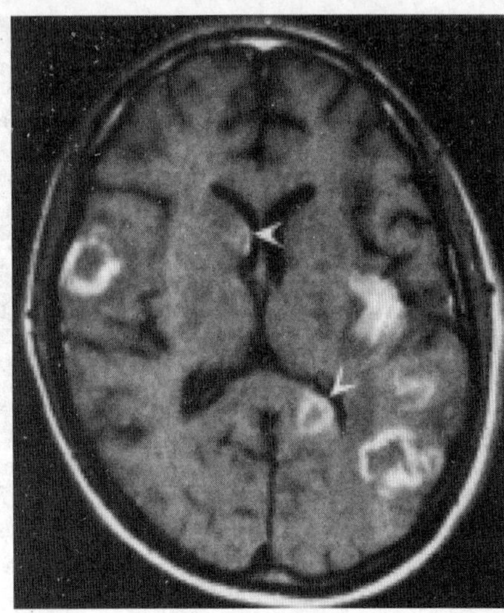

FIGURE 202-45 Central nervous system lymphoma. Postcontrast T1-weighted MRI scan in a patient with AIDS, altered mental status, and hemiparesis. Multiple enhancing lesions, some ring-enhancing, are present. The left sylvian lesion shows gyral and subcortical enhancement, and the lesions in the caudate and splenium (*arrowheads*) show enhancement of adjacent ependymal surfaces.

Both conventional and unconventional approaches have been employed in an attempt to treat HIV-related lymphomas. Systemic lymphoma is generally treated by the oncologist with combination chemotherapy. Earlier disappointing figures are being replaced with more optimistic results for the treatment of systemic lymphoma following the availability of more effective ART and the use of rituximab in CD20+ tumors. While there is some controversy regarding the use of antiretrovirals during chemotherapy, there is no question that their use overall in patients with HIV lymphoma has improved survival. Concerns regarding synergistic bone marrow toxicities with chemotherapy and ART are mitigated with the use of ART regimens that avoid bone marrow–toxic antiretrovirals. As in most situations in patients with HIV disease, those with higher CD4+ T-cell counts tend to fare better. Response rates as high as 72% with a median survival of 33 months and disease-free intervals up to 9 years have been reported. Treatment of primary CNS lymphoma remains a significant challenge. Treatment is complicated by the fact that this illness usually occurs in patients with advanced HIV disease. Palliative measures such as radiation therapy provide some relief. The prognosis remains poor in this group, with a 2-year survival of 29%.

Multicentric Castleman's disease (MCD) is a KSHV-associated lymphoproliferative disorder that is seen with an increased frequency in patients with HIV infection. While the incidence of Kaposi's sarcoma has decreased, the incidence of MCD has increased in the setting of ART. While not a true malignancy, MCD shares many features with lymphoma including generalized lymphadenopathy, hepatosplenomegaly, and systemic symptoms of fever, fatigue, and weight loss. Pulmonary symptoms may be seen in ~50% of patients. KS is present in 75–82% of cases. Lymph node biopsies reveal a predominance of interfollicular plasma cells and/or germinal centers with vascularization and an "onion skin" (hyaline vascular) appearance. Prior to the availability of ART, HIV-infected patients with multicentric Castleman's disease had a 15-fold increased risk of developing non-Hodgkin's lymphoma compared with HIV-infected patients in general. Treatment typically involves chemotherapy. Rituximab may be of benefit, but it has been associated with worsening of coexisting KS. The median survival of patients with treated multicentric Castleman's disease pre-ART was initially reported as 14 months. This has increased to a 2-year survival of more than 90% in the era of ART.

Evidence of infection with *human papillomavirus* (HPV), associated with *intraepithelial dysplasia of the cervix* or *anus*, is approximately twice as common in HIV-infected individuals as in the general population and can lead to intraepithelial neoplasia and eventually invasive cancer. In a series of studies, HIV-infected men were examined for evidence of anal dysplasia, and Papanicolaou (Pap) smears were found to be abnormal in 20–80%. These changes tend to persist and are generally not affected by ART, raising the possibility of a subsequent transition to a more malignant condition. While the incidence of an abnormal Pap smear of the cervix is ~5% in otherwise healthy women, the incidence of abnormal cervical smears in women with HIV infection is 30–60%, and *invasive cervical cancer* is included as an AIDS-defining condition. While only small increases in the absolute numbers of cervical or anal cancers have been seen as a consequence of HIV infection, the relative risk of these conditions when one compares HIV-infected to noninfected men and women is on the order of 10- to 100-fold. Given the high rates of dysplasia and relative risks for cervical and anal cancer, a comprehensive gynecologic and rectal examination, including Pap smear, is indicated at the initial evaluation and 6 months later for all patients with HIV infection. If these examinations are negative at both time points, the patient should be followed with yearly evaluations. If an initial or repeat Pap smear shows evidence of severe inflammation with reactive squamous changes, the next Pap smear should be performed at 3 months. If, at any time, a Pap smear shows evidence of squamous intraepithelial lesions, colposcopic examination with biopsies as indicated should be performed. The 2-year survival rate for HIV-infected patients with invasive cervical cancer is 64% compared with 79% in non-HIV-infected patients. In addition to rectal and cervical lesions, HPV can also lead to head and neck cancers. In one study of men who have sex with men, 25% were found to have oral HPV; high-risk HPV genotypes were three times more common in the HIV-infected men. The most common HPV genotypes in the general population and the genotypes upon which current HPV vaccines are based are 6, 11, 16, and 18. In the HIV-infected population other genotypes such as 58 and 53 are also prominent. This raises a concern about the level of effectiveness of the current HPV vaccines for HIV-infected patients. Despite this, it is recommended that patients with HIV infection be vaccinated against HPV.

IDIOPATHIC CD4+ T LYMPHOCYTOPENIA

A syndrome was recognized in 1992 characterized by an absolute CD4+ T-cell count of <300/μL or <20% of total T cells on a minimum of two occasions at least 6 weeks apart; no evidence of HIV-1, HIV-2, HTLV-1, or HTLV-2 on testing; and the absence of any defined immunodeficiency or therapy associated with decreased levels of CD4+ T cells. By mid-1993, ~100 patients had been described. After extensive multicenter investigations, a series of reports were published in early 1993, which together allowed a number of conclusions. Idiopathic CD4+ lymphocytopenia (ICL) is a very rare syndrome, as determined by studies of blood donors and cohorts of HIV-seronegative men who have sex with men. Cases were clearly identified as early as 1983. The definition of ICL based on CD4+ T-cell counts coincided with the ready availability of testing for CD4+ T cells in patients suspected of being immunodeficient. However, as a result of immune deficiency, certain patients with ICL develop some of the opportunistic diseases (particularly cryptococcosis, nontuberculous mycobacterial infections, and HPV disease) seen in HIV-infected patients. Approximately 10% of patients may exhibit an autoimmune disease. The syndrome is demographically, clinically, and immunologically unlike HIV infection and AIDS. Fewer than half of the reported ICL patients had risk factors for HIV infection, and there were wide geographic and age distributions. The fact that a significant proportion of initially diagnosed patients did have risk factors probably reflects a selection bias, in that physicians who take care of HIV-infected patients were more likely to monitor CD4+ T cells. Approximately half of the patients are women, compared with approximately one-third among HIV-infected individuals in the United States. Many patients with ICL remained clinically stable, and their condition may not deteriorate progressively as is common with seriously immunodeficient HIV-infected patients. Approximately 15% of patients with ICL experience spontaneous reversal of the CD4+ T lymphocytopenia. Immunologic abnormalities in ICL are somewhat different from those of HIV infection. ICL patients often have increases in CD4+ T-cell activation with decreases in CD8+ T cells and B cells. Furthermore, immunoglobulin levels are either normal or, more commonly, decreased in patients with ICL, compared with the usual hypergammaglobulinemia of HIV-infected individuals. Virologic studies of these patients have revealed no evidence of HIV-1, HIV-2, HTLV-1, or HTLV-2 or of any other mononuclear cell–tropic virus. Furthermore, there has been no epidemiologic evidence to suggest that a transmissible microbe was involved. The cases of ICL have been widely dispersed, with no clustering. Close contacts and sexual partners who were studied were clinically well and were serologically, immunologically, and virologically negative for HIV. ICL is a heterogeneous syndrome, and it is highly likely that there is no common cause; however, there may be common causes among subgroups of patients that are currently unrecognized.

Patients who present with laboratory data consistent with ICL should be worked up for underlying diseases that could be responsible for the immune deficiency. If no underlying cause is detected, no specific therapy should be initiated. However, if opportunistic diseases occur, they should be treated appropriately (see above). Depending on the level of the CD4+ T-cell count, patients should receive prophylaxis for the commonly encountered opportunistic infections.

TREATMENT

AIDS and Related Disorders

GENERAL PRINCIPLES OF PATIENT MANAGEMENT

The CDC guidelines call for the testing for HIV infection to be a part of routine medical care. It is recommended that the patient be informed of the intention to test, as is the case with other routine laboratory determinations, and be given the opportunity to "opt out." Such an approach is critical to the goal of identifying as many infected individuals as possible since 13% of the 1.2 million individuals in the United States who are HIV-infected are not aware of their status. In the setting of routine testing, although it is difficult, pretest counseling is an important part of the process. No matter how well prepared a patient is for adversity, the discovery of a diagnosis of HIV infection is a devastating event. Thus, physicians should be sensitive to this fact and, where possible, utilize pretest counseling to at least partially prepare the patient should the results demonstrate the presence of HIV infection. Following a diagnosis of HIV infection, the health care provider should be prepared to immediately activate support systems for the newly diagnosed patient and initiate ART. These supports should include individuals who can spend time talking to the newly diagnosed person and ensuring that he or she is emotionally stable and ready to begin therapy. Most communities have HIV support centers that can be of great help in these difficult situations.

The treatment of patients with HIV infection requires not only a comprehensive knowledge of the possible disease processes that may occur and up-to-date knowledge of and experience with ART, but also the ability to deal with the problems of a chronic, potentially life-threatening illness. A comprehensive knowledge of internal medicine is required to deal with the changing spectrum of illnesses associated with HIV infection, many of which are similar to a state of accelerated aging. The appropriate use of potent ART and other treatment and prophylactic interventions are of critical importance in providing each patient with the best opportunity to live a long and healthy life with HIV infection. In contrast to the earlier days of this epidemic, a diagnosis of HIV infection needs no longer be equated with having an inevitably fatal disease. In addition to medical interventions, the health care provider has a responsibility to provide each patient with appropriate counseling and education concerning their disease as part of a comprehensive care plan. Patients must be educated about the potential transmissibility of their infection and about the fact that while health care providers may refer to levels of the virus as "undetectable," this is only a reflection of the sensitivity of the assay being used to measure the virus, rather than a comment on the presence or absence of the virus. It is important for patients to be aware that the virus is still present in virtually all patients who have ever been diagnosed with HIV infection and capable of being transmitted in the absence of effective ART. Thus, there must be frank discussions concerning sexual practices and the sharing of syringes and other paraphernalia used in illicit drug use. The treating physician not only must be aware of the latest medications available for patients with HIV infection but also must educate patients concerning the natural history of their illness, listen to their concerns, and be sensitive to their fears. As with other diseases, therapeutic decisions should be made in consultation with the patient, when possible, and with the patient's proxy if the patient is incapable of making decisions. In this regard, it is recommended that all patients with HIV infection, and in particular those with CD4+ T-cell counts <200/μL, designate a trusted individual with durable power of attorney to make medical decisions on their behalf, if necessary.

Following a diagnosis of HIV infection, several examinations and laboratory studies should be performed to help determine the extent of disease and provide baseline standards for future reference (**Table 202-19**). In addition to routine chemistry, fasting lipid profile, aspartate aminotransferase, alanine aminotransferase, total and direct bilirubin, fasting glucose and hematology screening panels, Pap smear, urinalysis, and chest x-ray, one should also obtain a CD4+ T-cell count, a plasma HIV RNA level, an HIV resistance test, a rapid plasma reagin or VDRL test, an anti-*Toxoplasma* antibody titer, and serologies for hepatitis A, B, and C. A PPD test or IFN-γ release assay should be done and an MMSE performed and recorded. A pregnancy test should be done in women in whom the drug efavirenz is being considered, and HLA-B5701 testing should be done in all patients in whom the drug abacavir is being considered. Patients should be immunized with pneumococcal polysaccharide, with annual influenza shots, and, if seronegative for these viruses, with HPV, hepatitis A, and hepatitis B vaccines. The status of hepatitis C infection should be determined. In addition, patients should be counseled with regard to sexual practices and needle sharing, and counseling should be offered to people whom the patient knows, or suspects, may also be infected. Once these baseline activities are performed, short- and long-term medical management strategies should be developed based on the most recent information available and modified as new information becomes available. The field of HIV medicine is changing rapidly, and it is difficult to remain fully up to date. Fortunately, there

TABLE 202-19 Initial Evaluation of the Patient with HIV Infection

History and physical examination
Routine chemistry and hematology
AST, ALT, alkaline phosphatase, direct and indirect bilirubin
Lipid profile and fasting glucose
CD4+ T lymphocyte count
Plasma HIV RNA level
HIV resistance testing
HLA-B5701 screening
RPR or VDRL test
Anti-*Toxoplasma* antibody titer
Urinalysis
PPD skin test or IFN-γ release assay
Mini-Mental Status Examination
Serologies for hepatitis A, hepatitis B, and hepatitis C
Immunization with pneumococcal polysaccharide; influenza; HPV as indicated
Immunization with hepatitis A and hepatitis B if seronegative
Counseling regarding natural history and transmission
Help contacting others who might be infected

Abbreviations: ALT, alanine aminotransferase; AST, aspartate aminotransferase; PPD, purified protein derivative; RPR, rapid plasma reagin; VDRL, Venereal Disease Research Laboratory.

TABLE 202-20 HIV Disease Resources Available on the World Wide Web

www.hivinfo.nih.gov	HIVinfo a service of the U.S. Department of Health and Human Services, posts federally approved treatment guidelines for HIV and AIDS; provides information on federally funded and privately funded clinical trials and CDC publications and data
www.cdcnpin.org	Updates on epidemiologic data and prevention information from the CDC

Abbreviation: CDC, Centers for Disease Control and Prevention.

are a series of excellent sites on the Internet that are frequently updated, and they provide the most recent information on a variety of topics, including consensus panel reports on treatment (**Table 202-20**).

ANTIRETROVIRAL THERAPY

Combination antiretroviral therapy (ART), also referred to as highly active antiretroviral therapy (HAART), is the cornerstone of management of patients with HIV infection and should be initiated as soon as possible following a diagnosis of HIV infection. One exception to immediate initiation of ART is in the setting of cryptococcal or TB meningitis where several weeks of specific antimicrobial therapy prior to initiation of ART may decrease the risk of severe IRIS. Following the initiation of widespread use of ART in the United States in 1995–1996, marked declines were noted in the incidence of most AIDS-defining conditions (Fig. 202-34). Suppression of HIV replication is an important component in prolonging and improving the quality of life for the patient as well as minimizing the risk of transmission of HIV to others. Adequate suppression of HIV replication requires strict adherence to prescribed regimens of antiretroviral drugs. This has been facilitated by the coformulations of antiretrovirals and the development of once-daily and monthly regimens. Unfortunately, many of the most important questions related to the treatment of HIV disease currently lack definitive answers. Among the decisions that need to be made in the context of prescribing ART are selection of the best initial regimen, determining when a given regimen should be changed, and deciding what regimen should be selected when a change is made. The care provider and patient must come to a mutually agreeable plan based on the best available data. In an effort to facilitate this process, the U.S. Department of Health and Human Services makes available on the Internet *(https://clinicalinfo.hiv.gov/en/guidelines)* a series of periodically updated guidelines, including *"Guidelines for the Use of Antiretroviral Agents in HIV-Infected Adults and Adolescents"* and "*Guidelines for the Prevention of Opportunistic Infections in Persons Infected with Human Immunodeficiency Virus*." At present, an extensive clinical trials network, involving both clinical investigators and patient advocates, is in place attempting to develop improved approaches to therapy. Consortia comprising representatives of academia, industry, independent foundations, and the federal government are involved in the process of drug development, including a wide-ranging series of clinical trials. As a result, new therapies and new therapeutic strategies are continually emerging. New drugs are often available through expanded-access programs prior to official licensure. Given the complexity of this field, decisions regarding ART are best made in consultation with experts.

Currently available drugs for the treatment of HIV infection as part of a combination regimen fall into four categories: those that inhibit the viral reverse transcriptase enzyme (nucleoside and nucleotide reverse transcriptase inhibitors; nonnucleoside reverse transcriptase inhibitors), those that inhibit the viral protease enzyme (protease inhibitors), those that inhibit the viral integrase enzyme (integrase negative strand transfer inhibitors), and those that interfere with viral entry (fusion inhibitors; CCR5 antagonists; CD4 antagonists) (**Table 202-21; Fig. 202-46**). A typical initial regimen will include two nucleoside/nucleotide reverse transcriptase inhibitors (usually a tenofovir-based drug or abacavir + 3TC or FTC) plus a nonnucleoside reverse transcriptase inhibitor, an integrase inhibitor, or a protease inhibitor boosted with a pharmacokinetic enhancer (ritonavir or cobicistat). More recent studies have also supported the two-drug regimen of dolutegravir plus 3TC for initial therapy in hepatitis B–negative patients with baseline HIV RNA levels under 500,000 copies/mL. Numerous fixed-drug formulations combining two or more of these antiretroviral drugs have been licensed (**Table 202-22**). Prior to initiation of therapy and at any time a change in therapy due to treatment failure is being considered, drug resistance testing should be performed to help guide the selection of drugs to be used in combination. A summary of known resistance mutations for antiretroviral drugs is shown in **Fig. 202-47**.

While most patients with HIV infection will be infected with HIV-1, some patients, especially those with an epidemiologic link to West Africa, may be infected with HIV-2. While the principles of treatment are the same as those for persons infected with HIV-1, it is important to note that the nonnucleoside reverse transcriptase inhibitors enfuvirtide and fostemsavir are not active against HIV-2 and should not be used as part of ART regimens in HIV-2–infected individuals.

The FDA-approved reverse transcriptase inhibitors include the *nucleoside analogues* zidovudine, didanosine, zalcitabine, stavudine, lamivudine, abacavir, and emtricitabine; the *nucleotide analogues* tenofovir disoproxil and tenofovir alafenamide; and the *nonnucleoside reverse transcriptase inhibitors* nevirapine, delavirdine, efavirenz, etravirine, rilpivirine, long-acting rilpivirine, and doravirine (Table 202-21). These represent the first class of drugs licensed for the treatment of HIV infection. They are indicated for this use as part of combination regimens. It should be stressed that none of these drugs should be used as monotherapy for HIV infection due to the relative ease with which drug resistance may develop under such circumstances. Thus, when lamivudine, emtricitabine, or tenofovir is used to treat hepatitis B infection in the setting of HIV infection, one should ensure that the patient is also on additional antiretroviral medication. Similarly, when any of these three medications are discontinued, one needs to be vigilant for a flare of hepatitis B in coinfected patients. The reverse transcriptase inhibitors block the HIV replication cycle at the point of RNA-dependent DNA synthesis, the reverse transcription step. While the nonnucleoside reverse transcriptase inhibitors are quite selective for the HIV-1 reverse transcriptase, the nucleoside and nucleotide analogues inhibit a variety of DNA polymerases in addition to those of the HIV-1 reverse transcriptase. For this reason, serious side effects are more varied with the nucleoside analogues and include mitochondrial damage that can lead to hepatic steatosis and lactic acidosis as well as peripheral neuropathy and pancreatitis. The use of either of the thymidine analogues zidovudine and stavudine has been associated with a syndrome of hyperlipidemia, glucose intolerance/insulin resistance, and fat redistribution often referred to as *lipodystrophy syndrome* (discussed in "Diseases of the Endocrine System and Metabolic Disorders," above). For these reasons, the older drugs in this class, zidovudine, didanosine, zalcitabine, and stavudine are no longer recommend for use in the United States due to their side effect profiles. The nucleoside and nucleotide transcriptase inhibitors preferred for use in combination regimens according to the DHHS Panel on the use of antiretroviral drugs are lamivudine, emtricitabine, abacavir, tenofovir disoproxil, and tenofovir alafenamide. Given its renal toxicity, tenofovir disoproxil should be limited to use in patients with creatinine clearance (CrCl) >70 while tenofovir alafenamide should generally be limited to use in patients with CrCl >30. The preferred nonnucleoside reverse transcriptase inhibitors are efavirenz, rilpivirine, and doravirine. Of note, rilpivirine is approved for treatment only in ART-naïve patients with HIV RNA levels <100,000 copies/mL and is contraindicated in patients taking proton pump inhibitors.

TABLE 202-21 Antiretroviral Drugs Most Commonly Used in the Treatment of HIV Infection

DRUG	STATUS	INDICATION	DOSE IN COMBINATION	SUPPORTING DATA	TOXICITY
Nucleoside or Nucleotide Reverse Transcriptase Inhibitors					
Zidovudine (AZT, azidothymidine, *Retrovir, 3′azido-3′-deoxythymidine)	Licensed	Treatment of HIV infection in combination with other antiretroviral agents	200 mg q8h or 300 mg bid	19 vs 1 death in original placebo-controlled trial in 281 patients with AIDS or ARC	Anemia, granulocytopenia, myopathy, lactic acidosis, hepatomegaly with steatosis, headache, nausea, nail pigmentation, lipid abnormalities, lipoatrophy, hyperglycemia
		Prevention of maternal-fetal HIV transmission		In pregnant women with CD4+ T-cell count ≥200/µL, AZT PO beginning at weeks 14–34 of gestation plus IV drug during labor and delivery plus PO AZT to infant for 6 weeks decreased transmission of HIV by 67.5% (from 25.5% to 8.3%); n = 363	
Lamivudine (Epivir, 2′3′-dideoxy-3′-thiacytidine, 3TC)	Licensed	In combination with other antiretroviral agents for the treatment of HIV infection	150 mg bid 300 mg qd	In combination with AZT superior to AZT alone with respect to changes in CD4+ T-cell counts in 495 patients who were zidovudine-naïve and 477 patients who were zidovudine-experienced; overall CD4+ T-cell counts for the zidovudine group were at baseline by 24 weeks, while in the group treated with zidovudine plus lamivudine, they were 10–50 cells/µL above baseline; 54% decrease in progression to AIDS/death compared with AZT alone	Flare of hepatitis in HBV-co-infected patients who discontinue drug
Emtricitabine (FTC, Emtriva)	Licensed	In combination with other antiretroviral agents for the treatment of HIV infection	200 mg qd	Comparable to lamivudine in combination with stavudine and nevirapine/efavirenz	Hepatotoxicity in HBV-co-infected patients who discontinue drug, skin discoloration
Abacavir (Ziagen)	Licensed	For treatment of HIV infection in combination with other antiretroviral agents	300 mg bid	Abacavir + AZT + 3TC equivalent to indinavir + AZT + 3TC with regard to viral load suppression (~60% in each group with <400 HIV RNA copies/mL plasma) and CD4+ T-cell increase (~100/µL in each group) at 24 weeks	Hypersensitivity reaction In HLA-B5701+ individuals (can be fatal); fever, rash, nausea, vomiting, malaise or fatigue, and loss of appetite
Tenofovir disoproxil fumarate (Viread)	Licensed	For use in combination with other antiretroviral agents when treatment is indicated	300 mg qd	Reduction of ~0.6 log in HIV-1 RNA levels when added to background regimen in treatment-experienced patients	Renal, osteomalacia, flare of hepatitis in HBV-co-infected patients who discontinue drug
Tenofovir alafenamide (Vemlidy)	Licensed	In combination with emtricitabine and other antiretroviral agents for treatment of HIV-1 infection	25 mg qd	92% of patients treated in combination with emtricitabine, elvitegravir, and cobicistat had HIV-1 RNA levels <50 copies/mL	Nausea, less renal toxicity than tenofovir disoproxil fumarate
Non-Nucleoside Reverse Transcriptase Inhibitors					
Nevirapine (Viramune)	Licensed	In combination with other antiretroviral agents for treatment of progressive HIV infection	200 mg/d × 14 days then 200 mg bid *or* 400 mg extended release qd	Increase in CD4+ T-cell count, decrease in HIV RNA when used in combination with nucleosides	Skin rash, hepatotoxicity
Efavirenz (Sustiva)	Licensed	For treatment of HIV infection in combination with other antiretroviral agents	600 mg qhs	Efavirenz + AZT + 3TC comparable to indinavir + AZT + 3TC with regard to viral load suppression (a higher percentage of the efavirenz group achieved viral load <50 copies/mL, but the discontinuation rate in the indinavir group was unexpectedly high, accounting for most treatment "failures"); CD4 cell increase (~140/µL in each group) at 24 weeks	Rash, dysphoria, elevated liver function tests, drowsiness, abnormal dreams, depression, lipid abnormalities, potentially teratogenic
Etravirine (Intelence)	Licensed	In combination with other antiretroviral agents in treatment-experienced patients whose HIV is resistant to nonnucleoside reverse transcriptase inhibitors and other antiretroviral medications	200 mg bid	Higher rates of HIV RNA suppression to <50 copies/mL (56% vs 39%); greater increases in CD4+ T-cell count (89 vs 64 cells) compared to placebo when given in combination with an optimized background regimen	Rash, nausea, hypersensitivity reactions

(*Continued*)

TABLE 202-21 Antiretroviral Drugs Most Commonly Used in the Treatment of HIV Infection (Continued)

DRUG	STATUS	INDICATION	DOSE IN COMBINATION	SUPPORTING DATA	TOXICITY
Rilpivirine (Edurant)	Licensed	In combination with other drugs in previously untreated patients when treatment is indicated.	25 mg qd	Noninferior to efavirenz with respect to suppression at week 48 in 1368 treatment-naive individuals, except in patients with pretherapy HIV RNA levels >100,000 where it was inferior	Nausea, dizziness, somnolence, vertigo, less CNS toxicity and rash than efavirenz
Protease Inhibitors					
Ritonavir (Norvir)	Licensed	In combination with other antiretroviral agents for treatment of HIV infection when treatment is warranted	600 mg bid (also used in lower doses as pharmacokinetic booster)	Reduction in the cumulative incidence of clinical progression or death from 34% to 17% in patients with CD4+ T-cell count <100/μL treated for a median of 6 months	Nausea, abdominal pain, hyperglycemia, fat redistribution, lipid abnormalities, may alter levels of many other drugs, paresthesias, hepatitis
Atazanavir (Reyataz)	Licensed	For treatment of HIV infection in combination with other antiretroviral agents	400 mg qd or 300 mg qd + ritonavir 100 mg qd when given with efavirenz	Comparable to efavirenz when given in combination with AZT + 3TC in a study of 810 treatment-naïve patients; comparable to nelfinavir when given in combination with stavudine + 3TC in a study of 467 treatment-naïve patients	Hyperbilirubinemia, PR prolongation, nausea, vomiting, hyperglycemia, fat maldistribution, rash transaminase elevations, renal stones
Darunavir (Prezista)	Licensed	In combination with 100 mg ritonavir for combination therapy in treatment-experienced adults	600 mg + 100 mg ritonavir twice daily with food	At 24 weeks, patients with prior extensive exposure to antiretrovirals treated with a new combination including darunavir showed a –1.89-log change in HIV RNA levels and a 92-cell increase in CD4+ T cells compared with –0.48 log and 17 cells in the control arm	Diarrhea, nausea, headache, skin rash, hepatotoxicity, hyperlipidemia, hyperglycemia
Entry Inhibitors					
Enfuvirtide (Fuzeon)	Licensed	In combination with other agents in treatment-experienced patients with evidence of HIV-1 replication despite ongoing antiretroviral therapy	90 mg SC bid	In treatment of experienced patients, superior to placebo when added to new optimized background (37% vs 16% with <400 HIV RNA copies/mL at 24 weeks; + 71 vs + 35 CD4+ T cells at 24 weeks)	Local injection reactions, hypersensitivity reactions, increased rate of bacterial pneumonia
Maraviroc (Selzentry)	Licensed	In combination with other antiretroviral agents in adults infected with only CCR5-tropic HIV-1	150–600 mg bid depending on concomitant medications (see text)	At 24 weeks, among 635 patients with CCR5-tropic virus and HIV-1 RNA >5000 copies/mL despite at least 6 months of prior therapy with at least 1 agent from 3 of the 4 antiretroviral drug classes, 61% of patients randomized to maraviroc achieved HIV RNA levels <400 copies/mL compared with 28% of patients randomized to placebo	Hepatotoxicity, nasopharyngitis, fever, cough, rash, abdominal pain, dizziness, musculoskeletal symptoms
Ibalizumab (Trogarzo)	Licensed	In combination with other antiretroviral agents in patients with multidrug-resistant HIV-1	Single loading dose of 2000 mg followed by a maintenance dose of 800 mg every 2 weeks	At 25 weeks, 50% of patients with multi-drug resistant HIV-1 with HIV-1 RNA >1000 copies/mL treated with an optimized background of 1 active drug and ibalizumab achieved HIV RNA levels <200 copies/mL	Rash, diarrhea, nausea
Integrase Inhibitor					
Raltegravir (Isentress)	Licensed	In combination with other antiretroviral agents	400 mg bid	At 24 weeks, among 436 patients with 3-class drug resistance, 76% of patients randomized to receive raltegravir achieved HIV RNA levels <400 copies/mL compared with 41% of patients randomized to receive placebo	Nausea, headache, diarrhea, CPK elevation, muscle weakness, rhabdomyolysis
Elvitegravir (Available only in combination with cobicistat, tenofovir, and emtricitabine [Stribild])	Licensed	Fixed-dose combination	1 tablet daily	Noninferior to raltegravir or atazanavir/ritonavir in treatment-experienced patients.	Diarrhea, nausea, upper respiratory infections, headache
Dolutegravir (Tivicay)	Licensed	In combination with other antiretroviral agents	50 mg daily for treatment-naïve patients 50 mg twice daily for treatment-experienced patients or those also receiving efavirenz or rifampin	Noninferior to raltegravir, superior to efavirenz or darunavir/ritonavir	Insomnia, headache, hypersensitivity reactions, hepatotoxicity
Bictegravir (Available only in combination with tenofovir alafenamide and emtricitabine [Biktarvy])	Licensed	For treatment of HIV infection in adults	50 mg bictegravir/25 mg tenofovir alafenamide/200 mg emtricitabine qd	Noninferior to dolutegravir/tenofovir/emtricitabine and non-inferior to dolutegravir/abacavir/lamivudine	Nausea, diarrhea, headache

(*Continued*)

TABLE 202-21 Antiretroviral Drugs Most Commonly Used in the Treatment of HIV Infection (Continued)

DRUG	STATUS	INDICATION	DOSE IN COMBINATION	SUPPORTING DATA	TOXICITY
Cabotegravir (Vocabria)	Licensed	In combination with rilpivirine for treatment of HIV infection in adults	Oral lead-in of 30 mg + 25 mg rilpivirine for 1 month; followed by an initial injection of 600 mg (3 mL) IM + 900 mg (3 mL) rilpivirine IM; followed by monthly injections of 400 mg (2 mL) IM + 600 mg (2 mL) rilpivirine IM	Noninferior to abacavir/dolutegravir/lamivudine or dolutegravir + 2 nucleoside/tide reverse transcriptase inhibitors Noninferior to nonnucleoside reverse transcriptase inhibitor + 2 nucleoside/tide reverse transcriptase inhibitors or a protease inhibitor + 2 nucleoside/tide reverse transcriptase inhibitors or an integrase inhibitor and 2 nucleoside/tide reverse transcriptase inhibitors	Injection site reactions

*Initial trade names are provided. Generic forms may be available.

Abbreviations: ARC, AIDS-related complex; NRTIs, nonnucleoside reverse transcriptase inhibitors.

The HIV-1 protease inhibitors (saquinavir, indinavir, ritonavir, nelfinavir, amprenavir, fosamprenavir, lopinavir/ritonavir, atazanavir, atazanavir/cobicistat, tipranavir, darunavir, and darunavir/cobicistat) are an important part of the therapeutic armamentarium of antiretrovirals. While possessing antiviral properties of its own, ritonavir is typically used as a pharmacokinetic enhancer due to its high affinity for several isoforms of cytochrome P450 (3A4, 2D6) leading to large increases in the plasma concentrations of co-administered drugs metabolized by these pathways. As in the case of reverse transcriptase inhibitors, resistance to protease inhibitors can develop rapidly in the setting of monotherapy, and thus these agents should be used only as part of combination therapeutic regimens. Based on superior efficacy and side-effect profile, ritonavir-boosted darunavir in combination with emtricitabine and tenofovir (disoproxil or alafenamide) is the protease inhibitor strategy preferred for initial therapy in patients with CrCl >70 (tenofovir disoproxil) or >30 (tenofovir alafenamide) according to the DHHS Panel on the use of antiretroviral drugs.

Integrase strand transfer inhibitors act by blocking the action of the HIV integrase enzyme and thus preventing integration of the HIV provirus into the host cell genome. They are among the most potent and safest of the antiretroviral drugs and frequently part of initial combination regimens. The five licensed integrase inhibitors are raltegravir, cabotegravir, elvitegravir, dolutegravir, and bictegravir. Cabotegravir is an integrase inhibitor that is given in combination with rilpivirine as a monthly injection. Prior to initiation of the monthly injections, patients should initially be treated with oral preparations of the two drugs to be sure they are well tolerated. Elvitegravir is always given in combination with cobicistat, which acts to boost the concentrations of elvitegravir. Cobicistat also inhibits tubular secretion of creatinine, resulting in increases in serum creatinine, and is not recommended for patients with estimated creatinine clearances <70 mL/min. Dolutegravir has been associated with a slight increase (0.2 vs 0.1%) in the incidence of neural tube defects in infants exposed to dolutegravir at the time of conception. Bictegravir is available only in combination with tenofovir alafenamide and emtricitabine. When used as part of initial ART, integrase inhibitor–containing regimens have been associated with greater weight gain than nonnucleoside reverse transcriptase inhibitor– or protease inhibitor–containing regimens.

Entry inhibitors act by interfering with the binding of HIV to its receptor or co-receptor or by interfering with the process of fusion (see above). The first drug in this class to be licensed was the fusion inhibitor *enfuvirtide*, or T-20, followed by the CCR5 antagonist *maraviroc*. The anti-CD4 monoclonal antibody ibalizumab was licensed in 2018, and the small molecule fostemsavir in 2020. Given that maraviroc is effective only against CCR5-tropic viruses, a co-receptor tropism assay should be performed when use of this agent is being considered.

PRINCIPLES OF THERAPY

The principles of therapy for HIV infection have been articulated by a panel sponsored by the U.S. Department of Health and Human Services as a working group of the NIH Office of AIDS Research Advisory Council. These principles are summarized in **Table 202-23**. As noted in these guidelines, ART of HIV infection does not lead to eradication or cure of HIV. The possible exceptions are a limited number of individuals with HIV infection and cancer who received allogeneic stem cell transplants from donors who were homozygous for the CCR5Δ32 mutation (see above) and thus resistant to HIV infection.

Treatment decisions must consider the fact that one is dealing with a chronic infection that requires daily therapy. Patients initiating antiretroviral therapy must be willing to commit to life-long treatment and understand the importance of adherence to their prescribed regimen. The importance of adherence is illustrated by the observation that treatment interruption is associated with rapid increases in HIV RNA levels, rapid declines in CD4+ T-cell counts, and an increased risk of clinical progression. While it seems reasonable to assume that the complications associated with ART could be minimized by intermittent treatment regimens designed to minimize exposure to the drugs in question, all efforts to do so have paradoxically been associated with an increase in serious adverse events in the patients randomized to intermittent therapy, demonstrating that some "non-AIDS-associated" serious adverse events such as heart attack and stroke are linked to HIV replication. Thus, unless contraindicated for reasons of toxicity, patients started on ART should remain on ART.

At present, the U.S. Department of Health and Human Services Guidelines panel recommends that everyone with HIV infection be treated with ART and that therapy be initiated a soon as possible after diagnosis. Therapy has been associated with a decrease in disease progression in patients at all stages of HIV infection and leads to a decrease in the risk of transmission of infection. In addition, one may wish to administer a 6-week course of therapy to uninfected individuals immediately following a high-risk exposure to HIV. The combination of tenofovir and emtricitabine is also licensed for pre-exposure prophylaxis in individuals at high risk of HIV infection, as is an injectable, long-acting formulation of cabotegravir that may be even more effective. For patients diagnosed with an opportunistic infection and HIV infection at the same time and a CD4+ count >50 cells/μL, one may consider a 2- to 4-week delay in the initiation of antiretroviral therapy during which time treatment is focused on the opportunistic infection. This delay may decrease the severity of any subsequent immune reconstitution inflammatory syndrome by lowering the antigenic burden of the opportunistic infection. This is particularly true for patients with TB or cryptococcal infections of the central nervous system. For patients with advanced HIV infection (CD4+ <50 cells/μL), however, ART should be initiated as soon as possible.

Once the decision has been made to initiate therapy, the health care provider must decide which drugs to use as the first regimen. The decision regarding choice of drugs not only will affect the immediate response to therapy but also will have implications regarding options for future therapeutic regimens. The initial regimen is usually the most effective insofar as the virus has yet to be under any selective pressure to develop significant drug resistance. HIV is capable of rapidly developing resistance to any single agent, and therapy must be given as a multidrug combination. Given that patients can be infected with viruses that harbor drug resistance mutations, it is recommended that a viral genotype be done prior to the initiation of therapy to optimize the selection of antiretroviral agents. The combination regimens currently recommended for initial therapy in most treatment-naïve patients are listed in **Table 202-24**. It is currently debated whether treatment-naïve individuals with <50 copies/mL of HIV RNA benefit from ART. While these individuals are at low risk of disease progression in the short term, they do have evidence of persistent immune activation

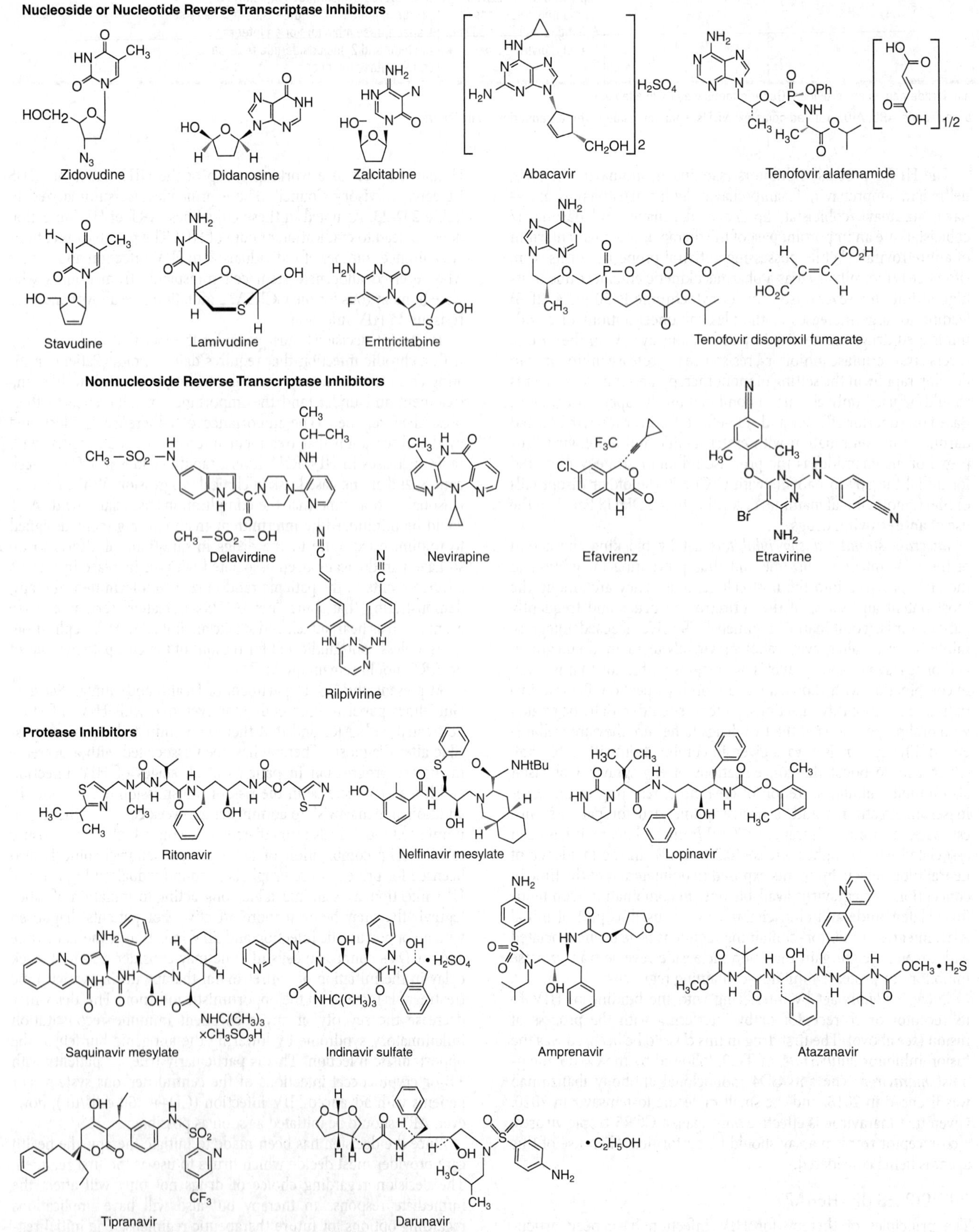

Nucleoside or Nucleotide Reverse Transcriptase Inhibitors
Zidovudine
Didanosine
Zalcitabine
Abacavir
Tenofovir alafenamide
Stavudine
Lamivudine
Emtricitabine
Tenofovir disoproxil fumarate
Nonnucleoside Reverse Transcriptase Inhibitors
Delavirdine
Nevirapine
Efavirenz
Etravirine
Rilpivirine
Protease Inhibitors
Ritonavir
Nelfinavir mesylate
Lopinavir
Saquinavir mesylate
Indinavir sulfate
Amprenavir
Atazanavir
Tipranavir
Darunavir

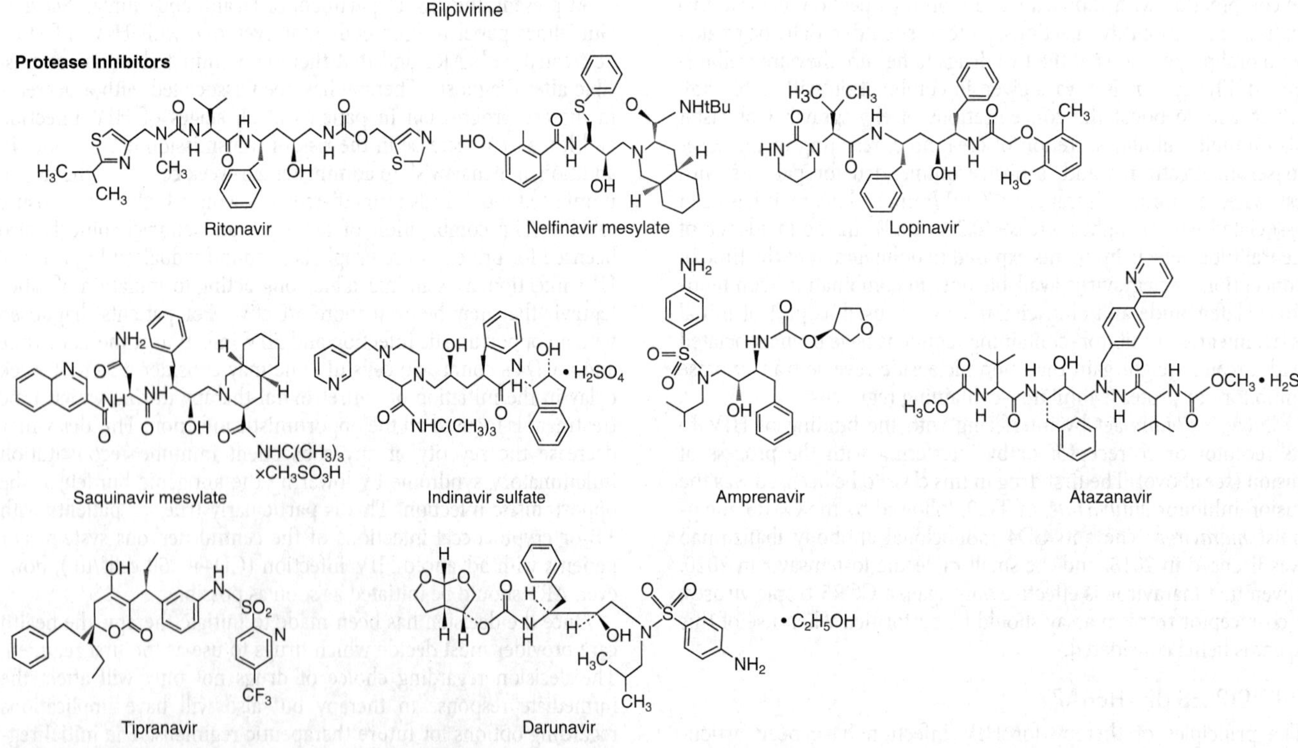

FIGURE 202-46 Molecular structures of antiretroviral agents.

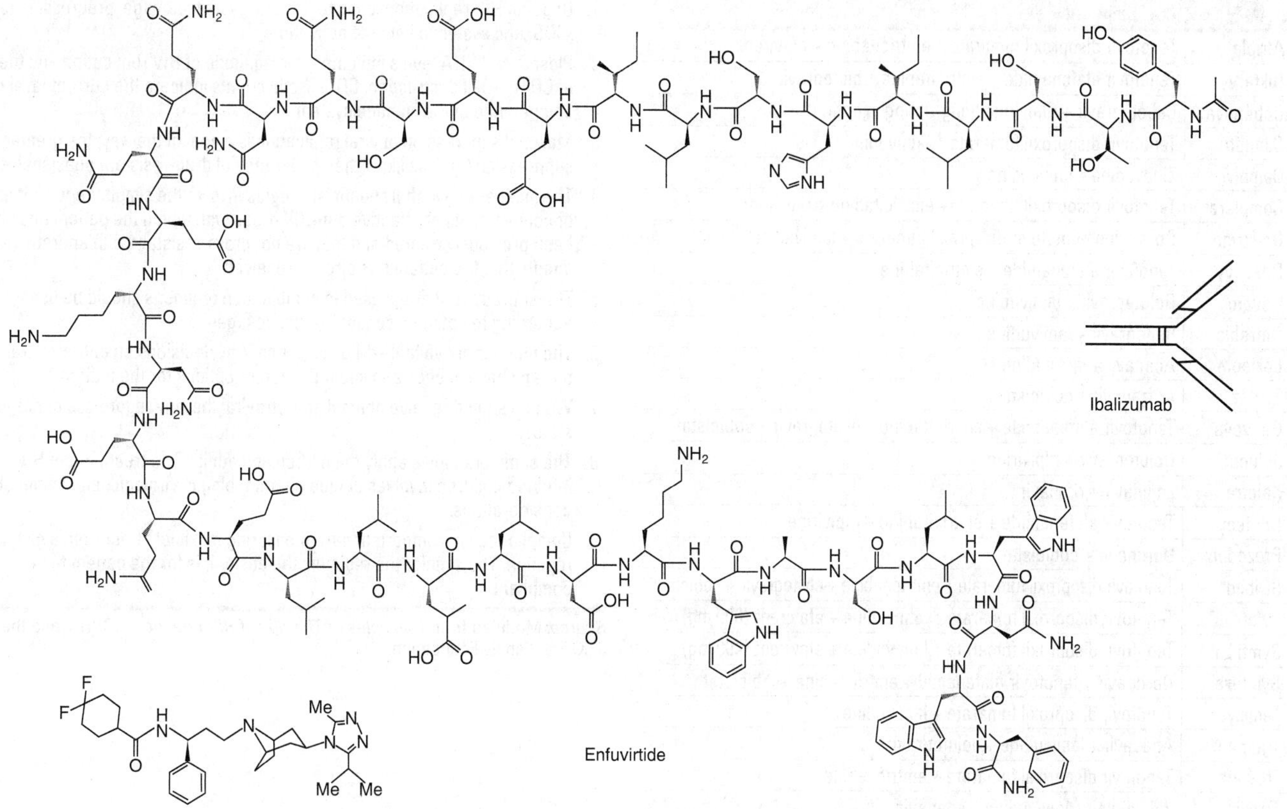

Entry Inhibitors

Ibalizumab

Enfuvirtide

Maraviroc

Integrase Inhibitors

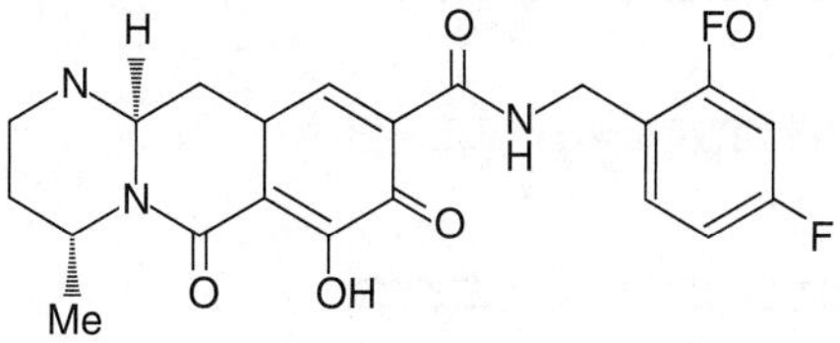

Elvitegravir

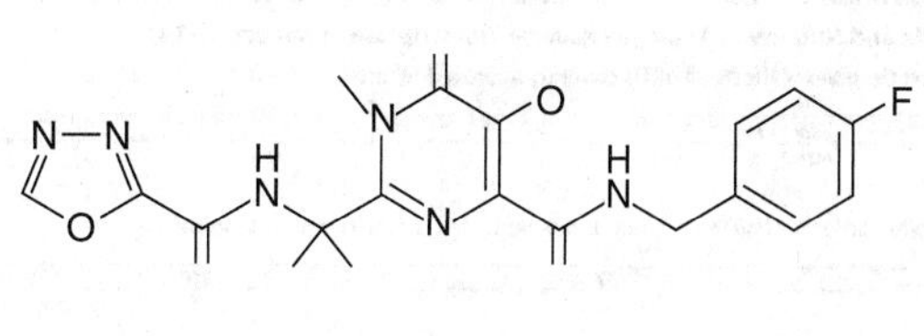

Raltegravir

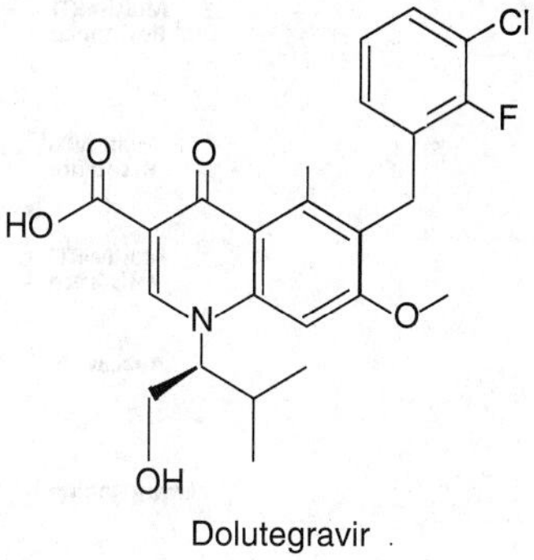

Dolutegravir

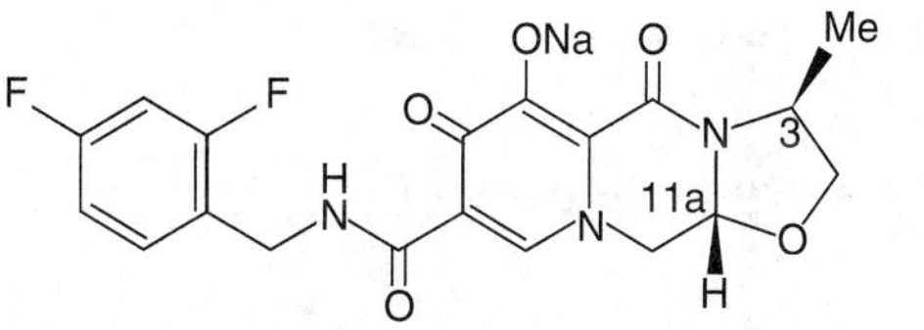

Cabotegravir

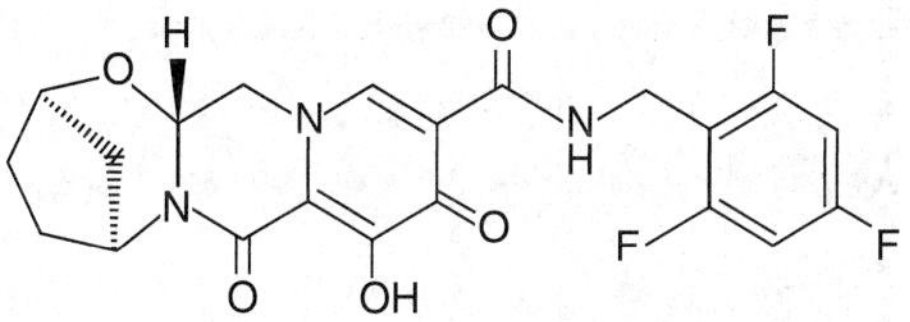

Bictegravir

FIGURE 202-46 (Continued)

that may have long-term consequences. Following the initiation of therapy, one should expect a rapid, at least 1-log (tenfold) reduction in plasma HIV RNA levels within 1–2 months and then a slower decline in plasma HIV RNA levels to <50 copies/mL within 6 months. During this same time there should be a rise in the CD4+ T-cell count of 100–150/cells μL that is also particularly brisk during the first month of therapy. Subsequently, one should anticipate a CD4+ T-cell count increase of 50–100 cells/year until numbers approach normal. Many clinicians feel that failure to achieve these endpoints is an indication for a change in therapy. Other reasons for a change in therapy include a persistently declining CD4+ T-cell count, a consistent increase in HIV RNA levels to >200 copies/mL, clinical deterioration, or drug toxicity (**Table 202-25**). As in the case of initiating therapy, changing therapy may have a lasting impact on future therapeutic options. When changing therapy because of treatment failure (clinical progression or worsening laboratory parameters), it is important to attempt to provide a regimen with at least two new active drugs. This decision can be guided by resistance testing (see below). In the patient in whom a change is made for reasons of drug toxicity, a simple replacement of one drug is reasonable. It should be stressed that in attempting to sort out a drug toxicity it may be advisable to hold all therapy for a period of time to distinguish between drug toxicity and disease progression. Drug toxicity will usually begin to show signs of reversal within 1–2 weeks. Prior to changing a treatment regimen because of drug failure, it is important to ensure that the patient has been adherent to the prescribed regimen. As in the case of initial therapy, the simpler the new therapeutic regimen, the easier it is for the patient to

TABLE 202-22 Combination Formulations of Antiretroviral Drugs

NAME	COMBINATION
Atripla*	Tenofovir disoproxil fumarate + emtricitabine + efavirenz
Biktarvy*	Tenofovir alafenamide + emtricitabine + bictegravir
Cabenuva*	Cabotegravir + rilpivirine (long-acting injection)
Cimduo	Tenofovir disoproxil fumarate + lamivudine
Combivir	Zidovudine + lamivudine
Complera*	Tenofovir disoproxil fumarate+ emtricitabine + rilpivirine
Delstrigo*	Doravirine +tenofovir disoproxil fumarate + lamivudine
Descovy	Tenofovir alafenamide + emtricitabine
Dovato*	Dolutegravir + lamivudine
Dutrebis	Raltegravir + lamivudine
Epzicom	Abacavir + lamivudine
Evotaz	Atazanavir + cobicistat
Genvoya*	Tenofovir alafenamide + emtricitabine + elvitegravir + cobicistat
Juluca*	Dolutegravir + rilpivirine
Kaletra	Lopinavir + ritonavir
Odefsey*	Tenofovir alafenamide + emtricitabine + rilpivirine
Prezcobix	Darunavir + cobicistat
Stribild*	Tenofovir disoproxil fumarate + emtricitabine + elvitegravir + cobicistat
Symfi*	Tenofovir disoproxil fumarate + lamivudine + efavirenz (600 mg)
Symfi Lo*	Tenofovir disoproxil fumarate + lamivudine + efavirenz (400 mg)
Symtuza*	Darunavir + tenofovir alafenamid + emtricitabine +cobicistat
Temixys	Tenofovir disoproxil fumarate + lamivudine
Triumeq*	Abacavir + lamivudine + dolutegravir
Truvada	Tenofovir disoproxil fumarate + emtricitabine
Trizivir	Zidovudine + lamivudine + abacavir

*Complete, once-daily, single-tablet regimens.

TABLE 202-23 Principles of Therapy of HIV Infection

1. Ongoing HIV replication leads to immune system damage, progression to AIDS, and systemic immune activation.
2. Plasma HIV RNA levels indicate the magnitude of HIV replication and the rate of CD4+ T-cell destruction. CD4+ T-cell counts indicate the current level of competence of the immune system.
3. Maximal suppression of viral replication is a goal of therapy; the greater the suppression the less likely the appearance of drug-resistant quasispecies.
4. The most effective therapeutic strategies involve the simultaneous initiation of combinations of effective anti-HIV drugs with which the patient has not been previously treated and that are not cross-resistant with antiretroviral agents that the patient has already received.
5. The antiretroviral drugs used in combination regimens should be used according to optimum schedules and dosages.
6. The number of available drugs is limited. Any decisions on antiretroviral therapy have a long-term impact on future options for the patient.
7. Women should receive optimal antiretroviral therapy regardless of pregnancy status.
8. The same principles apply to children and adults. The treatment of HIV-infected children involves unique pharmacologic, virologic, and immunologic considerations.
9. Compliance is an important part of ensuring maximal effect from a given regimen. The simpler the regimen, the easier it is for the patient to be compliant.

Source: Modified from *Principles of Therapy of HIV Infection*, USPHS, and the Henry J. Kaiser Family Foundation.

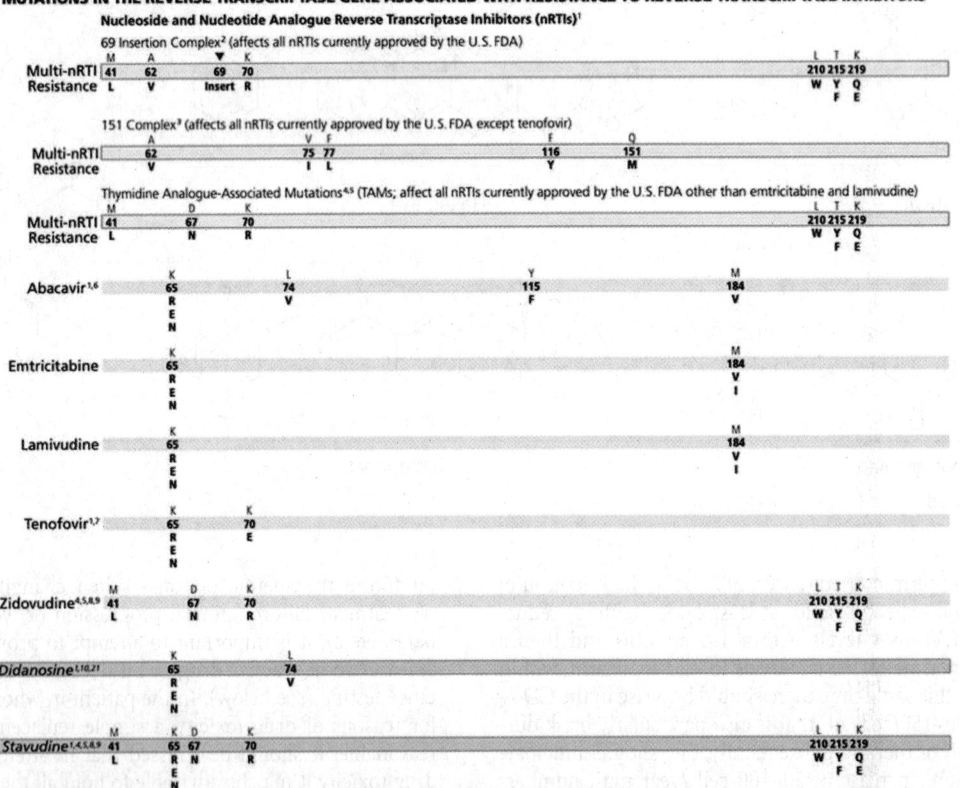

FIGURE 202-47 Amino acid substitutions conferring resistance to antiretroviral drugs. For each amino acid residue, the letter above the bar indicates the amino acid associated with wild-type virus and the letter(s) below indicate the substitution(s) that confer viral resistance. The number shows the position of the mutation in the protein. Mutations selected by protease inhibitors in Gag cleavage sites are not listed. HR1, first heptad repeat; NAMs, nRTI-associated mutations; nRTI, nucleoside reverse transcriptase inhibitor; NNRTI, nonnucleoside reverse transcriptase inhibitor; PI, protease inhibitor. Amino acid abbreviations: A, alanine; C, cysteine; D, aspartate; E, glutamic acid; F, phenylalanine; G, glycine; H, histidine; I, isoleucine; K, lysine; L, leucine; M, methionine; N, asparagine; P, proline; Q, glutamine; R, arginine; S, serine; T, threonine; V, valine; W, tryptophan; Y, tyrosine. *(Reprinted with permission from the International Antiviral Society—USA. AM Wensing et al: 2019 resistance mutations update. Top Antivir Med 27:111, 2019. Updated information [and thorough explanatory notes] available at www.iasusa.org.)*

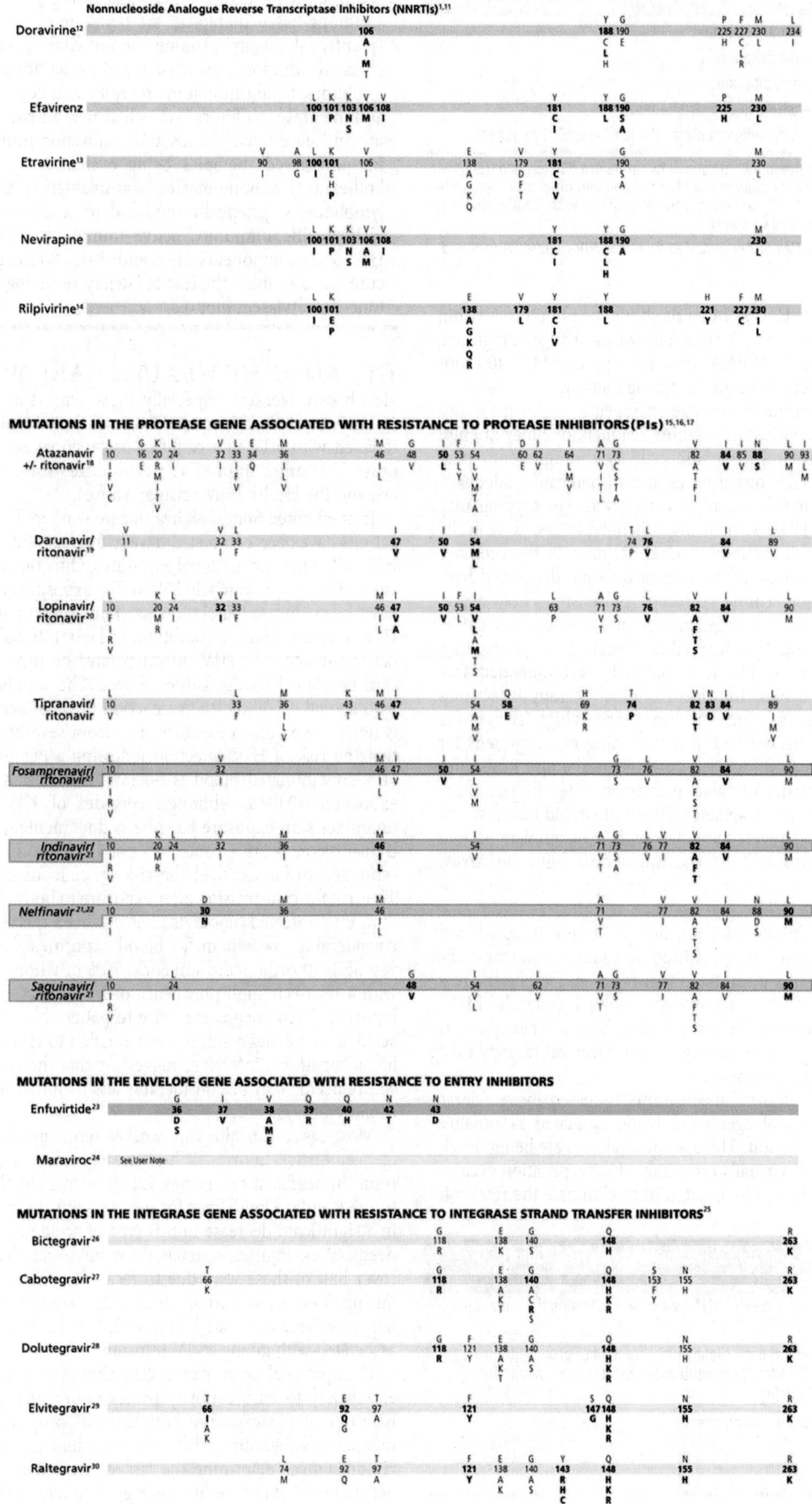

FIGURE 202-47 (Continued)

TABLE 202-24 Initial Combination Regimens Recommended for Most Treatment-Naïve Patients Regardless of HIV RNA Level or CD4 Count

Dolutegravir + tenofovir* + emtricitabine†
Raltegravir + tenofovir* + emtricitabine†
Bictegravir + tenofovir*+ emtricitabine†
Elvitegravir + cobicistat + tenofovir* + emtricitabine†
Dolutegravir + abacavir + lamivudine† (only for those HLA-B*5701 negative)

*Tenofovir alafenamide and tenofovir disoproxil fumarate are two forms of tenofovir approved by FDA. Tenofovir alafenamide has fewer bone and renal toxicities while tenofovir disoproxil fumarate is associated with lower lipid levels. †Lamivudine may substitute for emtricitabine and vice versa.

Source: Guidelines for the Use of Antiretroviral Agents in HIV-Infected Adults and Adolescents, USPHS.

be compliant. Plasma HIV RNA levels should be monitored within 2–4 weeks after initiation of ART or following a change in regimen, every 4–8 weeks until HIV RNA levels are suppressed to <200 copies/mL, and then every 3–6 months during therapy.

In order to determine an optimal therapeutic regimen for initial therapy or for a patient on a failing regimen, one may attempt to measure antiretroviral drug susceptibility through genotyping or phenotyping of HIV quasispecies and to determine adequacy of dosing through measurement of drug levels. Genotyping may be done through cDNA sequencing. Phenotypic assays typically measure the enzymatic activity of viral enzymes in the presence or absence of different concentrations of different drugs and have also been used to determine co-receptor tropism. These assays will generally detect quasispecies present at a frequency of ≥10%. Next-generation sequencing may allow detection of quasispecies at frequencies down to 1%. It is generally recommended that resistance testing be used in selecting initial therapy in settings where the risk of transmission of resistant virus is high (such as the United States and Europe) and in determining new regimens for patients experiencing virologic failure while on therapy. Resistance testing may be of particular value in distinguishing drug-resistant virus from poor patient compliance. Due to the rapid rate at which drug-resistant viruses revert to wild-type, it is recommended that resistance testing performed in the setting of drug failure be carried out while the patient is still on the failing regimen. Measurement of plasma drug levels can also be used to tailor an individual treatment. The inhibitory quotient, defined as the trough blood level/IC_{50} of the patient's virus, is used by some to determine the adequacy of dosing of a given treatment regimen. Despite the best of efforts there will still be patients with ongoing high levels of HIV replication while receiving the best available therapy. These patients will receive benefit from remaining on antiretroviral therapy even though it is not fully suppressive.

In addition to the licensed medications discussed above, a large number of experimental agents are being evaluated as possible therapies for HIV infection. Therapeutic strategies are being developed to interfere with virtually every step of the replication cycle of the virus (Fig. 202-3) and in an attempt to eliminate the reservoir of infected cells to "cure" HIV infection. In addition to directly acting antiviral drugs, other strategies, generically referred to as "immune-based therapies," are being developed as a complement to antiviral therapy. Among the antiviral agents in early clinical trials are additional nucleoside and nucleotide analogues, protease inhibitors, fusion inhibitors, receptor and co-receptor antagonists, and integrase inhibitors—as well as new antiviral strategies including antisense nucleic acids and maturation inhibitors. Among the immune-based therapies being evaluated are monoclonal antibodies, IFN-α, bone marrow transplantation, adoptive transfer of lymphocytes genetically modified to resist infection or enhance HIV-specific immunity, active immunotherapy with inactivated HIV or its components, IL-7, and IL-15. Strategies directed toward cure are examining the role of latency-reversing agents such as histone-deacetylase inhibitors.

TABLE 202-25 Indications for Changing Antiretroviral Therapy in Patients with HIV Infection[a]

Less than a 1-log drop in plasma HIV RNA by 4 weeks following the initiation of therapy
A reproducible significant increase (defined as threefold or greater) from the nadir of plasma HIV RNA level not attributable to intercurrent infection, vaccination, or test methodology
Persistently declining CD4+ T-cell numbers
Clinical deterioration
Side effects

[a]Generally speaking, a change should involve the initiation of at least two drugs felt to be effective in the given patient. The exception to this is when change is being made to manage toxicity, in which case a single substitution is reasonable.

Source: Guidelines for the Use of Antiretroviral Agents in HIV-Infected Adults and Adolescents, USPHS.

HIV AND THE HEALTH CARE WORKER

Health care workers, especially those who deal with large numbers of HIV-infected patients, have a small but definite risk of becoming infected with HIV as a result of professional activities (see "Occupational Transmission of HIV: Health Care Workers, Laboratory Workers, and the Health Care Setting," above).

In the United States, 58 health care workers for whom case investigations have been completed have had documented seroconversions to HIV following occupational exposures. Only one of these has occurred since 1999. Approximately 85% of the exposures resulting in infection have been due to percutaneous (puncture/cut injury) exposures to HIV-infected blood. In addition, at least 150 possible cases of occupationally acquired HIV infection have been reported among health care personnel in the United States. The number of these workers who actually acquired their infection through occupational exposures is not known. Taken together, data from several large studies suggest that the risk of HIV infection following a percutaneous exposure to HIV-contaminated blood is ~0.23%, and after a mucous membrane exposure, ~0.09%. Although episodes of HIV transmission after nonintact skin exposure have been documented, the average risk for transmission by this route has not been precisely quantified but is estimated to be less than the risk for mucous membrane exposures. The risk for transmission after exposure to body fluids or tissues other than HIV-infected blood also has not been quantified but is probably considerably lower than for blood exposures. A seroprevalence survey of 3420 orthopedic surgeons, 75% of whom practiced in an area with a relatively high prevalence of HIV infection and 39% of whom reported percutaneous exposure to patient blood, usually through an accident involving a suture needle, failed to reveal any cases of possible occupational infection, suggesting that the risk of infection with a suture needle may be considerably less than that with a blood-drawing (hollow-bore) needle.

Most cases of health care worker seroconversion occur as a result of needle-stick injuries. When one considers the circumstances that result in needle-stick injuries, it is immediately obvious that adhering to the standard guidelines for dealing with sharp objects would result in a significant decrease in this type of accident. In one study, 27% of needle-stick injuries resulted from improper disposal of the needle (over half of these were due to recapping the needle), 23% occurred during attempts to start an IV line, 22% occurred during blood drawing, 16% were associated with an IM or SC injection, and 12% were associated with giving an IV infusion.

Occupational exposures to HIV should be considered as a medical emergency to ensure timely postexposure management and administration of postexposure antiretroviral prophylaxis (PEP). Recommendations regarding PEP must take into account that a variety of circumstances determine the risk of transmission of HIV following occupational exposure. In this regard, several factors have been associated with an increased risk for occupational transmission of HIV infection, including deep injury, the presence of visible blood on the instrument causing the exposure, injury with a device that had been placed in the vein or artery of the source patient, and advanced

HIV disease in the source patient. Other important considerations when considering PEP in the health care worker include known or suspected pregnancy or breast-feeding, the possibility of exposure to drug-resistant virus, and the toxicities of different PEP regimens. Regardless of the decision to use PEP, the wound should be cleansed immediately and antiseptic applied. If a decision is made to offer PEP, U.S. Public Health Service guidelines recommend that PEP regimens contain three (or more) antiretroviral drugs administered for a 4-week duration for all occupational exposures to HIV. Detailed guidelines are available from the *Updated U.S. Public Health Service Guidelines for the Management of Occupational Exposures to HIV and Recommendations for Postexposure Prophylaxis* (CDC, 2015). The report emphasizes the importance of adherence to PEP when it is indicated, and close follow-up of exposed workers should be provided including counseling, baseline and follow-up HIV testing, and monitoring for drug toxicity. Follow-up appointments should begin within 72 h of an HIV exposure and may be concluded 4 months after exposure. For consultation on the treatment of occupational exposures to HIV and other bloodborne pathogens, the clinician managing the exposed patient can call the National Clinicians' Post-Exposure Prophylaxis Hotline (PEPline) at 888-448-4911. This service is available 24 hours a day at no charge. (Additional information on the Internet is available at *www.nccc.ucsf.edu*.) PEPline support may be especially useful in challenging situations, such as when drug-resistant HIV strains are suspected or if the health care worker is pregnant.

Health care workers can minimize their risk of occupational HIV infection by following the CDC guidelines of June 2015, which include adherence to universal precautions and assuming that blood and other body fluids from all patients are potentially infectious. Therefore, the following infection control precautions should be adhered to at all times: (1) routinely use barriers (such as gloves and/or goggles) when anticipating contact with blood or body fluids; (2) immediately wash hands and other skin surfaces after contact with blood or body fluids; and (3) carefully handle and dispose of sharp instruments during and after use. For further information contact the CDC at 800-CDC-INFO (232-4636) or see *www.cdc.gov/cdc-info/*. The risk of HBV infection following a needle-stick injury from a hepatitis antigen–positive patient is much higher than the risk of HIV infection (see "Transmission," above). There are multiple examples of needle-stick injuries where the patient was positive for both HBV and HIV and the health care worker became infected only with HBV. For these reasons, it is advisable, given the high prevalence of HBV infection in HIV-infected individuals, that all health care workers dealing with HIV-infected patients be immunized with the HBV vaccine.

TB is another infection common to HIV-infected patients that can be transmitted to the health care worker. For this reason, all health care workers should know their PPD status, have it checked yearly, and, where appropriate, receive 6 months of isoniazid treatment if their skin test converts to positive. In addition, all patients in whom a diagnosis of active pulmonary TB is being entertained should be placed immediately in respiratory isolation, pending results of the diagnostic evaluation. The emergence of drug-resistant organisms, including extensively drug-resistant TB strains, has made TB an increasingly important problem for health care workers. This is particularly true for the health care worker with preexisting HIV infection.

HIV PREVENTION

Many proven interventions, usually applied in combination, have a role in preventing the transmission of HIV (**Fig. 202-48**). Education, counseling, and behavior modification are the cornerstones of any HIV prevention strategy. A major problem in the United States and elsewhere is that many infections are passed on by those who do not know that they are infected. Of the ~1.2 million persons in the United States who are HIV-infected, it is estimated that ~13% do not know their HIV status and that a substantial proportion of all new infections are transmitted by those people. In this regard, the CDC has recommended that HIV testing become part of routine medical care and that all individuals between the ages of 13 and 64 years be tested at least one time. These individuals should be informed of the testing and be tested without the

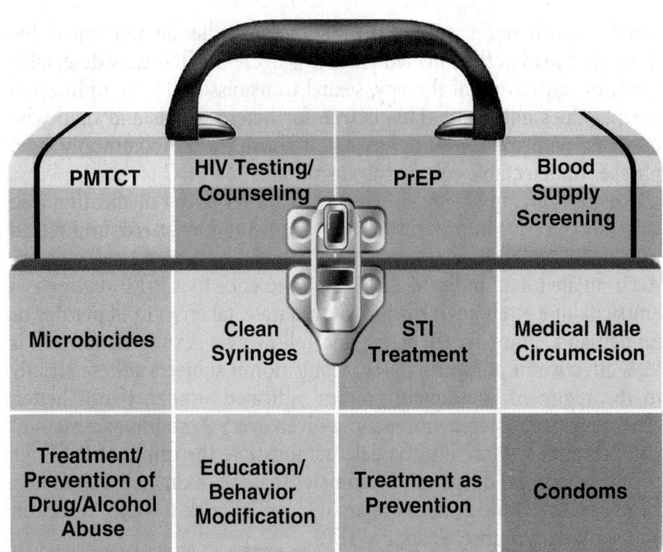

FIGURE 202-48 The HIV prevention "toolkit." See text for detailed description. PrEP, pre-exposure prophylaxis with antiretroviral drugs; PMTCT, prevention of mother-to-child transmission of HIV. *(From RW Eisinger et al Clin Infect Dis 69:2122, 2019.)*

need for written informed consent. Each individual can "opt out" of testing; however, testing should otherwise be routinely administered. Individuals who are practicing high-risk behavior should be tested more often and should use pre-exposure prophylaxis (PrEP) (see below). Partners engaged in monogamous sexual relationships who wish to be assured of safety should both be tested for HIV antibody. If both are negative, it must be understood that any divergence from monogamy puts both partners at risk; open discussion of the importance of honesty in such relationships should be encouraged.

When the HIV status of either partner is not known, or when one partner is positive, there are a number of options. *Use of condoms* can markedly decrease the chance of HIV transmission. It should be remembered that condoms are not 100% effective in preventing transmission of HIV infection, and there is a ~10% failure rate of condoms used for contraceptive purposes. Most condom failures result from breakage or improper usage, such as not wearing the condom for the entire period of intercourse. Latex condoms are preferable since virus has been shown to leak through natural skin condoms. Petroleum-based gels should never be used for lubrication of the condom, since they increase the likelihood of condom rupture.

Microbicides composed of gels or rings containing antiretroviral drugs have been shown to be variably efficacious in preventing acquisition of HIV infection in women engaging in vaginal intercourse. The considerable degree of variability in efficacy relates to the generally poor adherence of participants to the use of the intervention. One product, a vaginal ring that releases the antiretroviral drug dapivirine from the ring into the vagina slowly over 28 days, has been recommended by WHO as an additional prevention choice for women at substantial risk of HIV infection as part of combination prevention approaches.

Large, prospective clinical trials have clearly demonstrated that ART for people with HIV has an important role in HIV prevention. The initial results of the HPTN 052 clinical trial published in 2011 demonstrated a 96% reduction in HIV transmission risk among heterosexual HIV-discordant couples where the partner with HIV started ART immediately versus delayed ART initiation. The final results of HPTN 052, published in 2016, reported no HIV transmissions within these couples when the partner with HIV had a suppressed viral load (defined as having a viral load of <400 copies of HIV RNA per milliliter). Three subsequent studies reported similar results, with no genetically linked infections while the partner with HIV was virally suppressed even though couples were engaging in sex without a condom and not using PrEP. These three studies included >500 HIV-discordant heterosexual couples and >1100 HIV-discordant couples of men who have sex with men. Combined, these couples engaged in over 125,000 sex acts without a condom or PrEP over more than 2600 couple-years of observation. Collectively, the studies demonstrated that if the viral load of the infected partner is decreased to below detectable levels by antiretroviral therapy, sexual transmission to the uninfected partner does not occur. This is true for heterosexuals and men who have sex with men, leading, as noted above, to the commonly used phrase "undetectable equals untransmittable" or U=U.

Pre-exposure prophylaxis (PrEP) with antiretroviral medication also is highly effective in preventing HIV acquisition by at-risk uninfected men who have sex with men and heterosexual men and women. Accumulated data indicate that high adherence to a PrEP regimen of emtricitabine + tenofovir disoproxil fumarate, taken as 1 pill per day or on demand (immediately before and following a sexual encounter), is 99% effective in preventing HIV acquisition if subjects adhere strictly to the regimen. Subsequent studies indicated similar, if not better, efficacy with cabotegravir injections given every 2 months as a maintenance regimen. More limited data demonstrate the utility of PrEP for people who inject drugs. CDC estimates that approximately 1.2 million people in the United States are at "substantial" risk for HIV infection and should be counseled about PrEP.

Adult male circumcision, which has been shown to result in a 50–65% reduction in HIV acquisition in the circumcised subject, is currently being pursued, particularly in developing nations, as a component of HIV prevention (see above). The most effective way to prevent transmission of HIV infection among IDUs is to stop the use of injectable drugs. Unfortunately, that is extremely difficult to accomplish unless the individual enters a treatment program. For those who will not or cannot participate in a drug treatment program and who will continue to inject drugs, the avoidance of sharing of needles and other paraphernalia ("works") is the next best way to avoid transmission of infection. However, the cultural and social factors that contribute to the sharing of paraphernalia are complex and difficult to overcome. Under these circumstances, paraphernalia should be cleaned after each usage with a virucidal solution, such as undiluted sodium hypochlorite (household bleach). *Needle exchange programs* have been highly successful in decreasing HIV transmission among injection drug users without increasing the use of injection drugs. As noted, above, oral PrEP also is effective in preventing acquisition of HIV infections among IDUs. It is important for IDUs to be tested for HIV infection and counseled to avoid transmission to their sexual partners. Prevention of transmission through blood or blood products and prevention of mother-to-child transmission are discussed in "Transmission," above.

HIV VACCINES

There is currently no safe and effective vaccine approved for the prevention of HIV infection. Successful vaccines for other diseases are predicated on the assumptions that the body can mount an adequate immune response to the microbe or virus in question during natural infection and that the vaccine will mimic the natural response to infection. Even with serious diseases, such as smallpox, poliomyelitis, measles, and influenza among others, the body in the vast majority of cases clears the infectious agent and provides protection, which is usually life-long against future exposure against the same pathogen. Unfortunately, this is not the case with HIV infection since the natural immune response to HIV infection is unable to clear the virus from the body and cases of superinfection are not rare.

Some of the factors that contribute to the problematic nature of developing a preventive HIV vaccine are (1) the high mutability of the virus; (2) the fact that the infection can be transmitted by cell-free or cell-associated virus; (3) the fact that the HIV provirus integrates itself into the genome of the target cell and may remain in a latent form unexposed to the immune system; (4) the likely need for the development of effective mucosal immunity; and, importantly, (5) the difficulty that the immune system has in readily mounting broadly neutralizing antibodies in response to natural infection with HIV (see below).

Early attempts to develop a vaccine with the envelope protein gp120 aimed at inducing neutralizing antibodies in humans were unsuccessful; the elicited antisera failed to neutralize primary isolates of HIV. In this regard, two phase 3 trials were undertaken in the United States and Thailand using soluble gp120, and the vaccines failed to protect human volunteers from HIV infection. In addition, two separate vaccine trials aimed at eliciting CD8+ T-cell responses to prevent infection and, if unsuccessful in preventing infection, to control postinfection viremia, also failed at both goals. In 2009, a vaccine using a poxvirus vector prime expressing various viral proteins followed by an envelope protein boost was tested in a 16,000-person clinical trial (RV144) conducted in Thailand among predominantly low-HIV-prevalence heterosexuals. The vaccine provided the first positive, albeit very modest, signal ever reported in an HIV vaccine trial, showing 31% protection against acquisition of infection. Such a result is certainly not sufficient justification for clinical use of the vaccine; however, it served as an important first step in the direction of the development of a safe and effective vaccine against HIV infection.

Follow-up studies of RV144 indicate that nonneutralizing or weakly neutralizing antibody responses against certain constant epitopes in the otherwise highly variable V1–V2 region of the HIV envelope may be associated with the modest degree of protection observed in that clinical trial. Additional similar studies were undertaken in high-HIV-prevalence countries in sub-Saharan Africa as well as in the Americas and certain European countries in attempts to improve on the results of RV144 by a variety of approaches, including increasing the number of vaccine boosts with envelope protein, the use of mosaic antigens, and the addition of adjuvant. Unfortunately, two recent phase 3 studies of candidate vaccines failed to show efficacy. A third phase 3 trial is underway in the Americas and Europe with results expected in 2024.

An area of HIV vaccine research that is currently being actively pursued is the attempt to induce broadly neutralizing antibodies by developing as immunogens for vaccination certain epitopes on the HIV envelope that are the targets of naturally occurring broadly neutralizing antibodies during HIV infection (Fig. 202-30). It is curious that only about 20% of HIV-infected individuals develop broadly neutralizing antibodies in response to natural infection and they do so only after 2–3 years of ongoing infection. By the time these antibodies appear, they can neutralize a broad range of primary HIV isolates, but they appear to be ineffective against the autologous virus in the infected subject. Upon close examination, these broadly neutralizing antibodies manifest a high degree of somatic mutations that were accumulated over time and are responsible for their affinity maturation and broadly neutralizing capacity. The goal of current efforts is to develop the conformationally correct HIV envelope epitopes that, when used as immunogens, would direct the immune response of an uninfected individual to the production of broadly neutralizing antibodies over a reasonable time frame by sequential immunizations. It remains to be seen whether this approach will be feasible.

FURTHER READING

Bekker LG et al: The complex challenges of HIV vaccine development require renewed and expanded global commitment. Lancet 395:384, 2020.

Centers for Disease Control and Prevention (CDC): HIV risk and prevention. Available at *www.cdc.gov/hiv/risk/*.

Centers for Disease Control and Prevention (CDC): HIV prevention in the United States: Mobilizing to end the epidemic. Available at *www.cdc.gov/hiv/pdf/policies/cdc-hiv-prevention-bluebook.pdf*.

Cohn LB et al: Biology of the HIV-1 latent reservoir and implications for cure strategies. Cell Host Microbe 27:519, 2020.

Collins DR et al: CD8+ T cells in HIV control, cure and prevention. Nat Rev Immunol 20:471, 2020.

Eisinger RW et al: Ending the human immunodeficiency virus pandemic: Optimizing the prevention and treatment toolkits. Clin Infect Dis 69:2212, 2019.

Eisinger RW et al: HIV viral load and transmissibility of HIV infection: Undetectable equals untransmittable. JAMA 321:451, 2019.

Elliott T et al: Challenges of HIV diagnosis and management in the context of pre-exposure prophylaxis (PrEP), post-exposure prophylaxis (PEP), test and start and acute HIV infection: A scoping review. J Int AIDS Soc 22:e25419, 2019.

Fauci AS, Lane HC: Four decades of HIV/AIDS—much accomplished, much to do. N Engl J Med 383:1, 2020.

Haynes BF et al: Multiple roles for HIV broadly neutralizing antibodies. Sci Transl Med 11:eaaz2686, 2019.
Kazer SW: Evolution and diversity of immune responses during acute HIV Infection. Immunity 53:908, 2020.
Moir S, Fauci AS: B-cell responses to HIV infection. Immunol Rev 275:33, 2017.
Panel on Opportunistic Infections in Adults and Adolescents with HIV: Guidelines for the Prevention and Treatment of Opportunistic Infections in Adults and Adolescents with HIV. Available at *clinicalinfo.hiv.gov/en/guidelines/adult-and-adolescent-opportunistic-infection/whats-new-guidelines.*
Saez-Cirion A, Sereti I: Immunometabolism and HIV-1 pathogenesis: Food for thought. Nat Rev Immunol 21:5, 2021.
Thompson ME et al: Primary care guidance for persons with human immunodeficiency virus: 2020 update by the HIV Medicine Association of the Infectious Diseases Society of America. Clin Infect Dis Nov 6, 2020 [Epub ahead of print].
UN Joint Programme On HIV/AIDS (UNAIDS): 2021 UNAIDS Global AIDS Update – Confronting inequalities – Lessons for pandemic responses from 40 years of AIDS. Available at *https://www.unaids.org/en/resources/documents/2021/2021-global-aids-update.*
U.S. Department of Health and Human Services Panel on Antiretroviral Guidelines for Adults and Adolescents: Guidelines for the use of antiretroviral agents in adults and adolescents living with HIV. Available at *clinicalinfo.hiv.gov/en/guidelines/adult-and-adolescent-arv/whats-new-guidelines.*

Section 15 Infections Due to RNA Viruses

203 Viral Gastroenteritis

Umesh D. Parashar, Roger I. Glass

Acute infectious gastroenteritis is a common illness that affects persons of all ages worldwide. It is a leading cause of death among children in developing countries, accounting for an estimated 0.5 million deaths each year, and is responsible for up to 6–8% of all hospitalizations among children in industrialized countries, including the United States. Elderly persons, especially those with debilitating health conditions, also are at risk of severe complications and death from acute gastroenteritis. Among healthy young adults, acute gastroenteritis is rarely fatal but incurs substantial medical and social costs, including those of time lost from work.

Several enteric viruses have been recognized as important etiologic agents of acute infectious gastroenteritis (**Table 203-1, Fig. 203-1**). Although most viral gastroenteritis is caused by RNA viruses, the DNA viruses that are occasionally involved (e.g., adenovirus types 40 and 41) are included in this chapter. Illness caused by these viruses is characterized by the acute onset of vomiting and/or diarrhea, which may be accompanied by fever, nausea, abdominal cramps, anorexia, and malaise. As shown in **Table 203-2**, several features can help distinguish gastroenteritis caused by viruses from that caused by bacterial agents. However, the distinction based on clinical and epidemiologic parameters alone is often difficult, and laboratory tests are required to confirm the diagnosis.

HUMAN CALICIVIRUSES

Etiologic Agent The Norwalk virus is the prototype strain of a group of small (27–40 nm), nonenveloped, round, icosahedral viruses with relatively amorphous surface features on visualization by electron microscopy. Molecular cloning and characterization have demonstrated that the viruses have a single, positive-strand RNA genome ~7.5 kb in length and possess a single virion-associated protein—similar to that of typical caliciviruses—with a molecular mass of 60 kDa. On the basis of these molecular characteristics, these viruses are presently classified into two genera belonging to the family Caliciviridae, the *noroviruses* and the *sapoviruses* (previously called Norwalk-like viruses and Sapporo-like viruses, respectively), which are further classified into genogroups and genotypes. Of the 10 recognized norovirus genogroups in humans and animals, 35 different genotypes belonging to 5 genogroups (GI, GII, GIV, GVIII, and GIX) are known to infect humans.

Epidemiology Infections with the Norwalk and related human caliciviruses are common worldwide, and most adults have antibodies to these viruses. Antibody is acquired at an earlier age in developing countries—a pattern consistent with the presumed fecal–oral mode of transmission. Infections occur year-round, although, in temperate climates, a distinct increase has been noted in cold-weather months. Noroviruses may be the most common infectious agents of mild gastroenteritis in the community and affect all age groups, whereas sapoviruses primarily cause gastroenteritis in children. Noroviruses also cause traveler's diarrhea, and outbreaks have occurred among military personnel deployed to various parts of the world. The limited data available indicate that norovirus may be the second most common viral agent (after rotavirus) among young children and the most common agent among older children and adults. In the United States and some other developed countries, with the decline in severe rotavirus disease following implementation of a rotavirus vaccination program, norovirus has become the leading cause of medically attended gastroenteritis in young children. Noroviruses are also recognized as the major cause of epidemics of gastroenteritis worldwide. In the United States, ~50% of all reported outbreaks of gastroenteritis are caused by noroviruses.

Norovirus is transmitted predominantly by the fecal–oral route but is also present in vomitus. Because an inoculum with very few viruses can be infectious, transmission can occur by aerosolization, by contact with contaminated fomites, and by person-to-person contact. Viral shedding and infectivity are greatest during the acute illness, but challenge studies with Norwalk virus in volunteers indicate that viral antigen may be shed by asymptomatically infected persons and also by symptomatic persons before the onset of symptoms and for several weeks after the resolution of illness. Viral shedding can be prolonged in immunocompromised individuals.

Pathogenesis The exact sites and cellular receptors for attachment of viral particles have not been determined. Data suggest that

TABLE 203-1 Viral Causes of Gastroenteritis Among Humans

VIRUS	FAMILY	GENOME	PRIMARY AGE GROUP AT RISK	CLINICAL SEVERITY	DETECTION ASSAYS
Group A rotavirus	Reoviridae	Double-strand segmented RNA	Children <5 years	+ + +	EM, EIA (commercial), PAGE, RT-PCR
Norovirus	Caliciviridae	Positive-sense single-strand RNA	All ages	+ +	EM, RT-PCR
Sapovirus	Caliciviridae	Positive-sense single-strand RNA	Children <5 years	+	EM, RT-PCR
Astrovirus	Astroviridae	Positive-sense single-strand RNA	Children <5 years	+	EM, EIA, RT-PCR
Adenovirus (mainly types 40 and 41)	Adenoviridae	Double-strand DNA	Children <5 years	+/+ +	EM, EIA (commercial), PCR

Abbreviations: EIA, enzyme immunoassay; EM, electron microscopy; PAGE, polyacrylamide gel electrophoresis; PCR, polymerase chain reaction; RT-PCR, reverse-transcription PCR.

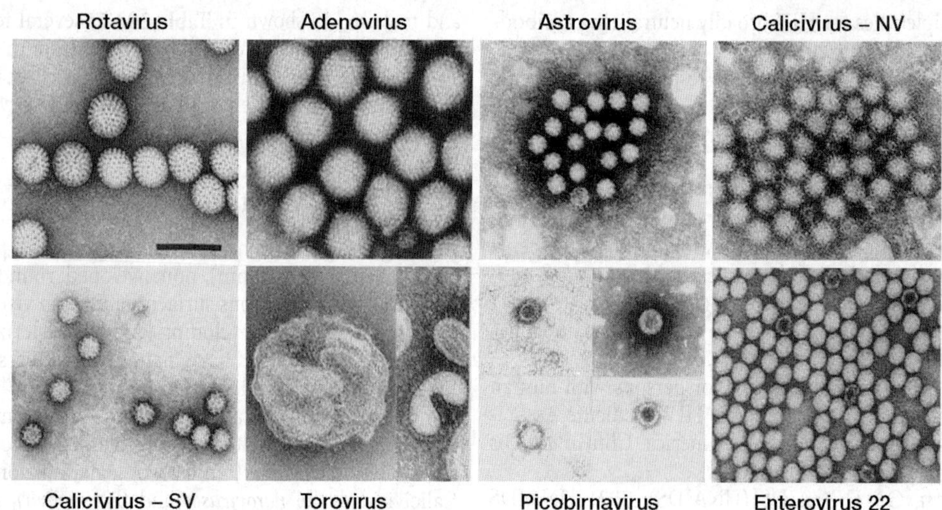

FIGURE 203-1 Viral agents of gastroenteritis. NV, norovirus; SV, sapovirus.

carbohydrates that are similar to human histo-blood group antigens (HBGA) and are present on the gastroduodenal epithelium of individuals with the secretor phenotype may serve as ligands for the attachment of Norwalk virus. Additional studies must more fully elucidate norovirus–carbohydrate interactions, including strain-specific variations. After the infection of volunteers, reversible lesions are noted in the upper jejunum, with broadening and blunting of the villi, shortening of the microvilli, vacuolization of the lining epithelium, crypt hyperplasia, and infiltration of the lamina propria by polymorphonuclear neutrophils and lymphocytes. The lesions persist for at least 4 days after the resolution of symptoms and are associated with malabsorption of carbohydrates and fats and a decreased level of brush-border enzymes. Adenylate cyclase activity is not altered. No histopathologic changes are seen in the stomach or colon, but gastric motor function is delayed, and this alteration is believed to contribute to the nausea and vomiting that are typical of this illness.

Clinical Manifestations Gastroenteritis caused by Norwalk and related human caliciviruses has a sudden onset following an average incubation period of 24 h (range, 12–72 h). The illness generally lasts 12–60 h and is characterized by one or more of the following symptoms: nausea, vomiting, abdominal cramps, and diarrhea. Vomiting is more prevalent among children, whereas a greater proportion of adults develop diarrhea. Constitutional symptoms are common, including headache, fever, chills, and myalgias. The stools are characteristically loose and watery, without blood, mucus, or leukocytes. White cell counts are generally normal; rarely, leukocytosis with relative lymphopenia may be observed. Death is a rare outcome and usually results from severe dehydration in vulnerable persons (e.g., elderly patients with debilitating health conditions).

Immunity Approximately 50% of persons challenged with Norwalk virus become ill and acquire short-term immunity against the infecting strain. In early human volunteer studies, immunity to Norwalk virus appeared to correlate inversely with level of antibody; i.e., persons with higher levels of preexisting antibody to Norwalk virus were more susceptible to illness on rechallenge. This paradoxical observation was later explained by data indicating that some individuals have a genetic

TABLE 203-2 Characteristics of Gastroenteritis Caused by Viral and Bacterial Agents

FEATURE	VIRAL GASTROENTERITIS	BACTERIAL GASTROENTERITIS
Setting	Incidence similar in developing and developed countries	More common in settings with poor hygiene and sanitation
Infectious dose	Low (10–100 viral particles) for most agents	High (>10^5 bacteria) for *Escherichia coli, Salmonella, Vibrio;* medium (10^2–10^5 bacteria) for *Campylobacter jejuni;* low (10–100 bacteria) for *Shigella*
Seasonality	In temperate climates, winter seasonality for most agents; year-round occurrence in tropical areas	More common in summer or rainy months, particularly in developing countries with a high disease burden
Incubation period	1–3 days for most agents; can be shorter for norovirus	1–7 days for common agents (e.g., *Campylobacter, E. coli, Shigella, Salmonella);* a few hours for bacteria producing preformed toxins (e.g., *Staphylococcus aureus, Bacillus cereus*)
Reservoir	Primarily humans	Depending on bacterial species, human (e.g., *Shigella, Salmonella*), animal (e.g., *Campylobacter, Salmonella, E. coli*), and water (e.g., *Vibrio*) reservoirs exist
Fever	Common with rotavirus and norovirus; uncommon with other agents	Common with agents causing inflammatory diarrhea (e.g., *Salmonella, Shigella*)
Vomiting	Prominent and can be the only presenting feature, especially in children	Common with bacteria producing preformed toxins; less prominent in diarrhea due to other agents
Diarrhea	Common; non-bloody in almost all cases	Prominent and occasionally bloody with agents causing inflammatory diarrhea
Duration	1–3 days for norovirus and sapovirus; 2–8 days for other viruses	1–2 days for bacteria producing preformed toxins; 2–8 days for most other bacteria
Diagnosis	This is often a diagnosis of exclusion in clinical practice. Commercial enzyme immunoassays are available for detection of rotavirus and adenovirus, but identification of other agents is limited to research and public health laboratories.	Fecal examination for leukocytes and blood is helpful in differential diagnosis. Culture of stool specimens, sometimes on special media, can identify several pathogens. Molecular techniques are useful epidemiologic tools but are not routinely used in most laboratories.
Treatment	Supportive therapy to maintain adequate hydration and nutrition should be given. Antibiotics and antimotility agents are contraindicated.	Supportive hydration therapy is adequate for most patients. Antibiotics are recommended for patients with dysentery caused by *Shigella* or diarrhea caused by *Vibrio cholerae* and for some patients with *Clostridium difficile* colitis.

predisposition to illness, with specific HBGA phenotypes influencing susceptibility to norovirus infection. Contemporary data show that functional antibodies that block norovirus binding to HBGAs correlate with protective immunity in human volunteer challenge and vaccination studies. Furthermore, initial studies have demonstrated that norovirus grown in vitro in the newly developed human intestinal enteroid (HIE) cell-based system can be neutralized by sera containing blocking antibodies.

Diagnosis Cloning and sequencing of the genomes of Norwalk and several other human caliciviruses have allowed the development of assays based on polymerase chain reaction (PCR) for detection of virus in stool and vomitus. Virus-like particles (VLPs) produced by expression of capsid proteins in a recombinant baculovirus vector have been used to develop enzyme immunoassays (EIAs) for detection of virus in stool or a serologic response to a specific viral antigen. These newer diagnostic techniques are considerably more sensitive than previous detection methods, such as electron microscopy, immune electron microscopy, and EIAs based on reagents derived from humans. However, given that these single-stranded RNA viruses show great antigenic and genetic diversity, no currently available single assay can detect all human caliciviruses. In addition, the assays are still cumbersome and are available primarily in research laboratories, although they are increasingly being adopted by public health laboratories for routine screening of fecal specimens from patients affected by outbreaks of gastroenteritis. Commercial EIA kits have limited sensitivity and usefulness in clinical practice and are of greatest utility in outbreaks, in which many specimens are tested and only a few need be positive to identify norovirus as the cause.

TREATMENT

Infections with Norwalk and Related Human Caliciviruses

The disease is self-limited, and oral rehydration therapy is generally adequate. If severe dehydration develops, IV fluid therapy is indicated. No specific antiviral therapy is available.

Prevention Epidemic prevention relies on situation-specific measures, such as control of contamination of food and water, exclusion of ill food handlers, and reduction of person-to-person spread through good personal hygiene and disinfection of contaminated fomites. The role of immunoprophylaxis is not clear, given the lack of long-term immunity from natural disease, but efforts to develop norovirus vaccines are ongoing. Vaccines based on VLPs are being tested in human volunteers. In a proof-of-concept trial, the efficacy of a monovalent GI.1 VLP vaccine was 47% among volunteers who received the vaccine intranasally and were then challenged with a homologous strain. In a second trial, norovirus disease severity was reduced in volunteers who received a bivalent G1.1/GII.4 VLP vaccine intramuscularly (with the GII.4 component including a consensus sequence from three different GII.4 strains) and were subsequently challenged with a GII.4 norovirus strain. Data from the first field efficacy study of this bivalent vaccine conducted in ~4700 healthy U.S. Navy recruits given one intramuscular injection of the bivalent vaccine were recently reported. While the primary endpoint of protection against homotypic infection could not be evaluated because only six total moderate/severe cases due to GI.1 or GII.4 norovirus strains occurred during the trial, the vaccine efficacy was 61.8% (95.01% confidence interval, 20.8–81.6%) for moderate/severe norovirus acute gastroenteritis due to any type. These initial data are encouraging; however, key issues to be further studied include the duration of protection and the level of heterotypic protection against antigenically distinct strains, particularly given the continuing and rapid natural evolution leading to the emergence of novel norovirus strains.

ROTAVIRUS

Etiologic Agent Rotaviruses are members of the family Reoviridae. The viral genome consists of 11 segments of double-strand RNA that is enclosed in a triple-layered, nonenveloped, icosahedral capsid 75 nm in diameter. Viral protein 6 (VP6), the major structural protein, is the target of commercial immunoassays and determines the group specificity of rotaviruses. Seven major groups of rotavirus (A through G) exist; human illness is caused primarily by group A and, to a much lesser extent, by groups B and C. Two outer-capsid proteins, VP7 (G-protein) and VP4 (P-protein), determine serotype specificity, induce neutralizing antibodies, and form the basis for binary classification of rotaviruses (G and P types). The segmented genome of rotavirus allows genetic reassortment (i.e., exchange of genome segments between viruses) during co-infection—a property that plays a role in viral evolution and that has been utilized in the development of reassortant animal/human rotavirus–based vaccines.

Epidemiology Worldwide, nearly all children are infected with rotavirus by 3–5 years of age. Neonatal infections are common but are often asymptomatic or mild, presumably because of protection by maternal antibody or breast milk. Compared with rotavirus disease in industrialized countries, disease in developing countries occurs at a younger age, is less seasonal, is more frequently caused by uncommon or multiple rotavirus strains, and is more often fatal. Moreover, because of suboptimal access to hydration therapy, rotavirus is a leading cause of diarrheal death among children in the developing world, with the highest mortality rates among children in sub-Saharan Africa and southern Asia (**Fig. 203-2**).

First infections after 3 months of age are likely to be symptomatic, and the incidence of disease peaks among children 4–23 months of age. Reinfections are common, but the severity of disease decreases with each repeat infection. Therefore, severe rotavirus infections are less common among older children and adults than among younger individuals. Nevertheless, rotavirus can cause illness in parents and caretakers of children with rotavirus diarrhea, immunocompromised persons, travelers, and elderly individuals and should be considered in the differential diagnosis of gastroenteritis among adults.

In tropical settings, rotavirus disease occurs year-round, with less pronounced seasonal peaks than in temperate settings, where rotavirus disease occurs predominantly during the cooler fall and winter months. Before the introduction of rotavirus vaccine in the United States, the rotavirus season each year began in the Southwest during the autumn and early winter (October through December) and migrated across the continent, peaking in the Northeast during late winter and spring (March through May). The reasons for this characteristic pattern are not clear but may be correlated with state-specific differences in birth rates, which could influence the rate of accumulation of susceptible infants after each rotavirus season. After the implementation of routine vaccination of U.S. infants against rotavirus in 2006, the characteristic prevaccine geotemporal pattern of U.S. rotavirus was dramatically altered, and these changes were accompanied by substantial declines in rotavirus detections by a national network of sentinel laboratories. In addition, a pattern of biennial increases in rotavirus activity has emerged during postvaccine seasons.

During episodes of rotavirus-associated diarrhea, virus is shed in large quantities in stool (10^7–10^{12}/g). Viral shedding detectable by EIA usually subsides within 1 week but may persist for >30 days in immunocompromised individuals; it may be detected for longer periods by sensitive molecular assays, such as PCR. The virus is transmitted predominantly through the fecal–oral route. Spread through respiratory secretions, person-to-person contact, or contaminated environmental surfaces has been postulated to explain the rapid acquisition of antibody in the first 3 years of life, regardless of sanitary conditions.

At least 10 different G serotypes of group A rotavirus have been identified in humans, but only 5 types (G1 through G4 and G9) are common. While human rotavirus strains that possess a high degree of genetic homology with animal strains have been identified, animal-to-human transmission appears to be uncommon.

Group B rotaviruses have been associated with several large epidemics of severe gastroenteritis among adults in China since 1982 and have also been identified in India. Group C rotaviruses have been associated with a small proportion of pediatric gastroenteritis cases in several countries worldwide.

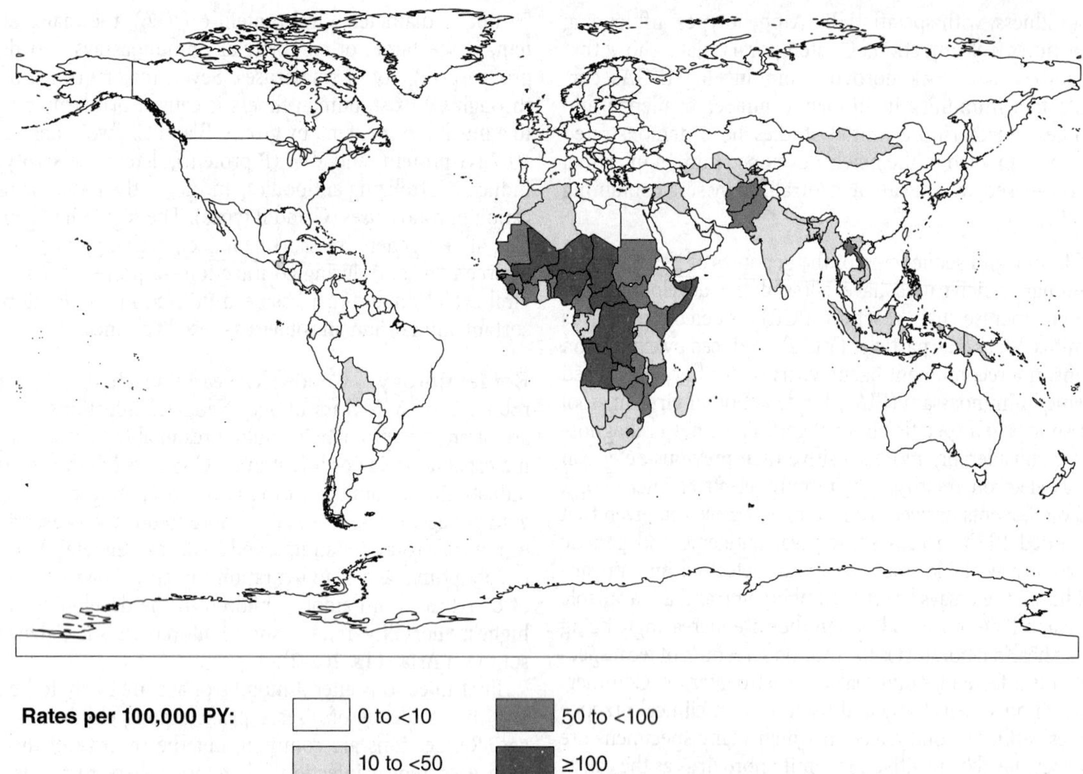

FIGURE 203-2 Rotavirus mortality rates by country, per 100,000 children <5 years of age. *(From JE Tate et al: Global, regional, and national estimates of rotavirus mortality in children <5 years of age, 2000-2013. Clin Infect Dis 62(Suppl 2):S96, 2016.)*

Pathogenesis Rotaviruses infect and ultimately destroy mature enterocytes in the villous epithelium of the proximal small intestine. The loss of absorptive villous epithelium, coupled with the proliferation of secretory crypt cells, results in secretory diarrhea. Brush-border enzymes characteristic of differentiated cells are reduced, and this change leads to the accumulation of unmetabolized disaccharides and consequent osmotic diarrhea. Studies in mice indicate that a nonstructural rotavirus protein, NSP4, functions as an enterotoxin and contributes to secretory diarrhea by altering epithelial cell function and permeability. In addition, rotavirus may evoke fluid secretion through activation of the enteric nervous system in the intestinal wall. Data indicate that rotavirus antigenemia and viremia are common among children with acute rotavirus infection, although the antigen and RNA levels in serum are substantially lower than those in stool.

Clinical Manifestations The clinical spectrum of rotavirus infection ranges from subclinical infection to severe gastroenteritis leading to life-threatening dehydration. After an incubation period of 1–3 days, the illness has an abrupt onset, with vomiting frequently preceding the onset of diarrhea. Up to one-third of patients may have a temperature of >39°C. The stools are characteristically loose and watery and only infrequently contain red or white cells. Gastrointestinal symptoms generally resolve in 3–7 days.

Respiratory and neurologic features in children with rotavirus infection have been reported, but causal associations have not been proven. Moreover, rotavirus infection has been associated with a variety of other clinical conditions (e.g., sudden infant death syndrome, necrotizing enterocolitis, intussusception, Kawasaki disease, and type 1 diabetes), but no causal relationship has been confirmed with any of these syndromes.

Rotavirus does not appear to be a major opportunistic pathogen in children with HIV infection. In severely immunodeficient children, rotavirus can cause protracted diarrhea with prolonged viral excretion and, in rare instances, can disseminate systemically. Persons who are immunosuppressed for bone marrow transplantation also are at risk for severe or even fatal rotavirus disease.

Immunity Protection against rotavirus disease is correlated with the presence of virus-specific secretory IgA antibodies in the intestine and, to some extent, the serum. Because virus-specific IgA production at the intestinal surface is short-lived, complete protection against disease is only temporary. However, each infection and subsequent reinfection confers progressively greater immunity; thus, severe disease is most common among young children with first or second infections. Immunologic memory is believed to be important in the attenuation of disease severity upon reinfection.

Diagnosis Illness caused by rotavirus is difficult to distinguish clinically from that caused by other enteric viruses. Because large quantities of virus are shed in feces, the diagnosis can usually be confirmed by a wide variety of commercially available EIAs or by techniques for detecting viral RNA, such as gel electrophoresis, probe hybridization, or PCR.

TREATMENT

Rotavirus Infections

Rotavirus gastroenteritis can lead to severe dehydration. Thus, appropriate treatment should be instituted early. Standard oral rehydration therapy is successful for most children who can take fluids by mouth, but IV fluid replacement may be required for patients who are severely dehydrated or are unable to tolerate oral therapy because of frequent vomiting. The therapeutic roles of probiotics, bismuth subsalicylate, enkephalinase inhibitors, and nitazoxanide have been evaluated in clinical studies but are not clearly defined. Antibiotics and antimotility agents should be avoided. In immunocompromised children with chronic symptomatic rotavirus disease, orally administered immunoglobulins or colostrum may result in the resolution of symptoms, but the best choices regarding agents and their doses have not been well studied, and treatment decisions are often empirical.

Prevention Efforts to develop rotavirus vaccines were pursued because it was apparent—given the similar rates in less developed and industrialized nations—that improvements in hygiene and sanitation were unlikely to reduce disease incidence. The first rotavirus vaccine

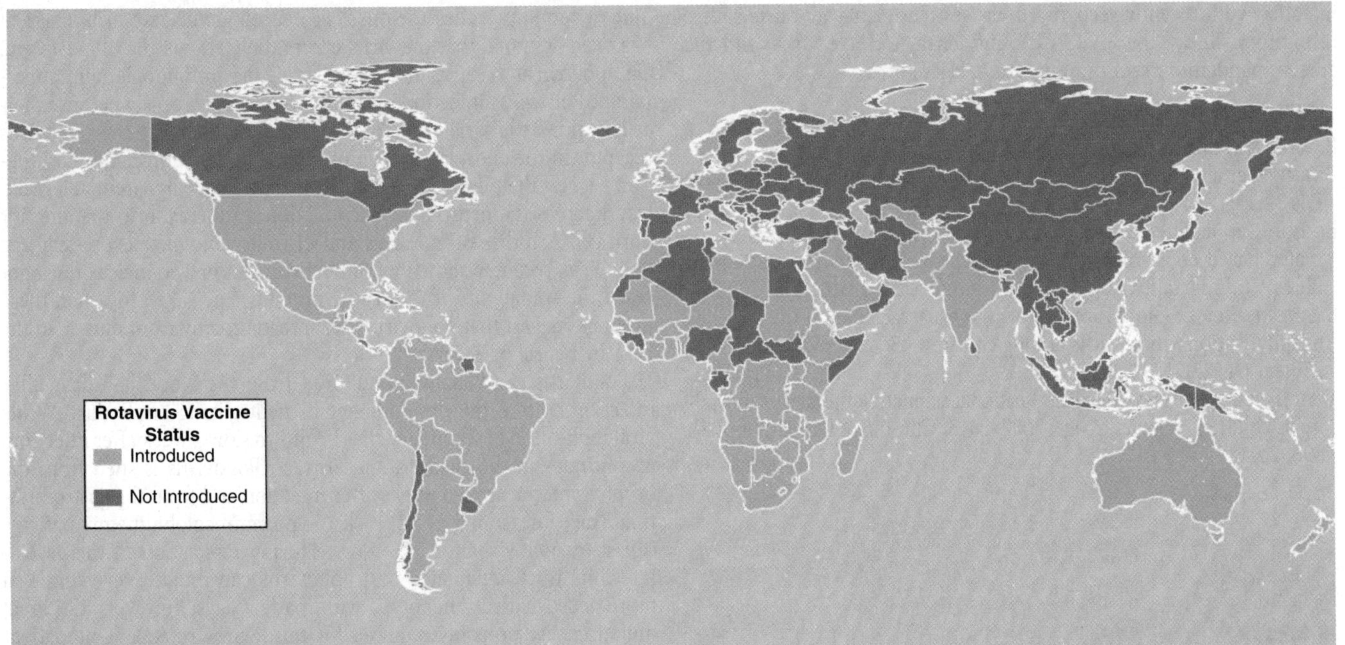

FIGURE 203-3 Countries that have implemented national rotavirus vaccination programs, December 31, 2019. *(Source: View-Hub, http://www.view-hub.org/viz/.)*

licensed in the United States in 1998 was withdrawn from the market within 1 year because it was linked with a low incidence of intussusception, a form of bowel obstruction.

In 2006, promising safety and efficacy (85–98% against severe rotavirus disease) data for two new rotavirus vaccines—RotaTeq (Merck, United States) and Rotarix (GlaxoSmithKline, Belgium)—were reported from large clinical trials conducted in North America, Europe, and Latin America. Both vaccines are now recommended for routine immunization of all U.S. infants, and their use has rapidly led to a >70–80% decline in rotavirus hospitalizations and emergency department visits at hospitals across the United States. Somewhat unexpectedly, rotavirus vaccination of young infants has also resulted in the added benefit of declines in rotavirus disease among children who miss vaccination and even among older children and adults who are not eligible for vaccination in some settings. The reason is likely to be a reduction in community transmission of rotavirus because of vaccination—i.e., herd protection. In April 2009, the World Health Organization (WHO) recommended the use of rotavirus vaccines in all countries worldwide. As of May 2020, nearly 100 countries, including several low-income countries in Africa and Asia, have incorporated rotavirus vaccine into their national childhood immunization programs (**Fig. 203-3**). Large declines in severe morbidity and mortality from childhood diarrhea have been documented in many countries. Postmarketing surveillance has identified a low risk of intussusception in some countries; however, the benefits of vaccination exceed the risks, and no changes in vaccine administration policy have been implemented.

The different epidemiology of rotavirus disease and the greater prevalence of co-infection with other enteric pathogens, of comorbidities, and of malnutrition in developing countries may adversely affect the performance of oral rotavirus vaccines, as is the case with oral vaccines against poliomyelitis, cholera, and typhoid in these regions. Therefore, evaluation of the efficacy of rotavirus vaccines in resource-poor settings of Africa and Asia was specifically recommended, and these trials have now been completed. As anticipated, the efficacy of rotavirus vaccines was moderate (50–65%) in these settings when compared with that in industrialized countries. Despite modest efficacy, routine use of rotavirus vaccines in low-income African countries with a heavy disease burden has yielded substantial public health benefits.

Several manufacturers in emerging markets, including India, China, Vietnam, Indonesia, and Brazil, are developing candidate rotavirus vaccines. Beginning in 2016, two Indian-made rotavirus vaccines—Rotavac (Bharat Biotech, India) and Rotasiil (Serum Institute, India)—were implemented in India's routine childhood immunization program, which has since expanded to all Indian states with a birth cohort of >25 million. In trials conducted in low-income countries, the efficacy of Rotavac and Rotasiil ranged from 36 to 66%, similar to the efficacy of multinational vaccines in these settings. In 2018, these two vaccines were prequalified by WHO, allowing their procurement with funding support from Gavi, the Vaccine Alliance, in low-income countries outside India.

OTHER VIRAL AGENTS OF GASTROENTERITIS

Enteric *adenoviruses* of serotypes 40 and 41 belonging to subgroup F are 70- to 80-nm viruses with double-strand DNA that cause ~2–12% of all diarrhea episodes in young children. Unlike adenoviruses that cause respiratory illness, enteric adenoviruses are difficult to cultivate in cell lines, but they can be detected with commercially available EIAs. Adenovirus types 31 and 42–49 have been linked to diarrhea in HIV-infected and other immunocompromised persons.

Astroviruses are 28- to 30-nm viruses with a characteristic icosahedral structure and a positive-sense, single-strand RNA. At least seven serotypes have been identified, of which serotype 1 is most common. Astroviruses are primarily pediatric pathogens, causing ~2–10% of cases of mild to moderate gastroenteritis in children. The availability of simple immunoassays to detect virus in fecal specimens and of molecular methods to confirm and characterize strains will permit more comprehensive assessment of the etiologic role of these agents.

Toroviruses are 100- to 140-nm, enveloped, positive-strand RNA viruses that are recognized as causes of gastroenteritis in horses (Berne virus) and cattle (Breda virus). Their role as a cause of diarrhea in humans is still unclear, but studies from Canada have demonstrated associations between torovirus excretion and both nosocomial gastroenteritis and necrotizing enterocolitis in neonates. These associations require further evaluation.

Picobirnaviruses are small, bisegmented, double-strand RNA viruses that cause gastroenteritis in a variety of animals. Their role as primary causes of gastroenteritis in humans remains unclear, but several studies have found an association between picobirnaviruses and gastroenteritis in HIV-infected adults.

Several other viruses (e.g., enteroviruses, reoviruses, pestiviruses, aichivirus, and parvovirus B) have been identified in the feces of patients with diarrhea, but their etiologic role in gastroenteritis has not been proven. Diarrhea has also been noted as a manifestation of infection with recently recognized viruses that primarily cause severe respiratory illness: the SARS-CoV, influenza A/H5N1 virus, and the current pandemic strain of influenza A/H1N1 virus.

FURTHER READING

Banyai K et al: Viral Gastroenteritis. Lancet 392:175, 2018.

Burke R et al: Current and new rotavirus vaccines. Curr Opin Infect Dis 32:435, 2019.

Burke R et al: The burden of norovirus in the United States, as estimated based on administrative data: Updates for medically attended illness and mortality, 2001–2015. Clin Infect Dis 14:ciaa438, 2020.

Burnett E et al: Global impact of rotavirus vaccination on diarrhea hospitalizations and deaths among children <5 years old: 2006-2019. J Infect Dis 222:1731, 2020.

Tate JE et al: Global, regional, and national estimates of rotavirus mortality in children <5 years of age, 2000–2013. Clin Infect Dis 62(Suppl 2): S96, 2016.

204 Enterovirus, Parechovirus, and Reovirus Infections

Jeffrey I. Cohen

ENTEROVIRUSES

CLASSIFICATION AND CHARACTERIZATION

Enteroviruses, members of the family Picornaviridae, are so designated because of their ability to multiply in the gastrointestinal tract. Despite their name, these viruses are not a prominent cause of gastroenteritis. Enteroviruses encompass more than 115 human serotypes: 3 serotypes of poliovirus, 23 serotypes of coxsackievirus A, 6 serotypes of coxsackievirus B, 29 serotypes of echovirus, enteroviruses 68–71, and multiple new enteroviruses (beginning with enterovirus 73) that have been identified by molecular techniques. Human enteroviruses have been reclassified into four species designated A–D. Echoviruses 22 and 23 have been reclassified as parechoviruses 1 and 2 on the basis of low nucleotide homology and differences in viral proteins. Enterovirus and parechovirus surveillance conducted in the United States by the Centers for Disease Control and Prevention (CDC) in 2014–2016 showed that the most common enteroviruses and parechoviruses were enterovirus D68 (55.9% of cases), followed in frequency by echovirus 30, coxsackievirus A6, echovirus 18, and coxsackievirus B3, which accounted for 75% of all isolates.

Human enteroviruses contain a single-stranded RNA genome surrounded by an icosahedral capsid comprising four viral proteins. These viruses have no lipid envelope and are stable in acidic environments, including the stomach. They are susceptible to chlorine-containing cleansers but resistant to inactivation by standard disinfectants (e.g., alcohol, detergents) and can persist for days at room temperature.

PATHOGENESIS AND IMMUNITY

Much of what is known about the pathogenesis of enteroviruses has been derived from studies of poliovirus infection. After ingestion, poliovirus is thought to infect epithelial cells in the mucosa of the gastrointestinal tract and then to spread to and replicate in the submucosal lymphoid tissue of the tonsils and Peyer's patches. The virus next spreads to the regional lymph nodes, a viremic phase ensues, and the virus replicates in organs of the reticuloendothelial system. In some cases, a second episode of viremia occurs and the virus replicates further in various tissues, sometimes causing symptomatic disease.

It is uncertain whether poliovirus reaches the central nervous system (CNS) during viremia or whether it also spreads via peripheral nerves. Since viremia precedes the onset of neurologic disease in humans, it has been assumed that the virus enters the CNS via the bloodstream. The poliovirus receptor is a member of the immunoglobulin superfamily. Poliovirus infection is limited to primates, largely because their cells express the viral receptor. Studies demonstrating the poliovirus receptor in the end-plate region of muscle at the neuromuscular junction suggest that, if the virus enters the muscle during viremia, it could travel across the neuromuscular junction up the axon to the anterior horn cells. Studies of monkeys and of transgenic mice expressing the poliovirus receptor show that, after IM injection, poliovirus does not reach the spinal cord if the sciatic nerve is cut. Taken together, these findings suggest that poliovirus can spread directly from muscle to the CNS by neural pathways.

Poliovirus can usually be cultured from the blood 3–5 days after infection, before the development of neutralizing antibodies. While viral replication at secondary sites begins to slow 1 week after infection, it continues in the gastrointestinal tract. Poliovirus is shed from the oropharynx for up to 3 weeks after infection and from the gastrointestinal tract for as long as 12 weeks; hypogammaglobulinemic patients can shed poliovirus for >20 years. During replication in the gastrointestinal tract, attenuated oral poliovirus can mutate, reverting to a more neurovirulent phenotype within a few days; however, additional mutations are probably required for full neurovirulence. One patient with hypogammaglobulinemia who had been infected 12 years earlier and was receiving IV immune globulin suddenly developed quadriplegia and respiratory muscle paralysis and died; analysis showed that the virus had reverted to a more wild-type sequence.

Humoral and secretory immunity in the gastrointestinal tract is important for the control of enterovirus infections. Enteroviruses induce specific IgM, which usually persists for <6 months, and specific IgG, which persists for life. Capsid protein VP1 is the predominant target of neutralizing antibody, which generally confers lifelong protection against subsequent disease caused by the same serotype but does not prevent infection or virus shedding. Enteroviruses also induce cellular immunity of uncertain significance. Patients with impaired cellular immunity are not known to develop unusually severe disease when infected with enteroviruses. In contrast, the severe infections in patients with agammaglobulinemia emphasize the importance of humoral immunity in controlling enterovirus infections. Disseminated enterovirus infections have occurred in hematopoietic cell transplant recipients. IgA antibodies are instrumental in reducing poliovirus replication in and shedding from the gastrointestinal tract. Breast milk contains IgA specific for enteroviruses and can protect humans from infection.

EPIDEMIOLOGY

Enteroviruses have a worldwide distribution. More than 50% of nonpoliovirus enterovirus infections and >90% of poliovirus infections are subclinical. When symptoms do develop, they are usually nonspecific and occur in conjunction with fever; only a minority of infections are associated with specific clinical syndromes. The incubation period for most enterovirus infections ranges from 2 to 14 days but usually is <1 week.

Enterovirus infection is more common in socioeconomically disadvantaged areas, especially in those where conditions are crowded and in tropical areas where hygiene is poor. Infection is most common among infants and young children; serious illness develops most often during the first few days of life and in older children and adults. In developing countries, where children are infected at an early age, poliovirus infection has less often been associated with paralysis; in countries with better hygiene, older children and adults are more likely to be seronegative, become infected, and develop paralysis. Passively acquired maternal antibody reduces the risk of symptomatic infection in neonates. Young children are the most frequent shedders of enteroviruses and are usually the index cases in family outbreaks. In temperate climates, enterovirus infections occur most often in the summer and fall; no seasonal pattern is apparent in the tropics.

Most enteroviruses are transmitted primarily by the fecal–oral or oral–oral route. Patients are most infectious shortly before and after the onset of symptomatic disease, when virus is present in the stool and throat. The ingestion of virus-contaminated food or water also can cause disease. Certain enteroviruses (such as enterovirus 70, which causes acute hemorrhagic conjunctivitis) can be transmitted by direct inoculation from the fingers to the eye. Airborne transmission is important for some viruses that cause respiratory tract disease, such as coxsackievirus A21. Enteroviruses can be transmitted across the placenta from mother to fetus, causing severe disease in the newborn. The transmission of enteroviruses through blood transfusions or insect bites has not been documented. Nosocomial spread of coxsackievirus and echovirus has taken place in hospital nurseries. Outbreaks of enteroviruses correlate with levels of preexisting immunity to specific serotypes and birth rates.

■ CLINICAL FEATURES

Poliovirus Infection Most infections with poliovirus are asymptomatic. After an incubation period of 3–6 days, ~5% of patients present with a minor illness (abortive poliomyelitis) manifested by fever, malaise, sore throat, anorexia, myalgias, and headache. This condition usually resolves in 3 days. About 1% of patients present with aseptic meningitis (nonparalytic poliomyelitis). Examination of cerebrospinal fluid (CSF) reveals lymphocytic pleocytosis, a normal glucose level, and a normal or slightly elevated protein level; CSF polymorphonuclear leukocytes may be present early. In some patients, especially children, malaise and fever precede the onset of aseptic meningitis.

PARALYTIC POLIOMYELITIS The least common presentation is that of paralytic disease. After one or several days, signs of aseptic meningitis are followed by severe back, neck, and muscle pain and by the rapid or gradual development of motor weakness. In some cases, the disease appears to be biphasic, with aseptic meningitis followed first by apparent recovery but then (1–2 days later) by the return of fever and the development of paralysis; this form is more common among children than among adults. Weakness is generally asymmetric, is proximal more than distal, and may involve the legs (most commonly); the arms; or the abdominal, thoracic, or bulbar muscles. Paralysis develops during the febrile phase of the illness and usually does not progress after defervescence. Urinary retention also may occur. Examination reveals weakness, fasciculations, decreased muscle tone, and reduced or absent reflexes in affected areas. Transient hyperreflexia sometimes precedes the loss of reflexes. Patients frequently report sensory symptoms, but objective sensory testing usually yields normal results. Bulbar paralysis may lead to dysphagia, difficulty in handling secretions, or dysphonia. Respiratory insufficiency due to aspiration, involvement of the respiratory center in the medulla, or paralysis of the phrenic or intercostal nerves may develop, and severe medullary involvement may lead to circulatory collapse. Most patients with paralysis recover some function weeks to months after infection. About two-thirds of patients have residual neurologic sequelae.

Paralytic disease is more common among older individuals, pregnant women, and persons exercising strenuously or undergoing trauma at the time of CNS symptoms. Tonsillectomy predisposes to bulbar poliomyelitis, and IM injections increase the risk of paralysis in the involved limb(s).

VACCINE-ASSOCIATED POLIOMYELITIS The risk of developing poliomyelitis after oral vaccination is estimated at 1 case per 2.5 million doses. The risk is ~2000 times higher among immunodeficient persons, especially persons with hypo- or agammaglobulinemia. Before 1997, an average of eight cases of vaccine-associated poliomyelitis occurred—in both vaccinees and their contacts—in the United States each year. With the change in recommendations first to a sequential regimen of inactivated poliovirus vaccine (IPV) and oral poliovirus vaccine (OPV) in 1997 and then to an all-IPV regimen in 2000, the number of cases of vaccine-associated polio declined. From 1997 to 1999, six such cases were reported in the United States; no cases have been reported since 1999.

POSTPOLIO SYNDROME The *postpolio syndrome* presents as new onset of weakness, fatigue, fasciculations, and pain with additional atrophy of the muscle group involved during the initial paralytic disease 20–40 years earlier. The syndrome is more common among women and with increasing time after acute disease. The onset is usually insidious, and weakness occasionally extends to muscles that were not involved during the initial illness. The prognosis is generally good; progression to further weakness is usually slow, with plateau periods of 1–10 years. The postpolio syndrome is thought to be due to progressive dysfunction and loss of motor neurons that compensated for the neurons lost during the original infection and not to persistent or reactivated poliovirus infection.

TABLE 204-1 Manifestations Commonly Associated with Enterovirus Serotypes

	SEROTYPE(S) OF INDICATED VIRUS	
MANIFESTATION	COXSACKIEVIRUS	ECHOVIRUS (E) AND ENTEROVIRUS (Ent)
Acute hemorrhagic conjunctivitis	A24	E70
Aseptic meningitis	A2, 4, 7, 9, 10; B1–5	E4, 6, 7, 9, 11, 13, 16, 18, 19, 30, 33; Ent70, 71
Encephalitis	A9; B1–5	E3, 4, 6, 7, 9, 11, 18, 25, 30; Ent71
Exanthem	A4, 5, 6, 9, 10, 16; B1, 3–5	E4–7, 9, 11, 16–19, 25, 30; Ent71
Generalized disease of the newborn	B1–5	E4–7, 9, 11, 14, 16, 18, 19
Hand-foot-and-mouth disease	A5–7, 9, 10, 16; B1, 2, 5	Ent71
Herpangina	A1–10, 16, 22; B1–5	E6, 9, 11, 16, 17, 25, 30; Ent71
Myocarditis, pericarditis	A4, 9, 16; B1–5	E6, 9, 11, 22
Paralysis	A4, 7, 9; B1–5	E2–4, 6, 7, 9, 11, 18, 30; EntD68, 70, 71
Pleurodynia	A1, 2, 4, 6, 9, 10, 16; B1–6	E1–3, 6, 7, 9, 11, 12, 14, 16, 19, 24, 25, 30
Pneumonia	A9, 16; B1–5	E6, 7, 9, 11, 12, 19, 20, 30; EntD68, 71

Other Enteroviruses An estimated 5–10 million cases of symptomatic disease due to enteroviruses other than poliovirus occur in the United States each year. Among neonates, enteroviruses are the most common cause of aseptic meningitis and nonspecific febrile illnesses. Certain clinical syndromes are more likely to be caused by certain serotypes (**Table 204-1**).

NONSPECIFIC FEBRILE ILLNESS (SUMMER GRIPPE) The most common clinical manifestation of enterovirus infection is a nonspecific febrile illness. After an incubation period of 3–6 days, patients present with an acute onset of fever, malaise, and headache. Occasional cases are associated with upper respiratory symptoms, and some cases include nausea and vomiting. Symptoms often last for 3–4 days, and most cases resolve in a week. While infections with other respiratory viruses occur more often from late fall to early spring, febrile illness due to enteroviruses frequently occurs in the summer and early fall.

GENERALIZED DISEASE OF THE NEWBORN Most serious enterovirus infections in infants develop during the first week of life, although severe disease can occur up to 3 months of age. Neonates often present with an illness resembling bacterial sepsis, with fever, irritability, and lethargy. Laboratory abnormalities include leukocytosis with a left shift, thrombocytopenia, elevated values in liver function tests, and CSF pleocytosis. The illness can be complicated by myocarditis and hypotension, fulminant hepatitis and disseminated intravascular coagulation, meningitis or meningoencephalitis, or pneumonia. It may be difficult to distinguish neonatal enterovirus infection from bacterial sepsis, although a history of a recent virus-like illness in the mother provides a clue.

ASEPTIC MENINGITIS AND ENCEPHALITIS In children and young adults, enteroviruses are the cause of up to 90% of cases of aseptic meningitis in which an etiologic agent can be identified. Patients with aseptic meningitis typically present with an acute onset of fever, chills, headache, photophobia, and pain on eye movement. Nausea and vomiting also are common. Examination reveals meningismus without localizing neurologic signs; drowsiness or irritability also may be apparent. In some cases, a febrile illness may be reported that remits but returns several days later in conjunction with signs of meningitis. Other systemic manifestations may provide clues to an enteroviral cause, including diarrhea, myalgias, rash, pleurodynia, myocarditis, and herpangina. Examination of the CSF invariably reveals pleocytosis; the CSF cell count shows a shift from neutrophil to lymphocyte predominance within 1 day of presentation, and the total cell count does not exceed 1000/μL. The CSF glucose level is usually normal (in contrast to the low CSF glucose level in mumps), with a normal or slightly elevated protein concentration. Partially treated bacterial meningitis may be particularly difficult to exclude in some instances. Enteroviral meningitis is more common in summer and fall in temperate climates, while viral meningitis of other etiologies is more common in winter and spring. Symptoms ordinarily resolve within a week, although CSF abnormalities can persist for several weeks. Enteroviral meningitis is often more severe in adults than in children. Neurologic sequelae are rare, and most patients have an excellent prognosis.

Enteroviral encephalitis is much less common than enteroviral aseptic meningitis. Occasional highly inflammatory cases of enteroviral meningitis may be complicated by a mild form of encephalitis that is recognized on the basis of progressive lethargy, disorientation, and sometimes seizures. Less commonly, severe primary encephalitis may develop. An estimated 10–35% of cases of viral encephalitis are due to enteroviruses. Immunocompetent patients generally have a good prognosis.

Patients with hypogammaglobulinemia, agammaglobulinemia, or severe combined immunodeficiency may develop chronic meningitis or encephalitis; about half of these patients have a dermatomyositis-like syndrome, with peripheral edema, rash, and myositis. They may also have chronic hepatitis. Patients may develop neurologic disease while receiving immunoglobulin replacement therapy. Echoviruses (especially echovirus 11) are the most common pathogens in this situation.

Paralytic disease due to enteroviruses other than poliovirus occurs sporadically and is usually less severe than poliomyelitis. Most cases are due to enterovirus 70 or 71 or to coxsackievirus A7 or A9. Guillain-Barré syndrome is also associated with enterovirus infection. While earlier studies suggested a link between enteroviruses and chronic fatigue syndrome, most recent studies have not demonstrated such an association.

ACUTE FLACCID MYELITIS Patients with acute flaccid myelitis present with fever or respiratory symptoms and progress within hours to a few days to flaccid paralysis in one or more limbs. The disease is much more frequent in children. Less commonly, the disease can affect cranial nerves and respiratory or bulbar muscles. Like polio and some other enteroviruses, the disease affects the anterior horn cells in the spinal cord; gray matter changes can be seen on MRI of the spinal cord. The CSF shows a lymphocytic pleocytosis and often a mildly elevated protein. Cases of acute flaccid myelitis have occurred in late summer or early fall since 2012. Several studies have shown antibodies to enteroviruses in the CSF; antibodies to enterovirus D68 are most frequently detected. While enterovirus D68 has been detected in respiratory, stool, and nasopharyngeal samples from patients with acute flaccid myelitis, the virus has been rarely detected in the CSF. Treatment is supportive, and most patients have persistent neurologic deficits.

PLEURODYNIA (BORNHOLM DISEASE) Patients with pleurodynia present with an acute onset of fever and spasms of pleuritic chest or upper abdominal pain. Chest pain is more common in adults, and abdominal pain is more common in children. Paroxysms of severe, knifelike pain usually last 15–30 min and are associated with diaphoresis and tachypnea. Fever peaks within an hour after the onset of paroxysms and subsides when pain resolves. The involved muscles are tender to palpation, and a pleural rub may be detected. The white blood cell count and chest x-ray results are usually normal. Most cases are due to coxsackievirus B and occur during epidemics. Symptoms resolve in a few days, and recurrences are rare. Treatment includes the administration of nonsteroidal anti-inflammatory agents or the application of heat to the affected muscles.

MYOCARDITIS AND PERICARDITIS Enteroviruses are estimated to cause up to one-third of cases of acute myocarditis. Coxsackievirus B and its RNA have been detected in pericardial fluid and myocardial tissue in some cases of acute myocarditis and pericarditis. Most cases of enteroviral myocarditis or pericarditis occur in newborns, adolescents, or young adults. More than two-thirds of patients are male. Patients often present with an upper respiratory tract infection that is followed by fever, chest pain, dyspnea, arrhythmias, and occasionally heart failure. A pericardial friction rub is documented in half of cases, and the electrocardiogram shows ST-segment elevations or ST- and T-wave abnormalities. Serum levels of myocardial enzymes are often elevated. Neonates commonly have severe disease, while older children and adults recover completely. Up to 10% of cases progress to chronic dilated cardiomyopathy. Chronic constrictive pericarditis also may be a sequela.

EXANTHEMS Enterovirus infection is the leading cause of exanthems in children in the summer and fall. While exanthems are associated with many enteroviruses, certain types have been linked to specific syndromes. Echoviruses 9 and 16 have frequently been associated with exanthem and fever. Rashes may be discrete or confluent, beginning on the face and spreading to the trunk and extremities. Echovirus 9 is the most common cause of a rubelliform (discrete) rash. Unlike the rash of rubella, the enteroviral rash occurs in the summer and is not associated with lymphadenopathy. Roseola-like rashes develop after defervescence, with macules and papules on the face and trunk. The Boston exanthem, caused by echovirus 16, is a roseola-like rash. A variety of other rashes have been associated with enteroviruses, including erythema multiforme **(see Fig. A1-24)** and vesicular, urticarial, petechial, bullous, or purpuric lesions. Enanthems also occur, including lesions that resemble the Koplik's spots seen with measles **(see Fig. A1-2)**.

HAND-FOOT-AND-MOUTH DISEASE (FIG. 204-1) After an incubation period of 4–6 days, patients with hand-foot-and-mouth disease present with fever, anorexia, and malaise; these manifestations are followed by the development of sore throat and vesicles **(see Fig. A1-22)** on the buccal mucosa and often on the tongue and then by the appearance of tender vesicular lesions on the dorsum of the hands, sometimes with involvement of the palms. The vesicles may form bullae and quickly ulcerate. About one-third of patients also have lesions on the palate, uvula, or tonsillar pillars, and one-third have a rash on the feet (including the soles) or on the buttocks. Generalized rashes also have been reported. The disease is highly infectious, with attack rates of close to 100% among young children. The lesions usually resolve in 1 week. Most cases are due to coxsackievirus A16 or enterovirus 71.

An epidemic of enterovirus 71 infection in Taiwan in 1998 resulted in thousands of cases of hand-foot-and-mouth disease or herpangina (see below). Severe complications included CNS disease, myocarditis, and pulmonary hemorrhage. About 90% of those who died were children ≤5 years old, and death was associated with pulmonary edema or pulmonary hemorrhage. CNS disease included aseptic meningitis, flaccid paralysis (similar to that seen in poliomyelitis), and rhombencephalitis with myoclonus and tremor or ataxia. The mean age of patients with CNS complications was 2.5 years, and MRI in cases with encephalitis usually showed brainstem lesions. Follow-up of children at 6 months showed persistent dysphagia, cranial nerve palsies, hypoventilation, limb weakness, and atrophy; at 3 years, persistent neurologic sequelae were documented, with delayed development and impaired cognitive function.

Yearly epidemics of enterovirus 71 infection have occurred in China since 2008, with thousands of cases and hundreds of deaths each year. Infections have been associated with fever, rash, brainstem encephalitis with myoclonic jerks, and limb trembling; some cases have progressed to seizures and coma. Lung findings include pulmonary edema and hemorrhage. While the level of creatine kinase MB is sometimes elevated, myocardial necrosis generally is not found.

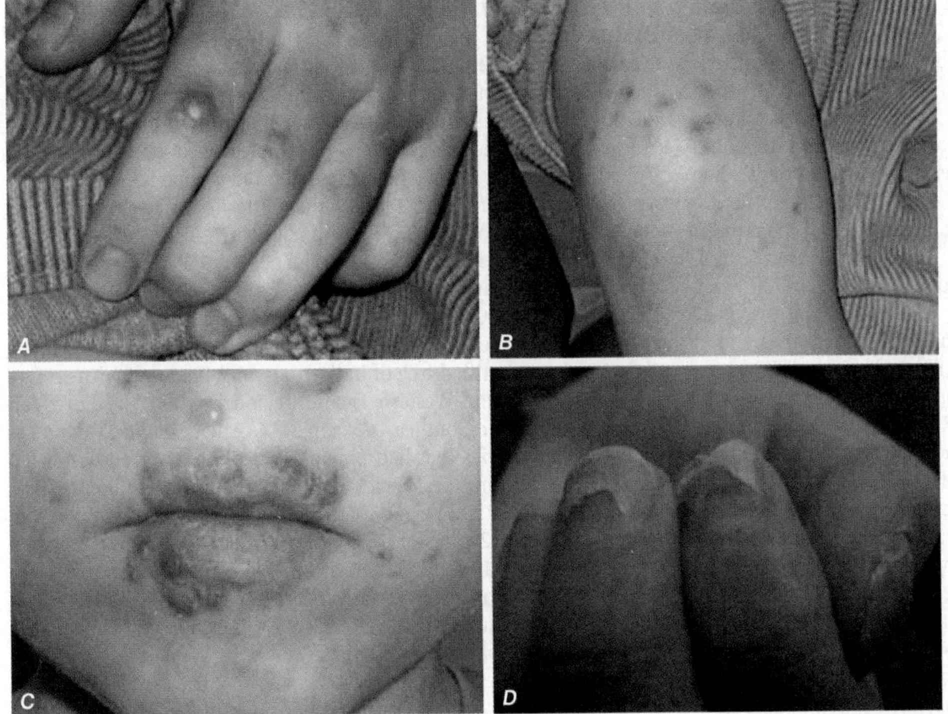

FIGURE 204-1 Vesicular eruptions of the hand (*A*), knee (*B*), and mouth (*C*) of a 6-year-old boy with coxsackievirus A6 infection. Several of his fingernails were shed 2 months later (***D***). *(Images reprinted courtesy of Centers for Disease Control and Prevention/Emerging Infectious Diseases.)*

Cyclic epidemics occur every 2–3 years in other Asian countries. However, the virus circulates at lower rates in the United States, Europe, and Africa. In the United States, hand-foot-and-mouth disease is most commonly associated with coxsackievirus A16. Between November 2011 and February 2012, outbreaks of hand-foot-and-mouth disease due to coxsackievirus A6 occurred in several U.S. states, and 19% of the affected persons were hospitalized.

HERPANGINA Herpangina is usually caused by coxsackievirus A and presents as acute-onset fever, sore throat, odynophagia, and grayish-white papulovesicular lesions on an erythematous base that ulcerate. The lesions can persist for weeks; are present on the soft palate, anterior pillars of the tonsils, and uvula; and are concentrated in the posterior portion of the mouth. In contrast to herpes stomatitis, enteroviral herpangina is not associated with gingivitis. Acute lymphonodular pharyngitis associated with coxsackievirus A10 presents as white or yellow nodules surrounded by erythema in the posterior oropharynx. The lesions do not ulcerate.

ACUTE HEMORRHAGIC CONJUNCTIVITIS Patients with acute hemorrhagic conjunctivitis present with an acute onset of severe eye pain, blurred vision, photophobia, and watery discharge from the eye. Examination reveals edema, chemosis, and subconjunctival hemorrhage and often shows punctate keratitis and conjunctival follicles as well (**Fig. 204-2**). Preauricular adenopathy is often found. Epidemics and nosocomial spread have been associated with enterovirus 70 and coxsackievirus A24. Outbreaks have been due to coxsackievirus A24 in China and India (2010), Japan (2011), and Thailand (2014). Systemic symptoms, including headache and fever, develop in 20% of cases, and recovery is usually complete in 10 days. The sudden onset and short duration of the illness help to distinguish acute hemorrhagic conjunctivitis from other ocular infections, such as those due to adenovirus and *Chlamydia trachomatis*. Paralysis has been associated with some cases of acute hemorrhagic conjunctivitis due to enterovirus 70 during epidemics.

OTHER MANIFESTATIONS Enteroviruses are an infrequent cause of childhood pneumonia and the common cold. From mid-August 2014 to January 2015, enterovirus D68 infection was confirmed in more than 1000 persons with mild to severe respiratory illnesses in 49 U.S. states. Nearly all reported cases were in children, many of whom had asthma. A prospective study of >300 children showed that prolonged shedding of enteroviruses in the stool was associated with development of islet cell autoantibodies and type 1 diabetes. Coxsackievirus B has been isolated at autopsy from the pancreas of a few children presenting with type 1 diabetes mellitus; however, most attempts to isolate the virus have been unsuccessful. Other diseases that have been associated with enterovirus infection include parotitis, bronchitis, bronchiolitis, croup, infectious lymphocytosis, polymyositis, acute arthritis, and acute nephritis.

DIAGNOSIS

Isolation of enterovirus in cell culture is the traditional diagnostic procedure. While cultures of stool, nasopharyngeal, or throat samples from patients with enterovirus diseases are often positive, isolation of the virus from these sites does not prove that it is directly associated with disease because these sites are frequently colonized for weeks in patients with subclinical infections. Isolation of virus from the throat is more likely to be associated with disease than is isolation from the stool since virus is shed for shorter periods from the throat. Cultures of CSF, serum, fluid from body cavities, or tissues are positive less frequently, but a positive result is indicative of disease caused by enterovirus. In some cases, the virus is isolated only from the blood or only from the CSF; therefore, it is important to culture multiple sites. Cultures are more likely to be positive earlier than later in the course of infection. Most human enteroviruses can be detected within a week after inoculation of cell cultures. Cultures may be negative because of the presence of neutralizing antibody, lack of susceptibility of the cells used, or inappropriate handling of the specimen. Coxsackievirus A may require inoculation into special cell-culture lines or into suckling mice.

Identification of the enterovirus serotype is useful primarily for epidemiologic studies and, with a few exceptions, has little clinical utility. It is important to identify serious infections with enterovirus during epidemics and to distinguish the vaccine strain of poliovirus from the other enteroviruses in the throat or in the feces. Stool and throat samples for culture as well as acute- and convalescent-phase serum specimens should be obtained from all patients with suspected

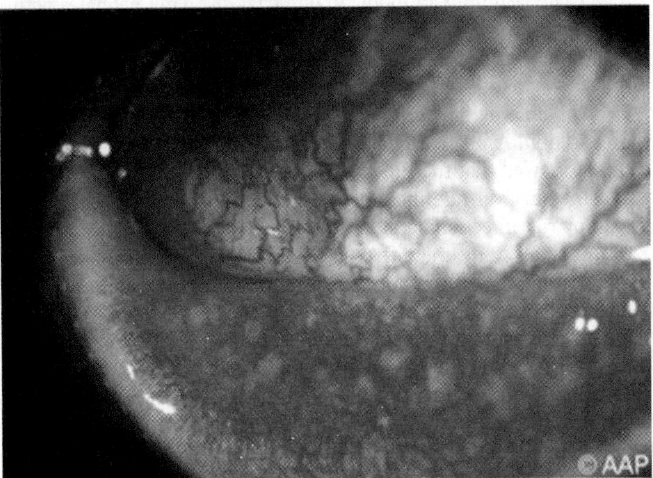

FIGURE 204-2 Acute hemorrhagic conjunctivitis due to enterovirus 70. *(Image reprinted courtesy of Jerri Ann Jenista, MD.)*

poliomyelitis. In the absence of a positive CSF culture, a positive culture of stool obtained within the first 2 weeks after the onset of symptoms is most often used to confirm the diagnosis of poliomyelitis. If poliovirus infection is suspected, two or more fecal and throat swab samples should be obtained at least 1 day apart and cultured for enterovirus as soon as possible. If poliovirus is isolated, it should be sent to the CDC for identification as either wild-type or vaccine virus.

Reverse-transcription polymerase chain reaction (PCR) has been used to amplify viral nucleic acid from CSF, serum, urine, stool, conjunctiva, throat swabs, and tissues. A pan-enterovirus PCR assay can detect all human enteroviruses. With the proper controls, PCR of the CSF is highly sensitive (70–100%) and specific (>80%) and is more rapid than culture. PCR of the CSF is less likely to be positive when patients present ≥3 days after the onset of meningitis or with enterovirus 71 infection; in these cases, PCR of throat or rectal swabs—although less specific than PCR of CSF—should be considered.

PCR of serum is also highly sensitive and specific in the diagnosis of disseminated disease. PCR may be particularly helpful for the diagnosis and follow-up of enterovirus disease in immunodeficient patients receiving immunoglobulin therapy, whose viral cultures may be negative. Antigen detection is less sensitive than PCR.

Serologic diagnosis of enterovirus infection is limited by the large number of serotypes and the lack of a common antigen. Demonstration of seroconversion may be useful in rare cases for confirmation of culture results, but serologic testing is usually limited to epidemiologic studies. Serum should be collected and frozen soon after the onset of disease and again ~4 weeks later. Measurement of neutralizing titers is the most accurate method for antibody determination; measurement of complement-fixation titers is usually less sensitive. Titers of virus-specific IgM are elevated in both acute and chronic infection.

TREATMENT

Enterovirus Infections

Most enterovirus infections are mild and resolve spontaneously; however, intensive supportive care may be needed for cardiac, hepatic, or CNS disease. IV, intrathecal, or intraventricular immunoglobulin has been used with apparent success in some cases for the treatment of chronic enterovirus meningoencephalitis and dermatomyositis in patients with hypogammaglobulinemia or agammaglobulinemia. The disease may stabilize or resolve during therapy; however, some patients decline inexorably despite therapy. IV immunoglobulin often prevents severe enterovirus disease in these patients. IV administration of immunoglobulin with high titers of antibody to the infecting virus has been used in some cases of life-threatening infection in neonates, who may not have maternally acquired antibody. In one trial involving neonates with enterovirus infections, immunoglobulin containing very high titers of antibody to the infecting virus reduced rates of viremia; however, the study was too small to show a substantial clinical benefit. The level of enteroviral antibodies varies with the immunoglobulin preparation. A phase 2 trial of pleconaril for neonatal enterovirus sepsis showed that the time to serum PCR negativity was reduced and the survival rate increased in newborns who had confirmed enterovirus infections and were treated with the drug, although in this small study, the differences did not reach significance; as of this writing, the drug is not available on a compassionate-use basis. Pocapavir and vapendavir are also being tested for enterovirus infections; resistance developed rapidly to OPV in a clinical trial of the drug. Glucocorticoids are contraindicated.

Good hand-washing practices and the use of gowns and gloves are important in limiting nosocomial transmission of enteroviruses during epidemics. Enteric precautions are indicated for 7 days after the onset of enterovirus infections. Inactivated enterovirus 71 vaccines have been licensed in China.

PREVENTION AND ERADICATION OF POLIOVIRUS

(See also Chap. 123) After a peak of 57,879 cases of poliomyelitis in the United States in 1952, the introduction of IPV in 1955 and of OPV in 1961 ultimately eradicated disease due to wild-type poliovirus in the Western Hemisphere. Such disease has not been documented in the United States since 1979, when cases occurred among religious groups who had declined immunization. In the Western Hemisphere, paralysis due to wild-type poliovirus was last documented in 1991.

In 1988, when ~350,000 cases of polio occurred in 125 countries, the World Health Organization adopted a resolution to eradicate poliomyelitis by the year 2000. Wild-type poliovirus type 2 and wild-type poliovirus type 3 were declared eradiated in 2015 and 2019, respectively. The Americas were certified free of indigenous wild-type poliovirus transmission in 1994, the Western Pacific Region in 2000, the European Region in 2002, and Southeast Asia in 2014. After a nadir of 496 cases in 2001, 21 countries that had previously been free of polio reported cases imported from 6 polio-endemic countries in 2002–2005. By 2006, polio transmission had been reduced in most of these 21 countries. In 2017, there were 22 cases of wild-type polio, the lowest ever reported for 1 year—all of these cases were from Pakistan and Afghanistan. In 2020, the number of cases of wild-type polio had risen to 140, all from the same two countries (**Table 204-2**). Polio is a source of concern for unimmunized or partially immunized travelers. While importation of poliovirus accounted for nearly 50% of cases in 2013 and also occurred in 2014, it has not been reported recently. Clearly, global eradication of polio is necessary to eliminate the risk of importation of wild-type virus. Outbreaks are thought to have been facilitated by suboptimal rates of vaccination, isolated pockets of unvaccinated children, poor sanitation and crowding, improper vaccine-storage conditions, and a reduced level of response to one of the serotypes in the vaccine. While the global eradication campaign has markedly reduced the number of cases of endemic polio, doubts have been raised as to whether eradication is a realistic goal, given the large number of asymptomatic infections and the political instability in developing countries.

Use of OPV, especially in areas with low vaccination rates, has been associated with vaccine-derived polio due to mutations that result in restoration of viral fitness and neurovirulence during prolonged replication in individuals or person-to-person transmission. Vaccine-derived polio was recognized in Egypt in 1983–1993, and hundreds of cases have been reported in many countries, including 385 cases in Nigeria in 2005–2012. Epidemics have been rapidly terminated after intensive vaccination with OPV. In 2005, a case of vaccine-derived polio occurred in an unvaccinated U.S. woman returning from a visit to

TABLE 204-2 Laboratory-Confirmed Cases of Poliomyelitis in 2020

COUNTRY	WILD-TYPE POLIO	VACCINE-DERIVED POLIO
Pakistan	84	135
Afghanistan	56	308
Chad	0	99
Democratic Republic of the Congo	0	81
Burkina Faso	0	65
Côte d'Ivoire	0	61
Sudan	0	58
Mali	0	51
South Sudan	0	50
Guinea	0	44
Ethiopia	0	36
Yemen	0	31
Somalia	0	14
Others	0	73[a]
Total	140	1106

[a]Others with <13 cases; Ghana, 12 cases; Sierra Leone, Niger 10 cases each; Togo, 9 cases; Nigeria, 8 cases; Cameroon, 7 cases; Central African Republic, 4 cases; Angola, Benin, 3 cases each; Madagascar, Congo, 2 cases each; Malaysia, Philippines, Tajikistan, 1 case each.

Central and South America. In the same year, an unvaccinated immunocompromised infant in Minnesota was found to be shedding vaccine-derived poliovirus; further investigation identified 4 of 22 infants in the same community who were shedding the virus. All 5 infants were asymptomatic. These outbreaks emphasize the need for maintaining high levels of vaccine coverage and continued surveillance for circulating virus. From 2010 to 2014, 60–70 cases of vaccine-derived polio were reported annually. In 2016, only 5 cases were reported (in Nigeria, Pakistan, and Laos). However, this number has been increasing each year, with 1106 cases of vaccine-derived polio in 2020 from 27 countries; about half of these cases were from the Eastern Mediterranean Region and half were from Africa (Table 204-2). From 2018 to March 2020, 92% of cases of vaccine-derived polio were due to type 2 virus. Cessation of vaccination with type 2 OPV is believed to be responsible for this increase in polio type 2. IPV is used in most industrialized countries and OPV in most developing countries, including those in which polio still is or recently was endemic. While IM injections of other vaccines (live or attenuated) can be given concurrently with OPV, unnecessary IM injections should be avoided during the first month after OPV vaccination because they increase the risk of vaccine-associated paralysis. Since 1988, an enhanced-potency inactivated poliovirus vaccine has been available in the United States.

After several doses of OPV alone, the seropositivity rate for individual poliovirus serotypes may still be suboptimal for children in developing countries; one or more supplemental doses of IPV can increase the rate of seropositivity for these serotypes. Against a given serotype, monovalent OPV containing only that serotype is more immunogenic than trivalent vaccine because of a lack of interference from other serotypes. Given the eradication of wild-type poliovirus type 2 and the establishment of OPV type 2 as the primary cause of vaccine-derived polio, bivalent OPV (types 1 and 3), which had been shown to be superior to trivalent OPV in inducing antibodies to types 1 and 3, replaced trivalent OPV vaccine in April 2016. However, outbreaks of vaccine-derived polio due to polio type 2 have required vaccination with monovalent OPV type 2. Two modified type 2 OPVs that are impaired for reversion to neurovirulence were safe and immunogenic in phase 2 clinical trials. Addition of at least one dose of trivalent IPV after immunization with bivalent OPV will reduce the risk of vaccine-derived polio associated with type 2 virus and enhance immunity to poliovirus types 1 and 3. Accordingly, in 2016, ~90% of countries included trivalent IPV in their immunization schedules. As the frequency of wild-type polio declines and reports of polio associated with circulating vaccine-derived viruses increase, the World Health Organization is investigating whether IPV can be produced from OPV strains that require less biocontainment, ultimately replacing OPV.

OPV and IPV induce antibodies that persist for at least 5 years. Both vaccines induce IgG and IgA antibodies. Compared with recipients of IPV, recipients of OPV shed less virus and less frequently develop reinfection with wild-type virus after exposure to poliovirus. Although IPV is safe and efficacious, OPV offers the advantages of ease of administration, lower cost, and induction of intestinal immunity resulting in a reduction in the risk of community transmission of wild-type virus. Because of progress toward global eradication of polio and the continued occurrence of cases of vaccine-associated polio, an all-IPV regimen was recommended in 2000 for childhood poliovirus vaccination in the United States, with vaccine administration at 2, 4, and 6–18 months and 4–6 years of age. The risk of vaccine-associated polio should be discussed before OPV is administered. Recommendations for vaccination of adults are listed in **Table 204-3**.

There are concerns about discontinuing vaccination in the event that endemic spread of poliovirus is eliminated. Among the reasons for these concerns are that poliovirus is shed from some immunocompromised persons for >25 years, that vaccine-derived poliovirus can circulate and cause disease, and that wild-type poliovirus is present in research laboratories and vaccine manufacturing facilities. Antivirals and monoclonal antibodies are in development to reduce or terminate shedding of poliovirus by long-term virus excretors. Pocapavir was shown to reduce shedding of OPV type 1 in a clinical trial, but rapid development of resistance with virus transmission, despite reduced shedding, indicates that combination therapy with other antivirals and/or monoclonal antibodies will be needed.

TABLE 204-3 Recommendations for Poliovirus Vaccination of Adults

1. Most adults in the United States have little risk for exposure to polioviruses, and most are immune as a result of vaccination during childhood. Vaccination with IPV is recommended for those at greater risk for exposure to polioviruses than the general population:
   a. travelers to areas or countries where polio is epidemic or endemic;
   b. members of communities or specific population groups with disease caused by wild-type polioviruses;
   c. laboratory workers who handle specimens that might contain polioviruses;
   d. health care workers who have close contact with patients who might be excreting wild-type polioviruses; and
   e. unvaccinated adults whose children will be receiving oral poliovirus vaccine.
2. Adults who are unvaccinated or whose vaccination status is unknown and who are at increased risk should receive three doses of IPV. Two doses of IPV should be administered at intervals of 4–8 weeks; a third dose should be administered 6–12 months after the second.
3. Adults who have had a primary series of polio vaccine and who are at increased risk should receive another dose of IPV. Currently, data do not indicate a need for more than a single lifetime booster dose with IPV for adults. However, adults who will be in a polio-infected or polio-exporting country for >4 weeks and whose booster dose of polio vaccine was administered >1 year earlier should receive an additional booster dose of vaccine before departing for that country.

Abbreviation: IPV, inactivated poliovirus vaccine.

Source: Modified from Centers for Disease Control and Prevention: MMWR Recomm Rep 46(RR-5):1, 2000; and Wallace et al: MMWR Morb Mortal Wkly Rep 63(27):591, 2014.

PARECHOVIRUSES

Human parechoviruses (HPeVs), like enteroviruses, are members of the family Picornaviridae. The 16 serotypes of HPeV commonly cause infections in early childhood. Infections with HPeV type 1 (HPeV-1) occur throughout the year, while other parechovirus infections occur more commonly in summer and fall. Infections with HPeVs present similarly to those due to enteroviruses and may cause generalized disease of the newborn, aseptic meningitis, encephalitis, seizures, transient paralysis, exanthems, respiratory tract disease, rash, hepatitis, and gastroenteritis. While HPeV-1 is the most common serotype and generally causes mild disease, deaths of infants in the United States have been associated with HPeV-1, HPeV-3, and HPeV-6. HPeVs can be isolated from the same sites as enteroviruses, including the nasopharynx, stool, and respiratory tract secretions. PCR using pan-enterovirus primers does not detect HPeVs, and while PCR assays are performed by the CDC and research laboratories, many commercial laboratories do not perform the test. Pleconaril is not active against parechoviruses.

REOVIRUSES

Reoviruses are double-stranded RNA viruses encompassing three serotypes. Serologic studies indicate that most humans are infected with reoviruses during childhood. Most infections either are asymptomatic or cause mild upper respiratory tract symptoms. Reovirus is considered a rare cause of mild gastroenteritis or meningitis in infants and children. Speculation regarding an association of reovirus type 3 with idiopathic neonatal hepatitis and extrahepatic biliary atresia is based on an elevated prevalence of antibody to reovirus in some affected patients and the detection of viral RNA by PCR in hepatobiliary tissues in some studies. New orthoreoviruses have been associated with human disease—e.g., Melaka and Kampar viruses with fever and acute respiratory disease in Malaysia and Nelson Bay virus with acute respiratory disease in a traveler from Bali.

FURTHER READING

Abedi GR et al: Enterovirus and parechovirus surveillance–United States, 2014-2016. MMWR Morb Mortal Wkly Rep 67:515, 2018.

Chard AN et al: Progress toward polio eradication-worldwide, January 2018-March 2020. MMWR Morb Mortal Wkly Rep 69:784, 2020.

Macklin GR et al: Evolving epidemiology of poliovirus serotype 2 following withdrawal of the serotype 2 oral poliovirus vaccine. Science 368:401, 2020.

McKay SL et al: Increase in acute flaccid myelitis—United States, 2018. Morb Mortal Wkly Rep 67:1273, 2018.

Murphy OC, Pardo CA: Acute flaccid myelitis: A clinical review. Semin Neurol 40:211, 2020.

Saez-Llorens et al: Safety and immunogenicity of two novel type 2 oral poliovirus vaccine candidates compared with monovalent type 2 oral poliovirus vaccine in children and infants: Two clinical trials. Lancet 397:27, 2021.

Schubert RD et al: Pan-viral serology implicates enteroviruses in acute flaccid myelitis. Nat Med 25:1748; 2019.

205 Measles (Rubeola)

Kaitlin Rainwater-Lovett, William J. Moss

DEFINITION

Measles is a highly contagious viral disease that is characterized by a prodromal illness of fever, cough, coryza, and conjunctivitis followed by the appearance of a generalized maculopapular rash. Before the widespread use of measles vaccines, it was estimated that measles caused >2 million deaths worldwide each year.

GLOBAL CONSIDERATIONS

Remarkable progress has been made in reducing global measles incidence and mortality rates through measles vaccination. In the Americas, intensive vaccination and surveillance efforts—based in part on the successful Pan American Health Organization strategy of periodic nationwide measles vaccination campaigns (supplementary immunization activities, or SIAs)—and high levels of routine measles vaccine coverage interrupted endemic transmission of measles virus. The World Health Organization's (WHO's) Region of the Americas was declared to have eliminated measles in September 2016—the first region in the world to do so. In the United States, high-level coverage with two doses of measles vaccine eliminated endemic measles virus transmission in 2000. Progress also has been made in reducing measles incidence and mortality rates in sub-Saharan Africa and Asia as a consequence of increasing routine measles vaccine coverage and provision of a second dose of measles vaccine through mass measles vaccination campaigns and childhood immunization programs. From 2000 to 2019, estimated global measles deaths decreased 62%, from 539,000 (95% confidence interval [CI], 357,200–911,900) to 207,500 (95% CI, 123,100–472,900). Measles vaccination prevented an estimated 25.5 million deaths over this period. However, a global measles resurgence in 2019 led to the loss of measles elimination status in the Region of the Americas and threatened elimination in the United States, highlighting the continual risk. In 2019, the 1282 measles cases reported in the United States were the highest since 1992.

The Measles and Rubella Initiative, a partnership led by the American Red Cross, the United Nations Foundation, UNICEF, the U.S. Centers for Disease Control and Prevention (CDC), and the WHO, is playing an important role in reducing global measles incidence and mortality rates. Since its inception in 2001, the Initiative has provided governments and communities in 88 countries with technical and financial support for routine immunization activities, mass vaccination campaigns, and disease surveillance systems.

ETIOLOGY

Measles virus is a spherical, nonsegmented, single-stranded, negative-sense RNA virus and a member of the *Morbillivirus* genus in the family Paramyxoviridae. Measles was originally a zoonotic infection, arising from animal-to-human transmission of an ancestral morbillivirus thousands of years ago, when human populations had attained sufficient size to sustain virus transmission. Although RNA viruses typically have high mutation rates, measles virus is considered to be an antigenically monotypic virus; i.e., the surface proteins responsible for inducing protective immunity have retained their antigenic structure across time and distance. The public health significance of this stability is that measles vaccines developed decades ago from a single strain of measles virus remain protective worldwide. Measles virus is killed by ultraviolet light and heat, and attenuated measles vaccine viruses retain these characteristics, necessitating a cold chain for vaccine transport and storage.

EPIDEMIOLOGY

Measles virus is one of the most highly contagious directly transmitted pathogens. Outbreaks can occur in populations in which <10% of persons are susceptible. Chains of transmission are common among household contacts, school-age children, and health care workers. There are no latent or persistent measles virus infections that result in prolonged contagiousness, nor are there animal reservoirs for the virus. Thus, measles virus can be maintained in human populations only by an unbroken chain of acute infections, which requires a continuous supply of susceptible individuals. Newborns become susceptible to measles virus infection when passively acquired maternal antibody is lost; when not vaccinated, these infants account for the bulk of new susceptible individuals.

Endemic measles has a typical temporal pattern characterized by yearly seasonal epidemics superimposed on longer epidemic cycles of 2–5 years or more. In temperate climates, annual measles outbreaks typically occur in the late winter and early spring. These annual outbreaks are probably attributable to social networks facilitating transmission (e.g., congregation of children at school) and environmental factors favoring the viability and transmission of measles virus. Measles cases continue to occur during interepidemic periods in large populations, but at low incidence. The longer epidemic cycles occurring every several years result from the accumulation of susceptible persons over successive birth cohorts and the subsequent decline in the number of susceptibles following an outbreak.

Secondary attack rates among susceptible household and institutional contacts generally exceed 90%. The average age at which measles occurs depends on rates of contact with infected persons, protective maternal antibody decline, and vaccine coverage. In densely populated urban settings with low-level vaccination coverage, measles is a disease of infants and young children. The cumulative incidence can reach 50% by 1 year of age, with a significant proportion of children acquiring measles before 9 months—the age of routine vaccination in many countries, in line with the schedule recommended by the WHO's Expanded Programme on Immunization. As measles vaccine coverage increases or population density decreases, the age distribution shifts toward older children. In such situations, measles cases predominate in school-age children. Infants and young children, although susceptible if not protected by vaccination, are not exposed to measles virus at a rate sufficient to cause a heavy disease burden in this age group. As vaccination coverage increases further, the age distribution of cases may be shifted into adolescence and adulthood; this distribution is seen in measles outbreaks in the United States and necessitates targeted measles vaccination programs for these older age groups. Some countries have a bimodal distribution, with measles cases predominantly in young infants and adults.

Persons with measles are infectious for several days before and after the onset of rash, when levels of measles virus in blood and body fluids are highest and when cough, coryza, and sneezing, which facilitate virus spread, are most severe. The contagiousness of measles before the onset of recognizable disease hinders the effectiveness of isolation measures. Viral shedding by children with impaired cell-mediated immunity can be prolonged.

Medical settings are well-recognized sites of measles virus transmission. Children may present to health care facilities during the prodrome, when the diagnosis is not obvious although the child is infectious and is likely to infect susceptible contacts. Health care workers can acquire measles from infected children and transmit measles virus to others. Nosocomial transmission can be reduced by maintenance of a high index of clinical suspicion, use of appropriate isolation precautions when measles is suspected, administration of measles vaccine to susceptible children and health care workers, and documentation of health care workers' immunity to measles (i.e., proof of receipt of two doses of measles vaccine or detection of antibodies to measles virus).

As efforts at measles control are increasingly successful, public perceptions of the risk of measles as a disease diminish and are replaced by concerns about possible adverse events associated with measles vaccine. As a consequence, numerous measles outbreaks have occurred because of opposition to vaccination on religious or philosophical grounds or unfounded fears of serious adverse events (see "Active Immunization," below, and **Chap. 3**).

PATHOGENESIS

Measles virus is transmitted primarily by respiratory droplets over short distances and, less commonly, by small-particle aerosols that remain suspended in the air for long periods. Airborne transmission appears to be important in certain settings, including schools, physicians' offices, hospitals, and enclosed public places. The virus can be transmitted by direct contact with infected secretions but does not survive for long on fomites.

The incubation period for measles is ~10 days to fever onset and 14 days to rash onset. This period may be shorter in infants and longer (up to 3 weeks) in adults. Infection is initiated when measles virus is deposited in the respiratory tract, oropharynx, or conjunctivae (**Fig. 205-1*A***). During the first 2–4 days after infection, measles virus proliferates locally in the respiratory mucosa, primarily in dendritic cells and lymphocytes, and spreads to draining lymph nodes. Virus then enters the bloodstream in infected lymphocytes, producing the primary viremia that disseminates infection throughout the reticuloendothelial system. Further replication results in secondary viremia that begins 5–7 days after infection and disseminates measles virus throughout the body. Replication of measles virus in the target organs, together with the host's immune response, is responsible for the signs and symptoms of measles that occur 8–12 days after infection and mark the end of the incubation period (**Fig. 205-1*B***).

IMMUNE RESPONSES

Host immune responses to measles virus are essential for viral clearance, clinical recovery, and the establishment of long-term immunity (**Fig. 205-1*C***). Early nonspecific (innate) immune responses during the prodromal phase include activation of natural killer cells and increased production of antiviral proteins. The adaptive immune responses consist of measles virus–specific antibody and cellular responses. The protective efficacy of antibodies to measles virus is illustrated by the immunity conferred to infants from passively acquired maternal antibodies and the protection of exposed, susceptible individuals after administration of anti–measles virus immunoglobulin. The first measles virus–specific antibodies produced after infection are of the IgM subtype, with a subsequent switch to predominantly IgG1 and IgG3 isotypes. The IgM antibody response is typically absent following reexposure or revaccination and serves as a marker of primary infection.

The importance of cellular immunity to measles virus is demonstrated by the ability of children with agammaglobulinemia (congenital inability to produce antibodies) to recover fully from measles and the contrasting picture for children with severe defects in T lymphocyte function, who often develop severe or fatal disease (**Chap. 351**). The initial predominant T_H1 response (characterized by interferon γ) is essential for viral clearance, and the later T_H2 response (characterized by interleukin 4) promotes the development of measles virus–specific antibodies that are critical for protection against reinfection.

The duration of protective immunity following wild-type measles virus infection is generally thought to be lifelong. Immunologic memory to measles virus includes both continued production of measles virus–specific antibodies and circulation of measles virus–specific CD4+ and CD8+ T lymphocytes.

However, the intense immune responses induced by measles virus infection are paradoxically associated with depressed responses to unrelated (non–measles virus) antigens, which persist for several weeks to months beyond resolution of the acute illness. This state of immune suppression enhances susceptibility to secondary infections with bacteria and viruses that cause pneumonia and diarrhea and is responsible for a substantial proportion of measles-related morbidity and deaths. Delayed-type hypersensitivity responses to recall antigens, such as tuberculin, are suppressed, and cellular and humoral responses to new antigens are impaired. Reactivation of tuberculosis and remission of autoimmune diseases after measles have been described and are attributed to this period of immune suppression. Importantly, measles results in depletion of circulating antibodies against previously encountered viruses and bacteria, impairing immunologic memory. This mechanism may explain why child morbidity and mortality can be increased for >2 years after measles.

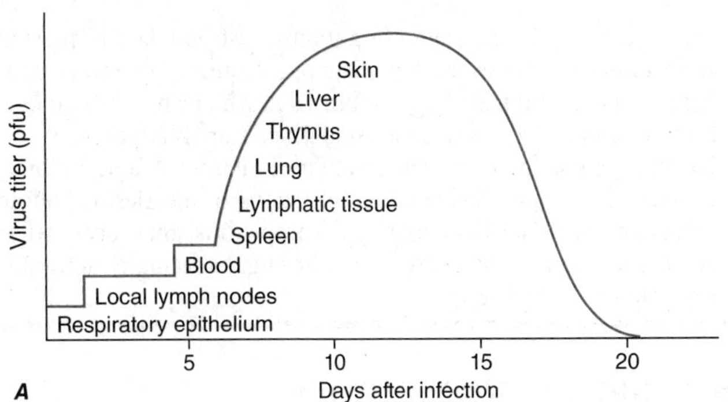

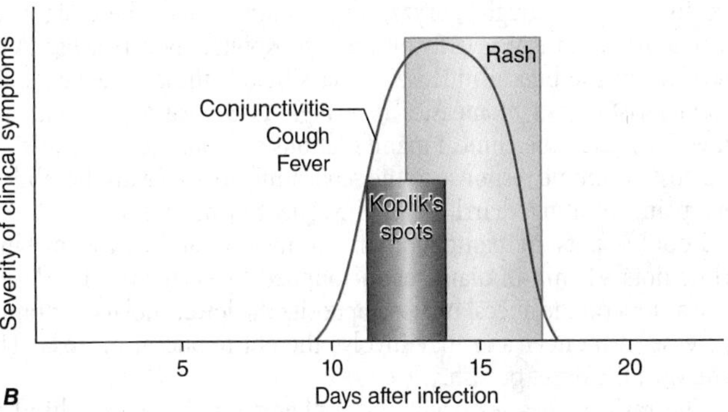

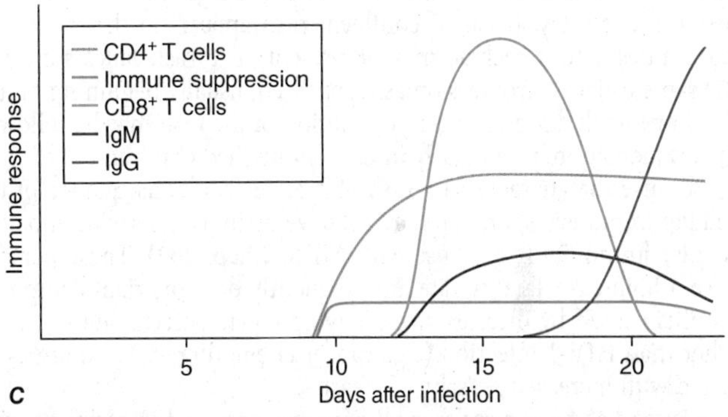

FIGURE 205-1 Measles virus infection: pathogenesis, clinical features, and immune responses. ***A.*** Spread of measles virus, from initial infection of the respiratory tract through dissemination to the skin. ***B.*** Appearance of clinical signs and symptoms, including Koplik's spots and rash. ***C.*** Antibody and T cell responses to measles virus. The signs and symptoms of measles arise coincident with the host immune response. *(Reproduced with permission from WJ Moss: Global measles elimination. Nat Rev Microbiology 4:900, 2006.)*

APPROACH TO THE PATIENT

Measles

Clinicians should consider measles in persons presenting with fever and generalized erythematous rash, particularly when measles virus is known to be circulating or the patient has a history of travel to endemic areas. Appropriate precautions must be taken to prevent nosocomial transmission. The diagnosis requires laboratory confirmation except during large outbreaks in which an epidemiologic link to a confirmed case can be established. Care is largely supportive and consists of the administration of vitamin A and antibiotics (see "Treatment," below). Complications of measles, including secondary bacterial infections and encephalitis, may occur after acute illness and require careful monitoring, particularly in immunocompromised persons.

CLINICAL MANIFESTATIONS

In most persons, the signs and symptoms of measles are highly characteristic (Fig. 205-1*B*). Fever and malaise beginning ~10 days after exposure are followed by cough, coryza, and conjunctivitis. These signs and symptoms increase in severity over 4 days. Koplik's spots (**see Fig. A1-2**) develop on the buccal mucosa ~2 days before the rash appears. The characteristic rash of measles (**see Fig. A1-3**) begins 2 weeks after infection, when the clinical manifestations are most severe, and signal the host's immune response to the replicating virus. Headache, abdominal pain, vomiting, diarrhea, and myalgia may be present.

Koplik's spots are pathognomonic of measles and consist of bluish white dots ~1 mm in diameter surrounded by erythema. The lesions appear first on the buccal mucosa opposite the lower molars but rapidly increase in number and may involve the entire buccal mucosa. They fade with the onset of rash.

The rash of measles begins as erythematous macules behind the ears and on the neck and hairline. The rash progresses to involve the face, trunk, and arms, with involvement of the legs and feet by the end of the second day. Areas of confluent rash appear on the trunk and extremities, and petechiae may be present. The rash fades slowly in the same order of progression as it appeared, usually beginning on the third or fourth day after onset. Resolution of the rash may be followed by desquamation, particularly in undernourished children.

Because the characteristic rash of measles is a consequence of the cellular immune response, it may not develop in persons with impaired cellular immunity (e.g., those with AIDS; **Chap. 202**). These persons have a high case–fatality rate and frequently develop giant cell pneumonitis caused by measles virus. T lymphocyte defects due to causes other than HIV-1 infection (e.g., cancer chemotherapy) also are associated with increased severity of measles.

A severe atypical measles syndrome was observed in recipients of a formalin-inactivated measles vaccine (used in the United States from 1963 to 1967 and in Canada until 1970) who were subsequently exposed to wild-type measles virus. The atypical rash began on the palms and soles and spread centripetally to the proximal extremities and trunk, sparing the face. The rash was initially erythematous and maculopapular but frequently progressed to vesicular, petechial, or purpuric lesions.

DIFFERENTIAL DIAGNOSIS

The differential diagnosis of measles includes other causes of fever, rash, and conjunctivitis, including rubella, Kawasaki disease, infectious mononucleosis, roseola, scarlet fever, Rocky Mountain spotted fever, enterovirus or adenovirus infection, and drug sensitivity. Rubella is a milder illness without cough and with distinctive lymphadenopathy. The rash of roseola (exanthem subitum) (**see Fig. A1-5**) appears after fever has subsided. The atypical lymphocytosis in infectious mononucleosis contrasts with the leukopenia commonly observed in children with measles.

DIAGNOSIS

Measles is readily diagnosed on clinical grounds by clinicians familiar with the disease, particularly during outbreaks. Koplik's spots are especially helpful because they appear early and are pathognomonic. Clinical diagnosis is more difficult (1) during the prodromal illness; (2) when the rash is attenuated by passively acquired antibodies or prior immunization; (3) when the rash is absent or delayed in immunocompromised children or severely undernourished children with impaired cellular immunity; and (4) in regions where the incidence of measles is low and other pathogens are responsible for the majority of illnesses with fever and rash. The CDC case definition for measles requires (1) a generalized maculopapular rash of at least 3 days' duration; (2) fever of at least 38.3°C (101°F); and (3) cough, coryza, or conjunctivitis.

Serology is the most common method of laboratory diagnosis. The detection of measles virus–specific IgM in a single specimen of serum or oral fluid is considered diagnostic of acute infection, as is a fourfold or greater increase in measles virus–specific IgG antibody levels between acute- and convalescent-phase serum specimens. Primary infection in the immunocompetent host results in antibodies that are detectable within 1–3 days of rash onset and reach peak levels in 2–4 weeks. Measles virus–specific IgM antibodies may not be detectable until 4–5 days or more after rash onset and usually fall to undetectable levels within 4–8 weeks of rash onset.

Several methods for measurement of antibodies to measles virus are available. Neutralization tests are sensitive and specific, and the results are highly correlated with protective immunity; however, these tests require propagation of measles virus in cell culture and thus are expensive and laborious. Commercially available enzyme immunoassays are most frequently used. Measles can also be diagnosed by isolation of the virus in cell culture from respiratory secretions, nasopharyngeal or conjunctival swabs, blood, or urine. Direct detection of giant cells in respiratory secretions, urine, or tissue obtained by biopsy provides another method of diagnosis.

For detection of measles virus RNA by reverse-transcription polymerase chain reaction amplification of RNA extracted from clinical specimens, primers targeted to highly conserved regions of measles virus genes are used. Extremely sensitive and specific, this assay may also permit identification and characterization of measles virus genotypes for molecular epidemiologic studies and can distinguish wild-type from vaccine virus strains.

TREATMENT

Measles

There is no specific antiviral therapy for measles. Treatment consists of general supportive measures, such as hydration and administration of antipyretic agents. Because secondary bacterial infections are a major cause of morbidity and death attributable to measles, effective case management involves prompt antibiotic treatment for patients who have clinical evidence of bacterial infection, including pneumonia and otitis media. *Streptococcus pneumoniae* and *Haemophilus influenzae* type b are common causes of bacterial pneumonia following measles; vaccines against these pathogens probably lower the incidence of secondary bacterial infections following measles.

Vitamin A is effective for the treatment of measles and can markedly reduce rates of morbidity and mortality. The WHO recommends administration of once-daily doses of 200,000 IU of vitamin A for 2 consecutive days to all children with measles who are ≥12 months of age. Lower doses are recommended for younger children: 100,000 IU per day for children 6–12 months of age and 50,000 IU per day for children <6 months old. A third dose is recommended 2–4 weeks later for children with evidence of vitamin A deficiency. While such deficiency is not a widely recognized problem in the United States, many American children with measles do, in fact, have low serum levels of vitamin A, and these children experience increased measles-associated morbidity. The Committee on Infectious Diseases of the American Academy of Pediatrics recommends that the administration of two consecutive daily doses of vitamin A be considered for children who are hospitalized with measles and its complications as well as for children with measles who are immunodeficient; who have ophthalmologic evidence of vitamin A deficiency, impaired intestinal absorption, or moderate to severe malnutrition; or who have recently immigrated from areas with high measles mortality rates. Parenteral and oral formulations of vitamin A are available.

Anecdotal reports have described the recovery of previously healthy pregnant and immunocompromised patients with measles pneumonia and of immunocompromised patients with measles encephalitis after treatment with aerosolized and IV ribavirin. However, the clinical benefits of ribavirin in measles have not been conclusively demonstrated in clinical trials.

COMPLICATIONS

Most complications of measles involve the respiratory tract and include the effects of measles virus replication itself and secondary bacterial infections. Acute laryngotracheobronchitis (croup) can occur during measles and may result in airway obstruction, particularly in young children. Giant cell pneumonitis due to replication of measles virus in the lungs can develop in immunocompromised children, including those with HIV-1 infection. Many children with measles develop diarrhea, which contributes to undernutrition.

Most complications of measles result from secondary bacterial infections of the respiratory tract that are attributable to a state of immune suppression lasting for several weeks to months, and perhaps even years, after acute measles. Otitis media and bronchopneumonia are most common and may be caused by *S. pneumoniae*, *H. influenzae* type b, or staphylococci. Recurrence of fever or failure of fever to subside with the rash suggests secondary bacterial infection.

Rare but serious complications of measles involve the central nervous system (CNS). Post-measles encephalomyelitis complicates ~1 in 1000 cases, affecting mainly older children and adults. Encephalomyelitis occurs within 2 weeks of rash onset and is characterized by fever, seizures, and a variety of neurologic abnormalities. The finding of periventricular demyelination, the induction of immune responses to myelin basic protein, and the absence of measles virus in the brain suggest that post-measles encephalomyelitis is an autoimmune disorder triggered by measles virus infection. Other CNS complications that occur months to years after acute infection are measles inclusion body encephalitis (MIBE) and subacute sclerosing panencephalitis (SSPE). In contrast to post-measles encephalomyelitis, MIBE and SSPE are caused by persistent measles virus infection. MIBE is a rare but fatal complication that affects individuals with defective cellular immunity and typically occurs months after infection. SSPE is a slowly progressive disease characterized by seizures and progressive deterioration of cognitive and motor functions, with death occurring 5–15 years after measles virus infection. SSPE most often develops in persons infected with measles virus at <2 years of age.

PROGNOSIS

Most persons with measles recover and develop long-term protective immunity to reinfection. Measles case–fatality proportions vary with the average age of infection, the nutritional and immunologic status of the population, measles vaccine coverage, and access to health care. Among previously vaccinated persons who do become infected, disease is less severe and mortality rates are significantly lower. In developed countries, <1 in 1000 children with measles dies. In endemic areas of sub-Saharan Africa, the measles case–fatality proportion may be 5–10% or even higher. Measles is a major cause of childhood deaths in refugee camps and in internally displaced populations, where case–fatality proportions have been as high as 20–30%.

PREVENTION

Passive Immunization Human immunoglobulin given shortly after exposure can attenuate the clinical course of measles. In immunocompetent persons, administration of immunoglobulin within 72 h of exposure usually prevents measles virus infection and almost always prevents clinical measles. Administered up to 6 days after exposure, immunoglobulin will still prevent or modify the disease. Prophylaxis with immunoglobulin is recommended for susceptible household and nosocomial contacts who are at risk of developing severe measles, particularly children <1 year of age, immunocompromised persons (including HIV-infected persons previously immunized with live attenuated measles vaccine), and pregnant women. Except for premature infants, children <6 months of age usually will be partially or completely protected by passively acquired maternal antibody. Infants born to women with vaccine-induced measles immunity become susceptible to measles at a younger age than infants born to women with acquired immunity from natural infection. If measles is diagnosed in a household member, all unimmunized children in the household should receive immunoglobulin. The recommended dose is 0.25 mL/kg given intramuscularly. Immunocompromised persons should receive 0.5 mL/kg. The maximal total dose is 15 mL. IV immunoglobulin contains antibodies to measles virus; the usual dose of 100–400 mg/kg generally provides adequate prophylaxis for measles exposures occurring as long as 3 weeks or more after IV immunoglobulin administration.

Active Immunization The first live attenuated measles vaccine was developed by passage of the Edmonston strain in chick embryo fibroblasts to produce the Edmonston B virus, which was licensed in 1963 in the United States. Further passage of Edmonston B virus produced the more attenuated Schwarz vaccine that currently serves as the standard in much of the world. The Moraten ("more attenuated Enders") strain, which was licensed in 1968 and is used in the United States, is genetically identical to the Schwarz strain.

Lyophilized measles vaccines are relatively stable, but reconstituted vaccine rapidly loses potency. Live attenuated measles vaccines are inactivated by light and heat and lose about half their potency at 20°C and almost all their potency at 37°C within 1 h after reconstitution. Therefore, a cold chain must be maintained before and after reconstitution. Antibodies first appear 12–15 days after vaccination, and titers peak at 1–3 months. Measles vaccines are often combined with other live attenuated virus vaccines, such as those for mumps and rubella (MMR) and for mumps, rubella, and varicella (MMR-V).

The recommended age of first vaccination varies from 6 to 15 months and represents a balance between the optimal age for seroconversion and the probability of acquiring measles before that age. The proportions of children who develop protective levels of antibody after measles vaccination approximate 85% at 9 months of age and 95% at 12 months. Common childhood illnesses concomitant with vaccination may reduce the level of immune response, but such illness is not a valid reason to withhold vaccination. Measles vaccines have been well tolerated and immunogenic in HIV-1-infected children and adults, although antibody levels may wane. Because of the potential severity of wild-type measles virus infection in HIV-1-infected children, routine measles vaccination is recommended except for those who are severely immunocompromised. Measles vaccination is contraindicated in individuals with other severe deficiencies of cellular immunity because of the possibility of disease due to progressive pulmonary or CNS infection with the vaccine virus.

The duration of vaccine-induced immunity is at least several decades, if not longer. Rates of secondary vaccine failure 10–15 years after immunization have been estimated at ~5%, but are probably lower when vaccination takes place after 12 months of age. Decreasing antibody concentrations do not necessarily imply a complete loss of protective immunity: a secondary immune response usually develops after reexposure to measles virus, with a rapid rise in antibody titers in the absence of overt clinical disease.

Standard doses of currently licensed measles vaccines are safe for immunocompetent children and adults. Fever to 39.4°C (103°F) occurs in ~5% of seronegative vaccine recipients, and 2% of vaccine recipients develop a transient rash. Mild transient thrombocytopenia has been reported, with an incidence of ~1 case per 40,000 doses of MMR vaccine.

Since the publication of a report in 1998 falsely hypothesizing that MMR vaccine may cause a syndrome of autism and intestinal inflammation, much public attention has focused on this purported association. The events that followed publication of this report led to diminished vaccine coverage in the United Kingdom and provide important lessons in the misinterpretation of epidemiologic evidence and the communication of scientific results to the public. The publication that incited the concern was a case series describing 12 children with a regressive developmental disorder and chronic enterocolitis; 9 of these children had autism. In 8 of the 12 cases, the parents associated onset of the developmental delay with MMR vaccination. This simple temporal association was misinterpreted and misrepresented as a possible causal relationship, first by the lead author of the study and then by elements of the media and the public. Subsequently, many comprehensive reviews and additional epidemiologic studies refuted evidence of a causal relationship between MMR vaccination and autism.

PROSPECTS FOR MEASLES ERADICATION

Progress in global measles control has renewed discussion of measles eradication. In contrast to poliovirus eradication, the eradication of measles virus will not entail challenges posed by prolonged shedding of potentially virulent vaccine viruses and environmental viral reservoirs. However, in comparison with smallpox eradication, higher levels of population immunity will be necessary to interrupt measles virus transmission, more highly skilled health care workers will be required to administer measles vaccines, and containment through case detection and ring vaccination will be more difficult for measles virus because of infectivity before rash onset. New tools, such as microneedle patches to deliver measles vaccine, will facilitate mass vaccination campaigns and vaccination of hard-to-reach children such as those residing in remote rural areas. Despite enormous progress, measles remains a leading vaccine-preventable cause of childhood mortality worldwide and continues to cause outbreaks in communities with low vaccination coverage rates in industrialized nations.

FURTHER READING

De Swart RL, Moss WJ: The immunological basis for immunization series: Module 7: Measles. Update 2020. Geneva: World Health Organization, 2020.

Griffin DE: Measles immunity and immunosuppression. Curr Opin Virol 46:9, 2020.

Mina MJ et al: Measles virus infection diminishes preexisting antibodies that offer protection from other pathogens. Science 366:599, 2019.

Moss WJ: Measles. Lancet 380:2490, 2017.

Moss WJ et al: Feasibility assessment of measles and rubella eradication. Vaccine 39:3544, 2021.

Phadke VK et al: Vaccine refusal and measles outbreaks in the US. JAMA 324:1344, 2020.

Strebel PM, Orenstein WA: Measles. N Engl J Med 381:349, 2019.

World Health Organization: Measles vaccines: WHO position paper—April 2017. Wkly Epidemiol Rec 92:205, 2017.

World Health Organization: Progress towards regional measles elimination—worldwide, 2000-2019. MMWR Morb Mortal Wkly Rep 69:1700, 2020.

206 Rubella (German Measles)

Laura A. Zimmerman, Susan E. Reef

Rubella was historically viewed as a variant of measles or scarlet fever. After an epidemic of rubella in Australia in the early 1940s, the ophthalmologist Norman Gregg noticed the occurrence of congenital cataracts among infants whose mothers had reported rubella during early pregnancy, and congenital rubella syndrome (CRS; see "Clinical Manifestations," below) was first described. Not until 1962 was a separate viral agent for rubella isolated.

ETIOLOGY

Rubella virus is a member of the Matonaviridae family and the only member of the genus *Rubivirus*. This single-strand RNA enveloped virus measures 40–80 nm in diameter. Its core protein is surrounded by a single-layer lipoprotein envelope with spike-like projections containing two glycoproteins, E1 and E2. There is only one antigenic type of rubella virus, and humans are its only known reservoir.

PATHOGENESIS AND PATHOLOGY

Although the pathogenesis of postnatal (acquired) rubella has been well documented, data on pathology are limited because of the mildness of the disease. Rubella virus is spread from person to person via respiratory droplets. Primary implantation and replication in the nasopharynx are followed by spread to the lymph nodes. Subsequent viremia occurs, which in pregnant women often results in infection of the placenta. Placental virus replication may lead to infection of fetal organs. The pathology of CRS in the infected fetus is well defined, with almost all organs found to be infected; however, the pathogenesis of CRS is only poorly delineated. In tissue, infections with rubella virus have diverse effects, ranging from no obvious impact to cell destruction. The hallmark of fetal infection is a chronic infection with persistence throughout fetal development in utero and for up to 1 year after birth.

Individuals with acquired rubella may shed virus from 7 days before rash onset to ~5–7 days thereafter. Both clinical and subclinical infections are considered contagious. Infants with CRS may shed large quantities of virus from bodily secretions, particularly from the throat and in the urine, up to 1 year of age. Outbreaks of rubella, including some in nosocomial settings, have originated with index cases of CRS. Thus, only individuals immune to rubella virus should have contact with infants who have CRS or who are congenitally infected with rubella virus but are not showing signs of CRS.

EPIDEMIOLOGY

The largest recent rubella epidemic in the United States took place in 1964–1965, when an estimated 12.5 million cases occurred, resulting in ~20,000 cases of CRS. Since the introduction of the routine rubella vaccination program in the United States in 1969, the number of rubella cases reported each year has dropped by >99%; the rate of vaccination coverage with rubella-containing vaccine (RCV) has been >90% among children 19–35 months old since 1996. In the United States, a goal for the elimination of rubella and CRS by 2000 was set in 1989. Interruption of endemic transmission of rubella virus was achieved by 2001. In 2004, a panel of experts agreed unanimously that rubella was no longer an endemic disease in the United States. The criteria used to document lack of endemic transmission included low disease incidence, high nationwide rubella antibody seroprevalence, outbreaks that were few and contained (i.e., small numbers of cases), and lack of endemic virus transmission (as assessed by genetic sequencing). Although interruption of endemic transmission has been sustained since 2001, rubella virus importations continue to occur, and cases continue to develop among susceptible persons. During 2010–2018, 47 cases of rubella were reported; 70% of these cases were in persons 20–49 years old—an age group that includes women of childbearing age. During this period, 13 cases of CRS were reported, all from foreign-born mothers. Therefore, health care providers should remain vigilant, considering the possibility of rubella virus infection in adults (especially those emigrating or returning from countries without rubella control programs) and recognizing the potential for CRS among their infants.

The Global Vaccine Action Plan 2011–2020 called for the elimination of rubella in five of the six World Health Organization (WHO) regions by 2020. Although rubella and CRS are no longer endemic in the WHO Region of the Americas, they remain important public health problems globally. The number of rubella cases reported worldwide in 2000 was ~700,000; this figure declined to 26,006 in 2018. However, the number of rubella cases may be underestimated because cases are often mild, patients may not seek care, cases may not be recognized or may not be reported, and, in some countries, cases are identified through measles surveillance systems that are not specific for rubella. Despite a continued increase in the number of countries with rubella vaccination programs, 31% of the world's children remained unvaccinated against rubella in 2018. In 2010, it was estimated that 105,000 cases of CRS occurred annually globally.

CLINICAL FEATURES

Acquired Rubella Acquired rubella commonly presents with a generalized maculopapular rash that usually lasts for up to 3 days (**Fig. 206-1**), although as many as 50% of cases may be subclinical or

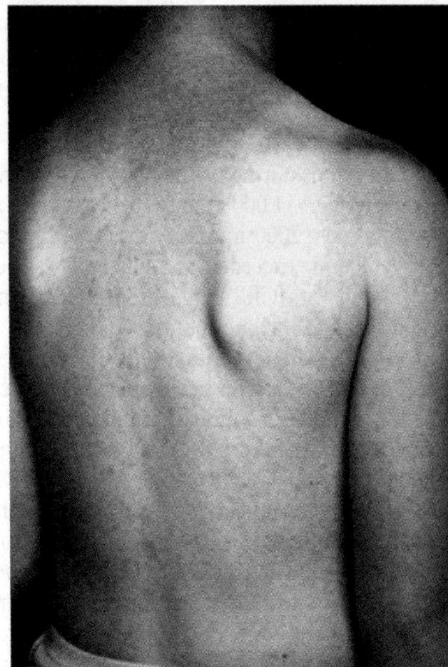

FIGURE 206-1 Mild maculopapular rash of rubella in a child.

without rash. When the rash occurs, it is usually mild and may be difficult to detect in persons with darker skin. In younger children, rash is usually the first sign of illness. However, in older children and adults, a 1- to 5-day prodrome often precedes the rash and may include low-grade fever, malaise, and upper respiratory symptoms. The incubation period is 14 days (range, 12–23 days).

Lymphadenopathy, particularly occipital and postauricular, may be noted during the second week after exposure. Although acquired rubella is usually thought of as a benign disease, arthralgia and arthritis are common in infected adults, particularly women. Thrombocytopenia and encephalitis are less common complications.

Congenital Rubella Syndrome The most serious consequence of rubella virus infection can develop when a woman becomes infected during pregnancy, particularly during the first trimester. The resulting complications may include miscarriage, fetal death, premature delivery, or live birth with congenital defects. Infants infected with rubella virus in utero may have myriad physical defects (**Table 206-1**), which most commonly relate to the eyes, ears, and heart. This constellation of severe birth defects is known as *CRS*. In addition to permanent manifestations, there are a host of transient physical manifestations, including thrombocytopenia with purpura/petechiae (e.g., dermal erythropoiesis, "blueberry muffin syndrome"). Some infants may be born with congenital rubella virus infection but have no apparent signs or symptoms of CRS and are referred to as "infants with congenital rubella virus infection only."

DIAGNOSIS

Acquired Rubella Clinical diagnosis of acquired rubella is difficult because of the mimicry of many illnesses with rashes, the varied clinical presentations, and the high rates of subclinical and mild disease. Illnesses that may be similar to rubella in presentation include scarlet fever, roseola, toxoplasmosis, fifth disease, measles, Zika, and illnesses with suboccipital and postauricular lymphadenopathy. Thus, laboratory documentation of rubella virus infection is considered the only reliable way to confirm acute disease.

TABLE 206-1 Common Transient and Permanent Manifestations in Infants with Congenital Rubella Syndrome

TRANSIENT MANIFESTATIONS	PERMANENT MANIFESTATIONS
Hepatosplenomegaly	Hearing impairment/deafness
Interstitial pneumonitis	Congenital heart defects (patent ductus arteriosus, pulmonary arterial stenosis)
Thrombocytopenia with purpura/ petechiae (e.g., dermal erythropoiesis or "blueberry muffin syndrome")	Eye defects (cataracts, cloudy cornea, microphthalmos, pigmentary retinopathy, congenital glaucoma)
Hemolytic anemia	Microcephaly
Bony radiolucencies	Central nervous system sequelae (mental and motor delay, autism)
Intrauterine growth retardation	
Adenopathy	
Meningoencephalitis	

Laboratory assessment of rubella virus infection is conducted by serologic and virologic methods. For acquired rubella, serologic diagnosis is most common and depends on the demonstration of IgM antibodies in an acute-phase serum specimen or a fourfold rise in IgG antibody titer between acute- and convalescent-phase specimens. To detect a rise in IgG antibody titer indicative of acute disease, the acute-phase serum specimen should be collected within 7–10 days after onset of illness and the convalescent-phase specimen ~14–21 days after the first specimen. The enzyme-linked immunosorbent assay IgM capture technique is considered most accurate for serologic diagnosis, but the indirect IgM assays also are acceptable. After rubella virus infection, IgM antibody may be detectable for up to 6 weeks. In case of a negative result for IgM in specimens taken earlier than day 5 after rash onset, serologic testing should be repeated.

Although uncommon, reinfection with rubella virus is possible, and IgM antibodies may be present. In this instance, IgG avidity testing is used in conjunction with IgG testing to distinguish primary rubella infection from reinfection. The detection of low-avidity antibodies in a patient's serum indicates recent infection. The presence of mature (high-avidity) IgG antibodies most likely indicates an infection occurring at least 2 months previously. Avidity testing may be particularly useful in diagnosing rubella in pregnant women and assessing the risk of CRS.

Rubella virus is typically detected in the nasopharynx during the prodromal period and for as long as 2 weeks after rash onset. However, since the secretion of virus in individuals with acquired rubella is maximal just before or up to 4 days after rash onset, this is the optimal time frame for collecting specimens for virus detection. Rubella is usually diagnosed by viral RNA detection in a reverse-transcriptase polymerase chain reaction (RT-PCR) assay; rubella virus isolation can also be used to diagnose rubella.

Congenital Rubella Syndrome The classic triad of CRS—clinical manifestations of cataracts, hearing impairment, and heart defects—is seen in ~10% of infants with CRS. Infants may present with different combinations of defects depending on when infection occurs during gestation. Hearing impairment is the most common single defect of CRS. However, as with acquired rubella, laboratory diagnosis of congenital infection is highly recommended, particularly because most features of the clinical presentation are nonspecific and may be associated with other intrauterine infections. Early diagnosis of CRS allows the prompt implementation of infection control measures and facilitates appropriate medical intervention for specific disabilities.

Diagnostic tests used to confirm CRS include serologic assays and virus detection. In an infant with congenital infection, serum IgM antibodies are normally present for up to 6 months but may be detectable for up to 1 year after birth. In some instances, IgM may not be detectable until 1 month of age; thus, infants who have symptoms consistent with CRS but who test negative shortly after birth should be retested at 1 month. A rubella serum IgG titer persisting beyond the time expected after passive transfer of maternal IgG antibody (i.e., a rubella titer that does not decline at the expected rate of a twofold dilution per month) is another serologic criterion used to confirm CRS.

In congenital infection, rubella virus is detected most commonly from throat swabs and less commonly from urine and cerebrospinal fluid. Infants with congenital rubella may excrete virus for up to 1 year, but specimens for virus isolation are most likely to be positive if obtained within the first 6 months after birth. Rubella virus in infants with CRS can also be detected by RT-PCR.

Rubella Diagnosis in Pregnant Women In the United States, screening for rubella IgG antibodies is recommended as part of routine prenatal care. Pregnant women with a positive IgG antibody serologic test are considered immune. Susceptible pregnant women should be vaccinated postpartum.

A susceptible pregnant woman exposed to rubella virus should be tested for IgM antibodies and, if positive, confirmed by testing for low-avidity IgG antibodies to determine whether she was infected during pregnancy. Pregnant women with evidence of acute infection must be clinically monitored, and gestational age at the time of maternal infection must be determined to assess the possibility of risk to the fetus. Among women infected with rubella virus during the first 10 weeks of gestation, the risk of delivering an infant with CRS is 90%. The risk of birth defects declines with infection later in gestation, and fetal defects are rarely associated with maternal rubella after the 16th week of gestation, although sensorineural hearing deficit may occur with infection as late as 20 weeks. Because of the potential for false-positive results, rubella IgM antibody testing is not recommended for pregnant women with no history of illness or contact with a rubella-like illness.

TREATMENT
Rubella

No specific therapy is available for rubella virus infection. Symptom-based treatment for various manifestations, such as fever and arthralgia, is appropriate. Immunoglobulin does not prevent rubella virus infection after exposure and therefore is not recommended as routine postexposure prophylaxis. Although immunoglobulin may modify or suppress symptoms, it can create an unwarranted sense of security: infants with congenital rubella have been born to women who received immunoglobulin shortly after exposure. Administration of immunoglobulin should be considered only if a pregnant woman who has been exposed to a person with rubella will not consider termination of the pregnancy under any circumstances. In such cases, IM administration of 20 mL of immunoglobulin within 72 h of rubella exposure may reduce—but does not eliminate—the risk of rubella.

PREVENTION

After the isolation of rubella virus in the early 1960s and the occurrence of a devastating rubella pandemic in 1964–1965, a vaccine for rubella was developed and licensed in 1969. The majority of rubella-containing vaccines (RCVs) used worldwide are combined measles and rubella (MR) or measles, mumps, and rubella (MMR) formulations. A tetravalent measles, mumps, rubella, and varicella (MMRV) vaccine is available but is not widely used. Available rubella-containing vaccines are live attenuated vaccine virus.

The public health burden of rubella virus infection is measured primarily through the occurrence of CRS cases among women who were infected during pregnancy. The 1964–1965 rubella epidemic in the United States resulted in >30,000 infections during pregnancy. CRS occurred in ~20,000 infants born alive, including >11,000 infants who were deaf, >3500 infants who were blind, and almost 2000 infants with intellectual disability. The medical cost of this epidemic exceeded $1.5 billion. It has been estimated that the cost for children with CRS ranges from $11,255 in low-income countries to $934,000 in high-income countries.

In some countries, there are few data to document the epidemiology of CRS, but clusters of CRS cases have been reported in developing countries. Before the introduction of routine immunization against rubella in the United States, the incidence of CRS was 0.1–0.2 case per 1000 live births during endemic periods and 1–4 cases per 1000 live births during epidemic periods. Where rubella virus is circulating and women of childbearing age are susceptible, CRS cases will continue to occur.

The most effective method of preventing acquired rubella and CRS is through vaccination with an RCV. One dose induces seroconversion in ≥95% of persons ≥1 year of age. Immunity is considered long-term and is probably lifelong. The most commonly used vaccine globally is the RA27/3 virus strain. The recommendation for routine rubella vaccination schedules in the United States is a first dose of MMR vaccine at 12–15 months of age and a second dose at 4–6 years. Other persons recommended to receive a dose of a rubella-containing vaccine include adolescents and adults without documented evidence of immunity, individuals in congregate settings (e.g., college students, military personnel, childcare and health care workers), international travelers, and susceptible women before and after pregnancy.

Because of the theoretical risk of transmission of live attenuated rubella vaccine virus to the developing fetus, women known to be pregnant should not receive RCV. In addition, pregnancy should be avoided for 28 days after receipt of RCV. In follow-up studies of ~3000 unknowingly pregnant women who received rubella vaccine, no infant was born with CRS. Receipt of RCV during pregnancy is not ordinarily a reason to consider termination of the pregnancy.

In 2018, 168 (87%) of the 194 member countries of the WHO recommend inclusion of RCV in the routine childhood vaccination schedule (**Fig. 206-2**). Goals for the elimination of rubella and CRS have

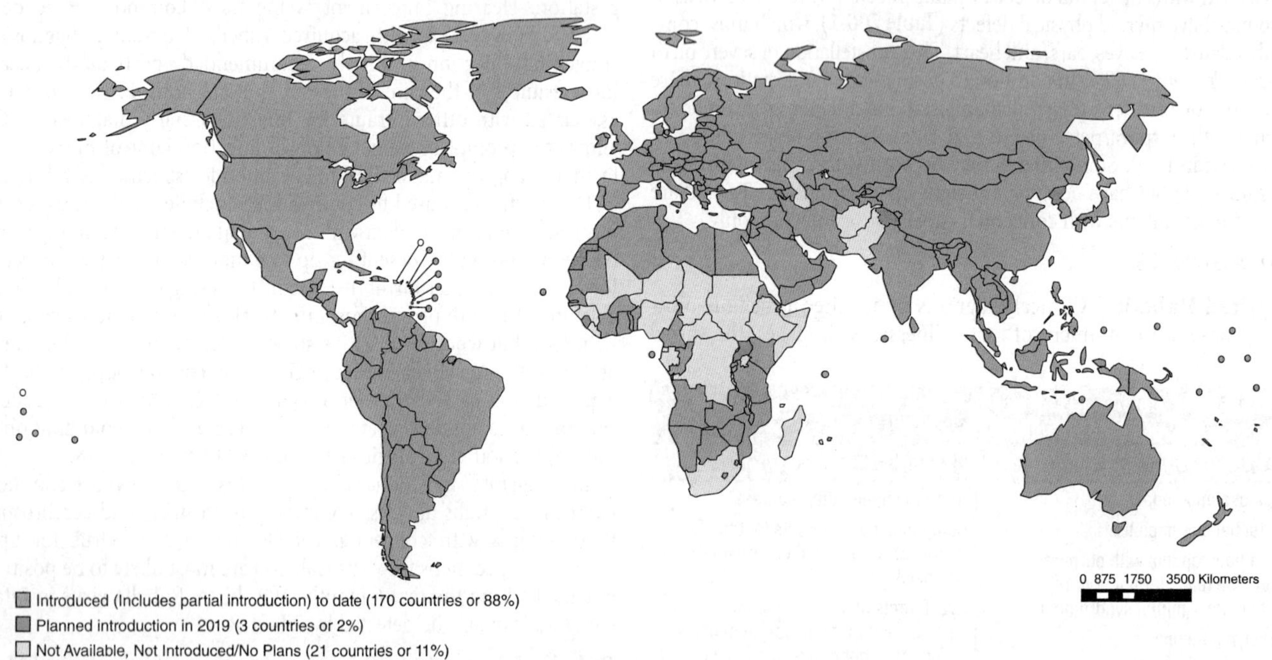

FIGURE 206-2 Countries using rubella vaccine in national childhood immunization schedules, 2018. Disclaimer—The boundaries and names shown and the designations used on this map do not imply the expression or any opinion whatsoever on the part of the World Health Organization concerning the legal status of any country, territory, city, or area nor of its authorities, or concerning the delimitation of its frontiers or boundaries. Dotted or dashed lines on maps represent approximate border lines for which there may not be full agreement. *(From the World Health Organization, WHO, 2019. All rights reserved.)*

been established in the WHO American, European, Southeast Asian, and Western Pacific regions. The African and Eastern Mediterranean regions have not yet set such goals.

FURTHER READING

Centers for Disease Control and Prevention: Control and prevention of rubella: Evaluation and management of suspected outbreaks, rubella in pregnant women, and surveillance for congenital rubella syndrome. MMWR Morb Mortal Wkly Rep 50:1, 2001.

Centers for Disease Control and Prevention: Notice to readers: Revised ACIP recommendation for avoiding pregnancy after receiving a rubella-containing vaccine. MMWR Morb Mortal Wkly Rep 50:1117, 2001.

Centers for Disease Control and Prevention: Rubella, in *Manual for the Surveillance of Vaccine-Preventable Diseases*, 5th ed, SW Roush et al (eds). Atlanta, Centers for Disease Control and Prevention, 2018, Chapter 14. Available at *https://www.cdc.gov/vaccines/pubs/surv-manual/index.html*. Accessed January 1, 2020.

Centers for Disease Control and Prevention: Rubella, in *Epidemiology and Prevention of Vaccine Preventable Diseases*, 13th ed, Jennifer Hamborsky et al (eds). Washington, DC, Public Health Foundation, 2015, Chapter 18. Available at *https://www.cdc.gov/vaccines/pubs/pinkbook/index.html*. Accessed December 4, 2017.

Grant GB et al: Progress toward rubella and congenital rubella syndrome control and elimination: Worldwide, 2000–2018. MMWR Morb Mortal Wkly Rep 68:855, 2019.

Reef S, Plotkin SA: Rubella vaccine, in *Vaccines*, SA Plotkin and WA Orenstein (eds). Philadelphia, Saunders, 2018, pp 970–1000.

Thompson K, Odahowski C: The costs and valuation of health impacts of measles and rubella risk management policies. Risk Anal 36:1357, 2016.

Vynnycky E et al: Using seroprevalence and immunisation coverage data to estimate the global burden of congenital rubella syndrome, 1996–2010: A systematic review. PLoS One 11:e0149160, 2016.

World Health Organization: Rubella, module 11, in *The Immunological Basis for Immunization Series*. Geneva, WHO, 2008. Available at *http://www.who.int/immunization/documents/ISBN9789241596848/en/index.html*. Accessed December 4, 2017.

World Health Organization: Rubella vaccines: WHO position paper. Wkly Epidemiol Rec 86:301, 2011. Available at *http://www.who.int/wer/2011/wer8629.pdf?ua=1*. Accessed December 4, 2017.

World Health Organization: Global Vaccine Action Plan 2011– 2020. Geneva, WHO, 2013. Available at *http://www.who.int/immunization/global_vaccine_action_plan/GVAP_doc_2011_2020/en/*. Accessed May 26, 2021.

207 Mumps

Jessica Leung, Mariel Marlow

Mumps is an acute, self-limited, systemic viral illness typically characterized by parotitis or other salivary gland swelling. Although mumps was once considered a universal childhood disease in the United States, routine mumps vaccination had led to a >99% reduction in cases by the early 2000s. However, since 2006, there has been an increase in mumps cases in this country, the majority among fully vaccinated persons. Mumps should be suspected in all patients with parotitis or mumps complications (see "Clinical Manifestations"), regardless of age, vaccination status, or travel history.

ETIOLOGIC AGENT

Mumps is an acute viral illness caused by a paramyxovirus from the *Rubulavirus* genus in the Paramyxoviridae family. This single-stranded, negative-sense, enveloped RNA virus is ~15.3 kb in size and encodes several minor proteins and seven major proteins. Mumps virus is rapidly inactivated by formalin, ether, chloroform, heat, and ultraviolet light. There is only one mumps virus serotype. One of the seven major encoded proteins, the small hydrophobic (SH) protein, exhibits hypervariability among strains; thus, the SH gene nucleotide sequence is used to genotype the virus for molecular epidemiologic purposes.

The 12 known genotypes of mumps virus are designated by the letters A to N (except E and M). In the United States, >98% of mumps virus specimens genotyped from 2015 through 2017 were genotype G. Most mumps vaccines licensed globally are composed of virus strains from genotype A, B, or N. The mumps virus strain (Jeryl Lynn) used in vaccines in the United States is genotype A.

EPIDEMIOLOGY

Mumps occurs worldwide and is endemic in many countries. In the absence of routine vaccination, the incidence of mumps is 100–1000 cases per 100,000 population, with epidemic peaks every 2–5 years. From 1999 through 2019, on average, >500,000 mumps cases were reported to the World Health Organization annually; however, global mumps incidence is challenging to estimate, as few countries routinely collect data on mumps incidence. Since 2018, mumps vaccine is routinely used in 122 countries. Mumps incidence has been reduced by 97–99% in countries with a routine two-dose measles, mumps, and rubella (MMR) vaccination schedule and by 87–88% in those with a one-dose vaccination program. However, since the mid-2000s, large mumps outbreaks have been reported among populations with high two-dose MMR coverage in countries with routine mumps immunization programs. Most outbreaks have occurred in settings with intense or frequent close contact, such as universities, close-knit communities, and correctional facilities, and most cases have occurred in fully vaccinated persons. Despite these outbreaks, mumps incidence is still much higher in countries that do not have routine mumps vaccination.

In the United States, prior to licensure of a vaccine for mumps in 1967, >100,000 mumps cases occurred annually. After the implementation of a one-dose mumps vaccination policy in 1977 and a subsequent two-dose policy in 1989, reported mumps cases declined to an annual average of ~300 by the early 2000s. However, since 2006, there has been an increase in mumps cases reported in the United States, with several peak years (**Fig. 207-1**). During the highest peak in cases, from January 2016 through June 2017, 150 mumps outbreaks and 9200 outbreak-associated cases were reported in a range of settings and groups, including schools, universities, athletic teams and facilities, church groups, workplaces, and large parties and events. While a majority of cases have occurred in fully vaccinated young adults in association with large university outbreaks, about one-third of cases have affected children or adolescents, most of whom were vaccinated. As of 2020, mumps is endemic in the United States, and there are no elimination goals for the disease.

Multiple factors are likely involved in being at risk for mumps infection among vaccinated persons. Following vaccination, these factors include (1) failure to develop an immune response, (2) the development of a low-level immune response that is insufficient for protection, (3) a decrease in immunity over time (waning immunity) after initial development of a vaccine-induced immune response, (4) lower levels of vaccine-induced antibodies to the circulating wild-type virus strains than to the vaccine virus strain, and (5) a lower frequency of subclinical immunologic boosting due to lack of exposure to wild-type virus during periods of low disease incidence.

PATHOGENESIS

Humans are the only known natural reservoir for mumps virus, which is transmitted through direct contact with respiratory droplets or saliva of an infected person. The average incubation period is 16–18 days, with a range of 12–25 days. A person is most infectious from 2 days before until 5 days after onset of parotitis or other salivary gland swelling. However, mumps virus has been detected in saliva as early as 7 days before onset and as late as 9 days after onset of these manifestations. Mumps virus has been isolated from urine and seminal fluid up to 14 days after onset of parotitis, although no studies have assessed transmissibility of the virus through these fluids.

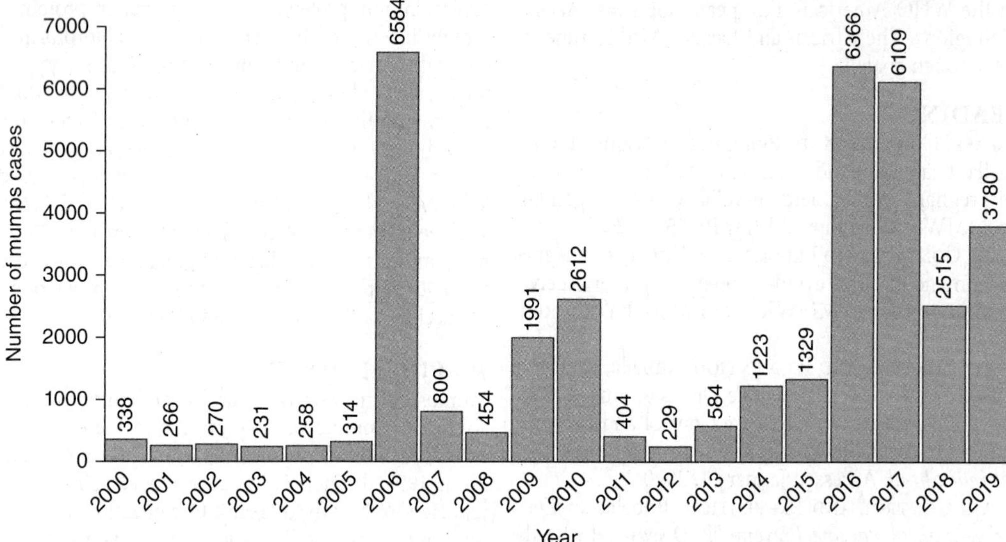

FIGURE 207-1 Reported mumps cases: United States, 2000–2019. *(Source: National Notifiable Diseases Surveillance System, 2000–2019 Annual Tables of Infectious Disease Data. Atlanta, GA, CDC Division of Health Informatics and Surveillance, 2019. Available at https://www.cdc.gov/nndss/infectious-tables.html.)*

Primary mumps virus replication likely occurs in the nasal mucosa or upper respiratory mucosal epithelium. Given the range of symptoms, it is assumed that, after infection of the respiratory mucosa, the virus spreads to regional lymph nodes. Mononuclear cells and cells within regional lymph nodes can become infected; such infection facilitates the development of viremia, which usually lasts 3–5 days. Viremia can result in a range of acute inflammatory reactions, most commonly in the salivary glands (resulting in parotitis) and the testes (resulting in orchitis). Other sites of virus dissemination include the kidneys (reflected in the frequency of viruria), the central nervous system (CNS), the pancreas, the heart, the ovaries, the mammary glands, the perilymphatic fluid within the cochlea, and (during pregnancy) the fetus.

Little is known about the pathology of mumps since the disease is rarely fatal. Affected salivary glands contain perivascular and interstitial mononuclear-cell infiltrates and exhibit hemorrhage with prominent edema. Serum and urine amylase levels may be elevated as a result of inflammation and tissue damage in the parotid gland. Necrosis of acinar and epithelial duct cells is evident in the salivary glands and in the germinal epithelium of the seminiferous tubules of the testes. The virus probably enters cerebrospinal fluid (CSF) through the choroid plexus or via transiting mononuclear cells during plasma viremia. Although relevant data are limited, in many cases, mumps encephalitis appears to be a para- or postinfectious process (as suggested by perivenous demyelination and perivascular mononuclear-cell inflammation) rather than the result of a direct cytotoxic effect caused by viral invasion of the CNS. However, although rare, primary mumps encephalitis does occur, as shown by mumps virus isolation from brain tissue. Infection of the perilymphatic fluid likely develops via retrograde penetration by the virus from the cervical lymph nodes following viremia, but infection could also occur via the CSF in cases of mumps CNS infection, given that the perilymph communicates with the CSF. Virus in the perilymph can result in infection of the cochlea and damage to the organ of Corti and the tectorial membrane, leading to transient or permanent deafness. Evidence of placental and intrauterine spread has been found in both early and late gestation. Virus frequently disseminates to the kidneys, but kidney involvement in mumps is almost always benign.

■ CLINICAL MANIFESTATIONS

While typically presenting with parotitis or other salivary gland swelling, mumps infection can range from asymptomatic or nonspecific respiratory symptoms to serious complications. Mumps can occur in a person who is fully vaccinated, but vaccinated persons are at a lower risk for mumps and mumps complications. Mumps infection is asymptomatic in ~20% of unvaccinated patients; the proportion asymptomatic among vaccinated persons is unknown.

Parotitis can be preceded by several days by a prodrome of low-grade fever, malaise, myalgia, headache, and anorexia. Parotitis typically lasts for 5 days (range, 3–7 days); most cases resolve within 10 days. Parotitis is generally bilateral and may not occur synchronously on both sides; unilateral involvement occurs in about one-third of cases. Swelling of the parotid gland is accompanied by tenderness and obliteration of the space between the earlobe and the angle of the mandible (**Figs. 207-2 and 207-3**). The patient frequently reports an earache and jaw pain and finds it difficult to eat, swallow, or talk. The orifice of the parotid duct is commonly red and swollen. The submaxillary and sublingual glands are involved less often than the parotid gland and are rarely involved alone. In ~6% of mumps cases, obstruction of lymphatic drainage secondary to bilateral salivary gland swelling may lead to presternal pitting edema, associated often with submandibular adenitis and rarely with the more life-threatening supraglottic edema.

The most frequent complications of mumps include orchitis, oophoritis, mastitis, pancreatitis, hearing loss, meningitis, and encephalitis. Complications can occur in the absence of parotitis and are more

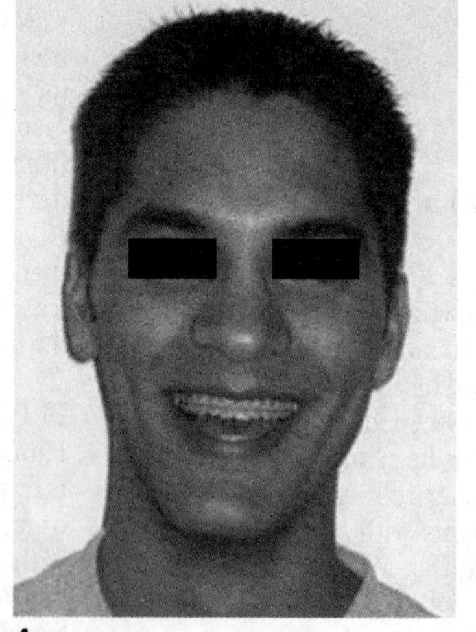

A

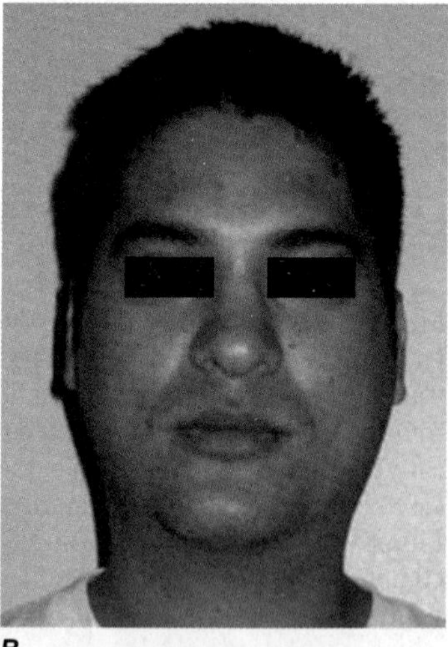

B

FIGURE 207-2 The same person before mumps acquisition (*A*) and on day 3 of acute bilateral parotitis (*B*). *(Courtesy of patient C.M. From JD Shanley: The resurgence of mumps in young adults and adolescents. Cleve Clin J Med 74:42, 2007. Reprinted with permission. Copyright © 2007 Cleveland Clinic Foundation. All rights reserved.)*

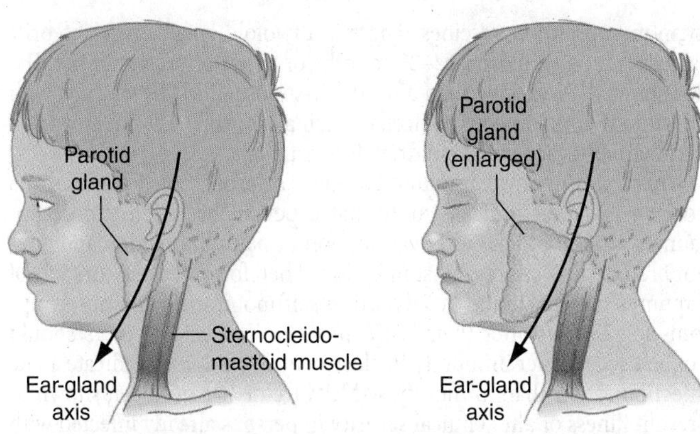

FIGURE 207-3 Schematic drawings of a normal parotid gland (left) and a parotid gland infected with mumps virus (right). An enlarged cervical lymph node is usually posterior to the imaginary line. *(Reproduced with permission from A Gershon et al: Krugman's Infectious Diseases of Children, 11th ed. Philadelphia, Elsevier, 2004.)*

common among adults than among children and among males than among females, likely due to rates of orchitis.

Orchitis (testicular inflammation), usually accompanied by fever, is the most common complication, developing in up to 30% of unvaccinated and 6% of vaccinated postpubertal males. This complication is rare in children. Orchitis typically occurs during the first week of parotitis but can develop up to 6 weeks after parotitis. Both testes are involved in ~10–30% of cases. The testis is painful and tender and can be enlarged to several times its normal size. Pain and swelling may last for 1 week, while tenderness may last for several weeks. Testicular atrophy develops in ~30–50% of affected testicles. The development of anti-sperm antibodies, reduced testosterone production, and impaired sperm mobility through oligospermia, azoospermia, or asthenospermia may lead to temporary sterility or subfertility. However, no studies have assessed the risk of permanent infertility in men with mumps orchitis.

Approximately 7% of unvaccinated and ≤1% of vaccinated postpubertal women develop oophoritis, which may be associated with lower abdominal pain and vomiting. The rate of mastitis in mumps has been estimated to be as high as 30% among unvaccinated postpubertal women and as low as ≤1% among vaccinated postpubertal women. Pancreatitis occurs in ~4% of unvaccinated and <1% of vaccinated mumps patients. Mumps pancreatitis, which may present as abdominal pain, is difficult to diagnose because an elevated serum amylase level can be associated with either parotitis or pancreatitis. However, serum lipase is elevated in pancreatitis and the presence of both elevated serum amylase and lipase can help determine if pancreatitis is present in addition to parotitis. Hearing loss associated with mumps infection can occur in up to 4% of unvaccinated and <1% of vaccinated mumps patients. Mumps-related hearing loss is usually sudden in onset, unilateral, and transient and may be associated with vestibular symptoms. Bilateral and permanent hearing loss are rare.

Mumps virus is highly neurotropic, with subclinical CNS involvement occurring in up to 55% of patients as manifested by CSF pleocytosis. However, symptomatic CNS infection is less common. Aseptic meningitis occurs in ≤1% of vaccinated patients and up to 10% of unvaccinated patients and is a self-limited manifestation without significant risk of death or long-term sequelae. Symptoms of aseptic meningitis, including stiff neck, headache, and drowsiness, typically appear ~5 days after parotitis. Encephalitis develops in ≤1% of patients, who present with high fever, marked changes in the level of consciousness, seizures, and focal neurologic symptoms. Electroencephalographic abnormalities may be seen. Permanent sequelae are sometimes identified in survivors, and adult infections more commonly have poor outcomes than do pediatric infections. The mortality rate associated with mumps encephalitis is ~1.5%. Other CNS problems occasionally associated with mumps include cerebellar ataxia, facial palsy, transverse myelitis, hydrocephalus, Guillain-Barré syndrome, flaccid paralysis, and behavioral changes.

Although rare and self-limited, myocarditis and endocardial fibroelastosis may represent severe complications of mumps infection; however, mumps-associated electrocardiographic abnormalities have been reported in up to 15% of cases. Other unusual complications include thyroiditis, nephritis, arthritis, hepatic disease, keratouveitis, and thrombocytopenic purpura. Abnormal renal function is common, but severe, life-threatening nephritis is rare.

Mumps infection in pregnant women is generally benign and is not more severe than in women who are not pregnant. Evidence suggesting an association between maternal mumps infection and an increased rate of spontaneous abortion or intrauterine fetal death is inconclusive.

Both mumps reinfection after natural infection and recurrent infection (in which parotid gland swelling resolves and then, weeks to months later, develops on the same or the other side) can occur. In the past, mumps reinfection was thought to be rare, but more recent data have suggested that it may be more common than previously thought.

Death due to mumps is exceedingly rare.

DIFFERENTIAL DIAGNOSIS

Mumps is the only cause of parotitis outbreaks, although an increase in parotitis cases may also result from increased influenza activity—specifically, infection with influenza A virus subtype H3N2. Other infectious causes of parotitis include parainfluenza virus types 1–3, Epstein-Barr virus, human herpesviruses 6A and 6B, herpes simplex viruses types 1 and 2, coxsackievirus A, adenovirus, parvovirus B19, echovirus, lymphocytic choriomeningitis virus, and HIV. Laboratory testing for sporadic parotitis cases caused by these infectious pathogens can help rule out mumps.

Parotitis can also develop in the setting of sarcoidosis, Sjögren's syndrome, Mikulicz's syndrome, Parinaud's oculoglandular syndrome, uremia, diabetes mellitus, laundry starch ingestion, malnutrition, cirrhosis, and some drug treatments. Unilateral parotitis can be caused by ductal obstruction, cysts, and tumors. In the absence of parotitis or other salivary gland enlargement, symptoms of other visceral-organ and/or CNS involvement may predominate, and a laboratory diagnosis is required. Other entities should be considered when manifestations consistent with mumps appear in organs other than the parotid. For example, testicular torsion may produce a painful scrotal mass resembling that seen in mumps orchitis. Orchitis can also be caused by bacterial infections in the prostate and urinary tract, sexually transmitted diseases such as chlamydia and gonorrhea, and other viral infections such as those with coxsackievirus, varicella, echovirus, and cytomegalovirus. Oophoritis can also be caused by sexually transmitted diseases such as chlamydia and gonorrhea. A number of viruses (e.g., enteroviruses) can cause aseptic meningitis that is clinically indistinguishable from that due to mumps virus.

LABORATORY DIAGNOSIS

If mumps is suspected, infection is confirmed by virologic methods, but serologic testing can aid in diagnosis. Especially in vaccinated patients, a negative virologic or serologic result in a person with clinical signs of mumps does not rule out mumps infection.

Virologic methods for confirming mumps include reverse transcription polymerase chain reaction (RT-PCR) and viral culture. RT-PCR is preferred because of its sensitivity, specificity, and timeliness. Mumps virus and viral RNA can be detected in blood, saliva, urine, and CSF. Buccal or oral swabs provide the best specimens for virus detection. The parotid gland should be massaged for 30 s prior to collection of the buccal/oral swab sample. As maximal viral shedding occurs within 5 days after symptom onset, specimens for mumps virologic testing ideally should be collected as close to parotitis onset as possible. The diagnostic yield of urine specimens increases over time up to 10 days after parotitis onset, but buccal specimens are more likely than urine specimens to result in virus detection at any time point.

Serologic methods that can aid in the diagnosis of mumps include detection of mumps-specific IgM antibodies or a fourfold rise between acute- and convalescent-phase IgG antibodies. In unvaccinated persons, IgM antibody is usually detectable within 5 days after onset, reaches a maximal level a week after onset, and remains elevated for weeks or months. Failure to detect mumps IgM in vaccinated patients is very common, as the IgM response is often undetectable, transient, or delayed in these individuals. Collection of specimens >3 days after onset may improve IgM detection. Use of IgG testing is generally not recommended, as IgG titers in vaccinated or previously infected patients may already be elevated at the time of acute-phase specimen collection, such that a fourfold rise is not detected in the convalescent-phase specimen.

TREATMENT
Mumps

Mumps is generally a benign, self-resolving illness. Therapy for parotitis and other clinical manifestations is symptom based and supportive. The administration of analgesics and the application of warm or cold compresses to the parotid area may be helpful. Testicular pain may be minimized by the local application of cold compresses and gentle support for the scrotum. Anesthetic blocks also may be used. Neither the administration of glucocorticoids nor incision of the tunica albuginea is of proven value in severe orchitis. Mumps immune globulin is not recommended for postexposure prophylaxis or treatment.

PREVENTION

Vaccination is the best prevention measure against mumps. Mumps vaccine is commonly included as part of the combination MMR vaccine or the combination measles–mumps–rubella–varicella (MMRV) vaccine. All mumps vaccines currently on the market are live attenuated virus vaccines. Strains used in mumps vaccines have included Jeryl Lynn, RIT-4385, Urabe Am9, Rubini, Leningrad-3 and Leningrad-Zagreb; Urabe- and Rubini-containing vaccines are no longer available. The Jeryl Lynn strain is the only strain used in mumps vaccines in the United States since 1967.

In the United States, children are recommended to receive the first MMR dose at 12—15 months of age and the second dose at 4—6 years. Adequate vaccination against mumps is defined as two doses of MMR for school-aged children (i.e., grades K–12) and for adults at high risk (i.e., health care workers, international travelers, and students at post-high school educational institutions) and one dose for preschool-aged children and adults not at high risk. During an outbreak, a second dose should be considered for children aged 1—4 years and adults who have received one dose. In 2017, after an increase in cases among persons with two MMR doses and a study demonstrating added benefit of a third MMR vaccine dose for individual protection, a third dose was recommended for use during outbreaks. The third dose of MMR vaccine is intended for groups whom public health authorities identify as at increased risk of acquiring mumps during an outbreak; public health authorities will inform providers of these groups at increased risk. As the duration of protection provided by a third dose of MMR vaccine is unknown and may be short term (<1 year), there is no recommendation for a routine third dose.

The effectiveness of MMR vaccine (in which the mumps component is based on the Jeryl Lynn strain) is estimated to be 80% (range, 49–92%) for one dose and 88% (range, 32–95%) for two doses. The effectiveness of the mumps component is lower than that of the measles component (two-dose effectiveness of 97%) and the rubella component (one-dose effectiveness of 97%). Incremental vaccine effectiveness of a third MMR dose—compared with two doses—during outbreaks is estimated at 78% (range, 61–88%).

In general, most recipients of mumps vaccine will seroconvert after vaccination and will have detectable antibodies to mumps virus; however, antibody levels start to decline soon after vaccination. Vaccine-induced neutralizing antibodies to wild-type strains may be lower in titer and may decline more rapidly than antibodies to the vaccine strain (Jeryl Lynn). However, most young adults given two vaccine doses in childhood appear to retain memory B cells.

Mumps vaccines are generally very safe. Urabe and Leningrad-Zagreb mumps strain vaccines have been associated with a slightly increased risk of aseptic meningitis, but there is no evidence of this risk for Jeryl Lynn mumps strain vaccines. There is a twofold greater risk of febrile seizures among children 12–23 months of age after receipt of the first dose of MMRV vaccine than after the first dose of MMR vaccine, with or without simultaneous varicella vaccination; this risk has not been found among vaccinated children 4–6 years of age.

There is no known immune correlate of protection for mumps; a positive IgG titer indicates only that a person has been exposed to mumps virus through either vaccination or natural infection and does not predict protection against infection. Therefore, all close contacts of a mumps patient should be advised to self-monitor for mumps symptoms for 25 days after their last exposure. Further, IgG titers should not be used to infer immunity in close contacts as it may indicate acute infection rather than immunity. MMR vaccine has not been shown to prevent illness or alter clinical severity in persons already infected with mumps virus and is not recommended as postexposure prophylaxis for immediate close contacts of mumps patients.

Acknowledgment

The authors acknowledge and thank Dr. Steve Rubin, the author of the previous edition of this chapter.

FURTHER READING

Marin M et al: Recommendation of the Advisory Committee on Immunization Practices for use of a third dose of mumps virus–containing vaccine in persons at increased risk for mumps during an outbreak. MMWR Morb Mortal Wkly Rep 67:33, 2018.

Masarani M et al: Mumps orchitis. J R Soc Med 99:573, 2006.

McClean HQ et al: Prevention of measles, rubella, congenital rubella syndrome, and mumps, 2013: Summary recommendations of the Advisory Committee on Immunization Practices (ACIP). MMWR Recomm Rep 62(RR-04):1, 2013.

Rota JS et al: Comparison of the sensitivity of laboratory diagnostic methods from a well-characterized outbreak of mumps in New York City in 2009. Clin Vaccine Immunol 20:391, 2013.

Rubin S et al: Molecular biology, pathogenesis and pathology of mumps virus. J Pathol 235:242, 2015.

World Health Organization: WHO immunological basis for immunization series. Module 16: Mumps update 2020. Available at *https://apps.who.int/iris/bitstream/handle/10665/338004/9789240017504-eng.pdf.*

208 Rabies and Other Rhabdovirus Infections

Alan C. Jackson

RABIES

Rabies is a rapidly progressive, acute infectious disease of the central nervous system (CNS) in humans and animals that is caused by infection with rabies virus. The infection is normally transmitted from animal vectors via a bite exposure. Rabies has encephalitic and paralytic forms that progress to death.

ETIOLOGIC AGENT

Rabies virus is a member of the family *Rhabdoviridae*. Two genera in this family, *Lyssavirus* and *Vesiculovirus*, contain species that cause human disease. Rabies virus is a lyssavirus that infects a broad range of mammals and causes serious neurologic disease when transmitted to humans. This single-strand RNA virus has a nonsegmented, negative-sense (antisense) genome that consists of 11,932 nucleotides and encodes 5 proteins: nucleocapsid protein, phosphoprotein, matrix protein, glycoprotein, and a large polymerase protein. Rabies virus variants, which can be characterized by distinctive nucleotide sequences, are associated with specific animal reservoirs. Six other non-rabies virus species in the *Lyssavirus* genus have been reported to cause a clinical picture similar to rabies. Vesicular stomatitis virus, a vesiculovirus, causes vesiculation and ulceration in cattle, horses, and other animals and causes a self-limited, mild, systemic illness in humans (see "Other Rhabdoviruses," below).

EPIDEMIOLOGY

Rabies is a zoonotic infection that occurs in a variety of mammals throughout the world except in Antarctica and on some islands. Rabies virus is usually transmitted to humans by the bite of an infected animal. Worldwide, endemic canine rabies is estimated to cause 59,000 human deaths annually. Most of these deaths occur in Asia and Africa, with rural populations and children disproportionally affected. Thus, in many resource-poor and resource-limited countries, canine rabies continues to be a threat to humans. However, in Latin America, rabies control efforts in dogs have been quite successful in recent years. Endemic canine rabies has been eliminated from the United States and most other resource-rich countries. Rabies is endemic in wildlife species, and a variety of animal reservoirs have been identified in different countries of the world (**Fig. 208-1**). Surveillance data from 2019 identified 4690 confirmed animal cases of rabies in the United States and Puerto Rico. Only 8.2% of these cases were in domestic animals, including 245 cases in cats, 66 in dogs, and 39 in cattle. In North American wildlife reservoirs, including bats, raccoons, skunks, and foxes, the infection is endemic, with involvement of one or more rabies virus variants in each reservoir species (**Fig. 208-2**). "Spillover" of rabies to other wildlife species and to domestic animals occurs. Bat rabies virus variants are present in every state except Hawaii and are responsible for most indigenously acquired human rabies cases in the United States. Raccoon rabies is endemic along the entire eastern coast of the United States. Skunk rabies is present in the midwestern states, with another focus in California. Rabies in foxes occurs in New Mexico, Arizona, and Alaska. In the United States there were two human rabies deaths in 2017, three in 2018, and none in 2019.

In Canada and Europe, epizootics of rabies in red foxes have been well controlled with the use of baits containing rabies vaccine. A similar approach, along with additional measures, is used in Canada to control incursions of raccoon rabies from the United States.

Rabies virus variants isolated from humans or other mammalian species can be identified by reverse-transcription polymerase chain reaction (RT-PCR) amplification and sequencing or by characterization with monoclonal antibodies. These techniques are helpful in human cases with no known history of exposure. Worldwide, most human rabies is transmitted from dogs in countries with endemic canine rabies and dog-to-dog transmission, and human cases can be imported by travelers returning from these regions. In North America, indigenously acquired human disease is usually associated with transmission from bats; there may be no known history of bat bite or other bat exposure in these cases. Most human cases are due to a bat rabies virus variant associated with silver-haired and tricolored bats. These are small bats whose bite may not be recognized, and the virus has adapted for replication at skin temperature and in cell types that are present in the skin.

Transmission from nonbite exposures is relatively uncommon. Aerosols generated in the laboratory or in caves containing millions of Brazilian free-tail bats have rarely caused human rabies. Transmission has resulted from corneal transplantation and also from solid-organ transplantation and a vascular conduit (for a liver transplant) from

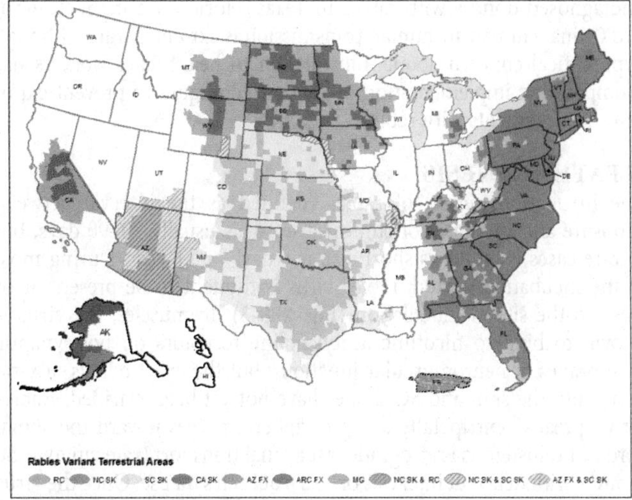

FIGURE 208-2 Distribution of the major rabies virus variants among wild terrestrial reservoirs in the United States and Puerto Rico, 2015-2019. Darker shading indicates counties with confirmed animal rabies cases in the past 5 years; lighter shading represents counties bordering enzootic counties without animal rabies cases that did not satisfy criteria for adequate surveillance. Small nonenzootic areas with no rabies cases reported in the past 15 years are shaded if they are in the vicinity of known-enzootic counties and do not satisfy criteria for adequate surveillance. ARC FX, Arctic fox rabies virus variant (RVV); AZ FX, Arizona fox RVV; CA SK, California skunk RVV; MG, Dog-mongoose RVV; NC SK, North central skunk RVV; RC, Eastern raccoon RVV; SC SK, South central skunk RVV. *(X Ma et al: Rabies surveillance in the United States during 2019. J Am Vet Med Assoc 258:1205, 2021.)*

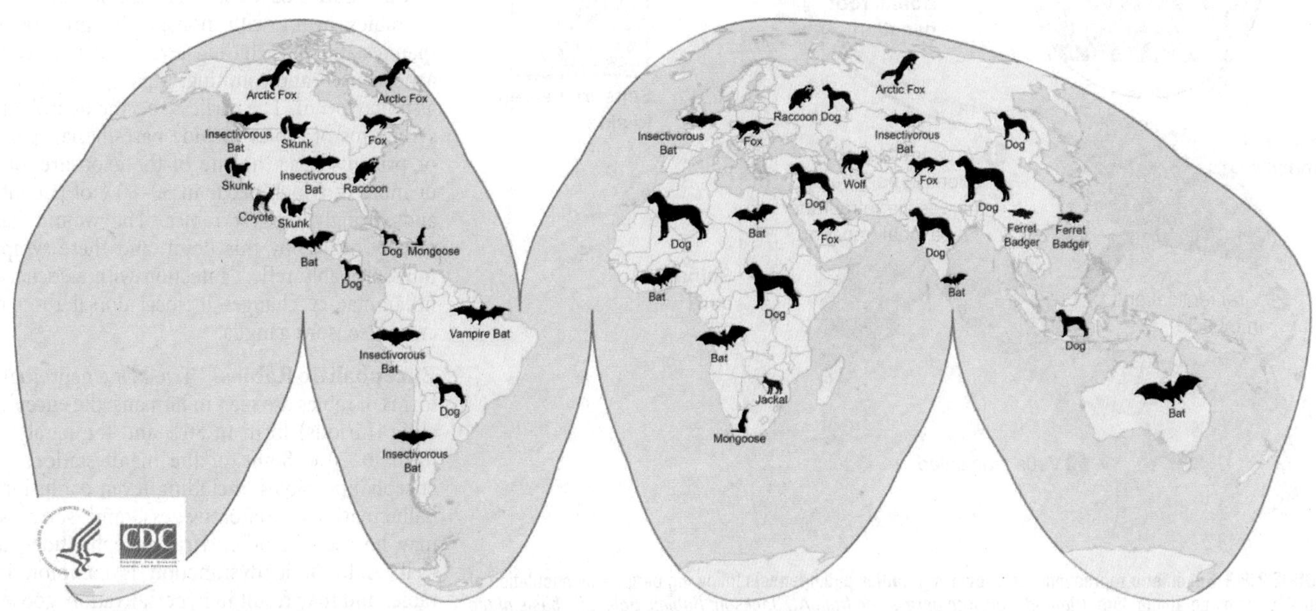

FIGURE 208-1 Distribution of global rabies vectors. *(Courtesy of the Centers for Disease Control and Prevention.)*

undiagnosed donors with rabies in Texas, Florida, Germany, Kuwait, and China. Human-to-human transmission is extremely rare, although hypothetical concern about transmission to health care workers has prompted the implementation of barrier techniques to prevent exposures from patients with rabies.

PATHOGENESIS

The incubation period of rabies (defined as the interval between exposure and the onset of clinical disease) is usually 20–90 days, but in rare cases is either as short as a few days or >1 year. During most of the incubation period, rabies virus is thought to be present at or close to the site of inoculation (**Fig. 208-3**). In muscles, the virus is known to bind to nicotinic acetylcholine receptors on postsynaptic membranes at neuromuscular junctions, but the exact details of viral entry into the skin and SC tissues have not yet been clarified. Rabies virus spreads centripetally along peripheral nerves toward the spinal cord or brainstem via retrograde fast axonal transport (rate, up to ~250 mm/d), with delays at intervals of ~12 h at each synapse. Once the virus enters the CNS, it rapidly disseminates to other regions of the CNS via fast axonal transport along neuroanatomic connections. Neurons are prominently infected in rabies; infection of astrocytes is unusual. After CNS infection becomes established, there is centrifugal spread along sensory and autonomic nerves to other tissues, including the salivary glands, heart, adrenal glands, and skin. Rabies virus replicates in acinar cells of the salivary glands and is secreted in the saliva of rabid animals that serve as vectors of the disease. There is no well-documented evidence for hematogenous spread of rabies virus.

Pathologic studies show mild inflammatory changes in the CNS in rabies, with mononuclear inflammatory infiltration in the leptomeninges, perivascular regions, and parenchyma, including microglial nodules called *Babes nodules*. Degenerative neuronal changes usually are not prominent, and there is little evidence of neuronal death; neuronophagia is observed occasionally. The pathologic changes are surprisingly mild in light of the clinical severity and fatal outcome of the disease. The most characteristic pathologic finding in rabies is the *Negri body* (**Fig. 208-4**). Negri bodies are eosinophilic cytoplasmic inclusions in brain neurons that are composed of rabies virus proteins and viral RNA. These inclusions occur in a minority of infected neurons, are commonly observed in Purkinje cells of the cerebellum and in pyramidal neurons of the hippocampus, and are less frequently seen in cortical and brainstem neurons. Negri bodies are not observed in all cases of rabies. The lack of prominent degenerative neuronal changes has led to the concept that neuronal dysfunction—rather than neuronal death—is responsible for clinical disease in rabies. The basis for behavioral changes, including the aggressive behavior of rabid animals, is not well understood but may be related to infection of serotonergic neurons in the brainstem.

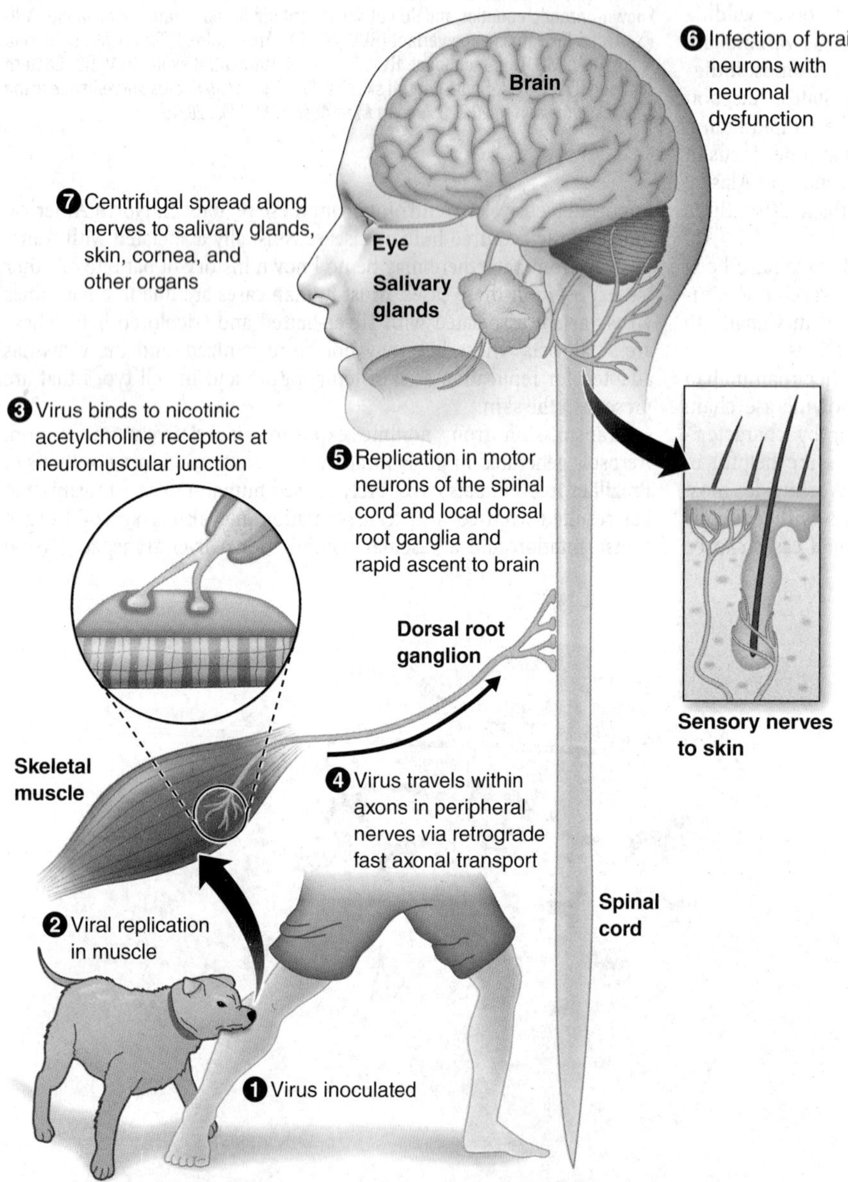

Brain
6 Infection of brain neurons with neuronal dysfunction
7 Centrifugal spread along nerves to salivary glands, skin, cornea, and other organs
Eye
Salivary glands
3 Virus binds to nicotinic acetylcholine receptors at neuromuscular junction
5 Replication in motor neurons of the spinal cord and local dorsal root ganglia and rapid ascent to brain
Dorsal root ganglion
Sensory nerves to skin
Skeletal muscle
4 Virus travels within axons in peripheral nerves via retrograde fast axonal transport
Spinal cord
2 Viral replication in muscle
1 Virus inoculated

FIGURE 208-3 Schematic representation of events in rabies pathogenesis following peripheral inoculation of rabies virus by an animal bite. *(Reproduced with permission from AC Jackson: Rabies: Scientific basis of the disease and its management, 3rd ed. Oxford, UK, Elsevier Academic Press, 2013.)*

CLINICAL MANIFESTATIONS

For rabies prevention, the emphasis must be on postexposure prophylaxis (PEP) initiated after a recognized exposure and before any symptoms or signs develop. Rabies should usually be suspected on the basis of the clinical presentation with or without a history of an exposure. The disease generally presents as atypical encephalitis with relative preservation of consciousness. Rabies may be difficult to recognize late in the clinical course when progression to coma has occurred. A minority of patients (~20%) present with acute flaccid paralysis. There are prodromal, acute neurologic, and comatose phases that usually progress to death despite aggressive therapy (**Table 208-1**).

Prodromal Features The clinical features of rabies begin with nonspecific prodromal manifestations, including fever, malaise, headache, nausea, and vomiting. Anxiety or agitation also may occur. The earliest specific neurologic symptoms of rabies include paresthesias, pain, or pruritus near the site of the exposure, one or more of which occur in 50–80% of patients and strongly suggest rabies. The wound has usually healed by this point, and these symptoms probably reflect infection with associated inflammatory changes in local dorsal root or cranial sensory ganglia.

Encephalitic Rabies Two acute neurologic forms of rabies are seen in humans: the encephalitic (furious) form in 80% and the paralytic form in 20%. Some of the manifestations of encephalitic rabies, including fever, confusion, hallucinations, combativeness, and seizures, may be seen in other viral encephalitides as well. Autonomic dysfunction is common in rabies and may result in hypersalivation, gooseflesh, cardiac arrhythmia, and priapism. In

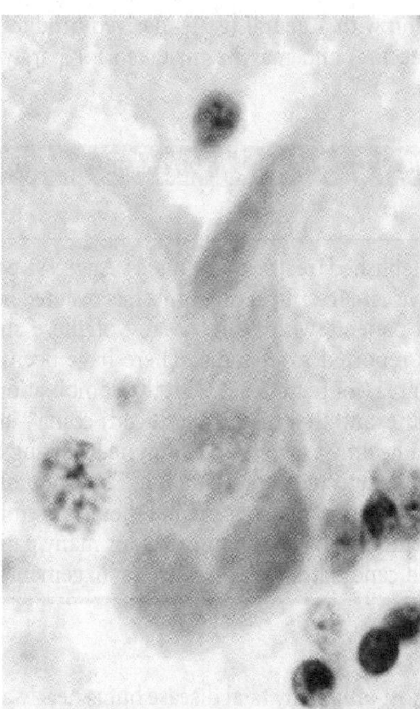

FIGURE 208-4 Three large Negri bodies in the cytoplasm of a cerebellar Purkinje cell from an 8-year-old boy who died of rabies after being bitten by a rabid dog in Mexico. *(Reproduced with permission from AC Jackson, E Lopez-Corella. N Engl J Med 335:568, 1996; © Massachusetts Medical Society.)*

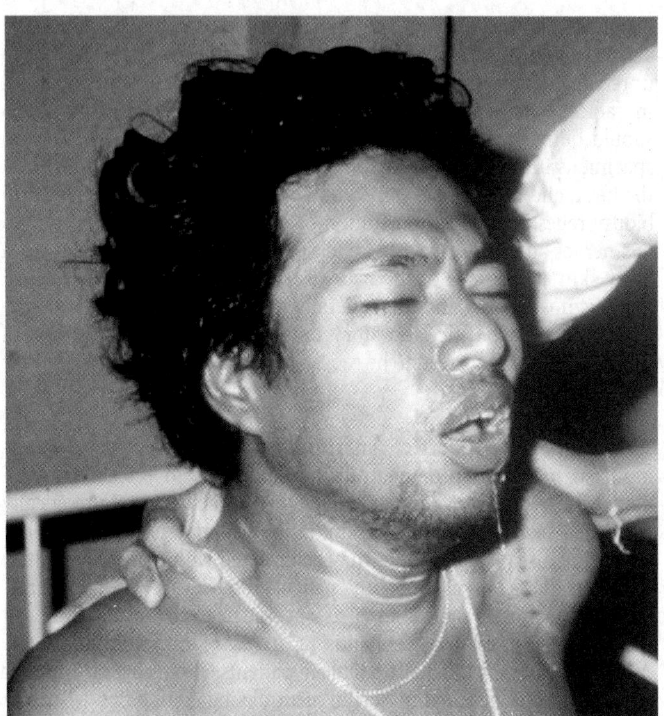

FIGURE 208-5 Hydrophobic spasm of inspiratory muscles associated with terror in a patient with encephalitic (furious) rabies who is attempting to swallow water. *(Copyright DA Warrell, Oxford, UK; with permission.)*

encephalitic rabies, episodes of hyperexcitability are typically followed by periods of complete lucidity that become shorter as the disease progresses. Rabies encephalitis is distinguished by early brainstem involvement, which results in the classic features of *hydrophobia* (involuntary, painful contraction of the diaphragm and accessory respiratory, laryngeal, and pharyngeal muscles in response to swallowing liquids) (**Fig. 208-5**) and *aerophobia* (the same features caused by stimulation from a draft of air). These symptoms are probably due to dysfunction of infected brainstem neurons that normally inhibit inspiratory neurons near the nucleus ambiguus, resulting in exaggerated defense reflexes that protect the respiratory tract. The combination of hypersalivation and pharyngeal dysfunction is responsible for the classic appearance of "foaming at the mouth." Brainstem dysfunction progresses rapidly, and coma—followed within days by death—is the rule unless the course is prolonged by supportive measures. With such measures, late complications can include cardiac and/or respiratory failure, disturbances of water balance (syndrome of inappropriate antidiuretic hormone secretion or diabetes insipidus), noncardiogenic pulmonary edema, and gastrointestinal hemorrhage. Cardiac arrhythmias may be due to dysfunction affecting vital centers in the brainstem or autonomic pathways or to myocarditis. Multiple-organ failure is common in patients treated aggressively in critical care units.

TABLE 208-1 Clinical Stages of Rabies

STAGE	TYPICAL DURATION	SYMPTOMS AND SIGNS
Incubation period	20–90 days	None
Prodrome	2–10 days	Fever, malaise, anorexia, nausea, vomiting; paresthesias, pain, or pruritus at the wound site
Acute Neurologic Disease		
Encephalitic (80%)	2–7 days	Anxiety, agitation, hyperactivity, bizarre behavior, hallucinations, autonomic dysfunction, hydrophobia
Paralytic (20%)	2–10 days	Flaccid paralysis in limb(s) progressing to quadriparesis with facial paralysis
Coma, death[a]	0–14 days	

[a]Recovery is rare.

Source: Adapted from MAW Hattwick: Rabies virus, in *Principles and Practice of Infectious Diseases,* GL Mandell et al (eds). New York, Wiley, 1979.

Paralytic Rabies About 20% of patients have paralytic rabies in which muscle weakness predominates and cardinal features of encephalitic rabies (hyperexcitability, hydrophobia, and aerophobia) are lacking. There is early and prominent flaccid muscle weakness, often beginning in the bitten extremity and spreading to produce quadriparesis and facial weakness. Sphincter involvement is common, sensory involvement is usually mild, and these cases are commonly misdiagnosed as Guillain-Barré syndrome. Patients with paralytic rabies generally survive a few days longer than those with encephalitic rabies, but multiple-organ failure nevertheless ensues.

LABORATORY INVESTIGATIONS

Most routine laboratory tests in rabies yield normal results or show nonspecific abnormalities. Complete blood counts are usually normal. Examination of cerebrospinal fluid (CSF) often reveals mild mononuclear-cell pleocytosis with a mildly elevated protein level. Severe pleocytosis (>1000 white cells/μL) is unusual and should prompt a search for an alternative diagnosis. Imaging is usually performed to exclude other diagnostic possibilities. CT head scans are usually normal in rabies. MRI brain scans may show signal abnormalities in the brainstem or other gray-matter areas, but these findings are variable and nonspecific. Electroencephalograms typically show only nonspecific abnormalities. Of course, important tests in suspected cases of rabies include those that may identify an alternative, potentially treatable diagnosis (see "Differential Diagnosis," below).

DIAGNOSIS

In North America, a diagnosis of rabies often is not considered until relatively late in the clinical course, even with a typical clinical presentation. This diagnosis should be considered in patients presenting with acute atypical encephalitis or acute flaccid paralysis, including those in whom Guillain-Barré syndrome is suspected. The absence of an animal-bite history is common in North America, particularly due to unrecognized bat exposures. The lack of hydrophobia is not unusual in rabies. Once rabies is suspected, rabies-specific laboratory tests should be performed to confirm the diagnosis. Diagnostically useful specimens include serum, CSF, fresh saliva, skin biopsy samples from the neck, and brain tissue (rarely obtained before death). Because skin biopsy relies on the demonstration of rabies virus antigen in cutaneous nerves at the base of hair follicles, samples are usually taken from hairy skin at the nape of the neck. Corneal impression smears are of low diagnostic yield and are generally not performed. Negative antemortem rabies-specific laboratory tests never exclude a diagnosis of rabies, and tests may need to be repeated after an interval for diagnostic confirmation.

Rabies Virus–Specific Antibodies In a previously unimmunized patient, serum neutralizing antibodies to rabies virus are diagnostic. However, because rabies virus infects immunologically privileged neuronal tissues, serum antibodies may not develop until late in the disease. Antibodies may be detected within a few days after the onset of symptoms, but some patients die without detectable antibodies. The presence of rabies virus–specific neutralizing antibodies in the CSF suggests rabies encephalitis, regardless of immunization status. A diagnosis of rabies is questionable in patients who recover from their illness without developing serum neutralizing antibodies to rabies virus.

RT-PCR Amplification Detection of rabies virus RNA by RT-PCR is highly sensitive and specific. This technique can detect virus in fresh saliva samples, skin biopsy specimens, CSF (less sensitive), and brain tissues. In addition, RT-PCR with genetic sequencing can distinguish among rabies virus variants, permitting identification of the probable source of an infection.

Direct Fluorescent Antibody Testing Direct fluorescent antibody (DFA) testing with rabies virus antibodies conjugated to fluorescent dyes is highly sensitive and specific for the detection of rabies virus antigen in tissues; the test can be performed quickly and applied to skin biopsy and brain tissue samples. In skin biopsy samples, rabies virus antigen may be detected in cutaneous nerves at the base of hair follicles.

DIFFERENTIAL DIAGNOSIS

The diagnosis of rabies may be difficult without a history of animal exposure, and no exposure to an animal (e.g., a bat) may be recalled. The presentation of rabies is usually quite different from that of acute viral encephalitis due to most other causes, including herpes simplex encephalitis and arboviral (e.g., West Nile) encephalitis. Early neurologic symptoms may occur at the site of the bite, and there may be early features of brainstem involvement with preservation of consciousness. Anti–*N*-methyl-D-aspartate receptor (anti-NMDA) encephalitis occurs in young patients (especially females) and is characterized by behavioral changes, autonomic instability, hypoventilation, and seizures. Many other antibodies are also associated with autoimmune encephalitis. Postinfectious (immune-mediated) encephalomyelitis may follow influenza, measles, mumps, and other infections; it may also occur as a sequela of immunization with rabies vaccines derived from neural tissues, which are now infrequently used and only in resource-limited and resource-poor countries. Rabies may present with unusual neuropsychiatric symptoms and may be misdiagnosed as a psychiatric disorder. Rabies hysteria (now classified as a somatic symptom disorder) may occur as a psychological response to the fear of rabies and is often characterized by a shorter incubation period than rabies, aggressive behavior, inability to communicate, and a long course with recovery.

As previously mentioned, paralytic rabies may mimic Guillain-Barré syndrome. In these cases, fever, bladder dysfunction, a normal sensory examination, and CSF pleocytosis favor a diagnosis of rabies. Conversely, Guillain-Barré syndrome may occur as a complication of rabies vaccination with a neural tissue–derived product (e.g., suckling mouse brain vaccine) and may be mistaken for paralytic rabies (i.e., vaccine failure).

TREATMENT
Rabies

There is no established treatment for rabies. Aggressive management with supportive care in critical care units has resulted in the survival of at least 30 patients with rabies. Many of these survivors have recently been reported from India. There have been many recent treatment failures (more than 55) with the combination of antiviral drugs, ketamine, and therapeutic (induced) coma—measures that were used in a healthy survivor in whom neutralizing antibodies to rabies virus were detected at presentation. Expert opinion is recommended before a course of experimental therapy is embarked upon. A palliative approach may be appropriate for many patients who are not considered candidates for aggressive management.

PROGNOSIS

Rabies is an almost uniformly fatal disease but is nearly always preventable after recognized exposures with appropriate postexposure therapy during the early incubation period (see below). All but 1 of 30 documented survivors of rabies received 1 or more doses of rabies vaccine before disease onset. The single survivor who had not received vaccine had neutralizing antibodies to rabies virus in serum and CSF at clinical presentation. Most patients with rabies die within several days of the onset of illness, despite aggressive care in a critical care unit.

PREVENTION

Postexposure Prophylaxis Since there is no effective therapy for rabies, it is extremely important to prevent the disease after an animal exposure. **Figure 208-6** shows the steps involved in making decisions about PEP. On the basis of the exposure history and local epidemiologic information, the physician must decide whether initiation of PEP is warranted. Healthy dogs, cats, or ferrets may be confined and observed for 10 days. PEP is not necessary if the animal remains healthy. If the animal develops signs of rabies during the observation period, it should be euthanized immediately; the head should be transported to the laboratory under refrigeration, rabies virus should be sought by DFA testing, and viral isolation should be attempted by cell culture and/or mouse inoculation. Any animal other than a dog, cat, or ferret should be euthanized immediately and the head submitted for laboratory examination. In high-risk exposures and in areas where canine rabies is endemic, rabies prophylaxis should be initiated without waiting for laboratory results. If the laboratory results prove to be negative, it may safely be concluded that the animal's saliva did not contain rabies virus, and immunization should be discontinued. If an animal escapes after an exposure, it must be considered rabid, and PEP must be initiated unless information from public health officials indicates otherwise (i.e., there is no endemic rabies in the area). Although controversial, the use of PEP may be warranted when a person (e.g., a small child or a sleeping adult) has been present in the same space as a bat and an unrecognized bite cannot be reliably excluded.

PEP includes local wound care and both active and passive immunization. It is important that current recommendations are followed very closely because minor deviations can lead to failure of prophylactic measures. Local wound care is essential and may greatly decrease the risk of rabies virus infection. Wound care should not be delayed, even if the initiation of immunization is postponed pending the results of the 10-day observation period. All bite wounds and scratches should be washed thoroughly with soap and water. Devitalized tissues should be debrided, tetanus prophylaxis given, and antibiotic treatment initiated whenever indicated.

Previously unvaccinated persons (but not those who have previously been immunized) should be passively immunized with rabies

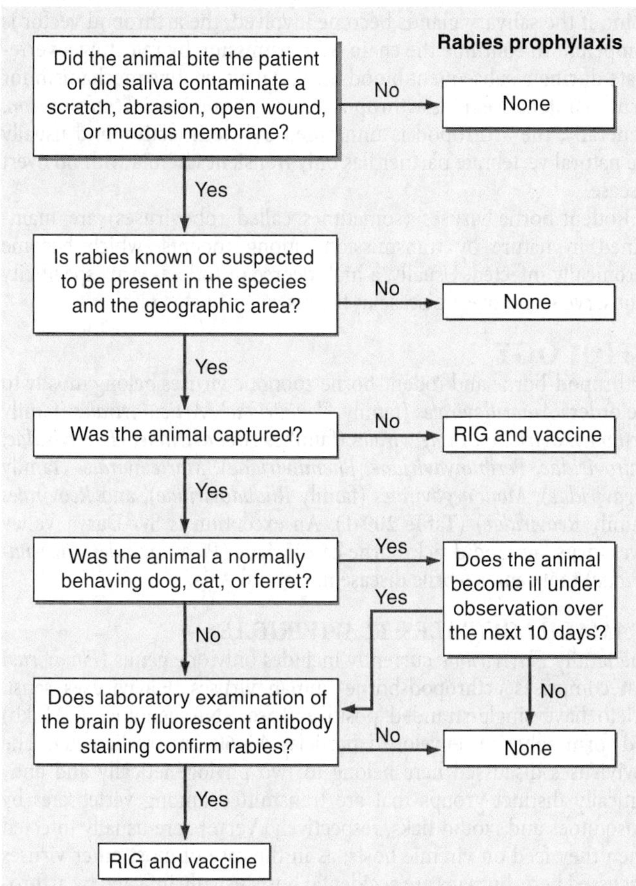

FIGURE 208-6 Algorithm for rabies postexposure prophylaxis. RIG, rabies immune globulin. *(Reproduced with permission from L Corey, in Harrison's Principles of Internal Medicine, 15th ed. E Braunwald et al [eds]: New York, McGraw-Hill, 2001.)*

immune globulin (RIG). If RIG is not immediately available, it should be administered no later than 7 days after the first vaccine dose. After day 7, endogenous antibodies are being produced, and passive immunization may actually be counterproductive. If anatomically feasible, the entire dose of RIG (20 IU/kg) should be infiltrated at the site of the bite, and any RIG remaining after infiltration of the bite site should be administered IM at a distant site. Recent recommendations by the World Health Organization indicate that under certain circumstances the remainder of the dose does not need to be administered after local infiltration of the wound(s). With multiple or large wounds, the RIG preparation may need to be diluted in order to obtain a sufficient volume for adequate infiltration of all wound sites. If the exposure involves a mucous membrane, the entire dose should be administered IM. Rabies vaccine and RIG should never be administered at the same site or with the same syringe. Commercially available RIG in the United States is purified from the serum of hyperimmunized human donors. These human RIG preparations are much better tolerated than are the equine-derived preparations still in use in some countries (see below). Serious adverse effects of human RIG are uncommon. Local pain and low-grade fever may occur.

Two purified inactivated rabies vaccines are available for rabies PEP in the United States. They are highly immunogenic and remarkably safe compared with earlier vaccines. Four 1-mL doses of rabies vaccine should be given IM in the deltoid area. (The anterolateral aspect of the thigh also is acceptable in children.) Gluteal injections, which may not always reach muscle, should not be given and have been associated with rare vaccine failures. Ideally, the first dose should be given as soon as possible after exposure; failing that, it should be given without further delay. The three additional doses should be given on days 3, 7, and 14; a fifth dose on day 28 is no longer recommended. Pregnancy is not a contraindication for immunization. Glucocorticoids and other immunosuppressive medications may interfere with the development of active immunity and should not be administered during PEP unless they are essential. Routine measurement of serum neutralizing antibody titers is not required, but titers should be measured 2–4 weeks after immunization in immunocompromised persons. Local reactions (pain, erythema, edema, and pruritus) and mild systemic reactions (fever, myalgias, headache, and nausea) are common; anti-inflammatory and antipyretic medications may be used, but immunization should not be discontinued. Systemic allergic reactions are uncommon, but anaphylaxis does occur rarely and can be treated with epinephrine and antihistamines. The risk of rabies development should be carefully considered before the decision is made to discontinue vaccination because of an adverse reaction.

Most of the burden of rabies PEP is borne by persons with the fewest resources. In addition to the rabies vaccines discussed above, vaccines grown in either primary cell lines (hamster or dog kidney) or continuous cell lines (Vero cells) are satisfactory and are available in many countries outside the United States. Less expensive vaccines derived from neural tissues are still used in a diminishing number of developing countries; however, these vaccines are associated with serious neuroparalytic complications, including postinfectious encephalomyelitis and Guillain-Barré syndrome. The use of these vaccines should be discontinued as soon as possible, and progress has been made in this regard. Worldwide, more than 10 million individuals receive postexposure rabies vaccine each year.

If human RIG is unavailable, purified equine RIG can be used in the same manner at a dose of 40 IU/kg. The incidence of anaphylactic reactions and serum sickness has been low with recent equine RIG products.

Preexposure Rabies Vaccination Preexposure rabies prophylaxis should be considered for people with an occupational or recreational risk of rabies exposures and also for certain travelers to rabies-endemic areas. The primary schedule consists of three doses of rabies vaccine given on days 0, 7, and 21 or 28. Serum neutralizing antibody tests help determine the need for subsequent booster doses. When a previously immunized individual is exposed to rabies, two booster doses of vaccine should be administered on days 0 and 3. Wound care remains essential. As stated above, RIG should not be administered to previously vaccinated persons.

OTHER RHABDOVIRUSES

OTHER LYSSAVIRUSES

A growing number of lyssaviruses other than rabies virus have been discovered to infect bat populations in Europe, Africa, Asia, and Australia. Six of these viruses have produced a very small number of cases of a human disease indistinguishable from rabies: European bat lyssaviruses 1 and 2, Australian bat lyssavirus, Irkut virus, and Duvenhage virus. Mokola virus, a lyssavirus that has been isolated from shrews with an unknown reservoir species in Africa, may also produce human disease indistinguishable from rabies.

VESICULAR STOMATITIS VIRUS

Vesicular stomatitis is a viral disease of cattle, horses, pigs, and some wild mammals. Vesicular stomatitis virus is a member of the genus *Vesiculovirus* in the family *Rhabdoviridae*. Outbreaks of vesicular stomatitis in horses and cattle occur sporadically in the southwestern United States. The animal infection is associated with severe vesiculation and ulceration of oral tissues, teats, and feet and may be clinically indistinguishable from the more dangerous foot-and-mouth disease. Epidemics are usually seasonal, typically beginning in the late spring, and are probably due to arthropod vectors. Direct animal-to-animal spread can also occur, although the virus cannot penetrate intact skin. Transmission to humans usually results from direct contact with infected animals (particularly cattle) and occasionally follows laboratory exposure. In human disease, early conjunctivitis is followed by an acute influenza-like illness with fever, chills, nausea, vomiting, headache, retrobulbar pain, myalgias, substernal pain, malaise, pharyngitis, and lymphadenitis. Small vesicular lesions may be present on the buccal mucosa or on the fingers. Encephalitis is very rare. The illness usually lasts 3–6 days, with complete recovery. Subclinical infections are common. A serologic diagnosis can be made on the basis of a rise in titer of complement-fixing or neutralizing antibodies. Therapy is symptom-based.

FURTHER READING

Fooks AR et al: Current status of rabies and prospects for elimination. Lancet 384:1389, 2014.

Fooks AR, Jackson AC (eds). *Rabies: Scientific Basis of the Disease and Its Management*, 4th ed. London, Elsevier Academic Press, 2020.

Jackson AC: Treatment of rabies. In: Post TW, ed. UpToDate. Waltham, Massachusetts: Wolters Kluwer, 2021. *www.uptodate.com.*

Letchworth GJ et al: Vesicular stomatitis. Vet J 157:239, 1999.

Manning SE et al: Human rabies prevention—United States, 2008: Recommendations of the Advisory Committee on Immunization Practices. MMWR Recomm Rep 57(RR-3):1, 2008.

World Health Organization: *WHO Expert Consultation on Rabies: Third Report* (WHO Technical Report Series No. 1012). Geneva, World Health Organization, 2018. Available at *apps.who.int/iris/bitstream/handle/10665/272364/9789241210218-eng.pdf.* Accessed June 17, 2021.

209 Arthropod-Borne and Rodent-Borne Virus Infections

Jens H. Kuhn, Ian Crozier

This chapter summarizes the major features of selected arthropod-borne and rodent-borne viruses. Numerous viruses of this category are transmitted in nature among animals without ever infecting humans. Other viruses incidentally infect humans, but few induce disease. In addition, some viruses are regularly introduced into human populations or spread among humans by arthropods (specifically, insects and ticks) or by chronically infected rodents. These zoonotic viruses are taxonomically diverse and therefore differ fundamentally from one another in terms of virion morphology, replication strategies, genomic organization, and genome sequence. Although a virus's classification in a taxon is enlightening regarding natural maintenance strategies, sensitivity to antiviral agents, and aspects of pathogenesis, the classification does not necessarily predict which clinical signs and symptoms (if any) the virus will cause in humans. Zoonotic viruses are evolving, and "new" zoonotic viruses are regularly discovered. The epizootiology and epidemiology of zoonotic viruses continue to change because of environmental alterations affecting vectors, reservoirs, wildlife, livestock, and humans. Zoonotic viruses are most numerous in the tropics but are also found in temperate and even frigid climates. The distribution and seasonal activity of zoonotic viruses may vary, and the rate at which they change is likely to depend largely on ecologic conditions (e.g., rainfall and temperature), which can affect the density of virus vectors and reservoirs and the development of infection.

Arthropod-borne viruses (arboviruses) infect their vectors after ingestion of blood meals from viremic, usually nonhuman vertebrates; some arthropods may also become infected by saliva-activated transmission. The arthropod vectors then develop chronic systemic infection as the viruses penetrate the gut and spread throughout the body to the salivary glands; such virus dissemination, referred to as *extrinsic incubation*, typically lasts 1–3 weeks in mosquitoes. At this point, if the salivary glands become involved, the arthropod vector is competent to continue the chain of transmission by infecting a vertebrate during a subsequent blood meal. An alternative mechanism for virus maintenance in its arthropod vector is *transovarial transmission*. Generally, the arthropod is unharmed by the infection and usually the natural vertebrate partner has only transient viremia with no overt disease.

Rodent-borne viruses (sometimes called roboviruses) are maintained in nature by transmission among rodents, which become chronically infected. Usually, a high degree of rodent–virus specificity is observed, and overt disease in the reservoir host is rare.

ETIOLOGY

Arthropod-borne and rodent-borne zoonotic viruses belong mostly to the orders *Amarillovirales* (family *Flaviviridae*), *Articulavirales* (family *Orthomyxoviridae*), *Bunyavirales* (families *Arenaviridae, Hantaviridae, Nairoviridae, Peribunyaviridae, Phenuiviridae*), *Martellivirales* (family *Togaviridae*), *Mononegavirales* (family *Rhabdoviridae*), and *Reovirales* (family *Reoviridae*) (**Table 209-1**). An exception is Syr-Darya Valley fever virus, an ixodid tick-borne cardiovirus (*Picornavirales*: *Picornaviridae*) that causes febrile disease in Central Asia.

AMARILLOVIRALES: FLAVIVIRIDAE

The family *Flaviviridae* currently includes only one genus (*Flavivirus*) that comprises arthropod-borne human viruses. Flaviviruses sensu stricto have single-stranded positive-sense RNA genomes (~11 kb) and form spherical enveloped particles 40–60 nm in diameter. The flaviviruses discussed here belong to two phylogenetically and antigenically distinct groups that are transmitted among vertebrates by mosquitoes and ixodid ticks, respectively. Vectors are usually infected when they feed on viremic hosts; as in the case of most other viruses discussed here, humans are accidental hosts usually infected by arthropod bites. Arthropods maintain flavivirus infections horizontally, although transovarial transmission has been documented. Under certain circumstances, flaviviruses can also be transmitted by aerosol or via contaminated food products; in particular, raw milk can transmit tick-borne encephalitis virus.

ARTICULAVIRALES: ORTHOMYXOVIRIDAE

The family *Orthomyxoviridae* includes two genera of medically relevant arthropod-borne viruses: *Quaranjavirus* and *Thogotovirus*. Quaranjaviruses are transmitted among birds by ixodid ticks, whereas thogotoviruses have a predilection for mammalian host reservoirs and can be transmitted by both ixodid ticks and mosquitoes.

BUNYAVIRALES: ARENAVIRIDAE

The members of the family *Arenaviridae* that infect humans are all assigned to the genus *Mammarenavirus*. The members of this genus are divided into two main phylogenetic branches: Old World viruses (the Lassa–lymphocytic choriomeningitis serocomplex) and New World viruses (the Tacaribe serocomplex). Mammarenaviruses form spherical, oval, or pleomorphic enveloped and spiked virions (~50–300 nm in diameter) that bud from the plasma membrane of the infected cell. The particles contain two genomic single-stranded RNAs (S, ~3.5 kb; and L, ~7.5 kb), encoding structural proteins in an ambisense orientation. Most mammarenaviruses persist in nature by chronically infecting rodents. The human Old World mammarenaviruses are maintained by murid rodents that often are persistently viremic and commonly transmit viruses vertically and horizontally. One Old World mammarenavirus associated with human infections is maintained by shrews. Human New World mammarenaviruses are found in cricetid rodents; horizontal transmission is typical, vertical infection may occur, and persistent viremia may be observed. Strikingly, each mammarenavirus is predominantly adapted to one particular type of rodent. Humans usually become infected through inhalation of or direct contact with infected rodent excreta or secreta (e.g., aerosols of rodents in harvesting machines, aerosolized dried rodent urine or feces in barns or houses, direct contact with rodents in traps). Person-to-person transmission of mammarenaviruses is uncommon.

TABLE 209-1 Zoonotic Arthropod- and Rodent-Borne Viruses That Infect Humans

VIRUS GROUP	VIRUS (ABBREVIATION)	MAJOR NONHUMAN HOST(S)[a]	VECTOR(S)	SYNDROME[b]
Alphaviruses (Barmah Forest serocomplex)	Barmah Forest virus (BFV)	Horses, possums	Biting midges (*Culicoides marksi*), mosquitoes (*Aedes camptorhynchus, A. normanensis, A. notoscriptus, A. vigilax, Culex annulirostris*)	A/R
Alphaviruses (eastern equine encephalitis serocomplex)	Eastern equine encephalitis virus (EEEV)	Freshwater swamp passeriform birds, but also opportunistic amphibians, other birds (emu, gallinaceous poultry, pheasants), reptiles, and mammals (goats, horses, pigs)	Mosquitoes (*Aedes, Coquillettidia, Culex* spp.; *Culiseta melanura, Mansonia perturbans, Psorophora* spp.)	E
	Madariaga virus (MADV)	Likely birds and reptiles	Mosquitoes (*Culex, Culiseta* spp.)	F/M, E
Alphaviruses (Semliki Forest serocomplex)	Chikungunya virus (CHIKV)	Bats, nonhuman primates	Mosquitoes (*Aedes, Culex* spp.)	A/R[c]
	Mayaro virus (MAYV)	Nonhuman primates, possums, rodents; possibly caimans, horses, sheep	Mosquitoes (predominantly *Haemagogus* spp., but also *Aedes, Culex, Mansonia, Psorophora, Sabethes*)	A/R
	O'nyong-nyong virus[d] (ONNV)	Unknown	Mosquitoes (in particular *Anopheles gambiae, A. funestus, Mansonia* spp.)	A/R
	Una virus (UNAV)	Birds, horses, rodents	Mosquitoes (*Aedes, Anopheles, Coquillettidia, Culex, Ochlerotatus, Psorophora* spp.)	F/M
	Ross River virus (RRV)	Macropods, rodents	Mosquitoes (*Aedes normanensis, A. vigilax, Culex annulirostris*)	A/R
	Semliki Forest virus (SFV)	Birds, rodents	Mosquitoes (*Aedes, Culex* spp.)	A/R
Alphaviruses (Venezuelan equine encephalitis serocomplex)	Everglades virus (EVEV)	Hispid cotton rats (*Sigmodon hispidus*)	Mosquitoes (*Culex cedecei*)	F/M, E
	Mucambo virus (MUCV)	Nonhuman primates, rodents	Mosquitoes (*Culex, Ochlerotatus* spp.)	F/M, E
	Tonate virus (TONV)	Birds, Suriname crested oropendolas (*Psarocolius decumanus*)	Mosquitoes (*Anopheles, Coquillettidia, Culex, Mansonia, Uranotaenia, Wyeomyia* spp.), sandflies (*Lutzomyia* spp.)	F/M, E
	Venezuelan equine encephalitis virus (VEEV)	Equids, rodents	Mosquitoes (*Aedes, Culex* spp., *Psorophora confinnis*)	F/M, E
Alphaviruses (western equine encephalitis serocomplex)	Sindbis virus[e] (SINV)	Typically birds, but also frogs and rats	Typically mosquitoes (*Culex, Culiseta* spp.), but tick isolation has been reported	A/R
	Western equine encephalitis virus (WEEV)	Equids, lagomorphs, passeriform birds, pheasants	Mosquitoes (*Aedes* spp., *Culex tarsalis, Culiseta* spp.)	E
Bandaviruses (Bhanja serocomplex)	Bhanja virus[f] (BHAV)	Cattle, four-toed hedgehog (*Atelerix albiventris*), goats, sheep, striped ground squirrels (*Xerus erythropus*)	Ixodid ticks (*Amblyomma, Dermacentor, Haemaphysalis, Hyalomma, Rhipicephalus* spp.)	E, F/M
	Heartland virus (HRTV)	Cattle, deer, elk, goats, raccoons, sheep?	Ixodid ticks (*Amblyomma americanum*)	F/M
	Severe fever with thrombocytopenia syndrome virus[g] (SFTSV)	Cats, cattle, chickens, dogs, goats, rodents, sheep?	Ixodid ticks (*Amblyomma testudinarium*, Haemaphysalis *concinna, H. flava, H. longicornis, Ixodes nipponensis, Rhipicephalus microplus*)	F/M, VHF
Bunyavirals (family and genus undetermined)	Bangui virus (BGIV)	Unknown	Unknown	F/M
Coltiviruses	Colorado tick fever virus (CTFV)	Bushy-tailed woodrats (*Neotoma cinerea*), Columbian ground squirrels (*Spermophilus columbianus*), deermice (*Peromyscus maniculatus*), golden-mantled ground squirrels (*Spermophilus lateralis*), least chipmunks (*Tamias minimus*), North American porcupines (*Erethizon dorsata*), yellow pine chipmunks (*Tamias amoenus*)	Ixodid ticks (predominantly *Dermacentor andersoni*)	E, F/M
	Eyach virus (EYAV)	Lagomorphs, rodents	Ixodid ticks (*Ixodes ricinus, I. ventalloi*)	E, F/M
	Salmon River virus (SRV)	Unknown	Ixodid ticks (*Ixodes* spp.)	E, F/M

(*Continued*)

TABLE 209-1 Zoonotic Arthropod- and Rodent-Borne Viruses That Infect Humans (Continued)

VIRUS GROUP	VIRUS (ABBREVIATION)	MAJOR NONHUMAN HOST(S)[a]	VECTOR(S)	SYNDROME[b]
Flaviviruses (mosquito-borne)	Dengue viruses 1–4 (DENV 1–4)	Nonhuman primates	Mosquitoes (predominantly *Aedes aegypti, A. albopictus*)	F/M, VHF
	Edge Hill virus (EHV)	Bandicoots, dogs, wallabies	Mosquitoes (*Aedes vigilax, Culex annulirostris*)	F/M
	Japanese encephalitis virus (JEV)	Ardeid wading birds (in particular herons), horses, pigs	Mosquitoes (*Culex* spp., in particular *C. tritaeniorhynchus*)	E
	Kokobera virus (KOKV)	Macropods, horses	Mosquitoes (*Culex* spp.)	A/R
	Murray Valley encephalitis virus[h] (MVEV)	Birds	Mosquitoes (predominantly *C. annulirostris*)	E
	Rocio virus (ROCV)	Rufous-collared sparrows (*Zonotrichia capensis*)	Mosquitoes (*Aedes, Culex, Psorophora* spp.)	E
	St. Louis encephalitis virus (SLEV)	Columbiform and passeriform birds (finches, sparrows)	Mosquitoes (predominantly *Culex* spp., in particular *C. nigripalpus, C. pipiens, C. quinquefasciatus, C. tarsalis*)	E
	Usutu virus (USUV)	Passeriform birds	Mosquitoes (*Culex* spp., in particular *C. pipiens*)	(E)
	Stratford virus (STRV)	Unknown	Mosquitoes (*A. vigilax*)	F/M
	West Nile virus (WNV)[i]	Passeriform birds (blackbirds, crows, finches, sparrows), small mammals, horses	Mosquitoes (*Culex* spp., in particular *C. pipiens, C. quinquefasciatus, C. restuans, C. tarsalis*)	E
	Yellow fever virus (YFV)	Nonhuman primates (*Alouatta, Ateles, Cebus, Cercopithecus, Colobus* spp.)	Mosquitoes (*Aedes* spp., in particular *Ae. aegypti*)	VHF
	Zika virus (ZIKV)	Nonhuman primates (*Macaca, Pongo* spp.)	Mosquitoes (*Aedes* spp.)	A/R, F/M
Flaviviruses (tick-borne)	Alkhurma hemorrhagic fever virus (AHFV)[j]	Unknown	Sand tampans (*Ornithodoros savignyi*)	VHF
	Karshi virus (KSIV)	Great gerbils (*Rhombomys opimus*)	Argasid ticks (*Ornithodoros capensis*), ixodid ticks (*Hyalomma asiaticum*)	E, F/M
	Kyasanur Forest disease virus (KFDV)[k]	Indomalayan vandeleurias (*Vandeleuria oleracea*), roof rats (*Rattus rattus*)	Ixodid ticks (predominantly *Haemaphysalis spinigera*)	VHF
	Omsk hemorrhagic fever virus (OHFV)	Migratory birds, rodents	Ixodid ticks (predominantly *Dermacentor* spp.)	VHF
	Powassan virus (POWV)	Red squirrels (*Tamiasciurus hudsonicus*), white-footed deermice (*Peromyscus leucopus*), woodchucks (*Marmota monax*), other small mammals	Ixodid ticks (in particular *Ixodes cookei*, other *Ixodes* spp., *Dermacentor* spp.)	E
	Tick-borne encephalitis virus (TBEV)	Passeriform birds, deer, eulipotyphla, goats, grouse, small mammals, rodents, sheep	Ixodid ticks (*Ixodes gibbosus, I. persulcatus, I. ricinus*; sporadically *Dermacentor, Haemaphysalis, Hyalomma* spp.)	E, F/M, (VHF)
Mammarenaviruses (Old World)	Lassa virus (LASV)	Natal mastomys (*Mastomys natalensis*), likely other rodents	None	F/M, VHF
	Lujo virus (LUJV)	Unknown	None	VHF
	Lymphocytic choriomeningitis virus (LCMV)	House mice (*Mus musculus*)	None	E, F/M, (VHF)
Mammarenaviruses (New World)	Chapare virus (CHAPV)	Unknown	None	VHF
	Guanarito virus (GTOV)	Short-tailed zygodonts (*Zygodontomys brevicauda*)	None	VHF
	Junín virus (JUNV)	Drylands lauchas (*Calomys musculinus*)	None	VHF
	Machupo virus (MACV)	Big lauchas (*Calomys callosus*)	None	VHF
	Sabiá virus (SBAV)	Unknown	None	VHF
	Whitewater Arroyo virus (WWAV)[l]	White-throated woodrats (*Neotoma albigula*)	None	(E)
Orbiviruses	Kemerovo virus (KEMV)	Birds, rodents	Ixodid ticks (*Ixodes persulcatus*)	E, F/M
	Lebombo virus (LEBV)	Unknown	Mosquitoes (*Aedes, Mansonia* spp.)	F/M
	Orungo virus (ORUV)	Camels, cattle, goats, nonhuman primates, sheep	Mosquitoes (*Aedes, Anopheles, Culex* spp.)	E, F/M
	Tribeč virus (TRBV)[m]	Bank voles (*Myodes glareolus*), birds, common pine voles (*Microtus subterraneus*), goats, hares	Ixodid ticks (*Ixodes persulcatus, I. ricinus*)	F/M

(*Continued*)

TABLE 209-1 Zoonotic Arthropod- and Rodent-Borne Viruses That Infect Humans (Continued)

VIRUS GROUP	VIRUS (ABBREVIATION)	MAJOR NONHUMAN HOST(S)[a]	VECTOR(S)	SYNDROME[b]
Orthobunyaviruses (Anopheles A serogroup)	Tacaiuma virus (TCMV)	Nonhuman primates	Mosquitoes (*Anopheles*, *Haemagogus* spp.)	F/M
Orthobunyaviruses (Bunyamwera serogroup)	Batai virus (BATV)[n]	Birds, camels, cattle, goats, rodents, sheep	Mosquitoes (*Aedes abnormalis*, *A. curtipes*, *Anopheles barbirostris*, *Culex gelidus*, other spp.)	F/M
	Bunyamwera virus (BUNV)	Birds, cows, goats, horses, sheep	Mosquitoes (*Aedes* spp.)	F/M
	Cache Valley virus (CVV)	Cattle, deer, foxes, horses, nonhuman primates, raccoons	Mosquitoes (*Aedes*, *Anopheles*, *Culiseta* spp.)	F/M
	Fort Sherman virus (FSV)	Cattle, goats, horses, sheep?	Mosquitoes?	F/M
	Germiston virus (GERV)	Rodents	Mosquitoes (*Culex* spp.)	F/M
	Guaroa virus (GROV)	Unknown	Mosquitoes (*Anopheles* spp.)	F/M
	Ilesha virus (ILEV)	Unknown	Mosquitoes (*Anopheles gambiae*)	F/M, (VHF)
	Maguari virus (MAGV)	Birds, cattle, horses, sheep, water buffalo	Mosquitoes (*Aedes*, *Anopheles*, *Culex*, *Psorophora*, *Wyeomyia* spp.)	F/M
	Ngari virus (NRIV)	Unknown	Mosquitoes (*Aedes*, *Anopheles* spp.)	F/M, VHF
	Shokwe virus (SHOV)	Rodents	Mosquitoes (*Aedes*, *Anopheles*, *Mansonia* spp.)	F/M
	Xingu virus (XINV)	Unknown	Unknown	F/M
Orthobunyaviruses (Bwamba serogroup)	Bwamba virus (BWAV)	Unknown	Mosquitoes (*Aedes*, *Anopheles*, *Mansonia* spp.)	F/M
	Pongola virus (PGAV)	Cattle, donkeys, goats, sheep	Mosquitoes (*Aedes*, *Anopheles*, *Mansonia* spp.)	F/M
Orthobunyaviruses (California serogroup)	California encephalitis virus (CEV)	Lagomorphs, rodents	Mosquitoes (*Aedes*, *Culex*, *Culiseta*, *Psorophora* spp.)	E, F/M
	Inkoo virus (INKV)	Cattle, foxes, hares, moose, rodents	Mosquitoes (*Aedes* spp.)	E, F/M
	Jamestown Canyon virus (JCV)	Bison, deer, elk, moose	Mosquitoes (*Aedes*, *Culiseta*, *Ochlerotatus* spp.)	E, F/M
	La Crosse virus (LACV)	Chipmunks, squirrels	Mosquitoes (*Ochlerotatus triseriatus*)	E, F/M
	Lumbo virus (LUMV)	Unknown	Mosquitoes (*Aedes pembaensis*)	E, F/M
	Snowshoe hare virus (SSHV)	Snowshoe hares, squirrels, other small mammals	Mosquitoes (*Aedes*, *Culiseta*, *Ochlerotatus* spp.)	E, F/M
	Ťahyňa virus (TAHV)	Cattle, dogs, eulipotyphla, foxes, hares, horses, pigs, rodents	Mosquitoes (*Aedes*, *Culex*, *Culiseta* spp.)	E, F/M
Orthobunyaviruses (group C serogroup)	Apeú virus (APEUV)	Bare-tailed woolly opossums (*Caluromys philander*) and other opossums; rodents; tufted capuchins (*Cebus apella*)	Mosquitoes (*Aedes*, *Culex* spp.)	F/M
	Caraparú virus (CARV)	Rodents, tufted capuchins (*C. apella*)	Mosquitoes (*Culex* spp.)	F/M
	Itaquí virus (ITQV)	Capuchins (*Cebus* spp.), opossums, rodents	Mosquitoes (*Culex* spp.)	F/M
	Madrid virus (MADV)	Capuchins (*Cebus* spp.), opossums, rodents	Mosquitoes (*Culex* spp.)	F/M
	Marituba virus (MTBV)	Capuchins (*Cebus* spp.), opossums, rodents	Mosquitoes (*Culex* spp.)	F/M
	Murutucú virus (MURV)	Capuchins (*Cebus* spp.), opossums, pale-throated sloths (*Bradypus tridactylus*), rodents	Mosquitoes (*Coquillettidia*, *Culex* spp.)	F/M
	Nepuyo virus (NEPV)	Bats (*Artibeus* spp.), rodents	Mosquitoes (*Culex* spp.)	F/M
	Oriboca virus (ORIV)	Capuchins (*Cebus* spp.), opossums, rodents	Mosquitoes (*Aedes*, *Culex*, *Mansonia*, *Psorophora* spp.)	F/M
	Ossa virus (OSSAV)	Rodents	Mosquitoes (*Culex* spp.)	F/M
	Restan virus (RESV)	Unknown	Mosquitoes (*Culex* spp.)	F/M
	Zungarococha virus (ZUNV)	Unknown	Unknown	F/M
Orthobunyaviruses (Guamá serogroup)	Catú virus (CATUV)	Bats, capuchins (*Cebus* spp.), opossums, rodents	Mosquitoes (*Culex* spp.)	F/M
	Guamá virus (GMAV)	Bats, capuchins (*Cebus* spp.), howlers (*Alouatta* spp.), marsupials, rodents	Mosquitoes (*Aedes*, *Culex*, *Limatus*, *Mansonia*, *Psorophora*, *Trichoprosopon* spp.)	F/M
Orthobunyaviruses (Mapputta serogroup)	Gan Gan virus (GGV)	Unknown	Mosquitoes (*Aedes*, *Culex* spp.)	A/R
	Trubanaman virus (TRUV)	Unknown	Mosquitoes (*Anopheles*, *Culex* spp.)	(A/R)

(*Continued*)

TABLE 209-1 Zoonotic Arthropod- and Rodent-Borne Viruses That Infect Humans (Continued)

VIRUS GROUP	VIRUS (ABBREVIATION)	MAJOR NONHUMAN HOST(S)[a]	VECTOR(S)	SYNDROME[b]
Orthobunyaviruses (Nyando serogroup)	Nyando virus (NDV)	Unknown	Mosquitoes (*Aedes, Anopheles* spp.), sandflies (*Lutzomyia* spp.)	F/M
Orthobunyaviruses (Simbu serogroup)	Iquitos virus (IQTV)	Unknown	Unknown	F/M
	Oropouche virus (OROV)	Marmosets (*Callithrix* spp.), pale-throated sloths (*B. tridactylus*)	Biting midges (*Culicoides paraensis*), mosquitoes (*Coquillettidia venezuelensis, Culex quinquefasciatus, Mansonia* spp., *Ochlerotatus serratus*)	F/M
	Shuni virus (SHUV)	Horses, livestock	Mosquitoes (*Culex theileri, Culicoides spp.*)	E
Orthobunyaviruses (Turlock serogroup)	Cristoli virus	Unknown	Mosquitoes?	E
Orthobunyaviruses (Wyeomyia serogroup)	Wyeomyia virus (WYOV)	Unknown	Mosquitoes (*Wyeomyia* spp.)	F/M
Orthobunyaviruses (other)	Tataguine virus (TATV)	Unknown	Mosquitoes (*Anopheles* spp.)	F/M
Orthohantaviruses (Old World)	Amur virus (AMRV)	Korean field mice (*Apodemus peninsulae*)	None	VHF
	Dobrava virus (DOBV)	Caucasus field mice (*Apodemus ponticus*), striped field mice (*Apodemus agrarius*), yellow-necked field mice (*Apodemus flavicollis*)	None	VHF
	Gōu virus (GOUV)	Brown rats (*Rattus norvegicus*), roof rats (*R. rattus*), Oriental house rats (*Rattus tanezumi*)	None	VHF
	Hantaan virus (HTNV)	Striped field mice (*A. agrarius*)	None	VHF
	Kurkino virus (KURV)	Striped field mice (*A. agrarius*)	None	VHF
	Muju virus (MUJV)	Korean red-backed voles (*Myodes regulus*)	None	VHF
	Puumala virus (PUUV)	Bank voles (*Myodes glareolus*)	None	(P), VHF
	Saaremaa virus (SAAV)	Striped field mice (*A. agrarius*)	None	VHF
	Seoul virus (SEOV)	Brown rats (*R. norvegicus*), roof rats (*R. rattus*)	None	VHF
	Sochi virus (SOCV)	Caucasus field mice (*A. ponticus*)	None	VHF
	Tula virus (TULV)	Common voles (*Microtus arvalis*), East European voles (*Microtus levis*), field voles (*Microtus agrestis*)	None	(P), VHF
Orthohantaviruses (New World)	Anajatuba virus (ANJV)	Fornes' colilargos (*Oligoryzomys fornesi*)	None	P
	Andes virus (ANDV)	Long-tailed colilargos (*Oligoryzomys longicaudatus*)	None	P
	Araraquara virus (ARAV)	Hairy-tailed akodonts (*Necromys lasiurus*)	None	P
	Araucária virus (ARAUV)	Black-footed colilargos (*Oligoryzomys nigripes*)	None	P
	Bayou virus (BAYV)	Marsh rice rats (*Oryzomys palustris*)	None	P
	Bermejo virus (BMJV)	Chacoan colilargos (*Oligoryzomys chacoensis*)	None	P
	Black Creek Canal virus (BCCV)	Hispid cotton rats (*S. hispidus*)	None	P
	Blue River virus (BRV)	White-footed deermice (*P. leucopus*)	None	P
	Caño Delgadito virus (CADV)	Alston's cotton rats (*Sigmodon alstoni*)	None	P
	Castelo dos Sonhos virus (CASV)	Brazilian colilargos (*Oligoryzomys eliurus*)	None	P
	Catacamas virus (CATV)	Coues' oryzomys (*Oryzomys couesi*)	None	P
	Choclo virus (CHOV)	Fulvous colilargos (*Oligoryzomys fulvescens*)	None	F/M, P
	Juquitiba virus (JUQV)	Black-footed colilargos (*O. nigripes*)	None	P
	Laguna Negra virus (LANV)	Little lauchas (*Calomys laucha*)	None	P
	Lechiguanas virus (LECV)	Flavescent colilargos (*Oligoryzomys flavescens*)	None	P
	Maciel virus (MCLV)	Dark-furred akodonts (*Necromys obscurus*)	None	P
	Maripa virus (MARV)	Unknown	None	P
	Monongahela virus (MGLV)	North American deermice (*P. maniculatus*)	None	P

(*Continued*)

TABLE 209-1 Zoonotic Arthropod- and Rodent-Borne Viruses That Infect Humans (Continued)

VIRUS GROUP	VIRUS (ABBREVIATION)	MAJOR NONHUMAN HOST(S)[a]	VECTOR(S)	SYNDROME[b]
	New York virus (NYV)	White-footed deermice (*P. leucopus*)	None	P
	Orán virus (ORNV)	Long-tailed colilargos (*O. longicaudatus*)	None	P
	Paranoá virus (PARV)	Unknown	None	P
	Pergamino virus (PRGV)	Azara's akodonts (*Akodon azarae*)	None	P
	Rio Mamoré virus (RIOMV)	Common bristly mice (*Neacomys spinosus*)	None	P
	Sin Nombre virus (SNV)	North American deermice (*P. maniculatus*)	None	P
	Tunari virus (TUNV)	Unknown	None	P
Orthonairoviruses (Crimean-Congo hemorrhagic fever virus group)	Crimean-Congo hemorrhagic fever virus (CCHFV)	Cattle, dogs, goats, hares, hedgehogs, mice, ostriches, sheep	Predominantly ixodid ticks (*Hyalomma* spp.)	VHF
Orthonairoviruses (Dugbe virus group)	Dugbe virus (DUGV)	Northern giant pouched rats (*Cricetomys gambianus*), Zébu cattle (*Bos primigenius*)	Biting midges (*Culicoides* spp.), ixodid ticks (*Amblyomma, Hyalomma, Rhipicephalus* spp.)	F/M
	Nairobi sheep disease virus[c] (NSDV)	Sheep	Ixodid ticks (*Haemaphysalis, Rhipicephalus* spp.), mosquitoes (*Culex* spp.)	F/M
Orthonairoviruses (Sakhalin virus group)	Avalon virus (AVAV)	European herring gulls (*Larus argentatus*)	Ixodid ticks (*Ixodes uriae*)	(Polyradiculoneuritis?)
Orthonairoviruses (Thiafora virus group)	Erve virus (ERVEV)	Greater white-toothed shrews (*Crocidura russula*)	?	(Thunderclap headache?)
Orthonairoviruses (other)	Issyk-Kul virus (ISKV)	Bats, birds	Biting midges (*Culicoides schultzei*), horseflies (*Tabanus agrestis*), mosquitoes (*Aedes caspius, Anopheles hyrcanus*), argasid ticks (*Argas vespertilionis, A. pusillus*), ixodid ticks (*Ixodes vespertilionis*)	F/M
	Söngl'ing virus (SGLV)	Unknown	Ixodid ticks (*Ixodes crenulatus, Ixodes persulcatus, Haemaphysalis concinna*, and *Haemaphysalis longicornis*)	F/M
	Tamdy virus (TAMV)	Gerbils, other mammals (including Bactrian camels), birds	Ixodid ticks (*Hyalomma* spp.)	F/M
Phleboviruses (Candirú serocomplex)	Alenquer virus (ALEV)	Unknown	Unknown	F/M
	Candirú virus (CDUV)	Unknown	Unknown	F/M
	Escharate virus (ESCV)	Unknown	Unknown	F/M
	Maldonado virus (MLOV)	Unknown	Unknown	F/M
	Morumbi virus (MRBV)	Unknown	Unknown	F/M
	Serra Norte virus (SRNV)	Unknown	Unknown	F/M
Phleboviruses (Punta Toro serocomplex)	Coclé virus (CCLV)	Unknown	Sandflies	F/M
	Punta Toro virus (PTV)	Unknown	Sandflies (*Lutzomyia* spp.)	F/M
Phleboviruses (sandfly fever serocomplex)	Chagres virus (CHGV)	Unknown	Sandflies (*Lutzomyia* spp.)	F/M
	Chios virus	Unknown	Unknown	E
	Granada virus (GRV)	Unknown	Sandflies	F/M
	Rift Valley fever virus (RVFV)	Cattle, sheep	Mosquitoes (*Aedes, Anopheles, Coquillettidia, Culex, Eretmapodites, Mansonia* spp.)	E, F/M, VHF
	Sandfly fever Cyprus virus (SFCV)	Unknown	Unknown	F/M
	Sandfly fever Ethiopia virus (SFEV)	Unknown	Sandflies	F/M
	Sandfly fever Naples virus (SFNV)	Unknown	Sandflies (*Phlebotomus papatasi, P. perfiliewi, P. perniciosus*)	F/M
	Sandfly fever Sicilian virus (SFSV)	Eulipotyphla, least weasels (*Mustela nivalis*), rodents	Sandflies (particularly *Phlebotomus papatasi*)	F/M
	Sandfly fever Turkey virus (SFTV)	Unknown	Sandflies (*Phlebotomus* spp.)	F/M
	Toscana virus (TOSV)	Unknown	Sandflies (*Phlebotomus papatasi, P. perfiliewi*)	E, F/M
Phleboviruses (Salehabad serocomplex)	Adria virus (ADRV)	Unknown	Sandflies	E

(*Continued*)

TABLE 209-1 Zoonotic Arthropod- and Rodent-Borne Viruses That Infect Humans (Continued)

VIRUS GROUP	VIRUS (ABBREVIATION)	MAJOR NONHUMAN HOST(S)[a]	VECTOR(S)	SYNDROME[b]
Phleboviruses (Uukuniemi serocomplex)	Tăchéng tick virus 2 (TcTV-2)	Unknown	Ixodid ticks (*Dermacentor marginatus, Dermacentor nuttalli, Dermacentor silvarum, Hyalomma asiaticum*)	E?
	Uukuniemi virus (UUKV)	Birds, cattle, rodents	Ixodid ticks (*Ixodes* spp.)	F/M
Quaranjaviruses	Quaranfil virus (QRFV)	Birds	Argasid ticks (*Argas arboreus*)	F/M
Seadornaviruses	Banna virus (BAV)	Cattle, pigs	Mosquitoes (*Aedes, Anopheles, Culiseta* spp.)	E
Thogotoviruses	Bourbon virus (BRBV)	Unknown	Ticks?	F/M
	Dhori virus (DHOV)[p]	Bats, camels, horses	Mosquitoes (*Aedes, Anopheles, Culex* spp.), argasid ticks (*Ornithodoros* spp.), ixodid ticks (*Dermacentor, Hyalomma* spp.)	E, F/M
	Thogoto virus (THOV)	Camels, cattle	Ixodid ticks (*Amblyomma, Hyalomma, Rhipicephalus* spp.)	E, F/M
Uukuviruses	Uukuniemi virus (UUKV)	Birds, cattle, rodents	Ixodid ticks (*Ixodes* spp.)	F/M
Vesiculoviruses	Chandipura virus (CHPV)	Hedgehogs	Mosquitoes (*Aedes aegypti*), sandflies (*Phlebotomus, Sergentomyia* spp.)	E, F/M
	Isfahan virus (ISFV)	Great gerbils (*Rhombomys opimus*)	Sandflies (*Phlebotomus papatasi*)	F/M
	Piry virus (PIRYV)	Gray four-eyed opossums (*Philander opossum*)	Mosquitoes (*Aedes, Culex, Toxorhynchites* spp.)	F/M
	Vesicular stomatitis Indiana virus (VSIV)	Cattle, horses, pigs	Sandflies (*Lutzomyia* spp.)	F/M
	Vesicular stomatitis New Jersey virus (VSNJV)	Cattle, horses, pigs	Biting midges (*Culicoides* spp.), chloropid flies, mosquitoes (*Culex, Mansonia* spp.), muscoid flies (*Musca* spp.), simuliid flies	F/M

[a]Mammalian names as listed in Wilson & Reeder's *Mammal Species of the World*, 3rd edition (*https://www.departments.bucknell.edu/biology/resources/msw3/*). [b]Abbreviations refer to the syndromes most associated with the viruses: A/R, arthritis/rash; E, encephalitis; F/M, fever/myalgia; P, pulmonary; VHF, viral hemorrhagic fever. Abbreviations are placed in parentheses when cases are either extremely rare or controversial. [c]In the older literature, chikungunya virus often is also listed as a causative agent of VHF. However, later studies revealed that, in most cases, people with "chikungunya hemorrhagic fever" were co-infected with one or more dengue viruses, an observation suggesting that the VHF was severe dengue. [d]Also known as Igbo-Ora virus. [e]Also known as Ockelbo virus (OCKV), Pogosta virus, and Karelian fever virus (KFV). [f]Also known as Palma virus (PALV). [g]Alternatives used in the literature are Huáiyángshān virus (HYSV) and Hénán fever virus (HNFV). [h]Also known as Alfuy virus (ALFV). [i]Also includes Kunjin virus (KUNV). [j]Also spelled Alkhumra hemorrhagic fever virus (AHFV) and known as Alkhurma/Alkhumra virus (ALKV). [k]Also known as Nánjiànyí(n) virus. [l]Whitewater Arroyo virus is often listed as a causative agent of VHF in the literature, but convincing data associating this virus with VHF have not been published. [m]Also known as Brezová virus, Cvilín virus, Kharagysh virus, Koliba virus, or Lipovník virus. [n]Also known as Čalovo virus (CVOV) or Chittoor virus (CHITV). [o]Also known as Ganjam virus (GV). [p]Also known as Astra virus and Batken virus (BKNV).

BUNYAVIRALES: HANTAVIRIDAE, NAIROVIRIDAE, PERIBUNYAVIRIDAE, AND PHENUIVIRIDAE

The members of all these families that infect humans form spherical to pleomorphic enveloped virions containing three genomic RNAs (S, ~1–2 kb; M, 3.6–5.3 kb; and L, 6.4–12.3 kb) of negative (hantavirids, nairovirids, peribunyavirids) or ambisense (phenuivirids) polarity. These bunyavirals mature into particles ~80–120 nm in diameter in the Golgi complex of infected cells and exit these cells by exocytosis.

Hantavirids that infect humans are classified in the genus *Orthohantavirus* and are maintained in nature by rodents that chronically shed virions. Old World orthohantaviruses are harbored by murid and cricetid rodents, and New World orthohantaviruses are maintained by cricetid rodents. As with mammarenaviruses, individual orthohantaviruses are usually specifically adapted to a particular type of rodent. However, orthohantaviruses do not cause chronic viremia in their rodent hosts and are transmitted only horizontally from rodent to rodent. Similar to mammarenaviruses, orthohantaviruses infect humans primarily through inhalation of or direct contact with rodent excreta or secreta, and person-to-person transmission is not a common event (with the notable exception of Andes virus). Although there is overlap, the human Old World orthohantaviruses are usually the etiologic agents of hemorrhagic fever with renal syndrome (HFRS), whereas the New World orthohantaviruses usually cause hantavirus pulmonary syndrome.

Nairovirids that infect humans are classified in the genus *Orthonairovirus*. Orthonairoviruses are maintained by ixodid ticks, which transmit these viruses vertically (transovarially and transstadially) to progeny tick generations and horizontally spread them through viremic vertebrate hosts. Humans are usually infected via a tick bite or during handling of infected vertebrates.

Peribunyavirids of one genus (*Orthobunyavirus*) infect humans. Orthobunyaviruses are largely mosquito-borne and rarely midge-borne and have viremic vertebrate intermediate hosts. Many orthobunyaviruses are transmitted transovarially to their mosquito hosts. Numerous orthobunyaviruses have been associated with human infection and disease. They have been considered as members of ~19 serogroups based on antigenic cross-reactions, but this grouping is undergoing revision through accumulation of new genomic data and phylogenetic analyses. Humans are infected by viruses in at least 10 serogroups.

Phenuivirids are transmitted vertically (transovarially) in their arthropod hosts and horizontally through viremic vertebrate hosts. Human phenuivirids are found in three genera: *Bandavirus*, *Phlebovirus*, and *Uukuvirus*. Bandaviruses and uukuviruses are transmitted by ticks, whereas viruses of the phlebovirus sandfly fever group are transmitted by sandflies. Phleboviruses are assigned to at least 10 serocomplexes; human pathogens are found in at least three of these serocomplexes.

MARTELLIVIRALES: TOGAVIRIDAE

The members of the family *Togaviridae* have linear, positive-stranded RNA genomes (~9.7–11.8 kb) and form enveloped icosahedral virions (~60–70 nm in diameter) that bud from the plasma membrane of the infected cell. The togavirids discussed here are all members of the genus *Alphavirus* and are transmitted to vertebrates by mosquitoes.

MONONEGAVIRALES: RHABDOVIRIDAE

Rhabdovirids have linear, typically nonsegmented, negative-sense RNA genomes (~11–15 kb) and form bullet-shaped to pleomorphic enveloped particles (100–430 nm long and 45–100 nm wide). Only the genus *Vesiculovirus* includes confirmed human arthropod-borne viruses, all of which are transmitted by insects (biting midges, mosquitoes, and sandflies). **The general properties of rhabdovirids are discussed in more detail in Chap. 208.**

■ *REOVIRALES: REOVIRIDAE*

The family *Reoviridae* was established for viruses with linear, multisegmented, double-stranded RNA genomes (~16–29 kb in total). These viruses produce particles that have icosahedral symmetry and are 60–80 nm in diameter. In contrast to all other virions discussed here, reovirions are not enveloped and thus are insensitive to detergent inactivation. Human arthropod-borne viruses are found within the genera *Coltivirus* (subfamily *Spinareovirinae*), *Orbivirus* (subfamily *Sedoreovirinae*), and *Seadornavirus* (subfamily *Sedoreovirinae*). Arthropod-borne coltiviruses possess 12 genome segments. Coltiviruses are transmitted by numerous tick types transstadially but not transovarially. Overall maintenance of the transmission cycle therefore involves viremic mammalian hosts infected by tick bites. Arthropod-borne orbiviruses have 10 genome segments and are transmitted by mosquitoes or ixodid ticks, whereas relevant seadornaviruses have 12 genome segments and are transmitted exclusively by mosquitoes.

EPIDEMIOLOGY

The distributions of arthropod-borne and rodent-borne viruses are restricted by the areas inhabited by their reservoir hosts and/or vectors. Consequently, a patient's geographic origin or travel history can provide important clues in the differential diagnosis. **Table 209-2** lists the approximate geographic distribution of most arthropod-borne and rodent-borne infections. Many of these diseases can be acquired in either rural or urban settings; the diseases include yellow fever, dengue without/with warning signs (previously called dengue fever), severe dengue (previously called dengue hemorrhagic fever and dengue shock syndrome), chikungunya virus disease, HFRS caused by Seoul virus, sandfly fever caused by sandfly fever Naples and Sicilian viruses, and Oropouche virus disease.

DIAGNOSIS

In patients with suspected viral infection, a recognized history of mosquito bite(s) has little diagnostic significance, but a history of tick bite(s) is more useful. Exposure to rodents is sometimes reported by people infected with mammarenaviruses or orthohantaviruses. Laboratory diagnosis is required in all cases, although epidemics occasionally provide enough clinical and epidemiologic clues for a presumptive etiologic diagnosis. For most arthropod-borne and rodent-borne viruses, acute-phase serum samples (collected within 3 or 4 days of onset) have yielded isolates. Paired serum samples have been used to demonstrate rising antibody titers. Intensive efforts to develop rapid tests for viral hemorrhagic fevers (VHFs) have resulted in reliable antigen-detection enzyme-linked immunosorbent assays (ELISAs), IgM-capture ELISAs, and multiplex polymerase chain reaction (PCR) assays. These tests can provide a diagnosis based on a single serum sample within a few hours and are particularly useful in patients with severe disease. More sensitive reverse-transcription PCR (RT-PCR) assays may yield diagnoses based on samples without detectable antigen and may also provide useful genetic information about the etiologic agent.

Orthohantavirus infections differ from other viral infections discussed here in that severe acute disease is immunopathologic; patients present with serum IgM that serves as the basis for a sensitive and specific test. At diagnosis, patients with encephalitides generally are no longer viremic or antigenemic and usually do not have virions in cerebrospinal fluid (CSF). In this situation, serologic methods for IgM determination and RT-PCR are highly valuable. Increasingly, IgM-capture ELISA is used for the simultaneous testing of serum and CSF. IgG ELISA or classic serology is useful in the evaluation of past exposure to viruses, many of which circulate in areas with minimal medical infrastructures and sometimes cause only mild or subclinical infections.

CLINICAL DISEASE SYNDROMES

There is a wide spectrum of possible human responses to infection with arthropod-borne or rodent-borne viruses, and knowledge of the outcome of most of these infections is limited. People infected with these viruses may not develop symptoms or signs of illness. If viral disease is recognized, it can usually be grouped into one of five broad syndromic categories: arthritis and rash, encephalitis, fever and myalgia, pulmonary disease, or VHF (**Table 209-3**). Although a useful clinical heuristic, it should be recognized that these categories often overlap in complex spectra of disease caused by arthropod-borne or rodent-borne viruses. Indeed, illness caused by many of these viruses is often best known by the most severe disease phenotypes, which are typically not the most common disease manifestation. For example, infections with West Nile virus and Venezuelan equine encephalitis virus are discussed here as encephalitides, but during epidemics, many patients present with much milder febrile syndromes. Similarly, Rift Valley fever virus is best known as a cause of VHF, but the attack rates for febrile disease are far higher, with encephalitis and blindness occurring occasionally as well. Lymphocytic choriomeningitis virus is classified here as a cause of fever and myalgia because this syndrome is the most common disease manifestation. Even when central nervous system (CNS) disease evolves during infection with this virus, neurologic manifestations are usually mild and preceded by fever and myalgia. However, this virus may also cause fetal microcephaly. Overlap between syndromic categories is further complicated by evolving nomenclature around their classification. For example, infection with any dengue virus (1, 2, 3, or 4) is considered as a cause of fever and myalgia because this syndrome, historically called "dengue fever," is by far the most common manifestation worldwide. However, severe manifestations of dengue virus infection have a complicated pathogenesis: the historical classification of disease as "dengue hemorrhagic fever" included a subset of patients with "dengue shock syndrome," which is of tremendous consequence for pediatric populations in certain areas of the world. Further complicating this overlap, recent World Health Organization revision of disease classification recommended a less descriptive but more pragmatic use of "dengue without warning signs," "dengue with warning signs," and "severe dengue" to describe the same spectrum and enhance clinical management and case reporting. Unfortunately, most of the known arthropod-borne or rodent-borne viral diseases have not been studied in detail with modern medical approaches. Thus, available data may be incomplete or biased. Data on geographic distribution are often difficult to interpret: Frequently, the literature is not clear as to whether the data pertain to the distribution of a particular virus or to the areas where human disease has been observed. In addition, the designations for viruses and viral diseases have changed multiple times over decades. Here, virus and taxon names are in line with the latest reports of the International Committee on Taxonomy of Viruses, and disease names are in accordance with the World Health Organization's International Classification of Diseases 11th revision (ICD-11). When needed for clarity or historical reference, other nomenclature will be specifically identified. In light of this syndromic approach, the reader should be aware that the variable clinical manifestations of particular viruses may be captured over a number of sections.

■ ARTHRITIS AND RASH

Arthritides are common clinical presentations (or manifestations) of several viral diseases, such as hepatitis B, parvovirus B19 infection, and rubella, and occasionally accompany infection due to adenovirids, enteroviruses, herpesvirids, or mumps virus. Two orthobunyaviruses—Gan Gan virus and Trubanaman virus—and the flavivirus Kokobera virus have been associated with single cases of polyarthritic disease. Arthropod-borne alphaviruses are also common causes of arthritides—usually acute febrile diseases accompanied by the development of a maculopapular rash. Rheumatic involvement includes arthralgia alone, periarticular swelling, and (less commonly) joint effusions. Most alphavirus infections are less severe and have fewer articular manifestations in children than in adults. In temperate climates, these ailments are summer diseases. No specific therapies or licensed vaccines exist. The most significant alphavirus arthritides are chikungunya virus disease, Ross River disease, Barmah Forest virus infection, and Sindbis virus infection. Also of interest is the emerging Zika virus infection. Less significant but historically notable are viruses that caused isolated

TABLE 209-2 Geographic Distribution of Zoonotic Arthropod-Borne or Rodent-Borne Viral Diseases

	TYPE OF DISEASE[b]						
AREA[a]	ARENAVIRAL	BUNYAVIRAL	FLAVIVIRAL	ORTHOMYXOVIRAL	REOVIRAL	RHABDOVIRAL	TOGAVIRAL
Africa	Lassa fever; Lujo virus infection	Bangui, Batai, Bhanja, Bunyamwera, and Bwamba virus infections; Crimean-Congo hemorrhagic fever; Dugbe, Germiston, Ilesha virus infections; Nairobi sheep disease virus infection; Ngari, Nyando, and Pongola virus infections; Rift Valley fever; sandfly fever; Shokwe, Shuni, Tataguine virus infections	Alkhurma hemorrhagic fever; dengue without/with warning signs/severe dengue; Usutu, West Nile virus infections; yellow fever; Zika virus disease	Dhori, Quaranfil, Thogoto virus infections	Lebombo, Orungo, Tribeč virus infections	—	Chikungunya virus disease; o'nyong-nyong fever; Semliki Forest, Sindbis virus infections
Central Asia	—	Bhanja, Issyk-Kul virus infections; Crimean-Congo hemorrhagic fever; sandfly fever; Ťahyňa, Tamdy virus infections	Far Eastern tick-borne encephalitis; Karshi, Powassan, West Nile virus infections	Dhori virus infections	—	Isfahan virus infection	Sindbis virus infection
Eastern Asia		Crimean-Congo hemorrhagic fever; hemorrhagic fever with renal syndrome; sandfly fever; severe fever with thrombocytopenia syndrome; Tăchéng tick virus 2 and Tamdy and Sōnglǐng virus infections	Dengue without/with warning signs/severe dengue; Far Eastern tick-borne encephalitis; Japanese encephalitis; Kyasanur Forest disease		Banna virus infection		
Southern Asia	—	Batai, Bhanja virus infections; Crimean-Congo hemorrhagic fever; hemorrhagic fever with renal syndrome; Nairobi sheep disease virus infection; sandfly fever	Dengue without/with warning signs/severe dengue; Japanese encephalitis; Kyasanur Forest disease; West Nile virus infection; Zika virus disease	Dhori, Quaranfil, Thogoto virus infections	—	Chandipura, Isfahan virus infections	Chikungunya virus disease
South-Eastern Asia	—	Batai virus infection; hemorrhagic fever with renal syndrome	Dengue without/with warning signs/severe dengue; Japanese encephalitis; West Nile virus infection; Zika virus disease	—	—	—	Chikungunya virus disease
Western Asia	—	Batai, Bhanja virus infections; Crimean-Congo hemorrhagic fever; hemorrhagic fever with renal syndrome; sandfly fever; Tamdy virus infection	Alkhurma hemorrhagic fever; Central European tick-borne encephalitis; dengue without/with warning signs/severe dengue; West Nile virus infection	Dhori, Quaranfil virus infections	—	—	Chikungunya virus disease
Latin/Central America and the Caribbean	Argentinian hemorrhagic fever; Bolivian hemorrhagic fever; "Brazilian hemorrhagic fever"; Chapare virus infection; lymphocytic choriomeningitis; Venezuelan hemorrhagic fever	Alenquer, Apeú, Bunyamwera, Cache Valley, Candirú, Caraparú, Catú, Chagres, Coclé, Echarate, Fort Sherman, Guamá, Guaroa virus infections; hantavirus pulmonary syndrome; Itaquí, Juquitiba, Madrid, Maguari, Maldonado, Marituba, Mayaro, Morumbi, Murutucú, Nepuyo, Oriboca virus infections; Oropouche virus disease; Ossa, Punta Toro, Restan, Serra Norte, Tacaiuma, Trinidad, Wyeomyia, Xingu, Zungarococha virus infections	Dengue without/with warning signs/severe dengue; Rocio viral encephalitis; St. Louis encephalitis; yellow fever; Zika virus disease		—	Piry fever; vesicular stomatitis fever	Chikungunya virus disease; Madariaga, Mayaro, Mucambo, Tonate, Una virus infections; Venezuelan equine encephalitis

(Continued)

TABLE 209-2 Geographic Distribution of Zoonotic Arthropod-Borne or Rodent-Borne Viral Diseases (Continued)

	TYPE OF DISEASE[b]						
AREA[a]	ARENAVIRAL	BUNYAVIRAL	FLAVIVIRAL	ORTHOMYXOVIRAL	REOVIRAL	RHABDOVIRAL	TOGAVIRAL
Northern America	Lymphocytic choriomeningitis; Whitewater Arroyo virus infection	Avalon, Cache Valley virus infections; California encephalitis; hantavirus pulmonary syndrome; Heartland, Nepuyo, snowshoe hare virus infections	Dengue without/with warning signs/severe dengue; Powassan virus disease; St. Louis encephalitis; West Nile virus infection; Zika virus disease	Bourbon virus infection	Colorado tick fever; Salmon River virus infection	Vesicular stomatitis fever	Eastern equine encephalitis; Everglades virus infection; western equine encephalitis
Europe	Lymphocytic choriomeningitis	Adria, Avalon, Bhanja, Cristoli virus infections; California encephalitis; Crimean-Congo hemorrhagic fever; Erve virus infection; hemorrhagic fever with renal syndrome; Inkoo virus infection; sandfly fever; snowshoe hare, Ťahyňa, Uukuniemi virus infections	Central European tick-borne encephalitis; dengue without/ with warning signs/ severe dengue; Omsk hemorrhagic fever; Powassan, Usutu, West Nile virus infections	Dhori, Thogoto virus infections	Eyach, Kemerovo, Tribeč virus infections	—	Chikungunya virus disease; Sindbis virus infection
Oceania	—	Gan Gan, Trubanaman virus infections	Dengue without/with warning signs/severe dengue; Edge Hill virus infection; Japanese encephalitis; Kokobera virus infection; Murray Valley encephalitis; Stratford, West Nile virus infections; Zika virus disease	—	—	—	Barmah Forest virus infection; Ross River disease; Sindbis virus infection

[a]Geographic names here and throughout the chapter are as recommended by the UN geoscheme (*https://unstats.un.org/unsd/methodology/m49/*). [b]Disease names according to the World Health Organization's International Classification of Diseases 11th revision (ICD-11; *https://icd.who.int/browse11/l-m/en*). Quotation marks indicate common usage in the absence of ICD-11 recognition. Diseases not acknowledged by the ICD-11 are designated as "virus infection(s)."

cases or epidemics: A large (>2 million cases), albeit isolated, epidemic was caused by o'nyong-nyong virus from 1959 to 1962 (o'nyong-nyong fever). Mayaro, Semliki Forest, and Una viruses caused isolated cases or limited and infrequent epidemics (30 to several hundred cases per year). Signs and symptoms of infections with these viruses often are similar to those observed with chikungunya virus disease.

Chikungunya Virus Disease Chikungunya virus is endemic in rural areas of Africa. Intermittent epidemics take place in towns and cities of both Africa and Asia. Yellow fever mosquitoes (*Aedes aegypti*) are the usual vectors for the disease in urban areas. In 2004, a massive epidemic began in the Indian Ocean region (specifically on the islands of Réunion and Mauritius) and was most likely spread by travelers. The Asian tiger mosquito (*Aedes albopictus*) was identified as the major vector of chikungunya virus during that epidemic. In 2013 and 2014, several thousand chikungunya virus infections were reported (with as many as 900,000 cases suspected) from Caribbean islands. The virus was carried to Italy, France, and the United States by travelers from the Caribbean. Chikungunya virus poses a threat to the continental United States as suitable vector mosquitoes are present in southern states.

The disease is most common among adults, in whom the clinical presentation may be dramatic. The abrupt onset of chikungunya virus disease follows an incubation period of 2–10 days. Fever (often severe) with a saddleback pattern and severe arthralgia are accompanied by chills and constitutional symptoms and signs, such as abdominal pain, anorexia, conjunctival injection, headache, nausea, and photophobia. Migratory polyarthritis mainly affects the small joints of the ankles, feet, hands, and wrists, but the larger joints may be involved. Rash may appear at the outset or several days into the illness; its development often coincides with defervescence, which occurs around day 2 or 3 of the disease. The rash is most intense on the trunk and limbs and may desquamate. Young children develop less prominent signs and are therefore less frequently hospitalized. Children also often develop a bullous rather than a maculopapular/petechial rash. Maternal–fetal transmission has been reported and, in some cases, has led to fetal death. Recovery may require weeks, and a significant portion of middle-aged to older patients develop chronic arthritis or arthralgia syndromes (typically involving the same joints) that may be disabling. This persistence of signs and symptoms may be especially common in patients who test positive for the human leukocyte antigen B27 subtype (HLA-B27). In addition to arthritis, petechiae are seen occasionally and epistaxis is not uncommon, but chikungunya virus should not be considered a VHF agent. A few patients develop leukopenia. Elevated activities of aspartate aminotransferase (AST) and concentrations of C-reactive protein have been described, as have mildly decreased platelet counts. Treatment of chikungunya virus disease relies on nonsteroidal anti-inflammatory drugs and sometimes chloroquine for refractory arthritis.

Ross River Disease and Barmah Forest Virus Infection Ross River virus and Barmah Forest virus cause diseases that are indistinguishable on clinical grounds alone (hence the previously common disease designation of "epidemic polyarthritis" for both infections). Ross River virus has caused epidemics in Australia, Papua New Guinea, and the South Pacific since the beginning of the 20th century. In 1979 and 1980, the virus swept through the Pacific Islands, causing >500,000 infections. From 1991 to 2011, the virus caused 92,559 infections or disease in rural and suburban areas of Australia. From 2014 to 2015, >10,000 cases were recorded in Australia. Ross River virus is predominantly transmitted by *Aedes normanensis*, *Aedes vigilax*, and *Culex annulirostris* mosquitoes. Wallabies and rodents are probably the main vertebrate hosts. Barmah Forest virus infections have been on the rise since the early 1990s. For instance, from 1991 to 2011, 21,815 cases of Barmah Forest virus infection were recorded in Australia, and new data indicate that the disease also occurs in Papua New Guinea. Barmah Forest virus is transmitted by both *Aedes* and *Culex* mosquitoes and has been isolated from biting midges. The vertebrate hosts remain to be determined, but serologic studies implicate horses and possums.

Of the human Barmah Forest and Ross River virus infections surveyed, 55–75% were asymptomatic; however, these viral diseases can

TABLE 209-3 Clinical Syndromes Caused by Zoonotic Arthropod-Borne or Rodent-Borne Viruses

SYNDROME	VIRUS
Arthritis and rash (A/R)	*Flaviviridae:* Kokobera and Zika viruses *Peribunyaviridae:* Gan Gan and Trubanaman viruses *Togaviridae:* Barmah Forest, chikungunya, Mayaro, o'nyong-nyong, Ross River, Semliki Forest, and Sindbis viruses
Encephalitis (E)	*Arenaviridae:* lymphocytic choriomeningitis and Whitewater Arroyo viruses *Flaviviridae:* Japanese encephalitis, Karshi, Murray Valley encephalitis, Powassan, Rocio, St. Louis encephalitis, tick-borne encephalitis, Usutu, and West Nile viruses *Orthomyxoviridae:* Dhori and Thogoto viruses *Peribunyaviridae:* California encephalitis, Cristoli, Inkoo, Jamestown Canyon, La Crosse, Lumbo, snowshoe hare, Shuni, and Ťahyňa viruses *Phenuiviridae:* Adria, Bhanja, Chios, Rift Valley fever, Tăchéng tick virus 2, and Toscana viruses *Reoviridae:* Banna, Colorado tick fever, Eyach, Kemerovo, Orungo, and Salmon River viruses *Rhabdoviridae:* Chandipura virus *Togaviridae:* eastern equine encephalitis, Everglades, Madariaga, Mucambo, Tonate, Venezuelan equine encephalitis, and western equine encephalitis viruses
Fever and myalgia (F/M)	*Arenaviridae:* Lassa and lymphocytic choriomeningitis viruses *Bunyavirales* (unclassified): Bangui virus *Flaviviridae:* dengue 1–4, Edge Hill, Karshi, tick-borne encephalitis, Stratford, and Zika viruses *Hantaviridae:* Choclo virus *Nairoviridae:* Dugbe, Issyk-Kul, Nairobi sheep disease, Sōnglǐng, Tamdy viruses *Orthomyxoviridae:* Bourbon, Dhori, and Thogoto viruses *Peribunyaviridae:* Apeú, Batai, Bunyamwera, Bwamba, Cache Valley, California encephalitis, Caraparú, Catú, Fort Sherman, Germiston, Guamá, Guaroa, Ilesha, Inkoo, Iquitos, Itaquí, Jamestown Canyon, La Crosse, Lumbo, Madrid, Maguari, Marituba, Nepuyo, Ngari, Nyando, Oriboca, Oropouche, Ossa, Pongola, Restan, Shokwe, snowshoe hare, Tacaiuma, Ťahyňa, Tataguine, Wyeomyia, Xingu, and Zungarococha viruses *Phenuiviridae:* Alenquer, Bhanja, Candirú, Chagres, Echarate, Heartland, Maldonado, Morumbi, Punta Toro, Rift Valley fever, sandfly fever Cyprus, sandfly fever Ethiopia, sandfly fever Naples, sandfly fever Sicilian, sandfly fever Turkey, Serra Norte, severe fever with thrombocytopenia syndrome, Toscana, and Uukuniemi viruses *Reoviridae:* Colorado tick fever, Eyach, Kemerovo, Lebombo, Orungo, Salmon River, and Tribeč viruses *Rhabdoviridae:* Chandipura, Isfahan, Piry, vesicular stomatitis Indiana, and vesicular stomatitis New Jersey viruses *Togaviridae:* Everglades, Madariaga, Mucambo, Tonate, Una, and Venezuelan equine encephalitis viruses
Pulmonary disease (P)	*Hantaviridae:* Anajatuba, Andes, Araucária, bayou, Bermejo, Black Creek Canal, Blue River, Caño Delgadito, Castelo dos Sonhos, Catacamas, Choclo, Juquitiba, Laguna Negra, Lechiguanas, Maciel, Monongahela, New York, Orán, Paranoá, Pergamino, Puumala, Rio Mamoré, Sin Nombre, Tula, and Tunari viruses
Viral hemorrhagic fever (VHF)	*Arenaviridae:* Chapare, Guanarito, Junín, Lassa, Lujo, lymphocytic choriomeningitis, Machupo, and Sabiá viruses *Hantaviridae:* Amur, Dobrava, gōu, Hantaan, Kurkino, Muju, Puumala, Saaremaa, Seoul, Sochi, and Tula viruses *Nairoviridae:* Crimean-Congo hemorrhagic fever virus *Peribunyaviridae:* Ilesha and Ngari viruses *Phenuiviridae:* Rift Valley fever and severe fever with thrombocytopenia syndrome viruses *Flaviviridae:* Alkhurma hemorrhagic fever, dengue 1–4, Kyasanur Forest disease, Omsk hemorrhagic fever, tick-borne encephalitis, and yellow fever viruses

be debilitating. The incubation period is 7–9 days, the onset of illness is sudden, and disease is usually ushered in by disabling symmetrical joint pain. Generally, a non-itchy, diffuse, maculopapular rash (more common in Barmah Forest virus infection) develops coincidentally or follows shortly, but, in some patients, rash can precede joint pain by several days. Constitutional symptoms (such as low-grade fever, asthenia, headache, myalgia, and nausea) are not prominent or are absent in many cases. Most patients are incapacitated for considerable periods (6 months or more) by joint involvement, which interferes with grasping, sleeping, and walking. Ankle, interphalangeal, knee, metacarpophalangeal, and wrist joints are most often involved, although elbows, shoulders, and toes may also be affected. Periarticular swelling and tenosynovitis are common, and one-third of patients have true arthritis (more common in Ross River disease). Myalgia and nuchal stiffness may accompany joint pains. Only half of all patients with arthritis can resume normal activities within 4 weeks, and 10% continue to limit their activities after 3 months. Occasionally, patients are symptomatic for 1–3 years but without progressive arthropathy.

In the diagnosis of either infection, clinical laboratory values are normal or variable. Tests for rheumatoid factor and antinuclear antibodies are negative, and the erythrocyte sedimentation rate is acutely elevated. Joint fluid contains 1000–60,000 mononuclear cells per μL, and viral antigen can usually be detected in macrophages. IgM antibodies are valuable in the diagnosis of this infection, although occasionally, such antibodies persist for years. Isolation of the virus from blood after mosquito inoculation or growth of the virus in cell culture is possible early in the illness. Because of the great economic impact of annual epidemics in Australia, an inactivated Ross River virus vaccine has been under advanced development; phase 3 trials were completed in 2015 with promising results, but the candidate vaccine has not yet been developed for the market. Nonsteroidal anti-inflammatory drugs, such as naproxen or acetylsalicylic acid, are effective for treatment.

Sindbis Virus Infection Sindbis virus is typically transmitted to birds by infected mosquitoes. Infections with northern European or southern African variants are particularly likely in rural environments. After an incubation period of <1 week, Sindbis virus infection begins with rash and arthralgia. Constitutional clinical signs are not marked, and fever is modest or lacking altogether. The rash, which lasts ~1 week, begins on the trunk, spreads to the extremities, and evolves from macules to papules that often vesiculate. The arthritis is polyarticular, migratory, and incapacitating, with resolution of the acute phase in a few days. The ankles, elbows, knees, phalangeal joints, wrists, and—to a much lesser extent—proximal and axial joints are involved. Persistence of joint pain and occasionally of arthritis is a major problem and may continue for months or even years despite lack of deformities.

Zika Virus Disease Zika virus is an emerging pathogen that is transmitted to nonhuman primates and humans by *Aedes* mosquitoes. The virus was discovered 1947 in a sentinel rhesus monkey (*Macaca mulatta*) and *Aedes africanus* mosquitoes in the Zika Forest in what was then the British Protectorate of Uganda. Human Zika virus infection was first documented during a yellow fever outbreak in 1954 in Nigeria. Later, Zika virus infections were recognized in South-Eastern Asia and Southern Asia. Prior to 2007, only 14 clinically identified cases of Zika virus disease had been reported. In recent years, the number of Zika virus infections reported has increased steadily and rapidly, with large, but generally mild, disease outbreaks on Yap Island, Micronesia (2007), and in Cambodia (2010), the Philippines (2012), and French Polynesia (2013–2014). Invasion of the New World was first reported on Easter Island, Chile (2014), and in Brazil (2015). An estimated 440,000 to 1.3 million cases had occurred in Brazil by the end of 2015. At the end of May 2017, Zika virus infections had been recorded on five continents in 85 countries, including Mexico and the United States. Beginning in 2018, the global activity of Zika virus declined rather rapidly for unknown reasons.

Phylogenetic analysis of all available African Zika virus isolates revealed two geographically overlapping clades (Western Africa and Eastern Africa). A descendant Asian lineage, represented by viruses collected from mosquitoes trapped in homes in Malaysia, was first reported in 1969. All Zika virus isolates causing human cases outside of Africa trace back to this Asian lineage.

Human infections are usually asymptomatic or benign and self-resolving and are most likely misdiagnosed as dengue without/with warning signs or influenza. Typically, Zika virus disease is characterized by low-grade fever, headache, and malaise. An itchy maculopapular rash, nonpurulent conjunctivitis, myalgia, and arthralgia usually accompany or follow those manifestations. Vomiting, hematospermia, and hearing impairments are relatively common clinical signs. In severe cases, Zika virus infection is associated with serious complications, such as Guillain-Barré syndrome or fetal microcephaly after congenital transmission. Other neurologic complications of Zika virus infection are encephalitis, meningoencephalitis, transverse myelitis, peripheral neuropathies, retinopathies, and neurologic birth defects. Although most human Zika virus infections are acquired after bites by infected female mosquitoes, transmission may also occur perinatally or via heterosexual or homosexual contact with an infected person, breastfeeding, or transfusion of blood products. Specifically worrisome is viral persistence in the testes, which can last up to at least 160 days, as sexual virus transmission be may be possible throughout that period. Unfortunately, antiviral treatments (curative or preventive) and licensed vaccines against Zika virus are not yet available.

■ ENCEPHALITIS

The major encephalitis viruses are found in the families *Flaviviridae, Peribunyaviridae, Rhabdoviridae,* and *Togaviridae*. However, individual agents of other families, including Dhori virus and Thogoto virus (*Orthomyxoviridae*) and Banna virus (*Reoviridae*), have been known to cause isolated cases of encephalitis as well. Arboviral encephalitides are seasonal diseases, commonly occurring in the warmer months. Their incidence varies markedly with time and place, depending on ecologic factors. The causative viruses differ substantially in terms of case-to-infection ratio (i.e., the ratio of clinical to subclinical infections), lethality, and residual disease. Humans are not important amplifiers of these viruses.

All the viral encephalitides discussed in this section have a similar pathogenesis. An infected arthropod ingests blood from a human and thereby initiates infection. The initial viremia is thought to originate from the lymphoid system. Viremia leads to multifocal entry into the CNS, presumably through infection of olfactory neuroepithelium, with passage through the cribriform plate, "Trojan horse" entry with infected macrophages, or infection of brain capillaries. During the viremic phase, there may be little or no recognizable disease except in tick-borne flavivirus encephalitides, which may manifest with clearly delineated phases of fever and systemic illness.

CNS lesions arise partly from direct neuronal infection and subsequent damage and partly from edema, inflammation, and other indirect effects. The usual pathologic features of arboviral encephalitides are focal necroses of neurons, inflammatory glial nodules, and perivascular lymphoid cuffing. Involved areas display the "luxury perfusion" phenomenon, with normal or increased total blood flow and low oxygen extraction. The typical patient presents with a prodrome of nonspecific constitutional signs and symptoms, including fever, abdominal pain, sore throat, and respiratory signs. Headache, meningeal signs, photophobia, and vomiting follow quickly. The severity of human infection varies from an absence of signs/symptoms to febrile headache, aseptic meningitis, and full-blown encephalitis. The proportions and severity of these manifestations vary with the infecting virus. Involvement of deeper brain structures may be signaled by lethargy, somnolence, and intellectual deficit (as disclosed by a mental status examination). More severely affected patients are obviously disoriented and may become comatose. Tremors, loss of abdominal reflexes, cranial nerve palsies, hemiparesis, monoparesis, difficulty swallowing, limb-girdle syndrome, and frontal lobe signs are all common. Spinal and motor neuron diseases are documented after West Nile virus and Japanese encephalitis virus infections. Seizures and focal signs may be evident early or may appear during the course of the disease. Some patients present with an abrupt onset of fever, convulsions, and other signs of CNS involvement. The acute encephalitis usually lasts from a few days to 2–3 weeks. The infections may be fatal, or recovery may be slow (with weeks or months before the return of maximal recoverable function) or incomplete (with persisting long-term deficits). Difficulty concentrating, fatigability, tremors, and personality changes are common during recovery.

The diagnosis of arboviral encephalitides depends on the careful evaluation of a febrile patient with CNS disease and the performance of laboratory studies to determine etiology. Clinicians should (1) consider empirical acyclovir treatment for herpesvirus meningoencephalitis and antibiotic treatment for bacterial meningitis until test results are received; (2) exclude intoxination and metabolic or oncologic causes, including paraneoplastic syndromes, hyperammonemia, liver failure, and anti-*N*-methyl-D-aspartate (NMDA) receptor encephalitis; and (3) rule out a brain abscess or a stroke. Leptospirosis, neurosyphilis, Lyme disease, cat-scratch disease, and more recently described viral encephalitides (e.g., Nipah virus infection), among others, should be considered if epidemiologically relevant. CSF examination usually shows a modest increase in leukocyte counts—in the tens or hundreds or perhaps a few thousand. Early in the process, a significant proportion of these leukocytes may be polymorphonuclear, but mononuclear cells are usually predominant later. CSF glucose concentrations are generally normal. There are exceptions to this pattern of findings: In eastern equine encephalitis, for example, polymorphonuclear leukocytes may predominate during the first 72 h of disease, and hypoglycorrhachia may be detected. In lymphocytic choriomeningitis, lymphocyte counts may be in the thousands, and glucose concentrations may be diminished. A humoral immune response is usually detectable at or near the onset of disease. Both serum (acute- or convalescent-phase) and CSF should be examined for IgM antibodies, and viruses should be detected by plaque-reduction neutralization assay and/or RT-PCR. Virus generally cannot be isolated from blood or CSF, although Japanese encephalitis virus has been recovered from CSF of patients with severe disease. RT-PCR analysis of CSF may yield positive results. Viral antigen is present in brain tissue, although its distribution may be focal. Electroencephalography usually shows diffuse abnormalities and is not directly helpful.

Experience with medical imaging is still evolving. Both computed tomography (CT) and magnetic resonance imaging (MRI) scans may be normal except for evidence of preexisting conditions or occasional diffuse edema. Imaging is generally nonspecific, as most patients do not present with pathognomonic lesions, but it can be used to rule out other suspected causes of disease. It is important to remember that imaging may yield negative results if done early in the disease course but may later detect abnormalities. For example, eastern equine encephalitis (focal abnormalities) and severe Japanese encephalitis (hemorrhagic bilateral thalamic lesions) have caused abnormalities detectable by medical imaging.

Comatose patients may require management of intracranial pressure elevations, inappropriate secretion of antidiuretic hormone, respiratory failure, or seizures. Specific therapies for these viral encephalitides are not available. The only practical preventive measures are vector management and personal protection against the arthropod transmitting the virus. For Japanese or Central European/Far Eastern tick-borne encephalitides, vaccination should be considered in certain circumstances (see relevant sections below).

Flavivirids The most significant flavivirus encephalitides are Central European/Far Eastern tick-borne encephalitides, Japanese encephalitis, St. Louis encephalitis, and West Nile virus infection. Murray Valley encephalitis and Rocio virus infection resemble Japanese encephalitis but are documented only occasionally in Australia and Brazil. Powassan virus has caused ~144 cases of often-severe disease (lethality, ~8%), frequently occurring among children in eastern Canada and the United States. Usutu virus has caused only individual cases of human infection, but such infections may be underdiagnosed.

CENTRAL EUROPEAN/FAR EASTERN TICK-BORNE ENCEPHALITIDES Tick-borne encephalitis viruses are currently subdivided into four groups: the western/European subtype (previously called central European encephalitis virus), the (Ural-)Siberian subtype (previously called Russian spring–summer encephalitis virus), the Far Eastern subtype, and the louping ill ("leaping" behavior described in ill sheep with severe neurologic manifestations) subtype (previously called louping ill virus, or, in Japan, Negishi virus). Small mammals, grouse, deer, and sheep are the vertebrate amplifiers for these viruses, which are transmitted by ticks. The risk of infection varies by geographic area and can be highly localized within a given area. Human infections usually follow outdoor activities resulting in tick bites or consumption of raw (unpasteurized) milk from infected goats or, less commonly, from infected cows or sheep. Milk seems to represent the main transmission route for louping ill subtype viruses, which cause disease very rarely. Several thousand infections with tick-borne encephalitis virus are recorded each year among people of all ages. Tick-borne encephalitis occurs between April and October, with a peak in June and July.

Western/European viruses classically caused bimodal disease. After an incubation period of 7–14 days, the illness begins with an influenza-like fever-myalgia phase (arthralgia, fever, headaches, myalgia, and nausea) that lasts for 2–4 days and is thought to correlate with viremia. A subsequent remission for several days is followed by the recurrence of fever and the onset of meningeal signs. The CNS phase (7–10 days before onset of improvement) varies from mild aseptic meningitis, which is more common among younger patients, to severe (meningo) encephalitis with coma, seizures, tremors, and motor signs. Spinal and medullary involvement can lead to typical limb-girdle paralysis and respiratory paralysis. Most patients with western/European virus infections recover (lethality, 1%), and only a minority of patients have significant deficits. However, the lethality from (Ural-)Siberian virus infections reaches 7–8%.

Infections with Far Eastern viruses generally run a more abrupt course. The encephalitic syndrome caused by these viruses sometimes begins without a remission from the fever-myalgia phase and has more severe manifestations than the western/European syndrome. Lethality is high (20–40%), and major sequelae—most notably, lower motor neuron paralyses of the proximal muscles of the extremities, trunk, and neck—are common, developing in approximately half of patients. Thrombocytopenia sometimes develops during the initial febrile illness, resembling the early hemorrhagic phase of some other tick-borne flavivirus infections, such as Kyasanur Forest disease. In the early stage of the illness, virus may be detected by PCR or isolated from the blood; however, after the onset of CNS manifestations, virus cannot typically be detected in or isolated from the CSF, and diagnosis requires detection of IgM antibodies in serum and/or CSF.

Diagnosis of Central European/Far Eastern tick-borne encephalitides primarily relies on serology and detection of viral genomes by RT-PCR. There is no specific therapy for infection. However, effective alum-adjuvanted, formalin-inactivated virus vaccines (FSME-IMMUN and Encepur) are produced in Austria, Germany, and Russia in chicken embryo cells. Two doses of the Austrian vaccine separated by an interval of 1–3 months appear to be effective in the field, and antibody responses are similar when vaccine is given on days 0 and 14. Because rare cases of postvaccination Guillain-Barré syndrome have been reported, vaccination should be reserved for people likely to experience rural exposure in an endemic area during the season of transmission. Cross-neutralization for the western/European and Far Eastern variants has been established, but there are no published field studies on cross-protection among formalin-inactivated vaccines.

Because 0.2–4% of ticks in endemic areas may be infected, the use of immunoglobulin prophylaxis of Central European/Far Eastern tick-borne encephalitides has been increased. Prompt administration of high titer specific immmunoglobulin is routine in some areas (e.g., Russia), but has been discontinued in many European countries because of concerns for antibody-mediated enhancement of infections and disease.

JAPANESE ENCEPHALITIS Japanese encephalitis is the most significant viral encephalitis in Asia. Each year ~68,000 cases and ~13,600–20,400 deaths are reported. Japanese encephalitis virus is found throughout Asia—including in the Russian Far East, Japan, China, India, Pakistan, and South-Eastern Asia—and causes occasional epidemics on western Pacific islands. The virus has been detected in the Torres Strait islands, and five human encephalitis cases have been identified on the nearby Australian mainland. The virus is particularly common in areas where irrigated rice fields attract the natural avian vertebrate hosts and provide abundant breeding sites for *Culex tritaeniorhynchus* mosquitoes, which transmit the virus to humans. Additional amplification by pigs, which suffer abortion, and horses, which develop encephalitis, may be significant as well. Vaccination of these additional amplifying hosts may reduce the transmission of the virus.

After an incubation period of 5–15 days, clinical signs of Japanese encephalitis range from nonspecific febrile illness (nausea, vomiting, diarrhea, cough) to aseptic meningitis, meningoencephalitis, acute flaccid paralysis, and severe encephalitis. Common findings are cerebellar signs, cranial nerve palsies, and cognitive and speech impairments. A Parkinsonian presentation and seizures are typical in severe cases. Case fatality in hospitalized patients is high (20–30%) and long-term neurologic dysfunction and disability are common in survivors. Effective vaccines are available. Vaccination is indicated for summer travelers to rural Asia, where the risk of acquiring Japanese encephalitis is considered to be about 1 per 5000 to 1 per 20,000 travelers per week if travel duration exceeds 3 weeks. Usually, two intramuscular doses of the vaccine are given 28 days apart, with the second dose administered at least 1 week prior to travel.

ST. LOUIS ENCEPHALITIS St. Louis encephalitis virus is transmitted between mosquitoes and birds. This virus causes a low-level endemic infection among rural residents of the central and Western United States, where *Culex tarsalis* mosquitoes serve as vectors. The more urbanized mosquitoes (*Culex pipiens* and *Culex quinquefasciatus*) have been responsible for epidemics resulting in hundreds or even thousands of cases in cities of the central and eastern United States. In this country, most cases occur in June through October, but sporadic cases of the disease have also been noted throughout the year in Latin/Central America and the Caribbean. The urban mosquitoes breed in accumulations of stagnant water and sewage with high organic content and readily feed on humans in and around houses at dusk. The elimination of open sewers and trash-filled drainage systems is expensive and may not be possible. However, screening of houses and implementation of personal protective measures may be effective approaches to the prevention of infection. The rural mosquito vector is most active at dusk and outdoors; bites can be avoided by modification of activities and use of repellents.

Most infections are subclinical; when present, disease severity increases with age. St. Louis encephalitis virus infections that result in aseptic meningitis or mild encephalitis are concentrated among children and young adults, whereas severe and fatal cases primarily affect the elderly. Infection rates are similar in all age groups; the pathophysiologic explanation for susceptibility to disease in older individuals is unexplained. After an incubation period of 4–21 days, patients typically present with a non-specific prodrome (fever, malaise, myalgia, headache) followed by rapid-onset CNS manifestations that include mcneurologic abnormalities. Common findings include, nuchal rigidity, hypotonia, hyperreflexia, myoclonus, and tremors are common. Severe cases can include cranial nerve palsies, hemiparesis, and seizures. Of interest, during and after the prodrome, patients often report dysuria and may have viral antigen in urine as well as pyuria. The overall lethality is generally ~7% but may reach 20% among patients >60 years of age. Recovery is slow. Emotional lability, difficulties with concentration and memory, asthenia, and tremors are commonly prolonged in older convalescent patients. The CSF of patients with St. Louis encephalitis usually contains tens to hundreds of leukocytes, with a lymphocytic predominance and a left shift. The CSF glucose concentration is normal in these patients.

WEST NILE VIRUS INFECTION West Nile virus is now the primary cause of arboviral encephalitis in the United States. From 1999 to 2018, 24,657 cases of neuroinvasive disease (e.g., meningitis, encephalitis, acute flaccid paralysis), with 2199 deaths, and 26,173 cases of nonneuroinvasive infection, with 131 deaths, were reported. West Nile virus was initially described as being transmitted among wild birds by *Culex* mosquitoes in Africa, Asia, and southern Europe. In addition, the virus has been implicated in severe and fatal hepatic necrosis in Africa. West Nile virus was introduced into New York City via diseased birds in 1999 and subsequently spread to other areas of the northeastern United States, causing die-offs among crows, exotic zoo birds, and other birds. The virus has continued to spread and is now found in almost all of the United States as well as in Canada, Mexico, South America, and the Caribbean islands. *C. pipiens* mosquitoes remain the major vectors in the northeastern United States, but mosquitoes of several other *Culex* species and Asian tiger mosquitoes (*A. albopictus*) are also involved. Jays compete with crows and other corvids as amplifiers and lethal targets in other areas of the country.

West Nile virus is a common cause of febrile disease without CNS involvement (incubation period, 3–14 days), but it occasionally causes aseptic meningitis and severe encephalitis, particularly among the elderly. The fever-myalgia syndrome caused by West Nile virus differs from that caused by other viruses in terms of the frequent—rather than occasional—appearance of a maculopapular rash concentrated on the trunk (especially in children) and the development of lymphadenopathy. Back pain, fatigue, headache, myalgia, retroorbital pain, sore throat, nausea and vomiting, and arthralgia (but not arthritis) are common accompaniments that may persist for several weeks. Overall, only 1 in 50 patients develops neuroinvasive disease, characterized typically, though with overlap, as meningitis, encephalitis, or acute flaccid paralysis syndromes. The risk of encephalitis, neurologic sequelae, and death is increased in elderly, diabetic, and hypertensive patients and patients with previous CNS insults. In addition to the more severe motor and cognitive sequelae, milder findings may include tremor, slight abnormalities in motor skills, and loss of executive functions. Intense clinical interest and the availability of laboratory diagnostic methods have made it possible to define a number of unusual clinical features. Such features include chorioretinitis, flaccid paralysis with histologic lesions resembling poliomyelitis, and initial presentation with fever and focal neurologic deficits in the absence of diffuse encephalitis. Immunosuppressed patients may have fulminant courses or develop persistent CNS infection. Virus transmission through both transplantation and blood transfusion has necessitated screening of blood and organ donors by nucleic-acid–based tests. Occasionally, pregnant women infect their fetuses with West Nile virus. Diagnosis rests upon detection of IgM antibodies in serum or CSF. Treatment is supportive only, and ventilatory support may be required for severe neuroinvasive disease. Although an equine vaccine is available, prevention of West Nile virus infection in humans relies on avoidance of mosquito bites, vector control, and safe handling of potentially infected carcasses.

Peribunyavirids • **CALIFORNIA ENCEPHALITIS** The isolation of California encephalitis virus established California serogroup orthobunyaviruses as causes of encephalitides. However, California encephalitis virus has been implicated in only a very few cases of encephalitis (California encephalitis sensu stricto), whereas its close relative, La Crosse virus, is the major cause of encephalitis in this serogroup (~80–100 cases per year in the United States). La Crosse encephalitis is most commonly reported from the upper midwestern United States but is also found in other areas of the central and eastern parts of the country, such as West Virginia, Tennessee, North Carolina, and Georgia. The serogroup includes 13 other viruses, some of which (e.g., Inkoo, Jamestown Canyon, Lumbo, snowshoe hare, and Ťahyňa viruses) also cause human disease (California encephalitis sensu lato, including La Crosse encephalitis). Transovarial infection is a strong component of transmission of the California serogroup viruses in *Aedes* and *Ochlerotatus* mosquitoes. The vector of La Crosse virus is the *Ochlerotatus triseriatus* mosquito. These mosquitos are infected by transovarial transmission, feeding on viremic chipmunks and other mammals, and by venereal transmission. *O. triseriatus* breeds in sites such as tree holes and abandoned tires and bites during daylight hours. The habits of this mosquito correlate with the risk factors for human cases: recreation in forested areas, residence at a forest's edge, and the presence of water-containing abandoned tires around the home. Intensive environmental modification based on these findings has reduced the incidence of disease in a highly endemic area in the midwestern United States.

Most humans are infected from July through September. Asian tiger mosquitoes (*A. albopictus*) efficiently transmit La Crosse virus to mice and also transmit the agent transovarially in the laboratory. This aggressive anthropophilic mosquito has the capacity to urbanize, and its possible impact on transmission of virus to humans is of concern. The prevalence of antibody to La Crosse virus in humans is 20% or higher in endemic areas, indicating that infection is common but often asymptomatic. CNS disease has been recognized primarily in children <15 years of age.

The illness from La Crosse virus varies from aseptic meningitis accompanied by confusion to severe and occasionally fatal encephalitis (lethality, <0.5%). The incubation period is ~3–7 days. Although there may be prodromal symptoms/signs, the onset of CNS disease is sudden, with fever, headache, and lethargy often with nausea and vomiting, convulsions (in half of patients), and coma (in one third of patients). Focal seizures, hemiparesis, tremor, aphasia, chorea, Babinski signs, and other evidence of significant neurologic dysfunction are common acutely, but residual sequelae are not, although approximately 10% of patients have recurrent seizures in the succeeding months. Other serious sequelae of La Crosse virus infection are rare, although a decrease in scholastic standing among children has been reported, and mild personality change has occasionally been suggested.

The blood leukocyte count is commonly elevated in patients with La Crosse virus infection, sometimes reaching 20,000 per μL, usually with a left shift. CSF leukocyte counts are typically 30–500 per μL, usually with a mononuclear cell predominance (although 25–90% of cells are polymorphonuclear in some patients). The blood protein concentration is normal or slightly increased, and the glucose concentration is normal. Specific virologic diagnosis based on IgM-capture assays of serum and CSF is efficient. The only human anatomic site from which virus has been isolated is the brain.

Treatment is supportive over a 1- to 2-week acute phase during which status epilepticus, cerebral edema, and inappropriate secretion of antidiuretic hormone are important concerns. A phase 2B clinical trial of intravenous (IV) ribavirin in children with La Crosse virus infection was discontinued during dose escalation because of adverse effects.

Jamestown Canyon virus has been implicated in several cases of encephalitis in adults (~30 cases per year since 2013), usually with a significant respiratory illness at onset. Human infection with this virus has been documented in Massachusetts, New York, Wisconsin, Ohio, Michigan, Ontario, and other areas of Northern America (both in the United States and Canada), where the vector mosquito (*Aedes stimulans*) feeds on its main host, the white-tailed deer (*Odocoileus virginianus*). Ťahyňa virus can be found in Africa, China, Central Europe, and Russia. The virus is a prominent cause of febrile disease but can also cause pharyngitis, pulmonary syndromes, aseptic meningitis, or meningoencephalitis.

Rhabdovirids • CHANDIPURA VIRUS INFECTION Chandipura virus is an emerging and increasingly significant human virus in India, where it is transmitted among hedgehogs by mosquitoes and sandflies. In humans, the disease begins as an influenza-like illness, with fever, headache, abdominal pain, nausea, and vomiting. These manifestations are followed by neurologic impairment and infection-related or autoimmune-mediated encephalitis. Chandipura virus infection is characterized by high lethality in children. Several hundred cases of infection are recorded in India every year. Infections with other arthropod-borne rhabdovirids (Isfahan, Piry, vesicular stomatitis Indiana, vesicular stomatitis New Jersey viruses) may imitate the early febrile stage of Chandipura virus infection.

Togavirids • EASTERN EQUINE ENCEPHALITIS This disease is encountered primarily in swampy foci along the east coast of the United States, with a few inland foci as far removed as Michigan. In recent years, virus activity appears to be increasing. Infected humans present for medical care from June through October. During this period, the bird–*Culiseta* mosquito cycle spills over into other vectors, such as *Aedes sollicitans* or *Aedes vexans* mosquitoes, which are more likely to feed on mammals. There is concern over the potential role of introduced Asian tiger mosquitoes (*A. albopictus*), which have been found to be infected with eastern equine encephalitis virus and are an effective experimental vector in the laboratory. Horses are a common target for the virus. Contact with unvaccinated horses may be associated with human disease, but horses probably do not play a significant role in amplification of the virus.

Most of those infected do not develop neurologic manifestations; however, after an incubation period of approximately 5–10 days, 2% (adults) and 6% (children) develop sudden and rapidly progressive encephalitis leading to profoundly altered mental status and coma that is highly lethal (at least 30–50%) and leaves survivors with frequent sequelae. Acute polymorphonuclear CSF pleocytosis, often occurring during the first 1–3 days of disease, is another indication of severity. In addition, leukocytosis with a left shift is a common feature. Extensive necrotic lesions and polymorphonuclear infiltrates are found at postmortem examination of the brain. A formalin-inactivated vaccine has been used to protect laboratory workers but is not generally available or applicable.

VENEZUELAN EQUINE ENCEPHALITIS Venezuelan equine encephalitis viruses are separated into epizootic viruses (subtypes IA/B and IC) and enzootic viruses (subtypes ID, IE, and IF). Closely related enzootic viruses are Everglades virus, Mucambo virus, and Tonate virus. Enzootic viruses are found primarily in humid tropical-forest habitats and are maintained between culicoid mosquitoes and rodents. These viruses cause acute febrile human disease but are not pathogenic for horses and do not cause epizootics. Everglades virus has caused encephalitis in humans in Florida. Extrapolation from the rate of genetic change suggests that Everglades virus may have been introduced into Florida <200 years ago. Everglades virus is most closely related to the ID-subtype viruses that appear to have given evolutionary rise to the epizootic variants active in South America.

Epizootic viruses have an unknown natural cycle but periodically cause extensive epizootics/epidemics in equids and humans in the Americas. These epizootics/epidemics are the result of high-level viremia in horses and mules, which transmit the infection to several types of mosquitoes. Infected mosquitoes in turn infect humans. Humans also have high-level viremia, but their role in virus transmission is unclear. Relatively restricted epizootics of Venezuelan equine encephalitis occurred repeatedly in South America at intervals of 10 years or less from the 1930s until 1969, when a massive epizootic, including tens of thousands of equine and human infections, spread throughout Central America and Mexico, reaching southern Texas in 1971. Genetic sequencing suggested that the virus from that outbreak originated from residual "un-inactivated" IA/B-subtype virus in veterinary vaccines. The outbreak was terminated in Texas with a live attenuated vaccine (TC-83) originally developed for human use by the U.S. Army; the epizootic virus was then used for further production of inactivated veterinary vaccines. No further major epizootic disease outbreaks occurred until 1995 and 1996, when large epizootics of Venezuelan equine encephalitis occurred in Colombia/Venezuela and Mexico, respectively. Of the >85,000 clinical cases, 4% (more children than adults) included neurologic symptoms/signs, and 300 cases ended in death. The viruses involved in these epizootics as well as previously epizootic IC viruses are close phylogenetic relatives of known enzootic ID viruses. This finding suggests that active evolution and selection of epizootic viruses are underway in South America.

During epizootics, extensive human infection is typical, with clinical disease occurring in 10–60% of infected individuals. Most infections result in notable acute febrile disease, whereas relatively few infections (5–15%) result in neurologic disease. A low rate of CNS invasion is supported by the absence of encephalitis among the many infections resulting from exposure to aerosols in the laboratory setting or from vaccination accidents.

The prevention of epizootic Venezuelan equine encephalitis depends on vaccination of horses with the attenuated TC-83 vaccine or with an inactivated vaccine prepared from that variant. Enzootic viruses are genetically and antigenically different from epizootic viruses, and protection against the former with vaccines prepared from the latter is relatively ineffective. Humans can be protected by immunization with similar vaccines prepared from Everglades virus, Mucambo virus, and Venezuelan equine encephalitis virus, but the use of the vaccines is restricted to laboratory personnel because of reactogenicity, possible fetal pathogenicity, and limited availability.

WESTERN EQUINE ENCEPHALITIS The primary maintenance cycle of western equine encephalitis virus in the western United States and Canada involves *Aedes*, *C. tarsalis*, and *Culiseta* mosquitoes and birds (principally sparrows and finches). Equids and humans become infected, and both suffer encephalitis without amplifying the virus in nature. St. Louis encephalitis virus is transmitted in a similar cycle in the same regions harboring western equine encephalitis virus; disease caused by the former occurs about a month earlier than that caused by the latter (July through October). Large epidemics of western equine encephalitis occurred in the western and central United States and Canada from the 1930s through the 1950s, but the disease subsequently has been uncommon. From 1964 through 2010, only 640 cases were reported in the United States. This decline in incidence may reflect, in part, the integrated approach to mosquito management employed in irrigation projects and, in part, the increasing use of agricultural pesticides. The decreased incidence of western equine encephalitis almost certainly reflects the increased tendency for humans to be indoors behind closed windows at dusk—the peak biting period of the major vector.

After an incubation period of ~5–10 days, western equine encephalitis virus causes a typical diffuse viral meningo-encephalitis, with an increased attack rate and increased morbidity among the young, particularly children <2 years of age. In addition, lethality is high among the young and the very elderly (3–7% overall). One third of individuals who have convulsions during the acute illness have subsequent seizure activity. Infants <1 year of age—particularly those in the first months of life—are at serious risk of motor and intellectual damage. Of those 5–9 years of age, twice as many males as females develop clinical encephalitis. This difference in incidence may be related to greater outdoor exposure of boys to the vector but may also be due in part to biologic differences. A formalin-inactivated vaccine has been used to protect laboratory workers but is not generally available.

FEVER AND MYALGIA

The fever and myalgia syndrome is the most common clinical presentation associated with zoonotic virus infection. Many of the viruses listed in Table 209-1 probably cause at least a few cases of this syndrome, but only some of these viruses have prominent associations with the syndrome and are of biomedical importance. The fever and myalgia syndrome typically begins with the abrupt onset of fever, chills, intense myalgia, and malaise. Patients may also report joint or muscle pains, but true arthritis is not found. Anorexia is characteristic and may be accompanied by nausea or even vomiting. Headache is common and may be severe, with photophobia and retroorbital pain. Physical findings are minimal and are usually confined to conjunctival injection with pain on palpation of muscles or the epigastrium. The duration of symptoms/signs is quite variable (generally 2–5 days), with a biphasic course in some instances. The spectrum of disease varies from subclinical to temporarily incapacitating. Less common findings include a nonpruritic maculopapular rash, epistaxis (not necessarily indicating a bleeding diathesis), and aseptic meningitis. Even in the presence of headache, meningismus, or photophobia, the lack of opportunity to examine the CSF in remote areas makes diagnosis difficult. Although pharyngitis or radiographic evidence of pulmonary infiltrates is found in some patients, the agents causing this syndrome are not primary respiratory pathogens.

The fever and myalgia syndrome is also the most nonspecific of the disease syndromes caused by arthropod-borne and rodent-borne viruses. Furthermore, the early stages of other syndromes discussed in this chapter may begin similarly and are encompassed in a broad differential diagnosis that includes community-acquired parasitic infections (e.g., malaria), bacterial infections (e.g., anicteric leptospirosis, rickettsial diseases), and other viral infections. The fever and myalgia syndrome is often described as "influenza-like," but the usual absence of cough and coryza makes influenza an unlikely confounder except at the earliest stages. Treatment is supportive, but acetylsalicylic acid is avoided because of the potential for exacerbated bleeding or Reye's syndrome. Complete recovery is the general outcome for people with this syndrome, although prolonged asthenia and nonspecific symptoms have been described in some patients, particularly after infection with lymphocytic choriomeningitis virus or dengue viruses 1–4.

Efforts to prevent viral infection are best based on vector control, which, however, may be expensive or impossible. For mosquito control, destruction of breeding sites is generally the most economically and environmentally sound approach. Emerging containment technologies include the release of genetically modified mosquitoes and the spread of *Wolbachia* bacteria to limit mosquito multiplication rates. Depending on the vector and its habits, other possible approaches include the use of screens or other barriers (e.g., permethrin-impregnated bed nets) to prevent the vector from entering dwellings, judicious application of arthropod repellents (such as *N,N*,-diethyltoluamide [DEET]) to the skin, use of long-sleeved (ideally permethrin-impregnated) clothing, and avoidance of the vectors' habitats and times of peak activity.

Bunyavirals Numerous bunyavirals cause fever and myalgia. Many of these viruses cause individual infections and usually do not result in epidemics. These viruses include arenavirids, such as lymphocytic choriomeningitis mammarenavirus; hantavirids, such as the orthohantavirus Choclo virus; nairovirids, such as the orthonairoviruses Dugbe virus, Nairobi sheep disease virus, and Sōngling virus; peribunyavirids, such as the viruses of the orthobunyavirus Anopheles A serogroup (e.g., Tacaiuma virus), the Bunyamwera serogroup (Bunyamwera, Batai, Cache Valley, Fort Sherman, Germiston, Guaroa, Ilesha, Ngari, Shokwe, and Xingu viruses), the Bwamba serogroup (Bwamba virus, Pongola virus), the Guamá serogroup (Catú virus, Guamá virus), the Nyando serogroup (Nyando virus), the Wyeomyia serogroup (Wyeomyia virus), and the ungrouped orthobunyavirus Tataguine virus; and phenuivirids, such as bandaviruses (Bhanja virus, Heartland virus) and the phlebovirus Candirú complex (Alenquer, Candirú, Echarate, Maldonado, Morumbi, and Serra Norte viruses).

ARENAVIRIDS Lymphocytic choriomeningitis is the only human mammarenavirus infection resulting predominantly in fever and myalgia. Lymphocytic choriomeningitis virus is transmitted to humans from the common house mouse (*Mus musculus*) by aerosols of excreta or secreta. The virus is maintained in the mouse mainly by vertical transmission from infected dams. Infected mice remain viremic and shed virus for life, with high concentrations of virus in all tissues. Infected colonies of pet hamsters also can serve as a link to humans. In addition, infections among scientists and animal caretakers can occur because the virus is widely used in immunology laboratories to study T-lymphocyte function and can silently infect cell cultures and passaged tumor lines. Moreover, patients may have a history of residence in rodent-infested housing or other exposure to rodents. An antibody prevalence of ~5–10% has been reported among adults from Argentina, Germany, and the United States.

Lymphocytic choriomeningitis differs from the general syndrome of fever and myalgia in that the onset is gradual. Conditions occasionally associated with the disease are orchitis, transient alopecia, arthritis, pharyngitis, cough, and maculopapular rash. An estimated one fourth of patients (or fewer) experience a febrile phase of 3–6 days. After a brief remission, many develop renewed fever accompanied by severe headache, nausea and vomiting, and meningeal signs lasting for ~1 week (the CNS phase). These patients virtually always recover fully, as do the rare patients with clear-cut signs of encephalitis. Recovery may be delayed by transient hydrocephalus. During the initial febrile phase, leukopenia and thrombocytopenia are common, and virus can usually be isolated from blood. During the CNS phase, the virus may be found in the CSF, and antibodies are present in the blood. The pathogenesis of lymphocytic choriomeningitis is thought to resemble manifestations following direct intracranial inoculation of the virus into adult mice. The onset of the immune response leads to T cell–mediated immunopathologic meningitis. During the meningeal phase, CSF mononuclear-cell counts range from the hundreds to the low thousands per microliter, and hypoglycorrhachia is found in one third of patients.

IgM-capture ELISA, immunochemistry, and RT-PCR are used in the diagnosis of lymphocytic choriomeningitis. IgM-capture ELISA of serum and CSF usually yields positive results; RT-PCR assays have been developed for probing CSF. In particular, patients who have fulminant infections transmitted by recent organ transplantation do not mount an immune response, so immunohistochemistry or RT-PCR is required for diagnosis. Infection should be suspected in acutely ill febrile patients with marked leukopenia and thrombocytopenia. In patients with aseptic meningitis, any of the following suggests lymphocytic choriomeningitis: a well-marked febrile prodrome, adult age, occurrence in the autumn, low CSF glucose levels, or CSF mononuclear-cell counts of >1000 per μL. In pregnant women, infection may lead to fetal invasion, with consequent congenital hydrocephalus, microcephaly, and/or chorioretinitis. Because the maternal infection may be mild, causing only a short febrile illness, antibodies to the virus should be sought in both the mother and the fetus under suspicious circumstances, particularly in TORCH (toxoplasmosis, rubella, cytomegalovirus, herpes simplex, and HIV-1/2)–negative neonatal hydrocephalus.

ORTHOBUNYAVIRUS GROUP C SEROGROUP Apeú, Caraparú, Itaquí, Madrid, Marituba, Murutucú, Nepuyo, Oriboca, Ossa, Restan, and Zungarococha viruses are among the most common causes of arboviral infection in humans entering South American jungles. These viruses cause acute febrile disease and are transmitted by mosquitoes in neotropical forests.

ORTHOBUNYAVIRUS SIMBU SEROGROUP Oropouche virus is transmitted in Central and South America by biting midges (*Culicoides paraensis*), which often breed to high density in cacao husks and other vegetable detritus found in towns and cities. Explosive epidemics involving thousands of patients have been reported from several towns in Brazil and Peru. Rash and aseptic meningitis have been detected in a number of patients. Iquitos virus, a recently discovered reassortant and close relative of Oropouche virus, causes disease that is easily mistaken for Oropouche virus disease; its overall epidemiologic significance remains to be determined.

PHLEBOVIRUS SANDFLY FEVER GROUP The phlebovirus sandfly fever group consists of numerous viruses that may cause human infection. Sandfly fever Cyprus virus, sandfly fever Ethiopia virus, sandfly fever Sicilian virus, and sandfly fever Turkey virus (and the encephalitis-causing Chios virus) are very closely related genetically and antigenically. In contrast, sandfly fever Naples virus is only distantly related genetically and antigenically to these viruses. Sandfly fever Naples virus has not been detected in sandflies, humans, or nonhuman vertebrates since the 1980s and therefore may be extinct. Sandfly fever Naples virus is the type virus of the species *Sandfly fever Naples phlebovirus*, which includes other human viruses, such as Granada virus and Toscana virus. Toscana virus is thus far the only phlebovirus transmitted by sandflies that is known to cause diseases affecting the central and peripheral nervous systems, such as encephalitis, meningitis, myositis, or polymyeloradiculopathy. *Phlebotomus* sandflies transmit the virus, probably by biting small mammals and humans. Female sandflies may be infected by the oral route as they take a blood meal and may transmit the virus to offspring when they lay their eggs after a second blood meal. This prominent transovarial transmission confounds virus control.

Sandfly fever is found in the circum-Mediterranean area, extending to the east through the Balkans into parts of China as well as into Western Asia. Sandflies are found in both rural and urban settings and are known for their short flight ranges and their small sizes; the latter enables them to penetrate standard mosquito screens and netting. Epidemics have been described in the wake of natural disasters and wars. After World War II, extensive spraying in parts of Europe to control malaria greatly reduced sandfly populations and transmission of sandfly fever Naples virus; the incidence of sandfly fever continues to be low.

A common pattern of disease in endemic areas consists of high attack rates among travelers and military personnel and little or no disease in the local population, who are protected after childhood infection. Toscana virus infection is common during the summer among rural residents and vacationers, particularly in Italy, Spain, and Portugal; a number of cases have been identified in travelers returning to Germany and Scandinavia. The disease may manifest as an uncomplicated febrile illness but is often associated with aseptic meningitis, with virus isolated from the CSF.

Coclé virus and Punta Toro virus are phleboviruses that are not part of the sandfly fever serocomplex but, like the members of this complex, are transmitted by sandflies. These two viruses cause a sandfly-fever-like disease in Latin American and Caribbean tropical forests, respectively, where the vectors rest on tree buttresses. Epidemics have not been reported, but antibody prevalence among inhabitants of villages in endemic areas indicates a cumulative lifetime exposure rate of >50% in the case of Punta Toro virus.

Flavivirids The most clinically significant flaviviruses that cause the fever and myalgia syndrome are dengue viruses 1–4. In fact, dengue without/with warning signs ("dengue," historically called "dengue fever"—to be distinguished from severe dengue) is probably the most prevalent arthropod-borne viral disease worldwide, with ~400 million infections occurring per year, of which ~100 million (25%) cause clinical illness. Dengue is endemic in >100 countries worldwide, including in Africa, the Americas, the eastern Mediterranean, South-Eastern Asia, and the western Pacific. More than half of the world's population is considered at risk, although Asia bears 70% of the global burden, with alarming increases over the past decade including, for example, >400,000 cases in 2019 in the Philippines. Year-round transmission of dengue viruses 1–4 occurs between latitudes 25°N and 25°S, but seasonal forays of the viruses into the United States and Europe have been documented. The principal vectors for all four viruses are yellow fever mosquitoes (*Ae. aegypti*). Through increasing spread of mosquitoes throughout the tropics and subtropics and international travel by infected humans, large areas of the world have become vulnerable to the introduction of dengue viruses 1–4. Thus, dengue and severe dengue (see "Viral Hemorrhagic Fever," below) are becoming increasingly common. For instance, conditions favorable to dengue viruses 1–4 transmission via yellow fever mosquitoes exist in Hawaii and the southern United States. The range of a lesser vector of dengue viruses 1–4 (*A. albopictus*) now extends from Asia to the continental United States, the Indian Ocean, parts of Europe, and Hawaii. Also anthrophilic, *Ae. aegypti* mosquitoes typically breed near human habitation, using relatively fresh water from sources such as water jars, vases, discarded containers, coconut husks, and old tires. These mosquitoes usually bite during the day. Bursts of dengue and severe dengue cases are to be expected in the southern United States, particularly along the Mexican border, where containers of water may be infested with yellow fever mosquitoes. Closed habitations with air-conditioning may inhibit transmission of many arboviruses, including dengue viruses 1–4.

After dengue virus infection and an incubation period averaging 4–7 days, three evolving phases are described: a febrile phase, a critical phase, and a recovery phase. The majority of patients presenting with fever and myalgia do not go through a critical phase, although early recognition of the critical phase consistent with severe dengue must be considered in all patients. (For further discussion of severe dengue—previously called "dengue hemorrhagic fever" and including dengue shock syndrome—see "Viral Hemorrhagic Fever," below.) In most patients, dengue begins with the typical sudden onset of fever, frontal headache, retroorbital pain, back pain, and severe myalgias. These symptoms gave rise to the colloquial designation of dengue as "break-bone fever." Often a transient macular rash appears on the first day, as do adenopathy, palatal vesicles, and scleral injection. The illness may last a week, with additional symptoms and clinical signs including anorexia, nausea or vomiting, and marked cutaneous hypersensitivity. Near the time of defervescence on days 3–5, a maculopapular rash begins on the trunk and spreads to the extremities and the face. Epistaxis and scattered petechiae are often noted in uncomplicated dengue without/with warning signs, and preexisting gastrointestinal lesions may bleed during the acute illness. A positive tourniquet test—i.e., the detection of 10 or more new petechiae in one square inch of the upper arm after a 5-min blood pressure cuff inflation to midway between systolic and diastolic pressure—may demonstrate microvascular fragility associated with dengue but is more likely to be associated with severe disease.

Laboratory findings of dengue without/with warning signs include leukopenia, thrombocytopenia, and, in many cases, modest elevations of serum aminotransferase concentrations without hepatic synthetic dysfunction. The diagnosis is made by IgM ELISA or paired serology during recovery or by antigen-detection ELISA or RT-PCR during the acute phase. Virus is readily isolated from blood in the acute phase if mosquito inoculation or mosquito cell culture is used.

Orthomyxovirids Bourbon virus was recently identified as the cause of a rare, severe, and sometimes fatal febrile disease of humans in the midwestern and southern United States.

Reovirids Several coltiviruses (Colorado tick fever, Eyach, and Salmon River viruses) and orbiviruses (Lebombo, Kemerovo, Orungo, and Tribeč viruses) can cause fever and myalgia in humans. With the exception of Lebombo and Orungo viruses, all are transmitted by ticks. The most significant reoviral arthropod-borne disease is Colorado tick fever. Several hundred patients with this disease are reported annually in the United States and Canada. The infection is acquired between March and November through the bite of an infected ixodid tick, the Rocky Mountain wood tick (*Dermacentor andersoni*), in mountainous western regions at altitudes of 1200–3000 m. Small mammals serve as amplifying hosts. The most common presentation is fever and myalgia, often with headache; meningoencephalitis is not uncommon, and hemorrhagic disease, pericarditis, myocarditis, orchitis, and pulmonary presentations have also been reported. Rash develops in a minority of patients. Leukopenia and thrombocytopenia are also noted. The disease usually lasts 7–10 days and is often biphasic. The most important differential diagnostic considerations since the beginning of the 20th century have been Rocky Mountain spotted fever (although Colorado tick fever is much more common in Colorado) and tularemia. Colorado tick fever virus replicates for several weeks in erythropoietic cells and can be found in erythrocytes. This feature, detected in erythroid smears stained by immunofluorescence, can be diagnostically helpful and is important during screening of blood donors.

PULMONARY DISEASE

Hantavirus pulmonary syndrome (HPS) was first described in 1993, but retrospective identification of cases by immunohistochemistry (1978) and serology (1959) supports the idea that HPS is a recently discovered rather than a truly new disease. The causative agents are orthohantaviruses of a distinct phylogenetic lineage that is associated with the cricetid rodent subfamily Sigmodontinae. Sin Nombre virus, which chronically infects North American deermice (*Peromyscus maniculatus*), is the most important agent of HPS in the United States. Several other related viruses (Anajatuba, Andes, Araraquara, Araucária, bayou, Bermejo, Black Creek Canal, Blue River, Caño Delgadito, Castelo dos Sonhos, Catacamas, Choclo, Juquitiba, Laguna Negra, Lechiguanas, Maciel, Maripa, Monongahela, New York, Orán, Paranoá, Pergamino, Rio Mamoré, and Tunari viruses) cause the disease in Northern America and South America. Andes virus is unusual in that it has been implicated in human-to-human transmission. HPS particularly affects rural residents living in dwellings permeable to rodent entry or people working in occupations that pose a risk of rodent exposure. Each type of rodent has its own particular habits; in the case of deermice, these behaviors include living in and around human habitation.

HPS begins with a prodrome of ~3–4 days (range, 1–11 days) comprising fever, malaise, myalgia, and—in many cases—gastrointestinal disturbances (such as abdominal pain, nausea, and vomiting). Dizziness is common, and vertigo is occasional. Severe prodromal symptoms/signs may bring some patients to medical attention, but most cases are recognized as the pulmonary phase begins. Typical signs are slightly lowered blood pressure, tachycardia, tachypnea, mild hypoxemia, thrombocytopenia, and early radiographic signs of pulmonary edema. Physical findings in the chest are often surprisingly scant. The conjunctival and cutaneous signs of vascular involvement seen in hantavirus VHFs (see "Viral Hemorrhagic Fever," below) are uncommon. During the next few hours, decompensation may progress rapidly to severe hypoxemia and respiratory failure.

The differential diagnosis of HPS includes abdominal surgical conditions and pyelonephritis as well as rickettsial disease, sepsis, meningococcemia, plague, tularemia, influenza, and relapsing fever. A specific diagnosis is best made by IgM antibody testing of acute-phase serum, which has yielded positive results even in the prodrome. Tests using a Sin Nombre virus antigen detect antibodies to the related HPS-causing orthohantaviruses. Occasionally, heterotypic viruses will react only in the IgG ELISA, but such a finding is highly suspicious given the very low seroprevalence of these viruses in normal populations. RT-PCR is usually positive when used to test blood clots obtained in the first 7–9 days of illness and when used to test tissues. This assay is useful in identifying the infecting virus in areas outside the home range of deermice and in atypical cases.

During the prodrome, the differential diagnosis of HPS is difficult, but by the time of presentation or within 24 h thereafter, a number of diagnostically helpful clinical features become apparent. Usually, cough is not present at the outset. Interstitial edema is evident on chest x-ray. Later, bilateral alveolar edema with a central distribution develops in the setting of a normal-sized heart; occasionally, the edema is initially unilateral. Pleural effusions are often seen. Thrombocytopenia, circulating atypical lymphocytes, and a left shift (often with leukocytosis) are almost always evident; thrombocytopenia is a particularly important early clue. Hemoconcentration, hypoalbuminemia, and proteinuria should also be sought for diagnosis. Although thrombocytopenia virtually always develops and prolongation of the partial thromboplastin time is the rule, clinical evidence of coagulopathy or laboratory indications of disseminated intravascular coagulation (DIC) are found in only a minority of severely ill patients. Patients with severe illness also have acidosis and elevated serum lactate concentrations. Mildly increased values in renal function tests are common, but patients with severe HPS often have markedly elevated serum creatinine concentrations. Some New World orthohantaviruses other than Sin Nombre virus (e.g., Andes virus) have been associated with greater kidney involvement, but few such cases have been studied.

Management of HPS during the first few hours after presentation is critical. The goal is to prevent severe hypoxemia by oxygen therapy, with intubation and intensive respiratory management if needed. During this period, hypotension and shock with increasing hematocrit invite aggressive fluid administration, but this intervention should be undertaken with great caution. Because of low cardiac output with myocardial depression and increased pulmonary vascular permeability, shock should be managed expectantly with vasopressors and modest infusion of fluid guided by pulmonary capillary wedge pressure. Mild cases can be managed by frequent monitoring and oxygen administration without intubation. Many patients require intubation to manage hypoxemia and shock. Extracorporeal membrane oxygenation is instituted in severe cases, ideally before the onset of shock. The procedure is indicated in patients who have a cardiac index of 2.3 L/min/m^2 or an arterial oxygen tension to fractional inspired oxygen (Pa_{O_2}:F_{IO_2}) ratio of <50 and who are unresponsive to conventional support. Lethality remains at ~30–40%, even with good management, but most patients surviving the first 48 h of hospitalization are extubated and discharged within a few days with no apparent long-term residua. The antiviral drug ribavirin inhibits orthohantaviruses in vitro but showed no marked effect on patients treated in an open-label study.

■ VIRAL HEMORRHAGIC FEVER

VHF is a syndromic constellation of findings based on vascular instability and decreased vascular integrity. A direct or indirect assault on the microvasculature leads to increased permeability and (particularly when platelet function is decreased) to actual disruption and local hemorrhage (a positive tourniquet sign). Blood pressure is decreased, and in severe cases, shock supervenes. Cutaneous flushing and conjunctival suffusion are examples of common, observable abnormalities in the control of local circulation. Hemorrhage occurs infrequently. In most patients, hemorrhage is an indication of widespread vascular damage rather than a life-threatening loss of blood volume. In some VHFs, specific organs may be particularly impaired. For instance, the kidneys are primary targets in HFRS, and the liver is a primary target in yellow fever and filovirus diseases. However, in all of these diseases, generalized circulatory disturbance appears centrally in clinical manifestations. The pathogenesis of VHF is poorly understood and varies among the viruses regularly implicated in the syndrome. In some viral infections, direct damage to the vascular system or even to parenchymal cells of target organs is an important factor; in other viral infections, soluble mediators are thought to play a major role in the development of hemorrhage or fluid redistribution.

The acute phase in most cases of VHF is associated with ongoing virus replication and viremia. VHFs begin with fever and myalgia, usually of abrupt onset. (Mammarenavirus infections are the exceptions, as they often develop gradually.) Within a few days, the patient presents for medical attention because of increasing prostration that is often accompanied by abdominal or chest pain, anorexia, dizziness, severe headache, hyperesthesia, photophobia, nausea or vomiting, and other gastrointestinal disturbances. Initial examination often reveals only an acutely ill patient with conjunctival suffusion, tenderness to palpation of muscles or abdomen, and borderline hypotension or postural hypotension (perhaps with tachycardia). Petechiae (often best visualized in the axillae), flushing of the head and thorax, periorbital edema, and proteinuria are common. AST activities are usually elevated at presentation or within a day or two thereafter. Hemoconcentration from vascular leakage, which is usually evident, is most marked in HFRS and in severe dengue. The seriously ill patient progresses to more severe clinical signs and develops shock and other findings typical of the causative virus. Shock, multifocal bleeding, and CNS involvement (encephalopathy, coma, seizures) are all poor prognostic signs.

One of the major diagnostic clues to VHF is travel to an endemic area within the incubation period for a given syndrome. Except in infections with Seoul virus, dengue viruses 1–4, and yellow fever virus, which have urban hosts/vectors, travel to a rural setting is especially suggestive of a diagnosis of VHF. In addition, several diseases considered in the differential diagnosis—falciparum malaria, shigellosis, typhoid fever, leptospirosis, relapsing fever, and rickettsial diseases—are treatable and potentially lethal.

Early recognition of VHF is important because of the need for virus-specific therapy and supportive measures. Such measures include prompt, atraumatic hospitalization; judicious fluid therapy that takes into account the patient's increased capillary permeability; administration of cardiotonic drugs; use of vasopressors to maintain blood pressure at levels that will support renal perfusion; treatment of the relatively common secondary bacterial (and the rarer fungal) infections; replacement of clotting factors and platelets as indicated; and the usual precautionary measures used in the treatment of patients with hemorrhagic diatheses. DIC should be treated only if clear laboratory evidence of its existence is found and if laboratory monitoring of therapy is feasible; there is no proven benefit of such therapy. The available evidence suggests that VHF patients have decreased cardiac output and will respond poorly to fluid loading, which is often practiced in the treatment of shock associated with bacterial sepsis. Specific therapy is available for several of the VHFs. Strict barrier nursing and other precautions against infection of medical staff and visitors are indicated when VHFs are encountered, except when the illness is due to dengue viruses 1–4, orthohantaviruses, Rift Valley fever virus, or yellow fever virus.

Novel VHF-causing agents are still being discovered. Besides the viruses listed below, the latest additions are the severe fever with thrombocytopenia syndrome bandavirus (which is continuing to cause VHF cases in China, Japan, the Republic of Korea, and Vietnam) and possibly the tibrovirus Bas-Congo virus (which has been associated with three cases of VHF in the Democratic Republic of the Congo). However, Koch's postulates have not yet been fulfilled to prove cause and effect in the case of Bas-Congo virus.

Bunyavirals The most significant VHF-causing bunyavirals are arenavirids (Junín, Lassa, and Machupo viruses), hantavirids, nairovirids (Crimean-Congo hemorrhagic fever virus), and phenuivirids (Rift Valley fever and severe fever with thrombocytopenia syndrome viruses). Other bunyavirals—e.g., the Garissa variant of Ngari virus and Ilesha virus (both orthobunyaviruses) or Chapare, Guanarito, Lujo, and Sabiá viruses (all mammarenaviruses)—have caused sporadic VHF outbreaks.

ARGENTINIAN AND BOLIVIAN HEMORRHAGIC FEVERS These severe diseases (with lethality reaching 15–30%) are caused by Junín virus and Machupo virus, respectively. Their clinical presentations are similar, but their epidemiology differs because of the distribution and behavior of the viruses' rodent reservoirs. Argentinian hemorrhagic fever has thus far been recorded only in rural areas of Argentina, whereas Bolivian hemorrhagic fever seems to be confined to rural Bolivia. Infection with the causative agents almost always results in disease, and all ages and both sexes are affected. Person-to-person or nosocomial transmission is rare but has occurred. The transmission of Argentinian hemorrhagic fever from convalescing men to their wives suggests the need for counseling of patients with mammarenavirus hemorrhagic fever concerning the avoidance of intimate contacts for several weeks after recovery. In contrast to the pattern in Lassa fever (see below), thrombocytopenia—often marked—is the rule, hemorrhage is common, and CNS dysfunction (e.g., marked confusion, tremors of the upper extremities and tongue, and cerebellar signs) is much more common in disease caused by Junín virus and Machupo virus. Some cases follow a predominantly neurologic course, with a poor prognosis.

The clinical laboratory is helpful in diagnosis since thrombocytopenia, leukopenia, and proteinuria are typical findings. Argentinian hemorrhagic fever is readily treated with convalescent-phase plasma given within the first 8 days of illness. In the absence of passive antibody therapy, IV ribavirin in the dose recommended for Lassa fever is likely to be effective in all South American VHFs caused by mammarenaviruses. A safe, effective, live attenuated vaccine exists for Argentinian hemorrhagic fever. After vaccination of >250,000 high-risk people in the endemic area, the incidence of this VHF decreased markedly. In experimental animals, this vaccine is cross-protective against Bolivian hemorrhagic fever.

LASSA FEVER Lassa virus is known to cause endemic and epidemic disease in Nigeria, Sierra Leone, Guinea, and Liberia, although it is probably more widely distributed in Western Africa. In countries where Lassa virus is endemic, Lassa fever can be a prominent cause of febrile disease. For example, in one hospital in Sierra Leone, laboratory-confirmed Lassa fever is consistently responsible for one fifth of admissions to the medical wards. In Western Africa alone, probably tens of thousands of Lassa virus infections occur annually. Lassa virus can be transmitted by close person-to-person contact. The virus is often present in urine during convalescence and has been detected in seminal fluid early in recovery. Nosocomial spread has occurred but is uncommon if proper sterile parenteral techniques are used. All ages and both sexes are affected; the incidence of disease is highest in the dry season, but transmission takes place year-round.

Among the VHF agents, only mammarenaviruses are typically associated with a gradual onset of illness, which begins after an incubation period of 5–16 days. Hemorrhage is seen in only ~15–30% of Lassa fever patients; a maculopapular rash is often noted in light-skinned patients. Effusions are common, and male-dominant pericarditis may develop late in infection. Lethality among pregnant women is higher than the usual 15–30% and is especially increased during the last trimester. Fetal lethality reaches 90%. Excavation of the uterus may increase survival rates of pregnant women, but data on Lassa fever and pregnancy are still sparse. These figures suggest that interruption of the pregnancy of women infected with Lassa virus should be considered. White blood cell counts are normal or slightly elevated, and platelet counts are normal or somewhat low. Deafness coincides with clinical improvement in ~20% of patients and is permanent and bilateral in some patients. Reinfection may occur but has not been associated with severe disease.

High-level viremia or high serum AST activity statistically predicts a fatal outcome. Data from randomized controlled trials is needed to identify the optimal LASV-specific treatment to accompany aggressive supportive and critical care. Observational studies of Lassa fever patients in the 1980's informed the current practice of treating patients with ribavirin (intravenous route preferred). This antiviral nucleoside analogue appears to be partially effective in reducing lethality from that documented among retrospective controls. However, possible side effects, such as reversible anemia (which usually does not require transfusion), dependent hemolytic anemia, and bone marrow suppression, need to be kept in mind. Ribavirin should be given by slow IV infusion in a dose of 32 mg/kg; this dose should be followed by 16 mg/kg every 6 h for 4 days and then by 8 mg/kg every 8 h for 6 days. Inactivated Lassa virus vaccines failed in preclinical studies, but several promising vaccine platforms are under experimental evaluation.

HEMORRHAGIC FEVER WITH RENAL SYNDROME HFRS is the most significant VHF today, with >100,000 cases of severe disease in Asia annually and thousands of mild infections in Europe. The disease is widely distributed in Eurasia. The major causative viruses are Puumala virus (Europe), Dobrava virus (the Balkans), and Hantaan virus (Eastern Asia). Amur, gōu, Kurkino, Muju, Saaremaa, Sochi, and Tula viruses also cause HFRS but much less frequently and in more geographically confined areas that are determined by the distribution of reservoir hosts. Seoul virus is an exception in that it is associated with brown rats (*Rattus norvegicus*); therefore, the virus has a worldwide distribution because of the migration of these rodents on ships. Despite the wide distribution of Seoul virus, only mild or moderate HFRS occurs in Asia, and human disease has been difficult to identify in many areas of the world. Most cases of HFRS occur in rural residents or vacationers; again, the exception is Seoul virus infection, which may be acquired in an urban, rural, or laboratory setting. Classic Hantaan virus infection in Korea and in rural China is most common in the spring and fall and is related to rodent density and agricultural practices. Human infection is acquired primarily through aerosols of rodent urine, although virus is also present in rodent saliva and feces. Patients with HFRS are not infectious.

Severe cases of HFRS evolve in four identifiable stages:

1. The *febrile* stage lasts 3 or 4 days and is identified by the abrupt onset of fever, headache, severe myalgia, thirst, anorexia, and often nausea and vomiting. Photophobia, retroorbital pain, and pain on ocular movement are common, and the vision may become blurred with ciliary body inflammation. Flushing over the face, the V area of the neck, and the back is characteristic, as are pharyngeal injection, periorbital edema, and conjunctival suffusion. Petechiae often develop in areas of pressure, the conjunctivae, and the axillae. Back pain and tenderness to percussion at the costovertebral angle reflect massive retroperitoneal edema. Laboratory evidence of mild to moderate DIC is present. Other laboratory findings of HFRS include proteinuria and active urinary sediment.
2. The *hypotensive* stage lasts from a few hours to 48 h and begins with falling blood pressure and sometimes shock. The relative bradycardia typical of the febrile phase is replaced by tachycardia.

Kinin activation is marked. The rising hematocrit reflects increasing vascular leakage. Leukocytosis with a left shift develops, and thrombocytopenia continues. Atypical lymphocytes—which, in fact, are activated $CD8^+$ and, to a lesser extent, $CD4^+$ T cells—circulate. Proteinuria is marked, and the urine's specific gravity falls to 1.010. Renal circulation is congested and compromised from local and systemic circulatory changes resulting in necrosis of tubules, particularly at the corticomedullary junction, and oliguria.

3. During the *oliguric* stage, hemorrhagic tendencies continue, probably in large part because of uremic bleeding defects. Oliguria persists for 3–10 days before the return of renal function marks the onset of the polyuric stage.
4. The *polyuric* stage (diuresis and hyposthenuria) carries the danger of dehydration and electrolyte abnormalities.

Mild cases of HFRS may be much less stereotypical. The presentation may include only fever, gastrointestinal abnormalities, and transient oliguria followed by hyposthenuria. Infections with Puumala virus, the most common cause of HFRS in Europe (*nephropathia epidemica*), result in a much-attenuated picture but the same general presentation. Bleeding manifestations are found in only 10% of patients, hypotension rather than shock is usually documented, and oliguria is present in only about half of patients. The dominant features may be fever, abdominal pain, proteinuria, mild oliguria, and sometimes blurred vision or glaucoma, followed by polyuria and hyposthenuria in recovery. Lethality is <1%.

HFRS should be suspected in patients with rural exposure in an endemic area. Prompt recognition of the disease permits rapid hospitalization and expectant management of shock and renal failure. Useful clinical laboratory parameters include leukocytosis, which may be leukemoid and is associated with a left shift; thrombocytopenia; and proteinuria. HFRS is readily diagnosed by an IgM-capture ELISA that is positive at admission or within 24–48 h thereafter. The isolation of orthohantaviruses is difficult, but RT-PCR of a blood clot collected early in the clinical course or of tissues obtained postmortem should give positive results. Such testing is usually undertaken if definitive identification of the infecting virus is required.

Mainstays of therapy are management of shock, reliance on vasopressors, modest crystalloid infusion, IV human serum albumin administration, timely renal replacement therapy to prevent overhydration that may result in pulmonary edema, and control of hypertension that increases the possibility of intracranial hemorrhage. Use of IV ribavirin has reduced lethality and morbidity in severe cases, provided treatment is begun within the first 4 days of illness. Lethality may be as high as 15% but, with proper therapy, lethality should be lower than 5%. Sequelae have not been definitively established.

CRIMEAN-CONGO HEMORRHAGIC FEVER (CCHF) This severe VHF has a wide geographic distribution, potentially emerging wherever virus-bearing ticks occur. Because of the propensity of CCHF virus-transmitting ticks to feed on domestic livestock and certain wild mammals, veterinary serosurveys are the most effective mechanism for the monitoring of virus circulation in a particular region. Human infections are acquired via tick bites or during the crushing of infected ticks. Domestic animals do not become ill but do develop viremia. Thus, risk of acquiring CCHF occurs during sheep shearing, animal slaughter, or contact with infected hides or carcasses from recently slaughtered infected animals. Nosocomial epidemics are common and are usually related to extensive blood exposure or needlesticks.

Although generally similar to other VHFs, CCHF causes extensive liver damage, resulting in jaundice in some patients. Clinical laboratory values indicate DIC, elevations in activities of AST and creatine phosphokinase, and elevated bilirubin concentrations. Generally, patients who do not survive have more distinct changes in the concentrations of these markers than do survivors, even in the early days of illness, and also develop leukocytosis rather than leukopenia. In addition, thrombocytopenia is more marked and develops earlier in patients who do not survive than in survivors. The mainstay of treatment is supportive care that may include support of organ dysfunction. The benefit of IV ribavirin for treatment remains debated and unproven. Clinical experience and retrospective comparison of patients with ominous clinical laboratory values support a contention that ribavirin may be efficacious, but a randomized clinical trial was not supportive of a benefit in lowering lethality rates. No human or veterinary vaccines are recommended.

RIFT VALLEY FEVER The natural range of Rift Valley fever virus was previously confined to sub-Saharan Africa, with circulation of the virus markedly enhanced by substantial rainfall. The El Niño Southern Oscillation phenomenon of 1997 facilitated subsequent spread of Rift Valley fever to the Arabian Peninsula, with epidemic disease in 2000. The virus has also been found in Madagascar and Egypt, where it caused major epidemics in 1977–1979, 1993, and thereafter. Rift Valley fever virus is maintained in nature by transovarial transmission in floodwater *Aedes* mosquitoes and presumably also has a vertebrate amplifier. Increased transmission during particularly heavy rains leads to epizootics characterized by high-level viremia in cattle, goats, or sheep. Numerous types of mosquitoes feed on these animals and become infected, thereby increasing the possibility of human infections. Remote sensing via satellite can detect the ecologic changes associated with high rainfall that predict the likelihood of Rift Valley fever virus transmission. High-resolution satellites can also detect the special depressions in floodwaters from which the mosquitoes emerge. The virus can be transmitted by contact with blood or aerosols from domestic animals. Therefore, transmission risk is high during birthing, and both abortuses and placentas need to be handled with caution. Risk is also high during animal slaughter but decreases thereafter as anaerobic glycolysis in postmortem tissues results in an acidic environment that rapidly inactivates bunyavirals in carcasses. Neither person-to-person nor nosocomial transmission of Rift Valley fever has been documented.

Rift Valley fever virus is unusual in that it causes several clinical syndromes. Most infections are manifested as the fever-myalgia syndrome. A small proportion of infections result in VHF with especially prominent liver involvement or encephalitis. Renal failure and DIC are also common features. Perhaps 10% of otherwise mild infections lead to retinal vasculitis, and some patients have permanently impaired vision. Funduscopic examination reveals edema, hemorrhages, and infarction of the retina as well as optic nerve degeneration. In a small proportion of patients (<1 in 200), retinal vasculitis is followed by viral encephalitis.

No proven therapy exists for Rift Valley fever. Both retinal disease and encephalitis occur after the acute febrile syndrome has resolved and serum neutralizing antibody has developed—but the immunopathophysiology is uncertain. Epidemic disease is best prevented by vaccination of livestock. The ability of this virus to propagate after introduction into Egypt suggests that other potentially receptive areas, including the United States, should develop response plans. Rift Valley fever, like Venezuelan equine encephalitis, is likely to be controlled only with adequate stocks of an effective live attenuated vaccine, but global stocks are unavailable. A formalin-inactivated vaccine confers immunity in humans; however, quantities are limited, and three injections are required. This vaccine is recommended for potentially exposed laboratory workers and for veterinarians working in sub-Saharan Africa. A new live attenuated vaccine, MP-12, is being tested in humans (phase 2 trials have been completed). The vaccine is safe and licensed for use in sheep and cattle. In addition, several vaccines are being developed specifically for use in animals.

SEVERE FEVER WITH THROMBOCYTOPENIA SYNDROME This tick-borne disease is caused by severe fever with thrombocytopenia syndrome bandavirus. Numerous human infections have been reported during the past few years from China, and several cases have also been detected in Japan, the Republic of Korea, and Vietnam. The clinical presentation ranges from mild nonspecific fever to severe VHF with high (>12%) lethality.

Flaviviruses The most significant flaviviruses that cause VHF are the mosquito-borne dengue viruses 1–4 and yellow fever virus. These viruses are widely distributed and cause tens to hundreds of thousands of infections each year. Alkhurma hemorrhagic fever virus (isolated infections every year), Kyasanur Forest disease virus (~10,000 cases over 60 years), and Omsk hemorrhagic fever virus (isolated infections every year with intermittent larger outbreaks) are geographically very restricted but prevalent tick-borne flaviviruses that cause VHF, sometimes with subsequent viral encephalitis. Tick-borne encephalitis virus has caused VHF in a few patients. There is currently no therapy for infection with these VHFs, but an inactivated vaccine has been used in India to prevent Kyasanur Forest disease.

SEVERE DENGUE Although most individuals infected with dengue virus 1, 2, 3, or 4 have either subclinical infection or fever and myalgia syndrome, some of these patients enter a critical phase—often as fever declines—and develop the criteria for severe dengue: plasma leakage severe enough to cause shock or respiratory distress, severe bleeding, or severe organ dysfunction. The complex determinants of risk for this progression include contributing host and viral factors but center most notably around the potential for immune-mediated enhancement of disease. Several weeks after convalescence from infection with dengue virus 1, 2, 3, or 4, the transient protection conferred by that infection against reinfection with a heterotypic dengue virus usually wanes. Heterotypic reinfection may result in classic dengue without/with warning signs or, less commonly, in severe dengue. In the past 20 years, yellow fever mosquitoes (*Ae. aegypti*) have progressively reinvaded Latin America and other areas, and frequent travel by infected individuals has introduced multiple variants of dengue viruses 1–4 from many geographic areas. Thus, the pattern of hyperendemic transmission of multiple dengue virus serotypes established in the Americas and the Caribbean has led to the emergence of severe dengue as a major problem. Among the millions of dengue viruses 1–4 infections, ~500,000 cases of severe dengue occur annually, with a lethality of ~2.5%. The induction of vascular permeability and shock depends on multiple factors, such as the presence or absence of enhancing and nonneutralizing antibodies, age (susceptibility to severe dengue drops considerably after 12 years of age), sex (females are more often affected than males), race (whites are more often affected than Black people), nutritional status, and timing and sequence of infections (e.g., dengue virus 1 infection followed by dengue virus 2 infection seems to be more dangerous than dengue virus 4 infection followed by dengue virus 2 infection). In addition, considerable heterogeneity exists among each dengue virus population. For instance, South-Eastern Asian dengue virus 2 variants have more potential to cause severe dengue than do other variants. Recent evidence points to a key role for the dengue virus NS1 protein in the vascular leak phenomenon associated with severe dengue.

In milder cases of severe dengue, restlessness, lethargy, thrombocytopenia (<100,000 per μL), and hemoconcentration are detected 2–5 days after the onset of typical dengue, usually at the time of defervescence. The maculopapular rash that often develops in dengue without/with warning signs may also appear in severe dengue. However, severe dengue is most notoriously identified as the consequence of a vascular leak syndrome leading to intravascular volume depletion, hypoalbuminemia, serosal effusions (pleural, ascitic), and, in severe cases, circulatory collapse (i.e., shock), often with an accompanying narrowed pulse pressure, hepatomegaly, and cyanosis. Recognizing this critical period early enough to initiate appropriate supportive care is crucial. (Shock typically lasts 2 or 3 days.) Bleeding tendencies (evidenced by a positive tourniquet test and petechiae) or overt bleeding in the absence of underlying causes (e.g., preexisting gastrointestinal lesions) may be detected but are less common in children. Organ involvement may include mild hepatic injury, CNS abnormalities (e.g., altered mental status, seizures), cardiac abnormalities (e.g., arrhythmias), renal disturbances (e.g., acute kidney injury), and ocular dysfunction.

A virologic diagnosis of severe dengue can be made by the usual means (nucleic acid amplification or antigen detection) in the first 5 days of infection, after which diagnosis rests on serologic testing. Combination testing—point-of-care rapid tests for NS1 antigen and IgM antibody assays—is increasingly used in the clinical setting. However, multiple flavivirus infections result in broad immune responses to several members of the genus, and this situation may result in a lack of virus specificity of the IgM and IgG immune responses. A secondary antibody response can be sought with tests against several flavivirus antigens to demonstrate the characteristic wide spectrum of reactivity.

Most patients with shock respond promptly to close monitoring, oxygen administration, and infusion of crystalloid or—in severe cases—colloid. Lethality varies greatly with case ascertainment and quality of treatment. However, most patients with severe dengue respond well to supportive therapy, and the overall lethality at an experienced center in the tropics is probably as low as 1%.

The key to control of both dengue without/with warning signs and severe dengue is the control of yellow fever mosquitoes, which also reduces the risk of urban yellow fever and chikungunya virus circulation. Control efforts have been handicapped by the presence of nondegradable tires and long-lived plastic containers in trash repositories—creating perfect mosquito breeding grounds upon filling with water during rainfall—and by insecticide resistance. Urban poverty and an inability of the public health community to mobilize the populace to respond to the need to eliminate mosquito breeding sites are also factors in lack of mosquito control. New approaches that may be considered in the future of vector control include the release of *Aedes* mosquitoes infected with *Wolbachia* or carrying dominant lethal genetic mutations that will be passed on to offspring. A tetravalent live attenuated dengue vaccine based on the attenuated yellow fever virus 17D platform (CYD-TDV, or Dengvaxia) was licensed in 2015 and registered in 20 countries for individuals 9–45 years of age. However, retrospective analysis of phase 3 trials in Latin America and Asia suggested protection from severe dengue only in previously seropositive individuals; indeed, the risk of severe dengue was actually increased in seronegative vaccine recipients over that in nonvaccinated seronegative individuals, a result suggesting that a "first serologic hit" from the vaccine predisposes naïve recipients to more severe natural dengue infection. Strategic revision to avoid vaccine-enhanced disease now includes prevaccination serologic screening aimed at the restriction of vaccination to seropositive individuals. At least two live attenuated candidate vaccines based on modified recombinant dengue viruses are being evaluated in phase 3 clinical studies; similar concerns about safety are being addressed.

YELLOW FEVER Yellow fever virus had caused major epidemics in Africa and Europe before its transmission by yellow fever mosquitoes (*Ae. aegypti*) was discovered in 1900. Urban yellow fever became established in the New World as a result of colonization with yellow fever mosquitoes—originally an African mosquito. Subsequently, different types of mosquitoes and nonhuman primates were found to maintain yellow fever virus in Africa and also in Central and South American jungles. Transmission to humans is incidental, occurring via bites from mosquitoes that have fed on viremic monkeys. After the identification of *Ae. aegypti* as the vector of yellow fever, containment strategies were aimed at increased mosquito control. Today, urban yellow fever transmission occurs only in some African cities, but the threat exists in the cities of South America, where reinfestation by yellow fever mosquitoes has taken place, and dengue viruses 1–4 transmission by these mosquitoes is common. Despite the existence of a highly effective and safe vaccine, several hundred jungle cases of yellow fever occur annually in South America, and 84,000–170,000 severe jungle and urban cases (resulting in 29,000–60,000 deaths) occurred in Africa in 2013 alone. In 2016, a large urban outbreak (Luanda, Angola) spilled over to generate local transmission in large cities in neighboring countries (e.g., Kinshasa, Democratic Republic of the Congo) as well as travel-related cases in China; the signal of a global threat that included exportation to Asia stimulated ongoing efforts to identify and vaccinate highest-risk populations in 40 targeted countries in Africa and South America, to reactively vaccinate people in outbreak settings, and to increase measures to prevent exportation.

Yellow fever is a typical VHF accompanied by prominent hepatic necrosis. After an incubation period of 3–6 days, patients present with a nonspecific febrile illness (fatigue, myalgia, backache, headaches, photophobia, anorexia, nausea or vomiting) associated with viremia typically lasting 3–4 days. After defervescence, 10–15% of patients develop recrudescent fever and "intoxication" characterized by severe dysfunction of the liver and other organs. Hepatic failure leads to the characteristic jaundice, bleeding (gastrointestinal tract, nasopharyngeal mucosa), abdominal pain with nausea and vomiting, and hyperammonemic encephalopathy; acute kidney injury leads to oliguria, azotemia, and marked albuminuria; and myocardial injury and encephalitis have been described. Abnormalities in liver function tests range from modest elevations of hepatic aminotransferase activities in mild cases to severe liver injury, hyperbilirubinemia, and the synthetic dysfunction of acute hepatic failure. Early leukopenia may become leukocytosis as disease progresses, and coagulation abnormalities are common. Treatment is supportive only. Although the majority of infections are subclinical, 50% of patients who enter the toxic phase die in the next 7–10 days.

Urban yellow fever can be prevented by the control of yellow fever mosquitoes. The continuing sylvatic cycles require vaccination of all visitors to areas of potential transmission with live attenuated variant 17D vaccine virus, which cannot be transmitted by mosquitoes. With few exceptions, reactions to the vaccine are minimal; immunity is provided within 10 days and lasts for at least 25–35 years. An egg allergy mandates caution in vaccine administration. Although there are no documented harmful effects of the vaccine on fetuses, pregnant women should be immunized only if they are definitely at risk of exposure to yellow fever virus. Because vaccination has been associated with several cases of encephalitis in children <6 months of age, it is contraindicated in this age group and not recommended for infants 6–8 months of age unless the risk of exposure is very high. Rare, serious, multisystemic adverse reactions (occasionally fatal), including vaccine-associated "viscerotropic" yellow fever, have been reported, particularly affecting the elderly, and the risk-to-benefit ratio should be weighed before vaccine administration to individuals ≥60 years of age. Nevertheless, the number of deaths of unvaccinated travelers with yellow fever exceeds the number of deaths from vaccination, and a liberal vaccination policy for travelers to involved areas should be pursued. Timely information on changes in yellow fever distribution and yellow fever vaccine requirements can be obtained from the U.S. Centers for Disease Control and Prevention (*http://www.cdc.gov/vaccines/vpd-vac/yf/default.htm*).

Acknowledgment

The authors gratefully acknowledge the major contributions of Clarence J. Peters and additional contributions by Rémie N. Charrel to this chapter in previous editions.

FURTHER READING

Centers for Disease Control and Prevention: Arbovirus catalog. Available at *https://wwwn.cdc.gov/arbocat/*. Accessed May 24, 2021.

Howley PM, Knipe DM (eds): *Fields Virology. Volume 1: Emerging Viruses*, 7th ed. Philadelphia, Wolters Kluwer/Lippincott Williams & Wilkins, 2020.

International Committee on Taxonomy of Viruses (ICTV): Virus taxonomy: The ICTV report on virus classification and taxon nomenclature. Available at *https://talk.ictvonline.org/ictv-reports/ictv_online_report/*. Accessed May 24, 2021.

Lvov DK et al: *Zoonotic Viruses of Northern Eurasia: Taxonomy and Ecology*. London, Elsevier/Academic Press, 2015.

Singh SK, Ruzek D (eds): *Viral Hemorrhagic Fevers*. Boca Raton, FL, CRC Press, 2013.

Vasilakis N, Gubler DJ (eds): *Arboviruses: Molecular Biology, Evolution and Control*. Haverhill, UK, Caister Academic Press, 2016.

WEBSITE

International Committee on Taxonomy of Viruses (ICTV). *https://talk.ictvonline.org/*. Accessed May 24, 2021.

210 Ebolavirus and Marburgvirus Infections

Jens H. Kuhn, Ian Crozier

Several viruses in the family *Filoviridae* cause severe and frequently fatal infections in humans. Introduction of filoviruses into human populations is an extremely rare event that most likely occurs by direct or indirect contact with reservoir hosts (known and unknown) or by contact with filovirus-infected, sick, or deceased mammals. Filoviruses are highly infectious but not exceptionally contagious. Human-to-human transmission takes place through direct person-to-person contact or exposure to infected body fluids or tissues; there is no evidence of aerosol or respiratory droplet transmission in natural outbreak settings. Infections manifest initially with a nonspecific influenza-like febrile illness that rapidly progresses to commonly include gastrointestinal manifestations and, in severe illness, coagulopathy, multiple-organ dysfunction syndrome, shock, and death. Although the prevalence and source remain controversial, serologic footprints of subclinical acute filoviral infections have been identified since the first descriptions of filovirus disease outbreaks. Filovirus disease survivors may be persistently infected in immune-privileged tissue compartments, commonly the male reproductive tract, central nervous system (CNS), and intraocular tissues and fluids. Historically, the prevention of filovirus infections has consisted primarily of tried-and-true epidemiologic approaches (e.g., isolation of cases, tracing of contacts, effective infection prevention and control, safe burial practices), and treatment has consisted only of limited supportive clinical care (often constrained by in-field capacity); indeed, filovirus-specific vaccines or therapeutic agents had not been rigorously evaluated in humans prior to the 2013–2016 outbreak of Ebola virus disease (EVD) that occurred in Western Africa. Building on the knowledge gained in Western Africa and during the 2018–2020 EVD outbreak in the Democratic Republic of the Congo, prevention and treatment strategies now include the widespread deployment of an effective Ebola virus–specific vaccine; the use of effective therapeutics based on virus-specific monoclonal antibodies (mAbs), which were identified in a first-of-its-kind randomized controlled trial; and the delivery of more advanced supportive care. Although these advances have essentially become new standards for prevention and treatment of EVD, the same cannot yet be said for other filovirus diseases.

Filoviruses are categorized as World Health Organization (WHO) Risk Group 4 pathogens. Consequently, all work with material suspected of containing replicating filoviruses should be conducted only in maximal containment (biosafety level 4) laboratories, or the viruses should be inactivated prior to analysis in biosafety level 2 laboratories. Experienced personnel handling these viruses must wear appropriate personal protective equipment (PPE; see "Control and Prevention," below) and follow rigorous standard operating procedures. In addition, when filovirus infections are suspected, the appropriate national authorities and WHO reference laboratories should be contacted immediately.

ETIOLOGY

The family *Filoviridae* includes six official and two proposed genera (**Table 210-1 and Fig. 210-1**). Human pathogens are found in two of these genera, *Ebolavirus* and *Marburgvirus*. Collectively, these pathogens cause filovirus disease (FVD; International Classification of Diseases, Eleventh Revision [ICD-11], code 1D60). FVD is subdivided into Ebola disease (EBOD; ICD-11, code 1D60.0), caused by four of six classified ebolaviruses (Bundibugyo virus, Ebola virus, Sudan virus, and Taï Forest virus), and Marburg disease (MARD; ICD-11, code 1D60.1), caused by the two marburgviruses, Marburg virus and Ravn virus.

TABLE 210-1 Current Filovirus Taxonomy

Realm *Riboviria*
- Kingdom *Orthornavirae*
  - Phylum *Negarnaviricota*
    - Subphylum *Haplovirictina*
      - Class *Monjiviricetes*
        - Order *Mononegavirales*
          - Family *Filoviridae*
            - Genus *Cuevavirus*
              - Species *Lloviu cuevavirus*
                - Virus: Lloviu virus (LLOV)
            - Genus *Dianlovirus*
              - Species *Mengla dianlovirus*
                - Virus: Měnglà virus (MLAV)
            - Genus *Ebolavirus*
              - Species *Bombali ebolavirus*
                - Virus: Bombali virus (BOMV)
              - Species *Bundibugyo ebolavirus*
                - Virus: Bundibugyo virus (BDBV)
              - Species *Reston ebolavirus*
                - Virus: Reston virus (RESTV)
              - Species *Sudan ebolavirus*
                - Virus: Sudan virus (SUDV)
              - Species *Tai Forest ebolavirus*
                - Virus: Taï Forest virus (TAFV)
              - Species *Zaire ebolavirus*
                - Virus: Ebola virus (EBOV)
            - Genus *Marburgvirus*
              - Species *Marburg marburgvirus*
                - Virus 1: Marburg virus (MARV)
                - Virus 2: Ravn virus (RAVV)
            - Genus *"Oblavirus"*
              - Species *"Oblavirus percae"*
                - Virus: Oberland virus (OBLV)
            - Genus *Striavirus*
              - Species *Xilang striavirus*
                - Virus: Xīlǎng virus (XILV)
            - Genus *"Tapjovirus"*
              - Species *"Tapjovirus bothropis"*
                - Virus: Tapajós virus (TAPV)
            - Genus *Thamnovirus*
              - Species *Huangjiao thamnovirus*
                - Virus: Huángjiāo virus (HUJV)
              - Species *"Thamnovirus kanderense"*
                - Virus: Kander virus (KNDV)
              - Species *"Thamnovirus percae"*
                - Virus: Fiwi virus (FIWIV)

Filoviruses that are known to infect humans are depicted in color. Officially proposed taxa are indicated by quotation marks.

Mammalian filoviruses have linear, nonsegmented, negative-sense RNA genomes that are ~19 kb in length. These genomes contain seven genes that encode seven structural proteins: nucleoprotein (NP), polymerase cofactor (VP35), matrix protein (VP40), glycoprotein ($GP_{1,2}$), transcriptional activator (VP30), ribonucleoprotein complex-associated protein (VP24), and large protein (L) that contains an RNA-directed RNA polymerase domain. Ebolaviruses, but not marburgviruses, additionally encode three nonstructural proteins of unknown function (sGP, ssGP, and Δ-peptide). Filovirions are unique among human virus particles in that they are predominantly pleomorphic filaments but also assume torus-like or 6-like shapes (width ~91–98 nm; average length <1 μm). These enveloped virions contain helical ribonucleoprotein capsids and are covered with $GP_{1,2}$ spikes (**Fig. 210-2**).

EPIDEMIOLOGY

The majority of recorded FVD outbreaks, including the 2013–2016 EVD outbreak, can be traced back to single index patients who transmitted the infection to others. Although small outbreaks may have been missed historically, the epidemiology of these transmission chains suggests that only ~50 natural host-to-human spillover events have occurred since the discovery of filoviruses in 1967. Outbreak frequency, size, and overall case–fatality rate are likely the result of complex interactions of the specific filovirus, the reservoir hosts (known and unknown), the susceptible human population (e.g., varying with age, unknown genetic determinants of susceptibility and disease severity, risk behavior), and the geographic setting (e.g., local public health capacity, socioeconomic conditions, cultural practices).

As of August 25, 2021, 35,311 human filovirus infections and 15,758 deaths had been recorded (**Fig. 210-3**). These numbers emphasize both the high case–fatality rate (number of deaths per number of sick people; 44.6%) and the overall low mortality rate (reflecting the impact on the healthy population) of filovirus infections. Of these totals, 28,652 infections and 11,325 deaths occurred during the 2013–2016 EVD (ICD-11 EBOD subcategory code 1D60.01) outbreak in Western Africa; this was the largest of all recorded FVD outbreaks. Natural FVD outbreaks had not been considered a global threat until regional and then global spread during this outbreak challenged that tenet. Filoviruses that are pathogenic in humans appear to be exclusively endemic to equatorial (Western, Middle, and Eastern) Africa (**Fig. 210-4**), although this distribution may change if natural or artificial environmental alterations lead to filovirus host migration and increased contacts between nonhuman hosts and humans.

Outbreaks have been contained when high-risk activities (e.g., ritual washing as part of burial practices) have been limited or been made safer with appropriate infection prevention and control. Of particular importance is accessibility to health care centers with staff trained and equipped (e.g., with PPE) for adequate prevention and control of infections, which have a crucial effect on overall case numbers. The incidence of FVD may have increased over the past two decades (Figs. 210-3 and 210-4), but debate continues as to whether this increase is due to increased filovirus activity, more frequent human interaction with filovirus hosts, or improvement in surveillance capabilities.

FVD outbreaks are associated with distinct meteorologic and geographic conditions and are probably associated with distinct hosts or reservoirs. The four ebolaviruses that cause disease in humans appear to be endemic in humid rainforests. EVD outbreaks in particular have often been associated with hunting in forests or contact with bushmeat (i.e., meat from apes, other nonhuman primates, duikers, or bush pigs). Ecologic studies indicate that Ebola virus may play a role in extensive and frequently fatal epizootics among wild ape populations. However, only one ebolavirus, Taï Forest virus, has been isolated from nonhuman primates in the wild. Marburgviruses, on the other hand, seem to infect hosts inhabiting arid woodlands. MARD outbreaks have almost always been epidemiologically linked to individuals visiting or working in natural or engineered caves or mines. A pteropodid (fruit) bat, the cave-dwelling Egyptian rousette (*Rousettus aegyptiacus*), serves as a natural and subclinically infected reservoir for both Marburg virus and Ravn virus. Although bats are suspected hosts for ebolaviruses as well, definitive proof is lacking. To date, the nonpathogenic Bombali virus is the only ebolavirus that has been isolated directly from bats. Ebola virus and Reston virus have been loosely connected to frugivorous and insectivorous bats by means of antibody or genome fragment detection, whereas the hosts of Bundibugyo virus, Sudan virus, and Taï Forest virus are enigmatic.

PATHOGENESIS

Human infections typically occur through direct exposure of skin lesions or mucosal surfaces to contaminated body fluids or material or by parenteral inoculation (e.g., via accidental needlesticks or reuse

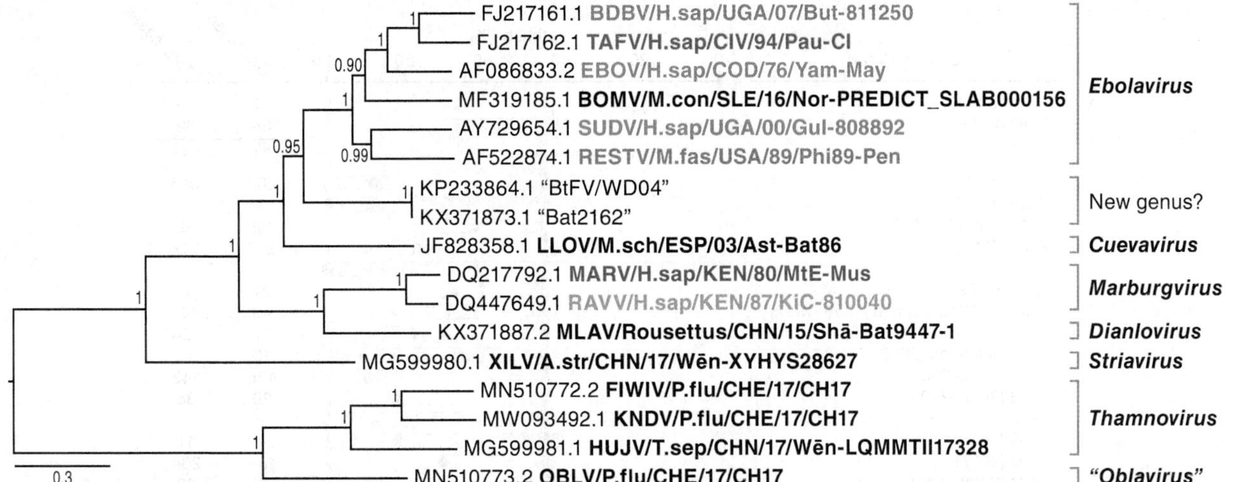

FIGURE 210-1 Filovirus phylogeny/evolution. Midpoint-rooted maximum-likelihood tree inferred by using filovirus large gene (*L*) sequences. Bootstrap values are shown at each node. The scale bar indicates nucleotide substitutions per site. Tips of branches are labeled with GenBank accession numbers followed by filovirus isolate designation. BDBV, Bundibugyo virus; BOMV, Bombali virus; EBOV, Ebola virus; FIWIV, Fiwi virus; HUJV, Huángjiāo virus; KNDV, Kander virus; LLOV, Lloviu virus; MARV, Marburg virus; MLAV, Měnglà virus; OBLV, Oberland virus; RAVV, Ravn virus; RESTV, Reston virus; SUDV, Sudan virus; TAFV, Taï Forest virus; XILV, Xīlǎng virus. *(Adapted and expanded from JH Kuhn et al:* Filoviridae, *in Fields Virology, Vol 1, 7th ed, PM Howley et al (eds). Philadelphia, Wolters Kluwer/Lippincott Williams & Wilkins, 2020, pp 449–503. Analysis courtesy of Nicholas Di Paola, PhD, USAMRIID, Fort Detrick, MD, USA. Figure courtesy of Jiro Wada, NIH/NIAID/DCR/IRF-Frederick, Fort Detrick, MD, USA.)*

of needles in poorly equipped hospitals). Numerous studies, both in vitro and in vivo (in several animal models of human disease), have illuminated aspects of FVD pathogenesis (Fig. 210-5). The $GP_{1,2}$ spikes on the surface of filovirions determine their cell and tissue tropism by engaging yet-unidentified cell-surface molecules and the intracellular filovirus receptor NPC intracellular cholesterol transporter 1.

One of the hallmarks of filovirus pathogenesis is a pronounced modulation and dysregulation of immune responses. The first targets of filovirions are local macrophages, monocytes, and dendritic cells. Several structural proteins of filovirions (i.e., VP35, VP40, and/or VP24) then suppress intrinsic and innate immune responses by, for example, inhibiting the type I interferon antiviral pathways. This immunomodulation ultimately enables a productive filovirus infection, resulting in very high viral titers (>10^6 plaque-forming units [PFU]/mL of serum in humans) with dissemination to most tissues. In tissues, filovirions infect additional phagocytic cells, including other macrophages (alveolar, peritoneal, and pleural macrophages; Kupffer cells in the liver; and microglia in the CNS), epithelial cells (e.g., adrenal cortical cells, hepatocytes), stromal cells (fibroblasts), and endothelial cells. Infection is cytolytic in some—but not all—infected cells (e.g., hepatocyte necrosis likely contributes to elevated aminotransferase activities, and hepatic synthetic dysfunction contributes to coagulopathy). Infection leads to the secretion of soluble signaling molecules (varying with the cell type) that most likely contribute to forward dysregulation of immune responses and ultimately to multiorgan dysfunction syndrome. For instance, infected macrophages react by secreting proinflammatory cytokines, a response that leads to further recruitment of macrophages to the site of infection. In contrast, infected dendritic cells are not activated to secrete cytokines, and expression of major histocompatibility class II antigens is partially suppressed, with consequently deficient antigen presentation. Immunosuppression also occurs in part by massive lymphoid depletion in lymph nodes, spleen, and thymus in the absence of effective humoral and cell-mediated immune responses, especially in lethal infections. Results from animal studies suggest that depletion is a direct consequence of considerable lymphocyte death; this explanation would also account for the severe lymphopenia that develops in patients. In addition to potential florid filovirus dissemination, another consequence may be susceptibility of FVD patients to secondary bacterial and fungal infections.

Other pathogenic hallmarks of filovirus infections include coagulopathy and endothelial dysfunction. Along with hepatic synthetic dysfunction, disseminated intravascular coagulation may contribute

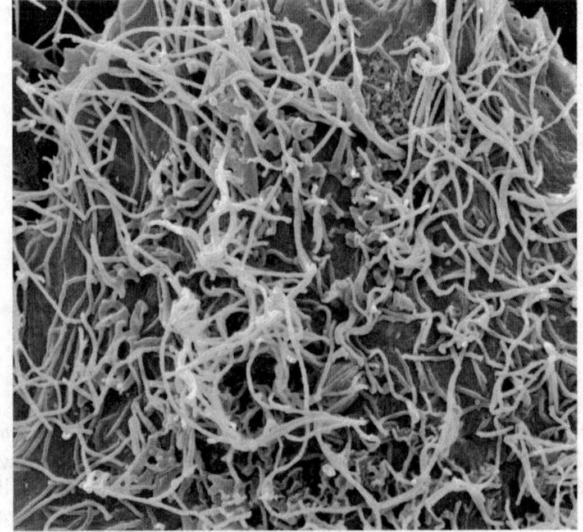
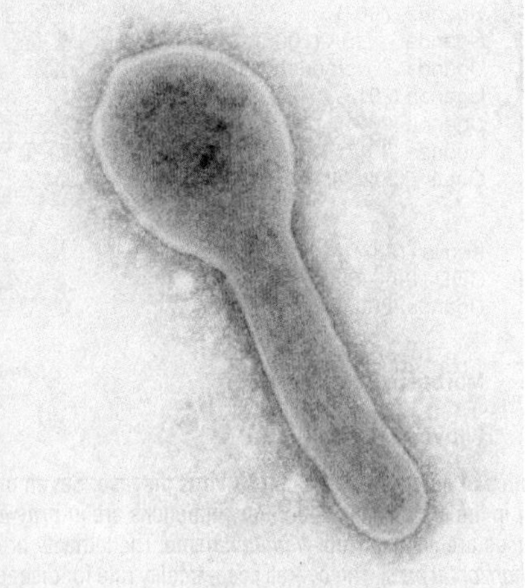

FIGURE 210-2 Ultrastructure of filovirions. ***Left:*** Colorized scanning electron micrograph of Ebola virus particles (*green*) attached to the surface of an infected grivet (*Chlorocebus aethiops*) Vero E6 producer cell (blue). ***Right:*** Colorized transmission electron micrograph of a Marburg virus particle collected from purified Vero E6 producer cell supernatant. *(Figure courtesy of John G. Bernbaum and Jiro Wada, NIH/NIAID/DCR/IRF-Frederick, Fort Detrick, MD, USA.)*

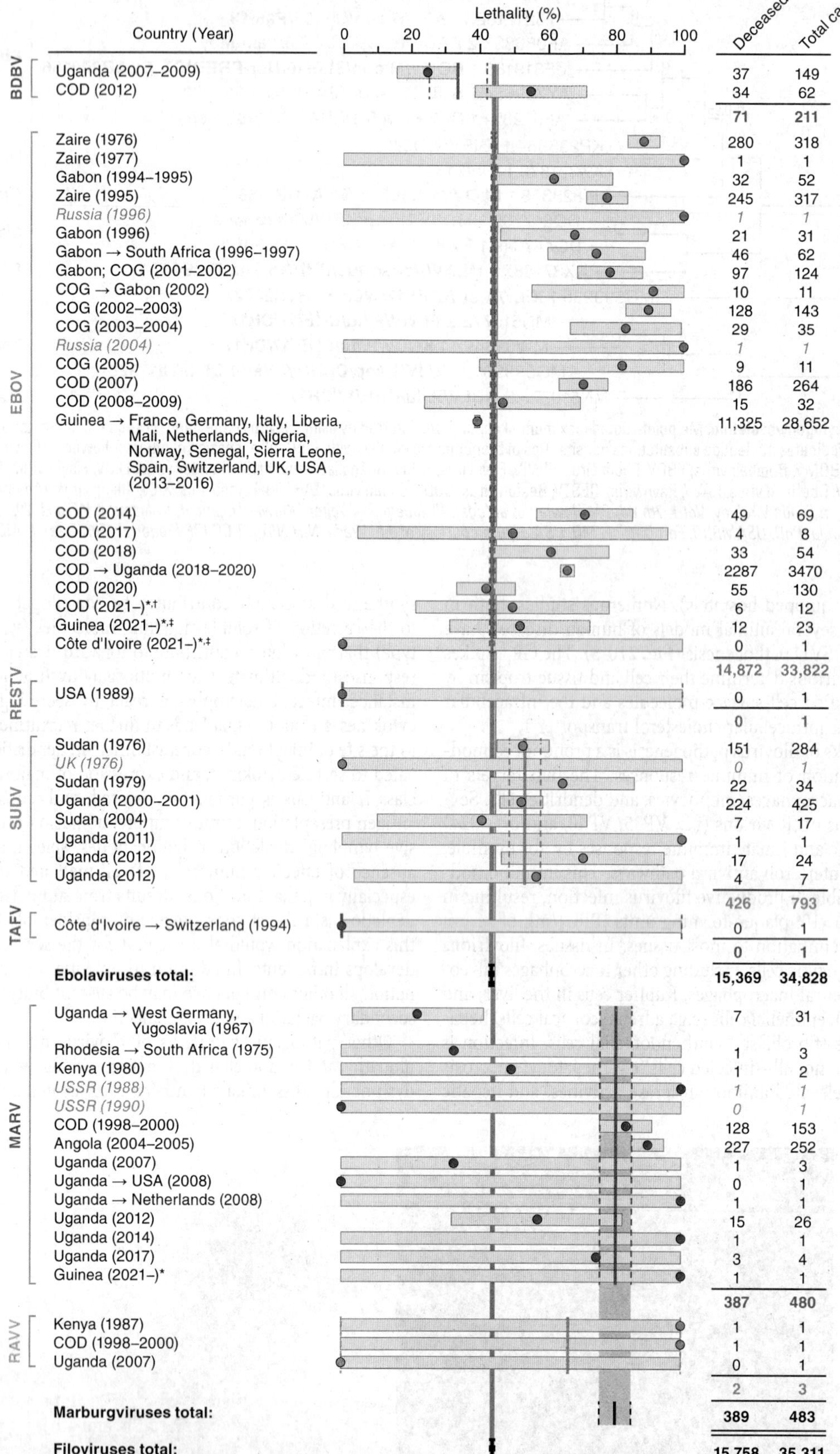

FIGURE 210-3 Characteristics of outbreaks of human filovirus disease. Seven of 12 classified filoviruses have caused infections in humans. ***Left column:*** Outbreaks are listed by virus in chronological order in the left column. Laboratory infections are in *gray italicized* text. International case exportations are indicated with *arrows*. ***Right column:*** Numbers of lethal cases and total cases are summarized. ***Middle column:*** The lethality or case–fatality rate (*colored dots*) for each outbreak is plotted on a 0–100% scale along with 99% confidence intervals (*gray horizontal bars*). The overall case–fatality rate for disease caused by a particular virus is delineated by *vertical colored lines*, with *vertical colored dashed lines* indicating the corresponding 99% confidence intervals. The overall case–fatality rates for all ebolavirus infections, all marburgvirus infections, and all filovirus infections are shown by (underlaid) *vertical gray bars*. BDBV, Bundibugyo virus; COD, Democratic Republic of the Congo (formerly Zaire); COG, Republic of the Congo; EBOV, Ebola virus; MARV, Marburg virus; RAVV, Ravn virus; RESTV, Reston virus; SUDV, Sudan virus; TAFV, Taï Forest virus; UK, United Kingdom; USSR, Union of Soviet Socialist Republics (today Russia). *, as of August 25, 2021. †, possibly connected to the 2018–2020 EVD outbreak. ‡, possibly connected to the 2013–2016 EVD outbreak. *(Adapted and expanded from JH Kuhn et al: Evaluation of perceived threat differences posed by filovirus variants. Biosecur Bioterror 9:361, 2011. Figure courtesy of Jiro Wada, NIH/NIAID/DCR/IRF-Frederick, Fort Detrick, MD, USA.)*

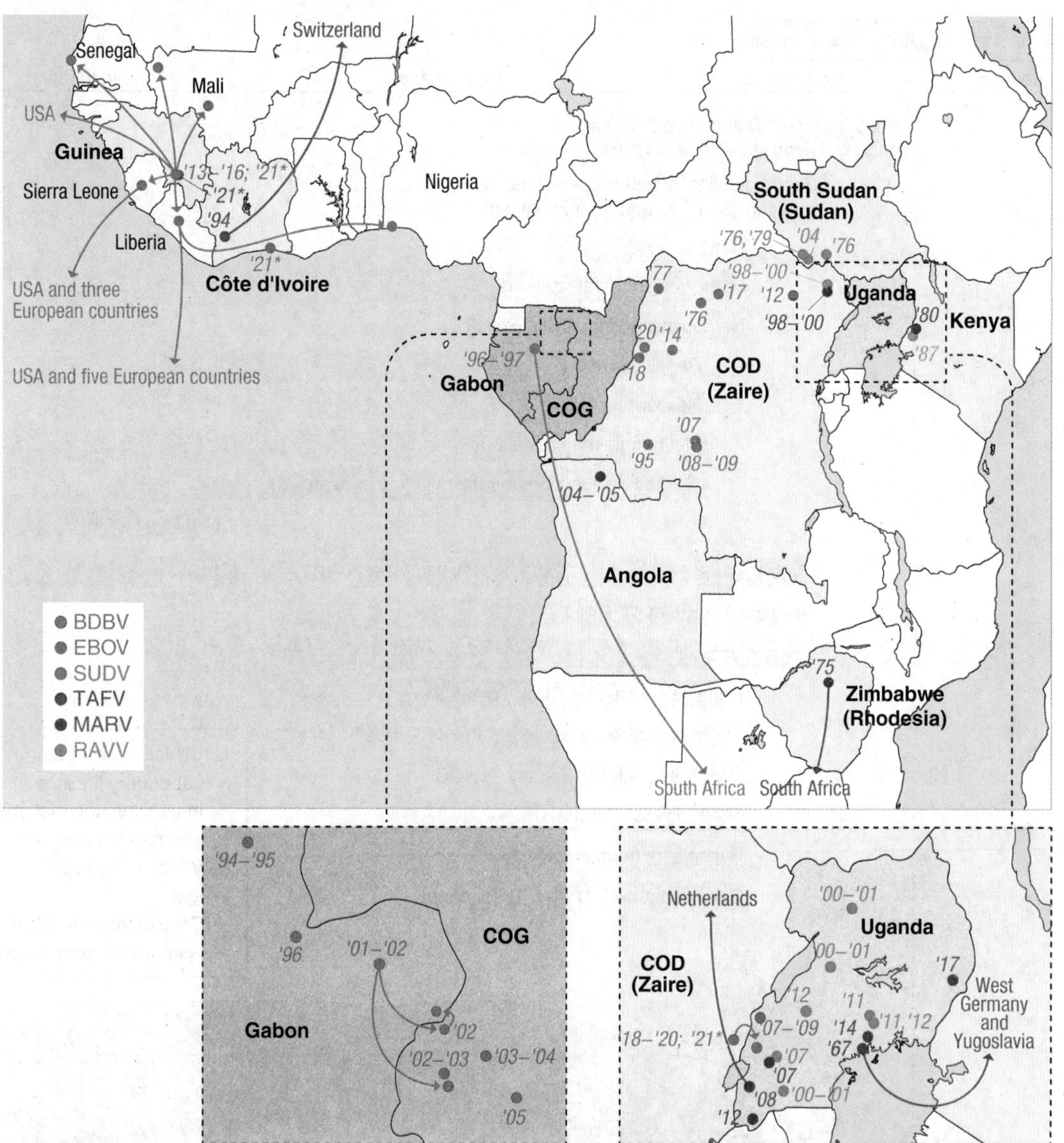

FIGURE 210-4 Geographic distribution of human filovirus disease outbreaks and years of occurrence. *Arrows* indicate international case exportations. BDBV, Bundibugyo virus; COD, Democratic Republic of the Congo (formerly Zaire); COG, Republic of the Congo; EBOV, Ebola virus; MARV, Marburg virus; RAVV, Ravn virus; SUDV, Sudan virus; TAFV, Taï Forest virus. *(Figure courtesy of Jiro Wada, NIH/NIAID/DCR/IRF-Frederick, Fort Detrick, MD, USA.)*

to the clotting dysfunction seen in filovirus-infected patients. Thrombocytopenia, increased concentrations of tissue factor, consumption of clotting factors, increased concentrations of fibrin degradation products (D-dimers), and declining concentrations of protein C are typical features of infection. Consequently, fibrin deposition and microthrombotic small-vessel occlusion and necrotic/hypoxic infarction may occur in some tissues, particularly in the gonads and less often in the kidneys and spleen. In addition, petechiae, ecchymoses, extensive visceral effusions, and other hemorrhagic signs are observed in internal organs, mucous membranes, and skin. Actual severe blood loss, however, is a rare event (although it frequently occurs during or after childbirth). Most likely, aberrance in cytokines or other factors, such as nitric oxide, and direct infection and activation of endothelial cells are responsible for upregulated permeability of blood-vessel endothelia. This upregulation leads to fluid redistribution; interstitial tissue edema and hypovolemic or septic shock are common developments.

Despite this long list of pathogenetic hallmarks, increasing evidence from humans suggests that effective filovirus-specific adaptive immune responses do develop, coinciding with control and clearance of viremia and subsequent clinical improvement in surviving patients. However, depending on the severity of illness (including organ dysfunction and late complications), clinical illness may be protracted and recovery incomplete.

CLINICAL MANIFESTATIONS

EBOD and MARD cannot be distinguished by clinical observation and for all practical purposes may be considered the same disease, although this situation may change as higher-resolution characterization of human FVD accrues. The incidence of clinical signs does not differ significantly among human infections caused by disparate filoviruses (with the exception of the possibly apathogenic Reston virus), although, apart from the patients in the 2013–2016 EVD outbreak, the numbers of thoroughly observed patients are very low. The incubation period is 2–25 days (most commonly 6–10 days), after which infected people develop a nonspecific influenza-like syndrome characterized by sudden onset of fever and chills, severe headaches, cough, myalgia, pharyngitis, arthralgia of the larger joints, development of a maculopapular rash, and other signs/symptoms. This stage is followed by a second phase (~5–7 days after disease onset and thereafter) initially involving the gastrointestinal tract (nausea and vomiting and/or diarrhea, sometimes with abdominal pain), respiratory tract (chest pain, cough), vascular system (postural hypotension, edema), and CNS (confusion, headache, coma). Common hemorrhagic manifestations include subconjunctival injection, petechial rash, gingival bleeding, and bleeding at injection sites; epistaxis, hematemesis, hematuria, and melena occur but are less common. Patients usually succumb to acute disease 4–14 days after infection, often with severe

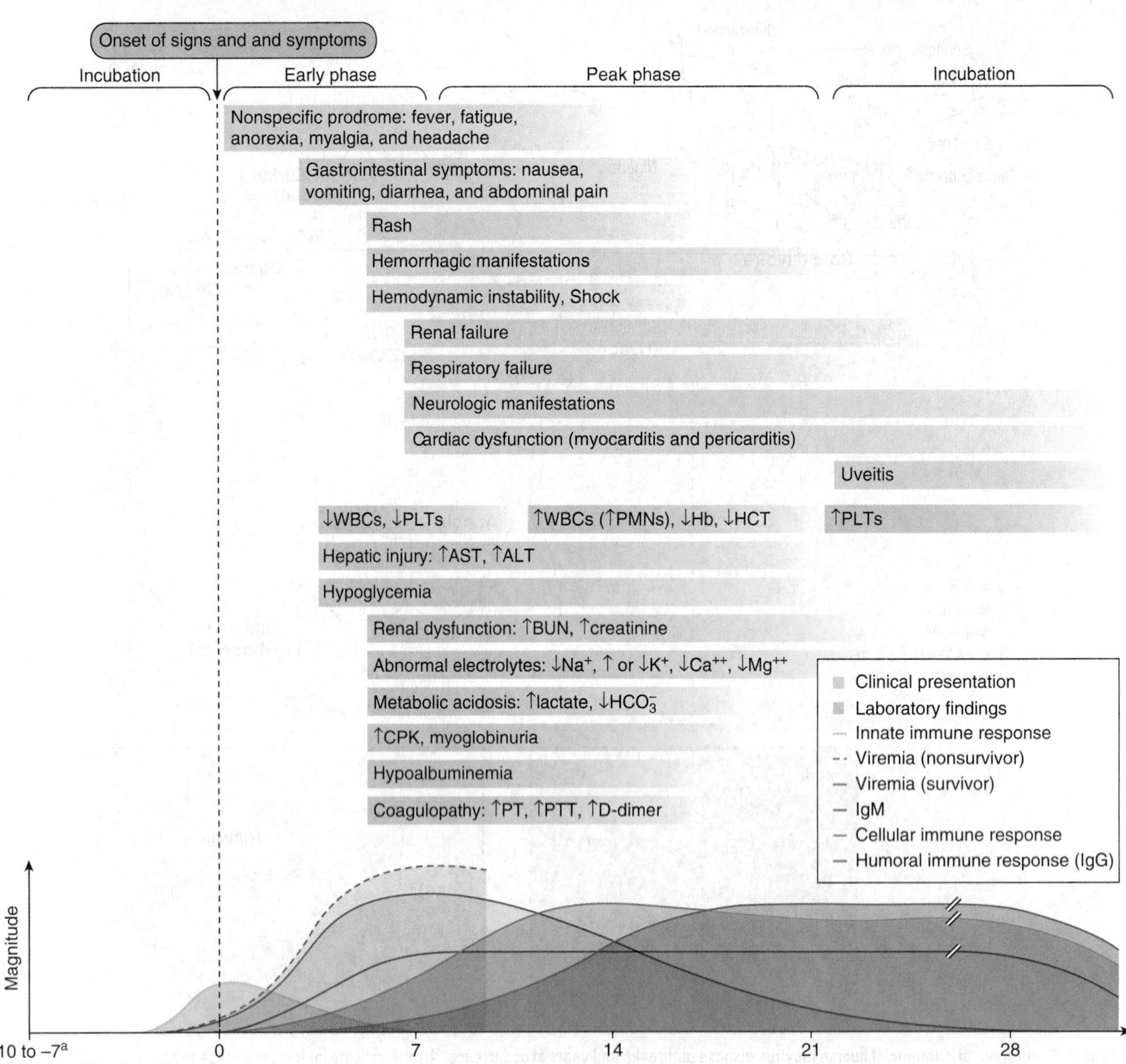

FIGURE 210-5 Ebola virus disease course. ALT, alanine aminotransferase; AST, aspartate aminotransferase; BUN, blood urea nitrogen; CPK, creatine phosphokinase; Hb, hemoglobin; HCT, hematocrit; PLTs, platelets; PMNs, polymorphonuclear leukocytes; PT, prothrombin time; PTT, partial thromboplastin time; WBCs, white blood cells. *(Adapted and expanded from JH Kuhn et al:* Filoviridae, *in Fields Virology, 7th ed, Vol. 1. Howley PM et al. (eds). Philadelphia, Wolters Kluwer/Lippincott Williams & Wilkins, 2020, pp 449–503. Figure courtesy of Jiro Wada, NIH/NIAID/DCR/IRF-Frederick, Fort Detrick, MD, USA.)*

multiorgan failure, including shock and acute renal failure or respiratory failure.

Typical laboratory findings are leukopenia (with cell counts as low as 1000 per μL) with a left shift prior to leukocytosis, thrombocytopenia (with counts as low as 50,000 per μL), increased activities of liver enzymes (aspartate aminotransferase > alanine aminotransferase, γ-glutamyltransferase), increased creatinine and urea concentrations with proteinuria, electrolyte derangement (hypokalemia or hyperkalemia, hyponatremia, hypocalcemia), hypoglycemia, hypoalbuminemia, prolonged prothrombin and partial thromboplastin times, and elevated creatine phosphokinase activities. Nonspecific markers of systemic inflammation (e.g., C-reactive protein concentrations) may be markedly elevated in severely ill patients.

DIAGNOSIS

Filovirus infections cannot be diagnosed on the basis of clinical presentation alone. Numerous diseases common in equatorial Africa need to be considered in the differential diagnosis of a febrile patient. Almost all of these diseases occur at a much higher incidence than filovirus infections and are much more likely differential diagnoses in non-outbreak settings; however, during and in peri-outbreak periods, the importance of accurate laboratory diagnosis to rule in or rule out filovirus infection cannot be diminished. The most important infectious diseases that closely mimic FVD are falciparum malaria and typhoid fever; also important are enterohemorrhagic *Escherichia coli* enteritis, gram-negative septicemia (including shigellosis), meningococcal septicemia, rickettsial infections, fulminant viral hepatitis, leptospirosis, measles, and other high-consequence viral infections (in particular, Lassa and yellow fevers). Noninfectious possibilities, including venomous snakebites, warfarin intoxication, and the many causes of acquired or inherited coagulopathy, also must be considered in the bleeding patient. An exposure history—including exposure to caves or mines; direct contact with bats, nonhuman primates, or bushmeat; direct contact with severely ill local residents; or admission to rural hospitals with patient-to-patient or patient-to-health-care-worker clusters of illness—should raise the index of suspicion.

If FVD is suspected on the basis of epidemiologic and/or clinical manifestations, infectious disease specialists and the proper public-health authorities (including WHO) should be notified immediately. Laboratory diagnosis of FVD is relatively straightforward but ideally requires maximal containment (biosafety level 4) capacity, which usually is not available in filovirus-endemic countries. Increasingly, laboratory diagnosis is performed with patient samples inactivated in mobile field "glove boxes" by on-site personnel trained in the safe use of diagnostic assays adapted for field use in lower-containment settings. Consequently, diagnostic samples should be collected and processed with great caution and with the use of appropriate PPE and strict barrier techniques. With adherence to established biosafety precautionary measures, samples should be sent in suitable transport media to national or international WHO reference laboratories. Acute-phase blood/serum is the preferred diagnostic specimen, because it usually contains high titers of filovirions and filovirion-specific antibodies.

The current assay of choice for the diagnosis of filovirus infection is reverse-transcription polymerase chain reaction (RT-PCR) targeting one or more filovirus genes; a typical detection limit is 1000–5000 PFU/mL of serum, depending on the assay. Safe, rapid-turnaround, and standardized in-field PCR-based approaches (e.g., the Cepheid GeneXpert platform) are increasingly deployed during outbreaks. Antigen-capture enzyme-linked immunosorbent assays (ELISAs) for the detection of filovirus genomes and filovirion proteins are in development and may be useful as rapid point-of-care diagnostic tests in the future. Direct IgM capture, direct IgG capture, or IgM-capture ELISA is used for the detection of filovirion-targeting antibodies from patients in the later stages of disease (i.e., those who have been able to mount a detectable antibody response), including survivors. All of these assays can be conducted on samples treated with guanidinium isothiocyanate (for RT-PCR), cobalt-60 irradiation (for ELISA), or other effective measures that render filoviruses noninfectious. Virus isolation in cell culture and plaque assays for quantification or diagnostic confirmation are relatively easy but must be performed in maximal-containment laboratories. If available, electron microscopic examination of inactivated samples or cultures can further support the diagnosis because filovirions have unique filamentous shapes (Fig. 210-2). Formalin-fixed skin biopsy samples and possibly skin swabs can be useful for safe postmortem diagnoses. In-field (or near in-field) rapid genome sequencing was first deployed to inform classic epidemiology in Western Africa during the 2013–2016 EVD outbreak and is likely to become a mainstay of outbreak control and response, even in challenging settings.

TREATMENT

Filovirus Infections

Treatment of patients with suspected or confirmed filovirus infection should be administered by health care workers who are using appropriate PPE and who have been well trained in the complex care of the FVD patient under restrictions appropriate for infection prevention and control (see "Control and Prevention," below). Treatment of FVD has historically been entirely supportive (and even that therapy has been limited by resource constraints) as the efficacy and safety of specific antiviral countermeasures had not been rigorously studied outside of animal models of disease. The 2013–2016 EVD outbreak in Western Africa highlighted the need to conduct rigorous, feasible, and ethically acceptable clinical research in the outbreak setting. Building on challenges and lessons learned in that setting, the first-of-its-kind Pamoja Tulinde Maisha (PALM) randomized clinical trial was conducted during the 2018–2020 EVD outbreak in the Democratic Republic of the Congo and identified two therapeutics based on Ebola virus–specific mAbs to improve survival rates. mAb114 (ansuvimab-zykl) and REG-EB3 (atoltivimab, maftivimab, and odesivimab-ebgn) were subsequently approved for the treatment of EVD in PCR-confirmed adults (including pregnant women) and children. Both are administered via carefully monitored single dose infusions to be initiated as soon as possible after diagnosis. In addition, the PALM trial demonstrated the will and capacity to deliver more advanced supportive and critical care accompanying specific therapeutics in the outbreak setting. Although evidence is lacking, consensus treatment strategies include those generally recommended for severe septicemia/sepsis/shock (**Chap. 304**) and should be applied with an emphasis on standard approaches—i.e., monitoring and response to respiratory dysfunction (e.g., oxygen), circulatory dysfunction (e.g., intravascular fluid repletion and vasopressor support), and CNS dysfunction (e.g., ruling out of reversible causes, notably hypoglycemia)—as well as the detection and management of acute kidney injury, hemorrhage, electrolyte derangements, and nutritional status and the prevention and treatment of secondary or co-infections. Pain management and administration of antipyretics, antiemetics, and antidiarrheal agents may be considered. Crucial strategies to improve outcomes in the most severely ill FVD patients include preventing organ dysfunction and providing safe and effective temporary organ support (e.g., mechanical ventilation and renal replacement) in order to expand the window for administration of medical countermeasures and development of effective endogenous immune responses.

COMPLICATIONS

Even in patients who have initial virologic or clinical improvement, complications in the second or third weeks of illness may include secondary infections, persistent renal dysfunction, neurologic compromise (e.g., Ebola-virus-related meningoencephalitis, cerebrovascular events, seizures), cardiac dysfunction (e.g., myocarditis, pericarditis), and venous thrombosis. Pregnancy and labor cause severe and frequently fatal complications in filovirus infections due to clotting factor consumption, fetal loss, and/or severe blood loss during birth.

A number of sequelae have been self-reported or historically described in survivors of FVD, including prolonged and sometimes incapacitating arthralgia and myalgia, asthenia, alopecia, visual problems (including uveitis), hearing loss, memory loss and neurocognitive dysfunction, mental health conditions (anxiety, depression, posttraumatic stress disorder), and reproductive problems. Well-controlled observational studies of EVD survivors were first conducted in the aftermath of the 2013–2016 West African EVD outbreak. Compared with their close-contact controls, Liberian EVD survivors had an increased incidence of headache, arthralgia and myalgia, memory loss, fatigue, and urinary frequency as well as abnormal results in abdominal, chest, neurologic, musculoskeletal, and ocular exams. Of individual and public health significance is the potential for persistence of filoviruses in immune-privileged tissue compartments (and their associated fluids) in FVD survivors, most commonly in the semen of male survivors (with the rare but documented potential for sexual transmission and reignition of outbreaks) and rarely in the CNS (causing recrudescent meningoencephalitis), the eye (causing recrudescent uveitis), and the placenta (causing transmission or placental insufficiency). True relapses that resemble the course of primary FVD are extremely rare but have been described.

PROGNOSIS

Among the most severe of acute viral diseases in humans, FVD generally has a poor prognosis, although with much greater heterogeneity than was historically assumed; i.e., the 90% case–fatality rate ascribed for many decades to EVD has required revision. With an incomplete evidence base, the outcome probably depends on factors that include the particular filovirus causing the infection (Fig. 210-3), host factors (age, immune status, unknown host genetic factors), virus exposure route and dose, viral load, the presence and severity of organ dysfunction, and—critically—the availability of filovirus-specific countermeasures and requisite supportive care. Continued advances in the latter countermeasures and supportive care will likely result in improved survival rates in EVD, but the long-term health and well-being of and survival outcomes for FVD survivors are unknown. It is also uncertain how increased access to filovirus-specific therapeutics and life-saving support will impact filovirus persistence in survivors; short- and long-term surveillance will be necessary to avoid individual consequences (e.g., relapse, recrudescent inflammatory syndromes) and public health consequences (e.g., reignition of outbreak transmission chains in the peri-outbreak or post-outbreak period).

Although remarkable progress has been made at the human EVD bedside, the same cannot yet be said for disease caused by filoviruses other than Ebola virus, either in acute disease or in convalescence.

CONTROL AND PREVENTION

Prevention of filovirus exposure in nature is difficult because the ecology of the viruses is not completely understood. To prevent marburgvirus infection, the most useful advice to people entering or living in areas where Egyptian rousettes can be found is to avoid direct or indirect contact with these animals. Prevention in nature is more difficult in the case of pathogenic ebolaviruses, largely because definite reservoirs have not yet been pinpointed. EBOD outbreaks have been associated not so much with bats as with hunting or consumption of nonhuman primates. The mechanism of introduction of ebolaviruses into nonhuman primate populations, if it occurs at all, is unclear. (Only one ebolavirus, Taï Forest virus, has unequivocally been detected in wild nonhuman primates.) Therefore, for now, to prevent ebolavirus infection, the only advice that can be offered to travelers and locals is to avoid contact with bushmeat, nonhuman primates, and bats. In any setting, the early local involvement of medical anthropologists is strongly advised to ensure proper communications and explanations that are not perceived as threatening or patronizing.

Biomedical prevention strategies have historically been limited to tried-and-true pillars of outbreak control, centering on the identification and isolation of cases, contact tracing, ensuring that health care workers and other response personnel have appropriate training and capacity in infection prevention and control, and preventing high-risk transmission events. Measures aimed at preventing and controlling infection, including relatively simple barrier nursing techniques, vigilant use of appropriate PPE, quarantine, and contact tracing, usually effectively terminate or at least contain FVD outbreaks. Isolation of infected people and their contacts and avoidance of direct person-to-person contact without appropriate PPE usually prevents further spread, as the virions are not transmitted through droplets or aerosols under natural conditions. Typical protective gear sufficient to prevent filovirus infections consists of disposable gloves, gowns, and shoe covers and a face shield and/or goggles. If available, N-95 or N-100 respirators may be used to further limit infection risk. Positive-air-pressure respirators should be considered for high-risk medical procedures, such as intubation or suctioning. Medical equipment used in the care of an infected patient, such as gloves or syringes, should never be reused. Because filovirions are enveloped, disinfection with detergents (e.g., 1% sodium deoxycholate, diethyl ether, or phenolic compounds) is relatively straightforward. Bleach solutions are recommended at 1:100 for surface disinfection and 1:10 for application to excreta or corpses. Whenever possible, potentially contaminated materials should be autoclaved, irradiated, or destroyed.

Emerging from research conducted during the 2013–2016 EVD outbreak in Western Africa, a vaccine based on a recombinant vesicular stomatitis Indiana virus expressing Ebola virus glycoprotein (rVSV-ZEBOV/Ervebo) was the first filovirus vaccine approved for use in the United States and the European Union. It is now widely deployed in a reactive-ring vaccination strategy, targeting close contacts and their contacts in EVD outbreak settings, and also used for vaccination of health care workers. Development and evaluation of other vaccine candidates continue toward complementary preventive approaches for non-outbreak or peri-outbreak settings, with emphasis on the durability of immune responses and increases in preventive breadth toward other filoviruses.

Even in the absence of high-level evidence, expert consensus informs the targeted use of Ebola-virus–specific vaccine or post-exposure prophylaxis to prevent infection or disease in health care workers considered to have had a high-risk Ebola virus exposure (e.g., after needlestick injury). For male survivors, abstinence from sexual activity with a partner for at least 12 months after disappearance of clinical signs is recommended, unless testing proves semen to be free of filoviruses. (The use of condoms is generally recommended for all sexual activities.) Reproductive tract and CNS tissues, including ocular tissues and fluids from survivors, should be handled with appropriate precautions until demonstrated to be filovirus-free. The role of filovirus-specific therapeutics in the prevention or treatment of filoviral persistence is unclear.

FURTHER READING

Cnops L et al: Essentials of filoviral load quantification. Lancet Infect Dis 16:e134, 2016.

Dudas G et al: Virus genomes reveal factors that spread and sustained the Ebola epidemic. Nature 544:309, 2017.

Hoenen T et al: Therapeutic strategies to target the Ebola virus life cycle. Nat Rev Microbiol 17:593, 2019.

Jacob ST et al: Ebola virus disease. Nat Rev Dis Primers 6:13, 2020.

Kuhn JH et al: *Filoviridae*, in *Fields Virology*, Vol 1, 7th ed, PM Howley et al (eds). Philadelphia, Wolters Kluwer/Lippincott Williams & Wilkins, 2020, pp 449–503.

Matz KM et al: Ebola vaccine trials: Progress in vaccine safety and immunogenicity. Expert Rev Vaccines 18:1229, 2019.

Mulangu S et al: A randomized, controlled trial of Ebola virus disease therapeutics. N Engl J Med 381:2293, 2019.

Regules JA et al: A recombinant vesicular stomatitis virus Ebola vaccine. N Engl J Med 376:330, 2017.

Section 16 Fungal Infections

211 Pathogenesis, Diagnosis, and Treatment of Fungal Infections

Michail S. Lionakis,
John E. Edwards Jr.

DEFINITION AND ETIOLOGY

In recent decades, human fungal infections have dramatically increased worldwide as a result of the AIDS pandemic, the widespread use of antibacterial agents, and the introduction of cytotoxic agents and precision medicine biologics for the treatment of autoimmune and neoplastic diseases and for use in patients undergoing solid organ transplantation or hematopoietic stem cell transplantation. Moreover, of great concern has been the recent rise in fungal infections caused by drug-resistant species, such as azole- and/or echinocandin-resistant *Candida glabrata* and *Candida auris* and azole-resistant *Aspergillus fumigatus*. Among the ~5 million fungal species, only a few cause human infections (**Table 211-1**).

Fungal infections are classified as *mucocutaneous* and *deep organ* infections on the basis of anatomic location and as *endemic* and *opportunistic* infections on the basis of epidemiology. Mucocutaneous infections can cause serious morbidity but are rarely fatal. Deep organ infections cause severe illness and often carry a high mortality rate. The endemic mycoses are caused by fungi that are not part of the normal human microbiota but are environmentally acquired. The opportunistic mycoses are caused by fungi (*Candida, Aspergillus*) that often are components of the human microbiota and whose ubiquity in nature renders them easily acquired by immunosuppressed hosts (Table 211-1). Opportunistic fungi cause serious infections when impaired host immune responses allow the organisms to transition from commensals to invasive pathogens. Endemic fungi typically cause self-limited disease in immunocompetent hosts but severe illness in immunosuppressed patients.

Fungi are morphologically classified as *yeast*, *mold*, and *dimorphic*. Yeasts are seen as round single cells or budding organisms. Molds grow as filamentous forms called *hyphae* both at room temperature and in tissue. *Aspergillus*, Mucorales, and dermatophytes that infect skin and nails are mold fungi. Variations exist within this classification system. For instance, when *Candida* infects tissue, both yeasts and filamentous forms (pseudohyphae) may be present (except in the cases of

TABLE 211-1 Major Fungal Infections, Associated At-Risk Patient Populations, and Diagnostic Tests

INFECTION (MOST COMMON FUNGAL GENERA AND SPECIES)	CLINICAL SYNDROME(S)	RISK FACTOR(S)	DIAGNOSTIC TEST(S)
Mold (Filamentous) Fungi			
Aspergillosis (*Aspergillus fumigatus, A. terreus, A. flavus, A. niger, A. nidulans*[a])	Pneumonia or disseminated infection ABPA Keratitis	Neutropenia, glucocorticoids, HSCT, post-influenza or COVID-19, BTK inhibition Atopic individuals Direct inoculation	*Culture* of BAL fluid: low sensitivity, nonspecific (colonization, contamination) *Histologic examination* of tissue[b]: acute-angle septate hyphae *Biomarkers:* GM (BAL > serum); serum BDG (nonspecific)
Mucormycosis (*Rhizopus, Rhizomucor, Mucor, Cunninghamella,* and *Lichtheimia* spp.)	Sinopulmonary infection Rhinocerebral infection Necrotizing skin infection	Neutropenia, HSCT Diabetic ketoacidosis Direct inoculation (e.g., tornado victims)	*Culture* of BAL fluid or sinus tissue: very low sensitivity *Histologic examination* of tissue: ribbon-like aseptate hyphae *Biomarkers:* Negative
Fusariosis (*Fusarium solani, F. oxysporum*)	Pneumonia or disseminated infection Keratitis	Neutropenia Direct inoculation	*Culture* of tissue or blood: one of the few molds recovered from blood *Histologic examination* of tissue: acute-angle septate hyphae *Biomarkers:* GM can be positive; BDG (nonspecific)
Scedosporiosis (*Scedosporium apiospermum*)	Pneumonia or disseminated infection	Neutropenia, glucocorticoids, HSCT	*Culture* of BAL: low sensitivity, nonspecific (colonization, contamination) *Histologic examination* of tissue: acute-angle septate hyphae *Biomarkers:* BDG can be positive
Phaeohyphomycosis (*Cladophialophora, Alternaria, Phialophora, Rhinocladiella, Exophiala,* and *Exserohilum* spp.)	Sinopulmonary, CNS, or disseminated infection Skin infection Allergic sinusitis	HSCT, neutropenia, glucocorticoids, healthy individuals (for CNS) Direct inoculation Atopic individuals	*Culture* of ordinarily sterile site *Histologic examination* of tissue: cell walls may appear dark brown or golden on H&E; Fontana-Masson may stain fungal melanin
Dermatophytosis (*Trichophyton, Microsporum,* and *Epidermophyton* spp.)	Skin and nail infections	Healthy individuals	*Culture* or *microscopic examination* of scrapings or clippings: chains of arthrospores (diagnostic)
Eumycetoma (*Madurella mycetomatis*)	Skin and subcutaneous infections	Healthy individuals	*Culture* and *macroscopic and histologic examination* of grains harvested from biopsy or aspiration
Yeast Fungi			
Mucosal candidiasis[c] (*Candida albicans, C. glabrata*)	Oropharyngeal or esophageal candidiasis Vulvovaginal candidiasis	AIDS, glucocorticoids Antibiotic use	*Culture* of mucosal surfaces *Histologic examination* of esophageal tissue or wet preparation (10% KOH) of vaginal discharge: yeast and/or pseudohyphae
Invasive candidiasis[c] (*C. albicans, C. glabrata, C. parapsilosis, C. tropicalis, C. auris*)	Candidemia Disseminated infection (spleen, liver, kidney, eye, heart, CNS)	Critical illness (ICU) Neutropenia, glucocorticoids	*Culture* of blood: low sensitivity *Histologic examination* of tissue: yeast and/or pseudohyphae *Biomarkers/other tests:* BDG (nonspecific); T2 magnetic resonance in whole blood
Cryptococcosis (*Cryptococcus neoformans, C. gattii*)	Pneumonia Osteomyelitis Meningoencephalitis	AIDS, glucocorticoids Sarcoidosis AIDS, AAbs to IFN-γ or GM-CSF, BTK or JAK inhibition	*Culture* of CSF, BAL fluid, blood *Microscopic examination* of tissue or CSF: encapsulated yeast (GMS, India ink, mucicarmine stain) *Biomarkers: Cryptococcus* Ag (serum, CSF) is sensitive and specific
Trichosporonosis[d] (*Trichosporon asahii, T. mucoides, T. asteroides*)	Superficial skin infection (white piedra) Disseminated infection (skin, eye)	Healthy individuals Neutropenia, glucocorticoids, HSCT, SOT	*Culture* of tissue or blood *Histologic examination* of tissue: yeasts, hyphae, and arthroconidia *Biomarkers:* BDG can be positive
Endemic Dimorphic Fungi			
Histoplasmosis (*Histoplasma capsulatum, H. duboisii* [in Africa])	Self-limited pneumonia Disseminated infection (liver, bone, bone marrow) Fibrosing mediastinitis	Healthy individuals AIDS, SOT, glucocorticoids, AAbs to IFN-γ, JAK or TNF-α inhibition	*Culture* of blood or tissue: low sensitivity; weeks needed for growth *Histologic examination* of tissue: yeast with narrow-based budding *Other tests: Histoplasma* Ag (urine > serum > BAL); BDG can be positive; serology (CF) can be useful in non-AIDS patients
Blastomycosis (*Blastomyces dermatitidis, B. gilchristii*)	Pneumonia Disseminated infection (skin, bone, mucosal surfaces, genitourinary tract)	Healthy individuals AIDS, glucocorticoids, TNF-α inhibition	*Culture* of BAL or tissue: low sensitivity; weeks needed for growth *Histologic examination* of tissue: yeast with broad-based budding *Other tests:* serology (CF, ID) has low sensitivity; *Blastomyces* Ag test cross-reacts with other endemic fungi; GM can be positive
Coccidioidomycosis (*Coccidioides immitis, C. posadasii*)	Self-limited pneumonia Disseminated infection (CNS, bone)	Healthy individuals AIDS, glucocorticoids, TNF-α inhibition	*Culture* is diagnostic[e] *Histologic examination:* spherules *Other tests:* serology (CF, ID); *Coccidioides* Ag test can be useful in CNS infection; BDG can be positive

(*Continued*)

TABLE 211-1 Major Fungal Infections, Associated At-Risk Patient Populations, and Diagnostic Tests (Continued)

INFECTION (MOST COMMON FUNGAL GENERA AND SPECIES)	CLINICAL SYNDROME(S)	RISK FACTOR(S)	DIAGNOSTIC TEST(S)
Paracoccidioidomycosis (*Paracoccidioides brasiliensis, P. lutzii*)	Pneumonia Disseminated infection (skin, bone, mucosal surfaces)	Healthy individuals AIDS, glucocorticoids	*Culture* of tissue: active disease; several weeks needed for growth *Histologic examination* of KOH preparations or tissue: yeast with budding in steering-wheel pattern *Other tests:* serology (ID, CF); *Paracoccidioides* Ag test
Sporotrichosis (*Sporothrix schenckii*)	Lymphocutaneous infection (ascending lymphangitis) Disseminated infection	Direct inoculation AIDS, glucocorticoids	*Culture* of tissue (diagnostic) *Histologic examination*: cigar-shaped yeast, often with surrounding asteroid body
Talaromycosis (*Talaromyces marneffei*)	Pneumonia Disseminated infection (skin, bone, mucosal surfaces)	Healthy individuals AIDS, glucocorticoids, AAbs to IFN-γ	*Culture* of tissue (diagnostic) *Histologic examination* of tissue: yeasts with transverse septa *Biomarkers:* GM is often positive
Adiaspiromycosis (*Emmonsia crescens, E. parva*)	Pneumonia	Occupational dust exposure	*Culture:* nonculturable *Histologic examination*: thick-walled adiaspore within granuloma
Emergomycosis (*Emergomyces africanus, E. pasteurianus*)	Disseminated infection (lungs, skin)	AIDS, SOT	*Culture* of infected tissue *Histologic examination* of tissue: yeast with narrow-based budding *Biomarkers: Histoplasma* Ag can be positive
Chromoblastomycosis (*Fonsecaea pedrosoi, F. monophora*)	Skin and subcutaneous tissue infections	Healthy individuals	*Culture* of infected tissue *Histologic examination* of scrapings (KOH) or tissue (GMS): sclerotic bodies (pathognomonic)
Other Fungi			
Pneumocystosis[f] (*Pneumocystis jirovecii*)	Pneumonia Disseminated infection (eye, CNS, skin, gastrointestinal tract)	AIDS, glucocorticoids, BTK inhibition AIDS	*Culture:* nonculturable *Histologic examination* (gold standard): special (GMS, Diff-Quik) or immunofluorescence stains *Biomarkers/other tests:* BDG (nonspecific); BAL fluid PCR (sensitive; can be positive in colonized individuals)

[a]*A. nidulans* is seen almost exclusively in chronic granulomatous disease. [b]GMS or PAS stains. [c]Some *Candida* species form pseudohyphae. [d]*Trichosporon* species are yeast-like fungi that also generate septate hyphae and arthroconidia. [e]*Coccidioides* is a laboratory hazard. It is important to notify the microbiology laboratory if this infection is suspected. [f]*Pneumocystis* is present in cyst and trophozoite forms.

Abbreviations: AAbs, autoantibodies; ABPA, allergic bronchopulmonary aspergillosis; Ag, antigen; BAL, bronchoalveolar lavage; BDG, β-D-glucan; BTK, Bruton's tyrosine kinase; CF, complement fixation; CNS, central nervous system; CSF, cerebrospinal fluid; GM, galactomannan; GM-CSF, granulocyte-macrophage colony-stimulating factor; GMS, Gomori methenamine silver; H&E, hematoxylin and eosin; HSCT, hematopoietic stem cell transplantation; ICU, intensive care unit; ID, immunodiffusion; IFN-γ, interferon γ; JAK, Janus kinase; KOH, potassium hydroxide; PAS, periodic acid–Schiff; PCR, polymerase chain reaction; SOT, solid organ transplantation; TNF-α, tumor necrosis factor α.

C. glabrata and *C. auris*, which form only yeasts in tissue); in contrast, *Cryptococcus* exists only in yeast form. *Dimorphic* is the term used to describe fungi that grow as yeasts or large spherical structures in tissue but as filamentous forms at room temperature in the environment (Table 211-1).

Patients acquire deep organ infection by molds and endemic dimorphic fungi via inhalation. Skin dermatophytes are primarily environmentally acquired, but human-to-human transmission may also occur. The commensal *Candida* invades deep tissues from sites of mucosal colonization, usually in the gastrointestinal tract.

In this chapter, we outline general principles of immunology, diagnosis, and treatment related to the most common human fungal infections.

■ PATHOGENESIS

In the past decade, our understanding of fungal recognition pathways and of tissue-specific innate and adaptive antifungal host defense mechanisms has markedly expanded. A major breakthrough has been the discovery and functional characterization of the C-type lectin receptor/spleen tyrosine kinase/caspase recruitment domain–containing protein 9 (CLR/SYK/CARD9) signaling pathway, which mediates fungal polysaccharide recognition and orchestrates proinflammatory mediator production, leukocyte recruitment, inflammasome activation, and Th17 cell differentiation upon fungal invasion. Human inherited CARD9 deficiency causes severe mucocutaneous and invasive fungal disease and is the only known primary immunodeficiency to feature fungus-specific infection susceptibility without a predisposition to other infections, autoimmunity, allergy, or cancer. Notably, CARD9-deficient patients develop infections by certain fungi in certain tissues, including (1) chronic mucocutaneous candidiasis linked to defective interleukin (IL) 17 responses; (2) infections of the central nervous system (CNS) caused by *Candida* (but also by *Aspergillus* and phaeohyphomycetes) and linked to impaired microglial-neutrophilic responses; and (3) deep dermatophytosis. Thus, the clinical use of SYK inhibitors for autoimmunity and cancer may cause opportunistic fungal disease. Human inherited deficiency of Toll-like receptor (TLR) signaling does not lead to spontaneous fungal disease, yet polymorphisms in TLR pathway molecules may increase the risk of fungal disease in critically ill or immunosuppressed persons, and TLR stimulation may boost protective CLR immunity, as has been shown with the TLR7 agonist imiquimod in chromoblastomycosis.

The development of clinically relevant animal models of mycoses and the phenotypic characterization of fungal infections that develop in patients with primary immunodeficiencies and in recipients of immune pathway–targeting biologics have led to the delineation of fungus-, cell-, and tissue-specific requirements for antifungal host defense (**Fig. 211-1**).

At the mucosal interface, IL-17-producing lymphoid cells play a critical role in protection by driving epithelial cell production of antimicrobial peptides that restrict mucosal *Candida* invasion. Indeed, AIDS patients are at risk for mucosal—but not invasive—candidiasis. Concordantly, inherited deficiency of IL-17 signaling caused by mutations in *IL17F, IL17RA, IL17RC*, or *TRAF3IP2* (encoding the IL-17 receptor adaptor ACT1) or pharmacologic inhibition of IL-17 signaling

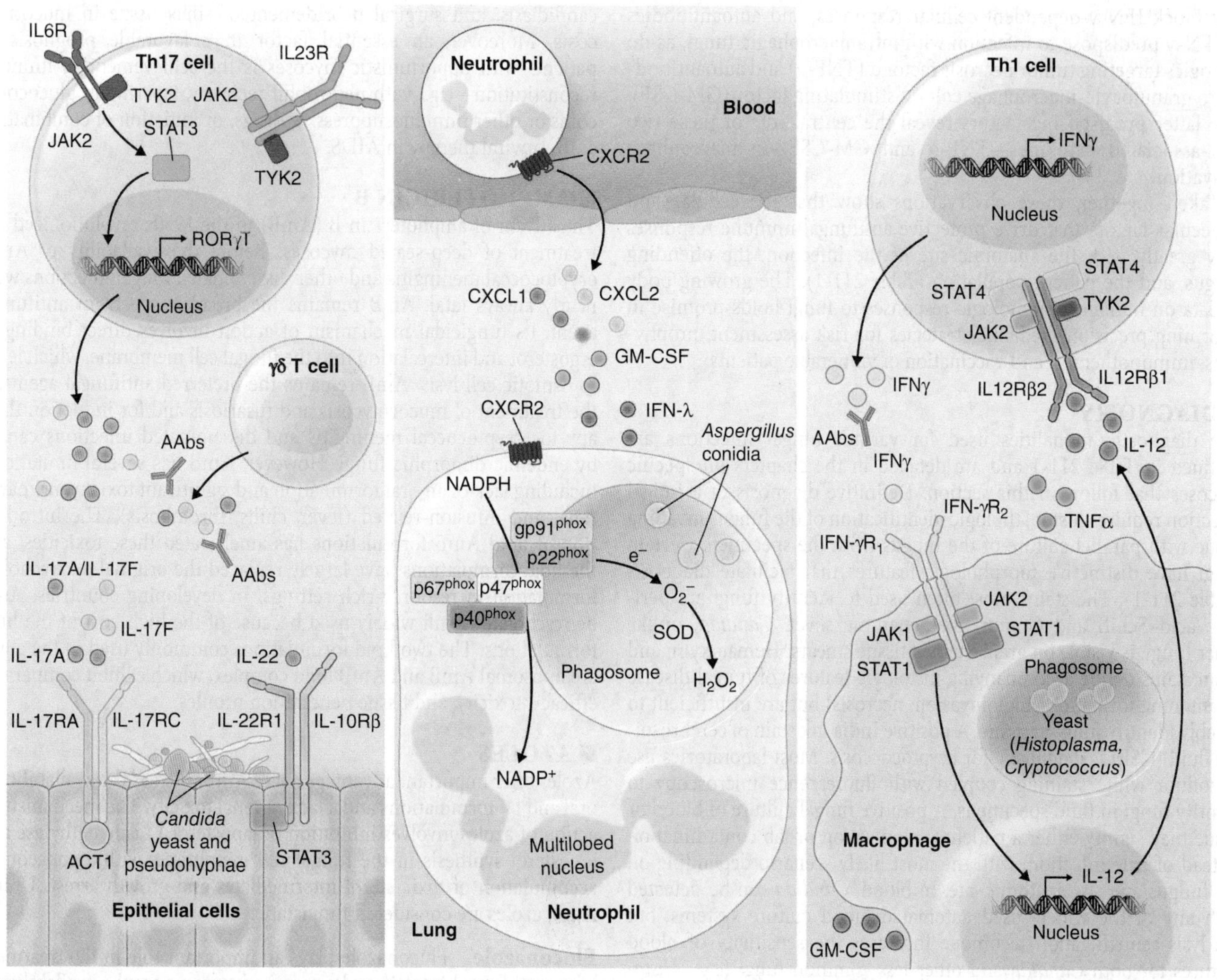

FIGURE 211-1 Host defense against fungi. ***Left:*** Production of IL-17A, IL-17F, and IL-22 by Th17 cells, Tc17 cells, γδ T cells, and innate lymphoid cells confers protection from mucosal *Candida* invasion. STAT3 promotes Th17 differentiation via RORγt induction. IL-17A and IL-17F bind to IL-17RA and IL-17RC on epithelial cells and signal via ACT1 to produce antimicrobial peptides that inhibit fungal growth. IL-22 binds to its receptor on epithelial cells and activates STAT3 to mediate epithelial proliferation and repair. ***Middle:*** Activation of CXCR2+ neutrophils recruited from blood in the *Aspergillus*-infected lung enables assembly of the five subunits of NADPH oxidase and superoxide generation that promotes fungal killing. Production of reactive oxygen species by neutrophils is facilitated by recruited monocyte-derived and plasmacytoid dendritic cells via type I and type III IFNs and GM-CSF. ***Right:*** The interaction of Th1 cells with macrophages is protective against intramacrophagic endemic dimorphic fungi, *Pneumocystis*, and *Cryptococcus*. Upon fungal uptake, macrophages produce IL-12 that binds to its receptor on T cells and activates STAT4, with consequent release of IFN-γ. IFN-γ binds to its receptor on macrophages and activates STAT1, thereby enabling fungal killing. TNF-α and GM-CSF are also critical for macrophage activation. AAbs, autoantibodies; IL, interleukin; IFN, interferon; JAK, Janus kinase; GM-CSF, granulocyte-macrophage colony-stimulating factor; NADPH, nicotinamide adenine dinucleotide phosphate; RORγt; RAR-related orphan receptor γ; SOD, superoxide dismutase; STAT, signal transducer and activator of transcription; TNF, tumor necrosis factor; TYK2, tyrosine kinase 2.

by biologics that target IL-12p40, IL-23p19, IL-17A, IL-17A/IL-17F, or IL-17RA causes mucosal—but not invasive—candidiasis. Other conditions that underlie a predisposition to chronic mucocutaneous candidiasis include primary immunodeficiencies due to mutations in *STAT3*, *STAT1*, *DOCK8*, *JNK1*, *IRF8*, *RORC*, and *CARD9*, all of which impair Th17 cells, as well as autoimmune polyendocrinopathy–candidiasis–ectodermal dystrophy (APECED) and thymoma, which feature autoantibodies to IL-17A, IL-17F, and IL-22. Of note, vaginal candidiasis (unlike oropharyngeal and esophageal candidiasis) develops in the setting of antibiotic treatment, not AIDS; this observation underscores the role of the microbiota in fungal control at the vaginal—but not the oral—mucosa.

On the other hand, neutrophils—but not lymphocytes—are critical for control of invasive infections caused by *Aspergillus* (and other inhaled molds) and *Candida* (Fig. 211-1). Indeed, patients with chemotherapy-induced neutropenia and patients undergoing allogeneic hematopoietic stem cell transplantation are at risk for invasive aspergillosis and candidiasis. Both oxidative and nonoxidative burst-dependent effector mechanisms are operational within neutrophils for fungal killing. Inherited deficiency in neutrophil superoxide generation due to mutations in the five subunits of the nicotinamide adenine dinucleotide phosphate (NADPH) oxidase complex causes chronic granulomatous disease, a prototypic primary immunodeficiency that carries a lifetime risk for invasive aspergillosis of ~40–50%; infrequently (i.e., in <5% of cases), chronic granulomatous disease predisposes to invasive candidiasis. The unexpected development of invasive mold infections in recipients of Bruton's tyrosine kinase (BTK) inhibitors has recently uncovered the critical role of BTK in promoting myeloid phagocyte-dependent antifungal effector functions.

Moreover, host defenses against fungi that reside within macrophages, such as *Cryptococcus*, *Pneumocystis*, and endemic dimorphic fungi, depend on the interplay of interferon γ (IFN-γ)–producing lymphoid cells and IL-12-producing macrophages that enable intramacrophagic fungal killing (Fig. 211-1). Indeed, AIDS patients and those receiving glucocorticoids, which affect lymphocytes and macrophages both quantitatively and qualitatively, are at risk for severe infections by these fungi. Accordingly, inherited impairment of the IL-12/IFN-γ signaling axis caused by mutations in *IL12RB1*, *IFNGR1*, *IFNGR2*, *STAT1*, *IRF8*, or *GATA2* underlies susceptibility to severe infection by intramacrophagic fungi (and other intramacrophagic pathogens, such as mycobacteria and salmonellae). In addition, the IFN-γ-targeting monoclonal antibody emapalumab, JAK inhibitors

patients, most centers now use newer azoles in such patients. Disadvantages of itraconazole include its poor CSF penetration, the use of cyclodextrin in its oral suspension and IV formulation, and its variable level of absorption in the capsule form, which requires monitoring of blood levels in patients receiving capsules for disseminated mycoses. Itraconazole is a potent CYP3A4 inhibitor; this characteristic leads to significant drug interactions. The drug causes hepatotoxicity and cardiac toxicity that may manifest as congestive heart failure.

Voriconazole Voriconazole is also available in oral and IV formulations, has far broader antifungal activity than fluconazole (including *C. glabrata*, *C. krusei*, *Aspergillus*, *Scedosporium*, and endemic dimorphic fungi—but not Mucorales), and penetrates into most body fluids (ocular fluid, CSF). It is the preferred agent for the treatment of aspergillosis and also has been used to treat scedosporiosis and as step-down (but not primary) therapy for coccidioidomycosis, blastomycosis, and histoplasmosis. Voriconazole is considerably more expensive than fluconazole, and, as with itraconazole, its use is associated with numerous interactions with drugs typically used in patients at risk for fungal infections. Hepatotoxicity, visual disturbances, and skin rashes (including photosensitivity) are relatively common, and long-term use requires skin cancer surveillance. A unique toxicity of voriconazole among azoles is fluorosis-associated periostitis. It is crucial to monitor drug levels because (1) voriconazole is metabolized in the liver by CYP2C9, CYP3A4, and CYP2C19; and (2) human genetic variation in CYP2C19 activity exists and can lead to significant interpatient variability in drug levels. Dosages should be reduced in patients with hepatic, but not renal, failure; however, because the IV formulation is prepared in cyclodextrin, it should be given with caution to patients with severe renal failure.

Posaconazole Posaconazole has broader activity than voriconazole, including activity against Mucorales. Both oral (suspension, tablet) and IV formulations are available. Posaconazole is approved by the FDA for antifungal prophylaxis in neutropenic leukemic patients and allogeneic hematopoietic stem cell transplant recipients as well as for treatment of oropharyngeal candidiasis, including infections refractory to fluconazole or itraconazole. Posaconazole has been reported to be effective salvage therapy for aspergillosis, mucormycosis, fusariosis, cryptococcosis, histoplasmosis, and coccidioidomycosis, although controlled clinical trials are lacking. The tablet formulation is not hampered by the suboptimal absorption that occurs with the suspension; the tablet also results in higher and more reliable blood levels of the drug. Posaconazole is less hepatotoxic than voriconazole and does not cause the skin, visual, or bone toxicity that occurs with voriconazole. However, the use of posaconazole is linked to significant P450-related drug interactions.

Isavuconazole The newest azole, isavuconazole, is available in oral and IV formulations and has broad antifungal activity similar to that of posaconazole. Isavuconazole is approved by the FDA for treatment of aspergillosis (on the basis of a randomized controlled trial that found it noninferior to voriconazole) and mucormycosis (on the basis of an open-label, noncomparative trial of 37 patients). Future experience will definitively determine its place in the antifungal armamentarium. Isavuconazole appears to be less hepatotoxic than voriconazole; it does not cause skin or visual toxicity, and it causes fewer P450-associated drug interactions than voriconazole.

ECHINOCANDINS

The echinocandins include the FDA-approved drugs caspofungin, anidulafungin, and micafungin, which are available solely as an IV formulation and inhibit β-1,3-glucan synthase, an enzyme that is crucial for fungal cell-wall synthesis but is not a constituent of human cells. The three echinocandins have comparable efficacy, toxicity, and tissue penetration profiles; are fungicidal for *Candida* and fungistatic for *Aspergillus*; and have no activity against other molds, *Cryptococcus*, or endemic dimorphic fungi. Their most common use to date is in candidal infections. These drugs offer three major advantages: minimal toxicity, minimal drug interactions, and activity against all *Candida* species. The minimal inhibitory concentrations (MICs) of echinocandins are higher against *Candida parapsilosis* than against other *Candida* species, but the higher MICs do not translate into less clinical efficacy against this species.

In controlled trials, caspofungin was as efficacious as AmB against candidemia and invasive candidiasis and as efficacious as fluconazole against candidal esophagitis. Caspofungin has also been efficacious as salvage therapy for aspergillosis. Anidulafungin is approved by the FDA as therapy for candidemia in nonneutropenic patients and for *Candida* esophagitis, abdominal infection, and peritonitis. In controlled trials, anidulafungin was noninferior and possibly superior to fluconazole against candidemia and invasive candidiasis and was as efficacious as fluconazole against candidal esophagitis. Micafungin is approved by the FDA for the treatment of candidal esophagitis and candidemia and for antifungal prophylaxis in hematopoietic stem cell transplantation. Moreover, micafungin yielded favorable results when used for the treatment of invasive aspergillosis and candidiasis in open-label trials.

FLUCYTOSINE (5-FLUOROCYTOSINE)

Flucytosine use has diminished as newer antifungal drugs have been developed. Its mechanism of action involves intrafungal conversion to 5-fluorouracil, which inhibits fungal DNA synthesis. The use of flucytosine in combination with AmB as induction therapy for cryptococcal meningitis is based on the drugs' synergistic interaction and favorable flucytosine CSF penetration that promotes a rapid decline of the cryptococcal burden in the CSF. Flucytosine is also used in combination with AmB for the treatment of candidal meningitis and endocarditis, although comparative trials with AmB monotherapy are lacking. Flucytosine monotherapy is not recommended as it is associated with the development of resistance. Flucytosine can cause bone marrow suppression and liver toxicity, which are intensified when the drug is used with AmB.

GRISEOFULVIN AND TERBINAFINE

Historically, griseofulvin was used for ringworm infection. Terbinafine, which inhibits squalene epoxidase and ergosterol synthesis, is now used for onychomycosis and ringworm infection and is as effective as itraconazole and more effective than griseofulvin in both conditions. Although active against other fungi, terbinafine penetrates poorly into tissues beyond the skin and nails and therefore is not preferred for systemic mycoses. Terbinafine carries a risk for hepatotoxicity.

TOPICAL ANTIFUNGAL AGENTS

A detailed discussion of topical agents for mucocutaneous mycoses is beyond the scope of this chapter; the reader is referred to **Chap. 219** and the dermatology literature. Azoles such as clotrimazole, miconazole, and ketoconazole are often used topically to treat common cutaneous mycoses as well as oropharyngeal and vaginal candidiasis. In vaginal candidiasis, oral fluconazole given once has the advantage of not requiring repeated intravaginal application. The polyenes nystatin and AmB have also been used topically for oropharyngeal and vaginal candidiasis. Agents from other classes that are used to treat these conditions include ciclopirox, haloprogin, terbinafine, naftifine, tolnaftate, and undecylenic acid.

FURTHER READING

Bennett JE: Introduction to mycoses, in *Mandell, Douglas, and Bennett's Principles and Practice of Infectious Diseases*, 9th ed, JE Bennett et al (eds). Philadelphia, Elsevier Saunders, 2020, pp 3082–3086.

Lionakis MS, Levitz SM: Host control of fungal infections: Lessons from basic studies and human cohorts. Annu Rev Immunol 36:157, 2018.

Pappas PG et al: Clinical mycology today: A synopsis of the mycoses study group education and research consortium (MSGERC) second biennial meeting, September 27–30, 2018, Big Sky, Montana, a proposed global research agenda. Med Mycol 58:569, 2020.

212 Histoplasmosis

Chadi A. Hage, L. Joseph Wheat

ETIOLOGY

Histoplasma capsulatum, a thermal dimorphic fungus, is the etiologic agent of histoplasmosis. In most endemic areas in North America, *H. capsulatum* var. *capsulatum* is the causative agent. In Central and South America, histoplasmosis is common and is caused by genetically different clades of *H. capsulatum* var. *capsulatum*. In Africa, *H. capsulatum* var. *duboisii* is also found. Yeasts of var. *duboisii* are larger than those of var. *capsulatum*.

Mycelia—the naturally infectious form of *Histoplasma*—have a characteristic appearance, with microconidial and macroconidial forms (**Fig. 212-1**). Microconidia are oval and are small enough (2–4 μm) to reach the terminal bronchioles and alveoli. Shortly after infecting the host, mycelia transform into the yeasts that are found inside macrophages and other phagocytes. The yeast forms are characteristically small (2–5 μm), with occasional narrow budding (**Fig. 212-2**). In the laboratory, mycelia are best grown at room temperature, whereas yeasts are grown at 37°C on enriched media.

EPIDEMIOLOGY

Histoplasmosis is the most prevalent endemic mycosis in North America. Although this fungal disease has been reported throughout the world, its endemicity is particularly notable in the Ohio and Mississippi river valleys of North America and in certain parts of Mexico, Central and South America (Brazil), Africa, and Asia. Histoplasmosis is increasingly reported outside of the traditionally known endemic areas. The geographic distribution of histoplasmosis is related to the humid and acidic nature of the soil in the endemic areas. Soil enriched with bird or bat droppings promotes the growth and sporulation of *Histoplasma*. Disruption of soil containing the organism leads to aerosolization of the microconidia and exposure of humans nearby. Activities associated with high-level exposure include spelunking, excavation, cleaning of chicken coops, demolition and remodeling of old buildings, and cutting of dead trees. Most cases seen outside of highly endemic areas represent imported disease, e.g., in Europe, histoplasmosis is diagnosed fairly often, mostly in emigrants from or travelers to endemic areas on other continents. The epidemiology of histoplasmosis is changing as a result of global climate changes and with the continued expansion of at-risk populations and the acceleration of intercontinental and international travel that brings this infection to areas of the world that are not known to be endemic. The population at risk for histoplasmosis continues to grow as a result of increasing numbers of patients receiving immunosuppressive therapies for autoimmune disorders, cancers, and organ transplants.

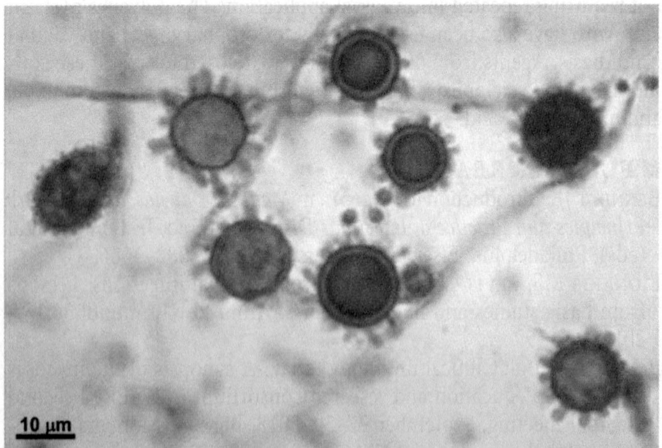

FIGURE 212-1 Spiked spherical conidia of *H. capsulatum* (lacto-phenol cotton blue stain) grown in the laboratory at room temperature.

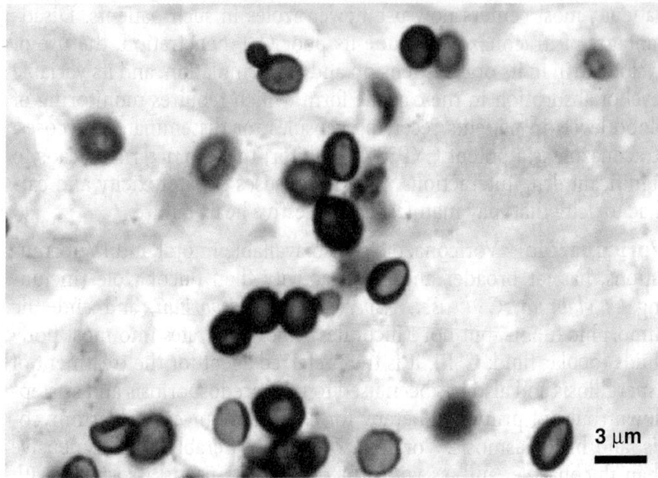

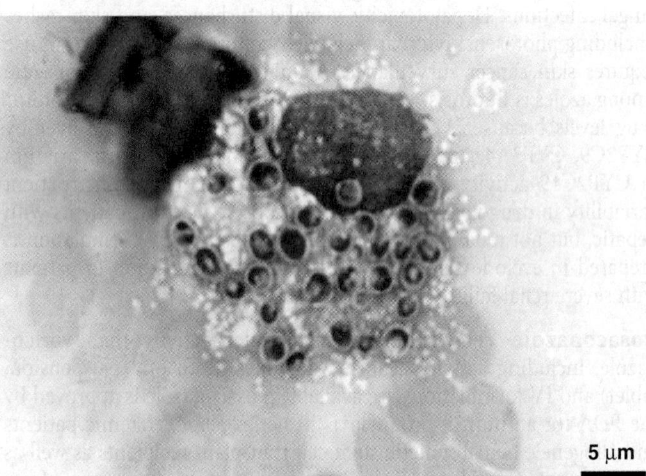

FIGURE 212-2 ***A.*** Small (2–5 μm) narrow budding yeasts of *H. capsulatum* from bronchoalveolar lavage fluid (Grocott's methenamine silver stain). ***B.*** Intracellular yeasts of *H. capsulatum* within an alveolar macrophage from a patient with AIDS and disseminated histoplasmosis (Giemsa stain).

PATHOGENESIS AND PATHOLOGY

Infection follows inhalation of microconidia (Fig. 212-1). Once they reach the alveolar spaces, microconidia are rapidly recognized and engulfed by alveolar macrophages, where they transform into yeasts (Fig. 212-2), a process that is integral to the pathogenesis of histoplasmosis and is dependent on the availability of calcium and iron inside the phagocytes. The yeasts are capable of multiplying inside resting macrophages. Neutrophils and then lymphocytes are attracted to the site of infection. Before the development of cellular immunity, yeasts use the phagosomes as a vehicle for translocation to local draining lymph nodes, whence they spread hematogenously throughout the reticuloendothelial system. Adequate cellular immunity develops ~2 weeks after infection. T cells produce interferon-γ to assist the macrophages in killing the organism and controlling the progression of disease. Interleukin 12 and tumor necrosis factor α (TNF-α) play an essential role in cellular immunity to *H. capsulatum*. In the immunocompetent host, macrophages, lymphocytes, and epithelial cells eventually organize and form granulomas that contain the organisms. These granulomas typically fibrose and calcify; calcified lung nodules, mediastinal lymph nodes, and hepatosplenic calcifications are frequently found in healthy individuals from endemic areas. In immunocompetent hosts, infection with *H. capsulatum* confers protective immunity to reinfection. In patients with impaired cellular immunity, the infection is not properly contained and can disseminate throughout the reticuloendothelial system. Progressive disseminated histoplasmosis (PDH) can involve multiple organs, most commonly the lungs, bone marrow,

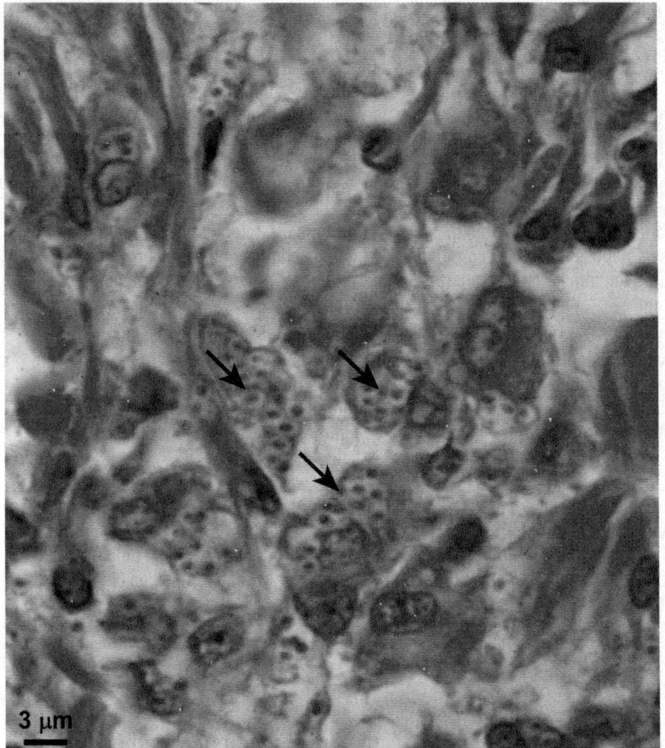

FIGURE 212-3 Intracellular yeasts (*arrows*) of *H. capsulatum* in a liver biopsy specimen (hematoxylin and eosin stain) from a patient who developed progressive disseminated histoplasmosis while receiving anti–tumor necrosis factor therapy for rheumatoid arthritis.

spleen, liver (**Fig. 212-3**), adrenal glands, and mucocutaneous membranes. Unlike latent tuberculosis, inactive histoplasmosis does not reactivate. In patients with mildly impaired immune systems, active infection may smolder and eventually worsen with further decline in immunity.

Structural lung disease (e.g., emphysema) impairs the clearance of pulmonary histoplasmosis leading to the development of chronic pulmonary disease. This chronic process is characterized by progressive inflammation, tissue necrosis, and fibrosis mimicking cavitary tuberculosis.

■ CLINICAL MANIFESTATIONS

The clinical spectrum of histoplasmosis ranges from asymptomatic infection to life-threatening illness. The attack rate and the extent and severity of the disease depend on the intensity of exposure, the immune status of the exposed individual, and the underlying lung architecture of the host.

In immunocompetent individuals with low-level exposure, most *Histoplasma* infections are either asymptomatic or mild and self-limited. Of adults residing in endemic areas, up to 75% have immunologic and/or radiographic evidence of previous infection without clinical manifestations. Asymptomatic lung nodules representing controlled histoplasmosis are frequently found on chest CT scans obtained during screening for lung cancer in smokers from endemic areas. When symptoms of acute histoplasmosis develop, they usually appear 1–4 weeks after exposure. Heavy exposure leads to a flulike illness with fever, chills, sweats, headache, myalgia, anorexia, dry cough, dyspnea, and chest pain. Chest radiographs usually show signs of pneumonitis with prominent hilar or mediastinal adenopathy. Pulmonary infiltrates may be focal with light exposure or diffuse with heavy exposure. Rheumatologic symptoms of arthralgia or arthritis, often associated with erythema nodosum, occur in 5–10% of patients with acute histoplasmosis. Pericarditis may also develop. These manifestations represent inflammatory responses to the acute pulmonary infection rather than extrapulmonary spread. Affected hilar or mediastinal lymph nodes may undergo necrosis and coalesce to form large mediastinal masses that can cause compression of great vessels, proximal airways, and the esophagus. These necrotic lymph nodes may also rupture and create fistulas between mediastinal structures (e.g., bronchoesophageal fistulas).

PDH is typically seen in immunocompromised individuals, who account for ~70% of cases. Common risk factors include AIDS (CD4+ T-cell count, <200/μL), extremes of age, the administration of immunosuppressive medications to prevent or treat rejection following transplantation (e.g., prednisone, mycophenolate, calcineurin inhibitors), and the use of methotrexate, anti-TNF-α agents, and other biologic response modifiers for autoimmune disorders. PDH may also occur in healthy individuals, some of whom may have rare undiagnosed genetic immunodeficiencies—workup for these conditions should be considered in healthy subjects with PDH.

The clinical spectrum of PDH ranges from an acute, rapidly fatal course—with diffuse interstitial or reticulonodular lung infiltrates causing respiratory failure, shock, coagulopathy, and multiorgan failure—to a subacute or chronic course with a focal organ distribution. Common manifestations include fever, weight loss, hepatosplenomegaly, and thrombocytopenia. Other findings may include meningitis or focal brain lesions, ulcerations of the oral mucosa, gastrointestinal ulcerations and bleeding, and adrenal insufficiency. Prompt recognition of this devastating illness is of paramount importance in patients with severe manifestations or with underlying immunosuppression, especially that due to AIDS (**Chap. 202**).

Chronic cavitary histoplasmosis is seen in smokers who have structural lung disease (e.g., bullous emphysema). This chronic illness is characterized by productive cough, dyspnea, low-grade fever, night sweats, and weight loss. Chest radiographs usually show upper-lobe infiltrates, cavitation, and pleural thickening—findings resembling those of tuberculosis. Without treatment, the course is slowly progressive.

Fibrosing mediastinitis is an uncommon but serious complication of histoplasmosis. In certain patients, acute infection is followed for unknown reasons by progressive fibrosis around the hilar and mediastinal lymph nodes, encasing mediastinal structures with potentially devastating consequences. Major manifestations include superior vena cava syndrome, obstruction of pulmonary vessels, and airway obstruction. Patients may experience recurrent pneumonia, hemoptysis, or respiratory failure. Fibrosing mediastinitis is fatal in up to one-third of cases.

In healed histoplasmosis, calcified mediastinal nodes or lung parenchymal nodules may erode through the walls of the airways and cause hemoptysis and expectoration of calcified material. This condition is called *broncholithiasis*.

The clinical features and management of histoplasmosis caused by the genetically different clades in Central and South America are similar to those of the disease in North America. African histoplasmosis caused by var. *duboisii* is clinically distinct and is characterized by frequent skin and bone involvement.

■ DIAGNOSIS

Recommendations for the diagnosis and treatment of histoplasmosis are summarized in **Table 212-1**. Once suspected, the diagnosis of histoplasmosis is usually straightforward as many diagnostic tools are now available in the United States. This is not the case in resource-limited endemic regions of Central America, South America, and Africa, where the diagnosis is often delayed, with consequently poor outcomes.

Fungal culture remains the gold standard diagnostic test for histoplasmosis. However, culture results may not be known for up to 1 month, and cultures are often negative in less severe cases. Cultures are positive in ~75% of patients with PDH and chronic pulmonary histoplasmosis. Cultures of bronchoalveolar lavage (BAL) fluid are positive in about half of patients with acute pulmonary histoplasmosis causing diffuse infiltrates and hypoxemia. In PDH, the culture yield is highest for BAL fluid, bone marrow aspirate, and blood. Cultures of sputum or bronchial washings are usually positive in chronic pulmonary histoplasmosis. Cultures are typically negative, however, in other forms of histoplasmosis.

Fungal stains of cytopathology or biopsy materials showing structures resembling *Histoplasma* yeasts are helpful in the diagnosis of PDH, yielding positive results in about half of cases. Yeasts can be seen in BAL fluid (Fig. 212-2) from patients with diffuse pulmonary infiltrates, in bone marrow biopsy samples, and in biopsy specimens

TABLE 212-1 Recommendations for the Diagnosis and Treatment of Histoplasmosis

TYPE OF HISTOPLASMOSIS	DIAGNOSTIC TESTS	TREATMENT RECOMMENDATIONS	COMMENTS
Acute pulmonary, moderate to severe illness or no improvement by the time of diagnosis	*Histoplasma* antigen (BAL fluid, serum, urine) Cytopathology on and fungal culture of BAL fluid *Histoplasma* serology (ID and CF), (EIA): IgG and IgM	Lipid AmB (3–5 mg/kg per day) ± glucocorticoids for 1–2 weeks; then itraconazole (200 mg bid) for 6–12 weeks. Monitor renal and hepatic function.	Patients with mild cases usually recover without therapy, but itraconazole should be considered if the patient's condition is not already improving by the time the diagnosis is established.
Chronic/cavitary pulmonary	*Histoplasma* serology (ID and CF), (EIA): IgG and IgM Fungal culture of sputum or BAL fluid	Itraconazole (200 mg qd or bid to achieve blood levels of 2–5 μg/ml) for at least 12 months. Monitor hepatic function.	Continue treatment until radiographic findings show no further improvement. Monitor for relapse after treatment is stopped.
Progressive disseminated	*Histoplasma* antigen (BAL fluid, serum, urine) *Histoplasma* serology (ID and CF), (EIA): IgG and IgM Fungal culture of blood or bone marrow aspirate Cytopathology on biopsy of affected organ	Lipid AmB (3–5 mg/kg per day) for 1–2 weeks; then itraconazole (200 mg qd or bid to achieve blood levels of 2–5 μg/ml) for at least 12 months. Monitor renal and hepatic function.	Liposomal AmB is preferred, but the AmB lipid complex may be used because of cost. Chronic antifungal maintenance therapy may be necessary if the degree of immunosuppression cannot be substantially reduced.
Central nervous system	*Histoplasma* antigen CSF *Histoplasma* serology (ID and CF), (EIA): IgG and IgM Fungal culture of CSF	Liposomal AmB (5 mg/kg per day) for 4–6 weeks; then itraconazole (200 mg qd or bid to achieve blood levels of 2-5 μg/ml) for at least 12 months. Monitor renal and hepatic function.	A longer course of lipid AmB is recommended because of the high risk of relapse. Itraconazole should be continued until CSF or MRI abnormalities clear.

Abbreviations: AmB, amphotericin B; BAL, bronchoalveolar lavage; CF, complement fixation; CSF, cerebrospinal fluid; EIA, enzyme immunoassay; ID, immunodiffusion.

of other involved organs (e.g., liver, adrenal glands). Occasionally, yeasts are seen within circulating phagocytes on blood smears from patients with severe PDH. However, staining artifacts and other fungal elements sometimes stain positively and may be misidentified as *Histoplasma* yeasts. Culture and pathology are no longer performed in most patients because diagnosis is more often established by antigen detection and/or serology, more rapidly and without subjecting the patient to invasive procedures.

The detection of *Histoplasma* antigen in body fluids is extremely useful in the diagnosis of PDH and acute diffuse pulmonary histoplasmosis. The sensitivity of this method is >95% in patients with PDH and >80% in patients with severe acute pulmonary histoplasmosis resulting from heavy exposure, if both urine and serum are tested. Antigen levels correlate with severity of illness in PDH and can be used to follow disease progression, as levels predictably decrease with effective therapy. Increased antigen levels also predict relapse. *Histoplasma* antigen can be detected in cerebrospinal fluid from patients with *Histoplasma* meningitis and in BAL fluid from those with pulmonary histoplasmosis. Cross-reactivity occurs with African histoplasmosis, blastomycosis, coccidioidomycosis, paracoccidioidomycosis, talaromycosis, and rarely aspergillosis.

Serologic tests, including immunodiffusion (ID), complement fixation (CF), and IgG and IgM enzyme immunoassay (EIA), are useful for the diagnosis of histoplasmosis, especially in immunocompetent patients. One month may be required for the detection of antibodies after the onset of infection by ID or CF, but antibodies may be detected earlier by more sensitive methods (EIA). IgM appears first then declines, and IgG appears later and increases during the infection. EIA for IgG and IgM antibodies provides a more accurate method for monitoring changes and antibody levels. Serologic tests are especially useful for the diagnosis of chronic pulmonary histoplasmosis. Limitations of ID and CF, however, include insensitivity early in the course of infection and reduced sensitivity in immunosuppressed patients, especially those receiving immunosuppression for organ transplantation. Also, antibodies may persist for several years after infection. Positive results from past infection may lead to a misdiagnosis of active histoplasmosis in a patient with another disease process.

TREATMENT

Histoplasmosis

Treatment is indicated for all patients with PDH or chronic pulmonary histoplasmosis as well as for most symptomatic patients with acute pulmonary histoplasmosis who have not improved by the time the diagnosis is established especially in those with diffuse infiltrates and difficulty breathing. In most other cases of pulmonary histoplasmosis, treatment is not recommended especially if the immune system of the host is intact, and the degree of exposure is not heavy. The symptoms usually are mild, subacute, and not progressive, and the illness resolves without therapy. Treatment should be considered if the symptoms are not improving within a month.

The preferred treatments for histoplasmosis (Table 212-1) include the lipid formulations of amphotericin B in severe cases and itraconazole in others. Liposomal amphotericin B is more effective and better tolerated than the deoxycholate formulation and is more effective in patients with AIDS and PDH. The deoxycholate formulation of amphotericin B is an alternative to a lipid formulation for patients at low risk for nephrotoxicity and if liposomal amphotericin B is not available. Posaconazole and isavuconazole are alternatives for patients who cannot take itraconazole. *Histoplasma* may develop resistance to fluconazole and voriconazole, and they are not the preferred alternative to itraconazole, especially in immunocompromised patients.

In severe cases requiring hospitalization, a lipid formulation of amphotericin B is used first, followed by itraconazole. In patients with meningitis, a lipid formulation of amphotericin B should be given for 4–6 weeks before switching to itraconazole. In immunosuppressed patients, the degree of immunosuppression should be reduced if possible, although immune reconstitution inflammatory syndrome (IRIS) may ensue. Antiretroviral treatment improves the outcome of PDH in patients with AIDS and is recommended; however, whether antiretroviral treatment should be delayed to avoid IRIS is unknown.

Blood levels of itraconazole should be monitored to ensure adequate drug exposure, with target concentrations of the parent drug and its hydroxy metabolites measuring 2–5 μg/mL. Drug interactions should be carefully assessed; itraconazole not only is cleared by cytochrome P450 metabolism but also inhibits cytochrome P450. This profile causes interactions with many other medications.

The duration of treatment for acute pulmonary histoplasmosis is 6–12 weeks, while that for PDH and chronic pulmonary histoplasmosis is at least 1 year. Antigen levels in urine and serum should be monitored during and for at least 1 year after therapy for PDH. Stable or rising antigen levels suggest treatment failure or relapse and should raise concerns regarding proper intake of itraconazole (capsule formulation with food), adherence to treatment, itraconazole serum concentrations, and drug interactions.

Lifelong itraconazole maintenance therapy is recommended for patients with persistently suppressed immunity but not for those with immune recovery—e.g., patients with AIDS who complete at least 1 year of itraconazole and show no signs of active infection including *Histoplasma* antigen levels <2 ng/mL respond well to antiretroviral treatment with CD4+ T-cell counts of at least 150/µL (preferably >250/µL) and HIV viral load <50 copies/mL. Similarly, maintenance therapy may not be necessary in other immunocompromised patients if the clinical findings have cleared, antigen levels are <2 ng/mL, and immunosuppression is substantially reduced.

Fibrosing mediastinitis, which represents a chronic fibrotic reaction to past mediastinal histoplasmosis rather than an active infection, does not respond to antifungal therapy. Often patients with mediastinal granuloma have chronic or progressive courses and receive treatment with itraconazole and corticosteroids to reduce disease progression.

■ FURTHER READING

AZAR MM et al: Clinical perspectives in the diagnosis and management of histoplasmosis. Clin Chest Med 38:403, 2017.

AZAR MM et al: Current concepts in the epidemiology, diagnosis, and management of histoplasmosis. Semin Respir Crit Care Med 41:13, 2020.

BAHR NC et al: Histoplasmosis infections worldwide: Thinking outside of the Ohio River valley. Curr Trop Med Rep 2:70, 2015.

HAGE CA et al: A multicenter evaluation of tests for diagnosis of histoplasmosis. Clin Infect Dis 53:448, 2011.

213 Coccidioidomycosis

Neil M. Ampel

■ DEFINITION AND ETIOLOGY

Coccidioidomycosis, commonly known as Valley fever (see "Epidemiology," below), is caused by dimorphic soil-dwelling fungi of the genus *Coccidioides*. Genetic analysis has demonstrated the existence of two species, *C. immitis* and *C. posadasii*. These species are indistinguishable with regard to the clinical disease they cause and their appearance on routine laboratory media. Thus, the organisms will be referred to simply as *Coccidioides* for the remainder of this chapter.

■ EPIDEMIOLOGY

Coccidioidomycosis is confined to the Western Hemisphere between the latitudes of 40°N and 40°S. In the United States, areas of high endemicity include the San Joaquin Valley of California (hence the sobriquet "Valley fever") and the south-central region of Arizona. However, infection may be acquired in other areas of the southwestern United States, including the southern coastal counties in California, southern Nevada, southwestern Utah, southern New Mexico, and western Texas (including the Rio Grande Valley). Cases where infection was acquired well outside the recognized endemic areas, including in eastern Washington state and in northeastern Utah, have been recently described, suggesting that the endemic region may be expanding. Outside the United States, coccidioidomycosis is endemic to northern Mexico as well as to localized regions of Central America. In South America, there are endemic foci in Colombia, Venezuela, northeastern Brazil, Paraguay, Bolivia, and north-central Argentina.

The risk of infection is increased by direct exposure to soil harboring *Coccidioides*. Because of difficulty in isolating *Coccidioides* from environmental sites, the precise characteristics of potentially infectious soil are not known. In the United States, several outbreaks of coccidioidomycosis have been associated with soil from archeologic excavations of Amerindian sites both within and outside of the recognized endemic region. These cases often involved alluvial soils in regions of relative aridity with moderate temperature ranges. When found, *Coccidioides* is isolated 2–20 cm below the surface; it is not found at greater depths, nor is it usually isolated from cultivated soil.

In endemic areas, most cases of coccidioidomycosis occur without obvious soil or dust exposure, and it is presumed that infection occurs through inhalation of airborne fungal particles. Climatic factors may increase the infection rate in these regions. In particular, periods of aridity following rainy seasons have been associated with marked increases in the number of symptomatic cases. From 2011–2017, there were 95,371 cases of coccidioidomycosis reported in the United States. During this time, there has been a general increase in the incidence of disease. In California, this increase has occurred both within the established endemic area of the San Joaquin Valley and in the areas contiguous to it. The factors associated with this increase have not been elucidated but likely include an influx of older individuals without prior coccidioidal infection into endemic areas, construction activity, increased reporting, and changing climatic conditions.

■ PATHOGENESIS, PATHOLOGY, AND IMMUNE RESPONSE

On agar media and in the environment, *Coccidioides* organisms exist as filamentous molds. Within this mycelial structure, individual filaments (*hyphae*) elongate and branch, some growing upward. Alternating cells within the hypha degenerate, leaving barrel-shaped viable elements called *arthroconidia*. Measuring ~2 µm by 5 µm, individual arthroconidia may dislodge and become airborne for extended periods. When inhaled by a susceptible host, their small size allows them to evade initial mechanical mucosal defenses and reach deep into the bronchial tree, where infection is initiated.

Once within a susceptible host, the arthroconidia enlarge, become rounded, and develop internal septations. The resulting structures, called *spherules* (**Fig. 213-1**), may attain sizes up to 200 µm and are unique to *Coccidioides*. The septations encompass uninuclear elements called *endospores*. Spherules may rupture and release packets of endospores that can themselves develop into spherules, thus

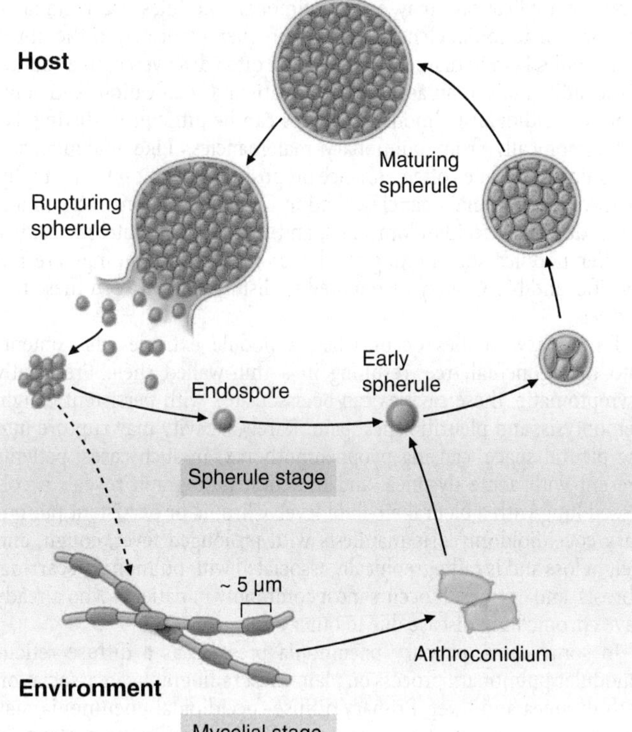

FIGURE 213-1 Life cycle of *Coccidioides*, including the mycelial phase in the environment and the spherule phase in the host.

propagating infection locally. If returned to artificial media or the soil, the fungus reverts to its mycelial stage.

Clinical observations and data from animal studies strongly support the critical role of a robust cellular immune response in the host's control of coccidioidomycosis. Necrotizing granulomas containing spherules are typically identified in patients with resolved pulmonary infection. In disseminated disease, granulomas are generally poorly formed or do not develop at all, and a polymorphonuclear leukocyte response occurs frequently. In patients who are asymptomatic or in whom the initial pulmonary infection resolves, delayed-type hypersensitivity to coccidioidal antigens has been routinely documented.

CLINICAL AND LABORATORY MANIFESTATIONS

After infection, 60% of individuals remain completely asymptomatic. The other 40% have symptoms that are related primarily to pulmonary infection, including fever, cough, and pleuritic chest pain. Symptoms generally occur from several days to 2 weeks after inhalation of infectious spores. The risk of symptomatic illness increases with age.

There are several manifestations of primary pulmonary coccidioidomycosis that are due to an immunologic response rather than directly to infection. Most prominent among these are cutaneous reactions. A diffuse, erythematous maculopapular rash, known as toxic erythema, has been noted in some cases. In addition, erythema nodosum (**see Fig. A1-39**)—typically over the lower extremities—and erythema multiforme (**see Fig. A1-24**)—usually in a necklace distribution—may occur. Lesions consistent with Sweet's syndrome have also been reported (**Chap. 19**). Cutaneous manifestations are especially common in women. Symmetrical arthralgias ("desert rheumatism") may also occur with or without cutaneous manifestations.

Primary pulmonary coccidioidomycosis is often misdiagnosed as community-acquired bacterial pneumonia. However, the diagnosis of primary pulmonary coccidioidomycosis is strongly suggested by the findings of rash and symmetrical arthralgias in a patient with an appropriate exposure history in a patient with pneumonia. The finding of any of the following is also strongly suggestive of coccidioidomycosis: a history of night sweats, marked fatigue, peripheral-blood eosinophilia, failure to improve with antibacterial therapy, and hilar or mediastinal lymphadenopathy on chest imaging.

In most patients, primary pulmonary coccidioidomycosis usually resolves without sequelae over several weeks. However, several pneumonic complications may arise. Pulmonary nodules are residua of primary pneumonia. Generally single, frequently located in the upper lobes, and ≤4 cm in diameter, nodules are often discovered on a routine chest radiograph in an asymptomatic patient. Calcification is uncommon. Coccidioidal pulmonary nodules can be difficult to distinguish radiographically from pulmonary malignancies. Like malignancies, coccidioidal nodules often enhance on positron emission tomography. However, unlike malignancies, routine CT often demonstrates multiple nodules in coccidioidomycosis, and there may be satellite lesions, smaller nodules surrounding the larger one. These findings are not specific, and biopsy may be required to distinguish between these two entities.

Pulmonary cavities occur when a nodule extrudes its contents into the bronchial tree, resulting in a thin-walled shell. Frequently asymptomatic, these cavities can be associated with persistent cough, hemoptysis, and pleuritic chest pain. Rarely, a cavity may rupture into the pleural space, causing pyopneumothorax. In such cases, patients present with acute dyspnea, and the chest radiograph reveals a collapsed lung with a pleural air-fluid level. Chronic or persistent pulmonary coccidioidomycosis manifests with prolonged fever, cough, and weight loss and is radiographically associated with pulmonary scarring, fibrosis, and cavities. It occurs most commonly in patients who already have chronic lung disease due to other etiologies.

In some cases, primary pneumonia presents as a diffuse reticulonodular pulmonary process on plain chest radiography in association with dyspnea and fever. Primary diffuse coccidioidal pneumonia may occur in settings of intense environmental exposure or profoundly suppressed cellular immunity (e.g., in patients with AIDS), with unrestrained fungal growth that is frequently associated with fungemia.

Clinical dissemination of infection outside the thoracic cavity occurs in <1% of infected individuals. Dissemination is more likely to occur in male patients, particularly those of African-American or Filipino ancestry, and in persons with depressed cellular immunity, including patients with HIV infection and peripheral-blood CD4+ T-cell counts of <250/μL, those receiving chronic glucocorticoid therapy, those with allogeneic solid-organ transplants, and those being treated with tumor necrosis factor α antagonists. Women who acquire new coccidioidal infection during the second or third trimester of pregnancy or postpartum also are at risk for disseminated disease. Common sites for dissemination include the skin, bones, joints, soft tissues, and meninges. Dissemination may follow symptomatic or asymptomatic pulmonary infection and may involve only one site or multiple anatomic foci. When it occurs, clinical dissemination is usually evident within the first 6 months after primary pulmonary infection.

Of the disseminated syndromes, coccidioidal meningitis is the most dire and, if untreated, is uniformly fatal. Patients usually present with a persistent headache, often accompanied by lethargy and confusion. Nuchal rigidity, if present, is not severe. Examination of cerebrospinal fluid (CSF) demonstrates lymphocytic pleocytosis with profound hypoglycorrhachia and elevated protein levels. CSF eosinophilia is occasionally observed. With or without appropriate therapy, patients may develop hydrocephalus, either communicating or noncommunicating, which presents clinically as a marked decline in mental status, often with gait disturbances.

DIAGNOSIS

Serology plays an important role in establishing a diagnosis of coccidioidomycosis. Several techniques are available, including the traditional tube-precipitin (TP) and complement-fixation (CF) assays, immunodiffusion TP and CF (IDTP and IDCF), and enzyme immunoassay (EIA) to detect IgM and IgG antibodies. TP and IgM antibodies are found in serum soon after infection and persist for weeks to months. They are not useful for gauging severity of disease. The CF and IgG antibodies occur later in the course of the disease and persist longer than TP and IgM antibodies. Rising CF titers are associated with clinical progression, and the presence of CF antibody in CSF is indicative of coccidioidal meningitis. Antibodies disappear over time in persons whose clinical illness resolves.

Because of its commercial availability, the coccidioidal EIA is frequently used as a screening tool for coccidioidal serology. There has been concern that the IgM EIA is occasionally falsely positive, particularly in asymptomatic individuals. In addition, while the sensitivity and specificity of the IgG EIA appear to be higher than those of the CF and IDCF assays, the optical density obtained in the EIA does not correlate with the serologic titer of either of the latter tests.

Coccidioides grows within 3–7 days at 37°C on a variety of artificial media, including blood agar. Therefore, it is always useful to obtain samples of sputum or other respiratory fluids and tissues for culture in suspected cases of coccidioidomycosis. The clinical laboratory should be alerted to the possibility of this diagnosis, since *Coccidioides* poses a significant laboratory hazard if it is inadvertently inhaled. The organism can also be identified directly. While treatment of samples with potassium hydroxide is rarely fruitful in establishing the diagnosis, examination of sputum or other respiratory fluids after Papanicolaou, Gomori methenamine silver, or calcofluor white staining reveals spherules in a significant proportion of patients with pulmonary coccidioidomycosis. For fixed tissues (e.g., those obtained from biopsy specimens), spherules with surrounding inflammation can be demonstrated with hematoxylin-eosin or Gomori methenamine silver staining.

A commercially available test for coccidioidal antigenuria and antigenemia has been developed and appears to be particularly useful in immunosuppressed patients with severe or disseminated disease. It appears to be useful when the CSF is assayed in cases of suspected coccidioidal meningitis. False-positive results may occur in cases of histoplasmosis or blastomycosis. Some laboratories offer genomic detection by polymerase chain reaction; this assay does not appear to be more sensitive than culture but can be more rapid.

TREATMENT
Coccidioidomycosis

Currently, two main classes of antifungal agents are useful for the treatment of coccidioidomycosis (**Table 213-1**). While once prescribed routinely, amphotericin B in all its formulations is now reserved for only the most severe cases of dissemination and for intrathecal or intraventricular administration to patients with coccidioidal meningitis in whom triazole antifungal therapy has failed. The original formulation of amphotericin B, which is dispersed with deoxycholate, is usually administered intravenously in doses of 0.7–1.0 mg/kg either daily or three times per week. The newer lipid-based formulations are associated with less renal toxicity but have not been demonstrated to lead to better improvement than the deoxycholate formulation in coccidioidomycosis. The lipid dispersions are administered intravenously at doses of 3–5 mg/kg daily or three times per week.

Triazole antifungals are the principal drugs now used to treat most cases of coccidioidomycosis. Clinical trials have demonstrated the usefulness of both fluconazole and itraconazole. Evidence indicates that itraconazole is more effective against bone and joint disease. Fluconazole has been the triazole of choice for the treatment of coccidioidal meningitis, but itraconazole also is effective. For both drugs, a minimal oral adult dosage of 400 mg/d should be used. The maximal dose of itraconazole is 200 mg three times daily, but higher doses of fluconazole may be given. The newer triazole antifungals, voriconazole and posaconazole, are useful for all types of clinical disease, including meningitis, and should be considered in cases where fluconazole or itraconazole therapy has failed. To date, isavuconazole has been used in limited circumstances in coccidioidomycosis. High-dose triazole therapy may be teratogenic during the first trimester of pregnancy; thus, if antifungal therapy is needed, amphotericin B should be considered in pregnant women during this period.

Most patients with focal primary pulmonary coccidioidomycosis do not require antifungal therapy. Patients for whom antifungal therapy should be considered include those with underlying cellular immunodeficiencies and those with prolonged symptoms and signs of extensive disease. Specific criteria include symptoms persisting for ≥2 months, night sweats occurring for >3 weeks, weight loss of >10%, a serum CF antibody titer of >1:16, and extensive pulmonary involvement apparent on chest radiography. When antifungal therapy is used, either fluconazole or itraconazole at 400 mg daily for up to 6 months is considered appropriate.

Diffuse pulmonary coccidioidomycosis represents a special situation. Because most patients with this form of disease are profoundly hypoxemic and critically ill, many clinicians favor beginning therapy with an amphotericin B formulation combined with an oral triazole antifungal. The triazole antifungal therapy is continued alone once clinical improvement occurs and should be continued for 6 months to 1 year.

The nodules that may follow primary pulmonary coccidioidomycosis do not require treatment. As noted above, these nodules are not easily distinguished from pulmonary malignancies by means of radiographic imaging. Close clinical follow-up and biopsy may be required to distinguish between these two entities. Most pulmonary cavities do not require therapy. Antifungal treatment should be considered in patients with persistent cough, pleuritic chest pain, and hemoptysis. Occasionally, pulmonary coccidioidal cavities become secondarily infected. This development is often manifested by an air-fluid level within the cavity. Bacterial flora or *Aspergillus* species are commonly involved, and therapy directed at these organisms should be considered. Surgery is sometimes required in cases of persistent productive cough and hemoptysis. In addition, cavities >4 cm in diameter are unlikely to resolve spontaneously, and surgical extirpation should be considered. Surgery is always required to reexpand the lung in cases of pyopneumothorax. For chronic pulmonary coccidioidomycosis, prolonged antifungal therapy—lasting for at least 1 year—is usually required, with monitoring of symptoms, radiographic changes, sputum cultures, and serologic titers.

Most cases of disseminated coccidioidomycosis require prolonged antifungal therapy. Duration of treatment is based on clinical improvement in conjunction with a significant decline in serum CF antibody titer. Such therapy routinely is continued for at least several years. Relapse occurs in 15–30% of individuals once therapy is discontinued.

Coccidioidal meningitis poses a special challenge. While most patients with this form of disease respond to treatment with oral triazoles, 80% experience relapse when therapy is stopped. Thus, lifelong therapy is recommended. In cases of triazole failure, intrathecal or intraventricular amphotericin B may be used. Installation requires considerable expertise and should be undertaken only by an experienced health care provider. Shunting of CSF in addition to appropriate antifungal therapy is required in cases of meningitis complicated by hydrocephalus. It is prudent to obtain expert consultation in all cases of coccidioidal meningitis.

TABLE 213-1 Clinical Presentations of Coccidioidomycosis, Their Frequency, and Recommended Initial Therapy for the Immunocompetent Host

CLINICAL PRESENTATION	FREQUENCY, %	RECOMMENDED THERAPY
Asymptomatic infection	60	None
Primary pneumonia (focal)	40	In most cases, none[a]
Diffuse pneumonia	<1	Amphotericin B followed by prolonged oral triazole therapy
Pulmonary sequelae	5	
Nodule		None
Cavity		In most cases, none[b]
Chronic pneumonia		Prolonged triazole therapy
Disseminated disease	≤1	
Skin, bone, joint, soft tissue disease		Prolonged triazole therapy[c]
Meningitis		Lifelong triazole therapy[d]

[a]Treatment is indicated for hosts with depressed cellular immunity as well as for those with prolonged symptoms and signs of increased severity, including night sweats for >3 weeks, weight loss of >10%, a complement-fixation titer of >1:16, and extensive pulmonary involvement on chest radiography. [b]Treatment (usually with the oral triazoles fluconazole and itraconazole) is recommended for persistent symptoms. [c]In severe cases, some clinicians would use amphotericin B as initial therapy. [d]Intraventricular or intrathecal amphotericin B is recommended in cases of triazole failure. Hydrocephalus may occur, requiring a cerebrospinal fluid shunt.

Note: See text for dosages and durations.

PREVENTION

There are no proven methods to reduce the risk of acquiring coccidioidomycosis among residents of an endemic region, but avoidance of direct contact with uncultivated soil or with visible dust-containing soil is a reasonable measure. For individuals with suppressed cellular immunity, the risk of developing symptomatic coccidioidomycosis is greater than that in the general population. Among those about to undergo allogeneic solid-organ transplantation, antifungal therapy is appropriate when there is evidence of active or recent coccidioidomycosis. Some transplant centers in the endemic region are providing universal antifungal prophylaxis for 6 months to 1 year after solid-organ transplantation. Several cases of donor-transmitted coccidioidomycosis have occurred during transplantation. If possible, donors from an endemic region should be screened for coccidioidomycosis before transplantation. Data on the use of antifungal agents for prophylaxis in other situations are limited. The administration of prophylactic antifungals is not recommended for HIV-1-infected patients who live in an endemic region. Most experts would administer a triazole antifungal to patients with a history of active coccidioidomycosis or a positive coccidioidal serology in whom therapy with tumor necrosis factor α antagonists is being initiated.

FURTHER READING

Benedict K et al: Surveillance for coccidioidomycosis–United States, 2011-2017. Morbid Mortal Wkly Rep 68:1, 2019.

Galgiani JN et al: 2016 Infectious Diseases Society of America (IDSA) clinical practice guideline for the treatment of coccidioidomycosis. Clin Infect Dis 63:e112, 2016.

Kahn A et al: Universal fungal prophylaxis and risk of coccidioidomycosis in liver transplant recipients living in an endemic area. Liver Transpl 21:353, 2015.

Kusne S et al: Coccidioidomycosis transmission through organ transplantation: A report of the OPTN Ad Hoc Disease Transmission Advisory Committee. Am J Transplant 16:3562, 2016.

Litvintseva AP et al: Valley fever: Finding new places for an old disease: *Coccidioides immitis* found in Washington state soil associated with recent human infection. Clin Infect Dis 60:e1, 2015.

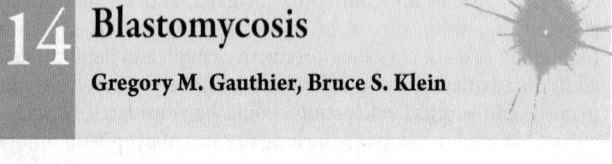

214 Blastomycosis

Gregory M. Gauthier, Bruce S. Klein

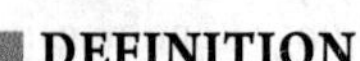

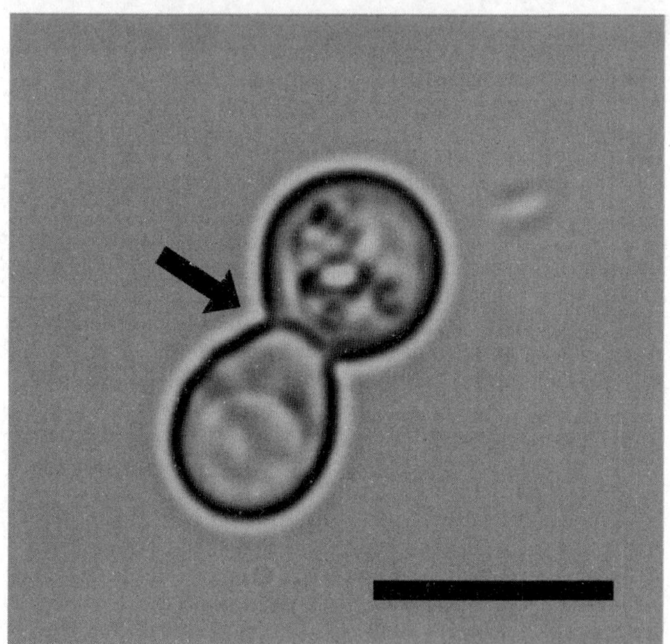

FIGURE 214-1 ***Blastomyces* yeast at 37°C,** with broad-based budding between mother and daughter cells (*arrow*). Bar = 10 μm. *(Gregory M. Gauthier, MD, MS)*

DEFINITION

Blastomycosis is a pyogranulomatous disease that follows the inhalation of *Blastomyces* conidia or hyphal fragments. Typically, *Blastomyces* causes pulmonary infection; however, a subset of patients will have disseminated disease that involves organs such as the skin, bone, brain, or genitourinary system. Blastomycosis is considered a primary fungal infection because it affects persons with either intact or impaired immune systems. A delay in diagnosis is common because blastomycosis mimics other diseases such as bacterial pneumonia, tuberculosis, and malignancy. Diagnosis involves culture- and nonculture-based tests. Amphotericin B formulations and triazoles are the drugs of choice for treatment.

ETIOLOGY

Blastomyces is a species complex comprising *B. dermatitidis*, *B. gilchristii*, *B. helicus*, *B. percursus*, *B. emzantsi*, *B. silverae*, and *B. parvus*. *B. silverae* and *B. parvus* are not known to commonly infect humans. *Blastomyces* species exhibit thermal dimorphism, which involves the ability to convert between hyphal and yeast morphologies in response to temperature. In the soil (22–25°C), *Blastomyces* grows as septate hyphae that produce infectious conidia. Among the *Blastomyces* species, *B. helicus* is unique because its hyphae grow in a coiled pattern and it does not sporulate under in vitro growth conditions. In organs and tissues (37°C), *Blastomyces* grows as a pathogenic yeast (Fig. 214-1) that elicits pyogranulomatous inflammation. The yeast form of all *Blastomyces* species grows as broad-based budding yeast cells, with subtle differences in size among the different species (4–29 μm).

EPIDEMIOLOGY

Although the majority of *Blastomyces* infections occur in North America, blastomycosis is a systemic fungal infection of global importance, with infections also occurring in Africa and Asia. In the United States, the traditional geographic range for *Blastomyces* includes the Mississippi and Ohio River basins, the St. Lawrence River basin, states bordering the Great Lakes, and southeastern states. In Canada, the traditional geographic range includes the provinces of Saskatchewan, Manitoba, Ontario, and Quebec. In North America, *B. dermatitidis* is located throughout the traditional geographic range. *B. gilchristii* is geographically restricted to Minnesota, Wisconsin, Canada, and areas along the St. Lawrence River. *B. dermatitidis* and *B. gilchristii* are thought to have diverged 1.9 million years ago during the Pleistocene epoch, with *B. gilchristii* restricted to formerly glaciated areas. *B. dermatitidis* is found in glaciated and nonglaciated areas. In the environment, *B. dermatitidis* and *B. gilchristii* are not uniformly distributed; rather, they grow in ecologic niches often referred to as *microfoci*, which are characterized by acidic, sandy soils that are found near water and that contain decaying organic matter such as vegetation or wood. *B. helicus* infections have been reported in the western United States (California, Montana, Idaho, Colorado, Nebraska, Texas) and Canada (Saskatchewan, Alberta); their ecologic niche has yet to be defined. The geographic range and ecologic niche for *B. parvus* and *B. silverae* are unknown.

Outside of North America, blastomycosis has been reported in Africa (more than 100 cases), India (fewer than 10 cases), and Israel. On the basis of morphologic analysis, nearly all clinical isolates of *Blastomyces* in Africa were originally thought to be *B. dermatitidis*. However, molecular phylogenetic analysis of human clinical isolates has demonstrated that multiple *Blastomyces* species exist in Africa, including *B. dermatitidis*, *B. gilchristii*, *B. percursus*, and *B. emzantsi*. A combination of internal transcribed spacer (ITS) sequencing, multilocus sequence typing (MLST), and whole-genome sequencing was used to identify a new species, *B. emzantsi*, and to differentiate *B. percursus* from other *Blastomyces* species. MLST has identified a *B. dermatitidis* isolate from Rwanda and *B. gilchristii* from Zimbabwe and South Africa. Analysis of 20 isolates from South Africa collected over a 40-year period identified them as either *B. emzantsi* or *B. percursus*. The geographic distribution and ecologic niche of the four *Blastomyces* species in Africa are unknown. In India, there have been fewer than 10 autochthonous cases of blastomycosis, with the majority identified by morphologic analysis. One autochthonous case (caused by *B. percursus*) with molecular confirmation has been reported from Israel.

Epidemiologic information about blastomycosis derives primarily from passive laboratory surveillance, retrospective studies, and outbreak investigations. The lack of sensitive skin testing and serologic testing, along with difficulty in isolating *Blastomyces* from the environment by culture or molecular methods, has limited an in-depth epidemiologic understanding of blastomycosis. In North America, blastomycosis is reportable in 5 U.S. states (Minnesota, Wisconsin, Michigan, Arkansas, and Louisiana) and two Canadian provinces (Manitoba, Ontario). The annual incidence of blastomycosis in the traditional endemic area ranges from 0.11 to 2.17 cases/100,000 persons. In older persons (Medicare beneficiaries, 1999–2008), the nationwide annual incidence of blastomycosis was 0.7/100,000, with the highest rates in the Midwest and Southern regions of the United States. In certain places, such as Vilas County, Wisconsin, and Kenora, Ontario, blastomycosis is hyperendemic, with annual incidence rates ranging from 40 to 117 cases/100,000 persons. Incidence data likely underestimate the true burden of infection because they are limited to persons with clinically apparent infection. Patients with asymptomatic or subclinical infections are undercounted.

Most *Blastomyces* infections are sporadic and can occur in either rural or urban areas. There have been at least 20 outbreaks of blastomycosis in the United States since the mid-1950s. Wisconsin, Minnesota, and North Carolina have had multiple outbreaks. The majority of outbreaks have been in rural areas, but several have occurred in urban settings. Activities associated with outbreaks include construction (of homes, cabins, factories, and roads), excavation of dirt, participation in water sports (canoeing, tubing on a river, and fishing), and exposure to a community compost pile or to beaver dams. *Blastomyces* infection is typically acquired from disturbed soil, which liberates infectious particles that are then inhaled into the lungs.

An investigation of a blastomycosis outbreak in Marathon County, Wisconsin (2009–2010) found that 45% of patients were of Hmong ethnicity. A retrospective study from the Marshfield Clinic in Wisconsin (1999–2014) found that 14.4% of patients with blastomycosis were of Asian ethnicity—a figure higher than was anticipated given that <2.5% of the population within the catchment area is Asian, including a large Hmong population. These findings suggest that persons of Hmong ethnicity have an increased risk of acquiring blastomycosis. A combination of whole-genome sequencing and immunologic analyses indicated that polymorphisms in the interleukin 6 (IL-6) gene in the Hmong population result in decreased IL-6 production, which in turn impairs development of IL-17-producing $CD4^+$ T lymphocytes. IL-17 is a critical cytokine for recruitment and activation of innate immune cells such as neutrophils and macrophages active against *Blastomyces*. Thus, alterations in IL-6 production may be responsible for the increased risk of blastomycosis in the Hmong population. Although data are limited, persons of Hmong ethnicity do not appear to be at increased risk for disseminated blastomycosis. Increased incidence rates of blastomycosis have also been reported in indigenous people of Canada and the United States. Compared with Caucasians, Asian and indigenous persons with blastomycosis tend to have fewer underlying medical conditions and to be younger.

PATHOGENESIS

A defining feature of the *Blastomyces* species complex is the ability to respond to shifts in temperature by switching between hyphal and yeast forms. In the soil, *Blastomyces* grows as mold cells with hyphae that produce conidia. Hyphal growth promotes environmental survival, genetic diversity through mating, and production of infectious conidia that facilitate transmission of *Blastomyces* from the environment to mammals, including humans. At 37°C (the core temperature of mammals), *Blastomyces* hyphae and conidia convert into pathogenic yeast that upregulate yeast phase–specific virulence factors and downregulate host immune defenses, thereby facilitating infection. Virulence traits that *Blastomyces* shares with *Histoplasma*, *Coccidioides*, *Sporothrix*, and *Paracoccidioides* are thermotolerance at 37°C, intracellular survival, and capacity to cause infection in persons with either healthy or impaired immune defenses. Although *Emergomyces* and *Talaromyces marneffei* (formerly *Penicillium marneffei*) exhibit thermal dimorphism, growth as yeast at 37°C, and intracellular survival, these dimorphic fungi tend to cause infection primarily in immunocompromised persons.

The morphologic switch from hyphae to yeast at 37°C is driven chiefly by temperature and is coupled with the uptake of exogenous cysteine. Cysteine uptake is required to complete the transition to the yeast form because it helps restart mitochondrial respiration, which ceases during the morphologic switch. Over the past two decades, knowledge about the genetic mechanisms that promote the temperature-dependent transition between hyphae and yeast has substantially increased. The discovery of dimorphism-regulating kinase 1 (*DRK1*), which encodes a group III hybrid histidine kinase that is part of the high-osmolarity glycerol (HOG) signaling pathway, provided genetic proof that that the transition to yeast is essential for virulence of the thermally dimorphic fungi. Disruption of *DRK1* by gene deletion or RNA interference resulted in *Blastomyces* cells that grew as hyphae at 37°C instead of yeast. Although viable at 37°C, these cells had altered cell-wall composition, failed to upregulate the *Blastomyces* adhesin 1 (*BAD1*, formerly WI-1) virulence factor, and were avirulent in a mouse model of lethal pulmonary infection. Subsequent studies of *Histoplasma* and *Talaromyces* demonstrated that the function of *DRK1* is conserved with regard to thermal dimorphism and virulence.

The temperature-dependent transition in the other direction—from yeast to hyphae—is regulated in part by a GATA-transcription factor encoded by siderophore biosynthesis repressor in *Blastomyces* (*SREB*), which influences neutral lipid metabolism. In addition, sensing of chitin by *NGT1* and *NGT2* N-acetylglucosamine transporters accelerates the conversion to hyphae following a drop in temperature from 37°C to 22°C. These two mechanisms are conserved in *Histoplasma capsulatum*.

As a primary fungal pathogen, *Blastomyces* is one of the few fungi that can infect immunocompetent persons. In its yeast form, *Blastomyces* evades and modulates immune defenses. Following disruption of soil, conidia that are aerosolized and inhaled into the lungs are phagocytosed by pulmonary macrophages, in which a subset of the conidia germinate as yeast and replicate during the early phases of infection. *Blastomyces* is also capable of replicating outside of macrophages. Upon conversion to the yeast phase, an essential virulence factor encoded by *BAD1* is upregulated. *BAD1* encodes a multifunctional 120-KDa cell-surface protein that facilitates yeast adherence to lung epithelial cells via interaction with heparin sulfate, attachment to host immune cells by binding to CR3 and CD14 complement receptors, and down-regulation of tumor necrosis factor alpha (TNF-α) in macrophages and neutrophils. In addition, the BAD1 protein impairs activation of CD4+ T lymphocytes, thereby decreasing the production of IL-17 and interferon gamma (IFN-γ). In vivo transcriptional profiling of *B. dermatitidis* yeast during pulmonary infection demonstrated that *BAD1* is the most highly upregulated gene. Deletion of *BAD1* renders *B. dermatitidis* avirulent in a murine model of pulmonary infection. Thus, BAD-1 is essential for virulence in *B. dermatitidis* and likely in *B. gilchristii* as well. In contrast, *BAD1* is absent from the sequenced genomes of *B. helicus*, *B. parvus*, *B. silverae*, B. *percursus*, and *B. emzantsi*.

Additional factors that contribute to the virulence of *Blastomyces* yeast include relative resistance to oxidative stress, upregulation of catalase and superoxide dismutase during infection, active uptake of zinc by a *PRA1*-encoded zincophore and transmembrane transporter (*ZRT1*), and cleavage of granulocyte-macrophage colony-stimulating factor by dipeptidyl peptidase IVA, which blocks activation of innate immune cells (macrophages, neutrophils) and their recruitment to the lung.

APPROACH TO THE PATIENT

Blastomycosis

On the basis of outbreak investigations, it is estimated that 50% of persons exposed to *Blastomyces* develop symptomatic infection after a 3-week to 3-month incubation period. The relatively long incubation period means that patients can be diagnosed with blastomycosis throughout the year. Blastomycosis has been referred to as the "the great pretender" because it can mimic infectious and noninfectious diseases. Blastomycotic pneumonia clinically and radiographically resembles community-acquired bacterial pneumonia, viral pneumonia, tuberculosis, and lung cancer. Patients often receive two or three courses of antibiotics before pulmonary blastomycosis is diagnosed. Without fungal stain and culture, cutaneous lesions can mimic skin cancer, sarcoidosis, and pyoderma gangrenosum. Rarely, blastomycosis can mimic laryngeal cancer. The most important aspect of the approach to a patient with a compatible illness is the consideration of *Blastomyces* as an etiologic agent in the differential diagnosis. This awareness facilitates early diagnosis and treatment, enhancing the potential for improved clinical outcomes. Clinical clues to blastomycosis, especially in persons who reside in or visit endemic regions, include pneumonia that does not improve with antibiotic treatment, pneumonia with extrapulmonary manifestations (e.g., skin lesions, osteomyelitis, central nervous system [CNS] involvement), and skin ulcers that do not respond to standard therapy. Blastomycosis should also be considered in persons from an endemic area who have unexplained respiratory failure or acute respiratory distress syndrome (ARDS). In addition, a detailed exposure history can elevate blastomycosis in the differential diagnosis. This history includes inquiries about a pet or family member with blastomycosis; these factors have been reported in 7.7–10% and 4–9% of patients, respectively.

CLINICAL MANIFESTATIONS

PULMONARY BLASTOMYCOSIS Pulmonary manifestations occur in 69–93% of patients with symptomatic blastomycosis and are the most common clinical feature of infection. Signs and symptoms can include fever, chills, productive or nonproductive cough, shortness of breath, hemoptysis, malaise, and decreased appetite. Pulmonary blastomycosis also can manifest as asymptomatic infection, a brief influenza-like illness, acute pneumonia, chronic pneumonia, or ARDS. Radiographic findings in the lungs include lobar consolidation, a mass lesion, interstitial infiltrates, nodule(s), a miliary pattern, cavitary disease, and diffuse involvement of multiple lobes. Hilar adenopathy, pleural effusion, and empyema are uncommon. No distinctive features differentiate blastomycosis from other pulmonary diseases. Diabetes, receipt of a solid organ transplant, immunosuppression, and multilobar pneumonia are risk factors for severe pulmonary blastomycosis. Approximately 4–15% of patients with pulmonary blastomycosis develop ARDS, which is characterized by a fulminant course and high mortality rates ranging from 40 to 89% in most studies. The mortality rate in ARDS is increased when the diagnosis is delayed.

DISSEMINATED BLASTOMYCOSIS Disseminated blastomycosis occurs in 15–48% of patients and has the potential to involve nearly any organ in the body. The most common site of dissemination is the skin, in which the infection can manifest as papules, ulcers, verrucous lesions, or abscesses. The second most common site is bone, with consequent osteomyelitis characterized by bone pain, soft tissue swelling, soft tissue abscess, and sinus tract formation. Typically, a single bone is involved; however, multifocal osteomyelitis can occur. The most common sites for osteomyelitis include the spine, long bones, and ribs. Dissemination to the CNS (e.g., manifesting as meningitis, an abscess, or a mass lesion), the larynx, or the genitourinary system (e.g., to the prostate or epididymis) occurs in fewer than 10%; the majority of the affected patients have concomitant involvement of other organs, such as the lung or the skin.

Factors that influence dissemination include the infecting *Blastomyces* species, the duration of pulmonary symptoms, and concomitant AIDS. Multiple studies from Wisconsin, a state in which *B. dermatitidis* and *B. gilchristii* are endemic, have demonstrated that *B. dermatitidis* is more likely to cause disseminated infection (31.4–47.8% of cases), whereas *B. gilchristii* tends to remain localized to the lung (90.7–92.2%). Surprisingly, immunosuppression has only a minimal influence on dissemination, an observation suggesting that *Blastomyces* virulence factors have a greater impact than host immune defenses. The frequency of disseminated blastomycosis among solid organ transplant recipients, persons receiving cancer chemotherapy, and patients undergoing pharmacologic immunosuppression is similar to that among patients with intact immune systems. Although patients treated with TNF-α antagonists are considered at risk for blastomycosis, the clinical manifestations and frequency of disseminated disease are unknown in this group because of a paucity of published data. Persons with AIDS and $CD4^+$ T lymphocyte counts of <100/μL are an exception: they are at increased risk for CNS dissemination. Blastomycosis in pregnancy is uncommon, is typically diagnosed in the second or third trimester (91%), and most frequently manifests as pneumonia (74%) or disseminated infection (48%). Transmission to the neonate by either the transplacental route or aspiration of infected vaginal secretions is rare. Persons infected with *B. helicus* can have localized pulmonary infection or disseminated disease; they are typically immunosuppressed (e.g., as a result of solid organ transplantation, chemotherapy, HIV infection, or lupus) and have a high mortality rate (71.4% in seven patients). In contrast to *B. dermatitidis* and *B. gilchristii*, *B. helicus* commonly causes fungemia. Infections with *B. percursus* and *B. emzantsi* are often of long duration (persisting for 4 weeks to 5 years) and can involve the lungs or become disseminated (skin, bone, brain).

DIAGNOSIS

Timely diagnosis of blastomycosis requires a high degree of clinical suspicion because its clinical and radiographic presentations mimic more common etiologies, such as community-acquired pneumonia, malignancy, and tuberculosis. Laboratory findings such as leukocytosis, mild anemia, increased C-reactive protein level, and elevated erythrocyte sedimentation rate are nonspecific. Once suspected, the diagnosis of blastomycosis is straightforward and involves microscopic examination of stained specimens, fungal culture, and antigen testing. The poor sensitivity of complement fixation (9%) and immunodiffusion (28%) renders serologic testing diagnostically dispensable. However, a recently developed serologic test designed to detect antibodies to BAD1 has a sensitivity of 87% and a specificity of 94–99%. This test is not yet commercially available.

A presumptive diagnosis of blastomycosis can be made by staining of clinical specimens and looking for broad-based budding yeast with a doubly refractile cell wall. Along with the broad-based budding pattern, yeast size (4–29 μm) allows *Blastomyces* to be distinguished from other fungi. An exception is *B. helicus*, which has the potential to be confused with *Histoplasma* because of its small-sized yeast. Respiratory tract specimens such as sputum, tracheal aspirate, and bronchoalveolar (BAL) fluid can be stained with calcofluor, 10% potassium hydroxide, or Papanicolaou stain. Purulent drainage can be stained in a similar manner. The sensitivity of staining of respiratory samples ranges from 50 to 90%. Tissue samples for histopathology should be stained with Gomori methenamine silver or periodic acid–Schiff stain and assessed for pyogranulomatous inflammation and broad-based budding yeast. Traditional stains, such as Gram's stain or hematoxylin and eosin, do not permit optimal visualization of *Blastomyces* yeast.

Growth of *Blastomyces* in cultures of respiratory tissue or body fluid samples provides a definitive diagnosis of blastomycosis but typically requires 5–28 days of incubation. Special media such as Sabouraud dextrose, potato dextrose, and brain–heart infusion are required because *Blastomyces* does not grow well on standard bacteriologic media. Most clinical microbiology laboratories incubate fungal cultures at 25–30°C, a temperature that results in hyphal growth of *Blastomyces*. Unfortunately, *Blastomyces* hyphae are not morphologically distinct enough to confirm diagnosis. Thus, fungal identification and diagnosis are commonly confirmed via chemiluminescent DNA probe or, less commonly, via conversion to yeast upon incubation at 37°C. Diagnosis can also be confirmed by polymerase chain reaction. Neither the chemiluminescent DNA probe nor morphologic analysis of yeast by light microscopy differentiates among the different species of *Blastomyces*. Moreover, some species, such as *B. emzantsi*, are difficult to convert to yeast at 37°C. The species of *Blastomyces* is not typically determined because DNA sequencing is required.

An antigen test that detects a conserved galactomannan component in the *Blastomyces* cell wall has supplanted serologic testing. This test can be performed on urine, blood, BAL fluid, and cerebrospinal fluid. The sensitivity of the antigen test is 85–93% for urine and 57–82% for serum. Infection burden appears to influence test sensitivity, with a lower burden of infection resulting in reduced sensitivity. The antigen test can detect *B. dermatitidis*, *B. gilchristii*, and *B. helicus*; however, its utility for detection of other *Blastomyces* species is unknown. Cross-reactions in the antigen test occur during infection with other dimorphic fungi, including *H. capsulatum* (96%), *Paracoccidioides* species (100%), and *T. marneffei* (70%). Among these, only *H. capsulatum* is found in the same endemic region as *Blastomyces*. Rare cross-reactions can occur with *Aspergillus* and *Cryptococcus* infections. Antigen levels in urine and blood decline with successful treatment, and their measurement can be used to monitor the response to antifungal therapy.

TREATMENT

Blastomycosis

Guidelines for the treatment of blastomycosis have been published by the Infectious Diseases Society of America, the American Thoracic Society, and the American Society of Transplantation. Although there are isolated reports of self-limited pulmonary blastomycosis, there are no criteria to determine which patients will experience a resolution of infection. Thus, treatment is recommended for all patients with blastomycosis in order to prevent progressive infection, respiratory failure, and disseminated disease. Antifungal selection is influenced by immune status, CNS involvement, pregnancy, medical comorbidities (e.g., congestive heart failure, prolonged QT interval), and drug–drug interactions. Antifungal drugs active against *Blastomyces* include amphotericin B (AmB) formulations and triazoles. The minimal amount of beta-(1,3)-glucan in the *Blastomyces* yeast cell wall renders echinocandins ineffective, and they should not be used to treat blastomycosis. Hematologic, hepatic, and renal function should be assessed prior to initiation of antifungal therapy, and possible drug–drug interactions should be evaluated. In addition, patients should be educated about proper administration of triazole antifungals. For example, itraconazole capsules require an acidic gastric environment for optimal absorption and should be taken with food and an acidic beverage to improve bioavailability; they cannot be used by persons taking antacids, H2 antagonists, or proton pump inhibitors. In contrast, itraconazole solution can be given to patients receiving gastric acid–lowering therapies and should be taken without food.

Treatment for blastomycosis is summarized in **Table 214-1**. For immunocompetent patients with pulmonary or disseminated blastomycosis of mild or moderate severity (e.g., treatable in the outpatient setting), itraconazole therapy for 6 months is recommended. For severe blastomycosis (e.g., that requiring hospitalization), induction therapy with lipid AmB for 7–14 days (or until clinical improvement), followed by itraconazole treatment for 6–12 months, is recommended. Although not well studied, combination antifungal therapy with lipid AmB and itraconzole can be considered for patients with severe pulmonary blastomycosis. In patients with ARDS, prednisone can be considered; however, the benefits of steroids are unclear. Osteomyelitis due to blastomycosis requires at least 12 months of antifungal therapy, and some patients may require surgical debridement. For blastomycosis involving the CNS, lipid AmB is administered for 4–6 weeks and is followed by treatment with itraconazole, voriconazole, or fluconazole for at least 12 months. Although fluconazole has excellent CNS penetration, its MIC against *B. dermatitidis* and *B. gilchristii* is higher than that of either itraconazole or voriconazole.

Immunosuppressed patients should be treated with 7–14 days of lipid AmB followed by 12 months of itraconazole. For patients requiring irreversible immunosuppression, indefinite suppressive azole therapy may be needed; however, in light of the heterogeneity of this patient population, a decision about suppressive therapy should be made on a case-by-case basis. The majority of solid organ transplant recipients do not require lifelong suppression because rates of relapse are low when treatment guidelines are followed.

For pregnant women, lipid AmB treatment for 6–8 weeks is recommended because, unlike the triazole antifungals, lipid AmB is not teratogenic. Fluconazole can cause craniofacial, skeletal, and cardiac defects in the developing fetus (Antley-Bixler-like syndrome); voriconazole and posaconazole also can result in skeletal abnormalities. Itraconazole increases the risk of spontaneous abortion. Before starting antifungal therapy, women of childbearing age with blastomycosis should have a pregnancy test.

Voriconazole, posaconazole, and isavuconazonium sulfate have potent activity against *B. dermatitidis* and *B. gilchristii* and can be considered as alternatives for persons who cannot tolerate itraconazole. These agents, along with itraconazole and AmB, also exhibit good activity against newly identified species of *Blastomyces*, such as *B. helicus*, *B. percursus*, and *B. emzantsi*. Fluconazole MICs against *B. percursus* and *B. emzantsi* are higher than those of other triazoles. Moreover, fluconazole appears to have poor activity against *B. helicus*, *B. parvus*, and *B. silverae*.

PROGNOSIS

Mortality rates for blastomycosis range from 5 to 13%; most deaths are associated with respiratory failure due to ARDS. The vast majority of patients who recover from pulmonary blastomycosis do not experience

TABLE 214-1 Treatment of Blastomycosis

PATIENT POPULATION	SEVERITY OF INFECTION	SITE OF INFECTION	THERAPY
Immunocompetent	Mild to moderate[a]	Lung	Itraconazole for 6–12 months[b]
		Disseminated	Itraconazole for 6–12 months[b] (≥12 months for osteomyelitis)
	Severe[c]	CNS	Lipid AmB (5 mg/kg daily[d,e] for 4–6 weeks) followed by itraconazole,[b] fluconazole (800 mg daily), or voriconazole (200–400 mg bid) for at least 12 months of treatment
		Lung	Lipid AmB (3–5 mg/kg daily[e,f] for 7–14 days) followed by itraconazole[b] for 6–12 months
		Disseminated	Lipid AmB (3–5 mg/kg daily[e,f] for 7–14 days) followed by itraconazole[b] for 12 months of treatment (≥12 months for osteomyelitis)
Immunocompromised	Any severity	CNS	Lipid AmB (5 mg/kg daily[d,e] for 4–6 weeks) followed by itraconazole,[b] fluconazole (800 mg daily), or voriconazole (200–400 mg bid) for at least 1 year of treatment[g]
		Lung or disseminated	Lipid AmB (3–5 mg/kg daily[e,f] for 7–14 days) followed by itraconazole[b] for 12 months[g]
Pregnant[h]	Any severity	Any site	Lipid AmB (3–5 mg/kg daily[e,f] for 6–8 weeks), with avoidance of azole antifungals

[a]Mild to moderate infections can typically be managed in the outpatient setting. [b]A loading dose of 200 mg PO tid for 3 days followed by 200 mg PO daily or bid, with dosing based on serum itraconazole levels. The goal for levels of total itraconazole (i.e., itraconazole plus hydroxyitraconazole) is 1–5 μg/mL. Liquid itraconazole has greater bioavailability than the capsule formulation. Liquid itraconazole and oral capsules are administered differently (see text for details). Serum itraconazole levels should be measured after steady state has been reached (2 weeks). Because of the drug's long half-life, blood for serum itraconazole determinations can be drawn regardless of the time of administration. In contrast, serum drug levels for voriconazole, posaconazole, and isavuconazole should be measured before a dose is administered when steady state has been reached (~1 week). [c]Severe blastomycosis requires hospitalization on a medical ward, an intermediate care unit, or an intensive care unit. [d]Lipid amphotericin B (AmB) is the preferred formulation because it has the best CNS penetration among AmB formulations. For patients with CNS blastomycosis that results in neurologic dysfunction, surgical intervention should be considered. [e]For patients with CNS blastomycosis, severe pulmonary blastomycosis, or severe disseminated blastomycosis, combination therapy with lipid AmB plus a triazole antifungal can be considered; however, this combination has not been formally studied. For patients with ARDS, adjunctive steroid therapy with prednisone (40–60 mg daily for 1–2 weeks) can be considered; however, the benefit of steroid administration is not well defined. [f]If lipid AmB is not available, then AmB deoxycholate (0.7–1. 0 mg/kg daily) can be substituted; however, this formulation is associated with higher rates of nephrotoxicity and infusion reactions than lipid AmB. [g]Consider lifelong suppression with itraconazole (200 mg daily) if immunosuppression cannot be reversed. This decision should be made on a case-by-case basis; not all immunosuppressed patients require lifelong suppressive therapy. In addition, lifelong antifungal suppression can be considered in patients who experience relapse after appropriate therapy. [h]All women of childbearing age should undergo pregnancy testing before initiation of therapy.

long-term loss of pulmonary function. Cutaneous blastomycosis typically results in scarring.

PREVENTION

Prevention of blastomycosis is challenging because most infections are sporadic and unpredictably acquired from the environment. However, substantial progress has been made in understanding vaccine-mediated immunity conferred by a live, attenuated vaccine strain that is deficient in BAD1. When injected subcutaneously into mice, the *B. dermatitidis* BAD1-null vaccine strain induces sterilizing immunity by activating T_H17 lymphocytes to protect against lethal pulmonary challenge. Major antigenic components of the vaccine include calnexin and *Blastomyces* endoglucanase-2, which may also be conserved in other pathogenic fungi, including *Histoplasma capsulatum*, *Coccidioides* species, *Aspergillus* species, *Fonsecaea pedrosoi*, and *Pseudogymnoascus destructans*. Neither the BAD1-null attenuated vaccine nor recombinant antigen-based vaccines are commercially available.

FURTHER READING

Chapman SW et al: Clinical practice guidelines for the management of blastomycosis: 2008 update by the Infectious Diseases Society of America. Clin Infect Dis 46:1801, 2008.

Limper AH et al: An official American Thoracic Society statement: Treatment of fungal infections in adult pulmonary and critical care patients. Am J Respir Crit Care Med 183:96, 2011.

Maphanga TG et al: Human blastomycosis in South Africa caused by *Blastomyces percursus* and *Blastomyces emzantsi* sp. Nov. 1967–2014. J Clin Microbiol 58:e01661, 2020.

215 Cryptococcosis

Arturo Casadevall

DEFINITION AND ETIOLOGY

Cryptococcus, a genus of yeast-like fungi, is the etiologic agent of cryptococcosis. Until recently, cryptococcal strains were separated into two species, *Cryptococcus neoformans* and *Cryptococcus gattii*, both of which can cause cryptococcosis in humans. The two varieties of *C. neoformans—grubii* and *neoformans*—correlate with serotypes A and D, respectively. *C. gattii*, although not divided into varieties, also is antigenically diverse, encompassing serotypes B and C. However, genome sequencing studies have now revealed tremendous diversity among isolates previously assigned to each species, leading to the proposal that each of the prior species classifications includes numerous new species. Hence, *C. neoformans* and *C. gattii* are now considered as species complexes. However, for clinical purposes, these species complexes cause indistinguishable disease referred to as cryptococcosis. Consequently, this chapter will continue to use the nomenclature *C. neoformans* and *C. gattii* with the understanding that these terms refer to species complexes.

EPIDEMIOLOGY

Cryptococcosis was first described in the 1890s but remained relatively rare until the mid-twentieth century, when advances in diagnosis and increases in the number of immunosuppressed individuals markedly raised its reported prevalence. Although serologic evidence of cryptococcal *infection* is common among immunocompetent individuals, cryptococcal *disease* (cryptococcosis) is relatively rare in the absence of impaired immunity. Individuals at high risk for disease due to *C. neoformans* include patients with hematologic malignancies, recipients of solid-organ transplants who require ongoing immunosuppressive therapy, persons whose medical conditions necessitate glucocorticoid therapy, and patients with advanced HIV infection and CD4+ T lymphocyte counts of <200/μL. In contrast, *C. gattii*–related disease is not associated with specific immune deficits and often occurs in immunocompetent individuals.

Cryptococcal infection is acquired from the environment. *C. neoformans* and *C. gattii* species complexes inhabit different ecologic niches. *C. neoformans* is frequently found in soils contaminated with avian excreta and can easily be recovered from shaded and humid soils contaminated with pigeon droppings. In contrast, *C. gattii* is not found in bird feces. Instead, it inhabits a variety of arboreal species, including several types of eucalyptus tree. *C. neoformans* strains are found throughout the world; however, var. *grubii* (serotype A) strains are far more common than var. *neoformans* (serotype D) strains among both clinical and environmental isolates. The geographic distribution of *C. gattii* was thought to be largely limited to tropical regions until an outbreak of cryptococcosis caused by a new serotype B strain began in Vancouver in 1999. This outbreak has extended into the United States, and *C. gattii* infections are being encountered increasingly in several states in the Pacific Northwest.

The global burden of cryptococcosis was estimated in 2012 at ~1 million cases, with >600,000 deaths annually, although the prevalence of this disease has declined since then with the greater availability of antiretroviral therapy (ART) for HIV. Thus cryptococci are important human pathogens. Since the onset of the HIV pandemic in the early 1980s, the overwhelming majority of cryptococcosis cases have occurred in patients with AIDS (**Chap. 202**). To comprehend the impact of HIV infection on the epidemiology of cryptococcosis, it is instructive to note that in the early 1990s there were >1000 cases of cryptococcal meningitis each year in New York City—a figure far exceeding that for all cases of bacterial meningitis. With the advent of effective ART, the incidence of AIDS-related cryptococcosis has been sharply reduced among treated individuals. Therefore, most cases of cryptococcosis now occur in resource-limited regions of the world. The disease remains distressingly common in regions where ART is not readily available (e.g., parts of Africa and Asia); in these regions, up to one-third of patients with AIDS have cryptococcosis. Among HIV-infected persons, those with a decreased percentage of memory B cells expressing IgM may be at greater risk for cryptococcosis.

PATHOGENESIS

Cryptococcal infection is acquired by inhalation of aerosolized infectious particles. The exact nature of these particles is not known; the two leading candidate forms are small desiccated yeast cells and basidiospores. Little is known about the pathogenesis of initial infection. Serologic studies have shown that cryptococcal infection is acquired in childhood, but it is not known whether the initial infection is symptomatic. Given that cryptococcal infection is common while disease is rare, the consensus is that pulmonary defense mechanisms in immunologically intact individuals are highly effective at containing this fungus. It is not clear whether initial infection leads to a state of immunity or whether most individuals are subject throughout life to frequent and recurrent infections that resolve without clinical disease. However, evidence indicates that some human cryptococcal infections lead to a state of latency in which viable organisms are harbored for prolonged periods, possibly in granulomas. Thus, the inhalation of cryptococcal cells and/or spores can be followed by either clearance or establishment of the latent state. The consequences of prolonged harboring of cryptococcal cells in the lung are not known, but evidence from animal studies indicates that the organisms' prolonged presence could alter the immunologic milieu in the lung and predispose to allergic airway disease.

Cryptococcosis usually presents clinically as chronic meningoencephalitis. The mechanisms by which the fungus undergoes extrapulmonary dissemination and enters the central nervous system (CNS) remain poorly understood. The mechanism by which cryptococcal cells cross the blood-brain barrier is a subject of intensive study. Current evidence suggests that both direct fungal-cell migration across the endothelium and fungal-cell carriage inside macrophages as "Trojan horse" invaders can occur. *Cryptococcus* species have well-defined virulence factors that include the expression of the polysaccharide capsule, the ability to make melanin, and the elaboration of enzymes (e.g.,

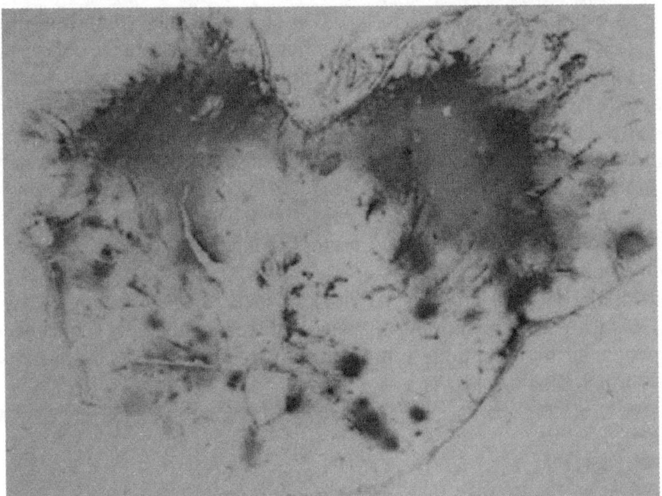

FIGURE 215-1 Cryptococcal antigen in human brain tissue, as revealed by immunohistochemical staining. Brown areas show polysaccharide deposits in the midbrain of a patient who died of cryptococcal meningitis. *(Reproduced with permission from SC Lee, A Casadevall, DW Dickson. Immunohistochemical localization of capsular polysaccharide antigen in the central nervous system cells in cryptococcal meningoencephalitis. Am J Pathol 148:1267, 1996.)*

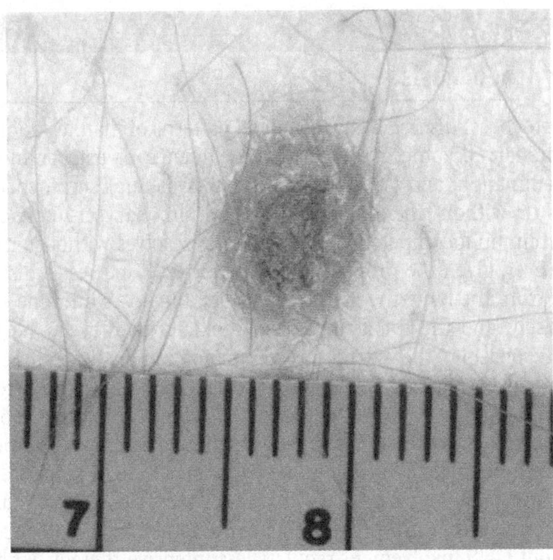

FIGURE 215-2 Disseminated fungal infection. A liver transplant recipient developed six cutaneous lesions similar to the one shown. Biopsy and serum antigen testing demonstrated *Cryptococcus*. Important features of the lesion include a benign-appearing fleshy papule with central umbilication resembling molluscum contagiosum. *(Photo courtesy of Dr. Lindsey Baden; with permission.)*

phospholipase and urease) that enhance the survival of fungal cells in tissue. Among these virulence factors, the capsule and melanin production have been most extensively studied. The cryptococcal capsule is antiphagocytic, and the capsular polysaccharide has been associated with numerous deleterious effects on host immune function. Cryptococcal infections can elicit little or no tissue inflammatory response. The immune dysfunction seen in cryptococcosis has been attributed to the release of copious amounts of capsular polysaccharide into tissues, where it probably interferes with local immune responses (**Fig. 215-1**). In clinical practice, the capsular polysaccharide is the antigen that is measured as a diagnostic marker of cryptococcal infection.

APPROACH TO THE PATIENT

Cryptococcosis

Cryptococcosis should be included in the differential diagnosis when any patient presents with findings suggestive of chronic meningitis. Concern about cryptococcosis is heightened by a history of headache and neurologic symptoms in a patient with an underlying immunosuppressive disorder or state that is associated with an increased incidence of cryptococcosis, such as advanced HIV infection or solid-organ transplantation.

■ CLINICAL MANIFESTATIONS

The clinical manifestations of cryptococcosis reflect the site of fungal infection. The spectrum of disease caused by *Cryptococcus* species consists predominantly of meningoencephalitis and pneumonia, but skin and soft tissue infections also occur; in fact, cryptococcosis can affect any tissue or organ. CNS involvement usually presents as signs and symptoms of chronic meningitis, such as headache, fever, lethargy, sensory deficits, memory deficits, cranial nerve paresis, vision deficits, and meningismus. Cryptococcal meningitis differs from bacterial meningitis in that many *Cryptococcus*-infected patients present with symptoms of several weeks' duration. In addition, classic characteristics of meningeal irritation, such as meningismus, may be absent in cryptococcal meningitis. Indolent cases can present as subacute dementia. Meningeal cryptococcosis can lead to sudden catastrophic vision loss.

Pulmonary cryptococcosis usually presents as cough, increased sputum production, and chest pain. Patients infected with *C. gattii* can present with granulomatous pulmonary masses known as *cryptococcomas*. Fever develops in a minority of cases. Like CNS disease, pulmonary cryptococcosis can follow an indolent course, and the majority of cases probably do not come to clinical attention. In fact, many cases are discovered incidentally during the workup of an abnormal chest radiograph obtained for other diagnostic purposes. Pulmonary cryptococcosis can be associated with antecedent diseases such as malignancy, diabetes, and tuberculosis.

Skin lesions are common in patients with disseminated cryptococcosis and can be highly variable, including papules, plaques, purpura, vesicles, tumor-like lesions, and rashes. The spectrum of cryptococcosis in HIV-infected patients is so varied and has changed so much since the advent of ART that a distinction between HIV-related and HIV-unrelated cryptococcosis is no longer pertinent. In patients with AIDS and solid-organ transplant recipients, the lesions of cutaneous cryptococcosis often resemble those of molluscum contagiosum (**Fig. 215-2; Chap. 196**).

■ DIAGNOSIS

A diagnosis of cryptococcosis requires the demonstration of yeast cells or cryptococcal antigen in normally sterile tissues. Visualization of the capsule of fungal cells in cerebrospinal fluid (CSF) mixed with India ink remains a useful rapid diagnostic technique. Cryptococcal cells in India ink have a distinctive appearance because their capsules exclude ink particles. However, the CSF India ink examination may yield negative results in patients with a low fungal burden. Cultures of CSF and blood that are positive for cryptococcal cells are diagnostic for cryptococcosis. In cryptococcal meningitis, CSF examination usually reveals evidence of chronic meningitis with mononuclear cell pleocytosis and increased protein levels. A particularly useful test is cryptococcal antigen (CRAg) detection in CSF and blood. The assay is based on serologic detection of cryptococcal polysaccharide and is both sensitive and specific. A major advance in recent years has been the introduction of rapid point-of-care CRAgs that provides results in minutes. A positive CRAg test provides strong presumptive evidence for cryptococcosis; however, because the result is often negative in pulmonary cryptococcosis, the test is less useful in the diagnosis of pulmonary disease and is of only limited usefulness in monitoring the response to therapy.

In areas of Africa where there is a high prevalence of HIV infection, routine screening of blood for CRAg in HIV-infected patients with low CD4+ T lymphocyte counts may identify individuals at high risk of cryptococcal disease who are candidates for antifungal therapy. CRAg screening has shown that a significant proportion of HIV-infected patients hospitalized with pneumonia in Thailand harbor cryptococcal infection. Inexpensive point-of-care CRAg tests are under development and could be of great diagnostic benefit in resource-limited regions.

TREATMENT
Cryptococcosis

Cryptococcal disease has two general patterns of manifestation: (1) pulmonary cryptococcosis, with no evidence of extrapulmonary dissemination; and (2) extrapulmonary (systemic) cryptococcosis, with or without meningoencephalitis. Pulmonary cryptococcosis in an immunocompetent host sometimes resolves without therapy. However, given the propensity of *Cryptococcus* species to disseminate from the lung, the inability to gauge the host's immune status precisely, and the availability of low-toxicity therapy in the form of fluconazole, the current recommendation is for pulmonary cryptococcosis in an immunocompetent individual to be treated with fluconazole (200–400 mg/d for 3–6 months). Extrapulmonary cryptococcosis without CNS involvement in an immunocompetent host can be treated with the same regimen, although amphotericin B (AmB; 0.5–1 mg/kg daily for 4–6 weeks) may be required for more severe cases. In general, extrapulmonary cryptococcosis without CNS involvement requires less intensive therapy, with the caveat that morbidity and death in cryptococcosis are associated with meningeal involvement. Thus, the decision to categorize cryptococcosis as "extrapulmonary without CNS involvement" should be made only after careful evaluation of the CSF reveals no evidence of cryptococcal infection. For CNS involvement in a host without AIDS or obvious immune impairment, most authorities recommend initial therapy with AmB (0.5–1 mg/kg daily) during an induction phase, which is followed by prolonged therapy with fluconazole (400 mg/d) during a consolidation phase. For cryptococcal meningoencephalitis without a concomitant immunosuppressive condition, the recommended regimen is AmB (0.5–1 mg/kg) plus flucytosine (100 mg/kg) daily for 6–10 weeks. Alternatively, patients can be treated with AmB (0.5–1 mg/kg) plus flucytosine (100 mg/kg) daily for 2 weeks and then with fluconazole (400 mg/d) for at least 10 weeks. Patients with immunosuppression are treated with the same initial regimens except that consolidation therapy with fluconazole is given for a prolonged period to prevent relapse.

Cryptococcosis in patients with HIV infection always requires aggressive therapy and is considered incurable unless immune function improves. Consequently, therapy for cryptococcosis in the setting of AIDS has two phases: induction therapy (intended to reduce the fungal burden and alleviate symptoms) and lifelong maintenance therapy (to prevent a symptomatic clinical relapse). Pulmonary and extrapulmonary cryptococcosis without evidence of CNS involvement can be treated with fluconazole (200–400 mg/d). In patients who have more extensive disease, flucytosine (100 mg/kg per day) may be added to the fluconazole regimen for 10 weeks, with lifelong fluconazole maintenance therapy thereafter. For HIV-infected patients with evidence of CNS involvement, most authorities recommend induction therapy with AmB. An acceptable regimen is AmB (0.7–1 mg/kg) plus flucytosine (100 mg/kg) daily for 2 weeks followed by fluconazole (400 mg/d) for at least 10 weeks and then by lifelong maintenance therapy with fluconazole (200 mg/d). Fluconazole (400–800 mg/d) plus flucytosine (100 mg/kg per day) for 6–10 weeks followed by fluconazole (200 mg/d) as maintenance therapy is an alternative. Newer triazoles like voriconazole and posaconazole are highly active against cryptococcal strains and appear to be clinically effective, but clinical experience with these agents in the treatment of cryptococcosis is limited. Lipid formulations of AmB can be substituted for AmB deoxycholate in patients with renal impairment. Neither caspofungin nor micafungin is effective against *Cryptococcus* species; consequently, neither drug has a role in the treatment of cryptococcosis. Cryptococcal meningoencephalitis is often associated with increased intracranial pressure, which is believed to be responsible for damage to the brain and cranial nerves. Appropriate management of CNS cryptococcosis requires careful attention to the management of intracranial pressure, including the reduction of pressure by repeated therapeutic lumbar puncture and the placement of shunts. Studies suggest that the addition of a short course of interferon γ to antifungal therapy in patients with HIV infection increases clearance of cryptococci from the CSF. In contrast, administration of dexamethasone was associated with reduced fungal clearance and increased mortality. Antifungal drug resistance has not been a major problem with cryptococcal strains, but there are increasing reports of drug-resistant strains, including some emerging during the prolonged therapy needed for cryptococcosis. Hence, cryptococcosis that is refractory to antifungal therapy should prompt an investigation into the susceptibility of the clinical isolates in question.

In HIV-infected patients with previously treated cryptococcosis who are receiving fluconazole maintenance therapy, it may be possible to discontinue antifungal drug treatment if ART results in immunologic improvement.

PROGNOSIS AND COMPLICATIONS

Even with antifungal therapy, cryptococcosis is associated with high rates of morbidity and death. For the majority of patients with cryptococcosis, the most important prognostic factors are the extent and the duration of the underlying immunologic deficits that predisposed them to develop the disease. Cryptococcosis is often curable with antifungal therapy in individuals with no apparent immunologic dysfunction, but in patients with severe immunosuppression (e.g., those with AIDS), the best that can be hoped for is that antifungal therapy will induce remission, which can then be maintained with lifelong suppressive therapy. Before the advent of ART, the median overall survival period for AIDS patients with cryptococcosis was <1 year. Cryptococcosis in patients with underlying neoplastic disease has a particularly poor prognosis. For CNS cryptococcosis, poor prognostic markers are a CSF assay positive for yeast cells on initial India ink examination (evidence of a heavy fungal burden), high CSF pressure, low CSF glucose levels, low CSF pleocytosis (<2/μL), recovery of yeast cells from extraneural sites, absence of antibody to capsular polysaccharide, a CSF or serum cryptococcal antigen level of ≥1:32, and concomitant glucocorticoid therapy or hematologic malignancy. A response to treatment does not guarantee cure since relapse of cryptococcosis is common even among patients with relatively intact immune systems. Complications of CNS cryptococcosis include cranial nerve deficits, vision loss, and cognitive impairment.

IMMUNE RECONSTITUTION INFLAMMATORY SYNDROME

The immune reconstitution inflammatory syndrome (IRIS) occurs when immunity rebounds in the setting of treated cryptococcosis (or an undiagnosed asymptomatic infection) and the immune response to cryptococcal antigens in tissue triggers an inflammatory response that can be difficult to distinguish from a relapsing infection. IRIS can occur when patients with AIDS and treated cryptococcosis are given ART that results in improved immunity. A major consideration for clinicians treating cryptococcosis in the setting of AIDS is when to begin ART, which can trigger rebounding immunity. Current recommendations are to start ART 4–6 weeks after initiation of antifungal therapy. Apart from the difficulties in distinguishing IRIS from cryptococcal relapse, the management of this syndrome is complex because it is caused by the desirable outcome of improving immunity, which is important in controlling cryptococcal infection and preventing relapses. The approach to the patient with IRIS must attempt to balance resurgent immunity against immune-mediated damage. Currently, management of IRIS is individualized and can involve the use of glucocorticoids to reduce inflammation.

PREVENTION

No vaccine is available for cryptococcosis. In patients at high risk (e.g., those with advanced HIV infection and CD4+ T lymphocyte counts of <200/μL), primary prophylaxis with fluconazole (200 mg/d) is effective in reducing the prevalence of disease. Since ART raises the CD4+ T lymphocyte count, it constitutes an immunologic form of prophylaxis.

FURTHER READING

Alanio A: Dormancy in *Cryptococcus neoformans*: 60 years of accumulating evidence. J Clin Invest 130:3353, 2020.

Boyer-Chammard T et al: Recent advances in managing HIV-associated cryptococcal meningitis. F1000Res 8:F1000 Faculty Rev-743, 2019.

Kwon-Chung KJ et al: The case for adopting the "species complex" nomenclature for the etiologic agents of cryptococcosis. mSphere 2:e00357, 2017.

Maziarz EK, Perfect JR: Cryptococcosis. Infect Dis Clin North Am 30:179, 2016.

Robertson EJ et al: *Cryptococcus neoformans* ex vivo capsule size is associated with intracranial pressure and host immune response in HIV-associated cryptococcal meningitis. J Infect Dis 209:74, 2014.

Srichatrapimuk S, Sungkanuparph S: Integrated therapy for HIV and cryptococcosis. AIDS Res Ther 13:42, 2016.

216 Candidiasis

Michail S. Lionakis, Shakti Singh, Ashraf S. Ibrahim, John E. Edwards, Jr.

The genus *Candida* encompasses >150 species, only a few of which cause disease in humans. With rare exceptions (although the exceptions are increasing in number), the human pathogens are *C. albicans*, *C. guilliermondii*, *C. krusei*, *C. parapsilosis*, *C. tropicalis*, *C. kefyr*, *C. lusitaniae*, *C. dubliniensis*, *C. glabrata*, and the emerging, multidrug-resistant, *C. auris*, which has been responsible for several outbreaks in health care facilities in recent years. Ubiquitous in nature, they inhabit the gastrointestinal tract (including the mouth and oropharynx), the female genital tract, and the skin in the majority of healthy persons. Although cases of candidiasis have been described since antiquity in debilitated patients, the advent of *Candida* species as common human pathogens dates to the introduction of modern therapeutic approaches that suppress normal host defense mechanisms. Of these relatively recent advances, the most important is the use of antibacterial agents that alter the normal human microbiota and allow nonbacterial species to become more prevalent in the commensal flora. With the introduction of antifungal agents, the causes of *Candida* infections shifted from an almost complete dominance of *C. albicans* to the common involvement of *C. glabrata* and the other species listed above. The non-*albicans* species now account for approximately half of all cases of candidemia and hematogenously disseminated candidiasis. Recognition of this change is clinically important since the various species differ in susceptibility and are increasingly resistant to the newer antifungal agents.

Candida is a small, thin-walled, ovoid yeast that measures 4–6 μm in diameter and reproduces by budding. Organisms of this genus occur in three forms in tissue: blastospores, pseudohyphae, and hyphae. *Candida* grows readily on simple media; lysis centrifugation enhances its recovery from blood. Species are identified by biochemical testing (currently with automated devices) or on special agar (e.g., CHROMagar).

EPIDEMIOLOGY

Candida are present in humans as commensals, in animals, in foods, and on inanimate objects. In developed countries, where contemporary medical therapeutics are commonly used, *Candida* species are now among the most common nosocomial pathogens. In the United States, these species are among the four most common pathogens isolated from the blood of hospitalized patients. In fact, in a recent point-prevalence study in the United States, *Candida* species were the most common organisms infecting the bloodstream of hospitalized patients. In regions where advanced medical care is not readily available, mucocutaneous *Candida* infections, such as thrush, are more common than deep-organ infections, which rarely occur. However, the incidence of deep-organ candidiasis is increasing steadily as advances in health care—such as therapy with broad-spectrum antibiotics, more aggressive treatment of cancer, and the use of immunosuppression for sustaining organ transplants—are implemented. In aggregate, the global incidence of infections due to *Candida* species has risen steadily over the past few decades.

C. auris is an emerging species of *Candida* that has spread rapidly in recent years to >30 countries and is a major public health concern. This concern stems from its occurrence in health care facilities, its ability to adhere to and persist long term in inanimate objects (in hospitals) and the human skin despite decolonization efforts, its association with substantial mortality, its propensity for misidentification as other *Candida* species, the incomplete understanding of its environmental reservoirs, and its multidrug resistance to the current antifungal therapeutic armamentarium, with some *C. auris* strains being resistant to all antifungal drug classes currently available for treatment. *C. auris* (*auris* meaning *ear* in Latin) was first identified in 2009 from the ear drainage of a patient with an ear infection in Japan. However, subsequent retrospective analysis of *Candida* strain collections identified the earliest known *C. auris* strain to date back to 1996 in South Korea. Notably, whole genome sequencing analysis of *C. auris* strains from South Asia, East Asia, South America, and South Africa found that although strains within each geographic region are closely related to each other, they are distinct compared to strains from other geographic regions. These findings indicate that *C. auris* emerged independently in multiple geographic locations around the same time; the epidemiologic reasons for this emergence remain poorly understood.

The presence of a central venous catheter and/or other invasive medical devices and recent residence in nursing homes are major risk factors for *C. auris* colonization and infection. Screening of selected patients who are in a hospital or nursing home where *C. auris* has been cultured and are at risk for dissemination from a colonization site may help implementing effective infection control measures. Hand hygiene with an alcohol-based hand sanitizer is recommended when hands are not visibly soiled, in which case washing with soap and water is preferred. Identifying the source of contamination, if possible, and using an Environmental Protection Agency (EPA)-registered hospital-grade disinfectant effective against *Clostridioides difficile* spores are desirable. If a patient develops an invasive or bloodstream infection, it is recommended that the health care facility informs the Centers for Disease Control and Prevention (CDC), or a similar agency in other countries and adheres to recommendations for infection control, including isolation of patients (contact or enhanced barrier precautions), use of proper personal protective coverings, enforcement of hospital environment hygiene, and communicating with other health care facilities if the patient is being transferred.

PATHOGENESIS

In the most severe form of *Candida* infection, the organisms disseminate hematogenously and form microabscesses and small macroabscesses in major organs. Although the exact mechanism is not known, *Candida* probably enters the bloodstream from mucosal surfaces after growing to large numbers as a consequence of bacterial suppression by antibacterial drugs and breaches in the integrity of the mucosal barrier; alternatively, in some instances, the organism may enter the bloodstream from the skin via central venous catheters. A change from the blastospore stage to the pseudohyphal and hyphal stages is generally considered integral to *Candida*'s penetration into tissue. However, *C. glabrata* and *C. auris* can cause life-threatening infection, even though they do not transform into pseudohyphae or hyphae. Adherence to both epithelial and endothelial cells is thought to be the first step in invasion and infection; several adhesins have been identified as well as a mucosal toxin, candidalysin. Biofilm formation also is considered important in pathogenesis. Numerous reviews of cases of hematogenously disseminated candidiasis have identified the predisposing factors or conditions associated with disseminated disease (**Table 216-1**).

Several genes that are involved in the pathogenesis of other *Candida* species—such as those responsible for biofilm formation, proteinases, lipases, phospholipases, hydrolases, adhesins, secreted aspartyl

TABLE 216-1 Well-Recognized Factors and Conditions Predisposing to Hematogenously Disseminated Candidiasis

Antibacterial agents	Abdominal and thoracic surgery
Indwelling intravenous catheters	Cytotoxic chemotherapy
Hyperalimentation fluids	Immunosuppressive agents for organ transplantation
Indwelling urinary catheters	Respirators
Parenteral glucocorticoids	Myeloperoxidase deficiency
Severe burns	Neutropenia
CARD9 deficiency (central nervous system)	Low birth weight (neonates)
	Diabetes

proteases, and transporters involved in azole resistance—are also present in *C. auris*. Unlike other *Candida* species, several *C. auris* strains exhibit aggregate-forming properties in vivo, which may enable immune evasion. In addition, *C. auris* shows a unique tolerance to high temperature and saline concentrations and can grow optimally at up to 42°C and in a 10% saline concentration, making it possible to exist and persist in harsh environments. Furthermore, *C. auris* has significantly greater affinity for abiotic surfaces such as plastic materials and medical devices, as well as human skin and nasal and ear cavities, which may account for its persistent colonization capabilities.

Innate immunity is the most important defense mechanism against hematogenously disseminated candidiasis, and the neutrophil is the most potent component of this defense. Macrophages also play an important host defense role. On the other hand, T_H17 lymphocytes contribute significantly to defense against mucocutaneous candidiasis as evidenced by several monogenic disorders of interleukin (IL) 17 receptor signaling that manifest with *chronic mucocutaneous candidiasis* (CMC) (see "Clinical Manifestations," below). Although many immunocompetent individuals have antibodies to *Candida*, the role of these antibodies in defense against the organism is not clear. Multiple genetic polymorphisms in host immune-related genes that predispose to both disseminated and focal candidiasis have been identified and may contribute to patient susceptibility.

CLINICAL MANIFESTATIONS

Mucocutaneous Candidiasis *Thrush* is characterized by white, adherent, painless, discrete or confluent patches in the mouth, on the tongue, or in the esophagus, occasionally with fissuring at the corners of the mouth. This form of disease caused by *Candida* can also occur at points of contact with dentures (called "denture sore mouth"). Organisms are identifiable in gram-stained scrapings from lesions. The occurrence of thrush in a young, otherwise healthy-appearing person should prompt an investigation for underlying HIV infection. More commonly, thrush is seen as a nonspecific manifestation of severe debilitating illness. Vulvovaginal candidiasis is accompanied by pruritus, pain, and vaginal discharge, which is usually thin but may contain whitish "curds" in severe cases. In contrast to oral thrush, HIV is not considered a major risk factor for vulvovaginal candidiasis. Instead, many women who receive antibiotics may develop vulvovaginal candidiasis. A subset of patients with recurrent vulvovaginitis may have a deficiency in the surface expression of Dectin-1, a major recognition factor for β-glucan on the surface of *Candida* and/or in the downstream adaptor molecule CARD9, which ultimately increases the propensity for recurrent mucocutaneous (including vaginal) infections.

Other *Candida* skin infections include *paronychia*, a painful swelling at the nail–skin interface; *onychomycosis*, a fungal nail infection rarely caused by this genus; *intertrigo*, an erythematous irritation with redness and pustules in the skin folds; *balanitis*, an erythematous-pustular infection of the glans penis; *erosio interdigitalis blastomycetica*, an infection between the digits of the hands or toes; *folliculitis*, with pustules developing most frequently in the area of the beard; *perianal candidiasis*, a pruritic, erythematous, pustular infection surrounding the anus; *mastitis*; and *diaper rash*, a common erythematous, pustular perineal infection in infants. *Generalized disseminated cutaneous candidiasis*, another form of infection that occurs primarily in infants,

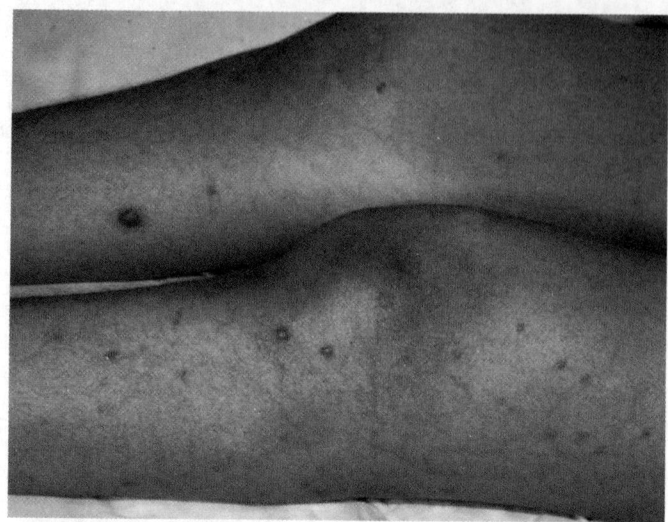

FIGURE 216-1 Macronodular skin lesions associated with hematogenously disseminated candidiasis. *Candida* organisms are usually but not always visible on histopathologic examination. The fungi grow when a portion of the biopsied specimen is cultured. Therefore, for optimal identification, both histopathology and culture should be performed. *(Image courtesy of Dr. Noah Craft and the Victor Newcomer collection at UCLA, archived by Logical Images, Inc.; with permission.)*

is characterized by widespread eruptions over the trunk, thorax, and extremities. The diagnostic macronodular lesions of hematogenously disseminated candidiasis (**Fig. 216-1**) indicate a high probability of dissemination to multiple organs as well as the skin. While the lesions are seen predominantly in immunocompromised patients treated with cytotoxic drugs, they may also develop in patients without neutropenia.

CMC is a heterogeneous infection of the hair, nails, skin, and mucous membranes that persists despite intermittent antifungal therapy. The onset of disease usually comes in infancy or within the first two decades of life, but in rare cases, it occurs in later life. The condition may be mild and limited to a specific area of the skin or nails, or it may take a severely disfiguring form (*Candida* granuloma) characterized by exophytic outgrowths on the skin. CMC is usually associated with specific immunologic dysfunction; most frequently reported is a failure of T lymphocytes to secrete type-17 cytokines in response to stimulation by *Candida* antigens in vitro. A subset of the affected patients has mutations in the IL-17 receptor, its adaptor molecule ACT1 (TRAF3IP2), or, more often, in STAT1, resulting in an insufficiency of IL-17 and IL-22 production.

Approximately half of patients with CMC have associated endocrine abnormalities either in the setting of gain-of-function mutations in *STAT1* or in the context of *a*utoimmune *p*oly*e*ndocrinopathy–*c*andidiasis–*e*ctodermal *d*ystrophy (APECED) syndrome. This syndrome is due to mutations in the autoimmune regulator (*AIRE*) gene and is most prevalent among Finns, Iranian Jews, and Sardinians. Conditions that usually follow the onset of the disease include hypoparathyroidism, adrenal insufficiency, autoimmune thyroiditis, chronic active hepatitis, autoimmune pneumonitis, alopecia, juvenile-onset pernicious anemia, intestinal malabsorption, and primary hypogonadism. In addition, dental enamel dysplasia, vitiligo, nail dystrophy, asplenia, and calcification of the tympanic membranes may occur. Patients with CMC rarely develop hematogenously disseminated candidiasis, reflecting their intact neutrophil function.

Deeply Invasive Candidiasis Deeply invasive *Candida* infections may or may not be due to hematogenous seeding. Deep esophageal infection may result from penetration by organisms from superficial esophageal erosions; joint or deep-wound infection from contiguous spread of organisms from the skin; kidney infection from catheter-initiated ascending spread of organisms through the urinary tract; infection of intraabdominal organs and the peritoneum from perforation of the gastrointestinal tract; and gallbladder infection from retrograde migration of organisms from the gastrointestinal tract into the biliary drainage system.

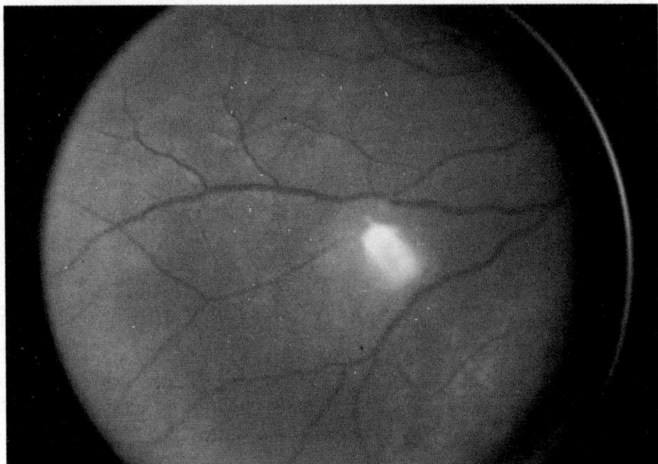

FIGURE 216-2 Hematogenous *Candida* endophthalmitis. A classic off-white lesion projecting from the chorioretina into the vitreous causes the surrounding haze. The lesion is composed primarily of inflammatory cells rather than organisms. Lesions of this type may progress to cause extensive vitreal inflammation and eventual loss of the eye. Partial vitrectomy, combined with IV and possibly intravitreal antifungal therapy, may be helpful in controlling the lesions. *(Image courtesy of Dr. Gary Holland; with permission.)*

However, more commonly, deeply invasive candidiasis results from hematogenous seeding of various organs as a complication of candidemia. Once the organism gains access to the intravascular compartment (either from the gastrointestinal tract or, less often, from the skin through the site of an indwelling intravascular catheter), it may spread hematogenously to a variety of deep organs. The brain, chorioretina (**Fig. 216-2**), heart, and kidneys are most commonly infected and the liver and spleen are less commonly affected in nonneutropenic hosts (but most often involved in neutropenic patients). In fact, nearly any organ can become involved, including the endocrine glands, pancreas, heart valves (native or prosthetic), skeletal muscle, joints (native or prosthetic), bones, and meninges. *Candida* organisms can also spread hematogenously to the skin and cause classic macronodular lesions (Fig. 216-1). Frequently, painful muscular involvement is evident beneath the area of affected skin. Chorioretinal involvement and skin involvement are highly significant since both findings are associated with a very high probability of abscess formation in multiple deep organs as a result of generalized hematogenous seeding. Ocular involvement (Fig. 216-2) may require specific treatment (e.g., partial vitrectomy or intraocular injection of antifungal agents) to prevent permanent blindness. An ocular examination is indicated for all patients with candidemia, whether or not they have ocular manifestations. *C. auris* invasive infections are similar to those of other *Candida* species, and are most frequently associated with recent surgical procedures, immunosuppression, invasive devices such as catheters or various support or drainage tubes, and extended hospital stays. In the majority of invasive infections, *C. auris* has been isolated from the blood, but invasion of the kidney or spleen, and its recovery from cerebrospinal, bile, peritoneal, and pleural fluids demonstrate its invasiveness and dissemination potential. *C. auris*-associated candidemia can be life-threatening, with a crude mortality rate of 30–60%.

DIAGNOSIS

The diagnosis of *Candida* infection is established by visualization of pseudohyphae or hyphae on wet mount (saline and 10% KOH), tissue Gram's stain, periodic acid–Schiff stain, or methenamine silver stain in the presence of inflammation. Absence of organisms on hematoxylin-eosin staining does not reliably exclude *Candida* infection. The most challenging aspect of diagnosis is determining which patients with *Candida* isolates have hematogenously disseminated candidiasis. For instance, recovery of *Candida* from sputum, urine, or peritoneal catheters may indicate mere colonization rather than deep-seated infection, and *Candida* isolation from the blood of patients with indwelling intravascular catheters may reflect inconsequential seeding of the blood from or growth of the organisms on the catheter. Despite extensive research into both antigen and antibody detection systems, there is currently no widely available and validated diagnostic test to distinguish patients with inconsequential seeding of the blood from those whose positive blood cultures represent hematogenous dissemination to multiple organs. Many studies have examined the utility of the β-glucan test; at present, its greatest utility is its negative predictive value (~90%). Meanwhile, the presence of ocular or macronodular skin lesions is highly suggestive of widespread infection of multiple deep organs. Despite extensive diagnostic tests for hematogenous dissemination, such as polymerase chain reaction and T2 technology, no test is fully validated or widely available at present. Matrix-assisted laser desorption–ionization–time-of-flight mass spectrometry (MALDI-TOF MS) is now being used extensively for detection and speciation and is useful for the correct diagnosis of *C. auris*.

C. auris is usually misdiagnosed in the microbiology laboratory, often leading to inappropriate treatment and delay in the implementation of appropriate infection control measures. Preliminary testing by culturing the fungus and examination of colony morphology may help in the initial identification, but this must be confirmed with more advanced diagnostic methods. For example, features such as budding yeast morphology, absence of hyphal growth or germ tubes, and growth at 40–42°C (unlike other *Candida* species) on CHROMagar that may appear white, pink, red, or purple could raise suspicion for *C. auris* (**Fig. 216-3**).

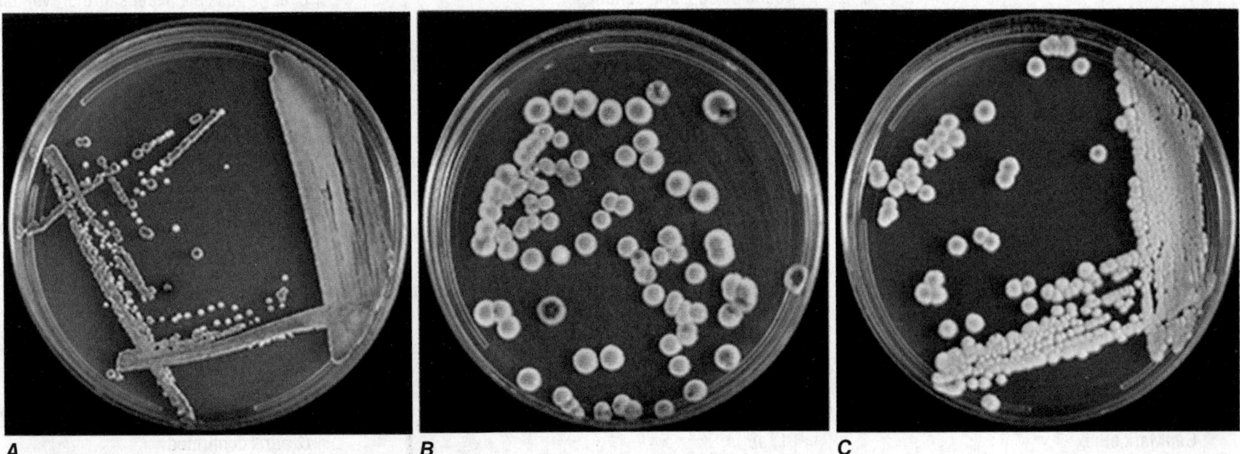

FIGURE 216-3 *C. auris* colony morphology and color on CHROMagar plates. A. *Candida* mixed culture: culture of *C. glabrata* (purple), *C. tropicalis* (navy blue), and *C. auris* (white, circled in red). **B.** *C. auris* showing multiple colony morphologies. **C.** *C. auris* after Salt SAB Dulcitol Broth enrichment. *(From CDC: Identification of Candida auris. 2019. Available at: www.cdc.gov/fungal/candida-auris/recommendations.html.)*

Several advanced molecular techniques accurately identify *C. auris* strains and therefore are being used for the follow-up testing and confirmation of the specimens that failed to be identified by traditional methods. MALDI-TOF equipment with upgraded libraries, such as Bruker Biotyper MALDI-TOF (CA System library version claim 4 or research use only [RUO] libraries versions 2014 [5627] and more recent), and using the bioMérieux VITEK MALDI-TOF MS (IVD v3.2 or RUO libraries with Saramis Ver 4.14 database and Saccharomycetaceae update), are the most common methods of *C. auris* identification. Other supplemental MALDI-TOF databases, such as MicrobeNet, that include additional *C. auris* strains from the four phylogenetic clades (i.e., South Asian, East Asian, South American, and South African) also can be used for the identification of *C. auris* strains. Sequencing of the D1–D2 region of the 28s rDNA or the internal transcribed region (ITS) of rDNA can also correctly identify *C. auris*. Recently, an automated, qualitative nucleic acid multiplex in vitro diagnostic test by GenMark called ePlex Blood Culture Identification Fungal Pathogen (BCID-FP) Panel was approved by the U.S. Food and Drug Administration for *C. auris* testing. Also, several polymerase chain reaction–based detection methods have been reported to identify *C. auris* in various specimens. **Table 216-2** outlines the typical decision-making steps in the diagnosis of *C. auris* by using different methods. A suspicious *C. auris* specimen is usually sent to a regional reference laboratory for further testing and confirmation of *C. auris*.

TREATMENT

Candida Infections

MUCOCUTANEOUS *CANDIDA* INFECTION

The treatment of mucocutaneous candidiasis is summarized in **Table 216-3**.

CANDIDEMIA AND SUSPECTED HEMATOGENOUSLY DISSEMINATED CANDIDIASIS

All patients with candidemia are treated with a systemic antifungal agent. A certain percentage of patients, including many of those who have candidemia associated with an indwelling intravascular catheter, probably have "benign" candidemia rather than deep-organ seeding. However, because there is no reliable way to distinguish benign candidemia from deep-organ infection, and because antifungal drugs less toxic than amphotericin B are available, antifungal treatment for candidemia—with or without clinical evidence of deep-organ involvement—has become the standard of practice.

TABLE 216-2 Typical Decision-Making Steps in the Diagnosis of *C. auris*

NO.	METHOD	DATABASE/SOFTWARE	INITIAL FINDING →		CONFIRMATION
1.	Bruker Biotyper MALDI-TOF	RUO libraries	*C. auris*		*C. auris*
		CA System library	*C. auris*		*C. auris*
2.	bioMérieux VITEK MS MALDI-TOF	RUO library	*C. auris*		*C. auris*
		IVD library	*C. auris*		*C. auris*
		Older IVD libraries	*C. haemulonii*		*C. auris* possible: Needs further workup
			C. lusitaniae		*C. auris* possible: Needs further workup
			No identification		*C. auris* possible: Needs further workup
3.	VITEK 2 YST	Software version 8.01	*C. auris*		*C. auris* confirmed
			C. haemulonii		*C. auris* possible: Needs further workup
			C. duobushaemulonii		*C. auris* possible: Needs further workup
			Candida spp. not identified		*C. auris* possible: Needs further workup
		Older versions	*C. haemulonii*		*C. auris* possible: Needs further workup
			C. duobushaemulonii		*C. auris* possible: Needs further workup
			Candida spp. not identified		*C. auris* possible: Needs further workup
4.	API 20C		*Rhodotorula glutinis*, if characteristic red color absent		*C. auris* possible: Needs further workup
			C. sake		*C. auris* possible: Needs further workup
			Candida spp. not identified		*C. auris* possible: Needs further workup
5.	BD Phoenix		*C. catenulata*		*C. auris* possible: Needs further workup
			C. haemulonii		*C. auris* possible: Needs further workup
			Candida spp. not identified		*C. auris* possible: Needs further workup
6.	MicroScan		*C. lusitaniae*	No hyphal growth present	Can rule out *C. lusitaniae, C. guilliermondii, and C. parapsilosis.* *C. auris* possible: Needs further workup
			C. guilliermondii		
			C. parapsilosis		
			C. lusitaniae	Hyphal growth present	Possibly *C. lusitaniae, C. guilliermondii, C. parapsilosis, or C. auris*: Needs further workup
			C. guilliermondii		
			C. parapsilosis		
			C. famata		*C. auris* possible: Needs further workup
			Candida spp. not identified		*C. auris* possible: Needs further workup
7.	RapID Yeast Plus		*C. parapsilosis* → Test on corneal agar	No hyphal growth present	Can rule out *C. parapsilosis. C. auris* possible: Needs further work-up
				Hyphal growth present	Possibly *C. parapsilosis or C. auris*: Needs further workup
			Candida spp. not identified		*C. auris* possible: Needs further workup
8.	GenMark ePlex BCID-FP Panel		*C. auris*		*C. auris* confirmed

IVD, in vitro diagnostic; RUO, research use only.

Source: Adapted from CDC: Identification of *Candida auris*. 2019. Available at: *www.cdc.gov/fungal/candida-auris/recommendations.html*

TABLE 216-3 Treatment of Mucocutaneous Candidal Infections

DISEASE	PREFERRED TREATMENT	ALTERNATIVES
Cutaneous	Topical azole	Topical nystatin
Vulvovaginal	Oral fluconazole (150 mg) or azole cream or suppository	Nystatin suppository
Oral (thrush)	Clotrimazole troches	Nystatin, fluconazole
Esophageal	Fluconazole tablets (100–200 mg/d) or itraconazole solution (200 mg/d)	Caspofungin, micafungin, or amphotericin B

In addition, if an indwelling intravascular catheter is present, it is best to remove or replace the device whenever feasible.

The drugs used for the treatment of candidemia and suspected disseminated candidiasis are listed in **Table 216-4**. Various lipid formulations of amphotericin B, three echinocandins, the azoles fluconazole and voriconazole, and in some instances, the newer triazoles—posaconazole and isavuconazole—are used; no agent within a given class has been clearly identified as superior to the others. Most institutions choose an agent from each class on the basis of their own specific microbial epidemiology, strategies to minimize toxicities, and cost considerations. An echinocandin is now considered the first choice of treatment if there is concern for resistance, which will be the case in nearly all hospitals. Echinocandin treatment continues until sensitivities or speciation is determined. In stable patients, many centers then switch to fluconazole if a sensitive strain is identified and there is no evidence of hematogenous dissemination. For hemodynamically unstable or neutropenic patients, initial treatment with broader-spectrum agents is desirable; these drugs include polyenes, echinocandins, or later-generation azoles such as voriconazole. Once the clinical response has been assessed and the pathogen specifically identified, the regimen can be altered according to the sensitivities. At present, the vast majority of *C. albicans* isolates are sensitive to fluconazole. Isolates of *C. glabrata* and *C. krusei* are less sensitive to fluconazole and more sensitive to polyenes and echinocandins. *C. parapsilosis* is less sensitive to echinocandins in vitro; however, this lesser sensitivity is considered clinically insignificant. Posaconazole has been approved for prophylaxis, including against *Candida*, in neutropenic patients. Itraconazole is rarely used for *Candida*, and isavuconazole has not been approved for this indication to date.

TABLE 216-5 Typical MICs of Available Antifungal Drugs for *C. auris*

DRUG	TENTATIVE RESISTANCE BREAKPOINTS[a]	MIC RANGE, µg/mL		
		MIC	MIC_{50}	MIC_{90}
Amphotericin B	≥2	0.06–8	0.5–1	2–4
Fluconazole	≥32	0.12–≥64	≥64	≥64
Itraconazole	N/A	0.032–2	0.06–0.5	0.25–1
Voriconazole	N/A	0.032–16	0.5–2	2–8
Posaconazole	N/A	0.015–16	0.016–0.5	0.125–2
Isavuconazole	N/A	0.015–4	0.125–0.25	0.5–2
Caspofungin	≥2	0.03–16	0.25–1	1–2
Anidulafungin	≥4	0.015–16	0.125–0.5	0.5–1
Micafungin	≥4	0.015–8	0.125–0.25	0.25–2

[a]Tentative resistance breakpoints per CDC (*www.cdc.gov/fungal/candida-auris/c-auris-antifungal.html*).

Abbreviations: MIC, minimum inhibitory concentration; N/A, not available.

Source: Adapted from CDC: Antifungal Susceptibility Testing and Interpretation. 2019. Available at: *www.cdc.gov/fungal/candida-auris/c-auris-antifungal.html*

Antifungal drug resistance is one of the hallmarks of *C. auris* infections. Some *C. auris* strains have multidrug resistance with elevated minimal inhibitory concentrations (MICs) to all three major antifungal classes—azoles, echinocandins, and polyenes—resulting in limited treatment options. A recent CDC study reported antifungal resistance in *C. auris* strains obtained from 54 patients in India, Pakistan, South Africa, and Venezuela: 93% were resistant to fluconazole, 35% to amphotericin B, and 7% to echinocandins; 41% of the tested strains were resistant to 2 antifungal classes, and, alarmingly, 4% of the tested strains were resistant to all 3 classes of antifungal drugs. Almost all *C. auris* strains that have been identified have elevated MICs for fluconazole with variable susceptibilities to other triazoles (**Table 216-5**), associated with mutations in *ERG11*-encoded lanosterol demethylase and/or overexpression of drug transporters/efflux pumps.

Due to the high rates of azole resistance among *C. auris* strains, the use of echinocandins is recommended as first-line therapy for *C. auris* infection. By contrast, the CDC discourages the use of antifungal drugs for the treatment of colonization of *C. auris* in the absence of invasive or bloodstream infection. A history of patient travel or residence in a healthcare or nursing facility with a known

TABLE 216-4 Agents for the Treatment of Disseminated Candidiasis

AGENT	ROUTE OF ADMINISTRATION	DOSE[a]	COMMENT
Amphotericin B deoxycholate	IV only	0.5–1.0 mg/kg daily	Mostly replaced by lipid formulations
Amphotericin B lipid formulations			Not approved as primary therapy by the U.S. Food and Drug Administration, but used commonly because they are less toxic than amphotericin B deoxycholate
Liposomal (AmBiSome, Abelcet)	IV only	3.0–5.0 mg/kg daily	
Lipid complex (ABLC)	IV only	3.0–5.0 mg/kg daily	
Colloidal dispersion (ABCD)	IV only	3.0–5.0 mg/kg daily	Associated with frequent infusion reactions
Azoles[b]			
Posaconazole	IV and oral	300 mg/d (IV) 200 mg tid (oral)	Approved for prophylaxis
Fluconazole	IV and oral	400 mg/d	Most commonly used
Voriconazole	IV and oral	400 mg/d	Multiple drug interactions Approved for candidemia in nonneutropenic patients
Echinocandins			Broad spectrum against *Candida* species; approved for disseminated candidiasis; less toxic than amphotericin B formulations
Caspofungin	IV only	50 mg/d	
Anidulafungin	IV only	100 mg/d	
Micafungin	IV only	100 mg/d	

[a]For loading doses and adjustments in renal failure, see Pappas PG et al: Clinical practice guidelines for the management of candidiasis: 2016 update by the Infectious Diseases Society of America. Clin Infect Dis 62:e1, 2016. The recommended duration of therapy is 2 weeks beyond the last positive blood culture and the resolution of signs and symptoms of infection. [b]Although ketoconazole is approved for the treatment of disseminated candidiasis, it has been replaced by the newer agents listed in this table. Posaconazole has been approved for prophylaxis in neutropenic patients and for oropharyngeal candidiasis.

TABLE 216-6 List of CDC-Recommended Echinocandin Doses for the Treatment of *C. auris* Infections

DRUG	ADULTS	CHILDREN (>2 MONTHS)	INFANTS (<2 MONTHS)
Caspofungin	Loading dose 70 mg IV, then 50 mg IV daily	Loading dose 70 mg/m² per day IV, then 50 mg/m² per day IV	25 mg/m² per day IV
Anidulafungin	Loading dose 200 mg IV, then 100 mg IV daily	Not approved for use in children	Not approved for use in children
Micafungin	100 mg IV daily	2 mg/kg per day IV with option to increase to 4 mg/kg per day IV in children 40 kg	10 mg/kg per day IV

Source: Adapted from CDC: Treatment and Management of Infections and Colonization. 2019.

Available at: *www.cdc.gov/fungal/candida-auris/c-auris-treatment.html*

outbreak of *C. auris* infection, as well as drug susceptibility data of identified strains, act as a guide for the effective choice of treatment of invasive and bloodstream infections. *C. auris* is known to develop antibiotic resistance during treatment. Therefore, the emergence of antifungal resistance should be closely monitored with follow-up cultures and repeat susceptibility testing. Antibiotic stewardship should be implemented to ameliorate the risk of development of drug resistance. Patients may remain colonized with *C. auris* during or after the successful treatment of invasive *C. auris* infection. Therefore, infection control measures should be implemented throughout patient care. **Table 216-6** outlines CDC-recommended echinocandin doses for the initial antifungal treatment for *C. auris* infections.

In cases of echinocandin resistance, liposomal amphotericin B (5 mg/Kg/d) can be considered. For neonates and infants (<2 months old), amphotericin B deoxycholate (1 mg/Kg/d) treatment can be initiated. If this fails, liposomal amphotericin B (5 mg/Kg/d) can be given. In very severe cases, if all treatment options fail, echinocandins per CDC recommendations can be given (Table 216-6). Other considerations for *C. auris* infection management can be referenced from the 2016 Infectious Diseases Society of America (IDSA) Clinical Practice Guideline for the Management of Candidiasis.

Some generalizations exist regarding the management of specific *Candida* infections. Recovery of *Candida* from sputum is almost never indicative of underlying pulmonary candidiasis and does not by itself warrant antifungal treatment. Similarly, *Candida* in the urine of a patient with an indwelling bladder catheter may represent colonization only, rather than bladder or kidney infection. However, the threshold for systemic treatment is lower in general in severely ill patients in this category since it is impossible to distinguish colonization from lower or upper urinary tract infection. If the isolate is *C. albicans*, most clinicians use oral fluconazole rather than a bladder washout with amphotericin B, which was more commonly used in the past. Caspofungin has been used with success; although echinocandins are poorly excreted into the urine, they may be an option, especially for non-*albicans* isolates. The doses and duration are the same as for disseminated candidiasis. The significance of the recovery of *Candida* from abdominal drains in postoperative patients is unclear, but again, the threshold for treatment is generally low because most of the affected patients have been subjected to risk factors predisposing them to disseminated candidiasis. In addition, there has been a considerable increase in the recognition and diagnosis of intraabdominal candidiasis.

Removal of the infected valve and long-term antifungal administration constitute appropriate treatment for *Candida* endocarditis. Although definitive studies are not available, patients usually are treated for weeks with a systemic antifungal agent (Table 216-4) and then given chronic suppressive therapy for months or years (sometimes indefinitely) with an oral azole (usually fluconazole at 400–800 mg/d).

Hematogenous *Candida* endophthalmitis is a special problem requiring ophthalmologic consultation. When lesions are expanding or are threatening the macula, an IV polyene combined with flucytosine (25 mg/kg four times daily) has been the regimen of choice, although comparative studies with other regimens have not yet been reported. As more data on the newer triazoles (e.g., voriconazole) and the echinocandins become available, new strategies involving these agents are developing, although it is important to note that echinocandins exhibit low penetration in ocular tissue. Of paramount importance is the decision to perform a partial vitrectomy. This procedure debulks the infection and can preserve sight, which may otherwise be lost due to vitreal scarring. All patients with candidemia should undergo ophthalmologic examination because of the relatively high frequency of this ocular complication (up to 15–20% in some case series). This examination can detect a developing eye lesion early in its course; in addition, identification of a lesion signifies a probability of ~90% of deep-organ abscesses and may prompt prolongation of therapy for candidemia beyond the recommended 2 weeks after the last positive blood culture. Although the basis for the consensus is a very small data set, the recommended treatment for *Candida* meningitis is a polyene (Table 216-4) plus flucytosine (25 mg/kg four times daily). Development of *Candida* meningoencephalitis in an otherwise immunocompetent individual should raise suspicion for deficiency in the C-type lectin receptor adaptor molecule CARD9 and should prompt genetic testing to rule out this monogenic disorder. Successful treatment of *Candida*-infected prosthetic material (e.g., an artificial joint) nearly always requires removal of the infected material followed by long-term administration of an antifungal agent selected on the basis of the isolate's sensitivity and the logistics of administration.

PROPHYLAXIS

The use of antifungal agents to prevent *Candida* infections has been controversial, but some general principles have emerged. Most centers administer prophylactic fluconazole (400 mg/d) to recipients of allogeneic hematopoietic stem cell transplantation. High-risk liver transplant recipients are also given fluconazole prophylaxis in most centers. The use of prophylaxis for neutropenic patients has varied considerably from center to center; many centers that elect to give prophylaxis to this population use either fluconazole (200–400 mg/d) or a lipid formulation of amphotericin B (AmBisome, 1–2 mg/d). Caspofungin (50 mg/d) also has been recommended. Some centers have used itraconazole suspension (200 mg/d). Posaconazole (200 mg three times daily) has been approved by the U.S. Food and Drug Administration for prophylaxis in neutropenic patients; it is gaining in popularity and may replace fluconazole.

Prophylaxis is sometimes given to surgical patients at very high risk for candidiasis. The widespread use of prophylaxis for nearly all patients in general surgical or medical intensive care units is not—and should not be—a common practice for three reasons: (1) the incidence of disseminated candidiasis is relatively low, (2) the cost–benefit ratio is suboptimal, and (3) increased resistance with widespread prophylaxis is a valid concern.

Prophylaxis for oropharyngeal or esophageal candidiasis in HIV-infected patients is not recommended unless there are frequent recurrences.

FURTHER READING

LIONAKIS MS, EDWARDS JE JR: *Candida* species, in *Mandell, Douglas, and Bennett's Principles of Infectious Diseases*, 9th ed. JE Bennett et al (eds). Philadelphia, Elsevier, 2020, pp 3087-3102.

PAPPAS PG et al: Invasive candidiasis. Nat Rev Dis Primers 62:e1, 2018.

PROCTOR DM et al: Integrated genomic, epidemiologic investigation of *Candida auris* skin colonization in a skilled nursing facility. Nature Medicine 27:1401, 2021.

TSAI SV et al: Burden of candidemia in the United States, 2017. Clin Infect Dis 71:e449, 2020.

217 Aspergillosis

David W. Denning

Aspergillosis is the collective term used to describe all disease entities caused by any one of ~50 pathogenic and allergenic species of *Aspergillus*. Only those species that grow at 37°C can cause invasive infection, although some species without this ability can cause allergic syndromes. Each common pathogenic species is actually a complex of many species (many of them cryptic) but is referred to as a single species here for simplicity. *A. fumigatus* is responsible for most cases of invasive aspergillosis, almost all cases of chronic aspergillosis, and most allergic syndromes. *A. flavus* is more prevalent in some hospitals and causes a higher proportion of cases of sinus infections, cutaneous infections, and keratitis than *A. fumigatus*. *A. niger* can cause invasive infection but more commonly colonizes the respiratory tract and causes external otitis. *A. terreus* causes only invasive disease, usually with a poor prognosis. *A. nidulans* occasionally causes invasive infection, primarily in patients with chronic granulomatous disease (CGD).

■ EPIDEMIOLOGY AND ECOLOGY

Aspergillus has a worldwide distribution, most commonly growing in decomposing plant materials (i.e., compost) and in bedding. This hyaline (nonpigmented), septate, branching mold produces vast numbers of conidia (spores) on stalks above the surface of mycelial growth. Aspergilli are found in indoor and outdoor air, on surfaces, and in water from surface reservoirs. Daily exposures vary from a few to many millions of conidia; high numbers of conidia are encountered in hay barns and other very dusty environments. The required size of the infecting inoculum is uncertain; however, only intense exposures (e.g., during construction work, handling of moldy bark or hay, or composting) are sufficient to cause disease—acute community-acquired pulmonary aspergillosis—in healthy immunocompetent individuals. Allergic syndromes may be exacerbated by continuous antigenic exposure arising from sinus or airway colonization or from nail infection. High-efficiency particulate air (HEPA) filtration is often protective against infection; thus, HEPA filters should be installed and monitored for efficiency in operating rooms and in areas of the hospital that house high-risk patients.

The incubation period of invasive aspergillosis after exposure is highly variable, extending in documented cases from 2 to 90 days. Thus, community acquisition of an infecting strain frequently manifests as invasive infection during hospitalization, although nosocomial acquisition is also common. Outbreaks usually are directly related to a contaminated air source or construction in the hospital.

Global aspergillosis incidence and prevalence have been estimated (**Table 217-1**). The frequency of different manifestations of aspergillosis varies considerably with geographic location; most notably, chronic granulomatous sinusitis is rare outside the Middle East and India. Fungal (mycotic) keratitis is particularly common in Nepal, Myanmar, Bhutan, and India but occurs globally. Chronic pulmonary aspergillosis follows pulmonary tuberculosis in ~6–13% of treated cases and also mimics pulmonary tuberculosis as smear-negative or "clinically diagnosed" tuberculosis. *Aspergillus* onychomycosis, usually of the toenail, has been reported in as low as <1% and as high as 35% of cases of onychomycosis and is more common in diabetes.

■ RISK FACTORS AND PATHOGENESIS

The primary risk factors for invasive aspergillosis are profound neutropenia, glucocorticoid use, and underlying respiratory disease; risk increases with longer duration of these conditions. Higher doses of glucocorticoids increase the risk of both acquisition of invasive aspergillosis and death from the infection. Neutrophil and/or phagocyte dysfunction also is an important risk factor, as evidenced by aspergillosis in CGD, advanced HIV infection, and relapsed leukemia. Invasive aspergillosis is increasingly recognized (if actively sought) in medical intensive care units (2–5%), those with severe influenza (8–25%), severe COVID-19 (13%) and patients in the hospital with chronic obstructive pulmonary disease (COPD; 1.3–3.9%). Extracorporeal membrane oxygenation therapy is a risk factor. Temporary abrogation of protective responses from glucocorticoid use or compensatory anti-inflammatory response syndrome is a significant risk factor. Many patients have some evidence of prior pulmonary disease—typically, a history of pneumonia or COPD. Many new immunomodulating agents, such as infliximab and ibrutinib, increase the risk of invasive aspergillosis, as do severe liver disease and high levels of stored iron in bone marrow.

TABLE 217-1 Disease Frequency and Diagnostic Sensitivity for Different Manifestations of Aspergillosis

	TYPE OF DISEASE		
PARAMETER	**INVASIVE**	**CHRONIC**	**ALLERGIC**
Incidence/100,000[a]	0.6–16	~10.4	?[b]
Prevalence/100,000[a]	—	1.4–126	286[c]
Global burden[a]	~850,000	~3,000,000	~10,000,000
Mortality rate without treatment	~100%	~50%	<1%
Respiratory Diagnostic Sensitivity[d]			
Culture[e]	✓	✓-✓✓[e]	✓-✓✓[e]
Microscopy	✓	✓	?
Antigen	✓✓✓	✓✓	✓✓✓
Real-time PCR	✓✓	✓✓	✓✓
Blood Diagnostic Sensitivity[d]			
Culture	×	×	×
Antigen	✓✓	✓	×
β-D-Glucan	✓✓	✓	?
Real-time PCR	✓✓	×	×
IgG antibody	✓	✓✓✓	✓✓✓
IgE antibody	×	✓✓	✓✓✓✓

[a]*http://www.gaffi.org/roadmap/.* [b]Allergic fungal disease can develop at any age, usually in adulthood; the annual frequency with which it occurs is not known. [c]Allergic bronchopulmonary aspergillosis and severe asthma with fungal sensitization. [d]Key for sensitivity: 1 check = limited (as the text indicates, 10–30% for culture); 2 checks = higher; 3 checks = >80%; and 4 checks = ~95%. [e]High-volume fungal culture increases sensitivity to the same level as PCR.

Abbreviation: PCR, polymerase chain reaction.

Patients with chronic pulmonary aspergillosis have a wide spectrum of underlying pulmonary disease, including tuberculosis, prior pneumothorax, or COPD. These patients are apparently immunocompetent, but natural killer and/or interleukin 12 or gamma interferon production defects are common. Their inflammatory immune (T_H1-like) response is suboptimal, and persistent inflammation is typical. Glucocorticoids accelerate disease progression.

Allergic bronchopulmonary aspergillosis (ABPA) usually complicates asthma and cystic fibrosis. Many genetic associations indicate a strong basis for the development of a T_H2-like and "allergic" response to *A. fumigatus*. Remarkably, high-dose glucocorticoid treatment for exacerbations of ABPA almost never leads to invasive aspergillosis. Fungal, and especially *Aspergillus*, sensitization is especially common in those with poorly controlled asthma. COPD exacerbations are linked to *Aspergillus* sensitization. Most patients with *Aspergillus* bronchitis have bronchiectasis, with or without cystic fibrosis.

Different genetic traits are associated with invasive, chronic, and allergic aspergillosis; the majority of people probably are not at risk for aspergillosis. Multiple gene variants appear to be necessary for susceptibility to each form of aspergillosis.

■ CLINICAL FEATURES AND APPROACH TO THE PATIENT

(Table 217-2)

Invasive Pulmonary Aspergillosis Both the frequency of invasive disease and the pace of its progression increase with greater degrees of immunocompromise. Invasive aspergillosis is arbitrarily

TABLE 217-2 Major Manifestations of Aspergillosis

	TYPE OF DISEASE			
ORGAN	INVASIVE (ACUTE AND SUBACUTE)	CHRONIC	SAPROPHYTIC	ALLERGIC
Lung	Angioinvasive (in neutropenia), nonangioinvasive, granulomatous	Chronic cavitary, chronic fibrosing, bronchitis, *Aspergillus* nodule	Aspergilloma (single), airway colonization	Allergic bronchopulmonary, severe asthma with fungal sensitization, extrinsic allergic alveolitis
Sinus	Acute invasive	Chronic invasive, chronic granulomatous	Maxillary fungal ball	Allergic fungal sinusitis, eosinophilic fungal rhinosinusitis
Brain	Abscess, hemorrhagic infarction, meningitis	Granulomatous, meningitis	None	None
Skin	Acute disseminated, locally invasive (trauma, burns, IV access)	External otitis, onychomycosis	None	None
Heart	Endocarditis (native or prosthetic), pericarditis	None	None	None
Eye	Keratitis, endophthalmitis	None	None	None described

classified as acute and subacute, with courses of ≤1 month and 1–3 months, respectively. More than 80% of cases of invasive aspergillosis involve the lungs, and most are community acquired. The most common clinical features are no symptoms at all, fever, cough (sometimes productive), nondescript chest discomfort, trivial hemoptysis, and shortness of breath. Although the fever often responds to glucocorticoids, the disease progresses. In ventilated patients, screening for *Aspergillus* antigen on tracheobronchial lavage fluid is necessary for diagnosis as radiology is not distinctive. The keys to early diagnosis in at-risk patients are a high index of suspicion, screening for circulating antigen (in leukemia), and urgent CT of the thorax. Invasive aspergillosis is one of the most common diagnostic errors revealed at autopsy.

Invasive Sinusitis The sinuses are involved in 5–10% of cases of invasive aspergillosis, especially affecting patients with leukemia and recipients of hematopoietic stem cell transplants. In addition to fever, the most common features are nasal or facial discomfort, blocked nose, and nasal discharge (sometimes bloody). Endoscopic examination of the nose reveals pale, dusky or necrotic-looking tissue in any location. CT or MRI of the sinuses is essential but does not distinguish invasive *Aspergillus* sinusitis from preexisting allergic or bacterial sinusitis early in the disease process.

Tracheobronchitis Occasionally, only the airways are infected by *Aspergillus*. The resulting manifestations seen on bronchoscopy range from acute or chronic bronchitis to ulcerative or pseudomembranous tracheobronchitis. These entities are particularly common among lung transplant recipients and patients on artificial ventilation. Obstruction with mucous plugs may occur and is called obstructing bronchial aspergillosis in immunocompromised patients and mucous impaction in other patients, such as those with ABPA.

***Aspergillus* Bronchitis** Recurrent chest infections that only partially improve with antibiotic treatment and are associated with significant breathlessness or coughing up of thick sputum plugs are typical features of *Aspergillus* bronchitis. Patients are not significantly immunocompromised and usually have bronchiectasis or cystic fibrosis. Occasional patients present with respiratory failure because of airway obstruction with mucus. Concurrent bacterial bronchitis is common. The diagnosis rests on recurrent detection of *Aspergillus* in the airway by microscopy, culture, or polymerase chain reaction (PCR). *Aspergillus* IgG is usually detectable.

Disseminated Aspergillosis In the most severely immunocompromised patients, *Aspergillus* disseminates from the lungs to multiple organs—most often to the brain but also to the skin, thyroid, bone, kidney, liver, gastrointestinal tract, eye (endophthalmitis), and heart valve. Aside from cutaneous lesions, the most common features are gradual clinical deterioration over 1–3 days, with low-grade fever and features of mild sepsis, and nonspecific abnormalities in laboratory tests. In most cases, at least one localization becomes apparent before death. Blood cultures are almost always negative.

Cerebral Aspergillosis Hematogenous dissemination to the brain is a devastating complication of invasive aspergillosis. Single or multiple lesions may develop. In acute disease, hemorrhagic infarction is most typical, and cerebral abscess is common. Rarer manifestations include meningitis, mycotic aneurysm, and cerebral granuloma (mimicking a brain tumor). Local spread from cranial sinuses also occurs. Postoperative infection develops rarely and is exacerbated by glucocorticoids, which are often given after neurosurgery. The presentation can be either acute or subacute, with mood changes, focal signs, seizures, and decline in mental status. MRI is the most useful immediate investigation; unenhanced CT of the brain is usually nonspecific, and contrast is often contraindicated because of poor renal function. Cerebral aspergillosis is disproportionately common in those on ibrutinib.

Endocarditis Most cases of *Aspergillus* endocarditis are prosthetic-valve infections resulting from contamination during surgery. Native-valve disease is reported, especially as a feature of disseminated infection and in persons using illicit IV drugs. Culture-negative endocarditis with large vegetations is the most common presentation; embolectomy occasionally reveals the diagnosis.

Cutaneous Aspergillosis Dissemination of *Aspergillus* occasionally results in cutaneous features, usually an erythematous or purplish nontender area that progresses to a necrotic eschar. Direct invasion of the skin occurs in neutropenic patients at the site of IV catheter insertion and in burn patients. Surgical, burn, and trauma wounds may become infected with *Aspergillus* (especially *A. flavus*).

Chronic Pulmonary Aspergillosis The hallmark of chronic cavitary pulmonary aspergillosis (**Fig. 217-1**) is one or more pulmonary cavities expanding over a period of months or years in association with pulmonary symptoms and systemic manifestations such as fatigue and weight loss. Often mistaken initially for tuberculosis, >90% of chronic cavitary pulmonary aspergillosis cases occur in patients with prior pulmonary disease (e.g., tuberculosis, atypical mycobacterial infection, sarcoidosis, rheumatoid lung disease, pneumothorax, bullae) or lung surgery. The onset is insidious, and systemic features (weight loss, fatigue) may be more prominent than pulmonary symptoms. An irregular internal cavity surface and thickened cavity walls are typical and indicative of disease activity. Irregular material, fluid level, and a well-formed fungal ball are seen in a minority of cavities. Multiple cavities are more common than a single cavity, and most cavities are in the upper lobes. Pleural thickening and pericavitary infiltrates are typical and most obvious if a positron emission tomography scan has been done as part of the workup. Chronic cavitary pulmonary aspergillosis is usually caused by *A. fumigatus*, but *A. niger* has been implicated, particularly in diabetic patients, as have other species, rarely. IgG antibodies to *Aspergillus* are detectable in ~90% of patients with chronic cavitary pulmonary aspergillosis. Some patients have concurrent infections—even without a fungal ball—with atypical mycobacteria and/or other bacterial pathogens. The most significant complication is life-threatening hemoptysis, which may be the presenting manifestation. If untreated, chronic cavitary pulmonary aspergillosis typically progresses (sometimes relatively rapidly) to

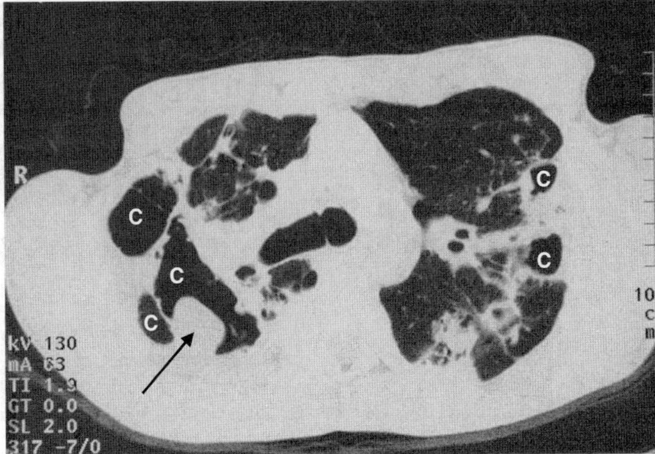

FIGURE 217-1 CT scan image of the chest in a patient with long-standing bilateral chronic cavitary pulmonary aspergillosis. This patient had a history of several bilateral pneumothoraces and had required bilateral pleurodesis in 1990. CT then demonstrated multiple bullae, and sputum cultures grew *A. fumigatus*. The patient had initially weakly and later strongly positive serum IgG *Aspergillus* antibody tests. This scan (2003) shows a mixture of thick- and thin-walled cavities in both lungs (each marked with *C*), with a probable fungal ball (*black arrow*) protruding into the large cavity on the patient's right side (*R*). There is also considerable pleural thickening bilaterally.

unilateral or upper-lobe fibrosis. This end-stage entity is termed *chronic fibrosing pulmonary aspergillosis* (destroyed lung).

Aspergilloma Aspergilloma (fungal ball) is a late manifestation of chronic cavitary pulmonary aspergillosis, but some patients are asymptomatic. The inside of a pulmonary cavity allows fungal growth that peels off, forming the layers of the fungal ball. Signs and symptoms associated with single (simple) aspergillomas are minor, including cough (sometimes productive), hemoptysis, wheezing, and mild fatigue. More significant signs and symptoms are associated with chronic cavitary pulmonary aspergillosis and should be treated as such. About 10% of fungal balls resolve spontaneously (by being coughed up), but the cavity may still be infected and the patient symptomatic.

***Aspergillus* Nodule** A recently recognized form of chronic pulmonary aspergillosis is the *Aspergillus* nodule, which may resemble early lung carcinoma and may cavitate. Nodules may be single or multiple and 5–50 mm in diameter. Larger mass lesions are rarely seen. Nodules are usually avid on positron emission tomography. IgG antibodies to *Aspergillus* are detectable in ~65% of patients with an *Aspergillus* nodule.

Chronic *Aspergillus* Sinusitis Three entities are subsumed under this broad designation: fungal ball of the sinus, chronic invasive sinusitis, and chronic granulomatous sinusitis. Fungal ball of the sinus is limited to the maxillary sinus (except in rare cases involving the sphenoid sinus) in which the sinus cavity is filled with a fungal ball. Maxillary disease is associated with prior upper-jaw root canal work and chronic (bacterial) sinusitis. About 90% of CT scans show focal hyperattenuation related to concretions; on MRI scans, the T2-weighted signal is decreased, whereas it is increased in bacterial sinusitis. Removal of the fungal ball is curative. No tissue invasion is demonstrable histologically or radiologically.

In contrast, chronic invasive sinusitis is a slowly destructive process that most commonly affects the ethmoid and sphenoid sinuses. Patients are usually but not always immunocompromised to some degree (e.g., as a result of diabetes or HIV infection). Imaging of the cranial sinuses shows opacification of one or more sinuses, local bone destruction, and invasion of local structures. The differential diagnosis is wide, including other infections. Apart from a history of chronic nasal discharge and blockage, loss of the sense of smell, and persistent headache, the usual presenting features are related to local involvement of critical structures. The orbital apex syndrome (blindness and proptosis) is characteristic. Facial swelling, cavernous sinus thrombosis, carotid artery occlusion, pituitary fossa, and brain and skull-base invasion are complications.

Chronic granulomatous sinusitis due to *Aspergillus* is most commonly seen in the Middle East and India and is often caused by *A. flavus*. It typically presents late, with facial swelling and unilateral proptosis. The prominent granulomatous reaction histologically distinguishes this disease from chronic invasive sinusitis, in which tissue necrosis with a low-grade mixed-cell infiltrate is typical. IgG antibodies to *A. flavus* are usually detectable.

Allergic Bronchopulmonary Aspergillosis In almost all cases, ABPA represents a hypersensitivity reaction to *A. fumigatus*; rare cases are due to other aspergilli and other fungi. ABPA occurs in ~2.5% of patients with asthma who are referred to secondary care, although it may be less common in the United States and more common in those from the Indian subcontinent. In cystic fibrosis, up to 15% of teenagers are affected. Episodes of bronchial obstruction with mucous plugs leading to coughing fits, "pneumonia," consolidation, and breathlessness are typical. Many patients report coughing up thick sputum casts, often brown in color. Eosinophilia commonly develops before systemic glucocorticoids are given. The cardinal diagnostic test is detection of *Aspergillus*-specific IgE (or a positive skin-prick test in response to *A. fumigatus* extract) together with an elevated serum level of total IgE (usually >1000 IU/mL). The presence of hyperattenuated mucus in airways is highly specific. Bronchiectasis is characteristic, and some patients develop chronic cavitary pulmonary aspergillosis.

Severe Asthma with Fungal Sensitization (SAFS) Many adults with severe asthma do not fulfill the criteria for ABPA and yet are allergic to fungi. Although *A. fumigatus* is a common allergen, numerous other fungi (e.g., *Cladosporium* and *Alternaria* species) are implicated by skin-prick testing and/or specific IgE testing. Serum total IgE concentrations are <1000 IU/mL, and bronchial-wall thickening is common. ABPA and SAFS are collectively referred to as *fungal asthma*.

Allergic Fungal Rhinosinusitis Like the lungs, the sinuses manifest allergic responses to *Aspergillus* and other fungi. The affected patients present with chronic (i.e., perennial) sinusitis that is relatively unresponsive to antibiotics. Many of these patients have nasal polyps, and all have congested nasal mucosae and sinuses full of mucoid material. The histologic hallmarks of allergic fungal sinusitis are local eosinophilia and Charcot-Leyden crystals. Removal of abnormal mucus and polyps, with local and occasionally systemic administration of glucocorticoids, usually leads to resolution. Persistent or recurrent signs and symptoms may require more extensive surgery (ethmoidectomy) and sometimes oral antifungal therapy. Recurrence is common, often after another bacterial or viral infection.

Superficial Aspergillosis *Aspergillus* can cause keratitis onychomycosis and otitis externa. The former may be difficult to diagnose early enough to save the patient's sight. Natamycin (5%) eye drops are the optimal therapy for fungal keratitis, often with surgery. Otitis externa usually resolves with debridement and local application of antifungal agents.

DIAGNOSIS

Several techniques are required to establish the diagnosis of any form of aspergillosis with confidence (Table 217-1).

Acute Invasive Aspergillosis Patients with acute invasive aspergillosis have a relatively heavy load of fungus in the affected organ; thus, antigen detection, PCR, microscopy, culture, and/or histopathology usually confirm the diagnosis. However, the pace of progression leaves only a narrow window for making the diagnosis without losing the patient, and some invasive procedures are not possible because of coagulopathy, respiratory compromise, and other factors. Many cases of invasive aspergillosis are missed clinically and are diagnosed only at autopsy. Histologic examination of affected tissue reveals either infarction, with invasion of blood vessels by many fungal hyphae, or acute necrosis, with limited inflammation and fewer hyphae. *Aspergillus* hyphae are hyaline, narrow, and septate, with branching at 45°; no yeast forms are present in infected tissue. Hyphae can be seen in cytology or microscopy preparations, which therefore provide a rapid means of presumptive diagnosis.

One *Aspergillus* antigen test relies on detection of galactomannan release from *Aspergillus* organisms during growth, the other a novel protein antigen. Respiratory sample antigen detection is more sensitive than serum and is critical in the intensive care unit patient in whom radiology is nonspecific. Positive serum antigen results usually precede clinical or radiologic features by several days. The sensitivity of antigen detection is reduced by antifungal therapy.

A positive culture supports the diagnosis, given that multiple other (rarer) fungi can mimic *Aspergillus* species histologically, but only 10–30% of patients with invasive aspergillosis have a positive culture. Bacterial agar is less sensitive than fungal media for culture; thus, if physicians do not request fungal culture, the diagnosis may be missed. High-volume fungal cultures enhance yield. A positive culture may represent noninvasive forms of aspergillosis or airway colonization. Both antigen detection and real-time PCR are faster and much more sensitive than culture of respiratory samples and blood.

Definitive confirmation of a diagnosis of invasive aspergillosis requires (1) a positive culture of a sample taken directly from an ordinarily sterile site (e.g., a brain abscess) or (2) positive results of both histologic testing and culture (or molecular confirmation of *Aspergillus* spp.) of a sample taken from an affected organ (e.g., sinuses or skin). Most diagnoses of invasive aspergillosis are inferred from fewer data, including the presence of the *halo sign* on a thoracic CT scan—a localized ground-glass appearance representing hemorrhagic infarction surrounds a nodule or consolidation. Halo signs are present for ~7 days early in the course of infection in neutropenic patients and are a good prognostic feature, reflecting an early diagnosis. Nodules with halo signs are a feature of COVID-19 and do not imply invasive aspergillosis with supportive evidence. Other characteristic radiologic features of invasive pulmonary aspergillosis include nodules and pleural-based infarction or cavitation, but nonspecific consolidation is common (Fig. 217-2).

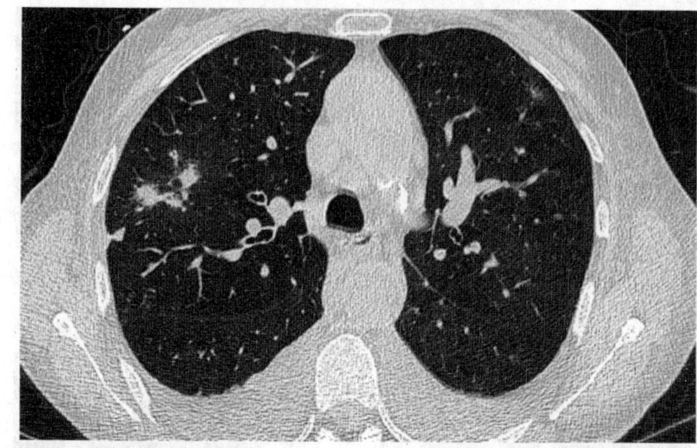

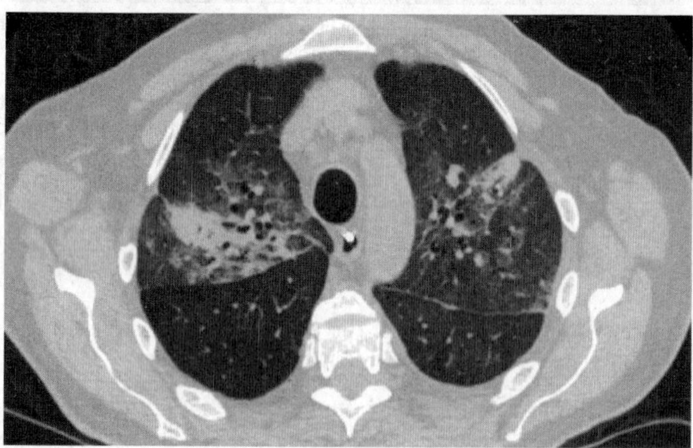

FIGURE 217-2 Markedly different appearances of invasive aspergillosis on CT scan of the thorax. ***A.*** Patient with myelodysplasia and moderate neutropenia showing small right-sided nodules with minimal surrounding ground glass and a separate area of ground glass only on the left laterally. ***B.*** Patient with multiple myeloma undergoing intensive chemotherapy with corticosteroids showing bilateral areas of consolidation and some nonspecific atelectasis with probable ground glass surrounding the right-sided lesion. The anterior component of the left-sided lesion is demarcated by the fissure.

Chronic Aspergillosis For chronic aspergillosis, *Aspergillus* antibody testing combined with characteristic imaging is sufficient for the diagnosis. Biopsy of *Aspergillus* nodules reveals hyphae surrounded by cells of chronic inflammation and sometimes granulomas. Antibody titers fall slowly with successful therapy. Cultures are infrequently positive but are important in checking for azole resistance. Real-time PCR of sputum is often strongly positive. Some patients with chronic pulmonary aspergillosis also have elevated titers of total serum IgE and *Aspergillus*-specific IgE.

ABPA, SAFS, and Allergic *Aspergillus* Sinusitis ABPA and SAFS are diagnosed serologically with elevated specific and total serum IgE levels or with skin-prick tests. Allergic *Aspergillus* sinusitis is usually diagnosed histologically, accompanied by *Aspergillus* IgE antibody.

TREATMENT

Aspergillosis

Antifungal drugs active against *Aspergillus* include voriconazole, itraconazole, posaconazole, isavuconazole, caspofungin, micafungin, and amphotericin B (AmB). Possible interactions with other drugs must be considered before azoles are prescribed. In addition, plasma azole concentrations vary substantially from one patient to another, and many authorities recommend monitoring levels to ensure that drug concentrations are adequate but not excessive, especially with itraconazole and voriconazole. Initial IV administration is preferred for acute invasive aspergillosis and oral administration for all other diseases that require antifungal therapy. Current recommendations are shown in **Table 217-3**.

Voriconazole, isavuconazole and posaconazole are the preferred agents for invasive aspergillosis; caspofungin, micafungin, and lipid-associated AmB are second-line agents. AmB is not active against *A. terreus* or *A. nidulans*; multi-azole resistance in *A. fumigatus* is present in <5% of isolates but is increasing, especially in Southeast Asia; and *A. niger* is resistant to itraconazole and isavuconazole. An infectious disease consultation is advised for patients with invasive disease, given the complexity of management. Immune reconstitution can complicate recovery. The duration of therapy for invasive aspergillosis varies from ~3 months to several years, depending on the patient's immune status and response to therapy. Relapse occurs if the response is suboptimal and immune reconstitution is not complete.

Voriconazole is currently the preferred oral agent for chronic aspergillosis with itraconazole or posaconazole as substitutes when failure, emergence of resistance, or adverse events occur. Because chronic cavitary pulmonary aspergillosis responds slowly, therapy for >6 months is necessary, and disease control may require years of treatment, whereas the duration of treatment for other forms of chronic and allergic aspergillosis requires case-by-case evaluation. Glucocorticoids should be used in chronic cavitary pulmonary aspergillosis only if covered by adequate antifungal therapy. Acute exacerbations of ABPA respond well to voriconazole, itraconazole, or a short course of glucocorticoids—long-term azole therapy usually helps minimize corticosteroid exposure and maintain remission. Antifungal response in *Aspergillus* bronchitis is gratifying, but relapse after 4 months of therapy is common.

Resistance in *A. fumigatus* to one or more azoles, although uncommon, is increasingly found globally. Resistance may be derived from azole fungicide use for crops. In addition, resistance arising from multiple mechanisms may develop during long-term treatment, and a positive culture during antifungal therapy is an indication for susceptibility testing.

TABLE 217-3 Treatment of Aspergillosis[a]

INDICATION	PRIMARY TREATMENT	PRECAUTIONS	SECONDARY TREATMENT	COMMENTS
Invasive disease[b]	Voriconazole, isavuconazole, posaconazole	Drug interactions (especially with rifampin and carbamazepine)[c]	AmB, caspofungin, posaconazole, micafungin	As primary therapy, voriconazole, isavuconazole, and posaconazole have a 20% higher response rate than AmB. Therapeutic drug monitoring is recommended for voriconazole.
Prophylaxis	Posaconazole tablet, itraconazole solution SUBA-itraconazole	Vincristine, cyclophosphamide interaction	Micafungin, aerosolized AmB	Some centers monitor plasma levels of itraconazole and posaconazole.
Single aspergilloma	Surgical resection	Multicavity disease: poor outcome of surgery, medical therapy preferable	Itraconazole, voriconazole, intracavity AmB	Single large cavities with an aspergilloma are best resected. Relapse reduced by pre- and peri-operative antifungal therapy.
Chronic pulmonary disease[b]	Voriconazole, itraconazole	Poor absorption of itraconazole capsules with proton pump inhibitors or H_2 blockers	Posaconazole, IV AmB, IV micafungin	Resistance may emerge during treatment, especially if plasma drug levels are subtherapeutic. Resistance is less common with voriconazole.
ABPA/SAFS ("fungal asthma")	Itraconazole	Some glucocorticoid interactions, including with inhaled formulations	Voriconazole, posaconazole	Long-term therapy is helpful in most cases. No evidence indicates whether therapy modifies progression to bronchiectasis/fibrosis.

[a]For information on duration of therapy and drug resistance in certain *Aspergillus* species, see text. [b]An infectious disease consultation is appropriate for these patients. [c]Online drug-interaction resource: *www.aspergillus.org.uk/content/antifungal-drug-interactions.*

Note: After loading doses, the oral dose is usually 200 mg bid for voriconazole and itraconazole, 100 mg bid for SUBA-itraconazole, 300 mg qd for posaconazole tablets, and 200 mg qd for isavuconazole. The IV dose of voriconazole for adults is 6 mg/kg twice at 12-h intervals (loading doses) followed by 4 mg/kg q12h; a larger dose is required for children and teenagers; a lower dose may be safer for persons >70 years of age. Plasma monitoring is helpful in optimizing the dosage. The IV dose of isavuconazole is 200 mg tid for 2 days (loading dose) followed by 200 mg qd. Caspofungin is given as a single loading dose of 70 mg and then at 50 mg/d; some authorities use 70 mg/d for patients weighing >80 kg, and lower doses are required with hepatic dysfunction. Micafungin is given as 50 mg/d for prophylaxis and as at least 150 mg/d for treatment; this drug has not yet been approved by the U.S. Food and Drug Administration (FDA) for this indication. AmB deoxycholate is given at a daily dose of 1 mg/kg if tolerated. Several strategies are available for minimizing renal dysfunction. Lipid-associated AmB is given at 3 mg/kg (AmBisome) or 5 mg/kg (Abelcet). Different regimens are available for aerosolized AmB, but none is FDA approved. Other considerations that may alter dose selection or route include age; concomitant medications; renal, hepatic, or intestinal dysfunction; and drug tolerability.

Abbreviations: ABPA, allergic bronchopulmonary aspergillosis; AmB, amphotericin B; SAFS, severe asthma with fungal sensitization.

Surgical treatment is important in several forms of aspergillosis, including fungal ball of the sinus and single aspergillomas, in which surgery is curative; invasive aspergillosis involving bone, heart valve, sinuses, and proximal areas of the lung (to avoid catastrophic hemoptysis); brain abscess; keratitis; and endophthalmitis. In allergic fungal sinusitis, removal of abnormal mucus and polyps, with local and occasionally systemic glucocorticoid treatment, usually leads to resolution. Persistent or recurrent signs and symptoms may require more extensive surgery (ethmoidectomy) and possibly antifungal therapy. Surgery is problematic in chronic cavitary pulmonary aspergillosis, usually resulting in serious complications. Bronchial artery embolization is preferred for problematic hemoptysis.

PROPHYLAXIS

In situations in which moderate or high risk is predicted (e.g., after induction therapy for acute myeloid leukemia), the need for antifungal prophylaxis for superficial and systemic candidiasis and for invasive aspergillosis is generally accepted. Fluconazole is commonly used in these situations but has no activity against *Aspergillus* species. Itraconazole solution of SUBA-itraconazole capsules provide enough bioavailability for modest efficacy, the latter with fewer adverse events. Posaconazole tablets are more effective in reducing infection rates and the need for empirical antifungal therapy. Some data support the use of IV micafungin in those with azole contraindications. No prophylactic regimen is completely successful.

OUTCOME

Invasive aspergillosis is curable if immune reconstitution occurs, whereas allergic and chronic forms are not. The mortality rate for invasive aspergillosis is 30–70% if the infection is treated but is 100% if the diagnosis is missed. Cerebral aspergillosis, *Aspergillus* endocarditis, and bilateral extensive invasive pulmonary aspergillosis have very poor outcomes, as does invasive infection in persons with late-stage AIDS or relapsed uncontrolled leukemia.

The mortality rate for chronic cavitary pulmonary aspergillosis is ~40% over 5 years and 50–60% over 10 years if the patient is actively treated with antifungal agents. After 12 months with no antifungal therapy, 70% of patients have deteriorated, and 10–35% have died. Therapy fails in ~30% of recipients of antifungal therapy and still more often if azole resistance is present.

Both ABPA and SAFS patients respond to antifungal therapy; ~60% respond to itraconazole and ~80% to voriconazole and posaconazole (if tolerated). Inhaled amphotericin B is effective in and tolerated by ~15% of patients. If the severity of asthma declines, the inhaled glucocorticoid dose can be reduced, and oral glucocorticoids can be stopped. Relapse after discontinuation is common but not universal.

FURTHER READING

GOH KJ et al: Sensitization to *Aspergillus* species is associated with frequent exacerbations in severe asthma. J Asthma Allergy 10:131-40, 2017.

LAMOTH F et al: Incidence of invasive pulmonary aspergillosis among critically ill COVID-19 patients. Clin Microbiol Infect 26:1706, 2020.

MULDOON EG et al: *Aspergillus* nodules; another presentation of chronic pulmonary aspergillosis. BMC Pulm Med 16:123, 2016.

SCHAUWVLIEGHE AFAD et al: Invasive aspergillosis in patients admitted to the intensive care unit with severe influenza: A retrospective cohort study. Lancet Respir Med 6:782, 2018.

ULLMAN AJ et al: Diagnosis and management of *Aspergillus* diseases: Executive summary of the 2017 ESCMID-ECMM-ERS guideline. Clin Microbiol Infect 24:e1ee38, 2018.

218 Mucormycosis

Brad Spellberg, Ashraf S. Ibrahim

Mucormycosis represents a group of life-threatening infections caused by fungi of the order Mucorales of the subphylum Mucoromycotina. Mucormycosis is highly invasive and relentlessly progressive, resulting in higher rates of morbidity and mortality than many other infections. The mortality rates from mucormycosis have declined in recent years as a result of early initiation of more effective antifungal therapies. However, mortality remains high overall, often driven by progression of the underlying predisposing condition.

TABLE 218-1 Taxonomy of Fungi Causing Mucormycosis (Subphylum Mucoromycotina, Order Mucorales)

FAMILY	GENUS (SPECIES LISTED FOR SOME)
Mucoraceae	*Rhizopus oryzae*
	Rhizopus delemar
	Rhizopus microsporus
	Rhizomucor
	Mucor
	Actinomucor
Lichtheimiaceae	*Lichtheimia* (formerly *Mycocladus*, formerly *Absidia*)
Cunninghamellaceae	*Cunninghamella*
Thamnidiaceae	*Cokeromyces*
Mortierellaceae	*Mortierella*
Saksenaceae	*Saksenaea*
	Apophysomyces
Syncephalastraceae	*Syncephalastrum*

ETIOLOGY

The fungal order Mucorales consists of seven families that are known to cause mucormycosis (**Table 218-1**). *Rhizopus oryzae* and *R. delemar* (both in the family Mucoraceae) are by far the most common causes of mucormycosis in the Western Hemisphere. Less frequently isolated species of the Mucoraceae that cause a similar spectrum of infections include *Rhizopus microsporus, Rhizomucor pusillus, Lichtheimia corymbifera* (formerly *Absidia corymbifera*), *Apophysomyces elegans*, and *Mucor* species. Increasing numbers of cases of mucormycosis due to infection by mold in the family Cunninghamellaceae have also been reported, particularly in highly immunocompromised patients. Other Mucorales can be the major cause of disease in certain geographic areas (e.g., *A. elegans* in India and *Mucor irregularis* in China) or in outbreaks following natural disasters (e.g., *Apophysomyces trapeziformis* outbreak following the 2011 tornado in Joplin, Missouri). Only rare case reports have demonstrated the ability of fungi in the remaining families of the Mucorales to cause mucormycosis.

PATHOGENESIS

The Mucorales are ubiquitous environmental fungi to which humans are constantly exposed. These fungi cause infection primarily in patients with uncontrolled diabetes, defects in phagocytic function (e.g., neutropenia or glucocorticoid treatment), and/or elevated levels of free iron, which supports fungal growth in serum and tissues. In the past, iron-overloaded patients with end-stage renal failure who were treated with deferoxamine had a high risk of developing rapidly fatal disseminated mucormycosis; deferoxamine is an iron chelator for the human host, but it serves as a fungal siderophore, directly delivering iron to the Mucorales. Furthermore, patients with diabetic ketoacidosis (DKA) are at high risk of developing rhinocerebral mucormycosis. The acidosis causes dissociation of iron from sequestering proteins, resulting in enhanced fungal survival and virulence. The ketoacid β-hydroxybutyrate also increases expression of host and fungal receptors that result in fungal adherence and penetration into tissues.

Nevertheless, the majority of diabetic patients who present with mucormycosis are not acidotic, and, even absent acidosis, hyperglycemia directly contributes to the risk of mucormycosis by at least four likely mechanisms: (1) hyperglycation of iron-sequestering proteins, disrupting normal iron sequestration; (2) upregulation of a mammalian cell receptor (GRP78) that binds to Mucorales, enabling tissue penetration (due to both a direct effect of hyperglycemia and increasing levels of free iron); (3) induction of poorly characterized defects in phagocytic function; and (4) enhanced expression of CotH, a Mucorales-specific protein that mediates host cell invasion by binding to GRP78 (due to hyperglycemia and the resulting free iron). More recently, the mucoricin toxin—with structural and functional similarities to ricin—was found to be responsible for host cell death and tissue necrosis. The toxin is a key virulence factor of Mucorales fungi and is a promising therapeutic target.

EPIDEMIOLOGY

Mucormycosis typically occurs in patients with diabetes mellitus, solid-organ transplantation or hematopoietic stem cell transplantation (HSCT), prolonged neutropenia or corticosteroid use, or malignancy. As mentioned, the majority of diabetic patients are not acidotic on presentation with mucormycosis. Furthermore, patients often have no previously recognized history of diabetes mellitus when they present with mucormycosis. In these instances, presentation for mucormycosis may result in the first clinical recognition of hyperglycemia, which often has been unmasked by recent glucocorticoid use. Thus, a high index of suspicion of mucormycosis must be maintained, even in the absence of a known history of diabetes, if hyperglycemia is present. In patients undergoing HSCT, mucormycosis develops at least as commonly during nonneutropenic as during neutropenic periods, probably because of glucocorticoid treatment of graft-versus-host disease. Mucormycosis can occur as isolated cutaneous or subcutaneous infection in immunologically normal individuals after traumatic implantation of soil or vegetation (e.g., due to natural disasters, motor vehicle accidents, or severe injuries in war zones) or in nosocomial settings via direct access through intravenous catheters, subcutaneous injections, or maceration of the skin by a moist dressing.

Patients receiving antifungal prophylaxis with either itraconazole or voriconazole may be at increased risk of mucormycosis. These patients typically present with disseminated mucormycosis, the most lethal form of disease. Breakthrough mucormycosis also has been described in patients receiving posaconazole, isavuconazole, or echinocandin prophylaxis.

Mucormycosis has also emerged as an important superinfection in COVID-19 patients, with patients in India being particularly heavily affected. Even before COVID-19, India was hyper-endemic for mucormycosis, with population-based case rates that were up to 70 times higher than the worldwide rate. Whether or not COVID-19 itself somehow predisposes to mucormycosis is not clear. Both in India and the rest of the world, the vast majority of excess cases of mucormycosis during the COVID-19 pandemic have likely been attributable to a combination of diabetes mellitus and corticosteroid use. In India, one-third of mucormycosis cases during the COVID-19 pandemic were in patients not infected with COVID-19, underscoring the high baseline rate there. Furthermore, the large majority of mucormycosis cases in COVID-19 patients in India and the rest of the world have been of the rhino-orbital-cerebral variety, and pulmonary infection has been rare, consistent with diabetes and corticosteroids predisposing to these cases.

CLINICAL MANIFESTATIONS

Mucormycosis presents as one of five well-defined clinical syndromes: rhino-orbital-cerebral, pulmonary, cutaneous, gastrointestinal, and disseminated disease. However, infection of any body site can occur. Patients with specific defects in host defense tend to develop specific syndromes. For example, patients with diabetes mellitus and/or DKA typically develop the rhino-orbital-cerebral form and much more rarely develop pulmonary or disseminated disease. In contrast, pulmonary mucormycosis occurs most commonly in leukemic patients who are receiving chemotherapy and in patients undergoing HSCT.

Rhino-Orbital-Cerebral Disease Rhino-orbital-cerebral mucormycosis continues to be the most common form of the disease worldwide. Most cases occur in patients with diabetes, although such cases are also described in the transplantation setting, often along with glucocorticoid-induced diabetes mellitus. The initial symptoms of rhino-orbital-cerebral mucormycosis are nonspecific and include eye or facial pain and facial numbness followed by the onset of conjunctival suffusion and swelling, and blurry vision. In contrast to the acute, bright red, periocular skin manifestations typical of acute bacterial orbital cellulitis, periorbital skin in patients with rhino-orbital-cerebral mucormycosis may take on a more dusky, subacute appearance. Fever may be absent in up to half of cases. White blood cell counts are typically elevated as long as the patient has functioning bone marrow. If untreated, infection usually spreads from the ethmoid sinus to the orbit, resulting in compromise of extraocular muscle function and proptosis, typically with chemosis. From the orbit, the fungus can spread contiguously or hematogenously to the frontal lobe of the brain and/or via venous drainage to the cavernous sinus. Onset of signs and symptoms in the contralateral eye, with resulting bilateral proptosis, chemosis, vision loss, and ophthalmoplegia, is ominous, suggesting the development of cavernous sinus thrombosis.

Upon visual inspection, infected tissue often has a normal appearance during the earliest stages of fungal spread, which can make diagnosis difficult; blind biopsies of normal-appearing sinus tissue are warranted when suspicion for mucormycosis is high. Tissue then progresses through an erythematous phase, with or without edema, before the onset of a violaceous appearance and finally the development of a black necrotic eschar. Infection can sometimes extend from the sinuses into the mouth and produce painful necrotic ulcerations of the hard palate, but this is a late finding that suggests extensive, well-established infection.

One common misperception about mucormycosis is that it is always rapidly progressive. In fact, the rate of progression is extremely variable and is possibly dependent on the immune status of the patient, the infectious inoculum, and the causative Mucorales species, some of which are more virulent and/or have faster growth rates than others. Patients may go from initial symptoms to death in days; alternatively, it can take months or even a year or more for lethal progression to occur.

Pulmonary Disease Pulmonary mucormycosis is the second most common manifestation. Symptoms include dyspnea, cough, and chest pain; fever is often but not invariably present. Angioinvasion results in necrosis, cavitation, and/or hemoptysis. Lobar consolidation, isolated masses, nodular disease, cavities, or wedge-shaped infarcts may be seen on chest radiography. High-resolution chest CT is the best method for determining the extent of pulmonary mucormycosis and may demonstrate evidence of infection before it is seen on chest x-ray. In the setting of cancer, where mucormycosis may be difficult to differentiate from aspergillosis, the presence of ≥10 pulmonary nodules, pleural effusion, or concomitant sinusitis makes mucormycosis more likely. It is important to distinguish mucormycosis from aspergillosis because treatments for these infections may differ. Indeed, voriconazole—the first-line treatment for aspergillosis—exacerbates mucormycosis in mouse and fly models of infection. Isavuconazole and posaconazole were noninferior to voriconazole for the treatment of aspergillosis in randomized controlled trials, and also have activity against Mucorales. Hence if there is doubt about whether infection is caused by a septated mold (e.g., *Aspergillus*) or a Mucorales, inclusion of isavuconazole or posaconazole in a treatment regimen is a reasonable consideration. Consideration must also be given to the possibility of dual infection with both a septated mold and Mucorales; dual infection is not infrequently encountered in highly compromised patients.

Cutaneous Disease Cutaneous mucormycosis may result from external implantation of the fungus or from hematogenous dissemination. External implantation–related infection has been described in the setting of soil exposure from trauma (e.g., in a motor vehicle accident, a natural disaster, or combat-related injuries), penetrating injury with plant material (e.g., a thorn), injections of medications (e.g., insulin), catheter insertion, contamination of surgical dressings, and use of tape to secure endotracheal tubes. Cutaneous disease can be highly invasive, penetrating into muscle, fascia, and even bone. Necrotizing fasciitis caused by mucormycosis carries a mortality rate approaching 80%. Necrotic cutaneous lesions in the setting of hematogenous dissemination also are associated with an extremely high mortality rate. However, with prompt, aggressive surgical debridement, isolated cutaneous mucormycosis has a favorable prognosis and a low mortality rate.

Gastrointestinal Disease In the past, gastrointestinal mucormycosis occurred primarily in premature neonates in association with disseminated disease and necrotizing enterocolitis. However, there has been a marked increase in case reports describing adults with neutropenia, glucocorticoid use, or other immunocompromising conditions. In addition, gastrointestinal disease has been reported as a nosocomial process following administration of medications mixed with contaminated wooden applicator sticks. Nonspecific abdominal pain and distention associated with nausea and vomiting are the most common symptoms. Gastrointestinal bleeding is common, and fungating masses may be seen in the stomach at endoscopy. The disease may progress to visceral perforation, with extremely high mortality rates.

Disseminated and Miscellaneous Forms of Disease Hematogenously disseminated mucormycosis may originate from any primary site of infection. The most common site of dissemination is the brain, but metastatic lesions may also be found in any other organ. Mortality rates for widely disseminated mucormycosis exceed 90%; however, these high rates are likely to be due in part to the underlying predisposing condition leading to the infection and the inability to surgically remove the infected foci.

Mucormycosis may affect any body site, including bones, mediastinum, trachea, kidneys, peritoneum (in association with dialysis), scalp (causing a kerion), and even isolated infection of teeth.

DIAGNOSIS

A high index of suspicion is required for diagnosis of mucormycosis. Unfortunately, autopsy series have shown that up to half of cases are diagnosed only postmortem. Because the Mucorales are environmental isolates, definitive diagnosis requires a positive culture from a sterile site (e.g., a needle aspirate, a tissue biopsy specimen, or pleural fluid) or histopathologic evidence of invasive mucormycosis. A probable diagnosis of mucormycosis can be established by culture from a nonsterile site (e.g., sputum or bronchoalveolar lavage) or the detection of Mucorales on the surface of histopathology samples (without visualization of evidence of invasion) when a patient has appropriate risk factors as well as clinical and radiographic evidence of disease. In such cases, given the urgency of administering therapy early, the patient should be treated while confirmation of the diagnosis is awaited.

Biopsy with histopathologic examination remains the most sensitive and specific modality for definitive diagnosis (**Fig. 218-1**). Biopsy reveals characteristic wide (≥6- to 30-μm), thick-walled, ribbon-like, aseptate hyphal elements that branch at right angles. Other fungi, including *Aspergillus, Fusarium*, and *Scedosporium* species, have septa, are thinner, and branch at acute angles. However, artificial septa may result from folding of tissue during processing (which may also alter the appearance of the angle of branching), which can make Mucorales appear to have septa. Thus, the width and the ribbon-like form of the fungus are the most reliable features distinguishing mucormycosis from other pathogenic molds. The Mucorales are visualized most effectively with periodic acid–Schiff or hematoxylin and eosin; in contrast to many other fungi, methenamine silver may not result in optimal staining. While histopathology can identify the Mucorales,

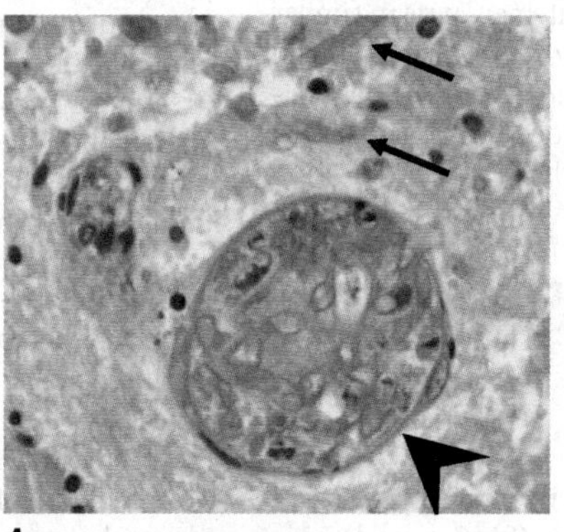

A

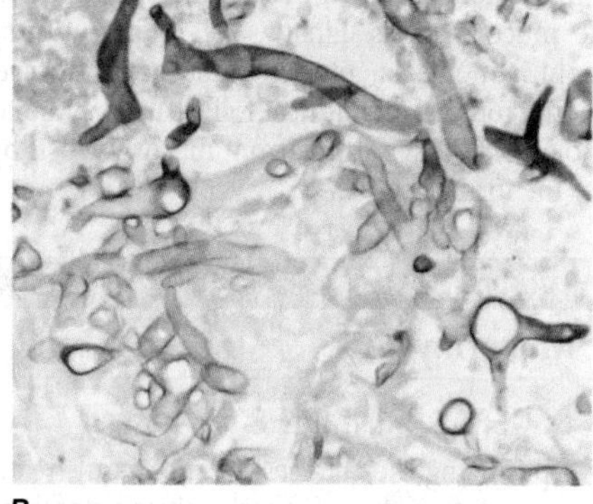

B

FIGURE 218-1 Histopathology sections of *Rhizopus delemar* in infected brain. *A.* Broad, ribbon-like, nonseptate hyphae in the parenchyma (*arrows*) and a thrombosed blood vessel with extensive intravascular hyphae (*arrowhead*) (hematoxylin and eosin). ***B.*** Extensive, broad, ribbon-like hyphae invading the parenchyma (Gomori methenamine silver).

that block IFN-γ-dependent cellular responses, and autoantibodies to IFN-γ predispose to infection with intramacrophagic fungi, as do biologics targeting tumor necrosis factor α (TNF-α) and autoantibodies to granulocyte-macrophage colony-stimulating factor (GM-CSF). The latter predisposing factors reveal the central role of these two Th1-associated cytokines—TNF-α and GM-CSF—in macrophage activation.

Taken together, these observations show that the cellular and molecular factors that drive protective antifungal immune responses vary greatly with the anatomic site of the infection, the offending fungus, and the patient population (Table 211-1). The growing body of data on human immunologic responses to fungi holds promise in informing precision medicine strategies for risk assessment, prophylaxis, immunotherapy, and vaccination of vulnerable patients.

DIAGNOSIS

The diagnostic modalities used for various fungal infections are outlined in Table 211-1 and are detailed in the chapters on specific mycoses that follow in this section. Definitive diagnosis of a fungal infection requires histopathologic identification of the fungus invading tissue with parallel culture of the fungus from the specimen. Certain fungi have distinctive morphologic features that facilitate diagnosis (Table 211-1). The stains most often used to identify fungi are periodic acid–Schiff and Gomori methenamine silver. *Candida*, unlike other fungi, is visible on gram-stained tissue smears. Hematoxylin and eosin stains define accompanying histologic features of fungal disease (granuloma formation, angioinvasion, necrosis) but are insufficient to reliably identify fungi in tissue. A positive India ink stain of cerebrospinal fluid (CSF) is diagnostic for cryptococcosis. Most laboratories use calcofluor white staining coupled with fluorescence microscopy to identify fungi in fluid specimens. A positive fungal culture of blood or tissue may signify either a patient's colonization or lab contamination instead of true infection, with the most likely scenario depending on the fungus and the anatomic site. In blood, *Candida* can be detected with any of the widely used automated blood culture systems, but the lysis-centrifugation technique increases the sensitivity of blood cultures for both *Candida* and other less common fungi (e.g., *Histoplasma*). Matrix-assisted laser desorption/ionization time-of-flight mass spectrometry (MALDI-TOF-MS) is now used extensively for detection and speciation of fungi recovered from culture.

The several available fungal-antigen and serologic tests vary in sensitivity and specificity. The most reliable of these tests are the antibody to *Coccidioides*, *Histoplasma* antigen, and cryptococcal polysaccharide antigen. Serologic tests are also available for other endemic dimorphic fungi (Table 211-1). The galactomannan test—especially in the bronchoalveolar lavage fluid—is useful for the diagnosis of aspergillosis; however, false-negative results are common, particularly in patients receiving antifungal prophylaxis, and false-positive results may occur with other fungal infections. The β-glucan test has a high negative predictive value for invasive candidiasis but lacks specificity. T2 magnetic resonance is now approved by the U.S. Food and Drug Administration (FDA) for detection of *Candida* in blood. Several polymerase chain reaction and nucleic acid hybridization assays exist for fungal detection but are not standardized and are not widely used in the clinic.

ANTIFUNGAL DRUGS

This section provides a brief overview of available agents for the treatment of fungal infections. Drug regimens and schedules are detailed in the chapters on specific mycoses that follow in this section. Since fungal organisms, like human cells, are eukaryotic, the identification of drugs that selectively kill or inhibit fungi but that are not toxic to human cells poses challenges. Indeed, far fewer antifungal than antibacterial agents have been introduced into clinical medicine.

Early initiation of appropriate antifungal therapy is a critical determinant of favorable outcome, as has been shown for candidemia, aspergillosis, and mucormycosis. In addition, source control of the infection is important—e.g., with removal of the central venous catheter in candidemia, drainage of abdominal abscesses in intraabdominal candidiasis, and surgical debridement of sinus tissue in mucormycosis. Moreover, an essential factor in a favorable prognosis in patients with opportunistic mycoses is the achievement of immune reconstitution—e.g., with neutrophil recovery, tapering of glucocorticoids or other immunosuppressive drugs, or initiation of combination antiretroviral therapy in AIDS.

AMPHOTERICIN B

The advent of amphotericin B (AmB) in the 1950s revolutionized the treatment of deep-seated mycoses. Before the availability of AmB, cryptococcal meningitis and other disseminated fungal infections were nearly always fatal. AmB remains the broadest-spectrum antifungal agent. Its fungicidal mechanism of action involves direct binding to ergosterol and intercalation into the fungal cell membrane, which leads to osmotic cell lysis. AmB remains the preferred antifungal agent for the treatment of mucormycosis and fusariosis and for induction therapy for cryptococcal meningitis and disseminated infections caused by endemic dimorphic fungi. However, AmB has several limitations, including lack of an oral formulation and significant toxicity, primarily renal and infusion-related (fever, chills, thrombosis). The introduction of lipid AmB formulations has ameliorated these toxicities, and the lipid formulations have largely replaced the original deoxycholate formulation in resource-rich settings. In developing countries, AmB deoxycholate is still widely used because of the high cost of the lipid formulations. The two lipid formulations commonly used in the clinic are liposomal AmB and AmB lipid complex, which exhibit comparable efficacy, toxicity, and tissue penetration profiles.

AZOLES

Azoles offer important advantages over AmB, such as the availability of oral and IV formulations and a lack of renal toxicity. The mechanism of action of azoles involves inhibition of lanosterol 14α-demethylase and ergosterol synthesis in the fungal cell membrane, with a consequent accumulation of toxic sterol intermediates and growth arrest. Unlike AmB, azoles are considered fungistatic.

Fluconazole Fluconazole plays an important role in the treatment of several fungal infections. Its major advantages are the availability of oral and IV formulations, a long half-life, penetration into most body fluids (ocular fluid, CSF, urine), and minimal toxicity. This drug rarely causes liver toxicity; high doses may result in alopecia, dry mouth, and a metallic taste. Notably, the administration of even low doses of fluconazole to pregnant women for the treatment of vaginal candidiasis was recently linked to miscarriage and stillbirth. Fluconazole has no activity against molds and most endemic dimorphic fungi and is less active than the newer azoles against *C. glabrata* and *C. krusei.*

Fluconazole is the preferred agent for the treatment of coccidioidal meningitis, although relapses may occur despite therapy. Fluconazole is also used as consolidation and maintenance therapy for cryptococcal meningitis and for the treatment of mucosal candidiasis. It is used for treating candidemia in patients who are not critically ill or immunosuppressed; in these patients, fluconazole was found to be as efficacious as AmB. Because of increasing rates of azole-resistant *Candida* strains, many clinicians opt to initiate therapy with an echinocandin, which is replaced by fluconazole once a susceptible *Candida* species is recovered. Fluconazole is effective as prophylaxis in recipients of high-risk liver and allogeneic bone marrow transplants, although many centers now use posaconazole in neutropenic patients, given its added spectrum against molds. Fluconazole prophylaxis in leukemic patients, in AIDS patients with low CD4+ T-cell counts, and in patients on surgical intensive care units is controversial.

Itraconazole Itraconazole is available in oral (capsule, suspension) and IV formulations and has broader antifungal activity—i.e., against molds and endemic dimorphic fungi. Itraconazole is the drug of choice for mild to moderate histoplasmosis and blastomycosis and has also been used to treat chronic coccidioidomycosis, phaeohyphomycosis, sporotrichosis, and mucocutaneous mycoses such as oropharyngeal candidiasis, tinea versicolor, tinea capitis, and onychomycosis. Although it is approved by the FDA for use in febrile neutropenic species can be identified only by culture. Several studies showed that polymerase chain reaction (PCR) of Mucorales-specific targets is useful in diagnosing mucormycosis. However, the U.S. Food and Drug Administration (FDA) has not approved any of these PCR-based assays for this purpose.

Unfortunately, cultures are positive in fewer than half of cases of mucormycosis. Nevertheless, the Mucorales are not fastidious organisms and tend to grow quickly (i.e., within 48–96 h) on culture media. The likely explanation for the low sensitivity of culture is that the Mucorales form long filamentous structures that are killed by tissue homogenization—the standard method for preparing tissue cultures in the clinical microbiology laboratory. Thus, the laboratory should be advised when a diagnosis of mucormycosis is suspected, and the tissue should be cut into sections and placed in the center of culture dishes rather than homogenized. Because there is also substantial variability among isolates in optimal growth temperature, growth at both room temperature and 37°C is advisable.

Imaging techniques often yield subtle findings that underestimate the extent of disease. For example, the most common finding on CT or MRI of the head or sinuses of a patient with rhino-orbital mucormycosis is sinusitis that is indistinguishable from bacterial sinusitis. While sinusitis is almost always seen on CT scans in patients with the rhino-orbital-cerebral disease, erosion through the sinus bones and into the orbit is rarely seen on CT even when it is clinically present. MRI is more sensitive (~80%) for detecting orbital and central nervous system (CNS) disease than is CT. High-risk patients should always undergo endoscopy and/or surgical exploration, with biopsy of the areas of suspected infection. If mucormycosis is suspected, initial empirical therapy with a polyene antifungal agent should be initiated while the diagnosis is being confirmed.

■ DIFFERENTIAL DIAGNOSIS

Other mold infections, including aspergillosis, scedosporiosis, fusariosis, and infections caused by the dematiaceous fungi (brown-pigmented soil organisms), can cause clinical syndromes identical to mucormycosis. Histopathologic examination usually allows distinction of the Mucorales from these other organisms, and a positive culture permits definitive species identification. As stated above, it is important to distinguish the Mucorales from these other fungi, as the preferred antifungal treatments differ (i.e., polyenes for the Mucorales vs expanded-spectrum triazoles for most septate molds). The entomophthoromycoses caused by *Basidiobolus* and *Conidiobolus* also can cause identical clinical syndromes. These fungi cannot be readily distinguished from the Mucorales by histopathology but can be reliably distinguished by culture. Fortunately, entomophthoromycoses are uncommon in developed countries and can be treated with polyenes; it is not urgent to distinguish them from mucormycosis.

In a patient with sinusitis and proptosis, orbital cellulitis and cavernous sinus thrombosis caused by bacterial pathogens (most commonly *Staphylococcus aureus*, but also streptococcal and gram-negative species) must be excluded. *Klebsiella rhinoscleromatis* is a rare cause of an indolent facial rhinoscleroma syndrome that may appear similar to mucormycosis. Finally, the Tolosa-Hunt syndrome causes painful ophthalmoplegia, ptosis, headache, and cavernous sinus inflammation; biopsies and clinical follow-up may be needed to distinguish the Tolosa-Hunt syndrome from mucormycosis by the lack of progression of the former entity.

TREATMENT

Mucormycosis

GENERAL PRINCIPLES

Optimizing the chances for successful treatment of mucormycosis requires four steps: (1) early initiation of therapy; (2) surgical debridement, when possible; (3) rapid reversal of underlying predisposing risk factors, if possible; and (4) proceeding to treat underlying malignancy, if present, without waiting to complete antifungal therapy first.

Early initiation of antifungal therapy requires maintaining a high index of suspicion for at-risk patients. Multiple studies have found that earlier initiation of polyene-based therapy improves survival of patients with mucormycosis. Because the disease can present subtly at first and confirmation of the diagnosis can take days, therapy often must be started empirically before the diagnosis is established. When there is a reasonable suspicion of mucormycosis, clinicians should not hesitate to initiate therapy with a lipid polyene as soon as possible since the toxicity of lipid polyenes (unlike that of amphotericin B [AmB] deoxycholate) is rarely substantial after one or two doses.

Blood vessel thrombosis and resulting tissue necrosis during mucormycosis can result in poor penetration of antifungal agents to the site of infection. Therefore, debridement of all necrotic tissues can help eradicate the disease. Surgery has been found (by logistic regression and in multiple case series) to be an independent variable for favorable outcome in patients with mucormycosis. However, these data are confounded by the fact that sicker patients are often unable to tolerate surgical procedures. Thus, a moderated approach where tissue is debrided when and to the extent it is safe to do so is advisable. Limited data from a retrospective study support the use of intraoperative frozen sections to delineate the margins of infected tissues, with sparing of tissues lacking evidence of infection.

Rapidly reversing hyperglycemia, acidosis, or iron overload and lowering corticosteroid doses are important to improving cure. Indeed, a recent study confirmed that resolution of acidosis in mice with DKA via the administration of sodium bicarbonate (used in the mice in lieu of insulin) improved survival. Administration of glucocorticoids predisposes animals to death from mucormycosis in experimental models. Similarly, iron administration to patients with active mucormycosis should be avoided as iron exacerbates infection in experimental models. Blood transfusion typically results in some liberation of free iron due to hemolysis, so a conservative approach to red blood cell transfusions is advisable.

One of the most common errors made in management of mucormycosis is the belief that mucormycosis must be eradicated before an underlying malignancy can be treated. This belief can result in halting or delaying treatment for the underlying disease (e.g., chemotherapy or transplantation) until the mucormycosis is cured. Three fallacies belie this concern. First, mucormycosis will not be definitively eradicated until near-normal immunity is restored; the antifungals provide a holding action and are unlikely to be curative until the underlying disease is treated. Second, modern antifungals can halt progression of mucormycosis temporarily, enabling aggressive chemotherapy or transplantation to be administered to cure the underlying disease. Finally, the primary driver of death in such patients is typically progression of the underlying disease due to failure to treat it appropriately.

Initially, some consideration can be given to moderating the level of aggressiveness of the chemotherapy and resulting duration and depth of neutropenia. The aggressiveness of immune suppression and antifungal therapy can then be adjusted during the course of treatment in response to changes in clinical status. Chemotherapy should be given sufficiently aggressively to attempt cure of the underlying disease. These patients are extremely complex, and multidisciplinary, team-based care is advisable.

ANTIFUNGAL THERAPY

Primary therapy for mucormycosis should be based on a polyene antifungal agent (**Table 218-2**), except perhaps in mild localized infection (e.g., isolated suprafascial cutaneous infection) that has been eradicated surgically in an immunocompetent patient. Lipid formulations of AmB are significantly less nephrotoxic than AmB deoxycholate, can be administered at higher doses, and are probably more effective for this purpose. Liposomal amphotericin B (LAmB) is preferred to amphotericin B lipid complex (ABLC) for management of brain infection on the basis of retrospective survival data and superior brain penetration; there is no clear efficacy advantage

TABLE 218-2 Antifungal Options for the Treatment of Mucormycosis[a]

DRUG	RECOMMENDED DOSAGE	ADVANTAGES AND SUPPORTING STUDIES	DISADVANTAGES
First-Line Antifungal Therapy			
AmB deoxycholate	1.0–1.5 mg/kg once per day	• >5 decades of clinical experience • Inexpensive • FDA approved for treatment of mucormycosis	• Highly toxic • Poor CNS penetration
LAmB	5–10 mg/kg once per day	• Less nephrotoxic than AmB deoxycholate • Better CNS penetration than AmB deoxycholate or ABLC • Better outcomes than with AmB deoxycholate in murine models and a retrospective clinical review	• Expensive
ABLC	5 mg/kg once per day	• Less nephrotoxic than AmB deoxycholate • Murine and retrospective clinical data suggest benefit of combination therapy with echinocandins	• Expensive • Possibly less efficacious than LAmB for CNS infection
Second-Line/Salvage Option			
Isavuconazole	200 mg of isavuconazole (372 mg of isavuconazonium sulfate), load q8h × 6 followed by once-daily dosing	• Efficacy similar to that of LAmB in mouse models • FDA approved for treatment of mucormycosis • May be a rational empirical option when septate mold vs mucormycosis is not yet established	• Much less clinical experience • Clinical study supporting approval was small and historically controlled
Posaconazole	200 mg four times per day	• In vitro activity against the Mucorales, with lower MICs than isavuconazole • Retrospective data for salvage therapy in mucormycosis	• Substantially lower blood levels than isavuconazole • No data on initial therapy for mucormycosis, and no evidence for combination therapy with posaconazole • Experience limited, potential use for salvage therapy
Combination Therapy[b]			
Echinocandin plus lipid polyene	Standard echinocandin doses	• Favorable toxicity profile • Synergistic in murine disseminated mucormycosis • Retrospective clinical data suggest superior outcomes for rhino-orbital-cerebral mucormycosis.	• Limited clinical data on combination therapy
Lipid polyene plus azole (posaconazole or isavuconazole)	Standard doses	• Favorable toxicity profile	• Limited efficacy data, with no available evidence of superiority vs monotherapy
Triple therapy (lipid polyene plus echinocandin plus azole)	Standard doses	• Maximal aggressiveness	• Limited efficacy data, with no available evidence for superiority vs monotherapy or dual therapy

[a]Primary therapy should generally include a polyene. Non-polyene-based regimens may be appropriate for patients who refuse polyene therapy or for relatively immunocompetent patients with mild disease (e.g., isolated suprafascial cutaneous infection) that can be surgically eradicated. [b]Prospective randomized trials are necessary to confirm the suggested benefit (from animal and small retrospective human studies) of combination therapy for mucormycosis. Dose escalation of any echinocandin is not recommended because of a paradoxical loss of benefit of combination therapy at echinocandin doses of ≥3 mg/kg per day.

Abbreviations: ABLC, AmB lipid complex; AmB, amphotericin B; CNS, central nervous system; FDA, U.S. Food and Drug Administration; LAmB, liposomal AmB; MIC, minimal inhibitory concentration.

Source: Modified from B Spellberg et al: Clin Infect Dis 48:1743, 2009.

of either agent for infections outside the brain, although LAmB may be less nephrotoxic than ABLC.

Starting dosages of 1 mg/kg per day for AmB deoxycholate and 5 mg/kg per day for LAmB and ABLC are commonly given to adults and children to treat mucormycosis. Dose escalation of LAmB to 7.5 or 10 mg/kg per day for CNS mucormycosis may be considered in light of the limited penetration of polyenes into the brain. Because of autoinduction of metabolism, which results in paradoxically lower drug levels, there is no advantage to escalating the LAmB dose above 10 mg/kg per day, and doses of 5 mg/kg per day are probably adequate for nonbrain infections. ABLC dose escalation above 5 mg/kg per day is not advisable given the lack of relevant data and the drug's potential toxicity.

In multiple studies, various combinations of lipid polyenes (both ABLC and LAmB) plus echinocandins (e.g., caspofungin, micafungin, and anidulafungin) improved survival rates among mice with disseminated mucormycosis (including CNS disease). Furthermore, combination lipid polyene–echinocandin therapy was associated with significantly better outcomes than polyene monotherapy in a retrospective clinical study involving patients with rhino-orbital-cerebral mucormycosis (including CNS disease). The effect of echinocandins appears to be to downmodulate the virulence of the fungus and reduce tissue necrosis and destruction from fungal invasion. On the basis of such data, some experts prefer combination lipid polyene–echinocandin therapy as a first-line option. However, at least one retrospective study did not find an advantage of any combination regimens (including polyene-azole, polyene-echinocandin, or others) in patients who primarily had malignancy as the underlying disease. Ultimately definitive randomized controlled trials are needed to establish whether the combination is superior in efficacy to monotherapy for mucormycosis. When used, echinocandins should be administered at standard, FDA-approved doses since dose escalation has resulted in paradoxical loss of efficacy in preclinical models.

In contrast to deferoxamine, the iron chelator deferasirox is fungicidal against clinical isolates of the Mucorales. In mice with DKA and disseminated mucormycosis, combination deferasirox–LAmB therapy resulted in synergistic improvement of survival rates and reduced the fungal burden in the brain. Unfortunately, a small randomized, double-blind, phase 2 safety clinical trial of adjunctive therapy with deferasirox (plus LAmB) documented excess mortality among patients treated with deferasirox. Of note, the study population included primarily patients with active malignancy, and few patients in the study had diabetes mellitus as their only risk factor.

Deferasirox is therefore contraindicated as therapy in patients with active malignancy, but its role in patients who have diabetes mellitus without malignancy (the setting in which its preclinical efficacy was optimal) remains uncertain.

Posaconazole and isavuconazole are the only FDA-approved azoles with reliable in vitro activity against the Mucorales. However, there are limited data regarding the efficacy of posaconazole monotherapy for mucormycosis, and in contrast to polyene-echinocandin therapy, there are no data to support the use of combination posaconazole-polyene regimens. Although the minimal inhibitory concentrations of isavuconazole against the Mucorales are four- to eightfold higher than those of posaconazole, blood levels may be higher with standard isavuconazole dosing than with posaconazole. Isavuconazole is FDA approved for the treatment of mucormycosis on the basis of a small, historically controlled study. Given this limited data set, many experts continue to think that lipid polyenes are first-line options and that isavuconazole, like posaconazole, is best reserved for oral stepdown therapy in patients whose condition has substantially improved on polyene-based therapy or for salvage therapy in patients who are intolerant of polyene-based regimens or whose infection is refractory to these regimens. As with posaconazole, no data support the use of combination isavuconazole-polyene regimens in lieu of polyene monotherapy or polyene-echinocandin combination regimens. Some experts use triple therapy with a polyene, echinocandin, and either posaconazole or isavuconazole for patients who have extensive disease or whose disease has progressed on prior therapy. Empirical, dual lipid polyene–azole therapy is a rational choice in a patient with likely invasive mold infections when septate molds and mucormycosis are both in the differential diagnosis and the etiologic agent has not yet been confirmed. Alternatively, initial therapy with isavuconazole monotherapy may be reasonable for a brief period of time in a stable patient if mucormycosis is felt to be possible, but less likely than a septated mold infection.

The roles of recombinant cytokines and neutrophil transfusions in the primary treatment of mucormycosis are not clear, although it is intuitive that earlier recovery of neutrophil counts should improve survival rates. Limited data from uncontrolled case series support the use of hyperbaric oxygen in centers with the appropriate technical expertise and facilities; its efficacy remains undefined. As mentioned previously, one study in mice with DKA found that administration of sodium bicarbonate improved survival from mucormycosis; however, because insulin was not administered to the mice, it is unclear whether the therapeutic effect is clinically relevant.

In general, antifungal therapy for mucormycosis should be continued until resolution of clinical signs and symptoms of infection and resolution of underlying immunosuppression. However, after several weeks of daily therapy in a patient who is clinically improving, it is reasonable to consider switching to thrice-weekly lipid polyene doses—with ultimate weaning down to twice-weekly doses—for maintenance therapy. For patients with mucormycosis who are receiving immunosuppressive medications, secondary antifungal prophylaxis is typically continued for as long as the immunosuppressive regimen is administered. Stepdown to azoles for chronic suppression is a reasonable alternative to continuing polyene therapy in this setting, with reinitiation of polyenes during periods of deep neutropenia.

One common source of error in the long-term management of mucormycosis is follow-up radiology. Analysis of data from the DEFEAT Mucor study indicated that early radiographic progression (within the first 2 weeks) did not predict long-term survival. Changing the therapeutic plan based on early radiographic changes can result in therapeutic errors. For example, it is common for CNS Mucorales to cavitate in the brain parenchyma over time. This does not necessarily reflect therapeutic failure, but rather may reflect increased immune reactivity to the fungus, particularly in patients recovering from neutropenia or with removal of immune suppression. Thus, it may not be advisable to obtain serial radiographic studies in the short term, and if such studies are obtained, caution should be used in reacting to their results. Greater emphasis should be placed on clinical response, particularly within the first 2–4 weeks after initiation of therapy.

PROGNOSIS

Over the past two decades, the prognosis of mucormycosis has substantially improved with aggressive antifungal therapy. Even CNS infection is often successfully treated. As mentioned, the key driver of outcome may be control of the patient's predisposing condition.

FURTHER READING

Cornely O et al: Global guideline for the diagnosis and management of mucormycosis: An initiative of the European Confederation of Medical Mycology in cooperation with the Mycoses Study Group Education and Research Consortium. Lancet Infect Dis 19:e405, 2019.

Pettrikos G et al: Epidemiology of mucormycosis in Europe. Clin Microbiol Infect 20(S3):67, 2014.

Spellberg B et al: Novel perspectives on mucormycosis: Pathophysiology, presentation, and management. Clin Microbiol Rev 18:556, 2005.

Spellberg B et al: Combination therapy for mucormycosis: Why, what, and how? Clin Infect Dis 54(S1):S73, 2012.

Spellberg B et al: Risk factors for mortality in patients with mucormycosis. Med Mycol 50:611, 2012.

219 Less Common Systemic Mycoses and Superficial Mycoses

Carol A. Kauffman

ENDEMIC MYCOSES (DIMORPHIC FUNGI)

Dimorphic fungi exist in discrete environmental niches as molds that produce conidia, which are their infectious form. In tissues and at temperatures of >35°C, the mold converts to the yeast form. **Other endemic mycoses—histoplasmosis, coccidioidomycosis, and blastomycosis—are discussed in Chaps. 212, 213, and 214, respectively.**

SPOROTRICHOSIS

Etiologic Agent, Epidemiology, and Pathogenesis *Sporothrix schenckii* complex is comprised of six closely related organisms; *S. schenckii* and *S. brasiliensis* are the species that cause most human infection. *Sporothrix* species are found worldwide in sphagnum moss, decaying vegetation, and soil. Sporotrichosis most commonly affects persons who participate in outdoor activities such as landscaping, gardening, and tree farming. Infected animals can transmit *S. schenckii* to humans. A large ongoing outbreak of sporotrichosis in Rio de Janeiro caused by *S. brasiliensis* has been traced to cats, which are highly susceptible to this infection. Sporotrichosis is primarily a localized infection of skin and subcutaneous tissues that follows traumatic inoculation of conidia. Osteoarticular sporotrichosis is uncommon, occurring most often in middle-aged men who abuse alcohol, and pulmonary sporotrichosis occurs almost exclusively in persons with chronic obstructive pulmonary disease who have inhaled the organism from the environment. Dissemination occurs almost entirely in markedly immunocompromised patients, especially those with AIDS.

Clinical Manifestations and Differential Diagnosis Days or weeks after inoculation, a papule develops at the site and then usually ulcerates but is not very painful. Similar lesions develop sequentially along the lymphatic channels proximal to the original

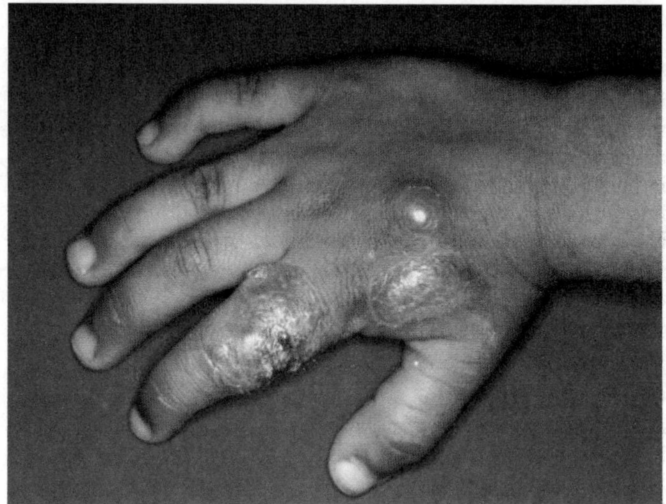

FIGURE 219-1 Several nodular lesions that developed after a young boy pricked his index finger with a thorn. A culture yielded *S. schenckii*. *(Courtesy of Dr. Angela Restrepo.)*

lesion (**Fig. 219-1**). Some patients develop a fixed cutaneous lesion that can be verrucous or ulcerative and that remains localized without lymphatic extension. The differential diagnosis of lymphocutaneous sporotrichosis includes nocardiosis, tularemia, nontuberculous mycobacterial infection (especially that due to *Mycobacterium marinum*), and leishmaniasis. Osteoarticular sporotrichosis can present as chronic synovitis or septic arthritis. Pulmonary sporotrichosis must be differentiated from tuberculosis and other fungal pneumonias. Numerous ulcerated skin lesions, with or without spread to visceral organs (including the central nervous system [CNS]), are characteristic of disseminated sporotrichosis.

Diagnosis *S. schenckii* usually grows readily as a mold on Sabouraud's agar when material from a cutaneous lesion is incubated at room temperature. Histopathologic examination of biopsy material shows a mixed granulomatous and pyogenic reaction, and tiny oval or cigar-shaped yeasts sometimes can be seen with special stains.

Treatment and Prognosis Guidelines for the management of the various forms of sporotrichosis have been published by the Infectious Diseases Society of America (**Table 219-1**). Itraconazole is the drug of choice for lymphocutaneous and cutaneous sporotrichosis. Fluconazole is less effective, voriconazole is not effective, and posaconazole has been used successfully in a small number of patients. Saturated solution of potassium iodide (SSKI) continues to be used for lymphocutaneous infection because it costs much less than itraconazole. However, SSKI is poorly tolerated because of adverse reactions, including metallic taste, salivary gland swelling, rash, and fever. High-dose terbinafine may be effective for lymphocutaneous infection. Treatment for lymphocutaneous sporotrichosis is continued for 2–4 weeks after all lesions have resolved, usually for a total of 3–6 months. The success rate for treatment of lymphocutaneous sporotrichosis is 90–100%.

Pulmonary and osteoarticular forms of sporotrichosis are treated with itraconazole for at least 1 year. Severe pulmonary infection and disseminated sporotrichosis, including that involving the CNS, should be treated initially with amphotericin B (AmB), with a switch to itraconazole after improvement has been noted. Lifelong suppressive therapy with itraconazole often is required for AIDS patients. These forms of sporotrichosis respond poorly to antifungal therapy.

PARACOCCIDIOIDOMYCOSIS

Etiologic Agent, Epidemiology, and Pathogenesis *Paracoccidioides brasiliensis* and the less frequently reported *Paracoccidioides lutzii* are thermally dimorphic fungi found in humid areas of Central and South America, especially in Brazil. A striking male-to-female ratio varies from 14:1 to as high as 70:1 in various reports. Most patients are middle-aged or elderly men from rural areas. Paracoccidioidomycosis develops after the inhalation of aerosolized conidia encountered in the environment. For most patients, disease rarely develops at the time of the initial infection but appears years later, presumably after reactivation of a latent infection.

TABLE 219-1 Suggested Treatment for Endemic Mycoses

DISEASE	FIRST-LINE THERAPY	ALTERNATIVES/COMMENTS
Sporotrichosis		
Cutaneous, lymphocutaneous	Itraconazole, 200 mg/d until 2–4 weeks after lesions resolve	SSKI, increasing doses[a] Terbinafine, 500 mg bid
Pulmonary, osteoarticular	Itraconazole, 200 mg bid for 12 months	Lipid AmB[b] for severe pulmonary disease until stable; then itraconazole
Disseminated, central nervous system	Lipid AmB[b] for 4–6 weeks	Itraconazole, 200 mg bid after AmB for 12 months AIDS patients: itraconazole maintenance, 200 mg/d until CD4+ T cell count is >200/μL for ≥12 months
Paracoccidioidomycosis		
Chronic (adult form)	Itraconazole, 100–200 mg/d for 6–12 months	Voriconazole, 200 mg bid for 6–12 months Posaconazole, 300 mg/d for 6–12 months TMP-SMX, 160/800 mg bid for 12–36 months
Acute (juvenile form)	AmB[c] or lipid AmB[b] until improvement	Itraconazole, 200 mg bid after AmB for 12 months Voriconazole or posaconazole at doses noted above may be used
Talaromycosis (Penicilliosis)		
Mild or moderate	Itraconazole, 200 mg bid for 12 weeks	Voriconazole, 200 mg bid
Severe	Lipid AmB[b] or AmB[c] until improvement	Itraconazole, 200 mg bid after AmB for 12 weeks
Maintenance therapy (AIDS)	200 mg/d until CD4+ T cell count is >100/μL for ≥6 months	

[a]The starting dosage is 5–10 drops tid in water or juice. The dosage is increased weekly by 10 drops per dose, as tolerated, up to 40–50 drops tid. [b]The dosage of lipid AmB is 3–5 mg/kg daily; the higher dosage should be used when the central nervous system is involved. [c]The dosage of AmB deoxycholate is 0.6–1.0 mg/kg daily.

Abbreviations: AmB, amphotericin B; SSKI, saturated solution of potassium iodide; TMP-SMX, trimethoprim-sulfamethoxazole.

Clinical Manifestations Two major syndromes are associated with paracoccidioidomycosis: the acute or juvenile form and the chronic or adult form. The acute form is uncommon, occurs mostly in persons <30 years old, and manifests primarily as disseminated infection of the reticuloendothelial system. Immunocompromised individuals also develop this type of rapidly progressive disease. The chronic form of paracoccidioidomycosis accounts for ~90% of cases and predominantly affects older men. The primary manifestations are progressive pulmonary disease, primarily in the lower lobes, with fibrosis and ulcerative and nodular mucocutaneous lesions that occur primarily in mucous membranes of the upper respiratory tract and that must be differentiated from leishmaniasis (**Chap. 226**) and squamous cell carcinoma (**Chap. 76**).

Diagnosis The diagnosis is established by growth of the mold form of *P. brasiliensis* in culture at room temperature. A presumptive diagnosis can be made by detection of the distinctive thick-walled yeast, which has multiple narrow-necked buds attached circumferentially, in purulent material or tissue biopsies.

Treatment and Prognosis Itraconazole is the treatment of choice for paracoccidioidomycosis (Table 219-1). Voriconazole and posaconazole also are effective. Sulfonamides have been used for years and are the least costly agents; however, the response is slower and the relapse rate higher. Seriously ill patients should be treated with AmB initially. Patients with paracoccidioidomycosis have an excellent response to therapy, but pulmonary fibrosis can be progressive in those with chronic disease.

■ TALAROMYCOSIS (PENICILLIOSIS)

Etiologic Agent, Epidemiology, and Pathogenesis *Talaromyces marneffei* (formerly *Penicillium marneffei*) is a thermally dimorphic fungus that is endemic in the soil in certain areas of Vietnam, Thailand, and other southeastern Asian countries. The epidemiology of talaromycosis is linked to bamboo rats that are infected with the fungus but rarely manifest disease. The disease occurs most often among persons living in rural areas in which the rats are found, but there is no evidence for transmission of the infection directly from rats to humans. Infection is rare in immunocompetent hosts, and most cases are reported in persons who have advanced AIDS. Infection results from the inhalation of conidia from the environment. The organism converts to the yeast phase in the lungs and then spreads hematogenously throughout the reticuloendothelial system.

Clinical Manifestations The clinical manifestations of talaromycosis mimic those of disseminated histoplasmosis and include fever, fatigue, weight loss, dyspnea, lymphadenopathy, hepatosplenomegaly, and skin lesions, which appear as papules that often umbilicate and resemble molluscum contagiosum (**Chap. 196**).

Diagnosis Talaromycosis is diagnosed by culture of *T. marneffei* from blood or from biopsy samples of skin, bone marrow, or lymph node. The organism usually grows within 1 week as a mold producing a distinctive red pigment that diffuses into the agar. Histopathologic examination of tissues and smears of blood or material from skin lesions shows oval or elliptical yeast-like organisms with central septation and can quickly establish a presumptive diagnosis.

Treatment and Prognosis For mild or moderate infection, itraconazole is the drug of choice; voriconazole can also be used. Severe infection should be treated with AmB until improvement occurs; then therapy can be changed to itraconazole (Table 219-1). For patients with AIDS, suppressive therapy with itraconazole is recommended until the CD4+ T cell count has been >100 cells/μL for at least 6 months. Disseminated talaromycosis is usually fatal if not treated. With treatment, the mortality rate is ~10%.

PHAEOHYPHOMYCOSES

Dematiaceous or brown-black fungi, the common soil organisms that cause phaeohyphomycoses, contain melanin, which causes the hyphae and conidia to be darkly pigmented. The term *phaeohyphomycosis* is used to describe any infection with a pigmented mold. This definition encompasses two specific syndromes—eumycetoma and chromoblastomycosis—as well as all other types of infections caused by these organisms. It is important to note that eumycetomas can be caused by hyaline molds as well as by brown-black molds and that only about half of all mycetomas are due to fungi. Actinomycetes cause the remainder (**Chap. 174**). Most dematiaceous fungi cause localized subcutaneous infections after direct inoculation, but disseminated infections and serious focal visceral infections do occur, especially in immunocompromised patients.

Etiologic Agents, Epidemiology, and Pathogenesis A large number of pigmented molds can cause human infection. Most are found in the soil or on plants, and some cause economically important plant diseases. *Alternaria*, *Exophiala*, *Curvularia*, and *Wangiella* species are among the more common molds reported to cause human infection. In 2012, *Exserohilum* species caused a large outbreak in the United States of severe and in some patients fatal CNS infections after the injection of methylprednisolone contaminated with this fungus. The most common cause of eumycetoma is *Madurella* species. *Fonsecaea*, *Phialophora*, and *Cladophialophora* species are responsible for most cases of chromoblastomycosis. Infections with dematiaceous molds are acquired by traumatic inoculation into the eye or through the skin, by inhalation, or by injection of contaminated medication. Melanin is a virulence factor for all the pigmented molds. Several organisms, specifically *Cladophialophora bantiana* and *Rhinocladiella mackenziei*, are neurotropic and likely to cause CNS infection. When a patient is immunocompromised or when a pigmented mold is injected directly into a deep structure, these organisms become opportunists, invading blood vessels and mimicking better-known opportunistic infections, such as aspergillosis. Eumycetoma and chromoblastomycosis are acquired by inoculation through the skin; these two syndromes are seen almost entirely in tropical and subtropical areas and occur mostly in rural laborers who are frequently exposed to the organisms.

Clinical Manifestations Dematiaceous molds are the most common cause of allergic fungal sinusitis and a less common cause of invasive fungal sinusitis. Keratitis occurs with traumatic corneal inoculation. Even in many immunocompromised patients, inoculation through the skin generally produces only localized nodular lesions at the entry site. However, other immunocompromised patients develop pneumonia, brain abscess, or disseminated infection. In the outbreak mentioned above, epidural injection of *Exserohilum*-contaminated glucocorticoids led to meningitis, basilar stroke, epidural abscess and phlegmon, vertebral osteomyelitis, and arachnoiditis.

Eumycetoma is a chronic subcutaneous and cutaneous infection that usually occurs on the lower extremities and is characterized by swelling, the development of sinus tracts, and the appearance of grains that are actually colonies of fungi discharged from the sinus tract. As the infection progresses, adjacent fascia and bony structures become involved. The disease is indolent and disfiguring, progressing slowly over years. Complications include fractures of infected bone and bacterial superinfection.

Chromoblastomycosis is an indolent subcutaneous infection characterized by nodular, verrucous, or plaque-like painless lesions that occur predominantly on the lower extremities and grow slowly over months to years. There is hardly ever extension to adjacent structures, as is seen with eumycetoma. Long-term consequences include bacterial superinfection, chronic lymphedema, and (rarely) the development of squamous cell carcinoma.

Diagnosis The specific diagnosis of infection with a pigmented mold is established by growth of the organism in culture, which is essential to differentiate infection with a hyaline mold (e.g., *Aspergillus* or *Fusarium*) from that due to a pigmented mold. A tentative clinical diagnosis of mycetoma can be made when a patient presents with a lesion characterized by swelling, sinus tracts, and grains. Histopathologic examination and culture are necessary to confirm that the etiologic agent is a mold and not an actinomycete. In chromoblastomycosis, the diagnosis rests on the histologic demonstration of sclerotic bodies (dark brown, thick-walled, septate fungal forms that resemble large yeasts) in the tissues; culture establishes which pigmented mold is causing the infection. PCR assays are increasingly used in the diagnosis of infection due to dematiaceous molds but are available only through fungal reference laboratories.

Treatment and Prognosis The choice of antifungal agent to treat disseminated and focal visceral infections with brown-black molds is based on the location and extent of the infection, in vitro test results, and clinical experience with the specific infecting organism. AmB is not effective against many of these organisms but has been used successfully against some species (**Table 219-2**). Itraconazole, voriconazole, or posaconazole can be used in the treatment of localized infections. Voriconazole is preferred when infections involve the CNS because this drug reaches adequate concentrations at that site. Voriconazole or posaconazole could be used for disseminated infection; these agents are available as both IV and well-absorbed oral formulations. Disseminated and focal visceral infections, especially those involving the CNS, are associated with high mortality rates.

Treatment of eumycetoma and chromoblastomycosis involves both surgical extirpation of the lesion and use of antifungal agents. Surgical

TABLE 219-2 Suggested Treatment for Phaeohyphomycoses and Opportunistic Infections

DISEASE	FIRST-LINE THERAPY	ALTERNATIVES/ COMMENTS
Phaeohyphomycoses	Voriconazole, 200 mg bid Itraconazole, 200 mg bid Posaconazole, 300 mg/d	Lipid AmB may be effective against some mold species.
Fusariosis	Voriconazole, 200–300 mg bid Lipid AmB, 5 mg/kg per day Posaconazole, 300 mg/d	Lipid AmB plus voriconazole or posaconazole is used by some physicians for initial therapy.
Scedosporiosis/ lomentosporiosis	Voriconazole, 200–300 mg bid Posaconazole, 300 mg/d	Not susceptible to AmB *Lomentospora prolificans* is resistant to almost all antifungal drugs.
Trichosporonosis	Voriconazole, 200–300 mg bid	Posaconazole, 300 mg/d

Abbreviation: AmB, amphotericin B.

removal of the lesions is most effective if performed before extensive spread has occurred. In chromoblastomycosis, cryosurgery and laser therapy have been used with variable success. Eumycetoma has been treated with itraconazole, voriconazole, posaconazole, and less commonly terbinafine with variable rates of success. Itraconazole, terbinafine, and flucytosine have been used to treat chromoblastomycosis, again with variable success. Chromoblastomycosis and eumycetoma are chronic indolent infections that are difficult to cure, and the cost of antifungal treatment can be prohibitively expensive.

OPPORTUNISTIC FUNGAL INFECTIONS

Three genera of hyaline (nonpigmented) molds, *Fusarium*, *Scedosporium*, and *Lomentospora*, and one yeast-like genus, *Trichosporon*, have become prominent pathogens among immunocompromised patients. Invasive infections caused by these hyaline molds mimic aspergillosis in their clinical manifestations and their histopathologic appearance in tissues. In the immunocompetent host, these fungi cause localized infections of skin, skin structures, and subcutaneous tissues, but their role as causes of infection in immunocompromised patients will be emphasized in this section.

■ FUSARIOSIS

Etiologic Agent, Epidemiology, and Pathogenesis *Fusarium* species, which are found worldwide in soil and on plants, have emerged as major opportunists in markedly immunocompromised patients. Most human infections follow inhalation of conidia, but ingestion and direct inoculation also can lead to disease. An outbreak of severe *Fusarium* keratitis among soft contact lens wearers was traced back to a particular brand of contact lens solution and individual contact lens cases that had been contaminated with this mold. Disseminated infection is reported most often in patients who have a hematologic malignancy, are neutropenic, have received a hematopoietic cell or solid-organ transplant, or have severe burn wounds.

Clinical Manifestations In immunocompetent persons, *Fusarium* species cause localized infections of various organs. These organisms are a common cause of fungal keratitis, which can extend into the anterior chamber of the eye, cause loss of vision, and require corneal transplantation. Onychomycosis due to *Fusarium* species, while basically an annoyance in immunocompetent patients, is a source of subsequent hematogenous dissemination and should be aggressively sought and treated in neutropenic patients. In profoundly immunocompromised patients, fusariosis is angioinvasive, and clinical manifestations mimic those of aspergillosis. Pulmonary infection is characterized by multiple nodular lesions. Sinus infection is likely to lead to invasion of adjacent structures. Disseminated fusariosis occurs primarily in neutropenic patients with hematologic malignancies and in allogeneic hematopoietic cell transplant recipients. Disseminated fusariosis differs from

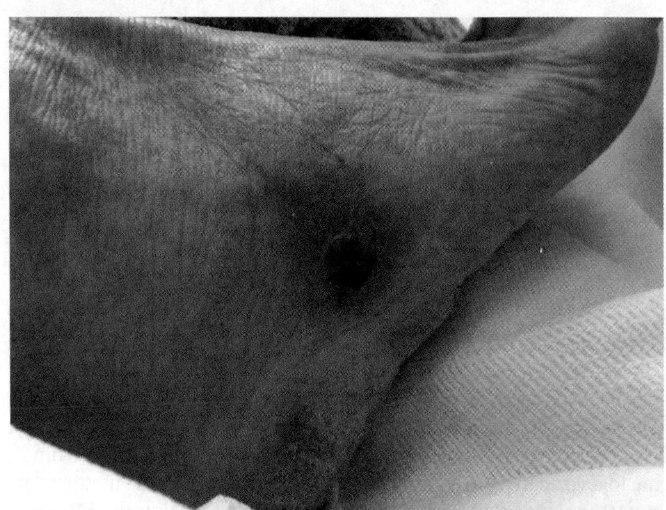

FIGURE 219-2 Painful necrotic foot lesion that developed over a week in a woman who had acute leukemia and who had been neutropenic for 2 months. *Fusarium* species were grown from a punch biopsy. *(Courtesy of Dr. Nessrine Ktaich.)*

disseminated aspergillosis in that skin lesions are extremely common with fusariosis; the lesions are nodular or necrotic, are usually painful, and appear over time in different locations (Fig. 219-2).

Diagnosis The diagnostic approach usually includes both documentation of the growth of *Fusarium* species from involved tissue and demonstration of invasion by histopathologic techniques that show septate hyphae in tissues. The organism is difficult to differentiate from *Aspergillus* species in tissues; thus, identification with culture is imperative. An extremely helpful diagnostic clue is growth in blood cultures, which are positive in as many as 50% of patients with disseminated fusariosis.

Treatment and Prognosis *Fusarium* species are resistant to many antifungal agents. A lipid formulation of AmB, voriconazole, or posaconazole is recommended. Many physicians use both a lipid formulation of AmB and either voriconazole or posaconazole because susceptibility information is not standardized and is not always predictive of clinical response. Serum drug levels should be monitored with either azole to ensure that absorption is adequate and with voriconazole to avoid toxicity. Mortality rates for disseminated fusariosis have been as high as 85%. With the improved antifungal therapy now available, mortality rates have fallen to ~50%. However, if neutropenia persists, the mortality rate approaches 100%.

■ SCEDOSPORIOSIS AND LOMENTOSPORIOSIS

Etiologic Agent, Epidemiology, and Pathogenesis *Scedosporium apiospermum* complex, which is composed of several related species, is reported more often as a cause of human infection than *Lomentospora prolificans,* formerly *Scedosporium prolificans,* but both are major pathogens in immunocompromised hosts, causing pneumonia, disseminated infection, and brain abscess. Organisms of the *S. apiospermum* complex are found worldwide in temperate climates in tidal flats, swamps, ponds, manure, and soil. *L. prolificans* also is found in soil but is more geographically restricted. Infection occurs predominantly through inhalation of conidia, but direct inoculation through the skin or into the eye also can occur.

Clinical Manifestations Among immunocompetent persons, *Scedosporium* and *Lomentospora* species are a prominent cause of eumycetoma. Keratitis as a result of accidental corneal inoculation is a sight-threatening infection. In patients who have hematologic malignancies (especially acute leukemia with neutropenia), recipients of solid-organ or hematopoietic cell transplants, and patients receiving glucocorticoids, these organisms are angioinvasive, causing pneumonia and widespread dissemination. Pulmonary infection mimics aspergillosis; nodules, cavities, and lobar infiltrates are common. Disseminated infection involves the skin, heart, brain, and many other organs. Skin lesions are not as common or as painful as those of fusariosis.

Diagnosis Diagnosis depends on the growth of *Scedosporium* or *Lomentospora* species from involved tissue and the histologic demonstration of septate hyphae invading tissues. Culture evidence is essential because these molds are difficult to differentiate from *Aspergillus* in tissues, and demonstration of tissue invasion is essential because these ubiquitous environmental molds can be mere contaminants or colonizers. *L. prolificans* can grow in blood cultures, but *S. apiospermum* usually does not.

Treatment and Prognosis *Scedosporium* and *Lomentospora* species are resistant to AmB, echinocandins, and some azoles. Voriconazole is the agent of choice for *S. apiospermum*, and posaconazole also can be used for this infection. *L. prolificans* is resistant in vitro to almost every available antifungal agent; the addition of agents such as terbinafine to a voriconazole regimen has been attempted because in vitro data suggest possible synergy against some strains of *L. prolificans*. Mortality rates for invasive *S. apiospermum* infection are ~50%, but those for invasive *L. prolificans* infection remain as high as 85–100%.

TRICHOSPORONOSIS

Etiologic Agent, Epidemiology, and Pathogenesis The genus *Trichosporon* contains many species, some of which cause localized infection of hair and nails. The major pathogen responsible for invasive infection is *Trichosporon asahii*. *Trichosporon* species grow as yeast-like colonies in vitro; in vivo, however, hyphae, pseudohyphae, and arthroconidia, in addition to yeast forms, can be seen. These yeasts are commonly found in soil, sewage, and water and in rare instances can colonize human skin and the human gastrointestinal tract. Most infections follow inhalation or entry via central venous catheters. Systemic infection occurs almost exclusively in immunocompromised hosts, including those who have hematologic malignancies, are neutropenic, have received a solid-organ or hematopoietic cell transplant, or are receiving glucocorticoids.

Clinical Manifestations Disseminated trichosporonosis resembles invasive candidiasis, and fungemia is often the initial manifestation of infection. Pneumonia, skin lesions, and sepsis are common. The skin lesions begin as papules or nodules surrounded by erythema and progress to central necrosis. A chronic form of infection mimics hepatosplenic candidiasis (chronic disseminated candidiasis).

Diagnosis The diagnosis of systemic *Trichosporon* infection is established by growth of the organism from involved tissues or from blood. Histopathologic examination of a skin lesion showing a mixture of yeast forms, arthroconidia, and hyphae can lead to an early presumptive diagnosis of trichosporonosis. The serum cryptococcal antigen latex agglutination test may be positive in patients with disseminated trichosporonosis, because *T. asahii* and *Cryptococcus neoformans* share polysaccharide antigens.

Treatment and Prognosis Rates of response to AmB have been disappointing, and many *Trichosporon* isolates are resistant in vitro. Voriconazole is the antifungal agent of choice. The mortality rates for disseminated *Trichosporon* infection have been as high as 70% but are decreasing with the use of voriconazole; however, patients who remain neutropenic are likely to succumb to this infection.

SUPERFICIAL CUTANEOUS INFECTIONS

Fungal infections of the skin and skin structures are caused by molds and yeasts that do not invade deeper tissues but rather cause disease merely by inhabiting the superficial layers of skin, hair follicles, and nails. These agents are the most common fungal infections of humans but only rarely cause serious infections.

YEAST INFECTIONS

Etiologic Agents, Epidemiology, and Pathogenesis *Malassezia* species, primarily *M. furfur* and M. *pachydermatis*, are lipophilic yeasts that generally cause only minor skin infections but, on occasion, can cause invasive infection. *Malassezia* species are part of the indigenous human microbiota found in the stratum corneum of the back, chest, scalp, and face—areas rich in sebaceous glands. The organisms do not invade below the stratum corneum and generally elicit little if any inflammatory response.

Clinical Manifestations *Malassezia* species cause tinea versicolor (also called *pityriasis versicolor*), folliculitis, and seborrheic dermatitis. Tinea versicolor presents as flat round scaly patches of hypo- or hyperpigmented skin on the neck, chest, or upper arms. The lesions are usually asymptomatic but can be pruritic. They can be mistaken for vitiligo, but the latter is not scaly. Folliculitis occurs on the back and chest and mimics bacterial folliculitis. Seborrheic dermatitis manifests as erythematous pruritic scaly lesions in the eyebrows, moustache, nasolabial folds, and scalp (dandruff). Seborrheic dermatitis can be severe in patients with advanced AIDS. Fungemia and disseminated infection occur rarely with *Malassezia* species, and almost always this occurs in premature neonates receiving parenteral lipid preparations through a central venous catheter.

Diagnosis *Malassezia* infections are diagnosed clinically in most cases. If scrapings are collected on a microscope slide on which a drop of potassium hydroxide has been placed, a mixture of budding yeasts and short septate hyphae is seen. In order to culture *Malassezia* from those patients in whom disseminated infection is suspected, sterile olive oil must be added to the medium.

Treatment and Prognosis Topical creams and lotions, including selenium sulfide shampoo, ketoconazole shampoo or cream, and terbinafine cream, are effective in treating *Malassezia* infections and are usually given for 2 weeks. Other more expensive antifungal creams are rarely needed. Mild topical steroid creams are sometimes used to treat seborrheic dermatitis. For extensive disease, oral itraconazole or fluconazole (200 mg daily) can be used for 5–7 days. The rare cases of fungemia caused by *Malassezia* species are treated with AmB or an azole, such as voriconazole, prompt removal of the catheter, and discontinuance of parenteral lipid infusions. *Malassezia* skin infections are benign and self-limited, although recurrences are the rule. The outcome of systemic infection depends on the host's underlying conditions, but most infected neonates do well.

DERMATOPHYTE (MOLD) INFECTIONS

Etiologic Agents, Epidemiology, and Pathogenesis The molds that cause skin infections in humans include the genera *Trichophyton*, *Microsporum*, and *Epidermophyton*. These organisms, which are not components of the normal skin microbiota, can live within the keratinized structures of the skin—hence the term *dermatophytes*. Dermatophytes occur worldwide, and infections with these organisms are extremely common. Some organisms cause disease only in humans and can be transmitted by person-to-person contact and by fomites, such as hairbrushes or wet floors, that have been contaminated by infected individuals. Several species cause infections in cats and dogs and can readily be transmitted from these animals to humans, and others are spread from contact with soil. The characteristic ring shape of cutaneous lesions is the result of the organisms' outward growth in a centrifugal pattern in the stratum corneum. Fungal invasion of the nail usually occurs through the lateral or superficial nail plates and then spreads throughout the nail; when hair shafts are invaded, the organisms can be found either within the shaft or surrounding it. Symptoms are caused by the inflammatory reaction elicited by fungal antigens and not by tissue invasion. Dermatophyte infections occur more commonly in males than in females, and progesterone has been shown to inhibit dermatophyte growth.

Clinical Manifestations Dermatophyte infection of the skin is often called *ringworm*. This term is confusing because worms are not involved. *Tinea*, the Latin word for *worm*, describes the serpentine nature of the skin lesions. Tinea is a less confusing term and can be used with the name of the body part affected—e.g., tinea capitis (head), tinea pedis (feet), tinea corporis (body), tinea cruris (crotch), and tinea unguium (nails, although infection at this site is more often termed *onychomycosis*).

Tinea capitis occurs most commonly in children 3–7 years old. Children with tinea capitis usually present with well-demarcated scaly patches in which hair shafts are broken off right above the skin; alopecia can result. Tinea corporis is manifested by well-demarcated, annular, pruritic, scaly lesions that undergo central clearing. Usually one or several small lesions are present. However, in some patients, tinea corporis can involve much of the trunk. The rash should be differentiated from contact dermatitis, eczema, and psoriasis. Tinea cruris is seen almost exclusively in men. The perineal rash is erythematous and pustular, has a discrete scaly border, is without satellite lesions, and is usually pruritic. The rash must be differentiated from intertriginous candidiasis, erythrasma, and psoriasis.

Tinea pedis also is more common among men than among women. It usually starts in the web spaces of the toes; peeling, maceration, and pruritus are followed by development of a scaly pruritic rash along the lateral and plantar surfaces of the feet. Hyperkeratosis of the soles of the feet often ensues. Tinea pedis has been implicated in lower-extremity cellulitis, as streptococci and staphylococci can gain entrance to the tissues through fissures between the toes. Onychomycosis affects toenails more often than fingernails and is most common among persons who have tinea pedis. The nail becomes thickened and discolored and may crumble; onycholysis almost always occurs. Onychomycosis is more common in older adults and in persons with vascular disease, diabetes mellitus, and trauma to the nails. Fungal infection must be differentiated from psoriasis, which can mimic onychomycosis but usually has associated skin lesions.

Diagnosis Many dermatophyte infections are diagnosed by their clinical appearance. If the diagnosis is in doubt, scrapings should be taken from the edge of a lesion with a scalpel blade, transferred to a slide to which a drop of potassium hydroxide is added, and examined under a microscope for the presence of hyphae. Cultures are indicated if an outbreak is suspected or the patient does not respond to therapy.

Treatment and Prognosis Dermatophyte infections usually respond to topical therapy. Lotions or sprays are easier than creams to apply to large or hairy areas. Particularly for tinea cruris, the affected area should be kept as dry as possible. When patients have extensive skin lesions, oral itraconazole or terbinafine can hasten resolution (**Table 219-3**). Terbinafine interacts with fewer drugs than itraconazole and is generally the first-line agent.

Onychomycosis generally does not respond to topical therapy, although efinaconazole topical solution applied to the affected nail for as long as a year has been shown to be beneficial in several trials. Itraconazole and terbinafine both accumulate in the nail plate and can be used to treat onychomycosis (Table 219-3). The major decision to be made with regard to therapy is whether the extent of nail involvement justifies the use of systemic antifungal agents that have adverse effects, may interact with other drugs, and are very costly. Treating for cosmetic reasons alone is discouraged. Relapses of tinea cruris and tinea pedis are common and should be treated as early as possible with topical creams to avoid development of more extensive disease. Relapses of onychomycosis follow treatment in 25–30% of cases.

TABLE 219-3 Suggested Oral Treatment for Extensive Tinea Infections and Onychomycosis

ANTIFUNGAL AGENT	SUGGESTED DOSAGE	COMMENTS
Extensive Tinea Infection		
Terbinafine	250 mg/d for 1–2 weeks	Adverse reactions minimal with short treatment period
Itraconazole[a]	200 mg/d for 1–2 weeks	Adverse reactions minimal with short treatment period except for drug interactions
Onychomycosis		
Terbinafine	250 mg/d for 3 months	Slightly superior to itraconazole; monitor for hepatotoxicity
Itraconazole[a]	200 mg/d for 3 months *or* 200 mg bid for 1 week each month for 3 months	Drug interactions frequent; monitor for hepatotoxicity; rarely causes hypokalemia, hypertension, edema; use with caution in patients with congestive heart failure

[a]Itraconazole capsules require food and gastric acid for absorption, whereas itraconazole solution is taken on an empty stomach.

FURTHER READING

Bonifaz A, Tirado-Sanchez A: Cutaneous disseminated and extracutaneous sporotrichosis: Current status of a complex disease. J Fungi 3:6, 2017.

De Almeida Junior JN, Hennequin C: Invasive *Trichosporon* infections: A systematic review on a re-emerging fungal pathogen. Front Microbiol 7:1629, 2016.

Nelson KE et al: Penicilliosis, in *Essentials of Clinical Mycology*, 2nd ed. CA Kauffman et al (eds). New York, Springer, 2011, pp 399–411.

Nucci M et al: Fusariosis. Semin Respir Crit Care Med 36:706, 2015.

Ramirez-Garcia A et al: *Scedosporium* and *Lomentospora*: An updated overview of underrated opportunists. Med Mycol 56(suppl 1): 102, 2018.

Revankar SG et al: A Mycoses Study Group international prospective study of phaeohyphomycosis: An analysis of 99 proven/probable cases. Open Forum Infect Dis 4:ofx200, 2017.

Shikanai-Yasuda MA et al: Brazilian guidelines for the clinical management of paracoccidioidomycosis. Rev Soc Bras Med Trop 50:715, 2017.

Theelan B et al: The *Malassezia* genus in skin and systemic diseases. Med Mycol 56:510, 2018.

Woo TE et al: Diagnosis and management of cutaneous tinea infections. Adv Skin Wound Care 32:350, 2019.

220 *Pneumocystis* Infections

Alison Morris, Henry Masur

DEFINITION AND DESCRIPTION

Pneumocystis is an opportunistic pathogen that is an important cause of pneumonia in immunocompromised hosts, particularly those with HIV infection (**Chap. 202**), organ transplants, or hematologic malignancies and those receiving high-dose glucocorticoids or certain immunosuppressive monoclonal antibodies. *Pneumocystis* was discovered in rodents in 1909 and was initially believed to be a protozoan. Because *Pneumocystis* cannot be cultured, our understanding of its biology has been limited, but molecular techniques have demonstrated that the organism is actually a fungus. Formerly known as *Pneumocystis carinii*, the species infecting humans has been renamed *Pneumocystis jirovecii*.

EPIDEMIOLOGY

Pneumocystis jirovecii pneumonia (PCP) came to medical attention in the early 1950s when pathologists in Czechoslovakia recognized *Pneumocystis* in the alveolar exudates of infants involved in nursery outbreaks of interstitial pneumonia, outbreaks that had been described in Europe since the 1920s. Among adults, PCP was rarely recognized until the populations of immunosuppressed adults increased due to the development of immunosuppressive therapies for solid-organ transplantation, bone marrow transplantation, cancer, and autoimmune disorders, and the development of better pulmonary diagnostic techniques such as bronchoscopy. In 1981, PCP was first reported in men who had sex with men and in intravenous (IV) drug users who had no obvious cause of immunosuppression. These cases were subsequently recognized as the first presentations of what came to be known as the acquired immunodeficiency syndrome (AIDS) (**Chap. 202**).

The incidence of PCP increased dramatically as the AIDS epidemic grew: without chemoprophylaxis or antiretroviral therapy (ART), 80–90% of patients with HIV/AIDS in North America and Western Europe ultimately developed one or more episodes of PCP. While its incidence declined with the introduction of anti-*Pneumocystis* prophylaxis and combination ART, PCP has continued to be a leading cause of AIDS-associated morbidity in the United States and Western Europe, particularly in individuals who do not know they are infected with HIV until they are profoundly immunosuppressed and in people living with HIV (PLWH) with CD4+ T lymphocyte counts of <200/μL who are not receiving ART or PCP prophylaxis.

PCP also develops in HIV-uninfected patients who are immunocompromised secondary to hematologic or malignant neoplasms, stem cell or solid-organ transplantation, and treatment with immunosuppressive medications. The incidence of PCP depends on the degree and duration of immunosuppression. PCP is increasingly reported among individuals receiving tumor necrosis factor α inhibitors and immunosuppressive monoclonal antibodies for autoimmune, rheumatologic, or neoplastic diseases. While clinical disease due to *Pneumocystis* in immunocompetent hosts has not been clearly documented, studies have shown that *Pneumocystis* organisms can colonize the airways of children and adults who are not immunocompromised. The relevance of these organisms to acute or chronic syndromes, such as chronic obstructive pulmonary disease (COPD), in immunocompetent patients is being investigated.

In some developing countries, the incidence of PCP among PLWH has been reported to be lower than that in industrialized countries. This lower incidence may be due to competing mortality from infectious diseases such as tuberculosis and bacterial pneumonia, which typically occur before patients become immunosuppressed enough to develop PCP. Geographic variations in *Pneumocystis* exposure and underdiagnosis attributable to lack of diagnostic resources also may explain the apparent lower frequency of PCP in some countries.

■ PATHOGENESIS AND PATHOLOGY

Life Cycle and Transmission The life cycle of *Pneumocystis* likely involves both sexual and asexual reproduction. The organism exists as a trophic form, a cyst, and a precyst. Studies in rodents show that immunocompetent animals can serve as reservoirs for respiratory transmission of *P. carinii* (the infecting species in rodents) to immunocompetent and immunosuppressed animals. Human *Pneumocystis* is thought to be transmitted by a respiratory route as well. *P. jirovecii*, like all pneumocystis species, is host-specific. Thus, humans are not infected, for example, by *P. carinii* (rodents) or *P. oryctolagi* (rabbits), but are only infected by *P. jirovecii*.

Serologic and molecular studies have demonstrated that most humans are exposed to *P. jirovecii* early in life. It was historically thought that *Pneumocystis* pneumonia usually developed from reactivation of latent infection. However, molecular evidence makes it clear that children and adults can develop PCP from primary infection or reinfection. It is difficult to prove whether reactivation of latent infection in fact occurs. The source of infection is thought to be either healthy or immunosuppressed individuals who themselves experienced recent infection or reinfection, or immunosuppressed persons with clinical PCP. Nosocomial outbreaks occur in inpatient and outpatient settings. The utility of droplet or airborne isolation for preventing transmission from patients with PCP to other immunosuppressed individuals has been debated; no clear evidence exists, although it seems prudent to isolate patients with active PCP from other immunosuppressed patients using at least droplet precautions.

Role of Immunity Defects in cellular and/or humoral immunity predispose to development of PCP. Such defects may be congenital, or they may be acquired as a result of HIV infection or of treatment with immunosuppressive drugs such as glucocorticoids, fludarabine, temozolomide, temsirolimus, cyclophosphamide, rituximab, or alemtuzumab. CD4+ T cells are critical in host defense against *Pneumocystis*. Among PLWH, the incidence of PCP is inversely related to the CD4+ T-cell count: at least 80% of cases occur at counts of <200/μL, and most of these cases develop at counts of <100/μL. HIV viral load is another factor that predisposes patients to PCP. CD4+ T-cell counts are less useful in predicting the risk of PCP in patients who are immunosuppressed for reasons other than HIV infection. Clinicians must recognize that PCP can occur at CD4+ T-cell counts >200/μL in any immunosuppressed population including persons with HIV infection. Such occurrences are especially common in patients who are immunosuppressed due to causes other than HIV infection, especially among patients who have undergone solid-organ transplantation, since CD4+ T-cell counts are not as sensitive and specific indicators of PCP as they are in PLWH.

Lung Pathology *Pneumocystis* has a unique tropism for the lung. Organisms are presumably inhaled into the alveolar space after being exhaled by another human. Clinically apparent pneumonia occurs only if an individual is immunocompromised. *Pneumocystis* proliferates in the lung, provoking a mononuclear cell response. The alveoli become filled with proteinaceous material, and alveolar damage results in increased alveolar-capillary injury and surfactant abnormalities. Stained lung sections typically show foamy, vacuolated alveolar exudates composed largely of viable and nonviable organisms (**Fig. 220-1*A***). Interstitial edema and fibrosis may develop, and organisms can be seen in the alveolar space with silver or other stains. Moreover, the organisms can be seen when tissue is subjected to colorimetric or immunofluorescent staining (**Fig. 220-1*B*–*1D***).

■ CLINICAL FEATURES

Clinical Presentation PCP presents as acute or subacute pneumonia that may initially be characterized by a vague sense of dyspnea alone but that subsequently manifests as fever and nonproductive cough with progressive shortness of breath. Patients may ultimately progress to respiratory failure and death. Extrapulmonary manifestations of PCP are rare but can include involvement of almost any organ, most notably the lymph nodes, spleen, and liver.

Physical Examination, Oxygen Saturation, and Imaging The physical examination findings in PCP are nonspecific. Patients have decreased oxygen saturation—at rest or with exertion—that, without treatment, progresses to severe hypoxemia. Patients may initially have a normal chest examination and no adventitious sounds, but later develop diffuse rales and signs of consolidation.

Laboratory Findings The results of routine laboratory tests are nonspecific in PCP. Serum levels of lactate dehydrogenase (LDH) are often elevated as a result of pulmonary damage; however, a normal LDH level does not rule out PCP, nor is an elevated LDH value specific for PCP. The peripheral white blood cell count may be elevated in relation to the patient's baseline values, but the increase is usually modest. Hepatic and renal function are typically normal.

Radiographic Findings Although the initial chest radiograph may be normal when patients have mild symptoms, the classic radiographic appearance of symptomatic PCP consists of diffuse bilateral interstitial infiltrates that are perihilar and symmetric (**Fig. 220-2*A***)—yet another finding that is not specific for PCP. The interstitial infiltrates can progress to alveolar filling (**Fig. 220-2*B***). High-resolution chest CT shows diffuse ground-glass opacities in virtually all patients with PCP, often before a routine chest radiograph becomes abnormal (**Fig. 220-2*C***). A normal chest CT essentially rules out the diagnosis of PCP. Pneumatoceles and pneumothoraces are characteristic chest radiographic findings, especially in patients with HIV infection (**Fig. 220-2*D***). A wide variety of atypical radiographic findings have been described, including asymmetric patterns, upper-lobe infiltrates, mediastinal adenopathy, nodules, cavities, and effusions.

■ DIAGNOSIS

The optimal sample for a specific microbiologic diagnostic examination depends on how ill the patient is and what resources are

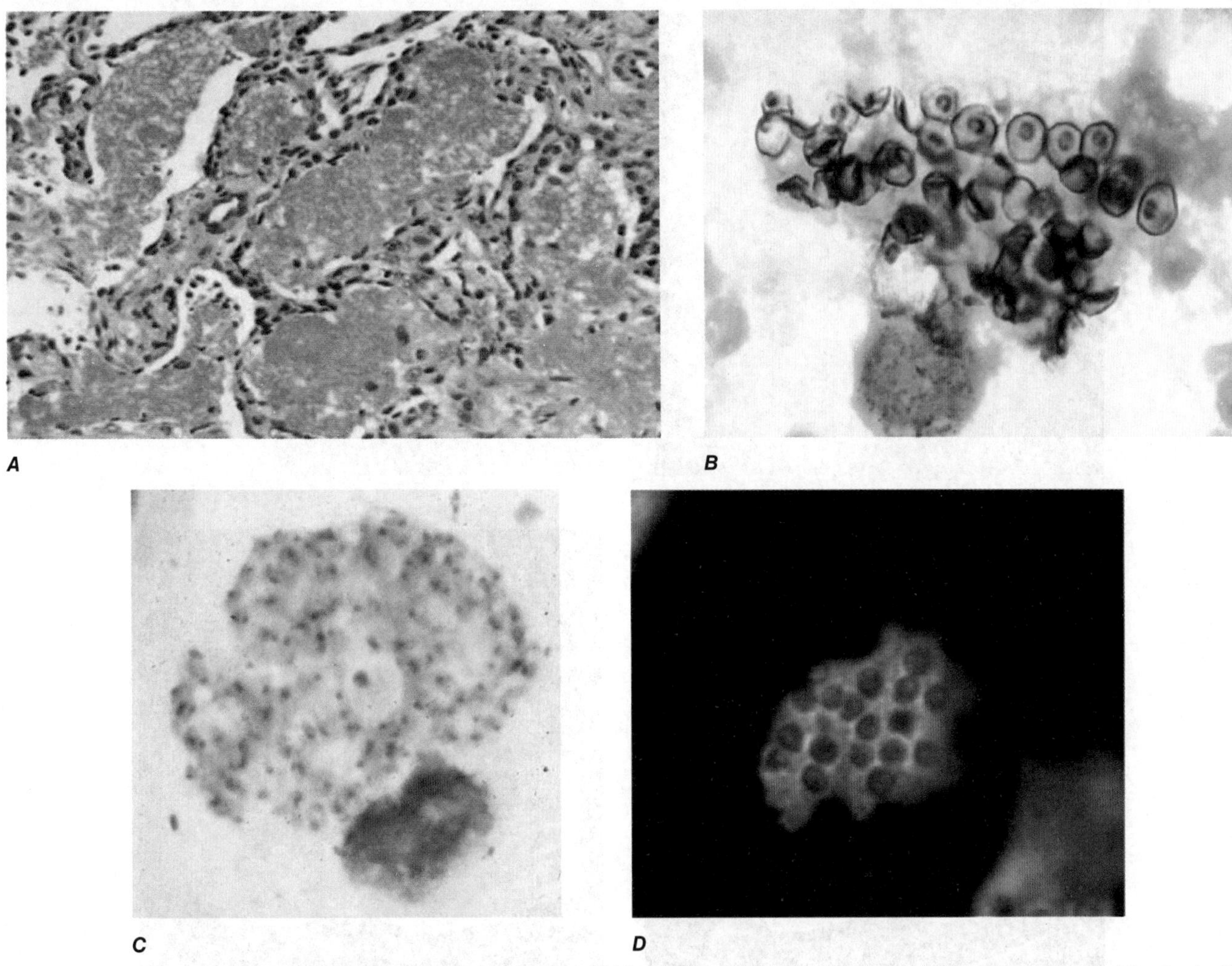

FIGURE 220-1 Direct microscopy of *Pneumocystis* pneumonia. *A.* Transbronchial lung biopsy stained with hematoxylin and eosin shows eosinophilic alveolar filling. ***B.*** Methenamine silver–stained bronchoalveolar lavage (BAL) fluid. ***C.*** Giemsa-stained BAL fluid. ***D.*** Immunofluorescent stain of BAL fluid.

available. Before the 1990s, diagnoses of PCP were usually established by open lung biopsy; later, transbronchial lung biopsy was employed. Hematoxylin and eosin staining of pulmonary tissue demonstrates a foamy alveolar infiltrate and a mononuclear interstitial infiltrate (Fig. 220-1*A*). This appearance is pathognomonic for PCP even though the organisms cannot be specifically identified with this stain. The diagnosis is typically established in lung tissue or pulmonary secretions by staining of the cyst—e.g., with methenamine silver (Fig. 220-1*B*), toluidine blue O, or Giemsa (Fig. 220-1*C*)—or by staining with a specific immunofluorescent antibody (Fig. 220-1*D*).

The demonstration of organisms in bronchoalveolar lavage (BAL) fluid is almost 100% sensitive and specific for PCP in patients with HIV infection and is almost as sensitive in patients with immunosuppression due to other processes. The organisms are identified in pulmonary secretions with the specific stains indicated above for lung biopsy. While expectorated sputum or throat swabs have very low sensitivity, an induced sputum sample obtained and interpreted by an experienced provider can be highly sensitive and specific; however, the sensitivity is dependent on both the characteristics of the patient and the experience of the center conducting the test and is widely variable (55–90%).

Many laboratories now offer polymerase chain reaction (PCR) testing of respiratory specimens for *Pneumocystis* in preference to direct microscopy of appropriately stained respiratory secretions. However, these PCR tests are so sensitive that it is difficult to distinguish patients with colonization (i.e., those whose acute lung disease is due to some other process but who have low levels of *Pneumocystis* DNA in the lungs) from those with acute pneumonia due to *Pneumocystis*. Such PCR tests on appropriate samples may be more useful for ruling out a diagnosis of PCP if they are negative than for definitively attributing the disease to *Pneumocystis*.

There has been considerable interest in serologic tests, such as assays for (1→3)-β-D-glucan, a component of the fungal cell wall. These levels are frequently elevated in patients with PCP. However, serum or BAL (1→3)-β-D-glucan levels are not perfectly sensitive or highly specific for PCP. There are increasing numbers of reports of serum PCR tests for *Pneumocystis*, but such tests are still in preliminary stages of development.

COURSE AND PROGNOSIS

Untreated, PCP is invariably fatal. Patients with HIV infection often have an indolent course that may present early as mild exercise intolerance or chest tightness without fever or cough and a normal or nearly normal posterior–anterior chest radiograph but progresses over days, weeks, or even a few months to fever, cough, diffuse alveolar infiltrates, and profound hypoxemia. Some patients with HIV infection and most patients with other types of immunosuppression have more acute disease that progresses over a few days to respiratory failure. Rare patients also develop distributive shock. A few unusual patients present with extrapulmonary manifestations in the skin or soft tissue, retina, brain, liver, kidney, or spleen. Extrapulmonary disease is nonspecific in presentation and can be diagnosed only by histology. When there is extrapulmonary clinical disease in a patient with PCP, the priority is to determine what other concurrent infectious or neoplastic process might be present, given the rarity of extrapulmonary pneumocystosis.

Factors that influence mortality risk of PCP include the patient's age and degree of immunosuppression as well as the presence of preexisting lung disease, a low serum albumin level, the need for mechanical ventilation, and the development of a pneumothorax. With advances in supportive critical care, the prognosis for patients with PCP who require intubation and respiratory support has improved and now

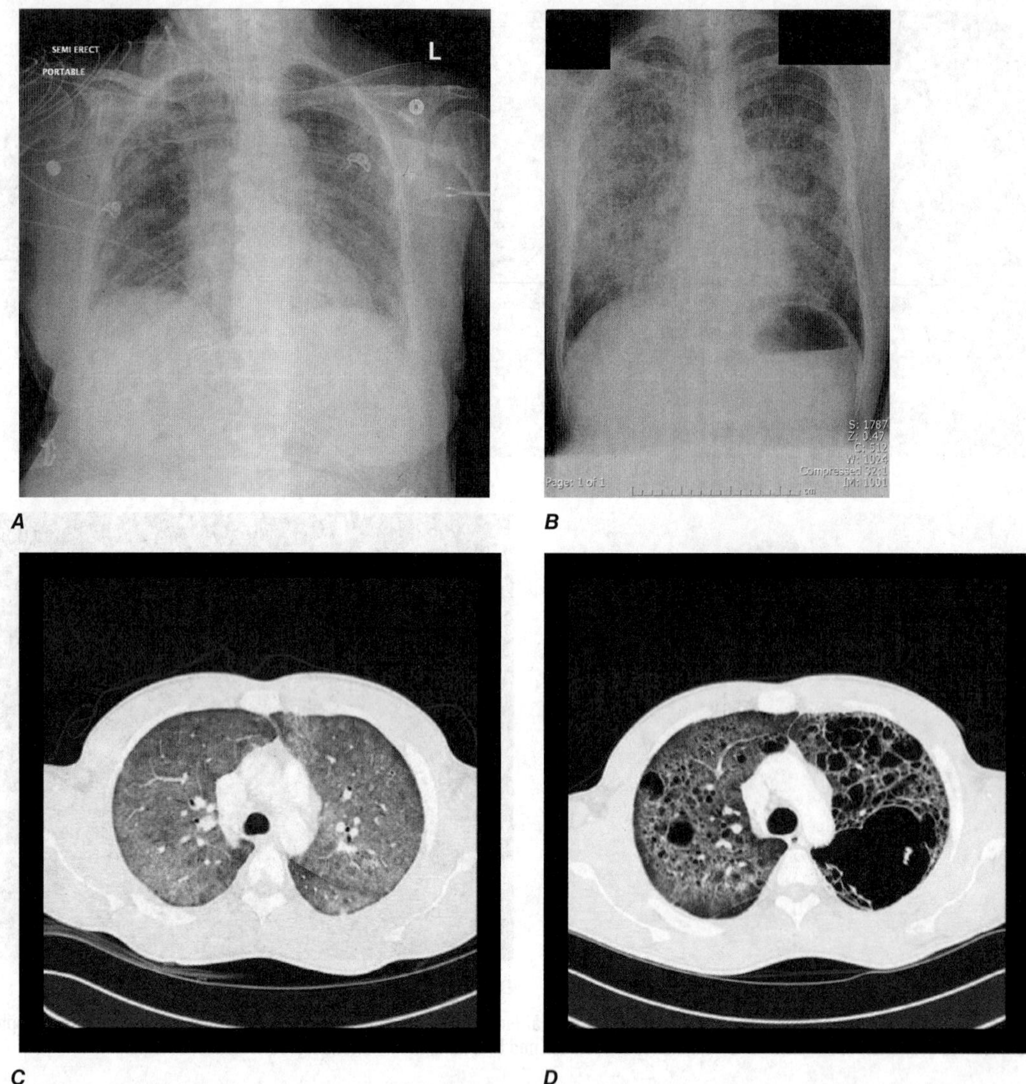

FIGURE 220-2 Radiographs in *Pneumocystis* pneumonia. ***A.*** Posterior–anterior chest radiograph showing symmetric interstitial infiltrates. ***B.*** Posterior–anterior chest radiograph showing symmetric alveolar infiltrates (courtesy of Alison Morris). ***C.*** CT image demonstrating symmetric interstitial infiltrates and ground-glass opacities. ***D.*** CT image showing symmetric interstitial infiltrates, ground-glass opacities, and pneumatoceles.

depends to a large extent on comorbidities and the prognosis of the underlying disease. Since patients typically do not respond to therapy for 4–8 days, supportive care for a minimum of 10 days is a reasonable consideration if such support is compatible with the patient's wishes and the prognosis of comorbidities. Patients whose condition continues to deteriorate after 3 or 4 days or has not improved after 7–10 days should be reevaluated to determine whether other infectious processes are present (either having been missed on initial evaluation or having developed during treatment), whether initial anti-*Pneumocystis* treatment has failed, or whether noninfectious processes (e.g., congestive heart failure, pulmonary emboli, pulmonary hypertension, drug toxicity, or a neoplastic process) are causing pulmonary dysfunction.

TREATMENT

P. jirovecii Pneumonia

The treatment of choice for PCP is trimethoprim-sulfamethoxazole (TMP-SMX), given either IV or PO for 14 days to non-HIV-infected patients with mild disease and for 21 days to all other patients (**Table 220-1**). TMP-SMX, which interferes with the organism's folate metabolism, is at least as effective as alternative agents and is better tolerated. TMP-SMX can cause leukopenia, hepatitis, rash, and fever as well as anaphylactic and anaphylactoid reactions. Patients with HIV infection have an unusually high incidence of hypersensitivity to TMP-SMX. Monitoring of serum drug levels is useful if renal function or toxicities are issues in order to enhance the likelihood that therapy will be effective and toxicity will be avoided. Maintenance of a 2-h post-dose serum sulfamethoxazole level of 100–150 μg/mL has been associated with a successful outcome. Resistance to TMP-SMX cannot be measured by organism growth inhibition in the laboratory because *Pneumocystis* cannot be cultured. However, mutations in the target gene for sulfamethoxazole that confer in vitro sulfa resistance when found in other organisms have been recognized in *Pneumocystis*. The clinical relevance of these mutations for the response to therapy is unknown. Sulfadiazine plus pyrimethamine, an oral regimen more often used for treatment of toxoplasmosis, also is highly effective.

Intravenous pentamidine or the combination of clindamycin plus primaquine is an option for patients who cannot tolerate TMP-SMX and for patients in whose treatment TMP-SMX appears to be failing. Pentamidine must be given IV over at least 60 min to avoid potentially lethal hypotension. Adverse effects can be severe and irreversible and include renal dysfunction, dysglycemia (life-threatening hypoglycemia that can occur days or weeks after initial infusion and be followed by hyperglycemia), neutropenia, and torsades des pointes. Clindamycin plus primaquine is effective, but primaquine can be given only by the oral route—a disadvantage for patients who cannot ingest or absorb oral drugs. Oral atovaquone is also a reasonable option for patients with mild disease who have no

TABLE 220-1 Treatment of *Pneumocystis* pneumonia[a]

DRUG(S)	DOSE, ROUTE	ADVERSE EFFECTS
First-Choice Agent		
TMP-SMX	TMP (5 mg/kg) plus SMX (25 mg/kg) q6–8h PO or IV (i.e., 2 double-strength tablets tid or qid)	Fever, rash, cytopenias, hepatitis, hyperkalemia
Alternative Agents		
Atovaquone	750 mg bid PO	Rash, fever, hepatitis
Clindamycin *plus* Primaquine	300–450 mg q6h PO or 600 mg q6–8h IV 15–30 mg qd PO	Hemolysis (G6PD deficiency), methemoglobinemia, neutropenia, rash
Pentamidine	3–4 mg/kg qd IV	Hypotension, azotemia, cardiac arrhythmias (torsades des pointes), pancreatitis, dysglycemias, hypocalcemia, neutropenia, hepatitis
Adjunctive Agent		
Prednisone or methylprednisolone	40 mg bid × 5 d, 40 mg qd × 5 d, 20 mg qd × 11 d; PO or IV	Peptic ulcer disease, hyperglycemia, mood alteration, hypertension

[a]Treatment can be administered for 14 days to non-HIV-infected patients with mild disease and for 21 days to all other patients.

Abbreviations: G6PD, glucose-6-phosphate dehydrogenase; TMP-SMX, trimethoprim-sulfamethoxazole.

impediments to absorbing an oral drug that requires a high-fat meal for optimal absorption. There is some evidence for activity of echinocandins against the cyst form (but not the trophozoite form) of pneumocystis, but the role for echinocandins as part of combination therapy is currently uncertain.

A major advance in therapy for PCP was the recognition that glucocorticoids could improve survival rates among PLWH with moderate to severe disease (room air PO_2 <70 mmHg or alveolar–arterial oxygen gradient ≥35 mmHg). Glucocorticoids appear to reduce the pulmonary inflammation that occurs after specific therapy is started and organisms begin to die, eliciting inflammation. Therapy with glucocorticoids should be the standard of care for patients with HIV infection and probably is also effective for patients with other immunodeficiencies. This treatment should be started for moderate or severe disease when therapy for PCP is initiated, even if the diagnosis is suspected but has not yet been confirmed. If PLWH or HIV-uninfected patients are receiving high-dose glucocorticoids when they develop PCP, there are theoretical advantages to either increasing the steroid dose (to reduce the inflammatory response to the dying organisms) or decreasing the steroid dose (to improve immune function), but there is no convincing evidence on which to base any specific strategy.

No definitive trials have defined the best therapeutic algorithm for patients in whom TMP-SMX treatment for PCP is failing. If no other treatable infectious or noninfectious processes are detected and pulmonary dysfunction appears to be due to PCP alone, many authorities would switch from TMP-SMX to either IV pentamidine or IV clindamycin plus oral primaquine. Some authorities would add the second drug or drug combination to TMP-SMX rather than switching regimens. If patients are not already receiving them, glucocorticoids should be added to the regimen; the dosage and regimen, which are usually chosen empirically, depend on what glucocorticoid regimen (if any) the patient was receiving when PCP therapy was begun.

For patients with HIV infection who present with PCP before the initiation of ART, ART should be started within the first 2 weeks of therapy for PCP in most situations. Immune reconstitution inflammatory syndrome (IRIS) can occur, and the decision to initiate ART thus requires considerable expertise in optimal timing relative to PCP recovery as well as for the other factors that are relevant when ART is initiated in any patient.

PREVENTION

The most effective method for preventing PCP is to eliminate the cause of immunosuppression by withdrawing immunosuppressive therapy or treating the underlying cause (e.g., HIV infection). Patients who are susceptible to PCP benefit from chemoprophylaxis during the period of susceptibility. For patients with HIV infection, CD4+ T-cell counts are a reliable marker of susceptibility, and counts below 200/μL are an indication to start prophylaxis (**Table 220-2**).

For patients who are immunosuppressed as a result of factors other than HIV infection, there is no laboratory parameter, including the CD4+ T-cell count, that predicts susceptibility to PCP with adequate positive and negative accuracy. The period of susceptibility is usually estimated on the basis of experience with the underlying disease and immunosuppressive regimen. Premature cessation of prophylaxis has been associated with clusters of cases in certain patient populations, such as solid-organ transplant recipients. Patients receiving a prolonged course of high-dose glucocorticoids appear to be particularly susceptible to PCP. The glucocorticoid exposure threshold that warrants chemoprophylaxis is controversial, but such preventive therapy should be strongly considered for any patient who is receiving more than the equivalent of 20 mg of prednisone daily for 30 days or who is receiving glucocorticoids in conjunction with other immunosuppressive agents. Clinical experience also suggests that chemoprophylaxis is useful for patients receiving certain immunosuppressive agents (e.g., tumor necrosis factor inhibitors, antithymocyte globulin, rituximab, and alemtuzumab). The duration of such chemoprophylaxis is empirically estimated based on prior clinical experience and immunologic factors that would plausibly relate to immunity such as CD4+ T-cell counts, recognizing that such estimates are not precise.

TMP-SMX is the most effective prophylactic drug; few patients experience a PCP breakthrough when they are reliably taking a recommended TMP-SMX chemoprophylactic regimen. Several TMP-SMX regimens have been used successfully. Regimens of one single-strength or double-strength tablet daily are the regimens with which there is the most experience, but one double-strength tablet two or three times weekly also has been recommended for various PLWH and non-HIV-infected populations of patients.

TABLE 220-2 Prophylaxis of *Pneumocystis* pneumonia

DRUG(S)	DOSE, ROUTE	COMMENTS
First-Choice Agent		
TMP-SMX	1 tablet (double- or single-strength) qd PO	Incidence of hypersensitivity is high. Rechallenge for non-life-threatening hypersensitivity; consider dose-escalation protocol.
Alternative Agents		
Dapsone	50 mg bid or 100 mg qd PO	Hemolysis is associated with G6PD deficiency.
Dapsone *plus* Pyrimethamine *plus* Leucovorin	50 mg qd PO 50 mg weekly PO 25 mg weekly PO	Leucovorin ameliorates cytopenias due to pyrimethamine.
Dapsone *plus* Pyrimethamine *plus* Leucovorin	200 mg weekly PO 75 mg weekly PO 25 mg weekly PO	Leucovorin ameliorates cytopenias due to pyrimethamine.
Pentamidine	300 mg monthly via Respirgard II nebulizer	Aerosol may cause bronchospasm. Pentamidine is probably less effective than TMP-SMX or dapsone regimens.
Atovaquone	1500 mg qd PO	Requires fatty meal for optimal absorption

Abbreviations: G6PD, glucose-6-phosphate dehydrogenase; TMP-SMX, trimethoprim-sulfamethoxazole.

For patients who cannot tolerate TMP-SMX (usually because of hypersensitivity or bone marrow suppression), alternative drugs include daily dapsone, weekly dapsone-pyrimethamine, atovaquone, and monthly aerosol pentamidine. Patients who develop hypersensitivity to TMP-SMX can sometimes tolerate the drug if a gradual dose-escalation protocol is used. Dapsone cross-reacts with sulfonamides in a substantial fraction of patients and is rarely useful in patients with a history of life-threatening reactions to TMP-SMX. Aerosolized pentamidine is highly effective, but it is not as effective as TMP-SMX and may not provide protection in areas of the lung that are not well ventilated. Atovaquone is also effective and well tolerated; however, this drug is available only as an oral preparation, and gastrointestinal absorption is unpredictable in patients with abnormal gastrointestinal motility or function.

FURTHER READING

Akgun KM, Miller RF: Critical care in human immunodeficiency virus–infected patients. Semin Respir Crit Care Med 37:303, 2016.

Buchacz K et al: Incidence of AIDS-defining opportunistic infections in a multicohort analysis of HIV-infected persons in the United States and Canada, 2000–2010. J Infect Dis 214:862, 2016.

Chen P et al: Anidulafungin as an alternative treatment for Pneumocystis jirovecii pneumonia in patients who cannot tolerate trimethoprim/sulfamethoxazole. Int J Antimicrob Agents 55:105820, 2020.

Le Gal S et al: *Pneumocystis* infection outbreaks in organ transplantation units in France: A nation-wide survey. Clin Infect Dis 70:2216, 2020.

Ma L et al: Genome analysis of three *Pneumocystis* species reveals adaptation mechanisms to life exclusively in mammalian hosts. Nat Commun 7:10740, 2016.

Panel on Opportunistic Infections in HIV-Infected Adults and Adolescents: Guidelines for the prevention and treatment of opportunistic infections in HIV-infected adults and adolescents: Recommendations from the Centers for Disease Control and Prevention, the National Institutes of Health, and the HIV Medicine Association of the Infectious Diseases Society of America. Available at *http://aidsinfo.nih.gov/contentfiles/lvguidelines/adult_oi.pdf*. Accessed June 22, 2021.

Zolopa A et al: Early antiretroviral therapy reduces AIDS progression/death in individuals with acute opportunistic infections: A multicenter randomized strategy trial. PLoS One 4:e5575, 2009.

Section 17 Protozoal and Helminthic Infections: General Considerations

221 Introduction to Parasitic Infections

Sharon L. Reed

The word *parasite* comes originally from the Greek *parasitos* (*para*, alongside of; and *sitos*, food), meaning someone who eats at another's table or lives at another's expense. Although the same is true of many bacteria and viruses, the designation *parasite* is reserved, by convention, for helminths and protozoa. These organisms are larger and more complex than bacteria, with a eukaryotic cell structure similar to that of human host cells. Historically, this similarity has made it difficult to find effective antiparasitic agents that do not cause unacceptable toxicity to human cells. Fortunately, intensive research and modern techniques have now provided suitable agents for safe and effective treatment of most parasitic infections. **See Chap. S12 for details on diagnostic procedures and Chap. 222 for details on treatment.**

Internal parasites of human beings are divided into two types: helminths (worms) and protozoa. *Helminths* are multicellular organisms that can often be seen with the naked eye (**Chap. 230**). There are two phyla: Platyhelminthes (flat worms) and Nemathelminthes (roundworms). Both phyla include some genera that mature in the gastrointestinal tract and others that migrate through the tissue after ingestion or skin penetration. **Tables S12-1 and S12-2** present the helminthic genera, their definitive and intermediate hosts, geographic distributions, and the parasitic stages in the human body.

The key to understanding which helminths use humans as definitive hosts is to remember that helminth ova develop into larvae, and larval stages develop into adults. Humans serve as the definitive host when they ingest helminth larvae, which develop into adults in the intestine and usually cause mild disease, often without any symptoms. (The exception is ingestion of the late-stage larvae of the somatic or tissue flukes, as shown in **Table S12-2**.) In contrast, if humans ingest helminth ova and serve as the intermediate host, the ova develop into larvae, which penetrate the intestine, migrate through the tissue, and invade organs where they mature into adults. Intermediate hosts with parasitic invasion of organs may experience severe disease.

Protozoa are microscopic single-celled organisms. Among the many differences between helminths and protozoans, the most important is the ability of protozoa (like bacteria) to multiply within the human body and cause overwhelming infections. A major mechanism promoting unrestrained growth is evasion of the host immune response either by antigenic variation (*Trypanosoma brucei*) or by survival inside host cells (e.g., *Plasmodium*, *Babesia*, *Cryptosporidium*, *Leishmania*, and *Toxoplasma*). In contrast, almost all helminths require stages in other hosts to complete their life cycles and multiply. As a result, except for *Strongyloides* and *Capillaria*, which can complete their life cycle in humans, increases in the burden of infection with helminths require repeated exogenous reinfections. Thus, permanent residents of endemic countries, who are exposed repeatedly, may have heavy severe infections, while most travelers with one or two exposures are unlikely to experience the full spectrum of chronic helminthic infections.

In contrast to helminthic infections, naïve patients with their first protozoal infection usually are the most severely affected because partial immunity often limits the number of parasites during recurrent infections. Protozoan replication to large numbers in the host also promotes the development of drug-resistant forms, especially in malaria (**Chap. 222**). Because protozoa belong to many different phyla, it is easier to understand the pathogenesis and management of protozoal infections when they are classified by the site of infection (intestinal protozoans, free-living amebae, and blood and tissue protozoans) (**Table S12-3**). Immunocompromised hosts are at risk of disseminated infection with a number of protozoa, including *Leishmania*, *Toxoplasma*, *Cryptosporidium*, *and Trypanosoma cruzi*, which are AIDS-defining illnesses. In contrast, *Strongyloides* is the only helminth to disseminate.

HELMINTHIC INFECTIONS

The Platyhelminthes (flatworms) are categorized as tapeworms (cestodes) and flukes (trematodes). Tapeworms are composed of a head or scolex bearing the holdfast organs and segments, which become gravid as they mature. Some tapeworms can reach lengths of many yards; the longest tapeworms develop in the intestine, where they rarely cause serious disease. In contrast, flukes are small leaf-shaped organisms whose size is not a measure of disease severity.

FLATWORMS

Cestodes Tapeworms cause either intestinal or somatic infection, depending on the species. *Intestinal* infections occur when the human host ingests larvae in the tissue of the intermediate host, whereas *somatic* infections occur when humans accidentally ingest ova excreted from the wild or domesticated definitive animal host.

INTESTINAL TAPEWORMS As shown in **Table S12-1**, humans acquire most intestinal tapeworms by eating the insufficiently cooked flesh of the intermediate host. Thus, *Taenia saginata* is commonly called the beef tapeworm, *Taenia solium* the pork tapeworm, and *Diphyllobothrium latum* the fish tapeworm. *Hymenolepis nana* is capable of completing its life cycle in the human intestine and is acquired by ingestion of infected grain beetles or of ova from infected humans or mice. None of these parasites causes significant damage, and infection is usually asymptomatic. There are two occasional exceptions. When people ingest *T. solium* ova from their own intestine or from another infected individual, it can cause somatic infection. *D. latum* avidly absorbs vitamin B_{12} in the intestine and can cause pernicious anemia in 1–2% of infected Scandinavians with a genetic predisposition.

SOMATIC TAPEWORMS There are three major causes of somatic tapeworm infections. Two species of *Echinococcus* cause echinococcosis. *E. granulosus* is acquired by accidental ingestion of ova from dogs infected when fed the infected tissues of sheep or other animals by sheepherders or hunters. *E. multilocularis* is transmitted primarily in sub-Arctic areas when humans ingest ova from foxes, dogs, or cats that have been infected through consumption of the tissues of infected rodents. Both species cause hydatid cysts when the eggs hatch into larvae, penetrate the intestine, and migrate into the liver or lung. Ingested *T. solium* ova cause somatic disease (cysticercosis) when the larvae penetrate the intestine, migrate into tissue, and form cysts (*cysterci*), usually in the muscles or central nervous system (CNS).

Trematodes Flukes also cause both intestinal and somatic infections (**Chap. 234 and Table S12-1**). Most fluke infections are localized to Asia, Africa, Southeast Asia, or the Pacific islands. Infection with intestinal flukes is usually asymptomatic, although heavy infections sometimes cause abdominal discomfort and mucous diarrhea. Liver flukes and lung flukes cause somatic infections when humans ingest a larval form from an intermediate host. Adults develop in the intestine, migrate into adjacent tissues, and cause disease. The major liver flukes (*Clonorchis sinensis*, *Opisthorchis* spp., and *Fasciola hepatica*) are causes of recurrent bacterial cholangitis (due to obstruction) or portal hypertension and cirrhosis. Only *F. hepatica* can be acquired worldwide; it is especially common in sheep-raising areas, where the animals ingest water plants (e.g., watercress). The lung flukes (*Paragonimus* spp.) occur globally except in Europe; most lesions occur as pulmonary cysts, although occasional lesions develop in the CNS or the abdominal cavity.

The blood flukes cause schistosomiasis, one of the most common and serious parasitic infections (**Chap. 234 and Table S12-1**). The major species are *Schistosoma mansoni*, *S. haematobium*, and *S. japonicum*. All are transmitted to humans when free-swimming larvae exit an infected snail in freshwater and penetrate the skin. Swimmer's itch sometimes follows skin penetration but is usually of short duration. The larvae then wander in the skin until they find a blood vessel and migrate to the target organ. *S. mansoni* and *S. japonicum* migrate to the mesentery vessels and eventually make their way to the liver, while *S. haematobium* targets the veins around the ureter and bladder. Extensive egg deposition by *S. mansoni* and *S. japonicum* and the immune reactions to the ova cause granuloma formation and, with many repeated exposures, portal vein obstruction and cirrhosis. The same process in the ureters and bladders during infection with *S. haematobium* eventually interferes with urine flow and leads to repeated urinary tract infections and kidney damage.

■ ROUNDWORMS

Nematodes Roundworms are nonsegmented bisexual organisms. The species that infect humans include intestinal and tissue groups. Humans may also acquire certain nonhuman mammalian roundworms that either can be limited to the skin or can migrate to tissues and cause serious disease (the larva migrans syndromes).

INTESTINAL ROUNDWORMS The major intestinal roundworms are *Ascaris lumbricoides*, *Necator americanus* (New World hookworms), *Ancylostoma duodenale* (Old World hookworms), *Trichuris trichiura* (whipworms), *Enterobius vermicularis* (pinworms), and *Strongyloides stercoralis*. Taken together, infections caused by intestinal roundworms are the most common infections in the world. *Ascaris*, hookworms, and *Trichuris* infect about 1.5 billion individuals, and at least 30–100 million have strongyloidiasis. These infections are most common in resource-poor developing countries, especially where people defecate outside and/or human feces is used as fertilizer ("night soil"). Infection is transmitted either by ingestion of ova (*A. lumbricoides*, *T. trichiura*, and *E. vermicularis*) or by active penetration of the skin by larvae (hookworms and *S. stercoralis*) (**Table S13-2**).

Intestinal roundworms cause serious health problems in residents of endemic regions with poor sanitation, but travelers are at low risk of developing significant disease from most of these parasites. Intestinal blockage and malnutrition from heavy *Ascaris* infections and anemia from heavy hookworm infections are now restricted to areas of heavy endemicity. Except in the case of *Strongyloides* and *Capillaria*, which can reproduce in the body, multiple exposures over time are necessary for the development of severe disease. *Strongyloides* infection persists over decades and can disseminate when the immune system is compromised. Although *Capillaria* remains localized to the intestine, infections can become so heavy that protein-losing enteropathy and malnutrition cause serious disease.

The life cycles of *Ascaris* and the hookworms involve migration through the heart and lungs before development into adults in the intestine. In particular, *Ascaris* occasionally causes eosinophilic pneumonia (Loeffler's syndrome) during heavy infections. Pinworms are the most common causes of intestinal roundworm infection persisting in the United States and other developed countries. The anal and perineal itching caused by pinworm migration out of the anus and subsequent egg deposition is well known to families throughout the world.

TISSUE ROUNDWORMS The major diseases caused by tissue roundworms are filariasis, angiostrongyliasis, gnathostomiasis, and trichinellosis. By far, the most important globally is filariasis; the thread-like filarial worms infect an estimated 120 million individuals in tropical and subtropical areas of the world. Four filarial species cause three distinct diseases: lymphatic filariasis (*Wuchereria bancrofti* and *Brugia malayi*), river blindness (*Onchocercus volvulus*), and loiasis (*Loa loa*, the African eye worm). Humans, the major reservoir, acquire these infections from bites of infected arthropods (**Table S12-2**). The larvae develop into adults, which remain static in tissue: the lymphatics for lymphatic filariasis and subcutaneous tissue for *O. volvulus* and *L. loa*. After adults mate, next-stage larvae are produced, and their migration causes additional damage.

Repeated bouts of migrating larvae and blocking of the lymphatics by adults are necessary to establish the syndrome of lymphatic filariasis; thus, it is unusual for the short-term traveler (<3 months' residence in an endemic region) to develop significant disease. In river blindness, the larvae produced by adult *O. volvulus* migrate through the skin and eye, causing skin damage and eventual blindness. Loiasis is a milder disease restricted to central and western Africa. Although both the adults and the larvae of *L. loa* migrate through the skin and eye, many infected individuals are asymptomatic, and the infection is often diagnosed only when an adult worm migrates across the subconjunctival tissue and is visible to the patient and the physician. Red lumps in the skin from heavy cutaneous migration are called *Calabar swellings*.

The other four major roundworm tissue infections are acquired by ingestion of larvae in undercooked food. The sources for trichinellosis are swine and other large mammals; for gnathostomiasis, freshwater fish and chicken; for ancylostomiasis, snails, fish, prawns, and crabs; and for Guinea worm, infected water fleas. Guinea worm infection (dracunculiasis, caused by *Dracunculus medinensis*) has been almost eradicated. *Trichinella spiralis* larvae penetrate the intestine and migrate widely, with a preference for skeletal tissue; the release of eosinophils and IgE causes muscle soreness and may cause palpebral swelling and other manifestations of generalized allergic reactions. *Angiostrongylus cantonensis* is the most common parasitic cause of eosinophilic meningitis. Ingested larvae penetrate the intestine and migrate to the brain and meninges, where they quickly die and attract massive numbers of eosinophils. Although complications can occur, most individuals recover spontaneously. *Gnathostoma spinigerum* larvae also penetrate the intestine and migrate, showing a preference for the skin, eyes, and meninges. Mechanical damage from the migration and inflammation produced by the resultant immune reaction can cause boil-like lesions on the skin, painful eye damage, and eosinophilic meningitis. Although eosinophilic meningitis caused by *G. spinigerum* is less common than that caused by *A. cantonensis*, it is often more severe and can result in paralysis or brain hemorrhage.

PROTOZOAL INFECTIONS

■ INTESTINAL PROTOZOA

Entamoeba histolytica is the one intestinal protozoan that causes invasive disease. This disease consists of dysentery or bloody diarrhea that must be differentiated from that due to bacteria such as *Salmonella*, *Campylobacter*, and *Shigella*. Although amebiasis usually has a slower onset with lower fever than these bacterial infections, *E. histolytica* can disseminate from the bloodstream to cause distant abscesses, particularly of the liver. The diagnosis cannot be made by identification of the characteristic cyst or trophozoites (**Chap. 223**) as they are identical to those of the noninvasive *E. dispar*, which is more common globally.

Cryptosporidium and *Giardia* are the most common water-borne protozoal infections. *Cryptosporidium* can cause major outbreaks because it is highly infectious and resistant to high levels of chlorine (**Chap. 229**). Without immune reconstitution, immunosuppressed patients, particularly those with AIDS, can develop severe, even fatal watery diarrhea. Infections caused by the remaining intestinal protozoans—*Giardia*, *Isospora*, *Cyclospora*, and microsporidia (**Chap. 229**)—have a much more indolent course, with intermittent diarrhea. Microsporidia, unique intracellular protozoa that form infectious spores, may cause limited gastrointestinal infection in immunocompetent hosts, but patients with AIDS can develop chronic diarrhea and wasting or disseminated infection to the biliary or respiratory tract.

■ FREE-LIVING AMOEBAS

The free-living amoebas *Acanthamoeba* and *Naegleria* are found worldwide in freshwater and brackish water (**Chap. 223 and Table S12-3**). Organisms of these two genera cause very different syndromes. In immunocompromised individuals, *Acanthamoeba* may cause invasive infection, with brain masses and skin lesions. However, all humans are susceptible to *Acanthamoeba* keratitis after trauma to the eye and exposure to contaminated water. In contrast, naeglerial meningitis, acquired in warm lakes or hot springs, causes sudden pyogenic and usually fatal meningitis. *Balamuthia*, reported only from the Americas, causes indolent meningoencephalitis, with both cerebrospinal fluid pleocytosis and a space-occupying lesion, in immunocompetent patients. Despite the availability of miltefosine, which is active in vitro against *Naegleria*, infection of the CNS is almost universally fatal.

■ BLOOD AND TISSUE PROTOZOANS

Plasmodium* and *Babesia Malaria, caused by six species of *Plasmodium*, carries higher mortality rates than any other parasitic infection (**Chap. 224**). All species are transmitted in tropical and subtropical areas by female *Anopheles* mosquitoes. *Plasmodium falciparum* is most common in sub-Saharan Africa, where it causes more than 80% of malaria infections and 90% of malarial deaths. Infection with *P. falciparum* may be particularly severe because the organism can invade any erythrocyte, reaches very high parasite loads, damages organs by adhering to vascular epithelium, and is the most likely *Plasmodium* species to be resistant to antimalarial drugs. *Plasmodium vivax*, the dominant cause of malaria outside sub-Saharan Africa, reaches lower levels of parasitemia and exhibits less drug resistance because it invades only reticulocytes with Duffy antigen. Many Africans, especially in the western part of the continent, lack the Duffy blood group; consequently, *Plasmodium ovale*, another cause of milder malaria, can compete successfully with *P. vivax*. Both *P. vivax* and *P. ovale* produce persistent liver forms, which must be treated with primaquine (**Chap. 222**). Because malaria can cause a variety of symptoms ranging from acute fever to coma, this diagnosis must be considered in any traveler or immigrant from a malarial area. *Babesia* also infects erythrocytes and may cause a nonspecific febrile illness or, in asplenic patients, severe infection. This parasite is carried by ixodid ticks and is geographically limited to the northeastern and midwestern United States, with only sporadic cases in Europe and other temperate areas.

Trypanosomes The three species of trypanosomes all have flagellated bloodstream forms, but they cause very different diseases. *T. cruzi*, the cause of Chagas disease, is transmitted in South and Central America in the feces of blood-sucking reduviid bugs (**Chap. 227**). After initial parasitemia, patients are often asymptomatic for years while the parasite multiplies intracellularly in muscle and ganglion cells. Although only a minority of patients go on to develop organ damage (megaesophagus and cardiomyopathy), all infected patients can spread the disease through transfusions, mother-to-child transmission, and organ transplants.

African trypanosomiasis is limited to sub-Saharan Africa, where it is transmitted by the bite of a tsetse fly. A history of a tsetse bite and the presence of a painful chancre are strong diagnostic clues (**Chap. 227**). Although the parasites causing this disease in western Africa (*Trypanosoma brucei gambiense*) and eastern Africa (*T. brucei rhodesiense*) look identical, they are genetically and clinically distinct. *T. b. gambiense* causes low-level parasitemia with cyclical fevers over months or years before CNS invasion, whereas *T. b. rhodesiense* causes high-level parasitemia, invades the CNS early on, and can lead to death within weeks of onset.

Leishmania Leishmaniasis is caused by more than 20 species of obligate intracellular protozoa transmitted by sandflies, which are present in almost 100 countries in tropical and temperate zones (**Chap. 226**). A wide spectrum of clinical symptoms result, ranging from self-healing, painless skin ulcers to mucocutaneous disease with destruction of the nose and palate to disseminated visceral leishmaniasis with hepatic and splenic involvement. The resulting disease depends on the infecting strain and the host immune response. Visceral leishmaniasis can present as an acute febrile illness, with the later development of hepatosplenomegaly, and is an AIDS-defining illness in HIV-infected patients. More than 90% of cases of visceral leishmaniasis occur in India, Bangladesh, Ethiopia, Sudan, and Brazil.

Toxoplasma *Toxoplasma gondii* is an obligate intracellular parasite that is found worldwide. Infection follows ingestion of oocysts in food or water contaminated by cat feces, ingestion of tissue cysts in undercooked meat, or transplacental transmission. After gastrointestinal invasion, tachyzoites can invade any nucleated cell and cause lifelong infection in most patients (**Chap. 228**). Clinical manifestations depend on the host's age and immune status at the time of infection. Congenital toxoplasmosis results from primary maternal infection; outcomes are most severe early in pregnancy and include visual, hearing, and cognitive impairments. Babies infected later in pregnancy may appear normal but can develop chorioretinitis decades later. Primary infection in immunocompetent hosts may be asymptomatic, may present as an infectious mononucleosis–like syndrome or may manifest as chorioretinitis during outbreaks. During immunosuppression by AIDS or organ transplantation, reactivation of latent cerebral infection can be fatal unless diagnosed and treated early.

APPROACH TO THE PATIENT

Parasitic Infection

A thorough history and physical examination are the keys to diagnosis of any disease and particularly of parasitic infections. Because many of the more serious parasitic infections are uncommon in the United States, a travel history, particularly to developing nations, is a critical component. The longer the stay in an area endemic for significant parasitic infections, the greater the risk, even for healthy travelers. In addition, other factors increase the chance of acquiring these infections. Notably, immunocompromise greatly increases the likelihood of developing some of the more serious parasitic infections. Even healthy travelers with adventure itineraries, extensive travel to rural areas, or involvement in war zones or refugee camps

TABLE 221-1 Parasitic Infections, by Organ System and Signs/Symptoms[a]

ORGAN SYSTEM, MAJOR SIGN(S)/SYMPTOM(S)	PARASITE(S)	GEOGRAPHIC DISTRIBUTION	COMMENTS
Skin			
Serpentine rash	Hookworm	Worldwide	Can cause anemia in heavy infections
	Strongyloides	Moist tropics and subtropics	Disseminated infection in immunocompromise
	Toxocara (animal roundworm)	Tropical and temperate zones	Cutaneous or visceral larva migrans
Itchy skin rash	*Onchocerca*	Mexico, Central/South America, Africa	Larvae detectable in skin snips and nodules
Painless ulcers	*Leishmania*	Tropics and subtropics	Amastigotes detectable in biopsies; may cause destructive mucocutaneous infection; AIDS-defining infection
Skin nodules	*Onchocerca*	Mexico, South America, Africa	Large nodules of adult worms
	Loa loa (African eye worm)	Western and central Africa	Migratory nodules
	Gnathostoma	Southeast Asia and China	Migratory nodules with eosinophilia
Painful nodules, especially involving feet	*Dracunculus* (Guinea worm)	Africa	Nearly eradicated
Central Nervous System			
Somnolence, seizures, coma	*Plasmodium falciparum*	Subtropics and tropics	Cerebral malaria, especially in children
	Trypanosoma brucei rhodesiense	Sub-Saharan eastern Africa	Painful chancre from tsetse fly bite; death in weeks to months
Space-occupying lesions, seizures	*Acanthamoeba*	Worldwide	Immunocompromised individuals
	Balamuthia	Americas	Indolent meningoencephalitis with brain mass
	Toxoplasma	Worldwide	Reactivation disease in immunocompromise; ring-enhancing lesions; AIDS-defining infection
	Taenia solium	Mexico, Central/South America, Africa	Cysticercosis; variable sized or calcified larval cysts on CT
	Schistosoma japonicum	Far East	Aberrant eggs can form brain or spinal cord masses.
	Schistosoma mansoni	Africa, Central/South America	Aberrant eggs can form brain or spinal cord masses.
Pyogenic meningitis	*Naegleria*	Worldwide	Motile trophozoites in fresh cerebrospinal fluid; pyogenic; rapid death
Eosinophilic meningitis	*Angiostrongylus* (rat lung worm)	Southeast Asia, Pacific, Caribbean	Most common cause globally of eosinophilic meningitis; spontaneous resolution
	Gnathostoma	Southeast Asia and China	Migratory nodules
Eyes			
Painful corneal ulcers	*Acanthamoeba*	Worldwide	Freshwater and brackish water; corneal trauma; long-wear contact lenses
Corneal opacification	*Onchocerca*	Mexico, Central/South America, Africa	Immune response to microfilaria in cornea
Congenital or adult visual loss	*Toxoplasma*	Worldwide	Primary infection in pregnancy and normal hosts; reactivation infection in immunocompromised
Retinal mass	*Toxocara*	Worldwide	Ocular larva migrans
Visible roundworm in eye	*Onchocerca*	Mexico, Central/South America, Africa	Worms may cross eye during migration.
	L. loa	Western and central Africa	Worms may cross eye during migration.
Pain, possible vision loss	*Gnathostoma*	Southeast Asia and China	Migratory skin nodules, eosinophilia
Lungs			
Pulmonary nodule/abscess	*Paragonimus*	Far East, Africa, Americas	Ectopic migration to abdomen or central nervous system
Cough, transient infiltrates, eosinophilia	Migrating helminths	Worldwide	Loeffler's syndrome from migrating *Ascaris*, hookworm, *Strongyloides*
Heart			
Pulmonary edema	*P. falciparum* (complication)	Tropics and subtropics	End-organ damage from severe malaria
Cardiomegaly, arrhythmias	*Trypanosoma cruzi*	Mexico, Central/South America	Late amastigote infection of myocardium; AIDS-defining infection
Gastrointestinal Tract			
Hepatosplenomegaly	Malaria (multiple episodes)	Tropics and subtropics	Splenomegaly with anemia and recurrent fever are hallmarks of malaria.
	S. mansoni	Africa, Central/South America	Portal obstruction with cirrhosis and late varices
	Leishmania donovani complex	Tropics and subtropics	Visceral leishmaniasis; AIDS-defining infection
Hepatomegaly	*Entamoeba histolytica*	Tropics	Acute with fever, right-upper-quadrant pain; or chronic with enlarged liver; hypoechoic abscess(es) on ultrasound or CT
	Echinococcus	Sheep-raising areas	Characteristic cysts of liver > lung
	Fasciola	Sheep-raising areas	Eosinophilia

(*Continued*)

TABLE 221-1 Parasitic Infections, by Organ System and Signs/Symptoms[a] (Continued)

ORGAN SYSTEM, MAJOR SIGN(S)/SYMPTOM(S)	PARASITE(S)	GEOGRAPHIC DISTRIBUTION	COMMENTS
Cholangitis	*Clonorchis*	China, Southeast Asia	Recurrent cholangitis and late cholangiocarcinoma
	Microsporidia	Worldwide	AIDS
	Cryptosporidium	Worldwide	AIDS-defining infection
Bloody diarrhea	*E. histolytica*	Tropics	Less fever than in diarrhea of bacterial etiology
	S. mansoni	Africa, Central/South America	Only in heavy, acute infection with fever and eosinophilia
	S. japonicum	Far East	Only in heavy, acute infection
Watery diarrhea	*Cryptosporidium*	Worldwide	Severe in immunocompromised patients
	Giardia	Worldwide	Foul-smelling stool with steatorrhea
	Isospora belli	Worldwide	Fever, abdominal pain, chronic diarrhea
	Microsporidia	Worldwide	Chronic diarrhea with AIDS
	Capillaria	Southeast Asia, Egypt	Malabsorption, wasting
Passage of large roundworm (>6 cm)	*Ascaris*	Worldwide	Patients may confuse the roundworm with an earthworm.
Small roundworms visible around anus	Pinworm	Worldwide	Anal itching; eggs rarely detected by ova and parasite (O&P) exam
	Trichuris	Worldwide	Rectal prolapse with heavy infection in children
Passage of tapeworm segments	*T. solium* or *Taenia saginata*	Worldwide	Usual reason for seeking medical care
	Diphyllobothrium latum	Worldwide	Pernicious anemia in genetically predisposed Scandinavians
Genitourinary System			
Itchy discharge	*Trichomonas vaginalis*	Worldwide	Common sexually transmitted disease of both sexes
Hematuria	*Schistosoma haematobium*	Africa	Hematuria with negative cultures, urinary tract infections, and late bladder cancer
Muscular System			
Myalgias, myositis	*Trichinella*	Worldwide	Palpebral swelling; high-level eosinophilia
Bloodstream			
Fever without localizing symptoms	*Plasmodium*	Tropics and subtropics	Consider in any patient from a malarious area.
	Babesia	New England, United States	Geographically limited; worse with splenectomy
	T. brucei rhodesiense, T. brucei gambiense	Sub-Saharan Africa	Limited to tsetse fly range; painful chancre; adenopathy and cyclical fevers; early (*rhodesiense*) or late (*gambiense*) central nervous system involvement
	Filariae	Asia, India	Periodic fever with eosinophilia, adenolymphangitis, chronic lymphangitis
	L. donovani complex	Tropics and subtropics	Hepatosplenomegaly, fever, wasting; AIDS-defining infection

[a]See also text and **Tables S12-1, S12-2, and S12-3** for vectors and routes of transmission.

are at increased risk. Immigrants from developing countries may seek care for symptoms or signs associated with parasitic infections.

Information on the patient's immunization history and adherence to appropriate malarial chemoprophylaxis is critical. The recent approval of the first parasitic vaccine against *P. falciparum* is very exciting, but it will be targeted only for children in high prevalence areas because of its modest efficacy. For example, typhoid fever is much less likely to be the cause of prolonged fever in an immunized individual. Similarly, hepatitis A or B is unlikely to be the cause of jaundice and fever in fully immunized patients. In this era of increasing drug resistance, even adherence to appropriate malarial chemoprophylaxis does not guarantee that fever is not malarial. Nevertheless, most travelers who acquire malaria have taken inadequate or no prophylaxis. Although these considerations do not prove that the symptoms are caused by parasites, they narrow the differential diagnosis.

There are many other important aspects of the history, including when symptoms began. Was the individual still in the endemic area at the time, or did the symptoms commence after return to the United States? If they started during travel, was any treatment received? Malaria must be the first consideration in a febrile patient returning from an endemic area. If the patient was well upon return from travel, the timing of symptom onset is a critical point. For example, if the chief manifestation is fever that began >10–14 days after departure from the endemic region, many tropical diseases can be ruled out, including dengue fever, chikungunya fever, and Zika virus infection. On the other hand, fever beginning several months or later after return makes malaria a likely diagnosis. Travelers' diarrhea, the most common complaint of travelers, is usually caused by bacteria or viruses and resolves in a short time with or without treatment. Travelers' diarrhea that persists for weeks is much more likely to be parasitic in origin.

Most patients who consult physicians after international travel either have troublesome symptoms or have been referred for symptoms or signs whose source was unclear to a referring caregiver. After a careful travel history including the individual's symptoms and the exact geographic zones visited, a thorough physical examination must be conducted. The symptoms, signs, and physical findings should help to establish possible diagnoses. **Table 221-1** breaks down the symptoms of major parasitic infections by organ system and geographic distribution, with comments on clinical and epidemiologic associations.

Acknowledgment
The author gratefully acknowledges the substantial contributions of Charles E. Davis, MD, to this chapter in the previous editions.

FURTHER READING

Ashley EA et al: Malaria. Lancet 391:1608, 2018.
Fink D et al: Fever in the returning traveler. BMJ 360:j5773, 2018.
Rupali P: Introduction to tropical medicine. Infect Dis Clin N Am 33:1, 2019.
Thwaites GE, Day NPJ: Approach to fever in the returning traveler. N Engl J Med 376:6, 2017.
Vos T et al: Global, regional, and national incidence, prevalence and years lived with disability for 328 diseases and injuries for 195 countries, 1990-2016: a systemic analysis for the Global Burden of Disease Study 2016. Lancet 390:1211, 2017.

222 Agents Used to Treat Parasitic Infections

Thomas A. Moore

Parasitic infections continue to afflict more than half of the world's population and impose a substantial health burden, particularly in underdeveloped nations, where they are most prevalent. The reach of some parasitic diseases, including malaria, has expanded over the past few decades as a result of factors such as deforestation, population shifts, global warming, and other climatic events. Although there have been significant advances in vaccine development and vector control, chemotherapy remains the single most effective means of controlling parasitic infections. Efforts to combat the spread of some diseases are hindered by the development and spread of drug resistance, the limited introduction of new antiparasitic agents, the proliferation of counterfeit medications, and, most recently, profiteering, which has dramatically increased the cost of once-affordable agents. However, there are good reasons to be optimistic. Ambitious global initiatives aimed at controlling or eliminating threats such as AIDS, tuberculosis, and malaria have demonstrated successes. The ongoing efforts of multinational partnerships to address the substantial burden imposed by neglected tropical diseases have generated mechanisms to develop and deploy effective antiparasitic agents. In addition, the development of vaccines against several tropical diseases continues.

This chapter deals exclusively with the agents used to treat infections due to parasites. Specific treatment recommendations for the parasitic diseases of humans are listed in subsequent chapters. Many of the agents discussed herein are approved by the U.S. Food and Drug Administration (FDA) but are considered investigational for the treatment of certain infections. Drugs marked in the text with an asterisk (*) are available through the Centers for Disease Control and Prevention (CDC) Drug Service (telephone: 404-639-3670; email: drugservice@cdc.gov; *www.cdc.gov/ncpdcid/dsr/*). Drugs marked with a dagger (†) are available only through their manufacturers; contact information for these manufacturers may be available from the CDC.

Table 222-1 presents a brief overview of each agent (including some drugs that are covered in other chapters), along with major toxicities, spectrum of activity, and safety for use during pregnancy and lactation.

Albendazole Like all benzimidazoles, albendazole acts by selectively binding to free β-tubulin in nematodes, inhibiting the polymerization of tubulin and the microtubule-dependent uptake of glucose. Irreversible damage occurs in gastrointestinal (GI) cells of the nematodes, resulting in starvation, death, and expulsion by the host. This fundamental disruption of cellular metabolism offers treatment for a wide range of parasitic diseases.

Albendazole is poorly absorbed from the GI tract, a feature that is advantageous for the treatment of intestinal helminths but not for that of tissue helminth infections (e.g., hydatid disease and neurocysticercosis), which requires that a sufficient amount of active drug reach the site of infection. Administration with a high-fat meal (~40 g) increases the drug's absorption by up to five-fold. The metabolite albendazole sulfoxide is responsible for the drug's therapeutic effect outside the gut lumen. Albendazole sulfoxide crosses the blood–brain barrier, reaching a level significantly higher than that achieved in plasma. The high concentrations of albendazole sulfoxide attained in cerebrospinal fluid (CSF) may explain the efficacy of albendazole in the treatment of neurocysticercosis.

Albendazole is extensively metabolized in the liver, but there are few data regarding the drug's use in patients with hepatic disease. Single-dose albendazole therapy in humans is largely without side effects (overall frequency, ≤1%). More prolonged courses (e.g., as administered for cystic and alveolar echinococcal disease) have been associated with liver function abnormalities and bone marrow toxicity. Thus, when prolonged use is anticipated, the drug should be administered in treatment cycles of 28 days interrupted by 14-day intervals off therapy. Prolonged therapy with full-dose albendazole (800 mg/d) should be approached cautiously in patients also receiving drugs with known effects on the cytochrome P450 system.

Amodiaquine Amodiaquine has been widely used in the treatment of malaria for >60 years. Like chloroquine (the other major 4-aminoquinoline), amodiaquine is now of limited use because of the spread of resistance. Amodiaquine interferes with hemozoin formation through complexation with heme. It is rapidly absorbed and acts as a prodrug after oral administration; the principal plasma metabolite, monodesethylamodiaquine, is the predominant antimalarial agent. Amodiaquine and its metabolites are all excreted in urine, but there are no recommendations concerning dosage adjustment in patients with impaired renal function. Agranulocytosis and hepatotoxicity can develop with repeated use; therefore, this drug should not be used for prophylaxis. Despite widespread resistance, amodiaquine is effective in some areas when combined with other antimalarial drugs (e.g., artesunate, sulfadoxine-pyrimethamine), particularly in children. Although on the World Health Organization's *List of Essential Medicines*, amodiaquine is not yet available in the United States.

Amphotericin B See Table 222-1 and **Chap. 211**.

Antimonials* Despite associated adverse reactions and the need for prolonged parenteral treatment, the pentavalent antimonial compounds (designated Sb^v) have remained the first-line therapy for all forms of leishmaniasis throughout the world, primarily because they are affordable and effective and have survived the test of time. Pentavalent antimonials are active only after bioreduction to the trivalent Sb(III) form, which inhibits trypanothione reductase, a critical enzyme involved in the oxidative stress management of *Leishmania* species. The fact that *Leishmania* species use trypanothione rather than glutathione (which is used by mammalian cells) may explain the parasite-specific activity of antimonials. The drugs are taken up by the reticuloendothelial system, and their activity against *Leishmania* species may be enhanced by this localization. Sodium stibogluconate is the only pentavalent antimonial available in the United States; meglumine antimoniate is used principally in francophone countries.

Resistance is a major problem in some areas. Although low-level unresponsiveness to Sb^v was identified in India in the 1970s, incremental increases in both the recommended daily dosage (to 20 mg/kg) and the duration of treatment (to 28 days) satisfactorily compensated for the growing resistance until around 1990. There has since been steady erosion in the capacity of Sb^v to induce long-term cure in patients with kala-azar who live in eastern India. Co-infection with HIV impairs the treatment response.

Sodium stibogluconate is available in aqueous solution and is administered parenterally. Antimony appears to have two elimination phases. When the drug is administered IV, the mean half-life of the first phase is <2 h; the mean half-life of the terminal elimination phase is

TABLE 222-1 Overview of Agents Used for the Treatment of Parasitic Infections

DRUGS BY CLASS	PARASITIC INFECTION(S)	ADVERSE EFFECTS	MAJOR DRUG–DRUG INTERACTIONS	PREGNANCY CLASS[a]	BREAST MILK
4-Aminoquinolines					
Amodiaquine	Malaria[b]	Agranulocytosis, hepatotoxicity	No information	Not assigned	Yes[c]
Chloroquine	Malaria[b]	*Occasional:* pruritus, nausea, vomiting, headache, hair depigmentation, exfoliative dermatitis, reversible corneal opacity *Rare:* irreversible retinal injury, nail discoloration, blood dyscrasias	Antacids and kaolin: reduced absorption of chloroquine Ampicillin: bioavailability reduced by chloroquine Cimetidine: increased serum levels of chloroquine Cyclosporine: serum levels increased by chloroquine	Not assigned[d]	Yes[c]
Piperaquine	Malaria[b]	*Occasional:* GI disturbances	None reported	Not assigned	Yes
8-Aminoquinolines					
Primaquine	Malaria[b]	*Frequent:* hemolysis in patients with G6PD deficiency *Occasional:* methemoglobinemia, GI disturbances *Rare:* CNS symptoms	Quinacrine: potentiated toxicity of primaquine	Contraindicated	Yes
Tafenoquine	Malaria[b]	*Frequent:* hemolysis in patients with G6PD deficiency, mild GI upset *Occasional:* methemoglobinemia, headache	No information	Not assigned	Yes
Aminoalcohols					
Halofantrine	Malaria[b]	*Frequent:* abdominal pain, diarrhea *Occasional:* ECG disturbances (dose-related prolongation of QTc and PR interval), nausea, pruritus; contraindicated in persons who have cardiac disease or who have taken mefloquine in the preceding 3 weeks	Concomitant use of agents that prolong QTc interval contraindicated	C	No information
Lumefantrine	Malaria[b]	*Occasional:* nausea, vomiting, diarrhea, abdominal pain, anorexia, headache, dizziness	Plasma levels increased by darunavir and nevirapine, decreased by etravirine	Not assigned	No information
Aminoglycosides					
Paromomycin	Amebiasis,[b] infection with *Dientamoeba fragilis*, giardiasis, cryptosporidiosis, leishmaniasis	*Frequent:* GI disturbances (oral dosing only) *Occasional:* nephrotoxicity, ototoxicity, vestibular toxicity (parenteral dosing only)	No major interactions	Oral: B Parenteral: not assigned[d]	No information
Amphotericin B Amphotericin B deoxycholate Amphotec (InterMune) Amphotericin B lipid complex, ABLC (Abelcet) Amphotericin B, liposomal (AmBisome)	Leishmaniasis,[e] amebic meningoencephalitis	*Frequent:* fever, chills, hypokalemia, hypomagnesemia, nephrotoxicity *Occasional:* vomiting, dyspnea, hypotension	Antineoplastic agents: renal toxicity, bronchospasm, hypotension Glucocorticoids, ACTH, digitalis: hypokalemia Zidovudine: increased myelo- and nephrotoxicity	B	No information
Antimonials	Leishmaniasis	*Frequent:* arthralgias/myalgias, pancreatitis, ECG changes (QT prolongation, T wave flattening or inversion)			
Pentavalent antimony[f]			No major interactions	Not assigned	Yes
Meglumine antimoniate			Antiarrhythmics and tricyclic antidepressants: increased risk of cardiotoxicity	Not assigned	No information
Artemisinin and derivatives	Malaria[g]	*Occasional:* neurotoxicity (ataxia, convulsions), nausea, vomiting, anorexia, contact dermatitis			
Arteether			No information	Not assigned	Yes[c]
Artemether			Artemether levels decreased by darunavir, etravirine, and nevirapine	C	Yes[c]
Artesunate[f]			Mefloquine: levels decreased and clearance accelerated by artesunate	C	Yes[c]
Dihydroartemisinin			Mefloquine: increased absorption	Not assigned	Yes[c]

(*Continued*)

TABLE 222-1 Overview of Agents Used for the Treatment of Parasitic Infections (Continued)

DRUGS BY CLASS	PARASITIC INFECTION(S)	ADVERSE EFFECTS	MAJOR DRUG–DRUG INTERACTIONS	PREGNANCY CLASS[a]	BREAST MILK
Atovaquone	Malaria,[b] babesiosis	*Frequent:* nausea, vomiting *Occasional:* abdominal pain, headache	Plasma levels decreased by rifampin, tetracycline, atazanavir, efavirenz, lopinavir/ritonavir; bioavailability decreased by metoclopramide	C	No information
Azoles Fluconazole Itraconazole Ketoconazole	Leishmaniasis	*Serious:* hepatotoxicity *Rare:* exfoliative skin disorders, anaphylaxis	Warfarin, oral hypoglycemics, phenytoin, cyclosporine, theophylline, digoxin, dofetilide, quinidine, carbamazepine, rifabutin, busulfan, docetaxel, vinca alkaloids, pimozide, alprazolam, diazepam, midazolam, triazolam, verapamil, atorvastatin, cerivastatin, lovastatin, simvastatin, tacrolimus, sirolimus, indinavir, ritonavir, saquinavir, alfentanil, buspirone, methylprednisolone, trimetrexate: plasma levels increased by azoles Carbamazepine, phenobarbital, phenytoin, isoniazid, rifabutin, rifampin, antacids, H_2-receptor antagonists, proton pump inhibitors, nevirapine: decreased plasma levels of azoles Clarithromycin, erythromycin, indinavir, ritonavir: increased plasma levels of azoles	C	Yes
Benzimidazoles					
Albendazole	Ascariasis, capillariasis, clonorchiasis, cutaneous larva migrans, cysticercosis,[b] echinococcosis,[b] enterobiasis, eosinophilic enterocolitis, gnathostomiasis, hookworm, lymphatic filariasis, microsporidiosis, strongyloidiasis, trichinellosis, trichostrongyliasis, trichuriasis, visceral larva migrans	*Occasional:* nausea, vomiting, abdominal pain, headache, reversible alopecia, elevated aminotransferases *Rare:* leukopenia, rash	Dexamethasone, praziquantel: plasma level of albendazole sulfoxide increased by ~50%	C	Yes[c]
Mebendazole	Ascariasis,[b] capillariasis, eosinophilic enterocolitis, enterobiasis,[b] hookworm,[b] trichinellosis, trichostrongyliasis, trichuriasis,[b] visceral larva migrans	*Occasional:* diarrhea, abdominal pain, elevated aminotransferases *Rare:* agranulocytosis, thrombocytopenia, alopecia	Cimetidine: inhibited mebendazole metabolism	C	No information
Thiabendazole	Strongyloidiasis,[b] cutaneous larva migrans,[b] visceral larva migrans[b]	*Frequent:* anorexia, nausea, vomiting, diarrhea, headache, dizziness, asparagus-like urine odor *Occasional:* drowsiness, giddiness, crystalluria, elevated aminotransferases, psychosis *Rare:* hepatitis, seizures, angioneurotic edema, Stevens-Johnson syndrome, tinnitus	Theophylline: serum levels increased by thiabendazole	C	No information
Triclabendazole	Fascioliasis, paragonimiasis	*Occasional:* abdominal cramps, diarrhea, biliary colic, transient headache	No information	Not assigned	Yes
Benznidazole	Chagas disease	*Frequent:* rash, pruritus, nausea, leukopenia, paresthesias	No major interactions	Not assigned	No information
Clindamycin	Babesiosis, malaria, toxoplasmosis	*Occasional:* pseudomembranous colitis, abdominal pain, diarrhea, nausea/vomiting *Rare:* pruritus, skin rashes	No major interactions	B	Yes[c]
Diloxanide furoate	Amebiasis	*Frequent:* flatulence *Occasional:* nausea, vomiting, diarrhea *Rare:* pruritus	None reported	Contraindicated	No information

(*Continued*)

TABLE 222-1 Overview of Agents Used for the Treatment of Parasitic Infections (Continued)

DRUGS BY CLASS	PARASITIC INFECTION(S)	ADVERSE EFFECTS	MAJOR DRUG–DRUG INTERACTIONS	PREGNANCY CLASS[a]	BREAST MILK
Eflornithine[h] (difluoromethylornithine, DFMO)	Trypanosomiasis	*Frequent:* pancytopenia *Occasional:* diarrhea, seizures *Rare:* transient hearing loss	No major interactions	Contraindicated	No information
Emetine and dehydroemetine[f]	Amebiasis, fascioliasis	*Severe:* cardiotoxicity *Frequent:* pain at injection site *Occasional:* dizziness, headache, GI symptoms	None reported	X	No information
Folate antagonists					
Dihydrofolate reductase inhibitors					
Pyrimethamine	Malaria,[b] isosporiasis, toxoplasmosis[b]	*Occasional:* folate deficiency *Rare:* rash, seizures, severe skin reactions (toxic epidermal necrolysis, erythema multiforme, Stevens-Johnson syndrome)	Sulfonamides, proguanil, zidovudine: increased risk of bone marrow suppression when used concomitantly	C	Yes
Proguanil and chlorproguanil	Malaria	*Occasional:* urticaria *Rare:* hematuria, GI disturbances	Atazanavir, efavirenz, lopinavir/ritonavir: plasma levels of proguanil decreased	C	Yes
Trimethoprim	Cyclosporiasis, isosporiasis	Hyperkalemia, GI upset, mild stomatitis	Methotrexate: reduced clearance Warfarin: effect prolonged Phenytoin: hepatic metabolism increased	C	Yes
Dihydropteroate synthetase inhibitors: sulfonamides Sulfadiazine Sulfamethoxazole Sulfadoxine	Malaria,[b] toxoplasmosis[b]	*Frequent:* GI disturbances, allergic skin reactions, crystalluria *Rare:* severe skin reactions (toxic epidermal necrolysis, erythema multiforme, Stevens-Johnson syndrome), agranulocytosis, aplastic anemia, hypersensitivity of the respiratory tract, hepatitis, interstitial nephritis, hypoglycemia, aseptic meningitis	Thiazide diuretics: increased risk of thrombocytopenia in elderly patients Warfarin: effect prolonged by sulfonamides Methotrexate: levels increased by sulfonamides Phenytoin: metabolism impaired by sulfonamides Sulfonylureas: effect prolonged by sulfonamides	B	Yes
Dihydropteroate synthetase inhibitors: sulfones					
Dapsone	Leishmaniasis, malaria, toxoplasmosis	*Frequent:* rash, anorexia *Occasional:* hemolysis, methemoglobinemia, neuropathy, allergic dermatitis, anorexia, nausea, vomiting, tachycardia, headache, insomnia, psychosis, hepatitis *Rare:* agranulocytosis	Rifampin: lowered plasma levels of dapsone	C	Yes
Fumagillin	Microsporidiosis	*Rare:* neutropenia, thrombocytopenia	None reported	No information	No information
Furazolidone	Giardiasis	*Frequent:* nausea/vomiting, brown urine *Occasional:* rectal itching, headache *Rare:* hemolytic anemia, disulfiram-like reactions, MAO inhibitor interactions	Risk of hypertensive crisis when administered for >5 days with MAO inhibitors	C	No information
Iodoquinol	Amebiasis,[b] balantidiasis, *D. fragilis* infection	*Occasional:* headache, rash, pruritus, thyrotoxicosis, nausea, vomiting, abdominal pain, diarrhea *Rare:* optic neuritis, peripheral neuropathy, seizures, encephalopathy	No major interactions	C	No information
Lactones					
Ivermectin	Ascariasis, cutaneous larva migrans, gnathostomiasis, loiasis, lymphatic filariasis, onchocerciasis,[b] scabies, strongyloidiasis,[b] trichuriasis	*Occasional:* fever, pruritus, headache, myalgias *Rare:* hypotension	No major interactions	C	Yes[c]
Moxidectin	Onchocerciasis	*Occasional:* fever, pruritus, headache, myalgias *Rare:* orthostatic hypotension, elevated transaminases	No major interactions	C	Yes[c]

(*Continued*)

TABLE 222-1 Overview of Agents Used for the Treatment of Parasitic Infections (Continued)

DRUGS BY CLASS	PARASITIC INFECTION(S)	ADVERSE EFFECTS	MAJOR DRUG–DRUG INTERACTIONS	PREGNANCY CLASS[a]	BREAST MILK
Macrolides					
Azithromycin	Babesiosis	*Occasional:* nausea, vomiting, diarrhea, abdominal pain *Rare:* angioedema, cholestatic jaundice	Cyclosporine and digoxin: levels increased by azithromycin Nelfinavir: increased levels of azithromycin	B	Yes
Spiramycin[h]	Toxoplasmosis	*Occasional:* GI disturbances, transient skin eruptions *Rare:* thrombocytopenia, QT prolongation in an infant, cholestatic hepatitis	No major interactions	Not assigned[d]	Yes[c]
Mefloquine	Malaria[b]	*Frequent:* lightheadedness, nausea, headache *Occasional:* confusion; nightmares; insomnia; visual disturbance; transient and clinically silent ECG abnormalities, including sinus bradycardia, sinus arrhythmia, first-degree AV block, prolongation of QTc interval, and abnormal T waves *Rare:* psychosis, convulsions, hypotension	Administration of halofantrine <3 weeks after mefloquine use may produce fatal QTc prolongation. Mefloquine may lower plasma levels of anticonvulsants. Levels are decreased and clearance is accelerated by artesunate. Mefloquine decreases plasma levels of ritonavir and possibly other protease inhibitors.	C	Yes
Melarsoprol[f]	Trypanosomiasis	*Frequent:* myocardial injury, encephalopathy, peripheral neuropathy, hypertension *Occasional:* G6PD-induced hemolysis, erythema nodosum leprosum *Rare:* hypotension	No major interactions	Not assigned	No information
Metrifonate	Schistosomiasis	*Frequent:* abdominal pain, nausea, vomiting, diarrhea, headache, vertigo, bronchospasm *Rare:* cholinergic symptoms	No major interactions	B	No
Miltefosine	Leishmaniasis,[b] primary amebic meningoencephalitis	*Frequent:* mild and transient (1–2 days) GI disturbances within first 2 weeks of therapy (resolve after treatment completion); motion sickness *Occasional:* reversible elevations of creatinine and aminotransferases	No major interactions	Not assigned	No information
Niclosamide	Intestinal cestode infections[b]	*Occasional:* nausea, vomiting, dizziness, pruritus	No major interactions	B	No information
Nifurtimox[f]	Chagas disease	*Frequent:* nausea, vomiting, abdominal pain, insomnia, paresthesias, weakness, tremors *Rare:* seizures (all reversible and dose-related)	No major interactions	Not assigned	No information
Nitazoxanide	Cryptosporidiosis,[b] giardiasis[b]	*Occasional:* abdominal pain, diarrhea *Rare:* vomiting, headache	Increases plasma levels of highly protein-bound drugs (e.g., phenytoin, warfarin)	B	No information
Nitroimidazoles					
Metronidazole	Amebiasis,[b] balantidiasis, dracunculiasis, giardiasis, trichomoniasis,[b] *D. fragilis* infection	*Frequent:* nausea, headache, anorexia, metallic aftertaste *Occasional:* vomiting, insomnia, vertigo, paresthesias, disulfiram-like effects *Rare:* seizures, peripheral neuropathy	Warfarin: effect enhanced by metronidazole Disulfiram: psychotic reaction Phenobarbital, phenytoin: accelerate elimination of metronidazole Lithium: serum levels elevated by metronidazole Cimetidine: prolonged half-life of metronidazole Oral solutions of antiretrovirals containing alcohol: disulfiram effect due to alcohol	B	Yes
Tinidazole	Amebiasis,[b] giardiasis, trichomoniasis	*Occasional:* nausea, vomiting, metallic taste	*See* metronidazole	C	Yes

(*Continued*)

TABLE 222-1 Overview of Agents Used for the Treatment of Parasitic Infections (Continued)

DRUGS BY CLASS	PARASITIC INFECTION(S)	ADVERSE EFFECTS	MAJOR DRUG–DRUG INTERACTIONS	PREGNANCY CLASS[a]	BREAST MILK
Oxamniquine	Schistosomiasis	*Occasional:* dizziness, drowsiness, headache, orange urine, elevated aminotransferases *Rare:* seizures	No major interactions	C	No information
Pentamidine isethionate	Leishmaniasis, trypanosomiasis	*Frequent:* hypotension, hypoglycemia, pancreatitis, sterile abscesses at IM injection sites, GI disturbances, reversible renal failure *Occasional:* hepatotoxicity, cardiotoxicity, delirium *Rare:* anaphylaxis	No major interactions	C	No information
Piperazine and derivatives					
Piperazine	Ascariasis, enterobiasis	*Occasional:* nausea, vomiting, diarrhea, abdominal pain, headache *Rare:* neurotoxicity, seizures	None reported	C	No information
Diethylcarbamazine[f]	Lymphatic filariasis, loiasis, tropical pulmonary eosinophilia	*Frequent:* dose-related nausea, vomiting *Rare:* fever, chills, arthralgias, headache	None reported	Not assigned[d]	No information
Praziquantel	Clonorchiasis,[b] cysticercosis, diphyllobothriasis, hymenolepiasis, taeniasis, opisthorchiasis, intestinal trematodes, paragonimiasis, schistosomiasis[b]	*Frequent:* abdominal pain, diarrhea, dizziness, headache, malaise *Occasional:* fever, nausea *Rare:* pruritus, singultus	No major interactions	B	Yes
Pyrantel pamoate	Ascariasis, eosinophilic enterocolitis, enterobiasis,[b] hookworm, trichostrongyliasis	*Occasional:* GI disturbances, headache, dizziness, elevated aminotransferases	No major interactions	C	No information
Pyronaridine	Malaria	*Occasional:* headache, nausea	None reported to date	B	Yes
Quinacrine[h]	Giardiasis[b]	*Frequent:* headache, nausea, vomiting, bitter taste *Occasional:* yellow-orange discoloration of skin, sclerae, urine; begins after 1 week of treatment and lasts up to 4 months after drug discontinuation *Rare:* psychosis, exfoliative dermatitis, retinopathy, G6PD-induced hemolysis, exacerbation of psoriasis, disulfiram-like effects	Primaquine: toxicity potentiated by quinacrine	C	No information
Quinine and quinidine	Malaria, babesiosis	*Frequent:* cinchonism (tinnitus, high-tone deafness, headache, dysphoria, nausea, vomiting, abdominal pain, visual disturbances, postural hypotension), hyperinsulinemia resulting in life-threatening hypoglycemia *Occasional:* deafness, hemolytic anemia, arrhythmias, hypotension due to rapid IV infusion	Carbonic anhydrase inhibitors, thiazide diuretics: reduced renal elimination of quinidine Amiodarone, cimetidine: increased quinidine levels Nifedipine: decreased quinidine levels; quinidine slows metabolism of nifedipine Phenobarbital, phenytoin, rifampin: accelerated hepatic elimination of quinidine Verapamil: reduced hepatic clearance of quinidine Diltiazem: decreased clearance of quinidine	X	Yes[c]
Quinolones					
Ciprofloxacin	Cyclosporiasis, isosporiasis	*Occasional:* nausea, diarrhea, vomiting, abdominal pain/discomfort, headache, restlessness, rash *Rare:* myalgias/arthralgias, tendon rupture, CNS symptoms (nervousness, agitation, insomnia, anxiety, nightmares, or paranoia); convulsions	Probenecid: increased serum levels of ciprofloxacin Theophylline, warfarin: serum levels increased by ciprofloxacin	C	Yes

(*Continued*)

TABLE 222-1 Overview of Agents Used for the Treatment of Parasitic Infections (Continued)

DRUGS BY CLASS	PARASITIC INFECTION(S)	ADVERSE EFFECTS	MAJOR DRUG–DRUG INTERACTIONS	PREGNANCY CLASS[a]	BREAST MILK
Suramin[f]	Trypanosomiasis	*Frequent:* immediate: fever, urticaria, nausea, vomiting, hypotension; delayed (up to 24 h): exfoliative dermatitis, stomatitis, paresthesias, photophobia, renal dysfunction *Occasional:* nephrotoxicity, adrenal toxicity, optic atrophy, anaphylaxis	No major interactions	Not assigned	No information
Tetracyclines	Balantidiasis, *D. fragilis* infection, malaria; lymphatic filariasis (doxycycline)	*Frequent:* GI disturbances *Occasional:* photosensitivity dermatitis *Rare:* exfoliative dermatitis, esophagitis, hepatotoxicity	Warfarin: effect prolonged by tetracyclines	D	Yes

[a]Based on U.S. Food and Drug Administration (FDA) pregnancy categories of A–D, X. [b]Approved by the FDA for this indication. [c]Not believed to be harmful. [d]Use in pregnancy is recommended by international organizations outside the United States. [e]Only AmBisome has been approved by the FDA for this indication. [f]Available through the CDC. [g]Only artemether (in combination with lumefantrine) and artesunate have been approved by the FDA for this indication. [h]Available through the manufacturer.

Abbreviations: ACTH, adrenocorticotropic hormone; AV, atrioventricular; CNS, central nervous system; ECG, electrocardiogram; G6PD, glucose 6-phosphate dehydrogenase; GI, gastrointestinal; MAO, monoamine oxidase.

nearly 36 h. This slower phase may be due to conversion of pentavalent antimony to a trivalent form that is the likely cause of the side effects often seen with prolonged therapy.

Artemisinin Derivatives* Artesunate, artemether, artemotil, and the parent compound artemisinin are sesquiterpene lactones derived from the wormwood plant *Artemisia annua*. These agents are at least 10-fold more potent in vivo than other antimalarial drugs and presently show no cross-resistance with known antimalarial drugs; thus they have become first-line agents for the treatment of severe falciparum malaria. The artemisinin compounds are rapidly effective against the asexual blood forms of *Plasmodium* species but are not active against intrahepatic forms. With the exception of artesunate, artemisinin and its derivatives are highly lipid soluble and readily cross both host and parasite cell membranes. One factor that explains the drugs' highly selective toxicity against malaria is that parasitized erythrocytes concentrate artemisinin and its derivatives to concentrations 100-fold higher than those in uninfected erythrocytes. The antimalarial effect of these agents results primarily from the active metabolite dihydroartemisinin; in the presence of heme or molecular iron, the endoperoxide moiety of dihydroartemisinin decomposes, generating free radicals and other metabolites that damage parasite proteins. The compounds are available for oral, rectal, IV, or IM administration, depending on the derivative. In the United States, IV artesunate is available for the treatment of severe, quinidine-unresponsive malaria through the CDC malaria hotline (770-488-7788 or 855-856-4713 [toll-free], M–F, 0800–1630 EST; 770-488-7100 after hours). Artemisinin and its derivatives are cleared rapidly from the circulation. Their short half-lives limit their value for prophylaxis and monotherapy. Side effects appear to be minor, although sinus bradycardia and transient first-degree heart block have been reported. Although seen in animal models, embryotoxicity and neurotoxicity have not been identified in humans despite active investigation. These agents should be used only in combination with another, longer-acting agent (e.g., artesunate-mefloquine, dihydroartemisinin-piperaquine). While artesunate is only available in the United States from the CDC drug service, a combined formulation of artemether and lumefantrine is widely available for the treatment of acute uncomplicated falciparum malaria acquired in areas where *Plasmodium falciparum* is resistant to chloroquine and antifolates.

Atovaquone Atovaquone is a hydroxynaphthoquinone that exerts broad-spectrum antiprotozoal activity via selective inhibition of parasite mitochondrial electron transport. This agent exhibits potent activity against toxoplasmosis and babesiosis when used with pyrimethamine and azithromycin, respectively. Atovaquone possesses a novel mode of action against *Plasmodium* species, inhibiting the electron transport system at the level of the cytochrome bc1 complex. The drug is active against both the erythrocytic and the exoerythrocytic stages of *Plasmodium* species; however, because it does not eradicate hypnozoites from the liver, patients with *P. vivax* or *P. ovale* infections must be given radical prophylaxis.

Malarone is a fixed-dose combination of atovaquone and proguanil used for malaria prophylaxis as well as for the treatment of acute, uncomplicated *P. falciparum* malaria. Malarone has been shown to be effective in regions with multidrug-resistant *P. falciparum*. Resistance to atovaquone develops rapidly via mutations in the parasite's mitochondrial cytochrome b complex. However, the mutations result in sterility of female parasites; thus atovaquone-resistant parasites cannot be transmitted to another person. This situation may explain why clinical resistance has yet to be reported.

The bioavailability of atovaquone varies considerably. Absorption after a single oral dose is slow, increases two- to three-fold with a fatty meal, and is dose-limited above 750 mg. The elimination half-life is increased in patients with moderate hepatic impairment. Because of the potential for drug accumulation, the use of atovaquone is generally contraindicated in persons with a creatinine clearance rate <30 mL/min. No dosage adjustments are needed in patients with mild to moderate renal impairment.

Azithromycin See Table 222-1 and **Chap. 144.**

Azoles See Table 222-1 and **Chap. 211.**

Benznidazole* This oral nitroimidazole derivative is used to treat Chagas disease, with cure rates of 80–90% recorded in acute infections. Benznidazole is believed to exert its trypanocidal effects by generating oxygen radicals to which the parasites are more sensitive than mammalian cells because of a relative deficiency in antioxidant enzymes. Benznidazole also appears to alter the balance between pro- and anti-inflammatory mediators by downregulating the synthesis of nitrite, interleukin (IL) 6, and IL-10 in macrophages. Benznidazole is highly lipophilic and readily absorbed. The drug is extensively metabolized; only 5% of the dose is excreted unchanged in the urine. Benznidazole is well tolerated; adverse effects are rare and usually manifest as GI upset or pruritic rash.

Chloroquine This 4-aminoquinoline has marked, rapid schizonticidal and gametocidal activity against blood forms of *P. ovale* and *P. malariae* and against susceptible strains of *P. vivax* and *P. falciparum*. It is not active against intrahepatic forms (*P. vivax* and *P. ovale*). Parasitized erythrocytes accumulate chloroquine in significantly greater concentrations than do normal erythrocytes. Chloroquine, a weak base, concentrates in the food vacuoles of intraerythrocytic parasites because of a relative pH gradient between the extracellular space and the acidic food vacuole. Once it enters the acidic food vacuole, chloroquine is rapidly converted to a membrane-impermeable protonated form and is trapped. Continued accumulation of chloroquine in the parasite's acidic food vacuoles results in drug levels that are 600-fold higher at this site than in plasma. The high accumulation of chloroquine results in an increase in pH within the food vacuole to a level above that required for the acid proteases' optimal activity, inhibiting parasite heme polymerase; as a result, the parasite is effectively killed with its own metabolic waste. Compared with susceptible strains, chloroquine-resistant plasmodia transport chloroquine out of intraparasitic compartments more rapidly and maintain lower chloroquine concentrations in their acid vesicles. Hydroxychloroquine, a congener of chloroquine, is equivalent to chloroquine in its antimalarial efficacy but is preferred to chloroquine for the treatment of autoimmune disorders because it produces less ocular toxicity when used in high doses.

Chloroquine is well absorbed. However, because it exhibits extensive tissue binding, a loading dose is required to yield effective plasma concentrations. A therapeutic drug level in plasma is reached 2–3 h after oral administration (the preferred route). Chloroquine can be administered IV, but excessively rapid parenteral administration can result in seizures and death from cardiovascular collapse. The mean half-life of chloroquine is 4 days, but the rate of excretion decreases as plasma levels decline, making once-weekly administration possible for prophylaxis in areas with sensitive strains. About one-half of the parent drug is excreted in urine, but the dose should not be reduced for persons with acute malaria and renal insufficiency.

Ciprofloxacin See Table 222-1 and **Chap. 144**.

Clindamycin See Table 222-1 and **Chap. 144**.

Dapsone See Table 222-1 and **Chap. 181**.

Dehydroemetine Emetine is an alkaloid derived from ipecac; dehydroemetine is synthetically derived from emetine and is considered less toxic. Both agents are active against *Entamoeba histolytica* and appear to work by blocking peptide elongation and thus inhibiting protein synthesis. Emetine is rapidly absorbed after parenteral administration, rapidly distributed throughout the body, and slowly excreted in the urine in unchanged form. Both agents are contraindicated in patients with renal disease.

Diethylcarbamazine* A derivative of the antihelminthic agent piperazine with a long history of successful use, diethylcarbamazine (DEC) remains the treatment of choice for lymphatic filariasis and loiasis and has also been used for visceral larva migrans. Although piperazine itself has no antifilarial activity, the piperazine ring of DEC is essential for the drug's activity. DEC's mechanism of action remains to be fully defined. Proposed mechanisms include immobilization due to inhibition of parasite cholinergic muscle receptors, disruption of microtubule formation, and alteration of helminthic surface membranes resulting in enhanced killing by the host's immune system. DEC enhances adherence properties of eosinophils. The development of resistance under drug pressure (i.e., a progressive decrease in efficacy when the drug is used widely in human populations) has not been observed, although DEC has variable effects when administered to persons with filariasis. Monthly administration provides effective prophylaxis against both bancroftian filariasis and loiasis.

DEC is well absorbed after oral administration, with peak plasma concentrations reached within 1–2 h. No parenteral form is available. The drug is eliminated largely by renal excretion, with <5% found in feces. If more than one dose is to be administered to an individual with renal dysfunction, the dose should be reduced commensurate with the reduction in creatinine clearance rate. Alkalinization of the urine prevents renal excretion and increases the half-life of DEC. Use in patients with onchocerciasis can precipitate a Mazzotti reaction, with pruritus, fever, and arthralgias. Like other piperazines, DEC is active against *Ascaris* species. Patients co-infected with this nematode may expel live worms after treatment.

Diloxanide Furoate Diloxanide furoate, a substituted acetanilide, is a luminally active agent used to eradicate the cysts of *E. histolytica*. After ingestion, diloxanide furoate is hydrolyzed by enzymes in the lumen or mucosa of the intestine, releasing furoic acid and the ester diloxanide; the latter acts directly as an amebicide.

Diloxanide furoate is given alone to asymptomatic cyst passers. For patients with active amebic infections, diloxanide is generally administered in combination with a 5-nitroimidazole such as metronidazole or tinidazole. Diloxanide furoate is rapidly absorbed after oral administration. When coadministered with a 5-nitroimidazole, diloxanide levels peak within 1 h and disappear within 6 h. About 90% of an oral dose is excreted in the urine within 48 h, chiefly as the glucuronide metabolite. Diloxanide furoate is contraindicated in pregnant and breast-feeding women and in children <2 years of age.

Eflornithine* Eflornithine (difluoromethylornithine, or DFMO) is a fluorinated analogue of the amino acid ornithine. Although originally designed as an antineoplastic agent, eflornithine has proven effective against some trypanosomatids.

Eflornithine has specific activity against all stages of infection with *Trypanosoma brucei gambiense*; however, it is inactive against *T. b. rhodesiense*. The drug acts as an irreversible suicide inhibitor of ornithine decarboxylase, the first enzyme in the biosynthesis of the polyamines putrescine and spermidine. Polyamines are essential for the synthesis of trypanothione, an enzyme required for the maintenance of intracellular thiols in the correct redox state and for the removal of reactive oxygen metabolites. However, polyamines are also essential for cell division in eukaryotes, and ornithine decarboxylase is similar in trypanosomes and mammals. The selective antiparasitic activity of eflornithine is partly explained by the structure of the trypanosomal enzyme, which lacks a 36-amino-acid C-terminal sequence found on mammalian ornithine decarboxylase. This difference results in a lower turnover of ornithine decarboxylase and a more rapid decrease of polyamines in trypanosomes than in the mammalian host. The diminished effectiveness of eflornithine against *T. b. rhodesiense* appears to be due to the parasite's ability to replace the inhibited enzyme more rapidly than *T. b. gambiense*.

Eflornithine is less toxic but more costly than conventional therapy. It can be administered IV or PO. The dose should be reduced in renal failure. Eflornithine readily crosses the blood–brain barrier; CSF levels are highest in persons with the most severe central nervous system (CNS) involvement.

Fumagillin† Originally discovered as an anti-angiogenic compound derived from the fungus *Aspergillus fumigatus*, fumagillin is a water-insoluble antibiotic that is active against microsporidia and is used topically to treat ocular infections due to *Encephalitozoon* species. When given systemically, fumagillin was effective but caused thrombocytopenia in all recipients in the second week of treatment; this side effect was readily reversed when administration of the drug was stopped. Fumagillin acts by binding to methionine aminopeptidase 2, thus inhibiting microsporidial replication by irreversibly blocking the active site.

Furazolidone This nitrofuran derivative is an effective alternative agent for the treatment of giardiasis and also exhibits activity against *Isospora belli*. Because it is the only agent active against *Giardia* that is available in liquid form, it is most often used to treat young children. Furazolidone undergoes reductive activation in *Giardia lamblia* trophozoites—an event that, unlike the reductive activation of metronidazole, involves an NADH oxidase. The killing effect correlates with the toxicity of reduced products, which damage important cellular components, including DNA. Although furazolidone had been thought to be largely unabsorbed when administered orally, the occurrence of systemic adverse reactions indicates that this is not the case. More than 65% of the drug dose can be recovered from the urine as colored metabolites. Omeprazole reduces the oral bioavailability of furazolidone.

Furazolidone is a monoamine oxidase (MAO) inhibitor; thus caution should be used in its concomitant administration with other drugs (especially indirectly acting sympathomimetic amines) and in the consumption of food and drink containing tyramine during treatment. However, hypertensive crises have not been reported in patients receiving furazolidone, and it has been suggested that—because furazolidone inhibits MAOs gradually over several days—the risks are small if treatment is limited to a 5-day course. Because hemolytic anemia can occur in patients with glucose-6-phosphate dehydrogenase

(G6PD) deficiency and glutathione instability, furazolidone treatment is contraindicated in mothers who are breast-feeding and in neonates.

Halofantrine This 9-phenanthrenemethanol is one of three classes of arylaminoalcohols first identified as potential antimalarial agents by the World War II Malaria Chemotherapy Program. Its activity is believed to be similar to that of chloroquine, although it is an oral alternative for the treatment of malaria due to chloroquine-resistant *P. falciparum*.

Halofantrine is thought to share one or more mechanisms with the 4-aminoquinolines, forming a complex with ferriprotoporphyrin IX and interfering with the degradation of hemoglobin. It has been shown to bind to plasmepsin, a hemoglobin-degrading enzyme unique to plasmodia.

Halofantrine exhibits erratic bioavailability, but its absorption is significantly enhanced when it is taken with a fatty meal. The elimination half-life of halofantrine is 1–2 days; it is excreted mainly in feces. Halofantrine is metabolized into *N*-debutyl-halofantrine by the cytochrome P450 enzyme CYP3A4. Grapefruit juice should be avoided during treatment because it increases both halofantrine's bioavailability and halofantrine-induced QT interval prolongation by inhibiting CYP3A4 at the enterocyte level. Halofantrine should not be given simultaneously with or <3 weeks after mefloquine because of the potential occurrence of a fatal prolongation of the QTc interval on electrocardiography.

Iodoquinol Iodoquinol (diiodohydroxyquin), a hydroxyquinoline, is an effective luminal agent for the treatment of amebiasis, balantidiasis, and infection with *Dientamoeba fragilis*. Its mechanism of action is unknown. It is poorly absorbed. Because the drug contains 64% organically bound iodine, it should be used with caution in patients with thyroid disease. Iodine dermatitis occurs occasionally during iodoquinol treatment. Protein-bound serum iodine levels may be increased during treatment and can interfere with certain tests of thyroid function. These effects may persist for as long as 6 months after discontinuation of therapy. Iodoquinol is contraindicated in patients with liver disease. Most serious are the reactions related to prolonged high-dose therapy (optic neuritis, peripheral neuropathy), which should not occur if the recommended dosage regimens are followed.

Ivermectin Ivermectin (22,23-dihydroavermectin) is a derivative of the macrocyclic lactone avermectin produced by the soil-dwelling actinomycete *Streptomyces avermitilis*. Ivermectin is active at low doses against a wide range of helminths and ectoparasites. It is the drug of choice for the treatment of onchocerciasis, strongyloidiasis, cutaneous larva migrans, and scabies. Ivermectin is highly active against microfilariae of the lymphatic filariases but has no macrofilaricidal activity. When ivermectin is used in combination with other agents such as DEC or albendazole for treatment of lymphatic filariasis, synergistic activity is seen. Although active against the intestinal helminths *Ascaris lumbricoides* and *Enterobius vermicularis*, ivermectin is only variably effective in trichuriasis and is ineffective against hookworms. Widespread use of ivermectin for treatment of intestinal nematode infections in sheep and goats has led to the emergence of drug resistance in veterinary practice; this development may portend problems in human medical use.

Data suggest that ivermectin acts by opening the neuromuscular membrane-associated, glutamate-dependent chloride channels. The influx of chloride ions results in hyperpolarization and muscle paralysis—particularly of the nematode pharynx, with consequent blockage of the oral ingestion of nutrients. As these chloride channels are present only in invertebrates, paralysis is seen only in the parasite.

Ivermectin is available for administration to humans only as an oral formulation. The drug is highly protein bound; it is almost completely excreted in feces. Both food and beer increase the bioavailability of ivermectin significantly. Ivermectin is distributed widely throughout the body; animal studies indicate that it accumulates at the highest concentration in adipose tissue and liver, with little accumulation in the brain. Few data exist to guide therapy in hosts with conditions that may influence drug pharmacokinetics.

Ivermectin is generally administered as a single dose of 150–200 μg/kg. In the absence of parasitic infection, the adverse effects of ivermectin in therapeutic doses are minimal. Adverse effects in patients with filarial infections include fever, myalgia, malaise, lightheadedness, and (occasionally) postural hypotension. The severity of such side effects is related to the intensity of parasite infection, with more symptoms in individuals with a heavy parasite burden. In onchocerciasis, skin edema, pruritus, and mild eye irritation may also occur. The adverse effects are generally self-limiting and only occasionally require symptom-based treatment with antipyretics or antihistamines. More severe complications of ivermectin therapy for onchocerciasis include encephalopathy in patients heavily infected with *Loa loa*.

Lumefantrine Lumefantrine (benflumetol), a fluorene arylaminoalcohol derivative synthesized in the 1970s by the Chinese Academy of Military Medical Sciences (Beijing), has marked blood schizonticidal activity against a wide range of plasmodia. This agent conforms structurally and in mode of action to other arylaminoalcohols (quinine, mefloquine, and halofantrine). Lumefantrine exerts its antimalarial effect as a consequence of its interaction with heme, a degradation product of hemoglobin metabolism. Although its antimalarial activity is slower than that of the artemisinin-based drugs, the recrudescence rate with the recommended lumefantrine regimen is lower. The pharmacokinetic properties of lumefantrine are reminiscent of those of halofantrine, with variable oral bioavailability, considerable augmentation of oral bioavailability by concomitant fat intake, and a terminal elimination half-life of ~4–5 days in patients with malaria.

Artemether and lumefantrine have synergistic activity, and the combined formulation of artemether and lumefantrine is effective for the treatment of falciparum malaria in areas where *P. falciparum* is resistant to chloroquine and antifolates.

Mebendazole This benzimidazole is a broad-spectrum antiparasitic agent widely used to treat intestinal helminthiases. Its mechanism of action is similar to that of albendazole; however, it is a more potent inhibitor of parasite malic dehydrogenase and exhibits a more specific and selective effect against intestinal nematodes than the other benzimidazoles.

Mebendazole is available only in oral form but is poorly absorbed from the GI tract; only 5–10% of a standard dose is measurable in plasma. The proportion absorbed from the GI tract is extensively metabolized in the liver. Metabolites appear in the urine and bile; impaired liver or biliary function results in higher plasma mebendazole levels in treated patients. No dose reduction is warranted in patients with renal function impairment. Because mebendazole is poorly absorbed, its incidence of side effects is low. Transient abdominal pain and diarrhea sometimes occur, usually in persons with massive parasite burdens.

Mefloquine Mefloquine is used for prophylaxis of chloroquine-resistant malaria; high doses can be used for treatment. Despite the development of drug-resistant strains of *P. falciparum* in parts of Africa and Southeast Asia, mefloquine remains an effective drug throughout most of the world. Cross-resistance of mefloquine with halofantrine and with quinine has been documented in limited areas. Like quinine and chloroquine, this quinoline is active only against the asexual erythrocytic stages of malarial parasites. Unlike quinine, however, mefloquine has a relatively poor affinity for DNA and, as a result, does not inhibit the synthesis of parasitic nucleic acids and proteins. Although both mefloquine and chloroquine inhibit hemozoin formation and heme degradation, mefloquine differs in that it forms a complex with heme that may be toxic to the parasite.

Mefloquine HCl is poorly water soluble and intensely irritating when given parenterally; thus it is available only in tablet form. Its absorption is adversely affected by vomiting and diarrhea but is significantly enhanced when the drug is administered with or after food. About 98% of the drug binds to protein. Mefloquine is excreted mainly in the bile and feces; therefore, no dose adjustment is needed in persons with renal insufficiency. The drug and its main metabolite are not appreciably removed by hemodialysis. No special chemoprophylactic dosage adjustments are indicated for the achievement of plasma concentrations in dialysis patients that are similar to those in healthy persons. Pharmacokinetic differences have been detected among various ethnic populations; however, these distinctions are of minor importance compared with host immune status and parasite sensitivity. In patients with impaired liver function, the elimination of mefloquine may be prolonged, leading to higher plasma levels.

Mefloquine should be used with caution by individuals participating in activities requiring alertness and fine-motor coordination because dizziness, vertigo, or tinnitus can develop and persist. If the drug is to be administered for a prolonged period, periodic evaluations are recommended, including liver function tests and ophthalmic examinations. Sleep abnormalities (insomnia, abnormal dreams) have occasionally been reported. Psychosis and seizures occur rarely; mefloquine should not be prescribed to patients with neuropsychiatric conditions. The development of acute anxiety, depression, restlessness, or confusion may be considered prodromal to a more serious event, and the drug should be discontinued.

Concomitant use of quinine, quinidine, or drugs producing β-adrenergic blockade may cause significant electrocardiographic abnormalities or cardiac arrest. Halofantrine must not be given simultaneously with or <3 weeks after mefloquine because a potentially fatal prolongation of the QTc interval on electrocardiography may occur. No data exist on mefloquine use after halofantrine use. Administration of mefloquine with quinine or chloroquine may increase the risk of convulsions. Mefloquine may lower plasma levels of anticonvulsants. Caution should be exercised with regard to concomitant antiretroviral therapy, because mefloquine has been shown to exert variable effects on ritonavir pharmacokinetics that are not explained by hepatic CYP3A4 activity or ritonavir protein binding. Vaccinations with attenuated live bacteria should be completed at least 3 days before the first dose of mefloquine.

Women of childbearing age who are traveling to areas where malaria is endemic should be warned against becoming pregnant and encouraged to practice contraception during malaria prophylaxis with mefloquine and for up to 3 months thereafter. However, in the case of unplanned pregnancy, use of mefloquine is not considered an indication for pregnancy termination. Analysis of prospectively monitored cases demonstrates a prevalence of birth defects and fetal loss comparable to background rates.

Melarsoprol* Melarsoprol has been used since 1949 for the treatment of human African trypanosomiasis. This trivalent arsenical compound is indicated for the treatment of African trypanosomiasis with neurologic involvement and for the treatment of early disease that is resistant to suramin or pentamidine. Melarsoprol, like other drugs containing heavy metals, interacts with thiol groups of several different proteins; however, its antiparasitic effects appear to be more specific. Trypanothione reductase is a key enzyme involved in the oxidative stress management of both *Trypanosoma* and *Leishmania* species, helping to maintain an intracellular reducing environment by reduction of disulfide trypanothione to its dithiol derivative dihydrotrypanothione. Melarsoprol sequesters dihydrotrypanothione, depriving the parasite of its main sulfhydryl antioxidant, and inhibits trypanothione reductase, depriving the parasite of the essential enzyme system that is responsible for keeping trypanothione reduced. These effects are synergistic. The selectivity of arsenical action against trypanosomes is due at least in part to the greater melarsoprol affinity of reduced trypanothione than of other monothiols (e.g., cysteine) on which the mammalian host depends for maintenance of high thiol levels. Melarsoprol enters the parasite via an adenosine transporter; drug-resistant strains lack this transport system.

Melarsoprol is always administered IV. A small but therapeutically significant amount of the drug enters the CSF. The compound is excreted rapidly, with ~80% of the arsenic found in feces.

Melarsoprol is highly toxic. The most serious adverse reaction is reactive encephalopathy, which affects 6% of treated individuals and usually develops within 4 days of the start of therapy, with an average case–fatality rate of 50%. Glucocorticoids are administered with melarsoprol to prevent this development. Because melarsoprol is intensely irritating, care must be taken to avoid infiltration of the drug.

Metrifonate Metrifonate has selective activity against *Schistosoma haematobium*. This organophosphorous compound is a prodrug that is converted nonenzymatically to dichlorvos (2,2-dichlorovinyl dimethylphosphate, DDVP), a highly active chemical that irreversibly inhibits the acetylcholinesterase enzyme. Schistosomal cholinesterase is more susceptible to dichlorvos than is the corresponding human enzyme. The exact mechanism of action of metrifonate is uncertain, but the drug is believed to inhibit tegumental acetylcholine receptors that mediate glucose transport.

Metrifonate is administered in a series of three doses at 2-week intervals. After a single oral dose, metrifonate produces a 95% decrease in plasma cholinesterase activity within 6 h, with a fairly rapid return to normal. However, 2.5 months are required for erythrocyte cholinesterase levels to return to normal. Treated persons should not be exposed to neuromuscular blocking agents or organophosphate insecticides for at least 48 h after treatment.

Metronidazole and Other Nitroimidazoles See Table 222-1 and Chap. 144.

Miltefosine In the early 1990s, miltefosine (hexadecylphosphocholine), originally developed as an antineoplastic agent, was discovered to have significant antiproliferative activity against *Leishmania* species, *T. cruzi*, and *T. brucei* parasites in vitro and in experimental animal models. Miltefosine is the first oral drug that has proved to be highly effective and comparable to amphotericin B against visceral leishmaniasis in India, where antimonial-resistant cases are prevalent. Miltefosine is also effective in previously untreated visceral infections. Cure rates in cutaneous leishmaniasis are comparable to those obtained with antimony. Miltefosine is also effective against the free-living ameba *Naegleria fowleri*.

The activity of miltefosine is attributed to interaction with cell signal transduction pathways and inhibition of phospholipid and sterol biosynthesis. Resistance to miltefosine has not been observed clinically. The drug is readily absorbed from the GI tract, is widely distributed, and accumulates in several tissues. The efficacy of a 28-day treatment course in Indian visceral leishmaniasis is equivalent to that of amphotericin B therapy; however, it appears that a shortened course of 21 days may be equally efficacious.

General recommendations for the use of miltefosine are limited by the exclusion of specific groups from the published clinical trials: persons <12 or >65 years of age, persons with the most advanced disease, breast-feeding women, HIV-infected patients, and individuals with significant renal or hepatic insufficiency.

Moxidectin Like ivermectin, moxidectin is a macrocyclic lactone that is an effective antihelminthic. In 2018, the FDA approved its use for the treatment of onchocerciasis. The primary mode of action of moxidectin is believed to be similar to that of ivermectin; however, there are likely different binding sites, as suggested by the identification of ivermectin-resistant helminths that are susceptible to moxidectin. The drug is well tolerated, with most adverse effects attributed to death of microfilariae. Some adverse effects occurred more commonly compared with ivermectin, including orthostatic hypotension (5% vs 2%) and elevated transaminases (1% vs 0.6%). In clinical trials, no clinically significant differences in the pharmacokinetics were observed with age, gender, weight, or renal impairment. The effect of hepatic dysfunction is unknown.

Niclosamide† Niclosamide is active against a wide variety of adult tapeworms but not against tissue cestodes. The drug uncouples oxidative phosphorylation in parasite mitochondria, thereby blocking the uptake of glucose by the intestinal tapeworm and resulting in the parasite's death. Niclosamide rapidly causes spastic paralysis of intestinal cestodes in vitro. Its use is limited by its side effects, the necessarily long duration of therapy, the recommended use of purgatives, and—most important—limited availability (i.e., on a named-patient basis from the manufacturer).

Niclosamide is poorly absorbed. Tablets are given on an empty stomach in the morning after a liquid meal the night before, and this dose is followed by another 1 h later. For treatment of hymenolepiasis, the drug is administered for 7 days. A second course is often prescribed. The scolex and proximal segments of the tapeworms are killed on contact with niclosamide and may be digested in the gut. However, disintegration of the adult tapeworm results in the release of viable ova, which theoretically can result in autoinfection. Although fears of the development of cysticercosis in patients with *Taenia solium* infections have proved unfounded, it is still recommended that a brisk purgative be given 2 h after the first dose.

Nifurtimox* This nitrofuran compound is an inexpensive and effective oral agent for the treatment of acute Chagas disease. Trypanosomes lack catalase and have very low levels of peroxidase; as a result, they are very vulnerable to by-products of oxygen reduction. When nifurtimox is reduced in the trypanosome, a nitro anion radical is formed and undergoes autooxidation, resulting in the generation of the superoxide anion O_2^-, hydrogen peroxide (H_2O_2), hydroperoxyl radical (HO_2), and other highly reactive and cytotoxic molecules. Despite the abundance of catalases, peroxidases, and superoxide dismutases that neutralize these destructive radicals in mammalian cells, nifurtimox has a poor therapeutic index. Prolonged use is required, but the course may have to be interrupted because of drug toxicity, which develops in 40–70% of recipients. Nifurtimox is well absorbed and undergoes rapid and extensive biotransformation; <0.5% of the original drug is excreted in urine.

Nitazoxanide Nitazoxanide is a 5-nitrothiazole compound used for the treatment of cryptosporidiosis and giardiasis; it is active against other intestinal protozoa as well. The drug is approved for use in children 1–11 years of age.

The antiprotozoal activity of nitazoxanide is believed to be due to interference with the pyruvate-ferredoxin oxidoreductase (PFOR) enzyme–dependent electron transfer reaction that is essential to anaerobic energy metabolism. Studies have shown that the PFOR enzyme from *G. lamblia* directly reduces nitazoxanide by transfer of electrons in the absence of ferredoxin. The DNA-derived PFOR protein sequence of *Cryptosporidium parvum* appears to be similar to that of *G. lamblia*. Interference with the PFOR enzyme–dependent electron transfer reaction may not be the only pathway by which nitazoxanide exerts antiprotozoal activity.

After oral administration, nitazoxanide is rapidly hydrolyzed to an active metabolite, tizoxanide (desacetyl-nitazoxanide). Tizoxanide then undergoes conjugation, primarily by glucuronidation. It is recommended that nitazoxanide be taken with food; however, no studies have been conducted to determine whether the pharmacokinetics of tizoxanide and tizoxanide glucuronide differ in fasted versus fed subjects. Tizoxanide is excreted in urine, bile, and feces, and tizoxanide glucuronide is excreted in urine and bile. The pharmacokinetics of nitazoxanide in patients with impaired hepatic and/or renal function have not been studied. Tizoxanide is highly bound to plasma protein (>99.9%). Therefore, caution should be used when administering this agent concurrently with other highly plasma protein–bound drugs that have narrow therapeutic indices, as competition for binding sites may occur.

Oxamniquine This tetrahydroquinoline derivative is an effective alternative agent for the treatment of *S. mansoni*, although susceptibility to this drug exhibits regional variation. Oxamniquine exhibits anticholinergic properties, but its primary mode of action seems to rely on ATP-dependent enzymatic drug activation generating an intermediate that alkylates essential macromolecules, including DNA. In treated adult schistosomes, oxamniquine produces marked tegumental alterations that are similar to those seen with praziquantel but that develop less rapidly, becoming evident 4–8 days after treatment.

Oxamniquine is administered orally as a single dose and is well absorbed. Food retards absorption and reduces bioavailability. About 70% of an administered dose is excreted in urine as a mixture of pharmacologically inactive metabolites. Patients should be warned that their urine might have an intense orange-red color. Side effects are uncommon and usually mild, although hallucinations and seizures have been reported.

Paromomycin (Aminosidine) First isolated in 1956, this aminoglycoside is an effective oral agent for the treatment of infections due to intestinal protozoa. Parenteral paromomycin appears to be effective against visceral leishmaniasis in India.

Paromomycin inhibits protozoan protein synthesis by binding to the 30S ribosomal RNA in the aminoacyl-tRNA site, causing misreading of mRNA codons. Paromomycin is less active against *G. lamblia* than standard agents; however, like other aminoglycosides, paromomycin is poorly absorbed from the intestinal lumen, and the high levels of drug in the gut compensate for this relatively weak activity. If absorbed or administered systemically, paromomycin can cause ototoxicity and nephrotoxicity. However, systemic absorption is very limited, and toxicity should not be a concern in persons with normal kidneys. Topical formulations are not generally available.

Pentamidine Isethionate This diamidine is an effective alternative agent for some forms of leishmaniasis and trypanosomiasis. It is available for parenteral and aerosolized administration. Although its mechanism of action remains undefined, it is known to exert a wide range of effects, including interaction with trypanosomal kinetoplast DNA; interference with polyamine synthesis by a decrease in the activity of ornithine decarboxylase; and inhibition of RNA polymerase, topoisomerase, ribosomal function, and the synthesis of nucleic acids and proteins.

Pentamidine isethionate is well absorbed, highly tissue bound, and excreted slowly over several weeks, with an elimination half-life of 12 days. No steady-state plasma concentration is attained in persons given daily injections; the result is extensive accumulation of pentamidine in tissues, primarily the liver, kidney, adrenal gland, and spleen. Pentamidine does not penetrate well into the CNS. Pulmonary concentrations of pentamidine are increased when the drug is delivered in aerosolized form, but not when it is delivered systemically.

Rapid (<1-h) infusion of intravenous pentamidine often results in hypotension. Because electrolyte disturbances and mild to moderate nephrotoxicity occur commonly, pentamidine should be used with caution with other nephrotoxic agents. Pancreatitis and QT prolongation may also occur; cumulative damage to pancreatic islet cells may result in drug-induced diabetes mellitus. Similarly, hypoglycemia can develop, although much less commonly when pentamidine is given by the inhaled route.

Piperaquine This bisquinoline was synthesized in the 1960s and used widely for malaria control in China. The development of artemisinin-based combination therapy led to its evaluation as a partner drug, and it is now combined with dihydroartemisinin. Piperaquine is highly lipophilic and has a prolonged half-life (~20 days), thus providing a period of posttreatment prophylaxis. The drug's mechanisms of action and resistance have not been well studied but are presumed to be similar to those of the other 4-aminoquinolines.

Piperazine The antihelminthic activity of piperazine is confined to ascariasis and enterobiasis. Piperazine acts as an agonist at extrasynaptic γ-aminobutyric acid (GABA) receptors, causing an influx of chloride ions in the nematode somatic musculature. Although the initial result is hyperpolarization of the muscle fibers, the ultimate effect is flaccid paralysis, leading to the expulsion of live worms. Patients should be warned, as this occurrence can be unsettling.

Praziquantel This heterocyclic pyrazinoisoquinoline derivative is highly active against a broad spectrum of trematodes and cestodes. It is the mainstay of treatment for schistosomiasis and is a critical part of community-based control programs.

All of the effects of praziquantel can be attributed either directly or indirectly to an alteration of intracellular calcium concentrations. Although the exact mechanism of action remains unclear, the major mechanism is disruption of the parasite tegument, causing tetanic contractures with loss of adherence to host tissues and, ultimately, disintegration or expulsion. Praziquantel induces changes in the antigenicity of the parasite by causing the exposure of concealed antigens. Praziquantel also produces alterations in schistosomal glucose metabolism, including decreases in glucose uptake, lactate release, glycogen content, and ATP levels.

Praziquantel exerts its parasitic effects directly and does not need to be metabolized to be effective. It is well absorbed but undergoes extensive first-pass hepatic clearance. Levels of the drug are increased when it is taken with food, particularly carbohydrates, or with cimetidine. Serum levels are reduced by glucocorticoids, chloroquine, carbamazepine, and phenytoin. Praziquantel is completely metabolized in humans, with 80% of the dose recovered as metabolites in urine within 4 days. It is not known to what extent praziquantel crosses the placenta, but retrospective studies suggest that it is safe in pregnancy.

Patients with schistosomiasis who have heavy parasite burdens may develop abdominal discomfort, nausea, headache, dizziness, and drowsiness. Symptoms begin 30 min after ingestion, may require spasmolytics for relief, and usually disappear spontaneously after a few hours.

Primaquine Phosphate Primaquine, an 8-aminoquinoline, has a broad spectrum of activity against all stages of plasmodial development in humans but has been used most effectively for eradication of the hepatic stage of these parasites. Despite its toxicity, it remains the drug of choice for radical cure of *P. vivax* infections. Primaquine must be metabolized by the host to be effective. It is, in fact, rapidly metabolized; only a small fraction of the dose of the parent drug is excreted unchanged. Although the parasiticidal activity of the three oxidative metabolites remains unclear, they are believed to affect both pyrimidine synthesis and the mitochondrial electron transport chain. The metabolites appear to have significantly less antimalarial activity than primaquine; however, their hemolytic activity is greater than that of the parent drug.

Primaquine causes marked hypotension after parenteral administration and therefore is given only by the oral route. It is rapidly and almost completely absorbed from the GI tract.

Patients should be tested for G6PD deficiency before they receive primaquine. The drug may induce the oxidation of hemoglobin into methemoglobin, regardless of the G6PD status of the patient. Primaquine is otherwise well tolerated.

Proguanil (Chloroguanide) Proguanil inhibits plasmodial dihydrofolate reductase and is used with atovaquone for oral treatment of uncomplicated malaria or with chloroquine for malaria prophylaxis in parts of Africa without widespread chloroquine-resistant *P. falciparum*.

Proguanil exerts its effect primarily by means of the metabolite cycloguanil, whose inhibition of dihydrofolate reductase in the parasite disrupts deoxythymidylate synthesis, thus interfering with a key pathway involved in the biosynthesis of pyrimidines required for nucleic acid replication. There are no clinical data indicating that folate supplementation diminishes drug efficacy; women of childbearing age for whom atovaquone/proguanil is prescribed should continue taking folate supplements to prevent neural tube birth defects.

Proguanil is extensively absorbed regardless of food intake. The drug is 75% protein bound. The main routes of elimination are hepatic biotransformation and renal excretion; 40–60% of the proguanil dose is excreted by the kidneys. Drug levels are increased and elimination is impaired in patients with hepatic insufficiency.

Pyrantel Pamoate Pyrantel is a tetrahydropyrimidine formulated as pamoate. This safe, well-tolerated, inexpensive drug is used to treat a variety of intestinal nematode infections but is ineffective in trichuriasis. Pyrantel pamoate is usually effective in a single dose. Its target is the nicotinic acetylcholine receptor on the surface of nematode somatic muscle. Pyrantel depolarizes the neuromuscular junction of the nematode, resulting in its irreversible paralysis and allowing the natural expulsion of the worm.

Pyrantel pamoate is poorly absorbed from the intestine; >85% of the dose is passed unaltered in feces. The absorbed portion is metabolized and excreted in urine. Piperazine is antagonistic to pyrantel pamoate and should not be used concomitantly.

Pyrantel pamoate has minimal toxicity at the oral doses used to treat intestinal helminthic infection. It is not recommended for pregnant women or for children <12 months old.

Pyrimethamine When combined with short-acting sulfonamides, this diaminopyrimidine is effective in malaria, toxoplasmosis, and isosporiasis. Unlike mammalian cells, the parasites that cause these infections cannot use preformed pyrimidines obtained through salvage pathways but rather rely completely on de novo pyrimidine synthesis, for which folate derivatives are essential cofactors. The efficacy of pyrimethamine is increasingly limited by the development of resistant strains of *P. falciparum* and *P. vivax*. Single amino acid substitutions to parasite dihydrofolate reductase confer resistance to pyrimethamine by decreasing the enzyme's binding affinity for the drug.

Pyrimethamine is well absorbed; the drug is 87% bound to human plasma proteins. In healthy volunteers, drug concentrations remain at therapeutic levels for up to 2 weeks; drug levels are lower in patients with malaria.

At the usual dosage, pyrimethamine alone causes little toxicity except for occasional skin rashes and, more rarely, blood dyscrasias. Bone marrow suppression sometimes occurs at the higher doses used for toxoplasmosis; at these doses, the drug should be administered with folinic acid.

Pyronaridine This potent antimalarial is a benzonaphthyridine derivative first synthesized by Chinese researchers in 1970. Like chloroquine, pyronaridine targets hematin formation, inhibiting the production of β-hematin by forming complexes with it, with consequent enhancement of hematin-induced hemolysis. However, this drug is more potent than chloroquine: for complete lysis, pyronaridine is required at only 1/100th of the concentration needed with chloroquine. It also inhibits glutathione-dependent heme degradation. Despite its similar mode of action, pyronaridine remains effective against chloroquine-resistant strains. When combined with artesunate, it is effective for the treatment of acute, uncomplicated infection caused by *P. falciparum* or *P. vivax* in areas of low transmission with evidence of artemisinin resistance.

Pyronaridine is readily absorbed, widely distributed throughout the body, metabolized by the liver, and excreted in urine and stool. Its use is contraindicated in patients with severe liver or kidney impairment. Pyronaridine inhibits both CYP2D6 and P-glycoprotein in vitro, and these effects may have clinical relevance for patients taking medications for cardiac disease (e.g., metoprolol and digoxin).

Quinacrine* Quinacrine is the only drug approved by the FDA for the treatment of giardiasis. Although its production was discontinued in 1992, quinacrine can be obtained from alternative sources through the CDC Drug Service. The antiprotozoal mechanism of quinacrine has not been fully elucidated. The drug inhibits NADH oxidase—the same enzyme that activates furazolidone. The differing relative quinacrine uptake rate between human cells and *G. lamblia* may explain the selective toxicity of the drug. Resistance correlates with decreased drug uptake.

Quinacrine is rapidly absorbed from the intestinal tract and is widely distributed in body tissues. Alcohol is best avoided because of a disulfiram-like effect.

Quinine and Quinidine When combined with another agent, the cinchona alkaloid quinine is effective for the oral treatment of both uncomplicated, chloroquine-resistant malaria and babesiosis. Quinine acts rapidly against the asexual blood stages of all forms of the human malaria parasites. For severe malaria, only quinidine (the dextroisomer of quinine) is available in the United States. Quinine concentrates in the acidic food vacuoles of *Plasmodium* species. The drug inhibits the nonenzymatic polymerization of the highly reactive, toxic heme molecule into the nontoxic polymer pigment hemozoin.

Quinine is readily absorbed when given orally. In patients with malaria, the elimination half-life of quinine increases according to the severity of the infection. However, toxicity is avoided by an increase in the concentration of plasma glycoproteins. The cinchona alkaloids are extensively metabolized, particularly by CYP3A4; only 20% of the dose is excreted unchanged in urine. The drug's metabolites are also excreted in urine and may be responsible for toxicity in patients with renal failure. Renal excretion of quinine is decreased when cimetidine is taken and increased when the urine is acidic. The drug readily crosses the placenta.

Quinidine is both more potent as an antimalarial and more toxic than quinine. Its use requires cardiac monitoring. Dose reduction is necessary in persons with severe renal impairment.

Spiramycin† This macrolide is used to treat acute toxoplasmosis in pregnancy and congenital toxoplasmosis. While the mechanism of action is similar to that of other macrolides, the efficacy of spiramycin in toxoplasmosis appears to stem from its rapid and extensive intracellular penetration, which results in macrophage drug concentrations 10–20 times greater than serum concentrations.

Spiramycin is rapidly and widely distributed throughout the body and reaches concentrations in the placenta up to five times those in serum. This agent is excreted mainly in bile. Indeed, in humans, the urinary excretion of active compounds represents only 20% of the administered dose.

Serious reactions to spiramycin are rare. Of the available macrolides, spiramycin appears to have the lowest risk of drug interactions. Complications of treatment are rare but, in neonates, can include life-threatening ventricular arrhythmias that disappear with drug discontinuation.

Sulfonamides See Table 222-1 and **Chap. 144.**

Suramin* This derivative of urea is the drug of choice for the early stage of African trypanosomiasis. The drug is polyanionic and acts by forming stable complexes with proteins, thus inhibiting multiple enzymes essential to parasite energy metabolism. Suramin appears to inhibit all trypanosome glycolytic enzymes more effectively than it inhibits the corresponding host enzymes.

Suramin is parenterally administered. It binds to plasma proteins and persists at low levels for several weeks after infusion. Its metabolism is negligible. This drug does not penetrate the CNS.

Tafenoquine Tafenoquine is an 8-aminoquinoline with causal prophylactic activity. Its prolonged half-life (2–3 weeks) allows longer dosing intervals when the drug is used for prophylaxis. Tafenoquine has been well tolerated in clinical trials. When tafenoquine is taken with food, its absorption is increased by 50% and the most commonly reported adverse event—mild GI upset—is diminished. Like primaquine, tafenoquine is a potent oxidizing agent, causing hemolysis in patients with G6PD deficiency as well as methemoglobinemia.

Tetracyclines See Table 222-1 and **Chap. 144.**

Thiabendazole Discovered in 1961, thiabendazole remains one of the most potent of the numerous benzimidazole derivatives. However, its use has declined significantly because of a higher frequency of adverse effects than is seen with other, equally effective agents.

Thiabendazole is active against most intestinal nematodes that infect humans. Although the exact mechanism of its antihelminthic activity has not been fully elucidated, it is likely to be similar to that of other benzimidazole drugs: namely, inhibition of polymerization of parasite β-tubulin. The drug also inhibits the helminth-specific enzyme fumarate reductase. In animals, thiabendazole has anti-inflammatory, antipyretic, and analgesic effects, which may explain its usefulness in dracunculiasis and trichinellosis. Thiabendazole also suppresses egg and/or larval production by some nematodes and may inhibit the subsequent development of eggs or larvae passed in feces. Despite the emergence and global spread of thiabendazole-resistant trichostrongyliasis among sheep, there have been no reports of drug resistance in humans.

Thiabendazole is available in tablet form and as an oral suspension. The drug is rapidly absorbed from the GI tract but can also be absorbed through the skin. Thiabendazole should be taken after meals. This agent is extensively metabolized in the liver before ultimately being excreted; most of the dose is excreted within the first 24 h. The usual dose of thiabendazole is determined by the patient's weight, but some treatment regimens are parasite specific. No particular adjustments are recommended in patients with renal or hepatic failure; only cautious use is advised.

Coadministration of thiabendazole to patients taking theophylline can result in an increase in theophylline levels by >50%. Therefore, serum levels of theophylline should be monitored closely in this situation.

Tinidazole This nitroimidazole is effective for the treatment of amebiasis, giardiasis, and trichomoniasis. Like metronidazole, tinidazole must undergo reductive activation by the parasite's metabolic system before it can act on protozoal targets. Tinidazole inhibits the synthesis of new DNA in the parasite and causes degradation of existing DNA. The reduced free-radical derivatives alkylate DNA, with consequent cytotoxic damage to the parasite. This damage appears to be produced by short-lived reduction intermediates, resulting in helix destabilization and strain breakage of DNA. The mechanism of action and side effects of tinidazole are similar to those of metronidazole, but adverse events appear to be less frequent and severe with tinidazole. In addition, the significantly longer half-life of tinidazole (>12 h) offers potential cure with a single dose.

Tribendimidine Tribendimidine, a diamidine derivative of aminophenylamidine amidantel, is a cholinergic agonist that is selective for the nicotinic acetylcholine receptors of nematode muscle. It is the first new antiparasitic agent to appear in the last three decades and has a broad spectrum of activity against a wide variety of helminths. The drug is highly effective against food-borne trematodes, with a similar cure rate to praziquantel. Clinical trials have demonstrated efficacy of a single dose alone or in combination with other helminthics against soil-transmitted helminth infections. The drug is an L-type nicotinic acetylcholine receptor agonist, and exhibits the same method of action as levamisole and pyrantel; therefore, it may not be effective in regions where resistance to these agents is widespread.

Triclabendazole While most benzimidazoles have broad-spectrum antihelminthic activity, they exhibit minimal or no activity against *Fasciola hepatica*. In contrast, the antihelminthic activity of triclabendazole is highly specific for *Fasciola* and *Paragonimus* species, with little activity against nematodes, cestodes, and other trematodes. Triclabendazole is effective against all stages of *Fasciola* species. The active sulfoxide metabolite of triclabendazole binds to fluke tubulin by assuming a unique nonplanar configuration and disrupts microtubule-based processes. Resistance to triclabendazole in veterinary use has been reported in Australia and Europe; however, no resistance has been documented in humans.

Triclabendazole is rapidly absorbed after oral ingestion; administration with food enhances its absorption and shortens the elimination half-life of the active metabolite. Both the sulfoxide and the sulfone metabolites are highly protein bound (>99%). Treatment with triclabendazole is typically given in one or two doses. No clinical data are available regarding dose adjustment in renal or hepatic insufficiency; however, given the short course of therapy and extensive hepatic metabolism of triclabendazole, dose adjustment is unlikely to be necessary. No information exists on drug interactions.

Trimethoprim-Sulfamethoxazole See Table 222-1 and **Chap. 144.**

FURTHER READING

Fehintola FA et al: Drug interactions in the treatment and chemoprophylaxis of malaria in HIV infected individuals in sub Saharan Africa. Curr Drug Metab 12:51, 2011.

Keiser J, Häberli C: Evaluation of commercially available anthelminthics in laboratory models of human intestinal nematode infections. ACS Infect Dis 7:1177, 2021.

Keiser J et al: Antiparasitic drugs for paediatrics: Systematic review, formulations, pharmacokinetics, safety, efficacy and implications for control. Parasitology 138:1620, 2011.

Kelesidis T, Falagas ME: Substandard/counterfeit antimicrobial drugs. Clin Microbiol Rev 28:443, 2015.

Milton P et al: Moxidectin: An oral treatment for human onchocerciasis. Expert Review of Anti-Infective Therapy 18:1067, 2020.

Pink R et al: Opportunities and challenges in antiparasitic drug discovery. Nat Rev Drug Discov 4:727, 2005.

223 Amebiasis and Infection with Free-Living Amebae

Rosa M. Andrade, Sharon L. Reed

AMEBIASIS

DEFINITION

Amebiasis is an infection caused by *Entamoeba histolytica*, an intestinal protozoan. Its spectrum of clinical syndromes ranges from asymptomatic colonization (90% of cases) to invasive amebiasis, which accounts for 10% of affected individuals. Invasive amebiasis frequently presents as intestinal colitis (dysentery or diarrhea) or as extraintestinal amebiasis, in which abscesses of the liver are more commonly found than involvement of the lungs or brain.

LIFE CYCLE AND TRANSMISSION

E. histolytica is acquired by ingestion of viable cysts from fecally contaminated water, food, or hands (Fig. 223-1). Food-borne exposure is the most prevalent form of transmission. It occurs when food handlers are shedding cysts or food is being grown with feces-contaminated soil, fertilizer, or water. Less common means of transmission include oral and anal sexual practices and—in rare instances—direct rectal inoculation through colonic irrigation devices. Motile trophozoites are released from cysts in the small intestine and, in most patients, remain as harmless commensals in the large bowel. After encystation, infectious cysts are shed in the stool and can survive for several weeks in a moist environment. In some patients, the trophozoites invade either the bowel mucosa, causing symptomatic colitis, or the bloodstream, causing distant abscesses of the liver, lungs, or brain. The trophozoites may not encyst in patients with active dysentery, and motile hematophagous trophozoites are frequently present in fresh stools. Trophozoites are rapidly killed by exposure to air or stomach acid and therefore cannot transmit infection.

EPIDEMIOLOGY

E. histolytica infection typically affects underdeveloped tropical regions with poor sanitation systems and hygiene, occurring often in children <5 years of age. This infection is widespread in the Indian subcontinent and Africa, parts of East Asia (Thailand), and Central and South America (Mexico and Colombia). According to the Global Burden of Disease 2016 study, amebiasis accounts for 26,748 all-age deaths, including 4567 children <5 years old.

In contrast, returning travelers, recent immigrants, men who have sex with men (MSM), military personnel, and inmates of institutions are the main groups at risk for amebiasis in developed countries. Data for 1997–2011 from the GeoSentinel Surveillance Network, which encompasses information from tropical medicine clinics on six continents, showed that, among long-term travelers (trip duration, >6 months), diarrhea due to *E. histolytica* was among the most

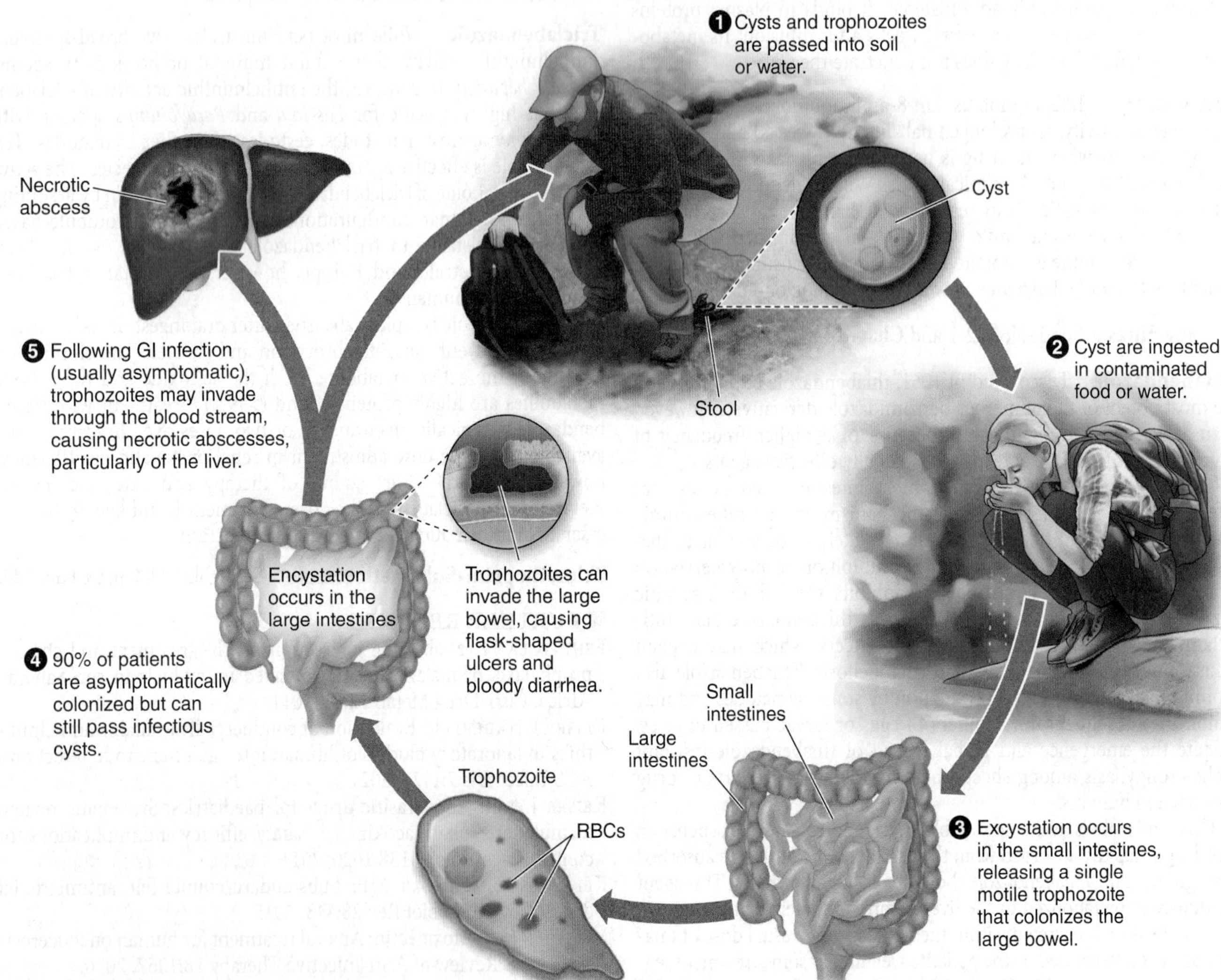
1 Cysts and trophozoites are passed into soil or water.
Cyst
Stool
2 Cyst are ingested in contaminated food or water.
Small intestines
Large intestines
3 Excystation occurs in the small intestines, releasing a single motile trophozoite that colonizes the large bowel.
Trophozoite
RBCs
4 90% of patients are asymptomatically colonized but can still pass infectious cysts.
Encystation occurs in the large intestines
Trophozoites can invade the large bowel, causing flask-shaped ulcers and bloody diarrhea.
5 Following GI infection (usually asymptomatic), trophozoites may invade through the blood stream, causing necrotic abscesses, particularly of the liver.
Necrotic abscess

FIGURE 223-1 Life cycle of *Entamoeba histolytica*. GI, gastrointestinal; RBCs, red blood cells.

common diagnoses. In fact, amebiasis may be considered an emerging infectious disease in developed countries such as Japan, where the number of reported cases among HIV-positive patients, and particularly among MSM, has increased.

Worldwide, *E. histolytica* is the second most common cause of death related to parasitic infection (after malaria). Invasive colitis and liver abscesses are tenfold more common among men than among women; this difference has been attributed to a disparity in complement-mediated killing and effects of testosterone on the secretion of interferon γ. The wide spectrum of clinical disease caused by *Entamoeba* is due in part to the differences between the two major infecting species, *E. histolytica* and *E. dispar*. *E. histolytica* has unique surface antigens, is genetically distinct, and possesses virulence properties that distinguish it from the morphologically identical *E. dispar*.

Most asymptomatic carriers, including MSM and patients with AIDS, harbor *E. dispar* and have self-limited infections. In this respect, *E. dispar* is dissimilar to other enteric pathogens such as *Cryptosporidium* and *Cystoisospora belli*, which can cause self-limited illnesses in immunocompetent hosts but devastating diarrhea in patients with AIDS. These observations indicate that *E. dispar* is incapable of causing invasive disease. Through genomic sequencing, new species of *Entamoeba* have been identified: *E. moshkowskii* and *E. bangladeshi*. These new species are microscopically indistinguishable from *E. histolytica*. Although *E. moshkovskii* causes diarrhea, weight loss, and colitis in mice, a prospective evaluation of children from the Mirpur community of Dhaka, Bangladesh, found that most children who had diarrheal diseases associated with *E. moshkovskii* were simultaneously infected with at least one other enteric pathogen. *E. bangladeshi nov.* sp., *Bangladesh* was first reported in 2012 in this Bangladeshi community; however, it has been isolated in South African subjects of all ages in recent years. Additional clinical and epidemiologic studies are needed to discern the true role of *E. bangladeshi* in the human host.

PATHOGENESIS AND PATHOLOGY

Both trophozoites and cysts are found in the intestinal lumen, but only trophozoites of *E. histolytica* invade tissue. The trophozoite is 20–60 μm in diameter and contains vacuoles and a nucleus with a characteristic central nucleolus. Trophozoites attach to colonic mucus and epithelial cells by Gal/GalNAc adherence lectin and release glycosidases and proteases that cause degradation of mucous polymers. Extracellular cysteine proteinases degrade collagen, elastin, IgA, IgG, and the anaphylatoxins C3a and C5a. After disruption of the mucous layer, trophozoites damage the mucosa by contact-dependent and contact-independent cytotoxicity. The contact-dependent cytotoxicity is attributable to induction of apoptotic cell death; trogocytosis-mediated cell death (ingestion of fragments of living cells); and lysis of inflammatory cells (neutrophils, monocytes, and lymphocytes), colonic cells, and hepatic cells through release of phospholipase A and pore-forming peptides. Contact-independent cytotoxicity follows production of inflammatory mediators, such as prostaglandin E2, by trophozoites, ultimately leading to increased ion permeability of intercellular tight junctions.

E. histolytica trophozoites are constantly exposed to reactive oxygen and nitrogen species arising from their own metabolism and from the host during tissue invasion. The ability to resist reactive oxygen species or reactive nitrogen species such as nitric oxide or *S*-nitrosothiols (e.g., *S*-nitrosoglutathione [GSNO] and *S*-nitrosocysteine [CySNO]) is also a virulence factor. Overexpression of hydrogen peroxide–regulatory motif-binding protein appears to increase *E. histolytica* cytotoxicity. Since *E. histolytica* lacks glutathione and glutathione reductase, it relies on its thioredoxin–thioredoxin reductase system to prevent, regulate, and repair the damage caused by oxidative stress. This antioxidant system is versatile: it has the ability to reduce reactive nitrogen species and use an alternative electron donor, such as nicotinamide adenine dinucleotide. Metronidazole, the current standard of therapy for amebiasis, seems to exert its antiparasitic effect through inhibition of this antioxidant system. Auranofin, a reprofiled drug approved by the U.S. Food and Drug Administration for rheumatoid arthritis, inhibits thioredoxin reductase and displays in vitro and in vivo efficacy against *E. histolytica* and *Giardia intestinalis*. Auranofin is currently undergoing clinical trials against *E. histolytica* and *Giardia* infections in Bangladesh.

Phagocytosis is a virulence factor that leads to a defective proliferation of *E. histolytica* if inhibited. Trophozoites use membrane-associated carbohydrate-binding proteins to phagocytose intestinal bacteria, especially gram-negative Enterobacteriaceae, for their nutrients. Interactions with commensal bacteria, such as *Escherichia coli*, can attenuate the virulence of *E. histolytica* by decreasing the expression of Gal/GalNAc lectin. In contrast, ingestion of enteropathogenic bacteria, such as enteropathogenic *E. coli* and *Shigella dysenteriae*, increases expression of the Gal/GalNAc lectin and enhances *E. histolytica* cysteine protease activity.

E. histolytica is capable of altering the commensal gut microbiota. In a cohort in northern India, adult patients who had had amebic dysentery for 5–7 days had significant decreases in intestinal *Bacteroides*, the *Clostridium coccoides* subgroup, the *Clostridium leptum* subgroup, *Lactobacillus*, *Campylobacter*, and *Eubacterium* but displayed increases in *Bifidobacterium*. During the first 2 years of life, the gut immune system and the microbiota mature rapidly. In one study, ~80% of children from the Bangladeshi community of Dhaka were found to be infected with *E. histolytica* by 2 years of age. Fecal anti–Gal/GalNAc lectin IgA was associated with protection from reinfection, while a high parasite burden in the first year of life was associated with the expansion of *Prevotella copri* in their gut microbiota and presence of diarrhea.

Antimicrobial peptides, such as cathelicidins, are an important component of innate immunity and are induced by *E. histolytica* upon intestinal invasion in a mouse model. In this model, cecal cathelicidin-related antimicrobial peptide mRNA increased by >4-fold at 3 days and >100-fold at 7 days. However, *E. histolytica* remained resistant to cathelicidin-mediated killing, probably because the antimicrobial peptide was digested by amebic cysteine proteinases.

IgA plays a critical role in acquired immunity to *E. histolytica*. A study in Bangladeshi schoolchildren revealed that an intestinal IgA response to Gal/GalNAc reduced the risk of new *E. histolytica* infection by 64%. Serum IgG antibody is not protective; titers correlate with the duration of illness rather than with the severity of disease. Indeed, Bangladeshi children with a serum IgG response were more likely than those without such a response to develop new *E. histolytica* infection. In infants from this same Bangladeshi community, passive immunity conferred by maternal parasite-specific IgA via breastfeeding resulted in a 39% reduced risk of infection and a 64% reduced risk of diarrheal disease from *E. histolytica* during the first year of life. However, this protection appeared to be species-specific, with little or no protection conferred from infections with other species such as *E. dispar* or *E. bangladeshi*.

This Bangladeshi cohort has furthered our understanding of the genetic susceptibility factors associated with *E. histolytica* disease. Heterozygosity of the major histocompatibility complex (MHC) class II allele DQB1*0601 was found to protect against amebic intestinal disease, which supports the role of antigen processing and CD4+ T cells in resistance to amebiasis. Adipocyte leptin receptors (LEPRs) are expressed on intestinal epithelial cells, prevent apoptosis, promote tissue repair, and may decrease neutrophil infiltration. In this cohort, a single amino acid substitution (Q223R) in LEPRs nearly quadrupled the risk for amebic intestinal disease in children and increased the risk for amebic liver abscesses in adults. Similarly, variations in the locus of cAMP-responsive element modulator/cullin 2 (CREM/CUL2) may increase the risk for diarrhea in children that acquired *E. histolytica* within their first year of life. Interestingly, both genetic variations, Q223R and CREM, are overrepresented in this geographical region. Furthermore, these CREM polymorphisms are also associated with susceptibility to inflammatory bowel disease, suggesting that CREM may regulate the homeostatic interactions between the gut microbiota and the intestinal immune response.

The earliest intestinal lesions are micro-ulcerations of the mucosa of the cecum, sigmoid colon, or rectum that release erythrocytes, inflammatory cells, and epithelial cells. A colonoscopy reveals small ulcers with heaped-up margins and normal intervening mucosa

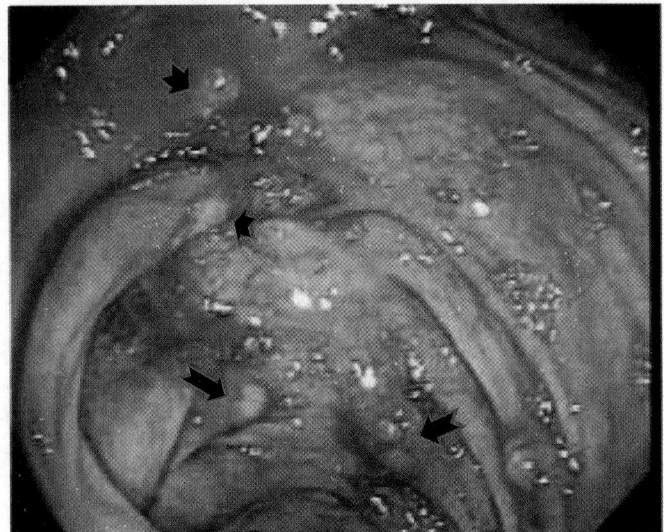

A

B

FIGURE 223-2 Endoscopic and histopathologic features of intestinal amebiasis. ***A.*** Appearance of ulcers on colonoscopy (*arrows*). ***B.*** Inflammatory infiltrate and *Entamoeba histolytica* trophozoites (*arrows*) in invasive amebic colitis (hematoxylin and eosin). *(Courtesy of the Department of Pathology and Gastroenterology, San Diego VA Medical Center.)*

(Fig. 223-2*A*). Submucosal extension of ulcerations under viable-appearing surface mucosa causes the classic "flask-shaped" ulcer containing trophozoites at the margins of dead and viable tissues. Although neutrophilic infiltrates may accompany early lesions in animals, human intestinal infection is marked by a paucity of inflammatory cells, probably in part because of the killing of neutrophils by trophozoites **(Fig. 223-2*B*)**. Treated ulcers characteristically heal with little or no scarring. Occasionally, however, full-thickness necrosis and perforation occur.

Rarely, intestinal infection results in the formation of a mass lesion, or *ameboma*, in the bowel lumen. The overlying mucosa is usually thin and ulcerated, while other layers of the wall are thickened, edematous, and hemorrhagic; this condition results in exuberant formation of granulation tissue with little fibrous-tissue response.

Amebic liver abscesses are age- and gender-dependent. Men 30–60 years of age are most commonly infected at a rate 10–12 times higher than women in the same age group. Studies in animal models have demonstrated that testosterone may increase susceptibility to amebic liver abscess by modulating the secretion of interferon γ by natural killer T cells, which are activated through *E. histolytica* lipopeptidophosphoglycan present on the surface of ameba trophozoites. Liver abscesses are always preceded by intestinal colonization, which may be asymptomatic. Blood vessels may be compromised early by wall lysis and thrombus formation. Trophozoites invade veins to reach the liver through the portal venous system. *E. histolytica* is resistant to complement-mediated lysis—a property critical to survival in the bloodstream. Inoculation of amebae into the portal system of hamsters results in an acute cellular infiltrate consisting predominantly of neutrophils. Later, the neutrophils are lysed by contact with amebae, and the release of neutrophil toxins may contribute to necrosis of hepatocytes. The liver parenchyma is replaced by necrotic material that is surrounded by a thin rim of congested liver tissue. Although the necrotic contents of a liver abscess are classically described as "anchovy paste," the fluid is variable in color; it is composed of bacteriologically sterile granular debris with few or no cells. Amebae, if seen, tend to be found near the capsule of the abscess.

■ CLINICAL SYNDROMES

Intestinal Amebiasis The most common type of amebic infection is asymptomatic cyst passage. Even in highly endemic areas, most patients harbor *E. dispar*.

Symptomatic amebic colitis develops 2–6 weeks after the ingestion of infectious cysts. A gradual onset of lower abdominal pain and mild diarrhea is followed by malaise, weight loss, and diffuse lower abdominal or back pain. Cecal involvement may mimic acute appendicitis. Patients with full-blown dysentery may pass 10–12 stools per day. The stools contain little fecal material and consist mainly of blood and mucus. In contrast to those with bacterial diarrhea, fewer than 40% of patients with amebic dysentery are febrile. Virtually all patients have heme-positive stools.

More fulminant intestinal infection, with severe abdominal pain, high fever, and profuse diarrhea, is rare and occurs predominantly in children. Patients may develop toxic megacolon, in which there is severe bowel dilation with intramural air. Patients receiving glucocorticoids are at risk for severe amebiasis. The association between severe amebiasis complications and glucocorticoid therapy emphasizes the importance of excluding amebiasis when inflammatory bowel disease is suspected. An occasional patient presents with only an asymptomatic or tender abdominal mass caused by an ameboma, which is easily confused with cancer on barium studies. A positive serologic test or biopsy can prevent unnecessary surgery in this setting.

Environmental enteropathy ("impoverished gut"; blunted small-intestinal villi with lamina propria inflammation) is observed in tropical developing areas with endemic enteric infections, such as amebiasis. It is associated with functional gastrointestinal impairment causing malnutrition and stunted growth in children within the first 2 years of life. Bangladeshi children with symptomatic *E. histolytica* infections were 2.9 times more likely to be malnourished and 4.7 times more likely to be short for their age than were children without symptomatic infections. These factors affect their cognitive development and may be linked to loss of productivity in adulthood.

Amebic Liver Abscess Extraintestinal infection by *E. histolytica* most often involves the liver. Of travelers who develop an amebic liver abscess after leaving an endemic area, 95% do so within 5 months. Young patients with an amebic liver abscess are more likely than older patients to present in the acute phase with prominent symptoms of <10 days' duration. Most patients are febrile and have right-upper-quadrant pain, which may be dull or pleuritic in nature and may radiate to the shoulder. Point tenderness over the liver and right-sided pleural effusion are common. Jaundice is rare. Although the initial site of infection is the colon, fewer than one-third of patients with an amebic abscess have active diarrhea. Older patients from endemic areas are more likely to have a subacute course lasting 6 months, with weight loss and hepatomegaly. About one-third of patients with chronic presentations are febrile. Thus, the clinical diagnosis of an amebic liver abscess may be difficult to establish because the symptoms and signs are often nonspecific. Since 10–15% of patients present only with fever, amebic liver abscess must be considered in the differential diagnosis of fever of unknown origin **(Chap. 20)**.

Complications of Amebic Liver Abscess Pleuropulmonary involvement, which is reported in 20–30% of patients, is the most frequent complication of amebic liver abscess. Manifestations include sterile effusions, contiguous spread from the liver, and rupture into the pleural space. Sterile effusions and contiguous spread usually resolve with medical therapy, but frank rupture into the pleural space requires drainage. A hepatobronchial fistula may cause cough productive of large amounts of necrotic material that may contain amebae. This dramatic complication carries a good prognosis. Abscesses that rupture into the peritoneum may present as an indolent leak or an acute abdomen and require both percutaneous catheter drainage and medical therapy. Rupture into the pericardium, usually from abscesses of the left lobe of the liver, carries the gravest prognosis; it can occur during medical therapy and requires surgical drainage.

Involvement of Other Extraintestinal Sites The genitourinary tract may become involved by direct extension of amebiasis from the colon or by hematogenous spread of the infection. Painful genital ulcers, characterized by a punched-out appearance and profuse discharge, may develop secondary to extension from either the intestine or the liver. Both of these conditions respond well to medical therapy. Cerebral involvement has been reported in fewer than 0.1% of patients in large clinical series. Symptoms and prognosis depend on the size and location of the lesion.

DIAGNOSTIC TESTS

Laboratory Diagnosis Stool examinations, serologic tests, and noninvasive imaging of the liver are the most important procedures in the diagnosis of amebiasis. Fecal findings suggestive of amebic colitis include a positive test for heme, a paucity of neutrophils, and amebic cysts or trophozoites. The definitive diagnosis of amebic colitis is made by the demonstration of hematophagous trophozoites of *E. histolytica*. Because trophozoites are killed rapidly by water, drying, or barium, it is important to examine at least three fresh stool specimens. Examination of a combination of wet mounts, iodine-stained concentrates, and trichrome-stained preparations of fresh stool and concentrates for cysts or trophozoites confirms the diagnosis in 75–95% of cases. Cultures of amebae are more sensitive but are not routinely available. If stool examinations are negative, sigmoidoscopy with biopsy of the edge of ulcers may increase the yield, but this procedure is dangerous during fulminant colitis because of the risk of perforation. Trophozoites in a biopsy specimen from a colonic mass confirm the diagnosis of ameboma, but trophozoites are rare in liver aspirates because they are found in the abscess capsule and not in the readily aspirated necrotic center. Accurate diagnosis requires experience, since the trophozoites may be confused with neutrophils and the cysts must be differentiated morphologically from those of *Entamoeba hartmanni*, *Entamoeba coli*, and *Endolimax nana*, which do not cause clinical disease and do not warrant therapy. Unfortunately, the cysts of *E. histolytica* cannot be distinguished microscopically from those of *E. dispar*, *E. moshkovskii*, or *E. bangladeshi*. Therefore, the microscopic diagnosis of *E. histolytica* can be made only by the detection of *Entamoeba* trophozoites that have ingested erythrocytes. More sensitive and specific tests in stool include enzyme immunoassay detection of the Gal/GalNAc lectin of *E. histolytica* and multiplex polymerase chain reaction (PCR) stool panels that include *E. histolytica*.

Serology is an important addition to the methods used for parasitologic diagnosis of invasive amebiasis. Enzyme-linked immunosorbent assays and agar gel diffusion assays are positive in >90% of cases with colitis, ameboma, or liver abscess. Positive results in conjunction with the appropriate clinical syndrome suggest active disease because serologic findings usually revert to negative within 6–12 months. Even in highly endemic areas such as South Africa, fewer than 10% of asymptomatic individuals have a positive amebic serology. The interpretation of the indirect hemagglutination test is difficult because titers may remain positive for as long as 10 years.

Up to 10% of patients with acute amebic liver abscess may have negative serologic findings; in suspected cases with an initially negative result, testing should be repeated in a week. In contrast to carriers of *E. dispar*, most asymptomatic carriers of *E. histolytica* develop antibodies. Thus, serologic tests are helpful in assessing the risk of invasive amebiasis in asymptomatic, cyst-passing individuals in nonendemic areas. Serologic tests also should be performed in patients with ulcerative colitis before the institution of glucocorticoid therapy to prevent the development of severe colitis or toxic megacolon owing to unsuspected amebiasis. Recently, a loop-mediated isothermal amplification (LAMP) assay was shown to be a potential alternative for direct detection of *E. histolytica* DNA in pus samples from amebic liver abscesses. LAMP is a relatively simple, rapid, and low-cost method of DNA amplification that could be a better alternative for diagnosis in developing countries. Routine hematology and chemistry tests usually are not very helpful in the diagnosis of invasive amebiasis. About three-fourths of patients with an amebic liver abscess have leukocytosis (>10,000 cells/μL); this condition is particularly likely if symptoms are acute or complications have developed. Invasive amebiasis does not elicit eosinophilia. Anemia, if present, is usually multifactorial. Even with large liver abscesses, liver enzyme levels are normal or minimally elevated. The alkaline phosphatase level is most often elevated and may remain so for months. Aminotransferase elevations suggest acute disease or a complication.

Radiographic Studies Radiographic barium studies are potentially dangerous in acute amebic colitis. Amebomas are usually identified first by a barium enema, but biopsy is necessary for differentiation from carcinoma.

Radiographic techniques such as ultrasonography, CT, and MRI are all useful for detection of the round or oval hypoechoic cyst. More than 80% of patients who have had symptoms for >10 days have a single abscess of the right lobe of the liver (Fig. 223-3). Approximately 50% of patients who have had symptoms for <10 days have multiple abscesses. Findings associated with complications include large abscesses (>10 cm) in the superior part of the right lobe, which may rupture into the pleural space; multiple lesions, which must be differentiated from pyogenic abscesses; and lesions of the left lobe, which may rupture into the pericardium. Because abscesses resolve slowly and may increase in size despite a clinical response to therapy, frequent follow-up ultrasonography may prove confusing. Complete resolution of a liver abscess within 6 months can be anticipated in two-thirds of patients, but 10% may have persistent abnormalities for a year.

Differential Diagnosis The differential diagnosis of intestinal amebiasis includes bacterial diarrheas (Chap. 133) caused by *Campylobacter* (Chap. 167); enteroinvasive *Escherichia coli* (Chap. 161); and species of *Shigella* (Chap. 166), *Salmonella* (Chap. 165), and *Vibrio* (Chap. 168). Because the typical patient with amebic colitis has less prominent fever than in these other conditions as well as heme-positive

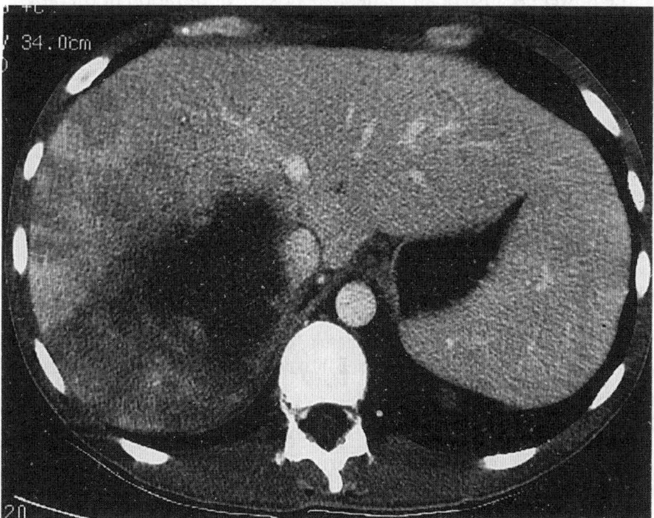

FIGURE 223-3 Abdominal CT scan of a large amebic abscess of the right lobe of the liver. *(Courtesy of the Department of Radiology, UCSD Medical Center, San Diego; with permission.)*

stools with few neutrophils, correct diagnosis requires bacterial cultures, microscopic examination of stools, and amebic serologic testing. As has been mentioned, amebiasis must be ruled out in any patient thought to have inflammatory bowel disease.

Because of the variety of presenting signs and symptoms, amebic liver abscess can easily be confused with pulmonary or gallbladder disease or with any febrile illness with few localizing signs, such as malaria **(Chap. 224)** or typhoid fever **(Chap. 165)**. The diagnosis should be considered in members of high-risk groups who have recently traveled outside the United States **(Chap. 124)** and in inmates of institutions. Once radiographic studies have identified an abscess in the liver, the most important differential diagnosis is between amebic and pyogenic abscess. Patients with pyogenic abscess typically are older and have a history of underlying bowel disease or recent surgery. Amebic serology is helpful, but aspiration of the abscess, with Gram's staining and culture of the material, may be required for differentiation of the two diseases.

TREATMENT
Amebiasis

INTESTINAL DISEASE (TABLE 223-1)

The drugs used to treat amebiasis can be classified according to their primary site of action. Luminal amebicides are poorly absorbed and reach high concentrations in the bowel, but their activity is limited to cysts and trophozoites close to the mucosa. Only two luminal drugs are available in the United States: iodoquinol and paromomycin. Indications for the use of luminal agents include eradication of cysts in patients with colitis or a liver abscess and treatment of asymptomatic carriers. The majority of asymptomatic individuals who pass cysts are colonized with *E. dispar*, which does not warrant specific therapy. However, it is prudent to treat asymptomatic individuals who pass cysts unless *E. dispar* colonization can be definitively demonstrated by specific antigen-detection tests.

Tissue amebicides reach high concentrations in the blood and tissue after oral or parenteral administration. The development of nitroimidazole compounds, especially metronidazole, was a major advance in the treatment of invasive amebiasis. Patients with amebic colitis should be treated with IV or oral metronidazole. Side effects include nausea, vomiting, abdominal discomfort, and a disulfiram-like reaction. Another, longer-acting imidazole compound, tinidazole, is likewise effective and is available in the United States. All patients should also receive a full course of therapy with a luminal agent, since metronidazole does not eradicate cysts. Resistance to metronidazole has been selected in the laboratory but has not been found in clinical isolates. Relapses are not uncommon and probably represent reinfection or failure to eradicate amebae from the bowel because of an inadequate dosage or duration of therapy.

AMEBIC LIVER ABSCESS

Metronidazole is the drug of choice for amebic liver abscess. Longer-acting nitroimidazoles (tinidazole and ornidazole) have been effective as single-dose therapy in developing countries. With early diagnosis and therapy, mortality rates from uncomplicated amebic liver abscess are <1%. There is no evidence that combined therapy with two drugs is more effective than the single-drug regimen. Studies of South Africans with liver abscesses demonstrated that 72% of patients without intestinal symptoms had bowel infection with *E. histolytica*; thus, all treatment regimens should include a luminal agent to eradicate cysts and prevent further transmission. Amebic liver abscess recurs rarely.

More than 90% of patients respond dramatically to metronidazole therapy with decreases in both pain and fever within 72 h. Indications for aspiration of liver abscesses are (1) the need to rule out a pyogenic abscess, particularly in patients with multiple lesions; (2) the lack of a clinical response in 3–5 days; (3) the threat of imminent rupture; and (4) the need to prevent rupture of left-lobe abscesses into the pericardium. There is no evidence that aspiration, even of large abscesses (up to 10 cm), accelerates healing. Percutaneous drainage may be successful even if the liver abscess has already ruptured. Surgery should be reserved for instances of bowel perforation and rupture into the pericardium.

TABLE 223-1 Drug Therapy for Amebiasis

INDICATION	THERAPY
Asymptomatic carriage	Luminal agent: iodoquinol (650-mg tablets), 650 mg tid for 20 days; *or* paromomycin (250-mg tablets), 500 mg tid for 10 days
Acute colitis	Metronidazole (250- or 500-mg tablets), 750 mg PO or IV tid for 5–10 days; *or* tinidazole, 2 g/d PO for 3 days ***plus*** Luminal agent as above
Amebic liver abscess	Metronidazole, 750 mg PO or IV for 5–10 days; *or* tinidazole, 2 g PO once; *or* ornidazole,[a] 2 g PO once ***plus*** Luminal agent as above

[a]Not available in the United States.

PREVENTION

Amebic infection is spread by ingestion of food or water contaminated with cysts. Since an asymptomatic carrier may excrete up to 15 million cysts per day, prevention of infection requires adequate sanitation and eradication of cyst carriage. In high-risk areas, infection can be minimized by the avoidance of unpeeled fruits and vegetables and the use of bottled water. Because cysts are resistant to readily attainable levels of chlorine, disinfection by iodination (tetraglycine hydroperiodide) is recommended. There is no effective prophylaxis.

INFECTION WITH FREE-LIVING AMEBAE

EPIDEMIOLOGY

There are multiple genera of free-living amebae, but the major human pathogens are *Acanthamoeba*, *Naegleria*, and *Balamuthia*. All of these parasites can cause serious central nervous system (CNS) infections, which are almost always fatal. *Acanthamoeba* and *Naegleria* are distributed throughout the world and have been isolated from a wide variety of fresh and brackish water, including water from taps, lakes, hot springs, swimming pools, heating and air-conditioning units, and hospital water networks, and even from the nasal passages of healthy children. Encystation may protect these protozoa from desiccation and food deprivation. The persistence of *Legionella pneumophila* in water supplies is attributable in part to chronic infection of free-living amebae, particularly *Acanthamoeba*. Recent in vitro studies have suggested that several pathogens that can resist phagosome-mediated killing may be able to survive within water systems in free-living amebae. These pathogens include *Pseudomonas aeruginosa*, nontuberculous *Mycobacteria* (both slow-growing species—e.g., those in the *Mycobacterium avium* complex, *M. kansasii*, and *M. gordonae*—and rapid-growing species—e.g., *M. chelonae and M. abscessus*), and viruses such as adenoviruses and echoviruses.

In contrast, the environmental niche of free-living amebae of the genus *Balamuthia* appears to be soil. A soil sample from a flowerpot was linked to a fatal infection in a child. Cases have been reported from all continents except Africa, but the majority of cases are from warm, dry areas of the southwestern United States and Latin America.

With better recognition of these pathogens, additional risk factors have been identified. Since 2010, five cases of *Naegleria fowleri* infection have been reported in northern U.S. states and have been associated with exposure to piped water, which represents a new ecologic niche. Since 2009, three clusters of *Balamuthia mandrillaris* infections have been associated with organ transplantation. *Acanthamoeba* species have caused large outbreaks of microbial keratitis associated with contact lens wear.

NAEGLERIA INFECTIONS

Primary amebic meningoencephalitis (PAM) is a fulminant CNS infection caused by the free-living ameba *N. fowleri*, which thrives in warm freshwater of lakes and rivers. In the United States, 138 cases of PAM were reported from 1962 through 2015. Although the number of infections reported annually has remained stable (0–8), recent changes in the epidemiology of PAM are a cause of concern. In 2010–2015, 24 cases of PAM were reported and confirmed by the Centers for Disease Control and Prevention (CDC). In 2010, a PAM case was reported for the first time from the northern state of Minnesota; this case was followed by additional cases from Minnesota, Indiana, and Kansas in 2011 and 2012. With climate change, other areas may be at risk because of higher temperatures. The remaining cases were reported mostly from southern states. Sixty-three percent of cases affected female patients, and the median age of patients was 11 years (range, 4–56 years). The majority of patients (19, or 79%) were exposed to recreational freshwater from lakes, reservoirs, rivers, streams, or ditches. The remaining five cases (21%) were due to tap-water exposure through nasal irrigation with a neti pot, playing on a backyard waterslide, and swimming in a poorly maintained pool.

PAM follows the aspiration of water contaminated with trophozoites or cysts or the inhalation of contaminated dust leading to invasion of the olfactory neuroepithelium. Infection is most common in otherwise healthy children or young adults, who often report swimming in lakes or heated swimming pools. In rare instances, cases occur when contaminated water is used for nasal irrigation. After an incubation period of 2–15 days, severe headache, high fever, nausea, vomiting, and meningismus develop. Photophobia and palsies of the third, fourth, and sixth cranial nerves are common. Rapid progression to seizures and coma may follow. The prognosis is uniformly poor: most patients die within a week.

The diagnosis of *Naegleria* infection should be considered in any patient who has purulent meningitis without evidence of bacteria on Gram's staining, antigen detection assay, and culture. Other laboratory findings resemble those for fulminant bacterial meningitis, with elevated intracranial pressure, high white blood cell counts (up to 20,000/μL), and elevated protein concentrations and low glucose levels in cerebrospinal fluid (CSF). Diagnosis depends on the detection of motile trophozoites in wet mounts of fresh spinal fluid. Antibodies to *Naegleria* species have been detected in healthy adults; thus, serologic testing is not useful in the diagnosis of acute infection. Diagnostic PCR and histochemical staining of biopsies are available through the CDC.

A number of antimicrobial agents have in vitro activity against *N. fowleri*, but the prognosis remains poor. The few survivors have been treated with different combinations of amphotericin B, azoles, azithromycin, and rifampin. The new antiparasitic agent miltefosine—an alkylphosphocholine compound used to treat breast cancer and visceral leishmaniasis—is active in vitro against *Naegleria*, *Acanthamoeba*, and *Balamuthia* and is available from the CDC. Of three patients who received miltefosine for *Naegleria* infection, one recovered completely, one survived with significant neurologic deficits, and one died. Since 2013, when miltefosine became available through the CDC, this drug has been administered to both of two surviving U.S. patients with PAM and to three (33%) of nine patients who died of PAM (CDC, unpublished data). Early diagnosis, prompt combination therapy including miltefosine, and aggressive management of neurologic complications, including therapeutic hypothermia, are important factors in better outcomes. A clinician whose patient may have PAM should contact the CDC Emergency Operations Center at (770) 488-7100 for assistance in diagnosis by PCR and treatment recommendations (which should include miltefosine).

ACANTHAMOEBA INFECTIONS

Granulomatous Amebic Encephalitis Infection with *Acanthamoeba* species follows a more indolent course than *Naegleria* infection and typically occurs in chronically ill or debilitated patients. Risk factors include lymphoproliferative disorders, chemotherapy, glucocorticoid therapy, lupus erythematosus, and AIDS. Infection usually reaches the CNS hematogenously from a primary focus in the sinuses, skin, or lungs. In the CNS, the onset is insidious, and the syndrome often mimics a space-occupying lesion. Altered mental status, headache, and stiff neck may be accompanied by focal findings such as cranial nerve palsies, ataxia, and hemiparesis. Cutaneous ulcers or hard nodules containing amebae are frequently detected in AIDS patients with disseminated *Acanthamoeba* infection.

Examination of the CSF for trophozoites may be diagnostically helpful, but lumbar puncture may be contraindicated because of increased intracerebral pressure. CT frequently reveals cortical and subcortical lesions of decreased density consistent with embolic infarcts. In other patients, multiple enhancing lesions with edema may mimic the CT appearance of toxoplasmosis (**Chap. 228**). Demonstration of the trophozoites and cysts of *Acanthamoeba* on wet mounts or in biopsy specimens establishes the diagnosis. Culture on nonnutrient agar plates seeded with *Escherichia coli* also may be helpful. Fluorescein-labeled antiserum is available from the CDC for the detection of protozoa in biopsy specimens. Granulomatous amebic encephalitis in patients with AIDS may have an accelerated course (with survival for only 3–40 days) because of the difficulty these individuals have in forming granulomas. Various antimicrobial agents have been used to treat *Acanthamoeba* infection, but miltefosine from the CDC should be included in combination therapy.

Keratitis The incidence of keratitis caused by *Acanthamoeba* has increased in the past 20 years, in part as a result of improved diagnosis. Earlier infections were associated with trauma to the eye and exposure to contaminated water. At present, most infections are linked to extended-wear contact lenses, and rare cases are associated with laser-assisted in situ keratomileusis (LASIK). Risk factors include the use of homemade saline, the wearing of lenses while swimming, and inadequate disinfection. Since contact lenses presumably cause microscopic trauma, early corneal findings may be nonspecific. The first symptoms usually include tearing and the painful sensation of a foreign body. Once infection is established, progression is rapid. The characteristic clinical sign is an annular, paracentral corneal ring representing a corneal abscess. Deeper corneal invasion and loss of vision may follow.

The differential diagnosis includes bacterial, mycobacterial, and herpetic infection. The irregular polygonal cysts of *Acanthamoeba* (**Fig. 223-4**) may be identified in corneal scrapings or biopsy material, and trophozoites can be grown on special media. Cysts are resistant to available drugs, and the results of medical therapy have been disappointing. Some reports have suggested partial responses to propamidine isethionate eyedrops. Severe infections usually require keratoplasty.

BALAMUTHIA INFECTIONS

Balamuthia mandrillaris is a free-living ameba that was first identified in 1986 as the cause of a fatal infection in a mandrill baboon at the Wild Animal Park in San Diego, California. The parasite has been isolated from soil and dust and is probably widespread in the environment. It is an important etiologic agent of granulomatous amebic encephalitis, cutaneous lesions, and sinus infections in humans. The potential risk factors for

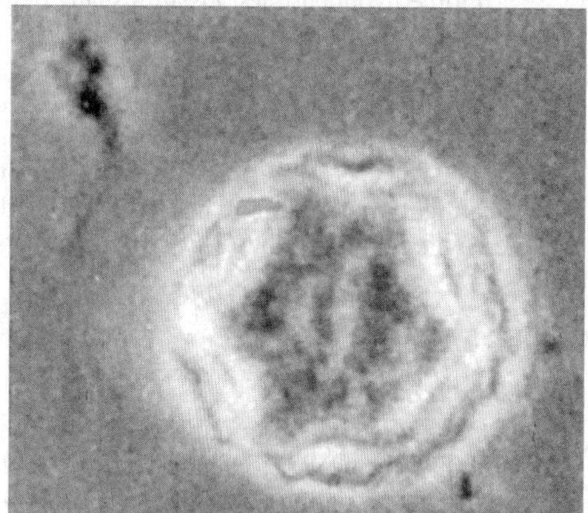

FIGURE 223-4 Double-walled cyst of *Acanthamoeba castellani*, as seen by phase-contrast microscopy. *(From DJ Krogstad et al, in A Balows et al [eds]: Manual of Clinical Microbiology, 5th ed. Washington, DC, American Society for Microbiology, 1991.)*

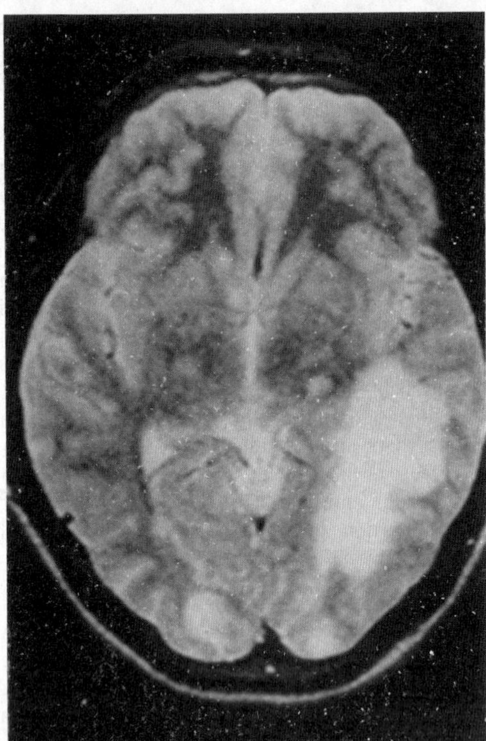

FIGURE 223-5 Brain MRI of amebic meningoencephalitis due to *Balamuthia mandrillaris*. A large lesion in the parieto-occipital lobe and other smaller lesions are seen. *(Courtesy of the Department of Radiology, UCSD Medical Center, San Diego.)*

granulomatous amebic encephalitis identified by the California Encephalitis Project include young age, immunocompromising conditions, and Hispanic ethnicity. The infection likely starts with percutaneous or mucous membrane exposure and then spreads hematogenously to the brain and other organs—a pattern that explains the risk for transmission through organ transplantation. In 2009–2010, two clusters of organ transplant–transmitted *B. mandrillaris* infections were detected by recognition of severe unexpected illness in multiple recipients from the same donor after an incubation period of 17–24 days.

Frequently, *Balamuthia* affects immunocompetent individuals, in whom the course is typically subacute, with focal neurologic signs, fever, seizures, and headaches leading to death within 1 week to several months after onset. Skin lesions may occur on the face, trunk, or extremities. In addition to dust inhalation, inoculation of trophozoites or cysts from stagnant water may occur through open wounds or mucous membranes. Diagnosis relies on examination of CSF, which reveals mononuclear or neutrophilic pleocytosis, elevated protein levels, and normal to low glucose concentrations. Amebae are rarely isolated from CSF. Multiple hypodense lesions are usually detected with imaging studies (**Fig. 223-5**). Fluorescent antibody and PCR assays are available from the CDC.

The five surviving patients in the United States have been treated with a variety of drugs, including pentamidine, flucytosine, sulfadiazine, and macrolides. The CDC recommends that miltefosine now be included, as for treatment of other free-living amebae. The differential diagnosis includes tuberculomas (**Chap. 178**) and neurocysticercosis (**Chap. 235**).

FURTHER READING

Amebiasis

Burgess SL et al: Gut microbiome communication with bone marrow regulates susceptibility to amebiasis. J Clin Invest 130:4019, 2020.

Debnath A et al: A high-throughput drug screen for *Entamoeba histolytica* identifies a new lead and target. Nat Med 18:956, 2012.

Gilchrist CA et al: Role of the gut microbiota of children in diarrhea due to the protozoan parasite *Entamoeba histolytica*. J Infect Dis 213:1579, 2016.

Ngobeni R et al: *Entamoeba* species in South Africa: Correlations with the host microbiome, parasite burdens, and first description of *Entamoeba bangladeshi* outside of Asia. J Infect Dis 216:1592, 2017.

Shirley DAT et al: A review of the global burden, new diagnostics, and current therapeutics for amebiasis. Open Forum Infect Dis 5:1, 2018.

Wojcik GL et al: Genome-wide association study reveals genetic link between diarrhea-associated *Entamoeba histolytica* infection and inflammatory bowel disease. mBio 9:e01668, 2018.

Free-Living Amebae

Bellini NK et al: The therapeutic strategies against *Naegleria fowleri*. Exp Parasitol 187:1, 2018.

Capewell LG et al: Diagnosis, clinical course, and treatment of primary amoebic meningoencephalitis in the United States, 1937–2013. J Pediatr Infect Dis Soc 4:e68, 2015.

Farnon EC et al: Transmission of *Balamuthia mandrillaris* by organ transplantation. Clin Infect Dis 63:878, 2016.

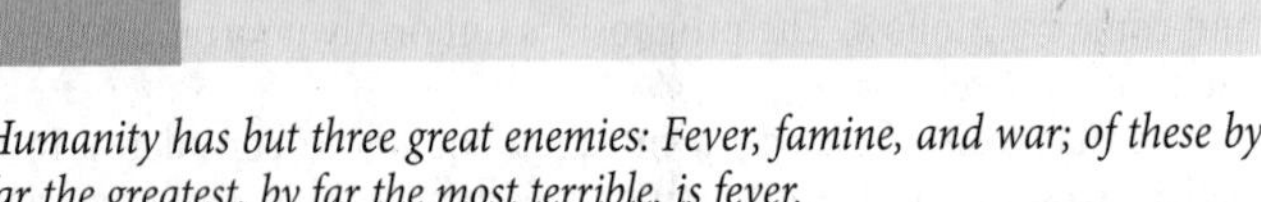

224 Malaria

Nicholas J. White, Elizabeth A. Ashley

Humanity has but three great enemies: Fever, famine, and war; of these by far the greatest, by far the most terrible, is fever.

—*William Osler, 1896*

Malaria is a protozoan disease transmitted by the bite of infected female *Anopheles* mosquitoes. The most important of the parasitic diseases of humans, malaria is transmitted in 87 countries containing 3 billion people. In 2019, it was estimated that there were 229 million cases and 409,000 deaths (i.e., ~1100 deaths each day). Mortality rates decreased dramatically between 2000 and 2015 as a result of highly effective control programs in several countries, but since then, progress has reversed and estimated global case numbers have risen steadily. Malaria was eliminated from the United States, Canada, Europe, and Russia >50 years ago, but its prevalence rose in many parts of the tropics between 1970 and 2000. In response to this rise, there has been substantial investment aimed at increasing access to accurate diagnosis, effective treatments, and insecticide-treated bed nets. An increasing number of countries that had low malaria transmission are now targeting malaria elimination. This ambitious goal is threatened by increasing resistance to antimalarial drugs and insecticides.

Malaria remains today, as it has been for centuries, a heavy burden on tropical communities, a threat to nonendemic countries, and a danger to travelers.

ETIOLOGY AND PATHOGENESIS

Six species of the genus *Plasmodium* cause nearly all malarial infections in humans. These are *P. falciparum*, *P. vivax*, two morphologically identical sympatric species of *P. ovale* (*curtisi* and *wallikeri*), *P. malariae*, and—in Southeast Asia—the monkey malaria parasite *P. knowlesi* (**Table 224-1**). Occasionally humans are also infected with the monkey parasites *P. simium* (South America) and *P. cynomolgi* (Southeast Asia). While almost all deaths are caused by falciparum malaria, *P. knowlesi* and *P. vivax* can also cause severe illness. Human infection begins when a female anopheline mosquito inoculates plasmodial *sporozoites* from its salivary glands during a blood meal (**Fig. 224-1**). These microscopic motile forms of the malaria parasite are carried rapidly via the bloodstream to the liver, where they invade hepatic parenchymal cells and begin a period of asexual reproduction. By this amplification process (known as *intrahepatic* or *preerythrocytic schizogony*), a single sporozoite may produce from 10,000 to >30,000 daughter merozoites. These few swollen infected liver cells eventually burst, discharging motile

TABLE 224-1 Characteristics of *Plasmodium* Species Infecting Humans

	FINDING FOR INDICATED SPECIES				
CHARACTERISTIC	***P. FALCIPARUM***	***P. VIVAX***	***P. OVALE***[a]	***P. MALARIAE***	***P. KNOWLESI***
Duration of intrahepatic phase (days)	5.5	8	9	15	5.5
Number of merozoites released per infected hepatocyte	30,000	10,000	15,000	15,000	20,000
Approximate duration of erythrocytic cycle (hours)	48	48	50	72	24
Red cell preference	Younger cells (but can invade cells of all ages)	Reticulocytes and cells up to 2 weeks old	Reticulocytes	Older cells	Younger cells
Morphology	Usually only ring forms; banana-shaped gametocytes	Irregularly shaped large rings and trophozoites; enlarged erythrocytes; Schüffner's dots	Infected erythrocytes, enlarged and oval with tufted ends; Schüffner's dots	Band or rectangular forms of trophozoites common	Resembles *P. falciparum* (early trophozoites) or *P. malariae* (later trophozoites, including band forms)
Pigment color	Black	Yellow-brown	Dark brown	Brown-black	Dark brown
Ability to cause relapses	No	Yes	Yes	No	No

[a]Genomic studies have revealed *P. ovale* to be two sympatric species: *P. ovale curtisi* and *P. ovale wallikeri*. which are morphologically very similar but may have different incubation periods and latencies.

merozoites into the bloodstream. The merozoites then invade red blood cells (RBCs) to become *trophozoites* and, in non-immune subjects, multiply six- to twentyfold every 48 h (*P. knowlesi*, 24 h; *P. malariae*, 72 h). When the parasites reach densities of ~50/μL of blood (~100 million parasites in total in the blood of an adult), the symptomatic stage of the infection begins. In *P. vivax* and *P. ovale* infections, a proportion of the intrahepatic forms do not divide immediately but remain inert for a period ranging from 2 weeks to ≥1 year. These dormant forms, or *hypnozoites*, are the cause of the relapses that characterize infection with these species.

Attachment of merozoites to erythrocytes is mediated via a complex interaction with several different binding ligands and specific erythrocyte surface receptors. *P. falciparum* merozoites bind via erythrocyte binding antigen 175 to glycophorin A and via EBL140 to glycophorin C. The other glycophorins (B and D) also contribute.

The merozoite reticulocyte-binding protein homologue 5 (PfRh5) plays a critical role binding to red cell basigin (CD147, EMMPRIN). *P. vivax* binds to receptors on developing erythrocytes. The Duffy blood-group antigen Fy^a or Fy^b plays an important role in invasion. Most West Africans and people with origins in that region are the Duffy-negative FyFy phenotype and are generally resistant to *P. vivax* malaria. *P. knowlesi* also invades Duffy-positive human RBCs preferentially. During the first few hours of intraerythrocytic development, the small "ring forms" of the different malaria species appear similar under light microscopy. As the trophozoites enlarge, species-specific characteristics become evident, malaria pigment (hemozoin) becomes visible, and the parasite assumes an irregular or ameboid shape. By the end of the intraerythrocytic life cycle, the parasite has consumed two-thirds of the RBC's hemoglobin and has grown to occupy most of the cell. It is now called a *schizont*. Multiple nuclear divisions have taken place (*schizogony* or *merogony*). The infected RBC then ruptures to release 6–30 daughter merozoites, each potentially capable of invading a new RBC and repeating the cycle. The disease in human beings is caused by the direct effects of the asexual parasite—RBC invasion and destruction—and by the host's reaction. Some of the blood-stage parasites develop into morphologically distinct, longer-lived sexual forms (*gametocytes*) that can transmit malaria. In falciparum malaria, a delay of several asexual cycles precedes this switch to gametocytogenesis. Female gametocytes typically outnumber males by 4:1.

After being ingested in the blood meal of a biting female anopheline mosquito, the male gametocyte exflagellates and divides rapidly into eight motile male gametes. These fuse with female gametocytes, undergoing two rounds of sexual division (meiosis) to form a zygote in the insect's midgut. This zygote matures into an ookinete, which penetrates and encysts in the mosquito's gut wall. The resulting oocyst expands by asexual division until it bursts to liberate myriad motile sporozoites, which then migrate in the hemolymph to the salivary gland of the mosquito to await inoculation into another human at the next feed, thus completing the life cycle.

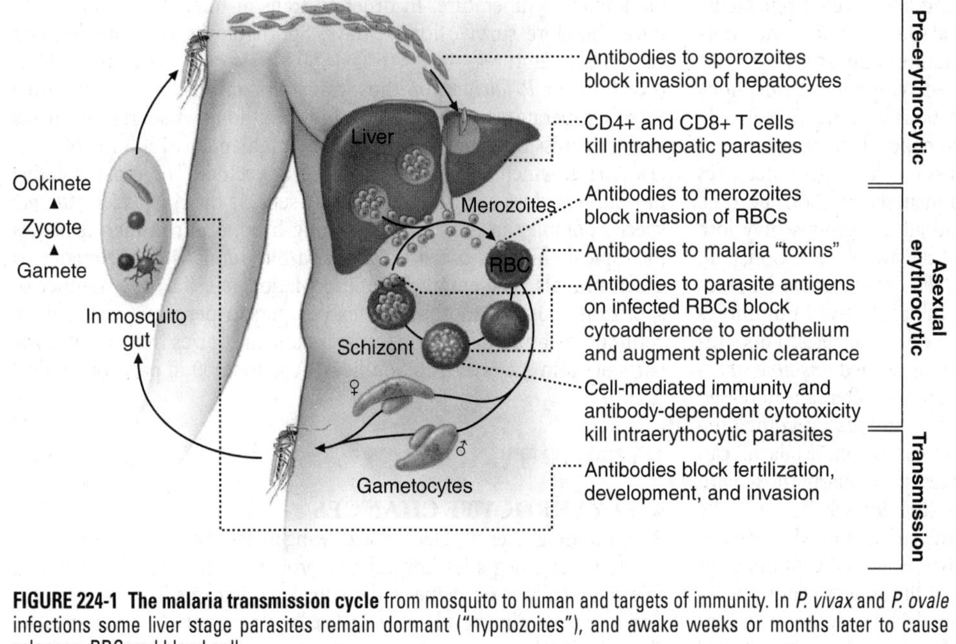

FIGURE 224-1 The malaria transmission cycle from mosquito to human and targets of immunity. In *P. vivax* and *P. ovale* infections some liver stage parasites remain dormant ("hypnozoites"), and awake weeks or months later to cause relapses. RBC, red blood cell.

EPIDEMIOLOGY

Malaria occurs throughout most of the tropical regions of the world (**Fig. 224-2**). *P. falciparum* predominates in Africa, New Guinea, and Hispaniola (i.e., the Dominican Republic and Haiti); *P. vivax* is more common in Central and

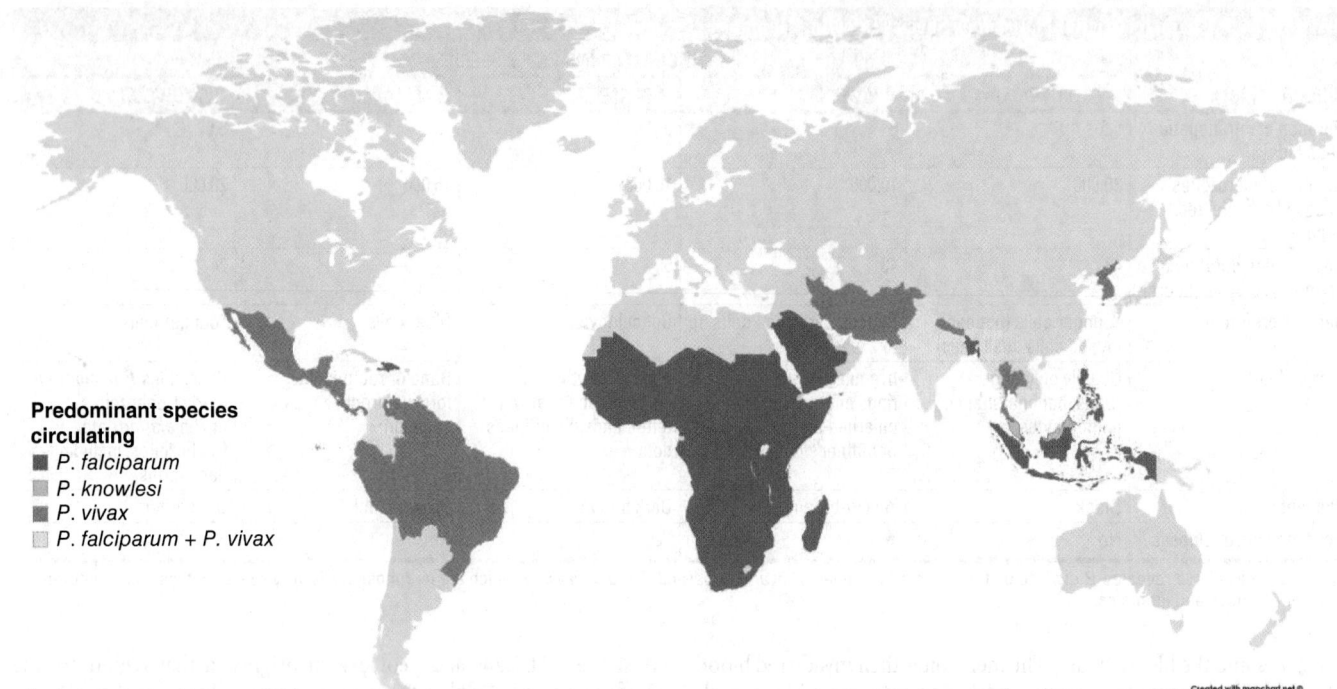

FIGURE 224-2 Malaria-endemic countries showing predominant *Plasmodium* species. *Plasmodium vivax* is common in the Horn of Africa and in Mauritania but relatively unusual elsewhere in the continent

South America and Southeast Asia. The prevalence of these two species is approximately equal on the Indian subcontinent and in Oceania. *P. malariae* is found in most endemic areas, especially throughout sub-Saharan Africa, but is much less common. *P. ovale* is relatively unusual outside of Africa and, where it is found, comprises <1% of isolates. *P. knowlesi* causes human infections commonly on the island of Borneo and, to a lesser extent, elsewhere in Southeast Asia, where the main hosts, long-tailed and pig-tailed macaques, are found.

The epidemiology of malaria is complex and may vary considerably even within relatively small geographic areas. Endemicity traditionally has been defined in terms of rates of microscopy-detected parasitemia or palpable spleens in children 2–9 years of age and has been classified as hypoendemic (<10%), mesoendemic (11–50%), hyperendemic (51–75%), and holoendemic (>75%). In holo- and hyperendemic areas (e.g., certain regions of tropical Africa or coastal New Guinea) where there is intense *P. falciparum* transmission, people may sustain one or more infectious mosquito bites per week and are infected repeatedly throughout their lives. In such settings, malaria morbidity and mortality are substantial during early childhood. Immunity against disease is hard won in these areas following repeated symptomatic infections in childhood, but, if the child survives, infections become increasingly likely to be asymptomatic. These asymptomatic older children and adults are a major source of malaria transmission. As control measures progress and urbanization expands, environmental conditions become less conducive to malaria transmission, and all age groups may lose protective immunity and become susceptible to illness. Constant, frequent, year-round infection is termed *stable transmission.* In areas where transmission is low, erratic, or focal, full protective immunity is not acquired, and symptomatic disease may occur at all ages. This situation usually exists in hypoendemic areas and is termed *unstable transmission.* Even in stable transmission areas, there is often an increased incidence of symptomatic malaria during the rainy season coinciding with increased mosquito breeding and transmission. Malaria can behave like an epidemic disease in some areas, particularly those with unstable malaria, such as northern India (the Punjab region), the Horn of Africa, Rwanda, Burundi, southern Africa, and Madagascar. Epidemics may occur when changes in environmental, economic, or social conditions (e.g., heavy rains following drought or migration—usually of refugees or workers—from a nonmalarious region to an area of high transmission) are compounded by failure to invest in national programs or by a breakdown in malaria control and prevention services caused by war or civil disorder. The recent socioeconomic and political crisis in Venezuela has led to a resurgence of malaria. Epidemics often result in high mortality rates among all age groups. The principal determinants of the epidemiology of malaria are the number (density), the human-biting habits, and the longevity of the anopheline mosquito vectors. More than 100 of the >400 anopheline species can transmit malaria, but the ~40 species that do so commonly vary considerably in their efficiency as malaria vectors. More specifically, the transmission of malaria is directly proportional to the density of the vector, the square of the number of human bites per day per mosquito, and the tenth power of the probability of the mosquito's surviving for 1 day. Mosquito longevity is particularly important as a determinant of malaria transmissibility because the portion of the parasite's life cycle that takes place within the mosquito—from gametocyte ingestion to subsequent inoculation (*sporogony*)—lasts 8–30 days, depending on ambient temperature. In order to transmit malaria, the mosquito must therefore survive for >7 days. Sporogony is not completed at cooler temperatures—i.e., <16°C (<60.8°F) for *P. vivax* and <21°C (<69.8°F) for *P. falciparum*; thus, transmission does not occur below these temperatures or at high altitudes, although malaria outbreaks and transmission have occurred in the highlands (>1500 m) of eastern Africa, which were previously free of vectors. The most effective mosquito vectors of malaria are those, such as the *Anopheles gambiae* species complex in Africa, that are long-lived, occur in high densities in tropical climates, breed readily, and bite humans in preference to other animals. The entomologic inoculation rate (i.e., the number of sporozoite-positive mosquito bites per person per year) is the most common measure of malaria transmission and varies from <1 in some parts of Latin America and Southeast Asia to >300 in parts of tropical Africa.

PATHOPHYSIOLOGY

■ ERYTHROCYTE CHANGES

After invading an erythrocyte, the growing malarial parasite progressively consumes and degrades intracellular proteins, principally hemoglobin. The potentially toxic heme is detoxified by lipid-mediated crystallization to biologically inert hemozoin (malaria pigment). The parasite also alters the RBC membrane by changing its transport properties, exposing cryptic surface antigens, and inserting new parasite-derived proteins. The RBC becomes more irregular in shape, more antigenic, and less deformable.

In *P. falciparum* infections, membrane protuberances appear on the erythrocyte's surface 12–15 h after cell invasion. These "knobs" extrude a high-molecular-weight, antigenically variant, strain-specific erythrocyte membrane adhesive protein (PfEMP1) that mediates attachment to receptors on venular and capillary endothelium (*cytoadherence*). Several vascular receptors have been identified; intercellular adhesion molecule 1 and endothelial protein C receptor are important in the brain, chondroitin sulfate B predominates in the placenta, and CD36 binds parasitized RBCs in most other organs. Erythrocytes containing more mature parasites stick inside and eventually block capillaries and venules. These infected RBCs may also adhere to uninfected RBCs (to form rosettes) and to other parasitized erythrocytes (agglutination). The processes of cytoadherence, rosetting, and agglutination are central to the pathogenesis of falciparum malaria. They result in the sequestration of infected RBCs in vital organs (particularly the brain), where they interfere with microcirculatory flow and metabolism. Sequestered parasites continue to develop out of reach of the principal host defense mechanism: splenic processing and filtration. As a consequence, only the younger ring forms of the asexual parasites circulate in the peripheral blood in falciparum malaria, and the level of peripheral parasitemia variably underestimates the true number of parasites within the body. In severe malaria, uninfected erythrocytes also become less deformable, which compromises their passage through the partially obstructed capillaries and venules and shortens their survival.

In the other human malarias, significant sequestration does not occur, and all stages of the parasite's development are evident on peripheral-blood smears. *P. vivax* and *P. ovale* show a marked predilection for young RBCs and *P. malariae* for old cells; these species produce a level of parasitemia that seldom exceeds 2%. In contrast, *P. falciparum* can invade erythrocytes of all ages and may be associated with very high parasite densities. Dangerously high parasite densities may also occur in *P. knowlesi* infections, with rapid increases as a result of the shorter (24-h) asexual life cycle.

HOST RESPONSE

Initially, the host responds to malaria infection by activating nonspecific defense mechanisms. Splenic immunologic and filtrative clearance functions are augmented, and the removal of both parasitized and uninfected erythrocytes is accelerated. The spleen also removes damaged ring-form parasites (a process known as "pitting") from within the red cell and returns the once-infected cells back to the circulation, where their survival is shortened. The parasitized cells escaping splenic removal are destroyed when the schizont ruptures. The material released induces monocyte/macrophage activation and the release of proinflammatory cytokines, which cause fever and other pathologic effects. Temperatures of ≥40°C (≥104°F) damage mature parasites; in untreated infections, the effect of such temperatures is to further synchronize the parasitic cycle, with eventual production of the regular fever spikes and rigors that originally characterized the different malarias. These regular fever patterns (*quotidian*, daily; *tertian*, every 2 days; *quartan*, every 3 days) are seldom seen today as patients receive prompt and effective antimalarial treatment.

The geographic distributions of the thalassemias, sickle cell disease, hemoglobins C and E, hereditary ovalocytosis, and glucose-6-phosphate dehydrogenase (G6PD) deficiency closely resemble that of falciparum malaria before the introduction of control measures. This similarity suggests that these genetic disorders confer protection against death from falciparum malaria. HbA/S heterozygotes (sickle cell trait) have a sixfold reduction in the risk of dying from severe falciparum malaria and are correspondingly protected from the bacterial infections that complicate malaria. Hemoglobin S–containing RBCs impair parasite growth at low oxygen tensions, and *P. falciparum*–infected RBCs containing hemoglobin S or C exhibit reduced cytoadherence because of reduced surface presentation of the adhesin PfEMP1. Parasite multiplication in HbA/E heterozygotes is reduced at high parasite densities. In Melanesia, children with α-thalassemia have more frequent malaria (both vivax and falciparum) in the early years of life, and this pattern of infection appears to protect them against severe disease. In Melanesian ovalocytosis, rigid erythrocytes resist merozoite invasion, and the intraerythrocytic milieu is hostile. G6PD deficiency provides some protection against severe *P. falciparum* infections but has a much stronger protective effect against *P. vivax* infections.

Nonspecific host defense mechanisms stop the infection's expansion, and the subsequent strain-specific immune response then controls the infection. Eventually, exposure to sufficient strains confers protection from high-level parasitemia and disease but not from infection. As a result of this state of infection without illness (*premunition*), asymptomatic parasitemia is very common among adults and older children living in regions with stable and intense transmission (i.e., holo- or hyperendemic areas) and also in parts of low-transmission areas. Parasitemia in asymptomatic infections fluctuates in density but often averages ~5000/mL—just below the level of microscopy detection but sufficient to generate transmissible densities of gametocytes. Immunity is mainly specific for both the species and the strain of infecting malarial parasite. Both humoral immunity and cellular immunity are necessary for protection, but the mechanisms of each are incompletely understood (Fig. 224-1). Immune individuals have a polyclonal increase in serum levels of IgM, IgG, and IgA, although much of this antibody is unrelated to protection. Antibodies to a variety of parasite antigens presumably act in concert to limit in vivo replication of the parasite. In *P. falciparum* infections, the variant surface adhesin PfEMP1 is the most important of these antigens. Passive transfer of maternal antibody contributes to the partial protection of infants from severe malaria in the first months of life. This complex immunity to disease declines when a person lives outside an endemic area for several months or longer.

Several factors retard the development of cellular immunity to malaria. These factors include the absence of major histocompatibility antigens on the surface of infected RBCs, which precludes direct T cell recognition; malaria antigen–specific immune unresponsiveness; and the enormous strain diversity of malarial parasites, along with the ability of the parasites to express variant immunodominant antigens on the erythrocyte surface that change during the course of infection. Parasites may persist in the blood for months or years (or, in the case of *P. malariae*, for decades) if treatment is not given. The complexity of the immune response in malaria, the sophistication of the parasites' evasion mechanisms, and the lack of a good in vitro correlate with clinical immunity have all slowed progress toward an effective vaccine.

CLINICAL FEATURES

Malaria is a common cause of fever in tropical countries. Clinical diagnosis is notoriously unreliable. The first symptoms of malaria are nonspecific; the lack of a sense of well-being, headache, fatigue, abdominal discomfort, and muscle aches followed by fever are all similar to the symptoms of a minor viral illness. In some instances, a prominence of headache, chest pain, abdominal pain, cough, arthralgia, myalgia, or diarrhea may suggest another diagnosis. Although headache may be severe in malaria, the neck stiffness and photophobia seen in meningitis do not occur. While myalgia may be prominent, it is not usually as severe as in dengue fever, and the muscles are not tender as in leptospirosis or typhus. Nausea, vomiting, and orthostatic hypotension are common. The classic malarial paroxysms, in which fever spikes, chills, and rigors occur at regular intervals, are unusual and at presentation suggest infection (often relapse) with *P. vivax* or *P. ovale*. The fever is usually irregular at first (that of falciparum malaria may never become regular). The temperature of nonimmune individuals and children often rises above 40°C (104°F), with accompanying tachycardia and sometimes delirium. Although childhood febrile convulsions may occur with any of the malarias, generalized seizures are associated specifically with falciparum malaria and may herald the development of encephalopathy (cerebral malaria). Many clinical abnormalities have been described in acute malaria, but most patients with uncomplicated infections have few abnormal physical findings other than fever, malaise, mild anemia, and (in some cases) a palpable spleen. Anemia is common among young children living in areas with stable transmission (e.g., much of West Africa), and increases in prevalence where resistance has compromised the efficacy of antimalarial drugs. Frequent vivax malaria relapse is an important cause of anemia in young children in some areas (e.g., on the island of New Guinea). In nonimmune individuals with acute malaria, the spleen takes several days to become palpable, but splenic enlargement is found in a high proportion of otherwise healthy individuals in malaria-endemic areas and reflects repeated infections. Slight enlargement of the liver is also common, particularly among young children. Mild jaundice is common among adults; it may develop in patients with otherwise uncomplicated malaria and usually resolves over 1–3 weeks. Malaria is not associated with a rash. Petechial hemorrhages in the skin or mucous membranes—features of viral hemorrhagic fevers and leptospirosis—develop only very rarely in severe falciparum malaria.

SEVERE FALCIPARUM MALARIA

Appropriately and promptly treated, uncomplicated falciparum malaria (i.e., that in which the patient can sit or stand unaided and can swallow medicines and food) carries a mortality rate of <0.1%. However, once vital-organ dysfunction occurs or the total proportion of erythrocytes infected increases to >2% (a level corresponding to >10^{12} parasites in an adult), mortality risk rises steeply, depending on the immunity of the host. The major manifestations of severe falciparum malaria are shown in **Table 224-2**, and features indicating a poor prognosis are listed in **Table 224-3**.

TABLE 224-2 Manifestations of Severe Falciparum Malaria

SIGNS	MANIFESTATIONS
Major	
Unarousable coma/cerebral malaria	Failure to localize or respond appropriately to noxious stimuli; coma persisting for >30 min after generalized convulsion
Acidemia/acidosis	Arterial pH of <7.25, base deficit >8 meq/L, or plasma bicarbonate level of <15 mmol/L; venous lactate level of >5 mmol/L; manifests as labored deep breathing, often termed "respiratory distress"
Severe normochromic, normocytic anemia	Hematocrit of <15% or hemoglobin level of <50 g/L (<5 g/dL) with parasitemia level of >10,000/μL[a]
Renal failure	Serum or plasma creatinine level of >265 μmol/L (>3 mg/dL); urine output (24 h) of <400 mL for adults or <12 mL/kg for children; no improvement with rehydration[b]
Pulmonary edema/adult respiratory distress syndrome	Noncardiogenic pulmonary edema, often aggravated by overhydration
Hypoglycemia	Plasma glucose level of <2.2 mmol/L (<40 mg/dL)
Hypotension/shock	Systolic blood pressure of <50 mmHg in children 1–5 years or <80 mmHg in adults; core/skin temperature difference of >10°C; capillary refill >2 s
Bleeding/disseminated intravascular coagulation	Significant bleeding and hemorrhage from the gums, nose, and gastrointestinal tract and/or evidence of disseminated intravascular coagulation
Convulsions	More than two generalized seizures in 24 h; signs of continued seizure activity, sometimes subtle (e.g., tonic-clonic eye movements without limb or face movement)
Other	
Hemoglobinuria[c]	Macroscopic black, brown, or red urine; not associated with effects of oxidant drugs and red blood cell enzyme defects (such as G6PD deficiency)
Extreme weakness	Prostration; inability to sit unaided[d]
Hyperparasitemia	Parasitemia level of >5% in nonimmune patients (>10% in any patient)
Jaundice	Serum bilirubin level of >50 mmol/L (>3 mg/dL) if combined with a parasite density of 100,000/μL or other evidence of vital-organ dysfunction

[a]This is nonspecific and may include patients with chronic anemia; a parasitemia threshold of 100,000/μL is more specific for acute malarial anemia. [b]In practice, urine output information is usually unavailable, so the plasma or serum creatinine alone is used. [c]Hemoglobinuria may also occur in uncomplicated malaria and in patients with G6PD deficiency, particularly if they take oxidant drugs such as primaquine. [d]In children who are normally able to sit.

Abbreviation: G6PD, glucose-6-phosphate dehydrogenase.

Cerebral Malaria Coma is a characteristic and ominous feature of falciparum malaria and, even with treatment, has been associated with death rates of ~20% among adults and 15% among children. Any obtundation, delirium, or abnormal behavior in falciparum malaria should be taken very seriously. The onset of coma may be gradual or sudden following a convulsion.

Cerebral malaria manifests as a diffuse symmetric encephalopathy; focal neurologic signs are unusual. Although some passive resistance to head flexion may be detected, signs of meningeal irritation are absent. The eyes may be divergent, and bruxism and a pout reflex are common, but other primitive reflexes are usually absent. The corneal reflexes are preserved, except in deep coma. Muscle tone may be either increased or decreased. The tendon reflexes are variable, and the plantar reflexes may be flexor or extensor; the abdominal and cremasteric reflexes are absent. Flexor or extensor posturing may be seen. On routine funduscopy, ~15% of patients have retinal hemorrhages; with pupillary dilation and indirect ophthalmoscopy, this figure increases to 30–40%. Other funduscopic abnormalities (**Fig. 224-3**) include discrete spots of retinal opacification (30–60%), papilledema (8% among children, rare among adults), cotton wool spots (<5%), and decolorization of a retinal vessel or segment of vessel (occasional cases). Convulsions, which are usually generalized and often repeated, occur in ~10% of adults and up to 50% of children with cerebral malaria. More covert seizure activity is common, particularly among children, and may manifest as repetitive tonic-clonic eye movements or even hypersalivation. Whereas adults rarely (<3% of cases) suffer neurologic sequelae, ~10% of children surviving cerebral malaria—especially those with hypoglycemia, severe anemia, repeated seizures, and deep coma—have residual neurologic deficits when they regain consciousness; hemiplegia, cerebral palsy, cortical blindness, deafness, and impaired cognition may all occur. The majority of these deficits improve markedly or resolve completely within 6 months. However, the prevalence of some other deficits increases over time; ~10% of children surviving cerebral malaria have a persistent language deficit. There may also be deficits in learning, planning and executive functions, attention, memory, and nonverbal functioning. The incidence of epilepsy is increased and life expectancy decreased among these children.

Hypoglycemia Hypoglycemia, an important and common complication of severe malaria, is associated with a poor prognosis and is particularly problematic in children and pregnant women. Hypoglycemia in malaria results from both a failure of hepatic gluconeogenesis and an increase in the consumption of glucose by the host and, to a much lesser extent, the malaria parasites. This may be compounded by quinine, a powerful stimulant of pancreatic insulin secretion, which is still widely used for the treatment of both severe and uncomplicated falciparum malaria. Hyperinsulinemic hypoglycemia is especially troublesome in pregnant women receiving quinine treatment. In severe disease, the clinical diagnosis of hypoglycemia is difficult: the usual physical signs (sweating, gooseflesh, tachycardia) are absent, and the neurologic impairment caused by hypoglycemia cannot be distinguished from that caused by malaria.

Acidosis Acidosis, resulting from accumulation of organic acids, is an important cause of death from severe malaria, which in adults is often compounded by coexisting renal impairment. Hyperlactatemia commonly coexists with hypoglycemia. In children, ketoacidosis may contribute. Hydroxyphenyllactic acid, α-hydroxybutyric acid, and β-hydroxybutyric acid concentrations are elevated. Acidotic breathing, sometimes called "respiratory distress," is a sign of poor prognosis. It is followed often by circulatory failure refractory to volume expansion or inotropic drug treatment and ultimately by respiratory arrest. Plasma concentrations of bicarbonate or lactate are the best biochemical prognosticators in severe malaria. Hypovolemia is not a major contributor to acidosis. Lactic acidosis is caused by the combination of anaerobic glycolysis in tissues where sequestered parasites interfere with

TABLE 224-3 Features Indicating a Poor Prognosis in Severe Falciparum Malaria

Clinical
Marked agitation
Hyperventilation (respiratory distress)
Low core temperature (<36.5°C; <97.7°F)
Bleeding
Deep coma
Repeated convulsions
Anuria
Shock
Laboratory
Biochemistry
Hypoglycemia (<2.2 mmol/L)
Hyperlactatemia (>5 mmol/L)
Acidemia (arterial pH <7.25, base deficit >8 meq/L, or serum HCO_3 <15 mmol/L)
Elevated serum creatinine (>265 μmol/L)
Elevated total bilirubin (>50 μmol/L)
Elevated liver enzymes (AST/ALT 3 times upper limit of normal)
Elevated muscle enzymes (CPK ↑, myoglobin ↑)
Elevated urate (>600 μmol/L)
Hematology
Leukocytosis (>12,000/μL)
Severe anemia (PCV <15%)
Coagulopathy
Low platelet count (<50,000/μL)
Prolonged prothrombin time (>3 s)
Prolonged partial thromboplastin time
Decreased fibrinogen (<200 mg/dL)
Parasitology
Hyperparasitemia
Increased mortality at >100,000/μL
High mortality at >500,000/μL
>20% of parasites identified as pigment-containing trophozoites and schizonts
>5% of neutrophils contain visible malaria pigment

Note: Increased risk of concomitant bacteremia in adults if >20% parasitemia.

Abbreviations: ALT, alanine aminotransferase; AST, aspartate aminotransferase; CPK, creatine phosphokinase; PCV, packed cell volume.

microcirculatory flow, lactate production by the parasites, and a failure of hepatic and renal lactate clearance.

Noncardiogenic Pulmonary Edema Adults with severe falciparum malaria may develop noncardiogenic pulmonary edema even after several days of antimalarial therapy. The pathogenesis of this variant of the adult respiratory distress syndrome is unclear. The mortality rate is >80%. Pulmonary edema can be precipitated by overly vigorous administration of IV fluid. Noncardiogenic pulmonary edema can also develop in otherwise uncomplicated vivax malaria, where recovery is usual.

Renal Impairment Acute kidney injury is common in severe falciparum malaria. The pathogenesis of renal failure is unclear but may be related to erythrocyte sequestration and agglutination interfering with renal microcirculatory flow and metabolism. Clinically and pathologically, this syndrome manifests as acute tubular necrosis. Acute renal failure may occur simultaneously with other vital-organ dysfunction (in which case the mortality risk is high) or may progress as other disease manifestations resolve. In survivors, urine flow resumes in a median of 4 days, and serum creatinine levels return to normal in a mean of 17 days (**Chap. 310**). Early dialysis or hemofiltration considerably improves the chances of survival, particularly in acute hypercatabolic renal failure. Oliguric renal failure is rare among children.

Hematologic Abnormalities Anemia results from accelerated RBC removal by the spleen, obligatory RBC destruction at parasite

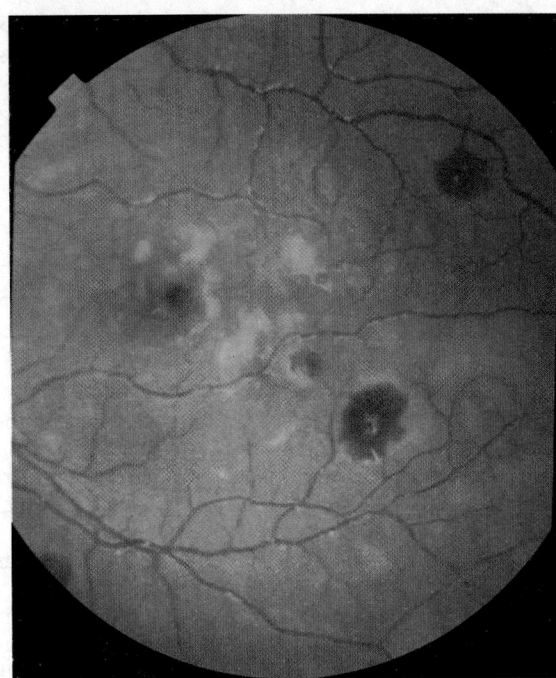

FIGURE 224-3 The eye in cerebral malaria: perimacular whitening and pale-centered retinal hemorrhages. *(Courtesy of N. Beare, T. Taylor, S. Harding, S. Lewallen, and M. Molyneux; with permission.)*

schizogony, and ineffective erythropoiesis. In severe malaria, the deformability of both infected and uninfected RBCs is reduced. The degree of reduced deformability correlates with prognosis and with the development of anemia. Splenic clearance of all RBCs is increased. In nonimmune individuals and in areas with unstable transmission, anemia can develop rapidly and transfusion is often required. A hemoglobin of ≤3g/dL on presentation is associated with increased mortality. Acute hemolytic anemia with massive hemoglobinuria ("blackwater fever") may occur. Hemoglobinuria may contribute to renal injury. Some patients with blackwater fever have G6PD deficiency, but in the majority of cases, it is unclear why massive hemolysis has occurred. In non-immune patients sudden hemolysis may follow many days after artesunate treatment of hyperparasitemia, usually as a result of relatively synchronous loss of once-parasitized "pitted" RBCs. As a consequence of repeated malarial infections, children in high-transmission areas are usually anemic and often develop severe anemia. This results from both shortened survival of uninfected RBCs and marked dyserythropoiesis. Anemia is a common consequence of antimalarial drug resistance, which results in repeated or continued infection.

Slight coagulation abnormalities are common in falciparum malaria, and mild thrombocytopenia is usual (a normal platelet count should question the diagnosis of malaria). Fewer than 5% of patients with severe malaria have significant bleeding with evidence of disseminated intravascular coagulation. Hematemesis from stress ulceration or acute gastric erosions also may occur rarely.

Liver Dysfunction Mild hemolytic jaundice is common in malaria. Severe jaundice is associated with *P. falciparum* infections; is more common among adults than among children; and results from hemolysis, hepatocyte injury, and cholestasis. Liver failure does not occur. When accompanied by other vital-organ dysfunction (often renal impairment), liver dysfunction carries a poor prognosis. Hepatic dysfunction contributes to hypoglycemia, lactic acidosis, and impaired drug metabolism. Occasional patients with falciparum malaria may develop deep jaundice (with hemolytic, hepatic, and cholestatic components) without evidence of other vital-organ dysfunction, in which case the prognosis is good.

Other Complications HIV/AIDS and malnutrition predispose to more severe malaria in nonimmune individuals. Malaria anemia is worsened by concurrent infections with intestinal helminths,

TABLE 224-4 Relative Incidence of Severe Complications of Falciparum Malaria

COMPLICATION	NONPREGNANT ADULTS	PREGNANT WOMEN	CHILDREN
Anemia	+	++	+++
Convulsions	+	+	+++
Hypoglycemia	+	+++	+++
Jaundice	+++	+++	+
Renal failure	+++	+++	–
Pulmonary edema	++	+++	+

Note: –, rare; +, infrequent; ++, frequent; +++, very frequent.

hookworm in particular. Approximately 6% of children diagnosed with severe malaria have concomitant bacteremia. In adults, the proportion is lower (<1%), except in those with very high parasite counts (>20% parasitemia). In areas of moderate and high malaria transmission, differentiating severe malaria from sepsis with incidental parasitemia in childhood is very difficult. In endemic areas, *Salmonella* spp. bacteremia has been associated specifically with *P. falciparum* infections. Chest infections and catheter-induced urinary tract infections are common among patients who are unconscious for >3 days. Aspiration pneumonia may follow generalized convulsions. The frequencies of complications of severe falciparum malaria are summarized in **Table 224-4**.

MALARIA IN PREGNANCY

Malaria in early pregnancy causes fetal loss. In areas of high malaria transmission, falciparum malaria in primi- and secundigravid women is associated with low birth weight (average reduction, ~170 g) and consequently increased infant mortality rates. In general, infected mothers in areas of stable transmission remain asymptomatic despite intense accumulation of parasitized erythrocytes in the placental microcirculation. Maternal HIV infection predisposes pregnant women to more frequent and higher-density malaria infections, predisposes their newborns to congenital malarial infection, and exacerbates the reduction in birth weight associated with malaria.

In areas with unstable transmission of malaria, pregnant women are prone to severe infections and are particularly likely to develop high *P. falciparum* parasitemias complicated by anemia, hypoglycemia, and acute pulmonary edema. Fetal distress, premature labor, and stillbirth or low birth weight are common results. Fetal death is usual in severe malaria. Congenital malaria occurs in <5% of newborns of infected mothers; its frequency and the level of parasitemia are related directly to the timing of maternal infection and the parasite density in maternal blood and in the placenta. *P. vivax* malaria in pregnancy is also associated with a reduction in birth weight (average, 110 g), but in contrast to falciparum malaria, this effect is more pronounced in multigravid than in primigravid women. About 300,000 women die in childbirth yearly, with most deaths occurring in low-income countries; maternal death from hemorrhage at childbirth is correlated with malaria-induced anemia.

MALARIA IN CHILDREN

Most of the >400,000 deaths from falciparum malaria each year are in young African children. Convulsions, coma, hypoglycemia, metabolic acidosis, and severe anemia are relatively common among children with severe malaria, whereas deep jaundice, oliguric acute kidney injury, and acute pulmonary edema are unusual. Severely anemic children may present with labored deep breathing, which in the past has been attributed incorrectly to "anemic congestive cardiac failure" but in fact is usually caused by metabolic acidosis, sometimes compounded by hypovolemia. In general, children tolerate antimalarial drugs well and respond rapidly to treatment.

TRANSFUSION MALARIA

Malaria can be transmitted by blood transfusion, needlestick injury, or organ transplantation. The incubation period in these settings is often short because there is no preerythrocytic stage of development, and thus there are no relapses of *P. vivax* and *P. ovale* infections. The clinical features and management of these cases are the same as for naturally acquired infections although primaquine is not needed for vivax or ovale malaria as there are no liver stages.

CHRONIC COMPLICATIONS OF MALARIA

HYPERREACTIVE MALARIAL SPLENOMEGALY

Chronic or repeated malarial infections produce hypergammaglobulinemia; normochromic, normocytic anemia; and, in certain situations, splenomegaly. Some residents of malaria-endemic areas in tropical countries exhibit an abnormal immunologic response to repeated infections that is characterized by massive splenomegaly, hepatomegaly, marked elevations in serum IgM and malarial antibody titers, hepatic sinusoidal lymphocytosis, and (in Africa) peripheral B-cell lymphocytosis. This syndrome has been associated with the production of cytotoxic IgM antibodies to CD8+ T lymphocytes, antibodies to CD5+ T lymphocytes, and an increase in the ratio of CD4+ to CD8+ T cells. These events may lead to uninhibited B cell production of IgM and the formation of cryoglobulins (IgM aggregates and immune complexes). This immunologic process stimulates lymphoid hyperplasia and clearance activity and eventually produces splenomegaly. Patients with hyperreactive malarial splenomegaly present with an abdominal mass or a dragging sensation in the abdomen and occasional sharp abdominal pains suggesting perisplenitis. There is usually anemia and some degree of pancytopenia (hypersplenism). In some cases, malaria parasites cannot be found in peripheral-blood smears by microscopy. Respiratory and skin infections are common and many patients die of overwhelming sepsis. Persons with hyperreactive malarial splenomegaly living in endemic areas should receive antimalarial chemoprophylaxis; the results are usually good. In nonendemic areas, antimalarial treatment is advised. Some cases have been mistaken for hematologic malignancy. However, in other cases refractory to therapy, clonal lymphoproliferation may develop and this can evolve into a malignant lymphoproliferative disorder.

QUARTAN MALARIAL NEPHROPATHY

Chronic or repeated infections with *P. malariae* (and possibly with other malarial species) may cause soluble immune complex injury to the renal glomeruli, resulting in the nephrotic syndrome. Other unidentified factors must contribute to this process since only a very small proportion of infected patients develop renal disease. The histologic appearance is that of focal or segmental glomerulonephritis with splitting of the capillary basement membrane. Subendothelial dense deposits are seen on electron microscopy, and immunofluorescence reveals deposits of complement and immunoglobulins and *P. malariae* antigens are often visible. A coarse-granular pattern of basement membrane immunofluorescent deposits (predominantly IgG3) with selective proteinuria carries a better prognosis than a fine-granular, predominantly IgG2 pattern with nonselective proteinuria. Quartan nephropathy is rarely reported nowadays. It usually responds poorly to treatment with either antimalarial agents or glucocorticoids and cytotoxic drugs.

BURKITT'S LYMPHOMA AND EPSTEIN-BARR VIRUS INFECTION

It is possible that malaria-related immune dysregulation provokes infection with lymphoma viruses. Childhood Burkitt's lymphoma is strongly associated with Epstein-Barr virus (EBV) and with high transmission of *P. falciparum*. Chronic *P. falciparum* malaria drives large numbers of EBV-infected cells through the lymph node germinal centers and deregulates activation-induced cytidine deaminase, resulting in DNA damage, c-myc translocations, and sometimes lymphoma.

DIAGNOSIS OF MALARIA

When a patient in or from a malarious area presents with fever, thick and thin blood smears should be prepared and *examined immediately* to confirm the diagnosis and identify the species of infecting parasite

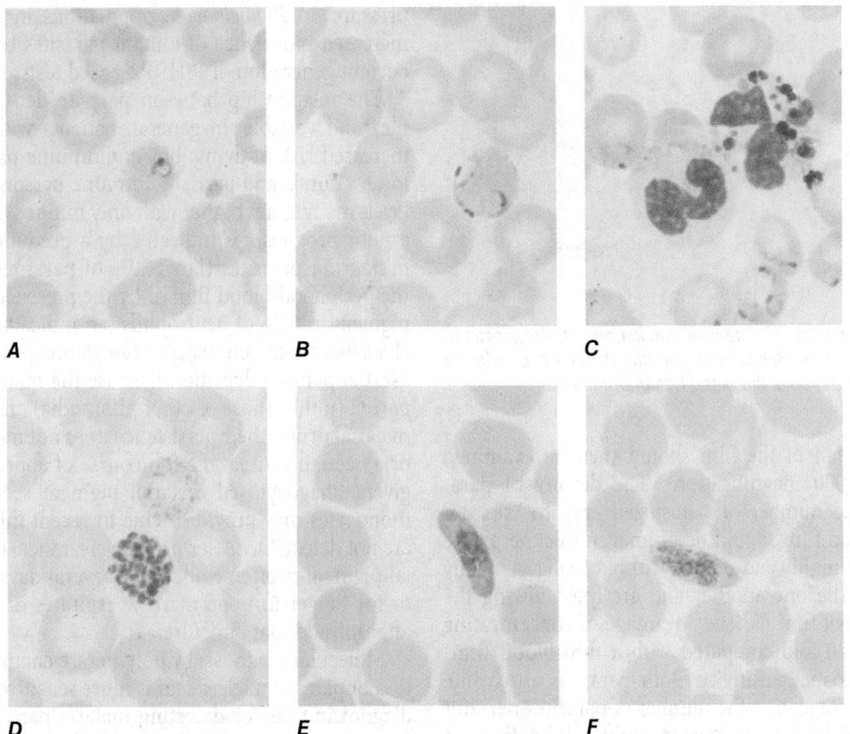

FIGURE 224-4 Thin blood films of *Plasmodium falciparum*. ***A.*** Young trophozoite. ***B.*** Old trophozoite. ***C.*** Trophozoites in erythrocytes and pigment in polymorphonuclear cells. ***D.*** Mature schizont. ***E.*** Female gametocyte. ***F.*** Male gametocyte. *(Reproduced from Bench Aids for the Diagnosis of Malaria Infections, 2nd ed, with the permission of the World Health Organization.)*

(**Figs. 224-4 through 224-9**). In general, if the blood smear is negative when examined by an experienced microscopist, the patient does not have malaria. If reliable microscopy is not available, a rapid test should be performed. Malaria is not a clinical diagnosis.

■ DEMONSTRATION OF THE PARASITE

The definitive diagnosis of malaria rests on the demonstration of asexual forms of the parasite in stained peripheral-blood smears. Of the Romanowsky stains, Giemsa at pH 7.2 is preferred; Field's, Wright's, or Leishman's stain can also be used. Staining of parasites with the fluorescent dye acridine orange allows more rapid diagnosis of malaria (but not speciation of the infection) in patients with low-level parasitemia.

Both thin (Figs. 224-4 and 224-5) and thick (Figs. 224-6, 224-7, 224-8, and 224-9) blood smears should be examined. The thin blood smear should be air-dried, fixed in anhydrous methanol, then

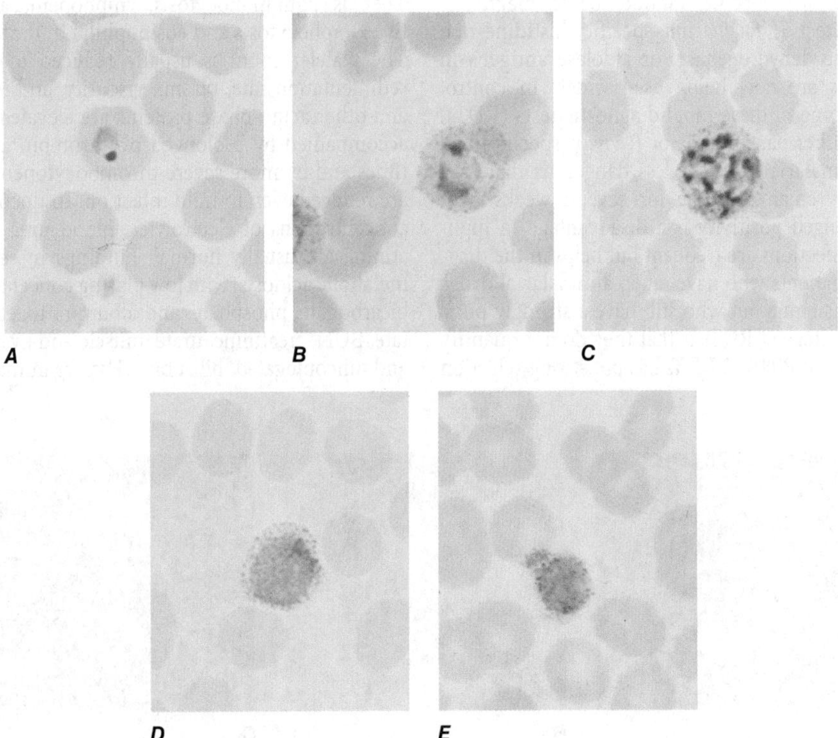

FIGURE 224-5 Thin blood films of *Plasmodium vivax*. ***A.*** Young trophozoite. ***B.*** Old trophozoite. ***C.*** Mature schizont. ***D.*** Female gametocyte. ***E.*** Male gametocyte. *(Reproduced from Bench Aids for the Diagnosis of Malaria Infections, 2nd ed, with the permission of the World Health Organization.)*

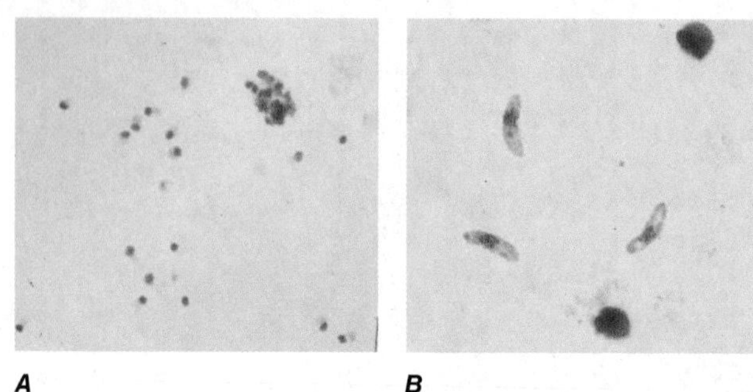

FIGURE 224-6 Thick blood films of *Plasmodium falciparum*. *A.* Trophozoites. ***B.*** Gametocytes. *(Reproduced from Bench Aids for the Diagnosis of Malaria Infections, 2nd ed, with the permission of the World Health Organization.)*

stained; the RBCs in the tail of the film should then be examined under oil immersion (×1000 magnification). The density of parasitemia is expressed as the number of parasitized erythrocytes per 1000 RBCs. The thick blood film should be of uneven thickness. The smear should be dried thoroughly and stained without fixing. As many layers of erythrocytes overlie one another and are lysed during the staining procedure, the thick film has the advantage of concentrating the parasites (by 40- to 100-fold compared with a thin blood film) and thus increasing diagnostic sensitivity. Both parasites and white blood cells (WBCs) are counted, and the number of parasites per unit volume is calculated from the total leukocyte count. Alternatively, a WBC count of 8000/μL is assumed. This figure is converted to the number of parasitized erythrocytes per microliter. A minimum of 200 WBCs should be counted under oil immersion. Interpretation of blood smears, particularly thick films, requires some experience because artifacts are common. Before a thick smear is judged to be negative, 100–200 fields should be examined. In high-transmission areas, the presence of up to 10,000 parasites/μL of blood may be tolerated without symptoms or signs in partially immune individuals. Thus, in these areas, the detection of low-density malaria parasitemia is sensitive but has low specificity in identifying malaria as the cause of illness. Because the prevalence of asymptomatic parasitemia is often high, low-density parasitemia is a common incidental finding in other conditions causing fever.

Rapid, simple, sensitive, and specific antibody-based diagnostic stick or card tests that detect *P. falciparum*–specific, histidine-rich protein 2 (PfHRP2), lactate dehydrogenase, or aldolase antigens in finger-prick blood samples are now being used widely in control programs (**Table 224-5**). Some of these rapid diagnostic tests (RDTs) carry a second antibody (either pan-malaria or *P. vivax*–specific) and so distinguish falciparum malaria from the less dangerous malarias. PfHRP2-based RDTs may remain positive for several weeks after acute infection. This prolonged positivity is a disadvantage in high-transmission areas where infections are frequent but helps in the diagnosis of severe malaria in patients who have taken antimalarial drugs and cleared peripheral parasitemia but who still have a strongly positive PfHRP2 test. A disadvantage of RDTs is that they do not quantify parasitemia. Widespread use of PfHRP2 RDTs has put strong selection pressure on *P. falciparum* populations in some areas, leading to an increased prevalence of mutant parasites that are not detected by the current generation of PfHRP2-based tests.

The relationship between parasite density and prognosis is complex and variable; in general, patients with >10^5 parasites/μL are at increased risk of dying, but nonimmune patients may die with much lower counts, and partially immune persons may tolerate parasitemia levels many times higher with only minor symptoms. In severe malaria, a poor prognosis is indicated by a predominance of more mature *P. falciparum* parasites (i.e., >20% of parasites with visible pigment) in the peripheral-blood film or by the presence of phagocytosed malarial pigment in >5% of neutrophils (an indicator of recent schizogony). In *P. falciparum* infections, gametocytemia peaks 1 week after the peak of asexual parasite densities. Because the mature gametocytes of *P. falciparum* (unlike those of other plasmodia) are not affected by most antimalarial drugs, their persistence does not mean there is drug resistance or a need to re-treat if a full course of appropriate treatment has been given. Phagocytosed malarial pigment seen inside peripheral-blood monocytes may provide a clue to recent infection if malaria parasites are not detectable. After parasite clearance, this intraphagocytic malarial pigment is often evident for several days in peripheral-blood films or for longer in bone marrow aspirates or smears of fluid expressed after intradermal puncture.

Molecular diagnosis by polymerase chain reaction (PCR) amplification of parasite nucleic acid is more sensitive than microscopy or rapid diagnostic tests for detecting malaria parasites and defining malarial species. While currently impractical in the standard clinical setting, PCR is used in reference centers in endemic areas. In epidemiologic surveys, ultrasensitive PCR detection has proved very useful in identifying asymptomatic infections as control and eradication programs drive parasite prevalences down to very low levels. Serologic diagnosis with either indirect fluorescent antibody or enzyme-linked immunosorbent assays is useful for screening of prospective blood donors and may prove useful as a measure of transmission intensity in future epidemiologic studies. Serology has no place in the diagnosis of acute illness.

LABORATORY FINDINGS IN ACUTE MALARIA

Normochromic, normocytic anemia is usual. The leukocyte count is generally normal, although it may be raised in very severe infections. There is slight monocytosis, lymphopenia, and eosinopenia, with reactive lymphocytosis and eosinophilia in the weeks after acute infection. The platelet count is usually reduced to ~10^5/μL. The erythrocyte sedimentation rate, plasma viscosity, and levels of C-reactive protein and other acute-phase proteins are elevated. Severe infections may be accompanied by prolonged prothrombin and partial thromboplastin times and by more severe thrombocytopenia. Antithrombin III levels are reduced even in mild infection. In uncomplicated malaria, plasma concentrations of electrolytes, blood urea nitrogen (BUN), and creatinine are usually normal. Findings in severe malaria may include metabolic acidosis, with low plasma concentrations of glucose, sodium, bicarbonate, phosphate, and albumin, together with elevations in lactate, BUN, creatinine, urate, muscle and liver enzymes, and conjugated and unconjugated bilirubin. Hypergammaglobulinemia is usual in

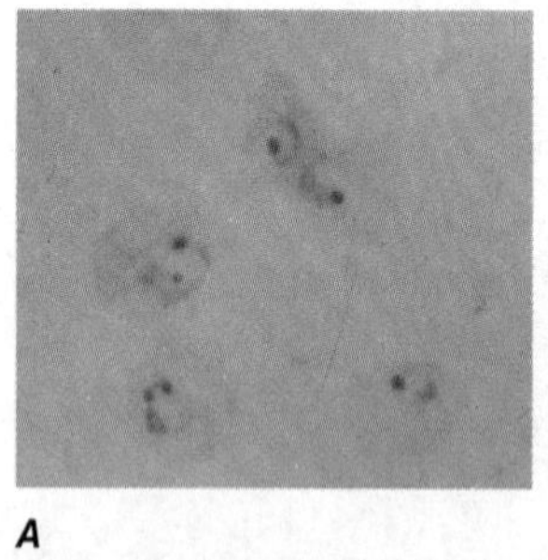

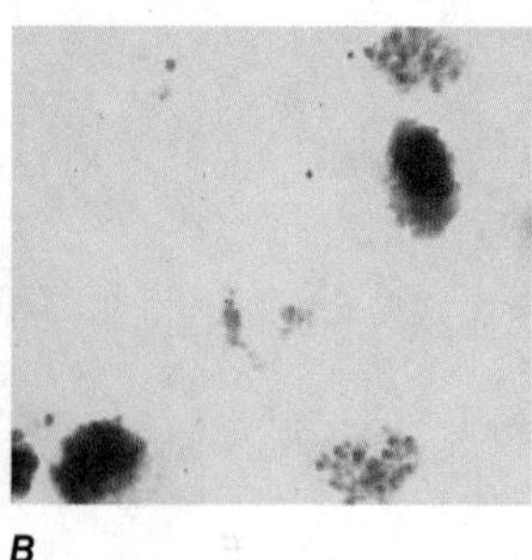

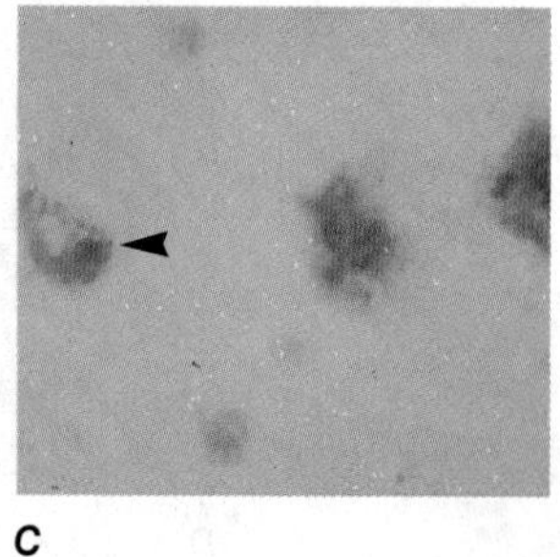

FIGURE 224-7 Thick blood films of *Plasmodium vivax*. *A.* Trophozoites. ***B.*** Schizonts. ***C.*** Gametocytes. *(Reproduced from Bench Aids for the Diagnosis of Malaria Infections, 2nd ed, with the permission of the World Health Organization.)*

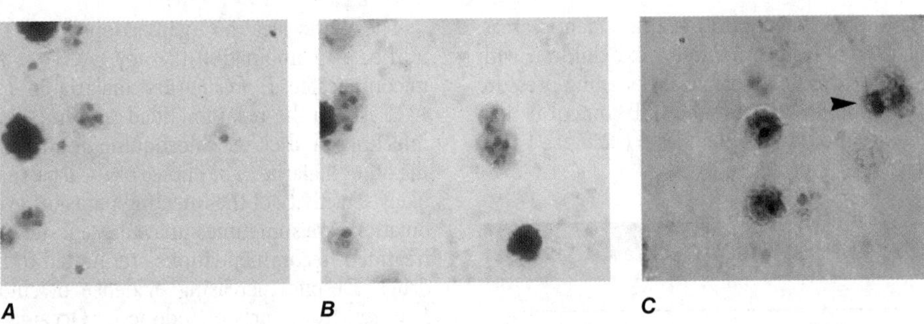

FIGURE 224-8 Thick blood films of *Plasmodium ovale*. *A*. Trophozoites. ***B*.** Schizonts. ***C*.** Gametocytes. *(Reproduced from Bench Aids for the Diagnosis of Malaria Infections, 2nd ed, with the permission of the World Health Organization.)*

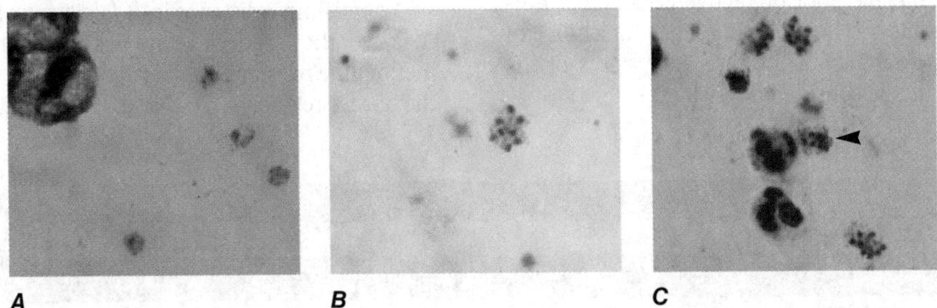

FIGURE 224-9 Thick blood films of *Plasmodium malariae*. *A*. Trophozoites. ***B*.** Schizonts. ***C*.** Gametocytes. *(Reproduced from Bench Aids for the Diagnosis of Malaria Infections, 2nd ed, with the permission of the World Health Organization.)*

TABLE 224-5 Standard Methods for the Diagnosis of Malaria[a]

METHOD	PROCEDURE	ADVANTAGES	DISADVANTAGES
Thick blood film[b]	Blood should be uneven in thickness but thin enough that the hands of a watch can be read through part of the spot. Stain dried, unfixed blood spot with Giemsa, Field's, or another Romanowsky stain. Count number of asexual parasites per 200 WBCs (or per 500 WBC at low densities). Count and report gametocytes separately.[c]	Sensitive (0.001% parasitemia); species specific; inexpensive	Requires experience (artifacts may be misinterpreted as low-level parasitemia); underestimates true count
Thin blood film[d]	Stain fixed smear with Giemsa, Field's, or another Romanowsky stain. Count number of RBCs containing asexual parasites per 1000 RBCs. In severe malaria, assess stage of parasite development and count neutrophils containing malaria pigment.[e] Count and report gametocytes separately.[c]	Rapid; species specific; inexpensive; in severe malaria, provides prognostic information[e]	Insensitive (<0.05% parasitemia); uneven distribution of *P. vivax*, as enlarged infected red cells concentrate at leading edge
PfHRP2 dipstick or card test	A drop of blood is placed on the stick or card, which is then immersed in washing solutions. Monoclonal antibody capture of parasitic antigens reads out as a colored band.	Robust and relatively inexpensive; rapid; sensitivity similar to or slightly lower than that of thick films (~0.001% parasitemia)	Detects only *Plasmodium falciparum*; remains positive for weeks after high-density infections[f]; does not quantitate *P. falciparum* parasitemia; evasion of detection by certain strains due to polymorphisms in *HRP2* gene
Plasmodium LDH dipstick or card test	A drop of blood is placed on the stick or card, which is then immersed in washing solutions. Monoclonal antibody capture of parasitic antigens reads out as two colored bands. One band is genus specific (all malarias), or *P. vivax* specific, and the other band is specific for *P. falciparum*.	Rapid; sensitivity similar to or slightly lower than that of thick films for *P. falciparum* (~0.001% parasitemia)	May miss low-level parasitemia with *P. vivax*, *P. ovale*, and *P. malariae* and may not speciate these organisms; does not quantitate *P. falciparum* parasitemia; lower sensitivity for detection of *P. knowlesi*, which may be misidentified as *P. falciparum*
Microtube concentration methods with acridine orange staining	Blood is collected in a specialized tube containing acridine orange, anticoagulant, and a float. After centrifugation, which concentrates the parasitized cells around the float, fluorescence microscopy is performed.	Sensitivity similar or superior to that of thick films (~0.001% parasitemia); ideal for processing large numbers of samples rapidly	Does not speciate or quantitate; requires fluorescence microscopy

[a]Malaria cannot be diagnosed clinically with accuracy, but treatment should be started on clinical grounds if laboratory confirmation is likely to be delayed. In areas of the world where malaria is endemic and transmission rates are high, low-level asymptomatic parasitemia is common in otherwise healthy people. Thus, malaria may not be the cause of a fever, although in this context, the presence of >10,000 parasites/μL (~0.2% parasitemia) does indicate that malaria is likely to be the cause. Antibody and polymerase chain reaction (PCR) tests have no role in the diagnosis of malaria except that PCR is increasingly used for genotyping and speciation in mixed infections and for detection of low-level parasitemia in asymptomatic residents of endemic areas. [b]Asexual parasites/200 WBCs × 40 = parasite count/μL (assumes a WBC count of 8000/μL). See Figs. 224-6 through 224-9. [c]*P. falciparum* gametocytemia may persist for days or weeks after clearance of asexual parasites. Gametocytemia without asexual parasitemia does not indicate active infection. [d]Parasitized RBCs (/1000) × hematocrit × 125.6 = parasite count/μL. See Figs. 224-4 and 224-5. [e]The presence of >100,000 parasites/μL (~2% parasitemia) is associated with an increased risk of severe malaria, but some patients have severe malaria with lower counts. At any level of parasitemia, the finding that >50% of parasites are tiny rings (cytoplasm thickness less than half of nucleus width) carries a relatively good prognosis. In a severely ill patient, the presence of visible pigment in >20% of parasites or of phagocytosed pigment in >5% of polymorphonuclear leukocytes (indicating massive recent schizogony) carries a worse prognosis. [f]Persistence of PfHRP2 is a disadvantage in high-transmission settings, where many asymptomatic people have positive tests, but can be used to diagnostic advantage in low-transmission settings when a sick patient has previously received unknown treatment (which, in endemic areas, often consists of antimalarial drugs). In this situation, a positive PfHRP2 test indicates that the illness is falciparum malaria, even if the blood smear is negative.

Abbreviations: LDH, lactate dehydrogenase; PfHRP2, *P. falciparum* histidine-rich protein 2; RBCs, red blood cells; WBCs, white blood cells.

immune and semi-immune subjects living in malaria-endemic areas. Urinalysis generally gives normal results. In adults and children with cerebral malaria, the mean cerebrospinal fluid (CSF) opening pressure at lumbar puncture is ~160 mm H_2O; usually the CSF content is normal or there is a slight elevation of total protein level (<1.0 g/L [<100 mg/dL]) and cell count (<20/μL).

TREATMENT

Malaria

Patients with severe malaria and those unable to take oral drugs should receive parenteral antimalarial therapy immediately (**Table 224-6**). Antimalarial drug susceptibility testing can be performed but is rarely available, has poor predictive value in an individual case, and yields results too slowly to influence the choice of treatment. If there is any doubt about the resistance status of the infecting organism, it should be considered resistant.

The World Health Organization (WHO) recommends artemisinin-based combination therapy (ACT) as first-line treatment for uncomplicated *P. falciparum* malaria in malaria-endemic areas. ACT is also the recommended first-line treatment for *P. knowlesi* infections, and either chloroquine or an ACT is recommended for the other malarias. The choice of ACT partner drug depends on the likely sensitivity of the infecting parasites. Artemisinin-based combinations are sometimes unavailable in temperate countries, where treatment recommendations are limited to the registered available drugs. Despite increasing evidence of chloroquine resistance in *P. vivax* (from parts of Indonesia, Oceania, eastern and southern Asia, and Central and South America), chloroquine remains an effective treatment for *P. vivax* malaria in many areas and for *P. ovale* and *P. malariae* infections everywhere.

Artemisinin resistance in *P. falciparum* has emerged in Southeast Asia over the past decade and has been followed by piperaquine and mefloquine resistance. ACTs are failing in Cambodia, Vietnam, and the border regions of Thailand. Significant artemisinin resistance is

TABLE 224-6 Regimens for the Treatment of Malaria[a]

TYPE OF DISEASE OR TREATMENT	REGIMEN(S)
Uncomplicated Malaria	
Known chloroquine-sensitive strains of *Plasmodium vivax, P. malariae, P. ovale, P. falciparum*[b]	Chloroquine (10 mg of base/kg stat followed by 5 mg/kg at 12, 24, and 36 h *or* by 10 mg/kg at 24 h and 5 mg/kg at 48 h) *or* Amodiaquine (10–12 mg of base/kg qd for 3 days)
Radical treatment for *P. vivax or P. ovale* infection (prevention of relapse)	In addition to chloroquine or amodiaquine or ACT, primaquine (0.5 mg of base/kg qd in Southeast Asia and Oceania [total dose 7 mg/kg] and 0.25 mg/kg elsewhere [total dose 3.5 mg/kg]) should be given for 14 days to prevent relapse.[c] In mild G6PD deficiency, 0.75 mg of base/kg should be given once weekly for 8 weeks. Primaquine should not be given in severe G6PD deficiency.
P. falciparum malaria[c]	Artesunate[d,e] (4 mg/kg qd for 3 days) *plus* sulfadoxine (25 mg/kg)/pyrimethamine (1.25 mg/kg) as a single dose ***or*** Artesunate[d] (4 mg/kg qd for 3 days) *plus* amodiaquine (10 mg of base/kg qd for 3 days)[d,e] *or* Artemether-lumefantrine[d] (1.5/9 mg/kg bid for 3 days with food) ***or*** Artesunate[d] (4 mg/kg qd for 3 days) *plus* mefloquine (24–25 mg of base/kg—either 8 mg/kg qd for 3 days or 15 mg/kg on day 2 and then 10 mg/kg on day 3)[f] ***or*** DHA-piperaquine[d] (target dose: 4/24 mg/kg qd for 3 days in children weighing <25 kg and 4/18 mg/kg qd for 3 days in persons weighing ≥25 kg) *or* Artesunate-pyronaridine[d] (4/12 mg/kg qd for 3 days)
Second-line treatment/treatment of imported malaria	Artesunate[e] (2 mg/kg qd for 7 days) *or* quinine (10 mg of salt/kg tid for 7 days) *plus 1 of the following 3:* 1. Tetracycline[f] (4 mg/kg qid for 7 days) 2. Doxycycline[f] (3 mg/kg qd for 7 days) 3. Clindamycin (10 mg/kg bid for 7 days) *or* Atovaquone-proguanil (20/8 mg/kg qd for 3 days with food)
Severe Falciparum Malaria[g,h]	
	Artesunate[e] (2.4 mg/kg stat IV followed by 2.4 mg/kg at 12 and 24 h and then daily if necessary; for children weighing <20 kg, give 3 mg/kg per dose) ***or, if unavailable,*** Artemether[e] (3.2 mg/kg stat IM followed by 1.6 mg/kg qd) ***or, if unavailable,*** Quinine dihydrochloride (20 mg of salt/kg[i] infused over 4 h, followed by 10 mg of salt/kg infused over 2–8 h q8h[j])

[a]In endemic areas where malaria transmission is low, except in pregnant women and infants, a single dose of primaquine (0.25 mg of base/kg) should be added as a gametocytocide to all falciparum malaria treatments to prevent transmission. This addition is considered safe, even in G6PD deficiency. [b]Very few areas now have chloroquine-sensitive *P. falciparum* malaria. [c]Recent large studies indicate that these total doses can be condensed into 7-day primaquine regimens. [d]In areas where the partner drug to artesunate is known to be effective. Fixed-dose co-formulated combinations are available. The World Health Organization recommends artemisinin combination regimens as first-line therapy for falciparum malaria in all tropical countries and advocates use of fixed-dose combinations. [e]Artemisinin derivatives are not readily available in some temperate countries. [f]Tetracycline and doxycycline should not be given to pregnant women or to children <8 years of age. [g]Oral treatment should be substituted as soon as the patient recovers sufficiently to take fluids by mouth. [h]Artesunate is the drug of choice when available. The data from large studies in Southeast Asia showed a 35% lower mortality rate than with quinine, and very large studies in Africa showed a 22.5% reduction in mortality rate compared with quinine. The doses of artesunate in children weighing <20 kg should be 3 mg/kg. [i]A loading dose should not be given if therapeutic doses of quinine have definitely been administered in the previous 24 h. [j]Infusions can be given in 0.9% saline and 5–10% dextrose in water. Infusion rates for quinine should be carefully controlled.

Abbreviations: ACT, artemisinin combination therapy; DHA, dihydroartemisinin; G6PD, glucose-6-phosphate dehydrogenase.

now prevalent throughout the Greater Mekong subregion and there is recent clear evidence for the emergence of artemisinin resistance in East Africa (Rwanda, Uganda). Falsified or substandard antimalarial drugs are sold in many Asian and African countries and may be the cause of treatment failures. Characteristics of antimalarial drugs are shown in **Table 224-7**.

SEVERE MALARIA

In large randomized controlled clinical trials, parenteral artesunate, a water-soluble artemisinin derivative, has reduced severe falciparum malaria mortality rates by 35% in Asian adults and children and by 22.5% in African children compared with quinine treatment. Artesunate therefore is now the drug of choice for all patients with severe malaria everywhere. Artesunate is given by IV injection but is also absorbed rapidly following IM injection. Artemether and the closely related drug artemotil (arteether) are oil-based formulations given by IM injection; they are erratically absorbed and do not confer the same survival benefit as artesunate. A rectal formulation of artesunate has been developed as a community-based pre-referral treatment for patients in the rural tropics who cannot take oral medications. Pre-referral administration of rectal artesunate has been shown to decrease mortality rates among severely ill children without access to immediate parenteral treatment. IV artesunate has been approved by the U.S. Food and Drug Administration for emergency use in severe malaria and can be obtained through the Centers for Disease Control and Prevention (CDC) Drug Service (see end of chapter for contact information). The antiarrhythmic quinidine gluconate was used to treat severe malaria in the United States previously, but manufacturing was discontinued in 2019; artesunate is much more effective and safer. Although parenteral quinine is steadily being replaced by parenteral artesunate in endemic areas, it still has a role in the very few cases of artemisinin-resistant severe falciparum malaria from Southeast Asia, where both artesunate and quinine are given together in full doses.

Severe falciparum malaria constitutes a medical emergency requiring intensive nursing care and careful management. Frequent evaluation of the patient's condition is essential. Adjunctive treatments such as high-dose glucocorticoids, urea, heparin, dextran, desferrioxamine, antibody to tumor necrosis factor α, high-dose phenobarbital (20 mg/kg), mannitol, or large-volume fluid or albumin boluses have proved either ineffective or harmful in clinical trials and should not be used. In acute renal failure or severe metabolic acidosis, hemofiltration or hemodialysis should be started as early as possible.

In severe malaria, parenteral antimalarial treatment should be started immediately. Artesunate, given by either IV or IM injection, is simple to administer, very safe, and rapidly effective. It does not require dose adjustments in liver dysfunction or renal failure. It should be used in pregnant women with severe malaria. If artesunate is unavailable and artemether or quinine is used, an initial loading dose must be given so that therapeutic concentrations are reached as soon as possible. Quinine causes dangerous hypotension if injected rapidly and so must be administered carefully by rate-controlled infusion only. If this approach is not possible, quinine may be given by deep IM injections into the anterior thigh. The optimal therapeutic range for quinine in severe malaria is not known with certainty, but total plasma concentrations of 8–15 mg/L for quinine are effective and do not cause serious toxicity. The systemic clearance and apparent volume of distribution of quinine are markedly reduced and plasma protein binding is increased in severe malaria, so that the blood concentrations attained with a given dose are higher. If the patient remains seriously ill or in acute renal failure for >2 days, maintenance doses of quinine should be reduced by 30–50% to prevent toxic accumulation of the drug. The initial dose should never be reduced. Convulsions should be treated promptly with IV (or rectal) benzodiazepines. The role of prophylactic anticonvulsants in children is uncertain. If respiratory support is not available, a full loading dose of phenobarbital (20 mg/kg) to prevent convulsions should *not* be given as it may cause respiratory arrest.

When the patient is unconscious, the blood glucose level should be measured every 4–6 h. All patients should receive a continuous infusion of dextrose, and blood concentrations ideally should be maintained above 4 mmol/L. Hypoglycemia (<2.2 mmol/L or 40 mg/dL) should be treated immediately with bolus glucose. The parasite count and hematocrit should be measured every 6–12 h. Anemia develops rapidly. There is uncertainty as to the thresholds for transfusion as there is some evidence that moderate anemia may be beneficial in a patient with severe malaria and vital organ dysfunction. It has been recommended that if the hematocrit falls to <20%, whole blood (preferably fresh) or packed cells should be transfused slowly, with careful attention to circulatory status. In areas with higher malaria transmission, where blood for transfusion is in short supply, a threshold of 15% is widely used. Renal function should be checked at least daily. Children presenting with very severe anemia (hemoglobin <4 g/dL) and acidotic breathing require immediate blood transfusion. Accurate assessment is vital. Management of fluid balance is difficult in severe malaria, particularly in adults, because of the thin dividing line between overhydration (leading to pulmonary edema) and underhydration (contributing to renal impairment). Fluid balance management is *different* from that in sepsis: fluid boluses are potentially dangerous in severe malaria. Nasogastric feeding should be delayed in nonintubated patients (for 60 h in adults and 36 h in children) to reduce the risk of aspiration pneumonia. As soon as the patient can take fluids, oral therapy should be substituted for parenteral treatment and a full 3-day course of ACT given. Mefloquine should be avoided as follow-on treatment for severe malaria because of the increased risk of post-malaria neurologic syndrome.

In areas of high transmission of both *P. falciparum* and *P. vivax* (the island of New Guinea), severe and potentially life-threatening anemia is common among children, and both species contribute. Elsewhere, severe vivax malaria may occur but is uncommon. Many patients have had comorbidities contributing to vital-organ dysfunction.

P. knowlesi can cause severe disease associated with high parasite densities. Acute kidney injury, respiratory distress, and shock have all been described, but cerebral malaria does not occur. Treatment for severe vivax and knowlesi malaria should follow the recommendations given for falciparum malaria.

UNCOMPLICATED MALARIA

P. falciparum and *P. knowlesi* infections should be treated with an artemisinin-based combination because of their propensity for high parasite densities and severe disease. Infections with sensitive strains of *P. vivax*, *P. malariae*, and *P. ovale* should be treated either with an ACT or oral chloroquine (total dose, 25 mg of base/kg). The ACT regimens now recommended are safe and effective in adults, children, and pregnant women. The rapidly eliminated artemisinin component is usually an artemisinin derivative (artesunate, artemether, or dihydroartemisinin) given for 3 days, and the partner drug is usually a more slowly eliminated antimalarial to which *P. falciparum* in the area is sensitive. Six ACT regimens are currently recommended by the WHO: artemether-lumefantrine, artesunate-mefloquine, dihydroartemisinin-piperaquine, artesunate-sulfadoxine-pyrimethamine, artesunate-amodiaquine, and artesunate-pyronaridine. In areas of low malaria transmission, a single dose of primaquine (0.25 mg/kg) should be added to ACT as a *P. falciparum* gametocytocide to reduce the transmissibility of the infection. This low dose of primaquine is safe even in G6PD deficiency. Pregnant women should not be given primaquine. Atovaquone-proguanil is highly effective everywhere, although it is seldom used in endemic areas because of its high cost and the propensity for rapid emergence of resistance. Recovery is slower after atovaquone-proguanil treatment than after ACT. Of great concern is the spread of artemisinin-resistant *P. falciparum* in the Greater Mekong subregion of Southeast Asia. Infections with these resistant parasites are cleared slowly from the blood, with parasite clearance half-lives over 5 hours and clearance times typically exceeding 3 days. Cure rates with ACT have fallen to unacceptably

TABLE 224-7 Properties of Antimalarial Drugs

DRUG(S)[a]	PHARMACOKINETIC PROPERTIES	ANTIMALARIAL ACTIVITY	MINOR TOXICITY	MAJOR TOXICITY
Quinine	Good oral and IM absorption (quinine); *Cl* and V_d reduced, but plasma protein binding (principally to α1 acid glycoprotein) increased (90%) in malaria; quinine $t_{1/2}$: 16 h in malaria, 11 h in healthy persons	Acts mainly on trophozoite blood stage; kills gametocytes of *P. vivax, P. ovale*, and *P. malariae* (but not *P. falciparum*); no action on liver stages	*Common:* cinchonism (tinnitus, high-tone hearing loss, nausea, vomiting, dysphoria, postural hypotension); ECG QT interval prolongation (usually by <10%). *Rare:* diarrhea, visual disturbance, rashes. *Note:* very bitter taste	*Common:* hypoglycemia. *Rare:* hypotension, blindness, deafness, cardiac arrhythmias, thrombocytopenia, hemolysis, hemolytic-uremic syndrome, vasculitis, cholestatic hepatitis, neuromuscular paralysis.
Chloroquine	Good oral absorption, very rapid IM and SC absorption; complex pharmacokinetics; enormous *Cl* and V_d (unaffected by malaria); blood concentration profile determined by distribution processes in malaria; $t_{1/2}$: 1–2 months. Active desethyl metabolite about 25% of parent drug concentrations	As for quinine, but acts slightly earlier in asexual cycle	*Common:* nausea, dysphoria, pruritus in dark-skinned patients, postural hypotension, ECG QT prolongation. *Rare:* accommodation difficulties, keratopathy, hypoglycemia, rash. *Note:* bitter taste but usually well tolerated	*Acute:* hypotensive shock (parenteral), cardiac arrhythmias, neuropsychiatric reactions. *Chronic:* retinopathy (cumulative dose, >100 g), skeletal and cardiac myopathy
Piperaquine	Adequate oral absorption, may be enhanced by fats; similar pharmacokinetics to chloroquine; $t_{1/2}$: 21–28 days	As for chloroquine; retains activity against multidrug-resistant *P. falciparum*, but resistance has emerged in Southeast Asia	Occasional epigastric pain, diarrhea, ECG QT prolongation	None identified
Amodiaquine	Good oral absorption; largely converted to active metabolite desethylamodiaquine; $t_{1/2}$: 4–5 days	As for chloroquine, but more active against chloroquine-resistant *P. falciparum*	Nausea (tastes better than chloroquine), dysphoria, headache, bradycardia, ECG QT prolongation	Agranulocytosis; hepatitis, mainly with prophylactic use; should not be used with efavirenz
Primaquine	Complete oral absorption; active metabolite produced mainly via CYP2D6; $t_{1/2}$: 5–7 h	Radical cure; eradicates hepatic forms of *P. vivax* and *P. ovale;* kills *P. falciparum* gametocytes development; kills developing liver stages of all species	Nausea, vomiting, diarrhea, abdominal pain, hemolysis, methemoglobinemia	Serious hemolytic anemia in severe G6PD deficiency; hemoglobinuria
Mefloquine	Adequate oral absorption; no parenteral preparation; $t_{1/2}$: 14–20 days (shorter in malaria)	As for quinine	Nausea, giddiness, dysphoria, fuzzy thinking, sleeplessness, nightmares, sense of dissociation	Neuropsychiatric reactions, convulsions, encephalopathy
Lumefantrine	Highly variable absorption related to fat intake; $t_{1/2}$: 3–4 days	As for quinine	None identified	None identified
Artemisinin and derivatives (artemether, artesunate)	Good oral absorption; good absorption of IM artesunate but slow and variable absorption of IM artemether; artesunate and artemether biotransformed to active metabolite dihydroartemisinin; all drugs eliminated very rapidly; $t_{1/2}$: <1 h	Broader stage specificity and more rapid than other drugs; no action on liver stages; kills all but fully mature gametocytes of *P. falciparum*	Reduction in reticulocyte count (but not anemia); neutropenia at high doses; in some cases, delayed anemia after treatment of severe malaria with hyperparasitemia	Anaphylaxis, urticaria, fever
Pyrimethamine	Good oral absorption, variable IM absorption; $t_{1/2}$: 4 days	For blood stages, acts mainly on mature forms; causal prophylactic	Well tolerated	Megaloblastic anemia, pancytopenia, pulmonary infiltration
Proguanil[b] (chloroguanide)	Good oral absorption; biotransformed to active metabolite cycloguanil; $t_{1/2}$: 16 h; biotransformation reduced by oral contraceptive use and in pregnancy	Causal prophylactic; not used alone for treatment	Well tolerated; mouth ulcers and rare alopecia	Megaloblastic anemia in renal failure
Atovaquone[b]	Highly variable absorption related to fat intake; $t_{1/2}$: 30–70 h	Acts mainly on trophozoite blood stage	None identified	None identified
Tetracycline, doxycycline[c]	Excellent absorption; $t_{1/2}$: 8 h for tetracycline, 18 h for doxycycline	Weak antimalarial activity; should not be used alone for treatment	Gastrointestinal intolerance, deposition in growing bones and teeth (tetracycline), photosensitivity, moniliasis, benign intracranial hypertension	Renal failure in patients with impaired renal function (tetracycline)
Pyronaridine	Rapid variable absorption, large V_d; $t_{1/2}$: 12–14 days	Acts mainly on trophozoite blood stage; kills gametocytes of *P. vivax, P. ovale*, and *P. malariae* (but not *P. falciparum*); no action on liver stages	Gastrointestinal intolerance, anemia, transient elevation of aminotransferases, hypoglycemia, headache	None identified
Arterolane	$t_{1/2}$: 3 h	Broad stage specificity; no action on liver stages; kills all but fully mature gametocytes of *P. falciparum*	Gastrointestinal intolerance, transient elevation of aminotransferases	None identified

[a]Several antimalarial drugs are formulated as different salts (e.g., phosphate, sulfate, hydrochloride) and are therefore prescribed as base equivalents. For example, chloroquine phosphate 250 salt contains 155 mg base equivalent. It is very important to check when prescribing that the correct dose is being given. [b]Atovaquone and proguanil are prescribed as a fixed-dose combination. This and proguanil alone should not be given if the estimated glomerular filtration rate is <30 mL/min. [c]Tetracycline and doxycycline should not be given to pregnant women or to children <8 years of age.

Abbreviations: Cl, systemic clearance; ECG, electrocardiogram; G6PD, glucose-6-phosphate dehydrogenase; V_d, total apparent volume of distribution.

low levels in some areas. Triple antimalarial combinations are under evaluation with promising results to date.

The 3-day ACT regimens are all well tolerated, although mefloquine is associated with increased rates of vomiting and dizziness. As second-line treatments for recrudescence following first-line therapy, a different ACT regimen may be given; another alternative is a 7-day course of either artesunate or quinine plus tetracycline, doxycycline, or clindamycin. Tetracycline and doxycycline are not recommended to treat pregnant women or children <8 years of age, however evidence for doxycycline toxicity in these groups is weak. Oral quinine is extremely bitter and regularly produces cinchonism comprising tinnitus, high-tone deafness, nausea, vomiting, and dysphoria. Clinical responses are slower than those following ACT. Adherence is poor with the required 7-day regimens of quinine.

Patients should be monitored for vomiting for 1 h after the administration of any oral antimalarial drug. If there is vomiting, the dose should be repeated. Symptom-based treatment, with acetaminophen (paracetamol) administration, lowers fever and thereby reduces the patient's propensity to vomit these drugs. Minor central nervous system reactions (nausea, dizziness, sleep disturbances) are common. The incidence of serious adverse neuropsychiatric reactions to mefloquine treatment is ~1 in 1000 in Asia but may be as high as 1 in 200 among Africans and white ethnic groups. All the antimalarial quinolines (chloroquine, amodiaquine, mefloquine, and quinine) exacerbate the orthostatic hypotension associated with malaria, and all are tolerated better by children than by adults. Pregnant women, young children, patients unable to tolerate oral therapy, and nonimmune individuals (e.g., travelers) with suspected malaria should be evaluated carefully and hospitalization considered. If there is any doubt as to the identity of the infecting malarial species, treatment for falciparum malaria should be given. A negative blood smear read by an experienced microscopist makes malaria very unlikely but does not rule it out completely; thick blood films should be checked again 1 and 2 days later to exclude the diagnosis. Nonimmune patients receiving treatment for malaria should have daily parasite counts performed until the thick films are negative for asexual parasite stages. If the level of parasitemia does not fall below 25% of the admission value in 72 h or if parasitemia has not cleared by 7 days (and adherence is assured), drug resistance is likely and the regimen should be changed.

To eradicate persistent liver stages and prevent relapse (radical treatment), primaquine (0.5 mg of base/kg in East Asia and Oceania and 0.25 mg/kg elsewhere) should be given once daily for 14 days to patients with *P. vivax* or *P. ovale* infection after laboratory tests for G6PD deficiency have proved negative. The same total dose may be given over 7 days. If the patient has a mild variant of G6PD deficiency, primaquine can be given in a dose of 0.75 mg of base/kg (maximum, 45 mg) once weekly for 8 weeks. Pregnant women with vivax or ovale malaria should not be given primaquine but should receive suppressive prophylaxis with chloroquine (5 mg of base/kg per week) until delivery, after which radical treatment can be given. The slowly eliminated 8-aminoquinoline tafenoquine has been registered in some countries. This allows radical cure to be given in a single dose. The consequent risk of protracted hemolysis in G6PD deficiency, including in female heterozygotes who may test as normal with current G6PD screens (which detect <30–40% of normal enzyme activity), requires that all patients should have a quantitative test of G6PD activity before receiving tafenoquine. Only those with >70% of normal activity should receive the drug. Radical curative efficacy is lower than with primaquine in Southeast Asia.

MANAGEMENT OF COMPLICATIONS

Acute Renal Failure If plasma levels of BUN or creatinine rise despite adequate rehydration, fluid administration should be restricted to prevent volume overload. As in other forms of hypercatabolic acute renal failure, renal replacement therapy is best performed early (**Chap. 310**). Hemofiltration and hemodialysis are more effective than peritoneal dialysis and are associated with lower mortality risk. Some patients with renal impairment pass small volumes of urine sufficient to allow control of fluid balance; these cases can be managed conservatively if other indications for dialysis do not arise. Renal function usually improves within days, but full recovery may take weeks.

Acute Pulmonary Edema (Acute Respiratory Distress Syndrome) This syndrome is caused by increased pulmonary capillary permeability. Patients should be positioned with the head of the bed at a 45° elevation and should be given oxygen and IV diuretics. Positive-pressure ventilation should be started early if the immediate measures fail (**Chap. 305**). Rarely, patients may require extracorporeal membrane oxygenation.

Hypoglycemia An initial slow injection of 20% dextrose (2 mL/kg over 10 min) should be followed by an infusion of 10% dextrose (0.10 g/kg per hour). The blood glucose level should be checked regularly thereafter as recurrent hypoglycemia is common, particularly among patients receiving quinine. In severely ill patients, hypoglycemia commonly occurs together with metabolic (lactic) acidosis and carries a poor prognosis.

Sepsis Hypoglycemia or gram-negative septicemia should be suspected when the condition of any patient suddenly deteriorates for no obvious reason during antimalarial treatment. In malaria-endemic areas where a high proportion of children are parasitemic, it is usually impossible to distinguish severe malaria from bacterial sepsis with confidence. These children should be treated with both antimalarials and broad-spectrum antibiotics with activity against nontyphoidal *Salmonella* species from the outset. Empirical antibiotics should also be given to adults with >20% parasitemia. Antibiotics should be considered for severely ill patients of any age who are not responding to antimalarial treatment or deteriorate unexpectedly.

Other Complications Patients who develop spontaneous bleeding should be given fresh blood and IV vitamin K. Convulsions should be treated with IV or rectal benzodiazepines and, if necessary, respiratory support. Aspiration pneumonia should be suspected in any unconscious patient with convulsions, particularly with persistent hyperventilation; IV antimicrobial agents and oxygen should be administered, and pulmonary toilet should be undertaken.

GLOBAL CONSIDERATIONS

The goal of global eradication of malaria remains a challenge. Success will require strong leadership, increased national commitment, and substantial international support. The two main tools used to control malaria are insecticide-treated bed nets (ITNs), previously shown to reduce all-cause mortality in African children by 20%, and the ACTs. New drugs are in development. One vaccine (the RTS,S/AS01 vaccine) which, in African children, provided 35–40% protection against falciparum malaria over 4 years of follow-up, has recently been recommended by WHO for widespread roll-out. Challenges to malaria eradication include the widespread distribution of *Anopheles* breeding sites, the enormous number of infected persons, the emergence and spread of resistance in *P. falciparum* to ACTs, increasing insecticide resistance and behavioral changes (to avoid ITN contact) in anopheline mosquito vectors, and inadequacies in human and material resources, infrastructure, and control programs. Newer ITNs combine pyrethroids with piperonyl butoxide, which increases mosquito susceptibility to pyrethroids by inhibiting CYP P450. Eliminating vivax malaria is further hindered by the lack of a simple, safe, radical curative regimen.

MALARIA PREVENTION

Malaria may be contained by judicious use of insecticides to kill the mosquito vector, rapid diagnosis, patient management, and—where effective and feasible—administration of intermittent preventive treatments, seasonal malaria chemoprevention, or chemoprophylaxis to high-risk groups such as pregnant women and young children. Focal elimination of *P. falciparum* can be accelerated safely by mass treatment with slowly eliminated antimalarials such as dihydroartemisinin-piperaquine. Despite the enormous investment in efforts to develop a malaria vaccine, no safe, highly effective, long-lasting vaccine is likely to be available for general use in the near future. The licensed recombinant protein sporozoite-targeted adjuvanted vaccine RTS,S/AS01 was only moderately efficacious in protecting African children from malaria in field trials, and protection wanes rapidly. The vaccine is being deployed in Ghana, Kenya, and Malawi as part of a large-scale pilot project and has just been approved by WHO for general deployment. An irradiated live sporozoite vaccine is in late-stage development, and research is ongoing to develop a vaccine to protect against placental malaria (targeting VAR2CSA). While there is great promise for one or several malaria vaccines on the more distant horizon, prevention and control measures will continue to rely on antivector and drug-use strategies for the foreseeable future.

PERSONAL PROTECTION AGAINST MALARIA

Simple measures to reduce the frequency of bites by infected mosquitoes in malarious areas are very important. These measures include the avoidance of exposure to mosquitoes at their peak feeding times (usually dusk to dawn) and the use of insect repellents containing 10–35% DEET (or, if DEET is unacceptable, 7% picaridin), suitable clothing, and ITNs or other insecticide-impregnated materials. Widespread use of bed nets treated with residual pyrethroids reduces the incidence of malaria in areas where vectors bite indoors at night.

CHEMOPROPHYLAXIS

(**Table 224-8**; *https://wwwnc.cdc.gov/travel/yellowbook/2020/travel-related-infectious-diseases/malaria*) Recommendations for malaria prophylaxis depend on knowledge of local patterns of drug sensitivity in

TABLE 224-8 Drugs Used in the Prophylaxis of Malaria[a]

DRUG	USAGE	ADULT DOSE	PEDIATRIC DOSE	COMMENTS
Atovaquone-proguanil (Malarone)	Prophylaxis in areas with chloroquine- or mefloquine-resistant *Plasmodium falciparum*	1 adult tablet PO[b]	5–8 kg: ½ pediatric tablet[c] daily ≥8–10 kg: ¾ pediatric tablet daily ≥10–20 kg: 1 pediatric tablet daily ≥20–30 kg: 2 pediatric tablets daily ≥30–40 kg: 3 pediatric tablets daily ≥40 kg: 1 adult tablet daily	Begin 1–2 days before travel to malarious areas. Take daily at the same time each day while in the malarious areas and for 7 days after leaving such areas. Atovaquone-proguanil is contraindicated in persons with severe renal impairment (creatinine clearance rate, <30 mL/min). In the absence of data, it is not recommended for children weighing <5 kg, pregnant women, or women breast-feeding infants weighing <5 kg. Atovaquone-proguanil should be taken with food or a milky drink.
Chloroquine phosphate (Aralen and generic)	Prophylaxis only in the very few areas with chloroquine-sensitive *P. falciparum*[c] or areas with *P. vivax* only	300 mg of base (500 mg of salt) PO once weekly	5 mg of base/kg (8.3 mg of salt/kg) PO once weekly, up to maximum adult dose of 300 mg of base	Begin 1–2 weeks before travel to malarious areas. Take weekly on the same day of the week while in the malarious areas and for 4 weeks after leaving such areas. Chloroquine may exacerbate psoriasis.
Doxycycline (many brand names and generic)	Prophylaxis in areas with chloroquine- or mefloquine-resistant *P. falciparum*[d]	100 mg PO qd (except in pregnant women; see Comments)	≥8 years of age: 2 mg/kg PO qd, up to adult dose	Begin 1–2 days before travel to malarious areas. Take daily at the same time each day while in the malarious areas and for 4 weeks after leaving such areas. Doxycycline is contraindicated in children aged <8 years and in pregnant women.
Hydroxychloroquine sulfate (Plaquenil)	An alternative to chloroquine for primary prophylaxis only in the very few areas with chloroquine-sensitive *P. falciparum*[d] or areas with *P. vivax* only	310 mg of base (400 mg of salt) PO once weekly	5 mg of base/kg (6.5 mg of salt/kg) PO once weekly, up to maximum adult dose of 310 mg of base	Begin 1–2 weeks before travel to malarious areas. Take weekly on the same day of the week while in the malarious areas and for 4 weeks after leaving such areas. Hydroxychloroquine may exacerbate psoriasis.
Mefloquine (Lariam and generic)	Prophylaxis in areas with chloroquine-resistant *P. falciparum*[d]	228 mg of base (250 mg of salt) PO once weekly	≤9 kg: 4.6 mg of base/kg (5 mg of salt/kg) PO once weekly 10–19 kg: ¼ tablet[e] once weekly 20–30 kg: ½ tablet once weekly 31–45 kg: ¾ tablet once weekly ≥46 kg: 1 tablet once weekly	Begin 1–2 weeks before travel to malarious areas. Take weekly on the same day of the week while in the malarious areas and for 4 weeks after leaving such areas. Mefloquine is contraindicated in persons allergic to this drug or related compounds (e.g., quinine and quinidine) and in persons with active or recent depression, generalized anxiety disorder, psychosis, schizophrenia, other major psychiatric disorders, or seizures. Use with caution in persons with psychiatric disturbances or a history of depression. Mefloquine is not recommended for persons with cardiac conduction abnormalities.
Primaquine	For prevention of malaria in areas with mainly *P. vivax*	30 mg of base (52.6 mg of salt) PO qd	0.5 mg of base/kg (0.8 mg of salt/kg) PO qd, up to adult dose; should be taken with food	Begin 1–2 days before travel to malarious areas. Take daily at the same time each day while in the malarious areas and for 7 days after leaving such areas. Primaquine is contraindicated in persons with G6PD deficiency. It is also contraindicated during pregnancy.
Primaquine	Used for presumptive antirelapse therapy (terminal prophylaxis) to decrease risk of relapses of *P. vivax* and *P. ovale*	30 mg of base (52.6 mg of salt) PO qd for 14 days after departure from the malarious area	0.5 mg of base/kg (0.8 mg of salt/kg), up to adult dose, PO qd for 14 days after departure from the malarious area	This therapy is indicated for persons who have had prolonged exposure to *P. vivax* and/or *P. ovale*. It is contraindicated in persons with G6PD deficiency as well as during pregnancy.

[a]Several antimalarial drugs are formulated as different salts (e.g., phosphate, sulfate, hydrochloride) and are therefore prescribed as base equivalents. For example, chloroquine phosphate 250 salt contains 155 mg base equivalent. It is very important to check when prescribing that the correct dose is being given. [b]An adult tablet contains 250 mg of atovaquone and 100 mg of proguanil hydrochloride. [c]A pediatric tablet contains 62.5 mg of atovaquone and 25 mg of proguanil hydrochloride. [d]Very few areas now have chloroquine-sensitive falciparum malaria. [e]One tablet contains 228 mg of base (250 mg of salt).

Abbreviation: G6PD, glucose-6-phosphate dehydrogenase.

Source: Centers for Disease Control and Prevention, *https://www.cdc.gov/malaria/travelers/index.html.*

Plasmodium species and the likelihood of acquiring malarial infection. Drugs effective against resistant *P. falciparum* should be used (atovaquone-proguanil [Malarone], doxycycline, or mefloquine). Chemoprophylaxis is never entirely reliable, and malaria should always be considered in the differential diagnosis of fever in patients who have traveled to endemic areas, even if they are taking prophylactic antimalarial drugs.

Pregnant women planning to visit malarious areas should be warned about the potential risks and advised to avoid all nonessential travel. All pregnant women who live in endemic areas should be encouraged to attend regular antenatal clinics. Mefloquine is the only drug advised for pregnant women traveling to areas with drug-resistant malaria; this drug is generally considered safe in the second and third trimesters of pregnancy; the data on first-trimester exposure, although limited, are reassuring. Chloroquine and proguanil are regarded as safe, but there are now very few regions where these drugs can be recommended for protection. The safety of other prophylactic antimalarial agents in pregnancy has not been established. Antimalarial prophylaxis has been shown to reduce mortality rates among children between the ages of 3 months and 4 years in malaria-endemic areas; however, it is not a logistically or economically feasible option in many countries. The alternative—to give intermittent preventive treatment (IPT) to pregnant women, and in some areas to infants as well, or seasonal malaria chemoprevention (SMC) to young children—is being implemented. Other strategies are being evaluated, such as intermittent screening and treatment.

IPT in pregnancy (IPTp) involves giving treatment doses of sulfadoxine-pyrimethamine at each antenatal visit (maximum, once monthly) in the second and third trimesters of pregnancy. Women with HIV infection who are taking trimethoprim-sulfamethoxazole as prophylaxis should not be given concomitant sulfadoxine-pyrimethamine. Dihydroartemisinin-piperaquine is being evaluated as an alternative. IPT in infancy (IPTi) involves giving treatment doses of sulfadoxine-pyrimethamine along with the immunizations included in the WHO's Expanded Program on Immunization at 2, 3, and 9 months of life. Seasonal malaria chemoprevention involves giving monthly treatment doses of amodiaquine and sulfadoxine-pyrimethamine to children aged between 3 and 59 months during the 3- to 4-month rainy season across the Sahel region of Africa. Children born to nonimmune mothers in malaria-endemic areas (usually expatriates moving to these areas) should receive prophylaxis from birth.

Travelers to a malaria endemic region should start taking antimalarial drugs 2 days to 2 weeks before departure so that any untoward reactions can be detected before travel and so that therapeutic antimalarial blood concentrations will be present if and when any infections develop (Table 224-8). Antimalarial prophylaxis should continue for 4 weeks after the traveler has left the endemic area, except if atovaquone-proguanil or primaquine has been taken; these drugs have significant activities against the liver stage of the infection (causal prophylaxis) and can be discontinued 1 week after departure from the endemic area. If suspected malaria develops while a traveler is abroad, obtaining a reliable diagnosis and antimalarial treatment locally is a top priority. Presumptive self-treatment for malaria with atovaquone-proguanil (for 3 consecutive days) or one of the artemisinin-based combinations can be considered under special circumstances; medical advice on self-treatment should be sought before departure for malaria-endemic areas and as soon as possible after illness begins. Every effort should be made to confirm the diagnosis.

Atovaquone-proguanil (Malarone; 3.75/1.5 mg/kg or 250/100 mg, daily adult dose) is a fixed-combination, once-daily prophylactic agent that is very well tolerated by adults and children. This combination is effective against all types of malaria, including multidrug-resistant falciparum malaria. Atovaquone-proguanil is best taken with food or a milky drink to optimize absorption. It is not recommended if the estimated glomerular filtration rate is <30 mL/min. There are insufficient data on safety in pregnancy.

Mefloquine (250 mg of salt weekly, adult dose) has been widely used for malarial prophylaxis because it is usually effective against multidrug-resistant falciparum malaria and is reasonably well tolerated. Mefloquine has been associated with rare episodes of psychosis and seizures at prophylactic doses; these reactions are more frequent at the higher doses used for treatment. More common side effects with prophylactic doses of mefloquine include mild nausea, dizziness, fuzzy thinking, disturbed sleep patterns, vivid dreams, dysphoria, and malaise. Mefloquine is contraindicated for use by travelers with known hypersensitivity and by persons with active or recent depression, anxiety disorder, psychosis, schizophrenia, another major psychiatric disorder, or seizures; it is not recommended for persons with cardiac conduction abnormalities, although the evidence that it is cardiotoxic is very weak. Confidence is increasing with regard to the safety of mefloquine prophylaxis during pregnancy; in studies in Africa, mefloquine prophylaxis was found to be effective and safe during pregnancy. Daily administration of doxycycline (100 mg daily, adult dose) is an effective alternative to atovaquone-proguanil or mefloquine. Doxycycline is generally well tolerated but may cause vulvovaginal thrush, diarrhea, and photosensitivity and is not recommended for prophylaxis in children <8 years old or pregnant women, although, evidence that it is harmful is lacking.

Chloroquine can no longer be relied upon to prevent *P. falciparum* infections in nearly all endemic areas but is still used to prevent and treat malaria due to the other human *Plasmodium* species and for *P. falciparum* malaria in Central American countries west and north of the Panama Canal and in Caribbean countries. Chloroquine-resistant *P. vivax* has been reported from parts of eastern Asia, Oceania, and Central and South America. High-level resistance in *P. vivax* is prevalent in Oceania and Indonesia. Chloroquine is generally well tolerated, although some patients cannot take it because of malaise, headache, visual symptoms (due to reversible keratopathy), gastrointestinal intolerance, alopecia, or pruritus. Chloroquine is considered safe in pregnancy. With chronic administration for >5 years, a characteristic dose-related retinopathy may develop, but this condition is rare at the doses used for antimalarial prophylaxis. Idiosyncratic or allergic reactions are also rare. Skeletal and/or cardiac myopathy is a potential problem with protracted prophylactic use, although it is more likely to occur at the high doses used in the treatment of rheumatoid arthritis. Neuropsychiatric reactions and skin rashes are unusual. Amodiaquine should not be used for weekly prophylaxis because continuous weekly use is associated with a high risk of agranulocytosis (~1 person in 2000) and hepatotoxicity (~1 person in 16,000). Chloroquine, amodiaquine, and piperaquine all cause moderate electrocardiograph QT prolongation but have not been associated with ventricular arrhythmias at therapeutic doses.

Primaquine (0.5 mg of base/kg or a daily adult dose of 30 mg taken with food), an 8-aminoquinoline compound, has proved safe and effective in the prevention of drug-resistant falciparum and vivax malaria in adults. Primaquine can be considered for adults (with the exception of pregnant women) who are intolerant to other recommended drugs. Abdominal pain can be prevented by taking primaquine with food. G6PD deficiency must be excluded before primaquine is prescribed. In the past, the dihydrofolate reductase inhibitors pyrimethamine and proguanil (chloroguanide) were administered widely, but the rapid selection of resistance in both *P. falciparum* and *P. vivax* has limited their use. Whereas antimalarial quinolines such as chloroquine (a 4-aminoquinoline) act only on the erythrocyte stage of parasitic development, the dihydrofolate reductase inhibitors (as well as atovaquone and primaquine) also inhibit preerythrocytic growth in the liver (causal prophylaxis) and development in the mosquito (sporontocidal activity). Proguanil is safe and well tolerated, although mouth ulceration occurs in ~8% of persons using this drug; it is considered safe for antimalarial prophylaxis in pregnancy. Prophylactic use of the combination of pyrimethamine and sulfadoxine is not recommended for weekly administration because of an unacceptable incidence of severe toxicity, principally exfoliative dermatitis and other skin rashes, agranulocytosis, hepatitis, and pulmonary eosinophilia (incidence, 1 in 7000; fatal reactions, 1 in 18,000).

Because of the increasing spread and intensity of antimalarial drug resistance (**Fig. 224-10**), the CDC recommends that travelers and

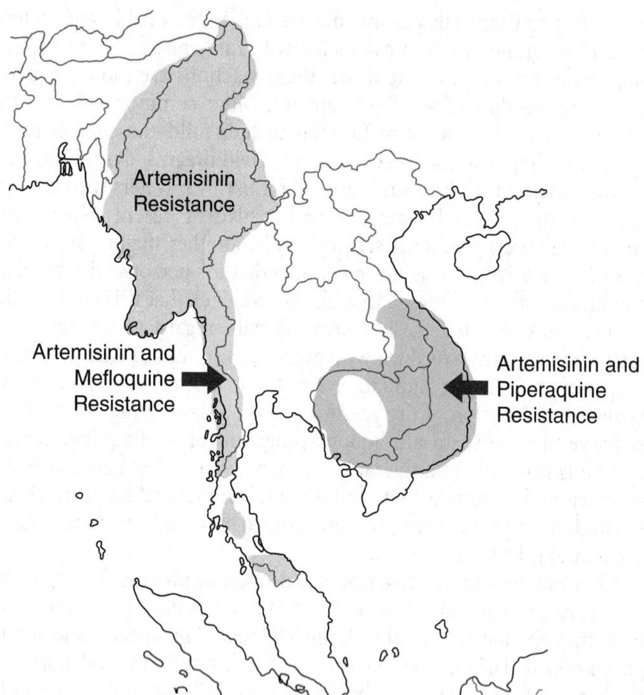

FIGURE 224-10 Current geographic extent of artemisinin resistance and artemisinin-based combination therapy partner drug resistance in *Plasmodium falciparum* in the Greater Mekong subregion.

their providers consider their destination, type of travel, and current medications and health risks when choosing antimalarial chemoprophylaxis. There is an increasingly appreciated problem of falsified and substandard antimalarial drugs (and other medicines) on the shelves of pharmacies in Southeast Asia and sub-Saharan Africa; hence, travelers should purchase their preventive drugs from a reputable source before going to a malarious country. Consultation for the evaluation of prophylaxis failures or treatment of malaria can be obtained from state and local health departments and the CDC Malaria Hotline (770-488-7788) or the CDC Emergency Operations Center (770-488-7100).

Acknowledgment

The authors gratefully acknowledge the substantial contributions of Joel G. Breman to this chapter in previous editions.

FURTHER READING

Dondorp AM et al: Artesunate versus quinine in the treatment of severe falciparum malaria in African children (AQUAMAT): An open-label, randomised trial. Lancet 376:1647, 2010.

Van Der Pluijm RW et al: Triple artemisinin-based combination therapies versus artemisinin-based combination therapies for uncomplicated *Plasmodium falciparum* malaria: A multicentre, open-label, randomised clinical trial. Lancet 395:1345, 2020. Erratum in: Lancet 395:1344, 2020.

World Health Organization: *Guidelines for the Treatment of Malaria*, 3rd ed. Geneva, World Health Organization, 2015. Available at *apps.who.int/iris/bitstream/10665/162441/1/9789241549127_eng.pdf.* Accessed December 8, 2017.

World Health Organization: Severe malaria. Trop Med Int Health 19(S1):i–vii, 2014. Available at *dx.doi.org/10.1111/tmi.12313_1.* Accessed December 8, 2017.

225 Babesiosis

Edouard Vannier, Jeffrey A. Gelfand

Babesiosis is an emerging infectious disease caused by protozoan parasites of the genus *Babesia* that invade and eventually lyse red blood cells (RBCs). Most cases occur in the United States during the summer months and are caused by *Babesia microti*, a species typically found in small rodents and transmitted by the deer tick, *Ixodes scapularis*. Symptoms are those of a flu-like illness. A single standard course of atovaquone plus azithromycin often is sufficient to achieve cure. Highly immunocompromised patients are at risk of persistent infection and antibiotic resistance and should be treated for a longer duration than immunocompetent patients. Adjunct exchange transfusion can be useful for severe cases. In the absence of vaccine and prophylaxis, persons at risk of severe babesiosis should minimize their exposure to ticks and, if possible, avoid endemic areas.

ETIOLOGY, EPIDEMIOLOGY, AND MODES OF TRANSMISSION

A few *Babesia* species have been implicated as etiologic agents of human babesiosis. These species use wild or domesticated mammals as reservoir hosts and are maintained in their enzootic cycle by ticks. Humans are incidental, dead-end hosts. Most cases of human babesiosis are reported from across the Northern Hemisphere, but the predominant etiologic agent varies by continent.

United States • Geographic Distribution *B. microti* is the etiologic agent of nearly all cases in the United States. Most cases (~95%) are reported from the Northeast and the upper Midwest, particularly from seven states: Massachusetts, Rhode Island, Connecticut, New York, New Jersey, Minnesota, and Wisconsin (**Fig. 225-1**). Aside from *B. microti*, other *Babesia* species seldom cause disease in the United States. Symptomatic infection with *Babesia duncani* and *B. duncani*–type organisms has been reported from Washington State, Oregon and California. Symptomatic infection with *Babesia divergens*–like organisms has been documented in Washington State but also in the central states of Arkansas, Missouri, Michigan, and Kentucky.

Incidence Babesiosis has been a nationally notifiable disease since January 2011. Cases are reported weekly by state health departments to the Centers for Disease Control and Prevention (CDC) via the National Notifiable Diseases Surveillance System. In 2018, a total of 2161 cases were reported from 28 of the 40 states in which babesiosis was notifiable. In 2008, when reporting to the CDC was yet to be instituted, 624 cases were made known to health departments in the seven highly endemic states; a decade earlier, this number was 230. The increase in incidence over time is best explained by a greater density of ticks in highly endemic areas as well as the steady expansion of the geographic range occupied by these ticks. Although *B. microti* and *Borrelia burgdorferi* (the agent of Lyme disease; **Chap. 186**) are maintained in their enzootic life cycle by the deer tick *I. scapularis*, the geographic expansion of babesiosis has lagged behind that of Lyme disease. This delay in geographic expansion likely reflects the poor ecologic fitness of *B. microti* compared with that of *B. burgdorferi* and is consistent with the observation that *B. burgdorferi* helps maintain *B. microti* in its enzootic cycle. Other factors contributing to the rise in incidence include greater exposure of residents to ticks due to forest fragmentation in suburban areas and more time spent in leisure activities in grassy or wooded areas. The seroprevalence of antibodies specific for *B. microti* has been as high as 9% among residents of highly endemic states, particularly in areas with the highest incidence of disease. Similar rates have been noted among blood donors in these highly endemic states, indicating that babesiosis is underreported and/or that asymptomatic infection is more common than is recognized.

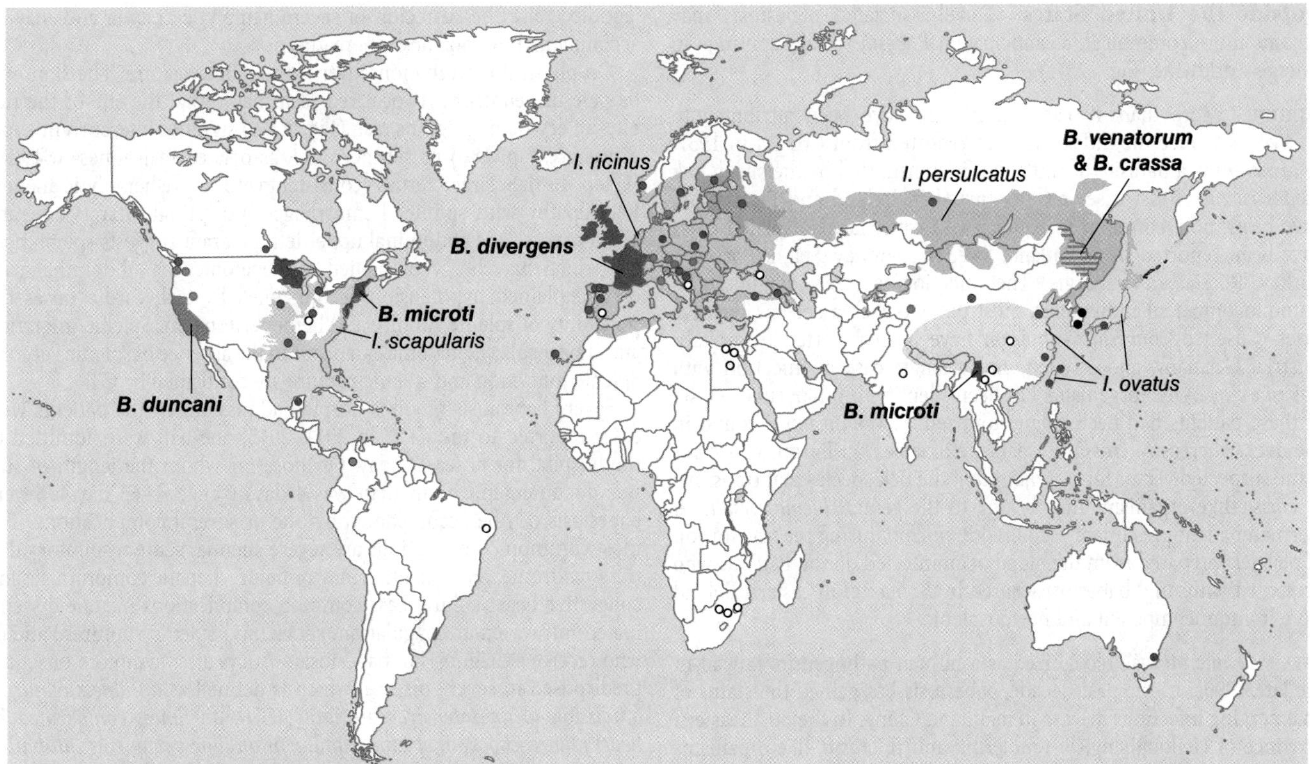

FIGURE 225-1 Geographic distribution of human babesiosis and associated tick vectors. Dark colors indicate areas where human babesiosis is endemic or sporadic (defined by ≥5 cases). Light colors indicate areas where tick vectors are present but human babesiosis is rare (<5 cases), undocumented, or absent. *Circles* depict single cases except in six locations (Colombia, Mexico, Montenegro, Poland, and the provinces of Gansu and Shandong in China) where all patients were diagnosed at one hospital or identified via survey in one location. Colors distinguish the etiologic agents: *red* for *Babesia microti, orange* for *B. duncani, blue* for *B. divergens, green* for *B. venatorum, pink* for *B. crassa, brown* for *B. bovis* and *B. bigemina, black* for *B. motasi*, and *yellow* for *Babesia* spp. XXB/Hang-Zhou. *White circles* depict cases caused by uncharacterized *Babesia* species. Asymptomatic infections and cases of travel-associated babesiosis are omitted.

Modes of Transmission • TICK BITE *B. microti* is acquired primarily during the blood meal of an *I. scapularis* tick. Only one-half (~45%) of patients recall a tick bite within the 8 weeks prior to symptom onset. Both nymphs and adult ticks can transmit *B. microti*; tick larvae are not infected because *B. microti* is not transmitted transovarially. Three-fourths of cases present from June through August because nymphs—the primary vector—are active from late spring to early summer. Patients who present in late summer or early fall have likely acquired *B. microti* from an adult female tick. *B. duncani* and *B. divergens*–like organisms are thought to be transmitted by *Dermacentor albipictus* and *Ixodes dentatus* ticks, respectively.

BLOOD TRANSFUSION More than 300 cases of transfusion-transmitted babesiosis due to *B. microti* have been reported. Most cases result from the transfusion of packed RBCs; a few have been caused by whole blood–derived platelets contaminated with RBCs. At the time of transfusion, the age of the refrigerated RBC units has been 4–42 days, a range indicating that *B. microti* remains viable throughout the RBC unit's shelf life. Transfusion-transmitted babesiosis occurs year-round because *B. microti* infection can persist for more than a year in untreated asymptomatic carriers. Given the seasonality of tick-borne babesiosis, three-quarters of cases of transfusion-transmitted babesiosis are diagnosed from June through November. Like that of tick-borne babesiosis, the incidence of transfusion-transmitted babesiosis has sharply risen in the past 15 years. Most cases (>85%) occur in residents of highly endemic areas, but transfusion-transmitted babesiosis does occur in nonendemic areas when contaminated blood products are imported from endemic areas or when asymptomatic *B. microti* carriers donate blood in nonendemic areas. *B. microti* is the pathogen most often identified by investigations of transfusion-transmitted illnesses. From 2010 to 2016, *B. microti* accounted for one-fourth of transfusion-related deaths caused by microbial infection. *B. duncani* has been implicated in three cases of transfusion-transmitted babesiosis; none ended in death. A fatal case of *B. divergens*–like infection in Arkansas is suspected to have been caused by packed RBC units imported from Missouri.

VERTICAL TRANSMISSION Passage of *B. microti* across the placenta has been documented but is rare. Most cases of neonatal babesiosis are acquired through blood transfusion or tick bite. Infants (<1 year of age) account for <1% of the annual number of cases of babesiosis reported to the CDC.

SOLID ORGAN TRANSPLANTATION This unusual mode of transmission has been highlighted in a single case report. Two patients received a diagnosis of babesiosis 8 weeks after transplantation of a kidney allograft obtained from a single donor who had received multiple transfusions shortly before his death. Corneas from the deceased donor were transplanted, but neither recipient was infected with *B. microti*; this outcome suggests that RBCs that had remained in the vasculature or fluids of the donated kidneys were the source of *B. microti*.

Risk Factors Most individuals (~80%) who present with symptoms of babesiosis are ≥50 years of age. Patients who are admitted to a hospital (median age, 68 years) are a decade older than those who are not (median age, 59 years). Although age >75 years is a risk factor for hospital admission, it is not a risk factor for severe babesiosis. Major risk factors for severe babesiosis include asplenia and immunosuppression. Asplenia can be congenital, functional (e.g., due to celiac disease or hemoglobinopathies such as sickle cell disease and thalassemia), or acquired (due to splenectomy). Immunosuppression often is iatrogenic and associated with conditions such as autoimmune disorders, chronic inflammatory disorders, malignancies, or transplantation. Immunosuppression can be inherent in comorbidities such as X-linked agammaglobulinemia, common variable hypogammaglobulinemia, and HIV/AIDS. Risk factors for transfusion-transmitted babesiosis include conditions that require blood transfusion, such as hematologic disorders, anemia of prematurity, bleeding during surgery, gastrointestinal disease, and cardiovascular surgery or another cardiovascular procedure.

Outside the United States Travel-associated babesiosis may become more common if, as anticipated, *Babesia* species continue to emerge worldwide (Fig. 225-1).

EUROPE More than 40 cases in Europe have been attributed to *B. divergens* since the index case was reported from Croatia in 1957. *B. divergens* is a parasite of cattle that is transmitted by the sheep tick *Ixodes ricinus*. Most cases have occurred in Ireland and France and have been more common in regions with cattle farms. Isolated cases have been reported from Finland, Sweden, Norway, Spain, Portugal, Turkey, Russia, and Georgia. The infection is rarely diagnosed in immunocompetent individuals; most patients lack a spleen. The five cases caused by *Babesia venatorum* have been reported from Italy, Austria, Germany, and Sweden, and a single case of infection with *Babesia crassa*–like organisms has been identified in Slovenia. All six of these patients had been splenectomized. *B. venatorum* is found in roe deer, whereas *B. crassa* is a parasite of sheep. In Europe, *I. ricinus* is the suspected vector for *B. venatorum*; the tick species that transmits *B. crassa*–like organisms may belong to the genus *Haemaphysalis*. A German patient presumably acquired *B. microti* during the transfusion of platelets prepared from the blood of an infected donor. Patients who presented with mild babesiosis caused by *B. microti* in eastern Poland were immunocompetent and normosplenic.

ASIA *B. microti* was recognized as a human pathogen in Taiwan in the late 1990s. In the past decade, babesiosis has gained the status of an emerging infectious disease in mainland China. In the northeastern province of Heilongjiang, *B. venatorum* and *B. crassa*–like organisms have caused mild disease in immunocompetent individuals, whereas antibodies specific for *B. microti* have been detected in blood donors. The taiga tick *Ixodes persulcatus* is a competent vector for *B. microti* and the presumed vector for *B. venatorum*. In this province, *B. crassa*–like organisms are found in *I. persulcatus* and *Haemaphysalis concinna* ticks. Isolated cases due to *B. divergens* have been reported from the eastern coastal province of Shandong and the north-central province of Gansu. A case of *B. venatorum* infection was documented in the northwestern Xinjiang Autonomous Region. Several cases of *B. microti* infection have been reported from the southwestern province of Yunnan; two of the patients involved were co-infected with *Plasmodium* species.

The single case of babesiosis in Japan was acquired through blood transfusion and was caused by a *B. microti* organism that defines the Kobe lineage. Two cases have been reported from South Korea; both occurred in splenectomized individuals and were caused by *Babesia motasi*–like organisms, which are parasites of sheep and goats. In one case, *Haemaphysalis longicornis* was the presumed vector.

REMAINDER OF THE WORLD One case of *B. microti* infection has been reported in New South Wales, Australia, and another in Manitoba, Canada, but serosurveys indicate that babesiosis is not endemic in these regions. Three cases of *B. microti* infection have occurred in the state of Yucatan in Mexico. Definitive evidence that *Babesia bovis* and *Babesia bigemina* can cause human illness has come from Uraba, a region of Colombia where cattle ranching is important and malaria is endemic. In Mozambique, *B. bovis* is presumed to have caused disease and occasionally death. In South Africa, two patients were diagnosed with babesiosis after visiting malaria-endemic areas in Namibia and Zimbabwe.

CLINICAL MANIFESTATIONS

United States • *B. MICROTI* INFECTION Symptoms typically appear 1–4 weeks after the bite of an infected tick but appear later—at 3–7 weeks (median, 37 days; range, 11–176 days)—after transfusion of contaminated blood products. Patients experience a gradual onset of fatigue and/or malaise that is followed within days by fever and one or more of the following: chills, sweats, headache, and myalgia. Fever is persistent or intermittent and has reached 40.9°C (105.6°F). Less common symptoms include anorexia, arthralgia, nausea, dry cough, neck stiffness, sore throat, emotional lability, and vomiting. Diarrhea, crampy abdominal pain, and joint swelling are rare. Dark urine and jaundice raise the suspicion of severe hemolytic anemia and may be accompanied by shortness of breath.

On physical examination, fever is the salient feature. The skin may be pale or yellowish. A focal red rash may reveal the site of the tick bite; an erythema migrans rash (**Fig. A1-8**) signifies intercurrent Lyme disease (**Chap. 186**) or southern tick-associated rash illness (STARI) (**Chap. 186**). Scleral icterus is consistent with severe hemolytic anemia. Retinopathy with splinter hemorrhages and retinal infarcts are rare. Tenderness of the abdominal upper left quadrant suggests splenomegaly, which may be accompanied by hepatomegaly. Abdominal pain or unexplained hypotension accompanied by tachycardia raises the possibility of splenic rupture and hemoperitoneum. Splenic infarction and subcapsular hematoma can occur in the absence of splenic rupture. Splenic infarction and splenic rupture are confirmed by CT.

Severe babesiosis requires hospital admission. Of the patients with cases reported to the CDC in 2011–2015, one-half were admitted to the hospital for at least 1 day. Of those for whom the length of stay was documented, the median was 4 days (range, 1–63 days). Severe babesiosis can be accompanied by one or several complications. The most common complications are severe anemia, acute respiratory distress syndrome, renal insufficiency or failure, hepatic compromise, and congestive heart failure. Less common complications include disseminated intravascular coagulation, shock, and splenic rupture. Patients who receive a diagnosis of babesiosis >7 days after symptom onset are predisposed to severe disease, which is defined as *an illness requiring admission to an intensive care unit (ICU); an illness complicated by heart failure, shock, or splenic rupture; or an illness requiring intubation or RBC exchange transfusion*. Among clinical features, diarrhea and nausea or vomiting are strong predictors of severe babesiosis as just defined. Asplenia and autoimmune disorders predispose to severe disease, but underlying cardiac conditions do not. Intercurrent Lyme disease does not increase the risk of severe disease but rather decreases the number and duration of symptoms evoked by babesiosis; the implication is that babesiosis may be overlooked if it is accompanied by intercurrent Lyme disease.

Despite therapy, babesiosis can be fatal. A review of 10,305 Medicare recipients who received a diagnosis of babesiosis between 2006 and 2013 revealed that 1% died within 30 days. Among inpatients, the fatality rate was 3%. Of the 7612 cases of babesiosis reported to the CDC in 2011–2015, 46 (0.6%) were fatal. Death rates are particularly high among immunocompromised patients (~20%) but are also elevated among patients who acquire *B. microti* through blood transfusion. In a series of 159 transfusion-transmitted cases reported from 1979 through 2009, the fatality rate was 17%. In a series of 77 cases identified by the American Red Cross Hemoviligance Program from 2010 through 2017, the fatality rate was 5%.

OTHER *BABESIA* INFECTIONS The eight documented cases of *B. duncani* infection reported in the United States were moderate to severe; one patient died. Symptoms were similar to those evoked by *B. microti*. All six patients infected with *B. divergens*–like organisms had severe illness and required hospitalization; three died.

Global Considerations Most cases of *B. divergens* infection in Europe have occurred in splenectomized individuals and have been severe. Symptoms develop suddenly and consist of fever (>41°C [>105.8°F]), shaking chills, drenching sweats, headache, myalgia, and lumbar and abdominal pain. Jaundice and hemoglobinuria are common. Without immediate therapy, patients often develop pulmonary edema and renal failure. All five patients infected with *B. venatorum* in Europe had been splenectomized; their illness ranged from mild to severe, and none died. The 32 cases of *B. venatorum* infection reported from northeastern China occurred in spleen-intact residents. The symptoms were similar to those evoked by *B. microti*, although chills were rare. Seven of the 32 patients were hospitalized for irregular fever (as high as 40°C). Only four patients were treated with clindamycin (without quinine), but all 32 patients recovered. Cases of *B. crassa*–like infection reported from northeastern China also occurred in spleen-intact residents. Fever, fatigue, and myalgia were less common than among patients infected with *B. microti*, but headache was as common and nausea or vomiting more common. No patient was admitted to the hospital. Only 3 of 31 patients were given clindamycin (without quinine), but in most cases, symptoms resolved. Cases of *B. motasi*–like infection in South Korea were severe; one patient died but the other recovered following clindamycin monotherapy.

PATHOGENESIS

Anemia Hemolytic anemia generates cell debris that may accumulate in the kidney and cause renal failure. Hemoglobin forms a complex with haptoglobin, but minute amounts of free hemoglobin are sufficient to promote systemic inflammation. Exposed to oxidative stress, RBCs are poorly deformable and filtered out by splenic macrophages as they attempt to pass through the red pulp. Erythrophagocytosis contributes to splenomegaly and splenic rupture and has led to hemophagocytic lymphohistiocytosis, a fatal condition. Anemia also results from erythropoiesis suppression by inflammatory cytokines such as interferon γ (IFN-γ) and interleukin (IL) 6. Persistent anemia, despite resolution of infection, has been attributed to autoantibodies that tag RBCs for clearance and may activate the complement system.

Inflammation The spleen not only clears parasitized RBCs but also provides protective immunity; thus, asplenia is a major risk factor for severe babesiosis. Protective immunity involves $CD4^+$ T cells, particularly Th1 cells, as revealed by high-grade persistent parasitemia in mice that are depleted of $CD4^+$ T cells or treated with an IFN-γ-neutralizing antibody. The importance of $CD4^+$ T cells is corroborated by the severity of babesiosis in patients with AIDS and in allograft recipients. Flulike symptoms such as fever, chills, and sweats likely result from an inflammatory response that has become systemic. Inflammatory cytokines such as tumor necrosis factor α (TNF-α) and IL-6 have been detected in the blood of a patient infected with *B. microti*. Excessive inflammation promotes pathology. In a mouse model of *B. duncani* infection, TNF-α was detected in the alveolar septa, and blockade of TNF-α rescued the animals from death caused by pulmonary edema. Even in the absence of pulmonary edema, as in mice infected with *B. microti*, TNF-α is detrimental to host defense, as indicated by faster parasite clearance in the absence of TNF receptor type 1. Although nearly every immunocompetent patient has antibody to *B. microti* detectable at the time of diagnosis, a role for humoral immunity is uncertain. Administration of rituximab for cancer or an autoimmune disorder predisposes to persistent or relapsing babesiosis; this observation indicates that B cells and presumably antibodies are critical for parasite clearance in some individuals.

DIAGNOSIS

Babesiosis should be considered for any patient who presents with symptoms compatible with babesiosis and who resides in an endemic area between late spring and early fall or has received transfused blood components, particularly packed RBCs, in the past 6 months. Given that one-tenth of patients with Lyme disease are infected with *B. microti*, and because co-infected patients usually experience an illness that lasts longer and is more severe than that caused by Lyme disease alone, babesiosis should be considered for any patient diagnosed with Lyme disease, particularly if symptoms worsen or do not abate within days or weeks of initiation of appropriate antibiotic therapy. Conversely, because one-half of patients diagnosed with babesiosis are infected with *B. burgdorferi*, a diagnosis of babesiosis should prompt a diagnostic evaluation for Lyme disease. Other tick-borne diseases, such as human granulocytotropic anaplasmosis and ehrlichiosis (**Chap. 187**), should also be considered.

Routine Laboratory Testing The complete blood count often is remarkable for anemia. An elevated reticulocyte count signifies stress-induced erythropoiesis. Low levels of haptoglobin or elevated levels of lactate dehydrogenase are consistent with hemolytic anemia. Severe anemia often is preceded by severe thrombocytopenia. The white blood cell (WBC) count is reduced, unchanged, or elevated. Elevated levels of alkaline phosphatase, aspartate aminotransferase, and alanine aminotransferase signify hepatocyte injury. Elevated total bilirubin levels result from hemolytic anemia but may denote hepatic compromise. Elevated levels of blood urea nitrogen and serum creatinine indicate renal compromise. Urinalysis may reveal excess urobilinogen, hemoglobinuria, and/or proteinuria. Given that babesiosis is an imitator of HELLP (hemolysis, elevated liver enzymes, and low platelet count) syndrome, a diagnosis of babesiosis should be considered for pregnant women who are at risk of tick exposure and have laboratory abnormalities that define this syndrome.

There is no consensus on the use of a particular laboratory parameter as a predictor of severe babesiosis. In a study of severe disease as defined above (see "Clinical Manifestations"), a total bilirubin level of >1.9 mg/dL was highly predictive of severe disease, whereas WBC counts of $<5 \times 10^3/\mu L$ were associated with a better prognosis. Parameters associated with severe disease also included parasitemia of >10% at diagnosis, WBC counts of $>10 \times 10^3/\mu L$, and creatinine levels of >1.2 mg/dL. An earlier study identified alkaline phosphatase levels of >125 IU/L and WBC counts of $>5 \times 10^3/\mu L$ as strong predictors of severe disease, in this case defined as a hospital stay of >2 weeks, an ICU stay of >2 days, or death. In that study, parasitemia of >4% at admission was associated with severe disease.

Specific Testing A definitive diagnosis of babesiosis is made by microscopic examination of Giemsa-stained thin blood smears (**Fig. 225-2**) or amplification of *Babesia* DNA in blood. *Babesia* trophozoites appear round, oval, or ameboid. The ring form is most common and lacks the central brownish (hemozoin) deposit typical of *Plasmodium falciparum* late-stage trophozoites (**see Fig. A2-1**). For travelers who have returned from *P. falciparum*–endemic areas and reside in a *Babesia*-endemic area, a negative result in the BinaxNOW malaria test readily rules out falciparum malaria when microscopy cannot. The presence of extracellular merozoites, particularly when parasitemia is high, and the absence of gametocytes and schizonts also distinguish

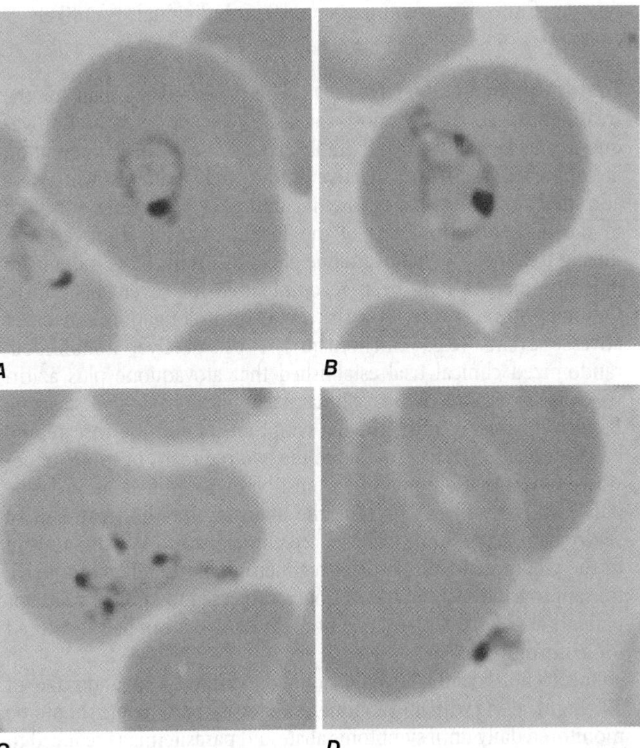

FIGURE 225-2 Giemsa-stained thin blood films showing *Babesia microti* parasites. *B. microti* is an obligate parasite of erythrocytes. Trophozoites may appear as ring forms (***A***) or as ameboid forms (***B***). ***C.*** Merozoites can be arranged in tetrads that are pathognomonic. ***D.*** Extracellular parasites can be noted, particularly when parasitemia is high. *(Reproduced with permission from E Vannier, PJ Krause: Human babesiosis. N Engl J Med 366:2397, 2012.)*

babesiosis from malaria. Merozoites are arranged in pairs and occasionally in tetrads (the "Maltese cross"). Tetrads are pathognomonic of babesiosis and can be seen in human erythrocytes infected with *B. microti*, *B. duncani*, *B. venatorum*, or *B. divergens*–like organisms. Parasitemia typically ranges from 0.1 to 10% in immunocompetent patients but has reached 30–40% in immunocompromised patients. If parasites cannot be identified by microscopy and babesiosis is still suspected, amplification of *Babesia* DNA is recommended. Most assays target the 18S rRNA gene, and the most sensitive use a fluorescent probe. Real-time polymerase chain reaction (PCR) assays detect as few as 1–10 parasites/μL of blood and are well suited for speciation of the causative agent.

A single positive serologic result is not sufficient to establish a diagnosis of babesiosis because antibodies can persist for >1 year after the illness has resolved and the parasite has been cleared. An indirect fluorescent antibody test is most commonly used. For *B. microti*, IgM titers of ≥1:64 and IgG titers of ≥1:1024 suggest active or recent infection. Antibodies to *B. microti* do not react with *B. duncani* or *B. divergens* antigen. Sera from patients infected with *B. venatorum* or *B. crassa*–like organisms react with *B. divergens* antigen.

TABLE 225-1 Treatment of Human Babesiosis

ADULTS	CHILDREN
Mild to Moderate *B. microti* Infection[a]	
Atovaquone (750 mg q12h PO) *plus* Azithromycin (500 mg/d PO on day 1, 250 mg/d PO thereafter)	Atovaquone (20 mg/kg q12h PO; maximum, 750 mg/dose) *plus* Azithromycin (10 mg/kg qd PO on day 1 [maximum, 500 mg], 5 mg/kg qd PO thereafter [maximum, 250 mg])
Severe *B. microti* Infection[b,c]	
Preferred[d] Atovaquone (750 mg q12h PO) *plus* Azithromycin (500 mg qd IV followed by 250–500 mg qd PO) **Alternative[e,f]** Clindamycin (600 mg q6h IV followed by 600 mg q8h PO) *plus* Quinine (650 mg q6–8h PO) Consider exchange transfusion	**Preferred** Atovaquone (20 mg/kg q12h PO; maximum, 750 mg/dose) *plus* Azithromycin (10 mg/kg qd IV followed by 10 mg/kg qd PO [maximum, 500 mg]) **Alternative** Clindamycin (7–10 mg/kg q6–8h IV followed by 7–10 mg/kg q6–8h PO [maximum, 600 mg/dose]) *plus* Quinine (8 mg/kg q8h PO; maximum, 650 mg/dose) Consider exchange transfusion
***B. divergens* Infection[g]**	
Immediate complete exchange transfusion *plus* Clindamycin (600 mg q6–8h IV) *plus* Quinine (650 mg q8h PO)	Immediate complete exchange transfusion *plus* Clindamycin (7–10 mg/kg q6–8h IV; maximum, 600 mg/dose) *plus* Quinine (8 mg/kg q8h PO; maximum, 650 mg/dose)

[a]Treat for 7–10 days. [b]Treat for 7–10 days, but extend duration if symptoms persist. [c]For severely immunocompromised patients, antimicrobial therapy should be given for at least 6 consecutive weeks, including 2 final weeks during which parasites are no longer detected on blood smear. [d]If the risk of QTc prolongation or allergy associated with use of azithromycin is a concern, clindamycin can be substituted for azithromycin. For severely immunocompromised patients, IV clindamycin can be added to atovaquone plus azithromycin at initiation of treatment. [e]Clindamycin plus quinine is no longer the preferred regimen because quinine often is discontinued due to QTc prolongation or other side effects, including tinnitus. This regimen can be considered for cases that respond poorly to atovaquone plus azithromycin. [f]Other alternative regimens have been used successfully, as documented in a limited number of case reports. If quinine toxicity is a concern, atovaquone can be substituted for quinine. For cases that respond poorly to atovaquone plus azithromycin, atovaquone-proguanil can be added to the two-drug regimen or can be substituted for atovaquone. [g]A few cases of *B. divergens* infection in Europe have been treated successfully with atovaquone plus azithromycin or atovaquone-proguanil plus azithromycin.

TREATMENT

Babesiosis

MILD TO MODERATE *B. MICROTI* ILLNESS

Mild to moderate babesiosis caused by *B. microti* should be treated with atovaquone plus azithromycin administered orally for 7–10 days. Dosages for adults and children are provided in **Table 225-1**. Symptoms usually abate within 48 h after initiation of therapy and resolve within 1–2 weeks. If symptoms persist despite therapy, testing for Lyme disease or other tick-borne diseases such as human granulocytotropic anaplasmosis is essential. Fatigue may persist for weeks to months but does not warrant, on its own, that treatment be extended or resumed. Parasite DNA can be detected for as long as 3 months, but follow-up PCR testing is not recommended because relapse of infection in immunocompetent individuals is unlikely.

SEVERE *B. MICROTI* ILLNESS

First-Line Antimicrobial Therapy The preferred regimen for the treatment of severe babesiosis caused by *B. microti* is oral atovaquone plus IV azithromycin (Table 225-1). Use of this combination is supported by a retrospective study of 40 patients who were admitted for severe babesiosis, including 11 who were admitted to the ICU. In all but one of the 40 patients, infection resolved during treatment with atovaquone plus azithromycin. Clindamycin plus quinine has long been recommended for severe babesiosis. Quinine, however, carries a risk for QTc prolongation and other adverse events (e.g., cinchonism). A prospective, nonblinded, randomized clinical trial established that atovaquone plus azithromycin is as effective as clindamycin plus quinine in clearing *B. microti* parasites and resolving symptoms of non-life-threatening babesiosis. No trial has compared the two regimens in severe babesiosis. Given that quinine often must be discontinued, atovaquone plus azithromycin has become the mainstay for the treatment of severe babesiosis. Some experienced clinicians add IV clindamycin to the recommended two-drug regimen (Table 225-1, footnote d); this approach, however, has not been subjected to clinical trial. For patients at risk of QTc prolongation, clindamycin can be substituted for azithromycin.

Intravenous azithromycin should be initiated at a dosage of 500 mg/d, along with atovaquone. Laboratory parameters should be monitored daily until symptoms abate and parasitemia is reduced to <4%. Thereafter, if the patient has a functional spleen and is immunocompetent, azithromycin can be administered orally and the dosage reduced to 250–500 mg/d. The regimen is administered for 7–10 days, but the duration should be extended if symptoms persist. If the patient is asplenic or immunocompromised, a higher dose of azithromycin (500 mg/d) should be considered. Given the risk of persistent or relapsing babesiosis in such patients, the regimen should be administered until symptoms have resolved and parasites are no longer seen on blood smear for 2 weeks.

Adjunct Exchange Transfusion Partial or complete RBC exchange (RCE) is recommended for patients with high-grade parasitemia (≥10%) or moderate- to high-grade parasitemia and any of the following: severe hemolytic anemia and/or pulmonary, renal, or hepatic compromise. Therapeutic apheresis should be performed in close consultation with a transfusion medicine specialist. The main purpose of RCE is to rapidly decrease parasitemia; it also corrects anemia and removes toxic by-products of hemolysis, particularly free hemoglobin and free heme. The criteria for RCE are not strictly defined and are based on single case reports and a few small case series. In one such study that was performed at a single institution and in which RCE reduced parasitemia by ~75%, age and pre-RCE parasitemia were predictors of post-RCE length of hospital stay. Post-RCE parasitemia, however, was not associated with post-RCE length of stay or mortality; this finding advocates against the use of repeat RCE to reduce parasitemia to an arbitrary level. Given that pre-RCE parasitemia did not predict mortality, the decision to use

RCE cannot be based solely on parasitemia at admission and should take the clinical status of the patient into consideration, particularly end-organ dysfunction such as renal compromise.

Severely Immunocompromised Patients Asplenia and use of rituximab for B-cell lymphoma or autoimmune disorder predispose to persistent or relapsing babesiosis. Other predisposing conditions include HIV/AIDS and immunosuppressive regimens for transplantation or malignancy. Antimicrobial therapy should be administered to patients with these conditions for at least 6 consecutive weeks, including 2 final weeks during which parasites are no longer seen on blood smear. Given the duration of treatment, atovaquone plus azithromycin is the preferred regimen. Azithromycin should be administered IV and should be initiated at a dosage of 500 mg/d. Laboratory parameters should be monitored daily until symptoms abate and parasitemia is reduced to <4%. Thereafter, azithromycin can be administered orally, but the dosage should not be <500 mg/d because lower dosages may promote antibiotic resistance. Once the patient is no longer severely ill, blood smears should be obtained at least weekly until treatment is completed. If the patient remains symptomatic but parasites are no longer observed on blood smear, real-time PCR should be used to monitor the infection. Once treatment is completed, close follow-up is recommended. If symptoms recur, blood smears and/or real-time PCR should be ordered.

Resistance to Antimicrobial Therapy Failure to respond to atovaquone plus azithromycin has been documented in highly immunocompromised patients infected with *B. microti*. Such resistance to atovaquone and azithromycin is explained by missense mutations in the parasite's mitochondrial cytochrome b gene (*cob*) and the apicoplast-encoded ribosomal protein subunit L4 gene (*rpl4*), respectively. Patients who are unresponsive to atovaquone plus azithromycin can be managed with clindamycin plus quinine (Table 225-1, footnote e). If quinine toxicity is a concern and the molecular basis of drug resistance unknown, clindamycin can be added to atovaquone plus azithromycin. An alternative approach is to substitute atovaquone-proguanil for atovaquone (Table 225-1, footnote f).

Splenic Rupture As a complication of babesiosis, splenic rupture typically occurs in young, healthy immunocompetent patients with low-grade parasitemia. If the patient is hemodymanically unstable or rapidly deteriorates, emergent splenectomy should be performed. If the patient is hemodynamically stable but bleeding persists, splenic arterial embolization should be considered. In the absence of hemoperitoneum, splenic rupture should be managed without surgery but with careful hemodynamic monitoring. Removal of the spleen leaves patients at risk for relapsing babesiosis or severe disease caused by other microorganisms.

OTHER *BABESIA* INFECTIONS

B. duncani and *B. divergens*–like infections typically have been treated with IV clindamycin (600 mg three or four times daily or 1200 mg twice daily) plus oral quinine (600–650 mg three times daily) for 7–10 days. If symptoms persist, antimicrobial therapy should be extended.

GLOBAL CONSIDERATIONS

In Europe, *B. divergens* infection is considered a medical emergency. The recommended approach is immediate, complete RCE combined with administration of clindamycin plus oral quinine (Table 225-1). Some cases have been cured with RCE and clindamycin monotherapy. Anemia may persist for >1 month and require blood transfusion. A severe case of *B. divergens* infection resolved during therapy with atovaquone plus azithromycin. A relapse in a spleen-intact individual was treated with atovaquone-proguanil plus azithromycin. The first-line therapy for *B. venatorum* infection in Europe has been IV or oral clindamycin plus quinine. In a patient intolerant to quinine, infection was cured after administration of atovaquone plus azithromycin. A pediatric case of mild *B. venatorum* infection in China was successfully treated by a standard course of atovaquone plus azithromycin.

PREVENTION

Given the increasing incidence and high mortality rate of transfusion-transmitted babesiosis, the U.S. Food and Drug Administration (FDA) has recommended that blood donated in 14 endemic states and the District of Columbia be screened for *B. microti* DNA with a nucleic acid test. In January 2019, the FDA approved the use of an ultrasensitive nucleic acid test that detects transcripts of the parasite's 18S rRNA gene. Screening of the blood supply, once implemented, likely will reduce if not prevent transfusion-transmitted babesiosis. At present, individuals with a history of babesiosis or asymptomatic *Babesia* infection confirmed by laboratory testing are indefinitely deferred from donating blood.

Given the lack of vaccine and prophylaxis, individuals who reside in endemic areas, especially those at risk of severe babesiosis, should wear protective clothing, apply tick repellents to the skin and permethrin to clothing, and limit outdoor activities where ticks abound from May through October. The skin should be thoroughly examined after outdoor activities and ticks carefully removed with tweezers. As babesiosis continues to spread into new areas and because climate change likely will shift the boundaries of these endemic areas, individuals at risk and physicians should remain aware of this once neglected disease.

FURTHER READING

Gray EB, Herwaldt BL: Babesiosis surveillance—United States, 2011–2015. MMWR Surveill Summ 68:1, 2019.

Kletsova EA et al: Babesiosis in Long Island: Review of 62 cases focusing on treatment with azithromycin and atovaquone. Ann Clin Microbiol Antimicrob 16:26, 2017.

Krause PJ et al: Persistent and relapsing babesiosis in immunocompromised patients. Clin Infect Dis 46:370, 2008.

Krause PJ et al: Clinical practice guidelines by the Infectious Diseases Society of America (IDSA): 2020 guideline on diagnosis and management of babesiosis. Clin Infect Dis 72:185, 2021.

Nixon CP et al: Adjunctive treatment of clinically severe babesiosis with red blood cell exchange: A case series of nineteen patients. Transfusion 59:2629, 2019.

Vannier E, Krause PJ: Human babesiosis. N Engl J Med 366:2397, 2012.

226 Leishmaniasis

Shyam Sundar

Encompassing a complex group of disorders, leishmaniasis is caused by unicellular eukaryotic obligatory intracellular protozoa of the genus *Leishmania* and primarily affects the host's reticuloendothelial system. *Leishmania* species produce widely varying clinical syndromes ranging from self-healing cutaneous ulcers to fatal visceral disease. These syndromes fall into three broad categories: visceral leishmaniasis (VL), cutaneous leishmaniasis (CL), and mucosal leishmaniasis (ML).

ETIOLOGY AND LIFE CYCLE

Leishmaniasis is caused by ~20 species of the genus *Leishmania* in the order Kinetoplastida and the family Trypanosomatidae (**Table 226-1**). Several clinically important species are of the subspecies *Viannia*. The organisms are transmitted by phlebotomine sandflies of the genus *Phlebotomus* in the "Old World" (Asia, Africa, and Europe) and the genus *Lutzomyia* in the "New World" (the Americas). Transmission may be anthroponotic (i.e., the vector transmits the infection from infected humans to healthy humans) or zoonotic (i.e., the vector transmits the infection from an animal reservoir to humans). Human-to-human transmission via shared infected needles has been documented in IV drug users in the Mediterranean region. In utero transmission to the fetus occurs rarely.

TABLE 226-1 Geographic Distribution and Characteristic Epidemiology of Leishmaniases

ORGANISM, ENDEMIC REGION	CLINICAL SYNDROME	SPECIES	VECTOR	RESERVOIR	TRANSMISSION	SETTING
***Leishmania donovani* Complex**						
South Asia	VL, PKDL	*L. donovani*	*Phlebotomus argentipes*	Humans	Anthroponotic	Rural, domestic
South Sudan, Sudan, South Sudan, Somalia, Ethiopia, Kenya, Uganda	VL, PKDL	*L. donovani*	*P. orientalis*, *P. martini*	Humans, rodents in Sudan, canines	Anthroponotic, occasionally zoonotic	Majority peridomestic, occasionally sylvatic
Mediterranean basin, Middle East, Central Asia, China	VL, CL	*L. infantum*	*P. perniciosus*, *P. ariasi*	Dogs, foxes, jackals	Zoonotic	Domestic, peridomestic
Middle East, Saudi Arabia, Yemen	VL	*L. donovani*	*P. perniciosus*, *P. ariasi*	Dogs, foxes, jackals	Zoonotic	Domestic, peridomestic
Central and South America	VL, CL	*L. infantum*[a]	*Lutzomyia longipalpis*	Foxes, dogs, opossums	Zoonotic	Domestic, peridomestic, periurban
Azerbaijan, Armenia, Georgia, Kazakhstan, Kyrgyzstan, Tajikistan, Turkmenistan, Uzbekistan	VL	*L. infantum*	*P. turanicus*	Humans, dogs, foxes	Anthroponotic, zoonotic	Domestic
L. tropica						
Western India to Turkey, parts of North and East Africa	CL, leishmaniasis recidivans	*L. tropica*	*P. sergenti*	Humans	Anthroponotic	Urban domestic, peridomestic
L. major						
Western and Central Asia, North and sub-Saharan Africa	CL	*L. major*	*P. papatasi*, *P. duboscqi*	Nile rats, rodents	Zoonotic	Sylvatic, peridomestic
Kazakhstan, Turkmenistan, Uzbekistan	CL	*L. major*	*P. papatasi*, *P. duboscqi*	Gerbils	Zoonotic	Rural
L. aethiopica						
Ethiopia, Uganda, Kenya	CL, DCL	*L. aethiopica*	*P. longipes*, *P. pedifer*	Hyraxes	Zoonotic	Sylvatic, peridomestic
Subspecies *Viannia*						
Peru, Ecuador	CL, ML	*L. (V.) peruviana*	*Lutzomyia verrucarum*, *L. peruensis*	Wild rodents	Zoonotic	Andean Valleys
Guyana, Surinam, French Guyana, Ecuador, Brazil, Colombia, Bolivia	CL, ML	*L. (V.) guyanensis*	*L. umbratilis*	Sloths, arboreal anteaters, opossums	Zoonotic	Tropical forest
Central America, Ecuador, Colombia	CL, ML	*L. (V.) panamensis*	*L. trapidoi*	Sloths	Zoonotic	Tropical forest and deforested areas
South and Central America	CL, ML	*L. (V.) braziliensis*	*Lutzomyia* spp., *L. umbratilis*, *Psychodopygus wellcomei*	Forest rodents, peridomestic animals	Zoonotic	Tropical forest and deforested areas
***L. mexicana* Complex**						
Central America and northern parts of South America	CL, ML, DCL	*L. amazonensis*	*L. flaviscutellata*	Forest rodents	Zoonotic	Tropical forest and deforested areas
	CL, ML, DCL	*L. mexicana*	*L. olmeca*	Variety of forest rodents and marsupials	Zoonotic	Tropical forest and deforested areas
	CL, DCL	*L. pifanoi*	*L. olmeca*	Variety of forest rodents and marsupials	Zoonotic	Tropical forest and deforested areas

[a]*L. infantum* is designated *L. chagasi* in the New World.

Abbreviations: CL, cutaneous leishmaniasis; DCL, diffuse cutaneous leishmaniasis; ML, mucosal leishmaniasis; PKDL, post–kala-azar dermal leishmaniasis; VL, visceral leishmaniasis.

Leishmania organisms occur in two forms: extracellular, flagellate promastigotes (length, 10–20 μm) in the sandfly vector and intracellular, nonflagellate amastigotes (length, 2–4 μm; **Fig. 226-1**) in vertebrate hosts, including humans. Promastigotes are introduced through the proboscis of the female sandfly into the skin of the vertebrate host. Neutrophils predominate among the host cells that first encounter and take up promastigotes at the site of parasite delivery. The infected neutrophils may undergo apoptosis and release viable parasites that are taken up by macrophages, or the apoptotic cells may themselves be taken up by macrophages and dendritic cells. The parasites multiply as amastigotes inside macrophages, causing cell rupture with subsequent invasion of other macrophages. While feeding on infected hosts, sandflies pick up amastigotes, which transform into the flagellate form in the flies' posterior midgut and multiply by binary fission; the promastigotes then migrate to the anterior midgut and can infect a new host when flies take another blood meal.

■ EPIDEMIOLOGY

Leishmaniasis occurs in 98 countries—most of them developing—in tropical and temperate regions (**Fig. 226-2**). More than 1.5 million cases occur annually, of which 0.7–1.2 million are CL (and its variations) and 200,000–400,000 are VL. More than 350 million people are

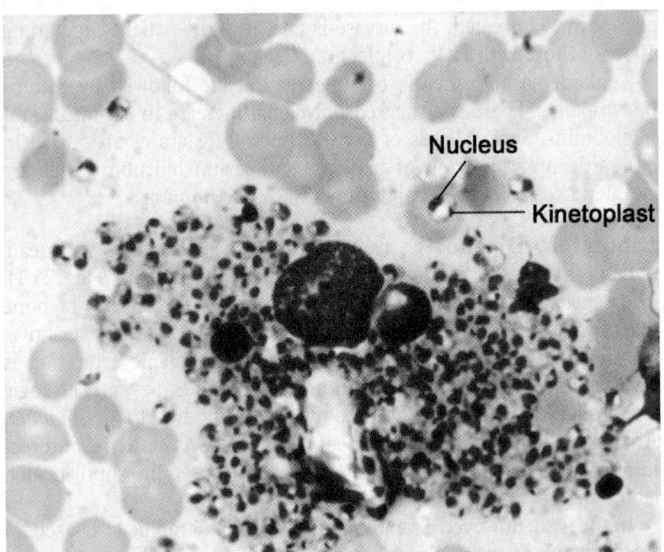

FIGURE 226-1 A macrophage with numerous intracellular amastigotes (2–4 μm) in a Giemsa-stained splenic smear from a patient with visceral leishmaniasis. Each amastigote contains a nucleus and a characteristic kinetoplast consisting of multiple copies of mitochondrial DNA. A few extracellular parasites are also visible.

at risk, with an overall prevalence of 12 million. The distribution of *Leishmania* is limited by the distribution of sandfly vectors.

VISCERAL LEISHMANIASIS

VL (also known as *kala-azar*, a Hindi term meaning "black fever") is caused by the *Leishmania donovani* complex, which includes *L. donovani* and *Leishmania infantum* (the latter designated *Leishmania chagasi* in the New World); these species are responsible for anthroponotic and zoonotic transmission, respectively. India and neighboring Bangladesh, Sudan and neighboring South Sudan, Ethiopia, and Brazil are the four largest foci of VL and account for 90% of the world's VL burden. Human leishmaniasis is on the increase worldwide except on the Indian subcontinent (India, Nepal, and Bangladesh), where a VL elimination program has been implemented, and VL incidence is markedly declining. More than 90% of the program sites in these three countries have reached the elimination target of the incidence of <1 in 10,000 persons. East Africa now has the distinction of being the largest focus of VL. Zoonotic VL is reported from all countries in the Middle East, Pakistan, and other countries from western Asia to China. Endemic foci also exist in the independent states of the former Soviet Union, mainly Georgia and Azerbaijan. In the Horn of Africa, Sudan, South Sudan, Ethiopia, Kenya, Uganda, and Somalia report VL. In Sudan and South Sudan, large outbreaks are thought to be anthroponotic, although zoonotic transmission also occurs. VL is rare in West and sub-Saharan Africa.

Mediterranean VL, long an established endemic disease due to *L. infantum*, has a large canine reservoir and was seen primarily in infants before the advent of HIV infection. In Mediterranean Europe, 70% of adult VL cases are associated with HIV co-infection. The combination is deadly because of the combined impact of the two infections on the immune system. IV drug users are at particular risk. Other forms of immunosuppression (e.g., that associated with organ transplantation) also predispose to VL. In the Americas, disease caused by *L. infantum* is endemic from Mexico to Argentina, but 90% of cases in the New World are reported from northeastern Brazil. After the introduction of highly active antiretroviral therapy, the incidence of HIV–VL co-infection declined significantly in Europe; however, ~30 and 5% of VL patients are co-infected with HIV in Ethiopia and India, respectively.

Immunopathogenesis The majority of individuals infected by *L. donovani* or *L. infantum* mount a successful immune response and control the infection, never developing symptomatic disease. Forty-eight hours after intradermal injection of killed promastigotes, these individuals exhibit delayed-type hypersensitivity (DTH) to leishmanial antigens in the leishmanin skin test (also called the Montenegro skin test). Results in mouse models indicate that the development of acquired resistance to leishmanial infection is controlled by the production of interleukin (IL) 12 by antigen-presenting cells and the subsequent secretion of interferon (IFN) γ, tumor necrosis factor (TNF) α, and other proinflammatory cytokines by the T helper 1 (T_H1) subset of T lymphocytes. The immune response in patients developing active VL is complex; in addition to increased production of multiple proinflammatory cytokines and chemokines, patients with active disease have markedly elevated levels of IL-10 in serum as well as enhanced IL-10 mRNA expression in lesional tissues. A direct role for IL-10 in the pathology of VL in humans is supported by studies demonstrating that IL-10 blockade can enhance IFN-γ responses in whole blood from VL patients. The main disease-promoting activity of IL-10 in VL may be to condition host macrophages for enhanced survival and growth of the parasite. IL-10 can render macrophages unresponsive to activation signals and inhibit killing of amastigotes by downregulating the production of TNF-α and nitric oxide. Multiple antigen-presentation

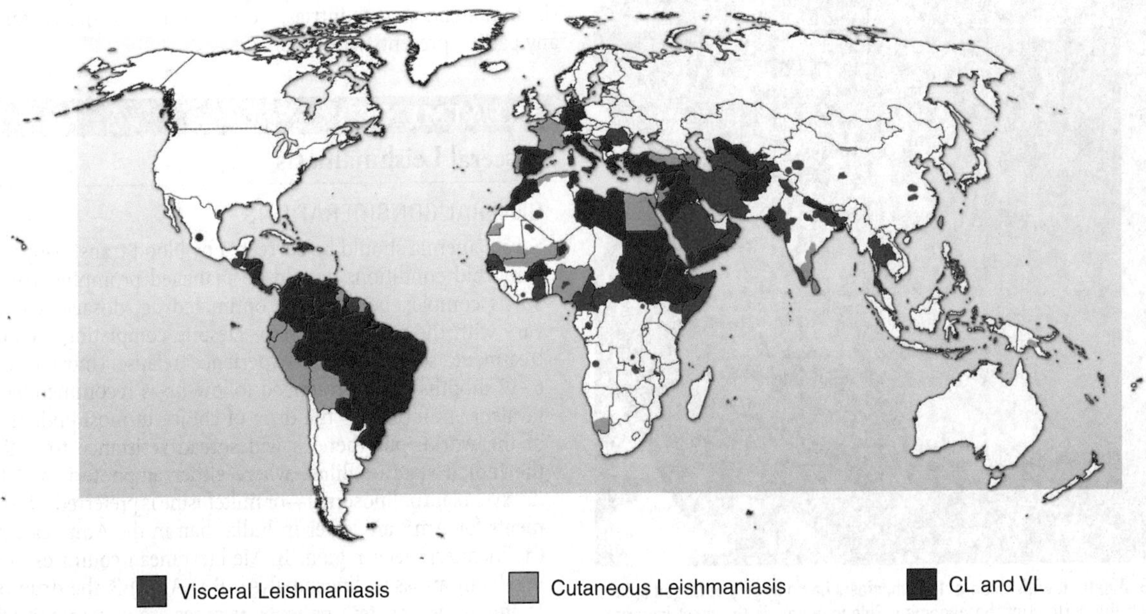

FIGURE 226-2 Worldwide distribution of human leishmaniasis. CL, cutaneous leishmaniasis; VL, visceral leishmaniasis.

functions of dendritic cells and macrophages are also suppressed by IL-10. Patients with such suppression do not have positive leishmanin skin tests, nor do their peripheral-blood mononuclear cells respond to leishmanial antigens in vitro. Organs of the reticuloendothelial system are predominantly affected, with remarkable enlargement of the spleen, liver, and lymph nodes in some regions. The tonsils and intestinal submucosa are also heavily infiltrated with parasites. Bone marrow dysfunction results in pancytopenia.

Clinical Features On the Indian subcontinent and in the Horn of Africa, persons of all ages are affected by VL. In endemic areas of the Americas and the Mediterranean basin, immunocompetent infants and small children as well as immunodeficient adults are affected especially often. The most common presentation of VL is an abrupt onset of moderate- to high-grade fever associated with rigor and chills. Fever may continue for several weeks with decreasing intensity, and the patient may become afebrile for a short period before experiencing another bout of fever. The spleen may be palpable by the second week of illness and, depending on the duration of illness, may become hugely enlarged (Fig. 226-3). Hepatomegaly (usually moderate in degree) soon follows. Lymphadenopathy is common in most endemic regions of the world except the Indian subcontinent, where it is rare. Patients lose weight and feel weak, and the skin gradually develops dark discoloration due to hyperpigmentation that is most easily seen in brown-skinned individuals. In advanced illness, hypoalbuminemia may manifest as pedal edema and ascites. Anemia appears early and may become severe enough to cause congestive heart failure. Epistaxis, retinal hemorrhages, and gastrointestinal bleeding are associated with thrombocytopenia. Secondary infections such as measles, pneumonia, tuberculosis, bacillary or amebic dysentery, and gastroenteritis are common. Herpes zoster, chickenpox, boils in the skin, and scabies may also occur. Untreated, the disease is fatal in most patients, including 100% of those with HIV co-infection.

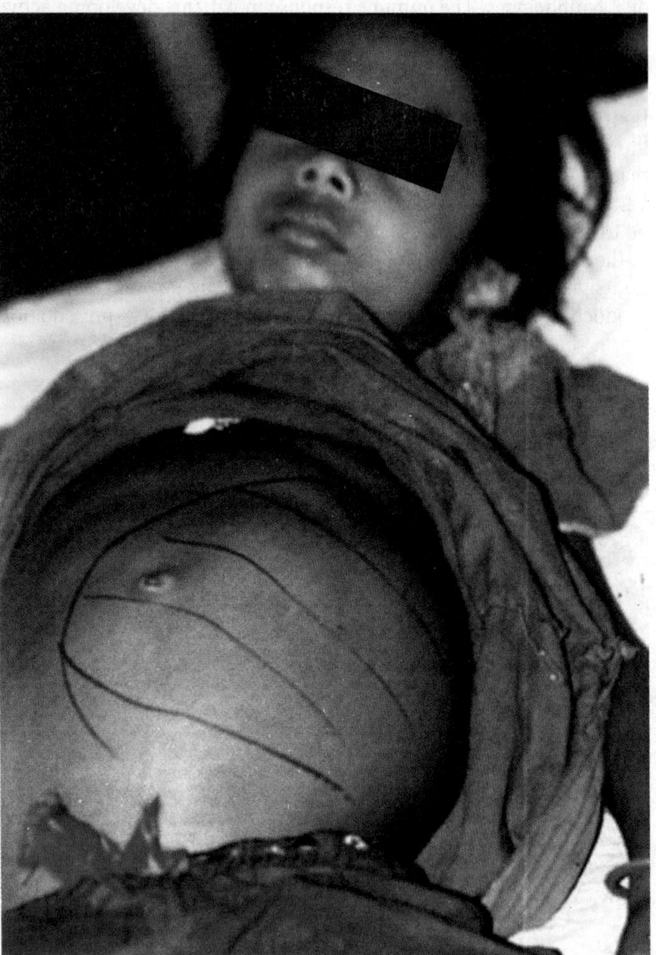

FIGURE 226-3 A patient with visceral leishmaniasis has a hugely enlarged spleen visible through the surface of the abdomen. Splenomegaly is the most important feature of visceral leishmaniasis.

Leukopenia and anemia occur early and are followed by thrombocytopenia. There is a marked polyclonal increase in serum immunoglobulins. Serum levels of hepatic aminotransferases are raised in a significant proportion of patients, and serum bilirubin levels are elevated occasionally. Renal dysfunction is uncommon.

Laboratory Diagnosis Demonstration of amastigotes in smears of tissue aspirates is the gold standard for the diagnosis of VL (Fig. 226-1). The sensitivity of splenic smears is >95%, whereas smears of bone marrow (60–85%) and lymph node aspirates (50%) are less sensitive. Culture of tissue aspirates increases sensitivity. Splenic aspiration is invasive and may be dangerous in untrained hands. Several serologic techniques are currently used to detect antibodies to *Leishmania.* An enzyme-linked immunosorbent assay (ELISA) and the indirect immunofluorescent antibody test (IFAT) are used in sophisticated laboratories.

In the field, however, a rapid immunochromatographic test based on the detection of antibodies to a recombinant antigen (rK39) consisting of 39 amino acids conserved in the kinesin region of *L. infantum* is used worldwide. The test requires only a drop of fingerprick blood or serum, and the result can be read within 15 min. Except in East Africa (where both its sensitivity and its specificity are lower), the sensitivity of the rK39 rapid diagnostic test (RDT) in immunocompetent individuals is ~98% and its specificity is ~90%. In Sudan, an RDT based on a new synthetic polyprotein, rK28, was more sensitive (96.8%) and specific (96.2%) than rK39-based RDTs. Since these antibody detection tests remain positive for years after cure, they cannot be used for measurement of cure or detection of relapse. Qualitative detection of leishmanial nucleic acid by polymerase chain reaction (PCR) or by loop-mediated isothermal amplification (LAMP) and quantitative detection by real-time PCR are highly sensitive; however, because the capacity to perform these tests is confined to specialized laboratories, they have yet to be used for routine diagnosis of VL in endemic areas. PCR can distinguish among the major species of *Leishmania* infecting humans.

Differential Diagnosis VL is easily mistaken for malaria. Other febrile illnesses that may mimic VL include typhoid fever, tuberculosis, brucellosis, schistosomiasis, and histoplasmosis. Splenomegaly due to portal hypertension, chronic myeloid leukemia, tropical splenomegaly syndrome, and (in Africa) schistosomiasis may also be confused with VL. Fever with neutropenia or pancytopenia in patients from an endemic region strongly suggests a diagnosis of VL; hypergammaglobulinemia in patients with long-standing illness strengthens the diagnosis. In nonendemic countries, a careful travel history is essential when any patient presents with fever.

TREATMENT

Visceral Leishmaniasis

GENERAL CONSIDERATIONS

Severe anemia should be corrected by blood transfusion, and other comorbid conditions should be managed promptly. Treatment of VL is complex because the optimal drug, dosage, and duration vary with the endemic region. Despite completing recommended treatment, some patients experience relapse (most often within 6–12 months), and prolonged follow-up is recommended. A pentavalent antimonial is the drug of choice in most endemic regions of the world, but there is widespread resistance to antimony in the Indian state of Bihar, where either amphotericin B (AmB)—deoxycholate or liposomal—or miltefosine is preferred. Dose requirements for AmB are lower in India than in the Americas, Africa, or the Mediterranean region. In Mediterranean countries, where cost is seldom an issue, liposomal AmB (LAmB) is the drug of choice. In immunocompetent patients, relapses are uncommon with AmB in its deoxycholate and lipid formulations. Antileishmanial therapy has recently evolved as new drugs and delivery systems have become available and resistance to antimonial compounds has emerged.

Except for AmB (deoxycholate and lipid formulations), antileishmanial drugs are available in the United States only from the Centers for Disease Control and Prevention Drug Service (telephone: 404-639-3670; email: drugservice@ cdc.gov; *www.cdc.gov/ncpdcid/dsr/*).

PENTAVALENT ANTIMONIAL COMPOUNDS

Two pentavalent antimonial (Sb^V) preparations are available: sodium stibogluconate (100 mg of Sb^V/mL) and meglumine antimoniate (85 mg of Sb^V/mL). The daily dose is 20 mg/kg by IV infusion or IM injection, and therapy continues for 28–30 days. Cure rates exceed 90% in Africa, the Americas, and most of the Old World but are <50% in Bihar, India, as a result of resistance. Adverse reactions to Sb^V treatment are common and include arthralgia, myalgia, and elevated serum levels of aminotransferases. Electrocardiographic changes are common. Concave ST-segment elevation is not significant, but prolongation of QTc to >0.5 s may herald ventricular arrhythmia and sudden death. Chemical pancreatitis is common but usually does not require discontinuation of treatment; severe clinical pancreatitis occurs in immunosuppressed patients.

AMPHOTERICIN B

AmB is currently used as a first-line drug in Bihar, India. In other parts of the world, it is used when initial antimonial treatment fails. Conventional AmB deoxycholate is administered in doses of 0.75–1.0 mg/kg on alternate days for a total of 15 infusions. Fever with chills is an almost universal adverse reaction to AmB infusions. Nausea and vomiting are also common, as is thrombophlebitis in the infused veins. Acute toxicities can be minimized by administration of antihistamines like chlorpheniramine and antipyretic agents like acetaminophen before each infusion. AmB can cause renal dysfunction and hypokalemia and, in rare instances, elicits hypersensitivity reactions, bone marrow suppression, and myocarditis, all of which can be fatal.

Several lipid formulations of AmB, developed to replace the deoxycholate formulation, are preferentially taken up by reticuloendothelial tissues. Because very little free drug is available to cause toxicity, a large amount of drug can be delivered over a short period. LAmB has been used extensively to treat VL in all parts of the world. With a terminal half-life of ~150 h, LAmB can be detected in the liver and spleen of animals for several weeks after a single dose. In addition to oral miltefosine (see below), this is the only drug approved by the U.S. Food and Drug Administration (FDA) for the treatment of VL; the regimen is 3 mg/kg daily on days 1–5, 14, and 21 (total dose, 21 mg/kg). However, the total-dose requirement for different regions of the world varies widely. In Asia, it is 10–15 mg/kg; in Africa, ~18 mg/kg; and in Mediterranean/American regions, ≥20 mg/kg. The daily dose is flexible (1–10 mg/kg). In a study in India, a single dose of 10 mg/kg cured infection in 96% of patients. This single-dose regimen is the preferred treatment in India, Bangladesh, and Nepal. Adverse effects of LAmB are usually mild and include infusion reactions, backache, and occasional reversible nephrotoxicity.

PAROMOMYCIN

Paromomycin (aminosidine) is an aminocyclitol-aminoglycoside antibiotic with antileishmanial activity. Its mechanism of action against *Leishmania* has yet to be established. Paromomycin is approved in India for the treatment of VL at an IM dose of 11 mg of base/kg daily for 21 days; this regimen produces a cure rate of 94.6%. However, the optimal dose has not been established in other endemic regions. Paromomycin is a relatively safe drug, but some patients develop hepatotoxicity, reversible ototoxicity, and (in rare instances) nephrotoxicity and tetany. Paromomycin, in combination with Sb^V, is used in sub-Saharan Africa.

MILTEFOSINE

Miltefosine, an alkylphosphocholine, is the first oral compound approved for the treatment of leishmaniasis in several endemic countries including the United States. This drug has a long half-life (150–200 h); its mechanism of action is not clearly understood. The recommended therapeutic regimens for patients on the Indian subcontinent are a daily dose of 50 mg for 28 days for patients weighing <25 kg, a twice-daily dose of 50 mg for 28 days for patients weighing ≥25 kg, and 2.5 mg/kg for 28 days for children 2–11 years of age. These regimens have resulted in a cure rate of 94% in India. However, recent studies from the Indian subcontinent indicate a decline in the cure rate. Doses in other regions remain to be established. Because of its long half-life, miltefosine is prone to induce resistance in *Leishmania*. Its adverse effects include mild to moderate vomiting and diarrhea in 40 and 20% of patients, respectively; these reactions usually clear spontaneously after a few days. Rare cases of severe allergic dermatitis, hepatotoxicity, and nephrotoxicity have been reported. Because miltefosine is expensive and is associated with significant adverse events, it is best administered as directly observed therapy to ensure completion of treatment and to minimize the risk of resistance induction. Because miltefosine is teratogenic in rats, its use is contraindicated during pregnancy and (unless contraceptive measures are strictly adhered to for at least 3 months after treatment) in women of childbearing age.

MULTIDRUG THERAPY

Multidrug therapy for leishmaniasis is likely to be preferred in the future. Its potential advantages in VL include (1) better compliance and lower costs associated with shorter treatment courses and decreased hospitalization, (2) less toxicity due to lower drug doses and/or shorter duration of treatment, and (3) a reduced likelihood that resistance to either agent will develop. In a study from India, one dose of LAmB (5 mg/kg) followed by miltefosine for 7 days, paromomycin for 10 days, or both miltefosine and paromomycin simultaneously for 10 days (in their usual daily doses) produced a cure rate of >97% (all three combinations). In Africa, a combination of Sb^V and paromomycin given for 17 days was as effective and safe as Sb^V given for 30 days. Studies are being conducted in East Africa to test combination chemotherapy with recently approved drugs such as miltefosine and LAmB.

Prognosis of Treated VL Patients Recovery from VL is quick. Within a week after the start of treatment, defervescence, regression of splenomegaly, weight gain, and recovery of hematologic parameters are evident. With effective treatment, no parasites are recovered from tissue aspirates at the posttreatment evaluation. Continued clinical improvement over 12 months is suggestive of cure. A small percentage of patients (with the exact figure depending on the regimen used) relapse but respond well to retreatment with AmB deoxycholate or lipid formulations.

VL in the Immunocompromised Host HIV/VL co-infection has been reported from 35 countries. Where both infections are endemic, VL behaves as an opportunistic infection in HIV-1-infected patients. HIV infection can increase the risk of VL development by several-fold in endemic areas. Co-infected patients usually show the classic signs of VL, but they may present with atypical features due to loss of immunity and involvement of unusual anatomic locations, e.g., infiltration of the skin, oral mucosa, gastrointestinal tract, lungs, and other organs. Serodiagnostic tests may be negative in up to 50% of patients. Parasites can be recovered from unusual sites such as bronchoalveolar lavage fluid and buffy coat. LAmB is the drug of choice for HIV/VL co-infection—both for primary treatment and for treatment of relapses. A total dose of 40 mg/kg, administered as 4 mg/kg on days 1–5, 10, 17, 24, 31, and 38, is considered optimal and is approved by the FDA, but most patients experience a relapse within 1 year. Pentavalent antimonials and AmB deoxycholate can also be used where LAmB is not accessible. Reconstitution of patients' immunity by antiretroviral therapy has led to a dramatic decline in the incidence of co-infection in the Mediterranean basin. In contrast, HIV/VL co-infection is on the rise in African and Asian countries. Ethiopia is worst affected: up to 30% of VL patients are also infected with HIV. Because restoration of the CD4+ T-cell count to >200/μL does decrease the frequency of relapse, antiretroviral therapy (in addition to antileishmanial therapy) is a cornerstone of the management of HIV/VL co-infection.

TABLE 226-2 Clinical, Epidemiologic, and Therapeutic Features of Post–Kala-Azar Dermal Leishmaniasis: East Africa and the Indian Subcontinent

FEATURE	EAST AFRICA	INDIAN SUBCONTINENT
Most affected country	Sudan and South Sudan	Bangladesh
Incidence among patients with VL	~50%	5–15%
Interval between VL and PKDL	During VL to 6 months	6 months to 3 years
Age distribution	Mainly children	Any age
History of prior VL	Yes	Not necessarily
Rashes of PKDL in presence of active VL	Yes	No
Treatment with sodium stibogluconate	2–3 months	2–4 months
Natural course	Spontaneous cure in majority of patients	Spontaneous cure in minority of patients

Abbreviations: PKDL, post–kala-azar dermal leishmaniasis; VL, visceral leishmaniasis.

Secondary prophylaxis with pentamidine or lipid AmB has been shown to delay relapses, but no regimen has been established as optimal.

Post–Kala-Azar Dermal Leishmaniasis On the Indian subcontinent and in Sudan and other East African countries, 2–50% of patients develop skin lesions concurrent with or after the cure of VL. Most common are hypopigmented macules, papules, and/or nodules or diffuse infiltration of the skin and sometimes of the oral mucosa. The African and Indian diseases differ in several respects; important features of post–kala-azar dermal leishmaniasis (PKDL) in these two regions are listed in **Table 226-2**, and disease in an Indian patient is depicted in **Fig. 226-4**.

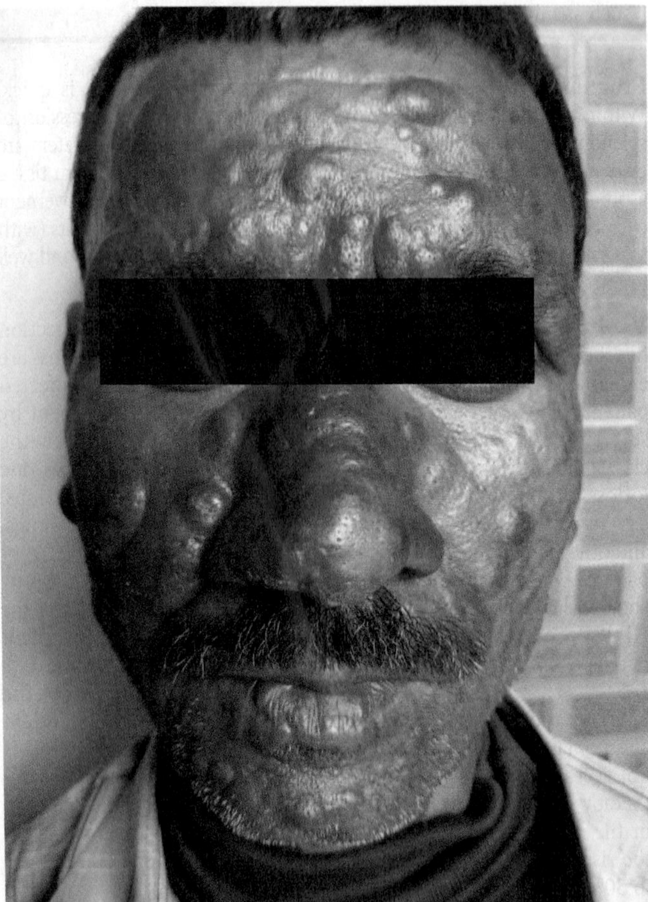

FIGURE 226-4 Post–kala-azar dermal leishmaniasis in an Indian patient. Note nodules of varying size involving the entire face. The face is erythematous, and the surface of some of the large nodules is discolored.

In PKDL, parasites are scanty in hypopigmented macules but may be seen and cultured more easily from nodular lesions. Cellular infiltrates are heavier in nodules than in macules. Lymphocytes are the dominant cells; next most common are histiocytes and plasma cells. In about half of cases, epithelioid cells—scattered individually or forming compact granulomas—are seen. The diagnosis is based on history and clinical findings, but rK39 and other serologic tests are positive in most cases. Indian PKDL was treated with prolonged courses (up to 120 days) of pentavalent antimonials. This prolonged course frequently led to noncompliance. The alternative—several courses of AmB spread over several months—is expensive and unacceptable for most patients. Except for cosmetic reasons, these patients do not have any physical limitation, and thus motivation for such long and arduous treatment is very low. This leads to either no or incomplete treatment. In the Indian subcontinent, the currently recommended regimen is oral miltefosine for 12 weeks, in the usual daily doses. This regimen cures most patients; however, its lower efficacy is now being reported in some studies. The efficacy of LAmB in combination with miltefosine in PKDL is being tested on the Indian subcontinent. In East Africa, a majority of patients experience spontaneous healing. In those with persistent lesions, the response to 60 days of treatment with a pentavalent antimonial is good.

CUTANEOUS LEISHMANIASIS

CL can be broadly divided into Old World and New World forms. Old World CL caused by *Leishmania tropica* is anthroponotic and is confined to urban or suburban areas throughout its range. Zoonotic CL is most commonly due to *Leishmania major*, which naturally parasitizes several species of desert rodents that act as reservoirs over wide areas of the Middle East, Africa, and central Asia. Local outbreaks of human disease are common. Major outbreaks currently affect Afghanistan, Syria, Iraq, Lebanon, and Turkey in association with refugees and population movement. CL is increasingly seen in tourists and military personnel on mission in CL-endemic regions of countries and as a co-infection in HIV-infected patients. *Leishmania aethiopica* is restricted to the highlands of Ethiopia, Kenya, and Uganda, where it is a natural parasite of hyraxes. New World CL is mainly zoonotic and is most often caused by *Leishmania mexicana, Leishmania (Viannia) panamensis*, and *Leishmania amazonensis*. A wide range of forest animals act as reservoirs, and human infections with these species are predominantly rural. As a result of extensive urbanization and deforestation, *Leishmania (Viannia) braziliensis* has adapted to peridomestic and urban animals, and CL due to this organism is increasingly becoming an urban disease. In the United States, a few cases of CL have been acquired indigenously in Texas.

Immunopathogenesis As in VL, the proinflammatory (T_H1) response in CL may result in either asymptomatic or subclinical infection. However, in some individuals, the immune response causes ulcerative skin lesions, the majority of which heal spontaneously, leaving a scar. Healing is usually followed by immunity to reinfection with that species of parasite.

Clinical Features A few days or weeks after the bite of a sandfly, a papule develops and grows into a nodule that ulcerates over weeks or months. The base of the ulcer, which is usually painless, consists of necrotic tissue and crusted serum, but secondary bacterial infection sometimes occurs. The margins of the ulcer are raised and indurated. Lesions may be single or multiple and vary in size from 0.5 to >3 cm (**Fig. 226-5**). Lymphatic spread and lymph gland involvement may be palpable and may precede the appearance of the skin lesion. There may be satellite lesions, especially in *L. major* and *L. tropica* infections. The lesions usually heal spontaneously after 2–15 months. Lesions due to *L. major* and *L. mexicana* tend to heal rapidly, whereas those due to *L. tropica* and parasites of subspecies *Viannia* heal more slowly. In CL caused by *L. tropica*, new lesions—usually scaly, erythematous papules and nodules—develop in the center or periphery of a healed sore, a condition known as *leishmaniasis recidivans*. Lesions of *L. mexicana* and *Leishmania (Viannia) peruviana* closely resemble those seen in the Old World; however, lesions on the pinna of the ear are common, chronic, and destructive in the former infections. *L. mexicana*

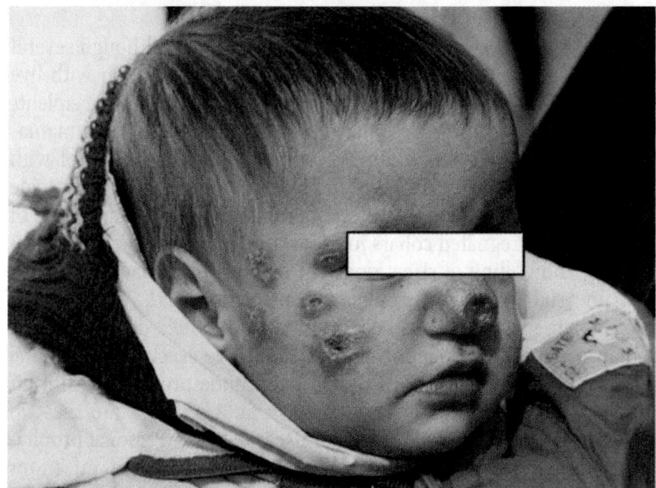

FIGURE 226-5 Cutaneous leishmaniasis in a Bolivian child. There are multiple ulcers resulting from several sandfly bites. The edges of the ulcers are raised. *(Courtesy of P. Desjeux, Retired Medical Officer, World Health Organization, Geneva, Switzerland.)*

is responsible for chiclero's ulcer, the so-called self-healing sore of Mexico. CL lesions on exposed body parts (e.g., the face and hands), permanent scar formation, and social stigmatization may cause anxiety and depression and may affect the quality of life of CL patients.

Differential Diagnosis A typical history (an insect bite followed by the events leading to ulceration) in a resident of or a traveler to an endemic focus strongly suggests CL. Cutaneous tuberculosis, fungal infections, leprosy, sarcoidosis, and malignant ulcers are sometimes mistaken for CL.

Laboratory Diagnosis Demonstration of amastigotes in material obtained from a lesion remains the diagnostic gold standard. Microscopic examination of slit skin smears, aspirates, or biopsies of the lesion is used for detection of parasites. Culture of smear or biopsy material may yield *Leishmania*. PCR is more sensitive than microscopy and culture and allows identification of *Leishmania* to the species level. This information is important in decisions about therapy because responses to treatment can vary with the species. Isoenzyme profiling is used to determine species for research purposes.

TREATMENT

Cutaneous Leishmaniasis

Although lesions heal spontaneously in the majority of cases, their spread or persistence indicates that treatment may be needed. One or a few small lesions due to "self-healing species" can be treated with topical agents. Systemic treatment is required for lesions over the face, hands, or joints; multiple lesions; large ulcers; lymphatic spread; New World CL with the potential for development of ML; and CL in HIV-co-infected patients.

A pentavalent antimonial is the first-line drug for all forms of CL and is used in a dose of 20 mg/kg for 20 days. The exceptions to this rule are CL caused by *Leishmania (Viannia) guyanensis*, for which pentamidine isethionate is the drug of choice (two injections of 4 mg of salt/kg separated by a 48-h interval), and CL due to *L. aethiopica*, which responds to paromomycin (16 mg/kg daily) but not to antimonials. Relapses usually respond to a second course of treatment. In Peru, topical imiquimod (5–7.5%) plus parenteral antimonials have been shown to cure CL more rapidly than antimonials alone. Azoles and triazoles have been used with mixed responses in both Old and New World CL but have not been adequately assessed for this indication in clinical trials. In *L. major* infection, oral fluconazole (200 mg/d for 6 weeks) resulted in a higher rate of cure than placebo (79% vs 34%) and also cured infection faster. Adverse effects include gastrointestinal symptoms and hepatotoxicity. Ketoconazole (600 mg/d for 28 days) is 76–90% effective in CL due to *L. (V.) panamensis* and *L. mexicana* in Panama and Guatemala. Miltefosine has been used in CL in doses of 2.5 mg/kg for 28 days. This agent is effective against *L. major* infections. In Colombia, where CL is due to *L. (V.) panamensis*, miltefosine was also effective, with a cure rate of 91%. For *L. (V.) braziliensis* infections, however, the results with miltefosine are less consistent. In Brazil, miltefosine cured 71% of patients with *L. (V.) guyanensis* infection. Other drugs, such as dapsone, allopurinol, rifampin, azithromycin, and pentoxifylline, have been used either alone or in combinations, but most of the relevant studies have had design limitations that preclude meaningful conclusions.

Small lesions (≤3 cm in diameter) may conveniently be treated weekly until cure with an intralesional injection of a pentavalent antimonial at a dose adequate to blanch the lesion (0.2–2.0 mL). An ointment containing 15% paromomycin sulfate, either alone or with 0.5% gentamicin or 12% methylbenzonium chloride, cured 70–82% of lesions due to *L. major* in 20 days and may be suitable for lesions caused by other species. Heat therapy with an FDA-approved radiofrequency generator and cryotherapy with liquid nitrogen have also been used successfully.

Diffuse Cutaneous Leishmaniasis (DCL) DCL is a rare form of leishmaniasis caused by *L. amazonensis* and *L. mexicana* in South and Central America and by *L. aethiopica* in Ethiopia and Kenya. DCL is characterized by the lack of a cell-mediated immune response to the parasite, the uncontrolled multiplication of which thus continues unabated. The DTH response does not develop, and lymphocytes do not respond to leishmanial antigens in vitro. DCL patients have a polarized immune response with high levels of immunosuppressive cytokines, including IL-10, transforming growth factor (TGF) β, and IL-4, and low concentrations of IFN-γ. Profound immunosuppression leads to widespread cutaneous disease. Lesions may initially be confined to the face or a limb but spread over months or years to other areas of the skin. They may be symmetrically or asymmetrically distributed and include papules, nodules, plaques, and areas of diffuse infiltration. These lesions do not ulcerate. The overlying skin is usually erythematous in pale-skinned patients. The lesions are teeming with parasites, which are therefore easy to recover. DCL does not heal spontaneously and is difficult to treat. If relapse and drug resistance are to be prevented, treatment should be continued for some time after lesions have healed and parasites can no longer be isolated. In the New World, repeated 20-day courses of pentavalent antimonials are given, with an intervening drug-free period of 10 days. Miltefosine has been used for several months with a good initial response. Combinations should be tried. In Ethiopia, a combination of paromomycin (14 mg/kg per day) and sodium stibogluconate (10 mg/kg per day) is effective.

■ MUCOSAL LEISHMANIASIS

The subgenus *Viannia* is widespread from the Amazon basin to Paraguay and Costa Rica and is responsible for deep sores and for ML (Table 226-1). In *L. (V.) braziliensis* infections, cutaneous lesions may be simultaneously accompanied by mucosal spread of the disease or followed by spread years later. ML is typically caused by *L. (V.) braziliensis* and rarely by *L. amazonensis*, *L. (V.) guyanensis*, and *L. (V.) panamensis*. Young men with chronic lesions of CL are at particular risk. Overall, ~3% of infected persons develop ML. Not every patient with ML has a history of prior CL. ML is almost entirely confined to the Americas. In rare cases, ML may also be caused by Old World species like *L. major*, *L. infantum* (*L. chagasi*), or *L. donovani*.

Immunopathogenesis and Clinical Features The immune response is polarized toward a T_H1 response, with marked increases of IFN-γ and TNF-α and varying levels of T_H2 cytokines (IL-10 and TGF-β). Patients have a stronger DTH response with ML than with CL, and their peripheral-blood mononuclear cells respond strongly to leishmanial antigens. The parasite spreads via the lymphatics or the bloodstream to mucosal tissues of the upper respiratory tract. Intense inflammation leads to destruction, and severe disability ensues.

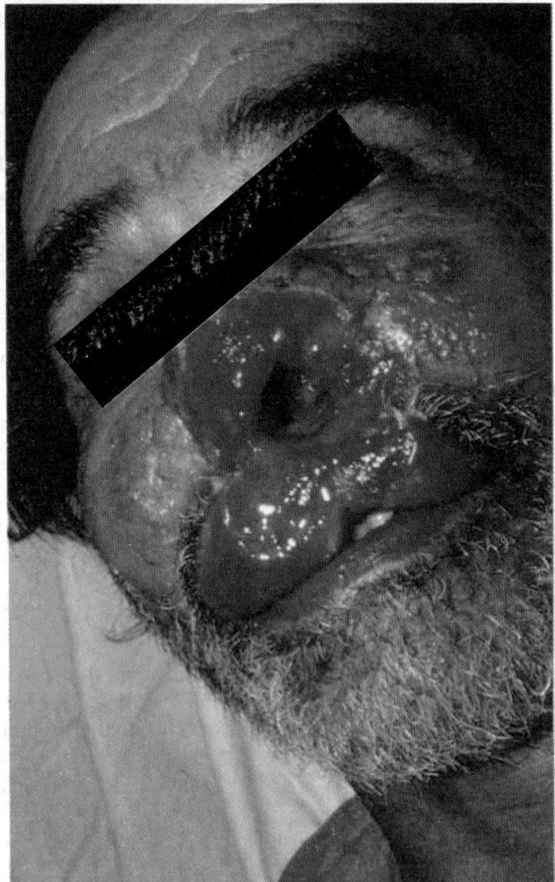

FIGURE 226-6 Mucosal leishmaniasis in a Brazilian patient. There is extensive inflammation around the nose and mouth, destruction of the nasal mucosa, ulceration of the upper lip and nose, and destruction of the nasal septum. *(Courtesy of R. Dietz, Universidade Federal do Espírito Santo, Vitória, Brazil.)*

Lesions in or around the nose or mouth (espundia; **Fig. 226-6**) are the typical presentation of ML. Patients usually provide a history of self-healed CL preceding ML by 1–5 years. Typically, ML presents as nasal stuffiness and bleeding followed by destruction of nasal cartilage, perforation of the nasal septum, and collapse of the nasal bridge. Subsequent involvement of the pharynx and larynx leads to difficulty in swallowing and phonation. The lips, cheeks, and soft palate may also be affected. Secondary bacterial infection is common, and aspiration pneumonia may be fatal. Despite the high degree of T_H1 immunity and the strong DTH response, ML does not heal spontaneously.

Laboratory Diagnosis Tissue biopsy is essential for identification of parasites, but the rate of detection is poor unless PCR techniques are used. The strongly positive DTH response fails to distinguish between past and present infection.

TREATMENT

Mucosal Leishmaniasis

The regimen of choice is a pentavalent antimonial agent administered at a dose of 20 mg of Sb^V/kg for 30 days. Patients with ML require long-term follow-up with repeated oropharyngeal and nasal examination. With failure of therapy or relapse, patients may receive another course of an antimonial but then become unresponsive, presumably because of resistance in the parasite. In this situation, AmB should be used. An AmB deoxycholate dose totaling 25–45 mg/kg is appropriate. There are no controlled trials of LAmB, but administration of 2–3 mg/kg for 20 days is considered adequate. Miltefosine (2.5 mg/kg for 28 days) cured 71% of ML patients in Bolivia. The more extensive the disease, the worse is the prognosis; thus, prompt, effective treatment and regular follow-up are essential.

PREVENTION OF LEISHMANIASIS

No vaccine is available for any form of leishmaniasis, although several candidates are in early phases of development. Inoculation with live *L. major* ("leishmanization") is practiced in Iran; 80% of recipients were protected, according to one report. Anthroponotic leishmaniasis is controlled by case finding, treatment, and vector control with insecticide-impregnated bed nets and curtains and residual insecticide spraying. Control of zoonotic leishmaniasis is more difficult. Use of insecticide-impregnated collars for dogs, treatment of infected domestic dogs, and culling of street dogs are measures that have been used with uncertain efficacy to prevent transmission of *L. infantum*. In Brazil, canine vaccines have been found to promote a decrease in the human and canine incidence of zoonotic VL. Two vaccines, Leishmune and Leish-Tec, are licensed in Brazil; Leishmune provides significant protection to vaccinated dogs. CaniLeish and LetiFend are the two licensed canine vaccines approved for use in Europe. Personal prophylaxis with bed nets and repellants may reduce the risk of CL infections in the New World.

FURTHER READING

Aronson NE, Joya CA: Cutaneous leishmaniasis: Updates in diagnosis and management. Infect Dis Clin North Am 33:101, 2019.

Burza S et al: Leishmaniasis. Lancet 392:951, 2018.

Chakravarty J, Sundar S: Current and emerging medications for the treatment of leishmaniasis. Expert Opin Pharmacother 10:1251, 2019.

Monge-Maillo B, López-Vélez R: Treatment options for visceral leishmaniasis and HIV coinfection. AIDS Rev 18:32, 2016.

van Griensven J, Diro E: Visceral leishmaniasis: Recent advances in diagnostics and treatment regimens. Infect Dis Clin North Am 33:79, 2019.

227 Chagas Disease and African Trypanosomiasis

François Chappuis, Yves Jackson

Myriads of protozoan parasites of the genus *Trypanosoma* infect plants and animals worldwide. Among these, three are of clinical significance for humans: *T. cruzi* causes Chagas disease, and *T. brucei gambiense* and *T. brucei rhodesiense* cause human African trypanosomiasis (HAT), which is also known as "sleeping sickness." Despite obvious differences in their geographic distribution, parasitic life cycle, clinical presentation, treatment, and outcome, these vector-borne diseases are archetypal examples of neglected tropical diseases. More broadly, these infectious diseases affect neglected populations of the lowest socioeconomic class who have limited access to care and who live either in remote rural areas of low- or middle-income tropical/subtropical countries or in urban areas of both endemic and nonendemic countries. The drugs to treat these conditions are several decades old, their availability is limited, and their efficacy and/or safety is suboptimal.

Other trypanosome species (e.g., *T. congolense* and *T. evansi*) predominantly cause nonhuman zoonoses and only occasionally cause illness in humans.

CHAGAS DISEASE (AMERICAN TRYPANOSOMIASIS)

DEFINITION

First described in 1909 by Carlos Chagas, Chagas disease (American trypanosomiasis) is a zoonosis caused by the flagellated protozoan *T. cruzi*. After a frequently asymptomatic acute phase, 30–40% of patients develop life-threatening chronic cardiomyopathy and/or digestive tract dysfunction over the course of decades. Acute reactivation may occur in immunocompromised patients. Chagas disease imposes an important human and social burden in Latin America and has recently spread outside its natural boundaries to become a global public health problem. A vast majority of affected individuals are unaware of being infected and do not have access to appropriate clinical management and counseling.

TRANSMISSION

Vectorial Transmission *T. cruzi* infection is primarily a zoonosis transmitted to a range of wild and domestic mammals by blood-sucking triatomine bugs. Sylvatic, peridomiciliary, and intradomiciliary vectorial cycles sometimes overlap. Over a large geographic area in the Americas (from northern Argentina to the southern United States), most human infections are intradomiciliary, arising from a triatomine bite during nighttime sleep. Feces released by triatomines during a blood meal contain the infective metacyclic form of *T. cruzi* that enters the human body through cutaneous breaks, mucosae, or conjunctivae. Despite recent laboratory research showing the potential for transmission by bedbugs, there is no evidence that bedbugs actually transmit *T. cruzi* to humans.

Nonvectorial Transmission Other modes of transmission can cause infection in both endemic and nonendemic regions. *T. cruzi* can be transmitted congenitally from mother to newborn, by transfusion of blood products, by tissue or organ transplantation, or by ingestion of contaminated food or drink. Congenital infection occurs in 1–10% of newborns of infected mothers. The risk of infection from contaminated blood products is low (1.7% overall, 13% for platelet recipients, and close to 0 for recipients of red blood cells and plasma). Transmission by infected organ and tissue transplants mostly affects heart, liver, and kidney recipients. Oral transmission is increasingly reported after ingestion of contaminated food (berries) or drinks (fruit or sugar cane juice) and occasionally causes outbreaks.

EPIDEMIOLOGY

An estimated 6 million people are infected by *T. cruzi*, including >1 million individuals with chronic cardiomyopathy. However, the true global burden of Chagas disease is in fact uncertain. The highest numbers of infected individuals reside in Argentina, Brazil, and Mexico; the prevalence is highest in Bolivia (6.1%), Argentina (3.6%), and Paraguay (2.1%). In highly endemic regions of these countries, the prevalence may exceed 40%. Formerly restricted to poor rural populations, the distribution of cases—and, to some extent, *T. cruzi* transmission—has progressively extended to cities in the context of rapid urbanization and rural migration. A recent history of migration from a rural area is the main risk factor in urban settings.

Overall, the prevalence and incidence of Chagas disease have sharply declined in recent decades because of improved housing and socioeconomic conditions as well as public health interventions, including regional vector-control initiatives, implementation of systematic screening of blood products, and improved detection of congenital transmission. Several countries have been declared free of domiciliary transmission as a result of sustained residual insecticide-spraying campaigns. This progress is threatened by adaptation of the vector to the periurban environment, its resurgence in areas where spraying has been discontinued, the development of resistance to pyrethroid insecticides, and the persistence of peridomiciliary transmission. A growing number of localized outbreaks are being reported in previously stable areas, with the Amazon basin particularly at risk.

Chagas disease distribution has recently expanded to nonendemic countries in the context of increased global travel, with cases reported more frequently in North America, Western Europe, Australia, and Japan. The United States harbors up to 300,000 cases, mostly among immigrants from Central America. In addition, sporadic vector-borne infections occur in the southern states. Western Europe has 68,000–123,000 cases, and Japan and Australia report a few thousand cases. Despite the implementation of blood bank screening and of some dedicated medical programs, only a small proportion of cases have been identified and properly managed to date. A low level of awareness among health care professionals and difficulties experienced by some groups in accessing care appear to be major drivers. At-risk migrant communities are frequently subject to factors that render them socially, legally, or economically vulnerable. Moreover, the cultural perception of Chagas as a disease embedded in poverty can create a social stigma that complicates its management at the community level. In contrast to immigrants, international tourists visiting endemic countries are at very low risk of being infected, whether by reduviid bug bites or by other routes, and reports of Chagas disease in travelers are rare.

PATHOLOGY

Several *T. cruzi* strains have been identified. These strains have partially overlapping transmission cycles and geographic distributions, but no definitive evidence supports an association of certain strains with specific clinical manifestations or with variation in disease severity. The rarity of digestive tract involvement north of the Amazon basin suggests that specific parasitic and host genetic factors may influence the disease course. The pathogenesis of Chagas disease results from the complex interactions between the pathogen and the host immune response. Many questions about the relative importance of these interactions, including the role of autoimmune mechanisms, remain unanswered. After local penetration of trypomastigotes, parasites rapidly enter the bloodstream and disseminate through the body, infecting a wide range of nucleated cells in which they differentiate into amastigotes (**Fig. 227-1**). The innate immune response triggered by parasite mucins and DNA leads to a predominantly T helper 1 response. The production of various proinflammatory cytokines and the activation of CD8+ T lymphocytes reduce parasitemia to a subpatent level within 4–8 weeks, a point marking the end of the acute phase.

Immune evasion mechanisms allow persistent low-intensity proliferation of amastigotes and their release into the bloodstream, with subsequent infection of potentially all types of nucleated cells—notably cardiac, skeletal, and smooth-muscle cells. Mechanisms that have been postulated to determine the pathogenic evolution toward cardiomyopathy include the parasites' persistence and the host's inability to downregulate the initial immune response, resulting in cell-mediated damage and an imbalance of T helper 1 and 2 responses with excessive production of proinflammatory cytokines. Secondary mechanisms, such as microcirculation abnormalities and dysautonomia, may also influence the progression of tissue damage.

In the myocardium, chronic inflammation results in cellular destruction and the development of fibrosis leading to a segmental loss of contractility and dilatation of the chambers, with the associated risk of left ventricle apical aneurism. Focal hypoperfusion and tissue damage are sources of ventricular arrhythmias, while scarring lesions mostly affect the conduction system. Autonomic cell destruction leads

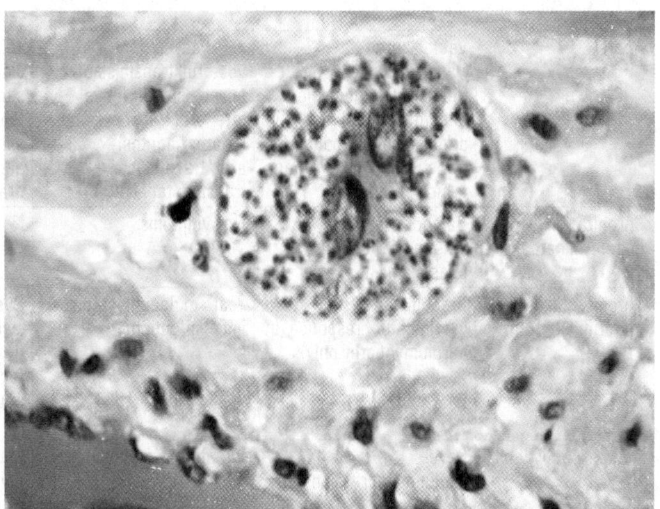

FIGURE 227-1 A cluster of *Trypanosoma cruzi* amastigotes with an inflammatory infiltrate in the placenta of a congenitally infected newborn infant.

to vagal and sympathetic denervation whose exact clinical significance remains to be clarified.

T. cruzi appears to have a direct toxic effect on digestive tract intramural autonomic ganglion cells. Over time, the loss of neural cells affects muscular tone, leading to motility disorders and ultimately to organ dilatation (megaviscera syndrome). The esophagus and colon are primarily affected, but lesions may occur along the whole digestive tract. Inadequate relaxation of the lower esophageal sphincter causes symptoms of achalasia, whereas damage to the colon ultimately mimics Hirschsprung's disease, with severe constipation and the risk of volvulus and toxic dilatation.

Factors reducing the cellular immune response, such as HIV infection, posttransplantation immunosuppressive therapies, or hematologic malignancies, may increase intracellular replication of amastigotes, with increased parasitemia (reactivation). Lesions develop predominantly in the central nervous system (CNS), the heart, and the skin. Among HIV-positive patients, the risk of reactivation is ~20% in the absence of antiretroviral therapies and occurs when the CD4+ T cell count falls to <100/μL. Clinically manifest *T. cruzi* reactivation is an AIDS-defining opportunistic infection.

CLINICAL MANIFESTATIONS

The clinical manifestations of *T. cruzi* infection vary greatly among individuals. The infection course is divided into two phases that are associated with different clinical features, duration, and prognosis (**Table 227-1**). The acute phase remains undetected and undiagnosed in most individuals. While 5–10% of these early infections spontaneously resolve without treatment, *T. cruzi* persists for life in the vast majority of individuals (the chronic phase); 60–70% of these individuals never develop apparent tissue damage (the indeterminate form), but the remaining 30–40% progress toward detectable organ damage of variable severity over decades (the determinate form). These chronic complications include cardiac (20–30%), digestive (5–20%), or mixed (5–10%) disorders. There is no predictor of evolution toward clinical manifestations during the chronic phase. In patients with cardiomyopathy, bundle branch blocks are usually the first signs and may cause no symptoms for years until more severe conduction system disease, arrhythmias, and left ventricular dysfunction occur. Advanced cardiac damage entails a worse prognosis than other cardiomyopathies—notably, ischemic heart disease.

APPROACH TO THE PATIENT

Chagas Disease (American Trypanosomiasis)

More than 90% of infections go undiagnosed, and cases are frequently identified at a late stage once chronic complications develop. The vast majority of *T. cruzi*–infected individuals are asymptomatic (i.e., in the indeterminate form of the chronic phase). An awareness of potential Chagas disease is important for general practitioners as well as for physicians from various specialties, including gastroenterologists, cardiologists, neurologists, obstetricians, pediatricians, and infectious disease specialists. Outside endemic areas, screening for Chagas disease should be proposed when any Latin American individual has evocative symptoms and signs, including abnormalities on electrocardiography (ECG) or increased risk of (1) *T. cruzi* infection (Chagas disease in the mother or other family members; origins in a highly endemic country or area; history of unscreened blood transfusion in Latin America); (2) transmission to others (e.g., via pregnancy or blood or organ donation); or (3) reactivation (current or pending immunosuppression). Screening of the relatives of an index case will probably identify additional cases.

DIAGNOSIS AND STAGING

Diagnostic Confirmation Diagnostic strategies depend on the clinical phase (**Table 227-2**). Detection of circulating parasites by microscopy of the blood with concentration (e.g., by the Strout method, microhematocrit) or by nucleic acid–based assay (polymerase chain reaction [PCR]) is the best diagnostic approach when the parasitemia level is high—i.e., during the acute phases, including reactivation. Once parasitemia becomes undetectable by microscopy (a point marking the end of the acute phase), diagnosis relies on immunologic tests that detect anti–*T. cruzi* IgG. The most common techniques include a conventional or recombinant enzyme-linked immunosorbent assay (ELISA) and immunofluorescence assays. Two positive serologic tests using different techniques and targeting different antigens confirm the diagnosis of Chagas disease during the chronic phase. In the presence of discordant serologic results, a third serologic test is warranted. Some of the immunochromatographic rapid diagnostic tests on the market have sufficient sensitivity and specificity to be used as first-line

TABLE 227-1 Characteristics of the Stages of *Trypanosoma cruzi* Infection

PHASE OR SETTING	CONTEXT	ONSET OF FIRST SYMPTOMS	CLINICAL MANIFESTATIONS	DURATION	PROGNOSIS
Acute (congenital)	~5% risk of maternal transmission to newborn	At birth or weeks after delivery	>90% asymptomatic; rare lymphadenopathy, hepatosplenomegaly, jaundice, respiratory distress, growth retardation	2–8 weeks	Favorable when infant is born alive; unknown rate of in utero or neonatal death
Acute	Vector-borne transmission; oral transmission (ingestion of contaminated food/drinks); blood product transfusion; tissue/organ transplantation	1–2 weeks after vectorial transmission; may be sooner (days) after oral transmission or later (months) after transfusion/transplantation	>90% asymptomatic or mild febrile illness; local swelling at inoculation site (eyelid [Romaña sign] or skin [chagoma]); polyadenopathy; splenomegaly; myocarditis, hepatitis, and encephalitis more frequent with oral transmission	4–8 weeks	Mortality: 0.1–5% with oral transmission or myocarditis/encephalitis
Chronic (indeterminate form)	Balanced immune response after acute phase subsides	No symptoms	Normal clinical examination and ECG result	Lifelong or until determinate phase	No attributable mortality
Chronic (determinate form)	Predominant inflammatory response (in cardiomyopathy only)	Years to decades after initial infection	Dyspnea, chest pain, palpitation, syncope, sudden death, stroke, dysphagia, regurgitation, constipation, fecaloma, volvulus, peripheral neuropathy	Chronic	5-year mortality: 2–63%, depending on extent of cardiac damage; most important causes of death: cardiac failure and sudden death, followed by stroke
Acute (reactivation)	Severe immunosuppression	Variable	Myocarditis, erythema nodosum, panniculitis, *Toxoplasma*-like focal brain lesion, meningoencephalitis	Variable	Mortality depends on rapidity of diagnosis and treatment and on underlying conditions

Abbreviation: ECG, electrocardiography.

TABLE 227-2 Diagnostic Procedures of Choice for Clinical Stages of *T. cruzi* Infection

STAGE	TECHNIQUE OF CHOICE	SAMPLE	DIAGNOSTIC CRITERIA
Acute	Microscopy after concentration, PCR	Peripheral blood, cerebrospinal or other body fluids	Positivity in one test
Acute (early congenital during first 9 months of life)	Microscopy after concentration, PCR	Cord or peripheral blood	Positivity in one test
Chronic (indeterminate and determinate forms)	Serology	Peripheral blood	Positivity in two tests with different techniques and antigens
Reactivation	Microscopy after concentration, PCR	Peripheral blood, cerebrospinal or other body fluids	Positivity with evidence of increasing parasitemia on serial samples or extremely high parasite load

Abbreviation: PCR, polymerase chain reaction.

screening tests where laboratory facilities are not easily accessible. If the rapid diagnostic test result is positive, at least one conventional serologic assay is necessary to confirm infection.

Diagnosis of congenital infection relies on examination of cord and/or peripheral blood by microscopy or PCR during the first days or weeks of life. A test conducted after 4 weeks of age is most accurate: PCR earlier in life may be falsely positive, likely because of the passage of *T. cruzi* DNA fragments from the mother to the child. If results are negative, serologic tests should be performed at 9 months of age, once maternal antibodies have been cleared.

During the chronic phase, the limited sensitivity (50–80%) of PCR restricts its usefulness for primary diagnosis; however, PCR can document therapeutic failure if it yields positive results after the completion of treatment. In the United States, the Centers for Disease Control and Prevention (CDC) provides reference laboratory testing (see contact information in the treatment section).

Disease Staging Once *T. cruzi* infection is confirmed, clinicians should assess the presence of complications and concomitant factors that may influence the course of the disease. The initial evaluation includes a thorough cardiac, neurologic, and digestive history and a clinical examination. Twelve-lead ECG with a 30-s strip is a good screening test for Chagas-associated cardiomyopathy. The most frequently found abnormalities are right bundle branch block, left anterior fascicular block, ventricular premature beats, repolarization disorders, Q waves, and low QRS voltage (**Fig. 227-2**). An abnormal ECG result or the presence of suggestive cardiac symptoms warrants further investigation. Echocardiography and the 24-h Holter test are the preferred methods for assessment of chamber dilatation, apical aneurysm, ventricular dysfunction, and arrhythmias. Depending on the findings, the workup can be supplemented by MRI or electrophysiologic studies. Gastroenterologic investigations are performed in patients with suggestive symptoms, such as dysphagia and severe constipation. Barium esophagraphy and enema are first-line diagnostic procedures, which can be supplemented by esophageal manometry. Megacolon is diagnosed when the sigmoid or descending colon diameter is ≥6.5 cm.

Comorbidities, including other cardiovascular risk factors, immunosuppressive conditions, and other chronic infections (e.g., with *Strongyloides stercoralis* or HIV) should be investigated.

TREATMENT

Chagas Disease (American Trypanosomiasis)

ETIOLOGIC TREATMENT

Only two drugs, benznidazole and nifurtimox (**Table 227-3**), have shown persistent efficacy against *T. cruzi* infection when administered for ≥30 days. While these drugs have been used since the early 1970s, many questions remain about their mode of action and efficacy at the different stages of infection. The treatment goal depends on the clinical stage; the overall objectives are to cure patients who

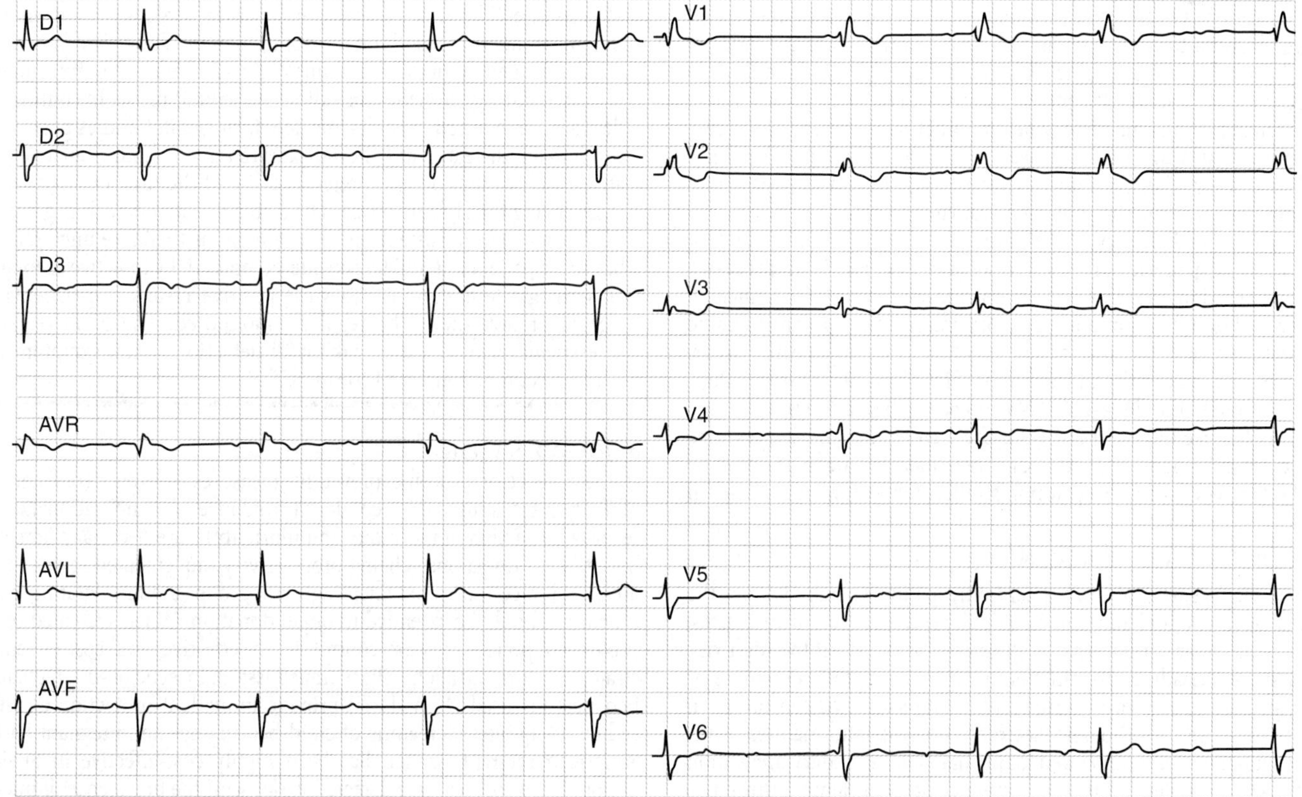

FIGURE 227-2 Electrocardiogram of a 43-year-old patient shows bradycardia with high-grade atrioventricular blocks.

TABLE 227-3 Chagas Treatment Regimens and Adverse Reactions to Benznidazole and Nifurtimox

DRUG	REGIMEN	DURATION	ADVERSE EVENTS IN ADULTS (FREQUENCY)	PREMATURE DISCONTINUATION (RATE)
Benznidazole	Age <12 years: 5–7.5 mg/kg per day in 2 doses Age >12 years: 5 mg/kg per day in 2 doses	30–60 days	Allergic dermatitis (29–50%), anorexia and weight loss (5–40%), paresthesia (0–30%), peripheral neuropathy (0–30%), nausea and vomiting (0–5%), leukopenia and thrombocytopenia (<1%)	7–20%
Nifurtimox	Age <10 years: 15–20 mg/kg per day in 3 or 4 doses Age 11–16 years: 12.5–15 mg/kg per day in 3 or 4 doses Age >16 years: 8–10 mg/kg per day in 3 or 4 doses	60–90 days	Anorexia and weight loss (50–81%), nausea and vomiting (15–50%), abdominal discomfort (12–40%), headaches (13–70%), dizziness and vertigo (12–33%), anxiety and depression (10–49%), insomnia (10–54%), myalgia (13–30%), peripheral neuropathy (2–5%), memory loss (6–14%), leukopenia (<1%)	6–44%

Source: From C Bern: Chagas' Disease. N Engl J Med 373:456, 2015. Copyright © 2015 Massachusetts Medical Society. Reprinted with permission from Massachusetts Medical Society.

have recent infection or reactivation, to reduce morbidity, and to prevent transmission at later stages. Treatment is most effective during the acute (including congenital) phase and the early chronic phase (i.e., in patients <18 years of age), with a 60–100% cure rate. The efficacy of treatment during the indeterminate form of the chronic phase in patients >18 years old is not known; however, treatment may protect against the development of cardiac damage later in life and eliminate the risk of vertical transmission when given before conception. In adults with chronic cardiomyopathy, benznidazole has no impact on disease progression and mortality risk. Neither benznidazole nor nifurtimox is effective against digestive complications. Treatment is contraindicated during pregnancy and in advanced renal or hepatic failure. Preferred regimens and drug tolerance vary with age. Adverse events are more frequent among adults, who are therefore at increased risk of premature treatment discontinuation (Table 227-3). As benznidazole seems better tolerated than nifurtimox in adults, it is the recommended first-line drug in this age range. Close (e.g., weekly) clinical and biological monitoring is necessary during treatment. While treatment is usually prescribed for 60 days, the optimal duration remains a matter of debate, with a growing interest in shorter courses.

Treatment should be undertaken for all children, women of child-bearing age, patients in the acute phase, and patients with reactivation. Given the uncertainties about the impact of treatment, the decision to treat patients >18 years old who have the indeterminate form of the chronic phase should be made on an individual basis after discussing the pros and cons with the patient. A negative pregnancy test is mandatory before initiating treatment as the recommended drugs have not been proven to be safe in pregnancy. The efficacy of second-line treatment (e.g., nifurtimox after failure with benznidazole) has not been evaluated to date.

The limited efficacy of current regimens and the understanding that living parasites are a driver of immunopathologic processes have fueled interest in novel therapeutic approaches. These include the addition of immunomodulatory interventions to antiparasitic treatment and the use of combinations of antiparasitic drugs. Drugs can be obtained through the CDC (Parasitic Diseases Public Inquiries line [404-718-4745] or parasites@cdc.gov), the CDC Drug Service (404-639-3670), or the CDC Emergency Operations Center (770-488-7100). In 2017, benznidazole was approved by the U.S. Food and Drug Administration for treatment of children 2–12 years of age.

NONETIOLOGIC TREATMENT

The management of Chagas cardiomyopathy generally follows the management guidelines for heart failure, conduction disturbances, or ventricular arrhythmia of other etiologies. Given the high risk of sudden death, early initiation of treatment with amiodarone or implantation of a cardioverter defibrillator should be considered in the presence of pathologic electrophysiologic abnormalities. Anticoagulation is recommended for primary and secondary prevention of cardioembolic events in the presence of an intramural thrombus or apical aneurysm. Strict control of other cardiovascular risk factors is warranted. Chagas cardiomyopathy is a prominent indication for heart transplantation in Latin America; some evidence indicates that the results are better than in cardiomyopathy of other etiologies. Posttransplantation immunosuppression requires close monitoring, given the high risk of reactivation.

Treatment of digestive dysmotility includes dietary counseling and meals rich in fiber and hydration, with smaller portions eaten more frequently. Drugs releasing the lower esophageal sphincter (e.g., nifedipine or isosorbide dinitrate before meals), pneumatic balloon dilatation, or laparoscopic myotomy improves upper gastrointestinal symptoms in the early stage. Use of botulinum toxin is effective but requires repeated injections. Laxatives and enemas alleviate chronic constipation in most patients. Surgery is indicated in patients with distressing symptoms that are refractory to medical treatment.

CLINICAL FOLLOW-UP

Defining the optimal cure after treatment remains very challenging and is a crucial topic of research. While the search for biomarkers (including through proteomics) to identify early indicators of treatment response holds some promise, serologic follow-up remains the cornerstone of posttreatment monitoring in the acute phase. In the chronic phase, there is no assay of proven value for documentation of response. The time needed for negative seroconversion after treatment indeed depends on the duration of infection. The interval is short (usually months, sometimes up to 2 years) when infection is treated during the acute (including congenital) phase. In contrast, decades are required in adults infected during childhood. A positive result in a posttreatment PCR indicates treatment failure, but a negative result cannot be interpreted because of the low sensitivity of PCR during the chronic phase. The status of patients with negative PCR results but persistent positive serology is therefore uncertain, but these patients should be considered potentially infective as long as serologic tests continue to yield positive results. All patients, treated or not, should be regularly monitored. The basic yearly assessment includes history-taking for detection of new symptoms, clinical examination, and 12-lead ECG.

■ PREVENTION

In the absence of a vaccine, preventive measures—primary (prevention of *T. cruzi* transmission), secondary (avoidance of complications), and tertiary (reduction of morbidity and mortality)—are necessary. Screening of blood donations is being progressively implemented in endemic areas and in countries to which high-risk groups are immigrating, and screening should be extended to organ donation. When sustained over prolonged periods, vector control is an effective and cost-effective strategy to curb intradomiciliary transmission. Insecticide-impregnated bed nets (as used for malaria) provide individual protection against reduviid bug bites. Screening of child-bearing-age and pregnant Latin American migrant women has been highly cost-effective in Spain, although the cost per case detected varies with the prevalence of infection in the targeted population. Early identification of cases through passive and active screening of the population at risk, along with provision of treatment, may reduce the risk of complications and secondary transmission, particularly congenital transmission. Finally, identification and treatment of cardiac complications and prevention of cardioembolic events at an early stage positively influence the disease course.

■ GLOBAL CONSIDERATIONS

With its geographic expansion, Chagas disease has become a global health issue, predominantly affecting vulnerable people on four continents. Yet, as with other neglected tropical diseases, progress against Chagas is limited by a lack of research and development and a lack of financial and political commitment. For example, the production and registration of existing drugs, and access to them, are still problematic in many countries, including the United States. Difficulties in research on and development of new drugs are compounded by the lack of financial incentives. The future of Chagas disease is likely to be influenced by global phenomena. Climatic changes, population aging, increasing prevalence of noncommunicable comorbidities (e.g., diabetes, hypertension) in low- and middle-income countries, and increasing use of immunosuppressive drugs are likely to impact the epidemiology, clinical course, and burden of Chagas disease. To tackle these challenges, clinical, public health, and policy interventions need to be scaled up and improved in areas of high or hidden prevalence (e.g., in the Chaco Region of Argentina, Bolivia, and Paraguay and in Mexico, Western Europe, and the United States, respectively).

HUMAN AFRICAN TRYPANOSOMIASIS (SLEEPING SICKNESS)

■ DEFINITION

HAT is a life-threatening illness caused by infection with extracellular protozoan parasites that are transmitted by tsetse flies in sub-Saharan Africa. *T. b. gambiense* and *T. b. rhodesiense* are the two pathogenic subspecies affecting humans; their epidemiologic and clinical features largely differ.

■ EPIDEMIOLOGY

The geographic range of HAT is restricted to sub-Saharan Africa in line with the distribution of its vector, the tsetse fly (*Glossina* species; Fig. 227-3). HAT due to *T. b. gambiense* is endemic in 24 countries of western and central Africa. Between 1999 and 2018, the number of reported cases fell by 97% (from 27,862 to 953) as a result of successful control measures based on systematic screening of populations at risk, diagnostic confirmation, and treatment of infected individuals. During the same period, the number of reported cases of HAT due to *T. b. rhodesiense* fell by 96% (from 619 to 24) in the 10 disease-endemic countries of eastern and southeastern Africa. However, the ratio of reported to unreported cases remains uncertain for disease caused by both species. In 2018, most cases of *T. b. gambiense* HAT were reported by the Democratic Republic of the Congo (DRC; 69%), whereas Malawi and Uganda reported most of the cases caused by *T. b. rhodesiense* (63 and 17%, respectively). The geographic distributions of *T. b. gambiense* and *T. b. rhodesiense* do not overlap, but the two species are present in distinct regions of Uganda. A roadmap for HAT elimination as a public health problem by 2020 has been mapped out by the World Health Organization (WHO) with two primary indicators: the number of cases reported annually (target: <2000; reached since 2018) and the area at risk reporting ≥1 case/10,000 people/year (target: reduction of 90% by 2016–2020 compared to the 2000–2004 baseline). The next goal set by WHO is the global elimination of transmission by 2030.

Humans are the predominant or exclusive reservoir of *T. b. gambiense*. Rare cases of vertical (in utero) or transfusional transmission have been reported, but almost all patients are infected by the bite of tsetse flies during their daily activities along or near rivers, where the flies live and reproduce. In contrast, *T. b. rhodesiense* causes zoonosis in a variety of wild and domesticated animals (e.g., antelopes and cattle, respectively), which act as reservoirs. Humans are infected by *T. b. rhodesiense* via tsetse bites in woodland savannah. Honey gatherers, game park rangers, poachers, and firewood collectors are particularly at risk. Imported cases of HAT are occasionally diagnosed among African immigrants and other travelers. While long-term travelers (>30 days) are at increased risk of *T. b. gambiense* HAT, most imported

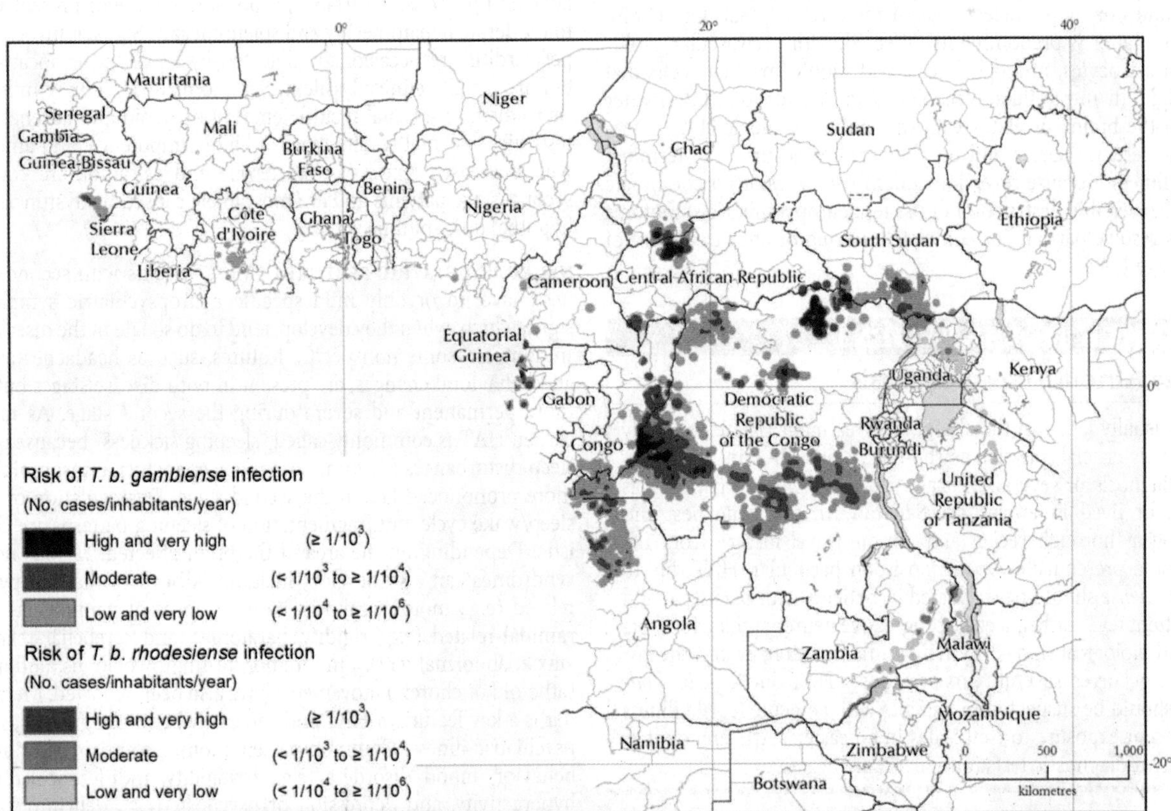

FIGURE 227-3 Areas at risk for human African trypanosomiasis, 2014–2018. *(Reproduced with permission from JR Franco et al: Monitoring the elimination of human African trypanosomiasis at continental and country level: Update to 2018. PLoS Negl Trop Dis 14:e0008261, 2020. © World Health Organization and Food and Agriculture Organization of the United Nations.)*

cases of *T. b. rhodesiense* HAT are seen in short-term travelers, typically following visits to game parks.

PATHOLOGY AND PATHOGENESIS

T. b. rhodesiense and *T. b. gambiense*, unlike other trypanosome species, can infect humans because they resist lytic factors in human serum—namely, apolipoprotein L-1 (*APOL1*). Human *APOL1* variants are prevalent in individuals of African ancestry, conferring protection against livestock trypanosome species, but at the cost of increasing the likelihood of chronic kidney disease. The serum resistance–associated protein is responsible for resistance in *T. b. rhodesiense*, whereas other mechanisms, notably involving the *T. b. gambiense*–specific glycoprotein (TgsGP) gene, are used by *T. b. gambiense.*

Trypanosomes are transmitted to humans by the tsetse bite, proliferate, and induce a local inflammatory reaction that is sometimes clinically apparent as a chancre. Trypanosomes then disseminate into the hematolymphatic system, with lymph nodes becoming enlarged after infiltration by mononuclear cells and lymphocytes. The degree of enlargement of the liver and spleen is usually mild to moderate, with infiltration by mononuclear cells as a prominent feature. Trypanosomes multiply in the blood, but their presence and density vary. This variation is mainly due to a cyclic immune-evasion process, whereby the parasite population can be decimated by the host's immune response until the reemergence of offspring parasites that express a different variant surface glycoprotein to which the immune system is temporarily blind. Each trypanosome genome encodes a repertoire of ~1000 variant surface glycoproteins between which the parasites can switch genetically. Trypanosomes also multiply in extravascular tissues during the first stage of illness. The skin, skeletal muscles, serous membranes (peritoneum, pleurae, and pericardium), and heart can be involved, with interstitial infiltration of mononuclear cells and vasculitis evident on microscopic examination. Myocarditis and pericarditis with myocardial degeneration and interstitial hemorrhage are common features of *T. b. rhodesiense* infection.

The CNS is invaded weeks to months (*T. b. rhodesiense*) or months to years (*T. b. gambiense*) after initial infection. This invasion corresponds to the second stage of HAT, which is defined by the presence of trypanosomes or mononuclear cells in the cerebrospinal fluid (CSF). The white matter is predominantly affected, with perivascular proliferation of astrocytes, microglial cells, and Mott's (morular) cells that contain IgM in intracellular vacuoles. The location of white-matter lesions in the brain correlates with the main neurologic clinical features. The cerebral cortex and neurons are spared until the terminal stages of illness. Because reversible inflammatory lesions predominate over the irreversible destruction of tissue, neuropsychiatric symptoms and signs resolve partially or completely during or after treatment of second-stage HAT.

APPROACH TO THE PATIENT

Human African Trypanosomiasis

HAT is usually lethal in the absence of treatment. Therefore, early diagnosis is crucial; physicians should include HAT in the differential diagnosis of several clinical syndromes when a patient has traveled or lived in at-risk sub-Saharan African countries, and obtaining a thorough recent and remote travel history from the patient is a prerequisite for diagnosis. In particular, HAT due to *T. b. gambiense* should be suspected in patients with persistent and intermittent fever or headaches, progressive neuropsychiatric disorders, and biological signs of systemic inflammation, even if the last exposure occurred several years previously. HAT due to *T. b. rhodesiense* should be suspected in patients with an acute febrile illness and a recent exposure to tsetse flies in an eastern African country, especially if diagnostic tests for malaria are negative.

CLINICAL MANIFESTATIONS

The clinical presentations of *T. b. gambiense* and *T. b. rhodesiense* HAT usually differ. *T. b. gambiense* HAT is a slowly evolving illness with a long incubation period (months to years) and a prolonged disease course. In contrast, *T. b. rhodesiense* HAT is an acute febrile illness with a short (<3-week) incubation period and a shorter (weeks to months) disease course. There are exceptions to this classical pattern. Acute forms of *T. b. gambiense* HAT have been reported, especially among travelers, and chronic forms of *T. b. rhodesiense* HAT occur in the southern range of its geographic distribution (e.g., Zambia and Malawi). Trypano-resistance (i.e., self-resolving first-stage infections) and trypano-tolerance (i.e., the long-term persistence of parasites [e.g., in the skin] without clinical features of disease) have been reported for *T. b. gambiense.* Concomitant HIV co-infection does not seem to predispose individuals to an increased risk of HAT, and the impact of the virus on the clinical presentation of HAT is not known.

T. b. gambiense The occurrence of trypanosomal chancre is reported in a sizeable proportion of travelers, but very rarely in patients living in endemic areas, where the nonpurulent, painful, and itchy nodule can easily be confused with the bite of another arthropod. The chancre spontaneously disappears in 1–3 weeks.

SYSTEMIC FEATURES After an asymptomatic incubation period that usually lasts for weeks or months but occasionally lasts for years, patients may present with irregular and remittent fever, sometimes accompanied by fatigue, malaise, and myalgia. Fever is more frequent among travelers than among natives, but the absence of fever in no way rules out the disease. Circinate or serpiginous rashes, commonly called trypanids, can occur on the trunk and on proximal parts of the extremities. Trypanids are almost impossible to detect on dark skin and have been reported only in Caucasians. Pruritus is a common but nonspecific symptom that affects up to half of patients during the second stage. Painless edema of the face and extremities occasionally occurs during the first phase.

Enlarged lymph nodes—a classical sign of HAT—are detected in 38–85% of patients at both disease stages. Cervical palpation is essential in patients with suspected HAT. The lateroposterior cervical group (Winterbottom sign) and the supraclavicular group are most commonly affected. Lymph nodes are movable, soft initially, harder later, and painless. A variable proportion of patients present with mild to moderate hepatomegaly and splenomegaly. Signs of myocarditis and pericarditis are occasionally detected by ECG and echocardiography but are usually clinically silent. Symptoms of HAT may mimic hypothyroidism or adrenal insufficiency, but thyroid and adrenal function tests yield normal results. Loss of libido, impotence, and amenorrhea, with decreased levels of testosterone and estradiol, are common in second-stage patients and are most likely caused by dysfunction of the hypothalamic–pituitary axis.

NEUROPSYCHIATRIC FEATURES Most patients with second-stage illness have no or only mild specific neuropsychiatric symptoms and signs, which, when they develop, tend to do so late in the disease course. In contrast, some nonspecific features, such as headaches and mood and behavioral changes, are present in both disease stages but become more permanent and severe during the second stage. As mentioned earlier, HAT is commonly called "sleeping sickness" because of various sleep disturbances (daytime somnolence, nocturnal insomnia) that are more pronounced late in the second stage. Dysregulation of the daily sleep/wake cycle and fragmentation of sleeping patterns are characteristic. Depending on the area of the brain affected, various neurologic syndromes can also develop, including disorders that are pyramidal-related (e.g., motor weakness, rare instances of hemiplegia), extrapyramidal-related (e.g., rigidity, paratonia), and cerebellar-related (e.g., ataxia, abnormal gait). Fine tremor, resting myoclonus, and abnormal (athetoid or choreic) movements have also been reported. Mental disorder is a key feature of HAT and can easily be misdiagnosed as primary psychiatric illness. Common presentations are antisocial or aggressive behavior, mood disorders (e.g., irritability, indifference), apathy or hyperactivity, and depression or psychosis (e.g., delirium, hallucinations). In the final stage of illness, decreased consciousness, dementia, and sometimes epilepsy are present, leading to coma, bed sores, aspiration pneumonia, or other bacterial infections and ultimately to death.

T. b. rhodesiense The clinical presentation of *T. b. rhodesiense* HAT can be similar to that of *T. b. gambiense* HAT in areas (e.g., Zambia, Malawi) that characteristically harbor specific parasite genotypes and host factors. The typical acute form with an incubation period of <3 weeks occurs in the northern range of the disease's distribution (e.g., Tanzania, Uganda) and in travelers. The initial trypanosomal chancre is clinically similar to that seen in *T. b. gambiense* HAT but is more common, especially among travelers.

SYSTEMIC FEATURES Fever can be high and occurs in both first- and second-stage patients, often in association with headaches and with diffuse myalgia and arthralgia. Pruritus and edema of the face and legs can be present. Lymphadenopathies have been reported in variable proportions in both disease stages and predominately affect the submandibular, axillary, and inguinal regions. Mild to moderate hepatomegaly and splenomegaly are documented in a minority of patients. Myocarditis and pericarditis appear to influence clinical course and outcome, even though clinical features of cardiac failure or arrhythmia have not been prominent findings in large case series. In contrast, conduction abnormalities, with various degrees of atrioventricular block, have been reported in travelers. Sepsis-like features, with disseminated intravascular coagulation and multiple-organ failure, can occur in the terminal stage.

NEUROPSYCHIATRIC FEATURES Neuropsychiatric symptoms and signs in *T. b. rhodesiense* HAT are reported with varying frequency but overall are similar to those described above for *T. b. gambiense* HAT. The notable exception in *T. b. rhodesiense* disease is a more rapid evolution toward coma and death.

DIAGNOSIS

The clinical and biological features of *T. b. gambiense* and *T. b. rhodesiense* HAT—anemia, thrombocytopenia, elevated levels of C-reactive protein and IgM—are not sufficiently specific, and current drug regimens are not sufficiently practical to allow the initiation of treatment solely on the basis of suspicion. Diagnostic confirmation is therefore mandatory in all patients.

T. b. gambiense The diagnosis of *T. b. gambiense* HAT is based on a three-step approach: screening, diagnostic confirmation, and staging.

SCREENING Immunologic (serologic) methods constitute the preferred screening tool. The card agglutination test for trypanosomiasis (CATT) has been used in most endemic areas for several decades. The test reagent contains stained, freeze-dried trypanosomes of selected variable-antigen types. If specific antibodies are present in the patient's blood or serum, agglutination can be seen with the naked eye. The sensitivity of the CATT on undiluted blood or serum is 69–100% (>90% in most studies), with some regional variation; its specificity is 84–99%. The CATT and associated equipment (e.g., a rotator) are manufactured and distributed by the Institute of Tropical Medicine in Antwerp, Belgium, but are not widely available outside endemic areas. In recent years, lateral flow tests have been developed and commercialized, first based on whole parasites and later on recombinant antigens. Their diagnostic performance appears similar to that of the CATT. Other serologic test formats (ELISA, immunofluorescence, indirect hemagglutination) are available in some reference laboratories in both endemic and nonendemic countries.

DIAGNOSTIC CONFIRMATION The microscopic observation of trypanosomes in the lymph, blood, or CSF confirms the diagnosis. Direct observation of motile trypanosomes on a wet preparation of lymph obtained by cervical lymph node puncture is simple and cheap but has limited sensitivity (50–65% in most studies). Trypanosomes can be found in the blood but often occur at low densities. Therefore, stained thin and thick blood smears have very low sensitivity. Sensitivity is improved (to 40–60% in most studies) with the microhematocrit centrifugation technique, which is based on microscopic examination of the buffy coat after centrifugation of four to six microhematocrit tubes. The most sensitive method (~90%) is the miniature anion-exchange centrifugation technique, which is based on the visualization of trypanosomes in eluate after the passage of a large volume (500 μL) of blood through an anion-exchange column and subsequent centrifugation.

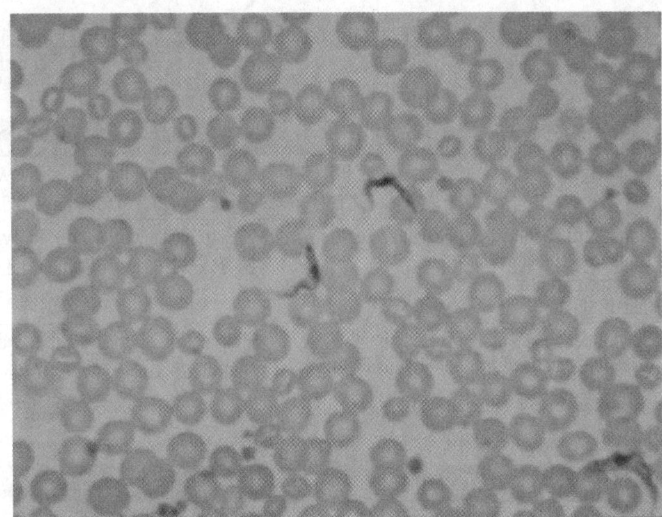

FIGURE 227-4 ***Trypanosoma brucei rhodesiense* in blood** (thin smear, Giemsa stain). *(Credit to the DPDx team, U.S. Centers for Disease Control and Prevention, Atlanta.)*

STAGING Staging is based on the examination of CSF obtained by lumbar puncture. Second-stage HAT is defined by the presence in CSF of a raised leukocyte count (>5/μL) and/or of trypanosomes. The latter can be detected in the cell-counting chamber or, preferably, after centrifugation of the CSF. Staging is no longer an obligatory step in settings where fexinidazole is used as first-line treatment for both first- and second-stage HAT patients, except for young children (<6 years or weighing <20 kg) and for patients with neuropsychiatric symptoms and signs consistent with severe HAT, i.e., mental confusion, abnormal behavior, logorrhea, anxiety, ataxia, tremor, motor weakness, speech impairment, abnormal gait or movements, or seizures (see "Treatment," below).

Several molecular methods based on PCR or loop-mediated isothermal amplification have been developed, mostly based on the detection of multiple-copy DNA targets of the Trypanozoon group (to which *T. brucei* belongs) or the single-copy TgsGP gene of *T. b. gambiense*. None of these methods have been fully validated for diagnostic purposes, and a positive result of their application to blood should be interpreted as suspected rather than confirmed HAT. Molecular methods applied to CSF (to detect biomarkers) have not proven more accurate than classical methods for staging and have yielded false-positive results in a substantial proportion of cases.

T. b. rhodesiense The diagnosis of *T. b. rhodesiense* HAT is usually simpler because parasites are more numerous in body fluids. They can occasionally be visualized in a chancre aspirate. In light of the lack of available serologic tests and the high sensitivity of parasite detection methods in blood, wet mounts, and thin/thick smears **(Fig. 227-4)**, the microhematocrit or other concentration techniques are used for both screening and confirmation. Because the modalities of treatment of *T. b. rhodesiense* are stage dependent, staging remains an obligatory step, and the definition and methods used are the same as for *T. b. gambiense* HAT.

TREATMENT
Human African Trypanosomiasis

The management of HAT is based on general supportive therapy (e.g., rehydration, pain management), treatment of concomitant infections (e.g., malaria, pneumonia), and antiparasitic treatment. The modalities of antitrypanosomal treatment depend on the *Trypanosoma* species, the stage of illness, and the presence of contraindications **(Table 227-4)**.

T. B. GAMBIENSE

Fexinidazole, a nitroimidazole compound, is the first effective oral treatment against HAT. It is administered with food for 10 days,

TABLE 227-4 Treatment of Human African Trypanosomiasis (HAT)

DISEASE AND STAGE	FIRST-LINE TREATMENT: DRUG(S) AND ROUTE	FIRST-LINE TREATMENT: DOSE AND DURATION	ALTERNATIVE TREATMENT
***T. b. gambiense* HAT**			
First stage	Fexinidazole PO	≥35 kg: 1800 mg for 4 days, followed by 1200 mg for 6 days 20–34 kg: 1200 mg for 4 days, followed by 600 mg for 6 days[a]	Pentamidine isethionate IM or IV[b]: 4 mg/kg per day for 7 days
Nonsevere second stage (6–99 leukocytes/μL in the cerebrospinal fluid [CSF])	Fexinidazole PO	≥35 kg: 1800 mg for 4 days, followed by 1200 mg for 6 days 20–34 kg: 1200 mg for 4 days, followed by 600 mg for 6 days[a]	Eflornithine: 200 mg/kg bid for 7 days *plus* Nifurtimox: 5 mg/kg tid for 10 days
Severe second stage (≥100 leukocytes/μL in the CSF)	Eflornithine IV + nifurtimox PO	Eflornithine: 200 mg/kg bid for 7 days Nifurtimox: 5 mg/kg tid for 10 days	Fexinidazole: ≥35 kg: 1800 mg for 4 days, followed by 1200 mg for 6 days 20–34 kg: 1200 mg for 4 days, followed by 600 mg for 6 days[a]
***T. b. rhodesiense* HAT**			
First stage	Suramin IV	4–5 mg/kg on day 1 followed by 5 weekly injections of 20 mg/kg (e.g., days 3, 10, 17, 24, 31)[c]	Pentamidine isethionate IM or IV[b]: 4 mg/kg per day for 7 days
Second stage	Melarsoprol IV	2.2 mg/kg per day for 10 days	—

[a] Fexinidazole should not be administered in children <6 years and weighing <20 kg. [b]For IV administration, slow infusion (60–120 min) should be used. [c]The maximal dose is 1 g per injection; the drug should be diluted in distilled water.

Sources: Control and surveillance of human African trypanosomiasis: Report of a WHO Expert Committee. WHO Technical Report Series 984, 2013; WHO interim guidelines for the treatment of gambiense human African trypanosomiasis. August 2019; *www.who.int/trypanosomiasis_african/resources/9789241550567/en/*.

divided into a 4-day loading phase and a 6-day maintenance phase. It is highly effective (>95% cure rate) in patients with first-stage and nonsevere second-stage HAT, the latter being defined as <100 leukocytes/μL in the CSF. Fexinidazole is associated with a lower cure rate (87%) in patients with severe second-stage (≥100 leukocytes/μL in the CSF) HAT. The most relevant adverse reactions reported in clinical trials are vomiting, headache, and neuropsychiatric disorders (e.g., insomnia, anxiety, agitation). Fexinidazole is contraindicated in patients with hepatic insufficiency or at increased risk of QT interval prolongation. In the absence of safety and efficacy data, it remains contraindicated in small children (<6 years and/or weighing <20 kg).

Pentamidine isethionate is highly effective (>95%) against first-stage *T. b. gambiense* HAT and is an excellent alternative to fexinidazole when the latter is contraindicated or not available. It is generally well tolerated and can therefore be administered in peripheral health care centers in endemic countries (Fig. 227-5). Hypotension after injection is common but generally mild. Hypoglycemia or hyperglycemia occasionally occurs, but permanent diabetes is very rare. Severe adverse events, such as acute pancreatitis and anaphylaxis, occur extremely rarely.

Nifurtimox-eflornithine combination therapy is very effective (>95% cure rate) and safe in patients with second-stage HAT, including patients with severe (≥100 leukocytes/μL in the CSF) illness. Common adverse reactions include gastrointestinal disturbances (nausea, vomiting, abdominal pain), headache, anorexia, and reversible bone marrow toxicity (anemia, leukopenia). Convulsions and psychosis are reported in <5% of patients.

T. B. RHODESIENSE

Suramin has been used for >90 years and remains the first-line treatment for first-stage *T. b. rhodesiense* HAT. Common adverse events are pyrexia and nephrotoxicity, which is usually mild and reversible but necessitates surveillance of albuminuria and renal function before each dose.

Because eflornithine is ineffective against *T. b. rhodesiense*, melarsoprol, an arsenic-based derivative, remains the only existing treatment for second-stage *T. b. rhodesiense* HAT. Reactive encephalopathy is a life-threatening adverse event that occurs in 5–18% of patients, with an associated mortality rate of 10–70%. The efficacy of concomitant high-dose prednisolone to prevent reactive encephalopathy in patients with *T. b. rhodesiense* HAT is not known. Other severe but less frequent adverse reactions to melarsoprol include exfoliative dermatitis, bloody diarrhea, peripheral neuropathy, renal dysfunction, and liver toxicity. Phlebitis is common, as is soft tissue necrosis if the drug is accidentally given paravenously.

PROGNOSIS

Provided that treatment guidelines are properly followed, >95% of patients with first-stage and second-stage *T. b. gambiense* HAT are definitively cured with fexinidazole, pentamidine, and nifurtimox-eflornithine combination therapy. The overall case-fatality rate is <1% except in very advanced cases. Because relapses can occur long after completion of treatment, follow-up visits are advised every 6 months for at least 2 years. If clinical features of HAT are present, both blood and CSF examinations are indicated. Patients with second-stage *T. b. rhodesiense* HAT are at a 5–10% risk of dying during or after melarsoprol treatment, but relapses are very rare.

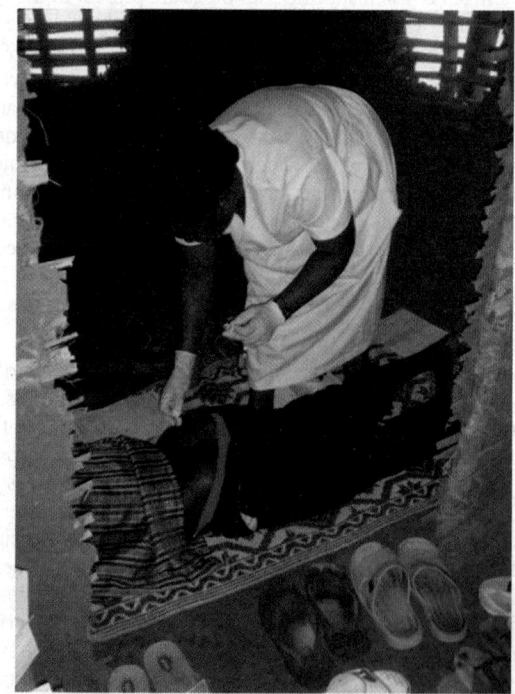

FIGURE 227-5 Intramuscular injection of pentamidine by a nurse in a village health center, Province Orientale, Democratic Republic of the Congo.

■ GLOBAL CONSIDERATIONS

The elimination of sleeping sickness as a public health problem has been achieved, thanks to increased control activities run by national control programs and nongovernmental medical organizations, improved funding, and the end of several civil wars (e.g., in Angola) in the past 20 years. Funding for research, development, and implementation of improved diagnostic (e.g., rapid diagnostic tests), therapeutic (e.g., oral drugs), and vector control tools remains crucial to sustain recent achievements and to move on to the next objective, i.e., the global elimination of transmission by 2030.

■ FURTHER READING

Bern C et al: Chagas disease in the United States: A public health approach. Clin Microbiol Rev 33:e00023-19, 2019.

Büscher P et al: Human African trypanosomiasis. Lancet 390:2397, 2017.

Lindner AK et al: New WHO guidelines for treatment of gambiense human African trypanosomiasis including fexinidazole: Substantial changes for clinical practice. Lancet Infect Dis 20:e38, 2020.

Pérez-Molina JA, Molina I: Chagas disease. Lancet 391:82, 2018.

Urech K et al: Sleeping sickness in travelers—Do they really sleep? PLoS Negl Trop Dis 5:e1358, 2011.

228 *Toxoplasma* Infections

Kami Kim

■ DEFINITION

Toxoplasmosis is caused by infection with the obligate intracellular parasite *Toxoplasma gondii*. Acute infection acquired after birth is typically asymptomatic, but some immunocompetent individuals can present with systemic or ocular disease. Acute infection is thought to result in the lifelong chronic persistence of cysts in the host's tissues. The classic presentation of toxoplasmosis is encephalitis in immunocompromised individuals (especially HIV-positive individuals) in whom latent infection has reactivated. Among the clinical manifestations of disease are lymphadenopathy, encephalitis, myocarditis, pneumonitis, and retinitis. Congenital toxoplasmosis is an infection of newborns that results from the transplacental passage of parasites from an infected mother to the fetus. These infants may be asymptomatic at birth, but many children later manifest signs and symptoms, including chorioretinitis, strabismus, epilepsy, and psychomotor retardation. Toxoplasmosis can also present as acute disease (typically chorioretinitis) associated with food- or waterborne sources.

■ ETIOLOGY

T. gondii is an intracellular coccidian that infects both birds and mammals. Up to a third of the world's population is thought to be infected latently with this organism. There are two distinct stages in the life cycle that are transmissible to humans (**Fig. 228-1**). Tissue cysts that contain bradyzoites are transmitted in undercooked meat. After an intermediate host (e.g., a human, mouse, sheep, pig) ingests the cyst, it is rapidly digested by the acidic-pH gastric secretions. Sporulated oocysts that contain sporozoites are products of the sexual cycle in feline intestines and acquired by ingestion of food or water contaminated with infected cat feces. Bradyzoites or sporozoites are released, enter the intestinal epithelium, and transform into rapidly dividing tachyzoites. The tachyzoites can infect and replicate in all mammalian cells except red blood cells. The parasite actively penetrates the cell and forms a parasitophorous vacuole. Parasite replication continues within the vacuole. After the parasites reach a critical mass, intracellular signaling within the host and the parasite result in parasite egress from the vacuole. The host cell is destroyed, and the released tachyzoites infect adjoining cells. Parasites can disseminate throughout the body as free tachyzoites or within phagocytic cells in the bloodstream or via lymphatics. Tachyzoites actively invade host cells and can cross epithelial and endothelial barriers.

The tachyzoite replication cycle within an infected organ causes cytopathology and clinical symptoms. Most tachyzoites are eliminated by the host's humoral and cell-mediated immune responses. Tissue cysts containing bradyzoites develop 7–10 days after systemic tachyzoite infection. These tissue cysts occur in various host organs but persist principally within the central nervous system (CNS) and muscle. The development of this chronic stage completes the asexual portion of the life cycle. Active infection in the immunocompromised host is usually due to the spontaneous release of encysted parasites that undergo rapid transformation into tachyzoites within the CNS that cannot be contained by the immune system.

The *sexual* stage in the life cycle takes place in the cat (the definitive host) and is defined by the formation of oocysts within the feline host intestine. This enteroepithelial cycle begins with the ingestion of the bradyzoite tissue cysts and, after several intermediate stages, culminates in the production of gametes. Gamete fusion produces a zygote, which envelops itself in a rigid wall and is secreted in the feces as an unsporulated oocyst. After 2–3 days of exposure to air at ambient temperature, the noninfectious oocyst sporulates to produce eight sporozoite progeny. The sporulated oocyst can be ingested by an intermediate host, such as a person emptying a cat's litter box or a pig

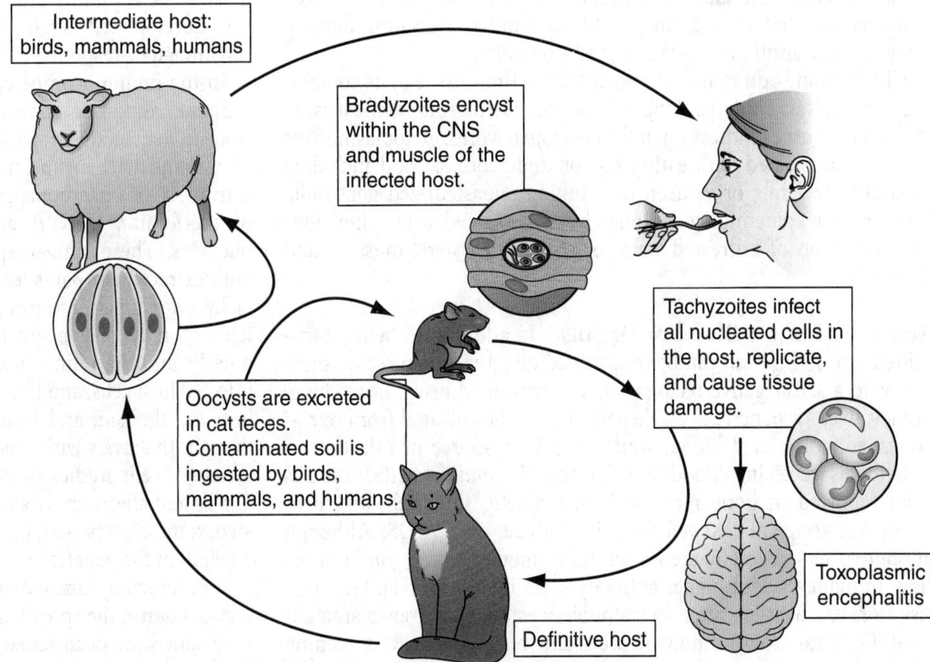

Intermediate host: birds, mammals, humans
Bradyzoites encyst within the CNS and muscle of the infected host.
Tachyzoites infect all nucleated cells in the host, replicate, and cause tissue damage.
Oocysts are excreted in cat feces. Contaminated soil is ingested by birds, mammals, and humans.
Toxoplasmic encephalitis
Definitive host

FIGURE 228-1 Life cycle of *Toxoplasma gondii*. The cat is the definitive host in which the sexual phase of the cycle is completed. Oocysts shed in cat feces can infect a wide range of animals, including birds, rodents, grazing domestic animals, and humans. The bradyzoites found in the muscle of food animals may infect humans who eat insufficiently cooked meat products, particularly lamb and pork. Although human disease can take many forms, congenital infection and encephalitis from reactivation of latent infection in the brains of immunosuppressed persons are the most important manifestations. CNS, central nervous system. *(Courtesy of Dominique Buzoni-Gatel, Institut Pasteur, Paris.)*

rummaging in a barnyard. It is in the intermediate host that *T. gondii* completes its life cycle.

Sporulated oocysts are environmentally hardy and very infectious; they are thought to be sources of waterborne outbreaks such as those reported in Victoria (British Columbia, Canada) and in South America. In the Northern Hemisphere, *T. gondii* strains are predominantly of three genotypes. Strains found in South and Central America are more virulent than those from the Northern Hemisphere, are frequently of the type I virulent genotype or atypical genotypes, and are more likely to be associated with symptomatic disease, usually ocular posterior uveitis. Ocular toxoplasmosis should be considered in a person from Central or South America with ocular symptoms and retinal abnormalities. Severe disease, including sepsis, fever of unknown origin, and pneumonia, has been reported and should be considered in a patient with travel history to South or Central America. There are no extensive data about the prevalence of *T. gondii* in Africa, but existing studies suggest *T. gondii* infection is common.

EPIDEMIOLOGY

T. gondii infects a wide range of mammals and birds. Its seroprevalence depends on the locale and the age of the population. Generally, hot arid climatic conditions are associated with a low prevalence of infection. In the United States and most European countries, the seroprevalence increases with age and exposure. In the United States, seroprevalence has steadily decreased, with 11% of individuals >6 years old having serologic evidence of *Toxoplasma* exposure in a 2011–2014 survey, with foreign-born Americans having a higher rate of seroprevalence. In most other regions of the world, the seroprevalence is higher, with a seroprevalence as high as 78% reported in Brazil. Perhaps because of increased awareness of foodborne infections, the prevalence of seropositivity has decreased worldwide over the past two decades.

TRANSMISSION

Oral Transmission Most cases of human *Toxoplasma* infection are thought to be acquired by the oral route. Transmission can be attributable to ingestion of sporulated oocysts from contaminated soil, food, or water. During acute feline infection, a cat may excrete as many as 100 million oocysts per day. These sporozoite-containing oocysts are highly infectious and may remain viable for many years in soil or water. Humans infected during an oocyst-transmitted infection develop stage-specific antibodies to the oocyst/sporozoite.

Children and adults also acquire infection from tissue cysts containing bradyzoites. Undercooking or insufficient freezing of meat is an important source of infection in the developed world. Toxoplasmososis has been associated with eating raw or undercooked food including ground beef, lamb, or venison or drinking unpasteurized goat milk. More recent epidemiologic studies have associated acute infections with ingestion of untreated water or shellfish (oysters, mussels, and clams).

Transmission via Blood or Organs In addition to being transmitted orally, *T. gondii* can be transmitted directly from a seropositive donor to a seronegative recipient in a transplanted heart, heart–lung, kidney, liver, or pancreas. Viable parasites can be cultured from refrigerated anticoagulated blood, which may be a source of infection in individuals receiving blood transfusions. *T. gondii* reactivation has been reported in bone marrow, hematopoietic stem cell, and liver transplant recipients as well as in individuals with AIDS. Although antibody titers generally are not useful in monitoring *T. gondii* infection, individuals with higher antibody titers may be at relatively high risk for reactivation after hematopoietic stem cell transplantation (HSCT). Thus, routine polymerase chain reaction (PCR) screening of blood from these patients may be in order, although not all centers routinely monitor HSCT patients for toxoplasmosis. Screening *Toxoplasma* serologies (donor and recipient) before transplantation may identify patients potentially at risk for reactivated toxoplasmosis. Finally, laboratory personnel can be infected after contact with contaminated needles or glassware or with infected tissue.

Transplacental Transmission On average, about one-third of all women who acquire infection with *T. gondii* during pregnancy transmit the parasite to the fetus; the remainder give birth to normal, uninfected babies. Of the various factors that influence fetal outcome, gestational age at the time of infection is the most critical (see below). Recrudescent maternal infection is rarely the source of congenital disease, although rare cases of transmission by immunocompromised women (e.g., those infected with HIV or those receiving high-dose glucocorticoids) have been reported. Thus, women who are seropositive before pregnancy usually are protected against acute infection and do not give birth to congenitally infected neonates.

There is essentially no risk for congenital infection if the mother becomes infected ≥6 months before conception. If infection is acquired <6 months before conception, the likelihood of transplacental infection increases as the interval between infection and conception decreases. Women with documented acute toxoplasmosis should be counseled to use appropriate measures to prevent pregnancy for 6 months after infection. In pregnancy, if the mother becomes infected during the first trimester, the incidence of transplacental infection is lowest (~15%), but the disease in the neonate is most severe. If maternal infection occurs during the third trimester, the incidence of transplacental infection is greatest (65%), but the infant is usually asymptomatic at birth. Infected infants who are normal at birth may have a higher incidence of learning disabilities and chronic neurologic sequelae than uninfected children. Only a small proportion (20%) of women infected with *T. gondii* develop clinical signs of infection. Often the diagnosis is first appreciated when routine postconception serologic tests show evidence of specific antibody.

PATHOGENESIS

Upon the host's ingestion of either tissue cysts containing bradyzoites or oocysts containing sporozoites, the parasites are released from the cysts by the digestive process. Bradyzoites are resistant to the effect of pepsin and invade the host's gastrointestinal tract. Within enterocytes (or other gut-associated cells), the parasites undergo morphologic transformation, giving rise to invasive tachyzoites. From the gastrointestinal tract, parasites disseminate to a variety of organs, particularly lymphatic tissue, skeletal muscle, myocardium, retina, placenta, and the CNS. At these sites, the parasite infects host cells, replicates, and invades the adjoining cells. In this fashion, the hallmarks of the infection develop: cell death and focal necrosis surrounded by an acute inflammatory response.

In the immunocompetent host, both the humoral and the cellular immune responses control infection; parasite virulence and tissue tropism may be strain specific. Tachyzoites are sequestered by a variety of immune mechanisms, including induction of parasiticidal antibody, activation of macrophages with radical intermediates, production of interferon γ (IFN-γ), and stimulation of CD8+ cytotoxic T lymphocytes. These antigen-specific lymphocytes are capable of killing both extracellular parasites and target cells infected with parasites. As tachyzoites are cleared from the acutely infected host, tissue cysts containing bradyzoites begin to appear, usually within the CNS, skeletal muscle, and the retina. *Toxoplasma* secretes signaling molecules into infected host cells, and these molecules modulate host gene expression, host metabolism, and host immune response. While it was initially thought that cysts with bradyzoites are not eliminated by the immune system, recent studies in the murine model indicate that both CD8+ T cells and alternatively activated macrophages are able to kill cysts in vivo; some cysts persist, however, and the ability to eliminate cysts may depend on the genetic background of the infected host.

Immunocompromised or fetal hosts lack the immune factors necessary to control the spread of tachyzoite infection. This altered immune state allows the persistence of tachyzoites and gives rise to progressive focal destruction in affected organs (i.e., necrotizing encephalitis, pneumonia, and myocarditis).

It is thought that all infected individuals have persistent infection with cysts containing bradyzoites, but this lifelong infection usually remains subclinical. Although bradyzoites are in a slow metabolic phase, bradyzoites can replicate, and cysts do rupture within the CNS.

These subclinical cycles of cyst ruptures followed by development of new bradyzoite-containing cysts are the probable source of recrudescent infection in immunocompromised individuals and the most likely stimulus for the persistence of antibody titers in the immunocompetent host. Although the concept is controversial, the persistence of toxoplasmosis has been hypothesized to be a contributing factor to a variety of neuropsychiatric conditions, including schizophrenia and bipolar disease. In rodents, chronic *T. gondii* infection clearly has significant effects on behavior, increasing predation. A role for parasite remodeling of the host epigenome has been hypothesized to play a role in long-lasting neuropsychiatric syndromes and is the subject of ongoing research.

PATHOLOGY

Cell death and focal necrosis due to replicating tachyzoites induce an intense mononuclear inflammatory response in any tissue or cell type infected. Tachyzoites rarely can be visualized by routine histopathologic staining of these inflammatory lesions. However, immunofluorescent staining with parasitic antigen–specific antibodies can reveal the organism. In contrast to the inflammatory process caused by tachyzoites, bradyzoite-containing cysts cause inflammation only at the early stages of development. Once the cysts reach maturity, the inflammatory process is blunted, and the cysts remain relatively immunologically quiescent within the brain matrix until they rupture.

Lymph Nodes During acute infection, lymph node biopsy demonstrates characteristic findings, including follicular hyperplasia and irregular clusters of tissue macrophages with eosinophilic cytoplasm. Granulomas rarely are evident in these specimens. Although tachyzoites are not usually visible, parasites can be demonstrated by subinoculation of infected tissue into mice, with resultant disease, or by PCR. PCR amplification of DNA fragments of *Toxoplasma* genes is effective and sensitive in establishing lymph node infection by tachyzoites.

Eyes In the eye, infiltrates of monocytes, lymphocytes, and plasma cells may produce uni- or multifocal lesions. Granulomatous lesions and retinochoroiditis can be observed in the posterior chamber after acute necrotizing retinitis. Other ocular complications include iridocyclitis, cataracts, and glaucoma. *T. gondii* is the most common cause of posterior uveitis in immunocompetent individuals.

Central Nervous System During CNS involvement, both focal and diffuse meningoencephalitis can be documented, with evidence of necrosis and microglial nodules. Necrotizing encephalitis in patients without AIDS is characterized by small diffuse lesions with perivascular cuffing in contiguous areas. In the AIDS population, polymorphonuclear leukocytes may be present in addition to monocytes, lymphocytes, and plasma cells. Cysts containing bradyzoites frequently are found contiguous with the necrotic tissue border. As a consequence of antiretroviral therapy (ART) for AIDS, the incidence of toxoplasmosis has decreased in the developed world. The incidence of toxoplasmosis in underresourced settings is not known due to lack of diagnostic infrastructure but is likely to be higher than in the United States.

Lungs and Heart Among patients with AIDS who die of toxoplasmosis, 40–70% have involvement of the lungs and heart. Interstitial pneumonitis can develop in neonates and immunocompromised patients. Thickened and edematous alveolar septa infiltrated with mononuclear and plasma cells are apparent. This inflammation may extend to the endothelial walls. Tachyzoites and bradyzoite-containing cysts have been observed within the alveolar membrane. Superimposed bronchopneumonia can be caused by other microbial agents. Cysts and aggregates of parasites in cardiac muscle tissue are evident in patients with AIDS who die of toxoplasmosis. Focal necrosis surrounded by inflammatory cells is associated with hyaline necrosis and disrupted myocardial cells. Pericarditis is associated with toxoplasmosis in some patients.

Gastrointestinal Tract Rare cases of human gastrointestinal tract infection with *T. gondii* have presented as ulcerations in the mucosa. Acute infection in certain strains of inbred mice (C57BL/6) results in lethal ileitis within 7–9 days. This inflammatory bowel disease has been recognized in several other mammalian species, including pigs and nonhuman primates.

Other Sites Pathologic changes during disseminated infection are similar to those described for the lymph nodes, eyes, and CNS. In patients with AIDS, the skeletal muscle, pancreas, stomach, and kidneys can be involved, with necrosis, invasion by inflammatory cells, and (rarely) tachyzoites detectable by routine staining. Large necrotic lesions may cause direct tissue destruction. In addition, secondary effects from acute infection of these various organs, including pancreatitis, myositis, and glomerulonephritis, have been reported.

HOST IMMUNE RESPONSE

Acute *Toxoplasma* infection evokes a cascade of protective immune responses in the immunocompetent host. *Toxoplasma* enters the host at the gut mucosal level and evokes a mucosal immune response that includes the production of antigen-specific secretory IgA. Titers of serum IgA antibody directed at the tachyzoite surface antigen p30/SAG1 are a useful marker for congenital and acute toxoplasmosis.

Within the host, *T. gondii* rapidly induces detectable levels of both IgM and IgG serum antibodies. Monoclonal gammopathy of the IgG class can occur in congenitally infected infants. IgM levels may be increased in newborns with congenital infection. The polyclonal IgG antibodies evoked by infection are parasiticidal in vitro in the presence of serum complement and are the basis for the Sabin-Feldman dye test. However, cell-mediated immunity is the major protective response evoked by the parasite during host infection. Macrophages are activated after phagocytosis of antibody-opsonized parasites. If the parasite is not phagocytosed and enters the macrophage, monocytes, or dendritic cells by active penetration, these "Trojan horses" represent a mechanism for transport and dissemination to distant organs. *Toxoplasma* stimulates a robust IL-12 response by human dendritic cells. The CD4+ and CD8+ T cell responses are antigen-specific and further stimulate the production of a variety of important lymphokines that expand the T cell and natural killer cell repertoire. *T. gondii* is a potent inducer of a T_H1 phenotype, with IL-12 and IFN-γ playing an essential role in the control of the parasites' growth in the host. Regulation of the inflammatory response is at least partially under the control of a T_H2 response that includes the production of IL-4 and IL-10 in seropositive individuals. Human T-cell clones of both the CD4+ and the CD8+ phenotypes are cytolytic against parasite-infected macrophages. These T-cell clones produce cytokines that are "microbistatic." IL-18, IL-7, and IL-15 upregulate the production of IFN-γ and may be important during acute and chronic infection. The effect of IFN-γ may be paradoxical, with stimulation of a host downregulatory response as well.

Although *T. gondii* infection is believed to be recrudescent in patients with AIDS or other immunocompromised states, antibody titers are not useful in establishing reactivation or in following the activity of infection. An absence of positive serologies suggests an alternative diagnosis, although AIDS patients may have borderline positive or low serologies. T cells from AIDS patients with reactivation of toxoplasmosis fail to secrete both IFN-γ and IL-2. This alteration in the production of these critical immune cytokines contributes to the persistence of infection. *Toxoplasma* infection frequently develops late in the course of AIDS (CD4+ count <100/μL), when the loss of T cell–dependent protective mechanisms, particularly CD8+ T cells, becomes most pronounced.

CLINICAL MANIFESTATIONS

In persons whose immune systems are intact, acute toxoplasmosis is usually asymptomatic and self-limited. This condition can go unrecognized in 80–90% of adults and children with acquired infection. The asymptomatic nature of this infection makes diagnosis difficult in mothers infected during pregnancy. In contrast, the wide range of clinical manifestations in congenitally infected children includes severe neurologic complications such as hydrocephalus, microcephaly, intellectual disability, and chorioretinitis. If prenatal infection is severe, multiorgan failure and subsequent intrauterine fetal death can occur.

In children and adults, chronic infection can persist throughout life, with little consequence to the immunocompetent host.

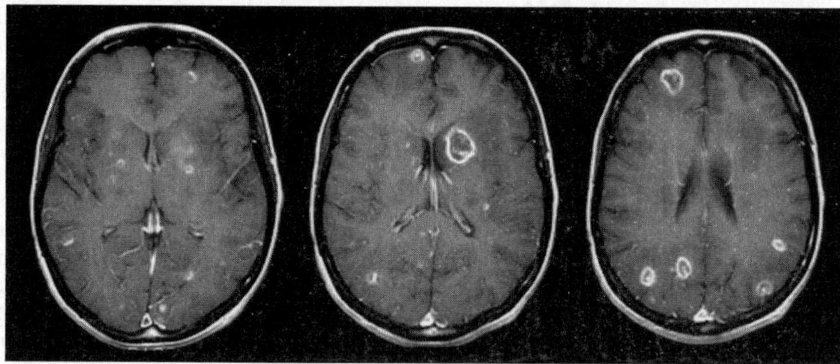

FIGURE 228-2 Toxoplasmic encephalitis in a 36-year-old patient with AIDS. The multiple lesions are demonstrated by MRI scanning (T1-weighted with gadolinium enhancement). *(Courtesy of Clifford Eskey, Dartmouth Hitchcock Medical Center, Hanover, NH; with permission.)*

Toxoplasmosis in Immunocompetent Patients The most common manifestation of acute toxoplasmosis is cervical lymphadenopathy. The nodes may be single or multiple, are usually nontender, are discrete, and vary in firmness. Lymphadenopathy also may be found in suboccipital, supraclavicular, inguinal, and mediastinal areas. Generalized lymphadenopathy occurs in 20–30% of symptomatic patients. Between 20% and 40% of patients with lymphadenopathy also have headache, malaise, fatigue, and fever (usually with a temperature of <40°C [<104°F]). A smaller proportion of symptomatic individuals have myalgia, sore throat, abdominal pain, maculopapular rash, meningoencephalitis, and confusion. Rare complications associated with infection in the normal immune host include pneumonia, myocarditis, encephalopathy, pericarditis, and polymyositis. Signs and symptoms associated with acute infection usually resolve within several weeks, although the lymphadenopathy may persist for some months. In one epidemic, toxoplasmosis was diagnosed correctly in only 3 of the 25 patients who consulted physicians. If toxoplasmosis is considered in the differential diagnosis, routine laboratory and serologic screening should precede node biopsy.

In North America and Europe, there are three predominant genotypes, but strains are more genetically diverse in Central and South America. Genotypes of *T. gondii* prevalent in South America are more virulent than those typically seen in North America or Europe. These genotypes may be associated with acute or recurrent ocular disease in immunocompetent individuals and have also been associated with pneumonitis and a fulminant sepsis picture in immunologically normal individuals. Thus, a detailed history, particularly regarding travel and countries of residence, is critical for establishing a diagnosis.

The results of routine laboratory studies are usually unremarkable except for minimal lymphocytosis, an elevated erythrocyte sedimentation rate, and a nominal increase in serum aminotransferase levels. Evaluation of cerebrospinal fluid (CSF) in cases with evidence of encephalopathy or meningoencephalitis shows an elevation of intracranial pressure, mononuclear pleocytosis (10–50 cells/mL), a slight increase in protein concentration, and (occasionally) an increase in the gamma globulin level. PCR amplification of the *Toxoplasma* DNA target sequence in CSF is specific for active toxoplasmosis, but not sensitive. The CSF of chronically infected individuals is normal.

Infection of Immunocompromised Patients Patients with AIDS and those receiving immunosuppressive therapy for lymphoproliferative disorders are at greatest risk for developing acute toxoplasmosis. Toxoplasmosis has also been reported after treatment with antibodies to tumor necrosis factor. The infection may be due either to reactivation of latent infection or to acquisition of parasites from exogenous sources such as blood or transplanted organs. In individuals with AIDS, >95% of cases of *Toxoplasma* encephalitis (TE) are believed to be due to recrudescent infection. In most of these cases, encephalitis develops when the CD4+ T-cell count falls below 100/μL. In immunocompromised hosts, the disease may be rapidly fatal if untreated. Thus, accurate diagnosis and initiation of appropriate therapy are necessary to prevent fulminant infection.

Toxoplasmosis is a principal opportunistic infection of the CNS in persons with AIDS. Although geographic origin may be related to frequency of infection, it has no correlation with the severity of disease in immunocompromised hosts. Individuals with AIDS who are seropositive for *T. gondii* are at high risk for encephalitis. Before the advent of current ART, about one-third of the 15–40% of adult AIDS patients in the United States who were latently infected with *T. gondii* developed TE. TE may still be a presenting infection in individuals who are unaware of their positive HIV status.

The signs and symptoms of acute toxoplasmosis in immunocompromised patients principally involve the CNS (Fig. 228-2). More than 50% of patients with clinical manifestations have intracerebral involvement. Clinical findings at presentation range from nonfocal to focal dysfunction. CNS findings include encephalopathy, meningoencephalitis, and mass lesions. Patients may present with altered mental status (75%), fever (10–72%), seizures (33%), headaches (56%), and focal neurologic findings (60%), including motor deficits, cranial nerve palsies, movement disorders, dysmetria, visual-field loss, and aphasia. Patients who present with evidence of diffuse cortical dysfunction develop evidence of focal neurologic disease as infection progresses. This altered condition is due not only to the necrotizing encephalitis caused by direct invasion by the parasite but also to secondary effects, including vasculitis, edema, and hemorrhage. The onset of infection can range from an insidious process over several weeks to an acute presentation with fulminant focal deficits, including hemiparesis, hemiplegia, visual-field defects, localized headache, and focal seizures.

Although lesions can occur anywhere in the CNS, the areas most often involved appear to be the brainstem, basal ganglia, pituitary gland, and corticomedullary junction. Brainstem involvement gives rise to a variety of neurologic dysfunctions, including cranial nerve palsy, dysmetria, and ataxia. With basal ganglion infection, patients may develop hydrocephalus, choreiform movements, and choreoathetosis. *Toxoplasma* usually causes encephalitis, and meningeal involvement is uncommon. CSF findings may be unremarkable or may include a modest increase in cell count and in protein—but not glucose—concentration.

Cerebral toxoplasmosis must be differentiated from other opportunistic infections or tumors in the CNS of AIDS patients. The differential diagnosis includes herpes simplex encephalitis, cryptococcal meningitis, progressive multifocal leukoencephalopathy, and primary CNS lymphoma. Involvement of the pituitary gland can give rise to panhypopituitarism and hyponatremia from inappropriate secretion of vasopressin (antidiuretic hormone). HIV-associated neurocognitive disorder (HAND) may present as cognitive impairment, attention loss, and altered memory. Brain biopsy in patients who have been treated for TE but who continue to exhibit neurologic dysfunction often fails to identify organisms.

Autopsies of *Toxoplasma*-infected patients have demonstrated the involvement of multiple organs, including the lungs, gastrointestinal tract, pancreas, skin, eyes, heart, and liver. *Toxoplasma* pneumonia can be confused with *Pneumocystis* pneumonia. Respiratory involvement usually presents as dyspnea, fever, and a nonproductive cough and may rapidly progress to acute respiratory failure with hemoptysis, metabolic acidosis, hypotension, and (occasionally) disseminated intravascular coagulation. Histopathologic studies demonstrate necrosis and a mixed cellular infiltrate. The presence of organisms is a helpful diagnostic indicator, but organisms can also be found in healthy tissue. Infection of the heart is usually asymptomatic but can be associated with cardiac tamponade or biventricular failure. Infections of the gastrointestinal tract and the liver have been documented.

Congenital Toxoplasmosis Between 400 and 4000 infants born each year in the United States are affected by congenital toxoplasmosis. Acute infection in mothers acquiring *T. gondii* during pregnancy is usually asymptomatic; most such women are diagnosed via prenatal serologic screening. Infection of the placenta leads to hematogenous infection of the fetus. As gestation proceeds, the proportion of fetuses that become infected increases, but the clinical severity of the infection declines. Although infected children may initially be asymptomatic, the persistence of *T. gondii* can result in reactivation and clinical disease—most frequently chorioretinitis—decades later. Factors associated with relatively severe disabilities include delays in diagnosis and in initiation of therapy, neonatal hypoxia and hypoglycemia, profound visual impairment (see "Ocular Infection," below), uncorrected hydrocephalus, and increased intracranial pressure. If treated appropriately, upward of 70% of children have normal developmental, neurologic, and ophthalmologic findings at follow-up evaluations. Treatment for 1 year with pyrimethamine, a sulfonamide, and folinic acid is tolerated with minimal toxicity (see "Treatment," below).

Ocular Infection Infection with *T. gondii* is estimated to cause 35% of all cases of chorioretinitis in the United States and Europe. It was formerly thought that the majority of cases of ocular disease were due to congenital infection. Ocular toxoplasmosis in immunocompetent individuals occurs more commonly than was previously appreciated and has been associated with outbreaks traced to oocyst contamination of soil or water in Victoria (British Columbia) and in South America. A variety of ocular manifestations are documented, including blurred vision, scotoma, photophobia, and eye pain. Macular involvement occurs, with loss of central vision, and nystagmus is secondary to poor fixation. Involvement of the extraocular muscles may lead to disorders of convergence and to strabismus. Ophthalmologic examination should be undertaken in newborns with suspected congenital infection. As the inflammation resolves, vision improves, but episodic flare-ups of chorioretinitis, which progressively destroy retinal tissue and lead to glaucoma, are common. The ophthalmologic examination reveals yellow-white, cotton-like patches with indistinct margins of hyperemia. As the lesions age, white plaques with distinct borders and black spots within the retinal pigment become more apparent. Lesions usually are located near the posterior pole of the retina; they may be single but are more commonly multiple. Congenital lesions may be unilateral or bilateral and show evidence of massive chorioretinal degeneration with extensive fibrosis. Surrounding these areas of involvement are a normal retina and vasculature. In patients with AIDS, retinal lesions are often large, with diffuse retinal necrosis, and include both free tachyzoites and cysts containing bradyzoites. Toxoplasmic chorioretinitis may be a prodrome to the development of encephalitis.

DIAGNOSIS

Tissue and Body Fluids The differential diagnosis of acute toxoplasmosis can be made by appropriate culture, serologic testing, and PCR (**Table 228-1**). PCR is the mainstay for detection of organisms in tissue or biological fluids. Although available only at specialized laboratories, the isolation of *T. gondii* from blood or other body fluids can be accomplished after subinoculation of the sample into the peritoneal cavity of mice. If no parasites are found in the mouse's peritoneal fluid 6–10 days after inoculation, its anti-*Toxoplasma* serum titer can be evaluated 4–6 weeks after inoculation. Isolation or PCR of *T. gondii* from the patient's body fluids reflects acute infection, whereas isolation from biopsied tissue is an indication only of the presence of tissue cysts and should not be misinterpreted as evidence of acute toxoplasmosis. Persistent parasitemia in patients with latent, asymptomatic infection is rare. Histologic examination of lymph nodes may suggest the characteristic changes described above. Demonstration of tachyzoites in lymph nodes establishes the diagnosis of acute toxoplasmosis. Histologic demonstration of cysts containing bradyzoites confirms prior infection with *T. gondii* but may represent latent rather than acute infection.

TABLE 228-1 Differential Laboratory Diagnosis of Toxoplasmosis

CLINICAL SETTING	ALTERNATIVE DIAGNOSIS	DISTINGUISHING CHARACTERISTICS
Mononucleosis syndrome	Epstein-Barr virus infection	Serology/PCR
	Cytomegalovirus infection	PCR/viral load/serology
	HIV infection	Serology/antigen/viral load
	Bartonella infection (cat-scratch disease)	Biopsy (PCR or culture)/serology
	Lymphoma	Biopsy
Congenital infection	Cytomegalovirus infection	PCR
	Herpes simplex virus infection	PCR
	Rubella virus infection	Serology
	Syphilis	Serology
	Listeriosis	Bacterial culture
Chorioretinitis in immunocompetent individual	Tuberculosis	Bacterial culture/PCR
	Syphilis	Serology
	Histoplasmosis	Serology/culture/antigen
Chorioretinitis in AIDS patient	Cytomegalovirus infection	Characteristic exam
	Syphilis	Serology
	Herpes simplex virus infection	PCR
	Varicella-zoster virus infection	PCR
	Fungal infection	PCR/culture
CNS lesions in AIDS patient	Lymphoma or metastatic tumor	Tissue biopsy
	Brain abscess	Culture/biopsy
	Progressive multifocal leukoencephalopathy	PCR for JC virus
	Fungal infection	Antigen/PCR/biopsy/culture
	Mycobacterial infection	PCR/biopsy/culture

Abbreviations: CNS, central nervous system; PCR, polymerase chain reaction.

Source: Reproduced with permission from JD Schwartzman: Toxoplasmosis, in *Principles and Practice of Clinical Parasitology.* Hoboken, Wiley, 2001.

Serology Because some diagnostic tests are only available at specialty labs, serologic testing has become the routine method of diagnosis. Diagnosis of acute infection with *T. gondii* can be established by detection of the simultaneous presence of IgG and IgM antibodies to *Toxoplasma* in serum. The presence of circulating IgA favors the diagnosis of an acute infection. The Sabin-Feldman dye test, the indirect fluorescent antibody test, and the enzyme-linked immunosorbent assay (ELISA) all satisfactorily measure circulating IgG antibody to *Toxoplasma.* Positive IgG titers (>1:10) can be detected as early as 2–3 weeks after infection. These titers usually peak at 6–8 weeks and decline slowly to a new baseline level that persists for life. Antibody avidity increases with time and can be useful in difficult cases during pregnancy for establishing when infection may have occurred. The serum IgM titer should be measured in concert with the IgG titer to better establish the time of infection; either the double-sandwich IgM-ELISA or the IgM-immunosorbent assay (IgM-ISAGA) should be used. Both assays are specific and sensitive, with fewer false-positive results than other commercial tests. The double-sandwich IgA-ELISA is more sensitive than the IgM-ELISA for detecting congenital infection in the fetus and newborn. Although a negative IgM result with a positive IgG titer indicates distant infection, IgM can persist for >1 year and should not necessarily be considered a reflection of acute disease. If acute toxoplasmosis is suspected, a more extensive panel of serologic tests can be performed. In the United States, testing is available at the Remington

 Laboratory for Specialty Diagnostics (formerly Toxoplasma Serology laboratory; *https://www.sutterhealth.org/pamf/services/lab-pathology/toxoplasma-serology-laboratory*).

Molecular Diagnostics Molecular approaches can directly detect *T. gondii* in biologic samples independent of the serologic response. Results obtained with PCR have suggested high sensitivity, specificity, and clinical utility in the diagnosis of TE. PCR technology is readily available. While very specific, depending on the body fluid type tested, the sensitivity of PCR of body fluids may be low, and diagnostic algorithms typically incorporate serologic testing of blood or body fluids. Real-time PCR, if available, can provide quantitative results. Isolates can be genotyped and polymorphic sequences can be obtained, with consequent identification of the precise strain. Molecular epidemiologic studies with polymorphic markers have been useful in correlating clinical signs and symptoms of disease with different *T. gondii* genotypes.

The Immunocompetent Adult or Child For the patient who presents with lymphadenopathy only, a positive IgM titer is an indication of acute infection—and an indication for therapy, if clinically warranted (see "Treatment," below). The serum IgM titer should be determined again in 3 weeks. An elevation in the IgG titer without an increase in the IgM titer suggests that infection is present but is not acute. If there is a borderline increase in either IgG or IgM, the titers should be reassessed in 3–4 weeks.

The Immunocompromised Host A presumptive clinical diagnosis of TE in patients with AIDS is based on clinical presentation, history of exposure (as evidenced by positive serology), and radiologic evaluation. To detect latent infection with *T. gondii*, HIV-infected persons should be tested for IgG antibody to *Toxoplasma* soon after HIV infection is diagnosed. When these criteria are used, the predictive value is as high as 80%. More than 97% of patients with AIDS and toxoplasmosis have IgG antibody to *T. gondii* in serum. IgM serum antibody usually is not detectable. Although IgG titers do not correlate with active infection, serologic evidence of infection virtually always precedes the development of TE. It is therefore important to determine the *Toxoplasma* antibody status of all patients infected with HIV. Antibody titers may range from negative to 1:1024 in patients with AIDS and TE. Fewer than 3% of patients have no demonstrable antibody to *Toxoplasma* at diagnosis of TE.

Patients with TE have focal or multifocal abnormalities demonstrable by CT or MRI. Neuroradiologic evaluation should include double-dose contrast CT of the head. By this test, single and frequently multiple contrast-enhancing lesions (<2 cm) may be identified. MRI usually demonstrates multiple lesions located in both hemispheres, with the basal ganglia and corticomedullary junction most commonly involved; MRI provides a more sensitive evaluation of the efficacy of therapy than does CT (Fig. 228-2). These findings are not pathognomonic of *Toxoplasma* infection, because 40% of CNS lymphomas are multifocal and 50% are ring-enhancing. For both MRI and CT scans, the rate of false-negative results is ~10%. The finding of a single lesion on an MRI scan increases the likelihood of primary CNS lymphoma (in which solitary lesions are four times more likely than in TE) and strengthens the argument for the performance of a brain biopsy. A therapeutic trial of anti-*Toxoplasma* medications is frequently used to assess the diagnosis. Treatment of presumptive TE with pyrimethamine plus sulfadiazine or clindamycin results in quantifiable clinical improvement in >50% of patients by day 3. Leucovorin is administered to prevent bone marrow toxicity. By day 7, >90% of treated patients show evidence of improvement. In contrast, if patients fail to respond or have lymphoma, clinical signs and symptoms worsen by day 7. Patients in this category require brain biopsy with or without a change in therapy. This procedure can now be performed by a stereotactic CT-guided method that reduces the potential for complications. Brain biopsy for *T. gondii* identifies organisms in 50–75% of cases. PCR amplification of CSF may also confirm toxoplasmosis or suggest alternative diagnoses (Table 228-1), such as progressive multifocal leukoencephalopathy (JC virus positive) or primary CNS lymphoma (Epstein-Barr virus positive).

CT and MRI with contrast are currently the standard diagnostic imaging tests for TE. As in other conditions, the radiologic response may lag behind the clinical response. Resolution of lesions may take from 3 weeks to 6 months. Some patients show clinical improvement despite worsening radiographic findings.

Congenital Infection The issue of concern when a pregnant woman has evidence of recent *T. gondii* infection is whether the fetus is infected. PCR analysis of the amniotic fluid for the B1 gene of *T. gondii* has replaced fetal blood sampling. Serologic diagnosis is based on the persistence of IgG antibody or a positive IgM titer after the first week of life (a time frame that excludes placental leak). The IgG determination should be repeated every 2 months. An increase in IgM beyond the first week of life is indicative of acute infection. Up to 25% of infected newborns may be seronegative and have normal routine physical examinations. Thus, assessment of the eye and the brain, with ophthalmologic testing, CSF evaluation, and radiologic studies, is important in establishing the diagnosis.

Ocular Toxoplasmosis The serum antibody titer may not correlate with the presence of active lesions in the fundus, particularly in cases of congenital toxoplasmosis. In general, a positive IgG titer (measured in undiluted serum if necessary) in conjunction with typical lesions establishes the diagnosis. If lesions are atypical and the serum antibody titer is in the low-positive range, the diagnosis is presumptive. The parasitic antigen–specific polyclonal IgG assay as well as parasite-specific PCR may facilitate the diagnosis. PCR of ocular samples has better yield than PCR of blood. Diagnosis may also be established by ocular fluid Western blot or comparison of ocular fluid antibody with blood antibody (Goldmann-Witmer coefficient). The clinical diagnosis of ocular toxoplasmosis can be supported in 60–90% of cases by laboratory tests, depending on the time of anterior chamber puncture and the panel of antibody analyses used.

TREATMENT

Toxoplasmosis

CONGENITAL INFECTION

Congenitally infected neonates are treated with daily oral pyrimethamine (1 mg/kg) and sulfadiazine (100 mg/kg) with folinic acid for 1 year. Depending on the signs and symptoms, prednisone (1 mg/kg per day) may be used for congenital infection. Some U.S. states and some countries routinely screen pregnant women (France, Austria) and/or newborns (Denmark, Massachusetts). Management and treatment regimens vary with the country and the treatment center. Most experts use spiramycin to treat pregnant women who have acute toxoplasmosis early in pregnancy and use pyrimethamine/sulfadiazine/folinic acid to treat women who seroconvert after 18 weeks of pregnancy or in cases of documented fetal infection. This treatment is somewhat controversial: clinical studies, which have included few untreated women, have not proven the efficacy of such therapy in preventing congenital toxoplasmosis. However, studies do suggest that treatment during pregnancy decreases the severity of infection. Many women who are infected in the first trimester elect termination of pregnancy. Those who do not terminate pregnancy are offered prenatal antibiotic therapy to reduce the frequency and severity of *Toxoplasma* infection in the infant. The optimal duration of treatment for a child with asymptomatic congenital toxoplasmosis is not clear, although most clinicians in the United States would treat the child for 1 year in light of cohort investigations conducted by the National Collaborative Chicago-Based, Congenital Toxoplasmosis Study.

INFECTION IN IMMUNOCOMPETENT PATIENTS

Immunologically competent adults and older children who have only lymphadenopathy do not require specific therapy unless they have persistent, severe symptoms. Patients with ocular toxoplasmosis are usually treated for 6 weeks with pyrimethamine plus either sulfadiazine or clindamycin and sometimes with prednisone.

Trimethoprim-sulfamethoxazole (TMP-SMX) can also be given if pyrimethamine cannot be obtained (5 mg/kg bid based on TMP). Treatment should be supervised by an ophthalmologist familiar with *Toxoplasma* disease. Ocular disease can be self-limited without treatment, but therapy is typically considered for lesions that are severe or close to the fovea or optic disc. Prolonged treatment with TMP-SMX prevents recurrences of ocular toxoplasmosis while on treatment and is often considered in individuals with frequent flares in a 1- to 2-year period. Whether treatment improves long-term visual outcomes is unclear.

INFECTION IN IMMUNOCOMPROMISED PATIENTS

Primary Prophylaxis Patients with AIDS should be treated for acute toxoplasmosis; in immunocompromised patients, toxoplasmosis is rapidly fatal if untreated. Despite their toxicity, the drugs used to treat TE were required for survival prior to ART. The incidence of TE has declined as the survival of patients with HIV infection has increased through the use of ART.

In Africa, many patients are diagnosed with HIV infection only after developing opportunistic infections. Hence, the optimal management of these opportunistic infections is important if the benefits of subsequent ART are to be realized. The incidence of TE in underresourced settings is unknown because serologic testing and imaging are not available. AIDS patients who are seropositive for *T. gondii* and who have a CD4+ T lymphocyte count of <100/μL should receive prophylaxis against TE.

Of the currently available agents, TMP-SMX appears to be an effective alternative for treatment of TE in resource-poor settings where the preferred combination of pyrimethamine plus sulfadiazine is not available. Pyrimethamine is very expensive in the United States, so many clinicians prescribe TMP-SMX if pyrimethamine cannot be obtained. The daily dose of TMP-SMX (one double-strength tablet) recommended for prophylaxis of *Pneumocystis jirovecii* pneumonia (PCP; formerly *Pneumocystis carinii*) is effective against TE. If patients cannot tolerate TMP-SMX, the recommended alternative is dapsone-pyrimethamine, which likewise is effective against PCP. Atovaquone with or without pyrimethamine also can be considered. Prophylactic monotherapy with dapsone, pyrimethamine, azithromycin, clarithromycin, or aerosolized pentamidine is probably insufficient. AIDS patients who are seronegative for *Toxoplasma* and are not receiving prophylaxis for PCP should be retested for IgG antibody to *Toxoplasma* if their CD4+ T-cell count drops to <100/μL. If seroconversion has taken place, then the patient should be given prophylaxis as described above.

Discontinuing Primary Prophylaxis Current studies indicate that prophylaxis against TE can be discontinued in patients who have responded to ART and whose CD4+ T lymphocyte count has been >200/μL for 3 months. Although patients with CD4+ T lymphocyte counts of <100/μL are at greatest risk for developing TE, the risk that this condition will develop when the count has increased to 100–200/μL has not been established. Thus, prophylaxis should be discontinued when the count has increased to >200/μL. Discontinuation of therapy reduces the pill burden; the potential for drug toxicity, drug interaction, or selection of drug-resistant pathogens; and cost. Prophylaxis should be recommenced if the CD4+ T lymphocyte count again decreases to <100–200/μL.

Individuals who have completed initial therapy for TE should receive treatment indefinitely unless immune reconstitution, with a CD4+ T-cell count of >200/μL, occurs as a consequence of combined ART (cART). Combination therapy with pyrimethamine plus sulfadiazine plus leucovorin is effective for this purpose. An alternative to sulfadiazine in this regimen is clindamycin or TMP-SMX.

Discontinuing Secondary Prophylaxis (Long-Term Maintenance Therapy) Patients receiving secondary prophylaxis for TE are at low risk for recurrence when they have completed initial therapy for TE, remain asymptomatic, and have evidence of restored immune function. Individuals with HIV infection should have a CD4+ T lymphocyte count of >200/μL for at least 6 months after cART. This recommendation is consistent with more extensive data indicating the safety of discontinuing secondary prophylaxis for other opportunistic infections during advanced HIV disease. A repeat MRI brain scan is recommended. Secondary prophylaxis should be reintroduced if the CD4+ T lymphocyte count decreases to <200/μL.

PREVENTION

All HIV-infected persons should be counseled regarding sources of *Toxoplasma* infection. The chances of primary infection with *Toxoplasma* can be reduced by not eating undercooked meat and by avoiding oocyst-contaminated material (i.e., a cat's litter box). Specifically, lamb, beef, pork, and venison should be cooked to an internal temperature of 63°C (145°F) measured in the thickest portion of the cut and rested for 3 minutes. Ground meat should be cooked to 71°C (145°F), whereas poultry should be cooked to 74°C (165°F). Hands should be washed thoroughly after work in the garden, and all fruits and vegetables should be washed. Ingestion of raw shellfish is a risk factor for toxoplasmosis, given that the filter-feeding mechanism of clams and mussels concentrates oocysts.

If the patient owns a cat, the litter box should be cleaned or changed daily, preferably by an HIV-negative, nonpregnant person; alternatively, patients should wash their hands thoroughly after changing the litter box. Litter boxes should be changed daily if possible, as freshly excreted oocysts will not have sporulated and will not be infectious. Patients should be encouraged to keep their cats inside and not to adopt or handle stray cats. Cats should be fed only canned or dried commercial food or well-cooked table food, not raw or undercooked meats. Patients need not be advised to part with their cats or to have their cats tested for toxoplasmosis. Blood intended for transfusion into *Toxoplasma*-seronegative immunocompromised individuals should be screened for antibody to *T. gondii.* Although such serologic screening is not routinely performed, seronegative women should be screened for evidence of infection several times during pregnancy if they are exposed to environmental conditions that put them at risk for infection with *T. gondii*. HIV-positive individuals should adhere closely to these preventive measures.

Acknowledgment

The author would like to acknowledge Dr. Lloyd Kasper for his numerous contributions to our understanding of the pathogenesis of toxoplasmosis and his essential role in preparation of this chapter for prior editions.

FURTHER READING

Cortés JA et al: Approach to ocular toxoplasmosis including pregnant women. Curr Opin Infect Dis 32:426, 2019.

Jones JL et al: *Toxoplasma gondii* infection in the United States, 2011–2014. Am J Trop Med Hyg 98:551 2018.

Peyron F et al: Congenital toxoplasmosis in France and the United States: One parasite, two diverging approaches. PLoS Negl Trop Dis 11:e0005222, 2017.

Schumacher AC et al: Toxoplasmosis outbreak associated with *Toxoplasma gondii*-contaminated venison–high attack rate, unusual clinical presentation, and atypical genotype. Clin Infect Dis 72:1557, 2021.

Wang ZD et al: Prevalence and burden of *Toxoplasma gondii* infection in HIV-infected people: A systematic review and meta-analysis. Lancet HIV 4:e177, 2017.

229 Protozoal Intestinal Infections and Trichomoniasis

Peter F. Weller

PROTOZOAL INFECTIONS

■ GIARDIASIS

Giardia duodenalis (also known as *G. lamblia* or *G. intestinalis*) is a cosmopolitan protozoal parasite that inhabits the small intestines of humans and other mammals. Giardiasis is one of the most common parasitic diseases in both developed and developing countries worldwide, causing both endemic and epidemic intestinal disease and diarrhea.

Life Cycle and Epidemiology (Fig. 229-1) Infection follows the ingestion of environmentally hardy cysts, which excyst in the small intestine, releasing flagellated trophozoites (Fig. 229-2) that multiply by binary fission. *Giardia* remains a pathogen of the proximal small bowel and does not disseminate hematogenously. Trophozoites remain free in the lumen or attach to the mucosal epithelium by means of a ventral sucking disk. As a trophozoite encounters altered conditions, it forms a morphologically distinct cyst, which is the stage of the parasite usually found in the feces. Trophozoites may be present and even predominate in loose or watery stools, but it is the resistant cyst that survives outside the body and is responsible for transmission. Cysts do not tolerate heating or desiccation, but they do remain viable for months in cold fresh water. The number of cysts excreted varies widely but can approach 10^7 per gram of stool.

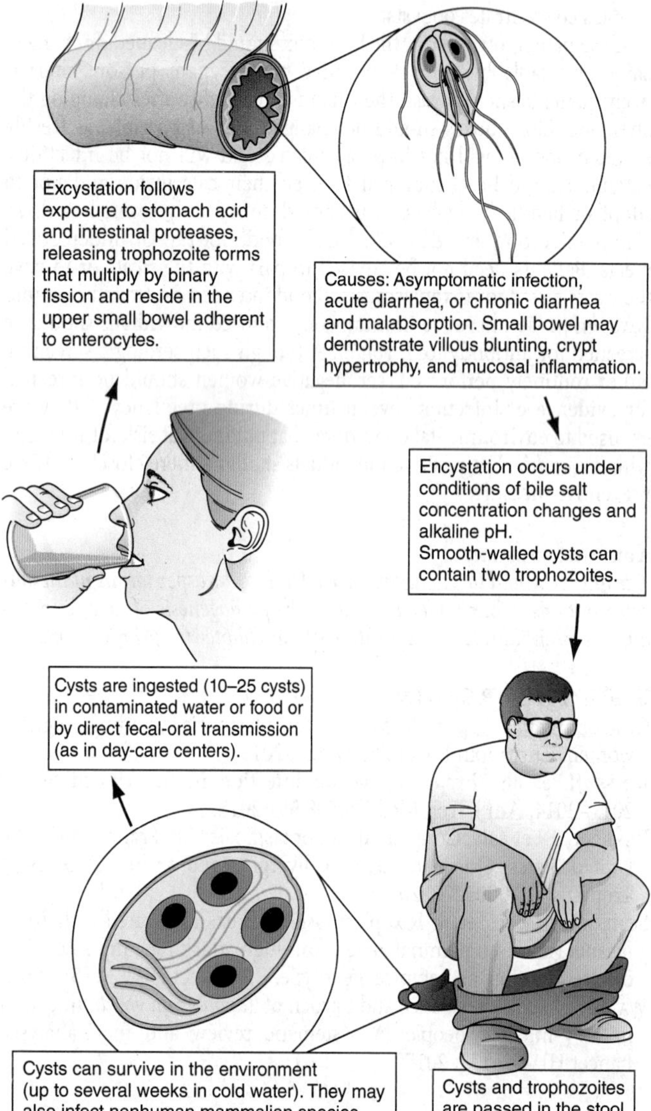

Excystation follows exposure to stomach acid and intestinal proteases, releasing trophozoite forms that multiply by binary fission and reside in the upper small bowel adherent to enterocytes.
Causes: Asymptomatic infection, acute diarrhea, or chronic diarrhea and malabsorption. Small bowel may demonstrate villous blunting, crypt hypertrophy, and mucosal inflammation.
Encystation occurs under conditions of bile salt concentration changes and alkaline pH. Smooth-walled cysts can contain two trophozoites.
Cysts are ingested (10–25 cysts) in contaminated water or food or by direct fecal-oral transmission (as in day-care centers).
Cysts can survive in the environment (up to several weeks in cold water). They may also infect nonhuman mammalian species.
Cysts and trophozoites are passed in the stool into the environment.

FIGURE 229-1 Life cycle of *Giardia*. *(Reproduced with permission from RL Guerrant et al [eds]: Tropical Infectious Diseases: Principles, Pathogens and Practice, 2nd ed, Elsevier, 2006.)*

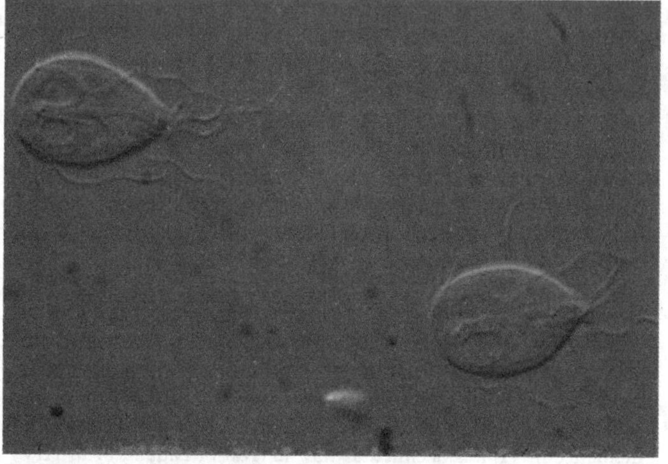

FIGURE 229-2 Flagellated, binucleate *Giardia* trophozoites.

Ingestion of as few as 10 cysts is sufficient to cause infection in humans. Because cysts are infectious when excreted, person-to-person transmission occurs where fecal hygiene is poor. Giardiasis is especially prevalent in day-care centers; person-to-person spread also takes place in other institutional settings with poor fecal hygiene and during anal–oral contact. If food is contaminated with *Giardia* cysts after cooking or preparation, foodborne transmission can occur. Waterborne transmission accounts for episodic infections (e.g., in campers and travelers) and for major epidemics in metropolitan areas. Surface water, ranging from mountain streams to large municipal reservoirs, can become contaminated with fecally derived *Giardia* cysts. The efficacy of water as a means of transmission is enhanced by the small infectious inoculum of *Giardia*, the prolonged survival of cysts in cold water, and the resistance of cysts to killing by routine chlorination methods that are adequate for controlling bacteria. Viable cysts can be eradicated from water by either boiling or filtration.

In the United States, *Giardia* (like *Cryptosporidium*; see below) is a common cause of waterborne epidemics of gastroenteritis. *Giardia* is common in developing countries, and infections may be acquired by travelers.

There are several recognized genotypes or assemblages of *G. duodenalis*. Human infections are due to assemblages A and B, whereas other assemblages are more common in other animals, including cats and dogs. Like beavers from reservoirs implicated in epidemics, dogs and cats have been found to be infected with assemblages A and B; this finding suggests both that these animals may have been infected from human sources and that they might be sources of further human infections.

Giardiasis, like cryptosporidiosis, creates a significant economic burden because of the costs incurred in the installation of water filtration systems required to prevent waterborne epidemics, in the management of epidemics that involve large communities, and in the evaluation and treatment of endemic infections.

Pathophysiology The reasons that some, but not all, infected patients develop clinical manifestations and the mechanisms by which *Giardia* causes alterations in small-bowel function are largely unknown. Although trophozoites adhere to the epithelium, they are not invasive but may elicit apoptosis of enterocytes, epithelial barrier dysfunction, and epithelial cell malabsorption and secretion. Consequent lactose intolerance and, in a minority of infected adults and children, significant malabsorption are clinical signs of the loss of epithelial brush-border enzyme activities. In most infections, the morphology of the bowel is unaltered; however, in chronically infected, symptomatic patients, the histopathologic findings (including flattened villi) and the clinical manifestations at times resemble those of tropical sprue and gluten-sensitive enteropathy. The pathogenesis of diarrhea in giardiasis is not known.

The natural history of *Giardia* infection varies markedly. Infections may be asymptomatic, transient, recurrent, or chronic. *G. duodenalis* parasites vary genotypically, and such variations might contribute to different courses of infection. Parasite as well as host factors may be important in determining the course of infection and disease. Both cellular and humoral responses develop in human infections, but their precise roles in disease pathogenesis and/or control of infection are unknown. Because patients with hypogammaglobulinemia suffer from prolonged, severe infections that are poorly responsive to treatment, humoral immune responses appear to be important. The greater susceptibilities of the young than of the old and of newly exposed persons than of chronically exposed populations suggest that at least partial protective immunity may develop.

Clinical Manifestations Disease manifestations of giardiasis range from asymptomatic carriage to fulminant diarrhea and malabsorption. Most infected persons are asymptomatic, but in epidemics, the proportion of symptomatic cases may be higher. Symptoms may develop suddenly or gradually. In persons with acute giardiasis, symptoms develop after an incubation period that lasts at least 5–6 days and usually 1–3 weeks. Prominent early symptoms include diarrhea, abdominal pain, bloating, belching, flatus, nausea, and vomiting. Although diarrhea is common, upper intestinal manifestations such as nausea, vomiting, bloating, and abdominal pain may predominate. The duration of acute giardiasis is usually >1 week, although diarrhea often subsides. Individuals with chronic giardiasis may present with or without having experienced an antecedent acute symptomatic episode. Diarrhea is not necessarily prominent, but increased flatus, loose stools, sulfurous belching, and (in some instances) weight loss occur. Symptoms may be continual or episodic and may persist for years. Some persons who have relatively mild symptoms for long periods recognize the extent of their discomfort only in retrospect. Fever, the presence of blood and/or mucus in the stools, and other signs and symptoms of colitis are uncommon and suggest a different diagnosis or a concomitant illness. Symptoms tend to be intermittent yet recurring and gradually debilitating, in contrast with the acute disabling symptoms associated with many enteric bacterial infections. Because of the less severe illness early on and the propensity for chronic infections, patients may seek medical advice late in the course of the illness; however, disease can be severe, resulting in malabsorption, weight loss, growth retardation in children, and dehydration. A number of extraintestinal manifestations have been described, such as urticaria, anterior uveitis, and arthritis; whether these are caused by giardiasis or concomitant processes is unclear.

Giardiasis can be severe in patients with hypogammaglobulinemia and can complicate other preexisting intestinal diseases, such as that occurring in cystic fibrosis. In patients with AIDS, *Giardia* can cause enteric illness that is refractory to treatment.

Diagnosis (Table 229-1) Giardiasis is diagnosed by detection of parasite antigens in the feces, by identification of cysts in the feces or of trophozoites in the feces or small intestines, or by nucleic acid amplification tests (NAATs). Cysts are oval, measure 8–12 μm × 7–10 μm, and characteristically contain four nuclei. Trophozoites are pear-shaped, dorsally convex, flattened parasites with two nuclei and four pairs of flagella (Fig. 229-2). The diagnosis is sometimes difficult to establish. Direct examination of fresh or properly preserved stools as well as concentration methods should be used. Because cyst excretion is variable and may be undetectable at times, repeated examination of stool, sampling of duodenal fluid, and biopsy of the small intestine may be required to detect the parasite. Tests for parasitic antigens in stool are at least as sensitive and specific as good microscopic examinations and are easier to perform. Newer NAATs are highly sensitive.

TREATMENT
Giardiasis

Cure rates with metronidazole (250 mg thrice daily for 5 days) are usually >90%. Tinidazole (2 g once by mouth) may be more effective than metronidazole. Nitazoxanide (500 mg twice daily for 3 days) is an alternative agent for treatment of giardiasis. Paromomycin, an oral aminoglycoside that is not well absorbed, can be given to symptomatic pregnant patients, although information is limited on how effectively this agent eradicates infection.

Almost all patients respond to therapy and are cured, although some with chronic giardiasis experience delayed resolution of symptoms after eradication of *Giardia*. For many of the latter patients, residual symptoms probably reflect delayed regeneration of intestinal brush-border enzymes. Continued infection should be documented by stool examinations before treatment is repeated. Patients who remain infected after repeated treatments should be evaluated for reinfection through family members, close personal contacts, and environmental sources as well as for hypogammaglobulinemia. In cases refractory to multiple treatment courses, prolonged therapy with metronidazole (750 mg thrice daily for 21 days) or therapy with varied combinations of multiple agents has been successful.

Prevention Giardiasis can be prevented by consumption of uncontaminated food and water and by personal hygiene during the provision of care for infected children. Boiling or filtering potentially contaminated water prevents infection.

CRYPTOSPORIDIOSIS

The coccidian parasite *Cryptosporidium* causes diarrheal disease that is self-limited in immunocompetent human hosts but can be severe in persons with AIDS or other forms of immunodeficiency. Two species of *Cryptosporidium*, *C. hominis* and *C. parvum*, cause most human infections.

Life Cycle and Epidemiology *Cryptosporidium* species are widely distributed in the world. Cryptosporidiosis is acquired by the consumption of oocysts (50% infectious dose: ~132 *C. parvum* oocysts in nonimmune individuals), which excyst to liberate sporozoites that

TABLE 229-1 Diagnosis of Intestinal Protozoal Infections

PARASITE	STOOL O+P	FECAL ACID-FAST STAIN	FECAL ANTIGEN IMMUNOASSAYS	FECAL NAATS	OTHER
Giardia	+		+	+	DFA
Cryptosporidium	±	+	+	+	DFA
Cystoisospora	±	+		+	
Cyclospora	±	+		+	
Dientamoeba	±		+	+	
Balantidium	+				
Microsporidia	–			+	Special fecal stains, tissue biopsies

Abbreviations: DFA, direct immunofluorescence assay; NAATs, nucleic acid amplification tests; O+P, conventional ova and parasites.

in turn enter and infect intestinal epithelial cells. The parasite's further development involves both asexual and sexual cycles, which produce forms capable of infecting other epithelial cells and of generating oocysts that are passed in the feces. *Cryptosporidium* species infect a number of animals, and *C. parvum* can spread from infected animals to humans. Since oocysts are immediately infectious when passed in feces, person-to-person transmission takes place in day-care centers and among household contacts and medical providers. Waterborne transmission (especially that of *C. hominis*) accounts for infections in travelers and for common-source epidemics. Oocysts are quite hardy and resist killing by routine chlorination. Both drinking water and recreational water (e.g., pools, waterslides) have been increasingly recognized as sources of infection.

Pathophysiology Although intestinal epithelial cells harbor cryptosporidia in an intracellular vacuole, the means by which secretory diarrhea is elicited remain uncertain. No characteristic pathologic changes are found by biopsy. The distribution of infection can be spotty within the principal site of infection, the small bowel. Cryptosporidia are found in the pharynx, stomach, and large bowel of some patients and at times in the respiratory tract. Especially in patients with AIDS, involvement of the biliary tract can cause papillary stenosis, sclerosing cholangitis, or cholecystitis.

Clinical Manifestations Asymptomatic infections can occur in both immunocompetent and immunocompromised hosts. In immunocompetent persons, symptoms develop after an incubation period of ~1 week and consist principally of watery nonbloody diarrhea, sometimes in conjunction with abdominal pain, nausea, anorexia, fever, and/or weight loss. In these hosts, the illness usually subsides after 1–2 weeks. In contrast, in immunocompromised hosts (especially those with AIDS and CD4+ T-cell counts <100/μL), diarrhea can be chronic, persistent, and remarkably profuse, causing clinically significant fluid and electrolyte depletion. Stool volumes may range from 1 to 25 L/d. Weight loss, wasting, and abdominal pain may be severe. Biliary tract involvement can manifest as mid-epigastric or right-upper-quadrant pain.

Diagnosis (Table 229-1) Evaluation starts with fecal examination for small oocysts, which are smaller (4–5 μm in diameter) than the fecal stages of most other parasites. Because conventional stool examination for ova and parasites (O+P) does not detect *Cryptosporidium*, specific testing must be requested. Detection is enhanced by evaluation of stools (obtained on multiple days) by several techniques, including modified acid-fast and direct immunofluorescent stains and enzyme immunoassays. NAATs are also useful. Cryptosporidia can also be identified by light and electron microscopy at the apical surfaces of intestinal epithelium from biopsy specimens of the small bowel and, less frequently, the large bowel.

TREATMENT

Cryptosporidiosis

Nitazoxanide, approved by the U.S. Food and Drug Administration (FDA) for the treatment of cryptosporidiosis, is available in tablet form for adults (500 mg twice daily for 3 days) and as an elixir for children. This agent has not been effective for the treatment of immunosuppressed patients or HIV-infected patients, in whom improved immune status due to antiretroviral therapy can lead to amelioration of cryptosporidiosis. Otherwise, treatment includes supportive care with replacement of fluids and electrolytes and administration of antidiarrheal agents. Biliary tract obstruction may require papillotomy or T-tube placement. Prevention requires minimizing exposure to infectious oocysts in human or animal feces. Use of submicron water filters may minimize acquisition of infection from drinking water.

CYSTOISOSPORIASIS

The coccidian parasite *Cystoisospora belli* causes human intestinal disease. Infection is acquired by the consumption of oocysts, after which the parasite invades intestinal epithelial cells and undergoes both sexual and asexual cycles of development. Oocysts excreted in stool are not immediately infectious but must undergo further maturation.

Although *C. belli* infects many animals, little is known about the epidemiology or prevalence of this parasite in humans. It is most common in tropical and subtropical countries. Acute infections can begin abruptly with fever, abdominal pain, and watery nonbloody diarrhea and can last for weeks or months. In patients who have AIDS or are immunocompromised for other reasons, infections often are not self-limited but rather resemble cryptosporidiosis, with chronic, profuse watery diarrhea. Eosinophilia, which is not found in other enteric protozoan infections, may be detectable. The diagnosis (Table 229-1) is usually made by detection of the large (~25 μm) oocysts in stool by modified acid-fast staining. Oocyst excretion may be low-level and intermittent; if repeated stool examinations are unrevealing, sampling of duodenal contents by aspiration or small-bowel biopsy (often with electron microscopic examination) may be necessary. NAATs are effective newer diagnostic tools.

TREATMENT

Cystoisosporiasis

Trimethoprim-sulfamethoxazole (TMP-SMX, 160/800 mg two times daily for 10 days; and, for HIV-infected patients, then continuing three times daily for 3 weeks) is effective. For patients intolerant of sulfonamides, pyrimethamine (50–75 mg/d) can be used. Relapses can occur in persons with AIDS and necessitate maintenance therapy with TMP-SMX (160/800 mg three times per week).

CYCLOSPORIASIS

Cyclospora cayetanensis, a cause of diarrheal illness, is globally distributed: illness due to *C. cayetanensis* has been reported in the United States, Asia, Africa, Latin America, and Europe. The epidemiology of this parasite has not yet been fully defined, but waterborne transmission and foodborne transmission (e.g., by basil, sweet peas, and imported raspberries) have been recognized. The full spectrum of illness attributable to *Cyclospora* has not been delineated. Some infected patients may be without symptoms, but many have diarrhea, flulike symptoms, and flatulence and belching. The illness can be self-limited, can wax and wane, or, in many cases, can involve prolonged diarrhea, anorexia, and upper gastrointestinal symptoms, with sustained fatigue and weight loss in some instances. Diarrheal illness may persist for >1 month. *Cyclospora* can cause enteric illness in patients infected with HIV.

The parasite is detectable in epithelial cells of small-bowel biopsy samples and elicits secretory diarrhea by unknown means. The absence of fecal blood and leukocytes indicates that disease due to *Cyclospora* is not caused by destruction of the small-bowel mucosa. The diagnosis (Table 229-1) can be made by detection of spherical 8- to 10-μm oocysts in the stool, although routine stool O+P examinations are not sufficient. Specific fecal examinations must be requested to detect the oocysts, which are variably acid-fast and are fluorescent when viewed with ultraviolet light microscopy. NAATs are proving to be sensitive. Cyclosporiasis should be considered in the differential diagnosis of prolonged diarrhea, with or without a history of travel by the patient to other countries.

TREATMENT

Cyclosporiasis

Cyclosporiasis is treated with TMP-SMX (160/800 mg twice daily for 7–10 days). HIV-infected patients may experience relapses after such treatment and thus may require longer-term suppressive maintenance therapy.

MICROSPORIDIOSIS

Microsporidia are obligate intracellular spore-forming protozoa that infect many animals and cause disease in humans, especially as opportunistic pathogens in AIDS. Microsporidia are members of a distinct phylum, Microspora, which contains dozens of genera and hundreds of species. The various microsporidia are differentiated by their developmental life cycles, ultrastructural features, and molecular taxonomy based on ribosomal RNA. The complex life cycles of the organisms result in the production of infectious spores (**Fig. 229-3**). Currently, at least 15 species of microsporidia, including the genera *Encephalitozoon, Tubulinosema, Pleistophora, Nosema, Vittaforma, Trachipleistophora, Anncaliia, Microsporidium*, and *Enterocytozoon*, are recognized as causes of human disease. Although some microsporidia are probably prevalent causes of self-limited or asymptomatic infections in immunocompetent patients, little is known about how microsporidiosis is acquired.

Microsporidiosis is most common among patients with AIDS, less common among patients with other types of immunocompromise, and rare among immunocompetent hosts. In patients with AIDS, intestinal infections with *Enterocytozoon bieneusi* and *Encephalitozoon intestinalis* are recognized to contribute to chronic diarrhea and wasting; these infections have been found in 10–40% of patients with chronic diarrhea. Both organisms have been found in the biliary tracts of patients with cholecystitis. *E. intestinalis* may also disseminate to cause fever, diarrhea, sinusitis, cholangitis, and bronchiolitis. In patients with AIDS, *Encephalitozoon hellem* has caused superficial keratoconjunctivitis as well as sinusitis, respiratory tract disease, and disseminated infection. Myositis due to *Pleistophora* has been documented. *Nosema, Vittaforma*, and *Microsporidium* have caused stromal keratitis associated with trauma in immunocompetent patients.

Microsporidia are small gram-positive organisms with mature spores measuring 0.5–2 μm × 1–4 μm. Diagnosis of microsporidial infections in tissue often requires electron microscopy, although intracellular spores can be visualized by light microscopy with hematoxylin and eosin, Giemsa, or tissue Gram's stain. For the diagnosis of intestinal microsporidiosis, modified trichrome or chromotrope 2R–based staining and Uvitex 2B or calcofluor fluorescent staining reveal spores in smears of feces or duodenal aspirates. NAATs are useful for diagnosis and speciation. Definitive therapies for microsporidial infections remain to be established. For superficial keratoconjunctivitis due to *E. hellem, E. cuniculi, E. intestinalis*, and *E. bieneusi*, topical therapy with fumagillin suspension has shown promise (**Chap. 222**). For enteric infections with *E. intestinalis* in HIV-infected patients, therapy with albendazole may be efficacious (**Chap. 222**).

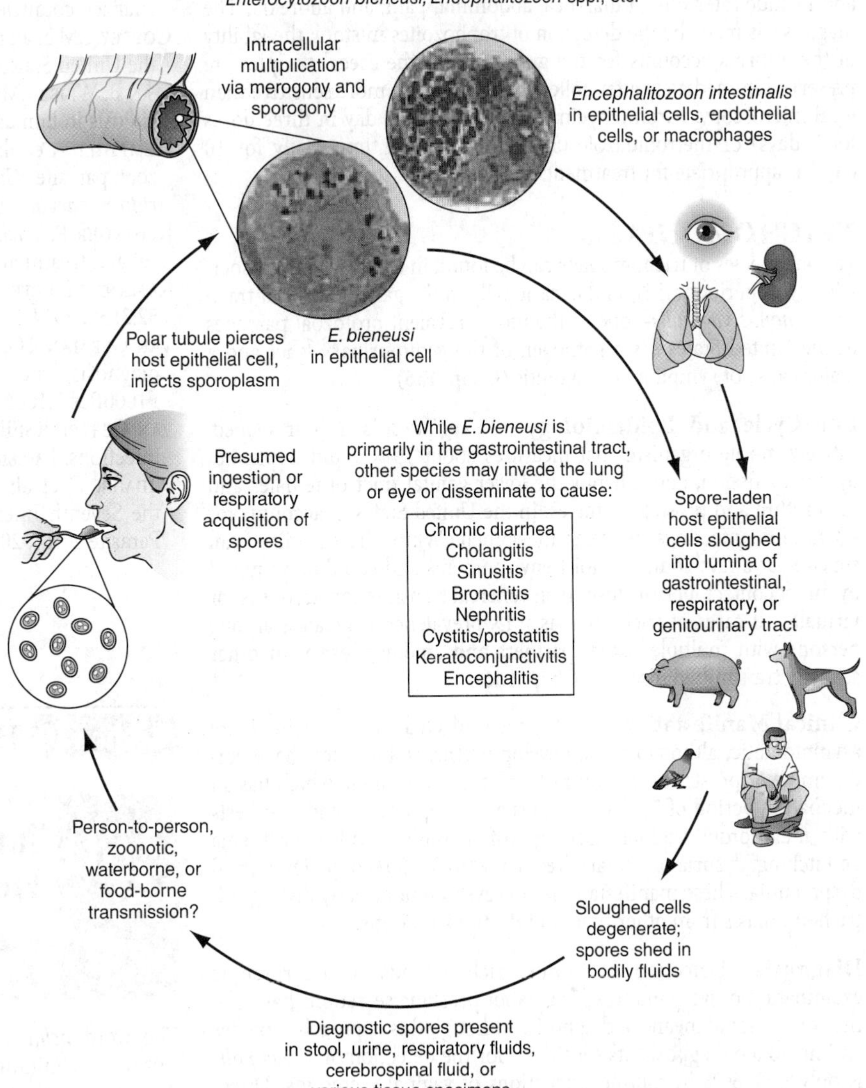

FIGURE 229-3 Life cycle of microsporidia. *(Reproduced with permission from RL Guerrant et al [eds]: Tropical Infectious Diseases: Principles, Pathogens and Practice, 2nd ed, Elsevier 2006.)*

OTHER INTESTINAL PROTOZOA

Balantidiasis *Balantidium coli* is a large ciliated protozoal parasite that can produce a spectrum of large-intestinal disease analogous to amebiasis. The parasite is widely distributed in the world. Since it infects pigs, cases in humans are more common where pigs are raised. Infective cysts can be transmitted from person to person and through water, but many cases are due to the ingestion of cysts derived from porcine feces in association with slaughtering, with use of pig feces for fertilizer, or with contamination of water supplies by pig feces.

Ingested cysts liberate trophozoites, which reside and replicate in the large bowel. Many patients remain asymptomatic, but some have persisting intermittent diarrhea, and a few develop more fulminant dysentery. In symptomatic individuals, the pathology in the bowel—both gross and microscopic—is similar to that seen in amebiasis, with varying degrees of mucosal invasion, focal necrosis, and ulceration. Balantidiasis, unlike amebiasis, only rarely spreads hematogenously to other organs. The diagnosis is made by detection of the trophozoite stage in stool or sampled colonic tissue. Tetracycline (500 mg four times daily for 10 days) is an effective therapeutic agent.

Blastocystosis *Blastocystis hominis* remains an organism of uncertain taxonomy and pathogenicity. Some patients who pass *B. hominis* in their stools are asymptomatic, whereas others have diarrhea and associated intestinal symptoms. Diligent evaluation reveals other potential bacterial, viral, or protozoal causes of diarrhea in some but not all patients with symptoms. Because the pathogenicity of *B. hominis* is uncertain and because therapy for *Blastocystis* infection is neither specific nor uniformly effective, patients with prominent intestinal symptoms should be fully evaluated for other infectious causes of diarrhea. If diarrheal symptoms associated with *Blastocystis* are prominent, either metronidazole (750 mg thrice daily for 10 days) or TMP-SMX (160 mg/800 mg twice daily for 7 days) can be used.

Dientamoebiasis *Dientamoeba fragilis* is unique among intestinal protozoa in that it has a trophozoite stage but not a cyst stage. How trophozoites survive to transmit infection is not known. When symptoms develop in patients with *D. fragilis* infection, they are generally mild and include intermittent diarrhea, abdominal pain, and anorexia. The diagnosis is made by the detection of trophozoites in stool; the lability of these forms accounts for the greater yield when fecal samples are preserved immediately after collection. NAATs are more sensitive than fecal microscopy. Paromomycin (25–35 mg/kg per day in three doses for 7 days) or metronidazole (500–750 mg three times daily for 10 days) is appropriate for treatment.

TRICHOMONIASIS

Various species of trichomonads can be found in the mouth (in association with periodontitis) and occasionally in the gastrointestinal tract. *Trichomonas vaginalis*—one of the most prevalent protozoal parasites in the United States—is a pathogen of the genitourinary tract and a major cause of symptomatic vaginitis (**Chap. 136**).

Life Cycle and Epidemiology *T. vaginalis* is a pear-shaped, actively motile organism that measures about 10 × 7 μm, replicates by binary fission, and inhabits the lower genital tract of females and the urethra and prostate of males. In the United States, it accounts for ~3 million infections per year in women. While the organism can survive for a few hours in moist environments and could be acquired by direct contact, person-to-person venereal transmission accounts for virtually all cases of trichomoniasis. Its prevalence is greatest among persons with multiple sexual partners and among those with other sexually transmitted diseases (**Chap. 136**).

Clinical Manifestations Many men infected with *T. vaginalis* are asymptomatic, although some develop urethritis and a few have epididymitis or prostatitis. In contrast, infection in women, which has an incubation period of 5–28 days, is usually symptomatic and manifests with malodorous vaginal discharge (often yellow), vulvar erythema and itching, dysuria or urinary frequency (in 30–50% of patients), and dyspareunia. These manifestations, however, do not clearly distinguish trichomoniasis from other types of infectious vaginitis.

Diagnosis Detection of motile trichomonads by microscopic examination of wet mounts of vaginal or prostatic secretions has been the conventional means of diagnosis. Although this approach provides an immediate diagnosis, its sensitivity for the detection of *T. vaginalis* is only ~50–60% in routine evaluations of vaginal secretions. Direct immunofluorescent antibody staining is more sensitive (70–90%) than wet-mount examinations. *T. vaginalis* can be recovered from the urethra of both males and females and is detectable in males after prostatic massage. NAATs are FDA approved and are highly sensitive and specific for urine and for endocervical and vaginal swabs from women.

TREATMENT

Trichomoniasis

Metronidazole (either a single 2-g dose or 500-mg doses twice daily for 7 days) or tinidazole (a single 2-g dose) is effective. All sexual partners must be treated concurrently to prevent reinfection, especially from asymptomatic males. In males with persistent symptomatic urethritis after therapy for nongonococcal urethritis, metronidazole therapy should be considered for possible trichomoniasis. Alternatives to metronidazole for treatment during pregnancy are not readily available. Reinfection often accounts for apparent treatment failures, but strains of *T. vaginalis* exhibiting high-level resistance to metronidazole have been encountered. Treatment of these resistant infections with higher oral doses, parenteral doses, or concurrent oral and vaginal doses of metronidazole or with tinidazole has been successful.

■ FURTHER READING

Buret AG et al: Update on *Giardia*: Highlights from the Seventh International *Giardia* and *Cryptosporidim* Conference. Parasite 27:49, 2020.

Carter BL et al: Health sequelae of human cryptosporidiosis in industrialized countries: A systematic review. Parasit Vectors 13:443, 2020.

Coffey CM et al: Evolving epidemiology of reported giardiasis cases in the United States, 1995-2016. Clin Infect Dis 72:764, 2021.

Han B, Weiss LM: Therapeutic targets for the treatment of microsporidiosis in humans. Expert Opin Ther Targets 22:903, 2018.

Hemphill A et al: Comparative pathobiology of the intestinal protozoan parasites *Giardia lamblia, Entamoeba histolytica* and *Cryptosporidium parvum*. Pathogens 8:116, 2019.

Kissinger P: *Trichomonas vaginalis*: A review of epidemiologic, clinical and treatment issues. BMC Infect Dis 15:307, 2015.

Ramanan P, Pritt BS: Extraintestinal microsporidiosis. J Clin Microbiol 52:3839, 2014.

Van German TO, Muzny CA: Recent advances in the epidemiology, diagnosis, and management of *Trichomonas vaginalis* infection. F1000Res 8:1666, 2019.

Van Gestel RSFE et al: A clinical guideline on *Dientamoeba fragilis* infections. Parasitology 146:1131, 2018.

Widmer G et al: Update on *Cryptosporidium* spp: Highlights from the Seventh International *Giardia* and *Cryptosporidim* Conference. Parasite 27:14, 2020.

Section 19 Helminthic Infections

230 Introduction to Helminthic Infections

Peter F. Weller

The word *helminth* is derived from the Greek *helmins* ("parasitic worm"). Helminthic worms are highly prevalent and, depending on the species, may exist as free-living organisms or as parasites of plant or animal hosts. The parasitic helminths have co-evolved with specific mammalian and other host species. Accordingly, most helminthic infections are restricted to nonhuman hosts, and only rarely do these zoonotic helminths accidentally cause human infections.

Helminthic parasites of humans belong to two phyla: Nemathelminthes, which includes nematodes (roundworms), and Platyhelminthes, which includes cestodes (tapeworms) and trematodes (flukes). Helminthic parasites of humans reside within the human body and hence are the cause of true infections. In contrast, parasites of other genera that reside only on mucocutaneous surfaces of humans (e.g., the parasites causing myiasis and scabies) are considered to represent infestations rather than infections.

Helminthic parasites differ substantially from protozoan parasites in several respects. First, protozoan parasites are unicellular organisms, whereas helminthic parasites are multicellular worms that possess differentiated organ systems. Second, helminthic parasites have complex life cycles that require sequential stages of development outside the human host. Thus, most helminths do not complete their replication within the human host; rather, they develop to a certain stage within the mammalian host and, as part of their obligatory life cycle, must mature further outside that host. During the "extra-human" stages of their life cycle, helminths exist either as free-living organisms or as parasites within another host species and thereafter mature into new developmental stages capable of infecting humans. Thus, with only two exceptions (*Strongyloides stercoralis* and *Capillaria philippinensis*, which are capable of internal human reinfections), increases in the number of adult helminths (i.e., the "worm burden") within the human host require repeated exogenous reinfections. In the case of protozoan parasites, a brief, even singular exposure (e.g., a single mosquito bite transmitting malaria) may lead rapidly to intense parasite loads and overwhelming infections; in contrast, for all but the two helminths noted above, increases in worm burden require multiple and usually ongoing exposures to infectious forms, such as ingestion of eggs of intestinal helminths or waterborne exposures to infectious cercariae of *Schistosoma mansoni*. This requirement is germane both to the consideration of helminthic infections in individuals and to ongoing global efforts to interrupt and/or minimize the acquisition of helminthic infections by humans.

Third, helminthic infections have a predilection toward stimulation of host immune responses that elicit eosinophilia within human tissues and blood. The many protozoan infections characteristically do not elicit eosinophilia in infected humans, with only three exceptions (two intestinal protozoan parasites, *Cystoisospora belli* and *Dientamoeba fragilis*, and tissue-borne *Sarcocystis* species). The magnitude of helminth-elicited eosinophilia tends to correlate with the extent of tissue invasion by larvae or adult helminths. For example, in several helminthic infections, including acute schistosomiasis (Katayama syndrome), paragonimiasis, and hookworm and *Ascaris* infections, eosinophilia is most pronounced during the early phases of infection, when migrations of infecting larvae and progression of subsequent developmental stages through the tissues are greatest. In established infections, local eosinophilia is often present around helminths in tissues, but blood eosinophilia may be intermittent, mild, or absent. In helminthic infections in which parasites are well contained within tissues (e.g., echinococcal cysts) or confined within the lumen of the intestinal tract (e.g., adult *Ascaris* or tapeworms), eosinophilia is usually absent.

NEMATODES

Nematodes are nonsegmented roundworms. Species of nematodes are remarkably diverse and abundant in nature. Among the many thousands of nematode species, few are parasites of humans. Most nematodes are free-living, and these species have variably evolved to survive in diverse ecologic niches, including saltwater, freshwater, or soil. The well-studied organism *Caenorhabditis elegans* is a free-living nematode. Nematodes can be either beneficial or deleterious parasites of plants. Parasitic nematodes have co-evolved with specific mammalian hosts and have no capacity to live their full life cycles in other hosts. Uncommonly, humans are exposed to infectious stages of nonhuman nematode parasites, and the resultant zoonotic nematode infections can elicit inflammatory and immune responses as larval forms migrate and die in the unsuitable human host. Examples include pulmonary coin lesions due to mosquito-transmitted infections with the dog heartworm *Dirofilaria immitis*; eosinophilic meningoencephalitis due to ingested eggs of the raccoon ascarid *Baylisascaris procyonis*; and eosinophilic meningitis due to ingestion of larvae of the rat lungworm *Angiostrongylus cantonensis*.

Nematode parasites of humans include worms that reside in the intestinal tract or localize in extraintestinal vascular or tissue sites. Roundworms are bisexual, with separate male and female forms (except for *S. stercoralis*, whose adult females are hermaphroditic in the human intestinal tract). Depending on the species, fertilized females release either larvae or eggs containing larvae. Nematodes have five developmental stages: an adult stage and four sequential larval stages. These parasites characteristically are surrounded by a durable outer cuticular layer. Nematodes have a nervous system; a muscular system, including muscle cells under the cuticle; and a developed intestinal tract, including an oral cavity and an elongated gut that ends in an anal pore. Adults may range in size from minute to >1 meter in length (with *Dracunculus medinensis*, for example, at the long end of this spectrum).

Humans acquire infections with nematode parasites by various routes, depending on the parasitic species. Ingestion of eggs passed in human feces is a major global health problem with many of the intestinal helminths (e.g., *Ascaris lumbricoides*). In other species, infecting larvae penetrate skin exposed to fecally contaminated soil (e.g., *S. stercoralis*, hookworms) or traverse the skin after the bite of infected insect vectors (e.g., filariae). Some nematode infections are acquired by consumption of specific animal-derived foods (e.g., trichinellosis from raw or undercooked pork or wild carnivorous mammals). As noted above, only two nematodes, *S. stercoralis* and *C. philippinensis*, can internally reinfect humans; thus, for all other nematodes, any increases in worm burden must be due to continued exogenous reinfections.

CESTODES

Tapeworms are the cestode parasites of humans. Adult tapeworms are elongated, segmented, hermaphroditic flatworms that reside in the intestinal lumen or, in their larval forms, may live in extraintestinal tissues. Tapeworms include a head (*scolex*) and a number of attached segments (*proglottids*). The worms attach to the intestinal tract via their scolices, which may possess suckers, hooks, or grooves. The scolex is the site of formation of new proglottids. Tapeworms do not have a functional gut tract; rather, each tapeworm segment passively and actively obtains nutrients through its specialized surface tegument. Mature proglottids possess both male and female sex organs, but insemination usually occurs between adjacent proglottids. Fertilized proglottids release eggs that are passed in the feces. When ingested by an intermediate host, an egg releases an oncosphere that penetrates the gut and develops further in tissues as a cysticercus. Humans acquire infection by ingesting animal tissues that contain cysticerci, and the resultant tapeworms develop and reside in the proximal small bowel (e.g., *Taenia solium*, *T. saginata*). Alternatively, if humans ingest eggs of these cestodes that have been passed in human or animal feces, oncospheres develop and can cause space-occupying extraintestinal cystic lesions in tissues; examples include cysticercosis due to *T. solium* and hydatid disease due to species of *Echinococcus*.

TREMATODES

Trematodes of medical importance include blood flukes, intestinal flukes, and tissue flukes. Adult flukes are often leaf-shaped flatworms. Oral and/or ventral suckers help adult flukes maintain their positions in situ. Flukes have an oral cavity but no distal anal pore. Nutrients are obtained both through their integument and by ingestion into the blind intestinal tract. Flukes are hermaphroditic except for blood flukes (schistosomes), which are bisexual. Eggs are passed in human feces (*Fasciola*, *Fasciolopsis*, *Clonorchis*, *Schistosoma japonicum*, *S. mansoni*), urine (*Schistosoma haematobium*), or sputum and feces (*Paragonimus*). Expelled eggs release miracidia—usually in water—that infect specific snail species. Within snails, parasites multiply and cercariae are released. Depending on the species, cercariae can penetrate the skin (schistosomes) or can develop into metacercariae that can be ingested with plants (e.g., watercress for *Fasciola*) or with fish (*Clonorchis*) or crabs (*Paragonimus*).

CONCLUSION

Many of the so-called neglected tropical diseases are due to helminthic infections. The health impacts of many helminthic infections are varied and are based on the frequent need for repeated exposures to increase the worm burdens in infected humans. In global regions where exposures to specific helminths occur even in childhood (e.g., fecally derived intestinal nematodes, mosquito-transmitted filariae, or waterborne snail-transmitted schistosomes), the morbidities in infected individuals can include nutritional, developmental, cognitive, and functional impairments. Ongoing global mass-treatment programs are currently aimed at diminishing the local prevalences of specific helminths and their consequent impacts on the health of local populations.

231 Trichinellosis and Other Tissue Nematode Infections

Peter F. Weller

Nematodes are elongated, symmetric roundworms. Parasitic nematodes of medical significance may be broadly classified as either predominantly intestinal or tissue nematodes. The intestinal nematodes are covered in **Chap. 232**. This chapter covers the tissue nematodes that cause trichinellosis, visceral and ocular larva migrans, cutaneous larva migrans, cerebral angiostrongyliasis, and gnathostomiasis. All of these zoonotic infections result from incidental exposure to infectious nematodes. The clinical symptoms of these infections are due largely to invasive larval stages that (except in the case of *Trichinella*) do not reach maturity in humans.

TRICHINELLOSIS

Trichinellosis develops after the ingestion of meat containing cysts of *Trichinella* (e.g., pork or other meat from a carnivore). Although most infections are mild and asymptomatic, heavy infections can cause severe enteritis, periorbital edema, myositis, and (infrequently) death.

Life Cycle and Epidemiology Nine species of *Trichinella* and 13 genotypes are recognized as causes of infection in humans. Two species are distributed worldwide: *T. spiralis*, which is found in a great variety of carnivorous and omnivorous animals, and *T. pseudospiralis*, which is found in mammals and birds. *T. nativa* is present in Arctic and subarctic regions and infects bears, foxes, and walruses; *T. nelsoni* is found in equatorial eastern Africa, where it is common among felid predators and scavengers such as hyenas and bush pigs; and *T. britovi* is found in Europe, western Africa, and western Asia among carnivores but not among domestic swine. *T. murrelli* is present in wild animals in North American and Japan. *T. papuae* is found in Papua New Guinea, Thailand, Taiwan, and Cambodia in domestic and feral pigs and in saltwater crocodiles and turtles. *T. zimbabwensis* is present in crocodiles in Tanzania. *T. patagoniensis* is found in cougars in South America.

After human consumption of trichinous meat, encysted larvae are liberated by digestive acid and proteases (**Fig. 231-1**). The larvae invade the small-bowel mucosa and mature into adult worms. After ~1 week, female worms release newborn larvae that migrate via the circulation to striated muscle. The larvae of all species except *T. pseudospiralis*, *T. papuae*, and *T. zimbabwensis* then encyst by inducing a radical transformation in the muscle cell architecture. Host immune responses may help to expel intestinal adult worms but have few deleterious effects on muscle-dwelling larvae.

Human trichinellosis classically has been caused by the ingestion of infected pork products and thus can occur in almost any location where the meat of domestic or wild swine is eaten. Increasingly, human trichinellosis has also been acquired from the meat of other animals, including dogs (in parts of Asia and Africa), horses (in Italy and France), and bears and walruses (in northern regions). Although cattle (being herbivores) are not natural hosts of *Trichinella*, beef has been implicated in outbreaks when contaminated or adulterated with trichinous pork. About 12 cases of trichinellosis are reported annually in the United States, but most mild cases probably remain undiagnosed. Recent U.S. and Canadian outbreaks have been attributable predominantly to consumption of wild game (especially bear and walrus meat).

Pathogenesis and Clinical Features Clinical symptoms of trichinellosis arise from the successive phases of parasite enteric invasion, larval migration, and muscle encystment (Fig. 231-1). Most light infections (those with <10 larvae per gram of muscle) are asymptomatic, whereas heavy infections (which can involve >50 larvae per gram of muscle) can be life-threatening. An initial enteric phase due to release of ingested muscle larvae may elicit diarrhea, abdominal pain, constipation, and nausea during the first weeks after infection.

Symptoms due to larval migration and muscle invasion begin to appear in the second week after infection. The migrating *Trichinella* larvae provoke a marked local and systemic hypersensitivity reaction, with fever and eosinophilia. Periorbital and facial edema is common, as are hemorrhages in the subconjunctivae, retina, and nail beds ("splinter" hemorrhages). A maculopapular rash, headache, cough, dyspnea, or dysphagia sometimes develops. Myocarditis with tachyarrhythmias or heart failure—and, less commonly, encephalitis or pneumonitis—may develop and accounts for most deaths of patients with trichinellosis.

Upon onset of larval encystment in muscle 2–3 weeks after infection, symptoms of myositis with myalgias, muscle edema, and weakness develop, usually overlapping with the inflammatory reactions to migrating larvae. The most commonly involved muscle groups include the extraocular muscles; the biceps; and the muscles of the jaw, neck, lower back, and diaphragm. Peaking ~3 weeks after infection, symptoms subside only gradually during a prolonged convalescence. Uncommon infections with *T. pseudospiralis*, whose larvae do not encapsulate in muscles, elicit a prolonged polymyositis-like illness.

Laboratory Findings and Diagnosis Blood eosinophilia develops in >90% of patients with symptomatic trichinellosis and may peak at a level of >50% 2–4 weeks after infection. Serum levels of muscle enzymes, including creatine phosphokinase, are elevated in most symptomatic patients. Patients should be questioned thoroughly

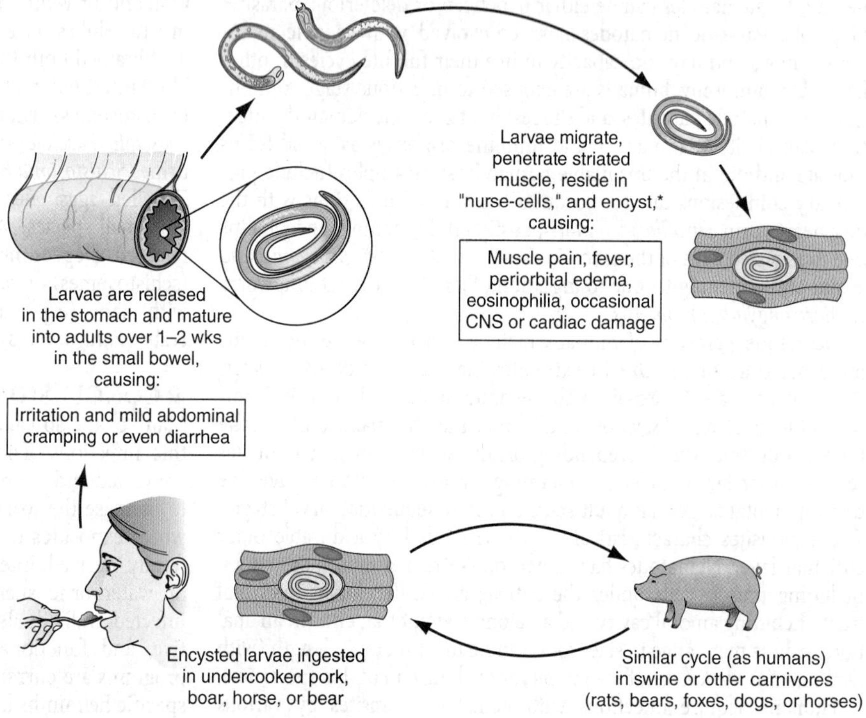
Larvae migrate, penetrate striated muscle, reside in "nurse-cells," and encyst,* causing:
Muscle pain, fever, periorbital edema, eosinophilia, occasional CNS or cardiac damage
Larvae are released in the stomach and mature into adults over 1–2 wks in the small bowel, causing:
Irritation and mild abdominal cramping or even diarrhea
Encysted larvae ingested in undercooked pork, boar, horse, or bear
Similar cycle (as humans) in swine or other carnivores (rats, bears, foxes, dogs, or horses)
*T. papuae, T. zimbabwensis, and T. pseudospiralis do not encyst.

FIGURE 231-1 Life cycle of *Trichinella spiralis* (cosmopolitan); *nelsoni* (equatorial Africa); *britovi* (Europe, western Africa, western Asia); *nativa* (Arctic); *murrelli* (North America); *papuae* (Papua New Guinea); *zimbabwensis* (Tanzania); and *pseudospiralis* (cosmopolitan). CNS, central nervous system. *(Reproduced with permission from RL Guerrant et al [eds]: Tropical Infectious Diseases: Principles, Pathogens and Practice, 2nd ed, Elsevier, 2006.)*

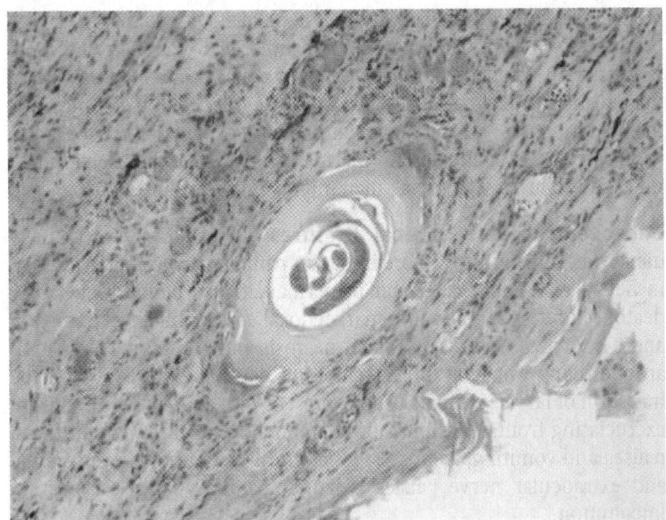

FIGURE 231-2 ***Trichinella*** **larva** encysted in a characteristic hyalinized capsule in striated muscle tissue. *(Photographs provided by Dr. Mary Wu Chang with permission of patient's mother.)*

about their consumption of pork or wild animal meat and about illness in other individuals who ate the same meat. A presumptive clinical diagnosis can be based on fevers, eosinophilia, periorbital edema, and myalgias after a suspect meal. A rise in the titer of parasite-specific antibody, which usually does not occur until after the third week of infection, confirms the diagnosis. Alternatively, a definitive diagnosis requires surgical biopsy of at least 1 g of involved muscle; the yields are highest near tendon insertions. The fresh muscle tissue should be compressed between glass slides and examined microscopically (**Fig. 231-2**) because larvae may be missed by examination of routine histopathologic sections alone.

TREATMENT

Trichinellosis

Most lightly infected patients recover uneventfully with bed rest, antipyretics, and analgesics. Glucocorticoids like prednisone (**Table 231-1**) are beneficial for severe myositis and myocarditis.

TABLE 231-1 Therapy for Tissue Nematode Infections

INFECTION	SEVERITY	TREATMENT
Trichinellosis	Mild	Supportive
	Moderate	Albendazole (400 mg bid × 8–14 days) *or*
		Mebendazole (200–400 mg tid × 3 days, then 500 mg tid × 10 days)
	Severe	Add glucocorticoids (e.g., prednisone, 1 mg/kg qd × 5 days)
Visceral larva migrans	Mild to moderate	Supportive
	Severe	Glucocorticoids (as above)
	Ocular	Not fully defined; albendazole (800 mg bid for adults, 400 mg bid for children) with glucocorticoids × 5–20 days has been effective
Cutaneous larva migrans		Ivermectin (single dose, 200 μg/kg) *or*
		Albendazole (200 mg bid × 3 days)
Angiostrongyliasis	Mild to moderate	Supportive
	Severe	Glucocorticoids (as above)
Gnathostomiasis		Ivermectin (200 μg/kg per day × 2 days) *or*
		Albendazole (400 mg bid × 21 days)

Mebendazole and albendazole are active against enteric stages of the parasite, but their efficacy against encysted larvae has not been conclusively demonstrated.

Prevention Larvae are usually killed by cooking pork until it is no longer pink or by freezing it at –15°C for 3 weeks. However, Arctic *T. nativa* larvae in walrus or bear meat are relatively resistant and may remain viable despite freezing.

■ VISCERAL AND OCULAR LARVA MIGRANS

Visceral larva migrans is a syndrome caused by nematodes that are normally parasitic for nonhuman host species. In humans, these nematode larvae do not develop into adult worms but instead migrate through host tissues and elicit eosinophilic inflammation. The most common form of visceral larva migrans is toxocariasis due to larvae of the canine ascarid *Toxocara canis*; the syndrome is due less commonly to the feline ascarid *T. cati* and even less commonly to the pig ascarid *Ascaris suum*. Rare cases with eosinophilic meningoencephalitis have been caused by the raccoon ascarid *Baylisascaris procyonis*.

Life Cycle and Epidemiology The canine roundworm *T. canis* is distributed among dogs worldwide. Ingestion of infective eggs by dogs is followed by liberation of *Toxocara* larvae, which penetrate the gut wall and migrate intravascularly into canine tissues, where most remain in a developmentally arrested state. During pregnancy, some larvae resume migration in bitches and infect puppies prenatally (through transplacental transmission) or after birth (through suckling). Thus, in lactating bitches and puppies, larvae return to the intestinal tract and develop into adult worms, which produce eggs that are released in the feces. Eggs must undergo embryonation over several weeks to become infectious. Humans acquire toxocariasis mainly by eating soil contaminated by puppy feces that contains infective *T. canis* eggs. Visceral larva migrans is most common among children who habitually eat dirt.

Pathogenesis and Clinical Features Clinical disease most commonly afflicts preschool children. After humans ingest *Toxocara* eggs, the larvae hatch and penetrate the intestinal mucosa, from which they are carried by the circulation to a wide variety of organs and tissues. The larvae invade the liver, lungs, central nervous system (CNS), and other sites, provoking intense local eosinophilic granulomatous responses. The degree of clinical illness depends on larval number and tissue distribution, reinfection, and host immune responses. Most light infections are asymptomatic and may be evidenced only by blood eosinophilia. Characteristic symptoms of visceral larva migrans include fever, malaise, anorexia and weight loss, cough, wheezing, and rashes. Hepatosplenomegaly is common. These features may be accompanied by extraordinary peripheral eosinophilia at levels that may approach 90%. Uncommonly, seizures or behavioral disorders develop. Rare deaths are due to severe neurologic, pneumonic, or myocardial involvement.

The ocular form of the larva migrans syndrome occurs when *Toxocara* larvae invade the eye. An eosinophilic granulomatous mass, most commonly in the posterior pole of the retina, develops around the entrapped larva. The retinal lesion can mimic retinoblastoma in appearance, and mistaken diagnosis of the latter condition can lead to unnecessary enucleation. The spectrum of eye involvement also includes endophthalmitis, uveitis, and chorioretinitis. Unilateral visual disturbances, strabismus, and eye pain are the most common presenting symptoms. In contrast to visceral larva migrans, ocular toxocariasis usually develops in older children or young adults with no history of pica; these patients seldom have eosinophilia or visceral manifestations.

Diagnosis In addition to eosinophilia, leukocytosis and hypergammaglobulinemia may be evident. Transient pulmonary infiltrates are apparent on chest x-rays of about one-half of patients with symptoms of pneumonitis. The clinical diagnosis can be confirmed by an enzyme-linked immunosorbent assay for toxocaral antibodies. Stool examination for parasite eggs is worthless in toxocariasis, since the larvae do not develop into egg-producing adults in humans.

TREATMENT
Visceral and Ocular Larva Migrans

The vast majority of *Toxocara* infections are self-limited and resolve without specific therapy. In patients with severe myocardial, CNS, or pulmonary involvement, glucocorticoids may be employed to reduce inflammatory complications. Available anthelmintic drugs, including mebendazole and albendazole, have not been shown conclusively to alter the course of larva migrans. Control measures include prohibiting dog excreta in public parks and playgrounds, deworming dogs, and preventing pica in children. Treatment of ocular disease is not fully defined, but the administration of albendazole in conjunction with glucocorticoids has been effective (Table 231-1).

■ CUTANEOUS LARVA MIGRANS

Cutaneous larva migrans ("creeping eruption") is a serpiginous skin eruption caused by burrowing larvae of animal hookworms, usually the dog and cat hookworm *Ancylostoma braziliense*. The larvae hatch from eggs passed in dog and cat feces and mature in the soil. Humans become infected after skin contact with soil in areas frequented by dogs and cats. Cutaneous larva migrans is prevalent among children and travelers in regions with warm humid climates, including the southeastern United States.

After larvae penetrate the skin, erythematous lesions form along the tortuous tracks of their migration through the dermal-epidermal junction; the larvae advance several centimeters in a day. The intensely pruritic lesions may occur anywhere on the body and can be numerous if the patient has lain on the ground. Vesicles and bullae may form later. The animal hookworm larvae do not mature in humans and, without treatment, will die after an interval ranging from weeks to a couple of months, with resolution of skin lesions. The diagnosis is made on clinical grounds. Skin biopsies only rarely detect diagnostic larvae. Symptoms can be alleviated by ivermectin or albendazole (Table 231-1).

■ ANGIOSTRONGYLIASIS

Angiostrongylus cantonensis, the rat lungworm, is the most common cause of human eosinophilic meningitis (Fig. 231-3).

Life Cycle and Epidemiology This infection occurs principally in Southeast Asia and the Pacific Basin but has spread to other areas of the world, including the Caribbean islands, countries in Central and South America, and the southern United States. *A. cantonensis* larvae produced by adult worms in the rat lung migrate to the gastrointestinal tract and are expelled with the feces. They develop into infective larvae in land snails and slugs. Humans acquire the infection by ingesting raw infected mollusks; vegetables contaminated by mollusk slime; or crabs, freshwater shrimp, and certain marine fish that have themselves eaten infected mollusks. The larvae then migrate to the brain.

Pathogenesis and Clinical Features The parasites eventually die in the CNS, but not before initiating pathologic consequences that, in heavy infections, can result in permanent neurologic sequelae or death. Migrating larvae cause marked local eosinophilic inflammation and hemorrhage, with subsequent necrosis and granuloma formation around dying worms. Clinical symptoms develop 2–35 days after the ingestion of larvae. Patients usually present with an insidious or abrupt excruciating frontal, occipital, or bitemporal headache. Neck stiffness, nausea and vomiting, and paresthesias are also common. Fever, cranial and extraocular nerve palsies, seizures, paralysis, and lethargy are uncommon.

Laboratory Findings Examination of cerebrospinal fluid (CSF) is mandatory in suspected cases and usually reveals an elevated opening pressure, a white blood cell count of 150–2000/μL, and an eosinophilic pleocytosis of >20%. The protein concentration is usually elevated and the glucose level normal. The larvae of *A. cantonensis* are only rarely seen in CSF. Peripheral-blood eosinophilia may be mild. The diagnosis is generally based on the clinical presentation of eosinophilic meningitis together with a compatible epidemiologic history.

TREATMENT
Angiostrongyliasis

Specific chemotherapy is not of benefit in angiostrongyliasis; larvicidal agents may exacerbate inflammatory brain lesions. Management consists of supportive measures, including the administration of analgesics, sedatives, and—in severe cases—glucocorticoids (Table 231-1). Repeated lumbar punctures with removal of CSF can relieve symptoms. In most patients, cerebral angiostrongyliasis has a self-limited course, and recovery is complete. The infection may be prevented by adequately cooking snails, crabs, and prawns and inspecting vegetables for mollusk infestation. Other parasitic or fungal causes of eosinophilic meningitis in endemic areas may

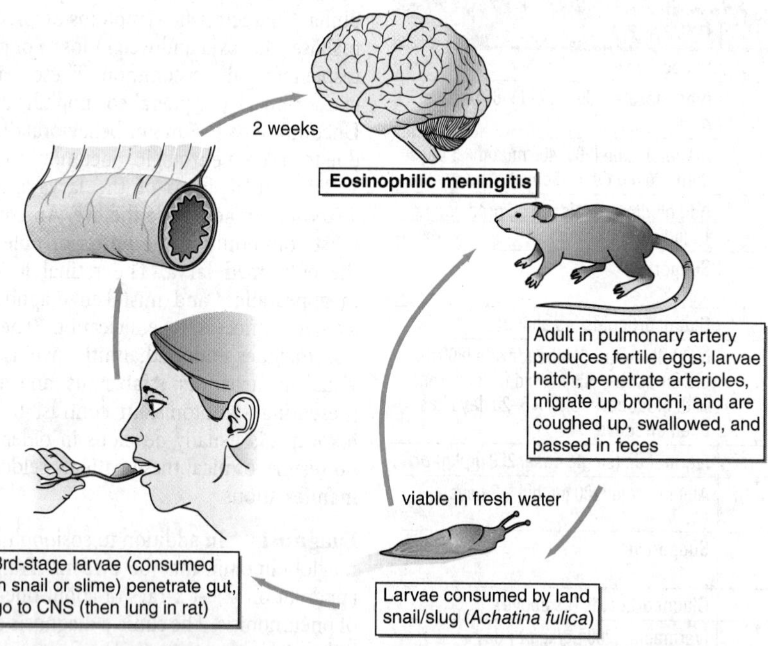
2 weeks
Eosinophilic meningitis
Adult in pulmonary artery produces fertile eggs; larvae hatch, penetrate arterioles, migrate up bronchi, and are coughed up, swallowed, and passed in feces
viable in fresh water
Larvae consumed by land snail/slug (Achatina fulica)
3rd-stage larvae (consumed in snail or slime) penetrate gut, go to CNS (then lung in rat)

FIGURE 231-3 Life cycle of *Angiostrongylus cantonensis* (rat lung worm) found in Southeast Asia and the Pacific Basin as well as on Caribbean islands, in countries of Central and South America, and in the southern United States. CNS, central nervous system. *(Reproduced with permission from RL Guerrant et al [eds]: Tropical Infectious Diseases: Principles, Pathogens and Practice, 2nd ed, Elsevier, 2006.)*

include gnathostomiasis (see below), paragonimiasis (Chap. 234), schistosomiasis (Chap. 234), neurocysticercosis (Chap. 235), and coccidioidomycosis (Chap. 213).

GNATHOSTOMIASIS

Infection of human tissues with larvae of *Gnathostoma spinigerum* can cause eosinophilic meningoencephalitis, migratory cutaneous swellings, or invasive masses of the eye and visceral organs.

Life Cycle and Epidemiology Human gnathostomiasis occurs in many countries and is notably endemic in Southeast Asia and parts of China and Japan. In nature, the mature adult worms parasitize the gastrointestinal tract of dogs and cats. First-stage larvae hatch from eggs passed into water and are ingested by *Cyclops* species (water fleas). Infective third-stage larvae develop in the flesh of many animal species (including fish, frogs, eels, snakes, chickens, and ducks) that have eaten either infected *Cyclops* or another infected second intermediate host. Humans typically acquire the infection by eating raw or undercooked fish or poultry. Raw fish dishes, such as *som fak* in Thailand and *sashimi* in Japan, account for many cases of human gnathostomiasis. Some cases in Thailand result from the local practice of applying frog or snake flesh as a poultice.

Pathogenesis and Clinical Features Clinical symptoms are due to the aberrant migration of a single larva into cutaneous, visceral, neural, or ocular tissues. After invasion, larval migration may cause local inflammation, with pain, cough, or hematuria accompanied by fever and eosinophilia. Painful, itchy, migratory swellings may develop in the skin, particularly in the distal extremities or periorbital area. Cutaneous swellings usually last ~1 week but often recur intermittently over many years. Larval invasion of the eye can provoke a sight-threatening inflammatory response. Invasion of the CNS results in eosinophilic meningitis with myeloencephalitis, a serious complication due to ascending larval migration along a large nerve tract. Patients characteristically present with agonizing radicular pain and paresthesias in the trunk or a limb, which are followed shortly by paraplegia. Cerebral involvement, with focal hemorrhages and tissue destruction, is often fatal.

Diagnosis and Treatment Cutaneous migratory swellings with marked peripheral eosinophilia, supported by an appropriate geographic and dietary history, generally constitute an adequate basis for a clinical diagnosis of gnathostomiasis. However, patients may present with ocular or cerebrospinal involvement without antecedent cutaneous swellings. In the latter case, eosinophilic pleocytosis is demonstrable (usually along with hemorrhagic or xanthochromic CSF), but worms are almost never recovered from CSF. Surgical removal of the parasite from subcutaneous or ocular tissue, though rarely feasible, is both diagnostic and therapeutic. Albendazole or ivermectin may be helpful (Table 231-1). At present, cerebrospinal involvement is managed with supportive measures and generally with a course of glucocorticoids. Gnathostomiasis can be prevented by adequate cooking of fish and poultry in endemic areas.

FURTHER READING

Centers for Disease Control and Prevention: Surveillance for trichinellosis—United States, 2015, Annual Summary. Atlanta, GA: U.S. Department of Health and Human Services, CDC, 2017.

Lupi O et al: Mucocutaneous manifestations of helminth infections. Nematodes. J Am Acad Dermatol 73:929, 2015.

Martins YC et al: Central nervous system manifestations of *Angiostrongylus cantonensis* infection. Acta Trop 141:46, 2015.

Rostami A et al: Meat sources of infection for outbreaks of human trichinellosis. Food Microbiol 64:65, 2017.

Rostami A et al: Human toxocariasis—A look at a neglected disease through an epidemiological "prism." Infect Genet Evol 74:104002, 2019.

Sitcar AD et al: Raccoon roundworm infection associated with central nervous system disease and ocular disease—six states, 2013–2015. Morbid Mortal Wkly Rep 65:930, 2016.

232 Intestinal Nematode Infections

Thomas B. Nutman, Peter F. Weller

More than a billion persons worldwide are infected with one or more species of intestinal nematodes. Table 232-1 summarizes biologic and clinical features of infections due to the major intestinal parasitic nematodes. These parasites are most common in regions with poor fecal sanitation, particularly in resource-poor countries in the tropics and subtropics, but they have also been seen with increasing frequency among immigrants and refugees to resource-rich countries. Although nematode infections are not usually fatal, they contribute to malnutrition and diminished work capacity. It is interesting that these helminth infections may protect some individuals from allergic disease. Humans may on occasion be infected with nematode parasites that ordinarily infect animals; these zoonotic infections produce diseases such as trichostrongyliasis, anisakiasis, capillariasis, and abdominal angiostrongyliasis.

Intestinal nematodes are roundworms; they range in length from 1 mm to many centimeters when mature (Table 232-1). Their life cycles are complex and highly varied; some species, including *Strongyloides stercoralis* and *Enterobius vermicularis*, can be transmitted directly from person to person, while others, such as *Ascaris lumbricoides* and the hookworms, require a soil phase for development. Because most helminth parasites do not self-replicate, the acquisition of a heavy burden of adult worms requires repeated exposure to the parasite in its infectious stage, whether larva or egg. Hence, clinical disease, as opposed to asymptomatic (or subclinical) infection, generally develops only with prolonged exposure in an endemic area and is typically related to infection intensity. In persons with marginal nutrition, intestinal helminth infections may impair growth and development. Eosinophilia and elevated serum IgE levels are features of many helminth infections and, when unexplained, should always prompt a search for intestinal helminths. Significant protective immunity to intestinal nematodes appears not to develop in humans, although the host immune response to these infections has not been elucidated in detail.

ASCARIASIS

A. lumbricoides is the largest intestinal nematode parasite of humans, reaching up to 40 cm in length. Most infected individuals have low worm burdens and are asymptomatic. Clinical disease arises from larval migration in the lungs or effects of the adult worms in the intestines.

Life Cycle Adult worms live in the lumen of the small intestine. Mature female *Ascaris* worms are extraordinarily fecund, each producing up to 240,000 eggs a day that pass with the feces. Ascarid eggs, which are remarkably resistant to environmental stresses, become infective after several weeks of maturation in the soil and can remain infective for years. After infective eggs are swallowed, larvae hatched in the intestine invade the mucosa, migrate through the circulation to the lungs, break into the alveoli, ascend the bronchial tree, and return—through swallowing—to the small intestine, where they develop into adult worms. The time between initial infection and egg production is typically between 2–3 months. Adult worms live for 1–2 years.

Epidemiology *Ascaris* is widely distributed in tropical and subtropical regions as well as in other humid areas in more temperate regions of the world. Transmission typically occurs through fecally contaminated soil and is due either to a lack of sanitary facilities or to the use of human feces as fertilizer. With their propensity for hand-to-mouth fecal carriage, younger children are most often affected. Infection outside endemic areas, though uncommon, can occur when eggs on transported vegetables are ingested.

Clinical Features During the lung phase of larval migration, ~9–12 days after egg ingestion, patients may develop an irritating

TABLE 232-1 Major Human Intestinal Parasitic Nematodes

FEATURE	PARASITIC NEMATODE				
	ASCARIS LUMBRICOIDES (ROUNDWORM)	*NECATOR AMERICANUS, ANCYLOSTOMA DUODENALE, ANCYLOSTOMA CEYLANICUM* (HOOKWORM)	*STRONGYLOIDES STERCORALIS*	*TRICHURIS TRICHIURA* (WHIPWORM)	*ENTEROBIUS VERMICULARIS* (PINWORM)
Global prevalence in humans (millions)	807	576	100	604	209
Endemic areas	Worldwide	Hot, humid regions	Hot, humid regions	Worldwide	Worldwide
Infective stage	Egg	Filariform larva	Filariform larva	Egg	Egg
Route of infection	Oral	Percutaneous	Percutaneous or autoinfective	Oral	Oral
Gastrointestinal location of worms	Jejunal lumen	Jejunal mucosa	Small-bowel mucosa	Cecum, colonic mucosa	Cecum, appendix
Adult worm size	15–40 cm	7–12 mm	2 mm	30–50 mm	8–13 mm (female)
Pulmonary passage of larvae	Yes	Yes	Yes	No	No
Incubation period[a] (days)	60–75	40–100	17–28	70–90	35–45
Longevity	1 year	*N. americanus*: 2–5 years *A. duodenale*: 6–8 years *A. ceylanicum*: 6–8 years[b]	Decades (owing to autoinfection)	5 years	2 months
Fecundity (eggs/day/worm)	240,000	*N. americanus*: 4000–10,000 *A. duodenale*: 10,000–25,000 *A. ceylanicum*: 5,000–15,000	5000–10,000	3000–7000	2000
Principal symptoms	Rarely, biliary obstruction or, in heavy infections, gastrointestinal obstruction	Iron-deficiency anemia in heavy infection	Gastrointestinal symptoms; malabsorption or sepsis in hyperinfection	Gastrointestinal symptoms or anemia in heavy infection	Perianal pruritus
Diagnostic stage	Eggs in stool	Eggs in fresh stool, larvae in old stool	Larvae in stool or duodenal aspirate; sputum in hyperinfection	Eggs in stool	Eggs from perianal skin on cellulose acetate tape
Treatment	Mebendazole Albendazole Ivermectin	Mebendazole Albendazole	Ivermectin Albendazole	Mebendazole Albendazole Ivermectin	Mebendazole Albendazole

[a]Time from infection to egg production by mature female worm. [b]Assumed but no evidence base in humans.

nonproductive cough and burning substernal discomfort that is aggravated by coughing or deep inspiration. Dyspnea and blood-tinged sputum are less common. Fever can occur. Eosinophilia develops during this symptomatic phase and subsides slowly over weeks. Chest imaging may reveal evidence of eosinophilic pneumonitis (Löffler's syndrome), with rounded infiltrates a few millimeters to several centimeters in size. These infiltrates may be transient and intermittent, clearing after several weeks. Where there is seasonal transmission of the parasite, seasonal pneumonitis with eosinophilia may develop in previously infected and sensitized hosts.

In established infections, adult worms in the small intestine usually cause no symptoms. In heavy infections, particularly in children, a large bolus of entangled worms can cause pain and small-bowel obstruction, sometimes complicated by perforation, intussusception, or volvulus. Single worms may cause disease when they migrate into aberrant sites. A large worm can enter and occlude the biliary tree, causing biliary colic, cholecystitis, cholangitis, pancreatitis, or (rarely) intrahepatic abscesses. Migration of an adult worm up the esophagus can provoke coughing and oral expulsion of the worm. In highly endemic areas, intestinal and biliary ascariasis can rival acute appendicitis and gallstones as causes of surgical acute abdomen.

Laboratory Findings Most cases of ascariasis can be diagnosed by microscopic detection of characteristic *Ascaris* eggs (65 × 45 μm) in fecal samples, although increasingly, polymerase chain reaction (PCR) of DNA extracted from stool is being used in research and some clinical settings. Occasionally, patients present after passing an adult worm—identifiable by its large size and smooth cream-colored surface—in the stool or, much less commonly, through the mouth or nose. During the early transpulmonary migratory phase, when eosinophilic pneumonitis occurs, larvae can be found in sputum or gastric aspirates before diagnostic eggs appear in the stool. The eosinophilia that is prominent during this early stage usually decreases to minimal levels in established infection. Adult worms may be visualized, occasionally serendipitously, on contrast studies of the gastrointestinal tract. A plain abdominal film may reveal masses of worms in gas-filled loops of bowel in patients with intestinal obstruction. Pancreaticobiliary worms can be detected by ultrasound and endoscopic retrograde cholangiopancreatography; the latter method also has been used to extract biliary *Ascaris* worms.

TREATMENT

Ascariasis

Ascariasis should always be treated to prevent potentially serious complications. Albendazole (400 mg once), mebendazole (100 mg twice daily for 3 days or 500 mg once), or ivermectin (150–200 μg/kg once) is effective. These medications are contraindicated in pregnancy, however. Mild diarrhea and abdominal pain are uncommon side effects of these agents. Partial intestinal obstruction should be managed with nasogastric suction, IV fluid administration, and instillation of piperazine through the nasogastric tube, but complete obstruction and its severe complications require immediate surgical intervention.

HOOKWORM

Three species (*Ancylostoma duodenale*, *Ancylostoma ceylanicum*, and *Necator americanus*) are responsible for most human hookworm infections. Most infected individuals are asymptomatic. Hookworm disease develops from a combination of factors—a heavy worm burden, a prolonged duration of infection, and an inadequate iron intake—and results in iron-deficiency anemia and, on occasion, hypoproteinemia.

Life Cycle Adult hookworms, which are ~1 cm long, use buccal teeth (*Ancylostoma*) or cutting plates (*Necator*) to attach to the small-bowel mucosa and suck blood (0.2 mL/d per *Ancylostoma* adult) and interstitial fluid. The adult hookworms produce thousands of eggs daily. The eggs are deposited with feces in soil, where rhabditiform larvae hatch and develop over a 1-week period into infectious filariform larvae. Infective larvae penetrate the skin and reach the lungs by way of the bloodstream. There they invade alveoli and ascend the airways before being swallowed and reaching the small intestine. The prepatent period from skin invasion to appearance of eggs in the feces is ~6–8 weeks, but it may be longer with *Ancylostoma* spp. Larvae of *Ancylostoma* spp., if swallowed, can survive and develop directly in the intestinal mucosa. Adult hookworms may survive over a decade but usually live ~6–8 years for *A. duodenale* and 2–5 years for *N. americanus*.

Epidemiology *A. duodenale* is prevalent in southern Europe, North Africa, and northern Asia, and *N. americanus* is the predominant species in the Western Hemisphere and equatorial Africa. *A. ceylanicum* is most prevalent in Southeast Asia. The species can overlap geographically, particularly in Southeast Asia. Age prevalence studies have shown a constant increase in hookworm prevalence over time; older children have the greatest intensity of hookworm infection; however, in rural areas where fields are fertilized with human feces, older working adults also may be heavily infected.

Clinical Features Most hookworm infections are clinically asymptomatic. Infective larvae may provoke pruritic maculopapular dermatitis ("ground itch") at the site of skin penetration as well as serpiginous tracks of subcutaneous migration (similar to those of cutaneous larva migrans; **Chap. 231**) in previously sensitized hosts. Larvae migrating through the lungs occasionally cause mild transient pneumonitis, but this condition develops less frequently in hookworm infection than in ascariasis. In the early intestinal phase, infected persons may develop epigastric pain (often with postprandial accentuation), inflammatory diarrhea, or other abdominal symptoms accompanied by eosinophilia. The major consequence of chronic hookworm infection is iron deficiency. Symptoms are minimal if iron intake is adequate, but marginally nourished individuals develop symptoms of progressive iron-deficiency anemia and hypoproteinemia, including weakness and shortness of breath.

Laboratory Findings The diagnosis is established by the finding of characteristic 40- by 60-μm oval hookworm eggs in the feces. Stool-concentration procedures may be required to detect light infections. Eggs of the three species are indistinguishable by light microscopy, whereas PCR has provided a significant improvement in species-specific diagnosis. In a stool sample that is not fresh, the eggs may have hatched to release rhabditiform larvae, which need to be differentiated from those of *S. stercoralis*. Hypochromic microcytic anemia, occasionally with eosinophilia or hypoalbuminemia, is characteristic of hookworm disease.

TREATMENT

Hookworm Infection

Hookworm infection can be treated with several safe and highly effective anthelmintic drugs, including albendazole (400 mg once) and mebendazole (500 mg once). Mild iron-deficiency anemia can often be treated with oral iron alone. Severe hookworm disease with protein loss and malabsorption necessitates nutritional support and oral iron replacement along with deworming. There is significant concern that the benzimidazoles (mebendazole and albendazole) are becoming much less effective against human hookworms.

Ancylostoma caninum* and *Ancylostoma braziliense *A. caninum*, the canine hookworm, has been identified as a cause of human eosinophilic enteritis, especially in northeastern Australia. In this zoonotic infection, adult hookworms attach to the small intestine (where they may be visualized by endoscopy) and elicit abdominal pain and intense local eosinophilia. Treatment with mebendazole (100 mg twice daily for 3 days) or albendazole (400 mg once) or endoscopic removal is effective. Both of these animal hookworm species can cause cutaneous larva migrans ("creeping eruption"; **Chap. 231**).

STRONGYLOIDIASIS

S. stercoralis is distinguished by its ability—unique among helminths (except for *Capillaria*; see below)—to replicate in the human host. This capacity permits ongoing cycles of autoinfection as infective larvae are internally produced. Infection with *S. stercoralis* can thus persist for decades without further exposure of the host to exogenous infective larvae. In immunocompromised hosts, large numbers of invasive *Strongyloides* larvae can disseminate widely and can be fatal.

Life Cycle In addition to a parasitic cycle of development, *Strongyloides* can undergo a free-living cycle of development in the soil (**Fig. 232-1**). This adaptability facilitates the parasite's survival in the absence of mammalian hosts. Rhabditiform larvae passed in feces can transform into infectious filariform larvae either directly or after a free-living phase of development. Humans acquire *S. stercoralis* when filariform larvae in fecally contaminated soil penetrate the skin or mucous membranes. The larvae then travel through the bloodstream to the lungs, where they break into the alveolar spaces, ascend the bronchial tree, are swallowed, and thereby reach the small intestine. There the larvae mature into adult worms that penetrate the mucosa of the proximal small bowel. The minute (2-mm-long) parasitic adult female worms reproduce by parthenogenesis; adult males do not exist. Eggs hatch in the intestinal mucosa, releasing rhabditiform larvae that migrate to the lumen and pass with the feces into soil. Alternatively, rhabditiform larvae in the bowel can develop directly into filariform larvae that penetrate the colonic wall or perianal skin and enter the circulation to repeat the migration that establishes ongoing internal reinfection. This autoinfection cycle allows strongyloidiasis to persist for decades.

Epidemiology *S. stercoralis* is spottily distributed in tropical areas and other hot, humid regions and is particularly common in Southeast Asia, sub-Saharan Africa, and Brazil. In the United States, the parasite is endemic in parts of the Southeast and is found in immigrants, refugees, travelers, and military personnel who have lived in endemic areas.

Clinical Features In uncomplicated strongyloidiasis, many patients are asymptomatic or have mild cutaneous and/or abdominal symptoms. Recurrent urticaria, often involving the buttocks and wrists, is the most common cutaneous manifestation. Migrating larvae can elicit a pathognomonic serpiginous eruption, *larva currens* ("running larva"). This pruritic, raised, erythematous lesion advances as rapidly as 10 cm/h along the course of larval migration. Adult parasites burrow into the duodenojejunal mucosa and can cause abdominal (usually midepigastric) pain, which resembles peptic ulcer pain except that it is aggravated by food ingestion. Nausea, diarrhea, gastrointestinal bleeding, mild chronic colitis, and weight loss can occur. Small-bowel obstruction may develop with early, heavy infection. Pulmonary symptoms are rare in uncomplicated strongyloidiasis. Eosinophilia is common, with levels fluctuating over time.

The ongoing autoinfection cycle of *S. stercoralis* is normally constrained by unknown factors of the host's immune system. Abrogation of host immunity, especially with glucocorticoid therapy and much less commonly with other immunosuppressive medications, leads to hyperinfection, with the generation of large numbers of filariform larvae. Colitis, enteritis, or malabsorption may develop. In disseminated strongyloidiasis, larvae may invade not only gastrointestinal tissues and the lungs but also the central nervous system, peritoneum, liver, and kidneys. Moreover, bacteremia may develop because of the passage of enteric flora through disrupted mucosal barriers. Gram-negative sepsis, pneumonia, or meningitis may complicate or dominate the clinical course. Eosinophilia is often absent in severely infected patients. Disseminated strongyloidiasis, particularly in patients with unsuspected

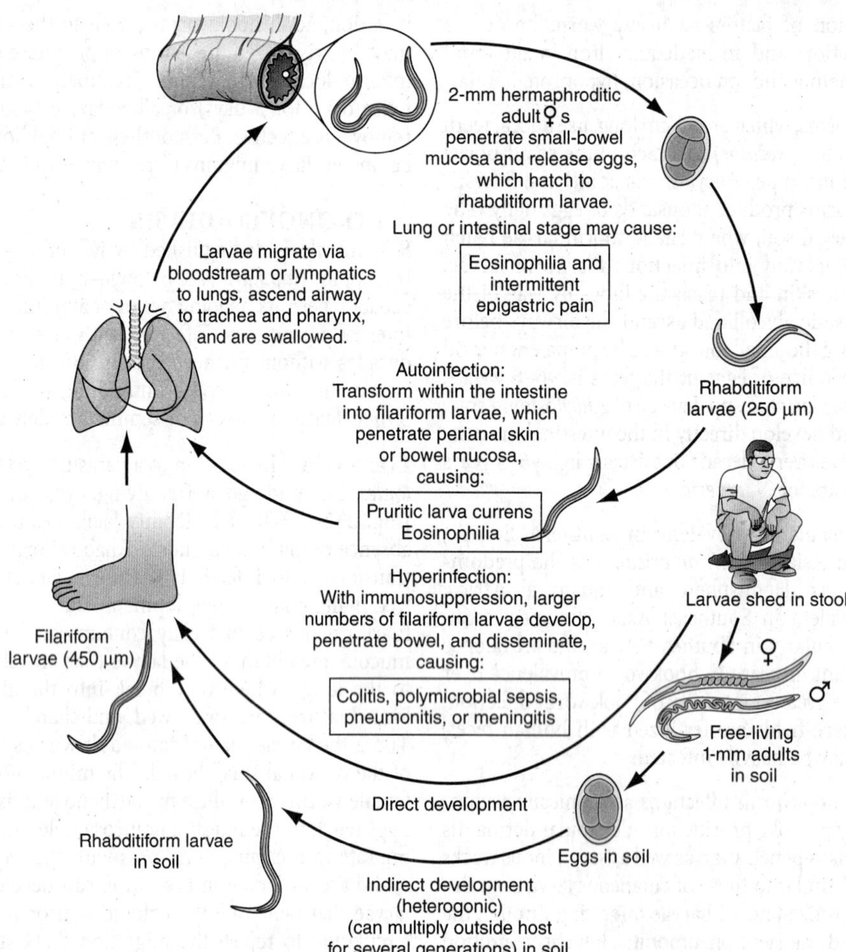

FIGURE 232-1 Life cycle of *Strongyloides stercoralis*. *(Reproduced with permission from RL Guerrant et al [eds]: Tropical Infectious Diseases: Principles, Pathogens and Practice, 2nd ed, Elsevier, 2006.)*

infection who are given glucocorticoids, can be fatal. Strongyloidiasis is a frequent complication of infection with human T-cell lymphotropic virus type 1 (HTLV-1), but disseminated strongyloidiasis is not common among patients infected with HIV-1.

Diagnosis In uncomplicated strongyloidiasis, the finding of rhabditiform larvae in feces is diagnostic. Rhabditiform larvae are ~250 μm long, with a short buccal cavity that distinguishes them from hookworm larvae. In uncomplicated infections, few larvae are passed and single stool examinations detect only about one-third of cases. Serial examinations and the use of the agar plate detection method improve the sensitivity of stool diagnosis. Again, PCR has begun to be used more widely and provides increased diagnostic specificity. In uncomplicated strongyloidiasis (but not in hyperinfection), microscopy-based stool examinations may be repeatedly negative. *Strongyloides* larvae may also be found by sampling of the duodenojejunal contents by aspiration or biopsy. An enzyme-linked immunosorbent assay for serum antibodies to antigens of *Strongyloides* is a sensitive method for diagnosing uncomplicated infections. Such serologic testing should be performed for patients whose geographic histories indicate potential exposure, especially those who exhibit eosinophilia and/or are candidates for glucocorticoid treatment of other conditions. In disseminated strongyloidiasis, filariform larvae should be sought in stool as well as in samples obtained from sites of potential larval migration, including sputum, bronchoalveolar lavage fluid, or surgical drainage fluid.

TREATMENT

Strongyloidiasis

Even in the asymptomatic state, strongyloidiasis must be treated because of the potential for subsequent dissemination and fatal hyperinfection. Ivermectin (200 μg/kg daily for 2 days) is consistently more effective than albendazole (400 mg daily for 3 days). For disseminated strongyloidiasis, treatment with ivermectin should be extended for at least 14 days or at least a week after parasites have been eradicated. In potentially immunocompromised hosts, the course of ivermectin should be repeated 2 weeks after initial treatment. Ivermectin has been successfully given parenterally (subcutaneously or intramuscularly) in those unable to take ivermectin orally.

TRICHURIASIS

Most infections with *Trichuris trichiura* are asymptomatic, but heavy infections may cause gastrointestinal symptoms. Like the other soil-transmitted helminths, whipworm is distributed globally in the tropics and subtropics and is most common among poor children from resource-poor regions of the world.

Life Cycle Adult *Trichuris* worms reside in the colon and cecum, the anterior portions threaded into the superficial mucosa. Thousands of eggs laid daily by adult female worms pass with the feces and mature in the soil. After ingestion, infective eggs hatch in the duodenum, releasing larvae that mature before migrating to the large bowel. The entire cycle takes ~3 months, and adult worms may live for several years.

Clinical Features Tissue reactions to *Trichuris* are mild. Most infected individuals have no symptoms or eosinophilia. Heavy infections may result in anemia, abdominal pain, anorexia, and bloody or mucoid diarrhea resembling inflammatory bowel disease. Rectal prolapse can result from massive infections in children, who often suffer from malnourishment and other diarrheal illnesses. Moderately heavy *Trichuris* burdens also contribute to growth retardation.

Diagnosis and Treatment The characteristic 50- by 20-μm lemon-shaped *Trichuris* eggs are readily detected on stool examination. Adult worms, which are 3–5 cm long, are occasionally seen on proctoscopy. PCR is being used increasingly in settings where it is available. Mebendazole (500 mg once) or albendazole (400 mg daily for 3 doses) is safe and modestly effective for treatment, with cure rates of 30–90%. Ivermectin (200 μg/kg daily for 3 doses) is also safe but is not quite as efficacious as the benzimidazoles.

■ ENTEROBIASIS (PINWORM)

E. vermicularis is more common in temperate countries than in the tropics. In the United States, ~40 million persons are infected with pinworms, with a disproportionate number of cases among children.

Life Cycle and Epidemiology *Enterobius* adult worms are ~1 cm long and dwell in the cecum. Gravid female worms migrate nocturnally into the perianal region and release up to 2000 immature eggs each. The eggs become infective within hours and are transmitted by hand-to-mouth passage. From ingested eggs, larvae hatch and mature into adults. This life cycle takes ~1 month, and adult worms survive for ~2 months. Self-infection results from perianal scratching and transport of infective eggs on the hands or under the nails to the mouth. Because of the ease of person-to-person spread, pinworm infections are common among family members.

Clinical Features Most pinworm infections are asymptomatic. Perianal pruritus is the cardinal symptom. The itching, which is often worse at night as a result of the nocturnal migration of the female worms, may lead to excoriation and bacterial superinfection. Heavy infections have been alleged to cause abdominal pain and weight loss. On rare occasions, pinworms invade the female genital tract, causing vulvovaginitis and pelvic or peritoneal granulomas. Eosinophilia is uncommon.

Diagnosis Since pinworm eggs are not released in feces, the diagnosis cannot be made by conventional fecal ova and parasite tests. Instead, eggs are detected by the application of clear cellulose acetate tape to the perianal region in the morning. After the tape is transferred to a slide, microscopic examination will detect pinworm eggs, which are oval, measure 55 × 25 μm, and are flattened along one side.

TREATMENT
Enterobiasis

Infected children and adults should be treated with mebendazole (100 mg once) or albendazole (400 mg once), with the same treatment repeated after 2 weeks. Treatment of household members is advocated to eliminate asymptomatic reservoirs of potential reinfection.

■ TRICHOSTRONGYLIASIS

Trichostrongylus species, which are normally parasites of herbivorous animals, occasionally infect humans, particularly in Asia and Africa. Humans acquire the infection by accidentally ingesting *Trichostrongylus* larvae on contaminated leafy vegetables. The larvae do not migrate in humans but mature directly into adult worms in the small bowel. These worms ingest far less blood than hookworms; most infected persons are asymptomatic, but heavy infections may give rise to mild anemia and eosinophilia. In stool examinations, *Trichostrongylus* eggs resemble hookworm eggs but are larger (85 × 115 μm). Treatment consists of mebendazole or albendazole (**Chap. 222**).

■ ANISAKIASIS

Anisakiasis is a gastrointestinal infection caused by the accidental ingestion in uncooked saltwater fish of nematode larvae belonging to the family Anisakidae. The incidence of anisakiasis in the United States has increased as a result of the growing popularity of raw fish dishes. Most cases occur in Japan, the Netherlands, and Chile, where raw fish—sashimi, pickled green herring, and ceviche, respectively—are national culinary staples. Anisakid nematodes parasitize large sea mammals such as whales, dolphins, and seals. As part of a complex parasitic life cycle involving marine food chains, infectious larvae migrate to the musculature of a variety of fish. Both *Anisakis simplex* and *Pseudoterranova decipiens* have been implicated in human anisakiasis, but an identical gastric syndrome may be caused by the red larvae of eustrongylid parasites of fish-eating birds.

When humans consume infected raw fish, live larvae may be coughed up within 48 h. Alternatively, larvae may immediately penetrate the mucosa of the stomach. Within hours, violent upper abdominal pain accompanied by nausea and occasionally vomiting ensues, mimicking an acute abdomen. The diagnosis can be established by direct visualization on upper endoscopy, outlining of the worm by contrast radiographic studies, or histopathologic examination of extracted tissue. Extraction of the burrowing larvae during endoscopy is curative. In addition, larvae may pass to the small bowel, where they penetrate the mucosa and provoke a vigorous eosinophilic granulomatous response. Symptoms may appear 1–2 weeks after the infective meal, with intermittent abdominal pain, diarrhea, nausea, and fever resembling the manifestations of Crohn's disease. Ingestion of *Anisakis*-derived proteins through consumption of fish meat containing *Anisakis* parasites can elicit allergic gastrointestinal and even anaphylactic responses.

The diagnosis may be suggested by barium or other radiographic upper gastrointestinal studies and confirmed by curative surgical resection of a granuloma in which the worm is embedded. Anisakid eggs are not found in the stool, since the larvae do not mature in humans. Serologic tests have been developed but are not widely available.

Anisakid larvae in saltwater fish are killed by cooking to 60°C, freezing at –20°C for 3 days, or commercial blast freezing, but usually not by salting, marinating, or cold smoking. No medical treatment is available; surgical or endoscopic removal should be undertaken.

■ CAPILLARIASIS

Intestinal capillariasis is caused by ingestion of raw fish infected with *Capillaria philippinensis*. Subsequent autoinfection can lead to a severe wasting syndrome. The disease occurs in the Philippines and Thailand and, on occasion, elsewhere in Asia. The natural cycle of *C. philippinensis* involves fish from fresh and brackish water. When humans eat infected raw fish, the larvae mature in the intestine into adult worms, which produce invasive larvae that cause intestinal inflammation and villus loss. Capillariasis has an insidious onset with nonspecific abdominal pain and watery diarrhea. If untreated, progressive autoinfection can lead to protein-losing enteropathy, severe malabsorption, and ultimately death from cachexia, cardiac failure, or superinfection. The diagnosis is established by identification of the characteristic peanut-shaped (20- × 40-μm) eggs on stool examination. Severely ill patients require hospitalization and supportive therapy in addition to prolonged anthelmintic treatment with albendazole (200 mg twice daily for 10 days; **Chap. 222**).

■ ABDOMINAL ANGIOSTRONGYLIASIS

Abdominal angiostrongyliasis is found in Latin America and Africa. The zoonotic parasite *Angiostrongylus costaricensis* causes eosinophilic ileocolitis after the ingestion of contaminated vegetation. *A. costaricensis* normally parasitizes the cotton rat and other rodents, with slugs and snails serving as intermediate hosts. Humans become infected by accidentally ingesting infective larvae in mollusk slime deposited on fruits and vegetables; children are at highest risk. The larvae penetrate the gut wall and migrate to the mesenteric artery, where they develop into adult worms. Eggs deposited in the gut wall provoke an intense eosinophilic granulomatous reaction, and adult worms may cause mesenteric arteritis, thrombosis, or frank bowel infarction. Symptoms may mimic those of appendicitis, including abdominal pain and tenderness, fever, vomiting, and a palpable mass in the right iliac fossa. Leukocytosis and eosinophilia are prominent. CT with contrast medium typically shows inflamed bowel, often with concomitant obstruction, but a definitive diagnosis is usually made surgically with partial bowel resection. Pathologic study reveals a thickened bowel wall with eosinophilic granulomas surrounding the *Angiostrongylus* eggs. In nonsurgical cases, the diagnosis rests solely on clinical grounds because larvae and eggs cannot be detected in the stool. Medical therapy for abdominal angiostrongyliasis is of uncertain efficacy. Careful observation and surgical resection for severe symptoms are the mainstays of treatment.

FURTHER READING

Bethony J et al: Soil-transmitted helminth infections: Ascariasis, trichuriasis, and hookworm. Lancet 367:1521, 2006.

Fox LM: Ivermectin: Uses and impact 20 years on. Curr Opin Infect Dis 19:588, 2006.

Hochberg NS, Hamer DH: Anisakidosis: Perils of the deep. Clin Infect Dis 51:806, 2010.

Horton J: Albendazole: A review of anthelmintic efficacy and safety in humans. Parasitology 121(Suppl):S113, 2000.

Loukas A et al: Hookworm infection. Nat Rev Dis Primers 2:16088, 2016.

Montressor A et al: The global progress of soil-transmitted helminthiases control in 2020 and World Health Organization targets for 2030. PLoS Negl Trop Dis 14:e0008505, 2020.

Nutman TB: Human infection with *Strongyloides stercoralis* and other related *Strongyloides* species. Parasitology 144:263, 2017.

O'Connell EM et al: *Ancylostoma ceylanicum* hookworm in Myanmar refugees, Thailand, 2012-2015. Emerg Infect Dis 24:1472, 2018.

233 Filarial and Related Infections

Thomas B. Nutman, Peter F. Weller

Filarial worms are nematodes that dwell in the subcutaneous tissues and the lymphatics. Eight filarial species infect humans (**Table 233-1**); of these, four—*Wuchereria bancrofti*, *Brugia malayi*, *Onchocerca volvulus*, and *Loa loa*—are responsible for most symptomatic filarial infections. Filarial parasites, which infect an estimated 170 million persons worldwide, are transmitted by specific species of mosquitoes or other arthropods and have a complex life cycle, including infective larval stages carried by insects and adult worms that reside in either lymphatic or subcutaneous tissues of humans. The offspring of adults are microfilariae, which, depending on their species, are 200–250 μm long and 5–7 μm wide, may or may not be enveloped in a loose sheath, and either circulate in the blood or migrate through the skin (Table 233-1). To complete the life cycle, microfilariae are ingested by the arthropod vector and develop over 1–2 weeks into new infective larvae. Adult worms live for many years, whereas microfilariae survive for 3–36 months. The bacterial endosymbiont *Wolbachia* has been found intracellularly in all stages of *Brugia*, *Wuchereria*, *Mansonella*, and *Onchocerca* species and has become a target for antifilarial chemotherapy.

Usually, infection is established only with repeated, prolonged exposures to infective larvae. Since the clinical manifestations of filarial diseases develop relatively slowly, these infections should be considered to induce chronic infections with possible long-term debilitating effects. In terms of the nature, severity, and timing of clinical manifestations, patients with filarial infections who are native to endemic areas and have lifelong exposure may differ significantly from those who are travelers or who have recently moved to these areas. Characteristically, filarial disease is more acute and intense in newly exposed individuals than in natives of endemic areas.

LYMPHATIC FILARIASIS

Lymphatic filariasis is caused by *W. bancrofti*, *B. malayi*, or *Brugia timori*. The threadlike adult parasites reside in afferent lymphatics or lymph nodes, where they may remain viable for more than two decades.

EPIDEMIOLOGY

W. bancrofti, the most widely distributed filarial parasite of humans, affects an estimated 110 million people and is found throughout the tropics and subtropics, including Asia and the Pacific Islands, Africa, areas of South America, and the Caribbean basin. Humans are the only definitive host for the parasite. Generally, the subperiodic form is found only in the Pacific Islands; elsewhere, *W. bancrofti* is nocturnally periodic. Nocturnally periodic forms of microfilariae are scarce in peripheral blood by day and increase at night, whereas subperiodic forms are present in peripheral blood at all times and reach maximal levels in the afternoon. Natural vectors for *W. bancrofti* are *Culex* mosquitoes in urban settings and *Anopheles* or *Aedes* mosquitoes in rural areas.

Brugian filariasis due to *B. malayi* occurs primarily in eastern India, Indonesia, Malaysia, and the Philippines. *B. malayi* also has two forms distinguished by the periodicity of microfilaremia. The more common nocturnal form is transmitted in areas of coastal rice fields, while the subperiodic form is found in forests. *B. malayi* naturally infects cats as

TABLE 233-1 Characteristics of the Filariae

ORGANISM	PERIODICITY	DISTRIBUTION	VECTOR	LOCATION OF ADULT	MICROFILARIAL LOCATION	SHEATH
Wuchereria bancrofti	Nocturnal	Cosmopolitan areas worldwide, including South America, Africa, southern Asia, Papua New Guinea, China, Indonesia	*Culex, Anopheles* (mosquitoes)	Lymphatic tissue	Blood	+
	Subperiodic	Eastern Pacific	*Aedes* (mosquitoes)	Lymphatic tissue	Blood	+
Brugia malayi	Nocturnal	Southeast Asia, Indonesia, India	*Mansonia, Anopheles* (mosquitoes)	Lymphatic tissue	Blood	+
	Subperiodic	Indonesia, Southeast Asia	*Coquillettidia, Mansonia* (mosquitoes)	Lymphatic tissue	Blood	+
Brugia timori	Nocturnal	Indonesia	*Anopheles* (mosquitoes)	Lymphatic tissue	Blood	+
Loa loa	Diurnal	West and Central Africa	*Chrysops* (deerflies)	Subcutaneous tissue	Blood	+
Onchocerca volvulus	None	South and Central America, Africa	*Simulium* (blackflies)	Subcutaneous tissue	Skin, eye	–
Mansonella ozzardi	None	South and Central America	*Culicoides* (midges)	Undetermined site	Blood	–
	None	Caribbean	*Simulium* (blackflies)	Undetermined site	Blood	–
Mansonella perstans	None	South and Central America, Africa	*Culicoides* (midges)	Body cavities, mesentery, perirenal tissue	Blood	–
Mansonella streptocerca	None	West and Central Africa	*Culicoides* (midges)	Subcutaneous tissue	Skin	–

well as humans. The distribution of *B. timori* is limited to the islands of southeastern Indonesia.

PATHOLOGY

The principal pathologic changes result from inflammatory damage to the lymphatics, which is typically caused by adult worms and not by microfilariae. Adult worms live in afferent lymphatics or sinuses of lymph nodes and cause lymphatic dilation and thickening of the vessel walls. The infiltration of plasma cells, eosinophils, and macrophages in and around the infected vessels, along with endothelial and connective tissue proliferation, leads to tortuosity of the lymphatics and damaged or incompetent lymph valves. Lymphedema and chronic stasis changes with hard or brawny edema develop in the overlying skin. These consequences of filarial infection are due both to the direct effects of the worms and to the host's inflammatory response to the parasite. Inflammatory responses are believed to cause the granulomatous and proliferative processes that precede total lymphatic obstruction. It is thought that the lymphatic vessel remains patent as long as the worm remains viable and that the death of the worm leads to enhanced granulomatous reactions and fibrosis. Lymphatic obstruction results, and despite collateralization, lymphatic function is compromised.

CLINICAL FEATURES

The most common presentations of the lymphatic filariases are asymptomatic (or subclinical) microfilaremia, hydrocele **(Fig. 233-1)**, acute adenolymphangitis (ADL), and chronic lymphatic disease. In areas where *W. bancrofti* or *B. malayi* is endemic, the overwhelming majority of infected individuals have few overt clinical manifestations of filarial infection despite the presence of circulating microfilariae in the peripheral blood. Although they may be clinically asymptomatic, virtually all persons with *W. bancrofti* or *B. malayi* microfilaremia have some degree of subclinical disease that includes microscopic hematuria and/or proteinuria, dilated (and tortuous) lymphatics (visualized by imaging), and—in men with *W. bancrofti* infection—scrotal lymphangiectasia (detectable by ultrasound). Despite these findings, the majority of individuals appear to remain clinically asymptomatic for years; in relatively few does the infection progress to either acute or chronic disease.

ADL is characterized by high fever, lymphatic inflammation (lymphangitis and lymphadenitis), and transient local edema. The lymphangitis is retrograde, extending peripherally from the lymph node draining the area where the adult parasites reside. Regional lymph nodes are often enlarged, and the entire lymphatic channel can become indurated and inflamed. Concomitant local thrombophlebitis can occur as well. In brugian filariasis, a single local abscess may form along the involved lymphatic tract and subsequently rupture to the surface. The lymphadenitis and lymphangitis can involve both the upper and lower extremities in both bancroftian and brugian filariasis, but involvement of the genital lymphatics occurs almost exclusively with *W. bancrofti* infection. This genital involvement can be manifested by funiculitis, epididymitis, and scrotal pain and tenderness. In endemic areas, another type of acute disease—dermatolymphangioadenitis (DLA)—is recognized as a syndrome that includes high fever, chills, myalgias, and headache. Edematous inflammatory plaques clearly demarcated from normal skin are seen. Vesicles, ulcers, and hyperpigmentation also may be noted. There is often a history of trauma, burns, irradiation, insect bites, punctiform lesions, or chemical injury. Entry lesions, especially in the interdigital area, are common. DLA is often diagnosed as cellulitis.

If lymphatic damage progresses, transient lymphedema can develop into lymphatic obstruction and the permanent changes associated with elephantiasis **(Fig. 233-2)**. Brawny edema follows early pitting edema, the subcutaneous tissues thicken, and hyperkeratosis occurs. Fissuring of the skin develops, as do hyperplastic changes. Superinfection of these poorly vascularized tissues becomes a problem. In bancroftian filariasis, in which genital involvement is common, hydroceles may develop (Fig. 233-1); in advanced stages, this condition may evolve into scrotal lymphedema and scrotal elephantiasis. Furthermore, if there is obstruction of the retroperitoneal lymphatics, increased renal lymphatic pressure leads to rupture of the renal lymphatics and the development of chyluria, which is usually intermittent and most prominent in the morning.

The clinical manifestations of filarial infections in travelers or transmigrants who have recently entered an endemic region are distinctive. Given a sufficient number of bites by infected vectors, usually over a 3- to 6-month period, recently exposed patients can develop acute lymphatic or scrotal inflammation with or without urticaria and localized angioedema. Lymphadenitis of epitrochlear, axillary, femoral, or inguinal lymph nodes is often followed by evolving retrograde lymphangitis. Acute attacks are short-lived and are not usually

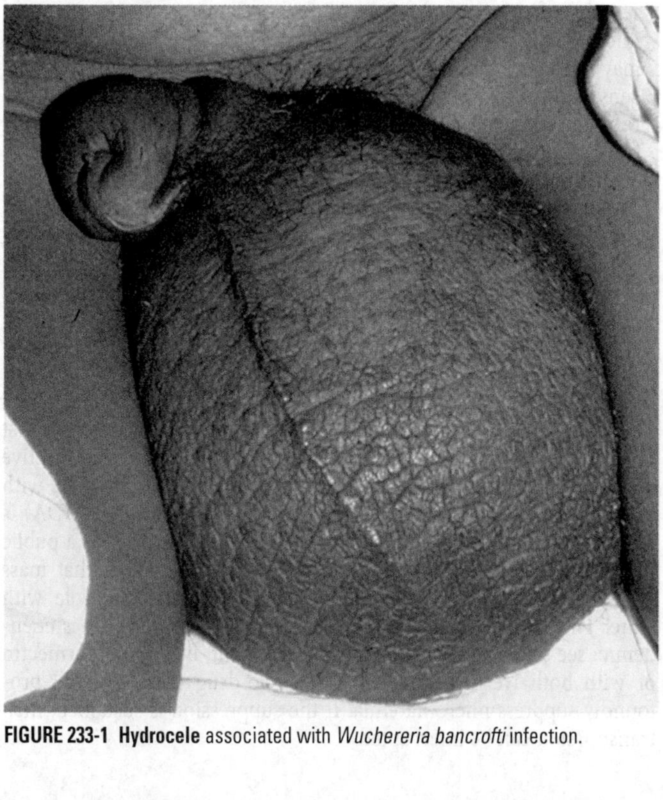

FIGURE 233-1 Hydrocele associated with *Wuchereria bancrofti* infection.

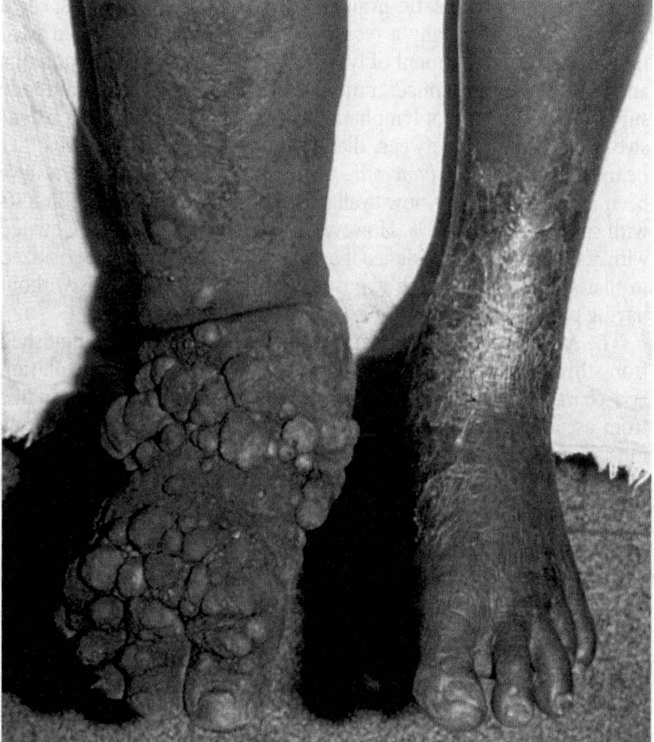

FIGURE 233-2 Elephantiasis of the lower extremity associated with *Wuchereria bancrofti* infection.

accompanied by fever. With prolonged exposure to infected mosquitoes, these attacks, if untreated, become more severe and lead to permanent lymphatic inflammation and obstruction.

DIAGNOSIS

A definitive diagnosis can be made only by detection of the parasites and hence can be difficult. Adult worms localized in lymphatic vessels or nodes are largely inaccessible. Microfilariae can be found in blood, in hydrocele fluid, or (occasionally) in other body fluids. Such fluids can be examined microscopically, either directly or—for greater sensitivity—after concentration of the parasites by the passage of fluid through a polycarbonate cylindrical-pore filter (pore size, 3 μm) or by the centrifugation of fluid fixed in 2% formalin (Knott's concentration technique). The timing of blood collection is critical and should be based on the periodicity of the microfilariae in the endemic region involved. Many infected individuals do not have microfilaremia, and definitive diagnosis in such cases can be difficult. Assays for circulating antigens of *W. bancrofti* permit the diagnosis of microfilaremic and cryptic (amicrofilaremic) infection. Two tests are commercially available: an enzyme-linked immunosorbent assay and a rapid-format immunochromatographic card test. Both assays have sensitivities of 93–100% and specificities approaching 100%. There are currently no tests for circulating antigens in brugian filariasis.

Polymerase chain reaction (PCR)–based assays for DNA of *W. bancrofti* and *B. malayi* in blood have been developed. A number of studies indicate that the sensitivity of this diagnostic method is equivalent to or greater than that of parasitologic methods.

In cases of suspected lymphatic filariasis, examination of the scrotum, the lymph nodes, or (in female patients) the breast by means of high-frequency ultrasound in conjunction with Doppler techniques may result in the identification of motile adult worms within dilated lymphatics. Worms may be visualized in the lymphatics of the spermatic cord in up to 80% of men infected with *W. bancrofti*. Live adult worms have a distinctive pattern of movement within the lymphatic vessels (termed the *filarial dance sign*). Radionuclide lymphoscintigraphic imaging of the limbs reliably demonstrates widespread lymphatic abnormalities in both subclinical microfilaremic persons and those with clinical manifestations of lymphatic pathology. Although of potential utility in the delineation of anatomic changes associated with infection, lymphoscintigraphy is unlikely to assume primacy in the diagnostic evaluation of individuals with suspected infection; it is principally a research tool, although it has been used more widely for assessment of lymphedema of any cause. Eosinophilia and elevated serum concentrations of IgE and antifilarial antibody support the diagnosis of lymphatic filariasis. There is, however, extensive cross-reactivity between filarial antigens and antigens of other helminths. Of note, *W. bancrofti*– and *B. malayi*–specific antigens have been identified and are now available for use in rapid diagnostic tests with specificities of >98%. However, seropositivity cannot be equated with active infection: residents of endemic areas can become sensitized to filarial antigens through exposure to infective mosquitoes without having patent filarial infections.

The ADL associated with lymphatic filariasis must be distinguished from thrombophlebitis, infection, and trauma. Retrograde evolution is a characteristic feature that helps distinguish filarial lymphangitis from ascending bacterial lymphangitis. Chronic filarial lymphedema must also be distinguished from the lymphedema of malignancy, postoperative scarring, trauma, chronic edematous states, and congenital lymphatic system abnormalities.

TREATMENT

Lymphatic Filariasis

With newer definitions of clinical syndromes in lymphatic filariasis and new tools to assess clinical status (e.g., ultrasound, lymphoscintigraphy, circulating filarial antigen assays, PCR), approaches to treatment based on infection status can be considered.

Orally administered diethylcarbamazine (DEC; 6 mg/kg daily for 12 days), which has both macro- and microfilaricidal properties, remains the drug of choice for the treatment of active lymphatic filariasis (defined by microfilaremia, antigen positivity, or adult worms on ultrasound), although albendazole (400 mg twice daily by mouth for 21 days) also has demonstrated macrofilaricidal efficacy. A 4- to 6-week course of oral doxycycline (targeting the intracellular *Wolbachia*) also has significant macrofilaricidal activity, as does DEC/albendazole used daily for 7 days. The addition of DEC to a 3-week course of doxycycline is efficacious in lymphatic filariasis.

Regimens that combine single doses of albendazole (400 mg) with either DEC (6 mg/kg) or ivermectin (200 μg/kg) all have a sustained microfilaricidal effect and are the mainstay of programs for the eradication of lymphatic filariasis in Africa (albendazole/ivermectin) and elsewhere (albendazole/DEC) (see "Prevention and Control," below). Recently, a regimen using single doses of the three major antifilarial drugs (albendazole/DEC/ivermectin) has been shown to sustain microfilarial clearance out to at least 2 years.

As has already been mentioned, a growing body of evidence indicates that, although they may be asymptomatic, virtually all persons with *W. bancrofti* or *B. malayi* microfilaremia have some degree of subclinical disease (hematuria, proteinuria, abnormalities on lymphoscintigraphy). Thus, early treatment of asymptomatic persons who have microfilaremia is recommended to prevent further lymphatic damage. For ADL, supportive treatment (including the administration of antipyretics and analgesics) is recommended, as is antibiotic therapy if secondary bacterial infection is likely. Similarly, because lymphatic disease is associated with the presence of adult worms, treatment with DEC is recommended for microfilaria-negative carriers of adult worms.

In persons with chronic manifestations of lymphatic filariasis, treatment regimens that emphasize hygiene, prevention of secondary bacterial infections, and physiotherapy have gained wide acceptance for morbidity control. These regimens are similar to those recommended for lymphedema of most nonfilarial causes and are known by a variety of names, including *complex decongestive physiotherapy* and *complex lymphedema therapy*. Hydroceles (Fig. 233-1) can be managed surgically. With chronic manifestations of lymphatic filariasis, drug treatment should be reserved for individuals who have evidence of active infection; however, a 6-week course of doxycycline has been shown to provide improvement in filarial lymphedema irrespective of disease activity.

Side effects of DEC treatment include fever, chills, arthralgias, headaches, nausea, and vomiting. Both the development and the severity of these reactions are directly related to the number of microfilariae circulating in the bloodstream. The adverse reactions may represent either an acute hypersensitivity reaction to the antigens being released by dead and dying parasites or an inflammatory reaction induced by the intracellular *Wolbachia* endosymbionts freed from their intracellular niche.

Ivermectin has a side effect profile similar to that of DEC when used in lymphatic filariasis. In patients infected with *L. loa* who have high levels of microfilaremia, DEC—like ivermectin (see "Loiasis," below)—can elicit severe encephalopathic complications. When used in single-dose regimens for the treatment of lymphatic filariasis, albendazole is associated with relatively few side effects.

PREVENTION AND CONTROL

To protect themselves against filarial infection, individuals must avoid contact with infected mosquitoes by using personal protective measures, including bed nets, particularly those impregnated with insecticides such as permethrin. Mass drug administration (MDA) is the current approach to elimination of lymphatic filariasis as a public health problem. The underlying tenet of this approach is that mass annual distribution of antifilarial chemotherapy—albendazole with either DEC (for all areas except those where onchocerciasis is coendemic; see section on onchocerciasis treatment, below) or ivermectin or with both ivermectin and DEC (triple-drug therapy)—will profoundly suppress microfilaremia. If the suppression is sustained, then transmission can be interrupted.

Created by the World Health Organization in 1997, the Global Programme to Eliminate Lymphatic Filariasis is based on mass administration of single annual doses of DEC plus albendazole in non-African regions and of albendazole plus ivermectin in Africa. Available information from late 2020 indicated that >792 million persons in 53 countries had thus far participated. Not only has lymphatic filariasis been eliminated in some defined areas, but collateral benefits—avoidance of disability and treatment of intestinal helminths and other conditions (e.g., scabies and louse infestation)—also have been noted. The strategy of the global program is being refined, and attempts are being made to integrate this effort with other mass-treatment strategies (e.g., deworming programs, malaria control, and trachoma control) in an integrated control strategy.

TROPICAL PULMONARY EOSINOPHILIA

Tropical pulmonary eosinophilia (TPE) is a distinct syndrome that develops in some individuals infected with the lymphatic-dwelling filarial species. The majority of cases have been reported from India, Pakistan, Sri Lanka, Brazil, Guyana, and Southeast Asia; the decreasing incidence of TPE in the past decade probably reflects global MDA efforts.

■ CLINICAL FEATURES

The main features include a history of residence in filaria-endemic regions, paroxysmal cough and wheezing (usually nocturnal and probably related to the nocturnal periodicity of microfilariae), weight loss, low-grade fever, lymphadenopathy, and pronounced blood eosinophilia (>3000 eosinophils/μL). Chest x-rays or CT scans may be normal but generally show increased bronchovascular markings. Diffuse miliary lesions or mottled opacities may be present in the middle and lower lung fields. Tests of pulmonary function show restrictive abnormalities in most cases and obstructive defects in half. Characteristically, total serum IgE levels (4–40 KIU/mL) and antifilarial antibody levels are markedly elevated.

■ PATHOLOGY

In TPE, microfilariae and parasite antigens are rapidly cleared from the bloodstream by the lungs. The clinical symptoms result from allergic and inflammatory reactions elicited by the cleared parasites. In some patients, trapping of microfilariae in other reticuloendothelial organs can cause hepatomegaly, splenomegaly, or lymphadenopathy. A prominent, eosinophil-enriched, intra-alveolar infiltrate is common, and with it comes the release of cytotoxic proinflammatory eosinophil granule proteins that may mediate some of the pathology seen in TPE. In the absence of successful treatment, interstitial fibrosis can lead to progressive pulmonary damage.

■ DIFFERENTIAL DIAGNOSIS

TPE must be distinguished from asthma, Löffler's syndrome, allergic bronchopulmonary aspergillosis, allergic granulomatosis with polyangiitis (eosinophilic granulomatosis with polyangiitis or Churg-Strauss syndrome), other systemic vasculitides (most notably, periarteritis nodosa), chronic eosinophilic pneumonia, and the hypereosinophilic syndromes (HESs).

TREATMENT
Tropical Pulmonary Eosinophilia

DEC is used at a daily dosage of 4–6 mg/kg for 14 days. Symptoms usually resolve within 3–7 days after the initiation of therapy. Relapse, which occurs in ~12–25% of cases (sometimes after an interval of several years), requires re-treatment.

ONCHOCERCIASIS

■ EPIDEMIOLOGY

Onchocerciasis ("river blindness") is caused by the filarial nematode *O. volvulus*, which infects an estimated 37 million individuals in 31 countries worldwide. The majority of individuals infected with *O. volvulus* live in the equatorial region of Africa extending from the Atlantic coast to the Red Sea. In the Americas, the only remaining countries with isolated foci are Venezuela and Brazil. The infection is also found in Yemen.

■ ETIOLOGY

Infection in humans begins with the deposition of infective larvae on the skin by the bite of an infected blackfly. The larvae develop into adults, which are typically found in subcutaneous nodules. About 7 months to 3 years after infection, the gravid female releases microfilariae that migrate out of the nodule and throughout the tissues, concentrating in the dermis. Infection is transmitted to other persons when a female fly ingests microfilariae from the host's skin and these microfilariae then develop into infective larvae. Adult *O. volvulus* females and males are ~40–60 cm and ~3–6 cm in length, respectively. The life span of adults can be as long as 18 years, with an average of ~9 years. Because the blackfly vector breeds along free-flowing rivers and streams (particularly in rapids) and generally restricts its flight to an area within several kilometers of these breeding sites, both biting and disease transmission are most intense in these locations.

■ PATHOLOGY

Onchocerciasis primarily affects the skin, eyes, and lymph nodes. In contrast to the pathology in lymphatic filariasis, the damage in onchocerciasis is elicited by microfilariae and not by adult parasites. In the skin, there are mild but chronic inflammatory changes that can result in loss of elastic fibers, atrophy, and fibrosis. The subcutaneous nodules (*onchocercomata*) consist primarily of fibrous tissues surrounding the adult worm, often with a peripheral ring of inflammatory cells surrounded by an endothelial layer (characterized as lymphatic in origin). In the eye, neovascularization and corneal scarring lead to corneal opacities and blindness. Inflammation in the anterior and posterior chambers frequently results in anterior uveitis, chorioretinitis, and optic atrophy. Although punctate opacities are due to an inflammatory reaction surrounding dead or dying microfilariae, the pathogenesis of most manifestations of onchocerciasis is still unclear.

■ CLINICAL FEATURES

Skin Pruritus and rash are the most common manifestations of onchocerciasis. The pruritus can be incapacitating; the rash is typically a papular eruption (Fig. 233-3) that is generalized rather than localized to a particular region of the body. Long-term infection results in exaggerated and premature wrinkling of the skin, loss of elastic fibers, and epidermal atrophy that can lead to loose, redundant skin and hypo- or

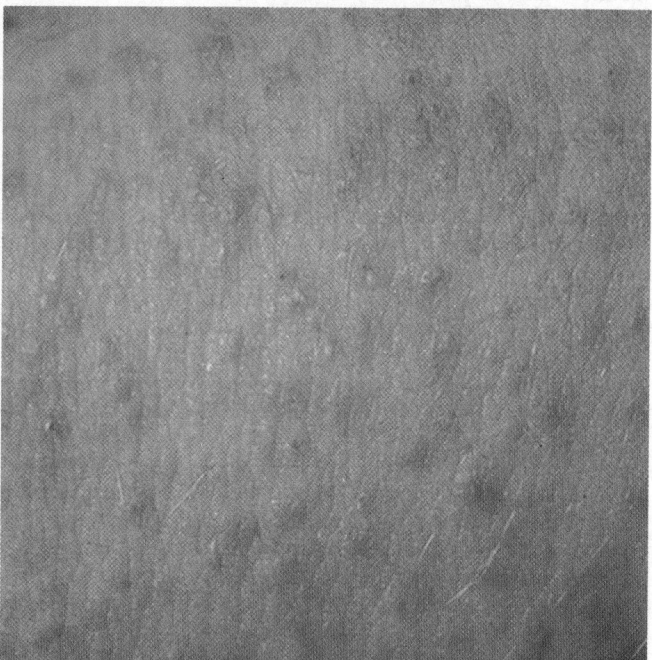

FIGURE 233-3 Papular eruption as a consequence of onchocerciasis.

hyperpigmentation. Localized eczematoid dermatitis can cause hyperkeratosis, scaling, and pigmentary changes. In an immunologically hyperreactive form of onchodermatitis (commonly termed *sowdah* or *localized onchodermatitis*), the affected skin darkens as a consequence of the profound inflammation that occurs as microfilariae in the skin are cleared.

Onchocercomata These subcutaneous nodules, which can be palpable and/or visible, contain the adult worm. They are most common over the coccyx and sacrum, the trochanter of the femur, the lateral anterior crest, and other bony prominences. Nodules vary in size and characteristically are firm and not tender. It has been estimated that, for every palpable nodule, there are four deeper nonpalpable ones.

Ocular Tissue Visual impairment is the most serious complication of onchocerciasis and usually affects only those persons with moderate or heavy infections. Lesions may develop in all parts of the eye. The most common early finding is conjunctivitis with photophobia. Punctate keratitis—acute inflammatory reactions surrounding dying microfilariae and manifested as "snowflake" opacities—is common among younger patients and resolves without apparent complications. Sclerosing keratitis occurs in 1–5% of infected persons and is the leading cause of onchocercal blindness. Anterior uveitis and iridocyclitis develop in ~5% of infected persons. Characteristic chorioretinal lesions develop as a result of atrophy and hyperpigmentation of the retinal pigment epithelium. Constriction of the visual fields and overt optic atrophy may occur.

Lymph Nodes Mild to moderate lymphadenopathy is common, particularly in the inguinal and femoral areas, where the enlarged nodes may hang down in response to gravity ("hanging groin"), sometimes predisposing to inguinal and femoral hernias.

Other Manifestations Some heavily infected individuals develop cachexia with loss of adipose tissue and muscle mass. A form of dwarfism, Nakalanga dwarfism, has been attributed to pituitary involvement in this infection. An association between onchocerciasis and epilepsy (including an epidemic form termed nodding syndrome) has gained attention recently. Among adults who become blind, there is a three- to fourfold increase in mortality rate.

DIAGNOSIS

Definitive diagnosis depends on the detection of an adult worm in an excised nodule or, more commonly, of microfilariae in a skin snip. Skin snips are obtained with a corneal-scleral punch or by lifting of the skin with the tip of a needle and excision of a small (1- to 3-mm) piece with a sterile scalpel blade. Both methods collect a blood-free skin biopsy sample extending to just below the epidermis. The biopsy tissue can be incubated in tissue culture medium or in saline on a glass slide or flat-bottomed microtiter plate. After incubation for 2–4 h (or occasionally overnight in light infections), microfilariae emergent from the skin can be seen by low-power microscopy or can be detected by PCR.

Eosinophilia and elevated serum IgE levels are common but, because these features are seen in many parasitic infections, are not diagnostic in themselves. Immunoassays to detect antibodies to *Onchocerca*-specific antigens are being used both in specialized laboratories and at the point of contact in rapid-diagnostic formats.

TREATMENT

Onchocerciasis

The main goals of therapy are to prevent the development of irreversible lesions and to alleviate symptoms. Chemotherapy is the mainstay of management. Ivermectin, a semisynthetic macrocyclic lactone active against microfilariae, is the first-line agent for the treatment of onchocerciasis. It is given orally in a single dose of 150 μg/kg, either yearly or semiannually. More frequent ivermectin administration (every 3 months) has been suggested to ameliorate pruritus and skin disease.

After treatment, most individuals have few or no reactions. Pruritus, cutaneous edema, and/or maculopapular rash occur in ~1–10% of treated individuals. In areas of Africa coendemic for *O. volvulus* and *L. loa*, however, ivermectin is contraindicated (as it is for pregnant or breast-feeding women) because of severe posttreatment encephalopathy, especially in patients who are heavily microfilaremic for *L. loa* (>30,000 microfilariae/mL). Although ivermectin treatment results in a marked drop in microfilarial density, its effect can be short-lived (<3 months in some cases). Thus, it is occasionally necessary to give ivermectin more frequently for persistent symptoms.

A 6-week course of doxycycline is macrofilaristatic, rendering female adult worms sterile for long periods.

PREVENTION

Vector control has been beneficial in highly endemic areas in which breeding sites are vulnerable to insecticide spraying, but most areas endemic for onchocerciasis are not suited to this type of control. Community-based administration of ivermectin every 6–12 months is being used to interrupt transmission in endemic areas. This measure, in conjunction with vector control, has already helped eliminate the infection in most of Latin America and has reduced the prevalence of disease in many endemic foci in Africa. No drug has proved useful for prophylaxis of *O. volvulus* infection.

LOIASIS

ETIOLOGY AND EPIDEMIOLOGY

Loiasis is caused by *L. loa* (the African eye worm), which is present in the rainforests of West and Central Africa. Adult parasites (females, 50–70 mm long and 0.5 mm wide; males, 25–35 mm long and 0.25 mm wide) live in subcutaneous tissues. Microfilariae circulate in the blood with a diurnal periodicity that peaks between 10:00 A.M. and 2:00 P.M.

CLINICAL FEATURES

Manifestations of loiasis in natives of endemic areas may differ from those in temporary residents or visitors. Among the indigenous population, loiasis is often an asymptomatic infection with microfilaremia. Infection may be recognized only after subconjunctival migration of an adult worm **(Fig. 233-4)** or may be manifested by episodic *Calabar swellings*—evanescent localized areas of angioedema and erythema developing on the extremities and less frequently at other sites. Nephropathy, encephalopathy, and cardiomyopathy can occur but are rare. In patients who are not residents of endemic areas, allergic symptoms predominate, episodes of Calabar swelling tend to be more frequent,

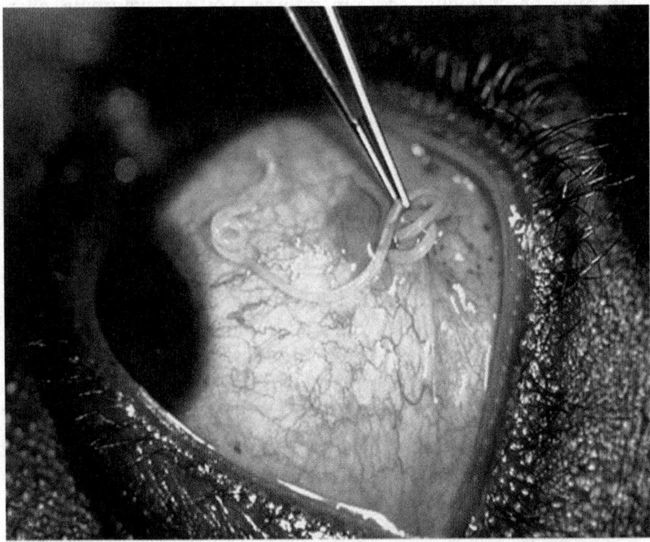

FIGURE 233-4 Adult *Loa loa* worm being surgically removed after its subconjunctival migration.

microfilaremia is less common, and eosinophilia and increased levels of antifilarial antibodies are characteristic.

PATHOLOGY

The pathogenesis of the manifestations of loiasis is poorly understood. Calabar swellings are thought to result from a hypersensitivity reaction to adult worm antigens.

DIAGNOSIS

Definitive diagnosis of loiasis requires the detection of microfilariae in the peripheral blood or the isolation of the adult worm from the eye (Fig. 233-4) or from a subcutaneous biopsy specimen collected from a site of swelling developing after treatment. PCR-based assays for the detection of *L. loa* DNA in blood are available in specialized laboratories and are highly sensitive and specific, as are some newer recombinant antigen–based serologic techniques. In practice, the diagnosis must often be based on a characteristic history and clinical presentation, blood eosinophilia, and elevated levels of antifilarial antibodies, particularly in travelers to an endemic region, who are often amicrofilaremic.

TREATMENT

Loiasis

DEC (8–10 mg/kg per day administered orally for 21 days) is effective against both the adult and the microfilarial forms of *L. loa*, but multiple courses are frequently necessary before loiasis resolves completely. In cases of heavy microfilaremia, allergic or other inflammatory reactions can take place during treatment, including central nervous system involvement with coma and encephalitis. Heavy infections can be treated initially with apheresis to remove the microfilariae and with glucocorticoids (40–60 mg of prednisone per day) followed by doses of DEC (0.5 mg/kg per day). If antifilarial treatment has no adverse effects, the prednisone dose can be tapered rapidly and the dose of DEC gradually increased to 8–10 mg/kg per day.

Albendazole or ivermectin is effective in reducing microfilarial loads, although neither is approved for this purpose by the U.S. Food and Drug Administration. Moreover, ivermectin is contraindicated in patients with >30,000 microfilariae/mL because this drug has been associated with severe adverse events (including encephalopathy and death) in heavily infected patients with loiasis in West and Central Africa. DEC (300 mg weekly) is an effective prophylactic regimen for loiasis.

STREPTOCERCIASIS

Mansonella streptocerca, found mainly in the tropical forest belt of Africa from Ghana to the Democratic Republic of the Congo, is transmitted by biting midges. The major clinical manifestations involve the skin and include pruritus, papular rashes, and pigmentation changes. Many infected individuals have inguinal adenopathy, although most are asymptomatic. The diagnosis is made by detection of the characteristic microfilariae in skin snips. Ivermectin at a single dose of 150 μg/kg leads to sustained suppression of microfilariae in the skin and is probably the treatment of choice for streptocerciasis.

MANSONELLA PERSTANS INFECTION

M. perstans, distributed across the center of Africa and in northeastern South America, is transmitted by midges. Adult worms reside in serous cavities—pericardial, pleural, and peritoneal—as well as in the mesentery and the perirenal and retroperitoneal tissues. Microfilariae circulate in the blood without periodicity. The clinical and pathologic features of the infection are poorly defined. Most patients appear to be asymptomatic, but manifestations may include transient angioedema and pruritus of the arms, face, or other parts of the body (analogous to the Calabar swellings of loiasis); fever; headache; arthralgias; and right-upper-quadrant pain. Occasionally, pericarditis and hepatitis occur. The diagnosis is based on the demonstration of microfilariae in blood or serosal effusions. Perstans filariasis is often associated with peripheral-blood eosinophilia and antifilarial antibody elevations.

With the identification of a *Wolbachia* endosymbiont in *M. perstans*, doxycycline (200 mg twice a day) for 6 weeks has been established as the first effective treatment for this infection.

MANSONELLA OZZARDI INFECTION

The distribution of *M. ozzardi* is restricted to Central and South America and certain Caribbean islands. Adult worms are rarely recovered from humans. Microfilariae circulate in the blood without periodicity. Although this organism has often been considered nonpathogenic, headache, articular pain, fever, pulmonary symptoms, adenopathy, hepatomegaly, pruritus, and eosinophilia have been ascribed to *M. ozzardi* infection. The diagnosis is made by detection of microfilariae in peripheral blood. Ivermectin is effective in treating this infection.

ZOONOTIC FILARIAL INFECTIONS

Dirofilariae that affect primarily dogs, cats, and raccoons occasionally infect humans incidentally, as do *Brugia* and *Onchocerca* parasites that affect small mammals. Because humans are an abnormal host, the parasites never develop fully. Pulmonary dirofilarial infection caused by the canine heartworm *Dirofilaria immitis* generally presents in humans as a solitary pulmonary nodule. Chest pain, hemoptysis, and cough are uncommon. Infections with *Dirofilaria repens* (from dogs) or *Dirofilaria tenuis* (from raccoons) can cause local subcutaneous nodules in humans. Zoonotic *Brugia* infection can produce isolated lymph node enlargement, whereas zoonotic *Onchocerca* species (particularly *O. lupi*) can cause subconjunctival masses. Eosinophilia levels and antifilarial antibody titers are not commonly elevated. Excisional biopsy is both diagnostic and curative. These infections usually do not respond to antifilarial chemotherapy.

DRACUNCULIASIS (GUINEA WORM INFECTION)

ETIOLOGY AND EPIDEMIOLOGY

The incidence of dracunculiasis, caused by *Dracunculus medinensis*, has declined dramatically because of global eradication efforts. However, between 2017 and 2020, there were increases in the number of human cases. At the end of 2020, there were a total of 27 human cases of Guinea worm disease across six African countries, with 12 cases in Chad, 11 cases in Ethiopia, and 1 each in South Sudan, Angola, Mali, and Cameroon.

Humans acquire *D. medinensis* when they ingest water containing infective larvae derived from *Cyclops*, a crustacean that is the intermediate host. Larvae penetrate the stomach or intestinal wall, mate, and mature. The adult male probably dies; the female worm develops over a year and migrates to subcutaneous tissues, usually in the lower extremity. As the thin female worm, ranging in length from 30 cm to 1 m, approaches the skin, a blister forms that, over days, breaks down and forms an ulcer. When the blister opens, large numbers of motile, rhabditiform larvae can be released into stagnant water; ingestion by *Cyclops* completes the life cycle.

CLINICAL FEATURES

Few or no clinical manifestations of dracunculiasis are evident until just before the blister forms, when there is an onset of fever and generalized allergic symptoms, including periorbital edema, wheezing, and urticaria. The emergence of the worm is associated with local pain and swelling. When the blister ruptures (usually as a result of immersion in water) and the adult worm releases larva-rich fluid, symptoms are relieved. The shallow ulcer surrounding the emerging adult worm heals over weeks to months. Such ulcers, however, can become secondarily infected, the result being cellulitis, local inflammation, abscess formation, or (uncommonly) tetanus. Occasionally, the adult worm does not emerge but becomes encapsulated and calcified.

DIAGNOSIS

The diagnosis is based on the findings developing with the emergence of the adult worm, as described above.

TREATMENT

Dracunculiasis

Gradual extraction of the worm by winding of a few centimeters on a stick each day remains the common and effective practice. Worms may be excised surgically. No drug is effective in treating dracunculiasis.

PREVENTION

Prevention, which remains the only real control measure, depends on the provision of safe drinking water.

FURTHER READING

Herrick JA et al: Infection-associated immune perturbations resolve one year following treatment for *Loa loa*. Clin Infect Dis 72:789, 2021.

Hopkins DR et al: Progress toward global eradication of dracunculiasis—January 2019–June 2020. Morb Mortal Wkly Rep 69:1563, 2020.

King CL et al: Single-dose triple-drug therapy for *Wuchereria bancrofti*—5-year follow-up. N Engl J Med 382:1956, 2020.

Mand S et al: Doxycycline improves filarial lymphedema independent of active filarial infection: A randomized controlled trial. Clin Infect Dis 55:621, 2012.

Taylor MJ et al: Lymphatic filariasis and onchocerciasis. Lancet 376:1175, 2010.

234 Schistosomiasis and Other Trematode Infections

Birgitte Jyding Vennervald

Trematodes, or flatworms, are a group of helminths that belong to the phylum Platyhelminthes. The adult flatworms share some common characteristics, such as macroscopic size (from one to several centimeters); dorsoventrally flattened, bilaterally symmetric bodies; and two suckers—oral and ventral. Except for schistosomes, which have separate sexes, all human parasitic trematodes are hermaphroditic. Their life cycles involve a mammalian/human definitive host, in which sexual reproduction by adult worms takes place, and an intermediate host (snails), in which asexual multiplication occurs. Some species of trematodes have more than one intermediate host.

Humans are infected either by direct penetration of intact skin (schistosomiasis) or by ingestion of raw freshwater fish, crustaceans, or aquatic plants with metacercariae—the infective larval stage.

Significant trematode infections of humans may be divided according to the location of the adult worms: blood, liver (biliary tree), intestines, or lungs (**Table 234-1**). Adult worms do not multiply within the mammalian host but can live for up to 30 years. Infections are often chronic.

Although it is relatively rare to encounter patients with trematode infections in the United States, many millions of people are infected worldwide. Both schistosomiasis and food-borne trematode infections are poverty-related chronic diseases with high morbidity and a significant public health impact. Various factors may increase the spread of the infections globally. Increasing temperatures may render new areas suitable for the intermediate host snails, and an increase in travel and migration may increase the number of patients with trematode infections—for example, in the United States.

TABLE 234-1 Major Human Trematode Infections

TREMATODE	TRANSMISSION ROUTE	GEOGRAPHIC DISTRIBUTION
Blood Flukes		
Intestinal schistosomiasis		
Schistosoma mansoni	Skin penetration by cercariae released from snails (*Biomphalaria* spp.)	Africa, Brazil, Venezuela, Surinam, the Caribbean (low risk)
Shistosoma japonicum	Skin penetration by cercariae released from snails (*Oncomelania* spp.)	China, Indonesia, Philippines
Schistosoma guineensis and *Schistosoma intercalatum*	Skin penetration by cercariae released from snails (*Bulinus* spp.)	Rain forest areas of Central Africa
Schistosoma mekongi	Skin penetration by cercariae released from snails (*Neotricula aperta*)	Several districts of Cambodia and Lao People's Democratic Republic (PDR)
Urogenital schistosomiasis		
Schistosoma haematobium	Skin penetration by cercariae released from snails (*Bulinus* spp.)	Africa, Middle East, Corsica (France)
Liver Flukes		
Clonorchis sinensis	Ingestion of metacercariae in freshwater fish	Asia, including Republic of Korea, China, Taiwan, Vietnam
Opisthorchis viverrini	Ingestion of metacercariae in freshwater fish	Northeast Thailand, Lao PDR, Cambodia, Vietnam
Opisthorchis felineus	Ingestion of metacercariae in freshwater fish	Former Soviet Union, Kazakhstan, Ukraine, Turkey
Fasciola hepatica	Ingestion of metacercariae on aquatic plants or in water	Worldwide
Fasciola gigantica	Ingestion of metacercariae on aquatic plants or in water	Africa, Asia
Intestinal Flukes		
Fasciolopsis buski	Ingestion of metacercariae on aquatic plants	Bangladesh, China, India, Indonesia, Lao PDR, Malaysia, Taiwan, Thailand, Vietnam
Echinostoma spp.	Ingestion of freshwater fish, frogs, mussels, snails	China, India, Indonesia, Japan, Malaysia, Russia, Republic of Korea, Philippines, Thailand
Heterophyes heterophyes, several other species	Ingestion of metacercariae in freshwater or brackish-water fish	Egypt, Greece, Islamic Republic of Iran, Italy, Japan, Republic of Korea, Sudan, Tunisia, Turkey
Lung Flukes		
Paragonimus westermani	Ingestion of metacercariae in crayfish or crabs	Tropical and subtropical areas of eastern and southern Asia and sub-Saharan Africa
Paragonimus kellicotti	Ingestion of metacercariae in crayfish or crabs	North America

APPROACH TO THE PATIENT

Trematode Infection

In the evaluation of a patient in whom trematode infection is suspected, certain questions are highly relevant and can assist in establishing a diagnosis: Where have you been? If you have traveled, when did you return? What activities have you been involved in (trekking, swimming, whitewater rafting)? What have you been eating (local dishes while traveling; raw, poorly cooked, or pickled freshwater fish or crustaceans)? Definitive diagnosis is based on detection of parasite eggs in stool, urine, sputum, and sometimes tissue samples or on serologic tests. The presence of eosinophilia and a history of travel to endemic areas should raise suspicion of trematode infection. The U.S. Centers for Disease Control and Prevention (CDC) can provide guidance with respect to diagnosis and treatment.

SCHISTOSOMIASIS

Human schistosomiasis is caused by six species of the parasitic genus *Schistosoma*: *S. mansoni, S. japonicum, S. mekongi, S. intercalatum*, and the recently described *S. guineensis* cause intestinal disease, and *S. haematobium* causes urogenital disease (Table 234-1). The infection may cause considerable intestinal, hepatic, and genitourinary morbidity. Avian schistosomes may penetrate human skin, but they die in subcutaneous tissue, producing only cutaneous manifestations.

■ ETIOLOGY

Schistosoma infection is contracted through contact with freshwater bodies harboring infected intermediate-host snails. Cercariae, the infective larval stage released from the snail, penetrate intact human skin within a few minutes after attaching to the skin. After penetration, the cercariae transform to schistosomula, which then enter a small vein or lymphatic vessel, circulate in the bloodstream through the lung capillaries, and are pumped via the heart to all parts of the body to reach the portal vein. There, the worms mature into adult males or females, pair, and migrate to their final location in the mesenteric or pelvic venous plexus.

The interval from cercarial penetration to sexual maturation and egg production, termed the *prepatent period*, lasts 5–7 weeks (up to 12 weeks for *S. haematobium*). The female worm then begins to produce eggs, which are excreted via feces or, for *S. haematobium*, urine. Approximately 50% of eggs are retained in tissue, where they are responsible for organ-specific morbidity (see "Pathogenesis," below). When excreted eggs reach water, they hatch and release a free-swimming larval stage (*miracidium*), which, after penetrating a host snail, undergoes several rounds of asexual multiplication. After ~4–6 weeks, infective cercariae are shed from the infected snails into the water. One snail, infected by one miracidium, can shed thousands of cercariae per day for several months; thus, the transmission potential of schistosomes is enormous.

The schistosome egg (**Fig. 234-1**) is the only stage of the parasites' life cycle that can be detected in humans, either in excreta or in tissue biopsies. The eggs are large and can easily be distinguished morphologically from other helminth eggs. *S. haematobium* eggs are ~140 mm long, with a terminal spine; *S. mansoni* eggs are ~150 mm long, with a lateral spine; and *S. japonicum* eggs are smaller, rounder, and ~90 mm long, with a small lateral spine or knob.

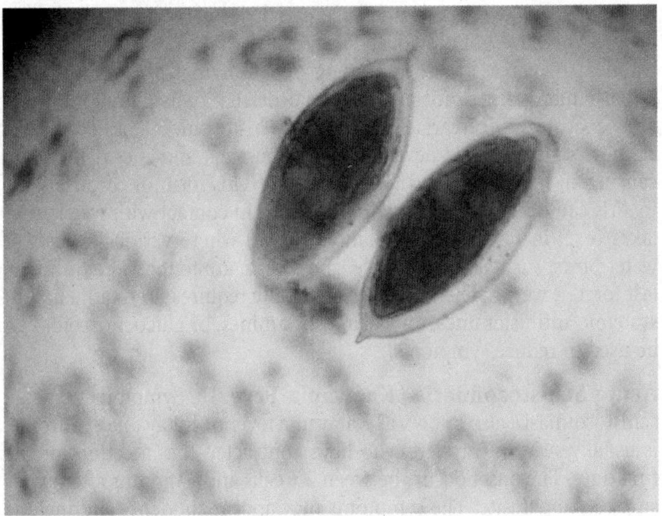

FIGURE 234-1 ***Schistosoma haematobium*** **eggs.**

Adult schistosomes are ~1–2 cm long. The male worm is flat, and the body forms a groove or gynecophoric canal in which the mature adult female is held like a sausage in a hotdog roll. Females are longer, thinner, and rounded. The females produce hundreds (African species) to thousands (Asian species) of eggs per day. Each ovum contains a ciliated miracidium larva, which secretes proteolytic enzymes that help the eggs to migrate into the lumen of the bladder (*S. haematobium*) or the intestine (other species). The lifespan of an adult schistosome averages 3–5 years but can be as long as 30 years. Schistosome worms feed on red blood cells; the debris is regurgitated in the host's blood, where it can be detected as circulating antigens (see "Diagnosis," below).

Adult schistosomes persist in the bloodstream for years and have evolved strategies of evading attack using immune effector mechanisms. This immune evasion is a result of several processes, such as binding of host proteins to the schistosome surface, which renders the parasite invisible to the host immune system.

The genome of schistosomes is relatively large (~300 Mb). Whole-genome sequences are available for *S. mansoni, S. japonicum*, and *S. haematobium*.

■ EPIDEMIOLOGY

Because of the complex life cycle of schistosomes, with snails as an intermediate host and humans as the final host, transmission is dependent on freshwater habitats that are suitable for the snails, are areas of human activity, and have climatic conditions favoring the survival of the snails and the development of the parasites inside the snail host. These requirements are reflected in the global distribution of schistosomiasis as well as in its microgeographic distribution within an endemic area. For *S. mansoni, S. haematobium, S. intercalatum* and *S. guineensis*, humans are the most important definitive host. *S. japonicum* and *S. mekongi* are zoonotic parasites, with a wide range of definitive hosts such as pigs, water buffaloes, and various rodents.

It is estimated that 229 million people are infected globally and at least 229 million people required preventive treatment in 2018. Schistosomiasis transmission has been reported from 78 countries, of which 52 endemic countries have moderate to high transmission (**Fig. 234-2**). More than 70% of infected people live in sub-Saharan Africa. Schistosomiasis is the most important of the neglected tropical diseases and is second only to malaria in public health impact. It is a poverty-related disease, and infection is prevalent in areas where adequate water supplies and sanitary facilities are lacking. In these areas, people come into contact with infested water through a variety of activities, including bathing, washing clothes, and collecting water for drinking or cooking. In some areas, adults have a high occupational risk of exposure; fishermen, canal cleaners, and workers in rice fields fall into this category. Among children, playing in water and swimming pose a risk. Large-scale irrigation and hydroelectric power operations can create suitable habitats for host snails and thus increase the risk of schistosomiasis transmission.

In general, children living in endemic areas initially acquire infection at ~3–4 years of age—i.e., when they are old enough to walk and come into contact with infested water. However, infection does occur in much younger children. As children grow older, the prevalence and intensity of infection increase, peaking around puberty. A characteristic feature of schistosomiasis infection in human populations is a convex age–prevalence curve, with low prevalence in very young children, higher prevalence in older children with a peak at 10–15 years of age, and declining prevalence in adults. The same pattern is observed between age and intensity of infection and is attributable to various factors. Generally, children have more frequent, prolonged, and extensive water contact than adults through activities like playing and swimming. Furthermore, several studies have indicated that acquired immunity to schistosomiasis develops slowly over several years, so that adults are reinfected to a much lesser extent than children. These factors, combined with progressive spontaneous death of adult worms from infections acquired during childhood, lead to lower levels of infection in the adult population.

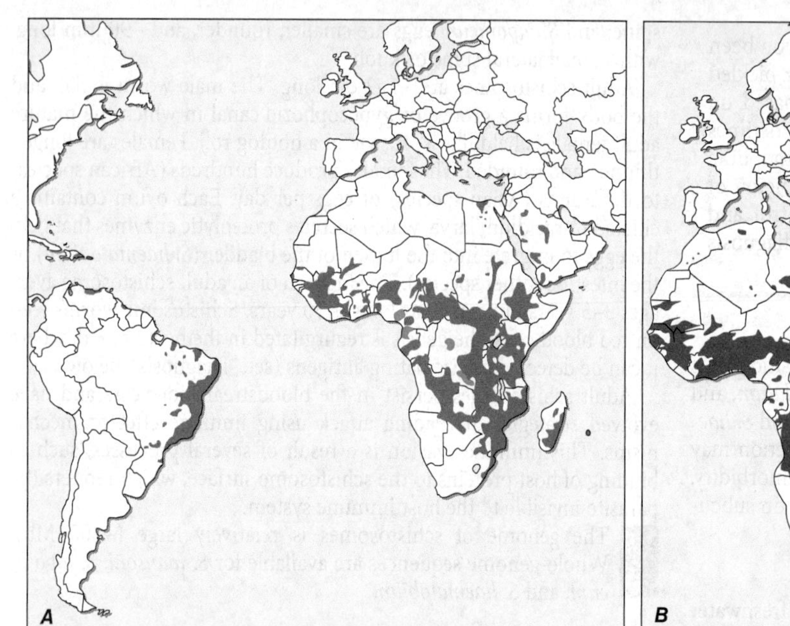

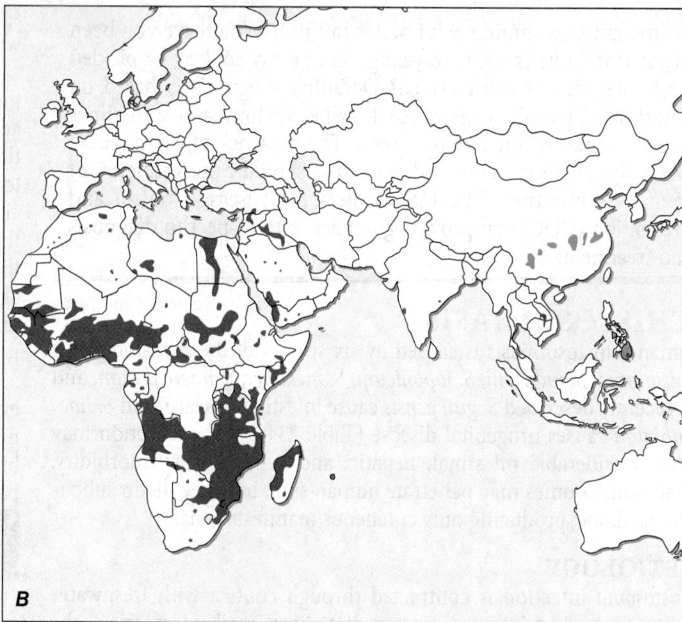

FIGURE 234-2 Global distribution of human schistosomiasis. ***A.*** *Schistosoma mansoni* infection (*dark blue*) is endemic in Africa, the Middle East, South America, and a few Caribbean countries. *S. intercalatum* infection (*green*) is endemic in sporadic foci in West and Central Africa. ***B.*** *Schistosoma haematobium* infection (*purple*) is endemic in Africa and the Middle East. The major endemic countries for *S. japonicum* infection (*green*) are China, the Philippines, and Indonesia. *Schistosoma mekongi* infection (*red*) is endemic in sporadic foci in Southeast Asia. *(Reprinted from CH King, AAF Mahmoud: Schistosomiasis and other trematode infections, in DL Kasper et al [eds], Harrison's Principles of Internal Medicine, 19th ed. New York, McGraw-Hill Education, 2015, pp 1423–1429.)*

■ PATHOGENESIS

Cercarial invasion may be associated with dermatitis arising from dermal and subdermal inflammatory reactions in response to dying cercariae that trigger innate immune responses. However, most manifestations of schistosomiasis—in the acute, established, and chronic phases of infection—are due to immunologic reactions to eggs retained in host tissues.

Around the time when oviposition commences, acute schistosomiasis (Katayama fever) may occur (see "Clinical Features," below). Antigen excess from eggs results in the formation of soluble immune complexes, which may be deposited in several tissues and initiate a serum sickness–like illness. All evidence suggests that schistosome eggs, and not adult worms, induce the organ-specific morbidity caused by schistosome infections. Approximately half of the eggs are not excreted via feces or urine but are trapped in intestinal or hepatic tissue (*S. mansoni*, *S. japonicum*, and *S. mekongi*) or in the bladder and urogenital system (*S. haematobium*). The eggs induce a granulomatous host immune response composed primarily of lymphocytes, eosinophils, and alternatively activated macrophages. The lymphocytes produce various T_H2 cytokines such as interleukins 4, 5, and 13. Later, in the chronic phase of infection, regulatory cytokines are responsible for immunomodulation or downregulation of host responses to schistosome eggs and play an important role in reducing the size of granulomas.

When *S. mansoni* or *S. japonicum* eggs are swept into the small portal branches of the liver via the portal vein, they lodge in the presinusoidal periportal tissues. The formation of granulomas around the eggs can cause significant enlargement of the spleen and liver. High-intensity infections in children are often accompanied by hepatosplenomegaly that generally decreases over time, partly because the number of eggs being deposited in the tissue gradually declines after the early teenage years as partial immunity to new infections develops and partly because of immunologic downregulation of the granulomatous response. However, in some infected individuals, egg-induced granulomatous responses lead to severe periportal fibrosis (*Symmers clay pipestem fibrosis*), with deposition of collagen around the portal vein, occlusion of the smaller portal branches, and severe, often irreversible, pathology. Occlusion of the portal branches may result in marked portal hypertension.

The signs and symptoms of *S. haematobium* infection relate to the worms' predilection for the veins of the urogenital plexus and result from deposition of eggs in the bladder, ureters, and genital organs. During established active infection, clusters of living eggs in the urogenital tissues can be found surrounded by intense inflammatory reactions and intense tissue eosinophilia. Movement of egg clusters into the lumen of the bladder is often followed by sloughing off of the epithelial surface, ulceration, and bleeding. Intense egg-induced tissue inflammation can result in bladder wall thickening and development of masses and pseudopolyps. Inflammation and granuloma formation around the ureteral ostia can lead to hydronephrosis.

Generally, late chronic-stage infections are characterized by accumulation of dead calcified eggs in tissue. Characteristic cervical lesions are found in *S. haematobium* infections, including active-stage lesions with intense tissue inflammation around live eggs and chronic-stage sandy patches with clusters of calcified eggs.

■ CLINICAL FEATURES

In general, disease manifestations of schistosomiasis occur in three stages—acute, active, and chronic—according to the duration and intensity of infection.

Cercarial Dermatitis ("Swimmer's Itch") Cercarial penetration of the skin may result in a maculopapular rash called cercarial dermatitis or "swimmer's itch." Cercarial dermatitis can develop in people who have not previously been exposed to schistosomiasis (e.g., travelers), whereas it is rare among people living in endemic areas. A particularly severe form of cercarial dermatitis is commonly seen after exposure to cercariae from avian schistosomes. These cercariae cannot complete their development in humans and die in the skin, causing an inflammatory allergic reaction. This form of cercarial dermatitis can occur in people who have been in contact with water from lakes (e.g., in Europe or the United States) where various species of water birds, such as ducks, geese, and swans, are found. The rash may last for 1–2 weeks. This condition normally requires no treatment, but systemic antihistamines, topical antihistamines, or glucocorticoids can be used to reduce symptoms.

Acute Schistosomiasis (Katayama Fever) Symptomatic acute schistosomiasis, also known as Katayama fever or Katayama syndrome, is usually seen in travelers who have contracted the infection for the first time. The onset occurs between 2 weeks and 3 months after exposure to the parasite. The symptoms may appear suddenly and include fever, myalgia, general malaise and fatigue, headache, nonproductive cough, and intestinal symptoms such as abdominal tenderness or pain. Various combinations of these symptoms are often accompanied by eosinophilia and transient pulmonary infiltrates. Many patients recover spontaneously from acute schistosomiasis after 2–10 weeks, but the illness follows a more severe clinical course in some individuals, with weight loss, dyspnea, diarrhea, and hepatomegaly. Severe cerebral or spinal cord manifestations may occur, and even light infections may cause severe illness. The syndrome can, in rare cases, be fatal.

Differential diagnosis includes many other febrile infectious diseases with acute onset, including malaria, salmonellosis, and acute hepatitis. Fever and eosinophilia occur in trichinosis, tropical eosinophilia, invasive ankylostomiasis, strongyloidiasis, visceral larva migrans, and infections with *Opisthorchis* and *Clonorchis* species. Katayama fever is rare in people chronically exposed to infection in areas endemic for *S. mansoni* or *S. haematobium*.

Intestinal Schistosomiasis (*S. mansoni, S. japonicum*) In intestinal schistosomiasis, adult worms are located in the mesenteric veins, and disease manifestations are associated with parasite eggs passing through or becoming trapped in intestinal tissue. This event induces mucosal granulomatous inflammation with microulcerations, superficial bleeding, and sometimes pseudopolyposis. The symptoms tend to be more pronounced with a high intensity of infection and include intermittent abdominal pain, loss of appetite, and sometimes bloody diarrhea. The clinical manifestations of *S. intercalatum, S. guineensis,* and *S. mekongi* infection are generally milder.

Hepatosplenic Schistosomiasis Hepatosplenic schistosomiasis is caused by schistosome eggs trapped in liver tissue and occurs in *S. mansoni* and *S. japonicum* infections. There are two distinct clinical entities: early inflammatory hepatosplenomegaly and late hepatosplenic disease with periportal fibrosis.

Early inflammatory hepatosplenic schistosomiasis is the main entity seen in children and adolescents. The liver is enlarged, especially the left lobe, and is smooth and firm. The spleen is enlarged, often extending below the umbilicus, and is firm or hard. Generally, ultrasonography shows no hepatic fibrosis. This form of hepatosplenic schistosomiasis may be found in up to 80% of infected children. Its severity is closely associated with the intensity of infection and may also be associated with concomitant chronic exposure to malaria.

Late hepatosplenic schistosomiasis with periportal or Symmers fibrosis may develop in young and middle-aged adults with long-standing, high-level exposure to infection. Patients with periportal fibrosis may excrete very few or no eggs in feces. During the early stage, the liver is enlarged, especially the left lobe; it is smooth and firm or hard. The spleen is enlarged, often massively, and is firm or hard. The patient may report a left hypochondrial mass with discomfort and anorexia. Ultrasonography reveals typical periportal fibrosis and dilation of the portal vein. Other complications include delayed growth and puberty, especially in *S. japonicum* infections, and severe anemia. Severe hepatosplenic schistosomiasis may lead to portal hypertension, but hepatic function usually remains normal, even in cases with marked periportal fibrosis and portal hypertension.

Ascites, attributable both to portal hypertension and to hypoalbuminemia, may be seen, especially in *S. japonicum* infection. Patients with severe hepatosplenic disease and portal hypertension may develop esophageal varices detectable by endoscopy or ultrasound. These patients may experience repeated bouts of hematemesis, melena, or both. Hematemesis is the most severe complication of hepatosplenic schistosomiasis, and death may result from massive loss of blood.

Urogenital Schistosomiasis (*S. haematobium*) The signs and symptoms of *S. haematobium* infection relate to the worms' predilection for the veins of the urogenital tract. Two stages of infection are recognized. An active stage occurring mainly in children, adolescents, and younger adults is characterized by egg excretion in the urine, with proteinuria and macroscopic or microscopic hematuria and deposition of eggs in the urinary tract. A chronic stage in older individuals is characterized by sparse or no urinary egg excretion despite urogenital tract pathology.

A characteristic sign in the active stage is painless, terminal hematuria. Dysuria and suprapubic discomfort or pain are associated with active urogenital schistosomiasis and may persist throughout the course of active infection. Eggs deposited in the bladder mucosa may give rise to an intense inflammatory response of the bladder wall, which may cause ureteric obstruction and lead to hydroureter and hydronephrosis. These early inflammatory lesions, including obstructive uropathy, can be visualized by ultrasonography.

As the infection progresses, the inflammatory component decreases and fibrosis becomes more prominent. The symptoms at this stage are nocturia, urine retention, dribbling, and incontinence. Cystoscopy reveals "sandy patches" composed of large numbers of calcified eggs surrounded by fibrous tissue and an atrophic mucosal surface. The ureters are less commonly involved, but ureteral fibrosis can cause irreversible obstructive uropathy that can progress to uremia.

Egg deposition may cause granulomas and lesions in the genital organs, most commonly in the cervix and vagina in women and the seminal vessels in men. The results may include dyspareunia, abnormal vaginal discharge, contact bleeding, and lower back pain in women and perineal pain, painful ejaculation, and hematospermia in men. Genital symptoms like bloody discharge and genital itch are associated with *S. haematobium* infection in school-aged girls living in schistosomiasis-endemic areas. Symptoms such as hematospermia and perineal discomfort have been described in travelers, and eggs have been demonstrated in seminal fluid. An association between female genital schistosomiasis and HIV infection has been demonstrated, but the impact of genital schistosomiasis on HIV transmission needs further elucidation.

S. haematobium has been classified by the International Agency for Research on Cancer (IARC) as definitely carcinogenic to humans (i.e., a group 1 carcinogen). Chronic *S. haematobium* infection is associated with squamous cell carcinoma of the urinary bladder.

Other Manifestations Worms and eggs can sometimes be located in ectopic sites, causing site-specific manifestations and symptoms. Neuroschistosomiasis is one of the most severe clinical forms of schistosomiasis and is caused by the inflammatory response around eggs in the cerebral or spinal venous plexus. *S. mansoni* and *S. haematobium* worms can end up in the spinal venous plexus, where they may cause transverse myelitis—an acute complication sometimes seen in travelers returning home with schistosomiasis. *S. japonicum* is mainly associated with granulomatous lesions in the brain, causing epileptic seizures, encephalopathy with headache, visual impairment, motor deficit, and ataxia. Pulmonary schistosomiasis is caused by portacaval shunting of eggs into the lung capillaries, where they induce granulomas in the perialveolar area. The consequences may be fibrosis, pulmonary hypertension, and cor pulmonale.

DIAGNOSIS

Anamnestic information on recent travels to endemic areas and exposure to freshwater bodies through recreational or other activities is important in the diagnosis of schistosomiasis in travelers. Information about exact geographic locations can facilitate identification of the relevant species of *Schistosoma*. Eosinophilia is a common finding and is often associated with helminthic infections such as schistosomiasis.

Detection of schistosome eggs in stool or urine is indicative of active infection and is the standard diagnostic method. The diagnosis is often based on the detection of eggs in a fixed small amount of excreta—e.g., 50 mg of stool or filtration of 10 mL of urine. This method is widely used among populations in endemic areas and allows quantitation of the level of infection (eggs per gram of feces or per 10 mL of urine). However, levels of egg excretion in people from nonendemic areas may be very low, in which case a larger sample and concentration methods (e.g., formol-ether concentration) may be needed.

Eggs can also be detected in rectal biopsies (both *S. mansoni* and *S. haematobium*) and occasionally in Pap smears and semen samples (*S. haematobium*). Polymerase chain reaction (PCR)–based detection of parasite DNA in stool or urine is more sensitive than parasitologic methods and is increasingly used. *Schistosoma* DNA can be detected in cerebrospinal fluid samples for diagnosis of neuroschistosomiasis.

Serology, with detection of specific antibodies to schistosomes, is useful in travelers but less so in people from endemic areas where transmission is ongoing. The serologic assays employed at the CDC are a Falcon assay screening test/enzyme-linked immunosorbent assay (FAST-ELISA) using *S. mansoni* adult microsomal antigen and a confirmatory species-specific immunoblot assay performed in light of the patient's travel history.

Schistosome proteoglycans—circulating anodic and cathodic antigens (CAAs and CCAs)—regurgitated into the bloodstream by the feeding worms can be detected in serum and urine by ELISA or monoclonal antibody–based lateral flow assays. The presence of CAA or CCA is an indication of active infection, and levels of these antigens correlate well with the intensity of infection. However, detection of CAAs and CCAs is not currently suitable for diagnosis in travelers, who are likely to have low levels of infection and very few worms, but promising results have been obtained using an ultrasensitive lateral flow assay. A commercially available point-of-care assay (Rapid Medical Diagnostics, Pretoria, South Africa) that detects CCA in urine is now widely used for screening of infected communities in relation to mass drug administration programs.

TREATMENT

Schistosomiasis

The drug of choice for treatment of schistosomiasis is praziquantel. It is administered orally, is available as 600-mg tablets, and is effective against all schistosome species infecting humans. The drug is safe and well tolerated. Standard regimens are shown in **Table 234-2**. In patients who are not cured by initial treatment, the same dose can be repeated at weekly intervals for 2 weeks. Since praziquantel does not affect the young migrating stages of the schistosomes, it may be necessary to repeat the dose 6–12 weeks later, especially if eosinophilia or symptoms persist despite treatment.

As a general principle, all patients with acute schistosomiasis should be treated with praziquantel. Glucocorticoids can be added in Katayama fever to suppress the hypersensitivity reaction. However, treatment for acute schistosomiasis or Katayama fever must be adjusted appropriately for each case, and in the most severe cases, management in an acute-care setting is necessary.

TABLE 234-2 Treatment of Schistosomiasis and Food-Borne Trematode Infections

INFECTION	DRUG OF CHOICE	ADULT DOSE[a]
Schistosoma mansoni, S. haematobium, S. intercalatum, S. guineensis	Praziquantel[b]	40 mg/kg PO in 2 divided doses for 1 day
S. japonicum, S. mekongi	Praziquantel	60 mg/kg PO in 3 divided doses for 1 day
Clonorchis sinensis, Opisthorchis viverrini, Opisthorchis felineus	Praziquantel	25 mg/kg PO tid for 2 consecutive days
Fasciola hepatica, Fasciola gigantica	Triclabendazole[c]	2 doses of 10 mg/kg PO given 12 h apart
Fasciolopsis buski	Praziquantel	75 mg/kg PO in 3 divided doses for 1 day
Echinostoma spp., *Heterophyes heterophyes*, several other species	Praziquantel	25 mg/kg PO tid
Paragonimus westermani, Paragonimus kellicotti	Praziquantel	25 mg/kg PO tid for 2 consecutive days
	Triclabendazole[c]	10 mg/kg PO once (or twice, 12–24 h apart)

[a]The pediatric dose is the same as the adult dose in all instances. [b]The safety of praziquantel in children <4 years old has not been established, although many children in this age group have been treated with praziquantel during mass drug-administration programs. [c]In February 2019, the U.S. Food and Drug Administration (FDA) approved triclabendazole for treatment of fascioliasis in patients at least 6 years of age.

Praziquantel is effective in cerebral *S. japonicum* infections, resulting in rapid dissipation of cerebral edema and resolution of cerebral masses. However, glucocorticoids and anticonvulsants are sometimes needed in neuroschistosomiasis.

The effect of antischistosomal treatment on disease manifestations depends on the stage and severity of the lesions. Early hepatosplenomegaly, mild or moderate fibrosis, and urinary bladder lesions seen during active infection resolve after chemotherapy. However, for late-stage manifestations (e.g., severe fibrosis with portal hypertension), praziquantel treatment is only one component of management, since the main complications are due to obstructive pathology. Management of portal hypertension and prevention of bleeding from esophageal varices should follow clinical guidelines for treatment of these conditions.

PREVENTION AND CONTROL

Schistosomiasis is contracted through direct contact with infested freshwater. Travelers should be made aware of the risk of infection if they come into contact with freshwater sources in schistosomiasis-endemic areas. For people living in rural areas where schistosomiasis is endemic, it may be very difficult, if not impossible, to avoid water contact—for example, during occupational activities such as fishing and working in rice fields. Schistosomiasis is a poverty-related disease, and access to safe water and good sanitary facilities may rarely be available. Because *S. japonicum* is a zoonotic parasite, preventive measures should target not only the human population but also animals such as water buffalo, which act as reservoirs for infection.

Praziquantel treatment of infected people, often during mass drug-administration programs, is a cornerstone of the management and control of schistosomiasis. Regular treatment will reduce the level of schistosomiasis morbidity in affected populations. However, treatment should be combined with other relevant strategies, such as control of the intermediate host snails, improved water-quality and sanitation facilities, and health education. Schistosomiasis control measures should be integrated into local health programs.

There have been intensive efforts to develop vaccines, but none is yet available. Two vaccine candidates are in clinical phase 1 trials and one is in phase 2 trials. Only one candidate, *S. haematobium* 28GST, has been tested in a clinical phase 3 trial in populations living in an endemic area. The vaccine candidate was immunogenic and well tolerated by infected children, but a sufficient efficacy was not reached.

FOOD-BORNE TREMATODE INFECTIONS

Food-borne trematode infections are a group of zoonotic diseases caused by hepatic, intestinal, and pulmonary parasitic flukes. These infections are contracted by ingestion of infective parasites in undercooked aquatic food or water plants. In 2015, an estimated 71 million people were infected with food-borne trematodes, and infections cause 2 million life-years lost to disability and death worldwide every year.

LIVER FLUKES

The most important liver flukes causing human infections are the related species *Opisthorchis viverrini* and *Opisthorchis felineus*, which cause opisthorchiasis; *Clonorchis sinensis*, which causes clonorchiasis; and *Fasciola hepatica* and *Fasciola gigantica*, which cause fascioliasis (Table 234-1).

Opisthorchiasis and Clonorchiasis *O. viverrini* is found mainly in northeastern Thailand, Laos, and Cambodia; *O. felineus* mainly in Europe and Asia, including the former Soviet Union; and *C. sinensis* in Asia, including Korea, China, Taiwan, Vietnam, Japan, and Asian regions of Russia. Parasite eggs excreted from infected humans or animals are ingested by a host snail (the first intermediate host), where they undergo several developmental stages. Cercariae are then released from the snail and penetrate freshwater fish (the second intermediate host), encysting as metacercariae in the muscles or under the scales. Humans become infected by eating raw or undercooked fish from endemic countries. After ingestion, the metacercariae excyst in gastric juices and migrate via the duodenum, the ampulla of Vater, and the extrahepatic biliary system to the intrahepatic bile ducts.

TABLE 234-3 Clinical Features of Food-Borne Trematode Infections

INFECTION	SYMPTOMS OR SIGNS		COMPLICATIONS
	EARLY OR ACUTE STAGE	ESTABLISHED OR CHRONIC STAGE	
Liver Flukes			
Clonorchis sinensis, *Opisthorchis viverrini*, *Opisthorchis felineus*	Often asymptomatic; sometimes hepatitis-like symptoms and high fever (especially with *O. felineus*)	Biliary colic, cholestatic jaundice, recurrent cholangitis and cholelithiasis; hepatomegaly, gallbladder enlargement, periductal fibrosis. Light infections are often asymptomatic and remain so for years.	Pancreatitis, cholangiocarcinoma[a]
Fasciola hepatica, *Fasciola gigantica*	Acute onset (1–4 weeks after infection) with high fever, weight loss, sometimes urticaria and liver tenderness	Biliary colic, cholestatic jaundice, recurrent cholangitis and cholelithiasis; thickening, enlargement, and fibrosis of biliary ducts; sometimes repeated relapses of acute symptoms	Pancreatitis. In rare cases: ectopic infections in the central nervous system, orbital area, gastrointestinal tract, lungs, and other organs. Rarely, fascioliasis can be fatal.
Intestinal Flukes			
Fasciolopsis buski, *Echinostoma* spp., *Heterophyes heterophyes*, several other species	Often asymptomatic; sometimes nonspecific gastrointestinal symptoms	Heavy infection may lead to ulceration of intestinal mucosa and malabsorption. Mild infections are often asymptomatic.	Malnutrition, anemia; rarely, ectopic infection in the central nervous system
Lung Flukes			
Paragonimus westermani, *Paragonimus kellicotti*	Often asymptomatic; sometimes insidious onset with anorexia and weight loss	Bronchitis-, asthma-, and tuberculosis-like symptoms and signs such as chronic cough, dyspnea, bloody ("rusty") sputum	Pulmonary cyst formation; ectopic infection in the central nervous system, eyes, skin, heart, abdominal and reproductive organs

[a]Carcinogenesis has not yet been established for *O. felineus*.

The clinical manifestations of infection with *Opisthorchis* species and *C. sinensis* are similar. Pathologic changes are typically seen in the bile ducts, liver, and gallbladder **(Table 234-3)**. Tissue damage and intense inflammation are caused by mechanical and chemical irritation and immune responses to worms or worm products, and chronic inflammation may result in the development of cholangiocarcinoma. Both *O. viverrini* and *C. sinensis* are classified by the IARC as definitely carcinogenic (class 1). Acute and light infections are mostly asymptomatic, but hepatitis-like signs and symptoms, with high fever and chills, have been reported, especially in *O. felineus* infections. In general, only heavily infected people have symptoms and severe complications (Table 234-3).

The diagnosis of these infections is based on microscopic identification of parasite eggs in stool specimens. The eggs of *Opisthorchis* are indistinguishable from those of *Clonorchis*.

Fascioliasis Fascioliasis occurs in many areas of the world and usually is caused by *Fasciola hepatica*, a common liver fluke of sheep and cattle. *F. hepatica* is found in more than 50 countries on all continents except Antarctica; *F. gigantica* is less widespread. The areas with the highest known rates of human *Fasciola* infection are in the Andean highlands of Bolivia and Peru. In other areas where fascioliasis is found, human cases are sporadic.

Unlike the other liver flukes, *Fasciola* species have no second intermediate host, as their infectious metacercariae adhere directly to aquatic plants. Humans usually acquire infection by ingesting aquatic plants, such as watercress, that contain viable metacercariae or by drinking water with free metacercariae.

After metacercariae have excysted in the duodenum, *Fasciola* species migrate through the intestinal wall into the body cavity, penetrate the liver capsule, and move through the liver into the bile ducts. This migration route is different from that of other liver flukes and gives rise to symptoms during the acute migratory phase; the parasites may cause tissue destruction, focal bleeding, and inflammation. Some migrating flukes may deviate from their usual route to cause ectopic infections. In the established latent stage of infection, the parasites may cause bile duct inflammation, resulting in thickening and expansion of the ducts, fibrosis, and ultimately biliary obstruction (Table 234-3). Although some infected people are asymptomatic in the latent phase, others may experience repeated relapses of acute manifestations.

The most widely used diagnostic approach is direct detection of *Fasciola* eggs by microscopic examination of stool or of duodenal or biliary aspirates. Eggs generally cannot be detected until 3–4 months after exposure, whereas antibodies to the parasite may become detectable 2–4 weeks after exposure. More than one stool specimen may be needed for diagnosis, especially in light infections.

■ INTESTINAL FLUKES

More than 70 species of intestinal flukes can cause human infection. These parasites are found in different geographic areas, with a relatively high prevalence in Southeast Asia. Humans are infected by ingestion of infective metacercariae attached to aquatic plants (*Fasciolopsis buski*) or encysted in freshwater fish. Flukes mature in the human intestines, and eggs are passed with feces. Mechanical irritation of the intestinal wall and inflammation may lead to nonspecific gastrointestinal symptoms such as diarrhea, constipation, and abdominal pain. Most individuals infected with intestinal flukes are asymptomatic, but heavy infections can be severe, with intestinal mucosal ulcerations and malabsorption (Table 234-3). The diagnosis is established by detection of eggs in stool samples. However, eggs from various intestinal trematodes are often morphologically similar, and it is very difficult to distinguish among species. A cautionary note: *Fasciola* eggs can be difficult to distinguish on the basis of morphologic criteria from the eggs of the intestinal fluke *F. buski*. The distinction has implications for therapy: infection with *F. buski* is treated with praziquantel, which is not effective against fascioliasis (Table 234-2).

■ LUNG FLUKES

Paragonimiasis is a parasitic lung infection caused by lung flukes of the genus *Paragonimus*. It is a food-borne parasitic zoonosis, with most cases reported from Asia and attributable to consumption of raw or undercooked freshwater crustaceans. *Paragonimus westermani* and related species (e.g., *Paragonimus africanus*) are endemic in West Africa, Central and South America, and Asia. The United States has one indigenous species of lung fluke, *Paragonimus kellicotti*.

Paragonimus species require two intermediate hosts: first, a freshwater snail; and second, a freshwater crustacean, such as a freshwater crab. Humans are infected by consuming raw or undercooked infected crustaceans containing *Paragonimus* metacercariae. *Paragonimus* infects other carnivores such as cats, dogs, foxes, rodents, and pigs in addition to humans. After ingestion, metacercariae quickly penetrate the duodenum and traverse the peritoneal cavity, diaphragm, and parietal pleura to mature into hermaphroditic worm pairs in the pleural spaces or lungs within 6–10 weeks. Adults cross-fertilize in cystic cavities in the pleural spaces or lungs within another 4–16 weeks and release unembryonated eggs into bronchioles. The eggs are then coughed up in bloody ("rusty") sputum and either discharged in sputum or swallowed and later excreted in feces. Unembryonated eggs are passed from the mammalian host into freshwater ecosystems, where they infect intermediate host snails.

The symptoms and signs of paragonimiasis are fever, cough, hemoptysis, and peripheral eosinophilia. Some patients with paragonimiasis and low parasite burdens may remain relatively asymptomatic for prolonged periods or may have recurrent attacks of cough, sputum production, fever, and night sweats that mimic tuberculosis. Infective metacercariae may migrate to extrapulmonary sites such as the brain (cerebral paragonimiasis).

Pulmonary paragonimiasis is diagnosed by detection of parasite ova in sputum and/or feces. Serology can be helpful in egg-negative cases and in cerebral paragonimiasis. Anamnestic information about the consumption of raw or undercooked freshwater crabs by immigrants, expatriates, and returning travelers—and, in the United States, the consumption of raw or undercooked crayfish from freshwater river systems where *P. kellicotti* is endemic—is important in patients presenting with fever, cough, hemoptysis, pleural effusions, and peripheral eosinophilia.

TREATMENT

Food-Borne Trematode Infections

Praziquantel and triclabendazole are the two drugs of choice; Table 234-2 summarizes the dosages recommended for the various trematode infections. All confirmed cases of human paragonimiasis should be treated with praziquantel (Table 234-2) to avoid the complications of extrapulmonary disease. Surgical management may be needed for pulmonary or cerebral lesions.

CONTROL AND PREVENTION

Drugs are currently the main method of controlling the morbidity associated with food-borne trematode infections, but integrated programs (including improved sanitation; food inspections; and information, education, and communication campaigns) are important for sustainable disease control. Collaboration with other sectors (e.g., agricultural, environmental, and educational) is necessary to tackle highly complex situations in which human behavior, biological factors, and agricultural practices all play a role.

FURTHER READING

Andrade G et al: Decline in infection-related morbidities following drug-mediated reductions in the intensity of *Schistosoma* infection: A systematic review and meta-analysis. PLoS Negl Trop Dis 11:e0005372, 2017.

Cucchetto G et al: High-dose or multi-day praziquantel for imported schistosomiasis? A systematic review. J Travel Med 26:taz050, 2019.

Fried B, Abruzzi A: Food-borne trematode infections of humans in the United States of America. Parasitol Res 106:1263, 2010.

Fürst T et al: Global burden of human food-borne trematodiasis: A systematic review and meta-analysis. Lancet Infect Dis 12:210, 2012.

Jordan P et al (eds): *Human Schistosomiasis*. CAB International, Wallingford, 1993.

Keiser J, Utzinger J: Food-borne trematodiases. Clin Microbiol Rev 22:466, 2009.

McManus DP et al: Schistosomiasis. Nat Rev Dis Primers 4:13, 2018.

Ross AG et al: Katayama syndrome. Lancet Infect Dis 7:218, 2007.

Sripa B et al: Update on pathogenesis of opisthorchiasis and cholangiocarcinoma. Adv Parasitol 102:97, 2018.

World Health Organization: *Female Genital Schistosomiasis: A Pocket Atlas for Clinical Health-Care Professionals*. Geneva, World Health Organization, 2015. Available at *http://brightresearch.org/wp-content/uploads/2016/05/FGS-pocket-atlas_eng.pdf*. WHO/HTM/NTD/2015.4, 2015. Accessed March 16, 2020.

235 Cestode Infections

A. Clinton White, Jr., Peter F. Weller

Cestodes, or tapeworms, are segmented flat worms. The adult worms reside in the gastrointestinal tract, but the larvae can be found in almost any organ. Human tapeworm infections can be divided into two major clinical groups. In one group, humans are the definitive hosts, with the adult tapeworms living in the gastrointestinal tract (*Taenia saginata*, *Diphyllobothrium*, and *Dipylidium caninum*). In the other, humans are intermediate hosts, with larval-stage parasites present in the tissues; diseases in this category include echinococcosis, sparganosis, and coenurosis. Humans may be the definitive and/or intermediate hosts for *Taenia solium*; both stages of *Hymenolepis nana* are found simultaneously in the human intestines.

The ribbon-shaped tapeworm attaches to the intestinal mucosa by means of sucking cups or hooks located on the scolex. Behind the scolex is a short, narrow neck from which proglottids (segments) form. As proglottids mature, they are displaced further back from the neck by the formation of new, less mature segments. The progressively elongating chain of attached proglottids, called the *strobila*, constitutes the bulk of the tapeworm. The length varies among species. In some, the tapeworm may consist of more than 1000 proglottids and may be several meters long. The mature proglottids are hermaphroditic and produce eggs, which are subsequently released. Because eggs of the different *Taenia* species are morphologically identical, only morphologic differences in the scolices or proglottids enable species-level diagnosis.

Most human tapeworms require at least one intermediate host for complete larval development. After ingestion of the eggs or proglottids by an intermediate host, the invasive larvae (oncospheres) are activated, escape the egg, and penetrate the intestinal mucosa. The oncosphere migrates to tissues and develops into an encysted form known as a *cysticercus* (single scolex), a *coenurus* (multiple scolices), or a *hydatid* (cyst with daughter cysts, each containing several protoscolices). The definitive host's ingestion of tissues containing a cyst enables a scolex to develop into a tapeworm.

TAENIASIS SAGINATA AND *TAENIASIS ASIATICA*

The beef tapeworm *T. saginata* occurs in all countries where raw or undercooked beef is eaten. It is most prevalent in sub-Saharan African and Middle Eastern countries. *Taenia asiatica* is closely related to *T. saginata* and is found in Asia, with pigs as intermediate hosts. The clinical manifestations and morphology of these two species are very similar and are therefore discussed together.

Etiology and Pathogenesis Humans are the only definitive host for the adult stage of *T. saginata* and *T. asiatica*. The tapeworms, which can reach 8 m in length with 1000–2000 proglottids, inhabit the upper jejunum. The scolex of *T. saginata* has four prominent suckers, whereas *T. asiatica* has an unarmed rostellum. Each gravid segment has 15–30 uterine branches (in contrast to 8–12 for *T. solium*). The eggs are indistinguishable from those of *T. solium*; they measure 30–40 μm, contain the oncosphere, and have a thick brown striated shell. Eggs deposited on vegetation can live for months or years until they are ingested by cattle or other herbivores (*T. saginata*) or pigs (*T. asiatica*). The embryo released after ingestion invades the intestinal wall and is carried to striated muscle or viscera, where it transforms into the cysticercus. When ingested in raw or undercooked meat, the cysticercus evaginates and forms a tapeworm in the human intestines. Over ~2 months, the adult worm matures and begins to produce eggs.

Clinical Manifestations Patients become aware of the infection most commonly by noting passage of proglottids in their feces. The proglottids of *T. saginata* are motile, and patients may experience perianal discomfort when proglottids are discharged. Mild abdominal pain or discomfort, nausea, change in appetite, weakness, and weight loss can occur.

Diagnosis The diagnosis is made by the detection of eggs or proglottids in the stool. Eggs may also be present in the perianal area; thus, if proglottids or eggs are not found in the stool, the perianal region should be examined with use of a cellophane-tape swab (as in pinworm infection; **Chap. 232**). Distinguishing *T. saginata* or *T. asiatica* from *T. solium* requires examination of mature proglottids or the scolex. Available serologic tests are not helpful diagnostically. Eosinophilia and elevated levels of serum IgE are usually absent.

TREATMENT
Taeniasis Saginata and *Taeniasis Asiatica*

A single dose of praziquantel (10 mg/kg) is highly effective. Niclosamide (adult dose, 2 g; 1 g for children weighing 11–34 kg) is also effective but is less available.

Prevention The major method of preventing infection is the adequate cooking of beef or pork viscera; exposure to temperatures as low as 56°C for 5 min will destroy cysticerci. Refrigeration or salting for long periods or freezing at –10°C for 9 days also kills cysticerci in beef. General preventive measures include inspection of beef and proper disposal of human feces.

■ *TAENIASIS SOLIUM* AND CYSTICERCOSIS

The pork tapeworm *T. solium* can cause two distinct forms of infection in humans: adult tapeworms in the intestine or larval forms in the tissues (cysticercosis). Humans are the only definitive hosts for *T. solium*; pigs are the usual intermediate hosts, although other animals may harbor the larval forms.

T. solium is found worldwide in areas where pigs are raised and have access to human feces. However, it is most prevalent in Latin America, sub-Saharan Africa, China, India, and Southeast Asia. Cysticercosis occurs in industrialized nations largely as a result of the immigration of infected persons from endemic areas.

Etiology and Pathogenesis The adult tapeworm generally resides in the upper jejunum. The scolex attaches by both sucking disks and two rows of hooklets. The adult worm usually lives for a few years. The mature tapeworm, usually ~3 m in length, may have as many as 1000 proglottids, each of which produces up to 50,000 eggs. Proglottids are released and excreted into the feces, and the eggs in these proglottids are infective for both humans and animals. After ingestion of eggs by the pig intermediate host, the invasive larvae are activated, escape the egg, penetrate the intestinal wall, and are carried via the bloodstream to many tissues; they are most frequently identified in striated muscle of the neck, tongue, and trunk. Within 60–90 days, the encysted larval stage develops. These cysticerci can survive for months to years. By ingesting undercooked pork containing cysticerci, humans acquire infections that lead to intestinal tapeworms. Infections that cause human cysticercosis follow the ingestion of *T. solium* eggs. Transmission is usually associated with close contact with a tapeworm carrier. The eggs are sticky and may be found under the fingernails of tapeworm carriers. Autoinfection may occur if an individual with an egg-producing tapeworm ingests eggs derived from his or her own feces.

Clinical Manifestations Intestinal infections with *T. solium* may be asymptomatic. Fecal passage of proglottids may be noted by patients. Other symptoms are infrequent.

In cysticercosis, the clinical manifestations are variable. Cysticerci can be found anywhere in the body but are most commonly detected in the brain, cerebrospinal fluid (CSF), skeletal muscle, subcutaneous tissue, or eye. The clinical presentation of cysticercosis depends on the number and location of cysticerci as well as on the extent of associated inflammatory responses or scarring. Neurologic manifestations are the most common (**Fig. 235-1**). Seizures are associated with inflammation surrounding cysticerci in the brain parenchyma. These seizures may be generalized, focal, or Jacksonian. Hydrocephalus results from CSF flow obstruction by cysticerci and accompanying inflammation or by CSF outflow obstruction from arachnoiditis. Symptoms of increased intracranial pressure, including headache, nausea, vomiting, changes in vision, dizziness, ataxia, or confusion, are often evident. Patients with hydrocephalus may develop papilledema or display altered mental status. When cysticerci develop at the base of the brain or in the subarachnoid space, they may cause chronic meningitis or arachnoiditis, communicating hydrocephalus, hemorrhages, or strokes.

Diagnosis The diagnosis of intestinal *T. solium* infection is made by the detection of eggs or proglottids, as described for *T. saginata*. More sensitive methods, including antigen-capture enzyme-linked immunosorbent assay (ELISA), polymerase chain reaction (PCR), and serology for tapeworm stage-specific antigens, are currently available only as research techniques. In cysticercosis, diagnosis can be difficult. A panel of international experts recently proposed revised diagnostic criteria (**Table 235-1**). Diagnostic certainty is possible only with definite demonstration of the parasite (absolute criteria). This task can be accomplished by histologic observation of the parasite in excised tissue, by funduscopic visualization of the parasite in the subretinal space of the eye, or by neuroimaging studies with definite evidence of a cystic lesion containing a characteristic scolex (Fig. 235-1). With improving resolution of neuroimaging studies, the scolex can now be identified in a large proportion of cases. In other instances, a clinical diagnosis is based on a combination of clinical presentation, radiographic studies, exposure history, and serodiagnosis.

Neuroimaging findings constitute the primary major diagnostic criteria (Fig. 235-1). Major findings include cystic lesions with or without enhancement (e.g., ring enhancement), one or more nodular calcifications (which may also have associated enhancement), focal enhancing lesions, or multilobulated cystic lesions in the subarachnoid space. Cysticerci in the brain parenchyma are usually 5–20 mm in diameter and rounded. Cystic lesions in the subarachnoid space or fissures may enlarge up to 6 cm in diameter and may be lobulated. For cysticerci within the subarachnoid space or ventricles, the walls may be very thin and the cyst fluid is often isodense with CSF. Thus, obstructive hydrocephalus or enhancement of the basilar meninges may be the only finding on CT in extraparenchymal neurocysticercosis. However, since these findings are less specific, they are considered only minor criteria. Cysticerci in the ventricles or subarachnoid space are more readily identified by MRI, especially with three-dimensional views (e.g., fast imaging employing steady-state acquisition [FIESTA] or three-dimensional constructive interference in steady state [3D CISS]). CT is more sensitive than MRI in identifying calcified lesions, whereas MRI is better for identifying cystic lesions, scolices, and enhancement. Spontaneous resolution, resolution after therapy with albendazole, or mobile cystic lesions within the ventricles are findings that can support the diagnosis of neurocysticercosis.

Prior exposure significantly modifies the interpretation of neuroimaging studies. Detection of specific antibodies to or antigens of *T. solium* are major exposure criteria. Antibody tests using unfractionated antigens (e.g., ELISAs using crude parasite antigen) have high rates of false-positive and false-negative results and should be avoided. An immunoblot assay using lentil lectin–purified glycoproteins is >99% specific and highly sensitive. However, patients with single intracranial lesions or with calcifications may be seronegative. With this assay, serum samples provide greater diagnostic sensitivity than CSF. All of the diagnostic antigens have been cloned, and assays using recombinant antigens are being developed. Antigen detection assays using monoclonal antibodies to detect parasite antigen in the blood or CSF may also facilitate diagnosis and patient follow-up. These assays are currently available commercially in Europe but not in the United States. More recently, real-time PCR has been employed for diagnosis and follow-up of extraparenchymal disease.

Other major clinical/exposure criteria for neurocysticercosis include the presence of cysticerci outside the central nervous system (CNS) (e.g., typical cigar-shaped calcifications in muscle) or exposure to a tapeworm carrier or a household member infected with *T. solium*. Minor clinical/exposure criteria include residence in an endemic area or clinical symptoms suggestive of neurocysticercosis (e.g., seizures or obstructive hydrocephalus).

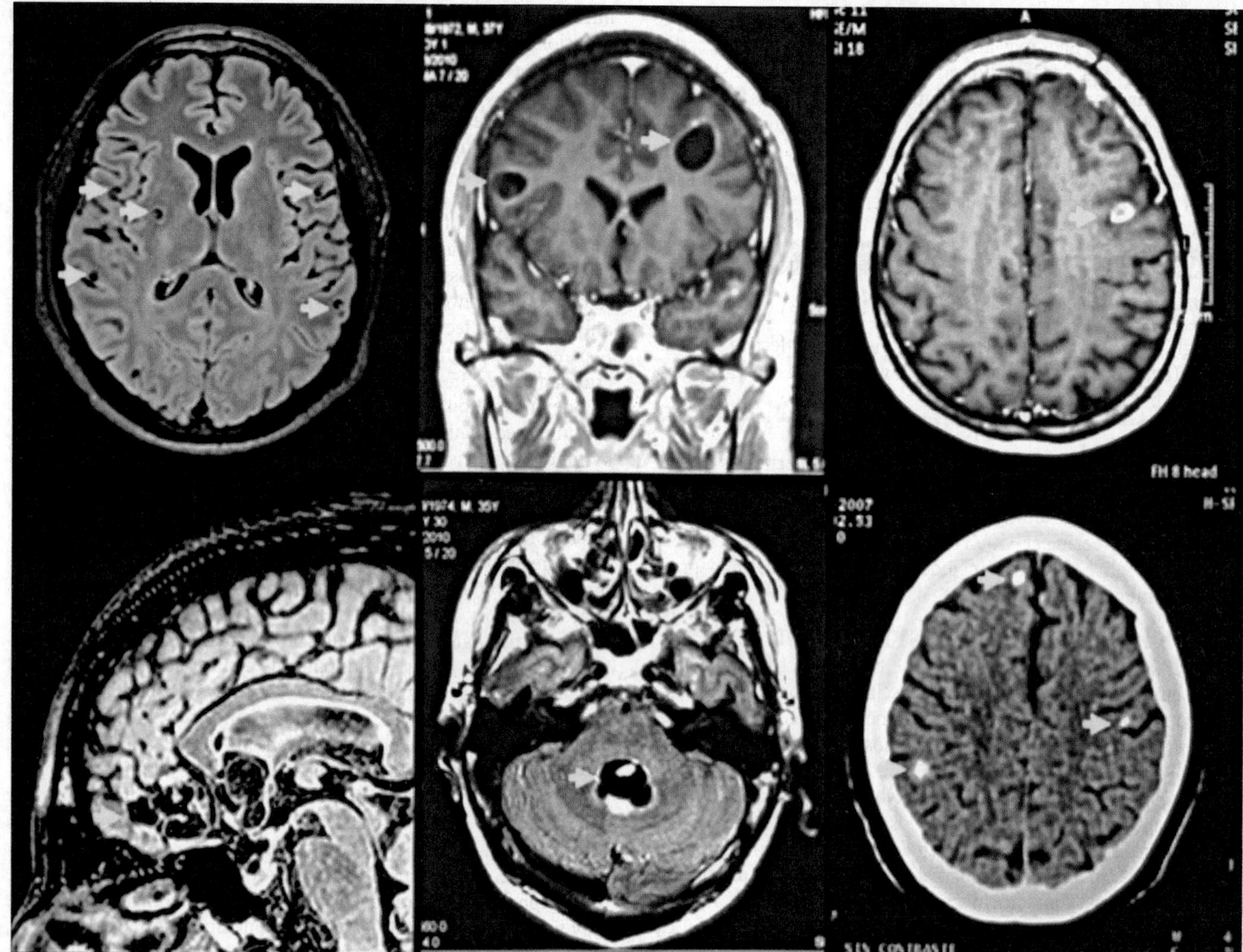

FIGURE 235-1 Neurocysticercosis is caused by *Taenia solium*. Neurologic infection can be classified on the basis of the location and viability of the parasites. ***Upper left:*** Parenchymal viable cysts (FLAIR MRI sequence). ***Upper center:*** Parenchymal viable cysts (postcontrast T1 MRI sequence). ***Upper right:*** Single enhancing lesion (postcontrast T1 MRI sequence). ***Bottom left:*** Extensive basal subarachnoid neurocysticercosis in the anterior fossa (FLAIR MRI sequence). ***Bottom center:*** Viable cyst in the fourth ventricle (FLAIR MRI sequence). ***Bottom right:*** Intraparenchymal brain calcifications (noncontrasted CT scan). Lesions are marked with *arrowheads*. FLAIR, fluid-attenuated inversion recovery. *(Modified with permission from A White, H Garcia: Curr Opin Infect Dis 31:377, 2018. Lippincott Williams & Wilkins.)*

Studies have demonstrated that clinical criteria may aid in diagnosis in selected cases. In patients from endemic areas who had single enhancing lesions presenting with seizures, a normal physical examination, and no evidence of systemic disease (e.g., no fever, adenopathy, or chest radiographic abnormalities), the constellation of rounded CT lesions 5–20 mm in diameter with no midline shift was almost always caused by neurocysticercosis.

A definite or probable diagnosis is made in accordance with the criteria and combinations of criteria listed in the footnote of Table 235-1. Patients may have CSF pleocytosis with a predominance of lymphocytes, neutrophils, or eosinophils. The protein level in CSF may be elevated; the glucose concentration is usually normal but may be depressed.

TREATMENT

Taeniasis Solium and Cysticercosis

Intestinal *T. solium* infection is treated with a single dose of praziquantel (10 mg/kg). However, praziquantel occasionally evokes an inflammatory response in the CNS if concomitant cryptic cysticercosis is present. Niclosamide (2 g) is also effective but is not widely available.

The initial management of neurocysticercosis should focus on symptom-based treatment of seizures or hydrocephalus. Seizures can usually be controlled with antiepileptic treatment. If parenchymal lesions resolve without development of calcifications and patients remain free of seizures, antiepileptic therapy can usually be discontinued after 2 years; less in patients with a single enhancing lesion. Placebo-controlled trials are clarifying the clinical advantage of antiparasitic drugs for parenchymal neurocysticercosis. Faster resolution of neuroradiologic abnormalities has been observed in most studies. The clinical benefits are less dramatic and consist mainly of shortening the period during which recurrent seizures occur and decreasing the number of patients who have many recurrent seizures. For the treatment of patients with brain parenchymal cysticerci, most authorities favor antiparasitic drugs, including albendazole (15 mg/kg per day for 8–28 days) and/or praziquantel (50–100 mg/kg daily in three divided doses for 15–30 days). A combination of albendazole and praziquantel (50 mg/kg per day) is more effective in patients with more than two cystic lesions. A longer course or combination therapy is needed in patients with multiple subarachnoid cysticerci. Both agents may exacerbate the inflammatory response around the dying parasite, thereby exacerbating seizures or hydrocephalus as well. Thus, patients receiving these drugs should be carefully monitored. High-dose glucocorticoids should be used during treatment. Because glucocorticoids induce first-pass metabolism of praziquantel and may decrease its antiparasitic effect, cimetidine should be co-administered to inhibit praziquantel metabolism.

For patients with hydrocephalus, the emergent reduction of intracranial pressure is the mainstay of therapy. In the case of obstructive

TABLE 235-1 Revised Diagnostic Criteria for Neurocysticercosis[a]

1. **Absolute criteria**
   a. Histologic demonstration of the parasite from biopsy of a brain or spinal cord lesion
   b. Visualization of subretinal cysticercus
   c. Conclusive demonstration of a scolex within a cystic lesion on neuroimaging studies
2. **Neuroimaging criteria**
   a. **Major neuroimaging criteria**
      Cystic lesions without a discernible scolex, typical small enhancing lesions, multilobulated cystic lesions in the subarachnoid space, typical parenchymal brain calcifications
   b. **Confirmative neuroimaging criteria**
      Resolution of cystic lesions spontaneously or after cysticidal drug therapy
      Migration of ventricular cysts documented on sequential neuroimaging studies
   c. **Minor neuroimaging criteria**
      Obstructive hydrocephalus or abnormal enhancement of basal leptomeninges
3. **Clinical/exposure criteria**
   a. **Major clinical/exposure criteria**
      Detection of specific anticysticercal antibodies (e.g., by enzyme-linked immunoelectrotransfer blot [EITB]) or cysticercal antigens by well-standardized immunodiagnostic tests
      Cysticercosis outside the central nervous system
      Evidence of a household contact with *T. solium* infection
   b. **Minor clinical/exposure criteria**
      Clinical manifestations suggestive of neurocysticercosis
      Individuals coming from or living in an area where cysticercosis is endemic

[a]Diagnosis is confirmed by one absolute criterion, by two major criteria or one major and one confirmatory neuroimaging criteria plus any clinical/exposure criterion, or by one major neuroimaging criterion plus two clinical/exposure criteria (including at least one major clinical/exposure criterion), together with the exclusion of other pathologies producing similar neuroimaging findings. A probable diagnosis is supported by one major neuroimaging criterion plus any two clinical/exposure criteria or by one minor neuroimaging criterion plus at least one major clinical/exposure criterion.

Source: Reproduced with permission from OH Del Brutto et al: Revised diagnostic criteria for neurocysticercosis. J Neurol Sci 372:202, 2017.

hydrocephalus, the preferred approach is removal of the cysticercus via neurosurgery. This should be performed via neuroendoscopy when the cysticerci are in the lateral or third ventricles. The fourth ventricular cysticerci can be approached by microdissection using an open craniotomy and a posterior approach or, in some cases, via neuroendoscopy. However, removal of the cysticercus is not always possible. An alternative approach is initially to perform a diverting procedure, such as ventriculoperitoneal shunting. Historically, shunts have usually failed, but failure rates may be lowered by administration of antiparasitic drugs and glucocorticoids. For patients with subarachnoid cysts or giant cysticerci, anti-inflammatory medications such as glucocorticoids are needed to reduce arachnoiditis and accompanying vasculitis. Most authorities recommend prolonged courses of antiparasitic drugs as well as shunting when hydrocephalus is present. Methotrexate and, in some cases, tumor necrosis factor inhibitors can be used as steroid-sparing agents in patients requiring prolonged therapy. In patients with diffuse cerebral edema and elevated intracranial pressure due to multiple inflamed lesions, glucocorticoids are the mainstay of therapy, and antiparasitic drugs should be avoided. For ocular and spinal medullary lesions, drug-induced inflammation may cause irreversible damage. Ocular disease should be managed surgically. Recent data suggest that either medical or surgical therapy can be used for spinal disease.

Prevention Measures for the prevention of intestinal *T. solium* infection consist of the application to pork of precautions similar to those described above for beef with regard to *T. saginata* infection. The prevention of cysticercosis involves minimizing the opportunities for ingestion of fecally derived eggs by means of good personal hygiene, effective fecal disposal, and treatment and prevention of human intestinal infections. Optimal eradication programs in endemic areas include mass chemotherapy administered to human and porcine populations and vaccinations of pigs. A vaccine for porcine infection is licensed in India and a few other countries.

ECHINOCOCCOSIS

Echinococcosis (also termed hydatidosis) is an infection caused in humans by the larval stage of *Echinococcus granulosus* sensu lato, *E. multilocularis*, or *E. vogeli*. *E. granulosus* sensu lato parasites produce cystic hydatid disease, with unilocular cystic lesions. These infections are prevalent in most areas where livestock is raised in association with dogs. Molecular evidence has demonstrated that *E. granulosus* strains belong to a range of genotypes and several species. Currently, human cystic hydatid disease is caused by organisms formerly termed *E. granulosus* that are now classified as *E. granulosus* sensu stricto (genotypes 1–3), *E. canadensis* (genotypes 6–8 and 10), and *E. ortleppi* (genotype 5). Other species—*E. equinus* (genotype 4) and *E. felidis* (lion strain)—have not been identified in human infections. Some classify genotypes 6 and 7 as a separate species—*E. intermedius*. *E. granulosus* sensu lato parasites are found on all continents, with areas of high prevalence in western China, central Asia, the Middle East, the Mediterranean region, eastern Africa, and parts of South America. *E. multilocularis*, which causes multilocular alveolar lesions that are locally invasive, is found in Alpine, sub-Arctic, or Arctic regions, including central and northern Europe; western China and central Asia; and isolated areas in North America. *E. vogeli* and *E. oligarthrus* cause neotropical echinococcosis (formerly termed polycystic hydatid disease) and are found only in South America.

Like other cestodes, echinococcal species have both intermediate and definitive hosts. The definitive hosts are canines that pass eggs in their feces. After the ingestion of eggs, cysts develop in the intermediate hosts—sheep, cattle, humans, goats, camels, and horses for the *E. granulosus* complex and mice and other rodents for *E. multilocularis*. When a dog (*E. granulosus*) or fox (*E. multilocularis*) ingests infected meat containing cysts, the life cycle is completed. Humans are an incidental dead-end host and not part of the transmission life cycle.

Etiology The small (5-mm-long) adult *E. granulosus* sensu lato worms live for 5–20 months in the jejunum of dogs. They have three proglottids: one immature, one mature, and one gravid. The gravid segments are shed to release eggs that are morphologically similar to *Taenia* eggs and are extremely hardy. After humans ingest the eggs, embryos escape from the eggs, penetrate the intestinal mucosa, enter the portal circulation, and are carried to various organs, most commonly the liver and lungs. Larvae of *E. granulosus* sensu lato develop into fluid-filled unilocular hydatid cysts that consist of an external membrane and an inner germinal layer. Daughter cysts develop from the inner aspect of the germinal layer, as do germinating cystic structures called *brood capsules*. New larvae, called *protoscolices*, develop in large numbers within the brood capsule. The cysts expand slowly over a period of years.

The life cycle of *E. multilocularis* is similar except that wild canines, such as foxes or wolves, serve as the main definitive hosts, and small rodents serve as the intermediate hosts. The larval form of *E. multilocularis*, however, is quite different in that it remains in the proliferative phase, the parasite is always multilocular, and vesicles without brood capsules or protoscolices progressively invade the host tissue by peripheral extension of processes from the germinal layer.

Clinical Manifestations Slowly enlarging echinococcal cysts generally remain asymptomatic until their expanding size or their space-occupying effect in an involved organ elicits symptoms. The liver and the lungs are the most common sites of these cysts. The liver is involved in about two-thirds of *E. granulosus* infections and in nearly all *E. multilocularis* infections. Because a period of years elapses before cysts enlarge sufficiently to cause symptoms, they may be discovered incidentally on a routine x-ray or ultrasound study.

Patients with hepatic echinococcosis who are symptomatic most often present with abdominal pain or a palpable mass in the right upper quadrant. Compression of a bile duct or leakage of cyst fluid into the biliary tree may mimic recurrent cholelithiasis, and biliary obstruction can result in jaundice. Rupture of or episodic leakage from a hydatid cyst may produce fever, pruritus, urticaria, eosinophilia, or anaphylaxis. Pulmonary hydatid cysts may rupture into the bronchial tree or pleural cavity and produce cough, salty phlegm, dyspnea, chest pain, or hemoptysis. Rupture of hydatid cysts, which can occur spontaneously or at surgery, may lead to multifocal dissemination of protoscolices, which can form additional cysts. Other presentations are due to the involvement of bone (invasion of the medullary cavity with slow bone erosion producing pathologic fractures), the CNS (space-occupying lesions), the heart (conduction defects, pericarditis), and the pelvis (pelvic mass).

The larval forms of *E. multilocularis* characteristically present as a slowly growing hepatic tumor, with progressive destruction of the liver and extension into vital structures. Clinical symptoms develop decades after initial infection. Patients commonly report upper-quadrant and epigastric pain. Liver enlargement and obstructive jaundice may be apparent. The lesions may infiltrate adjoining organs (e.g., diaphragm, kidneys, or lungs) or may metastasize to the spleen, lungs, or brain.

Diagnosis Radiographic and related imaging studies are important in detecting and evaluating echinococcal cysts. Plain x-rays will define pulmonary cysts of *E. granulosus*—usually as rounded masses of uniform density—but may miss cysts in other organs unless there is cyst wall calcification (as occurs in the liver). MRI, CT, and ultrasound reveal well-defined cysts with thick or thin walls. Imaging methods may reveal a fluid layer of different density, termed *hydatid sand*, that contains protoscolices. However, the most pathognomonic finding, if demonstrable, is that of daughter cysts within the larger cyst. This finding, like eggshell or mural calcification on CT, is indicative of *E. granulosus* infection and helps to distinguish the cyst from carcinomas, bacterial or amebic liver abscesses, or hemangiomas. In contrast, ultrasound or CT of alveolar hydatid cysts reveals indistinct solid masses with central necrosis and plaquelike calcifications.

A specific diagnosis of cystic hydatid disease can be made by the examination of aspirated fluids for protoscolices or hooklets, but diagnostic aspiration is not usually recommended because of the potential risk of fluid leakage resulting in either dissemination of infection or anaphylactic reactions. Serodiagnostic assays can be useful, although a negative test does not exclude the diagnosis of echinococcosis. Cysts in the liver elicit positive antibody responses in ~90% of cases, whereas up to 50% of individuals with cysts in the lungs are seronegative. Detection of antibody to specific echinococcal antigens by immunoblotting has the highest degree of specificity.

TREATMENT

Echinococcosis

Therapy for cystic echinococcosis is based on considerations of the size, location, and manifestations of cysts and the overall health of the patient. Surgery has traditionally been the principal definitive method of treatment. Currently, ultrasound staging is recommended for cystic echinococcosis (**Fig. 235-2**). Small CL, CE1, and CE3 lesions may respond to chemotherapy with albendazole. For CE1 lesions and uncomplicated CE3 lesions, PAIR (*p*ercutaneous *a*spiration, *i*nfusion of scolicidal agents, and *r*easpiration) is now recommended instead of surgery. PAIR is contraindicated for superficially located cysts (because of the risk of rupture) and for cysts communicating with the biliary tree. For prophylaxis of secondary peritoneal echinococcosis due to inadvertent spillage of fluid during PAIR, the administration of albendazole (15 mg/kg daily in two divided doses) should be initiated at least 2 days before the procedure and continued for at least 4 weeks afterward. Ultrasound- or CT-guided aspiration allows confirmation of the diagnosis by demonstration of protoscolices or hooks in the aspirate. After aspiration, contrast material should be injected to detect occult communications with the biliary tract. Alternatively, the fluid should be checked for bile staining visually and by dipstick. If no bile is found and no communication is visualized, the contrast material is reaspirated, with subsequent infusion of scolicidal agents (usually 95% ethanol; alternatively, hypertonic saline). This approach, when implemented by a skilled practitioner, yields rates of cure and relapse equivalent to those following surgery, with less perioperative morbidity and shorter hospitalization. In experienced hands, some CE2 lesions can be treated by modified catheter drainage. Daughter cysts within the primary cyst may need to be punctured separately.

Surgery remains the treatment of choice for complicated cystic echinococcosis (e.g., cysts communicating with the biliary tract), for most thoracic and intracranial cysts, and for areas where PAIR is not possible. For liver cysts, the preferred surgical approach is total cystectomy, in which the entire cyst and the surrounding fibrous tissue are removed. Recent studies demonstrate that many cysts can be safely removed by laparoscopic or robotic surgery. The risks posed by leakage of fluid during surgery or PAIR include anaphylaxis and dissemination of infectious protoscolices. The latter complication has been minimized by careful attention to the prevention of spillage of the cyst. Infusion of scolicidal agents is no longer recommended because of problems with hypernatremia, intoxication, or sclerosing cholangitis. Albendazole, which is active against *Echinococcus*, should be administered adjunctively, beginning several days before resection of the liver and continuing for several weeks for *E. granulosus*. Praziquantel (50 mg/kg daily for 2 weeks or weekly throughout the duration of albendazole) may hasten the death of the protoscolices. Medical therapy with albendazole alone for 12 weeks to 6 months results in cure in ~30% of cases and in improvement in another 50%. In many instances of treatment failure, *E. granulosus* infections are subsequently treated successfully with PAIR or additional courses of medical therapy. Response to treatment is best assessed by serial imaging studies, with attention to cyst size and consistency. Some cysts may not demonstrate complete radiologic resolution even though no viable protoscolices are present. Some of these cysts with partial radiologic resolution (e.g., CE4 or CE5) can be managed with observation only.

Surgical resection remains the treatment of choice for *E. multilocularis* infection. Complete removal of the parasite continues to offer the best chance for cure. Ongoing therapy with albendazole for at least 2 years after presumptively curative surgery is recommended. Positron emission tomography can be used to follow disease activity. Most cases are diagnosed at a stage at which complete resection is not possible; in these cases, albendazole treatment should be continued indefinitely, with careful monitoring. In some cases, liver transplantation has been used because of the size of the necessary liver resection. However, continuous immunosuppression favors the proliferation of *E. multilocularis* larvae and reinfection of the transplant. Thus, indefinite treatment with albendazole is required.

Prevention In endemic areas, echinococcosis can be prevented by administering praziquantel to infected dogs, by denying dogs access to viscera from infected animals, or by vaccinating sheep. Limiting the number of stray dogs is helpful in reducing the prevalence of infection among humans. In Europe, *E. multilocularis* infection has been associated with gardening; gloves should be used when working with soil. Praziquantel-impregnated bait has also been used to treat tapeworms in wild canines.

HYMENOLEPIASIS NANA

Infection with *H. nana*, the dwarf tapeworm, is the most common of all the cestode infections. *H. nana* is endemic in both temperate and tropical regions of the world. Infection is spread by fecal/oral contamination.

Etiology and Pathogenesis *H. nana* is the only cestode of humans that does not require an intermediate host. Both the larval

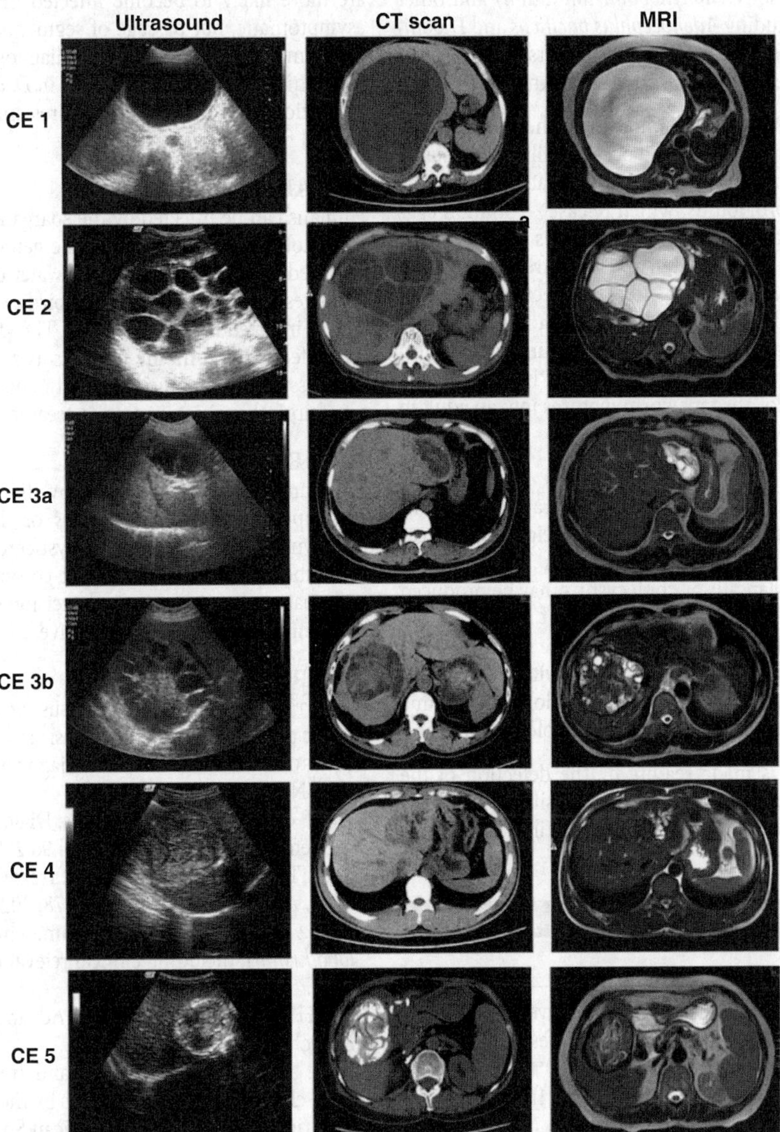

FIGURE 235-2 Management of cystic hydatid disease caused by *Echinococcus granulosus* should be based on viability of the parasite, which can be estimated from radiographic appearance. Staging is done by imaging studies including ultrasound, CT, or MRI and includes lesions classified as active, transitional, and inactive. *Active* cysts include types CL (with a cystic lesion and no visible cyst wall), CE1 (with a visible cyst wall and internal echoes [*snowflake sign*]), and CE2 (with a visible cyst wall and internal septation). *Transitional* cysts may have detached laminar membranes (CE3a) or may be partially collapsed (CE3b). *Inactive cysts* include types CE4 (a nonhomogeneous mass) and CE5 (a cyst with a thick calcified wall).

and adult phases of the life cycle take place in the same person. The adult—the smallest tapeworm parasitizing humans—is ~2 cm long and dwells in the proximal ileum. Proglottids, which are small and rarely seen in the stool, release spherical eggs 30–44 μm in diameter, each of which contains an oncosphere with six hooklets. The eggs are immediately infective and are unable to survive for >10 days in the external environment. When the egg is ingested by a new host, the oncosphere is freed and penetrates the intestinal villi, becoming a cysticercoid larva. Larvae migrate back into the intestinal lumen, attach to the mucosa, and mature into adult worms over 10–12 days. Eggs may also hatch before passing into the stool, causing internal autoinfection with increasing numbers of intestinal worms. Although the life span of adult *H. nana* worms is only ~4–10 weeks, the autoinfection cycle perpetuates the infection.

Clinical Manifestations *H. nana* infection, even with many intestinal worms, is usually asymptomatic. Heavy infection may be associated with diarrhea, abdominal pain, and weight loss.

Diagnosis Infection is diagnosed by the finding of eggs in the stool.

TREATMENT

Hymenolepiasis Nana

Praziquantel (25 mg/kg once) is the treatment of choice because it acts against both the adult worms and the cysticercoids in the intestinal villi. Nitazoxanide (500 mg bid for 3 days) may be used as an alternative.

Prevention Good personal hygiene and improved sanitation can eradicate the disease. Epidemics have been controlled by mass chemotherapy coupled with improved hygiene.

HYMENOLEPIASIS DIMINUTA

Hymenolepis diminuta, a cestode of rodents, occasionally infects small children, who ingest the larvae in uncooked cereal foods contaminated by fleas and other insects in which larvae develop. Infection is usually asymptomatic and is diagnosed by the detection of eggs in the stool. Treatment with praziquantel results in cure in most cases.

DIPHYLLOBOTHRIASIS

Dibothriocephalus latus (formerly *Diphyllobothrium latum*) and other diphyllobothriid species (including *Adenocephlus pacificus* and *Dibothriocephalus nihonkaiensis*) are found in the lakes, rivers, and deltas of the Northern Hemisphere, central Africa, and South America.

Etiology and Pathogenesis The adult worm—the longest tapeworm (up to 25 m)—attaches to the ileal and occasionally to the jejunal mucosa by its suckers, which are located on its elongated scolex. The adult worm has 3000–4000 proglottids, which release ~1 million eggs daily into the feces. If an egg reaches water, it hatches and releases a free-swimming embryo that can be eaten by small freshwater crustaceans (*Cyclops* or *Diaptomus* species). After an infected crustacean containing a developed procercoid is swallowed by a fish, the larva migrates into the fish's flesh and grows into a sparganum, or plerocercoid larva. Humans acquire the infection by ingesting infected raw or smoked fish. Within 3–5 weeks, the tapeworm matures into an adult in the human intestine.

Clinical Manifestations Most *Diphyllobothrium* infections are asymptomatic, although manifestations may include transient abdominal discomfort, diarrhea, vomiting, weakness, and weight loss. Occasionally, infection can cause acute abdominal pain and intestinal obstruction; in rare cases, cholangitis or cholecystitis may be produced by migrating proglottids.

Because the *D. latum* tapeworm absorbs large quantities of vitamin B_{12} and interferes with ileal B_{12} absorption, vitamin B_{12} deficiency can develop that uncommonly causes a megaloblastic anemia resembling pernicious anemia and may result in neurologic sequelae.

Diagnosis The diagnosis is made readily by the detection of the characteristic eggs in the stool. The eggs possess a single shell with an operculum at one end and a knob at the other. Mild to moderate eosinophilia may be detected.

TREATMENT
Diphyllobothriasis

Praziquantel (5–10 mg/kg once) is highly effective. Parenteral vitamin B_{12} should be given if B_{12} deficiency is manifest.

Prevention Infection can be prevented by heating fish to 54°C for 5 min or by freezing it at −18°C for 24 h. Placing fish in brine with a high salt concentration for long periods kills the eggs.

DIPYLIDIASIS

Dipylidium caninum, a common tapeworm of dogs and cats, may accidentally infect humans. Dogs, cats, and occasionally humans become infected by ingesting fleas harboring cysticercoids. Children are more likely to become infected than adults. Most infections are asymptomatic, but passage of segments in the stool or vague abdominal symptoms may occur. The diagnosis is made by the detection of proglottids or ova in the stool. As in *D. latus* infection, therapy consists of praziquantel. Prevention requires anthelminthic treatment and flea control for pet dogs or cats.

SPARGANOSIS

Humans can be infected by the sparganum, or plerocercoid larva, of a diphyllobothriid tapeworm of the genus *Spirometra*. Infection can be acquired by the consumption of water containing infected *Cyclops*; by the ingestion of infected snakes, birds, or mammals; or by the application of infected flesh as poultices. The worm migrates slowly in tissues, and infection commonly presents as a subcutaneous swelling. Periorbital tissues can be involved, and ocular sparganosis may destroy the eye. Surgical excision is used to treat localized sparganosis.

COENUROSIS

This rare infection of humans by the larval stage (coenurus) of the dog tapeworm *Taenia multiceps* or *T. serialis* results in a space-occupying cystic lesion. As in cysticercosis, involvement of the CNS and subcutaneous tissue is most common. Both definitive diagnosis and treatment require surgical excision of the lesion. Chemotherapeutic agents generally are not effective.

FURTHER READING

Brunetti E et al: Expert consensus for the diagnosis and treatment of cystic and alveolar echinococcosis in humans. Acta Trop 114:1, 2010.

Del Brutto OH et al: Revised diagnostic criteria for neurocysticercosis. J Neurol Sci 372:202, 2017.

Kern P et al: The echinococcoses: Diagnosis, clinical management and burden of disease. Adv Parasitol 96:259, 2017.

Nash TE et al: Natural history of treated subarachnoid neurocysticercosis. Am J Trop Med Hyg 102:78, 2020.

Scholz T et al: Update on the human broad tapeworm (genus *Diphyllobothrium*), including clinical relevance. Clin Microbiol Rev 22:146, 2009.

Wen H et al: Echinococcosis: Advances in the 21st century. Clin Microbiol Rev 32:e00075, 2019.

White AC Jr et al: Diagnosis and treatment of neurocysticercosis: 2017 clinical practice guidelines by the Infectious Diseases Society of America (IDSA) and the American Society of Tropical Medicine and Hygiene (ASTMH). Clin Infect Dis 66:1159, 2018.

Page numbers in **bold** indicate the start of the main discussion of the topic. Page numbers followed by "f" or "t" refer to the page location of figures and tables, respectively. Location entries starting with "A"(Atlases), "S" (Supplemental chapters), or "V" (Video chapters) indicate online-only chapter numbers; this content available to all *Harrison's* readers at *www.accessmedicine.com/harrisons*. Index entries that end with a "v" represent book page numbers where video content is referenced.

INDEX

INDEX

B

INDEX

INDEX

C

INDEX

INDEX

INDEX

INDEX

INDEX

INDEX

INDEX

INDEX

INDEX

INDEX

Q

INDEX

S

INDEX

INDEX